MARTINDALE
The Extra Pharmacopoeia

MARTINDALE

The Extra Pharmacopoeia

Twenty-ninth Edition

Edited by James E. F. Reynolds

Deputy Editor
Kathleen Parfitt

Assistant Editors
Anne V. Parsons
Sean C. Sweetman

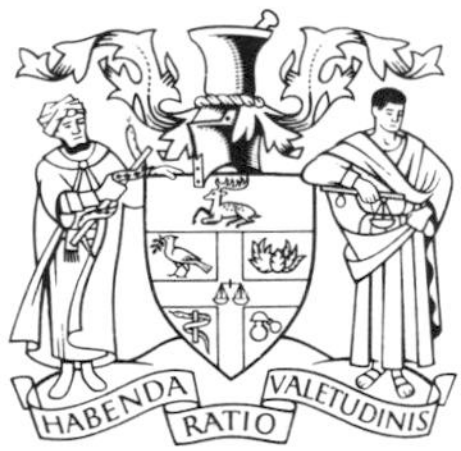

Published by direction of the Council of the Royal Pharmaceutical Society of Great Britain and prepared in the Society's Department of Pharmaceutical Sciences

London
THE PHARMACEUTICAL PRESS
1989

 Published by The Pharmaceutical Press, 1 Lambeth High Street, London SE1 7JN, England.

The first edition of the Extra Pharmacopoeia was published in July 1883. Squire's Companion was incorporated in the twenty-third edition in 1952. The twenty-eighth edition was published in December 1982. This current (twenty-ninth) edition was first published in February 1989, reprinted with corrections in January 1990, and reprinted in January 1992.

BRITISH LIBRARY CATALOGUING - IN-PUBLICATION DATA

The Extra pharmacopoeia.-29th ed.
1. Drugs. British pharmacopoeias.
I. Title.
615′.11′41

International Standard Book Number (ISBN): 0 85369 210 6. International Standard Serial Number (ISSN): 0263-5364.

Computer composition by Peter Peregrinus Ltd., Hitchin, Hertfordshire; phototypesetting output by Unwin Brothers Ltd., Old Woking, Surrey. Printed and bound in England by The Bath Press, Bath, Avon.

THE COUNCIL OF THE ROYAL PHARMACEUTICAL SOCIETY OF GREAT BRITAIN 1988–1989

DEPARTMENT OF PHARMACEUTICAL SCIENCES

Director: W. G. Thomas, MSc, PhD, FRPharmS

General Editor: A. Wade, BPharm, MPhil, FRPharmS

MARTINDALE EDITORIAL STAFF

Editor: J. E. F. Reynolds, PhD, FRPharmS, MIInfSc

Deputy Editor: Kathleen Parfitt, BSc, MRPharmS

Assistant Editors: Anne V. Parsons, BPharm, MRPharmS
S. C. Sweetman, BPharm, MRPharmS

Eileen J. Aitchison, BPharm, PhD, MRPharmS
Jacqueline O. Baines
P. S. Blake, BPharm, MRPharmS
A. G. Desson, BPharm, MSc, MRPharmS
Kathleen Eager, BPharm, MRPharmS
Wendy M. Farenden, BSc, MRPharmS
Anne M. P. Gilchrist, BSc, MSc, MRPharmS
Ann Harris, BPharm, PhD, MRPharmS
Susan L. Jefferson, BSc, MRPharmS
Julie M. McGlashan, BPharm, DipInfSc, MRPharmS
Rosalind McLarney, BPharm, DipInfSc, MRPharmS
J. Martin, BPharm, PhD, MRPharmS
Doris D. Moore

Contents

Preface

This edition of Martindale continues the tradition of its predecessors in aiming to provide unbiased concise reports on the actions and uses of most of the world's drugs and medicines to aid the practising pharmacist and physician. While the overall format of this edition remains similar to that of the 28th edition, its contents are the result of a complete revision and the changes resulting from that revision have been considerable.

Monographs have been reorganised into chapters that more accurately reflect current therapeutic practice and the needs of today's reader. The 105 chapters of the last edition have been reorganised into 72 mainly new or renamed chapters. Details have been provided on about 900 new compounds, mostly in the form of new monographs. Over 500 monographs have been deleted where they described substances for which there is little evidence of continued use or interest. Almost 500 other monographs have been deleted where the information could be better incorporated in monographs for related compounds; information on the substances that were the subjects of these deleted monographs can still be traced through the index. The overall effect has been an increase in the coverage of drugs in Martindale, but with a considerable saving of space that has allowed us to make some typographical improvements to assist the reader in locating sections of a monograph.

Abstracts of the relevant aspects of important or useful papers and other publications are still included, but we have written many more referenced reviews of important or contentious topics to back up our editorial text. We have also continued to increase the coverage of proprietary names. More manufacturers are identified for the proprietary names that are included, the directory of manufacturers having increased by 50%. We have also started to include the proprietary names for preparations containing more than one active ingredient and our coverage now extends to many of the English speaking countries.

Considerable changes have been made to Martindale the better to reflect developments in therapeutics in the last 5 or 6 years. Some of the developments have been successful, some have still to produce worthwhile results or remain to be evaluated. A distressing and dominant theme throughout much of the period of revision has been the continuing search for an effective treatment of AIDS. The much enlarged chapter on antiviral agents illustrates some of this work, but it also shows the improvements that there have been in the treatment of other viral diseases. A more optimistic theme has been the expected and growing yield of products from genetic engineering techniques.

A considerable proportion of Martindale is taken up with drugs used to treat infections. Notable features, in addition to developments in antiviral therapy, include the emergence of the fluorinated quinolones and imipenem in the treatment of bacterial infections; the establishment of praziquantel in the treatment of schistosomiasis and other fluke infections; the consolidation of metronidazole and the re-emergence of pentamidine in protozoal infections; and the emergence of the anthelmintic ivermectin for the treatment of onchocerciasis, commendably provided free of charge through a WHO scheme. The increase in cephalosporins seems to continue inexorably.

Advances in the cardiovascular group of drugs have been wide ranging and encouraging. This edition shows the greater benefit that can now be obtained with thrombolytic, anticoagulant, antiplatelet, and haemostatic therapy. ACE inhibitors have established themselves in the treatment of hypertension. Calcium channel blockers continue to appear and offer a range of cardiovascular activity. Improvements have also taken place in lipid regulation.

Developments have continued in the field of peptic ulcer therapy. There are more histamine H2 antagonists, but there is also increased interest in tripotassium dicitratobismuthate in the light of the involvement of *Campylobacter pylori*. Work still progresses on the use of prostaglandins in peptic ulcer and there are new approaches to treatment as with the proton pump inhibitor, omeprazole.

There are other areas where advances are less dramatic, as for instance with antineoplastic agents or antiparkinsonian drugs. Resistance is a continuing concern with antimalarial compounds. Some chapters indicate a decrease in the use of drugs such as the anxiolytic sedatives and hypnotics. A number of nonsteroidal anti-inflammatory drugs have been withdrawn, but our files show that many more are being considered at development stages. Some general anaesthetics have been withdrawn because of toxicity associated with the solvent or vehicle, emphasising the often unregarded importance of formulation to therapeutics.

Martindale is based on published information. It is not a book of standards. Inclusion of a substance or a preparation is not to be considered as a recommendation for use, nor does it confer any status on the substance or preparation. While considerable efforts have been made to check the material in Martindale, the publisher cannot accept any responsibility for errors and omissions. Also the reader is assumed to possess the necessary knowledge to interpret the information that Martindale provides.

Arrangement

PART 1 (pages 1–1535) contains monographs on about 4000 substances arranged in 72 chapters. These chapters generally bring together drugs that have similar uses or actions. Cross-references are used to guide the reader to drugs that may be of interest in related chapters. Most chapters now have an introduction which provides background information on that group of drugs. Some drugs such as the corticosteroids can be considered readily as a group with its members having many common actions; in such cases the introduction provides much of the information for that chapter.

PART 2 (pages 1537–1631) consists of a series of short monographs on some 800 drugs and ancillary substances arranged in the alphabetical order of their main titles. It includes monographs on new drugs, on drugs under investigation, on drugs not easily classified, and on obsolescent drugs still of interest. There are also some monographs on toxic substances, the effects of which may require drug therapy.

PART 3 (pages 1633–43) gives the composition of some 670 proprietary medicines that are advertised to the public in Great Britain and that are usually supplied on demand. The formulas are generally as described by the manufacturers. Herbal medicines have been omitted. This list should not be considered to be comprehensive; some such proprietary medicines are included in Parts 1 and 2, usually if the preparation contains one active ingredient or if proprietary names for similar preparations from other countries are already listed under the monographs. As in earlier editions of Martindale, the claims made for these products and their recommended doses are not included.

The number of 'counter' proprietary medicines continues to decline.

Indexes

DIRECTORY OF MANUFACTURERS. Throughout the text the names of manufacturers and distributors are abbreviated. Their full names are given in this directory together with the full address if it is available. This directory has considerably increased from about 3000 entries to 4600.

INDEX TO CLINICAL USES. This index is a guide to the uses described in the text; it should not be used otherwise and is not a comprehensive therapeutic index. It refers the reader to the chapters and monographs where the listed diseases are mentioned. The drugs under each disease heading are listed in alphabetical order and not in order of preference.

INDEX TO MARTINDALE IDENTITY NUMBERS. Each monograph in Martindale has an identity number which is used in our computer manipulation. These identity numbers are referred to in the databank (Martindale Online) and will mainly be of value to the user of the online service; however, they may also be of some value to the user of the book. The numbers have no structure and are not significant in themselves. The index lists the identity number followed by the relevant monograph title and the page on which it appears. Identity numbers for chapter introductions have also been included.

GENERAL INDEX. To make fullest use of the contents of Martindale the general index should always be consulted. The exhaustive index to the drugs, preparations, compounds, and pharmacological and therapeutic groups in the book has been compiled to exacting standards and this has resulted in an index of about 62 000 entries. As in previous editions, the index is arranged alphabetically 'word-by-word' rather than 'letter-by-letter'.

Nomenclature

MARTINDALE IDENTITY NUMBERS. Each monograph begins with an identity number which consists of a maximum of 6 figures followed by a check character. These numbers are used in our computer manipulation and their sole purpose is to identify monographs in Martindale. They are referred to in the databank and will mainly be of value to the user of the online or compact disc services; however, they may also be of value to the reader of the book.

TITLES AND SYNONYMS. The title of each monograph is in English, with preference being given to British Approved Names, United States Adopted Names, and International Nonproprietary Names. These 3 authorities are now shown where appropriate against our titles or synonyms. Names given as synonyms include commonly used abbreviated names; English, American, and Latin synonyms; names used in other languages when these may not be readily identifiable; manufacturers' code numbers; and chemical names. In some approved names it is now general policy to use 'f' for 'ph' in sulpha, 't' for 'th', and 'i' for 'y'; for this reason entries in alphabetical lists and indexes should be sought in alternative spellings if the expected spellings are not found. A table of contracted names for ions and groups used in approved names and titles is given on page xx.

CAS REGISTRY NUMBERS. Chemical Abstracts Service (CAS) registry numbers are provided, where available, for each monograph substance to help readers refer to other information systems. Numbers for various forms of the monograph substance are listed with the variation in form given in parenthesis.

Pharmacopoeias

The pharmacopoeias in which each substance appears are listed. Current copies of the pharmacopoeias and their addenda should be consulted for confirmation and for details of standards.

The pharmacopoeias covered include: Argentine, *Austrian, Belgian,* Brazilian, *British, British Veterinary, Chinese, Czechoslovakian, Egyptian, European, French, German,* Hungarian, *Indian, International, Italian, Japanese, Jugoslavian,* Mexican, *Netherlands,* Nordic, Polish, Portuguese, Roumanian, Russian, Spanish, *Swiss,* Turkish, and *United States* (including the *Formulary*). Those *italicised* in the above list either appeared as new editions or were revised by supplements since the last edition of Martindale, and have been examined for this 29th edition.

The abbreviations for these pharmacopoeias are included in the list of abbreviations used in Martindale, see page xvi which also includes details of the edition and/or supplement(s) consulted.

Atomic and Molecular Weights

Atomic weights are based on the table of Atomic Weights as revised in 1983 by the Commission on Atomic Weights and Isotopic Abundance, International Union of Pure and Applied Chemistry and based on the ^{12}C scale (see page xxx). Molecular weights are given corrected to one place of decimals or to four significant figures for relative weights of less than 100.

Pharmaceutical Information

Information on the chemical and physical properties of each substance is given where available and where it is likely to be of use or interest. Compared with earlier editions, this information has been much reduced and included only when it is certain that it applies to the form of substance being described in the monograph. Discrepancies in properties as described in the *B.P.* and *U.S.P.* are indicated.

PERCENTAGE STRENGTHS. Unless otherwise stated, solutions of solids in liquids are expressed as percentage w/v, of liquids in liquids as percentage v/v, and of gases in liquids as percentage w/w.

SOLUBILITY. The figures given for solubility in each monograph have generally been obtained from the major pharmacopoeias in which the substance is described, but should not be considered absolute. Unless otherwise indicated in the text, the figures are for solubility at 'ordinary room temperature' which is considered to be about 20°. Where solubilities are given in words, the following terms describe the indicated solubility ranges:

solubility	
very soluble	1 in less than 1
freely soluble	1 in 1 to 1 in 10
soluble	1 in 10 to 1 in 30
sparingly soluble	1 in 30 to 1 in 100
slightly soluble	1 in 100 to 1 in 1000
very slightly soluble	1 in 1000 to 1 in 10 000
practically insoluble	1 in more than 10 000

STORAGE. Substances and preparations should be stored under conditions which prevent contamination and diminish deterioration, and the conditions of storage given in the text indicate the precautions recommended in specific cases. Where authorities differ, we have included the most stringent storage requirement. The term 'a cool place' is generally used to describe a place in which the temperature does not exceed 15°. Unless otherwise specified, all injections should be stored in alkali-free containers.

TEMPERATURE. Temperatures are expressed in degrees Celsius (centigrade) unless otherwise indicated.

Pharmacological and Therapeutic Information

Information on the adverse effects, treatment of adverse effects, precautions, absorption and fate, and uses and administration of each substance is provided by concise statements and these are elaborated and expanded by referenced reviews and abstracts from papers and other publications.

This edition contains about 35 500 abstracts or reviews based on information in an ever widening range of publications. In making our selection, we have tried to include the key papers. Where there has been a large body of work, abstracts of some typical papers have been provided with perhaps a selection of references. However, room has also been made for the interesting letter or case report where it is felt that information on a rare effect or action may be useful to the reader.

Much information has been found in sources such as World Health Organization publications, government reports and legislation, and other official and standard publications. Manufacturers' literature has been considered in the light of other available information.

The risks of administering drugs in pregnancy are well known and the general principle is to give a drug only when the benefit to the individual mother outweighs the risk to the foetus. Where there is a clear risk it is noted under the Precautions or Adverse Effects heading but safety should not be inferred from the absence of a statement for any drug.

Interactions are described under the Precautions heading with detailed information being provided in the monograph for the drug that is being affected.

Doses

Doses are described under the Uses and Administration heading with as much detail as is necessary and available. Unless otherwise stated the doses represent the average range of quantities which are generally regarded as suitable for adults when administered by mouth. More information on doses and drug administration may be given in the abstracts and under the Preparations sections. Unless otherwise specified, glucose injection is 5% w/v, sodium chloride injection is 0.9% w/v, and water is purified water.

When doses for children are expressed as a range of quantities within specified age limits, the lower dose applies at the lower age and the higher dose at the higher age.

Formulas

Official preparations are included from current editions of the *British Pharmacopoeia* and the *United States Pharmacopoeia* and *National Formulary*. Preparations from the *British Pharmaceutical Codex 1973* are included if still relevant and not covered by the *British Pharmacopoeia*. Preparations have also been included from the *Australian Pharmaceutical Formulary and Handbook*. The synonyms sometimes included for these preparations may be official synonyms or synonyms that are or have been in common use.

Proprietary Preparations

In Parts 1 and 2, the information on proprietary preparations available in the *UK* is presented with each product being described in the proprietary preparations section of the monograph on its principal ingredient.

Lists of the proprietary names of single-ingredient preparations have been provided for a range of countries including the *UK*. Proprietary names of multi-ingredient preparations have also been included for some countries under the monograph for each of the significant active ingredients. Minor ingredients have not been included.

Readers should be aware that these lists are provided for the purposes of identification. They thus include the names of discontinued preparations as well as names for products registered but still to be marketed.

Acknowledgements

The Editor gratefully acknowledges the advice and assistance of the many experts who have suggested amendments to the text of Martindale. Special thanks are due to Heather M. Elliston, Margaret J. Gilmour, and P. Rowe for reading and commenting on drafts of this edition.

The Editor is grateful to the many organisations that have helped in providing information, including the British Pharmacopoeia Commission, the Medicines Division of the *UK* Department of Health, and the World Health Organization.

Martindale staff have been able to call freely on the expertise of other members of the Royal Pharmaceutical Society's staff. In particular the Editor is grateful to A. Wade, the General Editor, Anne B. Prasad and the editorial staff of the British National Formulary, and Pamela M. North and the staff of the library and information department.

Juliet Kahofer and Gail Neathercoat were assigned to work temporarily on Martindale and their efforts were invaluable. Thanks are also due to Janet M. Batson, P. Gotecha, Chloe Loewe and D. Shenton, who assisted for some of the period of revision, and to B. J. Yates the Society's publisher. Once again B. Tarry of Peter Peregrinus Ltd helped with some of the computer processing and this is gratefully acknowledged.

The contents of this 29th Edition were planned, written, checked, indexed, keyed, and proofed by the Martindale staff. It could not have been produced without that staff's commitment. The Editor welcomes this opportunity to record his gratitude and appreciation of the dedicated services of the clerical staff, Jacqueline O. Baines and Doris D. Moore, and of the editorial staff: Eileen J. Aitchison, P. S. Blake, A. G. Desson, Kathleen Eager, Wendy M. Farenden, Anne M. P. Gilchrist, Ann Harris, Susan L. Jefferson, Julie M. McGlashan, Rosalind McLarney, and J. Martin. Finally, the Editor is indebted to the Assistant Editors, Anne V. Parsons and S. C. Sweetman, and especially the Deputy Editor, Kathleen Parfitt, for invaluable assistance and support.

London
October 1988

Abbreviations

For abbreviations of the names of manufacturers or their distributors, see Directory of Manufacturers, p.1645.

≈—approximately equals.
α—alpha. Also used in radiation data for alpha particles.
A—ampere(s).
Å—ångström(s).
aa—*ana*, 'of each'.
ABPI—Association of the British Pharmaceutical Industry.
ADI—acceptable daily intake.
Afghan.—Afghanistan.
agg.—aggregate (in botanical names), including 2 or more species which resemble each other closely.
AIDS—acquired immune deficiency syndrome.
Ala—alanine.
Alg.—Algeria.
a.m.—*ante meridiem*, 'before noon'.
AMA—American Medical Association.
A.P.F.—Australian Pharmaceutical Formulary and Handbook, 1988.
Arg—arginine.
Arg.—Argentina, Argentine, *or* Argentinian.
Arg. P.—Argentinian Pharmacopoeia 1966 (Farmacopea Nacional Argentina, Quinta Edicion).
Asn—asparagine.
Asp—aspartic acid.
Aust.—Austria *or* Austrian.
Aust. P.—Austrian Pharmacopoeia 1981 (Österreichisches Arzneibuch).
Austral.—Australia.
β^+—beta particles: positrons.
β^-—beta particles: electrons.
B.—*Bacillus, Bacteroides,* or *Bordetella.*
BAN—British Approved Name.
BANM—British Approved Name Modified.
Barb.—Barbados.
Belg.—Belgium *or* Belgian.
Belg. P.—Belgian Pharmacopoeia 1982 (Pharmacopée Belge, Sixième Edition).
B.N.F.—British National Formulary.
Bol.—Bolivia.
Born.—Borneo.
B.P.—British Pharmacopoeia. Unless otherwise specified in the text, *B.P.* references are to the 1988 Edn.
b.p.—boiling point.
B.P. Vet.—British Pharmacopoeia (Veterinary) 1985.
B.P.C.—British Pharmaceutical Codex.
Bq—becqúerel(s).
Br.—British *or Brucella.*
Braz.—Brazil *or* Brazilian.
Braz. P.—Brazilian Pharmacopoeia 1977 (Farmacopéia Brasileira, 3ª Edição).
BS—British Standard (specification).
BSI—British Standards Institution.
Bulg.—Bulgaria.
BUN—Blood-urea-nitrogen.
B. Vet. C.—British Veterinary Codex.
°C—degrees Celsius (centigrade). Unless otherwise indicated in the text, temperatures are expressed in this thermometric scale.
C.—*Campylobacter, Candida,* or *Corynebacterium.*
Canad.—Canada.
CAS—Chemical Abstracts Service.
CCID50—cell-culture-infective dose 50 (the dose of the micro-organism which infects 50% of cell cultures inoculated).
Chin.—Chinese.
Chin. P.—Chinese Pharmacopoeia 1985.
CI—Colour Index.
Ci—curie(s).
CIA—Chemical Industries Association (UK).
Cl.—*Clostridium.*
CM—Chick-Martin (coefficient).
cm—centimetre(s).
cm^2—square centimetre(s).
cm^3—cubic centimetre(s).
CNS—central nervous system.
Col.—Colombia.
cP—centipoise(s).
CRM—Committee on the Review of Medicines (UK).
CSF—cerebrospinal fluid.
CSM—Committee on Safety of Medicines (UK).
cSt—centistokes.
Curac.—Curaçao.
Cys—cysteine.
Cz.—Czechoslovakia, Czechoslovak, *or* Czechoslovakian.
Cz. P.—Czechoslovak Pharmacopoeia 1987 (Československý Lékopis, Vydání čtvrté; Pharmacopoea Bohemoslovaca, Editio quarta).
D & C—designation applied in USA to dyes permitted for use in drugs and cosmetics.
d.c.—direct current.
Denm.—Denmark.
DHSS—Department of Health and Social Security (UK).
DNA—deoxyribonucleic acid.
Dom. Rep.—Dominican Republic.
D.P.F.—Dental Practitioners' Formulary.
D.T.F.—Drug Tariff Formulary: Drug Tariff, 1988 (National Health Service, Department of Health and Social Security, UK).
E.—*Escherichia.*
EC—electron capture.
ECG—electrocardiogram.
ECT—electroconvulsive therapy.
Ecuad.—Ecuador.
Ed.—editor(s) *or* edited by.
Edn—edition.
EEC—European Economic Community.
EEG—electro-encephalogram.
e.g.—*exempli gratia*, 'for example'.
Egypt. P.—Egyptian Pharmacopoeia, 3rd Edn, 1984.
EID50—egg-infective dose 50 (the dose of the micro-organism which infects 50% of the eggs inoculated).
El Salv.—El Salvador.
ENL—erythema nodosum leprosum.
ENT—ear, nose and throat.
ESR—erythrocyte sedimentation-rate.
et al.—*et alii*, 'and others': for three or more co-authors or co-workers.
Eur.—European.

Eur. P.—European Pharmacopoeia, 2nd Edn, Fascicules 1 to 11.
eV—electronvolt(s).
Ext. D & C—designation applied in USA to dyes permitted for use in external drug and cosmetic preparations.
°F—degrees Fahrenheit.
FAC—Food Additives and Contaminants Committee of the Ministry of Agriculture, Fisheries and Food (UK).
FAO—Food and Agriculture Organization of the United Nations.
FAO/WHO—Food and Agriculture Organization of the United Nations *and the* World Health Organization.
FDA—Food and Drug Administration of USA.
FdAC—Food Advisory Committee of the Ministry of Agriculture, Fisheries and Food (UK).
F D & C—designation applied in USA to dyes permitted for use in foods, drugs, and cosmetics.
FDD—Food and Drug Directorate of Canada.
FEV_1—forced expiratory volume in 1 second.
Fin.—Finland.
fL—femtolitre(s).
fl oz—fluid ounce(s).
f.p.—freezing point.
FPA—Family Planning Association (UK).
Fr.—France *or* French.
Fr. P.—French Pharmacopoeia 1982 (Pharmacopée Française, Xe Edition) and Supplements 1 to 3.
FSC—Food Standards Committee of the Ministry of Agriculture, Fisheries and Food (UK).
ft—foot (feet).
ft^2—square foot (feet).
γ—gamma. Also used in radiation data for gamma-radiation.
g—gram(s).
gal—gallon(s).
Ger.—W. Germany *or* W. German.
Ger. P.—West German Pharmacopoeia 1986 (Deutsches Arzneibuch, 9 Ausgabe).
GFR—glomerular filtration-rate.
Gib.—Gibraltar.
Gln—glutamine.
Glu—glutamic acid.
Gly—glycine.
GRAS—generally recognised as safe. A designation applied to food additives.
Guat.—Guatemala.
Gy—Gray.
H.—Haemophilus.
Hb—haemoglobin.
HDL—high-density lipoproteins.
His—histidine.
HIV—human immunodeficiency virus.
HLB—hydrophilic-lipophilic balance.
Hond.—Honduras.
Hung.—Hungary *or* Hungarian.
Hung. P.—VIth Hungarian Pharmacopoeia 1967 (Magyar Gyógyszerkönyv).
Hz—hertz.
IAEA—International Atomic Energy Agency.
ibid.—ibidem, 'in the same place (journal or book)'.
ICRP—International Commission on Radiological Protection.
ICRU—International Commission on Radiation Units and Measurements.
idem—'the same': used for the same authors and titles.
i.e.—*id est,* 'that is'.
Ig—immunoglobulin.
Ile—isoleucine.
in—inch(es)
in^2—square inch(es).
Ind.—India *or* Indian.
Ind. P.—Pharmacopoeia of India, 3rd Edn, 1985.
Indon.—Indonesia.
INN—International Nonproprietary Name.
Int.—International.
Int. P.—International Pharmacopoeia (Specifications for the Quality Control of Pharmaceutical Preparations, 2nd Edn, 1967, and 3rd Edn, 1981, Volume 1).
IQ—intelligence quotient.
i.r.—infra-red.
ISO—International Organization for Standardization.
IT—isomeric transition.
It.—Italian.
It. P.—Italian Pharmacopoeia 1985 (Farmacopea Ufficiale della Repubblica Italiana, Edizione) Nona.
Ital.—Italy.
iu—international unit(s).
IUB—International Union of Biochemistry.
IUD—intra-uterine device.
IUPAC—International Union of Pure and Applied Chemistry.
J—joule(s).
Jam.—Jamaica.
Jpn—Japan *or* Japanese.
Jpn P.—The Pharmacopoeia of Japan, 11th Edn, 1986.
Jug.—Jugoslav *or* Jugoslavian.
Jug. P.—Jugoslav Pharmacopoeia 1984 (Farmakopeja SFRJ; Pharmacopoea Jugoslavica, Editio Quarta).
K—kelvin.
kcal—kilocalorie(s).
keV—kiloelectronvolt(s).
kg—kilogram(s).
kJ—kilojoule(s).
Kleb.—Klebsiella.
Kor.—Korea.
kPa—kilopascal(s).
L.—Listeria.
lb—pound(s) avoirdupois.
LD50—a dose lethal to 50% of the specified animals or micro-organisms.
LDL—low-density lipoproteins.
Leu—leucine.
Lf—limit flocculation.
loc. cit.—*loco citato,* 'in the place cited'.
Lux.—Luxembourg.
Lys—lysine.
m—metre(s).
m^2—square metre(s).
m^3—cubic metre(s).
M—molar.
M.—Mycobacterium or *Mycoplasma.*
mA—milliampere(s).
Malay.—Malaysia.
MAOI—monoamine oxidase inhibitor.
max.—maximum.
MBC—minimum bactericidal concentration.
mCi—millicurie(s).
mEq—milliequivalent(s).
Met—methionine.
MeV—megaelectronvolt(s).
Mex.—Mexico *or* Mexican.
Mex. P.—Mexican Pharmacopoeia 1952 (Farmacopea Nacional de los Estados Unidos Mexicanos, Segunda Edicion).
mg—milligram(s).

MIC—minimum inhibitory concentration.
min—minute.
min.—minimum.
Mj—megajoule(s).
mL—millilitre(s).
mm—millimetre(s).
mm^2—square millimetre(s).
mm^3—cubic millimetre(s).
mmHg—millimetre(s) of mercury.
mmol—millimole.
mol—mole.
mol. wt—molecular weight.
Mon.—Monaco.
Mor.—Morocco.
mosmol—milliosmole.
m.p.—melting point.
Mrad—megarad.
MRC—Medical Research Council (UK).
mrem—millirӧntgen-equivalent-man.
μCi—microcurie(s).
μg—microgram(s).
μL—microlitre(s).
μm—micrometre(s).
N.—*Neisseria.*
nCi—nanocurie(s).
NCTC—National Collection of Type Cultures (Central Public Health Laboratory, London, England).
Neth.—The Netherlands.
Neth. P.—Netherlands Pharmacopoeia 1983 (Nederlandse Farmacopee, Negende Uitgave) and Supplements to 1985.
ng—nanogram(s).
NIH—National Institutes of Health (USA).
nm—nanometre(s).
Nord.—Nordic.
Nord. P.—Nordic Pharmacopoeia 1963 (Pharmacopoea Nordica) including all addenda published up to 1976.
Norw.—Norway.
NPU—National Pharmaceutical Union, now the National Pharmaceutical Association (NPA).
NRPB—National Radiological Protection Board, Harwell, Oxfordshire, England.
NZ—New Zealand.
OECD—Organisation for Economic Co-operation and Development.
OP—over proof.
o/w—oil-in-water.
oz—ounce(s).
P—probability.
Pa—pascal(s).
Parag.—Paraguay.
PBI—protein-bound iodine.
pCO—plasma partial pressure (concentration) of carbon dioxide.
p_aCO_2—arterial plasma partial pressure (concentration) of carbon dioxide.
per—'through'.
pg—picogram(s).
pH—the negative logarithm of the hydrogen ion concentration.
Phe—phenylalanine.
Pharm. Soc. Lab. Rep.—Royal Pharmaceutical Society's Laboratory Report.
Philipp.—Philippines.
pINN—Proposed International Nonproprietary Name.
pINNM—Proposed International Nonproprietary Name Modified.
pK_a—the negative logarithm of the dissociation constant.
p.m.—*post meridiem,* 'afternoon'.
pO_2—plasma partial pressure (concentration) of oxygen.
p_aO_2—arterial plasma partial pressure (concentration) of oxygen.
Pol.—Poland *or* Polish.
Pol. P.—Polish Pharmacopoeia 1965 (Farmakopea Polska IV).
Port.—Portugal *or* Portuguese.
Port. P.—Portuguese Pharmacopoeia 1946 (Farmacopeia Portuguesa IV) and Supplements 1961 and 1967.
ppm—parts per million.
Pr.—*Proteus.*
P.R.—Puerto Rico.
Pro—proline.
Ps.—*Pseudomonas.*
PSGB—The Pharmaceutical Society of Great Britain. Now the Royal Pharmaceutical Society of Great Britain.
q.s.—*quantum sufficit,* 'as much as suffices'.
q.v.—*quod vide,* 'which see'.
R—rӧntgen.
rad—radiation absorbed dose.
RCGP—Royal College of General Practitioners (UK).
REM sleep—rapid-eye-movement sleep.
rem—rӧntgen-equivalent-man.
rINN—Recommended International Nonproprietary Name.
rINNM—Recommended International Nonproprietary Name Modified.
RNA—ribonucleic acid.
Roum.—Roumanian.
Roum. P.—Roumanian Pharmacopoeia 1976 (Farmacopeea Românǎ. Editia A. IX-A).
Rus.—Russian.
Rus. P.—Russian Pharmacopoeia (State Pharmacopoeia of the USSR, Tenth Edition).
RW—Rideal-Walker (coefficient).
S.—*Salmonella* or *Serratia.*
S. Afr.—South Africa.
SCI—Society of Chemical Industry (UK).
Ser—serine.
SGOT—serum glutamic oxaloacetic transaminase (serum aspartate aminotransferase *now preferred*).
SGPT—serum glutamic pyruvic transaminase (serum alanine aminotransferase *now preferred*).
Sh.—*Shigella.*
SI—Statutory Instrument *or* Système International d'Unités (International System of Units).
SLE—systemic lupus erythematosus.
sp.—species (plural spp.).
sp. gr.—specific gravity.
Span.—Spanish.
Span. P.—Spanish Pharmacopoeia 1954 (Farmacopea Oficial Española, Novena Edicion).
St—stokes.
Staph.—*Staphylococcus.*
Str.—*Streptococcus.*
Suppl.—supplement(s).
Sv—sievert.
Swed.—Sweden.
Swiss P.—Swiss Pharmacopoeia 1987 (Pharmacopoea Helvetica, Editio Septima, Edition Française).
Switz.—Switzerland.
Tanz.—Tanzania.
TCID—tissue-culture-infective dose.
TCID50—tissue-culture-infective dose 50 (the dose of the micro-organism which infects 50% of tissue cultures inoculated).
Thai.—Thailand.
Thr—threonine.

TPN—total parenteral nutrition.
Trp—tryptophan.
Tun.—Tunisia.
Turk.—Turkey *or* Turkish.
Turk. P.—Turkish Pharmacopoeia 1974 (Türk Farmakopesi).
Tyr—tyrosine.
UK—United Kingdom.
UKAEA—United Kingdom Atomic Energy Authority.
UP—under proof.
Urug.—Uruguay.
US and *USA*—United States of America.
USAID—United States Agency for International Development.
USAN—United States Adopted Name.
U.S.N.F.—The United States 'National Formulary XVI', 1985, and Supplements 1 to 7.
U.S.P.—The United States Pharmacopeia XXI, 1985, and Supplements 1 to 7.
U.S.P. units—units defined in the United States Pharmacopeia.
USSR—Union of Soviet Socialist Republics.
u.v.—ultraviolet.
V—volt(s).
V.—*Vibrio.*
Val—valine.
var.—variety.
Venez.—Venezuela.
Viet.—Vietnam.
VLDL—very low-density lipoproteins.
vol.—volume(s).
v/v—volume in volume.
v/w—volume in weight.
WHO—World Health Organization.
w/o—water-in-oil.
wt—weight.
wt per mL—weight per millilitre.
w/v—weight in volume.
w/w—weight in weight.
Y.—*Yersinia.*

Contracted Names for Ions and Groups

Contracted Name	*Chemical Name*
acetonide	isopropylidene ether of a dihydric alcohol
aceturate	*N*-acetylglycinate
amsonate	4,4′-diaminostilbene-2,2′-disulphonate
axetil	1-acetoxyethyl
besylate (besilate)	benzenesulphonate
bunapsylate (bunapsilate)	3,7-di-*tert*-butylnaphthalene-1,5-disulphonate
camsylate (camsilate)	camphor-10-sulphonate
caproate	hexanoate
carbesilate	4-carboxybenzenesulphonate
closylate (closilate)	4-chlorobenzenesulphonate
cromacate	[(6-hydroxy-4-methyl-2-oxo-2*H*-chromen-7-yl)oxy]acetate
cromesilate	6,7-dihydroxycoumarin-4-methanesulphonate
cyclotate (ciclotate)	4-methylbicyclo[2.2.2]oct-2-ene-1-carboxylate
cypionate (cipionate)	3-cyclopentylpropionate
dibudinate	2,6-di-*tert*-butylnaphthalene-1,5-disulphonate
dibunate	2,6-di-*tert*-butyl-1-naphthalenesulphonate
diolamine	diethanolamine
edetate	ethylenediamine-*NNN′N′*-tetra-acetate
edisylate (edisilate)	ethane-1,2-disulphonate
embonate	4,4′-methylenebis(3-hydroxy-2-naphthoate) (=pamoate)
enanthate (enantate)	heptanoate
estolate	propionate dodecyl sulphate
esylate (esilate)	ethanesulphonate
fendizoate	2-[(2′-hydroxy-4-biphenylyl)-carbonyl]benzoate
gluceptate	glucoheptonate
hybenzate (hibenzate)	2-(4-hydroxybenzoyl)benzoate
hyclate	monohydrochloride hemi-ethanolate hemihydrate
isethionate (isetionate)	2-hydroxyethanesulphonate
lauryl sulphate (laurilsulfate)	dodecyl sulphate
megallate	3,4,5-trimethoxybenzoate
meglumine	*N*-methylglucamine
mesylate (mesilate)	methanesulphonate
napadisylate (napadisilate)	naphthalene-1,5-disulphonate
napsylate (napsilate)	naphthalene-2-sulphonate
olamine	ethanolamine
oxoglurate	2-oxoglutarate
pamoate	4,4′-methylenebis(3-hydroxy-2-naphthoate) (=embonate)
phenpropionate	3-phenylpropionate
pivalate	trimethylacetate
pivoxetil	1-(2-methoxy-2-methyl-propionyloxy)ethyl
pivoxil	(2,2-dimethyl-1-oxopropoxy)-methyl or (pivaloyloxy)methyl
polistirex	sulphonated styrene-divinylbenzene copolymer complex
proxetil	1-[(isopropoxycarbonyl)-oxy]ethyl
steaglate	stearoyloxyacetate
tebutate	*tert*-butylacetate
tenoate	2-thiophenecarboxylate
teprosilate	3-(theophyllin-7-yl)propane-sulphonate
theoclate (teoclate)	8-chlorotheophyllinate
tofesilate	2-(theophyllin-7-yl)ethane-sulphonate
tosylate (tosilate)	toluene-4-sulphonate
triclofenate	2,4,5-trichlorophenolate
trolamine	triethanolamine
troxundate	3,6,9-trioxaundecanoate

Weights and Measures

The International System of Units

The International System of Units (Système International d'Unités; SI) was established by resolutions of the Eleventh General Conference on Weights and Measures, 1960; some additions and changes have been made by later resolutions. The SI units are of 3 types: *base; supplementary;* and *derived.* The base units for the seven physical quantities which are regarded as dimensionally independent, are:

metre (m) (length)
kilogram (kg) (mass)
second (s) (time)
ampere (A) (electric current)
kelvin (K) (thermodynamic temperature)
mole (mol) (amount of substance)
candela (cd) (luminous intensity)

There are supplementary units for plane angle (radian=rad) and solid angle (steradian=sr).

The derived unit for any other physical quantity is that obtained by the dimensionally appropriate multiplication and division of the base units. Many of the derived units have special names and symbols. They include:

hertz	$Hz=s^{-1}$	frequency
newton	$N=m\ kg\ s^{-2}$	force
pascal	$Pa=m^{-1}\ kg\ s^{-2}$	pressure
joule	$J=m^2\ kg\ s^{-2}$	energy
watt	$W=m^2\ kg\ s^{-3}$	power
coulomb	$C=s\ A$	quantity of electricity, electric charge
volt	$V=m^2\ kg\ s^{-3}\ A^{-1}$	electric potential
ohm	$\Omega=m^2\ kg\ s^{-3}\ A^{-2}$	electric resistance
siemens	$S=m^{-2}\ kg^{-1}\ s^3\ A^2$	electric conductance
farad	$F=m^{-2}\ kg^{-1}\ s^4\ A^2$	electric capacitance
degree Celsius	°C=K	Celsius temperature
becquerel	$Bq=s^{-1}$	activity of a radioactive source
gray	$Gy=m^2\ s^{-2}$	absorbed dose of ionising radiation
sievert	$Sv=m^2\ s^{-2}$	dose equivalent

Certain decimal multiples and submultiples of SI units have special authorised names and symbols. They include:

litre* ($1\ L=10^{-3}\ m^3$)	L	volume
tonne** ($1\ t=10^3\ kg$)	t	mass

* The definition, adopted in 1964, of the litre as 1 cubic decimetre represents a decrease from its former value of 1.000028 cubic decimetres. The litre should not be used for measurements of high precision.

** For the ton see the equivalent tables below.

In addition there are units which although not part of SI will continue to be used in appropriate contexts, such as the minute (min), hour (h), day (d) (time); and electronvolt (eV) (energy) and units which although not part of SI will continue in use for a limited time. They include:

ångström	Å	length
curie	Ci	activity of a radioactive source
rad	rad	absorbed dose of ionising radiation
röntgen	R	exposure to ionising radiation

The use of other units not part of SI is generally deprecated; the values of some that may be encountered are defined in the equivalent tables below.

In the European Communities a directive (80/181/EEC, as amended) requires, with various exceptions, that SI units be used as legal units of measurements and specifies dates after which some non-SI units may not be used.

The following prefixes may be used to construct decimal submultiples and multiples of units.

Factor	Prefix	Symbol
10^{-18}	atto	a
10^{-15}	femto	f
10^{-12}	pico	p
10^{-9}	nano	n
10^{-6}	micro	μ
10^{-3}	milli	m
10^{-2}	centi	c
10^{-1}	deci	d
10	deca	da
10^2	hecto	h
10^3	kilo	k
10^6	mega	M
10^9	giga	G
10^{12}	tera	T
10^{15}	peta	P
10^{18}	exa	E

Thousandfold multiples are to be preferred, e.g. gram, milligram, microgram, nanogram; μg per mL, mg per litre; joule, kilojoule, megajoule.

Millimoles and Milliequivalents

The mole (mol) is the amount of substance of a system which contains as many elementary entities (atoms, molecules, ions, electrons, or other particles or specified groups of such particles) as there are atoms in 0.012 kilogram of carbon-12. A millimole is one thousandth this amount and for ions is the ionic mass (the sum of the relative atomic masses of the elements of an ion) expressed in milligrams. A milliequivalent is this quantity divided by the valency of the ion.

1 Millimole (mmol) = 10^{-3} mole

For ions, 1 millimole (mmol) = 1 milliequivalent (mEq) × valency of the ion.

The following terms, though not strictly correct, are still in common use:

ionic weight, for ionic mass
atomic weight, for relative atomic mass
molecular weight, for relative molecular mass.

CONCENTRATION

In the SI units, concentration may be expressed either as mass concentration (e.g. g per dm^3, conventionally expressed as g per litre) or as 'amount of substance' concentration (e.g. mol per litre). A solution containing one mole per dm^3 is described as a 1 molar (1M) solution.

SI Unit Equivalents of Imperial and other Units

LENGTH

1 ångström (Å)	$=10^{-10}$ metre
1 micron	$=10^{-6}$ metre
1 inch (in)	$=2.54\times10^{-2}$ metre
1 foot (ft)	$=3.048\times10^{-1}$ metre
1 yard (yd)	$=9.144\times10^{-1}$ metre

MASS

1 grain (gr)	$=6.47989\times10^{-2}$ gram
1 ounce (avoirdupois) (oz) (=437.5 grains)	$=2.83495\times10$ grams
1 ounce (apothecaries') (=480 grains)	$=3.11035\times10$ grams
1 pound (avoirdupois)	$=4.53592\times10^2$ grams
1 ton	$=1.01605\times10^3$ kg

AREA

1 square inch (in^2)	$=6.4516\times10^{-4}$ square metre
1 square foot (ft^2)	$=9.29030\times10^{-2}$ square metre
1 square yard (yd^2)	$=8.36127\times10^{-1}$ square metre

VOLUME

1 millilitre (mL)	=1 cubic centimetre
1 cubic inch (in^3)	$=1.63871\times10^{-5}$ cubic metre
1 cubic foot (ft^3)	$=2.83168\times10^{-2}$ cubic metre
1 cubic yard (yd^3)	$=7.64555\times10^{-1}$ cubic metre
1 minim (UK)	$=5.91939\times10^{-8}$ cubic metre
1 fluid ounce (UK) (fl oz)	$=2.8413\times10^{-5}$ cubic metre
1 pint	$=5.68261\times10^{-4}$ cubic metre
1 gallon (UK)	$=4.54609\times10^{-3}$ cubic metre
1 fluid ounce (US)	$=2.95735\times10^{-5}$ cubic metre
1 liquid pint (US)	$=4.73176\times10^{-4}$ cubic metre
1 gallon (US)	$=3.78541\times10^{-3}$ cubic metre

ENERGY

1 kilocalorie, thermochemical (kcal)	$=4.1840\times10^3$ joules
1 erg (erg)	$=10^{-7}$ joule
1 electronvolt (eV)	$=1.60219\times10^{-19}$ joule
1 British thermal unit (Btu)	$=1.05506\times10^3$ joules

PRESSURE

1 millimetre of mercury (mmHg)	$=1.33322\times10^2$ pascals
1 pound-force per square inch	$=6.89476\times10^3$ pascals
1 atmosphere (atm)	$=1.01325\times10^5$ pascals

VISCOSITY, DYNAMIC

1 poise (P)	$=10^{-1}$ pascal second

VISCOSITY, KINEMATIC

1 stokes (St)	$=10^{-4}$ square metre per second

TEMPERATURE

1 degree Fahrenheit (°F)	$=\frac{5}{9}$ kelvin

Imperial and other Equivalents of SI Units

LENGTH

1 metre (m)	$=10^{10}$ ångströms 10^6 microns 39.3701 inches 3.28084 feet 1.09361 yards
1 kilometre (km)	=0.621372 mile

MASS

1 gram (g)	=15.4324 grains 0.032151 ounce (apothecaries') 0.035274 ounce (avoirdupois)
1 kilogram (kg)	=35.274 ounces (avoirdupois) 2.20462 pounds

AREA

1 square metre (m^2)	=1550 square inches 10.7639 square feet 1.196 square yards

VOLUME

1 cubic metre (m^3)	$=6.10236\times10^4$ cubic inches 35.3147 cubic feet 1.30795 cubic yards
1 cubic centimetre* (cm^3)	=16.8934 minims (UK)
1 cubic decimetre (dm^3)	=35.1952 fluid ounces 1.75976 pints 0.21997 gallon (UK)

*The abbreviations 'cc', 'ccm', and 'cu cm' should not be used.

FORCE

1 newton (N)	$=10^5$ dynes 1.01972×10^{-1} kilogram-force 7.23301 poundals

ENERGY

1 joule (J)	$=2.39006\times10^{-4}$ kilocalorie, thermo chemical 10^7 ergs 6.2415×10^{18} electronvolts 9.47813×10^{-4} British thermal units

PRESSURE

1 pascal (Pa)	$=7.50064\times10^{-3}$ millimetre of mercury 1.45038×10^{-4} pound-force per square inch 9.86923×10^{-6} atmosphere

VISCOSITY, DYNAMIC

1 pascal second (Pa s)	=10.0 poises

VISCOSITY, KINEMATIC

1 square metre per second (m^2 s^{-1})	$=10^4$ stokes

TEMPERATURE

1 kelvin (K)	$=\frac{9}{5}$ degrees Fahrenheit

SI Unit Equivalents of Radiation Units

ACTIVITY OF A RADIOACTIVE SOURCE

1 curie (Ci) = 3.7×10^{10} becquerels

ABSORBED DOSE OF IONISING RADIATION

1 rad (rad) = 10^{-2} gray

ABSORBED DOSE RATE

1 rad per second (rad s^{-1}) = 10^{-2} gray per second

EXPOSURE TO IONISING RADIATIONS

1 röntgen (R) = 2.58×10^{-4} coulomb per kilogram

DOSE EQUIVALENT

1 rem (rem) = 10^{-2} sievert

Radiation Unit Equivalents of SI Units

ACTIVITY OF A RADIOACTIVE SOURCE

1 becquerel (Bq) = 2.7027×10^{-11} curie

ABSORBED DOSE OF IONISING RADIATION

1 gray (Gy) = 100 rads

EXPOSURE TO IONISING RADIATIONS

1 coulomb per kilogram (C kg^{-1}) = 3.876×10^{3} röntgens

DOSE EQUIVALENT

1 sievert (Sv) = 100 rems

Dissociation Constants

The pK_a values given are for some of the drugs and ancillary substances included in Parts 1 and 2. They are derived from official publications and published papers, but as they are largely unconfirmed they should be taken as approximate values only. The temperature is specified where it is known.

Substance	pK_a
Acebutolol	9.4
Acepromazine	9.3
Acetanilide (25°)	0.6
Acetarsol	3.7
	7.9
	9.3
Acetazolamide (25°)	7.2
	9.0
Acetic Acid, Glacial (25°)	4.8
Acetylcysteine (30°)	9.5
Aconitine (25°)	8.1
Acriflavine (25°)	9.1
Adrenaline (20°)	8.7
	10.2
	12.0
Ajmaline	8.2
Alclofenac	4.6
Alfentanil	6.5
Allobarbitone (25°)	7.8
Allopurinol	9.4
Alphaprodine (20°)	8.7
Alprazolam	2.4
Alprenolol (20°)	9.5
Amantadine	10.4
Ametazole (20°)	2.2
	9.6
Amethocaine (20°)	8.5
Amidephrine	9.1
Amidopyrine (20°)	5.1
Amiloride	8.7
Aminacrine (25°)	9.5
Aminobenzoic Acid (25°)	2.4
	4.9
Aminocaproic Acid (25°)	4.4
	10.8
Aminocephalosporanic Acid (35°)	2.0
	4.4
Aminodeacetoxycephalosporanic Acid (35°)	3.0
	4.9
Aminohippuric Acid	3.6
Aminophylline	5.0
Aminopterin	5.5
Aminosalicylic Acid (20°)	
(−NH_2)	1.8
(−COOH)	3.6
Amiodarone	5.6
Amitriptyline (25°)	9.4
Amoxycillin	2.4
	7.4
	9.6
Amphetamine (20°)	9.9
Amphotericin	5.5
	10.0
Ampicillin (25°) (−COOH)	2.5
(−NH_2)	7.3

Substance	pK_a
Amylobarbitone (25°)	7.9
Amylocaine (25°)	8.4
Anileridine	3.7
	7.5
Aniline (25°)	4.6
Anisindione	4.1
Antazoline (25°)	2.5
	10.1
Apomorphine (15°)	7.2
	8.9
Aprindine	10.1
Aprobarbitone (25°)	8.0
Arecoline (20°)	7.4
Arsthinol	9.5
Ascorbic Acid (25°)	4.2
	11.6
Aspirin (25°)	3.5
Atenolol (24°)	9.6
Atropine (20°)	9.9
Azathioprine	8.2
Baclofen	3.9
	9.6
Bamethan (25°)	9.0
	10.2
Barbitone (25°)	8.0
Bemegride	11.6
Benactyzine	6.6
Bendrofluazide (25°)	8.5
Benoxaprofen	3.5
Benzaldehyde (25°)	7.4
Benzocaine (20°)	2.5
Benzoic Acid (25°)	4.2
Benzphetamine	6.6
Benzquinamide	5.9
Benztropine (20°)	10.0
Benzylmorphine (20°)	8.1
Benzylpenicillin (25°)	2.8
Betahistine	3.5
	9.7
Betaine (25°)	1.8
Bethanidine	10.6
(20°)	12.0
Boric Acid (25°)	9.2
Brilliant Green (25°)	7.9
Bromazepam	2.9
	11.0
Bromocriptine	4.9
Bromodiphenhydramine (25°)	8.6
Brompheniramine	3.9
Bromvaletone	10.8
Brucine (25°)	2.3
	8.0
Bupivacaine	8.1
Buprenorphine	8.5
	10.0
Butacaine	9.0

Substance	pK_a
Butalbital (20°)	7.6
Butobarbitone (25°)	8.0
Cacodylic Acid (25°)	1.6
	6.2
Caffeine (40°)	0.6
(25°)	14.0
Capreomycin	6.2
	8.2
	10.1
	13.3
Captopril	3.7
	9.8
Carbachol	4.8
Carbenicillin	2.6
	2.7
	3.3
Carbenoxolone	6.7
	7.1
Carbinoxamine (25°)	8.1
Carbonic Acid (25°)	6.4
	10.3
Carbutamide (20°)	6.0
Cathine (25°)	9.4
Cefapirin	2.2
Cefoperazone	2.6
Cefoxitin (25°)	3.5
Cefuroxime	2.5
Cephacetrile	2.0
Cephalexin	2.5
	5.2
	7.3
Cephaloglycin	1.9
	4.6
	7.1
Cephaloridine (35°)	1.7
	3.4
Cephalothin (35°)	2.2
Cephazolin (35°)	2.5
Cephradine (35°)	2.5
	7.3
Chloral Hydrate	10.0
Chlorambucil	5.8
	8.0
Chloramphenicol	5.5
Chlorcyclizine (25°)	2.4
	7.8
Chlordiazepoxide (20°)	4.6
Chlormethiazole	3.2
Chlorocresol (20°)	9.2
Chloroprocaine	8.7
Chloropyrilene (25°)	8.4
Chloroquine (20°)	8.4
	10.8
Chlorothiazide (20°)	6.7
	9.5

Chlorpheniramine	4.0
	9.2
Chlorphentermine	9.6
Chlorpromazine (20°)	9.3
Chlorpropamide (20°)	5.0
Chlorprothixene	8.8
Chlortetracycline (25°)	3.3
	7.4
	9.3
Chlorthalidone	9.4
Chlorzoxazone (20°)	8.0
Ciclacillin (25°)	2.7
Cimetidine	6.8
	7.1
Cinchocaine (20°)	7.5
	8.3
Citric Acid (25°)	3.1
	4.7
	6.4
Clebopride	7.6
Clindamycin (25°)	7.7
Clofibrate	3.0
Clonazepam	1.5
	10.5
Clonidine	8.2
Clorazepate	3.5
	12.5
Clotrimazole	4.7
Cloxacillin (25°)	2.7
Cocaine (20°)	8.6
Codeine (20°)	8.2
Colchicine	1.7
	12.4
m-Cresol (25°)	10.1
o-Cresol (25°)	10.3
p-Cresol (25°)	10.3
Crystal Violet (25°)	9.4
Cyacetazide (20°)	2.3
	11.2
Cyanocobalamin	3.3
Cyclizine	2.4
	7.8
Cyclobarbitone (20°)	7.6
Cyclopentamine	10.5
	11.5
Cyclopentolate	7.9
Cycloserine	4.5
	7.4
Cyclothiazide	9.1
	10.5
Cytarabine	4.3
Dacarbazine	4.4
Dantrolene	7.5
Dapsone	1.3
	2.5
Daunorubicin	8.2
Debrisoquine	11.9
Dehydrocholic Acid	5.1
Demeclocycline (25°)	3.3
	7.2
	9.2
Demoxepam	4.5
	10.6
Deserpidine	6.7
Desipramine (24°)	10.2

Desmethylchlordiazepoxide	4.4
Dexamphetamine	9.9
Dexchlorpheniramine (20°)	9.0
Dextromethorphan	8.3
Dextromoramide (25°)	7.1
Dextropropoxyphene	6.3
Diamorphine (23°)	7.6
Diatrizoic Acid (20°)	3.4
Diazepam (20°)	3.3
Diazoxide	8.5
Dichlorphenamide	7.4
	8.6
Dicloxacillin (25°)	2.7
Dicoumarol	4.4
	8.0
Diethazine (20°)	9.1
Diethylcarbamazine (20°)	7.7
Dihydrocodeine (25°)	8.8
Dihydroergocornine (24°)	6.9
Dihydroergocristine (24°)	6.9
Dihydroergocryptine (24°)	6.9
Dihydroergotamine (24°)	6.8
Dihydrostreptomycin	7.8
Diltiazem	7.7
Dimethyl Sulphoxide	2.2
	2.8
Dinoprost	4.9
Diodone (20°)	2.8
Diphenhydramine (25°)	9.0
Diphenoxylate	7.1
Dipipanone (25°)	8.5
Dipyridamole	6.4
Disopyramide	8.4
	9.6
Dixyrazine (25°)	7.8
Dobutamine	9.5
Dopamine (20°)	8.8
	10.6
Doxepin	8.0
	9.0
Doxorubicin	8.2
	10.2
Doxycycline (20°)	3.5
	7.7
	9.5
Doxylamine	4.4
	9.2
Dronabinol	10.6
Droperidol	7.6
Emetine (25°)	7.4
	8.3
Ephedrine (25°)	9.6
Ergometrine (20°)	6.8
(25°)	7.2
Ergotamine (24°)	6.3
Erythromycin	8.9
Ethacrynic Acid (20°)	3.5
Ethambutol (20°)	6.3
	9.5
Ethanolamine (25°)	9.4
Ethebenecid (25°)	3.3
Ethoheptazine	8.5
Ethopropazine (20°)	9.6
Ethosuximide (20°)	9.5
Ethyl Biscoumacetate	3.1

Ethylenediamine (20°)	7.2
	10.0
Ethylmorphine (20°)	8.2
Ethylnoradrenaline (25°)	8.4
Etidocaine	7.7
Etilefrine (25°)	9.0
	10.2
Etomidate	4.2
Fencamfamin (25°)	8.7
Fenclofenac	5.5
Fenfluramine (25°)	9.1
Fenoprofen (25°)	4.5
Fenoterol	8.5
	10.0
Fentanyl	7.8
	8.4
Floxuridine	7.7
Flucloxacillin	2.7
Flucytosine	2.9
	10.7
Flufenamic Acid	3.9
Flumizole	10.7
Flunitrazepam	1.8
Fluopromazine (24°)	9.2
Fluorouracil	8.0
	13.0
Fluphenazine	3.9
	8.1
Flurazepam	1.9
	8.2
Folic Acid	4.7
	6.8
	9.0
Folinic Acid	3.1
	4.8
	10.4
Fomocaine	7.1
Formaldehyde (25°)	13.3
Formic Acid (25°)	3.8
Frusemide (20°)	3.9
Fumaric Acid (25°)	3.0
	4.5
Fusidic Acid	5.4
Gentamicin	8.2
Glibenclamide	5.3
Gliclazide	5.8
Glucose	12.1
Glutethimide	4.5
	9.2
Glycerophosphoric Acid (25°)	1.5
	6.2
Glycine (25°)	2.3
	9.8
Guanethidine (20°)	8.3
	11.4
Guanoxan	12.3
Haloperidol	8.3
Harmine (20°)	7.6
Heptabarbitone (20°)	7.4
Hexachlorophane	5.7
Hexetidine	8.3
Hexobarbitone (20°)	8.2
Hippuric Acid (25°)	3.8
Histamine (25°)	5.9
	9.7

Homatropine (20°)	9.9
Hydralazine	0.5
	7.1
Hydrastine (25°)	6.2
Hydrochlorothiazide	7.0
	9.2
Hydrocodone (20°)	8.3
Hydrocortisone Sodium Succinate	5.1
Hydroflumethiazide (20°)	8.5
	10.0
Hydromorphone (20°)	8.2
Hydroxyamphetamine (25°)	9.3
p-Hydroxybenzoic Acid	4.5
Hydroxyquinoline (20°)	5.0
	9.9
Hydroxyzine	2.1
	7.1
Hyoscine (23°)	7.6
Hyoscyamine (21°)	9.7
Hypochlorous Acid (17°)	7.4
Ibomal (20°)	7.7
Ibuprofen	4.4
	5.2
Idoxuridine	8.3
Imipramine (24°)	9.5
Imipramine Oxide (20°)	4.7
Indapamide	8.3
Indomethacin	4.5
Indoprofen	5.8
Indoramin	7.7
Iodipamide	3.5
Iprindole	8.2
Isocarboxazid	10.4
Isoniazid (20°)	1.8
	3.5
	10.8
Isoprenaline (20°)	8.6
	10.1
	12.0
Isoxsuprine	8.0
	9.8
Kanamycin	7.2
Ketamine	7.5
Ketobemidone (20°)	8.7
Labetalol	7.4
Lactic Acid (25°)	3.9
Levallorphan	4.5
	6.9
Levamisole	8.0
Levodopa (25°)	2.3
	8.7
	9.7
	13.4
Levorphanol (20°)	8.2
Lignocaine (25°)	7.9
Lincomycin	7.5
Liothyronine	8.5
Lithium Carbonate (20°)	6.5
	10.3
Loperamide	8.7
Loprazolam (24°)	6.0
Lorazepam (20°)	1.3
	11.5
Loxapine	6.6
Lysergide	7.5

Mandelic Acid (25°)	3.4
Maprotiline	10.5
Mazindol	8.6
Mebhydrolin	6.7
Mecamylamine	11.3
Mecillinam	3.4
	8.9
Meclozine (25°)	3.1
	6.2
Medazepam (20°)	4.4
(37°)	6.2
Mefenamic Acid	4.2
Meglumine (20°)	9.5
Mepacrine (20°)	7.7
	10.3
Mephentermine	10.4
Mepivacaine (20°)	7.7
Mepyramine (25°)	4.0
	8.9
Mercaptomerin	3.7
	5.1
Mercaptopurine (20°)	7.7
	11.0
Metaraminol	8.6
Metformin (32°)	2.8
	11.5
Methacycline (20°)	3.1
	7.6
	9.5
Methadone (20°)	8.3
Methapyrilene (25°)	3.7
	8.9
Methaqualone	2.5
Metharbitone (20°)	8.3
Methazolamide	7.3
Methdilazine	7.5
Methetoin	8.1
Methicillin (25°)	2.8
L-Methionine	2.3
	9.2
Methohexitone	8.3
Methotrexate	3.8
	4.8
	5.6
Methotrimeprazine	9.2
Methoxamine (25°)	9.2
Methoxyphenamine	10.1
Methyclothiazide	9.4
Methyl Hydroxybenzoate (22°)	8.4
Methyl Nicotinate (22°)	3.1
Methylamphetamine	10.1
Methyldopa (25°) (−COOH)	2.2
(−OH)	9.2
($-NH_2$)	10.6
(−OH)	12.0
Methylene Blue	3.8
Methylephedrine (25°)	9.3
Methylergometrine (24°)	6.7
Methylphenidate	8.8
Methylphenobarbitone (20°)	7.8
Methylprednisolone	2.6
	6.0
Methylthiouracil (20°)	8.2
Methyprylone	12.0
Methysergide (24°)	6.6

Metoclopramide	7.3
	9.0
Metolazone	9.7
Metoprolol	9.7
Metronidazole	2.5
Mexiletine	9.1
Mianserin	7.1
Miconazole	6.7
Midazolam	6.2
Minocycline	2.8
	5.0
	7.8
	9.5
Minoxidil	4.6
Molindone (25°)	6.9
Morphine (20°)	8.0
	9.9
Mustine (25°)	6.4
Nafcillin (25°)	2.7
Naftidrofuryl (30°)	8.2
Nalidixic Acid	6.0
Nalorphine (20°)	7.8
Naloxone	7.9
Naphazoline (20°)	10.9
Naphthol (20°)	8.8
Naproxen (25°)	4.2
Narceine (20°)	3.8
Narcotine	6.2
Nealbarbitone (20°)	7.2
Nefopam	9.2
Neostigmine	12.0
Nicotinamide (20°)	3.3
Nicotine (25°)	3.1
	7.9
Nicotinic Acid (25°) (−N=)	2.0
(−COOH)	4.8
Nicoumalone	4.7
Nifenalol	8.8
Nikethamide (20°)	3.5
Nitrazepam (20°)	3.2
	10.8
Nitrofurantoin (25°)	7.2
Noradrenaline (20°)	8.6
	9.8
	12.0
Norcodeine	5.7
Nordazepam	3.5
	12.0
Nordefrin (20°)	8.8
	9.8
Normethadone	9.2
Nortriptyline	9.7
Noscapine (20°)	6.2
Novobiocin (25°)	4.2
	9.1
Obidoxime (25°)	7.6
	8.3
Opipramol	3.8
Orciprenaline (25°) (−OH)	9.0
(−NH−)	10.1
(−OH)	11.4
Ornidazole	2.6
Orphenadrine	8.4
Oxacillin	2.8

Oxalic Acid (25°)	1.2
	4.2
Oxazepam (20°)	1.7
	11.6
Oxazolam	5.3
	11.9
Oxedrine (25°) (−OH)	9.3
(−NH−)	10.2
Oxpentifylline	0.3
Oxprenolol	9.5
Oxycodone (20°)	8.9
Oxyfedrine (20°)	7.5
Oxymorphone	4.8
	8.5
	9.3
Oxyphenbutazone (22°)	4.7
Oxypurinol	7.7
Oxytetracycline (25°)	3.3
	7.3
	9.1
Pamaquin	8.7
Papaverine (25°)	6.4
Paracetamol (25°)	9.5
Parachlorophenol (20°)	9.2
Parathiazine	8.9
	9.4
Pargyline	6.9
Pecazine (24°)	9.7
Pemoline	10.5
Pempidine	2.8
	11.0
Penicillamine	1.8
	7.9
	10.5
Pentazocine (20°)	8.5
	10.0
Pentobarbitone (20°)	8.0
Perphenazine (24°)	3.7
	7.8
Pethidine (20°)	8.7
Phenacetin	2.2
Phenadoxone (20°)	6.9
Phenazocine	8.5
Phenazone (25°)	1.5
Phencyclidine	8.5
Phendimetrazine	7.6
Phenethicillin (25°)	2.7
Phenformin (32°)	2.7
	11.8
Phenindamine (25°)	8.3
Phenindione	4.1
Pheniramine (25°)	4.2
	9.3
Phenmetrazine (25°)	8.4
Phenobarbitone (25°)	7.4
Phenol (25°)	10.0
Phenolphthalein (25°)	9.7
Phenolsulphonphthalein	7.9
Phenoxymethylpenicillin (25°)	2.7
Phentermine	10.1
Phentolamine	7.7
Phenylbutazone (20°)	4.4
Phenylephrine (20°) (−OH)	8.9
(−NH−)	10.1
Phenylmercuric Nitrate (20°)	3.3
Phenylmethylbarbituric Acid (25°)	7.7
Phenylpropanolamine (20°)	9.4
Phenyltoloxamine	9.1
Phenyramidol	5.9
Phenytoin (25°) (−OH)	8.3
Pholcodine (37°)	8.0
	9.3
Pholedrine (25°)	9.4
Phosphoric Acid (25°)	2.1
	7.2
	12.7
Physostigmine (25°)	1.8
	7.9
Pilocarpine (15°)	1.6
	7.1
Pimozide	7.3
	8.6
Pindolol	8.8
(24°)	9.7
Pipamazine	8.6
Piperazine (25°)	5.6
	9.8
Pirbuterol	3.0
	7.0
	10.3
Pirenzepine	2.1
	8.1
Pivampicillin	7.0
Pivmecillinam	8.9
Pizotifen	7.0
Polymyxin B	8.9
Practolol (20°)	9.5
Pralidoxime (25°)	8.0
Prazepam	2.7
Prazosin	6.5
Prilocaine (25°)	7.9
Probenecid (20°)	3.4
Procainamide (20°)	9.2
Procaine (25°)	9.0
Procarbazine	6.8
Prochlorperazine	3.7
	8.1
Proguanil (22.5°)	2.3
	10.4
Promazine (25°)	9.4
Promethazine (25°)	9.1
Propicillin (25°)	2.7
Propiomazine	6.6
Propionic Acid	4.9
Propoxycaine	8.6
Propranolol	9.5
Propyl Hydroxybenzoate (22°)	8.4
Propylhexedrine (25°)	10.7
Propylthiouracil (20°)	8.3
Prothipendyl (25°)	2.3
Pseudoephedrine	9.8
Pyrantel (20°)	11.0
Pyrazinamide	0.5
Pyridoxine (25°) (−N=)	5.0
(−OH)	9.0
Pyrimethamine (20°)	7.0
Pyrrobutamine (25°)	8.8
Quinalbarbitone (20°)	7.9
Quinethazone	9.3
	10.7
Quinidine (20°)	4.2
	8.8
Quinine (20°)	4.1
	8.5
Ranitidine	2.3
	8.2
Reserpine (25°)	6.6
Resorcinol (20°)	9.5
	10.1
Riboflavine (20°)	1.9
	10.2
Riboflavine Phosphate (Sodium Salt) (20°)	2.5
	6.5
	10.3
Rifampicin	1.7
	7.9
Rimiterol	8.7
	10.3
Rolitetracycline	7.4
Salbutamol	9.3
	10.3
Salicylamide (37°)	8.2
Salicylic Acid (25°)	3.0
	13.4
Salsalate (25°)	3.5
	9.8
Secbutobarbitone (20°)	8.0
Serotonin	9.1
	9.8
Sodium Calciumedetate (20°)	2.0
	2.7
	6.2
	10.3
Sodium Cromoglycate (20°)	2.5
Sodium Monofluorophosphate (20°)	2.5
	4.5
Sotalol	8.3
	9.8
Spectinomycin	7.0
	8.7
Spiramycin	8.0
Strychnine (25°)	2.3
	8.0
Sulfamerazine (25°)	7.1
Sulfametopyrazine	7.0
Sulfaquinoxaline (20°)	5.5
Sulindac	4.5
Sulphacetamide	1.8
	5.4
Sulphadiazine (25°)	6.5
Sulphadimethoxine (25°)	5.9
Sulphadimidine (25°)	7.4
Sulphaethidole	5.6
Sulphafurazole (25°)	4.9
Sulphaguanidine	11.3
	12.1
Sulphamethizole (25°)	5.3
Sulphamethoxazole (25°)	5.6
Sulphamethoxydiazine	7.0
Sulphamethoxypyridazine (25°)	7.2
Sulphamoxole	7.4
Sulphanilamide (20°)	10.4
Sulphaphenazole	6.5
Sulphapyridine (25°)	8.4

Sulphasalazine	0.6
	2.4
	9.7
	11.8
Sulphasomidine (27°)	7.5
Sulphathiazole (25°)	7.1
Sulphinpyrazone (22°)	2.8
Sulpiride	8.9
Sulthiame	10.0
Suprofen	3.9
Talbutal (20°)	7.9
Tartaric Acid (25°)	3.0
	4.4
Taurine (25°)	1.5
Temazepam	1.6
Terbutaline (20°)	8.7
	10.0
	11.0
Tetracycline (25°) (acidic)	3.3
(acidic)	7.7
(basic)	9.7
Tetramisole (20°)	7.8
Thebaine (20°)	8.2
Thenyldiamine (25°)	3.9
	8.9
Theobromine (25°)	<1
	10.0
Theophylline (25°)	<1
	8.6
Thiamine	4.8
	9.0
Thiamphenicol	7.2
Thiamylal	7.5
Thiopentone (20°)	7.6
Thiopropazate (24°)	7.3
Thioridazine (24°)	9.5
Thiouracil (25°)	7.5
Thonzylamine (25°)	2.1
	8.9
Thyroxine	2.2
	6.7
	10.0
Tiaprofenic Acid	3.0
Ticarcillin	2.5
	3.4
Tienilic Acid (25°)	2.7
Timolol	8.8
Tobramycin	6.7
	8.3
	9.9
Tocainide	7.8
Tolamolol	9.2
Tolazamide	3.5
	5.7
Tolazoline (20°)	10.6
Tolbutamide (25°)	5.3
Tolmetin	3.5
Tranexamic Acid (20°)	4.5
	10.5
Tranylcypromine	8.2
Triamterene	6.2
Trichlormethiazide	8.6
Trichloroacetic Acid (25°)	<1
Triethanolamine (25°)	7.8
Trifluoperazine (24°)	8.1
Trimethobenzamide	8.3
Trimethoprim	7.2
Trimustine (25°)	4.4
Tripelennamine (25°)	3.9
	9.0
Triprolidine	6.5
Trometamol (20°)	8.2
Tropacocaine (15°)	9.7
Tropicamide	5.2
Tuaminoheptane	10.5
Tubocurarine (22°)	8.0
	9.2
Urea (25°)	0.2
Valproic Acid	5.0
Vanillin (20°)	7.4
Viloxazine	8.1
Vinbarbitone (20°)	7.5
Vinblastine	5.4
	7.4
Vincristine	5.0
	7.4
Vindesine	5.4
	7.4
Viomycin	8.2
	10.3
Warfarin (20°)	5.0
Zimeldine	3.8

Determination of Body Surface Area from Height and Weight

Because of the variable relationship between the size and weight of patients it is sometimes more satisfactory to adjust dosage of medicaments to body surface area rather than to weight. The average normal body surface area for an adult man is 1.8 square metres. The following table sets out the relationship between the three functions, height (in centimetres), weight (in kilograms), and body surface area (in square metres). The values given are calculated from the formula of Dubois and Dubois (*Archs intern. Med.*, 1916, *17*, 863),

$$S = W^{0.425} \times H^{0.725} \times 71.84 \text{ (a constant)},$$

where S = surface area in square centimetres (expressed in the table as square metres), W = weight in kilograms, and H = height in centimetres.

Height cm	90	95	100	105	110	115	120	125	130	135	140	145	150	155	160	165	170	175	180	185	190	195
Weight kg																						
12.5	0.55	0.57	0.59	0.61																		
15	0.59	0.62	0.64	0.66	0.69	0.71																
17.5	0.63	0.66	0.68	0.71	0.73	0.76	0.78															
20	0.67	0.70	0.72	0.75	0.78	0.80	0.83	0.85	0.88													
22.5			0.76	0.79	0.82	0.84	0.87	0.89	0.92	0.95												
25				0.82	0.85	0.88	0.91	0.94	0.96	0.99	1.02	1.04										
27.5				0.86	0.89	0.92	0.95	0.97	1.00	1.03	1.06	1.08	1.11									
30					0.92	0.95	0.98	1.01	1.04	1.07	1.10	1.13	1.15	1.18								
32.5					0.95	0.98	1.02	1.05	1.08	1.11	1.14	1.16	1.19	1.22	1.25	1.28	1.31					
35						1.02	1.05	1.08	1.11	1.14	1.17	1.20	1.23	1.26	1.29	1.32	1.35					
37.5							1.08	1.11	1.14	1.17	1.21	1.24	1.27	1.30	1.33	1.36	1.39	1.42				
40								1.14	1.17	1.21	1.24	1.27	1.30	1.33	1.37	1.40	1.43	1.46				
42.5								1.17	1.21	1.24	1.27	1.30	1.34	1.37	1.40	1.43	1.46	1.50	1.53			
45									1.24	1.27	1.30	1.34	1.37	1.40	1.44	1.47	1.50	1.53	1.56			
47.5									1.26	1.30	1.33	1.37	1.40	1.44	1.47	1.50	1.53	1.57	1.60	1.63		
50									1.29	1.33	1.36	1.40	1.43	1.47	1.50	1.54	1.57	1.60	1.64	1.67	1.70	
52.5										1.36	1.39	1.43	1.46	1.50	1.53	1.57	1.60	1.64	1.67	1.70	1.74	1.77
55										1.38	1.42	1.46	1.49	1.53	1.56	1.60	1.63	1.67	1.70	1.74	1.77	1.80
57.5											1.45	1.48	1.52	1.56	1.59	1.63	1.66	1.70	1.74	1.77	1.80	1.84
60											1.47	1.51	1.55	1.59	1.62	1.66	1.70	1.73	1.77	1.80	1.84	1.87
62.5												1.54	1.58	1.61	1.65	1.69	1.72	1.76	1.80	1.83	1.87	1.91
65												1.56	1.60	1.64	1.68	1.72	1.75	1.79	1.83	1.86	1.90	1.94
67.5													1.63	1.67	1.71	1.74	1.78	1.82	1.86	1.90	1.93	1.97
70													1.65	1.69	1.73	1.77	1.81	1.85	1.89	1.92	1.96	2.00
72.5														1.72	1.76	1.80	1.84	1.88	1.91	1.95	1.99	2.03
75														1.74	1.78	1.82	1.86	1.90	1.94	1.98	2.02	2.06
77.5															1.81	1.85	1.89	1.93	1.97	2.01	2.05	2.09
80															1.83	1.87	1.92	1.96	2.00	2.04	2.08	2.12
82.5																1.90	1.94	1.98	2.02	2.06	2.10	2.14
85																	1.96	2.01	2.05	2.09	2.13	2.17
87.5																	1.99	2.03	2.07	2.12	2.16	2.20
90																		2.06	2.10	2.14	2.18	2.22
92.5																		2.08	2.12	2.17	2.21	2.25
95																			2.15	2.19	2.23	2.28
97.5																			2.17	2.22	2.26	2.30
100																				2.24	2.28	2.33
102.5																				2.26	2.31	2.35
105																					2.33	2.38
107.5																						2.40

Atomic Weights of the Elements— $^{12}C=12$

Atomic Number	Name	Symbol	Atomic Weight
89	Actinium	Ac	227.0278
13	Aluminium	Al	26.98154
95	Americium	Am	(243)
51	Antimony	Sb	121.75
18	Argon	Ar	39.948
33	Arsenic	As	74.9216
85	Astatine	At	(210)
56	Barium	Ba	137.33
97	Berkelium	Bk	(247)
4	Beryllium	Be	9.01218
83	Bismuth	Bi	208.9804
5	Boron	B	10.811
35	Bromine	Br	79.904
48	Cadmium	Cd	112.41
55	Caesium	Cs	132.9054
20	Calcium	Ca	40.078
98	Californium	Cf	(251)
6	Carbon	C	12.011
58	Cerium	Ce	140.12
17	Chlorine	Cl	35.453
24	Chromium	Cr	51.9961
27	Cobalt	Co	58.9332
29	Copper	Cu	63.546
96	Curium	Cm	(247)
66	Dysprosium	Dy	162.50
99	Einsteinium	Es	(252)
68	Erbium	Er	167.26
63	Europium	Eu	151.96
100	Fermium	Fm	(257)
9	Fluorine	F	18.998403
87	Francium	Fr	(223)
64	Gadolinium	Gd	157.25
31	Gallium	Ga	69.723
32	Germanium	Ge	72.59
79	Gold	Au	196.9665
72	Hafnium	Hf	178.49
2	Helium	He	4.002602
67	Holmium	Ho	164.9304
1	Hydrogen	H	1.00794
49	Indium	In	114.82
53	Iodine	I	126.9045
77	Iridium	Ir	192.22
26	Iron	Fe	55.847
36	Krypton	Kr	83.80
57	Lanthanum	La	138.9055
103	Lawrencium	Lr	(260)
82	Lead	Pb	207.2
3	Lithium	Li	6.941
71	Lutetium	Lu	174.967
12	Magnesium	Mg	24.305
25	Manganese	Mn	54.9380
101	Mendelevium	Md	(258)
80	Mercury	Hg	200.59
42	Molybdenum	Mo	95.94
60	Neodymium	Nd	144.24
10	Neon	Ne	20.179
93	*Neptunium	Np	237.0482
28	Nickel	Ni	58.69
41	Niobium	Nb	92.9064
7	Nitrogen	N	14.0067
102	Nobelium	No	(259)
76	Osmium	Os	190.2
8	Oxygen	O	15.9994
46	Palladium	Pd	106.42
15	Phosphorus	P	30.97376
78	Platinum	Pt	195.08
94	Plutonium	Pu	(244)
84	Polonium	Po	(209)
19	Potassium	K	39.0983
59	Praseodymium	Pr	140.9077
61	Promethium	Pm	(145)
91	*Protactinium	Pa	231.0359
88	*Radium	Ra	226.0254
86	Radon	Rn	(222)
75	Rhenium	Re	186.207
45	Rhodium	Rh	102.9055
37	Rubidium	Rb	85.4678
44	Ruthenium	Ru	101.07
62	Samarium	Sm	150.36
21	Scandium	Sc	44.95591
34	Selenium	Se	78.96
14	Silicon	Si	28.0855
47	Silver	Ag	107.8682
11	Sodium	Na	22.98977
38	Strontium	Sr	87.62
16	Sulphur	S	32.066
73	Tantalum	Ta	180.9479
43	Technetium	Tc	(98)
52	Tellurium	Te	127.60
65	Terbium	Tb	158.9254
81	Thallium	Tl	204.383
90	Thorium	Th	232.0381
69	Thulium	Tm	168.9342
50	Tin	Sn	118.710
22	Titanium	Ti	47.88
74	Tungsten	W	183.85
106	Unnilhexium	Unh	(263)
105	Unnilpentium	Unp	(262)
104	Unnilquadium	Unq	(261)
92	Uranium	U	238.0289
23	Vanadium	V	50.9415
54	Xenon	Xe	131.29
70	Ytterbium	Yb	173.04
39	Yttrium	Y	88.9059
30	Zinc	Zn	65.39
40	Zirconium	Zr	91.224

Values in parentheses are used for certain radioactive elements whose atomic weights cannot be quoted precisely without knowledge of origin; the value given is the atomic mass number of the most stable known isotope of that element. The atomic weight of elements marked (*) is that of the best known isotope.

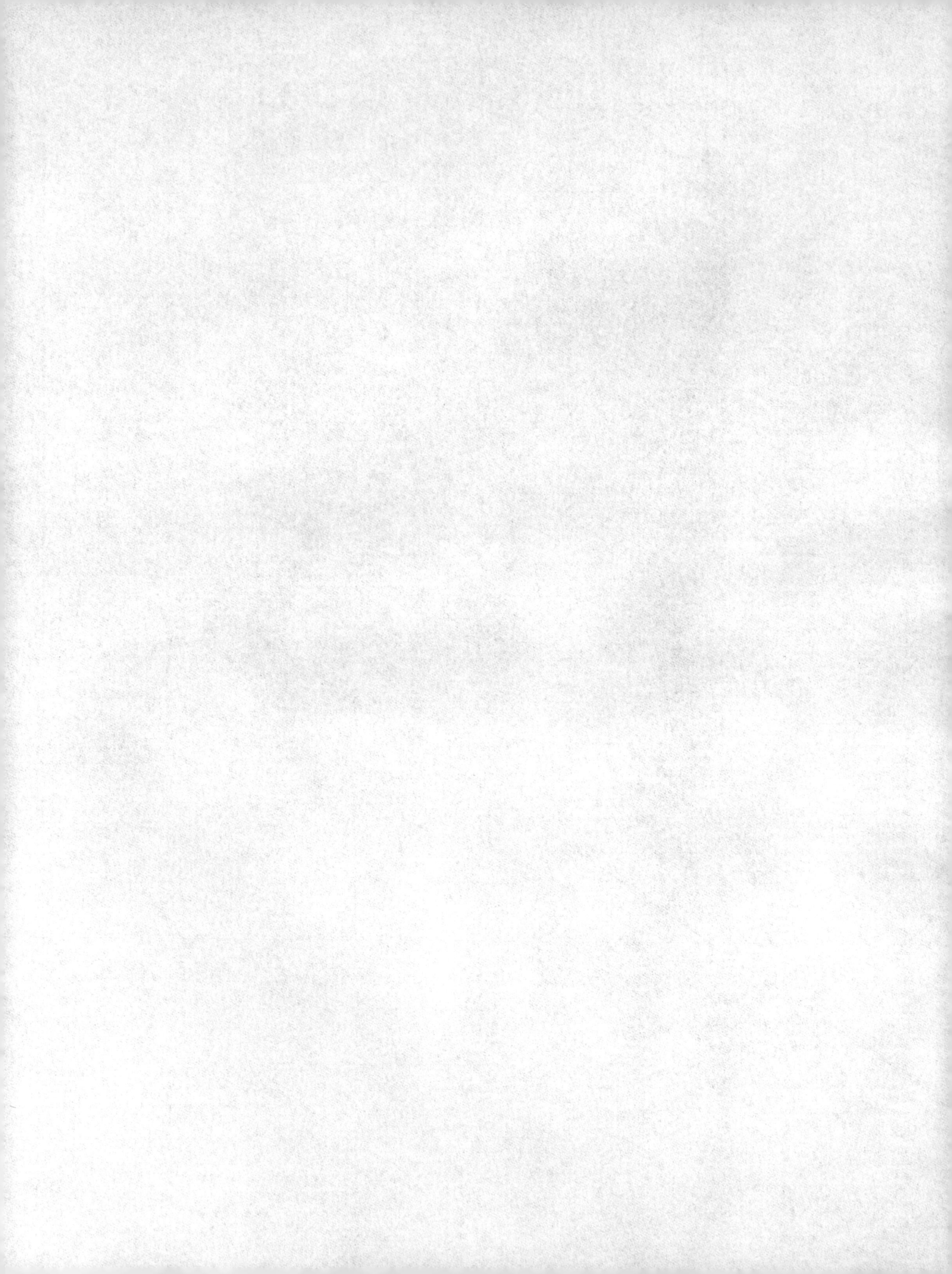

Part 1

Monographs on Drugs and Ancillary Substances

Analgesic and Anti-inflammatory Agents

2600-p

The majority of compounds described in this section are non-steroidal anti-inflammatory drugs (NSAIDs), agents which possess analgesic and anti-inflammatory properties and often antipyretic properties also. A few of the compounds included in this section reportedly possess only analgesic, anti-inflammatory, or antipyretic properties alone. Also included in this section are the gold compounds used in rheumatoid arthritis. Analgesics used for the relief of more severe types of pain than those described here are described in the section on Opioid Analgesics, p.1294. Other drugs used in the treatment of rheumatoid arthritis and described in other sections include chloroquine, p.508, corticosteroids, p.872, penicillamine, p.847, and sulphasalazine, p.1108. Some of the compounds in this section are used in the treatment of acute gout, but drugs used mainly in the treatment of gout are described under Antigout Agents, p.436.

Adverse Effects and Precautions

The commonest side-effects occurring during therapy with non-steroidal anti-inflammatory drugs are generally gastro-intestinal disturbances; these are usually mild and reversible but in some patients gastric ulcer and severe gastro-intestinal bleeding have been reported.

Some non-steroidal anti-inflammatory agents have been associated with nephrotoxicity or changes in renal function.

Chronic abuse of analgesics has been associated with nephropathy. Patients invariably have a history of regular ingestion of substantial or excessive doses over a period of years. In mild cases the condition is reversible if analgesics are withdrawn; in more severe cases renal function may continue to deteriorate despite the withdrawal of analgesics. The initial renal lesion is papillary necrosis and with continued analgesic use there are secondary atrophic changes in the renal cortex body. Phenacetin was originally considered to be the agent responsible for analgesic nephropathy, as it was present in all the various analgesic preparations implicated in the initial clinical reports. Nephropathy has however been reported in patients abusing analgesic preparations without phenacetin and less often in patients taking large quantities of single analgesics.

Because of their adverse gastro-intestinal effects non-steroidal anti-inflammatory agents should not be given to patients with peptic ulceration or a history of such disorders. Other general precautions to be observed include administration to patients with haemorrhagic disorders, history of allergy to aspirin, and impaired renal function. Although some of the drugs may often be given in normal dosage to elderly patients consideration should always be given to the possibility of altered pharmacokinetics and reduced renal function in such patients.

Notable interactions involving non-steroidal anti-inflammatory drugs include possible enhancement of the effects of oral anticoagulants and increased toxicity of lithium and methotrexate. The antihypertensive effects of some antihypertensive agents including beta-blockers and diuretics may be reduced.

Further details concerning the adverse effects and precautions of the individual drugs may be found under their respective monographs.

A review of suspected adverse drug reactions reported to the Committee on Safety of Medicines during 1985. Of 2603 reports received concerning non-steroidal anti-inflammatory drugs 364 described gastro-intestinal haemorrhage or perforation accounting for 21% of all suspected reactions and for 77% of all serious gastro-intestinal reactions. Other reports associated with the non-steroidal anti-inflammatory drugs were aplastic anaemia (19), thrombocytopenia (46), and anaphylaxis or anaphylactoid reactions (15).— *Br. med. J.*, 1986, *293*, 688.

Reviews of the comparative adverse effects of non-steroidal anti-inflammatory agents: *Drug & Ther. Bull.*, 1987, *25*, 81 and 103; P. D. Fowler, *Med. Toxicol.*, 1987, *2*, 338.

EFFECTS ON THE BLOOD. A review concerning the induction of haemolytic anaemia by non-steroidal anti-inflammatory drugs.— M. Sanford-Driscoll and L. C. Knodel, *Drug Intell. & clin. Pharm.*, 1986, *20*, 925.

EFFECTS ON THE GASTRO-INTESTINAL TRACT. Reviews and discussions on the adverse effects of non-steroidal anti-inflammatory drugs on the gastro-intestinal tract: *Br. med. J.*, 1986, *292*, 614; *ibid.*, 1190; K. W. Somerville and C. J. Hawkey, *Postgrad. med. J.*, 1986, *62*, 23; M. J. S. Langman, *Adverse Drug React. Bull.*, 1986, (Oct.), 448; R. Cockel, *Gut*, 1987, *28*, 515.

Some studies investigating the frequency of peptic ulceration or severe gastro-intestinal bleeding associated with non-steroidal anti-inflammatory drugs: M. J. S. Langman *et al.*, *Br. med. J.*, 1985, *290*, 347; D. St. J. Collier and J. A. Pain, *Gut*, 1985, *26*, 359; K. Somerville *et al.*, *Lancet*, 1986, *1*, 462; R. Walt *et al.*, *ibid.*, 489; S. S. Jick *et al.*, *ibid.*, 1987, *2*, 380; D. A. Henry *et al.*, *Br. med. J.*, 1987, *295*, 1227.

EFFECTS ON THE KIDNEYS. Reviews of nephrotoxicity and renal syndromes associated with non-steroidal anti-inflammatory agents: A. L. Linton, *Can. med. Ass. J.*, 1984, *131*, 189; T. I. Poirier, *Drug Intell. & clin. Pharm.*, 1984, *18*, 27; D. M. Clive and J. S. Stoff, *New Engl. J. Med.*, 1984, *310*, 563; M. L'E. Orme, *Br. med. J.*, 1986, *292*, 1621.

Some references to analgesic abuse and nephropathy: *Lancet*, 1982, *2*, 588; U. C. Dubach *et al.*, *New Engl. J. Med.*, 1983, *308*, 357; G. W. Hartman *et al.*, *J. Am. med. Ass.*, 1984, *251*, 1734; *ibid.*, 3123; J. M. Piper *et al.*, *New Engl. J. Med.*, 1985, *313*, 292; C. P. Armstrong and A. L. Blower, *Gut*, 1987, *28*, 527.

EFFECTS ON THE SKIN. A review of the diverse cutaneous reactions to non-steroidal anti-inflammatory drugs.— M. Bigby and R. Stern, *J. Am. Acad. Derm.*, 1985, *12*, 866.

A study of the ability of various non-steroidal anti-inflammatory drugs to produce phototoxic reactions. No phototoxic response was observed with benorylate, ibuprofen, indomethacin, and ketoprofen and although naproxen, piroxicam, and tiaprofenic acid were capable of producing photosensitive reactions it was considered that several hours of exposure to summer sunshine in the *UK* would be required to elicit such a response in clinical practice.— B. L. Diffey *et al.*, *Br. J. Rheumatol.*, 1983, *22*, 239.

INTERACTIONS. A review and discussion concerning drug interactions involving non-steroidal anti-inflammatory drugs. Particularly worrisome are the interactions with oral anticoagulants, captopril, lithium, methotrexate, and triamterene. Non-steroidal anti-inflammatory drugs may differ in their ability to interact with other drugs and details, where known, are presented of those most likely and least likely to interact.— P. D. Hansten and J. R. Horn, *Drug Interact. News.*, 1987, *7*, 7.

Reviews of the interaction between oral anticoagulants and non-steroidal anti-inflammatory drugs: T. Pullar and H. A. Capell, *Scott. med. J.*, 1983, *28*, 42; J. W. O'Callaghan *et al.*, *Can. med. Ass. J.*, 1984, *131*, 857.

For a review covering the interaction between diuretics and non-steroidal anti-inflammatory drugs, see under diuretics, p.974.

OVERDOSAGE. Reviews of poisoning after overdosage with non-steroidal anti-inflammatory drugs and methods of treatment of acute poisoning: M. Court and G. N. Volans, *Adverse Drug React. Ac. Pois. Rev.*, 1984, *3*, 1; J. A. Vale and T. J. Meredith, *Med. Toxicol.*, 1986, *1*, 12.

Absorption and Fate

Details of the pharmacokinetics of the individual drugs may be found under their respective monographs.

Some reviews of the pharmacokinetics of non-steroidal anti-inflammatory drugs: R. K. Verbeeck *et al.*, *Clin. Pharmacokinet.*, 1983, *8*, 297 (general); K. W. Woodhouse and H. Wynne, *ibid.*, 1987, *12*, 111 (in the elderly); J. H. Lin *et al.*, *ibid.*, 402 (protein binding).

Uses and Administration

The non-steroidal anti-inflammatory drugs have two main clinical properties. Administered as single doses or in short-term intermittent therapy they provide adequate analgesia for the symptomatic relief of mild to moderate pain in conditions such as headache and dysmenorrhoea. After longer-term use the anti-inflammatory properties become evident making them suitable for use in the symptomatic treatment of rheumatic disorders such as rheumatoid arthritis. Some of the non-steroidal anti-inflammatory agents also possess antipyretic properties and may be used in the control of fever.

The other main group of compounds discussed in this section are the gold compounds which are used as second-line agents in rheumatoid arthritis.

Further details concerning the indications and dosages for the individual drugs may be found under their respective monographs.

GOUT. A short review of the treatment of gout including the use of non-steroidal anti-inflammatory agents.— *Drug & Ther. Bull.*, 1985, *23*, 47.

PAIN. Some reviews and discussions on the use of analgesics for the control of pain: R. G. Twycross, *Postgrad. med. J.*, 1984, *60*, 876 (general); G. B. A. Veitch, *Pharm. J.*, 1984, *2*, 649 (counter-prescribing); K. M. Foley, *New Engl. J. Med.*, 1985, *313*, 84 (in cancer patients); R. G. Twycross, *Br. J. Hosp. Med.*, 1986, *36*, 244 (in terminal care).

RHEUMATOID ARTHRITIS. A discussion on the general management of rheumatoid arthritis. Rheumatoid arthritis is a common disease with a wide spectrum of disease severity but many patients have intermittent relapses and remissions with an overall pattern of slowly progressive joint destruction and deformity. Although many drugs alleviate symptoms, and some may slow the progress of the underlying disease, there is no uniformly accepted drug regimen, so that many different drugs are used, usually in combination. It is also important when considering therapeutic intervention that patients may require drug treatment for 30 or 40 years.

The choice of drugs for relief of pain depends upon the severity of symptoms. In mild cases an analgesic alone, such as paracetamol, may be all that is required but most patients have symptoms which need drugs with anti-inflammatory as well as analgesic properties. There is no 'best buy' in the non-steroidal anti-inflammatory drugs and individual responses of patients to different drugs vary greatly. Some, such as ibuprofen and ketoprofen, may have slightly weaker anti-inflammatory properties than others, but they have fewer side-effects and therefore may be considered before more powerful agents such as azapropazone, diclofenac, indomethacin, or naproxen. Slow-acting oral formulations or suppositories of non-steroidal anti-inflammatory drugs may be particularly effective for prolonged early-morning stiffness. Combinations of the non-steroidal anti-inflammatory drugs should not generally be used but it is reasonable to combine a short-acting drug, such as ibuprofen, during the day with a longer-acting drug, such as a suppository of indomethacin, at night. The acute joint inflammation is rapidly reduced with such non-steroidal anti-inflammatory drugs, the effect reaching a plateau after about one to two weeks.

Second-line drugs, often also called disease-modifying, remission-inducing, or slow-acting drugs are diverse agents with different structures and probably different modes of action. They are undoubtedly slow-acting, taking weeks or months to control acute joint inflammation, may modify the disease, but rarely do they induce remission. These second-line agents are reserved for patients with severe disease characterised by persistent inflammation failing to respond to non-steroidal anti-inflammatory drugs alone or for patients with progressive disease with X-ray changes, or more usually for patients with a combination of both features. Most patients requiring second-line drugs should also be taking a non-steroidal anti-inflammatory. Again the choice of a second-line agent is imprecise. The authors personal preference is for sulphasalazine as it appears to have fewer serious side-effects than the more conventional drugs such as gold and penicillamine; low-dose antimalarials are also well-tolerated and may be particularly useful in milder cases. It is important to use second-line agents for at least six months before abandoning treatment as ineffective.

Where traditional second-line drugs have been exhausted, third-line drugs (azathioprine, cyclophosphamide, or methotrexate) are now being used with increasing frequency.

The place of corticosteroids in rheumatoid arthritis is controversial. Intra-articular injections are used to treat acute flares of individual joints but should not be used more often than every six months. Steroids by mouth may still be used occasionally in special circumstances such as a severe arthritis in the elderly or disease failing to respond to second- or third-line drugs but the basic rule in patients with uncomplicated arthritis is to avoid steroids if at all possible.— D. G. I. Scott and J. S. Coppock, *Prescribers' J.*, 1987, *27 (1)*, 13. See also: D. G. I. Scott, *ibid.*, 20 (further discussion on the second-line agents chloroquine, hydroxychloroquine, and gold); B. McConkey and R. D. Situnayake, *ibid.*, 27 (sulphasalazine and dapsone as second-line agents); D. P. M. Symmons, *ibid.*, 32 (problems of prescribing for patients with gastro-intestinal disorders, or renal disease, or during pregnancy and lactation).

Further reviews and discussions on the management of rheumatoid arthritis: H. A. Bird, *Br. J. Hosp. Med.*, 1986, *35*, 374; V. Wright, *Br. med. J.*, 1986, *292*, 431; *Med. Lett.*, 1987, *29*, 21.

Juvenile rheumatoid arthritis. Outlines of the management of chronic arthritis in children.— A. W. Craft, *Prescribers' J.*, 1985, *25*, 75.

A further review and discussion concerning the treatment of children with juvenile rheumatoid arthritis noting a recent study (E.J. Brewer *et al.*, *New Engl. J. Med.*, 1986, *314*, 1269) that concluded that in the presence of a non-steroidal anti-inflammatory drug neither hydroxychloroquine nor penicillamine proved superior to a placebo. The reviewer considered that this report clearly emphasized the advisability of continuing to give non-steroidal anti-inflammatory drugs and weighing very carefully the benefits of and toxicity from other drugs such as hydoxychloroquine and penicillamine before prescribing them.— J. T. Cassidy, *New Engl. J. Med.*, 1986, *314*, 1312.

12308-x

Acemetacin *(BAN, rINN).*

Bay-f-4975; TVX-1322. *O*-[(1-*p*-Chlorobenzoyl-5-methoxy-2-methylindol-3-yl)acetyl]glycolic acid.
$C_{21}H_{18}ClNO_6$=415.8.

CAS — 53164-05-9.

Acemetacin is a non-steroidal anti-inflammatory agent that has been used in inflammatory and rheumatic disorders in doses of up to 60 mg three times daily by mouth.

Some references to acemetacin: H. Rechziegler and P. Zündorf, *Curr. med. Res. Opinion*, 1985, *9*, 701; R. Kronhagel, *Br. J. clin. Pract.*, 1986, *40*, 472.

Proprietary Names and Manufacturers
Rantudil *(Tropon, Ger.; Kowa, Jpn)*; Tilur *(Drossapharm, Switz.)*.

2602-w

Acetaminosalol *(rINN).*

Acetyl-*p*-aminosalol; Cétossalol; Phenetsal. 4-Acetamidophenyl salicylate.
$C_{15}H_{13}NO_4$=271.3.

CAS — 118-57-0.

Pharmacopoeias. In *Mex.*, *Port.*, and *Span.*

Acetaminosalol has antipyretic, anti-inflammatory, and analgesic properties. It has been used by mouth in rheumatic disorders.

2603-e

Acetanilide

Antifebrin. *N*-Phenylacetamide.
C_8H_9NO=135.2.

CAS — 103-84-4.

Pharmacopoeias. In *Fr.*, *Hung.*, *Mex.*, *Nord.*, *Port.*, and *Span.*

Acetanilide has analgesic and antipyretic properties. It has been replaced by safer analgesics.

2604-l

Acetylcresotinic Acid

o-Acetylcresotinic Acid. 2-Acetoxy-3-methylbenzoic acid.
$C_{10}H_{10}O_4$=194.2.

Acetylcresotinic acid has analgesic, antipyretic, and anti-inflammatory properties and has been given by mouth in the treatment of rheumatic disorders.

Proprietary Names and Manufacturers
Crésopirine *(Lemoine, Fr.)*.

2605-y

Alclofenac *(BAN, USAN, rINN).*

W-7320. (4-Allyloxy-3-chlorophenyl)acetic acid.
$C_{11}H_{11}ClO_3$=226.7.

CAS — 22131-79-9.

Adverse Effects and Precautions
Skin rashes are common and gastro-intestinal disturbances may occur.

Alclofenac should be given with caution to patients with impaired hepatic or renal function. Alclofenac may enhance the effects of oral anticoagulants, oral hypoglycaemics, and thyroxine.

Alclofenac appeared to be associated with a relatively high incidence of adverse reactions. Out of 230 reports of reactions notified to the Committee on Safety of Medicines 168 were for rash without systemic disturbance, 34 were for rash with systemic disturbance, and 7 were for gastro-intestinal haemorrhage or other symptoms.— D. Mansel-Jones (letter), *Lancet*, 1974, *1*, 97.

Two patients developed widespread cutaneous vasculitis within 5 to 7 days of commencing to take alclofenac 1 g two or three times daily. A third patient who developed symptoms 2 days after commencing to take 500 mg three times daily and who continued to take alclofenac for a week developed a widespread maculopapular eruption and recurrent episodes of purpura, haemoptysis, and haematuria, with evidence of renal involvement.— R. A. Billings *et al.*, *Br. med. J.*, 1974, *4*, 263.

From a study of about 1500 patients who had participated in trials of alclofenac in the UK the incidence of skin rash was 10.3% in those taking tablets and 2.1% in those taking capsules. There might be cross-sensitivity to penicillin, gold salts, or salicylates. Five cases of gastro-intestinal haemorrhage had occurred but the role of alclofenac could not be determined; 5 of 6 anaphylactoid reactions were attributable to alclofenac. Leucopenia had occurred in 2 patients, 1 with Felty's syndrome.— J. F. Hort, *Curr. med. Res. Opinion*, 1975, *3*, 333. See also S. S. Bedi, *Curr. med. Res. Opinion*, 1975, *3*, 309.

Angioedema occurred in a 44-year-old woman after taking alclofenac 1 g. She had been taking alclofenac intermittently for osteoarthritis for the previous 18 months, and had noted a rash on one other occasion.— N. G. Kounis, *Br. J. clin. Pract.*, 1975, *29*, 322.

A report of renal papillary necrosis in a 65-year-old woman who had taken aspirin 1.5 kg between 1971 and 1973 and alclofenac 2.2 kg between 1973 and 1975.— R. Gokal and D. R. Matthews, *Br. med. J.*, 1977, *2*, 1517.

Absorption and Fate
Alclofenac appears to be variably absorbed from the gastro-intestinal tract. Peak plasma concentrations are reached 1 to 4 hours after rectal or oral administration. The plasma half-life varies between 1.5 and 5.5 hours. It is excreted in urine mainly as glucuronide and as unchanged drug. Variable amounts are excreted in the faeces.

Some references to the pharmacokinetics of alclofenac: L. F. Wiggins, *Curr. med. Res. Opinion*, 1975, *3*, 241 (drug metabolites); G. M. Thomas *et al.*, *ibid.*, 264 (drug concentrations and protein binding); L. T. Sennello *et al.*, *Clin. Pharmac. Ther.*, 1978, *23*, 414 (drug absorption, half-life, and excretion).

Uses and Administration
Alclofenac has analgesic, antipyretic, and anti-inflammatory properties and has been used in rheumatic disorders in doses of 0.5 to 1 g three times daily by mouth. Following reports of toxicity it has been withdrawn from the market in several countries.

Proprietary Names and Manufacturers
Allopydin *(Jpn)*; Argun *(CEPA, Spain)*; Darkeyfenac *(Cuatrecasas-Darkey, Spain)*; Desinflam *(Sintyal, Arg.)*; Epinal *(Jpn)*; Mervan *(Continental Pharma, Belg.; Continental Pharma, Switz.)*; Mirvan *(Labaz, Neth.)*; Prinalgin *(Berk, S.Afr.; Berk Pharmaceuticals, UK)*; Vanadian *(Federico Bonet, Spain)*; Zubirol *(Abbott, Arg.)*; Zumaril *(Abbott, Ital.)*.

16021-j

Alminoprofen *(rINN).*

4-[(2-Methylallyl)amino]hydratropic acid.
$C_{13}H_{17}NO_2$=219.3.

CAS — 39718-89-3.

Alminoprofen is a non-steroidal anti-inflammatory agent that has been used in inflammatory and rheumatic disorders in doses of up to 900 mg daily by mouth.

Proprietary Names and Manufacturers
Minalfene *(Bouchara, Fr.)*.

2607-z

Aloxiprin *(BAN, rINN).*

A polymeric condensation product of aluminium oxide and aspirin.

CAS — 9014-67-9.

Pharmacopoeias. In *Br.* and *Cz.*

A fine white or slightly pink, odourless or almost odourless, powder. It contains 7.5 to 8.5% of aluminium and 79 to 87.4% of total salicylates.

Aloxiprin 600 mg is approximately equivalent to 500 mg of aspirin. Practically **insoluble** in water, alcohol, and ether; slightly soluble in chloroform. **Store** in well-closed containers.

Adverse Effects, Treatment, and Precautions

As for aspirin below

Aloxiprin, like aspirin (see p.5), because of the risk of Reye's syndrome, should not generally be given to children under the age of 12 years unless specifically indicated for conditions such as juvenile rheumatoid arthritis.

EFFECTS ON THE GASTRO-INTESTINAL TRACT. Aloxiprin appeared to be associated with less gastro-intestinal bleeding than plain aspirin though the reduction was not uniform in all subjects.— P. H. N. Wood *et al.*, *Br. med. J.*, 1962, *1*, 669.

INTERACTIONS. Reports of severe metabolic acidosis in 2 patients with normal renal and hepatic function while taking salicylates (aloxiprin or salsalate) concomitantly with carbonic anhydrase inhibitors (dichlorphenamide or acetazolamide). Such concomitant use should be minimised or avoided.— R. A. Cowan *et al.*, *Br. med. J.*, 1984, *289*, 347.

Absorption and Fate

Aloxiprin is hydrolysed in the gastro-intestinal tract to salicylate, the rate of breakdown being low in the acid conditions of the stomach and greater at the higher pH values of the intestine.

Uses and Administration

Aloxiprin has actions similar to those of aspirin, p.5. It is used as an analgesic and anti-inflammatory agent in rheumatic disorders in doses of up to 100 mg per kg body-weight daily in divided doses.

Preparations

Aloxiprin Tablets *(B.P.)*

Proprietary Preparations

Palaprin Forte *(Nicholas, UK)*. *Tablets*, scored, aloxiprin 600 mg.

Proprietary Names and Manufacturers

Lyman Tabs *(Lubapharm, Switz.)*; Palaprin Forte *(Nicholas, Austral.*; *Nicholas, Swed.*; *Nicholas, UK)*; Paloxin *(S.Afr.)*; Rumatral *(Wander, Switz.)*; Superpyrin *(Cz.)*; Tiatral *(Wander, Switz.)*.

12354-m

Amfenac Sodium *(BANM, USAN, rINNM)*.

AHR-5850; AHR-5850D. Sodium (2-amino-3-benzoylphenyl)acetate monohydrate.

$C_{15}H_{12}NNaO_3,H_2O$=295.3.

CAS — 51579-82-9 (amfenac); 61618-27-7 (sodium salt).

Amfenac sodium has analgesic and anti-inflammatory properties. It has been given by mouth in inflammatory and rheumatic disorders.

Some references to amfenac sodium: A. K. Jain *et al.*, *Pharmacotherapy*, 1986, *6*, 236 (postoperative dental pain).

Proprietary Names and Manufacturers

Fenazox *(Meiji, Jpn)*.

2609-k

Amidopyrine

Amidazofen; Amidopyrine-Pyramidon; Aminophenazone *(rINN)*; Aminopyrine; Dimethylaminoantipyrine; Dimethylaminophenazone. 4-Dimethylamino-1,5-dimethyl-2-phenyl-4-pyrazolin-3-one.

$C_{13}H_{17}N_3O$=231.3.

CAS — 58-15-1.

Pharmacopoeias. In *Arg.*, *Aust.*, *Belg.*, *Braz.*, *Cz.*, *Fr.*, *Hung.*, *Int.*, *It.*, *Jug.*, *Neth.*, *Nord.*, *Pol.*, *Port.*, *Roum.*, *Rus.*, *Span.*, and *Turk.*

Adverse Effects and Precautions

The risk of agranulocytosis in patients taking amidopyrine is sufficiently great to render this drug unsuitable for use. Onset of agranulocytosis may be sudden and unpredictable.

ALLERGY. Cross-sensitivity occurred between amidopyrine and aspirin in one patient. Amidopyrine produced a life-threatening asthmatic attack on one occasion.— E. Bartoli *et al.* (letter), *Lancet*, 1976, *1*, 1357.

The Boston Collaborative Drug Surveillance Program monitored consecutively 32 812 medical inpatients. Drug-induced anaphylaxis occurred in 1 of 1992 patients given amidopyrine.— J. Porter and H. Jick, *Lancet*, 1977, *1*, 587.

CARCINOGENICITY. Amidopyrine must be considered a potential carcinogen because it reacted readily with nitrous acid to form dimethylnitrosamine. The reaction was catalysed by thiocyanate present in the saliva particularly in smokers.— E. Boyland and S. A. Walker, *Arzneimittel-Forsch.*, 1974, *24*, 1181. See also *Lancet*, 1979, *1*, 283.

EFFECTS ON THE BLOOD. *Agranulocytosis*. From 960 patients treated with amidopyrine there were 11 cases of agranulocytosis—an incidence of 1.1%.— Association of Clinical Pathologists, *Lancet*, 1951, *1*, 389.

The AMA Registry of Adverse Reactions recorded 45 cases of agranulocytosis presumed or known to be due to amidopyrine and 25 in which another drug might have been involved in the period 1957–66. A hypersensitivity reaction was probably involved.— *Med. Lett.*, 1973, *15*, 4.

Four patients developed agranulocytosis while taking Chinese herbal medicines for relief of arthritis and back pain. The herbal medicines were found to contain both amidopyrine and phenylbutazone.— C. A. Ries and M. A. Sahud, *J. Am. med. Ass.*, 1975, *231*, 352.

Further reports and discussions of amidopyrine-induced agranulocytosis.— A. J. Barrett *et al.*, *Br. med. J.*, 1976, *2*, 850; S. Shapiro (letter), *Lancet*, 1984, *1*, 451 and 582; A. Herxheimer and J. S. Yudkin (letter), *ibid.*, 730; S. Shapiro (letter), *ibid.*, 1471.

Haemolytic anaemia. Amidopyrine had been implicated as a causative agent in immune haemolytic anaemia.— E. Beutler, *Pharmac. Rev.*, 1969, *21*, 73.

PORPHYRIA. Amidopyrine had been reported to precipitate attacks of porphyria.— *Drug & Ther. Bull.*, 1976, *14*, 55.

Amidopyrine was considered to be unsafe in patients with acute porphyria because it has been shown to be porphyrinogenic in *animals* or *in vitro* systems.— M.R. Moore and K.E.L. McColl, *Porphyrias, Drug Lists*, Glasgow, Porphyria Research Unit, University of Glasgow, 1987.

Absorption and Fate

Amidopyrine is absorbed from the gastro-intestinal tract. It has a half-life of about 1 to 4 hours.

Some references to the pharmacokinetics of amidopyrine: H. Oehne and E. Schmid, *Arzneimittel-Forsch.*, 1972, *22*, 2115 (rectal absorption and urinary excretion); R. Gradnik and L. Fleischmann, *Pharm. Acta Helv.*, 1973, *48*, 181 (metabolism); L. Fleischmann, *ibid.*, 192 (rectal absorption).

Uses and Administration

Amidopyrine has analgesic, anti-inflammatory, and antipyretic properties but owing to the risk of agranulocytosis its use is discouraged. It has also been used in the form of a variety of salts or complexes.

Amidopyrine is sometimes used in drug metabolism studies.

Proprietary Names and Manufacturers of Amidopyrine and its Salts or Complexes

Areumal *(Ecobi, Ital.)*; Baukal Suppositories *(Bruschettini, Ital.)*; Causyth *(Inverni della Beffa, Ital.)*; Depiral C *(Ital.)*; Farmidone *(Farmitalia, Ital.)*; Fenodone *(Ripari-Gero, Ital.)*; Fever *(Ital.)*; Ftalazone *(Terapeutico M.R., Ital.)*; Fugantil *(Ghimas, Ital.)*; Galenopyrin *(Keller, Switz.)*; Glucopirina *(Ganassini, Ital.)*; Hyparon *(Jpn)*; Inst *(Jpn)*; Isoftal *(Isola-Ibi, Ital.)*; Katareuma *(Lafare, Ital.)*; Latepyrine *(Landerlan, Spain)*; Malivan *(Recordati, Ital.)*; Metapirazone *(Ital.)*; Netsusarin *(Jpn)*; Nevrazon *(Panthox & Burck, Ital.)*; Nikartrone *(Pulitzer, Ital.)*; Piramidon *(Hoechst, Spain)*; Pirasco *(Ital.)*; Piraseptolo *(Lisapharma, Ital.)*; Piro Rectal *(Madaus Cerafarm, Spain)*; Piroreumal *(Medosan, Ital.)*; P.S.B.P. *(Vaillant-Defresne, Fr.)*; Reu-Bon *(Sifarma, Ital.)*; Reumanova *(Gibipharma, Ital.)*; Reumasedina *(Coli, Ital.)*; Reumo Termina *(Ital.)*; Reumoftal *(Chemil, Ital.)*; Reumotranc *(Ital.)*; Revulex *(Vaillant-Defresne, Switz.)*; Rosetin *(Benvegna, Ital.)*; Suppnon *(Jpn)*; Termidon *(Lepetit, Ital.)*; Tiomidone *(Edmond Pharma, Ital.)*.

12384-s

Antrafenine *(rINN)*.

2-[4-(ααα-Trifluoro-*m*-tolyl)piperazin-1-yl]ethyl *N*-(7-trifluoromethyl-4-quinolyl)anthranilate.

$C_{30}H_{26}F_6N_4O_2$=588.6.

CAS — 55300-29-3.

Antrafenine is an analgesic that has been given by mouth in rheumatic disorders. It was suspended from the market following colonic toxicity in *animal* studies.

Proprietary Names and Manufacturers

Stakane *(Dausse, Fr.)*.

2601-s

Aspirin *(BAN, USAN)*.

Acetylsal. Acid; Acetylsalicylic Acid; Acidum Acetylsalicylicum; Polopiryna; Salicylic Acid Acetate. *O*-Acetylsalicylic acid; 2-Acetoxybenzoic acid.

$C_9H_8O_4$=180.2.

CAS — 50-78-2.

NOTE. The use of the name Aspirin is limited; in some countries it is a trade-mark. Co-codaprin *(BAN)* is the name applied to compounded preparations of codeine phosphate and aspirin in the mass proportions 1 part to 50 parts.

Pharmacopoeias. In *Arg.*, *Aust.*, *Belg.*, *Br.*, *Braz.*, *Chin.*, *Cz.*, *Egypt.*, *Eur.*, *Fr.*, *Ger.*, *Hung.*, *Ind.*, *Int.*, *It.*, *Jpn*, *Jug.*, *Mex.*, *Neth.*, *Nord.*, *Pol.*, *Port.*, *Roum.*, *Rus.*, *Span.*, *Swiss*, *Turk.*, and *U.S.* Also in *B.P. Vet.*

Colourless or white crystals or white crystalline powder; odourless or almost odourless. **Soluble** 1 in 300 of water, 1 in 5 to 7 of alcohol, 1 in 17 of chloroform, and 1 in 10 to 20 of ether. **Store** in airtight containers. Aspirin is stable in dry air, but gradually hydrolyses in contact with moisture to acetic and salicylic acids.

Adverse Effects

The most common adverse effects occurring with therapeutic doses of aspirin are gastro-intestinal disturbances such as nausea, dyspepsia, and vomiting. Irritation of the gastric mucosa with erosion, ulceration, haematemesis and melaena may occur; slight blood loss may occur in about 70% of patients with most aspirin preparations, whether buffered, soluble, or plain, and often this is not accompanied by dyspepsia. Slight blood loss is not usually of clinical significance but may, in a few patients, cause iron-deficiency anaemia during long-term salicylate therapy.

Some persons, especially asthmatics, exhibit notable sensitivity to aspirin which may provoke various reactions including urticaria and other skin eruptions, angioedema, rhinitis, and severe, even fatal, paroxysmal bronchospasm and dyspnoea. Persons sensitive to aspirin may not tolerate therapeutic doses.

Aspirin increases the bleeding time, decreases platelet adhesiveness, and, in large doses, may cause hypoprothrombinaemia.

In children the use of aspirin has been implicated in some cases of Reye's syndrome, thus leading to severe restrictions on the indications for aspirin therapy in children. For further details see under Reye's Syndrome (below).

Mild chronic salicylate intoxication, or salicylism, usually occurs only after repeated administration of large doses. Symptoms include dizziness, tinnitus, deafness, sweating, nausea and vomiting, headache, and mental confusion, and may be controlled by reducing the dosage. Symptoms of more severe intoxication or of acute poisoning following overdosage include hyperventilation, fever, restlessness, ketosis, and respiratory alkalosis and metabolic acidosis. Depression of the central nervous system may lead to coma, cardiovascular collapse, and respiratory failure. In children drowsiness and metabolic acidosis commonly occur; hypoglycaemia may be severe.

In a report from the Boston Collaborative Drug Surveillance Program, adverse reactions attributed to aspirin occurred in 119 of 2391 hospitalised patients who received plain aspirin tablets. Minor gastro-intestinal disturbances occurred in 51 patients, tinnitus in 20, deafness in 8, gastro-intestinal bleeding in 23, and prolonged prothrombin times in 3. Drug fever, leucopenia, and epistaxis occurred in 2 each and sweating, purpura, dyspnoea, stomatitis, hypothermia, metabolic acidosis, and elevated serum concentrations of uric acid in 1 each. Other drugs administered concurrently could have contributed to the adverse reaction in 26 patients. Reactions occurred more often at higher doses and were more common in females.— R. R. Miller and H. Jick, *Am. J. med. Sci.*, 1977, *274*, 271.

ALLERGY. Intolerance to aspirin usually occurs in middle-aged adults and is more common in females. Manifestations of the aspirin-intolerance syndrome include vasomotor rhinitis, sinusitis, nasal polyps, bronchial asthma, angioedema, urticaria, and eosinophilia. Aspirin-induced prolongation of bleeding time and a tendency for diabetes may exist with it. Hypotension, shock, and syncope may occur. Salicylates other than aspirin are usually well tolerated but cross-reactivity with other analgesics, particularly indomethacin, and with tartrazine may occur. The mechanism underlying aspirin hypersensitivity is not known but an immunological basis seems unlikely.— M. A. Abrishami and J. Thomas, *Ann. Allergy*, 1977, *39*, 28.

In 11 patients hypersensitive to aspirin, reactions occurred in all when challenged with indomethacin, in 8 of 9 and 7 of 9 challenged respectively with mefenamic and flufenamic acids, and in 4 of 10 challenged with phenylbutazone. There were no reactions to benzydamine, chloroquine, paracetamol, or salicylamide.— A. Szczeklik *et al.*, *Br. med. J.*, 1975, *1*, 67.

An examination of published literature to estimate the rate of sensitivity reactions to aspirin and cross-sensitivity to other analgesics. The rate of aspirin sensitivity is lowest among non-allergic patients regardless of age, higher in adult patients with allergic rhinitis alone, and highest in adult patients with asthma although the true rates are unknown.— C. K. Kwoh and A. R. Feinstein, *Clin. Pharmac. Ther.*, 1986, *40*, 494.

See also under Effects on the Skin (below).

Desensitisation. Successful desensitisation was achieved in 16 of 18 patients (including 4 with aspirin-sensitive asthma). Incremental doses of aspirin (starting at 30 mg) were given at 2-hour intervals until an allergic response was obtained; the following day aspirin was re-administered at the dose that had caused the response and again incremental doses were given until finally a 650-mg dose could be tolerated.— S. I. Asad *et al.*, *Br. med. J.*, 1984, *288*, 745. Further reports of oral desensitisation procedures in aspirin-sensitive patients: D. D. Stevenson, *J. Asthma*, 1983, *20*, 31.

EFFECTS ON THE BLOOD. There were 787 reports of adverse reactions to aspirin reported to the Committee on Safety of Medicines between June 1964 and January 1973. These included 95 reports of blood disorders (17 fatal) including thrombocytopenia (26; 2 fatal), aplastic anaemia (13; 7 fatal), and agranulocytosis or pancytopenia (10; 2 fatal), gastro-intestinal haemorrhage (128; 64 fatal). There were 53 reports (26 fatalities) of analgesic nephropathy associated with preparations containing aspirin, phenacetin, and codeine.— M. F. Cuthbert, *Curr. med. Res. Opinion*, 1974, *2*, 600.

Aplastic anaemia. Reports of aspirin-induced aplastic anaemia.— M. Eldar *et al.* (letter), *S. Afr. med. J.*, 1979, *55*, 318.

Haemolytic anaemia. Aspirin, 4 to 12 g daily, had been reported to cause haemolytic anaemia in certain individuals with a deficiency of glucose-6-phosphate dehydrogenase. The reaction was not considered clinically significant under normal circumstances (e.g. in the absence of infection).— E. Beutler, *Pharmac. Rev.*, 1969, *21*, 73. See also A. Karaklis (letter), *Br. med. J.*, 1981, *283*, 731.

Further reports on the occurrence of aspirin-induced haemolytic anaemia in patients with glucose-6-phosphate dehydrogenase deficiency.— E. R. Burka, *Ann. intern. Med.*, 1966, *64*, 817; B. E. Glader, *J. Pediat.*, 1976, *89*, 1027; T. K. Chan *et al.*, *Br. med. J.*, 1976, *2*, 1227.

Thrombocytopenia. Reports on thrombocytopenia attributed to aspirin.— E. Thiel *et al.*, *Klin. Wschr.*, 1973, *51*, 754; I. H. Scheinberg (letter), *New Engl. J. Med.*, 1979, *300*, 678.

EFFECTS ON BLOOD GLUCOSE. The hypoglycaemic action of salicylates might be due to suppression of the release of fatty acids from adipose tissue. Plasma-salicylate concentrations of 200 to 300 μg per mL produced maximal hypoglycaemic activity. This effect was not significant in normal persons and salicylate poisoning had been complicated by hyperglycaemia and glycosuria.— V. Fang *et al.*, *J. pharm. Sci.*, 1968, *57*, 2111.

EFFECTS ON THE EYES. Transient myopia occurred in a patient following the ingestion of 2.7 g of aspirin.— J. H. Sandford-Smith, *Br. J. Ophthal.*, 1974, *58*, 698.

Aspirin 1.28 g affected colour discrimination in healthy subjects, but the effects were minor.— S. M. Luria *et al.*, *Br. J. clin. Pharmac.*, 1979, *7*, 585.

EFFECTS ON THE GASTRO-INTESTINAL TRACT. A review of the acute and chronic effects of aspirin on the stomach. Strong clinical and epidemiological evidence suggests that aspirin can induce gastric ulcer disease but the actual frequency is unclear; there does appear to be a relationship to dose. The evidence that increased aspirin intake causes gastro-intestinal bleeding is retrospective and epidemiologically inconclusive. All known non-steroidal anti-inflammatory drugs have the potential for causing acute damage to the gastric mucosa and comparative studies of acute gastric mucosal damage caused by such drugs consistently associate aspirin with the most severe lesions. However, aspirin-associated gastro-intestinal microbleeding and the appearance of superficial gastric mucosal haemorrhages and small erosions have no known clinical significance; the extent and degree of such changes have no proven value for predicting the frequency or severity of chronic gastric ulcer or overt gastro-intestinal bleeding.— D. Y. Graham and J. L. Smith, *Ann. intern. Med.*, 1986, *104*, 390.

EFFECTS ON HEARING. In 52 patients with rheumatoid arthritis, the daily dose of aspirin required to produce tinnitus varied from 3.6 to 10.8 g daily. The average serum-salicylate concentration was 295 μg per mL; tinnitus did not occur at concentrations less than 196 μg per mL. In 15 patients with pre-existing hearing loss tinnitus did not develop despite serum-salicylate concentrations ranging from 311 to 677 μg per mL.— E. Mongan *et al.*, *J. Am. med. Ass.*, 1973, *226*, 142.

The Boston Collaborative Drug Surveillance Program monitored consecutively 32 812 medical inpatients. Drug-induced deafness occurred in a dose-related manner in 32 of 2974 patients given aspirin.— J. Porter and H. Jick, *Lancet*, 1977, *1*, 587.

A report of a patient with high serum-salicylate concentrations 'hearing music'. Following reduction in the dosage of aspirin the condition ceased.— J. R. Allen (letter), *New Engl. J. Med.*, 1985, *313*, 642.

For reports of reversible and permanent deafness attributed to salicylate therapy, see J. Ballantyne, *J. Lar. Otol.*, 1972, *84*, 967; L. Jardini *et al.*, *Rheumatol. Rehabil.*, 1978, *17*, 233; R. R. Miller, *J. clin. Pharmac.*, 1978, *18*, 468.

EFFECTS ON THE HEART. Administration of aspirin 4 g daily markedly exacerbated anginal attacks in a 66-year-old man with Prinzmetal's variant angina.— K. Miwa *et al.* (letter), *Lancet*, 1979, *2*, 1382.

EFFECTS ON THE KIDNEYS. Although abuse of combined analgesic preparations containing aspirin has been implicated in the development of analgesic nephropathy, kidney damage associated with the therapeutic use of aspirin alone appears to be comparatively rare. Studies assessing renal function in patients who had received only aspirin over a prolonged period have found no real risk of renal damage (*Br. med. J.*, 1974, *1*, 593; A.F. Macklon *et al.*, *ibid.*, 597; B.R. Walker *et al.*, *New Engl. J. Med.*, 1977, *297*, 1405; S.M. Akyol *et al.*, *Br. med. J.*, 1982, *284*, 631; S.L. Bonney *et al.*, *Clin. Pharmac. Ther.*, 1986, *40*, 373). There have been some suggestions of nephrotoxicity occurring in patients with disorders such as systemic lupus erythematosus (R. P. Kimberly and P. H. Plotz, *New Engl. J. Med.*, 1977, *296*, 418; R. P. Kimberly *et al.*, *Am. J. Med.*, 1978, *64*, 804; R. P. Kimberly *et al.*, *Ann. intern. Med.*, 1978, *89*, 336) but such studies and findings have frequently been severely criticised.

EFFECTS ON THE LIVER. Aspirin-induced hepatotoxicity occurs more frequently in patients with rheumatoid arthritis and other connective tissue disorders than previously recognised. Increased concentrations of serum aminotransferases (SGOT, SGPT) appear to be correlated with salicylate concentrations greater than 250 to 350 μg per mL and with active rheumatoid disease. The effects are reversible on discontinuing aspirin or decreasing the dose.— S. A. Kanada *et al.*, *Am. J. Hosp. Pharm.*, 1978, *35*, 330.

For reports of hepatotoxicity associated with aspirin in patients with systemic lupus erythematosus or similar disorders, see W. E. Seaman *et al.*, *Ann. intern. Med.*, 1974, *80*, 1; J. D. Wolfe *et al.*, *ibid.*, 74; *ibid.*, 103; R. L. Travers and G. R. V. Hughes, *Br. med. J.*, 1978, *2*, 1532; B. G. Petty *et al.*, *J. Pediat.*, 1978, *93*, 881.

See also under Reye's Syndrome (below).

EFFECTS ON THE SKIN. Thirteen cases of toxic epidermal necrolysis had been reported associated with the use of aspirin or methyl salicylate.— E. D. Lowney *et al.*, *Archs Derm.*, 1967, *95*, 359.

In a retrospective study of fixed eruptions in 86 patients, confirmed by a positive challenge test in 84, aspirin was the agent responsible in 1 case.— K. Kauppinen and S. Stubb, *Br. J. Derm.*, 1985, *112*, 575.

Analysis, by the Boston Collaborative Drug Surveillance Program, of data on 15 438 patients hospitalised between 1975 and 1982 detected no allergic skin reactions attributed to aspirin among 984 recipients of the drug.— M. Bigby *et al.*, *J. Am. med. Ass.*, 1986, *256*, 3358.

OVERDOSAGE. The onset of symptoms of salicylate poisoning might be delayed for up to 24 hours. All children with suspected salicylate poisoning should be admitted to hospital and kept there at least 24 hours.— I. P. Brown, *Practitioner*, 1973, *211*, 553.

In a study of 73 adults with salicylate poisoning, diagnosis was delayed in those who had ingested salicylate for medical reasons compared with those who took an intentional overdose. Morbidity and mortality-rates were higher when diagnosis was delayed. It was suggested that diagnosis of salicylate intoxication should be considered in patients, and especially elderly patients, with unexplained encephalopathy, tachypnoea, or acid-base abnormalities.— R. J. Anderson *et al.*, *Ann. intern. Med.*, 1976, *85*, 745.

The main physiological effects resulting from acute salicylate poisoning include stimulation of the respiratory centre, uncoupling of oxidative phosphorylation mechanisms, altered glucose metabolism due to inhibition of Krebs cycle enzymes, stimulation of glyconeogenesis, increased tissue glycolysis, and stimulation of lipid metabolism. Other effects include inhibition of amino-acid metabolism and interference with haemostatic mechanisms. The principal manifestations of salicylate poisoning are respiratory alkalosis, metabolic acidosis, altered glucose metabolism, fluid and electrolyte losses, and hypermetabolism.— A. R. Temple, *Pediatrics*, 1978, *62*, *Suppl.*, 873.

Symptoms of mild salicylate poisoning in children include hyperpnoea, lethargy, vomiting, hyperthermia and hypocapnia. Symptoms of moderate poisoning include severe hyperpnoea, marked lethargy or excitability, and compensated metabolic acidosis while symptoms of severe poisoning include coma, uncompensated metabolic acidosis, and possibly convulsions. Inevitable symptoms include vomiting, hyperpnoea, and hyperthermia and salicylate poisoning should always be considered when these occur together in a child.— A. K. Done, *Pediatrics*, 1978, *62*, *Suppl.*, 890.

Asterixis as a manifestation of salicylate toxicity.— R. J. Anderson, *Ann. intern. Med.*, 1981, *95*, 188.

Reports of pulmonary oedema associated with salicylate intoxication.— P. R. Davis and R. E. Burch (letter), *Ann. intern. Med.*, 1974, *80*, 553; M. G. Tweeddale (letter), *ibid.*, *81*, 710; G. Hrnicek *et al.*, *J. Am. med. Ass.*, 1974, *230*, 866; T. W. Broderick *et al.*, *Am. J. Roentg.*, 1976, *127*, 865; J. Heffner *et al.*, *West. J. Med.*, 1979, *130*, 263; S. C. Sørensen (letter), *Lancet*, 1979, *1*, 1025; C. Thomas (letter), *ibid.*, 1294; A. Kahn and D. Blum (letter), *Lancet*, 1979, *2*, 1131.

PREGNANCY AND THE NEONATE. Salicylates readily cross the placenta and have been shown to be teratogenic in *animals*. Although some studies and anecdotal reports have implicated aspirin in the formation of congenital abnormalities, most large studies (D. Slone *et al.*, *Lancet*, 1976, *1*, 1373; S. Shapiro *et al.*, *ibid.*, 1375; K.A. Winship *et al.*, *Archs Dis. Childh.*, 1984, *59*, 1052) have failed to find any significant risk or evidence of teratogenicity. The ability of aspirin, however, to alter platelet function may be a potential risk and there have been a few reports of haemorrhagic disorders in infants whose mothers had consumed aspirin during pregnancy (W.A. Bleyer and R.T. Breckenridge, *J. Am. med. Ass.*, 1970, *213*, 2049; R.R. Haslam *et al.*, *J. Pediat.*, 1974, *84*, 556; M.J. Stuart *et al.*, *New Engl. J. Med.*, 1982, *307*, 909) although in a large study (E. Collins and G. Turner, *Lancet*, 1975, *2*, 338) no such evidence of neonatal haemorrhage was observed; evidence was found in this study though of increased perinatal mortality and of haemorrhagic complications in the mother.

For reports concerning the excretion of aspirin in breast milk and precautions for breast feeding see under Precautions.

REYE'S SYNDROME. Reye's syndrome is a disorder occurring almost exclusively in children and is characterised by acute encephalopathy and fatty degeneration of the liver. Many factors may be involved in its aetiology but it typically occurs after a viral infection such as chickenpox or influenza and may be precipitated by a chemical trigger. Several large studies, as well as individual case reports, have found an association between Reye's syndrome and the prior ingestion of aspirin (K.M. Starko *et al., Pediatrics*, 1980, *66*, 859; R.J. Waldman *et al., J. Am. med. Ass.*, 1982, *247*, 3089; T.J. Halpin *et al., ibid.*, *248*, 687; R.M. Rennebohm *et al., J. Pediat.*, 1985, *107*, 877; E.S. Hurwitz *et al., New Engl. J. Med.*, 1985, *313*, 849; M.F. Rogers *et al., Pediatrics*, 1985, *75*, 260; E.S. Hurwitz *et al., J. Am. med. Ass.*, 1987, *257*, 1905). Consequently, the use of aspirin in children as a general analgesic or antipyretic is no longer considered justified. Most authorities consider one of the few acceptable indications remaining for the use of aspirin in children to be juvenile rheumatoid arthritis although suggestions have been made that during periods of childhood epidemic diseases such as chickenpox or influenza an alternative non-steroidal anti-inflammatory agent should be used (*Am. J. Dis. Childh.*, 1985, *139*, 866).

Reviews and comments on the association of Reye's syndrome with aspirin: M. H. Bellman and S. M. Hall, *Archs Dis. Childh.*, 1983, *58*, 670; M. Tarlow, *Br. med. J.*, 1986, *292*, 1543; CSM Update, *ibid.*, 1590; R. D. Mann, *J. R. Coll. gen. Pract.*, 1986, *36*, 418; A. M. Glen-Bott, *Med. Toxicol.*, 1987, *2*, 161; E. A. Mortimer, *J. Am. med. Ass.*, 1987, *257*, 1941; *Lancet*, 1987, *2*, 429.

Treatment of Adverse Effects

In acute salicylate overdosage the stomach should be emptied by aspiration and lavage. Patients with mild intoxication should be encouraged to drink plenty of fluids. In patients with more severe intoxication forced alkaline diuresis may be required. Plasma electrolytes, especially potassium, and the acid-base balance should be monitored regularly. Encouraging results have been reported in some patients treated with repeated doses of oral suspensions of activated charcoal.

In the presence of cardiac or renal impairment or in very severe intoxication, haemodialysis or haemoperfusion may need to be considered.

Some guidelines for the management of poisoning with details of procedures for forced diuresis in adults. Forced diuresis is a metabolically invasive procedure and requires close supervision but forced alkaline diuresis may be considered in salicylate poisoning if the plasma concentration in adults is more than 750 mg per litre or more than 500 mg per litre if accompanied by metabolic acidosis. If the concentration is more than 900 mg per litre or more than 750 mg per litre accompanied by renal failure haemodialysis or haemoperfusion should be considered.— A. Vale *et al., Br. med. J.*, 1984, *289*, 366.

Studies in 40 patients with moderate or severe salicylate poisoning suggested that an intravenous regimen of forced diuresis using a solution containing sodium chloride 0.225%, sodium bicarbonate 0.315%, potassium chloride 0.15%, and fructose 2.5% was effective in reducing plasma-salicylate concentrations. The solution was infused at a rate of 2 litres per hour for 3 hours. Treatment with this regimen (forced cocktail diuresis) or forced alkaline diuresis with a regimen of saline, fructose, and sodium bicarbonate ameliorated symptoms in a few hours; forced water diuresis intravenously (with saline and fructose) or fluids by mouth required more than 24 hours. All 3 intravenous regimens produced a good diuresis, though it was delayed for up to 2 hours in some patients. Forced alkaline diuresis produced the most rapid fall in plasma-salicylate concentrations but was accompanied by a rise in arterial pH. Excretion of salicylate with the compound solution was less effective but there were no changes in arterial pH or blood-potassium concentrations. Potassium by mouth could be given later to treat delayed falls in plasma concentrations.— A. A. H. Lawson *et al., Q. J. Med.*, 1969, *38*, 31.

Sixteen patients with mild salicylate poisoning were treated, after gastric lavage, by oral fluids only. Of 28 with moderate poisoning 6 were treated by forced diuresis, 16 by forced alkaline diuresis, and 6 by alkali alone—sodium bicarbonate 225 mmol in 1.5 litres intravenously over 3 to 4 hours. Urinary recovery of salicylic acid after forced diuresis was of little value, was greater after forced alkaline diuresis, and was greatest after alkali alone. Mean urine pH in the 4 groups was 6.1, 6.5, 7.3, and 8.1 respectively; renal salicylate clearance was greatest in the fourth group; the alkali alone procedure did not cause fluid retention or significant biochemical abnormalities. The apparent fall of plasma-salicylate concentrations after forced alkaline diuresis was considered to be the result of haemodilution. Salicylate can be removed safely and effectively by alkali alone.— L. F. Prescott *et al., Br. med. J.*, 1982, *285*, 1383.

A report of the use of repeated oral doses of charcoal in the treatment of salicylate poisoning. In 5 patients with maximum plasma-salicylate concentrations of 425 to 655 mg per litre 2 to 8 hours after an aspirin overdosage, gastric lavage being performed in all on admission to hospital, forced alkaline diuresis produced an unsatisfactory response in the two on whom it was performed. All patients received activated charcoal (Medicoal) as an oral suspension in an initial dose of 75 g followed by further doses of 50 g, generally at 4-hour intervals, until symptoms were relieved. Compared with 6 control patients with mild poisoning given only oral fluids plasma-salicylate concentrations fell dramatically in all 5 patients following charcoal administration and this therapy appeared to be more effective than forced alkaline diuresis had been in previous patients. Further studies were necessary to assess the role of repeated oral charcoal in patients with severe poisoning due to aspirin.— R. J. Hillman and L. F. Prescott, *Br. med. J.*, 1985, *291*, 1472. A similar report of the beneficial use of repeated doses of activated charcoal (Carbomix) in 2 patients with plasma-salicylate concentrations in excess of 600 mg per litre who did not undergo alkaline diuresis. It was considered that Carbomix may not be as effective as Medicoal with mention being made that alternate doses of the two proprietaries were currently being employed to offset the apparent opposite effects each had in producing diarrhoea and constipation. It was considered, however, that the results of additional studies in progress were needed before alkaline diuresis was abandoned and repeated oral charcoal used routinely.— D. Boldy and J. A. Vale (letter), *ibid.*, 1986, *292*, 136.

Precautions

Aspirin should be cautiously employed, if at all, in patients prone to dyspepsia or known to have a lesion of the gastric mucosa. It should not be administered to patients with haemophilia or other haemorrhagic disorders or to those with an intolerance to aspirin (especially aspirin-sensitive asthmatics). Caution is necessary when renal or hepatic function is impaired. The use of aspirin in children under the age of 12 years is extremely limited because of the risk of Reye's syndrome (see under Adverse Effects and under Uses and Administration).

Some of the effects of aspirin on the gastro-intestinal tract are enhanced by alcohol. Aspirin may enhance the activity of coumarin anticoagulants and sulphonylurea hypoglycaemic agents. The haemorrhagic effects of aspirin on the gastric mucosa may be enhanced by anticoagulants. The activity of methotrexate may be markedly enhanced and its toxicity increased by administration with aspirin. Aspirin diminishes the effects of uricosuric agents such as probenecid and sulphinpyrazone.

INTERACTIONS. A review of potential drug interactions and adverse effects related to aspirin.— M. Suffness and B. S. Rose, *Drug Intell. & clin. Pharm.*, 1974, *8*, 694.

For the effect of aspirin on some other drugs, see under diuretics (p.974), propranolol (p.802), and warfarin (p.345).

Corticosteroids. In 4 patients taking salicylates and corticosteroids the serum-salicylate concentration rose when the corticosteroid was withdrawn or the dose reduced. One 5-year-old boy developed salicylism characterised by dyspnoea, lethargy, metabolic acidosis, and a serum-salicylate concentration of 880 µg per mL.— J. R. Klinenberg and F. Miller, *J. Am. med. Ass.*, 1965, *194*, 601.

Concurrent administration of corticosteroids or corticotrophin with aspirin or sodium salicylate was shown to lower the plasma-salicylate concentration.— M. Bardare *et al., Archs Dis. Childh.*, 1978, *53*, 381.

Further references: J. Edelman *et al., Br. J. clin. Pharmac.*, 1986, *21*, 301.

Diclofenac. Pretreatment with diclofenac sodium appeared to enhance renal excretion of salicylate. Acute administration of diclofenac had no effect on plasma-salicylate concentrations. Concurrent administration of aspirin resulted in a significant decrease in plasma concentrations of diclofenac.— F. O. Müller *et al., Int. J. clin. Pharmac. Biopharm.*, 1977, *15*, 397.

Paracetamol. In a study involving a total of 21 subjects administration of paracetamol with aspirin was noted to increase blood concentrations of unhydrolysed aspirin.— V. F. Cotty *et al., Toxic. appl. Pharmac.*, 1977, *41*, 7.

PREGNANCY AND THE NEONATE. Salicylates were excreted in breast milk and had caused macular rashes in breast-fed babies.— R. W. Smithells and D. M. Morgan, *Practitioner*, 1970, *204*, 14.

Aspirin appeared in breast milk in moderate amounts and could produce a bleeding tendency either by interfering with the function of the infant's platelets or by decreasing the amount of prothrombin in the blood. The risk was minimal if the mother took the aspirin just after nursing and if the infant had adequate store of vitamin K.— *Med. Lett.*, 1974, *16*, 25.

Serum-salicylate concentrations in a mother receiving aspirin 2.4 g daily for adult Still's disease and her 9-week-old breast-fed infant were 1.63 and 0.47 mmol per litre respectively. Because children under 12 years of age are rarely given aspirin due to the risk of Reye's syndrome appropriate warnings should be given to pregnant and breast-feeding women.— J. Unsworth *et al., Ann. rheum. Dis.*, 1987, *46*, 638.

Absorption and Fate

Absorption of non-ionised aspirin occurs in the stomach. Acetylsalicylates and salicylates are also readily absorbed from the intestine. Hydrolysis to salicylic acid occurs rapidly in the intestine and in the circulation. Salicylates are extensively bound to plasma proteins; aspirin to a lesser degree. Aspirin and salicylates are rapidly distributed to all body tissues; they appear in milk and cross the placenta. The rate of excretion of aspirin varies with the pH of the urine, increasing as the pH rises and being greatest at pH 7.5 and above. Aspirin is excreted as salicylic acid and as glucuronide conjugates and as salicyluric and gentisic acids.

Many studies have been performed to assess the pharmacokinetics of aspirin in patients of differing age and sex and with differing disease states but most have only investigated single doses. Although such studies have sometimes observed altered pharmacokinetics in such patients the direct relevance of these findings with regard to the clinical use of aspirin is not entirely clear. It has been considered that, in general, these differences are unlikely to be significant when only single or occasional doses of aspirin are employed as a simple analgesic or antipyretic. Suggestions have, however, been made that during long-term therapy with high doses in conditions such as rheumatoid arthritis females may require smaller doses than males and reduced doses may be necessary in the elderly.

Some references to the pharmacokinetics of aspirin: M. S. Roberts, *Eur. J. clin. Pharmac.*, 1983, *25*, 253 (single doses: young, elderly, or alcoholic males); Z. Trnavská and K. Trnavský, *ibid.*, 679 (single and multiple doses: males and females); P. C. Ho *et al., Br. J. clin. Pharmac.*, 1985, *19*, 675 (single doses: young and elderly, males and females); P. Netter *et al., Clin. Pharmac. Ther.*, 1985, *38*, 6 (single doses: young and elderly, males and females); P. R. Montgomery *et al., ibid.*, 1986, *39*, 571 (single doses: young and elderly, males and females); C. Jorup-Rönström *et al., Clin. Pharmacokinet.*, 1986, *11*, 250 (single doses: during viral hepatitis); J. O. Miners *et al., Br. J. clin. Pharmac.*, 1986, *22*, 135 (single doses: young males and females); R. R. Grigor *et al., J. Rheumatol.*, 1987, *14*, 60 (multiple doses: young and elderly, males and females, rheumatoid arthritis patients).

Uses and Administration

Aspirin has analgesic, anti-inflammatory, and antipyretic properties; it is an inhibitor of the enzyme cyclo-oxygenase which results in the inhibition of the biosynthesis of prostaglandins.

Aspirin is used for the relief of the less severe types of pain such as headache, dysmenorrhoea, myalgias, and toothache. It is also used in acute and chronic inflammatory disorders such as rheumatoid arthritis. In the treatment of minor febrile conditions, such as colds or influenza, aspirin is of value for the reduction of temperature and relief of the headache and the joint and muscle pains.

Aspirin is usually taken by mouth. Gastric irritation may be reduced by taking doses after food. Effervescent soluble tablets or enteric-coated tablets may be used. In some instances aspirin may be administered rectally by suppository.

The usual dose of aspirin by mouth as an analgesic and antipyretic is 0.3 to 0.9 g, which may be repeated every 4 to 6 hours according to clinical needs, up to a maximum of 4 g daily.

Plasma-salicylate concentrations of 150 to 300 μg per mL are required for optimal anti-inflammatory activity but may produce tinnitus; more serious adverse effects occur at concentrations above 300 μg per mL. Doses need to be adjusted individually to achieve these concentrations. Generally doses of about 4 to 8 g daily in divided doses are used for acute rheumatic disorders. Doses of up to 5.4 g daily in divided doses may be sufficient in chronic rheumatic disorders.

Indications for aspirin therapy in children, because of the risk of Reye's syndrome (see under Adverse Effects), are extremely limited. One of the few indications where aspirin therapy may still be considered is juvenile rheumatoid arthritis. Suggested doses for this condition have been up to 80 mg per kg body-weight daily in 5 or 6 divided doses with up to 130 mg per kg daily being employed during acute exacerbations.

Aspirin affects platelet function; by blocking synthesis of thromboxane A_2, platelet aggregation is inhibited. It may be used for the secondary prevention of myocardial infarction and stroke in patients with a history of such disorders but the optimum dose and duration of treatment remain to be firmly established. Large clinical studies have shown that doses of more than 300 to 325 mg daily are not necessary and some authorities have recommended much lower doses of about 75 to 100 mg daily. Aspirin may also be of value in the primary prevention of these disorders. Antiplatelet therapy is discussed below; thrombolytic therapy is discussed under streptokinase, p.1048.

ADMINISTRATION IN RENAL FAILURE. Aspirin could be administered to patients with renal failure by adjusting the dosage interval. A dosage interval of 4 hours is suitable for patients whose glomerular filtration-rates exceed 50 mL per minute; an interval of 4 to 6 hours is advisable for rates of 10 to 50 mL per minute; it should be avoided in those with a rate of less than 10 mL per minute. A dose supplement may be necessary to patients undergoing haemodialysis or peritoneal dialysis.— W. M. Bennett *et al.*, *Am. J. Kidney Dis.*, 1983, *3*, 155.

ANTIPLATELET THERAPY. *Action and dosage.* Aspirin is an inhibitor of the enzyme cyclo-oxygenase, the reaction being considered to be due to an irreversible acetylation process.

In blood platelets such enzyme inhibition prevents the synthesis of thromboxane A_2, a compound which is a vasoconstrictor, causes platelet aggregation and is thus potentially thrombotic. In blood vessel walls the enzyme inhibition prevents the synthesis of prostacyclin, which is a vasodilator, has anti-aggregating properties and is thus potentially anti-thrombotic. Aspirin therefore appears to have paradoxical biological effects. The duration of these effects, however, may be somewhat different with the effects on the vascular tissue generally being shorter lived than the effects on the platelets although the animal species studied, the type of blood vessel employed, and the prevailing experimental conditions may alter the results. The differing duration of effects may be explained by the fact that platelets are unable to re-synthesise cyclo-oxygenase thus resulting in no new thromboxane A_2 being produced until, after about 24 hours, more platelets are released by the bone marrow; as platelet activity in bone marrow may also be affected by aspirin it is generally considered that aspirin need not be given more frequently than once daily for inhibition of platelet aggregation to occur. In contrast to the effect on cyclo-oxygenase in platelets, re-generation of cyclo-oxygenase in the blood vessel wall does occur.

Although the balance between platelet thromboxanes and vascular prostacyclin has not yet been proved to be an important determinant in the pathogenesis of thrombosis, many pharmacological studies have been performed in an attempt to find a dose of aspirin that will inhibit the synthesis of thromboxane A_2 whilst sparing the effect on prostacyclin production. The results of such studies are often conflicting and confusing.

Nuotto *et al.* (*Eur. J. clin. Pharmac.*, 1983, *25*, 313) using aspirin in doses of 50, 100, 250, and 1000 mg daily found that all doses suppressed thromboxane formation after 14 days but did not study the effect on prostacyclin. Similarly, McLeod *et al.* (*Scand. J. Haemat.*, 1986, *36*, 379) found that doses of 50 to 100 mg daily significantly inhibited platelet function but that higher doses of up to 3900 mg daily produced no additional further changes. Studies by Weksler *et al.* (*New Engl. J. Med.*, 1983, *308*, 800) and by Roberts *et al.* (*Lancet*, 1986, *1*, 1153) have indicated that single doses of 40 to 80 mg and 50 mg respectively are capable of inhibiting platelet aggregation without having a significant or long-lasting effect on vascular prostacyclin. A dose of 40 mg every 48 hours was shown by Hanley *et al.* (*Br. med. J.*, 1982, *285*, 1299) to have similar effects, consistently reducing thromboxane synthesis to a degree which failed to support platelet aggregation and leading to only a short-lived reduction in vascular prostacyclin; these workers also showed that the same dose of 40 mg given every 72 hours, however, did not reduce thromboxane synthesis sufficiently. Doses of 20 mg daily have been investigated by Patrignani *et al.* (*J. clin. Invest.*, 1982, *69*, 1366) and by Cerletti *et al.* (*New Engl. J. Med.*, 1986, *314*, 316) with both sets of workers showing that such doses significantly prevent generation of thromboxane; the former study also indicated that such a dose did not affect vascular prostacyclin. Even doses as low as 1 mg daily have been studied by Sinzinger *et al.* (*New Engl. J. Med.*, 1984, *311*, 1052) and found to affect platelet sensitivity.

These pharmacological studies, therefore, do appear to indicate that aspirin in doses of 100 mg or less daily possesses an antithrombotic effect, this evidence also being supported by the successful use in clinical studies of doses of 100 mg daily to keep grafts patent following coronary bypass surgery (see below). It should, however, be noted that large-scale long-term clinical studies to assess the role of aspirin as an antiplatelet agent for the secondary prevention of myocardial infarction or stroke (see below) have not used doses of less than 300 mg daily and the optimum dose of aspirin as an antiplatelet agent perhaps remains to be established.

Cardiovascular and cerebrovascular disorders. Many studies have been conducted in patients with a history of myocardial infarction, stroke, transient ischaemic attacks, or unstable angina to elucidate whether antiplatelet drug therapy (usually aspirin, sulphinpyrazone, or aspirin with dipyridamole) can reduce the well-known risk of further cardiovascular or cerebrovascular events or of vascular death ocurring in such patients. In an overview (Antiplatelet Trialists' Collaboration, *Br. med. J.*, 1988, *296*, 320) of 25 such completed trials (a further 6 still being in progress) involving some 29 000 patients the authors stated that the two main purposes of the overview were firstly, and most obviously, to include far larger numbers of patients than had been included in individual trials, thus yielding results that were far less subject to random error, and secondly, to avoid the substantial systematic bias that may be engendered when many related trials have been performed and just a few become well known. The aim was to review the apparent effects of treatment on non-fatal myocardial infarction, non-fatal stroke, vascular death, and non-vascular death. In most cases the main results of the 25 trials were obtained from the principal investigators but it was noted that for some trials the data that was obtained differed slightly from that originally published (generally because of further follow-up).

The overview found extremely significant reductions in non-fatal myocardial infarctions and non-fatal strokes (in both instances the risk reduction being about 30%) such that it was considered that the significant reduction in vascular mortality (a risk reduction of about 15%) could be safely accepted as real. Overall, no apparent effect on non-vascular mortality was observed.

The observed benefit in patients with unstable angina was found to be somewhat greater than in patients with a history of myocardial infarction or cerebrovascular disease but the difference was not clearly significant and it was considered that there was no really clear evidence that antiplatelet therapy had a proportionally greater or lesser effect in any particular category of patient studied.

It was considered difficult to reliably estimate the absolute benefits of antiplatelet therapy but based upon crude estimates for various types of treatment it was suggested that in patients with some apparent risk of occlusive disease the expected benefit from antiplatelet therapy may well be comparable with the benefits to be expected from standard treatments, such as long-term β-blockade after myocardial infarction or diuretic treatment for moderately hypertensive elderly subjects, and that it would considerably exceed the yearly benefit to be expected from the treatment of moderate hypertension in middle age.

The three main antiplatelet therapies used in the 25 trials were aspirin, sulphinpyrazone, or aspirin with dipyridamole and the overview provided no good evidence that any one of the therapies was more or less effective than the others. All the trials that had employed aspirin used doses of 300 to 325 mg daily or 0.9 to 1.5 g daily and the low-dose studies appeared to have yielded results that were at least as good as those obtained with the higher doses. In the early trials high doses were used to facilitate biochemical checks on patient compliance.

For those with appropriate vascular disease there is clear evidence that antiplatelet treatment reduces the overall incidence of fatal or disabling vascular disease; the most convenient and least expensive type of antiplatelet agent, providing there are no contra-indications to its use, is low-dose aspirin, there being no good reason to use a dose higher than 300 to 325 mg daily, and there even being some other published pharmacological evidence demonstrating that much lower doses of about 100 mg daily have a substantial antithrombotic effect; no recommendations could be made on whether treatment should continue for one year, for several years, or even indefinitely.

The more recent large-scale ISIS-2 study (*Lancet*, 1988, *2*, 349) showed that aspirin 160 mg daily for 1 month, started immediately after admission for acute myocardial infarction, significantly reduced mortality. Even greater benefit was achieved when streptokinase was also given.

The role of aspirin in the primary prevention of cardiovascular and cerebrovascular disorders, in contrast to its role in the secondary prevention as discussed above, is far less clear. In two recent studies conducted in the *UK* (R. Peto *et al.*, *Br. med. J.*, 1988, *296*, 313) and the *USA* (The Steering Committee of the Physicians' Health Study Research Group, *New Engl. J. Med.*, 1988, *318*, 262) involving respectively about 5000 and 22 000 apparently healthy male physicians with no history of cardiovascular or cerebrovascular disorders, apparently conflicting results were found. Although in the *UK* study, where doses of aspirin were usually 500 mg daily, a significant reduction in the frequency of transient cerebral ischaemic attacks was found, no significant reduction in the incidence of non-fatal or fatal myocardial infarction was observed; disturbingly, an excess number of disabling or fatal strokes was also observed. In the *USA* study (the purpose of which was also to investigate the role of beta-carotene for the prevention of cancer) the component of the trial which employed aspirin 325 mg on alternate days was terminated early after the finding of a statistically extreme beneficial effect of aspirin in preventing non-fatal and fatal myocardial infarction. Again, however, there was an increased risk of moderate to severe or fatal haemorrhagic stroke in the aspirin groups. The conclusion of the authors of the *UK* study was that their results had provided no definite indication that treatment of apparently healthy people with aspirin had a beneficial effect whereas the conclusion from the *USA* study was that the benefit they had found in preventing myocardial ischaemia must be weighed against the hazards of gastrointestinal disorders and bleeding as well as against the observed risk of haemorrhagic stroke and that the decision of whether to use aspirin or not for such primary prevention must remain a matter for individual judgement.

Further reviews and comments concerning the use of aspirin in both primary and secondary prevention of myocardial infarction and stroke: M. Orme, *Br. med. J.*, 1988, *296*, 307; A. S. Relman, *New Engl. J. Med.*, 1988, *318*, 245; I. A. G. Reilly and G. A. FitzGerald, *Drugs*, 1988, *35*, 154; G. de Gaetano, *Lancet*, 1988, *1*, 1093.

In Kawasaki disease in children, aspirin has been used successfully to reduce or prevent thrombotic complications and coronary artery involvement that may result in myocardial infarction, although the doses reported to have been used appear to vary considerably (K.M. Goel *et al.*, *Lancet*, 1983, *1*, 1440; D.W. Denning, *ibid.*, *2*, 621; G. Koren *et al.*, *J. Am. med. Ass.*, 1985, *254*, 767; M. Terai *et al.*, *J. Pediat.*, 1985, *106*, 76; J.F.N. Taylor, *Br. med. J.*, 1987, *294*, 1112). The risk of Reye's syndrome (see under Adverse Effects) should always be considered before employing aspirin in children.

Postoperative Use. Aspirin has also been studied to assess its role in the prevention of thrombotic events associated with various forms of surgical procedures. Conflicting results with regard to the prevention of deep-vein thrombosis following chiefly orthopaedic surgery have been reported with some studies finding a beneficial effect (W.H. Harris *et al.*, *New Engl. J. Med.*, 1977, *297*, 1246; R. McKenna *et al.*, *Br. med. J.*, 1980, *280*, 514; R.D. Sautter *et al.*, *J. Am. med. Ass.*, 1983, *250*, 2649; M.J. Alfaro *et al.*, *Thromb. Haemostasis*, 1986, *56*, 53) whilst others reported essentially no changed effect on the incidence of postoperative events (Report of the Steering Committee of a Trial Sponsored by the MRC, *Lancet*, 1972, *2*, 441; M. Hume, *New Engl. J. Med.*, 1978, *298*, 1091; J.D. Stamatakis *et al.*, *Br. med. J.*, 1978, *1*, 1031).

The value of long-term treatment with aspirin to keep grafts patent following coronary by-pass surgery has however been demonstrated by several studies. Most reported beneficial effects using aspirin (about 325 mg three times daily) with dipyridamole (75 mg three times daily) (J.H. Chesebro *et al.*, *New Engl. J. Med.*, 1982, *307*, 73; *idem*, 1984, *310*, 209; B.G. Brown *et al.*, *Circulation*, 1985, *72*, 138; S.M. Raja *et al.*, *J. thorac. cardiovasc. Surg.*, 1985, *90*, 373) although some have reported good results using low-dose aspirin alone (100 mg daily) (R.L. Lorenz *et al.*, *Lancet*, 1984, *1*, 1261; W. Meister *et al.*, *Br. J. clin. Pharmac.*, 1984, *17*, 703).

Pregnancy and the neonate. A review and discussion on the possible place of low-dose aspirin in the prevention of toxaemia of pregnancy. There is a considerable body of evidence to support the concept that pregnancy-induced hypertension develops when an imbalance occurs between prostacyclin and thromboxane A_2 production and clinical studies have provided evidence for a therapeutic role for aspirin.

In a study involving 102 women regarded as being at high risk of developing pre-eclampsia because of previous complicated hypertensive pregnancies or of pre-existing hypertension (M. Beaufils *et al.*, *Lancet*, 1985, *1*, 840), treatment with aspirin 150 mg and dipyridamole 300 mg, each daily, resulted in no cases of pre-eclampsia in the treated group compared with 6 cases in the control group given no treatment. This study is, however, subject to some criticism on the grounds of its open nature and lack of a placebo control group. A more convincing report (H.C.S. Wallenburg *et al.*, *Lancet*, 1986, *1*, 1) describes a placebo-controlled study in 46 women identified at 28 weeks' gestation to be at risk. Of the 23 women who received placebo, 12 developed pregnancy-induced hypertension with one becoming eclamptic; of the 23 who received aspirin 60 mg daily none developed toxaemia. Less direct, but equally convincing, evidence is provided by studies of women with auto-immune disorders in pregnancy. A high prevalence of toxaemia occurs in women with lupus anticoagulant and treatment of such women with immunosuppresive doses of prednisone resulted in live births only when low-dose aspirin was included in the regimen (W.F. Lubbe and G.C. Liggins, *Am. J. Obstet. Gynec.*, 1985, *132*, 322). This study also showed that the occurrence of toxaemia was effectively eliminated by the early introduction of aspirin 75 mg daily whereas in another series of patients (D.W. Branch *et al.*, *New Engl. J. Med.*, 1985, *313*, 1322) toxaemia remained a serious complication when aspirin was used inconsistently, often being introduced relatively late.

Thus the evidence that antiplatelet treatment with low-dose aspirin is effective in preventing the development of toxaemia of pregnancy is compelling but further studies are required. The evidence is insufficient to justify the use in all primigravid women, but is strong enough to justify the use in women judged to be at risk (with factors such as pre-existing chronic hypertension, auto-immune disorders especially systemic lupus or lupus anticoagulant, or a history of recurring toxaemia in successive pregnancies). The question of aspirin dosage remains to be resolved; whether all women will be protected by 50 to 100 mg daily or whether some may need higher doses needs to be clarified.— W. F. Lubbe, *Drugs*, 1987, *34*, 515.

Further reviews concerning the use of aspirin for the prophylaxis of pre-eclampsia: *Lancet*, 1986, *1*, 18.

Encouraging results in 42 women with very bad obstetric histories treated with aspirin 75 mg daily from the first or second trimester until delivery. Nineteen women had a history of severe pregnancy-induced hypertension and intra-uterine growth retardation, 16 had systemic lupus erythematosus, and 7 had a history of severe foetal growth retardation not associated with the above 2 factors. After low-dose aspirin prophylaxis, 38 completed pregnancies occurred resulting in 35 live births. There were no maternal or neonatal complications attributable to aspirin. A controlled clinical study is now needed and low-dose aspirin should not be used indiscriminately until the benefits and safety have been properly evaluated.— M. G. Elder *et al.* (letter), *Lancet*, 1988, *1*, 410.

Miscellaneous conditions. A variety of other conditions with characteristics of abnormal blood clotting or platelet function have also been reported to respond to antiplatelet therapy involving the use of aspirin. Most of these beneficial effects, it should be noted though, are based on either anecdotal evidence or relatively small studies.

Beneficial results have been reported in *amaurosis fugax*, a recurrent transient uni-ocular loss of vision that can often be attributed to retinal-artery embolism (M.J.G. Harrison *et al.*, *Lancet*, 1971, *2*, 743; J. Mundall *et al.*, *ibid.*, 1972, *1*, 92; K.K.-Y. Wu, *Ann. intern. Med.*, 1978, *88*, 7).

Good responses have similarly been obtained in some patients with *polycythaemia vera* or *thrombocythaemia*, disorders again often showing abnormal platelet function (J.M. Levin and T.L. Ostrowski, *J. Am. med. Ass.*, 1974, *229*, 186; N.S. Gilbert, *ibid.*, *230*, 539; K.K.-Y. Wu, *Ann. intern. Med.*, 1978, *88*, 7).

Necrobiotic diabetic skin lesions have sometimes responded to aspirin with dipyridamole, the effect being attributed to an antiplatelet action (A. Eldor *et al.*, *New Engl. J. Med.*, 1978, *298*, 1033; B. Fjellner, *ibid.*, *299*, 1366).

Adjunctive therapy with aspirin has been reported to provide some benefit in patients with *thrombotic thrombocytopenic purpura* (E.C. Rossi *et al.*, *J. Am. med. Ass.*, 1974, *228*, 1141; E.L. Amorosi and S. Karpatkin, *Ann. intern. Med.*, 1977, *86*, 102; T.J. Myers *et al.*, *ibid.*, 1980, *92*, 149; E.B. Toffelmire *et al.*, *Can. med. Ass. J.*, 1984, *131*, 1371; J.B. Blitzer *et al.*, *Am. J. Haemat.*, 1987, *24*, 329).

Progression of *membranoproliferative glomerulonephritis* to end-stage renal disease occurred in fewer patients treated with aspirin and dipyridamole than in those given placebo (J.V. Donadio *et al.*, *New Engl. J. Med.*, 1984, *310*, 1421), again the rationale for the drug therapy stemming from the fact that platelet activation had been demonstrated to be a component of the disease.

Progression of another disorder, *peripheral occlusive arterial disease* of the lower extremities, has also been reported to be delayed by the administration of antiplatelet drug therapy involving the use of aspirin (H. Hess *et al.*, *Lancet*, 1985, *1*, 415 and 654).

Prophylaxis of migraine is another indication where some investigators have reported a beneficial effect of aspirin (B.P. O'Neill and J.D. Mann, *Lancet*, 1978, *2*, 1179; D.J. Dalessio, *J. Am. med. Ass.*, 1978, *239*, 52; A. Bamji, *Br. med. J.*, 1987, *294*, 772) although it is not always considered to be suitably free of side-effects for such a purpose (K.J. Zilkha, *Br. med. J.*, 1987, *294*, 427).

Preparations

Aspirin Capsules *(U.S.P.)*

Aspirin Delayed-release Capsules *(U.S.P.)*. The capsules or the contents are enteric-coated.

Aspirin Suppositories *(U.S.P.)*

Aspirin Tablets *(B.P.)*. Acetylsalicylic Acid Tablets

Aspirin Tablets *(U.S.P.)*

Aspirin Delayed-release Tablets *(U.S.P.)*. Enteric-coated aspirin tablets.

Buffered Aspirin Tablets *(U.S.P.)*

Dispersible Aspirin Tablets *(B.P.)*

NOTE. The *B.P.* directs that when Dispersible Aspirin Tablets are prescribed or demanded, no strength being stated, tablets containing 300 mg shall be dispensed or supplied.

Soluble Aspirin Tablets *(B.P.)*. Effervescent Aspirin Tablets

NOTE. The *B.P.* directs that when Soluble Aspirin Tablets are prescribed or demanded, no strength being stated, tablets containing 300 mg shall be dispensed or supplied.

Aspirin and Caffeine Tablets *(B.P.)*. Each tablet contains aspirin 350 mg and caffeine 30 mg.

Aspirin and Codeine Phosphate Tablets *(U.S.P.)*

Aspirin, Alumina, and Magnesia Tablets *(U.S.P.)*. Tablets containing aspirin, aluminium hydroxide, and magnesium hydroxide.

Aspirin, Codeine Phosphate, Alumina, and Magnesia Tablets *(U.S.P.)*. Tablets containing aspirin, codeine phosphate, aluminium hdroxide, and magnesium hydroxide.

Co-codaprin Tablets *(B.P.)*. Aspirin and Codeine Tablets. Tablets containing codeine phosphate and aspirin in the proportions, by weight, 1 part to 50 parts. Protect from light.

Dispersible Co-codaprin Tablets *(B.P.)*. Dispersible Aspirin and Codeine Tablets. Tablets containing codeine phosphate and aspirin in the proportions, by weight, 1 part to 50 parts in a suitable dispersible basis. Protect from light.

Proprietary Preparations

Antoin *(Cox, UK). Tablets*, dispersible, scored, aspirin 400 mg, codeine phosphate 5 mg, caffeine citrate 15 mg.

Aspav (formerly known as Soluble Aspirin and Papaveretum Tablets) *(Cox, UK). Tablets*, dispersible, aspirin 500 mg, papaveretum 10 mg.

Aspergum *(Plough, UK). Tablets*, chewing gum, aspirin 227 mg.

Caprin *(Sinclair, UK). Tablets*, sustained-release for intestinal release, aspirin 324 mg.

Claradin *(Nicholas, UK). Tablets*, soluble, aspirin 300 mg.

Codis *(Reckitt & Colman Pharmaceuticals, UK). Tablets*, soluble, aspirin 400 mg, codeine phosphate 8 mg (co-codaprin).

Hypon *(Calmic, UK). Tablets*, aspirin 325 mg, codeine phosphate 5 mg, caffeine 10 mg.

Laboprin *(Laboratories for Applied Biology, UK). Tablets*, scored, aspirin 300 mg, lysine 245 mg.

Migravess *(Bayer, UK). Tablets*, soluble, scored, aspirin 325 mg, metoclopramide hydrochloride 5 mg.

Tablets (Migravess Forte), soluble, scored, aspirin 450 mg, metoclopramide hydrochloride 5 mg.

Nu-seals Aspirin *(Lilly, UK). Tablets*, enteric-sealed, aspirin 300 and 600 mg.

Paynocil *(Beecham Research, UK). Tablets*, scored, aspirin 600 mg, glycine 300 mg.

Platet *(Nicholas, UK). Tablets*, effervescent, aspirin 100 mg.

Solmin *(Reckitt & Colman Pharmaceuticals, UK). Tablets*, dispersible, aspirin 300 mg, glycine 133 mg.

Solprin *(Reckitt & Colman Pharmaceuticals, UK). Tablets*, soluble, aspirin 300 mg.

Veganin *(Warner, UK). Tablets*, scored, aspirin 250 mg, codeine phosphate 6.8 mg, paracetamol 250 mg.

Proprietary Names and Manufacturers of Aspirin, its Salts, and its Complexes

AAS *(Arg.; Sterwin, Spain)*; Acentérine *(Switz.)*; Acenterine *(Belg.; Neth.)*; Acetard *(Benzon, Denm.; Benzon, Swed.)*; Acetophen *(Canad.)*; Acetyl *(Neth.)*; Acetylin *(Heyden, Ger.)*; Acetylo *(Switz.)*; Adiro *(Arg.; Belg.; Neth.; Bayer, Spain)*; Albyl *(Leo, Denm.; Nyco, Norw.; Leo, Swed.)*; Albyl-E *(Nyco, Norw.)*; Albyl-Selters *(Denm.; Swed.)*; Alcacyl *(Wander, Switz.)*; Alupir *(Farmacologico Milanese, Ital.)*; Aluprin *(Lemmon, USA)*; Apernyl *(Bayer, Ger.; Swed.)*; Aquaprin *(S.Afr.)*; Arthralgyl *(Nativelle, Switz.)*; Arthritis Pain Formula *(Whitehall, USA)*; A.S.A. *(Lilly, USA)*; ASA-Aspirin *(Smith Kline & French, Austral.)*; Asadrine C-200 *(Sabex, Canad.)*; Asagran *(Monsanto, UK)*; Asatard *(Ital.)*; Aspasol *(Vernleigh, S.Afr.)*; Aspegic *(Belg.; Synthelabo, Fr.; Lirca, Ital.; Neth.; S.Afr.; Synthelabo, Switz.)*; Aspergum *(Plough, UK)*; Aspidol *(Piam, Ital.)*; Aspilisina *(Roger, Spain)*; Aspinfantil *(Lasa, Spain)*; Aspirina *(Bayer, Ital.)*; Aspirine *(Bayer, Switz.)*; Aspirinetas *(Arg.)*; Aspirisucre *(Beecham Products, Fr.)*; Aspisol *(Fr.; Bayer, Ger.)*; Aspro *(Nicholas, Austral.; Nicholas, Ger.; Bouty, Ital.; Pan Química Farmac., Spain; Nicholas, Switz.; Nicholas, UK)*; Asrivo *(Switz.)*; ASS 500 Dolormin *(Engelhard, Ger.)*; Astrin *(Medic, Canad.)*; Astrix *(Faulding, Austral.)*;

Bamyl *(Hässle, Swed.)*; Bamyl S *(Hässle, Swed.)*; Bayaspirina *(Arg.)*; Bayer Aspirin *(Bayer, Denm.; Bayer, Swed.; Bayer, UK; Glenbrook, USA)*; Bebesan *(Switz.)*; Bi-prin *(Boots, Austral.)*; Breoprin *(Sterling Research, UK)*; Bufferin *(Astra, Austral.; Bristol-Myers Pharmaceuticals, UK; Bristol-Myers Products, USA)*; Calmantina *(Inexfa, Spain)*; Calmo Yer *(Yer, Spain)*; Caprin *(Sinclair, UK)*; Cardiprin *(Reckitt & Colman, Austral.)*; Casprium Retard *(Liade, Spain)*; Catalgine *(Théraplix, Fr.)*; Catalgix *(Rhone-Poulenc, Switz.)*; Cemirit *(Bayer, Ital.)*; Chefarine-N *(Neth.)*; Chu-Pax *(Multipax, UK)*; Claradin *(Nicholas, UK)*; Claragine *(Nicholas, Fr.)*; Codalgina Retard *(Spain)*; Codral Junior *(Austral.)*; Colfarit *(Bayer, Ger.; Bayer, Switz.)*; Contradol *(Merz, Ger.)*; Contrheuma *(Spitzner, Ger.)*; Coryphen *(Rougier, Canad.)*; Delgesic *(Karlspharma, Ger.; Remedia, S.Afr.)*; Disipal *(Gayoso Wellcome, Spain)*; Dispril *(Belg.; Reckitt & Colman, Norw.; Reckitt & Colman, Swed.; Switz.)*; Disprin *(Reckitt & Colman, Austral.; Reckitt & Colman, S.Afr.; Reckitt & Colman Pharmaceuticals, UK)*; Doléan pH 8 *(Riker 3M, Switz.)*; Dolean pH 8 *(Belg.; Ital.)*; Dolomega *(Almirall, Spain)*; Domupirina *(Medici Domus, Ital.)*; Easprin *(Parke, Davis, USA)*; Ecotrin *(Smith Kline & French, Austral.; Smith Kline & French, Canad.; Smith Kline & French, USA)*; Elsprin *(Austral.)*; Empirin *(Wellcome, USA)*; Encaprin *(Procter & Gamble, USA)*; Endydol *(Guidotti, Ital.)*; Enteretas *(Arg.)*; Enterosarin *(Belg.)*; Enterosarine *(Neth.; Switz.)*; Entrophen *(Frosst, Canad.)*; Flectadol *(Maggioni-Winthrop, Ital.)*; Globentyl *(Nyco, Denm.; Nyco, Norw.)*; Godamed *(Pfleger, Ger.)*; Halgon *(Ger.)*; Headstart *(Ciba-Geigy, Canad.)*; Helver Sal *(Bauxili, Spain)*; Hyprin *(Jpn)*; Idotyl *(Ferrosan, Denm.)*; Inyesprin *(Andromaco, Spain)*; Istopirine *(Hung.)*; Ivépirine *(Lucien, Fr.)*; Juvépirine *(Fr.)*; Kalcatyl *(DAK, Denm.)*; Kilios *(Carlo Erba, Ital.)*; Kynosina *(IRBI, Ital.)*; Lafena *(Cinfa, Spain)*; Levius *(Farmitalia Carlo Erba, UK)*; Licyl *(Norw.)*; Longasa *(Ital.)*; Magnecyl *(ACO, Swed.)*; Magnyl

(DAK, Denm.; NAF, Norw.); Mejoral *(Sterwin, Spain)*; Monobeltin *(Schwarz, Ger.)*; Neopirine-25 *(Canad.)*; Neutracétyl *(Fr.)*; Nova-Phase *(Canad.)*; Novasen *(Novopharm, Canad.)*; Novid *(Nyco, Norw.)*; Novosprin *(Austral.)*; Nuseals Aspirin *(Lilly, UK)*; Okal *(Puerto Galiano, Spain)*; Orravina *(Orravan, Spain)*;
Platet *(Nicholas, UK)*; Premaspin *(Laakefarmos, Swed.)*; Primaspan *(Belg.)*; Prodol *(Austral.)*; Provoprin *(Austral.)*; Pyracyl *(Ger.)*; Quinton *(Neopharmed, Ital.)*; Rectosalyl *(Bouty, Ital.)*; Reumyl *(Hässle, Denm.; Hässle, Swed.)*; Rhodine *(Belg.)*; Rhonal *(Arg.; Belg.; Canad.; Specia, Fr.; Jpn; Neth.; Rhone, Spain; Rhone-Poulenc, Switz.)*; Rhusal *(G.P. Laboratories, Austral.)*; Riane *(Vinas, Spain)*; Riphen *(Riva, Canad.)*; Rumasal *(Marshall's Pharmaceuticals, UK)*; Sal-Adult *(Beecham, Canad.)*; Salicilina *(Faes, Spain)*; Sal-Infant *(Beecham, Canad.)*; Salitison *(Jpn)*; Saspryl *(Inibsa, Spain)*; Sedalgin *(Austral.)*; Solmin *(Reckitt & Colman Pharmaceuticals, UK)*; Solprin *(Reckitt & Colman, Austral.; Reckitt & Colman Pharmaceuticals, UK)*; Solpyron *(Beecham-Wülfing, Ger.)*; Solusal *(Austral.)*; Solusprin *(Liade, Spain)*; Solvin *(Reckitt & Colman, Austral.)*; Soparine *(Belg.)*; Spiramon *(Robugen, Ger.)*; SRA *(Boots, Austral.)*; Supasa *(Nordic, Canad.)*; Superaspidin *(Landerlan, Spain)*; Tasprin-Sol *(Ticen, Eire)*; Temagin *(Beiersdorf, Ger.)*; Togal *(Manzoni, Ital.)*; Treuphalin *(Treupha, Switz.)*; Triaphen-10 *(Trianon, Canad.)*; Trineral *(Beiersdorf, Ger.)*; Verin *(Verex, USA)*; Winsprin *(Winthrop, Austral.)*; Zorprin *(Boots, USA)*.

The following names have been used for multi-ingredient preparations containing aspirin, its salts, and its complexes—217 Tablets *(Frosst, Canad.)*; 222 Tablets *(Frosst, Canad.)*; 282 Mep *(Frosst, Canad.)*; 282 Tablets *(Frosst, Canad.)*; 292 Tablets *(Frosst, Canad.)*; 293 Tablets *(Frosst, Canad.)*; 4-Way Tablets *(Bristol-Myers Products, USA)*; 692 Tablets *(Frosst, Canad.)*; A.C. & C. *(Pharmascience, Canad.)*; Alka-Seltzer *(Miles, Canad.; Bayer, UK; Miles Laboratories, USA)*; Alpha-Phed *(Metro Med, USA)*; Anacin *(Whitehall, USA)*; Anacin with Codeine *(Whitehall, Canad.)*; Analgesic Dellipsoids D6 *(Pilsworth, UK)*; Analgin *(Norton, UK)*; Ancasal *(Anca, Canad.)*; Anexsia with Codeine *(Beecham Laboratories, USA)*; Anexsia-D *(Beecham Laboratories, USA)*; Anodyne Dellipsoids D4 *(Pilsworth, UK)*; Antoin *(Cox, UK)*; Asasantine *(Boehringer Ingelheim, Canad.)*; Asco-Tin *(Faulding, Austral.)*; Ascriptin with Codeine *(Rorer, USA)*; Aspalgin *(Fawns & McAllan, Austral.)*; Aspav *(Cox, UK)*; Asprodeine *(Nicholas, Austral.)*; Axotal *(Adria, USA)*;
B-A-C *(Mayrand, USA)*; B-A-C 3 *(Mayrand, USA)*; Buff-A Comp *(Mayrand, USA)*; Bufferin with Codeine *(Bristol, USA)*; C-2 *(Wampole, Canad.)*; Cama *(Dorsey Laboratories, USA)*; Capedrin *(Key, Austral.)*; Codiphen *(G.P. Laboratories, Austral.)*; Codis *(Reckitt & Colman, Austral.; Reckitt & Colman Pharmaceuticals, UK)*; Codisprin; Codisprina; Codox *(Glaxo, Austral.)*; Codral *(Wellcome, Austral.)*; Congespirin *(Bristol-Myers Products, USA)*; Cordex *(Upjohn, Canad.; Upjohn, UK)*; Coricidin *(Schering, Canad.)*; Coricidin D *(Schering, Canad.)*; Coricidin with Codeine *(Schering, Canad.)*; Coryphen-Codeine *(Rougier, Canad.)*; Damason-P *(Mason, USA)*; Darvon Compound *(Lilly, USA)*; Darvon with A.S.A. *(Lilly, USA)*; Darvon-N Compound *(Lilly, Canad.)*; Darvon-N with A.S.A. *(Lilly, Canad.; Lilly, USA)*; Dasikon *(Beecham Laboratories, USA)*; Dasin *(Beecham Laboratories, USA)*; Decrin *(Nicholas, Austral.)*; Dexocodene *(Medo, UK)*; Dia-Gesic *(Central Pharmaceuticals, USA)*; Dolasan *(Lilly, UK)*; Dolene Compound-65 *(Lederle, USA)*; Doloxene Co *(Lilly, Austral.)*; Doloxene Compound *(Lilly, UK)*; Dolprn *(Bock, USA)*; Double-A *(Edwards, USA)*; Dristan Decongestant Tablets with Antihistamine *(Whitehall, UK)*; Ecuagesico; Empirin with Codeine *(Wellcome, USA)*; Equagesic *(Wyeth, Canad.; Wyeth, UK; Wyeth, USA)*; Excedrin *(Bristol-Myers Products, USA)*; Fiorinal *(Sandoz, Canad.; Sandoz, USA)*; Fiorinal with Codeine *(Sandoz, USA)*; Fiorinal-C *(Sandoz, Canad.)*; Histadyl and A.S.A. *(Lilly, USA)*; Hycodin *(Faulding, Austral.)*; Hyco-Pap *(Lasalle, USA)*; Hypon *(Calmic, UK)*;
Lortab ASA *(Russ, USA)*; Medro-Cordex *(Upjohn, UK)*; Mepro Compound *(Schein, USA)*; Meprogesic *(Quantum, USA)*; Midol *(Sterling, Canad.; Glenbrook, USA)*; Migravess *(Bayer, UK)*; Morphalgin *(Fawns & McAllan, Austral.)*; Myolgin *(Cox, UK)*; Napsalgesic *(Dista, UK)*; Norgesic *(Riker, Canad.; Riker, USA)*; Onadox-118 *(Duncan, Flockhart, UK)*; Orthoxicol Cold & Flu Caps *(Upjohn, Austral.)*; Oxycodan *(Technilab, Canad.)*; P-A-C *(Upjohn, USA)*; Paynocil *(Beecham Research, UK)*; Percodan *(Du Pont, Austral.; Du Pont, Canad.; Du Pont, USA)*; Persistin *(Fisons, USA)*; Phenaphen *(Robins, Canad.)*; Rheumalgesia Dellipsoids D5 *(Pilsworth, UK)*; Rheumatic Dellipsoids D10 *(Pilsworth, UK)*; Robaxisal *(Robins, Canad.; Robins, USA)*; Robaxisal-C *(Robins, Canad.)*; Robaxisal Forte *(Robins, UK)*; Safapryn *(Pfizer, UK)*; Safapryn-Co *(Pfizer, UK)*; Saleto *(Mallard, USA)*; SK-Oxycodone with Aspirin *(Smith Kline & French, USA)*; Solcode *(Reckitt & Colman, Austral.)*; Sol-Tercin *(Cox, UK)*; Soma Compound *(Wallace, USA)*; Soma Compound with Codeine *(Wallace, USA)*; Supac *(Mission Pharmacal, USA)*; Synalgos-DC *(Wyeth, USA)*; Talwin Compound *(Winthrop, Canad.; Winthrop-Breon, USA)*; Tecnal *(Technilab, Canad.)*; Tecnal C *(Technilab, Canad.)*; Tercin *(Cox, UK)*; Trancoprin *(Winthrop, UK)*; Ursinus *(Dorsey Laboratories, USA)*; Veganin *(Warner, Austral.; Parke, Davis, Canad.; Warner-Lambert, UK)*; Zactirin *(Wyeth, UK)*; Zactrin; Zamintol.

5293-j

Auranofin *(BAN, USAN, rINN)*.

SKF-D-39162. (1-Thio-β-D-glucopyranosato)(triethylphosphine)gold 2,3,4,6-tetra-acetate.
$C_{20}H_{34}AuO_9PS = 678.5$.

CAS — 34031-32-8.

Auranofin has a gold content of about 29%.

Adverse Effects and Treatment

The most common adverse effects of auranofin involve the gastro-intestinal tract with nausea, abdominal pain, and sometimes vomiting, but most often diarrhoea which can affect up to 50% of patients and may be severe enough to cause patients to withdraw from treatment. Other adverse effects are similar to those experienced with sodium aurothiomalate (p.40), although they appear to be less troublesome. As with other gold salts, treatment of adverse effects is generally symptomatic, see p.41.

EFFECTS ON THE GASTRO-INTESTINAL TRACT. Investigation of auranofin-induced diarrhoea in 6 patients indicated an association with a reversible defect in intestinal permeability.— R. Behrens *et al.*, *Gut*, 1986, *27*, 59.

EFFECTS ON THE KIDNEYS. In a retrospective review of 1283 patients who had received auranofin for treatment of rheumatoid arthritis 41 were found to have developed proteinuria. Treatment of proteinuria in the majority of patients consisted of discontinuing auranofin therapy. Long-term follow-up of 36 patients indicated that proteinuria had resolved in 31 patients within 2 years and in 29 patients within 1 year. Seven of 8 patients later rechallenged with auranofin had no relapses. In a further review of 2 comparative double-blind studies using gold compounds in the treatment of rheumatoid arthritis, proteinuria was found to have developed in 27% (23 of 85) of patients treated with sodium aurothiomalate, in 17% (42 of 247) of those treated with auranofin, and in 17% (36 of 210) of those receiving placebo.— W. A. Katz *et al.*, *Ann. intern. Med.*, 1984, *101*, 176.

Precautions

As for sodium aurothiomalate (p.41).

Absorption and Fate

Auranofin is rapidly though incompletely absorbed from the gastro-intestinal tract, only about 25% of a dose being considered to be bioavailable. It is bound to plasma proteins as well as to red blood cells. After several weeks' treatment the steady-state serum concentration is reported to be about 0.5 µg per mL.

Auranofin is principally excreted in the faeces due to its poor absorption, but equal amounts of the absorbed dose are excreted in the urine and in the faeces. Auranofin penetrates into synovial fluid.

Reviews: K. L. N. Blocka *et al.*, *Clin. Pharmacokinet.*, 1986, *11*, 133.

Uses and Administration

Auranofin has similar actions and uses to those of sodium aurothiomalate. It is given by mouth in progressive rheumatoid arthritis. The usual initial dose is 6 mg daily either as a single dose or in two divided doses. Treatment should be continued for 3 to 6 months to assess the response, and the dose may be increased, if necessary, to 3 mg three times daily.

Reviews of the actions and uses of auranofin: M. Chaffman *et al.*, *Drugs*, 1984, *27*, 378; J. C. Delafuente and T. G. Osborn, *Clin. Pharm.*, 1984, *3*, 121; V. Wright, *Br. med. J.*, 1984, *289*, 858; *Med. Lett.*, 1985, *27*, 89; J. L. Abruzzo *et al.*, *Ann. intern. Med.*, 1986, *105*, 274; *Drug & Ther. Bull.*, 1988, *26*, 69.

LUPUS. Clinical improvement in 19 of 23 patients with chronic discoid lupus erythematosus given auranofin.— K. Dalziel *et al.*, *Br. J. Derm.*, 1986, *115*, 211.

RHEUMATOID ARTHRITIS. Some references to the use of auranofin in rheumatoid arthritis: E. H. Giannini, *J. Pediat.*, 1983, *102*, 138 (children); R. G. Hull *et al.*, *Int. J. clin. Pharmacol. Res.*, 1984, *4*, 395 (comparison with sodium aurothiomalate); C. Bombardier *et al.*, *Am. J. Med.*, 1986, *81*, 565 (comparison with placebo); M. C. Hochberg, *Ann. intern. Med.*, 1986, *105*, 528 (comparison with penicillamine).

Proprietary Preparations

Ridaura *(Bridge, UK)*. *Tablets*, auranofin 3 mg.

Proprietary Names and Manufacturers

Ridaura *(Smith Kline & French, Austral.; Smith Kline & French, Canad.; Smith Kline & French, Denm.; Smith Kline Dauelsberg, Ger.; Smith Kline & French, Ital.; Smith Kline & French, Norw.; Smith Kline & French, S.Afr.; Smith Kline & French, Spain; Smith Kline & French, Swed.; Smith Kline & French, Switz.; Bridge, UK; Smith Kline & French, USA)*.

5294-z

Aurothioglucose *(USAN)*.

1-Aurothio-D-glucopyranose; Gold Thioglucose; (D-Glucosylthio)gold. (1-Thio-D-glucopyranosato)gold.
$C_6H_{11}AuO_5S = 392.2$.

CAS — 12192-57-3.

Pharmacopoeias. In *U.S.*

Adverse Effects, Treatment, and Precautions

As for sodium aurothiomalate, p.40.

Two cases of interstitial pneumonitis associated with aurothioglucose.— S. Miyachi (letter), *New Engl. J. Med.*, 1976, *295*, 506. See also: J. Heyd and A. Simmeran, *Postgrad. med. J.*, 1983, *59*, 368.

Uses and Administration

Aurothioglucose has similar actions and uses to those of sodium aurothiomalate. It is administered intramuscularly as a suspension in oil in an initial weekly dose of 10 mg increasing gradually to 50 mg weekly. Therapy is continued at weekly intervals until a total dose of 0.8 to 1 g has been given; if improvement has occurred at this stage with no signs of toxicity 50 mg may then be given at 3 or 4 week intervals. Children, 6 to 12 years, may be given one-quarter the adult dose.

Preparations

Sterile Aurothioglucose Suspension *(U.S.P.)*

Proprietary Names and Manufacturers

Aureotan *(Byk Gulden, Ger.; Byk Gulden, Switz.)*; Auromyose *(Nourypharma, Neth.)*; Gold-50 *(Essex, Austral.)*; Solganal *(Schering, USA)*.

12407-d

Aurotioprol

Sodium 3-aurothio-2-hydroxypropane-1-sulphonate.
$C_3H_6AuNaO_4S_2 = 390.2$.

CAS — 27279-43-2.

Pharmacopoeias. In *Fr.*

Aurotioprol is a gold compound used by intramuscular injection in the treatment of arthritic disorders.

Proprietary Names and Manufacturers

Allochrysine *(Sarbach, Fr.)*.

2610-w

Azapropazone *(BAN, rINN)*.

AHR-3018; Apazone *(USAN)*; Mi85; NSC-102824. 5-Dimethylamino-9-methyl-2-propylpyrazolo[1,2-*a*][1,2,4]benzotriazine-1,3(2*H*)-dione dihydrate.

$C_{16}H_{20}N_4O_2,2H_2O$=336.4.

CAS — 13539-59-8 (anhydrous).

Adverse Effects

Gastro-intestinal disturbances, allergic skin rashes and photosensitivity, oedema, and kidney impairment may occur. Gastro-intestinal bleeding and angioedema have been reported as have fibrosing alveolitis and haemolytic anaemia on isolated occasions.

EFFECTS ON THE BLOOD. Red cell antibodies and auto-immune haemolysis in patients treated with azapropazone. The Committee on Safety of Medicines in the *UK* has received 6 reports of Coombs positive haemolytic anaemia between January 1984 and March 1985 and the manufacturers 6 reports of auto-immune haemolysis over 10 years.— D. Chan-Lam *et al., Br. med. J.*, 1986, *293*, 1474.

Fatal haemolytic anaemia in a patient receiving azapropazone.— R. D. Montgomery (letter), *Br. med. J.*, 1987, *294*, 375.

See also under Effects on the Lung (below).

EFFECTS ON THE KIDNEY. Acute interstitial nephritis in one patient associated with azapropazone therapy.— R. Sipilä *et al.* (letter), *Mayo Clin. Proc.*, 1983, *58*, 209.

Reversible non-oliguric renal failure during treatment with azapropazone in one patient.— A. J. Goldstein and P. Grech (letter), *Br. med. J.*, 1986, *293*, 698.

Further reports of adverse effects on renal function associated with azapropazone: A. R. Morton *et al.* (letter), *Br. med. J.*, 1987, *294*, 375.

EFFECTS ON THE LUNG. A report of three patients with reversible pulmonary infiltration and haemolytic anaemia suggestive of an allergic or immune reaction. Since 1976 the Committee on Safety of Medicines in the *UK* has received 11 reports of allergic alveolitis, pulmonary fibrosis, or fibrosing alveolitis, and 18 reports of haemolytic anaemia in patients taking azapropazone.— M. K. Albazzaz *et al., Br. med. J.*, 1986, *293*, 1537.

EFFECTS ON THE SKIN. Two patients developed bullous skin eruptions when treated with azapropazone.— D. J. Barker and J. A. Cotterill (letter), *Lancet*, 1977, *1*, 90. See also D. J. Barker and J. A. Cotterill, *Acta derm.-vener., Stockh.*, 1977, *57*, 461.

PHOTOSENSITIVITY. A study of reports of photosensitivity associated with azapropazone forwarded to the WHO Collaborating Centre for International Drug Monitoring before September 1984. Of 154 reports, a causal relation was considered certain in 6, probable in 138, and possible in 10. The reports of photosensititiy accounted for 21% of the total number of reported adverse reactions.— S. Olsson *et al., Br. med. J.*, 1985, *291*, 939.

Precautions

Azapropazone should be given with caution to patients with acute gastritis or peptic ulceration, impaired renal function, or with a history of blood disorders. Reduced doses should be given to elderly patients (see under Uses and Administration, below).

Azapropazone may enhance the activity of coumarin anticoagulants and may increase blood-phenytoin concentrations.

ADMINISTRATION IN HEPATIC AND RENAL FAILURE. See under Uses and Administration (below).

INTERACTIONS. For the effect of azapropazone on other drugs see under chlorpropamide (p.388), methotrexate (p.638), phenytoin (p.408), and warfarin (p.345).

PORPHYRIA. Azapropazone was considered to be unsafe in patients with acute porphyria because it has been shown to be porphyrinogenic in *animals* or *in vitro* systems.— M.R. Moore and K.E.L. McColl, *Porphyrias, Drug Lists*, Glasgow, Porphyria Research Unit, University of Glasgow, 1987.

Absorption and Fate

Azapropazone is absorbed from the gastro-intestinal tract and peak plasma concentrations are reached about 5 hours after administration. It is excreted mainly in the urine, partly as unchanged drug.

Maximum plasma concentrations were reached 4 to 6 hours after administration of azapropazone by mouth. The plasma half-life was about 12 hours and the elimination half-life about 20 hours. About 95% of the dose was excreted in the urine of which 60% was unchanged azapropazone.— L. Klatt and F. W. Koss, *Arzneimittel-Forsch.*, 1973, *23*, 920. Similar conclusions were reached from a study of 6 subjects given a mean dose of azapropazone 8.4 mg per kg body-weight. When azapropazone 300 mg was given three times daily to these subjects a mean steady plasma concentration of 90 μg per mL was reached after 4 days, compared with a mean of about 45 μg per mL reached after a single dose of 600 mg. Little difference in plasma concentration was noted when the dose was given before or after food.— H. Leach, *Curr. med. Res. Opinion*, 1976, *4*, 35.

In 6 patients given azapropazone 600 mg by mouth peak plasma concentrations of 40 to 70 μg per mL occurred about 5 hours after administration.— H. E. Geissler *et al., Arzneimittel-Forsch.*, 1977, *27*, 1713.

A study of the determination of azapropazone and its metabolite 8-hydroxyazapropazone in plasma and urine using high performance liquid chromatography. No metabolite was detected in plasma following a single dose of azapropazone 600 mg by mouth in 3 healthy subjects although there were appreciable quantities in the urine. In 21 gouty patients receiving repeated high doses of azapropazone, 8-hydroxyazapropazone was present in some plasma samples, the amounts being 5 to 10% relative to the plasma concentration of azapropazone where this was greater than 100 μg per mL.— K. D. Rainsford, *J. Pharm. Pharmac.*, 1985, *37*, 341.

Further references.— K. M. Breuing *et al., Arzneimittel-Forsch.*, 1979, *29*, 971; H. Spahn *et al., Eur. J. clin. Pharmac.*, 1987, *32*, 303.

PROTEIN BINDING. Azapropazone was about 90% bound to human serum proteins *in vitro* at concentrations of 10 to 15 mg per 100 mL.— U. Jahn *et al., Arzneimittel-Forsch.*, 1973, *23*, 660.

Uses and Administration

Azapropazone has analgesic, anti-inflammatory, and antipyretic properties. It is used in various rheumatic disorders. The usual dose by mouth is 300 mg four times daily; or 600 mg twice daily.

Azapropazone also has uricosuric properties. In acute gout 2.4 g may be given in divided doses during the first 24 hours, followed by 1.8 g daily until the attack is resolving, then reduced to 1.2 g daily until symptoms have disappeared. In chronic gout the usual dose is 600 mg twice daily.

In elderly patients over the age of 65 years a reduced dose of 300 mg twice daily, possibly increased to a total of 900 mg daily if necessary, is recommended.

ADMINISTRATION IN HEPATIC AND RENAL FAILURE. Pharmacokinetic studies indicating a need for reduced dosage in hepatic and renal impairment. In patients with cirrhosis and moderate impairment of liver function a reduction to about half of the usual therapeutic dose may be necessary. In renal failure the dose should be reduced according to the degree of impairment of kidney function and protein binding in plasma.— K. -H. Breuing *et al., Eur. J. clin. Pharmac.*, 1981, *20*, 147.

Proprietary Preparations

Rheumox *(Robins, UK). Capsules,* azapropazone 300 mg.
Tablets (Rheumox 600), scored, azapropazone 600 mg.

Proprietary Names and Manufacturers

Cinnamin *(Jpn)*; Pentosol *(Spain)*; Prolix *(S.Afr.)*; Prolixan *(Belg.; Ferrosan, Denm.; Fr.; Siegfried, Ger.; Hung.; Ital.; Neth.; Siegfried, Switz.)*; Prolixana *(Leo, Swed.)*; Rheumox *(Continental Ethicals, S.Afr.; Robins, UK)*; Tolyprin *(DuPont, Ger.)*.

2611-e

Benorylate *(BAN)*.

Benorilate *(rINN)*; FAW-76; Fenasprate; Win-11450. 4-Acetamidophenyl *O*-acetylsalicylate.

$C_{17}H_{15}NO_5$=313.3.

CAS — 5003-48-5.

Pharmacopoeias. In *Br.*

A white or almost white, odourless or almost odourless, crystalline powder. Practically **insoluble** in water; sparingly soluble in alcohol and methyl alcohol; soluble in acetone and chloroform.

Adverse Effects, Treatment, and Precautions

As for aspirin, p.3, and paracetamol, p.32. It may cause nausea, indigestion, heartburn, and constipation; drowsiness, dizziness, diarrhoea, and skin rashes have also been reported. Some patients have experienced tinnitus and deafness associated with high blood-salicylate concentrations.

Benorylate, like aspirin (see p.5), because of the risk of Reye's syndrome, should not generally be given to children under the age of 12 years unless specifically indicated for conditions such as juvenile rheumatoid arthritis.

EFFECTS ON THE GASTRO-INTESTINAL TRACT. A 67-year-old woman with rheumatoid arthritis receiving benorylate suspension (20%) 5 mL four times daily experienced lower abdominal discomfort within 5 minutes of a dose, persisting for 5 to 10 minutes. When the dose was increased to 8 mL five times daily diarrhoea occurred within a few minutes of each dose. The symptoms ceased when benorylate was withdrawn.— A. J. Marshall and P. Sheridan (letter), *Br. med. J.*, 1973, *1*, 175.

EFFECTS ON HEARING. Eight of 11 patients given benorylate were unable to continue treatment because of loss of hearing, tinnitus, nausea, and disorientation. Some patients developed symptoms after the second dose. None of those who resumed treatment with half the dose [not quoted] were able to continue treatment.— R. E. Hope-Simpson (letter), *Br. med. J.*, 1973, *1*, 296.

Of 20 patients with rheumatoid arthritis given benorylate 4 g twice daily, 11 developed tinnitus and deafness after the second dose; 9 later developed the symptoms after the third dose when given 2 g three times daily. Mean total plasma-salicylate concentrations were 2.7 mmol per litre.— M. Aylward (letter), *Br. med. J.*, 1973, *2*, 118.

EFFECTS ON THE LIVER. Liver necrosis in one patient was attributed to benorylate and penicillamine that had been given for rheumatoid arthritis.— M. Sacher and H. Thaler (letter), *Lancet*, 1977, *1*, 481.

A 3-year-old child with cystic fibrosis and suspected juvenile chronic polyarthritis died following administration of benorylate in high therapeutic dosage accompanied by monitoring of blood-salicylate concentrations. Blood-paracetamol concentrations were very high and necropsy revealed liver changes typical of acute hepatocellular damage due to paracetamol poisoning. Paracetamol, as well as salicylate, blood concentrations should be monitored.— D. N. K. Symon *et al.* (letter), *Lancet*, 1982, *2*, 1153.

Absorption and Fate

Benorylate is absorbed virtually unchanged from the gastro-intestinal tract, although absorption may be prolonged. Following absorption, benorylate is rapidly metabolised to salicylate and paracetamol. It is excreted mainly as metabolites of salicylic acid and paracetamol in the urine. A small amount of the administered dose is excreted in the faeces. Benorylate has a longer duration of action than aspirin or paracetamol.

In 9 patients who had previously shown reactions to benorylate, doses of 4 g twice daily gave rise to total salicylate concentrations and free salicylate concentrations significantly higher than those achieved with soluble aspirin 1.2 g four times daily. In 12 further patients total and free salicylate concentrations were comparable after the above doses of benorylate and soluble aspirin. In some individuals benorylate appeared to interfere with the plasma binding of salicylate, but the high total salicylate concentrations in some patients after benorylate remained unexplained.— M. Aylward (letter), *Br. med. J.*, 1973, *3*, 347.

Salicylate absorption was significantly less with benorylate given in a dose providing 1.76 g of salicylic acid than with soluble aspirin equivalent to 1.84 g of salicylic acid in a study of 7 patients. Excretion was also slower with benorylate, approximately 55% of salicylate being excreted within 48 hours of the above dose compared with about 80% for soluble aspirin.— P. Duckworth and M. Earnshaw, *J. Hosp. Pharm.*, 1975, *33*, 83.

Studies on pharmacokinetics and distribution of benorylate in plasma and synovial fluid.— M. Aylward *et al.*, *Scand. J. Rheumatol.*, 1976, *Suppl.* 13, 9; M. Franke *et al.*, *ibid.*, 13.

Uses and Administration

Benorylate is the acetylsalicylic acid ester of paracetamol and it has analgesic, anti-inflammatory, and antipyretic properties. It is used in rheumatic disorders, in mild to moderate pain, and as an antipyretic. In active rheumatoid arthritis 4 g twice daily by mouth may be required. In osteoarthritis and other rheumatic conditions and for the relief of non-rheumatic pain lower doses of 2 g twice daily or 1.5 g three times daily are usually adequate.

In elderly patients reduced doses of 2 g twice daily or possibly 2 g in the morning and 4 g at night should be given.

In juvenile chronic polyarthritis an initial dose of 200 mg per kg body-weight daily has been given and should then be adjusted to produce blood-salicylate concentrations of about 250 μg per mL.

ADMINISTRATION. The bioavailability of benorylate was not significantly affected when the dose was taken in hot coffee.— N. A. Barrett *et al.*, *Rheumatol. Rehabil.*, 1978, *17*, 23.

ADMINISTRATION IN THE ELDERLY. A report of salicylate intoxication in an 82-year-old woman given benorylate 2 g four times daily; the serum-salicylate concentration after 8 days was 3.06 μmol per mL (425 μg per mL). When 5 other elderly patients and the orignal patient were given 1 g four times daily the concentration after 8 days ranged from 0.75 to 1.85 μmol per mL. The dose for elderly patients should not exceed 4 g daily.— T. R. O. Beringer, *Br. med. J.*, 1984, *288*, 1344.

OSTEOARTHRITIS. Reports on the use of benorylate in osteoarthrosis.— D. Kuntz *et al.*, *Scand. J. Rheumatol.*, 1976, *Suppl.* 13, 25; P. J. Cosgrove, *J. int. med. Res.*, 1977, *5*, 120; J. J. Hamill, *ibid.*, 265; B. Y. Marshall, *Clin. Trials J.*, 1978, *15* (3), 73; S. R. Mayhew, *Rheumatol. Rehabil.*, 1978, *17*, 29; P. A. Johnson, *Clin. Trials J.*, 1978, *15*, (3), 82; D. Woolf *et al.*, *Practitioner*, 1978, *221*, 791; C. Tranmer, *Rheumatol. Rehabil.*, 1978, *17*, 91; E. J. Valtonen, *Scand. J. Rheumatol.*, 1979, *Suppl.* 25, 9.

RHEUMATOID ARTHRITIS. Reports of the use of benorylate in rheumatoid arthritis and other rheumatic disorders: D. L. Beales *et al.*, *Br. med. J.*, 1972, *2*, 483; Report No. 178 of the General Practitioner Research Group, *Practitioner*, 1973, *210*, 291; V. Wright and I. Haslock (letter), *Br. med. J.*, 1973, *2*, 487; O. Vojtíšek *et al.*, *Arzneimittel-Forsch.*, 1973, *23*, 701; P. N. Sperryn *et al.*, *Ann. rheum. Dis.*, 1973, *32*, 157; M. H. F. Coigley, *Practitioner*, 1975, *215*, 348; K. Hingorani, *Scand. J. Rheumatol.*, 1976, *Suppl.* 13, 29; P. Doury and S. Pattin, *ibid.*, 33.

Juvenile chronic polyarthritis. In 12 children with active Still's disease benorylate 200 mg per kg body-weight daily (approximately twice the recommended analgesic dose) failed to produce adequate salicylate concentrations of 250 to 350 μg per mL in most patients. No side-effects were reported. It was recommended that the initial dose be 200 mg per kg daily, that the dose be adjusted to produce salicylate concentrations of 250 to 300 μg per mL, and that thereafter the dosage be maintained with occasional monitoring of the concentration in the blood.— R. H. Powell and B. M. Ansell, *Br. med. J.*, 1974, *1*, 145.

Preparations

Benorylate Oral Suspension *(B.P.).* Benorylate Mixture

Benorylate Tablets *(B.P.)*

Proprietary Preparations

Benoral *(Sterling Research, UK). Tablets*, benorylate 750 mg.
Granules, benorylate 2 g/sachet.
Suspension, benorylate 2 g/5 mL.

Proprietary Names and Manufacturers

Benoral *(Austral.; Sterling Research, UK)*; Benorile *(Rubio, Spain)*; Benortan *(Belg.; Denm.; Fin.; Fr.; Winthrop, Ger.; Iceland; Neth.; Winthrop, Switz.)*; Benotamol *(Arg.)*; Bentum *(Zambon, Ital.)*; Doline *(Ferrer, Spain)*; Duvium *(Inpharzam, Switz.)*; Salipran *(Bottu, Fr.)*; Vetedol *(Robert, Spain)*; Winolate *(Maggioni-Winthrop, Ital.; S.Afr.)*.

2612-l

Benoxaprofen *(BAN, USAN, rINN).*

Compound-90459; LRCL-3794. 2-[2-(4-Chlorophenyl)benzoxazol-5-yl]propionic acid.
$C_{16}H_{12}ClNO_3$=301.7.

CAS — 51234-28-7.

Adverse Effects

Benoxaprofen has been associated with a variety of adverse reactions and several fatalities have occurred mainly in elderly persons. Side-effects that have occurred with benoxaprofen include skin disorders, notably photosensitivity reactions but also erythema multiforme (the Stevens-Johnson syndrome), onycholysis and other nail disorders, gastro-intestinal disturbances including peptic ulceration and bleeding, blood disorders such as thrombocytopenia, cholestatic jaundice and other liver or biliary disorders, and renal failure.

Uses and Administration

Benoxaprofen has analgesic, anti-inflammatory, and antipyretic properties and was formerly given by mouth in rheumatoid arthritis and osteoarthritis but because of reports of adverse reactions and fatalities the manufacturers halted marketing worldwide. Before its withdrawal benoxaprofen was also shown to have a beneficial effect in psoriasis.

Proprietary Names and Manufacturers

Opren *(Dista, UK)*; Oraflex *(Lilly, USA)*.

12433-h

Benzpiperylone *(rINN).*

KB-95. 4-Benzyl-2-(1-methyl-4-piperidyl)-5-phenyl-4-pyrazolin-3-one.
$C_{22}H_{25}N_3O$=347.5.

CAS — 53-89-4.

Benzpiperylone is a non-steroidal anti-inflammatory agent that has been used in rheumatic disorders in doses of 300 mg three times daily by mouth.

Proprietary Names and Manufacturers

Benzometan *(Castejon, Spain)*; Humedil *(Cheminova, Spain)*.

2613-y

Benzydamine Hydrochloride *(BANM, USAN, rINNM).*

AF-864; Benzindamine Hydrochloride. 3-(1-Benzyl-1*H*-indazol-3-yloxy)-*NN*-dimethylpropylamine hydrochloride.
$C_{19}H_{23}N_3O,HCl$=345.9.

CAS — 642-72-8 (benzydamine); 132-69-4 (hydrochloride).

Pharmacopoeias. In *Chin.* and *Nord.*

Adverse Effects

Following topical application to the skin local reactions such as erythema or rash may occur and photosensitivity has been reported. Following use as mouth and throat preparations, numbness or stinging sensations of the oral mucosa have been reported.

After administration by mouth the most common side-effects with benzydamine are gastro-intestinal disturbances.

Uses and Administration

Benzydamine hydrochloride has analgesic, anti-inflammatory, and antipyretic properties. It is used topically on the skin in concentrations of 3% in rheumatic disorders and is also used as a mouth wash or mouth spray in concentrations of 0.15% for the relief of inflammatory conditions of the mouth and throat. It has also been given by mouth in doses of 50 mg three to four times daily.

A brief review of the efficacy of benzydamine (Difflam) preparations.— *Drug & Ther. Bull.*, 1986, *24*, 19.

Proprietary Preparations

Difflam *(Riker, UK). Cream*, benzydamine hydrochloride 3%.
Oral Rinse, mouth-wash, benzydamine hydrochloride 0.15%.
Spray, mouth and throat spray, benzydamine hydrochloride 0.15%.

Proprietary Names and Manufacturers

Afloben *(Esseti, Ital.)*; Andolex *(Riker, Denm.)*; A-Termadol *(Ital.)*; Bucco-Tantum *(Sauter, Switz.)*; Difflam *(Riker, Austral.; Riker, UK)*; Enzamin *(Jpn)*; Flogaton *(Radiumfarma, Ital.)*; Fulgium *(Liade, Spain)*; Ginesal *(Farmigea, Ital.)*; Imotryl *(Fr.)*; Multum *(Lampugnani, Ital.)*; Opalgyne *(Innothéra, Fr.)*; Rosalgin *(Farma-Lepori, Spain)*; Tamas *(Arg.)*; Tantum *(Arg.; Austral.; Riker, Canad.; Denm.; Giulini, Ger.; Angelini, Ital.; Neth.; Organon, S.Afr.; Syntex-Latino, Spain; Sauter, Switz.)*; Verax *(Tosi-Novara, Ital.)*.

2614-j

Bindazac *(BAN).*

AF-983; Bendazac *(USAN, rINN)*. (1-Benzyl-1*H*-indazol-3-yloxy)acetic acid.
$C_{16}H_{14}N_2O_3$=282.3.

CAS — 20187-55-7.

Bindazac has anti-inflammatory actions and is used topically in preparations containing 1 and 3% for the treatment of various skin disorders.

The lysine salt of bindazac is used in doses of up to 500 mg three times daily by mouth in the treatment of cataracts.

Hepatitis in 2 patients associated with oral bindazac therapy. The causal relationship was definite in the first patient and highly probable in the second.— J. A. Ballesteros *et al.* (letter), *Lancet*, 1987, *2*, 1030.

Reports of a beneficial effect of bindazac lysine by mouth in patients with cataracts: M. Testa *et al.* (letter), *Lancet*, 1982, *1*, 849; L. Bonomi *et al.*, *Curr. ther. Res.*, 1983, *33*, 727; N. Iuglio and G. Iuliano, *ibid.*, 1984, *35*, 119.

Proprietary Names and Manufacturers of Bindazac and its Salts

Bendalina *(Angelini, Ital.; Farma-Lepori, Spain)*; Hubersil *(Hubber, Spain)*; Versus *(Angelini, Ital.; Petersen, S.Afr.)*.

2616-c

Bucloxic Acid *(rINN).*

CB-804. 3-(3-Chloro-4-cyclohexylbenzoyl)propionic acid.
$C_{16}H_{19}ClO_3$=294.8.

CAS — 32808-51-8.

Bucloxic acid has analgesic, anti-inflammatory, and antipyretic properties. It has been used, as the calcium salt, in inflammatory and rheumatic disorders in doses of 400 mg two or three times daily by mouth.

Proprietary Names and Manufacturers of Bucloxic Acid and its Salts

Esfar *(Midy, Fr.)*.

2617-k

Bucolome *(rINN).*

5-Butyl-1-cyclohexylbarbituric acid.
$C_{14}H_{22}N_2O_3$=266.3.

CAS — 841-73-6.

Adverse Effects

Adverse effects occurring with bucolome include dry mouth, stomatitis, gastro-intestinal disorders, headache, drowsiness, ataxia, and, rarely, leucopenia and thrombocytopenia.

Uses and Administration

Bucolome has analgesic and anti-inflammatory properties. It has been used in inflammatory and rheumatic disorders in doses of up to 1.2 g daily by mouth.

Proprietary Names and Manufacturers

Paramidin *(Jpn)*; Sedalgol *(Berenguer-Beneyto, Spain)*.

2618-a

Bufexamac *(BAN, rINN).*

2-(4-Butoxyphenyl)acetohydroxamic acid.
$C_{12}H_{17}NO_3$=223.3.

CAS — 2438-72-4.

Adverse Effects

When given by mouth bufexamac may cause gastro-intestinal irritation, particularly in patients with a history of peptic ulcer.

Stinging and burning may occur after application of the cream; allergic reactions have been reported.

A report of allergic contact dermatitis with bufexamac.— G. Smeenk, *Dermatologica,* 1973, *147,* 334.

Uses and Administration

Bufexamac has analgesic, antipyretic, and anti-inflammatory properties. As a 5% cream bufexamac is applied topically, in a wide range of dermatoses. It has also been applied for the local treatment of rheumatic conditions. Bufexamac has also been given by mouth in doses of 0.75 to 1.5 g daily, for rheumatic disorders.

PHARMACOKINETICS. After administration by mouth of 125 to 500 mg of bufexamac, absorption was rapid and about 75% of the dose was excreted as a conjugate, probably the glucuronide. About 6% was excreted as a conjugate of 4-butoxyphenylacetic acid and less than 1% as free bufexamac or 4-butoxyphenylacetic acid. The peak rate of excretion was after 3 to 6 hours and excretion was complete within 24 hours.— D. R. Borham *et al., J. pharm. Sci.,* 1972, *61,* 164.

RHEUMATIC DISORDERS. References to the use of bufexamac in various rheumatic disorders: K. Pavelka and F. Wagenhauser, *Curr. ther. Res.,* 1970, *12,* 69 (orally and rectally in rheumatoid arthritis); B. S. Rose *et al., Curr. ther. Res.,* 1970, *12,* 150 (orally in rheumatoid arthritis); A. Mardjuadi and J. Dequeker, *Curr. med. Res. Opinion,* 1978, *5,* 401 (by local infiltration in acute periarthritis of the shoulder); M. Wauters, *Curr. ther. Res.,* 1978, *23,* 685 (intra-articularly in osteoarthritis of the knee).

SKIN DISORDERS. References to the use of bufexamac topically in various skin disorders.— J. Van Der Meersch, *Curr. ther. Res.,* 1974, *16,* 904; J. C. Valle-Jones, *Practitioner,* 1974, *213,* 383; Report No. 191 of the General Practitioner Research Group, *Practitioner,* 1975, *214,* 689; J. V. Christiansen *et al., Dermatologica,* 1977, *154,* 177; P. Wolf-Jürgensen, *Curr. med. Res. Opinion,* 1979, *5,* 779.

Proprietary Preparations

Parfenac *(Lederle, UK). Cream,* bufexamac, 5%.

Proprietary Names and Manufacturers

Droxaryl *(Belg.; Neth.)*; Feximac *(Nicholas, UK)*; Flogocid *(Continental Pharma, Switz.)*; Mofenar *(Federico Bonet, Spain)*; Norfemac *(Nordic, Canad.)*; Paraderm *(Lederle, Austral.)*; Parfenac *(Arg.; Austral.; Lederle, Canad.; Lederle, Fr.; Cyanamid-Novalis, Ger.; Lederle, Switz.; Lederle, UK)*; Parfenal *(Cyanamid, Ital.)*.

2619-t

Bumadizone Calcium *(rINNM).*

Calcium 2-(1,2-diphenylhydrazinocarbonyl)hexanoate hemihydrate.
$(C_{19}H_{21}N_2O_3)_2Ca,½H_2O$=699.9.

CAS — 3583-64-0 (bumadizone); 34461-73-9 (calcium salt, anhydrous).

Bumadizone calcium has analgesic and anti-inflammatory properties and is reported to be metabolised to phenylbutazone and oxyphenbutazone. It has been used in rheumatic disorders in doses of 220 mg two or three times daily by mouth initially and 110 mg two or three times daily for maintenance.

Proprietary Names and Manufacturers

Bumaflex *(Byk Liprandi, Arg.)*; Eumotol *(Valpan, Fr.; Byk Gulden, Ger.; Byk Gulden, Ital.; Byk Gulden, S.Afr.; Boehringer Mannheim, Spain; Byk Gulden, Switz.)*; Rheumatol *(Tosse, Ger.)*.

12475-l

Butibufen *(rINN).*

FF-106. 2-(4-Isobutylphenyl)butyric acid.
$C_{14}H_{20}O_2$=220.3.

CAS — 55837-18-8.

Butibufen is a non-steroidal anti-inflammatory agent that has been used by mouth as the sodium salt in inflammatory and rheumatic disorders.

Proprietary Names and Manufacturers of Butibufen and its Salts

Butilopan *(Juste, Spain)*.

2621-y

Calcium Succinate

$C_4H_4CaO_4,3H_2O$=210.2.

CAS — 140-99-8 (anhydrous); 5793-96-4 (trihydrate).

Calcium succinate has been given by mouth together with aspirin in rheumatic disorders but is of doubtful value.

Proprietary Names and Manufacturers

The following names have been used for multi-ingredient preparations containing calcium succinate— Berex *(Clinod, UK)*; Dolcin *(Clinod, UK)*; Rheumalgesia Dellipsoids D5 *(Pilsworth, UK)*.

2620-l

Carbaspirin Calcium *(USAN).*

Calcium Acetylsalicylate Carbamide; Calcium Carbaspirin; Carbasalate Calcium *(rINN)*. A 1:1 complex of calcium acetylsalicylate and urea.
$C_{19}H_{18}CaN_2O_9$=458.4.

CAS — 5749-67-7.

Carbaspirin calcium has analgesic, anti-inflammatory, and antipyretic properties and has been used similarly to aspirin in doses equivalent to 300 to 600 mg of aspirin, every 4 hours.

Proprietary Names and Manufacturers

Alcacyl *(Wander, Switz.)*; Ascal *(ACF, Neth.)*; Calurin *(Sandoz, USA)*; Iromin *(Ger.; Schmidgall, Switz.)*; Soluspan *(UPSA, Fr.)*.

The following names have been used for multi-ingredient preparations containing carbaspirin calcium— Fiogesic *(Sandoz, USA)*.

12531-b

Carprofen *(BAN, USAN, rINN).*

C-5720; Ro-20-5720/000. (±)-2-(6-Chlorocarbazol-2-yl)propionic acid.
$C_{15}H_{12}ClNO_2$=273.7.

CAS — 53716-49-7.

Carprofen is a non-steroidal anti-inflammatory agent that has been used in inflammatory and rheumatic disorders in usual doses of 150 to 300 mg daily by mouth. Photosensitivity reactions have been reported with carprofen.

Some references to carprofen: J. E. Ray *et al., J. clin. Pharmac.,* 1979, *19,* 635 (pharmacokinetics); F. Rubio *et al., J. pharm. Sci.,* 1980, *69,* 1245 (pharmacokinetics); B. Kirchheiner *et al., Curr. ther. Res.,* 1980, *28,* 875 (comparison with indomethacin); S. A. Cooper *et al., Clin. Pharmac. Ther.,* 1981, *29,* 237 (use for dental pain); J. F. Kelly *et al., ibid.,* 257 (pharmacokinetics); G. H. Stein *et al., Curr. ther. Res.,* 1983, *33,* 415 (comparison with aspirin in osteoarthrosis); A. Tursi *et al., Clin. Trials J.,* 1983, *20,* 319 (comparison with indomethacin in rheumatoid arthritis); S. Bianco *et al., J. int. med. Res.,* 1985, *13,* 294 (safety in asthmatic subjects).

Proprietary Names and Manufacturers

Imadyl *(Roche, Ger.; Roche, Switz.)*.

2623-z

Chlorthenoxazin *(BAN).*

Chlorthenoxazine *(rINN)*. 2-(2-Chloroethyl)-2,3-dihydro-4*H*-1,3-benzoxazin-4-one.
$C_{10}H_{10}ClNO_2$=211.6.

CAS — 132-89-8.

Chlorthenoxazin has analgesic, antipyretic, and anti-inflammatory properties. It has been used in rheumatic disorders in doses of up to 1.6 g daily by mouth.

Proprietary Names and Manufacturers

Apirogen *(Dessy, Ital.)*; Betix *(Saba, Ital.)*; Ossazin *(Ital.)*; Ossazone *(Brocchieri, Ital.)*; Ossipirina *(Radiumfarma, Ital.)*; Oxal *(Ital.)*; Reugaril *(Farber-Ref, Ital.)*; Reulin *(Isola-Ibi, Ital.)*; Reumital *(Farge, Ital.)*.

2624-c

Choline Magnesium Trisalicylate

A mixture of choline salicylate and magnesium salicylate.

CAS — 64425-90-7.

Choline magnesium trisalicylate has similar properties to aspirin (p.3). It is used in rheumatic disorders in doses equivalent to 1 or 1.5 g of salicylate twice daily by mouth; doses may also be given as a single daily dose if required. Each unit dose of 500 mg of salicylate is provided by approximately 293 mg of choline salicylate with 362 mg of magnesium salicylate (anhydrous).

Hepatoxicity in one patient associated with choline magnesium trisalicylate.— R. J. Cersosimo and S. J. Matthews, *Drug Intell. & clin. Pharm.,* 1987, *21,* 621.

Proprietary Preparations

Trilisate *(Napp, UK). Tablets,* scored, choline magnesium trisalicylate equivalent to salicylate 500 mg.

Proprietary Names and Manufacturers

Athrodest *(Krugmann, Ger.)*; Trilisate *(Purdue Frederick, Canad.; Napp, UK; Purdue Frederick, USA)*.

2625-k

Choline Salicylate *(BAN, rINN).*

(2-Hydroxyethyl)trimethylammonium salicylate.
$C_{12}H_{19}NO_4$=241.3.

CAS — 2016-36-6.

Pharmacopoeias. Br. includes Choline Salicylate Solution.

Choline Salicylate Solution *(B.P.)* is an aqueous solution containing 47.5 to 52.5% of choline salicylate. It is a clear colourless liquid.

Choline salicylate has similar properties to those of aspirin (p.3). It is used as a local analgesic. A 20% solution is employed in ear affections and an 8.7% gel in lesions of the mouth.

Choline salicylate is also given by mouth in the form of choline magnesium trisalicylate (see above).

A 21-month-old boy developed salicylate poisoning after the mother had rubbed the contents of 3 tubes of 'Bonjela' teething ointment on his gums over 48 hours.— A. S. Paynter and F. W. Alexander (letter), *Lancet,* 1979, *2,* 1132.

Preparations

Choline Salicylate Dental Gel *(B.P.)*
Choline Salicylate Ear Drops *(B.P.)*

Proprietary Preparations

Audax *(Napp, UK). Ear-drops,* choline salicylate 20%, glycerol 10%. For painful conditions of the ear.

Bonjela *(Reckitt & Colman Pharmaceuticals, UK). Oral gel,* choline salicylate 8.7%.

Teejel *(Napp, UK). Oral gel,* choline salicylate 8.7%.

Proprietary Names and Manufacturers

Applicaine Gel *(Nyal, Austral.)*; Arthropan *(Canad.; USA)*; Audax *(Ger.; Napp, UK)*; Bonjela *(Reckitt & Colman, Austral.; Reckitt & Colman Pharmaceuticals, UK)*; Mundisal *(Norw.)*; Ora-Sed Jel *(Rosken, Austral.)*;

Salicol *(Ital.)*; Seda-Gel *(Nelson, Austral.)*; Syrap *(Fr.)*; Teejel *(Belg.*; *Purdue Frederick, Canad.*; *Napp, UK)*.

2627-t

Cinchophen *(BAN, rINN)*.
Acifenokinolin; Phenylcinchoninic Acid; Quinophan. 2-Phenylquinoline-4-carboxylic acid.
$C_{16}H_{11}NO_2$=249.3.

CAS — 132-60-5.

Pharmacopoeias. In *Arg., Braz., Hung., Mex., Port.,* and *Span.*

Adverse Effects
Cinchophen may produce symptoms including vomiting, skin lesions, and angioedema. It may also cause severe hepatic symptoms such as acute hepatitis, jaundice, and yellow atrophy of the liver. The symptoms may not be immediately evident and may proceed even when the drug has been discontinued. Toxicity is unrelated to dosage or to previous medication and the fact that cinchophen medication has been given previously without ill effects is no guarantee that the next course of treatment will not cause jaundice.

Uses and Administration
Cinchophen, and the related compounds methylcinchophen and neocinchophen have analgesic and antipyretic properties. They were mainly used by mouth in the treatment of chronic gout but because of toxicity have been superseded by other analgesics.

12572-y

Cinmetacin *(rINN)*.
(1-Cinnamoyl-5-methoxy-2-methylindol-3-yl)acetic acid.
$C_{21}H_{19}NO_4$=349.4.

CAS — 20168-99-4.

Cinmetacin is a non-steroidal anti-inflammatory agent that has been used in rheumatic disorders in usual doses of 300 mg three times daily by mouth.

Some references to cinmetacin: E. Minchella and G. Vettori, *Curr. ther. Res.*, 1986, *40*, 312 (comparison with indomethacin).

Proprietary Names and Manufacturers
Cetanovo *(Llorens, Spain)*; Cindomet *(Chiesi, Ital.)*.

12578-t

Clidanac *(rINN)*.
TAI-284. 6-Chloro-5-cyclohexylindan-1-carboxylic acid.
$C_{16}H_{19}ClO_2$=278.8.

CAS — 28968-07-2; 34148-01-1.

Clidanac is an analgesic that has been used in doses of 15 mg two or three times daily by mouth.

Proprietary Names and Manufacturers
Indanal *(Takeda, Jpn)*.

15317-f

Clobuzarit *(BAN, rINN)*.
ICI-55897. 2-(4′-Chlorobiphenyl-4-ylmethoxy)-2-methylpropionic acid.
$C_{17}H_{17}ClO_3$=304.8.

CAS — 22494-47-9.

Clobuzarit has a penicillamine-like disease-modifying effect in rheumatoid arthritis. It was, however, withdrawn from study because of the development of the Stevens-Johnson syndrome.

A short comment that clobuzarit, a compound which appeared to have a penicillamine-like action in rheumatoid arthritis, was withdrawn by the manufacturers after 1800 patients had been enrolled in clinical trials, the major reason being the occurrence of the Stevens-Johnson syndrome in 4.— H. A. Bird (letter), *J. Rheumatol.*, 1983, *10*, 663.

12585-a

Clofexamide *(rINN)*.
ANP-246. 2-(4-Chlorophenoxy)-*N*-(2-diethylaminoethyl)acetamide.
$C_{14}H_{21}ClN_2O_2$=284.8.

CAS — 1223-36-5.

Clofexamide has been used with phenylbutazone in the form of clofezone (see below).

2628-x

Clofezone *(rINN)*.
ANP-3260. An equimolar combination of clofexamide and phenylbutazone.
$C_{14}H_{21}ClN_2O_2.C_{19}H_{20}N_2O_2.2H_2O$=629.2.

CAS — 60104-29-2.

Clofezone, a combination molecule containing phenylbutazone, has been used in rheumatic disorders in doses of 200 to 400 mg daily by mouth. It has also been used as a 5% ointment.

Proprietary Names and Manufacturers
Panas *(Jpn)*; Perclusone *(Boehringer, Arg.*; *Anphar-Rolland, Fr.*; *Mack, Illert., Ger.*; *Pierrel, Ital.*; *Mack, Switz.)*; Perclustop *(Uquifa, Spain)*.

2629-r

Clometacin *(rINN)*.
Clométacine. [3-(4-Chlorobenzoyl)-6-methoxy-2-methylindol-1-yl]acetic acid.
$C_{19}H_{16}ClNO_4$=357.8.

CAS — 25803-14-9.

Clometacin is an analgesic structurally related to indomethacin. It has been used for the relief of postoperative, traumatic, and rheumatic pain in doses of up to 900 mg daily in divided doses by mouth. There have been several reports of hepatotoxicity associated with its use.

Proprietary Names and Manufacturers
Dupéran *(Cassenne, Fr.)*.

2630-j

Clonixin *(USAN, rINN)*.
CBA-93626; Sch-10304. 2-(3-Chloro-*o*-toluidino)nicotinic acid.
$C_{13}H_{11}ClN_2O_2$=262.7.

CAS — 17737-65-4.

Clonixin has analgesic, anti-inflammatory, and antipyretic properties. It has been used as the lysine salt in doses of up to 250 mg four times daily. Clonixin has also been given as the lysine salt by intramuscular or intravenous injection.

Some references to clonixin: J. S. Finch and T. J. DeKornfeld, *J. clin. Pharmac.*, 1971, *11*, 371; K. D. Fitch *et al.*, *Aust. J. Sports Med.*, 1977, *9*, 56; H. Paredes *et al.*, *Curr. ther. Res.*, 1986, *40*, 86.

Proprietary Names and Manufacturers of Clonixin and its Salts
Dolalgial *(Pharmainvesti, Spain)*; Dorixina *(Roemmers, Arg.)*.

12590-z

Clopirac *(BAN, USAN, rINN)*.
BRL-13856; CP-172-AP. [1-(4-Chlorophenyl)-2,5-dimethylpyrrol-3-yl]acetic acid.
$C_{14}H_{14}ClNO_2$=263.7.

CAS — 42779-82-8.

Clopirac is a non-steroidal anti-inflammatory agent that has been given by mouth in rheumatic disorders.

Proprietary Names and Manufacturers
Clopiran *(Continental Pharma, Belg.)*.

2631-z

Cymene
p-Cymene; *p*-Cymol. 4-Isopropyl-1-methylbenzene; 4-Isopropyltoluene.
$C_{10}H_{14}$=134.2.

CAS — 25155-15-1; 99-87-6 (p-cymene).

Cymene is a local analgesic applied as a 30% ointment for the relief of pain in rheumatic conditions.

Proprietary Names and Manufacturers
Dolcymene *(Roland-Marie, Fr.*; *Semar, Spain)*.

1729-k

Diacerein *(rINN)*.
9,10-Dihydro-4,5-dihydroxy-9,10-dioxo-2-anthroic acid diacetate.
$C_{19}H_{12}O_8$=368.3.

CAS — 13739-02-1.

Diacerein is a non-steroidal anti-inflammatory agent that has been used in rheumatic disorders in doses of 50 to 100 mg daily by mouth.

Proprietary Names and Manufacturers
Artrodar *(Proter, Ital.)*; Fisiodar *(Gentili, Ital.)*.

2632-c

Diclofenac Sodium *(BANM, USAN, rINNM)*.
Diclophenac Sodium; GP-45840. Sodium [2-(2,6-dichloroanilino)phenyl]acetate.
$C_{14}H_{10}Cl_2NNaO_2$=318.1.

CAS — 15307-86-5 (diclofenac); 15307-79-6 (sodium salt).

Adverse Effects
As for ibuprofen, p.20.

Adverse reactions were observed in 1564 of 18 992 patients who received diclofenac sodium. Reactions included gastro-intestinal disturbances (1340), oedema (117), skin reactions (103), pruritus (20), dizziness (16), malaise (10), headache (9), drowsiness (9), jaundice (2), and bleeding tendency (1).— *Jpn med. Gaz.*, 1978, *15*, (July 20), 10.

A review of reported adverse reactions associated with diclofenac during 1973–7. A total of 447 reactions were reported in 194 patients, the most frequent being gastro-intestinal, followed by dermatological, and central nervous system effects.— A. G. Ciucci, *Rheumatol. Rehabil.*, 1980, *18*, *Suppl.* 2, 116.

ALLERGY. All of 11 aspirin-sensitive asthmatic patients developed reactions (rhinorrhoea, tightness of chest, wheezing, dyspnoea) after taking diclofenac in doses of 10 to 25 mg.— A. Szczeklik *et al.*, *Br. med. J.*, 1977, *2*, 231.

On 3 occasions ingestion of a single dose of diclofenac was followed within a few hours by rigors, vomiting, and pyrexia; on one of these the recorded blood pressure was 70/50 mmHg. The patient had taken a course of diclofenac ending 3 months before the first episode. He had also taken ibuprofen before each of the reactions.— S. Dux *et al.*, *Br. med. J.*, 1983, *286*, 1861.

EFFECTS ON THE BLOOD. Spontaneous bleeding in the elbow and haematoma of the forearm in a patient receiving diclofenac rectally; no evidence of bleeding was present about one week after withdrawal of therapy.— R. Michalevicz and U. Seligsohn (letter), *Arthritis Rheum.*, 1982, *25*, 599.

Severe bruising of the leg and spontaneous platelet aggregation in an elderly patient receiving diclofenac.— L. Parapia and J. A. Cox, *Br. med. J.*, 1984, *288*, 368.

Aplastic anaemia. The First Report of the International Agranulocytosis and Aplastic Anemia Study concerning the risks of agranulocytosis and aplastic anaemia and the relation to drug use with special reference to analgesics. Diclofenac sodium, taken 29 to 180 days previously, was significantly associated with aplastic anaemia, the estimated increase in risk being of the order of tenfold.— *J. Am. med. Ass.*, 1986, *256*, 1749.

Haemolytic anaemia. Severe reversible auto-immune haemolytic anaemia and thrombocytopenia developed in a patient within 10 days of starting diclofenac therapy.— M. R. Kramer *et al.*, *Scand. J. Haemat.*, 1986,

36, 118.

EFFECTS ON THE KIDNEY. Renal papillary necrosis in one patient following the use of diclofenac for about 5 years.— S. J. Scott *et al., Br. med. J.,* 1986, *292,* 1050.

Two cases of isolated minimal change nephropathy in patients taking diclofenac for about 3 months and 3 weeks respectively.— G. D. M. Beun *et al., Br. med. J.,* 1987, *295,* 182.

The nephrotic syndrome in one patient associated with diclofenac.— A. M. Yinnon *et al., Br. med. J.,* 1987, *295,* 556.

EFFECTS ON THE LIVER. A report of 3 patients in whom hepatic dysfunction occurred during treatment with diclofenac.— *Jpn med. Gaz.,* 1976, *13,* (Apr. 20), 10.

Acute hepatitis probably associated with diclofenac.— A. A. Dunk *et al., Br. med. J.,* 1982, *284,* 1605.

Fatal hepatitis in a patient who had received diclofenac.— E. G. Breen *et al., Gut,* 1986, *27,* 1390.

Further references: D. Schapira *et al., Postgrad. med. J.,* 1986, *62,* 63 (liver hypersensitivity reaction in 2 patients).

EFFECTS ON THE MUSCLES. Myoclonus occurred in a man who had taken diclofenac for 4 months and disappeared 48 hours after stopping the drug.— M. Alcalay *et al., Sem. Hôp. Paris,* 1979, *55,* 679.

EFFECTS ON THE SKIN. Diclofenac-induced bullous dermatosis in one patient; the eruptions subsided gradually after withdrawal of therapy and had disappeared after 5 weeks.— T. Ø. Gabrielsen *et al., Acta derm.-vener., Stockh.,* 1981, *61,* 439.

Implication of diclofenac in the causation of erythema multiforme (Stevens-Johnson syndrome) in one patient.— B. A. P. Morris and S. S. Remtulla, *Can. med. Ass. J.,* 1985, *133,* 665.

Precautions

As for ibuprofen, p.20.

Diclofenac sodium may cause increased blood concentrations of digoxin and lithium. Although studies have demonstrated a pharmacokinetic interaction between diclofenac and salicylates it has been stated that this has no clinical significance. It has also been reported that diclofenac, unlike some other non-steroidal anti-inflammatory agents, does not potentiate the effects of oral anticoagulants or hypoglycaemics.

INTERACTIONS. Deterioration in renal function in a patient attributed to the concomitant use of diclofenac and triamterene, both of which may have adverse effects on kidney function.— M. Härkönen and S. Ekblom-Kullberg (letter), *Br. med. J.,* 1986, *293,* 698.

For the effect of diclofenac on other drugs see under methotrexate (p.638).

PORPHYRIA. Diclofenac sodium was considered to be unsafe in patients with acute porphyria because it has been shown to be porphyrinogenic in *animals* or *in vitro* systems.— M.R. Moore and K.E.L. McColl, *Porphyrias, Drug Lists* , Glasgow, Porphyria Research Unit, University of Glasgow, 1987.

Absorption and Fate

Diclofenac is absorbed from the gastro-intestinal tract but is subject to first-pass metabolism. Peak plasma concentrations occur about 1 to 4 hours after ingestion of enteric-coated tablets. At therapeutic concentrations it is more than 99% bound to plasma proteins. The terminal plasma half-life is about 1 to 2 hours. Diclofenac is excreted primarily in the form of metabolites, mainly in the urine but also in the bile.

Plasma and synovial fluid concentrations of diclofenac.— P. D. Fowler *et al., Eur. J. clin. Pharmac.,* 1983, *25,* 389; P. D. Fowler *et al., ibid.,* 1986, *31,* 469.

Uses and Administration

Diclofenac sodium has analgesic, antipyretic, and anti-inflammatory properties; it is an inhibitor of prostaglandin synthetase (cyclo-oxygenase).

It is used for the relief of pain and inflammation in conditions such as rheumatoid arthritis, osteoarthritis, ankylosing spondylitis, acute gout, and following some surgical procedures. The usual dose by mouth is 75 to 150 mg daily in divided doses. It may also be given rectally as a suppository in a usual dose of 100 mg each evening. Diclofenac sodium may also be given by intramuscular injection in a dose of 75 mg once daily or, if required in severe conditions, 75 mg twice daily. It is also used intramuscularly in renal colic in a dose of 75 mg repeated once after 30 minutes if necessary. In children the suggested dose by mouth or rectally for juvenile chronic arthritis is 1 to 3 mg per kg body-weight daily in divided doses.

A review of the pharmacodynamic and pharmacokinetic properties, and the therapeutic efficacy of diclofenac sodium.— P. A. Todd and E. M. Sorkin, *Drugs,* 1988, *35,* 244.

ANKYLOSING SPONDYLITIS. A favourable report of the use of diclofenac in ankylosing spondylitis.— M. A. Khan, *J. Rheumatol.,* 1987, *14,* 118.

BILIARY AND RENAL COLIC. A short, but favourable, review of the use of diclofenac sodium by intramuscular injection for the relief of pain in biliary and renal colic.— *Drug & Ther. Bull.,* 1987, *25,* 85.

Studies on the use of diclofenac intramuscularly in colic: M. Broggini *et al., Br. med. J.,* 1984, *288,* 1042 (biliary); J. W. Hetherington and N. H. Philp, *ibid.,* 1986, *292,* 237 (renal); E. Grossi *et al., Curr. ther. Res.,* 1986, *40,* 876 (biliary); S. Lundstam *et al., ibid.,* 1987, *42,* 395 (biliary).

FEVER. A study confirming the antipyretic activity of diclofenac in adult patients with fever, usually associated with influenza.— R. Bettini *et al., J. int. med. Res.,* 1986, *14,* 95.

OSTEOARTHRITIS. Some references to the use of diclofenac in osteoarthritis: H. Berry *et al., Clin. Trials J.,* 1982, *19,* 349; T. Amundsen *et al., Curr. ther. Res.,* 1983, *33,* 793; M. J. Vandenburg *et al., Br. J. clin. Pract.,* 1984, *38,* 403; M. Aylward *et al., ibid.,* 1985, *39,* 135; G. Vetter, *ibid.,* 276; C. O. Dillard *et al., Curr. ther. Res.,* 1985, *37,* 259.

PAIN. Some studies on the use of diclofenac for analgesia: R. W. Matthews *et al., Br. dent. J.,* 1984, *157,* 357 (post-surgical dental pain); H. Dommerby and O. R. Rasmussen, *Acta oto-lar.,* 1984, *98,* 185 (postoperative pain); U. Lindgren and H. Djupsjö, *Acta orthop. scand.,* 1985, *56,* 28 (postoperative pain); D. R. Derbyshire and J. Richardson, *Br. J. Anaesth.,* 1987, *59,* 1327P (perioperative administration for postoperative pain); E. Wuolijoki *et al., Eur. J. clin. Pharmac.,* 1987, *32,* 249 (pre-operative administration for postoperative pain); N. B. A. Hodsman *et al., Anaesthesia,* 1987, *42,* 1005 (postoperative pain); E. Del Bene *et al., J. int. med. Res.,* 1987, *15,* 44 (migraine).

RENAL DISORDERS. In a placebo-controlled study involving 29 patients with glomerulonephritis but normal renal function, treatment with diclofenac 100 mg daily had a significant antiproteinuric effect. It was not known if this action affected the final outcome of the disease.— J. Laurent *et al., Am. J. Nephrol.,* 1987, *7,* 198.

See also under Biliary and Renal Colic (above).

RHEUMATOID ARTHRITIS. Some references to the use of diclofenac in rheumatoid arthritis: H. Berry *et al., Clin. Trials J.,* 1982, *19,* 248; T. Bendix *et al., Curr. ther. Res.,* 1983, *33,* 192; W. Eidsaunet *et al., ibid.,* 966; P. Humberto Lizarazo and M. Peņa Cortés, *ibid.,* *34,* 701; J. C. Huntwork, *ibid.,* 1986, *40,* 576.

Proprietary Preparations

Rhumalgan *(Lagap, UK). Tablets,* enteric-coated, diclofenac sodium 25 and 50 mg.

Voltarol *(Geigy, UK). Tablets* enteric-coated, diclofenac sodium 25 and 50 mg.

Tablets (Voltarol Retard), sustained-release, diclofenac sodium 100 mg.

Injection, diclofenac sodium 25 mg/mL, in ampoules of 3 mL.

Suppositories, diclofenac sodium 12.5 and 100 mg.

Proprietary Names and Manufacturers

Aflamin *(Ital.)*; Allvoran *(TAD, Ger.)*; Blesin *(Jpn)*; Delphimix *(Cyanamid-Lederle, Ger.)*; Dichronic *(Jpn)*; Diclo Attritin *(Atmos, Ger.)*; Diclo Phlogont *(Azuchemie, Ger.)*; Diclo Spondyril *(Dorsch, Ger.)*; Dicloreum *(Istituto Wassermann, Ital.)*; Dolobasan *(Sagitta, Ger.)*; Dolotren *(Faes, Spain)*; Duravolten *(Durachemie, Ger.)*; Effekton *(Efeka, Ger.)*; Flogofenac *(Ecobi, Ital.)*; Forgenac *(Zoja, Ital.)*; Inflamac *(Spirig, Switz.)*; Monoflam *(Brenner, Ger.)*; Myogit *(Pfleger, Ger.)*; Neriodin *(Jpn)*; Novapirina *(Zyma, Ital.)*; Olfen *(Mepha, Switz.)*; Panamor *(S.Afr.)*; Rheumavincin *(Schur, Ger.)*; Rhumalgan *(Lagap, UK)*; Seecoren *(Jpn)*; Silino *(Heilit, Ger.)*; Sofarin *(Jpn)*; Toryxil *(Baer, Ger.)*; Tsudohmin *(Jpn)*; Voltarène *(Geigy, Fr.; Geigy, Switz.)*; Voltaren *(Arg.; Geigy, Austral.; Belg.; Geigy, Canad.; Geigy, Denm.; Geigy, Ger.; Geigy, Ital.; Jpn; Neth.; Geigy, S.Afr.; Ciba, Spain; Geigy, Swed.)*; Voltarol *(Geigy, UK)*.

2633-k

Diethylamine Salicylate *(BAN).*

$C_{11}H_{17}NO_3$=211.3.

CAS — 4419-92-5.

Pharmacopoeias. In *Br.*

White or almost white, odourless or almost odourless crystals. **Soluble** 1 in less than 1 of water, 1 in 2 of alcohol, and 1 in 1.5 of chloroform. **Store** in well-closed containers. Protect from light. Avoid contact with iron or iron salts.

Diethylamine salicylate is used topically, usually at a concentration of 5 or 10%, in creams for rheumatic and muscular pain.

Preparations

Diethylamine Salicylate Cream *(B.P.)*

Proprietary Preparations

Algesal *(Duphar, UK). Cream,* diethylamine salicylate 10%.

Aradolene *(Rorer, UK). Cream,* diethylamine salicylate 5%, a water-soluble capsicum preparation 0.4%, rectified camphor oil 1.4%, menthol 2.5%.

Proprietary Names and Manufacturers

Algesal *(Charton, Canad.; Denm.; Farmades, Ital.; Neth.; Nyco, Norw.; S.Afr.; Latema, Swed.; Duphar, UK)*; Almyderm *(DAK, Denm.)*; Artrogota *(Parisis, Spain)*; Rubesal *(Hamilton, Austral.)*.

The following names have been used for multi-ingredient preparations containing diethylamine salicylate— Aradolene *(Rorer, UK)*; Feparil *(Madaus Cerafarm, Spain)*; Reparil Gel *(Bellon, Fr.; Madaus, Ger.; Ibi, Ital.; Madaus, S.Afr.; Madaus Switz.)*; Vascutonex *(Wellcome, UK)*.

2634-a

Difenamizole *(rINN).*

AP-14. 2-Dimethylamino-*N*-(1,3-diphenylpyrazol-5-yl)propionamide.

$C_{20}H_{22}N_4O$=334.4.

CAS — 20170-20-1.

Difenamizole is an analgesic which is claimed also to have anti-inflammatory and muscle-relaxing properties. It has been given by mouth in doses of 75 mg three times daily.

Hepatitis associated with difenamizole in 1 patient.— S. Imoto *et al.* (letter), *Ann. intern. Med.,* 1979, *91,* 129.

Proprietary Names and Manufacturers

Pasalin *(Takeda, Jpn)*.

12650-e

Difenpiramide

Diphenpyramide; Z-876. *N*-(2-Pyridyl)-2-(biphenyl-4-yl)acetamide.

$C_{19}H_{16}N_2O$=288.3.

CAS — 51484-40-3.

Difenpiramide has anti-inflammatory and analgesic properties and has been used in rheumatic disorders in doses of 250 mg three times daily by mouth.

Proprietary Names and Manufacturers

Difenax *(Zambeletti, Ital.)*.

2635-t

Diflunisal *(BAN, USAN, rINN).*

MK-647. 5-(2,4-Difluorophenyl)salicylic acid.

$C_{13}H_8F_2O_3$=250.2.

CAS — 22494-42-4.

Pharmacopoeias. In *Br.* and *U.S.*

A white to off-white, practically odourless, crystalline powder. *B.P.* **solubilities** are: practically insoluble in water; soluble in alcohol and ether. *U.S.P.* solubilities are: practically insoluble in water; freely soluble in alcohol and methyl alcohol; soluble in acetone and ethyl acetate; slightly soluble in chloroform. **Store** in well-closed containers. Protect from light.

Adverse Effects and Treatment

As for aspirin, p.3. The commonest side-effects occurring with diflunisal are gastro-intestinal disturbances, although the incidence may be slightly less than with aspirin. Peptic ulceration and gastro-intestinal bleeding have been reported. Skin rash, pruritus, dizziness, drowsiness, headache, and tinnitus may also occur.

EFFECTS ON THE BLOOD. Platelet aggregation in patients treated with diflunisal.— M. L. Ghosh and A. Tingle, *Curr. med. Res. Opinion*, 1980, *6*, 510.

EFFECTS ON THE GASTRO-INTESTINAL TRACT. A report of perforated duodenal ulcer after 7 days' treatment with diflunisal.— R. Talbot and H. Rees (letter), *Br. med. J.*, 1978, *2*, 1229.

Severe gastro-intestinal bleeding occurred in a 66-year-old woman following treatment with diflunisal.— A. K. Admani and D. M. N. F. Khaleque (letter), *Lancet*, 1979, *1*, 1247. Reports to the Committee on Safety of Medicines on diflunisal up to Feb 1979, included: gastro-intestinal haemorrhage (9), haematemesis (22), rectal haemorrhage (2), and melaena (13).— *ibid.*

Further reports of gastro-intestinal disturbances, haematemesis, and melaena.— B. Scott (letter), *Br. med. J.*, 1979, *1*, 489; A. M. Mason (letter), *Br. med. J.*, 1979, *1*, 888.

Studies which indicated that patients treated with diflunisal had fewer gastric lesions and less gastro-intestinal bleeding than patients treated with aspirin.— V. M. Tringham and P. Cochrane (letter), *Lancet*, 1979, *1*, 1409; M. Petrillo *et al.*, *ibid.*, 1979, *2*, 638.

EFFECTS ON THE KIDNEYS. A report of acute interstitial nephritis, presenting as acute oliguric renal failure, erythroderma, and eosinophilia following the use of diflunisal.— L. K. Chan, *Br. med. J.*, 1980, *280*, 84.

EFFECTS ON THE LIVER. A 64-year-old man developed cholestatic jaundice 5 days after starting to take diflunisal; the condition slowly regressed when diflunisal was withdrawn.— J. S. Warren, *Br. med. J.*, 1978, *2*, 736.

EFFECTS ON THE SKIN. Diflunisal was probably responsible for the Stevens-Johnson syndrome in 2 patients.— J. A. Hunter *et al.* (letter), *Br. med. J.*, 1978, *2*, 1088. Four severe cases of the Stevens-Johnson syndrome in patients taking diflunisal have been reported.— *Pharm. J.*, 1979, *1*, 318. A further report.— J. A. Grom *et al.*, *Hosp. Formul.*, 1986, *21*, 353.

OVERDOSAGE. A review of cases of diflunisal poisonings reported to the National Poisons Information Service of the *UK*. Of 43 reports 5 were classified as severe or fatal; one patient was dead when found, and one other died in hospital following a cardio-respiratory arrest but other drugs may also have contributed to the cause of death. It appeared that diflunisal overdose was not common. It has previously been stated that a dose of 15 g has caused death when no other drugs were involved and that 7.5 g has been ingested in a mixed drug overdose resulting in death. The treatment of a diflunisal overdose should involve gastric lavage and supportive care; the benefit of forced diuresis has not been established.— H. Court and G. N. Volans, *Adverse Drug React. Ac. Pois. Rev.*, 1984, *3*, 1.

Precautions

As for aspirin, p.5.

Diflunisal has been reported to significantly increase the plasma concentrations of indomethacin and paracetamol; it has been stated that the concomitant administration of diflunisal and indomethacin has been associated with fatal gastro-intestinal haemorrhage and therefore should not be used.

INTERACTIONS. *Antacids*. Concomitant administration of diflunisal and aluminium hydroxide reduced the bioavailability of diflunisal by about 40%.— R. Verbeeck *et al.*, *Br. J. clin. Pharmac.*, 1979, *7*, 519.

Aspirin. Aspirin 600 mg daily or 300 mg four times daily given in combination with diflunisal 250 mg twice daily had no significant effect on diflunisal plasma concentrations in 14 healthy subjects but aspirin 600 mg four times daily reduced diflunisal plasma concentrations. This was not considered to be clinically important.— P. Schulz *et al.*, *J. int. med. Res.*, 1979, *7*, 61.

Benzodiazepines. For the effect of diflunisal on oxazepam, see p.756.

Absorption and Fate

Diflunisal is well absorbed from the gastro-intestinal tract and peak plasma concentrations occur about 2 to 3 hours after ingestion of a single dose. It is extensively bound (more than 99%) to plasma protein and has an elimination half-life of about 8 to 12 hours. It is excreted mainly as glucuronide conjugates in the urine. Less than 5% of a single dose is excreted in the faeces. Diflunisal is excreted in breast milk with concentrations reported to be about 2 to 7% of those in plasma.

Uses and Administration

Diflunisal has analgesic, anti-inflammatory, and antipyretic properties; it inhibits prostaglandin synthetase. It is used as an analgesic for mild to moderate pain and for the relief of pain and inflammation in osteoarthritis and rheumatoid arthritis. The usual initial dose is 500 mg twice daily by mouth with doses of 250 to 500 mg twice daily being used for long-term therapy.

A review and discussion on non-steroidal anti-inflammatory agents as analgesics with some comments relevant to diflunisal. The onset of action of diflunisal is slightly slower than that of aspirin but the duration is more prolonged. As it needs to be taken twice daily it is less useful as an 'on demand' analgesic and more useful for a course of regular treatment.— E. C. Huskisson, *Prescribers' J.*, 1983, *23*, 10.

Reviews of the pharmacology, adverse effects, metabolism, and uses of diflunisal.— C. A. Stone *et al.*, *Br. J. clin. Pharmac.*, 1977, *4*, *Suppl.* 1, 19S; K. F. Tempero *et al.*, *ibid.*, 31S; *Drug & Ther. Bull.*, 1978, *16*, 101; R. N. Brogden *et al.*, *Drugs*, 1980, *19*, 84.

ADMINISTRATION IN RENAL FAILURE. Renal excretion of diflunisal was reduced in 17 patients with renal insufficiency compared with 5 healthy subjects. The impaired excretion was associated with increased diflunisal-glucuronide retention in the plasma. The plasma elimination half-life of 10.8 hours obtained in the healthy subjects was progressively prolonged with increasing degrees of renal function impairment.— P. J. De Schepper *et al.*, *Br. J. clin. Pharmac.*, 1977, *4*, 645P. Pharmacokinetic studies suggesting that in patients with a creatinine clearance of less than 10 mL per minute diflunisal should not be used, in those with a clearance of 15 to 50 mL per minute the dosage should be reduced or the interval between doses extended, and in those with higher clearance rates the normal doses may be given.— R. Verbeeck *et al.*, *ibid.*, 1979, *7*, 273.

OSTEOARTHRITIS. Some references to the use of diflunisal in osteoarthritis: R. White *et al.*, *Curr. med. Res. Opinion*, 1987, *10*, 436.

PAIN. Some references to the use of diflunisal as a postoperative analgesic: J. A. Forbes *et al.*, *J. clin. Pharmac.*, 1982, *22*, 89; G. H. Irvine *et al.*, *Br. dent. J.*, 1982, *152*, 18; R. Melzack *et al.*, *Curr. ther. Res.*, 1983, *34*, 929; J. J. Madsen *et al.*, *ibid.*, 1987, *42*, 319.

RHEUMATOID ARTHRITIS. Some references to the use of diflunisal in rheumatoid arthritis: T. S. Bocanegra *et al.*, *Curr. med. Res. Opinion*, 1985, *9*, 568.

Preparations

Diflunisal Tablets *(B.P.)*

Diflunisal Tablets *(U.S.P.)*

Proprietary Preparations

Dolobid *(Morson, UK)*. *Tablets*, diflunisal 250 and 500 mg.

Proprietary Names and Manufacturers

Adomal *(Malesci, Ital.)*; Algobid *(San Carlo, Ital.)*; Antadar *(Hubber, Spain)*; Artrodol *(AGIPS, Ital.)*; Diflonid *(Dumex, Denm.; Dumex, Swed.)*; Difludol *(Edmond Pharma, Ital.)*; Diflunil *(Schwarz, Ital.)*; Diflusan *(Von Boch, Ital.)*; Dolisal *(Guidotti, Ital.; Peru)*; Dolobid *(Merck Sharp & Dohme, Austral.; Frosst, Canad.; Merck Sharp & Dohme, Ital.; Merck Sharp & Dohme, S.Afr.; Merck Sharp & Dohme, Spain; Morson, UK; Merck Sharp & Dohme, USA)*; Dolobis *(Merck Sharp & Dohme-Chibret, Fr.)*; Donobid *(Costa Rica; Merck Sharp & Dohme, Denm.; Fin.; Merck Sharp & Dohme, Norw.; MSD, Swed.)*; Dopanone *(Greece)*; Dorbid *(Braz.)*; Flulisin *(Ripari-Gero, Ital.)*; Fluniget *(Chibret, Ger.)*; Fluodonil *(Herdel, Ital.)*; Flustar *(FIRMA, Ital.)*; Ilacen *(Hosbon, Spain)*; Noaldol *(Lampugnani, Ital.)*; Reuflos *(Scharper, Ital.)*; Unisal *(Merck Sharp & Dohme, Switz.)*.

2636-x

Diftalone *(USAN, rINN)*.

L-5418. Phthalazino[2,3-*b*]phthalazine-5,12(7*H*,14*H*)-dione.

$C_{16}H_{12}N_2O_2$=264.3.

CAS — 21626-89-1.

Diftalone has analgesic and anti-inflammatory properties and has been given by mouth in rheumatic disorders.

Some references to diftalone in osteoarthrosis: G. C. Pinheiro, *Curr. med. Res. Opinion*, 1976, *4*, 402; L. Mattara *et al.*, *Clin. Trials J.*, 1977, *14*, 30.

Some references to diftalone in rheumatoid arthritis: L. Brown *et al.*, *Clin. Trials J.*, 1977, *14*, 50; J. Vachtenheim, *ibid.*, 98; A. Šusta *et al.*, *ibid.*, 145; F. Chalem *et al.*, *J. int. med. Res.*, 1977, *5*, 18; P. Sfikakis and D. Charalambopoulos, *Acta ther.*, 1977, *3*, 237.

Studies on the absorption, metabolism, and excretion of diftalone.— G. Buniva *et al.*, *Int. J. clin. Pharmac. Biopharm.*, 1977, *15*, 460; L. T. Tenconi *et al.*, *ibid.*, 485; M. S. Benedetti *et al.*, *Arzneimittel-Forsch.*, 1977, *27*, 2364; J. C. Garnham *et al.*, *J. Pharm. Pharmac.*, 1978, *30*, 407.

Proprietary Names and Manufacturers

Retilon *(Lepetit, Spain)*.

16607-k

Diproqualone *(rINN)*.

3-(2,3-Dihydroxypropyl)-2-methyl-4(3*H*)-quinazolinone.

$C_{12}H_{14}N_2O_3$=234.3.

CAS — 36518-02-2.

Diproqualone is an analgesic that has been used as the camsylate in usual doses of 200 mg three times daily by mouth.

Proprietary Names and Manufacturers of Diproqualone and its Salts

The following names have been used for multi-ingredient preparations containing diproqualone and its salts— Algopriv *(Bouchard, Fr.; Interdelta, Switz.)*.

2637-r

Dipyrocetyl *(rINN)*.

Diacetsalicylic Acid; UCB-5080. *OO*-Diacetylpyrocatechol-3-carboxylic acid; 2,3-Diacetoxybenzoic acid.

$C_{11}H_{10}O_6$=238.2.

CAS — 486-79-3.

Pharmacopoeias. In *Cz.*

Dipyrocetyl is an analgesic, anti-inflammatory, and antipyretic agent that has been given in doses of up to 6 g daily, in divided doses, by mouth.

Proprietary Names and Manufacturers

Movirene *(Vesta, S.Afr.)*.

2638-f

Dipyrone *(BAN, USAN)*.

Aminopyrine-sulphonate Sodium; Analginum; Metamizole; Metamizole Sodium *(pINN)*; Methampyrone; Natrium Novaminsulfonicum; Noramidazophenum; Noraminophenazonum; Novamidazofen; Sodium Noramidopyrine Methanesulphonate; Sulpyrine. Sodium *N*-(2,3-dimethyl-5-oxo-1-phenyl-3-pyrazolin-4-yl)-*N*-methylaminomethanesulphonate monohydrate.

$C_{13}H_{16}N_3NaO_4S,H_2O$=351.4.

CAS — 68-89-3 (anhydrous); 5907-38-0 (monohydrate).

Pharmacopoeias. In *Arg., Aust., Braz., Chin., Cz., Egypt., Ger., Hung., Ind., Jpn, Jug., Nord., Pol., Roum., Rus., Swiss,* and *Turk.*

Adverse Effects and Precautions
As for amidopyrine, p.3.

ALLERGY. Cross-sensitivity between aspirin and dipyrone occurred in one patient. Dipyrone produced an exacerbation of dyspnoea, cyanosis, and respiratory arrest.— E. Bartoli *et al.* (letter), *Lancet,* 1976, *1,* 1357.

See also under Effects on the Skin (below).

EFFECTS ON THE BLOOD. The AMA Registry of Adverse Reactions recorded 40 cases of agranulocytosis presumed to be due to dipyrone and a further 22 possibly due to the drug in the period 1957–66. A hypersensitivity reaction was probably involved.— *Med. Lett.,* 1973, *15,* 4.

An analysis of blood dyscrasias reported to the Swedish Adverse Drug Reaction Committee for the 10-year period 1966–75 showed that agranulocytosis attributable to dipyrone had been reported on 38 occasions (12 fatal).— L. E. Bottiger *et al., Acta med. scand.,* 1979, *205,* 457.

A First Report by The International Agranulocytosis and Aplastic Anemia Study on the risks of agranulocytosis and aplastic anaemia with special reference to the use of analgesics. Analysis revealed that there was a significant regional variability in the rate-ratio estimate for agranulocytosis and dipyrone (0.9 in Budapest to 33.3 in Barcelona). Although a large relative increase in risk between agranulocytosis and use of dipyrone was found, the incidence was less than some previous reports had suggested.— *J. Am. med. Ass.,* 1986, *256,* 1749. Comment.— *Lancet,* 1986, *2,* 899. Correspondence.— R. Doll *et al.* (letter), *ibid.,* 1987, *1,* 101; J. -R. Laporte and X. Carné (letter), *ibid.,* 809.

EFFECTS ON THE SKIN. Dipyrone had been responsible for a case of drug-induced toxic epidermal necrolysis.— J. -C. Roujeau *et al., Lancet,* 1985, *1,* 609.

Analysis, by the Boston Collaborative Drug Surveillance Program, of data on 15 438 patients hospitalised between 1975 and 1982 detected 13 allergic skin reactions attributed to dipyrone among 3 279 recipients of the drug.— M. Bigby *et al., J. Am. med. Ass.,* 1986, *256,* 3358.

PORPHYRIA. Dipyrone was considered to be unsafe in patients with acute porphyria because it has been shown to be porphyrinogenic in *animals* or *in vitro* systems.— M.R. Moore and K.E.L. McColl, *Porphyrias, Drug Lists,* Glasgow, Porphyria Research Unit, University of Glasgow, 1987.

Uses and Administration
Dipyrone is the sodium sulphonate of amidopyrine (see p.3) and has similar properties. Its use is justified only in serious or life-threatening situations where no alternative antipyretic is available or suitable. It has been given by mouth in doses of 0.5 to 1 g up to three times daily. It has also been given by subcutaneous, intramuscular, or intravenous injection in doses of 0.5 to 1 g.

Proprietary Names and Manufacturers
Adolkin *(Kin, Spain)*; Alginodia *(Cilag, Arg.)*; Dolatets *(Pharmadrug, Ger.)*; Dolemicin *(Ale, Spain)*; Espyre *(Jpn)*; Lagalgin *(Lagap, Switz.)*; Lasain *(Lasa, Spain)*; Metilon *(Jpn)*; Minalgine *(Streuli, Switz.)*; Neo-Melubrina *(Hoechst, Spain)*; Nolotil *(Castejon, Spain)*; Novalgin *(Hoechst, Ger.; Hoechst, Neth.; Winthrop, S.Afr.)*; Novalgina *(Hoechst, Arg.; Albert-Farma, Ital.)*; Novalgine *(Hoechst, Belg.; Hoechst, Fr.; Hoechst, Switz.)*; Novaminsulfon *(Ger.)*; Novemina *(Lazar, Arg.)*; Optalgin *(Inibsa, Spain)*; Ortopirona *(Fides, Spain)*; Reflex Rectal *(Liade, Spain)*; Sulfonovin *(Ibsa, Switz.)*; Tapal *(Sterwin, Spain)*.

2639-d

Ditazole *(rINN).*

Diethamphenazole; S-222. 2,2′-[(4,5-Diphenyloxazol-2-yl)imino]diethanol monohydrate.
$C_{19}H_{20}N_2O_3,H_2O$=342.4.

CAS — 18471-20-0 (anhydrous).

Ditazole is an anti-inflammatory agent with an inhibitory effect on platelet aggregation. It has been used in the treatment of phlebitis, thrombosis, and similar disorders in doses of 400 mg two or three times daily.

Proprietary Names and Manufacturers
Ageroplas *(Serono, Ital.; Farma-Lepori, Spain)*.

19130-x

Emorfazone *(rINN).*

4-Ethoxy-2-methyl-5-morpholino-3(2*H*)-pyridazinone.
$C_{11}H_{17}N_3O_3$=239.3.

CAS — 38957-41-4.

Emorfazone is an analgesic and anti-inflammatory agent that has been used in rheumatic disorders in doses of about 100 to 200 mg.

Proprietary Names and Manufacturers
Pentoil *(Morishita, Jpn)*.

2640-c

Epirizole *(USAN, pINN).*

DA-398; Mepirizole. 4-Methoxy-2-(5-methoxy-3-methylpyrazol-1-yl)-6-methylpyrimidine.
$C_{11}H_{14}N_4O_2$=234.3.

CAS — 18694-40-1.

Pharmacopoeias. In *Jpn.*

Epirizole has analgesic and anti-inflammatory properties. It has been used by mouth in doses of up to 600 mg daily in divided doses.

Adverse effects occurred on 1583 occasions in 23 524 patients who received epirizole and included gastro-intestinal disturbances (1372), rash (71), stomatitis (50), dizziness (28), headache (26), oedema of fingers (16), anxiety (6), drowsiness (5), and tinnitus (2).— *Jpn med. Gaz.,* 1976, *13* (Mar. 20), 14.

Proprietary Names and Manufacturers
Analock *(Pfizer Taito, Jpn)*; Daicon *(Ibi, Ital.)*; Mebron *(Daiichi, Jpn; Ethimed, S.Afr.)*; Mepiral *(Robert, Spain)*; Mepirijust *(Hotta, Jpn)*.

2641-k

Etenzamide *(BAN).*

Aethoxybenzamidum; Ethenzamide *(rINN)*; Ethoxybenzamide; Ethylsalicylamide; HP-209. 2-Ethoxybenzamide.
$C_9H_{11}NO_2$=165.2.

CAS — 938-73-8.

Pharmacopoeias. In *Aust.* and *Jpn.*

Etenzamide has analgesic, anti-inflammatory, and antipyretic properties. It has been given in doses of up to 4 g daily in divided doses by mouth.

Proprietary Names and Manufacturers
Lucamid *(Lundbeck, Denm.)*; Trancalgyl *(Innothéra, Fr.)*.

3553-h

Etersalate *(rINN).*

Eterilate; Eterylate; Etherylate. 2-(4-Acetamidophenoxy)ethyl salicylate, acetate (ester).
$C_{19}H_{19}NO_6$=357.4.

CAS — 62992-61-4.

Etersalate has analgesic and anti-inflammatory properties. It has been given in doses of 750 mg three or four times daily by mouth as an analgesic and in doses of 1.5 g two or three times daily by mouth in rheumatic disorders.

Proprietary Names and Manufacturers
Daital *(Alter, Spain)*.

2642-a

Ethosalamide *(BAN).*

Etosalamide *(rINN)*; Salicylamide 2-ethoxyethyl ether. 2-(2-Ethoxyethoxy)benzamide.
$C_{11}H_{15}NO_3$=209.2.

CAS — 15302-15-5.

Ethosalamide has analgesic and antipyretic properties and was formerly used, usually in conjunction with paracetamol and caffeine.

Proprietary Names and Manufacturers
The following names have been used for multi-ingredient preparations containing ethosalamide— Antidol *(Lipomed, UK)*.

2643-t

Ethoxazene Hydrochloride *(USAN).*

Etoxazene Hydrochloride *(rINNM)*; *p*-Ethoxychrysoidine Hydrochloride; SN-612. 4-(4-Ethoxyphenylazo)benzene-1,3-diyldiamine hydrochloride.
$C_{14}H_{16}N_4O,HCl$=292.8.

CAS — 94-10-0 (ethoxazene); 2313-87-3 (hydrochloride).

Precautions
Ethoxazene is contra-indicated in patients with severe liver disease, uraemia, or chronic parenchymatous nephritis. It should be used with care in patients with gastro-intestinal disorders. Ethoxazene may colour the urine orange or red.

Uses and Administration
Ethoxazene hydrochloride is chemically related to phenazopyridine hydrochloride. It was formerly used to relieve pain in cystitis, urethritis, and pyelitis in doses of 100 mg three times daily before meals.

Proprietary Names and Manufacturers
Serenium *(Squibb, USA)*.

12707-l

Ethyl Salicylate

Ethyl 2-hydroxybenzoate.
$C_9H_{10}O_3$=166.2.

CAS — 118-61-6.

Ethyl salicylate has been used topically in concentrations of up to 4% for rheumatic and muscular pain.

Proprietary Names and Manufacturers
The following names have been used for multi-ingredient preparations containing ethyl salicylate— Aspellin *(Rorer, UK)*; Dubam *(Norma, UK)*.

12717-j

Etodolac *(BAN, USAN, rINN).*

AY-24236; Etodolic Acid. 1,8-Diethyl-1,3,4,9-tetrahydropyrano[3,4-*b*]indol-1-ylacetic acid.
$C_{17}H_{21}NO_3$=287.4.

CAS — 41340-25-4.

Adverse Effects
Reported side-effects with etodolac include gastro-intestinal disturbances, headache, drowsiness, dizziness, tinnitus, and skin rashes.

The safety profile of etodolac.— S. Ryder *et al., Curr. ther. Res.,* 1983, *33,* 948.

Precautions
Etodolac should not be used in patients with peptic ulceration or a history of such ulceration, or in patients sensitive to aspirin. It should be used with care in the presence of hepatic or renal failure and in patients receiving oral anticoagulants. The presence of metabolites in the urine may give rise to a false-positive reaction for bilirubin.

Absorption and Fate
Etodolac is absorbed from the gastro-intestinal tract with peak plasma concentrations being attained about 1 to 2 hours after ingestion. Etodolac is highly bound to plasma protein with the reported half-life being about 7 hours. It is excreted predominantly in the urine mainly as hydroxylated metabolites and glucuronide conjugates.

Uses and Administration
Etodolac has anti-inflammatory properties; it is

an inhibitor of prostaglandin synthetase.

Etodolac is used in rheumatoid arthritis in a usual dose by mouth of 200 mg twice daily; up to 600 mg daily may be given if necessary.

Reviews of the actions and uses of etodolac: S. Lynch and R. N. Brogden, *Drugs*, 1986, *31*, 288; *Drug & Ther. Bull.*, 1987, *25*, 11 and 28.

ADMINISTRATION IN THE ELDERLY. Pharmacokinetic data suggesting adjustment of dosage of etodolac in elderly patients is not necessary.— J. Scatina *et al.*, *Clin. Pharmac. Ther.*, 1986, *39*, 550.

ADMINISTRATION IN RENAL FAILURE. A study suggesting that the use of etodolac 200 mg twice daily in patients with chronic renal insufficiency would not result in adverse renal effects.— D. C. Brater *et al.*, *Clin. Pharmac. Ther.*, 1985, *38*, 674. See also: D. G. Shand *et al.*, *J. clin. Pharmac.*, 1986, *26*, 269.

RHEUMATOID ARTHRITIS. Some references to the use of etodolac in rheumatoid arthritis: G. V. Gordon and B. G. Polsky, *Curr. ther. Res.*, 1983, *33*, 89; G. B. Jacob *et al.*, *ibid.*, 703; R. A. del Toro and R. Concepcion, *Clin. Ther.*, 1983, *5*, 436; W. Edwards, *ibid.*, 495; G. Jacob *et al.*, *J. clin. Pharmac.*, 1986, *26*, 195; C. D. Waltham-Weeks, *Curr. med. Res. Opinion*, 1987, *10*, 540.

Proprietary Preparations

Lodine *(Ayerst, UK)*. *Capsules*, etodolac 200 mg. *Tablets*, etodolac 200 mg.

Proprietary Names and Manufacturers

Lodine *(Ayerst, UK)*; Ramodar *(Wyeth, UK)*.

2644-x

Etofenamate *(BAN, USAN, rINN).*

B-577; TV-485. 2-(2-Hydroxyethoxy)ethyl *N*-(ααα-trifluoro-*m*-tolyl)anthranilate.

$C_{18}H_{18}F_3NO_4$=369.3.

CAS — 30544-47-9.

Etofenamate has analgesic and anti-inflammatory properties. It is applied topically as a 5% gel or 10% cream for the relief of rheumatic and muscular pain.

Proprietary Names and Manufacturers

Afrolate *(Lafarquim, Spain)*; Bayrogel *(Bayropharm, Ital.)*; Flogoprofen *(Wasserman, Spain)*; Rheumon *(Tropon, Ger.*; *Bayer, Switz.)*; Zenavan *(Orfi, Spain)*.

2645-r

Famprofazone *(BAN, rINN).*

4-Isopropyl-2-methyl-3-[methyl(α-methylphenethyl)aminomethyl]-1-phenyl-3-pyrazolin-5-one.

$C_{24}H_{31}N_3O$=377.5.

CAS — 22881-35-2.

Famprofazone has analgesic and antipyretic properties and is claimed to have mild sympathomimetic properties. It has been used in doses of 25 to 50 mg up to three times daily by mouth, usually in conjunction with other analgesics.

Proprietary Names and Manufacturers

The following names have been used for multi-ingredient preparations containing famprofazone— Gewodin *(Gewo, Ger.)*.

3844-y

Feclobuzone *(rINN).*

AE-9. 4-Chlorobenzoic acid ester with 4-butyl-4(hydroxymethyl)-1,2-diphenyl-3,5-pyrazolidinedione.

$C_{27}H_{25}ClN_2O_4$=477.0.

CAS — 23111-34-4.

Feclobuzone is a non-steroidal anti-inflammatory agent that has been used in rheumatic disorders in doses of 200 mg one to three times daily by mouth.

Proprietary Names and Manufacturers

Rocador, Spain.

2646-f

Fenbufen *(BAN, USAN, rINN).*

CL-82204. 4-(Biphenyl-4-yl)-4-oxobutyric acid.

$C_{16}H_{14}O_3$=254.3.

CAS — 36330-85-5.

Adverse Effects and Precautions

The commonest side-effects of fenbufen are skin rashes with disorders such as erythema multiforme being reported. Other side-effects include gastro-intestinal disturbances and transient increases in values of liver function tests.

Fenbufen should be used with caution in patients with peptic ulceration.

Concomitant administration of fenbufen and aspirin may result in decreased serum concentrations of fenbufen and its metabolites.

EFFECTS ON THE GASTRO-INTESTINAL TRACT. Data suggesting that the incidence of peptic ulceration in patients receiving long-term fenbufen therapy is comparable to the background incidence for the population as a whole.— P. M. Cohen, *J. int. med. Res.*, 1986, *14*, 67.

EFFECTS ON THE LUNGS. Paratracheal and hilar lymphadenopathy together with pulmonary infiltration in a patient, believed to have been associated with the use of fenbufen.— C. R. Swinburn (letter), *Br. med. J.*, 1987, *294*, 375.

EFFECTS ON MENTAL STATE. Visual hallucinations with fenbufen.— D. E. Morris and R. L. Hardway, *Br. med. J.*, 1985, *290*, 822.

EFFECTS ON THE SKIN. The *UK* Committee on Safety of Medicines was still receiving large numbers of reports of adverse reactions to fenbufen when such reports were expected to have declined (*Current Problems, No. 23*, 1988). Fenbufen was the most commonly reported suspect drug on yellow cards in 1986 and 1987. More than 6000 such reports have been received, 80% concerning mucocutaneous reactions and most involving a generalised florid erythematous rash, often with pruritus. There were 178 reports of erythema multiforme, 30 of Stevens Johnson syndrome, and 2 fatalities.

Absorption and Fate

Fenbufen is absorbed from the gastro-intestinal tract. Fenbufen is strongly bound to plasma proteins. It is metabolised to active metabolites which are reported to have half-lives of 10 hours or more; further metabolism then occurs converting them to inactive compounds before excretion in the urine.

Some references to the pharmacokinetics of fenbufen: G. E. Van Lear *et al.*, *J. pharm. Sci.*, 1978, *67*, 1662; G. Cuisinaud *et al.*, *Eur. J. clin. Pharmac.*, 1979, *16*, 59; H. J. Rogers *et al.*, *Clin. Pharmac. Ther.*, 1981, *29*, 74; R. K. Verbeeck and S. M. Wallace (letter), *Eur. J. clin. Pharmac.*, 1983, *24*, 137.

Uses and Administration

Fenbufen has analgesic, anti-inflammatory, and antipyretic properties. It is used in rheumatic disorders such as rheumatoid arthritis and osteoarthrosis in doses of 900 mg daily by mouth; the dose may be either 450 mg in the morning and evening or 300 mg in the morning with 600 mg in the evening.

It is stated that a dosage modification in mild to moderate renal impairment is unnecessary since the pharmacokinetics of fenbufen are not altered significantly in the presence of renal insufficiency.

Reviews of fenbufen: R. N. Brogden *et al.*, *Drugs*, 1981, *21*, 1.

OSTEOARTHRITIS. Some references to fenbufen in osteoarthritis: R. Buxton *et al.*, *Curr. med. Res. Opinion*, 1978, *5*, 682; E. J. Valtonen, *Scand. J. Rheumatol.*, 1979, *Suppl.* 27, 1.

RHEUMATOID ARTHRITIS. Some references to fenbufen in rheumatoid arthritis: I. de Salcedo *et al.*, *Curr. ther. Res.*, 1975, *18*, 295; F. Chalem *et al.*, *ibid.*, 1977, *22*, 769; F. Ammitzbøll, *Scand. J. Rheumatol.*, 1979, *Suppl.* 23, 5 and 11; S. D. Deodhar and R. Sethi, *Curr. med. Res. Opinion*, 1979, *6*, 263; W. D. V. Burton and B. L. Hazleman, *Clin. Ther.*, 1983, *5*, 260; F. M. Khan, *ibid.*, 483; A. R. Khaled and N. P. Zissis, *Curr. ther. Res.*, 1986, *39*, 647.

Proprietary Preparations

Lederfen *(Lederle, UK)*. *Capsules*, fenbufen 300 mg. *Tablets*, fenbufen 300 and 450 mg.
Tablets (Lederfen F), effervescent, fenbufen 450 mg.

Proprietary Names and Manufacturers

Bufemid *(Braz.)*; Cincopal *(Cyanamid, Spain)*; Cinopal *(Lederle, Fr.*; *Cyanamid, Ital.*; *Lederle, S.Afr.*; *Lederle, Switz.)*; Lederfen *(Cyanamid-Lederle, Ger.*; *Lederle, UK)*.

12732-y

Fenbutamidol

An equimolecular combination of phenyramidol and oxyphenbutazone.

$C_{32}H_{34}N_4O_4$=538.6.

CAS — 25146-18-3.

Fenbutamidol has anti-inflammatory properties. It has been given by mouth and also applied topically.

Proprietary Names and Manufacturers

Febutolo *(ISM, Ital.)*.

2647-d

Fenclofenac *(BAN, USAN, rINN).*

RX-67408. [2-(2,4-Dichlorophenoxy)phenyl]acetic acid.

$C_{14}H_{10}Cl_2O_3$=297.1.

CAS — 34645-84-6.

Adverse Effects

Fenclofenac has been associated with adverse skin reactions, gastro-intestinal disturbances, and impaired hepatic and renal function.

In an open multicentre study 636 unwanted effects were reported by 229 out of 412 patients. Only 79 patients were withdrawn because of adverse effects and 13 of these subsequently took fenclofenac without further adverse effects. Side-effects were mainly gastro-intestinal disturbances (28.8%), central nervous system effects (27%), and dermatological effects (14.3%). Keratoconjunctivitis sicca and oedema of the legs were reported in a number of patients. Treatment was withdrawn in 4 patients with increased serum aminotransferases, 4 with increased blood-urea-nitrogen, and 1 with decreased platelet count.— R. B. Smith, *Proc. R. Soc. Med.*, 1977, *70*, *Suppl.* 6, 46.

EFFECTS ON THE KIDNEYS. A report of nephrotic syndrome in a patient taking fenclofenac.— D. V. Hamilton *et al.* (letter), *Br. med. J.*, 1979, *2*, 391.

Allergic interstitial nephritis associated with fenclofenac occurring again following inadvertent re-challenge.— M. J. Raftery *et al.*, *Br. med. J.*, 1985, *290*, 1178.

Absorption and Fate

Fenclofenac is absorbed from the gastro-intestinal tract with peak plasma concentrations occurring 2 to 4 hours after ingestion of a single dose. It is metabolised by hydroxylation and conjugation. It is about 96% bound to plasma proteins.

Uses and Administration

Fenclofenac has analgesic, anti-inflammatory, and antipyretic properties. It was formerly used in rheumatic disorders in doses of up to 1.2 g daily by mouth.

Proprietary Names and Manufacturers

Feclan; Flenac *(S.Afr.*; *Reckitt & Colman Pharmaceuticals, UK)*; Gidalon.

12737-a

Fenclozic Acid *(BAN, rINN).*

ICI-54450. [2-(4-Chlorophenyl)thiazol-4-yl]acetic acid.

$C_{11}H_8ClNO_2S$=253.7.

CAS — 17969-20-9.

Fenclozic acid has analgesic and anti-inflammatory properties. It was, however, withdrawn from study because of hepatotoxicity.

2648-n

Fendosal *(BAN, USAN, rINN).*
HP-129; P710129. 5-(4,5-Dihydro-2-phenyl-3*H*-benz[*e*]-indol-3-yl)salicylic acid.
$C_{25}H_{19}NO_3$=381.4.

CAS — 53597-27-6.

Fendosal has analgesic and anti-inflammatory properties. It has been studied as an analgesic in doses of 200 to 400 mg by mouth.

Some references to the use of fendosal as an analgesic: S. M. Bloomfield *et al., Clin. Pharmac. Ther.*, 1978, *23*, 390 (postpartum pain); S. A. Cooper *et al., ibid.*, 1980, *27*, 249 (postoperative pain); R. Okun, *Curr. ther. Res.*, 1982, *32*, 65 (postpartum pain); P. J. Desjardins *et al., Pharmacotherapy*, 1983, *3*, 52 (postoperative dental pain); J. A. Forbes *et al., ibid.*, 1984, *4*, 385 (postoperative dental pain).

Proprietary Names and Manufacturers
Alnovin *(Hoechst, USA).*

2649-h

Fenoprofen Calcium *(BANM, USAN, pINNM).*

53858 *(acid)*; 69323; Lilly-61169 *(sodium salt).*
Calcium (±)-2-(3-phenoxyphenyl)propionate dihydrate.
$(C_{15}H_{13}O_3)_2Ca,2H_2O$=558.6.

CAS — 31879-05-7 (fenoprofen); 34597-40-5 (calcium salt, anhydrous); 53746-45-5 (calcium salt, dihydrate).

Pharmacopoeias. In *Br.* and *U.S.*

A white or almost white odourless or almost odourless crystalline powder. Fenoprofen calcium (dihydrate) 1.1 g is approximately equivalent to 1 g of fenoprofen. Slightly **soluble** in water and chloroform; soluble 1 in 15 of alcohol. **Store** in airtight containers.

Adverse Effects

As for ibuprofen, p.20. The Stevens-Johnson syndrome (erythema multiforme) has been reported.

EFFECTS ON THE BLOOD. *Agranulocytosis.* Agranulocytosis occurred in a 55-year-old man who had started treatment with fenoprofen 8 weeks previously.— S. D. Simon and M. Kosmin (letter), *New Engl. J. Med.*, 1978, *299*, 490.

A report of pruritus and exfoliative rash following treatment with fenoprofen calcium in 1 patient, and associated with agranulocytosis.— P. J. Treusch *et al.* (letter), *J. Am. med. Ass.*, 1979, *241*, 2700.

Aplastic anaemia. Two cases, one a fatality, of aplastic anaemia associated with fenoprofen.— M. Ashraf *et al., Br. med. J.*, 1982, *284*, 1301.

Thrombocytopenia. Reports of thrombocytopenia associated with fenoprofen.— R. E. Simpson *et al.* (letter), *New Engl. J. Med.*, 1978, *298*, 629; M. E. Katz and P. Wang (letter), *Ann. intern. Med.*, 1980, *92*, 262.

EFFECTS ON THE KIDNEYS. Fenoprofen reduced renal function in 1 patient with systemic lupus erythematosus.— R. P. Kimberly *et al., Am. J. Med.*, 1978, *64*, 804. Severe renal papillary necrosis was associated with administration of fenoprofen calcium (total dose 36 g in 30 days), in a patient with systemic lupus erythematosus and urinary-tract infection.— F. E. Husserl *et al., J. Am. med. Ass.*, 1979, *242*, 1896.

Reversible renal failure and nephrotic syndrome developed in 2 patients who had been taking fenoprofen 1.8 to 2.4 g daily for up to a year. Renal biopsy in one patient revealed prominent interstitial nephritis.— J. H. Brezin *et al., New Engl. J. Med.*, 1979, *301*, 1271.

Further reports of reversible renal failure associated with fenoprofen: G. A. Curt *et al., Ann. intern. Med.*, 1980, *92*, 72; S. P. Handa (letter), *ibid.*, *93*, 508; J. Lorch *et al.* (letter), *ibid.*, 508; S. P. Handa, *Can. med. Ass. J.*, 1986, *135*, 1278.

EFFECTS ON THE LIVER. Cholestatic jaundice and hepatitis developed in a 68-year-old woman after treatment with fenoprofen 600 mg four times daily for 7 weeks.— D. J. Stennett *et al.* (letter), *Am. J. Hosp. Pharm.*, 1978, *35*, 901.

Cross hepatotoxicity between fenoprofen and naproxen in one patient.— M. Andrejak *et al., Br. med. J.*, 1987, *295*, 180.

OVERDOSAGE. A brief review of poisoning after fenoprofen overdosage with the comment that supportive therapy appears to be adequate and that the value of forced diuresis has not been established.— H. Court and G. N. Volans, *Adverse Drug React. Ac. Pois. Rev.*, 1984, *3*, 1.

Precautions

As for ibuprofen, p.20. Aspirin is reported to reduce plasma concentrations of fenoprofen.

INTERACTIONS. *Barbiturates.* Investigations in 18 subjects demonstrated that the administration of phenobarbitone might increase the rate of metabolism of fenoprofen.— L. Helleberg *et al., Br. J. clin. Pharmac.*, 1974, *1*, 371.

INTERFERENCE WITH DIAGNOSTIC TESTS. Reports of fenoprofen or flurbiprofen (but not ibuprofen) causing erroneously raised concentrations of tri-iodothyronine in certain thyroid function tests.— J. R. Gurney and R. J. Mills, *Br. med. J.*, 1986, *292*, 1560; J. Tillman *et al.* (letter), *ibid.*, *293*, 206; H. M. Thornes and D. Carr (letter), *Lancet*, 1986, *2*, 101.

Absorption and Fate

Fenoprofen is readily absorbed from the gastro-intestinal tract; peak plasma concentrations occur 1 to 2 hours after a dose; the half-life is about 3 hours. It is more than 99% bound to plasma proteins. About 90% of a dose is excreted in the urine in 24 hours, chiefly as the glucuronide and the glucuronide of hydroxylated fenoprofen. It has been detected in breast milk. Small amounts (about 2%) are excreted in the faeces.

Uses and Administration

Fenoprofen calcium has analgesic, anti-inflammatory, and antipyretic properties; it is an inhibitor of prostaglandin synthetase. It is used in the treatment of mild to moderate pain and in rheumatic disorders such as ankylosing spondylitis, osteoarthritis, and rheumatoid arthritis. The usual dose for pain is the equivalent of 200 mg of fenoprofen three or four times daily by mouth; doses of up to 600 mg may be given if necessary. In rheumatic disorders the usual dose is the equivalent of 300 to 600 mg of fenoprofen three or four times daily. It has been recommended that the total daily dose should not exceed 3 to 3.2 g.

A favourable report of the use of fenoprofen as an analgesic and antipyretic in patients with common non-bacterial upper-respiratory-tract infections.— P. B. Ryan *et al., Curr. ther. Res.*, 1987, *41*, 17.

OSTEOARTHRITIS. Some references to the use of fenoprofen in osteoarthrosis: J. A. Wojtulewski *et al., Br. med. J.*, 1974, *2*, 475; J. W. Brooke, *J. Rheumatol.*, 1976, *3*, *Suppl.* 2, 71; *idem, Curr. ther. Res.*, 1978, *23*, 538; W. Standel, *Clin. Trials J.*, 1978, *15*, 24; M. Thompson *et al., Curr. ther. Res.*, 1979, *26*, 779; R. A. Durance *et al., ibid.*, 791; D. J. Levinson and H. M. Rubinstein, *ibid.*, 1983, *34*, 280.

RHEUMATOID ARTHRITIS. Some references to the use of fenoprofen in rheumatoid arthritis: J. F. Fries and M. C. Britton, *Arthritis Rheum.*, 1973, *16*, 629; E. C. Huskisson *et al., Br. med. J.*, 1974, *1*, 176; M. Franke and G. Manz, *Curr. ther. Res.*, 1977, *21*, 43; J. D. Davis *et al., Clin. Pharmac. Ther.*, 1977, *21*, 52; J. E. Himes and I. F. Duff, *J. int. med. Res.*, 1977, *5*, 412; E. Semble *et al., Clin. Pharmac. Ther.*, 1980, *27*, 286.

Preparations

Fenoprofen Calcium Capsules *(U.S.P.).* Potency is expressed in terms of the equivalent amount of fenoprofen.

Fenoprofen Tablets *(B.P.).* Fenoprofen Calcium Tablets

Fenoprofen Calcium Tablets *(U.S.P.).* Potency is expressed in terms of the equivalent amount of fenoprofen.

Proprietary Preparations

Fenopron *(Dista, UK). Tablets*, fenoprofen 300 mg (as fenoprofen calcium).
Tablets, scored, fenoprofen 600 mg (as fenoprofen calcium).

Progesic *(Lilly, UK). Tablets*, fenoprofen 200 mg (as fenoprofen calcium).

Proprietary Names and Manufacturers

Fenopron *(Dista, Austral.; Dista, S.Afr.; Dista, UK)*; Fepron *(Belg.; Lilly, Ital.; Neth.)*; Feprona *(Lilly, Ger.)*; Nalfon *(Lilly, Canad.; Lilly, Denm.; Lilly, Spain; Switz.; Dista, USA)*; Nalgésic *(Lilly, Fr.)*; Progesic *(Lilly, UK).*

12747-x

Fentiazac *(BAN, USAN, rINN).*
BR-700; Wy-21894. [4-(4-Chlorophenyl)-2-phenylthiazol-5-yl]acetic acid.
$C_{17}H_{12}ClNO_2S$=329.8.

CAS — 18046-21-4.

Fentiazac has analgesic, anti-inflammatory, and antipyretic properties. It has been used in inflammatory and rheumatic disorders in usual doses of up to 200 mg once or twice daily by mouth. It has also been applied topically as a 5% cream.

Some references to fentiazac: J. Siquet, *Clin. Trials J.*, 1983, *20*, 305 (children with upper-respiratory-tract infection and inflammation); B. Bunde *et al., Curr. med. Res. Opinion*, 1983, *8*, 310 (rheumatoid arthritis); J. P. Famaey *et al., ibid.*, 675 (osteoarthritis); A. Schaerli and K. Bruelhart, *Curr. ther. Res.*, 1983, *34*, 285 (postoperative inflammation in children); V. D'Apuzzo and D. Zambelli, *ibid.*, 818 (postoperative inflammation in children); A. Catti, *J. int. med. Res.*, 1983, *11*, 298 (inflammatory disorders in children); F. Ginsberg and J. P. Famaey, *Curr. med. Res. Opinion*, 1985, *9*, 442 (tendinitis or bursitis).

Proprietary Names and Manufacturers
Domureuma *(Medici Domus, Ital.)*; Donorest *(Orfi, Spain)*; Fentac *(Sarget, Fr.)*; Flogene *(Polifarma, Ital.)*; Norvedan *(LPB, Ital.)*; Ragilon *(Beta, Arg.)*; Riscalon *(Boehringer Mannheim, Spain).*

2650-a

Feprazone *(BAN, rINN).*
DA-2370; Phenylprenazone; Prenazone. 4-(3-Methylbut-2-enyl)-1,2-diphenylpyrazolidine-3,5-dione.
$C_{20}H_{20}N_2O_2$=320.4.

CAS — 30748-29-9.

Adverse Effects
Gastro-intestinal disturbances, rashes, jaundice, nephropathy, blood disorders, oedema, headache, and tinnitus have been reported.

EFFECTS ON THE BLOOD. Thrombocytopenia and haemolytic anaemia associated with feprazone.— P. M. Bell and C. A. Humphrey, *Br. med. J.*, 1982, *284*, 17.

OVERDOSAGE. Some short comments on reports of poisonings following overdosage of feprazone.— H. Court and G. N. Volans, *Adverse Drug React. Ac. Pois. Rev.*, 1984, *3*, 1.

Precautions
Feprazone should be used with caution in patients with cardiac, hepatic, or renal insufficiency, in those with blood disorders, or in those with peptic ulceration or similar gastro-intestinal disorders. It has been stated that feprazone may potentiate the activity of oral anticoagulants, oral hypoglycaemics, methotrexate, and phenytoin.

Absorption and Fate
Feprazone is absorbed from the gastro-intestinal tract with peak plasma concentrations occurring 4 to 6 hours after ingestion. It has a plasma half-life of about 24 hours.

Uses and Administration
Feprazone has analgesic, anti-inflammatory, and antipyretic properties. It has been used in rheumatic disorders in initial doses of up to 600 mg daily in divided doses by mouth; maintenance doses of up to 400 mg daily have been given. Feprazone has also been used topically as an ointment containing 5%.

Proprietary Names and Manufacturers
Analud *(Arg.)*; Brotazona *(Escaned, Spain)*; Cocresol *(Areu, Spain)*; Danfenona *(Spain)*; Grisona *(Spain)*; Impremial *(Zambon, Spain)*; Methrazone *(WB Pharmaceuticals, UK: Boehringer Ingelheim, UK)*; Naloven *(Cruz, Spain)*; Nessazona *(Nessa, Spain)*; Nilatin *(Spain)*; Prenakes *(Albofarma, Spain)*; Prenazon *(Inexfa, Spain)*; Rangozona *(Mazuelos, Spain)*; Represil *(Llorens, Spain)*; Tabrien *(Spain)*; Zepelin *(De Angeli, Ital.; Switz.).*

2651-t

Floctafenine *(BAN, USAN, rINN).*
R-4318; RU-15750. 2,3-Dihydroxypropyl *N*-(8-trifluoromethyl-4-quinolyl)anthranilate.
$C_{20}H_{17}F_3N_2O_4$=406.4.
CAS — 23779-99-9.

Adverse Effects
Gastro-intestinal disturbances, dizziness, drowsiness, headache, dysuria, allergic reactions, and occasionally tinnitus have been reported with floctafenine.

Six of 16 healthy subjects taking floctafenine complained of 'hot urine' during early morning urination.— I. M. Baird (letter), *Br. J. clin. Pharmac.*, 1976, *3*, 936.

Absorption and Fate
Floctafenine is absorbed from the gastro-intestinal tract. It is metabolised in the liver to floctafenic acid. It is excreted mainly as glucuronide conjugates in the urine and bile.

Studies on the metabolism and excretion of floctafenine: J. Pottier *et al.*, *Drug Metab. & Disposit.*, 1975, *3*, 133; R. K. Lynn *et al.*, *J. clin. Pharmac.*, 1979, *19*, 20.

Uses and Administration
Floctafenine has analgesic properties. It is used in doses of up to 1.2 g daily, in divided doses, by mouth.

A study in 1 subject suggested that floctafenic acid was responsible for the analgesic activity of floctafenine.— N. Gerber *et al.*, *Fedn Proc.*, 1976, *35*, 565.

Some references to the use of floctafenine as an analgesic: S. Lipton *et al.*, *Curr. med. Res. Opinion*, 1975, *3*, 175 (postoperative pain); S. Lipton *et al.*, *Br. J. clin. Pract.*, 1975, *29*, 147 (postoperative pain); J. K. Stenport, *Curr. ther. Res.*, 1975, *18*, 303 (postoperative pain); S. Lipton *et al.*, *J. int. med. Res.*, 1975, *3*, 172 (postoperative pain); J. E. G. Walker and L. W. Kay, *Br. J. clin. Pract.*, 1976, *30*, 43 (postoperative pain); M. A. Hossain *et al.*, *Rheumatol. Rehabil.*, 1977, *16*, 260 (rheumatoid arthritis); M. E. Morris and I. W. D. Henderson, *Clin. Pharmac. Ther.*, 1978, *23*, 383 (postoperative pain); V. M. Rhind *et al.*, *J. int. med. Res.*, 1978, *6*, 11 (osteoarthritis).

Proprietary Names and Manufacturers
Idalon *(Roussel, Neth.)*; Idarac *(Roussel, Arg.; Houde, Belg.; Winthrop, Canad.; Diamant, Fr.; Albert-Roussel, Ger.; Roussel Maestretti, Ital.; Roussel, S.Afr.; Roussel, Spain).*

2652-x

Flufenamic Acid *(BAN, USAN, rINN).*
CI-440; INF-1837. *N*-(ααα-Trifluoro-*m*-tolyl)anthranilic acid.
$C_{14}H_{10}F_3NO_2$=281.2.
CAS — 530-78-9.

Adverse Effects
The commonest side-effects occurring with flufenamic acid are gastro-intestinal disturbances. Skin rash, depression, vertigo, tinnitus, leucopenia, and increased values for serum aminotransferases have occasionally been reported.

EFFECTS ON THE GASTRO-INTESTINAL TRACT. Acute proctocolitis associated with flufenamic acid.— S. Ravi *et al.*, *Postgrad. med. J.*, 1986, *62*, 773.

Precautions
As for mefenamic acid, p.27.

PORPHYRIA. Flufenamic acid was considered to be unsafe in patients with acute porphyria as it has been associated with acute attacks.— M.R. Moore and K.E.L. McColl, *Porphyrias, Drug Lists*, Glasgow, Porphyria Research Unit, University of Glasgow, 1987.

Absorption and Fate
Flufenamic acid is absorbed from the gastro-intestinal tract and peak plasma concentrations occur about two hours following ingestion. It is extensively bound to plasma proteins. It is metabolised by hydroxylation and conjugation and excreted in the urine and the faeces. It is excreted in bile and enterohepatic circulation has been suggested.

PREGNANCY AND THE NEONATE. A study in 10 nursing mothers and their infants, in the immediate post-partum period, indicated that only very small amounts of flufenamic acid were excreted into the breast milk and absorbed by the infant.— R. A. Buchanan *et al.*, *Curr. ther. Res.*, 1969, *11*, 533.

Uses and Administration
Flufenamic acid has analgesic, anti-inflammatory, and antipyretic properties. It is used in rheumatic disorders in usual doses of 400 to 600 mg daily by mouth in divided doses.

Proprietary Names and Manufacturers
Alfenamin *(Arg.)*; Ansatin *(Jpn)*; Arlef *(Parke, Davis, Austral.; Belg.; Fr.; Ger.; Ital.; Parke, Davis, S.Afr.; Switz.; Parke, Davis, UK)*; Meralen *(Merrell, UK)*; Parlef *(Arg.)*; Sastridex *(Lindopharm, Ger.)*; Surika *(Ger.).*

12760-k

Flunixin *(BAN, USAN, rINN).*
Sch-14714. 2-(2-Methyl-3-trifluoromethylanilino)nicotinic acid; 2-($\alpha^3,\alpha^3,\alpha^3$-Trifluoro-2,3-xylidino)nicotinic acid.
$C_{14}H_{11}F_3N_2O_2$=296.2.
CAS — 38677-85-9.

Flunixin has analgesic, anti-inflammatory, and antipyretic properties. It is used as the meglumine salt in veterinary medicine.

Proprietary Veterinary Names and Manufacturers
Finadyne *(Fisons, UK).*

16812-f

Flunoxaprofene *(rINN).*
Flunoxaprofen; RV-12424. (+)-2-(*p*-Fluorophenyl)-α-methyl-5-benzoxazoleacetic acid.
$C_{16}H_{12}FNO_3$=285.3.
CAS — 66934-18-7.

Flunoxaprofene has anti-inflammatory properties and has been given in rheumatic conditions in doses of 50 to 100 mg once or twice daily by mouth.

Some references to flunoxaprofene: F. Pupita *et al.*, *Curr. ther. Res.*, 1985, *37*, 70 (use in osteoarthritis); A. Forgione *et al.*, *ibid.*, 77 (use in osteoarthritis and effect on renal function); G. Quaglia *et al.*, *ibid.*, 1986, *39*, 66 (tolerability and pharmacokinetics); M. Testa *et al.*, *ibid.*, 1987, *42*, 182 (use for cataracts).

Proprietary Names and Manufacturers
Priaxim *(Ravizza, Ital.).*

18644-z

Flupirtine Maleate *(BANM, USAN, rINNM).*
D-9998; W-2964M. Ethyl 2-amino-6-(4-fluorobenzylamino)-3-pyridylcarbamate maleate.
$C_{15}H_{17}FN_4O_2.C_4H_4O_4$=420.4.
CAS — 75507-68-5.

Flupirtine maleate is an analgesic that has been given in usual doses of 100 mg three or four times daily by mouth; doses of up to 600 mg daily have been used where necessary.

Some references to flupirtine: *Arzneimittel-Forsch.*, 1985, *35*, 30-77; *Postgrad. med. J.*, 1987, *63*, *Suppl.* 3, 1-113.

Proprietary Names and Manufacturers
Katadolon *(Degussa, Ger.).*

12765-f

Fluproquazone *(BAN, USAN, rINN).*
46-790; RF-46-790; RF-46-790-n. 4-(4-Fluorophenyl)-1-isopropyl-7-methylquinazolin-2(1*H*)-one.
$C_{18}H_{17}FN_2O$=296.3.
CAS — 40507-23-1.

Fluproquazone is reported to have analgesic and anti-inflammatory properties.

Some references to fluproquazone: B. Von Graffenried and E. Nüesch, *Curr. ther. Res.*, 1979, *26*, 275; B. Maeglin *et al.*, *ibid.*, 284; U. Herrmann *et al.*, *Clin. Pharmac. Ther.*, 1980, *27*, 379; *Arzneimittel-Forsch.*, 1981, *31*, 871–940.

Proprietary Names and Manufacturers
Tormosyl *(Sandoz, Switz.).*

2653-r

Flurbiprofen *(BAN, USAN, rINN).*
2-(2-Fluorobiphenyl-4-yl)propionic acid.
$C_{15}H_{13}FO_2$=244.3.
CAS — 5104-49-4.
Pharmacopoeias. In *Br.*

A white or almost white crystalline powder. Practically **insoluble** in water; soluble 1 in 3 of alcohol, 1 in 4 of chloroform, and 1 in 4.5 of ether.

Adverse Effects
As for ibuprofen, p.20.

In 354 patients who had been treated in various centres with flurbiprofen, 83 had gastro-intestinal side-effects, 10 had dermatological side-effects, and 21 had side-effects affecting the CNS. There were 2 reports of thrombocytopenia and 1 of neutropenia; these were of uncertain significance.— J. W. Buckler *et al.*, XIII International Congress of Rheumatology, Japan, 1973, p. 181.

In a long-term study in 1220 patients with rheumatic disorders treated with flurbiprofen, side-effects reported were gastro-intestinal (452), central nervous system (198), skin (75), renal (43), haematological (29), respiratory (45), cardiovascular (28), and miscellaneous (46). Some patients had also received additional drugs. There were no alterations in haematological and biochemical investigations.— F. E. Sheldrake *et al.*, *Curr. med. Res. Opinion*, 1977, *5*, 106.

EFFECTS ON THE LIVER. A report of cholestatic jaundice probably due to flurbiprofen.— K. E. Kotowski and M. F. Grayson (letter), *Br. med. J.*, 1982, *285*, 377.

Precautions
As for ibuprofen, p.20.

INTERACTIONS. For the effect of flurbiprofen on some other drugs see under propranolol (p.802) and warfarin (p.345 for nicoumalone and phenprocoumon).

INTERFERENCE WITH DIAGNOSTIC TESTS. For reference to flurbiprofen interfering with thyroid function tests, see under fenoprofen calcium, p.17.

Absorption and Fate
Flurbiprofen is readily absorbed from the gastro-intestinal tract with peak plasma concentrations occurring about 90 minutes after ingestion. It is reported to be about 99% bound to plasma proteins and to have an elimination half-life of about 3 to 4 hours. It is metabolised mainly by hydroxylation and conjugation and excreted in urine.

In 19 fasting volunteers given flurbiprofen 50 mg mean peak concentrations of about 5.5 µg per mL were achieved in about 1½ hours; the half-life was about 3.9 hours. It was extensively bound (99%) to plasma proteins. Three hydroxylated or methoxylated metabolites were found in the urine. More than 95% of a dose was recovered in the urine in 24 hours including glucuronides of the metabolites.— S. S. Adams *et al.*, XIII International Congress of Rheumatology, Japan, 1973, p. 173.

Further references: N. Cardoe *et al.*, *Curr. med. Res. Opinion*, 1977, *5*, 21; S. Wanwimolruk *et al.*, *Br. J. clin. Pharmac.*, 1983, *15*, 91; C. Scaroni *et al.*, *Eur. J. clin. Pharmac.*, 1984, *27*, 367; L. Aarons *et al.*, *Br. J. clin. Pharmac.*, 1986, *21*, 155.

Uses and Administration
Flurbiprofen has analgesic, anti-inflammatory, and antipyretic properties; it is an inhibitor of prostaglandin synthetase.

Flurbiprofen is used in rheumatic disorders such as ankylosing spondylitis, osteoarthritis, and rheumatoid arthritis in usual doses of 150 to 200 mg daily by mouth in divided doses, increased to 300 mg daily in acute conditions if necessary.

Flurbiprofen is also used in the form of the sodium salt as 0.03% eye-drops to inhibit intraoperative miosis during ocular surgery. One drop is instilled into the eye every 30 minutes beginning 2 hours before surgery. Such eye-drops should not be used in patients with epithelial herpes simplex keratitis.

Reviews on the actions and uses of flurbiprofen: R. N. Brogden *et al.*, *Drugs*, 1979, *18*, 417.

Symposiums on flurbiprofen.— XIII International Congress of Rheumatology, Japan, 1973, pp. 137–187; *Curr. med. Res. Opinion*, 1975, *3*, *Suppl.* 4, 1–52; *ibid.*, 1977, *5*, 1–140.

ADMINISTRATION. A study in 30 patients with ankylosing spondylitis or coxarthrosis showed that twice daily dosage with flurbiprofen was as effective as three times daily dosage.— P. Doury and S. Pattin, *Curr. med. Res. Opinion*, 1977, *5*, 127.

A study involving patients with rheumatoid arthritis indicating the most effective therapeutic schedule for flurbiprofen given twice daily was giving the doses at the beginning and end of overnight sleep.— R. Pownall and N. J. Pickvance, *Br. J. clin. Pract.*, 1987, *41*, 689.

ANKYLOSING SPONDYLITIS. Some references to the use of flurbiprofen in ankylosing spondylitis: A. Calin and R. Grahame, *Br. med. J.*, 1974, *4*, 496; R. D. Sturrock and F. D. Hart, *Ann. rheum. Dis.*, 1974, *33*, 129; F. D. Hart, *Curr. med. Res. Opinion*, 1975, *3*, *Suppl.* 4, 39; R. Grahame and A. Calin, *Scand. J. Rheumatol.*, 1975, *4*, *Suppl.* 8, S11–22; F. D. Hart, *ibid*; A. Good and H. Mena, *Curr. med. Res. Opinion*, 1977, *5*, 117; H. R. Mena and R. F. Willkens, *Eur. J. clin. Pharmac.*, 1977, *11*, 263; P. L. Lomen *et al.*, *Am. J. Med.*, 1986, *80*, *Suppl.* 3A, 127.

BLOOD DISORDERS. Spontaneous platelet aggregation in a patient with polycythaemia rubra vera was unresponsive to aspirin but readily responsive to flurbiprofen.— C. Politis-Tsegos *et al.*, *Br. med. J.*, 1978, *1*, 1323.

HYPERCALCAEMIA. Hypercalcaemia in a patient with sarcoidosis was successfully treated on 2 occasions with flurbiprofen.— T. Littlewood *et al.*, *Br. med. J.*, 1983, *287*, 1762. See also R. C. Brown *et al.* (letter), *Lancet*, 1984, *2*, 37.

HYPOTENSION. Addition of flurbiprofen 50 mg twice daily to fludrocortisone therapy relieved the symptoms of an 18-year-old girl with idiopathic orthostatic hypotension, who had not responded to fludrocortisone 400 µg daily alone.— C. M. Perkins and M. R. Lee (letter), *Lancet*, 1978, *2*, 1058. Similar effects were observed in 5 patients, 4 of whom were also taking fludrocortisone.— S. J. Watt *et al.*, *Clin. Sci.*, 1980, *59*, (Sept.), 4P.

OCULAR SURGERY. A short review of the use of flurbiprofen sodium eye-drops for the inhibition of intra-operative miosis.— *Med. Lett.*, 1987, *29*, 58.

The use of eye-drops containing flurbiprofen 0.03% in addition to routine pre-operative mydriatic therapy resulted in less miosis in a group of 16 patients undergoing extracapsular cataract extraction than the use of placebo plus routine therapy in a similar group of 18 control patients. It was suggested that such prostaglandin synthesis inhibiting drugs may have a role in facilitating intra-ocular surgery by maintaining pupillary dilatation and lessening intra-operative complications.— R. H. Keates and K. A. McGowan, *Ann. Ophthal.*, 1984, *16*, 919.

A beneficial effect of flurbiprofen sodium 0.03% eye-drops for the control of ocular inflammation in patients with primary open-angle glaucoma treated with laser trabeculoplasty. Although the postoperative inflammation was well controlled in a high percentage of patients, flurbiprofen did not prevent an increase in postoperative intra-ocular pressure. It was considered that the study had provided a stimulus for the continued investigation of non-steroidal anti-inflammatory agents as an adjunct to ocular surgery.— R. N. Weinreb *et al.*, *Archs Ophthal., N.Y.*, 1984, *102*, 1629.

A study involving 20 patients undergoing cataract extraction and given flurbiprofen 100 mg twice daily by mouth for 10 days postoperatively suggested that flurbiprofen reduces the inflammatory response in the eye in the first few days after surgery and may therefore reduce the risk of severe and potentially disastrous reactions which sometimes occur.— D. W. Sabiston and I. G. Robinson, *Br. J. Ophthal.*, 1987, *71*, 418. A similar report.— M. F. Bizzotto *et al.*, *Drugs exp. & clin. Res.*, 1984, *10*, 421.

OSTEOARTHRITIS. Some references to the use of flurbiprofen in osteoarthritis: O. Kogstad, XIII International Congress of Rheumatology, Japan, 1973, p. 156; E. N. Glick and A. A. J. Goldberg, *ibid.*, p. 178; H. R. Mena *et al.*, *J. int. med. Res.*, 1976, *4*, 152; O. Frank, *Curr. med. Res. Opinion*, 1977, *5*, 91; N. Cardoe, *ibid.*, 99; E. C. Huskisson *et al.*, *Eur. J. Rheumatol. Inflamm.*, 1979, *2*, 69; J. P. Famaey and F. Ginsberg, *J. int. med. Res.*, 1983, *11*, 212; M. Bassiouni, *Br. J. clin. Pract.*, 1985, *39*, 393; M. Busson, *J. int. med. Res.*, 1986, *14*, 7.

PAIN. References to the beneficial effect of flurbiprofen in various types of pain: U. R. Krisna *et al.*, *Br. J. clin. Pharmac.*, 1980, *9*, 605 (dysmenorrhoea); R. A. Dionne *et al.*, *Curr. ther. Res.*, 1983, *34*, 15 (preoperative administration for postoperative pain); D. Maclean, *J. int. med. Res.*, 1983, *11*, *Suppl.* 2, 1 (dysmenorrhoea); G. J. Frank and R. H. Kefford, *ibid.*, 6 (dysmenorrhoea).

PERIODONTAL DISEASE. Studies in *dogs* showing that flurbiprofen decreased the resorption of alveolar bone and may have a place in the management of bone loss and periodontal disease.— R. C. Williams *et al.*, *Science*, 1985, *227*, 640.

RHEUMATOID ARTHRITIS. In a long-term study in 1220 patients with rheumatoid arthritis, osteoarthrosis, and other rheumatic disorders, flurbiprofen in doses of 75 to 400 mg daily was effective in relieving symptoms. Some patients had been followed for up to 5 years and some also received other drugs. Side-effects were responsible for withdrawal from the study in 117 patients who received flurbiprofen alone and 123 who received additional drugs.— F. E. Sheldrake *et al.*, *Curr. med. Res. Opinion*, 1977, *5*, 106.

Some further references to the use of flurbiprofen in rheumatoid arthritis: D. R. E. Barraclough *et al.*, *Med. J. Aust.*, 1974, *2*, 925; M. Nobunaga *et al.*, *Curr. med. Res. Opinion*, 1975, *3*, *Suppl.* 4, 45; H. A. Capel *et al.* (letter), *Br. J. clin. Pharmac.*, 1977, *4*, 623; H. R. Mena *et al.*, *J. clin. Pharmac.*, 1977, *17*, 56; *Curr. med. Res. Opinion*, 1977, *5*, 53-90; P. J. Rooney *et al.*, *Br. J. clin. Pharmac.*, 1978, *5*, 453; R. Marcolongo *et al.*, *Curr. ther. Res.*, 1983, *33*, 423; G. Cherie-Ligniere *et al.*, *J. int. med. Res.*, 1983, *11*, 85; M. Broggini *et al.*, *Curr. ther. Res.*, 1986, *40*, 587.

URINARY INCONTINENCE. In a double-blind crossover study in 30 women with detrusor instability flurbiprofen 50 mg three times daily significantly relieved frequency, urgency, and urge incontinence.— L. D. Cardozo *et al.*, *Br. med. J.*, 1980, *280*, 281. A similar report.— J. Palmer, *J. int. med. Res.*, 1983, *11*, *Suppl.* 2, 11.

Preparations

Flurbiprofen Tablets *(B.P.)*

Proprietary Preparations

Froben *(Boots, UK)*. *Capsules*, sustained-release, flurbiprofen 200 mg.
Tablets, flurbiprofen 50 and 100 mg.
Suppositories, flurbiprofen 100 mg.

Proprietary Names and Manufacturers

Ansaid *(Upjohn, Canad.)*; Cebutid *(Boots-Dacour, Fr.)*; Flugalin *(Galenika, Jug.)*; Flurofen *(Boots, Denm.)*; Froben *(Organon, Canad.; Thomae, Ger.; Boots-Formenti, Ital.; Boots, S.Afr.; Liade, Spain; Boots, Switz.; Boots, UK)*; Ocufen *(Allergan, USA)*.

15322-t

Fosfosal *(rINN)*.

UR-1521. 2-Phosphono-oxybenzoic acid.
$C_7H_7O_6P$=218.1.

CAS — 6064-83-1.

Fosfosal has analgesic, antipyretic, and anti-inflammatory properties. It has been given in usual doses of 1.2 g one to three times daily by mouth.

Some references to fosfosal: F. J. F. Tascón *et al.*, *Curr. ther. Res.*, 1987, *42*, 94 (rheumatoid arthritis).

Proprietary Names and Manufacturers
Disdolen *(Uriach, Spain)*.

2654-f

Glafenine *(rINN)*.

Glaphenine. 2,3-Dihydroxypropyl *N*-(7-chloro-4-quinolyl)anthranilate.
$C_{19}H_{17}ClN_2O_4$=372.8.

CAS — 3820-67-5.

Pharmacopoeias. In *Fr.*

Adverse Effects

Side-effects reported include gastro-intestinal disturbances, headache, drowsiness, fever, and renal failure. Allergic reactions may occur.

ALLERGY. Reports of anaphylaxis and other allergic reactions occurring with glafenine.— D. Chivrac *et al.*, *Nouv. Presse méd.*, 1974, *3*, 2578; C. Barral and M. Faivre, *ibid.*, 1975, *4*, 2797; J. L. Michaud and L. Doublet, *ibid.*, 1976, *5*, 716; G. J. A. Burgers *et al.*, *Ned. Tijdschr. Geneesk.*, 1976, *120*, 528; R. H. B. Meyboom, *ibid.*, 926; S. Weber *et al.* (letter), *Lancet*, 1982, *2*, 821.

EFFECTS ON THE KIDNEY. Reports of renal failure and interstitial nephritis often following overdosage with glafenine.— M. Gaultier *et al.*, *Nouv. Presse méd.*, 1972, *1*, 3125; D. Chevet *et al.*, *Thérapie*, 1974, *29*, 575; M. Gaultier *et al.*, *ibid.*, 579; J. Mirouze *et al.*, *ibid.*, 587; H. Duplay *et al.*, *ibid.*, 593; J. C. Renier *et al.*, *Nouv. Presse méd.*, 1975, *4*, 670.

EFFECTS ON THE LIVER. Acute reversible hepatitis in 2 patients after taking therapeutic doses of glafenine.— R. T. J. M. Ypma *et al.* (letter), *Lancet*, 1978, *2*, 480.

Absorption and Fate

Glafenine is absorbed from the gastro-intestinal tract with peak plasma concentrations occurring about 1 to 2 hours after ingestion. The half-life is reported to be about 75 minutes. It is metabolised to glafenic acid and excreted in the urine and bile.

Studies on the absorption, metabolism, and excretion of glafenine.— J. Rondelet *et al.*, *Thérapie*, 1966, *21*, 1573; R. Mallein *et al.*, *ibid.*, 1579; *idem*, 1976, *31*, 739.

Uses and Administration

Glafenine is an anthranilic acid derivative; it is an analgesic that has been used for the relief of all types of pain. For acute pain 400 mg by mouth has been given followed by 200 mg as required up to a total of 1 to 1.2 g daily. For less severe pain the initial dose has been 200 to 400 mg followed by 200-mg doses up to a total of 600 to 800 mg daily. It has also been given, as the hydrochloride, as 500-mg suppositories.

Proprietary Names and Manufacturers

Exidol *(Sopar, Belg.)*; Glifan *(Roussel Maestretti, Ital.)*; Glifanan *(Roussel, Arg.; Roussel, Belg.; Roussel, Fr.; Albert-Roussel, Ger.; Nippon Roussel, Jpn; Roussel, Neth.; Roussel, S.Afr.; Roussel, Spain; Roussel, Switz.)*; Osodent *(Cinfa, Spain)*; Privadol *(Roland-Marie, Fr.)*.

2655-d

Glucametacin *(rINN)*.

2-{2-[1-(4-Chlorobenzoyl)-5-methoxy-2-methylindol-3-yl]acetamido}-2-deoxy-D-glucose monohydrate.
$C_{25}H_{27}ClN_2O_8,H_2O$=537.0.

CAS — 52443-21-7(anhydrous).

Glucametacin has analgesic, anti-inflammatory, and antipyretic properties. It has been used in rheumatic disorders in doses of 280 to 420 mg daily in divided doses by mouth.

References to the use of glucametacin in rheumatic disorders: M. Giordano *et al.*, *Arzneimittel-Forsch.*, 1975, *25*, 435; P. Petera *et al.*, *Int. J. clin. Pharmac. Biopharm.*, 1977, *15*, 581; B. Colombo *et al.*, *Clin. Trials J.*, 1978, *15*, (3), 66; K. Chlud *et al.*, *Arzneimittel-Forsch.*, 1978, *28*, 1200; A. Romiti *et al.*, *Clin. Trials J.*, 1979, *16*, 108; G. Ibba *et al.*, *Curr. med. Res. Opinion*, 1983, *8*, 321.

Proprietary Names and Manufacturers
Euminex *(Lacer, Spain)*; Teoremac *(Farmades, Ital.)*.

2656-n

Glycol Salicylate

Ethylene Glycol Monosalicylate. 2-Hydroxyethyl salicylate.
$C_9H_{10}O_4$=182.2.

CAS — 87-28-5.

Glycol salicylate is an ingredient of a number of rubefacient creams. It is usually used in concentrations of up to 10%.

Proprietary Names and Manufacturers
The following names have been used for multi-ingredient preparations containing glycol salicylate— Algipan *(Wyeth, UK)*; Bayolin *(Bayer, UK)*; Butoroid Cream *(Faulding, Austral.)*; Cremalgex *(Norton, UK)*; Cremalgin *(Berk Pharmaceuticals, UK)*; Dubam *(Norma, UK)*.

12797-q

Gold Keratinate
Aurothiopolypeptide.

CAS — 9078-78-8.

A gold compound stated to contain 13% of Au.

Gold keratinate has been used by intramuscular injection in the treatment of arthritic disorders.

Proprietary Names and Manufacturers
Auro-Detoxin *(Beecham-Wülfing, Ger.).*

12839-n

Ibufenac *(BAN, USAN, rINN).*
(4-Isobutylphenyl)acetic acid.
$C_{12}H_{16}O_2$=192.3.

CAS — 1553-60-2.

Ibufenac has analgesic, anti-inflammatory, and antipyretic properties. It was formerly used in rheumatic disorders but was found to cause jaundice.

Proprietary Names and Manufacturers
Dytransin *(Boots, UK).*

2657-h

Ibuprofen *(BAN, USAN, rINN).*
RD-13621. 2-(4-Isobutylphenyl)propionic acid.
$C_{13}H_{18}O_2$=206.3.

CAS — 15687-27-1.

Pharmacopoeias. In *Br., Chin., Ind., Int., Jpn, Jug., Swiss,* and *U.S.*

A white or almost white powder or crystals with a characteristic odour. Practically **insoluble** in water; soluble 1 in 1.5 of alcohol, 1 in 1 of chloroform, 1 in 2 of ether, and 1 in 1.5 of acetone; soluble in aqueous solutions of alkali hydroxides and carbonates. **Store** in airtight containers.

Adverse Effects
The most frequent adverse effects occurring with ibuprofen are gastro-intestinal disturbances. Peptic ulceration and gastro-intestinal bleeding have been reported. Other side-effects include headache, dizziness, nervousness, skin rash, pruritus, tinnitus, oedema, depression, drowsiness, insomnia, and blurred vision and other ocular reactions. Hypersensitivity reactions, abnormalities of liver function tests, impairment of renal function including interstitial nephritis or the nephrotic syndrome, agranulocytosis, and thrombocytopenia have occasionally been observed.

A short review of the adverse effects of ibuprofen.— *Med. Lett.*, 1984, *26*, 63.

ALLERGY. There had been more reports of bronchospasm, some serious, with ibuprofen than with other non-steroidal anti-inflammatory drugs. It was not possible to assess whether this represented a real difference in incidence.— Committee on Safety of Medicines, *Current Problems Series No. 1*, Sept. 1975.

An urticarial rash, laboured breathing, laryngeal oedema, and tightness of the chest occurred in a 53-year-old man after a single dose of ibuprofen 400 mg. The patient had experienced a similar adverse reaction about 7 years previously after a single dose of aspirin.— G. J. Merritt and R. I. Selle, *Am. J. Hosp. Pharm.*, 1978, *35*, 1245.

A patient with systemic lupus erythematosus (SLE) developed a hypersensitivity reaction to ibuprofen, with fever, nausea and vomiting, abdominal pain, and elevated liver-function test values. A similar reaction occurred in a second patient who was found, 2 months later, to have SLE.— M. Sonnenblick and A. S. Abraham, *Br. med. J.*, 1978, *1*, 619.

Aseptic meningitis with nausea, vomiting, fever, rigors, and severe headache was reported in a 21-year-old woman with Raynaud's phenomenon and polyarthritis following administration of ibuprofen. The rapid onset of the symptoms suggested a hypersensitivity reaction.— R. F. Bernstein, *Ann. intern. Med.*, 1980, *92*, 206.

Further reports of hypersensitivity reactions to ibuprofen, sometimes in patients with systemic lupus erythematosus: B. Mandell *et al.* (letter), *Ann. intern. Med.*, 1976, *85*, 209 (fever); H. L. Widener and B. H. Littman, *J. Am. med. Ass.*, 1978, *239*, 1062 (aseptic meningitis); W. R. Finch and M. P. Strottman, *J. Am. med. Ass.*, 1979, *241*, 2616 (fever, headache, and hypotension); R. P. Lee *et al.*, *Can. med. Ass. J.*, 1983, *129*, 854 (hypotension and respiratory failure); J. P. Quinn *et al.*, *Neurology*, 1984, *34*, 108 (eosinophilic meningitis); D. R. Perera *et al.* (letter), *Ann. intern. Med.*, 1984, *100*, 619 (meningo-encephalitis); D. L. Bouland *et al.* (letter), *ibid.*, 1986, *104*, 731 (aseptic meningitis); J. G. Ayres *et al.* (letter), *Lancet*, 1987, *1*, 1082 (fatal asthma); B. G. Katona *et al.* (letter), *Lancet*, 1988, *1*, 59 (aseptic meningitis).

EFFECTS ON THE BLOOD. *Agranulocytosis.* Agranulocytosis and leucopenia leading to death 2 weeks after the cessation of medication was reported in an 82-year-old woman given ibuprofen and paracetamol to replace the long-term use of salicylates for the treatment of rheumatoid arthritis.— C. I. Gryfe and S. Rubenzahl (letter), *Can. med. Ass. J.*, 1976, *114*, 877.

Aplastic anaemia. Pure white-cell aplasia in a patient receiving ibuprofen.— S. W. Mamus *et al.*, *New Engl. J. Med.*, 1986, *314*, 624.

Haemolytic anaemia. Immunohaemolytic anaemia in a 69-year-old woman was considered due to ibuprofen; she had taken 400 mg three times daily for 8 months.— S. Korsager, *Br. med. J.*, 1978, *1*, 79.

Fatal haemolytic anaemia occurred in a man who had been treated with ibuprofen and oxazepam for 10 days before the onset of the acute illness.— J. B. Guidry *et al.*, *J. Am. med. Ass.*, 1979, *242*, 68.

Haemorrhagic disorders. A 33-year-old woman developed bruises on her limbs during the third week of treatment for a painful hip with ibuprofen 600 mg daily. Symptoms cleared on discontinuation of the drug.— T. Ward (letter), *Br. med. J.*, 1969, *4*, 430.

In 2 patients who were taking ibuprofen pre-operatively a significant increase in mediastinal bleeding occurred after coronary by-pass surgery.— M. Torosian *et al.*, *Ann. intern. Med.*, 1978, *89*, 325.

EFFECTS ON THE EYES. Of 40 patients treated with ibuprofen usually for rheumatoid arthritis, 2 developed toxic amblyopia due to ibuprofen. A further 3 had visual defects possibly related to ibuprofen.— L. M. T. Collum and D. I. Bowen, *Br. J. Ophthal.*, 1971, *55*, 472.

A 57-year-old woman developed toxic amblyopia after treatment for about 5 months with ibuprofen 1.2 g daily.— C. A. L. Palmer (letter), *Br. med. J.*, 1972, *3*, 765.

Visual disturbances were not encountered in 293 patients with rheumatic disorders treated with ibuprofen over a 5-year period. When ocular toxicity occurred it seemed to be early in treatment, rapidly progressive, and reversible.— M. Thompson (letter), *Br. med. J.*, 1972, *4*, 550. Similar findings.— J. W. Melluish *et al.*, *Archs Ophthal., N.Y.*, 1975, *93*, 781; J. Williamson and R. D. Sturrock, *Curr. med. Res. Opinion*, 1976, *4*, 128.

EFFECTS ON THE GASTRO-INTESTINAL TRACT. A 69-year-old man with a duodenal ulcer, but with no complications, developed gastro-intestinal bleeding one week after starting treatment with ibuprofen 200 mg three times daily. Death due to multiple factors occurred two days after surgery.— D. J. Holdstock (letter), *Lancet*, 1972, *1*, 541. See also: S. K. Vong (letter), *Pharm. J.*, 1986, *1*, 68; *ibid.*, 1987, *2*, 299.

Proctocolitis associated with ibuprofen in one patient.— S. Ravi *et al.*, *Postgrad. med. J.*, 1986, *62*, 773.

EFFECTS ON THE HAIR. Ingestion of ibuprofen was associated with thinning or loss of hair in 16 black patients. These patients also used preparations to straighten hair and it was suggested that ibuprofen might cause fragility or brittleness of the hair so that it breaks at the epidermal level when subjected to the straightening process.— H. C. Meyer (letter), *J. Am. med. Ass.*, 1979, *242*, 142.

EFFECTS ON THE KIDNEYS. Acute oliguric renal failure in a 65-year-old man was attributed to 6 days' treatment with ibuprofen 400 mg four times daily.— R. D. Brandstetter and D. D. Mar, *Br. med. J.*, 1978, *2*, 1194.

Impairment of renal function has been associated with ingestion of ibuprofen in patients with systemic lupus erythematosus.— R. P. Kimberly *et al.*, *Am. J. Med.*, 1978, *64*, 804; R. P. Kimberly *et al.*, *Arthritis Rheum.*, 1979, *22*, 281.

Reversible renal failure in an elderly patient probably caused by ibuprofen.— T. I. Poirier, *Drug Intell. & clin. Pharm.*, 1984, *18*, 27.

A report of a patient who developed the nephrotic syndrome without renal failure following the use of ibuprofen.— F. R. Justiniani (letter), *Ann. intern. Med.*, 1986, *105*, 303.

EFFECTS ON THE LIVER. A 12-year-old girl with juvenile rheumatoid arthritis suffered fever, hepatitis, and lymphocytopenia following treatment with ibuprofen. The symptoms resolved rapidly when ibuprofen was discontinued.— D. A. Stempel and J. J. Miller, *J. Pediat.*, 1977, *90*, 657.

A report of fatal fatty metamorphosis of the liver in a woman with mixed connective tissue disease who was treated with ibuprofen and ampicillin.— J. F. Bravo *et al.* (letter), *Ann. intern. Med.*, 1977, *87*, 200.

See also under Effects on the Skin, below.

EFFECTS ON MENTAL STATE. Paranoid psychosis probably associated with the use of ibuprofen in one patient.— J. D. Griffith *et al.*, *J. clin. Psychiat.*, 1982, *43*, 499.

EFFECTS ON THE MUSCLES. Muscle weakness and tenderness with rhabdomyolysis leading to respiratory failure developed in a patient 2 days after the initiation of ibuprofen therapy.— N. S. Ross and C. L. Hoppel, *J. Am. med. Ass.*, 1987, *257*, 62.

EFFECTS ON THE NERVOUS SYSTEM. Exacerbation of orofacial dyskinesia and the development of bilateral ballistic movements following the initiation of ibuprofen therapy.— R. Sandyk *et al.*, *Postgrad. med. J.*, 1987, *63*, 593.

EFFECTS ON THE SKIN. A report of erythema multiforme (Stevens-Johnson syndrome) and toxic hepatitis associated with ingestion of ibuprofen in 1 patient.— P. Sternlieb and R. M. Robinson, *N.Y. St. J. Med.*, 1978, *78*, 1239. At the time of this report there had been reported 17 other cases of ibuprofen-induced hepatotoxicity and 5 cases of serious dermatological problems in the category of erythema multiforme bullosum, including the variant known as Stevens-Johnson syndrome, as well as toxic epidermal necrolysis.— *idem* (letter), *Ann. intern. Med.*, 1980, *92*, 570.

Classical erythema nodosum rashes in one patient probably induced by ibuprofen.— A. R. Khan, *Br. med. J.*, 1984, *288*, 1048.

MENINGITIS. For reports of aseptic meningitis following administration of ibuprofen, see under Allergy, above.

OVERDOSAGE. A review of cases of ibuprofen overdose reported to the National Poisons Information Service of the *UK* in the 2 years following its introduction as an 'over-the-counter' medication. Although there was a substantial increase in the number of cases reported, no concurrent increases in severity of poisoning was demonstrated and in only 1 of 203 cases was ibuprofen thought to have caused serious problems. It was concluded that ibuprofen appeared to be much less toxic in acute overdose than either aspirin or paracetamol.— S. J. Perry *et al.*, *Hum. Toxicol.*, 1987, *6*, 173. See also.— H. Court and G. N. Volans, *Adverse Drug React. Ac. Pois. Rev.*, 1984, *3*, 1.

Precautions
Ibuprofen should be given with care to patients with asthma or bronchospasm, bleeding disorders, cardiovascular disease, peptic ulceration or a history of such ulceration, renal failure, and in those who are receiving coumarin anticoagulants. Patients who are sensitive to aspirin should generally not be given ibuprofen.

INFECTIONS. Activation of latent tuberculosis in a patient given ibuprofen and indomethacin.— M. Brennan (letter), *Can. med. Ass. J.*, 1980, *122*, 400.

INTERACTIONS. For the effect of ibuprofen on other drugs, see under digoxin (p.828), diuretics (p.974 and p.988), lithium carbonate (p.368), and phenytoin sodium (p.408).

PREGNANCY AND THE NEONATE. A study in 12 women indicating that in lactating women the ingestion of ibuprofen 400 mg every 6 hours would result in less than 1 mg of ibuprofen being excreted daily into breast milk.— R. J. Townsend *et al.*, *Am. J. Obstet. Gynec.*, 1984, *149*, 184.

Absorption and Fate
Ibuprofen is absorbed from the gastro-intestinal tract and peak plasma concentrations occur about 1 to 2 hours after ingestion. Ibuprofen is extensively bound to plasma proteins and has a half-life of about 2 hours. It is rapidly excreted in the urine mainly as metabolites and their conjugates. About 1% is excreted in urine as unchanged ibuprofen and about 14% as conjugated ibuprofen.

A study on the stereoselective disposition of ibuprofen enantiomers. It is known that only the S(+)-enantiomers of the anti-inflammatory agents derived from α-methylarylacetic acid inhibit prostaglandin synthesis and therefore the pharmacokinetics of ibuprofen cannot be adequately interpreted without study of the individual enantiomers.— E. J. D. Lee *et al.*, *Br. J. clin. Pharmac.*, 1985, *19*, 669. See also: A. J. Hutt and J. Caldwell, *Clin. Pharmacokinet.*, 1984, *9*, 371. Further references: G. J. Vangiessen and D. G. Kaiser, *J. pharm. Sci.*, 1975, *64*, 798; D. G. Kaiser *et al.*, *J. pharm. Sci.*, 1976, *65*, 269.

Studies on the protein binding of ibuprofen: L. Aarons *et al.*, *Eur. J. clin. Pharmac.*, 1983, *25*, 815; S. Wanwimolruk *et al.*, *Br. J. clin. Pharmac.*, 1983, *15*, 91.

Uses and Administration

Ibuprofen has analgesic, anti-inflammatory, and antipyretic properties; it is an inhibitor of prostaglandin synthetase.

Ibuprofen is used for the relief of mild to moderate pain in conditions such as dysmenorrhoea, migraine, postoperative pain, rheumatic disorders such as ankylosing spondylitis, osteoarthritis, and rheumatoid arthritis including juvenile rheumatoid arthritis, and in other musculoskeletal and joint disorders such as sprains and strains.

The usual dose by mouth is 1.2 to 1.8 g daily in divided doses although maintenance doses of 0.6 to 1.2 g daily may be effective in some patients. If necessary the dose may be increased to 2.4 g daily and some sources have suggested that up to 3.2 g daily may be given. If gastro-intestinal disturbances occur, ibuprofen should be given with food or milk.

A suggested dose for children is 20 mg per kg body-weight daily in divided doses with up to 40 mg per kg being given daily in juvenile rheumatoid arthritis if necessary; the maximum daily dose has been stated to be 500 mg for those weighing less than 30 kg.

Ibuprofen has also been given orally as the guaiacolate ester (methoxybutropate; metoxibutropate) and been used topically as the lactate.

Reviews of the actions and uses of ibuprofen.— M. Busson, *J. int. med. Res.*, 1986, *14*, 53.

ADMINISTRATION IN THE ELDERLY. A pharmacokinetic study involving healthy subjects aged 20 to 88 years and given a single dose of ibuprofen indicated that an ibuprofen dosage schedule of 3 or 4 times daily is unlikely to cause excessive accumulation in any individual, regardless of age.— D. J. Greenblatt *et al.*, *Arthritis Rheum.*, 1984, *27*, 1066.

ADMINISTRATION IN HEPATIC FAILURE. A study in 15 patients indicating minimal effects of alcoholic liver disease on the pharmacokinetics of ibuprofen.— R. P. Juhl *et al.*, *Clin. Pharmac. Ther.*, 1983, *34*, 104.

ADMINISTRATION IN RENAL FAILURE. Studies in 7 functionally anephric patients undergoing haemodialysis indicated that the pharmacokinetics of ibuprofen were not influenced by the disease state or by dialysis.— E. J. Antal *et al.*, *J. clin. Pharmac.*, 1986, *26*, 184. See also: H. O. Senekjian *et al.*, *Eur. J. Rheumatol. Inflamm.*, 1983, *6*, 155.

ANKYLOSING SPONDYLITIS. The use of ibuprofen in ankylosing spondylitis.— J. Nikolić and D. Lukačević, *Scand. J. Rheumatol.*, 1975, *4*, *Suppl.* 8, 20.

FEVER. Favourable reports of the use of ibuprofen as an antipyretic in children: G. Wilson *et al.*, *J. int. med. Res.*, 1984, *12*, 250; P. W. Kandoth *et al.*, *ibid.*, 292; A. Kotob, *ibid.*, 1985, *13*, 122; Amdekar Y.K. and R. Z. Desai, *Br. J. clin. Pract.*, 1985, *39*, 140; M. A. Phadke *et al.*, *ibid.*, 437.

GOUT. References to the use of ibuprofen in gouty arthritis: W. A. Franck and M. M. Brown, *Arthritis Rheum.*, 1976, *19*, 269; M. C. Schweitz *et al.*, *J. Am. med. Ass.*, 1978, *239*, 34.

OSTEOARTHRITIS. Some references to the use of ibuprofen in osteoarthrosis: L. Mattara *et al.*, *Clin. Trials J.*, 1977, *14*, 30; J. E. Giansiracusa *et al.*, *Sth. med. J.*, 1977, *70*, 49; L. S. Bain *et al.*, *Curr. med. Res. Opinion*, 1977, *4*, 665; C. Tranmer, *Rheumatol. Rehabil.*, 1978, *17*, 91; *Curr. med. Res. Opinion*, 1984, *9*, 41.

PAIN. Some references to the use of ibuprofen in dysmenorrhoea: D. R. Halbert and L. M. Demers, *J. reprod. Med.*, 1978, *21*, 219; R. M. Larkin *et al.*, *Obstet. Gynec.*, 1979, *54*, 456; W. Y. Chan *et al.*, *Am. J. Obstet. Gynec.*, 1979, *135*, 102; K. S. Gookin *et al.*, *Sth. med. J.*, 1983, *76*, 1361; S. Roy, *Obstet. Gynec.*, 1983, *61*, 628; I. Milsom and B. Andersch, *Br. J. Obstet. Gynaec.*, 1984, *91*, 1129; *idem*, *Int. J. Gynaecol. Obstet.*, 1985, *23*, 305.

Some references to the use of ibuprofen in headache: S. Diamond, *Headache*, 1983, *23*, 206; R. M. Noyelle *et al.*, *Pharm. J.*, 1987, *1*, 561.

Some references to the use ibuprofen for post-episiotomy pain: S. S. Bloomfield *et al.*, *Clin. Pharmac. Ther.*, 1974, *15*, 565; A. Sunshine *et al.*, *Clin. Pharmac. Ther.*, 1983, *34*, 254.

Some references to the use of ibuprofen for postoperative pain: R. A. Dionne *et al.*, *J. clin. Pharmac.*, 1983, *23*, 37; A. K. Jain *et al.*, *Pharmacotherapy*, 1986, *6*, 318; H. Owen *et al.*, *Br. J. Anaesth.*, 1986, *58*, 1371.

RHEUMATOID ARTHRITIS. Some references to the use of ibuprofen in rheumatoid arthritis: T. M. Chalmers, *Ann. rheum. Dis.*, 1969, *28*, 513; S. Sasaki, *Rheumatol. phys. Med.*, 1970, *Suppl.*, 32; C. D. Brooks *et al.*, *ibid.*, 48; M. Thompson and D. Bell, *ibid.*, 100; A. A. J. Goldberg *et al.*, *Practitioner*, 1971, *207*, 343; J. Dornan and W. J. Reynolds, *Can. med. Ass. J.*, 1974, *110*, 1370; W. J. Blechman *et al.*, *J. Am. med. Ass.*, 1975, *233*, 336; *Curr. med. Res. Opinion*, 1975, *3*, 475–606; A. Calin *et al.*, *J. Rheumatol.*, 1977, *4*, 153; K. Pavelka *et al.*, *J. int. med. Res.*, 1978, *6*, 355; E. J. Valtonen and M. Busson, *Scand. J. Rheumatol.*, 1978, *7*, 183; H. C. Burry and L. Witherington, *N.Z. med. J.*, 1979, *89*, 298; F. Montrone *et al.*, *Rheumatol. Rehabil.*, 1979, *18*, 114; J. P. Molnar and T. E. Moxley, *Curr. ther. Res.*, 1979, *26*, 581; N. H. Brodie *et al.*, *Br. J. clin. Pract.*, 1980, *34*, 279; J. J. Castles and J. L. Skosey, *Curr. ther. Res.*, 1980, *27*, 556; D. M. Grennan *et al.*, *Br. J. clin. Pharmac.*, 1983, *15*, 311; L. Aarons *et al.* (letter), *ibid.*, 387; J. Taborn *et al.*, *Curr. med. Res. Opinion*, 1985, *9*, 359.

SKIN DISORDERS. For a reference to the use of ibuprofen with minocycline in acne, see p.264.

Preparations

Ibuprofen Tablets *(B.P.)*

Ibuprofen Tablets *(U.S.P.)*

Proprietary Preparations

Apsifen *(Approved Prescription Services, UK)*. *Tablets*, ibuprofen 200 and 400 mg.
Tablets (Apsifen F), film-coated. ibuprofen 200, 400 and 600 mg.

Brufen *(Boots, UK)*. *Tablets*, ibuprofen 200 mg.
Tablets (Brufen 400), ibuprofen 400 mg.
Tablets (Brufen 600), ibuprofen 600 mg.
Syrup, ibuprofen 100 mg/5 mL.

Ebufac *(DDSA Pharmaceuticals, UK)*. *Tablets*, ibuprofen 200 and 400 mg.

Femafen *(Nicholas, UK)*. *Capsules*, sustained-release, ibuprofen 300 mg.

Fenbid *(Smith Kline & French, UK)*. *Spansules*, sustained-release capsules, ibuprofen 300 mg.

Ibumetin *(Benzon, UK)*. *Tablets*, ibuprofen 200, 400, and 600 mg.

Librofem *(Ciba, UK)*. *Tablets*, ibuprofen 200 mg.

Lidifen *(Berk Generics, UK)*. *Tablets*, ibuprofen 200 and 400 mg.

Migrafen *(Chatfield Laboratories, UK)*. *Tablets*, ibuprofen 200 mg.

Motrin *(Upjohn, UK)*. *Tablets*, ibuprofen 200, 400, 600, and 800 mg.

Novaprin *(Simpkin, UK)*. *Tablets*, ibuprofen 200 mg.

Nurofen *(Crookes Healthcare, UK)*. *Tablets*, ibuprofen 200 mg.

Pacifene *(Sussex, UK)*. *Tablets*, ibuprofen 200 mg.

Paxofen *(Steinhard, UK)*. *Tablets*, ibuprofen 200, 400, and 600 mg.

Proflex *(Ciba, UK)*. *Capsules*, sustained-release, ibuprofen 300 mg.
Tablets, ibuprofen 200 mg.

Relcofen *(Cox, UK)*. *Tablets*, ibuprofen 200 and 400 mg.

Seclodin *(Whitehall, UK)*. *Capsules*, ibuprofen 200 mg.

Suspren *(Nicholas, UK)*. *Capsules*, sustained-release, ibuprofen 300 mg.

Proprietary Names and Manufacturers of Ibuprofen and its Salts and Esters

Advil *(Whitehall, USA)*; Algiasdin *(Isdin, Spain)*; Algisan *(Prodes, Spain)*; Algofen *(Ital.)*; Amersol *(Horner, Canad.)*; Anco *(Kanoldt, Ger.)*; Andran *(Jpn)*; Anflagen *(Jpn)*; Antiflam *(Rolab, S.Afr.)*; Apsifen *(Approved Prescription Services, UK)*; Artrene *(IRBI, Ital.)*; Benflogin *(Angelini, Ital.)*; Betagesic *(Restan, S.Afr.)*; Bluton *(Jpn)*; Brufanic *(Jpn)*; Brufen *(Boots, Austral.; Belg.; Denm.; Boots-Dacour, Fr.; Kanoldt, Ger.; Boots-Formenti, Ital.; Jpn; Neth.; Boots, Norw.; Boots, S.Afr.; Spain; Boots, Swed.; Boots, Switz.; Boots, UK)*; Brufort *(Lampugnani, Ital.)*; Cuprofen *(Cupal, UK)*; Dolgit *(Dolorgiet, Ger.; Dolorgiet, Switz.)*; Donjust B *(Jpn)*; Ebufac *(DDSA Pharmaceuticals, UK)*; Emodin *(Arg.)*; Epobron *(Jpn)*; Femafen *(Nicholas, UK)*; Fenalgic *(Bottu, Fr.)*; Fenbid *(Smith Kline & French, UK)*; Flubenil *(Boots-Formenti, Ital.)*; Focus *(Angelini, Ital.)*; Haltran *(Upjohn, USA)*; IB-100 *(Jpn)*; Ibu-Attritin *(Atmos, Ger.)*; Ibucasen *(Casen Fisons, Spain)*; Ibufug *(Wolff, Ger.)*; Ibular *(Lagap, UK)*; Ibumetin *(Benzon, Denm.; Benzon, Norw.; Benzon, Swed.; Benzon, UK)*; Ibuprocin *(Jpn)*; Ibu-Slo *(Lipha, UK)*; Ibux *(Weiders, Norw.)*; Inabrin *(Upjohn, UK)*; Inflam *(Protea, Austral.)*; Inza *(Lennon, S.Afr.)*; Lamidon *(Jpn)*; Librofem *(Ciba, UK)*; Lidifen *(Berk Generics, UK)*; Liptan *(Jpn)*; Lisibudol *(Sigma Tau, Spain)*; Lunapain *(Lennon, S.Afr.)*; Maxagesic *(Leo, UK)*; Medipren *(McNeil Consumer, USA)*; Migrafen *(Chatfield Laboratories, UK)*; Moment *(Angelini, Ital.)*; Motrin *(Upjohn, Canad.; Upjohn, UK; Upjohn, USA)*; Mynosedin *(Jpn)*; Nagifen-D *(Jpn)*; Napacetin *(Jpn)*; Neobrufen *(Liade, Spain)*; Nobfelon *(Jpn)*; Nobgen *(Jpn)*; Novaprin *(Simpkin, UK)*; Novogent *(Temmler, Ger.)*; Novoprofen *(Novopharm, Canad.)*; Nuprin *(Upjohn, USA)*; Nurofen *(Boots-Formenti, Ital.; Crookes Healthcare, UK)*; Opturem *(Kade, Ger.)*; Pacifene *(Sussex, UK)*; Pantrop *(Jpn)*; Paxofen *(Steinhard, UK)*; Proflex *(Ciba, UK)*; Prontalgin *(SPA, Ital.)*; Rebugen *(Ital.)*; Relcofen *(Cox, UK)*; Roidenin *(Jpn)*; Rufen *(Boots, USA)*; Saren *(Bracco, Ital.)*; Seclodin *(Whitehall, UK)*; Staderm *(Torii, Jpn)*; Suspren *(Nicholas, UK)*; Trendar *(Whitehall, USA)*; Uniprofen *(Unimed, UK)*; Urem *(Kade, Ger.)*; Vesicum *(Hisamitsu, Jpn)*.

12841-a

Ibuproxam *(rINN)*.

4-Isobutylhydratropohydroxamic acid.
$C_{13}H_{19}NO_2$=221.3.

CAS — 53648-05-8.

Ibuproxam is a non-steroidal anti-inflammatory agent that has been used in rheumatic disorders in doses of up to 800 mg daily by mouth. It has also been applied topically as a 5% ointment.

Proprietary Names and Manufacturers
Deflogon *(Damor, Ital.)*; Ibudros *(Manetti Roberts, Ital.; Ferrer, Switz.)*; Nialen *(Novag, Spain)*.

16848-e

Imidazole Salicylate *(rINN)*.

Imidazole compounded with salicylic acid.
$C_{10}H_{10}N_2O_3$=206.2.

CAS — 36364-49-5.

Imidazole salicylate has anti-inflammatory properties and has been used in inflammatory and rheumatic disorders in doses of up to 1 g once or twice daily by mouth. It has also been given by intramuscular injection in doses of up to 1 g daily and has also been applied topically as a 5% gel.

Proprietary Names and Manufacturers
Selezen *(Italfarmaco, Ital.)*.

12850-t

Indobufen *(rINN)*.

K-3920. (±)-2-[4-(1-Oxo-isoindolin-2-yl)phenyl]butyric acid.
$C_{18}H_{17}NO_3$=295.3.

CAS — 63610-08-2.

Indobufen is an inhibitor of platelet aggregation and has been used in various thrombotic disorders in doses of 200 to 400 mg daily by mouth. It has also been given parenterally in similar doses.

Pharmacokinetics: L. M. Fuccella *et al.*, *Eur. J. clin. Pharmac.*, 1979, *15*, 323; V. Tamassia *et al.*, *ibid.*, 329.

A study on the effect of renal insufficiency on the pharmacokinetics of indobufen and suggesting the following oral doses according to creatinine clearance: creatinine clearance more than 80 mL per minute, 200 mg twice daily; 30 to 80 mL per minute, 100 mg twice daily; less than 30 mL per minute, 100 mg daily.— G. M. Savazzi *et al.*, *Curr. ther. Res.*, 1984, *36*, 119.

Proprietary Names and Manufacturers
Ibustrin *(Carlo Erba, Ital.)*.

2658-m

Indomethacin *(BAN, USAN).*

Indometacin *(rINN)*; Indometacinum. [1-(4-Chlorobenzoyl)-5-methoxy-2-methylindol-3-yl]acetic acid.

$C_{19}H_{16}ClNO_4$=357.8.

CAS — 53-86-1.

Pharmacopoeias. In *Belg., Br., Braz., Chin., Cz., Eur., Fr., Ind., Int., It., Jpn, Neth., Nord., Swiss,* and *U.S.*

A white to yellow-tan, odourless or almost odourless, crystalline powder. It exhibits polymorphism. Practically **insoluble** in water; soluble 1 in 50 of alcohol, 1 in 30 of chloroform, and 1 in 40 to 45 of ether. **Store** in well-closed containers. Protect from light.

Adverse Effects

The commonest adverse effects occurring with indomethacin are gastro-intestinal disturbances, headache, and dizziness. Gastro-intestinal ulceration and bleeding may also occur. Other adverse effects include depression, drowsiness, tinnitus, confusion, lightheadedness, insomnia, psychiatric disturbances, syncope, convulsions, coma, peripheral neuropathy, blurred vision and other ocular effects, oedema and weight gain, hypertension, haematuria, skin rashes, pruritus, urticaria, stomatitis, alopecia, and hypersensitivity reactions. Leucopenia, purpura, thrombocytopenia, aplastic anaemia, haemolytic anaemia, agranulocytosis, epistaxis, hyperglycaemia, hyperkalaemia, and vaginal bleeding have been reported. There have also been reports of hepatitis and jaundice or renal failure. Hypersensitivity reactions may also occur in aspirin-sensitive patients.

Indomethacin could cause green discoloration of the urine and a green discoloration of the faeces due to biliverdinaemia.— R. B. Baran and B. Rowles, *J. Am. pharm. Ass.*, 1973, *NS13*, 139.

ALLERGY. A fatal asthmatic attack occurred following the use of an indomethacin suppository in an aspirin-sensitive patient.— J. Timperman, *J. forens. Med.*, 1971, *18*, 30.

A patient sensitive to aspirin developed an urticarial reaction 30 minutes after taking his first dose of indomethacin.— J. I. Matthews and D. Stage (letter), *Ann. intern. Med.*, 1974, *80*, 771.

Severe dyspnoea occurred in a 43-year-old woman, with a history of allergy to penicillin and aspirin, after a single dose of indomethacin 50 mg.— N. M. Johnson *et al.* (letter), *Br. med. J.*, 1977, *2*, 1291.

EFFECTS ON THE BLOOD. An analysis of blood dyscrasias reported to the Swedish Adverse Drug Reaction Committee for the 5-year period 1966–70 showed that thrombocytopenia attributable to indomethacin had been reported on 6 occasions. It was estimated that reported figures represented one-third of the true frequency.— L. E. Böttiger and B. Westerholm, *Br. med. J.*, 1973, *3*, 339.

There were 1261 reports of adverse reactions to indomethacin reported to the Committee on Safety of Medicines between June 1964 and January 1973. These included 157 reports of blood disorders (25 fatal) including thrombocytopenia (35; 5 fatal), aplastic anaemia (17; no fatalities), and agranulocytosis or leucopenia (21; 3 fatal), gastro-intestinal haemorrhage (121; 25 fatal), and reports involving the CNS (chiefly headache, giddiness, vertigo, confusion, and visual abnormalities).— M. F. Cuthbert, *Curr. med. Res. Opinion*, 1974, *2*, 600.

Mention of 8 cases of fatal aplastic anaemia or agranulocytosis in one year probably due to indomethacin.— W. H. W. Inman, *Br. med. J.*, 1977, *1*, 1500.

A First Report from the International Agranulocytosis and Aplastic Anemia Study confirming a significant relationship between the use of indomethacin and agranulocytosis and aplastic anaemia.— *J. Am. med. Ass.*, 1986, *256*, 1749.

Further reports of aplastic anaemia associated with indomethacin.— A. T. Canada and E. R. Burka (letter), *New Engl. J. Med.*, 1968, *278*, 743; G. R. Fredrick and K. R. Tanaka (letter), *ibid.*, *279*, 1290.

EFFECTS ON THE ELECTROLYTES. Hyporeninaemia, hypoaldosteronism, and hyperkalaemia were associated with administration of indomethacin in 1 patient with glomerulonephritis.— S. Y. Tan *et al.*, *Ann. intern. Med.*, 1979, *90*, 783.

Severe hyperkalaemia with renal impairment associated in 3 patients with indomethacin therapy.— J. W. Findling *et al.*, *J. Am. med. Ass.*, 1980, *244*, 1127.

A study in 50 patients receiving indomethacin indicating that hyperkalaemia is a common and potentially dangerous complication of treatment.— A. Zimran *et al.*, *Br. med. J.*, 1985, *291*, 107.

Further reports of hyperkalaemia and hyporeninaemia associated with indomethacin.— E. P. MacCarthy *et al.*, *Med. J. Aust.*, 1979, *1*, 550; V. Beroniade *et al.* (letter), *Ann. intern. Med.*, 1979, *91*, 499; P. D. Mitnick *et al.*, *Clin. Pharmac. Ther.*, 1980, *28*, 680.

EFFECTS ON THE EYES. Decreased retinal sensitivity occurred in 34 patients who had been taking indomethacin, 22 of whom had presented with ocular complaints. Corneal deposits were observed in 6.— C. A. Burns, *Am. J. Ophthal.*, 1968, *66*, 825.

Five patients with rheumatic disorders developed ocular side-effects after prolonged treatment with indomethacin. The cornea was affected in 2 and the retina in 3. The effects were generally reversed after therapy had been discontinued for 1 year.— G. Palmeris *et al.*, *Ophthalmologica, Basel*, 1972, *164*, 339. There was no greater incidence of retinal malfunction in 18 patients receiving indomethacin than in 10 controls, some with similar diseases. Where abnormalities were present in both groups they were thought to be due to age and the disease.— R. E. Carr and I. M. Siegel, *Am. J. Ophthal.*, 1973, *75*, 302.

A further case of reversible indomethacin-induced retinopathy.— H. E. Henkes *et al.*, *Am. J. Ophthal.*, 1972, *73*, 846.

EFFECTS ON THE GASTRO-INTESTINAL TRACT. An elderly woman died 3 days after a massive haemorrhage from rectal ulceration following treatment with indomethacin suppositories, 100 mg twice daily, for about 3 weeks. She had previously developed analgesic nephropathy.— J. Walls *et al.* (letter), *Br. med. J.*, 1968, *2*, 52. Rectal bleeding occurred in a 15-year-old boy after several months of treatment with indomethacin 150 mg daily given as suppositories. Bleeding ceased when the indomethacin was withdrawn. Resumption of treatment with 50 mg daily caused very little rectal bleeding.— N. Levy and E. Gaspar (letter), *Lancet*, 1975, *1*, 577.

Gastric ulcers developed in 10 patients who had taken indomethacin by mouth and sometimes rectally for 2 to 24 months. The ulcers were prepyloric in 6 patients, and in 7 patients they had an appearance falsely suggestive of malignancy. Only one patient had a previous history of gastric ulceration. Withdrawal of indomethacin led to complete healing in 7 patients who had remained symptomless for periods of 4 months to 3 years.— R. T. Taylor *et al.*, *Br. med. J.*, 1968, *4*, 734. See also J. H. Swallow (letter), *ibid.*, 1969, *1*, 783; R. T. Taylor *et al.* (letter), *ibid.*, 1969, *2*, 53. Of 89 patients admitted to hospital with perforated duodenal ulcer, 11 were taking indomethacin; 8 were women aged over 60.— M. R. Thompson, *Br. med. J.*, 1980, *280*, 448. See also *idem* (letter), 1618.

Two cases of colonic perforation associated with short-term indomethacin therapy.— S. Coutrot *et al.* (letter), *Lancet*, 1978, *2*, 1055. Gastric perforation in a neonate might have been caused by indomethacin given for ductus arteriosus.— A. N. Campbell *et al.* (letter), *Lancet*, 1981, *1*, 1110. Intestinal perforations in 4 neonates receiving indomethacin via a naso-gastric tube for patent ductus arteriosus.— G. Alpan *et al.*, *J. Pediat.*, 1985, *106*, 277. A further report of multiple perforations of the small bowel in a 38-year-old man receiving indomethacin. Since January 1965 the Committee on Safety of Medicines in the *UK* has recorded 12 cases of intestinal perforation (7 deaths), 5 cases of intestinal ulceration (1 death), and 2 cases of intestinal ulceration and perforation (no deaths); it is not known how many of these cases were due to conventional formulations of indomethacin and how many were due to delayed-release preparations.— J. T. Stewart *et al.* (letter), *Br. med. J.*, 1985, *290*, 787.

EFFECTS ON THE KIDNEYS. Acute renal failure occurred in a woman with congestive heart failure 2 weeks after starting treatment with indomethacin. Renal function improved after indomethacin was withdrawn and deteriorated on rechallenge.— J. J. Walshe and R. C. Venuto, *Ann. intern. Med.*, 1979, *91*, 47.

Irreversible renal failure occurred in 6 children with steroid-resistant nephrosis, but normal renal function, treated with indomethacin.— C. Kleinknecht *et al.* (letter), *New Engl. J. Med.*, 1980, *302*, 691.

Oliguric acute renal failure associated with indomethacin in one patient with no previous kidney impairment.— N. E. Gary *et al.*, *Am. J. Med.*, 1980, *69*, 135.

Decrease in glomerular filtration-rate in 7 premature infants given indomethacin for patent ductus arteriosus. The dose was 200 µg per kg body-weight every 24 hours to a maximum of 600 µg per kg.— Z. Catterton *et al.*, *J. Pediat.*, 1980, *96*, 737. Another report of altered renal function.— R. F. Cifuentes *et al.*, *ibid.*, 1979, *95*, 583.

Further reports of acute renal failure associated with indomethacin therapy in patients with underlying renal disease.— J. L. Bernheim and Z. Korzets (letter), *Ann. intern. Med.*, 1979, *91*, 792; S. Y. Tan *et al.*, *J. Am. med. Ass.*, 1979, *241*, 2732.

Further reports of nephrotoxicity associated with indomethacin: H. Mitchell *et al.* (letter), *Lancet*, 1982, *2*, 558 (renal papillary necrosis); I. Boiskin *et al.* (letter), *Ann. intern. Med.*, 1987, *106*, 776 (reversible nephrotic syndrome); X. Chan (letter), *Lancet*, 1987, *2*, 340 (fatal renal failure).

EFFECTS ON THE LIVER. Toxic hepatitis, possibly due to indomethacin, caused the death of a 12-year-old boy who had been given 100 mg daily for rheumatoid disease.— W. M. Kelsey and M. Scharyj, *J. Am. med. Ass.*, 1967, *199*, 586.

Cholestatic hepatitis with biliverdinaemia developed in a 46-year-old man who had taken indomethacin 75 mg daily for 3 weeks. Symptoms subsided with conservative treatment and withdrawal of indomethacin.— F. F. Fenech *et al.*, *Br. med. J.*, 1967, *3*, 155.

EFFECTS ON MENTAL STATE. A psychotic episode characterised by paranoid delusions and perceptual abnormalities in a 65-year-old woman appeared to be associated with treatment with indomethacin.— M. W. P. Carney, *Br. med. J.*, 1977, *2*, 994. Further references: D. H. Ryan, *Br. med. J.*, 1985, *290*, 30 (hypomania).

EFFECTS ON THE NERVOUS SYSTEM. A 79-year-old man who had taken indomethacin 25 mg twice daily for a year developed loss of hearing and tremor.— *J. Am. med. Ass.*, 1973, *226*, 1471.

Brief case histories of 4 patients who developed peripheral neuropathy while taking indomethacin and in whom the condition slowly regressed when indomethacin was withdrawn.— O. E. Eade *et al.*, *Br. med. J.*, 1975, *2*, 66.

EFFECTS ON THE PANCREAS. A 69-year-old man developed acute pancreatitis after 3 months' treatment with indomethacin, 75 mg daily, for osteoarthritis. He was asymptomatic 24 days later.— M. Guerra, *J. Am. med. Ass.*, 1967, *200*, 552.

EFFECTS ON THE SKIN. A report of oral lichenoid eruption associated with the use of indomethacin by mouth or rectally. The condition was also induced by ibuprofen, fenclofenac, diflunisal, and flurbiprofen. Records showed 7 other patients in whom the eruption was associated with the use of non-steroidal anti-inflammatory agents. In 4 other patients ibuprofen, fenbufen, sulindac, or benoxaprofen was possibly implicated.— J. Hamburger and A. J. C. Potts, *Br. med. J.*, 1983, *287*, 1258.

Toxic epidermal necrolysis in one patient associated with indomethacin.— M. O'Sullivan *et al.*, *Br. J. Rheumatol.*, 1983, *22*, 47.

The rash and pruritus of dermatitis herpetiformis were exacerbated in 9 of 13 patients who took indomethacin in addition to their standard medication in a placebo-controlled double-blind crossover study investigating a subjective observation that non-steroidal anti-inflammatory drugs exacerbate the disease. One patient had an improvement and the other 3 no change while taking indomethacin.— C. E. M. Griffiths *et al.*, *Br. J. Derm.*, 1985, *112*, 443.

A report of 2 cases of benign mucous membrane pemphigoid apparently precipitated by indomethacin.— C. I. Harrington and A. G. Messenger (letter), *Br. J. Derm.*, 1986, *114*, 265.

Analysis, by the Boston Collaborative Drug Surveillance Program, of data on 15 438 patients hospitalised between 1975 and 1982 detected 1 allergic skin reaction attributed to indomethacin among 482 recipients of the drug.— M. Bigby *et al.*, *J. Am. med. Ass.*, 1986, *256*, 3358.

OVERDOSAGE. A review of poisoning with NSAIDs. In a report of 18 cases involving indomethacin (P. Queneau *et al.*, *Thérapie*, 1978, *33*, 645) the only symptoms were drowsiness and mild gastric irritation, findings which are supported by 31 cases reported to the National Poisons Information Service of the *UK* where 61% of patients remained asymptomatic.— H. Court and G. N. Volans, *Adverse Drug React. Ac. Pois. Rev.*, 1984, *3*, 1.

PREGNANCY AND THE NEONATE. For reports of adverse effects in neonates receiving indomethacin for patent ductus arteriosus, see under Effects on the Gastro-intestinal Tract and Effects on the Kidneys.

Precautions

Indomethacin should be administered with caution to patients with impaired renal function, and to those with bleeding disorders, epilepsy, parkinsonism, or psychiatric disorders. It should not be given to patients with peptic ulcer or a history of gastro-intestinal lesions or to those who are sensitive to aspirin.

INFECTIONS. The Canadian Food and Drug Directorate had received several reports that indomethacin had masked symptoms of infection or activated latent bacterial infection in the same way as corticosteroids.— R. A. Chapman, *Can. med. Ass. J.*, 1966, *95*, 1156.

Activation of latent tuberculosis in a patient given ibuprofen and indomethacin.— M. Brennan (letter), *Can. med. Ass. J.*, 1980, *122*, 400. Confirmation of an association between the reactivation of pulmonary tuberculosis and the use of non-steroidal anti-inflammatory agents.— H. O. Tomasson *et al.*, *ibid.*, 1984, *130*, 275.

Further references to masked infection: L. Solomon (preliminary communication), *Br. med. J.*, 1966, *1*, 961; J. C. Jacobs, *J. Am. med. Ass.*, 1967, *199*, 932; S. H. Block (letter), *ibid.*, 1972, *222*, 1062; *idem*, 1979, *241*, 2786.

INTERACTIONS. For the effect of indomethacin on other drugs see under captopril (p.470), digoxin (p.828), diuretics (p.974 and p.988), gentamicin (p.238), haloperidol (p.744), hydralazine (p.484), lithium carbonate (p.368), methotrexate (p.638), and propranolol (p.802).

Antacids. Studies in 12 healthy subjects suggested that the bioavailability of indomethacin was reduced by administration with an antacid containing aluminium hydroxide—magnesium carbonate and magnesium hydroxide.— R. L. Galeazzi, *Eur. J. clin. Pharmac.*, 1977, *12*, 65.

Aspirin. Chronic administration of aspirin 1.2 g three times daily reduced mean plasma concentrations of indomethacin by about 20% after single doses and by smaller amounts after multiple doses. After administration of single doses of both drugs together, mean plasma concentrations of indomethacin were reduced by about 8%. Chronic administration of indomethacin had no effect on plasma concentrations of salicylate following multiple doses of aspirin.— K. C. Kwan *et al.*, *J. Pharmacokinet. Biopharm.*, 1978, *6*, 451. Similar reports: R. Jeremy and J. Towson, *Med. J. Aust.*, 1970, *2*, 127; A. Rubin *et al.*, *Arthritis Rheum.*, 1973, *16*, 635.

Studies which did not demonstrate an effect of aspirin on plasma-indomethacin concentrations.— G. D. Champion *et al.*, *Clin. Pharmac. Ther.*, 1972, *13*, 239; P. M. Brooks *et al.*, *Br. med. J.*, 1975, *3*, 69; B. Lindquist *et al.*, *Clin. Pharmac. Ther.*, 1974, *15*, 247.

Frusemide. Plasma-indomethacin concentrations in 8 patients with rheumatoid arthritis were significantly reduced when frusemide 40 mg by mouth was administered concomitantly.— P. M. Brooks *et al.*, *Br. J. clin. Pharmac.*, 1974, *1*, 485.

PREGNANCY AND THE NEONATE. Convulsions in a breast-fed infant appeared to be associated with ingestion of indomethacin by the mother; the child had normal motor and mental development at the age of 1 year and seizures did not recur.— O. Eeg-Olofsson *et al.* (letter), *Lancet*, 1978, *2*, 215.

Absorption and Fate

Indomethacin is readily absorbed from the gastro-intestinal tract with peak plasma concentrations being reached about 2 hours after a dose. Indomethacin has a half-life of about 4.5 hours and about 99% is bound to plasma proteins. It is metabolised and undergoes enterohepatic circulation. Excretion of indomethacin and metabolites, as glucuronide conjugates, is predominantly in the urine with lesser amounts appearing in the faeces.

The elimination of indomethacin from plasma was biphasic and the half-life of the β-phase (terminal plasma half-life) varied between 2.6 and 11.2 hours.— G. Alvan *et al.*, *Clin. Pharmac. Ther.*, 1975, *18*, 364.

Deschlorobenzoylindomethacin and desmethylindomethacin were inactive metabolites of indomethacin.— W. O. A. Thomas *et al.*, *J. Pharm. Pharmac.*, 1979, *31*, *Suppl.*, 91P.

Uses and Administration

Indomethacin has analgesic, anti-inflammatory, and antipyretic properties; it is an inhibitor of prostaglandin synthetase.

It is used in rheumatic disorders such as ankylosing spondylitis, osteoarthritis, and rheumatoid arthritis, in acute gouty arthritis, and in some other acute musculoskeletal disorders. It may also be used in mild to moderate pain in conditions such as dysmenorrhoea.

The usual initial dose by mouth in rheumatic disorders is 25 mg two or three times daily with food, increased, if required, by 25 to 50 mg daily at weekly intervals to 150 to 200 mg daily. To alleviate night pain and morning stiffness, 100 mg may be administered by mouth, or rectally as a suppository, on retiring. In acute gouty arthritis a suggested dose is 50 mg three times daily and in dysmenorrhoea up to 75 mg daily has been suggested.

Indomethacin may also be used to close a patent ductus arteriosus in premature infants. It is given as a short course of therapy of three intravenous injections given at 12- to 24-hour intervals; each injection should be given over 5 to 10 seconds. The dose of indomethacin given depends upon the age of the neonate and the following have been suggested based upon the age at the first dose: less than 48 hours old, 200 µg per kg body-weight initially followed by two further doses of 100 µg per kg each; 2 to 7 days old, three doses of 200 µg per kg each; over 7 days old, 200 µg per kg initially followed by two further doses of 250 µg per kg each. If, 48 hours after this course of therapy the ductus remains open or re-opens a second course of therapy may be employed, but if this produces no response surgery may be necessary.

ADMINISTRATION IN RENAL FAILURE. A pharmacokinetic study in patients with end-stage renal disease concluding that although indomethacin is dialysable, no dosage adjustment is needed during periods of haemodialysis.— V. A. Skoutakis *et al.*, *Drug Intell. & clin. Pharm.*, 1986, *20*, 956.

BARTTER'S SYNDROME. A discussion of the pathophysiology of Bartter's syndrome and the use of prostaglandin synthetase inhibitors.— J. C. McGiff, *Ann. intern. Med.*, 1977, *87*, 369; S. Vaisrub, *J. Am. med. Ass.*, 1978, *239*, 137.

Indomethacin given in a dose of 7.5 mg daily gradually increased over 4 weeks to 20 mg daily in divided doses produced a beneficial response in a 33-month-old child with Bartter's syndrome.— J. M. Littlewood *et al.* (letter), *Lancet*, 1976, *2*, 795. After 1 year indomethacin was replaced by ketoprofen, gradually increased to 60 mg daily, and the improvement was maintained.— *idem*, *Archs Dis. Childh.*, 1978, *53*, 43.

Further reports on the use of indomethacin in Bartter's syndrome: L. Zancan *et al.* (letter), *Lancet*, 1976, *2*, 1354; P. V. Halushka *et al.*, *Ann. intern. Med.*, 1977, *87*, 281; A. J. M. Donker *et al.*, *Nephron*, 1977, *19*, 200; R. E. Bowden *et al.*, *J. Am. med. Ass.*, 1978, *239*, 117; T. A. Simatupang *et al.*, *Int. J. clin. Pharmac. Biopharm.*, 1978, *16*, 14; J. P. Rado *et al.*, *Int. J. clin. Pharmac. Biopharm.*, 1978, *16*, 22.

FEVER. Indomethacin, 25 to 50 mg every 6 to 8 hours, controlled fever due to Hodgkin's disease within 24 hours in all of 9 patients.— H. R. Silberman *et al.*, *J. Am. med. Ass.*, 1965, *194*, 597.

Indomethacin, 50 mg every 4 hours, controlled fever in 3 patients with Hodgkin's disease. A patient with fever due to acute granulocytic leukaemia was given 100 mg every 4 hours; prompt relief was obtained.— J. M. Kieley, *Mayo Clin. Proc.*, 1969, *44*, 272.

Further references: P. Engervall *et al.*, *Acta med. scand.*, 1986, *219*, 501.

HYPERCALCAEMIA. A brief discussión concerning the use of indomethacin in hypercalcaemia. In certain malignancies (excluding those associated with bony metastasis or parathyroid-hormone-secreting tumour where indomethacin is not effective) a trial of indomethacin may be warranted as high amounts of prostaglandins may have been produced.— G. T. Elliott and M. W. McKenzie, *Drug Intell. & clin. Pharm.*, 1983, *17*, 12.

Indomethacin 2 mg per kg body-weight daily in 4 to 6 divided doses was given to 5 patients with hypercalcaemia secondary to malignancy. There was a rapid reduction in serum-calcium concentration in 1 patient, a gradual fall in 2, and a slight fall in 1. These decreases might have been due to hydration.— A. Dindogru *et al.* (letter), *Lancet*, 1975, *2*, 365.

Further reports on the use of indomethacin in hypercalcaemia.— H. D. Brereton *et al.*, *New Engl. J. Med.*, 1974, *291*, 83; I. Blum (letter), *Lancet*, 1975, *1*, 866.

MALE INFERTILITY. For reference to the possible use of indomethacin in the treatment of male infertility, see J. Barkay *et al.*, *Fert. Steril.*, 1984, *42*, 406.

NEONATAL INTRAVENTRICULAR HAEMORRHAGE. Intraventricular haemorrhage is a well-recognised complication occurring in some extremely premature infants and some workers have investigated whether indomethacin given for patient ductus arteriosus had any effect on this cerebral bleeding. In a randomised study Ment and colleagues (*J. Pediat.*, 1985, *107*, 937) found that indomethacin 100 µg per kg body-weight intravenously every 12 hours for 5 doses resulted in a significant decrease in the incidence of ventricular haemorrhage (6 of 24 in the indomethacin group; 14 of 24 in the placebo group). However, in a similar study Rennie and others (*Archs Dis. Childh.*, 1986, *61*, 233) found no significant difference in the incidence of haemorrhage between infants given indomethacin and placebo.

OCULAR SURGERY. In a double-blind, placebo-controlled study of patients undergoing extracapsular cataract surgery the pre-operative instillation of indomethacin 0.5% eye-drops significantly reduced surgically-induced miosis which occurred despite the use of mydriatic drugs. Indomethacin was thought to act by inhibiting the prostaglandin synthesis caused by irritation of the iris during surgery.— H. C. J. Keulen-de Vos *et al.*, *Br. J. Ophthal.*, 1983, *67*, 94. See also: R. H. Keates and K. A. McGowan, *Ann. Ophthal.*, 1984, *16*, 1116.

OSTEOARTHRITIS. Some references to the use of indomethacin in osteoarthritis.— E. Zachariae, *Nord. Med.*, 1966, *75*, 384; M. Harth and D. C. Bondy, *Can. med. Ass. J.*, 1969, *101*, 311; R. Hodgkinson and D. Woolf, *Practitioner*, 1973, *210*, 392; D. Woolf *et al.*, *ibid.*, 1978, *221*, 791; A. Gordin *et al.*, *Curr. med. Res. Opinion*, 1985, *9*, 500.

PAIN. Some references to the use of indomethacin as an analgesic in various pain conditions: D. Holmlund and J. -G. Sjödin, *J. Urol.*, *Baltimore*, 1978, *120*, 676 (ureteric colic); M. G. Elder and L. Kapadia, *Br. J. Obstet. Gynaec.*, 1979, *86*, 645 (dysmenorrhoea); P. G. Reasbeck *et al.*, *Lancet*, 1982, *2*, 115 (postoperative); M. A. K. Mattila *et al.*, *Br. med. J.*, 1983, *287*, 1026 (postoperative); D. J. M. Keenan *et al.*, *ibid.*, 1335 (postoperative); N. Ebbehøj *et al.*, *Scand. J. Gastroenterol.*, 1985, *20*, 798 (acute pancreatitis); P. -E. Jönsson *et al.*, *Br. J. Urol.*, 1987, *59*, 396 (renal colic).

PATENT DUCTUS ARTERIOSUS. A review and discussion concerning the management of patent ductus arteriosus in premature infants. A major collaborative randomised study in the *US* (W.M. Gersony *et al.*, *J. Pediat.*, 1983, *102*, 895) has shown that there appears to be some merit in using intravenous indomethacin in those infants still with a notable patent ductus arteriosus after 36 to 48 hours of treatment with fluid restriction and diuretics and in whom there are no contra-indications (such as poor renal function, a bleeding tendency, or necrotising enterocolitis) to the use of indomethacin. Probably 25% of those treated with indomethacin will then eventually require surgical closure compared with about 66% if indomethacin is not used. If the ductus remains open after indomethacin therapy early surgical ligation should be undertaken, as good surgical results in the major cardiac centres justify fairly early referral. Although in some small randomised studies (J.M. Rennie *et al.*, *Archs Dis. Childh.*, 1986, *61*, 233) prophylactic administration of indomethacin resulted in a lower incidence of subsequent appreciable shunting, there were more complications, and the overall benefits of indomethacin used prophylactically in this manner must remain speculative.— E. D. Silove, *Archs Dis. Childh.*, 1986, *61*, 827.

Further reports and studies demonstrating a beneficial effect of indomethacin intravenously in premature infants with patent ductus arteriosus: M. L. Rigby *et al.*, *Archs Dis. Childh.*, 1984, *59*, 341; I. J. Smith *et al.*, *ibid.*, 537; M. Mellander *et al.*, *J. Pediat.*, 1984, *105*, 138; G. J. Peckman *et al.*, *ibid.*, 285; L. Mahony *et al.*, *ibid.*, 1985, *106*, 801.

PREGNANCY AND THE NEONATE. See under Neonatal Intraventricular Haemorrhage, Patent Ductus Arteriosus, and Premature Labour.

PREMATURE LABOUR. Indomethacin was given to 50 women with evidence of premature labour. The initial dose was 100 mg as a suppository, followed by 25 mg by mouth every 6 hours up to 24 hours after contractions ceased. Uterine contractions were stopped completely in 40 women. No adverse effects were noted in the infants and 38 mature and 12 premature infants were born. There were 4 neonatal deaths and 1 stillbirth, all in premature infants weighing less than 2000 g.— H. Zuckerman *et al.*, *Obstet. Gynec.*, 1974, *44*, 787.

The administration of nonsteroidal anti-inflammatory drugs (NSAID) to pregnant patients can lead to ductal constriction *in utero* and may lead to problems in establishing pulmonary blood flow after birth. Many obstetricians have changed their policy of using these compounds for delaying pre-term labour. Until more detailed evidence emerges from animal work, pregnancy should be regarded as a contra-indication to administration of NSAID. If there is no other appropriate therapy, then the period of treatment should be kept to a minimum since prolonged exposure seems to increase the hazard.— *Lancet*, 1980, *2*, 185. A view that the hazard of premature closure of the ductus arteriosus by nonsteroidal anti-inflammatory drugs should not rule out their chronic maternal administration in desperate cases of preterm labour.— H. van Kets *et al.* (letter), *ibid.*, 693.

A report on the perinatal outcome in 167 infants exposed to indomethacin used for tocolysis in gestations of less than 35 weeks. Maternal therapy with indomethacin usually consisted of 100 mg administered rectally and repeated after one or two hours if uterine contractions persisted together with 25 mg every 6 hours by mouth for 24 to 48 hours. Pre-term delivery occurred in 69 of the 167 cases (41.3%) and the overall perinatal mortality was 17 per 1000 (1.7%); no cases of premature closure of the ductus arteriosus or persistent foetal circulation were observed. It was considered that these results supported the view of other uncontrolled reports that a short course of indomethacin used for tocolysis in gestations of less than 34 weeks is without deleterious effects on the foetus or neonate. Prospective comparisons of indomethacin with beta-sympathomimetic agents should be undertaken.— D. K. L. Dudley and M. J. Hardie, *Am. J. Obstet. Gynec.*, 1985, *151*, 181. See also: J. R. Niebyl and F. R. Witter, *ibid.*, 1986, *155*, 747.

RENAL DISORDERS. A report of the use of indomethacin to produce medical nephrectomy. A patient with severe nephrotic syndrome, persisting despite terminal renal failure, became anuric shortly after receiving indomethacin; peritoneal dialysis then caused serum-protein values to return to normal. Indomethacin was discontinued after about 2 months and the patient, one year later, remained well still being anuric and maintained on regular haemodialysis. Further studies were needed to define the dosage of indomethacin required to induce a permanent or even a temporary medical nephrectomy and to specify the best indications for such a protocol.— A. Baumelou and M. Legrain, *Br. med. J.*, 1982, *284*, 234.

Beneficial response in 3 children with nephropathic cystinosis to indomethacin. Worthwhile clinical improvement was observed with marked effects on polyuria, polydipsia, and general well-being.— G. B. Haycock *et al.*, *Archs Dis. Childh.*, 1982, *57*, 934.

A report of the successful use of indomethacin to treat hereditary nephrogenic diabetes insipidus in a neonate. The antidiuretic effect of indomethacin resulted in a decrease in urine output, rehydration, and eventually increase in weight gain.— G. H. Rosen *et al.*, *Clin. Pharm.*, 1986, *5*, 254. A similar report of benefit with indomethacin in children.— S. Libber *et al.*, *J. Pediat.*, 1986, *108*, 305.

RHEUMATOID ARTHRITIS. Studies on the use of indomethacin in rheumatoid arthritis.—Report of Cooperating Clinics Committee of the American Rheumatism Association, *Clin. Pharmac. Ther.*, 1967, *8*, 11; P. Donnelly *et al.*, *Br. med. J.*, 1967, *1*, 69; V. Wright *et al.*, *Ann. rheum. Dis.*, 1969, *28*, 157; E. C. Huskisson and F. D. Hart, *Practitioner*, 1972, *208*, 248; N. Baber *et al.*, *Ann. rheum. Dis.*, 1979, *38*, 128; S. D. Deodhar and R. Sethi, *Curr. med. Res. Opinion*, 1979, *6*, 263; R. Ekstrand *et al.*, *Eur. J. clin. Pharmac.*, 1980, *17*, 437.

Preparations

Indomethacin Capsules *(B.P.)*
Indomethacin Capsules *(U.S.P.)*
Indomethacin Extended-release Capsules *(U.S.P.)*
Indomethacin Mixture *(B.P.C. 1973)*. Indomethacin Suspension. The mixture should not be diluted; where necessary doses should be measured in a graduated pipette.
Indomethacin Suppositories *(B.P.)*
Indomethacin Suppositories *(U.S.P.)*

Proprietary Preparations

Artracin *(DDSA Pharmaceuticals, UK)*. *Capsules*, indomethacin 25 and 50 mg.

Flexin Continus *(Napp, UK)*. *Tablets*, controlled-release, scored, indomethacin 75 mg.

Imbrilon *(Berk Pharmaceuticals, UK)*. *Capsules*, indomethacin 25 and 50 mg.
Suppositories, indomethacin 100 mg.

Indocid *(Morson, UK)*. *Capsules*, indomethacin 25 and 50 mg.
Capsules (Indocid R), sustained-release, indomethacin 75 mg.
Suspension, indomethacin 25 mg/5 mL.
Injection (Indocid PDA), indomethacin 1 mg (as sodium trihydrate). *Suppositories*, indomethacin 100 mg.

Indoflex *(Unimed, UK)*. *Capsules*, indomethacin 25 mg.

Indolar SR *(Lagap, UK)*. *Capsules*, sustained-release, indomethacin 75 mg.

Indomod *(Pharmacia, UK)*. *Capsules*, enteric-coated, sustained-release, indomethacin 25 and 75 mg.

Mobilan *(Galen, UK)*. *Capsules*, indomethacin 25 and 50 mg.

Proprietary Names and Manufacturers

Agilex *(Arg.)*; Algometacin *(Ital.)*; Amuno *(Chibret, Ger.; Merck Sharp & Dohme, Ger.)*; Arthrexin *(Alphapharm, Austral.; Lennon, S.Afr.)*; Articulen *(Rolab, S.Afr.)*; Artracin *(DDSA Pharmaceuticals, UK)*; Artrinovo *(Llorens, Spain)*; Artrivia *(Spain)*; Artrobase *(Ital.)*; Artrocid *(Rhone-Poulenc, Ital.)*; Boutycin *(Bouty, Ital.)*; Chrono-indocid *(Merck Sharp & Dohme-Chibret, Fr.)*; Cidalgon *(Ecobi, Ital.)*; Confortid *(Denm.; Dumex, Norw.; Dumex, Swed.; Dumex, Switz.)*; Durametacin *(Durachemie, Ger.)*; Elmetacin *(Luitpold, Switz.)*; Flamecid *(Bovit, S.Afr.)*; Flexin Continus *(Napp, UK)*; Flogoter *(Estedi, Spain)*;
IM-75 *(Arg.)*; Imbrilon *(Berk Pharmaceuticals, UK)*; Imet *(FIRMA, Ital.)*; Inacid *(Merck Sharp & Dohme, Spain)*; Indacin *(Jpn)*; Indium *(Ital.)*; Indocid *(Arg.; Merck Sharp & Dohme, Austral.; Belg.; Merck Sharp & Dohme, Canad.; Merck Sharp & Dohme, Denm.; Merck Sharp & Dohme-Chibret, Fr.; Ital.; Neth.; Merck Sharp & Dohme, Norw.; Merck Sharp & Dohme, S.Afr.; Merck Sharp & Dohme, Switz.; Morson, UK; Merck Sharp & Dohme, USA)*; Indocin *(Merck Sharp & Dohme, USA)*; Indoflex *(Unimed, UK)*; Indoftol *(Merck Sharp & Dohme, Spain)*; Indolar *(Lagap, UK)*; Indo-Lemmon *(Lemmon, USA)*; Indolgina *(Uriach, Spain)*; Indomee *(MSD, Swed.)*; Indomet *(Ketelhack Riker, Ger.)*; Indomod *(Pharmacia, UK)*; Indo-Phlogont *(Azuchemie, Ger.)*; Indoptic *(Chibret, Switz.)*; Indorektal *(Beiersdorf, Ger.)*; Indotard *(Benzon, Denm.)*; Indoxen *(Sigmatau, Ital.)*; Indren *(Cz.)*; Infrocin *(Col.)*;
Liometacen *(Chiesi, Ital.)*; Mederreumol *(Medea, Spain)*; Metacen *(Chiesi, Ital.)*; Metartril *(Ital.)*; Methabid *(Pharmador, S.Afr.)*; Mobilan *(Galen, UK)*; Neo-Decabutin *(Bicther, Spain)*; Novomethacin *(Novopharm, Canad.)*; Osmosin *(Merck Sharp & Dohme, UK)*; Peralgon *(Sarm, Ital.)*; Reusin *(Alfarma, Spain)*; Rheumacin *(Protea, Austral.)*; Rheumacin LA *(Generics, UK)*; Sadoreum *(Giustini, Ital.)*; Slo-Indo *(Generics, UK)*; Tannex *(Duncan, Flockhart, UK)*; Vonum *(Kanoldt, Ger.)*.

2659-b

Indoprofen *(BAN, USAN, rINN)*.

Isindone; K-4277. 2-[4-(1-Oxoisoindolin-2-yl)phenyl]propionic acid.
$C_{17}H_{15}NO_3$=281.3.

CAS — 31842-01-0.

Indoprofen has analgesic and anti-inflammatory properties and was formerly given by mouth in rheumatic disorders. Following reports of adverse reactions including reports of carcinogenicity in *animal* studies it was withdrawn from the market worldwide.

Proprietary Names and Manufacturers

Flosint *(Montedison, Arg.; Carlo Erba, Ital.; Chemfarma, S.Afr.; Farmitalia Carlo Erba, UK)*.

12870-d

Isonixin *(rINN)*.

2-Hydroxy-*N*-(2,6-dimethylphenyl)nicotinamide.
$C_{14}H_{14}N_2O_2$=242.3.

CAS — 57021-61-1.

Isonixin has analgesic and anti-inflammatory properties and has been used in rheumatic disorders in doses of 200 to 400 mg three or four times daily by mouth.

Proprietary Names and Manufacturers

Nixyn *(Organon, Spain)*; Nixyn Hermes *(Organon, Spain)*.

12872-h

Isoxepac *(BAN, USAN, rINN)*.

HP-549; P-720549. 6,11-Dihydro-11-oxodibenz[*b,e*]oxepin-2-ylacetic acid.
$C_{16}H_{12}O_4$=268.3.

CAS — 55453-87-7.

Isoxepac has been studied for its analgesic and anti-inflammatory properties.

Some references to isoxepac: L. S. Gerlis and J. M. Gumpel, *Rheumatol. Rehabil.*, 1981, *20*, 50 (rheumatoid arthritis); J. Scott and E. C. Huskisson, *ibid.*, 1982, *21*, 48 (rheumatoid arthritis); W. J. Honig *et al.*, *J. clin. Pharmac.*, 1982, *22*, 82 (postmeniscectomy pain).

Proprietary Names and Manufacturers

Hoechst, UK.

12873-m

Isoxicam *(BAN, USAN, rINN)*.

W-8495. 4-Hydroxy-2-methyl-*N*-(5-methylisoxazol-3-yl)-2*H*-1,2-benzothiazine-3-carboxamide 1,1-dioxide.
$C_{14}H_{13}N_3O_5S$=335.3.

CAS — 34552-84-6.

Isoxicam has analgesic, anti-inflammatory, and antipyretic properties. It has been given in rheumatic disorders such as rheumatoid arthritis and osteoarthritis in doses of 200 mg once daily by mouth but following reports of fatal skin reactions including phototoxicity, toxic epidermal necrolysis (Lyell's syndrome), and the Stevens-Johnson syndrome the manufacturers voluntarily suspended marketing worldwide.

A report of fatal toxic epidermal necrolysis attributed to isoxicam.— M. L. Fléchet *et al.* (letter), *Lancet*, 1985, *2*, 499.

The worldwide marketing of isoxicam was voluntarily suspended by the manufacturer following reports, mainly from France, of rare, but serious, vesiculo-bullous skin reactions. Investigations, particularly in France and Germany, attempting to clarify the relationship between the use of isoxicam and the occurrence of Lyell's syndrome have revealed a striking difference between the frequency in the two countries. It appears that a by-product generated in trace amounts during the synthesis of the isoxicam used in France may have been a key factor in the production of the skin reactions. It is anticipated that these findings may serve as a basis for re-establishing the availability of isoxicam.— C. F. George, *Br. J. clin. Pharmac.*, 1986, *22*, *Suppl.* 2, 107S.

Isoxicam: the evolving perspective. A series of papers presented at a symposium in May 1985.— *Br. J. clin. Pharmac.*, 1986, *22*, *Suppl.* 2, 107S-189S.

Proprietary Names and Manufacturers

Maxicam *(Parke, Davis, Philipp.)*; Pacyl *(Adenylchemie, Ger.)*; Vectren *(Substantia, Fr.)*.

2661-r

Kebuzone *(pINN).*
Ketophenylbutazone. 4-(3-Oxobutyl)-1,2-diphenylpyrazolidine-3,5-dione.
$C_{19}H_{18}N_2O_3$=322.4.

CAS — 853-34-9.

Pharmacopoeias. In *Cz.*

Kebuzone has analgesic and anti-inflammatory properties. It has been used in rheumatic disorders in doses of up to 1.2 g daily, in divided doses, by mouth.

Proprietary Names and Manufacturers
Chebutan *(Bioindustria, Ital.)*; Chepirol *(Esterfarm, Ital.)*; Chetopir *(Sarm, Ital.)*; Chetosol *(Ital.)*; Ejor *(Elea, Arg.)*; Gammachetone *(Tiber, Ital.)*; Kétazone *(Beytout, Fr.)*; Neo-Panalgyl *(Ital Suisse, Ital.)*; Neufenil *(Jpn).*

2662-f

Ketoprofen *(BAN, USAN, rINN).*

RP-19583. 2-(3-Benzoylphenyl)propionic acid.
$C_{16}H_{14}O_3$=254.3.

CAS — 22071-15-4.

Pharmacopoeias. In *Br.*

A white or almost white, odourless or almost odourless, crystalline powder. Practically **insoluble** in water; freely soluble in alcohol, chloroform, and ether.

Adverse Effects and Precautions

As for ibuprofen, p.20.

In an open study, ketoprofen caused side-effects requiring withdrawal of treatment in 256 of 4727 patients with rheumatic disorders. Gastro-intestinal effects occurred in 225 patients, including melaena/haematemesis in 7; also central nervous (37 patients), cardiovascular (2), and other side-effects (22). Side-effects not requiring withdrawal occurred in 665 of 4107 patients completing the study.— J. Mason and M. S. Bolton, *Br. J. clin. Pract.*, 1977, *31*, 127.

A report of the adverse effects observed during an extensive multicentre general practice study involving about 15 000 patients given ketoprofen as a controlled-delivery capsule.— G. G. De Bono and M. Pearlgood, *Br. J. clin. Pract.*, 1986, *40*, 421.

ALLERGY. Life-threatening asthma, urticaria, and angioneurotic oedema developed in 2 aspirin-sensitive patients after taking ketoprofen 50 mg by mouth.— P. Frith *et al.* (letter), *Lancet*, 1978, *2*, 847.

EFFECTS ON THE BLOOD. Mention of 1 case of fatal aplastic anaemia or agranulocytosis in one year probably due to ketoprofen.— W. H. W. Inman, *Br. med. J.*, 1977, *1*, 1500.

EFFECTS ON THE ELECTROLYTES. A 7-year-old girl with Bartter's syndrome developed symptoms attributable to pseudomotor cerebri after treatment with ketoprofen 20 mg per kg body-weight daily for 15 days. Retention of sodium and water, probably secondary to prostaglandin inhibition, was considered responsible.— D. Larizza *et al.* (letter), *New Engl. J. Med.*, 1979, *300*, 796.

EFFECTS ON THE EYES. A 45-year-old Nigerian woman with amyloidosis, twice developed painful swollen eyes with redness, on administration of ketoprofen.— E. M. Umez-Eronini (letter), *Lancet*, 1978, *2*, 737.

INTERACTIONS. For the effect of ketoprofen on methotrexate, see p.638.

MYASTHENIA GRAVIS. A brief report of a single dose of ketoprofen 50 mg by mouth precipitating a cholinergic crisis in a patient with well-controlled myasthenia gravis.— I. F. W. McDowell and J. B. McConnell, *Br. med. J.*, 1985, *291*, 1094.

PHOTOSENSITIVITY. Ketoprofen had been reported to cause photosensitivity reactions.— *Med. Lett.*, 1986, *28*, 51.

Absorption and Fate

Ketoprofen is readily absorbed from the gastro-intestinal tract; peak plasma concentrations occur about 0.5 to 1 hour after a dose. The plasma half-life is about 1 to 3 hours. Ketoprofen is extensively bound to plasma proteins. It is metabolised mainly by conjugation with glucuronic acid, and is excreted in the urine and to a lesser extent in the faeces.

Some references to the pharmacokinetics of ketoprofen: T. Ishizaki *et al.*, *Eur. J. clin. Pharmac.*, 1980, *18*, 407 (after oral, intramuscular, and rectal administration); J. D. McCrea *et al.*, *Curr. med. Res. Opinion*, 1986, *10*, 73 (plasma and synovial fluid profiles after controlled-release formulations); D. Debruyne *et al.*, *Clin. Pharmacokinet.*, 1987, *12*, 214 (after intravenous administration); M. Ollagnier *et al.*, *ibid.*, 367 (influence of circadian rhythm).

Uses and Administration

Ketoprofen has analgesic, anti-inflammatory, and antipyretic properties; it is an inhibitor of prostaglandin synthetase.

Ketoprofen is used in rheumatic disorders such as ankylosing spondylitis, osteoarthritis, and rheumatoid arthritis, in other various non-rheumatoid musculoskeletal and joint disorders, and in mild to moderate pain such as dysmenorrhoea. The usual dose by mouth is 50 to 100 mg twice daily with food; controlled-release formulations taken once daily may also be used. Ketoprofen may also be administered rectally as suppositories in a usual dose of 100 mg at night.

Ketoprofen has also been used both orally and topically as the lysinate.

Reviews of the actions and uses of ketoprofen.— *Med. Lett.*, 1986, *28*, 61.

ADMINISTRATION. *Controlled-release formulations.* Studies comparing the efficacy of controlled-release preparations with standard formulations of ketoprofen.— K. D. Morley *et al.*, *Curr. med. Res. Opinion*, 1984, *9*, 28; R. Marcolongo *et al.*, *Curr. ther. Res.*, 1984, *35*, 721; M. Teule, *ibid.*, 1986, *40*, 1129.

ADMINISTRATION IN THE ELDERLY. Pharmacokinetic data suggesting that controlled-release ketoprofen may be administered in standard doses (200 mg once daily) to elderly patients. A reduction in dosage should only be necessary in the presence of severe renal failure (creatinine clearance less than 20 mL per minute) or of liver disease.— M. J. Dennis *et al.*, *Br. J. clin. Pharmac.*, 1985, *20*, 567.

ANKYLOSING SPONDYLITIS. Some references to the use of ketoprofen in ankylosing spondylitis.— B. L. Treadwell and J. M. Tweed, *N.Z. med. J.*, 1975, *81*, 411; J. D. Jessop, *Rheumatol. Rehabil.*, 1976, *Suppl.*, 37.

OSTEOARTHRITIS. Some references to the use of ketoprofen in osteoarthritis: G. Fava *et al.*, *J. int. med. Res.*, 1977, *5*, 301; R. Franchi *et al.*, *Scand. J. Rheumatol.*, 1979, *Suppl.* 26, 1; J. Goulton, *Br. J. clin. Pract.*, 1979, *33*, 26.

PAIN. Some references to the use of ketoprofen in various pain syndromes: S. Gleeson and J. Sorbie, *Can. med. Ass. J.*, 1983, *129*, 842 (dysmenorrhoea); T. Kantor *et al.*, *J. clin. Pharmac.*, 1984, *24*, 228 (postpartum pain); D. Mehlisch *et al.*, *ibid.*, 486 (postoperative dental pain); G. Sacchetti *et al.*, *Drug Intell. & clin. Pharm.*, 1984, *18*, 403 (cancer pain); A. Himendra *et al.*, *Curr. med. Res. Opinion*, 1985, *9*, 436 (postoperative pain); M. Magrini *et al.*, *ibid.*, 454 (biliary colic); J.-G. Hébert, *Clin. Ther.*, 1986, *8*, 329 (dysmenorrhoea); D. Debruyne *et al.*, *Clin. Pharmacokinet.*, 1987, *12*, 214 (renal colic).

RHEUMATOID ARTHRITIS. Some references to the use of ketoprofen in rheumatoid arthritis: B. J. Cathcart *et al.*, *Ann. rheum. Dis.*, 1973, *32*, 62; S. B. Mills *et al.*, *Br. med. J.*, 1973, *4*, 82; D. W. Zutshi, *Rheumatol. Rehabil.*, 1973, *12*, 62; J. Chabot *et al.*, *Thérapie*, 1974, *29*, 417; M. Viara *et al.*, *Eur. J. clin. Pharmac.*, 1975, *8*, 205; E. F. El-Ghobarey *et al.*, *Curr. med. Res. Opinion*, 1976, *4*, 432; A. Calin *et al.*, *J. Rheumatol.*, 1977, *4*, 153; D. L. G. Howard, *Curr. ther. Res.*, 1978, *23*, 678; D. L. G. Howard, *J. int. med. Res.*, 1978, *6*, 300; J. Goulton and P. G. Baker, *Curr. med. Res. Opinion*, 1980, *6*, 423.

Preparations

Ketoprofen Capsules *(B.P.)*

Proprietary Preparations

Alrheumat *(Bayer, UK). Capsules*, ketoprofen 50 mg.
Orudis *(May & Baker, UK). Capsules*, ketoprofen 50 and 100 mg.
Suppositories, ketoprofen 100 mg.
Oruvail *(May & Baker, UK). Capsules*, sustained-release, ketoprofen 100 and 200 mg.

Proprietary Names and Manufacturers of Ketoprofen and its Salts
Alreumat *(Bayer, Denm.; Bayer, Swed.)*; Alreumun *(Arg.)*; Alrheumat *(Bayer, Swed.; Bayer, UK)*; Alrheumun *(Bayropharm, Ger.)*; Alrhumat *(Belg.; Switz.)*; Anaus *(Arg.)*; Arcental *(Spain)*; Artrosilene *(Dompè, Ital.)*; Bi-profenid *(Specia, Fr.)*; Capisten *(Jpn)*; Dexal *(Pulitzer, Ital.)*; Fastum *(Menarini, Ital.; Menarini, Spain)*; Flexen *(Lifepharma, Ital.)*; Iso-K *(San Carlo, Ital.)*; Kefenid *(SIT, Ital.)*; Ketalgin *(IBP, Ital.)*; Ketangel *(Angelini, Ital.)*; Ketartrium *(Esseti, Ital.)*; Keto *(Sigurtà, Ital.)*; Ketoartril *(IBYS, Spain)*; Ketofen *(Del Saz & Filippini, Ital.)*; Ketoprosil *(Liberman, Spain)*; Ketosolan *(Spyfarma, Spain)*; Kevadon *(Arg.)*; Lertus *(Arg.)*; Meprofen *(AGIPS, Ital.)*; Orudis *(May & Baker, Austral.; Rhône-Poulenc, Canad.; Rhone-Poulenc, Denm.; Rhône-Poulenc, Ger.; Farmitalia, Ital.; Jpn; Rhône-Poulenc, Norw.; May & Baker, S.Afr.; Rhone, Spain; Leo Rhodia, Swed.; May & Baker, UK; Wyeth, USA)*; Oruvail *(May & Baker, S.Afr.; May & Baker, UK)*; Profenid *(Arg.; Specia, Fr.; Rhone-Poulenc, Switz.)*; Profenil *(Lampugnani, Ital.)*; Remauric *(Spain)*; Reumoquin *(Inkey, Spain)*; Reuprofen *(Zoja, Ital.)*; Rofenid *(Belg.)*; Salient *(Biomedica Foscama, Ital.)*; Sinketol *(Locatelli, Ital.)*; Tafirol *(Tafir, Spain)*; Wasserprofen *(Wasserman, Spain).*

19403-g

Lefetamine *(pINN).*
(−)-*N*,*N*-Dimethyl-1,2-diphenylethylamine.
$C_{16}H_{19}N$=225.3.

CAS — 7262-75-1.

Lefetamine has analgesic properties and has been given in doses of up to 100 mg daily, in divided doses, by mouth.

Proprietary Names and Manufacturers
Santenol *(Coop. Farm., Ital.)*; Spa *(Santen, Jpn).*

2663-d

Lithium Salicylate

$C_7H_5LiO_3$=144.1.

CAS — 552-38-5.

Pharmacopoeias. In *Fr.* and *Span.*

Lithium salicylate has properties resembling those of sodium salicylate (see p.42) and has been used in rheumatic disorders. Its use cannot be recommended because of the pharmacological effect of the lithium ion.

12902-z

Lonazolac *(rINN).*
3-(4-Chlorophenyl)-1-phenylpyrazol-4-ylacetic acid.
$C_{17}H_{13}ClN_2O_2$=312.8.

CAS — 53808-88-1.

Lonazolac has analgesic and anti-inflammatory properties. It has been used, as the calcium salt, in rheumatic disorders in usual doses of up to 600 mg daily, in divided doses, by mouth.

Proprietary Names and Manufacturers
Argun L *(Merckle, Ger.)*; Arthro Akut *(Tosse, Ger.)*; Irritren *(Tosse, Ger.; Byk Gulden, Switz.).*

2664-n

Magnesium Salicylate *(USAN).*

$C_{14}H_{10}MgO_6,4H_2O$=370.6.

CAS — 18917-89-0 (anhydrous); 6150-94-3; 18917-95-8 (both tetrahydrate).

Pharmacopoeias. In *U.S.*

Store in airtight containers.

Magnesium salicylate has similar properties to aspirin (p.3). It is used in rheumatic disorders in usual doses equivalent to 1 g of salicylate three times daily by mouth.

Preparations

Magnesium Salicylate Tablets *(U.S.P.)*

Proprietary Names and Manufacturers

Analate *(Winston, USA)*; Arthrin *(Saron, USA)*; Causalin *(Amfre-Grant, USA)*; Efficin *(Adria, USA)*; Magan *(Adria, USA)*; Mobidin *(Ascher, USA)*; Triact *(Misemer, USA).*

The following names have been used for multi-ingredient preparations containing magnesium salicylate— Magsal *(US Pharmaceutical, USA)*; Mobigesic *(Ascher, USA).*

2717-r

Meclofenamic Acid *(BAN, USAN, rINN).*

CI-583; INF-4668. *N*-(2,6-Dichloro-*m*-tolyl)anthranilic acid.

$C_{14}H_{11}Cl_2NO_2$=296.2.

CAS — 644-62-2.

Pharmacopoeias. In *B.P. Vet.*

A white or almost white odourless crystalline powder. Practically **insoluble** in water; slightly soluble in alcohol and chloroform; sparingly soluble in ether.

2665-h

Meclofenamate Sodium *(BANM, USAN, rINNM).*

$C_{14}H_{10}Cl_2NNaO_2,H_2O$=336.1.

CAS — 6385-02-0.

Pharmacopoeias. In *U.S.*

A white to creamy white, odourless to almost odourless, crystalline powder. Freely **soluble** in water, the solution sometimes being somewhat turbid due to partial hydrolysis and absorption of carbon dioxide; soluble in methyl alcohol; slightly soluble in chloroform; practically insoluble in ether. **Store** in airtight containers. Protect from light.

Adverse Effects

As for mefenamic acid, below.

The commonest adverse effect in 2500 patients who received meclofenamate sodium in double-blind or long-term studies was gastro-intestinal disturbance. Diarrhoea occurred in 11.2% of patients in double-blind studies and 32.8% of patients in long-term studies (up to 3 years). Ulcers were detected in 22 patients during therapy and skin rashes occurred in 4% of patients. Transient increases in serum aminotransferases and BUN occurred in some patients.— S. N. Preston, *Curr. ther. Res.*, 1978, *23, Suppl.* 4S, S107.

EFFECTS ON THE BLOOD. *Agranulocytosis.* Agranulocytosis and suppression of erythropoiesis in one patient associated with the use of meclofenamate sodium.— A. J. Wishner and P. B. Milburn (letter), *J. Am. Acad. Derm.*, 1985, *13*, 1052.

Thrombocytopenia. Thrombocytopenia in an elderly patient associated with meclofenamate therapy.— J. Rodriguez (letter), *Drug Intell. & clin. Pharm.*, 1981, *15*, 999.

Precautions

As for ibuprofen, p.20.

Absorption and Fate

Meclofenamate sodium is readily absorbed when given by mouth; the free acid is absorbed more slowly. Peak plasma concentrations occur about 0.5 to 1 hour after ingestion of the sodium salt. Meclofenamic acid is over 99% bound to plasma proteins. The mean biological half-life of meclofenamate sodium is about 3 hours. It is metabolised by oxidation, hydroxylation, dehalogenation, and conjugation with glucuronic acid and excreted in urine mainly as metabolites. About 20 to 30% is recovered in the faeces.

Studies on the absorption and fate of sodium meclofenamate.— A. J. Glazko *et al.*, *Curr. ther. Res.*, 1978, *23, Suppl.* 4S, S22.

Uses and Administration

Meclofenamate sodium is an anthranilic acid derivative similar to mefenamic acid. It has analgesic, anti-inflammatory, and antipyretic properties; it is an inhibitor of prostaglandin synthetase. It is used in osteoarthritis and rheumatoid arthritis in doses equivalent to 200 to 400 mg daily of meclofenamic acid; daily doses are usually given in 3 to 4 divided doses.

The proceedings of a symposium on meclofenamate sodium.— *Curr. ther. Res.*, 1978, *23, Suppl.* 4S, S1–S152.

Further reviews: *Med. Lett.*, 1980, *22*, 111.

CEREBRAL OEDEMA. Evidence from *animal* studies and clinical use in one patient that meclofenamate sodium may be worth investigating for the reduction of cerebral and CNS oedema.— J. L. Ambrus *et al* (letter), *Lancet*, 1985, *2*, 148.

OSTEOARTHRITIS. Some references to the use of meclofenamate sodium in osteoarthritis: R. Willkens, *Curr. ther. Res.*, 1978, *23, Suppl.* 4S, S81; I. Schleyer, *ibid.*, S121.

RENAL DISORDERS. A patient who had lost his first renal transplant due to recurrence of corticosteroid-resistant idiopathic nephrotic syndrome obtained control of the disease in the second transplant by administration of meclofenamate 25 mg by mouth twice daily initially, progressively increased to 50 mg six times daily. An original initial dose of 50 mg every 6 hours had produced worsening of the oedema, despite the administration of frusemide. During the 2½ years of meclofenamate therapy the dose of methylprednisolone has been tapered from 20 to 8 mg daily without difficulty. Because of the potential side-effects of meclofenamate careful supervision is recommended.— V. E. Torres *et al.*, *Mayo Clin. Proc.*, 1984, *59*, 146. Comment.— C. F. Anderson, *ibid.*, 206. Further references: J. A. Velosa *et al.*, *ibid.*, 1985, *60*, 586.

RHEUMATOID ARTHRITIS. Some references to the use of meclofenamate sodium in rheumatoid arthritis: J. A. N. Rennie *et al.*, *Curr. med. Res. Opinion*, 1977, *4*, 580; J. Zuckner *et al.*, *Curr. ther. Res.*, 1978, *23, Suppl.* 4S, S66; C. V. Multz *et al.*, *ibid.*, S72; R. Wolf, *ibid.*, S113; E. M. Grace *et al.*, *Curr. med. Res. Opinion*, 1983, *8*, 417.

Preparations

Meclofenamate Sodium Capsules *(U.S.P.)*

Proprietary Names and Manufacturers of Meclofenamic Acid and Meclofenamate Sodium

Meclomen *(Warner, S.Afr.*; *Parke, Davis, Spain*; *Parke, Davis, Switz.*; *Parke, Davis, USA)*; Movens *(Inverni della Beffa, Ital.).*

2666-m

Mefenamic Acid *(BAN, USAN, rINN).*

CI-473; INF-3355. *N*-(2,3-Xylyl)anthranilic acid.

$C_{15}H_{15}NO_2$=241.3.

CAS — 61-68-7.

Pharmacopoeias. In *Br.* and *Jpn.*

A white to greyish-white, odourless or almost odourless, microcrystalline powder. Practically **insoluble** in water; slightly soluble in alcohol and chloroform; sparingly soluble in ether. **Store** in a well-closed container.

Adverse Effects

The commonest adverse effects occurring with mefenamic acid are gastro-intestinal disturbances. Peptic ulceration and gastro-intestinal bleeding have also been reported. Headache, drowsiness, dizziness, nervousness, and visual disturbances have been reported. There may be hypersensitivity reactions including skin rashes and urticaria, and occasionally allergic glomerulonephritis; asthma may be precipitated. Reported haematological effects include haemolytic anaemia, agranulocytosis, pancytopenia, thrombocytopenia or thrombocytopenic purpura, and bone-marrow aplasia.

Therapy should be discontinued if diarrhoea or skin rash occur.

A detailed review of the side-effects of mefenamic acid, flufenamic acid, and niflumic acid. Reports from different workers were very variable but although the side-effects were mainly gastro-intestinal a striking number of skin reactions were noted.— J. Strauss *et al.*, *Thérapie*, 1976, *31*, 325.

EFFECTS ON THE BLOOD. *Haemolytic anaemia.* Three patients who had taken mefenamic acid (1.5 g daily in 2 patients) for 1 to 2 years developed auto-immune haemolytic anaemia during therapy and all recovered completely and rapidly when the drug was withdrawn.— G. L. Scott *et al.*, *Br. med. J.*, 1968, *3*, 534.

Haemolytic anaemia in one patient attributed to mefenamic acid, though the possibility that gold had a combined or synergistic effect with mefenamic acid could not be excluded.— J. M. Jackson *et al.* (letter), *Br. med. J.*, 1970, *2*, 297.

A further report of auto-immune haemolytic anaemia induced by mefenamic acid.— J. -J. Farquet *et al.*, *Schweiz. med. Wschr.*, 1978, *108*, 1510.

Leucopenia. A report of 5 cases of symptomless leucopenia associated with mefenamic acid encountered over a six-month period of study.— A. Burns and R. E. Young (letter), *Lancet*, 1984, *2*, 46.

EFFECTS ON THE GASTRO-INTESTINAL TRACT. Reversible steatorrhoea occurred in a 65-year-old man who had been taking mefenamic acid 250 mg three times daily for about 2 years. Diarrhoea ceased 2 days after stopping mefenamic acid and the faecal fat output was normal 2 weeks later.— J. S. Marks and M. H. Gleeson, *Br. med. J.*, 1975, *4*, 442. Two further cases.— R. G. Chadwick *et al.* (letter), *ibid.*, 1976, *1*, 397.

Acute colitis in 2 patients associated with the use of mefenamic acid.— R. I. Hall *et al.*, *Br. med. J.*, 1983, *287*, 1182. Further reports of enteritis and colitis associated with the use of mefenamic acid.— M. S. Phillips *et al.* (letter), *ibid.*, 1626; A. L. Edwards *et al.* (letter), *ibid*; D. S. Rampton and P. J. Tapping (letter), *ibid.*, 1627; R. Williams and G. Glazer (letter), *ibid*; S. Ravi *et al.*, *Postgrad. med. J.*, 1986, *62*, 773.

EFFECTS ON THE KIDNEYS. Six elderly women who had been prescribed mefenamic acid 1 to 2 g daily for 2 to 6 weeks developed non-oliguric renal failure. Five of the women were admitted to hospital with a history of anorexia, nausea, and diarrhoea, followed by polyuria and dehydration; the sixth had received mefenamic acid after in-patient eye surgery, and had suffered nausea and vomiting, and polyuria. Four of the 6 patients also had rashes. Only one patient was known to have mild chronic renal failure; the remaining 5 had no history of renal disease, but 2 had maturity-onset diabetes well-controlled by diet alone, 2 had taken aspirin for many years, and 2 were taking diuretics; one patient had received tetracycline empirically one day before admission for urinary frequency. All made an uneventful recovery after intravenous fluid and electrolyte replacement, but renal function tests 2 to 4 weeks after admission showed persistent impairment of urinary concentrating ability and creatinine clearance, and at subsequent follow-up only 2 patients regained normal renal function; renal function remaining abnormal for their age in the other 4. Since mefenamic acid does not seem to have any advantage over other analgesics, and diarrhoea is a common side-effect, it is probably best avoided in the elderly and in patients with dehydration or pre-existing renal disease.— C. E. Robertson *et al.*, *Lancet*, 1980, *2*, 232. A report of allergic interstitial nephritis following mefenamic acid ingestion.— V. Venning *et al.* (letter), *ibid.*, 745. A report of a patient who developed glomerulonephritis with widespread vasculitis possibly associated with mefenamic acid.— S. Malik *et al.* (letter), *ibid.*, 746.

Non-oliguric renal failure, recurring on later inadvertent challenge, associated with the use of mefenamic acid.— P. L. Drury *et al.*, *Br. med. J.*, 1981, *282*, 865.

Further references: K. L. Woods and J. Michael (letter), *Br. med. J.*, 1981, *282*, 1471 (interstitial nephritis); L. R. I. Baker *et al.* (letter), *Postgrad. med. J.*, 1984, *60*, 82 (interstitial nephritis and renal failure); A. Taha *et al.*, *Br. med. J.*, 1985, *291*, 661 (non-oliguric renal failure).

EFFECTS ON THE LIVER. Mefenamic acid was associated with hepatitis in 1 patient.— S. Imoto *et al.* (letter), *Ann. intern. Med.*, 1979, *91*, 129.

EFFECTS ON THE NERVOUS SYSTEM. Extrapyramidal symptoms in a patient possibly induced by mefenamic acid.— A. Cremona-Barbaro (letter), *J. R. Soc. Med.*, 1983, *76*, 435.

Hyperacusis (severe hypersensitivity to noise) together with less severe symptoms of tinnitus and vertigo reported in association with mefenamic acid therapy.— D. L. Morris and A. Fletcher (letter), *Br. med. J.*, 1986, *293*, 823.

See also under Overdosage (below).

EFFECTS ON THE PANCREAS. Acute pancreatitis in one patient apparently precipitated by a course of mefenamic acid.— A. A. van Walraven *et al.* (letter), *Can. med. Ass. J.*, 1982, *126*, 894.

EFFECTS ON THE SKIN. Bullous pemphigoid, together with haemolytic anaemia and diarrhoea, in a patient and related to the use of mefenamic acid.— A. N. Shepherd *et al.*, *Postgrad. med. J.*, 1986, *62*, 67.

Fixed drug eruptions in 2 patients associated with the use of mefenamic acid.— C. L. Wilson and A. Otter (letter), *Br. med. J.*, 1986, *293*, 1243.

OVERDOSAGE. A short review of poisonings after overdosage with mefenamic acid.— H. Court and G. N. Volans, *Adverse Drug React. Ac. Pois. Rev.*, 1984, *3*, 1.

A report of status epilepticus in a 19-year-old woman 3 hours after the ingestion of mefenamic acid 12.5 g.— R. J. Young (letter), *Br. med. J.*, 1979, *2*, 672. Single convulsions occurred in 2 adolescent girls who had taken 25 or 50 g of mefenamic acid; plasma concentrations of mefenamic acid were 110 and 72 μg per mL compared with expected therapeutic concentrations of less than 10 μg per mL.— R. H. Robson *et al.* (letter), *Br. med. J.*, 1979, *2*, 1438. A report on the hazard of convulsions in patients with an overdose of mefenamic acid. Mefenamic acid should probably be avoided in epileptic patients.— M. Balali-Mood *et al.*, *Lancet*, 1981, *1*, 1354. Comment by the manufacturers that the suggestion that mefenamic acid should be avoided in patients with epilepsy cannot be accepted.— R. S. Kingswell (letter), *ibid.*, *2*, 307. A reply stating that grand mal convulsions were found in more than one-third of patients with a confirmed mefenamic acid overdosage and recent experience has shown that convulsions in poisoned patients are more likely to be due to mefenamic acid than to any other group of drugs.— L. F. Prescott *et al.* (letter), *ibid.*, 418.

Coma followed by grand mal convulsions in a case of mefenamic acid poisoning.— H. Gössinger *et al.* (letter), *Lancet*, 1982, *2*, 384.

Studies in healthy subjects indicating that early administration of charcoal in the ratio of 5 g to each 1 g of mefenamic acid ingested may be of value in reducing the toxicity of mefenamic acid after overdosage.— N. El-Bahie *et al.*, *Br. J. clin. Pharmac.*, 1985, *19*, 836.

Precautions

Mefenamic acid is contra-indicated in patients with peptic ulceration or inflammatory bowel disease. It should be used with caution in patients with impaired renal or liver function. It may enhance the effects of the coumarin anticoagulants.

Mefenamic acid has a marked tendency to induce tonic-clonic (grand mal) convulsions in overdosage; some sources have suggested that it should be avoided in epileptic subjects.

PORPHYRIA. Mefenamic acid was considered to be unsafe in patients with acute porphyria although there is conflicting experimental evidence on porphyrinogenicity.— M.R. Moore and K.E.L. McColl, *Porphyrias, Drug Lists*, Glasgow, Porphyria Research Unit, University of Glasgow, 1987.

Absorption and Fate

Mefenamic acid is absorbed from the gastro-intestinal tract. Peak plasma concentrations occur about 2 to 4 hours after ingestion. The half-life is reported to be 2 hours. Mefenamic acid is extensively bound to plasma proteins. Approximately 50% of a dose may be recovered in the urine within 48 hours, mainly as conjugated metabolites.

PREGNANCY AND THE NEONATE. Mefenamic acid given to nursing mothers was found in the breast milk in very small quantities.— R. A. Buchanan *et al.*, *Curr. ther. Res.*, 1968, *10*, 592.

Uses and Administration

Mefenamic acid has analgesic, anti-inflammatory, and antipyretic properties; it is an inhibitor of prostaglandin synthetase.

It is used for the relief of mild to moderate pain including headache, dental pain, postoperative and postpartum pain, and dysmenorrhoea; it is also used in rheumatic disorders such as osteoarthritis and rheumatoid arthritis. Mefenamic acid may also be used in menorrhagia. The usual dose by mouth is 500 mg three times daily. A suggested dose for children with Still's disease is 25 mg per kg body-weight daily in divided doses. Mefenamic acid has also been given to children as an antipyretic.

Some authorities suggest that treatment with mefenamic acid should not be continued for longer than 7 days.

ADMINISTRATION IN RENAL FAILURE. Four patients regularly undergoing haemodialysis were given mefenamic acid 500 mg by mouth 2 hours before a dialysis session. The mean drug recovery in the dialysate collected over 3 hours was 1.03 mg (0.2% of the dose). No dosage supplement during dialysis therefore appeared to be necessary.— L. -H. Wang *et al.*, *Clin. Pharmac. Ther.*, 1980, *27*, 292.

MENORRHAGIA. In 6 patients with menorrhagia mean blood loss was reduced from 119 to 60 mL when treated on the days of anticipated heavy loss with mefenamic acid 500 mg three times daily. A further patient with a mean loss of 158 mL due to an intra-uterine contraceptive device had the loss reduced to 49 and 80 mL on 2 occasions when she took mefenamic acid 500 mg thrice daily for 7 to 10 days starting on the first day of established bleeding.— A. B. M. Anderson *et al.*, *Lancet*, 1976, *1*, 774.

Further reports on the use of mefenamic acid to reduce menstrual blood loss in women with menorrhagia and women using intra-uterine contraceptive devices.— J. Guillebaud *et al.*, *Br. J. Obstet. Gynaec.*, 1978, *85*, 53.

See also under naproxen (p.29).

OSTEOARTHRITIS. Some references to the use of mefenamic acid in osteoarthritis: K. Barnard-Jones *et al.*, *Br. J. clin. Pract.*, 1986, *40*, 528.

PAIN. Some references to the use of mefenamic acid in dysmenorrhoea: M. O. Pulkkinen and H. -L. Kaihola, *Acta obstet. gynec. scand.*, 1977, *56*, 75; A. B. M. Anderson *et al.*, *Lancet*, 1978, *1*, 345; P. W. Budoff, *J. Am. med. Ass.*, 1979, *241*, 2713; A. F. Langrick, *Br. J. clin. Pract.*, 1983, *37*, 342; J. -G. Hébert *et al.*, *Clin. Ther.*, 1986, *8*, 329.

Some reference to the use of mefenamic acid for other types of pain: R. C. Peatfield *et al.*, *Cephalalgia*, 1983, *3*, 129 (migraine); R. H. Johnson *et al.*, *Acta neurol. scand.*, 1986, *73*, 490 (migraine); R. F. Harrison and M. Brennan, *Curr. med. Res. Opinion*, 1987, *10*, 375 (post-episiotomy pain).

RHEUMATOID ARTHRITIS. Some references to the use of mefenamic acid in rheumatoid arthritis: A. Stockman *et al.*, *Med. J. Aust.*, 1976, *2*, 819; R. D. G. Leslie, *J. int. med. Res.*, 1977, *5*, 161; M. E. Mavrikakis *et al.*, *Curr. med. Res. Opinion*, 1977, *4*, 535; M. E. Mavrikakis *et al.*, *Scott. med. J.*, 1978, *23*, 189; W. H. Stephens *et al.*, *Curr. med. Res. Opinion*, 1979, *5*, 754.

Preparations

Mefenamic Acid Capsules *(B.P.)*

Proprietary Preparations

Ponstan *(Parke, Davis, UK)*. *Capsules*, mefenamic acid 250 mg.
Tablets, dispersible, mefenamic acid 250 mg.
Tablets (Ponstan Forte), mefenamic acid 500 mg.
Paediatric suspension, mefenamic acid 50 mg/5 mL.

Proprietary Names and Manufacturers

Bafameritin-M *(Jpn)*; Bonabol *(Jpn)*; Citronamic *(Spain)*; Coslan *(Parke, Davis, Spain)*; Lysalgo *(SIT, Ital.)*; Mefalgic *(Rolab, S.Afr.)*; Mefedolo *(Biopharma, Ital.)*; Parkemed *(Parke, Davis, Ger.)*; Ponalar *(Adenylchemie, Ger.)*; Ponstan *(Parke, Davis, Austral.*; *Belg.*; *Parke, Davis, Canad.*; *Parke, Davis, S.Afr.*; *Parke, Davis, Switz.*; *Parke, Davis, UK)*; Ponstel *(Parke, Davis, USA)*; Ponstil *(Arg.)*; Ponstyl *(Substantia, Fr.)*; Pontal *(Jpn)*.

12947-v

Methyl Butetisalicylate

Methyl Diethylacetylsalicylate. Methyl *O*-(2-ethylbutyryl)salicylate.
$C_{14}H_{18}O_4$=250.3.

Methyl butetisalicylate has been applied topically as a 30% cream in rheumatic and similar disorders.

Proprietary Names and Manufacturers

Doloderm *(Montedison, Arg.*; *Bellon, Fr.*; *Rhone-Poulenc, Ital.*; *Rhone-Poulenc, Switz.)*.

2667-b

Methyl Salicylate *(BAN, USAN)*.

Methyl Sal.; Methylis Salicylas. Methyl 2-hydroxybenzoate.
$C_8H_8O_3$=152.1.

CAS — 119-36-8.

Pharmacopoeias. In *Arg.*, *Aust.*, *Belg.*, *Br.*, *Cz.*, *Egypt.*, *Eur.*, *Fr.*, *Ger.*, *Hung.*, *Ind.*, *It.*, *Jpn*, *Jug.*, *Mex.*, *Neth.*, *Pol.*, *Port.*, *Roum.*, *Rus.*, *Span.*, and *Swiss*. Also in *U.S.N.F.* Also in *B.P. Vet.*

Some pharmacopoeias allow in addition to synthetic methyl salicylate, that obtained from the leaves of *Gaultheria procumbens* (Ericaceae) and the bark of *Betula lenta* (Betulaceae). The source of the methyl salicylate must be indicated on the label.

A colourless or pale yellow or reddish liquid with a strong persistent characteristic aromatic odour. Very slightly **soluble** in water; soluble 1 in 7 of alcohol (70%); miscible with alcohol, chloroform, fatty oils, and essential oils. **Store** in airtight containers. Protect from light. Certain plastic containers, such as those made from polystyrene, are unsuitable for liniments or ointments containing methyl salicylate.

NOTE. The *B.P.* directs that methyl salicylate be dispensed or supplied when Oil of Wintergreen, Wintergreen, or Wintergreen Oil is prescribed or demanded, unless it is ascertained that Methyl Salicylate Liniment (*B.P.*) is required.

Adverse Effects and Treatment

As for aspirin, p.3. Doses of as little as 4 mL have caused death in infants.

Acute poisoning occurred in 2 men who drank about 90 mL and 30 mL respectively of wintergreen oil. The latter survived but the former died.— J. J. Canselmo, *J. Am. med. Ass.*, 1948, *136*, 651.

A 20-month-old child swallowed about 5 mL of wintergreen oil. Twenty-two hours later he was in a critical condition with poor chances of survival. The blood-salicylate concentration was 727 μg per mL. He recovered following an exchange blood transfusion, which reduced the salicylate concentration by 59%, and intravenous fluids.— J. T. Adams *et al.*, *J. Am. med. Ass.*, 1957, *165*, 1563.

Charcoal haemoperfusion in the successful treatment of poisoning with methyl salicylate.— J. A. Vale *et al.*, *Br. med. J.*, 1975, *1*, 5.

ALLERGY. A 6-year-old boy who was sensitive to aspirin developed generalised pustular psoriasis consequent upon walking in East Pennsylvanian woodland in April. The eruption was traced to inhaling pollen and chewing twigs of *B. lenta* and chewing the leaves of *G. procumbens*, all of which were a source of methyl salicylate.— W. B. Shelley, *J. Am. med. Ass.*, 1964, *189*, 985.

Urticaria and angioedema occurred on several occasions in an aspirin-sensitive patient following exposure to liniments, toothpaste, and candy containing methyl salicylate.— F. Speer, *Ann. Allergy*, 1979, *43*, 36.

Uses and Administration

Methyl salicylate is absorbed through the skin and is applied in liniments and ointments for the relief of pain in rheumatic conditions.

Preparations

Methyl Salicylate Compound Cream *(A.P.F.)*. Crem. Meth. Sal. Co. Methyl salicylate 25, eucalyptus oil 10, menthol 4, cetomacrogol emulsifying wax 20, water to 100.

Methyl Salicylate Liniment *(B.P.)*. Contains 25% methyl salicylate in arachis oil or other suitable fixed oil.

Methyl Salicylate Liniment *(A.P.F.)*. Methyl salicylate 25 mL, arachis oil to 100 mL.

Methyl Salicylate Liniment Compound *(A.P.F.)*. Methyl salicylate 25 mL, menthol 4 g, eucalyptus oil 10 mL, arachis oil to 100 mL.

Compound Methyl Salicylate Ointment *(B.P.C. 1973)*. Unguentum Methylis Salicylatis Compositum Forte; Analgesic Balsam. Methyl salicylate 50% w/w, menthol 10% w/w, with cajuput oil and cineole in white beeswax, wool fat, and water. Store in non-plastic containers which prevent evaporation.

Methyl Salicylate Ointment *(B.P.)*. Strong Methyl Salicylate Ointment. Contains 50% methyl salicylate in a suitable water-emulsifying basis. For extemporaneous preparations the following formula may be used: methyl salicylate 50 g, white beeswax 25 g, hydrous wool fat 25 g.

Proprietary Preparations

Aspellin *(Rorer, UK)*. *Liniment*, methyl and ethyl salicylate 0.54%, ammonium salicylate 1%, menthol 1.4%, camphor 0.6%.

Balmosa *(Pharmax, UK)*. *Cream*, methyl salicylate 4%, menthol 2%, camphor 4%, capsicum oleoresin 0.035%.

Bengué's Balsam *(Bengué, UK)*. *Ointment*, methyl salicylate 20%, menthol 20%.
Cream (Bengué's Balsam SG), methyl salicylate 15%, menthol 10%.

Dubam *(Norma, UK)*. *Spray*, methyl salicylate 1%, ethyl salicylate 4%, glycol salicylate 5%, methyl nicotinate 1.6%.

Proprietary Names and Manufacturers

Algoderm *(Inibsa, Spain)*.

The following names have been used for multi-ingredient preparations containing methyl salicylate— Analgesic Balm *(Parke, Davis, Austral.)*; Aspellin *(Rorer, UK)*; Balmosa *(Pharmax, UK)*; Bengué's Balsam *(Bengué, UK)*; Biogesic *(Everest, Canad.)*; Cremathurm *(Sinclair, UK)*; Deltoids *(Faulding, Austral.)*; Dencorub *(Carter-Wallace, Austral.)*; Dubam *(Norma, UK)*; Emsalin *(Drug Houses Austral., Austral.)*; Ger-O-Foam *(Geriatric Pharm. Corp., USA)*; Ho's Concentrated Liniment *(Bioglan, Austral.)*; Hotshot *(Robins, Austral.)*; Iodex with Methyl Salicylate *(Smith Kline & French, Austral.)*; Iodex with Wintergreen *(Menley & James, UK)*; Ivy-chex *(Bowman, USA)*; Liberol *(Multipax, UK)*; Meth-O-Sal *(Ingram & Bell, Canad.)*; Metsal *(Riker, Austral.)*; Monphytol *(Salmond & Spraggon, Austral.; Laboratories for Applied Biology, UK)*; Panalgesic *(Poythress, USA)*; Phytex *(Drug Houses Austral., Austral.)*; Ringworm Ointment *(Wellcome, Austral.)*; Solarub *(Nelson, Austral.)*; Thera-Gesic *(Mission Pharmacal, USA)*; Thermorub *(Key, Austral.)*; Tineafax Ointment *(Wellcome, Austral.)*.

2669-g

Metiazinic Acid *(rINN)*.

Methiazinic Acid; RP-16091. (10-Methylphenothiazin-2-yl)acetic acid.
$C_{15}H_{13}NO_2S=271.3$.

CAS — 13993-65-2.

Metiazinic acid has analgesic and anti-inflammatory properties and has been used in doses of 125 to 250 mg three times daily by mouth.

Gastro-intestinal disturbances, skin rashes, and dysuria have been reported and reddish-brown discoloration of urine may occur.

Proprietary Names and Manufacturers

Metian *(Spain)*; Novartril *(Andromaco, Spain)*; Roimal *(Kanto Isei, Jpn)*; Soridermal *(Belg.)*; Soripal *(Belg.; Specia, Fr.; Ital.; Torii, Jpn; Specia, Neth.; Spain)*.

2670-f

Mofebutazone *(rINN)*.

Monobutazone; Monophenylbutazone. 4-Butyl-1-phenylpyrazolidine-3,5-dione.
$C_{13}H_{16}N_2O_2=232.3$.

CAS — 2210-63-1.

Mofebutazone is a derivative of phenylbutazone (see p.36) with similar properties. It has been given by mouth and by intramuscular injection in rheumatic disorders.

Proprietary Names and Manufacturers

Chemiartrol *(Ital.)*; Mofesal *(Medice, Ger.)*; Monazone *(Meuse, Belg.)*; Monbutina *(Lafare, Ital.)*; Monoprine *(Sanico, Belg.)*; Reumatox *(Medosan, Ital.)*.

The following names have been used for multi-ingredient preparations containing mofebutazone— Clinit *(Kwizda, Switz.)*.

2671-d

Morazone Hydrochloride *(BANM, rINNM)*.

1,5-Dimethyl-4-(3-methyl-2-phenylmorpholinomethyl)-2-phenyl-4-pyrazolin-3-one hydrochloride.
$C_{23}H_{27}N_3O_2,HCl=413.9$.

CAS — 6536-18-1 (morazone); 50321-35-2 (hydrochloride).

Morazone hydrochloride has analgesic properties. It has been used, usually in conjunction with other analgesics, in doses of 75 to 150 mg by mouth. It has also been given by subcutaneous or intramuscular injection.

Proprietary Names and Manufacturers

Delimon Tablets *(Consolidated Chemicals, UK)*; Rosimon *(Vernleigh, S.Afr.)*; Rosimon-Neu *(Ravensberg, Ger.)*.

3845-j

Morniflumate *(USAN, rINN)*.

UP-164. 2-Morpholinoethyl 2-(α,α,α-trifluoro-*m*-toluidino)-nicotinate.
$C_{19}H_{20}F_3N_3O_3=395.4$.

CAS — 65847-85-0.

Morniflumate, the morpholinoethyl ester of niflumic acid (see p.31), has analgesic and anti-inflammatory properties. It has been used in inflammatory and rheumatic disorders in doses of 250 mg three times daily by mouth. It has also been given rectally as suppositories.

Proprietary Names and Manufacturers

Actol *(Upsamedica, Spain)*; Niflam *(Rhone-Poulenc, Ital.)*; Nifluril *(UPSA, Fr.; UPSA, Switz.)*.

12990-p

Nabumetone *(BAN, USAN, rINN)*.

BRL-14777. 4-(6-Methoxy-2-naphthyl)butan-2-one.
$C_{15}H_{16}O_2=228.3$.

CAS — 42924-53-8.

Adverse Effects

Side-effects reported with nabumetone include gastro-intestinal disturbances such as nausea, dyspepsia, abdominal pain, flatulence, and diarrhoea or constipation, headache, dizziness, sedation, and skin rashes and pruritus.

Precautions

Nabumetone should not be used in patients with peptic ulceration or severe hepatic impairment and should be used with caution in patients with renal impairment.

Absorption and Fate

Nabumetone is absorbed from the gastro-intestinal tract and rapidly metabolised in the liver to the principal active metabolite 6-methoxy-2-naphthylacetic acid. This metabolite is highly protein bound with a reported plasma half-life of between 12 and 36 hours. Excretion is predominantly in the urine.

Uses and Administration

Nabumetone has analgesic and anti-inflammatory properties; although it is a relatively weak inhibitor of prostaglandin synthesis itself, its active metabolite is a potent inhibitor. It is used in osteoarthritis and rheumatoid arthritis in a usual dose of 1 g by mouth taken as a single dose in the evening; if necessary 0.5 to 1 g may be given additionally in the morning. It has been recommended that a dose of 1 g daily should not be exceeded in elderly patients and that 500 mg daily may even be satisfactory in some cases.

A preliminary review of the pharmacodynamic and pharmacokinetic properties, and therapeutic efficacy of nabumetone in rheumatic diseases.— H. A. Friedel and P. A. Todd, *Drugs*, 1988, *35*, 504. A further review.— *Drug & Ther. Bull.*, 1988, *26*, 41.

OSTEOARTHRITIS. Some references to the use of nabumetone in osteoarthritis: J. Gillgrass and R. Grahame, *Pharmatherapeutica*, 1984, *3*, 592; E. J. Pisko *et al.*, *ibid.*, 1987, *5*, 90.

RHEUMATOID ARTHRITIS. Some references to the use of nabumetone in rheumatoid arthritis: A. M. Richards *et al.*, *N.Z. med. J.*, 1983, *96*, 1015.

Proprietary Preparations

Relifex *(Bencard, UK)*. *Tablets*, nabumetone 500 mg.

Proprietary Names and Manufacturers

Relifen *(Bencard, S.Afr.)*; Relifex *(Bencard, UK)*.

2672-n

Naproxen *(BAN, USAN, rINN)*.

RS-3540. (+)-2-(6-Methoxy-2-naphthyl)propionic acid.
$C_{14}H_{14}O_3=230.3$.

CAS — 22204-53-1.

Pharmacopoeias. In *Br.* and *U.S.* Also in *B.P. Vet.*

A white or almost white, odourless or almost odourless, crystalline powder. Practically **insoluble** in water; soluble 1 in 25 of alcohol, 1 in 15 of chloroform, 1 in 40 of ether, and 1 in 20 of methyl alcohol. **Store** in airtight containers. Protect from light.

2673-h

Naproxen Sodium *(BANM, USAN, rINNM)*.

RS-3650.
$C_{14}H_{13}NaO_3=252.2$.

CAS — 26159-34-2.

Pharmacopoeias. In *U.S.*

A white to creamy-white crystalline powder. **Soluble** in water and methyl alcohol; sparingly soluble in alcohol; very slightly soluble in acetone; practically insoluble in chloroform. **Store** in airtight containers.

Adverse Effects

As for ibuprofen, p.20.

ALLERGY. All of 11 aspirin-sensitive asthmatic patients developed reactions (rhinorrhoea, tightness of chest, wheezing, dyspnoea) after taking naproxen in doses of 40 to 80 mg.— A. Szczeklik *et al.*, *Br. med. J.*, 1977, *2*, 231.

Vasculitis and symptoms of nephritis and paralytic ileus occurred in a woman who had taken naproxen and aspirin for 3 years. Serum IgG, IgA, and IgE and circulating immune complex activity were raised. Symptoms resolved after naproxen and aspirin were discontinued and did not reappear when salicylate was restarted.— D. M. Grennan *et al.*, *N.Z. med. J.*, 1979, *89*, 48.

Pulmonary infiltrates probably due to a hypersensitivity reaction to naproxen in 3 patients.— A. J. Buscaglia *et al.*, *J. Am. med. Ass.*, 1984, *251*, 65. See also: D. A. Nader and R. F. Schillaci, *Chest*, 1982, *83*, 280; A. V. Londino *et al.* (letter), *J. Am. med. Ass.*, 1984, *252*, 1853.

Precipitation of status asthmaticus in an elderly patient following a single dose of naproxen.— R. V. Lewis (letter), *Lancet*, 1987, *1*, 1270.

EFFECTS ON THE BLOOD. Mention of 2 cases of fatal aplastic anaemia or agranulocytosis in one year probably due to naproxen.— W. H. W. Inman, *Br. med. J.*, 1977, *1*, 1500.

Aplastic anaemia in a 47-year-old man might have been caused by naproxen therapy.— R. Arnold and H. Heimpel (letter), *Lancet*, 1980, *1*, 321.

Further reports of adverse haematological effects associated with naproxen: J. A. Hughes and W. Sudell (letter), *Arthritis Rheum.*, 1983, *26*, 1054 (haemolytic anaemia); T. C. N. Lo and M. A. Martin, *Br. med. J.*, 1986, *292*, 1430 (auto-immune haemolytic anaemia); P. McNeil *et al.* (letter), *Med. J. Aust.*, 1986, *145*, 53 (aplastic anaemia); N. Nygard and G. Starkebaum (letter), *J. Am. med. Ass.*, 1987, *257*, 1732 (neutropenia).

EFFECTS ON THE EYES. Keratopathy, characterised by whorl-like corneal opacities, in a woman receiving naproxen; complete regression occurred after discontinuation of naproxen.— L. Szmyd and H. D. Perry, *Am. J. Ophthal.*, 1985, *99*, 598.

EFFECTS ON THE GASTRO-INTESTINAL TRACT. Reports mainly of melaena and sometimes of haematemesis: E. Beck (letter), *Br. med. J.*, 1974, *1*, 572; M. C. Hayes-Allen (letter), *ibid;* F. D. Hart (letter), *ibid.*, *2*, 51; S. G. F. Matts (letter), *ibid.*, 52.

Acute proctocolitis associated with the use of naproxen in one patient.— S. Ravi *et al.*, *Postgrad. med. J.*, 1986, *62*, 773.

EFFECTS ON THE KIDNEYS. Reversible renal failure and nephrotic syndrome developed in a patient who had been taking naproxen 250 mg twice daily for a year. Renal biopsy revealed prominent interstitial nephritis.— J. H. Brezin *et al.*, *New Engl. J. Med.*, 1979, *301*, 1271. Eight cases of genito-urinary disorders have been reported to the Committee on Safety of Medicines from recipients of at least 1 899 300 prescriptions.— J. H. Brezin (letter), *ibid.*, 1980, *302*, 1092.

Interstitial nephritis and renal insufficiency in an 18-year-old youth with rheumatoid arthritis were attributed to naproxen. Symptoms resolved when naproxen was discontinued.— K. C. Cartwright *et al.*, *Ariz. Med.*, 1979, *36*, 124.

Further reports of nephrotoxicity associated with naproxen: M. R. Quigley *et al.*, *Arthritis Rheum.*, 1982, *25*, 1016 (proteinuria); R. J. Caruana and E. L. Semble, *J. Rheumatol.*, 1984, *11*, 90 (renal papillary necrosis).

EFFECTS ON THE LIVER. Approximately 2 months after starting treatment with naproxen 250 mg twice daily a 35-year-old patient developed jaundice which disappeared when treatment was discontinued.— B. H. Bass (letter), *Lancet*, 1974, *1*, 998.

A report of jaundice and an enlarged liver associated with naproxen therapy in a 54-year-old woman. Dramatic improvement with return of liver-function tests to normal occurred within 4 weeks of discontinuation.— I. P. Law and H. Knight (letter), *New Engl. J. Med.*, 1977, *295*, 1201.

Jaundice occurred in a man who had been taking naproxen for one month. Histological findings after liver biopsy were consistent with drug-induced hepatitis.— R. M. M. Victorino *et al.*, *Postgrad. med. J.*, 1980, *56*, 368.

Cross hepatotoxicity in one patient between fenoprofen and naproxen.— M. Andrejak *et al.*, *Br. med. J.*, 1987, *295*, 180.

EFFECTS ON SEXUAL FUNCTION. Inhibition of ejaculation attributed to naproxen in one patient.— N. Wei and J. C. Hood (letter), *Ann. intern. Med.*, 1980, *93*, 933.

EFFECTS ON THE SKIN. Development of florid erythema nodosum in an elderly patient given naproxen.— C. E. H. Grattan and C. T. C. Kennedy, *Br. med. J.*, 1984, *288*, 114.

Naproxen-induced lichen planus in one patient 10 days after the commencement of therapy.— W. R. Heymann *et al.* (letter), *J. Am. Acad. Derm.*, 1984, *10*, 299.

A report of apparent pseudoporphyria associated with naproxen therapy in 5 patients.— A. M. Howard *et al.* (letter), *Lancet*, 1985, *1*, 819. A similar report.— P. M. Farr and B. L. Diffey (letter), *ibid.*, 1166.

Toxic pustular skin eruption in a patient taking naproxen.— S. R. Page and C. E. H. Grattan (letter), *Br. med. J.*, 1986, *293*, 510.

OVERDOSAGE. A study of the pharmacokinetics of naproxen following overdosage of healthy subjects with single doses of 1, 2, 3, or 4 g. An increase in the urinary-excretion rate was noted, with acceleration as naproxen-plasma concentrations rose to 100 to 200 μg per mL. Results indicated that the body can apparently handle doses of up to 4 g, without saturating any of its eliminating mechanisms, in a manner similar to doses in the therapeutic range. No side-effects were reported other than mild epigastric pain in 1 subject in the evening after receiving 3 g; clinical laboratory tests were normal.— R. Runkel *et al.*, *Clin. Pharmac. Ther.*, 1976, *20*, 269.

A patient reported to have ingested 25 g of naproxen suffered only mild transient gastro-intestinal distress. The serum concentration of naproxen 15 hours after ingestion was 414 μg per mL.— E. W. Fredell and L. J. Strand (letter), *J. Am. med. Ass.*, 1977, *238*, 938.

Precautions

As for ibuprofen, p.20.

Naproxen may interfere with some tests for 17-ketogenic steroids.

INTERACTIONS. For the effect of naproxen on other drugs, see lithium carbonate (p.368), methotrexate (p.638), and warfarin (p.345).

Antacids. The absorption of naproxen was altered by antacids. With sodium bicarbonate there was an earlier and increased peak plasma-naproxen concentration, whereas with magnesium oxide and aluminium hydroxide the peak was delayed and lower than with naproxen alone. Combination with a preparation of magnesium and aluminium hydroxides tended to reduce the time to peak plasma-naproxen concentration and to increase slightly the total amount absorbed.— E. J. Segre *et al.* (letter), *New Engl. J. Med.*, 1974, *291*, 582.

Aspirin. In 6 subjects given naproxen 500 mg and aspirin 1.2 g alone and concomitantly, plasma concentrations of naproxen were reduced when aspirin was given concomitantly; this appeared to be due to increased excretion of naproxen. Preliminary reports of clinical studies suggested that the interaction was not clinically significant.— E. Segre *et al.*, *Scand. J. Rheumatol.*, 1973, *Suppl.* 2, 37.

Probenecid. Probenecid increased plasma concentrations of naproxen and its 6-*O*-desmethyl metabolite in a study of 6 healthy subjects.— R. Runkel *et al.*, *Clin. Pharmac. Ther.*, 1978, *24*, 706.

INTERFERENCE WITH DIAGNOSTIC TESTS. A report of a false-positive 5-hydroxyindole test, a test used for carcinoid tumour, in a woman receiving naproxen.— P. J. Martin and L. Higginbotham, *Br. med. J.*, 1984, *288*, 1346.

PREGNANCY AND THE NEONATE. A study in a nursing mother receiving naproxen for rheumatoid arthritis and her breast-fed infant indicated that the amount of naproxen ingested in breast milk would be limited and would be unlikely to cause significant consequences in a suckling infant.— F. Jamali and D. R. S. Stevens (letter), *Drug Intell. & clin. Pharm.*, 1983, *17*, 910.

Absorption and Fate

Naproxen and naproxen sodium are readily absorbed from the gastro-intestinal tract. Absorption is claimed to be more rapid with the sodium salt. Peak plasma concentrations are attained 2 to 4 hours after ingestion. At therapeutic concentrations naproxen is more than 99% bound to plasma proteins and has a plasma half-life of about 13 hours. Approximately 95% of a dose is excreted in urine as naproxen and 6-*O*-desmethylnaproxen and their conjugates. Less than 3% of a dose has been recovered in the faeces. Naproxen crosses the placenta and is excreted in breast milk.

A study of naproxen concentrations in synovial fluid.— S. Javala *et al.*, *Scand. J. Rheumatol.*, 1977, *6*, 155.

Studies *in vitro* using plasma obtained from healthy subjects showed that a mean of 99.7% of naproxen was bound to plasma proteins but no correlation with α_1-acid glycoprotein or albumin concentration was found.— K. M. Piafsky and O. Borgå, *Clin. Pharmac. Ther.*, 1977, *22*, 545. Further studies on the protein binding of naproxen in patients with rheumatoid arthritis: S. Wanwimolruk *et al.*, *Br. J. clin. Pharmac.*, 1983, *15*, 91 (in synovial fluid and plasma); F. A. Van Den Ouweland *et al.*, *ibid.*, 1987, *23*, 189 (in serum).

Uses and Administration

Naproxen has analgesic, anti-inflammatory, and antipyretic properties; it is an inhibitor of prostaglandin synthetase.

Both naproxen and naproxen sodium are used in rheumatic disorders such as ankylosing spondylitis, osteoarthritis, and rheumatoid arthritis, in mild to moderate pain such as dysmenorrhoea, migraine, and some musculoskeletal disorders, and in acute gout.

In ankylosing spondylitis, osteoarthritis, and rheumatoid arthritis, the usual dose of naproxen or naproxen sodium is the equivalent of 500 mg to 1 g of naproxen daily in 2 divided doses. A dose of 10 mg per kg body-weight daily of naproxen in 2 divided doses has been used in children over 5 years of age with juvenile rheumatoid arthritis.

In painful conditions such as dysmenorrhoea the usual initial dose is the equivalent of 500 mg of naproxen followed by 250 mg every 6 or 8 hours. In acute gout an initial dose equivalent to 750 mg of naproxen followed by 250 mg every 8 hours has been suggested.

Rectal administration of naproxen is sometimes employed.

Naproxen has also been used orally as the piperazine salt.

A detailed review of the actions and uses of naproxen.— R. N. Brogden *et al.*, *Drugs*, 1979, *18*, 241.

ADMINISTRATION. A study suggesting that naproxen sodium appeared to be an improved form of naproxen for use as an analgesic, being more rapidly available and providing greater pain relief.— H. Sevelius *et al.*, *Br. J. clin. Pharmac.*, 1980, *10*, 259.

ADMINISTRATION IN THE ELDERLY. A suggestion, based upon pharmacokinetic studies, that a dosage reduction of 50% of naproxen in the elderly would appear to be prudent.— R. A. Upton *et al.*, *Br. J. clin. Pharmac.*, 1984, *18*, 207. A similar study suggesting that naproxen should be used at the lower end of the dosage range in elderly patients.— R. M. McVerry *et al.*, *Eur. J. clin. Pharmac.*, 1986, *31*, 463.

ADMINISTRATION IN HEPATIC FAILURE. Pharmacokinetic data suggesting that the dose of naproxen be reduced by at least 50% in patients with chronic alcoholic liver disease and also, in the absence of data to the contrary, in patients with other forms of hepatic disease.— R. L. Williams *et al.*, *Eur. J. clin. Pharmac.*, 1984, *27*, 291.

ADMINISTRATION IN RENAL FAILURE. No accumulation of naproxen was seen in a patient undergoing haemodialysis three times weekly and receiving naproxen 500 mg daily. Dialysis did not clear naproxen and a post-dialysis dose was considered to be unnecessary.— S. S. Weber *et al.*, *Am. J. Hosp. Pharm.*, 1979, *36*, 1567.

A study suggesting that no adjustment of naproxen dosage is needed in renal failure.— M. Anttila *et al.*, *Eur. J. clin. Pharmac.*, 1980, *18*, 263.

ANKYLOSING SPONDYLITIS. Some references to the use of naproxen in ankylosing spondylitis: H. F. H. Hill and A. G. S. Hill, *J. clin. Pharmac.*, 1975, *15*, 355; F. van Gerwen *et al.*, *Ann. rheum. Dis.*, 1978, *37*, 85; B. M. Ansell *et al.*, *Eur. J. Rheumatol. Inflamm.*, 1979, *2*, 45.

FEVER. As naproxen had previously been shown to be an effective antipyretic in neoplastic fever (a fever which cannot be ascribed to co-existent infection or other known causes) but to be ineffective in infectious fever in cancer patients (J.C. Chang and H.M. Gross, *Am. J. Med.*, 1984, *76*, 597) a further evaluation of its use in neoplastic fever was performed. Of 21 patients treated with naproxen, initially in a dose of 250 mg twice daily but increased to 1.5 g daily if necessary, 16 had a complete response with normalisation of temperature within 12 hours; an afebrile state was maintained in 15 of these patients whilst receiving naproxen. The usefulness of naproxen is limited, however, by a prompt relapse of fever in most patients when the drug is withdrawn. Studies should be performed to establish the value of other non-steroidal anti-inflammatory agents in the treatment of neoplastic fever, a condition in which standard antipyretic drugs are generally ineffective.— J. C. Chang and H. M. Gross, *J. clin. Oncol.*, 1985, *3*, 552. See also: S. K. Azeemuddin *et al.*, *Cancer*, 1987, *59*, 1966.

GOUT. Some references to the use of naproxen in acute gout: P. Cuq, *Scand. J. Rheumatol.*, 1973, *Suppl.* 2, 64; R. F. Willkens *et al.*, *J. clin. Pharmac.*, 1975, *15*, 363; R. A. Sturge *et al.*, *Eur. J. Rheumatol. Inflamm.*, 1979, *2*, 40.

MENORRHAGIA. Naproxen 500 mg in the morning and 250 mg in the afternoon for the first 2 days of a menstrual bleed and 250 mg twice daily for up to 7 days reduced the menstrual blood loss in 4 patients with primary menorrhagia. There was also a reduction in 5 patients with a blood loss of more than 80 mL per menstruation whose menorrhagia was associated with an intra-uterine device; there was no reduction in 5 similar women whose blood loss was less than 80 mL per menstruation.— G. Rybo *et al.* (letter), *Lancet*, 1981, *1*, 608.

In a double-blind crossover study involving 35 women with menorrhagia naproxen sodium (initial dose 550 mg followed by 275 mg every 6 hours for 5 days) and mefenamic acid (500 mg every 8 hours for 5 days) reduced excessive bleeding by an average of 47 and 46% respectively. It was believed that such treatment is useful for women with menorrhagia and a normal uterus or for menorrhagia associated with an intra-uterine contraceptive device.— P. Hall *et al.*, *Br. J. Obstet. Gynaec.*, 1987, *94*, 554.

OSTEOARTHRITIS. Some references to the use of naproxen in osteoarthritis: G. Binzus and G. Josenhans, *Scand. J. Rheumatol.*, 1973, *Suppl.* 2, 80; G. M. Cochrane, *ibid.*, 89; T. Kageyama, *ibid.*, 94; C. G. Barnes *et al.*, *J. clin. Pharmac.*, 1975, *15*, 347; W. Blechman *et al.*, *Ann. rheum. Dis.*, 1978, *37*, 80; J. T. Vainio and P. V. Lepistö, *Scand. J. Rheumatol.*, 1978, *Suppl.* 21, 25; A. Car *et al.*, *ibid.*, *Suppl.* 22, 63; S. R. Mayhew, *Rheumatol. Rehabil.*, 1978, *17*, 29; J. W. Melton *et al.*, *J. Rheumatol.*, 1978, *5*, 338; M. Thompson *et al.*, *Eur. J. Rheumatol. Inflamm.*, 1979, *2*, 25; T. Amundsen *et al.*, *Curr. ther. Res.*, 1983, *33*, 793; R. Willkens *et al.*, *ibid.*, *34*, 45; P. Janke *et al.*, *Pharmatherapeutica*, 1984, *3*, 663; *Curr. med. Res. Opinion*, 1984, *9*, 41; H. Berry and A. Nicholls, *ibid.*, 1985, *9*, 366; G. Vetter, *Br. J. clin. Pract.*, 1985, *39*, 276.

PAIN. Some references to the analgesic efficacy of naproxen in patients with postoperative pain or musculoskeletal disorders: J. Ruedy and W. McCullough, *Scand. J. Rheumatol.*, 1973, *Suppl.* 2, 56; D. L. Mahler *et al.*, *Clin. Pharmac. Ther.*, 1976, *19*, 18; G. Jaffé, *Curr. med. Res. Opinion*, 1976, *4*, 373; J. G. P. Williams and C. Engler, *Rheumatol. Rehabil.*, 1977, *16*, 265; U. Aromaa and K. Asp, *J. int. med. Res.*, 1978, *6*, 152; G. Sacchetti *et al.*, *ibid.*, 312; G. Martino *et al.*, *Arzneimittel-Forsch.*, 1978, *28*, 1657; T. A. Bouchier-Hayes and C. W. Jones, *Practitioner*, 1979, *223*, 706; D. Wheatley, *Curr. med. Res. Opinion*, 1979, *6*, 229; H. S. Filtzer, *Curr. ther. Res.*, 1980, *27*, 293; H. Sevelius *et al.*, *J. clin. Pharmac.*, 1980, *20*, 480; C. I. Backhouse *et al.*, *Rheumatol. Rehabil.*, 1980, *19*, 113; L. A. Andersen and P. C. Gotzsche, *Pharmatherapeutica*, 1984, *3*, 531; C. R. Brown *et al.*, *Curr. ther. Res.*, 1984, *35*, 511; P. G. McCulloch *et al.*, *Br. J. clin. Pract.*, 1985, *39*, 69; R. D. Ouellette *et al.*, *Curr. ther. Res.*, 1986, *39*, 839.

Some references to the use of naproxen or naproxen sodium in dysmenorrhoea: F. Pauls (letter), *Lancet*, 1978, *2*, 159; F. W. Hanson *et al.*, *Obstet. Gynec.*, 1978, *52*, 583; O. Ylikorkala *et al.* (letter), *Lancet*, 1979, *1*, 278; V. Buttram *et al.*, *Am. J. Obstet. Gynec.*, 1979, *134*, 575; M. R. Henzl *et al.*, *ibid.*, *135*, 455; A. F. Langrick, *Br. J. clin. Pract.*, 1983, *37*, 342; I. Milsom and B. Andersch, *Int. J. Gynaecol. Obstet.*, 1985, *23*, 305; R. H. DuRant *et al.*, *Am. J. Dis. Child.*, 1985, *139*, 489.

Several studies have been conducted to assess the role of naproxen in the treatment and prophylaxis of migraine. Two studies (E.S. Johnson *et al.*, *Cephalalgia*, 1985, *5*, 5; A. Pradalier *et al.*, *ibid.*, 107) both found naproxen to be an effective form of treatment for pain relief in an established attack of common migraine but Johnson and colleagues did not consider that the efficacy was established for classical migraine. Other studies in common or classical migraine (J. Sargent *et al.*, *Headache*, 1985, *25*, 320; K.M.A. Welch *et al.*, *Neurology*, 1985, *35*, 1304; D.K. Ziegler and D.J. Ellis, *Archs Neurol., Chicago*, 1985, *42*, 582) have indicated that prophylactic treatment with naproxen sodium 550 mg twice daily may be useful in reducing the number of attacks suffered.

RHEUMATOID ARTHRITIS. Some references to the use of naproxen in rheumatoid arthritis: H. Diamond *et al.*, *J. clin. Pharmac.*, 1975, *15*, 335; D. Myhal *et al.*, *ibid.*, 327; J. J. B. Flores and S. V. Rojas, *ibid.*, 373; S. H. Roth and G. Boost, *ibid.*, 378; H. Mathies and E. Wolff, *Arzneimittel-Forsch.*, 1975, *25*, 318; H. A. Capell *et al.*, *Curr. med. Res. Opinion*, 1976, *4*, 285; E. C. Huskisson *et al.*, *Br. med. J.*, 1976, *1*, 1048; J. J. Castles *et al.*, *Archs intern. Med.*, 1978, *138*, 362; H. Berry *et al.*, *Ann. rheum. Dis.*, 1978, *37*, 370; P. Lee *et al.*, *N.Z. med. J.*, 1978, *87*, 425; F. A. Wollheim *et al.*, *Rheumatol. Rehabil.*, 1978, *Suppl.*, 78; S. Luftschein *et al.*, *J. Rheumatol.*, 1979, *6*, 397; G. Katona *et al.*, *Curr. ther. Res.*, 1979, *25*, 493; A. G. Mowat *et al.*, *Eur. J. Rheumatol. Inflamm.*, 1979, *2*, 19; E. C. Huskisson *et al.*, *ibid.*, 33; H. Berry *et al.*, *ibid.*, 65; J. J. Castles and J. L. Skosey, *Curr. ther. Res.*, 1980, *27*, 556; W. Eidsaunet *et al.*, *ibid.*, 1983, *33*, 966; P. H. Lizarazo and M. Pẽna Cortés, *ibid.*, *34*, 701; A. M. Mowat *et al.*, *Br. J. clin. Pract.*, 1984, *38*, 95; J. Taborn *et al.*, *Curr. med. Res. Opinion*, 1985, *9*, 359; R. A. Mitchell *et al.*, *Br. J. clin. Pract.*, 1987, *41*, 560.

Some references to the use of naproxen in juvenile rheumatoid arthritis: A. -L. Mäkelä, *Scand. J. Rheumatol.*, 1977, *6*, 193; B. M. Ansell *et al.*, *Eur. J. Rheumatol. Inflamm.*, 1979, *2*, 79; H. Moran *et al.*, *Ann. rheum. Dis.*, 1979, *38*, 152; A. Nicholls *et al.*, *Curr. med. Res. Opinion*, 1982, *8*, 204.

Preparations

Naproxen Oral Suspension *(B.P.)*
Naproxen Suppositories *(B.P.)*
Naproxen Tablets *(B.P.)*
Naproxen Tablets *(U.S.P.)*
Naproxen Sodium Tablets *(U.S.P.)*

Proprietary Preparations

Laraflex *(Lagap, UK). Tablets*, scored, naproxen 250 and 500 mg.

Naprosyn *(Syntex, UK). Tablets*, scored, naproxen 250 and 500 mg.
Granules, sachets, naproxen 500 mg.
Suspension, naproxen 125 mg/5 mL.
Suppositories, naproxen 500 mg.

Synflex *(Syntex, UK). Tablets*, naproxen sodium 275 mg (equivalent to naproxen 250 mg).

Proprietary Names and Manufacturers of Naproxen and its Salts

Alganil *(Schwarz, Ital.)*; Aliviomas *(Alacan, Spain)*; Alprofen *(Cusi, Spain)*; Anaprox *(Syntex, Canad.; Syntex, USA)*; Antalgin *(Syntex-Latino, Spain)*; Apranax *(Laroche Navarron, Fr.; Syntex, Ger.; Syntex, Switz.)*; Artroxen *(Von Boch, Ital.)*; Axer Alfa *(Alfa Farmaceutici, Ital.)*; Denaxpren *(Smaller, Spain)*; Dysmenalgit *(Krewel, Ger.)*; Flanax *(Braz.; Mex.)*; Floginax *(Lifepharma, Ital.)*; Flògogin *(Tosi-Novara, Ital.)*; Floxalin *(Tiber, Ital.)*; Gibinap *(Gibipharma, Ital.)*; Gibixen *(Gibipharma, Ital.)*; Laraflex *(Lagap, UK)*; Laser *(Tosi-Novara, Ital.)*; Leniartril *(San Carlo, Ital.)*; Lundiran *(Llorente, Spain)*; Madaprox *(Madariaga, Spain)*; Nafasol *(Lennon, S.Afr.)*; Naixan *(Jpn)*; Napren *(Nyco, Norw.)*; Naprium *(Radiumfarma, Ital.)*; Naprius *(Magis, Ital.)*; Naprogesic *(Syntex, Austral.)*; Naprokes *(Albofarma, Spain)*; Naprorex *(Lampugnani, Ital.)*; Naprosyn *(Arg.; Syntex, Austral.; Syntex, Canad.; Syntex, Denm.; Ger.; Recordati, Ital.; Astra-Syntex, Norw.; Syntex, S.Afr.; Syntex-Latino, Spain; Astra-Syntex, Swed.; Syntex, Switz.; Syntex, UK; Syntex, USA)*; Naprosyne *(Belg.; Cassenne, Fr.; Neth.)*; Naproval *(Valles Mestre, Spain)*; Naxen *(Syncare, Canad.)*; Novonaprox *(Novopharm, Canad.)*; Numidan *(Coop. Farm., Ital.)*; Piproxen *(ISM, Ital.)*; Praxenol *(Biochimica Zanardi, Ital.)*; Prexan *(Lafare, Ital.)*; Primeral *(Master Pharma, Ital.)*; Proxen *(Syntex, Ger.; Berenguer-Beneyto, Spain; Grünenthal, Switz.)*; Proxine *(Giustini, Ital.)*; Rofanten *(Davur, Spain)*; Sobronil *(Septa, Spain)*; Synflex *(Recordati, Ital.; Syntex, S.Afr.; Syntex, UK)*; Ticoflex *(Aandersen, Ital.)*; Xenar *(Alfa Farmaceutici, Ital.)*.

2674-m

Nefopam Hydrochloride *(BANM, USAN, rINNM)*.

Benzoxazocine; Fenazoxine; R-738. 3,4,5,6-Tetrahydro-5-methyl-1-phenyl-1*H*-2,5-benzoxazocine hydrochloride.

$C_{17}H_{19}NO,HCl=289.8$.

CAS — 13669-70-0 (nefopam); 23327-57-3 (hydrochloride).

Adverse Effects

Side-effects occurring with nefopam include nausea, vomiting, sweating, drowsiness, insomnia, dizziness, lightheadedness, nervousness, blurred vision, headache, dry mouth, skin rashes, and tachycardia. Euphoria and convulsions have occasionally been reported. There may be pain at the site of injection.

ABNORMAL COLORATION. Dark pink discoloration of the urine in a healthy subject after taking nefopam.— S. J. Wroe *et al.*, *Br. med. J.*, 1986, *292*, 1672.

OVERDOSAGE. An account of a fatal overdose of nefopam, and details of 9 patients who recovered with routine supportive treatment. Treatment should be directed primarily to the prompt removal of ingested drug by gastric lavage, together with control of convulsions and hallucinations; diazepam appears to be effective for this purpose, and beta-adrenergic blockade might help to control the cardiovascular complications.— D. M. Piercy *et al.*, *Br. med. J.*, 1981, *283*, 1508.

Precautions

Nefopam is contra-indicated in patients with a history of convulsive disorders. It should be used with caution in patients with glaucoma, urinary retention, or impaired hepatic or renal function.

It has been recommended that nefopam should not be given to patients receiving monoamine oxidase inhibitors and should be used cautiously in those receiving tricyclic antidepressants.

PREGNANCY AND THE NEONATE. Studies in 5 healthy nursing mothers given nefopam for post-episiotomy pain indicated that a breast-fed infant would be exposed to less than 3% of the maternal dose ingested.— D. T. Y. Liu *et al.*, *Br. J. clin. Pharmac.*, 1987, *23*, 99.

Absorption and Fate

Nefopam is absorbed from the gastro-intestinal tract. Peak plasma concentrations occur 1 to 3 hours after administration by mouth and about 1.5 hours after intramuscular injection. About 73% is bound to plasma proteins. It has an elimination half-life of about 4 hours. It is extensively metabolised and excreted mainly in urine. Less than 5% of a dose is excreted unchanged in the urine. About 8% of a dose is excreted via the faeces.

Uses and Administration

Nefopam hydrochloride has analgesic properties. Its mechanism of action is unclear; prostaglandin synthesis is not inhibited. It also has some anticholinergic and sympathomimetic actions. It is used for the relief of acute and chronic pain. The usual dose by mouth is 30 to 90 mg three times daily; the suggested initial doses are 60 mg three times daily but 30 mg three times daily in elderly patients. Nefopam hydrochloride may also be given in doses of 20 mg by intramuscular injection, repeated every 6 hours if necessary; it is recommended that the patient should always be lying down when receiving the injection and should remain so for 15 to 20 minutes afterwards.

Reviews of the actions and uses of nefopam hydrochloride.— *Drug & Ther. Bull.*, 1979, *17*, 59; R. C. Heel *et al.*, *Drugs*, 1980, *19*, 249.

Some references to the use of nefopam for cancer pain: L. de T. de Boesinghe *et al.*, *Curr. ther. Res.*, 1976, *20*, 59; L. de T. de Boesinghe, *Curr. ther. Res.*, 1978, *24*, 646.

Some references to the use of nefopam hydrochloride for postoperative analgesia.— R. K. Ferguson and D. M. Turek, *Pharmatherapeutica*, 1977, *1*, 523; I. Tigerstedt *et al.*, *Br. J. Anaesth.*, 1977, *49*, 1133; W. T. Beaver and G. A. Feise, *J. clin. Pharmac.*, 1977, *17*, 579; D. Trop *et al.*, *Can. Anaesth. Soc. J.*, 1979, *26*, 296; G. Phillips and M. D. A. Vickers, *Br. J. Anaesth.*, 1979, *51*, 961; R. I. H. Wang and E. M. Waite, *J. clin. Pharmac.*, 1979, *19*, 395; S. S. Bloomfield *et al.*, *Clin. Pharmac. Ther.*, 1980, *27*, 502; M. Conway and S. Lipton, *Curr. med. Res. Opinion*, 1982, *7*, 580.

Proprietary Preparations

Acupan *(Riker, UK). Tablets*, nefopam hydrochloride 30 mg.
Injection, nefopam hydrochloride 20 mg/mL, in ampoules containing 1 mL.

Proprietary Names and Manufacturers

Acupan *(Arg.; Belg.; Riker, Fr.; Boehringer Biochemia, Ital.; Riker, S.Afr.; Federico Bonet, Spain; Riker 3M, Switz.; Riker, UK)*; Ajan *(Kettelhack Riker, Ger.)*; Dolitrone *(Lafarquim, Spain)*; Lenipan *(Chiesi, Ital.)*; Nefadol *(Zilliken, Ital.)*; Nefam *(Biagini, Ital.)*; Oxadol *(ISI, Ital.)*; Sinalgico *(Arg.)*.

2676-v

Nifenazone *(BAN, rINN)*.

N-(2,3-Dimethyl-5-oxo-1-phenyl-3-pyrazolin-4-yl)nicotinamide.

$C_{17}H_{16}N_4O_2=308.3$.

CAS — 2139-47-1.

Adverse Effects and Precautions

Nausea, dyspepsia, stomatitis, and agranulocytosis have been reported. Nifenazone should be given with caution to patients with peptic ulcer.

Blood dyscrasias in 4 patients being treated with nifenazone had been reported since early in 1964.— Committee on Safety of Drugs, *Adverse Reactions Series No. 3*, Aug. 1965.

Uses and Administration

Nifenazone has analgesic and anti-inflammatory properties. It has been used in rheumatic disorders in doses of 200 to 400 mg two or three times daily by mouth. It has also been applied topically in concentrations of 5%.

Proprietary Names and Manufacturers
Algotrex *(CT, Ital.)*; Dipiral *(Ital.)*; Dolongan *(SMB, Belg.)*; Neopiran *(Panthox & Burck, Ital.)*; Niapan *(Biosint, Ital.)*; Nicopyron *(Trommsdorff, Ger.)*; Nicoreumal *(SIT, Ital.)*; Niprazina *(ISOM, Ital.)*; Reumatosil *(Saba, Ital.)*; Supermidone *(Salfa, Ital.)*; Thylin *(Inibsa, Spain; Sinclair, UK)*.

2677-g

Niflumic Acid *(rINN)*.
UP-83. 2-(ααα-Trifluoro-*m*-toluidino)nicotinic acid.
$C_{13}H_9F_3N_2O_2$=282.2.

CAS — 4394-00-7.

Adverse Effects
Reported adverse effects include gastro-intestinal disturbances, signs of kidney impairment, and headache.

Fluoride associated osteosis with prolonged use of niflumic acid.— A. Prost *et al., Nouv. Presse méd.*, 1978, *7*, 754.

Uses and Administration
Niflumic acid has analgesic and anti-inflammatory properties. It has been used in inflammatory and rheumatic disorders in usual doses of about 250 mg three times daily by mouth. It has also been used topically as a 3% cream or ointment. It has been used rectally as suppositories in the form of morniflumate, morpholinoethyl ester (see p.28).

Proprietary Names and Manufacturers
Actol *(Holphar, Ger.; Upsamedica, Spain)*; Flaminon *(Squibb, Ital.; Squibb, S.Afr.)*; Flunir *(Oberlin, Fr.)*; Inflaryl *(Squibb, Belg.; Squibb, Neth.)*; Landruma *(Landerlan, Spain)*; Natik *(Celtia, Arg.)*; Niflam *(Rhone-Poulenc, Ital.)*; Nifluril *(UPSA, Fr.; UPSA, Switz.)*.

13017-k

Nimesulide *(BAN, rINN)*.
R-805. 4′-Nitro-2′-phenoxymethanesulphonanilide.
$C_{13}H_{12}N_2O_5S$=308.3.

CAS — 51803-78-2.

Nimesulide has analgesic, anti-inflammatory, and antipyretic properties. It has been given in doses of up to 200 mg twice daily by mouth.

Some references to nimesulide: M. Tomamichel and M. Reiner, *Clin. Trials J.*, 1983, *20*, 148 (Superficial phlebitis or deep thrombophlebitis); J. M. Pais and F. M. Rosteiro, *J. int. med. Res.*, 1983, *11*, 149 (dental inflammation); G. Cornaro, *Curr. ther. Res.*, 1983, *33*, 982 (dental inflammation); R. K. Rondel *et al., Curr. ther. Res.*, 1984, *35*, 123 (dysmenorrhoea); M. Reiner *et al., J. int. med. Res.*, 1984, *12*, 102 (fever); C. Milvio, *ibid.*, 327 (otitis media, sinusitis, rhinitis).

Proprietary Names and Manufacturers
Aulin *(Boehringer Biochemia, Ital.)*; Mesulid *(LPB, Ital.)*.

13020-l

Niprofazone *(rINN)*.
N-[(2,3-Dimethyl-5-oxo-1-phenyl-3-pyrazolin-4-yl)isopropylaminomethyl]nicotinamide.
$C_{21}H_{25}N_5O_2$=379.5.

CAS — 15387-10-7.

Niprofazone has analgesic, anti-inflammatory, and antipyretic properties. It has been given in doses of up to 2 g daily by mouth.

Proprietary Names and Manufacturers
Ravalgene *(Ravasini, Ital.)*.

13052-x

Oxametacin *(rINN)*.
Oxamethacin. 1-(4-Chlorobenzoyl)-5-methoxy-2-methylindole-3-acetohydroxamic acid.
$C_{19}H_{17}ClN_2O_4$=372.8.

CAS — 27035-30-9.

Oxametacin has analgesic, anti-inflammatory, and antipyretic properties. It has been used in rheumatic disorders in doses of up to 600 mg daily, in divided doses, by mouth.

Proprietary Names and Manufacturers
Dinulcid *(Pharmascience, Fr.)*; Flogar *(UCB, Belg.; ABC, Ital.)*; Restid *(UCB, Ital.; UCB, Spain)*.

13055-d

Oxaprozin *(BAN, USAN, rINN)*.
Wy-21743. 3-(4,5-Diphenyloxazol-2-yl)propionic acid.
$C_{18}H_{15}NO_3$=293.3.

CAS — 21256-18-8.

Oxaprozin has analgesic and anti-inflammatory properties. It has been studied in doses of 1.2 g once daily by mouth in patients with osteoarthritis and rheumatoid arthritis.

A detailed review of the actions and uses of oxaprozin.— P. A. Todd and R. N. Brogden, *Drugs*, 1986, *32*, 291.

3908-y

Oxipizone
Oxipizone is a non-steroidal anti-inflammatory agent which has been given in doses of 250 mg by mouth two or three times daily. It is the piperazine salt of oxyphenbutazone.

Proprietary Names and Manufacturers
Diflamil *(Spain)*.

2678-q

Oxyphenbutazone *(BAN, USAN, rINN)*.
G-27202; Hydroxyphenylbutazone. 4-Butyl-1-(4-hydroxyphenyl)-2-phenylpyrazolidine-3,5-dione monohydrate.
$C_{19}H_{20}N_2O_3,H_2O$=342.4.

CAS — 129-20-4 (anhydrous); 7081-38-1 (monohydrate).

Pharmacopoeias. In *Br., Egypt., Eur., Ind., It., Jug., Neth., Swiss,* and *U.S.*

A white to yellowish-white, odourless or almost odourless, crystalline powder. *B.P.* **Solubilities** are: practically insoluble in water; soluble 1 in 3 of alcohol, 1 in 20 of chloroform, 1 in 20 of ether; soluble in solutions of alkali hydroxides. *U.S.P.* solubilities are: practically insoluble in water; soluble 1 in 1.5 of alcohol, 1 in 4 of chloroform, and 1 in 15 of ether; freely soluble in acetone. **Store** in airtight containers.

Adverse Effects and Precautions
As for phenylbutazone, p.36.

EFFECTS ON THE BLOOD. An analysis of blood dyscrasias reported to the Swedish Adverse Drug Reaction Committee for the 5-year period 1966–70 showed that thrombocytopenia attributable to oxyphenbutazone had been reported on 2 occasions, aplastic anaemia on 10 occasions (5 fatal), and agranulocytosis on 3 occasions (1 fatal). It was estimated that reported figures represented one-third of the true frequency.— L. E. Böttiger and B. Westerholm, *Br. med. J.*, 1973, *3*, 339.

There were 421 reports of adverse reactions to oxyphenbutazone reported to the Committee on Safety of Medicines from June 1964 to Jan. 1973. These included 157 reports of blood disorders (74 fatal) including aplastic anaemia (63; 40 fatal), thrombocytopenia (38; 14 fatal), and agranulocytosis or pancytopenia (36; 15 fatal), and gastro-intestinal haemorrhage (16; 5 fatal). The incidence of reports and fatalities was about twice that for phenylbutazone.— M. F. Cuthbert, *Curr. med. Res. Opinion*, 1974, *2*, 600.

Aplastic anaemia or agranulocytosis were quoted as underlying or contributory causes of death in 376 death certificates in the year Oct. 1974 to Sept. 1975; adequate medical records were available for 269. Death was probably due to oxyphenbutazone in 11 cases. Mortality was estimated at 3.8 per 100 000 patients.— W. H. W. Inman, *Committee on Safety of Medicines, Br. med. J.*, 1977, *1*, 1500.

See also under phenylbutazone (p.36).

EFFECTS ON THE SKIN. Oxyphenbutazone might have been responsible for 2 cases of toxic epidermal necrolysis.— A. Lyell, *Br. J. Derm.*, 1967, *79*, 662. A further report associating oxyphenbutazone with toxic epidermal necrolysis in 2 patients.— J. -C. Roujeau *et al., Lancet*, 1985, *1*, 609.

Oxyphenbutazone was responsible for a fixed drug eruption in 1 patient and was strongly suspected in 2 further cases.— J. A. Savin, *Br. J. Derm.*, 1970, *83*, 546.

A report of contact dermatitis to oxyphenbutazone.— G. Krook, *Contact Dermatitis*, 1975, *1*, 385.

PORPHYRIA. Oxyphenbutazone was considered to be unsafe in patients with acute porphyria because it has been shown to be porphyrinogenic in *animals* or *in vitro* systems.— M.R. Moore and K.E.L. McColl, *Porphyrias, Drug Lists*, Glasgow, Porphyria Research Unit, University of Glasgow, 1987.

Absorption and Fate
As for phenylbutazone, p.36.

Uses and Administration
Oxyphenbutazone is a metabolite of phenylbutazone with similar analgesic, anti-inflammatory, and antipyretic properties (see p.36). Oxyphenbutazone was formerly used by mouth in rheumatic disorders such as ankylosing spondylitis, osteoarthritis, and rheumatoid arthritis but such use is no longer considered justified owing to the risk of severe haematological adverse effects.

Oxyphenbutazone has also been applied topically to the eye as an anti-inflammatory ointment in conditions such as episcleritis.

Oxyphenbutazone ointment was probably of value in the treatment of episcleritis but there was little evidence that it was useful in the treatment of other external eye diseases. There was no justification for inclusion of chloramphenicol in oxyphenbutazone ointment.— *Drug & Ther. Bull.*, 1979, *17*, 40. A reconsideration of oxyphenbutazone eye ointment following the withdrawal of systemic oxyphenbutazone preparations and concluding that it remains a useful and safe preparation for patients with episcleritis.— *ibid.*, 1984, *22*, 88.

Preparations
Oxyphenbutazone Eye Ointment *(B.P.)*
Oxyphenbutazone Tablets *(U.S.P.)*

Proprietary Preparations
Tanderil Eye Ointment *(Zyma, UK)*. *Eye ointment*, oxyphenbutazone 10%.

Tanderil Chloramphenicol Eye Ointment *(Zyma, UK)*. *Eye ointment*, oxyphenbutazone 10%, chloramphenicol 1%.

Proprietary Names and Manufacturers of Oxyphenbutazone and Derivatives
Artroflog *(Ital.)*; Artzone *(S.Afr.)*; Butaflogin *(Ital.)*; Butapirone *(Ital.)*; Buteril *(S.Afr.)*; Butilene *(Ital.)*; Butofen *(Arg.)*; Butolfen *(Spain)*; Californit *(Merckle, Ger.)*; Difmedol *(Ital.)*; Febutolo *(Spain)*; Fibutrox *(S.Afr.)*; Flogistin *(Ital.)*; Flogitolo *(Ital.)*; Flogodin *(Ital.)*; Imbun *(Ger.)*; Ipebutona *(Spain)*; Iridil *(Ital.)*; Isobutil *(Ital.)*; Naleran *(Arg.)*; Neo-Farmadol *(Ital.)*; Otone *(Lennon, S.Afr.)*; Oxalid *(USV Pharmaceutical Corp., USA)*; Oxibutol *(Spain)*; Oxybutazone *(ICN, Canad.)*; Phlogase *(Ger.)*; Phlogistol *(Ger.)*; Phlogont *(Azuchemie, Ger.)*; Piraflogin *(Ital.)*; Poliflogil *(Ital.)*; Rapostan *(Mepha, Switz.)*; Rheumapax *(Swed.; Switz.)*; Rumapax *(Denm.)*; Tandacote *(Geigy, UK)*; Tandearil *(Canad.; Geigy, USA)*; Tanderil *(Arg.; Geigy, Austral.; Belg.; Denm.; Geigy, Fr.; Dispersa, Ger.; Geigy, Ital.; Neth.; Norw.; S.Afr.; Padro, Spain; Dispersa, Switz.; Geigy, Switz.; Geigy, UK; Zyma, UK*; Validil *(Ital.)*.

The following names have been used for multi-ingredient preparations containing oxyphenbutazone and derivatives— Tandalgesic *(Geigy, UK)*; Tanderil-Alka *(Geigy, UK)*.

2679-p

Paracetamol *(BAN, rINN).*

Acetaminophen *(USAN)*; *N*-Acetyl-*p*-aminophenol; Paracetamolum. 4′-Hydroxyacetanilide; *N*-(4-Hydroxyphenyl)acetamide.

$C_8H_9NO_2$=151.2.

CAS — 103-90-2.

NOTE. Compounded preparations containing paracetamol have been given the following British Approved Names: Co-codamol, codeine phosphate and paracetamol in the mass proportions 2 parts to 125 parts; Co-dydramol, dihydrocodeine tartrate and paracetamol in the mass proportions 1 part to 50 parts; Co-proxamol, dextropropoxyphene hydrochloride and paracetamol in the mass proportions 1 part to 10 parts.

Pharmacopoeias. In *Aust., Belg., Br., Braz., Chin., Cz., Egypt., Eur., Fr., Ger., Ind., It., Jpn, Jug., Neth., Roum., Rus., Swiss, Turk.,* and *U.S.* Also in *B.P. Vet.*

A white odourless crystalline powder with a slightly bitter taste. **Soluble** 1 in 70 of water, 1 in 20 of boiling water, and 1 in 7 to 10 of alcohol; very slightly soluble in chloroform and ether. **Store** in airtight containers. Protect from light.

Adverse Effects

Side-effects of paracetamol are usually mild, though haematological reactions have been reported. Skin rashes and other allergic reactions occur occasionally.

Symptoms of paracetamol overdosage in the first 24 hours are pallor, nausea, vomiting, anorexia, and abdominal pain. Liver damage may become apparent 12 to 48 hours after ingestion. Abnormalities of glucose metabolism and metabolic acidosis may occur. In severe poisoning, hepatic failure may progress to encephalopathy, coma, and death. Acute renal failure with acute tubular necrosis may develop even in the absence of severe liver damage. Cardiac arrhythmias have been reported.

Liver damage is likely in adults who have taken 10 g or more of paracetamol. It is considered that excess quantities of a toxic metabolite (usually adequately detoxified by glutathione when normal doses of paracetamol are employed), become irreversibly bound to liver tissue.

ALLERGY. A report of a fixed drug eruption due to paracetamol.— H. T. H. Wilson, *Br. J. Derm.*, 1975, *92*, 213. See also: R. H. M. Thomas and D. D. Munro, *Br. J. Derm.*, 1986, *115*, 357.

Analysis, by the Boston Collaborative Drug Surveillance Program, of data on 15 438 patients hospitalised between 1975 and 1982 detected no allergic skin reactions attributed to paracetamol among 1600 recipients of the drug.— M. Bigby *et al.*, *J. Am. med. Ass.*, 1986, *256*, 3358.

Further reports of allergic reactions to paracetamol: B. H. C. Stricker *et al.*, *Br. med. J.*, 1985, *291*, 938 (bronchospasm and urticaria); J. A. Idoko *et al.* (letter), *Trans. R. Soc. trop. Med. Hyg.*, 1986, *80*, 175 (angioedema).

EFFECTS ON THE BLOOD. *Agranulocytosis.* A 78-year-old woman with osteoarthritis who took 2 to 3, and later 4, tablets of paracetamol daily for 6 to 7 months developed agranulocytosis from which she recovered. Paracetamol was considered the provocative agent.— T. W. Lloyd (letter), *Lancet*, 1961, *1*, 114.

Haemolytic anaemia. A report of haemolytic anaemia with episodes of massive haemolysis due to paracetamol in 1 patient.— E. Manor *et al.*, *J. Am. med. Ass.*, 1976, *236*, 2777.

Paracetamol did not cause haemolysis in Chinese patients with glucose-6-phosphate dehydrogenase deficiency.— T. K. Chan *et al.*, *Br. med. J.*, 1976, *2*, 1227.

A 30-year-old man developed thrombocytopenia associated with haemolytic anaemia after taking paracetamol 3 tablets daily for low-back pain during the previous month. His condition resolved spontaneously after a few days but recurred 8 months later after taking 8 tablets of paracetamol.— A. Kornberg and A. Polliack (letter), *Lancet*, 1978, *2*, 1159.

Pancytopenia. For reports of pancytopenia considered to be due to paracetamol, see S. B. Datta (letter), *Br. med. J.*, 1973, *3*, 173; G. K. Webster (letter), *Br. med. J.*, 1973, *3*, 353.

Thrombocytopenia. Reports of thrombocytopenia attributed to paracetamol.— R. C. Heading (letter), *Br. med. J.*, 1968, *3*, 743; E. V. Eisner and N. T. Shahidi, *New Engl. J. Med.*, 1972, *287*, 376; Y. Shoenfeld *et al.* (letter), *ibid.*, 1980, *303*, 47.

EFFECTS ON THE LIVER. A report of liver damage in a 16-year-old woman following ingestion of only 5.85 g of paracetamol.— E. Fernandez and A. C. Fernandez-Brito (letter), *New Engl. J. Med.*, 1977, *296*, 577.

A 59-year-old woman developed liver function abnormalities while taking about 3 g of paracetamol daily for one year for arthritis. The liver function tests returned to normal 5 weeks after withdrawing the paracetamol; the abnormalities recurred on administration of a test dose.— G. K. Johnson and K. G. Tolman, *Ann. intern. Med.*, 1977, *87*, 302.

Further reports of hepatic damage associated with ingestion of therapeutic doses of paracetamol.— D. M. Rosenberg and F. A. Neelon (letter), *Ann. intern. Med.*, 1977, *88*, 129; D. M. Rosenberg *et al.*, *Sth. med. J.*, 1977, *70*, 660; H. L. Bonkowsky *et al.*, *Lancet*, 1978, *1*, 1016; R. Olsson (letter), *Lancet*, 1978, *2*, 152.

Therapeutic doses of paracetamol were not considered to be implicated in liver damage.— J. Neuberger *et al.*, *J. R. Soc. Med.*, 1980, *73*, 701.

For reports of liver damage following paracetamol overdosage, see below.

OVERDOSAGE. Some reviews of overdosage with paracetamol: L. F. Prescott, *Drugs*, 1983, *25*, 290; M. Black, *Postgrad. med. J.*, 1983, *59*, *Suppl.* 4, 116; M. Black and J. Raucy, *Ann. intern. Med.*, 1986, *104*, 427.

A short comment that paediatric elixirs of paracetamol usually do not contain enough paracetamol to cause serious liver damage even if the whole bottle is ingested by a child. If a large dose (more than 150 mg per kg body-weight) is believed to have been taken a specific antidote should be given.— J. Henry and G. Volans, *Br. med. J.*, 1984, *289*, 486.

In 41 patients who had ingested overdoses of paracetamol, liver damage was the major complication and occurred in most patients who had ingested more than 15 g. Symptoms of acute overdosage included vomiting, anorexia, nausea, and epigastric pain. Maximum liver damage occurred after 2 to 4 days, the degree of damage being greater the larger the overdose. Jaundice might occur after 2 to 6 days. Profound hypoglycaemia and metabolic acidosis might complicate severe poisoning. One patient died of gastro-intestinal haemorrhage and acute massive necrosis of the liver. Acute tubular necrosis of the kidneys occurred in 1 patient who recovered.— A. T. Proudfoot and N. Wright, *Br. med. J.*, 1970, *3*, 557.

From studies in patients with paracetamol overdosage, it was found that severe hepatic lesions occurred when the plasma-paracetamol concentrations reached more than 300 µg per mL after 4 hours; none occurred in patients with concentrations of less than 120 µg per mL. There was no evidence of liver damage in 11 of 12 patients with plasma concentrations of less than 50 µg per mL at 12 hours, but hepatic necrosis developed in 16 of 18 with concentrations greater than 50 µg. The plasma half-life of unchanged paracetamol was raised from a mean of about 2 hours in 17 healthy adults given therapeutic doses to about 2.9 hours in 13 poisoned patients without liver damage and to about 7.6 hours in 17 patients who developed liver damage.— L. F. Prescott *et al.*, *Lancet*, 1971, *1*, 519.

Biochemical evidence of liver damage was found in 49 of 60 patients admitted to hospital after taking 13 to 100 g of paracetamol. Anorexia, nausea, and vomiting were seen on the first and second days and jaundice on the third or fourth. Serum-bilirubin concentrations of 40 µg or more per mL were observed in 19 patients, 17 of whom developed fulminant hepatic failure with hepatic encephalopathy which led to coma in 15 and death in 12. Gastro-intestinal haemorrhage requiring treatment occurred in 5, transient hypoglycaemia in 4, and renal failure in 6 patients. Liver specimens showed necrosis.— R. Clark *et al.*, *Lancet*, 1973, *1*, 66.

Analysis of 160 patients with fulminant hepatic failure due to paracetamol overdosage or other factors showed no relationship between paracetamol and renal failure. This lack of association was confirmed in 190 patients with less severe liver damage. Renal failure when it occurred in any of these patients was related to endotoxaemia.— S. P. Wilkinson *et al.*, *J. clin. Path.*, 1977, *30*, 141. There may be a not infrequent occurrence of acute tubular necrosis with renal failure in patients with relatively mild liver damage without hepatic encephalopathy following paracetamol overdosage. This usually occurred in patients who had taken large quantities of alcohol or other drugs which cause enzyme induction.— L. F. Prescott, in *Side-effects of Drugs Annual 2*, M.N.G. Dukes (Ed.), Oxford, Excerpta Medica, 1978, p. 79.

Reports and correspondence concerning the occurrence of paracetamol-induced acute renal failure in the absence of fulminant liver damage.— I. Cobden *et al.*, *Br. med. J.*, 1982, *284*, 21; L. F. Prescott *et al.* (letter), *ibid.*, 421; R. Gabriel (letter), *ibid.*, 505.

Reports and correspondence concerning metabolic acidosis associated with paracetamol poisoning: A. Zezulka and N. Wright, *Br. med. J.*, 1982, *285*, 851; H. F. Woods and H. Connor (letter), *ibid.*, 1208; J. A. Vale and T. J. Meredith (letter), *ibid;* M. Williams *et al.* (letter), *ibid;* C. Acomb *et al.* (letter), *Lancet*, 1985, *2*, 614; R. S. Heir and V. E. Allsup (letter), *ibid.*, 1182; R. J. Flanagan and T. G. K. Mant, *Hum. Toxicol.*, 1986, *5*, 179.

Treatment of Adverse Effects

Prompt treatment is essential in the management of paracetamol overdosage. Any patient who has ingested about 7.5 g or more of paracetamol in the preceeding 4 hours should undergo gastric lavage. Specific therapy with an antidote such as acetylcysteine or methionine may be necessary. Generally treatment is required if the blood-paracetamol concentration is higher than a line (the '200' line) drawn on semi-log/linear paper joining the points 200 mg per litre (1.32 mmol per litre) at 4 hours and 30 mg per litre (0.20 mmol per litre) at 15 hours; determination of the concentration before 4 hours is not considered to give a reliable measurement and administration of acetylcysteine or methionine more than 15 hours after the overdose is generally ineffective and may be associated with an excerbation of any liver abnormality.

Acetylcysteine may be given either intravenously or by mouth (see p.903 for details of dosages) or methionine may be given by mouth (see p.843 for details of dosages). Cysteamine (see p.837) was also formerly used.

The management of paracetamol poisoning is now well established. Patients who present to hospital within 4 hours of taking at least 10 g of paracetamol should undergo gastric lavage. Children under 6 years of age tend to swallow only small amounts of paracetamol, and gastric lavage is probably unnecessary. In neither adults nor children has the value of ipecacuanha been established and it may even induce symptoms indistinguishable from those that may occcur in the early stages of paracetamol poisoning. When four hours or more have elapsed since the overdose the plasma-paracetamol concentration should be measured. Specific treatment is required if the concentration falls above a line drawn between the points 200 mg per litre at 4 hours and 30 mg per litre at 15 hours after the overdose. Acetylcysteine should be given intravenously, or alternatively, methionine may be given by mouth unless the patient is vomiting or is unconscious; both agents are of little value more than 15 hours after the overdose. Patients at risk of hepatic failure should receive a glucose infusion intravenously to prevent hypoglycaemia and established hepatic or renal failure should be managed conventionally.— T. J. Meredith *et al.*, *Br. med. J.*, 1986, *293*, 345.

Further reviews on paracetamol overdosage and its management: L. F. Prescott, *Drugs*, 1983, *25*, 290; R. J. Flanagan, *Med. Toxicol.*, 1987, *2*, 93.

Precautions

Paracetamol should be given with care to patients with impaired kidney or liver function. Paracetamol should also be given with care to patients taking other drugs that affect the liver.

INTERACTIONS. A review of drug interactions involving paracetamol. The gastro-intestinal absorption of paracetamol may be delayed by drugs such as anticholinergic agents or opioid analgesics which decrease gastric emptying. The likelihood of toxicity may be increased by the concomitant use of enzyme-inducing agents such as alcohol or anti-epileptic drugs. Repeated doses of paracetamol increase somewhat the anticoagulant response to coumarins, and paracetamol may also increase chloramphenicol concentrations.— *Drug Interact. News.*, 1983, *3*, 55.

For reports of the effects of paracetamol on some other drugs, see under, aspirin (p.5), chloramphenicol (p.188), and warfarin sodium (p.345).

Absorption and Fate

Paracetamol is readily absorbed from the gastro-intestinal tract with peak plasma concentrations occurring about 30 minutes to 2 hours after ingestion. It is metabolised in the liver and excreted in the urine mainly as the glucuronide and sulphate conjugates. Less than 5% is excreted as unchanged paracetamol. The elimination half-life varies from about 1 to 4 hours. Plasma-protein binding is negligible at usual therapeutic concentrations but increases with increasing concentrations.

A minor hydroxylated metabolite which is usually produced in very small amounts by mixed-function oxidases in the liver and which is usually detoxified by conjugation with liver glutathione may accumulate following paracetamol overdosage and cause liver damage.

ABSORPTION. Peak plasma and saliva concentrations of paracetamol were found in 8 fasting volunteers within 50 minutes of the ingestion of paracetamol 1 g. The concentration reached varied with the formulation of the tablets taken.— J. P. Glynn and W. Bastain (letter), *J. Pharm. Pharmac.*, 1973, *25*, 420.

Studies on the rectal absorption of paracetamol.— S. Keinänen *et al.*, *Eur. J. clin. Pharmac.*, 1977, *12*, 77; J. J. Maron *et al.*, *Curr. ther. Res.*, 1976, *20*, 45; F. Moolenaar *et al.*, *Pharm. Weekbl. Ned., scient. Edn*, 1979, *1*, 25; R. Liedtke *et al.*, *Arzneimittel-Forsch.*, 1979, *29*, 1607.

METABOLISM. A study of paracetamol elimination kinetics in neonates, children, and adults. An adult pattern of metabolism was evident at 12 years of age but no significant differences were noted in the overall rate of elimination among the age groups studied despite the fact that infants and younger children had different major pathways for elimination. A higher percentage of a dose was excreted as the sulphate in neonates and younger children.— R. P. Miller *et al.*, *Clin. Pharmac. Ther.*, 1976, *19*, 284. Pharmacokinetics of paracetamol in children.— R. G. Peterson and B. H. Rumack, *Pediatrics*, 1978, *62, Suppl.*, 877.

Further studies on the effects of age on paracetamol metabolism and excretion.— R. H. Briant *et al.*, *J. Am. Geriat. Soc.*, 1976, *24*, 359; S. N. Alam *et al.*, *Pharmacologist*, 1976, *18*, 231; S. N. Alam *et al.*, *J. Pediat.*, 1977, *90*, 130; B. Fulton *et al.*, *Br. J. clin. Pharmac.*, 1979, *7*, 418P.

A comparison of the pharmacokinetics of paracetamol after administration by intravenous injection and by mouth, suggested that considerable 'first pass' inactivation took place in the gut wall or the liver.— M. D. Rawlins *et al.*, *Eur. J. clin. Pharmac.*, 1977, *11*, 283.

PREGNANCY AND THE NEONATE. Pharmacokinetic studies in 12 nursing mothers given a single dose of paracetamol suggested that maternal ingestion of paracetamol in usual therapeutic doses does not appear to present a risk to the nursing infant.— C. M. Berlin *et al.*, *Pediat. Pharmacol.*, 1980, *1*, 135. See also: E. L. Hurden *et al.*, *Archs Dis. Childh.*, 1980, *55*, 969.

Paracetamol metabolites in the neonate following maternal overdose at 36 weeks. The baby was delivered by Caesarean section and did not suffer liver damage; the mother was treated with acetylcysteine.— I. Roberts *et al.*, *Br. J. clin. Pharmac.*, 1984, *18*, 201.

The metabolism of paracetamol during pregnancy.— J. O. Miners *et al.*, *Br. J. clin. Pharmac.*, 1986, *22*, 359.

PROTEIN BINDING. Binding of paracetamol to plasma proteins did not occur with plasma concentrations of less than 60 μg per mL, corresponding to the usual therapeutic concentrations. After toxic doses of paracetamol up to 43% could be bound to plasma proteins.— B. G. Gazzard *et al.*, *J. Pharm. Pharmac.*, 1973, *25*, 964.

Uses and Administration

Paracetamol has analgesic and antipyretic properties but it has no useful anti-inflammatory properties.

The usual adult dose by mouth is 0.5 to 1 g every 4 to 6 hours up to a maximum of 4 g daily. Suggested doses in children are: 3 months to 1 year, 60 to 120 mg; 1 to 5 years, 120 to 250 mg; 6 to 12 years, up to 500 mg. These doses may be given 3 to 4 times daily as required.

Reviews of actions and uses of paracetamol.— J. Koch-Weser, *New Engl. J. Med.*, 1976, *295*, 1297; *Med. Lett.*, 1976, *18*, 73; B. Ameer and D. J. Greenblatt, *Ann. intern. Med.*, 1977, *87*, 202; C. H. Jackson *et al.*, *Can. med. Ass. J.*, 1984, *131*, 25.

ADMINISTRATION IN HEPATIC FAILURE. In a single-dose study, the metabolism of paracetamol, as judged by plasma half-life and plasma concentration of metabolites, was not depressed in patients with mild liver disease compared with normal subjects but was significantly impaired in those with severe liver disease. There were no significant differences in the overall 24-hour urinary excretion of paracetamol and its metabolites. There was no evidence that patients with liver disease were at increased risk of hepatotoxicity when given a single therapeutic dose of paracetamol.— J. A. H. Forrest *et al.*, *Eur. J. clin. Pharmac.*, 1979, *15*, 427.

Studies in subjects with chronic liver disease given paracetamol 4 g daily for up to 13 days showed that there was no contra-indication to the use of paracetamol in therapeutic doses in the presence of stable chronic liver disease.— G. D. Benson, *Clin. Pharmac. Ther.*, 1983, *33*, 95.

ADMINISTRATION IN RENAL FAILURE. Paracetamol could be administered to patients with renal failure by adjusting the dosage interval. A dosage interval of 4 hours is suitable for patients with a glomerular filtration-rate (GFR) above 50 mL per minute; an interval of 6 hours between doses is advisable for rates between 10 and 50 mL per minute. Where the rate is less than 10 mL per minute the dosage interval should be 8 hours. A dose supplement should be given to patients undergoing haemodialysis.— W. M. Bennett *et al.*, *Am. J. Kidney Dis.*, 1983, *3*, 155.

Preparations

Acetaminophen Capsules *(U.S.P.)*. Capsules containing paracetamol.

Acetaminophen, Aspirin, and Caffeine Capsules *(U.S.P.)*. Capsules containing paracetamol, aspirin, and caffeine.

Acetaminophen Elixir *(U.S.P.)*. An elixir containing paracetamol.

Paediatric Paracetamol Oral Solution *(B.P.)*. Paediatric Paracetamol Elixir. A solution containing paracetamol 2.4%. It should not be diluted.

Paracetamol Elixir CF *(A.P.F.)*. Paracetamol 120 mg, alcohol 0.7 mL, propylene glycol 0.5 mL, water 0.5 mL, glycerol to 5 mL.

Paracetamol Elixir Forte CF *(A.P.F.)*. Paracetamol 240 mg, alcohol 1 mL, propylene glycol 0.5 mL, water 0.5 mL, glycerol to 5 mL.

Paracetamol Oral Suspension *(B.P.)*

Acetaminophen and Codeine Phosphate Elixir *(U.S.P.)*. Elixir containing paracetamol and codeine phosphate.

Acetaminophen for Effervescent Oral Solution *(U.S.P.)*. It contains 5.63 to 6.88% of paracetamol.

Acetaminophen Oral Solution *(U.S.P.)*. An oral solution containing paracetamol.

Acetaminophen Oral Suspension *(U.S.P.)*. A suspension of paracetamol in a suitable aqueous vehicle.

Paracetamol Suppositories CF *(A.P.F.)*. Suppositories containing paracetamol 120 mg in macrogol basis.

Paracetamol Tablets *(B.P.)*

Acetaminophen Tablets *(U.S.P.)*. Tablets containing paracetamol.

Acetaminophen, Aspirin, and Caffeine Tablets *(U.S.P.)*. Tablets containing paracetamol, aspirin, and caffeine.

Acetaminophen and Diphenhydramine Citrate Tablets *(U.S.P.)*. Tablets containing paracetamol and diphenhydramine citrate.

Proprietary Preparations

Cafadol *(Typharm, UK)*. *Tablets*, scored, paracetamol 500 mg, caffeine 30 mg.

Calpol *(Calmic, UK)*. *Suspension* (Infant Suspension), paracetamol 120 mg/5 mL.
Suspension (Six Plus Suspension), paracetamol 250 mg/5 mL.

Coda-Med *(Dep, UK)*. *Tablets*, paracetamol 450 mg, codeine phosphate 8.1 mg, caffeine citrate 15 mg.

Disprol Paediatric *(Reckitt & Colman Pharmaceuticals, UK)*. *Suspension*, paracetamol 120 mg/5 mL. Disprol Junior also contains paracetamol 120 mg per soluble tablet or per 5 mL of suspension.

Hedamol *(Nicholas, UK)*. *Capsules*, paracetamol 500 mg, codeine phosphate 10.2 mg.

Lobak *(Sterling Research, UK)*. *Tablets*, scored, paracetamol 450 mg, chlormezanone 100 mg.

Medised *(Panpharma, UK)*. *Suspension*, paracetamol 120 mg, promethazine hydrochloride 2.5 mg/5 mL.

Medised *(Martindale Pharmaceuticals, UK)*. *Tablets*, scored, paracetamol 500 mg, promethazine hydrochloride 10 mg.

Medocodene *(Medo, UK)*. *Tablets*, scored, paracetamol 500 mg, codeine phosphate 8 mg (co-codamol).

Neurodyne *(Fisons, UK)*. *Capsules*, paracetamol 500 mg, codeine phosphate 8 mg (co-codamol).

Paldesic *(R.P. Drugs, UK)*. *Elixir*, paracetamol 120 mg/5 mL.

Panadeine *(Winthrop, UK)*. *Tablets*, scored, paracetamol 500 mg, codeine phosphate 8 mg (co-codamol).
Tablets (Panadeine Forte), paracetamol 500 mg, codeine phosphate 15 mg.
Tablets (Panadeine Soluble), effervescent, paracetamol 500 mg, codeine phosphate 8 mg (co-codamol).

Panadol *(Winthrop, UK)*. *Tablets*, paracetamol 500 mg.
Tablets (Panadol Caplets), paracetamol 500 mg.
Tablets (Panadol Soluble), scored, effervescent, paracetamol 500 mg.
Elixir , paracetamol 120 mg/5 mL.

Panaleve *(Leo, UK)*. *Elixir*, paracetamol 120 mg/5 mL.

Paraclear *(Nicholas, UK)*. *Tablets*, soluble, paracetamol 500 mg.
Tablets (Paraclear Junior), paracetamol 120 mg.

Paracodol *(Fisons, UK)*. *Tablets*, effervescent, paracetamol 500 mg, codeine phosphate 8 mg (co-codamol).

Paradeine *(Scotia, UK)*. *Tablets*, paracetamol 500 mg, codeine phosphate 10 mg, phenolphthalein 2.5 mg.

Parahypon *(Calmic, UK)*. *Tablets*, scored, paracetamol 500 mg, caffeine 10 mg, codeine phosphate 5 mg.

Parake *(Galen, UK)*. *Tablets*, paracetamol 500 mg, codeine phosphate 8 mg (co-codamol).

Paramax *(Beecham Research, UK)*. *Tablets*, scored, paracetamol 500 mg, metoclopramide hydrochloride 5 mg.
Sachets, paracetamol 500 mg, metoclopramide hydrochloride 5 mg.

Pardale *(Martindale Pharmaceuticals, UK)*. *Tablets*, scored, paracetamol 400 mg, codeine phosphate 9 mg, caffeine hydrate 10 mg.

Propain *(Panpharma, UK)*. *Tablets*, scored, paracetamol 400 mg, codeine phosphate 10 mg, diphenhydramine hydrochloride 5 mg, caffeine 50 mg.

Resolve *(Beecham Proprietaries, UK)*. *Granules*, paracetamol 500 mg/sachet.

Sinitol *(Nicholas, UK)*. *Capsules*, paracetamol 500 mg, pseudoephedrine 20 mg.

Solpadeine *(Sterling Research, UK)*. *Capsules*, paracetamol 500 mg, codeine phosphate 8 mg, caffeine 30 mg.
Tablets, effervescent, paracetamol 500 mg, codeine phosphate 8 mg, caffeine 30 mg.

Syndol *(Merrell, UK)*. *Tablets*, scored, paracetamol 450 mg, codeine phosphate 10 mg, doxylamine succinate 5 mg, caffeine 30 mg.

Tylex *(Ortho-Cilag, UK)*. *Capsules*, paracetamol 500 mg, codeine phosphate 30 mg.

Unigesic *(Unimed, UK)*. *Capsules*, paracetamol 500 mg, caffeine 30 mg.

Proprietary Names and Manufacturers

Acephen *(G & W, USA)*; Acetalgine *(Streuli, Switz.)*; Acetamol *(Gentili, Ital.)*; Aferadol *(Oberlin, Fr.)*; Alba-Temp *(Bart, USA)*; Alvedon *(Astra, Swed.)*; Anacin-3 *(Whitehall, USA)*; Anaflon *(Winthrop, Ger.)*; Anuphen *(USA)*; Atasol *(Horner, Canad.)*; Ben-u-ron *(Belg.*; *Bene, Ger.*; *Switz.)*; Bramcetamol *(Austral.)*; Calip *(Arg.)*; Calpol *(Wellcome, Ital.*; *Wellcome, S.Afr.*; *Calmic, UK)*; Calpon *(Austral.)*; Campain *(Canad.)*; Capital *(Carnrick, USA)*; Captin *(Krewel, Ger.)*; Ceetamol *(Protea, Austral.)*; Cetamol *(Eire)*; Cetapon *(Remedia, S.Afr.)*; Claradol *(Nicholas, Fr.)*; Claratal *(Nicholas, Austral.)*; Custodial *(Arg.)*; Dafalgan *(UPSA, Fr.)*; Datril *(Bristol-Myers Products, USA)*; Dirox *(Arg.)*; Disprol Paediatric *(Reckitt & Colman Pharmaceuticals, UK)*; Dolamin *(Austral.)*; Dolanex *(Lannett, USA)*; Doliprane *(Bottu, Fr.)*; Doloral *(Arg.)*; Dolorol *(Lennon, S.Afr.)*; Dolprone *(Bottu, Switz.)*; Dorcol Children's Fever and Pain Reducer *(Dorsey Laboratories, USA)*; Doregrippin *(Rentschler, Ger.)*; Dymadon *(Wellcome, Austral.)*; Efferalgan *(UPSA, Fr.*; *UPSA, Switz.)*; Enelfa *(Dolorgiet, Ger.)*; Ennagesic *(S.Afr.)*; Eu-Med *(Med Fabrik, Ger.)*; Exdol *(Frosst, Canad.)*; Fanalgic *(Mitchell, Denm.)*; Febrigesic *(Seatrace, USA)*; Fendon *(USA)*; Fevamol *(GS, S.Afr.)*; Fonafor *(Arg.)*; Gelocatil *(Gelos, Spain)*; Glenpar *(Ind.)*; Gynospasmine *(Vaillant-Defresne, Fr.)*; Kinderfinimal *(Neth.)*; Kinder-Finiweh *(Dentinox, Ger.)*; Korum *(USA)*; Liquiprin *(Norcliff Thayer, USA)*; Lyteca *(USA)*; Malgis *(Grémy-Longuet, Fr.)*; Melabon *(Lacer, Spain)*; Napamol *(Propan, S.Afr.)*; Nebs *(USA)*; Neuridal *(Beecham-Wülfing, Ger.)*; Nevral *(Ital.)*; Nina 120 *(Medichemie, Switz.)*;

Ophinal *(Kettelhack Riker, Ger.)*; Oraphen-PD *(USA)*; Pacemol *(Austral.)*; Painamol *(Be-Tabs, S.Afr.)*; Painaway *(Adcock Ingram, S.Afr.)*; Paldesic *(R.P. Drugs, UK)*; Pamol *(Marshall's Pharmaceuticals, UK)*; Panado *(Winthrop, S.Afr.)*; Panadol *(Winthrop, Austral.; Sterling, Canad.; Fin.; Maggioni-Winthrop, Ital.; Neth.; Sterwin, Spain; Winthrop, Switz.; Winthrop, UK; Glenbrook, USA)*; Panaleve *(Leo, UK)*; Panamax *(Winthrop, Austral.)*; Panasorb *(Winthrop, UK)*; Panodil *(Winthrop, Denm.; Iceland; Winthrop, Norw.; Sterling-Winthrop, Swed.)*; Panofen *(USA)*; Pantalgin *(UCB, Ger.)*; Paracet *(Austral.; Weiders, Norw.)*; Paraclear *(Nicholas, UK)*; Paralgin *(Fawns & McAllan, Austral.)*; Parapain *(Nicholas, Austral.)*; Paraprom *(S.Afr.)*; Parasin *(Nelson, Austral.)*; Paraspen *(Rosken, Austral.)*; Paratol *(High Noon, Pakistan)*; Parmol *(USV, Austral.)*; Pasolind *(Stada, Ger.)*; Phendex *(USA)*; Pinex *(A.L., Denm.; Apothekernes Laboratorium, Norw.)*; Placemol *(Austral.)*; Praecimed *(Molimin, Ger.)*; Proval *(USA)*; Puernol *(Formenti, Ital.; Switz.)*; Pyragesic *(SCS, S.Afr.)*; Pyralen *(S.Afr.)*;
Reliv *(ACO, Swed.)*; Repamol *(S.Afr.)*; Resolve *(Beecham Proprietaries, UK)*; Robigesic *(Robins, Canad.)*; Rounox *(Rougier, Canad.)*; Salzone *(Wallace Mfg Chem., UK)*; Schmerzex *(Roland, Ger.)*; Sedapyren *(S.Afr.)*; Servigesic *(Servipharm, Switz.)*; Setamol *(Pharmacia, Denm.)*; SK-APAP *(Smith Kline & French, USA)*; Summadol *(Selvi, Ital.)*; Tachipirina *(Angelini, Ital.)*; Tapar *(Parke, Davis, USA)*; Tempra *(Mead Johnson, Austral.; Belg.; Mead Johnson, Canad.; Mead Johnson Nutritional, USA)*; Tenasfen *(Arg.)*; Ticelgesic *(Ticen, Eire)*; Tivrin *(Canad.)*; Treupel *(Degussa, Ger.)*; Treuphadol *(Treupha, Switz.)*; Tricocetamol *(Vernleigh, S.Afr.)*; Tylenol *(Belg.; McNeil, Canad.; Johnson & Johnson, Fr.; Johnson & Johnson, Ger.; Johnson & Johnson, S.Afr.; Johnson & Johnson, Spain; Johnson & Johnson, Switz.; McNeil Consumer, USA)*; Tymol *(Reckitt & Colman, Austral.)*; Valadol *(Squibb, USA)*; Zolben *(Ciba, Spain; Geigy, Switz.)*.

The following names have been used for multi-ingredient preparations containing paracetamol—Acetaco *(Legere, USA)*; Actifed-A *(Wellcome, Canad.)*; Algisin *(Ram, USA)*; Allerest *(Pharmacraft, USA)*; Amacodone *(Trimen, USA)*; Amaphen *(Trimen, USA)*; Amaphen with Codeine *(Trimen, USA)*; Anexsia *(Beecham Laboratories, USA)*; Angesil Plus *(Drug Houses Austral., Austral.)*; Anoquan *(Mallard, USA)*; Apap with Codeine *(Ayerst, USA)*; Atasol *(Horner, Canad.)*; Atasol-15 *(Horner, Canad.)*; Atasol-30 *(Horner, Canad.)*; Bancap *(Forest Pharmaceuticals, USA)*; Benadryl Cold and Flu Tablets *(Parke, Davis, Austral.)*; Benylin Day and Night Cold Treatment *(Warner-Lambert, UK)*; Beta-Phed *(Metro Med, USA)*; Bex *(Nicholas, Austral.)*; Blanex *(Edwards, USA)*; Broncho-Grippol *(Charton, Canad.)*; Bucet *(UAD, USA)*; Budale *(Dales, UK)*;
Cafadol *(Typharm, UK)*; Capadex *(Fawns & McAllan, Austral.)*; Capital with Codeine *(Carnrick, USA)*; Carisoma Compound *(Pharmax, UK)*; Chlorzone *(Schein, USA)*; Codalan *(Lannett, USA)*; Codalgin *(Fawns & McAllan, Austral.)*; Coda-Med *(Dep, UK)*; Codamin *(Clark, Canad.)*; Codaminophen *(Clark, Canad.)*; Codral Pain Relief *(Wellcome, Austral.)*; Co-Gesic *(Central Pharmaceuticals, USA)*; Cold War *(Key, Austral.)*; Compal *(Reid-Rowell, USA)*; Comtrex *(Bristol-Myers Products, USA)*; Conar-A *(Beecham Laboratories, USA)*; Congespirin Aspirin Free *(Bristol-Myers Products, USA)*; Congesprin *(Bristol-Myers Products, USA)*; Coricidin Pediatric Drops *(Schering, Canad.)*; Coryban-D Cough Syrup *(Pfipharmecs, USA)*; Cosalgesic *(Cox, UK)*; Cotaminol *(Gen, Canad.)*; CoTylenol *(McNeil Consumer, USA)*; Cyclopane *(Alcon, Austral.)*; Damacet-P *(Mason, USA)*; Darvocet-N *(Lilly, USA)*; Decotan *(Gen, Canad.)*; Demerol Apap *(Winthrop-Breon, USA)*; Dextrogesic *(Unimed, UK)*; Dia-Gesic *(Central Pharmaceuticals, USA)*; Di-Gesic *(Dista, Austral.)*; Dimetapp Elixir-Plus *(Robins, Austral.)*; Dimetapp-A *(Robins, Canad.)*; Dimotapp P *(Robins, UK)*; Distalgesic *(Dista, UK)*; Dolacet *(Hauck, USA)*; Dolene AP-65 *(Lederle, USA)*; Dolprn *(Bock, USA)*; Dolvan *(Norma, UK)*; Double-A *(Edwards, USA)*; Dristan Advanced Formula *(Whitehall, Canad.; Whitehall, USA)*; Duradyne DHC *(Forest Pharmaceuticals, USA)*; Dymadon Co *(Wellcome, Austral.)*;
Empracet with Codeine Phosphate *(Wellcome, Canad.; Wellcome, USA)*; Emtec *(Technilab, Canad.)*; Esgic *(Forest Pharmaceuticals, USA)*; Espasmotex *(Arlo, USA)*; Excedrin *(Bristol-Myers Products, USA)*; Excedrin P.M. *(Bristol-Myers Products, USA)*; Exdol *(Frosst, Canad.)*; Femerital *(MCP Pharmaceuticals, UK)*; Fioricet *(Sandoz, USA)*; Fiorinal *(Sandoz, Austral.)*; Fortagesic *(Sterling Research, UK)*; G-1/G-2/G-3 Capsules *(Hauck, USA)*; Hedamol *(Nicholas, UK)*; Hycodaphen *(Ascher, USA)*; Hycomine Compound *(Du Pont, USA)*; Hyco-Pap *(Lasalle, USA)*; Hydrocet *(Carnrick, USA)*; Hydrogesic *(Edwards, USA)*; Hy-Phen *(Ascher, USA)*; Korigesic *(Trimen, USA)*; Lenoltec with Codeine *(Technilab, Canad.)*; Lobak *(Sterling Research, UK)*; Lorcet *(UAD, USA)*; Lortab *(Russ, USA)*; Maxigesic *(Mastar, USA)*; Medigesic Plus *(US Pharmaceutical, USA)*; Medised *(Martindale Pharmaceuticals, UK)*; Medocodene *(Medo, UK)*; Menoplex *(Fiske, USA)*; Mersyndol *(Merrell Dow, Austral.; Merrell Dow, Canad.)*; Midol *(Nyal, Austral.)*; Midol PMS *(Sterling, Canad.; Glenbrook, USA)*; Midrid *(Carnrick, UK)*; Midrin *(Carnrick, USA)*; Migralam *(Bart, USA)*; Migraleve *(International Laboratories, UK)*; Migralift *(International Laboratories, UK)*; Migranol *(Alcon, Austral.)*; Myolgin *(Cox, UK)*; Nembudeine *(Abbott, Austral.)*; Neo-Synephrine Antihistamine Cold Tablets *(Winthrop, Austral.)*; Neosynephrine Cold Tablets *(Winthrop, Austral.)*; Neurodyne *(Fisons, UK)*; Norcet *(Holloway, USA)*; Norgesic *(Riker, Austral.; Riker, UK)*; Novogesic *(Novopharm, Canad.)*; Nyquil *(Richardson-Vicks, Canad.)*; Oxycocet *(Technilab, Canad.)*;
Pacaps *(Lasalle, USA)*; Paedo-Sed *(Pharmax, UK)*; Pameton *(Winthrop, UK)*; Pamol Supps for Babies *(Marshall's Pharmaceuticals, UK)*; Panadeine *(Winthrop, Austral.; Winthrop, UK)*; Panadeine Co. *(Winthrop, UK)*; Panadol Elixir with Promethazine *(Winthrop, Austral.)*; Panamax Co. *(Winthrop, Austral.)*; Panquil *(Rosken, Austral.)*; Papzans Modified *(Bowman, USA)*; Paracodol *(Fisons, UK)*; Paradeine *(Scotia, UK)*; Paradex *(Protea, Austral.)*; Parafon Forte *(McNeil, Canad.; McNeil Pharmaceutical, USA)*; Parafon Forte C8 *(McNeil, Canad.)*; Paragesic *(Sandoz, UK)*; Parahypon *(Calmic, UK)*; Parake *(Galen, UK)*; Paralgin *(Norton, UK)*; Paramax *(Beecham Research, UK)*; Paramol *(Duncan, Flockhart, UK)*; Paraseltzer *(Sandoz, UK)*; Parazolidin *(Geigy, UK)*; Pardale *(Martindale Pharmaceuticals, UK)*; Paxalgesic *(Steinhard, UK)*; Paxidal *(Wallace Mfg Chem., UK)*; Pentalgin *(Fawns & McAllan, Austral.)*; Percocet *(Du Pont, Canad.; Du Pont, USA)*; Percodan *(Du Pont, Austral.)*; Percogesic *(Richardson-Vicks, USA)*; Pharma-Col *(Rosken, Austral.)*; Pharmidone *(Farmitalia Carlo Erba, UK)*; Phenaphen with Codeine *(Robins, USA)*; Phenate *(Mallard, USA)*; Pholcolix *(Parke, Davis, UK)*; Phrenilin *(Carnrick, USA)*; Phrenilin with Codeine *(Carnrick, USA)*; Prodismen *(Prosana, Austral.)*; Propacet *(Lemmon, USA)*; Propain *(Panpharma, UK)*; Propain HC *(Springbok, USA)*; Protid *(Lasalle, USA)*;
Repan *(Everett, USA)*; Rinurel Linctus *(Warner, UK)*; Rinurel Tablets *(Warner, UK)*; Robaxacet *(Robins, Canad.)*; Safapryn *(Pfizer, UK)*; Safapryn-Co *(Pfizer, UK)*; Saleto *(Mallard, USA)*; Saroflex *(Saron, USA)*; Seda-Gel Suspension *(Nelson, Austral.)*; Sedapap *(Mayrand, USA)*; Sigma Relief Cold Tablets *(Sigma, Austral.)*; Sinarest *(Pharmacraft, USA)*; Sine-Aid *(McNeil Consumer, USA)*; Singlet *(Lakeside, USA)*; Sinitol *(Nicholas, UK)*; Sinubid *(Parke, Davis, USA)*; Sinulin *(Carnrick, USA)*; Sinutab *(Warner, Austral.; Parke, Davis, Canad.; Warner-Lambert, UK)*; Sinuzets *(Boots, Austral.)*; SK-65 APAP *(Smith Kline & French, USA)*; SK-APAP with Codeine *(Smith Kline & French, USA)*; SK-Oxycodone with Acetaminophen *(Smith Kline & French, USA)*; Solpadeine *(Winthrop, Austral.; Sterling Research, UK)*; Sonalgin *(May & Baker, Austral.; May & Baker, UK)*; Stopayne *(Springbok, USA)*; Sudafed-Co *(Calmic, UK)*; Supac *(Mission Pharmacal, USA)*; Syndol *(Merrell, UK)*;
Talacen *(Winthrop-Breon, USA)*; Tandalgesic *(Geigy, UK)*; Teldrin *(Menley & James, USA)*; T-Gesic *(T.E. Williams, USA)*; Tinol *(Ticen, Eire)*; Triad *(UAD, USA)*; Triaminicin *(Ancalab, Canad.; Dorsey Laboratories, USA)*; Triogesic *(Sandoz, Austral.; Intercare, UK)*; Triolix *(Drug Houses Austral., Austral.)*; Triotussic *(Beecham Research, UK)*; Tuscodin *(Schering, Austral.)*; Two-Dyne *(Hyrex, USA)*; Tylenol No. 1 *(McNeil Consumer, USA)*; Tylenol with Codeine *(McNeil, Canad.)*; Tylenol Sinus Medication *(McNeil, Canad.)*; Tylex *(Ortho, UK)*; Tylox *(McNeil Pharmaceutical, USA)*; Uniflu *(Unigreg, UK)*; Unigesic *(Unimed, UK)*; Vanquish *(Glenbrook, USA)*; Veganin *(Parke, Davis, Canad.; Warner-Lambert, UK)*; Vicodin *(Knoll, USA)*; Wygesic *(Wyeth, USA)*; Zydone *(Du Pont, USA)*.

13084-v

Parsalmide *(rINN)*.
54106-CB; MY-41-6. 5-Amino-*N*-butyl-*O*-(prop-2-ynyl)salicylamide; 5-Amino-*N*-butyl-2-(prop-2-ynyloxy)benzamide.
$C_{14}H_{18}N_2O_2$=246.3.

CAS — 30653-83-9.

Parsalmide has analgesic and anti-inflammatory properties and has been given by mouth in rheumatic disorders.

Proprietary Names and Manufacturers
Parsal *(Midy, Ital.)*.

13096-s

Perisoxal *(pINN)*.
31252-S (citrate); Perixazole. 1-(5-Phenylisoxazol-3-yl)-2-piperidinoethanol.
$C_{16}H_{20}N_2O_2$=272.3.

CAS — 2055-44-9.

Perisoxal has analgesic properties and has been used as the citrate in doses of 100 to 200 mg three times daily by mouth.

Proprietary Names and Manufacturers of Perisoxal and its Salts
Isoxal *(Shionogi, Jpn)*.

2681-h

Phenacetin *(rINN)*.
Aceto-*p*-phenetidide; Acetophenetidin; Acetylphenetidin; Paracetophenetidin; Phenacetinum. *p*-Acetophenetidide; 4′-Ethoxyacetanilide; *N*-(4-Ethoxyphenyl)acetamide.
$C_{10}H_{13}NO_2$=179.2.

CAS — 62-44-2.

Pharmacopoeias. In *Arg., Aust., Belg., Braz., Cz., Eur., Fr., Ger., Hung., Int., It., Jpn, Jug., Mex., Neth., Nord., Pol., Port., Roum., Rus., Span., Swiss,* and *Turk.*

White glistening, crystalline scales or fine white crystalline powder. Very slightly **soluble** in water; soluble in alcohol and chloroform; slightly soluble in ether.

Phenacetin may cause methaemoglobinaemia, sulphaemoglobinaemia, and haemolytic anaemia. Methaemoglobinaemia may be treated as described under methylene blue (see p.844).

Prolonged administration of large doses of analgesic mixtures containing phenacetin has been associated with the development of renal papillary necrosis and appears to be associated also with the development of transitional-cell carcinoma of the renal pelvis.

Phenacetin could cause yellow discoloration of the urine or brown to black discoloration on standing due to excretion products.— R. B. Baran and B. Rowles, *J. Am. pharm. Ass.*, 1973, *NS13*, 139.

Phenacetin has analgesic and antipyretic properties. It was usually given with aspirin, caffeine, or codeine but is now little used due to adverse haematological effects and nephrotoxicity.

2684-v

Phenazone *(BAN, rINN)*.
Analgésine; Antipyrin; Antipyrine *(USAN)*; Azophenum; Fenazona; Phenazonum. 1,5-Dimethyl-2-phenyl-4-pyrazolin-3-one.
$C_{11}H_{12}N_2O$=188.2.

CAS — 60-80-0.

Pharmacopoeias. In *Arg., Aust., Belg., Br., Cz., Eur., Fr., Ger., Hung., Int., Jpn, Jug., Mex., Neth., Nord., Pol., Port., Roum., Rus., Span., Swiss, Turk.,* and *U.S.*

Colourless, odourless, or almost odourless, crystals or white crystalline powder with a slightly bitter taste. Very **soluble** in water, alcohol, and chloroform; and sparingly soluble in ether. **Store** in airtight containers.

2683-b

Phenazone and Caffeine Citrate

Antipyrino-Coffeinum Citricum; Migrenin.

Pharmacopoeias. In *Aust., Cz., Hung.,* and *Jpn.*

A powder usually containing phenazone 90%, caffeine 9%, and citric acid monohydrate 1%.

2682-m

Phenazone Salicylate

Antipyrin Salicylate; Salipyrin.

$C_{11}H_{12}N_2O,C_7H_6O_3=326.4$.

CAS — 520-07-0.

Pharmacopoeias. In *Arg., Aust., Fr., Port., Roum.,* and *Span.*

Adverse Effects

Phenazone is liable to give rise to skin eruptions and in susceptible individuals even small doses may have this effect. Large doses by mouth may cause nausea, drowsiness, coma and convulsions.

Phenazone could cause red discoloration of urine.— E. B. Baran and B. Rowles, *J. Am. pharm. Ass.*, 1973, *NS13*, 139.

ALLERGY. An immediate allergic reaction to phenazone and a latent leucopenic reaction.— D. Kadar and W. Kalow, *Clin. Pharmac. Ther.*, 1981, *28*, 820.

EFFECTS ON THE BLOOD. Phenazone had been shown to cause haemolytic anaemia in certain individuals with a deficiency of glucose-6-phosphate dehydrogenase.— T. A. J. Prankerd, *Clin. Pharmac. Ther.*, 1963, *4*, 334.

EFFECTS ON THE KIDNEYS. Recurrent acute renal failure was associated with phenazone in a 32-year-old male patient. A strong positive reaction was obtained in a phenazone skin test.— J. Ortuño and J. Botella, *Lancet*, 1973, *2*, 1473.

Precautions

Phenazone affects the metabolism of some other drugs and its metabolism is affected by other drugs that increase or reduce the activity of liver enzymes.

PORPHYRIA. Phenazone was considered to be unsafe in patients with acute porphyria because it has been shown to be porphyrinogenic in *animals* or *in vitro* systems.— M.R. Moore and K.E.L. McColl, *Porphyrias, Drug Lists*, Glasgow, Porphyria Research Unit, University of Glasgow, 1987.

Absorption and Fate

Phenazone is readily absorbed from the gastro-intestinal tract and is distributed throughout the body fluids. Peak plasma concentrations are usually attained in 1 to 2 hours. Less than 10% is bound to plasma proteins and it has a half-life of about 12 hours. Phenazone is metabolised in the liver; about 30 to 40% is metabolised to 4-hydroxyphenazone which is excreted in the urine as the glucuronide. About 5% is excreted unchanged and about 6% as norphenazone in the urine.

Because phenazone is metabolised primarily in the liver by microsomal mixed-function oxidases, it is widely used for drug metabolism studies. The half-life of phenazone is decreased by substances which induce liver microsomal enzymes and is also decreased by smoking and by hyperthyroidism. Phenazone half-life is increased by substances which inhibit liver microsomal enzymes and is also increased in older subjects and in patients with myxoedema and liver disorders. In addition, phenazone itself induces liver microsmal enzymes and may affect the metabolism of some other drugs.

Uses and Administration

Phenazone has analgesic and antipyretic properties and has been given by mouth; phenazone and caffeine citrate and phenazone salicylate have similarly been given by mouth as analgesics.

Topically, solutions containing 5% of phenazone have been used locally as ear drops in disorders such as acute otitis media.

Changes in the half-life of phenazone in the body (antipyrine half-life) are used as a test for the effect of other drugs or the effect of a disease state on the activity of drug-metabolising enzymes in the liver.

A short comment that there seems to be no justification for the inclusion of phenazone in local preparations used in treating acute otitis media. It is presumably included in such preparations because it is believed to have a local anti-inflammatory and therefore analgesic action. It would, however, seem unlikely that phenazone would have any action on the skin of the intact tympanic membrane and therefore on the pain which is due primarily to the stretching and distention of the membrane.— W. V. Carlin, *Br. med. J.*, 1987, *294*, 1333.

Preparations

Antipyrine and Benzocaine Otic Solution *(U.S.P.).* A solution of phenazone and benzocaine in glycerol. Store in airtight containers. Protect from light.

Antipyrine, Benzocaine, and Phenylephrine Hydrochloride Otic Solution *(U.S.P.).* A solution of phenazone, benzocaine, and phenylephrine hydrochloride in a suitable non-aqueous solvent. Store in airtight containers. Protect from light.

Proprietary Preparations

Auralgicin *(Fisons, UK). Ear-drops,* phenazone 5.5%, ephedrine hydrochloride 1%, benzocaine 1.4%, chlorbutol 1%, potassium hydroxyquinoline sulphate 0.1% in anhydrous glycerol. For acute otitis media.

Auraltone *(Fisons, UK). Ear-drops,* phenazone 5%, benzocaine 1%. For acute otitis media.

Proprietary Names and Manufacturers

Auralgan *(Ayerst, Canad.)*; Crema Antisolar Evanescente *(Imba, Spain)*; Spalt N *(Much, Swed.)*.

The following names have been used for multi-ingredient preparations containing phenazone—Asthma Dellipsoids D17 *(Pilsworth, UK)*; Aurafair *(Pharmafair, USA)*; Auralgan *(Ayerst, Austral.; Ayerst, Canad.; Ayerst, USA)*; Auralgicin *(Fisons, UK)*; Auraltone *(Fisons, UK)*; Breezeazy *(Cambridge Laboratories, Austral.)*; Felsol *(Bengué, UK)*; Lanceotic *(Lancet, UK : Kirby-Warrick, UK)*; Larylgan *(Ayerst, USA)*; Otipyrin *(Kramer, USA)*; Prednefrin *(Allergan, Austral.;)*; Prefrin Liquifilm *(Allergan, Austral.; Allergan, USA)*; Prefrin-Z *(Allergan, Austral.)*; Priatan *(Schering, Austral.)*; Sedaural *(Key, Austral.)*; Sedonan *(Sigma, Austral.; Napp, UK)*; Tympagesic *(Adria, USA)*.

2685-g

Phenazopyridine Hydrochloride *(BANM, USAN, rINNM).*

Chloridrato de Fenazopiridina; NC-150; W-1655. 3-Phenylazopyridine-2,6-diyldiamine hydrochloride.

$C_{11}H_{11}N_5,HCl=249.7$.

CAS — 94-78-0 (phenazopyridine); 136-40-3 (hydrochloride).

Pharmacopoeias. In *Braz.* and *U.S.*

A light or dark red to dark violet crystalline powder, odourless or with a slight odour.

Soluble 1 in 300 of cold water, 1 in 20 of boiling water, 1 in 59 of alcohol, 1 in 331 of chloroform, and 1 in 100 of glycerol; very slightly soluble in ether. **Store** in airtight containers.

REMOVAL OF STAINS. Phenazopyridine stains may be removed from fabric by soaking in a solution of sodium dithionite 0.25%.

Adverse Effects

Phenazopyridine hydrochloride has occasionally caused gastro-intestinal side-effects, headache, and rashes. Abnormalities in liver function, haemolytic anaemia, methaemoglobinaemia, and acute renal failure have also been reported, generally associated with overdosage or with therapeutic doses in patients with impaired renal function.

Abnormal coloration of body tissues or fluids may occur.

EFFECTS ON THE BLOOD. *Haemolytic anaemia.* Reports of haemolytic anaemia occurring in patients taking phenazopyridine.— M. S. Greenberg and H. Wong, *New Engl. J. Med.*, 1964, *271*, 431; E. P. Gabor *et al.*, *Can. med. Ass. J.*, 1964, *91*, 756; A. J. Eisinger and R. Jones (letter), *Lancet*, 1969, *1*, 151; H. C. Drysdale and M. D. Hellier (letter), *Br. med. J.*, 1978, *2*, 1021; C. J. T. Bateman (letter), *ibid.*, 1716; J. E. Mercieca *et al.* (letter), *Lancet*, 1982, *2*, 564.

See also under Overdosage (below).

Thrombocytopenia. Thrombocytopenia in one patient associated with the use of a combination product containing phenazopyridine and sulphamethoxazole. No report could be found of either drug causing thrombocytopenia or neutropenia when used alone.— J. T. Wilde and A. G. Prentice (letter), *Ann. intern. Med.*, 1986, *104*, 128.

EFFECTS ON THE CNS. Aseptic meningitis, characterised by distinct episodes of fever and confusion, in a patient was associated with the administration of phenazopyridine.— T. E. Herlihy (letter), *Ann. intern. Med.*, 1987, *106*, 172.

EFFECTS ON THE KIDNEYS. An 85-year-old woman developed a yellowish-orange pigmentation of the skin and urinary insufficiency after taking phenazopyridine hydrochloride. The drug was withdrawn and urinary output was restored the following day.— C. E. Eybel *et al.*, *J. Am. med. Ass.*, 1974, *228*, 1027.

See also under Overdosage (below).

Renal calculi. Vesical calculi composed of pure phenazopyridine were found in the urinary tract of a 67-year-old man who had been taking phenazopyridine hydrochloride 600 mg daily for 2 years.— W. P. Mulvaney *et al.*, *J. Am. med. Ass.*, 1972, *221*, 1511.

Phenazopyridine was deposited on ureteral stones already present in a 55-year-old man with chronic prostatitis who had taken phenazopyridine hydrochloride 200 mg three times daily for 5 months.— E. D. Crawford and W. P. Mulvaney, *J. Urol., Baltimore*, 1978, *119*, 280.

EFFECTS ON THE LIVER. Signs of liver disorder, considered to be a hypersensitivity reaction, occurred on 4 occasions in a woman given phenazopyridine.— B. W. D. Badley, *Br. med. J.*, 1976, *2*, 850.

Further reports of abnormalities of liver function following phenazopyridine.— J. W. Hood and W. N. Toth, *J. Am. med. Ass.*, 1966, *198*, 1366; A. J. Eisinger and R. Jones (letter), *Lancet*, 1969, *1*, 151; S. E. Goldfinger and S. Marx, *New Engl. J. Med.*, 1972, *286*, 1090.

EFFECTS ON THE SKIN. Analysis, by the Boston Collaborative Drug Surveillance Program, of data on 15 438 patients hospitalised between 1975 and 1982 detected 1 allergic skin reaction attributed to phenazopyridine hydrochloride among 113 recipients of the drug.— M. Bigby *et al.*, *J. Am. med. Ass.*, 1986, *256*, 3358.

OVERDOSAGE. A 13-month-old girl who ingested 2.5 to 3 g of phenazopyridine developed methaemoglobinaemia and haemolytic anaemia, and the haemoglobin concentration fell to 66 mg per mL. She recovered after treatment with methylene blue and blood transfusion.— B. L. Cohen and G. J. Bovasso, *Clin. Pediat.*, 1971, *10*, 537.

After taking phenazopyridine 2.4 g over a 24-hour period for acute loin pain an 18-year-old woman developed methaemoglobinaemia, haemolytic anaemia, and acute renal failure. She was given an intravenous injection of methylene blue 100 mg, with reversal of her methaemoglobinaemia and subsequent recovery.— D. M. Nathan *et al.*, *Archs intern. Med.*, 1977, *137*, 1636.

Further reports of acute renal failure attributed to overdosage with phenazopyridine hydrochloride.— D. A. Feinfeld *et al.*, *J. Am. med. Ass.*, 1978, *240*, 2661; N. Qureshi and R. W. Hedger (letter), *Ann. intern. Med.*, 1979, *90*, 443.

Treatment of Adverse Effects

Methaemoglobinaemia may be treated with methylene blue administered intravenously as a 1% solution in a dose of 1 to 2 mg per kg body-weight.

Precautions

Phenazopyridine hydrochloride is contra-indicated in patients with impaired renal function.

Absorption and Fate

Phenazopyridine hydrochloride is absorbed from the gastro-intestinal tract. It is excreted mainly in the urine; up to 65% may be excreted as unchanged phenazopyridine.

Following administration of phenazopyridine hydrochloride 200 mg three times daily to 6 healthy subjects, a mean of about 90% of the dose appeared in the urine within 24 hours, of which 41% was unchanged, 18% was *N*-acetyl-*p*-aminophenol, 24% was *p*-aminophenol, and about 7% was aniline. The amount of aniline released was in excess of the maximal allowable dose of 35 mg daily.— W. J. Johnson and A. Chartrand, *Toxic. appl. Pharmac.*, 1976, *37*, 371.

Uses and Administration

Phenazopyridine exerts an analgesic effect on the mucosa of the urinary tract and is used to provide symptomatic relief of pain and irritability in conditions such as cystitis, prostatitis, and urethritis. It is given by mouth in usual doses of 200 mg three times daily after food. If given in conjunction with an antibacterial agent for the treatment of urinary-tract infections it is recommended that phenazopyridine should be given for not more than 2 days. During administration the urine is tinged either orange or red and underclothes are apt to be stained.

Preparations

Phenazopyridine Hydrochloride Tablets *(U.S.P.)*

Proprietary Names and Manufacturers

Azodine *(Propan, S.Afr.)*; Giracid *(Switz.)*; Phenazo *(ICN, Canad.)*; Pyridacil *(Neth.; Cilag, Switz.)*; Pyridium *(Arg.; Warner, Austral.; Belg.; Parke, Davis, Canad.; Servier, Fr.; Gödecke, Ger.; Warner, S.Afr.; Spain; Parke, Davis, UK; Parke, Davis, USA)*; Pyronium *(Pro Doc, Canad.)*; Urogesic *(Edwards, USA)*; Uropyridin *(Jpn)*; Uropyrine *(Belg.)*; Vestin *(Spain)*.

The following names have been used for multi-ingredient preparations containing phenazopyridine hydrochloride— Azo Gantanol *(Roche, USA)*; Azo Gantrisin *(Roche, Canad.; Roche, USA)*; Azo-Sulfisoxazole *(Schein, USA)*; Azotrex *(Bristol, USA)*; Pyridium Plus *(Parke, Davis, USA)*; Thiosulfil-A *(Ayerst, USA)*; Uro Gantanol *(Roche, Canad.)*; Urobiotic *(Roerig, USA)*; Urogesic *(Edwards, USA)*; Uromide *(Consolidated Chemicals, UK)*.

2689-w

Phenicarbazide *(rINN)*.

Phenylsemicarbazide. 1-Phenylsemicarbazide.

$C_7H_9N_3O=151.2$.

CAS — 103-03-7.

Pharmacopoeias. In *Arg., Belg.,* and *Port.*

Phenicarbazide has analgesic properties. It has been given by mouth.

Proprietary Names and Manufacturers

The following names have been used for multi-ingredient preparations containing phenicarbazide— Antipyretic Dellipsoids D26 *(Pilsworth, UK)*.

2686-q

Phenylbutazone *(BAN, USAN, rINN)*.

Butadione; Fenilbutazona; Phenylbutazonum.

4-Butyl-1,2-diphenylpyrazolidine-3,5-dione.

$C_{19}H_{20}N_2O_2=308.4$.

CAS — 50-33-9.

Pharmacopoeias. In *Aust., Br., Braz., Chin., Cz., Eur., Fr., Ger., Hung., Ind., Int., It., Jpn, Jug., Neth., Nord., Pol., Port., Roum., Rus., Swiss, Turk.,* and *U.S.* Also in *B.P. Vet.*

A white or off-white, odourless or almost odourless, crystalline powder. *B.P.* **Solubilities** are: practically insoluble in water; sparingly soluble in alcohol; soluble 1 in 1.25 of chloroform and 1 in 15 of ether; soluble in aqueous solutions of alkali hydroxides. *U.S.P.* solubilities are: very slightly soluble in water; freely soluble in acetone and ether; soluble in alcohol. **Store** in airtight containers. Protect from light.

Adverse Effects

Nausea, vomiting, epigastric distress, diarrhoea, oedema due to salt retention, skin rashes, vertigo, headache, and blurred vision may occur. More serious reactions include gastric irritation with ulceration and gastro-intestinal bleeding, ulcerative stomatitis, hepatitis, jaundice, haematuria, nephritis, renal failure, and goitre. Salivary gland enlargement, hypersensitivity reactions, and severe generalised reactions including erythema multiforme (Stevens-Johnson syndrome), toxic epidermal necrolysis, and exfoliative dermatitis have been reported.

The most serious adverse effects of phenylbutazone are related to bone-marrow depression and include agranulocytosis and aplastic anaemia. Leucopenia, pancytopenia, haemolytic anaemia, and thrombocytopenia may also occur. These adverse haematological reactions have resulted in the indications for use of phenylbutazone being restricted in recent years (see under the uses and administration section, below). Blood disorders may develop soon after starting treatment or may occur suddenly after prolonged treatment. Blood-cell counts should be performed regularly but should not be relied upon to predict dysplasia. Patients should be told to discontinue the drug at the first signs of toxic effects and to report at once the appearance of symptoms such as fever, sore throat, stomatitis, skin rashes, and weight gain or oedema.

EFFECTS ON THE BLOOD. An analysis of blood dyscrasias reported to the Swedish Adverse Drug Reaction Committee for the 5-year period 1966–70 showed that thrombocytopenia attributable to phenylbutazone had been reported on 7 occasions (1 fatal), aplastic anaemia on 4 occasions (2 fatal), and agranulocytosis on 5 occasions (2 fatal). It was estimated that reported figures represented one-third of the true frequency.— L. E. Böttiger and B. Westerholm, *Br. med. J.*, 1973, *3*, 339.

There were 1276 reports of adverse reactions to phenylbutazone reported to the Committee on Safety of Medicines from June 1964 to January 1973. These included 398 reports of blood disorders (204 fatal) including aplastic anaemia (163; 121 fatal), thrombocytopenia (59; 18 fatal), agranulocytosis, leucopenia, or pancytopenia (95; 44 fatal), and gastro-intestinal haemorrhage (104; 27 fatal).— M. F. Cuthbert, *Curr. med. Res. Opinion*, 1974, *2*, 600.

Aplastic anaemia or agranulocytosis were quoted as underlying or contributory causes of death in 376 death certificates in the year October 1974 to September 1975; adequate medical records were available for 269. Death was probably due to phenylbutazone in 28 cases. Mortality was estimated at 2.2 per 100 000 patients.— W. H. W. Inman, *Committee on Safety of Medicines, Br. med. J.*, 1977, *1*, 1500.

A short review of the toxicity of phenylbutazone and oxyphenbutazone mentioning that in the *UK* between 1964 and 1982 the Committee on Safety of Medicines recorded 458 deaths due to bone marrow damage following treatment with these drugs and commenting that these figures almost certainly underestimate the problem.— *Drug & Ther. Bull.*, 1984, *22*, 5.

A First Report by The International Agranulocytosis and Aplastic Anemia Study concerning the risks of agranulocytosis and aplastic anaemia with special reference to analgesic use. The study confirmed the significant association of phenylbutazone and oxyphenbutazone with both disorders.— *J. Am. med. Ass.*, 1986, *256*, 1749.

EFFECTS ON THE CARDIOVASCULAR SYSTEM. A 64-year-old woman given phenylbutazone 100 mg three times daily, developed pericarditis and 15 days after the start of treatment her condition was critical. Prednisone, in a dosage of 10 mg three times daily, was life-saving.— J. Shafar, *Br. med. J.*, 1965, *2*, 795.

Four patients with polymyalgic disorders developed temporal arteritis during treatment with phenylbutazone or oxyphenbutazone, and one patient had partial loss of vision in one eye.— B. Wadman and I. Werner, *Lancet*, 1967, *1*, 597.

EFFECTS ON THE KIDNEYS. Reports of nephrotoxicity associated with phenylbutazone: J. H. Richardson and H. H. Alderfer, *New Engl. J. Med.*, 1963, *268*, 809 (acute renal failure); G. I. Russell *et al.*, *Br. med. J.*, 1978, *1*, 1322 (acute interstitial nephritis and renal failure); U. Kuhlmann *et al.*, *Schweiz. med. Wschr.*, 1978, *108*, 494 (interstitial nephritis); M. Greenstone *et al.*, *Br. med. J.*, 1981, *282*, 950 (nephrotic syndrome).

EFFECTS ON THE LIVER. Reports of toxic hepatitis attributed to phenylbutazone.— J. H. Fisher, *Can. med. Ass. J.*, 1960, *83*, 1211; J. M. Muscat-Baron and D. M. Freeman, *Br. J. clin. Pract.*, 1966, *20*, 437; D. J. Maberly and R. M. Greenhalgh, *Br. J. Derm.*, 1970, *82*, 618; K. G. Ishak *et al.*, *Am. J. dig. Dis.*, 1977, *22*, 611; T. R. Mayer, *Minn. Med.*, 1979, *62*, 349.

EFFECTS ON THE NERVOUS SYSTEM. Loss of taste sensitivity associated with phenylbutazone occurred in 3 patients, 2 of whom also received amidopyrine or isopropylaminophenazone.— H. Rollin, *Ann. Otol. Rhinol. Lar.*, 1978, *87*, 37.

EFFECTS ON THE SKIN. Phenylbutazone taken for 7 to 35 days before the eruption, might have been responsible for 6 cases, 2 fatal, of toxic epidermal necrolysis in Britain.— A. Lyell, *Br. J. Derm.*, 1967, *79*, 662. Three cases of toxic epidermal necrolysis associated with phenylbutazone.— J. Kvasnička *et al.*, *Br. J. Derm.*, 1979, *100*, 551.

A report of generalised pustular psoriasis in 2 patients precipitated by oxyphenbutazone and phenylbutazone respectively.— H. Reshad *et al.*, *Br. J. Derm.*, 1983, *108*, 111.

Analysis, by the Boston Collaborative Drug Surveillance Program, of data on 15 438 patients hospitalised between 1975 and 1982 detected 2 allergic skin reactions attributed to phenylbutazone among 172 recipients of the drug.— M. Bigby *et al.*, *J. Am. med. Ass.*, 1986, *256*, 3358.

LUPUS ERYTHEMATOSUS. Phenylbutazone was implicated in the development of systemic lupus erythematosus in 2 patients.— M. A. Ogryzlo, *Can. med. Ass. J.*, 1956, *75*, 980.

Although phenylbutazone had been either implicated or suspected in drug-associated systemic lupus erythematosus it was a rare reaction and the evidence was weak.— G. R. V. Hughes, *Adverse Drug React. Bull.*, 1987, (Apr.), 460.

OVERDOSAGE. A brief review and comments concerning poisoning after overdosage with phenylbutazone. If either a child or an adult is believed to have taken an overdose, gastric lavage (or emesis in children) should be urgently performed, even in the absence of symptoms. It is doubtful whether active treatments such as haemoperfusion or exchange transfusion were of any benefit in cases where they were employed.— H. Court and G. N. Volans, *Adverse Drug React. Ac. Pois. Rev.*, 1984, *3*, 1.

Precautions

Phenylbutazone is contra-indicated in patients with blood disorders or active gastro-intestinal disorders such as peptic ulcer and also in patients with a history of any such disorders. It is also contra-indicated in patients with cardiovascular or thyroid disease, in those with severe impairment of hepatic or renal function, and in those with a history of aspirin allergy.

It should be used with caution in elderly patients. Courses of treatment should be kept as short as possible and haematological monitoring performed (see under the uses and administration section, below).

Phenylbutazone may enhance the effects of some anticoagulants, oral hypoglycaemics, phenytoin, and some sulphonamides.

INTERACTIONS. The plasma half-life of phenylbutazone was reduced from a mean of 78.1 hours to 57.2 hours by pretreatment with drugs which increased liver microsomal enzyme activity. Barbiturates, chlorpheniramine, promethazine, and prednisone induced microsomal activity.— A. J. Levi *et al.*, *Lancet*, 1968, *1*, 1275.

Plasma concentrations of phenylbutazone were increased in 5 patients when methylphenidate 20 mg was given daily for 3 days; in 3 patients the concentration of oxyphenbutazone rose. In 2 of 4 patients given a single 400-mg dose of phenylbutazone the half-life was prolonged by methylphenidate.— P. G. Dayton *et al.*, *Pharmacologist*, 1969, *11*, 272.

For the effect of phenylbutazone on other drugs, see chlorpropamide (p.388), levodopa (p.1017), phenytoin sodium (p.408), and warfarin (p.345).

PORPHYRIA. Phenylbutazone was considered to be unsafe in patients with acute porphyria although there is conflicting experimental evidence on porphyrinogenicity.— M.R. Moore and K.E.L. McColl, *Porphyrias, Drug Lists*, Glasgow, Porphyria Research Unit, University of Glasgow, 1987.

Absorption and Fate

Phenylbutazone is readily absorbed from the gastro-intestinal tract with peak plasma concentrations occurring about 2 hours after ingestion. At therapeutic plasma concentrations phenylbutazone is 98% bound to plasma proteins; at higher concentrations the fraction bound decreases. It is extensively metabolised in the liver by oxidation and by conjugation with glucuronic acid. Oxyphenbutazone and γ-hydroxyphenbutazone are formed by oxidation but only small amounts appear in urine, the remainder being further metabolised. About 1% of a dose is excreted in the urine as unchanged phenylbutazone, and about 10% is excreted in bile, mainly as metabolites. The mean elimination half-life is about 70 hours but it is subject to large variations.

Phenylbutazone crosses the placenta and appears in breast milk.

Reviews of the pharmacokinetics of phenylbutazone: J. Aarbakke, *Clin. Pharmacokinet.*, 1978, *3*, 369.

Uses and Administration

Phenylbutazone has analgesic, antipyretic, and anti-inflammatory properties; however, because of its toxicity it is not employed as a general analgesic or antipyretic. Although phenylbutazone is effective in almost all rheumatic disorders including ankylosing spondylitis, acute gouty arthritis, osteoarthritis, rheumatoid arthritis, and Reiter's disease, it should only be used in acute rheumatic disorders where less toxic drugs have failed. In the *UK* the use of phenylbutazone is restricted to the treatment in hospital of ankylosing spondylitis.

In acute rheumatic disorders phenylbutazone may be given initially in doses of up to 600 mg daily; this should be given in divided doses with meals. This high initial dose should be given for as short a period as possible and if no improvement occurs within 1 week the drug should be discontinued. When improvement has been obtained the dosage should be reduced to the smallest dose that will provide relief of symptoms. Maintenance dosage should not exceed 400 mg daily and 100 to 200 mg daily may be adequate. Again, maintenace therapy should only be continued for the shortest period possible.

A dose of 400 mg initially, followed by 100 mg every 4 hours until articular inflammation subsides has been suggested for the treatment of acute gouty arthritis; therapy may usually only be required for 2 to 4 days and should not exceed 7 days in duration.

Blood counts should be made weekly during initial therapy and repeated at frequent intervals if medication is continued over a prolonged period. Irrespective of the blood count, medication should be stopped at the first appearance of toxic symptoms.

Preparations

Phenylbutazone Capsules *(U.S.P.)*

Phenylbutazone Tablets *(B.P.)*

Phenylbutazone Tablets *(U.S.P.)*

Proprietary Preparations

Butacote *(Geigy, UK). Tablets,* enteric coated, phenylbutazone 100 and 200 mg.

Butazolidin *(Geigy, UK). Tablets,* phenylbutazone 100 and 200 mg.

Butazone *(DDSA Pharmaceuticals, UK). Tablets,* phenylbutazone 100 and 200 mg.

Proprietary Names and Manufacturers of Phenylbutazone and some Derivatives

Algoverine *(Canad.)*; Artrizin *(Denm.; Norw.)*; Artropan *(Ital.)*; Azolid *(USV Pharmaceutical Corp., USA)*; Butacal *(Austral.)*; Butacote *(Geigy, Switz.; Geigy, UK)*; Butadion *(Streuli, Switz.)*; Butadiona *(Miquel, Spain)*; Butagesic *(Canad.)*; Butalan *(Austral.)*; Butalgin *(Fawns & McAllan, Austral.)*; Butalgina *(Esteve, Spain)*; Butaphen *(Switz.)*; Butapirazol *(Pol.)*; Butarex *(Austral.)*; Butartril *(Ital.)*; Butazina *(Vis, Ital.)*; Butazolidin *(Geigy, Austral.; Geigy, Canad.; Denm.; Geigy, Ger.; Neth.; Norw.; Geigy, S.Afr.; Geigy, Swed.; Switz.; Geigy, UK; Geigy, USA)*; Butazolidina *(Arg.; Geigy, Ital.; Padro, Spain)*; Butazolidine *(Belg.; Ciba, Fr.; Geigy, Switz.)*; Butazone *(Protea, Austral.; S.Afr.; DDSA Pharmaceuticals, UK)*; Butial *(Spain)*; Butoroid *(Faulding, Austral.)*; Butoz *(Austral.)*; Butrex *(SCS, S.Afr.)*; Buzon *(Austral.)*; Dibuzon *(Switz.)*; Diossidone *(Ital.)*; Ditrone *(Hosbon, Spain)*; Elmedal *(Switz.)*; Ethibute *(Ethigel, UK)*; Exrheudon *(Neos-Donner, Ger.)*; Fenibutasan *(Santos, Spain)*; Fenilbutina *(Ital.)*; Flexazone *(Berk Pharmaceuticals, UK)*; Glycyl *(Belg.)*; Inflazone *(Lennon, S.Afr.)*; Intrabutazone *(Organon, Canad.)*; Kadol *(Midy, Ital.)*; Malgesic *(Canad.)*; Megazone *(Doms, Fr.)*; Mepha-Butazon *(Switz.)*; Nadozone *(Canad.)*; Novobutazone *(Novopharm, Canad.)*; Oppazone *(Oppenheimer, UK)*; Panazone *(S.Afr.)*; Phenbutazone *(Canad.)*; Pirarreumol-P *(Spain)*; Praecirheumin *(Ger.)*; Rectofasa *(Sabater, Spain)*; Reumilene *(Ital.)*; Rheumaphen *(Ger.)*; Sintobutina *(Spain)*; Spondyril *(Dorsch, Ger.)*; Tetnor *(R.P. Drugs, UK)*; Tibutazone *(Ticen, Eire)*; Ticinil *(De Angeli, Ital.)*; Ticinil Calcio *(De Angeli, Ital.; Switz.)*; Todalgil *(Wasserman, Spain)*.

The following names have been used for multi-ingredient preparations containing phenylbutazone and some derivatives— Alka Butazolidin *(Geigy, Canad.)*; Alkabutazone *(ICN, Canad.)*; Alka-phenylbutazone *(Pro Doc, Canad.)*; Butazolidin Alka *(Geigy, UK)*; Butazolidin Ampoules with Xylocaine *(Geigy, UK)*; Butoroid Cream *(Faulding, Austral.)*; Delta-Butazolidin *(Geigy, UK)*; Neo-Zoline-M *(Neolab, Canad.)*; Parazolidin *(Geigy, UK)*; Phenylone Plus *(Medic, Canad.)*.

2698-e

Phenylbutazone Piperazine

Pyrazinobutazone.

$C_{23}H_{30}N_4O_2=394.5$.

CAS — 4985-25-5.

Phenylbutazone piperazine has the actions and uses of phenylbutazone (see p.36). It has been used by mouth in initial doses of up to 600 mg daily, or occasionally 900 mg daily, in divided doses; maintenance doses have generally been 300 mg daily. It has also been applied topically in concentrations of 5%.

Proprietary Names and Manufacturers

Carudol *(Boehringer Sohn, Arg.; Belg.; Boehringer Ingelheim, Fr.; Boehringer Ingelheim, Ital.; Fher, Spain; Wild, Switz.)*; Clavezona *(Finadiet, Arg.)*; Dartranol *(Cheminova, Spain)*; Ranoroc *(Biotherax, Ger.)*; Unifalgan *(Unifa, Arg.)*.

2690-m

Phenyramidol Hydrochloride *(BANM, USAN).*

Fenyramidol Hydrochloride *(rINNM)*; IN-511. 1-Phenyl-2-(2-pyridylamino)ethanol hydrochloride; α-(2-Pyridylaminomethyl)benzyl alcohol hydrochloride.

$C_{13}H_{14}N_2O,HCl=250.7$.

CAS — 553-69-5 (phenyramidol); 326-43-2 (hydrochloride).

Adverse Effects

Gastro-intestinal disturbances, drowsiness, skin rashes, and a fall in blood pressure have been reported.

Precautions

Phenyramidol may enhance the effects of coumarin anticoagulants, hypoglycaemic agents, and phenytoin.

Uses and Administration

Phenyramidol hydrochloride has analgesic and muscle relaxant properties. It has been used in doses of 400 to 800 mg up to 4 times daily by mouth.

Proprietary Names and Manufacturers

Anabloc *(IRBI, Ital.)*; Analexin *(Biotrading, Ital.)*; Aramidol *(ABC, Ital.)*; Cabral *(Kali-Chemie, Ger.)*; Firmalgil *(FIRMA, Ital.)*; Miodar *(ISM, Ital.)*; Vilexin *(Vitrum, Swed.)*.

9592-e

Picolamine Salicylate

NOTE. Picolamine is *rINN*.

Picolamine salicylate has been applied topically for its analgesic properties in the treatment of muscular pain and minor abrasions.

Proprietary Names and Manufacturers

Algiospray *(Robert, Spain)*; Algospray *(Boots-Dacour, Fr.)*; Pangesic *(Novag, Spain)*.

19662-h

Piketoprofen *(rINN).*

m-Benzoyl-*N*-(4-methyl-2-pyridyl)hydratropamide.

$C_{22}H_{20}N_2O_2=344.4$.

CAS — 60576-13-8.

Piketoprofen has analgesic and anti-inflammatory properties and has been used topically in concentrations of about 2% in rheumatic disorders.

Proprietary Names and Manufacturers

Calmatel *(Almirall, Spain)*.

3911-p

Pinazone

Pinazone is a non-steroidal anti-inflammatory agent. It has been reported to cause blood dyscrasias including, rarely, agranulocytosis. It has been used in the treatment of rheumatic and other inflammatory disorders in usual doses of 250 mg by mouth three times daily. It has also been given by the rectal route.

Pinazone is the piperazine salt of feprazone.

Proprietary Names and Manufacturers

Lubetrone *(Valles Mestre, Spain)*; Reuflodol *(Infar Nattermann, Spain)*.

2691-b

Pipebuzone *(rINN).*

4-Butyl-4-(4-methylpiperazin-1-ylmethyl)-1,2-diphenylpyrazolidine-3,5-dione.

$C_{25}H_{32}N_4O_2=420.6$.

CAS — 27315-91-9.

Pipebuzone has analgesic, anti-inflammatory, and antipyretic properties and has been given by mouth in inflammatory and rheumatic disorders.

Proprietary Names and Manufacturers

Élarzone *(Eurorga, Fr.)*.

3846-z

Piperylone *(pINN).*

4-Ethyl-1-(1-methyl-4-piperidyl)-3-phenyl-3-pyrazolin-5-one.

$C_{17}H_{23}N_3O=285.4$.

CAS — 2531-04-6.

Piperylone has analgesic and antipyretic properties and has been given as the malate in doses of 100 mg by mouth.

Proprietary Names and Manufacturers of Piperylone and its Salts

The following names have been used for multi-ingredient preparations containing piperylone and its salts— Theraflu *(Sandoz, Switz.)*.

13126-f

Pirazolac *(BAN, USAN, rINN).*

ZK-76604. 4-(4-Chlorophenyl)-1-(4-fluorophenyl)pyrazol-3-ylacetic acid.

$C_{17}H_{12}ClFN_2O_2=330.7$.

CAS — 71002-09-0.

Pirazolac has analgesic, anti-inflammatory, and antipyretic properties and is being studied for use by mouth in rheumatic disorders.

Some references to pirazolac: D. Symmons *et al., Curr. med. Res. Opinion*, 1985, *9*, 542 (dose study in rheumatoid arthritis); M. Kurowski *et al., Eur. J. clin. Pharmac.*, 1986, *31*, 307 (pharmacokinetics).

Proprietary Names and Manufacturers

Schering, Ger.

2692-v

Piroxicam *(BAN, USAN, rINN).*

CP-16171. 4-Hydroxy-2-methyl-*N*-(2-pyridyl)-2*H*-1,2-benzothiazine-3-carboxamide 1,1-dioxide.

$C_{15}H_{13}N_3O_4S=331.4$.

CAS — 36322-90-4.

Pharmacopoeias. In *U.S.*

An off-white to light tan or light yellow, odourless powder. It forms a monohydrate that is yellow. Very slightly **soluble** in water, dilute acids, and most organic solvents; slightly soluble in alcohol and aqueous alkaline solutions. **Store** in airtight containers. Protect from light.

Adverse Effects

Gastro-intestinal disturbances are the commonest

side-effects occurring with piroxicam. Peptic ulceration and gastro-intestinal bleeding have been reported. Other side-effects which have been reported include headache, dizziness, blurred vision, tinnitus, skin rashes and pruritus, and oedema.

A report of the adverse reactions associated with piroxicam received by the Medicines Safety Centre in South Africa including two reactions, paraesthesia and hair loss, not previously recorded in the literature.— D. Gerber, *Drug Intell. & clin. Pharm.*, 1987, *21*, 707.

ALLERGY. A report of cross-sensitivity between piroxicam and tartrazine (present in methylprednisolone tablets).— R. M. Oksas (letter), *Drug Intell. & clin. Pharm.*, 1985, *19*, 478.

See also under Effects on the Kidneys (below).

EFFECTS ON THE BLOOD. Fatal aplastic anaemia in a patient following long-term use of piroxicam.— S. H. Lee *et al.* (letter), *Lancet*, 1982, *1*, 1186.

A report of severe thrombocytopenic purpura in one patient associated with piroxicam.— H. Bjørnstad and Ø. Vik, *Br. J. clin. Pract.*, 1986, *40*, 42.

EFFECTS ON THE ELECTROLYTES. Reversible hyperkalaemic hyperchloraemic acidosis in a patient receiving piroxicam.— L. A. Grossman and S. Moss (letter), *Ann. intern. Med.*, 1983, *99*, 282. A further report of severe hyperkalaemia during piroxicam therapy.— K. P. Miller *et al.*, *Archs intern. Med.*, 1984, *144*, 2414.

Comment on heart failure in 6 patients receiving piroxicam and the suggestion that piroxicam may be even more likely to cause appreciable fluid retention than some other non-steroidal anti-inflammatory drugs.— R. W. Fowler and K. G. Arnold, *Br. med. J.*, 1983, *287*, 835.

See also under Effects on the Kidneys (below).

EFFECTS ON THE GASTRO-INTESTINAL TRACT. The gastro-intestinal toxicity attributable to piroxicam has recently aroused much interest. Several case reports and data from some drug monitoring centres (K.H. Fok *et al.*, *Br. med. J.*, 1985, *290*, 117; A.G. Morgan *et al.*, *ibid*, 564; B. Beermann, *ibid.*, 789; P. Meyer and I. Thijs, *ibid.*; C.P. Armstrong and A.L. Blower, *ibid.*, 1987, *294*, 772; *idem*, 1290) have suggested that piroxicam has an unusually high incidence of gastro-intestinal side-effects including the induction of peptic ulcer or perforation of an existing ulcer, haematemesis, and melaena. These reports and data have, however, either been criticised or new data presented refuting the above suggestions (R.D. Montgomery, *Br. med. J.*, 1985, *290*, 564; W.H.W. Inman and N.S.B. Rawson, *ibid.*, 932; A.C. Rossi *et al.*, *ibid.*, 1987, *294*, 147; E.A. Bortnichak *et al.*, *ibid.*, 1289; A. Calin, *ibid.*; M. Biour *et al.*, *Lancet*, 1987, *2*, 340). Although the commonest side-effects of piroxicam are indeed gastro-intestinal it would appear from the present evidence that the overall incidence of such reactions is not appreciably higher with piroxicam than with other non-steroidal anti-inflammatory agents.

EFFECTS ON THE KIDNEYS. A report of 2 patients, who as a result of hypersensitivity to piroxicam, developed acute nephropathy with characteristic features of Henoch-Schönlein purpura.— K. M. Goebel and W. Mueller-Brodmann, *Br. med. J.*, 1982, *284*, 311.

Piroxicam-induced acute renal failure and hyperkalaemia in one patient.— M. A. Frais *et al.* (letter), *Ann. intern. Med.*, 1983, *99*, 129.

Nephrotoxicity associated with piroxicam in 2 patients. In the first patient, severe reversible azotaemia with hyperkalaemia resolved after discontinuation of piroxicam; in the second, acute interstitial nephritis and the nephrotic syndrome developed necessitating treatment with corticosteroids.— P. D. Mitnick and W. J. Klein, *Archs intern. Med.*, 1984, *144*, 63.

EFFECTS ON THE LIVER. A report of a patient who presented with features of acute hepatocellular injury after taking piroxicam 40 mg daily for 3 days; the liver disorder progressed to subacute hepatic necrosis and the patient died.— S. M. Lee *et al.*, *Br. med. J.*, 1986, *293*, 540.

EFFECTS ON THE PANCREAS. A report of pancreatitis associated with piroxicam.— O. L. Haye (letter), *Ann. intern. Med.*, 1986, *104*, 895.

EFFECTS ON THE SKIN. Comment on the 29 reports of photosensitivity eruptions associated with piroxicam that had been received by the Adverse Drug Reaction Reporting System of the American Academy of Dermatology. The reaction appeared to be a phototoxic rather than a photo-allergic one.— R. S. Stern (letter), *New Engl. J. Med.*, 1983, *309*, 186.

A report of fatal pemphigus vulgaris in a patient taking piroxicam.— R. L. Martin *et al.* (letter), *New Engl. J. Med.*, 1983, *309*, 795.

Mention that piroxicam had been responsible for 2 cases of drug-induced toxic epidermal necrolysis.— J. -C. Roujeau *et al.*, *Lancet*, 1985, *1*, 609.

See also under Effects on the Blood and Effects on the Kidneys (both above).

OVERDOSAGE. Brief details of 16 patients who were considered to have taken an overdosage of piroxicam alone reported to the National Poisons Information Service of the *UK*. Thirteen patients (including 5 children) experienced no symptoms after doses estimated to be up to 300 to 400 mg; 2 patients complained of dizziness and blurred vision after 200 to 300 mg; the last patient who claimed to have taken 600 mg presented in coma, regained consciousness within one hour, and had recovered fully within 24 hours.— H. Court and G. N. Volans, *Adverse Drug React. Ac. Pois. Rev.*, 1984, *3*, 1.

Precautions

Piroxicam should not be used in patients with a history of gastro-intestinal haemorrhage or ulcers or aspirin sensitivity. It should be used with caution in patients with impaired renal function and in patients with cardiovascular disorders where oedema may worsen the condition.

Concomitant administration of piroxicam and aspirin has been reported to result in lowered plasma-piroxicam concentrations.

INTERACTIONS. For the effect of piroxicam on some other drugs see lithium carbonate (p.368) and warfarin sodium (p.345).

PORPHYRIA. Piroxicam was considered to be unsafe in patients with acute porphyria because it has been shown to be porphyrinogenic in *animals* or *in vitro* systems.— M.R. Moore and K.E.L. McColl, *Porphyrias, Drug Lists*, Glasgow, Porphyria Research Unit, University of Glasgow, 1987.

PREGNANCY AND THE NEONATE. A study in 2 nursing women indicated that piroxicam was present in breast milk at about 1% of the concentration in maternal serum; in one infant who was breast fed no piroxicam could be detected in the serum.— M. Østensen, *Eur. J. clin. Pharmac.*, 1983, *25*, 829.

Absorption and Fate

Piroxicam is well absorbed from the gastro-intestinal tract. It is metabolised in the liver by hydroxylation and conjugation with glucuronic acid and excreted predominantly in the urine with smaller amounts in the faeces. Less than 5% of the dose is excreted unchanged. Piroxicam is extensively bound to plasma proteins (about 99%) and has a long plasma half-life of approximately 50 hours.

A review of the pharmacokinetics of piroxicam.— E. H. Wiseman, *Eur. J. Rheumatol. Inflamm.*, 1978, *1*, 338.

The pharmacokinetics of piroxicam were studied following single and multiple-doses by mouth. A plasma half-life of about 45 hours was observed. Enterohepatic recirculation of piroxicam was suggested by the presence of multiple peaks in plasma-concentration curves.— D. C. Hobbs and T. M. Twomey, *J. clin. Pharmac.*, 1979, *19*, 270.

Further references: C. J. Richardson *et al.*, *Eur. J. clin. Pharmac.*, 1987, *32*, 89.

Uses and Administration

Piroxicam has analgesic, anti-inflammatory, and antipyretic properties. It is used in rheumatic disorders such as ankylosing spondylitis, osteoarthritis, and rheumatoid arthritis in a usual dose by mouth of 20 mg daily in single or divided doses with a range of 10 to 30 mg daily. In acute musculoskeletal conditions an initial dose of 40 mg daily may be given for 2 days followed by 20 mg daily for 1 to 2 weeks. Piroxicam is also used in acute gout, the usual dose being 40 mg daily for 5 to 7 days.

Piroxicam may also be used in children aged 6 years or over with juvenile chronic arthritis. The usual dose is 5 mg daily in those weighing less than 15 kg, 10 mg daily in those weighing 16 to 25 kg, 15 mg daily in those weighing 26 to 45 kg, and 20 mg daily in those weighing 46 kg or over.

A review of the actions and uses of piroxicam.— R. N. Brogden *et al.*, *Drugs*, 1984, *28*, 292.

A symposium on piroxicam: *The Rheumatological Disease Process: Focus on Piroxicam*, Royal Society of Medicine, London, 1985.

ADMINISTRATION IN THE ELDERLY. A study providing no evidence to suggest that the pharmacokinetics of piroxicam are grossly different in the elderly arthritic patient compared with younger subjects.— A. D. Woolf *et al.*, *Br. J. clin. Pharmac.*, 1983, *16*, 433. A similar study indicating that elderly patients receiving piroxicam 20 mg once daily are not exposed to undue risk related to pharmacokinetic considerations.— A. Darragh *et al.*, *Eur. J. clin. Pharmac.*, 1985, *28*, 305.

ANKYLOSING SPONDYLITIS. Some references to the use of piroxicam in ankylosing spondylitis: I. Radi *et al.*, *Eur. J. Rheumatol. Inflamm.*, 1978, *1*, 349; H. Müller-Fassbender and M. Schattenkirchner, in *Piroxicam*, W.M. O'Brien and E.H. Wiseman (Ed.), London, The Royal Society of Medicine, 1978, p. 83; O. A. Sydnes, *Br. J. clin. Pract.*, 1981, *35*, 40.

GOUT. Reports of the use of piroxicam in acute gout: P. Widmark, *Eur. J. Rheumatol. Inflamm.*, 1978, *1*, 346; G. Tausch and R. Eberl, *ibid.*, 365; J. E. Murphy, *J. int. med. Res.*, 1979, *7*, 507; S. B. Olupitan, *Curr. ther. Res.*, 1984, *36*, 833.

OSTEOARTHRITIS. Reports on the use of piroxicam in osteoarthritis: H. Telhag, *Eur. J. Rheumatol. Inflamm.*, 1978, *1*, 352; T. M. Zizic *et al.*, in *Piroxicam*, W.M. O'Brien and E.H. Wiseman (Ed.), London, The Royal Society of Medicine, 1978, p. 71; J. L. Abruzzo *et al.*, *Clin. Pharmac. Ther.*, 1979, *25*, 211; P. Dessain *et al.*, *J. int. med. Res.*, 1979, *7*, 335; C. H. Hybbinette, *Br. J. clin. Pract.*, 1981, *35*, 30; O. Kogstad, *ibid.*, 45; P. Janke *et al.*, *Curr. med. Res. Opinion*, 1983, *8*, 434; J. -M. Björkenheim *et al.*, *J. int. med. Res.*, 1985, *13*, 263; G. R. Kraag *et al.*, *J. Rheumatol.*, 1985, *12*, 328; R. Marcolongo *et al.*, *Clin. Rheumatol.*, 1985, *4*, 267.

PAIN. Reports of a beneficial response to piroxicam in patients with dysmenorrhoea: L. Wilhelmsson *et al.*, *Acta obstet. gynec. scand.*, 1985, *64*, 317; T. Saltveit, *ibid.*, 635; B. O. Osinusi and E. A. Bamgboye, *Curr. ther. Res.*, 1986, *39*, 715; E. M. Akinluyi, *ibid.*, 1987, *41*, 609; N. Iyagba and A. Agboola, *ibid.*, *42*, 48; S. Costa *et al.*, *ibid.*, 156.

Reports of the use of piroxicam in musculoskeletal disorders and sports injuries: C. M. Williamson, *Curr. med. Res. Opinion*, 1983, *8*, 622; V. Edwards *et al.*, *J. int. med. Res.*, 1984, *12*, 46; S. B. Olupitan, *Curr. ther. Res.*, 1984, *36*, 819; *idem*, 826; T. M. Reyes *et al.*, *ibid.*, 1986, *39*, 39.

PSYCHIATRIC DISORDERS. A report of a beneficial effect with piroxicam in a patient with panic disorders.— J. A. Goldstein (letter), *J. clin. Psychiat.*, 1986, *47*, 277.

RHEUMATOID ARTHRITIS. Some references to the use of piroxicam in rheumatoid arthritis: J. R. Ward *et al.*, in *Piroxicam*, W.M. O'Brien and E.H. Wiseman (Ed.), London, The Royal Society of Medicine, 1978, p. 31; J. Box *et al.*, *ibid.*, p. 41; J. C. Steigerwald, *ibid.*, p. 47; M. Weintraub *et al.*, *ibid.*, p. 53; G. Tausch *et al.*, *ibid.*, p. 59; P. Mäkisara and P. Nuotio, *ibid.*, p. 65; J. C. Steigerwald, *Eur. J. Rheumatol. Inflamm.*, 1978, *1*, 360; Z. Balogh *et al.*, *Curr. med. Res. Opinion*, 1979, *6*, 148; E. J. Pisko *et al.*, *Curr. ther. Res.*, 1980, *27*, 852; R. Finstad, *Br. J. clin. Pract.*, 1981, *35*, 35; J. M. Mbuyi-Muamba and J. Dequecker, *Curr. med. Res. Opinion*, 1983, *8*, 612; J. S. Goodwin *et al.*, *J. Am. med. Ass.*, 1983, *250*, 2485; I. G. De La Torre, *Curr. ther. Res.*, 1984, *35*, 130.

Preparations

Piroxicam Capsules *(U.S.P.)*

Proprietary Preparations

Feldene *(Pfizer, UK)*. *Capsules*, piroxicam 10 and 20 mg.
Tablets, dispersible, scored, piroxicam 10 mg.
Tablets, dispersible, piroxicam 20 mg.
Suppositories, piroxicam 20 mg.

Larapam *(Lagap, UK)*. *Capsules*, piroxicam 10 and 20 mg.

Proprietary Names and Manufacturers

Antiflog *(FIRMA, Ital.)*; Artroxicam *(Coli, Ital.)*; Baxo *(Toyama, Jpn)*; Dexicam *(OFF, Ital.)*; Doblexan *(Organon, Spain)*; Felden *(Pfizer, Denm.*; *Mack, Illert., Ger.*; *Pfizer, Norw.*; *Pfizer, Swed.*; *Pfizer, Switz.)*; Feldene *(Pfizer, Austral.*; *Pfizer, Canad.*; *Pfizer, Fr.*; *Pfizer, Ital.*; *Pfizer Taito, Jpn*; *Pfizer, S.Afr.*; *Pfizer, Spain*; *Pfizer, UK*; *Pfizer, USA)*; Flogobene *(Farge, Ital.)*; Impronta1 *(Fides, Spain)*; Lampoflex *(Lampugnani, Ital.)*; Larapam *(Lagap, UK)*; Lusoxicam *(Medinfar, Port.)*; Nirox *(Medici, Ital.)*; Novopirocam *(Novopharm, Canad.)*; Piroftal *(Bruschettini, Ital.)*; Polipirox *(Herdel, Ital.)*; Remoxicam *(Alkaloid, Jug.)*; Reucam *(CT, Ital.)*; Reudene *(ABC, Ital.)*; Reumagil *(Lenza, Ital.)*; Riacen *(Chiesi, Ital.)*; Roxene *(Ital Suisse, Ital.)*; Roxenil *(Caber, Ital.)*; Roxicam *(Wilson, Pakistan)*; Roxiden *(Pulitzer, Ital.)*; Sasulen *(Andreu, Spain)*; Vitaxicam *(Robert, Spain)*; Zacam *(Prophin, Ital.)*.

2693-g

Pirprofen *(BAN, USAN, rINN)*.
Su-21524. 2-[3-Chloro-4-(3-pyrrolin-1-yl)phenyl]propionic acid.
$C_{13}H_{14}ClNO_2$=251.7.
CAS — 31793-07-4.

Adverse Effects
Gastro-intestinal disturbances including gastro-intestinal bleeding, visual and hearing disturbances, and headache have been reported.

Uses and Administration
Pirprofen has analgesic and anti-inflammatory properties. It is used in rheumatic disorders in usual doses by mouth of 600 to 800 mg daily in divided doses; up to 1.2 g daily in divided doses may be given if necessary.

A detailed review of the actions and uses of pirprofen.— P. A. Todd and R. Beresford, *Drugs*, 1986, *32*, 509.

Following administration of pirprofen 100 and 200 mg to 10 subjects on 2 separate occasions pirprofen was rapidly and almost completely absorbed, peak concentrations of 8.9 to 15 µg per mL (average 12 µg per mL) and 14 to 38 µg per mL (average 23 µg per mL) respectively being obtained after an average of about 1 or 2 hours; the apparent elimination half-lives were 5.6 to 10 hours (average 6.8 hours) and 5.9 to 8.2 hours (average 6.5 hours) respectively. In 7 subjects who received pirprofen 1 hour after a substantial meal as well as in the fasting state, peak plasma concentrations were achieved after an average of about 3 hours, the delay not being statistically significant, and the apparent elimination half-lives were 4.7 to 7.7 hours (average 6.3 hours) and 5.9 to 7.8 hours (average 6.9 hours) respectively. In 8 subjects who received 600 mg daily, as 200 mg three times daily or 150 mg four times daily, average blood concentrations of 11 and 10 µg per mL respectively were found on the morning of the sixth day, 12 hours after the last dose. Absorption and excretion studies following administration of a radioactively labelled dose of 200 mg to 6 subjects indicated that at peak concentrations nearly all the drug in plasma was unchanged; about 80% was excreted in the urine within 24 hours with less than 5% as pirprofen, the major metabolite being the acyl glucuronide; about 8% of the dose was excreted in the faeces.— R. C. Luders *et al.*, *Clin. Pharmac. Ther.*, 1977, *21*, 721.

ADMINISTRATION IN THE ELDERLY. Results of a relatively small pharmacokinetic study suggesting no modification of pirprofen dosage would be necessary in elderly patients without overt hepatic or renal impairment.— L. Rooney *et al.*, *Eur. J. clin. Pharmac.*, 1985, *29*, 73.

Proprietary Names and Manufacturers
Rangasil *(Ciba, Fr.)*; Rengasil *(Ciba, Belg.; Ciba, Denm.; Brunnengräber, Ger.; Ciba, Ital.; Geigy, Switz.)*.

3847-c

Pranoprofen *(rINN)*.
α-Methyl-5*H*-[1]-benzopyrano[2,3-*b*]pyridine-7-acetic acid.
$C_{15}H_{13}NO_3$=255.3.
CAS — 52549-17-4.

Pranoprofen is a non-steroidal anti-inflammatory agent that has been given in doses of 75 mg three times daily by mouth.

Proprietary Names and Manufacturers
Niflan *(Yoshitomi, Jpn)*.

13160-n

Pranosal *(rINN)*.
3-(2,5-Dimethylpyrrolidin-1-yl)propyl salicylate.
$C_{16}H_{23}NO_3$=277.4.
CAS — 17716-89-1.

Pranosal has been used as the salicylate as a topical analgesic in concentrations of 5% in rheumatic and other disorders.

Proprietary Names and Manufacturers of Pranosal and its Esters
Pyradol *(Gallier, Fr.)*.

13174-q

Proglumetacin Maleate *(BANM, rINNM)*.
CR-604; Protacine Maleate. 3-{4-[2-(1-*p*-Chlorobenzoyl-5-methoxy-2-methylindol-3-ylacetoxy)ethyl]piperazin-1-yl}propyl 4-benzamido-*NN*-dipropylglutaramate dimaleate.
$C_{46}H_{58}ClN_5O_8,2C_4H_4O_4$=1076.6.
CAS — 57132-53-3 (proglumetacin); 59209-40-4 (maleate).

Proglumetacin maleate has analgesic and anti-inflammatory properties. It has been used in rheumatic disorders in doses of up to 450 mg daily, in divided doses, by mouth.

Some references to proglumetacin: F. M. Guardiola *et al.*, *Curr. med. Res. Opinion*, 1982, *8*, 14 (rheumatic disorders); S. Bozsoky and Z. Zahumenszky, *ibid.*, 89 (rheumatoid arthritis); J. E. Santo *et al.*, *ibid.*, 1983, *8*, 524 (rheumatoid arthritis); V. Pipitone *et al.*, *Clin. Trials J.*, 1983, *20*, 39 (rheumatoid arthritis).

Proprietary Names and Manufacturers
Afloxan *(Merck Sharp & Dohme, Ital.)*; Protaxil *(Abello, Spain)*; Protaxon *(Opfermann, Ger.)*; Proxil *(Rottapharm, Ital.)*.

3166-j

Propacetamol *(pINN)*.
N,N-Diethylglycine ester with paracetamol.
$C_{14}H_{20}N_2O_3$=264.3.
CAS — 66532-85-2.

Propacetamol is a pro-drug of paracetamol (see p.32) being hydrolysed to parcetamol in the plasma. It has been given as the hydrochloride in doses of 1 to 2 g two to four times daily by intramuscular or intravenous injection.

Proprietary Names and Manufacturers of Propacetamol and its Salts
Pro-dafalgan *(UPSA, Fr.)*.

2696-s

Propyphenazone *(BAN, rINN)*.
Isopropylantipyrine; Isopropylantipyrinum. 4-Isopropyl-2,3-dimethyl-1-phenyl-3-pyrazolin-5-one.
$C_{14}H_{18}N_2O$=230.3.
CAS — 479-92-5.
Pharmacopoeias. In *Aust.*, *It.*, and *Swiss.*

Propyphenazone has analgesic properties. It has been given in doses of up to about 250 mg three times daily by mouth.

Propyphenazone was considered to be unsafe in patients with acute porphyria because it has been shown to be porphyrinogenic in *animals* or *in vitro* systems.— M.R. Moore and K.E.L. McColl, *Porphyrias, Drug Lists*, Glasgow, Porphyria Research Unit, University of Glasgow, 1987.

Proprietary Names and Manufacturers
Baukal *(Bruschettini, Ital.)*; Budirol *(Castejon, Spain)*; Causyth *(Inverni della Beffa, Ital.)*; Cibalgina *(Ciba, Spain)*.

The following names have been used for multi-ingredient preparations containing propyphenazone— Saridone *(Roche, UK)*.

13180-v

Proquazone *(BAN, USAN, rINN)*.
43-715; RU-43-715-n. 1-Isopropyl-7-methyl-4-phenylquinazolin-2(1*H*)-one.
$C_{18}H_{18}N_2O$=278.4.
CAS — 22760-18-5.

Proquazone has analgesic, anti-inflammatory, and antipyretic properties. It is given by mouth in rheumatic disorders in usual doses of 400 to 900 mg daily in divided doses; up to 1.2 g daily may be given if necessary.

A detailed review of the pharmacodynamics and pharmacokinetics of proquazone and of its effectiveness in rheumatic diseases and pain states.— S. P. Clissold and R. Beresford, *Drugs*, 1987, *33*, 478.

Proprietary Names and Manufacturers
Biarison *(Sandoz, Denm.; Sandoz, Ger.; Wander, Neth.; Sandoz, Spain; Wander, Switz.)*.

2697-w

Protizinic Acid *(rINN)*.
2-(7-Methoxy-10-methylphenothiazin-2-yl)propionic acid.
$C_{17}H_{17}NO_3S$=315.4.
CAS — 13799-03-6.

Adverse Effects
Gastro-intestinal disturbances, dysuria, and skin rashes have been reported.

Following ingestion of about 8 g of protizinic acid and about 6 g of aspirin a 17-year-old girl developed fatal malignant hyperthermia. She had no history of myopathy and examination of her parents and siblings revealed no abnormalities. The following 3 causes were considered possible: the overdosage might have triggered a genetic predisposition; the protizinic acid had enhanced aspirin-induced hyperthermia; the effect was due to the neuroleptic effect of massive protizinic acid overdose.— G. Ginies *et al.*, *Thérapie*, 1976, *31*, 755.

Uses and Administration
Protizinic acid has analgesic and anti-inflammatory properties. It has been used in rheumatic disorders in doses of 600 to 800 mg daily, in divided doses, by mouth.

Proprietary Names and Manufacturers
Pirocrid *(Théraplix, Fr.; Mochida, Jpn)*.

2660-x

Ramifenazone *(rINN)*.
Isopropylaminophenazone; Isopyrin. 4-Isopropylamino-2,3-dimethyl-1-phenyl-3-pyrazolin-5-one.
$C_{14}H_{19}N_3O$=245.3.
CAS — 3615-24-5.

NOTE. The name Isopyrin has also been applied to isoniazid.

Ramifenazone has analgesic, anti-inflammatory, and antipyretic properties. It has been given by mouth and applied topically in conjunction with phenylbutazone.

Proprietary Names and Manufacturers
The following names have been used for multi-ingredient preparations containing ramifenazone— Tomanol *(Byk Gulden, Ger.)*.

13214-f

Rimazolium Methylsulphate
MZ-144; Rimazolium Metilsulfate *(rINN)*. 3-Ethoxycarbonyl-6,7,8,9-tetrahydro-1,6-dimethyl-4-oxo-4*H*-pyrido-[1,2-*a*]pyrimidinium methyl sulphate.
$C_{14}H_{22}N_2O_7S$=362.4.

CAS — 35615-72-6 (rimazolium); 28610-84-6 (methylsulphate).

Rimazolium methylsulphate has analgesic properties. It has been given in usual doses of 300 mg three or four times daily by mouth.

References: M. Haataja *et al., Curr. ther. Res.*, 1977, *22*, 784; M. Haataja and H. Saarimaa, *ibid.*, 1978, *23*, 277; M. Haataja *et al., ibid.*, *24*, 284; S. Fink and K. O. Nielsen, *ibid.*, 900; E. Ihasz, *Therapia hung.*, 1980, *28*, 22.

Proprietary Names and Manufacturers
Dolcuran *(Beta, Arg.)*; Probon *(Chinoin, Hung.)*; Rimagina *(Medipolar, Fin.)*.

2622-j

Salamidacetic Acid
Carbamoylphenoxyacetic acid; Salicylamide *O*-acetic acid. (2-Carbamoylphenoxy)acetic acid.
$C_9H_9NO_4$=195.2.

CAS — 25395-22-6 (salamidacetic acid); 3785-32-8 (sodium salt).

Salamidacetic acid has analgesic, anti-inflammatory, and antipyretic properties. It has been given, as the sodium salt, in rheumatic disorders, by mouth and parenterally. It has also been used topically as the diethylamine salt in concentrations of 10%.

Proprietary Names and Manufacturers of Salamidacetic Acid and its Salts
Akistin *(Truw, Ger.)*; Neosalid *(Bruco, Ital.)*.

2700-l

Salicylamide *(BAN, USAN, rINN)*.
2-Hydroxybenzamide.
$C_7H_7NO_2$=137.1.

CAS — 65-45-2.

Pharmacopoeias. In *Aust., Belg., Hung., Pol., Roum., Rus.* and *U.S.*

A white practically odourless crystalline powder. Slightly **soluble** in water and chloroform; soluble in alcohol and propylene glycol; freely soluble in ether and solutions of alkalis.

Adverse Effects, Treatment, and Precautions
As for aspirin, p.3.

Gross urticaria in 2 infants followed the use of a teething jelly containing salicylamide 8%.— B. Bentley-Philips (letter), *Br. J. Derm.*, 1968, *80*, 341.

Absorption and Fate
Salicylamide is readily absorbed from the gastro-intestinal tract and distributed to all body tissues. It is rapidly excreted in the urine, mainly as the glucuronide and sulphate conjugates.

Uses and Administration
Salicylamide has some analgesic, anti-inflammatory, and antipyretic properties. Doses of up to 1.5 g three times daily have been given by mouth but salicylamide is now little used.

Proprietary Names and Manufacturers
Amid-Sal *(Glenwood, USA)*; Salamide *(Austral.)*; Salimed *(Medo, UK)*; Salizell *(Ger.)*; Sinedol *(Corvi, Ital.)*; Urtosal *(Lifepharma, Ital.)*.

The following names have been used for multi-ingredient preparations containing salicylamide— Achrocidin *(Lederle, Canad.)*; Analgesic Dellipsoids D6 *(Pilsworth, UK)*; Anodyne Dellipsoids D4 *(Pilsworth, UK)*; Citra Forte Capsules *(Boyle, USA)*; Codalan *(Lannett, USA)*; D & M Tablets *(Cambridge Laboratories, Austral.)*; Delimon *(Consolidated Chemicals, UK)*; Espasmotex *(Arlo, USA)*; Intralgin *(Riker, UK)*; Korigesic *(Trimen, USA)*; Os-Cal-Gesic *(Marion Laboratories, USA)*; Saleto *(Mallard, USA)*; Salimed Compound *(Medo, UK)*; Sedu-Caps-D *(Lederle, Austral.*; Sinulin *(Carnrick, USA)*.

9315-y

Salol
Phenyl salicylate.
$C_{13}H_{10}O_3$=214.2.

CAS — 118-55-8.

Pharmacopoeias. In *Aust., Fr., Mex., Nord., Pol., Port., Rus.,* and *Span.*

Salol when given by mouth has mild analgesic and antipyretic properties. It was formerly used as an intestinal antiseptic, but effective doses were toxic owing to the liberation of phenol.
Salol has been used topically as a sunscreen agent. It has also been used as an enteric coating for some oral dosage forms.

It had been stated that sensitisation reactions to salicylates were rare. Salol, however, in the author's personal experience has been reported by a great number of individuals to produce irritation. It was unknown if this is due to salol itself or to its hydrolysis products phenol and salicylic acid. Many of the reports could have been due to the nature of the vehicle used for salol.— G. A. Groves, *Aust. J. Pharm.*, 1975, *56*, 601.

Proprietary Names and Manufacturers
Sola-Stick *(Hamilton, Austral.)*.

The following names have been used for multi-ingredient preparations containing salol— Lip-Sed Cold Sore Lotion *(Rosken, Austral.)*; Trac Tabs *(Hyrex, USA)*; Urised *(Webcon, USA)*; Uroblue *(Geneva, USA)*.

2702-j

Salsalate *(BAN, USAN, rINN)*.
Salicyl Salicylate; Salicylosalicylic Acid; Salicylsalicylic Acid; Salysal; Sasapyrine. *O*-(2-Hydroxybenzoyl)salicylic acid.
$C_{14}H_{10}O_5$=258.2.

CAS — 552-94-3.

Pharmacopoeias. In *Br.*

An odourless or almost odourless white or almost white powder. Very slightly **soluble** in water; soluble 1 in 6 of alcohol, 1 in 8 of chloroform, and 1 in 12 of ether. Store in a well-closed container.

Adverse Effects, Treatment, and Precautions
As for aspirin, p.3.

EFFECTS ON THE GASTRO-INTESTINAL TRACT. Small-bowel ulcerations in a patient associated with salsalate, one of the newer forms of salicylates that bypass the stomach for bioabsorption.— M. A. Souza Lima, *Archs intern. Med.*, 1985, *145*, 1139.

EFFECTS ON THE KIDNEYS. A report of the minimal-change nephrotic syndrome in one patient associated with salsalate.— M. Vallès and J. L. Tovar (letter), *Ann. intern. Med.*, 1987, *107*, 116.

INTERACTIONS. Reports of severe metabolic acidosis in 2 patients with normal renal and hepatic function while taking salicylates (aloxiprin or salsalate) concomitantly with carbonic anhydrase inhibitors (dichlorphenamide or acetazolamide). Such concomitant use should be minimised or avoided.— R. A. Cowan *et al., Br. med. J.*, 1984, *289*, 347.

Absorption and Fate
Salsalate is absorbed mainly from the small intestine. Following absorption it is slowly hydrolysed to 2 molecules of free salicylic acid.

References to the pharmacokinetics of salsalate: L. I. Harrison *et al., J. clin. Pharmac.*, 1981, *21*, 401; S. H. Dromgoole *et al., Clin. Pharmac. Ther.*, 1983, *34*, 539; S. H. Dromgoole *et al., J. pharm. Sci.*, 1984, *73*, 1657.

Uses and Administration
Salsalate has analgesic, antipyretic, and anti-inflammatory properties similar to those of aspirin (see p.5). It is used in rheumatic disorders in doses of up to 1 g three or four times daily by mouth with food.

ADMINISTRATION IN RENAL FAILURE. Based on short-term pharmacokinetic studies in 5 patients with chronic renal failure undergoing haemodialysis the following dosage schedule was suggested: the initial dose could be similar to that for patients with normal renal function (1.5 g by mouth); the maintenance dose between dialysis treatments be reduced to about 750 mg twice daily; an additional dose of 500 mg after haemodialysis be given. Further multiple-dose studies were needed.— M. E. Williams *et al., Clin. Pharmac. Ther.*, 1986, *39*, 420.

RHEUMATIC DISORDERS. Studies of the use of salsalate in rheumatic disorders: S. P. Liyanage and P. K. Tambar, *Curr. med. Res. Opinion*, 1978, *5*, 450; R. G. Regalado, *ibid.*, 454; O. N. Ré, *J. int. med. Res.*, 1979, *7*, 90.

Preparations
Salsalate Capsules *(B.P.)*

Proprietary Preparations
Disalcid *(Riker, UK). Capsules,* salsalate 500 mg.

Proprietary Names and Manufacturers
Arcylate *(USA)*; Atisuril *(Kali-Farma, Spain)*; Disalcid *(Riker, UK; Riker, USA)*; Disalgesic *(Kettelhack Riker, Ger.)*; Mono-Gesic *(Central Pharmaceuticals, USA)*; Nobegyl *(Denm.)*; Umbradol *(Salvat, Spain)*.
The following names have been used for multi-ingredient preparations containing salsalate— Persistin *(Fisons, USA)*.

2703-z

Simetride *(pINN)*.
1,4-Bis[(2-methoxy-4-propylphenoxy)acetyl]piperazine.
$C_{28}H_{38}N_2O_6$=498.6.

CAS — 154-82-5.

Simetride has analgesic, anti-inflammatory, and antipyretic properties. It has been given by mouth as an analgesic.

Proprietary Names and Manufacturers
The following names have been used for multi-ingredient preparations containing simetride— Kyorin AP2 *(Kyorin, Jpn)*.

5296-k

Sodium Aurothiomalate *(BAN, rINN)*.
Gold Sodium Thiomalate *(USAN)*; Sodium Aurothiosuccinate.

CAS — 12244-57-4 (xNa, anhydrous); 39377-38-3 (2 Na monohydrate).

Pharmacopoeias. In *Br., Ind., Jpn,* and *U.S.*

Sodium aurothiomalate *B.P.* is a fine, pale yellow, hygroscopic powder with a slight odour. It consists mainly of the disodium salt of (aurothio)succinic acid ($C_4H_3AuNa_2O_4S$ = 390.1) and has a gold content of 44.5 to 46.0% calculated on the dried material. Very **soluble** in water. A 10% solution in water has a pH of 6.0 to 7.0. The *B.P.* injection is **sterilised** by filtration.
Gold sodium thiomalate *U.S.P.* is a white to yellowish-white, odourless or almost odourless solid. It consists of a mixture of the monosodium and disodium salts of gold thiomalic acid-[(aurothio)succinic acid] ($C_4H_4AuNaO_4S$ = 368.1 and $C_4H_3AuNa_2O_4S$ = 390.1) and these salts have a gold content of 44.8 to 49.6%, and 49.0 to 52.5% calculated on the dried glycerol-free material. Very **soluble** in water; insoluble in alcohol, ether, and in most organic solvents. A 10% solution in water has a pH of 5.8 to 6.5.
Store in airtight containers. Protect from light.

Heating a clear commercial solution of sodium aurothiomalate injection at 100° or submitting it to light of 350 nm produced a yellow discoloration. Solutions sterilised by autoclaving were yellow, while solutions sterilised by filtration were clear. The yellow solution was associated with a different activity from the clear as measured by the effect on platelet aggregation.— D. A. Harvey *et al.* (letter), *Lancet*, 1983, *1*, 470.

Adverse Effects
Reports show a wide range for the incidence of adverse effects of sodium aurothiomalate. However, authorities consider that with careful treatment about one third of patients will experience adverse effects. The most common

effects involve the skin and mucous membranes with pruritus (an early sign of intolerance) and stomatitis (often with a metallic taste) being the most prominent. Other reactions affecting the skin and mucous membranes include erythema, maculopapular eruptions, erythema multiforme, urticaria, eczema, seborrhoeic dermatitis, lichenoid eruptions, alopecia, exfoliative dermatitis, glossitis, pharyngitis, vaginitis, photosensitivity reactions, and pigmentation (chrysiasis).

Toxic effects on the blood include thrombocytopenia, leucopenia, agranulocytosis, and aplastic anaemia and may be fatal.

Effects on the kidneys include mild transient proteinuria which may lead to heavy proteinuria, haematuria, and nephrosis.

Other effects reported include pulmonary fibrosis, toxic hepatitis, peripheral neuritis, encephalitis, psychoses, fever, and gastro-intestinal disorders including enterocolitis. Vasomotor or nitritoid reactions, with weakness, flushing, palpitations, and dyspnoea, may occur following injection of sodium aurothiomalate; local irritation may also follow injection, and sometimes there is initial exacerbation of the arthritic condition. Gold deposits may occur in the eyes.

A number of the adverse effects of gold have an immunogenic component.

A review of the adverse reactions of parenteral and oral gold preparations.— E. C. S. Tozman and N. L. Gottlieb, *Med. Toxicol.*, 1987, *2*, 177.

Herpes zoster occurred in 5 of 159 patients receiving gold salts for rheumatoid arthritis.— A. G. Fam *et al.* (letter), *Ann. intern. Med.*, 1981, *94*, 712.

An association between decreased powers of sulphoxidation and sodium aurothiomalate toxicity.— R. Madhock *et al.*, *Br. med. J.*, 1987, *294*, 483.

ALLERGY. Confirmation of earlier findings by G.S. Panayi *et al.* (*Br. med. J.*, 1978, *2*, 1326) of an association between the presence of HLA-DRw2 and DRw3 antigens and the toxicity of sodium aurothiomalate and penicillamine during treatment for rheumatoid arthritis. In a study of 91 patients with rheumatoid arthritis, 71 had toxic reactions to sodium aurothiomalate, penicillamine, or both. There was a highly significant association between the presence of antigens and the development of proteinuria during therapy with aurothiomalate and a similar trend in patients given penicillamine.— P. H. Wooley *et al.*, *New Engl. J. Med.*, 1980, *303*, 300. Further references to an immunological link between sodium aurothiomalate and its adverse effects: J. Bretza *et al.*, *Am. J. Med.*, 1983, *74*, 945; H. G. Nusslein *et al.*, *Arthritis Rheum.*, 1984, *27*, 833; P. L. C. Van Riel *et al.*, *Archs intern. Med.*, 1984, *144*, 1401. See also below under Effects on the Blood.

Small amounts of nickel were detected in sodium aurothiomalate injection and accounted for a hypersensitivity reaction in one patient.— R. A. Fulton *et al.*, *Ann. rheum. Dis.*, 1982, *41*, 100.

EFFECTS ON THE BLOOD. Thrombocytopenia in 23 patients being treated with gold salts. An immunological basis was demonstrated.— J. S. Coblyn *et al.*, *Ann. intern. Med.*, 1981, *95*, 178.

Fatal consumption coagulopathy in 4 children after the second injection of either sodium aurothioglucose or sodium aurothiomalate.— J. C. Jacobs *et al.* (letter), *J. Pediat.*, 1984, *105*, 674.

A discussion on eosinophilia being used as a marker for gold toxicity.— R. T. Foster, *Can. J. Hosp. Pharm.*, 1985, *38*, 150.

EFFECTS ON THE CARDIOVASCULAR SYSTEM. Reports of nitritoid or vasomotor reactions to sodium aurothiomalate: W. R. Austad (letter), *J. Am. med. Ass.*, 1970, *211*, 2158; N. L. Gottlieb and H. E. Brown, *Arthritis Rheum.*, 1977, *20*, 1026.

EFFECTS ON THE EYES. Symptomless ocular chrysiasis in 13 of 15 patients currently receiving sodium aurothiomalate injections and in 1 of 6 who had previously received therapy.— A. J. Bron *et al.*, *Am. J. Ophthal.*, 1979, *88*, 354.

EFFECTS ON THE GASTRO-INTESTINAL TRACT. A case report of enterocolitis due to sodium aurothiomalate and a review of the 27 other cases associated with gold therapy reported to date.— C. W. Jackson *et al.*, *Gut*, 1986, *27*, 452.

EFFECTS ON THE KIDNEYS. Twenty-one patients developed proteinuria while being treated with sodium aurothiomalate for rheumatoid arthritis in a standard intramuscular regimen consisting of 10 mg as a test dose then 50 mg weekly to response and 50 mg fortnightly or monthly for maintenance. The severity of the proteinuria varied greatly and in 11 it increased for 4 months after treatment was stopped. Eight patients were considered to have developed the nephrotic syndrome. The median duration of proteinuria was 11 months, resolving in all 21 patients when treatment was withdrawn; at 24 months 3 patients were still experiencing proteinuria and it was not until 39 months that all were free of the condition. Renal biopsy indicated several types of kidney damage.— C. L. Hall *et al.*, *Br. med. J.*, 1987, *295*, 745.

Further references to gold nephropathy: D. S. Silverberg *et al.*, *Arthritis Rheum.*, 1970, *13*, 812; G. Robbins and M. B. McIllmurray, *Postgrad. med. J.*, 1980, *56*, 366; L. J. Merle, *Clin. Pharmac. Ther.*, 1980, *28*, 216.

See also under Allergy and under auranofin (p.8).

EFFECTS ON THE LIVER. References to case reports of hepatotoxicity with sodium aurothiomalate: M. Favreau *et al.*, *Ann. intern. Med.*, 1977, *87*, 717; S. Prichanond and J. L. Skosey (letter), *Ann. intern. Med.*, 1978, *88*, 579; F. K. Ghishan *et al.*, *J. Pediat.*, 1978, *93*, 1042; D. L. Howrie and J. C. Gartner, *J. Rheumatol.*, 1982, *9*, 727; J. Edelman *et al.*, *ibid.*, 1983, *10*, 510.

EFFECTS ON THE LUNGS. Pulmonary fibrosis was reported in 1 patient after she had received a total dose of sodium aurothiomalate of 655 mg for the treatment of rheumatoid arthritis. Improvement followed during 1 year after stopping treatment with gold, but lung function deteriorated when treatment was restarted.— D. M. Geddes and J. Brostoff, *Br. med. J.*, 1976, *1*, 1444. Reversible gold-induced lung damage in a 41-year-old woman resembled adenocarcinoma; she recovered following withdrawal of gold and administration of prednisolone, although she was left with a pronounced restrictive lung disorder.— D. W. James *et al.*, *ibid.*, 1978, *1*, 1523.

Other reports of lung damage: R. H. Winterbauer *et al.*, *New Engl. J. Med.*, 1976, *294*, 919; D. Geddes and J. Brostoff (letter), *ibid.*, *295*, 506; G. S. Alarcón and E. Gotuzzo (letter), *ibid.*, 507.

EFFECTS ON THE NERVOUS SYSTEM. References to case reports of sodium aurothiomalate adversely affecting the nervous system: D. J. Dick and D. Raman, *Scand. J. Rheumatol.*, 1982, *11*, 119 (Guillain-Barré syndrome); U. Schlumpf *et al.*, *Arthritis Rheum.*, 1983, *26*, 825 (Guillain-Barré syndrome and neuropathy with myokymia); R. P. Perry and E. S. Jacobsen, *J. Rheumatol.*, 1984, *11*, 233 (encephalopathy); M. M. Cerinic *et al.*, *Br. med. J.*, 1985, *290*, 1042 (polyneuropathy in a child); M. Cohen *et al.*, *ibid.*, 1179 and 1987 (acute disseminated encephalomyelitis).

EFFECTS ON THE SKIN. *Erythema nodosum.* A woman with pemphigus vulgaris developed erythema nodosum after sodium aurothiomalate injections.— R. L. Stone *et al.*, *Archs Derm.*, 1973, *107*, 602.

Lichen planus and pityriasis rosea. In 37 patients who suffered skin eruptions during chrysotherapy, the most frequent clinical eruptions resembled non-specific dermatitis, lichen planus, and pityriasis rosea.— N. S. Penneys *et al.*, *Archs Derm.*, 1974, *109*, 372.

Toxic epidermal necrolysis. Toxic epidermal necrolysis which appeared in a woman with arthropathy had been blamed on gold, but might have been idiopathic.— A. Lyell, *Br. J. Derm.*, 1967, *79*, 662.

PREGNANCY AND THE NEONATE. Gold has been detected in the foetus (I. Rocker and W.J. Henderson, *Lancet*, 1976, *2*, 1246) and there are reports of possible teratogenic effects (J.G. Rogers *et al.*, *Aust. Paediat. J.*, 1980, *16*, 194), but there are also reports of safe use during pregnancy. Gold has been detected in breast milk and found bound to the red blood cells of breast-fed babies (C.J. Needs and P.M. Brooks, *Br. J. Rheumatol.*, 1985, *24*, 291).— M. A. Byron, *Br. med. J.*, 1987, *294*, 236.

Treatment of Adverse Effects

The treatment of the adverse effects of gold is usually symptomatic and most effects resolve when gold therapy is withdrawn. In severe cases a chelating agent such as dimercaprol (p.840) may be employed.

Precautions

Gold therapy is contra-indicated in exfoliative dermatitis, systemic lupus erythematosus, and severe renal or hepatic disorders. Patients with a history of haematological disorders or who have previously shown toxicity to heavy metals should not be given gold salts, nor should any severely debilitated patient.

It is recommended that patients with diabetes mellitus and those with congestive heart failure should be adequately controlled before gold is given. Conditions such as proteinuria, pruritus, and rash arising during treatment should be allowed to resolve before gold treatment is continued. Patients with a history of urticaria, eczema, or colitis should be treated with caution.

It is generally recommended that gold salts should not be given to pregnant patients or to patients who are breast-feeding.

Concurrent administration of gold salts with other therapy capable of inducing blood disorders should be undertaken with caution if at all.

Patients should be warned to report the appearance of sore throat or tongue, metallic taste, pruritus, rash, buccal ulceration, easy bruising, purpura, bleeding, pyrexia, indigestion, diarrhoea, or unexplained malaise.

The urine should be tested for albumin before each injection and the blood should be examined for signs of depressed haemopoiesis. Annual chest X-rays should be carried out.

Of 60 patients with rheumatoid arthritis 30% developed gold reactions compared with an incidence of only 17.7% in 41 patients also suffering from Sjögren's syndrome. Despite statements in the literature gold therapy was not contra-indicated in patients with Sjögren's syndrome.— M. H. Gordon *et al.*, *Ann. intern. Med.*, 1975, *82*, 47.

For a discussion on the effects of previous therapy with gold salts or penicillamine affecting the other's toxicity, see under penicillamine (p.849).

PORPHYRIA. Sodium aurothiomalate was considered to be unsafe in patients with acute porphyria because it has been shown to be porphyrinogenic in *animals* or *in vitro* systems.— M.R. Moore and K.E.L. McColl, *Porphyrias, Drug Lists*, Glasgow, Porphyria Research Unit, University of Glasgow 1987.

Absorption and Fate

Sodium aurothiomalate is absorbed readily after intramuscular injection and becomes bound to plasma proteins. With doses of 50 mg weekly the steady-state serum concentration of gold is about 3 to 5 µg per mL. It is widely distributed and accumulates in the body; concentrations in synovial fluid have been shown to be similar to or slightly less than those in plasma.

Sodium aurothiomalate is mainly excreted in the urine, with smaller amounts in the faeces. The serum half-life of gold clearance is about 5 or 6 days but after a course of treatment, gold may be found in the urine for up to 1 year or more owing to its presence in deep body compartments. Gold has been detected in the foetus following administration of sodium aurothiomalate to the mother. Gold has also been detected in the breast fed child whose mother has received sodium aurothiomalate.

A review of the clinical pharmacokinetics of oral and injectable gold compounds.— K. L. N. Blocka *et al.*, *Clin. Pharmacokinet.*, 1986, *11*, 133.

Some references to the pharmacokinetics of gold salts: N. L. Gottlieb *et al.*, *Arthritis Rheum.*, 1974, *17*, 171; M. Harth, *Clin. Pharmac. Ther.*, 1974, *15*, 354; R. C. Gerber *et al.*, *J. Lab. clin. Med.*, 1974, *83*, 778; A. Lorber, *Clin. Pharmacokinet.*, 1977, *2*, 127; A. Lorber *et al.*, *Clin. Pharmac. Ther.*, 1980, *27*, 267.

PREGNANCY AND THE NEONATE. Gold was detected in foetal liver and kidney and in the placenta; the mother had been receiving sodium aurothiomalate.— I. Rocker and W. J. Henderson (letter), *Lancet*, 1976, *2*, 1246.

Analysis of the milk of a 35-year-old woman who was receiving sodium aurothiomalate and of the urine of her 15-month-old breast-fed daughter demonstrated that gold is secreted in the milk of mothers receiving gold salts and that small but significant amounts are absorbed into the infant's circulation.— R. A. F. Bell and I. M. Dale, *Arthritis Rheum.*, 1976, *19*, 1374.

Uses and Administration

Sodium aurothiomalate and other gold salts are used mainly for their anti-inflammatory effect in active progressive rheumatoid arthritis. They are generally reserved for use as 'second-line' agents in

patients whose symptoms are unresponsive to non-steroidal anti-inflammatory agents.
Sodium aurothiomalate therapy should only be undertaken where facilities are available to carry out the tests specified under Precautions.

Sodium aurothiomalate is given by deep intramuscular injection. Initially 10 mg is given to test the patient's tolerance. If satisfactory, this is followed by doses of 50 mg at weekly intervals until signs of remission occur, when the dosage interval is increased to 2 weeks until full remission occurs; the dosage interval is then further increased gradually to every 6 weeks. If no major improvement has been observed after a total of 1 g has been given, and in the absence of toxicity, 100 mg may be given weekly for 6 weeks; should there be no response at this dose other forms of therapy should be tried.
For children with progressive juvenile chronic arthritis the suggested initial weekly dose is 1 mg per kg body-weight (maximum 50 mg weekly). Treatment should be continued for 6 months, and if an improvement is obtained maintenance therapy may then be continued with the same dosage at fortnightly or monthly intervals for 1 to 5 years.

A review of the possible mode of action of gold compounds.— P. Bresloff, *Adv. Drug Res.*, 1977, *11*, 1.

RHEUMATOID ARTHRITIS. Reviews of gold compounds in rheumatoid arthritis: G. D. Champion, *Med. J. Aust.*, 1984, *140*, 73; M. D. Smith and P. M. Brooks, *ibid.*, 77.

For further reviews and discussions concerning the role of gold compounds in the management of rheumatoid arthritis, see p.1.

A critical evaluation of 17 published studies carried out since 1940 on long-acting agents in the treatment of rheumatoid arthritis. Both gold and cyclophosphamide appeared to retard the radiographic progression of joint damage but there was insufficient evidence for a similar beneficial effect with penicillamine, chloroquine, hydroxychloroquine, azathioprine, or methotrexate.— L. Iannuzzi *et al.*, *New Engl. J. Med.*, 1983, *309*, 1023.

Results of a study to assess the outcome in 112 consecutive patients with rheumatoid arthritis treated for 20 years at one centre; a policy of active treatment including the use of gold salts, chloroquine, corticosteroids, penicillamine, or cytotoxic drugs had been pursued. Of 68 patients still alive and available for follow-up after 20 years, 19 were in functional classes I or II (leading a normal life), 29 were in class III, and 20 were in classes IV or V (severely disabled). The mortality (37 patients dead) was higher than would be expected in the general population and agreed with other studies showing that rheumatoid arthritis causes a highly significant excess of deaths. When the results after 10 years were analysed (D.L. Scott *et al.*, *J.R. Coll. Physns*, 1983, *17*, 79) it appeared that adequate therapy favourably influenced disease progression but during the second decade, therapy appeared to have become ineffective. The results therefore suggested that the beneficial effects of therapy extend over only a few years and do not influence long-term outcome. The concept of 'remission-inducing' drugs is fallacious and although early treatment rather than waiting until advanced changes have occurred may be advantageous, the prognosis of rheumatoid arthritis is not good.— D. L. Scott *et al.*, *Lancet*, 1987, *1*, 1108.

Preparations

Gold Sodium Thiomalate Injection *(U.S.P.)*

Sodium Aurothiomalate Injection *(B.P.)*

Proprietary Preparations

Myocrisin *(May & Baker, UK)*. *Injection*, sodium aurothiomalate 5, 10, 20, and 50 mg.

Proprietary Names and Manufacturers

Auro Lecit *(Wasserman, Spain)*; Aurosulfo *(Manzoni, Ital.)*; Miocrin *(Rubio, Spain)*; Myochrysine *(Rhône-Poulenc, Canad.; Merck Sharp & Dohme, USA)*; Myocrisin *(May & Baker, Austral.; Rhone-Poulenc, Denm.; Rhône-Poulenc, Norw.; May & Baker, S.Afr.; Leo Rhodia, Swed.; May & Baker, UK)*; Tauredon *(Byk Gulden, Ger.; Byk Gulden, Switz.)*.

2704-c

Sodium Gentisate *(rINN)*.

Gentisato Sodico; Natrii Gentisas. Sodium 2,5-dihydroxybenzoate dihydrate.
$C_7H_5NaO_4,2H_2O=212.1$.

CAS — 490-79-9 (gentisic acid); 4955-90-2 (sodium gentisate, anhydrous).

Pharmacopoeias. In *Cz.*, *Fr.*, and *Span.*

Gentisic acid has been used in the form of piperazine digentisate in rheumatic disorders in doses of up to 2.5 g daily by mouth.

Two cases of granulocytopenia occurred during treatment of acute rheumatism with sodium gentisate in doses of 10 g daily for 3 or 4 weeks.— R. G. Benians, *Br. med. J.*, 1953, *2*, 1142.

Proprietary Names and Manufacturers of Gentisic Acid and Related Substances
Gentiazina *(Lafare, Ital.)*.

2705-k

Sodium Salicylate *(BAN, USAN)*.

Natrii Salicylas. Sodium 2-hydroxybenzoate.
$C_7H_5NaO_3=160.1$.

CAS — 54-21-7.

Pharmacopoeias. In *Arg., Aust., Belg., Br., Cz., Egypt., Eur., Fr., Ger., Hung., Ind., Int., It., Jpn, Jug., Mex., Neth., Nord., Pol., Port., Roum., Rus., Span., Swiss, Turk.*, and *U.S.* Also in *B.P. Vet.*

Colourless crystals, crystalline flakes, or white or faintly pink powder, odourless or with a faint characteristic odour.
Soluble 1 in 1 of water and 1 in 11 of alcohol; freely soluble in glycerol; very soluble in boiling water and boiling alcohol; practically insoluble in ether. Concentrated aqueous solutions are liable to deposit crystals of the hexahydrate on standing. **Store** in airtight containers. Protect from light.

Adverse Effects, Treatment, and Precautions

As for aspirin, p.3.

Retinal haemorrhages were reported in a 60-year-old woman taking sodium salicylate 6 g daily by mouth for 2 months and in a 10-year-old girl taking sodium salicylate, 4 g daily by mouth, for 40 days. In both cases the haemorrhages were gradually resolved after the treatment was stopped.— A. Mortada and I. Abboud, *Br. J. Ophthal.*, 1973, *57*, 199.

Absorption and Fate

As for aspirin, p.5. The rate of absorption of sodium salicylate is probably greater than for aspirin and may be reduced by the concomitant administration of alkalis.

Uses and Administration

Sodium salicylate has analgesic, anti-inflammatory, and antipyretic properties similar to those of aspirin (see p.5). It has been used in rheumatic disorders in doses of up to about 5 g daily, in divided doses, by mouth, but aspirin is generally preferred.

PAIN. In a double-blind placebo-controlled crossover study in 24 patients with postoperative dental pain doses of sodium salicylate 537 mg and 1074 mg did not produce any significant analgesic effect. The poor efficacy of sodium salicylate as compared to aspirin may be due to its weak inhibitory effect on PGE_2 and $PGF_{2\alpha}$.— R. A. Seymour *et al.*, *Br. J. clin. Pharmac.*, 1984, *17*, 161.

Preparations

Sodium Salicylate Mixture *(B.P.)*. Sodium Salicylate Oral Solution. A solution containing sodium salicylate 5%. For extemporaneous preparations the following formula may be used: sodium salicylate 500 mg, sodium metabisulphite 10 mg, concentrated orange peel infusion 0.5 mL, double-strength chloroform water 5 mL, water to 10 mL. It should be recently prepared.

Strong Sodium Salicylate Mixture *(B.P.)*. Strong Sodium Salicylate Oral Solution. A solution containing sodium salicylate 10%. For extemporaneous preparations the following formula may be used: sodium salicylate 1 g, sodium metabisulphite 10 mg, concentrated peppermint emulsion 0.25 mL, double-strength chloroform water 5 mL, water to 10 mL. It should be recently prepared.

Sodium Salicylate Tablets *(U.S.P.)*

Proprietary Names and Manufacturers

Ancosal *(Austral.)*; Bidocyl *(Leo, Swed.)*; Ensalate *(Reckitt & Colman, Austral.)*; Entérosalicyl *(Fr.)*; Enterosalicyl *(Ital.; Neth.)*; Enterosalil *(Arg.)*; Entrosalyl *(Cox, UK)*; Idocyl *(Swed.)*; Kerasalicyl *(Ital.)*; Rhumax *(Prosana, Austral.)*; S-60 *(Ondee, Canad.)*; Saliglutin *(Switz.)*; Salisod *(Ital.)*; Salitine *(Switz.)*.

The following names have been used for multi-ingredient preparations containing sodium salicylate or another salt of salicylic acid — Drixine Cough Suppressant *(Essex, Austral.)*; Pabalate *(Robins, USA)*; pHisoDan *(Sterling, Canad.)*; pHisodan *(Winthrop, Austral.)*; Polaramine Compound *(Essex, Austral.)*; Tussirex *(Scot-Tussin, USA)*.

2706-a

Sulindac *(BAN, USAN, rINN)*.

MK-231. (*Z*)-[5-Fluoro-2-methyl-1-(4-methylsulphinylbenzylidene)inden-3-yl]acetic acid.
$C_{20}H_{17}FO_3S=356.4$.

CAS — 38194-50-2.

Pharmacopoeias. In *Br.* and *U.S.*

A yellow, odourless or almost odourless, crystalline powder. *B.P.* **solubilities** are: very slightly soluble in water and ether; sparingly soluble in alcohol; soluble in chloroform. *U.S.P.* solubilities are: practically insoluble in water and light petroleum; slightly soluble in alcohol, acetone, chloroform, and methyl alcohol; very slightly soluble in isopropyl alcohol and ethyl acetate. **Store** in well-closed containers. Protect from light.

Adverse Effects

As for indomethacin, p.22.

A report of 4 patients and a short review of 8 previously reported cases of serious adverse reactions to sulindac; reactions included fever and skin, liver, CNS, lymph node, bone-marrow, and lung involvement.— G. D. Park *et al.*, *Archs intern. Med.*, 1982, *142*, 1292.

Serious adverse reactions in 2 patients after taking sulindac. One patient developed toxic hepatitis and the Stevens-Johnson/toxic epidermal necrolysis syndrome which resulted in death; the other patient developed acute pancreatitis.— S. M. Klein and M. A. Khan, *J. Rheumatol.*, 1983, *10*, 512.

ALLERGY. Hypersensitivity reactions to sulindac: F. E. Smith and P. J. Lindberg, *J. Am. med. Ass.*, 1980, *244*, 269 (pneumonitis); M. Fein (letter), *Ann. intern. Med.*, 1981, *95*, 245 (pneumonitis); Z. K. Ballas and S. T. Donta, *Archs intern. Med.*, 1982, *142*, 165 (aseptic meningitis); D. J. Sprung, *Ann. intern. Med.*, 1982, *97*, 564 (generalised lymphadenopathy); C. Fordham von Reyn, *ibid.*, 1983, *99*, 343 (aseptic meningits).

EFFECTS ON THE BLOOD. *Agranulocytosis.* Agranulocytosis associated with sulindac administration.— K. R. Romeril *et al.* (letter), *Lancet*, 1981, *2*, 523.

Aplastic anaemia. Aplastic anaemia was associated with sulindac therapy in a 54-year-old man.— J. L. Miller (letter), *Ann. intern. Med.*, 1980, *92*, 129. A similar case.— L. Bennett *et al.* (letter), *ibid.*, 874.

Fatal aplastic anaemia in one patient and transitory erythroblastopenia in a second, were associated with sulindac administration.— M. A. Sanz *et al.* (letter), *Lancet*, 1980, *2*, 802.

Haemolytic anaemia. Two cases of severe immune haemolytic anaemia, one fatal, apparently related to the use of sulindac.— F. P. Johnson *et al.*, *Archs intern. Med.*, 1985, *145*, 1515.

Thrombocytopenia. A report of leucopenia and thrombocytopenia, associated with elevation of liver enzymes, in a 37-year-old man taking sulindac.— J. E. Stambaugh *et al.* (letter), *Lancet*, 1980, *2*, 594.

Further reports of thrombocytopenia associated with sulindac: A. M. Shojania and S. D. Rusen, *Can. med. Ass. J.*, 1981, *125*, 1313; G. N. Karachalios and J. G. Parigorakis (letter), *Ann. intern. Med.*, 1986, *104*, 128.

EFFECTS ON THE ENDOCRINE SYSTEM. Reversible gynaecomastia associated with sulindac therapy in one patient.— A. Kapoor (letter), *J. Am. med. Ass.*, 1983, *250*, 2284.

Reversible secondary hypothyroidism in an elderly patient taking sulindac.— R. P. Iyer and G. K. Duckett, *Br. med. J.*, 1985, *290*, 1788.

EFFECTS ON THE KIDNEYS. The nephrotic syndrome was associated with the use of sulindac in a 57-year-old woman with psoriasis and arthritis.— S. Lomvardias *et al.* (letter), *New Engl. J. Med.*, 1981, *304*, 424.

Sulindac-induced renal failure, interstitial nephritis, and nephrotic syndrome in one patient.— A. Whelton *et al.* (letter), *J. Am. med. Ass.*, 1983, *249*, 2892.

EFFECTS ON THE LIVER. A report of hepatotoxicity in a patient receiving sulindac and a limited review of previous reports.— A. G. Gallanosa and D. A. Spyker, *Clin. Toxicol.*, 1985, *23*, 205.

Severe but reversible hepatotoxicity developed in an 18-year-old woman about 2 weeks after she had started taking sulindac 200 mg twice daily.— R. J. Anderson (letter), *New Engl. J. Med.*, 1979, *300*, 735. A similar report.— P. B. Wolfe (letter), *Ann. intern. Med.*, 1979, *91*, 656.

Further reports of adverse hepatic reactions associated with sulindac: Y. Giroux *et al.*, *Can. J. Surg.*, 1982, *25*, 334 (cholestatic jaundice); S. J. Whittaker *et al.*, *Gut*, 1982, *23*, 875 (cholestatic jaundice); E. A. Fagan *et al.*, *ibid.*, 1983, *24*, 1199 (jaundice); L. J. Wood *et al.*, *Aust. N.Z. J. Med.*, 1985, *15*, 397 (cholestatic hepatitis).

EFFECTS ON MENTAL STATE. Paranoid psychosis began in a patient 4 hours after the first dose of sulindac, and resolved within 48 hours of the last dose.— R. Kruis and R. Barger (letter), *J. Am. med. Ass.*, 1980, *243*, 1420.

Delirium in one patient associated with sulindac.— T. L. Thornton (letter), *J. Am. med. Ass.*, 1980, *243*, 1630.

EFFECTS ON THE NERVOUS SYSTEM. Acute deterioration of parkinsonism in one patient following the introduction of sulindac therapy.— R. Sandyk and M. A. Gillman, *Ann. Neurol.*, 1985, *17*, 104.

A report of a case of encephalopathy associated with sulindac.— M. Y. Neufeld and A. D. Korczyn, *Hum. Toxicol.*, 1986, *5*, 55.

EFFECTS ON THE PANCREAS. Pancreatitis associated with sulindac in one patient.— J. Goldstein *et al.* (letter), *Ann. intern. Med.*, 1980, *93*, 151.

Further reports of pancreatitis associated with sulindac: A. D. Siefkin (letter), *Ann. intern. Med.*, 1980, *93*, 932; E. L. Lilly, *J. Am. med. Ass.*, 1981, *246*, 2680; A. N. Memon, *Ann. intern. Med.*, 1982, *97*, 139.

EFFECTS ON THE SKIN. Toxic epidermal necrolysis occurred in a patient taking sulindac 400 mg daily.— L. Levitt and R. W. Pearson, *J. Am. med. Ass.*, 1980, *243*, 1262.

An unusual pernio-like reaction in a patient shortly after starting sulindac therapy.— J. L. Reinertsen (letter), *Arthritis Rheum.*, 1981, *24*, 1215.

Mention that sulindac has been associated with photosensitivity reactions.— *Med. Lett.*, 1986, *28*, 51.

Precautions

As for indomethacin, p.23.

INTERACTIONS. For the effect of sulindac on other drugs see under diuretics (p.974), lithium carbonate (p.368), and warfarin (p.345).

Absorption and Fate

Sulindac is absorbed from the gastro-intestinal tract. It is metabolised by reversible reduction to the sulphide metabolite, which appears to be the biologically active form, and by irreversible oxidation to the sulphone metabolite. Peak plasma concentrations of the sulphide metabolite are achieved in about 2 to 4 hours. The mean half-life of sulindac is about 7 to 8 hours and of the sulphide metabolite about 16 to 18 hours. Sulindac and the sulphide metabolite are both highly bound to plasma protein. About 50% is excreted in the urine mainly as the sulphone metabolite and its glucuronide conjugate, with smaller amounts of sulindac and its glucuronide conjugate. Sulindac and its metabolites are also excreted in bile and undergo extensive enterohepatic circulation.

An account of the pooled results from 5 separate clinical studies involving a total of 56 healthy subjects. Following administration of sulindac 100 to 400 mg by mouth about 90% was absorbed, some being oxidised irreversibly into the sulphone and some reduced reversibly into the sulphide (which appeared to be the biologically active form). The sulphide had an apparent terminal half-life of about 18 hours none being excreted into the urine. In the urine, sulphone and its conjugate constituted nearly 30% of the dose administered whereas sulindac and its glucuronide constituted about 20%; unidentified metabolites were responsible for about 25%. Faecal recovery accounted for about 25% of the dose, this high figure being explained by enterohepatic recycling.— D. E. Duggan *et al.*, *Clin. Pharmac. Ther.*, 1977, *21*, 326. See also *idem*, *Biochem. Pharmac.*, 1978, *27*, 2311.

Further references to the pharmacokinetics of sulindac: M. R. Dobrinska *et al.*, *Biopharm. Drug Disposit.*, 1983, *4*, 347 (biliary excretion and enterohepatic recycling); C. A. Dujovne *et al.*, *Clin. Pharmac. Ther.*, 1983, *33*, 172 (enterohepatic recycling); H. A. Strong *et al.*, *ibid.*, 1985, *38*, 387 (metabolism and metabolites).

Uses and Administration

Sulindac has analgesic, anti-inflammatory, and antipyretic properties; it is an inhibitor of prostaglandin synthetase. It is used in rheumatic disorders such as ankylosing spondylitis, osteoarthritis, and rheumatoid arthritis, and also in the short-term management of conditions such as bursitis and tendinitis and acute gouty arthritis. The usual dose by mouth is between 100 and 200 mg twice daily taken with food.

Reviews of sulindac: T. Y. Shen and C. A. Winter, *Adv. Drug Res.*, 1977, *12*, 89; R. N. Brogden *et al.*, *Drugs*, 1978, *16*, 97.

Symposium on sulindac.— *Eur. J. Rheumatol. Inflamm.*, 1978, *1*, 3–68.

ADMINISTRATION IN THE ELDERLY. Pharmacokinetic data obtained from patients receiving sulindac 150 mg twice daily provided no evidence for lowering the recommended dose of sulindac in patients over the age of 65 years.— D. S. Sitar *et al.*, *Clin. Pharmac. Ther.*, 1985, *38*, 228.

ADMINISTRATION IN HEPATIC FAILURE. Pharmacokinetic studies demonstrating significantly raised plasma concentrations of the active sulphide metabolite of sulindac in patients with alcoholic liver disease compared to healthy subjects.— R. P. Juhl *et al.*, *Clin. Pharmac. Ther.*, 1983, *34*, 104.

ADMINISTRATION IN RENAL FAILURE. The dose of sulindac should be reduced by 50% in patients with a glomerular filtration-rate of less than 10 mL per minute.— W. M. Bennett *et al.*, *Am. J. Kidney Dis.*, 1983, *3*, 155.

Evidence for a reduction in renal synthesis of prostacyclin in patients with chronic glomerular disease and the view that sulindac, a selective cyclo-oxygenase inhibitor which does not inhibit renal prostaglandin E_2 and prostacyclin synthesis, may be a suitable substitute for other non-steroidal anti-inflammatory drugs in patients with mild impairment of renal function.— G. Ciabattoni *et al.*, *New Engl. J. Med.*, 1984, *310*, 279.

In a study in 15 healthy subjects, sulindac was not found to be specifically renal sparing at the clinical doses used, and caution should continue to be excercised with its use in situations in which impairment of renal function with NSAIDs may be expected.— D. G. Roberts *et al.*, *Clin. Pharmac. Ther.*, 1985, *38*, 258.

ANKYLOSING SPONDYLITIS. Some references to the use of sulindac in ankylosing spondylitis: R. Eberl, *Scand. J. Rheumatol.*, 1975, *4*, *Suppl.* 8, S 04–05; M. Gadomski *et al.*, *ibid.*, S 02–05; A. Calin and M. Britton, *J. Am. med. Ass.*, 1979, *242*, 1885.

GASTRO-INTESTINAL DISORDERS. A report of a beneficial response to sulindac in a 19-year-old man with familial polyposis coli.— R. A. F. Gonzaga *et al.* (letter), *Lancet*, 1985, *1*, 751.

OSTEOARTHRITIS. Some references to the use of sulindac in osteoarthritis: B. Brackertz and M. Busson, *Br. J. clin. Pract.*, 1978, *32*, 77; M. Thompson *et al.*, *Curr. ther. Res.*, 1979, *26*, 779; R. Willkens *et al.*, *ibid.*, 1983, *34*, 45; A. K. Admani and S. Verma, *Curr. med. Res. Opinion*, 1983, *8*, 315; P. Janke *et al.*, *ibid.*, 434; W. J. C. Currie *et al.*, *Br. J. clin. Pract.*, 1984, *38*, 176; M. J. Vandenburg *et al.*, *ibid.*, 403; A. Chubick *et al.*, *Curr. ther. Res.*, 1987, *41*, 692.

RESPIRATORY DISORDERS. A beneficial response to sulindac 100 mg twice daily in 5 patients with cough due to angiotensin-converting-enzyme inhibitors.— M. G. Nicholls and N. L. Gilchrist (letter), *Lancet*, 1987, *1*, 872.

RHEUMATOID ARTHRITIS. Some references to the use of sulindac in rheumatoid arthritis: T. C. Highton and R. Jeremy, *Scand. J. Rheumatol.*, 1975, *4*, *Suppl.* 8, S 02–06; P. M. G. Reynolds *et al.*, *Curr. med. Res. Opinion*, 1977, *4*, 485; F. Bachmann and W. Hartl, *Dt. med. Wschr.*, 1977, *102*, 1772; E. C. Huskisson and J. Scott, *Ann. rheum. Dis.*, 1978, *37*, 89; E. C. Huskisson, *Eur. J. Rheumatol. Inflamm.*, 1978, *1*, 12; J. Borrachero del Campo, *ibid.*, 16; I. Caruso *et al.*, *ibid.*, 58; H. C. Burry and L. Witherington, *N.Z. med. J.*, 1979, *89*, 298; P. H. Lizarazo and M. Peña Cortés, *Curr. ther. Res.*, 1983, *34*, 701; H. H. McIlwain *et al.*, *ibid.*, 1987, *41*, 679.

Preparations

Sulindac Tablets *(B.P.)*

Sulindac Tablets *(U.S.P.)*

Proprietary Preparations

Clinoril *(Merck Sharp & Dohme, UK)*. *Tablets*, sulindac 100 and 200 mg.

Proprietary Names and Manufacturers

Aflodac *(Janus, Ital.)*; Algocetil *(Francia Farm., Ital.)*; Arthrocine *(Merck Sharp & Dohme-Chibret, Fr.)*; Artribid *(Port.)*; Citireuma *(CT, Ital.)*; Clinoril *(Arg.; Frosst, Austral.; Belg.; Frosst, Canad.; Denm.; Merck Sharp & Dohme, Ital.; Neth.; Merck Sharp & Dohme, Norw.; Merck Sharp & Dohme, S.Afr.; MSD, Swed.; Merck Sharp & Dohme, Switz.; Merck Sharp & Dohme, UK; Merck Sharp & Dohme, USA)*; Clisundac *(Lagap, Ital.)*; Imbaral *(Ger.)*; Lyndak *(Tiber, Ital.)*; Reumofil *(Ausonia, Ital.)*; Sudac *(Errekappa, Ital.)*; Sulartrene *(Brocchieri, Ital.)*; Sulen *(Farmacologico Milanese, Ital.)*; Sulic *(Crosara, Ital.)*; Sulindal *(Merck Sharp & Dohme, Spain)*; Sulinol *(ICT-Lodi, Ital.)*; Sulreuma *(Von Boch, Ital.)*.

13292-y

Suprofen *(BAN, USAN, rINN).*

R-25061; Sutoprofen. 2-[4-(2-Thenoyl)phenyl]propionic acid.

$C_{14}H_{12}O_3S = 260.3$.

CAS — 40828-46-4.

Suprofen has analgesic, anti-inflammatory, and antipyretic properties. It was formerly given by mouth in mild to moderate pain and in osteoarthritis and rheumatoid arthritis but following reports of adverse renal reactions marketing was suspended worldwide.

Description of a unique clinical syndrome of flank pain and acute renal failure associated with suprofen; the syndrome is unlike other nephrotoxic syndromes related to non-steroidal anti-inflammatory drugs.— D. Hart *et al.*, *Ann. intern. Med.*, 1987, *106*, 235.

Some comments and discussion concerning the 308 cases of changes in renal function associated with suprofen reported to the Food and Drug Administration of the *USA*.— S. M. Wolfe (letter), *New Engl. J. Med.*, 1987, *316*, 1025; C. L. Ellis and J. J. Anisko (letter), *ibid*; R. Temple (letter), *ibid.*, 1026.

Further reports of nephrotoxicity associated with suprofen: N. E. Henann and J. R. Morales, *Drug Intell. & clin. Pharm.*, 1986, *20*, 860 (one patient; acute renal failure); K. Abreo and J. LaBarre (letter), *Ann. intern. Med.*, 1986, *105*, 799 (one patient; acute renal failure); N. S. Davis *et al.* (letter), *ibid.*, 976 (one patient; acute renal failure); S. Snyder and B. P. Teehan (letter), *ibid.*, 1987, *106*, 776 (one patient; allergic interstitial nephritis); N. E. Henann and J. R. Morales (letter), *Drug Intell. & clin. Pharm.*, 1987, *21*, 69 (one patient; acute renal failure).

Proprietary Names and Manufacturers

Erdol *(Herdel, Ital.)*; Masterfen *(Dompè, Ital.)*; Sufenid *(Italfarmaco, Ital.)*; Supranol *(Johnson & Johnson, S.Afr.)*; Suprol *(Cilag, Ital.; Cilag, Switz.; Ortho-Cilag, UK; McNeil Pharmaceutical, USA)*; Surfrex *(Janssen, Belg.)*.

2707-t

Suxibuzone *(rINN).*

4-Butyl-4-hydroxymethyl-1,2-diphenylpyrazolidine-3,5-dione hydrogen succinate (ester).

$C_{24}H_{26}N_2O_6 = 438.5$.

CAS — 27470-51-5.

Suxibuzone is a derivative of phenylbutazone (see p.36) and has been used in rheumatic disorders in doses of up to 300 mg three times daily by mouth. It has also been applied topically at a concentration of about 7%. Concern over safety and toxicity has led to its withdrawal from the market in some countries.

Proprietary Names and Manufacturers
Calibene *(Delalande, Belg.)*; Danalon OM *(Johnson, Arg.)*; Danilon *(Esteve, Spain)*; Flamilon *(Om, Switz.)*; Flogos *(Gentili, Ital.)*; Solurol *(Delalande, Ger.)*.

3848-k

Talniflumate *(USAN, rINN).*

BA-7602-06. Phthalidyl 2-(α,α,α-trifluoro-*m*-toluidino)nicotinate.
$C_{21}H_{13}F_3N_2O_4$=414.3.

CAS — 66898-62-2.

Talniflumate, an ester of niflumic acid (see p.31) has analgesic and anti-inflammatory properties. It has been used in inflammatory and rheumatic disorders in doses of up to about 1.5 g daily, in divided doses, by mouth.

Proprietary Names and Manufacturers
Somalgen *(Bago, Arg.)*.

13305-h

Tenoxicam *(BAN, USAN, rINN).*

Ro-12-0068. 4-Hydroxy-2-methyl-*N*-(2-pyridyl)-2*H*-thieno[2,3-*e*][1,2]thiazine-3-carboxamide 1,1-dioxide.
$C_{13}H_{11}N_3O_4S_2$=337.4.

CAS — 59804-37-4.

Tenoxicam has analgesic and anti-inflammatory properties. It is used in rheumatic disorders in usual doses of 10 to 20 mg daily by mouth.

A detailed review of the actions and uses of tenoxicam.— J. P. Gonzalez and P. A. Todd, *Drugs*, 1987, *34*, 289.

Proprietary Names and Manufacturers
Mobiflex *(Roche, UK)*; Tilcotil *(Roche, Denm.; Roche, Fr.)*.

3915-l

Tetrydamine *(USAN).*

POLI-67; Tetridamine *(rINN)*. 4,5,6,7-Tetrahydro-2-methyl-3-(methylamino)-2*H*-indazole.
$C_9H_{15}N_3$=165.2.

CAS — 17289-49-5.

Tetrydamine has been applied topically as a douche for its analgesic and anti-inflammatory properties in the treatment of vaginitis. The maleate has been used similarly.

Proprietary Names and Manufacturers
Fomene *(Funk, Spain)*; Tesos *(Elmu, Spain)*.

2708-x

Thurfyl Salicylate

Tetrahydrofurfuryl salicylate.
$C_{12}H_{14}O_4$=222.2.

CAS — 2217-35-8.

Thurfyl salicylate has been used topically at concentrations of up to 14%, in creams for rheumatic and muscular pain.

Proprietary Names and Manufacturers
The following names have been used for multi-ingredient preparations containing thurfyl salicylate— Transvasin *(Reckitt & Colman, Austral.; Lloyd Hamol, Reckitt & Colman Pharmaceuticals, UK)*.

2709-r

Tiaprofenic Acid *(BAN, rINN).*

FC-3001; RU-15060. 2-(5-Benzoyl-2-thienyl)propionic acid.
$C_{14}H_{12}O_3S$=260.3.

CAS — 33005-95-7.

Adverse Effects

Side-effects reported with tiaprofenic acid have been mainly gastro-intestinal disturbances including nausea, vomiting, abdominal pain, diarrhoea or constipation, and occasionally bleeding or perforation. Other reactions have included headache and drowsiness and skin reactions such as rashes, pruritus, urticaria or angioedema, photosensitivity, and alopecia.

EFFECTS ON THE LIVER. Disturbance of liver function in one patient related to tiaprofenic acid. Although no other published reports of hepatic problems with tiaprofenic acid were found two cases of abnormal hepatic function and two of hepatitis had been reported to the Committee on Safety of Medicines in the *UK*.— R. Coladangelo (letter), *Lancet*, 1986, *1*, 803.

Precautions

As for ibuprofen, p.20.

INTERACTIONS. For the effect of tiaprofenic acid on nicoumalone, see under warfarin p.345.

INTERFERENCE WITH DIAGNOSTIC TESTS. Interference by tiaprofenic acid with the assay for urinary oxo-and oxogenic-steroids, a test used for the investigation of adrenal disease. In one patient grossly elevated steroid concentrations were found which were shown to be due to tiaprofenic acid reacting with a reagent.— L. L. Ng *et al., Postgrad. med. J.*, 1985, *61*, 739.

Absorption and Fate

Tiaprofenic acid is readily absorbed from the gastro-intestinal tract. It has a short half-life of about 2 hours and is highly bound to plasma proteins (about 98%). Tiaprofenic acid is excreted predominantly in the urine with smaller amounts being excreted in the bile.

Some references to the pharmacokinetics of tiaprofenic acid: F. Jamali *et al., J. pharm. Sci.*, 1985, *74*, 953; N. N. Singh *et al., ibid.*, 1986, *75*, 439.

Uses and Administration

Tiaprofenic acid has analgesic, anti-inflammatory, and antipyretic properties; it is an inhibitor of prostaglandin synthetase. It is used for the relief of pain and in rheumatic disorders such as ankylosing spondylitis, osteoarthritis, and rheumatoid arthritis. The usual dose by mouth is 600 mg daily; this may be given in 2 or 3 divided doses or once daily as a sustained-release preparation. A suggested dose in severe renal impairment is 200 mg twice daily.

A detailed review of the actions and uses of tiaprofenic acid.— E. M. Sorkin and R. N. Brogden, *Drugs*, 1985, *29*, 208.

Proceedings of a symposium on the therapeutic aspects of tiaprofenic acid. The closing remarks included the statement that tiaprofenic acid continues to be a promising agent and should be included in the range of anti-inflammatory drugs needed to cover the range of patients encountered.— *Drugs*, 1988, *35, Suppl.* 1, 1–111.

ADMINISTRATION IN THE ELDERLY. Studies indicating no significantly altered pharmacokinetics of tiaprofenic acid in elderly patients: G. A. C. Hosie and J. Hosie, *Br. J. clin. Pharmac.*, 1987, *24*, 93; J. Hosie and G. A. C. Hosie, *Eur. J. clin. Pharmac.*, 1987, *32*, 93.

Proprietary Preparations

Surgam *(Roussel, UK). Capsules*, sustained-release, tiaprofenic acid 300 mg.
Tablets, tiaprofenic acid 200 and 300 mg.
Sachets, tiaprofenic acid 300 mg.

Proprietary Names and Manufacturers

Surgam *(Roussel, Canad.; Roussel, Fr.; Albert-Roussel, Ger.; Roussel, S.Afr.; Roussel, Switz.; Roussel, UK)*; Surgamic *(Roussel, Spain)*; Surgamyl *(Roussel, Denm.; Roussel Maestretti, Ital.)*; Tioprofen *(Scharper, Ital.)*.

2710-j

Tiaramide Hydrochloride *(BANM, USAN, rINNM).*

NTA-194; Tiaperamide Hydrochloride. 5-Chloro-3-{2-[4-(2-hydroxyethyl)piperazin-1-yl]-2-oxoethyl}benzothiazolin-2-one hydrochloride.
$C_{15}H_{18}ClN_3O_3S,HCl$=392.3.

CAS — 32527-55-2 (tiaramide); 35941-71-0 (hydrochloride).

Tiaramide hydrochloride has analgesic and anti-inflammatory properties. It has been given in doses of 100 mg three times daily by mouth.
It has also been studied as an oral anti-asthmatic agent.

Some references to the anti-asthmatic properties of tiaramide: N. Del Bono *et al., Curr. ther. Res.*, 1981, *30*, 578; K. E. Berkin and J. W. Kerr, *Br. J. clin. Pharmac.*, 1982, *14*, 505; J. E. Harvey *et al., Allergy*, 1985, *40*, 198.

Proprietary Names and Manufacturers
Deflal *(Toho, Jpn)*; Inlet *(Jpn)*; Solantal *(Fujisawa, Jpn)*.

2711-z

Tinoridine Hydrochloride *(rINNM).*

Tienoridine Hydrochloride; Y-3642 (tinoridine). Ethyl 2-amino-6-benzyl-4,5,6,7-tetrahydrothieno[2,3-*c*]pyridine-3-carboxylate hydrochloride.
$C_{17}H_{20}N_2O_2S,HCl$=352.9.

CAS — 24237-54-5 (tinoridine); 25913-34-2 (hydrochloride).

Adverse Effects
Gastro-intestinal disturbances, drowsiness, vertigo, pruritus, urticaria, skin eruptions, and changes in liver function tests may occur.

Uses and Administration
Tinoridine hydrochloride has analgesic, anti-inflammatory, and antipyretic properties. It has been used in rheumatic disorders in doses equivalent to 50 to 100 mg of tinoridine three times daily.

Some references to tinoridine: F. Cataldo *et al., Curr. ther. Res.*, 1983, *33*, 123 (use in children).

Proprietary Names and Manufacturers
Dimaten *(Promeco, Arg.)*; Nonflamin *(Yoshitomi, Jpn)*.

2712-c

Tolfenamic Acid *(BAN, rINN).*

N-(3-Chloro-*o*-tolyl)anthranilic acid.
$C_{14}H_{12}ClNO_2$=261.7.

CAS — 13710-19-5.

Adverse Effects
Gastro-intestinal disturbances, dysuria, headache, pruritus, sweating, skin rashes, and oedema have been reported.

Pulmonary infiltrations induced by tolfenamic acid in 6 patients.— C. Strömberg *et al.* (letter), *Lancet*, 1987, *2*, 685.

Uses and Administration
Tolfenamic acid has analgesic, anti-inflammatory, and antipyretic properties. It has been given in inflammatory and rheumatic disorders in doses of 100 to 200 mg three times daily by mouth.

Studies on the pharmacokinetics of tolfenamic acid: P. J. Pentikäinen *et al., Eur. J. clin. Pharmac.*, 1984, *27*, 349 (considerable biliary excretion); J. Stenderup *et al., Eur. J. clin. Pharmac.*, 1985, *28*, 573 (no dose adjustments necessary in alcoholic cirrhosis).

MIGRAINE. In a comparative double-blind, crossover study, 20 women with classic and common migraine took tolfenamic acid 200 mg, ergotamine tartrate 1 mg, aspirin 500 mg, or placebo, followed by an analgesic of choice after 2 hours if required. Tolfenamic acid was as effective as ergotamine tartrate in reducing the intensity and duration of attacks and had fewer side-effects.— H. Hakkarainen *et al., Lancet*, 1979, *2*, 326.

A 4-phase double-blind placebo-controlled crossover study, in 7 patients with common migraine, on the effect of metoclopramide pretreatment on the absorption of tolfenamic acid. Rectal administration of metoclopramide 20 mg as suppositories accelerated the absorption of tolfenamic acid between attacks and prevented the migraine-induced delay in absorption during attacks.— R. A. Tokola and P. J. Neuvonen, *Br. J. clin. Pharmac.*, 1984, *17*, 67.

Results of a double-blind placebo-controlled crossover study involving 31 patients indicated that the prophylactic effect of tolfenamic acid 300 mg daily in migraine was at least as good as that of propranolol 120 mg daily.— B. Mikkelsen *et al.*, *Acta neurol. scand.*, 1986, *73*, 423.

PAIN. Tolfenamic acid 100 mg and rimazolium methylsulphate 300 mg were considered to be of similar efficacy when used three times daily in the treatment of 60 patients with postoperative or post-traumatic pain. Response was considered to be good in 70% of the 30 patients who received tolfenamic acid and side-effects reported included restless legs (1), gastric irritation (1), nausea (1), and fatigue (2).— M. Haataja *et al.*, *Curr. ther. Res.*, 1978, *24*, 284.

Results of a double-blind placebo-controlled study involving 122 evaluable women, indicated that adminsitration of tolfenamic acid 200 mg three times daily for 7 days immediately after insertion of an intra-uterine device and during the next 3 menstrual periods, reduced the incidence of associated cramps and excessive bleeding. Four of the women who received tolfenamic acid experienced dyspepsia and diarrhoea.— O. Ylikorkala *et al.*, *Lancet*, 1978, *2*, 393.

RHEUMATIC DISORDERS. Studies on the use of tolfenamic acid in rheumatoid arthritis and other rheumatic disorders.— A. Kajander *et al.*, *Scand. J. Rheumatol.*, 1976, *5*, 158; K. Sørensen and L. V. Christiansen, *ibid.*, 1977, *Suppl.* 20;; L. Nyfos, *ibid.*, 1979, *Suppl.* 24, 5; V. Rejholec *et al.*, *ibid.*, 9 and 13.

Proprietary Names and Manufacturers
Clotam *(GEA, Denm.*; *Medica, Fin.*; *Tobishi, Jpn).*

2713-k

Tolmetin Sodium *(BANM, USAN, rINNM).*

McN-2559-21-98. Sodium (1-methyl-5-*p*-toluoylpyrrol-2-yl)acetate dihydrate.
$C_{15}H_{14}NNaO_3,2H_2O=315.3$.

CAS — 26171-23-3 (tolmetin); 35711-34-3 (sodium salt, anhydrous); 64490-92-2 (sodium salt, dihydrate).

Pharmacopoeias. In *U.S.*

A light yellow to light orange crystalline powder. Freely **soluble** in water and in methyl alcohol; slightly soluble in alcohol; very slightly soluble in chloroform.

Adverse Effects and Precautions

As for ibuprofen, p.20.

ALLERGY. Reports of allergic reactions or anaphylactic shock in patients taking tolmetin sodium.— C. Restivo and H. E. Paulus, *J. Am. med. Ass.*, 1978, *240*, 246 (2 patients); S. Ahmad (letter), *New Engl. J. Med.*, 1980, *303*, 1417 (1 patient); M. E. Moore and D. P. Goldsmith, *Archs intern. Med.*, 1980, *140*, 1105 (1 patient); A. C. Rossi and D. E. Knapp (letter), *New Engl. J. Med.*, 1982, *307*, 499 (brief review); C. D. Ponte and R. Wisman (letter), *Drug Intell. & clin. Pharm.*, 1985, *19*, 479.

Aseptic meningitis occurred in a patient with systemic lupus erythematosus given tolmetin. She had earlier experienced a similar but milder reaction with ibuprofen.— G. B. Ruppert and W. F. Barth, *J. Am. med. Ass.*, 1981, *245*, 67.

EFFECTS ON THE BLOOD. A fatal case of agranulocytosis in a 52-year-old woman was associated with tolmetin of which she had taken 400 mg three times daily for 5 weeks. The patient had previously been taking other anti-inflammatory and analgesic drugs for some years.— J. Sakai and M. W. Joseph (letter), *New Engl. J. Med.*, 1978, *298*, 1203.

Thrombocytopenia in a child receiving tolmetin.— J. M. Lockhart, *Arthritis Rheum.*, 1982, *25*, 1144.

EFFECTS ON THE KIDNEYS. Interstitial nephritis in a woman given tolmetin.— S. M. Katz *et al.*, *J. Am. med. Ass.*, 1981, *246*, 243.

A report of the nephrotic syndrome induced by tolmetin.— G. P. Chatterjee, *J. Am. med. Ass.*, 1981, *246*, 1589.

See also under Interference with Diagnostic Tests (below).

INTERFERENCE WITH DIAGNOSTIC TESTS. The urine of 5 patients receiving tolmetin gave false positive reactions for protein when tested by the standard sulphosalicylic acid method.— G. E. Ehrlich and G. F. Wortham, *Clin. Pharmac. Ther.*, 1975, *17*, 467. A similar report.— L. C. Knodel *et al.* (letter), *J. Am. med. Ass.*, 1986, *255*, 324.

PREGNANCY AND THE NEONATE. A study in one nursing mother indicating that only a negligible amount of tolmetin would be ingested by a breast-fed infant.— R. Sagraves *et al.* (letter), *Drug Intell. & clin. Pharm.*, 1985, *19*, 55.

Absorption and Fate

Tolmetin is almost completely absorbed from the gastro-intestinal tract. Peak plasma concentrations are attained about 30 to 60 minutes after ingestion. It is extensively bound to plasma proteins and has a biphasic plasma half-life of about 1 to 2 hours and 5 hours respectively. It is excreted in the urine as an inactive dicarboxylic acid metabolite and its glucuronide and as tolmetin glucuronide with small amounts of unchanged drug.

Some studies on the absorption and fate of tolmetin.— M. L. Selley *et al.*, *Clin. Pharmac. Ther.*, 1975, *17*, 599; D. D. Sumner *et al.*, *Drug Metab. & Disposit.*, 1975, *3*, 283; W. A. Cressman *et al.*, *J. pharm. Sci.*, 1975, *64*, 1965; W. A. Cressman *et al.*, *Clin. Pharmac. Ther.*, 1976, *19*, 224; M. L. Selley *et al.*, *ibid.*, 1978, *24*, 694; J. M. Grindel *et al.*, *ibid.*, 1979, *26*, 122; D. E. Furst *et al.*, *J. clin. Pharmac.*, 1983, *23*, 557; S. Wanwimolruk *et al.*, *Br. J. clin. Pharmac.*, 1983, *15*, 91.

Uses and Administration

Tolmetin sodium has analgesic, anti-inflammatory, and antipyretic properties; it is an inhibitor of prostaglandin synthetase. It is used in rheumatic disorders such as ankylosing spondylitis, osteoarthritis, and rheumatoid arthritis. The usual initial dose is the equivalent of 400 mg of tolmetin three times daily by mouth; maintenance doses of 600 to 1800 mg daily in divided doses have been used. Tolmetin sodium has also been used in juvenile chronic polyarthritis in doses equivalent to 15 to 30 mg of tolmetin per kg body-weight daily.

Reviews of the actions and uses of tolmetin: R. N. Brogden *et al.*, *Drugs*, 1978, *15*, 429.

ANKYLOSING SPONDYLITIS. Some references to the use of tolmetin sodium in ankylosing spondylitis.— F. Wagenhäuser, *Scand. J. Rheumatol.*, 1975, *4*, *Suppl.* 8, S 10-08; W. Standel, *ibid.*, S 10-09; M. Schattenkirchner and U. Schattenkirchner, *ibid.*, S 10-11; G. Manz, *ibid.*, S 10-10.

OSTEOARTHRITIS. Some references to the use of tolmetin sodium in osteoarthrosis.— R. Rau *et al.*, *Scand. J. Rheumatol.*, 1975, *4*, *Suppl.* 8, S 10-12; F. O. Müller *et al.*, *S. Afr. med. J.*, 1977, *51*, 794; S. P. Liyanage and C. E. Steele, *Curr. med. Res. Opinion*, 1977, *5*, 299; J. J. Cannella *et al.*, *Curr. ther. Res.*, 1979, *25*, 447; S. Kaplan and R. Salzman, *ibid.*, 508; S. Y. Andelman and A. Miyara, *ibid.*, *26*, 44; N. W. Shepherd and C. E. Steele, *Practitioner*, 1981, *225*, 1696; W. O'Brien, *Curr. ther. Res.*, 1986, *40*, 780.

RHEUMATOID ARTHRITIS. Some references to the use of tolmetin sodium in rheumatoid arthritis.— L. S. Bain *et al.*, *Br. J. clin. Pract.*, 1975, *29*, 208; J. H. Brown *et al.*, *J. clin. Pharmac.*, 1975, *15*, 455; M. Aylward *et al.*, *Curr. med. Res. Opinion*, 1976, *4*, 158; N. Cardoe and C. E. Steele, *ibid.*, 1977, *4*, 688; M. Alward *et al.*, *ibid.*, 695; A. M. Freeman *et al.*, *ibid.*, *5*, 262; G. M. Clark *et al.*, *Curr. ther. Res.*, 1977, *21*, 697; J. I. McMillen, *ibid.*, *22*, 266; K. Pavelka and A. Susta, *ibid.*, 1978, *24*, 83; B. M. Ansell *et al.*, *Rheumatol. Rehabil.*, 1978, *17*, 150.

Preparations

Tolmetin Sodium Capsules *(U.S.P.).* Store in airtight containers.

Tolmetin Sodium Tablets *(U.S.P.)*

Proprietary Preparations

Tolectin *(Ortho-Cilag, UK). Capsules*, tolmetin 400 mg (as tolmetin sodium).

Proprietary Names and Manufacturers

Artrocaptin *(Estedi, Spain)*; Index *(Edmond Pharma, Ital.)*; Midocil *(Pensa, Spain)*; Reutol *(Errekappa, Ital.)*; Tolectin *(Belg.*; *McNeil, Canad.*; *Cilag-Chemie, Denm.*; *Cilag, Ger.*; *Cilag, Ital.*; *Neth.*; *Johnson & Johnson, S.Afr.*; *Cilag, Switz.*; *Ortho-Cilag, UK*; *McNeil Pharmaceutical, USA)*; Tolmex *(Biopharma, Ital.).*

2714-a

Tribuzone *(pINN).*

Trimetazone; Trimethazone. 4-(4,4-Dimethyl-3-oxopentyl)-1,2-diphenylpyrazolidine-3,5-dione.
$C_{22}H_{24}N_2O_3=364.4$.

CAS — 13221-27-7.

Pharmacopoeias. In *Cz.*

Tribuzone has analgesic and anti-inflammatory properties. It has been used in inflammatory and rheumatic disorders in doses of 250 mg two to four times daily by mouth.

Proprietary Names and Manufacturers
Benetazon *(Spofa, Cz.).*

9593-l

Triethanolamine Salicylate *(BANM).*

Trolamine Salicylate *(pINNM).*

NOTE. Trolamine is *USAN.*

Triethanolamine salicylate has analgesic and anti-inflammatory properties and is used topically in a concentration of 10%.

Proprietary Names and Manufacturers
Aspercreme *(Thompson, USA)*; Bioglan Analgesic Cream *(Bioglan, Austral.)*; Mobisyl *(Ascher, USA)*; Myoflex *(Adria, Canad.*; *Adria, USA)*; Royflex *(Roy, Canad.).*

The following names have been used for multi-ingredient preparations containing triethanolamine salicylate— Radox Rub *(Nicholas, Austral.).*

13379-x

Triflusal *(rINN).*

UR-1501. 2-Acetoxy-4-trifluoromethylbenzoic acid.
$C_{10}H_7F_3O_4=248.2$.

CAS — 322-79-2.

Triflusal is an inhibitor of platelet aggregation. It has been used for the prophylaxis of thrombo-embolic disorders in doses of 300 mg daily by mouth and in maintenance therapy in usual doses of 300 to 600 mg daily.

References: J. Garcia-Rafanell and J. Morell, *Thérapie*, 1977, *32*, 337; -M. L. Rutllant *et al.*, *Curr. ther. Res.*, 1977, *22*, 510; R. M. Masso *et al.*, *ibid.*, 1979, *25*, 791.

Proprietary Names and Manufacturers
Disgren *(Uriach, Spain).*

2715-t

Viminol Hydroxybenzoate *(rINNM).*

Diviminol Hydroxybenzoate; Z-424 *(viminol)*. 1-[1-(2-Chlorobenzyl)pyrrol-2-yl]-2-(di-*sec*-butyl)aminoethanol 4-hydroxybenzoate.
$C_{21}H_{31}ClN_2O,C_7H_6O_3=501.1$.

CAS — 21363-18-8 (viminol); 21466-60-4; 23784-10-3 (both hydroxybenzoate).

Viminol hydroxybenzoate has analgesic and antipyretic properties. It has been given in doses equivalent to up to 400 mg of viminol daily, in divided doses, by mouth.

Studies on the analgesic action of viminol.— P. Procacci *et al.*, *Curr. ther. Res.*, 1969, *11*, 647; L. Martinetti *et al.*, *J. clin. Pharmac.*, 1970, *10*, 390; M. Moroni *et al.*, *Int. J. clin. Pharmac. Biopharm.*, 1978, *16*, 513; D. Foschi *et al.*, *Curr. ther. Res.*, 1985, *37*, 269.

Proprietary Names and Manufacturers
Dividol *(Zambon, Ital.*; *Zambon, Spain)*; Lenigesial *(Inpharzam, Ger.).*

2716-x

Zomepirac Sodium *(BANM, USAN, rINNM).* McN-2783-21-98. Sodium [5-(4-chlorobenzoyl)-1,4-dimethylpyrrol-2-yl]acetate dihydrate.
$C_{15}H_{13}ClNNaO_3,2H_2O$=349.7.

CAS — 33369-31-2 (zomepirac); 64092-48-4 (sodium salt, anhydrous); 64092-49-5 (sodium salt, dihydrate).

Pharmacopoeias. In *U.S.*

Zomepirac sodium has analgesic and anti-inflammatory properties. It was formerly given by mouth but was withdrawn from the market following reports of adverse reactions.

Reports of adverse effects associated with zomepirac: S. K. Fellner *et al.*, *Archs intern. Med.*, 1981, *141*, 1846 (acute renal failure); S. R. Ross *et al.*, *Ann. Allergy*, 1982, *48*, 233 (bronchospasm); K. A. Corre and R. J. Rothstein, *ibid.*, 299 (anaphylactic reaction); S. J. Ratner, *Ann. intern. Med.*, 1982, *96*, 793 (acute renal failure); P. J. Mease *et al.*, *ibid.*, *97*, 454 (interstitial nephritis and renal failure); P. S. Driver *et al.*, *Drug Intell. & clin. Pharm.*, 1982, *16*, 616 (anaphylactic-like reaction); V. T. Smith, *J. Am. med. Ass.*, 1982, *247*, 1172 (anaphylactic shock, acute renal failure, and disseminated intravascular coagulation); J. T. McCarthy *et al.*, *Mayo Clin. Proc.*, 1982, *57*, 351 (acute renal failure); S. C. Boike *et al.*, *Drug Intell. & clin. Pharm.*, 1983, *17*, 56 (acute renal failure); S. E. Warren and C. Mosley, *J. Am. med. Ass.*, 1983, *249*, 396 (acute renal failure); W. H. Lisker (letter), *ibid.*, 1706 (acute renal failure); R. Kiani and M. Kushner, *ibid.*, 2812 (serum sickness); K. M. Olsen *et al.*, *Clin. Pharm.*, 1984, *3*, 85 (agranulocytosis); D. M. Cummings *et al.*, *ibid.*, 198 (interstitial nephritis).

Preparations

Zomepirac Sodium Tablets *(U.S.P.)*

Proprietary Names and Manufacturers

Zomax *(Ortho-Cilag, UK; McNeil Pharmaceutical, USA).*

Anthelmintics

750-g

Anthelmintics are used to treat helminth or worm infections. The worms that cause infection in man generally fall either into the phylum Platyhelminthes, which includes the cestodes or tapeworms and the trematodes or flukes, or into the phylum Nematoda which includes the nematodes or roundworms.

Cestodes (tapeworms) are flat segmented worms and include
**Diphyllobothrium latum*—broad fish tapeworm
Echinococcus granulosus and *E. multilocularis*—causing hydatid disease
Hymenolepis nana—dwarf tapeworm
**Taenia saginata*—beef tapeworm
**Taenia solium*—pork tapeworm
The larvae of *Taenia solium* cause cysticercosis.
Trematodes (flukes) are generally flat, leaf-shaped, unsegmented worms and include
Clonorchis sinensis—Chinese liver fluke
Fasciola hepatica—liver fluke
Fasciolopsis buski—intestinal fluke
Heterophyes heterophyes—intestinal fluke
Metagonimus yokogawi—intestinal fluke
Opisthorchis felineus and *O. viverrini*—liver flukes
Paragonimus westermani—Oriental lung fluke
Schistosoma spp.—causing schistosomiasis (bilharziasis)
Schistosoma haematobium
Schistosoma intercalatum
Schistosoma japonicum
Schistosoma mansoni.

Nematodes are round unsegmented worms; those chiefly infecting the **intestine** include
Ancylostoma duodenale—Old World hookworm
**Ascaris lumbricoides*—common roundworm
Capillaria philippinensis
**Enterobius vermicularis*—threadworm, pinworm
Necator americanus—New World hookworm
Strongyloides stercoralis—sometimes called threadworm in USA
Trichostrongylus spp.
**Trichuris trichiura* —whipworm
Nematodes chiefly infecting the **tissues**, including the filarial worms, are
Brugia malayi—causing lymphatic filariasis
Dracunculus medinensis —guinea-worm
Loa loa—eye worm
Mansonella perstans—causing perstans filariasis
Mansonella streptocerca—causing streptocerciasis
Onchocerca volvulus—causing river blindness (onchocerciasis)
**Toxocara canis* and *T. cati*
**Trichinella spiralis*
Wuchereria bancrofti—causing lymphatic filariasis.
*NOTE. Infections due to the helminths marked with an asterisk may occur in Great Britain and other temperate climates; infections due to the other helminths are generally limited to tropical or localised areas, but may occur in travellers who have visited those areas.

Treatment
The following list is a guide to the principal anthelmintics used for specific worm infections, although choice in many parts of the world may reflect cost and availablilty. The drugs following each worm are in alphabetical order and not in order of preference.

CESTODE (TAPEWORM) INFECTIONS
Diphyllobothrium latum—niclosamide, praziquantel
Echinococcus spp.—mebendazole
Hymenolepis nana—niclosamide, praziquantel
Taenia spp.—niclosamide, praziquantel
cysticercosis—praziquantel

TREMATODE (FLUKE) INFECTIONS
Clonorchis sinensis—praziquantel
Fasciola hepatica—bithionol, praziquantel
Fasciolopsis buski—niclosamide, praziquantel, tetrachloroethylene
Opisthorchis spp.—praziquantel
Paragonimus westermani—bithionol, praziquantel
Schistosoma haematobium—metriphonate, praziquantel
Schistosoma japonicum—praziquantel
Schistosoma mansoni—oxamniquine, praziquantel

NEMATODE INFECTIONS (INTESTINAL)
Ancylostoma duodenale—bephenium, mebendazole, pyrantel, tetrachloroethylene
Ascaris lumbricoides—levamisole, mebendazole, piperazine, pyrantel
Capillaria philippinensis—mebendazole, thiabendazole
Enterobius vermicularis—mebendazole, piperazine, pyrantel, viprynium
Necator americanus—as for *Ancylostoma duodenale*, above
Strongyloides stercoralis—mebendazole, thiabendazole
Trichostrongylus spp.—pyrantel, thiabendazole
Trichuris trichiura—mebendazole, oxantel.

NEMATODE INFECTIONS (TISSUES)
Brugia malayi—diethylcarbamazine
Dracunculus medinensis—niridazole, thiabendazole
Loa loa—diethylcarbamazine
Mansonella spp.—diethylcarbamazine
Onchocerca volvulus—diethylcarbamazine, ivermectin
Toxocara spp.—diethylcarbamazine, thiabendazole
Trichinella spiralis—mebendazole, thiabendazole

Wuchereria bancrofti—diethylcarbamazine

For the use of paromomycin in tapeworm infections and metronidazole in guinea-worm infections, see the respective monographs.

Many of the drugs in this section are used in veterinary medicine.

WHO reports on various parasitic infections and their management: Intestinal Protozoan and Helminthic Infections, *Tech. Rep. Ser. Wld Hlth Org. No. 666*, 1981; Lymphatic Filariasis, *Tech. Rep. Ser. Wld Hlth Org. No. 702*, 1984; The Control of Schistosomiasis, *Tech. Rep. Ser. Wld Hlth Org. No. 728*, 1985; Prevention and Control of Intestinal Parasitic Infections, *Tech. Rep. Ser. Wld Hlth Org. No. 749*, 1987; Onchocerciasis, *Tech. Rep. Ser. Wld Hlth Org. No. 752*, 1987.

Reviews of anthelmintics: M. Katz, *Drugs*, 1986, *32*, 358.

Drug and dosage guidelines for the treatment of worm infections.— *Med. Lett.*, 1986, *28*, 9.

751-q

Alantolactone

Alant Camphor; Elecampane Camphor; Helenin; Inula Camphor. (3a*R*,5*S*,8a*S*,9a*R*)-3a,5,6,7,8,8a,9,9a-Octahydro-5,8a-dimethyl-3-methylenenaphtho[2,3-*b*]furan-2(3*H*)-one.
$C_{15}H_{20}O_2$=232.3.

CAS — 546-43-0.

A terpene obtained from the roots of *Inula helenium* (Compositae).

Alantolactone was formerly used in the treatment of roundworm (*Ascaris*), threadworm, hookworm, and whipworm infection.

752-p

Albendazole *(BAN, USAN, rINN).*

SKF-62979. Methyl 5-propylthio-1*H*-benzimidazol-2-ylcarbamate.
$C_{12}H_{15}N_3O_2S$=265.3.

CAS — 54965-21-8.

Adverse Effects and Precautions
As for Mebendazole, p.57.

Albendazole was well tolerated in a placebo-controlled study in 870 patients with intestinal helminthiasis, 457 of whom received albendazole, the majority as a single 400-mg dose. The following side-effects were reported: dizziness (3 patients), headache (8), epigastric pain (30), dry mouth (1), fever (1), pruritus (2), vomiting (2), and diarrhoea (8). They were not significantly different from the side-effects in the placebo group.— J. F. Rossignol and H. Maisonneuve, *Trans. R. Soc. trop. Med. Hyg.*, 1983, *77*, 707.

Although generally well-tolerated, the following adverse reactions were reported in studies involving 30 patients given *high-dose* therapy with albendazole for the treatment of cystic echinococcosis [hydatid disease]: raised serum-transaminase levels (2 patients); reduced leucocyte counts (1); gastro-intestinal symptoms (1); allergic conditions (1); and loss of hair (1). Treatment was stopped in a further patient with alveolar echinococcosis because of depressed bone-marrow activity. Close supervision is required to prevent serious complications during the treatment of echinococcosis with benzimidazole carbamates.— A. Davis *et al.*, *Bull. Wld Hlth Org.*, 1986, *64*, 383.

EFFECTS ON THE LIVER. Abnormalities of liver function tests developed during therapy in 7 of 40 patients with hydatid disease given albendazole 10 mg per kg body-weight daily. Six had a hepatocellular abnormality with moderately severe hepatitis in one; the seventh patient developed obstructive jaundice 3 days after starting treatment, but albendazole was considered unlikely to have been the cause. Liver function recovered rapidly in all patients on withdrawal of albendazole. Careful monitoring of liver function before and during therapy is required.— D. L. Morris and P. G. Smith, *Trans. R. Soc. trop. Med. Hyg.*, 1987, *81*, 343.

Absorption and Fate
Albendazole is poorly absorbed from the gastro-intestinal tract, but rapidly undergoes extensive first-pass metabolism. The principal metabolite albendazole sulphoxide has anthelmintic activity and a plasma half-life of about 8.5 hours; it is excreted in the urine together with other metabolites including albendazole sulphone and the 2-amino sulphoxide and 2-amino sulphone.

A study of the pharmacokinetics of albendazole in healthy subjects and patients being treated for hydatid disease. Albendazole appeared to be metabolised extremely rapidly since it could not be detected in plasma. Plasma concentrations of the active metabolite albendazole sulphoxide were extremely variable between individuals, probably because of variable absorption. Following an oral dose of 400 mg in 14 subjects, peak plasma concentrations of the sulphoxide ranged from 0.04 to 1.14 µg per mL at 1 to 4 hours. Similar concentrations were found in 5 patients with hydatid disease given albendazole 10 mg per kg body-weight daily, when allowance was made for differences in dosage regimen; bile and hydatid cyst fluid concentrations of sulphoxide were lower than those in plasma samples at the same times. Binding of albendazole sulphoxide to plasma protein has been noted to be about 70%. Since concentrations of the metabolite were low in bile, this route of excretion would appear to be quantitatively of minor importance. The major urinary metabolite was albendazole sulphoxide; in 4 healthy subjects 0.09 to 0.88% of the total dose of albendazole was excreted as the sulphoxide over 24 hours. The effect of fat (olive oil and milk) on absorption of albendazole in 4 healthy subjects was variable; in one, absorption was increased about 3.5 times, but there was little change in the other 3.— S. E. Marriner *et al.*, *Eur. J. clin. Pharmac.*, 1986, *30*, 705.

A study on the penetration of albendazole sulphoxide into hydatid cysts *in vitro* and *in vivo*. In patients with hydatid cysts given 3 doses of albendazole 5 mg per kg body-weight every 12 hours, before operation, mean concentrations of albendazole sulphoxide in serum and cyst fluid at operation were 341.6 and 61 ng per mL respectively; mean concentrations in patients given albendazole 10 mg per kg daily for 4 weeks or more before operation were 785.2 and 165 ng per mL. Overall a dose of 10 mg per kg daily was considered capable of achieving cyst fluid concentrations in excess of 100 ng per mL in most patients, which is at the lower end of effective concentrations *in vitro*.— D. L. Morris *et al.*, *Gut*, 1987, *28*, 75.

Further references to pharmacokinetic studies of albendazole: B. Penicaut *et al.*, *Bull. Soc. Path. exot.*, 1983, *76*, 698 (single 400-mg dose); A. G. Saimot *et al.*, *Lancet*, 1983, *2*, 652 (in patients with hydatid disease).

Uses and Administration

Albendazole is a benzimidazole anthelmintic structurally related to mebendazole (see p.57) and is similarly active against most nematode and some cestode worms.

Albendazole is given by mouth, usually as a single dose, in the treatment of single or mixed intestinal nematode infections. The usual dose for adults and children aged 2 years or over with ascariasis, enterobiasis, hookworm infections, or trichuriasis is 400 mg as a single dose. In strongyloidiasis, 400 mg is given daily for 3 consecutive days.

Albendazole has also been given in higher doses in the treatment of hydatid disease.

A review of the properties of albendazole and its use in the treatment of intestinal helminthiasis. In intestinal nematode infections, albendazole as a single dose of 400 mg appears to be a safe and effective treatment of enterobiasis, ascariasis, hookworm infections caused by *Necator americanus* or *Ancylostoma duodenale*, and trichuriasis; effectiveness against massive trichuriasis remains questionable. Strongyloidiasis requires treatment for 3 days. Albendazole is also effective against the larval migrating stages of *N. americanus* and is ovicidal in ascariasis, hookworm infections, and trichuriasis. Thus, unlike the closely related benzimidazole mebendazole, a single oral dose of albendazole is effective against most intestinal nematode infections; it may be of value in mass chemotherapy control programmes.

In intestinal cestode infections, some effect has been noted in patients with taeniasis due to *Taenia saginata* given a single 400-mg dose of albendazole, but 400 mg daily for 3 consecutive days was poorly effective against *Hymenolepis nana* infection. It is being extensively investigated by the WHO for the treatment of hydatid disease.

Albendazole has been unsuccessful in the treatment of trematode infections. It has been reported to be of no benefit against the liver flukes *Clonorchis sinensis* and *Fasciola hepatica* or against *Schistosoma mansoni*.— J.-F. Rossignol and H. Maisonneuve, *Gastroenterol. clin. biol.*, 1984, *8*, 569.

CUTANEOUS LARVA MIGRANS. Beneficial results with albendazole 400 mg daily for 5 consecutive days in the treatment of cutaneous larva migrans.— J. P. Coulaud *et al.*, *Bull. Soc. Path. exot.*, 1982, *75*, 534.

HYDATID DISEASE. A brief discussion on albendazole in the treatment of hydatid disease.— *Lancet*, 1984, *2*, 675. Comment and the view that toxicity had been played down. Albendazole must be suspected of having toxic effects similar to those of mebendazole.— P. A. Braithwaite (letter), *ibid.*, 1160.

Encouraging preliminary results with albendazole 5 to 7 mg per kg body-weight twice daily, in 30-day courses separated by 2-week intervals, in the treatment of hydatid disease.— A. G. Saimot *et al.*, *Lancet*, 1983, *2*, 652. Incontrovertible evidence of failure of scolicidal activity by albendazole in a patient given 30 mg per kg body-weight daily.— M. C. A. Puntis and L. E. Hughes (letter), *ibid.*, 1255. A warning from the manufacturers that daily doses of albendazole 10 mg per kg body-weight should not be exceeded. *Animal* chronic toxicity studies certainly do not support the clinical doses of 30 mg per kg daily.— B. Dickson (letter), *ibid.*, 1984, *1*, 57.

Albendazole 10 mg per kg body-weight daily in divided doses was given for 1-month courses to 32 patients with hydatid cysts caused by *Echinococcus granulosus*; 14 received 1 course, 15 received 2 courses, and 3 received 3 courses. Clinical response was seen in 13 patients, but this could not be taken as objective evidence of remission. Using computed tomography or ultrasound, virtual disappearance of cysts was detected in 5 of the 20 evaluable patients and diminution in cyst size in 10; 5 patients had no evidence of response to treatment. Six patients developed abnormalities of liver function during therapy. A further patient had a low white blood cell count at the end of treatment which was probably unrelated to albendazole. Although very careful and frequent monitoring of liver function tests, white blood cell and platelet counts, and urine for proteinuria is advised at present, albendazole is considered to be the current treatment of choice in inoperable hydatid disease and possibly in those with recurrent or multiple cysts.— D. L. Morris *et al.*, *J. Am. med. Ass.*, 1985, *253*, 2053.

Studies *in vitro* demonstrating that albendazole sulphoxide, the main metabolite of albendazole, significantly reduced the viability of *Echinococcus granulosus* scoleces derived from *sheep* and man and is probably responsible for the activity of this drug.— J. B. Chinnery and D. L. Morris, *Trans. R. Soc. trop. Med. Hyg.*, 1986, *80*, 815; D. L. Morris and D. Taylor (letter), *Lancet*, 1986, *2*, 1035.

Further references to beneficial results with albendazole in hydatid disease: G. B. A. Okelo, *Trans. R. Soc. trop. Med. Hyg.*, 1986, *80*, 193; S. Mansueto *et al.* (letter), *ibid.*, 1987, *81*, 168.

For reviews, comments, and further studies on hydatid disease and its treatment with benzimidazoles including albendazole, see Mebendazole, p.58.

INTESTINAL NEMATODE INFECTIONS. In a multicentre double-blind placebo-controlled study in 870 patients with single or mixed intestinal nematode and cestode infections, albendazole was shown to be effective against the 4 major soil-transmitted helminthiases—ascariasis, hookworm infections caused by *Necator americanus* and *Ancylostoma duodenale*, trichuriasis, and strongyloidiasis. In adults, albendazole 400 mg was effective against *Ascaris lumbricoides, Ancylostoma duodenale, Necator americanus*, and light infections with *Trichuris trichuria*; 400 mg daily for 3 consecutive days was effective against *Strongyloides stercularis*. Children were given half the adult dose which was much less effective. Only 5 of 17 patients with *Hymenolepis nana* infection given albendazole 400 mg daily for 3 consecutive days were cured.— J. F. Rossignol and H. Maisonneuve, *Trans. R. Soc. trop. Med. Hyg.*, 1983, *77*, 707. In an open multicentre study in 1455 similar patients a single 400-mg dose of albendazole in adults and children was well tolerated and effective against the 4 major species of intestinal nematodes: *Enterobius vermicularis, Ascaris lumbricoides, Necator americanus*, and *Trichuris trichuria* (light infections).— J. P. Coulaud and J. F. Rossignol, *Acta trop.*, 1984, *41*, 87.

Results indicating that albendazole has larvicidal activity against pre-intestinal stages of *Necator americanus*. A single 400-mg dose given by mouth 6 days after the forearm was exposed to *N. americanus* larvae prevented patent infection in 8 of 21 healthy subjects and reduced egg output in the remainder; 8 untreated subjects all developed infection.— B. L. Cline *et al.*, *Am. J. trop. Med. Hyg.*, 1984, *33*, 387.

Further references to albendazole in the treatment of intestinal nematode infections: P. Pene *et al.*, *Am. J. trop. Med. Hyg.*, 1982, *31*, 263 (single and mixed infections); C. Viravan *et al.*, *S. E. Asian J. trop. med. publ. Hlth*, 1982, *13*, 654 (hookworm infections); S. Chitchang *et al.*, *J. med. Ass. Thailand*, 1983, *66*, 45 (hookworm infections); R. C. Misra *et al.*, *Curr. ther. Res.*, 1983, *33*, 758 (single and mixed infections); S. Ramalingam *et al.*, *Am. J. trop. Med. Hyg.*, 1983, *32*, 984 (single and mixed infections); S. K. Chandiwana *et al.*, *Cent. Afr. J. Med.*, 1983, *29*, 213 (single and mixed infections); S. Bassily *et al.*, *Ann. trop. Med. Parasit.*, 1984, *78*, 81 (ancylostomiasis and ascariasis); D. A. P. Bundy *et al.*, *Trans. R. Soc. trop. Med. Hyg.*, 1985, *79*, 641 (multiple and single dose regimens in children with trichuriasis); P. K. Misra *et al.*, *Curr. med. Res. Opinion*, 1985, *9*, 516 (single and mixed infections in children); A. J. Gazder and J. Roy, *Curr. ther. Res.*, 1987, *41*, 324 (single and mixed infections in children).

OPISTHORCHIASIS. Beneficial results were achieved with albendazole 400 mg twice daily by mouth for 3 or 7 days in patients with *Opisthorchis viverrini* infection, including some also infected with intestinal nematodes, although an optimum dosage regimen remains to be determined. The authors comment that, although praziquantel has been shown to be the most effective drug in treating opisthorchiasis, albendazole has the advantage of activity against intestinal nematodes.— S. Pungpark *et al.*, *S. E. Asian J. trop. med. publ. Hlth*, 1984, *15*, 44.

Proprietary Names and Manufacturers

Alben; Zeben; Zentel *(Smith Kline & French, Fr.)*.

12371-b

Amoscanate *(rINN)*.
C-9333-Go/CGP-4540; GO-9333; Nithiocyamine. 4-*p*-Nitroanilinophenyl isothiocyanate.
$C_{13}H_9N_3O_2S$=271.3.

CAS — 26328-53-0.

Amoscanate is an isothiocyanate anthelmintic which has been tried in the treatment of hookworm infections. In China it has been widely used against schistosomiasis due to *Schistosoma japonicum*.

Adverse effects reported have included gastro-intestinal effects and giddiness.

References to the use of amoscanate in the treatment of hookworm infections: B. J. Vakil *et al.*, *Trans. R. Soc. trop. Med. Hyg.*, 1977, *71*, 247; B. V. Ashok *et al.*, *Br. J. clin. Pharmac.*, 1977, *4*, 463.

References to the use of amoscanate in the treatment of schistosomiasis.— Report of a WHO Expert Committee on the control of schistosomiasis, *Tech. Rep. Ser. Wld Hlth Org. No. 728*, 1985.

Proprietary Names and Manufacturers
Ciba-Geigy, Switz.

753-s

Amphotalide *(rINN)*.
M&B-2948A; RP-6171. *N*-[5-(4-Aminophenoxy)pentyl]-phthalimide.
$C_{19}H_{20}N_2O_3$=324.4.

CAS — 1673-06-9.

Amphotalide was formerly used in the treatment of schistosomiasis, particularly infections due to *Schistosoma haematobium*.

755-e

Antimony Potassium Tartrate *(USAN)*.
Antim. Pot. Tart.; Brechweinstein; Kalii Stibyli Tartras; Potassium Antimonyltartrate; Stibii et Kalii Tartras; Tartar Emetic; Tartarus Stibiatus. Dipotassium bis{*μ*-[2,3-dihydroxybutanedioato(4-)-$O^1,O^2:O^3,O^4$]}-diantimonate(2-) trihydrate; Dipotassium bis[*μ*-tartrato(4-)]diantimonate(2-) trihydrate.
$C_8H_4K_2O_{12}Sb_2,3H_2O$=667.9.

CAS — 11071-15-1 (anhydrous); 28300-74-5 (trihydrate).

Pharmacopoeias. In *Aust., Braz., Chin., Egypt., Fr., It., Mex., Nord., Pol., Port., Span.* and *U.S.* In some pharmacopoeias the monograph substance is described as $C_4H_4KO_7Sb,1/2H_2O$ (=333.9).

Odourless, colourless, transparent crystals or white powder. The crystals effloresce on exposure to air and do not readily rehydrate even when exposed to high humidity.

Soluble 1 in 12 of water, 1 in 3 of boiling water, and 1 in 15 of glycerol; insoluble in alcohol. Solutions in water are acid to litmus.

Incompatible with acids and alkalis, salts of heavy metals, albumin, soap, and tannins. **Store** in well-closed containers.

Antimony potassium tartrate is a trivalent antimony compound with similar properties to antimony sodium tartrate (see below). It is less soluble and more irritant than the sodium salt.

Reference to the topical application of antimony potassium tartrate in the treatment of cutaneous leishmaniasis acquired in Texas.— T. L. Gustafson *et al.*, *Am. J. trop. Med. Hyg.*, 1985, *34*, 58.

Proprietary Names and Manufacturers
Contra Pulmonia y Catarros *(Miguez, Spain)*.

756-l

Antimony Sodium Tartrate *(USAN)*.
Antim. Sod. Tart.; Sodium Antimonyltartrate; Stibium Natrium Tartaricum. Disodium bis{*μ*-[2,3-dihydroxybutanedioato(4-)-$O^1,O^2:O^3,O^4$]}diantimonate(2-); Disodium bis{*μ*-[L-(+)-tartrato(4-)]}diantimonate(2-).
$C_8H_4Na_2O_{12}Sb_2$=581.6.

CAS — 34521-09-0.

Pharmacopoeias. In *Chin.* (as $C_4H_4NaO_7Sb$ = 308.8) and *U.S.*

Colourless, transparent, odourless crystals or white powder. The crystals effloresce on exposure to air.
Freely **soluble** in water; insoluble in alcohol. **Incompatible** with acids and alkalis, salts of heavy metals, albumin, soap, and tannins. **Store** in well-closed containers.

Adverse Effects and Treatment

Antimony sodium tartrate and other trivalent antimonials are more toxic than pentavalent antimonials such as sodium stibogluconate, possibly because they are excreted much more slowly. The most serious adverse effects are on the heart and liver. There are invariably ECG changes during treatment, but hypotension, bradycardia, and cardiac arrhythmias are more serious. Sudden death or cardiovascular collapse may occur at any time. Elevated liver enzyme values are common; liver damage with hepatic failure and death is most likely in patients with pre-existing hepatic disease.
Adverse effects immediately after intravenous administration of trivalent antimonials, in particular the tartrates, have included coughing, chest pain, pain in the arms, vomiting, abdominal pain, fainting, and collapse, especially after rapid injection. Extravasation during injection is extremely painful because of tissue damage. An anaphylactoid reaction characterised by an urticarial rash, husky voice, and collapse has been reported after the sixth or seventh intravenous injection of a course of treatment.
Numerous less immediate adverse effects have occurred including gastro-intestinal disturbances, muscular and joint pains, arthritis, pneumonia, dyspnoea, headache, dizziness, weakness, pruritus, skin rashes, facial oedema, fever, haemolytic anaemia, and kidney damage.
Large doses of antimony compounds taken by mouth have an emetic action. Continuous treatment with small doses of antimony may give rise to symptoms of subacute poisoning similar to those of chronic arsenical poisoning.
Treatment of severe poisoning with antimony compounds is similar to that for arsenic poisoning (see p.1544); dimercaprol may be of benefit.
In Great Britain the recommended exposure limit of antimony is 0.5 mg per m^3 (long-term). In the *US* the permissible and the recommended exposure limits are 0.5 mg per m^3.

The pharmacology and toxicology of antimony.— K. L. Stemmer, *Pharmac. Ther.*, 1976, *1*, 157.

Precautions

Trivalent antimony therapy has generally been superseded by less toxic treatment. It is contra-indicated in the presence of pneumonia, heart, liver, and kidney disease. Intravenous injections should be administered very slowly and stopped if coughing, vomiting, or substernal pain occurs; extravasation should be avoided. Antimony sodium tartrate caused severe pain and tissue necrosis and was therefore not given by intramuscular or subcutaneous injection.

Absorption and Fate

Antimony sodium tartrate is poorly absorbed from the gastro-intestinal tract.
Like most trivalent compounds of antimony it is slowly excreted, mainly in the urine, following parenteral administration. Antimony accumulates in the body during treatment and persists for several months afterwards. Trivalent antimony has a greater affinity for cell proteins than for plasma proteins.

Uses and Administration

Antimony sodium tartrate and other trivalent antimony compounds were used in the treatment of the protozoal infection leishmaniasis until the advent of the less toxic pentavalent compounds (see sodium stibogluconate, p.677). They continued to be used in the treatment of schistosomiasis, but have now generally been superseded by less toxic and more easily administered drugs such as praziquantel.
Antimony sodium tartrate was formerly used as an emetic and expectorant.
Other trivalent antimony compounds include antimony lithium thiomalate (anthiolimine), antimony potassium tartrate (above), sodium antimonylgluconate, stibocaptate (p.67), and stibophen (p.67).

758-j

Areca

Areca Nuts; Arecae Semen; Arekasame; Betel Nuts; Noix d'Arec.

Pharmacopoeias. In *Chin.* and *Jpn.*

The dried ripe seeds of *Areca catechu* (Palmae) containing arecoline.

Areca was formerly used in the treatment of tapeworm infection.
It has sialagogue properties and is used in eastern countries as a masticatory. An increased incidence of oral leucoplakia and oral carcinoma has been reported in persons in the habit of chewing areca (betel nuts).

A review of areca.— K. N. Arjungi, *Arzneimittel-Forsch.*, 1976, *26*, 951.

In addition to arecoline, areca contained smaller amounts of the related alkaloid guvacoline and the amino acids arecaidine and guvacine. Guvacine and, to a lesser extent, arecaidine were competitive inhibitors of γ-aminobutyric acid uptake *in vitro*.— G. A. R. Johnston *et al.* (letter), *Nature*, 1975, *258*, 627.

Increased oral cancer associated with the chewing of 'quids' composed of areca, lime, and, occasionally, tobacco leaf, might be associated with the arecaidine content.— J. Ashby *et al.* (letter), *Lancet*, 1979, *1*, 112. Criticisms.— B. G. Burton-Bradley (letter), *ibid.*, *2*, 903.

CNS symptoms in 2 patients were due to withdrawal from betel-nut chewing, a custom almost universal among people living under traditional conditions in Papua New Guinea and other Asian and Melanesian countries. Syndromes associated with the practice range from habituation to addiction and psychosis.— D. M. Wiesner (letter), *Med. J. Aust.*, 1987, *146*, 453.

Severe extrapyramidal symptoms developed in 2 chronic schizophrenics after chewing betel nuts.— M. P. Deahl (letter), *Br. med. J.*, 1987, *294*, 841.

759-z

Arecoline Hydrobromide

Methyl 1,2,5,6-tetrahydro-1-methylnicotinate hydrobromide.
$C_8H_{13}NO_2,HBr$=236.1.

CAS — 63-75-2 (arecoline); 300-08-3 (hydrobromide).

Pharmacopoeias. In *Arg.*, *Hung.*, *Nord.*, *Pol.*, *Port.*, and *Span.*

Arecoline is an alkaloid present in Areca (see above); it has a parasympathomimetic action similar to that of pilocarpine. It has been used in veterinary medicine as a purgative and taenifuge. It is not taenicidal.

A review of programmes to control echinococcosis (hydatidosis; hydatid disease) caused by *Echinococcus granulosus*. Programmes in New Zealand, Tasmania, Cyprus, and Argentina have all relied on administration of arecoline to *dogs* to identify those infected.— M. A. Gemmell *et al.*, *Bull. Wld Hlth Org.*, 1986, *64*, 333.

ALZHEIMER'S DISEASE. Reference to arecoline in the treatment of Alzheimer's disease. Although some benefit has been reported from studies in *animals* and humans, its extremely short half-life makes the use of arecoline impractical.— E. Hollander *et al.*, *Br. med. Bull.*, 1986, *42*, 97.

761-s

Ascaridole

Ascaridol. 1-Isopropyl-4-methyl-2,3-dioxabicyclo[2.2.2]-oct-5-ene.
$C_{10}H_{16}O_2$=168.2.

CAS — 512-85-6.

The active principle of chenopodium oil. It is an unstable liquid which is liable to explode when heated or when treated with organic acids.

Ascaridole has the same actions as chenopodium oil (see p.50).

762-w

Bephenium Hydroxynaphthoate *(BAN, USAN, rINN).*

Naphthammonum. Benzyldimethyl(2-phenoxyethyl)ammonium 3-hydroxy-2-naphthoate.
$C_{28}H_{29}NO_4$=443.5.

CAS — 7181-73-9 (bephenium); 3818-50-6 (hydroxynaphthoate).

Pharmacopoeias. In *Br.*, *Braz.*, *Egypt.*, *Ind.*, *Int.*, *Rus.*, and *U.S.* Also in *B.P. Vet.*

A yellow to greenish-yellow odourless or almost odourless crystalline powder.
Practically **insoluble** in water; soluble 1 in 50 of alcohol. **Store** in airtight containers.

Adverse Effects

Nausea, diarrhoea, vomiting, headache, and vertigo have occasionally been reported.

Absorption and Fate

Only a small fraction of a dose of bephenium hydroxynaphthoate is absorbed from the gastro-intestinal tract.

Uses and Administration

Bephenium hydroxynaphthoate is an effective anthelmintic against hookworms of the species *Ancylostoma duodenale*, but is less effective against *Necator americanus*. It also has activity against *Ascaris* (roundworms) and *Trichostrongylus* worms.
A single oral dose of granules, equivalent to 2.5 g of bephenium, is usually effective in removing hookworms of the species *Ancylostoma duodenale*. Children weighing less than 10 kg or under 2 years old may be given the equivalent of 1.25 g of bephenium. The dose should be given, suspended in water or other suitable liquid. In the presence of severe infection, treatment may be repeated after 3 days.

Preparations

Bephenium Granules *(B.P.).* Bephenium Hydroxynaphthoate Granules

Bephenium Hydroxynaphthoate for Oral Suspension *(U.S.P.)*

Proprietary Preparations

Alcopar *(Wellcome, UK). Granules,* bephenium 2.5 g (as hydroxynaphthoate), in 5-g sachets.

Proprietary Names and Manufacturers

Alcopar *(Wellcome, Fr.; Wellcome, UK)*; Alcopara *(USA)*; Bephenate *(IBYS, Spain).*

763-e

Betanaphthol

β-Naftol; Naphthol. Naphth-2-ol.
$C_{10}H_8O$=144.2.

CAS — 135-19-3.

Pharmacopoeias. In *Aust.*, *Cz.*, *Hung.*, *Jug.*, *Nord.*, *Pol.*, *Port.*, *Span.*, and *Swiss.*

Adverse Effects

Symptoms of overdosage include vomiting, diarrhoea, haemolysis, lens opacities, oliguria, and convulsions. Nephritis has followed absorption from intact skin.

Uses and Administration

Betanaphthol was formerly used as an anthelmintic in hookworm and tapeworm infections, but it has been superseded by less toxic and more efficient drugs. It is excreted chiefly as the glucuronide and gives a reddish tint to the urine.
Betanaphthol has a potent parasiticidal effect and was used as an ointment in the treatment of scabies, ringworm, and other skin diseases.
Betanaphthyl benzoate was used similarly.

The absorption of betanaphthol from a paste containing 20%, with sulphur and soft soap, ranged from 5 to 41% of the amount applied to 10 patients. It was recommended that betanaphthol paste be applied to areas not larger than 150 cm^2, only to patients capable of metabolising betanaphthol, and be left on the skin for not more than 1 hour twice daily. A high output of urine was necessary, preferably alkaline, and treatment should not be given during pregnancy.— H. G. W. M. Hemels, *Br. J. Derm.*, 1972, *87*, 614.

2210-k

Bithionol *(BAN, rINN).*
Bitionol. 2,2′-Thiobis(4,6-dichlorophenol).
$C_{12}H_6Cl_4O_2S$=356.1.

CAS — 97-18-7.

Pharmacopoeias. In *Arg. Fr.* includes bithionol oxide for veterinary use.

Adverse Effects
Adverse effects in patients taking bithionol by mouth include anorexia, nausea, vomiting, abdominal discomfort, diarrhoea, salivation, dizziness, headache, and skin rashes.
Photosensitivity reactions have occurred in persons using soap containing bithionol. Cross-sensitisation with other halogenated disinfectants has also occurred.

Uses and Administration
Bithionol is a chlorinated bis-phenol with bactericidal and anthelmintic properties. It is active against most trematodes (flukes) although in general, and with the exception of fascioliasis, praziquantel is now the treatment of choice for trematode infections. A dose of 30 to 50 mg per kg body-weight by mouth on alternate days for 10 to 15 doses may be given in the treatment of fascioliasis and paragonimiasis.
Bithionol is no longer used topically as a bactericide because of photosensitivity reactions and its use in cosmetics is prohibited in many countries.

References to the use of bithionol in the treatment of paragonimiasis: T. S. Singh *et al.*, *Trans. R. Soc. trop. Med. Hyg.*, 1986, *80*, 967.

Proprietary Names and Manufacturers
Bitin *(Tanabe, Jpn).*

764-l

Bitoscanate *(rINN).*
Hoechst-16842. Phenylene-1,4-bisisothiocyanate.
$C_8H_4N_2S_2$=192.3.

CAS — 4044-65-9.

Bitoscanate is an isothiocyanate anthelmintic which has been used in the treatment of hookworm infections.
Adverse effects have included gastro-intestinal disturbances and dizziness.

Proprietary Names and Manufacturers
Jonit.

765-y

Bromonaphthol
1-Bromonaphth-2-ol.
$C_{10}H_7BrO$=223.1.

CAS — 34369-04-5 (1-bromonaphthol).

Bromonaphthol has been used in the treatment of hookworm infections (*Ancylostoma* and *Necator*) and against whipworms.

Proprietary Names and Manufacturers
Wormin *(Toyama, Jpn).*

12457-w

Brotianide *(BAN, rINN).*
Bay-4059Va; FBA-4059. 2-Bromo-6-(4-bromophenylthiocarbamoyl)-4-chlorophenyl acetate; 2-Acetoxy-3,4′-dibromo-5-chlorothiobenzanilide.
$C_{15}H_{10}Br_2ClNO_2S$=463.6.

CAS — 23233-88-7.

Brotianide is a veterinary anthelmintic used in the treatment of liver-fluke infection.

12466-e

Bunamidine Hydrochloride *(BANM, USAN, rINNM).*
NSC-106571. N^1,N^1-Dibutyl-4-hexyloxy-1-naphthamidine hydrochloride.
$C_{25}H_{38}N_2O,HCl$=419.0.

CAS — 3748-77-4 (bunamidine); 1055-55-6 (hydrochloride).

Pharmacopoeias. In *B.P. Vet.*

A white, odourless or almost odourless, crystalline powder. Slightly **soluble** in water; soluble 1 in 2 of alcohol, and 1 in 2 of chloroform; practically insoluble in ether.

Bunamidine hydrochloride is a veterinary anthelmintic, administered as tablets in the treatment of tapeworm infections in dogs and cats.

Proprietary Veterinary Names and Manufacturers
Scolaban *(Coopers Animal Health, UK).*

766-j

Cambendazole *(BAN, USAN, rINN).*
MK-905. Isopropyl 2-(thiazol-4-yl)-1*H*-benzimidazol-5-ylcarbamate.
$C_{14}H_{14}N_4O_2S$=302.4.

CAS — 26097-80-3.

Cambendazole is a benzimidazole anthelmintic structurally related to thiabendazole (see p.68); it has been used in the treatment of strongyloidiasis. It is also used in veterinary practice.

Cambendazole was teratogenic in *rats*.— P. Delatour and Y. Richard, *Thérapie*, 1976, *31*, 505.

STRONGYLOIDIASIS. Parasitological cure was obtained in all of 40 Brazilian patients with strongyloidiasis after a single dose of cambendazole 5 mg per kg body-weight by mouth. Side-effects, reported by 4 patients, were considered negligible and included dizziness (3 patients), nausea (2), abdominal discomfort (2), headache (2), anorexia (1), and vomiting 3 hours after the dose (1).— S. A. Bicalho *et al.*, *Am. J. trop. Med. Hyg.*, 1983, *32*, 1181.

Proprietary Veterinary Names and Manufacturers
Ascapilla *(Univet, UK)*; Porcam *(Merck Sharp & Dohme, UK).*

768-c

Chenopodium Oil
Aetheroleum Chenopodii; Esencia de Quenopodio Vermifuga; Oil of American Wormseed; Wurmsamenöl.

CAS — 8006-99-3.

Pharmacopoeias. In *Arg.*, *It.*, *Mex.*, *Port.*, *Span.*, and *Turk.*

Distilled with steam from the fresh flowering and fruiting plants, excluding roots, of *Chenopodium ambrosioides* var. *anthelminticum*. It contains ascaridole.

NOTE. Chenopodium oil may explode when heated.

Chenopodium oil was formerly used as an anthelmintic for the expulsion of roundworms (*Ascaris*) and hookworms. It is toxic and has caused numerous fatalities.

It was recommended that chenopodium herb be prohibited for use as a flavouring agent.— *Report on the Review of Flavourings in Food*, FAC/REP/22, London, HM Stationery Office, 1976.

12565-j

Ciclobendazole *(BAN, rINN).*
Cyclobendazole *(USAN)*; R-17147. Methyl 5-(cyclopropylcarbonyl)-1*H*-benzimidazol-2-ylcarbamate.
$C_{13}H_{13}N_3O_3$=259.3.

CAS — 31431-43-3.

Ciclobendazole is a benzimidazole anthelmintic structurally related to mebendazole (see p.57). It has been tried in the treatment of intestinal nematode infections.

References: A. Degrémont and E. Stahel, *Schweiz. med. Wschr.*, 1978, *108*, 1430; R. Guggenmoos *et al.*, *Tropenmed. Parasit.*, 1978, *29*, 423.

Proprietary Names and Manufacturers
Janssen, Belg.; Cilag, Switz.

12579-x

Clioxanide *(BAN, USAN, rINN).*
CI-633; CN-59567; SYD-230. 2-(4-Chlorophenylcarbamoyl)-4,6-di-iodophenyl acetate.
$C_{15}H_{10}ClI_2NO_3$=541.5.

CAS — 14437-41-3.

Clioxanide has been used as a veterinary anthelmintic.

1984-s

Closantel *(BAN, USAN, rINN).*
R-31520; R-34828 (sodium salt). 5′-Chloro-4′-(4-chloro-α-cyanobenzyl)-3,5-di-iodosalicyl-*o*-toluidide.
$C_{22}H_{14}Cl_2I_2N_2O_2$=663.1.

CAS — 57808-65-8; 61438-64-0 (sodium salt).

Closantel is an anthelmintic used in veterinary medicine.

Proprietary Veterinary Names and Manufacturers
Janssen, UK.

769-k

Cucurbita
Abóbora; Kürbissame; Melon Pumpkin Seeds; Pepo; Semence de Courge.

Pharmacopoeias. In *Port.* which permits other species of *Cucurbita*.

The fresh seeds of *Cucurbita maxima* (Cucurbitaceae).

Cucurbita has been used for the expulsion of tapeworms (*Taenia*).

770-w

Desaspidin *(rINN).*
3′-[(5-Butyryl-2,4-dihydroxy-3,3-dimethyl-6-oxocyclohexa-1,4-dien-1-yl)methyl]-2′,6′-dihydroxy-4′-methoxybutyrophenone.
$C_{24}H_{30}O_8$=446.5.

CAS — 114-43-2.

A phloroglucinol derivative obtained from the Finnish broad buckler-fern, *Dryopteris austriaca* (Polypodiaceae). It has also been found in the American aspidium, or marginal fern, *D. marginalis*, but *not* in Swiss and Austrian samples of *D. austriaca*.

Desaspidin has been used as an anthelmintic against the fish tapeworm, *Diphyllobothrium latum*.

12639-c

Diamphenethide *(BAN).*
Diamfenetide *(rINN)*. β,β′-Oxybis(aceto-*p*-phenetidide).
$C_{20}H_{24}N_2O_5$=372.4.

CAS — 36141-82-9.

Pharmacopoeias. In *B.P. Vet.*

A white to pale buff-coloured powder. Practically **insoluble** in water and in ether; slightly soluble in alcohol, chloroform, and methyl alcohol.

Diamphenethide is an anthelmintic used for the control of liver fluke in sheep.

Proprietary Veterinary Names and Manufacturers
Coriban *(Coopers Animal Health, UK).*

771-e

Dichlorophen *(BAN, rINN).*
Di-phenthane-70; G-4. 2,2′-Methylenebis(4-chlorophenol).
$C_{13}H_{10}Cl_2O_2$=269.1.

CAS — 97-23-4.

Pharmacopoeias. In *Aust.*, *Br.*, and *Fr.* Also in *B.P. Vet.*

A white or slightly cream-coloured powder with a not more than slightly phenolic odour.
Practically **insoluble** in water; soluble 1 in 1 of alcohol and 1 in less than 1 of ether.

Adverse Effects

Dichlorophen may cause nausea, vomiting, gastro-intestinal colic, and diarrhoea. In some patients it has produced an urticarial rash. Jaundice has occurred after a large dose.
Contact allergic dermatitis and photosensitivity have been associated with topical use.

Precautions

The use of dichlorophen as an anthelmintic is contra-indicated in the presence of impaired liver function and in conditions in which purgation is undesirable, such as during the last few months of pregnancy, in acute fevers, or in severe heart disease.

Uses and Administration

Dichlorophen is an anthelmintic used in the treatment of infection by tapeworms but has generally been superseded by niclosamide.
It has been given by mouth in various treatment schedules, often as a 6-g dose on 2 successive days.
Dichlorophen also has antifungal and antibacterial activity and has been used topically in the treatment of fungal infections and as a germicide in soaps and cosmetics. The use of dichlorophen in cosmetics and toiletries is controlled.

Preparations

Dichlorophen Tablets *(B.P.)*

Proprietary Names and Manufacturers

Anthiphen *(May & Baker, S.Afr.; May & Baker, UK)*; Ovis *(Warner, Ger.)*; Plath-Lyse *(Génévrier, Fr.)*; Wespuril *(Spitzner, Ger.)*.

The following names have been used for multi-ingredient preparations containing dichlorophen—Mycota Spray *(Crookes Healthcare, UK)*.

772-1

Diethylcarbamazine Citrate *(BANM, USAN, rINNM).*

Diethylcarbam. Cit.; Diethylcarbamazine Acid Citrate; Diethylcarbamazini Citras; Ditrazini Citras; RP-3799. *NN*-Diethyl-4-methylpiperazine-1-carboxamide dihydrogen citrate.
$C_{10}H_{21}N_3O,C_6H_8O_7=391.4$.

CAS — 90-89-1 (diethylcarbamazine); 1642-54-2 (citrate).

Pharmacopoeias. In *Arg.*, *Br.*, *Braz.*, *Chin.*, *Cz.*, *Egypt.*, *Eur.*, *Fr.*, *Ind.*, *Int.*, *Jpn*, *Neth.*, *Nord.*, *Rus.*, *Swiss*, and *U.S.* Also in *B.P. Vet.*

A white, crystalline, slightly hygroscopic powder, odourless or with a slight odour. M.p. about 138° with decomposition.
Very **soluble** in water; soluble 1 in 35 of alcohol; practically insoluble in acetone, chloroform, and ether. A 6.29% w/v solution is iso-osmotic with serum. Solutions for injection are **sterilised** by autoclaving. **Store** in airtight containers. Solutions should be protected from light.

Studies on sustained-release tablet formulations of diethylcarbamazine.— S. K. Baveja *et al.*, *Int. J. Pharmaceut.*, 1984, *19*, 229; S. K. Baveja *et al.*, *ibid.*, 1985, *24*, 355.

Adverse Effects

Adverse effects directly attributable to diethylcarbamazine include anorexia, nausea and vomiting, headache, dizziness, and drowsiness, but are seldom severe enough to cause discontinuance of treatment; convulsions and coma may occur in overdosage. Allergic reactions following the death of microfilariae, larvae, or adult worms are especially prominent in onchocerciasis and in *Brugia malayi* infections; eye changes may occur during the treatment of onchocerciasis. Reactions may be modified by the concomitant administration of antihistamines or corticosteroids. Encephalitis may occur in patients with loiasis and is probably due to massive lysis of microfilariae.

Seven patients, whose general condition was poor, lapsed into irreversible coma after being given diethylcarbamazine, 225 to 900 mg in 3 to 8 days, for onchocerciasis. Death followed 1 to 4 days later.— A. P. Oomen (letter), *Trans. R. Soc. trop. Med. Hyg.*, 1969, *63*, 548.

Reactions occurring during diethylcarbamazine treatment of lymphatic filariasis are basically of 2 types: pharmacological dose-dependent responses and a response of the infected host to the destruction and death of parasites. The first type are direct effects of the drug and include weakness, dizziness, lethargy and sleepiness, anorexia, nausea, and vomiting. They occur equally frequently in infected and non-infected recipients, begin within 1 to 2 hours of taking diethylcarbamazine, and persist for a few hours. The second type are attributable to the filaricidal action of diethylcarbamazine and are thought to be immunological reactions to disintegrating microfilariae and dead adult worms; they are less likely to occur and less severe in bancroftian than in brugian filariasis. They may be systemic or local, both with and without fever. Systemic reactions may occur a few hours after the first oral dose of diethylcarbamazine and generally do not last for more than 3 days. They include headache, aches in other parts of the body, joint pain, dizziness, anorexia, malaise, urticaria, vomiting, and sometimes attacks of bronchial asthma in asthmatic patients. Fever and systemic reactions are positively associated with microfilaraemia. Systemic reactions are reduced if diethylcarbamazine is given in spaced doses or in repeated small doses. They eventually cease spontaneously and interruption of treatment is rarely necessary; symptomatic treatment with antipyretics or analgesics may be helpful. Local reactions tend to occur later in the course of treatment, from 3 days up to 4 weeks after the first oral dose, and last longer; they also disappear spontaneously and interruption of treatment is not necessary. Local reactions include lymphadenitis, lymphangitis, abscess, ulceration, and transient lymphoedema. They are probably related to the presence of adult or immature worms or fourth-stage larvae in the tissues.— Fourth Report of the WHO Expert Committee on Filariasis, *Tech. Rep. Ser. Wld Hlth Org. No. 702*, 1984.

A series of events including dermal, ocular, and systemic components, known collectively as the Mazzotti reaction, occurs minutes to hours after the administration of diethylcarbamazine to most patients with onchocerciasis. Clinical manifestations can be severe, dangerous, and debilitating and limit the widespread use of the drug in onchocerciasis. None of the reactions is due to direct drug toxicity since they only occur when microfilariae are killed. The same reaction may occur to varying degrees with other microfilaricidal drugs.
Systemic reactions include increased itching, rash, headache, aching muscles, joint pain, painful swollen and tender lymph nodes, fever, tachycardia and hypotension, and vertigo. They mostly begin within the first 24 hours after treatment, but increased itching may begin within minutes. Levels of pruritus, fever, adenopathy, and hypotension are correlated with the intensity of infection; severity of the reaction also depends on the dose of diethylcarbamazine used and hence the extent and rapidity of microfilarial killing. Intravenous hydrocortisone and intravenous fluids are needed to control severe reactions and paracetamol or aspirin to control fever and musculoskeletal pain. The local use of corticosteroids and mydriatics is indicated for acute uveitis.
Ocular reactions, such as transient conjunctival hyperaemia and limbitis, often with excessive watering and photophobia develop in most patients in the first few hours after diethylcarbamazine treatment. Microfilariae migrate from the periocular tissues into the cornea and die during the next 2 to 4 days, together with those present before treatment. An inflammatory infiltrate forms around the dead microfilariae producing lesions of punctate keratitis that remain for some weeks before resolving completely. Microfilariae in the anterior chamber may increase in numbers transiently, but later decrease. In the posterior segment, transient retinal pigment epithelial defects have been detected in many patients during the first days of diethylcarbamazine treatment. Optic neuritis also occurs and leads to visual field loss.
Other changes include initial eosinopenia and later persistent eosinophilia, early neutrophilia and lymphocytopenia, elevations in liver enzyme values, and proteinuria.
The incidence and intensity of the Mazzotti reaction is usually a function of the severity of infection which suggests that it is related to microfilarial killing. There has been speculation that, as in the Jarisch-Herxheimer reaction, activation of complement may be the trigger, but numerous other inflammatory mediators and pathways may be involved.— Third Report of the WHO Expert Committee on Onchocerciasis, *Tech. Rep. Ser. Wld Hlth Org. No. 752*, 1987.

EFFECTS ON THE KIDNEY. A report of significant proteinuria in patients with moderate onchocerciasis receiving diethylcarbamazine topically or by mouth for periods of 4 to 6 months.— B. M. Greene *et al.* (letter), *Lancet*, 1980, *1*, 254. Similar findings.— J. L. Ngu *et al.* (letter), *ibid.*, 710.

Precautions

Treatment with diethylcarbamazine should be closely supervised since allergic reactions are common and may be severe, especially in patients with both onchocerciasis and loiasis. Patients with onchocerciasis should be monitored for eye changes.

In patients taking diethylcarbamazine citrate, the sensitivity of filarial skin tests using extracts of *Wuchereria bancrofti* was reduced.— J. C. Katiyar *et al.* (letter), *Trans. R. Soc. trop. Med. Hyg.*, 1974, *68*, 169. Similar results with skin tests using *Brugia malayi*.— P. K. Murthy *et al.*, *Indian J. med. Res.*, 1978, *68*, 428, per *Trop. Dis. Bull.*, 1979, *76*, 1029.

The use of diethylcarbamazine 2 mg per kg body-weight as a provocative day test for the detection of microfilariae of nocturnally periodic *Wuchereria bancrofti* in the blood, was not suitable in the presence of onchocerciasis or loiasis.— J. E. McMahon *et al.*, *Bull. Wld Hlth Org.*, 1979, *57*, 759.

ADMINISTRATION IN RENAL FAILURE. For a study on the effects of renal impairment on the pharmacokinetics of diethylcarbamazine, see under Absorption and Fate (below).

PREGNANCY AND THE NEONATE. Results of *animal* studies suggesting that the uterine hypermotility induced by diethylcarbamazine is mediated via prostaglandin synthesis and might explain the mechanism of the abortifacient action previously reported (V.S.V. Subbu and A.R. Biswas, *Indian J. med. Res.*, 1971, *59*, 646).— C. A. Joseph and A. F. Dixon, *J. Pharm. Pharmac.*, 1984, *36*, 281.

Absorption and Fate

Diethylcarbamazine citrate is readily absorbed from the gastro-intestinal tract and also through the skin and conjunctiva. It is widely distributed in tissues and is excreted in the urine unchanged and as the *N*-oxide metabolite. Urinary excretion and hence plasma half-life is dependent on urinary pH.

A pharmacokinetic study in 6 patients with onchocerciasis indicating that diethylcarbamazine is absorbed quickly and almost completely from the gastro-intestinal tract and, in contrast to its disposition in *rats*, is eliminated by both renal and extrarenal routes with relatively small amounts being excreted as the *N*-oxide metabolite. Following a single radioactively labelled dose of diethylcarbamazine citrate 0.5 mg per kg body-weight, administered by mouth as an aqueous solution, peak plasma concentrations of 100 to 150 ng per mL were achieved in 1 to 2 hours, followed by a sharp decline, then a marked secondary rise 3 to 6 hours after dosing followed by a steady decline. The half-life ranged from 9 to 13 hours. Urinary excretion of diethylcarbamazine and diethylcarbamazine *N*-oxide was complete within 96 hours; between 4 and 5% of the dose was recovered in the faeces. Disposition kinetics were similar in 5 healthy subjects given a single 50-mg tablet of diethylcarbamazine citrate. Peak plasma concentrations were initially 80 to 200 ng per mL, with a secondary rise 3 to 9 hours after dosing, the terminal half-life ranged from 5 to 13 hours, and urinary excretion of unchanged diethylcarbamazine and the *N*-oxide was complete within 48 hours.— G. Edwards *et al.*, *Clin. Pharmac. Ther.*, 1981, *30*, 551.

The effect of urinary pH on the pharmacokinetics of diethylcarbamazine citrate was assessed in 5 healthy subjects given 50 mg by mouth. When an alkaline urinary pH was maintained the elimination half-life of diethylcarbamazine and the area under the plasma concentration versus time curve were significantly increased compared with values when an acidic urinary pH was maintained; half-life was increased from 4.0 to 9.6 hours. Cumulative urinary recovery of diethylcarbamazine was significantly reduced from 62.3% of the administered dose in 48 hours for acidic urine to 5.1% for alkaline urine. There was no consistent change in the excretion of diethylcarbamazine *N*-oxide. Renal clearance was also significantly reduced with alkaline urine. Thus, under alkaline conditions accumulation of diethylcarbamazine might predispose to toxicity whereas under acidic urine conditions a therapeutically effective plasma concentration might not be maintained. With a largely vegetarian diet alkaline urine is often formed and acidic urine is usual when the diet is rich in animal protein. It might be possible to manipulate urinary pH in order to produce more effective dosage regimens.— G. Edwards *et al., Br. J. clin. Pharmac.*, 1981, *12,* 807. Results in patients with onchocerciasis indicating that alkalinisation of the urine during courses of diethylcarbamazine therapy, in an attempt to decrease the dose of diethylcarbamazine required and hence the severity of adverse effects, is unlikely to be of practical value.— K. Awadzi *et al., ibid.*, 1986, *21,* 669.

Further references.— G. H. Rée *et al., Trans. R. Soc. trop. Med. Hyg.*, 1977, *71,* 542.

ADMINISTRATION IN RENAL FAILURE. Results in patients with chronic renal impairment and healthy subjects, given a single 50-mg dose of diethylcarbamazine citrate by mouth, indicating that the plasma half-life of diethylcarbamazine is prolonged and its 24-hour urinary excretion considerably reduced in those with moderate and severe degrees of renal failure. Mean plasma half-lives in 7 patients with severe renal failure (creatinine clearance less than 25 mL per minute), 5 patients with moderate renal failure (creatinine clearance between 25 and 60 mL per minute), and 4 healthy subjects were 15.1, 7.7, and 2.7 hours, respectively. The patient with the longest plasma half-life of 32 hours did not have the poorest renal function, but it was considered likely that the abnormally slow elimination of diethylcarbamazine was due to the high urine pH (7) resulting from sodium bicarbonate therapy. A further patient with a half-life longer than expected also had a less acidic urine.— K. K. Adjepon-Yamoah *et al., Br. J. clin. Pharmac.*, 1982, *13,* 829.

Uses and Administration

Diethylcarbamazine citrate is an anthelmintic used in the treatment of filarial infections including lymphatic filariasis due to *Wuchereria bancrofti* (bancroftian filariasis), *Brugia malayi* (malayan filariasis), and *B. timori* (timorian filariasis); loiasis due to *Loa loa*, and onchocerciasis due to *Onchocerca volvulus*. It has also been tried in *Mansonella* infections, including perstans filariasis and streptocerciasis, with variable results. Diethylcarbamazine is effective against both the microfilariae and adult worms of *W. bancrofti*, *B. malayi*, and *Loa loa*, but only against the microfilariae of *O. volvulus*. Thus, in onchocerciasis treatment with diethylcarbamazine is followed by a course of suramin to kill the adult worms.

Diethylcarbamazine has also been used in the treatment of toxocariasis.

Diethylcarbamazine citrate is usually administered by mouth as tablets. In the treatment of filarial infections due to *W. bancrofti, B. malayi, O. volvulus,* and *Loa loa* 6 mg per kg body-weight daily in 3 divided doses for 3 weeks may be given (but see under Lymphatic Filariasis and Onchocerciasis, below, for WHO-recommended dosage regimens). In order to reduce the incidence and severity of allergic reactions due to the destruction of microfilariae, particularly in the treatment of onchocerciasis and malayan filariasis an initial dosage of 1 mg per kg daily is recommended, gradually increased to 6 mg per kg daily over 3 days.

In the prophylaxis of bancroftian and malayan filariasis a dose of 50 mg monthly has been recommended, and in the prophylaxis of loiasis a dose of 4 mg per kg body-weight for 3 successive days each month.

Diethylcarbamazine citrate has also been given by intramuscular injection in veterinary medicine.

A review of the actions and uses of diethylcarbamazine.— C. D. Mackenzie and M. A. Kron, *Trop. Dis. Bull.*, 1985, *82,* R1.

ADMINISTRATION. Diethylcarbamazine was first used as the chloride, but is now produced as the dihydrogen citrate which contains only half its weight as base. In reporting doses it is therefore important to indicate whether they refer to a specific salt or to the base; unless otherwise stated, it can generally be assumed that the dose refers to the citrate.— Fourth Report of the WHO Expert Committee on Filariasis, *Tech. Rep. Ser. Wld Hlth Org. No. 702,* 1984.

ADMINISTRATION IN RENAL FAILURE. For a study on the effects of renal impairment on the pharmacokinetics of diethylcarbamazine, see under Absorption and Fate (above).

LOIASIS. *Loa loa* is a filarial parasite limited to and highly endemic in equatorial West and Central Africa. It is transmitted by tabanid flies (deerflies) of the genus *Chrysops* and is the necessary intermediate host in which microfilariae from the blood develop into infective larvae. Man is the only significant reservoir of human loiasis. *Loa loa* causes chronic infection characterised by microfilariaemia, occasional angioedematous swelling, and often by migration of adult worms in subcutaneous tissues and across the eye. Much of the information about the infection has been based on isolated case reports with little long-term follow-up.

In a detailed study of 20 patients who had acquired loiasis while temporarily resident in Central or West Africa, clinical manifestations were markedly different from those seen in long-term residents of endemic areas. Only 3 of the 20 had detectable microfilariaemia, but there was often a state of marked immunological hyperresponsiveness with very high titres of antibody to filariae, increased serum-IgE concentrations, and profound hypereosinophilia; allergic symptoms such as pruritus and angioedema were frequent and severe. Other complications in the patients under study included endomyocardial fibrosis in 1, haematuria in 5, and proteinuria in 1. All 20 patients were treated with diethylcarbamazine 5 to 10 mg per kg body-weight daily for 21 days. In the absence of microfilariaemia the full dose was administered from day 1, whereas those with microfilariaemia were hospitalised and the full dose reached gradually over 3 days. Although 9 patients required more than one course of diethylcarbamazine, those followed up for more than 12 months have shown no further evidence of infection. Significant reactions developed in most of the patients as a result of treatment with diethylcarbamazine and included pruritus in 16, subcutaneous nodules in 13, and haematuria (present only after initiation of therapy) in 4.

In view of the increasing numbers of travellers and temporary residents in endemic areas of Africa and because loiasis can have very serious sequelae, early recognition of its features, of the value of a therapeutic trial of diethylcarbamazine, and of the importance of successful therapy is imperative. Evaluation of the feasibilty of chemoprophylaxis with diethylcarbamazine or with other drugs is also urgently needed.— T. B. Nutman *et al., J. infect. Dis.*, 1986, *154,* 10.

Beneficial results with apheresis followed by treatment with diethylcarbamazine in a patients with membranous glomerulopathy believed to be caused by loiasis with high microfilariaemia.— L. Abel *et al., Br. med. J.*, 1986, *292,* 24.

LYMPHATIC FILARIASIS. The term lymphatic filariasis includes infection with 3 closely related nematode worms widely distributed in many parts of the tropics and subtropics. The commonest is *Wuchereria bancrofti, Brugia malayi* is restricted to Asia, and *B. timori* is confined to Indonesia. All 3 are transmitted to man by the bites of infected mosquitoes and have similar life-cycles. Adult worms live in lymphatic vessels while the embryos or microfilariae circulate in peripheral blood and are available to infect mosquito vectors when they come to feed. WHO has estimated that 905 million people are at risk of infection and that more than 90 million are actually infected, the majority with *W. bancrofti*. Only a small proportion of infected individuals show clinical signs. The underlying process, lymphatic or lymphangitic inflammation may progress to characteristic lymphatic obstruction with elephantiasis, hydrocoele, and chyluria. Immunological hyperresponsiveness to filarial antigens in certain individuals living in endemic areas produces syndromes such as tropical pulmonary eosinophilia. Control of lymphatic filariasis has depended on the mass administration of diethylcarbamazine to affected populations, in some areas with striking success, whereas programmes have failed elsewhere because of poor compliance.— *Lancet*, 1985, *1,* 1135. Further comment on lymphatic filariasis. Diethylcarbamazine is still the only drug available for treatment of individuals and for control campaigns. Although it is cheap, moderately nontoxic, and kills all stages of the parasite, including the microfilariae which infect the mosquitoes and developing and adult worms which cause the lesions, it has several serious disadvantages for control campaigns: repeated doses are necessary over long periods, often for a year or more, and unpleasant side-effects occur in heavily infected individuals when worms die en masse in the circulation and in the lymphatics. In onchocerciasis only the microfilariae are killed by diethylcarbamazine and treatment is almost always associated with a severe reaction, the Mazzotti reaction, whereas in bancroftian filariasis reactions to diethylcarbamazine are mainly associated with the death of the adult and developing worms in the lymphatics although there are also general reactions with fever, dizziness, and nausea due to the death of microfilariae. The search for new antifilarial drugs which kill only adult worms has been unsuccessful. Some of the benzimidazoles and isothiocyanates have shown promise, but none of them is likely to replace diethylcarbamazine for the treatment of lymphatic filariasis. However, ivermectin, which kills microfilariae in onchocerciasis without producing severe Mazzotti reactions or ocular damage, has also shown promise in lymphatic filariasis.— *ibid.*, 1987, *1,* 1409.

Diethylcarbamazine has been the drug of choice for treating lymphatic filariasis for 35 years and attempts to find alternative drugs have been unsuccessful. An important goal for the immediate future is therefore to determine the most acceptable dosage schedules of diethylcarbamazine within the limits of toxicity, efficacy, and feasibility.

The mechanism of action of diethylcarbamazine against lymphatic filarial parasites is not clear. Therapeutic concentrations of diethylcarbamazine have no significant effect on the microfilariae of any species *in vitro*, but *in vivo* it causes a rapid disappearance of microfilariae from the circulation. Its microfilaricidal action depends on the proper function of the humoral and cellular immune mechanism of the host; most of the microfilariae from the blood are destroyed by the reticuloendothelial cells of the liver. Surviving microfilariae are able to develop in the insect host even after exposure to repeated courses of diethylcarbamazine. In man, diethylcarbamazine has a considerable macrofilaricidal action although sometimes not all the adult worms are killed, even after repeated courses of diethylcarbamazine, and a proportion of patients continue to experience periodic attacks of adenolymphangitis, a sign of active infection with adult worms.

Treatment of individual cases of lymphatic filariasis aims to destroy the parasite and to eliminate, reduce, or prevent morbidity. The most generally accepted dose of diethylcarbamazine for the treatment of bancroftian filariasis is 6 mg per kg body-weight daily by mouth for 12 days, preferably in divided doses after meals. Various dosage schedules are used in different countries for brugian filariasis, ranging from 3 to 6 mg per kg daily (total dose, 18 to 72 mg per kg). Repeated courses are usually necessary to ensure complete parasitological cure. In African patients with bancroftian filariasis, who may also be infected with *Onchocerca volvulus* and/or *Loa loa*, special care must be taken since the action of diethylcarbamazine on these parasites may cause a serious reaction. The treatment of microfilaria carriers with diethylcarbamazine reduces the incidence of chronic disease. Patients with the chronic clinical manifestations of transient lymphoedema, small developing hydrocoele, or chyluria usually respond well to treatment with diethylcarbamazine, although repeated courses are often necessary to eliminate all adult worms. Those with early elephantiasis and some patients with elephantiasis of several years' duration may respond favourably to diethylcarbamazine, but patients with a large hydrocoele and/or elephantiasis with deformities often show no improvement. Diethylcarbamazine is also beneficial in occult filariasis and is the drug of choice for tropical pulmonary eosinophilia, although pulmonary function returns to normal only if damage to the lungs is not extensive.

Chemotherapeutic control of filariasis in the community is at present based on the use of diethylcarbamazine and generally aims to reduce morbidity by treating clinical cases of filariasis and to reduce transmission by treating people with microfilariaemia. The interruption of transmission is the ultimate objective although, given the longevity of the adult worms and the limited resources in most endemic countries, it may be unrealistic to aim for total elimination of filariasis; only a few countries have achieved this goal. Infants, pregnant women, or persons with obvious debilitating disorders are normally excluded from diethylcarbamazine control programmes. In general, mass treatment is preferable in highly endemic areas whereas in areas of low endemicity, selective treatment of those found to be microfilaria-positive, after large-scale screening of the community, may be more suitable. Diethylcarbamazine may be administered as tablets in the dosage regimens used for individual cases (see above); in bancroftian filariasis diethylcarbamazine has also been given weekly, monthly, or even yearly with successful results. Alternatively, common salt medicated with 1 to 4 g of diethylcarbamazine per kg has been used for filariasis control in some endemic areas of *Wuchereria bancrofti* and *Brugia malayi*. In China, diethylcarbamazine-medicated salt has been distributed to more than 18 million people with no observed adverse effects and with satisfactory results.

Further studies with diethylcarbamazine should include: determination of the effect of prolonged treatment with diethylcarbamazine-medicated salt on adult filarial worms and on the prevention of clinical manifestations; determination of the usefulness of prophylactic treatment with diethylcarbamazine in preventing lymphatic filarial infection by killing or damaging developing larvae in man. Newer filaricides tried in the treatment of lymphatic filariasis include levamisole and mebendazole, which are not recommended; centperazine and furapyrimidone, under study in India and China, respectively; and flubendazole and ivermectin, both of which are active against *O. volvulus*.— Fourth Report of the WHO Expert Committee on Filariasis, *Tech. Rep. Ser. Wld Hlth Org. No. 702*, 1984.

Further references to diethylcarbamazine in the treatment and control of lymphatic filariasis: F. Partono, *Trans. R. Soc. trop. Med. Hyg.*, 1984, *78*, 9 (Indonesia); F. Partono *et al.*, *ibid.*, 370 (timorian filariasis in Indonesia); C. H. Zhong, *Practitioner*, 1984, *228*, 702 (bancroftian filariasis in China); F. Partono, *Trans. R. Soc. trop. Med. Hyg.*, 1985, *79*, 44 (elephantiasis in an Indonesian community with timorian filariasis).

For a description of the reactions associated with the use of diethylcarbamazine in the treatment of lymphatic filariasis and attributed to its filaricidal action, see under Adverse Effects (above).

ONCHOCERCIASIS. Onchocerciasis or 'river blindness' is caused by the nematode worm *Onchocerca volvulus* transmitted by a small biting fly of the genus *Simulium* [blackfly]. Victims suffer from a chronic itchy dermatosis and those most severely affected, from blindness. The majority of the 20 to 50 million people infected live in Africa. There is no reservoir of the infection in animals. Following the bite of an infected *Simulium* fly, infective larvae enter the wound and develop in about a year to become adult worms in the subcutaneous tissue; they may live for up to 20 years. Fertilised female worms produce larvae called microfilariae which migrate into the skin and may be taken up by a *Simulium* fly during feeding. Microfilariae live for about a year and the serious pathological process caused by the disease is a sequel to their death. Microfilariae in the eyes cause the most serious effects including sclerosing keratitis, chronic iridocyclitis, and the posterior segment lesions choroidoretinitis and optic atrophy; there may be secondary effects such as cataract and glaucoma. Up to a tenth of the population in some parts of Africa is blind because of onchocerciasis.

Efforts to control the disease have been greatly hampered by a lack of acceptably non-toxic drugs to kill the parasites and their young and WHO has been compelled to undertake long-term vector control by applying insecticides to the rivers in which the larval stages develop. Unfortunately transmission has not been completely arrested. The effectiveness of the control programme would be enormously enhanced by mass treatment with antiparasitic chemotherapy to reduce immediately the reservoir of infection, but neither of the drugs in widespread use, diethylcarbamazine and suramin, is suitable. Diethylcarbamazine is effective against microfilariae, but their death is often associated with a severe allergic reaction, the Mazzotti reaction, the control of which has proved pharmacologically intractable; also, diethylcarbamazine has no effect on the adult worms and thus microfilariae can return as a result of continued production by the females. Suramin, by intravenous injection, will kill the adult worms and accelerate the death of microfilariae but may cause a fatal generalised disease to which there is no antidote. Trials with metriphonate, mebendazole, and levamisole have not proved successful but recently ivermectin, a broad-spectrum antiparasitic drug originally used in veterinary medicine, has been shown to have a prolonged microfilaricidal action without causing the severe Mazzotti reaction associated with diethylcarbamazine. It seems to have no effect on adult worms but when combined with vector control measures ivermectin should greatly enhance the prospects of eradication of onchocerciasis; periodic mass treatment alone would probably eliminate serious ocular lesions.— D. Bell, *Br. med. J.*, 1985, *1*, 1450. It was hoped that a suitable preparation of ivermectin could be made available, at least for limited use, before the end of 1987.— *WHO Drug Inf.*, 1987, *1*, 83.

The use of diethylcarbamazine in the treatment of onchocerciasis has important limitations. Firstly, treatment is only suppressive since only the microfilariae are killed; adult worms are essentially unaffected, repopulation of the skin and eye occurs, and repeated administration of the drug at intervals is necessary for as long as the adult female worms are fertile. Secondly, severe and sometimes dangerous systemic reactions (Mazzotti reactions) occur, especially in heavily infected patients. Thirdly, aggravation of existing ocular lesions or precipitation of new lesions may occur.

It has not proved possible to develop entirely safe dosage schedules for diethylcarbamazine, but the following regimen for an adult weighing 50 to 60 kg has been extensively used: a low starting dose of 25 or 50 mg (0.5 or 1 mg per kg body-weight) should be given for the first one or two days. The maintenance dose should be 100 mg (2 mg per kg) twice daily for 5 to 7 days so that the total amount given is about 1.3 g (30 mg per kg) for an adult; longer treatment is unnecessary and not recommended. Long-term suppressive therapy with low intermittent doses of diethylcarbamazine has not been successful. Drugs administered concomitantly with diethylcarbamazine in an attempt to prevent or reduce the severity of the Mazzotti reaction have included dexamethasone, betamethasone, triamcinolone, prednisone, methysergide, cyproheptadine, promethazine, aspirin, indomethacin, and diazepam. Only corticosteroids have been shown to be beneficial and even they only partially suppress the itching or ocular reactions. Typically, betamethasone or dexamethasone 4 mg daily for an adult is started 1 or 2 days before the first dose of diethylcarbamazine is given and is continued or tapered off on an individual basis after 3 days of treatment with diethylcarbamazine. Aspirin may reduce fever and musculoskeletal pain during the Mazzotti reaction and antihistamines may decrease pruritus and help with insomnia.

Diethylcarbamazine has also been administered topically, but the safety and efficacy of applying diethylcarbamazine lotion to the skin has not been confirmed. Diethylcarbamazine eye-drops have not been found useful for the treatment of ocular onchocerciasis.

Induction of local pruritus and rash by a single small dose of diethylcarbamazine, usually 50 mg for an adult, is indicative of the parasite's presence and has been used as a provocative test, the Mazzotti test, to help diagnose onchocerciasis. However, because of the dangers of inducing the Mazzotti reaction, even in lightly infected patients, the test should only be used in individuals without detectable parasites in skin, eyes, or blood.

Recommended indications for the treatment of onchocerciasis have become more stringent as the sight-threatening side-effects of chemotherapy have become better known: it is now recognised that the standard drugs, diethylcarbamazine, and probably also suramin, although they may benefit anterior segment eye lesions, can worsen or provoke lesions in the posterior segment of the eye, particularly in patients with intra-ocular microfilariae. The major indication for chemotherapy with diethylcarbamazine and suramin, the only macrofilaricide available for use against *Onchocerca volvulus*, is onchocerciasis severe enough to threaten sight; severe onchodermatitis may also justify treatment. Patients should be hospitalised or under close medical supervision. Treatment should begin with diethylcarbamazine (as above) given under corticosteroid cover, followed by a course of suramin. Care must be taken in patients from endemic onchocerciasis areas with other parasitic diseases, since the drugs used to treat diseases such as loiasis or lymphatic filariasis (diethylcarbamazine), schistosomiasis (metriphonate), and trypanosomiasis (suramin) have an effect on *O. volvulus* and adverse reactions due to the killing of the *Onchocerca* parasite may occur during treatment of the primary condition.

It is hoped that the present unsatisfactory treatment of onchocerciasis will be improved by the availability of ivermectin if it lives up to the promise of early clinical trials.— Third Report of the WHO Expert Committee on Onchocerciasis, *Tech. Rep. Ser. Wld Hlth Org. No. 752*, 1987.

A reminder that since onchocerciasis is still endemic over large areas of West and East Africa and Central and South America, all doctors treating patients who have travelled to these countries should be alert to the early signs and symptoms of the disease.— C. A. Pearson (letter), *Lancet*, 1986, *2*, 805.

A diagnostic 'patch test' for onchocerciasis using topical diethylcarbamazine.— P. Stingl *et al.*, *Trans. R. Soc. trop. Med. Hyg.*, 1984, *78*, 254.

For comparative studies of diethylcarbamazine and ivermectin in the treatment of onchocerciasis, see Ivermectin, p.55.

For a description of the Mazzotti reaction associated with the administration of diethylcarbamazine to patients with onchocerciasis, see under Adverse Effects (above).

For the effect of urinary pH on the pharmacokinetics of diethylcarbamazine and the failure of alkalinisation of urine to allow a reduction of the dose in patients with onchocerciasis, see under Absorption and Fate (above).

TOXOCARIASIS. Toxocaral visceral larva migrans is generally benign and self-limiting, but larval invasion of the eye with subsequent loss of vision is possible. Diethylcarbamazine greatly reduces the number of larvae recovered from the tissues of *mice* infected experimentally, whereas thiabendazole is less effective. However, both drugs are reported to relieve symptoms and shorten convalescent time in patients with visceral larva migrans.— P. M. Schantz and L. T. Glickman, *New Engl. J. Med.*, 1978, *298*, 436.

Authorities in the *USA* have recommended diethylcarbamazine 2 mg per kg body-weight three times daily for 7 to 10 days, or thiabendazole, as the drug of choice for the treatment of visceral larva migrans.— *Med. Lett.*, 1986, *28*, 9.

Diethylcarbamazine, 3 mg per kg body-weight three times daily for 21 days was used successfully in 21 patients with eye infections due to *Toxocara canis* or *T. cati*, which without such diagnosis would have been confused with the presence of retinoblastoma requiring removal of the affected eye.— A. W. Woodruff, *Trans. R. Soc. trop. Med. Hyg.*, 1973, *67*, 755.

An 11-year-old girl with mild self-limiting eosinophilic meningitis due to *Toxocara canis* was treated with diethylcarbamazine 8 mg per kg body-weight [daily] for 10 days because of the risk of ocular lesions or recurrence in the CNS. She continued to be asymptomatic 9 months after presentation.— I. M. Gould *et al.*, *Br. med. J.*, 1985, *291*, 1239.

Preparations

Diethylcarbamazine Citrate Tablets *(U.S.P.)*

Diethylcarbamazine Tablets *(B.P.)*. Diethylcarbam. Tab. Tablets containing diethylcarbamazine citrate.

Proprietary Preparations

Banocide *(Wellcome, UK)*. *Tablets*, scored, diethylcarbamazine citrate, 50 mg.

Proprietary Names and Manufacturers

Banocide *(Wellcome, UK)*; Filarcidan *(Cidan, Spain)*; Filarex; Hetrazan *(Lederle, Austral.*; *Lederle, Canad.*; *Cyanamid-Lederle, Ger.)*; Loxuran; Notézine *(Specia, Fr.)*.

773-y

Diphenan *(rINN)*.

Carbaurine. 4-Benzylphenyl carbamate.

$C_{14}H_{13}NO_2$=227.3.

CAS — 101-71-3.

Diphenan was formerly used as an anthelmintic for the expulsion of threadworms (*Enterobius*).

774-j

Diphezyl

Difezil. (3-Acetyl-5-chloro-2-hydroxybenzyl)dimethyl(2-phenoxyethyl)ammonium 3-hydroxy-2-naphthoate.

$C_{30}H_{30}ClNO_6$=536.0.

CAS — 34987-38-7.

Diphezyl has been tried as an anthelmintic for hookworm and whipworm infections.

775-z

Dithiazanine Iodide *(BANM, rINN)*.

3,3′-Diethylthiadicarbocyanine Iodide. 3-Ethyl-2-[5-(3-ethylbenzothiazol-2(3*H*)-ylidene)penta-1,3-dienyl]benzothiazolium iodide.

$C_{23}H_{23}IN_2S_2$=518.5.

CAS — 7187-55-5 (dithiazanine); 514-73-8 (iodide).

Dithiazanine iodide is an anthelmintic that has been used against whipworms and strongyloid worms. It stains the stools a bluish-green colour.

Proprietary Names and Manufacturers

Ossiurene *(Ital.)*.

776-c

Dymanthine Hydrochloride *(USAN)*.

Dimantine Hydrochloride *(rINNM)*; GS-1339; NSC-5547. *NN*-Dimethyloctadecylamine hydrochloride.

$C_{20}H_{43}N,HCl$=334.0.

CAS — 124-28-7 (dymanthine); 1613-17-8 (hydrochloride).

Dymanthine hydrochloride is an anthelmintic reported to be effective against hookworm (*Ancylostoma* and *Neca-*

tor), roundworms (*Ascaris*), dwarf tapeworms, threadworms (*Enterobius*), and whipworms. The citrate and embonate have also been used.

777-k

Embelia
Vidang.

CAS — 550-24-3 (embelic acid).

The dried fruits of *Embelia ribes* and *E. robusta* (= *E. tsjeriamcottam*) (Myrsinaceae), containing about 2.5% of embelic acid (embelin).

Embelia has been used in India and other eastern countries for the expulsion of tapeworms.

2490-a

Epsiprantel *(BAN, rINN).*
BRL-38705. 2-Cyclohexylcarbonyl-1,2,3,4,6,7,8,12b-octahydropyrazino[2,1-*a*][2]benzazepin-4-one.
$C_{20}H_{26}N_2O_2$=326.4.

CAS — 98123-83-2.

Epsiprantel is an anthelmintic closely related to praziquantel.

Proprietary Names and Manufacturers
Beecham Research, UK.

12729-a

Febantel *(BAN, USAN, rINN).*
Bay-h-5757; BAY-Vh-5757. 2′-[2,3-Bis(methoxycarbonyl)guanidino]-5′-phenylthio-2-methoxyacetanilide; Dimethyl [2-[2-(2-methoxyacetamido)-4-(phenylthio)phenyl]imidocarbonyl]dicarbamate.
$C_{20}H_{22}N_4O_6S$=446.5.

CAS — 58306-30-2.

Febantel is an anthelmintic used in veterinary practice.

Proprietary Veterinary Names and Manufacturers
Amatron *(Coopers Animal Health, UK)*; Bayverm *(Bayer Agrochem, UK).*

778-a

Fenbendazole *(BAN, USAN, rINN).*
Hoe-881V. Methyl 5-phenylthio-1*H*-benzimidazol-2-ylcarbamate.
$C_{15}H_{13}N_3O_2S$=299.3.

CAS — 43210-67-9.

Fenbendazole is a benzimidazole anthelmintic structurally related to mebendazole (see p.57). It is mainly used in veterinary practice.

Proprietary Veterinary Names and Manufacturers
Panacur *(Hoechst Animal Health, UK).*

12756-r

Flubendazole *(BAN, USAN, rINN).*
Fluoromebendazole; R-17889. Methyl 5-(4-fluorobenzoyl)-1*H*-benzimidazol-2-ylcarbamate.
$C_{16}H_{12}FN_3O_3$=313.3.

CAS — 31430-15-6.

Flubendazole, a benzimidazole anthelmintic, is an analogue of mebendazole (see p.57) and has similar actions and uses.
For the treatment of enterobiasis (threadworm infections), flubendazole 100 mg is given by mouth as a single dose, repeated if necessary after 2 to 3 weeks. For ascariasis, hookworm infections, and trichuriasis 100 mg is given twice daily for 3 days.
Flubendazole is also used in veterinary practice.

Flubendazole was as effective as mebendazole in the treatment of *Ascaris* and hookworm infections, but slightly less effective against trichuriasis, in a double-blind study in 127 patients.— H. Feldmeier *et al., Acta trop.*, 1982, *39*, 185.

In a study in 169 Indian schoolchildren infected with *Trichuris trichuria*, flubendazole given as single doses of 200 mg, 500 mg, or 600 mg or as 2 doses of 300 mg on 2 consecutive days reduced egg output in each case by more than 90%, whereas cure-rates were 47.6, 17.3, 18.8, and 65.1% respectively. In the 122 children also infected with *Ascaris lumbricoides*, any of the dosages was highly effective with egg reduction-rates of 98.7 to 99.6% and cure-rates of 90.0 to 97.0%. Erratic migration of *Ascaris* was not seen.— S. P. Kan, *Trans. R. Soc. trop. Med. Hyg.*, 1983, *77*, 688.

CYSTICERCOSIS. Clinical improvement in 12 of 13 patients with neurocysticercosis following treatment with flubendazole given by mouth in a dose of 40 mg per kg body-weight daily in 2 divided doses for 10 days. Nine patients also received prednisone 10 mg three times daily starting one day before flubendazole and continuing until the day after treatment was finished, to protect against immunological reactions in the brain due to the death of parasites. However, allergic reactions were not seen in any of the patients and the high oral doses of flubendazole were well tolerated.— E. Tellez-Giron *et al., Am. J. trop. Med. Hyg.*, 1984, *33*, 627.

HYDATID DISEASE. For reference to the use of flubendazole in the treatment of hydatid disease, see mebendazole (p.58).

ONCHOCERCIASIS. Results from a double-blind controlled comparison suggest that flubendazole is safer and more effective than diethylcarbamazine in the treatment of onchocerciasis. Flubendazole is very poorly absorbed from the gastro-intestinal tract and was therefore given by injection. Eight patients with onchocerciasis received flubendazole 750 mg by intramuscular injection weekly for 5 weeks and 9 received diethylcarbamazine citrate, 50 mg as a test dose, then 100 mg twice daily for 14 days. Patients were followed up for 12 months. Skin microfilaria counts initially fell more rapidly with diethylcarbamazine, but by the end of 12 months were significantly lower in the flubendazole group. Similarly, at the end of 6 months intra-ocular microfilariae were present in only one patient given flubendazole, but had returned to pretreatment levels in the diethylcarbamazine group. Flubendazole had a profound effect on onchocercal embryogenesis but, unlike mebendazole, no demonstrable microfilaricidal activity. Pruritus, rash, and lymphadenopathy, adverse effects thought to be most directly associated with microfilarial killing, occurred only in those given diethylcarbamazine. Ocular complications were common in those given diethylcarbamazine but occurred in only one patient given flubendazole. However, intramuscular flubendazole caused a severe inflammatory reaction at the injection site and 2 of the 10 patients initially assigned to the flubendazole group withdrew from the study before the second injection.— A. Dominguez-Vazquez *et al., Lancet*, 1983, *1*, 139. Despite intensive efforts, preparation of a satisfactory reformulation for flubendazole to avoid the marked local reaction at the injection site has not proved possible.— Third Report of the WHO Expert Committee on Onchocerciasis, *Tech. Rep. Ser. Wld Hlth Org. No. 752*, 1987..

Proprietary Names and Manufacturers
Fluvermal *(Janssen, Fr.).*

779-t

Furapromidium
F-30066. *N*-Isopropyl-3-(5-nitro-2-furyl)acrylamide.
$C_{10}H_{12}N_2O_4$=224.2.

CAS — 1951-56-0.

Furapromidium was a schistosomicide reported to be effective against *Schistosoma japonicum* and in the treatment of clonorchiasis.

12815-c

Haloxon *(BAN, rINN).*
Bis(2-chloroethyl) 3-chloro-4-methylcoumarin-7-yl phosphate.
$C_{14}H_{14}Cl_3O_6P$=415.6.

CAS — 321-55-1.

Pharmacopoeias. In *B.P. Vet.*

A white or almost white, odourless or almost odourless powder. M.p. 88° to 93°. Practically **insoluble** in water; soluble 1 in 9 of alcohol, 1 in 4 of acetone, and 1 in 2 of chloroform.

Haloxon is an organophosphorus compound used as an anthelmintic in veterinary medicine.

Proprietary Veterinary Names and Manufacturers
Equilox *(Crown, UK).*

780-l

Hexachloroethane

C_2Cl_6=236.7.

CAS — 67-72-1.

Pharmacopoeias. In *Aust.* and *Nord.*

Hexachloroethane has been used in veterinary medicine as an anthelmintic.
It is a chlorinated hydrocarbon used in industry as a solvent. In Great Britain the recommended exposure limits of hexachloroethane vapour are 50 mg per m^3 (long-term), total inhalable dust 10 mg per m^3 (long-term), and respirable dust 5 mg per m^3 (long-term). In the *US* the permissible exposure limit is 10 mg per m^3.

781-y

Hexachloroparaxylene
Chloxyle; Hetol; Hexachloroparaxylol. 1,4-Bis(trichloromethyl)benzene.
$C_8H_4Cl_6$=312.8.

CAS — 68-36-0.

Hexachloroparaxylene has been used in China and the USSR as an anthelmintic, principally to treat the liver fluke infections clonorchiasis and opisthorchiasis. In general it has been superseded by praziquantel.
Adverse effects reported with hexachloroparaxylene have included gastro-intestinal disturbances, cardiac arrhythmias, and haemolysis.

783-z

Hycanthone Mesylate
Hycanthone Mesilate *(rINNM)*; Hydroxylucanthone Methanesulphonate; Win-24933. 1-(2-Diethylaminoethylamino)-4-hydroxymethylthioxanthen-9-one methanesulphonate.
$C_{20}H_{24}N_2O_2S,CH_3SO_3H$=452.6.

CAS — 3105-97-3 (hycanthone); 23255-93-8 (mesylate).

NOTE. Hycanthone is *USAN*.

Pharmacopoeias. In *Braz.*

Hycanthone, an active metabolite of lucanthone, has been used as a schistosomicide in the individual or mass treatment of infection with *Schistosoma haematobium* and *S. mansoni*. It has been given as the mesylate by deep intramuscular injection as a single dose containing the equivalent of 1.5 mg of hycanthone per kg body-weight, up to a maximum of 100 mg. A dose of 3 mg per kg was used when hycanthone was first introduced and was more effective, however such doses have been associated with a high incidence of severe nausea and vomiting and with liver damage that has sometimes proved fatal.
Owing to its toxicity and concern about possible carcinogenicity, mutagenicity, and teratogenicity, hycanthone has been largely replaced by other agents such as praziquantel in the treatment of schistosomiasis.

Proprietary Names and Manufacturers
Etrenol *(Winthrop, UK).*

15323-x

Imcarbofos *(USAN, rINN).*
CL-217658. Tetraethyl {(2-methoxy-*p*-phenylene)bis-[imino(thiocarbonyl)]}diphosphoramidate.
$C_{17}H_{30}N_4O_7P_2S_2$=528.5.

CAS — 66608-32-0.

Imcarbofos is an organophosphorus compound for use as a veterinary anthelmintic.

Proprietary Names and Manufacturers
American Cyanamid, USA.

784-c

Iodothymol
Thymolan. 6-Iodothymol.
$C_{10}H_{13}IO$=276.1.

CAS — 2364-44-5.

NOTE. The name iodothymol has also been applied to thymol iodide.

Iodothymol is an anthelmintic which has been used in the treatment of hookworm infections.

12874-b

Ivermectin *(BAN, USAN, rINN).*

A mixture of ivermectin component B_{1a} (5-*O*-demethyl-22,23-dihydroavermectin A_{1a}; $C_{48}H_{74}O_{14}$ = 875.1) and ivermectin component B_{1b} (5-*O*-demethyl-25-de(1-methylpropyl)-22,23-dihydro-25-(1-methylethyl)avermectin A_{1a}; $C_{47}H_{72}O_{14}$ = 861.1).

CAS — 70161-11-4 (component B_{1a}); 70209-81-3 (component B_{1b}); 70288-86-7 (mixture).

Ivermectin is a semisynthetic derivative of one of the avermectins, a group of macrocyclic lactones produced by *Streptomyces avermitilis*. It is an antiparasitic agent with a broad spectrum of activity against nematode worms and ectoparasites in *animals* and is widely used in veterinary practice.

More recently ivermectin has shown promise in the treatment of onchocerciasis in man. It has a more prolonged therapeutic effect than diethylcarbamazine and reactions during the treatment of onchocerciasis have been reported to be less severe. Ivermectin has been given by mouth as a single dose of 12 mg (about 200 µg per kg body-weight).

Reviews of ivermectin including its mode of action and veterinary use.— W. C. Campbell *et al.*, *Science*, 1983, *221*, 823; W. C. Campbell, *Parasitology Today*, 1985, *1*, 10.

LYMPHATIC FILARIASIS. In a preliminary study of ivermectin in filariasis due to *Wuchereria bancrofti*, a single dose of 50 or 100 µg per kg body-weight by mouth cleared the blood of microfilariae within 3 days. They had reappeared in most patients by the third month.— S. Diallo *et al.* (letter), *Lancet*, 1987, *1*, 1030.

ONCHOCERCIASIS. Ivermectin shows great promise as a single-dose oral agent in the treatment of onchocerciasis in man and as means of controlling disease and transmission in populations living in endemic areas. The predominant effect of ivermectin in onchocerciasis is the rapid elimination of microfilariae from the skin after a single oral dose, followed by their gradual disappearance from the eye. The microfilaricidal effect is thought to result from enhancement of both the presynaptic release of gamma-aminobutyric acid (GABA) and the postsynaptic GABA-binding to a chloride channel-linked receptor, leading to muscular paralysis and subsequent death of the microfilariae by immune or other mechanisms. Macrofilaricidal activity has been shown in some animal filarial species, but as yet there is no evidence for such an effect against *Onchocerca volvulus*. However, adult female worms isolated from ivermectin-treated subjects do show evidence of a suppressive effect on the release of microfilariae, probably of several months' duration. Retreatment at intervals of 6 to 18 months will probably be the ideal schedule in endemic areas with substantial ongoing transmission. No major toxicity has been observed so far with ivermectin. Systemic reactions have been less severe and less frequent than with diethylcarbamazine, the principal reactions noted being fever, rash, and lymph-node pain or swelling. Ocular reactions have been minimal, although ivermectin therapy has not yet been tested in those with advanced ocular disease.— Third Report of the WHO Expert Committee on Onchocerciasis, *Tech. Rep. Ser. Wld Hlth Org. No. 752*, 1987.

For further details of onchocerciasis and its treatment, see diethylcarbamazine citrate (p.53).

Reviews of ivermectin in the control of onchocerciasis: M. A. Aziz, *Rev. infect. Dis.*, 1986, *8*, 500; *WHO Drug Inf.*, 1987, *1*, 43.

In preliminary studies, ivermectin in single oral doses ranging from 30 to 200 µg per kg body-weight proved to be an effective slow microfilaricide with a prolonged therapeutic effect in patients with onchocerciasis of varying severity (M.A. Aziz *et al.*, *Lancet*, 1982, *2*, 171; M.A. Aziz *et al.*, *ibid.*, 1456; J.P. Coulaud *et al.*, *ibid.*, 1984, *2*, 526; K. Awadzi *et al.*, *ibid.*, 921 and *Ann. trop. Med. Parasit.*, 1985, *79*, 63). Systemic and ocular reactions were milder than those seen with diethylcarbamazine, probably because of its slow action on microfilariae. In double-blind placebo-controlled studies in patients with moderate to heavy infection with *Onchocerca volvulus* and with eye involvement, ivermectin given as a single oral dose of 12 mg (about 200 µg per kg) has been compared with standard treatment with diethylcarbamazine and appears to be better tolerated, safer, and more effective (M. Lariviere *et al.*, *Lancet*, 1985, *2*, 174; B.M. Greene *et al.*, *New Engl. J. Med.*, 1985, *313*, 133; S. Diallo *et al.*, *Trans. R. Soc. trop. Med. Hyg.*, 1986, *80*, 927; K.Y. Dadzie, *et al.*, *Br. J. Ophthal.*, 1987, *71*, 78). On analysing the ocular response to treatment Dadzie *et al.* concluded that ivermectin exerts a slow microfilaricidal effect on the eye, but, unlike diethylcarbamazine, does not produce any serious inflammatory reaction likely to cause functional deficit. It may thus be suitable for mass treatment, although they considered that further studies in patients with very heavy ocular infection with *O. volvulus* are needed.

Results from field experiments suggesting that ivermectin could be effective in interrupting transmission of *Onchocerca volvulus*. Three months after a single oral dose of ivermectin 200 µg per kg body-weight, patients infected vector flies at a significantly lower rate than those who had received an 8-day course of diethylcarbamazine or placebo. Reduced infectivity was still evident after 6 months.— E. W. Cupp *et al.*, *Science*, 1986, *231*, 740.

PREGNANCY AND THE NEONATE. Ivermectin should not be given to pregnant women. In *animal* studies it has been found to be neither teratogenic nor foetotoxic in *rats* and *rabbits*, but in *mice* it produced cleft palate in foetuses and occasional unexplained maternal deaths. Suckling neonatal *rats* exhibited enhanced sensitivity to the toxic effects of ivermectin, due to exposure via maternal milk after birth when the blood-brain barrier in this species is not complete.— M. A. Aziz, *Rev. infect. Dis.*, 1986, *8*, 500. Comment. Even if the potential for such toxicity exists in humans, the therapeutic dose is likely to be well below the threshold for its expression. Nevertheless, in the current state of knowledge ivermectin should not be administered to pregnant or lactating women or to young children. Despite this important reservation, ivermectin remains a compound of outstanding promise.— *WHO Drug Inf.*, 1987, *1*, 43.

Proprietary Names and Manufacturers
Mectizan *(Merck Sharp & Dohme, USA).*

Proprietary Veterinary Names and Manufacturers
Eqvalan *(Merck Sharp & Dohme, UK)*; Ivomec *(Merck Sharp & Dohme, UK).*

785-k

Kainic Acid *(rINN).*
Digenic Acid. 2-(2-Carboxy-4-isopropenylpyrrolidin-3-yl)acetic acid monohydrate.
$C_{10}H_{15}NO_4,H_2O$=231.2.

CAS — 487-79-6 (anhydrous).

Pharmacopoeias. In *Jpn.*

Obtained from the dried red alga *Digenea simplex.*

Kainic acid is an anthelmintic which was used in roundworm (*Ascaris*) infection.

Mention of kainic acid, a cyclic analogue of glutamate and potent neurotoxin, and its use to provide a model for the investigation of Huntington's disease.— C. D. Marsden, *Lancet*, 1982, *2*, 1141.

Proprietary Names and Manufacturers
Digenin *(Jpn).*

786-a

Kamala
Camala; Glandulae Rottlerae.

CAS — 12624-07-6.

Pharmacopoeias. In *Port.*

The trichomes and glands from the fruits of *Mallotus philippinensis* (Euphorbiaceae).

Kamala produces purgation and has been used in the treatment of tapeworm infection.

787-t

Kousso
Brayera; Cousso; Cusso; Flos Koso; Kosoblüte.

Pharmacopoeias. In *Port.* and *Span.*

The dried panicles of the fertilised pistillate flowers of *Brayera anthelmintica* (=*Hagenia abyssinica*) (Rosaceae).

Kousso has been used as an anthelmintic, particularly for the expulsion of tapeworms, but there is little evidence that it dislodges the heads.

788-x

Levamisole Hydrochloride *(BANM, USAN, rINNM).*

ICI-59623; *l*-Tetramisole Hydrochloride; NSC-177023; R-12564; RP-20605. (−)-(*S*)-2,3,5,6-Tetrahydro-6-phenylimidazo[2,1-*b*]thiazole hydrochloride.
$C_{11}H_{12}N_2S,HCl$=240.8.

CAS — 14769-73-4 (levamisole); 16595-80-5 (hydrochloride).

Pharmacopoeias. In *Br.*, *Chin.*, *Cz.*, *Fr.*, and *Swiss.* Also in *B.P. Vet.*

A white to pale cream-coloured, odourless or almost odourless, crystalline powder. Levamisole hydrochloride 1.18 g is approximately equivalent to 1 g of levamisole. **Soluble** 1 in 2 of water and 1 in 5 of methyl alcohol; practically insoluble in ether.

Adverse Effects
When given in single doses for the treatment of ascariasis or other worm infections, levamisole is generally well tolerated and side-effects are usually limited to nausea, vomiting, abdominal pain, dizziness, and headache.

When levamisole is used as an immunostimulant and given for longer periods, adverse effects are more frequent and diverse and, in common with other immunomodulators, may sometimes result from exacerbation of the primary underlying disease. Adverse effects associated especially with the more prolonged administration of levamisole in diseases like rheumatoid arthritis or cancer have included: hypersensitivity reactions such as fever, an influenza-like syndrome, arthralgia, muscle pain, skin rashes, and cutaneous vasculitis; central nervous system effects such as fatigue, headache, confusion, insomnia, dizziness, excitation, and convulsions; haematological abnormalities such as agranulocytosis, leucopenia, and thrombocytopenia; and gastro-intestinal disturbances, including an abnormal taste in the mouth.

A review from the manufacturers of 46 controlled studies in which 2635 cancer patients received adjuvant levamisole treatment. Most patients received levamisole on 3 consecutive days every 2 weeks (1102 patients) or on 2 consecutive days every week (1156 patients), usually in a daily dose of 150 mg. Levamisole can cause several side-effects, such as skin rash, nausea, vomiting, metallic or bitter taste in the mouth, which although troublesome are relatively trivial and may regress during therapy or disappear on cessation of therapy. The only serious and potentially life-threatening side-effect of levamisole is agranulocytosis, a symptom complex characterised by a drastic decrease in, or even a total absence of, granulocytes and less than 20% neutrophils. It is considered to be an idiosyncratic-allergic phenomenon and is often revealed by non-specific symptoms such as malaise, chills, and a 'flu-like' syndrome. Agranulocytosis should not be confused with leucopenia in which the bone marrow is essentially normal, 'flu-like' and other symptoms are generally absent, and the condition regresses with continued therapy, without progressing to agranulocytosis. A total of 38 patients developed agranulocytosis and of these 36 had received weekly treatment. Several contracted possible life-threatening infections and 2 died of septic shock. A dosage schedule of 2.5 mg per kg body-weight on 3 consecutive days every fortnight appears to provide optimal therapeutic efficacy and safety when levamisole is used as an adjunct to cancer chemotherapy.— W. K. Amery and B. S. Butterworth, *Int. J. Immunopharmacol.*, 1983, *5*, 1.

EFFECTS ON THE LIVER. Elevated aspartate aminotransferase concentrations in 2 of 11 patients given levamisole for recurrent pyoderma suggested liver toxicity, a very rarely occurring side-effect.— P. Papageorgiou *et al.*, *J. clin. Lab. Immunol.*, 1982, *8*, 121.

Precautions

The use of levamisole should be avoided in patients with advanced liver or kidney disease, and in patients with pre-existing blood disorders.

The appearance of side-effects in 9 of 10 patients with rheumatoid arthritis and Sjögren's syndrome while being treated with levamisole led to abandonment of the study. Levamisole should be given with caution, if at all, in patients with Sjögren's syndrome.— G. Balint *et al.*, *Br. med. J.*, 1977, *2*, 1386.

The presence of HLA B27 in seropositive rheumatoid arthritis is an important predisposing factor to the development of agranulocytosis during treatment with levamisole; it is recommended that the use of levamisole in this group should be avoided. Although the incidence of agranulocytosis did not appear to be reduced by any of the treatment schemes used, the use of a single dose per week, with blood counts 10 hours after drug intake, allowed high risk patients to be detected early.— H. Mielants and E. M. Veys, *J. Rheumatol.*, 1978, *5*, *Suppl.* 4, 77.

Absorption and Fate

Levamisole is rapidly absorbed from the gastro-intestinal tract and eliminated from the plasma. It is extensively metabolised in the liver and elimination is virtually complete, via the urine and faeces, within 2 days of a dose.

A study of the pharmacokinetics of levamisole in 10 healthy fasting subjects. Concentrations of levamisole in plasma and urine were measured using a new gas chromatographic method; the urinary metabolite *p*-hydroxylevamisole was measured using high performance liquid chromatography. Following a single dose of 150 mg by mouth levamisole was rapidly absorbed, with a mean peak plasma concentration of 716.7 ng per mL being achieved at 1.52 hours, and rapidly eliminated, with a plasma elimination half-life of 5.6 hours. The amount of unchanged drug excreted in the urine was inversely correlated with urinary pH. A mean of only 3.2% of the administered dose was excreted unchanged in the urine within 24 hours, suggesting the importance of clearance by other routes, most probably by hepatic metabolism. Amounts of *p*-hydroxylevamisole recovered in the urine, before and after hydrolysis of the urine samples, indicated that *p*-hydroxylation is a relatively important route of metabolism of levamisole and that the *p*-hydroxylated metabolite is excreted mainly in conjugation with glucuronic acid. Other than the absorption rate, which was about twice as rapid in the 3 women as in the 7 men, there was no marked difference between the sexes in the pharmacokinetics of levamisole.— E. Kouassi *et al.*, *Biopharm. Drug Disposit.*, 1986, *7*, 71.

Further references: M. Luyckx *et al.*, *Eur. J. Drug Metab. Pharmacokinet.*, 1982, *7*, 247.

Uses and Administration

Levamisole hydrochloride is the active laevo-isomer of tetramisole hydrochloride. It is used as an anthelmintic and for its effects on the immune system.

Levamisole is active against intestinal nematode worms and appears to act by paralysing susceptible worms which are subsequently eliminated from the intestines. It produces a depolarising type of neuromuscular blockade in vertebrate muscle, but a ganglion-stimulating effect in nematodes has been proposed. Levamisole is especially effective in the treatment of ascariasis (roundworm infection). It is also used in hookworm infections (ancylostomiasis and necatoriasis) and has shown some effect against *Enterobius vermicularis* (pinworm; threadworm), *Trichuris trichuria*, *Strongyloides stercoralis*, and *Trichostrongylus colubriformis*. Doses are expressed in terms of the equivalent amount of levamisole. The usual dose is 120 to 150 mg of levamisole by mouth as a single dose; children have been given 3 mg per kg body-weight as a single dose. In severe hookworm infection a second dose one or 7 days after the first, has been suggested.

Levamisole affects the immune response. The term 'immunostimulant' has often been used; it is appropriate only in so far as restoration of a depressed response is concerned; stimulation above normal levels does not seem to occur. Levamisole influences host defences by modulating cell-mediated immune responses; it restores depressed T-cell functions. Levamisole has been tried in a wide variety of disorders involving the immune response, including bacterial and viral infections, rheumatic disorders, and as an adjunct in patients with malignant disease.

The immunostimulant properties of levamisole have been used therapeutically with varying success in the treatment of recurrent aphthous stomatitis, bacterial infections, malignant neoplasms, renal disorders, rheumatic disorders, and viral infections (see below).

Results in numerous other disorders with an immune component, including amyotrophic lateral sclerosis, Crohn's disease, and ulcerative colitis, diabetes mellitus, multiple sclerosis, and systemic lupus erythematosus, have been disappointing.

Reviews and discussions on the immunomodulating properties of levamisole.— P. A. J. Janssen, *Prog. Drug Res.*, 1976, *20*, 347; J. Symoens and M. Rosenthal, *J. reticuloendoth. Soc.*, 1977, *21*, 175; *Lancet*, 1979, *2*, 291; W. K. Amery (letter), *ibid.*, 528; G. Renoux, *Drugs*, 1980, *20*, 89.

A review of levamisole in the treatment of parasitic infections. Levamisole was a treatment of choice for ascariasis and was active against hookworms although the most effective treatment regimen had not been determined. With rare exceptions drug trials had shown little or no activity against whipworms and pinworms and activity against *Strongyloides* required confirmation. There was limited information on the activity of levamisole against filarial infections. Beneficial results had been reported with levamisole in the treatment of the protozoal infections toxoplasmosis and cutaneous leishmaniasis, but required confirmation.— M. J. Miller, *Drugs*, 1980, *20*, 122.

APHTHOUS STOMATITIS. A review of levamisole in the treatment of recurrent aphthous stomatitis, a disease of the oral mucous membranes characterised by periodic recurrent oral ulcerations. Where ocular and genital lesions are also present, a diagnosis of Behçet's syndrome can be made. Beneficial results have been reported with levamisole in open studies, but results of double-blind studies have been conflicting. Nevertheless there have been patients with severe recurrent aphthous stomatitis refractory to all other modes of treatment who have responded to levamisole. Dosage has been with 150 mg daily in divided doses given for 3 days at the first sign of ulceration, followed by 11 days without treatment.— M. F. Miller, *Drugs*, 1980, *20*, 131. The view that levamisole has not always been shown to be effective in the treatment of recurrent aphthous stomatitis and is not indicated because of its adverse systemic effects.— J. S. Rennie *et al.*, *Br. dent. J.*, 1985, *159*, 361.

Levamisole was not considered to be of any help in the treatment of Behçet's disease.— J. J. H. Gilkes, *Practitioner*, 1978, *221*, 822. The successful treatment of Behçet's syndrome in 3 patients with levamisole 150 mg by mouth once a week.— H. A. Lavery and J. H. M. Pinkerton (letter), *Br. J. Derm.*, 1985, *113*, 372.

ASCARIASIS. A cure-rate of 92% was achieved in 453 children with roundworm (*Ascaris*) infection treated with a single dose of levamisole compared with 66% in 461 treated with piperazine citrate 150 mg per kg body-weight with a maximum of 3.5 g. The dose of levamisole was: 10 to 20 kg, 50 mg; 20 to 40 kg, 100 mg; over 40 kg, 150 mg. Levamisole was considered suitable for mass treatment.— M. J. Miller *et al.*, *Sth. med. J.*, 1978, *71*, 137. In an area of Burma endemic for ascariasis, mass chemotherapy with levamisole every 6 months reduced the intensity of infection in children and adults, whereas annual treatment reduced intensity in adults only.— Thein Hlaing *et al.*, *Trans. R. Soc. trop. Med. Hyg.*, 1987, *81*, 140.

Levamisole cured infection with *Lagochilascaris*, an unusual nematode parasite of man, in two Colombian patients. In one, earlier treatment with thiabendazole and mebendazole had been ineffective.— D. Botero and M. D. Little, *Am. J. trop. Med. Hyg.*, 1984, *33*, 381.

BACTERIAL INFECTIONS. Treatment with levamisole has been tried in various chronic or recurrent bacterial infections associated with depressed cellular immunity of the host.

Earlier reports of benefit with levamisole in the treatment of the hyperimmunoglobulin E recurrent-infection syndrome or Job's syndrome (A. Rebora *et al.*, *Br. J. Derm.*, 1980, *102*, 49; L. Businco *et al.*, *Archs Dis Childh.*, 1981, *56*, 60), a disorder characterised by high levels of circulating IgE, a leucocyte chemotactic defect, and recurrent skin and sinopulmonary bacterial infections, were not substantiated in a subsequent double-blind study in 8 patients. Despite restoration of normal chemotactic responsiveness, those given levamisole tended to have more serious infectious complications than those given placebo.— H. Donabedian *et al.*, *New Engl. J. Med.*, 1982, *307*, 290.

Further references: M. Renoux and G. Renoux (letter), *Lancet*, 1977, *1*, 372 (brucellosis; adjunct to antibiotic therapy); M. Raptpoulou-Gigi *et al.*, *J. Immunopharmac.*, 1980, *2*, 85 (brucellosis); D. Djawari and O. P. Hornstein, *Dermatologica*, 1980, *161*, 116 (recurrent chronic pyoderma); P. Papageorgiou *et al.*, *J. clin. Lab. Immunol.*, 1982, *8*, 121 (recurrent chronic pyoderma).

See also Tuberculosis (below).

BEHÇET'S SYNDROME. See Aphthous Stomatitis (above).

LYMPHATIC FILARIASIS. Levamisole is not recommended for use either alone or in combination with diethylcarbamazine or mebendazole in the treatment of lymphatic filariasis. It has been tried at a dose of 100 mg twice daily for 10 days, but compared with diethylcarbamazine was a less effective filaricide, produced more severe reactions as well as its own toxic effects, and was more expensive.— Lymphatic Filariasis, Fourth Report of the WHO Expert Committee on Filariasis, *Tech. Rep. Ser. Wld Hlth Org. No. 702*, 1984.

MALIGNANT NEOPLASMS. A review of 20 studies on the use of levamisole in the treatment of malignant disease and the conclusion that, although cancer immunotherapy was still a relatively experimental treatment approach, there was evidence for a favourable therapeutic effect when used as an adjunct to conventional chemotherapy. Levamisole itself is not a remission-inducing agent since it does not directly act on cancer cells and its use alone has no rationale. However, it could be helpful as adjunctive treatment in patients at risk of recurrent disease after they have undergone primary antineoplastic therapy. In view of the possibility of adverse haematological effects, intermittent administration of levamisole was recommended.— F. Spreafico, *Drugs*, 1980, *20*, 105.

A review by the manufacturers of 46 controlled studies of adjuvant levamisole treatment in 2365 patients with cancer indicating that the safest and most effective dosage schedule appeared to be 2.5 mg per kg body-weight given on 3 consecutive days every other week [see also under Adverse Effects, above]. With this regimen 18 of 20 studies reported better results in patients treated with levamisole than in controls.— W. K. Amery and B. S. Butterworth, *Int. J. Immunopharmacol.*, 1983, *5*, 1.

Some references to studies of levamisole as an adjunct to the treatment of various malignant neoplasms; results have been inconsistent and generally disappointing:
breast: *Lancet*, 1980, *2*, 824 (increased recurrence rate); P. Klefström *et al.*, *Cancer*, 1985, *55*, 2753 (benefit, especially in postmenopausal women).
lung: W. K. Amery, *Cancer Treat. Rep.*, 1978, *62*, 1677 (beneficial); S. Davis *et al.*, *Cancer*, 1982, *50*, 646 (no benefit).
melanoma: L. E. Spitler and R. Sagebiel, *New Engl. J. Med.*, 1980, *303*, 1143 (no benefit).
ovary: S. K. Khoo *et al.*, *Cancer*, 1984, *54*, 986 (no benefit).

ONCHOCERCIASIS. Levamisole has been used in association with mebendazole in the treatment of onchocerciasis (see under Mebendazole, p.59), but results have been variable.

RENAL DISORDERS. Some favourable results with levamisole in children with the nephrotic syndrome: P. Tanphaichitr *et al.*, *J. Pediat.*, 1980, *96*, 490; P. Niaudet *et al.*, *Acta paediat. scand.*, 1984, *73*, 637; K. P. Mehta *et al.*, *Archs Dis. Childh.*, 1986, *61*, 153. Brief comment on the mechanism of action of levamisole.— P. F. W. Miller (letter), *ibid.*, 718.

RHEUMATIC DISORDERS. Although levamisole has been of benefit in the second-line treatment of rheumatoid arthritis and related disorders its use has been limited by the frequency of serious adverse effects. Tolerance has been improved by reducing the dose originally used (150 mg daily or on 3 days each week) to 150 mg or 2.5 mg per kg body-weight once a week, but efficacy may be reduced. Because of the risk of agranulocytosis, blood counts should be monitored during treatment.

Some references to the use of levamisole in rheumatic disorders: Multicentre Study Group, *Lancet*, 1978, *2*, 1007 (150 mg daily compared with 150 mg three times a week); *idem*, *J. Rheumatol.*, 1978, *5*, *Suppl.* 4, 5 (50 or 150 mg once a week); E. C. Huskisson and J. G. Adams, *Drugs*, 1980, *20*, 100 (a review); Multicentre Study Group, *Ann. rheum. Dis.*, 1982, *41*, 159 (50 or 150 mg once a week); E. M. Veys *et al.*, *Adv. Inflamm. Res.*, 1986, *11*, 301 (comparison with penicillamine and gold salts).

TUBERCULOSIS. Levamisole 150 mg daily on 2 consecutive days a week for 3 months enhanced the recovery of 50 patients with active pulmonary tuberculosis who were receiving standard antituberculous therapy, when compared with 50 similar patients who received only antituberculous drugs.— A. N. Singh *et al.*, *J. Ass. Physns India*, 1983, *31*, 405.

VIRAL INFECTIONS. A review of levamisole in the treatment of viral infections. Early promising results in herpes simplex infection and warts, infections associated with evidence of immune depression, have not been confirmed in controlled studies. The value of levamisole in viral hepatitis remains an open question and there is no good evidence of efficacy in any other viral infection at present.— A. S. Russell, *Drugs*, 1980, *20*, 117.

Possible drug toxicity and an apparent lack of efficacy with levamisole in the treatment of 5 patients with AIDS.— N. Surapaneni *et al.* (letter), *Ann. intern. Med.*, 1985, *102*, 137.

Proprietary Preparations

Ketrax (Available only in certain countries) *(ICI Pharmaceuticals, UK)*. *Tablets*, levamisole 40 mg (as the hydrochloride).
Syrup, levamisole 40 mg/5 mL (as the hydrochloride).

Proprietary Names and Manufacturers

Ascaridil *(Janssen, Belg.)*; Askamex; Decaris *(Janssen, Belg.; Janssen, Denm.)*; Ergamisol *(Janssen, Ital.)*; Immunol *(Sarm, Ital.)*; Ketrax *(ICI Pharmaceuticals, UK)*; Levimon; Meglum; Newkentax; Solaskil *(Specia, Fr.)*; Stimamizol.

789-r

Lucanthone Hydrochloride *(BANM, USAN, rINNM)*.

79-T61; BW-57-233; Lucanth. Hydrochlor.; Lucanthoni Hydrochloridum; NSC-14574. 1-(2-Diethylaminoethylamino)-4-methylthioxanthen-9-one hydrochloride.
$C_{20}H_{24}N_2OS,HCl=376.9$.

CAS — 479-50-5 (lucanthone); 548-57-2 (hydrochloride).

Pharmacopoeias. In *Int.* and *Turk.*

Lucanthone hydrochloride is a schistosomicide formerly given by mouth in the treatment of schistosomiasis. It was replaced by its active metabolite hycanthone (p.54) which was better tolerated and more potent, but hycanthone in turn has largely been superseded by less toxic and more effective drugs such as praziquantel (p.64).

Proprietary Names and Manufacturers
Nilodin *(Wellcome, UK)*.

790-j

Male Fern

Aspidium; Farnwurzel; Felce Maschio; Feto Macho; Filix Mas; Fougère Mâle; Helecho Macho; Rhizoma Filicis Maris.

Pharmacopoeias. In *Arg.*, *Fr.*, *Int.*, *Mex.*, *Nord.*, *Port.*, *Roum.*, *Rus.*, *Span.*, and *Turk.*
Int. and *Mex.* allow also *Dryopteris marginalis.*

The rhizome, frond-bases, and apical bud of *Dryopteris filix-mas* agg. (Polypodiaceae), collected late in the autumn, divested of the roots and dead portions and carefully dried, retaining the internal green colour. It contains not less than 1.5% of filicin. During storage the green colour of the interior gradually disappears, often after a lapse of 6 months, and such material is unfit for medicinal use. **Store** in airtight containers. Protect from light.

Filicin is the mixture of ether-soluble substances obtained from male fern. Its activity is chiefly due to flavaspidic acid, a phloroglucinol derivative.

Adverse Effects

Male fern is highly toxic but poorly absorbed; severe toxicity may occur if its absorption is increased, for example in the presence of fatty foods. Adverse effects include headache, nausea and vomiting, severe abdominal cramp, diarrhoea, dyspnoea, albuminuria, and hyperbilirubinaemia. Other adverse effects include dizziness, tremors, convulsions, visual disturbances including blindness (possibly permanent), stimulation of uterine muscle, coma, respiratory failure, bradycardia, and cardiac failure. Fatalities have occurred.

The treatment of poisoning with male fern is symptomatic, following its removal from the stomach by aspiration and lavage.

Absorption and Fate

Filicin is variably absorbed from the gastro-intestinal tract and is excreted partly unchanged in the urine.

Uses and Administration

Male fern is an effective anthelmintic for the expulsion of tapeworms and was formerly administered as male fern extract (aspidium oleoresin), in a draught, sometimes by duodenal tube. However, it has been superseded by other less toxic and more easily administered agents.

It was recommended by the Food Additives and Contaminants Committee that male fern rhizome be prohibited for use in foods as a flavouring agent.— *Report on the Review of Flavourings in Food*, FAC/REP/22, Ministry of Agriculture, Fisheries and Food, London, HM Stationery Office, 1976.

791-z .

Mebendazole *(BAN, USAN, rINN)*.

R-17635. Methyl 5-benzoyl-1*H*-benzimidazol-2-ylcarbamate.
$C_{16}H_{13}N_3O_3=295.3$.

CAS — 31431-39-7.

Pharmacopoeias. In *Cz.*, *Ind.*, and *U.S.*

A white to slightly yellow powder. Practically **insoluble** in water, alcohol, chloroform, ether, and dilute mineral acids; freely soluble in formic acid.

Adverse Effects

Since mebendazole is poorly absorbed from the gastro-intestinal tract at the usual therapeutic doses, side-effects have generally been restricted to gastro-intestinal disturbances such as transient abdominal pain and diarrhoea. However, adverse effects have been reported more frequently with the high doses tried in the treatment of hydatid disease and have included allergic reactions, raised liver enzyme values, leucopenia, and alopecia.

Two of over 100 patients, treated with mebendazole in *normal doses* for 3 days, complained of slight headache and dizziness. There were no reports of gastro-intestinal side-effects or of skin rashes.— S. K. K. Seah, *Can. med. Ass. J.*, 1976, *115*, 777.

Respiratory symptoms with cough and fever had been reported in 8 of 133 Kenyan patients receiving mebendazole in *high doses* for hydatid disease. Glomerulonephritis, histologically confirmed in 6, was possibly a result of immune complexes liberated into the circulation.— *Br. med. J.*, 1979, *2*, 563.

Although generally well tolerated, the following adverse reactions were reported in studies involving 139 patients given *high-dose* therapy with mebendazole for the treatment of echinococcosis [hydatid disease]: raised serum-transaminase levels (22 patients); reduced leucocyte counts (25); reduced haemoglobin level (3); gastro-intestinal symptoms, including severe abdominal pain, nausea and/or vomiting (22); allergic conditions, including fever, skin eruptions, and/or pruritus (4); CNS symptoms, including dizziness, vertigo, and/or headache (6); and loss of hair (7). These adverse reactions do not include disease-related complications. Treatment was stopped temporarily or permanently in 7 patients because of suspected adverse reactions. Close supervision is required to prevent serious complications during the treatment of echinococcosis with benzimidazole carbonates.— A. Davis *et al.*, *Bull. Wld Hlth Org.*, 1986, *64*, 383.

EFFECTS ON THE BLOOD. A report of severe reversible granulocytopenia in 2 patients with hydatid disease during high-dose mebendazole therapy and the suggestion that blood cell counts should be monitored frequently during the first month of treatment.— M. H. Levin *et al.*, *J. Am. med. Ass.*, 1983, *249*, 2929.

Precautions

Mebendazole is teratogenic in *rats*.

Patients receiving high doses of mebendazole, such as those with hydatid disease, should be supervised closely.

ADMINISTRATION IN LIVER FAILURE. For reports of increased plasma concentrations of mebendazole in patients with cholestasis receiving high doses for the treatment of hydatid disease, see under Absorption and Fate (below).

INTERACTIONS. For the effect of the concomitant administration of other drugs on plasma concentrations of mebendazole in patients receiving high-dose therapy for hydatid disease, see under Absorption and Fate, below.

PREGNANCY AND THE NEONATE. Since mebendazole is teratogenic in *rats*, the *UK* manufacturers have stated that it is contra-indicated in pregnant women. The *US* manufacturers and others (*Med. Lett.*, 1987, *29*, 61; R. Wise, *Br. med. J.*, 1987, *294*, 42) have advised caution or avoidance.

Lactation ceased in a nursing mother after she was given mebendazole for roundworm infection.— T. S. Rao (letter), *N.Z. med. J.*, 1983, *96*, 589.

Absorption and Fate

Mebendazole is poorly absorbed from the gastro-intestinal tract and undergoes extensive first-pass elimination, being metabolised in the liver, eliminated in the bile as unchanged drug and metabolites, and excreted in the faeces. Only about 2% of a dose is excreted unchanged or as metabolites in the urine.

Mebendazole is highly protein-bound.

Findings from pharmacokinetic studies, carried out in cooperation with the Swiss Echinococcosis Study Group, on mebendazole given long term in high oral doses for the treatment of hydatid disease.

There was a large intra- and interindividual variation in plasma concentrations in patients on long-term therapy. Bioavailability was enhanced in 3 healthy subjects when mebendazole was given with a standard breakfast; plasma concentrations were also higher in a patient with cholestasis.— G. J. Münst *et al.*, *Eur. J. clin. Pharmac.*, 1980, *17*, 375. Mebendazole was extensively metabolised in the liver. Biliary elimination of mebendazole and its metabolites, almost entirely as conjugates, is a major route of disposition and was compromised in a patient with cholestasis and impaired hepatic drug metabolising capacity.— F. Witassek *et al.*, *ibid.*, 1983, *25*, 81. The drug metabolism enzyme system (microsomal function) of the liver, as measured by the aminopyrine breath test, and cholestasis are major determinants of plasma concentrations of mebendazole.— F. Witassek and J. Bircher, *ibid.*, 85. Mebendazole is highly bound to albumin. Plasma concentrations 4 hours after the morning dose exhibited the best correlation with the average 24-hour concentration and were significantly correlated with the drug concentration in cyst fluid; free mebendazole concentration in cyst fluid was almost identical with free drug concentration in plasma.— P. J. Luder *et al.*, *ibid.*, 1985, *28*, 279. Confirmation from a retrospective analysis of the lack of relationship between dose and plasma concentration of mebendazole and of interindividual variation in plasma concentrations, emphasising the need for repeated monitoring. Several patients appeared to have subtherapeutic plasma concentrations, if 250 nmol per litre measured 4 hours after the morning dose is accepted as the lower limit of the therapeutic range. The concomitant administration of phenytoin or carbamazepine appeared to lower plasma concentrations, presumably as a result of enzyme induction; valproic acid had no such effect. Although plasma concentrations of mebendazole were raised when the enzyme inhibitor cimetidine was given concomitantly, the increase was too small to be of therapeutic relevance. Co-administration of ursodeoxycholic acid did not improve systemic bioavailability of mebendazole.— P. J. Luder *et al.*, *ibid.*, 1986, *31*, 443.

Investigation of the variable efficacy of mebendazole in the treatment of larval echinococcal infections [hydatid disease] has been hampered by limited knowledge of its clinical pharmacokinetics owing to the lack of an intravenous dosage form. A solution of radiolabelled mebendazole suitable for intravenous injection has recently been formulated and a tracer dose of 1.18 μg given intravenously and orally to 5 subjects previously treated with mebendazole for cystic hydatid disease. After intravenous administration, mebendazole was rapidly distributed and rapidly eliminated, the average distribution half-life, elimination half-life, and rate of clearance being 0.2 hour, 1.12 hour, and 1.063 litres per minute respectively. After oral administration, mebendazole was rapidly absorbed and rapidly eliminated, the average time to peak plasma concentration and average elimination half-life being 0.42 hour and 0.94 hour respectively; bioavailability was about 22% and oral rate of clearance 0.846 litre per minute. Other studies, in which longer half-lives of 2 to 8 hours were observed, used large oral doses of mebendazole (about 500 mg) and probably measured absorption half-life rather than elimination half-life.

About 50% of the dose was eliminated in the urine during the 24 hours following intravenous and oral dosage. The major unconjugated metabolite of mebendazole detected in the urine was 2-amino-5(6) [α-hydroxybenzyl]benzimidazole, with smaller amounts of 2-amino-5(6)-benzoylbenzimidazole and very small amounts of mebendazole and methyl-5(6) [α-hydroxybenzyl]benzimidazole carbamate.

Absorption of mebendazole from the gastro-intestinal tract was almost complete and overall the results indicate that the poor bioavailability of mebendazole observed at therapeutic dose levels is due to a combination of high first-pass elimination and the very low solubility of the compound. Modification of the dose form rather than administration of large doses may be a more rational method of increasing plasma concentrations in the treatment of extra-intestinal infections.— M. Dawson *et al.*, *Br. J. clin. Pharmac.*, 1985, *19*, 79.

In a study in healthy subjects of different dose forms, bioavailability of mebendazole, as judged by urinary excretion of mebendazole and its unconjugated metabolites, was slightly enhanced when 500 mg was administered by mouth as gelatin capsules containing mebendazole dispersed in olive oil, compared with that following the administration of commercially available tablets or 2% suspension. Following oral administration, 1.33 to 1.85% of the dose was excreted in the urine; about 86% of that excreted appeared as 2-amino-5(6)[α-hydroxybenzyl]benzimidazole. Mebendazole was not absorbed following rectal administration as suppositories.— M. Dawson and T. R. Watson, *Br. J. clin. Pharmac.*, 1985, *19*, 87.

Further references: A. Bekhti *et al.*, *Br. J. clin. Pharmac.*, 1986, *21*, 223 (correlation between serum-mebendazole concentrations and hepatic drug metabolising activity).

Uses and Administration

Mebendazole, a benzimidazole carbamate derivative, is an anthelmintic with activity against most nematode and some cestode worms (see p.47); activity against some larval stages and ova has also been demonstrated. It appears to act by irreversibly inhibiting glucose uptake by susceptible worms, resulting in depletion of the worm's energy sources, glycogen and adenosine triphosphate (ATP), and their slow death.

Unlike the related anthelmintic thiabendazole, mebendazole is poorly absorbed from the gastro-intestinal tract and is used principally in the treatment of the intestinal nematode infections ascariasis (roundworm infection), enterobiasis (threadworm infections), hookworm infections (ancylostomiasis and necatoriasis), and trichuriasis (whipworm infection); it is useful in mixed infections. During treatment with mebendazole, migration of worms with expulsion through the mouth and nose has occurred in some patients heavily infected with *Ascaris*. Mebendazole is also used in the treatment of capillariasis.

Mebendazole also has activity against the adult and larval forms of some cestode worms and has been tried in high doses in the treatment of hydatid disease.

Mebendazole is given by mouth. The usual dose for adults and children aged 2 years or over with enterobiasis is 100 mg as a single dose, repeated if necessary after 2 to 3 weeks; for ascariasis, hookworm infections, and trichuriasis the usual dose is 100 mg twice daily for 3 days.

Recommendations by authorities in the *USA* for the treatment of parasitic infections. Mebendazole is an alternative to thiabendazole in the treatment of *Angiostrongylus cantonensis* infection (100 mg twice daily for 5 days); the drug of choice in *Ascaris lumbricoides* (roundworm) infection (100 mg twice daily for 3 days); the drug of choice in *Capillaria philippinensis* infection (200 mg twice daily for 20 days); an alternative to pyrantel embonate in *Enterobius vermicularis* (pinworm) infection (a single 100-mg dose, repeated after 2 weeks); an alternative to surgical removal in gnathostomiasis (200 mg every 3 hours for 6 days); the drug of choice in hookworm infections due to *Ancylostoma duodenale* or *Necator americanus* (100 mg twice daily for 3 days); an alternative to diethylcarbamazine followed by suramin in *Onchocerca volvulus* infection (1 g twice daily for 28 days); an alternative to corticosteroids plus thiabendazole in trichinosis (200 to 400 mg three times daily for 3 days, then 400 to 500 mg three times daily for 10 days); the drug of choice in *Trichuris trichiura* (whipworm) infection (100 mg twice daily for 3 days); and an alternative to diethylcarbamazine or thiabendazole in visceral larva migrans (200 to 400 mg daily for 5 days). In hydatid disease due to *Echinococcus granulosus*, mebendazole can be tried when surgery is contra-indicated or cysts rupture spontaneously during surgery; in infection due to *E. multilocularis*, surgical excision is the only reliable treatment although there have been recent reports of encouraging results with high doses of mebendazole given long term.— *Med. Lett.*, 1986, *28*, 9.

After treatment of 85 children with mebendazole 100 mg twice daily for 3 days the overall cure-rate for ascaris infection was 100%, for trichuris 94%, for hookworm 82%, and for hymenolepis 39%. Infection with *Giardia lamblia* cysts was eliminated in 10 of 25 children.— J. G. P. Hutchison *et al.*, *Br. med. J.*, 1975, *2*, 309.

A study in children in rural Papua New Guinea on re-infection with intestinal worms after treatment with mebendazole 100 mg twice daily for 3 days. Initially about two-thirds of the children were infected with *Ascaris lumbricoides* and *Trichuris trichiura* and nearly all with *Necator americanus*; *T. trichiura* egg counts were low on the whole. The results indicated that in areas with comparable transmission-rates, annual treatment with a course of anthelmintic would keep hookworm levels low and an additional dose at mid-year would also considerably reduce ascariasis.— J. Shield *et al.*, *Papua New Guin. med. J.*, 1984, *27*, 89.

Results from a double-blind placebo-controlled study in Indonesia indicating that a single dose of mebendazole is effective, inexpensive, and convenient in mass treatment for the control of soil-transmitted intestinal nematode infections, especially in highly infected communities. Of 156 subjects, 105 of whom were children, ascariasis was present in 105, trichuriasis in 105, and hookworm infection in 88; mixed infections were seen in 138. Mebendazole was given as a single 500-mg dose and, overall, parasitological cure-rates of 93.4, 77.6, and 91.1% and egg reduction-rates of 99.0, 92.8, and 98.3% were obtained for ascariasis, trichuriasis, and hookworm infections, respectively.— K. Abadi, *Am. J. trop. Med. Hyg.*, 1985, *34*, 129.

Further references to the successful use of single doses of mebendazole for the treatment of intestinal nematode infections: M. A. Muttalib *et al.*, *J. trop. Med. Hyg.*, 1981, *84*, 159 (a single 200-mg dose in children with ascariasis and trichuriasis); S. P. Kan, *Am. J. trop. Med. Hyg.*, 1983, *32*, 118 (single doses of 100 to 600 mg in children with trichuriasis and ascariasis).

ADMINISTRATION IN RENAL FAILURE. Lack of effect of haemodialysis on plasma concentrations and protein binding of mebendazole in a patient with renal failure receiving mebendazole therapy for echinococcosis [hydatid disease].— H. Allgayer *et al.*, *Eur. J. clin. Pharmac.*, 1984, *27*, 243.

DIABETES MELLITUS. Mebendazole 100 to 300 mg daily for one month decreased plasma-glucose concentrations and improved metabolic control in 6 insulin-dependent and 6 non-insulin-dependent diabetics, apparently by increasing insulin secretion. The effects might be transient.— S. Caprio *et al.*, *Diabetologia*, 1984, *27*, 52.

DRACONTIASIS. In 12 patients with guinea-worm infection given mebendazole 200 mg four times daily for 6 days (repeated if necessary) there was rapid relief of pain and inflammation, and the worm was fragmented and extruded.— A. Z. Shafei, *J. trop. Med. Hyg.*, 1976, *79*, 197. An unfavourable report.— O. O. Kale, *Am. J. trop. Med. Hyg.*, 1975, *24*, 600.

HYDATID DISEASE. A review of the chemotherapy of hydatid disease. In the *UK*, hydatid disease is relatively uncommon and most cases are likely to be due to *Echinococcus granulosus*, a common parasite of *dogs* and *sheep*, as primary and secondary hosts respectively. In man, 70% of primary cysts are hepatic and 15% occur in the lungs. *E. multilocularis* is a more aggressive form unlikely to be seen in the indigenous *UK* population. Surgical removal of hydatid cysts may entail relatively major surgery and postoperative problems are not uncommon. Recurrent disease occurs in over 10% of cases and mortality rises with repeated surgery.

Mebendazole was the first drug to show any effect in hydatid disease although results have often been disappointing even after treatment with 40 mg per kg body-weight daily for months or even years. This is possibly due to the extremely poor absorption of mebendazole resulting in low plasma and minimal cyst concentrations. Allergic reactions, prolonged fevers, reversible neutropenia, and glomerulonephritis have been associated with the use of mebendazole. Flubendazole has also been used in hydatid disease, but subcutaneous or intramuscular injections have produced equally discouraging blood concentrations. Albendazole is much better absorbed than mebendazole and preliminary results have been encouraging.— D. L. Morris, *J. antimicrob. Chemother.*, 1983, *11*, 494. Further comment on hydatid disease and its treatment. Given its apparent effectiveness, tolerance, and pharmacokinetics, albendazole appears to be a leading candidate for continuing clinical investigations.— P. M. Schantz, *J. Am. med. Ass.*, 1985, *253*, 2095. See also *Lancet*, 1987, *1*, 21.

Comment from the manufacturers that although there is some evidence that after high doses by mouth mebendazole can be detected in plasma in low concentrations, it is not reasonable to treat hydatid disease which requires significant blood and cyst fluid concentrations, by mouth with a drug developed specifically to be poorly absorbed from the gastro-intestinal tract. Alternative compounds and routes of administration are to be studied.— A. L. Macnair (letter), *Br. med. J.*, 1980, *280*, 1055.

A report at the end of the first phase of a WHO programme of co-ordinated studies on the treatment of echinococcosis [hydatid disease] with benzimidazolecarbamates, launched in 1981 because individual studies undertaken since 1977 had given inconsistent results.

A total of 121 patients with cystic (*Echinococcus granulosus*) echinococcosis were treated with mebendazole, flubendazole, or albendazole by mouth. Mebendazole was given to 85 patients in doses ranging from 13.0 to 136.4 mg per kg body-weight daily (1 to 10 g daily) the most frequently used dose being 50 mg per kg daily; as a rule patients were treated for 3 months but in some, especially those with liver localisation or multiple cysts, treatment was extended to 6 months or more. Flubendazole was given to 6 patients in a fixed daily dose of 1.5 to 4 g daily (37.5 to 54.5 mg per kg daily; mode, 50 mg per kg daily) for 3 to 6 months. Albendazole was given to 30 patients in a daily dose of 800 mg in adults and 250 or 400 mg in children (range, 9.8 to 15.4 mg per kg daily; mode, 12.5 mg per kg daily); treatment cycles of 30 days were repeated 2 or 3 times with 2-week intervals between courses. Treatment with mebendazole was fully successful in 8 of 85 patients (9%) and partially successful in 4 others (5%). Flubendazole was effective in one patient with lung echinococcosis, but not in the remaining 5 who had liver or other organ involvement. Albendazole was fully successful in 5 of 30 patients (17%) and partially successful in 4 others (13%). Overall, treatment was more successful in those with localisation of cysts in the lungs than in the liver or other organs. It was concluded that mebendazole is not an optimal compound in the treatment of cystic echinococcosis. Further studies on new drugs or new formulations and methods of administration of existing benzimidazoles are needed and in the meantime chemotherapy of cystic echinococcosis should be restricted to inoperable cases.

A total of 54 patients with *Echinococcus multilocularis* infection were treated with mebendazole in daily doses ranging from 26.8 to 169.5 mg per kg (1.5 to 10 g), the mode being 41.7 mg per kg; treatment and observation

had continued for up to 12 years. In the majority of patients with alveolar echinococcosis (70%), the condition was stabilised and improvement seen, although a definite reduction in the size of the lesion was observed in only 4 patients (7%). It was concluded that mebendazole is indicated in most cases of alveolar echinococcosis, irrespective of surgery, although further studies are needed to clarify the optimal regimen. Studies are also underway with albendazole in 20 patients.
Overall, treatment was well tolerated by most patients although close supervision is required in order to prevent serious complications. Treatment was stopped temporarily or permanently in 8 of 195 patients (4%) because of suspected adverse reactions [see also under Adverse Effects, for details of the adverse reactions encountered].— A. Davis *et al.*, *Bull. Wld Hlth Org.*, 1986, *64*, 383.

Some references to experience with high-dose mebendazole therapy in the treatment of hydatid disease.— A. D. M. Bryceson *et al.*, *Trans. R. Soc. trop. Med. Hyg.*, 1982, *76*, 510 (inoperable hydatid disease in 11 patients; mebendazole 40 to 200 mg per kg body-weight daily for 16 to 48 weeks; results difficult to assess); D. N. Bhattacharyya and J. R. Harries, *ibid.*, 1984, *78*, 78 (multiple pulmonary hydatid cysts with myopathy in 1 patient; successful treatment with mebendazole 200 mg per kg body-weight daily); T. Karpathios *et al.*, *Archs Dis. Childh.*, 1984, *59*, 894 (multiple ruptured hydatid cysts in 2 children; successful treatment with mebendazole 100 mg per kg body-weight for up to 12 weeks).

For pharmacokinetic studies of mebendazole in patients being treated for hydatid disease, see Absorption and Fate (above).

LOIASIS. Beneficial preliminary results with mebendazole in the treatment of loiasis. *Loa loa* parasitaemia was reduced or eliminated in 4 patients given mebendazole 100 mg three times daily by mouth for 45 days.— M. Van Hoegaerden and F. Flocard (letter), *Lancet*, 1985, *1*, 1278.

LYMPHATIC FILARIASIS. Mebendazole has shown antifilarial activity in *animals* and has undergone trials in man. No adverse reactions were produced in patients suffering from *Brugia malayi* and *Wuchereria bancrofti* infections treated with mebendazole 500 mg three times daily for 21 days and follow-up of the few patients treated so far has suggested a macrofilaricidal action. However, the use of mebendazole at the high doses required for filariasis is not recommended because its absorption is erratic, it is teratogenic in some *animals* and cannot be safely used in women, it can be toxic in large doses, and it is expensive. Neither is the use of levamisole in combination with mebendazole recommended.— Lymphatic Filariasis, Fourth Report of the WHO Expert Committee on Filariasis, *Tech. Rep. Ser. Wld Hlth Org. No. 702*, 1984.

ONCHOCERCIASIS. The standard treatment of onchocerciasis, with diethylcarbamazine and suramin, remains unsatisfactory and alternative drugs are sought which ideally should kill or permanently sterilise the adult worms of *Onchocerca volvulus*, without causing severe allergic reactions in the recipients from microfilaricidal action. Compounds tested more recently include the benzimidazoles. Benzimidazoles have an unusual effect on embryogenesis in various *Onchocerca* spp. In general they do not kill microfilariae and therefore, unlike diethylcarbamazine, do not initiate the cascade of events leading to a Mazzotti reaction, but appear to 'sterilise' the adult females, at least temporarily, and allow a gradual attrition in the numbers of microfilariae. However, benzimidazoles are very poorly absorbed orally and need to be given in much larger than conventional doses.
Mebendazole has been the benzimidazole most widely tested and produces a prolonged reduction in microfilarial skin-snip counts. It has also been used in combination with levamisole although results have varied; some studies have shown no advantage whereas others have suggested that combined treatment might possibly be more effective than mebendazole alone. Mebendazole has three serious disadvantages when used at the prolonged high-dose level needed for treating onchocerciasis: it is teratogenic in some *animals*; idiosyncratic neutropenia can develop and death from septicaemia has been reported in a patient with hydatid disease given high doses; it seems to have a moderate microfilaricidal effect and produces a mild Mazzotti-type of reaction.— H. R. Taylor, *Bull. Wld Hlth Org.*, 1984, *62*, 509. Reference to the current status of benzimidazoles in the treatment of onchocerciasis. Mebendazole is unsuitable for prolonged use at the high oral doses required because of its inconsistent effects on *O. volvulus*, its toxicity, and potential teratogenicity. Flubendazole is inactive orally and it has proved impossible to prepare a satisfactory formulation for injection. Both thiabendazole and albendazole are ineffective.— Third Report of the WHO Expert Committee on Onchocerciasis, *Tech. Rep. Ser. Wld Hlth Org. No. 752*, 1987.

Mebendazole, alone or in combination with levamisole, was as effective as diethylcarbamazine and produced fewer systemic side-effects and ocular complications in a double-blind study in 40 male patients with onchocerciasis. The following 4 drug regimens were employed: mebendazole 1 g twice daily for 28 days, levamisole 150 mg weekly for 5 weeks, the mebendazole and levamisole regimens together, or diethylcarbamazine citrate 100 mg twice daily for 28 days. Diethylcarbamazine produced the more rapid fall in skin microfilaria counts but on follow-up at 6 months those receiving mebendazole alone or with levamisole showed similar or slightly greater reductions. Levamisole alone had no significant effect on microfilaria counts and used in combination with mebendazole seemed to offer no advantage over mebendazole alone.— A. R. Rivas-Alcalá *et al.*, *Lancet*, 1981, *2*, 485. At 12-month follow-up, the reduction in microfilarial levels had been maintained in those given mebendazole, but not in those given diethylcarbamazine.— *idem* (letter), 1043.

PERSTANS FILARIASIS. Three of 4 patients infected with microfilariae resembling *Mansonella perstans* (*Dipetalonema perstans*) were successfully treated with mebendazole 100 mg three times daily and levamisole 100 mg twice daily for 10 days.— H. C. Bernberg *et al.*, *Trans. R. Soc. trop. Med. Hyg.*, 1979, *73*, 233.

Following the successful use of mebendazole in a patient with symptomatic *Mansonella perstans* (*Dipetalonema perstans*) filariasis which had not responded to diethylcarbamazine, a total of 9 patients with *M. perstans* filariasis have been treated with mebendazole 100 mg twice daily by mouth. Five were cured following treatment for 30 days, one received a second course after which only a few circulating microfilariae were seen, and two were given mebendazole for 7 weeks and were free of microfilariae, one of them after 4 weeks. The ninth patient, a 6-year-old child, had to discontinue treatment because of severe side-effects (high fever and angioedema) with recurrence of symptoms when the dose was halved. Mild side-effects, including rashes and pruritus, were seen quite frequently in some other patients.— M. Wahlgren and I. Frolov (letter), *Trans. R. Soc. trop. Med. Hyg.*, 1983, *77*, 422.

STRONGYLOIDIASIS. Thiabendazole is the drug of choice in the treatment of strongyloidiasis, since it is absorbed and acts against the tissue stages as well as the intestinal parasites, but side-effects are frequent. Mebendazole is poorly absorbed and doses of 200 mg three times daily for 3 days were unsuccessful in treating 2 patients with strongyloidiasis in whom thiabendazole was contra-indicated. However, subsequent treatment with mebendazole 1 g on the first day, followed by 500 mg daily for 20 consecutive days was effective and well-tolerated.— S. Mravak *et al.*, *Acta trop.*, 1983, *40*, 93.

Persistent *Strongyloides stercoralis* infection in a blind loop of the bowel of a 55-year-old man was eradicated by mebendazole 1.5 g daily for 14 days, after treatment with 3 courses of thiabendazole had failed.— K. H. Wilson and C. A. Kauffman, *Archs intern. Med.*, 1983, *143*, 357.

TAENIASIS. Cure of 10 patients with *Taenia saginata* or *T. solium* infection with mebendazole 300 mg twice daily for 3 days.— A. P. Chavarria *et al.*, *Am. J. trop. Med. Hyg.*, 1977, *26*, 118. See also P. V. Arambulo *et al.*, *Acta trop.*, 1978, *35*, 281.

TOXOCARIASIS. Toxocariasis, due to *Toxocara canis*, in a 23-year-old woman who had had symptoms for 2 years was treated successfully with mebendazole 1 g three times daily (50 mg per kg body-weight daily) for 21 days.— A. Bekhti (letter), *Ann. intern. Med.*, 1984, *100*, 463.

TRICHINOSIS. Long-term high-dose treatment with mebendazole was successful in a patient chronically ill with trichinosis unresponsive to corticosteroid therapy. Mebendazole 400 mg every 6 hours was given for 25 days; a Herxheimer-like reaction occurred after 6 days, but treatment was continued without further incident. A second course of mebendazole, begun at a dosage of 1.2 g daily and continued until a total of 37 g had been given, was needed for complete resolution of the generalised symptoms and death of the encysted *Trichinella*.— M. L. Levin, *Am. J. trop. Med. Hyg.*, 1983, *32*, 980.

Preparations

Mebendazole Tablets *(U.S.P.)*

Proprietary Preparations

Vermox *(Janssen, UK)*. *Tablets*, scored, chewable, mebendazole 100 mg.
Suspension, mebendazole 100 mg/5mL.

Proprietary Names and Manufacturers

Anelmin; Antiox *(Janssen, Belg.)*; Bantenol *(Janssen, Spain)*; Benda; Bendosan; Damaben; Elmetin; Fugacar *(Janssen, Belg.)*; Hawkben; Lomper *(Esteve, Spain)*; Mebasol; Meben; Mebendacin; Mebendan *(Mabo, Spain)*; Mebenda-P; Mebutar; Medazole; Nemasole; Oxitover *(Llorente, Spain)*; Sufil *(Cusi, Spain)*; Thelmox *(Remedica, Cyprus)*; Totamin; Vagaka; Vercid; Vermoran; Vermox *(Janssen, Austral.*; *Janssen, Belg.*; *Janssen, Canad.*; *Janssen, Denm.*; *Janssen, Ger.*; *Janssen, Ital.*; *Neth.*; *Janssen, Norw.*; *NZ*; *Janssen, S.Afr.*; *Janssen Pharmaceutica, Swed.*; *Janssen, Switz.*; *Janssen, UK*; *Janssen, USA)*; Vorme; Wormin *(Cadila, Ind.)*; Wormox; Zadomen.

12952-h

Methyridine *(BAN)*.

Metyridine *(pINN)*. 2-(2-Methoxyethyl)pyridine.
$C_8H_{11}NO = 137.2$.

CAS — 114-91-0.

Methyridine is an anthelmintic which has been used in veterinary medicine for the treatment of roundworm infections.

3594-e

Metriphonate *(BAN)*.

Metrifonate *(rINN)*; Trichlorfon; Trichlorphon.
Dimethyl 2,2,2-trichloro-1-hydroxyethylphosphonate.
$C_4H_8Cl_3O_4P = 257.4$.

CAS — 52-68-6.

Pharmacopoeias. In *Cz.*

CAUTION. *Metriphonate is very toxic when inhaled, swallowed, or spilled on the skin. It can be removed from the skin by washing with soap and water. Contaminated material should be immersed in a 2% aqueous solution of sodium hydroxide for several hours.*

Adverse Effects, Treatment, and Precautions

Metriphonate is generally well tolerated, but may cause nausea, vomiting, abdominal pain, diarrhoea, headache, dizziness, and weakness.
It is an organophosphorus compound and because of its anticholinesterase properties depresses plasma-cholinesterase concentrations. Patients treated with metriphonate should not be given depolarising muscle relaxants such as suxamethonium for at least 48 hours. The administration of metriphonate should be avoided in those recently exposed to insecticides or other agricultural chemicals with anticholinesterase activity.
For a description of the toxic effects of organophosphorus compounds and the treatment of acute poisoning, see under organophosphorus pesticides (p.1344).

A summary of toxicological and pharmacological information on metriphonate.— B. Holmstedt *et al.*, *Arch. Tox.*, 1978, *41*, 3.

A few hours after a dose of metriphonate 7.5, 10, or 12.5 mg per kg body-weight in children with schistosomiasis, plasma cholinesterase was almost completely inhibited, regardless of the dose, and erythrocyte cholinesterase was inhibited by 40 to 60%, depending on the dose. Plasma cholinesterase recovered more rapidly and after 14 days was about 75% of normal. Doses were given up to 3 times at 14-day intervals and 4 weeks after the last dose plasma cholinesterase was nearly normal whereas erythrocyte cholinesterase returned to normal 8 to 15 weeks after the last dose.— P. Pleština *et al.*, *Bull. Wld Hlth Org.*, 1972, *46*, 747.

A report of apparent clinical organophosphate poisoning in an 8-year-old child after receiving a single dose of metriphonate 250 mg (10 mg per kg body-weight) for the treatment of *Schistosoma haematobium* infection. Symptoms included profuse vomiting, salivation, and sweating, small pupils, fasciculation, and bradycardia. Serum pseudocholinesterase was markedly depressed. He made a good recovery after intravenous atropine and rehydration.— V. P. Jamnadas and J. E. P. Thomas, *Cent. Afr. J. Med.*, 1979, *25*, 130.

PREGNANCY AND THE NEONATE. In an area where *Schistosoma haematobium* was hyperendemic, a woman not known to be pregnant was treated twice with metriphonate during the second month of pregnancy. She subsequently gave birth to a baby with massive hydrocephalus and a large meningeomyelocele. The baby died one hour after delivery. It had previously been considered that schistosomiasis was more of a risk to pregnancy than the potential risks of metriphonate. Although a cause and effect relationship cannot be established with this single case it suggests caution when using metriphonate during pregnancy.— M. H. Monson and K. Alexander (letter), *Trans. R. Soc. trop. Med. Hyg.*, 1984, *78*, 565. Extensive toxicological studies have demonstrated a wide margin of safety for metriphonate. Mutagenic activity has not been established, carcinogenicity studies in *animals* were negative, and embryotoxicity and teratogenicity have not been found in laboratory tests. Nevertheless, administration of metriphonate during pregnancy is not recommended.— The Control of Schistosomiasis, *Tech. Rep. Ser. Wld Hlth Org. No. 728*, 1985.

Residues in the body and diet. Temporary maximum acceptable daily intake of metriphonate: 5 µg per kg body-weight. Further work was required on carcinogenicity and further studies were desirable on the spontaneous conversion of metriphonate to dichlorvos and on the possible intermediaries involved.— Report of the 1975 Joint FAO/WHO Meeting on Pesticide Residues in Food, *Tech. Rep. Ser. Wld Hlth Org. No. 592*, 1976.

For background toxicological data, see 1971 Evaluations of some Pesticide Residues in Food, *Pestic. Residue Ser. Wld Hlth Org. No. 1*, 1972.

Uses and Administration

Metriphonate is an organophosphorus compound and is converted in the body to the active metabolite dichlorvos (see p.1347), an anticholinesterase.

Metriphonate has anthelmintic activity, principally against *Schistosoma haematobium*. It is given by mouth in the treatment of urinary schistosomiasis due to *S. haematobium*. Three doses of 7.5 to 10 mg per kg body-weight may be given at intervals of 2 weeks. Single doses of 10 mg per kg at intervals of 3, 6, or 12 months have also been used.

Metriphonate has also been used as an insecticide.

CYSTICERCOSIS. Rapid improvement in a patient with a large number of subcutaneous nodules of cysticercosis following treatment with metriphonate. It was given in a single daily dose of 635 mg (10 mg per kg body-weight) by mouth for 6 days and the course repeated after one month. Some evidence of anticholinesterase activity developed during treatment, especially during the first course, when atropine was given to relieve symptoms of dizziness, nausea, facial flushing, and abdominal pain.— E. H. Tschen *et al.*, *Archs Derm.*, 1981, *117*, 507.

ONCHOCERCIASIS. Metriphonate 100 mg daily for 14 days or as four doses of 10 mg per kg body-weight either on alternate days or at weekly intervals exhibited moderate activity against the microfilariae but none against the adult *Onchocerca volvulus* in 10 patients with onchocerciasis.— O. O. Kale, *Bull. Wld Hlth Org.*, 1982, *60*, 109. Trials with metriphonate in the treatment of onchocerciasis have not proved successful.— D. Bell, *Br. med. J.*, 1985, *1*, 1450. Metriphonate is primarily microfilaricidal, but less effective and less consistent than diethylcarbamazine. It also precipitates a Mazzotti reaction.— Third Report of the WHO Expert Committee on Onchocerciasis, *Tech. Rep. Ser. Wld Hlth Org. No. 752*, 1987.

SCHISTOSOMIASIS. The report of a WHO Expert Committee on the control of schistosomiasis. Metriphonate is an organophosphorus ester active only against *Schistosoma haematobium*. It is rapidly absorbed, metabolised, and excreted. Its metabolite, dichlorvos, is a cholinesterase inhibitor that acts directly; this is the active compound and metriphonate acts as a slow-release formulation. The standard dosage regimen in the treatment of *S. haematobium* infection is 7.5 to 10 mg per kg body-weight of metriphonate given on three occasions at intervals of 2 weeks. Single doses of 10 mg per kg at intervals of 3, 6, or 12 months have also been suggested but so far have not been evaluated sufficiently in the field. Cure-rates with metriphonate in schistosomiasis control programmes range from 40 to more than 80%, with a 90% reduction in egg counts among those not cured. In one group of clinical trials, the cure-rate at 6 months following treatment with 1, 2, or 3 doses of metriphonate was 28, 65, and 84% respectively. Tolerance of metriphonate is good and cholinergic side-effects are rare, generally mild, and disappear within a few hours. Occupational groups recently exposed to organophosphate insecticides should be treated with metriphonate only when blood cholinesterase concentrations are shown to be normal.— The Control of Schistosomiasis, *Tech. Rep. Ser. Wld Hlth Org. No. 728*, 1985.

Beneficial results with a single dose of metriphonate 10 mg per kg body-weight in the treatment of children with *Schistosoma haematobium* infection: A. El Kholy *et al.*, *Am. J. trop. Med. Hyg.*, 1984, *33*, 1170; S. A. Tswana and P. R. Mason, *ibid.*, 1985, *34*, 746.

For further details on schistosomiasis and its control and a report indicating the superiority of praziquantel over metriphonate, see praziquantel (p.65).

Proprietary Names and Manufacturers

Bilarcil *(Bayer, Ger.)*.

12977-e

Morantel Tartrate *(BANM, USAN, pINNM)*.

CP-12009-18; UK-2964-18. (*E*)-1,4,5,6-Tetrahydro-1-methyl-2-[2-(3-methyl-2-thienyl)vinyl]pyrimidine hydrogen tartrate.

$C_{12}H_{16}N_2S,C_4H_6O_6$=370.4.

CAS — 20574-50-9 (morantel); 26155-31-7 (tartrate).

Morantel is an analogue of pyrantel. The tartrate is used as a veterinary anthelmintic.

Proprietary Veterinary Names and Manufacturers

Paratect *(Pfizer, UK)*.

13000-p

Naphthalophos *(BAN)*.

Bay-9002; Naftalofos *(USAN, rINN)*; Phthalophos. Diethyl naphthalimido-oxyphosphonate.

$C_{16}H_{16}NO_6P$=349.3.

CAS — 1491-41-4.

Naphthalophos is an organophosphorus compound which has been used as a veterinary anthelmintic.

2190-g

Netobimin *(BAN, USAN, rINN)*.

Sch-32481. 2-{3-Methoxycarbonyl-2-[2-nitro-5-(propylthio)phenyl]guanidino}ethanesulphonic acid.

$C_{14}H_{20}N_4O_7S_2$=420.5.

CAS — 88255-01-0.

Netobimin is an anthelmintic used in veterinary medicine.

Proprietary Veterinary Names and Manufacturers

Hapadex *(Kirby-Warrick, UK)*.

13009-k

Niclofolan *(BAN, rINN)*.

Bayer-9015; Menichlopholan. 5,5′-Dichloro-3,3′-dinitrobiphenyl-2,2′-diol.

$C_{12}H_6Cl_2N_2O_6$=345.1.

CAS — 10331-57-4.

Niclofolan is an anthelmintic with activity against trematodes (flukes), but it appears to have been overtaken by praziquantel.

793-k

Niclosamide *(BAN, USAN, rINN)*.

Bay-2353; Phenasale. 2′,5-Dichloro-4′-nitrosalicylanilide; 5-Chloro-*N*-(2-chloro-4-nitrophenyl)-2-hydroxybenzamide.

$C_{13}H_8Cl_2N_2O_4$=327.1.

CAS — 50-65-7.

Pharmacopoeias. In *Br.*, *Chin.*, *Cz.*, *Egypt.*, *Fr.*, *Ind.*, *Int.*, *It.*, and *Nord. Int.*, *Jug.*, and *Nord.* include the monohydrate. Also in *B.P. Vet.*

A cream-coloured odourless or almost odourless powder. Practically **insoluble** in water; slightly soluble in alcohol; very slightly soluble in chloroform and in ether. **Protect** from light.

Adverse Effects

Gastro-intestinal disturbances may occur occasionally with niclosamide. Lightheadedness and pruritus have been reported less frequently.

Absorption and Fate

Niclosamide is not significantly absorbed from the gastro-intestinal tract.

Uses and Administration

Niclosamide is an anthelmintic which is active against most tapeworms, including the beef tapeworm (*Taenia saginata*), the pork tapeworm (*T. solium*), the fish tapeworm (*Diphyllobothrium latum*), the dwarf tapeworm (*Hymenolepis nana*), and the dog tapeworm (*Dipylidium caninum*).

Niclosamide is administered in tablets, which must be chewed thoroughly before swallowing and washed down with the minimum amount of water. For infections with pork tapeworm a single 2-g dose is given after a light breakfast. Niclosamide is not active against the larval form (cysticerci) and some have recommended the use of a saline laxative about 2 hours after the dose to expel the killed worms and minimise the possibility of the migration of ova of *T. solium* into the stomach, with the consequent risk of cysticercosis. An anti-emetic has been given before treatment to reduce this risk.

For infections with beef or fish tapeworms the 2-g dose of niclosamide may be divided, with 1 g taken after breakfast and 1 g an hour later.

In dwarf-tapeworm infections an initial dose of 2 g is given on the first day followed by 1 g daily for 6 days.

Children aged 2 to 6 years are given half the above doses and those under 2 years of age are given one-quarter the above doses.

Unless expulsion of the worm is aided by a laxative, portions are voided in a partially digested form after treatment with niclosamide; the scolex is rarely identifiable.

Niclosamide has also been given in the treatment of infection with the intestinal fluke *Fasciolopsis buski* in a single 2-g dose.

Niclosamide is used as a molluscicide for the treatment of water in schistosomiasis control programmes.

A brief review of niclosamide and its use in the treatment of tapeworm infections.— R. D. Pearson and E. L. Hewlett, *Ann. intern. Med.*, 1985, *102*, 550.

Comment on the treatment of *Taenia solium* infections with niclosamide, including arguments against the routine use of laxatives.— F. Richards and P. M. Schantz, *Lancet*, 1985, *1*, 1264.

USE AS A MOLLUSCICIDE. Mention of the use of niclosamide as a molluscicide against *Bulinus* snails. Stagnant and running water was treated with niclosamide 1 mg per litre of water.— J. Massoud *et al.*, *Bull. Wld Hlth Org.*, 1982, *60*, 577. See also Report of a WHO Expert Committee on the control of schistosomiasis, *Tech. Rep. Ser. Wld Hlth Org. No. 728*, 1985.

Preparations

Niclosamide Tablets *(B.P.)*

Proprietary Preparations

Yomesan *(Bayer, UK)*. *Tablets*, chewable, niclosamide 500 mg.

Proprietary Names and Manufacturers
Cestocida; Copharten; Niclocide *(Miles Pharmaceuticals, USA)*; Rotape-Tab; Sulqui; Taenia-Passin; Tepacide; Trédémine *(Bellon, Fr.)*; Vermmide; Yomesan *(Arg.; Bayer, Austral.; Canad.; Bayer, Denm.; Bayer, Ger.; Bayer, Ital.; Neth.; Bayer, S.Afr.; Bayer, Swed.; Bayer, UK*; Yomésane *(Bayer, Switz.)*.

794-a

Niridazole *(BAN, USAN, rINN)*.

BA-32644; NSC-136947. 1-(5-Nitrothiazol-2-yl)imidazolidin-2-one.
$C_6H_6N_4O_3S$=214.2.

CAS — 61-57-4.

Pharmacopoeias. In *It.*

Adverse Effects

Common side-effects with niridazole include anorexia, nausea, vomiting, diarrhoea, abdominal pain, abnormal taste, dizziness, and headache.

Less frequent, but more serious, are effects on the CNS including insomnia, anxiety, agitation, confusion, hallucinations, and convulsions; they have occurred especially in patients with impaired liver function such as those with severe hepato-intestinal schistosomiasis.

Allergic reactions have been reported and may be associated with destruction of parasites; they have included skin rashes, fever, and peripheral eosinophilia. Other adverse effects reported occasionally with niridazole include ECG abnormalities. Haemolysis may occur in persons with a deficiency of glucose-6-phosphate dehydrogenase. The urine may be coloured a deep brown because of the presence of niridazole metabolites.

The possible carcinogenic and mutagenic potential of niridazole in man has not yet been resolved. It has been shown to be a potent carcinogen in *mice* (H.K. Urman *et al., Cancer Letts*, 1975, *1*, 69) and tumorigenic effects have been demonstrated in *mice* and *hamsters* (Report of a WHO Expert Committee on Schistosomiasis, *Tech. Rep. Ser. Wld Hlth Org. No. 643*, 1980). Niridazole is also a mutagen in bacteria (T. Connor *et al., Mutat. Res.*, 1974, *26*, 456) and several studies in *mice* have revealed that it exerts a mutagenic effect on the male germinal epithelium and have indicated a cytotoxic action on spermatogonia, spermatids, and spermatozoa (WHO, 1980). More recently niridazole was found to produce reversible oligospermia in a study of 20 men being treated for schistosomiasis (A.H. El-Beheiry *et al., Arch. Androl.*, 1982, *8*, 297).

A study on the incidence of side-effects with niridazole in 100 in-patients and out-patients with urinary schistosomiasis and the influence of dosing interval.— I. Abdu-Aguye and L. Sambo-Donga, *Hum. Toxicol.*, 1986, *5*, 275.

Precautions

Niridazole should not be given to patients with epilepsy, severe heart disease, or a history of mental disturbance. Great care is necessary in patients with impaired liver function or with liver damage due to heavy infection with *Schistosoma mansoni*. Niridazole should be used with caution in patients with glucose-6-phosphate dehydrogenase deficiency.

It has been contra-indicated in pregnancy by some authorities because of its mutagenic potential (see Adverse Effects, above).

Absorption and Fate

Niridazole is slowly absorbed from the gastro-intestinal tract over 10 to 15 hours and is rapidly metabolised during its first pass through the liver. Metabolites are present in much greater concentrations than unchanged drug in peripheral blood and are bound to plasma proteins. Schistosomicidal activity is due to the unchanged niridazole in the blood; high concentrations are reached in the portal blood. Niridazole is eliminated mainly as dark brown metabolites, almost equally in the urine and in the faeces via the bile.—

A study of the pharmacokinetics of niridazole and 6 metabolites in 4 patients treated for schistosomiasis.— C. I. Valencia *et al., J. Pharmac. exp. Ther.*, 1984, *230*, 133.

Uses and Administration

Niridazole is a nitrothiazole derivative with a broad spectrum of antimicrobial activity. It is a schistosomicide particularly active against *Schistosoma haematobium*, but has generally been replaced by less toxic drugs such as praziquantel (p.64) in the treatment of schistosomiasis. Niridazole also has antiprotozoal activity and was formerly used in the treatment of amoebiasis. It is active *in vitro* against a variety of bacteria.

Niridazole is now used principally in the treatment of dracontiasis (guinea worm infection) where its action may be related to an anti-inflammatory rather than an anthelmintic effect. It has been given by mouth in a dose of 25 mg per kg body-weight daily, up to a maximum of 1.5 g daily, for 10 days.

Evidence from clinical studies that niridazole had immunosuppressant activity.— B. M. Jones *et al., Br. med. J.*, 1977, *2*, 792; L. T. Webster *et al., New Engl. J. Med.*, 1975, *292*, 1144.

Results indicating that niridazole had uricosuric properties.— M. Weintraub *et al., Clin. Pharmac. Ther.*, 1977, *22*, 568.

ANTIBACTERIAL ACTIVITY. In a study *in vitro* niridazole and some other nitrothiazole derivatives were very active against anaerobic bacteria and moderately active against some aerobic bacteria including *Escherichia coli* and *Salmonella* spp.— H. Hof *et al., J. antimicrob. Chemother.*, 1984, *14*, 31.

Further references to the antibacterial activity of niridazole *in vitro*: H. Hof *et al., Antimicrob. Ag. Chemother.*, 1982, *22*, 332 (anaerobic and microaerophilic bacteria); A. M. Freydiere *et al., ibid.*, 1984, *25*, 145 (*Campylobacter fetus* subsp. *jejuni*; more active than metronidazole); H. Hof *et al., ibid.*, *26*, 498 (microaerophilic *Campylobacter jejuni* and *Campylobacter coli*); H. Hof *et al., J. antimicrob. Chemother.*, 1985, *16*, 205 (infections in *mice* with *Salmonella typhimurium* and *Bacteroides fragilis*); R. M. Bannatyne *et al., Antimicrob. Ag. Chemother.*, 1986, *29*, 923 (*Salmonella*).

ANTIPROTOZOAL ACTIVITY. References to the antiprotozoal activity of niridazole *in vitro*: P. F. L. Boreham *et al., J. antimicrob. Chemother.*, 1985, *16*, 589 (*Giardia intestinalis*); N. Yarlett *et al., ibid.*, 1987, *19*, 767 (*Trichomonas vaginalis*).

DRACONTIASIS. Niridazole, usually given in a dose of 25 mg per kg body-weight daily for 10 days, has been reported to have a marked effect on the emerging adult female worms in patients with dracontiasis (R. Muller, *Bull. Wld Hlth Org.*, 1979, *57*, 683); it is thought to act by lessening the intense host tissue reaction, thus allowing the worms to be removed more quickly, rather than by a direct effect on the worms. On completion of a series of field studies Kale *et al.* (*Ann. trop. Med. Parasit.*, 1983, *77*, 151) concluded that niridazole, metronidazole, and thiabendazole were generally better than placebo and had a place in the treatment of dracontiasis. Authorities in the *USA* have recommended niridazole as the drug of choice (*Med. Lett.*, 1986, *28*, 9).

TUNGIASIS. A single oral dose of niridazole 30 mg per kg body-weight given once or repeated after one week was effective in the treatment of tungiasis (infection with the human flea *Tunga penetrans*) in a double-blind placebo-controlled Nigerian study in 155 children. Of those given one dose of niridazole, alleviation of local pruritus and total lysis of the gravid fleas occurred within 2 weeks and healing of the ulcer crater took about 3 weeks. Results were similar in those given 2 doses of niridazole, except that healing occurred within 2 weeks.— M. A. Ade-Serrano *et al., Ann. trop. Med. Parasit.*, 1982, *76*, 89.

Proprietary Names and Manufacturers

Ambilhar *(Ciba, Fr.; Ciba, S.Afr.; Ciba, Switz.; Ciba, UK)*; Yarocen *(Medimpex, Hung.)*.

13027-t

Nitroscanate *(BAN, USAN, rINN)*.
CGA-23654; GS-23654. 4-(4-Nitrophenoxy)phenyl isothiocyanate.
$C_{13}H_8N_2O_3S$=272.3.

CAS — 19881-18-6.

Nitroscanate is an isothiocyanate anthelmintic used in veterinary practice.

Proprietary Veterinary Names and Manufacturers
Lopatol *(Ciba-Geigy Agrochemicals, UK)*.

13029-r

Nitroxynil *(BAN)*.
Nitroxinil *(rINN)*. 4-Hydroxy-3-iodo-5-nitrobenzonitrile.
$C_7H_3IN_2O_3$=290.0.

CAS — 1689-89-0 (nitroxynil); 27917-82-4 (eglumine salt).

Pharmacopoeias. In *B.P. Vet.* Also in *Fr.* for veterinary use.

A yellow odourless or almost odourless powder. Practically **insoluble** in water; slightly soluble in alcohol; soluble 1 in 60 of ether; freely soluble in solutions of alkali hydroxides. Solutions of the eglumine salt of nitroxynil are **sterilised** by autoclaving. **Protect** from light.

Nitroxynil is a veterinary anthelmintic used in the treatment of liver-fluke infections in cattle and sheep. It is administered by subcutaneous injection as the eglumine salt.

Proprietary Veterinary Names and Manufacturers
Trodax *(RMB Animal Health, UK)*.

795-t

Oxamniquine *(BAN, USAN, rINN)*.

UK-4271. 1,2,3,4-Tetrahydro-2-isopropylaminomethyl-7-nitro-6-quinolylmethanol.
$C_{14}H_{21}N_3O_3$=279.3.

CAS — 21738-42-1.

Pharmacopoeias. In *Braz.* and *U.S.*

A yellow-orange crystalline solid. Sparingly **soluble** in water; soluble in acetone, chloroform, and methyl alcohol. A 1% suspension has a pH of 8.0 to 10.0. **Store** in well-closed containers.

Adverse Effects

Oxamniquine caused severe pain at the injection site when administered intramuscularly and is no longer given by this route.

It is generally well tolerated following administration by mouth, although dizziness with or without drowsiness occurs in at least a third of patients, beginning up to 3 hours after a dose and usually lasting for up to 6 hours. Other common side-effects include headache and gastro-intestinal effects such as nausea, vomiting, and diarrhoea.

Allergic-type reactions including urticaria, pruritic skin rashes, and fever may occur. Liver enzyme values have been raised transiently in some patients. Epileptiform convulsions have been reported, especially in patients with a history of convulsive disorders. Hallucinations and excitement have occurred rarely.

A reddish discoloration of urine, probably due to a metabolite of oxamniquine, has been reported.

Of 106 patients treated in Egypt with oxamniquine for schistosomiasis 40 developed a characteristic fever 1 to 3 days after the completion of the course and lasting 2 to 5 days. Six of the 40 patients also developed a typical Löffler-like syndrome with fever, pronounced peripheral blood eosinophilia and scattered pulmonary infiltrates.— G. I. Higashi and Z. Farid, *Br. med. J.*, 1979, *2*, 830.

Although a modest post-treatment rise in temperature has been reported occasionally from several areas, fever is not a common side-effect of oxamniquine, except in Egypt where it appears to be characteristic. The cause is not known. Increased immune complexes and excretion of antigens occurred in only half the cases, there is no evidence that Egyptian patients metabolise the drug differently to produce a pyrogenic metabolite, and the effect has not been seen in other areas where a similar high-dose regimen is used.— R. Foster, *Trans. R. Soc. trop. Med. Hyg.*, 1987, *81*, 55.

EFFECTS ON THE NERVOUS SYSTEM. In 37 patients with *Schistosoma mansoni* infection treated successfully with oxamniquine, dizziness and drowsiness were most common but the only significant adverse effect was the development of EEG abnormalities in 6 of 34 patients whose pretreatment EEG was normal. Of the 3 patients with pre-existing EEG abnormalities one suffered a grand mal seizure during therapy as previously reported (J.S. Keystone, *Am. J. trop. Med. Hyg.*, 1978, *27*, 360), one did not suffer seizures, and the third received phenytoin prophylaxis during oxamniquine therapy. It was considered prudent to administer anticonvulsant drugs prior to initiating oxamniquine therapy in patients with a history of seizure disorder. Since completion of this study a patient with no history of seizures suffered a grand mal seizure 2 hours after each of the second and third doses of oxamniquine.— S. Krajden *et al.*, *Am. J. trop. Med. Hyg.*, 1983, *32*, 1344.

The main neuropsychiatric side-effects seen in 180 Brazilian patients with *Schistosoma mansoni* infection treated with single oral doses of oxamniquine were: drowsiness (50.6%), dizziness (41.1%), headache (16.1%), temporary amnesia (2.2%), behavioural disturbances (1.7%), chills (1.1%), and seizures (1.1%). An EEG was performed before and after treatment in 20 patients; there were alterations in 3 but they were not associated with neuropsychiatric changes.— S. A. de Carvalho *et al.*, *Revta Inst. Med. trop. S Paulo*, 1985, *27*, 132.

Precautions

Oxamniquine should be used with caution in epileptics or patients with a history of epilepsy. Patients should be warned that oxamniquine can cause dizziness or drowsiness and if affected they should not drive or operate machinery.

Absorption and Fate

Oxamniquine is readily absorbed following administration by mouth. Peak plasma concentrations are achieved 1 to 3 hours after a dose and the plasma half-life is 1 to 2.5 hours.

It is extensively metabolised to inactive metabolites, principally the 6-carboxy derivative, which are excreted in the urine. About 70% of a dose of oxamniquine is excreted as the 6-carboxy metabolite within 12 hours of administration; traces of 2-carboxy metabolite have also been detected in the urine.

A study of the pharmacokinetics of oxamniquine in Sudanese subjects, including 9 patients with advanced hepatosplenic schistosomiasis and 5 controls, following a single 1-g oral dose. In the 9 patients peak plasma concentrations ranged from 300 to 2252 ng per mL (mean, 1267 ng per mL) 1 to 3 hours after the dose compared with 1205 to 2619 ng per mL (mean, 1983 ng per mL) after 1 to 2 hours in the 5 healthy subjects. Mean plasma half-lives for patients and controls were 151.2 and 111.0 minutes, respectively. There were no significant differences in time to reach peak concentration or plasma half-lives. It seemed that elimination of oxamniquine may be non-linear and, although the mean peak plasma concentration was 36% lower in patients than in controls, the higher dosage requirements noted in Sudanese patients were unlikely to be due to lower plasma concentrations. There was no correlation between severity of the disease and pharmacokinetic values.— T. K. Daneshmend and M. A. Homeida, *J. antimicrob. Chemother.*, 1987, *19*, 87.

Further references to the pharmacokinetics of oxamniquine: G. O. Kokwaro and G. Taylor, *J. Pharm. Pharmac.*, 1985, *37*, *Suppl.*, 41P.

Uses and Administration

Oxamniquine is an anthelmintic with schistosomicidal activity against *Schistosoma mansoni*, but not against other *Schistosoma* spp. It causes worms to shift from the mesenteric veins to the liver where the male worms are retained; the female worms return to the mesentery, but can no longer release eggs.

Oxamniquine is given by mouth, preferably after food, in the treatment of schistosomiasis due to *S. mansoni*. Dosage depends on the geographical origin of the infection and total doses range from 15 to 60 mg per kg body-weight given over 1 to 3 days (see below for further details).

A review of clinical experience with oxamniquine in the treatment of schistosomiasis.— R. Foster, *Trans. R. Soc. trop. Med. Hyg.*, 1987, *81*, 55.

The report of a WHO Expert Committee on the control of schistosomiasis. Oxamniquine is a tetrahydroquinoline active only against *Schistosoma mansoni* infection. The adult male worms are more susceptible to oxamniquine than the female worms. The precise mode of action is not known, but worm death has been seen to be associated with the formation of large subtegumental vesicles. Early developmental stages of *S. mansoni* are also vulnerable to oxamniquine. Distinct differences in response to oxamniquine occur in schistosoma strains of South American and African origin. A single dose of 15 mg per kg body-weight is adequate for adults in South America, the Caribbean islands, and West Africa; infections in children are less responsive and a single total dose of 20 mg per kg or two doses of 10 mg per kg in one day, separated by an interval of 3 to 8 hours, is recommended for patients under 14 years of age in South America and the Caribbean.

In Africa no distinction is made between doses for adults and children. In East and Central Africa (Kenya, Madagascar, Malawi, Rwanda/Burundi, Tanzania, Zambia) and the Arabian peninsular a total dose of 30 mg per kg, given as 15 mg per kg twice daily for one day or once daily for two consecutive days, is required. In Sudan, Uganda, and Zaire a total dose of 40 mg per kg is necessary. In Egypt, South Africa, and Zimbabwe a total dose of 60 mg per kg, given as 15 mg per kg twice daily for two days, or 20 mg per kg daily for three consecutive days, is required. Ethiopia occupies an intermediate position between East Africa and Egypt, both geographically and in terms of dosage.

Oxamniquine has been widely used for the treatment of rural communities with *S. mansoni* infection. After the appropriate therapeutic dose of oxamniquine, cure-rates of at least 60%, and often more than 90%, can be expected. Egg excretion in those not cured will be reduced by over 80%, and usually by over 90%, one year after treatment.

Oxamniquine is well tolerated, especially if given after a meal and side-effects have not limited its use in large-scale treatment programmes.— The Control of Schistosomiasis, *Tech. Rep. Ser. Wld Hlth Org. No. 728*, 1985.

Studies on the mode of action of oxamniquine and related schistosomicidal drugs, including hycanthone and lucanthone.— L. Pica-Mattoccia and D. Cioli, *Am. J. trop. Med. Hyg.*, 1985, *34*, 112.

An 11-year evaluation of successful disease control with oxamniquine in a rural area of Brazil where severe schistosomiasis mansoni is endemic. Systematic treatment of infected populations was considered a practical and potent method to prevent and cure disease caused by *Schistosoma mansoni* in Brazil.— A. C. Sleigh *et al.*, *Lancet*, 1986, *1*, 635.

For further details on schistosomiasis and its control and a comparative study of oxamniquine and praziquantel, see praziquantel (p.65).

Preparations

Oxamniquine Capsules *(U.S.P.)*

Proprietary Preparations

Vansil *(Pfizer, UK)*. *Capsules*, oxamniquine 250 mg.

Proprietary Names and Manufacturers

Mansil *(Pfizer, USA)*; Vansil *(Pfizer, Fr.; Pfizer, UK; Pfizer, USA)*.

796-x

Oxantel Embonate *(BANM, rINNM).*

CP-14445-16; Oxantel Pamoate *(USAN)*. *(E)*-3-[2-(1,4,5,6-Tetrahydro-1-methylpyrimidin-2-yl)vinyl]phenol 4,4′-methylenebis(3-hydroxy-2-naphthoate).

$C_{13}H_{16}N_2O,C_{23}H_{16}O_6$=604.7.

CAS — 36531-26-7 (oxantel); 68813-55-8 (embonate); 42408-84-4 (embonate).

A pale yellow crystalline powder. Oxantel embonate 2.8 g is approximately equivalent to 1 g of oxantel. Practically **insoluble** in water.

Adverse Effects

Nausea, vomiting, abdominal pain, and diarrhoea may occasionally occur.

Absorption and Fate

Oxantel embonate is only slightly absorbed from the gastro-intestinal tract. Urinary excretion indicates that up to 8% of a therapeutic dose may be absorbed.

Uses and Administration

Oxantel embonate is an analogue of pyrantel embonate with anthelmintic activity against whipworm (*Trichuris*). It is given together with pyrantel embonate to treat mixed intestinal nematode infections that include whipworm.

In the treatment of trichuriasis a dose of 10 to 15 mg of oxantel per kg body-weight daily for 2 to 3 days has been recommended. Single doses are effective only in light infections. Unlike its analogue pyrantel, oxantel is not effective in ascariasis. However, the combination of pyrantel and oxantel has been used successfully as a wide-spectrum anthelmintic, being effective against *Ascaris*, *Enterobius*, *Trichuris*, and hookworm.— Report of a WHO Scientific Group on Intestinal Protozoan and Helminthic Infections, *Tech. Rep. Ser. Wld Hlth Org. No. 666*, 1981.

Trichuris trichiura was eliminated from 20 of 26 children and adults given oxantel 10 mg per kg body-weight as a single dose, from 23 of 25 given 15 mg per kg, and from 10 of 10 given 20 mg per kg.— E. G. Garcia, *Am. J. trop. Med. Hyg.*, 1976, *25*, 914.

Proceedings of a symposium on trichuriasis and mixed intestinal nematode infections and the use of combined oxantel-pyrantel preparations.— *Drugs*, 1978, *15*, *Suppl.* 1, 63–110.

Proprietary Names and Manufacturers

Pfizer, USA.

13060-x

Oxfendazole *(BAN, USAN, rINN).*

RS-8858. Methyl 5-phenylsulphinyl-1*H*-benzimidazol-2-ylcarbamate.

$C_{15}H_{13}N_3O_3S$=315.3.

CAS — 53716-50-0.

Pharmacopoeias. In *Cz.* Also in *B.P. Vet.*

A white or almost white powder with a slight characteristic odour. Practically **insoluble** in water; slightly soluble in acetone, chloroform, ether, and methyl alcohol. **Protect** from light.

Oxfendazole is a benzimidazole anthelmintic structurally related to mebendazole (see p.57). It is used in veterinary practice.

Proprietary Veterinary Names and Manufacturers

Synanthic *(Syntex, UK)*; Systamex *(Coopers Animal Health, UK)*.

13062-f

Oxibendazole *(BAN, USAN, rINN).*

SKF-30310. Methyl 5-propoxy-1*H*-benzimidazol-2-ylcarbamate.

$C_{12}H_{15}N_3O_3$=249.3.

CAS — 20559-55-1.

Oxibendazole is a benzimidazole anthelmintic structurally related to mebendazole (see p.57). It is used in veterinary practice.

Proprietary Veterinary Names and Manufacturers

Dio *(Alan Hitchins, UK)*; Equidin *(Univet, UK)*; Equitac *(Smith Kline Animal Health, UK)*; Loditac *(Smith Kline Animal Health, UK)*.

13071-d

Oxyclozanide *(BAN, rINN).*

ICI-46683. 3,3′,5,5′,6-Pentachloro-2′-hydroxysalicylanilide.

$C_{13}H_6Cl_5NO_3$=401.5.

CAS — 2277-92-1.

Pharmacopoeias. In *Cz.* and *Nord.* Also in *B.P. Vet.*

A cream-coloured, odourless, powder. Very slightly **soluble** in water; soluble 1 in 20 of alcohol and 1 in 5 of acetone; slightly soluble in chloroform.

Oxyclozanide is a veterinary anthelmintic used in the control of liver-fluke infections in cattle and sheep.

Proprietary Veterinary Names and Manufacturers
Zanil *(Coopers Animal Health, UK).*

13079-p

Pararosaniline Embonate *(rINN).*
CI-403A; CN-15573-23A; NSC-107529; Pararosaniline Pamoate *(USAN)*; PS-1286; TAC Pamoate; Tris-(aminophenyl)carbonium Pamoate. 4-[(4-Aminophenyl)(4-iminocyclohexa-2,5-dien-1-ylidene)methyl]aniline 4,4′-methylenebis(3-hydroxy-2-naphthoate) (2:1) dihydrate.
$(C_{19}H_{18}N_3)_2,C_{23}H_{14}O_6,2H_2O$ = 999.1.

CAS — 569-61-9 (pararosaniline); 7232-51-1 (embonate, dihydrate).

Pararosaniline embonate is a schistosomicide with activity against *Schistosoma mansoni, S. haematobium* , and *S. japonicum.*

Proprietary Names and Manufacturers
Parke, Davis, USA.

13081-h

Parbendazole *(BAN, USAN, rINN).*
SKF-29044. Methyl 5-butyl-1*H*-benzimidazol-2-ylcarbamate.
$C_{13}H_{17}N_3O_2$=247.3.

CAS — 14255-87-9.

Parbendazole is a benzimidazole anthelmintic structurally related to mebendazole (see p.57). It is used in veterinary practice.

Proprietary Veterinary Names and Manufacturers
Helmatac *(Smith Kline Animal Health, UK)*; Topclip Wormer Pellets *(Ciba-Geigy Agrochemicals, UK).*

797-r

Pelletierine Tannate
Punicine Tannate.

Pharmacopoeias. In *Arg.*

A mixture of the tannates of the alkaloids obtained from the bark of the root and stems of the pomegranate, *Punica granatum* (Punicaceae). *Arg. P.* allows other varieties.

Pelletierine tannate has a specific action on tapeworms but is ineffective against other intestinal parasites. Its highly toxic nature prohibits its use.

798-f

Phenothiazine *(rINN).*

$C_{12}H_9NS$=199.3.

CAS — 92-84-2.

Pharmacopoeias. In *Arg., Aust., Fr., It.,* and *Nord.*

Phenothiazine is too toxic for use in human medicine. It has been used as an anthelmintic in veterinary medicine.

Many derivatives of phenothiazine are used in human medicine, particularly as antihistamines and tranquillisers.

13108-x

Phthalofyne *(USAN).*
Ftalofyne *(rINN)*; Methylparafynol Phthalate; Methylpentynol Phthalate; Methylpentynyl Phthalate; NSC-25614. 3-Methylpent-1-yn-3-yl hydrogen phthalate.
$C_{14}H_{14}O_4$=246.3.

CAS — 131-67-9.

Phthalofyne is a veterinary anthelmintic.

13112-c

Picadex
Piperazine Carbon Disulphide Complex. A polymer of the equimolecular complex of piperazine and carbon disulphide.
$(C_5H_{10}N_2S_2)_n$=162.3×*n*.

CAS — 99-00-3 ($C_5H_{10}N_2S_2$).

Picadex is an anthelmintic which has been used in veterinary medicine.

799-d

Piperazine Adipate *(BAN).*

Piperaz. Adip.; Piperazini Adipas; Piperazinum Adipicum.
$C_4H_{10}N_2,C_6H_{10}O_4$=232.3.

CAS — 142-88-1.

Pharmacopoeias. In *Aust., Br., Cz., Egypt., Eur., Fr., Ger., Ind., Int., It., Jpn, Jug., Neth., Nord., Pol., Roum., Rus., Swiss,* and *Turk.* Also in *B.P. Vet.*

A white crystalline powder. Piperazine adipate 120 mg is approximately equivalent to 100 mg of piperazine hydrate. **Soluble** 1 in 18 of water; practically insoluble in alcohol. **Store** in well-closed containers.

801-n

Piperazine Citrate *(BAN, USAN).*

Hydrous Tripiperazine Dicitrate; Piperazini Citras.
$(C_4H_{10}N_2)_3,2C_6H_8O_7,xH_2O$=642.7 (anhydrous substance).

CAS — 144-29-6 (anhydrous); 41372-10-5 (hydrate).

Pharmacopoeias. In *Aust., Br., Chin., Egypt., Eur., Fr., Ger., Ind., Int., It., Neth., Swiss, Turk.,* and *U.S.* Also in *B.P. Vet.*

A white, odourless, or almost odourless, crystalline or granular powder. It contains a variable amount of water. Piperazine citrate 125 mg is approximately equivalent to 100 mg of piperazine hydrate. **Soluble** 1 in 1.5 of water; practically insoluble in alcohol and ether. A 10% solution in water has a pH of about 5. **Store** in well-closed containers.

802-h

Piperazine Hydrate *(BAN).*

Diethylenediamine; Hexahydropyrazine; Piperazidine; Piperazine; Piperazini Hydras; Piperazinum Hydricum. Piperazine hexahydrate.
$C_4H_{10}N_2,6H_2O$=194.2.

CAS — 110-85-0 (anhydrous); 142-63-2 (hexahydrate).

Pharmacopoeias. In *Aust., Br., Cz., Eur., Fr., Ger., Ind., It., Jug., Neth., Pol., Port., Roum., Span.,* and *Swiss. Braz.* and *U.S.* include anhydrous piperazine ($C_4H_{10}N_2$ = 86.14).

Colourless deliquescent crystals. M.p. about 43°. The dosage of the salts of piperazine is usually expressed in terms of piperazine hydrate; 100 mg of piperazine hydrate is approximately equivalent to 120 mg of piperazine adipate, to 125 mg of piperazine citrate, and to 104 mg of piperazine phosphate.
Freely **soluble** in water and alcohol; very slightly soluble in ether. A 5% solution in water has a pH of 10.5 to 12.0. **Store** in airtight containers. Protect from light.

A decrease in the content of piperazine in syrups on storage was attributed to interaction with fructose and glucose formed by hydrolysis of sucrose. A syrup prepared with sorbitol lost no potency when stored at 25° for 14 months.— A. Nielsen and P. Reimer, *Arch. Pharm. Chemi, scient. Edn,* 1975, *3,* 73.

803-m

Piperazine Phosphate *(BAN).*

Piperazini Phosphas.
$C_4H_{10}N_2,H_3PO_4,H_2O$=202.1.

CAS — 14538-56-8 (anhydrous); 18534-18-4 (monohydrate).

Pharmacopoeias. In *Br., Chin., Ind.,* and *Int.* Also in *B.P. Vet.*

A white odourless or almost odourless crystalline powder. Piperazine phosphate 104 mg is approximately equivalent to 100 mg of piperazine hydrate. **Soluble** 1 in 60 of water; practically insoluble in alcohol. A 1% solution in water has a pH of 6.0 to 6.5.

Adverse Effects

Serious adverse effects are rare with piperazine and are generally evidence of overdosage or impaired excretion. Nausea, vomiting, diarrhoea, abdominal pain, headache, and urticaria occasionally occur. Severe neurotoxicity has been reported with symptoms including somnolence, dizziness, nystagmus, muscular incoordination and weakness, ataxia, myoclonic contractions, choreiform movements, tremor, convulsions, and loss of reflexes.
Transient visual disturbances such as blurred vision have occurred occasionally and there were reports of cataract formation after treatment with piperazine although they do not appear to have been substantiated.
Hypersensitivity reactions have occurred in some individuals, especially in those sensitised during occupational exposure.

A study in 2 healthy subjects indicated that mononitrosation of piperazine can occur in the stomach to produce the potential carcinogen *N*-mononitrosopiperazine; the more potent *N,N*-dinitrosopiperazine was not found (B.T.D. Bellander *et al., Lancet,* 1981, *2,* 372). However, potentially carcinogenic *N*-nitroso compounds are very widely distributed in food, drink, and many other products, but there is no direct proof of a causal role in the aetiology of a specific human disease (S.R. Tannenbaum, *ibid.,* 1983, *1,* 629). For further reference to *N*-nitroso compounds and nitrosamines, see under Adverse Effects in Sodium Nitrite (p.854).

ALLERGY. A 55-year-old man, with a history of eczema and respiratory symptoms due to occupational exposure to piperazine, developed pruritus and respiratory symptoms on patch testing with piperazine.— S. Fregert, *Contact Dermatitis,* 1976, *2,* 61.

A 37-year-old man with a contact allergy to ethylenediamine (obtained from applications of Tri-Adcortyl cream) developed a cross-sensitivity reaction on 3 occasions to piperazine.— S. Wright and R. R. M. Harman, *Br. med. J.* 1983, *287,* 463.

EFFECTS ON THE BLOOD. A 4-year-old African boy developed haemolytic anaemia. He, but no other member of the family, had a deficiency of glucose-6-phosphate dehydrogenase. No cause for the haemolysis was found except that 2 days previously he had taken Pripsen (piperazine and senna).— N. Buchanan *et al.* (letter), *Br. med. J.,* 1971, *2,* 110.

EFFECTS ON THE LIVER. A reaction resembling viral hepatitis occurred on 2 occasions in a 25-year-old woman after the administration of piperazine; it appeared to be a hypersensitivity reaction.— A. N. Hamlyn *et al., Gastroenterology,* 1976, *70,* 1144.

Precautions

Piperazine is contra-indicated in patients with liver disease, epilepsy or renal failure and should be given with care to patients with latent epilepsy, neurological disturbances, or impaired renal function.
The anthelmintic effect of piperazine may be antagonised by pyrantel.

INTERACTIONS. Caution has been advised in patients receiving phenothiazines because of the possibility that piperazine might enhance their adverse effects. Convulsions developed in a child given chlorpromazine following treatment with piperazine several days earlier and in *animals* given the two drugs (B.M. Boulos and L.E. Davis, *New Engl. J. Med.,* 1969, *280,* 1245). However, Armbrecht (*ibid.,* 1970, *282,* 1490) was unable to confirm the interaction in *animals* and, following a further *animal* study, Sturman (*Br. J. Pharmac.*, 1974, *50*, 153) concluded that enhancement of the effect of chlorpromazine would only be clinically significant when high concentrations of piperazine were reached in the body.

PREGNANCY AND THE NEONATE. Although there is no new evidence the Committee on the Review of Medicines (CRM) in the *UK* has requested manufacturers to caution against the use of piperazine in pregnancy unless immediate treatment is deemed essential. Piperazine has been taken off the market in some European countries because of general concern about its safety, but the CRM concluded that the incidence of serious adverse reactions was low and that with appropriate warnings products containing piperazine could be available from pharmacies without a prescription.— *Pharm. J.*, 1988, *240*, 367.

Absorption and Fate

Piperazine is readily absorbed from the gastro-intestinal tract and is excreted in the urine, partly as metabolites. The rate at which different individuals excrete piperazine has been reported to vary widely.

Following the administration of piperazine citrate by mouth, between 15 and 75% was recovered from the urine. Urinary excretion was maximal between 2 and 6 hours and nearly completed in 24 hours.— S. Hanna and A. Tang, *J. pharm. Sci.*, 1973, *62*, 2024.

Uses and Administration

Piperazine is an anthelmintic effective against the intestinal nematodes *Ascaris lumbricoides* (roundworm) and *Enterobius vermicularis* (pinworm, threadworm). The mechanism of action is not fully understood, but piperazine produces a flaccid muscle paralysis in susceptible worms which are then easily dislodged from their position by the movement of the gut and are expelled in the faeces.

Piperazine is usually administered as the citrate or phosphate, but dosage is generally stated in terms of the hexahydrate, piperazine hydrate.

For the treatment of roundworm infection, a single dose equivalent to 4 g of piperazine hydrate is given by mouth, preferably in the morning; children may be given the equivalent of 120 mg per kg body-weight up to a maximum of 4 g. Some authorities have suggested the equivalent of 75 mg per kg daily, to a maximum of 3.5 g, on 2 successive days.

For elimination of threadworms, treatment should be continued for 7 days. Adults and children over 12 years of age are given the equivalent of 2 g of the hydrate once daily, children aged 5 to 12 the equivalent of 1.5 g daily, those aged 2 to 4 the equivalent of 750 mg daily, and those under 2 the equivalent of 50 to 75 mg per kg body-weight daily. A second course after a 7-day interval may be required.

Suppositories containing piperazine sebacate are used in some countries.

The adipate and dihydrochloride are used in veterinary medicine.

Preparations of Piperazine and its Salts

Piperazine Citrate Elixir *(B.P.)*. Piperazine Citrate Oral Solution. Store at a temperature not exceeding 25°. Protect from light.

Piperazine Citrate Syrup *(U.S.P.)*. Store in airtight containers.

Piperazine Citrate Tablets *(U.S.P.)*. Store in airtight containers.

Piperazine Phosphate Tablets *(B.P.)*

Proprietary Preparations of Piperazine and its Salts

Antepar *(Wellcome, UK)*. *Tablets*, scored, piperazine hydrate 500 mg (as piperazine phosphate). *Elixir*, piperazine hydrate 750 mg/5 mL (as piperazine hydrate and piperazine citrate).

Ascalix *(Wallace Mfg Chem., UK)*. *Syrup*, piperazine hydrate 750 mg/5 mL (as piperazine citrate). Also available as 4 g/20-mL sachet and 4 g/30-mL bottle.

Pripsen *(Reckitt & Colman Pharmaceuticals, UK)*. *Oral powder*, piperazine phosphate 4 g and sennosides 15.3 mg/sachet.

Proprietary Names and Manufacturers of Piperazine and its Salts

Adelmitex *(Liberman, Spain)*; Adipalit *(Lipha, Ital.)*; Adiver; Aloxin Forte; Antelmina *(Clin Midy, Fr.)*; Antepar *(Wellcome, UK; Wellcome, USA)*; Anthelcolin; Anticucs *(Camps, Spain)*; Antivermine; Ascalix *(Wallace Mfg Chem., UK; Wallace, USA)*; Ascapel; Ascarinex; Ascarzan; Bioxurin; Citrazine; Diatesurico; Divermex; Dr. Ronwins Worm Elixir; Ectodyne *(Regent, UK)*; Entacyl *(Allen & Hanburys, Canad.; Duncan, Flockhart, UK)*; Escovermine *(Streuli, Switz.)*; Evilon; Fugapar *(Carol, Spain)*; Helmezine *(Allen & Hanburys, UK)*; Helmizin; Hitepar *(High Noon, Pakistan)*; Ismiverm; Jetsan; Lombrifher *(Fher, Spain)*; Lombrikal Piperazina; Lombrimade; Mimedran *(Esteve, Spain)*; Minizin; Mintrex; Nématorazine *(Millot, Fr.)*; Neox *(Rocador, Spain)*; Oxiustip; Oxurasin; Oxyvermin; Parabel; Parixon; Piavermit; Pip-a-ray *(Vernleigh, S.Afr.)*; Pipenin; Piperacina Midy; Piperacyl; Piperasol; Piperiod; Piperol *(Vaillant-Defresne, Fr.)*; Pipersan; Piperverm; Pipralen *(Lennon, S.Afr.)*; Piprazyl; Piprelix; Razinate; Rotape Worm; Starworm; Tasnon *(Tropon, Ger.)*; Upixon; Uvilon *(Bayer, Ital.)*; Vermenter; Vermex; Vermicompren *(E. Merck, Ger.)*; Vermigon; Vermiquimpe *(Quimpe, Spain)*; Vermizin; Vinoverm; Wormelix *(SCS, S.Afr.)*; Wurmex; Wurmsirup Siegfried.

The following names have been used for multi-ingredient preparations containing piperazine and its salts— Pripsen *(Reckitt & Colman Pharmaceuticals, UK)*.

804-b

Pomegranate Bark

Granado; Granati Cortex; Granatrinde; Granatum; Grenadier; Melograno; Pomegranate; Pomegranate Root Bark; Romeira.

Pharmacopoeias. In *Chin.*, *Port.*, and *Span.*

NOTE. Pomegranate Rind, the dried pericarp separated from the fruit of the pomegranate, contains gallotannic acid but no alkaloids.

The dried bark of the stem and root of *Punica granatum* (Punicaceae) containing about 0.4 to 0.9% of alkaloids (see Pelletierine Tannate, p.63).

Pomegranate bark has been used for the expulsion of tapeworms.

It was recommended by the Food Additives and Contaminants Committee that pomegranate root be prohibited for use in foods as a flavouring agent.— *Report on the Review of Flavourings in Food*, FAC/REP/22, Ministry of Agriculture Fisheries and Food, London, HM Stationery Office, 1976.

13161-h

Praziquantel *(BAN, USAN, rINN)*.

EMBAY-8440. 2-Cyclohexylcarbonyl-1,2,3,6,7,11b-hexahydropyrazino[2,1-*a*]isoquinolin-4-one.

$C_{19}H_{24}N_2O_2$=312.4.

CAS — 55268-74-1.

Pharmacopoeias. In *Chin.* and *U.S.*

White or practically white crystalline powder; odourless or with a faint characteristic odour. Very slightly **soluble** in water; freely soluble in alcohol and in chloroform. **Store** in well-closed containers. Protect from light.

Adverse Effects

Praziquantel is generally well tolerated and side-effects are usually mild and transient. Headache, dizziness, drowsiness, abdominal discomfort, and nausea have been reported most frequently; there may also be vomiting and diarrhoea. Allergic-type reactions such as fever, urticaria, and pruritic skin rashes may occur; they may be due to death of the infecting parasites. Raised liver enzyme values have been reported rarely.

Most patients given praziquantel for the treatment of cerebral cysticercosis suffer adverse nervous system effects, including headache, hyperthermia, seizures, and intracranial hypertension, which are thought to result from an inflammatory response to dead and dying parasites in the central nervous system. The concomitant administration of corticosteroids is advised in such patients. See also under Cysticercosis in Uses and Administration (below).

A retrospective survey from China on the side-effects of praziquantel involving 25 693 patients treated for *Schistosoma japonicum* infection.— M. G. Chen *et al.*, *S. E. Asian J. trop. med. publ. Hlth*, 1983, 14, 495.

EFFECTS ON THE GASTRO-INTESTINAL TRACT. A report of unexpectedly frequent and intense episodes of colicky abdominal pain and bloody diarrhoea in a small community in Zaire shortly after treatment for *Schistosoma mansoni* infection with single doses of praziquantel 40 mg per kg body-weight by mouth.— A. M. Polderman *et al.*, *Trans. R. Soc. trop. Med. Hyg.*, 1984, *78*, 752. A similar syndrome in 4 of 20 patients with *Schistosoma japonicum* infection given praziquantel. The abdominal pain occurring in these patients was very different from the mild abdominal discomfort much more commonly reported with praziquantel therapy.— G. Watt *et al.* (letter), *ibid.*, 1986, *80*, 345.

Precautions

Patients should be warned that praziquantel may cause dizziness or drowsiness and if affected they should not drive or operate machinery during or for 24 hours after treatment.

Praziquantel is excreted in breast milk and mothers should not breast feed during or for 72 hours after treatment.

Absorption and Fate

Praziquantel is rapidly absorbed after administration by mouth, even when taken with a meal; more than 80% of a dose is reported to be absorbed. Peak plasma concentrations are achieved 1 to 3 hours after a dose, but there is a pronounced first-pass effect and praziquantel undergoes rapid and extensive metabolism in the liver being hydroxylated to metabolites that are thought to be inactive. The plasma elimination half-life of praziquantel is 1 to 1.5 hours and that of the metabolites about 4 hours.

It is excreted in the urine, mainly as metabolites, about 80% of the dose being eliminated within 4 days and more than 90% of this in the first 24 hours.

Praziquantel is excreted in breast milk.

References to the absorption and fate of praziquantel: G. Leopold *et al.*, *Eur. J. clin. Pharmac.*, 1978, *14*, 281; K. U. Bühring *et al.*, *Eur. J. Drug Metab. Pharmacokinet.*, 1978, *3*, 179; K. Patzschke *et al.*, *ibid.*, 1979, *4*, 149.

Uses and Administration

Praziquantel is an anthelmintic with a broad spectrum of activity against trematodes (flukes) and cestodes (tapeworms). It is administered by mouth.

Praziquantel is active against all species of *Schistosoma* pathogenic to man. In the treatment of schistosomiasis it is given on one day as three doses of 20 mg per kg body-weight with food at intervals of 4 to 6 hours; alternatively 40 mg per kg may be given as a single dose. See below for further details of dosage in schistosomiasis, other trematode infections, and cestode infections.

Reviews of praziquantel: R. D. Pearson and R. L. Guerrant, *Ann. intern. Med.*, 1983, *99*, 195 and 574 (correction); C. P. Conlon and C. J. Ellis, *J. antimicrob. Chemother.*, 1985, *15*, 1.

ADMINISTRATION IN RENAL FAILURE. Severe renal insufficiency could be one of the final consequences of *Schistosoma haematobium* infection. Investigation in a uraemic patient with *S. haematobium* infection undergoing haemodialysis indicated that the pharmacokinetics of praziquantel were not affected by the underlying kidney disease and that the use of usual doses in the treatment of such patients was possible.— P. O. Pehrson *et al.*, *Trans. R. Soc. trop. Med. Hyg.*, 1983, *77*, 687.

CESTODE (TAPEWORM) INFECTIONS. In the *USA* praziquantel has been recommended, in a single dose of 10 to 20 mg per kg body-weight, as an alternative to niclosamide in the treatment of tapeworm infections due to

Diphyllobothrium latum (fish tapeworm), *Taenia saginata* (beef tapeworm), *Taenia solium* (pork tapeworm), and *Dipylidium caninum* (dog tapeworm); as the drug of choice in a single dose of 25 mg per kg in the treatment of *Hymenolepis nana* (dwarf tapeworm) infection; and as the drug of choice in a dose of 50 mg per kg daily in three divided doses for 14 days in the treatment of *Cysticercus cellulosae* infection (cysticercosis). In cysticercosis, corticosteroids should be given for 2 to 3 days before and during praziquantel therapy.— *Med. Lett.*, 1986, *28*, 9.

Cysticercosis. A review of recent advances in the diagnosis and treatment of cerebral cysticercosis. Cysticercosis is caused by infection with the cysticercus or larval form of *Taenia solium*, the pork tapeworm, and is particularly common in Mexico and other parts of Central and South America, Africa, India, China, Eastern Europe, and Indonesia. Humans acquire the adult tapeworm by eating undercooked pork, but can become infected with the cysticercus by ingesting food contaminated with tapeworm eggs. Cysticerci can lodge anywhere in the body, especially in the brain and skeletal muscle. Signs and symptoms of infection depend on where they are located, although most of the morbidity and mortality arises from CNS involvement.
Surgical intervention was considered virtually the only form of treatment, but praziquantel has been used recently with promising results. Most patients with cerebral cysticercosis are currently treated with praziquantel 50 mg per kg body-weight daily in three divided doses for 15 days. Prolonged administration may be associated with an increase in side-effects due directly to the drug. Corticosteroids have frequently been employed to suppress exacerbations of symptoms associated with treatment.
Although issues such as optimal doses, duration of therapy, and whether the concomitant use of steroids is warranted still need to be addressed, there is no doubt that praziquantel represents a major advance in the treatment of cerebral cysticercosis. Nevertheless, the introduction of simple, preventive health practices in endemic areas would be even more effective in controlling this disease.— T. E. Nash and F. A. Neva, *New Engl. J. Med.*, 1984, *311*, 1492.

Beneficial results with praziquantel 50 mg per kg body-weight daily for 15 days in 26 patients with cysticercosis of the brain parenchyma. Corticosteroids were not given.— J. Sotelo *et al.*, *New Engl. J. Med.*, 1984, *310*, 1001. Criticism and the view that corticosteroids should be given concomitantly.— L. D. deGhetaldi *et al.* (letter), *ibid.*, *311*, 732; F. Ciferri (letter), *ibid.*, 733; M. A. Goldberg (letter), *ibid.* Reply and agreement that corticosteroids should be given.— J. Sotelo *et al.* (letter), *ibid.*, 734.

Comment on the cerebrospinal fluid (CSF) reaction syndrome during treatment of neurocysticercosis with praziquantel and a report of 3 patients with a delayed reaction. An 'immediate' reaction has occurred in 92 to 100% of patients on praziquantel alone and in 11 to 16% of those on concurrent corticosteroids (F. Ciferri, *New Engl. J. Med.*, 1984, *311*, 733). A 'delayed' reaction has been reported only twice, but was seen in 3 patients during the past year. In each case a cluster of acute CNS reactions developed within about 2 weeks of finishing treatment with praziquantel; the sudden and unexpected development of papilloedema in 2 patients was a striking feature. Tolerance of praziquantel treatment appears to be no guarantee that a delayed CSF reaction syndrome will not develop. The syndrome can be treated successfully with corticosteroids or conservatively. Continuing the administration of corticosteroids during and perhaps after the full course of praziquantel may prevent the late reaction.— F. Ciferri (letter), *Lancet*, 1988, *1*, 642.

Further references to the successful use of praziquantel in the treatment of cysticercosis: D. Botero and S. Castano, *Am. J. trop. Med. Hyg.*, 1982, *31*, 811 (subcutaneous infection and neurocysticercosis in 35 patients; prednisone was given to minimise cerebral reactions to the death of parasites); L. D. deGhetaldi *et al.*, *Ann. intern. Med.*, 1983, *99*, 179 (cerebral cysticercosis; biphasic administration of dexamethasone and praziquantel in one patient); R. M. Norman and C. Kapadia, *Pediatrics*, 1986, *78*, 291 (cerebral cysticercosis; a 13-month-old infant given praziquantel 50 mg per kg body-weight daily for 14 days together with dexamethasone before and during therapy).

Lack of benefit with systemic praziquantel in a patient with intra-ocular cysticercosis.— P. Kestelyn and H. Taelman, *Br. J. Ophthal.*, 1985, *69*, 788. Praziquantel is contra-indicated by the manufacturers in the treatment of ocular cysticercosis because of the risk of irreparable lesions resulting from destruction of the parasite within the eye.

Hydatid disease. Although it has been suggested that praziquantel is unlikely to be effective in the treatment of hydatid disease, studies *in vitro* (D.L. Morris *et al.*, *J. antimicrob. Chemother.*, 1986, *18*, 687) have shown it to be a rapid and effective scolicidal agent against *Echinococcus granulosus*.

SCHISTOSOMIASIS. Schistosomiasis (bilharziasis) is a trematode infection caused by schistosomes or blood flukes. It is widely distributed and at least 200 million people are thought to be infected. The three species principally responsible are *Schistosoma mansoni*, the most widespread, occurring in Africa, the Middle East, the Caribbean, and South America; *S. haematobium* in Africa and the Middle East; and *S. japonicum* in the Far East. *S. intercalatum* is limited to Africa and *S. mekongi* to Southeast Asia.
Infection is transmitted to man by exposure to water containing larvae (cercariae) released by infected freshwater snails, the intermediate host. The larvae penetrate the skin and immature parasites (schistosomula) travel via the lymph and blood vessels to the lungs and liver and onto the veins of the intestinal or bladder walls where as adult worms they may reside for years. The worms do not multiply but produce eggs, a large proportion of which remain within the tissues, especially in the intestines, liver, and urinary tract. Some eggs are excreted in the urine or faeces and on reaching fresh water hatch into free-swimming miracidia which penetrate into snails living in the water to complete the cycle.
Penetration of the skin by the larvae results in inflammatory skin reactions and severe itching. This may be followed several weeks later by acute schistosomiasis, a serum sickness-like syndrome known in Japan as Katayama fever. It is most common and most severe in *S. japonicum* infection, less common in *S. mansoni* infection, and very rare in *S. haematobium* infection. The pathogenesis of chronic schistosomiasis is correlated with the extent of the worm burden, the number of eggs in the tissues, and the extent of the inflammatory reaction to them. Tissue damage is continuous and progressive. After many, mainly asymptomatic years, the results of progressive fibrotic tissue damage become evident. *S. mansoni* and *S. japonicum* infections commonly involve the intestines, liver, and spleen and *S. haematobium* infections the urinary tract. Manifestations of infection with *S. intercalatum* are similar to those of *S. mansoni* and those with *S. mekongi* are similar to those of *S. japonicum*. Other parts of the body such as the lungs and CNS may also be affected.
Methods of mass control of schistosomiasis include the provision of adequate water supplies and sanitation, destruction of the snails with molluscicides, and chemotherapy.

The report of a WHO Expert Committee on the control of schistosomiasis. Eradication of schistosomiasis or elimination of its transmission are long-term objectives, but the immediate aim is to control morbidity which is caused by the eggs deposited in the tissues. Thus reduction or elimination of the adult worms will reduce the risk of morbidity developing; this is the primary objective of chemotherapy. High cure-rates are achieved after treatment with all the new antischistosomal drugs and, even if egg excretion persists, the intensity of infection and the risk of developing disease are greatly reduced. Only three of the many drugs with antischistosomal activity, metriphonate, oxamniquine, and praziquantel, can be considered for large-scale chemotherapy.
Praziquantel is effective against *Schistosoma mansoni*, *S. haematobium*, *S. japonicum*, *S. mekongi*, *S. intercalatum*, and *S. mattheei*. Its mechanism of action cannot yet be explained at the molecular level, but is known to be associated with strong muscular contraction and tegumental vesicle formation. A single dose of 40 mg per kg body-weight of praziquantel is recommended for *S. haematobium*, *S. intercalatum*, or *S. mansoni* infections; up to 60 mg per kg may be required in certain areas for *S. mansoni* or mixed infections. The present recommended regimen for *S. japonicum* infections is 2 doses of 30 mg per kg (total dose 60 mg per kg) given with a 4-hour interval. In the field the cure-rate for *S. haematobium* infection is usually between 80 and 95% and the reduction in egg count in those not cured is usually 90 to 95% one year after treatment. A lower cure-rate has been seen in combined *S. mansoni* and *S. haematobium* infections. Cure-rates for *S. mansoni*, *S. intercalatum*, *S. japonicum*, and *S. mekongi* infections have generally been more than 60% after one year with a reduction in egg count of 95% or more in those not cured. About 1 million people have been treated with praziquantel to date. It is well tolerated, the main side-effects being abdominal discomfort, diarrhoea, dizziness, and sleepiness; fever and skin rash have been less frequent. All side-effects are less frequent when used for *S. haematobium* infection. Fainting, hallucinations, psychotic symptoms, and excitement have been observed for up to 15 days after treatment of *S. japonicum* infection and although the very rapid elimination of praziquantel from the body suggests that the drug is unlikely to be responsible, the relationship between these clinical manifestations and cerebral infection due to *S. japonicum* has not been fully evaluated.
Metriphonate is active only against *S. haematobium* and cure-rates have ranged from 40 to more than 80%, with a 90% reduction in egg counts in those not cured [for further details of metriphonate, see p.60].
Oxamniquine is active only against *S. mansoni* infection and cure-rates of at least 60%, and often more than 90%, can be expected. Egg excretion in those not cured is reduced by over 80% and usually by over 90% one year after treatment [for further details of oxamniquine, see p.62].
Other drugs under development include amoscanate [see p.48] which has been widely used in China.
The possibility of drug resistance occurring has been recognised. Resistance to oxamniquine and hycanthone can be induced experimentally and is genetically transmitted. In Brazil, strains of *S. mansoni* have been isolated from patients not completely cured by repeated standard doses of oxamniquine or hycanthone. All the resistant strains of *S. mansoni* are susceptible to praziquantel.
In conclusion, metriphonate, oxamniquine, and praziquantel were considered safe, highly effective, and easily administered orally at the community level and to provide the basis for a feasible strategy for morbidity control. Treatment reduces the prevalence and intensity of infection, prevents or reduces pathological manifestations in infected individuals, and is generally considered the most cost-effective way of achieving schistosomiasis control.— The Control of Schistosomiasis, *Tech. Rep. Ser. Wld Hlth Org. No. 728*, 1985. A single treatment with an antischistosomal drug should never be expected to achieve a permanent cure or to prevent infection. In general a planned assessment of the treatment programme is required after 6 months or 1 year in populations with a high prevalence of schistosomiasis.— *Bull. Wld Hlth Org.*, 1986, *64*, 23. Praziquantel has transformed the treatment of schistosomiasis since it is effective, often in a single dose, against all strains of *Schistosoma* and is extremely well tolerated. However, older drugs are still widely used including metriphonate against *S. haematobium* infection and oxamniquine against *S. mansoni* infection. Antimony salts, stibocaptate, hycanthone, and niridazole have been largely superseded because of their greater toxicity.— *WHO Drug Inf.*, 1987, *1*, 162.

In the *USA*, praziquantel has been recommended as the drug of choice for the treatment of schistosomiasis due to *Schistosoma haematobium*, *S. japonicum*, *S. mansoni*, and *S. mekongi*, in each case in a dose of 20 mg per kg body-weight three times daily for one day. Oxamniquine has been suggested as an alternative to praziquantel for *S. mansoni* infection.— *Med. Lett.*, 1986, *28*, 9.

Some reviews and discussions on schistosomiasis: *Lancet*, 1985, *2*, 1166 (control projects); K. M. De Cock, *Gut*, 1986, *27*, 734 (hepatosplenic schistosomiasis); *Lancet*, 1987, *1*, 1015 (immunity to schistosomiasis); *ibid.*, *2*, 194 (immunopathology).

Studies on various aspects of schistosomiasis: possible immunity to re-infection after the treatment of *Schistosoma mansoni* infection.— R. F. Sturrock *et al.*, *Trans. R. Soc. trop. Med. Hyg.*, 1983, *77*, 363; D. G. Colley *et al.*, *ibid.*, 1986, *80*, 952; R. F. Sturrock *et al.*, *ibid.*, 1987, *81*, 303.
Schistosomiasis in expatriates returning to Britain from the tropics.— A. D. Harries *et al.*, *Lancet*, 1986, *1*, 86.
Rapid detection of acute schistosomiasis with a circulating antigen assay.— E. G. Hayunga *et al.*, *Lancet*, 1986, *2*, 716.

A 2-year follow-up of a double-blind study in children infected with *Schistosoma haematobium* indicating that a single dose of praziquantel 40 mg per kg body-weight had superior all-round efficacy to treatment with single doses of niridazole 25 mg per kg together with metriphonate 10 mg per kg or metriphonate 10 mg per kg alone.— R. N. N. Pugh and C. H. Teesdale, *Trans. R. Soc. trop. Med. Hyg.*, 1984, *78*, 55. Praziquantel 40 mg per kg body-weight produced a greater reduction in symptoms and egg output than oxamniquine 15 mg per kg in a study involving 166 children infected with *Schistosoma mansoni*.— J. B. Rugemalila *et al.*, *J. trop. Med. Hyg.*, 1984, *87*, 231.

The condition of 3 patients with acute schistosomiasis deteriorated markedly during treatment with praziquantel or niridazole. The cause was not clear, but it seems advisable to delay treatment until after the acute phase of the disease or to cover treatment with a corticosteroid.— A. D. Harries and G. C. Cook, *J. Infect.*, 1987,

14, 159.

Further reports of the successful use of praziquantel in the treatment of schistosomiasis: Z. Farid and C. K. Wallace (letter), *Ann. intern. Med.*, 1983, *99*, 883 (*S. haematobium*; 30 mg per kg body-weight as a single oral dose in Egyptian children); Z. Farid *et al.* (letter), *ibid.*, 1984, *101*, 882 (*S. mansoni*; 3 doses of 20 mg per kg in one day in Egyptian children); B. Keittivuti *et al.*, *Trans. R. Soc. trop. Med. Hyg.*, 1984, *78*, 477 (*S. mekongi*; 2 doses of 30 mg per kg 6 hours apart in Cambodian refugees); G. Watt *et al.*, *Lancet*, 1986, *2*, 529 (*S. japonicum*; 3 doses of 20 mg per kg at 4-hour intervals on the same day in cerebral infection in the Philippines); C. N. Chunge *et al.* (letter), *Trans. R. Soc. trop. Med. Hyg.*, 1987, *81*, 170 (*S. mansoni*; a single dose of 30 mg per kg in an area in Kenya of low intensity infection); G. C. Cook and A. D. M. Bryceson (letter), *Lancet*, 1988, *1*, 127 (*S. mansoni*; longstanding infection 23 and 32 years after moving to the *UK* from Uganda).

For the use of praziquantel in *Schistosoma haematobium* infection and chronic renal failure, see Administration in Renal Failure, above.

TREMATODE (FLUKE) INFECTIONS. In the *USA* praziquantel has been recommended, in a dose of 25 mg per kg body-weight three times daily for one day, as the treatment of choice for fluke infections due to *Clonorchis sinensis* (Chinese liver fluke), the intestinal flukes *Fasciolopsis buski*, *Heterophyes heterophyes*, and *Metagonimus yokogawai*, and *Opisthorchis viverrini* (liver fluke). It has also been recommended as an alternative to bithionol in *Fasciola hepatica* (sheep liver fluke) infection in a dose of 25 mg per kg three times daily for 5 to 8 days and as the drug of choice in *Paragonimus westermani* (lung fluke) infection in a dose of 25 mg per kg three times daily for 2 days.— *Med. Lett.*, 1986, *28*, 9.

Clonorchiasis. The Chinese liver fluke which causes clonorchiasis belongs to the genus *Opisthorchis* (see Opisthorchiasis, below), but is still generally termed *Clonorchis sinensis*.

Complete cure was achieved in 20 Korean patients with clonorchiasis given praziquantel 25 mg per kg body-weight three times daily for 2 days; cure was almost complete in 33 patients given 25 mg per kg three times daily on a single day and either regimen was recommended (C.-T. Soh, *Arzneimittel-Forsch.*, 1984, *34*, 1156). Similar results were reported from a study in Taiwan (C.-Y. Chen and W.-C. Hsieh, *ibid.*, 1160) and single-day treatment was effective in a Chinese study involving 50 patients given 25 mg per kg three times daily, 20 mg per kg three times daily, or 40 mg per kg as a single dose (Q.-H. Kuang *et al.*, *ibid.*, 1162). Following the treatment of 2958 Koreans infected with *Clonorchis sinensis* with either praziquantel 40 mg per kg as a single dose, 30 mg per kg twice daily for one day, or 30 mg per kg three times daily for one day cure-rates of 87.1, 94.9, or 91.4%, respectively, were achieved (S.-H. Lee, *ibid.*, 1227); considering the efficacy, side-effects, and cost of praziquantel a single dose of 40 mg per kg was recommended for mass treatment under field conditions.

Fascioliasis. Human fascioliasis, infection caused by the sheep liver fluke *Fasciola hepatica*, is usually mild. Praziquantel 25 mg per kg body-weight three times a day for one or two days has been reported to be effective. Severe infection in a 28-year-old Yemenite woman was treated successfully with praziquantel 25 mg per kg three times a day by mouth for one day (R.H. Schiappacasse *et al.*, *J. infect. Dis.*, 1985, *152*, 1339). However, good therapeutic results were not achieved with praziquantel in 10 Egyptian patients (H.F. Farag *et al.*, *J. trop. Med. Hyg.*, 1986, *89*, 79). Following treatment egg counts dropped to zero in only 2 patients; they received 40 mg per kg as a single dose by mouth on 2 successive days. The other patients received either 40 mg per kg as a single dose (3 patients), 40 mg per kg on 2 successive days (2), or 75 mg per kg in 3 divided doses on 2 successive days (3). In the *USA* (*Med. Lett.*, 1986, *28*, 9), praziquantel 25 mg per kg three times a day for 5 to 8 days has been advised.

Fasciolopsiasis. Praziquantel in a dose of 25 mg per kg body-weight three times daily for one day has been recommended as the treatment of choice for fasciolopsiasis (*Med. Lett.*, 1986, *28*, 9). However, single doses of 15 mg per kg, 25 mg per kg, or 40 mg per kg all yielded a cure-rate of 100% in a study in 72 primary school children in Thailand who were harbouring *Fasciolopsis buski* (T. Harinasuta *et al.*, *Arzneimittel-Forsch.*, 1984, *34*, 1214); a single dose of 15 mg per kg at bedtime was therefore recommended for the treatment of fasciolopsiasis, although it was suggested that lower doses might be tried.

Opisthorchiasis. Praziquantel 25 mg per kg three times daily for one day has been recommended as the treatment of choice for *Opisthorchis viverrini* infection (*Med. Lett.*, 1986, *28*, 9). In a study from Thailand (D. Bunnag *et al.*, *Arzneimittel-Forsch.*, 1984, *34*, 1173) cure-rates of 100% were achieved with praziquantel 25 mg per kg three times daily for 1 or 2 days; single doses of 40 mg per kg or 50 mg per kg (in heavily infected patients) produced cure-rates of 91 and 97% respectively. A 100% cure-rate was also achieved in 108 Southeast Asian refugees who were carriers of *Clonorchis sinensis* (78) and *Opisthorchis viverrini* (30) when they were treated in France with praziquantel given in 3 doses of 25 mg per kg 4 to 6 hours apart (P. Ambroise-Thomas *et al.*, *ibid.*, 1177).

Paragonimiasis. Praziquantel in a dose of 25 mg per kg body-weight three times daily (at 4-hour intervals) for 2 consecutive days was the most effective of 4 dosage regimens and produced a cure-rate of 100% in a study from Thailand of patients infected with *Paragonimus heterotremus*, the clinical manifestations of which are similar to those of *P. westermani* infection (S. Vanijanonta *et al.*, *Arzneimittel-Forsch.*, 1984, *34*, 1186). The drug was generally well tolerated but, as with cerebral cysticercosis, it was noted that serious side-effects may occur in patients with cerebral paragonimiasis. A patient in the *USA* (C.T. Pachucki *et al.*, *New Engl. J. Med.*, 1984, *311*, 582), infected with a *Paragonimus* spp. after eating raw crayfish, was treated successfully with praziquantel 25 mg per kg three times daily for 2 days; this dosage regimen has been recommended in the *USA* as the treatment of choice for *Paragonimus westermani* infection (*Med. Lett.*, 1986, *28*, 9).

Schistosomiasis. See above.

Proprietary Names and Manufacturers

Biltricide *(Bayer, Ger.; Bayer, S.Afr.; Miles Pharmaceuticals, USA)*; Cesol *(E. Merck, Ger.)*; Livera; Pontel; Praquantel; Prazi; Prazite; Pyquiton *(Chin.)*; V Day Prazide.

13165-g

Pretamazium Iodide *(BAN, rINN)*.

66-269. 4-(Biphenyl-4-yl)-3-ethyl-2-[4-(pyrrolidin-1-yl)styryl]thiazolium iodide.

$C_{29}H_{29}IN_2S = 564.5$.

CAS — 24840-59-3.

An anthelmintic.

805-v

Pyrantel Embonate *(BANM, rINNM)*.

CP-10423-16; Pirantel Pamoate; Pyrantel Pamoate *(USAN)*. 1,4,5,6-Tetrahydro-1-methyl-2-[(*E*)-2-(2-thienyl)vinyl]pyrimidine 4,4′-methylenebis(3-hydroxy-2-naphthoate).

$C_{11}H_{14}N_2S, C_{23}H_{16}O_6 = 594.7$.

CAS — 15686-83-6 (pyrantel); 22204-24-6 (embonate).

Pharmacopoeias. In *Chin.*, *Jpn*, and *U.S.*

A yellow to tan-coloured solid. Pyrantel embonate 2.9 g is approximately equivalent to 1 g of pyrantel. Practically **insoluble** in water and methyl alcohol; soluble in dimethyl sulphoxide; slightly soluble in dimethylformamide. **Store** in well-closed containers. Protect from light.

Adverse Effects

The side-effects of pyrantel embonate are generally mild and transient. The most frequent are gastro-intestinal effects such as nausea and vomiting, anorexia, abdominal pain, and diarrhoea. Other adverse effects reported include headache, dizziness, drowsiness, insomnia, skin rashes, and elevated liver enzyme values.

Precautions

Pyrantel embonate should be used with caution in patients with impaired liver function. The anthelmintic effect of pyrantel may be antagonised by piperazine.

Absorption and Fate

Only a small proportion of a dose of pyrantel embonate is absorbed from the gastro-intestinal tract. Up to about 7% is excreted as unchanged drug and metabolites in the urine but over half of the dose is excreted unchanged in the faeces.

Uses and Administration

Pyrantel embonate is an anthelmintic effective against intestinal nematodes including roundworms (*Ascaris*), threadworms (*Enterobius*), *Trichostrongylus*, and hookworms, although it is possibly less effective against *Necator americanus* hookworms than against *Ancylostoma duodenale*. Pyrantel is not active against whipworm (*Trichuris trichiura*). It appears to act by paralysing susceptible worms which are then dislodged by peristaltic activity.

Single or mixed infections due to susceptible worms are treated with a single oral dose equivalent to 10 mg of pyrantel per kg body-weight; infections with *Ascaris* alone may only require 5 mg per kg. In hookworm infections due to *Necator*, 10 mg per kg daily for 3 days or 20 mg per kg daily for 2 days may be necessary.

Pyrantel embonate is used concomitantly with oxantel embonate when infection includes whipworms.

Pyrantel base and pyrantel tartrate have been used as veterinary anthelmintics.

In the *USA* pyrantel embonate has been recommended as the treatment of choice for *Enterobius vermicularis* (pinworm) infection, as an alternative to mebendazole for *Ascaris lumbricoides* (roundworm) and hookworm (*Ancylostoma duodenale, Necator americanus*) infection, and as an alternative to thiabendazole for *Trichostrongylus* infection.— *Med. Lett.*, 1986, *28*, 9.

Preparations

Pyrantel Pamoate Oral Suspension *(U.S.P.)*

Proprietary Preparations

Combantrin *(Pfizer, UK)*. *Tablets*, pyrantel 125 mg (as embonate).

Proprietary Names and Manufacturers

Anthel *(Alphapharm, Austral.)*; Anthelcide; Antiminth *(Pfizer, USA)*; Ascantrine; Aut *(Elea, Arg.)*; Bantel; Cobantril *(Pfizer, Switz.)*; Combantrin *(Pfizer, Arg.; G.P. Laboratories, Austral.; Pfizer, Belg.; Pfizer, Canad.; Pfizer, Fr.; Pfizer, Ital.; Pfizer, Neth.; Pfizer, S.Afr.; Pfizer, UK; Pfizer, USA)*; Early Bird *(Austral.)*; Helmex *(Pfizer, Ger.)*; Lombriareu *(Areu, Spain)*; Medicomtrin; Nemocid; Pantrin; Pirantel; Pirapam; Proca; Pyrabon; Pyrantin; Pyrantrin; Pyrapam; Pyrasan; Pyrasil; Scanminth; Trilombrin *(Pfizer, Spain)*; Vermdrite; Vermisan; Wormetrin.

13206-f

Rafoxanide *(BAN, USAN, rINN)*.

MK-990. 3′-Chloro-4′-(4-chlorophenoxy)-3,5-di-iodosalicylanilide.

$C_{19}H_{11}Cl_2I_2NO_3 = 626.0$.

CAS — 22662-39-1.

Pharmacopoeias. In *B.P. Vet.*

A greyish-white to brown powder. Practically **insoluble** in water; soluble 1 in 25 of acetone, 1 in 40 of chloroform and 1 in 35 of ethyl acetate; slightly soluble in methyl alcohol. **Store** in a well-closed container. Protect from light.

Rafoxanide is an anthelmintic used for the treatment and control of liver fluke in sheep and cattle.

Proprietary Veterinary Names and Manufacturers
Flukanide *(Merck Sharp & Dohme, UK)*.

806-g

Santonica

Flos Cinae; Semen Cinae; Semen Contra; Wormseed; Wormwood Flowers; Zitwerblüte.

Pharmacopoeias. In *Rus.* and *Span.*

The dried unexpanded flowerheads of *Artemisia cina* and other species of *Artemisia* (Compositae) containing not less than 2% of santonin.

Santonica is a source of santonin.

807-q

Santonin

Santoninum. (3*S*,3a*S*,5a*S*,9b*S*)-3a,5,5a,9b-Tetrahydro-3,5a,9-trimethylnaphtho[1,2-*b*]furan-2,8(3*H*,4*H*)-dione.
$C_{15}H_{18}O_3$=246.3.

CAS — 481-06-1.

Pharmacopoeias. In *Arg., Int., Jpn, Mex., Nord., Port., Rus., Span.,* and *Turk.*

A crystalline lactone obtained from the dried unexpanded flowerheads of *Artemisia cina* and other species of *Artemisia* (Compositae).

Santonin was formerly used as an anthelmintic in the treatment of roundworm (*Ascaris*) infection, but has been superseded by other less toxic anthelmintics.

810-h

Stibocaptate *(BAN).*

Antimony Sodium Dimercaptosuccinate; Ro-4-1544/6; Sb-58; Sodium Stibocaptate *(rINN)*; TWSb/6. Antimony sodium *meso*-2,3-dimercaptosuccinate. The formula varies from $C_{12}H_{11}NaO_{12}S_6Sb_2$ = 806.1 to $C_{12}H_6Na_6O_{12}S_6Sb_2$ = 916.0.

CAS — 3064-61-7 ($C_{12}H_6Na_6O_{12}S_6Sb_2$).

Stibocaptate is a trivalent antimony compound with properties similar to those of antimony sodium tartrate (p.48), but reputed to be better tolerated. It has been given by intramuscular injection in the treatment of schistosomiasis, but has generally been replaced by less toxic drugs such as praziquantel.

Proprietary Names and Manufacturers

Astiban *(Roche, Switz.).*

811-m

Stibophen

Estibofeno; Fouadin; Stibophenum. Bis[4,5-dihydroxybenzene-1,3-disulphonato(4−)-O^4,O^5]antimonate(5−) pentasodium heptahydrate.
$C_{12}H_4Na_5O_{16}S_4Sb,7H_2O$=895.2.

CAS — 15489-16-4 (heptahydrate).

Pharmacopoeias. In *Int., It., Jug.,* and *Turk.*

Stibophen is a trivalent antimony compound with properties similar to those of antimony sodium tartrate (p.48). It was formerly administered by intramuscular injection in the treatment of schistosomiasis and has also been given in leishmaniasis.

Proprietary Names and Manufacturers

Fantorin *(Glaxo, Ind.).*

812-b

Stilbazium Iodide *(BAN, USAN, rINN).*

BW-61-32. 1-Ethyl-2,6-bis[4-(pyrrolidin-1-yl)styryl]-pyridinium iodide.
$C_{31}H_{36}IN_3$=577.6.

CAS — 3784-99-4 (iodide).

Stilbazium iodide is an anthelmintic reported to be effective against roundworms (*Ascaris*), threadworms (*Enterobius*), and, to some extent, whipworms. It stains the stools red.

813-v

Tetrachloroethylene *(BAN, USAN).*

Perchloroethylene; Tetrachloroethylenum.
C_2Cl_4=165.8.

CAS — 127-18-4.

Pharmacopoeias. In *Arg., Br., Braz., Egypt., Fr., Ind., Int., Nord., Turk.,* and *U.S.*

A colourless, mobile liquid with a characteristic ethereal odour; it usually contains thymol 0.01% w/w or alcohol 0.5 to 1%. Wt per mL 1.620 to 1.626 g. B.p. 118° to 122°.

Practically **insoluble** in water; soluble in alcohol; miscible with chloroform, ether, light petroleum, and most fixed and volatile oils. It is slowly decomposed by light and by various metals in the presence of moisture. **Store** in airtight containers. Protect from light.

Adverse Effects and Treatment

As for Carbon Tetrachloride, p.1425. Symptoms, especially following administration by mouth when used therapeutically, are less severe.

Dependence may follow habitual inhalation of small quantities of tetrachloroethylene vapour.

In Great Britain the recommended exposure limits of tetrachloroethylene are 100 ppm (long-term); 150 ppm (short-term). In the *US* the permissible exposure limit is 100 ppm.

Toxic epidermal necrolysis had been reported after the ingestion of tetrachloroethylene.— B. Potter *et al., Archs Derm.*, 1960, *82*, 903.

A 68-year-old launderette worker was anaesthetised and suffered erythema and 30% superficial burns after spilling a container of tetrachloroethylene over his clothes. The defatting property of tetrachloroethylene would lead to cracking of damaged skin.— B. Morgan (letter), *Br. med. J.*, 1969, *2*, 513.

A 25-year-old man became unconscious after exposure to the vapour of tetrachloroethylene which he was using for cleansing the interior of a tank. He recovered consciousness within 30 minutes of removal from the tank and his subsequent clinical progress was uneventful except for fatigue when resuming work about 3 days later. Elevated serum aspartate aminotransferase (SGOT) and urobilinogen concentrations were indicative of slight liver damage. There was no specific treatment for tetrachloroethylene poisoning. Sympathomimetic drugs should not be used to counter hypotension because of the danger of inducing ventricular fibrillation.— R. D. Stewart, *J. Am. med. Ass.*, 1969, *208*, 1490.

Intoxication resembling drunkenness in a 62-year-old factory worker exposed to tetrachloroethylene 500 ppm in his work.— J. K. McMullen (letter), *Br. med. J.*, 1976, *2*, 1563.

Disorders resembling vinyl chloride disease (coldness, stiffness, burning pain, and discoloration of the hands on exposure to cold; sclerotic changes of the hands, forearms, and face; an immune complex vasculitis) had occurred after exposure to tetrachloroethylene.— N. Rowell, *Practitioner*, 1977, *219*, 820. Mention of recurrent parotitis complicating a connective tissue disorder similar to vinyl chloride disease in a 29-year-old man exposed occupationally to tetrachloroethylene.— J. Watkinson, *Br. med. J.*, 1985, *291*, 1094.

Tetrachloroethylene, *Environmental Health Criteria 31*, Geneva, Wld Hlth Org., 1984.

Comments on the hazards of working in an environment containing tetrachloethylene fumes.— F. W. Lunau, *Br. med. J.*, 1984, *288*, 1818; J. R. Bennett (letter), *ibid.*, *289*, 255; H. K. Wilson and D. Gompertz (letter), *ibid.*

ABUSE. Coma, cardiac arrhythmias, and death have followed sniffing of tetrachloroethylene.— *Med. Lett.*, 1985, *27*, 77.

Precautions

In general tetrachloroethylene should not be given to patients with roundworm (*Ascaris*) as well as hookworm infection, since by stimulating the roundworms it may initiate migration within the bowel causing obstruction; treatment for roundworms should therefore precede tetrachloroethylene therapy. It should not be administered to alcoholics or to patients with impaired liver function, severe debility or anaemia, or inflammation or ulceration of the gastro-intestinal tract.

Laxatives, alcohol, and fats may enhance the toxic effects of tetrachloroethylene.

Obstructive jaundice in a 6-week old infant was considered to be caused by tetrachloroethylene in the breast milk of her mother who was exposed at intervals to vapours from a dry-cleaning plant.— P. C. Bagnell and H. A. Ellenberger, *Can. med. Ass. J.*, 1977, *117*, 1047.

Absorption and Fate

Tetrachloroethylene is slightly absorbed from the gastro-intestinal tract; absorption is increased in the presence of alcohol and fats or oils. It is absorbed following inhalation and after direct contact with the skin. It is excreted in expired air.

Metabolites of tetrachloroethylene, mainly trichloroacetic acid, have been found in the urine following occupational exposure.

For a report of the excretion of tetrachloroethylene in breast milk, see Precautions (above).

Uses and Administration

Tetrachloroethylene is a chlorinated hydrocarbon. It is an effective anthelmintic against hookworms (*Ancylostoma* and *Necator*) and is still widely used in endemic areas. It has also been used in the treatment of intestinal fluke infections.

Tetrachloroethylene is given by mouth on an empty stomach, usually as a suspension or in gelatin capsules, in a single dose of 0.1 mL per kg body-weight to a maximum of 5 mL.

Tetrachloroethylene is widely used as a solvent in industry.

Tetrachloroethylene in a single dose of 0.1 mL per kg body-weight (maximum, 5 mL) has been recommended as an alternative to praziquantel in the treatment of the intestinal flukes *Fasciolopsis buski*, *Heterophyes heterophyes*, and *Metagonimus yokogawai*.— *Med. Lett.*, 1986, *28*, 9.

Following a comparative study in children infected with *Fasciolopsis buski* it was concluded that tetrachloroethylene is effective treatment. However, because of its potential for causing anaphylactic reactions, especially where there are heavy worm burdens, it should be administered under clinical supervision, preferably with prior antihistamine treatment. The broad-spectrum anthelmintics thiabendazole, mebendazole, levamisole, and pyrantel embonate were not effective.— G. H. Rabbani *et al., Trans. R. Soc. trop. Med. Hyg.*, 1985, *79*, 513.

Preparations

Tetrachloroethylene Capsules *(U.S.P.)*

Proprietary Names and Manufacturers

Perklone *(ICI Mond, UK).*

814-g

Tetramisole Hydrochloride *(BANM, USAN, rINNM).*

ICI-50627; McN-JR-8299-11; R-8299. (±)-2,3,5,6-Tetrahydro-6-phenylimidazo[2,1-*b*]thiazole hydrochloride.
$C_{11}H_{12}N_2S,HCl$=240.8.

CAS — 5036-02-2 (tetramisole); 5086-74-8 (hydrochloride).

Pharmacopoeias. In *Cz., Ind.,* and *Nord.* Also in *B.P. Vet.* and in *Fr.* for veterinary use.

A white to pale cream-coloured, odourless or almost odourless, crystalline powder.

Soluble 1 in 5 of water, and 1 in 10 of methyl alcohol; very slightly soluble in ether.

Tetramisole hydrochloride is an anthelmintic used in veterinary practice. It is a racemic mixture and the laevo-isomer, levamisole hydrochloride (p.55), accounts for most of its activity.

Proprietary Veterinary Names and Manufacturers

Nilverm *(Coopers Animal Health, UK).*

815-q

Thenium Closylate *(BAN, USAN).*

611-C-65; NSC-106569; Thenium Closilate *(rINN)*. Dimethyl(2-phenoxyethyl)(2-thenyl)ammonium 4-chlorobenzenesulphonate.
$C_{21}H_{24}ClNO_4S_2$=454.0.

CAS — 16776-64-0 (thenium); 4304-40-9 (closylate).

Pharmacopoeias. In *B.P. Vet.*

A white, odourless or almost odourless, crystalline powder. Slightly **soluble** in water; soluble 1 in 25 of alcohol and 1 in 35 of chloroform; readily soluble in hot water, any excess forming an oily layer.

Thenium closylate is a veterinary anthelmintic used for the treatment of canine hookworm infections; it is generally used in conjunction with piperazine.

816-p

Thiabendazole *(BAN, USAN).*

E233; MK-360; Tiabendazole *(rINN).* 2-(Thiazol-4-yl)-1*H*-benzimidazole.

$C_{10}H_7N_3S$=201.3.

CAS — 148-79-8.

Pharmacopoeias. In *Br., Braz., Egypt., Ind., It., Jug., Nord.,* and *U.S.* Also in *B.P. Vet.*

A white to cream-coloured, odourless or almost odourless, powder.

Practically **insoluble** in water; slightly soluble in alcohol, in chloroform, and in ether; dissolves in dilute mineral acids.

Adverse Effects

Dizziness and gastro-intestinal disturbances, especially anorexia, nausea, and vomiting, are common during treatment with thiabendazole. Other adverse effects occurring occasionally include pruritus, skin rashes, headache, fatigue, drowsiness, hyperglycaemia, disturbance of colour vision (xanthopsia), leucopenia, tinnitus, effects on the liver, crystalluria, and bradycardia and hypotension. There have also been reports of erythema multiforme, including fatal Stevens-Johnson syndrome, toxic epidermal necrolysis, convulsions, and effects on mental state.

Fever, chills, angioedema, and lymphadenopathy have been reported, but may possibly represent allergic response to dead parasites rather than to thiabendazole.

The urine of some patients taking thiabendazole may have a characteristic odour similar to that following the ingestion of asparagus; it is attributed to the presence of a thiabendazole metabolite.

Some references to adverse effects of thiabendazole: W. J. Cunliffe and S. Shuster (letter), *Lancet,* 1967, *1,* 579 (severe muscle aches on exercising); R. H. Lloyd-Mostyn (letter), *Br. med. J.,* 1968, *3,* 557 (acute psychiatric reaction); H. M. Robinson and C. S. Samorodin, *Archs Derm.,* 1976, *112,* 1757 (bullous erythema multiforme and toxic epidermal necrolysis); P. Tchao and T. Templeton, *J. Pediat.,* 1983, *102,* 317 (grand mal seizures); D. Rex *et al., Gastroenterology,* 1983, *85,* 718 (intrahepatic cholestasis and sicca complex).

For toxicological data, see 1971 and 1972 Evaluations of some Pesticide Residues in Food, *Pestic. Residue Ser. Wld Hlth Org. Nos 1,* 1972 and *2,* 1973, respectively..

Precautions

Thiabendazole is contra-indicated in patients with a history of hypersensitivity and should be discontinued at the first sign of hypersensitivity. It should be used with caution in patients with hepatic or renal impairment. Thiabendazole causes drowsiness in some patients and those affected should not take charge of vehicles or machinery where loss of attention could cause accidents.

ADMINISTRATION IN RENAL FAILURE. Thiabendazole and its 5-hydroxy metabolite did not accumulate in an anephric patient on haemodialysis and haemoperfusion and receiving treatment for severe strongyloidiasis. However, the potentially toxic conjugated glucuronide and sulphate metabolites did accumulate. The clearance of all 3 metabolites was poor by haemodialysis; haemoperfusion was much more efficient although for rapid removal the haemoperfusion columns should be changed every hour.— L. Bauer *et al., J. clin. Pharmac.,* 1982, *22,* 276.

INTERACTIONS. For the effect of thiabendazole on serum concentrations of theophylline during treatment with aminophylline, see Theophylline, p.1530.

PREGNANCY AND THE NEONATE. Thiabendazole has been reported to be teratogenic in *rats* and *mice* (J.L. Schardein, *Chemically Induced Birth Defects,* New York, Dekker, 1985) and although toxicity in pregnancy is not known, it has been recommended (*Med. Lett.,* 1987, *29,* 61) that thiabendazole should only be used when there is no suitable alternative. The *UK* manufacturers have stated (1986) that thiabendazole should not be used during pregnancy or lactation.

RESIDUES IN THE DIET. Maximum acceptable daily intake of thiabendazole in the diet: 50 µg per kg body-weight.— Report of the 1975 Joint FAO/WHO Meeting on Pesticide Residues in Food, *Tech. Rep. Ser. Wld Hlth Org. No. 592,* 1976.

Absorption and Fate

Thiabendazole is readily absorbed from the gastro-intestinal tract and reaches peak concentrations in the plasma after 1 to 2 hours. It is metabolised to 5-hydroxythiabendazole and is excreted principally in the urine as glucuronide or sulphate conjugates; about 90% is recovered in the urine within 48 hours of ingestion, but only 5% in the faeces. Absorption may occur from preparations applied to the skin or eyes.

References: D. J. Tocco *et al., Toxic. appl. Pharmac.,* 1966, *9,* 31.

Uses and Administration

Thiabendazole, a benzimidazole derivative, is an anthelmintic with activity against most nematode worms (see p.47); activity against some larval stages and ova has also been demonstrated. The mode of action is not certain, but thiabendazole may inhibit the fumarate-reductase system of worms thereby interfering with their source of energy.

Thiabendazole is used in the treatment of cutaneous larva migrans (creeping eruption), dracontiasis (guinea worm infection), strongyloidiasis, and visceral larva migrans (toxocariasis). It has also been given for angiostrongyliasis, anisakiasis, capillariasis, and trichostrongyliasis and can provide symptomatic relief during the invasion stage of trichinosis. Thiabendazole is also active against *Ascaris lumbricoides* (roundworm), *Enterobius vermicularis* (pinworm, threadworm), *Necator americanus* and *Ancylostoma duodenale* (hookworms), and *Trichuris trichiuria* (whipworm), but should not be used as primary therapy for these worm infections; the treatment of mixed infections including ascariasis is not recommended since thiabendazole may cause the worms to migrate and live *Ascaris* have been reported in the mouth and nose.

Thiabendazole is given by mouth, with meals, usually in a dose of 25 mg per kg body-weight twice daily for 2 or 3 days, although the duration depends on the type of infection; the daily dose should not exceed 3 g. For those unable to tolerate 2 doses daily, 25 mg per kg may be given after the largest meal on day 1 and repeated 24 hours later after a similar meal on day 2. For mass treatment, a single dose of 50 mg per kg after the evening meal is suggested although the incidence of adverse effects may be higher than with 2 doses of 25 mg per kg.

In cutaneous larva migrans, 25 mg per kg may be given twice daily for 2 days, repeated after 2 days if necessary; topical treatment with a cream containing up to 15% of thiabendazole or a 10% suspension intended for oral use has also been advocated.

In dracontiasis, 25 to 50 mg per kg may be given twice daily for one day; in massive infection a further 50 mg per kg may be given after 5 to 8 days.

In strongyloidiasis, 25 mg per kg may be given twice daily for 2 days or 50 mg per kg as a single dose; when the infection is disseminated treatment for at least 5 days may be necessary.

In visceral larva migrans, 25 mg per kg may be given twice daily for 7 days.

Thiabendazole also has some antifungal activity. In the *UK* and *EEC,* regulations control the use of thiabendazole as a fungicidal preservative for bananas and citrus fruit; its use for this purpose has been questioned.

Recommendations by authorities in the *USA* for the treatment of parasitic infections. Thiabendazole is the drug of choice in the treatment of angiostrongyliasis (*Angiostrongylus cantonensis,* 25 mg per kg body-weight twice daily for 3 days; *A. costaricensis,* 25 mg per kg three times daily for 3 days); an alternative to surgical removal in anisakiasis (25 mg per kg twice daily for 3 days); an alternative to mebendazole in capillariasis (25 mg per kg daily for 30 days); the drug of choice in cutaneous larva migrans (25 mg per kg twice daily for 2 to 5 days); an alternative to niridazole or metronidazole in dracontiasis (25 mg per kg daily for 3 days); the drug of choice in strongyloidiasis (25 mg per kg twice daily for 2 days or for at least 5 days in disseminated infection); the drug of choice, together with corticosteroids for severe symptoms, in trichinosis (25 mg per kg twice daily for 5 days); the drug of choice in trichostrongyliasis (25 mg per kg twice daily for 2 days); and an alternative to diethylcarbamazine in visceral larva migrans (25 mg per kg twice daily for 5 days).— *Med. Lett.,* 1986, *28,* 9.

ADMINISTRATION IN RENAL FAILURE. For a report of the use of thiabendazole in an anephric patient, see Precautions, above.

DRACONTIASIS. Thiabendazole 25 mg per kg body-weight daily for 3 days has been recommended by authorities in the *USA* (*Med. Lett.,* 1986, *28,* 9) as an alternative to niridazole or metronidazole in the treatment of infection with *Dracunculus medinensis* (guinea worm). All 3 compounds have marked anti-inflammatory properties and probably act by lessening the intense host tissue reaction, thus allowing the emerging worms to be removed more quickly, rather than by a direct anthelmintic effect (R. Muller, *Bull. Wld Hlth Org.,* 1979, *57,* 683). In a field study in Nigeria (O.O. Kale *et al., Ann. trop. Med. Parasit.,* 1983, *77,* 151), thiabendazole 50 or 100 mg per kg body-weight daily for 2 days was as effective as metronidazole in patients with dracontiasis and both drugs were significantly better than placebo. Side-effects, notably gastro-intestinal effects and dizziness, were much more common in those given thiabendazole, but both drugs were considered to have a place in treatment.

FUNGAL INFECTIONS. A patient with keratitis due to *Aspergillus flavus* was successfully treated with thiabendazole eye-drops. After approximately 14 days' treatment with a 4% suspension instilled every 2 hours, smear and culture of corneal scrapings yielded no fungal growth.— M. P. Upadhyay *et al., Br. J. Ophthal.,* 1980, *64,* 30.

Marked improvement was noted 6 weeks after the initiation of treatment with thiabendazole 3 g daily in divided doses in a patient with chromomycosis involving one leg extensively. Dosage was reduced to 2 g daily after 10 weeks and thiabendazole was discontinued after 8 months, when only scars and thickening of the skin were noticeable.— J. E. Ollé-Goig and J. Domingo, *Trans. R. Soc. trop. Med. Hyg.,* 1983, *77,* 773. See also M. A. Bayles (letter), *Br. J. Derm.,* 1974, *91,* 715.

GAPEWORM INFECTION. A woman with asthmatic symptoms caused by infection with the nematode *Syngamus laryngeus* [gapeworm], following a visit to the Caribbean, was treated successfully with thiabendazole 1.5 g twice daily for 2 days.— W. -D. Leers *et al., Can. med. Ass. J.,* 1985, *132,* 269. See also G. A. C. Grell *et al., Br. med. J.,* 1978, *2,* 1464.

SCABIES. Of 40 patients with scabies 32 had a satisfactory response after topical treatment with thiabendazole 10% suspension; 6 needed a second course of treatment, and 2 received triamcinolone.— E. Hernǎndez-Pérez, *Archs Derm.,* 1976, *112,* 1400.

STRONGYLOIDIASIS. Thiabendazole is considered to be the drug of choice for the treatment of *Strongyloides stercoralis* infection by authorities in the *USA*.— *Med. Lett.,* 1986, *28,* 9.

Nematode worms of the *Strongyloides* spp. are widely distributed, although most human infections are due to *S. stercoralis* which is confined to the tropics. Of 602 ex-prisoners of war in the Far East, 88 had strongyloid infection 23 to 33 years after repatriation; creeping eruption was common and gastro-intestinal symptoms rare. Treatment with thiabendazole 25 mg per kg body-weight twice daily for 3 days was generally effective. Many undiagnosed cases of strongyloidiasis must exist among ex-prisoners of war and, since a severe and often fatal 'hyperinfective' form of the disease with massive larval tissue invasion may occur in infected patients immunosuppressed by drugs such as corticosteroids, or disease, it is important to identify and treat them.— G. V. Gill and D. R. Bell, *Br. med. J.,* 1979, *2,* 572. A further study confirming the persistence of strongyloidiasis in ex-prisoners of war. In view of the difficulty of diagnosis and the danger of overwhelming infection, those patients who were prisoners of war in south-east Asia and are about to receive immunosuppressants should probably first be treated prophylactically with thiabendazole.— D. I. Grove, *Br. med. J.*, 1980, *280*, 598. The prophylactic use of thiabendazole in individuals who may have latent infection, but whose stool examination yields negative results is contentious.— E. M. Proctor *et al.*, *Can. med. Ass. J.*, 1985, *133*, 876.

In a study of the toxicity and effectiveness of thiabendazole in treating strongyloidiasis in 43 ex-prisoners of war who had been infected about 35 years previously, side-effects were frequent and sometimes severe, and the infection was not always eradicated.— D. I. Grove, *Trans. R. Soc. trop. Med. Hyg.*, 1982, *76*, 114.

A 17-year-old English girl contracted strongyloidiasis, possibly by walking barefoot in her local park, and was treated successfully with thiabendazole 1.5 g twice daily for 3 days.— V. Sprott *et al.*, *Br. med. J.*, 1987, *294*, 741.

Strongyloides cf. *fuelleborni* is associated with the fatal condition known as swollen belly syndrome in Papua New Guinea. Thiabendazole 25 mg per kg body-weight twice daily for 3 days was effective in treating *S. fuelleborni*-like infections in 88 asymptomatic children aged from 1 to 124 months. Side-effects were reported in 26 children, but did not prevent completion of treatment.— G. Barnish and J. Barker, *Trans. R. Soc. trop. Med. Hyg.*, 1987, *81*, 60.

Preparations

Thiabendazole Eye-drops. Thiabendazole 4 g, hydroxyethylcellulose 1 g, benzalkonium chloride 20 mg, disodium edetate 50 mg, sorbitol solution 1 mL, water to 100 mL. Sterile thiabendazole is added aseptically to the previously sterilised eye-drop vehicle. For *Fusarium* and *Aspergillus* infection of the eye.—A. Baker, *J. Hosp. Pharm.*, 1972, *30*, 45.

Thiabendazole Oral Suspension *(U.S.P.)*. pH 3.4 to 4.2. Store in airtight containers.

Thiabendazole Tablets *(B.P.)*. They should be chewed before swallowing.

Thiabendazole Tablets *(U.S.P.)*. They should be chewed before swallowing. Store in airtight containers.

Proprietary Preparations

Mintezol *(Merck Sharp & Dohme, UK)*. *Tablets*, chewable, thiabendazole 500 mg.

Proprietary Names and Manufacturers

Foldan *(Arg.)*; Lombristop *(Septa, Spain)*; Mintezol *(Merck Sharp & Dohme, Austral.; Canad.; S.Afr.; Switz.; Merck Sharp & Dohme, UK; Merck Sharp & Dohme, USA)*; Minzolum *(Merck Sharp & Dohme, Ger.)*; Nomoxiur *(Cronofar, Spain)*; Tiabenda *(Cidan, Spain)*; Triasox *(Andreu, Spain)*.

13328-s

Thiophanate *(BAN)*.

4,4′-*o*-Phenylenebis(ethyl 3-thioallophanate).
$C_{14}H_{18}N_4O_4S_2$=370.4.

CAS — 23564-06-9.

Thiophanate is an anthelmintic used in veterinary practice.

Proprietary Veterinary Names and Manufacturers
Helminate *(Micro-Biologicals, UK)*; Nemafax *(RMB Animal Health, UK)*.

3230-g

Triclabendazole *(rINN)*.

5-Chloro-6-(2,3-dichlorophenoxy)-2-(methylthio)benzimidazole.
$C_{14}H_9Cl_3N_2OS$=359.7.

CAS — 68786-66-3.

Triclabendazole is a benzimidazole anthelmintic active against the liver fluke *Fasciola hepatica*. It is used in veterinary practice.

References: D. P. Britt, *Trans. R. Soc. trop. Med. Hyg.*, 1986, *80*, 334.

Proprietary Veterinary Names and Manufacturers
Fasinex *(Ciba-Geigy Agrochemicals, UK)*.

819-e

Viprynium Embonate *(BAN)*.

Pyrvinium Embonate; Pyrvinium Pamoate *(USAN)*; Viprynium Pamoate. Bis{6-Dimethylamino-2-[2-(2,5-dimethyl-1-phenylpyrrol-3-yl)vinyl]-1-methylquinolinium} 4,4′-methylenebis(3-hydroxy-2-naphthoate).

$C_{52}H_{56}N_6,C_{23}H_{14}O_6$=1151.4.

CAS — 3546-41-6.

NOTE. Pyrvinium Chloride is *rINN*.

Pharmacopoeias. In *Braz.*, *Cz.*, *Jug.*, and *U.S.*

A bright orange or orange-red to almost black crystalline powder. Viprynium embonate 7.5 mg is approximately equivalent to 5 mg of viprynium.
Practically **insoluble** in water and ether; very slightly soluble in methyl alcohol; slightly soluble in chloroform and methoxyethanol; freely soluble in glacial acetic acid. **Store** in airtight containers. Protect from light.

Adverse Effects
Viprynium occasionally causes nausea, vomiting, and diarrhoea. Allergic reactions and photosensitivity have been reported.
Viprynium stains the stools bright red and may stain clothing if vomiting occurs.

Absorption and Fate
Viprynium embonate is not significantly absorbed from the gastro-intestinal tract.

References: T. C. Smith *et al.*, *Clin. Pharmac. Ther.*, 1976, *19*, 802.

Uses and Administration
Viprynium embonate is an effective anthelmintic in the treatment of threadworm (*Enterobius*) infection, but has generally been superseded by other drugs such as mebendazole, piperazine, or pyrantel.
It has been administered by mouth in a single dose equivalent to 5 mg of viprynium per kg body-weight, repeated after 2 to 3 weeks if necessary.

Preparations

Pyrvinium Pamoate Oral Suspension *(U.S.P.)*. Contains viprynium embonate. pH 6 to 8.

Pyrvinium Pamoate Tablets *(U.S.P.)*. Contain viprynium embonate.

Proprietary Names and Manufacturers
Antioxiur *(Cheminova, Spain)*; Molevac *(Parke, Davis, Ger.; Parke, Davis, Switz.)*; Neo-Oxypaat *(Katwijk, Neth.)*; Oxialum *(Kairon, Spain)*; Pamovin *(Frosst, Canad.)*; Pamoxan *(Uriach, Spain)*; Polyquil *(Parke, Davis, Spain)*; Povan *(Parke, Davis, USA)*; Povanyl *(Substantia, Fr.)*; Pyr-Pam *(ICN, Canad.)*; Pyrvin *(Benzon, Denm.)*; Tru *(Elea, Arg.)*; Vanquin *(Parke, Davis, Austral.; Belg.; Parke, Davis, Canad.; Parke, Davis, Denm.; Parke, Davis, Ital.; Parke, Davis, Neth.; Parke, Davis, Norw.; Parke, Davis, Swed.; Parke, Davis, UK)*; Vermitiber *(Tiber, Ital.)*.

Anti-arrhythmic Agents

7770-x

Anti-arrhythmic agents (formerly described as cardiac depressants) may be divided broadly into those that act on ventricular and supraventricular arrhythmias, such as quinidine (p.85), those that act mainly on ventricular arrhythmias, such as lignocaine (p.1217), and those that act on supraventricular arrhythmias, such as verapamil (p.89). The most frequently used classification is that devised by Vaughan Williams (E.M. Vaughan Williams, *Pharmac. Ther.*, 1975, *1*, 115; B.N. Singh and E.M. Vaughan Williams, *Cardiovasc. Res.*, 1972, *6*, 109) and subsequently modified by Harrison (D.C. Harrison, *Drugs*, 1986, *31*, 93). This uses the mode of action of anti-arrhythmic agents as the basis of the classification:
class I includes drugs which directly interfere with depolarisation of the cardiac membrane (membrane-stabilising agents) by blocking the fast inward current of sodium into cardiac cells; they also have local anaesthetic properties, and are subdivided according to their effect on the action potential duration (APD); class Ia prolong APD and include quinidine (p.85), procainamide (p.82), and disopyramide (p.75); class Ib shorten APD and include lignocaine (p.1217), mexiletine (p.80), tocainide (p.88), and phenytoin (p.406); class Ic have no effect on APD and include flecainide (p.78), encainide (p.78), and lorcainide (p.80);
class II includes drugs with antisympathetic properties, such as propranolol (p.798) and bretylium (p.74);
class III includes drugs that prolong the duration of the cardiac action potential, such as amiodarone (p.71);
class IV includes drugs that block the slow inward calcium current (calcium-channel blockers) such as verapamil (p.89) although not all drugs that fall into the broad general category of calcium-channel blockers share the same specific properties.
It has been suggested that alinidine (p.71) which has a direct negative chronotropic action may represent a fifth class of anti-arrhythmic agents.
Many of the drugs classified in the above manner may have more than one type of anti-arrhythmic action.

Reviews of anti-arrhythmic drugs.— W. S. Hillis and B. Whiting, *Br. med. J.*, 1983, *286*, 1332; J. C. Somberg, *Am. J. Cardiol.*, 1984, *54*, 8B; K. A. Muhiddin and P. Turner, *Postgrad. med. J.*, 1985, *61*, 665; P. F. Nestico *et al.*, *Drugs*, 1988, *35*, 286.

ADVERSE EFFECTS. Report of a possible link between the use of anti-arrhythmic agents and cardiac arrest in some patients.— J. N. Ruskin *et al.*, *New Engl. J. Med.*, 1983, *309*, 1302. While agreeing that anti-arrhythmic drugs have the potential to worsen or provoke ventricular arrhythmias, the authors point out that a high proportion of patients in whom these arrhythmias occur have had earlier cardiac arrests or previously recognised arrhythmias and are probably not representative.— L. A. Cobb and W. D. Weaver (letter), *ibid.*, 1984, *310*, 1122.

A survey of the outcome of poisoning with anti-arrhythmic agents indicated that although the incidence of poisoning with anti-arrhythmics was low, mortality was high due to cardiac disturbances.— K. Hruby and J. Missliwetz, *Int. J. clin. Pharmac. Ther. Toxic.*, 1985, *23*, 253.

A study of the incidence of adverse reactions to anti-arrhythmic agents used to treat ventricular arrhythmias indicated that the risk-benefit ratio would only be acceptable in patients at a significant risk from symptomatic arrhythmias.— T. W. Nygaard *et al.*, *J. Am. med. Ass.*, 1986, *256*, 55.

Further references to the adverse effects of anti-arrhythmic drugs: J. B. Schwartz *et al.*, *Drugs*, 1981, *21*, 23.

CLASSIFICATION. Classification of anti-arrhythmic agents.— E. M. Vaughan Williams, *Pharmac. Ther.*, 1975, *1*, 115; B. N. Singh and E. M. Vaughan Williams, *Cardiovasc. Res.*, 1972, *6*, 109; E. M. Vaughan Williams, *J. clin. Pharmac.*, 1984, *24*, 129.

A suggested classification of anti-arrhythmic drugs according to the cardiac tissue which each affects. Thus drugs which act on the sino-atrial node include beta-blockers, Class IV anti-arrhythmics and cardiac glycosides; Class I and Class III anti-arrhythmics act on the ventricles, and drugs acting on atrial arrhythmias include Class Ia, Ic, and III anti-arrhythmic agents and beta-blockers. Class Ia and III anti-arrhythmics act on accessory pathways and drugs acting on the atrioventricular node include Class Ic and IV anti-arrhythmics, beta-blockers, and cardiac glycosides. Other factors which will influence the clinical choice of treatment will include the nature of the arrhythmias and any underlying disease, anticipated adverse effects, and drug interactions.— J. K. Aronson, *Br. med. J.*, 1985, *290*, 487. Criticism including additions to the clinical classification suggested and comment on the rational choice of treatment.— D. Ward and J. Camm (letter), *ibid.*, 1077.

A modification of the Vaughan-Williams classification of anti-arrhythmic agents.— D. C. Harrison, *Drugs*, 1986, *31*, 93.

Further references: E. M. Vaughan Williams, *Anti-arrhythmic Agents*, London, Academic Press, 1980.

USES. A brief review of the treatment of supraventricular tachycardias.— D. E. Ward, *Br. med. J.*, 1984, *288*, 344.

A review of the management of acute arrhythmias.— W. T. Brownlee, *Br. J. Hosp. Med.*, 1985, *33*, 138.

Further references to the use of anti-arrhythmic agents: D. P. Zipes, *New Engl. J. Med.*, 1981, *304*, 475; J. A. Kastor *et al.*, *ibid.*, 1004; *Med. Lett.*, 1986, *28*, 111.

Pregnancy and the neonate. Reviews of the use of anti-arrhythmic drugs during pregnancy and breast feeding.— H. H. Rotmensch *et al.*, *Ann. intern. Med.*, 1983, *98*, 487; H. H. Rotmensch *et al.*, *Drugs*, 1987, *33*, 623.

7776-m

Acecainide Hydrochloride *(USAN, rINNM)*.
ASL-601; *N*-Acetylprocainamide Hydrochloride; NAPA.
4′-[(2-Diethylaminoethyl)carbamoyl]acetanilide hydrochloride.
$C_{15}H_{23}N_3O_2,HCl=313.8$.

CAS — 32795-44-1 (acecainide); 34118-92-8 (hydrochloride).

Acecainide is the acetylated form of procainamide (see p.82) and has anti-arrhythmic activity although it is less potent than procainamide. It has a longer duration of action and causes adverse effects less frequently than procainamide.

A brief review of acecainide. The haemodynamic and cardiac effects of acecainide differ in several respects from procainamide and it is less potent than procainamide. Effective plasma concentrations are reported to be between 9.4 and 19.5 µg per mL with adverse effects becoming more prevalent above 10 µg per mL. The elimination is significantly reduced in patients with renal failure, and the clearance of acecainide has been reported to correlate with creatinine clearance. In clinical trials acecainide was effective in only a few patients for the treatment of ventricular arrhythmias and chronic premature ventricular contraction. The oral dose of acecainide is 0.5 to 2.5 g every 6 to 8 hours adjusted to the needs of individual patients. Adverse effects are dose-related but appear to be less severe than those of procainamide. In particular, patients rarely develop positive anti-nuclear antibody titres or drug-induced lupus erythematosus. At present there is little evidence to suggest that acecainide has widely applicable anti-arrhythmic action.— D. L. D. Keefe *et al.*, *Drugs*, 1981, *22*, 363.

A review of the pharmacokinetics of acecainide. Acecainide is well absorbed following oral administration and has a plasma half-life of 4.3 to 15.1 hours in patients with normal renal function. About 10% of acecainide is bound to plasma proteins. The major route of excretion is via the kidneys, between 59 and 87% as unchanged acecainide. A small proportion of the dose is de-acetylated to procainamide.— S. J. Connolly and R. E. Kates, *Clin. Pharmacokinet.*, 1982, *7*, 206.

USE IN CARDIAC DISORDERS. Reports of the efficacy of acecainide in the treatment of cardiac arrhythmias: J. Kluger *et al.*, *Am. J. Cardiol.*, 1980, *45*, 1250; D. M. Roden *et al.*, *Am. J. Cardiol.*, 1980, *46*, 463; A. J. Atkinson *et al.*, *Clin. Pharmac. Ther.*, 1983, *33*, 565; T. M. Ludden *et al.*, *Pharmacotherapy*, 1985, *5*, 11.

ADVERSE EFFECTS. *Lupus erythematosus.* Acecainide induced antinuclear antibodies and anti-sDNA antibodies only after a much longer period of treatment than that at which these serological changes appeared with procainamide.— R. Lahita *et al.*, *New Engl. J. Med.*, 1979, *301*, 1382.

In patients with procainamide-induced lupus subsequently treated with acecainide, there was a remission of symptoms or no recurrence of symptoms in most patients.— J. Kluger *et al.*, *Ann. intern. Med.*, 1981, *95*, 18.

Proprietary Names and Manufacturers
American Critical Care, USA.

18724-z

Adenosine
6-Amino-9-β-D-ribofuranosyl-9*H*-purine.
$C_{10}H_{13}N_5O_4=267.2$.

CAS — 58-61-7.

Adenosine is an endogenous nucleoside which is under study as an anti-arrhythmic agent. Adenosine phosphate and triphosphate have been tried in a variety of conditions and are described in the section on vasodilators (see p.1492).

A discussion on the pharmacology of adenosine, an endogenous nucleoside formed mainly as a degradation product of adenosine triphosphate, and on its possible pathophysiological roles.— *Lancet*, 1985, *2*, 927. See also A. H. Watt and P. A. Routledge, *Br. med. J.*, 1986, *293*, 1455.

Studies on the pharmacological effects of adenosine in healthy subjects: A. H. Watt and P. A. Routledge, *Br. J. clin. Pharmac.*, 1985, *20*, 503 (stimulation of respiration); *idem*, 1986, *21*, 533 (transient bradycardia and subsequent sinus tachycardia); C. Sylvén *et al.*, *Br. med. J.*, 1986, *293*, 227 (provocation of angina pectoris-like pain); P. G. Reid *et al.*, *Br. J. clin. Pharmac.*, 1987, *23*, 331 (stimulation of respiration by adenosine, but not by its metabolite inosine).

Adenosine 50 to 250 µg per kg body-weight intravenously successfully terminated resistant supraventricular tachycardia in 3 seriously ill neonates and one 10-year-old child, in each case within 20 seconds of injection.— B. Clarke *et al.*, *Lancet*, 1987, *1*, 299.

Adenosine was considered to have an important role as a diagnostic and therapeutic agent in the emergency management of regular broad complex tachycardias following a study in 26 patients who were given incremental intravenous doses of 50 µg per kg body-weight, to a maximum of 250 µg per kg, during episodes of tachycardia. The ability of adenosine to block atrioventricular conduction allows diagnosis and treatment for most supraventricular tachycardias, and the short half-life and absence of negative inotropic effects make it moderately safe (unlike verapamil) if administered during ventricular tachycardia.— M. J. Griffith *et al.*, *Lancet*, 1988, *1*, 672. A note that the adenosine injection used was prepared as a 0.2% aqueous solution of adenosine base in 0.9% sodium chloride and presented as 20 mg adenosine per 10-mL ampoule. The injection is sterilised by filtration.— C. J. Cairns and C. Clarke (letter), *ibid.*, 1105.

For reference to the use of adenosine triphosphate in the treatment of paroxysmal supraventricular tachycardia, see p.1492.

7777-b

Ajmaline *(BAN)*.
Ajmalina; Ajmalinum; Rauwolfine. An alkaloid obtained from the root of *Rauwolfia serpentina* (Apocynaceae).
(17*R*,21*R*)-Ajmalan-17,21-diol.
$C_{20}H_{26}N_2O_2=326.4$.

CAS — 4360-12-7.

Pharmacopoeias. In *Aust.*, *Cz.*, *Fr.*, *It.*, *Jpn*, and *Neth.* *Aust.*, *Fr.*, and *Neth.* also include the monohydrate (Ajmaline Monohydrate).

A white or slightly yellowish, odourless or almost odourless, crystalline powder. Practically **insoluble** in water; freely soluble in alcohol, chloroform, and glacial acetic acid; sparingly soluble in ether and methyl alcohol. **Protect** from light.

7778-v

Ajmaline Monoethanolate *(BAN).*

Ajmalinum Monoaethanolum.
$C_{20}H_{26}N_2O_2,C_2H_6O=372.5$.

CAS — 60991-48-2.

Pharmacopoeias. In *Aust., Fr., It.,* and *Neth.*

A white or slightly yellowish crystalline powder with a slight odour characteristic of alcohol. Practically **insoluble** in water; freely soluble in alcohol, chloroform, and glacial acetic acid; sparingly soluble in ether and methyl alcohol. **Protect** from light.

Adverse Effects

Ajmaline depresses the conductivity of the heart, and at high doses can cause heart block. At very high doses it may produce a negative inotropic effect. High doses may also cause cardiac arrhythmias, coma, and death. Adverse neurological effects have been reported including eye twitching, convulsions, and respiratory depression. Hepatotoxicity and agranulocytosis may occasionally occur.

Precautions

As for Quinidine, p.86.

INTERACTIONS. Concurrent oral administration of quinidine with ajmaline gave considerably increased plasma concentrations of ajmaline in 4 healthy subjects; the elimination half-life of ajmaline was increased about twofold. The pharmacokinetics of quinidine did not seem to be affected by the presence of ajmaline.— R. Hori *et al., J. Pharm. Pharmac.*, 1984, *36*, 202.

MYASTHENIA GRAVIS. Under experimental conditions ajmaline has been shown to interfere with neuromuscular transmission. It should therefore be used with caution in patients with myasthenia.— Z. Argov and F. L. Mastaglia, *New Engl. J. Med.*, 1979, *301*, 409.

Uses and Administration

Ajmaline is a class I anti-arrhythmic agent (p.70). It is used in the treatment of cardiac arrhythmias in usual maintenance doses of 200 to 300 mg daily by mouth. It can also be administered by intramuscular or slow intravenous injection. It has also been used as the hydrochloride and as the aminoethyl phosphate.

A brief review of ajmaline. Ajmaline has two principal uses: it is used to diagnose Wolff-Parkinson-White syndrome and as a provocative test of the AV conduction system in patients suspected of having paroxysmal heart block. However, further study and confirmation is necessary before ajmaline can be used widely to detect latent heart block. Ajmaline is administered by slow intravenous injection over 3 minutes under well-controlled hospital conditions. The advantage of ajmaline is that it has a short duration of action and is generally well tolerated.— D. L. D. Keefe *et al., Drugs*, 1981, *22*, 363. See also: J. B. Schwartz *et al., Drugs*, 1981, *21*, 23.

Proprietary Names and Manufacturers of Ajmaline and its Salts

Aritmina *(Byk Gulden, Ital.)*; Cardiorythmine *(Eutherapie, Belg.; Servier, Fr.; Servier, Switz.)*; Gilurytmal *(Nativelle, Belg.; Giulini, Denm.; Giulini, Ger.; Giulini, Neth.; Lacer, Spain; Giulini, Swed.; Kali-Chemie, Switz.)*; Normorytmina *(Chemil, Ital.)*; Ritmas *(Toyo Jozo, Jpn)*; Ritmos *(Inverni della Beffa, Ital.)*; Ritmosedina *(Inverni della Beffa, Ital.)*; Rythmaton *(Nippon Kayaku, Jpn)*.

7779-g

Alinidine *(BAN, rINN).*

ST-567; ST-567-BR (hydrobromide). *N*-Allyl-2,6-dichloro-*N*-(2-imidazolin-2-yl)aniline.
$C_{12}H_{13}Cl_2N_3=270.2$.

CAS — 33178-86-8.

Alinidine resembles clonidine in chemical structure, but has been reported to differ in pharmacological action. It causes bradycardia probably due to a direct effect on the heart. It has been suggested that its properties may represent a fifth class of anti-arrhythmic action (see p.70).

ABSORPTION AND FATE. A study of alinidine pharmacokinetics following acute and chronic dosing. Alinidine was rapidly absorbed following oral administration with peak plasma concentrations occurring at 1.8 hours. Comparison with data from intravenous administration indicated 100% bioavailability. The elimination half-life was 4.2 hours following intravenous administration. During chronic dosing, steady-state plasma concentrations were attained from day 2 and there was no evidence of further accumulation. Small amounts of clonidine were detected in the plasma and urine, reaching mean plasma concentrations of 0.8 to 1.0 ng per mL during chronic dosing with alinidine 40 mg twice daily. It was considered unlikely that the formation of clonidine would be responsible for the observed pharmacodynamic effects of alinidine, but it was suggested that clonidine could be responsible for drowsiness and dry mouth occurring during treatment.— D. W. G. Harron *et al., Br. J. clin. Pharmac.*, 1982, *13*, 821.

ACTION. Evidence that alinidine may represent a new, fifth class of anti-arrhythmic action.— J. S. Millar and E. M. Vaughan Williams, *Lancet*, 1981, *1*, 1291. Comment.— H. Nawrath (letter), *ibid.*, *2*, 209.

A study in 6 healthy subjects suggested that a reduction in sympathetic activity could be partly responsible for the hypotensive action of alinidine.— D. P. Nicholls *et al., Br. J. clin. Pharmac.*, 1984, *18*, 215. Further references to the mode of action of alinidine.— K. Weerasuriya and J. Hamer (letter), *ibid.*, 1981, *11*, 398; B. Stanek *et al., Eur. J. clin. Pharmac.*, 1983, *24*, 31; D. W. G. Harron *et al., Br. J. clin. Pharmac.*, 1983, *16*, 451; B. E. Jaski and P. W. Serruys, *Am. J. Cardiol.*, 1985, *56*, 270.

USES. A study in healthy subjects indicating that alinidine may be of value in patients with angina or tachyarrhythmias. Although chemically related to clonidine its effect more closely resembled that of propranolol, since it reduced exercise tachycardia which clonidine did not. Unlike propranolol, however, alinidine did not induce beta-blockade. In a dose of 80 mg alinidine reduced an exercise-induced tachycardia to the same extent as propranolol 40 mg; the 80-mg dose also significantly reduced arterial blood pressure in the standing and supine positions, and produced drowsiness and dry mouth. It was considered that 40 mg may be the preferred dose of alinidine on oral administration since this dose reduced heart-rate without adverse effects.— D. W. G. Harron *et al., Lancet*, 1981, *1*, 351.

Comment on a possible exacerbation of angina by alinidine. Patients given 20 or 40 mg three times daily complained of precordial pain with a lower heart-rate at the same work-load as before treatment.— W. Ebm and H. Zilcher (letter), *Lancet*, 1981, *1*, 611.

Treatment with alinidine 40 mg three times daily reduced the number of anginal attacks and the amount of glyceryl trinitrate consumed in a placebo-controlled study involving 14 men with stable angina. Clinical symptoms and exercise tolerance improved in most but not all patients despite decreases in heart-rate and systolic blood pressure. One patient with impaired left ventricular function had to be withdrawn from the study because of deterioration in his clinical condition.— T. Meinertz *et al., Clin. Pharmac. Ther.*, 1983, *34*, 770.

Further references: M. L. Simoons and P. G. Hugenholtz, *Eur. Heart J.*, 1984, *5*, 227.

Proprietary Names and Manufacturers

Boehringer Ingelheim, UK.

7780-f

Amiodarone Hydrochloride *(BANM, rINNM).*

51087N; L-3428 (amiodarone); SKF-33-134-A (amiodarone). 2-Butylbenzofuran-3-yl 4-(2-diethylaminoethoxy)-3,5-di-iodophenyl ketone hydrochloride.
$C_{25}H_{29}I_2NO_3,HCl=681.8$.

CAS — 1951-25-3 (amiodarone); 19774-82-4 (hydrochloride).

Pharmacopoeias. In *Chin.*

Incompatibility has been reported with aminophylline, heparin, and sodium chloride solutions.

An investigation of the physicochemical and analytical characteristics of amiodarone, including studies of the solubility of amiodarone hydrochloride in a range of solvents, u.v., i.r., and mass spectrometry, high-performance liquid chromatography, and the partition coefficient. Amiodarone hydrochloride was found to be freely soluble in chloroform, sparingly soluble in alcohol, and very slightly soluble in water. The melting point was found to be 159°C and the pK_a was 6.56.— M. Bonati *et al., J. pharm. Sci.*, 1984, *73*, 829.

The drop size delivered by an intravenous infusion set was found to decrease with increasing concentrations of amiodarone such that the volume of a solution of amiodarone 1200 mg in glucose 5% 500 mL delivered over unit time was reduced by about 30% compared to glucose controls. The reduction in drop size was attributed to a reduction in surface tension caused by the inclusion of Tween 80 in the formulation.— P. A. Capps and A. L. Robertson, *Pharm. J.*, 1985, *1*, 14. A reduction in drop size of diluted amiodarone injection due to surfactant properties of the proprietary preparation may result in a reduction in the expected delivery rates of amiodarone when the infusion is controlled by drip rate. Amiodarone should be administered either by a volumetric infusion pump or adjustment made by a factor of 3/2 when a normal adult giving set is employed.— U. M. Chouhan and E. Lynch (letter), *ibid.*, *2*, 466.

ADSORPTION. There was a rapid fall in the concentration of solutions of amiodarone hydrochloride by 10% in 3 hours followed by a steady decrease to 60% of the initial concentration after 5 days storage in flexible polyvinyl chloride bags at ambient temperature. When amiodarone solutions were perfused through polyvinyl chloride giving sets the concentration had fallen to 82% after 15 minutes. Similar losses were not observed from solutions stored in glass or rigid polyvinyl chloride bottles, and the losses were attributed to the presence of the plasticizer, di-2-ethylhexylphthalate.— S. J. Weir *et al., Am. J. Hosp. Pharm.*, 1985, *42*, 2679. Correction.— *ibid.*, 1986, *43*, 900.

INCOMPATIBILITY. Precipitation was observed in the intravenous lines of 2 patients receiving amiodarone and heparin injections concomitantly through a common central venous line.— C. J. Cairns (letter), *Pharm. J.*, 1986, *1*, 68.

Adverse Effects

Adverse cardiovascular effects associated with amiodarone include severe bradycardia and conduction disturbances. Severe hypotension may follow intravenous administration particularly, though not exclusively, at rapid infusion rates. Amiodarone may also give rise to ventricular tachyarrhythmias.

Amiodarone is reported to reduce the peripheral transformation of thyroxine (T_4) to tri-iodothyronine (T_3) and to increase the formation of reverse-T_3. It can affect thyroid function and may induce hypo- or hyperthyroidism.

There have been reports of severe pulmonary toxicity including pulmonary fibrosis and interstitial pneumonitis. These effects may be reversible on withdrawal of amiodarone but are potentially fatal.

Amiodarone can adversely affect the liver. There may be abnormal liver function tests and cirrhosis; fatalities have been reported.

Prolonged treatment with amiodarone causes the development of benign yellowish-brown corneal microdeposits, sometimes associated with coloured haloes of light; these are reversible on stopping therapy. Photosensitivity reactions are also common and more rarely slate-grey discoloration of the skin may also occur. Generally sunscreen agents are ineffective at preventing this reaction.

Other adverse effects reported include peripheral neuropathy, tremor, nausea, vomiting, a metallic taste, nightmares, headaches, and sleeplessness.

Adverse effects due to amiodarone therapy were recorded in 82% of 80 patients during follow-up periods of up to 51 months; adverse effects were sufficiently severe to necessitate withdrawing amiodarone in 18% of patients. Lung toxicity characterised as interstitial pneumonitis occurred in 5% of patients. Three patients taking 600 mg or more of amiodarone daily plus digoxin developed sinus node arrest, and four patients developed incessant ventricular tachycardia. Among other more common though less serious adverse effects observed were: neurological effects in 24% of patients, gastro-intestinal effects in 34%, dermatological effects in 14%, and neuromuscular effects in 14%. Increases in liver enzymes were found in 14 out of 35 patients assessed. Although some of the adverse effects were improved or abolished by reducing the dose of amiodarone, many reactions occurred at the minimum dose required to control arrhythmias. It was concluded that while amiodarone is effective in many patients whose arrhythmias are refractory to other drugs its usefulness is limited by frequent and potentially serious toxicity.— B. McGovern *et al.*, *Br. med. J.*, 1983, *287*, 175. For a contrary view that most adverse reactions occur at plasma concentrations in excess of those required to control arrhythmias see under Uses, p.73.

EFFECTS ON THE CARDIOVASCULAR SYSTEM. *Cardiac arrhythmias.* A report of incessant, polymorphic ventricular tachycardia in one patient within a week of treatment with amiodarone for paroxysmal ventricular tachycardia.— D. C. Westveer *et al.*, *Ann. intern. Med.*, 1982, *97*, 561. Comment that disturbance of atrioventricular conduction is unusual during an early stage of therapy with amiodarone.— K. Nademanee and B. N. Singh (letter), *ibid.*, 1983, *98*, 110.

Sinus bradycardia and a 12-second period of sinus arrest developed in a patient 20 days after the start of treatment with amiodarone and 10 days after the discontinuation of digoxin.— W. M. Brodine and J. De Santis (letter), *Br. med. J.*, 1982, *285*, 1047.

Atrial fibrillation with a ventricular rate up to 230 beats per minute was associated with amiodarone administration in a patient with Wolff-Parkinson-White syndrome and a history of myocardial infarction. It was suggested that the myocardial infarction may have damaged the atrioventricular node which would have been further impaired by amiodarone administration thus allowing conduction through an accessory pathway and the resultant increase in ventricular rate.— B. D. Sheinman and T. Evans, *Br. med. J.*, 1982, *285*, 999.

Life-threatening ventricular tachyarrhythmias resembling torsades de pointes were attributed to amiodarone therapy in 2 patients.— C. R. Kumana *et al.*, *Hum. Toxicol.*, 1985, *4*, 169.

Hypotension. Severe hypotension in 3 out of 8 patients receiving amiodarone 300 mg in 10 minutes by intravenous infusion was attributed to the rapid infusion rate.— M. Koblic *et al.* (letter), *Br. med. J.*, 1983, *286*, 1825.

EFFECTS ON THE ENDOCRINE SYSTEM. There was evidence of abnormalities of carbohydrate and lipid metabolism associated with amiodarone treatment in 3 patients with normal thyroid function.— A. Politi *et al.*, *Br. med. J.*, 1984, *288*, 285.

Gynaecomastia. A report of gynaecomastia in a 41-year-old man during treatment with amiodarone. Gynaecomastia regressed when amiodarone was withdrawn and recurred when treatment with amiodarone was restarted.— D. Antonelli *et al.* (letter), *New Engl. J. Med.*, 1986, *315*, 1553.

Thyroid function. A brief review of the seemingly contradictory effects of amiodarone — hyperthyroidism and hypothyroidism — with reference to recent work on the mechanism of amiodarone-associated thyrotoxicosis.— *Lancet*, 1987, *2*, 24.

Amiodarone contains 75 mg of iodine in each 200 mg tablet and although the rate of de-iodination is comparatively low, significant amounts of iodine are released. In practice fewer than 2% of patients receiving amiodarone develop overt thyroid disease. Clinical hyperthyroidism seems to occur predominantly in patients with goitre or active auto-immune thyroid disease. Amiodarone complicates the interpretation of thyroid function tests: the serum concentration of tri-iodothyronine (T_3), or ideally of free T_3, is the most helpful test in confirming a diagnosis of hyperthyroidism. The clinical diagnosis of thyrotoxicosis may be difficult as amiodarone masks many of the signs of hyperthyroidism. The most useful pointers to hyperthyroidism in patients taking amiodarone are loss of weight, asthenia, restlessness, and recurrence of arrhythmias; low grade fever, a rapid erythrocyte sedimentation rate, and shortening of the Q-T interval may also be seen.— W. J. McKenna *et al.*, *Br. med. J.*, 1983, *287*, 1654. A discussion of the evaluation of thyroid function in patients taking amiodarone in which it is suggested that several biological variables should be considered in patients in whom thyroid complications are suspected. Hyperthyroidism was considered to be unlikely in patients with normal serum concentrations of total and free thyroxine (T_4). When either total or free T_4, or both, are elevated, a thyrotrophin releasing hormone test should be performed.— Y. Abramovici *et al.* (letter), *ibid.*, 1984, *288*, 327.

Hypothyroidism occurred in 10 patients and hyperthyroidism in 1 patient out of 100 patients taking amiodarone studied by Jaggarao *et al.* (*Postgrad. med. J.*, 1982, *58*, 693). Raised free thyroxine index was noted in 25% of patients studied, although they remained euthyroid. It was concluded that amiodarone need not be withdrawn in patients with high thyroxine but normal tri-iodothyronine concentrations. The mechanism of this effect was also discussed by Martino *et al.* (*Ann. intern. Med.*, 1984, *101*, 28) who found hyperthyroidism in 9.6% of patients taking amiodarone living in an area of low-iodine intake in Tuscany compared with 2% of patients living in Massachusetts in an area of adequate iodine intake. In contrast, hypothyroidism was more frequent in Massachusetts at 22% than in Tuscany at 5%.

Antithyroid microsomal antibodies were detectable in 6 out of 14 patients taking amiodarone after 30 days of treatment, but in none of 23 patients on placebo. These results and increases in thyroid stimulating hormone suggested that amiodarone had a toxic effect on the thyroid even over relatively short treatment periods, although the effect appeared to be reversible.— E. Monteiro *et al.*, *Br. med. J.*, 1986, *292*, 227. See also: J. A. Amico *et al.*, *Archs intern. Med.*, 1984, *144*, 487.

EFFECTS ON THE EYES. Slit-lamp examination showed corneal abnormalities in 103 out of 105 patients being treated with amiodarone, although no decrease in visual acuity attributable to the drug was observed. The density of the corneal deposits was dependent on dosage, and deposits disappeared over a period of 3 to 7 months in 16 patients after amiodarone was withdrawn. It was considered that ophthalmological surveillance was not required in asymptomatic patients on long-term amiodarone therapy.— D. V. Ingram *et al.*, *Br. J. Ophthal.*, 1982, *66*, 676.

A report of a sicca syndrome with diminished tear and saliva production in a 65-year-old man 4 months after starting treatment with amiodarone. Sjögren's syndrome could not be firmly diagnosed.— E. J. Dickinson and R. L. Wolman (letter), *Br. med. J.*, 1986, *293*, 510.

Optic neuropathy associated with amiodarone therapy in 13 patients.— L. A. Feiner *et al.*, *Mayo Clin. Proc.*, 1987, *62*, 702.

EFFECTS ON THE GENITAL SYSTEM. Scrotal pain associated with epididymal enlargement developed in 6 out of 56 men treated with amiodarone. Symptoms occurred 7 to 15 months after the start of treatment and resolved within 10 weeks despite continuation of full amiodarone dosage in 4 patients.— J. P. Gasparich *et al.* (letter), *Lancet*, 1984, *2*, 1211.

High concentrations of amiodarone and desethylamiodarone were found in necropsy samples of testis from 5 patients, one of whom had complained of scrotal and groin pain before death. A further patient receiving amiodarone 400 mg daily complained of brown discoloration of sweat and semen which persisted when the dose was reduced to 200 mg daily. Amiodarone and desethylamiodarone were both detected in the semen.— P. C. Adams *et al.* (letter), *Lancet*, 1985, *1*, 341.

EFFECTS ON THE LIVER. Irreversible neuropathy and severe hepatitis progressing to cirrhosis was attributed to amiodarone therapy in a 68-year-old man. Liver enzyme concentrations fell when amiodarone was withdrawn, but the patient died from liver failure 5 months after stopping amiodarone.— P. K. Lim *et al.*, *Br. med. J.*, 1984, *288*, 1638.

Asymptomatic elevated aminotransferase concentrations persisted for several months after amiodarone was withdrawn. Histological abnormalities of liver tissue closely resembled those associated with active alcoholic hepatitis with fibrosis.— J. B. Simon *et al.*, *New Engl. J. Med.*, 1984, *311*, 167.

Further reports of fatal cirrhosis of the liver in patients taking amiodarone.— K. Tordjman *et al.* (letter), *Ann. intern. Med.*, 1985, *102*, 411; H. M. Rinder *et al.* (letter), *New Engl. J. Med.*, 1986, *314*, 318.

EFFECTS ON THE LUNGS. Pulmonary infiltration and bone marrow depression were associated with amiodarone treatment in a 71-year-old man.— A. J. Wright and R. G. Brackenridge, *Br. med. J.*, 1982, *284*, 1303. Comment that there was insufficient evidence for a diagnosis of bone-marrow depression.— C. J. T. Bateman (letter), *ibid.*, *285*, 60.

Amiodarone-induced pneumonitis was considered to be immunologically mediated and not dose-dependent in a report of 5 patients.— A. Venet *et al.* (letter), *Lancet*, 1984, *1*, 962.

In the *UK* the CSM had received 46 reports of alveolitis or pulmonary fibrosis attributed to amiodarone by July 1985, of which 4 were fatal. Pulmonary alveolitis may be mistaken for deterioration of an underlying cardiac condition.— *Br. med. J.*, 1986, *292*, 50.

Further reports of pulmonary toxicity associated with amiodarone treatment: S. A. Riley *et al.*, *Br. med. J.*, 1982, *284*, 161; F. E. Marchlinski *et al.*, *Ann. intern. Med.*, 1982, *97*, 839; J. Morera *et al.*, *Eur. J. clin. Pharmac.*, 1983, *24*, 591; D. L. Wood *et al.*, *Mayo Clin. Proc.*, 1985, *60*, 601.

EFFECTS ON THE NERVOUS SYSTEM. Of 10 patients treated with amiodarone for more than 2 years, 3 patients had evidence of peripheral neuropathy. Initial results suggested that neuropathy correlated with high doses and high serum concentrations of amiodarone.— A. G. Fraser and I. N. F. McQueen (letter), *Br. med. J.*, 1983, *287*, 612.

EFFECTS ON THE SKIN. A study of 10 patients taking amiodarone indicated that amiodarone photosensitivity was due to a phototoxic rather than a photo-allergic mechanism and that the wavelengths responsible range from the long UV into the visible portion of the spectrum. The common sunscreen agents are likely to be of little value and topical preparations of zinc and titanium oxide would seem to be the most suitable agents. Dosage reduction could also be indicated.— J. Ferguson *et al.* (letter), *Lancet*, 1984, *2*, 414. See also: C. B. Zachary *et al.*, *Br. J. Derm.*, 1984, *110*, 451; J. Ferguson *et al.*, *ibid.*, 1985, *113*, 537; J. Boyle (letter), *ibid.*, 1986, *115*, 253.

Acute cutaneous vasculitis was associated with amiodarone therapy in a 72-year-old patient.— I. D. Starke and C. Barbatis (letter), *Br. med. J.*, 1985, *291*, 940.

Fatal toxic epidermal necrolysis (Lyell's disease) occurred in a patient 10 days after receiving amiodarone 400 mg daily for cardiac arrhythmias.— P. L. Bencini *et al.* (letter), *Archs Derm.*, 1985, *121*, 838.

Alopecia. A report of total hair loss associated with amiodarone administration. An improvement in the quantity of scalp hair was noted 2 months after amiodarone was withdrawn, and after 8 months the patient had regained all her hair.— A. Samanta *et al.* (letter), *Br. med. J.*, 1983, *287*, 503.

OVERDOSAGE. The only abnormal clinical sign about 12 hours after an overdose with amiodarone 8 g by mouth in a 20-year-old patient was profuse perspiration. Apart from slight bradycardia observed during the second and third days, no cardiovascular effects were seen. Thyroid and hepatic function were not affected. The elimination half-life was 31.5 hours.— M. Bonati *et al.*, *J. Toxicol. clin. Toxicol.*, 1983, *20*, 181.

Treatment of Adverse Effects

In overdosage by mouth the stomach should be emptied by aspiration and lavage.

A beta-adrenoceptor stimulant (for example, isoprenaline) or glucagon, has been recommended for bradycardia. Corticosteroids have been recommended for the treatment of pulmonary toxicity.

Report of 3 patients in whom pyridoxine appeared to protect against amiodarone-induced photosensitivity.— G. Kaufmann (letter), *Lancet*, 1984, *1*, 51. In a study in 46 patients to assess the efficacy of pyridoxine in preventing amiodarone-induced photosensitivity, results indicated that pyridoxine may *enhance* photosensitivity. There was an unexpectedly high response rate to placebo treatment.— J. P. Mulrow *et al.*, *Ann. intern. Med.*, 1985, *103*, 68 (see also under Effects on the Skin, above).

Precautions

Amiodarone should not be given to patients with bradycardia or with impairment of atrioventricular conduction. It may be used with caution in patients with heart failure. The use of amiodarone should be avoided in patients with iodine sensitivity, disorders of the thyroid gland, or with a history of thyroid disorders; amiodarone can induce spurious results from some thyroid-function tests. Patients taking amiodarone should avoid exposure to sunlight.

Liver function tests should be carried out regularly in patients on long-term therapy.

Intravenous injections of amiodarone should be given slowly: if prolonged or repeated infusions are envisaged, the use of a central venous catheter should be considered.

Amiodarone should be used with caution with other agents liable to induce bradycardia, such as beta-blockers or calcium-channel blockers, and with other anti-arrhythmic drugs. The effects of warfarin and other oral anticoagulants may be enhanced by concomitant administration of amiodarone, and plasma concentrations of digoxin may be raised.

For the problems of controlling the delivery rate of amiodarone by intravenous infusion, see p.71.

For comments on thyroid function tests in patients taking amiodarone see under Adverse Effects on thyroid function, above.

INTERACTIONS. A review of drug interactions with amiodarone.— F. I. Marcus, *Am. Heart J.*, 1983, *106*, 924.

The administration of amiodarone has been reported to enhance the effects of a number of drugs, including those listed below and for which further details are provided under their individual monographs: aprindine (p.74), digoxin (p.827), flecainide (p.79), phenytoin (p.408), quinidine (p.86), warfarin (p.345).

PREGNANCY AND THE NEONATE. The view that amiodarone is contra-indicated in women who are breast-feeding.— P. C. Rubin, *Br. med. J.*, 1986, *293*, 1415; R. L. Nation and N. Hotham, *Med. J. Aust.*, 1987, *146*, 308.

For reports of the use of amiodarone during pregnancy, see under Uses, below.

Absorption and Fate

Amiodarone is absorbed variably and erratically from the gastro-intestinal tract and is reported to have a half-life of between 25 and 100 days during long-term administration.

Amiodarone is extensively distributed to body tissues and accumulates notably in muscle and fat; it has been reported to be 96% bound to plasma proteins. A steady state is reached after about a month. There is very little urinary excretion of amiodarone or its metabolites but they have been detected in the faeces. Amiodarone is reported to cross the placenta and to appear in breast milk. On stopping prolonged amiodarone therapy a pharmacological effect is evident for a month or more.

Following intravenous injection the maximum effect is achieved within 1 to 30 minutes and persists for 1 to 3 hours.

A review of the clinical pharmacokinetics of amiodarone. The available evidence suggests that the absorption of amiodarone from the gastro-intestinal tract is erratic and unpredictable, with bioavailability ranging from 22 to 86%. There is evidence to suggest an hepatic first-pass effect in *rats*. The only metabolite to be positively identified is desethylamiodarone (DEA), and this has been shown to accumulate to steady-state concentrations comparable to those of amiodarone, although the clinical significance of this observation is unclear. Generally, little or no amiodarone or its metabolites have been detected in the urine after single- or multiple-dose administration. During long-term oral administration, steady-state plasma concentrations were not reached for at least 30 days. Amiodarone half-lives during the washout period after long-term therapy have ranged from 14 to 107 days: this is longer than that reported after most single-dose studies and more consistent with the rate of disappearance of therapeutic effects. A plasma concentration range between 1.0 and 2.5 µg per mL seems to be generally associated with therapeutic response. Both amiodarone and DEA have been shown to cross the placenta and to be excreted in breast milk.— R. Latini *et al.*, *Clin. Pharmacokinet.*, 1984, *9*, 136.

Amiodarone 175 mg per hour by intravenous infusion for 2 hours then 50 mg per hour for 46 hours produced plasma concentrations below the provisional therapeutic range of 1.0 to 2.5 µg per mL in at least 3 of 8 patients between 3 and 16 hours after the start of the infusion.— A. H. Watt *et al.*, *Br. J. clin. Pharmac.*, 1986, *21*, 525.

Further references to the pharmacokinetics of amiodarone: D. W. Holt *et al.*, *Am. Heart J.*, 1983, *106*, 840; T. A. Plomp *et al.*, *Arzneimittel-Forsch.*, 1984, *34*, 513.

Uses and Administration

Amiodarone is a class III anti-arrhythmic agent (see p.70). It is used in the control of ventricular and supraventricular arrhythmias, where other drugs cannot be used, including arrhythmias associated with Wolff-Parkinson-White syndrome. It has also been used in the treatment of angina pectoris, but less toxic alternatives are generally preferred.

Amiodarone is given as the hydrochloride in initial doses of 200 mg three times daily for a week, then is gradually reduced to a usual maintenance dosage of 200 mg to 400 mg daily, according to the patient's response. Some patients may require loading doses of up to 1600 mg daily and maintenance doses of up to 600 mg daily, but consideration should be given to potential adverse effects, and patients should be given the minimum effective dose.

Amiodarone hydrochloride may be given intravenously where facilities for close monitoring of cardiac function and resuscitation are available. It is given by intravenous infusion usually in concentrations of 5 mg per kg body-weight in 250 mL of glucose injection, infused over 20 minutes to 2 hours, and repeated two or three times in 24 hours to a maximum of 1.2 g in up to 500 mL of glucose injection daily. Repeated infusions are preferably made through a central venous catheter. In emergencies it may also be given in doses of 5 mg per kg body-weight (doses of about 300 to 450 mg) given over a period of 30 seconds to 3 minutes; a second injection should not be given until at least 15 minutes after the first.

A review of amiodarone.— J. W. Mason, *New Engl. J. Med.*, 1987, *316*, 455 and 760 (correction).

ADMINISTRATION. The mean steady-state serum-amiodarone concentrations in 17 patients ranged between 0.65 and 5.7 nmol per mL and correlated with the prescribed daily dose. Results of the study indicated that serum concentrations between 1.5 and 4.0 nmol per mL may control arrhythmias without leading to dose-dependent adverse effects. Adverse effects of amiodarone therapy on thyroid function appeared to be independent of serum-amiodarone concentrations.— M. Stäubli *et al.*, *Eur. J. clin. Pharmac.*, 1983, *24*, 485.

A discussion of the various parameters which may be used to assist in dosage adjustments during amiodarone therapy. Changes in the QT interval may be a useful indicator of drug effect in some patients, although correlation with anti-arrhythmic effect can be poor, and interpretation difficult. The measurement of reverse tri-iodothyronine concentrations was also considered unlikely to be a reliable index. There were indications that plasma-amiodarone concentration monitoring could be useful.— W. J. McKenna and D. M. Krikler, *Br. Heart J.*, 1984, *51*, 241.

In a study involving 127 patients being treated with amiodarone it was concluded that it was necessary to maintain serum-amiodarone concentrations above 1.0 µg per mL to minimise the chance of recurrence of arrhythmias. Most adverse effects occurred at a mean amiodarone concentration in excess of 2.5 µg per mL. The results suggested that hepatic, neuromuscular, and ocular disturbances were serum concentration-dependent whereas pulmonary toxicity, cutaneous manifestations, cardiovascular and gastro-intestinal complaints may occur at low serum-amiodarone concentrations in susceptible patients.— H. H. Rotmensch *et al.*, *Ann. intern. Med.*, 1984, *101*, 462. For a contrary view that many adverse reactions occur at doses required to abolish arrhythmias see under Adverse Effects, p.71.

For recommendations of adjustments to the infusion rate which are necessary to take acccount of surface active effects of amiodarone injection, see p.71.

In children and neonates. A review of the use of amiodarone for the treatment of cardiac arrhythmias in children.— P. Coumel *et al.*, *PACE*, 1983, *6*, 930.

Brief report of the successful treatment of a case of foetal cardiac arrhythmias with amiodarone. It was considered that transplacental treatment with amiodarone should only be considered as a last resort until more information about its possible effects on the foetal thyroid has been obtained.— J. W. Wladimiroff and P. A. Stewart, *Br. J. Hosp. Med.*, 1985, *34*, 134.

CARDIAC ARRHYTHMIAS. A review of amiodarone. Amiodarone is an effective agent for treating troublesome supraventricular and some serious ventricular arrhythmias. It is particularly effective for paroxysmal atrial fibrillation, supraventricular arrhythmias associated with the Wolff-Parkinson-White syndrome, and in the suppression of ventricular arrhythmias complicating hypertrophic cardiomyopathy. Its place in the treatment of arrhythmias during acute myocardial infarction is still uncertain, but it has been found to be effective in patients with refractory ventricular tachycardia or fibrillation. Life-threatening arrhythmias should initially be treated in hospital where resuscitation facilities are available. Each patient should receive the minimum effective maintenance dose; in patients with non-life-threatening arrhythmias the need for continuing treatment should periodically be reassessed. Patients with disorders of the thyroid, lung, or liver are at particular risk of adverse effects.— W. J. McKenna *et al.*, *Br. med. J.*, 1983, *287*, 1654.

The anti-arrhythmic effect of amiodarone has been confirmed by several studies in a wide variety of supraventricular arrhythmias. It has been particularly valuable in the prevention of atrial arrhythmias unresponsive to other drugs. Similar beneficial effects have been recorded in patients with sustained ventricular arrhythmias of all types. There is some evidence that amiodarone can improve survival prospects in patients with recurrent ventricular fibrillation and "failed sudden death". However, objective evidence of therapeutic action cannot be obtained by electrophysiological testing, and there is a delay of several weeks before a therapeutic effect is achieved. Unwanted effects necessitating withdrawal of therapy have arisen in up to 22% of patients. Total elimination of amiodarone may take weeks, so adverse effects may persist for some time after drug withdrawal. It is now evident that adverse effects are common and occasionally fatal. In view of its complex pharmacokinetics, electrophysiology, and adverse effects, it has been recommended that amiodarone be reserved for patients with arrhythmias not responsive to other anti-arrhythmic drugs.— *Lancet*, 1983, *2*, 1123.

The observation of an anti-arrhythmic effect within 3 hours of the first oral dose of amiodarone in 2 patients by Mattison and Rodger (*Br. med. J.*, 1982, *285*, 939) was attributed by Norrell (*ibid.*, 1358) to a possible transient but rapid fixation of amiodarone to cardiac receptors. This rapid onset of effect after oral therapy had been previously described.

For a report of a symposium on the therapeutic role of amiodarone in cardiology, see: *Br. J. clin. Pract.*, 1986, *40, Suppl.* 44, 1-163.

Studies of the anti-arrhythmic effects of amiodarone.— L. Rakita and S. M. Sobol, *J. Am. med. Ass.*, 1983, *250*, 1293; K. Nademanee *et al.*, *Ann. intern. Med.*, 1983, *98*, 577; M. Komajda *et al.*, *Annls Cardiol. Angeiol.*, 1985, *34*, 269; T. Peter *et al.*, *Eur. Heart J.*, 1985, *6*, 151; W. M. Smith *et al.*, *Am. J. Cardiol.*, 1986, *57*, 1288.

PREGNANCY AND THE NEONATE. Normal infants were delivered to 2 women after amiodarone administration during pregnancy; one patient took amiodarone throughout her pregnancy and the other for the final 17 weeks. Relatively high placental concentrations of amiodarone and desethylamiodarone were measured in both patients.— D. J. Robson *et al.*, *Postgrad. med. J.*, 1985, *61*, 75.

Following treatment with amiodarone during pregnancy in a woman with recurrent ventricular tachycardia, both mother and infant had iodine levels 10 to 40 times higher than normal. However, the infant was healthy and there was no evidence of thyroid dysfunction.— E. Rey *et al.*, *Can. med. Ass. J.*, 1987, *136*, 959.

Further references: W. J. McKenna *et al.*, *Am. J. Cardiol.*, 1983, *51*, 1231; D. Pitcher *et al.* (letter), *Lancet*, 1983, *1*, 597.

PSORIASIS. Psoriatic lesions disappeared 6 weeks after a patient with chronic psoriasis started treatment with amiodarone for ventricular fibrillation, and recurred 2 months after treatment was stopped. The improvement was attributed to the phototoxic effect of amiodarone.— C. P. Lau *et al.* (letter), *Br. med. J.*, 1986, *293*, 510.

Proprietary Preparations

Cordarone X *(Labaz Sanofi, UK)*. *Tablets*, scored, amiodarone hydrochloride 100 and 200 mg.
Injection, amiodarone hydrochloride 50 mg/mL, in ampoules of 3 mL.

Proprietary Names and Manufacturers

Amiodar *(Midy, Ital.)*;
Atlansil *(Roemmers, Arg.)*; Cardilor *(Remedica, Cyprus)*; Corbionax *(Millot-Solac, Fr.)*; Cordarex *(Labaz, Ger.)*; Cordarone *(Reckitt & Colman, Austral.; Ayerst, Canad.; Sandoz, Denm.; Labaz, Fr.; Sigmatau, Ital.; Neth.; Labaz, Switz.; Wyeth, USA)*; Cordarone X *(Reckitt & Colman, S.Afr.; Labaz Sanofi, UK)*; Coronovo *(Labinca, Arg.)*; Ortacrone *(Pharmainvesti, Spain)*; Ritmocardyl *(Bago, Arg.)*; Rythmarone *(Leurquin, Fr.)*; Trangorex *(Labaz, Spain)*.

7781-d

Aprindine Hydrochloride *(BANM, USAN, rINNM)*.

AC-1802; Compound 83846; Compound 99170 *(aprindine)*. *N*-(3-Diethylaminopropyl)-*N*-indan-2-ylaniline hydrochloride; *NN*-Diethyl-*N'*-indan-2-yl-*N'*-phenyltrimethylenediamine hydrochloride.
$C_{22}H_{30}N_2$,HCl=359.0.

CAS — 37640-71-4 (aprindine); 33237-74-0 (hydrochloride).

Adverse Effects and Precautions

Aprindine has adverse effects and precautions similar to those of mexiletine, p.80. Neurological effects are generally dose-related. There have been reports of agranulocytosis which may be fatal. Hepatitis and cholestatic jaundice have occasionally been reported.

A brief review of the adverse effects of aprindine. Adverse effects are relatively common with both intravenous and oral formulations. Most may be controlled by a decrease in dosage and neurological effects are minimal or absent with serum concentrations less than 1 μg per mL. Vertigo may be troublesome and usually responds to meclozine. Agranulocytosis usually occurs between the 4th and 16th week of therapy and may be quite severe. Reversible granulocytopenia has also been observed. The incidence of agranulocytosis appears to be between 0.1 and 1%. Hepatitis is much less common and generally reversible with discontinuation of treatment.— J. B. Schwartz *et al.*, *Drugs*, 1981, *21*, 23.

Adverse effects were assessed in 27 patients on long-term therapy with aprindine. Aprindine was discontinued due to seizures in 2 patients, and agranulocytosis, confusion, or recurrence of ventricular tachycardia each in 1 patient after 2 to 58 months of therapy. Two deaths occurred in patients with underlying heart disease. In other patients, aprindine was deemed to be safe and effective with most patients experiencing only tolerable ataxia and tremor.— J. L. Bauman *et al.*, *Drug Intell. & clin. Pharm.*, 1983, *17*, 435.

EFFECTS ON THE BLOOD. The Netherlands Centre for Monitoring of Adverse Drug Reactions had received 8 reports of agranulocytosis attributed to the use of aprindine. Two patients died during the acute phase of the agranulocytosis; in the remaining cases recovery began 1 to 4 weeks after aprindine had been withdrawn.— R. van Leeuwen and R. H. B. Meyboom (letter), *Lancet*, 1976, *2*, 1137.

EFFECTS ON THE LIVER. Alterations in liver function tests occurred in 2 patients within 3 weeks of starting aprindine therapy. Liver biopsy in one patient showed mild diffuse hepatitis. There was rapid resolution of liver changes on withdrawing aprindine. The reintroduction of aprindine in 1 patient was associated with the reappearance of signs of liver dysfunction but these resolved over 3 weeks even though aprindine therapy was continued.— H. F. Herlong *et al.*, *Ann. intern. Med.*, 1978, *89*, 359.

EFFECTS ON MENTAL STATE. Psychosis in one patient attributed to treatment with aprindine.— G. P. Jacobs and I. H. Pores, *Am. Heart J.*, 1980, *100*, 347.

INTERACTIONS. Steady-state plasma-aprindine concentrations increased in 2 patients after the initiation of *amiodarone* therapy and coincided with the appearance of adverse effects.— W. Southworth *et al.* (letter), *Am. Heart J.*, 1982, *104*, 323.

Absorption and Fate

Aprindine is readily absorbed from the gastro-intestinal tract. It has a long plasma half-life, usually between 20 and 27 hours, and is extensively bound to plasma proteins. It is excreted in the urine and the bile.

METABOLISM AND PHARMACOKINETICS. Studies of the pharmacokinetics of aprindine: L. Dodion *et al.*, *Thérapie*, 1974, *29*, 221; J. P. Van Durme *et al.*, *Eur. J. clin. Pharmac.*, 1974, *7*, 343; F. Hagemeijer, *Eur. J. clin. Pharmac.*, 1975, *9*, 21; P. L. Malini *et al.*, *Int. J. clin. Pharmac. Biopharm.*, 1979, *17*, 396.

Uses and Administration

Aprindine is a class I anti-arrhythmic agent (see p.70) with actions similar to those of quinidine (p.87). Aprindine is used for the treatment of ventricular tachyarrhythmias and for supraventricular arrhythmias, especially in Wolff-Parkinson-White syndrome. It is given as the hydrochloride in usual doses of 50 to 100 mg daily. If necessary initial doses of 150 to 200 mg daily may be given under strict surveillance for the first 2 to 3 days; initial doses of 50 mg daily are recommended for the elderly. Therapy should be monitored by ECG during initial stabilisation of the dose and intermittently thereafter. It has also been given by intravenous infusion at an initial dose of 200 mg administered at a rate of between 2 and 10 mg per minute.

CARDIAC DISORDERS. A review of the long-acting anti-arrhythmic agent, aprindine, in the treatment of ventricular arrhythmias of various aetiologies.— P. Danilo, *Am. Heart J.*, 1979, *97*, 119. See also: D. P. Zipes *et al.*, *Am. Heart J.*, 1980, *100*, 1055.

In a study of 30 patients treated with aprindine, good control of arrhythmias with minor or no adverse effects was achieved in 17 patients after a period of up to 60 months. Neurological adverse effects including grand mal seizure necessitated the withdrawal of aprindine from 3 patients. In one patient treatment was withdrawn because of recurrence of arrhythmias. There were 6 deaths.— B. Strasberg *et al.*, *Archs intern. Med.*, 1983, *143*, 2131.

Proprietary Names and Manufacturers

Amidonal *(Madaus, Ger.)*; Fibocil *(Lilly, USA)*; Fiboran *(Christiaens, Belg.*; *Pharmacia, Denm.*; *Fournier Frères, Fr.*; *Neth.*; *Rhone, Spain)*.

855-z

Bretylium Tosylate *(BAN, USAN)*.

Bretylium Tosilate *(rINN)*. (2-Bromobenzyl)ethyldimethylammonium toluene-4-sulphonate.

$C_{11}H_{17}BrN,C_7H_7O_3S=414.4$.

CAS — 59-41-6 (bretylium); 61-75-6 (tosylate).

Adverse Effects, Treatment, and Precautions

The most common adverse effect following administration of bretylium is hypotension which may be severe. Bretylium may cause a transient initial increase in blood pressure and a worsening of cardiac arrhythmias due to a release of noradrenaline. Nausea and vomiting may occur particularly during rapid intravenous infusion. Intramuscular injection of bretylium can lead to local tissue necrosis and muscle atrophy, which can be avoided by limiting the volume and varying the site of the injection (see Uses). Care should be taken when administering bretylium to patients with impaired renal function and to patients with severe aortic stenosis or pulmonary hypertension who may be unable to increase cardiac output in response to the fall in peripheral resistance produced by bretylium. Bretylium may exacerbate arrhythmias caused by digitalis toxicity. If sympathomimetics are required to reverse bretylium-induced hypotension, great care should be exercised since their effects may be enhanced.

Seven patients with recent cardiac infarction, 3 with and 4 without left ventricular failure, received bretylium tosylate 5 to 10 mg per kg body-weight intravenously. Initial transient tachycardia, hypertension and late sustained bradycardia, hypotension with decreased vascular resistance, and increased calf blood flow and venous capacitance occurred in all 7 patients. Bretylium should be used cautiously in patients with hypotension as it might cause a significant reduction in arterial pressure.— K. Chatterjee *et al.*, *J. Am. med. Ass.*, 1973, *223*, 757.

Absorption and Fate

Bretylium tosylate is incompletely absorbed from the gastro-intestinal tract. It is not metabolised in the body and is largely excreted unchanged in the urine. The half-life is reported to be between 4 and 17 hours in patients with normal renal function and is prolonged in patients with impaired renal function. Bretylium is dialysable.

A review of the pharmacokinetics of bretylium.— W. G. Rapeport, *Clin. Pharmacokinet.*, 1985, *10*, 248.

Uses and Administration

Bretylium tosylate is a quaternary ammonium agent with class II and class III anti-arrhythmic activity (see p.70); it blocks adrenergic transmission by preventing noradrenaline release from adrenergic nerve endings. It suppresses ventricular fibrillation and ventricular arrhythmias, but the exact mode of action has yet to be determined. It was originally used in the treatment of hypertension but because of poor gastric absorption and the development of tolerance during long-term therapy it has been superseded by other drugs. It is given parenterally under electrocardiographic monitoring to control ventricular arrhythmias resistant to standard treatment; a delay of up to 2 hours may occur before the onset of the anti-arrhythmic activity therefore it should only be used if the arrhythmia is resistant to more rapidly acting agents. The patient should be supine or closely observed for postural hypotension. A suggested dose by intramuscular or slow intravenous injection is 5 to 10 mg per kg body-weight as a 5% (50 mg per mL) solution, repeated in 1 to 2 hours if the arrhythmia persists, and subsequently given every 6 to 8 hours for up to about 3 to 5 days. The site of intramuscular injections should be varied on repeated injection and not more than 5 mL should be given into any one site. Nausea and vomiting during intravenous administration can be avoided by administering the injection over not less than 8 minutes: the injection can be diluted to 10 mg per mL with glucose injection or sodium chloride injection. Alternatively an intravenous infusion of 1 to 2 mg per minute has been recommended.

In immediately life-threatening ventricular arrhythmias or ventricular fibrillation a suggested dose is 5 mg per kg as a 5% (50 mg per mL) solution by rapid intravenous injection, in association with other resuscitative measures and cardioversion, increased to 10 mg per kg if the ventricular fibrillation persists, and repeated as necessary. A more rapid response has been reported in patients with ventricular fibrillation than with other arrhythmias.

ADMINISTRATION IN RENAL FAILURE. Preliminary data from 3 subjects, one healthy and 2 with renal disease, indicate that bretylium accumulates with progressive renal impairment and is removed by haemodialysis. Appropriate adjustment of dosage should be made.— J. Adir *et al.* (letter), *New Engl. J. Med.*, 1979, *300*, 1390.

Bretylium could be given in usual doses to patients with a glomerular filtration-rate greater than 50mL per minute but patients with a glomerular filtration-rate of between 10 and 50 mL per minute should be given 25 to 50% of the usual dose. Bretylium should be avoided in patients with a glomerular filtration-rate of less than 10 mL per minute.— W. M. Bennett *et al.*, *Am. J. Kidney Dis.*, 1983, *3*, 155.

CARDIAC ARRHYTHMIAS. A detailed review of the actions and uses of bretylium in cardiac arrhythmias. The onset of anti-arrhythmic effect is fastest after intravenous bolus injection; by this route it can facilitate cardioversion and suppress recurrent ventricular fibrillation within minutes. After intramuscular administration the onset of anti-arrhythmic action may be delayed by 20 minutes to an hour. In some patients the full anti-arrhythmic effects of bretylium require several hours to develop. Anti-arrhythmic effects of a single dose last for 6 to 12 hours.— J. Koch-Weser, *New Engl. J. Med.*, 1979, *300*, 473.

Comment on the anti-arrhythmic properties of bretylium tosylate. Hypotension can be a troublesome side-effect. Another problem is that against some ventricular arrhythmias it takes 20 to 40 minutes to act, though against ventricular fibrillation it acts very quickly.— L. H. Opie, *Lancet*, 1980, *1*, 861.

Mention of the use of bretylium to restore sinus rhythm in hypothermia.— *Med. Lett.*, 1986, *28*, 123. See also G. Kochar *et al.* (letter), *Ann. intern. Med.*, 1986, *105*, 624.

Further reviews of the use of bretylium in cardiac arrhythmias: *Med. Lett.*, 1986, *28*, 111.

Proprietary Preparations

Bretylate *(Wellcome, UK)*. *Injection*, bretylium tosylate 50 mg/mL, in ampoules of 2 mL.

Proprietary Names and Manufacturers

Bretylate *(Wellcome, Austral.*; *Belg.*; *Wellcome, Canad.*; *Wellcome, Fr.*; *Neth.*; *Wellcome, UK)*; Bretylol *(Boots, S.Afr.*; *American Critical Care, USA)*.

7782-n

Bunaftine Citrate *(rINNM)*.

N-Butyl-*N*-(2-diethylaminoethyl)-1-naphthamide dihydrogen citrate.

$C_{21}H_{30}N_2O,C_6H_8O_7=518.6$.

CAS — 32421-46-8 (bunaftine).

Bunaftine is used for the treatment of cardiac arrhythmias; it is reported to have class III anti-arrhythmic activity (see p.70). Bunaftine is given by mouth as the citrate in doses equivalent to bunaftine 400 to 800 mg daily. Bunaftine hydrochloride is given by intramuscular injection in doses of 200 to 400 mg daily, and by slow intravenous infusion of 200 mg.

An investigation of the effect of bunaftine on the right atrial action potential in patients with recurrent attacks of paroxysmal atrial tachycardia indicated that bunaftine is a class III anti-arrhythmic agent.— R. Fenici *et al.*, *Br. Heart J.*, 1977, *39*, 787.

Proprietary Names and Manufacturers of Bunaftine and its Salts

Bunamide *(Menarini, Spain)*; Meregon *(Malesci, Ital.)*.

15315-x

Cibenzoline *(BAN, rINN).*
Cifenline *(USAN)*; Ro-22-7796; UP-339-01. (±)-2-(2,2-Diphenylcyclopropyl)-2-imidazoline.
$C_{18}H_{18}N_2$=262.4.

CAS — 53267-01-9.

Cibenzoline is an anti-arrhythmic agent. It possesses Class I activity but also has some Class III and Class IV properties. It is used in the treatment and prevention of ventricular and supraventricular arrhythmias. Cibenzoline succinate is given by mouth in a dose equivalent to cibenzoline base 130 mg initially, then 4 to 6 mg per kg body-weight or 260 to 390 mg daily. Cibenzoline may also be given parenterally at an initial dose of 1 mg per kg cibenzoline base over 2 minutes followed by either 8 mg per kg over 24 hours by infusion or by oral therapy.

A report of false-positive proteinuria results with bromphenol reagent strips in patients receiving cibenzoline.— J. L. Kovacs *et al., J. clin. Pharmac.*, 1984, *24*, 127.

ABSORPTION AND FATE. The elimination half-life of cibenzoline ranged from 7.3 to 8.7 hours in a study in 4 healthy subjects. Oral clearance ranged from 380 to 575 mL per minute. Maximum plasma concentrations were reported to be proportional to the dose.— K. -C. Khoo *et al., J. clin. Pharmac.*, 1984, *24*, 283.

The renal and non-renal clearance of cibenzoline was found to decrease with increasing age in healthy subjects. The mean elimination half-life was 7 hours in the 20- to 30-year age group and 10.5 hours in the 70- to 80-year age group. The reduction in renal clearance was considered to be related to the decrease in creatinine clearance with increasing age. The results suggested that older patients may need lower doses than younger patients to maintain therapeutic plasma-cibenzoline concentrations.— R. K. Brazzell *et al., Clin. Pharmac. Ther.*, 1984, *36*, 613.

Further references to the pharmacokinetics of cibenzoline.— R. K. Brazzell *et al., J. clin. Pharmac.*, 1985, *25*, 418 (intravenous route); M. Canal *et al., ibid.*, 197 (in patients with renal impairment); J. W. Massarella *et al., ibid.*, 1986, *26*, 125 (after repetitive dosing).

ADVERSE EFFECTS. Cibenzoline therapy was associated with severe hypoglycaemia in a 67-year-old patient.— D. E. Hilleman *et al., Drug Intell. & clin. Pharm.*, 1987, *21*, 38.

USES. Beneficial results of cibenzoline treatment in 16 of 20 patients with refractory ventricular arrhythmias which were maintained in 14 patients after a follow-up period of 6 to 15 months. Side-effects comprising transient light-headedness and dry mouth were reported in 6 patients.— S. M. Mohiuddin *et al., Drug Intell. & clin. Pharm.*, 1984, *18*, 499.

Further references: K. F. Browne *et al., J. Am. Coll. Cardiol.*, 1984, *3*, 857; G. Cocco *et al., Eur. Heart J.*, 1984, *5*, 108; A. Waleffe *et al., ibid.*, 1985, *6*, 253; D. S. Miura *et al., Am. Heart J.*, 1985, *109*, 827; N. Wasty *et al., ibid.*, *110*, 1181; R. C. Klein *et al., Am. J. Cardiol.*, 1986, *57*, 592; S. T. Rothbart and S. Saksena, *ibid.*, 941.

Proprietary Names and Manufacturers of Cibenzoline and its Salts
Cipralan *(UPSA, Fr.)*;

16585-b

Clofilium Phosphate *(USAN, rINN).*
LY-150378. [4-(*p*-Chlorophenyl)butyl]-diethylheptylammonium phosphate.
$C_{21}H_{36}ClN,H_3PO_4$=436.0.

CAS — 68379-03-3.

Clofilium is an anti-arrhythmic agent reported to have a prolonged duration of action.

The electrophysiological effects of intravenous infusion of clofilium in total doses of between 20 and 240 µg per kg body-weight were studied in 22 patients with ventricular arrhythmias and in 3 patients with paroxysmal supraventricular arrhythmias. Clofilium produced increases in Q-T interval, atrial effective refractory period, and ventricular refractory period without altering conduction time. Clofilium produced no changes in the frequency or complexity of premature ventricular complexes, but was shown to abolish the ability to induce ventricular tachycardia by programmed stimulation. No adverse effects were noted, and there were no changes in blood pressure or laboratory parameters.— E. V. Platia and P. R. Reid, *Clin. Pharmac. Ther.*, 1984, *35*, 193.
Further references: H. L. Greene *et al., Am. Heart J.*, 1983, *106*, 492.

Proprietary Names and Manufacturers
Lilly, USA.

7783-h

Disopyramide *(BAN, USAN, rINN).*

SC-7031. 4-Di-isopropylamino-2-phenyl-2-(2-pyridyl)butyramide.
$C_{21}H_{29}N_3O$=339.5.

CAS — 3737-09-5.

Pharmacopoeias. In *Br.*

A white odourless or almost odourless powder. Slightly **soluble** in water; soluble 1 in 10 of alcohol, 1 in 5 of chloroform, and 1 in 5 of ether.

7784-m

Disopyramide Phosphate *(BANM, USAN, rINNM).*

SC-13957.
$C_{21}H_{29}N_3O,H_3PO_4$=437.5.

CAS — 22059-60-5.

Pharmacopoeias. In *Br.* and *U.S.*

A white or almost white odourless powder. Disopyramide phosphate 1.3 g is approximately equivalent to 1 g of disopyramide. *B.P.* **solubilities** are: 1 in 20 of water and 1 in 50 of alcohol; practically insoluble in chloroform. *U.S.P.* solubilities are: freely soluble in water, slightly soluble in alcohol, practically insoluble in chloroform and in ether. A 5% solution has a pH of 4.0 to 5.0. **Store** in airtight containers. Protect from light.

The manufacturers of disopyramide reported that an oral liquid preparation of disopyramide could be formulated using disopyramide phosphate capsules and cherry syrup. The preparation has a recommended shelf-life of 4 weeks when stored at ambient room temperature.— L. K. Mathur *et al., Am. J. Hosp. Pharm.*, 1982, *39*, 309 and 793 (correction).

Adverse Effects

The adverse effects most commonly associated with disopyramide therapy relate to its antimuscarinic properties and are dose-related. They include dry mouth, blurred vision, urinary hesitancy, impotence, and constipation. The most serious effect is urinary retention. Gastro-intestinal effects are less common, but nausea, bloating, and abdominal pain may occur. Other adverse effects reported include skin rashes, hypoglycaemia, dizziness, fatigue, muscle weakness, headache, and urinary frequency. Insomnia and depression have also been associated with disopyramide administration. There have been rare reports of psychosis, cholestatic jaundice, elevated liver enzymes, thrombocytopenia, and agranulocytosis. Like other anti-arrhythmic agents, disopyramide has cardiac depressant properties, and may induce cardiac arrhythmias particularly ventricular tachycardia, heart block, conduction disturbances, heart failure, and hypotension.

Over-rapid intravenous injection of disopyramide may cause profuse sweating and severe cardiovascular depression.

In overdose cardiovascular and antimuscarinic effects are pronounced, and there may be apnoea, loss of consciousness, loss of spontaneous respiration and asystole.

A 75-year-old woman with atrial fibrillation suffered a grand mal convulsion followed by respiratory arrest after receiving disopyramide 150 mg intravenously over a period of 10 minutes. On recovery she complained of a dry mouth and blurred vision and it was considered that the convulsion was caused by the anticholinergic action of disopyramide, although it may have been due to a direct stimulant action.— N. M. Johnson *et al.* (letter), *Lancet*, 1978, *2*, 848.

During long-term therapy with disopyramide in 40 patients, 28 (70%) had one or more adverse effects. Xerostomia occurred in 15 (38%), constipation in 12 (30%), blurred vision in 11 (28%), urinary hesitancy in 9 (23%), nausea in 9 (23%), impotence in 2 (5%), and dyspareunia in one patient (3%). In addition 3 of the 9 patients with pre-existing compensated congestive heart failure had worsening of heart failure due to disopyramide. Adverse effects were sufficiently severe for disopyramide to be discontinued in 7 patients, and for dosage reductions in another 7.— J. L. Bauman *et al., Am. Heart J.*, 1986, *111*, 654.

ALLERGY. Worsening of ventricular arrhythmia and an anaphylactoid reaction occurred in a 58-year-old man after a single dose of disopyramide 300 mg by mouth. Two hours after the dose he complained of a swollen tongue and difficulty in breathing. He became cyanotic and was given diphenhydramine 25 mg intravenously, which resulted in improvement of his respiratory status.— J. G. Porterfield *et al.* (letter), *New Engl. J. Med.*, 1980, *303*, 584.

EFFECTS ON THE BLOOD. Granulocytopenia was associated on 2 occasions with the use of disopyramide phosphate in a 61-year-old man.— M. E. Conrad *et al.* (letter), *J. Am. med. Ass.*, 1978, *240*, 1857.

EFFECTS ON THE EYES. Acute closed-angle glaucoma developed in a patient on the 7th day of treatment with disopyramide 100 mg three times daily for 6 days then 200 mg three times daily for another 6 days. After treatment with pilocarpine, physostigmine, and then surgery the patient was returned to treatment with disopyramide 100 mg four times daily.— G. E. Trope and V. M. D. Hind (letter), *Lancet*, 1978, *1*, 329.

A report of a 16-year-old girl who suffered severe blurred vision and pupillary dilatation after high doses of disopyramide; the ocular side-effects were probably a result of the anticholinergic properties of the drug.— J. Frucht *et al., Br. J. Ophthal.*, 1984, *68*, 890.

EFFECTS ON THE HEART. Manifestations of acute congestive heart failure occurred in 16 of 100 patients receiving disopyramide by mouth. It was concluded that disopyramide exerts a profound negative myocardial inotropic effect and that recurrence of congestive heart failure may be precipitated in as many as 50% of those receiving disopyramide. The likelihood of this complication in patients without a history of heart failure is probably less than 5%.— P. J. Podrid *et al., New Engl. J. Med.*, 1980, *302*, 614.

A possible association between cardiac dysrhythmias and treatment with disopyramide in 5 patients with heart disease.— E. L. Kinney *et al.* (letter), *New Engl. J. Med.*, 1980, *302*, 1146.

In a comparative study with lignocaine, intravenous disopyramide was found to have a potent coronary constrictive activity which might be hazardous under some circumstances.— V. Kötter *et al., Am. J. Cardiol.*, 1980, *46*, 469.

Reductions in stroke volume by 28% and cardiac output by 21% were noted in 7 subjects immediately after an intravenous infusion of disopyramide 2 mg per kg body-weight over 5 minutes. There were no marked changes in blood pressure or in cerebral blood flow.— C. G. Maidment *et al.* (letter), *Br. J. clin. Pharmac.*, 1981, *11*, 310.

EFFECTS ON THE LIVER. A report of severe hepatocellular damage in a patient shortly after the start of disopyramide treatment. Disseminated intravascular coagulation developed simultaneously, and both problems gradually subsided 14 days after cessation of disopyramide therapy.— P. T. Doody, *Sth. med. J.*, 1982, *75*, 496.

Reports of cholestatic jaundice and raised liver enzymes associated with disopyramide treatment: T. Meinertz *et al.* (letter), *Lancet*, 1977, *2*, 828; N. Riccioni *et al.* (letter), *ibid.*, 1362; A. Craxi *et al.* (letter), *Ann. intern. Med.*, 1980, *93*, 150; A. M. Tonkin *et al.* (letter), *Chest*, 1980, *77*, 125; M. E. Edmonds and A. M. Hayler (letter), *Eur. J. clin. Pharmac.*, 1980, *18*, 285; G. L. Bakris *et al., Mayo Clin. Proc.*, 1983, *58*, 265.

EFFECTS ON MENTAL STATE. Agitation and distress leading to paranoia and auditory hallucinations developed in a patient given disopyramide. Withdrawal of the disopyramide produced a rapid and complete recovery.— R. H. Falk *et al.* (letter), *Lancet*, 1977, *1*, 858. See also: P. L. Padfield *et al.* (letter), *ibid.*, 1152.

EFFECTS ON THE NERVOUS SYSTEM. Peripheral neuropathy affecting the feet and severe enough to prevent walking was associated with disopyramide in a 72-year-old patient. There was gradual improvement on withdrawal of disopyramide with the patient being symptom-free after 4 months.— K. D. Dawkins and J. Gibson (letter), *Lancet*, 1978, *1*, 329.

EFFECTS ON SEXUAL FUNCTION. Impotence occurred in a patient taking disopyramide. When the plasma concentration of disopyramide was reduced from 14 to 3 μg per mL the impotence was abolished without clinical deterioration.— D. J. McHaffie *et al.* (letter), *Lancet*, 1977, *1*, 859.

EFFECTS ON THE URINARY TRACT. *Urinary retention.* A report of 9 cases of urinary retention associated with disopyramide therapy and a review of the literature. It was observed that urinary retention secondary to disopyramide therapy was most likely to develop in male patients over the age of 65 in whom there was some pre-existing renal dysfunction: there was an increased risk in patients with evidence of prostatic hypertrophy.— L. H. Danziger and J. R. Horn, *Archs intern. Med.*, 1983, *143*, 1683.

Further case reports of urinary retention.— S. H. Large and C. H. Todd (letter), *Lancet*, 1977, *2*, 1362; G. R. Donald (letter), *ibid*; L. E. Alves *et al.*, *Archs intern. Med.*, 1984, *144*, 2099.

HYPOGLYCAEMIA. Disopyramide produced a decrease in blood glucose concentrations in 2 controlled studies in healthy subjects. Although there were no clinical symptoms of hypoglycaemia in these subjects it was considered that the effect could be clinically significant in patients with renal or hepatic impairment.— I. Strathman *et al.*, *Drug Intell. & clin. Pharm.*, 1983, *17*, 635.

There have been several reports of hypoglycaemia occurring in patients during disopyramide therapy.— I. J. Goldberg *et al.*, *Am. J. Med.*, 1980, *69*, 463; S. F. Quevedo *et al.*, *J. Am. med. Ass.*, 1981, *245*, 2424; M. Rubin *et al.*, *N.Y. St. J. Med.*, 1983, *83*, 1057; J. M. Nappi *et al.*, *West. J. Med.*, 1983, *138*, 95; J. T. Stapleton and M. W. Gillman, *Sth. med. J.*, 1983, *76*, 1453.

OVERDOSAGE. A 2-year-old boy suffered hypotension, cardiac arrhythmias, and convulsions and died 28 hours after ingestion of 600 mg of disopyramide.— A. Hutchison and H. Kilham, *Med. J. Aust.*, 1978, *2*, 335.

See also under Treatment of Adverse Effects, below.

Treatment of Adverse Effects

In overdosage by mouth the stomach should be emptied by aspiration and lavage. Treatment is generally symptomatic and supportive. The ECG should be monitored until symptoms subside.

Isoprenaline infusion is reported to be beneficial in severe hypotension; since cardiovascular collapse can occur abruptly without warning, it is recommended that the patient be prepared for an isoprenaline infusion as soon as disopyramide overdosage is suspected.

Other supportive measures include correction of hypokalaemia and acidosis, assisted respiration, and electrical pacing.

Haemodialysis or charcoal haemoperfusion may be of value especially if kidney function is compromised.

A report of 5 cases of fatal overdosage with disopyramide. The most common clinical finding appeared to be an early loss of consciousness following an episode of respiratory arrest. Four of the patients initially responded to resuscitation but subsequently deteriorated rapidly, with cardiac arrhythmias and loss of spontaneous respiration; in 4 of the cases post-mortem examination demonstrated pulmonary congestion secondary to left ventricular failure.— A. M. Hayler *et al.*, *Lancet*, 1978, *1*, 968. *In vitro* data suggested that haemodialysis might be of value in enhancing the elimination of toxic concentrations of disopyramide.— A. Karim (letter), *ibid.*, *2*, 214. Further comment.— J. R. Horn and M. L. Hughes (letter), *ibid*.

Recommendations, based on *animal* experiments, for the management of disopyramide overdosage: monitor arterial blood pressure continuously, preferably with an indwelling cannula, to provide immediate warning of cardiovascular collapse which may be sudden and without obvious ECG abnormalities; if disopyramide overdose is suspected set up an intravenous infusion containing a pressor agent immediately the patient is admitted to hospital, so that, in the event of a cardiovascular crisis, treatment can be initiated promptly. Isoprenaline appears to be superior to the other drugs used in this situation. Sudden cardiac arrhythmias may occur and may well be exacerbated by cardiodepressant drugs such as procainamide or quinidine—attention to raising the blood-potassium concentration, correcting acidosis, and the cautious use of isoprenaline are more likely to prove effective. Reports suggest that, due to high endocardial threshold, patients may be refractory to transvenous ventricular pacing—isoprenaline appears to be the drug most likely to be effective when symptomatic bradycardia follows disopyramide poisoning.— A. M. Hayler *et al.* (letter), *Med. J. Aust.*, 1979, *1*, 234.

Pyridostigmine 180 to 540 mg daily prevented antimuscarinic adverse effects of disopyramide in each of 17 patients and abolished or reduced them in 10 additional patients. In a group of 89 patients who were not given pyridostigmine, antimuscarinic adverse effects occurred in 29%. Pyridostigmine treatment allowed a measurable increase in tolerated disopyramide blood concentrations and dosages administered.— S. L. Teichman *et al.*, *J. cardiovasc. Pharmac.*, 1985, *7*, 108.

Precautions

Disopyramide is contra-indicated in patients with complete heart block. It should be used with extreme caution in patients with incomplete heart block, pre-existing conductive tissue disease, and uncompensated heart failure. If disopyramide is used to treat atrial tachycardia it may be necessary to pre-treat with digoxin; see quinidine, (p.86). Hypokalaemia should be corrected before treatment with disopyramide is initiated since the effectiveness of disopyramide may be diminished. Care should be taken in patients susceptible to hypoglycaemia, including those with congestive heart failure, renal or hepatic impairment, and patients taking beta-blockers or alcohol.

Disopyramide should also be used with caution in association with other cardiac depressants including beta-blockers and other class I anti-arrhythmic agents and it is recommended that facilities for cardiac monitoring and defibrillation should be available when the injection is used. Hypotension is a special risk following intravenous administration of disopyramide; it should be injected slowly.

Dosage reduction is necessary in patients with renal or hepatic impairment and in patients with heart failure.

Owing to its antimuscarinic properties, disopyramide should be avoided in patients with glaucoma or a tendency to urinary retention and also in patients with myasthenia gravis due to the risk of precipitating a myasthenic crisis; the effects of other antimuscarinic agents are enhanced by concomitant disopyramide therapy. The metabolism of disopyramide may be increased by the concurrent use of drugs which induce liver enzymes including phenytoin, phenobarbitone, and rifampicin.

For recommended dosage reductions in the elderly and in patients with abnormal renal or hepatic function, see under Uses, p.77.

INTERACTIONS. The metabolism of disopyramide was shown to be accelerated by concurrent administration of *rifampicin* or *phenytoin*.— M. -L. Aitio *et al.*, *Br. J. clin. Pharmac.*, 1981, *11*, 279.

Alcohol. A study of the effects of ethanol ingestion on the clearance of disopyramide in healthy subjects showed that although the half-life and total body clearance were not affected, the renal clearance was increased in those subjects in whom ethanol increased urine output. There was also evidence to suggest that ethanol inhibited the metabolism of disopyramide.— H. Olsen *et al.*, *Eur. J. clin. Pharmac.*, 1983, *25*, 103.

Anti-arrhythmic agents. Data indicating that cardiac toxicity from disopyramide may add to the toxicity of lignocaine, phenytoin, procainamide, or other class I anti-arrhythmic agents.— G. Ellrodt and B. N. Singh, *Heart & Lung*, 1980, *9*, 469.

See also Lignocaine Hydrochloride, p.1218.

A small but significant increase in peak serum-disopyramide concentrations was caused by concurrent administration of quinidine in 16 healthy subjects and a reciprocal small decrease in peak quinidine concentrations was observed. There was no change in elimination half-life of either drug.— B. J. Baker *et al.*, *Am. Heart J.*, 1983, *105*, 12.

Anticoagulants. For the effect of disopyramide on warfarin, see Warfarin Sodium, p.345.

Beta-blockers. Bradycardia with unconsciousness and severe hypotension in one patient and fatal bradycardia and asystole in a second patient after the intravenous injection of disopyramide 20 minutes after practolol intravenously.— A. D. Cumming and C. Robertson, *Br. med. J.*, 1979, *2*, 1264. A similar report.— D. Gelipter and M. Hazell (letter), *ibid.*, 1980, *280*, 52.

The clearance of disopyramide was found to be decreased by almost 20% during concomitant treatment with atenolol.— J. Bonde *et al.*, *Eur. J. clin. Pharmac.*, 1985, *28*, 41.

Cardiac glycosides. For reports of an interaction with digoxin, see p.827.

Electrolytes. Possible enhancement of the toxic effects of disopyramide on the heart by hyperkalaemia.— B. D. Maddux and R. B. Whiting, *Chest*, 1980, *78*, 654.

PREGNANCY AND THE NEONATE. Uterine contractions occurred 1 to 2 hours after successive oral doses of disopyramide were given to a woman who was 8 months pregnant.— R. F. Leonard *et al.*, *New Engl. J. Med.*, 1978, *299*, 84.

Disopyramide 200 mg every 8 hours was used to treat bigeminy and paroxysmal ventricular tachycardia from the 26th week of pregnancy in a 27-year-old woman. Labour was spontaneous and normal and no evidence of congenital abnormality or growth retardation was found.— E. J. Shaxted and P. J. Milton, *Curr. med. Res. Opinion*, 1979, *6*, 70.

For reports of the excretion of disopyramide in breast milk, see Absorption and Fate, below.

Absorption and Fate

Disopyramide is readily and almost completely absorbed from the gastro-intestinal tract, peak plasma concentrations being attained about 0.5 to 3 hours after oral administration.

Disopyramide is partially metabolised in the liver; the major metabolite is mono-*N*-dealkylated disopyramide which retains some anti-arrhythmic and antimuscarinic activity. The major route of excretion is through the kidney, approximately 50% as the unchanged drug, 20% as the *N*-dealkylated metabolite, and 10% as other metabolites. About 10% is excreted in the faeces. The clearance of disopyramide does not appear to be influenced by urinary pH.

The therapeutic plasma concentration range is generally accepted as 2 to 4 μg per mL. Within this range, protein binding is reported to be 50 to 65%, but the degree of binding varies with the plasma concentration and this limits the usefulness of plasma concentration monitoring as a guide to therapy. Estimations of the plasma half-life of disopyramide range from about 4 to 10 hours.

Disopyramide crosses the placental barrier and it is excreted in breast milk.

A review of the pharmacokinetics of disopyramide.— L. A. Siddoway and R. L. Woosley, *Clin. Pharmacokinet.*, 1986, *11*, 214.

In a study of 9 patients 3 to 14 days after myocardial infarction, bioavailability and half-life of disopyramide were unchanged by ischaemic heart disease and age, but the volume of distribution was reduced by 25%, and there was a reduction in drug clearance. Nevertheless, no alteration in the dosage was deemed necessary.— S. M. Bryson *et al.*, *Br. J. clin. Pharmac.*, 1982, *13*, 417.

Significant changes in the pharmacokinetics of disopyramide in the acute phase of myocardial infarction were shown following oral but not intravenous administration. The absorption of oral disopyramide was delayed resulting in low plasma concentrations in the acute phase of infarction, but the extent of gastro-intestinal absorption was not apparently affected.— P. J. Pentikäinen *et al.*, *Eur. J. clin. Pharmac.*, 1985, *28*, 45. See also: C. R. Kumana *et al.*, *Br. J. clin. Pharmac.*, 1982, *14*, 529; A. J. Jounela *et al.*, *Int. J. clin. Pharmac. Ther. Toxic.*, 1982, *20*, 276; P. L. Weissberg *et al.*, *Ther. Drug Monit.*, 1982, *4*, 277.

BIOAVAILABILITY. Each of 8 healthy subjects received the following single doses of different disopyramide preparations in randomised sequence: disopyramide 300 mg (Rythmodan capsules), disopyramide 300 mg, as the phosphate (Norpace capsules), and disopyramide 2 mg per kg body-weight as a bolus intravenous injection over 2 minutes. The mean half-life after injection was 7.79 hours. Absorption from Rythmodan capsules was significantly faster than from Norpace capsules, peak serum concentrations being achieved after 1.69 and 2.80 hours respectively with half-lives of 7.96 and 8.91 hours. Although the bioavailability of Norpace was significantly higher than that of Rythmodan it was not considered that this should normally be of any clinical significance. Urinary excretion of disopyramide after intravenous injection was almost complete within 24 hours and about 58% of the dose was excreted unchanged over about 72 hours; about 51 and 55% of an oral dose of Rythmodan and Norpace were excreted respectively.— S. M. Bryson *et al.*, *Br. J. clin. Phar-*

mac., 1978, *6*, 409.

In a study involving 19 patients disopyramide was given either as capsules containing 200 mg three times a day or as controlled-release tablets of 300 mg administered twice a day. Both formulations produced plasma concentrations within the suggested therapeutic range and there was no difference in fluctuation in plasma concentration or bioavailability.— K. Arnman *et al.*, *Eur. J. clin. Pharmac.*, 1983, *24*, 199.

Further references to the bioavailability of disopyramide: E. Lien and O. M. Bakke, *Br. J. clin. Pharmac.*, 1983, *16*, 71; M. J. Zema, *Ther. Drug Monit.*, 1984, *6*, 192.

METABOLISM. Mono-*N*-dealkylated disopyramide produced no substantial cardiac effects after a single dose in healthy subjects, but produced greater antimuscarinic effects than disopyramide.— W. -T. Chiang *et al.*, *Clin. Pharmac. Ther.*, 1985, *38*, 37.

PLASMA CONCENTRATION. A study of plasma concentrations of disopyramide in myocardial infarction patients. The most important clinical implication was the finding that despite a loading dose of 400 mg of disopyramide by mouth, between 18 and 170 hours were needed for most of them to achieve trough plasma concentrations surpassing the lower end of a range of 3.3 to 7.5 μg per mL.— K. F. Ilett *et al.*, *Clin. Pharmac. Ther.*, 1979, *26*, 1.

PREGNANCY AND THE NEONATE. Disopyramide was detected in human breast milk in concentrations similar to those in plasma. It was estimated the the infant would receive a dose of less than 2 mg per kg body-weight per day which was considered to be clinically insignificant.— D. B. Barnett *et al.*, *Br. J. clin. Pharmac.*, 1982, *14*, 310. In a similar study the ratio of disopyramide in breast milk and serum was 0.4. No disopyramide was detected in the infant's serum and no adverse effects were evident.— D. MacKintosh and N. Buchanan (letter), *ibid.*, 1985, *19*, 856. Serum-disopyramide concentrations of 0.4 and 0.3 nmol per mL were found in an infant whose mother was taking disopyramide 200 mg twice daily. Disopyramide concentrations in samples taken immediately before and 3.5 hours after a dose were 3.7 and 5.5 nmol per mL in maternal serum and 1.7 and 2.9 nmol per mL in breast milk respectively, giving milk to plasma ratios of 0.46 and 0.53. The amount of disopyramide likely to be ingested by the infant was 1.15 mg per day. Transient symptoms of restlessness were considered unlikely to be caused by disopyramide.— K. Hoppu *et al.* (letter), *ibid.*, 1986, *21*, 553.

PROTEIN BINDING. A study of the binding characteristics of disopyramide in normal plasma and a discussion on the large variation in binding behaviour in earlier studies.— B. M. David *et al.* (letter), *Br. J. clin. Pharmac.*, 1980, *9*, 614.

In a study of the effect of age on plasma protein binding of disopyramide, disopyramide binding was lowest in neonate patients and highest in geriatric patients.— D. W. Holt *et al.* (letter), *Br. J. clin. Pharmac.*, 1983, *16*, 344.

Increases in disopyramide plasma binding were shown in 20 patients with acute myocardial infarction which were maximal at 5 and 12 days after infarction. The increases were dependent on both drug and α_1-acid glycoprotein concentration.— B. M. David *et al.*, *Br. J. clin. Pharmac.*, 1983, *15*, 435. See also: J. L. Caplin *et al.*, *Eur. J. clin. Pharmac.*, 1985, *28*, 253.

Further studies of protein binding of disopyramide and its dealkylated metabolite: J. E. Bredesen *et al.*, *Br. J. clin. Pharmac.*, 1982, *14*, 673; J. E. Bredesen and P. Kierulf, *Br. J. clin. Pharmac.*, 1984, *18*, 779; K. M. Giacomini and T. F. Blaschke, *Clin. Pharmacokinet.*, 1984, *9*, *Suppl.* 1, 42; E. Pike *et al.*, *ibid.*, 84; L. M. Shaw *et al.*, *ibid.*, 98.

Uses and Administration

Disopyramide is a class Ia anti-arrhythmic agent (see p.70) with a depressant action on the heart similar to that of quinidine (p.87). It also has antimuscarinic and negative inotropic properties.

Disopyramide is mainly used for the prevention and treatment of ventricular arrhythmias; it has also been used for the treatment of supraventricular arrhythmias. It may be given by mouth as either the base or the phosphate although the dose is generally expressed in terms of the base. A dose of 100 to 150 mg is given every 6 hours adjusted according to the patient's response. Alternatively a sustained-release preparation can be used, enabling 12-hourly dosage intervals. The daily dose is normally between 300 and 800 mg. An initial loading dose of 200 to 300 mg may be given.

Disopyramide may be given by slow intravenous injection of the phosphate in doses equivalent to 2 mg of the base per kg body-weight to a maximum of 150 mg, at a rate not exceeding 30 mg per minute, followed by 200 mg by mouth immediately on completion of the injection and every 8 hours for 24 hours with subsequent maintenance doses usually in the range of 500 to 750 mg daily; if the arrhythmia recurs on completion of the intravenous injection it may be repeated, but a total intravenous dose of 4 mg per kg (maximum, 300 mg) should not be exceeded in the first hour, nor should the total by both intravenous and oral routes exceed 800 mg in 24 hours. Alternatively, the initial intravenous injection may be followed by the intravenous infusion of 0.4 mg of base per kg per hour (or 20 to 30 mg per hour) to a maximum of 800 mg daily. Patients receiving disopyramide intravenously or in high oral doses should be monitored by ECG.

An optimum dosage regimen for children has not been fully established, but the following oral doses have been used: under 1 year, 10 to 30 mg per kg body-weight per day; age 1 to 4 years, 10 to 20 mg per kg per day; age 4 to 12 years, 10 to 15 mg per kg per day; age 12 to 18 years, 6 to 15 mg per kg per day.

A detailed review of disopyramide, including its pharmacodynamic and pharmacokinetic properties and its therapeutic use in cardiac arrhythmias.— R. N. Brogden and P. A. Todd, *Drugs*, 1987, *34*, 151.

ADMINISTRATION. Disopyramide 0.5 mg per kg body-weight by intravenous injection over 5 minutes repeated 2 to 3 times at intervals of not less than 5 minutes over an hour was administered in conjunction with a continuous intravenous infusion of 1 mg per kg per hour for 3 hours, then 0.4 mg per kg per hour for 15 hours with monitoring of cardiac function, to 10 patients with ventricular arrhythmias. This regimen was well tolerated, rapidly produced therapeutic serum concentrations, and reduced arrhythmias in 6 patients.— C. P. Reddy *et al.*, *Clin. Pharmac. Ther.*, 1984, *35*, 610.

For lowered plasma concentrations of disopyramide following myocardial infarction, see under Absorption and Fate, above.

ADMINISTRATION IN THE ELDERLY. The clearance of disopyramide was reduced in elderly non-smoking patients compared with young subjects, but the reduction was less marked in elderly patients who smoked more than 20 cigarettes daily. It was recommended that the dose of disopyramide should be reduced by approximately 30% in elderly non-smokers.— J. Bonde *et al.*, *Br. J. clin. Pharmac.*, 1985, *20*, 453.

See also under Absorption and Fate, above.

ADMINISTRATION IN HEPATIC FAILURE. The results of an investigation into the influence of a decrease in hepatic function on the pharmacokinetics of disopyramide suggested that the dosage of disopyramide should be reduced by 25% when it is given intravenously to patients with decreased hepatic function.— J. Bonde *et al.*, *Eur. J. clin. Pharmac.*, 1986, *31*, 73.

The observation of a dramatic reduction in plasma protein binding of disopyramide in patients with liver cirrhosis suggested that the therapeutic range of plasma-disopyramide concentration in cirrhosis should be approximately 50% lower than in patients with normal hepatic function.— H. Echizen *et al.*, *Clin. Pharmac. Ther.*, 1986, *40*, 274.

ADMINISTRATION IN RENAL FAILURE. Indications that therapeutic concentrations of disopyramide are not appreciably dialysed.— M. J. Sevka *et al.*, *Clin. Pharmac. Ther.*, 1981, *29*, 322. See also A. D. Blair *et al.*, *ibid.*, 234.

The dosage interval should be adjusted when disopyramide is administered to patients with renal failure. In patients with a glomerular filtration-rate greater than 50 mL per minute no increase is necessary; for rates between 10 and 50 mL per minute the dosage interval should be increased to 12 to 24 hours, and for rates below 10 mL per minute to 24 to 40 hours. A supplementary dose may be necessary for patients undergoing haemodialysis.— W. M. Bennett *et al.*, *Am. J. Kidney Dis.*, 1983, *3*, 155.

Results of a study of the pharmacokinetics of disopyramide in patients with chronic renal failure suggesting that the dosage of disopyramide should be reduced when plasma creatinine concentrations are greater than 250 μmol per litre and creatinine clearance is lower than 30 mL per minute.— B. Francois *et al.*, *Eur. J. Drug Metab. Pharmacokinet.*, 1983, *8*, 85.

CARDIAC DISORDERS. A review of anti-arrhythmic agents, including disopyramide, giving details of its uses and adverse effects. Disopyramide has properties and some side-effects akin to those of quinidine but some of its electrophysiological properties more closely resemble those of lignocaine, and it may help in the treatment of ventricular tachycardia where quinidine has failed. It is as effective as quinidine in reducing recurrence after electrical cardioversion and has fewer side-effects, but it is less impressive against atrial arrhythmias, except for the Wolff-Parkinson-White syndrome. Disopyramide is one of several agents used intravenously for lignocaine failure, but the risk of cardiac depression (hypotension) is greater than with lignocaine, possibly due to a mild calcium antagonist action. Like quinidine, disopyramide occasionally precipitates ventricular fibrillation and *torsade de pointes*, and when there is cardiomegaly a high first dose can cause collapse. Although the antimuscarinic effect of disopyramide makes it particularly useful in the management of arrhythmias associated with sinus bradycardia, the sick-sinus syndrome may be a contra-indication (unexpectedly, bundle-branch block is not). Disopyramide is not effective in digitalis toxicity, and its use in association with quinidine, digoxin or methyldopa is inadvisable in the sick sinus syndrome. Intravenous disopyramide can substantially reduce cardiac output in beta-blocked patients; there is no interaction with lignocaine.— L. H. Opie, *Lancet*, 1980, *1*, 861.

A review of disopyramide. Disopyramide is as effective as quinidine or procainamide in the treatment of patients with ventricular premature depolarisations. It is also effective in selected patients with recurrent ventricular tachycardia; the available data suggests that its effectiveness in such patients can be predicted by invasive electrophysiological drug testing. The therapeutic spectrum of disopyramide in treating patients with supraventricular arrhythmias is also similar to that of quinidine and procainamide. Disopyramide may suppress sinus node function especially in patients with sinus pauses or sino-atrial exit block. Although it lengthens the infranodal conduction time, disopyramide can be used to treat patients with bundle branch block. The available data also suggests that it may be used safely in patients with first-degree or type I second-degree atrio-ventricular block. However, the safety of disopyramide treatment in patients with bundle branch block or atrio-ventricular nodal disease who have metabolic or electolyte abnormalities is unknown. Disopyramide can precipitate ventricular tachycardia or fibrillation. Its use is contra-indicated in patients with severe heart failure and it should be used with great caution in patients with compensated congestive heart failure.— F. Morady *et al.*, *Ann. intern. Med.*, 1982, *96*, 337.

Further reviews of disopyramide: J. Koch-Weser, *New Engl. J. Med.*, 1979, *300*, 957.

A preliminary study indicating beneficial response in patients with hypertrophic obstructive cardiomyopathy to treatment with disopyramide.— C. Pollick, *New Engl. J. Med.*, 1982, *307*, 997.

Arrhythmias. A view that disopyramide at a dose of 2 mg per kg body-weight intravenously initially followed by up to 1 g a day intravenously or by mouth may be used as an alternative to lignocaine for the treatment of haemodynamically significant ventricular arrhythmias and arrhythmias where R-on-T phenomenon are detected, or where sustained ventricular tachycardia has been detected or treated by cardioversion.— W. T. Brownlee, *Br. J. Hosp. Med.*, 1985, *33*, 138.

In a study of 156 patients with post-operative atrial tachycardia in whom sinus rhythm was not restored by digoxin given intravenously, disopyramide was administered as a loading dose of 2 mg per kg body-weight intravenously initially followed by oral or parenteral maintenance doses. Sinus rhythm was restored in 75 patients within 12 hours of starting disopyramide, and in a further 44 patients treated with disopyramide either alone or combined with digoxin within 1 to 13 days. Adverse effects were seen in 30 patients including 1:1 atrioventricular conduction in 4 patients and ventricular tachycardia in 1 patient.— T. P. Gavaghan *et al.*, *Aust. N.Z. J. Med.*, 1985, *15*, 27.

References to beneficial reponses of arrhythmias to disopyramide: A. M. Tonkin *et al.*, *Aust. N.Z. J. Med.*, 1982, *12*, 271 (arrhythmias in a coronary care unit); B. Trimarco *et al.*, *Curr. ther. Res.*, 1983, *33*, 472 (ventricular arrhythmias); P. Fechter *et al.*, *Eur. J. clin. Pharmac.*, 1983, *25*, 729 (comparison with propranolol in ventricular arrhythmias).

Myocardial infarction. The effectiveness of disopyramide in reducing the mortality after myocardial infarction is controversial. Zainal *et al.* (*Lancet*, 1977, *2*, 887) showed a dramatic reduction in mortality in a study of patients with suspected myocardial infarction treated on open wards and recommended that disopyramide should regularly be given prophylactically to such patients. Their study was, however, strongly criticised on the grounds that only 30 patients were included and on other aspects of the trial design (C.T. Dollery *et al.*, *ibid.*, 1185; R. Greenbaum, *ibid.*; A. Pottage *et al.*, *ibid.*, 1185 and 1362). Subsequent trials by Wilcox *et al.* (*Lancet*, 1980, *2*, 765) and Nicholls *et al.* (*Lancet*, 1980, *2*, 936) involving 158 and 68 patients respectively treated with disopyramide did not show any reduction in mortality compared with controls. These results were confirmed by the *UK* Rythmodan Multicentre Study Group trial (*Postgrad. med. J.*, 1984, *60*, 98) involving 1985 patients; in addition patients with cardiac failure or hypotension at entry to this study did not fare worse on disopyramide but patients with a conduction defect did.

Reports of reductions in the frequency of cardiac arrhythmias after myocardial infarction in patients treated with disopyramide.— C. R. Kumana *et al.*, *Br. J. clin. Pharmac.*, 1982, *14*, 519; R. A. C. Allen-Narker *et al.*, *ibid.*, 1984, *18*, 725.

For reports of alterations in the pharmacokinetics of disopyramide after myocardial infarction, see Absorption and Fate p.76.

PREGNANCY AND THE NEONATE. For reports of the use of disopyramide during pregnancy, see Precautions p.76.

RESTLESS LEG SYNDROME. Disopyramide, initially 100 mg three times daily followed by a maintenance dose of 100 to 150 mg at night alone or in combination with an antidepressant agent was recommended for the treatment of restless leg syndrome in non-depressed and depressed patients respectively.— W. Blättler and M. Mühlemann, *Schweiz. med. Wschr.*, 1982, *112*, 115.

Preparations

Disopyramide Capsules *(B.P.)*

Disopyramide Phosphate Capsules *(B.P.)*. Potency is expressed in terms of the equivalent amount of disopyramide.

Disopyramide Phosphate Capsules *(U.S.P.)*. Potency is expressed in terms of the equivalent amount of disopyramide.

Disopyramide Phosphate Extended-release Capsules *(U.S.P.)*

Proprietary Preparations

Dirythmin SA *(Astra, UK)*. *Durules*, sustained-release tablets, disopyramide 150 mg (as phosphate).

Rythmodan *(Roussel, UK)*. *Capsules*, disopyramide 100 and 150 mg.
Injection, disopyramide 10 mg (as phosphate)/mL, in ampoules of 5 mL.

Rythmodan Retard *(Roussel, UK)*. *Tablets*, sustained-release, scored, disopyramide 250 mg (as phosphate).

Proprietary Names and Manufacturers of Disopyramide and Disopyramide Phosphate

Dicorynan *(Roussel, Spain)*; Dirythmin *(Astra, UK)*; Dirytmin *(Hässle, Norw.; Hässle, Swed.)*; Diso-Duriles *(Astra, Ger.)*; Durbis *(Roussel, Denm.; Roussel, Norw.; Roussel, Swed.)*; Norpace *(Searle, Austral.; Searle, Canad.; Searle, Denm.; Fin.; Searle, Ger.; Gib.; Hong Kong; Israel; Jordan; Kenya; Malay.; Mex.; Neth.; Nigeria; Norw.; NZ; Philipp.; Puerto Rico; Searle, S.Afr.; Singapore; Searle, Switz.; Taiwan; Tanzania; Thai.; Searle, UK; Searle, USA; Zambia)*; Norpaso *(Searle, Arg.)*; Ritmodan *(Roussel Maestretti, Ital.)*; Ritmoforine *(Neth.)*; Rythmodan *(Roussel, Austral.; Roussel, Canad.; Roussel, Fr.; Neth.; Roussel, S.Afr.; Switz.; Roussel, UK)*; Rythmodul *(Albert-Roussel, Ger.)*.

7785-b

Encainide Hydrochloride *(BANM, USAN, rINNM)*.

MJ-9067-1. (±)-2′-[2-(1-Methyl-2-piperidyl)ethyl]-*p*-anisanilide hydrochloride.
$C_{22}H_{28}N_2O_2,HCl = 388.9$.

CAS — 37612-13-8; 66778-36-7 (both encainide); 66794-74-9 (hydrochloride).

Adverse Effects and Precautions

Encainide may cause neurological effects including tremor, ataxia, headache, blurred vision and dizziness, and gastro-intestinal disturbances, all of which tend to be dose related. Cardiac effects occur more rarely but may be serious. There may be worsening of pre-existing ventricular arrhythmias, and hypotension and ECG changes have also been reported.

For recommended dosage reductions in patients with renal failure, see under Uses, below.

Uses and Administration

Encainide is a class Ic anti-arrhythmic agent (see p.70) and is used for the treatment of ventricular arrhythmias. It has also been tried in patients with supraventricular arrhythmias. Part of its activity appears to be due to cardio-active metabolites. Encainide is given by mouth as the hydrochloride and doses are titrated according to the patient's response. The initial dose is 25 mg every 8 hours increased, if necessary, after an interval of 3 to 5 days to 35 mg every 8 hours and after a further 3 to 5 days to 50 mg every 8 hours. Up to 75 mg four times a day has been given for life-threatening arrhythmias, but a dose of 200 mg daily should not normally be exceeded. Dosage may need to be reduced in patients with renal impairment.

Encainide hydrochloride has also been given intravenously.

Reviews of encainide: *Med. Lett.*, 1987, *29*, 50; R. N. Brogden and P. A. Todd, *Drugs*, 1987, *34*, 519; R. L. Woosley *et al.*, *New Engl. J. Med.*, 1988, *318*, 1107.

ADMINISTRATION IN RENAL FAILURE. The elimination of encainide and its active metabolites was substantially reduced in 7 patients with severe renal failure compared with healthy subjects. A reduction in the elimination half-life of encainide was attributed to an increase in protein binding from 70% to 81% in patients with renal failure and an associated reduction in the volume of distribution. It was recommended that the dose of encainide should be reduced by at least 50% in patients with severe renal failure.— R. H. Bergstrand *et al.*, *Clin. Pharmac. Ther.*, 1986, *40*, 64.

CARDIAC DISORDERS. A review of the use of encainide for the treatment of benign and potentially lethal ventricular arrhythmias. Overall, the data from multicentre placebo-controlled trials showed that about 80% of patients obtain at least a 75% decrease in ventricular premature complex frequency and suppression of ventricular tachycardia. The lowest effective dose had been shown to be 25 mg three times a day, with increasing efficacy demonstrated with doses up to 150 to 200 mg daily. Efficacy was maintained during long-term therapy with no evidence of late adverse effects.— J. Morganroth, *Am. J. Cardiol.*, 1986, *58*, 74C.

Reports of studies of encainide in ventricular arrhythmias.— H. J. Duff *et al.*, *Am. J. Cardiol.*, 1985, *56*, 887 (arrhythmias associated with myocardial infarction); P. Dumoulin *et al.*, *Am. Heart J.*, 1985, *110*, 575 (use in premature ventricular complexes); J. F. Caron *et al.*, *J. Am. Coll. Cardiol.*, 1985, *5*, 1457 (comparison with disopyramide); J. Morganroth *et al.*, *ibid.*, 1986, *7*, 9 (comparison with quinidine); J. Morganroth *et al.*, *Am. J. Cardiol.*, 1986, *57*, 769 (comparison with placebo); M. H. Sami, *ibid.*, *58*, 25C (long-term therapy); T. Tordjman *et al.*, *ibid.*, 87C (use in ventricular arrhythmias).

Use in atrial arrhythmias.— K. -P. Kunze *et al.*, *J. Am. Coll. Cardiol.*, 1986, *7*, 1121; J. F. Strasberger *et al.*, *Am. J. Cardiol.*, 1986, *58*, 49C; P. E. Pool, *ibid.*, 55C.

EFFECT OF METABOLITES. A patient whose arrhythmia did not respond to treatment with encainide had a prolonged half-life of 7.8 hours and the *O*-demethylated metabolite was not detected until doses of 500 mg daily were given. It was suggested that the *O*-demethylated metabolite may contribute to the anti-arrhythmic and electrocardiographic effects of encainide.— D. M. Roden *et al.*, *New Engl. J. Med.*, 1980, *302*, 877.

Encainide was found to have a mean half-life of 1.16 hours in 13 patients after 6-months treatment, and was almost completely eliminated from the body during dosing intervals of 6 to 8 hours. The major metabolites of encainide have considerably longer half-lives and probably contribute substantially to the anti-arrhythmic efficacy of long-term encainide therapy and may be responsible for the qualitative differences in electrophysiological effect seen during short- and long-term administration of oral encainide.— R. E. Kates *et al.*, *Clin. Pharmac. Ther.*, 1982, *31*, 427. See also: J. W. Mason, *Am. J. Cardiol.*, 1986, *58*, 18C.

Proprietary Names and Manufacturers

Enkaid *(Bristol-Myers Products, USA)*;

12753-a

Flecainide Acetate *(BANM, USAN, rINNM)*.

R-818. *N*-(2-Piperidylmethyl)-2,5-bis(2,2,2-trifluoroethoxy)benzamide acetate.
$C_{17}H_{20}F_6N_2O_3,C_2H_4O_2 = 474.4$.

CAS — 54143-55-4 (flecainide); 54143-56-5 (acetate).

Adverse Effects

The most common adverse effects caused by flecainide affect the central nervous system and include dizziness, blurred vision, and light-headedness. Nausea, headache, tremor, and paraesthesia may also occur. These effects are generally transient and respond to dosage reduction. Cardiovascular effects are less common, but can be serious and sometimes fatal. Ventricular tachyarrhythmias have been reported, particularly in patients with a history of ventricular tachyarrhythmias and taking high doses of flecainide.

A review of the adverse effects of flecainide found that while effects on the central nervous system were fairly common during flecainide therapy, symptoms could generally be managed by reduction of dosage. Flecainide prolongs QRS and PR duration, and although a prolongation of up to 30% is generally well tolerated, there is a potential for atrioventricular and intranodal block. Flecainide may also depress sinus node function in patients with pre-existing sinus node abnormalities. The incidence of severe ventricular arrhythmias approaches 20% in patients with severe ventricular dysfunction and a history of sustained ventricular tachycardia who are taking doses of flecainide greater than 400 mg a day. Resuscitation was reported to be more difficult to accomplish than it had been in earlier episodes, or unsuccessful. Patients with a history of sustained ventricular tachycardia and a reduced ejection fraction who are taking relatively high doses of flecainide and who have relatively high plasma-flecainide concentrations appear to be at a particular risk of serious ventricular arrhythmias and death.— D. M. Roden and R. L. Woosley, *New Engl. J. Med.*, 1986, *315*, 36.

Report of the non-cardiac adverse effects from one short-term and 3 longer term studies. The most common adverse effects during both short-and long-term studies were dizziness and visual disturbances which occurred in about 30% of patients. Headache and nausea both occurred in about 10% of patients. Other adverse effects reported include dyspnoea, chest pain, asthenia, fatigue, and tremor. Therapy was discontinued due to non-cardiac adverse effects in 10% of patients in the short-term trial, and in 6% of those in the chronic studies.— G. D. Gentzkow and J. Y. Sullivan, *Am. J. Cardiol.*, 1984, *53*, 101B.

A brief report of a patient who developed painful eye movement during treatment with flecainide. The pain resolved when treatment was withdrawn, but recurred when flecainide was restarted, and was accompanied by lateral rectus spasm, a facial rash, and positive anti-nuclear factor, suggestive of lupus erythematosus.— M. Skander and P. E. T. Isaacs, *Br. med. J.*, 1985, *291*, 450.

The adverse cardiovascular effects of flecainide were found to be associated with higher plasma-flecainide concentrations than those routinely observed during flecainide dosing.— D. M. Salerno *et al.*, *Clin. Pharmac. Ther.*, 1986, *40*, 101.

Dysarthria and visual hallucinations were associated with elevated plasma concentration of flecainide (2500 ng per mL) in 1 patient. A serial rise and fall in plasma-bilirubin concentration during flecainide therapy also suggested possible direct hepatotoxicity.— E. Ramhamadany *et al.*, *Postgrad. med. J.*, 1986, *62*, 61.

OVERDOSAGE. A report of life-threatening ventricular tachycardia in a healthy young woman after she took a massive overdose of flecainide.— B. R. Winkelmann and H. Leinberger, *Ann. intern. Med.*, 1987, *106*, 807.

Failure of haemoperfusion to reduce flecainide intoxication in a patient with terminal renal failure and undergoing haemodialysis.— J. Braun *et al.*, *Med. Toxicol.*, 1987, *2*, 463.

Precautions

Flecainide should be used with extreme caution in patients with sinus node dysfunction or conduction abnormalities. It has some negative inotropic activity and may precipitate or aggravate heart failure in patients with compromised left ventricular function. Flecainide has been shown to increase the endocardial pacing threshold and should be used with caution in patients with pacemakers. Electrolyte imbalances should be corrected before flecainide therapy is started. Reduction of dosage may be necessary in patients with impaired renal function, and in the elderly. Concomitant administration with other anti-arrhythmic agents may increase the incidence of cardiac arrhythmias.

ADMINISTRATION IN RENAL FAILURE. Renal flecainide clearance was reduced and elimination half-life increased in patients with renal impairment compared with patients with normal renal function.— J. Braun *et al.*, *Eur. J. clin. Pharmac.*, 1987, *31*, 711.

For a report of flecainide intoxication in a patient with chronic renal failure, see under Overdosage in Adverse Effects, above.

INTERACTIONS. There was an increase in plasma-flecainide concentrations in each of 8 patients when *amiodarone* was added to their treatment regimen.— P. Shea *et al.*, *J. Am. Coll. Cardiol.*, 1986, *7*, 1127.

Pretreatment with *cimetidine* delayed maximum plasma-flecainide concentrations and increased the total amount of flecainide absorbed in a study in 8 healthy subjects. There was no change in elimination half-life or renal clearance of flecainide. The most likely mechanism was considered to be a decrease in biotransformation of flecainide.— T. B. Tjandra-Maga *et al.*, *Br. J. clin. Pharmac.*, 1986, *22*, 108.

Absorption and Fate

Flecainide is almost completely absorbed after oral administration and does not undergo extensive first-pass hepatic metabolism. The bioavailability has been reported as 90 to 95%. The plasma half-life is about 20 hours, and flecainide is about 40% bound to plasma proteins. Flecainide is excreted in the urine as the unchanged drug and its metabolites. Excretion may be reduced in patients with congestive heart failure or renal failure.

In a study of 8 healthy subjects, the elimination of flecainide was found to be inversely proportional to urinary pH. The mean elimination half-life ranged from 10.7 hours at urinary pH 5.0 to 17.6 hours at pH 8.— A. Johnston *et al.*, *Br. J. clin. Pharmac.*, 1985, *20*, 333. See also: K. A. Muhiddin *et al.*, *ibid.*, 1984, *17*, 447.

The serum protein binding was found to range from 37 to 58% with a mean of 48% in healthy subjects. A correlation was found between the fraction of flecainide bound and the serum α_1-acid glycoprotein concentration, the subjects' age, and serum albumin concentration.— A. Johnston *et al.*, *Br. J. clin. Pharmac.*, 1982, *13*, 606P.

The plasma protein binding of flecainide fell from 61% to 53% in 11 patients after myocardial infarction, possibly due to displacement of flecainide from binding sites by endogenous substances.— J. L. Caplin *et al.*, *Eur. J. clin. Pharmac.*, 1985, *28*, 253.

Uses and Administration

Flecainide is a class Ic anti-arrhythmic agent (see p.70) used for the treatment of ventricular arrhythmias and tachycardias. Treatment should be carefully monitored during the initial stages and plasma concentration measurement may be helpful: a suggested therapeutic concentration range is 200 to 1000 ng per mL. Doses may need to be reduced in patients with renal impairment. Flecainide is given by mouth as the acetate in a usual initial dose of 100 mg every 12 hours. The usual maximum dose is 200 mg every 12 hours, although doses of 600 mg a day have been used cautiously. The dose may be adjusted after 3 to 5 days and reduced once control has been achieved. Flecainide may also be administered as an intravenous injection. For rapid control flecainide acetate 2 mg per kg body-weight is administered over 10 to 30 minutes, to a maximum dose of 150 mg. If long-term parenteral therapy is necessary therapy is initiated by intravenous injection of 2 mg per kg over 30 minutes, as above, then continued by intravenous infusion of 1.5 mg per kg over the first hour, and 0.1 to 0.25 mg per kg per hour thereafter.

A review of flecainide. Flecainide has been shown to depress cardiac conduction particularly in the His-Purkinje system. It has also been shown to depress conduction in accessory pathways, with retrograde conduction being the most profoundly affected. Haemodynamic studies in healthy subjects, patients with heart failure, patients with coronary artery disease, and patients with recent myocardial infarctions have differed in their results of the effects of flecainide on heart-rate. In most studies flecainide administration produced a negative inotropic effect, but, apart from significant increases in pulmonary wedge pressures, blood pressure seemed to be unaffected.

In several open studies, orally administered flecainide brought about a greater than 90% suppression of ventricular ectopic beats in about 80% of patients, and a greater than 80% suppression of ventricular tachycardia in about 83% of patients. Intravenous infusions of flecainide gave similar results in a slightly greater proportion of patients. Flecainide has also been used successfully in patients with Wolff-Parkinson-White syndrome and in others with arrhythmias involving anomalous pathways. Flecainide was reported to be more effective than quinidine, tocainide, disopyramide, and mexiletine in the suppression of ventricular arrhythmias, and as effective as propafenone in the treatment of repetitive ventricular ectopic beats. However, generally small numbers of patients have been involved in comparative studies.— B. Holmes and R. C. Heel, *Drugs*, 1985, *29*, 1.

A review of flecainide concluded that it had been shown to be more potent and better tolerated than currently available anti-arrhythmic drugs in patients with non-sustained ventricular arrhythmias and nearly normal left ventricular function. Arrhythmias that are not associated with an increased risk of sudden death can be effectively suppressed with flecainide, but patients with recurrent sustained ventricular tachycardia or ventricular fibrillation associated with a substantial risk of sudden death are at high risk of serious adverse reactions to flecainide therapy. In patients with severe left ventricular dysfunction, both the underlying heart disease and the accumulation of flecainide in the plasma due to heart failure may contribute to an increased risk of aggravation of arrhythmias.— D. M. Roden and R. L. Woosley, *New Engl. J. Med.*, 1986, *315*, 36.

Further reviews of flecainide: *Lancet*, 1984, *1*, 85.

Studies of the electrophysiological effects of flecainide.— K. J. Hellestrand *et al.*, *Br. Heart J.*, 1982, *48*, 140; K. A. Muhiddin and A. Johnston, *Br. J. clin. Pharmac.*, 1982, *14*, 588P; P. W. Serruys *et al.*, *ibid.*, 1983, *16*, 51.

Flecainide was shown to have negative inotropic activity which was appreciably greater in patients with heart failure, although overall differences were small.— V. Legrand *et al.*, *Eur. Heart J.*, 1985, *6*, 664.

The results of a study of 43 patients receiving flecainide indicated that a therapeutic range of plasma-flecainide concentrations of 381 to 710 ng per mL would include at least a 50% probability of efficacy with no more than a 10% probability of adverse cardiovascular effects.— D. M. Salerno *et al.*, *Clin. Pharmac. Ther.*, 1986, *40*, 101.

ADMINISTRATION IN RENAL FAILURE. For reference to reduced clearance of flecainide in patients with impaired renal function, see under Precautions, above.

CARDIAC ARRHYTHMIAS. Flecainide has compared favourably with other anti-arrhythmic agents in several studies. Flecainide was found to be more effective in suppressing chronic stable ventricular ectopic depolarisations than *quinidine* in a small study by Salerno *et al.* (*Ann. intern. Med.*, 1983, *98*, 455). In a multicentre study involving 280 patients (The Flecainide-Quinidine Research Group, *Circulation*, 1983, *67*, 1117), flecainide caused greater than 80% suppression of premature ventricular contractions in 85% of patients compared with 57% of patients on quinidine, and was also more effective than quinidine in suppressing couplets and ventricular tachycardia. Oral flecainide twice daily was also found to be more effective than *disopyramide* given 4 times a day in suppressing the occurrence and severity of premature ventricular complexes in patients with chronic and symptomatic arrhythmias in a study by Kjekshus *et al.* (*Am. J. Cardiol.*, 1984, *53*, 72B) with 60% of patients on flecainide achieving at least 80% suppression compared with 32% during the disopyramide treatment period. Dubner *et al.* (*Am. Heart J.*, 1985, *109*, 523) reported flecainide to be more effective than *amiodarone* in suppressing chronic, stable ventricular ectopic beats.

A study of the long-term administration of flecainide to 47 out of 60 patients with chronic ventricular arrhythmias who responded favourably during an initial trial period. Flecainide was considered to be highly effective in suppressing ventricular arrhythmias in a high proportion of patients, although there was evidence to suggest an arrhythmogenic effect in some patients.— G. Vanhaleweyk *et al.*, *Eur. Heart J.*, 1984, *5*, 814. A similarly favourable study in which 90% of successfully treated patients were controlled with 300 mg of flecainide or less daily to maintain trough plasma-flecainide concentrations of 0.2 to 1.0 μg per mL.— L. N. Horowitz *et al.*, *Am. J. Cardiol.*, 1986, *57*, 1299.

Further references to the use of flecainide in ventricular arrhythmias.— H. Abitbol *et al.*, *Am. Heart J.*, 1983, *105*, 227; T. Meinertz *et al.*, *Am. J. Cardiol.*, 1984, *54*, 91; D. Flowers *et al.*, *Am. J. Cardiol.*, 1985, *55*, 79; R. Lal *et al.*, *Ann. intern. Med.*, 1986, *105*, 493.

Sinus rhythm was restored in 18 out of 24 patients with atrial fibrillation within 24 hours of the first intravenous dose of flecainide 1 to 2 mg per kg body-weight.— J. -J. Goy *et al.* (letter), *Eur. J. clin. Pharmac.*, 1985, *27*, 737.

In a study involving 13 children, flecainide 2 mg per kg body-weight by intravenous infusion terminated supraventricular tachycardias in 11 out of 12 children within 12 minutes of the start of the infusion. Successful long-term prophylaxis was achieved in 11 of the 13 children with flecainide administered by mouth. One child developed pro-arrhythmic adverse effects, and another complained of nausea, both during flecainide infusion.— J. A. Till *et al.*, *Archs Dis. Childh.*, 1987, *62*, 247.

PAIN. Beneficial results with flecainide in the control of severe pain associated with malignant infiltration of nerves.— R. Dunlop *et al.* (letter), *Lancet*, 1988, *1*, 420.

Proprietary Preparations

Tambocor *(Riker, UK)*. *Tablets*, scored, flecainide acetate 100 mg.
Injection, flecainide acetate 10 mg/mL, in ampoules of 15 mL.

Proprietary Names and Manufacturers

Almarytm *(Selvi, Ital.)*; Flecaine *(Riker, Fr.)*; Tambocor *(Riker, Arg.; Riker, Austral.; Riker, Denm.; Kettelhack Riker, Ger.; Riker, Norw.; Riker, Swed.; Riker 3M, Switz.; Riker, UK; Riker, USA)*.

16819-g

Gallopamil Hydrochloride *(BANM, rINNM)*.

D-600 (gallopamil); Methoxyverapamil Hydrochloride.
5-[*N*-(3,4-Dimethoxyphenethyl)-*N*-methylamino]-2-(3,4,5-trimethoxyphenyl)-2-isopropylvaleronitrile hydrochloride.
$C_{28}H_{40}N_2O_5,HCl=521.1$.

CAS — 16662-47-8 (gallopamil).

Gallopamil is a calcium-channel blocking agent with anti-arrhythmic activity and is chemically related to verapamil. It is used for the prophylaxis and treatment of chronic cardiac insufficiency, angina pectoris, and atrial tachyarrhythmias. Gallopamil hydrochloride is given by mouth in doses of 25 to 50 mg every 6 to 12 hours up to a maximum total dose of 200 mg daily.

In a multicentre study involving 455 patients over a 1-year period, gallopamil was reported to improve subjective and objective symptoms of angina pectoris and caused no severe adverse effects. The most frequently used dosage was gallopamil 50 mg two or three times daily, and full effectiveness was usually reached 4 weeks after the start of therapy. Therapeutic success was defined as good in 73% of cases. The most frequent adverse effects were gastric discomfort, bradycardia, and atrioventricular prolongation: therapy was discontinued in 4 patients due to cardiac adverse reactions.— M. Sućić and J. Schiemann, *Arzneimittel-Forsch.*, 1984, *34*, 1587.

Proprietary Names and Manufacturers
Procorum *(Minden, Ger.)*.

7786-v

Hydroquinidine Hydrochloride

Dihydrochinidin Hydrochloride; Dihydroquinidine Hydrochloride; Hydroconchinine Hydrochloride.
(8*R*,9*S*)-10,11-Dihydro-6′-methoxycinchonan-9-ol hydrochloride.
$C_{20}H_{26}N_2O_2,HCl=362.9$.

CAS — 1435-55-8 (hydroquinidine); 1476-98-8 (hydrochloride).

Pharmacopoeias. In Fr.

Hydroquinidine is an anti-arrhythmic agent with actions and uses similar to those of quinidine (see p.85). It is given as the hydrochloride in usual maintenance doses of 450 to 600 mg daily in divided doses.

Study of the bioavailability and pharmacokinetics of hydroquinidine administered as a sustained-release capsule.— B. Flouvat *et al.*, *Thérapie*, 1984, *39*, 337.

Proprietary Names and Manufacturers
Algiquin *(Berenguer-Beneyto, Spain)*; Lentoquine *(Berenguer-Beneyto, Spain)*; Sérécor *(Houdé, Fr.)*.

19340-q

Indecainide Hydrochloride *(USAN)*.
LY-135837; Ricainide. 9-[3-(Isopropylamino)propyl]fluorene-9-carboxamide hydrochloride.
$C_{20}H_{24}N_2O,HCl=344.9$.

CAS — 73681-12-6 (hydrochloride); 74517-78-5 (indecainide).

Indecainide is an anti-arrhythmic agent reported to have class Ic activity.

In a dose-ranging study in 19 patients with premature ventricular complex frequency from 30 to 2197 per hour, 16 patients responded to indecainide and continued treatment for a mean of 6 months. Ventricular tachycardia was also suppressed completely in 14 of these patients and there was greater than 98% reduction in the remaining 2 patients. Therapeutic plasma-indecainide concentrations ranged from 300 to 900 µg per mL. Blurred vision and dizziness were reported in 2 patients during the initial phase of the study and mild CNS symptoms occurred in 5 patients on long-term therapy.— J. Morganroth *et al.*, *J. clin. Pharmac.*, 1984, *24*, 414.

Report of the intravenous use of indecainide.— L. N. Horowitz *et al.*, *Am. Heart J.*, 1985, *110*, 784.

Proprietary Names and Manufacturers
Lilly, USA.

7787-g

Lorajmine Hydrochloride *(USAN, rINNM)*.
Chloroacetylajmaline Hydrochloride; Win-11831. Ajmaline 17-chloroacetate hydrochloride.
$C_{22}H_{27}ClN_2O_3,HCl=439.4$.

CAS — 47562-08-3 (lorajmine); 40819-93-0 (hydrochloride).

Pharmacopoeias. In *It.*

Lorajmine is an anti-arrhythmic agent which is related to ajmaline (p.70). It is given as the hydrochloride in maintenance doses of 200 to 400 mg daily. It is also given by slow intravenous injection or by infusion.

Proprietary Names and Manufacturers
Ritmos Elle *(Inverni della Beffa, Ital.)*; Viaductor *(Servier, Fr.)*.

7788-q

Lorcainide Hydrochloride *(BANM, USAN, rINNM)*.

Isocainide Hydrochloride; R-15889; Socainide Hydrochloride. 4′-Chloro-*N*-(1-isopropyl-4-piperidyl)-2-phenylacetanilide hydrochloride.
$C_{22}H_{27}ClN_2O,HCl=407.4$.

CAS — 59729-31-6 (lorcainide); 58934-46-6 (hydrochloride).

Adverse Effects and Precautions
The most common and troublesome adverse effects of lorcainide during oral therapy are sleep disturbances which may be accompanied by vivid dreams, sweating, and sensations of heat. During intravenous administration transient dizziness, blurred vision, and paraesthesia have been reported. Cardiovascular effects are rare, and are usually associated with depression of cardiac conduction. Lorcainide should be used cautiously in patients with sinus node dysfunction.

Uses and Administration
Lorcainide is a class Ic anti-arrhythmic agent (see p.70). It is given by mouth as the hydrochloride in doses of 100 mg twice daily increasing as necessary to a usual maximum dose of 400 mg daily. It may be given by intravenous infusion at a rate of 10 mg per minute, preferably under ECG control. An initial dose of 2 mg per kg body-weight has been recommended.

A review of lorcainide. The actions of lorcainide result in slowing of cardiac conduction, prolongation of the refractory period, and a slight increase in action potential duration. There is a log-linear relationship between QRS duration and plasma-lorcainide concentration. A slight increase in heart-rate has been seen after intravenous administration. Sinus node function may be significantly depressed in patients with sino-atrial node dysfunction and lorcainide should also be used with caution in patients with bundle branch block. Pharmacokinetic studies show that lorcainide is about 85% bound to plasma protein and has a half-life of about 8 hours. The therapeutic plasma concentration range is about 150 to 400 ng per mL. A wide dosage range may be required to produce a given plasma concentration in different patients, and dosage must be adjusted according to individual response. Lorcainide administered orally undergoes saturable first-pass hepatic elimination resulting in dose-dependent bioavailability. Lorcainide is almost completely metabolised in the liver and the half-life can be prolonged in cirrhosis and congestive heart failure. Norlorcainide, the *N*-dealkylated metabolite, has some anti-arrhythmic activity and accumulates during prolonged administration, with a half-life of 27 hours. Lorcainide has been shown to be effective in the treatment of premature ventricular contractions and other ventricular arrhythmias. Some beneficial effects have also been seen in Wolff-Parkinson-White syndrome. Initial short-term comparisons suggest that lorcainide is a useful alternative to lignocaine in acute myocardial infarction, premature ventricular contractions, and ventricular tachycardia and to mexiletine and aprindine in ventricular arrhythmias. The most troublesome adverse effects during oral treatment are disturbed sleep with insomnia and vivid dreams, which occur particularly during the early stages of treatment and usually respond to a benzodiazepine. Adverse cardiovascular effects are uncommon.— C. E. Eiriksson and R. N. Brogden, *Drugs*, 1984, *27*, 279. See also.— J. B. Schwartz *et al.*, *Drugs*, 1981, *21*, 23.

Pharmacokinetics of lorcainide: E. Jähnchen *et al.*, *Clin. Pharmac. Ther.*, 1979, *26*, 187; T. Meinertz *et al.*, *ibid.*, 196; U. Klotz *et al.*, *ibid.*, 221; U. Klotz *et al.*, *Int. J. clin. Pharmac. Biopharm.*, 1979, *17*, 152.

CARDIAC DISORDERS. Clinical studies of the therapeutic effectiveness of lorcainide: R. A. Winkle *et al.*, *Am. J. Cardiol.*, 1984, *53*, 544; B. Chesnie *et al.*, *J. Am. Coll. Cardiol.*, 1984, *3*, 1531; G. Schmidt *et al.*, *Eur. J. clin. Pharmac.*, 1985, *27*, 633; M. I. Anastasiou-Nana *et al.*, *Am. Heart J.*, 1985, *110*, 1168; R. Stroobandt and H. Kesteloot, *Acta cardiol.*, 1985, *40*, 637; J. C. Somberg *et al.*, *Am. Heart J.*, 1986, *111*, 648.

Comparison with lignocaine.— J. L. Anderson *et al.*, *J. Am. Coll. Cardiol.*, 1985, *5*, 333. See also: R. D. Blevins *et al.*, *Am. Heart J.*, 1986, *111*, 447.

Proprietary Names and Manufacturers
Remivox *(Janssen, Belg.; Janssen, Ger.)*.

7789-p

Mexiletine Hydrochloride *(BANM, rINNM)*.

Kö-1173. 1-Methyl-2-(2,6-xylyloxy)ethylamine hydrochloride.
$C_{11}H_{17}NO,HCl=215.7$.

CAS — 31828-71-4 (mexiletine); 5370-01-4 (hydrochloride).

Pharmacopoeias. In *Br., Chin.,* and *U.S.*

A white or almost white, odourless, crystalline powder. Freely **soluble** in water and in methyl alcohol; sparingly soluble in chloroform; insoluble in ether. A 10% solution in water has a pH of 4.0 to 5.5; the *B.P.* injection has a pH of 5.0 to 6.0. Solutions for injection are **sterilised** by autoclaving. **Store** in airtight containers.

Adverse Effects
Mexiletine has a narrow therapeutic ratio: many adverse effects of mexiletine are dose-related and will respond to dosage reduction but may be severe enough to necessitate discontinuation of therapy. Toxicity is commonly seen with oral or parenteral loading doses when plasma concentrations are high.
The most common adverse effects are nausea and vomiting. Effects on the nervous system include tremor, confusion, light-headedness, dizziness, blurred vision, and other visual disturbances. The most frequent cardiovascular effects are hypotension, sinus bradycardia, atrioventricular dissociation, and atrial fibrillation. Other adverse effects which have been reported include skin rashes, abnormal liver function tests and, at overdose, convulsions.

No pattern of serious unexpected adverse reactions could be discerned from reports received by the CSM after long-term therapy, apart from rare reports of hepatic disorders and blood dyscrasias.— *Br. med. J.*, 1986, *292*, 50.

EFFECTS ON THE BLOOD. Thrombocytopenia was reported in a patient 4 days after starting treatment with mexiletine. Platelet count had returned to normal within 10 days of discontinuing the drug. There was no evidence of platelet antibody formation.— G. P. Fasola *et al.* (letter), *Ann. intern. Med.*, 1984, *100*, 162. A report of pseudothrombocytopenia associated with mexiletine in which it was suggested that antibodies were reacting with platelets anticoagulated with edetic acid causing agglutination and spuriously low platelet counts.— G. Girmann *et al.* (letter), *ibid.*, 767.

OVERDOSAGE. A 22-year-old man who had ingested 4.4 g of mexiletine died. Symptoms included paraesthesia of the tongue, nausea, convulsions, cyanosis, rigidity, bradycardia, and an unrecordable blood pressure. The ECG showed complete heart block; ventricular asystole was unresponsive to isoprenaline, adrenaline, electrical pacing, and cardiac massage. The blood-mexiletine concentration post mortem was 34 to 37 µg per mL compared with the therapeutic range of 1 to 2 µg per mL.— P. Jequier *et al.* (letter), *Lancet*, 1976, *1*, 429.

Treatment of Adverse Effects
Adverse cardiovascular effects of mexiletine will call for symptomatic therapy. Hypotension associated with bradycardia may be reversed with atropine. It has been reported that *animal* studies indicate that toxic neurological effects of mexiletine may respond to diazepam.

Precautions
Mexiletine should be used with special caution in patients with sinus node dysfunction, conduction defect, bradycardia, hypotension, cardiogenic shock, or cardiac or hepatic failure. ECG and blood pressure monitoring should be carried out during treatment.
Absorption of mexiletine may be delayed by concurrent administration of opiates, and after myocardial infarction. Plasma concentrations of mexiletine may be reduced by the concurrent administration of drugs which induce hepatic enzymes such as phenytoin and rifampicin.

INTERACTIONS. A review and discussion of drug interactions with mexiletine. Drugs that induce hepatic mixed-function oxidases will increase the elimination rate of mexiletine and decrease its plasma concentration by about 50%. This may be a particular problem with *phenytoin* which is also used for its anti-arrhythmic effect.
Several beneficial interactions of mexiletine with other anti-arrhythmic agents are of clinical importance since the efficacy of mexiletine used alone is limited. However, combinations of mexiletine with *quinidine* or *beta-blockers* can increase its efficacy and reduce adverse effects. It is probably necessary to use reduced doses of mexiletine in these combinations.— J. T. Bigger, *Am. Heart J.*, 1984, *107*, 1079.

Evidence that *metoclopramide* enhances and *atropine* decreases the rate of mexiletine absorption without altering the relative oral bioavailability.— L. M. H. Wing *et al.*, *Br. J. clin. Pharmac.*, 1980, *9*, 505.

Plasma concentrations of mexiletine were reduced in 3 patients and 6 healthy subjects by concurrent administration of *phenytoin*. The suggested mechanism for the interaction was induction of hepatic mixed-function oxidase by phenytoin.— E. J. Begg *et al.*, *Br. J. clin. Pharmac.*, 1982, *14*, 219.

Administration of *rifampicin* was shown markedly to enhance the elimination of mexiletine in a study in 8 healthy subjects. The suggested mechanism was increased metabolism due to induction of hepatic enzymes by rifampicin.— P. J. Pentikäinen *et al.*, *Eur. J. clin. Pharmac.*, 1982, *23*, 261.

Short-term administration of *cimetidine* to 6 healthy subjects had no demonstrable effect on the disposition of a single oral dose of mexiletine.— A. Klein *et al.*, *Clin. Pharmac. Ther.*, 1985, *37*, 669.

For a report of mexiletine reducing the elimination of caffeine, see p.1522.

PREGNANCY AND THE NEONATE. A normal male child was born to a woman given mexiletine with propranolol for the control of ventricular dysrhythmias during the third trimester of pregnancy. During the first 6 hours after delivery the child had a heart-rate of only 90 beats per minute, probably due to the propranolol; it was normal thereafter. At delivery the concentration of mexiletine in the infant's serum was the same as in the mother's. The infant was breast fed and determinations on the second day and the sixth week after birth indicated that mexiletine is excreted in breast milk, but in an insufficient quantity to be measureable in the serum of the breast-fed infant. Though caution should still be exercised, mexiletine appears safe in pregnancy, and breast feeding can proceed normally.— A. D. Timmis *et al.* (letter), *Lancet*, 1980, *2*, 647. See also: A. M. Lewis *et al.*, *Postgrad. med. J.*, 1981, *57*, 546.

Absorption and Fate

Mexiletine is readily and almost completely absorbed from the gastro-intestinal tract.

Mexiletine is metabolised in the liver to a number of metabolites. It is excreted in the urine, mainly in the form of its metabolites with a small proportion of unchanged mexiletine; the clearance of mexiletine is increased in acid urine.

Mexiletine is widely distributed throughout the body and is about 60 to 70% bound to plasma proteins. It has a plasma half-life of 10 hours in healthy subjects but this may be prolonged in patients with heart disease. Its therapeutic effect has been correlated with plasma concentrations of 0.75 to 2 µg per mL, but the margin between therapeutic and toxic concentrations is narrow, and severe toxicity may occur within this range.

A study of the pharmacokinetics of mexiletine given in various doses by mouth or intravenously to 156 patients, 153 of whom had ischaemic heart disease, revealed great inter-patient variation. The mean plasma elimination half-life after a single intravenous dose of mexiletine 200 mg in 10 patients was 13.24 hours compared with 11.31 hours after chronic oral therapy in 30 patients. From 2 to 48% (mean 14%) of the total daily dose was excreted unchanged in the urine during the 48 hours after the last dose. In 149 patients, 79% of plasma concentrations within the range of 0.75 to 2 µg per mL were effective but 5.5% were associated with severe side-effects including hypotension, with or without bradycardia, atrio-ventricular dissociation, vomiting, tremor, and toxic confusional states. A dose of 10 to 14 mg per kg body-weight daily achieved plasma concentrations in this therapeutic range in 72% of patients. Significant increases in plasma concentration did not occur after the third day when maintenance doses of mexiletine were given.— N. P. S. Campbell *et al.*, *Br. J. clin. Pharmac.*, 1978, *6*, 103.

Use of a slow-release tablet of mexiletine to maintain plasma concentrations within the therapeutic range with a 12-hourly dosage regimen.— D. M. Boyle *et al.*, *Br. J. clin. Pharmac.*, 1980, *9*, 293P. See also: D. W. Holt *et al.*, *Clin. Ther.*, 1983, *5*, 268.

EFFECTS OF HEART DISEASE. A study of the pharmacokinetics of mexiletine in 58 patients. Large interindividual variations in the serum concentration were found. The pharmacokinetics were not significantly altered in patients with congestive heart failure.— S. Vozeh *et al.*, *Eur. J. clin. Pharmac.*, 1982, *23*, 445.

Low serum concentrations of mexiletine were produced by oral dosing in the acute phase of myocardial infarction due to delayed gastro-intestinal absorption in 7 patients. In addition the elimination half-life of mexiletine was prolonged from 11.75 hours to 15 hours.— P. J. Pentikäinen *et al.*, *Eur. J. clin. Pharmac.*, 1983, *25*, 773.

EFFECTS OF RENAL FAILURE. The pharmacokinetics of mexiletine were not significantly modified in patients with chronic renal failure when the creatinine clearance was above 10 mL per minute. However in patients with a creatinine clearance below 10 mL per minute the steady-state plasma concentration and half-life were increased.— D. El Allaf *et al.*, *Br. J. clin. Pharmac.*, 1982, *14*, 431.

Only 2.8% of the daily oral dose of mexiletine was cleared daily by continuous ambulatory peritoneal dialysis in a patient with chronic renal failure.— D. R. P. Guay *et al.* (letter), *Br. J. clin. Pharmac.*, 1985, *19*, 857.

EXCRETION. A study of the effects of spontaneous changes in urinary pH in healthy subjects given subtherapeutic doses of mexiletine confirmed that at high urinary pH excretion and clearance of mexiletine is low and the plasma concentration is raised. Urinary pH may partly account for inter-individual differences in the pharmacokinetics of mexiletine. Urinary pH measurements may be useful during mexiletine therapy and any factors likely to cause large variations in the urinary pH, such as antacids, should be avoided.— A. Johnston *et al.*, *Br. J. clin. Pharmac.*, 1979, *8*, 349.

In a study of 5 healthy subjects, urinary acidification produced a large and consistent increase in the renal clearance of mexiletine, although the total plasma clearance and half-life was affected in only 2 subjects. Changes in mexiletine disposition cannot be predicted accurately from urine pH measurements due to the large individual variations.— B. G. Mitchell *et al.*, *Br. J. clin. Pharmac.*, 1983, *16*, 281.

PREGNANCY AND THE NEONATE. In a patient taking mexiletine 200 mg every 8 hours the mean breast milk to plasma concentration ratio was 1.45. The mean peak concentration of mexiletine was 724 ng per mL in blood and 959 ng per mL in milk.— A. M. Lewis *et al.*, *Postgrad. med. J.*, 1981, *57*, 546.

Uses and Administration

Mexiletine is a class Ib anti-arrhythmic agent (see p.70) with actions similar to those of lignocaine (p.1219), to which it is structurally related. Unlike lignocaine it is suitable for oral administration.

Mexiletine is used for the prevention and treatment of ventricular arrhythmias particularly after myocardial infarction. It is given by mouth as the hydrochloride in initial doses of 400 mg followed by 200 to 250 mg three to four times daily, starting 2 hours after the loading dose. The usual maintenance dosage of mexiletine is 600 to 800 mg daily in divided doses. Higher doses may be necessary in patients after myocardial infarction to overcome delayed absorption. Use of a controlled-release preparation allows 12-hourly administration.

Mexiletine may be given by slow intravenous injection of the hydrochloride in doses of 100 to 250 mg at a rate of 25 mg per minute, followed by an infusion at a rate of 250 mg over 1 hour, 250 mg over the next 2 hours, and then at about 0.5 mg per minute for maintenance, according to the patient's response; when appropriate the patient may be transferred to oral therapy with doses of 200 to 250 mg of the hydrochloride 3 or 4 times daily. Alternatively, an initial intravenous dose of 200 mg at a rate of 25 mg per minute, may be followed by an oral dose of 400 mg on completion of the injection, with subsequent oral therapy as before.

ADMINISTRATION IN CHILDREN. The dose of mexiletine in children should be titrated according to the concentration in plasma. In a 2-week-old girl and a 20-month-old boy high doses of 25 and 15 mg per kg body-weight respectively were needed to produce therapeutic concentrations in plasma.— D. W. Holt *et al.*, *Br. med. J.*, 1979, *2*, 1476.

ADMINISTRATION IN RENAL FAILURE. For reference to the effect of renal failure on the pharmacokinetics of mexiletine, see Absorption and Fate, above.

CARDIAC DISORDERS. Reviews of mexiletine: *Med. Lett.*, 1986, *28*, 65; R. W. F. Campbell, *New Engl. J. Med.*, 1987, *316*, 29.

For the effect of cardiac disease on the pharmacokinetics of mexiletine, see Absorption and Fate, above.

Arrhythmias. Mexiletine hydrochloride 250 mg intravenously controlled *supraventricular tachycardia* in 1 patient who had not responded to other drugs. Subsequent maintenance was with mexiletine by mouth. Beneficial results were also achieved in another 5 patients. All 6 suffered short-lived dizziness, vomiting, and hypotension from the initial parenteral dose but the first two side-effects could be controlled by the intravenous injection of prochlorperazine 12.5 mg given 5 minutes before the mexiletine injection.— H. H. Salem (letter), *Lancet*, 1977, *2*, 94. See also S. D. Slater *et al.* (letter), *Br. med. J.*, 1980, *281*, 1072.

In 4 patients with *ventricular tachycardia* refractory to previous standard drug therapy, including mexiletine, the addition of propranolol 240 mg daily to the highest dose of mexiletine that failed to produce adverse effects resulted in either greater than 80% suppression of ventricular premature depolarisations or the absence of ventricular tachycardia or both. Follow-up for 12 to 23 months has indicated that maintenance treatment has produced excellent control.— E. B. Leahey *et al.*, *Br. med. J.*, 1980, *281*, 357.

The long-term efficacy of mexiletine in the treatment of ventricular arrhythmias refractory to other drug therapy has been the subject of several studies. In 107 of 313 patients in whom mexiletine was found to be effective and well tolerated during short-term evaluation, Stein *et al.* (*Am. Heart J.*, 1984, *107*, 1091) reported an annual mortality of 4.2%, with 19 deaths during an average follow-up period of 22.8 months, and non-fatal recurrence of arrhythmias in 14 patients, or 4.9% a year. Treatment was discontinued in 13 patients, and the remaining 61 patients (57%) continued on mexiletine therapy for up to 70 months. Effective anti-arrhythmic therapy was achieved during long-term treatment in 13 of 52 patients in a study reported by Rutledge *et al.* (*J. Am. Coll. Cardiol.*, 1985, *6*, 780). In 6 other patients who responded initially, 5 had intolerable adverse reactions at between 0.83 and 63.2 weeks and sudden death occurred in 1 patient. In a comparative study (K. Nademanee *et al.*, *Am. Heart J.*, 1985, *110*, 923) mexiletine was as effective as, or marginally better than, procainamide at suppressing premature ventricular contractions, but was found to have limited efficacy in controlling life-threatening ventricular arrhythmias: only 3 of 25 patients were successfully treated with long-term therapy. In the 21 patients who either could not tolerate or did not respond to mexiletine, early control of arrhythmias was achieved by amiodarone in all but one patient. Poole *et al.* (*ibid.*, 1986, *112*, 322) reported that of 32 out of 51 patients discharged from hospital on mexiletine therapy, only 6 continued taking mexiletine long-term; 6 patients had fatal recurrent arrhythmias, 5 had non-fatal arrhythmias, 7 had non-arrhythmia related deaths, and 8, intolerable adverse effects. Thus, mexiletine may be effective in the treatment of some patients with resistant ventricular arrhythmias, but adverse effects may limit the usefulness of mexiletine in long-term therapy.

Further references to mexiletine in ventricular arrhythmias: B. Trimarco *et al.*, *Curr. ther. Res.*, 1983, *33*, 472; P. E. Fenster and C. D. Hanson, *Clin. Pharmac. Ther.*, 1983, *34*, 136; P. E. Fenster and K. B. Kern, *ibid.*, 777; M. E. Assey *et al.*, *Sth. med. J.*, 1985, *78*, 565.

Combined therapy. A review of clinical studies into the use of mexiletine in combination with other anti-arrhythmic agents. Favourable responses have been reported with mexiletine used in combination with propranolol, amiodarone, disopyramide, or quinidine.— *Drug Interact. News.*, 1986, *6*, 5.

Myocardial infarction. In a study involving 344 high-risk patients mexiletine therapy reduced the prevalence of ventricular arrhythmias following myocardial infarction, but no favourable trend in mortality was observed (D.A. Chamberlain *et al.*, *Lancet*, 1980, *2*, 1324). In an attempt to prevent ventricular arrhythmias occurring during the first hours after acute myocardial infarction, Halinen *et al.*, (*Eur. Heart J.*, 1984, *5*, 675) evaluated the use of a combined intravenous and oral loading dose of mexiletine followed by oral maintenance dosage during the 48 hours following suspected infarction in a study of 99 patients. The incidence of ventricular arrhythmias was smaller in the mexiletine group than in the placebo group, and suppression was seen within the first hour of analysis. There were no serious adverse effects attributable to mexiletine, although serum-mexiletine concentrations tended to be low throughout the study. The IMPACT Research Group (*J. Am. Coll. Cardiol.*, 1984, *4*, 1148) reported a reduction in the risk of arrhythmias during the first 4 months after discharge from hospital in a study of sustained-release mexiletine in 630 patients, although the observed reduction in mortality did not reach statistical significance. Bell *et al.*, (*Br. Heart J.*, 1982, *48*, 285) concluded that administration of prophylactic mexiletine in home coronary care could be both safe and practicable.

PAIN. A beneficial response to mexiletine 50 mg three times a day by mouth in a patient with Dercum's disease, a condition involving painful fatty deposits.— P. Petersen *et al.*, *Br. med. J.*, 1984, *288*, 1880.

Mexiletine relieved the symptoms of chronic painful diabetic neuropathy when compared with placebo in a double-blind crossover study in 16 patients.— A. Dejgård *et al.*, *Lancet*, 1988, *1*, 9.

PREGNANCY AND THE NEONATE. For reports of patients treated with mexiletine during pregnancy see Precautions, above.

Preparations

Mexiletine Capsules *(B.P.)*. Mexiletine Hydrochloride Capsules

Mexiletine Hydrochloride Capsules *(U.S.P.)*

Mexiletine Injection *(B.P.)*. Mexiletine Hydrochloride Injection

Proprietary Preparations

Mexitil *(Boehringer Ingelheim, UK). Capsules*, mexiletine hydrochloride 50 and 200 mg.
Injection, mexiletine hydrochloride 25 mg/mL, in ampoules of 10 mL.

Mexitil PL *(Boehringer Ingelheim, UK). Perlongets*, sustained-release capsules, mexiletine hydrochloride 360 mg.

Proprietary Names and Manufacturers

Mexitil *(Boehringer Ingelheim, Austral.; Belg.; Boehringer Ingelheim, Canad.; Boehringer Ingelheim, Denm.; Boehringer Ingelheim, Fr.; Boehringer Ingelheim, Ger.; Boehringer Ingelheim, Ital.; Boehringer Ingelheim, Norw.; NZ; Boehringer Ingelheim, S.Afr.; Boehringer Ingelheim, Spain; Boehringer Ingelheim, Swed.; Boehringer Ingelheim, Switz.; Boehringer Ingelheim, UK; Boehringer Ingelheim, USA)*; Mexitilen *(Boehringer Sohn, Arg.)*.

12978-l

Moricizine *(USAN)*.

EN-313; Ethmosine; Ethmozine; Etmozin; Moracizine *(rINN)*. Ethyl [10-(3-morpholinopropionyl)phenothiazin-2-yl]carbamate.
$C_{22}H_{25}N_3O_4S$=427.5.

CAS — 31883-05-3.

Moricizine is a phenothiazine compound with Class Ib anti-arrhythmic activity.

A brief review of moricizine.— J. C. Somberg, *Am. J. Cardiol.*, 1984, *54*, 8B. See also.— J. B. Schwartz *et al.*, *Drugs*, 1981, *21*, 23.

A study of the efficacy, safety, haemodynamic effects, and pharmacokinetics of high doses of moricizine (15 mg per kg body-weight daily) in 10 patients with ventricular arrhythmias.— D. M. Salerno *et al.*, *Clin. Pharmac. Ther.*, 1987, *42*, 201. Further reports of moricizine in ventricular arrhythmias: C. M. Pratt *et al.*, *Am. Heart J.*, 1983, *106*, 85; J. Morganroth, *ibid.*, 1985, *110*, 1188; D. S. Miura *et al.*, *ibid.*, 1986, *111*, 661; K. Gear *et al.*, *Am. J. Cardiol.*, 1986, *57*, 947; C. M. Pratt *et al.*, *Am. J. Med.*, 1986, *80*, 626.

ADVERSE EFFECTS. Fever was associated with moricizine administration in 2 patients. The fever abated within 48 hours of withdrawing moricizine and recurred within 24 hours of rechallenge in both patients. Results suggested a similarity to the neuroleptic malignant syndrome which has been attributed to other phenothiazine derivatives.— D. S. Miura *et al.*, *J. clin. Pharmac.*, 1986, *26*, 153.

Proprietary Names and Manufacturers

Endo, Canad.; Du Pont, USA.

12992-w

Nadoxolol Hydrochloride *(rINNM)*.

LL-1530. 3-Hydroxy-4-(1-naphthyloxy)butyramide oxime hydrochloride.
$C_{14}H_{16}N_2O_3$,HCl=296.8.

CAS — 54063-51-3 (nadoxolol); 35991-93-6 (hydrochloride).

Nadoxolol hydrochloride is an agent used for its anti-arrhythmic properties in the treatment of extrasystoles; doses of 0.75 to 1.5 g daily have been given, increased if necessary up to 2.25 g daily.

Proprietary Names and Manufacturers

Bradyl 250 *(Lafon, Fr.)*.

16955-j

Pirmenol Hydrochloride *(USAN, rINNM)*.

CI-845. ±-*cis*-2,6-Dimethyl-α-phenyl-α-2-pyridyl-1-piperidinebutanol hydrochloride.
$C_{22}H_{30}N_2O$,HCl=375.0.

CAS — 61477-94-9; 68252-19-7 (pirmenol).

Pirmenol is an anti-arrhythmic agent reported to have Class I activity.

Study of the disposition of intravenous pirmenol.— S. W. Sanders *et al.*, *J. clin. Pharmac.*, 1983, *23*, 113.

Brief review of the clinical pharmacokinetics of pirmenol.— A. M. Gillis and R. E. Kates, *Clin. Pharmacokinet.*, 1984, *9*, 375.

A brief review.— J. C. Somberg, *Am. J. Cardiol.*, 1984, *54*, 8B.

Suppression of premature ventricular complexes (PVC) occurred in 8 of 11 patients treated with pirmenol 100 to 600 mg daily during the initial stages of a long-term study. Treatment continued successfully in 5 patients for a mean duration of 642 ± 90 days with a mean PVC suppression of 98%. Adverse effects were mild but moderately frequent and included dry mouth, bitter taste, difficulty in urinating, constipation, hot flushes, and mild fatigue. Plasma-pirmenol concentrations appeared generally to correlate with efficacy.— E. M. Hampton *et al.*, *Eur. J. clin. Pharmac.*, 1986, *31*, 15. Further references to the anti-arrhythmic use of pirmenol: L. K. Toivonen *et al.*, *Eur. Heart J.*, 1985, *6*, 737; *idem, J. cardiovasc. Pharmac.*, 1986, *8*, 156; *idem, Br. Heart J.*, 1986, *55*, 176; L. K. Toivonen, *Clin. Cardiol.*, 1986, *9*, 369; A. R. Eastey *et al.*, *Am. J. Cardiol.*, 1986, *58*, 86.

Proprietary Names and Manufacturers

Parke, Davis, USA.

7790-n

Prajmalium Bitartrate *(BAN, rINN)*.

GT-1012; NPAB. *N*-Propylajmalinium hydrogen tartrate.
$C_{23}H_{33}N_2O_2$,$C_4H_5O_6$=518.6.

CAS — 35080-11-6 (prajmalium); 2589-47-1 (bitartrate).

Adverse Effects, Treatment, and Precautions

The adverse cardiovascular effects of prajmalium are similar to those of quinidine.

Cholestatic jaundice associated with pruritus, chills, and eosinophilia was attributed to an allergic reaction to prajmalium in a patient 20 days after the start of treatment.— H. H. Rotmensch *et al.*, *Postgrad. med. J.*, 1980, *56*, 738.

EFFECTS ON MENTAL STATE. Confusion and disorientation in time and place occurred on 2 occasions in a 67-year-old man given prajmalium bitartrate 100 mg daily for the control of supraventricular tachycardia; the confusion rapidly disappeared when prajmalium was withdrawn.— J. B. Lessing and I. J. Copperman, *Br. med. J.*, 1977, *2*, 675.

Uses and Administration

Prajmalium is an anti-arrhythmic agent which is the *N*-propyl derivative of ajmaline (p.70). It is given as the bitartrate in the treatment of cardiac arrhythmias in maintenance doses of 20 mg to 40 mg daily in divided doses.

CARDIAC DISORDERS. Evidence that prajmalium bitartrate 20 mg every 4 hours by mouth for 3 doses is an alternative to intravenous lignocaine in the treatment of ventricular arrhythmias after acute myocardial infarction.— W. -D. Bussmann *et al.*, *Am. Heart J.*, 1980, *99*, 589.

The beneficial action of prajmalium bitartrate in suppressing premature ventricular complexes was comparable to that of disopyramide in a study of 13 patients. Both drugs produced a significant reduction in ventricular ectopic activity.— M. Chiariello *et al.*, *Eur. J. clin. Pharmac.*, 1983, *24*, 35.

Proprietary Names and Manufacturers

Neo Aritmina *(Byk Gulden, Ital.)*; Neo-Gilurytmal *(Giulini, Ger.; Lacer, Spain; Kali-Chemie, Switz.)*.

7791-h

Procainamide Hydrochloride *(BANM, USAN, rINNM)*.

Novocainamidum; Procainamidi Chloridum; Procainamidi Hydrochloridum. 4-Amino-*N*-(2-diethylaminoethyl)benzamide hydrochloride.
$C_{13}H_{21}N_3O$,HCl=271.8.

CAS — 614-39-1 (hydrochloride); 51-06-9 (procainamide).

Pharmacopoeias. In *Arg., Aust., Br., Braz., Chin., Cz., Egypt., Eur., Fr., Ind., Int., It., Jpn, Jug., Nord., Pol., Rus., Swiss, Turk.,* and *U.S.*

A white to tan-coloured, odourless, hygroscopic, crystalline powder. *B.P.* **solubilities** are: 1 in 0.25 of water and 1 in 2 of alcohol; slightly soluble in chloroform; practically insoluble in ether. *U.S.P* solubilities are: very soluble in water, soluble in alcohol, slightly soluble in chloroform, and very slightly soluble in ether. A 10% solution in water has a pH of 5.0 to 6.5; the injection has a pH of 4.0 to 6.0. Solutions are **sterilised** by autoclaving. **Store** in airtight containers.

STABILITY. The concentration of procainamide decreased substantially when diluted with glucose 5% in sodium chloride 0.9% injection and stored under different conditions of lighting and temperature for between 24 hours and 7 days.— Y. -C. Lee *et al.*, *Am. J. Hosp. Pharm.*, 1981, *38*, 183.

The concentration of procainamide in solution decreased even under refrigeration when glucose was present. The interaction was attributed to the formation of a complex between procainamide and glucose.— D. M. Baaske *et al.* (letter), *Am. J. Hosp. Pharm.*, 1980, *37*, 1050.

Adverse Effects

Cardiac effects occur particularly during intravenous administration of procainamide and in overdose. Rapid intravenous infusion may result in severe hypotension, ventricular fibrillation, and asystole. High plasma concentrations are also associated with impaired cardiac conduction.

Hypersensitivity reactions to procainamide are common. Procainamide is a frequent cause of drug-induced systemic lupus erythematosus (SLE) and the incidence has been reported to be as high as 30% of patients taking procainamide over prolonged periods. Antinuclear antibodies may be detected in a high proportion of patients, but they do not necessarily develop the symptoms of SLE that include arthralgia, pleurisy, pericarditis, and fever. Agranulocytosis, eosinophilia, neutropenia, and thrombocytopenia have been reported. Other symptoms of hypersensitivity not necessarily related to SLE may also occur including hepatomegaly, angioedema, skin rashes, pruritus, and hypergammaglobulinaemia.

Anorexia, nausea, vomiting, a bitter taste, and diarrhoea are more common with higher oral doses. Effects on the central nervous system such as mental depression, dizziness, and psychosis with hallucinations, have been reported.

Out of 488 hospitalised patients in the Boston Collaborative Drug Surveillance Program who had received procainamide, 45 experienced acute adverse effects attributed to the drug. Life-threatening reactions included heart block in 3, tachyarrhythmias in 2, and bradycardia and/or hypotension in 2. Other reactions included gastro-intestinal upsets in 19, pyrexia in 8, bradycardia and hypotension in 5, tachyarrhythmias in 3, heart block in 1, eosinophilia in 1 and urticaria in 1 patient.— D. H. Lawson and H. Jick, *Br. J. clin. Pharmac.*, 1977, *4*, 507.

Blurred vision, constipation, dry mouth, and urinary retention which occurred in a patient 48 hours after the institution of combined oral and intravenous procainamide therapy in a total dose of 6.32 g daily, were attributed to the antimuscarinic effects of procainamide.— M. D. Prendergast and T. J. Nasca (letter), *J. Am. med. Ass.*, 1984, *251*, 2926.

Repeated episodes of torsades de pointes degenerating into ventricular fibrillation were attributed to elevated plasma concentrations of *N*-acetylprocainamide in a patient being treated with procainamide. Haemodialysis using a dialyser with high-clearance characteristics successfully reversed arrhythmias.— K. P. V. Nguyen *et al.*

(letter), *Ann. intern. Med.*, 1986, *104*, 283.

EFFECTS ON THE BLOOD. Pancytopenia occurred in a 73-year-old woman taking procainamide hydrochloride.— A. Z. Bluming *et al.*, *J. Am. med. Ass.*, 1976, *236*, 2520.

The blood of a 67-year-old man who had received procainamide 1 g daily for 3 years was found to have *anticoagulant substances* which caused a slightly elevated whole-blood clotting time and a significantly prolonged plasma thrombin time and partial thromboplastin time, while prothrombin time, plasma fibrinogen and serum fibrinogen-fibrin antigen concentrations were normal. When procainamide was withdrawn the circulating anticoagulant effect was gradually reduced.— D. K. Galanakis *et al.*, *J. Am. med. Ass.*, 1978, *239*, 1873.

A report of bone marrow granulomas and neutropenia in a 77-year-old man after receiving procainamide for 50 days.— J. Riker *et al.*, *Archs intern. Med.*, 1978, *138*, 1731.

Three cases of immune haemolytic anaemia were diagnosed in a study of 100 patients taking procainamide. Haemolysis resolved when procainamide was withdrawn.— S. Kleinman *et al.*, *New Engl. J. Med.*, 1984, *311*, 809.

Agranulocytosis or severe neutropenia developed in 8 patients taking sustained-release procainamide. Of these, 5 had undergone open-heart surgery, representing 4.4% of patients treated with open-heart surgery and postoperative procainamide.— A. G. Ellrodt *et al.*, *Ann. intern. Med.*, 1984, *100*, 197.

Further reports of procainamide adversely affecting the blood: S. Fleet (letter), *Ann. intern. Med.*, 1984, *100*, 616 (fatal agranulocytosis); D. J. Christensen *et al.* (letter), *ibid.*, 918 (agranulocytosis and thrombocytopenia); D. J. Meisner *et al.*, *Archs intern. Med.*, 1985, *145*, 700 (thrombocytopenia).

EFFECTS ON THE LIVER. A report of fever, chills and granulomatous hepatitis in a 63-year-old man with myocardial infarction who had received lignocaine followed by procainamide. Fever subsided and serum-liver-enzyme concentrations returned to normal 24 hours after withdrawal of procainamide.— H. H. Rotmensch *et al.*, *Ann. intern. Med.*, 1978, *89*, 646.

EFFECTS ON MENTAL STATE. Acute psychosis occurred in a 74-year-old patient after 3 days' treatment with procainamide 3 g daily by mouth. Plasma-procainamide concentrations were mildly elevated and paranoid behaviour ceased 48 hours after procainamide was discontinued.— D. S. P. Schubert *et al.* (letter), *Can. med. Ass. J.*, 1984, *131*, 1188.

EFFECTS ON THE MUSCLES. Severe generalised myopathy occurred in a patient after treatment with procainamide for 4 days. Blood-procainamide concentrations were above the normal therapeutic range at 48 µg per mL, and the patient improved when procainamide was stopped.— C. A. Lewis *et al.*, *Br. med. J.*, 1986, *292*, 593.

EFFECTS ON THE NERVOUS SYSTEM. Cerebellar ataxia was associated with elevated serum-procainamide concentrations in a patient taking procainamide 2 g every 6 hours by mouth. The symptoms had completely resolved 3 days after procainamide was discontinued, and did not return when treatment was restarted at a dose of 2 g every 8 hours, giving a serum-procainamide concentration of 17 µg per mL.— A. B. Schwartz *et al.*, *Archs intern. Med.*, 1984, *144*, 2260.

LUPUS ERYTHEMATOSUS. A discussion of recent developments in drug-associated systemic lupus erythematosus with reference to procainamide.— *Adverse Drug React. Bull.*, 1987, Apr., 460.

In a study of 20 patients on long-term procainamide treatment all 11 slow acetylators had developed antinuclear antibodies after about 5 months but only 3 of 9 rapid acetylators. Of 7 patients who developed the lupus syndrome 4 were slow and 3 were rapid acetylators. The syndrome developed after about 12 and 54 months of treatment respectively. Acetylation appeared to offer some protection against the induction of antinuclear antibody and the lupus syndrome.— R. L. Woosley *et al.*, *New Engl. J. Med.*, 1978, *298*, 1157.

Evidence is suggestive that procainamide itself, rather than its active metabolite *N*-acetylprocainamide (acecainide), leads to the development of antinuclear antibodies and ultimately lupus erythematosus. First, acetylprocainamide has been associated with little or no lupus erythematosus reaction, and second, slow acetylators are far more likely to experience lupus erythematosus. Should these findings be substantiated it would seem reasonable to prescribe acetylprocainamide.— R. E. Bernstein (letter), *Lancet*, 1979, *2*, 1076.

Slow acetylators showed some trend to a higher frequency and to a shorter time for development of antinuclear antibodies than rapid acetylators, in a study of 35 patients, but the difference between the phenotypes was marginal.— P. Ylitalo *et al.*, *Eur. J. clin. Pharmac.*, 1983, *25*, 791.

Further studies and comments on lupus erythematosus and procainamide, including the role of acetylation and the possibility of a lower incidence with the acetylated metabolite acetylprocainamide (acecainide): H. G. Bluestein *et al.*, *Lancet*, 1979, *2*, 816; P. F. J. Ryan *et al.* (letter), *ibid.*, 1248.

Treatment of Adverse Effects

In overdosage by mouth the stomach should be emptied by aspiration and lavage.

Severe hypotension may be treated by placing the patient in the supine position with the feet raised. If necessary an intravenous infusion of noradrenaline acid tartrate may be given; injection of phenylephrine hydrochloride or dopamine has also been suggested.

Systemic lupus erythematosus will normally respond to withdrawal of procainamide but corticosteroids may be required.

Studies in 4 healthy men showed that the renal excretion of procainamide was not affected by changes in pH.— W. Meyer *et al.*, *Eur. J. clin. Pharmac.*, 1974, *7*, 287.

DIALYSIS. Following ingestion of an estimated excess of 7 g of procainamide over her maintenance dose a 67-year-old woman with heart disease developed severe hypotension, renal insufficiency, and life-threatening cardiac toxicity. She recovered after haemodialysis which doubled procainamide clearance and increased *N*-acetylprocainamide clearance fourfold.— A. J. Atkinson *et al.*, *Clin. Pharmac. Ther.*, 1976, *20*, 585. In a patient undergoing chronic haemodialysis, *N*-acetylprocainamide accumulated to toxic concentrations while plasma-procainamide concentrations remained within the therapeutic range. Haemoperfusion provided excellent *N*-acetylprocainamide clearance producing a fall of 19 µg per mL over 4 hours.— G. L. Braden *et al.*, *Ann. intern. Med.*, 1986, *105*, 64. The reduction of toxic concentrations of *N*-acetylprocainamide by continuous arteriovenous haemofiltration or haemodiafiltration in 2 patients with renal failure receiving procainamide.— D. T. Domoto *et al.*, *ibid.*, 1987, *106*, 550. Critical comment.— P. D. Mitnick (letter), *ibid.*, *107*, 424. Reply.— D. T. Domoto (letter), *ibid.*

Precautions

Procainamide is contra-indicated in patients with moderately severe heart block, and should be used with caution in those with myocardial damage or severe organic heart disease. It may cause ventricular tachycardia in patients with atrial fibrillation. Procainamide should preferably not be used in patients with myasthenia gravis or systemic lupus erythematosus.

Accumulation of procainamide may occur in patients with heart failure, renal insufficiency, or impaired hepatic function.

Regular blood tests should be carried out in patients receiving procainamide, and screening for lupus erythematosus and serum antinuclear factor should be carried out before and regularly during therapy.

Procainamide may enhance the effects of antihypertensive agents, other anti-arrhythmic drugs, and neuromuscular blocking agents, and diminish those of parasympathomimetic agents, such as neostigmine. There is cross-sensitivity between procaine and procainamide.

Grave hypotension may follow intravenous administration of procainamide; it should be injected slowly under ECG control.

Decreases in left ventricular performance in 14 patients with primary myocardial disease given procainamide 7.5 mg per kg body-weight intravenously were directly related to procainamide blood concentrations. This effect may be clinically significant in patients with severe heart failure.— P. Geleris *et al.*, *Eur. J. clin. Pharmac.*, 1980, *18*, 311.

ADMINISTRATION IN THE ELDERLY. Reduced renal clearance of procainamide in the elderly.— M. M. Reidenberg *et al.*, *Clin. Pharmac. Ther.*, 1980, *28*, 732.

ADMINISTRATION IN RENAL FAILURE. Lethal accumulation of *N*-acetylprocainamide, an active metabolite of procainamide, occurred in 4 patients with severe renal dysfunction and heart disease who were given conventional doses of procainamide.— P. H. Vlasses *et al.*, *Drug Intell. & clin. Pharm.*, 1984, *18*, 493.

INTERACTIONS. *Alcohol.* The half-life of procainamide was decreased and the total body clearance and acetylation rate increased when alcohol was present.— H. Olsen and J. Mørland, *Br. J. clin. Pharmac.*, 1982, *13*, 203.

Antibiotics. Trimethoprim was shown to increase procainamide and *N*-acetylprocainamide-serum concentrations by competing for renal tubular secretion.— P. H. Vlasses *et al.*, *Clin. Pharmac. Ther.*, 1986, *39*, 233.

Cardiac glycosides. Confirmation of reports that serum-*digoxin* concentration rises during concomitant quinidine administration. No such rise occurred when procainamide was given.— E. B. Leahey *et al.*, *Ann. intern. Med.*, 1980, *92*, 605.

Gastro-intestinal agents. Cimetidine reduced the renal clearance of procainamide by almost a half in healthy subjects.— A. Somogyi and B. Heinzow (letter), *New Engl. J. Med.*, 1982, *307*, 1080. See also C. D. Chistian *et al.*, *Clin. Pharmac. Ther.*, 1984, *36*, 221.

A study in healthy subjects indicating that concurrent administration of ranitidine and procainamide may lead to a reduction in the renal clearance of procainamide and also a possible effect on gastro-intestinal absorption.— A. Somogyi and F. Bochner, *Br. J. clin. Pharmac.*, 1984, *18*, 175.

INTERFERENCE WITH DIAGNOSTIC TESTS. A review of drug interference with plasma-procainamide assays concluded that *chlordiazepoxide* and *sulphonamides* are potential sources of interference in the determination of procainamide by colorimetric methods, although the use of such methods is declining. Procainamide estimation by HPLC is subject to interference by *caffeine* and by *metronidazole*, and the estimation of *N*-acetylprocainamide by HPLC is subject to interference by *sulphathiazole* and by a metabolite of *quinidine*.— S. Yosselson-Superstine, *Clin. Pharmacokinet.*, 1984, *9*, 67.

PREGNANCY AND THE NEONATE. There was evidence of accumulation of procainamide and *N*-acetylprocainamide in the breast milk of a woman taking procainamide 500 mg four times a day. However, it was considered that the amount ingested by an infant would not be expected to yield clinically significant plasma concentrations.— W. B. Pittard and H. Glazier, *J. Pediat.*, 1983, *102*, 631.

Absorption and Fate

Procainamide is readily absorbed from the gastro-intestinal tract and has a very short half-life of 2.5 to 4 hours in healthy subjects. Absorption is subject to individual variation.

Procainamide is partly acetylated in the liver and its acetylated metabolite, *N*-acetylprocainamide or acecainide (see p.70) also has anti-arrhythmic properties, together with a longer half-life of 6 to 7 hours. The rate of acetylation of procainamide is genetically determined. Procainamide is excreted in the urine, 40 to 70% as unchanged procainamide, with the remainder as *N*-acetylprocainamide and other metabolites. *N*-Acetylprocainamide may represent a significant fraction of the total drug in the circulation.

Procainamide is widely distributed throughout the body and is only about 15 to 20% bound to plasma proteins. The therapeutic effect of procainamide has been correlated with plasma concentrations of about 4 to 8 µg per mL, progressively severe toxicity being noted at concentrations above 12 µg per mL. Plasma concentrations may be elevated in cardiac or renal insufficiency. Procainamide crosses the placental barrier and is excreted in breast milk.

A review of the clinical pharmacokinetics of procainamide.— E. Karlsson, *Clin. Pharmacokinet.*, 1978, *3*, 97.

A study of the pharmacokinetics of procainamide derived from clinical data from hospital inpatients receiving procainamide for the treatment of various cardiac arrhythmias showed that mild congestive heart failure was associated with only minor effects on procainamide kinetics, although this did not discount the possibility of a greater influence of more severe heart failure. Total clearance at 18.8 litres per hour in patients was about one third lower than previously reported. There was also a suggestion that bioavailability of a sustained-release preparation may be reduced by 15 to 20% compared with conventional solid dosage formulations.— T. H. Grasela and L. B. Sheiner, *Clin. Pharmacokinet.*, 1984, *9*, 545.

For altered pharmacokinetics of procainamide in children, see under Uses, below.

BIOAVAILABILITY. The administration of a sustained-release procainamide preparation resulted in similar steady-state serum concentrations of procainamide and *N*-acetylprocainamide when compared with equivalent total doses of immediate-release capsules.— P. H. Vlasses *et al.*, *Ann. intern. Med.*, 1983, *98*, 613.

Tablet matrices of a sustained-release preparation of procainamide recovered from the stools of a patient with diarrhoea over an 18-hour period contained 3.5 g of procainamide. The patient had correspondingly low plasma-procainamide concentrations.— R. L. Woosley *et al.*, *J. clin. Pharmac.*, 1984, *24*, 295.

THERAPEUTIC DRUG MONITORING. Assessment of the acetylator phenotype of individual patients is of little value when procainamide therapy is guided by plasma-concentration monitoring to achieve similar procainamide concentrations in all subjects regardless of phenotype.— D. W. J. Clark, *Drugs*, 1985, *29*, 342.

Peak and trough plasma-procainamide concentrations could be accurately predicted following the administration of a sustained-release preparation of procainamide in healthy subjects using 2 methods, each based on *in vitro* dissolution data and pharmacokinetic values from immediate-release preparations.— D. M. DiPersio and M. S. S. Chow, *Clin. Pharm.*, 1985, *4*, 186.

A reminder that interpretation of plasma-procainamide concentrations is complicated by the presence of an active metabolite which may account for a considerable part of its therapeutic effect.— *Lancet*, 1985, *2*, 309.

Saliva concentrations. Therapeutic drug monitoring in saliva including details of studies on saliva-procainamide concentrations. Due to variability in the saliva-plasma ratio it is impossible to predict plasma concentrations from salivary drug concentration, but since saliva concentrations seem to reflect the drug concentrations at an active cardiac site, they may be clinically more relevant.— M. Danhof and D. D. Breimer, *Clin. Pharmacokinet.*, 1978, *3*, 39.

Marked intra- and inter-individual variation of *N*-acetylprocainamide (acecainide) salivary concentrations were observed in the elderly. The results indicated that salivary concentrations would be of no clinical value for monitoring therapy.— R. L. Galeazzi *et al.*, *Clin. Pharmac. Ther.*, 1981, *29*, 440.

Uses and Administration

Procainamide is a class Ia anti-arrhythmic agent (see p.70); it has properties similar to those of quinidine (p.87).

Procainamide is generally only used for the acute control of arrhythmias: the short duration of action and high incidence of adverse effects limit its usefulness for long-term maintenance therapy. Procainamide is preferred to quinidine for intravenous therapy since hypotension is less severe. It is used for the treatment of ventricular arrhythmias particularly those resistant to lignocaine. It is also used to maintain sinus rhythm after cardioversion of atrial fibrillation, and for the prevention of supraventricular and ventricular arrhythmias, and the treatment of arrhythmias associated with surgery or anaesthesia. Therapeutic effect is generally associated with plasma concentrations of 4 to 8 µg per mL.

The dose required will depend on the age, renal function, and underlying cardiac condition of the patient: an adult with normal renal function generally requires 50 mg per kg body-weight per day in divided doses.

For ventricular arrhythmias, procainamide hydrochloride 250 to 500 mg is given by mouth every 3 to 6 hours. A loading dose of 1 g may be given if necessary. Doses of up to 1 g every 2 hours may be required to control some arrhythmias.

If the oral route is not suitable, procainamide hydrochloride may be given intramuscularly. A suggested intramuscular dose is 0.5 to 1 g every four to eight hours; in general the intramuscular dose required is similar to that given orally.

In emergency and under continuous ECG and blood pressure monitoring, procainamide hydrochloride may be given intravenously. The injection should be diluted in a 5% solution of glucose to permit better control of the speed of injection, and should be given in doses of 100 mg every 5 minutes at a rate not exceeding 25 to 50 mg per minute until the arrhythmia has been suppressed or a maximum dose of 1 g has been reached. A response may be obtained after 100 to 200 mg has been given and more than 500 or 600 mg is not generally required. Alternatively, procainamide may be administered by continuous infusion of 500 to 600 mg over 25 to 30 minutes. Therapeutic plasma concentrations may then be maintained by giving an infusion in a 5% solution of glucose, at a rate of 2 to 6 mg per minute. When transferring to oral therapy, a period of about 3 to 4 hours should elapse between the last intravenous dose and the first oral dose.

Procainamide is generally not recommended for use in children: however a dose of 50 mg per kg body-weight daily in 4 to 6 divided doses has been suggested.

In order to prolong its duration of action procainamide hydrochloride is also given in the form of a long-acting preparation for maintenance therapy.

ADMINISTRATION IN CHILDREN. In a study in 5 children treated with procainamide for various cardiac arrhythmias the mean elimination half-life was found to be 1.7 hours, and the plasma clearance was higher than that reported in adults. The data suggested unusually rapid elimination of procainamide in children compared with adults and continuous intravenous infusion may be needed to maintain therapeutic plasma-procainamide concentrations.— S. Singh *et al.*, *Clin. Pharmac. Ther.*, 1982, *32*, 607.

Procainamide was used successfully to treat foetal supraventricular tachycardia refractory to digoxin or propranolol. The concentration of procainamide in the serum of the neonate after delivery was only one-quarter that in the mother.— D. A. Dumesic *et al.*, *New Engl. J. Med.*, 1982, *307*, 1128.

ADMINISTRATION IN THE ELDERLY. For reference to a reduction in renal clearance of procainamide in the elderly, see under Precautions, above.

ADMINISTRATION IN HEPATIC FAILURE. In 20 healthy subjects and 20 patients with chronic liver disease given a single dose of procainamide hydrochloride 500 mg by mouth about 64 and 33% respectively of the administered dose was excreted in the urine within 6 hours. Decreased procainamide acetylation in the patients compared with the control group was not correlated with the severity of liver disease whereas decreased procainamide hydrolysis and increased procainamide-derived aminobenzoic acid acetylation appeared to be related to the degree of hepatic impairment. It was suggested that the decrease in excretion of procainamide and its metabolites in the urine of the patients with liver disease could be due to an impairment in oral absorption since renal function was within the normal range but the variations in acetylation and hydrolysis were related to hepatic function.— P. du Souich and S. Erill, *Clin. Pharmac. Ther.*, 1977, *22*, 588.

ADMINISTRATION IN RENAL FAILURE. The normal half-life of 2.5 to 4.9 hours was increased to 5.3 to 5.9 hours in end-stage renal failure. The interval between doses should be adjusted to 4 hours in patients with a glomerular filtration-rate above 50 mL per minute, to 6 to 12 hours in those with a glomerular filtration-rate of 10 to 50 mL per minute, and to 8 to 24 hours in those with a glomerular filtration-rate of less than 10 mL per minute. Patients on haemodialysis require a dosage supplement to ensure adequate therapeutic plasma concentrations.— W. M. Bennett *et al.*, *Am. J. Kidney Dis.*, 1983, *3*, 155.

Insignificant quantities of procainamide and *N*-acetylprocainamide were removed by continuous ambulatory peritoneal dialysis (CAPD). The mean procainamide half-life was approximately 24 hours and *N*-acetylprocainamide remained elevated for up to 72 hours following a single oral dose.— C. Yonce *et al.*, *Clin. Pharmac. Ther.*, 1984, *35*, 285.

See also Precautions, above.

Preparations

Procainamide Hydrochloride Capsules *(U.S.P.)*

Procainamide Hydrochloride Injection *(U.S.P.)*

Procainamide Injection *(B.P.)*. A sterile solution of procainamide hydrochloride in Water for Injections.

Procainamide Tablets *(B.P.)*. Tablets containing procainamide hydrochloride.

Proprietary Preparations

Procainamide Durules *(Astra, UK)*. *Tablets*, sustained-release, procainamide hydrochloride 500 mg.

Pronestyl *(Squibb, UK)*. *Tablets*, scored, procainamide hydrochloride 250 mg.
Injection, procainamide hydrochloride 100 mg/mL, in vials of 10 mL.

Proprietary Names and Manufacturers

Biocoryl *(Uriach, Spain)*; Novocamid *(Hoechst, Ger.)*; Procaïnamide Duriles *(Astra, Switz.)*; Procainamid Duriles *(Ger.)*; Procainamid Retard *(Collett, Denm.)*; Procainamide Durettes *(Neth.)*; Procainamide Durules *(Astra, Austral.; Astra, UK)*; Procamide *(Belg.; Simes, Ital.)*; Procan SR *(Parke, Davis, Canad.; Parke, Davis, USA)*; Procapan *(USA)*; Pronestyl *(Arg.; Squibb, Austral.; Belg.; Squibb, Canad.; Squibb, Denm.; Fr.; Ital.; Neth.; Novo, Norw.; Squibb, S.Afr.; Squibb, Swed.; Squibb, Switz.; Squibb, UK; Princeton, USA)*; Rhythmin *(Sidmak, USA)*.

13177-w

Propafenone Hydrochloride *(BANM, rINNM)*.

Fenopraine (propafenone); SA-79; WZ-884642; WZ-884643. 2′-(2-Hydroxy-3-propylaminopropoxy)-3-phenylpropiophenone hydrochloride.
$C_{21}H_{27}NO_3,HCl = 377.9$.

CAS — 34183-22-7; 54063-53-5 (propafenone).

Adverse Effects and Precautions

Propafenone can cause disturbances in cardiac conduction which can result in bradycardia, heart block, and sinus arrest. In common with other anti-arrhythmic agents, propafenone may induce arrhythmias in some patients.

Among the most common adverse effects are gastro-intestinal intolerance, a bitter or metallic taste, dizziness, blurred vision, and fatigue. Convulsions, increased liver enzymes, and impotence have also been reported.

Propafenone may aggravate heart failure and should be avoided in patients with moderate or severe conduction disturbances or heart block. It should be given with caution to patients with cardiac insufficiency, severe bradycardia, or pronounced hypotension. Patients should be closely monitored particularly at the start of therapy and if a change in dosage is necessary, especially in those with conduction disorders or left ventricular dysfunction.

Fatal exacerbation of ventricular tachycardia was associated with propafenone therapy in a 63-year-old man.— A. W. Nathan *et al.*, *Postgrad. med. J.*, 1984, *60*, 155.

Symptoms of lupus erythematosus and raised antinuclear antibody titres were associated with propafenone therapy on 2 occasions in a 63-year-old woman.— J. Guindo *et al.* (letter), *Ann. intern. Med.*, 1986, *104*, 589.

INTERACTIONS. For reference to propafenone enhancing the effect of warfarin, see p.345.

Uses and Administration

Propafenone hydrochloride is a class Ic anti-arrhythmic agent (see p.70) with some negative inotropic and beta-adrenoceptor blocking activity. It is given by mouth as the hydrochloride in doses of 450 to 900 mg daily. It may also be given by slow intravenous injection or by infusion.

A review of the actions and uses of propafenone. Propafenone is well absorbed after oral administration but undergoes extensive but apparently saturable first-pass hepatic metabolism. The resulting dose-related bioavailability leads to a non-linear relationship between dosage and plasma concentrations. Propafenone has been used to treat ventricular arrhythmias, atrial fibrillation and flutter, paroxysmal atrio-ventricular nodal re-entrant tachycardia, and reciprocating tachycardias associated with pre-excitation syndromes. The predominant action is blockade of the fast, inward sodium current, but propafenone also has beta-blocking, negative inotropic, and weak calcium-channel blocking activity. Propafenone reduces the conduction velocity throughout the heart, and prolongs intra-atrial conduction time, atrial and ventricular effective refractory periods, and corrected sinus node recovery time. In patients with Wolff-Parkinson-White syndrome, propafenone reduces conduction and increases refractoriness in the accessory pathways. Propafenone is well tolerated in most patients although aggravation of arrhythmias and heart block may be seen early in therapy.— L. A. Siddoway and R. L. Woosley, *Cardiovasc. Rev. & Rep.*, 1986, *7*, 153.

A further review of propafenone.— D. W. G. Harron and R. N. Brogden, *Drugs*, 1987, *34*, 617.

A study of 71 patients with a variety of ventricular and supraventricular arrhythmias demonstrated that the class I anti-arrhythmic effect of propafenone was very significant and surpassed that of the more conventional drugs, particularly quinidine. The beta-adrenergic inhibitory effect was useful when there was an adrenergic component to arrhythmias as in those occurring with emotion or exercise, although this effect was deleterious in patients with vagally-related atrial arrhythmias. The clinical effects of propafenone were seen within 1 hour of oral administration and the anti-arrhythmic effects lasted for 6 to 8 hours. Gastro-intestinal intolerance, dizziness, and fatigue were reported in 25% of patients and were dose-related. Adverse cardiac effects included bundle branch block, sinus bradycardia, sino-atrial block, and episodes of vagally-mediated atrial fibrillation.— P. Coumel *et al.*, *Am. J. Cardiol.*, 1984, *54*, 60D.

Propafenone was found to be as effective as quinidine for treatment of ventricular arrhythmias and was well tolerated in a study of 29 patients.— H. Dinh *et al.*, *Clin. Pharmac. Ther.*, 1984, *35*, 235.

Propafenone, 300 mg every 8 hours was compared with disopyramide, 200 mg every 8 hours, in the treatment of 16 patients with frequent and complex premature ventricular contractions (PVCs). Propafenone was found to be more effective than disopyramide for reducing the frequency of PVCs and suppressing complex forms and nonsustained ventricular tachycardia, and also produced fewer adverse effects.— F. Naccarella *et al.*, *Am. Heart J.*, 1985, *109*, 833.

In a study of propafenone therapy in 45 patients with ventricular arrhythmias refractory to conventional therapy, propafenone was effective and well tolerated in 30 patients and ineffective in 8. Treatment was discontinued in 4 patients because of constipation, rash, nausea, and light-headedness: in 3 patients complex ventricular activity became worse. During long-term follow-up of the 30 patients who responded, propafenone was effective and well tolerated in 22 and discontinued in 7 because of adverse effects and in 1 who developed ventricular tachycardia.— S. C. Hammill *et al.*, *Mayo Clin. Proc.*, 1986, *61*, 98.

Further references to propafenone in ventricular arrhythmias: F. Naccarella *et al.*, *Am. J. Cardiol.*, 1984, *54*, 1008; P. J. Podrid and B. Lown, *J. Am. Coll. Cardiol.*, 1984, *4*, 117; S. W. Rabkin *et al.*, *Can. med. Ass. J.*, 1984, *131*, 601; E. N. Shen *et al.*, *Ann. intern. Med.*, 1986, *105*, 655.

Proprietary Names and Manufacturers

Normorytmin *(Knoll, Arg.)*; Rythmol *(Biosédra, Fr.)*; Rytmonorm *(Knoll, Denm.*; *Knoll, Ger.*; *Knoll, Ital.*; *Knoll-Made, Spain*; *Knoll, Switz.)*.

13197-j

Quinalbital

Chinalbitale.

$C_{20}H_{26}N_2O_2,C_{11}H_{18}N_2O_3=552.7$.

Quinalbital is the hydroquinidine salt of amylobarbitone and has been used in the treatment of cardiac disorders.

Proprietary Names and Manufacturers

Amoquine *(Houde, Belg.)*; Amosedil *(Roussel Maestretti, Ital.)*.

7771-r

Quinidine *(BAN)*.

Chinidinum; Quinidina. (8*R*,9*S*)-6′-Methoxycinchonan-9-ol dihydrate; (+)-(α*S*)-α-(6-Methoxy-4-quinolyl)-α-[(2*R*,4*S*,5*R*)-(5-vinylquinuclidin-2-yl)]methanol dihydrate.

$C_{20}H_{24}N_2O_2,2H_2O=360.5$.

CAS — 56-54-2 (anhydrous); 63717-04-4 (dihydrate); 72402-50-7 (±).

Pharmacopoeias. In *Roum.*

An isomer of quinine, obtained from the bark of species of *Cinchona* and their hybrids. The *U.S.P.* (under Quinidine Gluconate) also allows quinidine obtained from *Remijia pedunculata*, or prepared from quinine. It contains up to 20% of hydroquinidine, a closely allied base with similar chemical, physical, and physiological properties.

7772-f

Quinidine Bisulphate *(BANM)*.

$C_{20}H_{24}N_2O_2,H_2SO_4=422.5$.

CAS — 747-45-5; 6151-39-9 (tetrahydrate).

Pharmacopoeias. In *Br.*

Colourless, odourless crystals. The *B.P.* specifies not more than 15% of hydroquinidine bisulphate (dihydroquinidine bisulphate). Quinidine bisulphate 234 mg is approximately equivalent to 200 mg of quinidine. **Soluble** 1 in 8 of water and 1 in 3 of alcohol; practically insoluble in ether. A 1% solution in water has a pH of 2.6 to 3.6. **Store** in well-closed containers. Protect from light.

7773-d

Quinidine Gluconate *(BANM, USAN)*.

Quinidinium Gluconate.

$C_{20}H_{24}N_2O_2, C_6H_{12}O_7=520.6$.

CAS — 7054-25-3.

Pharmacopoeias. In *Braz.* and *U.S.*

A white odourless powder. It contains not more than 20% of hydroquinidine gluconate (dihydroquinidine gluconate). Quinidine gluconate 289 mg is approximately equivalent to 200 mg of quinidine. Freely **soluble** in water; slightly soluble in alcohol. **Protect** from light.

7774-n

Quinidine Polygalacturonate

Quinidine poly(D-galacturonate) hydrate.

$C_{20}H_{24}N_2O_2,(C_6H_{10}O_7)_x,xH_2O$.

CAS — 27555-34-6 (anhydrous); 65484-56-2 (hydrate).

7775-h

Quinidine Sulphate *(BANM)*.

Chinidini Sulfas; Chinidinsulfate; Chinidinum Sulfuricum; Quinidine Sulfate *(USAN)*; Quinidini Sulfas.

$(C_{20}H_{24}N_2O_2)_2,H_2SO_4,2H_2O=783.0$.

CAS — 50-54-4 (anhydrous); 6591-63-5 (dihydrate).

Pharmacopoeias. In *Arg., Aust., Belg., Br., Braz., Chin., Cz., Egypt., Eur., Fr., Ger., Hung., Ind., Int., It., Japn, Jug., Mex., Neth., Nord., Pol., Port., Roum., Span., Swiss, Turk.*, and *U.S.*

White, or almost white, odourless, needle-like crystals, or fine crystalline powder, darkening on exposure to light. The *B.P.* specifies not more than 15% of hydroquinidine sulphate (dihydroquinidine sulphate); the *U.S.P.* specifies not more than 20%. Quinidine sulphate 217 mg is approximately equivalent to 200 mg of quinidine. Slightly **soluble** in water; soluble in boiling water, alcohol, and chloroform; practically insoluble in acetone and in ether. A 1% solution in water has a pH of 6.0 to 6.8. **Store** in well-closed containers. Protect from light.

Adverse Effects

Quinidine and its salts cause both cardiac and extracardiac adverse effects. They commonly cause gastro-intestinal irritation with nausea, vomiting, and diarrhoea.

Hypersensitivity similar to that occurring with quinine may also occur and should be tested for in each patient by the administration of a test dose (see Uses). Reactions include respiratory difficulties, urticaria, pruritus, skin rashes, purpura, thrombocytopenia and other blood dyscrasias, and, rarely, fever and anaphylaxis. Granulomatous hepatitis and a lupus-like syndrome have been reported.

Quinidine may give rise to cinchonism (see Quinine, p.518) with tinnitus, impaired hearing, visual disturbances, headache, confusion, vertigo, vomiting, and abdominal pain; it is usually associated with large doses, but in idiosyncratic subjects may occur with small doses.

Quinidine may induce hypotension; this is a special risk with parenteral administration.

In quinidine overdosage, the cardiac symptoms of intoxication predominate. Quinidine is cumulative in action and inappropriately high plasma concentrations may induce ECG changes, heart block, asystole, ventricular tachycardia, ventricular fibrillation, syncope, and sometimes death.

In a Boston Collaborative Drug Surveillance Program study of 652 consecutively monitored hospital in-patients taking quinidine, adverse reactions attributable to quinidine occurred in 91. Detailed analysis of the adverse reactions in the 91 patients indicated that gastro-intestinal reactions occurred in 51; arrhythmias occurred in 16; drug fever in 11 (with associated hepatic granulomas in 1); skin reactions in 6; symptoms of cinchonism in 6; and auto-immune haemolytic anaemia in one patient was considered probably attributable to quinidine. Quinidine given alone had a 30% incidence of adverse reactions; when given with other agents, most frequently digitalis, the incidence was lower (11 to 17%), but the reason for this was not clear.— I. S. Cohen *et al.*, *Prog. cardiovasc. Dis.*, 1977, *20*, 151.

EFFECTS ON THE BLOOD. *Agranulocytosis and thrombocytopenia.* Leucopenia and thrombocytopenia were associated with quinidine therapy in a 70-year-old woman; the serum had both antiplatelet and antileucocyte activity.— O. Castro and I. Nash (letter), *New Engl. J. Med.*, 1977, *296*, 572.

An analysis of blood dyscrasias reported to the Swedish Adverse Drug Reaction Committee for the 10-year period 1966-75 showed that thrombocytopenia attributable to quinine or quinidine had been reported on 43 occasions.— L. E. Böttiger *et al.*, *Acta med. scand.*, 1979, *205*, 457.

Drug-induced blood disorders requiring hospital treatment were identified in 26 patients from an average population of over 200 000 during a 10-year survey. Of 15 cases of thrombocytopenia, 9 were associated with quinidine therapy. The reaction occurred within a few weeks of starting therapy in a quarter of patients.— D. A. Danielson *et al.*, *J. Am. med. Ass.*, 1984, *252*, 3257.

Aplastic anaemia. Pancytopenia and marrow aplasia occurred in a 66-year-old man who was taking quinidine sulphate 300 mg four times daily. Studies *in vitro* suggested that both a transient serum factor and quinidine were responsible for the aplasia.— J. G. Kelton *et al.*, *New Engl. J. Med.*, 1979, *301*, 621.

EFFECTS ON THE ENDOCRINE SYSTEM. Mean plasma-insulin concentrations increased and mean plasma-glucose concentrations decreased in 8 healthy subjects and 10 patients with malaria given quinidine intravenously. Profound hypoglycaemia occurred in one patient with cerebral malaria and acute renal failure. Hypoglycaemia may occur in any severely ill fasting patient given parenteral quinidine.— R. E. Phillips *et al.*, *Br. med. J.*, 1986, *292*, 1319.

EFFECTS ON THE EYES. Corneal deposits resembling those found in keratopathy developed in a patient who had been taking quinidine for 2 years. Symptoms had improved and both corneas had cleared completely within 2 months of stopping the drug.— G. W. Zaidman (letter), *Am. J. Ophthal.*, 1984, *97*, 247.

EFFECTS ON THE HEART. Five of 42 patients treated with quinidine, up to 1.5 g daily, suffered ventricular fibrillation or ventricular tachycardia. Another patient with acute cardiac infarction and ventricular ectopic beats developed ventricular tachycardia during quinidine treatment. Common to all these patients were enlargement of the left ventricle and ventricular ectopic beats, conditions which could, on treatment with quinidine, trigger ventricular arrhythmias.— W. Bleifeld and S. Effert (letter), *New Engl. J. Med.*, 1972, *286*, 667.

Prolongation of the QT interval correlating with the plasma-quinidine concentration was seen in each of 14 patients being treated for falciparum malaria, although no cardiotoxicity was observed.— N. J. White *et al.*, *Lancet*, 1981, *2*, 1069.

Quinidine and other class Ia anti-arrhythmic agents may cause *torsade de pointes* by prolonging the QT interval.— L. H. Opie, *Lancet*, 1984, *1*, 496.

EFFECTS ON THE JOINTS. Reversible, symmetrical polyarthritis was attributed to quinidine therapy on three occasions in 1 patient. No abnormalities in immunological variables were found.— P. Kertes and D. Hunt, *Br. med. J.*, 1982, *284*, 1373.

EFFECTS ON THE LIVER. Hypersensitivity reactions developed in 32 of 487 patients receiving quinidine. Of these, 10 had biochemical and clinical manifestations of liver involvement. Liver biopsies carried out in 4 patients all showed granulomatous hepatitis.— D. Geltner *et al.*, *Gastroenterology*, 1976, *70*, 650.

A report of reversible granulomatous hepatitis as a manifestation of quinidine hypersensitivity, which recurred on rechallenge. The patient also had fever, urticaria, and mild thrombocytopenia.— D. A. Bramlet *et al.*, *Archs intern. Med.*, 1980, *140*, 395.

Cholestatic jaundice without evidence of extrahepatic bile duct obstruction was associated with quinidine therapy in 1 patient.— D. B. Hogan *et al.* (letter), *Can. med. Ass. J.*, 1984, *130*, 973.

In a retrospective survey of drug-induced hepatitis over a 10-year period, quinidine was the most common offending agent accounting for one third of all diagnosed cases. Quinidine-induced hepatitis was found to be easily recognised because it is frequently preceded by fever and is sometimes accompanied by gastro-intestinal symptoms, rash, and thrombocytopenia which resolve when the drug is discontinued. The histopathological findings consisted of portal and parenchymal, acute and chronic hepatitis combined with granulomas. Hepatitis was found to be reversible in the patients studied.— H. Knobler *et al.*, *Archs intern. Med.*, 1986, *146*, 526.

EFFECTS ON THE SKIN. Exacerbation of psoriasis was associated with quinidine therapy in 1 case. Psoriasis persisted despite PUVA therapy during quinidine administration, but began to clear 1 week after quinidine was stopped.— W. B. Harwell (letter), *J. Am. Acad. Derm.*, 1983, *9*, 278.

Eczematous dermatitis was attributed to quinidine photosensitivity in 2 patients. Both patients showed marked sensitivity to u.v.-A radiation which subsided, together with the symptoms, when quinidine was discontinued.— J. L. Marx *et al.*, *Archs Derm.*, 1983, *119*, 39.

LUPUS ERYTHEMATOSUS. A report of drug-induced lupus erythematosus which occurred 6 months after starting therapy with quinidine sulphate 300 mg four times a day. The diagnosis was confirmed by a positive antinuclear antibody test and symptoms resolved within 3 months once quinidine was discontinued.— S. G. West *et al.*, *Ann. intern. Med.*, 1984, *100*, 840.

Two patients who had previously developed lupus-like symptoms including arthralgia, myalgia, malaise, rash, and elevated antinuclear antibody titres associated with procainamide therapy experienced a recurrence of symptoms when treatment with quinidine was substituted.— P. Amadio *et al.* (letter), *Ann. intern. Med.*, 1985, *102*, 419.

Report of 5 cases of systemic lupus erythematosus associated with quinidine therapy. Short-term treatment with oral prednisolone was necessary to treat debilitating polyarthritis. There was no recurrence of symptoms at 1.5 to 7 years.— C. J. Lavie *et al.*, *Archs intern. Med.*, 1985, *145*, 446.

Treatment of Adverse Effects

The treatment of quinidine intoxication is largely based on general supportive measures and symptomatic treatment of cardiac dysfunction. The stomach should be emptied by gastric lavage or emesis if appropriate. Respiratory support may be necessary and metabolic acidosis should be corrected but since renal excretion is greatest in acid urine, excessive alkalinisation should be avoided. The management of cardiac toxicity remains controversial. The administration of sodium lactate has been advocated but reports of clinical experience are scarce. Correction of hypokalaemia may be undesirable as hypokalaemia has been reported to reduce cardiac toxicity, but administration of potassium salts may be necessary if hypokalaemia is severe. Hypotension is corrected using intravenous fluid replacement and sympathomimetic drugs. Isoprenaline may also be used to treat bradycardia and ventricular arrhythmias. Ventricular arrhythmias caused by quinidine may be difficult to control: among the treatments which have been suggested are lignocaine, phenytoin, propranolol, and bretylium. Temporary pacing and mechanical support of the circulation have also been recommended.

Measures to enhance the excretion of quinidine are generally ineffective. Acidification of the urine may be undertaken, but forced acid diuresis is not considered to increase the amount of drug excreted to a clinically significant extent. Dialysis and charcoal haemoperfusion are probably only effective when renal or hepatic function is compromised.

A report of the management of acute quinidine intoxication in a 16-year-old girl. Profound hypotension, resistant to standard therapeutic measures, responded favourably to an intra-aortic balloon pump.— C. Shub *et al.*, *Chest*, 1978, *73*, 173.

For comments on the limited role of dialysis and diuresis in eliminating drugs that are extensively protein bound and largely metabolised in the liver, see Quinine, p.519.

Precautions

Quinidine sulphate is contra-indicated in patients who have previously experienced hypersensitivity to quinidine or in patients with complete heart block or acute infection with fever. It should be used with extreme caution in patients with incomplete heart block, pre-existing conductive tissue disease, and uncompensated heart failure. It should be avoided in patients with myasthenia gravis as it can exacerbate the symptoms and may reduce the effectiveness of parasympathomimetic drugs.

When quinidine is used to treat atrial flutter or fibrillation, the reduction in A-V block may result in ventricular tachycardia. This can be avoided by prior digitalisation. However, quinidine is contra-indicated in digitalis overdosage as concomitant administration of quinidine with digoxin results in markedly increased plasma concentrations of digoxin.

Quinidine may enhance the effects of oral anticoagulants, beta blockers, and some neuromuscular blocking agents. Drugs with enzyme-inducing effects such as phenobarbitone, phenytoin, and rifampicin may enhance the metabolism of quinidine leading to reduced plasma concentrations. Some cardiac arrhythmias due to quinidine overdosage may be enhanced by noradrenaline and related drugs. Drugs and foods which increase urinary pH including carbonic anhydrase inhibitors and some antacids may reduce the excretion of quinidine.

An initial test dose of quinidine should always be given to detect hypersensitivity.

ADMINISTRATION IN THE ELDERLY. Evidence that reduced doses of quinidine are needed in the elderly.— D. E. Drayer *et al.*, *Clin. Pharmac. Ther.*, 1980, *27*, 72.

ADMINISTRATION IN CARDIAC AND RENAL FAILURE. For references to alterations in the kinetics of quinidine in patients with cardiac disease and renal failure, see under Uses, below.

ADMINISTRATION IN HEPATIC FAILURE. Indications of a significantly longer quinidine half-life in patients with cirrhosis. Maintenance quinidine dosage may have to be reduced in those with moderate to severe hepatic cirrhosis. Owing to decreased plasma protein binding in cirrhosis, total quinidine concentration measurements underestimate free quinidine concentrations in most cirrhotic patients.— K. M. Kessler *et al.*, *Am. Heart J.*, 1978, *96*, 627.

INTERACTIONS. Quinidine may enhance the effects of hypotensive or beta-blocking agents (danger in sick-sinus syndrome).— L. H. Opie, *Lancet*, 1980, *1*, 861.

Anticoagulants. A study of the factors affecting the protein binding of quinidine. Of greatest potential clinical impact was the decrease in protein binding of quinidine in patients given heparin.— K. M. Kessler *et al.*, *Clin. Pharmac. Ther.*, 1979, *25*, 204.

For the effect of quinidine on coumarin anticoagulants, see Warfarin Sodium, p.345.

Anti-arrhythmic agents and calcium-channel blockers. Torsades de pointes associated with a prolongation of the QT interval was reported in 2 patients treated with quinidine and *amiodarone*. A prolonged QT interval and increased plasma-quinidine concentrations were subsequently noted when amiodarone was administered to a healthy subject who had been given quinidine for 6 days previously.— R. Tartini *et al.*, *Lancet*, 1982, *1*, 1327.

A report of a reduction of the serum-quinidine concentration in a patient taking quinidine and *nifedipine*. Incremental increases of quinidine dose up to 20 mg per kg body-weight per day failed to result in significant elevations of the serum concentration. After discontinuation of nifedipine the serum-quinidine concentration doubled.— J. A. Green *et al.*, *Clin. Pharm.*, 1983, *2*, 461. A further report.— J. A. Farringer *et al.*, *Am. Heart J.*, 1984, *108*, 1570.

A report of severe hypotension in 3 patients receiving quinidine gluconate by mouth following intravenous administration of *verapamil*. Results of radioligand-binding studies *in vitro* suggest that this interaction may be due to an additive blockade of alpha-adrenergic receptors.— A. S. Maisel *et al.*, *New Engl. J. Med.*, 1985, *312*, 167.

For reports of interactions between quinidine and *ajmaline* see p.71, and between quinidine and *disopyramide* see p.76.

Beta-blockers. Sinus bradycardia developed in a patient taking quinidine when timolol eye-drops were added to his therapy. The symptoms did not occur when either drug was administered separately, but recurred on rechallenge with both drugs given concomitantly.— Y. Dinai *et al.*, *Ann. intern. Med.*, 1985, *103*, 890.

Cardiac glycosides. For a discussion of the interaction between quinidine and digoxin, see Digoxin, p.827.

Gastro-intestinal agents. After cimetidine treatment in healthy subjects the elimination half-life of quinidine was increased by 55%, the maximum plasma concentration was increased by 21%, and the time to peak was increased by 33%. The clearance was decreased by a mean of 37%. Pharmacokinetic changes were accompanied by increases in the pharmacodynamic response.— B. G. Hardy *et al.*, *Am. J. Cardiol.*, 1983, *52*, 172.

The plasma-quinidine concentration was increased, the total body clearance of quinidine was decreased by about 25%, and the half-life was increased by 22.6% in 9 healthy subjects when quinidine, 400 mg by mouth was administered during a period of cimetidine administration. The most likely mechanism for the interaction was considered to be a decrease in the metabolism of quinidine caused by cimetidine.— K. W. Kolb *et al.*, *Ther. Drug Monit.*, 1984, *6*, 306.

The serum-quinidine concentration in 1 patient increased by about 50% when therapy with cimetidine 300 mg every 6 hours was commenced. A reduction in the dose of quinidine was necessary to avoid toxic serum concentrations on a second occasion.— J. A. Farringer *et al.*, *Clin. Pharm.*, 1984, *3*, 81.

INTERFERENCE WITH DIAGNOSTIC TESTS. Quinidine might interfere with fluorimetric estimations of urinary catecholamines.— J. Millhouse, *Adverse Drug React. Bull.*, 1974, Dec., 164.

The administration of quinidine could interfere with measurements of urinary 17-hydroxycorticosteroids.— J. M. Rosenberg and I. S. Kampa, *Drug Intell. & clin. Pharm.*, 1973, *7*, 33.

Concurrent administration of anti-arrhythmic agents such as disopyramide, procainamide, and propranolol may interfere with HPLC methods for the determination of quinidine in plasma. Other drugs which may interfere with quinidine assays include quinine, primaquine, chlordiazepoxide, and triamterene.— S. Yosselson-Superstine, *Clin. Pharmacokinet.*, 1984, *9*, 67.

MYASTHENIA GRAVIS. An athletic 80-year-old man given quinidine and digoxin for atrial fibrillation developed obvious and frightening symptoms of myasthenia gravis. He was subsequently found to be hyperthyroid and noted marked improvement in his muscle strength within 4 days of stopping quinidine and taking propylthiouracil. The possibility of co-existing myasthenia gravis must be carefully excluded before using drugs that can depress the skeletal muscle motor endplate in patients with thyroid disease, since they are known to have an increased incidence of myasthenia gravis.— S. S. Stoffer *et al.* (letter), *Archs intern. Med.*, 1980, *140*, 283.

PREGNANCY AND THE NEONATE. A report on the administration of quinidine sulphate to one woman throughout pregnancy. Concentrations in the infant's serum at delivery were similar to the mother's although amniotic fluid concentrations were raised. Quinidine diffused freely into the mother's milk and, although the infant would have received a dose far below the therapeutic dose, she was advised not to breast feed because of potential quinidine accumulation in the immature newborn liver.— L. M. Hill and G. D. Malkasian, *Obstet. Gynec.*, 1979, *54*, 366.

Absorption and Fate

Quinidine is rapidly absorbed from the gastro-intestinal tract, peak plasma concentrations being achieved about 1.5 hours after oral administration of quinidine sulphate and about 4 hours after quinidine gluconate; its bioavailability is variable, owing to first-pass metabolism in the liver.

Quinidine is metabolised in the liver to a number of metabolites, at least some of which are pharmacologically active. It is excreted in the urine, mainly in the form of its metabolites with about 20% as unchanged quinidine. Quinidine metabolism can be increased by agents that induce liver enzymes.

Quinidine is widely distributed throughout the body and is 80 to 90% bound to plasma proteins. It has a plasma half-life of about 6 to 8 hours. Its therapeutic effect has been correlated with plasma concentrations within about 2 to 5 or 6 µg per mL, according to the assay technique used, progressively severe toxicity being noted at higher concentrations.

Quinidine crosses the placental barrier and is excreted in milk.

A review of the clinical pharmacokinetics of quinidine. After intravenous administration the mean elimination half-life of quinidine ranges from 5 to 12 hours. Between 15 and 40% of quinidine clearance is accounted for by renal excretion of unchanged quinidine. The bioavailability following oral administration is influenced by first-pass hepatic metabolism and has been found to be 70% or greater. During multiple dosing, steady-state concentrations are reached after 24 to 48 hours. The use of sustained-release preparations, which can be administered every 8 to 12 hours reduce interdose fluctuations in plasma concentrations. Unpredictable variations in absorption kinetics occur within the same individual and indicate the need to monitor serum concentrations during maintenance therapy. Quinidine is extensively bound to plasma proteins, predominantly albumin, with between 5 and 25% of unbound drug in the serum. The method of serum collection can influence the results of protein binding studies. Among the factors which can influence the kinetics of quinidine are age, dose, and the presence of congestive heart failure or hepatic disease.— H. R. Ochs *et al.*, *Clin. Pharmacokinet.*, 1980, *5*, 150.

ABSORPTION AND BIOAVAILABILITY. A controlled 4-way crossover study in 13 subjects of quinidine sulphate given by mouth as solution, capsules, and tablets, and quinidine gluconate given intramuscularly. Considerable intersubject and intrasubject variability was noted in the biological half-life of quinidine (ranging from 1.16 to 15.75 hours) regardless of dosage form or route. Any differences in the bioavailability of the different dosage forms could be biased by this, and in this study, following correction for the half-life variability only the tablet was significantly less bioavailable than the injection.— W. D. Mason *et al.*, *J. pharm. Sci.*, 1976, *65*, 1325.

Studies of the bioavailability of different quinidine formulations have shown that considerable variations in pharmacokinetic parameters occur depending upon the formulation and the salt used.— W. A. Mahon *et al.*, *Clin. Pharmac. Ther.*, 1976, *19*, 566. Comparison of quinidine sulphate, bisulphate, polygalacturonate and arabogalactansulphate.— G. M. Frigo *et al.*, *Br. J. clin. Pharmac.*, 1977, *4*, 449. Bioavailability of an enteric-coated formulation.— D. Fremstad *et al.*, *Eur. J. clin. Pharmac.*, 1979, *16*, 107. Therapeutic inequivalence of 2 sustained-release formulations of quinidine gluconate.— M. C. Meyer *et al.*, *J. clin. Pharmac.*, 1982, *22*, 131. Comparison of 2 long-acting forms.— A. Leizorovicz *et al.*, *Br. J. clin. Pharmac.*, 1984, *17*, 729. Comparison of 3 sustained-release formulations.— W. A. Mahon *et al.*, *Clin. Pharmacokinet.*, 1987, *13*, 118.

METABOLISM AND ELIMINATION. The clearance of orally administered quinidine was found to be more rapid in children than in adolescents and healthy adults in a study of 13 patients aged between 4 and 22 years. There was a reasonably good correlation between the clearance of quinidine and age. The serum half-life found in children under 12 years was 2 to 3 hours and it was suggested that the use of sustained-release preparations would help reduce fluctuations in serum concentrations and improve compliance. Higher doses may be necessary in children, and careful monitoring of serum-quinidine concentrations and clinical response was recommended.— S. J. Szefler *et al.*, *Pediatrics*, 1982, *70*, 370.

PROTEIN BINDING. Results of *in vitro* protein binding studies suggested that in neonates and young infants the binding of quinidine to serum proteins was substantially reduced.— A. S. Pickoff *et al.*, *Develop. Pharmac. Ther.*, 1981, *3*, 108.

Survivors of cardiac arrest were shown to have decreased quinidine free-drug fraction when compared with healthy subjects. The decrease could not be correlated with α-1-glycoprotein concentrations.— K. M. Kessler *et al.*, *Am. Heart J.*, 1984, *107*, 665.

Further references to the protein binding of quinidine: M. Pérez-Mateo and S. Erill, *Eur. J. clin. Pharmac.*, 1977, *11*, 225; D. J. Edwards *et al.*, *J. pharm. Sci.*, 1984, *73*, 1264.

THERAPEUTIC DRUG MONITORING. *Plasma concentrations.* In a comparison of an enzyme immunoassay with HPLC for quinidine in plasma it was found that higher results were obtained with the enzyme immunoassay technique. This was probably due to cross-reactivity with quinidine metabolites. Although the immunoassay was considered to be sufficiently sensitive to be used for clinical quinidine-concentration monitoring it was considered that the HPLC technique would be necessary for pharmacokinetic studies, and in patients with renal or hepatic disease in whom abnormal accumulation of metabolites may occur.— H. R. Ha *et al.* (letter), *Br. J. clin. Pharmac.*, 1981, *11*, 312.

A multiple dose study in 4 healthy subjects showed that an increase in the dose of quinidine may result in a disproportionate increase in steady-state plasma concentrations in some individuals.— J. Russo *et al.*, *J. clin. Pharmac.*, 1982, *22*, 264.

A discussion of the reliability of plasma-quinidine concentration monitoring. Early recommendations for the range of therapeutic plasma concentrations were based on assays which did not differentiate between quinidine and its metabolites. Although it was not possible to recommend an optimum quinidine concentration, the lower limit of anti-arrhythmic activity is usually about 2 µg per mL.— F. Follath *et al.*, *Clin. Pharmacokinet.*, 1983, *8*, 63.

A report of high total quinidine concentrations in serum caused by increased binding to alpha-1-acid glycoprotein in a patient after myocardial infarction and cardiac surgery. The limitations of serum assays in determining unbound drug concentrations when protein binding is altered from normal were stressed.— D. Garfinkel *et al.*, *Ann. intern. Med.*, 1987, *107*, 48.

Saliva concentrations. Concentrations of quinidine in saliva and serum were compared after a single dose of quinidine and at steady-state. It was found that saliva-quinidine concentrations at steady-state were not linearly related to serum concentrations although there was excellent linear correlation after a single dose. The use of saliva concentrations for therapeutic quinidine monitoring cannot be recommended.— P. K. Narang *et al.*, *Clin. Pharmac. Ther.*, 1983, *34*, 695.

Uses and Administration

Quinidine is a class Ia anti-arrhythmic agent (see p.70); it prolongs the refractory period of cardiac muscle, decreases its excitability, prolongs the action potential, and decreases the conduction velocity. It also has antimuscarinic and alpha-adrenergic blocking properties.

The use of quinidine as an anti-arrhythmic agent has largely been superseded by less toxic agents. Quinidine was formerly used for the conversion of atrial fibrillation, but it has been superseded for this purpose by cardioversion. It is used to maintain sinus rhythm after cardioversion of atrial fibrillation, and for the prevention of supraventricular and ventricular arrhythmias. It has also been used in conjunction with digoxin for the treatment of recurrent atrial flutter, but see Precautions (above). Quinidine may be used as an alternative to quinine in the treatment of malaria.

Quinidine sulphate is given by mouth in usual doses of 200 to 400 mg three or four times daily. Doses of up to 600 mg every 2 to 4 hours have been given for the treatment of supraventricular tachycardias to a maximum of 3 to 4 g a day; these higher doses should only be given with frequent monitoring of the electrocardiogram and plasma concentration. An initial test dose of 200 mg should always be given to detect hypersensitivity.

Quinidine is also given by mouth as the bisulphate, the gluconate, and the polygalacturonate. Sustained-release formulations are generally preferred as the plasma concentration profile is smoother and doses can be given at 8- to 12-hourly intervals.

Quinidine has been given intramuscularly or by slow intravenous injection, but absorption from the intramuscular route is erratic and incomplete, and the intravenous route is considered to be very hazardous owing to the risk of severe hypotension and is normally only undertaken in hospital. Suggested parenteral doses of quinidine gluconate are: intramuscularly, 600 mg initially then 400 mg repeated every 2 to 6 hours if necessary; by intravenous infusion 800 mg diluted to a volume of 50 mL with 5% glucose injection and given at a rate of 1 mL per minute with electrocardiogram and blood-pressure monitoring.

ADMINISTRATION. A re-evaluation of intravenous quinidine, and the view that, contrary to general opinion, well-controlled and monitored intravenous infusions of quinidine at appropriate slow rates are safe and reliable. Because quinidine is rapidly and extensively distributed to tissues, potentially toxic serum concentrations are not likely to be reached during a slow, controlled infusion of a therapeutic dose at a rate of 300 to 400 µg per kg body-weight per minute. If untoward ECG or haemodynamic effects do develop in susceptible individuals during the infusion, they can be reversed readily by stopping the infusion.— E. Woo and D. J. Greenblatt, *Am. Heart J.*, 1978, *96*, 829.

Evidence that administration of quinidine sulphate after food does not influence total systemic availability but slows the appearance in serum of unbound quinidine, and is associated with a lower incidence of side-effects compared with administration in the fasting state.— E. Woo and D. J. Greenblatt, *Clin. Pharmac. Ther.*, 1980, *27*, 188.

Quinidine gluconate was administered by intravenous infusion at a rate of 400 to 500 µg per kg body-weight per minute to 100 patients with ventricular or supraventricular tachyarrhythmias. There were reductions in blood pressure in all patients and 37 received sodium chloride infusion to maintain preload. Hypotension responded to dosage reduction in 14 patients. Quinidine was discontinued in 10 patients because hypotension persisted despite dosage reduction and saline administration, but severe or sustained hypotension did not occur. It was concluded that loading doses of quinidine could be safely administered intravenously to most patients, even those with intraventricular conduction delays or moderate heart failure, if preload is adequately maintained and continuous electrocardiographic monitoring is performed.— C. D. Swerdlow *et al.*, *Am. J. Med.*, 1983, *75*, 36.

ADMINISTRATION IN THE ELDERLY. For reference to a reduction of dosage in the elderly, see under Precautions, above.

ADMINISTRATION IN CARDIAC AND RENAL FAILURE. Plasma-quinidine half-lives were similar in 7 patients with congestive heart failure (median 8.2 hours), 8 patients with renal failure (6.6 hours), and 9 controls (7.2 hours). One patient with heart failure showed virtually no fall in plasma-quinidine concentration over a 10-hour period.— K. M. Kessler *et al.*, *New Engl. J. Med.*, 1974, *290*, 706.

A significantly smaller distribution volume accounted for the significantly higher plasma-quinidine concentration in 9 patients with congestive heart failure compared to 8 control subjects after the intravenous administration of quinidine gluconate.— C. T. Ueda and B. S. Dzindzio, *Clin. Pharmac. Ther.*, 1978, *23*, 158. See also *idem*, *Br. J. clin. Pharmac.*, 1981, *11*, 571.

Serum-quinidine concentrations were found to be significantly elevated in patients undergoing haemodialysis compared with non-azotaemic patients.— D. E. Drayler *et al.*, *Clin. Pharmac. Ther.*, 1978, *24*, 31.

Decreased plasma protein binding of quinidine during haemodialysis.— K. M. Kessler and G. O. Perez, *Clin. Pharmac. Ther.*, 1981, *30*, 121.

In a patient undergoing peritoneal dialysis, overall elimination of quinidine was unchanged, but there was evidence of accumulation of metabolites.— K. Hall *et al.*, *Am. Heart J.*, 1982, *104*, 646.

Quinidine may be administered in normal doses to patients with renal failure. A dose supplement should be given to patients undergoing haemodialysis or peritoneal dialysis.— W. M. Bennett *et al.*, *Am. J. Kidney Dis.*, 1983, *3*, 155.

ADMINISTRATION IN HEPATIC FAILURE. For reference to recommended dosage reductions in patients with hepatic disorders, see under Precautions, above.

CARDIAC DISORDERS. In a study of 19 patients with ventricular arrhythmias the use of quinidine in combination with procainamide in smaller doses was more effective and better tolerated than either drug alone at the maximum tolerated dose.— S. G. Kim *et al.*, *Am. J. Cardiol.*, 1985, *56*, 84.

HICCUP. For details of a protocol for the control of hiccups which eventually leads to oral administration of quinidine, see Chlorpromazine Hydrochloride, p.725.

MALARIA. Quinidine was administered in a dose of 10 mg per kg body-weight orally every 8 hours for seven days to 14 patients with falciparum malaria. All patients were cured; in 12 who were followed up for 35 days after the start of treatment, there was no recrudescence of *P. falciparum* infection, although *P. vivax* appeared in the blood of 6 patients 12 to 28 days after the end of the quinidine course. No cardiotoxicity was observed.— N. J. White *et al.*, *Lancet*, 1981, *2*, 1069.

A study of the effectiveness, pharmacokinetics, and toxicity of intravenous quinidine in the treatment of severe falciparum malaria in 14 patients. Patients received quinidine gluconate in a loading dose equivalent to quinidine 15 mg per kg body-weight, by intravenous infusion over 4 hours; subsequent doses equivalent to 7.5 mg per kg of base were given every 8 hours for 7 days by intravenous infusion over 4 hours or, when patients were well enough to swallow, as quinidine sulphate by mouth in similar doses. Two of the 5 patients with cerebral malaria died; the remaining 3 were fully conscious 42 to 90 hours after the commencement of treatment. In all 12 survivors quinidine cleared the parasitaemia in a mean of 49.4 hours and relieved fever in a mean of 69.5 hours. Follow-up for 35 days in 11 patients, showed that 9 had no recurrence of fever or parasitaemia; re-infection with *Plasmodium falciparum* could not be excluded in the 2 remaining patients. Mean elimination half-life of quinidine was 12.8 hours; the mean plasma-quinidine concentration after the loading dose was 9.4 µg per mL, but concentrations varied considerably between patients. Twelve patients had no evidence of cardiovascular toxicity at any stage. Two comatose patients became hypotensive during infusion of the loading dose, in one case when the total dose was inadvertently given over 2 ½ hours; in both patients the blood pressure rose again within 30 minutes when the infusion was stopped and intravenous saline was given. The available data suggest that in life-threatening *P. falciparum* infections, including cerebral malaria, parenteral quinidine is effective, and clears the parasitaemia as rapidly as quinine.— R. E. Phillips *et al.*, *New Engl. J. Med.*, 1985, *312*, 1273.

Further references to quinidine in the treatment of malaria: H. B. Ris *et al.*, *Schweiz. med. Wschr.*, 1983, *113*, 254; J. M. Agosti *et al.* (letter), *Ann. intern. Med.*, 1985, *103*, 307.

Preparations of Quinidine Salts

Quinidine Gluconate Injection *(U.S.P.)*. Contains 76 to 84 mg of quinidine gluconate in each mL.

Quinidine Sulfate Capsules *(U.S.P.)*

Quinidine Sulfate Extended-release Tablets *(U.S.P.)*

Quinidine Sulfate Tablets *(U.S.P.)*

Quinidine Sulphate Tablets *(B.P.)*

Proprietary Preparations of Quinidine Salts

Kiditard *(Delandale, UK)*. *Capsules*, sustained-release, quinidine bisulphate 250 mg.

Kinidin Durules *(Astra, UK)*. *Tablets*, sustained-release, quinidine bisulphate 250 mg.

Proprietary Names and Manufacturers of Quinidine and its Salts

Biquin *(Astra, Canad.)*; Cardioquin *(Purdue Frederick, Canad.; Neth.; Swed.; Purdue Frederick, USA)*; Cardioquine *(Belg.; Sarget, Fr.; Berenguer-Beneyto, Spain; Switz.)*; Chinidina *(Carlo Erba, Ital.)*; Chinidin-Duriles *(Astra, Ger.)*; Chinteina *(Lafare, Ital.)*; Cin-Quin *(Rowell, USA)*; Duraquin *(Parke, Davis, USA)*; Galactoquin *(Mundipharma, Ger.)*; Galatturil-Chinidina *(Ital.)*; Gluquine *(Vernleigh, S.Afr.)*; Kiditard *(Belg.; Neth.; Delandale, UK)*; Kinichron *(Biochimica, Switz.)*; Kinidin *(DAK, Denm.; ACO, Swed.; Hässle, Swed.)*; Kinidin Duretter *(Hässle, Denm.; Hässle, Norw.; Hässle, Swed.)*; Kinidin Durules *(Astra, Austral.; Astra, UK)*; Kinidin-Duriles *(Astra, Switz.)*; Kinidine *(Canad.)*; Kinidine Durettes *(Belg.; Neth.)*; Kinilentin *(Leo, Denm.)*; Kinitard *(Cilag, Ital.)*; Longachin *(Nativelle, Ital.)*; Longacor *(Nativelle, Fr.; Ital.; Rovi, Spain; Nativelle, Switz.)*; Naticardina *(Chinoin, Ital.)*; Natisédine *(Sabex, Canad.; Nativelle, Fr.: Lipomed, UK; Neth.; Nativelle, Switz.)*; Natisedina *(Nativelle, Ital.)*; Neochinidin *(Brocchieri, Ital.)*; Optochinidin *(Boehringer Mannheim, Ger.)*; Prosedyl *(Rougier, Canad.)*; Quinaglute *(Berlex, Canad.; Berlex, S.Afr.; Berlex, USA)*; Quinalan *(Lannett, USA)*; Quinate *(Rougier, Canad.)*; Quincardina *(Ital.)*; Quincardine *(Austral.)*; Quini Durules *(Pfizer, Arg.)*; Quinicardina *(Nativelle, Ital.; Berenguer-Beneyto, Spain)*; Quinicardine *(Nativelle, Fr.: Lipomed, UK; Spain; Switz.)*; Quinidex *(Robins, Austral.; Robins, Canad.; Robins, USA)*; Quinidis *(USV, Austral.)*; Quinidoxin *(Wellcome, Austral.)*; Quinidurule *(Astra, Fr.)*; Quinilent *(Dominguez, Arg.)*; Quinobarb *(Welcker-Lyster, Canad.)*; Quinora *(Key, USA)*; Ritmocor *(Malesci, Ital.)*; Sedoquin *(Belg.)*; SK-Quinidine Sulfate *(Smith Kline & French, USA)*; Solfachinid *(Bouty, Ital.)*; Systodin *(Buchler, Ger.; Nyco, Norw.)*.

7793-b

Tocainide Hydrochloride *(BANM, rINNM)*.

W-36095. 2-Aminopropiono-2′,6′-xylidide hydrochloride.

$C_{11}H_{16}N_2O,HCl = 228.7$.

CAS — 41708-72-9 (tocainide); 35891-93-1 (hydrochloride).

NOTE. Tocainide is *USAN*.

Pharmacopoeias. In *U.S.*

A fine, white, odourless powder. Freely **soluble** in water and alcohol; practically insoluble in chloroform and ether.

Adverse Effects

Adverse effects associated with tocainide are mainly neurological or on the gastro-intestinal tract. Nausea and vomiting may occur, particularly in the initial stages of therapy. Effects on the central nervous system include tremor, dizziness, lightheadedness, ataxia, blurred vision, paraesthesia, and various mental changes.

Other adverse effects reported include skin rash, lupus erythematosus, sweating, and tinnitus.

As with other anti-arrhythmic agents, tocainide can cause various cardiac arrhythmias and disturbances of conduction. Bradycardia and hypotension may occur after intravenous administration of tocainide. Interstitial pneumonitis and pulmonary fibrosis have been associated with tocainide therapy.

Several serious blood dyscrasias have been associated with tocainide therapy including agranulocytosis, aplastic anaemia, and thrombocytopenia. Some fatalities have occurred.

EFFECTS ON THE BLOOD. Fatal agranulocytosis developed 4 weeks after the start of tocainide therapy in a 62-year-old man.— K. Volosin *et al.*, *Am. Heart J.*, 1985, *109*, 1392.

A report of 2 cases of aplastic anaemia associated with tocainide administration.— M. A. Gertz *et al.* (letter), *New Engl. J. Med.*, 1986, *314*, 583.

EFFECTS ON THE LIVER. Evidence of toxic hepatitis was found in a patient who developed an urticarial rash and confusion within 3 weeks of starting tocainide therapy.— D.L. Farquhar and N.M. Davidson, *Scott. med. J.*, 1984, *29*, 238.

Granulomatous hepatitis occurred in a patient a month after starting treatment with tocainide. Symptoms, including fever and a diffuse rash, disappeared when tocainide was discontinued and liver function tests returned to normal.— L. E. Tucker (letter), *J. Am. med. Ass.*, 1986, *255*, 3362.

EFFECTS ON THE LUNGS. Interstitial pneumonitis developed in 2 patients during tocainide therapy. Both patients recovered on withdrawal of therapy, but one required corticosteroids initially to control the symptoms.— G. M. Perlow *et al.* (letter), *Ann. intern. Med.*, 1981, *94*, 489.

EFFECTS ON MENTAL STATE. Confusion and paranoid symptoms were associated with tocainide therapy in 2 patients. Both patients had impaired renal function, and the plasma-tocainide concentration was found to be above the normal therapeutic range in 1 patient.— C. W. F. Clarke and E. O. El-Mahdi, *Postgrad. med. J.*, 1985, *61*, 79.

A report of paranoid psychosis occurring in 2 patients after treatment with tocainide; the symptoms rapidly regressed when tocainide was withdrawn.— P. Currie and D. R. Ramsdale, *Br. med. J.*, 1984, *288*, 606.

Psychosis and leucopenia was associated with the use of tocainide in one elderly patient.— D. J. Harrison and C. G. Wathen (letter), *Br. med. J.*, 1984, *288*, 1010.

OVERDOSAGE. Fatal overdose occurred in a 70-year-old man after taking tocainide 16 g by mouth. Postmortem tocainide concentrations were 384.8 µmol per mL in the blood and 2860 µmol per mL in the urine. Toxic effects included convulsions, complete heart block, multiple ventricular ectopic beats, profound hypotension, evidence of ischaemic cardiac changes, and multiple episodes of asystole which was eventually unresponsive to cardiac pacing.— C. W. F. Clarke and E. O. El-Mahdi, *Br. med. J.*, 1984, *288*, 760.

Precautions

Tocainide should not be used in patients with second or third degree atrioventricular block, in the absence of a pacemaker. It should be used with caution in patients with uncompensated heart failure and in patients receiving other anti-arrhythmic agents. Blood counts should be monitored particularly during the first 12 weeks of therapy and periodically thereafter. Tocainide should be given with caution to patients with impaired renal or hepatic function.

ADMINISTRATION IN RENAL AND HEPATIC FAILURE. The elimination of tocainide was found to be impaired in patients with renal dysfunction. The mean plasma half-life ranged from 16.6 to 42.7 hours in patients with end-stage renal failure undergoing haemodialysis, and from 13.2 to 22.0 hours in patients with severe renal dysfunction. The mean half-life of tocainide during dialysis was 8.5 hours and dialysis was calculated to have removed 25% of the drug present in the body.— U. Wiegers *et al.*, *Eur. J. clin. Pharmac.*, 1983, *24*, 503.

A study of 6 patients with severe liver disease and renal dysfunction suggested that the half-life of tocainide was prolonged in some patients, the increase correlating better with abnormality of renal function than with any biochemical marker of liver disease. However, abnormalities of distribution resulted in elevated plasma-tocainide concentrations persisting for several hours; this abnormality appeared to be most marked in patients with the greatest degree of liver dysfunction.— D. Oltmanns *et al.*, *Eur. J. clin. Pharmac.*, 1983, *25*, 787.

The renal elimination of tocainide was found to be significantly reduced in 20 patients with impaired renal function after a single dose. Disturbances of urine pH could cause clinically significant alterations in tocainide excretion in patients with mild to moderate renal insufficiency, although this factor becomes less important as renal function decreases.— J. Braun *et al.*, *Eur. J. clin. Pharmac.*, 1985, *28*, 665.

Absorption and Fate

Tocainide is readily and almost completely absorbed from the gastro-intestinal tract.

Tocainide is metabolised to a number of apparently inactive metabolites, and 30 to 50% of the dose is excreted in the urine unchanged.

Tocainide is widely distributed throughout the body and is reported to be about 10% bound to plasma proteins. It has a plasma half-life of about 10 to 15 hours; renal clearance is reduced in alkaline urine. Its therapeutic effect has been correlated with plasma concentrations of about 4 to 10 µg per mL.

Differences in the pharmacokinetics of the R(−) and S(+) enantiomers of tocainide have been reported although the clinical significance is unknown.— B. Edgar *et al.*, *Br. J. clin. Pharmac.*, 1984, *17*, 216P; A. J. Sedman *et al.* (letter), *ibid.*, 113; A. H. Thomson *et al.*, *ibid.*, 1986, *21*, 149.

EFFECTS OF HEART DISEASE. In a study of 28 patients after myocardial infarction the average plasma half-life of tocainide was 13.6 hours which matched that reported in healthy subjects.— R. A. Ronfeld *et al.*, *Clin. Pharmac. Ther.*, 1982, *31*, 384.

The pharmacokinetics of tocainide were not found to be significantly altered in patients with acute myocardial infarction complicated by mild left ventricular failure.— B. MacMahon *et al.*, *Br. J. clin. Pharmac.*, 1985, *19*, 429.

EFFECTS OF RENAL AND HEPATIC DISEASE. For references to the effects of renal and hepatic disease on the kinetics of tocainide, see under Precautions, above.

PROTEIN BINDING. Evidence that tocainide is about 50% bound to plasma proteins in the clinical range.— D. Lalka *et al.*, *Clin. Pharmac. Ther.*, 1976, *19*, 757.

Tocainide was not significantly bound. The free fraction in serum ranged from 0.78 to 0.96 in healthy subjects and from 0.80 to 0.90 in trauma patients.— A. T. Elvin *et al.* (letter), *Br. J. clin. Pharmac.*, 1982, *13*, 872.

Uses and Administration

Tocainide is a class Ib anti-arrhythmic agent (see p.70) with actions similar to those of lignocaine (p.1219) to which it is structurally related. Unlike lignocaine, it is suitable for oral administration.

Tocainide is indicated for the prevention and treatment of symptomatic ventricular arrhythmias: in the *UK* its use is restricted to the treatment of life-threatening symptomatic ventricular arrhythmias associated with severely compromised left ventricular function not responsive to other treatment. For treatment of chronic arrhythmias and as maintenance therapy after control of arrhythmias by intravenous therapy, 1.2 g of tocainide hydrochloride is given by mouth daily divided in 2 or 3 doses, the dose being adjusted according to the patient's tolerance and response. Doses above 2.4 g daily are not normally required. For rapid control of acute arrhythmias, tocainide hydrochloride 500 to 750 mg is given by slow intravenous injection or by infusion over 15 to 30 minutes, followed immediately by 600 to 800 mg by mouth. Doses may need to be reduced in patients with renal or hepatic insufficiency.

A review of the pharmacokinetics, toxicology, and electrophysiological and clinical effects of tocainide. Lignocaine continues to be the drug of choice for short-term treatment of serious ventricular arrhythmias. Tocainide is a primary amine analogue of lignocaine which is suitable for long-term oral therapy. In an uncontrolled evaluation, 71% of patients with ventricular arrhythmias resistant to conventional therapy had some initial response to tocainide and 89% of responders tolerated long-term treatment. In studies of patients after myocardial infarction tocainide appeared to decrease the frequency of ventricular arrhythmias but the effect on mortality has not been evaluated. Tocainide has little or no effect on atrial fibrillation or flutter. Patients with prolonged QT intervals not associated with drug therapy and those whose arrhythmias are sensitive to lignocaine may be especially suitable for tocainide therapy. The frequency of adverse effects is increased at plasma concentrations above 10 µg per mL and it was recommended that dosage adjustments should be made at not less than 3 to 4 day intervals to avoid accumulation. Adverse effects may be reduced by taking tocainide with meals. The most serious non-cardiac adverse effect was haematological abnormalities including potentially fatal agranulocytosis. This adverse effect has led to the approved indications for tocainide therapy to be severely curtailed in the *UK*. It was concluded that tocainide therapy should be reserved for use in patients considered to be at risk of substantial morbidity from their arrhythmias.— D. M. Roden and R. L. Woosley, *New Engl. J. Med.*, 1986, *315*, 41.

Further reviews of tocainide: B. Holmes *et al.*, *Drugs*, 1983, *26*, 93; G. R. Hasegawa, *Drug Intell. & clin. Pharm.*, 1985, *19*, 514 and 682 (correction); S. P. Kutalek *et al.*, *Ann. intern. Med.*, 1985, *103*, 387; J. Morganroth *et al.*, *Am. Heart J.*, 1985, *110*, 856.

ADMINISTRATION. A recommendation that patients who had received lignocaine intravenously to steady-state after acute myocardial infarction could be safely transferred to tocainide prophylaxis without a loading dose by giving 600 mg every 6 hours during the first 12 hours before proceeding to maintenance therapy. To ensure continuity of anti-arrhythmic activity the first dose of tocainide should be given during the 6 hours preceding cessation of lignocaine infusion.— D. W. Holt *et al.*, *Br. J. clin. Pharmac.*, 1982, *14*, 586P. See also J. W. Upward *et al.*, *Eur. J. clin. Pharmac.*, 1983, *25*, 589.

ADMINISTRATION IN RENAL AND HEPATIC FAILURE. For references to the effect of renal or hepatic dysfunction on the kinetics of tocainide, see under Precautions, above.

CARDIAC DISORDERS. Studies comparing tocainide with other anti-arrhythmic agents: R. A. C. Allen-Narker *et al.*, *Br. J. clin. Pharmac.*, 1984, *18*, 725 (comparison with disopyramide); J. Morganroth *et al.*, *Am. J. Cardiol.*, 1984, *54*, 1253 (comparison with lignocaine); J. Morganroth *et al.*, *ibid.*, 1985, *56*, 581 (comparison with quinidine).

Studies of the effectiveness of tocainide in controlling ventricular arrhythmias after myocardial infarction: R. W. F. Campbell *et al.*, *Br. Heart J.*, 1983, *49*, 557; D. L. Keefe *et al.*, *Am. J. Cardiol.*, 1986, *57*, 527.

MUSCULAR DISORDERS. Tocainide 400 mg three times daily had a beneficial effect on the muscular stiffness and weakness brought about by cooling, in 7 patients with paramyotonia congenita. An eighth patient aged 78 years was treated for only one day since he complained of nausea; his ECG showed no disturbances. Two patients experienced transient dizziness, anxiety, and tremor on the second day of treatment; the other 5 had no side-effects.— K. Ricker *et al.*, *J. Neurol. Neurosurg. Psychiat.*, 1980, *43*, 268.

Preparations

Tocainide Hydrochloride Tablets *(U.S.P.)*

Proprietary Preparations

Tonocard *(Astra, UK)*. *Tablets*, tocainide hydrochloride 400 and 600 mg.

Injection, tocainide hydrochloride 50 mg/mL, in vials of 15 mL.

Proprietary Names and Manufacturers

Taquidil *(Roemmers, Arg.)*; Tonocard *(Astra, Austral.; Astra, Canad.; Hässle, Denm.; Hassle, Fin.; Hässle, Norw.; Astra, NZ; Hässle, Swed.; Astra, UK; Merck Sharp & Dohme, USA)*; Xylotocan *(Astra, Ger.; Astra, Switz.)*.

7794-v

Verapamil Hydrochloride *(BANM, USAN, rINNM)*.

CP-16533-1 (verapamil); D-365 (verapamil); Iproveratril Hydrochloride; Verapamili Chloridum. 5-[*N*-(3,4-Dimethoxyphenethyl)-*N*-methylamino]-2-(3,4-dimethoxyphenyl)-2-isopropylvaleronitrile hydrochloride.

$C_{27}H_{38}N_2O_4,HCl = 491.1$.

CAS — 52-53-9 (verapamil); 152-11-4 (hydrochloride).

Pharmacopoeias. In *Br.*, *Chin.*, *Eur.*, *Ind.*, *Jpn*, *Jug.*, and *Nord.*

A white or almost white, odourless or almost odourless, crystalline powder. **Soluble** 1 in 20 of water; sparingly soluble in alcohol; freely soluble in chloroform; practically insoluble in ether. A 5% solution in water has a pH of 4.5 to 6.5. Solutions are **sterilised** by autoclaving. **Store** in well-closed containers. Protect from light.

Precipitation of verapamil was observed when verapamil was administered into an intravenous line containing sodium bicarbonate solution in saline.— D. Bar-Or *et al.* (letter), *Ann. intern. Med.*, 1982, *97*, 619. The precipitation of verapamil hydrochloride by sodium bicarbonate injection was attributed to the high pH of the solution: verapamil will precipitate at a pH greater than 7.— M. R. Cutie (letter), *ibid.*, 1983, *98*, 672.

Studies of the compatibility of verapamil hydrochloride injection with a range of commonly used additives.— M. R. Cutie, *Am. J. Hosp. Pharm.*, 1983, *40*, 1205. Correction.— *ibid.*, 1984, *41*, 450.

Precipitation was observed when verapamil hydrochloride and nafcillin sodium were administered through a common intravenous line.— R. Tucker and J. F. Gentile (letter), *Ann. intern. Med.*, 1984, *101*, 880.

Adverse Effects

Treatment with verapamil is generally well tolerated, but adverse effects connected with verapamil's pharmacological effects on cardiac conduction can arise and may be particularly severe in patients with hypertrophic cardiomyopathies. Adverse effects on the heart include bradycardia, depression of atrioventricular or sinoatrial nodal function, atrioventricular block, worsening heart failure, and transient asystole. These effects are more common with parenteral than with oral therapy.

The most troublesome non-cardiac adverse effect is constipation. Nausea may occur but is less frequently reported. Other adverse effects which may occur include hypotension, dizziness, flushing, and headaches. Some cases of abnormal liver function have been reported.

A review of the adverse effects with calcium-channel blockers. Negative inotropic effects and disturbances in cardiac conduction were predominant after verapamil, while adverse effects due to vasodilation were seen more frequently with nifedipine.— R. Krebs, *Hypertension*, 1983, *5*, *Suppl.* 2, 125.

Sudden respiratory failure was believed to have been precipitated by intravenous verapamil therapy in a patient with Duchenne's muscular dystrophy.— F. Zalman *et al.*, *Am. Heart J.*, 1983, *105*, 510.

ALLERGY. A woman prescribed verapamil felt increasingly unwell from the first dose, and complained of increasing nausea, mild headache, and aching joints. On the eighth day of therapy she complained of slightly itchy and sore eyes, and a severe headache, and was then noted to have a generalised red urticarial rash which was markedly worse in areas exposed to sunlight. She recovered on discontinuation of verapamil and 4 days of corticosteroid and antihistamine therapy.— *Med. J. Aust.*, 1979, *2*, 204.

EFFECTS ON THE CARDIOVASCULAR SYSTEM. Asystole was reported in 1 infant and severe bradycardia in another following intravenous administration of verapamil 0.1 mg per kg body-weight.— D. Radford, *Archs Dis. Childh.*, 1983, *58*, 465.

Report of the sudden death, without any warning symptoms, of a patient with hypertrophic cardiomyopathy 4 days after starting treatment with verapamil. Death was caused by complete atrioventricular block which was attributed to verapamil.— B. Perrot *et al.*, *Br. Heart J.*, 1984, *51*, 352.

Hypotension. Sustained hypotension requiring treatment with vasopressors was associated with the second of two intravenous injections of verapamil 5 mg and 10 mg respectively in a patient on long-term beta-blocker therapy.— R. A. Tucker and W. F. Serote, *Drug Intell. & clin. Pharm.*, 1984, *18*, 239.

EFFECTS ON THE ENDOCRINE SYSTEM. Hyperprolactinaemia and galactorrhoea in 1 patient associated with verapamil therapy.— L. E. Gluskin *et al.*, *Ann. intern. Med.*, 1981, *95*, 66. For further reports see.— E. L. Fearrington *et al.* (letter), *Am. J. Cardiol.*, 1983, *51*, 1466.

Verapamil 240 mg daily by mouth in divided doses had no substantial effect on pituitary-testicular or pituitary-thyroid function in a study in 8 patients. However 2 patients developed abnormally elevated serum-prolactin concentrations while taking verapamil.— C. G. Semple *et al.*, *Br. J. clin. Pharmac.*, 1984, *17*, 179.

Verapamil 5 mg per hour by intravenous infusion had no effect on calcitonin secretion in 15 healthy subjects.— J. A. Amado *et al.*, *Postgrad. med. J.*, 1987, *63*, 23.

EFFECTS ON THE LIVER. Asymptomatic hepatotoxicity was reported in a patient within 2 weeks of starting treatment with verapamil, and again after 3 days on rechallenge. Liver function tests returned to normal when verapamil was withdrawn on both occasions.— S. J. Brodsky *et al.*, *Ann. intern. Med.*, 1981, *94*, 490.

Hepatic injury associated with jaundice and diffuse abdominal pain was reported in a patient 2 weeks after starting treatment with verapamil 120 mg daily. There was clinical evidence to suggest that a hypersensitivity reaction was involved.— P. Guarascio *et al.*, *Br. med. J.*, 1984, *288*, 362.

Further reports of verapamil adversely affecting the liver: E.H. Stern *et al.* (letter), *New Engl. J. Med.*, 1982, *306*, 612; D. T. Nash and T. D. Feer, *J. Am. med. Ass.*, 1983, *249*, 395.

EFFECTS ON THE NERVOUS SYSTEM. A report of 3 patients who complained of unusual perceptual symptoms, described as painful coldness and numbness or bursting feelings, especially in the legs, in association with verapamil therapy.— C. R. Kumana and W. A. Mahon (letter), *Lancet*, 1981, *1*, 1324.

A myoclonic, dystonic movement disorder was apparently induced by verapamil in a 70-year-old man.— C. B. Hicks and K. Abraham (letter), *Ann. intern. Med.*, 1985, *103*, 154.

EFFECTS ON SEXUAL FUNCTION. Impotence was associated with verapamil therapy in 3 out of 14 men. In one patient normal sexual function returned when verapamil was discontinued and a recurrence of impotence was reported when verapamil therapy was re-instituted.— B. D. King *et al.*, *Archs intern. Med.*, 1983, *143*, 1248.

OVERDOSAGE. A 19-year-old woman who ingested 3.2 g of verapamil developed bradycardia, hypotension, and cyanosis of the hands and feet. Because of a history of cardiac arrhythmias sympathomimetic agents were considered to be contra-indicated. She was treated, after gastric lavage, with 10 mL of 10% calcium gluconate given intravenously over 5 minutes; sinus rhythm was restored; later nodal bradycardia with an intraventricular conduction defect responded to further calcium gluconate and the patient recovered.— C. M. Perkins,

Br. med. J., 1978, *2*, 1127.

A 39-year-old woman who had ingested at least 1200 mg verapamil up to 18 hours before hospital admission had an unrecordable blood pressure, bradycardia of 48 beats per minute, and ECG abnormalities. The maximum recorded plasma-verapamil concentration was over 3.5 µg per mL. The response to calcium gluconate infusion was negligible save for a reduction of an intraventricular conduction abnormality. Isoprenaline was found to be the most effective agent for treating the bradycardia and myocardial depression. The patient's physical condition improved although she sustained cerebral anoxic damage during the period of prolonged hypotension.— B. J. Crump *et al.* (letter), *Lancet*, 1982, *2*, 939. A report of fatal verapamil overdosage in a 17-year-old girl despite an initial response to atrioventricular sequential pacing together with continuous infusion of isoprenaline and calcium gluconate. The serum-verapamil concentration was 3 µg per mL 12 hours after admission and the serum-norverapamil concentration was 2.5 µg per mL.— G. M. Orr *et al.* (letter), *ibid.*, 1218.

Haematemesis and gastric ulceration were reported in a 22-year-old man after ingestion of 3200 mg of verapamil. Gastroscopy showed multiple acute superficial ulcers and signs of recent haemorrhage. The patient recovered uneventfully.— A. R. O. Miller and C. J. Ingamells (letter), *Br. med. J.*, 1984, *288*, 1346.

Treatment of Adverse Effects

In overdosage by mouth the stomach should be emptied by aspiration and lavage. Treatment of cardiovascular effects is supportive and symptomatic.

Intravenous infusion of calcium salts has been recommended as a specific antagonist to verapamil and may reverse the haemodynamic and electrophysiological effects: calcium gluconate in a dose of 10 to 20 mL of a 10% solution has been suggested.

Atropine or a beta-adrenoceptor agonist, for example, isoprenaline, has been recommended for prolonged atrioventricular conduction and heart block; electrical pacing may also be required. Patients with hypertrophic cardiomyopathy should not be treated with beta-adrenergic agonists: alpha-adrenergic agonists, for example phenylephrine, are recommended in these patients. Hypotension may be treated by placing the patient in the supine position with the feet raised; infusions of dopamine, dobutamine, and noradrenaline may be given if necessary.

Should prolonged atrioventricular conduction occur with verapamil, atropine is the antagonist of choice, though theoretically calcium gluconate might help.— *Br. med. J.*, 1981, *282*, 89.

Calcium chloride, 1 g by intravenous injection brought about an immediate haemodynamic improvement and the appearance of junctional tachycardia after hypotension and severe bradycardia following the intravenous administration of verapamil four hours after a dose of propranolol. The vasodilatory effects of calcium chloride were considered to be outweighed by the reversal of the actions of verapamil.— D. L. Morris and N. Goldschlager, *J. Am. med. Ass.*, 1983, *249*, 3212.

Restoration of sinus rhythm and normal blood pressure was achieved approximately 90 minutes after 2 slow intravenous infusions of 4-aminopyridine 10 mg given 5 minutes apart in a patient following accidental overdosage of verapamil. Prior administration of calcium laevulinate and isoprenaline had increased the blood pressure only slightly.— P. M. ter Wee *et al.*, *Hum. Toxicol.*, 1985, *4*, 327.

Severe faecal impaction in an 80-year-old man was associated with verapamil therapy and was treated successfully with calcium given intravenously. He was given 2 ampoules (1.36 mEq each) of calcium chloride, each diluted in 50 mL of 5% glucose in water and infused over 30 minutes.— D.J. Ward *et al.* (letter), *New Engl. J. Med.*, 1982, *307*, 1709.

For further reports of overdosage and its management, see under Overdosage, above.

Precautions

Verapamil is contra-indicated in hypotension associated with cardiogenic shock, in marked bradycardia, in partial or complete atrioventricular block, and in uncompensated heart failure. It is also contra-indicated in the sick-sinus syndrome unless a pacemaker is fitted. Verapamil may precipitate or worsen existing heart failure. There is an increased incidence of adverse cardiac effects in patients with hypertrophic cardiomyopathy and in those with impaired nodal conduction. In patients with atrial flutter or fibrillation and an accessory pathway with anterograde conduction, for example Wolff-Parkinson-White syndrome, verapamil may induce severe ventricular tachycardia, although it may be used to treat paroxysmal supraventricular tachycardia.

Reduced dosage of verapamil may be required in patients with impaired liver function owing to the risk of reduced metabolism.

Severe toxicity has followed the concomitant use of verapamil and beta-adrenoceptor blocking agents, particularly by the intravenous route. However beta-blockers have been used in combination with oral verapamil in the treatment of angina. Intravenous verapamil is contra-indicated in digitalis toxicity, but verapamil and digitalis may be given together by mouth in the absence of digitalis toxicity or atrioventricular block. Verapamil can also cause increases in the plasma concentration of digoxin. For further details see under Interactions, below.

Discussion of the use of calcium-channel blockers in patients with hypertrophic cardiomyopathy. Potential major adverse effects of verapamil treatment include depression in sino-atrial activity and atrioventricular conduction, marked hypotension, and, rarely, pulmonary oedema.— B. H. Lorell, *Am. J. Med.*, 1985, *78, Suppl.* 2B, 43.

Three of 5 patients with the Wolff-Parkinson-White syndrome developed ventricular fibrillation minutes after the intravenous administration of verapamil 5 to 10 mg. The remaining 2 patients developed ventricular arrhythmias resulting in severe hypotension that responded to cardioversion. The authors suggest that the use of intravenous verapamil is contra-indicated in patients with atrial fibrillation and pre-excited ventricular complexes.— B. McGovern *et al.*, *Ann. intern. Med.*, 1986, *104*, 791. See also.— R. W. Harper *et al.*, *Am. J. Cardiol.*, 1982, *50*, 1323; S. Gulamhusein *et al.*, *Am. Heart J.*, 1983, *106*, 145.

Although intravenous verapamil is effective in the acute termination of supraventricular tachycardia it has also been used for broad-complex tachycardia when the diagnosis is in doubt. After reviewing the effects of intravenous verapamil in patients with ventricular tachycardia it was concluded that verapamil is ineffective and potentially hazardous in most such patients. Since the true diagnosis in most patients with broad-complex tachycardia will be ventricular tachycardia, verapamil should not be used to treat broad-complex tachycardia unless a supraventricular origin has been established.— A. C. Rankin *et al.*, *Lancet*, 1987, *2*, 472.

ADMINISTRATION IN THE ELDERLY. For a reference to reduced clearance of verapamil in elderly hypertensive patients, see under Absorption and Fate, below.

ADMINISTRATION IN HEPATIC FAILURE. For references to the effect of impaired hepatic function on the kinetics of verapamil, see under Uses, below.

INTERACTIONS. Review of the interactions of calcium-channel blockers with other drugs. Verapamil is known to have intrinsic depressant effects on myocardial contractility, but this tends to be offset by a reflex increase in heart-rate resulting from peripheral vasodilation. The concurrent use of beta-blockers reduces the reflex increase in heart-rate thus allowing the negative inotropic effect of verapamil to remain unopposed, resulting in combined cardiodepressant effects. The combined inhibitory effects of verapamil and beta-blockers on the atrioventricular node represents another potential site of interaction. However, this combination has been recommended recently, particularly for the treatment of angina. While most patients do not manifest important adverse interactions, some are at greater risk of developing adverse effects and predisposing factors include: impaired left ventricular function, arrhythmias, aortic stenosis, the use of large doses or the intravenous administration of either drug, and possibly treatment with agents which decrease alpha-adrenergic vasomotor tone, for example methyldopa. Prescribers should be alert for hypotension or reduced cardiac performance.

Verapamil appears to impair both renal and non-renal elimination of digoxin and additive effects may be seen on atrioventricular conduction rates. Clinical experience indicates that combined therapy with digitalis glycosides and calcium-channel blockers is generally well tolerated although patients should be monitored for evidence of increased digitalis effect, and patients with pre-existing impairment of atrioventricular conduction or digitalis toxicity may be particularly at risk from depression of the cardiac conduction system.

Other potential interactions include a possible improvement in glucose tolerance in patients with non-insulin-dependent diabetes affecting dosage requirements for antidiabetic drugs, additive negative inotropic effects with disopyramide, and theoretical inhibition of the effects of verapamil by adrenaline, isoprenaline, theophylline, and caffeine.— *Drug Interact. News.*, 1982, *2*, 27.

Anti-arrhythmic agents. For reports of an interaction between verapamil and *quinidine*, see Quinidine, p.86.

Antibiotics. In a study in 4 patients receiving rifampicin, isoniazid, and ethambutol for tuberculosis, plasma concentrations of verapamil following a single dose of verapamil 40 mg by mouth were undetectable in 3; two of these were given a repeat dose 4 weeks after discontinuing treatment with isoniazid and ethambutol, with the same result. It was suggested that this decrease in plasma-verapamil concentrations could be due to hepatic enzyme induction by *rifampicin*.— K. H. Rahn *et al.* (letter), *New Engl. J. Med.*, 1985, *312*, 920.

A daily dose of verapamil 1920 mg was required to control supraventricular tachycardia in a patient taking rifampicin. When ethambutol was substituted for the rifampicin, the plasma-verapamil concentration showed an almost 4-fold increase and the verapamil dosage was subsequently reduced without recurrence of the arrhythmias.— R. A. Barbarash, *Drug Intell. & clin. Pharm.*, 1985, *19*, 559.

Antiepileptics. For a report of verapamil enhancing the toxicity of carbamazepine, see carbamazepine (p.401).

Beta-blockers. A 46-year-old man developed symptomatic bradycardia associated with Wenckebach type atrioventricular block while receiving verapamil 80 mg three times a day when his dose of metoprolol was increased from 50 mg to 100 mg twice a day for angina.— J. N. H. Eisenberg and G. D. G. Oakley, *Postgrad. med. J.*, 1984, *60*, 705.

A report of complete heart block associated with the administration of verapamil and atenolol by mouth in a patient with no evidence of cardiomyopathy or conduction disorders.— S. J. Hutchison *et al.*, *Br. med. J.*, 1984, *289*, 659. See also.— I. N. Findlay *et al.* (letter), *ibid.*, 1074; J. C. McGourty and J. H. Silas (letter), *ibid.*, 1624.

Severe bradycardia in a 64-year-old patient was attributed to an interaction between verapamil and timolol eye-drops. Sinus rhythm and a heart-rate of 78 beats per minute were restored when verapamil was replaced by nifedipine.— S. D. Pringle and C. J. MacEwen, *Br. med. J.*, 1987, *294*, 155.

Calcium salts. Atrial fibrillation re-occurred in a patient maintained on verapamil when treatment was started with calcium adipinate and calciferol. The effect was attributed to an increase in extracellular calcium concentration.— D. Bar-Or and G. Yoel, *Br. med. J.*, 1981, *282*, 1585.

Cardiac glycosides. For reports of the interaction between verapamil and digoxin, see Digoxin p.828.

Cyclosporin. A report of increased blood concentrations of cyclosporin associated with the concomitant administration of verapamil.— A. Lindholm and S. Henricsson (letter), *Lancet*, 1987, *1*, 1262.

Gastro-intestinal agents. Verapamil undergoes considerable first-pass hepatic elimination and several studies have been undertaken to ascertain whether the pharmacokinetics of verapamil in common with other extensively metabolised drugs would be affected by concurrent administration of cimetidine. Smith *et al.* (*Clin. Pharmac. Ther.*, 1984, *36*, 551) found no alteration in verapamil kinetics after intravenous administration, but found an apparent increase in bioavailability of oral verapamil from 26.3% to 49.3% which was attributed to slight changes in verapamil clearance. Wing *et al.* (*Br. J. clin. Pharmac.*, 1985, *19*, 385), in a study of similar design, found that cimetidine had no effect on verapamil kinetics and similar results were obtained by Abernethy *et al.* (*Clin. Pharmac. Ther.*, 1985, *38*, 342) although cimetidine was only administered for 12 hours prior to verapamil administration in this study. However Loi *et al.* (*ibid.*, *37*, 654) reported a reduction in intravenous verapamil clearance by 21% and an increase of 50% in the elimination half-life.

Several problems arise in interpreting these results: firstly, only single doses of verapamil were studied, although verapamil can influence its own kinetics during prolonged administration. Secondly, where individual results are given it can be seen that there was considerable interpatient variation. Finally, despite the increase in bioavailability seen by Smith *et al.*, there were no associated changes in the electrophysiological effects measured. Thus the clinical significance of any potential interaction between cimetidine and verapamil remains unclear.

General anaesthetics. For references to adverse reactions during general anaesthesia in patients given verapamil, see halothane (p.1118).

Lithium carbonate. For references to the effects of verapamil on lithium, see lithium carbonate (p.368).

Theophylline. For reference to theophylline toxicity associated with the concomitant administration of verapamil, see theophylline (p.1529).

PORPHYRIA. Verapamil was considered to be unsafe in patients with acute porphyria because it has been shown to be porphyrinogenic in *animals* or *in-vitro* systems.— M.R. Moore and K.E.L. McColl, *Porphyrias, Drug Lists*, Glasgow, Porphyria Research Unit, University of Glasgow, 1987.

PREGNANCY AND THE NEONATE. For a report of the excretion of verapamil in breast milk, see under Absorption and Fate, below.

SURGICAL PROCEDURES. A warning that verapamil can cause a decrease in lower oesophageal sphincter pressure which is maximal 30 minutes after commencing an intravenous infusion.— B. R. Cotton and G. Smith, *Br. J. Anaesth.*, 1984, *56*, 37.

Absorption and Fate

Verapamil is approximately 90% absorbed from the gastro-intestinal tract, but is subject to very considerable first-pass metabolism in the liver and the bioavailability is only 20 to 30%.

Verapamil exhibits bi- or tri-phasic elimination kinetics and is reported to have a terminal plasma half-life of 2.8 to 7.4 hours following a single oral dose, increasing to 4.5 to 12.0 hours after repeated doses. The plasma half-life of verapamil is 2 to 8 hours after intravenous administration. Verapamil acts within 5 minutes of intravenous administration and in 1 to 2 hours after oral administration with a peak plasma concentration at about 2 hours. Correlation has been found between plasma concentrations and response.

Verapamil is about 90% bound to plasma proteins. It is extensively metabolised in the liver to a number of metabolites of which norverapamil has been shown to have some activity. It is mainly excreted by the kidneys in the form of its metabolites but about 16% is also excreted in the bile into the faeces. Less than 4% is excreted unchanged.

A review of the pharmacokinetics of verapamil.— S. R. Hamann *et al.*, *Clin. Pharmacokinet.*, 1984, *9*, 26.

METABOLISM AND PHARMACOKINETICS. A study of the disposition kinetics of verapamil and its active metabolite, norverapamil, in patients with chronic atrial fibrillation. In the atrial fibrillation patients the half-life of verapamil was 4.9 (±3.0) hours after intravenous administration; norverapamil was not present in blood after intravenous administration. Following oral administration the half-life of verapamil was 7.2 (±4.2) hours and the half-life of norverapamil was 9.3 (±4.5) hours. It was concluded that the disappearance of verapamil in the plasma is more rapid following intravenous than oral administration, and the accumulation of norverapamil is greater than that of verapamil and may be important in influencing the clinical effect.— R. E. Kates *et al.*, *Clin. Pharmac. Ther.*, 1981, *29*, 257.

Total verapamil clearance was found to be decreased in elderly hypertensive patients compared with that in young patients, and the elimination half-life was prolonged.— D. R. Abernethy *et al.*, *Ann. intern. Med.*, 1986, *105*, 329.

Verapamil was noted to have a prolonged half-life under steady-state conditions compared with that seen after single doses by Freedman *et al.* (*Clin. Pharmac. Ther.*, 1981, *30*, 644) and Shand *et al.* (*ibid.*, 701) resulting in the accumulation of verapamil and norverapamil. It was postulated that this could be due to saturation of hepatic metabolism. In an investigation Schwartz *et al.* (*Br. J. clin. Pharmac.*, 1985, *19*, 512) found no evidence of a change in hepatic blood flow during chronic drug administration compared with that before the start of treatment, but Meredith *et al.* (*ibid.*, *20*, 101) showed that acute verapamil administration was associated with a significant increase in apparent liver blood flow which fell again during continued administration. A similar increase was found in effective renal plasma flow, and it was considered that these changes in blood flow could account in part for the differences in pharmacokinetics during acute and chronic administration.

A series of studies have been carried out to determine whether differences in the pharmacokinetics of the *d*- and *l*-isomers of verapamil could account for observed differences in the plasma concentration-response curve following oral and intravenous administration. Eichelbaum *et al.* (*Br. J. clin. Pharmac.*, 1984, *17*, 453) found that, after intravenous administration, there were pronounced differences in the pharmacokinetics and protein binding of the 2 isomers; the volume of distribution and total systemic clearance of *l*-verapamil were much higher than those of the *d*-isomer although the terminal half-life was similar. After oral administration of a mixture of *d*- and *l*-verapamil, plasma concentrations of the *d*-isomer were found to be substantially higher than those of the *l*-isomer (Vogelgesang *et al.*, *ibid.*, *18*, 733) suggesting stereospecific first-pass hepatic metabolism; following oral dosing total verapamil concentrations thus consist of a smaller proportion of the more potent *l*-isomer accounting for the apparent lower potency of verapamil when given orally. Echizen *et al.* (*Clin. Pharmac. Ther.*, 1985, *38*, 71) subsequently showed that *l*-verapamil was 3.3 times more potent than the racemic mixture and 11 times more potent than *d*-verapamil. Thus the authors conclude that the cardiac effects of verapamil are related not to the total plasma-verapamil concentration but to the concentration of the *l*-isomer, and conventional plasma concentration monitoring will be of little value in establishing therapeutic plasma concentrations during multiple oral dosing.

PREGNANCY AND THE NEONATE. *Breast feeding.* Verapamil concentrations in breast milk similar to those found in plasma were reported by Inoue *et al.* (*Eur. J. clin. Pharmac.*, 1984, *26*, 657) in a woman taking verapamil 80 mg four times a day. The maximum concentration measured in breast milk was 300 ng per mL. However, the average concentration in milk found by Anderson (*ibid.*, 1983, *25*, 279) was 23% of that in serum in a report of a patient taking 80 mg three times daily. The serum concentration of verapamil in the child was 2.1 ng per mL during treatment and undetectable 38 hours after the last maternal dose. In another patient taking the same dose, the average steady-state concentrations of verapamil and norverapamil in milk were, respectively, 60% and 16% of the concentration in plasma (P. Anderson, *ibid.*, 1987, *31*, 625). No verapamil or norverapamil could be detected in the plasma of the infant.

PROTEIN BINDING. A study of verapamil protein binding in patients and in healthy subjects. Verapamil was found to be approximately 90% bound to plasma proteins in a concentration-independent manner over the clinically observed plasma concentration range. This binding was not affected by similar concentrations of the metabolite, norverapamil, nor by end-stage renal failure or the postoperative state in coronary bypass graft patients. Changes noted in patients with reduced creatinine clearance and those undergoing cardiac catheterisation were not considered likely to be of clinical importance.— D. L. Keefe *et al.*, *Clin. Pharmac. Ther.*, 1981, *29*, 21.

Verapamil was found to be bound to α_1-acid glycoprotein as well as albumin. The concentration of α_1-acid glycoprotein appeared to be the major contributory factor in individual variation in protein binding.— F. X. McGowan *et al.*, *Clin. Pharmac. Ther.*, 1983, *33*, 485.

Uses and Administration

Verapamil is a calcium-channel blocker and is classified as a class IV anti-arrhythmic agent (see p.70). It is used in the control of supraventricular tachyarrhythmias, and in the management of classical and variant angina pectoris. Verapamil may be used to treat paroxysmal supraventricular tachycardia associated with Wolff-Parkinson-White syndrome but should be used with caution if atrial flutter or fibrillation is present. It is also used in the treatment of hypertension.

Verapamil may be given intravenously or by mouth as the hydrochloride for the control of supraventricular arrhythmias. When given intravenously a dose of 5 to 10 mg is injected over a period of 30 seconds; if necessary, a further 5 mg may be injected 5 to 10 minutes after the first. In the *USA* it is recommended that the injection should be given over 2 to 3 minutes with a further dose of 10 mg given after 30 minutes if required. Suggested intravenous doses for children are: neonates, 0.75 to 1 mg; infants, 0.75 to 2 mg; children aged 1 to 5 years, 2 to 3 mg; children aged 6 to 15 years, 2.5 to 5 mg. Smaller doses may be adequate and the injection should be stopped when a response has been obtained. Intravenous injections should be given under continuous ECG monitoring, particularly in infancy.

Oral doses for the treatment of supraventricular arrhythmias are 40 to 120 mg three times daily, according to the severity of the condition and the patient's response. Suggested oral doses for children are: up to 2 years of age, 20 mg two or three times daily; 2 years and over, 40 to 120 mg two or three times daily according to age and response.

In the management of angina pectoris, verapamil hydrochloride is given by mouth in doses of 120 mg three times daily; some patients with angina of effort may respond to 80 mg three times daily, but this lower dose is not likely to be effective in angina at rest or Prinzmetal's variant angina.

In the treatment of hypertension the dose of verapamil is generally 160 mg twice daily with a range of 240 mg to 480 mg daily. A dose of up to 10 mg per kg body-weight daily in divided doses has been suggested for children.

Sustained-release oral preparations are available for use in the treatment of angina and hypertension.

Reviews and comments on the actions and therapeutic uses of the calcium-channel blockers.— E. M. Antman *et al.*, *Ann. intern. Med.*, 1980, *93*, 875; *Drug & Ther. Bull.*, 1984, *22*, 65; S. H. Snyder and I. J. Reynolds, *New Engl. J. Med.*, 1985, *313*, 995; J. Kenny, *Br. med. J.*, 1985, *291*, 1150.

Investigations of the haemodynamic effects of verapamil in patients with coronary heart disease: B. Silke *et al.*, *Br. J. clin. Pharmac.*, 1985, *19*, 539P; A. L. Soward *et al.*, *Drugs*, 1986, *32*, 66.

Verapamil inhibited platelet aggregation due to adrenaline *in vitro*, but much greater concentrations were required to inhibit the aggregatory response to adenosine diphosphate. The aggregatory response to adrenaline was also altered *in vivo* after 4 days' dosing with verapamil, but results suggested that the changes were mediated by a different mechanism.— C. R. Jones *et al.*, *Br. J. clin. Pharmac.*, 1985, *20*, 191.

ADMINISTRATION IN CHILDREN. Verapamil was considered to be the drug of first choice for the treatment of severely symptomatic paroxysmal tachycardia in infants and children. There should be continuous ECG monitoring during and after drug treatment.— J. L. Wilkinson, *Archs Dis. Childh.*, 1983, *58*, 945.

Reviews of the use of verapamil and other calcium-channel blocking agents in children.— C. J. Porter *et al.*, *Pediatrics*, 1983, *71*, 748; C. Cho and A. W. Pruitt, *Am. J. Dis. Child.*, 1986, *140*, 360.

Both intravenous verapamil and intravenous digoxin were found to be effective in stopping paroxysmal supraventricular tachycardia in children with Wolff-Parkinson-White syndrome. Treatment with verapamil terminated the arrhythmia more rapidly than digoxin, and caused fewer adverse effects. Oral treatment was more successful in young infants without cardiac defects than in older children, some of whom had cardiac anomalies.— E. Shahar *et al.*, *Archs Dis. Childh.*, 1983, *58*, 207. See also.— R. P. Leitner *et al.*, *Aust. paediat. J.*, 1983, *19*, 40.

ADMINISTRATION IN THE ELDERLY. For a report that the pharmacokinetics of verapamil are altered in the elderly, see Absorption and Fate, above.

ADMINISTRATION IN HEPATIC FAILURE. In an investigation of verapamil kinetics in patients with liver disease and patients in intensive care, good correlation was found between calculated apparent hepatic blood flow and systemic verapamil clearance.— B. G. Woodcock *et al.*, *Clin. Pharmac. Ther.*, 1981, *29*, 27. In patients with liver cirrhosis steady-state plasma concentrations of verapamil were double those seen in patients with normal liver function following intravenous administration and 5 times the normal concentration when given by mouth. A steady-state plasma concentration will not be reached until about 56 hours after therapy has started.— A. Somogyi *et al.*, *Br. J. clin. Pharmac.*, 1981, *12*, 51.

ADMINISTRATION IN RENAL FAILURE. Verapamil could be given in normal doses to patients with renal failure.—

W. M. Bennett *et al.*, *Am. J. Kidney Dis.*, 1983, *3*, 155. See also J. Mooy *et al.*, *Eur. J. clin. Pharmac.*, 1985, *28*, 405.

ASTHMA. In 8 adults both nebulised verapamil (about 3 mg) and nebulised sodium cromoglycate (about 12 mg) significantly inhibited exercise-induced asthma compared with saline. A combination of the two drugs was superior to sodium cromoglycate alone but not to verapamil alone. There was considerable intrasubject variability in response to both drugs.— K. R. Patel, *Br. med. J.*, 1983, *286*, 606.

Further references to verapamil in asthma: S. E. Brown, *Thorax*, 1983, *38*, 840; A. Fennerty *et al.*, *Postgrad. med. J.*, 1983, *59*, *Suppl.* 3, 74; A. L. Boner *et al.*, *Archs Dis. Childh.*, 1987, *62*, 264.

BITES AND STINGS. Results of a study in *mice* suggesting that verapamil could delay the lethal effects of box-jelly-fish (*Chironex fleckeri*) cardiotoxin.— J. W. Burnett and G. J. Calton, *Med. J. Aust.*, 1983, *2*, 192.

CANCER CHEMOTHERAPY. For a reference to the reversal of doxorubicin resistance in human ovarian cancer cells by verapamil, see under Doxorubicin Hydrochloride, p.625.

CARDIOVASCULAR DISORDERS. *Angina pectoris.* A short review of the efficacy of calcium-channel blocking agents in vasospastic or Prinzmetal's angina.— G. Ambrosio, *Postgrad. med. J.*, 1983, *59*, *Suppl.* 3, 26.

Brief review of the use of calcium-channel blocking agents in angina pectoris.— I. N. Findlay and H. J. Dargie, *Pharm. J.*, 1985, *1*, 445. See also: W. H. Frishman and S. Charlap, *Archs intern. Med.*, 1983, *143*, 1407.

Despite some initial reports of severe adverse effects arising from the combination of verapamil with a beta-blocking agent (M.E. Benaim, *Br. med. J.*, 1972, *2*, 169; C.B. Boothby *et al.*, *ibid.*, 349), the combination has been found to be effective in the treatment of angina in both short-term (M. Bassan *et al.*, *Br. med. J.*, 1982, *284*, 1067) and in long-term studies (J.C. McGourty *et al.*, *Postgrad. med. J.*, 1985, *61*, 229). McGourty *et al.* reported mild heart failure to be the most frequent adverse effect, affecting 15% of patients. Withdrawal of one drug was necessary in 14% of patients mainly due to cardiac effects. In a review and discussion of the use of calcium-channel blockers in combination with beta-blockers, Leon *et al.* (*Am. J. Cardiol.*, 1985, *55*, 69B) concluded that verapamil had the greatest therapeutic efficacy in this combination but also the highest frequency of harmful adverse cardiac effects compared with nifedipine. It was recommended that close clinical monitoring for adverse effects is necessary if this drug combination is used.

For reports of adverse effects due to the use of beta-blockers with verapamil, see Interactions under Precautions, above.

Arrhythmias. A detailed review of the actions and uses of calcium antagonists, including verapamil. Verapamil inhibits the action potential of the upper and middle nodal regions of the heart where the slow inward calcium-ion-mediated current contributes to depolarisation. Thus, by blocking slow-channel conduction in the atrioventricular node, verapamil inhibits one limb of the re-entry circuit which is believed to underlie most paroxysmal supraventricular tachycardias. This also explains the reduction of ventricular rate in atrial flutter and fibrillation, but verapamil has negligible effects on ventricular arrhythmias probably because its first action is to cause atrioventricular block, this undesirable effect developing before it can influence ventricular arrhythmias.— L. H. Opie, *Lancet*, 1980, *1*, 806.

Discussion of the treatment of atrial fibrillation and flutter. The use of intravenous verapamil has become increasingly popular to reduce the ventricular rate during atrial fibrillation. The advantages over digitalis include a rapid onset of action and a direct action on the atrioventricular node which persists to a greater extent during exercise and stress. However, intravenous verapamil has less predictable effects on the anomalous atrioventricular bypass tract and is not recommended in patients with pre-excitation and atrial fibrillation especially when antegrade conduction occurs primarily by the accessory pathway. The use of oral verapamil in this situation remains controversial and other drugs may be preferred.— H. O. Klein and E. Kaplinsky, *Drugs*, 1986, *31*, 185. See also: W. T. Brownlee, *Br. J. Hosp. Med.*, 1985, *33*, 138.

Verapamil 80 mg three times a day by mouth for 5 days did not reduce the incidence of supraventricular tachycardia compared with placebo in a trial involving 141 patients undergoing myocardial revascularisation.— D. B. Williams *et al.*, *J. thorac. cardiovasc. Surg.*, 1985, *90*, 592.

Verapamil 5 mg by intravenous injection followed by an intravenous infusion of 5 mg per hour was reported to be effective in the treatment of supraventricular tachycardia of recent onset in 10 post-operative patients.— T. J. Iberti *et al.*, *Crit. Care Med.*, 1986, *14*, 283.

For a warning that verapamil should not be used to treat broad-complex tachycardia unless a supraventricular origin has been established, see under Precautions, above.

Hypertension. Verapamil was considered to have a place in the treatment of hypertension in doses of 240 to 720 mg when other agents have failed or are contra-indicated. The main drawbacks to its use are its negative inotropic activity which can precipitate heart failure, and its depressant effect on the atrioventricular node. Its action on conducting tissues may make it a particularly useful drug for treating hypertension in patients with episodic supraventricular arrhythmias.— S. A. Smith and W. A. Littler, *J. clin. Hosp. Pharm.*, 1985, *10*, 113.

Further reviews of the use of verapamil and other calcium-channel blockers in hypertension.— *Lancet*, 1983, *2*, 22; B. M. Massie, *Am. J. Cardiol.*, 1985, *56*, 97H; Y. W. F. Lam *et al.*, *Drug Intell. & clin. Pharm.*, 1986, *20*, 187.

Clinical studies of the use of verapamil in hypertension.— R. S. Hornung *et al.*, *Am. Heart J.*, 1984, *108*, 554 (compared with propranolol); I. Wigler *et al.*, *Int. J. clin. Pharmac. Ther. Toxic.*, 1984, *22*, 162 (long-term therapy); J. Escudero *et al.*, *Am. J. Cardiol.*, 1986, *57*, 54D (compared with atenolol); B. N. Singh *et al.*, *ibid.*, 99D (in mild to moderate hypertension compared with propranolol).

Hypertrophic obstructive cardiomyopathy. Verapamil was given in a daily dose of 480 to 720 mg to 22 patients with hypertrophic obstructive cardiomyopathy. After an average of 15 months (4 to 24 months) of treatment significant reductions were obtained in the QRS amplitude in the electrocardiogram and in heart volume. Follow-up catheterisation in 10 patients showed a decrease in left ventricular muscle mass in 7 patients and an increase in 3; coronary artery diameter decreased in 7 patients, increased in 1 and was unchanged in 2. Treatment with verapamil was considered to be superior to therapy with beta-blockers.— M. Kaltenbach *et al.*, *Br. Heart J.*, 1979, *42*, 35.

Several studies have shown that verapamil can reduce left ventricular outflow tract obstruction, increase exercise capacity, and reduce symptoms in patients with hypertrophic cardiomyopathy. Treatment is well tolerated and withdrawal in 2% of patients has been reported due to adverse effects that were not life-threatenting. However, serious complications can occur through verapamil's haemodynamic and electrophysiological actions. Verapamil is generally only used if other treatment, including the use of beta-blocking agents, is unsuccessful or contra-indicated, but verapamil has advantages in patients with bronchospastic respiratory disorders and in nonobstructive hypertrophic cardiomyopathy. Since there is insufficient evidence to show that verapamil modifies the disease process, and additionally since it does not possess any ventricular anti-arrhythmic activity, its use as a prophylactic agent in asymptomatic or minimally symptomatic patients was not recommended by the authors. Verapamil provides an important alternative or additive form of therapy in selected patients.— R. Rosing and S. E. Epstein, *Ann. intern. Med.*, 1982, *96*, 670.

See also under Precautions, above.

Myocardial infarction. The Danish Study Group on Verapamil in Myocardial Infarction reported the results of a multicentre study involving 1436 patients, on the influence of the early administration of verapamil on mortality and incidence of re-infarction in patients with myocardial infarction. No differences were found in the mortality rates in patients who received verapamil within 6 hours of the onset of symptoms, although a reduction in mortality was noted in patients with a duration of symptoms between 6 and 24 hours; overall, there was no significant difference between the death-rates in the verapamil-treated and placebo-treated groups. There was no difference in the incidence of re-infarction between the two groups. A high incidence of atrio-ventricular blocks in the verapamil group during the first week of treatment was not associated with an increased mortality-rate.— *Eur. Heart J.*, 1984, *5*, 516. See also.— *Am. J. Cardiol.*, 1984, *54*, 24E.

CEREBROVASCULAR DISORDERS. Beneficial responses were observed in acute neurological deficits due to moyamoya disease, a vaso-occlusive disease of the intracranial circulation, in 2 children after intravenous administration of verapamil.— M. J. McLean *et al.* (letter), *Lancet*, 1985, *1*, 163.

Migraine. In a study involving 12 patients with either classic or common migraine verapamil 80 mg four times a day reduced the mean frequency of migraines from 6.7 to 3.8 per patient per month. The effects were seen within the first month and persisted throughout the 3 months of the study. The loss of migraine prodrome in 1 patient was considered to be a potential disadvantage, but generally there were no major adverse effects to the treatment.— G. D. Solomon *et al.*, *J. Am. med. Ass.*, 1983, *250*, 2500.

Verapamil 80 mg three times a day produced subjective improvement in 9 patients and objective improvement in 8 of 14 patients with migraine during a double-blind cross-over study. Both frequency and duration of migraine attacks were reduced in responsive patients, and verapamil was equally effective in preventing both common and classic migraine. Six patients with severe migraine who did not respond during the trial subsequently became headache-free on treatment with higher doses of calcium-channel blockers. The only adverse effect reported was constipation which was generally mild, but severe enough in 1 patient to necessitate withdrawal after 6 weeks of therapy with verapamil.— H. G. Markley *et al.*, *Neurology*, 1984, *34*, 973.

MUSCULAR DISORDERS. A 35-year-old man with long-standing and disabling muscle pain of unknown origin had a dramatic response to verapamil 60 mg three times daily and obtained complete relief with a dose of 120 mg three times daily. His 39-year-old sister who had the same condition obtained a similar response to 120 mg three times daily which was reduced to 60 mg four times daily owing to tachycardia and extrasystoles, with no return of pain.— J. Walton (letter), *Lancet*, 1981, *1*, 993. A similar report.— K. Midtbø, *Curr. ther. Res.*, 1981, *30*, 917.

In a study involving 8 boys with Duchenne muscular dystrophy (DMD) verapamil produced beneficial effects on muscle function compared with placebo. However, since the effect appeared to be slight, and because of the danger of heart block, it was concluded that the use of verapamil in DMD did not seem justified.— A. E. H. Emery *et al.* (letter), *Lancet*, 1982, *1*, 559.

For a report of respiratory failure attributed to verapamil in a patient with Duchenne muscular dystrophy, see Adverse Effects, above.

PSYCHIATRIC DISORDERS. Verapamil has been studied as a possible alternative to lithium therapy in manic patients. There is evidence that lithium salts affect calcium metabolism (R.D. Franks *et al.*, *Archs gen. Psychiat.*, 1982, *39*, 1074) and share some of the properties of calcium-channel blockers (S.L. Dubovsky *et al.*, *Am. J. Psychiat.*, 1982, *139*, 502). A beneficial response to verapamil therapy was reported in a manic patient by Dubovsky *et al.* In a study of 12 patients with mild to moderate mania, Giannini *et al.* (*ibid.*, 1984, *141*, 1602) reported that verapamil 80 mg four times a day was as effective in relieving symptoms as lithium carbonate, and suggested that verapamil could provide a practical alternative to lithium especially for patients refractory to lithium or unable to tolerate its adverse effects. Subsequently the same team (A.J. Giannini *et al.*, *J. clin. Pharmac.*, 1985, *25*, 307) compared the effectiveness of verapamil 80 mg four times a day with clonidine 17 µg per kg body-weight in 20 manic patients previously unresponsive to lithium carbonate. The results suggested that verapamil may have had superior antimanic effects and may be a more suitable therapeutic alternative than clonidine in lithium-resistant patients. The antimanic effect of verapamil was confirmed by Dubovsky *et al.*, (*Psychiatry Res.*, 1986, *18*, 309) in a double-blind cross-over study in which improvement was seen in 5 out of 7 severely manic patients. Price and Giannini (*J. clin. Psychiat.*, 1986, *47*, 213) have also reported an improvement of psychiatric symptoms in a patient with severe premenstrual tension when treatment with verapamil 50 mg three times a day was started for an unrelated cardiac disorder.

Preparations

Verapamil Injection *(B.P.).* Verapamil Hydrochloride Injection

Verapamil Tablets *(B.P.).* Verapamil Hydrochloride Tablets

Proprietary Preparations

Berkatens *(Berk Pharmaceuticals, UK). Tablets*, verapamil hydrochloride 40, 80, 120, and 160 mg.

Cordilox *(Abbott, UK). Tablets*, verapamil hydrochloride 40, 80, 120, and 160 mg.
Injection, verapamil hydrochloride 2.5 mg/mL, in ampoules of 2 mL.

Securon *(Knoll, UK). Tablets*, verapamil hydrochloride 40 mg.
Tablets, scored, verapamil hydrochloride 80, 120, and 160 mg.

Securon SR *(Knoll, UK). Tablets*, sustained-release, scored, verapamil hydrochloride 240 mg.

Comment on the use of sustained-release verapamil (Securon SR) to treat mild to moderate hypertension.— *Drug & Ther. Bull.*, 1987, *25*, 47.

Univer *(Rorer, UK). Capsules*, sustained-release, verapamil hydrochloride 120, 180, and 240 mg.

Proprietary Names and Manufacturers

Azupamil *(Azuchemie, Ger.)*; Berkatens *(Berk Pharmaceuticals, UK)*; Calan *(Searle, USA)*; Cardiagutt *(Engelhard, Ger.)*; Cardibeltin *(Schwarz, Ger.)*; Cardimil *(S.Afr.)*; Cavartil *(GEA, Swed.)*; Cordilox *(Schering, Austral.; Abbott, UK)*; Durasoptin *(Durachemie, Ger.)*; Geangin *(GEA, Denm.; GEA, Norw.)*; Hexasoptin *(Durascan, Denm.)*; Isoptin *(Schering, Austral.; Searle, Canad.; Knoll, Denm.; Knoll, Ger.; Knoll, Ital.; Neth.; Knoll, Norw.; Knoll, S.Afr.; Knoll, Swed.; Knoll, Switz.; Knoll, USA)*; Isoptine *(Belg.; Biosédra, Fr.)*; Isoptino *(Knoll, Arg.)*; Manidon *(Knoll-Made, Spain)*; Praecicor *(Molimin, Ger.)*; Securon *(Knoll, UK)*; Univer *(Rorer, UK)*; Vasolan *(Jpn)*; Verakard *(Nyco, Norw.)*; Veraloc *(Erco, Denm.; Orion, Swed.)*; Veramex *(Labaz, Ger.)*; Veramil *(Orion, Eire)*; Veroptinstada *(Stadapharm, Ger.)*; Verpamil *(Orion, Switz.)*.

Antibacterial Agents

1-z

In this section are antimicrobial agents used principally in the treatment and prophylaxis of bacterial infections. They include antibiotics, sulphonamides, urinary antimicrobial agents such as nalidixic acid, and the quinolones; in practice the term 'antibiotics' often encompasses all of these agents. Antibacterial agents described elsewhere include metronidazole (p.666) which, as well as being an antiprotozoal agent, is used in the treatment of anaerobic bacterial infections, and antimycobacterial agents (p.546) which are used principally in the treatment of tuberculosis and leprosy. Immunological approaches to the treatment and prophylaxis of bacterial infections are discussed under Immunological Agents, p.1155.

In addition, disinfectants (p.949) and preservatives (p.1355) are used to kill or inhibit the growth of micro-organisms.

Antimicrobial Action

Antibiotics have traditionally been divided into *bacteriostatic* antibiotics which reversibly inhibit the growth of susceptible micro-organisms and *bactericidal* antibiotics which kill the organisms *in vitro*. Given in high therapeutic doses, the aminoglycosides, cephalosporins, penicillins, and polymyxins are generally bactericidal by this criterion, whereas chloramphenicol, erythromycin, the sulphonamides, and the tetracyclines are usually bacteriostatic. However, an antibiotic which is bactericidal in a certain concentration may become bacteriostatic at lower concentrations.

As a guide to the sensitivity of any specific micro-organism to an antibiotic, the *minimum inhibitory concentration* (MIC) is utilised. This is the lowest concentration of antibiotic which will inhibit the growth of a given strain of micro-organism under controlled conditions, and is usually expressed in terms of μg of antibiotic per mL of medium. Similarly, the *minimum bactericidal concentration* (MBC) may also be used. This is the lowest concentration of antibiotic that totally suppresses growth of organisms when subcultured onto antibiotic-free media. The MIC of a bactericidal antibiotic is usually within one or two dilutions of its MBC. *Break points*, concentrations of antibiotic which inhibit sensitive but not resistant organisms, are also used.

A discussion on the inhibitory effects of antibiotics at concentrations below their MICs (subinhibitory concentrations).— G. N. Rolinson, *J. antimicrob. Chemother.*, 1977, *3*, 111.

A brief discussion of the potentiation of phagocytosis of pathogenic bacteria by exposure to low (sub-MIC) concentrations of antibiotics.— C. G. Gemmell, *J. antimicrob. Chemother.*, 1984, *13*, 407.

Antibiotics may enhance or depress host defences. Susceptibility testing *in vitro*, which does not pay any attention to host defence mechanisms, in no way describes the full potential of an antibiotic in the infected patient.— F. D. Daschner, *J. antimicrob. Chemother.*, 1985, *16*, 135.

A discussion of terminology and methodology in the study of antibiotic interactions including definition of the following recommended terms: synergism, addition, antagonism, and indifference.— J. M. T. Hamilton-Miller, *J. antimicrob. Chemother.*, 1985, *15*, 655.

Testing Bacteria for Sensitivity to Antibiotic Action

Two principal methods are available for testing bacteria for sensitivity to antibiotic action. The dilution method is reasonably precise but fairly time consuming and one test determines only the action of one antibiotic on a given bacterial strain. It is used for the determination of the minimum inhibitory concentration or more usually the minimum bactericidal concentration when there is a severe infection such as endocarditis or where slowly growing organisms such as *Mycobacterium tuberculosis* or *Actinomyces israelii* are to be tested. The disk diffusion method is less exact, but is able to test simultaneously the inhibitory effect of several antibiotics on a given strain; it is mainly used for routine diagnostic procedures.

In the broth dilution method doubling dilutions of a given antibiotic are made in broth and inoculated with a broth culture of the bacterial strain under investigation. After overnight incubation, the highest dilution at which no bacterial growth occurs is taken as the end-point of the titration. This is the minimum inhibitory concentration (MIC). A similar method may be used for determining the minimum bactericidal concentration (MBC); any tubes with no growth are subcultured and those which show no growth on antibiotic-free medium demonstrate bactericidal activity. An agar dilution method is also available.

In the disk diffusion method the whole surface of a culture plate is inoculated with the strain of organism under investigation and filter paper disks containing specified concentrations of various antibiotics are laid on the surface of the plate. After incubation the zone of inhibition of growth surrounding each disk is measured. Disks of low or high potency are used according to the clinical conditions and special features of each individual case.

A general review of laboratory tests used to guide antimicrobial therapy.— J. E. Rosenblatt, *Mayo Clin. Proc.*, 1987, *62*, 799.

Factors influencing the assay of antimicrobial drugs in clinical samples by the agar plate diffusion method.— J. de Louvois, *J. antimicrob. Chemother.*, 1982, *9*, 253. See also C. Krasemann and G. Hildenbrand, *J. antimicrob. Chemother.*, 1980, *6*, 181.

Comment on sensitivity testing and various *in-vitro* factors which affect the results. The composition and pH of the test media, the incubation conditions such as time, temperature, and atmosphere, and the criteria used for interpretation are all factors that can influence the test results. In addition the inoculum size of several different organisms including *Haemophilus influenzae*, *Pseudomonas aeruginosa*, and *Klebsiella* for beta-lactam antimicrobial agents may influence the results of the susceptibility tests; this is known as the inoculum effect.— S. R. Erickson *et al.* (letter), *Drug Intell. & clin. Pharm.*, 1984, *18*, 530.

The use of serum bactericidal-activity testing to monitor antibiotic therapy.— J. S. Wolfson and M. N. Swartz, *New Engl. J. Med.*, 1985, *312*, 968. See also *Lancet*, 1986, *2*, 200. Comment on the role of the microbiology laboratory in the treatment of infective endocarditis and the problems of assessing bactericidal activity.— C. W. Stratton, *J. antimicrob. Chemother.*, 1987, *20*, *Suppl.* A, 41.

Interpretation of antimicrobial sensitivity tests.— *Med. Lett.*, 1986, *28*, 2.

Resistance

Resistance of a micro-organism to an antibiotic may be natural (inherent or intrinsic) or acquired. The emergence of antibiotic-resistant bacteria is closely linked to the extent that antibiotics are used in man and in items of his diet; resistant strains may appear rapidly or slowly depending on the organism, the amount and type of antibiotic used, and the way in which it is used.

Resistance may develop by *selection* of resistant strains during the use of an antibiotic. It may be acquired by random *mutation* which can occur rapidly as a single step or more gradually in a step-wise manner. Resistance may also be transferred from one organism to another and this is discussed in more detail below.

Several mechanisms may be responsible for the resistance of organisms to antibiotics. It may occur due to altered drug target (such as penicillin-binding proteins) within the cells, or by exclusion of the antibiotic from the target either by decreased cell-wall permeability or destruction of the drug. Some examples of these mechanisms include trimethoprim-resistant organisms with a modified target enzyme which no longer binds the drug, the intrinsic resistance of Gram-negative bacilli to benzylpenicillin due to the impermeability of the cell wall to the antibiotic, and the *inhibition of uptake* of antibiotic in bacteria resistant to tetracycline. *Inactivating enzymes* produced by bacteria are also responsible for resistance and are very important clinically. Beta-lactamases such as penicillinase are a group of enzymes which hydrolyse the beta-lactam ring of penicillins and cephalosporins; they are produced by many bacteria including Gram-positive bacteria such as *Staphylococcus aureus*, which, in general, produce a large amount of extracellular beta-lactamase, and Gram-negative organisms which produce relatively small amounts of beta-lactamase located between the inner and outer cell membranes. Chloramphenicol and the aminoglycosides are also inactivated by enzymes. Another mechanism of resistance is due to the phenomenon of *tolerance*. Tolerant strains of bacteria can be detected by measuring minimum inhibitory concentrations (MICs) and minimum bactericidal concentrations (MBCs) since in such organisms the MBC will be considerably greater than the MIC.

Organisms resistant to one antibiotic may become resistant to another and this is termed *cross-resistance*. There is often complete cross-resistance between structurally related antibiotics such as the tetracyclines.

Resistance may be acquired by the *transfer* of genetic material from one organism to another. This may be achieved by *transduction* which involves the transfer by bacteriophage (bacterial virus) of DNA carrying genes for resistance, or by *conjugation*, when genetic material in the form of extrachromosomal particles of DNA (known as plasmids) is passed from one bacterium to another while they are in contact. These transferable resistance plasmids, termed *R-plasmids* or *R-factors*, consist of 2 parts, one coding for drug resistance and the other for transfer (the resistance transfer factor). The 2 parts may be linked to form a single unit which transfers intact to the recipient bacterium. Resistance may also be rapidly disseminated due to transposable genetic elements (*transposons*) which can 'jump' (transpose) from one plasmid to another or between bacterial chromosomes and plasmids. The transfer of bacterial resistance may occur in the intestinal tract and R-plasmids are the major source of acquired antibiotic resistance in enterobacteria. Some transference has been observed in burns and in peritoneal dialysis fluid. Transfer also appears to occur outside the body, probably in sewage and other very contaminated surface water.

Resistance to several antibiotics is termed multiple or multiply resistance and may be transferred from one bacterial species to another. Plasmids may confer resistance by specifying the production of enzymes such as the beta-lactamases or by bringing about permeability changes in the bacterial cell wall. Fortunately, it appears that if the antibiotics involved are witheld, transferable resistance can be lost spontaneously within weeks or months of its appearance.

General reviews and discussions on microbial resistance to antibiotics: S. B. Levy, *Lancet*, 1982, *2*, 83; *Bull. Wld Hlth Org.*, 1983, *61*, 383; R. W. Lacey, *Lancet*, 1984, *2*, 1022; P. J. Sanderson, *Br. med. J.*, 1984, *289*, 638; L. J. V. Piddock and R. Wise, *J. antimicrob. Chemother.*, 1985, *16*, 279.

A series of articles on antibiotic resistance in bacteria.— *Br. med. Bull.*, 1984, *40*, 1–106.

The proceedings of a symposium on bacterial resistance.— *J. antimicrob. Chemother.*, 1986, *18*, *Suppl.* C, 1–260.

Reviews and discussions on antibiotic resistance in specific organisms: L. D. Sabath, *Ann. intern. Med.*, 1982, *97,* 339 (*Staphylococcus aureus* resistant to beta-lactam antibiotics); J. D. Sleigh, *Br. med. J.*, 1983, *287,* 1651 (*Serratia marcescens*); B. E. Britigan *et al.*, *New Engl. J. Med.*, 1985, *312,* 1683 (*Neisseria gonorrhoeae*); *Lancet*, 1985, *2,* 189 (methicillin-resistant *Staphylococcus aureus*); D. L. Dworzack, *Drug Intell. & clin. Pharm.*, 1986, *20,* 562 (Gram-negative bacteria; a risk of using broad-spectrum beta-lactam antibiotics); G. J. Cuchural and F. P. Tally, *ibid.*, 567 (*Bacteroides fragilis*); C. W. Stratton and F. Tausk, *J. antimicrob. Chemother.*, 1987, *19,* 413 (*Pseudomonas aeruginosa*); S. A. Hoffmann and R. C. Moellering, *Ann. intern. Med.*, 1987, *106,* 757 (enterococci).

MECHANISMS OF RESISTANCE. A review of antibiotic resistance resulting from decreased drug accumulation. This includes the intrinsic resistance of Gram-negative bacteria attributed to relatively impermeable outer membranes and capsules surrounding many clinically important micro-organisms, the plasmid-mediated tetracycline resistance, and chromosomal mutations in envelope components which affect the accumulation of aminoglycosides, beta-lactams, chloramphenicol, cycloserine, fosfomycin, peptide antibiotics, and tetracycline.— I. Chopra, *Br. med. Bull.*, 1984, *40,* 11.

The role of porins in bacterial antibiotic resistance.— L. Gutmann *et al.*, *Ann. intern. Med.*, 1984, *101,* 554.

A review of resistance due to alterations in the antibiotic target site including: altered penicillin-binding proteins, the target of beta-lactam antibiotics; altered DNA gyrase, a target of inhibitors of replication such as novobiocin, and oxolinic and nalidixic acids; altered RNA polymerase, a target of inhibitors of transcription such as ansamycins [rifamycins] including rifampicin; and altered ribosomes, the target of inhibitors of translation such as aminoglycosides, spectinomycin, and erythromycin.— P. E. Reynolds, *Br. med. Bull.*, 1984, *40,* 3.

Penicillin-binding proteins and the intrinsic resistance to beta-lactams in Gram-positive cocci.— R. Fontana, *J. antimicrob. Chemother.*, 1985, *16,* 412.

Transposons and transposable multiresistance.— B. Wiedemann *et al.*, *J. antimicrob. Chemother.*, 1985, *16,* 416. See also H. -K. Young, *ibid.*, 679; R. Schmitt, *ibid.*, 1986, *18, Suppl.* C, 25; J. Grinsted, *ibid.*, 77.

R-plasmid transfer.— R. Thompson, *J. antimicrob. Chemother.*, 1986, *18, Suppl.* C, 13.

Antibiotic tolerance among clinical isolates of bacteria.— E. Tuomanen *et al.*, *Antimicrob. Ag. Chemother.*, 1986, *30,* 521. See also L. D. Sabath *et al.*, *Lancet*, 1977, *1,* 443.

Beta-lactamases. The beta-lactamases produced by Gram-negative bacteria and their role in resistance to beta-lactam antibiotics.— R. B. Sykes and M. Matthew, *J. antimicrob. Chemother.*, 1976, *2,* 115.

Clinical and genetic perspectives on beta-lactamases.— J. -C. Pechère and R. Levesque, *J. antimicrob. Chemother.*, 1983, *12,* 529.

Inducible beta-lactamases and non-hydrolytic resistance mechanisms.— C. C. Sanders, *J. antimicrob. Chemother.*, 1984, *13,* 1. See also N. A. C. Curtis *et al.*, *ibid.*, 1986, *17,* 51.

Beta-lactamases hydrolyse the amide bond in the beta-lactam ring of penicillins and cephalosporins producing derivatives with no antibacterial properties. They are the major determinants of resistance to beta-lactam antibiotics of most bacterial pathogens; the genetic determinants for many beta-lactamases can be transferred from one bacterial cell to another even across boundaries of species and genera. Among the Gram-positive bacteria, staphylococci are the principal pathogens which produce beta-lactamase. Four enzyme types, designated A to D, can be identified serologically but are otherwise indistinguishable. The wide variety of beta-lactamases produced by Gram-negative bacteria has led to a number of classification schemes. Richmond and Sykes divided the beta-lactamases into 5 classes: class I consists of beta-lactamases with a high rate of hydrolysis of cephalosporins (cephalosporinases) and includes the chromosomally determined beta-lactamases of the most of the Enterobacteriaceae and pseudomonas, except for those of *Proteus* and *Klebsiella* which are more active against penicillins and make up classes II and IV, respectively; class III is made up of the plasmid-determined TEM-type beta-lactamases; and class V is a heterogeneous group containing the oxacillin-hydrolysing and carbenicillin-hydrolysing beta-lactamases. This classification is, however, difficult to utilise. Matthew *et al.* (*J. gen. Microbiol.*, 1975, *88,* 169) showed that specific beta-lactamases could be identified by flat-bed isoelectric focusing (IEF) in polyacrylamide gel and this technique made it possible to identify the active proteins using crude cell extracts even when several beta-lactamases co-existed within the same bacterial cell. This method revealed the presence of beta-lactamases in virtually all Gram-negative bacteria studied. The nomenclature of beta-lactamases has been a source of considerable confusion and several investigators have applied different terms to the same enzymes. A particular problem arises when beta-lactamases are labelled as host-specific such as with the PSE beta-lactamases which were initially thought to be pseudomonas specific.— A. A. Medeiros, *Br. med. Bull.*, 1984, *40,* 18.

Absorption and Fate

Antibiotics which are well absorbed from the alimentary tract may be given by mouth. However, the instability of many other antibiotics to acid makes their parenteral administration necessary. For patients with a severe infection, parenteral administration is usually the most effective and rapid means of producing an antimicrobial concentration of antibiotic in the blood and other tissues. Intramuscular injection is the commonest route, but some antibiotics which are painful and irritant when injected into muscle are usually administered intravenously. Alternatively, antibiotics such as the penicillins may be given intramuscularly with a local anaesthetic to reduce pain. The intravenous route is preferred for life-threatening infections.

The efficacy with which an orally administered antibiotic is absorbed is not necessarily reflected in its plasma concentration since some compounds are rapidly removed from circulation by the liver and appear in relatively high concentration in the bile. Reabsorption of an antibiotic which has been preferentially concentrated in bile may prolong its therapeutic activity. Chelation of the tetracycline antibiotics with aluminium, calcium, magnesium, and possibly other cations may delay or prevent their absorption after administration by mouth in conjunction with antacid preparations given to reduce gastric upset.

The absorption of many antibiotics given by mouth is affected by food and it is common practice to give many of them before meals.

Binding to plasma proteins decreases the concentration of free antibiotic available. There is, however, controversy over the significance of the effect of protein binding on activity.

Penetration of an antibiotic into infected tissue depends on local vascularity. Diffusion into abscesses or exudates in body cavities may be slow and severely limited.

Chloramphenicol is one of the few antibiotics that can enter the cerebrospinal fluid when the meninges are normal although with many antibiotics penetration is facilitated when the meninges are inflamed. In infections of the CNS, adequate concentrations of some antibiotics may only be achieved by intrathecal injection.

Although sex-linked differences in drug kinetics exist for some antibiotics such as cephradine, chloramphenicol, gentamicin, kanamycin, penicillin, rifampicin, and tetracycline, in general they do not call for dosage modification.— J. F. Giudicelli and J. P. Tillement, *Clin. Pharmacokinet.*, 1977, *2,* 157.

ADMINISTRATION IN THE ELDERLY. Pharmacokinetics of antimicrobial agents in the elderly.— B. Ljungberg and I. Nilsson-Ehle, *Rev. infect. Dis.*, 1987, *9,* 250.

ADMINISTRATION IN LIVER DISORDERS. A discussion on the pharmacokinetics of beta-lactam antibiotics in liver disease. Although hepatic dysfunction can alter the hepatic clearance, protein binding, volume of distribution, and renal clearance of these agents, the observed alterations are not great enough to require dosage modification unless there is concurrent renal impairment. This is because the half-lives of beta-lactam antibiotics in liver disease are still less than the recommended dosing intervals and thus significant accumulation does not occur. Liver disease may, however, affect the biliary concentrations of beta-lactams, but there is no consensus that this would affect the clinical outcome in the treatment of infections.— J. D. Turnidge and W. A. Craig, *J. antimicrob. Chemother.*, 1983, *11,* 499.

ADMINISTRATION IN RENAL FAILURE. Reviews and discussions on the pharmacokinetics of antibiotics during peritoneal dialysis: C. A. Johnson *et al.*, *Am. J. Kidney Dis.*, 1984, *4,* 3; D. K. Scott and D. E. Roberts, *Pharm. J.*, 1985, *1,* 621; T. W. Paton *et al.*, *Clin. Pharmacokinet.*, 1985, *10,* 404; A. J. Bint, *J. antimicrob. Chemother.*, 1987, *20,* 626.

DIFFUSION INTO BODY TISSUES AND FLUIDS. A method for calculating the tissue penetration of antibiotics following intravenous administration.— G. N. Rolinson, *J. antimicrob. Chemother.*, 1984, *13,* 593.

Penetration of antimicrobial agents into the cerebrospinal fluid.— A. J. Tuchman *et al.*, *Sth. med. J.*, 1984, *77,* 1443.

A discussion on the penetration of antibiotics into bone.— S. P. F. Hughes and F. M. Anderson, *J. antimicrob. Chemother.*, 1985, *15,* 517.

A reveiw of the pharmacokinetics of antimicrobial agents administered to the eye.— T. S. Lesar and R. G. Fiscella, *Drug Intell. & clin. Pharm.*, 1985, *19,* 642.

Penetration of antibiotics into the respiratory tract.— J. Symonds, *Br. med. J.*, 1987, *294,* 1181.

A discussion of the penetration of antimicrobial drugs into cardiac valves and endocarditic lesions.— F. D. Daschner and U. Frank, *J. antimicrob. Chemother.*, 1987, *20,* 776.

DRUG ABSORPTION. The effect of food on the absorption of antimicrobial agents.— P. G. Welling and F. L. S. Tse, *J. antimicrob. Chemother.*, 1982, *9,* 7.

DRUG EXCRETION. The excretion of antibiotics in the bile.— J. S. Dooley *et al.*, *Gut*, 1984, *25,* 988.

PREGNANCY AND THE NEONATE. A brief review of the excretion of antibiotics in breast milk.— J. T. Wilson *et al.*, *Clin. Pharmacokinet.*, 1980, *5,* 1.

Reviews and discussions of the pharmacokinetics of antimicrobial agents during pregnancy: A. Philipson, *J. antimicrob. Chemother.*, 1983, *12,* 101; A. W. Chow and P. J. Jewesson, *Rev. infect. Dis.*, 1985, *7,* 287.

Pharmacokinetics of antibiotics in the newborn.— J. de Louvois, *J. antimicrob. Chemother.*, 1987, *20,* 623.

PROTEIN BINDING. A review of the protein binding of beta-lactam antibiotics. Protein binding is a very important property of an antibiotic, determining both the microbiologically active fraction and the degree of penetration into tissue fluids. The implication of protein binding studies is that, if other aspects of an antibiotic's properties are equal, a low-bound agent should be preferable to a high-bound agent; clinical studies to support this do not, however, appear to have been performed. Serum half-life and lipid solubility are among the other factors which are important in determining penetration into extravascular tissues.— R. Wise, *J. antimicrob. Chemother.*, 1983, *12,* 1 and 105. See also D. N. Gerding and L. R. Peterson, *ibid.*, 1985, *15,* 136.

A review of binding of antibiotics by non-albumin proteins.— J. M. T. Hamilton-Miller, *J. antimicrob. Chemother.*, 1984, *13,* 303.

Choice of Antibiotic

Before choosing an antibiotic it is advisable to consider whether such treatment is essential and whether a single antibiotic, several antibiotics, or antibiotic therapy in conjunction with surgery should be used. Consideration should also be given to the length of the course of treatment, particularly if a response does not occur as expected, and alternative treatments must be considered for any patient who does not respond.

Ideally, the choice of antibiotic is made on the results of sensitivity tests which should be interpreted with reference to the response achieved with the indicated treatment in similar conditions. When it is necessary to treat patients before sensitivity tests have been carried out, therapy should be broad enough to cover the pathogens that are suspected of causing the infection, based on the site of infection and the condition of the patient; the known local patterns of bacterial resistance should also be taken into account. Sensitivity tests should still be done, as results can confirm the choice or indicate a change.

The severity, site, and type of infection and the state of the patient influence the choice of an antibiotic and its route of administration. The parenteral route of administration is the most reliable in patients with severe infections and intravenous or more direct routes produce peak antibiotic concentrations rapidly. Oral administration is convenient but should usually only be used when reliable absorption and a rapid effect are not essential. A few antibiotics are administered topically; it is advisable that those that are so used should preferably not be those given systemically.

The chosen antibiotic must be as safe as possible and a balance has to be achieved between toxicity, effectiveness, and duration of treatment.

General reviews on the choice of antimicrobial agents: *Med. Lett.*, 1986, *28*, 33; *Drug & Ther. Bull.*, 1986, *24*, 33; C. J. Wilkowske and P. E. Hermans, *Mayo Clin. Proc.*, 1987, *62*, 789; R. Wise, *Lancet*, 1987, *2*, 1251; A. M. Geddes, *ibid.*, 1988, *1*, 286.

Reviews of newer antibiotics and their areas of appropriate use: C. R. Pennington and J. Crooks, *Br. med. J.*, 1983, *286*, 1732; J. W. Stone and A. J. Davies, *Br. J. Hosp. Med.*, 1986, *36*, 119; H. C. Neu, *J. infect. Dis.*, 1987, *155*, 403.

A review of the treatment of anaerobic infections.— *Med. Lett.*, 1984, *26*, 87.

ABSCESS, ABDOMINAL. Patients with pyogenic liver abscesses have been successfully treated with needle aspiration under ultrasound guidance and appropriate antibiotic treatment such as metronidazole in association with gentamicin, cephradine, or ampicillin (M.R. Perera *et al.*, *Lancet*, 1980, *2*, 629; L.A. Berger and D.R. Osborne, *ibid.*, 1982, *1*, 132). Most liver abscesses will respond to a long course of suitable antimicrobials, but for abscesses at other sites within the abdomen some type of drainage is still essential (*Lancet*, 1982, *1*, 889). vanSonnenberg *et al.* (*J. Am. med. Ass.*, 1982, *247*, 190) reported effective treatment with percutaneous abscess drainage in 40 of 45 abdominal abscesses, and operative drainage was avoided in 34 of the 40 patients. Similar results have been obtained in other studies using percutaneous drainage and antibiotics (S.G. Gerzof *et al.*, *New Engl. J. Med.*, 1981, *305*, 653). However, a retrospective study of patients with pyogenic liver abscesses indicated that some will not respond well to intravenous antibiotics with or without percutaneous aspiration, and surgery will be necessary in some patients (S.J. McCorkell and N.L. Niles, *Lancet*, 1985, *1*, 803). Factors such as duration of symptoms and the presence of underlying diseases will affect the response to treatment; the role of anaerobes in pyogenic liver abscesses must also be emphasised. The empirical therapy of these infections requires antimicrobial agents that are active against the expected enteric pathogens, both aerobic and anaerobic, such as gentamicin in association with clindamycin, although cefoxitin, chloramphenicol, carboxypenicillins, acylaminopenicillins, third-generation cephalosporins, and metronidazole may also be appropriate in various combinations. Broad-spectrum antibiotic therapy should be narrowed only when it is certain that all significant pathogens have been identified (D.A. Herbert *et al.*, *Lancet*, 1985, *1*, 1384).

ABSCESS, BRAIN. Treatment of brain abscess is both medical and surgical. Choice of antibiotics is ideally based on the analysis of pus from the primary source and/or the cerebral lesion. As soon as pus is removed, the patient should be treated with large doses of intravenous antibiotic, which may be changed when bacteriological results become available. Abscesses of sinusitic origin, predominantly caused by anaerobic streptococci, should be treated with penicillin and chloramphenicol or metronidazole. Otitic abscesses frequently yield mixed cultures, including *Bacteroides* and *Proteus* spp., and a similar regimen with the possible addition of ampicillin or gentamicin has been recommended. Traumatic and postoperative abscesses, nearly always due to *Staphylococcus aureus*, are best treated with fusidic acid, but if an additional agent seems desirable the choice should fall on erythromycin, lincomycin, or clindamycin; flucloxacillin penetrates brain abscesses poorly. Abscesses of metastatic origin may be caused by streptococci or a mixture of bacteria, and multiple broad-spectrum therapy including penicillin should be used until culture results are available.— *Lancet*, 1988, *1*, 219.

Further references: J. de Louvois, *J. antimicrob. Chemother.*, 1983, *12*, 205; A. J. Strong and H. R. Ingham, *Br. J. Hosp. Med.*, 1983, *30*, 396.

ABSCESS, LUNG. For comment on the treatment of anaerobic lung abscess with benzylpenicillin or clindamycin, see under Benzylpenicillin Sodium p.135.

ACTINOMYCOSIS. Untreated actinomycosis is usually fatal, but a combination of surgery and antibiotics is usually curative; a prolonged course of treatment is necessary in view of the avascular fibrosis surrounding the lesions. Most authors recommend parenteral penicillin for at least 4 weeks followed by oral penicillin for 3 to 6 months. Tetracycline, erythromycin, cephalosporins, and nalidixic acid have all been reported as successful alternatives.— M. D. Stringer and A. E. P. Cameron, *Br. J. Hosp. Med.*, 1987, *38*, 125.

For the use of benzylpenicillin and phenoxymethylpenicillin in the treatment of actinomycosis, see under Benzylpenicillin Sodium p.136.

ADMINISTRATION. Comment on the choice between topical and systemic therapy.— R. Lancaster, *Prescribers' J.*, 1983, *23*, 47.

Discussion on the oral or parenteral route of administration for antibiotics in serious infections.— J. Symonds, *Archs Dis. Childh.*, 1984, *59*, 501.

A discussion on parenteral antibiotics and the view that substantial sums of money could be saved by slightly greater use of intramuscular antibiotics.— *Lancet*, 1984, *1*, 660. Comment on the potential for intramuscular or subcutaneous infusions.— B. M. Wright (letter), *ibid.*, 1130.

A discussion of out-patient intravenous antibiotic therapy.— D. N. Williams *et al.*, *J. antimicrob. Chemother.*, 1984, *14*, 102. See also D. M. Poretz *et al.*, *J. Am. med. Ass.*, 1982, *248*, 336; S. J. Rehm and A. J. Weinstein, *Ann. intern. Med.*, 1983, *99*, 388.

ADMINISTRATION IN THE ELDERLY. Rational antibiotic therapy in the elderly.— P. P. Lamy and F. B. Palumbo, *Hosp. Formul.*, 1985, *20*, 454.

ADMINISTRATION IN INFANTS AND CHILDREN. Reviews of the use of antibiotics in infants and children: K. H. Rhodes and C. M. Johnson, *Mayo Clin. Proc.*, 1983, *58*, 158.

Comments on antibiotic prescribing practices in older children and the problem of determining dosages. Several techniques may be used including by weight, by percentage of adult dose, by surface area, and by pharmacokinetic calculations. However, if, for example, body-weight is used in an older child the dose calculated may, absurdly, be greater than the adult dose. There are enormous variations in the doses prescribed for children and in how these doses are determined.— C. Block and D. Engelhard (letter), *Lancet*, 1983, *1*, 868.

Administration of antibiotics in children who require courses of injectable drugs is usually achieved by injection of the drugs into an indwelling intravenous cannula. This avoids multiple intramuscular injections and allows the child to remain ambulant.— R. J. Purvis, *Prescribers' J.*, 1983, *23*, 25.

Comment on the distress, at times terror, of many children given repeated intramuscular injections of antibiotics, and the view that a return to the more frequent use of the intramuscular route on the grounds of financial expediency should be vigorously opposed by all paediatricians.— J. M. Littlewood and M. G. Miller (letter), *Lancet*, 1984, *1*, 911.

The widespread use of intravenous antibiotic treatment in paediatric wards has been questioned (*Archs Dis. Childh.*, 1983, *58*, 161). Intravenous administration usually offers the quickest and most reliable means of establishing therapeutic antibiotic concentrations at the site of infection and avoids uncertainties related to incomplete absorption from the gastro-intestinal tract; intramuscular injection is unsuitable for large doses and impaired absorption may occur in patients with poor peripheral circulation. However, intravenous treatment involves problems of controlling and supervising drug administration, the restriction imposed on children, and the possibility of cannula-related sepsis. Once a clinical response to parenteral antibiotics has been established it becomes important to consider whether a child's interests are best served by changing to oral treatment. This decision about the best route must take into account the site and severity of infection, the known or likely pathogen and its antibiotic susceptibility as well as the pharmacology of the antibiotic used.— J. Symonds, *Archs Dis. Childh.*, 1984, *59*, 501.

A report on the duration of antibiotic courses for neonates, suggesting that antibiotics can be stopped after 48 to 72 hours if no organisms are grown on culture, without apparently increasing morbidity.— D. Isaacs *et al.*, *Archs Dis. Childh.*, 1987, *62*, 727.

ADMINISTRATION IN RENAL FAILURE. Recommendations for the use of antimicrobial agents in patients with renal insufficiency: J. Fabre *et al.*, *Clin. Pharmacokinet.*, 1980, *5*, 441; W. M. Bennett *et al.*, *Am. J. Kidney Dis.*, 1983, *3*, 155; R. E. Van Scoy and W. R. Wilson, *Mayo Clin. Proc.*, 1983, *58*, 246.

ANIMAL BITES. A review of pet-associated illness. An animal bite should be treated with prompt wound irrigation and cleansing with soap and water. When appropriate, tetanus prophylaxis should be administered. Recommendations regarding the use of prophylactic antibiotics are not established, and the potential of bites for infection varies with less than 5% of dog bites and up to 50% of cat bites becoming infected; the increased rate in cat bites is attributed to difficulty in effectively irrigating the puncture wounds that typically occur from these bites. Controlled studies using prophylactic antibiotics in the treatment of dog bites have shown no significant difference in the incidence of subsequent wound infections. However, prophylactic treatment with a cephalosporin, penicillinase-resistant penicillin, or tetracycline should be considered for bites with a high risk of infection such as bites with puncture wounds, wounds to the hand, and wounds in compromised hosts. *Pasteurella multocida* is the predominant pathogen in infections developing within the first 24 hours of a bite and causes redness and pain within hours. Penicillin, the antibiotic of choice for this organism, should be administered for infections evident within 24 hours if Gram-negative rods are present; tetracycline is an alternative for patients allergic to penicillin. For infections developing more than 24 hours after a bite, treatment should be guided by the results of a Gram stain: a penicillinase-resistant penicillin should be given if Gram-positive cocci or a mixed infection is found, pending culture results, and additional antimicrobial coverage is necessary for Gram-negative organisms.— D. L. Elliot *et al.*, *New Engl. J. Med.*, 1985, *313*, 985. Erythromycin and co-trimoxazole are possible alternatives to penicillins for the prophylactic treatment of animal bites. In overtly infected patients, drugs active against anaerobes, preferably metronidazole, should be added to the initial therapy.— *Lancet*, 1983, *2*, 553.

ANTHRAX. For comments on the treatment of anthrax, see under Benzylpenicillin Sodium, p.136.

ARTHRITIS, BACTERIAL. Reviews of bacterial arthritis and its management: S. H. Norris, *J. antimicrob. Chemother.*, 1983, *12*, 203 (in children); D. L. Goldenberg and J. I. Reed, *New Engl. J. Med.*, 1985, *312*, 764; *Lancet*, 1986, *2*, 721.

Experience with short-duration treatment in children with acute suppurative osteoarticular infections.— G. A. Syrogiannopoulos and J. D. Nelson, *Lancet*, 1988, *1*, 37.

For a detailed review of the empirical treatment of bacterial arthritis, see under Osteomyelitis in Flucloxacillin Sodium, p.232.

For the treatment of Lyme arthritis, see under Lyme Disease, below.

BILIARY-TRACT INFECTIONS. Reviews of antibiotic treatment of biliary infection: J. S. Dooley *et al.*, *Gut*, 1984, *25*, 988; R. Munro and T. C. Sorrell, *Drugs*, 1986, *31*, 449.

BRUCELLOSIS. For details of the WHO recommendations for the treatment of brucellosis, see under Doxycycline Hydrochloride, p.218.

CYSTIC FIBROSIS. For comment on the use of antibiotics in patients with cystic fibrosis, see under Respiratory-tract Infections, below.

DIARRHOEA. A brief review of acute diarrhoea and its treatment. The first priority is to maintain hydration. The cause of acute diarrhoea is often not infectious and, when it is, many infections are due to a virus or other organism not susceptible to anti-infective medication. In general, antimicrobial therapy should only be used when a susceptible organism has been identified and where it is likely to shorten the course of the illness.— *Drug & Ther. Bull.*, 1983, *21*, 101. A review of bacterial diarrhoea including the specific treatment of bacterial pathogens and the symptomatic relief of all forms of diarrhoea.— S. L. Gorbach, *Lancet*, 1987, *2*, 1378.

The most common cause of travellers' diarrhoea, usually a self-limited illness of several days' duration, is infection with enterotoxigenic *Escherichia coli*. Various drugs such as doxycycline, co-trimoxazole, trimethoprim, or norfloxacin taken prophylactically can prevent travellers' diarrhoea, but for most people the risks of such use probably outweigh the benefits. Bismuth salicylate has also been used prophylactically. Travellers to areas where hygiene is poor should be advised to avoid uncooked foods, unwashed salads, unpeeled fruit, and unboiled tap water including ice. Prompt treatment of travellers' diarrhoea with co-trimoxazole or ciprofloxacin has produced beneficial results. Symptomatic treatment with loperamide hydrochloride has also been used.— *Med. Lett.*, 1987, *29*, 53. See also *Lancet*, 1982, *1*, 777; A. M. Geddes, *Br. med. J.*, 1983, *287*, 513.

For details of oral rehydration therapy in the management of acute diarrhoea, see p.1024.

See also under Enteric Infections, below, for the treatment of diarrhoea due to specific pathogens.

For mention of antibiotic-associated colitis, see under Effects on the Gastro-intestinal Tract, in Hazards of Antibiotic Therapy, p.104.

EAR INFECTIONS. See under Otitis Media, below.

ENDOCARDITIS. Over 80% of cases of infective endocarditis are due to streptococcal and staphylococcal infections and therefore the Working Party of the British Society for Antimicrobial Chemotherapy (BSAC) has recommended that treatment of very ill patients should be started with a combination of a penicillin, usually benzylpenicillin, and an aminoglycoside, usually gentamicin, as soon as one blood sample has been taken for culture; flucloxacillin should be added to the regimen where there is a strong possibility of staphylococcal infections, for example in drug addicts or patients with skin sepsis (*Lancet*, 1985, *2*, 815). Several controversies exist in the treatment of streptococcal and staphylococcal endocarditis, including single against combined antibiotic therapy, continuous infusion against bolus doses, the duration of therapy, and the role of surgery (J. Francis and S.W.B. Newsom, *J. antimicrob. Chemother.*, 1986, *18*, 554). Several workers have commented on the need to continue treatment for an adequate period namely 4 or preferably 6 weeks. A potent cause of failure of treatment is ill-advised shortening of the period of treatment and the use of inferior oral regimens (C.M. Oakley and J.H. Darrell, *Lancet*, 1984, *1*, 690). A change to oral therapy should be carefully monitored using back-titration techniques and is only appropriate with drugs that are absorbed predictably by mouth such as amoxycillin (R.H. George *et al.*, *ibid.*, 1018); part oral treatment is considered by some to be highly desirable in paediatric practice (R.J.D. Moy *et al.*, *Archs Dis. Childh.*, 1986, *61*, 394).

For streptococcal endocarditis due to organisms that are fully sensitive to penicillin, the BSAC has recommended treatment with benzylpenicillin in association with gentamicin, both given by intravenous injection. After 14 days the gentamicin should be stopped and the benzylpenicillin may then be replaced with amoxycillin administered by mouth for another 14 days; probenecid may also be administered concurrently. If, however, the minimum bactericidal concentration (MBC) of benzylpenicillin is greater than 1 µg per mL then the gentamicin must be given with the penicillin for not less than 4 weeks (*Lancet*, 1985, *2*, 815). The BSAC has also suggested that netilmicin should be considered as an alternative to gentamicin in elderly patients or where there is impaired renal function, but Freeman and Gould (*ibid.*, 1250) pointed out that netilmicin cannot always be substituted for gentamicin because synergy between penicillins and netilmicin does not occur with *Streptococcus faecium* [*Enterococcus faecium*]. A regimen of penicillin in association with streptomycin has been used by other workers, particularly in the *USA* (W.R. Wilson, *J. antimicrob. Chemother.*, 1987, *20*, *Suppl.* A, 147). In patients genuinely allergic to the penicillins the BSAC has advised initial treatment with vancomycin plus gentamicin, but, in view of the potential toxicity of both drugs some workers have suggested cephalothin as a non-toxic substitute for penicillin (R.C. Spencer and K.G. Kristinsson, *Lancet*, 1985, *2*, 1250). However, about 10% of penicillin-sensitive patients will also be allergic to cephalosporins, which precludes any recommendation to give cephalosporins to these patients (N.A. Simmons, *ibid.*).

Enterococci are isolated from 10 to 15% of patients with endocarditis and may prove difficult to treat because *Streptococcus faecalis* [*Enterococcus faecalis*] is relatively resistant to most antibiotics. Synergy between the penicillins or vancomycin and streptomycin or gentamicin has been demonstrated *in vitro* and in *animals* and therefore combination antimicrobial therapy is used routinely to treat this disease. However, controversy exists over the length of treatment and over which aminoglycoside to use. Wilson *et al.* (*Ann. intern. Med.*, 1984, *100*, 816) proposed that the duration of symptoms may be relevant to the duration of therapy and that 4 weeks of therapy may be sufficient in patients who have had symptoms for less than 3 months. However, the duration of symptoms may be difficult to determine and, therefore, 6 weeks of therapy is usually preferred (W.M. Scheld and G.L. Mandell, *ibid.*, 904).

For staphylococcal endocarditis due to *Staphylococcus aureus* the BSAC has recommended flucloxacillin by intravenous injection in association with fusidic acid administered by mouth or gentamicin given intravenously. Treatment should be continued for at least 4 weeks, but gentamicin should seldom be given for more than 14 days and netilmicin should be considered as an alternative (*Lancet*, 1985, *2*, 815). The inclusion of fusidic acid in the regimen has been criticised (R. Freeman and F.K. Gould, *ibid.*, 1250) and antagonism between penicillins and fusidic acid has been demonstrated *in vitro* and clinically in one patient (S.J. Hudson, *ibid.*, 1249). However, the BSAC recommended the combination because they have obtained good results with it (N.A. Simmons, *ibid.*, 1250) and other workers have also used the combination successfully (R.J.D. Moy *et al.*, *Archs Dis. Childh.*, 1986, *61*, 394). Others have suggested cephalosporins to treat *Staph. aureus* endocarditis (D. Webb and H. Thadepalli, *Curr. ther. Res.*, 1983, *34*, 311; R.L. Greenman *et al.*, *Antimicrob. Ag. Chemother.*, 1984, *25*, 16).

For patients with staphylococcal endocarditis who are allergic to penicillins or when the organism is resistant to methicillin/flucloxacillin, the BSAC has recommended vancomycin alone. However, there is some controversy over whether vancomycin should be used alone or with other antibiotics. Despite variable results *in vitro* (A.S. Bayer and J.O. Morrison, *Antimicrob. Ag. Chemother.*, 1984, *26*, 220), some workers have advocated the use of vancomycin with rifampicin. Morris and Tenney (*Ann. intern. Med.*, 1983, *99*, 283) found that the combination of vancomycin and rifampicin was effective in one patient with methicillin-resistant *Staph. aureus* endocarditis after treatment failure with vancomycin alone, although antagonism had been demonstrated *in vitro* with the 2 drugs. Karchmer *et al.* (*ibid.*, *98*, 447) found that the addition of rifampicin, an aminoglycoside, or both to vancomycin therapy for *Staph. epidermidis* endocarditis was associated with a 90% cure-rate compared with 50% with vancomycin alone. They advocated that rifampicin be combined with vancomycin to treat endocarditis caused by methicillin-resistant *Staph. epidermidis*; gentamicin was not recommended for routine use because of the increased potential for adverse reactions. However, there is the possibility of development of resistance to rifampicin during therapy (B. Chamovitz *et al.*, *J. Am. med. Ass.*, 1985, *253*, 2867). With *Staph. aureus* infections, some workers prefer the use of vancomycin in association with gentamicin with careful monitoring for potential toxicity, because of the antagonism between vancomycin and rifampicin that has been reported *in vitro* (E. Smyth and L. Pomeroy (*J. antimicrob. Chemother.*, 1987, *19*, 699).

For staphylococcal endocarditis due to *Staph. epidermidis* the BSAC has recommended the same treatment regimens as for *Staph. aureus* endocarditis, provided that the *Staph. epidermidis* is shown to be sensitive (*Lancet*, 1985, *2*, 815); they noted, however, that despite sensitivity *in vitro* eradication of the infection is frequently impossible and valve replacement will be necessary.

The persistence or recurrence of fever during treatment of endocarditis with appropriate antibiotic treatment has been found to be mainly due to extensive cardiac infection, systemic and pulmonary embolism, or drug hypersensitivity, rather than resistance of the infecting organism. Thus, if a definite microbiological diagnosis has been made and appropriate bactericidal antibiotic therapy instituted, prolonged or recurrent fever is not an indication to change the antibiotics unless there is drug hypersensitivity or unequivocal microbiological evidence of another infection; prompt surgical intervention will, however, probably be necessary and delay may be fatal (A. Douglas *et al.*, *Lancet*, 1986, *1*, 1341; see also editorial comment, *ibid.*, *2*, 202).

A meeting of the British Society for Antimicrobial Chemotherapy to review the present status of infective endocarditis.— *J. antimicrob. Chemother.*, 1987, *20*, *Suppl.* A, 1–192.

ENTERIC INFECTIONS. A review of the treatment of bacterial diarrhoea due to specific pathogens including *Shigella*, *Salmonella*, and *Campylobacter* spp., *Escherichia coli*, *Yersinia enterocolitica*, *Vibrio cholerae* and other pathogenic vibrios.— S. L. Gorbach, *Lancet*, 1987, *2*, 1378.

A review of chemoprophylaxis for diarrhoeal diseases in young children, concluding that there was little evidence for its effectiveness in reducing morbidity or mortality. It could contribute to the widespread emergence and dissemination of antimicrobial resistance.— I. De Zoysa and R. G. Feachem, *Bull. Wld Hlth Org.*, 1985, *63*, 295.

See also Diarrhoea, above.

Campylobacter enteritis. A discussion on diarrhoea caused by *Campylobacter* spp., with comment on the use of erythromycin and other antimicrobial agents.— S. Levin and L. Goodman, *J. Am. med. Ass.*, 1985, *253*, 1303. See also C. A. M. McNulty, *J. antimicrob. Chemother.*, 1987, *19*, 281.

For mention of campylobacter enteritis, see under Peptic Ulcer, below.

Cholera. Patients with mild to moderate vibrio gastro-enteritis generally require no therapy other than oral fluid replacement with a glucose-electrolyte solution. Patients with severe gastro-enteritis, dehydration, and shock should receive vigorous fluid replacement, preferably intravenously (J.G. Morris and R.E. Black, *New Engl. J. Med.*, 1985, *312*, 343). Antimicrobial therapy has been shown to decrease the duration and volume of diarrhoea in cholera and may also decrease the duration of other vibrio diarrhoeas (P.A. Blake, *Ann. intern. Med.* 1983, *99*, 558). Drugs which are considered suitable for *Vibrio cholerae* infections include tetracycline, doxycycline, or alternatively co-trimoxazole or chloramphenicol (*Drug & Ther. Bull.*, 1983, *21*, 101; *Med. Lett.*, 1986, *28*, 33), but multiple drug resistance may be a problem. Hospital outbreaks of cholera transmitted through close person-to-person contact have been controlled by isolation of infected patients, administration of antibacterial chemoprophylaxis to all at-risk patients and their accompanying relatives, and by reducing overcrowding (F.S. Mhalu *et al.*, *Lancet*, 1984, *2*, 82).

Cryptosporidiosis. Comment on *Cryptosporidium* and diarrhoea.— J. G. Bissenden, *Br. med. J.*, 1986, *293*, 287.

See also under Spiramycin, p.296.

Salmonellosis. Antibacterial drugs do not shorten the course of acute diarrhoea caused by salmonellae other than *Salmonella typhi* and *S. paratyphi* and both absorbable and non-absorbable antibiotics may prolong carriage of the organism. Antimicrobial treatment is, however, necessary for patients with severe salmonella gastro-enteritis, typhoid, or paratyphoid, and should also be considered when a patient with some underlying debility such as an immunocompromised patient develops salmonella enteritis. The choice between co-trimoxazole, ampicillin/amoxycillin, and chloramphenicol depends on the sensitivity of the organism (*Drug & Ther. Bull.*, 1983, *21*, 101; S.L. Gorbach, *Lancet*, 1987, *2*, 1378). Drug resistance in salmonellae, particularly multiple resistant strains, is a serious clinical problem in both developing and developed countries (*Lancet*, 1982, *1*, 1391; H. Goossens *et al.*, *ibid.*, *2*, 769).

Shigellosis. Infections with strains of *Shigella dysenteriae* type 1 that are resistant to several drugs continue to wreak havoc in developing countries. *Sh. dysenteriae* 1 strains isolated recently from various geographical locations have been resistant to older antimicrobial agents such as tetracycline, chloramphenicol, streptomycin, and sulpha drugs, and it is considered that these drugs should no longer be used for treating dysentery due to *Sh. dysenteriae* 1. Resistance to co-trimoxazole, nalidixic acid, and ampicillin has varied and their use should be based on *in-vitro* susceptibility tests. Drugs offer only short-term solutions. The organism very quickly becomes resistant and there is the risk of normal gut flora acquiring resistance.— M. J. Albert (letter), *Lancet*, 1985, *2*, 948.

Comment on the drugs used in the treatment of shigella enteritis and the repeated emergence of resistant strains. The new quinolones have been shown to have excellent activity against shigella *in vitro* and these agents could be useful in the struggle against resistance in severe shigellosis.— L. A. Jewes, *J. antimicrob. Chemother.*, 1987, *19*, 557.

Yersiniosis. The predominant form of *Yersinia enterocolitica* infection in man is an enteric illness with or without mesenteric adenitis. Most forms of mild, uncomplicated enteritis do not require antibiotic treatment, in contrast with other forms. Drugs like trimethoprim, co-trimoxazole, tetracycline, and chloramphenicol remain the drugs of first choice for the treatment of yersiniosis by virtue of their good intracellular activity. However, the gap in their spectrum, with about 15% of organisms showing resistance, and the clinical failures, possibly due to insufficient intracellular concentration, inactivation of the drug in the presence of pus in abscesses, and inadequate length of treatment, do cause problems. The quinolones, with high tissue concentrations and intracellular activity, may have a possible role in yersiniosis.— J. A. A. Hoogkamp-Korstanje, *J. antimicrob. Chemother.*, 1987, *20*, 123.

Yersinia enterocolitica infection in children.— D. J. E. Marriott *et al.*, *Med. J. Aust.*, 1985, *143*, 489.

For further comment on the treatment of yersiniosis, see under Tetracycline Hydrochloride, p.319.

EYE INFECTIONS. General reviews: D. L. Easty, *Practitioner*, 1980, *224*, 593.

Investigation of the microbial flora of patients with acute bacterial infection of the external eye, including acute bacterial conjunctivitis, corneal ulceration, blepharitis, dacryocystitis, and discharging sockets revealed that *Staphylococcus aureus*, *Streptococcus pneumoniae*, and *Haemophilus influenzae* were the main pathogens. All these pathogens were sensitive to chloramphenicol which remained the most effective topical antibiotic with the least overall resistance of 6%; tetracycline was the next most effective. Gentamicin was the antibiotic of choice for infections due to *Pseudomonas aeruginosa* and coliform bacilli.— D. V. Seal *et al.*, *Br. J. Ophthal.*, 1982, *66*, 357.

A review of 49 patients with orbital cellulitis and guidelines for treatment. Aggressive parenteral antibiotic therapy is usually required, together with judicious surgical intervention.— D. J. Bergin and J. E. Wright, *Br. J. Ophthal.*, 1986, *70*, 174. See also *Lancet*, 1986, *2*, 497.

Management of bacterial corneal ulcers. Treatment should be started with a broad combination of antibiotics while awaiting culture results.— R. Maske *et al.*, *Br. J. Ophthal.*, 1986, *70*, 199.

For reference to the prophylaxis and treatment of neonatal conjunctivitis, see Neonatal Conjunctivitis, under Pregnancy and the Neonate, below.

For the treatment of adult gonococcal conjunctivitis, see Gonorrhoea in Sexually Transmitted Diseases, below. For the treatment of trachoma, see under Trachoma, below.

IMMUNOCOMPROMISED PATIENTS. The management of pneumonias in immunocompromised patients.— H. Masur *et al.*, *J. Am. med. Ass.*, 1985, *253*, 1769. See also D. C. Flenley, *Postgrad. med. J.*, 1983, *59*, 1; W. R. Wilson *et al.*, *Mayo Clin. Proc.*, 1985, *60*, 610.

For reference to regimens used to prevent colonisation and infection in high-risk patients by the selective decontamination of the gastro-intestinal tract, see Colistin Sulphomethate Sodium, p.205.

AIDS. Reviews of the treatment of opportunistic infections in patients with the acquired immune deficiency syndrome (AIDS): J. Cohen, *Br. J. Hosp. Med.*, 1984, *31*, 250; I. V. D. Weller, *Br. med. J.*, 1987, *295*, 200; L. S. Young, *Lancet*, 1987, *2*, 1503.

Neutropenia. A review of empirical antibiotic therapy in the febrile neutropenic cancer patient with special reference to the efficacy and impact of monotherapy. Traditionally, combinations of 2 or 3 antibiotics have been considered necessary to provide effective coverage and synergistic activity against the array of potential Gram-positive and Gram-negative pathogens in such patients. Before the mid-1960s Gram-positive bacteria, particularly *Staphylococcus aureus*, were the predominant pathogens in neutropenic cancer patients, but by the early 1970s aerobic Gram-negative bacilli, especially *Pseudomonas aeruginosa*, *Escherichia coli*, and *Klebsiella pneumoniae*, were increasingly isolated. Early empirical antibiotic regimens were formulated to provide coverage against both Gram-positive and Gram-negative organisms and most included an antistaphylococcal penicillin or cephalosporin with an aminoglycoside and an antipseudomonal carboxypenicillin. In the late 1970s the introduction of the extended-spectrum ureidopenicillins, especially piperacillin and azlocillin, offered improved activity against *Ps. aeruginosa* as well as *Klebsiella* spp., enterococci, and anaerobes. Empirical use of bactericidal broad-spectrum antibiotics as soon as the neutropenic patient became febrile reduced documented mortality from Gram-negative bacteraemias from 60% in the 1960s to 10 to 30% in the 1980s. No particular combination regimen was shown to be clearly superior. Despite their improved activity, the ureidopenicillins have not been effective for empirical monotherapy, but there is mounting evidence that the initial empirical management of the febrile, neutropenic cancer patient can be successfully accomplished with a single antibiotic, especially a broad-spectrum cephalosporin such as ceftazidime. Newer antimicrobial compounds, such as the carbapenems and quinolones, are also being evaluated. Regardless of whether a single antibiotic or a combination of antibiotics is used for initial management, continued attention must be directed to even subtle changes in the clinical and microbiological status of the patient. Appropriate modifications of therapy, particularly as the duration of neutropenia increases, must be made and are as important as the choice of initial therapy.— J. W. Hathorn *et al.*, *Antimicrob. Ag. Chemother.*, 1987, *31*, 971.

Further references: S. S. Frøland, *Scand. J. infect. Dis.*, 1984, *43*, *Suppl*, 7; L. S. Young, *J. antimicrob. Chemother.*, 1985, *16*, 4; *idem*, *New Engl. J. Med.*, 1986, *315*, 580; R. E. Marcus and J. M. Goldman, *Br. med. J.*, 1986, *293*, 406.

For a review of antibiotic regimens for the treatment of febrile episodes in neutropenic patients, see under Piperacillin Sodium, p.287.

LEGIONNAIRES' DISEASE. Management of an epidemic of legionnaires' disease in Stafford. Once the diagnosis was confirmed, the final regimen included erythromycin 1 g every 6 hours in every case, given intravenously initially for the very ill and then orally. Intravenous rifampicin was given in addition to patients whose condition was causing concern, or who failed to respond to erythromycin alone.— K. Rashed *et al.*, *Lancet*, 1986, *1*, 197.

For further reference to the treatment of legionnaires' disease, see under Erythromycin, p.225, and Rifampicin, p.576.

LEPTOSPIROSIS. Treatment of leptospirosis with antibiotics is controversial; there have been many reports of treatment, but little satisfactory evidence that antibiotics alter the course or outcome of the disease. The general consensus favours parenteral penicillin in large doses for severe illnesses and amoxycillin for oral treatment (R.J.C. Hart *et al.*, *Br. med. J.*, 1984, *288*, 1983). A tetracycline such as doxycycline has been used as an alternative treatment (B.F. Kingscote, *Can. med. Ass. J.*, 1985, *133*, 879; *Med. Lett.*, 1986, *28*, 33).

See also under Benzylpenicillin Sodium, p.136.

LISTERIOSIS. A report of epidemic listeriosis and evidence for its transmission by food. In adults *Listeria monocytogenes* is an uncommon cause of bacterial meningitis and a rare cause of sepsis, endocarditis, peritonitis, or focal abscess. In neonates it is the third most common cause of bacterial meningitis. In addition, perinatal infections can cause abortion, stillbirth, and a devastating septic illness called 'granulomatosis infantisepticum'.— W. F. Schlech *et al.*, *New Engl. J. Med.*, 1983, *308*, 203.

A brief review of perinatal listeriosis. Treatment of suspected neonatal listeriosis usually begins before firm bacteriological confirmation with a combination of ampicillin or penicillin with gentamicin or kanamycin. Perinatal listeriosis has been prevented by treating listeric septicaemia in the mother, during pregnancy, with ampicillin. Success in managing this condition appears to depend on the degree of foetal or neonatal infection at the time of presentation.— J. A. D. Spencer, *Br. med. J.*, 1987, *295*, 349.

See also under Ampicillin Trihydrate, p.120.

LYME DISEASE. Lyme disease is a seasonal infectious disease found in the United States, Europe, and Australia, caused by the spirochaete *Borrelia burgdorferi*, and transmitted primarily by ixodes ticks. The usual initial manifestation, which occurs days to weeks after the spirochaete enters the body, is erythema chronicum migrans, a characteristic rapidly expanding erythematous rash. Skin lesions are often accompanied by malaise, fatigue, headache, fever, stiff neck, myalgias, arthralgias, or lymphadenopathy; abdominal pain and vomiting may also occur. About 15% of patients develop neurological problems, about 8% heart problems, and about 60% develop arthritis. Tetracycline or phenoxymethylpenicillin are given by mouth for the early treatment of Lyme disease (A. Parke, *Br. med. J.*, 1987, *294*, 525). Intravenous benzylpenicillin has been used for established infection or treatment of neurological sequelae (see p.136); for neurological Lyme disease resistant to penicillin, cephalosporins such as ceftriaxone or cefotaxime may be effective (G.S. Pal *et al.*, *Lancet*, 1988, *1*, 50). There has been a report of congenital heart disease in a neonate born to a woman who developed Lyme disease during the first trimester of pregnancy and it has been recommended that such women should be treated promptly with penicillin or, if allergic, erythromycin (P.A. Schlesinger *et al.*, *Ann. intern. Med.*, 1985, *103*, 67).

MELIOIDOSIS. Tetracycline and chloramphenicol have been the mainstays of treatment for melioidosis which is caused by *Pseudomonas pseudomallei*. There have been reports of the successful use of co-trimoxazole (C.K. Chan *et al.*, *Can. med. Ass. J.*, 1984, *131*, 1365) and So *et al.*, (*Trans. R. Soc. trop. Med. Hyg.*, 1984, *78*, 456) referred to their successful use of ceftazidime in a patient with lung abscesses caused by a multi-resistant strain of *Ps. pseudomallei*.

MENINGITIS. Prompt treatment is essential for bacterial meningitis and antimicrobial drugs should not be withheld until laboratory studies are completed. The organisms most commonly responsible for bacterial meningitis are *Haemophilus influenzae*, *Streptococcus pneumoniae*, and *Neisseria meningitidis*. Benzylpenicillin is usually recommended for treatment of meningitis in adults, because of its effectiveness against possible pneumococcal or meningococcal meningitis, although ampicillin may be used to cover *H. influenzae*; chloramphenicol, cefuroxime, cefotaxime, or ceftriaxone can be used to treat meningitis due to penicillinase-producing strains of *H. influenzae*. When the cerebrospinal fluid from an adult showns Gram-negative rods cefotaxime or ceftriaxone may be used, although *Pseudomonas aeruginosa* infection requires the use of carbenicillin, ticarcillin, mezlocillin, piperacillin, azlocillin, or ceftazidime in association with an aminoglycoside. In children more than one month old *H. influenzae* is the most common cause of bacterial meningitis and chloramphenicol and ampicillin are usually used; in some parts of the *USA* 20% or more of *H. influenzae* strains are resistant to ampicillin and rare strains are resistant to chloramphenicol, thus both chloramphenicol and ampicillin should be given initially until the results of cultures and susceptibility tests are known. Cefuroxime, cefotaxime, and ceftriaxone are effective alternatives. In neonates meningitis and sepsis are often caused by Gram-negative enteric organisms, group B streptococci, or *Listeria monocytogenes* and treatment is usually with ampicillin plus an aminoglycoside such as gentamicin; ampicillin plus cefotaxime or ceftriaxone is an alternative regimen.— *Med. Lett.*, 1986, *28*, 33.

Comment on the lack of activity of the cephalosporins against *Listeria monocytogenes*. Caution may be necessary when using a cephalosporin as the sole initial antibiotic for the treatment of meningitis.— C. J. Hall *et al.* (letter), *Lancet*, 1985, *2*, 608.

Further reviews of the treatment of bacterial meningitis: H. P. Lambert, *Br. med. J.*, 1983, *286*, 741; M. Whitby and R. Finch, *Drugs*, 1986, *31*, 266.

For the treatment of meningitis caused by *Staphylococcus aureus*, see under Flucloxacillin Sodium, p.231.

MOUTH INFECTIONS. A review of dental infections, their treatment and prophylaxis. The organisms most often encountered in oral infections are *Streptococcus viridans*, a variety of anaerobes, and facultative streptococci. Penicillin continues to be the most effective drug in combating these pathogens, and erythromycin is considered the drug of second choice. Other drugs that might be useful include other penicillins, the cephalosporins, the aminoglycosides in association with penicillin, and clindamycin.— W. Guralnick, *Br. dent. J.*, 1984, *156*, 440. Metronidazole is also considered useful for the treatment of anaerobic infections.— L. P. Samaranayake (letter), *ibid.*, *157*, 84.

For comment on the topical and systemic use of tetracyclines in periodontal disease, see under Tetracycline Hydrochloride, p.320.

MYCOBACTERIAL INFECTIONS. See the section on Antimycobacterial Agents for main coverage of the treatment of tuberculosis (p.546), atypical mycobacterial infections (p.553), and leprosy (p.551).

OSTEOMYELITIS. For a detailed review of the empirical treatment of osteomyelitis, see under Flucloxacillin Sodium, p.232.

OTITIS MEDIA. An outline of acute and chronic inflammatory middle ear disease and its management. Acute otitis media is predominantly a disease of children; the key point in treatment is whether or not to use antibacterial therapy, but whatever the treatment the patient should be followed up until eardrum and hearing return to normal. Chronic otitis media presents most commonly as secretory otitis media or 'glue-ear', but chronic suppurative otitis media is potentially more damaging; both require specialist management.— J. Fry and J. W. Stephenson, *Prescribers' J.*, 1984, *24*, 15.

A review of the management of acute otitis media. The commonest pathogens in American studies have been *Streptococcus pneumoniae* and *Haemophilus influenzae* (in children under 5 years); viruses may sometimes be implicated. Treatment aims to relieve pain and distress, to eliminate bacterial infection, and to avoid later complications such as chronic middle ear disease and hearing loss. The necessity for antibiotic treatment has not been demonstrated conclusively in published studies, but in Britain an antibiotic is given almost routinely to children with acute otitis media and when clinical signs suggest a bacterial infection an antibiotic will probably speed resolution and avoid complications. Antibiotics used have included penicillin, penicillin/sulphonamide combinations, ampicillin, amoxycillin, co-trimoxazole, cefaclor, and erythromycin. The optimum length of treatment is not known.

To summarise, most children with pink or injected eardrums and pain recover spontaneously and need only an analgesic and continuing observation and review. When the eardrum is, or becomes, red or yellow and bulging, bacterial otitis media is likely and should be treated with amoxycillin or co-trimoxazole. Oral decongestants and antihistamines do not help symptoms and may cause unwanted effects.— *Drug & Ther. Bull.*, 1984, *22*, 53. See also B. L. True and D. K. Helling, *Drug Intell. & clin. Pharm.*, 1986, *20*, 666; J. Wilmott, *Practitioner*, 1987, *231*, 1101.

A review of the pathogenesis and management of secretory otitis media in childhood.— A. R. Maw, *Br. med. Bull.*, 1987, *43*, 950.

A report of a new treatment strategy for the treatment of acute otitis media in children. It was suggested that in general treatment could be limited to nose drops and analgesics for the first 3 to 4 days.— F. L. van Buchem *et al.*, *Br. med. J.*, 1985, *290*, 1033. Criticisms and the view that early antibiotic therapy is important.— J. E. Osborne *et al.* (letter), *ibid.*, 1743; J. Siegler (letter), *ibid.*, 1744. Reply.— F. L. van Buchem *et al.* (letter), *ibid.*

PELVIC INFLAMMATORY DISEASE. Pelvic inflammatory disease (PID) is infection involving the uterus, fallopian tubes, peritoneum and adjacent structures, or any extension from those organs. The tubes are usually primarily involved, but the disease may extend to the ovaries and pelvic peritoneum. The majority of infections of the upper genital tract are sexually transmitted. In Europe most cases of PID are probably caused by *Chlamydia trachomatis. Neisseria gonorrhoeae* is also an important pathogen and is potentially the most destructive to subsequent reproductive function. Other organisms which may be involved include *Mycoplasma hominis* and anaerobic organisms especially anaerobic cocci and *Bacteroides fragilis*. In order to minimise the residual tubal damage in an acute case of PID it is important to treat the woman adequately and it is often necessary to commence treatment with broad-spectrum antibiotic coverage before bacteriological results are available. Appropriate therapy includes an antibiotic effective against chlamydia such as a tetracycline or erythromycin, and an antibiotic against gonococci such as procaine penicillin, ampicillin, or amoxycillin; in areas with a high frequency of penicillin-resistant gonococci, spectinomycin or cefotaxime should be used. Metronidazole should also be given, prior to obtaining cultures, to cover the possibility of infection with *B. fragilis*.— M. A. R. Thomson, *Prescribers' J.*, 1987, *27* (2), 22. In the *USA*, recommendations for the treatment of pelvic inflammatory disease have included cefoxitin plus doxycycline or clindamycin plus gentamicin (for further details, see Cefoxitin Sodium, p.159).— *Med. Lett.*, 1988, *30*, 5.

A suitable regimen for severely ill patients with acute salpingitis would be spectinomycin 4 to 6 g six hourly for 24 hours with doxycycline 100 mg twice daily for 7 days and daily for a further 14 days, and rectal metronidazole 500 mg twice daily for 10 days. An alternative regimen comprises penicillin 7.2 to 12 g daily in divided doses, switching after 72 hours to a tetracycline such as doxycycline 100 mg twice daily or erythromycin 500 mg four times daily for 7 to 10 days; gentamicin 2 to 5 mg per kg body-weight daily in divided doses is also given, together with rectal metronidazole 500 mg twice daily for 10 days. Cephalosporins have a lesser role as they are not effective against chlamydia, although penicillinase-producing *N. gonorrhoeae* may be managed with cefoxitin 1 to 2 g given intramuscularly every 6 hours.— S. L. Stanton, *Br. med. J.*, 1987, *295*, 621.

Further references: D. A. Grimes *et al.*, *J. Am. med. Ass.*, 1986, *256*, 3223; P. Wølner-Hanssen *et al.*, *ibid.*, 3262.

PEPTIC ULCER. Comment on campylobacter enteritis and the role of *Campylobacter pylori* (*Campylobacter pyloridis*) in peptic ulceration. Strains of *C. pylori* are highly sensitive *in vitro* to beta-lactams, unlike most other campylobacteria, and also to erythromycin, gentamicin, chloramphenicol, ciprofloxacin, and rifampicin. They are also moderately sensitive to bismuth salts and *in vivo C. pylori* has been eradicated with bismuth salts or amoxycillin. Relapse is a problem and a combination of bismuth salt plus a high dose of antibiotic such as pivampicillin or amoxycillin might be required.— C. A. M. McNulty, *J. antimicrob. Chemother.*, 1987, *19*, 281.

See also under Tripotassium Dicitratobismuthate, p.1111.

PERITONITIS. A report of a working party of the British Society for Antimicrobial Chemotherapy on the diagnosis and management of peritonitis in continuous ambulatory peritoneal dialysis (CAPD). *Staphylococcus epidermidis* causes about half the episodes of confirmed peritonitis and many other organisms causing peritonitis in CAPD such as alpha-haemolytic streptococci, 'diphtheroids', and *Staph. aureus* are also skin bacteria. The Enterobacteriaceae and *Pseudomonas aeruginosa* together account for almost a fifth of the infecting organisms. CAPD-associated peritonitis should be treated promptly with antibiotics. Drugs should be given by the intraperitoneal route, rather than orally or intravenously, since precise therapeutic and non-toxic concentrations can be delivered to the site of infection; with many antibiotics adequate serum concentrations are achieved within a few hours of intraperitoneal administration. CAPD should be continued as usual with antibiotics added to the dialysis fluid. In the severely ill patient, an intravenous or intraperitoneal loading dose may be given to ensure prompt therapeutic concentrations.

The initial antibiotic regimen for CAPD peritonitis must be effective against both Gram-positive and Gram-negative pathogens. For the initial empirical treatment of peritonitis a combination of vancomycin and an aminoglycoside such as gentamicin, netilmicin, or tobramycin is recommended. Once the pathogen and its sensitivity are known, either vancomycin or the aminoglycoside should be discontinued. As an alternative to the above regimen cefuroxime or ceftazidime may be used. The optimum length of treatment remains controversial but the working party recommend continuation for at least 5 days after resolution of clinical signs and symptoms and clearing of the effluent; usually a total of 7 to 10 days is adequate.

For peritonitis due to *Ps. aeruginosa*, a combination of an antipseudomonal penicillin such as azlocillin or ticarcillin and an aminoglycoside is recommended; ceftazidime may be used as an alternative drug but this too should be combined with an aminoglycoside. Failure to respond promptly is an indication for early catheter removal. Flucloxacillin or vancomycin are recommended for *Staph. aureus* infections, ampicillin or vancomycin for *Enterococcus faecalis* (*Streptococcus faecalis*) infections, and vancomycin for diphtheroids. For fungal peritonitis a series of rapid exchanges should be carried out to eliminate gross turbidity and then the catheter should be removed. Amphotericin given intravenously is the antifungal agent of choice although flucytosine, miconazole, and ketoconazole have also been used. If cultures prove negative and there is no response after 3 to 5 days of empirical treatment a full clinical and microbiological review is indicated, which should include a search for mycobacteria.— *Lancet*, 1987, *1*, 845. Comment on the effect of peritoneal dialysate in decreasing the activity of some antibiotics.— C. F. Craddock (letter), *ibid.*, 1320.

Futher references: P. Fenton, *J. antimicrob. Chemother.*, 1984, *13*, 411; D. K. Scott and D. E. Roberts, *Pharm. J.*, 1985, *1*, 621.

PLAGUE. A report by the Public Health Laboratory Service Communicable Disease Surveillance Centre on the occurrence and control of plague. Treatment with streptomycin, tetracycline, or chloramphenicol is highly effective in all forms of human disease if recognised early.— *Br. med. J.*, 1983, *287*, 118.

PREGNANCY AND THE NEONATE. For a guide to antibiotics used in the treatment of common infections in pregnancy and their possible adverse effects, see R. Wise, *Br. med. J.*, 1987, *294*, 42. See also *Med. Lett.*, 1987, *29*, 61.

In the management of syphilis in pregnancy, pregnant women should be treated with either benzathine penicillin or procaine penicillin in the dosage schedules recommended for nonpregnant patients at the same stage of the disease. Penicillin-allergic patients should be treated with erythromycin, although the efficacy of such regimens is not well established. Infants should be treated at birth if the treatment of the mother was inadequate or unknown, if a drug other than penicillin (e.g. erythromycin) was used, or if clinical and serological follow-up of the infant cannot be ensured. For early congenital syphilis (up to 2 years of age) in infants with abnormal cerebrospinal fluid, benzylpenicillin or procaine penicillin should be given for 10 days; in infants with normal cerebrospinal fluid, a single dose of benzathine penicillin may be given.— WHO Expert Committee on Venereal Diseases and Treponematoses, Sixth Report, *Tech. Rep. Ser. Wld Hlth Org. No. 736*, 1986, p.127. See also G. Buttigieg, *Br. J. Hosp. Med.*, 1985, *33*, 28.

Urogenital infections, during pregnancy, due to *Chlamydia trachomatis* should be treated with erythromycin, and the male partner(s) should receive concurrent treatment with a tetracycline.— WHO Expert Committee on Venereal Diseases and Treponematoses, Sixth Report, *Tech. Rep. Ser. Wld Hlth Org. No. 736*, 1986, p.124.

See also under Sexually Transmitted Diseases and Urinary-tract Infections, below.

Neonate. The treatment of neonatal sepsis depends on the time of onset. Early-onset sepsis, occurring within the first 48 hours of life, is usually treated with penicillin or ampicillin and an aminoglycoside, because group B streptococcal infection and infection with Gram-negative organisms are currently the most commonly identified causes. Late-onset sepsis, occurring after 48 hours, is usually due to Gram-negative organisms, although staphylococcal infections may also be a common cause. Treatment may include flucloxacillin in association with gentamicin, or a third-generation cephalosporin such as ceftazidime, although the routine use of third-generation cephalosporins for suspected sepsis may be inappropriate because of their inactivity against enterococci (M.M. Placzek and A. Whitelaw, *Archs Dis. Childh.*, 1983, *58*, 728; D. Isaacs and A.R. Wilkinson, *ibid.*, 1987, *62*, 204) and their potential for rapidly developing resistance (N. Modi *et al.*, *ibid.*, 148).

In the prevention of early-onset group B streptococcal infections, antibiotics such as benzylpenicillin have been administered to neonates within one hour of birth, but variable results have been achieved as this does not prevent infection acquired *in utero* and probably has little effect on the incidence of late-onset disease (D.J. Lloyd *et al.*, *Lancet*, 1979, *1*, 713; J.D. Siegel *et al.*, *ibid.*, 1982, *1*, 1426; S.P. Pyati *et al.*, *New Engl. J. Med.*, 1983, *308*, 1383). Intrapartum administration of antibiotics such as ampicillin until delivery, as well as antibiotics given to the neonate for 48 hours after delivery, has been shown to almost eliminate transmission of group B streptococci from colonised mothers to their infants (K.M. Boyer and S.P. Gotoff, *New Engl. J. Med.*, 1986, *314*, 1665) and selective chemoprophylaxis in those mothers whose infants have a very high risk of infection is justified (*Lancet*, 1986, *1*, 247).

Further references: *Drug & Ther. Bull.*, 1981, *19*, 13; J. D. Siegel and G. H. McCracken, *New Engl. J. Med.*, 1981, *304*, 642; *Lancet*, 1981, *2*, 181.

Neonatal conjunctivitis. Bacterial causes of neonatal conjunctivitis (ophthalmia neonatorum) include staphylococci, streptococci, haemophilus, Gram-negative aerobic bacilli, and *Neisseria gonorrhoeae*. Eye infections due to *Chlamydia trachomatis* may be unrecognised because signs often develop after the baby has been discharged from hospital, usually appearing 5 to 14 days after delivery. The approach to management must vary according to local patterns of infection. Babies with sticky eyes yielding no bacteria on culture usually respond to simple measures such as cleansing and irrigation with sterile saline. Topical antibiotics are required if bacteria are cultured or seen in large numbers on microscopy. Chloramphenicol 0.5% and neomycin 0.5% ointments are widely used and effective in most acute bacterial infections, although neomycin has the disadvantage of being inactive against streptococci. Systemic antibiotics are recommended for both gonococcal and chlamydial ophthalmia.— *Lancet*, 1984, *2*, 1375.

The prevention and treatment of conjunctivitis of the newborn at the primary health care level. Gonococcal conjunctivitis has to be treated with both systemic and topical antimicrobial agents. In areas where the prevalence of penicillin-resistant gonococci is less than 1% systemic treatment with benzylpenicillin is justifiable, but where the prevalence of penicillin resistance is more than 1% or is unknown, cefotaxime is recommended; possible alternative agents include spectinomycin or kanamycin. For topical treatment tetracycline hydrochloride 1% ointment is the preferred medication, but erythromycin 0.5% eye ointment can be used. Infants known to have been exposed to gonorrhoea at birth should be given treatment similar to that for known gonococcal infection.

Infants with presumed chlamydial or other nongonococcal conjunctivitis should be treated with tetracycline hydrochloride 1% ointment or erythromycin 0.5% ointment; infants with presumed chlamydial conjunctivitis should also be given erythromycin by mouth.

Conjunctivitis of the newborn is best prevented by treatment of infected pregnant women, but systematic detection and treatment of infected mothers is not available in many areas and therefore the application of prophylactic measures to the newborn child is often the only means of reducing the incidence of this disease. Prophylaxis involves cleaning of the infant's eyes followed by application of an antiseptic or antimicrobial agent to the conjunctivae as soon as possible after birth. In areas where the risk of gonococcal infection is high, silver nitrate 1% eye-drops or tetracycline hydrochloride 1% eye ointment can be used. However, in areas where the risk of gonococcal infection is low but chlamydial infection is frequent, the prophylactic use of tetracycline hydrochloride 1% eye ointment or erythromycin 0.5% ointment is preferable.— *Conjunctivitis of the newborn*, World Health Organization, Geneva, 1986.

Further references to the prophylaxis and treatment of neonatal conjunctivitis: J. D. Oriel, *J. antimicrob. Chemother.*, 1984, *14*, 209; E. M. Zola, *Drug Intell. & clin. Pharm.*, 1984, *18*, 692; WHO Expert Committee on Venereal Diseases and Treponematoses, Sixth Report *Tech. Rep. Ser. Wld Hlth Org. No. 736*, 1986, p.122.

RELAPSING FEVER. Comment on the treatment of relapsing fever with erythromycin stearate, tetracycline, or procaine penicillin, and the problem of the Jarisch-Herxheimer reaction.— T. Butler, *Ann. intern. Med.*, 1985, *102*, 397.

RESPIRATORY-TRACT INFECTIONS. A review of the treatment of respiratory-tract infections.— S. R. Smith *et al.*, *J. clin. Hosp. Pharm.*, 1985, *10*, 243.

The role of antibiotics given by inhalation in chronic chest disease.— D. Maxwell, *J. antimicrob. Chemother.*, 1983, *11*, 203.

Penetration of systemic antibiotics into the respiratory tract.— J. Symonds, *Br. med. J.*, 1987, *294*, 1181.

For reference to the treatment of respiratory-tract infections in immunocompromised patients, see Immunocompromised Patients, above.

Bronchitis. Most physicians include an antibiotic in their treatment regimen for exacerbations of chronic bronchitis and a broad-spectrum antibiotic active against *Haemophilus influenzae* and *Streptococcus pneumoniae* is usually recommended. The majority of studies, however, have found no benefit from antibiotic treatment although, following a recent study (N.R. Anthonisen *et al.*, *Ann. intern. Med.*, 1987, *106*, 196) in which amoxycillin, co-trimoxazole, and doxycycline were compared with placebo, the researchers felt that antibiotics were justified in exacerbations characterised by increased dyspnoea, sputum production, and purulence. Nevertheless the question of the need for antibiotic treatment remains unanswered and, while it seems appropriate to use antibiotics in an acute exacerbation, some restraint should be exercised in less severe episodes since up to 50% of exacerbations respond to placebo.— *Lancet*, 1987, *2*, 23. See also N. C. Thomson, *Prescribers' J.*, 1987, *27* (2), 15.

Cystic fibrosis. A review of the management of cystic fibrosis. Mortality and morbidity are generally determined by the severity of pulmonary involvement. Management of the pulmonary disorder is based on clearing secretions from the lungs and on preventing or controlling infection. Physiotherapy is the mainstay for clearing secretions. Antimicrobial drugs should be used in therapeutic dosage and for adequate periods in the treatment of active infection, but views about their prophylactic use differ. *Staphylococcus aureus* is the most common pathogen in patients with mild to moderate pulmonary damage; occasionally the pathogen is *Haemophilus influenzae*. *Pseudomonas aeruginosa* is very frequently present in patients with severe pulmonary damage, sometimes in association with *Staph. aureus* or *H. influenzae*.— M. B. Mearns, *Archs Dis. Childh.*, 1985, *60*, 272.

Lung infection with *Pseudomonas aeruginosa* has emerged as one of the greatest challenges in the management of cystic fibrosis. Antibiotics seldom eradicate the organism but they do curtail the numbers, usually with improvement in general health and delayed deterioration of lung function. Antibiotic treatment of pseudomonal chest infection is difficult largely because antibacterial activity is not easily achieved in respiratory secretions, and therefore high peak serum concentrations are required. Mucoid strains of *Ps. aeruginosa* are common in cystic fibrosis and their mucopolysaccharide slime is a barrier to antibacterial activity, because of the inability of antibiotics to reach lethal concentrations within the cell. The viscosity of bronchial secretions and fibrotic bronchopulmonary changes further hamper penetration of antibiotics to the site of infection. Also there is unusually rapid elimination of many antibiotics in cystic fibrosis including antipseudomonal penicillins such as azlocillin, aminoglycosides, and ceftazidime. High doses of antibiotics in cystic fibrosis are rational in the context of their pharmacokinetics in these patients. Nevertheless, there is as yet no persuasive evidence that high-dose antipseudomonal regimens free the patients from recurrent pseudomonal lung infection or contribute substantially to the quality of life in cystic fibrosis.— *Lancet*, 1985, *1*, 1020.

For further comment on the use of antibiotics including nebulised antibiotics in the management of exacerbations of pulmonary infection in cystic fibrosis, see under Carbenicillin Sodium p.141.

Epiglottitis. Comment on the management of adult epiglottitis including the use of antibiotics, such as ampicillin and chloramphenicol or second- or third-generation cephalosporins, for presumed *Haemophilus influenzae* infection.— A. S. Baker and R. D. Eavey, *New Engl. J. Med.*, 1986, *314*, 1185. See also M. F. MayoSmith *et al.*, *ibid.*, 1135.

Legionnaires' disease. See Legionnaires' Disease, above.

Pertussis. For comment on the treatment of pertussis, see under Erythromycin, p.226.

Pharyngitis. Treatment of bacterial pharyngitis is usually directed against the group A beta-haemolytic streptococcus, *Streptococcus pyogenes*, because eradication of this organism from the pharynx has been shown to prevent subsequent acute rheumatic fever; rheumatic fever has, however, become increasingly rare in developed countries and greater emphasis has been placed on relief of the acute symptoms. An abrupt onset of febrile pharyngitis in a child, especially during the winter months, is typical of streptococcal infection and empirical antibiotic therapy should be used, accompanied by culture of a throat swab. Intramuscular benzathine penicillin is optimum treatment but uncomfortable for the patient. Oral penicillin still seems clinically to be sufficiently effective, but if the rate of relapse following penicillin therapy continues to increase then an oral cephalosporin or erythromycin may become preferable. In an older person, especially if there is an accompanying rash, erthromycin is a better initial choice since it covers both group A streptococci and *Corynebacterium haemolyticum*; *C. haemolyticum* is now known to be an important cause of pharyngitis in patients in the second and third decades of life.— *Lancet*, 1987, *1*, 1241.

Further references to the management of streptococcal pharyngitis: M. A. Gerber and M. Markowitz, *Pediatr. infect. Dis. J.*, 1985, *4*, 518; H. C. Dillon, *Pediatr. infect. Dis. J.*, 1987, *6*, 123.

See also under Rheumatic Fever Prophylaxis, in Prophylactic Use of Antibiotics, below.

Pneumonia. The British Thoracic Society research committee, in association with the PHLS [Public Health Laboratory Service] Communicable Diseases Surveillance Centre have studied community-acquired, radiologically confirmed pneumonia requiring admission to hospital. There are indications that early treatment is important in preventing mortality and does not compromise diagnosis except in pneumococcal infection. Pneumonia in previously fit individuals should be treated immediately, probably with a penicillin effective against *Streptococcus pneumoniae* and erythromycin to cover mycoplasma and legionella. When influenza A is prevalent in the community an antistaphylococcal agent should be added. Although legionella occurs sporadically the principal causal agent associated with death from pneumonia is still *Str. pneumoniae*.— C. K. Connolly and B. Harrison (letter), *Br. med. J.*, 1985, *290*, 1586.

Any antibiotic for community-acquired pneumonia must provide effective cover for pneumococcal infection and initial therapy should be with a penicillin such as ampicillin. Erythromycin is a suitable alternative for penicillin-sensitive patients and is also suitable for atypical infections. An antistaphylococcal penicillin such as flucloxacillin, oxacillin, or nafcillin should be added to primary therapy if pneumonia is post-influenzal. Less satisfactory alternatives for treating community-acquired pneumonia include oral cephalosporins, co-trimoxazole, and tetracyclines. For patients who are more than mildly ill intravenous therapy may be required. Atypical pneumonias, including mycoplasma, psittacosis and Q fever pneumonias, are best treated with either tetracycline or erythromycin. Other causes of atypical pneumonia that are not susceptible to penicillins include *Branhamella catarrhalis* which may be treated with erythromycin, co-trimoxazole, or amoxycillin plus clavulanic acid, and *Legionella pneumophila* which may be treated with erythromycin.

For nosocomial pneumonia broad-spectrum antimicrobial therapy is essential as aerobic Gram-negative bacillary infection features prominently and 2 or more pathogens are found in over half the cases. Initial therapy is with a third-generation cephalosporin, with addition of an aminoglycoside in severe infection. Where pseudomonal infection is likely such as in immunocompromised or granulocytopenic patients and those being managed on an intensive-care unit, an antipseudomonal cephalosporin or penicillin plus an aminoglycoside should be used. The quinolones, monobactams, and carbapenems will probably make an increasing impact on the empirical treatment of this type of pneumonia.

Community-acquired aspiration pneumonia, usually due to oropharyngeal anaerobes, can be treated with clindamycin or benzylpenicillin; an alternative approach, in patients who are not seriously ill, is high-dose ampicillin with metronidazole both given by mouth. In hospital-acquired aspiration pneumonia a wide range of Gram-negative bacilli, *Staphylococcus aureus*, and also anaerobes including *Bacteroides fragilis* are implicated, and an appropriate regimen would be an aminoglycoside plus clindamycin or penicillin or a cephamycin such as cefoxitin.— J. T. Macfarlane, *Lancet*, 1987, *2*, 1446.

Further references: J. A. Innes, *Br. med. J.*, 1987, *295*, 1083 (community-acquired pneumonia); *Drug & Ther. Bull.*, 1988, *26*, 13 (community-acquired pneumonia); *Lancet*, 1988, *1*, 741 (childhood pneumonia).

Psittacosis. The causative organism of psittacosis is *Chlamydia psittaci*. It is usually transmitted to man by direct or indirect contact with infected birds and the primary site of infection in man is the lung. The clinical presentation of the disease can vary widely from a mild 'flu-like' illness to a fulminating toxic state with multiple organ involvement. Most patients will have a cough, although this is not always prominent. Tetracyclines are considered to be the treatment of choice and early therapy may be life saving; alternative agents including chloramphenicol, sulphadiazine, and high-dose penicillin are less effective. Erythromycin and rifampicin have also been used.— J. T. Macfarlane and A. D. Macrae, *Br. med. Bull.*, 1983, *39*, 163. Comment that human-to-human transmission of *Chlamydia* causing respiratory infection is common. Strains differing from the known serotypes of *C. psittaci* and *C. trachomatis*, and designated as TWAR (Taiwan acute respiratory) strains, might be responsible.— *Lancet*, 1988, *1*, 974.

RICKETTSIAL INFECTIONS. Therapy of the rickettsioses is based on the use of specific antibiotics including the tetracyclines, such as doxycycline, and chloramphenicol. Louse-borne typhus, and perhaps scrub typhus may be treated with a single dose of doxycycline, but other rickettsioses such as murine typhus, Rocky Mountin spotted fever, and perhaps other tick-borne rickettsioses of the spotted fever group and Q fever require antibiotic therapy over a period of several days; chronic Q fever infections and endocarditis will require more prolonged therapy.— WHO Working Group on Rickettsial Diseases, *Bull. Wld Hlth Org.*, 1982, *60*, 157.

The use of antibiotics in the treatment of Q fever.— A. M. Geddes, *Br. med. J.*, 1983, *287*, 927.

See also Pneumonia in Respiratory-tract Infections, above.

SEPTICAEMIA. Bacteraemia requires prompt treatment without waiting for results of laboratory tests. Choice of drugs depends on the probable source of infection, Gram-stained smears of appropriate clinical specimens, and the immune status of the patient; it should also reflect current patterns of bacterial resistance in the community and the hospital. For bacteraemia in an adult when the infecting organism is not known, some workers recommend concurrent use of a penicillinase-resistant penicillin or a cephalosporin with gentamicin, tobramycin, netilmicin, or amikacin. Since such combinations may not be effective against enterococci, ampicillin or benzylpenicillin may be added to the regimen, particularly when the urinary tract is considered a likely source of the infection or when endocarditis is suspected. For infections likely to involve anaerobes, such as intra-abdominal infections or pelvic infections in women, additional coverage with clindamycin, metronidazole, cefoxitin, chloramphenicol, ticarcillin with clavulanic acid, or imipenem is indicated. When methicillin-resistant staphylococci are suspected, treatment with vancomycin should be considered. The third-generation cephalosporins or imipenem can be effective for treatment of bacteraemia caused by many strains of Gram-negative bacilli, including some resistant to gentamicin and tobramycin. Whether one or more of these new beta-lactams will eventually replace the aminoglycosides for Gram-negative coverage is not yet clear. They do not have the ototoxicity or nephrotoxicity of the aminoglycosides, but many infectious disease experts are reluctant to recommend frequent or routine use of these new agents because of their high cost and the potential for emergence of resistance.— *Med. Lett.*, 1986, *28*, 33. See also *Drug & Ther. Bull.*, 1986, *24*, 33.

For the treatment of neonatal sepsis, see Pregnancy and the Neonate, above.

Catheter-related infections. A discussion of infection associated with intravenous catheters. Once infected, an intravenous catheter should be removed and cultured, however inconvenient. Although in many patients removal of the catheter alone will cure the associated infection, antibiotics are frequently given at the same time and are sometimes clearly justified particularly if another catheter is required. The choice of antibiotic will be governed by the sensitivity or likely sensitivity of the organism isolated from skin site, catheter tip, or blood.— S. J. Eykyn, *J. antimicrob. Chemother.*, 1984, *14*, 203. Comment that, at least for Broviac and Hickman catheters, administration of antibiotics through the catheter often results in cure of the infection particularly if the colonisation is by a single bacterial strain rather than multiple strains. As long as blood is cultured whenever there is fever, and antibiotics are administered promptly, it is justifiable to attempt to eradicate colonisation rather than remove the infected catheter.— N. C. Weightman *et al.* (letter), *ibid.*, 1985, *16*, 275.

Toxic shock syndrome. The number of cases of toxic shock syndrome (TSS) reported before 1980 was small and the cases were often non-menstrual. However once TSS and its association with menstruation and tampon use became the subject of widespread publicity, physicians were stimulated to look for and report cases. The incubation period can be remarkably short, frequently 12 to 24 hours. In addition, surgical and nonsurgical lesions associated with TSS and from which *Staphylococcus aureus* is isolated can be small and can appear uninfected at the time when the patient is desperately ill. Therapy should include adequate fluid support, antibiotics effective against *Staph. aureus*, and, when appropriate, local measures such as incision and drainage.— A. L. Reingold, *J. Am. med. Ass.*, 1983, *249*, 932. The pathogenesis of TSS is still not understood but it often results from a localised infection with a strain of *Staph. aureus* that produces what is now called toxic shock toxin-1 (previously termed staphylococcal enterotoxin F and pyrogenic exotoxin C); lately, staphylococcal enterotoxin B has been assocated with non-menstrual TSS. The absence of bacteraemia in almost all reported cases of TSS provides further indirect evidence for the role of a toxin in the disease. It thus follows that treatment of TSS is primarily supportive. Antistaphylococcal antibiotics, together with removal of tampon or other drainage procedure, will eradicate the organism and thus prevent further elaboration of toxin. There is, however, no evidence that antibiotics will materially alter the clinical course of the disease, although they may prevent recurrences.— S. J. Eykyn, *Lancet*, 1988, *1*, 100.

Clinical and bacteriological observations of a toxic shock-like syndrome due to *Streptococcus pyogenes*.— L. A. Cone *et al.*, *New Engl. J. Med.*, 1987, *317*, 146.

Further references: *Ann. intern. Med.*, 1982, *96*, 831–996; A. W. Chow *et al.*, *Can. med. Ass. J.*, 1984, *130*, 425; A. S. Naidu *et al.* (letter), *Lancet*, 1986, *2*, 1454.

SEXUALLY TRANSMITTED DISEASES. Reviews on the treatment of sexually transmitted diseases: A. E. Washington, *Drugs*, 1984, *28*, 355; B. T. Goh, *Prescribers' J.*, 1987, *27* (5), 18; *Med. Lett.*, 1988, *30*, 5.

For comments on the treatment of pelvic inflammatory disease, see Pelvic Inflammatory Disease, above.

Chancroid. For the treatment of chancroid (*Haemophilus ducreyi* infection) the WHO recommends erythromycin 500 mg four times daily by mouth for 7 days or co-trimoxazole 960 mg twice daily by mouth for 5 days. Limited data suggest that adequate cure rates can also be obtained with thiamphenicol 2 to 5 g by mouth for 2 consecutive days or with single-dose regimens of ceftriaxone 250 mg intramuscularly, spectinomycin 2 g intramuscularly, or co-trimoxazole 3.84 g by mouth. Treatment failures have, however, been observed with co-trimoxazole in some areas.— WHO Expert Committee on Venereal Diseases and Treponematoses, Sixth Report, *Tech. Rep. Ser. Wld Hlth Org. No. 736*, 1986, p.130. A review from the Centers for Disease Control, USA concluding that erythromycin, co-trimoxazole, ceftriaxone, or the combination of amoxycillin with clavulanic acid could currently be relied on to treat chancroid successfully. However, there was significant geographical variability in the susceptibility of *H. ducreyi* to co-trimoxazole and limited experience with ceftriaxone and amoxycillin/clavulanic acid.— G. P. Schmid, *J. Am. med. Ass.*, 1986, *255*, 1757.

Further references: *Lancet*, 1982, *2*, 747; A. R. Ronald and F. A. Plummer, *Ann. intern. Med.*, 1985, *102*, 705.

Chlamydial infections. For the treatment of uncomplicated urethral, endocervical, or rectal infections due to *Chlamydia trachomatis* in adults the WHO recommends doxycycline or tetracycline hydrochloride both given by mouth for 7 days. Erythromcyin may be used as an alternative regimen for patients in whom tetracyclines are contra-indicated, such as pregnant women. Chlamydial lymphogranuloma due to lymphogranuloma venereum (LGV) biovars of *C. trachomatis* should be treated with tetracycline for 2 weeks. Alternative regimens include doxycycline, erythromycin, or sulphamethoxazole all given by mouth for 2 weeks.— WHO Expert Committee on Venereal Diseases and Treponematoses, Sixth Report, *Tech. Rep. Ser. Wld Hlth Org. No. 736*, 1986, p.124.

See also under Trachoma, below.

For the treatment of neonatal conjunctivitis due to *Chlamydia trachomatis*, see Pregnancy and the Neonate, above.

Further references: *Br. med. Bull.*, 1983, *39*, 107–208; W. R. Bowie, *Drugs*, 1984, *27*, 459; *Morb. Mortal.*, 1985, *34*, *Suppl.*, 53S; T. A. Bell and J. T. Grayston, *Ann. intern. Med.*, 1986, *104*, 524; L. L. Sanders *et al.*, *J. Am. med. Ass.*, 1986, *255*, 1750; S. M. Lisby and M. C. Nahata, *Clin. Pharm.*, 1987, *6*, 25; G. L. Gilbert, *Med. J. Aust.*, 1987, *146*, 205.

Gonorrhoea. For the treatment of uncomplicated urogenital infections due to gonococci the WHO recommends three groups of treatment regimen depending on resistance and geographical location. In areas in which gonococci are known to have maintained chromosomal sensitivity to antimicrobial agents and where beta-lactamase-producing gonococci comprise less than 1%, the WHO recommends single-dose regimens with amoxycillin, ampicillin, benzylpenicillin, or procaine penicillin, all given in association with probenecid, or treatment with doxycycline hydrochloride or tetracycline hydrochloride for 7 days. In areas where chromosomal gonococcal resistance has reduced the efficacy of antimicrobial agents such as benzylpenicillin, tetracycline, and co-trimoxazole to below 95%, and in areas where the prevalence of beta-lactamase-producing gonococci exceeds 5%, the WHO recommends single-dose regimens with cefotaxime, ceftriaxone, or spectinomycin, or cefoxitin given in association with probenecid. The third group of regimens show considerable geographical variation in their efficacy. They are active against beta-lactamase-producing gonococci, but are not recommended for pregnant women. These regimens include single-dose treatment with kanamycin or thiamphenicol, or co-trimoxazole given for 3 days, however, the co-trimoxazole regimen is often ineffective in localities where it has been used regularly for the treatment of gonorrhoea.

For rectal infections procaine penicillin in association with probenecid, cefotaxime, cefoxitin in association with probenecid, ceftriaxone, spectinomycin, kanamycin, or co-trimoxazole have been recommended, and for pharyngeal infections procaine penicillin with probenecid, tetracycline, ceftriaxone, or co-trimoxazole have been recommended, depending on the sensitivity of *N. gonorrhoeae* in the particular area. For disseminated infection benzylpenicillin which may be followed by amoxycillin or ampicillin, tetracycline hydrochloride, cefotaxime, cefoxitin, ceftriaxone, or spectinomycin have been recommended.

Treatment regimens recommended for adult conjunctivitis due to *N. gonorrhoeae* include parenteral cefoxitin, spectinomycin, or, in areas where the prevalence of penicillin-resistant strains is known to be less that 1%, benzylpenicillin. The eyes should be irrigated immediately with saline or buffered ophthalmic solutions, and irrigation repeated at hourly intervals until the discharge is eliminated; it is advisable to apply a topical antibiotic preparation each time the eyes are cleaned.— WHO Expert Committee on Venereal Diseases and Treponematoses, Sixth Report, *Tech. Rep. Ser. Wld Hlth Org. No. 736*, 1986, p.118.

For the prophylaxis and treatment of neonatal conjunctivitis due to *Neisseria gonorrhoeae*, see Pregnancy and the Neonate, above.

Further references to the treatment of gonorrhoea and the problem of resistant gonococci: E. W. Hook and K. K. Holmes, *Ann. intern. Med.*, 1985, *102*, 229; R. J. Rice and S. E. Thompson, *J. Am. med. Ass.*, 1986, *255*, 1739; C. R. Philpot and J. W. Tapsall, *Med. J. Aust.*, 1987, *146*, 254.

Syphilis. For the treatment of early syphilis, that is primary, secondary, and latent infections of not more than 2 years' duration, the WHO recommends benzathine penicillin as a single dose or procaine penicillin given daily for 10 days; in penicillin-allergic patients, tetracycline hydrochloride or erythromycin should be given for 15 days. Late syphilis, that is latent syphilis of more than 2 years' duration, or of indeterminate duration, late benign syphilis, cardiovascular syphilis, and neurosyphilis, require longer periods of treatment and the WHO recommends procaine penicillin for 15 days or, in the case of cardiovascular syphilis and neurosyphilis, for 20 days. Benzathine penicillin may be used as an alternative regimen, and tetracycyline hydrochloride or erythromycin should be used for patients who are allergic to penicillin.— WHO Expert Committee on Venereal Diseases and Treponematoses, Sixth Report, *Tech. Rep. Ser. Wld Hlth Org. No. 736*, 1986, p.126.

Further references: M. W. Adler, *Br. med. J.*, 1984, *288*, 551.

For the treatment of syphilis in pregnancy, see Pregnancy and the Neonate, above.

SKIN DISORDERS. A review of topical antibiotics and antiseptics for skin disorders. Topical antibiotics are useful for short-course treatment of impetigo, infected eczema, and other skin infection such as folliculitis; neomycin remains the drug of choice in impetigo. However, topical antibiotics encourage the emergence of bacterial resistance and can cause contact allergy, and should, therefore, not be used for longer than a week or two. Antibiotics of value in systemic use, such as gentamicin and fusidic acid, are best not used topically. Few studies have compared oral with topical antibiotics, or antibiotics with antiseptics in the management of skin infections. An oral antibiotic such as flucloxacillin is usually advised for widespread impetigo and infected eczema, some deep boils, or an antibiotic such as penicillin for cellulitis; an oral antibiotic is also used for less severe infections in immunocompromised patients and diabetics.— *Drug & Ther. Bull.*, 1987, *25*, 97.

A review of skin and soft-tissue infections and their treatment.

Impetigo is the most superficial skin infection and is especially contagious. In the *UK* it is usually caused by *Staphylococcus aureus*, but in West Indian and Asian immigrants *Streptococcus pyogenes* is more likely. Where the pathogen is *Staph. aureus* an antistaphylococcal penicillin such as flucloxacillin, oxacillin, cloxacillin, dicloxacillin or nafcillin is indicated; erythromycin is a suitable alternative in penicillin-allergic patients. Topical antibiotics are widely used but drug resistance has been encountered with tetracyclines, gentamicin, and fusidic acid; mupirocin has also proved topically effective against impetigo and other specific infections including those caused by methicillin-resistant *Staph. aureus*, but again resistant strains have been reported.

Erysipelas is a rapidly spreading infection of the skin complicated by lymphatic involvement and is largely caused by *Str. pyogenes*, although other beta-haemolytic streptococci and *Staph. aureus* occasionally produce a similar picture. Penicillin is usually indicated, but staphylococcal erysipelas should be treated with a penicillinase-resistant penicillin; erythromycin is an acceptable alternative in penicillin-hypersensitive patients.

Cellulitis is a more deep-seated spreading infection largely caused by *Str. pyogenes* or *Staph. aureus*. The principles of treatment are similar to those for erysipelas although parenteral therapy is needed more often. *Haemophilus influenzae* is an occasional cause of localised cellulitis and as resistant organisms may be a problem with ampicillin or chloramphenicol, cefuroxime seems preferable.

Folliculitis and *furunculosis* are usually due to *Staph. aureus*. Antibiotics are required only in the presence of systemic symptoms or spreading cellulitis; the drug of choice is an antistaphylococcal penicillin such as flucloxacillin or erythromycin as an alternative agent for penicillin-allergic patients. Recurrent furunculosis can be controlled with antiseptic soaps and shampoos containing chlorhexidine or hexachlorophane; mupirocin is also effective for localised staphylococcal sepsis.

For patients with *burns*, sepsis remains the major fatal complication. Prophylactic and especially topical antibiotics encourage resistance and may be toxic. Silver sulphadiazine cream has a broad spectrum and is especially active against Gram-negative bacteria although resistance can occur; mafenide acetate is also used. An essential element of management is removal of devitalised tissue, preferably before it has been heavily colonised. Infections with *Str. pyogenes* or *Staph. aureus* require aggressive treatment: for streptococcal infection penicillin is usually given with flucloxacillin to cover other beta-lactamase producing organisms; for staphylococcal infection a penicillinase-resistant penicillin is used; and for *Pseudomonas aeruginosa* infection an aminoglycoside plus an antipseudomonal beta-lactam antibiotic is used.

Staph. aureus can also cause the toxin-mediated condition, *staphylococcal scalded skin syndrome* (SSSS) which is an exfoliative dermatitis. Fluid and protein loses should be corrected and antistaphylococcal antibiotics such as flucloxacillin should be prescribed to eliminate the primary focus of infection.— R. Finch, *Lancet*, 1988, *1*, 164.

Acne. The mainstay in the management of moderate or severe acne is long-term, low-dose oral antibiotic therapy with either erythromycin or tetracyclines such as tetracycline or oxytetracycline; for maximum benefit treatment must be continued for at least 6 months. The place of topical antibiotics is less certain.— *Lancet*, 1982, *2*, 1138.

Further references to the treatment of acne vulgaris, with particular discussion on topical antibiotics: E. A. Eady *et al.*, *Br. J. Derm.*, 1982, *107*, 235; *idem*, *J. antimicrob. Chemother.*, 1982, *10*, 89; W. J. Cunliffe, *Prescribers' J.*, 1987, *27* (4), 23.

For a detailed review of the treatment of acne vulgaris, see under Tetracycline Hydrochloride, p.321.

Eczema. The treatment of atopic eczema in childhood.— D. J. Atherton, *Prescribers' J.*, 1986, *26*, 140. See also T. J. David and G. C. Cambridge, *Archs Dis. Childh.*, 1986, *61*, 20.

Ulcers. Management of ulcers of the leg with comments on the use of systemic and topical antibiotics.— T. J. Ryan, *Prescribers' J.*, 1987, *27* (4), 11.

TRACHOMA. References to the treatment and control of trachoma: C. R. Dawson *et al.*, *Guide to Trachoma Control*, World Health Organization, Geneva, 1981; S. Darougar and B. R. Jones, *Br. med. Bull.*, 1983, *39*, 117.

For the topical and systemic treatment of trachoma with tetracyclines, see under Tetracycline Hydrochloride, p.322.

For the treatment of other chlamydial infections, see Sexually Transmitted Diseases, above.

URINARY-TRACT INFECTIONS. General reviews and discussions on the aetiology of urinary-tract infections and the use of antimicrobial agents in their treatment: *Med. Lett.*, 1981, *23*, 69; C. M. Kunin, *Am. J. Med.*, 1981, *71*, 849; T. F. Keys and R. S. Edson, *Mayo Clin. Proc.*, 1983, *58*, 165; W. Brumfitt and J. M. T. Hamilton-Miller, *J. antimicrob. Chemother.*, 1984, *13*, *Suppl.* B, 121.

Reviews of the use of *single-dose therapy* in the management of uncomplicated urinary-tract infection: J. D. Anderson, *J. antimicrob. Chemother.*, 1980, *6*, 170;

Lancet, 1981, *1*, 26; J. T. Philbrick; J. P. Bracikowski, *Archs intern. Med.*, 1985, *145*, 1672; R. R. Bailey, *N.Z. med. J.*, 1985, *98*, 327; J. A. Whitworth, *Med. J. Aust.*, 1986, *144*, 136.

Reviews of the treatment of urinary-tract infections in *infants and children*: A. W. Asscher, *Prescribers' J.*, 1982, *22*, 19; P. L. Ogra and H. S. Faden, *J. Pediat.*, 1985, *106*, 1023.

Although treatment of asymptomatic bacteriuria reduced the infection in 110 schoolgirls compared with 98 controls followed-up for a mean period of 4 years, there was no significant difference in clinical outcome. Kidney scars that were associated with infection appeared to develop before the age of 5 years. It might be more beneficial to study these younger girls.— Cardiff-Oxford Bacteriuria Study Group, *Lancet*, 1978, *1*, 889.

A later 5-year study by the Newcastle Covert Bacteriuria Research Group (*Archs Dis. Childh.*, 1981, *56*, 585) had similar results to the Cardiff-Oxford Bacteriuria Study Group and found that when kidneys are radiologically normal, covert bacteriuria does not lead to renal damage even if no treatment is given. They concluded that until a reliable, non-radiological technique to detect renal scarring is available, screening schoolgirls for covert bacteriuria should not be recommended. However, the adequacy of the treatment used in some of these studies has been questioned (G.C. Arneil, *Br. med. J.*, 1985, *290*, 1925) and the view that untreated urinary-tract infections do not lead to further damage and scarring is contrary to the findings of J.M. Smellie *et al.* (*Br. med. J.*, 1985, *290*, 1957) who found that vesicoureteric reflux and urinary-tract infections are major contributory factors to the development of new renal scarring in children. They recommended that, to minimise the possibility of the formation of new scars in either normal or previously scarred kidneys, a child presenting with symptomatic urinary-tract infection for the first time, even if over 5 years of age, or one who suffers further infections after earlier presentation should receive prompt antibacterial treatment. This should be followed by prophylactic chemotherapy until the underlying cause of the infection has been determined. It has also been pointed out that scarring can now be detected using ultrasound techniques (G.A. Arneil, *Br. med. J.*, 1985, *290*, 1925).

Reviews of urinary-tract infection in the *elderly*: M. J. Bendall, *J. antimicrob. Chemother.*, 1984, *13*, *Suppl.* B, 69; W. G. Erwin and R. J. Anderson, *Hosp. Formul.*, 1985, *20*, 339.

References to the significance of bacteriuria in old age: A. S. Dontas *et al.*, *New Engl. J. Med.*, 1981, *304*, 939; G. R. Nordenstam *et al.*, *ibid.*, 1986, *314*, 1152.

References to urinary-tract infections associated with indwelling bladder catheters: R. Platt *et al.*, *New Engl. J. Med.*, 1982, *307*, 637; R. P. Stark and D. G. Maki, *New Engl. J. Med.*, 1984, *311*, 560.

Reviews of the management of *epididymitis*: *Lancet*, 1987, *2*, 1310.

Reviews of the treatment of chronic bacterial *prostatitis*: *Lancet*, 1983, *1*, 393; P. M. Hanus and L. H. Danziger, *Clin. Pharm.*, 1984, *3*, 49.

Reviews of dysuria in *women* and its treatment: A. L. Komaroff, *New Engl. J. Med.*, 1984, *310*, 368; B. Chattopadhyay, *J. antimicrob. Chemother.*, 1985, *16*, 680; *Lancet*, 1985, *1*, 1199; L. Cardozo, *Br. med. J.*, 1986, *293*, 1419.

From the re-evaluation of diagnostic criteria for coliform infection of the lower urinary-tract in symptomatic women it appeared that the presence of 100 coliforms or more per mL of urine, with pyuria may be the optimal predictive criteria for bladder infection.— W. E. Stamm *et al.*, *New Engl. J. Med.*, 1982, *307*, 463. Correction.— W. E. Stamm *et al.* (letter), *ibid.*, 1983, *308*, 463. Criticism. The increase in sensitivity is not cost effective and the specificity of the test is reduced. The sampling error involved with the use of such small quantities precludes any meaningful analysis.— G. W. Smith *et al.* (letter), *ibid.*, *309*, 1393. Comments.— *Lancet*, 1982, *2*, 694; N. B. Eastwood (letter), *ibid.*, 927.

Pregnancy and the neonate. Reviews on the management of bacteriuria in pregnancy: R. R. Bailey, *Drugs*, 1984, *27*, 183 (single-dose treatment); G. D. V. Hankins and P. J. Whalley, *Clin. Obstet. Gynec.*, 1985, *28*, 266; S. J. Pedler and A. J. Bint, *Drugs*, 1987, *33*, 413.

Prophylactic Use of Antibiotics

There are few occasions when the prophylactic use of antibiotics is justifiable. Patients at risk of developing endocarditis, including those with valvular heart disease or other cardiac abnormalities and those with a history of endocarditis or rheumatic fever, should be given antibiotics prophylactically when about to undergo dental operations, tonsillectomy, or other procedure liable to lead to bacteraemia. The antibiotic should be administered so that adequate blood and tissue concentrations are achieved throughout the procedure. Penicillins such as amoxycillin, phenoxymethylpenicillin, or benzylpenicillin, with or without an aminoglycoside, may be used or erythromycin or vancomycin in penicillin-allergic patients.

Patients who have had rheumatic fever may require prolonged prophylaxis against recurrent streptococcal infection. Phenoxymethylpenicillin given every day by mouth or a monthly intramuscular injection of benzathine penicillin may provide reasonable prophylaxis.

Antibiotics are sometimes given prophylactically to immunocompromised patients who are at special risk of acquiring infection.

The prophylactic use of antibiotics in surgery has been recommended in patients undergoing gastro-intestinal operations and in other types of surgery including cardiovascular, gynaecological, and orthopaedic operations. Antibiotics frequently used include cephalosporins, penicillins, and aminoglycosides. They should be injected immediately before, and if necessary, during the operation so that adequate concentrations are present. When anaerobic organisms are likely to be a problem, metronidazole (see p.669) may be used.

A review of the prophylactic use of antimicrobial agents.— R. E. Van Scoy and C. J. Wilkowske, *Mayo Clin. Proc.*, 1983, *58*, 241.

DIARRHOEA PROPHYLAXIS. For brief comments on the prophylactic use of antibiotics to prevent travellers' diarrhoea and in controlling cholera outbreaks, see under Diarrhoea and Enteric Infections in Choice of Antibiotic, p.96 and p.97.

ENDOCARDITIS PROPHYLAXIS. Reviews and discussions on prophylaxis of infective endocarditis: *Lancet*, 1984, *1*, 603; J. Delaye *et al.*, *Eur. Heart J.*, 1985, *6*, 826; G. K. Morris, *Br. med. J.*, 1985, *290*, 1532; *Drug & Ther. Bull.*, 1985, *23*, 53; D. Kaye, *Ann. intern. Med.*, 1986, *104*, 419; *Med. Lett.*, 1987, *29*, 109; S. Lang and A. Morris, *Drugs*, 1987, *34*, 279.

All authorities agree that it is important to provide antibiotic prophylaxis to cover certain procedures associated with predictable bacteraemia in patients with known or suspected susceptible heart lesions. Viridans streptococci are still the most frequent cause of infective endocarditis. Procedures which may result in bacteraemia include tonsillectomy or adenoidectomy and surgery or instrumentation of the genito-urinary or gastro-intestinal tracts, however dental treatment is the most common. To obtain most benefit from antibiotic prophylaxis it is essential that there should be maximum compliance by patients and dentists with simple recommendations. Earlier recommendations were usually complex and involved parenteral regimens which were painful for the patient and often difficult to arrange. It was against this background that an alternative simpler approach was suggested in the *UK* and guidelines were laid down by the Infective Endocarditis Working Party of the British Society for Antimicrobial Chemotherapy (BSAC). Similar procedures are now followed in many European countries (D.C. Shanson, *J. antimicrob. Chemother.*, 1987, *20*, *Suppl.* A, 119).

The Working Party of the BSAC (*Lancet*, 1982, *2*, 1323) has laid down the following recommendations for antibiotic prophylaxis of infective endocarditis: for prophylaxis of patients with prosthetic valves or other susceptible patients undergoing dental treatment in general dental practice the Working Party has recommended single-dose treatment with amoxycillin by mouth one hour before the operation; patients who are allergic to penicillins or patients who have received penicillins in the preceding month should be given erythromycin stearate by mouth 1 to 2 hours before the dental procedure followed by a second dose 6 hours later. The Working Party has, however, subsequently proposed that if prophylaxis is required twice in a month, amoxycillin should be given on both occasions (N.A. Simmons *et al.*, *Lancet*, 1986, *1*, 1267). The Working Party recommended that patients who are to have a general anaesthetic should receive amoxycillin intramuscularly before induction and a further dose by mouth 6 hours later. However, they subsequently amended this recommendation (N.A. Simmons *et al.*, *Lancet*, 1986, *1*, 1267) allowing 2 further regimens as alternatives: these regimens are amoxycillin given by mouth 4 hours before anaesthesia and again as soon as possible after the operation, or amoxycillin given by mouth together with probenecid 4 hours before the operation. The alternative regimens are considered more appropriate for use in general dental practice than parenteral administration. Patients who are to be given a general anaesthetic who have been given penicillins in the previous month, or who have a prosthetic valve, and patients who have had one or more attacks of endocarditis should be referred to hospital. The BSAC (*Lancet*, 1982) has recommended that they should be given amoxycillin in association with gentamicin both given intramuscularly immediately before induction of anaesthesia or 15 minutes before the dental procedure, and a further dose of amoxycillin by mouth 6 hours later. Patients to be given a general anaesthetic who are allergic to penicillins should also be referred to hospital and should be given vancomycin by intravenous infusion followed by gentamicin intravenously before induction of anaesthesia.

The BSAC has also recommended similar prophylaxis for genito-urinary surgery or instrumentation under general anaesthesia in patients with sterile urine; prophylaxis should be directed against faecal streptococci. They have recommended the use of amoxycillin in association with gentamicin both given intramuscularly immediately before induction and a further dose of amoxycillin given 6 hours later by mouth or intramuscularly; for patients allergic to penicillins the Working Party has recommended vancomycin followed by gentamicin given intravenously. The Working Party has not recommended any prophylaxis for uncomplicated vaginal delivery, minor obstetric and gynaecological procedures such as cervical dilatation and curettage of the uterus, and the insertion or removal of intra-uterine contraceptive devices, except in patients with prosthetic valves who should receive the same prophylaxis as for genito-urinary surgery. Similarly routine prophylaxis has not been recommended for patients undergoing some gastro-intestinal procedures such as endoscopy, colonoscopy, proctoscopy, sigmoidoscopy, or barium enema, although patients with prosthetic valves should receive prophylaxis effective against faecal streptococci as recommended for genito-urinary surgery. Prophylactic antibiotics should be given to susceptible patients undergoing tonsillectomy or adenoidectomy similarly to dental patients under general anaesthesia, although since patients will have pain on swallowing the second dose of amoxycillin should be given intramuscularly or in liquid form by mouth.

Other workers have commented on the BSAC recommendations including O'Connor and Axon (*Lancet*, 1983, *1*, 237) who suggested that the simpler regimen of amoxycillin by mouth could be used for patients with prosthetic valves undergoing gastro-intestinal endoscopy, and Holbrook (*Br. med. J.*, 1985, *290*, 317) who commented on the occurrence of streptococci tolerant to penicillin and that a second dose of amoxycillin 8 hours after the first may well give time for host defences to operate by prolonging the period during which the bacteria are inhibited.

The American Heart Association (AHA) has proposed slightly different regimens for prophylaxis of dental procedures and upper respiratory-tract surgical procedures (S.T. Shulman *et al.*, *Circulation*, 1984, *70*, 1123A). For standard prophylaxis the Committee on Rheumatic Fever and Infective Endocarditis of the Council on Cardiovascular Disease in the Young has proposed administration of phenoxymethylpenicillin by mouth 1 hour before the procedure and 6 hours later, or benzylpenicillin given intravenously or intramuscularly for patients unable to take oral antibiotics. When maximal protection is required, as in patients with prosthetic valves, ampicillin plus gentamicin both given intravenously or intramuscularly half an hour before the procedure have been recommended, followed by phenoxymethylpenicillin given by mouth 6 hours later or, alternatively, the parenteral regimen may be repeated once 8 hours later. For penicillin-allergic patients, the AHA has recommended an oral regimen of erythromycin given one hour before the procedure and 6 hours later, and a parenteral regimen of vancomycin given by slow intravenous infusion. For genito-urinary/gastro-intestinal tract procedures prophylaxis with ampicillin and gentamicin given intramuscularly or intravenously has been recommended, or vancomycin plus gentamicin for patients allergic to penicillin. For minor or repetitive procedures in low-risk patients amoxycillin may be given by mouth.

INFECTION PROPHYLAXIS, HYPOSPLENISM. In the absence of splenic phagocytic function asplenic patients or hyposplenic patients, such as those with sickle-cell anaemia, have impaired immunity to blood-borne bacterial and protozoal infections (A. Ferguson, *Br. med. J.*, 1982, *285*, 1375; S.C. Davies and P.E. Hewitt, *Br. J. Hosp. Med.*, 1984, *31*, 440). Pneumococci are a major cause of infection and meningococci and *Haemophilus*

influenzae are amongst the other organisms associated with fulminant infection. Prophylactic penicillin and pneumococcal vaccine have been recommended for asplenic patients (*Lancet*, 1985, *2*, 928); penicillin is usually given by mouth in a dose of 125 mg twice daily, however, there are problems of compliance associated with long-term therapy and so a long-acting preparation such as benzathine penicillin has been tried although the pain of intramuscular injection has limited its use (B. Modell and M. Petrou, *Archs Dis. Childh.*, 1983, *58*, 1026; A.B. John *et al.*, *Br. med. J.*, 1984, *288*, 1567).
There are problems associated with the length of treatment necessary, the increasing resistance of pneumococci to penicillin, and the penicillin-sensitivity of other organisms which can cause post-splenectomy sepsis (*Lancet*, 1985, *2*, 928). The patients at risk after splenectomy can be divided into 3 groups: firstly, infants less than 2 years old, susceptible to Gram-negative organisms as well as pneumococci, who should receive penicillin prophylaxis and probably coverage for Gram-negative organisms as well; secondly, patients requiring splenectomy for underlying disease who should receive pneumococcal vaccine before the operation and prophylactic penicillin for an indefinite period with routine revaccination every 3 years; and thirdly, patients with splenectomy related to trauma who can receive pneumococcal vaccine alone (J.P. Hatch *et al.*, *Can. med. Ass. J.*, 1983, *129*, 851). There have, however, been reports of fatal post-splenectomy pneumococcal sepsis despite prophylaxis with penicillin and pneumococcal vaccine (D.I.K. Evans, *Lancet*, 1984, *1*, 1124; F. Brivet *et al.*, *ibid.*, *2*, 356; D.I.K. Evans, *J. clin. Path.*, 1985, *38*, 309).
The risk of infection remains life-long so cases will continue to occur, and the best hope for a successful outcome is early recognition and urgent treatment (S.D. Scott, *Lancet*, 1987, *2*, 569). To reduce the case-fatality it has been proposed that patients should be given a 'splenectomy warning' card to carry at all times and a stock of amoxycillin 500 mg tablets (or an alternative if they are hypersensitive to penicillin) with instructions to take 2 tablets with the first symptom of illness or fever, and to seek medical advise urgently. This should delay the development of overwhelming sepsis while a medical assessment is made. Amoxycillin is considered preferable to phenoxymethylpenicillin because of better oral absorption and activity against other organisms that may cause fatal post-splenectomy sepsis, such as *H. influenzae* and meningococci (A.S. Duncombe *et al.*, *Lancet*, 1987, *1*, 570).
For children with sickle-cell anaemia, prophylaxis with phenoxymethylpenicillin potassium 125 mg twice daily by mouth has been demonstrated to significantly reduce the incidence of pneumococcal septicaemia (M.H. Gaston *et al.*, *New Engl. J. Med.*, 1986, *314*, 1593). Babies with sickle-cell disease should receive penicillin prophylaxis by 4 months of age at the latest, in order to decrease the morbidity and mortality associated with pneumococcal infections. Pneumococcal vaccine does not provide protection for young children because of their suboptimal immune response and because the vaccine does not contain all the serotypes that can cause infection in these young children (*Lancet*, 1986, *2*, 1432).

MENINGITIS PROPHYLAXIS. Although vaccines have been used to prevent infections due to *Haemophilus influenzae* and meninogococci (see p.1163 and p.1169), appropriate vaccines are not available for all types of these pathogens and they may not be effective in children under 2 years of age. Consequently prophylaxis against meningitis in contacts of patients infected with these organisms has largely been implemented using antimicrobial agents. Sulphonamides such as sulphadiazine (p.303) have been used for eradication of nasopharyngeal carriage and prophylaxis against meningococcal meningitis, but many strains are now resistant and therefore unless sulphonamide-sensitivity has been demonstrated, rifampicin (p.576) is considered to be the agent of choice with minocycline (p.263) being used as a reserve agent. Chemoprophylaxis against *Haemophilus influenzae* is still controversial and not so widely accepted, however, rifampicin appears to be effective in eradicating nasal carriage and some authorities in the *US* recommend its use in certain patients at risk (p.576).
As antimicrobial agents used to treat meningitis often do not eliminate carriage of the causative organism it is generally recommended that the index patient should also receive prophylaxis following treatment.

NEONATAL CONJUNCTIVITIS PROPHYLAXIS. For the prevention of conjunctivitis of the newborn, see under Pregnancy and the Neonate in Choice of Antibiotic, p.99.

RHEUMATIC FEVER PROPHYLAXIS. Acute rheumatic fever as a consequence of preceding group A streptococcal upper-respiratory-tract infection can usually be prevented by accurate diagnosis of streptococcal tonsillopharyngitis, followed by therapy with penicillin or, in allergic patients, with erythromycin (S.T. Shulman *et al.*, *Circulation*, 1984, *70*, 1118A). However, the occurrence of rheumatic fever has declined in developed countries and some clinicians feel that the use of antibiotics should be determined by the incidence of rheumatic fever in their particular area (A. Shuper and M. Mimouni, *Can. med. Ass. J.*, 1984, *131*, 278). Howie and Foggo (*J. R. Coll. gen. Pract.*, 1985, *35*, 223) carried out a retrospective study of 58 children classified as having had rheumatic fever and they concluded that the prescribing of antibiotics for streptococcal sore throats made little contribution to the low incidence of rheumatic fever. However, Krober *et al.*, (*J. Am. med. Ass.*, 1985, *253*, 1271) demonstrated a significant clinical improvement in children with group A beta-haemolytic streptococcal infection who received early treatment with phenoxymethylpenicillin compared with placebo. Although a delay in treatment of up to a few days was not considered to place the patient at risk of developing rheumatic fever, they suggested that the clinical benefits of early treatment of streptococcal sore throats, which included shorter duration of symptoms and reduced contagious period, should be taken into consideration when making the decision of early or delayed treatment of these patients. Some workers feel that therapy need not be initiated if rapid latex agglutination tests are negative or that therapy can be discontinued in those patients who have negative throat cultures (V.A. Fulginiti, *J. Am. med. Ass.*, 1985, *254*, 907; H.W. Fink, *ibid.*), whereas others would continue therapy despite negative throat cultures (M. Soman, *ibid.*).
When antibiotic therapy is given to prevent acute rheumatic fever, penicillin is considered the drug of choice. For many years benzathine penicillin has been used, thus avoiding problems of patient compliance. However, the injection is painful and there is a risk of hypersensitivity reactions; in developed countries treatment has shifted in favour of oral therapy (A.L. Bisno, *J. Am. med. Ass.*, 1985, *254*, 538; J.W. Bass, *ibid.*, 1986, *256*, 740).
Once a patient has had an attack of rheumatic fever, continuous antibiotic prophylaxis is required because of the high risk of recurrence. The precise duration of prophylactic treatment is uncertain, although it is generally recommended that antibiotic administration should be continued until late childhood (*Lancet*, 1985, *2*, 647).

See also under Respiratory-tract Infections, Pharyngitis, in Choice of Antibiotic, p.100.

SUPPRESSION OF INTESTINAL FLORA. For reference to regimens used to prevent colonisation and infection in high-risk patients by the selective decontamination of the gastro-intestinal tract, see Colistin Sulphomethate Sodium, p.205.

SURGICAL INFECTION PROPHYLAXIS. When considering a surgical patient for antibiotic prophylaxis it must be decided whether the surgical field is contaminated with bacteria. If there is an area of cellulitis, an abscess, or a fistula or if a perforated viscus or an established infection is present before operation, prophylaxis is inappropriate as antibiotics in therapeutic doses are required. It must also be decided whether the bacterial contamination is likely to be exogenous or endogenous. Exogenous sepsis is usually staphylococcal unless the wound is in the groin or near the perineum. Prophylactic antibiotics play no part in preventing such infections, but this form of sepsis may be minimised by aseptic techniques, adequate preparation of the skin, and control of the environment of the operating theatre. Perioperative antibiotic cover is indicated, however, for replacement of joints, heart valves, and arteries with synthetic grafts, because although the risk of sepsis in such patients is low, the morbidity and mortality of 'implant sepsis' are high. In endogenous sepsis the bacteria originate from the female genital tract, the lower urinary tract, and the intestine. This form of sepsis is not influenced by preparation of the skin or the environment, and perioperative antibiotics play an important part in preventing infection. The principle of antibiotic prophylaxis is to provide a concentration of antibiotic in the circulation and tissues that will kill any bacteria introduced into the operative field. The antibiotic should be effective against the predominant pathogenic bacteria and given in a dose that provides a serum concentration at least 4 times greater than the minimum inhibitory concentration of these organisms for the duration of the operation. It is preferable to choose a non-toxic antibiotic, with low protein binding, which is not usually used as first-line treatment for serious infections. Controversy remains over the most appropriate route of administration of the antibiotic. Topical application into the wound at the end of an operation is not recommended because this does not give adequate peroperative serum concentrations; similarly intraperitoneal antibiotics are not advised for prophylaxis. Antibiotics may, however, be given by local infiltration into the site of surgical incision before operation, as high concentrations of antibiotic are maintained in both the wound and in the circulation. Some surgeons give combinations of agents such as neomycin with metronidazole or erythromycin by mouth before colorectal surgery on the premise that this will 'sterilise' the colon. However, this is only a theoretical concept as although counts of faecal bacteria in the colon may be reduced, disturbance of the normal ecology of the colon has disadvantages, and several studies have shown that systemic antibiotic administration is at least as effective and is safer than giving oral antibiotics.— M. R. B. Keighley, *Br. med. J.*, 1983, *286*, 1844.

Recommendations from the *USA* for antimicrobial prophylaxis in surgery; a single dose of a parenteral antimicrobial given within 30 minutes of an operation usually provides adequate tissue concentrations throughout the procedure. When surgery is delayed or prolonged, a second, intra-operative dose is advisable, unless the prophylactic agent has an extended serum half-life. Postoperative doses of prophylactic drugs are generally unnecessary and potentially harmful. An effective prophylactic regimen should be directed against the most likely infecting organisms, but need not eradicate every potential pathogen. For most procedures, a first-generation cephalosporin such as cephazolin, cephalothin, cefapirin, or cephradine should be effective; cephazolin has the advantage of a longer serum half-life and causes less pain with intramuscular injection. For colorectal surgery and appendectomy, cefoxitin is preferred because it is more active against bowel anaerobes including *Bacteroides fragilis*. Single-dose prophylaxis with second-generation cephalosporins that have extended serum half-lives such as cefotetan, ceforanide, cefonicid, or cefuroxime has no advantage over single-dose cephazolin or cefoxitin prophylaxis unless the surgery is protracted.— *Med. Lett.*, 1987, *29*, 91.

A review from the *UK* of surgical infection prophylaxis. The choice of drug can only be decided by comparative clinical studies, but a knowledge of the nature of the likely contaminants is essential. The selected antibiotic must be capable of diffusing into the tissues and should have a reasonably long elimination half-life. Antimicrobial drugs are usually given intravenously at induction of anaesthesia, but intra-incisional placement of the drug before skin closure is an acceptable alternative that provides a high local concentration of the antibiotic. The number of doses which should be given is still controversial, but prolonged use is not justified. For clean operations, with no prosthesis inserted, antibiotics are not considered to be necessary, but for clean operations with prosthesis inserted or clean cardiac or neurosurgical operations, 1 to 3 parenteral doses of flucloxacillin and/or an aminoglycoside have been used. For potentially contaminated operations including those on the gastric/biliary or urinary tracts, caesarean section, or lung resection, 1 to 3 parenteral doses of a beta-lactam antibiotic have been used, and for lower intestinal or uterus/vagina operations metronidazole is given in addition to the beta-lactam antibiotic; an aminoglycoside may be used in place of the beta-lactam for lower intestinal operations. In contaminated operations antibiotics may be required for longer: for perforated peptic ulcer, 1 to 3 parenteral doses of a beta-lactam antibiotic have been used; for perforated appendix, 3 or more parenteral doses of beta-lactam with metronidazole are required; and for perforated intestine, 3 or more parenteral doses of beta-lactam or aminoglycoside, both in association with metronidazole, are used.— A. V. Pollock, *Lancet*, 1988, *1*, 225.

Further references: P. O'Brien and P. McDonald, *Med. J. Aust.*, 1985, *143*, 149; A. B. Kaiser, *New Engl. J. Med.*, 1986, *315*, 1129; M. R. B. Keighley, *Br. med. Bull.*, 1988, *44*, 374.
References to the prophylactic use of antibiotics for specific surgical procedures: *Lancet*, 1985, *1*, 378 (joint surgery); *ibid.*, *2*, 701 (cardiac surgery); T. R. Beam, *Antibiotics Chemother.*, 1985, *33*, 114 (cardiac surgery); M. Farrington, *J. antimicrob. Chemother.*, 1986, *18*, 656 (coronary artery bypass surgery); A. P. R. Wilson *et al.*, *Thorax*, 1986, *41*, 396 (cardiothoracic surgery); *Lancet*, 1986, *1*, 537 (cardiac pacemaker insertion); E. M. Brown, *J. antimicrob. Chemother.*, 1987, *20*, 143 (hysterectomy); L. Danziger and E. Hassan, *Drug Intell. & clin. Pharm.*, 1987, *21*, 406 (gastro-intestinal surgery).

See under Flucloxacillin Sodium, p.232, for the use of beta-lactamase-stable penicillins and other antibiotics in cardiothoracic surgery. See under Metronidazole, p.670, for the prophylactic use of metronidazole and related nitroimidazoles in surgical procedures where anaerobic organisms are likely pathogens.

Hazards of Antibiotic Therapy

Most antibiotics given by mouth in large enough doses may cause gastro-intestinal irritation. Severe and sometimes fatal pseudomembranous colitis has occurred, especially with clindamycin and lincomycin and also with ampicillin and amoxycillin. Antibiotics may interfere with the absorption of essential food factors such as vitamins by provoking diarrhoea; they may also reduce the numbers of micro-organisms synthesising vitamin K in the intestines.

Supra-infection is usually attributable to the suppression of antibiotic-susceptible micro-organisms which normally provide natural competition to prevent the unlimited multiplication of antibiotic-resistant micro-organisms. The administration of broad-spectrum antibiotics, especially by mouth, may result in supra-infection with *Candida* and other yeasts, filamentous fungi, or resistant Gram-negative bacteria, affecting the mouth, gastro-intestinal tract, or upper respiratory tract. If supra-infection occurs the antibiotic should be withdrawn and other measures to which the supra-infection responds should be substituted.

Compounds may cause pain when given by intramuscular injection and thrombophlebitis when given intravenously.

Allergy and hypersensitivity reactions to antibiotics are particularly troublesome with the penicillins, streptomycin, and sulphonamides. The topical application of neomycin and other antibiotics increases the risk of inducing sensitisation, and allergic reactions in a previously sensitised person may be severe and life-threatening. They often take the form of an urticarial rash and angioedema, and may involve bronchospasm and cardiovascular failure. Adrenaline, antihistamines, and corticosteroids are used to treat severe or persistent toxic symptoms. Allergic contact dermatitis has been reported in persons who regularly handle antibiotics. The topical use of antibiotics is also associated with an increased incidence of bacterial resistance.

Tetracycline has a tendency to be concentrated in developing teeth and bones. The aminoglycosides, polymyxins, tetracyclines, and lincosamides are liable to cause apnoea by blocking neuromuscular transmission if given in large doses, especially if introduced into the peritoneal cavity. Many antibiotics cause damage to the kidneys; a few may damage the eighth cranial nerve or the bone marrow, especially if abnormally high serum concentrations result from impaired excretion. Antibiotics which readily diffuse across the placenta, such as tetracyclines, may be toxic to the foetus if given during pregnancy. The inability of premature and newborn infants to conjugate some antibiotics in the liver may be a factor in toxicity.

A brief analysis of adverse effects of antimicrobial agents reported to the Committee on Safety of Drugs and the Committee on Safety of Medicines between 1964 and 1985.— *Br. med. J.*, 1986, *293*, 1163.

Antibiotics, especially those that exert their effect on the bacterial cell wall, have the potential to release endotoxins from Gram-negative bacteria and could therefore induce or exacerbate shock in bacteraemic patients.— *Lancet*, 1985, *2*, 594.

A discussion on the pathogenesis of the Jarisch-Herxheimer reaction which occurs commonly after treatment of syphilis or relapsing fever with antibiotics.— T. Butler, *Ann. intern. Med.*, 1985, *102*, 397.

ALLERGY. Proceedings of a conference on immediate hypersensitivity reactions to beta-lactam antibiotics.— *Ann. intern. Med.*, 1987, *107*, 204.

EFFECTS ON THE BLOOD. Reviews and discussions on hypoprothrombinaemia and platelet dysfunction caused by antimicrobial agents, particularly beta-lactam antibiotics: C. R. Smith and J. J. Lipsky, *J. antimicrob. Chemother.*, 1983, *11*, 496; *Lancet*, 1983, *1*, 510; H. Ferres and B. Nunn (letter), *ibid.*, *2*, 226; F. R. Sattler *et al.*, *Ann. intern. Med.*, 1986, *105*, 924; L. M. Babiak and M. J. Rybak, *Drug Intell. & clin. Pharm.*, 1986, *20*, 833; J. J. Lipsky, *J. antimicrob. Chemother.*, 1988, *21*, 281.

Case reports and discussion on neutropenia associated with beta-lactam antibiotics.— C. F. Kirkwood *et al.*, *Clin. Pharm.*, 1983, *2*, 569.

EFFECTS ON THE GASTRO-INTESTINAL TRACT. References to the effects of antimicrobial agents on the bacterial flora of the gastro-intestinal tract: H. Sakata *et al.*, *Antimicrob. Ag. Chemother.*, 1986, *29*, 225; S. T. Chambers *et al.*, *J. antimicrob. Chemother.*, 1987, *19*, 685.

Antibiotic-associated colitis. A review of pseudomembranous colitis which is most commonly attributed to antibiotic therapy. Antibiotic-associated pseudomembranous colitis usually develops as a result of overgrowth and toxin production by *Clostridium difficile* when the normal colonic microflora has been disturbed. *Cl. difficile* produces toxin A (enterotoxin) and toxin B (cytotoxin); toxin C has also been described. Pseudomembranous colitis has occasionally been associated with the overgrowth of *Campylobacter jejuni*, *Staphylococcus aureus*, or *Cl. perfringens*. Most cases of antibiotic-associated pseudomembranous colitis occur 4 to 9 days after the start of antibiotic therapy, although onset is delayed for up to 6 weeks after completion of treatment in 25 to 40% of patients and can occur after a single dose. Oral administration accounts for 50 to 80% of reported cases and usually involves a single agent. When pseudomembranous colitis follows parenteral therapy antibiotic combinations are commonly implicated. Most antibiotics have now been associated with the development of pseudomembranous colitis although those that cause least upset to the colonic microflora are less likely to be implicated. Changing prescribing patterns probably account for the recent decrease in cases attributed to clindamycin; the cephalosporins have shown a corresponding rise and now account for about 30% of cases. Ampicillin and amoxycillin together also account for about 30% of cases while other penicillins are much less frequently involved.— R. P. Bolton and D. F. M. Thomas, *Br. J. Hosp. Med.*, 1986, *35*, 37.

Further references: M. H. Gross, *Clin. Pharm.*, 1985, *4*, 304; G. P. Young *et al.*, *Med. J. Aust.*, 1986, *144*, 303.

For reference to the treatment of antibiotic-associated colitis, see Vancomycin Hydrochloride, p.335.

EFFECTS ON IMMUNE FUNCTION. A brief discussion of the effects of antimicrobial agents on host defence mechanisms.— J. M. Oleske, *J. antimicrob. Chemother.*, 1984, *13*, 413.

EFFECTS ON THE KIDNEY. A review of the nephrotoxicity of antimicrobial agents.— G. B. Appel and H. C. Neu, *New Engl. J. Med.*, 1977, *296*, 663, 722, and 784.

Antibiotic damage to damaged kidneys.— *Lancet*, 1978, *2*, 558.

EFFECTS ON THE LIVER. A short discussion on antimicrobial agents and hepatotoxicity.— *Br. med. J.*, 1980, *280*, 1486.

EFFECTS ON THE NERVOUS SYSTEM. References to the neurotoxicity of antimicrobial agents: S. R. Snavely and G. R. Hodges, *Ann. intern. Med.*, 1984, *101*, 92.

EFFECTS ON THE NEUROMUSCULAR SYSTEM. Case reports and a discussion of antibiotic-induced paralysis.— C. B. Pittinger *et al.*, *Anesth. Analg.*, 1970, *49*, 487.

INTERACTIONS. A review of the interactions of antibiotics with other drugs.— M. J. Wood, *J. antimicrob. Chemother.*, 1987, *20*, 628.

Oral contraceptives. A brief review of the effects of antimicrobial agents on the efficacy of oral contraceptives.— *Drug & Ther. Bull.*, 1987, *25*, 5.

PREGNANCY AND THE NEONATE. Reviews and discussions on the safety of antimicrobial agents in pregnancy: A. W. Chow and P. J. Jewesson, *Rev. infect. Dis.*, 1985, *7*, 287; H. Knothe and G. A. Dette, *Infection*, 1985, *13*, 49; R. Wise, *Br. med. J.*, 1987, *294*, 42; *Med. Lett.*, 1987, *29*, 61.

Antibiotics in Food

The use of antibiotics for the treatment of bovine mastitis or other infections in animals, the feeding of antibiotics to young farm stock to accelerate growth, or the employment of antibiotics in various ways as food preservatives or to control diseases of plants may result in possible hazards to human health due to traces of antibiotics being present in food; such uses are therefore controlled in many countries. Hazards may include direct toxic effects, hypersensitivity reactions, and the production of antibiotic resistance in pathogenic organisms transmissible to man.

For a discussion of the uses of antibiotics in animal husbandry with a consideration of the hazards to public health, see *Report of the Joint Committee on the Use of Antibiotics in Animal Husbandry and Veterinary Medicine*, [Swann Report], London, HM Stationery Office, 1969.

A discussion of controls on the use of antibiotics in animal husbandry.— J. Wingfield and G. E. Appelbe, *Pharm. J.*, 1984, *2*, 717.

Recommendations on the use of human food from animals treated with antibiotics. In order to ensure that there were no antibiotic residues in human food derived from animals treated for diseases an interval should be allowed between the last treatment and the time of slaughter. Usually 48 hours was sufficient for the elimination of the antibiotic but this might not be so and manufacturers should state on the label the interval that was required. Eggs from poultry receiving therapeutic amounts of antibiotics should not be sold for human consumption.— *Tech. Rep. Ser. Wld Hlth Org. No. 260*, 1963.

Generally, antibiotics should only be considered for use as direct food additives if they did not affect microbial spoilage of food so as to result in danger to the consumer, were not of therapeutic importance, and did not give rise to cross-resistance or affect the clinical use of other antibiotics. Information should be obtained on the effects on the normal body flora of an antibiotic suggested for use as an intentional food additive. The usual standards of food hygiene should not be permitted to diminish because of the use of an antibiotic as a food additive.— Twelfth Report of the Joint FAO/WHO Expert Committee on Food Additives, *Tech. Rep. Ser. Wld Hlth Org. No. 430*, 1969.

In surveys conducted over the past 10 years by the Working Party on Veterinary Residues in Animal Products, antimicrobial activity was detected infrequently in meat and kidney but the bacteriological tests used did not always allow identification of the substances present. Residues of sulphadimidine could, however, be quantified and were sometimes found in concentrations that were beyond the maximum acceptable, especially in pig kidneys.— *Lancet*, 1987, *2*, 1225.

ANTIBIOTIC RESIDUES IN MILK

When antibiotics are administered parenterally in full therapeutic doses some excretion occurs in the milk. A much more important cause of the presence of antibiotics in cows' milk is intramammary injection via the teat canal for the treatment of mastitis. Antibiotics used for this purpose include procaine penicillin, cloxacillin, cephalonium, cephoxazole, dihydrostreptomycin, erythromycin, neomycin, spiramycin, and the tetracyclines. There are guidelines both on the time that should elapse after the antibiotic treatment of cows before milk should be collected for human consumption, and on the concentrations of antibiotic residues permitted in milk.

A detailed review of the risk of primary sensitisation, and of the hazard to penicillin-allergic patients, of low concentrations of penicillins in milk resulting from their use in the treatment of bovine mastitis. It was concluded that no immunological benefits were likely to accrue from further lowering of acceptable levels of penicillin in milk.— J. M. Dewdney and R. G. Edwards, *J. R. Soc. Med.*, 1984, *77*, 866.

Comment on outbreaks of serious group C streptococcal disease in which unpasteurised milk had been implicated as a cause. The average penicillin content of milk had fallen from 0.01 to 0.00018 μg per mL in the years 1961 to 1983 reflecting the more rigorous control of penicillin content. Under current statutory controls of penicillin concentrations in retailed milk, pasteurisation remains the sole means of protection against serious group C streptococcal disease.— M. R. Millar and T. J. J. Inglis (letter), *Lancet*, 1985, *1*, 694.

ANTIBIOTIC SUPPLEMENTS FOR ANIMAL FEEDS

Small quantities of certain antibiotics are added to the feed of young animals with the object of stimulating the rate of growth. Antibiotics which have been permitted in the European Economic Community (EEC) include avoparcin, bacitracin zinc, bambermycin, monensin sodium, nosiheptide, spiramycin, tylosin, and virginiamycin. Carbadox, nitrovin, and olaquindox are also used as growth promoters, although the use of carbadox is prohibited in the *UK*.

In the *UK* control is implemented by means of

the Medicines (Medicated Animal Feeding Stuffs) Regulations 1988.

The administration of antibiotics to farm livestock at subtherapeutic concentrations posed certain hazards to human and animal health. There was evidence to show that enteric bacteria of animal origin were commonly ingested by man and an infection by an organism with multiple drug resistance could endanger the life of the patient. Further, transfer of resistance from nonpathogenic to pathogenic organisms could occur. It was recommended that the use without prescription of antibiotics in animal feeding stuffs should be restricted to those antibiotics which had little or no application as therapeutic agents in man or animals and which would not impair the efficacy of a prescribed therapeutic drug through the development of resistant strains of organisms.— *Report of the Joint Committee on the Use of Antibiotics in Animal Husbandry and Veterinary Medicine* [Swann Report], London, HM Stationery Office, 1969. See also *Ten Years on from Swann*, D.W. Jolly *et al.* (Ed.), London, The Association of Veterinarians in Industry, 1981.

There has been concern that the addition of subtherapeutic amounts of broad-spectrum antibiotics as growth promotors to animal feeds may result in the emergence of increasing numbers of antibiotic-resistant bacteria that threaten human health. These concerns have led to the removal of therapeutic antibiotics from subtherapeutic use in England and other countries of the EEC, but not in the *USA*. To date, all cases of animal-to-human spread of disease from resistant bacteria have originated in livestock in which antibiotic use has been either at therapeutic levels or ill-defined. Holnberg *et al.* (*New Engl. J. Med.*, 1984, *311*, 617), however, reported an outbreak of infection in 18 people attributed to a multiply-resistant strain of *Salmonella newport* which appeared to have been transmitted in contaminated meat from cattle fed subtherapeutic amounts of chlortetracycline. This report also showed that probable inappropriate use of antibiotics by the people involved increased the disease potential of the resistant *Salmonella* once ingested. Every animal or person taking an antibiotic, whether in therapeutic or subtherapeutic amounts, becomes a factory producing resistant strains of bacteria through selection of existing and newly emerging resistant organisms.— S. B. Levy, *New Engl. J. Med.*, 1984, *311*, 663.

Antibiotic Groups

Although antibiotics are a very diverse class of compounds they are often classified and discussed in groups. They may be classified according to their mode of action or spectrum of antimicrobial activity but generally antibiotics with similar chemical structures are grouped together.

The Aminoglycosides

The aminoglycosides are a closely-related group of bactericidal antibiotics derived from bacteria of the order Actinomycetales or, more specifically, the genus *Streptomyces* (framycetin, kanamycin, neomycin, paromomycin, streptomycin, and tobramycin) and the genus *Micromonospora* (gentamicin and sissomicin). They are polycationic compounds which are generally used as the sulphate and contain 2-deoxystreptamine (or streptose in streptomycin) with cyclic amino-sugars attached by glycosidic linkages. They have also been termed aminoglycosidic aminocyclitols.

The aminoglycosides have broadly similar toxicological features. Ototoxicity is a major limitation to their use; streptomycin and gentamicin are generally considered to be more toxic to the vestibular branch of the eighth cranial nerve and neomycin and kanamycin to be more toxic to the auditory branch. Other adverse effects common to the group include nephrotoxicity, neuromuscular blocking activity, and allergy, including cross-reactivity.

The pharmacokinetics of the aminoglycosides are very similar. Little is absorbed from the gastro-intestinal tract but they are generally well-distributed in the body after parenteral administration although penetration into the cerebrospinal fluid is poor. They are excreted unchanged in the urine by glomerular filtration.

The aminoglycosides have a similar antimicrobial spectrum and appear to act by interfering with bacterial protein synthesis, possibly by binding irreversibly to the 30S portion of the bacterial ribosome. They are most active against Gram-negative rods. *Staphylococcus aureus* is susceptible to the aminoglycosides but otherwise most Gram-positive bacteria, and also anaerobic bacteria, are naturally resistant. They show enhanced activity with penicillin against some enterococci and streptococci. Bacterial resistance to streptomycin may occur by mutation whereas with the other aminoglycosides it is usually associated with the plasmid-mediated production of inactivating enzymes which are capable of phosphorylation, acetylation, or adenylation.

Streptomycin was the first aminoglycoside to become available commercially and was isolated from a strain of *Streptomyces griseus* in 1944. Its use is now restricted mainly to the treatment of tuberculosis when it is always administered in association with other antituberculous drugs because of the rapid development of resistance. *Dihydrostreptomycin*, a reduction product of streptomycin, is only rarely used because of its toxicity. The *neomycin* complex of antibiotics were the next to be isolated; neomycin itself is mainly a mixture of the B and C isomers and neomycin B is considered to be identical with *framycetin.* Because of their toxicity they are not given systemically. The same applies to *paromomycin* which may be used in the treatment of intestinal amoebiasis. *Kanamycin* is less toxic than neomycin and can be used systemically. However, it is not active against *Pseudomonas aeruginosa* and has generally been replaced by gentamicin and other newer aminoglycosides, although it has been used in penicillin-resistant gonorrhoea and streptomycin-resistant tuberculosis.

Gentamicin was isolated from *Micromonospora purpurea* in 1963 and, being active against *Ps. aeruginosa* and *Serratia marcescens*, is widely used in the treatment of life-threatening infections. *Tobramycin* is one of several components of the nebramycin complex of aminoglycosides produced by *Streptomyces tenebrarius*. It has an antimicrobial spectrum very similar to that of gentamicin and is reported to be more active against *Ps. aeruginosa*. *Amikacin*, a semisynthetic derivative of kanamycin, has a side-chain rendering it less susceptible to inactivating enzymes. It has a spectrum of activity like that of gentamicin but Gram-negative bacteria resistant to gentamicin, tobramycin, and kanamycin are often sensitive. *Sissomicin* is closely related structurally to gentamicin, and *netilmicin* is the *N*-ethyl derivative of sissomicin. Netilmicin may be active against some gentamicin-resistant strains of bacteria although not to the same extent as amikacin. Other aminoglycosides recently introduced or under investigation include *isepamicin, micronomicin*, and *pentisomicin.*

Because of their potential toxicity and antimicrobial spectrum, aminoglycoside antibiotics should in general only be used for the treatment of serious infections. Doses must be carefully regulated to maintain plasma concentrations within the therapeutic range but avoiding accumulation, especially in patients with renal impairment. Neomycin and framycetin, which are considered too toxic to be given parenterally, have been given by mouth to suppress the intestinal flora. The topical use of neomycin and gentamicin has been associated with allergic reactions and the emergence of resistant bacteria. Gentamicin or tobramycin are the antibiotics of choice in the treatment of life-threatening infections due to aminoglycoside-sensitive organisms and are often used in association with other antibacterial agents. With the continuing emergence of resistant strains, amikacin and netilmicin should be reserved for severe infections resistant to gentamicin and the other aminoglycosides.

The Cephalosporins and related Beta-Lactams

The cephalosporins are semisynthetic antibiotics derived from cephalosporin C a natural antibiotic produced by the mould *Cephalosporium acremonium.* The active nucleus, 7-aminocephalosporanic acid, is very closely related to the penicillin nucleus, 6-aminopenicillanic acid, and consists of a beta-lactam ring fused with a 6-membered dihydrothiazine ring and having an acetoxymethyl group at position 3. Cephalosporin C has a side-chain at position 7 derived from D-α-aminoadipic acid. Chemical modification of positions 3 and 7 has resulted in a series of antibiotics with different characteristics. Substitution at the 7-amino group tends to affect antibacterial action whereas at position 3 it may have more of an effect on pharmacokinetic properties.

The cephalosporins are bactericidal and, similarly to the penicillins, they act by inhibiting synthesis of the bacterial cell wall. The most widely used system of classification of cephalosporins is by generations and is based on the general features of their antibacterial activity, but may depend to some extent on when they were introduced.

Cephalothin (see p.176) was one of the first cephalosporins to become available and is representative of the **first-generation** cephalosporins. It has good activity against a wide spectrum of Gram-positive bacteria including penicillinase-producing, but not methicillin-resistant staphylococci; enterococci are however resistant. Its activity against Gram-negative bacteria is modest. Cephalothin is not absorbed from the gastro-intestinal tract and must be administered parenterally although intramuscular administration is painful. *Cephacetrile* and *cefapirin* are also administered parenterally, and like cephalothin retain the 3-acetoxy group of the parent compound cephalosporin C. *Cephazolin* is a widely used parenteral first-generation cephalosporin which is reported to be less painful on intramuscular injection than cephalothin. *Cephaloridine* was the first of this group to be used in the *UK* but is now rarely used due to its nephrotoxicity. Other parenteral first-generation cephalosporins include *cefazaflur*, *cefazedone*, and *ceftezole*. *Cephradine* is absorbed from the gastro-intestinal tract and can be administered both by mouth and by injection. *Cefroxadine* (the oxymethyl derivative of cephradine), *cefadroxil, cefatrizine, cephaloglycin, cephalexin* and its pivaloyloxymethyl ester *pivcephalexin* are all administered only by mouth. All of these agents have a very similar spectrum of antimicrobial activity to cephalothin. *Cefaclor* has similar activity to cephalothin against Gram-positive cocci, but because of its greater activity against Gram-negative bacteria, particularly *Haemophilus influenzae*, it is often classified as a second-generation agent. The first-generation agents generally penetrate into the CSF only poorly.

Cephamandole (see p.179) was the first available **second-generation** cephalosporin. It has similar or slightly less activity than cephalothin against Gram-positive bacteria. It has, however, greater stability to hydrolysis by beta-lactamases produced by Gram-negative bacteria and has enhanced activity against many of the Enterobacteriaceae and *Haemophilus influenzae*. *Cefuroxime* has a similar spectrum of activity to cephamandole although it is even more resistant to hydrolysis by beta-lactamases. *Cefuroxime axetil* is the recently developed acetoxyethyl ester of cefuroxime which can be administered by mouth. The other agents classified as second-generation cephalosporins are all administered parenterally and include *cefonicid, ceforanide*, and *cefotiam*; these all have spectra of activity comparable to cephamandole.

The **third-generation** cephalosporins, sometimes referred to as **extended-spectrum** cephalosporins are even more stable to hydrolysis by beta-lactamases than cephamandole and cefuroxime. Compared to the earlier generations of cephalosporins they have a wider spectrum and greater potency of activity against Gram-negative organisms including most clinically important Enterobacteriaceae. Their activity against Gram-positive organisms is, however, generally less than that of the first-generation agents. *Cefotaxime* (see p.151) was the first of this group to become available and it has relatively modest activity against *Pseudomonas aeruginosa*. *Cefmenoxime*, *ceftizoxime*, and *ceftriaxone* are all very similar to cefotaxime in their antimicrobial activity. These agents are all administered parenterally and differ mainly in their pharmacokinetic characteristics. *Latamoxef* is an **oxacephalosporin** which differs from the true cephalosporins in that the S atom of the 7-aminocephalosporanic acid nucleus is replaced by an O atom. It differs from cefotaxime mainly in its enhanced activity against *Bacteroides fragilis*. *Ceftazidime* (see p.162) is typical of a group of parenteral third-generation cephalosporins with enhanced activity against *Ps. aeruginosa*. *Cefoperazone* is similar in its activity to ceftazidime. *Cefpiramide* is structurally related to cefoperazone and has comparable activity although not all workers have been able to confirm its good antipseudomonal activity. Although *cefsulodin* is classified as a third-generation cephalosporin its activity against Gram-negative bacteria is confined to *Ps. aeruginosa*; its activity against Gram-positive organisms and against anaerobes is comparable to that of ceftazidime.

Many more cephalosporins are under development, structural modifications being made to broaden their spectrum of action yet further or to enhance activity against specific organisms; agents that can be administered by mouth are also being studied. Most of these new cephalosporins cannot yet be classified into a generation. Those described in this chapter are *cefempidone*, *cefepime*, *cefetamet*, *cefixime*, *cefodizime*, *cefpimizole*, *cefpirome*, *cefteram* and its pivaloyloxymethyl ester, and *cefuzonam*. *Flomoxef* is an oxacephalosporin. Other cephalosporins under investigation include: *cefedrolor*, *cefmepidium*, *cefpodoxime*, *ceftiofur* (*CM-31916*) and its hydrochloride (*U-642794A*) and sodium (*U-64279E*) salts, *ceftiolene*, *CGP-31523A*, *CM-40874*, *DN-9550*, and *E-0702*.

Cephamycins A, B, and C are beta-lactam antibiotics produced naturally by *Streptomyces* spp. and are structurally related to cephalosporin C. The semisynthetic **cephamycins** in use are chemical modifications of cephamycin C. They differ from the cephalosporins by the addition of a 7-α-methoxy group to the 7-aminocephalosporanic acid nucleus. Steric hindrance by this methoxy group is considered to be responsible for their greater stability to beta-lactamases. Due to their similarity to cephalosporins they are generally included in the same classification. *Cefoxitin* (see p.158) and *cefmetazole* are classified with the second-generation cephalosporins. The most significant difference from agents such as cephamandole is their good activity against *B. fragilis*. *Cefbuperazone* and *cefotetan* are classified with the third-generation agents; their activity is generally similar to that of cefotaxime but again they have greater activity against *B. fragilis*. All these cephamycins must be administered by the parenteral route. *Cefminox* is a new cephamycin antibiotic.

Some cephalosporins including cefazaflur, cefmenoxime, cefmetazole, cefoperazone, ceforanide, cefotetan, cephamandole, and latamoxef have an *N*-methylthiotetrazole side-chain which, in some of them, has been implicated in the development of adverse effects (see Cephamandole Sodium, p.179). These include hypoprothrombinaemia and other adverse effects on haemostasis which may result in clinical bleeding and the occurrence of a disulfiram-like reaction to alcohol. More recently it has been suggested that the sulphydryl group in the *N*-methylthiotetrazole side-chain may be specifically responsible for these effects, since hypoprothrombinaemia has been reported to occur after administration of ceftriaxone, an agent with a sulphydryl group but no *N*-methylthiotetrazole side-chain.

Imipenem was the first of the **carbapenem** group of antibiotics to become available; it is the *N*-formimidoyl derivative of thienamycin which is produced by *Streptomyces cattleya*. It is bactericidal, and, similarly to the cephalosporins, acts by inhibiting synthesis of the bacterial cell wall. It has a very broad spectrum of antimicrobial activity including Gram-positive and Gram-negative aerobic and anaerobic organisms; it has good activity against both *Ps. aeruginosa* and *B. fragilis*. Imipenem is administered parenterally in association with *cilastatin*, a dehydropeptidase I inhibitor which inhibits the renal metabolism of imipenem. *Sch-29482* is a carbapenem which has been extensively studied *in vitro*.

The **monobactams** were first identified as monocyclic beta-lactams isolated from bacteria; they are now produced synthetically. *Aztreonam* was the first commercially available monobactam. It too is bactericidal with a similar action on bacterial cell-wall synthesis to the cephalosporins. Its antimicrobial activity, however, differs from imipenem and the newer cephalosporins in that it is restricted to Gram-negative aerobic organisms. It has good activity against *Ps. aeruginosa*. Aztreonam must be administered by the parenteral route. Other monobactams under investigation are *carumonam* (see p.142), *oximonam*, *pirazmonam*, and *tigemonam*.

A new classification of cephalosporins; agents may be classified in groups I to IV according to their antimicrobial activity, and each group is divided into three sub-groups according to the pharmacological properties of the drug.— J. D. Williams, *Drugs*, 1987, *34*, *Suppl.* 2, 15.

Reviews and discussions of the actions and uses of cephalosporins and cephamycins: H. C. Neu, *Lancet*, 1982, *2*, 252; *idem*, *Ann. intern. Med.*, 1982, *97*, 408; P. Garzone *et al.*, *Drug Intell. & clin. Pharm.*, 1983, *17*, 507 and 615; *Med. Lett.*, 1983, *25*, 57; S. J. Eykyn, *Prescribers' J.*, 1983, *23*, 58; S. L. Barriere and J. F. Flaherty, *Clin. Pharm.*, 1984, *3*, 351; R. Kemp, *Med. J. Aust.*, 1984, *141*, 437; I. M. Gould and R. Wise, *Br. med. J.*, 1985, *290*, 878; *Drug & Ther. Bull.*, 1986, *24*, 101; R. L. Thompson, *Mayo Clin. Proc.*, 1987, *62*, 821; R. Wise, *Lancet*, 1987, *2*, 1251.

For proceedings of a seminar on the cephalosporin antibiotics, see *Drugs*, 1987, *34*, *Suppl.* 2, 1–258.

Adverse reactions and interactions with newer cephalosporin and cephamycin antibiotics.— S. R. Norrby, *Med. Toxicol.*, 1986, *1*, 32.

The Chloramphenicols

Chloramphenicol is an antibiotic which was first isolated from cultures of *Streptomyces venezuelae* in 1947 but is now produced synthetically. It has a relatively simple structure and is a derivative of dichloroacetic acid with a nitrobenzene moiety. Chloramphenicol was the first broad-spectrum antibiotic to be discovered; it acts by interfering with bacterial protein synthesis and is mainly bacteriostatic. Its range of activity is similar to that of tetracycline and includes Gram-positive and Gram-negative bacteria, rickettsias, and chlamydias. The sensitivity of *Salmonella typhi*, *Haemophilus influenzae*, and *Bacteroides fragilis* to chloramphenicol provides the principal indications for its use.

After one or two years' use chloramphenicol was found to have a serious and sometimes fatal depressant effect on the bone marrow. The 'grey syndrome', another potentially fatal adverse effect, was reported later in newborn infants. As a result of this toxicity the use of chloramphenicol has been restricted in many countries; it should only be given when there is no suitable alternative and never for minor infections.

Chloramphenicol is active when given by mouth and, unlike most other antibiotics, it diffuses into the cerebrospinal fluid even when the meninges are not inflamed. The majority of a dose is inactivated in the liver, only a small proportion appearing unchanged in the urine.

Chloramphenicol is used for typhoid fever in many countries although resistance is sometimes a problem. For *Haemophilus influenzae* infections, especially meningitis, the emergence of ampicillin-resistant strains led to a reappraisal of the use of chloramphenicol. Some workers consider that ampicillin and chloramphenicol should both be given to patients with meningitis until the sensitivity of the infecting organisms is known, however, the newer cephalosporins have challenged this use. Chloramphenicol is also effective against many anaerobic bacteria and may be valuable in such conditions as cerebral abscess where anaerobes such as *Bacteroides fragilis* are often involved, although metronidazole may be preferred.

Chloramphenicol sodium succinate is used parenterally and the palmitate, which is almost tasteless, is given in oral suspensions. Ophthalmic preparations of chloramphenicol are used widely for a variety of infections.

Thiamphenicol is a semisynthetic derivative of chloramphenicol in which the nitro group on the benzene ring has been replaced by a methylsulphonyl group, resulting, in general, in a loss of activity *in vitro*. It has been claimed that thiamphenicol is less toxic than chloramphenicol and there have been fewer reports of aplastic anaemia but reversible bone-marrow depression may occur more frequently. Unlike chloramphenicol, thiamphenicol is not metabolised in the liver to any extent and is excreted largely unchanged in the urine. It has been used similarly to chloramphenicol in some countries.

Azidamfenicol is another analogue of chloramphenicol which has been used topically in the treatment of eye infections.

Fusidic Acid

Fusidic acid is an antibiotic which is derived from strains of the fungus *Fusidium coccineum*. It has a steroid structure and is related to cephalosporin P, an antibiotic produced by *Cephalosporium acremonium* which also produces cephalosporin C from which the cephalosporin antibiotics are derived. Fusidic acid has a narrow spectrum of antibacterial activity but is very active against *Staphylococcus aureus*, including penicillinase-producing and some methicillin-resistant strains. Unfortunately resistance to fusidic acid is readily acquired and it is often given in conjunction with other antibiotics; the topical use of fusidic acid in a hospital environment has been associated with an increased incidence of resistance.

It penetrates well into most body tissues and fluids, apart from the cerebrospinal fluid, a property of value in infectious conditions such as abscesses and osteomyelitis. Fusidic acid is used in the treatment of staphylococcal infections, especially those resistant to other antibiotics. The sodium salt, sodium fusidate, is given by mouth and is also used in topical preparations; fusidic acid itself is available as a suspension for oral use and as a cream or gel. For severe staphylococcal infections the antibiotic is given intravenously as diethanolamine fusidate.

The Lincosamides

Lincomycin is an antibiotic produced by a strain of *Streptomyces lincolnensis* and was first described in 1962; *clindamycin* is the 7-chloro-7-deoxy derivative of lincomycin.

Although not related structurally to erythromycin and the other macrolide antibiotics, the lincosamides have similar antimicrobial activity and act at the same site on the bacterial ribosome to suppress protein synthesis.

The lincosamides are bacteriostatic or bactericidal depending on the concentration and are active mainly against Gram-positive bacteria, and against *Bacteroides* spp. Clindamycin and lincomycin have qualitatively similar activity but clindamycin is more active than lincomycin *in vitro*. Cross-resistance occurs between the lincosamide, streptogramin, and macrolide groups of antibiotics.

The lincosamides have been used, like erythromycin, as an alternative to penicillin but reports of the occurrence of severe and sometimes fatal pseudomembranous colitis in association with lincomycin and clindamycin have led to the recommendation that they should only be used in severe infections when there is no suitable alternative.

Both lincomycin and clindamycin can be given orally and parenterally but clindamycin is much better absorbed from the gastro-intestinal tract and less affected by the presence of food in the stomach. They both penetrate well into bone and have been used successfully in osteomyelitis. They have also been used topically in the treatment of severe acne vulgaris.

The main indication for the use of lincosamides is now in the treatment of severe anaerobic infections although metronidazole (see p.669) or some beta-lactams may be a more suitable choice in such infections.

Pirlimycin is a lincosamide antibiotic under investigation.

The Macrolides

The macrolides are a large group of antibiotics mainly derived from *Streptomyces* spp. and having a common macrocyclic lactone ring to which one or more sugars are attached. They are all weak bases and only slightly soluble in water. Their properties are very similar and in general they have low toxicity and the same spectrum of antimicrobial activity with cross-resistance between individual members of the group. The macrolide antibiotics are bacteriostatic or bactericidal, depending on the concentration and the type of micro-organism, and are thought to interfere with bacterial protein synthesis. Their antimicrobial spectrum is similar to that of benzylpenicillin but they are also active against such organisms as *Legionella pneumophila*, *Mycoplasma pneumoniae*, and some rickettsias and chlamydias.

Erythromycin was discovered in 1952 and is the only macrolide antibiotic to be used widely. It is destroyed by gastric acid and must therefore be given as enteric-coated formulations or as one of its more stable salts or esters such as the stearate or ethyl succinate. Hepatotoxicity has been reported after the administration of erythromycin, most commonly as the estolate. Erythromycin lactobionate or gluceptate may be given intravenously and the ethyl succinate has been given intramuscularly. Erythromycin is used as an alternative to penicillin, especially in patients who are allergic to penicillin, and, similarly to tetracycline, in the treatment of infections due to *Mycoplasma pneumoniae* and *Chlamydia trachomatis*, and in acne vulgaris. It is also used in the treatment of infections caused by *Legionella pneumophila*.

The other macrolide antibiotics include *spiramycin* which has been used extensively in Europe and has been claimed to be effective in the treatment of toxoplasmosis. High tissue concentrations are achieved and maintained for longer than with the other macrolides.

Oleandomycin has been used orally and parenterally as the phosphate. Its ester, *triacetyloleandomycin*, is better absorbed from the gastro-intestinal tract but, like erythromycin estolate, has proved hepatotoxic. *Josamycin*, *kitasamycin*, and *midecamycin* have been used in Europe and/or Japan.

More recent macrolide antibiotics include *miocamycin*, the diacetyl derivative of midecamycin, *rokitamycin*, and *roxithromycin*, a macrolide with a longer half-life than erythromycin. These agents all appear to have similar properties to erythromycin. *Rosaramicin*, unlike the other macrolides mentioned, is obtained from a *Micromonospora* spp. *A-56268* (*TE-031*) is a macrolide under investigation.

Tylosin is a macrolide antibiotic used in veterinary medicine.

The **streptogramin** group of antibiotics are also derived from *Streptomyces* spp. and include *mikamycin*, *pristinamycin*, and *virginiamycin*. They consist of two components, which act synergistically and they are therefore also known as synergistins. One of the components is structurally related to the macrolides, and they have a similar spectrum of antimicrobial activity to erythromycin. For further discussion of the streptogramins, see Virginiamycin, p.337.

Cross-resistance is often observed between the macrolide, lincosamide (see above), and streptogramin groups of antibiotics.

The Penicillins

Penicillin was the first antibiotic to be used therapeutically and was originally obtained, as a mixture of penicillins known as F, G, X, and K, from the mould *Penicillium notatum*. Better yields were achieved using *P. chrysogenum* and benzylpenicillin (penicillin G) was selectively produced by adding the precursor phenylacetic acid to the fermentation medium. The term 'penicillin' is now used generically for the entire group of natural and semisynthetic penicillins. Penicillins are still widely used; they are generally well tolerated, apart from hypersensitivity reactions, and are usually bactericidal by virtue of their inhibitory action on the synthesis of the bacterial cell wall.

They all have the same ring structure and are monobasic acids which readily form salts and esters; 6-aminopenicillanic acid, the penicillin nucleus, consists of a fused thiazolidine ring and a beta-lactam ring with an amino group at the 6-position.

The earlier or so-called 'natural' penicillins were produced by adding different side-chain precursors to fermentations of the *Penicillium* mould; *benzylpenicillin*, with a phenylacetamido side-chain at the 6-position, and *phenoxymethylpenicillin* (penicillin V), with a phenoxyacetamido side-chain, were 2 of the first and are still widely used. Benzylpenicillin can be considered the parent compound of the penicillins and is active mainly against Gram-positive bacteria and *Neisseria* spp. It is inactivated by penicillinase-producing bacteria and because of its instability in gastric acid it is usually injected. Long-acting preparations include *procaine penicillin* and *benzathine penicillin* which slowly release benzylpenicillin after injection. Phenoxymethylpenicillin is acid-stable and therefore given by mouth but it is also inactivated by penicillinase. It is generally used for relatively mild infections.

When no side-chain precursor is added to the fermentation medium 6-aminopenicillanic acid itself is obtained. A range of penicillins has been synthesised from 6-aminopenicillanic acid by substitution at the 6-amino position in an effort to improve on the instability of benzylpenicillin to gastric acid and penicillinases, to widen its antimicrobial spectrum, and to reduce its rapid rate of renal excretion. Two phenoxypenicillins in which the side-chain is α-phenoxypropionamido (*phenethicillin*) or α-phenoxybutyramido (*propicillin*) are more stable to acid than benzylpenicillin but offer no advantage over phenoxymethylpenicillin.

Methicillin has a 2,6-dimethoxybenzamido group at the 6-position and was the first penicillin found to be resistant to destruction by staphylococcal penicillinase. However, it is not acid-resistant and has to be injected. The isoxazolyl penicillins, *cloxacillin*, *dicloxacillin*, *flucloxacillin*, and *oxacillin*, are resistant to penicillinase and gastric acid. They have very similar chemical structures and differ mainly in their absorption characteristics. *Nafcillin* is a similar penicillinase-resistant antibiotic but is irregularly absorbed when taken by mouth.

Ampicillin has a D(−)-α-aminophenylacetamido side-chain and a broader spectrum of activity than benzylpenicillin; although generally less active against Gram-positive bacteria, some Gram-negative organisms including *Escherichia coli*, *Haemophilus influenzae*, and *Salmonella* spp. are sensitive although resistance is being reported increasingly. *Pseudomonas* spp. are not sensitive. Ampicillin is acid-stable and can be given by mouth but is destroyed by penicillinase. *Amoxycillin*, with a D(−)-α-aminohydroxyphenylacetamido side-chain, only differs from ampicillin by the addition of a hydroxyl group, but is better absorbed from the gastro-intestinal tract. A number of pro-drugs including *bacampicillin*, *hetacillin*, *metampicillin*, *pivampicillin*, and *talampicillin* are also said to be better absorbed and are hydrolysed to ampicillin *in vivo*.

Carbenicillin, with an α-carboxyphenylacetamido side-chain, has marked activity against *Pseudomonas aeruginosa* and some *Proteus* spp. but otherwise is generally less active than ampicillin. It has to be given by injection and large doses are required. *Carfecillin* and *carindacillin* are the phenyl and indanyl esters of carbenicillin respectively and are hydrolysed to carbenicillin *in vivo* when taken by mouth. *Sulbenicillin* has an α-phenylsulphoacetamido side-chain and ticarcillin an α-carboxythienylacetamido side-chain and both have similar activity to carbenicillin; *ticarcillin* appears to be more active against *Ps. aeruginosa*. The ureidopenicillins *azlocillin* and *mezlocillin*, and the closely-related *piperacillin* and *apalcillin* are reported to be more active than carbenicillin against *Ps. aeruginosa* and to have a wider range of activity.

Temocillin, a 6-α-methoxy derivative of ticarcillin, is resistant to many beta-lactamases and is active against most Gram-negative aerobic bacteria except *Ps. aeruginosa* and *Acinetobacter* spp.

Mecillinam is a penicillanic acid derivative with a substituted amidino group in the 6-position. Unlike the 6-aminopenicillanic acid derivatives it is active mainly against Gram-negative bacteria, although *Ps. aeruginosa*, *H. influenzae*, and *Bacteroides* spp. are considered resistant. Mecillinam is not active orally and is given by mouth as *pivmecillinam* which is hydrolysed to mecillinam on absorption.

The beta-lactamase inhibitors *clavulanic acid* and *sulbactam* are used to extend the antimicrobial range of certain beta-lactam antibiotics.

The Polymyxins

The polymyxins are basic antibiotics produced by the growth of different strains of *Bacillus polymyxa* (=*B. aerosporus*). They are cyclic polypeptides, have a molecular weight of about 1000, and readily form salts with acids.

Two similar antibacterial substances were originally isolated independently in 1947 in Great Britain and the *USA*, the British material being named 'aerosporin' and the American, 'polymyxin'. At least 3 other antibacterial substances were subsequently isolated from different strains of *B. polymyxa* and it was agreed that the generic name 'polymyxin' should be applied to this group of antibiotics, aerosporin becoming polymyxin A and the other original polymyxin becoming polymyxin D; the 3 later-discovered related substances were named polymyxin B, C, and E, respectively. 'Aerosporin' is now a proprietary name for polymyxin B sulphate and the name colistin is used for polymyxin E.

Only *polymyxin B* and *colistin* are used clinically. They have similar bactericidal activity against Gram-negative bacteria, especially *Pseudomonas*, but are potentially nephrotoxic and neurotoxic and have largely been replaced by other less toxic antibiotics such as gentamicin, the antipseudomonal penicillins, or the cephalosporins. Polymyxin B and colistin are not absorbed when taken by mouth and the sulphates have been used in gastro-intestinal infections. Polymyxin B sulphate or colistin sulphomethate sodium may be administered parenterally for the treatment of pseudomonal infections resistant to other antibiotics; *sulphomyxin sodium*, a sulphomethylated form of polymyxin B was formerly available for intramuscular injection. Both polymyxin B and colistin are used topically.

The Quinolones

The quinolonecarboxylic acids or 4-quinolones are a group of synthetic antibacterial agents structurally related to nalidixic acid. The term 4-quinolone has been used as a generic name for the common 4-oxo-1,4-dihydroquinoline skeleton. Under this system nalidixic acid, a naphthyridene derivative, is an 8-aza-4-quinolone, cinoxacin, a cinnoline derivative, is a 2-aza-4-quinolone, and pipemidic and piromidic acids, pyrido-pyrimidine derivatives, are 6,8-diaza-4-quinolones.

Nalidixic acid, introduced into clinical use in 1963, is active against Gram-negative bacteria but has little activity against *Pseudomonas* and Gram-positive organisms. Because bactericidal concentrations can only be achieved in urine its use has generally been limited to the treatment of urinary-tract infections.

Modification of the structure of nalidixic acid has produced related antibacterial agents such as *oxolinic acid, piromidic acid, cinoxacin*, and *flumequine*. Although some of these have a greater activity *in vitro* against Gram-negative organisms and activity against some Gram-positive organisms, none has been considered to represent a significant clinical advance over nalidixic acid. Addition of a piperazinyl radical at position 7, as in *pipemidic acid*, appears to confer some activity against *Pseudomonas*. Addition of the 7-piperazinyl group and a fluorine atom at position 6 has produced a group of antibacterial agents termed the fluorinated piperazinyl quinolones or the fluoroquinolones. These agents, which include *norfloxacin, enoxacin, ciprofloxacin, pefloxacin, ofloxacin*, and *amifloxacin* have a greater intrinsic antibacterial activity than nalidixic acid and a broader antibacterial spectrum that includes *Pseudomonas* and Gram-positive cocci. Other fluoroquinolones including *CI-934, difloxacin hydrochloride (Abbott-56619)*, and *fleroxacin* are also under investigation.

The fluoroquinolones are very active against aerobic Gram-negative bacilli and cocci including the Enterobacteriaceae, *Haemophilus influenzae*, and *Neisseria gonorrhoeae* and are also active against *Pseudomonas aeruginosa*. They are, however, less active against Gram-positive organisms such as staphylococci and streptococci. Activity against anaerobic bacteria is generally poor.

Like nalidixic acid, other 4-quinolone antibacterial agents are bactericidal and appear to interfere with DNA synthesis by inhibiting DNA gyrase (topoisomerase) activity. Cross-resistance among the 4-quinolones occurs but cross-resistance with other antibacterial agents appears to be rare as resistance is not transferable on plasmids. The fluoroquinolones are usually active against multiple-resistant Gram-negative bacilli, methicillin-resistant *Straphylococcus aureus* and beta-lactamase-producing *Neisseria gonorrhoeae*.

The fluoroquinolones appear to be rapidly absorbed when given by mouth and to have relatively long half-lives. Achievable serum and tissue concentrations in excess of the MICs of most Gram-negative and some Gram-positive organisms indicate that the fluoroquinolones are of potential use in the treatment of systemic as well as urinary-tract infections. They may be used to treat a variety of infections due to susceptible organisms including those of the respiratory, urinary, and gastro-intestinal tracts, and gonorrhoea and septicaemia.

Reviews of the actions and uses of the 4-quinolones: J. T. Smith, *Pharm. J.*, 1984, *2*, 299; J. S. Wolfson and D. C. Hooper, *Antimicrob. Ag. Chemother.*, 1985, *28*, 581; D. C. Hooper and J. S. Wolfson, *ibid.*, 716; *Lancet*, 1986, *1*, 837 and 1228.

The Sulphonamides

The sulphonamides are analogues of *p*-aminobenzoic acid. The first sulphonamide of clinical importance was *Prontosil*, an azo dye which is metabolised *in vivo* to *sulphanilamide*. It was synthesised in Germany in 1932 and first used as a chemotherapeutic agent in 1935. Many sulphonamides have since been synthesised; they differ only slightly in their antimicrobial activity, the choice of sulphonamide being determined principally by pharmacokinetic properties. The sulphonamides have been classified according to their rate of excretion as short-, medium- or intermediate-, long-, and ultra-long-acting. The **short-acting** sulphonamides are excreted in the urine in high concentrations and have therefore been of particular use in the treatment of urinary-tract infections. The solubility in urine of earlier short-acting sulphonamides, such as *sulphapyridine*, and their acetyl metabolites is low and hence crystalluria has been reported frequently. Of the short-acting sulphonamides most commonly used *sulphadiazine* also has low solubility in urine whereas *sulphadimidine* and *sulphafurazole* and their acetyl conjugates are very soluble. Three short-acting sulphonamides (triple sulphonamides) have been given together to reduce the risk of crystalluria, as the constituent sulphonamides can co-exist in solution in urine without affecting each other's solubility. Preparations of mixed sulphonamides have, however, generally been replaced by the more soluble sulphonamides. The **medium-acting** sulphonamides such as *sulphamethoxazole*, the **long-acting** sulphonamides such as *sulphadimethoxine, sulphamethoxydiazine*, and *sulphamethoxypyridazine*, and the **ultra-long-acting** sulphonamides such as *sulfadoxine* and *sulfametopyrazine* do not attain such high concentrations in the urine and rarely cause crystalluria. Sulphonamides which are slowly excreted from the body do appear, however, to have been more commonly implicated in the development of reactions such as the Stevens-Johnson syndrome. Although, theoretically, the ultra-long-acting sulphonamides may not be suitable for the treatment of urinary-tract infections, due to their low urinary concentrations, sulfametopyrazine has been used as single-dose treatment.

The sulphonamides are usually bacteriostatic, and interfere with folic acid synthesis of susceptible organisms; their broad spectrum of antimicrobial activity has, however, been limited by the development of resistance. The clinical use of sulphonamides has therefore been greatly reduced; in general they are indicated only in the treatment of urinary-tract infections and in the prophylaxis of meningococcal meningitis where susceptibility to sulphonamides has been demonstrated. Sulphonamides such as *sulphaguanidine, succinylsulphathiazole*, and *phthalylsulphathiazole* are poorly absorbed from the gastro-intestinal tract and have been used for the treatment of gastro-intestinal infections although they are now rarely indicated. *Silver sulphadiazine* and *mafenide acetate* are applied topically for their antibacterial action in patients with burns. *Sulphasalazine* (see p.1108) a conjugate of 5-aminosalicylic acid (mesalazine) and sulphapyridine is used in the treatment of inflammatory bowel diseases and in rheumatoid arthritis.

Groups of drugs structurally related to the sulphonamides include the thiazides and carbonic anhydrase inhibitors (p.973) which are used for their diuretic activity, and the sulphonylureas (p.386) which are used for their hypoglycaemic activity.

Trimethoprim is a diamino pyrimidine which also inhibits folic acid synthesis but at a different stage in the metabolic pathway to that inhibited by the sulphonamides. It has a similar spectrum of antimicrobial activity to sulphonamides and often demonstrates synergy *in vitro* with these agents. Trimethoprim was initially available only in combination with sulphonamides, most commonly with sulphamethoxazole as co-trimoxazole. It is now used alone particularly in the treatment of infections of the urinary and respiratory tracts. Analogues of trimethoprim include *brodimoprim, metioprim*, and *tetroxoprim*.

Co-trimoxazole has generally replaced the use of sulphonamides alone in the treatment of systemic infections. It is also used in the treatment and prophylaxis of infections, most commonly pneumonia, caused by the protozoan *Pneumocystis carinii* in immunocompromised patients including those with AIDS and those receiving immunosuppressant drugs. Other sulphonamides which have been used in combination with trimethoprim include sulphadiazine (see *co-trimazine*), sulfametopyrazine, sulfametrole, sulphadimidine, sulphamethoxypyridazine, and sulphamoxole (see *co-trifamole*). Sulphadiazine has been used in combination with tetroxoprim (see co-tetroxazine).

Sulphonamides have also been used in association with the diaminopyrimidine, pyrimethamine (see p.515) in the treatment or prophylaxis of some protozoal infections. Commonly used combinations are sulfadoxine and pyrimethamine for malaria, and sulphadiazine and pyrimethamine for the treatment of toxoplasmosis.

The Tetracyclines

The tetracyclines are a group of antibiotics, originally derived from certain *Streptomyces* spp., having the same tetracyclic nucleus, naphthacene, and similar properties. Unlike the penicillins and aminoglycosides they are usually bacteriostatic at the concentrations achieved in the body but act similarly to the aminoglycosides by interfering with protein synthesis in susceptible organisms.

Tetracyclines all have a broad spectrum of activity which includes Gram-positive and Gram-negative bacteria, chlamydias, rickettsias, mycoplasmas, and spirochaetes, but the emergence of resistant strains and the development of other antimicrobial agents has reduced their value. Adverse effects have also restricted their usefulness. Gastro-intestinal disturbances are common and other important toxic effects include deposition in bones and teeth, precluding their use in late pregnancy and young children; anti-anabolic effects, especially in patients with renal impairment; fatty changes in the liver, associated with the intravenous administration of tetracyclines; and photosensitivity, especially with demeclocycline. Allergic reactions are relatively uncommon. Intramuscular injections are painful and tetracyclines are preferably given by mouth. Because of these adverse effects tetracyclines should be avoided in pregnant women, children, and, apart from doxycycline and possibly minocycline, patients with renal failure.

The first tetracycline to be introduced was *chlortetracycline* in 1948 and, like chloramphenicol which was discovered about the same time, it was found to have a broad spectrum of activity and to be active by mouth unlike benzylpenicillin or streptomycin the only other antibiotics then in use. The discovery of chlortetracycline was followed closely by that of *oxytetracycline* and then *tetracycline*, a reduction product of chlortetracycline which may be produced semisynthetically. All 3 have very similar properties although chlortetracycline is less well absorbed, and oxytetracycline may cause less staining of teeth. *Demeclocycline*, demethylated chlortetracycline, has a longer half-life then tetracycline. However, phototoxic reactions have been reported most frequently with demeclocycline. It has been used with some success in patients with the syndrome of inappropriate secretion of antidiuretic hormone.

The 4 tetracyclines mentioned so far (chlortetracycline, oxytetracycline, tetracycline, and demeclocycline) are all natural products that have been isolated from *Streptomyces* spp. The more recent tetracyclines, clomocycline, methacycline, doxycycline, and minocycline are semisynthetic derivatives. *Lymecycline* and *rolitetracycline* are more water-soluble tetracyclines and have been used parenterally. *Methacycline*, like demeclocycline, has a longer half-life than tetracycline and has been given twice daily. *Doxycycline* and *minocycline*, 2 more recent semisynthetic tetracycline derivatives, are both more active *in vitro* than tetracycline against many species. More importantly, minocycline is active against some tetracycline-resistant bacteria including strains of staphylococci. Both antibiotics are well absorbed and, unlike the other tetracyclines, absorption is not significantly affected by the presence of food. They can be given in lower doses than the older members of the group and, having long half-lives, doxycycline is usually given once daily and minocycline twice daily. Doxycycline does not accumulate significantly in patients with renal impairment and can, therefore, be given to such patients; some workers consider that minocycline can also be used. Both doxycycline and minocycline are more lipid-soluble than the other tetracyclines and they penetrate well into tissues. The use of minocycline is, however, limited by its vestibular side-effects.

Because of the emergence of resistant organisms and the discovery of agents with narrower antimicrobial spectra, tetracyclines are not generally the antibiotics of choice in Gram-positive or Gram-negative infections. However they have a place in the treatment of chlamydial infections such as trachoma, rickettsial infections such as typhus, mycoplasmal infections such as atypical pneumonia, and in acute exacerbations of chronic bronchitis, leptospirosis, Lyme disease, relapsing fever, non-specific urethritis, brucellosis, plague, and cholera; low doses are used in the long-term treatment of severe acne. The tetracyclines have also been useful in the treatment of penicillin-allergic patients suffering from venereal diseases, anthrax, or actinomycosis.

Miscellaneous Antibacterial Agents

Vancomycin has a glycopeptide structure; it acts by interfering with bacterial cell wall synthesis and is very active against Gram-positive cocci. Intravenous vancomycin is reserved for the treatment of severe staphylococcal infections and for the treatment and prophylaxis of endocarditis when other antibiotics cannot be used either because of patient sensitivity or bacterial resistance. It is the treatment of choice for infections caused by methicillin-resistant staphylococci. Vancomycin hydrochloride is poorly absorbed when taken by mouth; it is used in the treatment of pseudomembranous colitis. *Teicoplanin* is a glycopeptide with very similar properties to vancomycin.

Fosfomycin is a derivative of phosphonic acid; it is active against a range of Gram-positive and Gram-negative bacteria and is administered by mouth or parenterally. Other phosphonic acid derivatives include *alafosfalin* and *fosmidomycin*.

The rifamycins also known as ansamycins or rifomycins are a group of antibiotics isolated from a strain of *Nocardia mediterranei* (*Streptomyces mediterranei*). Rifamycins described in this chapter include *rifamycin sodium*, a rifamycin rarely used as it has been superseded by more effective antibiotics, and a new rifamycin, *rifaximin*. The spectrum of activity of the rifamycins includes *Mycobacterium* spp. and the main antibiotic in this group, *rifampicin*, (see p.570), and two new drugs, *rifabutin* (see p.570) and *rifapentine* (see p.577) are described under Antimycobacterial Agents.

Spectinomycin is an aminocyclitol antibiotic with some similarities to streptomycin; it is not an aminoglycoside. Spectinomycin is active against a wide range of bacteria but its clinical use is restricted to the treatment of gonorrhoea.

Mupirocin is an antibiotic produced by *Pseudomonas fluorescens* with activity against most strains of staphylococci and streptococci and also some Gram-negative bacteria. It is applied topically.

Urinary antimicrobial agents such as *nitrofurantoin*, and also *hexamine* which has generally been given as the hippurate or mandelate, may be used in the treatment and prophylaxis of infections of the lower urinary tract. They are concentrated in the urine, but do not usually achieve antimicrobial concentrations in the blood, and therefore other agents such as ampicillin, co-trimoxazole or trimethoprim, or the 4-quinolones are preferred in the treatment of infections of the urinary tract.

12323-t

Acrosoxacin *(BAN)*.

Rosoxacin *(USAN, rINN)*; Win-35213. 1-Ethyl-1,4-dihydro-4-oxo-7-(4-pyridyl)quinoline-3-carboxylic acid.
$C_{17}H_{14}N_2O_3$=294.3.

CAS — 40034-42-2.

Adverse Effects and Precautions

As for Norfloxacin, p.274.

Dizziness, drowsiness, and visual disturbances may occur relatively frequently and patients should be advised not to drive or operate machinery if affected.

Uses and Administration

Acrosoxacin is a 4-quinolone antibacterial agent with actions similar to those of norfloxacin (p.275). It is active against *Neisseria gonorrhoeae* and is given by mouth in the treatment of gonorrhoea as a single dose of 300 mg, preferably on an empty stomach.

ANTIMICROBIAL ACTION. Studies of the antimicrobial activity of acrosoxacin.— R. A. Dobson *et al., Antimicrob. Ag. Chemother.*, 1980, *18*, 738; A. D. Seth, *J. antimicrob. Chemother.*, 1981, *7*, 331; D. Felmingham *et al., Drugs exp. & clin. Res.*, 1983, *9*, 157.

CHANCROID. Of 40 men with chancroid given acrosoxacin 150 mg twice daily for 3 days, 38 (95%) were cured at follow-up 1 month after therapy. Treatment with a single 300 mg dose of acrosoxacin was less effective and produced a cure in only 14 of 23 men. None of the treatment failures were caused by organism resistance.— D. A. Haase *et al., Antimicrob. Ag. Chemother.*, 1986, *30*, 39.

GONORRHOEA. Although acrosoxacin 300 mg daily appears to be effective in the treatment of uncomplicated pharyngeal or anogenital gonorrhoea in men and women it had been suggested that it should only be used where the bacteria are resistant, or the patient hypersensitive, to penicillin (*Drug & Ther. Bull.*, 1982, *20*, 10). However, some now consider that other agents may prove to be better alternatives in these circumstances. The incidence of adverse effects with acrosoxacin is relatively high and cns effects such as giddiness, drowsiness, and headache have been experienced by more than 50% of patients in some studies. Furthermore while some workers have found acrosoxacin to be of similar efficacy to spectinomycin in women (O.V. Calubiran *et al., Br. J. vener. Dis.*, 1982, *58*, 231), others have found it to be less effective in men (W.O. Harrison *et al., Lancet*, 1984, *1*, 566; K. Panikabutra *et al.. Br. J. vener. Dis.*, 1984, *60*, 231; A. Siboulet *et al., Eur. J. sex. transm. Dis.*, 1985, *2*,, 151). Cure-rates for acrosoxacin in other studies have generally been lower than those obtained with ampicillin or other penicillins (B. Romanowski *et al., Antimicrob. Ag. Chemother.*, 1984, *25*, 455). Acrosoxacin also appears to be less active against non-penicillinase than penicillinase producing strains of *Neisseria gonorrhoea* (K.B. Lim *et al., Br. J. vener. Dis.*, 1984, *60*, 157) and resistant gonococci have been reported to emerge during therapy by some workers (M.E. Macaulay, *Lancet*, 1982, *1*, 171; C. Jones and L. Cohen, *ibid.*, 855). Acrosoxacin has failed to eliminate co-existing cervical or urethral infections with *Chlamydia trachomatis* (D.A. Hicks *Eur. J. sex. transm. Dis.*, 1985, *2*, 103) and has also been reported to be ineffective in the treatment of non-gonococcal urethritis caused by *C. trachomatis* and *Ureaplasma urealyticum* (D.A. Hawkins *et al., Genitourinary Med.*, 1985, *61*, 51). The incidence of postgonococcal urethritis after treatment with acrosoxacin has been reported to be similar to that after penicillin therapy (R.J. Walsh *et al., Br. J. vener. Dis.*, 1983, *59*, 242).

Proprietary Preparations

Eradacin *(Sterling Research, UK)*. *Capsules*, acrosoxacin 150 mg.

Proprietary Names and Manufacturers

Eracin *(Winthrop, Belg.)*; Eradacil *(Winthrop, Austral.; Winthrop, S.Afr.; Sterwin, Spain)*; Eradacin *(Sterling Research, UK)*; Winuron *(Winthrop, Ger.)*.

12334-f

Alafosfalin *(BAN, rINN)*.

Alaphosphin; Ro-03-7008. (1*R*)-1-(L-Alaninamido)ethylphosphonic acid.
$C_5H_{13}N_2O_4P$=196.1.

CAS — 60668-24-8.

Alafosfalin is a phosphonic acid antibiotic and has antibacterial activity against many Gram-negative and some Gram-positive organisms; it has no significant activity against *Pseudomonas* and *Proteus* spp. It appears to enhance the activity of some beta-lactam antibiotics.

A brief review of phosphonic acid antibiotics. Alafosfalin prevents the formation of cross-links in the bacterial cell wall, has a broad antibacterial spectrum, and is synergistic *in vitro* with inhibitors of cell-wall biosynthesis such as the beta-lactams. It has not, however, been used clinically for several reasons, including the rapid development of bacterial resistance, high inoculum effect, pH-dependent activity, hydrolysis before entry into the circulation, and low urinary recovery.— M. Neuman, *J. antimicrob. Chemother.*, 1984, *14*, 309.

References: *Lancet*, 1978, *1*, 314; J. G. Allen *et al., Antimicrob. Ag. Chemother.*, 1979, *15*, 684; F. R. Atherton *et al., ibid.*, 696; H. B. Maruyama *et al., ibid.*, *16*, 444; J. G. Allen and L. J. Lees, *ibid.*, 1980, *17*, 973; P. G. Welling *et al., J. antimicrob. Chemother.*, 1980, *6*, 373; F. R. Atherton *et al., Antimicrob. Ag. Chemother.*, 1981, *20*, 470; M. Arisawa *et al., ibid.*, 1982, *21*, 706; M. J. Hall *et al., J. antimicrob. Chemother.*, 1983, *11*, 427.

Proprietary Names and Manufacturers

Roche, UK.

310186-j

Amifloxacin *(BAN, rINN)*.

Win-49375; Win-49375-3 *(mesylate)*. 6-Fluoro-1,4-dihydro-1-methylamino-4-oxo-7-(4-methylpiperazin)-1-ylquinoline-3-carboxylic acid.
$C_{16}H_{19}FN_4O_3$=334.4.

CAS — 86393-37-5; 88036-80-0 (mesylate).

NOTE. Amifloxacin Mesylate is *USAN*.

Amifloxacin is a fluorinated 4-quinolone antimicrobial agent with similar actions to norfloxacin, p.274.

Some references to the antibacterial activity of amifloxacin: D. J. Pohlod and L. D. Saravolatz, *Antimicrob. Ag. Chemother.*, 1984, *25*, 377; N. V. Jacobus *et al., ibid.*, *26*, 104; K. D. Thompson *et al., ibid.*, 275; I. Garcia *et al., ibid.*, 421; J. F. John and J. A. Twitty, *ibid.*, 781; J. B. Cornett *et al., ibid.*, 1985, *27*, 4; A. Iravani *et al., ibid.*, 449; S. M. Smith, *ibid.*, 1986, *29*, 325; C. H. Fenlon and M. H. Cynamon, *ibid.*, 386.

Proprietary Names and Manufacturers

Sterling Research, UK; Sterling, USA.

184-z

Amikacin *(BAN, USAN, rINN)*.

Amicacina. 6-*O*-(3-Amino-3-deoxy-α-D-glucopyranosyl)-4-*O*-(6-amino-6-deoxy-α-D-glucopyranosyl)-1-*N*-[(2*S*)-4-amino-2-hydroxybutyryl]-2-deoxy-D-streptamine.

$C_{22}H_{43}N_5O_{13}$=585.6.

CAS — 37517-28-5.

Pharmacopoeias. In *It.* and *U.S.*

A semisynthetic derivative of kanamycin A. A white crystalline powder containing not less than 900 µg of amikacin per mg, calculated on the anhydrous basis. Sparingly **soluble** in water. A 1% solution in water has a pH of 9.5 to 11.5. **Store** in airtight containers.

3-k

Amikacin Sulphate *(BANM, rINNM).*

Amikacin Sulfate *(USAN)*; BB-K8.

$C_{22}H_{43}N_5O_{13},2H_2SO_4$=781.8.

CAS — 39831-55-5.

Pharmacopoeias. In *Chin.* and *Jpn.*

1.3 g of monograph substance is approximately equivalent to 1 g of amikacin.

Solutions for injection may darken from colourless to pale yellow but this does not indicate a loss of potency.

Incompatibility or loss of activity has been reported between amikacin sulphate and some penicillins and cephalosporins (see Gentamicin Sulphate, p.236), amphotericin, chlorothiazide sodium, erythromycin gluceptate, heparin, nitrofurantoin sodium, phenytoin sodium, thiopentone sodium, and warfarin sodium, and, depending on the composition and strength of the vehicle, tetracyclines, vitamins of the B group with vitamin C, and potassium chloride.

The effect of freezing and thawing on the stability of amikacin sulphate intravenous infusions.— C. J. Holmes *et al., Am. J. Hosp. Pharm.*, 1982, *39*, 104.

Units

50 600 units of amikacin are contained in approximately 50.9 mg of amikacin base in one ampoule of the first International Standard Preparation (1983).

Adverse Effects, Treatment, and Precautions

As for Gentamicin Sulphate, p.236. Peak plasma concentrations of amikacin greater than 30 µg per mL or trough concentrations greater than 10 µg per mL should be avoided.

EFFECTS ON THE EAR. For reference to studies indicating that amikacin may be more cochleotoxic than gentamicin, see Gentamicin Sulphate, p.237.

EFFECTS ON THE KIDNEY. For reference to studies suggesting that the nephrotoxic potential of amikacin is similar to that of gentamicin, see Gentamicin Sulphate, p.237.

INTERACTIONS. For reference to the inactivation of amikacin by antipseudomonal penicillins *in vivo*, see Gentamicin Sulphate, p.238.

For the effect of indomethacin on amikacin, see Gentamicin Sulphate, p.238.

OVERDOSAGE. There was no evidence of nephrotoxicity or ototoxicity in a 60-year-old woman following the accidental administration of amikacin 9 g by intravenous infusion over 6 hours. Haemodialysis started 12 hours after administration of amikacin did not influence amikacin clearance.— P. W. L. Ho *et al., Ann. intern. Med.*, 1979, *91*, 227. See also J. P. Flandrois *et al., Infection*, 1979, *7*, 190.

For reference to the reduction of excessive plasma-amikacin concentrations by complexation with ticarcillin, see Gentamicin, Treatment of Adverse Effects, p.238.

Antimicrobial Action

Amikacin is bactericidal and has a mode of action and antimicrobial spectrum similar to that of gentamicin (see p.239). It is reported to be degraded by fewer of the aminoglycoside-inactivating enzymes produced by bacteria than other aminoglycosides and is active against some strains of Gram-negative bacteria which are resistant to gentamicin, tobramycin, and kanamycin, including *Pseudomonas aeruginosa*. Minimum inhibitory concentrations ranging from 0.5 to 16 µg per mL have been reported for Gram-negative bacteria.

For reference to a comparative study of the antimicrobial activity of 11 aminoglycosides including amikacin, and for studies of the activity of amikacin against *Aeromonas, Citrobacter*, and *Yersinia* spp., see Gentamicin Sulphate, p.239.

ACTIVITY AGAINST MYCOBACTERIA. Some aminoglycosides, including amikacin have been reported to be active *in vitro* against some atypical *Mycobacterium* spp. Of 16 strains of *M. marinum* tested, amikacin and kanamycin inhibited 89 and 62% respectively at a concentration of 2.5 µg per mL; gentamicin, however, inhibited only 44% of strains at 10 µg per mL (W.J. Sanders and E. Wolinsky, *Antimicrob. Ag. Chemother.*, 1980, *18*, 529). Swenson *et al.* (*ibid.*, 1985, *28*, 807) have tested a range of antimicrobial agents against 258 clinical isolates of *M. fortuitum* (3 biovariants) and *M. chelonae* (2 subspecies). Amikacin had the greatest activity against all 5 subgroups; tobramycin had good activity against one subgroup of each strain only. However, since no one agent was active against all isolates it was recommended that susceptibility to amikacin, tobramycin, cefoxitin, erythromycin, doxycycline, and sulphamethoxazole be determined in order to select a suitable therapeutic regimen for infections caused by these organisms. Dibekacin was more active than amikacin, streptomycin, and kanamycin against *M. avium-intracellulare* complex in human peripheral blood mononuclear cells (R.T. Nozawa *et al., ibid.*, 1984, *26*, 841). Horsburgh *et al.* (*ibid.*, 1987, *31*, 969) reported that isolates of this complex from patients both with and without AIDS were rarely susceptible to amikacin, streptomycin, and kanamycin although the concentrations of amikacin used were low. Synergy against *M. avium-intracellulare* complex has been shown when kanamycin or streptomycin were combined with either ethambutol, isoniazid, or rifampicin (B.L. Zimmer *et al., ibid.*, 1982, *22*, 148).

For reference to the activity of amikacin against *Mycobacterium leprae* infection in *mice*, see Gentamicin Sulphate, p.239.

ACTIVITY AGAINST NOCARDIA. Amikacin *in vitro* inhibited 44% of 27 strains of *Nocardia asteroides* at concentrations less than 0.25 µg per mL and inhibited all 27 strains at 1 µg per mL.— J. R. Dalovisio and G. A. Pankey, *Antimicrob. Ag. Chemother.*, 1978, *13*, 128. Amikacin was the most effective of 7 aminoglycosides tested *in vitro* against *Nocardia asteroides*.— J. A. Garcia-Rodriguez *et al.* (letter), *J. antimicrob. Chemother.*, 1979, *5*, 610. Amikacin was the most active of 13 antimicrobial agents tested *in vitro* against 26 strains of *Nocardia asteroides*. The MIC of amikacin was in the range of 0.125 to 32 µg per mL.— M. E. Gombert, *Antimicrob. Ag. Chemother.*, 1982, *21*, 1011.

ACTIVITY WITH OTHER ANTIMICROBIAL AGENTS. For reference to the effect of other agents on the antimicrobial activity of aminoglycosides *in vitro*, see Gentamicin Sulphate, p.239.

References to studies showing synergy between amikacin and other antimicrobial agents against various organisms: antipseudomonal penicillins.— J. A. Moody *et al., Antimicrob. Ag. Chemother.*, 1984, *26*, 256; M. E. Gombert and T. M. Aulicino, *J. antimicrob. Chemother.*, 1986, *17*, 323; S. H. Guenthner *et al.* (letter), *ibid.*, *18*, 550.
cefotaxime.— M. J. Maslow *et al., J. antimicrob. Chemother.*, 1985, *16*, 227.
imipenem.— M. E. Gombert and T. M. Aulicino, *Antimicrob. Ag. Chemother.*, 1983, *24*, 810; C. I. Bustamante *et al., ibid.*, 1987, *31*, 632.
trimethoprim.— T. L. Parsley *et al., Antimicrob. Ag. Chemother.*, 1977, *12*, 349; S. H. Zinner *et al., Eur. J. clin. Microbiol.*, 1982, *1*, 144.
various beta-lactam agents.— R. N. Jones and R. R. Packer, *Antimicrob. Ag. Chemother.*, 1982, *22*, 985; S. C. Aronoff and J. D. Klinger, *ibid.*, 1984, *25*, 279; R. H. Glew and R. A. Pavuk, *ibid.*, *26*, 378.

See also under Activity against Mycobacteria, above.

A study investigating the antagonistic effects of amikacin and benzylpenicillin against enterococci.— C. Thauvin *et al., Antimicrob. Ag. Chemother.*, 1985, *28*, 78.

For reference to the ability of different tests for synergy or antagonism between amikacin and cefsulodin to predict for therapeutic outcome, see Cefsulodin, p.161.

Resistance

Amikacin-resistant strains of Gram-negative bacteria have been reported; cross-resistance with other aminoglycoside antibiotics may occur. For the mechanisms of resistance of bacteria to aminoglycosides, see Gentamicin Sulphate, p.240.

Amikacin is active against many strains of Gram-negative bacteria resistant to other aminoglycosides such as gentamicin and tobramycin. Fear of the emergence of resistance to amikacin has led many authorities to reserve this drug for use only in infections caused by Gram-negative bacteria resistant to the other aminoglycosides. In the *USA*, however, where there appears to be a high incidence of gentamicin resistance, several centres have adopted amikacin as the aminoglycoside for routine use. Gerding and Larson (*Am. J. Med.*, 1985, *79, Suppl.* 1A, 1) have analysed the changes in the incidence of aminoglycoside resistance in 14 centres in the *USA* where amikacin has replaced gentamicin for a period of at least 12 months. During gentamicin usage, resistance to gentamicin, tobramycin, and amikacin was observed in 8.4, 6.0, and 1.4% of isolates of Gram-negative bacteria respectively. After the period of amikacin usage the corresponding figures were 7.0, 5.3, and 1.7% respectively. The marginal increase in amikacin-resistant strains was due to an increase in resistance among *Pseudomonas aeruginosa*. In one further centre, gentamicin was re-introduced for 12 months followed again by a 12-month period of amikacin use. During gentamicin use resistance to gentamicin and tobramycin rose but fell again during amikacin use. The incidence of amikacin-resistance decreased from 3.2 to 2.8% in this centre in the first and second periods of amikacin use.

Contrary to these findings, however, some studies have demonstrated an increase in the incidence of Gram-negative bacteria (A.S. Cross *et al., Archs intern. Med.*, 1983, *143*, 2075; J.F. Levine *et al., J. infect. Dis.*, 1985, *151*, 295) and in the proportion of *Ps. aeruginosa* (J.M. Martinez-Forde *et al., Lancet*, 1982, *2*, 719) showing resistance to amikacin after an increase in its use. There have also been reports of amikacin resistance in Enterobacteriaceae and *Ps. aeruginosa* which appears to be plasmid-mediated and transferable by conjugation (G.T. Van Nhieu *et al., Antimicrob. Ag. Chemother.*, 1986, *29*, 833; V. Krcméry and J. Havlik, *J. antimicrob. Chemother.*, 1986, *18*, 429). Thus a policy of restricted use of amikacin appears to be prudent.

Absorption and Fate

As for Gentamicin Sulphate, p.241.

After intramuscular injection of amikacin sulphate peak plasma concentrations equivalent to about 20 µg of amikacin per mL are achieved one hour after a 500-mg dose, reducing to about 2 µg per mL 10 hours after injection. A plasma concentration of 38 µg per mL has been reported after the intravenous infusion of 500 mg over 30 minutes, reduced to 18 µg per mL one hour later. Amikacin has been detected in body tissues and fluids after injection; it crosses the placenta but does not readily penetrate into the cerebrospinal fluid.

A plasma half-life of about 2 hours has been reported in patients with normal renal function. Most of a dose is excreted by glomerular filtration in the urine within 24 hours.

A comparison of the pharmacokinetics, efficacy, and toxicity of amikacin and gentamicin in patients with serious infections. It appeared that amikacin may have pharmacokinetic advantages over gentamicin.— S. E. Holm *et al., J. antimicrob. Chemother.*, 1983, *12*, 393. A comparative study of the pharmacokinetics of amikacin, gentamicin, and tobramycin. Although there was no difference in predictability of pharmacokinetic parameters between the 3 agents, amikacin achieved minimum therapeutic plasma concentrations more reliably.— A. Dyas *et al., ibid.*, 371.

Studies of the pharmacokinetics of amikacin in morbidly obese patients: L. A. Bauer *et al., Eur. J. clin. Pharmac.*, 1983, *24*, 643; R. A. Blouin *et al., Clin. Pharm.*, 1985, *4*, 70.

ADMINISTRATION IN INFANTS AND CHILDREN. The pharmacokinetics of amikacin in the newborn were comparable with those of kanamycin and mean serum-amikacin concentrations of 17 to 20 µg per mL had been recorded 30 minutes after 7.5 mg per kg body-weight given intramuscularly. Measurements made after several days' administration to 11 infants showed a mean peak serum-amikacin concentration of 21.1 µg per mL after intramuscular injection. Reduced concentrations were measured in 5 of the 11 after several intravenous injections and were associated with a birth-weight of 1.92 kg or less. Amikacin diffused into the CSF in concentrations ranging from 0.8 to 9.2 µg per mL 1 to 12 hours after 7.5 mg per kg given intramuscularly (mean 4.4 µg per mL).— J. B. Howard *et al., Antimicrob. Ag. Chemother.*, 1976, *10*, 205. See also M. G. Myers *et al., ibid.*, 1977, *11*, 1027 (pharmacokinetics in hypoxaemic and premature neonates); J. M. Lanao *et al., Eur. J. clin. Pharmac.*, 1982, *23*, 155 (pharmacokinetics during development from neonate to child).

DIFFUSION INTO BODY TISSUES AND FLUIDS. Studies of the concentrations of amikacin reached in the bile: R. H. Bermúdez *et al.*, *Antimicrob. Ag. Chemother.*, 1981, *19*, 352; J. F. Hansbrough *et al.*, *ibid.*, *20*, 515; J. L. LeFrock *et al.*, *J. clin. Pharmac.*, 1984, *24*, 247.

Studies of the diffusion of amikacin into bronchial secretions of patients with cystic fibrosis: J. Levy *et al.*, *J. antimicrob. Chemother.*, 1982, *10*, 227; E. Autret *et al.*, *Eur. J. clin. Pharmac.*, 1986, *31*, 79.

Studies of the penetration of amikacin through the blood-brain barrier: D. J. Briedis and H. G. Robson, *Antimicrob. Ag. Chemother.*, 1978, *13*, 1042 (healthy subjects); R. Yogev and W. M. Kolling, *ibid.*, 1981, *20*, 583 (hydrocephalic children with suspected ventriculitis).

Uses and Administration

Amikacin is a semisynthetic aminoglycoside antibiotic derived from kanamycin and is used similarly to gentamicin (see p.242) in the treatment of severe Gram-negative infections. It is given as the sulphate, and is generally reserved for the treatment of severe infections caused by susceptible bacteria which are resistant to gentamicin and tobramycin. As with gentamicin, amikacin may be used with penicillins and with cephalosporins; the injections should be given separately.

A suggested dose for adults and children is the equivalent of 15 mg of amikacin per kg bodyweight daily in equally divided doses every 8 or 12 hours by intramuscular injection, up to a maximum of 1.5 g daily in adults. Neonates may be given a loading dose equivalent to amikacin 10 mg per kg followed by 15 mg per kg daily in two divided doses. The same doses may be given by slow intravenous injection over 2 to 3 minutes or by intravenous infusion. In adults, 500 mg in 100 to 200 mL of sodium chloride 0.9% or glucose 5% injection or other suitable diluent has been infused over 30 to 60 minutes; for infants, infusions over 1 to 2 hours have been suggested. Treatment should preferably not continue for longer than 7 to 10 days, the total dose given to adults should not exceed 15 g, and peak plasma concentrations greater than 30 µg per mL or trough plasma concentrations greater than 10 µg per mL should be avoided. In patients with impaired renal function doses should be reduced or the intervals between them prolonged. In all patients, dosage should be adjusted according to plasma-amikacin concentrations (see under Uses, Administration, in Gentamicin Sulphate, p.242).

Amikacin has been given by intrathecal injection in conjunction with systemic administration. A 0.25% solution has been instilled into body cavities in adults.

A review of the actions and uses of amikacin.— R. D. Meyer, *Ann. intern. Med.*, 1981, *95*, 328.

For proceedings of a symposium on aminoglycosides with particular reference to amikacin sulphate, see *Am. J. Med.*, 1985, *79*, *Suppl.* 1A, 1–76.

See also under Gentamicin Sulphate, p.242, for general reviews of the aminoglycoside antibiotics.

For reference to the possible increase in bacterial resistance to amikacin after the introduction of amikacin as the aminoglycoside for routine use, see Resistance, above.

A 76-year-old man with a retroperitoneal *Nocardia asteroides* abscess did not respond to treatment with co-trimoxazole for 6.5 weeks and surgical drainage. Subsequent treatment with amikacin resulted in a cure after 7 weeks. Ornidazole was also given in the last 5 weeks but was considered unlikely to have contributed to the therapeutic success.— B. Meier *et al.*, *Antimicrob. Ag. Chemother.*, 1986, *29*, 150.

ATYPICAL MYCOBACTERIAL INFECTIONS. On the basis of experience with 123 patients with non-pulmonary infections caused by *Mycobacterium fortuitum* and *M. chelonei*, and of previous studies of the antimicrobial susceptibility of almost 250 isolates of the *M. fortuitum* complex, suggestions for the management of these infections were made. All patients with abscess formation or significant deep infections require surgical incision and drainage. For patients with serious infections, initial empirical parenteral therapy with amikacin 15 mg per kg body-weight daily and cefoxitin 200 mg per kg daily up to a maximum of 12 g daily, in association with probenecid by mouth should be given. The duration of therapy and subsequent dosing depend on the susceptibility of the organism isolated; it may be possible to administer parenteral cefoxitin alone after 4 to 8 weeks, or to change to oral therapy with a sulphonamide, doxycycline, minocycline, or erythromycin after a minimum of 2 to 6 weeks of parenteral therapy. In the treatment of less serious disease empirical oral therapy with a sulphonamide alone or in association with erythromycin may be suitable.— R. J. Wallace *et al.*, *J. infect. Dis.*, 1985, *152*, 500. See also J. N. Kuritsky *et al.*, *Ann. intern. Med.*, 1983, *98*, 938.

For further reference to the treatment of atypical mycobacterial infections including mention of the use of amikacin, see the section on Antimycobacterial Agents, p.553.

MENINGITIS. For reference to the use of amikacin sulphate in the treatment of meningitis, see Gentamicin Sulphate, p.244.

NEUTROPENIA. For reference to the use of amikacin sulphate in the treatment of febrile episodes in neutropenic patients see under Septicaemia in Gentamicin Sulphate, p.244.

OSTEOMYELITIS. The administration of amikacin via an implantable pump appeared to be a useful adjunct to surgical debridement and intravenous antibiotics in the treatment of 14 patients with osteomyelitis.— C. R. Perry *et al.*, *Am. J. Med.*, 1986, *80*, *Suppl.* 6B, 222.

PERITONITIS. For reference to the use of amikacin sulphate in the treatment of peritonitis associated with continuous ambulatory peritoneal dialysis, see Gentamicin Sulphate, p.244.

SEPTICAEMIA. For reference to the use amikacin sulphate in the treatment of septicaemia and septic shock, see Gentamicin Sulphate, p.244.

TUBERCULOSIS. Amikacin has been shown to be active *in vitro* against *Mycobacterium tuberculosis* and in *animal* models of tuberculosis. However, there appears to be complete cross-resistance of *M. tuberculosis* to amikacin and kanamycin, and studies in 4 patients with pulmonary tuberculosis resistant to conventional regimens indicated that amikacin had only very low activity. Amikacin therefore probably has no role in the treatment of this disease.— B. W. Allen *et al.*, *Tubercle*, 1983, *64*, 111.

URINARY-TRACT INFECTIONS. Report of a study involving 54 girls with first episodes of lower urinary-tract infections caused by *Escherichia coli*, suggested that a single intramuscular dose of amikacin 7.5 mg per kg bodyweight (maximum dose 240 mg) may be as effective as a 10-day course of sulphafurazole by mouth.— L. Wallen *et al.*, *J. Pediat.*, 1983, *103*, 316.

Preparations

Amikacin Sulfate Injection *(U.S.P.)*. Prepared using amikacin and sulphuric acid. pH 3.5 to 5.5.

Proprietary Preparations

Amikin *(Bristol-Myers Pharmaceuticals, UK). Injection*, amikacin 250 mg (as sulphate)/mL in vials of 2 mL. *Paediatric injection*, amikacin 50 mg (as sulphate)/mL in vials of 2 mL.

Proprietary Names and Manufacturers

Amikin *(Bristol-Myers, Austral.; Bristol, Canad.; Eire; Bristol, S.Afr.; Bristol-Myers Pharmaceuticals, UK; Bristol, USA)*; Amikine *(Bristol, Switz.)*; Amiklin *(Bristol, Fr.)*; Amukin *(Belg.; Neth.)*; BB-K8 *(Bristol Italiana Sud, Ital.; Mex.)*; Biclin *(Bristol-Myers, Spain)*; Biklin *(Arg.; Bristol-Myers, Denm.; Grünenthal, Ger.; Jpn; Bristol, Swed.)*; Chemacin *(CT, Ital.)*; Kaminax *(Ausonia, Ital.)*; Kanbine *(Septa, Spain)*; Likacin *(Lisapharma, Ital.)*; Lukadin *(San Carlo, Ital.)*; Mikavir *(Salus, Ital.)*; Pierami *(Pierrel, Ital.)*; Sifamic *(SIFI, Ital.)*.

4-a

Amoxycillin *(BAN)*.

Amoxicillin *(rINN)*; BRL-2333. (6*R*)-6-[α-D-(4-Hydroxyphenyl)glycylamino]penicillanic acid.
$C_{16}H_{19}N_3O_5S$=365.4.
CAS — 26787-78-0.

5-t

Amoxycillin Sodium *(BANM)*.

Amoxicillin Sodium *(rINNM)*. The sodium salt of amoxycillin.
$C_{16}H_{18}N_3NaO_5S$=387.4.
CAS — 34642-77-8.

Pharmacopoeias. In *It.*

1.06 g of monograph substance is approximately equivalent to 1 g of amoxycillin. Each g of monograph substance represents about 2.6 mmol of sodium.

It is recommended that reconstituted solutions of amoxycillin sodium for injection should be administered immediately after preparation. Amoxycillin sodium should not be mixed with blood products or other proteinaceous fluids such as protein hydrolysates.

The stability of amoxycillin sodium in intravenous fluids.— B. Cook *et al.*, *J. clin. Hosp. Pharm.*, 1982, *7*, 245.

Stability of aqueous solutions of amoxycillin sodium in the frozen and liquid states.— J. Concannon *et al.*, *Am. J. Hosp. Pharm.*, 1986, *43*, 3027.

For a review on the stability of aminopenicillins in solution, see p.116.

6-x

Amoxycillin Trihydrate *(BANM)*.

Amoxicillin *(USAN)*; Amoxicillin Trihydrate *(rINNM)*; Amoxicillinum Trihydricum. The trihydrate of amoxycillin.
$C_{16}H_{19}N_3O_5S,3H_2O$=419.5.
CAS — 61336-70-7.

Pharmacopoeias. In *Br., Chin., Cz., Egypt., Eur., Fr., Ind., It., Neth., Swiss*, and *U.S.*

A white or almost white almost odourless crystalline powder. 1.15 g of monograph substance is approximately equivalent to 1 g of amoxycillin. Slightly **soluble** in water, alcohol, methyl alcohol; practically insoluble in chloroform, ether, and fixed oils. It dissolves in dilute solutions of acids and of alkali hydroxides. A 0.2% solution in water has a pH of 3.5 to 6.0. **Store** at a temperature not exceeding 30° in airtight containers.

Adverse Effects

As for Ampicillin, p.116.

The incidence of diarrhoea is less with amoxycillin than ampicillin.

ALLERGY. See Effects on the Skin, below.

For reference to a comparative study of hypersensitivity reactions to amoxycillin and cefaclor, see Cefaclor, p.142.

EFFECTS ON THE BLOOD. Neutropenia, occurring 13 to 23 days after onset of treatment, was associated with the administration of amoxycillin by mouth in 3 patients. It was considered to be immune-mediated.— B. Rouveix *et al.*, *Br. med. J.*, 1983, *287*, 1832.

A report of pancytopenia in a 79-year-old man given amoxycillin 250 mg three times daily for 10 days followed by co-trimoxazole 960 mg twice daily for 11 days, both given by mouth. Results of bone-marrow culture studies implicated a direct toxic effect of amoxycillin.— A. E. Irvine *et al.*, *Br. med. J.*, 1985, *290*, 968.

EFFECTS ON THE GASTRO-INTESTINAL TRACT. Pseudomembranous colitis in a 5-week-old infant developed soon after administration of amoxycillin by mouth for an upper respiratory-tract infection. Amoxycillin was replaced by intravenous ampicillin when blood and mucus appeared in the stool. The infant died on the eighth day of the illness. *Clostridium difficile* and toxin were isolated from the gastro-intestinal tract at necropsy.— S. A. Richardson *et al.*, *Br. med. J.*, 1981, *283*, 1510.

Non-pseudomembranous colitis, presenting with abdominal pain and bloody diarrhoea, was associated with the administration of amoxycillin by mouth in 4 patients.— M. Iida *et al.*, *Endoscopy*, 1985, *17*, 64. See also.— R. B. Toffler *et al.*, *Lancet*, 1978, *2*, 707.

For reference to the ability of amoxycillin to select for resistant strains of *Escherichia coli* in the gastro-intestinal tract, see under Uses, Urinary-tract Infections, below.

EFFECTS ON THE LIVER. For mention of raised liver enzyme values after administration of amoxycillin in association with clavulanic acid, see under Uses, Urinary-tract Infections.

EFFECTS ON THE NERVOUS SYSTEM. Auditory and visual hallucinations occurred in a 60-year-old woman with pneumonia who was receiving amoxycillin 250 mg by mouth three times daily. Symptoms ceased on substitution of erythromycin for amoxycillin.— D. J. Oliver, *Practitioner*, 1984, *228*, 884.

EFFECTS ON THE SKIN. Photosensitivity reactions had been reported with amoxycillin.— K. Stone, *Aust. J. Pharm.*, 1985, *66*, 415.

Analysis, by the Boston Collaborative Drug Surveillance Program, of data on 15 438 patients hospitalised between 1975 and 1982 detected 63 allergic skin reactions attributed to amoxycillin among 1225 recipients of the drug. This was the highest incidence of skin reactions among the drugs studied.— M. Bigby *et al.*, *J. Am. med. Ass.*, 1986, *256*, 3358.

Stevens-Johnson syndrome developed in a 60-year-old man 5 days after beginning a course of amoxycillin by mouth. He recovered a few days after withdrawal of the drug.— N. J. Davidson and W. J. Windebank, *Br. med. J.*, 1986, *292*, 380.

Precautions

As for Ampicillin, p.117.

For a reference to impaired absorption in patients with coeliac disease, see below under Absorption and Fate.

ADMINISTRATION IN RENAL FAILURE. For reference to the precautions to be observed in renal failure, see under Uses, Administration in Renal Failure.

INTERACTIONS. *Allopurinol*. For a report of an increased incidence of skin rashes in patients taking amoxycillin and allopurinol concurrently, see Ampicillin Trihydrate p.117.

Oral contraceptives. Of 38 cases of failure of oral contraceptive steroids in women receiving antibiotics reported to the Committee on the Safety of Medicines, 2 had taken amoxycillin.— D. J. Back *et al.*, *Drugs*, 1981, *21*, 46.

PREGNANCY AND THE NEONATE. For the precautions to be observed during pregnancy, see under Uses, Pregnancy and the Neonate, p.114.

Antimicrobial Action and Resistance

Amoxycillin is bactericidal, is effective against the same range of organisms as ampicillin (see p.117), and has a similar mode of action. It has been reported that amoxycillin predominantly inhibits side-wall synthesis in susceptible bacteria while ampicillin mainly inhibits cross-wall synthesis. Amoxycillin has been reported to be slightly more active than ampicillin against some streptococci and *Salmonella* spp. but less active against *Shigella* spp. Synergy occurs between amoxycillin and clavulanic acid against bacteria usually resistant to amoxycillin due to the production of certain beta-lactamases, (see Clavulanic Acid p.197).

Amoxycillin is inactivated by penicillinase and complete cross-resistance has been reported between amoxycillin and ampicillin.

For reference to the activity of amoxycillin against *Actinomyces* spp., see under Actinomycosis in Uses, below.

ACTIVITY WITH OTHER ANTIMICROBIAL AGENTS. *Aminoglycosides*. The bactericidal activity of amoxycillin was generally enhanced *in vitro* against strains of *Enterococcus faecalis* over the first 6 hours when used with a sub-inhibitory concentration of an aminoglycoside antibiotic to which the strain was sensitive. A similar effect was obtained against one strain of each of *Str. salivarius* and *Str. bovis* when amoxycillin was used with gentamicin sulphate.— M. J. Basker and R. Sutherland, *J. antimicrob. Chemother.*, 1977, *3*, 273.

Clavulanic acid. Amoxycillin inhibited 8 of 13 strains of *Mycobacterium fortuitum* at a concentration of 32 µg per mL *in vitro*. In combination with potassium clavulanate the MIC was decreased several-fold against most strains.— M. H. Cynamon and G. S. Palmer, *Antimicrob. Ag. Chemother.*, 1983, *23*, 935. A combination of amoxycillin 2 µg per mL and potassium clavulanate 1 µg per mL inhibited all 15 strains of *M. tuberculosis in vitro*. Amoxycillin alone at a concentration of 8 µg per mL inhibited only 4 strains.— *idem*, *24*, 429.

Dicloxacillin. Synergy was demonstrated *in vitro* between amoxycillin and dicloxacillin against clinical isolates of *Staphylococcus aureus*, including some beta-lactamase-producing strains.— R. T. Yousef *et al.*, *Pharmazie*, 1985, *40*, 650.

Fosfomycin. Studies *in vitro* indicating a synergistic interaction between amoxycillin and fosfomycin.— N. A. Carlone *et al.*, *Drugs exp. & clin. Res.*, 1984, *10*, 47.

RESISTANCE. For reports of increasing resistance of urinary pathogens to amoxycillin, and of selection of intestinal bacteria resistant to amoxycillin, see under Uses, Urinary-tract Infections.

Absorption and Fate

Amoxycillin trihydrate is resistant to inactivation by the acid of gastric secretions and is rapidly absorbed when given by mouth. It is more completely absorbed than ampicillin and is reported to produce peak antibiotic plasma concentrations that are up to 2½ times as high as those from the same dose of ampicillin. Peak plasma-amoxycillin concentrations of about 5 µg per mL have been observed 1 to 2 hours after a dose of 250 mg, with detectable amounts present for up to 8 hours. Doubling the dose can produce double the concentration. The presence of food in the stomach does not appear to diminish absorption significantly.

Amoxycillin is given by injection as the sodium salt and a peak plasma concentration of about 14 µg of amoxycillin per mL has been reported to occur one hour after the intramuscular injection of a dose equivalent to 500 mg of amoxycillin. However, in general, similar concentrations are achieved with intramuscular and oral administration.

Up to 20% is bound to plasma proteins in the circulation and plasma half-lives of about one hour have been reported. The half-life may be longer in neonates and the elderly because of incomplete renal function. Amoxycillin is widely distributed at varying concentrations in body tissues and fluids. Amoxycillin diffuses across the placenta; little appears to be excreted in breast milk. It penetrates well into purulent and mucoid sputum and middle ear fluid, but only low concentrations have been found in ocular fluid. Little amoxycillin passes into the CSF unless the meninges are inflamed.

Amoxycillin is metabolised to a limited extent to penicilloic acid which is excreted in the urine. About 60% of an oral dose of amoxycillin is excreted unchanged in the urine in 6 hours by glomerular filtration and tubular secretion. Urinary concentrations above 300 µg per mL have been reported after a dose of 250 mg. Probenecid retards renal excretion. High concentrations have been reported in bile. Amoxycillin is removed by haemodialysis to some extent.

The absorption and fate of amoxycillin is not altered by administration with clavulanic acid.

A comparison of the pharmacokinetics of amoxycillin after oral, intramuscular, and intravenous administration.— D. A. Spyker *et al.*, *Antimicrob. Ag. Chemother.*, 1977, *11*, 132.

Studies of the pharmacokinetics of amoxycillin when administered in association with clavulanic acid: D. Adam *et al.*, *Antimicrob. Ag. Chemother.*, 1982, *22*, 353 (healthy subjects); U. B. Schaad *et al.*, *ibid.*, 1983, *23*, 252 (paediatric patients; intravenous infusion); I. Nilsson-Ehle *et al.*, *J. antimicrob. Chemother.*, 1985, *16*, 491 (healthy subjects); U. B. Schaad *et al.*, *ibid.*, 1986, *17*, 341 (paediatric patients).

ADMINISTRATION IN RENAL FAILURE. For reference to the pharmacokinetics of amoxycillin in renal failure, see under Uses, Administration in Renal Failure.

DIFFUSION INTO BODY TISSUES AND FLUIDS. Amoxycillin was given in a dose of 500 mg four times daily to 22 patients with pneumonia or acute exacerbations of chronic bronchitis. The mean sputum concentrations at 2 to 3 and 6 hours after a dose were 0.52 and 0.53 µg per mL respectively. Corresponding serum concentrations were 11 and 3.5 µg per mL. The mean concentration in saliva at 2 hours was 0.32 µg per mL. Clinical response occurred more rapidly when the sputum concentration exceeded 0.25 µg per mL but elimination of the organism was related to the pathogen rather than the concentration of amoxycillin.— S. M. Stewart *et al.*, *Thorax*, 1974, *29*, 110. In patients with acute exacerbations of chronic bronchitis sputum concentrations of amoxycillin increased proportionally with dose. Results in 30 patients with chronic bronchitis indicated that amoxycillin penetrated best into sputum containing about 50% pus.— A. Ingold, *Br. J. Dis. Chest*, 1975, *69*, 211. In a study involving 19 patients with chronic bronchitis given amoxycillin 500 mg by mouth followed by 6 further doses of 250 mg at 2-hourly intervals, the mean concentration of drug in the sputum up to 3 hours after the fifth dose was 0.4 µg per mL. Amoxycillin could not be detected at all, however, in 5 patients during this period. Sputum concentrations were 4 to 6% of those in the serum, and were higher the more purulent the sputum.— R. W. Light; F. A. Wyle, *Curr. ther. Res.*, 1983, *33*, 436. See also under Uses, Respiratory-tract Infections.

In a study of 22 children with chronic otitis media, mean concentrations of 6.2 and 1.48 µg per mL of antibiotic were achieved in the middle-ear fluid 1 to 2 hours after 1-g oral doses of amoxycillin and ampicillin respectively. Serum concentrations were not significantly different.— J. J. Klimek *et al.*, *J. infect. Dis.*, 1977, *135*, 999.

Mean CSF concentrations of amoxycillin in 12 healthy subjects given 33 mg per kg body-weight by intravenous infusion were 350 and 360 ng per mL, ½ and 3½ hours respectively after administration. Higher concentrations were achieved with the same dose of ampicillin given to a further 9 healthy subjects.— N. Clumeck *et al.*, *Antimicrob. Ag. Chemother.*, 1978, *14*, 531. In the presence of meningeal inflammation in 13 patients with tuberculous meningitis, concentrations of amoxycillin in the CSF ranged from 0.1 to 1.5 µg per mL 2 hours after administration of 1 g by mouth and represented about 1 to 21% of the concurrent serum concentrations. Following administration of 2 g intravenously, as the sodium salt, concentrations in the CSF ranged from 2.9 to 40 µg per mL at 1.5 hours and from 2.6 to 27 µg per mL at 4 hours and represented about 8 to 93% and 47 to 475% respectively of the concurrent serum concentrations.— L. J. Strausbaugh *et al.*, *Antimicrob. Ag. Chemother.*, 1978, *14*, 899. See also J. C. Craft *et al.*, *Antimicrob. Ag. Chemother.*, 1979, *16*, 346 (the effect of probenecid on amoxycillin concentrations in the CSF in bacterial meningitis).

In a study of 30 patients given an intravenous injection of amoxycillin 1 g in association with clavulanic acid 200 mg, both components of the preparation penetrated rapidly into peritoneal fluid, high concentrations being achieved 15 to 20 minutes after administration. The concentration of amoxycillin in peritoneal fluid exceeded 5 µg per mL for about 2 hours, and that of clavulanic acid exceeded 1 µg per mL for 2.5 to 3.5 hours. The mean percentage penetration into peritoneal fluid compared with serum concentrations was 84% and 66% respectively. The half-lives for both drugs in the serum and peritoneal fluid were similar, and the ratio of amoxycillin to clavulanic acid in both body fluids did not alter significantly from the initial proportions in the injected preparation.— R. Wise *et al.*, *J. antimicrob. Chemother.*, 1983, *11*, 57. Similar results; the concentration of amoxycillin in peritoneal fluid was maintained above 10 µg per mL for at least 2 hours after the injection, and that of clavulanic acid reached a maximum of about 4.2 µg per mL after one hour.— E. T. Houang *et al.*, *Antimicrob. Ag. Chemother.*, 1985, *28*, 165.

DRUG ABSORPTION. The absorption of amoxycillin was delayed in patients with coeliac disease.— R. L. Parsons *et al.*, *J. antimicrob. Chemother.*, 1975, *1*, 39.

A study in 12 healthy subjects indicating that the absorption of amoxycillin from the gastro-intestinal tract is saturable. It was estimated that approximately 2.3 g was the maximum that could be absorbed from the gastro-intestinal tract and excreted in the urine following a single dose.— J. Sjövall *et al.*, *Clin. Pharmac. Ther.*, 1985, *38*, 241.

A diet high in dietary fibre might increase the rate of absorption of amoxycillin and decrease the total amount absorbed according to a study in 10 healthy subjects.— M. Lutz *et al.*, *Clin. Pharmac. Ther.*, 1987, *42*, 220.

For reference to a comparative study of the absorption of amoxycillin and bacampicillin, see Bacampicillin Hydrochloride p.128.

METABOLISM. About 24% of a dose of amoxycillin 250 mg was metabolised and about 33% of a 500-mg dose. After 6 hours, 63% of a 250-mg dose, given to 10 healthy subjects, was recovered unchanged in the urine and 20% was excreted as penicilloic acid.— M. Cole *et al.*, *Antimicrob. Ag. Chemother.*, 1973, *3*, 463.

There was no evidence of active metabolites of amoxycillin in the urine of healthy subjects following administration of amoxycillin trihydrate.— M. C. Cole and B. Ridley (letter), *J. antimicrob. Chemother.*, 1978, *4*, 580.

Uses and Administration

Amoxycillin is the 4-hydroxy analogue of ampicillin, and is used in a similar variety of infections (see p.119), although it should not be used in shigellosis. Amoxycillin has been used as an alternative to chloramphenicol in the treatment of infections caused by *Salmonella* spp. and in the eradication of their carrier states. It is given by mouth, as the trihydrate. The usual dose is the equivalent of 250 to 500 mg of amoxycillin three times daily. Children up to 10 years of age may be given the equivalent of 125 to 250 mg three times daily; under 20 kg body-weight a dose of 20 to 40 mg per kg daily has been suggested.

Higher doses of amoxycillin, often in short courses, have been investigated in many conditions. Amoxycillin is given as a single dose of 3 g, often with probenecid 1 g, in the treatment of uncomplicated gonorrhoea in areas where gonococci have maintained sensitivity. This regimen, followed by a course of a tetracycline, has also been used for the treatment of pelvic inflammatory disease or sexually transmitted diseases where the aetiological agent is unknown. A single dose of 3 g may also be used for the treatment of uncomplicated acute urinary-tract infections and for the prophylaxis of endocarditis in susceptible patients about 1 hour before procedures such as dental extractions; children may be given half the adult dose. A high dose regimen of amoxycillin 3 g twice daily may be used in patients with severe or recurrent infections of the respiratory tract.

Amoxycillin is administered by injection as amoxycillin sodium and in moderate infections the equivalent of 500 mg of amoxycillin may be given intramuscularly every 8 hours. If pain is experienced the injection can be prepared using a 0.5% solution of procaine hydrochloride or a 1% solution of lignocaine hydrochloride. In severe infections the equivalent of 1 g of amoxycillin may be given every 6 hours by slow intravenous injection over 3 to 4 minutes or by infusion over 30 to 60 minutes. Children up to 10 years of age may be given the equivalent of 50 to 100 mg per kg body-weight daily by injection in divided doses. Doses may need to be adjusted in renal failure.

Amoxycillin may be administered as a combination preparation with clavulanic acid as the potassium salt (see p.197). Clavulanic acid is a beta-lactamase inhibitor that widens amoxycillin's antibacterial spectrum to organisms usually resistant due to their production of beta-lactamases. The combination should, however, be reserved for the treatment of infections caused by such amoxycillin-resistant organisms. It is administered by mouth in a ratio of amoxycillin (as the trihydrate), 2 or 4 parts to 1 part of clavulanic acid, or intravenously in a ratio of 5 parts of amoxycillin (as the sodium salt), to 1 part of clavulanic acid. Doses of the combination are calculated on amoxycillin content.

For comparative reviews and reports of aminopenicillins, see Ampicillin Trihydrate p.119.

Reviews and discussions on the actions and uses of a combination of amoxycillin trihydrate with potassium clavulanate: R. N. Brogden *et al.*, *Drugs*, 1981, *22*, 337; *Med. Lett.*, 1984, *26*, 99; G. E. Stein and M. J. Gurwith, *Clin. Pharm.*, 1984, *3*, 591; M. D. Reed and J. L. Blumer, *ibid.*, 653; B. R. Smith and J. L. LeFrock, *Drug Intell. & clin. Pharm.*, 1985, *19*, 415; *ibid.*, 475.

Experience of the treatment of soft-tissue infections caused by beta-lactamase-producing organisms with amoxycillin 500 mg (as the trihydrate) in combination with clavulanic acid 250 mg (as the potassium salt) usually given every 8 hours by mouth for 7 days. The infections treated included gynaecological sepsis (11 patients), abdominal or biliary sepsis (10), and cellulitis (4). All patients had clinical cure or improvement.— A. P. Ball *et al.*, *J. antimicrob. Chemother.*, 1982, *10*, 67.

A study of the use of a combination of amoxycillin and fosfomycin.— T. Barreca *et al.*, *Drugs exp. & clin. Res.*, 1984, *10*, 55.

ACTINOMYCOSIS. A study of the sensitivity of *Actinomyces* spp. to amoxycillin and benzylpenicillin *in vitro* and the use of amoxycillin in 10 patients with actinomycosis. MICs for amoxycillin against 89 *Actinomyces* spp. isolates did not exceed 0.8 μg per mL whereas those for benzylpenicillin ranged from 0.05 to 6.0 μg per mL. Of 86 clinical isolates from patients with cervicofacial actinomycosis, 85 were *A. israelii*, and one *A. viscosus*; the 3 isolates from type collections were *A. israelii*, *A. viscosus*, and *A. naeslundii*. In 10 patients with actinomycosis the lesion was drained surgically and amoxycillin 500 mg four times daily taken by mouth until clinical resolution occurred. All of the patients responded well, amoxycillin being discontinued by the end of 5 weeks; in 2 patients amoxycillin could be discontinued after only 3 weeks.— M. V. Martin, *Br. dent. J.*, 1984, *156*, 252. See also.— A. E. Holmes *et al.* (letter), *ibid.*, 1982, *153*, 212.

ADMINISTRATION IN RENAL FAILURE. A study of the pharmacokinetics of amoxycillin given by mouth to 19 patients on peritoneal dialysis.— R. H. Jones, *J. Infect.*, 1979, *1*, 235.

For patients undergoing haemodialysis 1 g of amoxycillin could be injected at the end of the dialysis session and repeated every 12 to 36 hours.— G. Humbert *et al.*, *Antimicrob. Ag. Chemother.*, 1979, *15*, 28. See also E. L. Francke *et al.*, *Clin. Pharmac. Ther.*, 1979, *26*, 31.

The normal half-life for amoxycillin of 0.9 to 2.3 hours was increased to 5 to 20 hours in end-stage renal failure. The interval between doses should be extended from 6 hours to up to 12 hours in patients with a glomerular filtration-rate (GFR) of 10 to 50 mL per minute, and to up to 16 hours in those with a GFR of less than 10 mL per minute. High doses are needed in end-stage renal failure to maintain adequate urinary concentrations for urinary-tract infections. Supplements should be given to patients undergoing haemodialysis.— W. M. Bennett *et al.*, *Am. J. Kidney Dis.*, 1983, *3*, 155.

A study of the pharmacokinetics of amoxycillin given by mouth or intravenously in association with clavulanic acid to 6 healthy subjects with normal renal function, 17 patients with varying degrees of renal impairment, and 12 maintained on haemodialysis. The clearance of amoxycillin decreased about 10-fold and that of clavulanic acid about 3-fold as the glomerular filtration-rate (GFR) decreased from greater than 75 to between 5 and 10 mL per minute; the ratio of amoxycillin to clavulanic acid in plasma increased from 5 to 13 over this range of renal function. In the patients on haemodialysis the mean half-lives on and off dialysis were 2.4 and 12.6 hours respectively for amoxycillin, and 1.2 and 3.8 hours for clavulanic acid. In normal volunteers the half-lives for amoxycillin and clavulanic acid were 2.0 and 1.3 hours respectively. In view of the greater attenuation of the pharmacokinetics of amoxycillin than clavulanic acid, the dosage in renal failure should be adjusted according to the pharmacokinetics of clavulanic acid to prevent underdosing of this component. It was recommended that the standard oral and intravenous doses of the combination could be given at 4, 8, or 12 hour intervals in patients with GFRs greater than 75, between 35 and 75, and between 10 and 35 mL per minute respectively; these doses should not result in excessive accumulation of amoxycillin.— F. F. Horber *et al.*, *Antimicrob. Ag. Chemother.*, 1986, *29*, 614.

BILIARY-TRACT INFECTIONS. Amoxycillin has been reported to achieve high concentrations in the bile and has therefore been suggested for use in infections of the biliary-tract. Dooley (*Gut*, 1984, *25*, 988) considered that when given by mouth it should be of use in the treatment of such infections in non-jaundiced patients; its value in jaundiced patients is less certain. Amoxycillin 250 mg three times daily was one of several regimens suggested for the treatment of recurrent cholangitis. Munro and Sorrell (*Drugs*, 1986, *31*, 449) also suggested it as a possible drug to be used in a dose of 500 mg three times daily in association with metronidazole as oral therapy for acute cholecystitis, after intravenous therapy or in patients with uncomplicated disease who are not severely ill.

ENDOCARDITIS. A Working Party of the British Society for Antimicrobial Chemotherapy recommended that endocarditis caused by penicillin-sensitive streptococci be treated initially with benzylpenicillin and gentamicin both given intravenously (*Lancet*, 1985, *2*, 815). After 14 days the gentamicin should be stopped and the benzylpenicillin may be replaced with amoxycillin 0.5 to 1.0 g three times daily by mouth for a further 14 days. Probenecid may be administered concurrently. Following a retrospective study of 26 cases of bacterial endocarditis, Moy *et al.* (*Archs Dis. Childh.*, 1986, *61*, 394) suggested that streptococcal endocarditis in children could be treated with intravenous benzylpenicillin and gentamicin for 3 weeks followed by amoxycillin by mouth for a further 3 weeks. They favoured amoxycillin rather than phenoxymethylpenicillin because of its more predictable absorption. However, they emphasised the need for monitoring of bactericidal titres.

Prophylaxis. Prophylaxis against infective endocarditis is recommended for susceptible patients during various surgical or instrumentation procedures that may give rise to bacteraemia. Endocarditis is most often caused by oral streptococci. Regimens recommended for dental procedures aim to maintain adequate antibiotic concentrations for 6 to 9 hours after the procedure. Although it has generally been considered that bactericidal concentrations of amoxycillin are required for prophylaxis, experiments in *animals* (M.P. Glauser *et al. Lancet*, 1983, *1*, 237) suggest that this may not be necessary provided that the inoculum of bacteria is small, and that mechanisms apart from killing of bacteria may be responsible for its effect. A Working Party of the British Society for Antimicrobial Chemotherapy (BSAC) (*Lancet*, 1982, *2*, 1323 and *ibid.*, 1986, *1*, 1267) have recommended that patients undergoing dental extractions or scaling, or surgery involving the gingival tissues who require prophylaxis and are not allergic to penicillins should receive a single dose of amoxycillin 3 g by mouth one hour before the operation. Children under 10 years of age may receive half the adult dose, and those under 5, a quarter of the adult dose. Most authorities consider one dose to be sufficient, but Kumana *et al.* (*Br. med. J.*, 1986, *293*, 1532) concluded from a study involving 50 subjects that if a second dose was indicated it should be given 4 hours after the procedure.

In patients who have received penicillins in the previous month prophylaxis with erythromycin stearate had been recommended by the BSAC due to the possibility of carriage of oral streptococci with a reduced sensitivity to amoxycillin. Although Harrison *et al.* (*J. antimicrob. Chemother.*, 1985, *15*, 501) demonstrated the emergence of resistant streptococci after repeated weekly doses of amoxycillin 3 g by mouth in healthy subjects, they considered that the serum concentrations of amoxycillin obtained after administration of this dose would greatly exceed the MBCs for these strains. Furthermore, they had also observed the development of resistant streptococci with repeated doses of erythromycin stearate (G.A.J. Harrison *et al.*, *ibid.*, 471), but to a greater extent. MacGregor and Hart (*ibid.*, 1986, *18*, 113) also concluded that the emergence of resistant strains of oral streptococci after a single dose of amoxycillin 3 g was unlikely to pose a significant problem. Therefore the BSAC now state that amoxycillin can be given twice in a month, although every effort should be made to complete dental treatment in one or 2 sessions. They consider there to be no value in the culturing of mouth swabs to search for resistant strains.

For patients at risk of endocarditis receiving dental treatment under general anaesthesia the BSAC recommends prophylaxis with intramuscular amoxycillin 1 g before induction of anaesthesia followed by 0.5 g by mouth 6 hours later. Alternatively, they recommend that amoxycillin 3 g be given by mouth 4 hours before induction and repeated as soon as possible after the operation as proposed by Cannon *et al.* (*ibid.*, 1984, *13*, 285). Amoxycillin 3 g with probenecid 1 g both given by mouth 4 hours before general anaesthesia as suggested by Shanson *et al.* (*ibid.*, 629) is also recommended. Shanson (*Br. med. J.*, 1985, *290*, 711) considered that this regimen might be expected to provide adequate prophylaxis against endocarditis even if a large inoculum of tolerant streptococci entered the blood stream.

For patients at special risk of endocarditis who are to be given dental treatment in hospital, the BSAC recommends administration of amoxycillin 1 g and gentamicin 120 mg both given intramuscularly, immediately before induction if they are to have a general anaesthetic, or, if not, 15 minutes before the dental procedure. This is followed by amoxycillin 500 mg by mouth 6 hours later. Children under 10 years of age may be given amoxycillin in half the adult dose, and gentamicin 2 mg per kg body-weight.

The regimens for prophylaxis against endocarditis during dental procedures recommended by a Working Party of the European Society of Cardiology (J. Delaye *et al.*, *Eur. Heart J.*, 1985, *6*, 826) are very similar to those recommended by the BSAC.

The BSAC also recommend prophylaxis for patients

undergoing genito-urinary surgery or instrumentation under general anaesthesia, for patients with prosthetic values undergoing obstetric and gynaecological procedures, and for patients undergoing gastro-intestinal procedures. They recommend a regimen similar to that given to patients at special risk from dental procedures, although they state that the amoxycillin dose after the procedure may be given by mouth or by intramuscular injection. It is stated that for all these procedures prophylaxis should be effective against faecal streptococci. O'Connor and Axon (*Lancet*, 1983, *1*, 237), however, considered that during upper gastro-intestinal endoscopy such organisms were only occasionally isolated and therefore amoxycillin 3 g by mouth 1 hour before the procedure should provide adequate cover. The American Heart Association (S.T. Shulman *et al.*, *Circulation.*, 1984, *70*, 1123A) only recommend the use of amoxycillin for the prophylaxis of endocarditis for minor or repetitive gastro-intestinal or genito-urinary procedures in low-risk patients. It should be given in a dose of 3 g by mouth 1 hour before the procedure followed by 1.5 g six hours later. Children may be given 50 mg per kg followed by 25 mg per kg.

The BSAC recommend the use of intramuscular amoxycillin 1 g before induction of anaesthesia followed by 500 mg intramuscularly 6 hours later, in patients undergoing surgery or instrumentation of the upper respiratory tract under general anaesthesia. Patients with prosthetic valves should also receive intramuscular gentamicin 120 mg with the first amoxycillin dose.

For patients allergic to penicillins the BSAC recommends erythromycin stearate if oral therapy is indicated, or vancomycin if parenteral therapy is required.

See also under Prophylactic Use of Antibiotics, p.102.

ENTERIC INFECTIONS. *Combination with clavulanic acid.* A report of the successful treatment of *Yersinia enterocolitica* infections with intravenous amoxycillin in combination with clavulanic acid in 4 thalassaemic children.— C. Kattamis *et al.*, *J. antimicrob. Chemother.*, 1984, *14*, 303.

INFECTIONS PROPHYLAXIS, HYPOSPLENISM. For comment on the use of amoxycillin in post-splenectomy patients, see under Prophylactic Use of Antibiotics, p.102.

LEPTOSPIROSIS. For reference to the use of amoxycillin in the treatment of leptospirosis, see Benzylpenicillin Sodium, p.136.

MOUTH INFECTIONS. In a study of 60 patients with acute dento-alveolar abscess, treatment with two doses of amoxycillin 3 g given 8 hours apart was as effective as phenoxymethylpenicillin 250 mg four times daily for 5 days. Surgical drainage was also performed whenever possible.— M. A. O. Lewis *et al.*, *Br. dent. J.*, 1986, *161*, 299.

OTITIS MEDIA. Report of a multicentre double-blind study involving 84 children with acute otitis media, suggesting little difference between a 3- or 10-day course of amoxycillin on either the speed of resolution of symptoms and signs, or on the frequency of recurrences and complications.— D. M. Chaput de Saintonge *et al.*, *Br. med. J.*, 1982, *284*, 1078. In a study involving 274 children with acute otitis media, a course of amoxycillin 750 mg by mouth twice daily was as effective as 125 mg three times daily for 7 days in resolving symptoms and signs. The frequency of recurrence during 1 year of follow-up and of hearing loss recorded 1 and 6 months after entry to the study were similar in the 2 groups.— J. Bain *et al.*, *ibid.*, 1985, *291*, 1243.

Report of a study of an estimated 4860 children seen by general practitioners in the Netherlands for acute otitis media over a 17-month period. All were treated initially with nose drops and analgesics. Those with persistent discharge after 14 days were referred to a specialist and given a course of amoxycillin. The condition was severe (persistent high temperature and/or severe pain after 3 to 4 days) in a further 126 children who were randomised to receive either myringotomy, amoxycillin 250 mg three times daily by mouth for 7 days, or a combination of the two. In the 100 children who could be assessed, the duration of discharge, restoration of the tympanic membrane, and clinical course were all least satisfactory in the patients treated with myringotomy alone. The data, however, did not warrant the conclusion that myringotomy and antibiotics combined give better results than antibiotics alone. Bacteriological studies in patients with a severe clinical course and with a persistent discharge showed a predominance of infection with haemolytic streptococci, and only a few with *Haemophilus influenzae*.— F. L. van Buchem *et al.*, *Br. med. J.*, 1985, *290*, 1033.

Amoxycillin was compared in the treatment of otitis media with effusion with amoxycillin plus decongestant and antihistamine in a placebo-controlled study involving 474 infants and children. The dose of amoxycillin was 40 mg per kg body-weight daily by mouth in three divided doses for 2 weeks. Children with acute otitis media or with systemic illness were not included in the study. Of 158 patients receiving both active medications, 50 (32%) had no effusion 4 weeks after commencing treatment. The corresponding figures for those receiving amoxycillin alone were 46 of 160 (29%) and for those receiving two placebo treatments, 22 of 156 (14%). There was a recurrence of effusion, however, in about half of the patients within 4 weeks of the end of treatment. Thus it was concluded that there was no advantage in addition of the decongestant-antihistamine preparation to treatment with amoxycillin; but due to the low rates of cure guidelines were given as to when any treatment is warranted for this condition.— E. M. Mandel *et al.*, *New Engl. J. Med.*, 1987, *316*, 432.

Two hundred and sixty-six children with acute otitis media were treated by mouth with either amoxycillin 750 mg twice daily for 2 days, erythromycin 250 mg four times daily or 500 mg twice daily for 5 days, or cephradine 250 mg twice daily for 5 days. From assessment of symptoms at one week, 92% were considered resolved or better, and there was no difference between treatments.— P. N. Jenner *et al.*, *Br. J. clin. Pract.*, 1987, *41*, 820.

Combination with clavulanic acid. In a double-blind study involving 133 infants and children with otitis media, amoxycillin in combination with potassium clavulanate was similar in efficacy to cefaclor, both in resolution of otalgia and fever, and of middle-ear effusion.— P. H. Kaleida *et al.*, *Pediatr. infect. Dis.*, 1987, *6*, 265.

PREGNANCY AND THE NEONATE. There appeared to be no significant risk to the foetus from amoxycillin when administered during pregnancy although there was the possibility of sensitising the foetus during the second and third trimesters. If an antimicrobial agent had to be used during pregnancy, amoxycillin was recommended for the treatment of asymptomatic bacteriuria or simple cystitis, bronchitis, or the prophylaxis of endocarditis.— R. Wise, *Br. med. J.*, 1987, *294*, 42.

RESPIRATORY-TRACT INFECTIONS. *Asthma.* A double-blind study of 60 asthmatic patients with 71 exacerbations of their disease, indicated that the addition of a course of amoxycillin 500 mg three times daily by mouth to conventional therapy did not appear to influence the rate of improvement. *Haemophilus influenzae* or *Streptococcus pneumoniae* was cultured from only 4 sputum specimens on admission (2 each from patients receiving amoxycillin or placebo), and from 5 specimens on discharge (2 in the amoxycillin-treated group and 3 in the placebo group). Their isolation could not, however, be related clinically to infection.— V. A. L. Graham *et al.*, *Lancet*, 1982, *1*, 418.

Bronchiectasis. Amoxycillin 3 g twice daily by mouth for 7 days was administered to 17 patients with bronchiectasis. Clinical and spirometric improvement was observed in 11 of 12 patients who were producing purulent sputum from which *Haemophilus influenzae* could be cultured. The mean peak serum and sputum concentrations measured in 9 patients on day 7 were 34.9 and 1.7 µg per mL respectively; trough concentrations in 3 patients were 0.5 and and 0.25 µg per mL respectively.— P. J. Cole *et al.*, *J. antimicrob. Chemother.*, 1983, *11*, 109.

A beneficial effect was obtained in patients with bronchiectasis associated with cystic fibrosis given amoxycillin and flucloxacillin both at a dose of 1 g per 20 kg body-weight twice daily by mouth.— R. K. Knight (letter), *Lancet*, 1983, *2*, 970 and 1258.

References to the need for prolonged or high doses of amoxycillin in bronchiectasis, and of its administration by nebuliser: R. A. Stockley and S. L. Hill (letter), *Lancet*, 1984, *2*, 977; D. C. Currie *et al.* (letter), *Br. med. J.*, 1987, *295*, 119.

Combination with clavulanic acid. Report of 20 patients with bronchopulmonary infections caused by beta-lactamase-producing *Branhamella catarrhalis*, treated with amoxycillin 500 mg with clavulanic acid 125 mg three times daily by mouth for 5 days. *B. catarrhalis* was no longer isolated from sputum within 3 days in all patients. A recurrence occurring 2 to 4 weeks later in 2 patients was cleared by a further course of treatment.— P. E. Thornley *et al.*, *Drugs*, 1986, *31*, *Suppl.* 3, 113. An adequate duration of therapy with a similar dosage of amoxycillin and clavulanic acid appeared to be 5 days for lower respiratory-tract infections caused by *B. catarrhalis* and 7 days for those caused by *Haemophilus influenzae*. The majority of isolates produced beta-lactamase.— R. J. Wallace *et al.*, *Antimicrob. Ag. Chemother.*, 1985, *27*, 912.

Twenty patients with acute exacerbations of chronic bronchitis were treated with amoxycillin 1 g in association with clavulanic acid 250 mg (as potassium salt) twice daily by mouth for 10 days; 10 patients received the drugs intravenously for the first 3 days. The infections were caused by various organisms only some of which were beta-lactamase-producing. By the end of treatment, 15 had a negative sputum culture, but 7 days later 5 of these patients had a purulent relapse, or re-infection with beta-lactamase-producing strains of *Branhamella catarrhalis*.— F. P. V. Maesen *et al.*, *J. antimicrob. Chemother.*, 1987, *19*, 373.

SEPTICAEMIA. *Combination with clavulanic acid.* Experience of amoxycillin with clavulanic acid administered intravenously for the treatment of severe bacterial infections, including septicaemia, caused by beta-lactamase-producing organisms.— S. Mehtar and A. P. Ball, *J. antimicrob. Chemother.*, 1985, *15*, 765.

SEXUALLY TRANSMITTED DISEASES. *Chancroid. Combination with clavulanic acid.* Report of a double-blind study of the efficacy of amoxycillin in association with clavulanic acid in the treatment of chancroid in Nairobi, Kenya. Sixy-eight men had genital ulcers from which *Haemophilus ducreyi* could be cultured; all strains were beta-lactamase-producing. Patients were given amoxycillin 500 mg, amoxycillin 500 mg with clavulanic acid 125 mg, or amoxycillin 500 mg with clavulanic acid 250 mg, all given three times daily by mouth for 7 days. Of 12 patients given amoxycillin alone, treatment failed in all 9 who returned for follow-up; therefore this arm of the study was subsequently discontinued. Of 33 patients who received combination therapy with the lower dose of clavulanic acid (7 of whom had failed to respond to amoxycillin alone) all 28 who were followed up were clinically cured or improved. One patient, however, was still culture-positive for *H. ducreyi* and was given alternative treatment. Of 30 treated with the combination with the higher dose of clavulanic acid, 27 returned for follow-up, and 26 had responded to therapy. Complete ulcer healing occurred after a mean interval of 12 and 10 days respectively from the onset of therapy, and all buboes (inflamed lymph nodes) resolved within 4 weeks. Twenty-seven men with ulcers of unknown aetiology were also treated with one of the 3 regimens and all responded to therapy.— M. V. Fast *et al.*, *Lancet*, 1982, *2*, 509.

Treatment with amoxycillin 500 mg in association with clavulanic acid 250 mg, both given every 8 hours by mouth for 3 days was considered successful in 42 of 44 patients with chancroid caused by *Haemophilus ducreyi*. Cure rates were 24, 57, 73, and 94% on days 3, 7, 10, and 14 after commencement of treatment respectively. All buboes responded to treatment. Treatment with one or 2 doses of amoxycillin 3 g with clavulanic acid 350 mg was not successful.— J. O. Ndinya-Achola *et al.*, *Genitourinary Med.*, 1986, *62*, 202.

Gonorrhoea. Combination with clavulanic acid. A study of the use of various regimens involving amoxycillin with clavulanic acid in the treatment of uncomplicated gonorrhoea. A regimen of amoxycillin 250 mg with clavulanic acid 125 mg, and probenecid 1 g all given by mouth, and intramuscular procaine penicillin 4.5 g was the most effective, producing cure rates of 96.6 and 100% for penicillinase-producing and non-penicillinase-producing strains of *Neisseria gonorrhoeae* respectively. This regimen was also favoured because of its efficacy against incubating syphilis. A regimen of 2 doses of amoxycillin 3 g with clavulanic acid 250 mg given 4 hours apart was considered to be a suitable alternative.— K. B. Lim *et al.*, *Ann. Acad. Med. Singapore*, 1986, *15*, 258.

SURGICAL INFECTION PROPHYLAXIS. For the prophylactic use of amoxycillin and ampicillin in children undergoing tonsillectomy see Ampicillin, p.121.

Cardiac surgery. For the prophylactic use of amoxycillin in cardiac surgery, see Flucloxacillin Sodium (p.232).

ULCERS. *Peptic ulcer.* Evidence suggesting that treatment with both tripotassium dicitratobismuthate and a systemic antibiotic, such as amoxycillin, may be required to eradicate *Campylobacter pyloridis*, a bacterium associated with gastritis and peptic ulceration.— C. S. Goodwin *et al.*, *J. clin. Path.*, 1986, *39*, 353. See also C. A. M. McNulty, *Practitioner*, 1987, *231*, 176.

URINARY-TRACT INFECTIONS. Report of a double-blind study of 110 elderly patients with acute urinary-tract infections with pyuria and generalised illness. They were treated with either amoxycillin (52 patients) or cephradine (58) both given in a dosage of 500 mg by mouth every 8 hours for 7 days. Immediately after the course of therapy 38 patients (73%) receiving amoxycillin and 49 (84%) receiving cephradine were considered to be cured, but the difference was not significant. Of the 14 infections associated with amoxycillin failure, 10 were due to amoxycillin-resistant *Escherichia coli*. After a further week, only about half of the patients from each group were free from infection. In the group who had taken amoxycillin, infections were caused by a variety of enterobacteria most of which were resistant to amoxycillin. Amoxycillin had a greater propensity than cephradine to selection of intestinal *E. coli* resistant to itself and also to trimethoprim, tetracycline, and chloramphenicol. This could not be explained by greater use since cephradine had been more widely used in the past few years in that district. The amoxycillin-resistant *E. coli* also persisted longer in the intestine than those resistant to cephradine. The selection by amoxycillin of resistant strains was suprising in view of its good gastro-intestinal absorption, although it is less well absorbed than cephradine. Amoxycillin also selected for Gram-negative bacilli in saliva whereas cephradine did not; however, neither drug had a significant effect on the numbers of salivary *Candida* spp. or selected for resistance of aerobic skin flora. It was concluded that the selection of resistance in intestinal *E. coli* by amoxycillin would limit its usefulness in the treatment of urinary-tract infections. The authors had observed a resistance rate of about 40% in *E. coli* isolated from urine specimens recently referred to their laboratory.— R. W. Lacey *et al., Lancet*, 1983, *2*, 529. Studies of urine specimens collected from general or hospital practice indicating a decline in sensitivity of urinary pathogens, including *E. coli* to amoxycillin.— R. N. Grüneberg, *J. antimicrob. Chemother.*, 1984, *14*, 17; S. R. Marper and P. Noone (letter), *ibid.*, 1985, *15*, 251.

Single-dose therapy. Carlson and Mulley (*Ann. intern. Med.*, 1985, *102*, 244) described an analysis model for the management of acute dysuria with amoxycillin or co-trimoxazole. They used in their analysis for amoxycillin 4 clinical studies comparing its use as a single- or multiple-dose regimen. The single-dose regimen appeared to be slightly less effective but was preferred, mainly because of the lower incidence of adverse effects. The analysis did, however, find co-trimoxazole to be preferable to amoxycillin. Philbrick and Bracikowski (*Archs intern. Med.*, 1985, *145*, 1672) analysed 6 studies comparing the use of a single dose of amoxycillin 3 g with a multiple-dose regimen of amoxycillin or another antibiotic, for the treatment of uncomplicated urinary-tract infections in women. Five of these concluded that there was no difference in cure rates between the 2 regimens, but all involved too few patients to detect any significant difference. On pooling data from 3 of these studies they found a significantly lower cure rate after single-dose (69%) than multiple-dose (84%) therapy. None of the studies included sufficient data to detect differences in the incidence of adverse effects. In a multicentre study of 210 women with similar infections Tolkoff-Rubin *et al.* (*Antimicrob. Ag. Chemother.*, 1984, *25*, 626) concluded that initial treatment should be with amoxycillin 3 g by mouth as a single dose. If, 4 to 7 days later the patient is asymptomatic but cultures are positive, a 10-day course of amoxycillin 500 mg three times daily can be given; patients who are still symptomatic and who have bacteriuria should be treated with a 6-week course.

Combination with clavulanic acid. An increasing prevalence of urinary pathogens showing resistance to amoxycillin has been observed (see above). Therefore amoxycillin has been administered in association with the beta-lactamase inhibitor clavulanic acid; this combination has been shown to be active *in vitro* against a higher proportion of urinary pathogens than amoxycillin alone (W. Brumfitt and J.M.T. Hamilton-Miller, *Lancet*, 1983, *2*, 566; S.R. Marper and P. Noone, *J. antimicrob. Chemother.*, 1985, *15*, 251). These observations have been supported by reports of the efficacy of the combination in adults (A.M.A. Abbas *et al.*, *Br. J. clin. Pract.*, 1984, *38*, 49) and children (L.G.A. Roomi *et al.*, *Archs Dis. Childh.*, 1984, *59*, 256) with urinary-tract infections caused by amoxycillin-resistant organisms or which had failed to respond to amoxycillin alone.
Iravani and Richard (*Antimicrob. Ag. Chemother.*, 1986, *29*, 107) have reported on a double-blind study of women with acute urinary-tract infections treated with amoxycillin 250 mg in combination with clavulanic acid 125 mg (as the potassium salt), (51 patients), or with cefaclor 250 mg (53), both given by mouth every 8 hours for 10 days. Short-term and long-term cure (urine culture sterile up to 1 and 4 weeks after completion of treatment respectively) was recorded in 49 and 40 patients in both groups. Relapses occurred in 4 and 11 patients, and re-infection in 7 and 2 patients receiving the combination or cefaclor respectively. Compared with cefaclor, treatment with amoxycillin and clavulanic acid was associated with a greater selection of rectal isolates of *Escherichia coli* resistant to amoxycillin (as determined by the use of ampicillin discs). In patients treated with the combination who developed recurrent infections within 12 weeks of completion of treatment, the prevalence of urinary pathogens resistant to amoxycillin increased by 30% compared with those causing initial infections. The prevalence of organisms resistant to both the combination and to cefaclor also increased in this group of patients. This increase in resistance was not observed to a significant extent in patients with recurrent infections who had been treated with cefaclor. Transient elevation of liver transaminase enzyme values occurred in 12 and 3 patients receiving amoxycillin with clavulanic acid and cefaclor respectively.
There have been several other studies comparing the use of amoxycillin with clavulanic acid in urinary-tract infections with other agents. Karachalios (*Antimicrob. Ag. Chemother.*, 1985, *28*, 693) observed similar cure and recurrence rates after 10-day courses of the combination or co-trimoxazole. Matts *et al.* (*Br. J. clin. Pract.*, 1985, *39*, 179) however, found the combination to produce a clinical cure in a shorter time than co-trimoxazole when both were given for 7 days. Amoxycillin 250 mg with clavulanic acid 125 mg or cephalexin 250 mg both given three times daily for 7 days were equally effective in the treatment of pregnant women with bacteriuria (S.J. Pedler and A.J. Bint, *Antimicrob. Ag. Chemother.*, 1985, *27*, 508).
Brumfitt and Hamilton-Miller (*Lancet*, 1983, *2*, 566) however, did emphasise the importance of accurate disc testing of isolates of urine samples to permit the treatment of less resistant infections with amoxycillin alone.

WOUND INFECTIONS. In a placebo-controlled study involving 71 patients with non-invasive wound infections, addition of treatment with a combination of amoxycillin and clavulanic acid by mouth for 5 days to routine cleansing with Chlorinated Lime and Boric Acid Solution *B.P.* (Eusol), did not influence the outcome when judged clinically, but did significantly increase the elimination of susceptible organisms.— W. K. J. Huizinga *et al., J. Infect.*, 1986, *13*, 11.

Preparations

Amoxicillin Capsules *(U.S.P.).* Capsules containing amoxycillin trihydrate.

Amoxycillin Capsules *(B.P.).* Capsules containing amoxycillin trihydrate.

Amoxicillin for Oral Suspension *(U.S.P.).* A dry mixture of amoxycillin trihydrate for reconstitution.

Amoxycillin Oral Suspension *(B.P.).* Amoxycillin Mixture; Amoxycillin Syrup. A dry mixture of amoxycillin trihydrate for reconstitution.

Amoxicillin Tablets *(U.S.P.).* Chewable tablets containing amoxycillin trihydrate.

Amoxicillin and Clavulanate Potassium for Oral Suspension *(U.S.P.).* Amoxycillin trihydrate and potassium clavulanate. pH of the suspension 4.8 to 6.6.

Amoxicillin and Clavulanate Potassium Tablets *(U.S.P.).* Tablets (chewable or nonchewable) containing amoxycillin trihydrate and potassium clavulanate.

Proprietary Preparations

Almodan *(Rorer, UK). Capsules*, amoxycillin 250 and 500 mg [manufacturers state as the sodium salt].
Syrup, powder for reconstitution, amoxycillin 125 and 250 mg (as trihydrate)/5 mL when reconstituted with water.
Injection, powder for reconstitution, amoxycillin 250 mg, 500 mg and 1 g (as sodium salt).

Amoxidin *(Lagap, UK). Capsules*, amoxycillin 250 and 500 mg (as trihydrate).

Amoxil *(Bencard, UK). Capsules*, amoxycillin 250 and 500 mg (as trihydrate).
Tablets, dispersible, amoxycillin 500 mg (as trihydrate).
Sugar-free syrup (Syrup SF), powder for reconstitution, amoxycillin 125 and 250 mg (as trihydrate)/5 mL when reconstituted with water.
Paediatric suspension, powder for reconstitution, amoxycillin 125 mg (as trihydrate)/1.25 mL when reconstituted with water.
Sugar-free oral powder (Sachets SF), amoxycillin 750 mg and 3 g (as trihydrate)/sachet. To be dispersed in water before administration.
Injection, powder for reconstitution, amoxycillin 0.25, 0.5, and 1 g (as sodium salt).

Augmentin *(Beecham Research, UK). Tablets*, amoxycillin 250 mg (as trihydrate), clavulanic acid 125 mg (as potassium salt).
Tablets, dispersible, amoxycillin 250 mg (as trihydrate), clavulanic acid 125 mg (as potassium salt).
Junior suspension, powder for reconstitution, amoxycillin 125 mg (as trihydrate), clavulanic acid 62 mg (as potassium salt)/5 mL when reconstituted with water.
Paediatric suspension, powder for reconstitution, amoxycillin 125 mg (as trihydrate), clavulanic acid 31 mg (as potassium salt)/5 mL when reconstituted with water.
Injection, powder for reconstitution, amoxycillin 500 mg (as sodium salt), clavulanic acid 100 mg (as potassium salt).
Injection, powder for reconstitution, amoxycillin 1 g (as sodium salt), clavulanic acid 200 mg (as potassium salt).

Proprietary Names and Manufacturers of Amoxycillin, Amoxycillin Salts, and Amoxycillin Trihydrate

Actimoxi *(Clariana, Spain)*; Acuotricina *(Andreu, Spain)*; Agerpen *(CEPA, Spain)*; Agram *(Inava, Fr.)*; Alfamox *(Alfa Farmaceutici, Ital.)*; Alfida *(Esteve, Spain)*; Almodan *(Rorer, UK)*; AM 73 *(Ital.)*; Amodex *(Gerbiol, Fr.)*; Amoflamisan *(Mazuelos, Spain)*; Amolin *(Jpn)*; Amox *(Salus, Ital.; High Noon, Pakistan; Berenguer-Beneyto, Spain)*; Amoxaren *(Areu, Spain)*; Amoxibacter *(Rubio, Spain)*; Amoxibiotic *(Lagap, Ital.)*; Amoxican *(Canad.)*; Amoxicum *(Wasserman, Spain)*; Amoxidal *(Arg.)*; Amoxidel *(Delagrange, Spain)*; Amoxidin *(Lagap, UK)*; Amoxi-Gobens *(Normon, Spain)*; Amoxil *(Beecham, Austral.; Ayerst, Canad.; Bencard, S.Afr.; Bencard, UK; Beecham Laboratories, USA)*; Amoxilay *(Ralay, Spain)*; Amoxillat *(Azuchemie, Ger.)*; Amoxillin *(Esseti, Ital.; Apothekernes Laboratorium, Norw.)*; Amoximedical *(Medical, Spain)*; Amoxina *(Magis, Ital.)*; Amoxine *(Negma, Fr.)*; Amoxipen *(Gibipharma, Ital.)*; Amoxipenil *(Arg.; Hortel, Spain)*; Amoxypen *(Grünenthal, Ger.)*; Amoxyvinco *(Reig Jofré, Spain)*; Amplimox *(Ausonia, Ital.)*; Apamox *(Spain)*; Apo-Amoxi *(Apotex, Canad.)*; Ardine *(Antibioticos, Spain)*; Aspenil *(Chemil, Ital.)*; Axibiot *(Galepharma, Spain)*; Becabil *(Carol, Spain)*; Bimoxi *(Jorba, Spain)*; Bioxidona *(Faes, Spain)*; Bolchipen *(Cruz, Spain)*; Borbalan *(Spyfarma, Spain)*; Bristamox *(Bristol, Fr.; Bristol, Swed.)*; Brondix *(Pentafarm, Spain)*; Cabermox *(Caber, Ital.)*; Cidanamox *(Cidan, Spain)*; Cilamox *(Sigma, Austral.)*; Clamox *(Fin.)*; Clamoxyl *(Belg.; Beecham-Sevigne, Fr.; Beecham-Wülfing, Ger.; Jpn; Neth.; Beecham, Spain; Beecham, Switz.)*; Co-Amoxin *(Smaller, Spain)*; Dacala *(Tafir, Spain)*; Damoxicil *(Elmu, Spain)*; Delacillin *(Jpn)*; Diacibrone *(Valles Mestre, Spain)*; Dobriciclin *(Crisol, Spain)*; Draximox *(Novo, Denm.)*; Dura AX *(Durachemie, Ger.)*; Edoxil *(Hubber, Spain)*; Efpenix *(Jpn)*; Eupen *(Uriach, Spain)*; Flemoxin *(Neth.)*; Fullcilina *(Arg.)*; Gramidil *(Leurquin, Fr.)*; Halitol *(Septa, Spain)*; Hiconcil *(Belg.; Allard, Fr.; Jpn)*; Himino Max *(Jpn)*; Hipen *(Cadila, Ind.)*; Hosboral *(Hosbon, Spain)*; Ibiamox *(Ibi, Ital.)*; Imacillin *(Astra, Denm.; Astra, Norw.; Astra, Swed.)*; Inexbron *(Inexfa, Spain)*; Isimoxin *(ISI, Ital.)*; Kapoxi *(Spain)*; Larocilin *(Arg.)*; Larotid *(Beecham Laboratories, USA)*; Lisoxil *(Fibos, Spain)*;
Majorpen *(Cyanamid, Ital.)*; Maxiampil *(Inkey, Spain)*; Mediamox *(Valles Mestre, Spain)*; Metifarma *(Igoda, Spain)*; Mopen *(FIRMA, Ital.)*; Morgenxil *(Morgens, Spain)*; Moxacin *(Commonwealth Serum Laboratories, Austral.)*; Moxal *(Rhone-Poulenc, Ital.)*; Moxaline *(Belg.)*; Moxilean *(Canad.)*; Moxipin *(Gamir, Spain)*; Moxypen *(Lennon, S.Afr.)*; Novabritine *(Belg.)*; Novagcilina *(Novag, Spain)*; Novamoxin *(Novopharm, Canad.)*; Olmopen *(Searle, Spain)*; Overal Ilfi *(Lusofarmaco, Ital.)*; Pamocil *(Aandersen, Ital.)*; Paradroxil *(Bristol Italiana Sud, Ital.)*; Pasetocin *(Jpn)*; Penamox *(Arg.; Canad.)*; Piramox *(Radiumfarma, Ital.)*; Polymox *(Canad.; Bristol, USA)*; Precopen *(Fides, Spain)*; Quimiopen *(Roger, Spain)*; Raudopen *(Alter, Spain)*; Raylina *(Spain)*; Reloxyl *(Cheminova, Spain)*; Remisan *(Vir, Spain)*; Robamox *(USA)*; Salvapen *(Salvat, Spain)*; Sawacillin *(Jpn)*; Sigamopen *(Siegfried, Ger.)*; Silamox *(Karlspharma, Ger.)*; Simoxil *(Ital Suisse, Ital.)*; Simplamox *(ISF, Ital.)*; Sintedix *(Spain)*; Sintopen *(Mitim, Ital.)*; Sintoplus *(Ital.)*; Suamoxil *(Cantabria, Spain)*; Sumox *(Reid-Provident, USA)*; Superpeni *(Roussel, Spain)*; Teramox *(Tilfarma, Spain)*; Tolodina *(Estedi, Spain)*; Trimox *(Squibb, USA)*; Utimox *(Parke, Davis, USA)*; Velamox *(Zambeletti, Ital.)*; Wassermox *(Wasserman, Spain)*; Widecillin *(Jpn)*; Wymox *(Wyeth, USA)*; Zamocillin *(Inpharzam, Ger.)*; Zamocilline *(Arsac, Fr.)*; Zimox *(Carlo Erba, Ital.)*.

The following names have been used for multi-ingredient preparations containing amoxycillin, amoxycillin salts, and amoxycillin trihydrate— Augmentan *(Beecham-Wülfing, Ger.)*; Augmentin *(Beecham, Austral.; Beecham-Sevigne, Fr.; Beecham, S.Afr.; Beecham, Switz.; Beecham Research, UK; Beecham Laboratories, USA)*; Clavulin *(Beecham, Canad.)*; Hiconcil-NS *(Bristol, S.Afr.)*; Suprapen *(Bencard, S.Afr.)*.

7-r

Amphomycin *(BAN, USAN).*
Amfomycin *(pINN).* A polypeptide antibiotic produced by the growth of *Streptomyces canus.*

CAS — 1402-82-0.

Amphomycin has an antibacterial action against Gram-positive bacteria, especially cocci, and was formerly used mainly as the calcium salt in ointments with neomycin and hydrocortisone in the treatment of impetigo and infected dermatitis.

Proprietary Names and Manufacturers
Amphocortin *(USA)*; Ecomytrin *(Warner, UK).*

8-f

Ampicillin *(BAN, USAN, rINN).*

Aminobenzylpenicillin; Ampicillinum; Ampicillinum Anhydricum; Anhydrous Ampicillin. (6*R*)-6-(α-D-Phenylglycylamino)penicillanic acid.
$C_{16}H_{19}N_3O_4S$=349.4.

CAS — 69-53-4.

Pharmacopoeias. In *Br., Braz., Eur., Fr., Ind., It., Jpn, Neth., Swiss,* and *Turk. Egypt., Int.,* and *U.S.* permit anhydrous or the trihydrate. Also in *B.P. Vet.*

A white, odourless or almost odourless, crystalline powder.

Sparingly **soluble** in water; practically insoluble in alcohol, acetone, chloroform, ether, and fixed oils. It dissolves in dilute solutions of acids and of alkali hydroxides. The *B.P.* specifies that a 0.25% solution in water has a pH of 3.5 to 5.5. The *U.S.P.* specifies that a 1% solution in water has a pH of 3.5 to 6.0. **Store** at a temperature not exceeding 30° in airtight containers.

9-d

Ampicillin Sodium *(BANM, USAN, rINNM).*

Ampicillinnatrium; Ampicillinum Natricum. The sodium salt of ampicillin.
$C_{16}H_{18}N_3NaO_4S$=371.4.

CAS — 69-52-3.

Pharmacopoeias. In *Br., Braz., Chin., Cz., Egypt., Ind., Int., It., Jpn, Jug., Nord., Roum.,* and *Turk. U.S.P.* has Sterile Ampicillin Sodium. Also in *B.P. Vet.*

A white to off-white, odourless or almost odourless, crystalline or amorphous, hygroscopic powder. 1.06 g of monograph substance is approximately equivalent to 1 g of ampicillin. Each g of monograph substance represents about 2.7 mmol of sodium.

Soluble 1 in 2 of water and 1 in 50 of acetone; slightly soluble in chloroform; practically insoluble in ether, liquid paraffin, and fixed oils. A 10% solution in water has a pH of 8 to 10.

Store at a temperature not exceeding 25° in well-closed containers.

The **stability** of solutions of ampicillin sodium is dependent on many factors including concentration, pH, temperature, and the nature of the vehicle.

Stability decreases significantly in the presence of glucose, fructose, invert sugar, dextrans, and lactate. Sodium Chloride Intravenous Infusion is reported to be a suitable vehicle. It is recommended that reconstituted solutions of ampicillin sodium for injection should be administered immediately after preparation, and should not be frozen. Ampicillin sodium should not be mixed with blood products or other proteinaceous fluids such as protein hydrolysates.

Ampicillin sodium has been reported to be **incompatible** with aminoglycosides, tetracyclines, and other antimicrobial agents including clindamycin phosphate, erythromycin ethyl succinate, erythromycin lactobionate, lincomycin hydrochloride, metronidazole, and polymyxin B sulphate. Incompatibility or loss of activity has also been reported with chlorpromazine hydrochloride, dopamine hydrochloride, heparin sodium, hydralazine hydrochloride, hydrocortisone sodium succinate, metoclopramide, prochlorperazine edisylate, prochlorperazine mesylate, sodium bicarbonate, and certain fluids for parenteral nutrition including fat emulsions.

STABILITY IN SOLUTION. The rate of degradation of penicillins increases with rise in temperature, and inactivation is also promoted by conditions of high or low pH. In general, penicillins have a good degree of stability within a pH range of 5.5 to 7.5. The initial slow decomposition leads to a gradual fall in pH however, which in turn increases the rate of degradation, and eventually a precipitate may form.

In addition to undergoing hydrolysis in aqueous solution by hydroxyl ion catalysis, the aminopenicillins such as ampicillin degrade by a process of self-aminolysis or dimerisation, a reaction which is subject to general base catalysis by side-chain amino groups of other molecules, and in the case of amoxycillin, also by phenoxide ions. The rate of dimerisation increases with penicillin concentration, and this constitutes the predominant route of degradation in relatively concentrated solutions. Ampicillin and amoxycillin lose activity rapidly in these solutions, which are best used immediately after preparation.— B. Lynn, *Br. J. intraven. Ther.*, 1981, *2*, 22.

For a report on the stability of ampicillin in various carbohydrate solutions, see Benzylpenicillin Sodium, p.131.

10-c

Ampicillin Trihydrate *(BANM, rINNM).*

Ampicillin; Ampicillinum Trihydricum. The trihydrate of ampicillin.
$C_{16}H_{19}N_3O_4S,3H_2O$=403.5.

CAS — 7177-48-2.

Pharmacopoeias. In *Br., Braz., Cz., Eur., Fr., Ind., It., Jug., Neth., Nord., Roum.,* and *Swiss.* In *Jpn* under the title Ampicillin. *Egypt., Int.,* and *U.S.* permit anhydrous or the trihydrate under the title Ampicillin. Also in *B.P. Vet.*

A white odourless or almost odourless crystalline powder. A 0.25% solution in water has a pH of 3.5 to 5.5. 1.15 g of monograph substance is approximately equivalent to 1 g of ampicillin.

Slightly **soluble** in water; practically insoluble in alcohol, chloroform, ether, and fixed oils. It dissolves in dilute solutions of acids and of alkali hydroxides. **Store** at a temperature not exceeding 30° in airtight containers.

STABILITY IN SOLUTION. For a study on the penicillin content and stability of diluted antibiotic syrups, see Phenoxymethylpenicillin Potassium, p.282.

Adverse Effects

As for Benzylpenicillin Sodium, p.132.

Allergic reactions occur in sensitised persons. Skin rashes are among the most common side-effects and are either urticarial or maculopapular; the urticarial reactions are typical of penicillin hypersensitivity while the erythematous maculopapular eruptions are characteristic of ampicillin and often appear more than 7 days after commencing treatment. Most patients with infectious mononucleosis develop a skin rash when treated with ampicillin, and patients with lymphatic leukaemia also appear to have a higher incidence of skin rashes.

Gastro-intestinal adverse effects particularly diarrhoea and also nausea and vomiting occur quite frequently, usually following administration by mouth. Pseudomembranous colitis has also been reported. Supra-infections with non-susceptible organisms may occur particularly with prolonged use.

Non-allergic fever was observed on the 3rd to 8th day of treatment in 11 of 110 patients with scarlet fever treated with ampicillin.— J. Ström (letter), *Br. med. J.*, 1973, *1*, 419. From an analysis of 148 reported episodes of drug fever 46 were caused by antimicrobial agents and of these 2 were due to ampicillin.— P. A. Mackowiak and C. F. LeMaistre, *Ann. intern. Med.*, 1987, *106*, 728.

ALLERGY. For mention of possible allergic reactions associated with ampicillin see Effects on the Kidney and Effects on the Skin, below. See also, above, for reference to drug fever. For other allergic reactions associated with penicillins, see Benzylpenicillin Sodium, p.132.

EFFECTS ON THE BLOOD. Reversible neutropenia associated with ampicillin therapy in 3 children.— K. Kumar and A. Kumar, *Drug Intell. & clin. Pharm.*, 1981, *15*, 802.

A report of neutropenia and thrombocytopenia in one patient following administration of ampicillin.— G. S. Hughes (letter), *Ann. intern. Med.*, 1983, *99*, 573.

EFFECTS ON THE EAR. Ampicillin administered intravenously in high doses has been associated with loss of hearing in children treated for meningitis (F.E. Jones and D.R. Hanson, *Develop. Med. Child Neurology*, 1977, *19*, 593; M. Koskiniemi *et al.*, *Acta paediat. scand.*, 1978, *67*, 17). However, other workers who have found hearing loss in similar patients could not confirm an association between ototoxicity and ampicillin (H. Dahnsjö *et al.*, *Acta paediat. scand.*, 1976, *65*, 733).

EFFECTS ON THE GASTRO-INTESTINAL TRACT. Of 83 children treated with ampicillin for otitis media 24 experienced loose or watery stools and 6 of these children discontinued therapy because of diarrhoea; ampicillin was less well tolerated than either amoxycillin or co-trimoxazole given to 180 similar children (H.M. Feder, *Antimicrob. Ag. Chemother.*, 1982, *21*, 426). Ampicillin administered by mouth had been found to cause remarkable changes in the faecal flora of children; considerable suppression of *Bifidobacterium*, *Streptococcus*, and *Lactobacillus* species occurred and *Escherichia coli* organisms were frequently replaced by *Klebsiella* spp. Similar effects were also found in patients receiving ampicillin intravenously. Suppression of the normal flora promoted overgrowth of resistant organisms which might lead to serious secondary infections (H. Sakata *et al.*, *Antimicrob. Ag. Chemother.*, 1986, *29*, 225). Although many antibiotics have been implicated in the development of pseudomembranous colitis, ampicillin has been reported to be one of the drugs most frequently associated with the disease (M.H. Gross, *Clin. Pharm.*, 1985, *4*, 304; S.L. Gorbach, *Lancet*, 1987, *2*, 1378). Antibiotics which upset the colonic microflora are most likely to cause the development of pseudomembranous colitis as a result of overgrowth and toxin production by *Clostridium difficile* (R.P. Bolton and D.F.M. Thomas, *Br. J. Hosp. Med.*, 1986, *35*, 37). Ampicillin and other penicillins have also been associated with non-pseudomembranous colitis (R.B. Toffler *et al.*, *Lancet*, 1978, *2*, 707; M. Iida *et al.*, *Endoscopy*, 1985, *17*, 64), and diarrhoea associated with ampicillin and other antibiotics has been reported due to *C. perfringens* enterotoxin (S.P. Borriello *et al.*, *Lancet*, 1984, *1*, 305).

EFFECTS ON THE KIDNEY. Reports of acute interstitial nephritis associated with ampicillin administration: H. G. Rennke *et al.* (letter), *New Engl. J. Med.*, 1980, *302*, 691 (1 patient); A. L. Linton *et al.*, *Ann. intern. Med.*, 1980, *93*, 735 (3 patients; possibly due to an immunological disturbance).

EFFECTS ON THE NERVOUS SYSTEM. Ampicillin has been reported to penetrate the brain less readily and to have a lower neurotoxicity than other penicillins (S. Ricci *et al.*, *Drugs Today*, 1986, *22*, 283). However, seizures occurred in 2 patients with underlying cerebral dysfunction who received therapy including ampicillin (M. Serdaru *et al.*, *Lancet*, 1982, *2*, 617) and seizures have also been associated with high serum-concentrations of ampicillin in 3 patients with renal insufficiency (S. Iwarson *et al.*, *J. antimicrob. Chemother.*, 1978, *4*, 229; T. Hodgman *et al.*, *Sth. med. J.*, 1984, *77*, 1323). It has been suggested that ampicillin should be given with caution to epileptic patients and that the dosage should be modified in patients with severe renal failure (M. Serdaru *et al.*, *Lancet*, 1982, *2*, 617; T. Hodgman *et al.*, *Sth. med. J.*, 1984, *77*, 1323).

EFFECTS ON THE SKIN. The Boston Collaborative Drug Surveillance Program found that skin reactions attributable to ampicillin occurred in 59 of 1775 patients (3.3%) who received the drug between 1975 and 1982 (M. Bigby *et al.*, *J. Am. med. Ass.*, 1986, *256*, 3358), although higher incidences had previously been reported (*Br. med. J.*, 1973, *1*, 7; J. Porter and H. Jick, *Lancet*, 1980, *1*, 1037). The skin reactions have been reported to appear about 4 to 14 days after beginning treatment with ampicillin, but they usually occur 8 to 10 days after the first exposure to the drug (J.R.W. Harris *et al.*, *Br. med. J.*, 1972, *1*, 687; *ibid.*, 1973, *1*, 7; J. Ström, *ibid.*, 419; J. Porter and H. Jick, *Lancet*, 1980, *1*, 1037). It has been reported that rashes are less likely to occur following administration by mouth compared with the parenteral route (*Br. med. J.*, 1973, *1*, 7) and polymer-free ampicillin is associated with fewer skin reactions (A.C. Parker and J. Richmond, *Br. med. J.*, 1976, *1*, 998). The incidence of rashes has also been reported to be higher in females than in males (*Br. med. J.*, 1973, *1*, 7) and higher in patients with some viral infections or lymphoid proliferation such as glandular fever, cytomegalovirus mononucleosis, or lymphatic leukaemia (H.P. Lambert *et al.*, *Br. med. J.*, 1972, *1*, 688; *ibid.*, 1973, *1*, 7); skin reactions to ampicillin have also been reported in patient with AIDS (F.X. Real *et al.*, *Ann. intern. Med.*,1984, *101*, 883; Z. Ackerman and M. Levy, *Postgrad. med. J.*, 1987, *63*, 55).

Although some rashes associated with ampicillin therapy can be attributed to penicillin allergy, there is controversy over whether or not the maculopapular rash might be associated with an allergic response. Bierman *et al.* (*J. Am. med. Ass.*, 1972, *220*, 1098) found negative skin-test results in 34 patients who developed a maculopapular rash to ampicillin, and other workers have reported a gradual disappearance of the rash and no adverse effects in patients who have continued with ampicillin treatment after the development of a rash. This may suggest a toxic rather than an allergic cause, and therefore some workers feel that the appearance of a maculopapular rash with ampicillin treatment is not a contra-indication for future treatment with ampicillin or another penicillin (*Br. med. J.*, 1973, *1*, 7; B. Sokoloff, *Pediatrics*, 1977, *59*, 637). However, positive intracutaneous reactions to penicillin have been observed in patients with a history of 'toxic' ampicillin rash and there is therefore a risk of anaphylactic reactions (W.G. van Ketel, *Br. J. Derm.*, 1984, *110*, 112). It may also be difficult to distinguish between maculopapular and allergic urticarial rashes and so some workers feel that skin-testing for hypersensitivity to penicillin should be used (A.B. Campbell and L.F. Soyka, *Pediatrics*, 1977, *59*, 638). There appears to be complete cross-sensitisation between ampicillin and amoxycillin (W.G. van Ketel, *Br. J. Derm.*, 1984, *110*, 112) and the incidence of rash attributable to the 2 drugs is similar (J. Porter and H. Jick, *Lancet*, 1980, *1*, 1037).

Other skin reactions reported to be associated with ampicillin therapy include photosensitivity reactions (K. Stone, *Aust. J. Pharm.*, 1985, *66*, 415) and toxic epidermal necrolysis (H. Tagami *et al.*, *Archs Derm.*, 1983, *119*, 910).

For a possible increase in the incidence of ampicillin-associated skin reactions due to concurrent administration of allopurinol, see under Precautions, Interactions, below.

Precautions

As for Benzylpenicillin Sodium, p.133.

Ampicillin should preferably not be given to patients with infectious mononucleosis since they are especially susceptible to ampicillin-induced skin rashes; patients with lymphatic leukaemia and patients with hyperuricaemia being treated with allopurinol may also be at increased risk of developing skin rashes.

Ampicillin may decrease the efficacy of oestrogen-containing oral contraceptives and it may also affect the absorption of other drugs due to its effect on the gastro-intestinal flora.

Of 63 patients with cystic fibrosis 10 (16%) experienced significant hypersensitivity reactions to penicillins and 3 of these were due to ampicillin with or without cloxacillin. Exposure to penicillins in the presence of a hyperimmune state might lead to this unusual high incidence of penicillin hypersensitivity.— T. J. McDonnell and M. X. FitzGerald (letter), *Lancet*, 1984, *1*, 1301.

The view that ampicillin should be avoided when treating tonsillitis because infectious mononucleosis may often present as tonsillitis and in this case, the use of ampicillin could result in a characteristic maculopapular rash in 65 to 95% of the patients. The patients may, in addition, be mistakenly branded 'penicillin allergic'.— A. D. Green (letter), *Br. med. J.*, 1986, *293*, 1030.

Hypersensitivity reactions to ampicillin, sulphasalazine, and other drugs occurred in a patient after developing AIDS. He had previously been repeatedly exposed to penicillins and sulphonamides without adverse effects.— Z. Ackerman and M. Levy, *Postgrad. med. J.*, 1987, *63*, 55.

For the suggestion that ampicillin should be used with caution in epileptic patients, see under Effects on the Nervous System, in Adverse Effects, above.

For the effect of liver diseases and biliary obstruction on the bioavailability of ampicillin, see under Absorption and Fate, p.119.

For the effect of pregnancy on the disposition of ampicillin and the possible risks to breast-fed neonates of mothers receiving ampicillin, see under Absorption and Fate, Pregnancy and the Neonate, p.119.

For reference to the precautions to be observed in renal failure, see under Uses, Administration in Renal Failure, p.120.

For mention of ampicillin acting as a selector for antibiotic resistance, see under Resistance, p.118.

INTERACTIONS. *Allopurinol.* The Boston Collaborative Drug Surveillance Program (BCDSP) monitored 4686 patients who had received ampicillin treatment, 252 of whom had also received concurrent therapy with allopurinol. An increased frequency of rashes occurred in patients who received both ampicillin and allopurinol (13.9%) compared with those who received ampicillin alone (5.7%). Similar results also occurred in 923 patients who received either amoxycillin in association with allopurinol or amoxycillin alone; rashes occurred in 22 and 5.9% of the patients, respectively. The data were, however, insufficient to determine whether the increased risk could be ascribed to allopurinol itself or to the presence of hyperuricaemia.— H. Jick and J. B. Porter, *J. clin. Pharmac.*, 1981, *21*, 456. The observed risk of rash for aminopenicillins without allopurinol was 10.1% of 3738 patients, the observed risk for aminopenicillins in association with allopurinol was 7.2% of 180 patients, and for allopurinol without an aminopenicillin 3.0% of 624 patients. Thus the excess of rashes observed by the BCDSP in patients concomitantly treated with ampicillin and allopurinol could not be confirmed.— R. Hoigné *et al.* (letter), *New Engl. J. Med.*, 1987, *316*, 1217.

Aminoglycosides. For the effects of beta-lactam antibiotics, including ampicillin, on the activity of aminoglycosides, see under Gentamicin Sulphate, Incompatibility, p.236.

Beta-blockers. For the effect of ampicillin on the bioavailability of atenolol administered by mouth, see Atenolol, p.783.

Chloramphenicol. Eight of 11 children treated for *Haemophilus influenzae* meningitis with ampicillin and chloramphenicol had long-term sequelae compared with 4 of 32 given ampicillin alone and 4 of 22 given chloramphenicol alone. An increased risk was suggested for this combination.— J. Lindberg *et al.*, *Pediatrics*, 1977, *60*, 1.

See also under Antimicrobial Action (below).

Chloroquine. In a study in 7 healthy subjects the bioavailability of ampicillin given by mouth was significantly reduced when ampicillin was administered in association with chloroquine phosphate. The action of chloroquine on the gastro-intestinal tract was thought to delay and reduce the absorption of ampicillin and it was suggested that concurrent oral administration of ampicillin and chloroquine should be avoided, or alternatively the 2 drugs could be administered at least 2 hours apart.— H. M. Ali, *J. antimicrob. Chemother.*, 1985, *15*, 781.

Oral contraceptives. Ampicillin has been reported to decrease oral contraceptive efficacy and there have been isolated cases of contraceptive failure in women taking ampicillin (J. Dossetor, *Br. med. J.*, 1975, *4*, 467). It has been suggested that suppression of intestinal bacteria might interupt the enterohepatic circulation of the oestrogen resulting in reduced circulating oestrogen concentration (*Drug Interact. News.*, 1985, *5*, 7; *Drug & Ther. Bull.*, 1987, *25*, 5). However, in a study of 7 women taking oral contraceptives ampicillin was found to have no significant effect on mean plasma concentrations of ethinyloestradiol or levonorgestrel, although in 2 of the women lower concentrations of ethinyloestradiol were noted during ampicillin therapy (D.J. Back *et al.*, *Br. J. clin. Pharmac.*, 1982, *14*, 43). Large interindividual variations in the plasma concentrations achieved with oral contraceptives occur (D.J. Back *et al.*, *Drugs*, 1981, *21*, 46) and therefore it would seem prudent for women to taken additional contraceptive precautions during antibiotic therapy (*Drugs & Ther. Bull.*, 1987, *25*, 5).

INTERFERENCE WITH DIAGNOSTIC TESTS. Metabolites of ampicillin in both the blood and urine reacted with ninhydrin causing interference with chromatograms for amino acids.— S. F. Cahalane and C. Mullins (letter), *Lancet*, 1975, *1*, 812.

Ampicillin had been reported to interfere with diagnostic tests for serum-albumin and glucose.— S. Yosselson-Superstine, *Am. J. Hosp. Pharm.*, 1982, *39*, 848 and 1479.

Antimicrobial Action

Ampicillin is bactericidal and has a similar mode of action to that of benzylpenicillin (see p.133), although it has a broader spectum of activity. It resembles benzylpenicillin in its action against Gram-positive organisms, including *Streptococcus pneumoniae*, and other streptococci but, apart perhaps from *Enterococcus faecalis*, it is slightly less potent than benzylpenicillin. *Listeria monocytogenes* is also highly sensitive. Ampicillin also has activity similar to benzylpenicillin against other organisms including many anaerobes and *Actinomyces* spp.

Ampicillin is an aminopenicillin with an amino group side chain attached to the basic penicillin structure, which enables ampicillin to penetrate the outer membrane of some Gram-negative bacteria. It is therefore more active than benzylpenicillin against some Gram-negative bacilli including some strains of *Bordetella pertussis*, *Haemophilus influenzae* and some Enterobacteriaceae such as *Escherichia coli*, *Proteus mirabilis*, *Salmonella* and *Shigella* spp.; many of these organisms are, however, becoming increasingly resistant to ampicillin mainly due to beta-lactamase production. Gram-negative cocci such as *Branhamella catarrhalis*, *Neisseria gonorrhoeae*, *and N. meningitidis* are usually sensitive to ampicillin providing that the organisms do not produce beta-lactamase.

Minimum inhibitory concentrations for sensitive Gram-positive organisms have been reported to range from 0.02 to 6 μg per mL and for Gram-negative organisms from 0.02 to 8 μg per mL. It is inactive against most strains of *Pseudomonas aeruginosa*.

Synergy against some beta-lactamase-producing organisms may occur between ampicillin and beta-lactamase inhibitors such as clavulanic acid or sulbactam, and also penicillinase-stable antibiotics such as cloxacillin. Synergy has also been demonstrated between ampicillin and aminoglycosides. Other antimicrobial agents including other beta-lactam antibiotics have exhibited variable amounts of synergy, antagonism, or indifference.

Ampicillin susceptibility was only slightly reduced in mutants of *Escherichia coli*, *Proteus mirabilis*, and *Enterobacter cloacae* lacking the outer membrane protein(s) porin, which constitutes a pore for the permeation route of small hydrophilic substances. This suggested that, in addition to the pore, ampicillin used another pathway, possibly passive diffusion through the phospholipid bilayer, for its outer membrane permeation.— T. Sawai *et al.*, *Antimicrob. Ag. Chemother.*, 1982, *22*, 585.

Ampicillin 10 mg daily by mouth administered with 2 litres of fluid daily for 3 days resulted in urinary concentrations of 0.5 to 4 μg per mL which were about one-fifth to one-half the MIC for *Escherichia coli.* The subinhibitory concentrations of ampicillin caused elongation of *E. coli* and inhibited the adherence of the organisms to epithelial cells of the urine sediment and resulted at least in a temporary bacteriological cure (S.B. Redjeb *et al.*, *Antimicrob. Ag. Chemother.*, 1982, *22*, 1084). However, the possibility that concentrations of drugs below the MIC might induce the development of resistance more rapidly and allow amplification of any R-plasmids present in the bacteria might override use in the clinical situation (B.A. Hales and S.G.B. Amyes, *J. antimicrob. Chemother.*, 1985, *16*, 671).

In a study of the sensitivity of isolates from urine specimens containing significant numbers of organisms and obtained from general practice, it appeared that there had been a continuation of the decline in ampicillin sensitivity that had been previously reported. Of 293 consecutive isolates, 70.6% were fully sensitive to ampicillin with 69.2, 80.6, 100, 100, and 0% sensitive to *Escherichia coli*, *Proteus* spp., staphylococci or micrococci, faecal streptococci, and *Klebsiella* spp., respectively.— S. R. Marper and P. Noone (letter), *J. antimicrob. Chemother.*, 1985, *15*, 251.

ACTIVITY WITH OTHER ANTIMICROBIAL AGENTS. Synergy has been demonstrated between ampicillin and various aminoglycosides against a variety of organisms *in vitro*, including: netilmicin or sissomicin against enterococci (C. Watanakunakorn and C. Glotzbecker, *J. antimicrob Chemother.*, 1978, *4*, 539); gentamicin, tobramycin, kanamycin, or amikacin against group B streptococci (M.D. Cooper *et al.*, *Antimicrob. Ag. Chemother.*, 1979, *15*, 484); and gentamicin or streptomycin against ampicillin-tolerant lactobacilli (A.S. Bayer *et al.*, *ibid.*, 1980, *17*, 359). Synergy has also been reported between ampicillin and fosfomycin against *Salmonella* and *Shigella* spp. (E. J. Perea *et al.*, *Antimicrob. Ag. Chemother.*, 1978, *13*, 705).

The activity of ampicillin against beta-lactamase-producing organisms has been enhanced by beta-lactamase inhibitors such as clavulanic acid or sulbactam (C.N.

Simpson *et al., J. Antimicrob. Chemother.*, 1984, *14*, 133; J.F. Plouffe, *Antimicrob. Ag. Chemother.*, 1982, *21*, 519). Synergism has also occurred between ampicillin and penicillinase-resistant penicillins such as dicloxacillin or nafcillin against beta-lactamase-producing organisms (J. Mizoguchi *et al., Antimicrob. Ag. Chemother.*, 1979, *16*, 439; R. Yogev *et al., ibid.*, 1980, *17*, 461). However, many beta-lactam combinations have been shown to produce only an indifferent or additive effect or occasionally synergy or antagonism (S.J. Pedler and A.J. Bint, *Br. med. J.*, 1984, *288*, 1022), and varied effects have been found with ampicillin and some cephalosporins such as cefotaxime (S.H. Landesman *et al., Antimicrob. Ag. Chemother.*, 1981, *19*, 794; J.A.A. Hoogkamp-Korstanje, *J. antimicrob. Chemother.*, 1985, *16*, 327; J.-R. Laponte *et al., Antimicrob. Ag. Chemother.*, 1986, *29*, 594). Several workers have noted disparity between different *in vitro* methods for determining synergy between ampicillin and cephalosporins, possibly due to the different drug concentrations used and the differences in affinity of the drugs to various penicillin binding proteins (PBPs). It has been suggested that at low concentrations ampicillin tends to bind to PBP1b whereas some cephalosporins primarily bind to PBP3 and the actions on different targets could result in a complementary or synergistic effect. However, when the concentrations of the drugs are far above the MIC for the organisms both ampicillin and cephalosporins also bind to other PBPs which could result in a competitive interaction (J.A.A. Hoogkamp-Korstanje, *J. antimicrob. Chemother.*, 1985, *16*, 327). Both synergy and antagonism have also been reported when ampicillin has been used in association with mecillinam, although synergy has been reported for many organisms possibly due to the different mechanism of action of mecillinam (I. Trestman *et al., Antimicrob. Ag. Chemother.*, 1979, *16*, 283; R. Hone and M. Foley, *J. antimicrob. Chemother.*, 1980, *6*, 410; L. Verbist, *ibid.*, 1985, *16*, 719; J.E. Mortensen *et al., Curr. ther. Res.*, 1986, *39*, 328).

Conflicting results have been obtained using ampicillin in association with chloramphenicol against *Haemophilus influenzae* type b (V. Rocco and G. Overturf, *Antimicrob. Ag. Chemother.*, 1982, *21*, 349). Indifferent or mixed results have been reported (F.S. Cole *et al., ibid.*, 1979, *15*, 415) as well as antagonism of the bactericidal activity of ampicillin by chloramphenicol (A.M.R. Mackenzie, *J. antimicrob. Chemother.*, 1979, *5*, 693). This antagonism does not appear to affect the action of chloramphenicol against *H. influenzae* (V. Schauf *et al., Antimicrob. Ag. Chemother.*, 1983, *23*, 364). However, inhibition of the bactericidal action of ampicillin by chloramphenicol, at concentrations close to those that might be achieved in the CSF during treatment for meningitis, has been reported for ampicillin-susceptible chloramphenicol-resistant strains of *H. influenzae* (A.M.R. Mackenzie and F.T.H. Chan, *Antimicrob. Ag. Chemother.*, 1986, *29*, 565). This might represent a clinical risk in the initial treatment of meningitis.

Antagonism between ampicillin and chloramphenicol has also occurred for meningeal isolates of group B streptococci (J.L. Weeks *et al., Antimicrob. Ag. Chemother.*, 1981, *20*, 281), and mainly antagonism but also some synergy has occurred against *Neisseria meningitidis* (W.E. Feldman and T. Zweighaft, *Antimicrob. Ag. Chemother.*, 1979, *15*, 240). Antagonism between the two drugs has been demonstrated for *Escherichia coli in vitro*, but a paradoxical synergistic effect occurred *in rats* (K.S. Kim *et al., Antimicrob. Ag. Chemother.*, 1984, *26*, 689). Chloramphenicol, erythromycin, doxycycline, and rifampicin have been found to antagonise the bactericidal action of ampicillin against *Listeria monocytogenes* (R.L. Penn *et al., Antimicrob. Ag. Chemother.*, 1982, *22*, 289; D.L. Winslow *et al., ibid.*, 1983, *23*, 555). However, synergy has also been reported between ampicillin and rifampicin against *L. monocytogenes* (C.U. Tuazon *et al., ibid.*, 1982, *21*, 525) and rifampicin has shown no evidence of antagonism or synergy with ampicillin against *H. influenzae* (T. Jadavji *et al., Antimicrob. Ag. Chemother.*, 1984, *26*, 91). The activity of ampicillin *in vitro* has been reported to be diminished by clindamycin, against *Staphylococcus aureus* (P. D. Meers, *Lancet*, 1973, *2*, 573).

For further reference to synergy between ampicillin and sulbactam, see under Sulbactam, p.299.

Resistance

Ampicillin is inactivated by beta-lactamases and beta-lactamase-producing strains of staphylococci, streptococci, *Branhamella catarrhalis, Haemophilus* spp., *Neisseria gonorrhoeae, Escherichia coli, Proteus, Klebsiella, Salmonella,* and *Shigella* spp. are resistant. Resistance not due to beta-lactamases has been reported in some strains of *E. coli, Bacteroides, Shigella,* and *Salmonella* spp. Further details on the mechanisms of resistance are provided under benzylpenicillin (p.134).

A review of the mechanisms of resistance to beta-lactam antibiotics in Gram-negative bacteria.— L. J. V. Piddock and R. Wise, *J. antimicrob. Chemother.*, 1985, *16*, 279.

Ampicillin usage has been reported to act as a selector for the transfer of trimethoprim resistance (D.J. Platt *et al., Lancet*, 1986, *2*, 928). It has also been noted that children with severe protracted diarrhoea due to multiresistant adherent *Escherichia coli* are more likely to have previously been treated with ampicillin compared with children with diarrhoea due to sensitive strains of *E. coli* (J. Lacroix *et al., Am. J. Dis. Childh.*, 1984, *138*, 693). Prophylactic administration of ampicillin to 10 chronically ill children resulted in an increase of ampicillin-resistant, and often multiple-resistant, Enterobacteriaceae biotypes in the faeces of the patients. The broad spectrum activity of ampicillin against the anaerobic flora of the intestinal tract appeared to decrease colonisation resistance (D. van der Waaij *et al., J. antimicrob. Chemother.*, 1986, *18*, *Suppl.* C, 155). However, Davies and Maesen (*J. Antimicrob. Chemother.*, 1986, *17*, 543) were unable to substantiate the claim of van Saene (*J. Drug Res.*, 1983, *8*, 2031) that aminopenicillins prescribed for patients with purulent respiratory infection frequently give rise to new infections with resistant organisms. Davies and Maesen consider that the effects of antimicrobial agents such as aminopenicillins or oropharyngeal colonisation resistance, however important they may be in some patients with severely compromised defences, should not be considered among the most important criteria for the selection of antimicrobial agents for the treatment of respiratory infections in ambulant general practice patients.

RESISTANCE OF BACTEROIDES. Of 60 strains of *Bacteroides fragilis* 56 were resistant to ampicillin.— O. A. Okubadejo *et al., Br. med. J.*, 1973, *2*, 212. Beta-lactamases are produced by a majority of resistant isolates of the *B. fragilis* group and other *Bacteroides* spp. With the addition of sulbactam to ampicillin all of 157 isolates of *Bacteroides* spp. were susceptible at a break point of 16 µg per mL for ampicillin.— H. M. Wexler and S. M. Finegold, *J. antimicrob. Chemother.*, 1987, *19*, 143.

RESISTANCE OF BRANHAMELLA. Of 81 isolates of *Branhamella catarrhalis* 41 produced beta-lactamase and were usually unresponsive to ampicillin (D.T. McLeod *et al., Br. med. J.*, 1983, *287*, 1446). The production of beta-lactamase by a large proportion of isolates of *B. catarrhalis* made ampicillin and amoxycillin inappropriate choices of antibiotic in the treatment of these infections (N.J. Slevin *et al., Lancet*, 1984, *1*, 782).

RESISTANCE OF ENTEROCOCCI. A report of *Enterococcus faecalis* in a 75-year-old man with endocarditis, that exhibited tolerance to ampicillin with an MIC of 1.6 µg per mL and an MBC of over 100 µg per mL.— M. McDonald *et al.* (letter), *Lancet*, 1980, *2*, 321.

RESISTANCE OF ESCHERICHIA. Of 232 strains of enteropathogenic *Escherichia coli* 86 (37%) were resistant to ampicillin at a concentration of 8 µg per mL (R.J. Gross *et al., Br. med. J.*, 1982, *285*, 472). Resistance to ampicillin was prevalent in enterotoxigenic *E. coli* and other bacterial enteropathogens and ampicillin should probably no longer be used in the empirical treatment of acute diarrhoea (J.R. Carlson *et al., Antimicrob. Ag. Chemother.*, 1983, *24*, 509). See also above.

RESISTANCE OF GONOCOCCI. Intrinsic ampicillin resistance in *Neisseria gonorrhoeae* was demonstrated to arise by a series of mutations in multiple genes. The step-wise resistance required the combined effects of a series of mutations, none of which conferred resistance independently.— F. Jones *et al., Antimicrob. Ag. Chemother.*, 1985, *28*, 21. See also under Benzylpenicillin Sodium, p.134.

RESISTANCE OF HAEMOPHILUS. There has been increasing resistance to ampicillin in *Haemophilus* spp.; resistance to *H. influenzae* type b has usually been reported to range from about 5 to 20%, but an incidence of over 30% has been reported from some areas (J. Philpott-Howard, *J. antimicrob. Chemother.*, 1984, *13*, 199; D. Hansman, *Med. J. Aust.*, 1985, *142*, 536; W.F. Schlech *et al., J. Am. med. Ass.*, 1985, *253*, 1749; M. Powell *et al., Br. med. J.*, 1987, *295*, 176; A.J. Howard, *ibid.*, 608). A high incidence of resistance has also been reported for *H. parainfluenzae, H. haemolyticus, H. parahaemolyticus*, and other *Haemophilus* spp. (A.P. Gillett *et al., Br. med. J.*, 1978, *2*, 278). Resistance of *H. influenzae* can be mediated by several mechanisms, the most important of which is plasmid-mediated production of TEM-1 beta-lactamase. These plasmids are probably derived from enterobacteria and resistance can be readily transferred from *H. influenzae* to *H. parainfluenzae, Escherichia coli*, or capsulate *H. influenzae*. In addition many of the genes conferring resistance have become integrated by transposition into the chromosomal DNA (J. Philpott-Howard, *J. antimicrob. Chemother.*, 1984, *13*, 199). A novel plasmid-mediated beta-lactamase has also been found which was not detected by an assay for TEM-1 beta-lactamase and caused failure of treatment with ampicillin (L.G. Rubin *et al., Lancet*, 1981, *2*, 1008). This new beta-lactamase, designated ROB-1 has been found to be produced by animal pathogens and it has been suggested that there is potential for spread of this form of ampicillin resistance from an animal reservoir to human pathogens (A.A. Medeiros *et al., Antimicrob. Ag. Chemother.*, 1986, *29*, 212).

Resistance of beta-lactamase-negative isolates of *H. influenzae* type b has also been demonstrated (S.M. Markowitz, *Antimicrob. Ag. Chemother.*, 1980, *17*, 80; S.M. Bell and D. Plowman, *Lancet*, 1980, *1*, 279; T.R. Parr and L.E. Bryan, *Antimicrob. Ag. Chemother.*, 1984, *25*, 747). Non-beta-lactamase resistance to ampicillin is considered to be mainly due to altered penicillin binding proteins, which are chromosomally mediated; alteration in permeability also appears to have a role (P.M. Mendelman *et al., Antimicrob. Ag. Chemother.*, 1984, *26*, 235).

Resistance to ampicillin occurs frequently enough in *H. influenzae* type b to exclude the use of ampicillin alone in the initial treatment of meningitis (H.P. Lambert, *Br. J. Hosp. Med.*, 1983, *29*, 128). Chloramphenicol has been used in association with ampicillin, however, clinical isolates of *H. influenzae* resistant to both ampicillin and chloramphenicol have been reported (P. MacMahon *et al., Br. med. J.*, 1982, *284*, 1229; M.A. Catry and M.V. Vaz Pato, *ibid.*, 1983, *287*, 1471; H. Guiscafré *et al., Archs Dis. Childh.*, 1986, *61*, 691; Z.A. Karrar *et al., J. Infect.*, 1987, *14*, 61) and multiple resistant organisms have also occurred (I. Braveny and K. Machka, *Lancet*, 1980, *2*, 752). Chloramphenicol may also antagonise the action of ampicillin (see Antimicrobial Action, Activity with other Antimicrobial Agents, above).

RESISTANCE OF SALMONELLAE. Ampicillin showed low activity against *Salmonella* spp. and other enteropathogens; a concentration of 128 µg per mL was required to inhibit 90% of 50 strains tested.— J. R. Carlson *et al., Antimicrob. Ag. Chemother.*, 1983, *24*, 509.

RESISTANCE OF SHIGELLAE. Both transferable and non-transferable types of resistance to ampicillin have been detected in strains of *Shigella sonnei* (J.T. Smith *et al., Antimicrob. Ag. Chemother.*, 1974, *6*, 418). In England and Wales the incidence of resistance of *Shigella* spp. to ampicillin at a concentration of 8 µg per mL increased from 2% in 1974 to 47.6% in the first half of 1983; this rapid increase in resistance might be the result of uncontrolled use of antibiotics in certain developing countries (R.J. Gross *et al., Br. med. J.*, 1984, *288*, 784). Resistance to ampicillin was reported in 60% or more of clinical isolates obtained during an epidemic of dysentery in India, when resistance to other commonly used drugs also occurred (S.C. Pal, *Lancet*, 1984, *1*, 1462; B.D. Chatterjee and S.N. Sanyal, *ibid.*, *2*, 574).

RESISTANCE OF STREPTOCOCCI. *Pneumococci*. Higher MICs for ampicillin were generally observed for *Streptococcus pneumoniae* strains with resistance or intermediate resistance to benzylpenicillin, although ampicillin had been found to have better activity than benzylpenicillin against a few penicillin-resistant isolates.— J. Michel *et al., Antimicrob. Ag. Chemother.*, 1983, *23*, 397.

Absorption and Fate

Ampicillin is relatively stable in the acid gastric secretion and is moderately well absorbed from the gastro-intestinal tract after oral administration. Food can interfere with the absorption of ampicillin so doses should be taken 30 minutes to an hour before meals. Peak concentrations in plasma are obtained in about 1 to 2 hours and following a dose of 500 mg by mouth are reported to range from 2 to 6 µg per mL.

Ampicillin is given by injection as the sodium salt and following the intramuscular administration of 500 mg peak plasma concentrations occur within about 1 hour and are reported to range from 7 to 14 µg per mL.

Ampicillin is widely distributed and therapeutic concentrations can be achieved in ascitic, pleural, and joint fluids. It diffuses across the placenta into the foetal circulation and concentrations can be detected in the milk of nursing mothers. There is little diffusion into the cerebrospinal fluid except when the meninges are inflamed, when higher concentrations can be achieved. About 20% is bound to plasma proteins and the plasma half-life is about 1 to 2 hours, but this may be increased in neonates and the elderly; in renal failure half-lives of 7 to 20 hours have been reported.

Renal clearance of ampicillin is slower than that of benzylpenicillin and occurs partly by glomerular filtration and partly by tubular secretion. About 20 to 40% of an orally administered dose is excreted unchanged in the urine in 6 hours; urinary concentrations range from 0.25 to 1 mg per mL following a dose of 500 mg. Following parenteral administration about 60 to 80% is excreted in the urine within 6 hours. A high concentration is reached in bile and some is excreted in the faeces. Renal elimination is retarded by the concomitant use of probenecid.

A review of the pharmacokinetics of the penicillins.— M. Barza and L. Weinstein, *Clin. Pharmacokinet.*, 1976, *1*, 297.

For the pharmacokinetics of ampicillin administered with sulbactam, see under Sulbactam, p.299.

Although the absorption of oral ampicillin is impaired in the presence of food, concurrent administration of a lactobacillus preparation to reduce ampicillin-associated diarrhoea does not appear to interfere with the bioavailability of oral ampicillin (R.L. Yost and V.P. Gotz, *Antimicrob. Ag. Chemother.*, 1985, *28*, 727). Coeliac disease does not seem to affect the absorption of ampicillin, however, absorption may be reduced in infants and children with acute shigellosis (P.G. Welling and F.L.S. Tse, *J. clin. Hosp. Pharm.*, 1984, *9*, 163). Absorption of ampicillin administered as pivampicillin may also be reduced in patients who have undergone intestinal bypass (J.P. Kampmann *et al.*, *Clin. Pharmacokinet.*, 1984, *9*, 168). There appears to be little impairment in ampicillin absorption in patients with partial gastrectomy or with gastric achlorhydria, but absorption seems to be impaired in patients with obstructive jaundice (J.A. Davies and J.M. Holt, *J. antimicrob. Chemother.*, 1975, *1*, *Suppl.* (Sept.), 69). Amoxycillin or the ester prodrugs of ampicillin are better absorbed than ampicillin (C.R. Pennington and J. Crooks, *Br. med. J.*, 1983, *286*, 1732; V.J. Stella *et al.*, *Drugs*, 1985, *29*, 455).

The renal clearance of ampicillin in healthy subjects is independent of the plasma concentration (J. Sjövall *et al.*, *Br. J. clin. Pharmac.*, 1985, *19*, 191), and large interindividual variations in serum-ampicillin concentrations have been noted in patients treated with a constant-rate intravenous infusion of ampicillin 150 mg per kg body-weight daily (E. Bouvet *et al.*, *Br. med. J.*, 1980, *280*, 1164). The plasma clearance of ampicillin has been found to be significantly reduced and the half-life and the area under the plasma-concentration time curve significantly increased in elderly patients compared with young subjects; half-lives of 6.7 and 1.7 hours, respectively, have been reported. The changes in drug handling in the elderly have been attributed to a decrease in renal elimination of ampicillin (E.J. Triggs *et al.*, *Eur. J. clin. Pharmac.*, 1980, *18*, 195). However, other workers have found that although ampicillin clearance correlates to renal function, in healthy elderly subjects the reduction in renal function is not necessarily enough to reduce the drug clearance (J. Sjövall *et al.*, *Br. J. clin. Pharmac.*, 1986, *21*, 171). In patients with renal failure there is decreased renal tubular secretion as well as decreased glomerular filtration of ampicillin and a dosage adjustment method probably needs to involve both (R. Hori *et al.*, *Clin. Pharmac. Ther.*, 1983, *34*, 792). In patients with liver disease such as cirrhosis, primary hepatocellular carcinoma, or hepatosplenic schistosomiasis there appears to be a greater metabolic clearance of ampicillin and this might affect the therapeutic efficacy of the drug. In patients with viral hepatitis, however, the bioavailability of ampicillin appears to be similar to that in healthy subjects (G.P. Lewis and W.J. Jusko, *Clin. Pharmac. Ther.*, 1975, *18*, 475; H.M. Ali *et al.*, *J. Antimicrob. Chemother.*, 1985, *15*, 737).

DIFFUSION INTO BODY TISSUES AND FLUIDS. Ampicillin penetrates relatively poorly into bronchial secretions; it achieves sputum concentrations about 10% of simultaneous serum concentrations after oral administration, though penetration may be 2 or 3 times greater in the presence of inflammation. It is important to use sufficiently high doses if oral ampicillin is used in the treatment of lower-respiratory-tract infections, as subtherapeutic concentrations not only lead to treatment failure but predispose to development of bacterial resistance to ampicillin. Amoxycillin is absorbed twice as efficiently from the gastro-intestinal tract and penetrates mucoid sputum more effectively than ampicillin, though penetration of both drugs into purulent bronchial secretion is similar.— J. Symonds, *Archs Dis. Childh.*, 1984, *59*, 501.

METABOLISM. In studies in healthy subjects about 21% of a dose of ampicillin 250 or 500 mg has been reported to be metabolised. After 12 hours about 26% of a 500-mg dose has been recovered in the urine as unchanged drug and about 7% excreted as metabolites mainly penicilloic acid (M. Cole *et al.*, *Antimicrob. Ag. Chemother.*, 1973, *3*, 463; J. Haginaka and J. Wakai, *J. Pharm. Pharmac.*, 1987, *39*, 5). Ampicillin is metabolised to 5*R*,6*R*-penicilloic acid and 5*S*,6*R*-penicilloic acid in man (A.E. Bird *et al.*, *J. Pharm. Pharmac.*, 1983, *35*, 138), but piperazine-2,5-dione has also been detected in human urine following administration of ampicillin by mouth (J. Haginaka and J. Wakai, *J. Pharm. Pharmac.*, 1986, *38*, 225).

PREGNANCY AND THE NEONATE. The disposition of ampicillin has been shown to be altered in pregnancy, sometimes resulting in less than adequate antibacterial concentrations, and therefore higher doses may be required especially for severe infections (B.M. Assael *et al.*, *Br. J. clin. Pharmac.*, 1979, *8*, 286). Ampicillin is poorly protein bound which results in higher concentrations in foetal tissues and amniotic fluid than would occur with highly protein bound penicillins; high foetal to maternal peak serum concentrations ratios of between 0.3 and 0.9 had been reported for ampicillin (A.W. Chow and P.J. Jewesson, *Rev. infect. Dis.*, 1985, *7*, 287). In a study of 42 women, administration of ampicillin 500 mg every 6 hours by mouth resulted in concentrations of 0.4 to 5.1 µg per mL in the amniotic fluid collected between 3.25 and 5.75 hours after the third dose and 0.24 to 2 µg per mL in cord sera collected at delivery after 2 to 13 doses (T.E. Blecher *et al.*, *Br. med. J.*, 1966, *1*, 137).

Ampicillin is excreted in very small amounts in breast milk and a concentration of 70 ng per mL was detected 2 hours after administration of ampicillin 500 mg to a nursing mother. The amount likely to be taken by the suckling infant was considered to be well below the normal paediatric dose (B.E. Takyi, *J. Hosp. Pharm.*, 1970, *28*, 317), however, there is a potential risk of diarrhoea or candidiasis in the neonate (A.W. Chow and P.J. Jewesson, *Rev. infect. Dis.*, 1985, *7*, 287).

The half-life of ampicillin in neonates may be increased due to immature kidney function. In a study involving 42 newborn infants a single dose of ampicillin 50 mg per kg body-weight by intragastric tube resulted in a mean serum concentration of 2.7 µg per mL within 30 minutes of administration increasing to a maximum mean concentration of 20.2 µg per mL at 4 hours. Serum concentrations of about 13 µg per mL were obtained at 10 hours after the dose, but then the concentrations decreased at a more rapid rate (A. Sabra *et al.*, *Curr. ther. Res.*, 1973, *15*, 866).

Uses and Administration

Ampicillin is used in the treatment of a variety of infections due to susceptible organisms, including respiratory-tract infections, urinary-tract infections, gonorrhoea, enteric infections, meningitis, and septicaemia. Susceptibility tests should be carried out because of the increasing resistance of bacteria to ampicillin. If beta-lactamase-producing-organisms are present, ampicillin can be administered with a beta-lactamase inhibitor such as sulbactam (see p.298) or a penicillinase-resistant antibiotic such as cloxacillin or flucloxacillin. It may also be administered in association with an aminoglycoside to increase the spectrum of organisms covered; it is advisable to administer the injections separately.

The dosage of ampicillin will depend on the severity of the disease, the age of the patient and their renal function; the dose should be reduced in renal failure. Ampicillin is usually administered by mouth as the trihydrate and by injection as the sodium salt. Doses are expressed in terms of the equivalent amount of ampicillin. The usual dose by mouth is 0.25 to 1 g of ampicillin every 6 hours. It is recommended that ampicillin be taken ½ to 1 hour before or 2 hours after food. Children may be given half the adult dose.

Ampicillin 2 to 3.5 g administered, in association with probenecid 1 g, as a single dose by mouth, may be used in the treatment of uncomplicated gonorrhoea, in areas where gonococci have maintained sensitivity. The dose may need to be repeated for females.

Ampicillin is administered by injection in usual doses of 500 mg every 4 to 6 hours intramuscularly, or it may be given by slow intravenous injection over 3 to 5 minutes or by infusion. Higher parenteral doses of ampicillin 150 to 300 mg per kg body-weight daily in divided doses are administered intravenously by infusion or alternatively by slow intravenous injection for treatment of serious infections such as meningitis. Children are given parenteral doses of ampicillin 100 to 400 mg per kg daily in divided doses. Solutions of ampicillin sodium given by infusion should be administered within one hour of preparation. Intramuscular injections are painful and have been prepared using a local anaesthetic solution.

Ampicillin sodium may also be administered by other routes usually as a supplement to systemic therapy. Intraperitoneal or intrapleural injections are given in a dose of ampicillin 500 mg dissolved in 5 to 10 mL of Water for Injection. For intra-articular injection ampicillin 500 mg may be dissolved in up to 5 mL of Water for Injection or a solution of procaine hydrochloride 0.5% may be used.

In meningitis, systemic treatment may be supplemented with intrathecal injections of ampicillin. The usual daily intrathecal dose is ampicillin 5 mg for infants up to 2 years of age, 10 mg for children up to 12 years of age, and 20 mg for adults; these doses should be given once daily. Ampicillin prepared for intrathecal use should be dissolved in sodium chloride injection 0.9% immediately before use to give a solution containing 10 mg per mL.

The Committee on Infectious Diseases and Immunization of the Canadian Paediatric Society has compared the efficacy and safety of ampicillin and other aminopenicillins including amoxycillin, bacampicillin, ciclacillin, and pivampicillin. There is no evidence that any one of the aminopenicillins is superior to any other in the treatment of infections for which oral administration is indicated, except that amoxycillin is ineffective in shigellosis. However, diarrhoea occurs more frequently in patients receiving ampicillin compared with amoxycillin or pivampicillin. The relative costs of the drugs and the frequency of their adverse effects should be considered when choosing an aminopenicillin, and amoxycillin appears to be the most suitable of the aminopenicillins for oral use in children (*Can. med. Ass. J.*, 1984, *131*, 1223). Amoxycillin and the ester prodrugs of ampicillin have improved intestinal absorption with correspondingly superior bioavailability characteristics, however, the ampicillin esters appear to confer no advantage over amoxycillin (C.R. Pennington and J. Crooks, *Br. med. J.*, 1983, *286*, 1732; V.J. Stella *et al.*, *Drugs*, 1985, *29*, 455).

ADMINISTRATION. A recommendation that ampicillin administered by mouth should be given with at least 100 mL of water while the patient is in an upright sitting position to avoid oesophagitis or oesphageal ulceration.— S. K. Vong and R. K. Parekh (letter), *Pharm. J.*, 1987, *1*, 5.

ADMINISTRATION IN INFANTS AND CHILDREN. A suggested dose of ampicillin for neonates of more than 37 weeks' gestation was 50 mg per kg body-weight given intramuscularly or intravenously, by very slow bolus injection, every 12 hours for the first 48 hours of life, every 8 hours from the 3rd day to 2 weeks, then every 6 hours. For immature infants (those of less than 37 weeks' gestation) this dose should be given every 12 hours for the first week of life, every 8 hours from then to 4 weeks of age, and every 6 hours thereafter (P.A. Davies, *Br. Med. J.*, 1978, *2*, 676). A similar dosage using ampicillin 100 mg per kg every 24 hours administered in divided doses every 4 to 6 hours when given intravenously by slow bolus injection, or every 8 hours when given intramuscularly or orally, has also been recommended for neonates, without adjusting for gestational or postnatal age (H.B. Valman, *Br. med. J.*, 1980, *280*, 457). For severe infections in neonates a higher daily dose of ampicillin administered intravenously has been suggested: 0 to 1 week of age, 150 to 200 mg per kg in 2 or 3 divided doses; 1 to 4 weeks, 200 mg per kg in 3 or 4 divided doses; over 4 weeks, 250 to 300 mg per kg in 4 to 6 divided doses. A dose of ampicillin 300 to 400 mg per kg daily in 6 divided doses has been suggested for severe infections in children (K.H. Rhodes and C.M. Johnson, *Mayo Clin. Proc.*, 1983, *58*, 158). Neonates requiring intensive care often have immature organs and multiple problems and therefore the dose of antibiotic should be adjusted according to serum concentrations.

Administration of ampicillin and gentamicin to neonates by continuous intravenous infusion in parenteral nutrition solutions.— H. Colding *et al.*, *Archs Dis. Childh.*, 1982, *57*, 602.

ADMINISTRATION IN RENAL FAILURE. Ampicillin can be administered to patients with renal failure by adjusting the dosage interval. A dosage interval of 6 hours is suitable for patients whose glomerular filtration-rates exceed 50 mL per minute; an interval of 6 to 12 hours is advisable for rates of between 10 and 50 mL per minute. Where the rate is less than 10 mL per minute, the dosage interval should be 12 to 16 hours. High doses are needed in end-stage renal disease to maintain adequate urinary concentrations for urinary-tract infections. A dose supplement should be given to patients undergoing haemodialysis.— W. M. Bennett *et al.*, *Am. J. Kidney Dis.*, 1983, *3*, 155. In patients with renal failure there is decreased renal tubular secretion resulting in reduced urinary excretion of ampicillin. Dosage adjustment based on creatinine clearance does not seem appropriate for patients receiving drugs which are excreted via tubular secretion and a dosage adjustment method that involves both glomerular and renal tubular functions may be required.— R. Hori *et al.*, *Clin. Pharmac. Ther.*, 1983, *34*, 792.

A suggested dosage for ampicillin given to anephric patients with relatively normal hepatic function was 7.5 mg per kg body-weight every 6 hours.— R. E. Van Scoy and W. R. Wilson, *Mayo Clin. Proc.*, 1983, *58*, 246.

For comment on the administration of ampicillin in association with sulbactam in patients with renal failure, see under Sulbactam, Uses and Administration, p.299.

For the administration of ampicillin in patients undergoing peritoneal dialysis, see Peritonitis, below.

Administration with sulbactam. For reference to the use of ampicillin administered in association with sulbactam, see Sulbactam, Uses and Administration, p.299.

AIDS. Bacteraemia due to *Listeria monocytogenes* occurred in 2 of 226 patients with the acquired immune deficiency syndrome (AIDS). The infection was successfully treated with ampicillin 12 g daily administered intravenously for 2 weeks, but both patients developed a generalised skin rash. Although no CNS involvement occurred in these 2 patients, cultures of the CSF should be carried out in patients with listeria infections and the duration of treatment should be extended to 4 weeks if evidence of CNS infection is found.— F. X. Real *et al.* (letter), *Ann. intern. Med.*, 1984, *101*, 883.

DIARRHOEA. For a comparison of ampicillin and furazolidone in the treatment of acute traveller's diarrhoea, see under Furazolidone, p.665.

See also under Enteric Infections, below.

ENDOCARDITIS. Ampicillin has been used for bacterial infections due to group B streptococci or enterococci (*Med. Lett.*, 1986, *28*, 33) and ampicillin 12 g daily administered intravenously for 4 to 6 weeks in association with gentamicin 1 mg per kg body-weight given intravenously every 8 hours has been suggested as a treatment for bacterial endocarditis due to some viridans streptococci or enterococci (K. King and J.L. Harkness, *Med. J. Aust.*, 1986, *144*, 588). However, benzylpenicillin and an aminoglycoside are usually recommended for streptococcal or enterococcal endocarditis (W.R. Wilson *et al.*, *Ann. intern. Med.*, 1984, *100*, 816; *Lancet*, 1985, *2*, 815; K. King and J.L. Harkness, *Med. J. Aust.*, 1986, *144*, 588). Ampicillin has also been used for the treatment of endocarditis due to some Enterobacteriaceae, following the results of *in vitro* sensitivity tests (K. King and J.L. Harkness, *Med. J. Aust.*, 1986, *144*, 588).

For the use of ampicillin in association with chloramphenicol and gentamicin for the treatment of pericarditis due to *Haemophilus influenzae* type b, see Pericarditis, below.

Prophylaxis. For patients at risk of developing bacterial endocarditis during dental or respiratory-tract surgical procedures, the American Heart Association has recommended a special parenteral regimen for use when maximum protection is desired, as in patients with prosthetic valves. The regimen consists of ampicillin 1 to 2 g plus gentamicin 1.5 mg per kg body-weight both administered intramuscularly or intravenously half-an-hour before the procedure, followed by phenoxymethylpenicillin 1 g administered by mouth 6 hours later or the parenteral regimen repeated once 8 hours later; for children, ampicillin 50 mg per kg and gentamicin 2 mg per kg per dose has been recommended (S.T. Shulman *et al.*, *Circulation*, 1984, *70*, 1123A). However, the Working Party of the British Society for Antimicrobial Chemotherapy has recommended the use of amoxycillin plus gentamicin for special-risk patients (*Lancet*, 1982, *2*, 1323).

For patients at risk of bacterial endocarditis undergoing genito-urinary or gastro-intestinal surgery or instrumentation where there is a risk of bacteraemia, the American Heart Association have recommended a similar regimen using ampicillin 2 g plus gentamicin 1.5 mg per kg both given intramuscularly or intravenously one-half to one hour before the procedure; these doses can be repeated 8 hours later. For minor or repetitive procedures in low-risk patients an oral regimen using amoxycillin has been recommended (S.T. Shulman *et al.*, *Circulation*, 1984, *70*, 1123A). However, the British Working Party has again recommended the use of amoxycillin plus gentamicin (*Lancet*, 1982, *2*, 1323). The routine use of antibiotic prophylaxis for minor obstetric and gynaecological procedures is not usually recommended because these procedures rarely cause infective endocarditis; it may be prudent to give prophylaxis to patients with prosthetic valves because the prognosis may be worse in such patients (*Lancet*, 1982, *2*, 1323; S.T. Shulman *et al.*, *Circulation*, 1984, *70*, 1123A). There has, however, been a report of a woman with a ventricular septal defect who developed infective endocarditis after insertion of an intra-uterine contraceptive device. It has, therefore, been suggested that all women attending for such procedures should be examined for signs of cardiac abnormalities, and if any doubt exists a cardiological opinion should be obtained, or if insertion of the device is carried out, full antibiotic cover with gentamicin and ampicillin should be used (M.D. Gammage *et al.*, *Br. med. J.*, 1984, *289*, 1516).

See also under Prophylactic Use of Antibiotics, p.102.

ENTERIC INFECTIONS. Ampicillin 1 or 2 g given four times daily for 2 weeks may be used for acute enteric infections and the same dose may be given for 4 to 12 weeks in the carrier state. However, resistant organisms are now a problem.

Shigellosis is usually a self-limiting disease which does not always require antibiotic therapy, although patients with severe colitis benefit from appropriate therapy. A single dose of ampicillin 4 g administered intravenously has been shown to reduce the mean duration of fever and the duration of positive stool cultures compared with placebo (I. Kabir *et al.*, *Antimicrob. Ag. Chemother.*, 1986, *29*, 645), and ampicillin 4 g given as a single dose by mouth has been found to be as effective as conventional regimens given for 5 days (R.H. Gilman *et al.*, *J. infect. Dis.*, 1981, *143*, 164). However, resistance of shigellae to ampicillin has become quite common (F.A. Barada and R.L. Guerrant, *Antimicrob. Ag. Chemother.*, 1980, *17*, 961) and a high prevalence of resistance to ampicillin among bacterial enteropathogens particularly *Salmonella* and *Shigella* spp. and enterotoxigenic *Escherichia coli* strains has been demonstrated *in vitro* suggesting that ampicillin should probably no longer be used in the empirical treatment of acute diarrhoea (J.R. Carlson *et al.*, *Antimicrob. Ag. Chemother.*, 1983, *24*, 509). During an epidemic of dysentery in West Bengal the clinical response to ampicillin and other anti-shigella drugs such as co-trimoxazole was not very satisfactory and resistance to these drugs was subsequently demonstrated *in vitro* (R. Bose *et al.*, *Lancet*, 1984, *2*, 1160). In an epidemic of dysentery in Burma, however, isolates of *Shigella dysenteriae* type 1 were found to be sensitive to ampicillin, but resistant to some other antibacterial agents (Tin-Aye *et al.*, *Lancet*, 1985, *1*, 1442). Resistance to nalidixic acid, co-trimoxazole, and ampicillin has varied and their use should be based on *in vitro* susceptibility tests (M.J. Albert, *Lancet*, 1985, *2*, 948).

Ampicillin has been used in the management of neonatal typhoid fever, although the duration of diarrhoea or carrier state does not appear to be shortened by treatment with oral antibiotics (K.C. Chin *et al.*, *Archs Dis. Childh.*, 1986, *61*, 1228). Many *Salmonella* strains are resistant to ampicillin and ampicillin is considered to be inferior to chloramphenicol in the treatment of salmonellal infections. However, the use of pivmecillinam in association with pivampicillin has shown promising results against salmonellal infections (B.M. Limson *et al.*, *J. antimicrob. Chemother.*, 1982, *9*, 405).

EYE INFECTIONS. Treatment of *Pasteurella multocida* endophthalmitis with subconjunctival, parenteral, and intravitreal administration of ampicillin. Sterilisation of the eye was achieved, but the visual outcome was poor due to the severity of the endophthalmitis at the time of presentation.— M. E. Hoffman *et al.*, *Br. J. Ophthal.*, 1987, *71*, 609.

GONORRHOEA. A single dose of ampicillin 1 g with sulbactam 500 mg administered intramuscularly in association with probenecid administered by mouth produced clinical and bacteriological cure in 36 (81.8%) of 44 patients with gonorrhoea due to beta-lactamase-positive *Neisseria gonorrheae*; a further 6 patients were cured when the regimen was repeated once and the final 2 patients were cured with 3 doses. The use of ampicillin and sulbactam without probenecid in 7 patients yielded poor results which were not unexpected because of the low dose of ampicillin used. Results using the single-dose regimen might be improved if the ampicillin component of the regimen is increased.— T. Odugbemi, *Curr. ther. Res.*, 1987, *41*, 542.

For reference to the use of ampicillin in the treatment of disseminated gonococcal infection, see under Benzylpenicillin Sodium, Sexually Transmitted Diseases, p.137.

GRANULOMA INGUINALE. Ampicillin 500 mg every 6 hours for 14 days has been found effective.— *Br. med. J.*, 1981, *282*, 461.

HEPATIC ENCEPHALOPATHY. Ampicillin has been reported to reduce gastric ammonia concentrations in patients with hepatic encephalopathy (S. Meyers and C.S. Lieber, *Gastroenterology*, 1976, *70*, 244) and it has been suggested as a possible alternative to neomycin treatment (C.L. Fraser and A.I. Arieff, *New Engl. J. Med.*, 1985, *313*, 865).

LISTERIOSIS. The incidence of perinatal listeriosis seems to be increasing steadily, but this may partly reflect increased awareness of the condition. Ampicillin is considered to be the treatment of choice for listeriosis in pregnancy; erythromycin may be used in penicillin-sensitive patients (*Lancet*, 1985, *2*, 364). Prompt antibiotic treatment of the pregnant mother may be life-saving for the neonate (V.W. Krause *et al.*, *Can. med. Ass. J.*, 1982, *127*, 36). For both the pregnant mother and the newborn infant, ampicillin may be given in association with kanamycin or gentamicin, or, where meningitis is present, with chloramphenicol, and treatment is usually continued for 2 to 3 weeks; a suggested initial dose for ampicillin is 200 to 400 mg per kg body-weight intravenously (*Lancet*, 1980, *1*, 911).

Ampicillin alone or with chloramphenicol or gentamicin has been used to treat adult listeriosis, but the prognosis is generally poor and appears to depend on the underlying disease (S. Iwarson *et al.*, *J. antimicrob. Chemother.*, 1978, *4*, 229; Y. Samra *et al.*, *Postgrad. med. J.*, 1984, *60*, 267).

See also Meningitis, below.

LYME DISEASE. Treatment with ampicillin and prednisolone resolved the systemic symptoms of Lyme disease in a 10-year-old girl.— D. E. Dateman *et al.*, *Br. med. J.*, 1987, *294*, 548.

MENINGITIS. Ampicillin is considered the treatment of choice for listeria meningitis and doses of ampicillin 200 to 400 mg per kg body-weight every 24 hours in 4 to 6 divided doses have been used in association with gentamicin (M. Whitby and R. Finch, *Drugs*, 1986, *31*, 266). Although synergy has been demonstrated between an aminoglycoside and a penicillin *in vitro*, the clinical superiority of combination therapy over ampicillin or penicillin alone has not been shown and some clinicians have reservations about the toxicity of aminoglycosides and their poor penetration into the CNS. Winslow *et al.* (*Antimicrob. Ag. Chemother.*, 1983, *23*, 555) demonstrated that the bactericidal activity of ampicillin against *Listeria monocytogenes* is delayed until after 48 hours of incubation and they speculated that if there is any benefit in adding aminoglycosides to a penicillin, it is probably only during the first 24 to 48 hours of treatment. They have also demonstrated antagonism between ampicillin and chloramphenicol, rifampicin, doxycycline, or erythromycin, against *L. monocytogenes in vitro* and they suggested that these combinations should be avoided in listeria infections. However, other workers have demonstrated some synergy between rifampicin and ampicillin (R.L. Hull, *Drug Intell. & clin. Pharm.*, 1984, *18*, 78).

For group B streptococcal meningitis benzylpenicillin or ampicillin in association with gentamicin have been recommended (M. Whitby and R. Finch, *Drugs*, 1986, *31*, 266) although the clinical relevance of the aminoglycoside is again uncertain (H.P. Lambert, *Br. J. Hosp. Med.*, 1983, *29*, 128). Other workers have suggested the use of benzylpenicillin or ampicillin alone for the treatment of group B streptococcal infections (*Med. Lett.*, 1986, *28*, 33). Ampicillin has also been used in association with gentamicin in the treatment of meningitis due to *Escherichia coli* and *Campylobacter jejuni* (M. Whitby and R. Finch, *Drugs*, 1986, *31*, 266; H. Goossens *et al.*, *Lancet*, 1986, *2*, 146), and with sulbactam in the treatment of meningococcal meningitis (A.I. Dutse *et al.*, *Curr. ther. Res.*, 1987, *41*, 128).

Ampicillin has been used for the treatment of meningitis caused by *Haemophilus influenzae* but the increasing prevalence of beta-lactamase-producing organisms has meant that some authorities recommend the use of ampicillin in association with chloramphenicol and some the use of chloramphenicol alone (H.P. Lambert, *Br. med. J.*, 1983, *286*, 741; A. Mulhall *et al.*, *Lancet*, 1983, *1*, 284; *Med. Lett.*, 1986, *28*, 33). Once susceptibility has been established, ampicillin has been administered in doses of 200 mg per kg every 24 hours in divided doses every 3 to 4 hours (M. Whitby and R. Finch, *Drugs*, 1986, *31*, 266). An ampicillin-resistant strain has been isolated during treatment of meningitis originally attributed to sensitive strains, and ampicillin resistance should be borne in mind before discontinuing chloramphenicol in severe *H. influenzae* infection even if initial cultures suggest sensitivity to ampicillin (P. MacMahon and P. Ramberan, *Lancet*, 1980, *1*, 1080). Meningitis due to *H. influenzae* type b resistant to both ampicillin and chloramphenicol has also been reported (P. MacMahon *et al.*, *Br. med. J.*, 1982, *284*, 1229; H. Guiscafré *et al.*, *Archs Dis. Childh.*, 1986, *61*, 691) and this, together with the adverse effects of chloramphenicol, has increased the need for alternative therapy (J.M. Gairi *et al.*, *Archs Dis. Childh.*, 1986, *61*, 1245; B.L. Congeni, *Antimicrob. Ag. Chemother.*, 1984, *25*, 40). Cephalosporins such as cefuroxime, cefotaxime, or ceftriaxone are considered to be suitable alternatives (R.G. Finch, *Br. med. J.*, 1984, *289*, 941; *Med. Lett.*, 1986, *28*, 33). Beneficial results have also been obtained by the addition of rifampicin to ampicillin therapy for *H. influenzae* type b meningitis refractory to conventional treatment despite sensitivity *in vitro* (M.A. Lewis and B.L. Priestley, *Br. med. J.*, 1986, *292*, 448; C.I. Haines and M. Patfield, *ibid.*, 900).

For the empirical treatment of meningitis in neonates which is often caused by gram-negative enteric organisms, group B streptococci, or *L. monocytogenes* , ampicillin has been used in association with gentamicin or tobramycin (A.P. Ball, *Pharm. J.*, 1984, *2*, 14; *Med. Lett.*, 1986, *28*, 33). Cephalosphorins such as cefotaxime or ceftazidime are considered suitable alternatives, although *L. monocytogenes* is not susceptible to these drugs and therefore the addition of ampicillin may be required (M. Whitby and R. Finch, *Drugs*, 1986, *31*, 266). In infants and children the major pathogens are *H. influenzae*, *Neisseria meningitidis*, and *Streptococcus pneumoniae* and although both ampicillin and chloramphenicol have been used alone, due to the increase in resistant organisms, they are usually given together until the results of susceptibility tests are known (J.H. Joncas *et al.*, *Can. med. Ass. J.*, 1985, *132*, 1006; M. Whitby and R. Finch, *Drugs*, 1986, *31*, 266; *Med. Lett.*, 1986, *28*, 33). Other alternatives for the treatment of childhood meningitis include cefuroxime, ceftriaxone, or cefotaxime (J. Pfenninger *et al.*, *Archs Dis. Childh.*, 1982, *57* 539; B.L. Congeni, *Antimicrob. Ag. Chemother.*, 1984, *25*, 40; J.M. Gairi *et al.*, *Archs Dis. Childh.*, 1986, *61*, 1245), but many specialists are reluctant to recommend a single agent and ampicillin in association with cefotaxime is considered a suitable alternative (J.H. Joncas *et al.*, *Can. med. Ass. J.*, 1985, *132*, 1006). For meningitis in adults benzylpenicillin is often used, but some workers prefer ampicillin in case *H. influenzae* is present (*Med. Lett.*, 1986, *28*, 33).

See also Listeriosis, above.

OTITIS MEDIA. For the use of ampicillin or its esters in the treatment of otitis media, see Choice of Antibiotic, p.98.

PELVIC INFLAMMATORY DISEASE. Aminopenicillins and tetracyclines were the most frequently prescribed single-drug treatments for pelvic inflammatory disease in the *USA* during the period 1980 to 1983. However, due to the polymicrobial nature of the disease most authorities feel that no single antibiotic is effective against all the implicated organisms (D.A. Grimes *et al.*, *J. Am. med. Ass.*, 1986, *256*, 3223). For the treatment of outpatients with pelvic inflammatory disease a single dose of ampicillin trihydrate 3.5 g plus probenecid 1 g by mouth, followed by doxycycline hydrochloride 100 mg twice daily by mouth is one of the regimens considered suitable, although the Centers for Disease Control recommends cefoxitin in association with doxycycline (P. Wølner-Hanssen *et al.*, *ibid.*, 3262). Beneficial results in the treatment of mixed aerobic and anaerobic pelvic infections have also been obtained with ampicillin used in association with sulbactam, with additional doxycycline used when chlamydial infection is present (W.R. Crombleholme *et al.*, *Am. J. Obstet. Gynec.*, 1987, *165*, 507).

See also under Choice of Antibiotic, p.98.

PERICARDITIS. A report of the intravenous use of ampicillin with chloramphenicol and gentamicin in a 4½-year-old boy with pericarditis due to *Haemophilus influenza* type B, and ampicillin with chloramphenicol in a similar 9-month-old boy. Use of parenterally administered antibiotics with early surgical pericardial drainage or partial pericardiectomy should reduce associated morbidity and mortality in this condition.— D. A. Fyfe *et al.*, *Mayo Clin. Proc.*, 1984, *59*, 415.

PERITONITIS. Ampicillin could be administered intraperitoneally in patients undergoing continuous ambulatory peritoneal dialysis. A loading dose of 500 mg per litre followed by maintenance doses of 50 mg per litre have been used in some units; a maintenance dose of 25 mg per litre could be used in rapid exchange peritoneal dialysis.— D. K. Scott and D. E. Roberts, *Pharm. J.*, 1985, *1*, 621.

The British Society for Antimicrobial Chemotherapy has recommended the use of ampicillin for the treatment of peritonitis caused by *Enterococcus faecalis* in patients undergoing continuous ambulatory peritoneal dialysis; vancomycin is considered to be a suitable alternative. Ampicillin may be administered as a loading dose of 1 g given either intravenously or preferably by the intraperitoneal route and then as a maintenance dose of 125 mg per litre intraperitoneally.— *Lancet*, 1987, *1*, 845.

For the initial empirical treatment of peritonitis, see under Choice of Antibiotic, Peritonitis, p.99.

PREGNANCY AND THE NEONATE. In a study of the prevention of early-onset neonatal group B streptococcal disease, *intrapartum* chemoprophylaxis with ampicillin resulted in a dramatic reduction in transmission of group B streptococci from colonised mothers to their infants. Colonisation with group B streptococci occurred in 40 of 79 neonates whose mothers were untreated compared with 8 of 85 neonates whose mothers had received ampicillin 2 g intravenously followed by 1 g every 4 hours until delivery; the infants of treated mothers also received ampicillin 50 mg per kg body-weight intramuscularly every 12 hours for 4 doses. Bacteraemia occurred in 5 neonates (6.3%) in the control group, but in none of the infants whose mothers received prophylaxis. Selective *intrapartum* ampicillin prophylaxis in women with positive prenatal cultures for group B streptococci who have certain perinatal risk factors could prevent early-onset neonatal group B streptococcal disease.— K. M. Boyer and S. P. Gotoff, *New Engl. J. Med.*, 1986, *314*, 1665. See also K. M. Boyer *et al.*, *J. infect. Dis.*, 1983, *148*, 810. The acceptability, safety, and effectiveness of selective prophylaxis for early-onset neonatal group B streptococcal disease remains to be seen. It may limit unnecessary use of antibiotics but will not, of course, protect infants without the recognised risk factors.— *Lancet*, 1984, *1*, 1056. See also under Benzylpenicillin Sodium p.137.

Ampicillin is considered probably safe for administration during pregnancy although in the second and third trimesters there is the possibility of sensitising the foetus. As little information is available for ampicillin prodrugs, it seems reasonable to avoid these drugs and use the parent ampicillin. Providing the organisms are sensitive, ampicillin may be administered during pregnancy for the treatment of asymptomatic bacteriuria or simple cystitis, and for acute bacterial bronchial infection; ampicillin had also been administered intravenously for acute pyelonephritis. During lactation the concentrations of ampicillin reaching the infant are considered to be extremely low and unlikely to affect the child.— R. Wise, *Br. med. J.*, 1987, *294*, 42. Ampicillin is excreted in breast milk and there is the potential for diarrhoea or candidiasis in the neonate.— A. W. Chow and P. J. Jewesson, *Rev. infect. Dis.*, 1985, *7*, 287. See also under Absorption and Fate, above.

For a comparison of ampicillin used in association with gentamicin, with vancomycin used in association with cefotaxime, for the treatment of neonatal necrotising enterocolitis, see under Vancomycin Hydrochloride, p.336.

See also under Administration for a reference to the administration of ampicillin to neonates in parenteral nutrition solutions.

RESPIRATORY-TRACT INFECTIONS. *Bronchitis.* The increase in resistance of *Haemophilus influenzae* to ampicillin has reduced its value in the treatment of bronchitis (G. Anderson, *Postgrad. med. J.*, 1983, *59*, *Suppl.* 3, 179). Similarly a high proportion of *Branhamella catarrhalis* organisms that have previously responded to treatment with ampicillin now produce beta-lactamase making ampicillin treatment inappropriate (D.T. McLeod *et al.*, *Br. med. J.*, 1986, *292*, 1103). The addition of a beta-lactamase inhibitor should, in theory, help to restore the efficacy of the penicillin.

Epiglottitis. Ampicillin has been used to treat acute epiglottitis in adults, but consideration needs to be given to ampicillin-resistant strains of *Haemophilus influenzae*, and chloramphenicol or a suitable third-generation cephalosporin should be included in the initial antimicrobial coverage.— M. F. MayoSmith *et al.*, *New Engl. J. Med.*, 1986, *314*, 1135.

Pertussis. A heavy growth of *Bordetella pertussis* was eradicated from the sputum of an adult after 36 hours of treatment with ampicillin (C.D. Ribeiro, *Lancet*, 1981, *1*, 951). However, other workers have found no detectable effect *in vivo*, although the organisms are sensitive to ampicillin *in vitro* (J. Broomhall and A. Herxheimer, *Archs Dis. Childh.*, 1984, *59*, 185).

For comment on the use of antibacterial agents, including ampicillin, in patients infected with *B. pertussis*, see under Erythromycin, p.226.

Pneumonia. High-dose intravenous ampicillin plus erythromycin given immediately after hospital admission was considered suitable for initial antibiotic therapy of adults with severe community-acquired pneumonia of unknown cause; during an influenza virus epidemic an additional antistaphylococcal agent such as flucloxacillin should be included.— M. A. Woodhead and J. T. Macfarlane (letter), *Br. med. J.*, 1985, *290*, 1745.

From a double-blind study of 90 patients with community-acquired pneumonia, ampicillin 2 g or cephamandole 2 g, both administered intravenously over 30 minutes every 6 hours for a mean of 4 days, were equally effective in the initial treatment of pneumonia. Failure of treatment occurred in 5 of 42 patients in the ampicillin group and 6 of 48 in the cephamandole group. A change to oral antibiotic therapy after 3 or 4 days of parenteral therapy did not appear to increase the risk of relapse of pneumonia.— D. J. Weber *et al.*, *Antimicrob. Ag. Chemother.*, 1987, *31*, 876.

Beneficial results with ampicillin administered in association with sulbactam in the treatment of 20 patients with lobar pneumonia.— V. O. Oviasu and A. D. Obasohan, *Curr. ther. Res.*, 1987, *41*, 99.

SEPTICAEMIA. Recovery of a 70-year-old woman with *Campylobacter fetus* bacteraemia treated with ampicillin 2 g administered intravenously 4 times daily for 15 days.— P. Francioli *et al.*, *Archs intern. Med.*, 1985, *213*, 289.

SKIN DISORDERS. Comment on the use of ampicillin to treat patients with acne who are not responding to tetracycline therapy.— W. J. Cunliffe, *Prescribers' J.*, 1987, *27*, (4), 23.

SURGICAL INFECTION PROPHYLAXIS. Ampicillin has been used to reduce the incidence of post-operative infections particularly in major gynaecological surgery. For hysterectomy an appropriate regimen is ampicillin 1 g administered intravenously immediately before the operation and every 6 hours for 24 hours, in association with metronidazole 500 mg administered intravenously before the operation and again 12 hours later (P. O'Brien and P. MacDonald, *Med. J. Aust.*, 1985, *143*, 149). Single-dose peri-operative prophylaxis with ampicillin 500 mg intravenously administered in association with either sulbactam 500 mg intravenously or metronidazole 1 g by suppository has also been demonstrated to reduce post-operative wound infections and febrile morbidity in abdominal hysterectomy (E.T. Houang *et al.*, *J. antimicrob. Chemother.*, 1984, *14*, 529). Ampicillin has been used pre-operatively to decrease septic complications after emergency caesarean section in high risk patients and it has also been shown to decrease the incidence of infection after appendectomy (*Med. Lett.*, 1985, *27*, 105). However, cephalosporins are generally preferred for most surgical procedures in which skin flora or the normal flora of the gastro-intestinal or genito-urinary tracts are the most likely pathogens (A.B. Kaiser, *New Engl. J. Med.*, 1986, *315*, 1129). Ampicillin plus the beta-lactamase inhibitor sulbactam have been of benefit in patients undergoing colorectal surgery and they did not adversely affect the faecal flora (L. Kager, *et al.*, *Antimicrob. Ag. Chemother.*, 1982, *22*, 208).

Beneficial results have been obtained with ampicillin and amoxycillin administered to children during the first week after tonsillectomy. Ampicillin sodium 0.5 or 1.0 g was administered intravenously following the removal of the tonsils and at 6-hourly intervals until discharge from hospital, usually within 24 hours following the operation; amoxycillin trihydrate 125 or 250 mg was then administered three times daily (S.A. Telian *et al.*, *Archs Otolar.*, 1986, *112*, 610).

Intra-incisional instillation of ampicillin just before closure of the wound has been found to reduce wound infection in a variety of abdominal procedures. However, topical agents cannot be relied upon to give satisfactory serum concentrations as they only give protection at the wound, and they are just as likely as systemic antibiotics to induce allergy or the emergence of resistant strains

(O.J.A. Gilmore and R.G. Sprignall, *Br. J. Hosp. Med.*, 1983, *29*, 440). The use of topical ampicillin has also been shown to give no benefit in colorectal surgery when systemic prophylaxis with ampicillin and metronidazole is also administered (P. Juul *et al.*, *Dis. Colon Rectum*, 1985, *28*, 804).

URINARY-TRACT INFECTIONS. Ampicillin is one of the drugs used for the treatment of acute urinary-tract infections in women (W.R. Cattell, *Prescribers' J.*, 1983, *23*, 81). Its use has, however, been compromised by a high incidence of resistant organisms (W. Brumfitt *et al.*, *Br. J. Hosp. Med.*, 1983, *30*, 381), although resistance mostly occurs in patients with complicated or recurrent disease. Amoxycillin or the ester pro-drugs of ampicillin, or mecillinam, are considered to be kinetically preferable to ampicillin when administered by mouth (A.P. Ball, *Pharm. J.*, 1984, *2*, 14).

For mention of the use of ampicillin in association with sulbactam for the treatment of urinary-tract infections due to ampicillin-resistant organisms, see under Sulbactam, p.299.

Preparations

Ampicillin Capsules *(B.P.)*. Capsules containing ampicillin or ampicillin trihydrate.

Ampicillin Capsules *(U.S.P.)*. Capsules containing ampicillin or ampicillin trihydrate.

Ampicillin and Probenecid Capsules *(U.S.P.)*. Capsules containing ampicillin trihydrate and probenecid.

Ampicillin Injection *(B.P.)*. Ampicillin Sodium Injection

Sterile Ampicillin *(U.S.P.)*. Ampicillin trihydrate suitable for parenteral use.

Sterile Ampicillin for Suspension *(U.S.P.)*. Ampicillin trihydrate suitable for parenteral use.

Sterile Ampicillin Sodium *(U.S.P.)*

Ampicillin Oral Suspension *(B.P.)*. Ampicillin Mixture; Ampicillin Syrup. A dry mixture of ampicillin or ampicillin trihydrate for reconstitution.

Ampicillin for Oral Suspension *(U.S.P.)*. A dry mixture of ampicillin or ampicillin trihydrate for reconstitution.

Ampicillin and Probenecid for Oral Suspension *(U.S.P.)*. A dry mixture of ampicillin trihydrate and probenecid for reconstitution.

Ampicillin Tablets *(U.S.P.)*. Tablets (chewable or non-chewable) containing ampicillin or ampicillin trihydrate.

Paediatric Ampicillin Tablets *(B.P.)*. Tablets containing ampicillin or ampicillin trihydrate.

Proprietary Preparations

Amfipen *(Brocades, UK)*. *Capsules*, ampicillin 250 and 500 mg.
Syrup, powder for reconstitution, ampicillin 125 mg/5 mL when reconstituted with water.
Syrup forte, powder for reconstitution, ampicillin 250 mg/5 mL when reconstituted with water.
Injection, powder for reconstitution, ampicillin 250 and 500 mg (as sodium salt).

Ampiclox *(Beecham Research, UK)*. *Injection*, powder for reconstitution, ampicillin 250 mg (as sodium salt), cloxacillin 250 mg (as sodium salt).

Ampiclox Neonatal *(Beecham Research, UK)*. *Suspension*, powder for reconstitution, ampicillin 60 mg (as trihydrate), cloxacillin 30 mg (as sodium salt)/0.6 mL when reconstituted with water.
Injection, powder for reconstitution, ampicillin 50 mg (as sodium salt), cloxacillin 25 mg (as sodium salt).

Ampilar *(Lagap, UK)*. *Capsules*, ampicillin 250 and 500 mg (as trihydrate).
Syrup, powder for reconstitution, ampicillin 125 mg (as trihydrate)/5 mL when reconstituted with water.
Syrup forte, powder for reconstitution, ampicillin 250 mg (as trihydrate)/5 mL when reconstituted with water.

Britcin *(DDSA Pharmaceuticals, UK)*. *Capsules*, ampicillin 250 and 500 mg (as trihydrate).

Flu-Amp *(Generics, UK)*. *Capsules*, ampicillin 250 mg (as trihydrate), flucloxacillin 250 mg (as sodium salt).

Magnapen *(Beecham Research, UK)*. *Capsules*, ampicillin 250 mg (as trihydrate), flucloxacillin 250 mg (as sodium salt).
Syrup, powder for reconstitution, ampicillin 125 mg (as trihydrate), flucloxacillin 125 mg (as magnesium salt)/5 mL when reconstituted with water.
Injection (500 mg), powder for reconstitution, ampicillin 250 mg (as sodium salt), flucloxacillin 250 mg (as sodium salt).
Injection (1 g), powder for reconstitution, ampicillin 500 mg (as sodium salt), flucloxacillin 500 mg (as sodium salt).

Penbritin *(Beecham Research, UK)*. *Capsules*, ampicillin 250 and 500 mg (as trihydrate).
Syrup, powder for reconstitution, ampicillin 125 mg (as trihydrate)/5 mL when reconstituted with water.
Syrup forte, powder for reconstitution, ampicillin 250 mg (as trihydrate)/5 mL when reconstituted with water.
Paediatric suspension , powder for reconstitution, ampicillin 125 mg (as trihydrate)/1.25 mL when reconstituted with water.
Injection, powder for reconstitution, ampicillin 250 and 500 mg (as sodium salt).

Vidopen *(Berk Pharmaceuticals, UK)*. *Capsules*, ampicillin 250 and 500 mg (as trihydrate).
Syrup, powder for reconstitution, ampicillin 125 mg (as trihydrate)/5 mL when reconstituted with water.
Syrup forte, powder for reconstitution, ampicillin 250 mg (as trihydrate)/5 mL when reconstituted with water.

Proprietary Names and Manufacturers of Ampicillin, Ampicillin Salts, and Ampicillin Trihydrate

A-Cillin *(USA)*; Adobacillin *(Jpn)*; Aletmicina *(Arg.)*; Alpen *(USA)*; Alpen-N *(USA)*; Amblosin *(Hoechst, Ger.; Spain)*; Amcill *(Canad.; Parke, Davis, USA)*; Amcill-S *(USA)*; Amfipen *(Neth.; Switz.; Brocades, UK)*; Ampen *(Medosan, Ital.)*; Amperil *(USA)*; Ampibel *(Belg.)*; Ampi-Biopharma *(Spain)*; Ampibiotic *(Ottolenghi, Ital.)*; Ampibronc Capsules *(Ital.)*; Ampicil *(Fr.; Ausonia, Ital.; Spain)*; Ampicillat *(Azuchemie, Ger.)*; Ampicilline *(Mepha, Switz.)*; Ampiciman *(Liberman, Spain)*; Ampicin *(Bristol, Canad.; Spain)*; Ampicina *(Ital.)*; Ampicur *(Urca, Spain)*; Ampifen *(Fisons, Ital.)*; Ampi-Framan *(Oftalmiso, Spain)*; Ampigal *(Bicther, Spain)*; Ampikel *(Dreikehl, Spain)*; Ampil *(GMP, S.Afr.)*; Ampilag *(Lagap, Switz.)*; Ampilan *(Ibirn, Ital.)*; Ampiland *(Landerlan, Spain)*; Ampilar *(Lagap, UK)*; Ampilean *(Organon, Canad.)*; Ampilisa *(Lisapharma, Ital.)*; Ampilux *(Allergan, Ital.)*; Ampinebiot *(Spain)*; Ampinova *(Spain)*; Ampinoxi *(Spain)*; Ampi-Oral *(Cheminova, Spain)*; Ampiorus *(Spain)*; Ampipenix *(Jpn)*; Ampi-Rol *(Rolab, S.Afr.)*; Ampisint *(Proter, Ital.)*; Ampi-Tablinen *(Beiersdorf, Ger.)*; Ampitex *(Neopharmed, Ital.)*; Ampivax *(Ital.)*; Ampi-Vial *(Esteve, Spain)*; Ampixilon *(Wasserman, Spain)*; Ampi-Zoja *(Zoja, Ital.)*; Amplibios *(Ital.)*; Amplicid *(Ital.)*; Amplimedix *(Medix, Spain)*; Amplipen *(Ital.)*; Amplipenyl *(ISF, Ital.)*; Ampliscocil *(Ital.)*; Amplital *(Farmitalia, Ital.)*; Amplizer *(OFF, Ital.)*; Anhypen *(Gist-Brocades, Denm.)*; Anidropen *(Ital.)*; Antibiopen *(Antibioticos, Spain)*; Anticyl *(San Carlo, Ital.)*; Apo-Ampi *(Apotex, Canad.)*; Argocillina *(Beta, Ital.)*; Austrapen *(Commonwealth Serum Laboratories, Austral.)*;
Bemicina *(Spain)*; Benusel Oral *(Spain)*; Binotal *(Bayer, Ger.; Ital.; Bayer, S.Afr.; Bayer, Spain)*; Bio-ampi *(Ital.)*; Biocellina *(Ital.)*; Bionacillin *(Jpn)*; Biosan *(Canad.)*; Bonapicillin *(Jpn)*; Bristin *(Austral.)*; Britapen *(Beecham, Spain)*; Britcin *(DDSA Pharmaceuticals, UK)*; Cilleral *(Spain)*; Cimexillin *(Cimex, Switz.)*; Citicil *(CT, Ital.)*; Cuxacillin *(TAD, Ger.)*; Cymbi *(Ger.)*; D-Amp *(Dunhall, USA)*; Deripen *(Ger.)*; Diancina *(Septa, Spain)*; Doca *(Organon, Swed.)*; Doktacillin *(Astra, Denm.; Astra, Norw.; Astra, Swed.)*; Domicillin *(Jpn)*; Dotirol *(Arg.)*; DuraAmpicillin *(Ger.)*; Espectrosira *(Spain)*; Espimin-Cilina *(Spyfarma, Spain)*; Eurocillin *(Borromeo, Ital.)*; Famicillin *(S.Afr.)*; Farmampil *(Ital.)*; Fidesbiotic *(Spain)*; Fortapen *(Belg.)*; Fuerpen *(Spain)*; Germicillina *(Ital.)*; Geycillina *(Ital.)*; Globipen Balsamico *(Andromaco, Spain)*; Gobemicina *(Normon, Spain)*; Gramcillina *(Caber, Ital.)*; Grampenil *(Arg.)*; Guicitrina *(Spain)*;
Helvecillin *(Switz.)*; Hostes *(Arg.)*; Iwacillin *(Jpn)*; Lampocillina *(Salus, Ital.)*; Lifeampil *(Spain)*; Marisilan *(Jpn)*; Maxicilina *(Antibioticos, Spain)*; Medicillin-D *(S.Afr.)*; Morepen *(Spain)*; Napicil *(Ital.)*; NC Cilin *(Jpn)*; Negmapen *(Negma, Fr.)*; Novoexpectro *(Spain)*; Nuvapen *(CEPA, Spain)*; Omnipen *(Wyeth, USA)*; Omnipen-N *(Wyeth, USA)*; Overcillina *(Ital.)*; Panbiotic *(Rhone-Poulenc, Ital.)*; Panestes *(Davur, Spain)*; Pénicline *(Delagrange, Fr.)*; Pen A *(USA)*; Pen Ampil *(Ital.)*; Pen A/N *(USA)*; Penampil *(Nuovo, Ital.)*; Penberin *(Bergamon, Ital.)*; Pen-Bristol *(Grünenthal, Ger.)*; Penbristol *(Bristol, Switz.)*; Penbritin *(Arg.; Beecham, Austral.; Belg.; Canad.; Neth.; Beecham, S.Afr.; Beecham, Switz.; Beecham Research, UK; USA)*; Penbritine *(Fr.)*; Penbrock *(Ger.)*; Penimaster *(Liade, Spain)*; Penimic *(Jpn)*; Penimul *(IBE, Spain)*; Peninovel *(Spain)*; Penisint B.G. *(Boniscontro & Gazzone, Ital.)*; Penisintex *(Jorba, Spain)*; Penorsin *(Spain)*; Penrite *(Columbia, S.Afr.)*; Pensyn *(USA)*; Pentrex *(Bristol, S.Afr.)*; Pentrexil *(Bristol Italiana Sud, Ital.)*; Pentrexyl *(Belg.; Bristol-Myers, Denm.; Bristol, Norw.; Bristol-Myers, Spain; Bristol, Swed.; Bristol-Myers Pharmaceuticals, UK)*; Pentrexyl-K *(Arg.)*; Petercillin *(Lennon, S.Afr.)*; Pharcillin *(Jpn)*; Platocillina *(Crosara, Ital.)*; Plumericin *(Spain)*; Poenbiotico *(Arg.)*; Polycillin *(Bristol, USA)*; Prestacilina *(Spain)*; Principen *(Arg.; Squibb, Ital.; Squibb, USA)*; Principen/N *(USA)*; Quimetam *(Spain)*; Racenacillin *(Jpn)*; Radiocillina *(Radiumfarma, Ital.)*; Resan *(Alacan, Spain)*; Rivocillin *(Switz.)*; Rosampline *(Rosa-Phytopharma, Fr.)*; Roscillin *(Ind.)*; Saicil *(Ital.)*; Semicillin *(Hung.)*; Sernabiotic *(Ital.)*; Servicilline *(Servipharm, Switz.)*; Sesquicillina *(ITA, Ital.)*; Sintopenyl *(Ital.)*; SK-Ampicillin *(Smith Kline & French, USA)*; SK-Ampicillin-N *(Smith Kline & French, USA)*; Spectracil *(Schwulst, S.Afr.)*; Sumipanto *(Spain)*; Supen *(Reid-Provident, USA)*; Suractin *(Ger.)*; Synpenin *(Jpn)*; Synthecillin *(S.Afr.)*; Tauglicolcillina *(Ibi, Ital.)*; Togram *(Morgens, Spain)*; Tokiocillin *(Jpn)*; Tolimal *(Arg.)*; Totacilina *(Ital.)*; Totacillin *(Jpn; Beecham Laboratories, USA)*; Totacillin-N *(Beecham Laboratories, USA)*; Totalciclina *(Benvegna, Ital.)*; Totapen *(Bristol, Fr.)*; Trafarbiot *(Spain)*; Trifacilina *(Arg.)*; Ukapen *(Spret-Mauchant, Fr.)*; Ultrabion *(Sabater, Spain)*; Urebion Ampicillina *(Spain)*; Valmingina *(Valles Mestre, Spain)*; Viacilina-A *(Arg.)*; Vidopen *(Berk Pharmaceuticals, UK)*.

The following names have been used for multi-ingredient preparations containing ampicillin, ampicillin salts, and ampicillin trihydrate— Ampicin-PRB *(Bristol, Canad.)*; Ampiclox *(Beecham, S.Afr.; Beecham Research, UK)*; Ampicyn *(Protea, Austral.)*; Flu-Amp *(Generics, UK)*; Magnapen *(Beecham Research, UK)*; Nuvapen Retard *(Spain)*; Orbecilina *(Arg.)*; Penbritin KS *(Beecham Research, UK)*; Pentrex-F *(Bristol, S.Afr.)*; Polycillin-PRB *(Bristol, USA)*; Principen with Probenecid *(Squibb, USA)*; Pro-Biosan *(ICN, Canad.)*; Unasyn *(Roerig, USA)*.

15329-m

Apalcillin Sodium *(USAN, pINNM)*.

PC-904; WY-44417 (apalcillin). (6*R*)-6-[(*R*)-2-(4-Hydroxy-1,5-naphthyridin-3-ylcarboxamido)-2-phenylacetamido]penicillanic acid, sodium salt.
$C_{25}H_{22}N_5NaO_6S = 543.5$.

CAS — 63469-19-2 (apalcillin); 58795-03-2 (sodium salt).

1.04 g of monograph substance is approximately equivalent to 1 g of apalcillin. Each g of monograph substance represents about 1.8 mmol of sodium.

Apalcillin sodium is a semi-synthetic penicillin derivative with actions and uses similar to piperacillin sodium, (see p.285). It is administered by intravenous infusion in doses equivalent to apalcillin 2 to 3 g three times daily.

ADVERSE EFFECTS AND PRECAUTIONS. Twenty-one healthy subjects were given intravenous apalcillin in a dose of 75, 150, or 225 mg per kg body-weight daily. The abnormalities in platelet aggregation that occurred were considered to be similar to those observed with piperacillin and mezlocillin. There were also abnormalities in other indices of haemostasis. Maculopapular skin rashes were observed in 7 subjects, which resolved on discontinuation of the drug.— L. O. Gentry *et al.*, *Antimicrob. Ag. Chemother.*, 1985, *27*, 683.

ANTIMICROBIAL ACTION. Studies *in vitro* of the antimicrobial action of apalcillin indicate a similar range of activity to piperacillin, including activity against anaerobic organisms. It does, however, appear to be slightly more active against *Pseudomonas aeruginosa* and *Acinetobacter calcoaceticus*. Its activity against *Ps. aeruginosa* appears comparable to that of some of the new cephalosporins including cefpiramide and ceftazidime.
References: G. P. Bodey *et al.*, *Antimicrob. Ag. Chemother.*, 1978, *13*, 14; H. Noguchi *et al.*, *ibid.*, 745; H. C. Neu and P. Labthavikul, *ibid.*, 1982, *21*, 906; H. Wexler *et al.*, *ibid.*, 1984, *25*, 162; A. L. Barry *et al.*, *ibid.*, 669; G. E. Hollick *et al.*, *ibid.*, *26*, 408; R. J. Fass and V. L. Helsel, *ibid.*, 660; J. D. Allan *et al.*, *ibid.*, 1985, *27*, 782.

Activity with other antimicrobial agents. Synergistic action against *Pseudomonas aeruginosa* has been observed *in vitro* between combinations of apalcillin and tobramycin or amikacin (H.C. Neu and P. Labthavikul, *Antimicrob. Ag. Chemother.*, 1982, *21*, 906) or gentamicin (J.D. Allan *et al.*, *ibid.*, 1985, *27*, 782). Allan *et al.*, and also Gombert and Aulicino using amikacin (*J. antimicrob Chemother.*, 1986, *17*, 323), demonstrated synergy against some other Gram-negative aerobes. Allan *et al.* observed antagonism between apalcillin and cefoxitin against some strains of *Enterobacter cloacae* and *Ps. aeruginosa*.

ABSORPTION AND FATE. The pharmacokinetics of apalcillin and piperacillin were compared in a crossover study involving 10 healthy subjects. The mean concentration of apalcillin in the serum 5 minutes after completion of the intravenous infusion, was 218.6 µg per mL, and declined to 59.2, 7.1, and 0.9 µg per mL after 1, 4, and 8 hours respectively. The decline of serum-piperacillin concentrations was slightly more rapid, falling from 201.3 to 1.0 µg per mL in the 6 hours following the infusion. The half-lives for apalcillin and piperacillin were 75.8 and 55.5 minutes respectively; 86 and 48% of the 2 drugs were bound to plasma proteins. Only 18.4% of apalcillin was excreted unchanged in the urine over 24 hours in contrast with 71.2% of piperacillin. However, an additional 18.1% of the apalcillin dose was excreted in the urine as metabolites, identified as stereoisomeric penicilloic acids.— H. Lode *et al.*, *Antimicrob. Ag. Chemother.*, 1984, *25*, 105.

Biliary elimination of apalcillin as assessed in 30 patients appeared to compare favourably with other beta-lactam agents.— J. M. Brogard *et al.*, *Antimicrob. Ag. Chemother.*, 1984, *26*, 428.

Further studies of the absorption and fate of apalcillin: E. Bergogne-Berezin *et al.*, *J. antimicrob. Chemother.*, 1984, *14*, 67 (pharmacokinetics and penetration into bronchial secretions after intermittent and continuous infusion); D. Raoult *et al.*, *ibid.*, 1985, *15*, 123 (penetration into the CSF).

Proprietary Names and Manufacturers
Lumota *(Thomae, Ger.)*.

12387-l

Apramycin *(BAN, USAN, rINN)*.
EL-857/820; Lilly 47657; Nebramycin Factor 2. 4-*O*-[(3-Amino-6-(4-amino-4-deoxy-α-D-glucopyranosyloxy)-8-hydroxy-7-methylaminoperhydropyrano[3,2-*b*]pyran-2-yl]-2-deoxystreptamine.
$C_{21}H_{41}N_5O_{11}$=539.6.

CAS — 37321-09-8.

An antibiotic produced by *Streptomyces tenebrarius*.

Apramycin is an aminoglycoside antibiotic used as the sulphate in veterinary practice.

For reference to the emergence of apramycin- and gentamicin-resistant strains of *Salmonella typhimurium* associated with the intensive use of apramycin in animal husbandry, see Gentamicin Sulphate, p.240.

Proprietary Veterinary Names and Manufacturers
Apralan *(RMB Animal Health, UK)*.

12394-e

Arsanilic Acid *(BAN, rINN)*.
Aminarsonic Acid; AS-101. 4-Aminophenylarsonic acid.
$C_6H_8AsNO_3$=217.1.

CAS — 98-50-0.

13241-h

Sodium Arsanilate *(BANM, rINNM)*.
Anhydrous Sodium Aminarsonate; Sodium Anilarsinate. Sodium hydrogen 4-aminophenylarsonate.
$C_6H_7AsNNaO_3$=239.0.

CAS — 127-85-5.

Pharmacopoeias. Fr. includes the anhydrous substance and the trihydrate.

Arsanilic acid and sodium arsanilate are used in veterinary medicine in pigs and poultry. They are used for the prophylaxis and treatment of enteric infections due to *Escherichia coli* and also as growth-promoting agents.

Poor activity of arsanilic acid against *Campylobacter* spp. isolated from *pigs*.— C. J. Gebhart *et al.*, *Antimicrob. Ag. Chemother.*, 1985, *27*, 55.

Proprietary Veterinary Names and Manufacturers of Arsanilic Acid and Sodium Arsanilate
Arsenol *(Micro-Biologicals, UK)*; Piglet Gen-Gro *(Ceva, UK)*.

1960-n

Aspoxicillin *(rINN)*.
TA-058. (2*S*,5*R*,6*R*)-6-{(2*R*)-2-[(2*R*)-2-amino-3-(methylcarbamoyl)propionamido]-2-(*p*-hydroxyphenyl)acetamido}-3,3-dimethyl-7-oxo-4-thia-1-azabicyclo[3.2.0]-heptane-2-carboxylic acid.
$C_{21}H_{27}N_5O_7S$=493.5.

CAS — 63358-49-6.

Aspoxicillin is a semisynthetic penicillin antibiotic.

Proprietary Names and Manufacturers
Tanabe, Jpn.

12404-x

Astromicin Sulphate *(pINNM)*.
Abbott-44747; Astromicin Sulfate *(USAN)*; Fortimicin A Sulphate; KW-1070. 4-Amino-1-(2-amino-*N*-methylacetamido)-1,4-dideoxy-3-*O*-(2,6-diamino-2,3,4,6,7-pentadeoxy-β-L-*lyxo*-heptopyranosyl)-6-*O*-methyl-L-*chiro*-inositol sulphate.
$C_{17}H_{35}N_5O_6,2H_2SO_4$=601.7.

CAS — 55779-06-1 (astromicin); 72275-67-3 (sulphate); 66768-12-5 (xH_2SO_4).

An antibiotic produced by *Micromonospora* spp.

Astromicin sulphate is an aminoglycoside antibiotic with actions and uses similar to gentamicin (see p.236). It is administered parenterally.

References to the antimicrobial action of astromicin: C. Thornsberry *et al.*, *Antimicrob. Ag. Chemother.*, 1981, *19*, 122; K. Yamashita *et al.*, *ibid.*, *20*, 33; N. Moreau *et al.*, *ibid.*, 1984, *26*, 857.

Proprietary Names and Manufacturers
Fortimicin *(Kyowa, Jpn)*.

11-k

Avoparcin *(BAN, USAN, rINN)*.
Compound 254. A glycopeptide antibiotic produced by *Streptomyces candidus* or by any other means.

CAS — 37332-99-3.

It is used as a food additive in veterinary practice to promote growth.

Proprietary Veterinary Names and Manufacturers
Avotan *(Cyanamid, UK)*.

12410-a

Azalomycin *(BAN, rINN)*.
A mixture of related macrolide antibiotics produced by *Streptomyces hygroscopicus* var. *azalomyceticus*. Azalomycins B, F, and M have been identified.

CAS — 54182-65-9; 11003-23-9 (azalomycin B); 11003-24-0 (azalomycin F); 28380-24-7 (azalomycin M).

Azalomycin was formerly used in the treatment of vaginitis due to *Trichomonas* spp. or *Candida albicans*.

Proprietary Names and Manufacturers
Sankyo, Jpn.

12-a

Azidamfenicol *(BAN, rINN)*.
Azidamphenicol; Azidoamphenicol; Bayer 52910. 2-Azido-*N*-[(α*R*,β*R*)-β-hydroxy-α-hydroxymethyl-4-nitrophenethyl]acetamide.
$C_{11}H_{13}N_5O_5$=295.3.

CAS — 13838-08-9.

Azidamfenicol is an antibiotic which is related structurally to chloramphenicol (see p.186) and has been used as eye-drops.

Proprietary Names and Manufacturers
Leukomycin-N *(Bayer, Ger.)*; Thilocanfol *(Thilo, Ger.)*.

13-t

Azidocillin *(BAN, rINN)*.
Azidobenzylpenicillin; BRL-2534; SPC-297D. (6*R*)-6-(D-2-Azido-2-phenylacetamido)penicillanic acid.
$C_{16}H_{17}N_5O_4S$=375.4.

CAS — 17243-38-8.

Azidocillin has actions and uses similar to those of benzylpenicillin (see p.131). It is acid-stable and absorbed from the gastro-intestinal tract. It has been given sometimes as the sodium or potassium salt in doses of 750 mg twice daily or 500 mg three times daily.

In a study in 16 children azidocillin 500 mg produced similar free serum-antibiotic concentrations to 250 mg of ampicillin. The half-life of azidocillin was 0.54 hours compared with 1.39 hours for ampicillin while plasma binding was 84 and 18% for azidocillin and ampicillin respectively.— M. F. Michel *et al.*, *Chemotherapy, Basle*, 1973, *18*, 77.

Further references to azidocillin: U. Forsgren, *Antimicrob. Ag. Chemother.*, 1968, 449 (*in vitro* activity against *Haemophilus influenzae*); O. Wasz-Höckert *et al.*, *Scand. J. infect. Dis.*, 1970, *2*, 125 (transplacental diffusion); C. Simon *et al.*, *Arzneimittel-Forsch.*, 1976, *26*, 424 (use in pertussis); B. A. Watts *et al.*, *J. antimicrob. Chemother.*, 1977, *3*, 331 (*in vitro* activity against *Neisseria gonorrhoeae*); O. Wieser and H. Weuta, *Br. J. clin. Pract.*, 1980, *34*, 101 (use in bronchitis).

Proprietary Names and Manufacturers of Azidocillin and its Salts
Astracilina *(Astra, Arg.)*; Globacillin *(Astra, Denm.*; *Astra, Norw.*; *Astra, Swed.)*; Longatren *(Bayer, Ital.)*; Nalpen *(Beecham-Wülfing, Ger.*; *Bencard, Neth.)*; Syncillin *(Tropon, Ger.)*.

14-x

Azlocillin Sodium *(BANM, USAN, rINNM)*.
BAY-e-6905. Sodium (6*R*)-6-[D-2-(2-oxoimidazolidine-1-carboxamido)-2-phenylacetamido]penicillanate.
$C_{20}H_{22}N_5NaO_6S$=483.5.

CAS — 37091-66-0 (azlocillin); 37091-65-9 (sodium salt).

Pharmacopoeias. U.S. includes Sterile Azlocillin Sodium.

1.05 g of monograph substance is approximately equivalent to 1 g of azlocillin. Each g of monograph substance represents about 2.1 mmol of sodium. A 10% solution in water has a pH of 6 to 8.

A 5% solution of azlocillin sodium is reported to be **stable** for up to 24 hours at 25°; a 10% solution is reported to be stable for 6 hours at 25°, and for 24 hours at 5°. However, it is recommended that reconstituted solutions of azlocillin sodium for injection should be administered immediately after preparation.

Incompatibility or loss of activity has been reported with aminoglycosides and tetracyclines.

Adverse Effects
As for Carbenicillin Sodium, p.139. As azlocillin sodium has a lower sodium content than carbenicillin sodium, hypernatraemia and hypokalaemia are less likely to occur.

An evaluation of the adverse effects to azlocillin sodium in 631 patients given multiple doses for the treatment of systemic or urinary-tract infections. There were a total of 183 systemic adverse reactions, 135 of which were classified as probably or possibly related to azlocillin administration; these resulted in withdrawal of the drug in 31 patients. Twenty patients experienced 24 local reactions including thrombophlebitis, pain or stinging on injection, and local skin reactions. Hypersensitivity reactions described in 28 instances were rashes, urticaria, oedema, pruritus, fever, wheezing, dyspnoea, and hypotension. Gastro-intestinal reactions including nausea, vomiting, diarrhoea, abdominal cramps, and taste disturbance were reported in 29 patients, but there was no report of pseudomembranous colitis. Abnormal coagulation was noted in 32 instances, with clinically severe bleeding in 6. Eosinophilia and mild, transient leucopenia are also observed. There were 11 cases of raised serum transaminases (SGOT or SGPT) most of which were mild, and all were reversible on termination of therapy. Hypokalaemia in 3 patients could be corrected by potassium supplements; there was also one case of hypernatraemia. Three of 6 cases of renal dysfunction were considered to be possibly related to administration of azlocillin, but 2 of these patients were also receiving an aminoglycoside or cephalosporin, and one had chronic pyelonephritis. Other adverse reactions reported after administration of azlocillin were one instance of convulsions, and 3 cases of chest discomfort on rapid intravenous infusion.— M. F. Parry, *J. antimicrob. Chemother.*, 1983, *11*, *Suppl.* B, 223.

Reports of transient, asymptomatic, decreases in serum-uric acid concentrations during treatment with azlocillin sodium.— H. M. Faris and D. W. Potts (letter), *Ann. intern. Med.*, 1983, *98*, 414; J. A. Ernst and E. R. Sy, *Antimicrob. Ag. Chemother.*, 1983, *24*, 609.

ALLERGY. For comparison of the incidence of allergic reactions to antipseudomonal penicillins in patients with cystic fibrosis, see Piperacillin Sodium, p.285.

EFFECTS ON THE BLOOD. Prolongation of bleeding time in 3 patients on intravenous azlocillin therapy.— B. A. C. Dijkmans *et al.* (letter), *J. antimicrob. Chemother.*, 1980, *6*, 554.

Precautions

As for Carbenicillin Sodium, p.139.

INTERACTIONS. For the effect of azlocillin on the elimination of cefotaxime in patients with normal and impaired renal function, see under Cefotaxime Sodium, p.152.

See also under Antimicrobial Action, below.

INTERFERENCE WITH DIAGNOSTIC TESTS. In a study *in vitro* of the effects of various antibiotics on tests for glycosuria, azlocillin in the urine could give falsely elevated readings with a test using a copper-reduction method (Clinitest). It had no effect however on glucose oxidase methods (Diastix and Tes-Tape) of estimating glycosuria.— W. A. Parker and M. E. MacCara, *Am. J. Hosp. Pharm.*, 1984, *41*, 125. See also.— M. LeBel *et al.*, *Drug Intell. & clin. Pharm.*, 1984, *18*, 617.

Antimicrobial Action

Azlocillin has a similar antimicrobial action to carbenicillin (p.139), although it is active against a wider range of Gram-negative organisms. Its activity *in vitro* against Enterobacteriaceae is generally less than that of mezlocillin or piperacillin, but it has comparable activity to piperacillin against *Pseudomonas aeruginosa.*

Studies of the antibacterial activity of azlocillin *in vitro*: D. Stewart and G. P. Bodey, *Antimicrob. Ag. Chemother.*, 1977, *11*, 865; K. P. Fu and H. C. Neu, *Antimicrob. Ag. Chemother.*, 1978, *13*, 930; A. R. White *et al.*, *Antimicrob. Ag. Chemother.*, 1980, *18*, 182; M. F. Parry, *J. antimicrob. Chemother.*, 1983, *11*, *Suppl.* B, 15; C. C. Sanders, *ibid.*, 21; H. Grimm, *ibid.*, 43.

ACTIVITY WITH OTHER ANTIMICROBIAL AGENTS. Both azlocillin and mezlocillin have been reported to be synergistic *in vitro* with aminoglycosides against *Pseudomonas aeruginosa*, and various Gram-negative bacteria (C.W. Norden and M.A. Shaffer, *Antimicrob. Ag. Chemother.*, 1982, *21*, 62; N.-X. Chin and H.C. Neu, *J. antimicrob Chemother.*, 1983, *11*, *Suppl.* B, 33; H. Giamarellou *et al.*, *Antimicrob. Ag. Chemother.*, 1984, *25*, 534; J.A. Moody *et al.*, *ibid.*, *26*, 256; M.E. Gombert and T.M. Aulicino, *J. antimicrob. Chemother.*, 1986, *17*, 323; S.H. Guenthner *et al.*, *ibid.*, *18*, 550), and also against *Staphylococcus aureus* (S.H. Zinner *et al.*, *Antimicrob. Ag. Chemother.*, 1981, *20*, 463). No antagonism appears to have been reported, but the incidence of synergy is variable.

The combined activity of azlocillin or mezlocillin with other beta-lactam agents is, however, more unpredictable. Studies have reported synergism with many cephalosporins against a range of bacteria, but there have also been cases of antagonism against some strains (N.A. Kuck *et al.*, *Antimicrob. Ag. Chemother.*, 1981, *19*, 634; H.C. Neu and P. Labthavikul, *J. antimicrob. Chemother.*, 1982, *9*, *Suppl.* A, 101; D.H. Wu *et al.*, *Antimicrob. Ag. Chemother.*, 1984, *26*, 519; J.R. Rodríguez *et al.*, *Curr. Ther. Res.*, 1984, *36*, 902). Antagonism has been reported to occur more often with cefoxitin (H. Grimm, *J. antimicrob. Chemother.*, 1982, *9*, *Suppl.* A, 31), an inducer of beta-lactamases, although Bansal and Thadepalli (*Antimicrob. Ag. Chemother.*, 1983, *23*, 166) reported synergy but no antagonism between cefoxitin and mezlocillin. The activity of mezlocillin has also been shown to be enhanced by a range of isoxazolyl penicillins (C.W. Norden and M. Shaffer, *J. antimicrob. Chemother.*, 1983, *11*, 377).

Clavulanic acid has been shown to increase the activity of azlocillin and mezlocillin *in vitro* against bacterial strains resistant to these drugs due to production of certain beta-lactamases (S.B. Calderwood *et al.*, *Antimicrob. Ag. Chemother.*, 1982, *22*, 266; M.B. Bansal *et al.*, *ibid.*, 1984, *26*, 606; C.N. Simpson *et al.*, *J. antimicrob. Chemother.*, 1984, *14*, 133).

Azlocillin has also been shown to be synergistic with ciprofloxacin *in vitro* against some bacterial strains, although there was also a small incidence of antagonism (J.A. Moody *et al.*, *Antimicrob. Ag. Chemother.*, 1985, *28*, 849; S.H. Zinner and M.N. Dudley, *J. antimicrob. Chemother.*, 1986, *18*, *Suppl.* D, 49).

The antipseudomonal activity of azlocillin was enhanced by the mucolytic agent, mesna, in one *in vitro* study (D.P. Heaf *et al.*, *Archs. Dis. Childh.*, 1983, *58*, 824).

Resistance

As for Carbenicillin Sodium, p.140.

A report of the emergence of isolates of *Pseudomonas aeruginosa* resistant to azlocillin during treatment of 2 patients with the drug; these isolates did not, however, show cross-resistance to carbenicillin. The reduced susceptibility to azlocillin was considered to be due to enhanced synthesis of a specific beta-lactamase.— K. Shannon *et al.* (letter), *Lancet*, 1982, *1*, 1466. See also S. J. Eykyn, *J. antimicrob. Chemother.*, 1982, *9*, 395.

A survey of the incidence of resistant strains of *Pseudomonas aeruginosa* to a range of antipseudomonal beta-lactams in 24 hospitals from February to April 1982. The incidence of strains resistant to azlocillin, taken as those with an MIC greater than 32 µg per mL, was 3.9%; many of these strains showed multiresistance to several of the beta-lactams. Resistance to azlocillin was considered to be due to the production of plasmid- or chromosomally- mediated beta-lactamases.— R. J. Williams *et al.*, *J. antimicrob. Chemother.*, 1984, *14*, 9.

Absorption and Fate

Azlocillin sodium is not absorbed from the gastro-intestinal tract to any significant extent. When administered intravenously, it exhibits non-linear pharmacokinetics, doubling of a dose resulting in more than double the plasma concentration. Between 20 and 46% of azlocillin in the circulation is bound to plasma proteins. Azlocillin is reported to have a dose-dependent plasma half-life which is usually about 1 hour. The half-life is prolonged in neonates and in patients with renal failure.

Azlocillin is widely distributed in body tissues and fluids. It diffuses across the placenta into the foetal circulation and is excreted in small amounts in breast milk. There is little diffusion into the CSF except when the meninges are inflamed.

Azlocillin is reported to be metabolised to a limited extent. About 50 to 70% of a dose is excreted unchanged in the urine by glomerular filtration and tubular secretion within 24 hours of administration, hence achieving high concentrations. Azlocillin is partly excreted in the bile where it is also found in high concentrations.

Serum concentrations are enhanced if probenecid is administered concomitantly.

Azlocillin is removed to some extent by haemodialysis.

A review of the pharmacokinetics of azlocillin sodium.— T. Bergan, *J. antimicrob. Chemother.*, 1983, *11*, *Suppl.* B, 101.

The pharmacokinetics of azlocillin in premature and mature neonates on the second to the twenty-sixth day of life. The elimination half-life was 2.5 and 2.6 hours in the two groups respectively.— G. Heimann, *J. antimicrob. Chemother.*, 1983, *11*, *Suppl.* B, 127.

A study in 2 healthy subjects and 11 patients of the pharmacokinetics of azlocillin after administration of 2 g by intravenous injection immediately followed by an intravenous infusion of 8 g. During the 4-hour infusion, the median serum-azlocillin concentration in the patients rose from 180 to 317 µg per mL at 3 hours, and reached 287 µg per mL at the end of the infusion. At 2, 4, and 6 hours after the infusion had stopped the median serum concentrations were 94, 43, and 11 µg per mL respectively. Thus, moderately high serum concentrations were maintained for a prolonged time, and the local and systemic tolerance was described as good. It was suggested that this high-dose regimen could be repeated after 12 hours.— K. G. Naber and D. Adam, *J. antimicrob. Chemother.*, 1983, *11*, *Suppl.* B, 115.

Several authors studying the pharmacokinetics of azlocillin sodium in patients with cystic fibrosis have suggested that it is more rapidly eliminated in such patients (T. Bergan and H. Michalsen, *Arzneimittel-Forsch.*, 1979, *29*, 1955; N. Martini *et al.*, *J. clin. Hosp. Pharm.*, 1984, *9*, 303; R.A. Woolf *et al.*, *Clin. Pharm.*, 1985, *4*, 664), although Bosso *et al.*, *Antimicrob. Ag. Chemother.*, 1984, *25*, 630) did not agree. None of these studies, however, had a control group, and all reached their conclusions by comparing their results with published studies in healthy subjects.

References to the pharmacokinetics of azlocillin after intravenous administration: L. Coppens and J. Klastersky, *Antimicrob. Ag. Chemother.*, 1979, *15*, 396; F. A. Delgado *et al.*, *J. antimicrob. Chemother.*, 1983, *11*, *Suppl.* B, 79.

For reference to the pharmacokinetics of azlocillin sodium in renal failure, see below under Uses, Administration in Renal Failure.

DIFFUSION INTO BODY TISSUES AND FLUIDS. References to studies of the diffusion of azlocillin into body tissues and fluids: D. A. Kafetzis *et al.*, *J. antimicrob. Chemother.*, 1983, *12*, 157 (diffusion into foetal tissues).

Uses and Administration

Azlocillin sodium is a ureidopenicillin which is used primarily for the treatment of infections known or suspected to be caused by *Pseudomonas aeruginosa.* It is used particularly for septicaemia, and infections of the respiratory and urinary tracts. It is commonly administered in association with an aminoglycoside; however they should not be administered in the same infusion as they have been shown to be incompatible. It has also been given in association with a cephalosporin.

Azlocillin sodium is administered intravenously. A 10% solution in a suitable diluent is given by slow injection over at least 5 minutes for doses of 2 g or less; higher doses should be infused over 20 to 30 minutes.

The usual dosage of azlocillin sodium is the equivalent of 2 to 4 g of azlocillin every 4 to 8 hours. For life-threatening infections, the equivalent of 5 g every 8 hours or 4 g every 4 hours should be given. The usual maximum daily dose is 24 g.

The following doses may be used for children: premature infants, 50 mg per kg body-weight twice daily; neonates less than 7 days old, 100 mg per kg twice daily; infants between 7 days and 1 year, 100 mg per kg three times daily; children up to 14 years, 75 mg per kg three times daily. Doses of up to 450 mg per kg daily have been used in children with cystic fibrosis.

Reviews of the actions and uses of azlocillin sodium: G. M. Eliopoulos and R. C. Moellering, *Ann. intern. Med.*, 1982, *97*, 755; *Med. Lett.*, 1982, *24*, 113.

ADMINISTRATION IN RENAL FAILURE. Most authorities recommend that the dosage of azlocillin sodium need only be adjusted in patients with severe renal impairment, usually considered as a glomerular filtration-rate (GFR) of less than 30 mL per minute. Bennett *et al.* (*Am. J. Kidney Dis.*, 1983, *3*, 155) stated that the half-life in patients with normal renal function ranged from 0.8 to 1.5 hours and was increased to 5 to 6 hours in end-stage renal disease. They have therefore suggested that in patients with a GFR between 10 and 50 mL per minute the dosage interval be increased from 4 to 6 hours to 6 to 8 hours, and in those with a GFR of less than 10 mL per minute, azlocillin sodium be administered every 8 hours. The manufacturers recommend similar dosage adjustments but suggest a dosage interval of 12 hours in those whose renal function is most severely impaired. For patients on haemodialysis, 12-hourly dosage with an additional dose either before or after each dialysis has been suggested.

Further references: A. Whelton *et al.*, *J. antimicrob. Chemother.*, 1983, *11*, *Suppl.* B, 89 (slower removal of azlocillin by peritoneal dialysis than by haemodialysis); *idem*, 97 (nomogram for administration of azlocillin in renal impairment).

For reference to the administration of azlocillin sodium by the intraperitoneal route in patients undergoing continuous ambulatory peritoneal dialysis, see under Peritonitis, below.

BILIARY-TRACT INFECTIONS. For reference to the use of

azlocillin sodium for the treatment of infections of the biliary tract, see Mezlocillin Sodium, p.261.

MENINGITIS. Reports of the use of intravenous azlocillin sodium in the treatment of pseudomonal meningitis: C. J. Ellis and P. H. Walter, *Br. med. J.*, 1979, *2*, 767.

For reference to the use of azlocillin in the treatment of pseudomonal meningitis, see Ticarcillin Sodium, p.325.

NEUTROPENIA. For reference to the use of azlocillin sodium in empiric antibiotic regimens in neutropenic patients with febrile episodes, see Piperacillin Sodium, p.287.

PERITONITIS. The British Society for Antimicrobial Chemotherapy (*Lancet*, 1987, *1*, 845) have recommended the use of the antipseudomonal penicillins, azlocillin or ticarcillin, in association with an aminoglycoside for the treatment of peritonitis due to *Pseudomonas aeruginosa* in patients on continuous ambulatory peritoneal dialysis (CAPD). Ceftazidime may be substituted for the penicillin. If the patient does not respond promptly the catheter should be removed. Azlocillin and ticarcillin may be given as a loading dose of 2 g by intravenous or intraperitoneal administration, followed by an intraperitoneal maintenance dose of 0.25 g per litre of dialysis fluid. The maximum safe blood concentration of either drug was considered to be 300 µg per mL. The aminoglycoside is administered by the same routes. Leigh (*ibid.*, 1142), in commenting on these recommendations considered that piperacillin could also be used in association with an aminoglycoside. In a review of antibiotics used for CAPD-related peritonitis, Scott and Roberts (*Pharm. J.*, 1985, *1*, 621) listed intraperitoneal doses of antipseudomonal penicillins that had been used in some units. For azlocillin, a loading dose of 1 g intravenously followed by an intraperitoneal maintenance dose of 0.25 to 1 g per litre of dialysis fluid; for ticarcillin an intraperitoneal loading dose of 1 g per litre followed by a maintenance dose of 0.1 g per litre; for piperacillin a maintenance dose of 0.5 g per litre, and for mezlocillin a maintenance dose of 1 g per litre.

PREGNANCY AND THE NEONATE. For reference to the use of azlocillin sodium in pregnancy, see Piperacillin Sodium, p.287.

RESPIRATORY-TRACT INFECTIONS. *Cystic fibrosis.* For reference to the use of azlocillin sodium in the treatment of pseudomonal chest infections in patients with cystic fibrosis, see Carbenicillin Sodium, p.141.

SURGICAL INFECTION PROPHYLAXIS. *Biliary-tract surgery.* For reference to the use of azlocillin sodium for the prophylaxis of infection during surgical procedures of the biliary tract, see Mezlocillin Sodium, p.261.

URINARY-TRACT INFECTIONS. Studies indicating azlocillin sodium to be as effective as ticarcillin sodium in the treatment of urinary-tract infections including those caused by *Pseudomonas aeruginosa*.— C. E. Cox, *J. antimicrob. Chemother.*, 1983, *11*, *Suppl.* B, 183; W. P. Reed and D. L. Palmer, *ibid.*, 189.

Preparations

Sterile Azlocillin Sodium *(U.S.P.)*

Proprietary Preparations

Securopen *(Bayer, UK). Injection*, powder for reconstitution, azlocillin 0.5, 1, and 2 g (as sodium salt). *Intravenous infusion*, powder for reconstitution, azlocillin 5 g (as sodium salt).

Proprietary Names and Manufacturers

Azlin *(Miles Pharmaceuticals, USA)*; Securopen *(Bayer, Austral.; Bayer, Fr.; Bayer, Ger.; Bayer, Ital.; Neth.; Bayer, Norw.; Bayer, Spain; Bayer, Switz.; Bayer, UK)*.

13266-e

Aztreonam *(BAN, USAN, rINN).*

Azthreonam; SQ-26776. (*Z*)-2-{2-Aminothiazol-4-yl-[(2*S*,3*S*)-2-methyl-4-oxo-1-sulphoazetidin-3-ylcarbamoyl]methyleneamino-oxy}-2-methylpropionic acid.

$C_{13}H_{17}N_5O_8S_2$=435.4.

CAS — 78110-38-0.

Pharmacopoeias. U.S. includes Sterile Aztreonam.

Solutions for injection are prepared with the aid of arginine to enhance stability. They may develop a slight pink tint on standing, but this does not affect potency.

Aztreonam has been reported to be **incompatible** with metronidazole (R.G. Bell *et al.*, *Am. J. Hosp. Pharm.*, 1986, *43*, 1444) and nafcillin (C.M. Riley and L.C. Lipford, *ibid.*, 2221). Several studies have reported compatibility with various other antibiotics.

Lack of effect of aztreonam on the activity of gentamicin after incubation *in vitro*.— T. S. J. Elliott *et al.* (letter), *J. antimicrob. Chemother.*, 1984, *14*, 668. Similar results with aztreonam and tobramycin.— *idem* (letter), 1986, *17*, 680.

Studies indicating stability of intravenous admixtures of aztreonam with other antimicrobial agents under specified storage conditions: M. J. James and C. M. Riley, *Am. J. Hosp. Pharm.*, 1985, *42*, 1095 (with ampicillin); *idem*, 1984 (with clindamycin phosphate); *ibid.*, 1986, *43*, 925 (with cephazolin).

Adverse Effects

The adverse effects of aztreonam are similar to those of other beta-lactam antibiotics. Allergic reactions, including skin rashes, urticaria, eosinophilia, and rarely anaphylaxis, may occur in patients receiving aztreonam. Gastro-intestinal effects include diarrhoea, nausea, vomiting, and an abnormal taste.

Phlebitis or thrombophlebitis have been reported after the intravenous administration of aztreonam, and pain or swelling after intramuscular injection.

Administration of aztreonam may result in the overgrowth of non-susceptible organisms, and there is the possibility that pseudomembranous colitis may develop.

Other adverse effects that have been reported with aztreonam include increases in liver enzymes, and abnormalities in haematological parameters.

An evaluation of the efficacy and safety of aztreonam in 1771 patients treated with multiple doses of the drug. Pain and phlebitis at the intravenous site occurred in 2.4% of patients, and rash in 1.5%. Of a total of 2117 patients treated with single or multiple doses of the drug 134 had a history of allergy to penicillins or cephalosporins, and only one had a possible IgE-mediated urticaria. Nausea occurred in 0.8% of the 1771 patients, diarrhoea in 0.7% (one patient having *Clostridium difficile*-associated diarrhoea), and other adverse gastro-intestinal effects in 0.3%. The incidence of marked deviations in haematological parameters was 7%, and was similar to the comparative drugs cephamandole and aminoglycosides. The incidence of marked elevations of liver function test results was also similar to that for the control drugs. Elevations in the range of 2 to 3 times the upper limit of normal or baseline occurred in up to 4 to 6% and returned towards baseline values during or after treatment. Marked elevations of serum creatinine occurred in 5% of patients in association with aztreonam, compared with 13% of patients receiving aminoglycosides and 7% given cephamandole. Superinfections, most commonly with enterococci, were reported in 9.7% of patients treated with aztreonam.— S. A. Henry and C. B. Bendush, *Am. J. Med.*, 1985, *78*, *Suppl.* 2A, 57.

ALLERGY. Studies in *rabbits* and in healthy subjects suggesting that aztreonam displays very low immunological cross-reactivity with other beta-lactam antibiotics and may be only weakly immunogenic.— N. F. Adkinson *et al.*, *Antimicrob. Ag. Chemother.*, 1984, *25*, 93. Studies in healthy subjects also suggested little or no cross-reactivity between IgE antibodies to penicillin and aztreonam.— A. Saxon *et al.*, *J. infect. Dis.*, 1984, *149*, 16.

See also Respiratory-tract Infections, Cystic Fibrosis, under Uses, below.

EFFECTS ON THE BLOOD. Aztreonam appeared to be free of significant interference with coagulation and platelet function in 10 healthy subjects given 2 g every 6 hours intravenously for 21 doses. No patient had abnormal bleeding or an increased tendency to bruise. The detection of an increase in bleeding time depended on the method of statistical analysis employed. There were no defects in platelet function or significant abnormalities in tests of coagulation. Studies *in vitro* could demonstrate only minimal changes in platelet aggregation and only at very high concentrations.— T. A. Tartaglione *et al.*, *Antimicrob. Ag. Chemother.*, 1986, *30*, 73.

EFFECTS ON THE GASTRO-INTESTINAL TRACT. The effect of aztreonam on gastro-intestinal microbial flora was studied in 18 patients with haematological malignancies given intravenous aztreonam in a dose of either 1 or 2 g every 8 hours for 7 to 9 days. Aztreonam had little effect on the predominant throat flora. In contrast, there was a marked decrease in facultative anaerobic Gram-negative bacilli in the stools. Strict anaerobes in the stools were variably affected.— P. G. Jones *et al.*, *Antimicrob. Ag. Chemother.*, 1984, *26*, 941. Of 45 patients treated intravenously with aztreonam, enterococcal superinfection requiring further antimicrobial therapy occurred in 5 patients, and colonisation with enterococci in 3. All patients had enterococci isolated from the urinary tract; 7 had an indwelling catheter, and one a nephrostomy tube. One patient had developed enterococcal bacteraemia following colonisation of the urinary tract.— P. H. Chandrasekar *et al.*, *Antimicrob. Ag. Chemother.*, 1984, *26*, 280.

Precautions

It is recommended that aztreonam be administered with caution to patients known to be hypersensitive to other beta-lactam antibiotics although the incidence of cross-sensitivity appears to be low.

Modification of dosage may be required in patients with renal impairment.

Because of the possibility of increased prothrombin time during therapy with aztreonam, caution has been recommended in patients also receiving anticoagulant therapy.

For studies investigating cross-sensitivity between aztreonam and other beta-lactam antibiotics, see above under Adverse Effects.

ADMINISTRATION IN RENAL FAILURE. For reference to the precautions to be observed in renal failure, see under Administration in Renal Failure in Uses, below.

INTERACTIONS. The pharmacokinetic interaction of aztreonam with other antibiotics was investigated in 5 separate single-dose studies in 48 healthy subjects. Aztreonam 1 g was administered by intravenous infusion simultaneously with cephradine 1 g, clindamycin 600 mg, gentamicin 80 mg, metronidazole 500 mg, or nafcillin 500 mg through separate lines. There was no major pharmacokinetic interaction between aztreonam and these agents.— W. A. Creasey *et al.*, *J. clin. Pharmac.*, 1984, *24*, 174.

For the effect of other antimicrobial agents on the antibacterial activity of aztreonam, see Activity with other Antimicrobial Agents under Antimicrobial Action, below.

INTERFERENCE WITH DIAGNOSTIC TESTS. Aztreonam did not interfere with the determination of creatinine in serum as measured by the Jaffé reaction.— M. LeBel *et al.*, *Drug Intell. & clin. Pharm.*, 1983, *17*, 908.

At some concentrations, aztreonam interfered with the measurement of urinary glucose by a copper reduction reaction (Clinitest).— M. LeBel *et al.*, *Drug Intell. & clin. Pharm.*, 1984, *18*, 617.

Antimicrobial Action

Aztreonam is bactericidal and acts similarly to the penicillins by inhibiting synthesis of the bacterial cell wall. The activity of aztreonam is restricted to Gram-negative aerobic organisms, including beta-lactamase-producing strains, with poor or no activity against Gram-positive aerobes or anaerobic organisms. It is active against most Enterobacteriaceae including *Citrobacter* and *Enterobacter* spp., *Escherichia coli, Klebsiella, Proteus, Providencia, Salmonella, Serratia, Shigella,* and *Yersinia* spp. Most of these organisms are inhibited *in vitro* by a concentration of aztreonam of 4 µg or less per mL. Aztreonam is active against *Pseudomonas aeruginosa* with MICs ranging upwards from less than 1 µg per mL. It is inactive against most other *Pseudomonas* spp. Aztreonam has good activity against *Haemophilus influenzae* and *Neisseria gonorrhoeae*; most strains are inhibited by concentrations of less than 1 µg per mL.

A review of aztreonam including its antimicrobial activity. Bacteria inhibited by 8 µg per mL of aztreonam or less may be regarded as sensitive; those inhibited by 16 µg per mL as having intermediate susceptibility, and those with an MIC of 32 µg per mL or more as resistant. In comparisons with other antibiotics, the activity of aztreonam against the Enterobacteriaceae was generally similar to that of cefotaxime and ceftazidime, and greater than that of cefoperazone, cefoxitin, gentamicin, tobramycin, or piperacillin. Reported MICs of aztreonam against *Enterobacter* spp. are widely variable. Among other Gram-negative bacilli, *Acinetobacter* spp. have generally been reported to be resistant to aztreonam as have *Alcaligenes dentrificans* and *faecalis*, *Ach-*

romobacter and *Flavobacterium* spp.
Although aztreonam is generally inactive against anaerobic bacteria, limited activity has been reported against *Clostridium, Eubacterium, Peptostreptococcus*, and *Peptococcus* spp., and greater activity against *Fusobacterium* spp.
The stability of aztreonam to hydrolysis by beta-lactamases is similar to that of third-generation cephalosporins. However enzymes have been isolated from certain strains of *Klebsiella pneumoniae* and *Pseudomonas aeruginosa* which do hydrolyse aztreonam. Aztreonam has been noted to inhibit chromosomal beta-lactamases, but not to induce the production of these enzymes.— R. N. Brogden and R. C. Heel, *Drugs*, 1986, *31*, 96.

A study *in vitro* indicating specific binding of aztreonam and related monobactams to penicillin-binding protein (PBP) 3 in *Escherichia coli* and other susceptible organisms. Aztreonam had a moderate affinity for PBP1a and poor affinities for PBP1b, PBP2, PBP4, and PBP5/6. Aztreonam did not bind to any essential PBP of a representative strain of *Staphylococcus aureus* or of *Bacteroides fragilis*.— N. H. Georgopapadakou *et al., Antimicrob. Ag. Chemother.*, 1982, *21*, 950.

A review of structure-activity relationships among the monobactams. The monobactam nucleus exhibits weak antibacterial activity and thus molecular substitution around the central nucleus is required. Side-chain structure-activity relationships in monobactams parallel those of the penicillins and cephalosporins.— D. P. Bonner and R. B. Sykes, *J. antimicrob. Chemother.*, 1984, *14*, 313.

ACTIVITY AGAINST ENTEROBACTERIACEAE. The MIC of aztreonam for 14 isolates of *Citrobacter diversus* ranged from less than 0.06 to 16 µg per mL; taking a breakpoint of 8 µg per mL, 79% were susceptible. For 27 isolates of *C. freundii*, however, the MIC ranged from less than 0.06 to 64 µg per mL, only 52% being susceptible.— G. Samonis *et al., Antimicrob. Ag. Chemother.*, 1987, *31*, 829.

Aztreonam, ceftazidime, and cefotaxime were the most active of a range of antibiotics tested *in vitro* against clinical isolates of *Salmonella* spp. from 4 different countries, including some chloramphenicol-resistant strains. Aztreonam and cefotaxime were found to be slightly superior to ceftazidime against multi-resistant organisms. The MIC of aztreonam against these organisms was up to 0.39 µg per mL.— H. Goossens *et al., J. antimicrob. Chemother.*, 1984, *13*, 559. See also under Enteric Infections in Uses, below.

The MIC of aztreonam against 75 faecal isolates of *Yersinia* spp. ranged from 0.5 to 8 µg per mL. Taking a breakpoint of 2 µg per mL, 41% of strains were considered susceptible. Activity was similar to that of cefuroxime, but less than that of ciprofloxacin, the aminoglycosides tested, cefotaxime, ceftazidime, or piperacillin.— A. M. Lewis and B. Chattopadhyay (letter), *J. antimicrob. Chemother.*, 1987, *19*, 406.

ACTIVITY AGAINST GONOCOCCI. The MIC of aztreonam against 100 beta-lactamase-negative strains of *Neisseria gonorrhoeae* ranged from 0.004 µg or less per mL to 0.5 µg per mL; the range for 42 beta-lactamase-positive strains was 0.032 to 0.063 µg per mL. These values compared favourably with the second- and third-generation cephalosporins tested.— M. Y. Khan *et al., Antimicrob. Ag. Chemother.*, 1983, *23*, 477. See also D. A. Strandberg *et al., Curr. ther. Res.*, 1983, *34*, 955.

ACTIVITY AGAINST HAEMOPHILUS. A study of the antimicrobial susceptibility of 83 strains of *Haemophilus influenzae*, resistant to ampicillin and chloramphenicol, isolated from paediatric patients and paediatric carriers. The MIC of aztreonam was in the range 0.12 to 0.5 µg per mL, and along with the newer cephalosporins it was one of the most active agents tested.— J. Campos and S. Garcia-Tornel, *J. antimicrob. Chemother.*, 1987, *19*, 297.

ACTIVITY AGAINST PSEUDOMONAS. The activity of aztreonam against *Pseudomonas aeruginosa* generally appears to be slightly less than that of ceftazidime and imipenem. It is active against some gentamicin- and carbenicillin-resistant strains (W.W.S. Ng *et al., Antimicrob. Ag. Chemother.*, 1985, *27*, 872), although a degree of cross-resistance with tobramycin has been observed (S.C. Aronoff and J.D. Klinger, *J. antimicrob. Chemother.*, 1985, *15*, 545). Isolates of *Ps. aeruginosa* from cystic fibrosis patients and those without cystic fibrosis were similarly susceptible to aztreonam (B. Gordts *et al., ibid.*, 1984, *14*, 25) although some isolates were resistant to aztreonam. In a study of isolates from neutropenic cancer patients (K.V.I. Rolston *et al., ibid.*, 1987, *19*, 193), aztreonam was less active than agents, particularly the 4-quinolones, which were not in clinical use in the institution, and MICs from 0.25 to 64 µg per mL were reported. Zar and Kany (*Antimicrob. Ag. Chemother.*, 1985, *27*, 1) tested 37 strains of *Ps. aeruginosa* isolated from patients with endocarditis against a range of antibiotics. Two of the isolates were resistant to aztreonam, assuming a breakpoint of 16 µg per mL; bactericidal activity was observed in about half of the strains at this concentration. There were no tolerant strains.

ACTIVITY WITH OTHER ANTIMICROBIAL AGENTS. Synergy between aztreonam and aminoglycosides has been observed *in vitro* with varying frequency. A greater proportion of strains of amikacin-resistant *Pseudomonas aeruginosa* and *Ps. cepacia* isolated from children with cystic fibrosis were susceptible to aztreonam when combined with amikacin (S.C. Aronoff and J.D. Klinger, *Antimicrob. Ag. Chemother.*, 1984, *25*, 279). Amikacin increased the killing rate of aztreonam against some Gram-negative bacteria although it had little effect on the serum bactericidal activity (Y. Van Laethem *et al., ibid.*, *26*, 224). Buesing and Jorgensen (*ibid.*, *25*, 283) noted synergy with amikacin against 71% of multiply-resistant isolates of Enterobacteriaceae and *Ps. aeruginosa*, and Stutman *et al.* (*ibid.*, 212) reported synergy with tobramycin against 62% of *Ps. aeruginosa* isolates. Stutman *et al.* tested aztreonam in combination with a range of antibiotics against paediatric clinical isolates of Enterobacteriaceae, *Ps. aeruginosa*, and Gram-positive cocci. Combinations with ampicillin, clindamycin, piperacillin, ticarcillin, or nafcillin were generally either indifferent or additive, although occasional synergy with clindamycin was observed against enteric organisms. Wu *et al.* (*ibid.*, *26*, 519) found similar results with combinations of aztreonam and azlocillin or piperacillin against *Ps. aeruginosa*.
The activity of aztreonam may be reduced by inducers of beta-lactamases such as imipenem (N.M. Ampel *et al., J. antimicrob. Chemother.*, 1984, *13*, 398) and cefoxitin (J.-E. Brorson and P. Larsson, *et al., ibid.*, *14*, 667). Chloramphenicol has also been reported to antagonise the action of aztreonam against some strains of *Klebsiella pneumoniae* (T.H. Brown and R.H. Alford, *Antimicrob. Ag. Chemother.*, 1984, *25*, 405).

Resistance

Aztreonam is stable to hydrolysis by beta-lactamases produced by a wide range of organisms.

Isolation of a multiply-resistant strain of *Enterobacter cloacae* after treatment of a patient with aztreonam and nafcillin. It was considered that aztreonam was responsible for the development of resistance.— D. L. Dworzack *et al.* (letter), *Clin. Pharm.*, 1984, *3*, 467. Criticism.— B. L. Ashby (letter), *ibid.*, 1985, *4*, 23. Reply.— D. L. Dworzack *et al., ibid.*

A study *in vitro* of a clinical isolate of *Enterobacter cloacae* resistant to aztreonam, indicating that resistance was mainly due to lack of penetration across the outer membrane.— K. Bush *et al., Antimicrob. Ag. Chemother.*, 1985, *27*, 555.

For reference to the stability of aztreonam to beta-lactamases, see above under Antimicrobial Action.

Absorption and Fate

Aztreonam is poorly absorbed from the gastro-intestinal tract. Absorption after intramuscular injection is good, peak plasma concentrations being achieved within one hour. Aztreonam has a plasma elimination half-life of approximately 2 hours, and about 56% in the circulation is bound to plasma proteins. It is widely distributed in body tissues and fluids. It crosses the placenta and enters the foetal circulation; small amounts are excreted in breast milk.
Aztreonam undergoes partial metabolism to several inactive metabolites; the principal metabolite is SQ-26992 and is formed by opening of the beta-lactam ring. Aztreonam is excreted predominantly in the urine; about 60 to 70% of a dose appears as unchanged drug with only small quantities of metabolites. Both unchanged drug and metabolites are excreted in the faeces in only small amounts.

A study of the pharmacokinetics of aztreonam after single intramuscular or intravenous doses administered to healthy subjects. After intramuscular administration of 0.5 or 1 g, mean peak serum concentrations of 22.0 and 46.5 µg per mL respectively were achieved after about 1 hour. Maximum urinary concentrations of 0.5 and 1.2 mg per mL respectively were measured over the first 2 hours after the dose. Mean peak serum concentrations after a 3-minute intravenous infusion of aztreonam 0.5 or 1 g were 58.2 and 125 µg per mL respectively. Urinary concentrations in the first 2 hours after the dose were 1.4 and 3.0 mg per mL. A total of 68% of an intravenous dose was excreted in the urine within 24 hours.— E. A. Swabb *et al., Antimicrob. Ag. Chemother.*, 1982, *21*, 944.

Peak serum concentrations of approximately 0.15 µg per mL were obtained about 2 hours after administration of a 500-mg dose of aztreonam by mouth as a solution and as capsules to 15 healthy subjects. After a 3-minute intravenous infusion of the same dose the peak concentration was 57 µg per mL. The oral preparations had a bioavailability of less than 1%.— E. A. Swabb *et al., Antimicrob. Ag. Chemother.*, 1983, *23*, 548.

Further references to the pharmacokinetics of aztreonam: E. A. Swabb *et al., Antimicrob. Ag. Chemother.*, 1983, *23*, 125 (pharmacokinetics after multiple intravenous or intramuscular doses); B. E. Scully *et al., ibid.*, *24*, 18 (pharmacokinetics after 30-minute intravenous infusions); P. G. Jones *et al., ibid.*, 1984, *26*, 455 (pharmacokinetics in patients with haematological malignancies); D. M. Janicke *et al., ibid.*, 1985, *27*, 16 (pharmacokinetics in patients with Gram-negative infections; protein binding of 30% reported); W. A. Creasey *et al., Br. J. clin. Pharmac.*, 1985, *19*, 233 (absence of an effect of age, apart from decreasing renal function, on pharmacokinetics).

See also under Drug Metabolism, below.

ADMINISTRATION IN INFANTS AND CHILDREN. Pharmacokinetic results from children with cystic fibrosis suggesting that administration of aztreonam every 4 to 6 hours may be required in these patients.— M. D. Reed *et al., Clin. Pharmac. Ther.*, 1985, *37*, 223.

See also under Uses, below.

ADMINISTRATION IN LIVER DISORDERS. The mean half-life of aztreonam was increased from 1.9 hours in 6 healthy subjects to 2.2 and 3.2 hours in groups of 6 patients with primary biliary cirrhosis and alcoholic cirrhosis respectively. Dosage adjustment may be required in patients with alcoholic cirrhosis.— C. M. MacLeod *et al., Antimicrob. Ag. Chemother.*, 1984, *26*, 493.

ADMINISTRATION IN RENAL FAILURE. For reference to the pharmacokinetics of aztreonam in renal failure, see under Administration in Renal Failure in Uses, below.

DIFFUSION INTO BODY TISSUES AND FLUIDS. Eleven adult patients with meningeal inflammation were given a single intravenous infusion of aztreonam 2 g over 5 minutes. Aztreonam penetrated the CSF but in a variable manner which appeared to be related to the degree of meningeal inflammation. Concentrations of aztreonam in the CSF obtained 2 to 4 hours after injection in 4 patients with viral meningitis ranged from 0.76 to 1.77 µg per mL and represented a percentage penetration of 2.5 to 14% relative to serum concentrations. In 3 patients with bacterial meningitis, however, CSF concentrations 2 to 8 hours after injection were 2.54 to 7.83 µg per mL representing a penetration of 5 to 24%.— R. L. Greenman *et al., J. antimicrob. Chemother.*, 1985, *15*, 637. In a similar study, the penetration of aztreonam into the CSF was considered adequate to inhibit most Enterobacteriaceae in patients with both uninflamed and inflamed meninges. Aztreonam was detected in the CSF 1 hour after the infusion, and peak concentrations were obtained after 4 to 5 hours. Concentrations of aztreonam in the CSF were about 4 times greater in patients with inflamed as compared with uninflamed meninges.— R. J. Duma *et al., Antimicrob. Ag. Chemother.*, 1984, *26*, 730. See also J. Modai *et al., ibid.*, 1986, *29*, 281.

Further studies of the diffusion of aztreonam into body tissues and fluids: R. Wise *et al., Antimicrob. Ag. Chemother.*, 1982, *22*, 969 (cantharides-induced blister fluid); P. O. Madsen *et al., ibid.*, 1984, *26*, 20 (prostatic tissue); D. L. Bechard *et al., ibid.*, 1985, *27*, 263 (bronchial secretions); B. I. Davies *et al., J. antimicrob. Chemother.*, 1985, *15*, 375 (sputum); C. M. MacLeod *et al., Antimicrob. Ag. Chemother.*, 1986, *29*, 710 (synovial fluid and bone); T. R. Beam *et al., ibid.*, *30*, 505 (tissues obtained during thoracic and gynaecological surgery); G. Haroche *et al., J. antimicrob. Chemother.*, 1986, *18*, 195 (aqueous humour); I. McKay *et al.* (letter), *ibid.*, 1987, *20*, 617 (prostatic tissue).

DRUG EXCRETION. Aztreonam was excreted in the urine of healthy subjects by glomerular filtration and tubular secretion. Concomitant administration of probenecid increased plasma-aztreonam concentrations and increased its half-life.— E. A. Swabb *et al., Clin. Pharmac. Ther.*, 1983, *33*, 609.

After intravenous injection of aztreonam 1 g to 10 patients following cholecystectomy, maximum biliary concentrations ranged from 9.7 to 88.2 µg per mL and were obtained 2.4 hours after the dose. Peak concentrations in 4 patients with total biliary-tract obstruction were approximately one-third of these values, and cumulative 12-hour biliary excretion accounted for 0.18% of the dose.— O. V. Martinez *et al.*, *Antimicrob. Ag. Chemother.*, 1984, *25*, 358. See also R. E. Condon *et al.*, *ibid.*, 1986, *29*, 1101 (concentrations in abdominal tissues and bile).

DRUG METABOLISM. The pharmacokinetics of radioactively-labelled aztreonam in 6 healthy subjects. Aztreonam did not undergo extensive metabolism; the predominant metabolite was SQ-26992, resulting from the hydrolytic opening of the beta-lactam ring. Whereas aztreonam had a half-life of 1.8 hours, the half-life of SQ-26992 was 25.8 hours. The excretion of aztreonam and SQ-26992 in urine represented a mean of about 66 and 7% of the dose, respectively, and in faeces about 1 and 3%. The excretion of aztreonam in urine was nearly complete by about 6 hours; SQ-26992 however was excreted for at least 48 hours.— E. A. Swabb *et al.*, *Antimicrob. Ag. Chemother.*, 1983, *24*, 394.

PREGNANCY AND THE NEONATE. Measurement of aztreonam concentrations in placenta, amniotic fluid, and foetal circulation.— R. Hayashi *et al.*, *Clin. Pharmac. Ther.*, 1984, *35*, 246.

Peak aztreonam concentrations in breast milk were less than 1% of those in serum after both intramuscular and intravenous administration.— P. M. Fleiss *et al.*, *Br. J. clin. Pharmac.*, 1985, *19*, 509.

For the pharmacokinetics of aztreonam in neonates, see under Administration in Infants and Children in Uses, below.

Uses and Administration

Aztreonam is a monobactam or monocyclic beta-lactam antibiotic used for the treatment of infections caused by susceptible Gram-negative aerobic organisms. To broaden its spectrum of activity for the empirical treatment of infections, it may be used in conjunction with other antibiotics. Concurrent use of an aminoglycoside may be of benefit in serious *Pseudomonas aeruginosa* infections.

Aztreonam is administered by deep intramuscular injection, or intravenously by slow injection over 3 to 5 minutes or infusion over 20 to 60 minutes. It is given in doses ranging from 1 to 8 g daily administered in divided doses every 6 to 12 hours according to the severity of the infection. Single doses over 1 g should be administered by the intravenous route. A single intramuscular dose of 1 g has been recommended for the treatment of gonorrhoea or cystitis.

SQ-82531, a prodrug of aztreonam to be administered by mouth is under investigation.

Reviews of the actions and uses of aztreonam: D. R. P. Guay and C. Koskoletos, *Clin. Pharm.*, 1985, *4*, 516; R. N. Brogden and R. C. Heel, *Drugs*, 1986, *31*, 96; *Drug & Ther. Bull.*, 1987, *25*, 86; *Med. Lett.*, 1987, *29*, 45; R. J. Duma, *Ann. intern. Med.*, 1987, *106*, 766.

For proceedings of a symposium on aztreonam, see *J. antimicrob. Chemother.*, 1981, *8*, *Suppl.* E, 1 to 148.

Good clinical and bacteriological results were obtained with intramuscular or intravenous aztreonam in 'difficult-to-treat' Gram-negative infections in 55 patients. Infections included those of the urinary and respiratory tracts, soft tissues and bones, and intra-abdominal infections. Of 18 patients whose infections had been treated unsuccessfully with amikacin, and who had pathogens multiresistant to aminoglycosides, cefotaxime, and antipseudomonal penicillins, 15 were cured with aztreonam. Treatment of *Pseudomonas aeruginosa* infections was also satisfactory.— H. Giamarellou *et al.*, *Antimicrob. Ag. Chemother.*, 1984, *26*, 245.

Further studies of the use of aztreonam in the treatment of serious Gram-negative infections: A. Torres and C. H. Ramírez-Ronda, *Curr. ther. Res.*, 1984, *36*, 875; P. H. Joubert and C. Teichler, *ibid.*, 1987, *41*, 1; Y. Van Laethem *et al.*, *ibid.*, 244.

ADMINISTRATION IN INFANTS AND CHILDREN. Twenty-nine infants and children received a single intravenous dose of aztreonam 30 mg per kg body-weight over 3 minutes. The half-life was inversely proportional to age: it was 5.71 hours in neonates under 7 days of age and weighing less than 2.5 kg, 2.56 hours in those under 7 days but over 2.5 kg, and 2.43 hours in those between 1 week and 1 month of age. In infants up to 2 years old the half-life of aztreonam was 1.70 hours and 1.67 hours in children between 2 and 12 years. These data suggest a dosage interval of 8 to 12 hours in neonates and 6 to 8 hours in infants and children over one month of age.— H. R. Stutman *et al.*, *Antimicrob. Ag. Chemother.*, 1984, *26*, 196. Six premature neonates of more than 7 days of age were treated for suspected or proven Gram-negative infections with intravenous aztreonam in association with either erythromycin or vancomycin. Pharmacokinetic studies confirmed the suitability of a dosage regimen of 30 mg per kg body-weight every 12 hours in such patients. Five of the patients showed a prompt improvement in their clinical condition.— M. R. Miller *et al.*, *Pharm. J.*, 1987, *2*, R20.

References to the treatment of paediatric infections with aztreonam: M. W. Kline *et al.*, *Curr. ther. Res.*, 1986, *39*, 625.

ADMINISTRATION IN RENAL FAILURE. The manufacturers of aztreonam have recommended that patients with renal impairment be given a usual initial dose followed by a maintenance dose adjusted according to the creatinine clearance (CC) of the patient: those with a CC of 10 to 30 mL per minute half the initial dose, those with a CC of less than 10 mL per minute one-quarter of the initial dose. A supplementary dose of one-eighth of the initial dose should be given to patients on haemodialysis after each dialysis session.

A study of the pharmacokinetics of aztreonam in 5 healthy subjects and in 20 patients with varying degrees of renal impairment. The mean half-life of aztreonam increased from 1.8 hours in healthy subjects to 8.4 hours in functionally anephric patients. Serum clearance decreased in parallel to the reduction in the creatinine clearance, whereas non-renal clearance was relatively constant. The mean cumulative urinary excretion of aztreonam in 48 hours decreased from 59.8 to 13.0%, whereas that of its metabolite SQ-26992 remained fairly constant between 3.4 and 6.3%. SQ-26992 was undetectable in the serum of healthy subjects but was measurable in patients with renal insufficiency.

The mean half-life of aztreonam in patients on haemodialysis was 8.4 hours between dialysis and 2.5 hours during dialysis.

From these results, guidelines were suggested for modifying the dosage regimen of aztreonam in patients with renal failure. The dosage interval could be increased or the dose decreased by a factor of 2, 3, or 4 for patients with creatinine clearance in the ranges 30 to 80 mL per minute, 10 to 29 mL per minute, or less than 10 mL per minute respectively. If the dose reduction method is used, patients should be given a usual initial loading dose. Patients on haemodialysis should be given a supplemental dose of half their maintenance dose after each dialysis session.— J. P. Fillastre *et al.*, *Clin. Pharmacokinet.*, 1985, *10*, 91. See also J. C. L. Mihindu *et al.*, *Antimicrob. Ag. Chemother.*, 1983, *24*, 252; H. Mattie and A. Matze-van der Lans, *J. antimicrob. Chemother.*, 1986, *17*, 215.

The pharmacokinetics of aztreonam after administration to patients with end-stage renal disease undergoing haemodialysis or continuous ambulatory peritoneal dialysis (CAPD). A mean of 38.2% of a dose was removed by haemodialysis. After CAPD only 10% of an intravenous dose was recovered in the peritoneal dialysate whereas 60 to 70% was available in the systemic circulation after peritoneal administration.— J. S. Gerig *et al.*, *Kidney Int.*, 1984, *26*, 308.

ENTERIC INFECTIONS. Successful treatment of *Salmonella hadar* carrier-state in an 82-year-old patient with cholelithiasis, following administration of aztreonam 2 g intravenously every 6 hours for 16 days. The MIC and MBC of aztreonam against the isolate was 0.13 µg per mL.— J. Righter and E. F. Vaughan-Neil (letter), *J. antimicrob. Chemother.*, 1984, *13*, 403.

GONORRHOEA. Cure in patients with gonorrhoea treated with a single intramuscular dose of either aztreonam 1 g or spectinomycin 2 g. The infections were mainly in urethral sites, but rectal and endocervical sites were also included. Only one isolate of *Neisseria gonorrhoeae* produced beta-lactamase.— A. Gottlieb and J. Mills, *Antimicrob. Ag. Chemother.*, 1985, *27*, 270. See also R. C. Spencer and M. D. Talbot, *Curr. med. Res. Opinion*, 1985, *9*, 591 (including successful treatment of pharyngeal sites).

NEUTROPENIA. Aztreonam in association with vancomycin was effective therapy for the treatment of febrile episodes in neutropenic cancer patients, with or without addition of amikacin.— P. G. Jones *et al.*, *Am. J. Med.*, 1986, *81*, 243.

PERITONITIS. Use of intraperitoneal aztreonam in association with intraperitoneal cloxacillin or vancomycin, for the treatment of peritonitis in patients on continuous ambulatory peritoneal dialysis (CAPD). Aztreonam was administered in a dose of 500 mg per litre in the first exchange after recognition of a cloudy effluent, and 250 mg per litre in the following bags. Treatment with aztreonam alone was continued in 31 episodes of Gram-negative infection among 26 patients; this included infections with *Escherichia coli*, *Pseudomonas*, *Acinetobacter*, and *Klebsiella* spp. The microbiological response was cure in 24 episodes, cure with relapse in 2, cure with superinfection in 2, and failure in 3 (with resistance to aztreonam in 2). Clinically, 26 cures, 1 part response, and 4 failures were observed. These results compared favourably with historical controls treated with aminoglycosides and/or co-trimoxazole.— M. Dratwa *et al.* (letter), *Lancet*, 1987, *2*, 213.

PREGNANCY AND THE NEONATE. For reference to the use of aztreonam in neonates, see under Administration in Infants and Children, above.

RESPIRATORY-TRACT INFECTIONS. *Bronchitis.* A study in 36 patients with acute purulent exacerbations of chronic bronchitis concluded that treatment with aztreonam alone is unsatisfactory since many such patients harbour *Streptococcus pneumoniae* in their bronchial secretions, even when they are not easily detectable on smears and cultures. The results suggested that infections with *Haemophilus influenzae* may respond satisfactorily, but that *Branhamella catarrhalis* and *Pseudomonas aeruginosa* infections may have a poorer response.— B. I. Davies *et al.*, *J. antimicrob. Chemother.*, 1985, *15*, 375.

Cystic fibrosis. Beneficial response in 14 of 15 cystic fibrosis patients, aged 11 to 33 years, with chronic *Pseudomonas aeruginosa* lung infections to treatment with aztreonam 150 mg per kg body-weight daily in association with tobramycin 10 to 20 mg per kg daily. Both drugs were administered in 3 daily doses as bolus intravenous injections. All patients had a history of hypersensitivity reactions to other beta-lactams, but no allergic reactions were observed on treatment with aztreonam. The fifteenth patient did not complete treatment because of phlebitis at the injection site.— T. Jensen *et al.* (letter), *Lancet*, 1987, *1*, 1319.

Pneumonia. A study involving 80 patients with community- or hospital-acquired pneumonia. All patients received clindamycin due to the possibility of mixed infection with aerobic and anaerobic organisms. In addition they received intravenous treatment with either aztreonam or tobramycin. Clinically and bacteriologically, results were comparable in the 2 groups. In the aztreonam group there were 3 bacteriological failures, one each of infections with *Pseudomonas aeruginosa*, *Serratia marcescens*, and *Enterobacter aerogenes*. In the tobramycin group, one patient with a *Klebsiella pneumoniae* infection was considered to be a bacteriological failure.— J. R. Rodríguez *et al.*, *Antimicrob. Ag. Chemother.*, 1985, *27*, 246.

SEPTICAEMIA. One hundred patients with suspected or proven aerobic Gram-negative infections complicated by bacteraemia were treated with either aztreonam or an aminoglycoside (gentamicin or tobramycin). Initially, concomitant therapy with penicillin, clindamycin, vancomycin, or metronidazole was administered if there was a possibility of the presence of Gram-positive or anaerobic organisms. The urinary tract was the most common origin of septicaemia, and *Escherichia coli* was the most frequent infecting organism. Clinical efficacy in 57 evaluable patients was similar in both groups. The most important drug-related adverse effects were nephrotoxicity in patients receiving aminoglycosides, and enterococcal superinfection, particularly of the urinary tract, in patients receiving aztreonam.— F. Gudiol *et al.*, *J. antimicrob. Chemother.*, 1986, *17*, 661.

A study in 74 patients concluded that aztreonam 1 g every 8 hours or 2 g every 12 hours is effective treatment for Gram-negative septicaemia. Superinfections, especially with *Enterococcus faecalis*, were however a possibility, and an additional antibiotic should be administered if a mixed infection is suspected.— D. Pierard *et al.*, *Antimicrob. Ag. Chemother.*, 1986, *29*, 359.

A comparison of parenteral therapy with aztreonam or ceftazidime for proven or suspected Gram-negative septicaemia in patients with severe underlying diseases. Twenty-two of 25 patients in the aztreonam group, and 18 of 22 in the ceftazidime group were considered to be clinically cured. There were however, no strains of *Pseudomonas aeruginosa* isolated from blood cultures, and only a small number of cases of pneumonia or abscess. Superinfections occurred in 7 and 3 patients in the 2 groups respectively; in 5 patients treated with aztreonam, superinfection was with Gram-positive cocci.— H. Lagast *et al.*, *Am. J. Med.*, 1986, *80*, *Suppl.* 5C, 79.

SUPPRESSION OF INTESTINAL FLORA. As aztreonam is active against Gram-negative organisms with little effect on anaerobic bacteria, it has been suggested as a possible agent for the selective decontamination of the gastro-intestinal tract to prevent infection in immunocompromised patients. Although a study in 10 healthy subjects has shown it to be effective when administered by mouth (D. van der Waaij, *Rev. infect. Dis.*, 1985, *7*, *Suppl.* 4, S628), its use may be limited by inactivation, which has been observed *in vitro* in the faeces from one patient (E.M. Veringa and D. van der Waaij, *J. antimicrob. Chemother.*, 1984, *14*, 605).

URINARY-TRACT INFECTIONS. Of 35 patients with serious urinary-tract infections treated with aztreonam, 1 g every 8 hours by intravenous infusion or intramuscularly, 23 had unqualified cures, 6 had cures with relapse, and 6 had cures with re-infection; corresponding figures for 17 treated with gentamicin, 1 mg per kg body-weight every 8 hours by intravenous infusion or intramuscularly, were 9, 1, and 4; whereas there were no failures in the aztreonam group, there were 3 in the gentamicin group. Higher doses were given if bacteraemia was suspected and lower doses in patients with creatinine clearances below 30 mL per minute. The most important determinant of outcome appeared to be the presence of urological abnormalities, and not the antibiotic given or the infecting organism. All of a further 11 patients, all with renal failure or gentamicin-resistant isolates, treated with aztreonam, were cured without relapse or re-infection, although 7 had major urological abnormalities. In 14 of the 46 aztreonam-treated patients urinary colonisation with group D streptococci occurred, compared with only 1 of the 17 gentamicin-treated patients.— F. R. Sattler *et al.*, *Lancet*, 1984, *1*, 1315.

Further references to the use of aztreonam for the treatment of urinary-tract infections; re-infection with enterococci during treatment may be a problem: D. W. Webb and F. A. Wyle, *Curr. ther. Res.*, 1984, *36*, 113; J. H. Phipps *et al.* (letter), *J. antimicrob. Chemother.*, 1985, *16*, 678; K. G. Naber *et al.*, *ibid.*, 1986, *17*, 517; F. Rusconi *et al.*, *Antimicrob. Ag. Chemother.*, 1986, *30*, 310.

Preparations

Aztreonam for Injection *(U.S.P.)*. A dry mixture of sterile Aztreonam (*U.S.P.*) and arginine.

Sterile Aztreonam *(U.S.P.)*

Proprietary Preparations

Azactam *(Squibb, UK)*. *Injection*, powder for reconstitution, aztreonam 0.5, 1, and 2 g.
Intravenous infusion, powder for reconstitution, aztreonam 2 g.

Proprietary Names and Manufacturers

Azactam *(Squibb, Denm.*; *Heyden, Ger.*; *Squibb, Ital.*; *Squibb, Swed.*; *Squibb, UK*; *Squibb, USA)*; Dynabiotic *(Pfizer, Ger.)*; Primbactam *(Menarini, Ital.)*.

15-r

Bacampicillin Hydrochloride *(BANM, USAN, rINNM)*.

Carampicillin; EPC-272. 1-(Ethoxycarbonyloxy)ethyl (6*R*)-6-(α-D-phenylglycylamino)penicillanate hydrochloride.

$C_{21}H_{27}N_3O_7S$, HCl=502.0.

CAS — 50972-17-3 (bacampicillin); 37661-08-8 (hydrochloride).

Pharmacopoeias. In *U.S.*

1.44 g of monograph substance is approximately equivalent to 1 g of ampicillin. A 2% solution in water has a pH of 3.0 to 4.5. **Store** in airtight containers.

Adverse Effects and Precautions

As for Ampicillin Trihydrate, p.116. Diarrhoea has been reported to occur less frequently with bacampicillin hydrochloride.

Report of a study demonstrating no significant alteration in immunological parameters of patients treated with bacampicillin by mouth.— A. Scordamaglia *et al.*, *J. antimicrob. Chemother.*, 1987, *19*, 791.

EFFECTS ON THE GASTRO-INTESTINAL TRACT. Oesophagitis in one patient associated with the administration of bacampicillin.— M. Meloni *et al.*, *Ital. J. Gastroenterol.*, 1983, *15*, 122.

Bacampicillin 400 mg administered to 6 healthy subjects by mouth every 8 hours for 7 days, induced only minor changes in the oropharyngeal microflora, causing a decrease in the numbers of *Streptococcus salivarius* and fusobacteria in most subjects; consequently there was no increase in the numbers of resistant bacterial strains. This may be explained by the absence of detectable concentrations of bacampicillin in the saliva. Bacampicillin was not detected in the faeces either, and produced no significant changes in the numbers of aerobic or anaerobic organisms in the intestinal microflora or in the numbers of resistant bacterial strains.— C. E. Nord and A. Heimdahl, *J. antimicrob. Chemother.*, 1986, *18*, *Suppl.* C, 159.

Antimicrobial Action

Bacampicillin has the antimicrobial action of ampicillin *in vivo* (see p.117). It possesses no intrinsic activity and requires to be hydrolysed to ampicillin.

Absorption and Fate

Bacampicillin is more rapidly and completely absorbed from the gastro-intestinal tract than ampicillin, to which it is hydrolysed in the intestinal wall and plasma. Peak plasma-ampicillin concentrations are obtained about 30 to 60 minutes after administration by mouth, and are approximately twice those obtained after an equivalent dose of ampicillin. The absorption of bacampicillin hydrochloride tablets does not appear to be affected by the presence of food in the stomach. About 75% of a dose is excreted in the urine as ampicillin within 8 hours.

A review of the absorption and fate of bacampicillin.— J. Sjövall, *J. antimicrob. Chemother.*, 1981, *8*, *Suppl.* C, 41.

DRUG ABSORPTION. In a crossover study in 9 patients given approximately equimolar doses of bacampicillin or amoxycillin by mouth a mean of 65% and 73% of the dose respectively were absorbed but this difference was less important than the significant interindividual variation in absorption. Amoxycillin was absorbed significantly more slowly than bacampicillin, resulting in different plasma-concentration profiles but the differences in absorption characteristics did not justify a preference for either drug. Both drugs are absorbed rather unpredictably and this should be kept in mind when the mode of administration of amoxycillin or ampicillin to patients is chosen.— P. L. Meenhorst *et al.*, *J. antimicrob. Chemother.*, 1984, *14*, 267.

Results suggesting that bacampicillin hydrochloride can be administered in a microcapsule suspension with sufficient microcapsule film thickness to reduce the bitter taste and still retain good bioavailability.— J. Sjövall *et al.*, *J. pharm. Sci.*, 1984, *73*, 141.

Uses and Administration

Bacampicillin hydrochloride has the actions and uses of ampicillin (see p.119) to which it is rapidly hydrolysed after administration. It is given in doses of 400 to 800 mg two to three times daily by. mouth. Children over 5 years of age may be given 200 mg three times daily.

Reviews of the actions and uses of bacampicillin: *Med. Lett.*, 1981, *23*, 49; *Drug & Ther. Bull.*, 1981, *19*, 78; R. T. Scheife and H. C. Neu, *Pharmacotherapy*, 1982, *2*, 313.

For comparative reviews and reports of aminopenicillins, see Ampicillin Trihydrate, p.119.

An analysis of data from 16 controlled comparative studies of the use of bacampicillin in the treatment of infections of the ear, nose, throat, and urinary tract, or in acute exacerbations of chronic bronchitis. A dosage of 400 to 800 mg twice daily was considered effective in most infections, although 1200 mg twice daily may be required for severe exacerbations of chronic bronchitis.— M. Blomqvist and S. Å. Hedström, *J. int. med. Res.*, 1987, *15*, 32.

GONORRHOEA. Report of a study of 203 patients treated for uncomplicated gonorrhoea with a single dose of bacampicillin 1.6 g in association with probenecid 1 g both given by mouth. At follow-up 5 to 9 days later, 94 of 99 males (94.9%) and 101 of 104 females (97.1%) were cured, as defined by negative culture and absence of symptoms. All 7 males with rectal infections were cured. No beta-lactamase-producing strains of *Neiserria gonorrhoeae* were isolated.— B. Romanowski, *Can. J. publ. Hlth*, 1985, *76*, 98.

RESPIRATORY-TRACT INFECTIONS. References to the use of bacampicillin in various infections of the respiratory system:; R. L. Renton *et al.*, *Clin. Trials J.*, 1984, *21*, 207 (acute bronchitis); R. Pauwels and J. J. Detiège, *J. int. med. Res.*, 1986, *14*, 110 (respiratory-tract and ear infections).

Preparations

Bacampicillin Hydrochloride for Oral Suspension *(U.S.P.)*

Bacampicillin Hydrochloride Tablets *(U.S.P.)*

Proprietary Preparations

Ambaxin *(Upjohn, UK)*. *Tablets*, scored, bacampicillin hydrochloride, 400 mg.

Proprietary Names and Manufacturers

Albaxin *(Upjohn, Ital.)*; Ambacamp *(Upjohn, Ger.)*; Ambaxin *(Upjohn, UK)*; Ambaxino *(Upjohn, Spain)*; Amplibac *(Schwarz, Ital.)*; Bacacil *(Arg.*; *Pfizer, Ital.*; *Mack, Switz.)*; Bacampicin *(Upjohn, Switz.)*; Bacampicine *(Upjohn, Fr.)*; Penglobe *(Arg.*; *Belg.*; *Astra, Canad.*; *Lundbeck, Denm.*; *Astra, Fr.*; *Astra, Ger.*; *Bracco, Ital.*; *Neth.*; *Essex, Spain*; *Astra, Swed.)*; Spectrobid *(Roerig, USA)*; Velbacil *(Pfizer, Spain)*.

17-d

Bacitracin *(BAN, USAN, rINN)*.

Bacitracinum.

CAS — 1405-87-4.

Pharmacopoeias. In *Arg.*, *Belg.*, *Br.*, *Braz.*, *Chin.*, *Cz.*, *Egypt.*, *Eur.*, *Ind.*, *Int.*, *It.*, *Jug.*, *Mex.*, *Nord.*, *Port.*, *Swiss*, *Turk.*, and *U.S.*

The *B.P.* states that bacitracin consists of one or more of the antimicrobial polypeptides produced by certain strains of ***Bacillus licheniformis*** and by *B. subtilis* var. Tracy. The *U.S.P.* states that it is a polypeptide produced by the growth of an organism of the *licheniformis* group of *Bacillus subtilis*.

It is a white to pale buff hygroscopic powder, odourless or with a slight odour. The *B.P.* specifies a potency of not less than 60 units per mg calculated on the dried substance, and the *U.S.P.* a potency of not less than 40 units per mg. *B.P.* **solubilities** are: freely soluble in water and in alcohol; practically insoluble in chloroform and in ether. *U.S.P.* solubilities are: freely soluble in water; soluble in alcohol, methyl alcohol, and glacial acetic acid, the solution in the organic solvents usually showing some insoluble residue; insoluble in acetone, chloroform, and ether. The *B.P.* states that a 1% solution has a pH of 6 to 7, and the *U.S.P.* that a solution containing 10 000 units per mL has a pH of 5.5 to 7.5.

Bacitracin is precipitated from solutions and inactivated by salts of many of the heavy metals. Solutions in water deteriorate rapidly at room temperature. **Store** at a temperature of 8° to 15° in airtight containers.

16-f

Bacitracin Zinc *(BANM, USAN, rINNM)*.

Bacitracins Zinc Complex; Bacitracinum Zincum; Zinc Bacitracin.

CAS — 1405-89-6.

Pharmacopoeias. In *Br.*, *Eur.*, *Ind.*, *It.*, *Swiss*, and *U.S.* Also in *B.P. Vet.*

The zinc complex of bacitracin.

A white or pale yellowish-grey or tan hygroscopic powder, odourless or with a slight odour.

B.P. **solubilities** are: slightly soluble in water and in alcohol; very slightly soluble in ether; practically insoluble in chloroform. *U.S.P.* solubilities are: sparingly soluble in water. A saturated solution in water has a pH of 6.0 to 7.5. **Store** in a cool place in airtight containers.

STABILITY. Bacitracin zinc was more stable than bacitracin and could be stored for 18 months at temperatures up to 40° without appreciable loss. Lozenges of bacitracin zinc and ointments and tablets containing bacitracin zinc with neomycin were more stable than the corresponding bacitracin preparations. Bacitracin zinc was less bitter than bacitracin and the taste was more readily disguised.— H. M. Gross *et al.*, *Drug Cosmet. Ind.*, 1954, *75*, 612.

The deterioration of bacitracin which occurred in solution was probably a process of oxidation initiated by light. Solutions in which the air had been replaced by nitrogen showed a loss in activity not greater than 10% after 3 months' storage in diffused light.— V. Würtzen, *Dansk Tidsskr. Farm.*, 1954, *28*, 34.

Bacitracin was stable in anhydrous bases such as paraffins, white wax, or wool fat. It was not affected by the addition of hydroquinone, ascorbyl palmitate, cetyl alcohol, calamine, zinc oxide, or benzocaine. It was slowly inactivated in bases containing stearyl alcohol, cholestrol, polyoxyethylene derivatives, and sodium lauryl sulphate. It was rapidly inactivated in bases containing water, macrogols, propylene glycol, glycerol, cetylpyridinium chloride, benzalkonium chloride, ichthammol, phenol, and tannic acid.— J. M. Plaxco and W. J. Husa, *J. Am. pharm. Ass., scient. Edn*, 1956, *45*, 141.

There was no significant loss of potency when bacitracin powder was added to 3 commercially available 0.5% hypromellose solutions in plastic squeezy bottles (Lacril, pH 5.9; Tearisol, pH 7.3; Isoptotears, pH 7.4) and the resulting solutions of bacitracin 9600 units per mL kept at 25° for 7 days.— E. Osborn *et al.*, *Am. J. Ophthal.*, 1976, *82*, 775.

Stability of bacitracin solution frozen in glass vials or plastic syringes.— P. F. Souney *et al.*, *Am. J. Hosp. Pharm.*, 1987, *44*, 1125.

Units

One unit of bacitracin is contained in 0.01351 mg of the second International Standard Preparation (1964) of bacitracin zinc which contains 74 units per mg.

Adverse Effects

When administered by intramuscular injection, bacitracin can be nephrotoxic. Nephrotoxicity may also occur after local application over the site of abdominal operations or after instillation into infected cavities. Local application of bacitracin has been associated with severe allergic disorders.

ALLERGY. A 50-year-old woman suffered an anaphylactic allergic reaction after the application of an ointment containing bacitracin to a skin-graft donor site.— M. A. Vale *et al.* (letter), *Archs Derm.*, 1978, *114*, 800.

Antimicrobial Action and Resistance

Bacitracin interferes with bacterial cell wall synthesis and is active against many Gram-positive bacteria including staphylococci, streptococci, clostridia and *Corynebacterium diphtheriae*; it is also active against *Treponema pallidum* and some Gram-negative cocci.

Acquired bacterial resistance to bacitracin rarely occurs, but resistant strains of *Staphylococcus aureus* have been detected.

Exposure to bacitracin 200 units per mL for one hour killed 90% of 48 clinical isolates of coagulase-negative staphylococci. Such a bactericidal concentration may be used for short-term topical prophylaxis in neurosurgical procedures.— P. R. Fischer *et al.*, *Antimicrob. Ag. Chemother.*, 1984, *25*, 502.

Absorption and Fate

Bacitracin is not appreciably absorbed from the gastro-intestinal tract. When administered by intramuscular injection it is rapidly absorbed; doses of 200 to 300 units per kg body-weight every 6 hours produce plasma concentrations of up to 2 units per mL. About 30% of a single injected dose is excreted in the urine within 24 hours. Bacitracin readily diffuses into the pleural and ascitic fluids but little passes into the cerebrospinal fluid.

The half-life of bacitracin in serum was 1.5 hours and 9 to 31% was excreted in the urine.— C. M. Kunin, *Ann. intern. Med.*, 1967, *67*, 151.

Uses and Administration

Bacitracin and bacitracin zinc are mainly used in the topical treatment of infections due to susceptible organisms. They may be administered in lozenges, ointments, dusting-powders, aerosol sprays, ear and eye preparations, and solutions for bladder irrigation, often in conjunction with other antibiotics such as neomycin and polymyxin B, or with hydrocortisone. Absorption from open wounds and from the bladder or peritoneal cavity may lead to adverse effects.

Bacitracin is only rarely administered by mouth or parenterally by intramuscular injection.

Bacitracin zinc is used as an additive for animal feeding stuffs.

Bacitracin methylene disalicylate is used in veterinary medicine.

ANTIBIOTIC-ASSOCIATED COLITIS. For the use of bacitracin by mouth in the treatment of antibiotic-associated colitis, see Vancomycin Hydrochloride, p.335.

CONTROL OF EPIDEMIC MRSA. Although bacitracin ointment has been applied to the nose of subjects colonised with methicillin-resistant *Staphylococcus aureus* (J.P. O'Keefe *et al.*, *New Engl. J. Med.*, 1985, *312*, 858), two studies have found it ineffective in eradicating nasal carriage (T.P. McAnally *et al.*, *Antimicrob. Ag. Chemother.*, 1984, *25*, 422; V.L. Yu *et al.*, *New Engl. J. Med.*, 1986, *315*, 91).

SURGICAL INFECTION PROPHYLAXIS. See under Antimicrobial Action, above.

Preparations

Bacitracin Ophthalmic Ointment *(U.S.P.)*

Bacitracin Ointment *(U.S.P.)*. It may contain a suitable anaesthetic. Preferably to be stored at a temperature maintained thermostatically between 15° and 30°.

Bacitracin Zinc Ointment *(U.S.P.)*. Preferably to be stored at a temperature maintained thermostatically between 15° and 30°.

Bacitracin Zinc and Polymyxin B Sulfate Ophthalmic Ointment *(U.S.P.)*

Bacitracin Zinc and Polymyxin B Sulfate Ointment *(U.S.P.)*. Protect from light.

Bacitracin and Polymyxin B Sulfate Topical Aerosol *(U.S.P.)*

Sterile Bacitracin *(U.S.P.)*. Bacitracin suitable for parenteral use.

Sterile Bacitracin Zinc *(U.S.P.)*. Bacitracin zinc suitable for parenteral use.

Other official preparations containing bacitracin are described under polymyxin B sulphate and neomycin sulphate.

For proprietary preparations of bacitracin and bacitracin zinc, see under hydrocortisone, polymyxin B sulphate, and neomycin sulphate.

Proprietary Names and Manufacturers of Bacitracin and Bacitracin Zinc

Baciguent *(Upjohn, Canad.; Upjohn, USA)*; Bacitin *(Pharmascience, Canad.)*.

The following names have been used for multi-ingredient preparations containing bacitracin and bacitracin zinc— Ak-Spore Ophthalmic Ointment *(Akorn, USA)*; Cicatrene; Cicatrex; Cicatrin *(Wellcome, Austral.; Wellcome, Canad.; Calmic, UK)*; Cortisporin Ointment *(Wellcome, Canad.; Wellcome, USA)*; Dispray Antibiotic Powder Spray *(Stuart, UK)*; Hydroderm *(Merck Sharp & Dohme, UK)*; Mycitracin *(Upjohn, Austral.)*; Nemdyn *(Hamilton, Austral.)*; Neo-Polycin *(Merrell Dow, USA)*; Neosporin Aerosol *(Wellcome, Canad.)*; Neosporin Ointment *(Wellcome, Austral.; Wellcome, Canad.; Wellcome, USA)*; Neosporin Ophthalmic Ointment *(Wellcome, Austral.; Wellcome, Canad.; Wellcome, USA)*; Neosporin Powder *(Wellcome, Canad.)*; Neotracin *(Cilag, Austral.)*; Ocu-Cort *(Ocumed, USA)*; Ocumycin *(Pharmafair, USA)*; Ocu-Spor B *(Ocumed, USA)*; Ocutricin HC Ointment *(Pharmafair, USA)*; Ocutricin Ointment *(Pharmafair, USA)*; Ototrips *(Consolidated Chemicals, UK)*; Plegettes *(Hamilton, Austral.)*; Polybactrin *(Wellcome, Austral.; Calmic, UK)*; Polyfax *(Calmic, UK)*; Polysporin *(Wellcome, Canad.; Wellcome, USA)*; Rikospray Antibiotic *(Riker, UK)*; Spersin Ointment *(Sigma, Austral.)*; Topisporin *(Pharmafair, USA)*; Tribiotic *(Riker, UK)*.

12416-n

Bambermycin *(BAN, pINN)*.

Bambermycins *(USAN)*; Flavophospholipol. An antibiotic complex containing mainly moenomycin A and moenomycin C and which may be obtained from cultures of *Streptomyces bambergiensis*.

CAS — 11015-37-5.

Bambermycin is used in feedstuffs for pigs, poultry, and cattle as a growth promotor.

Proprietary Veterinary Names and Manufacturers

Flavomycin *(Fisons, UK)*.

2485-r

Baquiloprim *(BAN, rINN)*.

138OU. 5-(8-Dimethylamino-7-methyl-5-quinolylmethyl)pyrimidin-2,4-diyldiamine.

$C_{17}H_{20}N_6$=308.4.

CAS — 102280-35-3.

Baquiloprim is an antibacterial agent for use in veterinary medicine.

Proprietary Veterinary Names and Manufacturers

Coopers Animal Health, UK.

18-n

Bekanamycin Sulphate *(rINNM)*.

Aminodeoxykanamycin Sulfate; Bekanamycini Sulfas; Kanamycin B Sulphate; KDM; NK-1006. 6-*O*-(3-Amino-3-deoxy-α-D-glucopyranosyl)-2-deoxy-4-*O*-(2,6-diamino-2,6-dideoxy-α-D-glucopyranosyl)-D-streptamine sulphate.

$C_{18}H_{37}N_5O_{10},2.5H_2SO_4$=728.7.

CAS — 4696-76-8 (bekanamycin); 70550-99-1 (sulphate).

Pharmacopoeias. In *Jpn.*

1.5 g of monograph substance is approximately equivalent to 1 g of bekanamycin.

Bekanamycin is an aminoglycoside antibiotic structurally related to kanamycin and with actions and uses similar to those of gentamicin (see p.236). It has been administered intramuscularly, intravenously, by mouth, or by inhalation as the sulphate.

In the treatment of gonorrhoea, a single intramuscular injection of bekanamycin 1.2 g produced a cure-rate of 93%, equivalent to the cure-rate following kanamycin 2g. Pain at the injection site occurred in some patients.— A. Guerrieri *et al.*, *Clin. Med.*, 1975, *82*, (Jan.), 25.

Proprietary Names and Manufacturers

Coltericin *(Argentia, Arg.)*; Kanendomicina *(Iquinosa, Spain)*; Kanendomycin *(Meiji, Jpn)*; Kanendos *(Crinos, Ital.)*; Stereocidin *(Crinos, Ital.)*.

19-h

Benethamine Penicillin *(BAN, rINN)*.

Benzyl(phenethyl)ammonium (6*R*)-6-(2-phenylacetamido)penicillanate.

$C_{15}H_{17}N,C_{16}H_{18}N_2O_4S$=545.7.

CAS — 751-84-8.

Benethamine penicillin is a poorly soluble derivative of benzylpenicillin with similar actions and uses (see p.131), although it is not recommended for chronic, severe, or deep-seated infections. After deep intramuscular injection it forms a depot from which it is slowly absorbed and hydrolysed to benzylpenicillin. Effective concentrations of benzylpenicillin are maintained for up to 5 days. Benethamine penicillin is usually given in conjunction with benzylpenicillin sodium and procaine penicillin to produce both an immediate and a prolonged effect.

Preparations

Fortified Benethamine Penicillin Injection *(B.P.C. 1973)*. Benethamine Penicillin with Benzylpenicillin Sodium and Procaine Penicillin Injection; Triple Penicillin Injection. To be reconstituted before use. Store in a cool place and use within 7 days, or within 14 days when stored at 2° to 10°; if stored at temperatures approaching 20°, it should be used within 4 days.

Proprietary Preparations

Triplopen *(Glaxo, UK)*. *Injection*, powder for reconstitution, benethamine penicillin 475 mg, procaine penicillin 250 mg, benzylpenicillin sodium 300 mg. *Dose*. The contents of 2 vials as a single dose or of 1 vial daily or every 2 or 3 days.

Proprietary Names and Manufacturers

Benapen *(S.Afr.)*.

20-a

Benzathine Penicillin *(BAN)*.

Benzathine Benzylpenicillin *(rINN)*; Benzathini Benzylpenicillinum; Benzethacil; Benzilpenicillina Benzatinica; Benzylpenicillinum Benzathinum; Penicillin G Benzathine *(USAN)*; Penzaethinum G. *NN'*-Dibenzylethylenediammonium bis-[(6*R*)-6-(2-phenylacetamido)penicillanate].
$C_{16}H_{20}N_2(C_{16}H_{18}N_2O_4S)_2$=909.1.

CAS — 1538-09-6 (anhydrous); 5928-83-6 (monohydrate); 41372-02-5 (tetrahydrate).

Pharmacopoeias. In *Arg., Aust., Br., Braz., Cz., Egypt., Eur., Fr., Ger., Ind., Int., It., Jug., Neth., Pol., Port., Swiss, Turk.,* and *U.S.* Also in *B.P. Vet.*

A white, odourless, crystalline powder. Benzathine penicillin 900 mg is approximately equivalent to 720 mg of benzylpenicillin (1.2 million units).

Soluble 1 in 5000 to 6000 of water, 1 in 65 of alcohol; practically insoluble in chloroform and ether. The pH of a 0.05% solution in equal quantities of water and dehydrated alcohol is 4.0 to 6.5.

Store at a temperature not exceeding 30° in airtight containers. Protect from light and moisture. Aqueous suspensions are most stable when buffered to pH 5.5 to 7.5 and stored at low temperatures. Injections of benzathine penicillin stored at 2° to 8° should be used within 7 days of preparation if unbuffered or within 14 days if buffered.

Adverse Effects and Precautions

As for Benzylpenicillin, p.132.

Non-allergic reactions similar to those reported after administration of procaine penicillin, p.291, have been reported rarely with benzathine penicillin.

Benzathine penicillin should not be injected intravascularly since ischaemic reactions may occur.

Absorption and Fate

When benzathine penicillin is given by intramuscular injection, it forms a depot from which it is slowly released and hydrolysed to benzylpenicillin. Peak plasma concentrations are produced in about 24 hours, and effective concentrations of benzylpenicillin are maintained for up to 4 weeks. However, plasma concentrations are lower than those following an equivalent dose of benzylpenicillin. Due to the slow absorption from the site of injection, benzylpenicillin has been detected in the urine for up to 12 weeks after a single dose.

Benzathine penicillin is stable in the presence of gastric juice, however its absorption from the gastro-intestinal tract is variable, and the amounts that are absorbed are smaller than those from the same dose of a soluble penicillin. Maximum concentrations of penicillin in the blood are also produced less rapidly than after a corresponding dose of a soluble salt of penicillin but effective blood concentrations persist for a longer time — up to 6 hours.

Benzathine penicillin 37.5 mg per kg body-weight given intramuscularly to 125 neonates produced peak serum concentrations of 1.23 µg per mL at 13 to 24 hours and concentrations decreased to 0.65 µg per mL by the fourth day. More than 100 µg per mL of penicillin was present in the urine of some infants throughout the first week of life.— J. O. Klein *et al., J. Pediat.*, 1973, *82*, 1065.

In 12 children given benzathine penicillin intramuscularly (450 mg for those weighing less than 27 kg; 900 mg for those of 27 kg or more) mean serum concentrations of penicillin at 24 hours were 0.15 to 0.16 µg per mL, and 0.31 µg per mL in 13 children given benzathine penicillin 675 mg with procaine penicillin 300 mg. At 10 days all subjects had concentrations of at least 0.01 µg per mL. At 18 days only 8 of 12 samples from those given benzathine penicillin had detectable penicillin, and only 6 of 12 samples for those given the combination preparation. Monthly administration of either preparation may be inadequate for the prophylaxis of streptococcal infections.— C. M. Ginsburg *et al., Pediatrics*, 1982, *69*, 452.

DIFFUSION INTO BODY FLUIDS AND TISSUES. A single intramuscular injection of benzathine penicillin 75 mg per kg body-weight was given to 59 infants born to mothers with syphilis. A mean peak serum concentration of 2.54 µg per mL occurred at 24 hours after the dose and at least 0.42 µg per mL of penicillin was found at 120 hours. Peak concentrations of penicillin in the CSF, noted between 12 and 24 hours, only ranged from 0.012 to 0.21 µg per mL and were not adequate for neonates with possible neurosyphilis.— M. E. Speer *et al., J. Pediat.*, 1977, *91*, 996.

In a study involving 33 patients with latent syphilis treated with intramuscular benzathine penicillin 1.8 or 3.6 g weekly for 3 weeks, with or without probenecid 500 mg four times daily by mouth continuously, CSF-penicillin concentrations greater than 18 ng per mL (considered to be the minimum effective concentration) were achieved in 2 patients only. These were 2 of 6 patients receiving the higher dose in association with probenecid.— J. Ducas and H. G. Robson, *J. Am. med. Ass.*, 1981, *246*, 2583.

Uses and Administration

Benzathine penicillin has the same antimicrobial action as benzylpenicillin (see p.133), but because of the relatively low blood concentrations of benzylpenicillin produced, its use should be restricted to micro-organisms that are highly susceptible to benzylpenicillin. In acute infections, and when bacteraemia is present, the initial treatment should be with benzylpenicillin by injection.

Benzathine penicillin is used for the treatment of syphilis, including that occurring in pregnant women. For early syphilis, a single dose of 1.8 g by deep intramuscular injection is given. In late syphilis, this dose is given at weekly intervals for a total of 3 doses. Benzathine penicillin is not usually recommended for the treatment of neurosyphilis because of reports of inadequate penetration into the CSF. Neonates may be given a single intramuscular injection of 37.5 mg per kg body-weight for the treatment of congenital syphilis provided there is no evidence of infection in the CSF.

Benzathine penicillin is also used for the treatment of other treponemal infections, such as yaws, pinta, and endemic syphilis (bejel), and may also be used in the treatment of streptococcal infections, particularly of the upper respiratory tract. For such infections it is usually given as a single intramuscular dose of 900 mg. Children may be given intramuscular doses of 225 to 675 mg according to body-weight. To prevent recurrences of acute rheumatic fever 900 mg may be given intramuscularly every 4 weeks; doses of 450 mg or 900 mg have been recommended for children.

Benzathine penicillin should not be used in the treatment of gonorrhoea.

For mild infections in adults, benzathine penicillin has been given by mouth in a dose of 450 mg every 6 to 8 hours although phenoxymethylpenicillin is usually preferred. Children have been given half the adult dose.

INFECTION PROPHYLAXIS, HYPOSPLENISM. Beneficial results with intramuscular benzathine penicillin used in the prevention of pneumococcal infection in children with homozygous sickle cell disease.— A. B. John *et al., Br. med. J.*, 1984, *288*, 1567.

See also under Prophylactic Use of Antibiotics, p.102.

LYME DISEASE. Benzathine penicillin 1.8 g administered weekly for 3 weeks by intramuscular injection to patients with established Lyme arthritis resulted in complete resolution of arthritis in 7 of 20 patients within a mean of 4 weeks from the beginning of treatment. In contrast, the remaining 13 patients, including 4 who withdrew from the study following the first penicillin injection due to the pain of injection, and an additional 20 patients who received placebo, required a mean of 17 to 18 weeks for resolution of their arthritis attack; they also experienced an average of 6 months of active arthritis during a mean follow-up period of 33 months.— A. C. Steere *et al., New Engl. J. Med.*, 1985, *312*, 869.

See also under Benzylpenicillin Sodium, p.136.

PHARYNGITIS. From a retrospective study of 33 cases of pharyngitis caused by *Corynebacterium haemolyticum*, treatment with a single intramuscular dose of benzathine penicillin 900 mg or erythromycin 250 mg four times daily by mouth for 10 days was clinically and microbiologically effective in most patients.— R. A. Miller *et al., Ann. intern. Med.*, 1986, *105*, 867.

For reference to the use of a combination of benzathine penicillin and rifampicin for the eradication of group A streptococci in chronic pharyngeal carriers, see Rifampicin, p.576.

PREGNANCY AND THE NEONATE. For reference to the use of benzathine penicillin in the neonate, see under Benzylpenicillin Sodium, p.137.

RHEUMATIC FEVER PROPHYLAXIS. Penicillin was considered the drug of choice to prevent acute rheumatic fever. For primary prevention, the American Heart Association recommend that group A streptococcal infections of the upper respiratory tract should be treated with benzathine penicillin given intramuscularly in a single dose of 450 mg for patients weighing 27 kg or less, or 900 mg for patients weighing more than 27 kg; benzathine penicillin in association with procaine penicillin might also be satisfactory. Alternatively phenoxymethylpenicillin 125 to 250 mg given 3 or 4 times daily by mouth for 10 days in children or adults was considered suitable provided that the patients completed the full course of treatment (S.T. Shulman *et al., Circulation*, 1984, *70*, 1118A). Bass (*J. Am. med. Ass.*, 1986, *256*, 740) considered the optimum dosage of phenoxymethylpenicillin for children to be 250 mg twice daily for 10 days although it could be given 3 or 4 times daily in the first 24 to 48 hours to assure an early bacteriological cure and render the patient noncontagious as early as possible. However, due to the low incidence of rheumatic fever in developed countries, controversy existed over whether or not to treat streptococcal sore throats (J.G.R. Howie and B.A. Foggo, *J. R. Coll. gen. Pract.*, 1985, *35*, 223) and also whether to continue treatment after negative throat cultures had been obtained (M. Soman, *J. Am. med. Ass.*, 1985, *254*, 907; V.A. Fulginiti, *ibid.*). For prevention of recurrent attacks the American Heart Association recommended benzathine penicillin 900 mg given intramuscularly every 4 weeks. The use of oral agents was considered appropriate for patients at lower risk of rheumatic recurrences; phenoxymethylpenicillin 125 or 250 mg twice daily or sulphadiazine 0.5 or 1 g daily were considered to be equally effective (S.T. Shulman *et al., Circulation*, 1984 *70*, 1118A).

See also under Prophylactic Use of Antibiotics, p.103, and under Absorption and Fate, above.

SYPHILIS. Syphilis is usually treated with benzathine penicillin or procaine penicillin. Benzathine penicillin 1.8 g intramuscularly is given as a single dose for early syphilis and at weekly intervals for 3 weeks for late syphilis. Procaine penicillin 600 mg daily by intramuscular injection is given for 10 days in early syphilis and for 15 days in late syphilis; treatment is given for 20 days in cardiovascular syphilis. In the treatment of neurosyphilis adequate concentrations of penicillin must be obtained in the CSF. Therefore, therapy is usually with intravenous benzylpenicillin 1.2 to 2.4 g every 4 hours for 10 days, or procaine penicillin 600 mg daily by intramuscular injection for 20 days. Some authorities, however, have recommended that procaine penicillin be given in a dose of 2.4 g daily in association with probenecid 500 mg four times daily by mouth, both given for 10 days (WHO Expert Committee on Venereal Diseases and Treponematoses, *Tech. Rep. Ser. Wld Hlth Org. No. 736*, 1986; *Med. Lett.*, 1986, *28*, 23; P. Manu and W. Varade, *Lancet*, 1982, *2*, 924). Caution is usually recommended in the use of benzathine penicillin for neurosyphilis although some authors (P.G. Cuddy, *Drug Intell. & clin. Pharm.*, 1982, *16*, 205) have considered it to have a useful role provided it is used in specific situations.

Syphilis occurring during pregnancy can be treated with benzathine penicillin or procaine penicillin in the usual doses as given above. Alternatively, a regimen of benzylpenicillin 600 mg every 8 hours for 5 days followed by procaine penicillin 1 g daily for 10 days has been used (G. Buttigieg, *Br. J. Hosp. Med.*, 1985, *33*, 28).

Congenital syphilis in infants up to 2 years of age with abnormal CSF may be treated with benzylpenicillin 30 mg per kg body-weight given by intramuscular or intravenous injection daily in 2 divided doses for a minimum of 10 days. Alternatively procaine penicillin 50 mg per kg may be given intramuscularly in a single daily dose for 10 days. In infants with normal cerebrospinal fluid benzathine penicillin 37.5 mg per kg is given intramuscularly as a single dose.

Non-venereal treponematoses. Benzathine penicillin is the drug of choice for the treatment of non-venereal treponematoses (endemic syphilis, pinta, and yaws) since it is widely available in most countries. Latent and active cases and their contacts should be given 900 mg as a single intramuscular dose; children under 10 years of age should receive 450 mg.— WHO Expert Committee on Venereal Diseases and Treponematoses, *Tech. Rep. Ser. Wld Hlth Org. No. 736*, 1986.

Preparations

Fortified Benzathine Penicillin Injection *(B.P.C. 1973).* Benzathine Penicillin with Benzylpenicillin Potassium and Procaine Penicillin Injection

Sterile Penicillin G Benzathine *(U.S.P.)*

Sterile Penicillin G Benzathine Suspension *(U.S.P.)*

Sterile Penicillin G Benzathine and Penicillin G Procaine Suspension *(U.S.P.)*

Penicillin G Benzathine Oral Suspension *(U.S.P.)*

Penicillin G Benzathine Tablets *(U.S.P.)*

Proprietary Preparations

Penidural *(Wyeth, UK). Suspension,* benzathine penicillin 229 mg/5 mL.
Oral drops, benzathine penicillin 115 mg/mL.

Proprietary Names and Manufacturers

Benzetacil *(Antibioticos, Spain)*; Benzetacil L-A *(Arg.)*; Bicillin *(Wyeth, Austral.*; *Wyeth, USA)*; Bicillin LA *(Wyeth, Canad.*; *Wyeth, S.Afr.)*; Brevicilina Simple *(Spain)*; Cepacilina *(CEPA, Spain)*; Diaminocillina *(Farmitalia, Ital.)*; Extencilline *(Specia, Fr.)*; LPG *(Austral.)*; Megacillin Suspension *(Frosst, Canad.)*; Penadur *(Belg.*; *Wyeth, Switz.)*; Pen-di-Ben *(Arg.)*; Penidural *(Austral.*; *Neth.*; *NZ*; *Wyeth, UK)*; Penilente-LA *(Novo, S.Afr.)*; Peniroger *(Roger, Spain)*; Permapen *(Pfipharmecs, USA)*; Pipercilina *(Urca, Spain)*; Provipen Benzatina *(Sabater, Spain)*; Tardocillin *(Bayer, Ger.)*; Tardopenil *(Spain)*; Wycillina A.P. *(Carlo Erba, Ital.)*.

The following names have been used for multi-ingredient preparations containing benzathine penicillin— Bicillin All Purpose *(Wyeth, Austral.)*; Bicillin A-P *(Wyeth, Canad.)*; Bicillin C-R *(Wyeth, USA)*.

21-t

Benzathine Phenoxymethylpenicillin

Penicillin V Benzathine *(USAN)*; Phenoxymethylpenicillini Dibenzylaethylendiaminum. *NN'*-Dibenzylethylenediammonium bis[(6*R*)-6-(2-phenoxyacetamido)penicillanate].
$(C_{16}H_{18}N_2O_5S)_2,C_{16}H_{20}N_2=941.1$.

CAS — 5928-84-7 (anhydrous); 63690-57-3 (tetrahydrate).

Pharmacopoeias. In *Aust.* and *U.S.* In *Jug.* as the tetrahydrate.

An almost white powder with a characteristic odour. Benzathine phenoxymethylpenicillin 1.3 g is approximately equivalent to 1 g of phenoxymethylpenicillin. **Soluble** 1 in 3200 of water, 1 in 330 of alcohol, 1 in 42 of chloroform, 1 in 910 of ether, and 1 in 37 of acetone. A 3% suspension in water has a pH of 4.0 to 6.5. **Store** in airtight containers.

Benzathine phenoxymethylpenicillin has properties and uses similar to those of benzylpenicillin see (p.131) but it is acid-stable and is absorbed from the gastro-intestinal tract. It is given by mouth in doses of 250 to 500 mg every 6 hours in the treatment of mild to moderate infections caused by susceptible Gram-positive organisms.

Preparations

Penicillin V Benzathine Oral Suspension *(U.S.P.)*. A suspension containing benzathine phenoxymethylpenicillin. Store in a refrigerator.

Proprietary Names and Manufacturers

Benoral *(Galepharma, Spain)*; Cilicaine V *(Sigma, Austral.)*; Falcopen-V *(Faulding, Austral.)*; Kelacilline *(Belg.)*; Meropenin *(Astra, Swed.)*; Minervacil *(Byk, Neth.)*; Monocillin *(Chassot, Switz.)*; Oracilline *(Rhone-Poulenc, Belg.*; *Théraplix, Fr.)*; Ospen *(Sandoz, Ger.*; *Sandoz, Switz.)*; Penorline *(Allard, Fr.)*; Phenocillin *(Streuli, Switz.)*; PVF *(Frosst, Canad.)*; Stabicilline *(Vifor, Switz.)*; Vicalin *(Austral.)*; Vicin *(Knoll, Austral.)*.

181-l

Benzylpenicillin *(rINN).*

Crystalline Penicillin G; Penicillin; Penicillin G. (2*S*,5*R*,6*R*)-3,3-Dimethyl-7-oxo-6-phenylacetamido-4-thia-1-azabicyclo[3.2.0]heptane-2-carboxylic acid; (6*R*)-6-(2-Phenylacetamido)penicillanic acid.
$C_{16}H_{18}N_2O_4S=334.4$.

CAS — 61-33-6.

The name benzylpenicillin is commonly used to describe either benzylpenicillin potassium or benzylpenicillin sodium as these are the forms in which benzylpenicillin is used.

In *Martindale*, benzylpenicillin means either the potassium or sodium salt.

182-y

Benzylpenicillin Potassium *(BAN, rINNM).*

Benzylpenicillin; Benzylpenicillinum Kalicum; Crystalline Penicillin G; Penicillin; Penicillin G; Penicillin G Potassium *(USAN).*
$C_{16}H_{17}KN_2O_4S=372.5$.

CAS — 113-98-4.

Pharmacopoeias. In *Arg., Aust., Belg., Br., Chin., Cz., Eur., Fr., Ger., Hung., Int., It., Jpn, Jug., Mex., Neth., Pol., Port., Roum., Rus., Span., Swiss, Turk.*, and *U.S.* Also in *B.P. Vet. Egypt.* and *Ind.* include Benzylpenicillin which may be either the potassium or sodium salt.

The potassium salt of 6-phenylacetamidopenicillanic acid, an antimicrobial acid produced by growing certain strains of *Penicillium notatum* or related organisms or obtained by any other means.

A white or almost white, moderately hygroscopic, crystalline powder, odourless or with a faint characteristic odour. Each g of monograph substance represents about 2.7 mmol of potassium.

Very **soluble** in water; practically insoluble in chloroform, ether, fixed oils, and liquid paraffin. The *B.P.* specifies that a 10% solution in water has a pH of 5.5 to 7.5; the *U.S.P.* specifies that a 6% solution has a pH of 5.0 to 7.5 while a 6% solution of the injection has a pH of 6.0 to 8.5. **Store** at a temperature not exceeding 30° in airtight containers.

Stability and **incompatibility**, as for Benzylpenicillin Sodium (below).

22-x

Benzylpenicillin Sodium *(BAN, rINNM).*

Benzylpenicillin; Crystalline Penicillin G; Penicillin; Penicillin G; Penicillin G Sodium *(USAN).*
$C_{16}H_{17}N_2NaO_4S=356.4$.

CAS — 69-57-8.

Pharmacopoeias. In *Arg., Aust., Belg., Br., Braz., Chin., Eur., Fr., Ger., Hung., Int., It., Jug., Mex., Neth., Nord., Pol., Port., Roum., Rus., Span., Swiss,* and *Turk.* Also in *B.P. Vet. U.S.* includes Sterile Penicillin G Sodium. *Egypt.* and *Ind.* include Benzylpenicillin which may be either the potassium or sodium salt.

The sodium salt of 6-phenylacetamidopenicillanic acid, an antimicrobial acid produced by growing certain strains of *Penicillium notatum* or related organisms or obtained by any other means.

A white to slightly yellow, moderately hygroscopic, crystalline powder, odourless or with a faint characteristic odour. Each g of monograph substance represents about 2.8 mmol of sodium.

Very **soluble** in water; practically insoluble in chloroform, ether, fixed oils, and liquid paraffin. The *B.P.* specifies a 10% solution in water has a pH of 5.5 to 7.5; the *U.S.P.* specifies a 6% solution of Sterile Penicillin G Sodium has a pH of 5.0 to 7.5 while that of a 6% solution of the injection has a pH range of 6.0 to 7.5. **Store** at a temperature not exceeding 30° in airtight containers. Benzylpenicillin sodium or potassium is hydrolysed in aqueous solutions by degradation of the β-lactam ring and hydrolysis is accelerated by increased temperature or alkaline conditions; inactivation also occurs under acid conditions. Degradation products include penillic, penicillenic, and penicilloic acids which lower the pH and cause a progressive increase in the rate of deterioration. By buffering solutions to pH 5.5 to 7.5 deterioration is retarded. Dilute solutions are more stable than concentrated ones.

Incompatibilities with benzylpenicillin potassium or sodium have been reported in many studies (including B.B. Riley, *J. Hosp. Pharm.*, 1970, *28*, 228; B. Lynn and A. Jones, *Advances in Antimicrobial and Antineoplastic Chemotherapy*, Vol. I, pt 2, Munich, Urban and Schwarzenberg, 1972, p.701; L. Landersjö *et al., Acta pharm. suec.*, 1977, *14*, 293). The pH of the admixture solution is an important factor affecting the stability of benzylpenicillin and therefore the use of buffered or unbuffered benzylpenicillin solutions may affect its compatibility with other drugs.

Benzylpenicillin has been reported to be incompatible with metal ions and some rubber products. Its stability may be affected by ionic and nonionic surfactants, oxidising and reducing agents, alcohols, glycerol, glycols, macrogols and other hydroxy compounds, some paraffins and bases, some preservatives for example chlorocresol or thiomersal, carbohydrate solutions in an alkaline pH, fat emulsions, blood and blood products, and viscosity modifiers. Benzylpenicillin has been reported to be incompatible with acidic drugs such as ascorbic acid, metaraminol tartrate, oxytetracycline hydrochloride, or tetracycline hydrochloride; alkaline drugs such as aminophylline, pentobarbitone sodium, sodium bicarbonate, or thiopentone sodium; sympathomimetic amines such as noradrenaline acid tartrate; and aminothiol compounds such as cysteine. Incompatibility or loss of activity has also been reported with aminacrine hydrochloride, chlorpromazine hydrochloride, heparin sodium, hydroxyzine hydrochloride, iodine and iodides, magnesium sulphate, metoclopramide hydrochloride, phenytoin sodium, procaine hydrochloride, prochlorperazine salts, promazine hydrochloride, promethazine hydrochloride, thiamine hydrochloride, trometamol, and several other antimicrobial agents including amphotericin, cephaloridine, cephalothin sodium, erythromycin ethyl succinate, lincomycin hydrochloride, metronidazole, streptomycin sulphate, and vancomycin hydrochloride; incompatibilities have also been reported with gentamicin sulphate or tobramycin sulphate in human serum.

STABILITY IN SOLUTION. There was a linear relationship between the degradation-rate of benzylpenicillin and ampicillin and the concentration (up to 10%) of aqueous solutions of glucose, fructose, sucrose, dextran, sorbitol, mannitol, and glycerol to which they were added. The rate-accelerating effect was directly proportional to hydroxide ion concentration up to pH about 10.5 and it proceeded through a nucleophilic pathway with the intermediate formation of penicilloyl esters. These esters might contribute to the allergic reactions which occurred with penicillin and their formation could be reduced or avoided by adjusting the pH of these penicillin-containing solutions to between 6 and 6.5. Trace amounts of ferrous ions have been found to catalyse the fructose-accelerated degradation of benzylpenicillin and ampicillin by accelerating penicilloyl ester formation but this could be eliminated by the addition of edetate or citrate.— H. Bundgaard and C. Larsen, *Arch. Pharm. Chemi, scient. Edn.*, 1978, *6*, 184.

Discrepancies between published results for the stability of benzylpenicillin potassium or sodium depended on the use of buffered or unbuffered material. Unbuffered benzylpenicillin appeared to be stable in sodium chloride 0.9% injection or glucose 5% injection for 16 hours at room temperature; thereafter loss of activity was more rapid in glucose than in saline solution. Buffered benzylpenicillin appeared to be stable in several intravenous solutions for at least 24 hours at room temperature. Benzylpenicillin potassium in sodium chloride 0.9% or glucose 5% solutions frozen at −20° for up to 30 days and then thawed at room temperature or thawed rapidly in a microwave oven appeared to retain its activity.— B. Lynn, *Br. J. intraven. Ther.*, 1981, *2*, 22.

Benzylpenicillin 6 µg per mL in peritoneal dialysate solutions lost approximately 25% of activity when stored at room temperature for 24 hours; the pH of the dialysate solutions was 5.2.— D. L. Sewell and T. A. Golper, *Antimicrob. Ag. Chemother.*, 1982, *21*, 528.

A study of the degradation of benzylpenicillin eye-drops containing benzylpenicillin sodium 300 mg, sodium chloride 800 mg, sodium citrate 500 mg, phenylmercuric acetate 2 mg, and water to 100 mL, and similar eye-drops containing benzylpenicillin sodium 150 mg per 100 mL. When stored at 2 to 8°, a shelf-life of 30 days was suggested and for unopened bottles a shelf-life of 6 weeks might be appropriate.— T. Deeks *et al.*, *Pharm. J.*, 1984, *2*, 233. See also E. Osborn *et al.*, *Am. J. Ophthal.*, 1976, *82*, 775.

Benzylpenicillin sodium 1.2 g in solution was added to 50 mL minibags containing glucose 5% in water and the benzylpenicillin was found to be stable when stored at −20° for up to 39 days. During subsequent refrigeration at 5° there appeared to be a progressive decline in the potency and after 31 days approximately 10% of the antibiotic had decomposed in one batch although the observed loss was not significant for a second batch.— S. Rayani and F. Jamali, *Can. J. Hosp. Pharm.*, 1985, *38*, 162.

Unbuffered 2% aqueous solutions of benzylpenicillin and various other penicillins including carbenicillin, flucloxacillin, methicillin, mezlocillin, phenoxymethylpenicillin, temocillin,, and ticarcillin stored at 37° for 7 days were found to contain the degradation product *N*-formylpenicillamine. The extent of formation of this product ranged from negligible amounts produced by the amino and ureido compounds such as amoxycillin or mezlocillin to 15% for benzylpenicillin, and yields of 46 and 35% for methicillin and flucloxacillin, respectively. Storage of 4 important degradation products of benzylpenicillin at pH 5 for up to 6 hours demonstrated that the penicilloic, penilloic, and penillic acids of benzylpenicillin produced a small amount of penicillamine and no *N*-formylpenicillamine. However, benzylpenicillenic acid produced no penicillamine but rapidly produced *N*-formylpenicillamine.— A. E. Bird *et al.*, *J. Pharm. Pharmac.*, 1986, *38*, 913.

Units

One unit of penicillin was contained in 0.0005988 mg of the second International Standard Preparation (1952) of benzylpenicillin sodium which contained 1670 units per mg. The International Standard was discontinued in 1968 since penicillin can now be characterised completely by chemical tests.

Benzylpenicillin potassium 600 mg or benzylpenicillin sodium 600 mg have generally been considered to be approximately equivalent to 1 million units (1 mega unit).

Adverse Effects

The most common adverse effects associated with benzylpenicillin are allergic reactions and of these skin rashes occur most frequently. Administration of benzylpenicillin to a hypersensitive patient may occasionally result in anaphylactic shock with collapse and sometimes death occurring within minutes; angioedema or bronchospasm may also occur. A generalised sensitivity reaction with urticaria, fever, joint pains, and eosinophilia can develop within a few hours to several weeks after starting penicillin treatment. Other allergic reactions include exfoliative dermatitis and other skin reactions, interstitial nephritis, and vasculitis.

Haemolytic anaemia and leucopenia have been reported usually following high intravenous doses of benzylpenicillin; prolongation of bleeding time and defective platelet function has also been observed.

Sensitivity reactions to penicillins are considered to be due mainly to breakdown products or metabolites of penicillin, and possibly penicillin itself, acting as haptens which when combined with proteins and other macromolecules produce potential antigens (see under Allergy, below). As the hypersensitivity is related to the basic penicillin structure, patients who are allergic to benzylpenicillin must be assumed to be allergic to all penicillins; sensitised patients may also react to the cephalosporins.

Convulsions and other signs of toxicity to the central nervous system may occur with very high doses of benzylpenicillin, particularly when administered intravenously or to patients with renal failure; encephalopathy may also follow intrathecal administration. Disturbances of blood electrolytes may follow the administration of large doses of the potassium and sodium salts of benzylpenicillin. Transient increases in liver enzyme values have been reported rarely in patients receiving benzylpenicillin.

Some patients with syphilis may experience a Jarisch-Herxheimer reaction shortly after starting treatment with penicillin which is probably due to the release of endotoxins from the killed treponemes. Symptoms include fever, chills, headache, and reactions at the site of the lesions. The reaction can be dangerous in cardiovascular syphilis or where there is a serious risk of increased local damage such as with optic atrophy.

Benzylpenicillin may produce diarrhoea, nausea, and heartburn, usually following administration by mouth. A sore mouth or tongue, or a black, hairy tongue have occasionally been reported.

Tests for hypersensitivity may be used to determine those patients most likely to develop serious allergic reactions to penicillins. Skin tests are used to evaluate the current risk of immediate or accelerated IgE-mediated reactions, the most serious being anaphylaxis. Both the major and minor determinants of penicillin hypersensitivity should be used; the major determinant is available as Penicilloyl-polylysine (see p.943) and a minor-determinant mixture consisting of benzylpenicillin and its derivatives, including penicilloic acid and benzylpenicilloylamine can be used, although if this is not available a solution of benzylpenicillin may be substituted. The skin tests are usually carried out with very dilute solutions, as scratch tests followed, if negative, by intradermal tests. Adrenaline should be available in case an anaphylactic reaction develops. Both false-positive and false-negative results may occur. Patients with a true positive result have a significant risk of developing a serious reaction and up to two-thirds of these patients are likely to experience some form of reaction.

A number of *in vitro* tests including the radioallergosorbent test (RAST), the lymphocyte transformation test, haemagglutination assays, basophil degranulation, and the histamine release test have been developed.

Desensitisation has been attempted in patients allergic to penicillin when treatment with penicillin has been considered essential. However, desensitisation may be hazardous and should only be carried out if the patient can be monitored continuously and adrenaline and resuscitation equipment are immediately available. Desensitisation involves the administration of very small doses of penicillin given at relatively short intervals, such as 15 to 60 minutes, and gradually increased to therapeutic concentrations. Once the therapeutic doses have been reached the treatment should not be interrupted. Desensitisation has been accomplished using intradermal, subcutaneous, intravenous, and oral routes. Some workers consider the oral route to be safer than the parenteral route, although no comparative studies have been carried out; several penicillins including benzylpenicillin, carbenicillin, and phenoxymethylpenicillin have been successfully used for oral desensitisation (T.J. Sullivan *et al.*, *J. Allergy & clin. Immunol.*, 1982, *69*, 275; G.D. Wendel *et al.*, *New Engl. J. Med.*, 1985, *312*, 1229). Other workers prefer the intravenous route because of better dosage control and more rapid cessation of therapy if necessary (P.R. Ziaya *et al.*, *J. Am. med. Ass.*, 1986, *256*, 2561).

ALLERGY. The overall incidence of allergic reactions to penicillin has been reported to vary between 0.7 and 10% and anaphylactic reactions to occur in about 0.015 to 0.04% of patients treated (O. Idsøe *et al.*, *Bull. Wld Hlth Org.*, 1968, *38*, 159); anaphylaxis usually occurs after parenteral administration but has also been reported after taking penicillin by mouth (J. Simmonds *et al.*, *Br. med. J.*, 1978, *2*, 1404). An incidence of 1.85% for allergic skin reactions attributable to benzylpenicillin has been reported by the Boston Collaborative Drug Surveillance Program (M. Bigby *et al.*, *J. Am. med. Ass.*, 1986, *256*, 3358).

All penicillins contain the 6-aminopenicillanic acid nucleus from which the major and minor antigenic determinants are derived and therefore patients giving a clear history of allergy to any penicillin must usually be assumed to be allergic to all penicillins. Some patients may, however, have been incorrectly labelled "allergic to penicillin" (L. Beeley, *Br. med. J.*, 1984, *288*, 511). In a study of 2100 patients 78 of them were considered to be allergic to penicillin; of these 78 patients, 28 were re-exposed to penicillin, but only 4 experienced a further reaction (N.T.A. Oswald, *Br. med. J.*, 1983, *287*, 265).

Allergy to penicillin gives rise to a wide variety of clinical syndromes. Immediate reactions include anaphylaxis, angioedema, urticaria, and some maculopapular rashes. Late reactions include serum sickness-like reactions, haemolytic anaemia, and acute interstitial nephritis (L. Beeley, *Br. med. J.*, 1984, *288*, 511). Benzylpenicillin has been reported as a possible aetiological agent in other hypersensitivity reactions including hypersensitivity myocarditis (C.P. Taliercio *et al.*, *Mayo Clin. Proc.*, 1985, *60*, 463), hypersensitivity vasculitis (T. Hannedouche and J.P. Fillastre, *J. antimicrob. Chemother.*, 1987, *20*, 3), and systemic lupus erythematosus (S.J. Pearce, *Adverse Drug React. Bull.*, 1982, Jun., 344). Benzylpenicillin also causes other adverse reactions which are less clearly immunological such as some cases of neutropenia (see under Effects on the Blood, below).

An allergic response to penicillin is considered to be due, at least in part, to formation of protein conjugates of penicillin or its degradation products *in vivo* or by breakdown *in vitro* before administration. Most allergic reactions to penicillins are due to antibodies specific for the penicilloyl group which is known as the major determinant of penicillin hypersensitivity. However, other penicillin breakdown products such as penicilloic acid, which are quantitatively less important and known as minor determinants, are often responsible for immediate IgE-mediated hypersensitivity reactions such as anaphylaxis. In addition to protein conjugates, penicillin polymers formed by reaction of penicillins with themselves or with their degradation products, and products formed by reaction of penicillins with some pharmaceutical excipients such as carbohydrates have also been suggested as capable of eliciting reactions (H. Bundgaard, *J. clin. Hosp. Pharm.*, 1980, *5*, 73). Patients given freshly prepared benzylpenicillin solutions, by bolus injection to avoid the formation of degradation products, have been shown to have significantly lower concentrations of penicillin-specific IgG antibodies and sensitised lymphocytes, compared with patients given benzylpenicillin which has been stored in solution or administered by intravenous infusion for up to 24 hours (K.A. Neftel *et al.*, *Lancet*, 1982, *1*, 986). However, other authors have found that despite administration of fresh penicillin solutions as very rapid intravenous infusions or bolus doses some patients still developed neutropenia; this might reflect the possibility of a dose-related rather than pure immunological reaction (I. Anagnou, *Lancet*, 1984, *1*, 452; M.S. Al-Hadramy *et al.*, *J. antimicrob. Chemother.*, 1986, *17*, 251).

For comment on crossreactivity with penicillamine, see under Penicillamine, Precautions, p.849.

Antibiotics in foods. Of 245 patients suffering from chronic recurrent urticaria 59 patients (24%) demonstrated penicillin hypersensitivity through intracutaneous tests. A diet free of milk and milk products produced a favourable effect in 22 of 42 patients (52.3%) with positive skin tests whereas only 2 of 40 patients (5%) with negative skin tests showed good results. A rather high percentage of patients with chronic urticaria were found to be allergic to penicillin and in many of these patients the chronic urticaria appeared to be caused mainly by penicillin allergy and maintained by small amounts of penicillin in food.— W. J. Boonk and W. G. Van Ketel, *Br. J. Derm.*, 1982, *106*, 183.

EFFECTS ON THE BLOOD. *Neutropenia.* Neutropenia has been widely reported in patients receiving high doses of beta-lactam antibiotics, although patients with minor infections on short courses of oral antibiotics are in little danger. Warning signs of neutropenia include fever, rash, and eosinophilia, but monitoring of the leucocyte count is recommended in patients on long-term treatment with high doses (*Lancet*, 1985, *2*, 814). An incidence of from 0.1 to more than 15% has been reported in patients on high doses of penicillins or cephalosporins, the majority of cases occurring in patients treated for 10 days or more (K.A. Neftel *et al.*,

J. infect. Dis., 1985, *152*, 90). It has been suggested that the development of neutropenia appears to be related to the total dose of penicillin received (M.S. Al-Hadramy *et al.*, *J. antimicrob. Chemother.*, 1986, *17*, 251). There is controversy over the mechanisms responsible for beta-lactam-induced neutropenia. Some authors have proposed a direct toxic effect (G.M. Corbett *et al.*, *New Engl. J. Med.*, 1982, *307*, 1642; K.A. Neftel *et al.*, *J. infect. Dis.*, 1985, *152*, 90) whereas others have postulated an immune mechanism (M.F. Murphy *et al.*, *Br. J. Haemat.*, 1983, *55*, 155; B. Rouveix *et al.*, *Br. med. J.*, 1983, *287*, 1832). Murphy *et al.* (*Lancet*, 1985, *2*, 1306) suggested that the mechanism of neutropenia appeared to be similar to that of penicillin-induced haemolytic anaemia, at least in some patients, and that the relative contribution of immune and toxic factors may vary from patient to patient.

EFFECTS ON THE CARDIOVASCULAR SYSTEM. See Allergy, above, and Overdosage, below.

EFFECTS ON THE NERVOUS SYSTEM. The Boston Collaborative Drug Surveillance Program monitored consecutively 32 812 medical inpatients. Drug-induced convulsions occurred in 5 of 3901 patients given penicillins. Four were given benzylpenicillin intravenously and 1 was given oxacillin intravenously.— J. Porter and H. Jick, *Lancet*, 1977, *1*, 587.

OVERDOSAGE. Haemodialysis has been used to treat penicillin intoxication, however, one patient who was receiving regular haemodialysis for analgesic nephropathy developed intoxication with severe central nervous system symptoms following large doses of benzylpenicillin. The patient was successfully treated with combined charcoal haemoperfusion and haemodialysis; it appeared that charcoal haemoperfusion was more efficient than dialysis in removing penicillin.— C. J. Wickerts *et al.*, *Br. med. J.*, 1980, *280*, 1254.

The recovery of a woman who was accidentally given benzylpenicillin 1.2 g intrathecally in mistake for 12 mg. Intravenous phenytoin and diazepam did not control the seizures which developed 45 minutes later, therefore she was paralysed, intubated, ventilated, and given thiopentone sodium by infusion. A neurosurgeon drained off 50 mL of CSF and replaced it with 40 mL of physiological saline. A further 40 mL of CSF was drained off 12 hours later, and 30 hours after the overdose the thiopentone infusion was stopped. Despite infusion of dopamine the patient remained severely hypotensive for a further 4 days; 36 hours after the thiopentone withdrawal several focal seizures and one grand mal seizure were controlled with intravenous clonazepam and sodium valproate by mouth. She remained unresponsive for 10 days; at 2 weeks she was speaking a little and beginning to feed herself; at 3 weeks she was walking unaided and her performance on simple verbal and arithmetic tests was better than on admission, but her short-term memory was poorer.— C. Marks and B. H. Cummins (letter), *Lancet*, 1981, *1*, 658.

A report of cardiac arrest in an 11-month-old boy who accidentally received over 300 mg per kg body-weight of benzylpenicillin, administered as the potassium salt, by an intravenous bolus dose; the ventricular arrhythmias were consistent with hyperkalaemia.— J. L. Stumpf (letter), *Drug Intell. & clin. Pharm.*, 1987, *21*, 292.

TESTS FOR HYPERSENSITIVITY. A review of the technique and usefulness of penicillin skin testing.— G. L. Sussman *et al.*, *Can. med. Ass. J.*, 1986, *134*, 1353.

In a study involving 740 patients, many with histories of apparent allergic reactions to beta-lactam antibiotics, 469 patients (63%) were found to be skin-test positive; skin testing was carried out using penicilloyl-polylysine, benzylpenicillin, and benzylpenicilloic acid. The prevalence of positive skin tests was related to the time that had elapsed between clinical allergic reactions and skin testing; 13 of 14 patients (93%) tested 6 to 12 months after a reaction were positive, whereas only 22% of the patients tested 10 years or more after a reaction were skin-test positive. None of 83 history-positive, skin-test negative patients, who received beta-lactam antibiotics promptly after immunologic assessment experienced immediate allergic reactions although 2 patients developed mild generalised urticaria 3 and 5 days after initiation of intravenous therapy. However, an allergic reaction did occur in a 7-year-old boy given penicillin by mouth 6 months after negative penicillin skin tests, which emphasised the unreliability of skin test results if significant time has elapsed before beginning therapy.— T. J. Sullivan *et al.*, *J. Allergy & clin. Immunol.*, 1981, *68*, 171.

Further references: C. Smolders, *Can. J. Hosp. Pharm.*, 1987, *40*, 69.

Precautions

Patients known to be hypersensitive to penicillin should be given an antibiotic of another class. However, sensitised patients may also react to the cephalosporins. Penicillin should be given with caution to patients with a history of allergy, especially to other drugs. Care is necessary if very high doses of penicillin are given, especially if renal function is poor, because of the risk of neurotoxicity. The intrathecal route should be avoided. Care is also necessary if large doses of the potassium or sodium salts are given to patients with impaired renal function or congestive heart failure and high doses of benzylpenicillin potassium should be used with caution in patients receiving potassium-containing drugs or potassium-sparing diuretics. Renal and haematological systems should be monitored during prolonged and high-dose therapy. Because of the Jarisch-Herxheimer reaction care is also necessary when treating some patients with syphilis.

Contact with penicillin should be avoided since skin sensitisation may occur.

One of the dangers of penicillin therapy is the emergence of supra-infection by resistant species such as *Pseudomonas*, or *Candida* which do not respond to penicillin therapy.

Interactions. Probenecid prolongs the half-life of benzylpenicillin by competing with it for renal tubular secretion. Some other drugs including some non-steroidal anti-inflammatory agents also appear to compete with benzylpenicillin for renal tubular secretion (J. Kampmann *et al.*, *Clin. Pharmac. Ther.*, 1972, *13*, 516). Benzylpenicillin may also interact with bacteriostatic antimicrobial agents (see under Antimicrobial Action, below).

Benzylpenicillin may interfere with some diagnostic tests such as those for urinary glucose using copper sulphate, and some tests for urinary or serum proteins. Benzylpenicillin may interfere with tests that use bacteria, for example the Guthrie test for phenylketonuria using *Bacillus subtilis* organisms. Various methods have been used to avoid antibiotic inhibition of this test including treatment with acids and/or alkalis (G. Bracco and S. Pagliardini, *Lancet*, 1983, *1*, 1331), autoclaving, or taking the blood sample before administration of a dose of antibiotic (P. Clemens *et al.*, *ibid.*, 1985, *2*, 778).

Several penicillins including benzylpenicillin have been reported to inactivate the aminoglycosides in human serum in a reaction that is dependent on temperature, concentration, and time.— R. J. Tindula *et al.*, *Drug Intell. & clin. Pharm.*, 1983, *17*, 906.

For further comments on the effects of beta-lactam antibiotics, including benzylpenicillin, on aminoglycosides, see under Gentamicin Sulphate, Incompatibility, p.236.

ADMINISTRATION IN RENAL FAILURE. For reference to the precautions to be observed in renal failure, see under Uses, Administration in Renal Failure, p.136.

NEUTROPENIA. Patients with bone-marrow failure, usually as a consequence of cytotoxic drug therapy, commonly receive large doses of beta-lactam antibiotics; care is required with such treatment. Controversy exists regarding the optimum duration of antibiotic therapy in patients with neutropenia: some workers recommend that the antibiotics be continued until the neutrophil count recovers, whereas others favour a limited course because of the risks of secondary infection if antibiotics are continued for longer than a week. Beta-lactam antibiotics have also been reported to prolong neutropenia in patients with acute myeloid leukaemia, and if these findings are confirmed the clinician will have to weigh the risks of delaying marrow recovery against those of failing to control a potentially fatal infection.— *Lancet*, 1985, *2*, 814.

Antimicrobial Action

Benzylpenicillin has a mainly bactericidal action against many Gram-positive bacteria and some Gram-negative cocci, and against some spirochaetes and actinomycetes.

It is considered to act through interference with the final stage of synthesis of the bacterial cell wall. The action depends upon benzylpenicillin's ability to reach and bind to certain membrane-bound proteins known as penicillin-binding proteins (PBPs) that are located beneath the cell wall. These proteins are involved in maintaining cell wall structure, in cell wall synthesis, and in cell division, and appear to possess transpeptidase and carboxypeptidase activity. Bacterial surface enzymes called autolysins also appear to be involved in the lethal effect of penicillins particularly for Gram-positive bacteria. In Gram-negative bacilli, osmotic rupture of cells may occur once the cell wall is weakened. Benzylpenicillin can also produce morphological changes *in vitro* including the formation of long filaments or abnormally shaped cells. Bacteria that are not growing and dividing are generally not killed by benzylpenicillin.

Its action is inhibited by penicillinase and other beta-lactamases that are produced during the growth of certain micro-organisms.

The sensitivity of bacteria to benzylpenicillin varies widely, even among the genera that are normally susceptible, especially as the incidence of beta-lactamase-producing organisms is increasing.

The following pathogenic organisms are usually sensitive to benzylpenicillin in the concentrations commonly achieved in the body during treatment: Gram-positive aerobes and anaerobes including *Bacillus anthracis*, *Clostridium* spp. (except *Cl. difficile*), *Corynebacterium diphtheriae*, *Erysipelothrix rhusiopathiae*, *Listeria monocytogenes*, some staphylococci (non-beta-lactamase-producing), and some streptococci but not enterococci or some viridans streptococci; Gram-negative cocci including *Branhamella catarrhalis*, *Neisseria meningitidis* (meningococci), and *Neisseria gonorrhoeae* (gonococci), although increasing resistance is occurring in *Branhamella catarrhalis* and gonococci. Gram-negative bacilli are generally less susceptible to benzylpenicillin, however, *Pasteurella multocida*, *Streptobacillus moniliformis*, *Spirillum minus*, and some strains of *Haemophilus* spp. are usually susceptible; many Gram-negative anaerobes are also sensitive to benzylpenicillin including some *Bacteroides* spp. (except *B. fragilis*) and *Fusobacterium* spp. Other organisms that are usually sensitive include *Actinomyces*, *Borrelia*, *Leptospira*, and *Treponema* spp. The minimum inhibitory concentrations of benzylpenicillin for these organisms have been reported to range from 0.006 to 2 μg per mL; bactericidal concentrations are generally considered to be 5 to 10 times greater, but tolerance may develop (see Resistance, below).

Among pathogenic micro-organisms usually insensitive to benzylpenicillin are *Acinetobacter* spp. and most Gram-negative bacilli including *Pseudomonas* spp. and *Enterobacteriaceae*, although some of these organisms such as some strains of *Proteus mirabilis* may be inhibited by high concentrations of benzylpenicillin. Other organisms which are insensitive include mycobacteria, fungi (though not *Actinomyces*), mycoplasmas, rickettsias, and most viruses.

Benzylpenicillin may exhibit synergy with other antimicrobial agents particularly the aminoglycosides. Its activity may be enhanced by clavulanic acid and similar drugs that inhibit beta-lactamase activity, and both enhancement and antagonism have been demonstrated between beta-lactam combinations. Antagonism has been reported to occur with some bacteriostatic agents, such as chloramphenicol, that interfere with active bacterial growth necessary for benzylpenicillin to achieve its effect. However, the clinical relevance of this is not clear.

See also p.107 for a brief discussion on the penicillin group of antibiotics.

Benzylpenicillin was active *in vitro* against *Campylobacter pyloridis*.— C. A. M. McNulty *et al.*, *Antimicrob. Ag. Chemother.*, 1985, *28*, 837.

ACTIVITY WITH OTHER ANTIMICROBIAL AGENTS. Synergy between beta-lactam compounds and aminoglycosides has been attributed to enhanced penetration of the aminoglycoside secondary to beta-lactam induced cell wall destruction (J.E. Kapusnik and S.L. Barriere, *Drug Interact. News.*, 1982, *2*, 35; I. Brook *et al.*, *Antimicrob. Ag. Chemother.*, 1984, *25*, 71). Synergism has been demonstrated between benzylpenicillin and gentamicin, or other aminoglycosides, against some Gram-positive organisms and some Gram-negative anaerobic organisms including lactobacilli, *Bacteroides* spp., and some streptococci (A.S. Bayer *et al.*, *Antimicrob. Ag. Chemother.*, 1980, *17*, 359; I. Brook *et al.*, *ibid.*, 1984, *25*, 71; K. Lam and A.S. Bayer, *ibid.*, *26*, 260), but studies *in vitro* have not always reflected the action *in vivo* (A. Bouvet *et al.*, *Antimicrob. Ag. Chemother.*, 1985, *28*, 607; I. Brook and R.I. Walker, *J. antimicrob. Chemother.*, 1985, *15*, 31). There have been reports of synergy between benzylpenicillin and gentamicin or netilmicin against enterococci (J. Carrizosa and M.E. Levison, *Antimicrob. Ag. Chemother.*, 1981, *20*, 405; J.J. Rahal and M.S. Simberkoff, *J. antimicrob. Chemother.*, 1986, *17*, 585), however, high level resistance of enterococci to gentamicin has increased, preventing synergy with penicillin (P.J. Sanderson, *Br. med. J.*, 1984, *289*, 638); antagonism has been reported between penicillin and amikacin against enterococci (C. Thauvin *et al.*, *Antimicrob. Ag. Chemother.*, 1985, *28*, 78).

When beta-lactamase-producing organisms are present, beta-lactamase inhibitors such as clavulanic acid may enhance the activity of benzylpenicillin as has been demonstrated against *Bacteroides* spp. (A. Eley and D. Greenwood, *J. antimicrob. Chemother.*, 1986, *18*, 325).

Combinations of beta-lactam antibiotics have shown synergy and antagonism. Synergy may occur because beta-lactamase inhibition by one agent prevents the hydrolysis of the other, or because each antibiotic binds to different target proteins. Antagonism of beta-lactam combinations *in vitro* may result from induction of beta-lactamases by one of the antimicrobials or because competition for, or alteration of, cell protein-binding sites may occur (J.E. Kapusnik and S.L. Barriere, *Drug Interact. News.*, 1982, *2*, 35). The final effect of beta-lactam combinations depends on the particular combination used and the characteristics of the organism concerned. Since antagonism between penicillins and cephalosporins may have clinical importance, it has been suggested that beta-lactam combinations should be avoided until clinical studies have shown a definite advantage over a single beta-lactam or a beta-lactam plus an aminoglycoside (S.J. Pedler and A.J. Bint, *Br. med. J.*, 1984, *288*, 1022).

Antagonism has been reported *in vitro* between benzylpenicillin and several other antimicrobial agents including chloroquine phosphate against *Staphylococcus aureus* (M.A. Toama *et al.*, *J. pharm. Sci.*, 1978, *67*, 23), erythromycin against *Listeria monocytogenes* (R.L. Penn *et al.*, *Antimicrob. Ag. Chemother.*, 1982, *22*, 289), and polymyxin B against *Proteus mirabilis* (I.J. Sud and D.S. Feingold, *ibid.*, 1978, *14*, 916). Bacteriostatic drugs such as chloramphenicol might antagonise the bactericidal action of penicillin, and clinical studies have demonstrated no benefit in giving chloramphenicol plus benzylpenicillin compared with chloramphenicol alone to treat children with bacterial meningitis or severe pneumonia (F. Shann *et al.*, *Lancet*, 1985, *2*, 681; *idem*, 684). However, some authors have found additive effects or limited synergy *in vitro* between penicillin and tetracycline or erythromycin against *Chlamydia trachomatis* (S.J. How *et al.*, *J. antimicrob. Chemother.*, 1985, *15*, 533).

Additive or synergistic effects were found with benzylpenicillin and probenecid against *Neisseria gonorrhoeae in vitro*. Probenecid appeared to potentiate the action of benzylpenicillin, in addition to its own pharmacological effects.— B. W. Catlin, *Antimicrob. Ag. Chemother.*, 1984, *25*, 676.

Resistance

Susceptible Gram-positive bacteria may develop resistance through the induction of beta-lactamases, including penicillinases. These enzymes are liberated extracellularly and hydrolyse the beta-lactam ring of the antibiotic. This resistance is usually plasmid-mediated and can be transferred from one bacterium to another. Resistance can also be acquired through chromosomal mutation; this has led for example to changes in the penicillin-binding proteins (PBPs).

Many Gram-negative organisms are intrinsically resistant by virtue of the inability of benzylpenicillin to penetrate their outer membranes. Intrinsic resistance can also be due to structural differences in the target penicillin-binding proteins. Gram-negative bacteria often produce small amounts of beta-lactamases which are present within the cell membranes. Beta-lactamase production can be altered by induction, mutation, or by the acquisition of resistance plasmids (R-plasmids). Resistance plasmids and also transposons containing genetic information for resistance to antibiotics can be transferred between bacteria by conjugation causing resistance to multiple drugs.

Some organisms, usually Gram-positive cocci such as staphylococci or streptococci, may be inhibited but not killed by benzylpenicillin and in such cases the minimum bactericidal concentration (MBC) is much greater than the minimum inhibitory concentration (MIC); this is known as tolerance.

Many organisms are showing increased resistance to benzylpenicillin particularly because of beta-lactamase production and these include a high proportion of staphylococci and *Branhamella catarrhalis*. The incidence of penicillinase-producing *Neisseria gonorrhoeae* (PPNG) has increased, but reduced sensitivity of gonococci to benzylpenicillin is also due to alterations in the penicillin-binding proteins. Altered penicillin-binding proteins have also developed in *Streptococcus pneumoniae* and resistance appears to be increasing. Resistant strains of other species usually sensitive to benzylpenicillin have emerged among *Bacillus anthracis* and *Corynebacterium diphtheriae*.

Failure of treatment with benzylpenicillin, in a 46-year-old man with a pleural effusion due to haemolytic group B streptococci sensitive to penicillin, was considered to be due to an enzyme (not a beta-lactamase) probably from the cell wall of the patient's leucocytes.— P. Barnes and P. M. Waterworth, *Br. med. J.*, 1977, *1*, 991. Four of 22 samples of human pus inactivated up to 90% of added penicillin within 1 hour *in vitro*. It was considered due to an enzyme in the pus, possibly an amidase; beta-lactamase was not detected.— J. de Louvois and R. Hurley, *ibid.*, 998.

Comment on penicillin-tolerant bacteria and the view that laboratories should be prepared to measure MICs and MBCs of isolates from serious infections where delayed or poor response to therapy is unexplained. Disk sensitivity tests alone may be misleading.— *Lancet*, 1980, *1*, 856.

Beta-lactamase-producing strains of *Bacteroides* spp. and *Staph. aureus* were present in the tonsils of 23 and 24 of 50 children with chronic recurrent tonsillitis, respectively. It was considered that these beta-lactamase-producing organisms might protect penicillin-susceptible group A β-haemolytic streptococci resulting in the failure of penicillin treatment.— I. Brook *et al.* (letter), *Lancet*, 1981, *1*, 332.

Penicillin-binding proteins (PBPs) essential for growth of *Escherichia coli* and several other Gram-negative rods have been identified as PBP 1, 2, and 3; other PBPs (PBP 4, 5, and 6) are considered non-essential because they are saturated by antibiotic concentrations far above the MIC and also mutants defective in these proteins grow normally. Beta-lactam antibiotics that specifically bind one or more of the essential PBPs have been considered the most useful for inhibiting bacterial growth. However, both enterococci and methicillin-resistant *Staphylococcus aureus* strains have been found to synthesise a PBP which appears to be non-essential for normal growth, but which under certain conditions can take over the functions of all other PBPs, thus becoming the only one essential for growth. This protein has a low sensitivity to many beta-lactams and has been named 'low-affinity PBP'. Cells overproducing this protein have been shown to grow in the presence of penicillin concentrations saturating all PBPs except the low-affinity PBP, and to stop growing in the presence of the minimal concentration of antibiotic saturating this protein. Although only Gram-positive cocci have been demonstrated to possess this novel mechanism of resistance to beta-lactams, it is possible that the target for growth inhibition could shift to otherwise non-essential PBPs in other bacteria as well.— R. Fontana, *J. antimicrob. Chemother.*, 1985, *16*, 412.

RESISTANCE OF ANAEROBIC ORGANISMS. Penicillin resistance has increased among the non-fragilis *Bacteroides* spp. and concentrations of 12.5, 50, and 100 µg per mL were required to inhibit 50, 70, and 90% of 43 strains tested. This resistance was related to the production of beta-lactamase and 59% of 559 strains tested were positive for beta-lactamase production. Penicillin resistance among some *Clostridium* spp., except *Cl. perfringens*, was also noted particularly for *Cl. innocuum* and *Cl. clostridiiforme*.— R. S. Edson *et al.*, *Mayo Clin. Proc.*, 1982, *57*, 737. Further comment on the increasing resistance of *Bacteroides* spp. to benzylpenicillin and similar beta-lactam agents.— H. M. Wexler and S. M. Finegold, *J. antimicrob. Chemother.*, 1987, *19*, 143.

Bacteroides fragilis. Of 60 strains of *Bacteroides fragilis* 59 were resistant to benzylpenicillin.— O. A. Okubadejo *et al.*, *Br. med. J.*, 1973, *2*, 212.

RESISTANCE OF GONOCOCCI. Antimicrobial resistance among gonococci results either from chromosomal mutations causing progressive increases in resistance or from the emergence of plasmid-mediated penicillinase-producing strains. The first penicillinase-producing strains of *Neisseria gonorrhoeae* (PPNG) appeared in the Philippines and in West Africa in 1976, although different plasmids were responsible for the resistance in the 2 areas. Beta-lactamase-producing strains have now spread to most countries of the world. In East and South-East Asia and sub-Saharan Africa, one-third to one-half of the gonococcal isolates are penicillinase-producing strains; in most industrialised countries the proportion of PPNG is about 1%, although in the *USA* and the *UK* beta-lactamase-producing strains continue to increase (WHO Expert Committee on Venereal Diseases and Treponematoses, *Tech. Rep. Ser. Wld Hlth Org. No. 736*, 1986). In the *USA* 1.8% of all cases of gonorrhoea reported to the Centers for Disease Control (CDC) during 1986 were caused by PPNG, which represented a 90% increase over the PPNG cases reported in 1985. Most of the cases occurred in hyperendemic areas, but PPNG is spreading to previously unaffected areas. Once antibiotic-resistant gonorrhoea has become endemic, the CDC recommends that all patients with a presumptive diagnosis of gonorrhoea should be treated with either ceftriaxone or spectinomycin (*J. Am. med. Ass.*, 1987, *257*, 1579).

Penicillin resistance among non-PPNG existed long before the emergence of PPNG. Unlike PPNG this form of resistance results from mutations at several chromosomal loci and alterations to the gonococcal cell envelope. Resistant non-PPNG have penicillin-binding proteins with a reduced affinity for penicillin, but other mechanisms may also be involved. Mutations at a series of loci on the chromosome result in small additive increases in penicillin resistance and eventually produce isolates with clinically significant resistance. Mutations at some loci, however, result in increased resistance not only to penicillin, but also to other antibiotics, for example erythromycin, tetracycline, and chloramphenicol. Antibiotic-resistant non-PPNG are becoming more common and may prove to be a more difficult problem than PPNG, as there is no simple rapid screening test for them and they are more likely to be resistant to a range of antibiotics (C.S.F. Easmon, *J. antimicrob. Chemother.*, 1985, *16*, 409). Outbreaks of gonorrhoea have occurred in which non-penicillinase-producing gonococcal strains exhibited relatively high resistance to penicillin (MIC 2 to 4 µg per mL) and to certain other antimicrobial agents, resulting in treatment failures after standard penicillin therapy (B.E. Britigan *et al.*, *New Engl. J. Med.*, 1985, *312*, 1683).

RESISTANCE OF MENINGOCOCCI. A strain of *Neisseria meningitidis* has been isolated with a beta-lactamase-producing plasmid and a transfer plasmid identical in size to plasmids found in penicillinase-producing *N. gonorrhoeae* (PPNG). The isolate was probably of urogenital origin and demonstrates the spread of plasmids from the gonococcus to *N. meningitidis*.— J. R. Dillon *et al.*, *Lancet*, 1983, *1*, 779.

RESISTANCE OF STAPHYLOCOCCI. Three general types of resistance to the penicillins and cephalosporins by staphylococci have been described. The first is drug inactivation due to beta-lactamases which are usually inducible enzymes. The epidemiological increase in the number of penicillinase-producing staphylococci has progressively limited the usefulness of benzylpenicillin. The second form of resistance is intrinsic, which is due to some mechanism other than inactivation of the antibiotic, and accounts for methicillin-resistant *Staphylococcus aureus*. Intrinsic resistance is partly associated with differences in the affinity of beta-lactams for penicillin-binding proteins but the phenotypic expression of resistance is affected by chemical and physical factors. The third form of resistance is tolerance to the killing action of the antibiotic so that the MBC is 32 or more times greater than the MIC. The tolerance phenomenon appears to be due to decreased autolytic activity and persistence of an inhibitor of the bacterial autolysins. A bacteriophage may play a role in transferring the tolerance trait from one strain to another.— L. D. Sabath, *Ann. intern. Med.*, 1982, *97*, 339. Further comment on intrinsic resistance.— S. J. Seligman (letter), *ibid.*, 931.

Few strains of *Staphylococcus aureus* are now sensitive to penicillin, even if they are acquired in the community setting, and therefore beta-lactamase-resistant antibiotics should always be used unless the results of susceptibility tests show sensitivity to penicillin.— J. N. Sheagren, *New Engl. J. Med.*, 1984, *310*, 1437.

There is evidence of widespread background resistance to benzylpenicillin and commonly used antibiotics in

Staphylococcus epidermidis.— A. J. Davies and A. Dyas (letter), *J. antimicrob. Chemother.*, 1985, *15*, 127.

RESISTANCE OF STREPTOCOCCI. Tolerance to benzylpenicillin has been reported in clinical isolates of group B streptococci (A. Broadbent, *J. antimicrob. Chemother.*, 1984, *13*, 396), group C streptococci (D. Portnoy *et al.*, *Antimicrob. Ag. Chemother.*, 1981, *20*, 235), and group G streptococci (J.T. Noble *et al.*, *Lancet*, 1980, *2*, 982), and has occurred frequently enough to justify careful susceptibility testing including determination of MBCs (K.V.I. Rolston *et al.*, *J. antimicrob. Chemother.*, 1984, *13*, 389). Penicillin-tolerant viridans streptococci have also been isolated (J. Dankert and J. Hess, *Lancet*, 1982, *2*, 1219) and therapeutic problems in patients with endocarditis due to penicillin-tolerant viridans streptococci (A.W. Anderson and J.G. Cruickshank, *Br. med. J.*, 1982, *285*, 854) and penicillin-tolerant group C streptococci (D. Portnoy *et al.*, *Can. med. Ass. J.*, 1980, *122*, 69) have been reported.

Pneumococci. Resistance of *Streptococcus pneumoniae* to benzylpenicillin appears to be increasing (P.J. Sanderson, *Br. med. J.*, 1984, *289*, 638) and highly penicillin-resistant strains of pneumococci have been shown to have altered penicillin-binding proteins (S. Handwerger and A. Tomasz, *Antimicrob. Ag. Chemother.*, 1986, *30*, 57). The prevalence of resistant strains has been reported to range from 1 to 16%. However, in a study in Spain, pneumococci were isolated from the nasopharynx of 159 (48.7%) of 326 healthy children aged 4 to 5 years, and 57 of the strains (35.9%) showed decreased susceptibility to benzylpenicillin indicating an important reservoir of resistant pneumococci in the community (J.L. Pérez *et al.*, *J. antimicrob. Chemother.*, 1987, *19*, 278). Resistant pneumococci have been divided into intermediate, or relative, resistance with MICs of benzylpenicillin ranging from 0.1 to 1.0 μg per mL (A.J. Saah *et al.*, *J. Am. med. Ass.*, 1980, *243*, 1824) and full resistance. Intermediate resistance is considered unlikely to cause therapeutic problems in the treatment of pneumonia (M. Gratten *et al.*, *Lancet*, 1980, *2*, 192). Although the death of a patient infected with a pneumococcus of intermediate resistance has been reported, this death could not be attributed solely to the failure of penicillin therapy (C. Feldman *et al.*, *New Engl. J. Med.*, 1985, *313*, 615). Treatment of patients with meningitis associated with intermediate-resistant pneumococci may be a problem because of the relatively poor concentrations of benzylpenicillin achieved in the CSF even with inflamed meninges (M. Gratten *et al.*, *Lancet*, 1980, *2*, 192); the death of such a patient has occurred (G.M. Caputo *et al.*, *Ann. intern. Med.*, 1983, *98*, 416). Pneumococci fully resistant to penicillin, with MICs as high as 16 μg per mL, and resistant to several other antibiotics have also been reported (M.R. Jacobs *et al.*, *New Engl. J. Med.*, 1978, *299*, 735; J.I. Ward and R.C. Moellering, *Antimicrob. Ag. Chemother.*, 1981, *20*, 204; F.K. Gould *et al.*, *J. Infect.*, 1987, *15*, 77) and deaths have occurred in patients with pneumonia due to these resistant pneumococci (C. Feldman *et al.*, *New Engl. J. Med.*, 1985, *313*, 615; R. Pallares *et al.*, *ibid.*, 1987, *317*, 18). Multiple resistant pneumococci showing resistance to tetracycline, clindamycin, erythromycin, and co-trimoxazole, but susceptible to benzylpenicillin have also been reported (K.P. Klugman *et al.*, *Br. med. J.*, 1986, *292*, 730).

Absorption and Fate

Benzylpenicillin rapidly appears in the blood following intramuscular injection of water-soluble salts, and maximum concentrations are usually reached in 15 to 30 minutes; peak plasma concentrations of about 12 μg per mL have been reported after single doses of 600 mg.

When given by mouth, benzylpenicillin is inactivated fairly rapidly by the acid gastric secretions and only up to about 30% is absorbed, mainly from the duodenum; maximum plasma-penicillin concentrations usually occur in about an hour. In order to attain plasma-penicillin concentrations after oral administration comparable to those following intramuscular injection, up to 5 times as much benzylpenicillin may be necessary. Absorption varies greatly in different individuals and is better in patients with achlorhydria, and in infants and elderly patients with reduced gastric acidity. Food decreases the absorption of benzylpenicillin and oral doses are best given no later than half an hour before and no earlier than 2 to 3 hours after a meal.

Benzylpenicillin is widely distributed at varying concentrations in body tissues and fluids. It appears in pleural, pericardial, peritoneal, and synovial fluids but diffuses only to a small extent into abscess cavities, avascular areas, the eye, the middle ear, and the CSF. Inflamed tissue is, however, more readily penetrated. Benzylpenicillin diffuses across the placenta into the foetal circulation, and small amounts appear in the milk of nursing mothers.

The plasma half-life is about 30 minutes although it may be longer in neonates and the elderly because of incomplete renal function. In renal failure the half-life may be increased to about 10 hours. Approximately 60% is reported to be bound to plasma protein.

Benzylpenicillin is metabolised to a limited extent and the penicilloic acid derivative has been recovered in the urine. Benzylpenicillin is rapidly excreted in the urine, principally by tubular secretion and about 20% of a dose given by mouth appears unchanged in the urine; about 60 to 90% of a dose of aqueous benzylpenicillin given intramuscularly appears in the urine mainly within the first hour. Significant concentrations are achieved in bile, but in patients with normal renal function only small amounts are excreted via the bile.

Tubular excretion is inhibited by probenecid (see p.440), which is sometimes given to increase plasma-penicillin concentrations.

A review of the pharmacokinetics of the penicillins.— M. Barza and L. Weinstein, *Clin. Pharmacokinet.*, 1976, *1*, 297.

A study of protein binding of penicillins to human serum albumin.— H. Zia *et al.*, *Can. J. pharm. Sci.*, 1980, *15*, 14.

Benzylpenicillin and 3 cephalosporin antibiotics penetrated human polymorphonuclear leucocytes poorly, probably reflecting the limited lipid solubility of these drugs. These antibiotics would therefore not inactivate organisms that survive intracellularly after ingestion by phagocytic cells.— R. C. Prokesch and W. L. Hand, *Antimicrob. Ag. Chemother.*, 1982, *21*, 373.

Probenecid inhibits the renal transport of penicillin, but it also interferes with the active transport of penicillin and other organic acids from the CSF via the choroid plexus. Probenecid may, therefore, be of benefit in maintaining the concentration of penicillin in the CSF in the treatment of meningitis.— *Lancet*, 1984, *2*, 499.

ADMINISTRATION IN RENAL FAILURE. The half-life of benzylpenicillin could be increased from 0.5 to 6 to 20 hours in end-stage renal disease.— W. M. Bennett *et al.*, *Am. J. Kidney Dis.*, 1983, *3*, 155.

The plasma-protein binding of benzylpenicillin had been reported to be decreased in patients with poor renal function.— M. M. Reidenberg and D. E. Drayer, *Clin. Pharmacokinet.*, 1984, *9*, *Suppl.* 1, 18.

Haemodialysis. Benzylpenicillin is removed by haemodialysis; the half-life has been decreased by 45% at a dialysis rate of 30 to 50 mL per minute.— M. Barza and L. Weinstein, *Clin. Pharmacokinet.*, 1976, *1*, 297.

In patients undergoing haemodialysis, with a dialysis clearance calculated as 42 mL per minute, the half-life of benzylpenicillin has been reported to be 2.3 hours.— C. -s. C. Lee and T. C. Marbury, *Clin. Pharmacokinet.*, 1984, *9*, 42.

DIFFUSION INTO BODY TISSUES AND FLUIDS. For a report of the diffusion of benzylpenicillin and cloxacillin into the atrium and diseased valve of patients undergoing open-heart surgery for valvular diseases, see under Cloxacillin Sodium, p.203.

Uses and Administration

Benzylpenicillin is used in the treatment of a variety of infections due to susceptible organisms, including abscesses, actinomycosis, anthrax, leptospirosis, Lyme disease, skin infections including erysipelas, wound infections, gas gangrene, tetanus, gonorrhoea, syphilis, yaws, pinta, rat-bite fever, diphtheria, pneumococcal pneumonia, scarlet fever, tonsillitis, Vincent's infection, rheumatic fever, some types of subacute bacterial endocarditis, meningitis, otitis media, and osteomyelitis.

Benzylpenicillin is also used prophylactically before dental and surgical procedures in patients at risk of developing endocarditis and to prevent a recurrence of rheumatic fever.

Whenever possible, cultural identification of the infecting organism and sensitivity tests should be carried out, but treatment should be started immediately in severe infections that are suspected to be caused by organisms normally sensitive to benzylpenicillin. For infections such as bacterial endocarditis, a second antibiotic, usually an aminoglycoside, may be given in addition to benzylpenicillin to enhance the antibacterial activity. Due to the increase in beta-lactamase-producing organisms, beta-lactamase-resistant penicillins or cephalosporins are often used until the absence of beta-lactamase is demonstrated. Once the results of the sensitivity tests are known the dosage and frequency of administration can be adjusted or another antibiotic used if necessary.

Benzylpenicillin is administered as the potassium or sodium salt. Doses are expressed in terms of the equivalent amount of benzylpenicillin. The dose of benzylpenicillin should be sufficient to achieve an optimum bactericidal concentration in the blood as rapidly as possible. For some of the infections listed above doses of 0.6 to 2.4 g daily in 2 to 4 divided doses by intramuscular or intravenous injection may be adequate, but doses of 3 to 12 g daily given intravenously, often by infusion, are more usual, particularly for severe infections such as endocarditis or meningitis; higher doses of 24 g or more daily may be used. In subacute bacterial endocarditis and osteomyelitis treatment should be continued for at least 4 to 6 weeks.

The plasma concentration of benzylpenicillin may be increased by concurrent administration of probenecid (see p.440). If high plasma-penicillin concentrations are not required then treatment with parenteral penicillin might be more easily carried out using slow-release forms such as benzathine penicillin or procaine penicillin.

Infants and children from 1 month to 12 years may be given 10 to 20 mg per kg body-weight daily in divided doses, which may be increased to 40 mg per kg daily in meningitis; doses of up to 240 mg per kg daily have been given in severe infections. Neonates may be given 30 mg per kg daily; this may be increased to 90 mg per kg daily in meningitis.

High doses should be administered slowly to avoid irritation of the central nervous system and electrolyte imbalance; it has been recommended that intravenous doses of benzylpenicillin above 1.2 g should be administered at not more than 300 mg per minute.

Intrathecal injections are hazardous and are best avoided unless absolutely necessary. For adults a dose of 6 mg has been used; a maximum dose of 12 mg daily should not be exceeded. For infants and children an intrathecal dose of 0.1 mg per kg has been used.

For subconjunctival injection, 300 or 600 mg of benzylpenicillin may be dissolved in 0.5 to 1.0 mL of Water for Injections, or another suitable solvent such as lignocaine 2% with adrenaline 1 in 100 000.

Benzylpenicillin is sometimes given by mouth in a dose ranging from 0.25 to 7.5 g daily, administered on an empty stomach, in the treatment of infections of moderate severity but one of the acid-resistant penicillins, such as phenoxymethylpenicillin, is preferred.

ABSCESS, LUNG. Benzylpenicillin has been considered the drug of choice for the treatment of anaerobic lung abscess (J.G. Bartlett and S.L. Gorbach, *Ann. intern. Med.*, 1983, *98*, 546), but there have been reports of increasing resistance to penicillin in anaerobes (H.R. Ingham *et al.*, *Lancet*, 1980, *2*, 748; D.R. Snydman *et al.*, *J. antimicrob. Chemother.*, 1980, *6*, 519; R.S. Edson *et al.*, *Mayo Clin. Proc.*, 1982, *57*, 737). Levison *et al.* (*Ann. intern. Med.*, 1983, *98*, 466) demonstrated a suboptimal response in patients with anaerobic lung abscess treated with benzylpenicillin intravenously followed by phenoxymethylpenicillin by mouth, but no failures or relapses in patients treated with clindamycin given intravenously and then by mouth. There were, however, criticisms of the study and it was suggested that inadequate doses of penicillin had been used (R.L.

Ruffalo and S.M. Garabedian-Ruffalo (*ibid.*, *99*, 125). Despite this, Levison *et al.*, as well as other case reports, have demonstrated superior results with clindamycin, and clindamycin may, therefore, be preferred to penicillin for the initial treatment of seriously ill patients and as a substitute drug for patients who have had an unfavourable or delayed response to penicillin. For the patient who is not seriously ill, penicillin may still be judged, by some, as the better drug in terms of cost and its long, favourable record (J.G. Bartlett and S.L. Gorbach, *Ann. intern. Med.*, 1983, *98*, 546). A test for beta-lactamase production may provide the most clinically relevant information regarding the choice of antibiotic (R.L. Ruffalo and S.M. Garabedian-Ruffalo, *Ann. intern. Med.*, 1983, *99*, 125).

ACTINOMYCOSIS. A 36-year-old man with septicaemia and a liver abscess due to a strain of *Actinomyces* was successfully treated with benzylpenicillin, without the need for surgical drainage. Initially benzylpenicillin 7.2 g intravenously was administered daily together with probenecid 500 mg three times daily. However, due to the development of a skin rash, probenecid was discontinued after 13 days and the dose of benzylpenicillin was increased to 14.4 g daily given by continuous intravenous infusion. The patient's condition improved rapidly and benzylpenicillin was discontinued after 62 days. The cure achieved in this patient might have been influenced by the *Actinomyces* strain, which could have been the less pathogenic *A. bovis* rather than *A. israelii*.— W. F. van Marion *et al.*, *Infection*, 1982, *10*, 287.

Pneumonia due to *Actinomyces meyeri* in a 13-year-old boy was successfully treated with benzylpenicillin administered intravenously for 4 weeks followed by phenoxymethylpenicillin given by mouth for a further 3 months.— A. M. Allworth *et al.*, *Med. J. Aust.*, 1986, *145*, 33.

ADMINISTRATION. A report of clinical improvement following reduction in the dose of benzylpenicillin in an 83-year-old man with an α-haemolytic streptococcal infection. This paradoxical effect had been demonstrated *in vitro* and was known as the 'Eagle effect' whereby the rate of killing of organisms was markedly reduced rather than increased above an optimal concentration. Where serum bactericidal activity is low and clinical response poor despite high serum-antibiotic concentrations and a low MIC for the infecting organism, a reduction in antibiotic dosage should be considered.— L. R. Griffiths and H. T. Green (letter), *J. antimicrob. Chemother.*, 1985, *15*, 507. A similar paradoxical effect occurred in an infant with congenital heart disease who had a non-haemolytic streptococcus infection. It appeared that this effect might be overcome by using a combination of penicillin and an aminoglycoside even though initial tests might show no advantage to such a regimen.— R. H. George and A. Dyas (letter), *ibid.*, 1986, *17*, 684.

ADMINISTRATION IN INFANTS AND CHILDREN. A suggested dose of benzylpenicillin for neonates of more than 37 weeks' gestation was 30 mg per kg body-weight given intramuscularly or intravenously, by very slow bolus injection, every 12 hours for the first 48 hours of life, every 8 hours from the 3rd day to 2 weeks, then every 6 hours. For immature infants (those of less than 37 weeks' gestation) this dose should be given every 12 hours for the first week of life, every 8 hours from then to 4 weeks of age, and every 6 hours thereafter (P.A. Davies, *Br. med. J.*, 1978, *2*, 676). Other authors have suggested a similar dosage regimen for severe infections in neonates, with daily intravenous doses of 60 to 90 mg per kg in 2 or 3 divided doses for neonates aged 0 to 1 week, 90 to 150 mg per kg in 3 or 4 divided doses for those aged 1 to 4 weeks, and 150 to 180 mg per kg in 4 to 6 divided doses for infants over 4 weeks. For severe infections in children a suggested intravenous dose for benzylpenicillin was 120 to 180 mg per kg daily in 4 to 6 divided doses, up to a total daily dose of 6 to 12 g in older children (K.H. Rhodes and C.M. Johnson, *Mayo Clin. Proc.*, 1983, *58*, 158). A dosage for infants which is not adjusted for gestational age or postnatal age has also been used: benzylpenicillin 150 mg per kg has been given daily in divided doses every 8 hours if administered intramuscularly or every 4 to 6 hours if administered intravenously by slow bolus injection (H.B. Valman, *Br. med. J.*, 1980, *280*, 457). However, neonates requiring intensive care often have immature organs and multiple problems and therefore the dose of antibiotic should be adjusted according to serum concentrations.

ADMINISTRATION IN RENAL FAILURE. Benzylpenicillin can be administered to patients with renal failure by adjusting the dosage interval. A dosage interval of 6 to 8 hours is suitable for patients whose glomerular filtration-rates exceed 50 mL per minute; an interval of 8 to 12 hours between doses is advisable for rates of between 10 and 50 mL per minute. Where the rate is less than 10 mL per minute, the dosage interval should be 12 to 16 hours and a dose of over 6 g per day should be avoided. A dose supplement should be given to patients undergoing haemodialysis, but is unnecessary for patients undergoing peritoneal dialysis.— W. M. Bennett *et al.*, *Am. J. Kidney Dis.*, 1983, *3*, 155.

Benzylpenicillin has been used in patients undergoing continuous ambulatory peritoneal dialysis. A loading dose of benzylpenicillin 600 mg given intravenously or intraperitoneally followed by a maintenance dose of 30 mg per litre intraperitoneally has been used.— D. K. Scott and D. E. Roberts, *Pharm. J.*, 1985, *1*, 621.

ANIMAL BITES. Early treatment with antibiotics has been recommended for serious wounds caused by animal bites, in patients at obvious risk. Penicillin will cover *Pasteurella* spp. but most *Staphylococcus aureus* strains require a penicillinase-resistant penicillin (*Lancet*, 1983, *2*, 553). A rapid response to benzylpenicillin was achieved in 2 patients with lion or tiger bites infected with *Pasteurella multocida*; the patients also received gentamicin and cloxacillin sodium or chloramphenicol sodium succinate (D.R. Burdge *et al.*, *J. Am. med. Ass.*, 1985, *253*, 3296). Human bites appear to have a greater potential for causing deep necrotising infection than animal bites and broad spectrum antibiotics are necessary until the culture and sensitivity reports are available. Treatment with penicillin plus a penicillinase-resistant penicillin, such as cloxacillin, has been considered satisfactory, however, some workers have used flucloxacillin or a cephalosporin alone, and other workers have recommended using a penicillinase-resistant penicillin in association with an aminoglycoside (B. Kirkpatrick and R. Wise, *Br. med. J.*, 1986, *293*, 1522).

ANTHRAX. Penicillin is considered to be the drug of choice for the treatment of anthrax; tetracycline has been used as an alternative drug. In mild uncomplicated cutaneous anthrax phenoxymethylpenicillin potassium 7.5 mg per kg body-weight administered by mouth every 6 hours for 5 to 7 days is considered sufficient; for more extensive disease procaine penicillin 10 mg per kg administered intramuscularly every 12 hours for 5 to 7 days is recommended. Pulmonary anthrax should be treated immediately; benzylpenicillin 50 mg per kg in the first hour administered by continuous intravenous drip, followed by benzylpenicillin 200 mg per kg every 24 hours has been used successfully when therapy was begun early, however, even with appropriate antibiotics the prognosis is usually extremely poor. Erythromycin may be used as an alternative agent. Intestinal anthrax or meningeal anthrax could be treated with the regimen described for pulmonary anthrax in addition to supportive measures. Once septicaemia has developed a fatal outcome is likely due to toxin release. Benzylpenicillin 10 mg per kg administered intramuscularly every 12 hours for 5 to 7 days has been used prophylactically if contaminated meat has been ingested or if *Bacillus anthracis* has been inadvertently injected beneath the skin. Combined penicillin and vaccine prophylaxis has been used for pulmonary anthrax prophylaxis.— G. B. Knudson, *Milit. Med.*, 1986, *151*, 71.

ARTHRITIS, BACTERIAL. For the use of benzylpenicillin in the treatment of disseminated gonococcal infection, the symptoms of which often include polyarthritis and tenosynovitis, see Sexually Transmitted Diseases, Gonorrhoea, below.

DENTAL PROPHYLAXIS. For the prophylactic use of benzylpenicillin before dental procedures in patients at special risk, see under Endocarditis, below.

ENDOCARDITIS. A report of a Working Party of the British Society for Antimicrobial Chemotherapy on the antibiotic treatment of streptococcal and staphylococcal endocarditis. Since two-thirds of endocarditis cases are streptococcal, the recommended combination for the early stage of endocarditis is a penicillin, usually benzylpenicillin, and an aminoglycoside, usually gentamicin, but where there is a strong possibility of staphylococcal infection, for example drug addicts or patients with skin sepsis, flucloxacillin should be added to the regimen. For streptococcal endocarditis, if the MBC for benzylpenicillin is 1 μg or less per mL then benzylpenicillin 7.2 g daily by intravenous injection in 6 divided doses should be given with gentamicin in initial doses of 80 mg twice daily by intravenous injection; subsequent dosage of gentamicin depends upon blood concentrations. Netilmicin could be considered as an alternative to gentamicin in elderly patients or when there is impaired renal function. After 14 days the gentamicin should be stopped and the benzylpenicillin may then be replaced with amoxycillin 0.5 to 1.0 g three times daily by mouth for another 14 days. Probenecid may also be administered concurrently. If the MBC is greater than 1 μg per mL, the gentamicin must be given with the penicillin for not less than 4 weeks. In patients genuinely allergic to the penicillins an initial treatment with vancomycin plus gentamicin is advised.— *Lancet*, 1985, *2*, 815. Care should be taken when using benzylpenicillin at the recommended dosage of 7.2 g daily in the presence of reduced renal function, which is not uncommon in endocarditis; blood concentrations should be monitored.— D. S. Reeves (letter), *ibid.*, 1420. Although the recommendations of the Working Party appear sensible some workers disagree with the suggested dosage schedule. Penicillin 12 g daily given by slow continuous infusion in association with gentamicin is a successful alternative and the higher dose might also be considered for enterococcal infection.— J. Francis and S. W. B. Newsom, *J. antimicrob. Chemother.*, 1986, *18*, 554. See also W. R. Wilson, *ibid.*, 1987, *20*, *Suppl.* A, 147.

For the treatment of staphylococcal endocarditis, see under Flucloxacillin Sodium, p.231.

Endocarditis due to penicillin-tolerant lactobacilli has been reported. The use of penicillin in association with gentamicin therefore seems appropriate treatment for endocarditis due to *Lactobacillus* spp. until the results of serum bactericidal testing are available.— A. J. Davies *et al.*, *J. Infect.*, 1986, *12*, 169.

See also under Choice of Antibiotic (p.96).

Prophylaxis. The American Heart Association has recommended a standard regimen for prophylaxis in patients at risk of endocarditis undergoing dental procedures or surgery of the upper respiratory tract. The regimen consists of phenoxymethylpenicillin by mouth, but in patients unable to take antibiotics by mouth, benzylpenicillin 1.2 g intravenously or intramuscularly 30 to 60 minutes prior to the procedure and 600 mg six hours later is recommended; children may be given benzylpenicillin 30 mg per kg body-weight prior to and 15 mg per kg after the procedure (S.T. Shulman *et al.*, *Circulation*, 1984, *70*, 1123A). However, the Working Party of the British Society for Antimicrobial Chemotherapy recommends a different regimen using amoxycillin either by mouth or parenterally (*Lancet*, 1982, *2*, 1323; N.A. Simmons *et al.*, *ibid.*, 1986, *1*, 1267). Prophylaxis with a combination of parenteral amoxycillin, ampicillin, or penicillin in association with gentamicin is recommended for patients at particularly high risk of endocarditis such as those with prosthetic valves (*Lancet*, 1982, *2*, 1323; S.T. Shulman *et al.*, *Circulation*, 1984, *70*, 1123A; J. Etienne *et al.*, *Lancet*, 1986, *2*, 511).

Testing of the MBC was the only reliable method of determining penicillin resistance in viridans streptococci and endurance and tolerance should be considered when penicillin prophylaxis for bacterial endocarditis fails.— Y. Holloway *et al.* (letter), *Lancet*, 1980, *1*, 589.

See also under Prophylactic Use of Antibiotics, p.102.

EYE INFECTIONS. For reference to the use of benzylpenicillin in the prophylaxis and treatment of neonatal conjunctivitis, see Pregnancy and the Neonate, below.

INFECTION PROPHYLAXIS, HYPOSPLENISM. For the prophylactic use of benzylpenicillin or phenoxymethylpenicillin in asplenic or hyposplenic patients, see under Prophylactic Use of Antibiotics, p.102.

LEPTOSPIROSIS. Treatment of leptospirosis with antibiotics is controversial and there has been little satisfactory evidence that they alter the course or outcome of the disease. Penicillin has been given in large parenteral doses for severe illnesses or amoxycillin has been used for treatment by mouth (R.J.C. Hart *et al.*, *Br. med. J.*, 1984, *288*, 1983). Doses of benzylpenicillin 7.2 to 9.6 g daily for 5 days, then 1.44 g daily for a further 5 days for severe infections, or amoxycillin 500 mg three times daily for 5 days for mild infections have been recommended (*J. R. Coll. gen. Pract.*, 1985, *35*, 36). Other antibiotics such as streptomycin or tetracycline have also been used in the treatment of leptospirosis, but newer drugs such as ceftizoxime or cefotaxime have been reported to be more effective *in vitro* than benzylpenicillin, ampicillin, streptomycin, or tetracycline (S. Oie *et al.*, *Antimicrob. Ag. Chemother.*, 1983, *24*, 905). It used to be thought that antimicrobial agents were of benefit only if given early in the course of the disease, however, in a double-blind placebo-controlled study intravenous benzylpenicillin was shown to be beneficial in patients with severe leptospirosis, even when given late in the course of illness (G. Watt *et al.*, *Lancet*, 1988, *1*, 433).

LYME DISEASE. Beneficial effects have been obtained with benzylpenicillin in the treatment of Lyme disease, a seasonal infectious disease caused by the spirochaete *Borrelia burgdorferi* which is transmitted primarily by ixodes ticks. Benzylpenicillin administered by mouth had been shown to shorten the duration of the characteristic skin lesion, erythema chronicum migrans, and often prevented or attenuated subsequent arthritis (A.C.

Steere *et al.*, *Ann. intern. Med.*, 1980, *93*, 1). However, for early Lyme disease, phenoxymethylpenicillin or tetracycline administered by mouth has produced better results than treatment with benzylpenicillin (A.C. Steere *et al.*, *Ann. intern. Med.*, 1983, *99*, 22). For neurological abnormalities of Lyme disease or related diseases benzylpenicillin 12 g daily administered intravenously in divided doses for 10 to 14 days has been found to be effective (B. Sköldenberg *et al.*, *Lancet*, 1983, *2*, 75; A.C. Steere *et al.*, *Ann. intern. Med.*, 1983, *99*, 767) and this regimen has also been of benefit to patients with established Lyme arthritis (A.C. Steere *et al.*, *New Engl. J. Med.*, 1985, *312*, 869). Some workers have used benzylpenicillin in higher doses or for longer duration to treat neurological abnormalities due to *Borrelia burgdorferi* infections (A. Kahan *et al.*, *Lancet*, 1985, *2*, 148). However, other workers have found that patients with lesions that have been present for a long time do not respond to benzylpenicillin treatment (J. Kohler *et al.*, *Lancet*, 1986, *2*, 35).

MENINGITIS. Benzylpenicillin is considered the drug of choice for meningitis caused by *Neisseria meningitidis* or *Streptococcus pneumoniae* (M. Whitby and R. Finch, *Drugs*, 1986, *31*, 266; *Med. Lett.*, 1986, *28*, 33), although there have been reports of tolerant or resistant organisms (P.J. Sanderson, *Br. med. J.*, 1984, *289*, 638). In the management of an outbreak of meningococcal meningitis general practitioners were encouraged to administer parenteral benzylpenicillin before arranging for hospital admission (K.A.V. Cartwright *et al.*, *Lancet*, 1986, *2*, 558). A standard therapy of benzylpenicillin 120 mg per kg body-weight daily given intravenously in divided doses has been recommended (M. Whitby and R. Finch, *Drugs*, 1986, *31*, 266) or alternatively a dosage range of benzylpenicillin 1.2 to 2.4 g every 4 hours has been suggested; children could be given 150 mg per kg daily administered in divided doses every 4 hours (H.P. Lambert, *Br. med. J.*, 1983, *286*, 741). For penicillin-hypersensitive patients chloramphenicol is a suitable alternative and cephalosporins such as cefuroxime or cefotaxime can also be considered, although penicillin-allergic patients may also have allergic reactions to cephalosporins (*Med. Lett.*, 1986, *28*, 33). For group B streptococcal meningitis benzylpenicillin or ampicillin together with gentamicin have been recommended (M. Whitby and R. Finch, *Drugs*, 1986, *31*, 266) despite doubts about clinical relevance of the aminoglycoside (H.P. Lambert, *Br. J. Hosp. Med.*, 1983, *29*, 128) and other authors have suggested benzylpenicillin or ampicillin alone for the treatment of group B streptococcal infections (*Med. Lett.*, 1986, *28*, 33).

Probenecid interferes with the active transport of penicillin and other organic acids from the CSF. It has therefore been suggested that probenecid be used to maintain the concentration of penicillin in the CSF, although this has not been widely adopted in the treatment of meningitis (*Lancet*, 1984, *2*, 499).

Several cases of presumed perinatal transmission of *Streptococcus pneumoniae* from mother to neonate have been described. The greatest susceptibility to pneumococcal meningitis occurs in the first year of life and the young age of patients with fatal pneumococcal meningitis may reflect inadequate acquired immunity. It has been suggested that any infant whose mother acquires clinical pneumococcal infection should receive penicillin prophylaxis and microbiological surveillance (P.J. Shaw *et al.*, *Lancet*, 1984, *2*, 47).

See also Choice of Antibiotic, p.98.

MOUTH INFECTIONS. Penicillin had been effective in combatting the organisms, such as viridans streptococci, a variety of anaerobes, and facultative streptococci, which were most often encountered in oral infections (V.L. Sutter *et al.*, *Antimicrob. Ag. Chemother.*, 1983, *23*, 483; W. Guralnick, *Br. dent. J.*, 1984, *156*, 440). With drainage, it was considered an adequate treatment for most orodental infections likely to involve oral anaerobic bacteria including orofacial infections of dental origin, gingivitis, peritonsillar abscess, perimandibular space infections, Vincent's angina, and suppurative venous thrombosis of the jugular vein or other infections following head and neck surgery. However, since the incidence of penicillin-resistant anaerobes had increased metronidazole plus penicillin, or treatment with clindamycin, cefoxitin, or chloramphenicol might be preferred for serious or refractory infections (*Med. Lett.*, 1984, *26*, 87).

OSTEOMYELITIS. Acute pyogenic osteomyelitis is predominantly caused by *Staphylococcus aureus*, the vast majority of which are now resistant to benzylpenicillin (S.C. Glover and A.M. Geddes, *J. antimicrob. Chemother.*, 1981, *8*, 347). A penicillinase-resistant penicillin such as flucloxacillin is therefore generally preferred. However, if the organisms are sensitive, benzylpenicillin may be used in a dose of 1.2 g administered intravenously every 4 hours. Benzylpenicillin has also been used for anaerobic infections, administered either alone or in association with metronidazole (A.S. Dickie, *Drugs*, 1986, *32*, 458).

PREGNANCY AND THE NEONATE. There appears to be no significant risk to the foetus from benzylpenicillin, phenoxymethylpenicillin, or probably the long-acting penicillins when administered during pregnancy, although there is the possibility of sensitising the foetus during the second and third trimesters. If an antimicrobial agent has to be used during pregnancy the following drugs are recommended, assuming that the patient is not allergic to the drug, or that the infecting bacteria are not resistant: for pharyngitis and tonsillitis associated with systemic infection, benzylpenicillin intravenously, procaine penicillin intramuscularly, or phenoxymethylpenicillin by mouth; for lobar pneumonia, benzylpenicillin; for streptococcal endocarditis, benzylpenicillin in association with gentamicin; and for gonorrhoea or syphilis, penicillin-based treatment.— R. Wise, *Br. med. J.*, 1987, *294*, 42.

For the use of benzylpenicillin in the treatment of syphilis in pregnant women, see under Benzathine Penicillin, Syphilis, p.130.

For the prophylactic use of benzylpenicillin before first-trimester abortions or emergency caesarean section, see under Surgical Infection Prophylaxis, below.

Neonate. Early-onset sepsis in the neonate is usually caused by infection with group B streptococci or Gram-negative organisms, although Gram-negative organisms are far more likely to cause late-onset than early-onset sepsis. Treatment of early-onset sepsis is usually with benzylpenicillin or ampicillin and an aminoglycoside, but despite early treatment with penicillin, 50% or more of the babies still die and therefore the use of prophylactic antibiotics has been tried (D. Isaacs and A.R. Wilkinson, *Archs Dis. Childh.*, 1987, *62*, 204). Administration of benzylpenicillin 15 or 30 mg intramuscularly within one hour of delivery has been found significantly to reduce early-onset group B streptococcal infections in the newborn compared with infants who only received tetracycline ophthalmic ointment; single-dose benzylpenicillin does not prevent infection acquired *in utero* and probably has little effect on the incidence of late-onset disease (J.D. Siegel *et al.*, *Lancet*, 1982, *1*, 1426). However, unselective prophylaxis involves many infants receiving benzylpenicillin unnecessarily and so attempts have been made to identify risk factors which include prematurity and prolonged rupture of membranes (*Lancet*, 1984, *1*, 1056). Over a 3-year study period, low birth-weight infants given benzylpenicillin 30 to 60 mg per kg body-weight daily administered intravenously or intramuscularly within 2 hours of birth, and continued for 10 days if group B streptococci were isolated, resulted in no deaths from infection with these organisms (D.J. Lloyd *et al.*, *Lancet*, 1979, *1*, 713). However, this study was uncontrolled and there may have been fluctuations in the incidence of group B streptococcal infections during the study period (R.S. Ramamurthy *et al.*, *Lancet*, 1979, *2*, 246; B.F. Anthony, *ibid.*, 751). In contrast, benzylpenicillin 60 mg per kg given intramuscularly within 90 minutes of birth and then every 12 hours for 72 hours did not prevent early-onset streptococcal disease in neonates weighing 2 kg or less (S.P. Pyati *et al.*, *New Engl. J. Med.*, 1983, *308*, 1383). The presence of group B streptococci in the urine of pregnant women appears to be associated with primary rupture of the membranes and preterm delivery, and treatment of such women with penicillin may reduce the frequency of preterm labour (A.C. Thomsen *et al.*, *Lancet*, 1987, *1*, 591).

For the intrapartum chemoprophylaxis of early-onset neonatal group B streptococcal disease, see under Ampicillin Trihydrate, p.121.

For the treatment of gonococcal conjunctivitis of the newborn, in areas where the prevalence of penicillin-resistant gonococci is less than 1%, the WHO recommends that the neonate should be admitted to hospital and benzylpenicillin 60 mg per kg body-weight be given intravenously or intramuscularly in 3 divided doses [daily] for 7 days in association with hourly conjunctival irrigation with saline or buffered ophthalmic solutions, and application of a topical antibiotic preparation, until the discharge is eliminated. When hospitalisation is not practical, treatment must be given on an outpatient basis and benzylpenicillin 30 mg per kg daily administered intramuscularly in 2 divided doses for 3 days, in association with tetracycline hydrochloride 1% or erythromycin 0.5% eye ointment applied topically for 10 days is recommended. Where there is a risk of penicillin resistance, the benzylpenicillin should be replaced by systemic administration of cefotaxime or kanamycin (WHO Expert Committee on Venereal Diseases and Treponematoses, *Tech. Rep. Ser. Wld Hlth Org. No. 736*, 1986, p.122). Similar regimens have been used by other workers, although some have used systemic benzylpenicillin with only saline irrigations to the eye (*Lancet*, 1984, *2*, 1375; *Med. Lett.*, 1986, *28*, 23).

For infants exposed to gonorrhoea at birth, in areas where gonococcal strains are sensitive to penicillin, the WHO recommends prophylactic treatment with benzylpenicillin given intramuscularly or intravenously in a single dose of 30 mg for full-term infants or 12 mg for low birth-weight infants; ocular prophylaxis is also necessary. In areas with a high prevalence of penicillin-resistant gonococci, systemic administration of cefotaxime or kanamycin might be considered (WHO Expert Committee on Venereal Diseases and Treponematoses, *Tech. Rep. Ser. Wld Hlth Org. No. 736*, 1986, p.123). Infants born to mothers with gonorrhoea have a high risk of becoming infected and full treatment for gonococcal infection has also been recommended. Systematic detection and treatment of infected pregnant women is the ideal method of preventing conjunctivitis of the newborn, but if this is not available ocular prophylaxis with silver nitrate 1% eye-drops or tetracycline 1% eye ointment is recommended in areas where the risk of gonococcal infection is high (*Conjunctivitis of the newborn: prevention and treatment at the primary health care level*, Geneva, World Health Organization, 1986, pp.12-17).

Congenital syphilis in infants up to 2 years of age could be treated with benzylpenicillin 30 mg per kg body-weight given by intramuscular or intravenous injection daily in 2 divided doses for a minimum of 10 days. Alternatively procaine penicillin 50 mg per kg could be given intramuscularly in a single daily dose for 10 days. In infants with normal cerebrospinal fluid some workers may administer benzathine penicillin 37.5 mg per kg intramuscularly as a single dose.— Report of a WHO Expert Committee on Venereal Diseases and Treponematoses, *Tech. Rep. Ser. Wld Hlth Org. No. 736* 1986, p.128.

RESPIRATORY-TRACT INFECTIONS. Penicillin has been used for pneumococcal infections, but sensitivity needs to be confirmed because levels of resistance appear to be increasing (P.J. Sanderson, *Br. med. J.*, 1984, *289*, 638; R. Pallares *et al.*, *New Engl. J. Med.*, 1987, *317*, 18). Bacterial pneumonia in children is usually caused by *Streptococcus pneumoniae* or *Haemophilus influenzae* and parenteral penicillin has been used for the standard treatment (*Bull. Wld Hlth Org.*, 1984, *62*, 47), although children are often treated with chloramphenicol as well to cover *H. influenzae*. However, in a study involving 748 children with severe pneumonia treatment with chloramphenicol alone was found to be as effective as chloramphenicol plus benzylpenicillin (F. Shann *et al.*, *Lancet*, 1985, *2*, 684).

For the use of benzylpenicillin in the treatment of pneumonia due to *Actinomyces meyeri* see Actinomycosis, above.

For the use of benzylpenicillin in the treatment of anaerobic lung abscess see Abscess, Lung, above.

For the use of benzylpenicillin in association with sodium calciumedetate for the treatment of respiratory-tract infection due to *Pseudomonas aeruginosa*, see under Sodium Calciumedetate, p.853.

RHEUMATIC FEVER PROPHYLAXIS. For the use of benzylpenicillin in the prevention of acute rheumatic fever, see Benzathine Penicillin, p.130.

SEPTICAEMIA. Of 14 children with occult pneumococcaemia, meningitis developed in 3 children despite treatment with penicillin in 2 of the children. All children with bacteraemia due to *Streptococcus pneumoniae* should be treated with intravenous penicillin in doses to cover meningitis.— T. Äärimaa *et al.*, *Archs Dis. Childh.*, 1982, *57*, 392.

SEXUALLY TRANSMITTED DISEASES. *Gonorrhoea*. Benzylpenicillin is used in the treatment of disseminated gonococcal infection, in areas where gonococci have maintained sensitivity to penicillin. Benzylpenicillin 6 g daily has been given intravenously in divided doses for 3 days, followed by ampicillin or amoxycillin 500 mg administered 4 times daily by mouth to complete 10 days of therapy; for more serious complications such as meningitis or endocarditis, the dose and duration of treatment with benzylpenicillin should be increased (E.W. Hook and K.K. Holmes, *Ann. intern. Med.*, 1985, *102*, 229; *Med. Lett.*, 1986, *28*, 23; WHO Expert Committee on Venereal Diseases and Treponematoses, *Tech. Rep. Ser. Wld Hlth Org. No. 736*, 1986). Most strains of gonococci in disseminated infection still appear to be very sensitive to benzylpenicillin (*Lancet*, 1984, *1*, 832), however, there have been reports of beta-lactamase producing organisms (R.Z. Rinaldi *et al.*, *Ann. intern. Med.*, 1982, *97*, 43; P. Ruutu *et al.*, *J. Am. med. Ass.*, 1984, *251*, 1836) and also chromosomally mediated, beta-lactamase-negative, penicillin-resistant organisms (K.W. Strader *et al.*, *Ann. intern. Med.*, 1986, *104*, 365). Therefore the local *in-vitro* susceptibility patterns of *Neisseria gonorrhoeae* need to be evaluated and all isolates need to be tested for beta-lactamase production and screened for chromosomally mediated resistance (W.R. Bowie *et al.*, *Can. med. Ass. J.*, 1986, *135*, 489). Some experts are of the opinion that beta-lactamase stable antibiotics should be used in preference to benzylpenicillin in all environments until the sensitivity of the infecting organism has been determined (WHO Expert Committee on Venereal Diseases and Treponematoses, *Tech. Rep. Ser. Wld Hlth Org. No. 736*, 1986).

For the treatment of adults with gonococcal conjunctivitis, in areas where the prevalence of penicillin-resistant strains is known to be less than 1%, the WHO recommends administration of benzylpenicillin 6 g daily by intramuscular injection for 5 days, as well as hourly irrigation of the eyes with saline or buffered ophthalmic solutions and topical application of an antibiotic preparation (WHO Expert Committee on Venereal Diseases and Treponematoses, *Tech. Rep. Ser. Wld Hlth Org. No. 736*, 1986). Once penicillin-resistant strains have emerged a change in treatment policy for gonococcal conjunctivitis from penicillin to one of the newer cephalosporins or spectinomycin should be considered (P. Kestelyn and A. Meheus, *Br. J. Ophthal.*, 1986, *70*, 875).

See also Pregnancy and the Neonate, above, and Choice of Antibiotic, p.101.

Syphilis. For the use of benzylpenicillin in the treatment of congenital syphilis see under Pregnancy and the Neonate, above. See also under Benzathine Penicillin, Syphilis, p.130 for mention of benzylpenicillin in the treatment of neurosyphilis.

SURGICAL INFECTION PROPHYLAXIS. Benzylpenicillin 600 mg intravenously has been used pre-operatively in women with a history of pelvic inflammatory disease undergoing first-trimester abortion (*Med. Lett.*, 1985, *27*, 105). However, in a study of 474 women prophylactic treatment with benzylpenicillin 1.2 g administered intramuscularly half an hour before and 3 hours after the procedure followed by pivampicillin 350 mg three times daily for 4 days, did not significantly alter the frequency of bacteraemia when compared with placebo (L. Heisterberg *et al.*, *Dan. med. Bull.*, 1985, *32*, 73).

Beneficial results have been obtained with benzylpenicillin used intra-incisionally for prophylaxis of surgical wound infection (D. Lindsey *et al.*, *J. antimicrob. Chemother.*, 1984, *14*, 196). However, topical antibiotics can induce allergy and the emergence of resistant strains just like systemically administered agents. In addition, intra-incisional antibiotics only give protection at the wound site as satisfactory serum concentrations cannot be relied upon (O.J.A. Gilmore and R.G. Sprignall, *Br. J. Hosp. Med.*, 1983, *29*, 440).

In rural developing countries where tetanus is common and active immunisation little practised, pre-operative metronidazole or penicillin might be used for patients undergoing emergency operations who have not been immunised against tetanus; the duration of antibiotic cover depends on the contamination risk.— *Lancet*, 1984, *2*, 964.

See also Wound Infections, below, and Prophylactic use of Antibiotics, p.103.

WHIPPLE'S DISEASE. Parenteral benzylpenicillin or procaine penicillin for 2 weeks followed by an antibiotic given by mouth, such as phenoxymethylpenicillin, has been used to treat Whipple's disease [intestinal dystrophy] (*Med. J. Aust.*, 1974, *1*, 646). If there is CNS involvement, however, reassessment of the antibiotic regimen, particularly with regard to its ability to penetrate the blood-brain barrier, is necessary; chloramphenicol has been used in association with benzylpenicillin to control CNS disease (M. Feldman *et al.*, *Ann. intern. Med.*, 1980, *93*, 709). Whipple's disease was once thought to be only a gut infection, but has now been shown to be a systemic disease and Whipple bacilli have been located in the gut, eye, heart, lungs, synovial membrane, and CNS. Due to the number of relapses reported in patients with Whipple's disease some workers have suggested that even though most of the patients who present with Whipple's disease do not have CNS manifestations, all of the patients have CNS involvement and therefore all patients with Whipple's disease should be treated for 1 year with antibiotics that penetrate the blood-brain barrier. Treatment protocols considered suitable include co-trimoxazole alone or parenteral penicillin and streptomycin followed by co-trimoxazole by mouth (R.D. Keinath *et al.*, *Gastroenterology*, 1985, *88*, 1867).

WOUND INFECTIONS. For injuries prone to clostridial infection such as extensive muscle damage, impaired blood supply, heavy bacterial contamination associated with a foreign body, agricultural injuries, or perineal injuries, it was considered essential that benzylpenicillin be administered immediately. Penicillin had also been used for cellulitis or acute streptococcal gangrene (O.J.A. Gilmore and R.G. Sprignall, *Br. J. Hosp. Med.*, 1983, *29*, 440). For penetrating intestinal injuries benzylpenicillin 600 mg given intravenously on admission and then every 4 hours for 12 hours, in association with doxycycline hydrochloride 300 mg administered intravenously as a single dose, was found to be equally effective as a similar regimen given for 5 days; treatment with cefoxitin achieved similar results except that cefoxitin appeared to be more effective in eliminating anaerobes (E.P. Dellinger *et al.*, *Archs Surg.*, 1986, *121*, 23). Benzylpenicillin 1.8 to 2.4 g every 4 hours intravenously combined with appropriate surgical drainage or removal of prosthetic devices was also found to be effective therapy for neurosurgical infections due to the anaerobic organism *Propionibacterium acnes* (P.J. Collignon *et al.*, *Med. J. Aust.*, 1986, *145*, 408).

See also Animal Bites, and Surgical Infection Prophylaxis, above.

Preparations

Penicillin G Potassium Capsules *(U.S.P.)*

Penicillin Eye-drops *(B.P.C. 1959)*. Benzylpenicillin Eye-drops

Benzylpenicillin Injection *(B.P.)*. Benzylpenicillin potassium or benzylpenicillin sodium.

Penicillin G Potassium for Injection *(U.S.P.)*

Sterile Penicillin G Potassium *(U.S.P.)*

Penicillin G Sodium for Injection *(U.S.P.)*

Sterile Penicillin G Sodium *(U.S.P.)*

Penicillin Lozenges *(B.P.C. 1973)*. Benzylpenicillin Lozenges

Penicillin G Potassium for Oral Solution *(U.S.P.)*

Penicillin G Potassium Tablets for Oral Solution *(U.S.P.)*

Penicillin G Potassium Tablets *(U.S.P.)*

Proprietary Preparations

Crystapen *(Glaxo, UK)*. *Injection* (unbuffered), powder for reconstitution, benzylpenicillin sodium 300 and 600 mg.

Injection (buffered), powder for reconstitution, benzylpenicillin sodium 3 and 6 g.

Proprietary Names and Manufacturers of Benzylpenicillin Salts

Abbocillin-G *(Austral.)*; Cidan-Cilina *(Cidan, Spain)*; Cilipen *(Hortel, Spain)*; Coliriocilina *(Medical, Spain)*; Crisocilin-G *(Spain)*; Cristapen *(Arg.)*; Crystapen *(Glaxo, Austral.; Glaxo, Canad.; NZ; S.Afr.; Glaxo, UK)*; Crystapen G *(Austral.; Glaxo, UK)*; Dermosa Cusi Penicilina *(Spain)*; Falapen *(Canad.)*; Gonopen *(NZ)*; Hyasorb *(USA)*; Lasacilina *(Spain)*; Liademycin *(Liade, Spain)*; M-Cillin B *(Misemer, USA)*; Megacillin *(Frosst, Canad.)*; Natricilin *(Spain)*; Novopen *(Novopharm, Canad.; Novo, S.Afr.)*; P-50 *(Horner, Canad.)*; Paclin G *(USA)*; Penibiot *(Galepharma, Spain)*; Penicilina Klari *(Clariana, Spain)*; Penifasa '450' Simple *(Spain)*; Penilevel *(Level, Spain)*; Penimiluy *(Spain)*; Peniroger *(Roger, Spain)*; Pentids *(Squibb, USA)*; Pfizerpen *(Roerig, USA)*; P.G.A. *(Canad.)*; Sanciline *(Spain)*; SK-Penicillin G *(Smith Kline & French, USA)*; Sodiopen *(CEPA, Spain)*; Spécilline G *(Specia, Fr.)*; Sugracillin *(USA)*; Tabillin *(Boots, UK)*; Unicilina Potasica *(Antibioticos, Spain)*; Unicilina Sodica *(Antibioticos, Spain)*.

The following names have been used for multi-ingredient preparations containing benzylpenicillin salts— Bicillin *(Brocades, UK)*; Bicillin All Purpose *(Wyeth, Austral.)*; Bicillin A-P *(Wyeth, Canad.)*; Crystamycin *(Glaxo, UK)*; Triplopen *(Glaxo, UK)*.

12442-m

Bicozamycin *(rINN)*.

Bicyclomycin; CGP-3543E; FR-1881. 6-Hydroxy-5-methylene-1-(1,2,3-trihydroxy-2-methylpropyl)-2-oxa-7,9-diazabicyclo[4.2.2]deca-8,10-dione.

$C_{12}H_{18}N_2O_7$=302.3.

CAS — 38129-37-2.

An antibiotic obtained from strains of *Streptomyces sapporonensis*.

Bicozamycin is an antibiotic reported to be effective *in vitro* against bacterial enteropathogens. It is poorly absorbed from the gastro-intestinal tract and has been given by mouth for treatment of acute diarrhoea associated with enteric infections.

ANTIMICROBIAL ACTION. A study comparing the activity *in vitro* of bicozamycin against enteropathogenic micro-organisms with that of other antibiotics. MICs of bicozamycin against various organisms were as follows: for 114 strains of *Campylobacter jejuni*, 1.56 to 100 μg per mL; for 86 strains of *Escherichia coli*, 6.25 to greater than 100 μg per mL; for 105 strains of *Salmonella* spp., 12.5 to 100 μg per mL; for 86 strains of *Shigella* spp., 3.12 to 100 μg per mL; and for 43 strains of *Yersinia enterocolitica*, 12.5 to 100 μg per mL.— R. Vanhoof *et al.*, *J. antimicrob. Chemother.*, 1982, *10*, 343. In a further comparative study of the activity of bicozamycin against bacterial enteropathogens, bicozamycin inhibited all the test strains at an intermediate to low level, with MICs against 90% of strains ranging from 16 to greater than 128 μg per mL.— J. R. Carlson *et al.*, *Antimicrob. Ag. Chemother.*, 1983, *24*, 509.

Bicozamycin was bacteriostatic *in vitro* against most Gram-negative anaerobes tested, including *Bacteroides* spp., at concentrations below 400 μg per mL. Strains of anaerobic cocci and *Clostridium difficile* were almost uniformly resistant.— B. Watt and F. V. Brown, *J. antimicrob. Chemother.*, 1983, *12*, 549.

DIARRHOEA. In a double-blind placebo-controlled study involving 148 patients with travellers' diarrhoea in association with one or more signs of enteric disease, bicozamycin given in a dose of 500 mg four times daily by mouth for 3 days appeared to be effective treatment. Causative organisms included toxigenic *Escherichia coli*, *Shigella* and *Salmonella* spp. Since bicozamycin is poorly absorbed from the gastro-intestinal tract, it should not be used if typhoid fever or bacteraemic salmonellosis is suspected.— C. D. Ericsson *et al.*, *Ann. intern. Med.*, 1983, *98*, 20. This course of bicozamycin temporarily reduced total counts of faecal Gram-negative bacteria, predominantly *E. coli*, but did not lead to the emergence of resistance in susceptible species. Bicozamycin resistance was not associated with cross-resistance to other antimicrobial agents; transferable resistance has not been demonstrated.— P. S. Harford *et al.*, *Antimicrob. Ag. Chemother.*, 1983, *23*, 630.

Proprietary Names and Manufacturers

Fujisawa, Jpn; Ciba-Geigy, Switz.

16546-x

Brodimoprim *(rINN)*.

2,4-Diamino-5-(4-bromo-3,5-dimethoxybenzyl)pyrimidine.

$C_{13}H_{15}BrN_4O_2$=339.2.

CAS — 56518-41-3.

Brodimoprim is closely related structurally to trimethoprim (see p.328), and has antibacterial activity.

ABSORPTION AND FATE. The pharmacokinetics of brodimoprim in serum and skin-blister fluid. The mean terminal half-life in serum after administration of a single 400-mg dose by mouth to 8 healthy subjects was 25.9 hours.— T. Kalager *et al.*, *Chemotherapy, Basle*, 1985, *31*, 405.

USES AND ADMINISTRATION. Disappointing results with brodimoprim following administration by mouth in 10 patients with acute purulent exacerbations of chronic bronchitis.— F. P. V. Maesen *et al.* (letter), *J. antimicrob. Chemother.*, 1984, *13*, 299.

A study of 60 patients with acute respiratory-tract infections found treatment with brodimoprim or doxycycline by mouth to be equally effective. Although fever fell more rapidly in those treated with doxycycline, more patients in the brodimoprim group had viral infections.— H. A. Salmi *et al.*, *Drugs exp. & clin. Res.*, 1986, *12*, 349.

For reference to a comparative study of the *in-vitro*

antimicrobial activity of brodimoprim, metioprim, and trimethoprim, see Metioprim, p.260.

Proprietary Names and Manufacturers
Roche, Switz.

15310-z

Butikacin *(BAN, USAN, rINN).*
UK-18892. 6-*O*-(3-Amino-3-deoxy-α-D-glucopyranosyl)-4-*O*-(6-amino-6-deoxy-α-D-glucopyranosyl)-N^1-[(2*S*)-4-amino-2-hydroxybutyl]-2-deoxy-D-streptamine.
$C_{22}H_{45}N_5O_{12}$=571.6.

CAS — 59733-86-7.

Butikacin is an aminoglycoside antibiotic with activity similar to that of amikacin.

Proprietary Names and Manufacturers
Pfizer, UK.

4901-j

Calcium Sulphaloxate *(BANM).*
Calcium Sulfaloxate *(rINNM).* Calcium 4′-[(hydroxymethylcarbamoyl)sulphamoyl]phthalanilate.
$(C_{16}H_{14}N_3O_7S)_2Ca$=824.8.

CAS — 14376-16-0 (sulphaloxic acid); 59672-20-7 (calcium salt).

Calcium sulphaloxate is a sulphonamide with properties similar to sulphamethoxazole, p.306. It is given for its antibacterial action in the gastro-intestinal tract. Approximately 95% is claimed to remain unabsorbed in the intestine.

The usual adult dose is 1 g three times daily by mouth; children may be given half the adult dose.

Proprietary Preparations

Enteromide *(Consolidated Chemicals, UK). Tablets,* calcium sulphaloxate 500 mg.

Proprietary Names and Manufacturers
Enteromide *(Consolidated Chemicals, UK)*; Intestin-Euvernil *(Heyden, Ger.).*

12522-m

Carbadox *(BAN, USAN, pINN).*
GS-6244. Methyl 3-(quinoxalin-2-ylmethylene)carbazate N^1N^4-dioxide.
$C_{11}H_{10}N_4O_4$=262.2.

CAS — 6804-07-5.

Carbadox is an antibacterial agent which has been used in veterinary practice for treating swine dysentery and enteritis and for promoting growth. However, its use has been prohibited in the *UK* following reports of carcinogenicity.

Demonstration of the mutagenicity of quinoxaline-di-*N*-oxides, including carbadox, in the *Salmonella* microsomal system.— L. Beutin *et al., Antimicrob. Ag. Chemother.*, 1981, *20*, 336.

Proprietary Veterinary Names and Manufacturers
Pfizer, UK.

24-f

Carbenicillin Sodium *(BANM, rINNM).*

α-Carboxybenzylpenicillin Sodium; BRL-2064; Carbenicillin Disodium *(USAN)*; Carbenicillinnatrium; CP-15-639-2. The disodium salt of (6*R*)-6-(2-carboxy-2-phenylacetamido)penicillanic acid.
$C_{17}H_{16}N_2Na_2O_6S$=422.4.

CAS — 4697-36-3 (acid); 4800-94-6 (disodium salt).

Pharmacopoeias. In *Br., Braz., Cz., Ind., It., Jpn, Jug.,* and *Nord. Nord.* includes an injection grade. *U.S.* includes Sterile Carbenicillin Disodium.

A white or almost white, hygroscopic powder. 1.1 g of monograph substance is approximately equivalent to 1 g of carbenicillin. Each g of monograph substance represents about 4.7 mmol of sodium. **Soluble** 1 in 1.2 of water and 1 in 25 of alcohol; practically insoluble in chloroform and ether. A 10% solution in water has a pH of 6 to 8. **Store** at a temperature not exceeding 5° in well-closed containers.

Aqueous solutions of carbenicillin sodium are reported to be **stable** for up to 24 hours at room temperature, and for up to 72 hours in a refrigerator; however, it is recommended that reconstituted solutions of carbenicillin sodium for injection should be administered immediately after preparation. Carbenicillin sodium should not be mixed with blood products or other proteinaceous fluids such as protein hydrolysates.

Carbenicillin sodium has been reported to be **incompatible** with aminoglycosides, tetracyclines, and other antimicrobial agents including amphotericin, chloramphenicol sodium succinate, colistin sulphomethate sodium, erythromycin, and lincomycin hydrochloride. Incompatibility or loss of activity has also been reported with bleomycin sulphate, fat emulsions, promethazine hydrochloride, and vitamins of the B group with vitamin C.

Adverse Effects

As for Benzylpenicillin Sodium, p.132.

Purpura and haemorrhage have been reported. Pain at the injection site and phlebitis may occur. Electrolyte disturbances, particularly hypokalaemia or hypernatraemia, may follow the administration of large doses of carbenicillin sodium.

ALLERGY. The Boston Collaborative Drug Surveillance Program monitored consecutively 32 812 medical inpatients. Drug-induced anaphylaxis occurred in 1 of 113 patients given carbenicillin.— J. Porter and H. Jick, *Lancet*, 1977, *1*, 587.

For comparison of the incidence of allergic reactions to antipseudomonal penicillins in patients with cystic fibrosis, see Piperacillin Sodium, p.285.

EFFECTS ON THE BLOOD. Prolongation of bleeding time and bleeding from mucous membranes have been associated with carbenicillin treatment (P.D. McClure *et al., Lancet*, 1970, *2*, 1307; J.O. Ballard *et al., Antimicrob. Ag. Chemother.*, 1984, *25*, 153). Alteration in platelet function has been reported (C.H. Brown *et al., New Engl. J. Med.*, 1974, *291*, 265) and seems to be most apparent in patients with renal insufficiency or in those undergoing surgical procedures. The potential for bleeding with carbenicillin has not always been appreciated because of its wide use in neutropenic patients; haemorrhage in these patients has invariably been attributed to the thrombocytopenia associated with the underlying haematological malignancy or chemotherapy (F.R. Sattler *et al., Ann. intern. Med.*, 1986, *105*, 924). Carbenicillin, like other penicillins, has also been associated with neutropenia in a few patients (C.F. Kirkwood *et al., Clin. Pharm.*, 1983, *2*, 569).

EFFECTS ON ELECTROLYTE HOMOEOSTASIS. Carbenicillin has been reported to be associated with excessive urinary loss of magnesium resulting in hypomagnesaemia.— D. P. Brenton and T. E. Gordon, *Br. J. Hosp. Med.*, 1984, *32*, 60.

EFFECTS ON THE KIDNEYS AND URINARY BLADDER. Reports of adverse effects on the urinary tract associated with carbenicillin administration: N. E. Møller (letter), *Lancet*, 1978, *2*, 946 (haemorrhagic cystitis in 7 children and haematuria in 1 child); G. B. Appel *et al., Archs intern. Med.*, 1978, *138*, 1265 (acute interstitial nephritis in 1 patient).

EFFECTS ON THE LIVER. Increases in serum aspartate aminotransferase (SGOT) values have been reported following intramuscular and intravenous injections of carbenicillin, but liver damage has not always been apparent (A.K. Knirsch and F.J. Gralla, *New Engl. J. Med.*, 1970, *282*, 1081; D.W. Gump, *ibid.*, 1489). However, mild, reversible, anicteric hepatitis has been reported in 4 patients (F.M. Wilson *et al., J. Am. med. Ass.*, 1975, *232*, 818).

EFFECTS ON THE NERVOUS SYSTEM. Individual reports of seizures associated with carbenicillin treatment in patients with renal impairment: N. A. Kurtzman *et al., J. Am. med. Ass.*, 1970, *214*, 1320; A. Whelton *et al., J. Am. med. Ass.*, 1971, *218*, 1942.

Precautions

As for Benzylpenicillin Sodium, p.133.

Carbenicillin sodium should be given with caution to patients on a restricted sodium diet.

Carbenicillin sodium has been shown to be incompatible with gentamicin and some other aminoglycosides *in vitro* and they should therefore be administered separately.

INTERACTIONS. For reference to the *in vitro* and *in vivo* inactivation of aminoglycosides by carbenicillin see Gentamicin Sulphate p.236 and p.238.

Antimicrobial Action

Carbenicillin has a bactericidal mode of action similar to that of benzylpenicillin. The most important feature of carbenicillin is its activity against *Pseudomonas aeruginosa*, although some strains have shown resistance. Its activity against *Ps. aeruginosa* and some other organisms can be enhanced by gentamicin (see p.239) and other aminoglycosides. Carbenicillin is also active against most strains of indole-positive *Proteus* spp. but not against penicillinase-producing strains of *Pr. mirabilis*. It is comparable with ampicillin against other Gram-negative bacteria; sensitive organisms include some Enterobacteriaceae, for example some strains of *Escherichia coli* or *Enterobacter* spp., *Haemophilus influenzae*, and *Neisseria* spp. *Klebsiella* spp. are usually insensitive. Its activity against Gram-positive micro-organisms is less than that of benzylpenicillin. Anaerobic organisms are generally susceptible to carbenicillin, including *Bacteroides fragilis* although high concentrations are required.

Many susceptible organisms are inhibited by carbenicillin 0.1 to 32 µg per mL, but some organisms, particularly strains of *Ps. aeruginosa* and *B. fragilis* may require relatively high concentrations of 128 µg or more per mL.

An inoculum effect was found *in vitro* with carbenicillin or cephamandole against isolates of *H. influenzae* type b, especially ampicillin-resistant strains.— V. P. Syriopoulou *et al., Antimicrob. Ag. Chemother.*, 1979, *16*, 510.

ACTIVITY WITH OTHER ANTIMICROBIAL AGENTS. Enhanced activity has been demonstrated *in vitro* between carbenicillin, or other antipseudomonal penicillins including piperacillin or ticarcillin, and aminoglycosides such as gentamicin, tobramycin, or amikacin against isolates of *Pseudomonas aeruginosa* (P. Chanbusarakum and P.R. Murray, *Antimicrob. Ag. Chemother.*, 1978, *14*, 505; G. Masuda *et al., ibid.*, 1980, *17*, 334). The addition of rifampicin to penicillin-aminoglycoside regimens in 4 seriously ill patients with *Ps. aeruginosa* infections also produced beneficial results (V.L. Yu *et al., Antimicrob. Ag. Chemother.*, 1984, *26*, 575). Synergy has been demonstrated between carbenicillin and aminoglycosides against other organisms including gentamicin-resistant Gram-negative bacteria (W. Farrell *et al., J. antimicrob. Chemother.*, 1979, *5*, 23), *Serratia marcescens* (M.Y.C. Lin *et al., ibid.*, 37), and *Staphylococcus aureus* (C. Watanakunakorn and C. Glotzbecker, *ibid.*, 151).

Clavulanic acid has been found to enhance the action of carbenicillin against *Bacteroides fragilis* (C.N. Simpson *et al., J. antimicrob. Chemother.*, 1984, *14*, 133) and synergy has been demonstrated between carbenicillin and cefoxitin against *B. fragilis* (M.B. Bansal and H. Thadepalli, *Antimicrob. Ag. Chemother.*, 1983, *23*, 166). However, antagonism has been reported between carbenicillin, or other antipseudomonal penicillins, and cefoxitin against *Enterobacteriaceae* and *Ps. aeruginosa*; this antagonism was considered to be due to induction of beta-lactamases by cefoxitin (C.C. Sanders *et al., Antimicrob. Ag. Chemother.*, 1982, *21*, 968).

Other agents which have been reported to enhance the action of carbenicillin include mecillinam against *Bacteroides* spp. (I. Trestman *et al., Antimicrob. Ag. Chemother.*, 1979, *16*, 283), and some antineoplastic drugs including mitomycin, bleomycin, doxorubicin, or fluorouracil against *Proteus vulgaris* (Y. Ueda *et al., ibid.*, 1983, *23*, 374) and mitomycin against *Staphylococcus aureus*, although antagonism has occurred between carbenicillin and plicamycin against *Staph. aureus* (J.Y. Jacobs *et al., ibid.*, 1979, *15*, 580). Synergy has been demonstrated between carbenicillin and chelating agents for example edetic acid against *Ps. aeruginosa* (G.F. Gerberick and P.A. Castric, *Antimicrob. Ag. Chemother.*, 1980, *17*, 732). Acetylcysteine with carbenicillin or ticarcillin has been shown to have additive or enhanced activity against *Ps. aeruginosa* (M.F. Parry and H.C. Neu, *J. clin. Microbiol.*, 1977, *5*, 58).

Resistance

Carbenicillin is inactivated by penicillinases and some other beta-lactamases, although it is more stable to the beta-lactamases (cephalosporinases) produced by some Gram-negative organisms including *Pseudomonas* and some *Proteus* spp. Resistance to carbenicillin may develop in *Pseudomonas aeruginosa* during treatment with carbenicillin or other beta-lactams. This resistance may be intrinsic where there are changes in cell wall permeability or penicillin-binding proteins or it may be due to plasmid-mediated beta-lactamase production that may be transferred to and from certain strains of Enterobacteriaceae.

RESISTANCE OF BACTEROIDES. In a study of the susceptibility of 228 strains of the *Bacteroides fragilis* group, 13% were resistant to carbenicillin at a break point of 128 µg per mL. Resistance to this drug at concentrations higher than 512 µg per mL may be explained by the presence of a new beta-lactamase in *B. fragilis* species.— A. E. C. C. de Almeida and M. de Uzeda, *Antimicrob. Ag. Chemother.*, 1987, *31*, 617.

RESISTANCE OF PSEUDOMONAS. Of 1866 clinical isolates of *Pseudomonas aeruginosa* obtained from hospitals all over the *UK* during a 3-month period in 1982, 9.6% were considered to be resistant to carbenicillin with a minimum inhibitory concentration (MIC) greater than 128 µg per mL. Both carbenicillin and gentamicin, the original antipseudomonal agents, appeared to have largely retained their activity and cross-resistance between the 2 drugs was rare with only 25 isolates being insusceptible to both gentamicin 2 µg per mL and carbenicillin 128 µg per mL (R.J. Williams *et al.*, *J. antimicrob. Chemother.*, 1984, *14*, 9). A higher incidence of resistance has, however, been reported in some hospitals (A.L. Barry *et al.*, *Antimicrob. Ag. Chemother.*, 1984, *25*, 669). Mucoid strains of *Ps. aeruginosa* isolated from the sputum of patients with cystic fibrosis appear to be more resistant to carbenicillin than non-mucoid strains (J.R.W. Govan, *J. antimicrob. Chemother.*, 1976, *2*, 215).

Strains with a high level of resistance to carbenicillin are generally resistant to ticarcillin (J.D. King *et al.*, *J. clin. Path.*, 1980, *33*, 297), piperacillin, and azlocillin. This resistance may be due to extra-chromosomal beta-lactamases which hydrolyse the penicillins and also to other resistance mechanisms such as reduced permeability (A.J. De Neeling *et al.*, *J. antimicrob. Chemother.*, 1987, *19*, 703). Development of resistance to beta-lactam antibiotics including carbenicillin, azlocillin, or ticarcillin may occur during therapy for *Ps. aeruginosa* infections. In one study increased resistance to both carbenicillin and azlocillin occurred after treatment with ticarcillin. In contrast, treatment with azlocillin resulted in isolates with reduced susceptibility to azlocillin, but little change in susceptibility for carbenicillin (K. Shannon *et al.*, *Lancet*, 1982, *1*, 1466). In another study, during treatment with ceftazidime a high-level resistance to carbenicillin developed as well as an increased MIC for ceftazidime. Furthermore the MIC did not always fall to pretreatment levels after cessation of therapy (S.S. Pedersen *et al.*, *J. antimicrob. Chemother.*, 1986, *17*, 505).

Carbenicillin is destroyed by penicillinase and other beta-lactamases, but has been found to be relatively resistant to hydrolysis by some beta-lactamases produced by some Gram-negative bacteria such as *Haemophilus influenzae* (S. Kattan *et al.*, *J. antimicrob. Chemother.*, 1975, *1*, 79). *Ps. aeruginosa* strains characteristically produce a chromosomal inducible beta-lactamase which does not hydrolyse carbenicillin, and resistance to this antibiotic often depends on plasmids coding for constitutive beta-lactamases (M. Jouvenot *et al.*, *ibid.*, 1983, *12*, 451). Resistance in strains of *Ps. aeruginosa*, *Enterobacter*, and *Serratia* spp. and in certain species of *Proteus*, *Providencia*, and *Citrobacter*, which produce chromosomally-mediated inducible cephalosporinases, is also thought to be due to non-hydrolytic mechanisms. Induction (or 'derepression') of these beta-lactamases produces simultaneous resistance to the broad-spectrum penicillins including carbenicillin, ticarcillin, mezlocillin, azlocillin, and piperacillin, the monobactams, most of the second and third generation cephalosporins, and the cephamycins. This resistance appears to be mediated by the enzymes via a barrier mechanism which traps the drug in a biologically inactive complex with the enzyme, thus preventing access to target proteins. Once bound, it is only slowly, if at all, hydrolysed. Differences between beta-lactam antibiotics in the number and types of target proteins may explain why the beta-lactamase barrier does not affect all of this class of drugs with the same efficiency (C.C. Sanders, *J. antimicrob. Chemother.*, 1984, *13*, 1).

Absorption and Fate

Carbenicillin is not absorbed from the gastro-intestinal tract. An intramuscular injection of 1 g produces a peak plasma concentration of about 20 to 30 µg per mL after about 1 hour; an intramuscular injection of 2 g has been reported to produce a plasma concentration of 47 µg per mL after 1 hour. An intravenous injection of 1 g produces a plasma concentration of about 70 to 140 µg per mL after 15 minutes, falling to about 3 to 4 µg per mL after 4 hours; after 5 g by intravenous injection, plasma concentrations of more than 300 µg per mL are achieved in 15 minutes. The intermittent intravenous infusion of 24 to 30 g of carbenicillin over 24 hours produces plasma concentrations of greater than 100 µg per mL.

The half-life of carbenicillin is reported to be about 1 to 1.5 hours; it is increased in patients with renal failure, especially if there is hepatic impairment, and also in neonates. Carbenicillin is approximately 50% bound to plasma proteins. Distribution of carbenicillin in the body is similar to that of other penicillins. Small amounts have been detected in human milk. There is little diffusion into the cerebrospinal fluid except when the meninges are inflamed. Relatively high concentrations have been reported in bile.

Carbenicillin is excreted principally by renal tubular secretion and glomerular filtration. Following intramuscular injection of 1 g, about 80% of the dose appears unchanged in the urine, in concentrations of 2 to 4 mg per mL, within 6 hours. Following intravenous injection of 1 g, urinary concentrations of 5 to 10 mg per mL have been reported.

Administration of probenecid increases and prolongs the serum concentrations of carbenicillin.

A comparative study of the pharmacokinetics of carbenicillin, piperacillin, and ticarcillin.— B. R. Meyers *et al.*, *Antimicrob. Ag. Chemother.*, 1980, *17*, 608.

In a study of 14 neonates given carbenicillin 100 mg per kg body-weight intramuscularly, peak serum concentrations of 147 µg per mL were achieved in babies of normal birth-weight and 174 µg per mL in those of low birth-weight. The average 12-hourly excretion was 36% of the administered dose in neonates of low birth-weight and 61% in those of normal weight and excretion correlated with creatinine clearance. Serum half-life was 2.7 hours in neonates of normal weight and 4.0 hours in those of low weight.— C. D. Morehead *et al.*, *Antimicrob. Ag. Chemother.*, 1972, *2*, 267.

The half-life of carbenicillin in patients with end-stage renal disease has been reported to range from 10 to 20 hours (W.M. Bennett *et al.*, *Am. J. Kidney Dis.*, 1983, *3*, 155). Significant amounts of carbenicillin are removed by haemodialysis and half-lives have been reduced by 53 to 70% (T.A. Hoffman *et al.*, *Ann. intern. Med.*, 1970, *73*, 173). A dialysis half-life of 4.5 hours has been reported with a dialysis clearance of 35 mL per minute. (C.-s.C. Lee and T.C. Marbury, *Clin. Pharmacokinet.*, 1984, *9*, 42). Carbenicillin is also removed by peritoneal dialysis (D.K. Scott and D.E. Roberts, *Pharm. J.*, 1985, *1*, 621).

DIFFUSION INTO BODY TISSUES AND FLUIDS. Carbenicillin diffused into interstitial fluid. This diffusion was related to the amount of protein binding.— J. S. Tan and S. J. Salstrom, *Antimicrob. Ag. Chemother.*, 1977, *11*, 698.

Relatively poor penetration of carbenicillin into the cerebrospinal fluid in 3 patients with meningoventriculitis.— G. Mombelli *et al.*, *J. antimicrob. Chemother.*, 1982, *10*, 249.

For reference to the diffusion of carbenicillin into sputum and the elimination of antipseudomonal penicillins in patients with cystic fibrosis, see Uses, Respiratory-tract Infections, below.

METABOLISM. Only about 2% of a 500 mg intramuscular dose of carbenicillin, given to 6 healthy subjects, was metabolised and recovered in the urine as penicilloic acid within 12 hours. About 82% of the dose was excreted unchanged.— M. Cole *et al.*, *Antimicrob. Ag. Chemother.*, 1973, *3*, 463.

Uses and Administration

Carbenicillin is used in the treatment of infections due to *Pseudomonas aeruginosa*, when large doses are given intravenously. It has also been administered intramuscularly or intravenously in the treatment of serious infections due to non-penicillinase producing strains of *Proteus* spp. and to some strains of *Escherichia coli*. Indications include general systemic infections, respiratory-tract infections, and urinary-tract infections.

Carbenicillin is often used with gentamicin (see p.242) since the 2 antibiotics have been shown to be synergistic, and the emergence of *Pseudomonas* resistance may be reduced when patients are treated with the 2 antibiotics; it is advisable to administer the injections separately as some inactivation may occur *in vitro*.

Carbenicillin is administered as the disodium salt. Doses are expressed in terms of the equivalent amount of carbenicillin. For severe systemic infections the usual adult dose is 20 to 30 g of carbenicillin daily in divided doses by intravenous infusion or injection, usually every 4 to 6 hours; doses of up to 40 g daily have been used. Carbenicillin should be injected slowly over 3 to 4 minutes and infusions should be given rapidly over 30 to 40 minutes since infusion over longer periods may not produce therapeutic concentrations. The concomitant administration of probenecid 1 g three times daily by mouth may lead to higher and more prolonged serum concentrations of carbenicillin but caution is recommended in patients with impaired renal function. Doses of carbenicillin may need to be reduced in renal failure.

In the treatment of urinary-tract infections the usual dose is 4 to 8 g of carbenicillin daily in divided doses by intramuscular injection. Probenecid should not be used.

The usual recommended dose for children is 50 to 100 mg per kg body-weight daily intramuscularly and 250 to 500 mg per kg daily intravenously, according to the severity of the infection.

If the pain following intramuscular injection is troublesome carbenicillin can be administered in a 0.5% solution of lignocaine hydrochloride.

As an adjunct to systemic use, carbenicillin may be given by intra-articular injection in a dose of 500 mg to 1 g daily and by intrapleural injection in a dose of 1 g daily; 125 mg in 0.5 mL of lignocaine and adrenaline injection has been recommended for subconjunctival use. The equivalent of carbenicillin 250 to 500 mg dissolved in 3 to 5 mL of water may be nebulised and inhaled 4 times daily. A 0.2% solution of carbenicillin has been suggested for local irrigation.

ADMINISTRATION. A review of the choice of nebulisers and compressors for delivery of carbenicillin aerosol.— S. P. Newman *et al.*, *Eur. J. resp. Dis.*, 1986, *69*, 160.

See also Respiratory-tract Infections, below.

ADMINISTRATION IN INFANTS AND CHILDREN. The suggested dose of carbenicillin for infants of more than 37 weeks' gestation was 100 mg per kg body-weight given intramuscularly or intravenously, by very slow bolus injection, every 12 hours for the first 48 hours of life, every 8 hours from the 3rd day to 2 weeks, then every 6 hours. For immature infants (those of less than 37 weeks' gestation) this dose should be given every 12 hours for the 1st week of life, every 8 hours from then to 4 weeks of age, and every 6 hours thereafter.— P. A. Davies, *Br. med. J.*, 1978, *2*, 676. For severe infections in neonates a suggested daily dose of carbenicillin administered intravenously was: 0 to 1 week, 200 to 250 mg per kg body-weight in 2 to 3 divided doses; 1 to 4 weeks, 300 to 400 mg per kg in 3 to 4 divided doses; over 4 weeks, 400 to 500 mg per kg in 4 to 6 divided doses. For severe infections in children a suggested intravenous dose was 400 to 500 mg per kg in 6 divided doses.— K. H. Rhodes and C. M. Johnson, *Mayo Clin. Proc.*, 1983, *58*, 158. Neonates requiring intensive care often have immature organs and multiple problems and therefore the dose of antibiotic should be adjusted according to serum concentrations.

ADMINISTRATION IN RENAL FAILURE. After a loading dose of 4 to 6 g carbenicillin could be given in a dose of 4 to 5 g every 4 hours to patients with a creatinine clearance (CC) of 40 to 80 mL per minute, 2 to 4 g every 6 to 12 hours to those with a CC of 20 to 30 mL per minute, and 2 g every 12 hours to those with a CC of 5 to 10 mL per minute. In haemodialysis 2 g could be given every 12 to 24 hours and 2 g after dialysis. In peritoneal dialysis, 2 g could be given every 6 to 12 hours; doses of 100 to 200 mg were used in each 2 litres of dialysate.— J. S. Cheigh, *Am. J. Med.*, 1977, *62*, 555.

Carbenicillin could be administered to patients with renal failure by adjusting the dosage interval. A dosage interval of 8 to 12 hours is suitable for patients whose glomerular filtration-rates exceed 50 mL per minute; an interval of 12 to 24 hours is advisable for rates of between 10 and 50 mL per minute. Where the rate is less than 10 mL per minute, the dosage interval should be 24 to 48 hours. A dose supplement should be given to patients undergoing haemodialysis or peritoneal dialysis.— W. M. Bennett *et al.*, *Am. J. Kidney Dis.*, 1983, *3*, 155.

In patients with renal insufficiency carbenicillin should be given in a usual first dose and then adjusted according to assay results; the patient should be monitored for toxicity and efficacy of treatment. The dose should not exceed 30 g daily corrected for the estimated percentage of normal renal function. In anephric patients a suggested dose was 15 to 30 mg per kg body-weight every 6 hours.— R. E. Van Scoy and W. R. Wilson, *Mayo Clin. Proc.*, 1983, *58*, 246.

NEUTROPENIA. For reference to the use of carbenicillin sodium for febrile episodes in neutropenic patients, see Piperacillin Sodium, p.287.

PREGNANCY AND THE NEONATE. For reference to the use of carbenicillin sodium in pregnancy, see Piperacillin Sodium, p.287.

RESPIRATORY-TRACT INFECTIONS. *Cystic fibrosis.* Cystic fibrosis patients chronically infected with *Pseudomonas aeruginosa* are usually treated with intravenous chemotherapy when there is evidence of an acute deterioration. Therapy consists of 10 to 14 days treatment with an aminoglycoside, such as gentamicin, tobramycin, or netilmicin, in association with an antipseudomonal penicillin or cephalosporin such as carbenicillin, ticarcillin, azlocillin, or ceftazidime. There appears to be no evidence from clinical studies of the superiority of any one of these penicillins (M.E. Hodson, *Postgrad. med. J.*, 1984, *60*, 225), even though activity *in vitro* may differ (A. Penketh *et al.*, *Thorax*, 1984, *39*, 299). Ticarcillin has been shown to have increased activity of the order of 2 to 4 times over carbenicillin against *Ps. aeruginosa in vitro*, and azlocillin and piperacillin have been shown to have lower minimum inhibitory concentrations than ticarcillin, although their bactericidal:inhibitory concentration ratios are greater than ticarcillin (H.W. Kelly and C. Lovato, *Drug Intell. & clin. Pharm.*, 1984, *18*, 772). Some workers consider that piperacillin should not be used in cystic fibrosis patients because of a reported higher incidence of adverse effects (see Piperacillin Sodium, p.285).

Aminoglycosides and antipseudomonal penicillins do not penetrate sputum readily; carbenicillin does not exceed one-fifth of its concentration in blood and therefore high peak serum concentrations are required. The penetration of newer, more active antipseudomonal penicillins is similar. Some workers have suggested that antipseudomonal penicillins such as azlocillin appear to be eliminated with abnormal rapidity in patients with cystic fibrosis and doses 2 to 3 times greater than conventional ones may be necessary. Ceftazidime also undergoes accelerated clearance in cystic fibrosis patients and so too do aminoglycosides. Although high antibiotic doses appear rational in the context of pharmacokinetics there is, as yet, no persuasive evidence that high-dose antipseudomonal regimens free the patient from recurrent pseudomonal lung infection or contribute to the quality of life in cystic fibrosis (*Lancet*, 1985, *1*, 1020). The continued use of antibiotics including carbenicillin and aminoglycosides might even contribute to the persistence of infection and to the appearance of mucoid strains (L.L. Kulczycki *et al.*, *J. Am. med. Ass.*, 1978, *240*, 30). Antibiotic therapy has been reported to be associated with an increase in resistant bacteria, although the presence of resistant bacteria in the sputum does not appear to adversely affect the outcome of therapy. There appears to be no correlation between the change in concentration of bacteria in the sputum and improved pulmonary function, and factors such as physiotherapy may contribute to the beneficial response achieved with hospitalisation and intravenous antibiotics (F.J. McLaughlin *et al.*, *J. antimicrob. Chemother.*, 1983, *11*, *Suppl.* B, 195).

Beneficial results have been demonstrated using aerosol gentamicin and carbenicillin in young adult cystic-fibrosis patients chronically infected with *Ps. aeruginosa* (M.E. Hodson *et al.*, *Lancet*, 1981, *2*, 1137), and also with inhaled tobramycin and ticarcillin (M.A. Wall, *ibid.*, 1983, *1*, 1325). The drugs are administered using a nebuliser; carbenicillin has been given in a dose of 0.5 to 1 g twice daily. The treatment is expensive and time consuming and carbenicillin is sticky in solution causing furniture in the room to become tacky (M.B. Mearns, *Archs Dis. Childh.*, 1985, *60*, 272). There is also some concern about the safety of aerosol therapy, in that the antibiotic solutions may become a source of infecting resistant organisms, aerosol use may potentiate the development of resistant strains of organisms, and the use of aerosol antibiotics could lead to an increased incidence of hypersensitivity reactions (H.W. Kelly and C. Lovato, *Drug Intell. & clin. Pharm.*, 1984, *18*, 772). For mention of other antibiotics used to treat respiratory infections in cystic fibrosis, see Choice of Antibiotic, p.100. See also Resistance, Pseudomonas, above.

Preparations

Carbenicillin Injection *(B.P.).* Carbenicillin sodium to be reconstituted before use.

Sterile Carbenicillin Disodium *(U.S.P.)*

Proprietary Preparations

Pyopen *(Beecham Research, UK). Injection,* powder for reconstitution, carbenicillin 1 and 5 g (as sodium salt).

Proprietary Names and Manufacturers

Anabactyl *(Ger.)*; Carbapen *(Commonwealth Serum Laboratories, Austral.)*; Fugacillin *(Astra, Denm.; Norw.; Swed.)*; Geopen *(Pfizer, Ital.; Roerig, USA)*; Microcillin *(Ger.)*; Pyocianil *(Farmitalia, Ital.)*; Pyopen *(Arg.; Austral.; Belg.; Ayerst, Canad.; Beecham Products, Fr.; Ital.; Jpn; Neth.; Beecham, S.Afr.; Beecham, Spain; Switz.; Beecham Research, UK; Beecham Laboratories, USA)*; Rexcilina *(Spain)*.

25-d

Carfecillin Sodium *(BANM, pINNM).*

BRL-3475; Carbenicillin Phenyl Sodium *(USAN).* Sodium (6*R*)-6-(2-phenoxycarbonyl-2-phenylacetamido)penicillanate.

$C_{23}H_{21}N_2NaO_6S$=476.5.

CAS — 27025-49-6 (carfecillin); 21649-57-0 (sodium salt).

1.3 g of monograph substance is approximately equivalent to 1 g of carbenicillin. Each g of monograph substance represents about 2.1 mmol of sodium.

Adverse Effects and Precautions

As for Carbenicillin Sodium, p.139. Nausea and diarrhoea have been reported.

Antimicrobial Action and Resistance

As for Carbenicillin Sodium, p.139.

Absorption and Fate

Carfecillin sodium is absorbed from the gastro-intestinal tract and is rapidly hydrolysed to carbenicillin and phenol. Following a dose of 1 g of carfecillin sodium plasma concentrations of 5 to 10 µg per mL of carbenicillin and urine concentrations of up to 1 mg per mL of carbenicillin may be achieved. Doubling the dose of carfecillin does not result in double the serum-carbenicillin concentration. The phenol moiety is excreted in the urine as conjugates.

A study of the pharmacokinetics of carfecillin sodium.— P. J. Wilkinson *et al.*, *Br. med. J.*, 1975, *2*, 250.

Uses and Administration

Carfecillin sodium is given by mouth in doses of 0.5 to 1 g three times daily for the treatment of urinary-tract infections due to *Pseudomonas* spp. and other sensitive bacteria including *Proteus* spp. Children from 2 to 10 years may be given half the adult dose; a recommended dose range is 30 to 60 mg per kg body-weight daily. Serious infections should be treated initially with parenteral carbenicillin sodium. Therapeutic urinary-carbenicillin concentrations may not be achieved in patients with severe renal impairment.

It is not used for the treatment of systemic infections since attainable plasma-carbenicillin concentrations are too low to be effective.

URINARY-TRACT INFECTIONS. References to the use of carfecillin sodium: D. A. Leigh and K. Simmons, *J. antimicrob. Chemother.*, 1976, *2*, 293; J. Borowski *et al.*, *ibid.*, 175.

Proprietary Preparations

Uticillin *(Beecham Research, UK). Tablets,* carfecillin sodium 500 mg.

Proprietary Names and Manufacturers

Gripenin-O *(Jpn)*; Pencina *(Switz.)*; Safepen *(Beecham, Spain)*; Uricillina *(Ibi, Ital.)*; Urocarf *(Schwarz, Ital.)*; Uticillin *(Jpn; S.Afr.; Beecham Research, UK)*.

26-n

Carindacillin Sodium *(BANM, pINNM).*

Carbenicillin Indanyl Sodium *(USAN)*; CP-15464-2. Sodium (6*R*)-6-[2-(indan-5-yloxycarbonyl)-2-phenylacetamido]penicillanate.

$C_{26}H_{25}N_2NaO_6S$=516.6.

CAS — 35531-88-5 (carindacillin); 26605-69-6 (sodium salt).

Pharmacopoeias. In *U.S.*

A white to off-white powder. **Soluble** in water and alcohol. A 10% solution in water has a pH of 5 to 8. 1.4 g of monograph substance is approximately equivalent to 1 g of carbenicillin. Each g of monograph substance represents about 1.9 mmol of sodium. **Store** in airtight containers.

Adverse Effects and Precautions

As for Carbenicillin Sodium, p.139.

Side-effects that have most frequently been reported with carindacillin sodium include bitter taste, nausea, vomiting, and diarrhoea.

EFFECTS ON THE GASTRO-INTESTINAL TRACT. Reports of pseudomembranous colitis associated with carindacillin sodium: T. F. O'Meara and R. A. Simmons (letter), *Ann. intern. Med.*, 1980, *92*, 440; H. A. Saadah (letter), *ibid.*, *93*, 645.

Antimicrobial Action and Resistance

As for Carbenicillin Sodium, p.139.

Carindacillin has a lower MIC for Gram-positive organisms and *Klebsiella pneumoniae* than carbenicillin *in vitro* but due to the rapid metabolism of the ester this is not observed *in vivo*.

Absorption and Fate

Carindacillin sodium is rapidly but incompletely absorbed from the gastro-intestinal tract. It is rapidly hydrolysed to carbenicillin and indanol. Peak plasma-carbenicillin concentrations ranging from 7 to 17 µg per mL have been reported about 1.5 hours after a dose of 1 g of carindacillin sodium. Doubling the dose of carindacillin does not result in double the serum-carbenicillin concentration. Low concentrations of carindacillin may be detected in the plasma. A dose of 1 g maintains a urine-carbenicillin concentration of 1 mg per mL for about 3 hours. The indanol moiety is excreted in the urine as glucuronide and sulphate conjugates.

References to the pharmacokinetics of carindacillin sodium: J. L. Bran *et al.*, *Clin. Pharmac. Ther.*, 1971, *12*, 525; R. R. Bailey *et al.*, *Postgrad. med. J.*, 1972, *48*, 422; K. Butler *et al.*, *J. infect. Dis.*, 1973, *127*, *Suppl.*, S97; A. K. Knirsch *et al.*, *ibid.*, S105.

Uses and Administration

Carindacillin sodium is given by mouth usually in doses equivalent to 382 to 764 mg of carbenicillin four times daily for the treatment of urinary-tract infections or prostatitis due to *Pseudomonas* spp. and other sensitive bacteria including *Proteus* spp. Serious infections should be treated initially with parenteral carbenicillin sodium. Therapeutic urinary-carbenicillin concentrations may not be attained after administration of carindacillin sodium to patients with severe renal impairment.

It is not used for the treatment of systemic infections since attainable plasma-carbenicillin concentrations are too low to be effective.

A report of the successful use of carindacillin sodium 1 g four times a day in patients with acute or chronic prostatitis.— R. A. Oliveri *et al.*, *Curr. ther. Res.*, 1979, *25*, 415. See also P. M. Hanus and L. H. Danziger, *Clin. Pharm.*, 1984, *3*, 49.

Preparations

Carbenicillin Indanyl Sodium Tablets *(U.S.P.)*. Tablets containing carindacillin sodium.

Proprietary Names and Manufacturers

Carindapen *(Pfizer, Ger.)*; Geocillin *(Roerig, USA)*; Geopen *(Pfizer, Austral.; Pfizer, Canad.; Pfizer, Denm.; Pfizer, Ital.; Pfizer, Switz.)*; Geopen-U *(Jpn)*; G.U.-Pen *(Pfizer, Belg.; Pfizer, Neth.)*; Unipen *(Pfizer, Spain)*.

18916-d

Carumonam Sodium *(BANM, USAN, rINNM)*.

AMA-1080 *(carumonam)*; Ro-17-2301 *(carumonam)*; Ro-17-2301/006 *(sodium salt)*. (*Z*)-(2-Aminothiazol-4-yl){[(2*S*,3*S*)-2-carbamoyloxymethyl-4-oxo-1-sulphoazetidin-3-yl]carbamoyl}methyleneamino-oxyacetic acid, disodium salt.

$C_{12}H_{12}N_6Na_2O_{10}S_2$=510.4.

CAS — 87638-04-8 (carumonam); 86832-68-0 (sodium salt).

Carumonam sodium is a monobactam antibiotic with a spectrum of antimicrobial action *in vitro* similar to that of aztreonam (see p.125).

Studies of the antimicrobial action of carumonam: A. Imada *et al.*, *Antimicrob. Ag. Chemother.*, 1985, *27*, 821; W. W. S. Ng *et al.*, *ibid.*, 872; R. J. Fass and V. L. Helsel, *ibid.*, *28*, 834; R. Wise *et al.*, *J. antimicrob. Chemother.*, 1985, *15*, 193; D. A. Bremner, *ibid.*, *16*, 457; K. Matsuda *et al.*, *ibid.*, 539; C. A. Bensons *et al.*, *Antimicrob. Ag. Chemother.*, 1986, *29*, 155; B. R. Smith *et al.*, *ibid.*, 346; K. E. Aldridge and C. V. Sanders, *Curr. ther. Res.*, 1986, *40*, 515; M. Nakao *et al.*, *J. antimicrob. Chemother.*, 1986, *17*, 433; H. C. Neu *et al.*, *ibid.*, *18*, 35; E. E. Stobberingh *et al.*, *ibid.*, 345; A. Pascual *et al.* (letter), *ibid.*, 1987, *19*, 701.

Studies of the absorption and fate of carumonam: E. Weidekamm *et al.*, *Antimicrob. Ag. Chemother.*, 1984, *26*, 898 (pharmacokinetic studies in healthy subjects); C. A. M. McNulty *et al.*, *ibid.*, 1985, *28*, 425 (pharmacokinetics and tissue penetration); F. Horber *et al.*, *ibid.*, 1986, *29*, 116 (pharmacokinetics and dosage recommendations in patients with renal insufficiency).

Proprietary Names and Manufacturers
Takeda, Jpn.

27-h

Cefaclor *(BAN, USAN, pINN)*.

99638. (7*R*)-3-Chloro-7-(α-D-phenylglycylamino)-3-cephem-4-carboxylic acid monohydrate.

$C_{15}H_{14}ClN_3O_4S,H_2O$=385.8.

CAS — 53994-73-3 (anhydrous); 70356-03-5 (monohydrate).

Pharmacopoeias. In *U.S.*

A 2.5% aqueous suspension has a pH of 3.0 to 4.5. **Store** in airtight containers.

Adverse Effects and Precautions

As for Cephalexin, p.173.

ADMINISTRATION IN RENAL FAILURE. For reference to the precautions to be observed in renal failure, see under Administration in Renal Failure in Absorption and Fate and Uses, below.

ALLERGY. A cluster of hypersensitivity reactions occurred in 8 children receiving cefaclor for the treatment of persistent otitis media; 6 were taking cefaclor for the second time. A generalised pruritic rash and arthritis appeared from 5 to 19 days after the initiation of treatment with cefaclor and generally disappeared within 4 to 5 days of discontinuation. Signs of erythema multiforme developed in 6 of the children and purpura in 4.— D. L. Murray *et al.* (letter), *New Engl. J. Med.*, 1980, *303*, 1003.

Of 2026 children who received 4841 courses of cefaclor or amoxycillin by mouth, hypersensitivity reactions were observed in 54 of 1017 (5.3%) assigned to cefaclor, and 37 of 1009 (3.7%) assigned to amoxycillin. Five serum-sickness reactions and 6 cases of erythema multiforme occurred in those treated with cefaclor, but none of these reactions occurred in those given amoxycillin. Urticaria was reported in 24 and 8 patients in the 2 groups respectively. The incidence of non-hypersensitivity reactions was similar in the 2 groups.— L. R. Levine, *Pediatr. infect. Dis.*, 1985, *4*, 358.

A report from Japan of a relatively high incidence of anaphylactic reactions to cefaclor.— R. Hama and K. Mori (letter), *Lancet*, 1988, *1*, 1331.

EFFECTS ON THE GASTRO-INTESTINAL TRACT. A comparison of changes in the faecal flora after administration of cefaclor or cefixime by mouth to healthy subjects.— S. M. Finegold *et al.*, *Antimicrob. Ag. Chemother.*, 1987, *31*, 443.

For reference to a study comparing the effects of cefaclor, and a combination of amoxycillin and clavulanic acid on the urogenital and rectal flora, see under Urinary-tract Infections in Amoxycillin, p.115.

EFFECTS ON THE LIVER. Cholestatic jaundice and haematuria in a 3-year-old boy was considered to be a hypersensitivity reaction to cefaclor.— M. Bosio, *J. Toxicol. clin. Toxicol.*, 1983, *20*, 79.

Antimicrobial Action and Resistance

Cefaclor is bactericidal and has antimicrobial activity similar to that of cephalexin (see p.174) but is reported to be more active against Gram-negative bacteria including *Escherichia coli, Klebsiella pneumoniae, Neisseria gonorrhoeae,* and *Proteus mirabilis*, and especially against *Haemophilus influenzae*. It is active against some beta-lactamase-producing strains of *H. influenzae*. It may be less resistant to staphylococcal penicillinase than cephalexin or cephradine and a marked inoculum effect has been reported *in vitro*.

A study of the sensitivity of 28 strains of *Branhamella catarrhalis* to a range of antibiotics. For 17 non-beta-lactamase-producing strains 90% were inhibited by 0.031 μg per mL of cefaclor; the corresponding concentration for 11 beta-lactamase-producing strains was greater than 256 μg per mL.— E. E. Stobberingh *et al.*, *J. antimicrob. Chemother.*, 1984, *13*, 55.

A study of the susceptibility of isolates of *Haemophilus influenzae* from 21 microbiology laboratories in Wales to a range of antibiotics. Taking resistance to cefaclor as an MIC of more than 4 μg per mL, 1.6% of strains tested were resistant to this agent.— A. J. Howard (letter), *Br. med. J.*, 1987, *295*, 608.

Absorption and Fate

Cefaclor is absorbed from the gastro-intestinal tract but plasma concentrations are slightly lower than those achieved with cephalexin or cephradine. Doses of 250 and 500 mg by mouth produce peak plasma concentrations of about 6 and 13 μg per mL respectively at 0.5 to 1 hour. The presence of food may delay the absorption of cefaclor, but the total amount absorbed is unchanged. Half-lives ranging from 30 minutes to 1 hour have been reported.

Cefaclor appears to be widely distributed in the body; it crosses the placenta and is excreted in low concentrations in breast milk. It is rapidly excreted by the kidneys; up to 85% of a dose appears unchanged in the urine within 8 hours, the greater part within 2 hours. High concentrations of cefaclor are achieved in the urine within 8 hours of a dose; peak concentrations of 600 and 900 μg per mL have been reported after doses of 250 and 500 mg respectively. Probenecid delays excretion.

The pharmacokinetics of cefaclor were studied in 28 children aged 4 to 63 months who were treated for impetigo, pharyngitis or otitis media. The mean serum concentrations of cefaclor 30 minutes after administration of cefaclor 10 mg per kg body-weight were 10.8 μg per mL in fasting children and 6.7 μg per mL in those who received the antibiotic and milk concomitantly; corresponding concentrations after 15 mg per kg were 13.1 and 10.9 μg per mL respectively. Although peak serum concentrations of cefaclor were smaller in non-fasting children the overall absorption of cefaclor was similar for both groups. Serum half-lives of cefaclor ranged from 36 to 46 minutes after 15 mg per kg and from 55 to 60 minutes after 10 mg per kg. Mean concentrations of cefaclor in saliva up to 6 hours after administration of 15 mg per kg were similar to the corresponding serum concentrations.— G. H. McCracken *et al.*, *J. antimicrob. Chemother.*, 1978, *4*, 515.

In 10 neonates given cefaclor by mouth in a dose of 7.5 mg per kg body-weight every 6 hours, a mean peak serum concentration of 7.7 μg per mL was achieved one hour after the initial dose. Urine concentrations in the first 6 hours after the dose ranged from 100 to 600 μg per mL.— K. C. Chin *et al.*, *Curr. med. Res. Opinion*, 1981, *7*, 168.

ADMINISTRATION IN RENAL FAILURE. The pharmacokinetics of cefaclor were studied in 17 patients with end-stage renal disease (creatinine clearance of less than 5 mL per minute). A mean peak plasma concentration of 48.3 μg per mL was obtained in 6 fasting patients after a 1-g dose and occurred within 4 hours of administration; the mean plasma half-life was 2.3 hours. A haemodialysis session of 5.5 hours starting 2 hours after the same dose reduced the mean half-life to 1.6 hours and about 35% of the dose was recovered in the dialysate. There was no evidence of drug accumulation in 5 patients who received cefaclor 500 mg every 6 hours for 36 hours and plasma concentrations were maintained between 10.6 and 16 μg per mL.— S. J. Berman *et al.*, *Antimicrob. Ag. Chemother.*, 1978, *14*, 281.

Fifteen anephric patients on maintenance haemodialysis three times a week were given cefaclor 500 mg by mouth every 8 hours for 11 days. A mean peak serum concentration of 24.9 μg per mL (corrected for a weight of 70 kg) was obtained about one hour after the initial dose. The mean half-life was 1.5 hours during haemodialysis, and 2.9 hours without dialysis. Haemodialysis appeared to approximately double the clearance of cefaclor, and it was recommended that the usual dose be repeated after each dialysis session. There was no evidence of accumulation of cefaclor during multiple dosing.— D. A. Spyker *et al.*, *Antimicrob. Ag. Chemother.*, 1982, *21*, 278.

See also under Administration in Renal Failure in Uses (below).

PROTEIN BINDING. Cefaclor was about 50% bound to plasma proteins *in vitro*.— F. P. Tally *et al.*, *J. antimicrob. Chemother.*, 1979, *5*, 159.

Uses and Administration

Cefaclor, a cephalosporin antibiotic, is administered by mouth similarly to cephalexin (see p.174), in the treatment of mild to moderate susceptible infections. Its greater activity against *Haemophilus influenzae*, however, may make it more useful than cephalexin for certain infections. The usual dose is 250 mg every 8 hours although up to 4 g daily has been given. A suggested dose for children is 20 mg per kg body-weight daily increased if necessary to 40 mg per kg daily but not exceeding a total daily dose of 1 g. A common dosage regimen is: children over 5 years, 250 mg three times daily; 1 to 5 years, 125 mg three times daily; under 1 year, 62.5 mg three times daily.

ADMINISTRATION IN RENAL FAILURE. The normal half-life for cefaclor of 0.75 hour was increased to 2.8 hours in end-stage renal failure. In patients with a glomerular filtration-rate (GFR) of 10 to 50 mL per minute 50 to 100% of the normal dose could be given and in those with a GFR of less than 10 mL per minute the dose should be reduced to 33%. A dose supplement should be given to patients undergoing haemodialysis.— W. M. Bennett *et al.*, *Am. J. Kidney Dis.*, 1983, *3*, 155.

See also under Absorption and Fate (above).

GONORRHOEA. Cefaclor 3 g in association with probenecid 1 g, both given by mouth, appeared to be an effective treatment for gonorrhoea caused by both penicillinase-producing and non-penicillinase-producing *Neisseria gonorrhoeae*.— K. Panikabutra *et al.*, *Br. J. vener. Dis.*, 1983, *59*, 298.

Further references to the treatment of gonorrhoea with cefaclor: R. R. Willcox *et al.*, *Curr. med. Res. Opinion*, 1982, *7*, 601.

IMPETIGO. Of 73 children aged 1 to 13 years with staphylococcal bullous impetigo who were evaluated after receiving cefaclor 30 mg per kg body-weight daily in 3 or 4 divided doses for 5 to 10 days, 66 were cleared of lesions and of 5 who were considered to have improved 3 were cleared after a further 4 days of therapy.— B. M. Gray *et al.*, *Antimicrob. Ag. Chemother.*, 1978, *13*, 988.

OTITIS MEDIA. In a review of otitis media (*Drug & Ther. Bull.*, 1984, *22*, 53), cefaclor was considered to be the only oral cephalosporin with sufficient activity against *Haemophilus* for the treatment of this condition, but studies demonstrating its clinical efficacy were stated to be few. In another review B.L. True and D.K. Helling, *Drug Intell. & clin. Pharm.*, 1986, *20*, 666) cefaclor was listed among those agents suitable for second-line therapy of otitis media. There have been several studies comparing the efficacy of cefaclor with other antibiotics in general practice. In a double-blind study involving 223 children under 12 years of age, Feldman *et al.* (*Archs Dis. Childh.*, 1982, *57*, 594) concluded that 10-day courses of cefaclor or co-trimoxazole were equally effective. In a single-blind study involving 150 children aged 6 months to 6 years (W.R.B. John and J.C. Vallé-Jones, *Practitioner*, 1983, *227*, 1805) half were treated with cefaclor and half with amoxycillin, both given by mouth in a dose of 125 mg three times daily for 7 days. The cure rates were 87 and 57% respectively. Both these studies, however, classified efficacy only by assessment of clinical signs or symptoms; no bacteriological studies were performed.

In a double-blind study evaluating 96 children aged 3 to 10 years who presented with otitis media to 14 general practitioners in 4 health centres, Jones and Bain (*J. R. Coll. gen. Pract.*, 1986, *36*, 356) concluded that 3- and 7-day courses of cefaclor 125 mg three times daily by mouth were equally effective both in terms of resolution of signs and symptoms, and in prevention of recurrences of middle-ear infections. Again, no bacteriological studies were performed. Two children in the 3-day group whose ear-ache recurred on the fifth day and who were prescribed an alternative antibiotic, were, however, excluded from the analysis.

PREGNANCY AND THE NEONATE. For reference to the use of cefaclor during pregnancy, see under Urinary-tract Infections in Cephalexin, p.175.

RESPIRATORY-TRACT INFECTIONS. *Bronchitis.* In a double-blind study of 80 patients with acute exacerbations of chronic bronchitis, cefaclor or amoxycillin, both given by mouth in a dose of 500 mg every 8 hours for 10 days, were considered to be equally effective, as assessed by resolution of symptoms, conversion from purulent to mucoid sputum, and decrease in sputum weight. There was considerable variation in serum and sputum concentrations for both agents.— M. R. Law *et al.*, *J. antimicrob. Chemother.*, 1983, *11*, 83.

A study of 19 patients with acute exacerbations of chronic bronchitis, all treated with conventional therapy including hydration, bronchodilators, diuretics, and oxygen. The addition of a course of cefaclor 500 mg three times daily by mouth for 8 days was no more effective than placebo in improving clinical and functional indices although it did decrease sputum volume and purulence. Many patients may not require antibiotics for exacerbations of chronic bronchitis.— F. Manresa *et al.* (letter), *Lancet*, 1987, *2*, 394.

Pharyngitis. In a study involving 104 children with Group A streptococcal pharyngitis, the failure rate appeared to be lower after treatment with cefaclor than after phenoxymethylpenicillin by mouth. Both drugs were given three times daily for 10 days.— M. Stillerman, *Pediatr. infect. Dis.*, 1986, *5*, 649.

URINARY-TRACT INFECTIONS. Of 33 evaluable women with acute uncomplicated urinary-tract infection given a single dose of cefaclor 2 g by mouth, 26 were considered cured 1 to 3 days later; after 4 weeks however, only 10 of the 30 who returned were cured. Of 27 evaluable patients given 250 mg every 8 hours for 10 days, 24 were cured within 3 days, and 18 of the 22 who returned at 4 weeks.— R. N. Greenberg *et al.*, *Am. J. Med.*, 1981, *71*, 841.

Further references to the use of cefaclor in the treatment of infections of the urinary tract: M. J. Gurwith *et al.*, *Antimicrob. Ag. Chemother.*, 1983, *24*, 716; A. Kumar and Y. Shah, *Curr. ther. Res.*, 1984, *35*, 932; J. A. Boscia *et al.*, *J. Am. med. Ass.*, 1987, *257*, 1067.

For reference to a comparative study of cefaclor and a combination of amoxycillin and clavulanic acid in the treatment of urinary-tract infections, see Amoxycillin, p.115.

For references to a comparative study of cefaclor, cephalexin, and cefuroxime axetil for the treatment of urinary-tract infections, see Cefuroxime Axetil, p.171.

Preparations

Cefaclor Capsules *(U.S.P.)*

Cefaclor for Oral Suspension *(U.S.P.)*

Proprietary Preparations

Distaclor *(Dista, UK)*. *Capsules*, cefaclor 250 mg. *Suspension*, granules for reconstitution, 125 and 250 mg/5mL when reconstituted with water.

Proprietary Names and Manufacturers

Alfatil *(Lilly, Fr.)*; Ceclor *(Lilly, Austral.; Lilly, Canad.; Lilly, S.Afr.; Lilly, Spain; Lilly, Switz.; Lilly, USA)*; Distaclor *(Dista, UK)*; Kefolor *(Lilly, Denm.; Lilly, Swed.)*; Panacef *(Lilly, Ital.)*; Panoral *(Lilly, Ger.)*.

28-m

Cefadroxil *(BAN, USAN, pINN)*.

BL-S578; MJF-11567-3. (7*R*)-7-(α-D-4-Hydroxyphenylglycylamino)-3-methyl-3-cephem-4-carboxylic acid monchydrate.

$C_{16}H_{17}N_3O_5S,H_2O$=381.4.

CAS — 50370-12-2 (anhydrous); 66592-87-8 (monohydrate).

Pharmacopoeias. In *It.* and *U.S.*

A 5% solution in water has a pH of 4 to 6. **Store** in airtight containers.

Adverse Effects and Precautions

As for Cephalexin, p.173.

ADMINISTRATION IN RENAL FAILURE. For reference to the precautions to be observed in renal failure, see under Administration in Renal Failure in Absorption and Fate and Uses, below.

EFFECTS ON THE LIVER. For a report of cholestatic jaundice associated with the administration of cefadroxil and cephazolin, see Cephazolin Sodium, p.183.

Antimicrobial Action and Resistance

As for Cephalexin, p.174.

A study of the activity *in vitro* of cefadroxil against 749 clinically-significant bacterial isolates.— M. W. Casewell and S. G. L. Bragman, *J. antimicrob. Chemother.*, 1987, *19*, 597.

Absorption and Fate

Cefadroxil is well absorbed from the gastro-intestinal tract. After doses of 500 mg and 1 g by mouth, peak plasma concentrations of about 16 and 30 μg per mL respectively are obtained after 1.5 to 2 hours. Although peak concentrations are similar to those of cephalexin, plasma concentrations are more sustained. Administration with food does not appear to affect the absorption of cefadroxil. About 20% of cefadroxil in the circulation is reported to be bound to plasma proteins. The half-life of cefadroxil is about 1.5 hours and is prolonged in patients with impaired renal function.

Cefadroxil is widely distributed to body tissues and fluids.

More than 90% of a dose of cefadroxil may be excreted unchanged in the urine within 24 hours by glomerular filtration and tubular secretion; peak urinary concentrations of greater than 1 mg per mL have been reported after a dose of 500 mg.

A review of the absorption and fate of cefadroxil. The pharmacokinetic profile of cefadroxil differs from those of cephalexin and cephradine in its more prolonged duration of activity and significantly lower rate of excretion; thus plasma and urine concentrations are higher over an extended period of time. This allows administration of cefadroxil once or twice daily.

Cefadroxil has been shown to be water-soluble and to have a fair degree of lipid solubility. Concentrations of cefadroxil are detectable in the tonsils, lungs, liver, gall bladder, bone, muscle, synovial capsule, prostate and gynaecological tissues, and in most body fluids, transudates, and exudates such as the pleural fluid, bile, sputum, amniotic fluid, breast milk, and aqueous humour. Cefadroxil crosses the placenta.

Like cephalexin and cephradine, cefadroxil is not metabolised in the body. After administration of equivalent doses, concentrations of cefadroxil in the urine are initially lower than those of cephalexin; at later time intervals, however, they are higher. Haemodialysis has been reported to decrease plasma-cefadroxil concentrations by 75%.— B. Tanrisever and P. J. Santella, *Drugs*, 1986, *32, Suppl.* 3, 1.

A comparative study of the pharmacokinetics of cefadroxil, cefaclor, cephalexin, and cephradine after oral administration to infants and children.— C. M. Ginsburg, *J. antimicrob. Chemother.*, 1982, *10, Suppl.* B, 27.

ADMINISTRATION IN RENAL FAILURE. A study of the pharmacokinetics of cefadroxil in 25 subjects with varying degrees of renal function, including 5 patients on haemodialysis. In renal insufficiency, peak serum concentrations were higher and occurred later, the half-life was longer, and urinary elimination and renal clearance were decreased. The elimination of cefadroxil was increased during haemodialysis, the half-life being 21.7 and 3.4 hours off and on dialysis respectively. These authors use a dose of 1 g at the end of each dialysis session and a further 1-g dose every 72 hours.— A. Leroy *et al.*, *J. antimicrob. Chemother.*, 1982, *10, Suppl.* B, 39.

See also under Administration in Renal Failure in Uses, below.

Uses and Administration

Cefadroxil is the para-hydroxy derivative of cephalexin, p.174, and is used similarly in the treatment of mild to moderate susceptible infections. It is administered by mouth, and doses are expressed in terms of the anhydrous substance. Usually, 1 to 2 g is given daily as a single dose or in 2 divided doses. The following doses have been suggested for children: 500 mg twice daily for those over 6 years of age, 250 mg twice daily for children aged 1 to 6 years, and 25 mg per kg body-weight daily in divided doses for infants under 1 year.

Series of papers on cefadroxil and its use in the treatment of various infections: *J. antimicrob. Chemother.*, 1982, *10, Suppl.* B, 1–160; *Drugs*, 1986, *32, Suppl.* 3, 1–56.

An evaluation of the efficacy and safety of cefadroxil in the treatment of infections in 395 paediatric patients aged 2 days to 15 years, involved in 15 clinical studies. Cefadroxil, in the form of a suspension, was administered to most patients in a dose of 30 to 50 mg per kg body-weight daily in 2 divided doses. Children with acute otitis media received 100 mg per kg daily in 2 divided doses, and those with urinary-tract infections, 25 mg per kg once daily. Overall, 378 patients (96%) were considered to be clinically cured; 15 patients failed treatment, and relapses occurred in 3 patients, 2 with pharyngotonsillitis and one with cystitis. Bacteriologically, 360 of 375 pathogens were eradicated. Adverse effects were reported in 37 (9%) patients, and were either allergic skin reactions or gastro-intestinal effects. Of the 5 patients with diarrhoea, 2 who had received cefadroxil 100 mg per kg daily discontinued therapy because of the severity of the effect. There were no clinically significant changes in haematocrit, or renal or hepatic function during treatment or follow-up periods.— H. Puhakka and E. Virolainen, *Drugs*, 1986, *32, Suppl.* 3, 21.

ADMINISTRATION IN RENAL FAILURE. The normal half-life for cefadroxil of 1.4 hours was increased to 20 to 25 hours in end-stage renal failure. The interval between doses should be extended from 8 hours to 12 to 24 hours in patients with a glomerular filtration-rate (GFR) of 10 to 50 mL per minute and to 24 to 48 hours in patients with a GFR of less than 10 mL per minute. A dose supplement should be given to patients undergoing haemodialysis.— W. M. Bennett *et al.*, *Am. J. Kidney Dis.*, 1983, *3*, 155. The view that the normal dosage interval should be 12 or 24 hours and that a 12-hour dosage interval may still be used even in patients with a creatinine clearance-rate as low as 25 mL per minute.— G. R. McKinney (letter), *Ann. intern. Med.*, 1980, *93*, 784. Reply.— R. A. Parker and W. M. Bennett (letter), *ibid.*

See also Absorption and Fate, above.

PHARYNGITIS. In a study involving 150 children with Group A beta-haemolytic streptococcal pharyngitis, cefadroxil given once daily by mouth was at least as effective as phenoxymethylpenicillin given three times daily in producing both bacteriological eradication and improvement in clinical symptoms.— M. E. Pichichero *et al.*, *Antimicrob. Ag. Chemother.*, 1987, *31*, 903.

Preparations

Cefadroxil Capsules *(U.S.P.)*

Cefadroxil for Oral Suspension *(U.S.P.)*

Cefadroxil Tablets *(U.S.P.)*

Proprietary Preparations

Baxan *(Bristol-Myers Pharmaceuticals, UK). Capsules,* cefadroxil equivalent to anhydrous cefadroxil 500 mg. *Suspension,* powder for reconstitution, cefadroxil equivalent to anhydrous cefadroxil 125, 250, and 500 mg/5 mL when reconstituted with water.

Proprietary Names and Manufacturers

Baxan *(Bristol-Myers Pharmaceuticals, UK)*; Bidocef *(Ciba, Ger.)*; Cefadril *(AGIPS, Ital.)*; Cefamox *(Bristol, Swed.)*; Cefroxil *(Fides, Spain)*; Ceoxil *(Magis, Ital.)*; Cephos *(CT, Ital.)*; Crenodyn *(Panthox & Burck, Ital.)*; Droxicef *(Alfa Farmaceutici, Ital.)*; Duracef *(Mead Johnson, Belg.; Bristol Italiana Sud, Ital.; Bristol, S.Afr.; Bristol-Myers, Spain; Ciba, Switz.)*; Duricef *(Bristol, Canad.; Mead Johnson Pharmaceutical, USA)*; Kefroxil *(Wharton, Ital.)*; Longacef *(Chiesi, Ital.)*; Oracefal *(Bristol, Fr.)*; Oradroxil *(Lampugnani, Ital.)*; Ultracef *(Bristol, USA)*.

29-b

Cefapirin Sodium *(BANM, pINNM).*

BL-P1322; Cephapirin Sodium *(USAN)*. Sodium (7*R*)-7-[2-(4-pyridylthio)acetamido]cephalosporanate; Sodium (7*R*)-3-acetoxymethyl-7-[2-(4-pyridylthio)acetamido]-3-cephem-4-carboxylate.

$C_{17}H_{16}N_3NaO_6S_2$=445.4.

CAS — 21593-23-7 (cefapirin); 24356-60-3 (sodium salt).

Pharmacopoeias. In *It. U.S.* includes Sterile Cephapirin Sodium.

A white to off-white crystalline powder, odourless or with a slight odour. 1.05 g of monograph substance is approximately equivalent to 1 g of cefapirin. Each g of monograph substance represents about 2.2 mmol of sodium.

Very **soluble** in water; insoluble in most organic solvents. A 1% solution in water has a pH of 6.5 to 8.5.

Aqueous solutions of up to 40% cefapirin sodium are reported to be **stable** for 12 hours at 25°, 10 days at 4°, and 60 days at −15°. Solutions of up to 10% cefapirin sodium in 0.9% sodium chloride or 5% glucose are reported to be stable for 24 hours at 25°, 10 days at 4°, and 60 days at −15°.

Solutions of cefapirin sodium may become yellow on storage, but slight discoloration does not affect potency.

Cefapirin sodium has been reported to be **incompatible** with aminoglycosides, tetracyclines, and other antimicrobial agents including erythromycin gluceptate, nitrofurantoin, polymyxin B sulphate, and sulphadiazine sodium. Incompatibility or loss of activity has also been reported with adrenaline hydrochloride, aminophylline, ascorbic acid, noradrenaline acid tartrate, phenytoin sodium, and thiopentone sodium.

Adverse Effects and Precautions

As for Cephalothin Sodium, p.176. Thrombophlebitis associated with intravenous administration may be less of a problem with cefapirin.

ADMINISTRATION IN RENAL FAILURE. For reference to the precautions to be observed in renal failure, see under Uses, Administration in Renal Failure, below.

ALLERGY. From an analysis of 148 reported episodes of drug fever, 46 were caused by antimicrobial agents and of these one was due to cefapirin.— P. A. Mackowiak and C. F. LeMaistre, *Ann. intern. Med.*, 1987, *106,* 728.

INTERFERENCE WITH ASSAY PROCEDURES. For precautions to be observed when assaying cefapirin in whole blood, see Cephalothin Sodium, p.177.

INTERFERENCE WITH DIAGNOSTIC TESTS. When present in urine in concentrations of 3.5 mg per mL or more, cefapirin interfered with the detection of urine-glucose by the copper-reduction (Clinitest) method, but not by the glucose-oxidase (Tes-Tape or KetoDiastix) methods.— J. D. Haas and M. A. Raebel, *Am. J. Hosp. Pharm.*, 1984, *41,* 1186.

Antimicrobial Action and Resistance

As for Cephalothin Sodium, p.177.

All 24 strains of *Actinobacillus actinomycetemcomitans* tested were inhibited by a concentration of 6.25 µg per mL of cefapirin *in vitro*. The MBCs of 12 strains ranged from 0.1 to 1.6 µg per mL. When cefapirin was tested in combination with trimethoprim against 8 strains, synergism was noted in 2 strains and antagonism in 1.— R. Yogev *et al., Antimicrob. Ag. Chemother.*, 1986, *29,* 179.

Absorption and Fate

Cefapirin is poorly absorbed from the gastro-intestinal tract and is given by intramuscular or intravenous injection as the sodium salt. Plasma concentrations of 16 to 24 µg per mL have been reported 30 minutes after a dose of 1 g given intramuscularly. About 50% of a dose is bound to plasma proteins and the plasma half-life is about 36 minutes. Cefapirin has been reported to cross the placenta and small amounts have been detected in breast milk.

Similarly to cephalothin, high concentrations are excreted in the urine and about 40% of a dose appears as the less active deacetylated metabolite. About 1% may be excreted in bile.

A review of the absorption and fate of cefapirin.— C. H. Nightingale *et al., J. pharm. Sci.*, 1975, *64,* 1899.

In a study of 5 healthy subjects given 1 g of cefapirin sodium intravenously, the average serum-cefapirin concentration was 73 µg per mL 15 minutes after injection and fell to zero at 6 hours; the serum half-life was 21 minutes. During the first 6 hours 72% of the dose was excreted in the urine in an average concentration of 2.6 mg per mL. Negligible amounts were excreted in the next 6 hours. Another 5 subjects given 1 g intramuscularly achieved serum concentrations of 24 µg per mL after 30 minutes falling to 0.2 µg per mL at 6 hours; the serum half-life was 47 minutes. About 53% was excreted in the urine within 6 hours in an average concentration of 1.3 mg per mL. A further 6% was excreted in the next 6 hours. All subjects complained of moderate pain after intramuscular injection.— J. Axelrod *et al., J. clin. Pharmac.*, 1972, *12,* 84.

Cefapirin was metabolised to desacetylcefapirin in healthy subjects. Although plasma concentrations of the metabolite ranged from 0.3 to 2.5 µg per mL compared with cefapirin concentrations of 1.7 to 63.6 µg per mL over the same period following 1 g intravenously, about 45% of the dose was excreted in the urine as desacetylcefapirin over 6 hours and about 49% as cefapirin. It was considered that cefapirin underwent renal metabolism. The plasma half-life of cefapirin was about 0.5 hours and that of desacetylcefapirin 0.43 hours. The metabolite had 54% of the activity of the parent compound against *Sarcina lutea*.— B. E. Cabana *et al., Antimicrob. Ag. Chemother.*, 1976, *10,* 307.

An investigation of the renal excretion of cefapirin suggested that active tubular reabsorption of the drug occurs as well as tubular secretion.— A. Arvidsson *et al., Clin. Pharmac. Ther.*, 1979, *25,* 870. See also A. Arvidsson *et al., Br. J. clin. Pharmac.*, 1983, *15,* 339.

Further references to the absorption and fate of cefapirin: R. C. Gordon *et al., Curr. ther. Res.*, 1971, *13,* 398 (pharmacokinetics in children); M. Barza *et al., Antimicrob. Ag. Chemother.*, 1976, *10,* 421 (comparison of pharmacokinetics with cephamandole and cephalothin); D. J. Schurman *et al., Curr. ther. Res.*, 1976, *20,* 194 (diffusion into bone and synovial fluid).

ADMINISTRATION IN RENAL FAILURE. For reference to the pharmacokinetics of cefapirin in renal failure, see under Administration in Renal Failure in Uses, below.

PREGNANCY AND THE NEONATE. The pharmacokinetics of cefapirin in 30 pregnant women. After a single intramuscular dose of 1 g the mean concentration of drug in maternal serum was 17.68, 10.90, 1.49, and 0.64 µg per mL 0.5, 2, 4, and 6 hours after the dose, respectively. The mean peak concentration of cefapirin in amniotic fluid was 13.00 µg per mL 6 hours after the dose; mean peak concentration in cord serum was 10.43 µg per mL at 4 hours.— G. Creatsas *et al., Curr. med. Res. Opinion*, 1980, *7,* 43.

Uses and Administration

Cefapirin sodium is a cephalosporin antibiotic with actions and uses similar to those of cephalothin (see p.178).

The usual adult dose is the equivalent of 0.5 to 1 g of cefapirin every 4 to 6 hours by intramuscular injection or intravenously by slow injection over 3 to 5 minutes or by intermittent infusion. In severe infections up to 12 g daily may be given. A suggested dose for children over 3 months of age is 40 to 80 mg per kg body-weight daily in 4 divided doses. For the prophylaxis of infection during surgery, cefapirin sodium is administered parenterally in a dose equivalent to 1 to 2 g given half to one hour prior to the operation, repeated during lengthy procedures, and continued postoperatively every 6 hours for 24 hours. In certain cases it may be continued for up to 5 days.

Reduced doses may be necessary in patients with impaired renal function.

ADMINISTRATION IN RENAL FAILURE. The normal half-life for cefapirin of 0.6 to 0.8 hours was increased to 2.4 to 2.7 hours in end-stage renal failure. The interval between doses should be extended from 6 hours to 6 to 8 hours in patients with a glomerular filtration-rate (GFR) of between 10 and 50 mL per minute and to 12 hours in those with a GFR of less than 10 mL per minute. A dose supplement should be given to patients undergoing haemodialysis.— W. M. Bennett *et al., Am. J. Kidney Dis.*, 1983, *3,* 155.

References to the administration of cefapirin sodium in patients undergoing haemodialysis: R. V. McCloskey *et al., Antimicrob. Ag. Chemother.*, 1972, *1,* 90; S. J. Berman *et al., Antimicrob. Ag. Chemother.*, 1978, *13,* 4.

ENDOCARDITIS. Of 10 patients with endocarditis caused by staphylococci or streptococci and treated with cefapirin, 8 were considered to be cured. In most cases cefapirin was given in a dose of 2 g intravenously every 4 hours for 4 to 6 weeks; in 1 of the 8 successfully treated patients high-dose penicillin and streptomycin was substituted for cefapirin after 19 days. Cefapirin was well-tolerated and no phlebitis was encountered at the infusion sites.— K. H. Burch *et al., Sth. med. J.*, 1983, *76,* 448.

SURGICAL INFECTION PROPHYLAXIS. In a study in 128 women who had undergone caesarean section, irrigation with 2 g of cefapirin or cefoxitin in one litre of sodium chloride 0.9% after delivery of the placenta was equally effective in decreasing the overall rate of infectious complications when compared with sodium chloride 0.9% irrigation alone.— D. K. Levin *et al., Am. J. Obstet. Gynec.*, 1983, *147,* 273.

Preparations

Sterile Cephapirin Sodium *(U.S.P.)*. Cefapirin sodium suitable for parenteral use.

Proprietary Names and Manufacturers

Ambrocef *(Lusofarmaco, Ital.)*; Ambrotina *(Lusofarmaco, Ital.)*; Brisfirina *(Bristol-Myers, Spain)*; Brisporin *(Bristol Italiana Sud, Ital.)*; Bristocef *(Bristol, Ger.)*; Céfaloject *(Bristol, Fr.)*; Cefadyl *(Bristol, Canad.; Bristol, USA)*; Cefatrexil *(Ciba-Geigy, Arg.)*; Cefatrexyl *(Bristol-Myers, Austral.; Mead Johnson, Belg.; Jpn; Bristol, NZ; Bristol, Switz.)*; Piricef *(CT, Ital.)*.

30-x

Cefatrizine *(BAN, USAN, pINN).*

BL-S640; S-640P; SKF-60771. (7*R*)-7-(α-D-4-Hydroxyphenylglycylamino)-3-(1*H*-1,2,3-triazol-4-ylthiomethyl)-3-cephem-4-carboxylic acid.

$C_{18}H_{18}N_6O_5S_2$=462.5.

CAS — 51627-14-6.

Pharmacopoeias. Jpn includes a monograph for Propylene Glycol Cefatrizine.

Cefatrizine is a cephalosporin antibiotic with actions and uses similar to those of cephalexin (see p.173). It is given by mouth in doses of up to 3 g daily.

Cefatrizine is often formulated in combination with propylene glycol.

ANTIMICROBIAL ACTION. The antimicrobial activity of cefatrizine was comparable *in vitro* with that of cephalexin, except that it appeared to be more effective against strains of *Enterobacter, Haemophilus,* and *Proteus.* It was not inactivated by beta-lactamases from 14 strains of *Salmonella typhimurium* and it was active against ampicillin-resistant *H. influenzae*.— C. C. Blackwell *et al., Antimicrob. Ag. Chemother.*, 1976, *10,* 288.

Cefatrizine had similar activity *in vitro* to cefaclor, and was generally more active than cephalexin, cephaloglycin, or cephradine against most Gram-positive cocci as well as against Gram-negative bacteria. Cefatrizine was also active against several indole-positive *Proteus* species.— S. Shadomy *et al., Antimicrob. Ag. Chemother.*, 1977, *12,* 609.

Further references to the antimicrobial action of cefatrizine: H. C. Neu and K. P. Fu, *Antimicrob. Ag. Chemother.*, 1979, *15*, 209; M. B. Pellegrino *et al.*, *Curr. ther. Res.*, 1986, *40*, 191; B. Dainelli *et al.*, *ibid.*, 1987, *42*, 335.

ABSORPTION AND FATE. Peak serum-concentrations of cefatrizine were lower and occurred slightly later than those of cephalexin when both drugs were administered by mouth in a dose of 500 mg; serum-cefatrizine concentrations, however, declined more slowly. After intramuscular administration, the half-lives of cefatrizine and cephazolin were 86 and 118 minutes respectively.— P. Actor *et al.*, *Antimicrob. Ag. Chemother.*, 1976, *9*, 800.

Further references to the absorption and fate of cefatrizine: B. Bernard *et al.*, *Antimicrob. Ag. Chemother.*, 1977, *12*, 231 (maternal-foetal transfer); M. Pfeffer *et al.*, *ibid.*, 1983, *24*, 915 (bioavailability).

USES AND ADMINISTRATION. A summary of clinical studies carried out in a total of 802 adults and children to evaluate the efficacy of cefatrizine in a variety of bacterial infections. Overall cure-rates were, for genito-urinary tract infections 90%, respiratory-tract infections 79%, infections of the skin and skin structures 96%, and for gastro-intestinal infections 83%. Adverse effects were considered to be mild, and were limited to gastro-intestinal disturbances, allergic reactions, and transient abnormalities in haematological parameters.— P. J. Santella and B. Tanrisever, *Drugs exp. & clin. Res.*, 1985, *11*, 441.

Further references to the use of cefatrizine: L. J. Baraff *et al.*, *Curr. ther. Res.*, 1977, *21*, 187; J. R. Dalovisio *et al.*, *ibid.*, 1978, *23*, 417; B. S. Ribner *et al.*, *ibid.*, *24*, 614.

Proprietary Names and Manufacturers
Biotrixina *(Biotrading, Ital.)*; Cefaperos *(Allard, Fr.)*; Cefatrix *(Biochimica Zanardi, Ital.)*; Cefotrizin *(FIRMA, Ital.)*; Cetrazil *(Giustini, Ital.)*; Cetrizina *(Magis, Ital.)*; Faretrizin *(Lafare, Ital.)*; Ipatrizina *(IPA, Ital.)*; Kefoxina *(CT, Ital.)*; Lampotrix *(Von Boch, Ital.)*; Latocef *(Del Saz & Filippini, Ital.)*; Miracef *(Tosi-Novara, Ital.)*; Novacef *(Locatelli, Ital.)*; Orosporina *(San Carlo, Ital.)*; Runicef *(Bergamon, Ital.)*; Tricef *(Tiber, Ital.)*; Trixidine *(Farmades, Ital.)*; Trixilan *(Pulitzer, Ital.)*; Trizina *(Francia Farm., Ital.)*; Zanitrin *(Bristol Italiana Sud, Ital.)*; Zinaf *(Crosara, Ital.)*; Zitrix *(Gibipharma, Ital.)*.

31-r

Cefazaflur Sodium *(USAN, pINNM).*
SKF-59962. Sodium (7*R*)-3-(1-methyl-1*H*-tetrazol-5-ylthiomethyl)-7-(2-trifluoromethylthioacetamido)-3-cephem-4-carboxylate.
$C_{13}H_{12}F_3N_6NaO_4S_3$=492.5.

CAS — 58665-96-6 (cefazaflur); 52123-49-6 (sodium salt).

Cefazaflur sodium is a cephalosporin antibiotic with similar antibacterial activity to that of cephalothin sodium (see p.177).

Antimicrobial action of cefazaflur.— G. W. Counts *et al.*, *Antimicrob. Ag. Chemother.*, 1977, *11*, 708; N. Aswapokee and H. C. Neu, *ibid.*, 1979, *15*, 444.

In 7 healthy subjects given cefazaflur 1 g by intramuscular injection, the mean peak serum concentration was about 25 µg per mL after 30 minutes.The apparent serum half-life was about 50 minutes. Cefazaflur was rapidly eliminated in the urine; about 90% of the dose was recovered after 6 hours and about 93% after 24 hours. Side-effects included slight local pain (1 subject), discomfort after injection (3), and eosinophilia (1).— C. Harvengt *et al.*, *J. clin. Pharmac.*, 1977, *17*, 128.

Proprietary Names and Manufacturers
Smith Kline & French, USA.

15311-c

Cefazedone Sodium *(BANM, rINNM).*
EMD-30087. (7*R*)-7-[2-(3,5-Dichloro-4-oxo-1-pyridyl)acetamido]-3-(5-methyl-1,3,4-thiadiazol-2-ylthiomethyl)-3-cephem-4-carboxylic acid, sodium salt.
$C_{18}H_{14}Cl_2N_5NaO_5S_3$=570.4.

CAS — 56187-47-4 (cefazedone); 63521-15-3 (sodium salt).

1.04 g of monograph substance is approximately equivalent to 1 g of cefazedone. Each g of monograph substance represents about 1.8 mmol of sodium.

Cefazedone sodium is a cephalosporin antibiotic. It is administered intramuscularly or intravenously in a dose of up to the equivalent of cefazedone 6 g daily in two or three divided doses.

For a series of papers on cefazedone, see *Arzneimittel-Forsch.*, 1979, *29*, 361–462.

Further references: D. von Kobyletzki *et al.*, *Arzneimittel-Forsch.*, 1979, *29*, 1763; D. Adam *et al.*, *ibid.*, 1901; A. D. Russell and D. T. Rogers (letter), *J. antimicrob. Chemother.*, 1980, *6*, 288.

Proprietary Names and Manufacturers
Refosporin *(E. Merck, Ger.)*.

16565-d

Cefbuperazone Sodium *(rINNM).*
BMY-25182; T-1982 *(both cefbuperazone)*. Sodium 7-[(2*R*,3*S*)-2-(4-ethyl-2,3-dioxopiperazin-1-ylcarboxamido)-3-hydroxybutyramido]-7-methoxy-3-(1-methyl-1*H*-tetrazol-5-ylthiomethyl)-3-cephem-4-carboxylate.
$C_{22}H_{28}N_9NaO_9S_2$=649.6.

CAS — 76610-84-9 (cefbuperazone).

NOTE. Cefbuperazone is *USAN*.

1.04 g of monograph substance is approximately equivalent to 1 g of cefbuperazone. Each g of monograph substance represents about 1.5 mmol of sodium.

Cefbuperazone sodium is a cephamycin antibiotic which is administered parenterally.

ADVERSE EFFECTS AND PRECAUTIONS. Cefbuperazone has a methylthiotetrazole side-chain. For the possible adverse effects, and the precautions to be taken with agents containing this group, see under Cephamandole Sodium, p.179.

ANTIMICROBIAL ACTION. A comparison of the antimicrobial action of cefbuperazone with cefmetazole, cefoxitin, cephazolin, and cefoperazone. It was less active than the other antibiotics against *Staphylococcus* spp. but at least four times as potent against Gram-negative bacteria including *Escherichia coli*, *Klebsiella pneumoniae*, *Serratia marcescens*, and some *Proteus* spp. It was as active or slightly less so than cefoperazone, but more active than the other agents against *Proteus morganii*, *Citrobacter freundii*, and *Enterobacter* spp. It was also less active than cefoperazone against *Haemophilus influenzae*. Cefbuperazone was the most active agent against *Bacteroides fragilis*.— M. Tai *et al.*, *Antimicrob. Ag. Chemother.*, 1982, *22*, 728. See also N. J. Khan *et al.*, *ibid.*, 1984, *26*, 585.

Activity against anaerobes. There have been many studies comparing the *in-vitro* activity of cefbuperazone against anaerobic bacteria with that of other antimicrobial agents. It is active against a wide range of these organisms, although it is not active against *Clostridium difficile*. In general its activity against *Bacteroides fragilis* is comparable to that of cefotetan, latamoxef, and cefoxitin, but greater than that of other third-generation cephalosporins. It is resistant to the beta-lactamase produced by *B. fragilis*, but does not appear to be active against cefoxitin-resistant strains. It is less active against other members of the *B. fragilis* group and against other *Bacteroides* spp. One study has shown it to be synergistic with cefoxitin against some strains of *B. fragilis*. References:; E. J. C. Goldstein and D. M. Citron, *Antimicrob. Ag. Chemother.*, 1985, *27*, 162; R. H. Prabhala *et al.*, *ibid.*, 640; H. Wexler *et al.*, *ibid.*, 674; S. D. Shafran *et al.*, *ibid.*, 749; V. E. Del Bene *et al.*, *ibid.*, 817; M. J. Ohm-Smith *et al.*, *ibid.*, 958; M. B. S. Dias *et al.*, *ibid.*, 968.

ABSORPTION AND FATE. From a study in 13 patients undergoing cholecystectomy it was concluded that after an intravenous injection of 1 g, concentrations in the bile were higher than the MICs for most likely pathogens. Although cefbuperazone concentrations in hepatic bile were lower in 5 patients with obstructive jaundice they were still considered adequate.— H. Tanaka *et al.*, *J. antimicrob. Chemother.*, 1987, *20*, 417.

USES AND ADMINISTRATION. For a series of studies on the *in vitro* activity and clinical uses of cefbuperazone, see *Chemotherapy, Tokyo*, 1982, *30*, *Suppl.* 3, 1—986.

Proprietary Names and Manufacturers
Bristol-Myers Products, USA.

1014-v

Cefempidone *(BAN, pINN).*
GR-50692; TA-5901. (*Z*)-7-[2-(2-Amino-1,3-thiazol-5-yl)-2-(2-oxopyrrolidin-3-yloxyimino)acetamido]-3-pyridiniomethyl-3-cephem-4-carboxylate.
$C_{22}H_{21}N_7O_6S_2$=543.6.

CAS — 103238-57-9.

Cefempidone is a cephalosporin antibiotic.

Proprietary Names and Manufacturers
Glaxo, UK.

18856-b

Cefepime *(USAN, pINN).*
BMY-28142. (*Z*)-7-[2-(2-Aminothiazol-4-yl)-2-methoxyiminoacetamido]-3-(1-methylpyrrolidiniomethyl)-3-cephem-4-carboxylate.
$C_{19}H_{24}N_6O_5S_2$=480.6.

CAS — 88040-23-7.

Cefepime is a cephalosporin antibiotic.

Studies of the antibacterial activity of cefepime *in vitro* and in *animals*: N. J. Khan *et al.*, *Antimicrob. Ag. Chemother.*, 1984, *26*, 585; R. E. Kessler *et al.*, *ibid.*, 1985, *27*, 207; G. P. Bodey *et al.*, *ibid.*, 265; M. G. Täuber *et al.*, *ibid.*, 340; A. Tsuji *et al.*, *ibid.*, 515; A. Vuye and J. Pijck, *ibid.*, 574; P. C. Fuchs *et al.*, *ibid.*, 679; K. S. Kim and A. S. Bayer, *ibid.*, *28*, 51; D. A. Conrad *et al.*, *ibid.*, 58; G. A. Jacoby and L. Sutton, *ibid.*, 703; A. M. Clarke *et al.*, *J. antimicrob. Chemother.*, 1985, *15*, 305; J. C. H. Steele *et al.*, *ibid.*, *16*, 463; H. C. Neu *et al.*, *ibid.*, *17*, 441; K. V. I. Rolston *et al.*, *ibid.*, 453; H. W. Van Landuyt *et al.*, *Antimicrob. Ag. Chemother.*, 1986, *29*, 362; J. A. Moody *et al.*, *Curr. ther. Res.*, 1986, *39*, 230.

Proprietary Names and Manufacturers
Bristol-Myers Products, USA.

3412-l

Cefetamet *(USAN, rINN).*
LY-097064; Ro-15-8074. (*Z*)-7-[2-(2-Aminothiazol-4-yl)-2-methoxyiminoacetamido]-3-methyl-3-cephem-4-carboxylic acid.
$C_{14}H_{15}N_5O_5S_2$=397.4.

CAS — 65052-63-3.

Cefetamet is a cephalosporin antibiotic.

Studies of the antibacterial activity of cefetamet *in vitro*: M. Peeters and P. Piot, *J. antimicrob. Chemother.*, 1985, *16*, 469; M. G. Thomas and S. D. R. Lang, *Antimicrob. Ag. Chemother.*, 1986, *29*, 945; R. Wise *et al.*, *ibid.*, 1067; H. C. Neu *et al.*, *ibid.*, *30*, 423; R. J. Fass and V. L. Helsel, *ibid.*, 429; R. N. Jones *et al.*, *ibid.*, 961; C. S. F. Easmon *et al.*, *J. antimicrob. Chemother.*, 1987, *19*, 761; W. R. Bowie *et al.*, *Antimicrob. Ag. Chemother.*, 1987, *31*, 470; P. Y. Chau *et al.*, *ibid.*, 473; N. M. Le Saux *et al.*, *ibid.*, 1153.

Proprietary Names and Manufacturers
Roche, Switz.

12006-g

Cefixime *(BAN, USAN, rINN).*
CL-284635; FK-027; FR-17027. (*Z*)-7-[2-(2-Aminothiazol-4-yl)-2-(carboxymethoxyimino)acetamido]-3-vinyl-3-cephem-4-carboxylic acid.
$C_{16}H_{15}N_5O_7S_2$=453.5.

CAS — 79350-37-1.

Cefixime is a cephalosporin antibiotic which is administered by mouth. It has good *in-vitro* activity against aerobic Gram-negative bacteria and most streptococci.

For proceedings of a symposium on cefixime, see *Pediatr. infect. Dis. J.*, 1987, *6*, 949—1009.

Cefixime had a similar range of activity against *Enterobacteriaceae* to ceftizoxime, but was generally less active. It did not inhibit *Pseudomonas* or *Acinetobacter* spp. or most anaerobes. It was less active than ceftizoxime against streptococci and had poor activity against *Staphylococcus* spp.— H. C. Neu *et al.*, *Antimicrob. Ag. Chemother.*, 1984, *26*, 174.

Twelve healthy subjects were each given cefixime 50, 100, 200, and 400 mg by mouth in the fasting state. Mean peak plasma concentrations of 1.02, 1.46, 2.63, and 3.85 μg per mL were obtained 2.7, 3.4, 3.9, and 4.3 hours after the four doses, respectively. The half-life was about 3 hours for all doses, and between 16 and 21% of the administered dose was excreted in the urine in 24 hours.— D. C. Brittain *et al.*, *Clin. Pharmac. Ther.*, 1985, *38*, 590.

In a study involving 528 patients with acute uncomplicated urinary-tract infections, treatment by mouth for 10 days with cefixime 400 mg once a day or 200 mg twice daily, or with co-trimoxazole 960 mg twice daily was equally effective. However, a high incidence of adverse gastro-intestinal effects with cefixime 400 mg once daily led to discontinuation of this arm of the study.— J. Levenstein *et al.*, *S. Afr. med. J.*, 1986, *70*, 455.

A comparison of changes in the faecal flora after administration of cefixime or cefaclor by mouth to healthy subjects.— S. M. Finegold *et al.*, *Antimicrob. Ag. Chemother.*, 1987, *31*, 443.

Further references to cefixime: D. R. P. Guay *et al.*, *Antimicrob. Ag. Chemother.*, 1986, *30*, 485 (pharmacokinetics in patients with renal insufficiency); W. R. Bowie *et al.*, *ibid.*, 590 (activity *in vitro* against *Neisseria gonorrhoeae*); M. Powell and J. D. Williams, *ibid.*, 1987, *31*, 1841 (activity *in vitro* against *Haemophilus influenzae*).

Proprietary Names and Manufacturers

Fujisawa, Jpn; Lederle, USA.

15312-k

Cefmenoxime Hydrochloride *(USAN, rINNM).*

Abbott-50192; SCE-1365 (cefmenoxime). (*Z*)-(7*R*)-7-[2-(2-Aminothiazol-4-yl)-2-methoxyiminoacetamido]-3-[(1-methyl-1*H*-tetrazol-5-yl)thiomethyl]-3-cephem-4-carboxylic acid hydrochloride.

$(C_{16}H_{17}N_9O_5S_3)_2,HCl=1059.6.$

CAS — 65085-01-0 (cefmenoxime); 75738-58-8 (hydrochloride).

1.04 g of monograph substance is approximately equivalent to 1 g of cefmenoxime.

Adverse Effects and Precautions

As for Cephalothin Sodium, p.176.

The most frequently reported adverse effects associated with cefmenoxime therapy are mild hypersensitivity, gastro-intestinal, and local reactions, and the most frequently reported abnormal laboratory parameters are transiently elevated liver function enzymes and haematological abnormalities. Abnormalities in concentrations of serum creatinine and blood-urea-nitrogen have also been observed.

Cefmenoxime has an *N*-methylthiotetrazole side-chain, and coagulopathy and disulfiram-like alcohol intolerance have been reported rarely.— D. M. Campoli-Richards and P. A. Todd, *Drugs*, 1987, *34*, 188.

For further reference to the possible adverse effects and the precautions to be taken with agents possessing a methylthiotetrazole side-chain, see under Cephamandole Sodium, p.179.

ADMINISTRATION IN RENAL FAILURE. For reference to the precautions to be observed in renal failure, see under Administration in Renal Failure in Uses, below.

EFFECTS ON THE BLOOD. Intravenous injections of cefmenoxime 1 or 2 g were administered twice daily for 7 days to 40 patients with complicated urinary-tract infections. Prolonged coagulation time was observed in one patient on the lower dose and 2 on the higher dose; one patient on the higher dose also had a decreased concentration of factor IX. These abnormalities were not observed in patients given vitamin K_2 on the first day of cefmenoxime administration. No effect on bleeding time, or clinical bleeding was observed in any patient.— H. Washida *et al.*, *Curr. ther. Res.*, 1986, *39*, 359.

INTERACTIONS. For a possible interaction with alcohol, see above.

Antimicrobial Action and Resistance

As for Cefotaxime Sodium, p.152.

Cefmenoxime has a spectrum of antibacterial activity and beta-lactamase stability which is similar to those of cefotaxime, ceftizoxime, and ceftriaxone. As with these other cephalosporins, it has also been reported to be active *in vitro* against *Branhamella catarrhalis* and *Yersinia enterocolitica*. *Chlamydia trachomatis* and most strains of *Nocardia asteroides* are, however, resistant. An inoculum effect has been observed for many organisms. Synergism between cefmenoxime and aminoglycosides has been demonstrated against widely variable percentages of tested strains of Gram-negative bacteria. Synergism between cefmenoxime and piperacillin has also been reported.— D. M. Campoli-Richards and P. A. Todd, *Drugs*, 1987, *34*, 188.

Absorption and Fate

Cefmenoxime is administered parenterally as the hydrochloride salt. It is well absorbed after intramuscular injection, peak plasma concentrations being obtained after about 45 minutes. The half-life of cefmenoxime is about 1 hour and is prolonged in renal impairment. About 77% of cefmenoxime in the circulation is bound to plasma proteins.

Cefmenoxime is widely distributed in body tissues and fluids; it passes into the CSF particularly when the meninges are inflamed. It diffuses across the placenta and has been detected in breast milk.

It is excreted chiefly in the urine; about 70 to 80% is recovered unchanged in the first 24 hours.

A review of the absorption and fate of cefmenoxime.— D. M. Campoli-Richards; P. A. Todd, *Drugs*, 1987, *34*, 188.

A study of the pharmacokinetics of cefmenoxime after intramuscular injection or intravenous injection or infusion.— G. R. Granneman *et al.*, *Antimicrob. Ag. Chemother.*, 1982, *21*, 141.

ADMINISTRATION IN RENAL FAILURE. For reference to the pharmacokinetics of cefmenoxime in renal failure, see under Administration in Renal Failure in Uses, below.

DIFFUSION INTO BODY TISSUES AND FLUIDS. Studies of the diffusion of cefmenoxime into the CSF: K. V. I. Rolston *et al.*, *J. antimicrob. Chemother.*, 1983, *12*, 519 (across non-inflamed meninges); G. Humbert *et al.*, *ibid.*, 1986, *18*, 503 (in patients with bacterial meningitis).

DRUG EXCRETION. Concomitant administration of probenecid increased the half-life and the mean peak plasma concentration of cefmenoxime in a study in 10 healthy subjects. It would appear that tubular secretion is the predominant mechanism of elimination.— L. T. Sennello *et al.*, *Antimicrob. Ag. Chemother.*, 1983, *23*, 803.

After intravenous administration of cefmenoxime 0.5 or 1 g to 19 patients undergoing cholecystectomy, concentrations in the bile were considered to be therapeutic for *Enterobacteriaceae* commonly associated with biliary-tract infections.— B. R. Smith *et al.*, *Antimicrob. Ag. Chemother.*, 1983, *23*, 941.

Uses and Administration

Cefmenoxime hydrochloride is a cephalosporin antibiotic with actions and uses similar to those of cefotaxime sodium (see p.154). It is administered by intramuscular injection, or intravenously by injection or infusion. Doses are expressed in terms of the equivalent amount of cefmenoxime. The usual dose is 1 to 4 g daily in 2 to 4 divided doses, although up to 12 g daily has been given in life-threatening infections. Children have been given 40 to 80 mg per kg body-weight daily in 2 to 4 divided doses; higher doses have been used in severe infections.

A review of the actions and uses of cefmenoxime. Cefmenoxime has been shown to be effective in the treatment of bacterial infections of a wide range of body systems. It has been compared with other antibiotics particularly for the treatment of infections of the urinary and respiratory tracts, in gonorrhoea, in postoperative infections, and in infections in immunocompromised patients.

Three large double-blind studies have demonstrated cefmenoxime to be superior to both cefotiam and cephazolin in the treatment of chronic or complicated urinary-tract infections as assessed clinically. However, since the susceptibility of the infecting organisms was not a criterion for inclusion into the studies, these results may reflect the antibacterial spectra of the drugs rather than their comparative clinical efficacies. Cefmenoxime has been studied alone or in combination with an aminoglycoside, an antipseudomonal penicillin such as azlocillin or piperacillin, or cefsulodin for the treatment of infections in immunocompromised patients including those with granulocytopenia.

Children are usually given a dose equivalent to cefmenoxime 40 to 80 mg per kg body-weight daily administered intravenously in 3 or 4 divided doses. Up to 160 mg per kg daily has been given to children with refractory or severe infections, and up to 200 mg per kg daily for meningitis. The intramuscular preparation is not recommended for use in infants and children.

In common with several other third-generation cephalosporins, cefmenoxime cannot be considered a drug of choice for infections caused by Gram-positive cocci, or be recommended for the treatment of known or suspected pseudomonal infections. Its relatively low *in-vitro* activity against *Bacteroides fragilis* and enterococci may limit its use in infections caused by mixed aerobic and anaerobic bacteria.— D. M. Campoli-Richards and P. A. Todd, *Drugs*, 1987, *34*, 188.

Studies of the use of cefmenoxime for the treatment of a variety of infections: M. E. Gombert *et al.*, *Antimicrob. Ag. Chemother.*, 1984, *25*, 510 (in adults); G. F. Tansino *et al.*, *ibid.*, 1985, *28*, 508 (in children).

ADMINISTRATION IN INFANTS AND CHILDREN. For reference to doses of cefmenoxime used in infants and children, see above.

ADMINISTRATION IN RENAL FAILURE. The half-life of cefmenoxime increased with decreasing renal function. Dosage modification was considered necessary only in patients with a creatinine clearance (CC) of 40 mL per minute or less. For patients with a CC of between 2 and 40 mL per minute a dose of 1 to 2 g could be given every 12 hours. For a CC of below 2 mL per minute 1 to 2 g every 24 hours could be given. A supplemental dose of 0.5 to 1.0 g after haemodialysis was recommended.— R. E. Polk *et al.*, *Antimicrob. Ag. Chemother.*, 1984, *26*, 322. From a similar study the following dosage modifications for cefmenoxime in patients with renal function impairment were recommended: for a CC of 80 to 120 mL per minute, cefmenoxime 70 to 200 mg per kg body-weight daily in divided doses every 4 to 6 hours; for a CC of 50 to 79 mL per minute, cefmenoxime 45 to 135 mg per kg daily in divided doses every 6 to 8 hours; for a CC of 10 to 49 mL per minute, cefmenoxime 20 to 85 mg per kg daily in divided doses every 8 hours; and for a CC of less than 10 mL per minute, cefmenoxime 10 to 35 mg per kg daily in divided doses every 12 hours. Patients on haemodialysis could be given 7.5 to 15 mg per kg every 24 hours, with a supplemental dose of 3.5 to 7.5 mg per kg after each dialysis session.— J. G. Gambertoglio *et al.*, *ibid.*, 845.

Cefmenoxime was administered in a dose of 15 mg per kg body-weight by 30-minute intravenous infusion to 6 patients on continuous ambulatory peritoneal dialysis (CAPD). The mean half-life was 5.5 hours. Approximately 8 and 6% of the administered dose was eliminated by renal clearance and peritoneal clearance respectively. Thus cefmenoxime may be administered to patients on CAPD in doses recommended for renal failure; administration once daily was suggested.— D. A. Sica *et al.*, *Eur. J. clin. Pharmac.*, 1986, *30*, 713.

Further references: K. Konishi, *Antimicrob. Ag. Chemother.*, 1986, *30*, 901.

GONORRHOEA. A comparative study of intramuscular cefmenoxime 1 g and intramuscular procaine penicillin 4.8 g in association with probenecid 1 g by mouth in the treatment of gonorrhoea caused by non-beta-lactamase-producing *Neisseria gonorrhoeae*. Of 50 men treated with cefmenoxime there was one case of reinfection in a patient with urethritis; the single rectal and 2 pharyngeal infections were considered to be cured. Of 49 patients treated with procaine penicillin and probenecid, one pharyngeal infection was not cured.— S. R. Obaid *et al.*, *Antimicrob. Ag. Chemother.*, 1983, *23*, 349.

PNEUMONIA. Cefmenoxime hydrochloride 1 g every 6 hours, increased to 2 g every 6 to 8 hours if necessary, gave a satisfactory response in 22 of 30 elderly patients with pneumonia complicated by underlying disease. Four patients responded favourably, but suffered a subsequent recurrence of symptoms, and response was unsatisfactory in 2 patients, both of whom died despite subsequent antibiotic therapy; the remaining 2 patients were withdrawn from the study because of rapid clinical deterioration. Cefmenoxime is a candidate for further study in nosocomial pneumonias.— D. P. Reitberg *et al.*, *J. antimicrob. Chemother.*, 1984, *14*, 81.

URINARY-TRACT INFECTIONS. For reference to the use of cefmenoxime in urinary-tract infections, see above.

Combination with cefsulodin. Beneficial effect of intravenous treatment with cefmenoxime in association with cefsulodin for complicated urinary-tract infections caused by *Pseudomonas aeruginosa* alone or with other organisms.— T. Doi *et al.*, *Chemotherapy, Basle*, 1986, *32*, 299.

Proprietary Names and Manufacturers

Bestcall *(Takeda, Jpn)*; Cemix *(Takeda, Fr.)*; Tacef *(Takeda, Ger.)*.

12540-v

Cefmetazole *(rINN).*
CS-1170; SKF-83088; U-72791A *(sodium salt). (7S)*-7-[2-(Cyanomethylthio)acetamido]-7-methoxy-3-(1-methyl-1*H*-tetrazol-5-ylthiomethyl)-3-cephem-4-carboxylic acid.
$C_{15}H_{17}N_7O_5S_3$=471.5.

CAS — 56796-20-4; 56796-39-5 (sodium salt).

NOTE. Cefmetazole Sodium is *USAN.*

Pharmacopoeias. Jpn includes Cefmetazole Sodium.

Cefmetazole is a cephamycin antibiotic with actions and uses similar to cefoxitin sodium (see p.158). It is administered by the intravenous or intramuscular route usually in doses of up to 4 g daily in divided doses every 12 hours. It may be administered as the sodium salt.

ADVERSE EFFECTS AND PRECAUTIONS. Cefmetazole is a cephamycin antibiotic containing a methylthiotetrazole side-chain. For the possible adverse effects, and the precautions to be taken with agents containing this group, see under Cephamandole Sodium, p.179.

ANTIMICROBIAL ACTION. Like cefoxitin, cefmetazole was a potent inducer *in vitro* of the beta-lactamases of *Enterobacter cloacae* and *Serratia marcescens.* Both drugs antagonised the activity of several third-generation cephalosporins against these bacteria.— K. Okonogi *et al., J. antimicrob. Chemother.,* 1985, *16,* 31.

Synergy was observed between cefmetazole and fosfomycin against methicillin-resistant *Staphylococcus aureus* both *in vitro* and in *mice.*— Y. Utsui *et al., Antimicrob. Ag. Chemother.,* 1986, *30,* 917.

Studies of the *in-vitro* activity of cefmetazole against anaerobic bacteria including *Bacteroides fragilis*: F. Soriano *et al.* (letter), *J. clin. Path.,* 1982, *35,* 1166; T. Kesado *et al., Antimicrob. Ag. Chemother.,* 1984, *25,* 131; M. J. Ohm-Smith and R. L. Sweet, *ibid.,* 1987, *31,* 1434; N. A. Cornick *et al., ibid.,* 2010.

The MIC of cefmetazole for 46 strains of *Mycobacterium fortuitum* ranged from 4 to 64 μg per mL. For 20 strains of *M. chelonei* the MIC ranged from 8 to greater than 128 μg per mL.— M. J. Casal *et al., Antimicrob. Ag. Chemother.,* 1985, *27,* 282.

ABSORPTION AND FATE. The pharmacokinetics of cefmetazole in patients with impaired renal function. Cefmetazole is excreted primarily in the urine in healthy subjects; as renal function decreased, so urinary excretion decreased.— M. Ohkawa *et al., Antimicrob. Ag. Chemother.,* 1980, *18,* 386.

Concentrations of cefmetazole in plasma and tissue after infiltration into and around the projected incision site for appendectomy.— J. R. Rodriguez *et al., Antimicrob. Ag. Chemother.,* 1984, *26,* 787.

The pharmacokinetics of cefmetazole in 7 healthy subjects. After intramuscular injection of a dose of 30 mg per kg body-weight, a mean peak plasma concentration of 90.1 μg per mL was obtained after 0.7 hour. The mean half-lives after intramuscular and intravenous administration were 1.3 and 1.8 hours respectively.— J. Rodriguez-Barbero *et al., Antimicrob. Ag. Chemother.,* 1985, *28,* 544.

Proprietary Names and Manufacturers
Cefmetazon *(Sankyo, Jpn)*; Cemetol *(Antibioticos, Spain).*

18922-r

Cefminox Sodium *(pINNM).*
MT-141. Sodium 7-{2-[(S)-2-amino-2-carboxyethyl]thioacetamido}-7-methoxy-3-(1-methyl-1*H*-tetrazol-5-ylthiomethyl)-3-cephem-4-carboxylate.
$C_{16}H_{20}N_7NaO_7S_3$=541.6.

CAS — 75481-73-1 (cefminox).

1.04 g of monograph substance is approximately equivalent to 1 g of cefminox. Each g of monograph substance represents about 1.8 mmol of sodium.

Cefminox sodium is a cephamycin antibiotic.

Studies *in vitro* of the antibacterial activity of cefminox: S. Inouye *et al., Antimicrob. Ag. Chemother.,* 1984, *26,* 722; T. Tsuruoka *et al., J. antimicrob. Chemother.,* 1985, *15,* 159; T. Kasai *et al., ibid.,* 701.

Proprietary Names and Manufacturers
Meiji, Jpn.

18923-f

Cefodizime *(rINN).*
HR-221. (Z)-7-[2-(2-Aminothiazol-4-yl)-2-methoxyiminoacetamido]-3-(5-carboxymethyl-4-methylthiazol-2-ylthiomethyl)-3-cephem-4-carboxylic acid.
$C_{20}H_{20}N_6O_7S_4$=584.7.

CAS — 69739-16-8.

Cefodizime is a cephalosporin antibiotic.

Studies *in vitro* of the antibacterial activity of cefodizime: R. N. Jones *et al., Antimicrob. Ag. Chemother.,* 1981, *20,* 760; V. I. Ahonkhai *et al., ibid.,* 1982, *22,* 715; M. Y. Khan *et al., ibid.,* 1983, *23,* 477; B. E. Scully *et al., ibid.,* 907; A. Pascual *et al.* (letter), *J. antimicrob. Chemother.,* 1987, *19,* 701.

Studies *in vitro* indicating potentiation by cefodizime of human neutrophil bactericidal activity: M. T. Labro *et al., J. antimicrob. Chemother.,* 1986, *18,* 233; M. T. Labro *et al., ibid.,* 1987, *19,* 331.

Concentrations of cefodizime in serum and blister fluid after intravenous and intramuscular administration to healthy subjects.— H. C. Korting *et al., Antimicrob. Ag. Chemother.,* 1987, *31,* 1822.

Proprietary Names and Manufacturers
Hoechst, Ger.

16566-n

Cefonicid Sodium *(BANM, USAN).*

Cefonicide Sodium *(rINNM)*; SKF-D-75073-Z *(monosodium salt)*; SKF-D-75073-Z_2. The disodium salt of 7-[(*R*)-mandelamido]-3-(1-sulphomethyl-1*H*-tetrazol-5-ylthiomethyl)-3-cephem-4-carboxylic acid.
$C_{18}H_{16}N_6Na_2O_8S_3$=586.5.

CAS — 61270-58-4 (cefonicid); 61270-78-8 (disodium salt); 71420-79-6 (monosodium salt).

Pharmacopoeias. U.S. includes Sterile Cefonicid Sodium.

1.08 g of monograph substance is approximately equivalent to 1 g of cefonicid. Each g of monograph substance represents about 3.4 mmol of sodium.

A 5% solution in water has a pH of 3.5 to 6.5. Aqueous solutions of cefonicid sodium are reported to be **stable** for 24 hours at room temperature and for 72 hours at 5°.

Solutions of cefonicid sodium may become yellow on storage, but slight discoloration does not affect potency.

Adverse Effects and Precautions

As for Cephalothin Sodium, p.176.

The most frequently reported adverse effects with cefonicid are local reactions on injection. Pain, discomfort and burning may occur on intramuscular injection; this pain has been considered as mild to moderate, lasting in the range of 10 minutes to 2 hours, and equivalent qualitatively to that experienced after injection of procaine penicillin. Pain and phlebitis have been noted after intravenous injection. Other adverse effects that have been reported after administration of cefonicid include hypersensitivity reactions, such as fever, rash, pruritus, and a flu-like syndrome; haematological effects such as eosinophilia, thrombocytosis, leucopenia, neutropenia, and a positive Coombs' test; abnormal liver function tests; and, rarely, alterations in renal function with transient increases in serum creatinine or blood urea nitrogen.— E. Saltiel and R. N. Brogden, *Drugs,* 1986, *32,* 222.

ADMINISTRATION IN RENAL FAILURE. For reference to the precautions to be observed in renal failure, see under Administration in Renal Failure in Uses, below.

Antimicrobial Action and Resistance

Cefonicid sodium has a similar antimicrobial action and pattern of resistance to cephamandole (see p.180), although it is generally less active against Gram-positive cocci.

Cefonicid generally has a similar antimicrobial action to cephamandole although it appears to be less active against Gram-positive cocci and more active against *Neisseria gonorrhoeae* and *Haemophilus influenzae.* It has poor activity against *Branhamella catarrhalis* and *Nocardia asteroides;* although it has been reported to demonstrate some inhibitory activity against *Listeria monocytogenes* its killing activity is negligible. Tolerance to cefonicid has been noted in some strains of streptococci and staphylococci and a marked inoculum effect has been reported for both Gram-positive and Gram-negative bacteria.— E. Saltiel and R. N. Brogden, *Drugs,* 1986, *32,* 22.

Absorption and Fate

Cefonicid is administered parenterally as the sodium salt. After intramuscular administration of a dose of 1 g peak plasma concentrations ranging from 67 to 126 μg per mL have been achieved after 1 to 2 hours. More than 90% of cefonicid in the circulation is bound to plasma proteins. Cefonicid has a half-life of approximately 4.5 hours, which is prolonged in patients with renal failure.

Therapeutic concentrations of cefonicid have been reported in a wide range of body tissues and fluids.

Up to 99% of a dose of cefonicid is excreted unchanged in the urine within 24 hours. The excretion of cefonicid is decreased by the concomitant administration of probenecid.

A review of the absorption and fate of cefonicid.— E. Saltiel and R. N. Brogden, *Drugs,* 1986, *32,* 222.

The pharmacokinetics of cefonicid after administration of 7.5 mg per kg body-weight by intravenous infusion over 5 minutes, to 5 healthy subjects. Peak plasma concentrations were achieved immediately, and ranged from 95 to 156 μg per mL; concentrations fell to a mean of 8.2 μg per mL, and less than 2.5 μg per mL at 12 and 24 hours respectively. Urinary concentrations were variable but averaged more than 100 μg per mL for 12 hours after the dose.— S. L. Barriere *et al., Antimicrob. Ag. Chemother.,* 1982, *21,* 935. See also D. Pitkin *et al., Clin. Pharmac. Ther.,* 1981, *30,* 587.

ADMINISTRATION IN RENAL FAILURE. For reference to the pharmacokinetics of cefonicid in renal failure, see under Administration in Renal Failure in Uses, below.

DIFFUSION INTO BODY TISSUES AND FLUIDS. Concentrations of cefonicid in the tissues and fluids of the heart after administration for prophylaxis during open-heart surgery: R. P. Sterling *et al., Antimicrob. Ag. Chemother.,* 1983, *23,* 790; M. N. Dudley *et al., ibid.,* 1984, *26,* 347.

Uses and Administration

Cefonocid sodium is a cephalosporin antibiotic used similarly to cephamandole in the treatment of susceptible infections (see p.181). It is administered by deep intramuscular injection, or intravenously by slow injection or by infusion. Doses are expressed in terms of the equivalent amount of cefonicid. The usual dose is cefonicid 1 g once daily. For uncomplicated urinary-tract infections a dose of 0.5 g once daily is recommended; up to 2 g once daily has been given in severe infections. More than 1 g should not be injected intramuscularly into a single site.

For patients with impaired renal function a loading dose of 7.5 mg per kg body-weight is recommended followed by reduced maintenance doses according to the creatinine clearance and the severity of the infection. A dose supplement is not required following dialysis.

Cefonicid sodium is also used for surgical infection prophylaxis. A single dose of 1 g given one hour prior to surgical incision is usually sufficient, but may be administered daily for a further 2 days in prosthetic arthroplasty or open-heart surgery.

A review of the actions and uses of cefonicid. Studies, mostly in small numbers of patients, have demonstrated its efficacy in the treatment of infections of the urinary tract, respiratory tract, skin, soft tissues, and bone, in gonorrhoea, and in surgical infection prophylaxis. When given in a single intramuscular dose of 1 g, sometimes in association with probenecid 1 g by mouth, to patients with gonorrhoea it has been shown to be of similar efficacy to procaine penicillin plus probenecid. However, it has not been compared with other cephalosporins in gonococcal infections and low cure-rates have been noted with cefonicid in rectal and pharyngeal infections. A small study in patients with endocarditis has suggested that it should not be used in patients with serious staphylococcal infections. It should also not be used in patients with meningitis because of insufficient informa-

tion on its penetration into the CSF.
The characteristic property of cefonicid which distinguishes it from other second-generation cephalosporins is its high protein binding and long half-life, resulting in relatively high serum concentrations for 12 to 24 hours; therefore administration is usually only required once daily.— E. Saltiel and R. N. Brogden, *Drugs*, 1986, *32*, 222.

Further reviews of the actions and uses of cefonicid: M. N. Dudley *et al.*, *Clin. Pharm.*, 1984, *3*, 23; *Med. Lett.*, 1984, *26*, 71; T. A. Tartaglione and R. E. Polk, *Drug Intell. & clin. Pharm.*, 1985, *19*, 188.

Further references to the use of cefonicid: R. J. Wallace *et al.*, *Antimicrob. Ag. Chemother.*, 1982, *21*, 231 (comparison with cephamandole in the treatment of community-acquired pneumonia); R. E. Pontzer *et al.*, *ibid.*, 1983, *23*, 814 (single-dose use in urinary-tract infections); D. H. Gremillion *et al.*, *ibid.*, 944 (skin and soft-tissue infections); M. J. Kunkel *et al.*, *Curr. ther. Res.*, 1986, *39*, 223 (a range of mild to moderately severe infections).

ADMINISTRATION IN RENAL FAILURE. The mean half-life of cefonicid was 10.3, 20.6, and 68.1 hours for patients whose creatinine clearance (CC) values were in the ranges 40 to 79, 10 to 39, or less than 5 mL per minute, respectively.
Patients with impaired renal function could be given a loading dose of 15 mg per kg body-weight followed by maintenance doses of: 15 mg per kg every 24 hours for a CC of 60 to 79 mL per minute; 10 mg per kg every 24 hours for a CC of 40 to 59 mL per minute; 7.5 mg per kg every 24 hours for a CC of 20 to 39 mL per minute; 7.5 mg per kg every 48 hours for a CC of 10 to 19 mL per minute; and 5 mg per kg every 72 hours for a CC of less than 5 mL per minute.— R. T. Phelps and J. E. Conte, *Antimicrob. Ag. Chemother.*, 1986, *29*, 913.
See also A. D. Blair *et al.*, *Clin. Pharmac. Ther.*, 1984, *35*, 798; J. -P. Fillastre *et al.*, *J. antimicrob. Chemother.*, 1986, *18*, 203.

SURGICAL INFECTION PROPHYLAXIS. For comments on the use of cefonicid for surgical infection prophylaxis, see under Ceforanide, p.151.

Preparations

Sterile Cefonicid Sodium *(U.S.P.)*

Proprietary Names and Manufacturers

Cefodie *(ISF, Ital.)*; Monocid *(Smith Kline & French, Ital.; Smith Kline & French, Spain; Smith Kline & French, USA)*.

187-a

Cefoperazone Sodium *(BANM, USAN, rINNM)*.

CP-52640-2; CP-52640-3 *(cefoperazone dihydrate)*; T-1551 *(cefoperazone or sodium salt)*.
Sodium (7*R*)-7-[(*R*)-2-(4-ethyl-2,3-dioxopiperazin-1-ylcarboxamido)-2-(4-hydroxyphenyl)acetamido]-3-[(1-methyl-1*H*-tetrazol-5-yl)thiomethyl]-3-cephem-4-carboxylate.
$C_{25}H_{26}N_9NaO_8S_2$=667.7.

CAS — 62893-19-0 (cefoperazone); 62893-20-3 (sodium salt).

Pharmacopoeias. U.S. includes Sterile Cefoperazone Sodium.

1.03 g of monograph substance is approximately equivalent to 1 g of cefoperazone. Each g of monograph substance represents about 1.5 mmol of sodium.
A 25% solution in water has a pH of 4.5 to 6.5.
Aqueous solutions of cefoperazone sodium 300 mg per mL are reported to be **stable** for 24 hours at 15° to 25°, for 5 days at 2° to 8°, and for 5 weeks at −20° to −10°.

Incompatibility or loss of activity has been reported between cefoperazone sodium and aminoglycosides, perphenazine, or pethidine hydrochloride.

Adverse Effects and Precautions

As for Cephalothin Sodium, p.176.
Hypoprothrombinaemia has been reported in patients treated with cefoperazone sodium and has rarely been associated with bleeding episodes. Prothrombin time should be monitored in patients at risk of hypoprothrombinaemia and vitamin K administered if necessary.
A disulfiram-like interaction with alcohol may occur, and patients receiving cefoperazone sodium should therefore avoid alcohol during and for at least several days after treatment.

For the possible effect of cefoperazone on the immune system, see under Antimicrobial Action, below.

ADMINISTRATION IN LIVER DISORDERS AND IN RENAL FAILURE. For reference to the precautions to be observed in liver disorders and in renal failure, see under Uses and Administration, below.

EFFECTS ON THE BLOOD. Coagulopathies, including an increase in the prothrombin time and bleeding time, and a decrease in the platelet count, have been reported in patients receiving cefoperazone sodium. In some cases these have been associated with episodes of clinical bleeding (S.W. Parker *et al.*., *Lancet*, 1984, *1*, 1016; P. Cristiano, *Drug Intell. & clin. Pharm.*, 1984, *18*, 314; S. Meisel, *ibid.*, 316; J.C. Osborne, *Ann. intern. Med.*, 1985, *102*, 721), which have resolved on administration of vitamin K, platelet products, and in some cases also red blood cells. Cohen and Washton (*Ann. intern. Med.*, 1987, *106*, 778) observed the effect of cefoperazone sodium on the prothrombin time in 894 patients most of whom received a dose of 2 g twice daily. The results in 695 evaluable patients were as follows: prothrombin time was abnormal in 12 patients (1.7%) before therapy; was changed by less than 2 seconds during therapy in 17 (2.4%), and by more than 2 seconds in 33 (4.7%); and was unchanged during therapy in 644 (92.6%). Clinical bleeding occurred in 4 of the patients in whom prolonged prothrombin time developed. Prolongation of prothrombin time could be correlated with increased age, and with renal impairment. Although the manufacturers recommend the monitoring of prothrombin time in patients at risk of hypoprothrombinaemia, and administration of vitamin K if required, some workers advocate the use of prophylactic vitamin K in patients at risk (J. Murdoch and K. Warrian, *Can. J. Hosp. Pharm.*, 1986, *39*, 110). Cefoperazone appears to have little or no effect on platelet function (M.R. Weitekamp *et al.*, *J. antimicrob. Chemother.*, 1985, *16*, 95; F.R. Sattler *et al.*, *Ann. intern Med.*, 1986, *105*, 924).
For a discussion on the possible mechanisms of cefoperazone-induced hypoprothrombinaemia, including the role of vitamin K deficiency, and of the methylthiotetrazole side-chain of cefoperazone, see Cephamandole Sodium, p.179.

EFFECTS ON THE GASTRO-INTESTINAL TRACT. Although many studies have not indicated an unusually high incidence of adverse gastro-intestinal effects after administration of cefoperazone sodium, there have been a few reports that suggest this. Norrby and Alestig (*Lancet*, 1981, *2*, 1417) observed adverse gastro-intestinal reactions, mainly diarrhoea, in 6 of 10 healthy subjects given an intravenous injection of cefoperazone 2 g over 3 minutes; this may have been due to the high concentrations of cefoperazone in the bile as a result of rapid administration. Carlberg *et al.* (*J. antimicrob. Chemother.*, 1982, *10*, 483), however, reported moderate or severe diarrhoea in 12 of 52 patients treated with cefoperazone sodium and administered as a 30-minute intravenous infusion; *Clostridium difficile* and its toxin was isolated from the faeces of 5 of these. An additional 11 patients reported stools which were looser than normal, and *Cl. difficile* and toxin was detected in 3 of these. Alestig *et al.* (*ibid.*, 1983, *12*, 163) studied the faecal flora of 29 of these patients. They noted a suppression of Enterobacteriaceae, aerobic and anaerobic cocci, and *Bacteroides* spp., and an increase in the numbers of enterococci and *Clostridia* spp.; one patient was colonised by *Pseudomonas* spp. Mulligan *et al.* (*Antimicrob. Ag. Chemother.*, 1982, *22*, 226) observed a similar change in the faecal flora of 4 patients on cefoperazone therapy.

EFFECTS ON THE KIDNEY. In a study of 19 patients given cefoperazone, renal tolerance appeared to be good. Patients with pre-existing renal impairment could be given the antibiotic in normal doses, with or without concomitant frusemide, with no signs of renal impairment. There were, however, slight changes in some parameters of renal function in a few patients, and it was considered that, as with most other cephalosporins, a nephrotoxic potential probably does exist.— B. Trollfors *et al.*, *J. antimicrob. Chemother.*, 1982, *9*, 485.

EFFECTS ON THE LIVER. Severe liver damage as an allergic reaction to cefoperazone.— A. Von Wolf *et al.*, *Z. Gastroent.*, 1985, *23*, 198.

INTERACTIONS. *Alcohol.* In 3 of 4 healthy subjects who took alcoholic beverages 36 hours after a dose of cefoperazone, alcohol intolerance occurred. In one subject the syndrome developed on 3 separate occasions.— D. S. Reeves and A. J. Davies (letter), *Lancet*, 1980, *2*, 540. See also F. G. McMahon (letter), *J. Am. med. Ass.*, 1980, *243*, 2397.
For a discussion of the possible mechanism of this interaction, see Cephamandole Sodium, p.180.

INTERFERENCE WITH ASSAY PROCEDURES. Cefoperazone sodium did not appear to interfere with theophylline assay by high-performance liquid chromatography.— R. H. Gannon and R. M. Levy, *Am. J. Hosp. Pharm.*, 1984, *41*, 1185.

INTERFERENCE WITH DIAGNOSTIC TESTS. In concentrations of up to 1.5 mg per mL cefoperazone did not interfere with the measurement of serum creatinine using the Jaffé reaction.— M. LeBel *et al.*, *Drug Intell. & clin. Pharm.*, 1983, *17*, 908.

PREGNANCY AND THE NEONATE. For precautions to be observed with cefoperazone sodium in pregnancy, see Cephamandole Sodium, p.180.

Antimicrobial Action

Cefoperazone has similar antimicrobial activity to ceftazidime (see p.162), although it is slightly less active against some Enterobacteriaceae. It has good activity against *Pseudomonas aeruginosa*, but is less active than ceftazidime.

Studies of the antimicrobial activity of cefoperazone.— A. King *et al.*, *J. antimicrob. Chemother.*, 1981, *8*, 107; C. Thornsberry and R. N. Jones, *Drugs*, 1981, *22*, *Suppl.* 1, 3.

Cefoperazone, unlike the other third-generation cephalosporins tested, produced a concentration-dependent inhibition of neutrophil chemotaxis *in vitro*.— A. Fietta *et al.*, *Antimicrob. Ag. Chemother.*, 1983, *23*, 930.

The antibacterial activity *in vitro* of the metabolite cefoperazone A, ranged from slightly below to 16-fold less than that of cefoperazone.— R. N. Jones and A. L. Barry, *Antimicrob. Ag. Chemother.*, 1983, *24*, 293. For reference to the formation of cefoperazone A *in vitro* and *in vivo*, see under Absorption and Fate, below.

A study comparing the bactericidal activities of cefoperazone, cefotaxime, and latamoxef after 2-g intravenous doses of the drugs to healthy subjects. All 3 agents had very good activity against *Escherichia coli*; latamoxef and cefotaxime were also extremely active against *Klebsiella pneumoniae*. Cefoperazone was considered to have adequate activity against these organisms provided that they do not produce a Richmond-Sykes class I beta-lactamase. Against *Staphylococcus aureus* cefoperazone had good bactericidal activity, and latamoxef and cefotaxime poor activity. Bactericidal activity against *Pseudomonas aeruginosa* was generally poor for all three agents, although greatest with cefoperazone. It was considered that none of these antibiotics would produce sufficient activity against this organism to be useful as single-agent therapy for suspected septicaemia in granulocytopenic cancer patients.— W. McNamee *et al.*, *J. antimicrob. Chemother.*, 1984, *14*, 491. A comparison of the serum bactericidal activity of ceftizoxime, cefoperazone, cefotaxime, and latamoxef against strains of *Escherichia coli* and *Staphylococcus aureus* in 6 healthy subjects. Cefotaxime resulted in reliable activity for only 8 hours. The other three drugs produced good activity for 12 hours; the highest titres were produced by latamoxef, then ceftizoxime, then cefoperazone. The bactericidal titre of a drug takes into account its antibacterial activity, the free drug concentration, and its half-life.— S. L. Barriere *et al.*, *Antimicrob. Ag. Chemother.*, 1985, *28*, 55. See also under Activity against Pseudomonas, below.

An *in vitro* study in *Proteus* and *Providencia* spp. suggesting that cefoperazone, a cephalosporin with a relatively high hydrophobic character, may cross through the outer membrane via both a nonporin and a porin pathway. This was in contrast to first- and second-generation cephalosporins tested which are more hydrophilic.— J. Mitsuyama *et al.*, *Antimicrob. Ag. Chemother.*, 1987, *31*, 379.

ACTIVITY AGAINST ANAEROBIC ORGANISMS. A study of the antimicrobial susceptibilities of anaerobic bacteria isolated from female genital-tract infections. The activity of cefoperazone against these organisms was often unpredictable. In general it lacked the high degree of activity and breadth of spectrum associated with clindamycin, chloramphenicol, metronidazole, and imipenem.— G. B. Hill and O. M. Ayers, *Antimicrob. Ag. Chemother.*, 1985, *27*, 324. See also M. W. Drulak and A. W. Chow, *ibid.*, 1981, *20*, 683.

Bacteroides. See under Resistance, below.

Clostridia. Cefoperazone sodium inhibited *in vitro* 5, 80, and 100% of 20 isolates of *Clostridium difficile* at concentrations of 16, 32, and 64 μg per mL, respectively. It was more active than either cefotaxime or latamoxef against this organism.— R. A. Greenfield *et al.*, *Antimicrob. Ag. Chemother.*, 1982, *21*, 846.

ACTIVITY AGAINST ENTEROBACTERIACEAE. In an *in vitro* study the MIC for 7 isolates of *Yersinia enterocolitica* ranged from 1 to 4 μg per mL.— V. I. Ahonkhai *et al.* (letter), *J. antimicrob. Chemother.*, 1982, *9*, 411.

An *in vitro* study indicating low beta-lactamase-inducing activity of cefoperazone in a strain of *Enterobacter cloacae*.— S. Minami *et al.*, *Antimicrob. Ag. Chemother.*, 1983, *24*, 123.

Taking a breakpoint of susceptibility of 16 μg per mL, cefoperazone was active *in vitro* against 71% of 14 strains of *Citrobacter diversus*, and 45% of 27 strains of *C. freundii*.— G. Samonis *et al.*, *Antimicrob. Ag. Chemother.*, 1987, *31*, 829.

For reference to the activity of cefoperazone against *Escherichia coli* and *Klebsiella pneumoniae*, see above.

ACTIVITY AGAINST GONOCOCCI. The MIC of cefoperazone was in the range 0.005 to 0.3 μg per mL for both penicillin-susceptible and penicillinase-producing isolates of *Neisseria gonorrhoeae*. This activity *in vitro* was less than the other third-generation cephalosporins tested.— S. B. Kerbs *et al.*, *Antimicrob. Ag. Chemother.*, 1983, *23*, 541. See also C. S. F. Easmon *et al.*, *Eur. J. sex. transm. Dis.*, 1985, *2*, 147.

ACTIVITY AGAINST LISTERIA. In an *in vitro* study the MIC of cefoperazone for 11 isolates of *Listeria monocytogenes* ranged from 8 to 16 μg per mL.— V. I. Ahonkhai *et al.* (letter), *J. antimicrob. Chemother.*, 1982, *9*, 411.

ACTIVITY AGAINST PNEUMOCOCCI. The MIC of cefoperazone was in the range of 0.03 to 0.125 μg per mL for 20 penicillin-susceptible strains of *Streptococcus pneumoniae*, 0.5 to 2.0 μg per mL for 14 strains with intermediate resistance to penicillin, and 1 to 8 μg per mL for 20 penicillin-resistant strains.— J. I. Ward and R. C. Moellering, *Antimicrob. Ag. Chemother.*, 1981, *20*, 204.

ACTIVITY AGAINST PSEUDOMONAS. Although serum-cefoperazone concentrations were higher than those of ceftazidime after administration of the same dose to 10 healthy subjects, ceftazidime had the greater serum bactericidal activity against *Pseudomonas aeruginosa*.— Y. Van Laethem *et al.*, *J. antimicrob. Chemother.*, 1983, *12*, 475. The minimum concentrations of cefoperazone required to inhibit 90% of strains of various *Pseudomonas* spp. isolated from cancer patients in a *US* hospital were as follows: *Ps. aeruginosa*, 128 μg per mL, *Ps. fluorescens*, 16 μg per mL, *Ps. maltophilia*, 64 μg per mL, and *Ps. putida*, 64 μg per mL. These values were 2- to 8-fold higher than those for ceftazidime, except for *Ps. maltophilia* when the values were the same. In general, agents, including cefoperazone and ceftazidime, that were already being used at this institution were less active *in vitro* against these organisms than some of the newer agents tested, particularly the 4-quinolone derivatives.— K. V. I. Rolston *et al.*, *ibid.*, 1987, *19*, 193. See also above, and under Resistance, below.

ACTIVITY AGAINST STAPHYLOCOCCI. See above.

ACTIVITY WITH OTHER ANTIMICROBIAL AGENTS. A strong synergistic interaction has been demonstrated *in vitro* against 5 to 70% of strains of *Pseudomonas aeruginosa* between cefoperazone and an aminoglycoside, depending on the particular aminoglycoside (amikacin, gentamicin, sissomicin, or tobramycin) tested (J.A.A. Hoogkamp-Korstanje *et al.*, *J. antimicrob. Chemother.*, 1981, *8*, 101). Van Laethem *et al.* (*Antimicrob. Ag. Chemother.*, 1983, *23*, 435) studied the serum bactericidal activity against *Ps. aeruginosa* and *Klebsiella pneumoniae* of a combination of amikacin and cefoperazone in 10 healthy subjects, and considered that this combination may be preferable to cefoperazone alone because of its greater killing rate in killing-curve studies, and in order to prevent emergence of resistant strains.

A combination of cefoperazone and fosfomycin was synergistic *in vitro* against 85% of 20 strains of *Ps. aeruginosa*; on further addition of tobramycin this was increased to 100% of strains (K. Takahashi and H. Kanno, *Antimicrob. Ag. Chemother.*, 1984, *26*, 789). Among the penicillins, synergism has been reported against Gram-negative bacilli when cefoperazone is combined with ticarcillin (H.M. Miles *et al.*, *Drugs*, 1981, *22*, *Suppl.* 1, 15) and against a range of Gram-positive and Gram-negative bacteria with piperacillin (F.D. Daschner and P. Hoffmann, *Arzneimittel-Forsch.*, 1982, *32*, 364). In the latter study there were also a few instances of antagonism. Synergism between cefoperazone and aztreonam has been reported against a few strains each of *Kleb. pneumoniae*, *Ps. aeruginosa*, and *Serratia marcescens*, but was not confirmed by serum bactericidal studies in healthy volunteers (Y. Van Laethem *et al.*, *Antimicrob. Ag. Chemother.*, 1984, *26*, 224).

Several studies have reported that the activity of cefoperazone against Gram-negative bacteria, particularly members of the Enterobacteriaceae, or against the *Bacteroides fragilis* group resistant to cefoperazone because of production of beta-lactamase, is increased by addition of a beta-lactamase inhibitor such as clavulanic acid or sulbactam (K.P. Fu and H.C. Neu, *J. antimicrob. Chemother.*, 1981, *7*, 287; P.K.W. Yu and J.A. Washington, *Antimicrob. Ag. Chemother.*, 1981, *20*, 63; M.A. Crosby and D.W. Gump, *ibid.*, 1982, *22*, 398; J.P. Maskell *et al.*, *J. antimicrob. Chemother.*, 1984, *13*, 23; M.B.S. Dias *et al.*, *ibid.*, 1986, *18*, 467).

Chloramphenicol has been shown to interfere with the bactericidal activity of cefoperazone against *Kleb. pneumoniae* (T.H. Brown and R.H. Alford, *Antimicrob. Ag. Chemother.*, 1984, *25*, 405).

A combination of cefoperazone with the antineoplastic agents bleomycin, fluorouracil, or mitomycin showed synergism *in vitro* against *Proteus vulgaris* whereas a combination of cefoperazone and carboquone was antagonistic against *Kleb. pneumoniae* and *Ps. aeruginosa* (Y. Ueda *et al.*, *ibid.*, 1983, *23*, 374).

Resistance

As for Cefotaxime Sodium, p.153.

Cefoperazone is more susceptible than cefotaxime to hydrolysis by certain beta-lactamases.

RESISTANCE OF BACTEROIDES. Report of a study of the susceptibility of clinical isolates of the *Bacteroides fragilis* group from 8 centres in the *USA*. Taking a breakpoint of 16 μg per mL, 57, 54, and 54% of isolates were resistant to cefoperazone in the 3 years from 1981 to 1983 respectively. Taking a breakpoint of 32 μg per mL, the resistance rates were 33, 32, and 27%.— F. P. Tally *et al.*, *Antimicrob. Ag. Chemother.*, 1985, *28*, 675.

RESISTANCE OF PSEUDOMONAS. An *in vitro* study of clinical isolates of *Pseudomonas aeruginosa* from Hong Kong indicating that although cefoperazone was more active than cefotaxime, ceftriaxone, and latamoxef against carbenicillin-susceptible isolates, it was less active than these agents against isolates resistant to carbenicillin. Ceftazidime, however, had good activity against all isolates. This cross-resistance between cefoperazone and carbenicillin may be due to the production of a beta-lactamase.— P. Y. Chau *et al.*, *J. antimicrob. Chemother.*, 1983, *12*, 337. Of 1866 clinical isolates of *Ps. aeruginosa* from hospitals in the *UK*, 4.3% were resistant to cefoperazone (MIC of greater than 16 μg per mL). Among a small number of isolates producing plasmid-mediated beta-lactamases, cross-resistance between carbenicillin and cefoperazone was usually observed. Resistance to cefoperazone was also due to chromosomally determined, inducible, beta-lactamases.— R. J. Williams *et al.*, *ibid.*, 1984, *14*, 9. Resistant mutants of *Ps. aeruginosa* were produced *in vitro* after incubation with cefoperazone. These mutants showed cross-resistance to a range of other beta-lactam antibiotics, and although they produced a cephalosporinase, the significance of this in the mechanism of resistance is unknown.— R. H. K. Eng *et al.*, *ibid.*, 1986, *17*, 717. See also D. Greenwood and A. Eley, *Antimicrob. Ag. Chemother.*, 1982, *21*, 204.

For reference to a comparative study of the susceptibility of cephalosporins to carbenicillin-resistant *Ps. aeruginosa*, see Cefsulodin Sodium, p.161.

Absorption and Fate

Cefoperazone is administered parenterally as the sodium salt. After intramuscular administration of doses equivalent to cefoperazone 1 or 2 g, peak plasma concentrations of 65 and 97 μg per mL have been reported after 1 to 2 hours. The half-life of cefoperazone is about 2 hours, and 82 to 93% in the circulation is bound to plasma proteins.

Cefoperazone is widely distributed in body tissues and fluids. It diffuses across the placenta, and is excreted in breast milk in low concentrations.

Cefoperazone is excreted principally in the bile where it rapidly achieves high concentrations. Up to 30% of a dose is excreted in the urine within 12 to 24 hours. Urinary excretion is primarily by glomerular filtration, and this proportion may be increased in patients with hepatic or biliary disease.

A review of the absorption and fate of cefoperazone.— W. A. Craig and A. U. Gerber, *Drugs*, 1981, *22*, *Suppl.* 1, 35.

After administration of cefoperazone 2 g by intravenous infusion over 30 minutes to 7 healthy subjects, mean serum-cefoperazone concentrations were 256 μg per mL at the end of the infusion, and 108, 20, 11, 4.2, and 0.25 μg per mL at 1, 4, 6, 8, and 12 hours after the end of the infusion, respectively. No drug could be detected at 24 hours. The mean half-life of cefoperazone was 1.6 hours. Urine concentrations ranged from 0.25 to 3.00 mg per mL in the first 8 hours, and most of the excretion took place in the first 4 hours after the infusion. The urinary recovery was 29.3%.— S. Srinivasan *et al.*, *Antimicrob. Ag. Chemother.*, 1981, *19*, 298.

Further studies of the pharmacokinetics of cefoperazone: A. W. Maksymiuk *et al.*, *Antimicrob. Ag. Chemother.*, 1981, *19*, 1037 (in patients with neoplastic diseases); B. Kemmerich *et al.*, *ibid.*, 1983, *23*, 429 (comparison with cefotaxime and latamoxef).

ADMINISTRATION IN LIVER DISORDERS AND IN RENAL FAILURE. For reference to the pharmacokinetics of cefoperazone in liver disorders and in renal failure, see under Uses and Administration, below.

DIFFUSION INTO BODY TISSUES AND FLUIDS. In a review of the pharmacokinetics of newer cephalosporins it was considered that the high protein binding of cefoperazone may contribute to its low CSF penetration and thus it could not be recommended for the treatment of meningitis.— J. T. Noble and M. Barza, *Drugs*, 1985, *30*, 175. Studies of the diffusion of cefoperazone into the CSF: D. Cable *et al.*, *Antimicrob. Ag. Chemother.*, 1983, *23*, 688 (adults and children with meningitis); W. N. Rosenfeld *et al.*, *ibid.*, 866 (neonates with meningitis); N. J. Owens *et al.*, *Curr. ther. Res.*, 1983, *33*, 513 (adults with non-inflamed meninges).

Further studies of the diffusion of cefoperazone into various tissues and fluids: R. E. Bawdon *et al.*, *Antimicrob. Ag. Chemother.*, 1982, *22*, 999 (pelvic tissues in patients undergoing abdominal hysterectomy); R. R. Muder *et al.*, *ibid.*, 1984, *25*, 473 (skeletal muscle and wound drainage in patients undergoing head and neck surgery); H. Yamada *et al.*, *ibid.*, 1985, *27*, 93 (pleural fluid).

DRUG EXCRETION. A study of cefoperazone concentrations in bile and gall-bladder wall in 4 patients with cholelithiasis, and one with obstructive jaundice.— T. Nakamura *et al.*, *Antimicrob. Ag. Chemother.*, 1980, *18*, 980.

In 6 patients undergoing cholecystectomy who received intravenous cefoperazone, biliary excretion was decreased, and urinary excretion increased compared with healthy subjects; this was attributed to a disturbance in hepatobiliary function. In one patient cefoperazone A was detected in the serum, bile, and urine. This was considered to indicate *in-vivo* metabolism of cefoperazone, although previously cefoperazone A was thought to be a degradation product formed *in vitro* during storage of samples at −20°. Biological activity of cefoperazone A was 3 to 5% of the parent drug.— B. Kemmerich *et al.*, *J. antimicrob. Chemother.*, 1983, *12*, 27.

For further reference to the antibacterial activity of cefoperazone A, see Antimicrobial Action, above.

DRUG METABOLISM. See Drug Excretion, above.

PREGNANCY AND THE NEONATE. Results of a pharmacokinetic study in 25 full-term and premature neonates indicating that during the first few days of life, serum-cefoperazone concentrations are higher, half-life is prolonged, and a greater proportion of the drug is excreted via the renal route.— W. N. Rosenfeld *et al.*, *Antimicrob. Ag. Chemother.*, 1983, *23*, 866. The half-life of cefoperazone in full-term infants aged 9 to 21 days appeared to be shorter than in those aged 1 to 2 days and longer than in adults. Absorption after intramuscular administration was rapid, and blood concentrations were comparable to those after intravenous administration.— M. Varghese *et al.*, *ibid.*, 1985, *28*, 149.

In a study involving 12 pregnant women, serum-cefoperazone concentrations were lower immediately postpartum than 4 months later. The total body clearance of cefoperazone was increased early in the puerperium, and doses may need to be adjusted accordingly.— D. Charles and B. Larsen, *Antimicrob. Ag. Chemother.*, 1986, *29*, 873. Similar results in 12 parturient women.— B. Gonik *et al.*, *ibid.*, *30*, 874.

Uses and Administration

Cefoperazone sodium is a cephalosporin antibiotic used similarly to ceftazidime (see p.164) in the treatment of susceptible infections, although it is not recommended for the treatment of meningitis because of poor penetration into the CSF. It is administered by deep intramuscular injection or intravenously by intermittent or continuous infusion. If pain following intramuscular injection is a problem cefoperazone sodium may be administered in a 0.5% solution of lignocaine hydrochloride. Doses are expressed in terms of the equivalent amount of cefoperazone. The usual dose for adults is 2 to 4 g daily in two divided doses. In severe infections, up to 12 g daily in two to four divided doses may be given.

If cefoperazone sodium is given in association with an aminoglycoside, the drugs should be administered separately.

Reviews of the actions and uses of cefoperazone sodium.— *Drugs*, 1981, *22*, 423; *Med. Lett.*, 1983, *25*, 29; J. A. Lyon, *Drug Intell. & clin. Pharm.*, 1983, *17*, 7.

International symposium on cefoperazone sodium.— *Drugs*, 1981, *22*, *Suppl.* 1, 1-124.

ADMINISTRATION IN INFANTS AND CHILDREN. Studies of the use of cefoperazone sodium in the treatment of paediatric infections. It was usually given in doses equivalent to cefoperazone 50 to 200 mg per kg body-weight daily in 2 to 4 divided doses: R. Chiong-Kho *et al.*, *Curr. ther. Res.*, 1985, *37*, 203; X. Navarro *et al.*, *ibid.*, 1986, *40*, 839; A. Barillari *et al.*, *ibid.*, 1987, *41*, 57.

ADMINISTRATION IN LIVER DISORDERS. As a consequence of the decrease in extrarenal clearance of cefoperazone in 6 patients with hepatocellular diseases, there was a marked increase in the urinary excretion of the drug to up to 90%. The mean half-life was 4.3 hours in these patients.— B. Cochet *et al.* (letter), *Br. J. clin. Pharmac.*, 1981, *11*, 389.

Although mild to moderate impairment of cefoperazone excretion occurred in 6 patients with severe liver disease compared with 6 healthy subjects, dosage modification may only be necessary in the presence of concomitant renal insufficiency. A mean increase in volume of distribution was apparently due to ascites in 5 patients and to decreased protein binding.— J. A. Boscia *et al.*, *Antimicrob. Ag. Chemother.*, 1983, *23*, 385.

A study of the pharmacokinetics of cefoperazone in 6 patients with hepatosplenic schistosomiasis. These patients had portal hypertension but only mild abnormalities of liver function tests. Pharmacokinetic parameters of cefoperazone were not significantly different from 4 healthy subjects, although a few patients had a slightly prolonged half-life.— J. A. Boscia *et al.*, *J. antimicrob. Chemother.*, 1983, *12*, 407.

A suggestion from experience with one patient that patients with concomitant hepatic and renal insufficiency may not require adjustment of cefoperazone dosage; serum-cefoperazone concentrations should be obtained to verify this.— J. H. Brasfield (letter), *Clin. Pharm.*, 1986, *5*, 550.

ADMINISTRATION IN RENAL FAILURE. The half-life of cefoperazone was 2.1 hours in end-stage renal disease compared to between 1.6 and 2.4 hours in patients with normal renal function. Thus no adjustment in dosage is required in renal impairment. In patients on haemodialysis, however, a dose supplement should be given.— W. M. Bennet *et al.*, *Am. J. Kidney Dis.*, 1983, *3*, 155.

A study in 5 patients given cefoperazone 1 g by intravenous infusion over 20 minutes indicating that end-stage renal failure managed by continuous ambulatory peritoneal dialysis did not influence the serum kinetics of intravenous cefoperazone. However, measurable cefoperazone concentrations were not achieved in the peritoneal effluent indicating that intravenously administered cefoperazone may not reach concentrations adequate for the treatment of peritonitis. Intraperitoneal administration of 1 g in 1 litre of dialysis fluid gave a mean peak plasma concentration of 33.2 μg per mL with a time to peak of 1.9 hours. Plasma-cefoperazone concentrations sufficient for the systemic treatment of bacterial infections were reached in less than 20 minutes after intraperitoneal administration and were maintained for at least 6 hours.— E. Keller *et al.*, *Clin. Pharmac. Ther.*, 1984, *35*, 208. Similar findings indicating that cefoperazone could be safely administered in normal doses, either intraperitoneally or intravenously, to patients in renal failure.— J. E. Hodler *et al.*, *Eur. J. clin. Pharmac.*, 1984, *26*, 609.

Cefoperazone has been administered intravenously in a dose of 1 to 2 g every 12 hours for the treatment of bacterial peritonitis in patients on continuous ambulatory peritoneal dialysis.— D. K. Scott and D. E. Roberts, *Pharm. J.*, 1985, *1*, 621.

BILIARY-TRACT INFECTIONS. Satisfactory results with cefoperazone in the treatment of biliary-tract infections.— K. Mashimo, *Drugs*, 1981, *22*, *Suppl.* 1, 100.

GONORRHOEA. Treatment of gonorrhoea with a single intramuscular dose of cefoperazone 500 mg.— C. S. F. Easmon *et al.*, *Eur. J. sex. transm. Dis.*, 1985, *2*, 147.

In a single intramuscular dose of 1 g, cefoperazone was as effective as spectinomycin for the treatment of urethral and rectal gonorrhoea caused by non-beta-lactamase-producing *Neisseria gonorrhoeae*. It was effective in 6 of 9 patients with pharyngeal gonorrhoea.— E. W. Hook *et al.*, *Antimicrob. Ag. Chemother.*, 1986, *30*, 619.

IMMUNOCOMPROMISED PATIENTS. For the use of cefoperazone sodium in the treatment of febrile episodes in immunocompromised patients, see under Septicaemia, below.

PELVIC INFECTIONS. In a study of 102 women with pelvic infections, a good clinical response was obtained in 47 of 51 patients treated with intravenous cefoperazone, and in 48 of 51 given intravenous therapy with clindamycin in association with gentamicin.— L. C. Gilstrap *et al.*, *Antimicrob. Ag. Chemother.*, 1986, *30*, 808.

PERITONITIS. See Administration in Renal Failure, above.

RESPIRATORY-TRACT INFECTIONS. Patients with acute bacterial infections of the lower respiratory tract, mainly acquired in the community, were treated intravenously with either cefoperazone 2 g every 12 hours (39 patients) or cephamandole 1 g every 6 hours (34). The majority of infections were due to *Haemophilus influenzae* and *Streptococcus pneumoniae*. In all cases these pathogens were eradicated. However, one patient each with *H. influenzae* and *Str. pneumoniae* pneumonia treated with cefoperazone, developed superinfection, in one case with *Acinetobacter* and in another with *Pseudomonas aeruginosa*. Of 2 patients with *Ps. aeruginosa* pneumonia, both treated with cefoperazone, one was cured both clinically and bacteriologically. The other patient, who was a clinical failure, and the patient with *Ps. aeruginosa* superinfection both died despite treatment with ticarcillin and tobramycin.— T. M. File *et al.*, *J. antimicrob. Chemother.*, 1983, *11*, 75.

Bronchitis. In a study of 48 patients with moderate to severe, acute, purulent exacerbations of chronic bronchitis, intramuscular cefoperazone 1 g twice daily for 10 days was considered adequate therapy for most patients. However, 5 of 25 patients given this dose, and 9 of 23 given 2 g twice daily, had recurrences or reinfections in the week following treatment.— B. I. Davies *et al.*, *J. antimicrob. Chemother.*, 1982, *9*, 149.

Cystic fibrosis. Intravenous treatment with either cefoperazone or ticarcillin in association with methicillin and tobramycin appeared equally effective in improving symptoms of 18 cystic fibrosis patients with 25 episodes of acute exacerbations of pulmonary infections. Both treatments, however, were associated with the emergence of resistant *Pseudomonas* spp.— C. V. Jewett *et al.*, *J. Pediat.*, 1985, *106*, 669.

SEPTICAEMIA. Report of a study of 85 non-neutropenic cancer patients with presumed bacteraemia, and 44 neutropenic febrile patients. Patients were treated intravenously with either cefoperazone 6 g twice daily or cefoperazone 2 g twice daily in association with amikacin 0.5 g twice daily. A previous study (Y. Van Laethem *et al.*, *Antimicrob. Ag. Chemother.*, 1983, *23*, 435) in healthy subjects had shown these regimens to have equivalent serum bactericidal activity. In non-neutropenic patients the overall response rate to empirical therapy with cefoperazone was 88%; 10 of 12 Gram-negative bacteraemic patients were cured. Cefoperazone plus amikacin resulted in a response rate of 88% and cured 14 of 15 patients with bacteraemia. In neutropenic patients the overall response rate was 77% with cefoperazone alone and 73% with cefoperazone plus amikacin; the cure rates for Gram-negative bacteraemias were 8 of 11 and 6 of 12 patients respectively. In conclusion, this study supports to some extent the use of cefoperazone monotherapy for suspected Gram-negative sepsis in cancer patients. In all patients with bacteraemias due to Gram-positive organisms, therapy could be safely adjusted when the susceptibility of the pathogen was established. However, there were only 3 infections due to *Pseudomonas aeruginosa* in this series, and one failed to respond. If the resistance of Gram-negative bacilli to cefoperazone becomes more common these conclusions may need to be reconsidered.— M. Piccart *et al.*, *Antimicrob. Ag. Chemother.*, 1984, *26*, 870.

For the view that the activity of cefoperazone against *Pseudomonas aeruginosa* is inadequate for it to be used as single agent therapy in neutropenic cancer patients, see under Antimicrobial Action, above.

For further reference to the use of cefoperazone sodium in the treatment of septicaemia, see under Cefotaxime Sodium, p.155.

SURGICAL INFECTION PROPHYLAXIS. *Appendectomy*. For reference to the use of cefoperazone for the prevention of sepsis in patients undergoing appendectomy, see Latamoxef Disodium, p.255.

TYPHOID FEVER. A study in 25 patients suggesting that cefoperazone may be as effective as choloramphenicol for the treatment of typhoid fever. Cefoperazone may be appropriate for disease caused by strains of *Salmonella typhi* resistant to currently recommended agents.— J. W. Pape *et al.*, *J. infect. Dis.*, 1986, *153*, 272.

URINARY-TRACT INFECTIONS. In a multicentre study, patients with clinical or bacteriological evidence of acute urinary-tract infection were treated with intramuscular or intravenous cefoperazone sodium, usually in a dose equivalent to cefoperazone 2 g every 12 hours, or up to a maximum of 4 g every 12 hours. Of 49 evaluable patients, the primary pathogen was eradicated in 45; in 26 of these, however, there was eventual reappearance of the infection. Of the 55 pathogens evaluated, all 33 isolates of *Escherichia coli*, all 4 of *Enterococcus faecalis (Streptococcus faecalis)*, but only 4 of 8 of *Pseudomonas aeruginosa* were eliminated. The MIC values for *Ps. aeruginosa* were relatively low, but all the failures were in patients with complicated infections; thus the failure of cefoperazone treatment in these patients may reflect the underlying complication or perhaps inadequate duration of therapy.— T. M. File *et al.*, *J. antimicrob. Chemother.*, 1982, *9*, 223.

Further references: E. Wespes *et al.*, *Curr. ther. Res.*, 1982, *31*, 543; P. Van Erps and L. J. Denis, *ibid.*, 1983, *33*, 524.

Preparations

Sterile Cefoperazone Sodium *(U.S.P.)*

Proprietary Names and Manufacturers

Bioperazone *(Von Boch, Ital.)*; Céfobis *(Pfizer, Switz.)*; Cefazone *(FIRMA, Ital.)*; Cefobid *(Pfizer, Canad.; Pfizer, Hong Kong; Pfizer, Ital.; Pfizer, Spain; Roerig, USA)*; Cefobine *(Pfizer, Belg.; Pfizer, Fr.)*; Cefobis *(Pfizer, Fr.; Pfizer, Ger.)*; Cefogram *(Gibipharma, Ital.)*; Cefoneg *(Tosi-Novara, Ital.)*; Cefoper *(Malesci, Ital.)*; Cefosint *(Proter, Ital.)*; Cefosyntex *(Francia Farm., Ital.)*; Dardum *(Lisapharma, Ital.)*; Faracef *(Lafare, Ital.)*; Mediper *(Medici, Ital.)*; Perocef *(Pulitzer, Ital.)*; Prontokef *(Master Pharma, Ital.)*; Tomabef *(Aandersen, Ital.)*; Zoncef *(AGIPS, Ital.)*.

12541-g

Ceforanide *(BAN, USAN, rINN)*.

BL-S786. 7-[2-(α-Amino-*o*-tolyl)acetamido]-3-(1-carboxymethyl-1*H*-tetrazol-5-ylthiomethyl)-3-cephem-4-carboxylic acid.

$C_{20}H_{21}N_7O_6S_2$=519.6.

CAS — 60925-61-3.

Pharmacopoeias. U.S. includes Sterile Ceforanide.

A 5% suspension in water has a pH of 2.5 to 4.5. The *U.S.P.* injection has a pH of 5.5 to 8.5. Solutions of ceforanide in water or sodium chloride 0.9% injection are reported to be stable for 48 hours at 25°, 14 days at 4°, and 90 days at −15°. Solutions of ceforanide may initially appear cloudy, but clear on standing.

Adverse Effects and Precautions

As for Cephalothin Sodium, p.176.

ADMINISTRATION IN RENAL FAILURE. For reference to the precautions to be observed in renal failure, see under Administration in Renal Failure in Uses, below.

INTERFERENCE WITH DIAGNOSTIC TESTS. Ceforanide interfered with serum and urine creatinine determinations by some methods using the Jaffé reaction, and at concentrations readily achieved in patients with all levels of renal function.— D. R. P. Guay *et al.*, *Am. J. Hosp. Pharm.*, 1983, *40*, 435.

Antimicrobial Action and Resistance

Ceforanide has a similar antimicrobial action and pattern of resistance to cephamandole (see p.180).

A review of ceforanide including its antimicrobial action. Its activity against streptococci is reported to be similar to that of cephamandole, but it appears to be less active against staphylococci. Although it is active against a similar spectrum of Enterobacteriaceae to cephamandole it has poor activity against *Citrobacter freundii*, *Enterobacter*, indole-positive *Proteus*, *Providencia* spp., and *Serratia marcescens*.— D. M. Campoli-Richards *et al.*, *Drugs*, 1987, *34*, 411.

Absorption and Fate

Ceforanide is administered parenterally as the lysine salt. After intramuscular administration of the equivalent of 0.5 or 1 g of ceforanide, peak plasma concentrations of about 38 and 70 µg per mL respectively have been obtained after 1 hour. About 80% of ceforanide in the circulation is bound to plasma proteins. Ceforanide has a half-life of approximately 3 hours, which is prolonged in patients with renal failure.

Ceforanide is widely distributed in the body, and therapeutic concentrations have been reported in various tissues and fluids.

About 85% of a dose of ceforanide is excreted unchanged in the urine within 12 hours; high urine concentrations have been reported.

Reports of the pharmacokinetics of ceforanide: M. Pfeffer *et al., J. pharm. Sci.*, 1980, *69*, 398; E. H. Estey *et al., Clin. Pharmac. Ther.*, 1981, *30*, 398; S. Ripa *et al., Antimicrob. Ag. Chemother.*, 1982, *21*, 323.

A study of the pharmacokinetics of ceforanide in infants and children aged 1 month to 17 years. The relationship of half-life with age was curvilinear; mean values for half-life were 2.18 hours in infants aged 1 to 6 months, decreasing to 1.5 hours in those aged 1 to 2 years, and then increasing to 2.3 hours in children over 10 years of age.— A. S. Dajani *et al., Antimicrob. Ag. Chemother.*, 1982, *21*, 282.

ADMINISTRATION IN RENAL FAILURE. For reference to the pharmacokinetics of ceforanide in renal failure, see under Administration in Renal Failure in Uses, below.

DIFFUSION INTO BODY TISSUES AND FLUIDS. Studies of the diffusion of ceforanide into body tissues and fluids: L. D. Mullany *et al., Antimicrob. Ag. Chemother.*, 1982, *21*, 416 (cardiac tissues in patients undergoing open-heart surgery); W. J. Cady *et al., Drug Intell. & clin. Pharm.*, 1983, *17*, 645 (bone and synovial fluid in patients undergoing total joint arthroplasty).

DRUG EXCRETION. In a study in 8 healthy subjects, probenecid had no effect on the plasma concentrations or the urinary excretion of ceforanide. It was suggested that either tubular secretion plays a less important role in the excretion of ceforanide than previously postulated (F.H. Lee *et al., Antimicrob. Ag. Chemother.*, 1980, *17*, 188), or that its physical properties prevent probenecid from affecting its excretion.— J. F. Jovanovich *et al., Antimicrob. Ag. Chemother.*, 1981, *20*, 530.

A study suggesting that ceforanide reaches high concentrations in the bile, although these were reduced in patients with obstructed biliary tracts.— D. E. Kenady and M. D. Ram, *Antimicrob. Ag. Chemother.*, 1983, *23*, 706.

PREGNANCY AND THE NEONATE. Results from an uncontrolled study suggesting decreased plasma concentrations and half-life of ceforanide during the puerperium.— L. D. Thrupp *et al., Curr. ther. Res.*, 1983, *34*, 130.

Uses and Administration

Ceforanide is a cephalosporin antibiotic used similarly to cephamandole in the treatment of susceptible infections (see p.181). It is given as the lysine salt but doses are expressed in terms of the equivalent amount of ceforanide. It is administered by deep intramuscular injection, or intravenously by slow injection or by infusion, in doses of 0.5 to 1 g twice daily. Children may be given 20 to 40 mg per kg body-weight daily in two divided doses.

Doses should be reduced for patients with impaired renal function.

Ceforanide is also used for surgical infection prophylaxis, and a dose of 0.5 to 1 g intravenously or intramuscularly one hour prior to surgical incision is recommended. Prophylactic administration is not usually required after the surgical procedure ends, and should be discontinued within 24 hours except in prosthetic arthroplasty or open-heart surgery when it may be continued for 2 days.

A review of the actions and uses of ceforanide. In non-comparative and comparative studies, mostly in small groups of patients, ceforanide has been shown to be clinically and bacteriologically effective in pneumonia due to *Streptococcus pneumoniae* and *Haemophilus influenzae*, in skin and soft tissue infections and endocarditis usually due to staphylococci and non-enterococcal streptococci, and in uncomplicated urinary-tract infections due to susceptible organisms. A few of these successfully treated infections were complicated by bacteraemia. Ceforanide has also shown promising results in a few patients with osteomyelitis, and in paediatric patients with infections of various body sites, excluding the central nervous system.— D. M. Campoli-Richards *et al., Drugs*, 1987, *34*, 411.

Further reviews of the actions and uses of ceforanide: *Med. Lett.*, 1984, *26*, 91; T. A. Tartaglione and R. E. Polk, *Drug Intell. & clin. Pharm.*, 1985, *19*, 188.

ADMINISTRATION IN RENAL FAILURE. The half-life for ceforanide of 2.2 to 3.0 hours was increased to 25 hours in end-stage renal failure. Ceforanide could be administered to patients with renal failure by adjusting the dosage interval. A dosage interval of 12 hours is suitable for patients whose glomerular filtration-rate (GFR) exceeds 50 mL per minute; an interval of 24 to 48 hours between doses is advisable for a GFR of 10 to 50 mL per minute. Where the GFR is less than 10 mL per minute, the dosage interval should be 48 to 72 hours. A dose supplement should be given to patients undergoing haemodialysis.— W. M. Bennett *et al., Am. J. Kidney Dis.*, 1983, *3*, 155.

Further references: J. R. Hess *et al., Antimicrob. Ag. Chemother.*, 1980, *17*, 251; S. S. Hawkins *et al., Clin. Pharmac. Ther.*, 1981, *30*, 468.

ENDOCARDITIS. Experience with ceforanide in the treatment of 17 intravenous drug abusers with endocarditis; 15 patients who completed therapy were cured of their original infection. Tolerance to ceforanide was observed frequently especially among streptococcal isolates, although adequate serum bactericidal titres and microbiological cure was achieved with many of these organisms.— R. H. Cooper *et al., Antimicrob. Ag. Chemother.*, 1981, *19*, 256. Beneficial results were achieved with ceforanide 1 g every 12 hours by intramuscular injection in the treatment of intravenous drug abusers with staphylococcal endocarditis and were comparable to those achieved with a standard intravenous regimen of cefapirin 2 g intravenously every 4 hours.— R. L. Greenman *et al., ibid.*, 1984, *25*, 16.

PNEUMONIA. Ceforanide and cephazolin were similarly effective in treating community-acquired bacterial pneumonia in 54 patients, although neither agent was effective in clearing *Haemophilus influenzae* from the sputum.— R. J. Wallace *et al., Antimicrob. Ag. Chemother.*, 1981, *20*, 648.

Further references: C. A. Perlino and R. Jurado, *Curr. ther. Res.*, 1981, *30*, 271 (comparison with procaine penicillin in the treatment of pneumococcal pneumonia).

SURGICAL INFECTION PROPHYLAXIS. The role of the second-generation cephalosporins, ceforanide, cefuroxime, and cefonicid in surgical infection prophylaxis. Although all these agents appear to be effective for most procedures where surgical prophylaxis is indicated, studies do not suggest any advantage over older first- or second-generation agents.— R. P. Rapp and D. Blue, *Drug Intell. & clin. Pharm.*, 1985, *19*, 214.

References to surgical infection prophylaxis with ceforanide; Cardiovascular surgery.— W. Karney *et al., Antimicrob. Ag. Chemother.*, 1983, *24*, 85; R. Platt *et al., Ann. intern. Med.*, 1984, *101*, 770. Vaginal hysterectomy.— J. A. Jacobson *et al., Antimicrob. Ag. Chemother.*, 1982, *22*, 643. Wound excision.— L. M. Miller *et al., Curr. ther. Res.*, 1987, *41*, 946.

Preparations

Ceforanide for Injection *(U.S.P.)*. A dry mixture of sterile ceforanide and L-lysine.

Sterile Ceforanide *(U.S.P.)*

Proprietary Names and Manufacturers

Precef *(Bristol, USA)*.

32-f

Cefotaxime Sodium *(BANM, USAN, rINNM)*.

CTX; HR-756; RU-24756. Sodium (7*R*)-7-[(*Z*)-2-(2-aminothiazol-4-yl)-2-(methoxyimino)acetamido]cephalosporanate; Sodium (7*R*)-3-acetoxymethyl-7-[(*Z*)-2-(2-aminothiazol-4-yl)-2-(methoxyimino)acetamido]-3-cephem-4-carboxylate.

$C_{16}H_{16}N_5NaO_7S_2$=477.5.

CAS — 63527-52-6 (cefotaxime); 64485-93-4 (sodium salt).

Pharmacopoeias. In *U.S.*

An odourless, white to slightly cream-coloured powder. 1.05 g of monograph substance is approximately equivalent to 1 g of cefotaxime. Each g of monograph substance represents about 2.09 mmol of sodium.

Freely **soluble** in water; practically insoluble in organic solvents. A 10% solution has a pH of between 4.5 and 6.5; the pH of Cefotaxime Sodium Injection (*U.S.P.*) is between 5.0 and 7.5. Variations in colour of the freshly prepared solution do not necessarily indicate changes in potency or safety. **Store** in airtight containers. It is recommended that it should be stored away from heat and protected from light.

Cefotaxime sodium has been reported to be **incompatible** with alkaline solutions such as sodium bicarbonate. It should be administered separately from aminoglycosides or metronidazole.

STABILITY. A study of the stability of cefotaxime sodium in solutions at various pH values and in intravenous admixtures. Stability was optimum at a pH of about 4.3 to 6.2. Solutions in glucose 5% or sodium chloride 0.9% injections were stable for at least 1, 22, and 112 days at 24°, 4° and −10°, respectively.— V. Das Gupta, *J. pharm. Sci.*, 1984, *73*, 565.

The degradation kinetics of cefotaxime in aqueous solution.— H. Fabre *et al., J. pharm. Sci.*, 1984, *73*, 611.

Degradation of cefotaxime sodium in the presence of haemolysis was not fully inhibited when the blood samples were stored at low temperatures. Cefotaxime sodium was, however, found to be stable in nonhaemolysed samples which could be stored deep frozen without significant changes in concentrations. It is essential to prevent haemolysis when taking blood for measurement of cefotaxime concentrations.— M. Freeman *et al., J. clin. Pharmac.*, 1984, *24*, 403.

Adverse Effects and Precautions

As for Cephalothin Sodium, p.176.

In a review by the manufacturers of the safety and efficacy of cefotaxime in 87 studies involving 2505 patients, there were 124 (4.95%) adverse effects directly attributed to cefotaxime. The most frequent side-effects were rashes which appeared in 2.24% of the patients, followed by phlebitis (0.48%), diarrhoea (0.44%), and candidiasis (0.28%). Rare but clinically important adverse effects were leucopenia and eosinophilia; one case each of thrombocytopenia and collapse after injection were also reported.— J. P. W. Young *et al., J. antimicrob. Chemother.*, 1980, *6*, *Suppl.* A, 293. On analysis of data from multidose studies, adverse effects were reported in 290 (8.4%) of 3463 patients given cefotaxime. The most frequent side-effect was injection-site reactions which occurred in 4.4% of patients, followed by skin reactions (1.6%), and gastro-intestinal effects (1.4%). Other side-effects reported included allergic reactions, fever, eosinophilia, and leucopenia.— S. J. Childs and J. W. Kosola, *Clin. Ther.*, 1982, *5*, *Suppl.* A, 97. See also R. H. Parker and S. -y. Park, *J. antimicrob. Chemother.*, 1984, *14*, *Suppl.* B, 331.

ADMINISTRATION IN RENAL FAILURE. For the precautions to be observed in renal failure, see under Administration in Renal Failure, in Uses, below.

EFFECTS ON THE BLOOD. There have been reports of neutropenia associated with cefotaxime therapy (T. Ohsawa and F. Furukawa, *Drug intell. & clin. Pharm.*, 1983, *17*, 739; B. Rouveix *et al., Br. med. J.*, 1983, *287*, 1832) and based on data accumulated from clinical studies the incidence appears to be about 0.2% (C.F. Kirkwood *et al., Clin. Pharm.*, 1983, *2*, 569). In 5 reported cases neutropenia occurred after a mean duration of therapy of 22 days (range 9 to 37 days) and a mean total dose of 171 g (K.A. Neftel *et al., J. infect. Dis.*, 1985, *152*, 90). Transient eosinophilia has also been reported (G.K. Daikos *et al., J. antimicrob. Chemother.*, 1980, *6*, *Suppl.* A, 255; P.M. Shah *et al., ibid.*, 269).

EFFECTS ON THE GASTRO-INTESTINAL TRACT. Gastro-intestinal side-effects such as diarrhoea, colitis, nausea, and vomiting have been reported to occur in about 1.7% of patients treated with cefotaxime; pseudomembranous colitis has been reported rarely (A.A. Carmine *et al., Drugs*, 1983, *25*, 223). Some workers have reported that cefotaxime has less effect on the intestinal flora than other third-generation cephem antibiotics (K. Sunakawa *et al., J. antimicrob. Chemother.*, 1984, *14*, *Suppl.* B, 317), but clostridial-toxin-positive antibiotic-associated diarrhoea has occurred in patients receiving cefotaxime (R.C.B. Slack *et al., ibid.*, 77) and other workers found the emergence of *Clostridium difficile* in 2 of 6 healthy subjects given a single intravenous dose of cefotaxime (N.S. Ambrose *et al., ibid.*, 1985, *15*, 319). Nolan *et al.* (*Lancet*, 1985, *2*, 888) reported an increase in the incidence of pseudomembranous colitis associated with increased prescribing of cefotaxime and in 3 cases it was the only antibiotic used. This might indicate a more frequent association of pseudomembranous colitis with cefotaxime than has hitherto been suspected. Other workers have also noted a similar association between pseudomembranous colitis and cefotaxime or other cephalosporins, and Slack and Finch (*Lancet*, 1985, *2*, 1358) suggested that, in relation to amounts prescribed, the risk of *Cl. difficile*-associated diarrhoea may be twice as great for the newer cephalosporins than with ampicillin. However, Kelly *et al.* (*ibid.*, 1986, *1*, 102) felt that the observed prominence of cefotaxime merely reflected prescribing patterns and that the outbreak in their hospital resulted from the infectious nature of *Cl. difficile* colitis.

EFFECTS ON THE SKIN. Erythema multiforme occurred in a cancer patient during treatment with cefotaxime 1 g three times daily administered intravenously. The rash responded to withdrawal of the antibiotic.— S. T. Green *et al.* (letter), *Postgrad. med. J.*, 1986, *62*, 415.

For the incidence of skin rashes associated with cefotaxime administration, see above.

INTERACTIONS. *Azlocillin.* When cefotaxime was given in association with azlocillin, the mean terminal half-life of cefotaxime increased from 1.12 to 1.36 hours in patients with normal renal function and from 2.82 to 4.78 hours in patients with advanced renal failure. It was recommended that in patients given cefotaxime with azlocillin the dosage interval of cefotaxime should be increased to 12 hours and the dose reduced to two-thirds of normal if the glomerular filtration-rate is 20 to 40 mL per minute; if the glomerular filtration-rate is less than this, the dose should be reduced to half the usual single dose while maintaining the dosage interval of 12 hours.— D. Kampf *et al.*, *Clin. Pharmac. Ther.*, 1984, *35*, 214.

Mezlocillin. The clearance of cefotaxime was greatly reduced when given with mezlocillin; mean clearance values for cefotaxime were 256.7 and 149.9 mL per minute when administered alone and with mezlocillin, respectively. The dosage of cefotaxime may require adjustment if the drug is given with mezlocillin.— J. Flaherty *et al.*, *Clin. Pharmac. Ther.*, 1985, *37*, 196.

INTERFERENCE WITH ASSAY PROCEDURES. For precautions to be observed when assaying cefotaxime in whole blood, see Cephalothin Sodium, p.177. See also under Stability, above.

Interference of cefotaxime with theophylline assay by high-performance liquid chromatography.— R. H. Gannon and R. M. Levy, *Am. J. Hosp. Pharm.*, 1984, *41*, 1185.

INTERFERENCE WITH DIAGNOSTIC TESTS. Cefotaxime interfered with the growth of *Bacillus subtilis* in the Guthrie test for phenylketonuria, at concentrations of cefotaxime below peak therapeutic serum concentrations.— P. Clemens *et al.* (letter), *Lancet*, 1985, *2*, 778.

Antimicrobial Action

Cefotaxime has a bactericidal action similar to cephamandole, but a broader spectrum of activity. It is highly stable to hydrolysis by most beta-lactamases and has greater activity against Gram-negative bacteria than first- or second-generation cephalosporins. However, it generally has slightly less activity than first-generation cephalosporins against Gram-positive organisms.

Among Gram-negative bacteria it is active *in vitro* against many Enterobacteriaceae including *Citrobacter* and *Enterobacter* spp., *Escherichia coli*, *Klebsiella* spp., both indole-positive and indole-negative *Proteus*, *Providencia*, *Salmonella*, *Serratia*, and *Shigella* spp. Other susceptible Gram-negative organisms include *Haemophilus influenzae*, *Neisseria gonorrhoeae*, and *N. meningitidis*. Some strains of *Pseudomonas* are susceptible, but resistance may develop during treatment. It is active against Gram-positive organisms including staphylococci and streptococci, but enterococci, *Listeria monocytogenes*, and methicillin-resistant *Staph. aureus* are usually resistant. Cefotaxime is active against some anaerobic bacteria but some strains of *Bacteroides fragilis* and *Clostridium* spp. are resistant.

Minimum inhibitory concentrations for susceptible organisms have been reported to range from about 0.03 to 16 μg per mL.

The activity of cefotaxime may be enhanced by aminoglycosides such as gentamicin; synergy has been demonstrated *in vitro* against Gram-negative bacteria including *Pseudomonas aeruginosa*. The desacetyl metabolite of cefotaxime also has some antibacterial activity.

Third-generation cephalosporins may be defined as having high stability to beta-lactamases, particularly those produced by coliforms, high potency against most of these coliforms, and moderate to good activity against *Pseudomonas aeruginosa*. Clinical experience has been largely with cefotaxime, ceftazidime, and latamoxef. Their spectrum of activity is very wide but does contain important gaps: their activity does not adequately cover rarer causes of hospital infections such as *Acinetobacter* spp. and the less common *Pseudomonas* spp., all are less active against Gram-positive bacteria and inactive against enterococci and listeria, and many anaerobic cocci, *Bacteroides*, and some *Clostridia* spp. are relatively resistant. With these gaps in their antibiotic spectrum, the new cephalosporins cannot be relied on as single drug antibiotic treatment for serious undefined sepsis (I.M. Gould and R. Wise, *Br. med. J.*, 1985, *290*, 878). In addition, emergence of multiple beta-lactam resistance and sometimes therapeutic failures have occurred during therapy with many of the newer beta-lactam antibiotics including cefotaxime, due to induction of Richmond-Sykes type I beta-lactamases (C.C. Sanders, *J. antimicrob. Chemother.*, 1984, *13*, 1).

In a study of 431 bacterial isolates cefotaxime was about 100 times more active than cefuroxime or cefoxitin against *Escherichia coli*, *Klebsiella aerogenes*, and *Proteus mirabilis* and 40 times more active against *Salmonella typhimurium*. Against species usually reported to be cephalosporin-resistant cefotaxime was about 1000 times more active against *Proteus morganii* and *Providencia stuartii* and 100 to 300 times more active against *Pr. vulgaris*, *Pr. rettgeri*, and *Serratia marcescens*; it was much more active than cefuroxime against *Enterobacter* spp. Against *Pseudomonas aeruginosa* cefotaxime was 4 times more active than carbenicillin and against *Haemophilus influenzae* it was 30 times more active than cefuroxime. Differences in activity against *Bacteroides fragilis* and Gram-positive cocci were less marked. Mean MICs for cefotaxime included 0.027 μg per mL for *H. influenzae*, 0.048 μg per mL for indole-positive *Proteus* spp., 0.066 μg per mL for *E. coli*, 0.14 μg per mL for *Serratia marcescens*, and 13.69 μg per mL for *Ps. aeruginosa*.— J. M. T. Hamilton-Miller *et al.*, *J. antimicrob. Chemother.*, 1978, *4*, 437.

In a comparative study of cefotaxime and a number of cephalosporins and penicillins against 659 isolates, cefotaxime was found to have a wide spectrum of activity. It was the most active beta-lactam antibiotic against Enterobacteriaceae and MICs against *Neisseria gonorrhoeae* and *Haemophilus influenzae* were similar to those with ampicillin. The activity of cefotaxime was comparable to that of carbenicillin against *Pseudomonas aeruginosa* but less active than piperacillin or amikacin. It was more active than carbenicillin against *Bacteroides fragilis* but less active than cefoxitin. Synergy was exhibited with gentamicin against some strains of indole-positive *Proteus* and *Ps. aeruginosa*. Cefotaxime was less active than cephalothin or cephamandole against *Staph. aureus*.— H. C. Neu *et al.*, *Antimicrob. Ag. Chemother.*, 1979, *15*, 273.

Further references to the antibacterial activity of cefotaxime compared with other cephalosporins and penicillins: R. Wise *et al.*, *Antimicrob. Ag. Chemother.*, 1978, *14*, 807; F. A. Drasar *et al.*, *J. antimicrob. Chemother.*, 1978, *4*, 445; G. W. Counts and M. Turck, *Antimicrob. Ag. Chemother.*, 1979, *16*, 64; E. Schrinner *et al.*, *J. antimicrob. Chemother.*, 1980, *6*, *Suppl.* A, 25; J. H. Jorgensen *et al.*, *Antimicrob. Ag. Chemother.*, 1980, *17*, 937; S. Masuyoshi *et al.*, *ibid.*, *18*, 1.

For further reference to studies comparing the bactericidal activity of some third-generation cephalosporins, see under Cefoperazone Sodium, p.148.

The desacetyl metabolite of cefotaxime had about one-tenth the activity of cefotaxime *in vitro* against the common Enterobacteriaceae but was somewhat more active than cephazolin, cefuroxime, or cefoxitin. The metabolite had no useful activity against *Ps. aeruginosa* and was less active than cefotaxime or cefoxitin against *Staph. aureus* or *Bacteroides fragilis*.— R. Wise *et al.*, *Antimicrob. Ag. Chemother.*, 1980, *17*, 84.

Cefotaxime has been found to be relatively poor at penetrating into epithelial cells which may cause discrepancy between clinical response and activity *in vitro*. This is particularly relevant for bacteria which are able to penetrate and survive inside cells such as salmonellae, shigellae, and enteroinvasive *Escherichia coli* (P.R. Chadwick and A.R. Mellersh, *J. antimicrob. Chemother.*, 1987, *19*, 211). McKendrick *et al.* (*ibid.*, 1980, *6*, *Suppl.* A, 277) reported a lack of clinical improvement in 2 patients with typhoid fever due to sensitive *S. typhi* strains treated with cefotaxime, despite the production of sterile blood cultures 48 hours after starting treatment. Discrepancy between the activity of cefotaxime against *Yersinia enterocolitica in vitro* and in a *mouse* model has also been observed (M.R. Scavizzi *et al.*, *Antimicrob. Ag. Chemother.*, 1987, *31*, 523).

Cefotaxime has been shown to stimulate host defence systems. It enhanced the bactericidal activity of human neutrophils against *Staphylococcus aureus in vitro* without altering phagocytosis. This activity appeared to be linked to an enhancement of superoxide anion production by the neutrophils.— M. T. Labro *et al.*, *J. antimicrob. Chemother.*, 1986, *18*, 233. See also M. T. Labro *et al.*, *ibid.*, 1987, *19*, 331.

ACTIVITY AGAINST BRANHAMELLA. All of 54 clinical isolates of *Branhamella catarrhalis* were susceptible to cefotaxime; 90% of beta-lactamase-positive and beta-lactamase-negative isolates were inhibited by 0.5 and 0.06 μg per mL, respectively.— F. Ahmad *et al.*, *Antimicrob. Ag. Chemother.*, 1984, *26*, 424. See also E. E. Stobberingh *et al.*, *J. antimicrob. Chemother.*, 1984, *13*, 55.

ACTIVITY AGAINST EIKENELLA. All of 28 strains of *Eikenella corrodens* tested were uniformly susceptible to cefotaxime with a minimum inhibitory concentration of 1.0 μg or less per mL.— E. J. C. Goldstein *et al.*, *Antimicrob. Ag. Chemother.*, 1980, *18*, 832.

ACTIVITY AGAINST ENTEROBACTERIACEAE. Reports of the activity of cefotaxime against various Enterobacteriaceae: A. P. Panwalker *et al.*, *Antimicrob. Ag. Chemother.*, 1980, *18*, 877 (*Klebsiella* spp.); H. Goossens *et al.*, *J. antimicrob. Chemother.*, 1984, *13*, 559 (*Salmonella* spp.); C. J. J. Mulder *et al.*, *ibid.*, 1985, *15*, 115 (*Escherichia coli*); A. M. Lewis and B. Chattopadhyay (letter), *ibid.*, 1987, *19*, 406 (*Yersinia* spp.); J. A. A. Hoogkamp-Korstanje, *ibid.*, *20*, 123 (*Yersinia enterocolitica*).

For comment on the poor penetration of cefotaxime into epithelial cells and the possible discrepancy between activity *in vitro* against various Enterobacteriaceae and clinical response, see above.

ACTIVITY AGAINST GONOCOCCI. Penicillinase-producing *Neisseria gonorrhoeae* isolates were extremely susceptible to cefotaxime *in vitro*; both penicillin-susceptible and penicillinase-producing strains, were inhibited by 0.0006 to 0.08 μg per mL. These results may not, however, correlate with clinical efficacy.— S. B. Kerbs *et al.*, *Antimicrob. Ag. Chemother.*, 1983, *23*, 541.

Further references: P. Piot *et al.*, *J. antimicrob. Chemother.*, 1980, *6*, *Suppl.* A, 47.

ACTIVITY AGAINST HAEMOPHILUS. Cefotaxime and latamoxef were highly active against all isolates of *Haemophilus influenzae* tested, irrespective of beta-lactamase production.— J. H. Jorgensen *et al.*, *Antimicrob. Ag. Chemother.*, 1980, *17*, 516. Cefotaxime, ceftriaxone, and ceftizoxime were very active against all of 169 clinical isolates of *H. influenzae*; for all 3 drugs the minimum inhibitory concentration for 90% of isolates was 0.02 μg or less per mL.— R. M. Bannatyne *et al.*, *J. antimicrob. Chemother.*, 1985, *15*, 187. Cefotaxime and its metabolite desacetylcefotaxime showed excellent activity against 83 strains of *H. influenzae* resistant to ampicillin and chloramphenicol.— J. Campos and S. Garcia-Tornel, *ibid.*, 1987, *19*, 297.

Cefotaxime was the most active of 6 cephalosporins tested against 30 strains of *Haemophilus ducreyi* including 27 beta-lactamase-producing strains. All the strains were inhibited by cefotaxime 0.016 μg or less per mL.— M. J. Sanson-Le Pors *et al.*, *J. antimicrob. Chemother.*, 1983, *11*, 271. The susceptibility of *H. ducreyi* to cefotaxime appeared to have decreased during an 8-year period from 1978 to 1985 in Amsterdam.— A. W. Sturm, *ibid.*, 1987, *19*, 187.

ACTIVITY AGAINST LEPTOSPIRA. In tests for minimum bactericidal concentration (MBC) against 5 *Leptospira* strains, cefotaxime and ceftizoxime were found to be more effective than benzylpenicillin, streptomycin, tetracycline, ampicillin, or cefmetazole. The MBC for cefotaxime ranged from 0.1 to 12.5 μg per mL and for ceftizoxime from 0.2 to 25 μg per mL.— S. Oie *et al.*, *Antimicrob. Ag. Chemother.*, 1983, *24*, 905.

ACTIVITY AGAINST MENINGOCOCCI. All but one of 150 strains of *Neisseria meningitidis* were inhibited by cefotaxime 0.008 μg per mL. These concentrations are much lower than those for cefuroxime, cefoxitin, or benzylpenicillin. When account is taken of the concentrations of 0.3 to 15 μg per mL of cefotaxime found in CSF, and the MICs for *Haemophilus influenzae* of up to 0.06 μg per mL and for *Streptococcus pneumoniae* of up to 0.016 μg per mL, cefotaxime may be the drug of first choice in the treatment of bacterial meningitis outside, and possibly in, the neonatal period.— W. M. Brown and R. J. Fallon (letter), *Lancet*, 1979, *1*, 1246.

ACTIVITY AGAINST PNEUMOCOCCI. Cefotaxime has good activity against penicillin-resistant *Streptococcus pneumoniae*; minimum inhibitory concentrations ranging from 0.125 to 4 μg per mL have been reported (J.I. Ward and R.C. Moellering, *Antimicrob. Ag. Chemother.*, 1981, *20*, 204; C.E. Cherubin *et al.*, *ibid.*, 553; J. Linares *et al.*, *J. antimicrob. Chemother.*, 1984, *13*, 353).

ACTIVITY AGAINST PSEUDOMONAS. Cefotaxime has some activity against *Pseudomonas aeruginosa* isolates. In one study 78% of 53 clinical isolates were susceptible to cefotaxime at a concentration of 62.5 μg per mL (V.L. Yu *et al.*, *Antimicrob. Ag. Chemother.*, 1980, *17*, 96). However, cefotaxime cannot really compete with cephalosporins with antipseudomonal activity such as ceftazidime (B. Van Klingeren *et al.*, *J. antimicrob. Chemother.*, 1980, *6*, 674). Variable clinical results have been obtained using cefotaxime to treat pseudomonal infections and it has been suggested that cefotaxime may be of value in treating urinary-tract infections because high concentrations are achieved at this site. The inactivity of the desacetyl metabolite against *Pseudomonas* spp. is important particularly when the dosage interval is increased in renal impairment as relative concentrations of this metabolite are increased (M.W. McKendrick *et al.*, *J. antimicrob. Chemother.*, 1981, *7*, 405; O.A. Okubadejo and R.P. Bax, *ibid.*, 1982, *9*, 86).

ACTIVITY WITH OTHER ANTIMICROBIAL AGENTS. Synergy has been demonstrated *in vitro* between cefotaxime and aminoglycosides particularly against Gram-negative organisms including *Pseudomonas aeruginosa* (P.R. Murray, *Antimicrob. Ag. Chemother.*, 1980, *17*, 474) although, in general, combinations of third-generation cephalosporins with aminoglycosides demonstrate synergy less frequently than broad-spectrum penicillin-aminoglycoside combinations (J.E. Kapusnik and S.L. Barriere, *Drug Interact. News.*, 1982, *2*, 35). Nevertheless enhanced activity of cefotaxime has been reported with amikacin against Enterobacteriaceae including multiple-resistant strains, and also multiple-resistant *Pseudomonas aeruginosa* (J. Klastersky *et al.*, EORTC International Antimicrobial Therapy Project Group, *J. antimicrob. Chemother.*, 1980, *6*, *Suppl.* A, 55; S.H. Zinner *et al.*, *Antimicrob. Ag. Chemother.*, 1981, *20*, 463; R.H. Glew and R.A. Pavuk, *ibid.*, 1984, *26*, 378; M.J. Maslow *et al.*, *J. antimicrob. Chemother.*, 1985, *16*, 227). Gentamicin has been reported to enhance the activity of cefotaxime against group G streptococci (K. Lam and A.S. Bayer, *Antimicrob. Ag. Chemother.*, 1984, *26*, 260) and also against enterococci to some extent, although not sufficiently to substitute for proven therapy (A.M. Elliott *et al.*, *Antimicrob. Ag. Chemother.*, 1983, *24*, 847). Synergy with tobramycin against *Ps. aeruginosa* has been demonstrated (L. Mintz and W.L. Drew, *ibid.*, 1981, *19*, 332), although a limited effect has been found by other workers; urinary recovery of cefotaxime may also be significantly decreased by tobramycin (H. Lagast *et al.*, *ibid.*, 1981, *20*, 539; M.G. Bergeron *et al.*, *ibid.*, 1986, *29*, 379).
Synergy has also been reported between cefotaxime and fosfomycin against staphylococci, enterococci, and *Pseudomonas* spp. (H. Portier *et al.*, *J. antimicrob. Chemother.*, 1984, *14*, *Suppl.* B, 277; A. Carvajal, *ibid.*, 1985, *16*, 677) and between cefotaxime and ciprofloxacin against Gram-negative anaerobic bacteria including *Bacteroides fragilis* (J.L. Whiting *et al.*, *Antimicrob. Ag. Chemother.*, 1987, *31*, 1379).
Variable results have been obtained with cefotaxime and other beta-lactam antibiotics such as azlocillin, piperacillin, and temocillin (H. Knothe, *J. antimicrob. Chemother.*, 1980, *6*, *Suppl.* A, 31; H.C. Neu and K.P. Fu, *Antimicrob. Ag. Chemother.*, 1980, *18*, 582; C.H. Ramírez-Ronda *et al.*, *Curr. ther. Res.*, 1984, *35*, 64; L. Verbist and J. Verhaegen, *Antimicrob. Ag. Chemother.*, 1984, *25*, 142). An enhanced action has been reported between cefotaxime and mecillinam against 5 strains of *Enterobacter cloacae*; this appeared to be due to a protective effect of mecillinam preventing the selection of cefotaxime-resistant mutants with derepressed beta-lactamases (E. Yourassowsky *et al.*, *Curr. ther. Res.*, 1987, *41*, 578). Some synergy has also been reported between cefotaxime and ampicillin against *Haemophilus* isolates (J.-R. Lapointe *et al.*, *Antimicrob. Ag. Chemother.*, 1986, *29*, 594) and with benzylpenicillin, ampicillin, or piperacillin against neonatal meningitis pathogens using chequerboard titration. However, in time-kill evaluations using concentrations representative for cerebrospinal fluid, the killing kinetics of *Escherichia coli* were unaffected by the drug combinations and there was a delayed killing-rate of group B streptococci when cefotaxime was combined with benzylpenicillin or ampicillin; the rate of killing of *Listeria monocytogenes* by benzylpenicillin was increased when combined with cefotaxime, but cefotaxime had no effect on the killing-rate of ampicillin or piperacillin (J.A.A. Hoogkamp-Korstanje, *J. antimicrob. Chemother.*, 1985, *16*, 327). Beta-lactam combinations have also been shown to be inferior *in vitro* to aminoglycoside-beta-lactam combinations against *Ps. aeruginosa* (S.L. Barriere, *Clin. Pharm.*, 1986, *5*, 24).
Cefotaxime and its desacetyl metabolite interact synergistically against some organisms; enhanced activity has been reported against *Bacteroides* spp. (R.N. Jones, *J. antimicrob. Chemother.*, 1984, *14*, *Suppl.* B, 39) and against some organisms causing meningitis (R.N. Jones and A.L. Barry, *ibid.*, 1987, *19*, 843). Beta-lactamases do not seem to be involved in the biochemical interaction of desacetylcefotaxime and cefotaxime when they are tested in combination. Moreover, these enzymes do not explain the different intrinsic antibacterial activities of the 2 compounds (R. Labia *et al.*, *ibid.*, 1984, *14*, *Suppl.* B, 45). For mention of synergy and antagonism occurring between cefotaxime and its desacetyl metabolite, see under Cephalothin Sodium, p.177.
Antagonism has been reported between cefotaxime and chloramphenicol against *Klebsiella pneumoniae* (T.H. Brown and R.H. Alford, *Antimicrob. Ag. Chemother.*, 1984, *25*, 405).

SUSCEPTIBILITY TEST METHODS. Diffusion disk susceptibility testing with cefotaxime indicated that a 30-μg disk provided data for the susceptibility of *Ps. aeruginosa*, but produced very large zones of inhibition against Enterobacteriaceae. A 5-μg disk appeared to provide the most useful susceptibility data for *Staph. aureus* and Enterobacteriaceae.— N. Aswapokee *et al.*, *Antimicrob. Ag. Chemother.*, 1979, *16*, 164. The use of both 5- and 30-μg disks for different genera is impracticable; the 30-μg disk alone is sufficient.— P. C. Fuchs *et al.*, *ibid.*, 1980, *18*, 88.

Resistance

As for Cephalothin Sodium, p.178, although cefotaxime is considerably less susceptible to hydrolysis by Gram-negative beta-lactamases. Resistance has been reported in some strains of *Enterobacter*, *Serratia*, and *Pseudomonas* spp. This resistance may develop during treatment with cefotaxime and is thought to be due to derepression of chromosomally mediated beta-lactamases.

The mechanism of resistance of Gram-negative bacteria to beta-lactam antibiotics, although mediated mostly by beta-lactamases, cannot simply be described as the hydrolytic function of the enzyme. Resistance depends on a complex interaction involving the amount of drug available at the target site, which depends mainly on the permeability of the outer membrane to the antibiotic molecules; the penicillin-binding proteins (PBPs) and the number of lethal target sites; the amount of beta-lactamase; and the respective affinities of the drug for both the PBPs and the beta-lactamases. Usually one of the factors is predominant: with the lactamase-labile drugs it is hydrolysis, but with the stable ones it is affinity together with permeability.— B. Wiedemann, *J. antimicrob. Chemother.*, 1986, *18*, *Suppl.* B, 31. With the development of the beta-lactamase stable antibiotics, a non-hydrolytic mechanism of resistance has been proposed. The enzymes responsible for this mechanism of resistance are Richmond-Sykes type I beta-lactamases which are primarily chromosomally-mediated, inducible cephalosporinases, which are found in strains of *Pseudomonas aeruginosa*, *Enterobacter* and *Serratia* spp., and other bacteria. Induction (or derepression) of these beta-lactamases produces simultaneous resistance to broad-spectrum penicillins, monobactams, cephamycins, and most of the second- and third-generation cephalosporins including cefotaxime, ceftazidime, cefoperazone, and latamoxef. Although many of these antibiotics are not good substrates for the enzymes they can be rapidly bound by the enzyme. Once bound the drug is only slowly (if at all) hydrolysed, but is trapped in a biologically inactive complex with the enzyme preventing access to target proteins.— C. C. Sanders, *ibid.*, 1984, *13*, 1. See also H. Vu and H. Nikaido, *Antimicrob. Ag. Chemother.*, 1985, *27*, 393.

RESISTANCE OF BACTEROIDES. A high level of resistance to cefotaxime has been reported for *Bacteroides fragilis* isolates; in one study of 749 isolates, 54 and 35% were resistant at breakpoints of 16 and 32 μg per mL, respectively (F.P. Tally *et al.*, *Antimicrob. Ag. Chemother.*, 1983, *23*, 536). Hydrolysis by beta-lactamases is a major mechanism in the resistance and an increase in the susceptibility of strains to cefotaxime occurs in the presence of clavulanic acid (R. Wise, *J. antimicrob. Chemother.*, 1979, *5*, 115; J.P. Maskell *et al.*, *ibid.*, 1984, *13*, 23; T. Kesado *et al.*, *Antimicrob. Ag. Chemother.*, 1984, *25*, 131). Due to the enzymatic degradation of the drug by *Bacteroides* strains, the presence of *Bacteroides* spp. in mixed cultures with *Escherichia coli* has allowed growth of the *E. coli* which would be killed in pure culture (F.Soriano and M.C. Ponte, *Antimicrob. Ag. Chemother.*, 1984, *26*, 39).

RESISTANCE OF CLOSTRIDIUM. In a study of the susceptibility of 20 isolates of *Clostridium difficile in vitro*, 75 and 100% of isolates were inhibited by cefotaxime in concentrations of 64 and 128 μg per mL, respectively. It appeared that cefotaxime would not necessarily inhibit growth of *Cl. difficile*, so that toxin elaboration and production of diarrhoea or colitis would be possible. The relationship between minimum inhibitory concentration and the propensity to produce *Cl. difficile*-induced diarrhoeal diseases needs to be clarified.— R. A. Greenfield *et al.*, *Antimicrob. Ag. Chemother.*, 1982, *21*, 846.

RESISTANCE OF ENTEROBACTERIACEAE. A report on the effect of antibiotic use on the incidence of cephalosporin resistance in 2 Australian hospitals; one hospital used almost 3 times the amount of cephalosporins used by the other hospital. The overall resistance of Enterobacteriaceae to cefotaxime was 4% in the hospital using large amounts of cephalosporins compared with 0.7% in the other hospital; resistance of *Enterobacter*, *Serratia*, and indole-positive *Proteus* spp. was more frequently seen in the hospital that used the greater quantities of cephalosporins. Resistant *Enterobacter cloacae* replaced initially sensitive strains in 4 patients given cefotaxime.— R. A. V. Benn and R. J. Kemp, *J. antimicrob. Chemother.*, 1984, *14*, *Suppl.* B, 71. See also C. H. Tancrede *et al.*, *ibid.*, 53.

Enterobacter. For reference to the selection of strains of *Enterobacter cloacae* resistant to cefuroxime, cefotaxime, and ceftazidime in a neonatal unit, see under Cefuroxime Sodium, Uses, Pregnancy and the Neonate, p.173.

Klebsiella. A report of transferable enzymatic resistance to third-generation cephalosporins during a nosocomial outbreak of multiresistant *Klebsiella pneumoniae*. The isolates had a relatively low level of resistance to third-generation cephalosporins with the minimum inhibitory concentrations for cefotaxime ranging from 0.5 to 4 μg per mL compared with reference values of 0.01 to 0.12 μg per mL; the isolates remained sensitive to cephamycins. Cefotaxime or ceftriaxone were effective in treating cases of uncomplicated urinary-tract infections but failed in major infections at other sites. The beta-lactamase inhibitors clavulanic acid or sulbactam restored normal activity to cefotaxime against the multiresistant strains.— C. Brun-Buisson *et al.*, *Lancet*, 1987, *2*, 302. See also D. Sirot *et al.*, *J. antimicrob. Chemother.*, 1987, *20*, 323.

RESISTANCE OF PSEUDOMONAS. Reports on the antipseudomonal activity of cefotaxime *in vitro* indicate that between one- and two-thirds of isolates are resistant. Combination with amikacin or cefsulodin may reduce the risk of selecting cefotaxime-resistant strains of *Pseudomonas aeruginosa*.— A. Bauernfeind and C. Petermüller (letter), *J. antimicrob. Chemother.*, 1980, *6*, 671.
From a survey of antibiotic resistance in *Pseudomonas aeruginosa*, 19% of 1866 clinical isolates from 24 British hospitals were insensitive to cefotaxime using a resistance break point of 16 μg per mL. Furthermore cefotaxime is rapidly metabolised to derivatives which lack antipseudomonal activity.— R. J. Williams *et al.*, *J. antimicrob. Chemother.*, 1984, *14*, 9.

TOLERANCE. A report of tolerance, defined as an MIC/MBC ratio of 32 or greater, to cefotaxime in a group C streptococcal isolate.— K. V. I. Rolston *et al.*, *J. antimicrob. Chemother.*, 1984, *13*, 389.

Absorption and Fate

Cefotaxime is administered by injection as the sodium salt. It is rapidly absorbed after intramuscular injection and mean peak serum concentrations of 11.9 and 25.3 μg per mL have been reported about 30 minutes after the equivalent of 0.5 and 1 g of cefotaxime, respectively. Immediately after the intravenous injection of 0.5, 1, or 2 g of cefotaxime mean peak serum concentrations of 38, 102, and 215 μg per mL, respectively, have been achieved with concentrations ranging from 1 to 3.27 μg per mL after 4 hours. The elimination half-life of cefotaxime is about one hour, but is increased in neonates and in patients with severe renal failure. About 40% of cefotaxime in the circulation is reported to be bound to plasma proteins.
Cefotaxime is widely distributed in body tissues

and fluids; therapeutic concentrations have been achieved in the cerebrospinal fluid when the meninges are inflamed. It diffuses across the placenta and is excreted in breast milk.

Cefotaxime is partially metabolised to desacetylcefotaxime, which has some activity, and to inactive metabolites. Cefotaxime is eliminated mainly by the kidneys and about 40 to 60% of a dose has been recovered unchanged in the urine within 24 hours; a further 20% is excreted as the desacetyl metabolite. Probenecid competes for renal tubular secretion with cefotaxime resulting in higher and prolonged plasma concentrations of cefotaxime and its desacetyl metabolite. Cefotaxime is also excreted in bile.

The pharmacokinetics of cefotaxime and its metabolites and the role of renal tubular secretion in their elimination.— R. M. J. Ings *et al.*, *J. Pharmacokinet. Biopharm.*, 1985, *13*, 121.

Pharmacokinetic studies of cefotaxime: F. Esmieu *et al.*, *J. antimicrob. Chemother.*, 1980, *6*, *Suppl.* A, 83; H. C. Neu *et al.*, *Clin. Pharmac. Ther.*, 1980, *27*, 677; R. Lüthy *et al.*, *Antimicrob. Ag. Chemother.*, 1981, *20*, 567.

For a report of a comparative study of the pharmacokinetics of cefotaxime and ceftizoxime, see under Ceftizoxime Sodium, p.167.

ADMINISTRATION IN INFANTS AND CHILDREN. In a study of 33 paediatric patients aged 5 months to 12 years the pharmacokinetics of cefotaxime were similar to those reported for adults, with mean elimination half-lives ranging from 63 to 91 minutes.— D. A. Kafetzis *et al.*, *Antimicrob. Ag. Chemother.*, 1981, *20*, 487.

ADMINISTRATION IN LIVER DISORDERS. The pharmacokinetics of cefotaxime and its desacetyl metabolite were found to be altered in 9 patients with advanced hepatic cirrhosis compared with results in healthy subjects. In the early distribution phase, the serum concentrations of cefotaxime were higher and the concentrations of desacetylcefotaxime were lower indicating a reduction in the transformation to desacetylcefotaxime in patients with complete and decompensated liver cirrhosis. The mean elimination half-life of cefotaxime was calculated to be 138.1 minutes (range 69.3 to 245.8 minutes) which is longer than reported values for patients with normal renal and liver function of 48 to 96 minutes. The biological half-life of desacetylcefotaxime was also prolonged. The mean total clearance of cefotaxime was reduced although there was notable variation between individual patients. The decrease in elimination of cefotaxime and desacetylcefotaxime may be due to the altered metabolic function of the liver as well as to cirrhosis-linked alterations of the renal elimination mechanisms.— G. Höffken *et al.*, *Chemotherapy, Basle*, 1984, *30*, 7. In contrast, in a study of 18 patients there was virtually no difference in blood concentrations or half-lives between patients with moderate or advanced cirrhosis. The half-life of cefotaxime in patients with cirrhosis did not differ from that reported in healthy subjects, although the half-life of the desacetyl metabolite was slightly prolonged in patients with moderate liver cirrhosis. W. Graninger *et al.*, *J. antimicrob. Chemother.*, 1984, *14*, *Suppl.* B, 143.

ADMINISTRATION IN RENAL FAILURE. A study of the pharmacology of cefotaxime involving 34 patients with various degrees of renal impairment and 6 patients with acute hepatocellular damage. Cefotaxime clearance was markedly depressed only when renal function fell below a creatinine clearance of 10 mL per minute. In 9 patients with severe renal failure the mean serum half-life of cefotaxime and its desacetyl metabolite were 2.6 and 10.0 hours, respectively, compared with 1.0 and 1.5 hours in 4 patients with normal renal function. Hepatic dysfunction in 6 patients reduced desacetyl metabolite formation, but did not affect overall cefotaxime elimination, which depended on renal function. A reduction in dosage would appear prudent when the creatinine clearance is 5 mL or less per minute to avoid accumulation of the parent compound and metabolite.— R. Wise *et al.*, *Antimicrob. Ag. Chemother.*, 1981, *19*, 526. See also G. R. Matzke *et al.*, *Clin. Pharmac. Ther.*, 1985, *38*, 31.

The pharmacokinetics of intravenous and intraperitoneal cefotaxime in chronic ambulatory peritoneal dialysis (CAPD). Instillation of cefotaxime in CAPD fluid may permit rapid absorption to achieve therapeutic serum concentrations.— H. C. Albin *et al.*, *Clin. Pharmac. Ther.*, 1985, *38*, 285. See also K. L. Heim *et al.*, *Antimicrob. Ag. Chemother.*, 1986, *30*, 15.

See also under Administration in Renal Failure and Peritonitis, in Uses, below.

DIFFUSION INTO BODY TISSUES AND FLUIDS. Following intravenous administration, cefotaxime penetrates into the cerebrospinal fluid (CSF) in sufficient amounts to achieve therapeutic concentrations in patients with meningitis (B.H. Belohradsky *et al.*, *Lancet*, 1980, *1*, 61). The degree of penetration into the CSF usually increases with meningeal inflammation, but consistent therapeutic concentrations have been achieved both early and late in the course of treatment. In a study of 13 children with meningitis, cefotaxime 40 mg per kg body-weight administered intravenously every 6 hours for about 14 days achieved mean concentrations of cefotaxime in the CSF of 6.0 and 1.2 µg per mL after treatment for 36 to 48 hours and 14 days, respectively; mean CSF concentrations of the desacetyl metabolite were 4.6 and 1.1 µg per mL, respectively (B.I. Asmar *et al.*, *Antimicrob. Ag. Chemother.*, 1985, *28*, 138). Similar results have been found by other workers using doses of 2 g every 8 hours intravenously, or 200 mg per kg daily by intravenous infusion, in adults, and 50 mg per kg by intravenous infusion over 30 minutes in infants and children (G. Humbert *et al.*, *J. antimicrob. Chemother.*, 1984, *13*, 487; P. Peretti *et al.*, *ibid.*, *14*, *Suppl.* B, 117; J.M. Trang *et al.*, *Antimicrob. Ag. Chemother.*, 1985, *28*, 791). In neurosurgical patients without meningitis, intravenous administration of a single dose of cefotaxime 30 mg per kg usually infused over 30 minutes, resulted in low or undetectable CSF concentrations and the prophylactic use of cefotaxime in neurosurgery could therefore not be recommended (A. Karimi *et al.*, *J. antimicrob. Chemother.*, 1980, *6*, *Suppl.* A, 119). However, other workers have found that administration of cefotaxime 2 g every 8 hours for 3 doses to neurosurgical patients without meningitis produced CSF concentrations of 0.5 to 8.0 µg per mL which were considered high enough to inhibit most common Gram-negative and Gram-positive isolates, indicating that the drug might be useful for bacterial prophylaxis in neurosurgery (W.Sachsenheimer and A. Kühner, *Eur. J. clin. Microbiol.*, 1984, *3*, 36).

A study of the penetration of cefotaxime into respiratory secretions in 17 patients undergoing bronchoscopy. Cefotaxime 2 g administered intravenously every 6 hours for 4 doses resulted in mean serum concentrations of 63.6, 23.1, and 7.8 µg of cefotaxime per mL, and 13.1, 9.3, and 5.1 µg of desacetylcefotaxime per mL in samples collected a mean of 45.0, 79.6, and 165.0 minutes afer the last dose; concentrations in bronchial secretions were, 5.0, 1.7, and not detectable for cefotaxime, and 9.6, 5.8, and 6.2 µg per mL for desacetylcefotaxime, respectively. The relatively high concentrations of desacetylcefotaxime in the bronchial secretions may be accounted for by metabolism of cefotaxime via enzymatic proteins present in respiratory secretions. In addition, the metabolite has a longer half-life than the parent compound and thus accumulates to a greater extent.— R. B. Fick *et al.*, *Antimicrob. Ag. Chemother.*, 1987, *31*, 815.

Reports on the penetration of cefotaxime into various body tissues and fluids: W. C. Shyu *et al.*, *Curr. ther. Res.*, 1984, *35*, 727 (bile); R. Krausse *et al.*, *Arzneimittel-Forsch.*, 1984, *34*, 1787 (bile); H. -M. Just *et al.*, *J. antimicrob. Chemother.*, 1984, *14*, 431 (heart valves, subcutaneous and muscle tissue); G. L. Benveniste and R. G. Morris (letter), *Lancet*, 1985, *1*, 588 (pancreatic juice).

PREGNANCY AND THE NEONATE. Following intravenous injection of cefotaxime 1 g to 12 healthy breast-feeding mothers, peak milk concentrations obtained 2 or 3 hours after injection ranged from 0.22 to 0.52 µg per mL. Milk to serum ratios at 1, 2, and 3 hours after the dose averaged 0.027, 0.091, and 0.17, respectively. The maternal-foetal transfer of cefotaxime was also investigated in 14 healthy women at 15 to 24 weeks' gestation undergoing abortion; 10 women received a single intravenous dose of 1 g and 4 women received 1 g every 6 hours for 2 to 4 doses. Cefotaxime was detected in all placental samples studied; a peak placental concentration of 1.89 µg per g occurred in a sample obtained 2 hours after maternal single dose administration. Antibiotic concentrations in the amniotic fluid ranged from not detectable to 1.0 µg per mL after single doses and 1.8 to 3.3 µg per mL after multiple doses. Cefotaxime concentrations in foetal serum ranged from not detectable to 6.5 µg per mL and from 0.8 to 6.7 µg per mL after single and multiple doses, respectively. The half-life of cefotaxime in foetal serum was calculated as 2.3 hours after single-dose administration. Cefotaxime produces low milk-antibiotic concentrations which, because of the high activity of cefotaxime, might affect the oropharyngeal flora of the infant. It crosses the placenta and produces bactericidal concentrations in foetal tissues and body fluids.— D. A. Kafetzis *et al.*, *J. antimicrob. Chemother.*, 1980, *6*, *Suppl.* A, 135.

A study of the pharmacokinetics of cefotaxime in newborn infants aged 1 to 7 days. The mean elimination half-lives in low and average birth-weight infants were 4.6 and 3.4 hours, respectively.— G. H. McCracken *et al.*, *Antimicrob. Ag. Chemother.*, 1982, *21*, 683. There were no significant differences in the elimination half-life of cefotaxime or formation of the desacetyl metabolite between full-term infants and premature infants; mean elimination half-lives ranged from 4.04 to 4.56 hours.— J. Baird-Lambert *et al.*, *J. antimicrob. Chemother.*, 1984, *13*, 471. See also J. Crooks *et al.*, *ibid.*, 1984, *14*, *Suppl.* B, 97.

A study of the pharmacokinetics of cefotaxime in the early puerperium. Twelve healthy parturient women received cefotaxime 1 g by intravenous injection 2 or 3 days postpartum and again 4 months later. In the early days postpartum the mean serum-drug concentrations measured 0.25 to 4 hours after administration were 56.0 to 57.8% of the values obtained 4 months later. There was an increased apparent volume of distribution for cefotaxime and the rate of clearance also increased significantly in the early postpartum period compared with 4 months postpartum. The lower concentrations in the serum obtained immediately postpartum may necessitate dosage alterations; it may be appropriate to increase the frequency of drug administration.— D. Charles and B. Larsen, *Antimicrob. Ag. Chemother.*, 1986, *29*, 873.

Uses and Administration

Cefotaxime is a third-generation cephalosporin antibiotic used in the treatment of infections due to susceptible organisms including meningitis, septicaemia, peritonitis, and infections of the genito-urinary and respiratory tracts, skin and soft tissue, and bones and joints. It is given as the sodium salt by intramuscular or intravenous injection or by intravenous infusion administered over 20 to 60 minutes. Doses are expressed in terms of the equivalent amount of cefotaxime. It is usually given in doses of 2 to 6 g daily in 2 or 3 divided doses. In severe infections up to 12 g may be given daily in 3 to 6 divided doses; pseudomonal infections usually require more than 6 g daily. Children may be given 100 to 150 mg of cefotaxime per kg body-weight (50 to 100 mg per kg for neonates) daily in 2 to 4 divided doses, increased to 200 mg per kg daily if necessary. Doses of cefotaxime should be reduced in severe renal failure. If pain following intramuscular injection is a problem, cefotaxime may be administered in a 1.0% solution of lignocaine hydrochloride.

In the treatment of gonorrhoea a single 1-g dose of cefotaxime by intramuscular or intravenous injection has been suggested.

Cefotaxime is also used for surgical infection prophylaxis; 1 g is administered 30 to 90 minutes before surgery and, if necessary, continued in the immediate postoperative period, usually for no longer than 24 hours.

Cefotaxime may be administered in association with an aminoglycoside as synergy may occur against some Gram-negative organisms. It has sometimes been used with another beta-lactam antibiotic to broaden the spectrum of activity. Cefotaxime has also been used in association with metronidazole in the treatment of mixed aerobic-anaerobic infections. The drugs should be administered separately.

A detailed review of cefotaxime.— A. A. Carmine *et al.*, *Drugs*, 1983, *25*, 223.

Proceedings of symposia on cefotaxime: *J. antimicrob. Chemother.*, 1980, *6*, *Suppl.* A, 1–303; *ibid.*, 1984, *14*, *Suppl.* B, 1–344; *Drugs*, 1988, *35*, *Suppl.* 2, 1–231.

ADMINISTRATION IN INFANTS AND CHILDREN. For severe infections in children cefotaxime could be given intravenously in a dose of 180 mg per kg body-weight daily in 4 to 6 divided doses. In neonates a suggested daily dose was: 0 to 1 week, 100 mg per kg in 2 divided doses; 1 to 4 weeks, 150 mg per kg in 3 divided doses; and over 4 weeks, 150 to 180 mg per kg in 4 to 6 divided doses.— K. H. Rhodes and C. M. Johnson, *Mayo Clin. Proc.*, 1983, *58*, 158.

ADMINISTRATION IN RENAL FAILURE. A recommendation that the dose of cefotaxime be reduced from 1 g twice daily to 500 mg twice daily in the severely compromised patient with renal failure, when the creatinine clearance is less than 5 mL per minute.— R. Wise and N. Wright (letter), *Lancet*, 1981, *1*, 1106.

Cefotaxime could be administered to patients with renal failure by adjusting the dosage interval. A dosage interval of 6 to 8 hours is suitable for patients whose glomerular filtration-rate exceeds 50 mL per minute; an interval of 8 to 12 hours between doses is advisable for rates of between 10 and 50 mL per minute. Where the rate is less than 10 mL per minute, the dosage interval should be 12 to 24 hours. A dose supplement should be given to patients undergoing haemodialysis.— W. M. Bennett *et al.*, *Am. J. Kidney Dis.*, 1983, *3*, 155.

See also under Peritonitis, below.

For a suggested reduction in dosage of cefotaxime in patients with renal failure who are also receiving azlocillin, see under Interactions in Precautions, above.

LEPTOSPIROSIS. Beneficial results with cefotaxime in the treatment of a patient with leptospirosis.— I. Thangkhiew (letter), *Antimicrob. Ag. Chemother.*, 1987, *31*, 1656.

LYME DISEASE. Neurological Lyme disease in a 52-year-old man unresponsive to intravenous benzylpenicillin responded to treatment with cefotaxime 2 g three times daily given intravenously in association with prednisolone 40 mg daily.— G. S. Pal *et al.* (letter), *Lancet*, 1988, *1*, 50.

MENINGITIS. Cefotaxime has been suggested as an alternative to conventional treatment for meningitis due to both Gram-positive and Gram-negative organisms including *Streptococcus pneumoniae*, *Haemophilus influenzae*, *Neisseria meningitidis*, and *Escherichia coli* (H. Lecour *et al.*, *J. antimicrob. Chemother.*, 1984, *14*, *Suppl.* B, 195), especially if resistance to aminoglycosides, penicillins, and chloramphenicol continues to increase (R.F. Jacobs *et al.*, *J. Pediat.*, 1985, *107*, 129). Cefotaxime 150 mg per kg body-weight daily administered intravenously in divided doses every 8 hours has been used in neonatal meningitis and cefotaxime with ampicillin has been suggested as an alternative to ampicillin and gentamicin for the empirical treatment of neonatal meningitis (M. Whitby and R. Finch, *Drugs*, 1986, *31*, 266). Cefotaxime 50 mg per kg administered intravenously 4 times daily alone or in association with ampicillin has been used successfully in childhood meningitis (B.H. Belohradsky *et al.*, *Lancet*, 1980, *1*, 61; P. Bégué *et al.*, *J. antimicrob. Chemother.*, 1984, *14*, *Suppl.* B, 161; J.-R. Lapointe *et al.*, *ibid.*, 167; T.G. Wells *et al.*, *ibid.*, 181). However, when cefotaxime, or another third-generation cephalosporin such as ceftriaxone, is used alone for the treatment of meningitis, the lack of activity of cephalosporins against *Listeria monocytogenes* and reduced activity against many Gram-positive organisms should be borne in mind (P.B. Iannini and M.J. Kunkel, *J. Am. med. Ass.*, 1982, *248*, 1878; K.H. Rhodes and C.M. Johnson, *Mayo Clin. Proc.*, 1983, *58*, 158; C.J. Hall *et al.*, *Lancet*, 1985, *2*, 608). Widespread use of these agents may also promote emergence of drug resistance more rapidly than has been the case with the aminoglycoside antibiotics (C.S. Bryan *et al.*, *Am. J. Dis. Childh.*, 1985, *139*, 1086).

Cefotaxime and some other cephalosporins with high intrinsic activity, broad antibacterial range, and a high degree of beta-lactamase resistance, appear promising in the treatment of ampicillin- and chloramphenicol-resistant *H. influenzae* meningitis, although individual susceptibility testing remains essential in choosing the correct drug (H.P. Lambert, *Br. J. Hosp. Med.*, 1983, *29*, 128); there have been several reports of successful treatment with cefotaxime (H. Guiscafré *et al.*, *Archs Dis. Childh.*, 1986, *61*, 691; A.P. Fraise *et al.*, *ibid.*, 1134; Z.A. Karrar *et al.*, *J. Infect.*, 1987, *14*, 61). Some workers have recommended that in the treatment of invasive *H. influenzae* type b disease, ampicillin and chloramphenicol should be replaced with a third-generation cephalosporin such as cefotaxime or ceftriaxone (J.M. Gairi *et al.*, *Archs Dis. Childh.*, 1986, *61*, 1245; D. Hansman, *Med. J. Aust.*, 1987, *146*, 111). However, other workers feel that cefotaxime should be reserved for treatment of infections with multiple-resistant strains (Z.A. Karrar *et al.*, *J. Infect.*, 1987, *14*, 61).

The incidence of meningitis caused by enteric Gram-negative bacteria is increased in patients more than 60 years old, and in those who have had neurosurgery or who have a compromised immune response. When Gram-negative rods are present in the CSF of an adult, many workers now begin therapy with cefotaxime or ceftriaxone which are active against most strains of Gram-negative bacilli except *Pseudomonas aeruginosa* or *Acinetobacter* spp. In severely ill patients an aminoglycoside may be added to the treatment (*Med. Lett.*, 1986, *28*, 33). Intravenous doses of cefotaxime 8 to 12 g daily have been reported to give CSF concentrations of the order of 5 µg per mL which is greater than the minimal bactericidal concentration for most strains of *E. coli* and *Klebsiella* spp. (H.P. Lambert, *Br. J. Hosp. Med.*, 1983, *29*, 128).

See also under Choice of Antibiotic, p.98.

PELVIC INFLAMMATORY DISEASE. In a study of 16 female patients with pelvic inflammatory disease cefotaxime 1 g administered by intravenous infusion over 30 minutes every 8 hours for 5 days or cefotaxime 1.5 g every 6 hours for 5 days produced excellent results in the 5 patients with gonococcal pelvic inflammatory disease. However, of the 11 patients with nongonococcal disease 4 had a suboptimal response.— T. P. Monson *et al.*, *Antimicrob. Ag. Chemother.*, 1981, *20*, 847.

PERITONITIS. Cefotaxime has been used in patients undergoing continuous ambulatory peritoneal dialysis (CAPD). A loading dose of 1 g intravenously and a maintenance dose of 125 to 250 mg per litre intraperitoneally, or 1 g intravenously every 8 to 12 hours, has been used in some units (D.K. Scott and D.E. Roberts, *Pharm. J.*, 1985, *1*, 621). However, in the treatment of CAPD-associated peritonitis the British Society for Antimicrobial Chemotherapy recommends that drugs be administered by the intraperitoneal route so that precise therapeutic and non-toxic concentrations can be delivered directly to the site of the infection. They recommend that a loading dose of 1 g may be given intravenously or intraperitoneally in the severely ill patient and that a maintenance dose of 250 mg per litre should be given intraperitoneally (*Lancet*, 1987, *1*, 845). Neville *et al.* (*Lancet*, 1987, *I*, 1320) reported an increase in the incidence of methicillin resistance in coagulase-negative staphylococci isolated from infected peritoneal dialysis fluid from 46 to 75% when cefotaxime was used as first-line therapy for CAPD peritonitis. This led to an unacceptable failure rate and netilmicin and vancomycin had to be used in place of the cephalosporin. For comparison of the antimicrobial activities of various cephalosporins and the problems associated with the use of a cephalosporin as first-line therapy for peritonitis, see under Cefuroxime Sodium, p.172. See also under Choice of Antibiotic, p.99.

A study of short-term antibiotic therapy in 37 patients with localised or generalised peritonitis including patients with appendicitis and diverticulitis; 28 of the patients were operated on as an emergency. Four-day courses using either cefotaxime 2 g with metronidazole 500 mg, both given intravenously 3 times daily, or clindamycin 600 mg intravenously 3 times daily in association with tobramycin 4.5 mg per kg body-weight daily in 3 divided doses, were found to be equally effective with 86% of patients cured.— S. Biron *et al.*, *J. antimicrob. Chemother.*, 1984, *14*, *Suppl.* B, 213.

PREGNANCY AND THE NEONATE. For the use of cefotaxime in patients undergoing caesarean section, see under Surgical Infection Prophylaxis, below.

Neonate. For the treatment of gonococcal conjunctivitis of the newborn the WHO recommends that the neonate be admitted to hospital and cefotaxime 50 mg per kg body-weight daily be given by intramuscular injection in 4 divided doses for 3 days, or alternatively kanamycin may be used; if the prevalence of penicillin-resistant strains is less than 1% benzylpenicillin is recommended. Systemic therapy should be accompanied by hourly conjunctival irrigation with saline or buffered ophthalmic solutions, and application of a topical antibiotic preparation, until the discharge is eliminated. When hospitalisation is not practical, treatment must be given on an outpatient basis and cefotaxime 100 mg per kg as a single intramuscular dose is recommended together with tetracycline hydrochloride 1% or erythromycin 0.5% eye ointment administered hourly for the first 24 hours, every 3 hours for the second 24 hours, and then every 6 hours for 8 further days.

For infants exposed to gonorrhoea at birth, the WHO recommends prophylactic treatment with benzylpenicillin, providing gonococcal strains have remained sensitive. For areas with a high prevalence of chromosomally-resistant gonococci or penicillinase-producing *Neisseria gonorrhoeae*, cefotaxime 100 mg per kg intramuscularly might be considered, or alternatively kanamycin may be used (WHO Expert Committee on Venereal Diseases and Treponematoses, *Tech. Rep. Ser. Wld Hlth Org. No. 736*, 1986, p.122).

In the treatment of neonatal arthritis, septicaemia, or meningitis due to *N. gonorrhoeae* some workers have used cefotaxime 25 to 50 mg per kg every 8 to 12 hours for 10 to 14 days, as an alternative to treatment with benzylpenicillin (*Med. Lett.*, 1986, *28*, 23).

In a study of neonatal necrotising enterocolitis during the period 1984-5, cefotaxime 150 mg per kg body-weight daily in association with vancomycin 30 to 45 mg per kg daily, both given by intravenous infusion to 44 infants, reduced the risk of infective peritonitis compared with 46 similar infants who received ampicillin and gentamicin during 1982-3. There were also no deaths in the group treated with cefotaxime and vancomycin compared with 9 deaths in the ampicillin/gentamicin group. The better outcome might be due to the greater suppression of aerobic faecal flora in the cefotaxime/vancomycin-treated patients.— D. W. Scheifele *et al.*, *J. antimicrob. Chemother.*, 1987, *20*, 421.

RESPIRATORY-TRACT INFECTIONS. The successful use of cefotaxime for ampicillin-resistant *Haemophilus influenzae* chest infections.— S. W. B. Newsom *et al.* (letter), *Lancet*, 1981, *1*, 667.

Pneumonia. Successful treatment of uncomplicated pneumococcal pneumonia in 19 patients who received cefotaxime 1 g intramuscularly every 12 hours for a minimum of 5 days.— S. G. Jenkinson *et al.*, *J. antimicrob. Chemother.*, 1980, *6*, *Suppl.* A, 177.

In a study of 39 patients with pneumonia, 34 of whom also had serious underlying disease, satisfactory bacteriological and clinical responses were observed in 85% of 41 episodes treated with cefotaxime 3 to 12 g daily; most patients received 1 g every 4 hours mainly by intravenous infusion for a mean of 7.2 days. Four episodes of pulmonary superinfections due to cefotaxime-resistant Gram-negative bacilli, usually *Pseudomonas*, developed in patients being assisted by mechanical ventilation and 3 of these cases were fatal. Cefotaxime appeared suitable for the treatment of pneumonia due to susceptible organisms.— C. J. Schleupner and J. C. Engle, *Antimicrob. Ag. Chemother.*, 1982, *21*, 327.

Further references: P. Hänninen *et al.*, *J. antimicrob. Chemother.*, 1980, *6*, *Suppl.* A, 181; D. T. Mullaney and J. F. John, *Antimicrob. Ag. Chemother.*, 1982, *21*, 421; J. A. Garcia-Rodriguez and A. C. Gomez-Garcia, *J. antimicrob. Chemother.*, 1984, *14*, *Suppl.* B, 301.

For reference to a comparative report of cefotaxime, ceftizoxime, and latamoxef in the treatment of pneumonia, see Ceftizoxime Sodium, p.167.

Prophylaxis. In a study involving 164 multiple trauma patients requiring mechanical ventilation, the addition of systemic cefotaxime to a selective gastro-intestinal and/or oropharyngeal decontamination regimen using non-absorbable antibiotics, reduced the incidence of early pneumonia; respiratory-tract infections occurred in only 5 of 63 patients (8%) who received prophylactic cefotaxime, whereas 49 of 101 patients who did not receive systemic antibiotic prophylaxis developed lower respiratory-tract infections. Cefotaxime 50 to 100 mg per kg body-weight daily was given immediately on arrival and was discontinued when no potentially pathogenic micro-organisms were isolated from the oropharynx or respiratory tract.— C. P. Stoutenbeek *et al.*, *J. Trauma*, 1987, *27*, 357.

See also Suppression of Intestinal Flora under Uses in Colistin Sulphomethate Sodium, p.205.

SEPTICAEMIA. The third-generation cephalosporins, cefotaxime, ceftizoxime, cefoperazone, ceftriaxone, and ceftazidime, can be effective for treatment of bacteraemia caused by many strains of Gram-negative bacilli, including some resistant to gentamicin and tobramycin. Whether the cephalosporins will replace the aminoglycosides for suspected Gram-negative sepsis is not yet clear. In contrast to the aminoglycosides, these cephalosporins, with the exception of cefoperazone and ceftazidime, have limited activity against *Pseudomonas aeruginosa*, but appear to be at least as effective as the aminoglycosides for treatment of other Gram-negative infections. Although the cephalosporins do not have the ototoxicity and nephrotoxicity of the aminoglycosides, many experts are reluctant to recommend the routine use of the cephalosporins because of their high cost and the potential for emergence of resistance. However, some consultants prefer a cephalosporin to an aminoglycoside when meningitis or renal failure may be present. These cephalosporins have also been used in association with an aminoglycoside in an attempt to increase effectiveness and prevent or delay emergence of resistance (*Med. Lett.*, 1986, *28*, 33).

Beneficial results have been obtained with cefotaxime in the treatment of septicaemia, including those patients with granulocytopenia, although its use as an alternative to aminoglycosides may be limited by its modest activity against *Pseudomonas aeruginosa* (M. Armengaud *et al.*, *J. antimicrob. Chemother.*, 1980, *6*, *Suppl.* A, 263; P.H. Karakusis *et al.*, *Antimicrob. Ag. Chemother.*, 1982, *21*, 119; K. Rolston *et al.*, *J. antimicrob Chemother.*, 1985, *15*, 91). Cefotaxime has been found to be at least as effective as nafcillin plus tobramycin for serious bacterial infections in patients who were not neutropenic (C.R. Smith *et al.*, *Ann. intern. Med.*, 1984, *101*, 469) and cefotaxime has been reported to be superior to benzylpenicillin in association with gentamicin in severe paediatric infections (I.E. Haffejee, *J. antimicrob. Chemother.*, 1984, *14*, *Suppl.* B, 147). An 86% response rate has also been reported with cefotaxime plus amikacin in the treatment of febrile episodes in 108 patients with haematological malignancies (P. Martino *et al.*,

Infection, 1985, *13*, 125). However, the European Organization for Research on Treatment of Cancer (EORTC) Antimicrobial Therapy Project Group found that cefotaxime in association with amikacin resulted in only a 37% response rate in febrile granulocytopenic patients (J. Klastersky *et al.*, *Antimicrob. Ag. Chemother.*, 1986, *29*, 263).

SEXUALLY TRANSMITTED DISEASES. *Gonorrhoea*. In a study of the treatment of uncomplicated gonococcal urethritis in 211 male patients, a single dose of cefotaxime 500 mg intramuscularly was found to be safe and effective.— S. Hard *et al.*, *J. antimicrob. Chemother.*, 1980, *6, Suppl.* A, 289.

Of 118 patients infected with beta-lactamase-producing *Neisseria gonorrhoeae* treated intramuscularly with cefotaxime 500 mg diluted in 2 mL of a 1% solution of lignocaine, 95 patients returned for assessment. There were no failures to eradicate genital or rectal infection but 3 of 4 patients with pharyngeal infection failed to respond.— D. Barlow and I. Phillips, *J. antimicrob. Chemother.*, 1984, *14, Suppl.* B, 291.

In a study of 590 male and female patients with gonorrhoea given cefotaxime 1 g intramuscularly as a single injection, 10 (1.7%) failed to respond. The highest failure rate occurred in patients with oropharyngeal infection; 3 of 26 (11.5%) failed to respond. Of 541 patients with urethral or urogenital infection 7 (1.3%) did not respond, but all of 103 cases of rectal infection responded to treatment.— E. Stolz *et al.*, *J. antimicrob. Chemother.*, 1984, *14, Suppl.* B, 295.

Further references to cefotaxime in gonorrhoea: M. L. Simpson *et al.*, *Antimicrob. Ag. Chemother.*, 1981, *19*, 798.

For recommendations by the World Health Organization of the use of cefotaxime in the treatment of gonorrhoea, see under Ceftriaxone Sodium, p.170.

For the use of cefotaxime in the treatment of gonococcal conjunctivitis of the newborn, see Pregnancy and the Neonate, above.

SURGICAL INFECTION PROPHYLAXIS. Cefotaxime 4 g daily resulted in complete recovery in 48 of 50 women with severe chorioamniotitis who underwent emergency caesarean section; the other two patients died. Antimicrobial chemotherapy was started during surgery with an intravenous injection of cefotaxime 2 g. Cefotaxime 2 g was then given morning and evening for about 10 days, firstly by intravenous injection and then intramuscularly as soon as there was recovery from postoperative ileus.— A. M. Sangaret *et al.*, *J. antimicrob. Chemother.*, 1984, *14, Suppl.* B, 285. In a study of 100 patients undergoing caesarean section, a single dose of cefotaxime 1 g was administered to all patients after cord clamping and 50 patients received a further 2 doses 6 and 12 hours postoperatively. There were no significant differences between the single-dose and triple-dose groups in terms of febrile morbidity or postoperative endometritis which occurred in 14 and 10% of patients receiving the single dose, and 20 and 14% of patients receiving the triple dose, respectively.— B. Gonik *et al.*, *Obstet. Gynec.*, 1985, *65*, 189.

In a double-blind placebo-controlled study of patients undergoing gastroduodenal, biliary tract, or small bowel surgery, cefotaxime was superior to cefoxitin or cephazolin in preventing infection. The drugs were administered as a 2-g dose given intravenously 30 to 60 minutes pre-operatively and as 1-g doses 6 and 12 hours later. Postoperative wound infection or intra-abdominal sepsis developed in 14 of 29 (48%) of patients who received placebo, and in 8 of 24 (33%), 7 of 37 (19%), and 2 of 35 (6%) of patients who received cephazolin, cefoxitin, and cefotaxime, respectively.— T. J. Louie *et al.*, *J. antimicrob. Chemother.*, 1984, *14, Suppl.* B, 255.

Further references to the use of cefotaxime for surgical infection prophylaxis: T. B. Hargreave *et al.*, *Br. med. J.*, 1982, *284*, 1008 (prostatic surgery); S. Roy and J. Wilkins, *J. antimicrob. Chemother.*, 1984, *14, Suppl.* B, 217 (vaginal or abdominal hysterectomy); P. J. McDonald *et al.*, *ibid.*, 223 (vaginal or abdominal hysterectomy); H. Botto *et al.*, *ibid.*, 231 (prostatic surgery); D. Sykes and P. K. Basu, *ibid.*, 237 (biliary surgery); J. P. Favre *et al.*, *ibid.*, 247 (colonic and rectal surgery); W. -Y. Lau, *Antimicrob. Ag. Chemother.*, 1985, *28*, 639 (appendectomy).

TYPHOID FEVER. Beneficial results were achieved with cefotaxime 1 g twice daily intravenously increased to 2 g twice daily if necessary after 4 days in the treatment of typhoid fever. Two-thirds of the patients (31 of 45) responded within 7 days of treatment, but many required a dosage of 4 g daily to achieve defervescence. Three patients who relapsed and 5 patients who were found to be excreting *Salmonella typhi* during the 7-day observation period after completion of drug therapy were successfully treated with co-trimoxazole.— S. C. Park *et al.*, *Clin. Ther.*, 1985, *7*, 448. A report of failure to respond to cefotaxime therapy in a 33-year-old woman with typhoid fever. Twenty hours after starting therapy with cefotaxime 2 g every 8 hours, blood cultures were still positive and the regimen was changed to amoxycillin.— P. M. Shah *et al.*, *J. antimicrob. Chemother.*, 1980, *6*, *Suppl.* A, 269. See also under Antimicrobial Action, p.152.

URINARY-TRACT INFECTIONS. Cefotaxime has been shown to be highly active against urinary bacterial pathogens including Enterobacteriaceae, *Staphylococcus epidermidis*, and *Streptococcus agalactiae*, but inactive against *Acinetobacter anitratus*, *Enterococcus faecalis*, and *Pseudomonas* spp. (P.L. Turgeon *et al.*, *Curr. ther. Res.*, 1987, *41*, 670). Single-dose therapy with cefotaxime 50 mg per kg body-weight intramuscularly has been found to be as effective as conventional 10-day treatment with co-trimoxazole, nalidixic acid, nitrofurantoin, cephalexin, or gentamicin in the treatment of acute urinary-tract infections in children (H.A. Repetto and G.J.F. MacLoughlin, *J. antimicrob Chemother.*, 1984, *14, Suppl.* B, 307). Similar results have been achieved in adults with cystitis without complicating factors given cefotaxime 0.5 or 1.0 g as a single dose. Beneficial results have also been achieved with cefotaxime 0.5 g to 1.0 g given 2 or 3 times daily for 10 days to patients with more complicated urinary tract infections including pyelonephritis (P. Porpaczy, *J. antimicrob. Chemother.*, 1984, *14, Suppl.* B, 311).

Further references: K. G. Naber *et al.*, *J. antimicrob. Chemother.*, 1986, *17*, 517 (comparison with aztreonam); B. M. Jones *et al.*, *ibid.*, 739 (comparison with pefloxacin).

VENTRICULITIS. Successful use of cefotaxime 5 mg administered intraventricularly using a Pudenz reservoir every 24 hours for 6 days, followed by 1 mg daily for 4 days in the treatment of ventriculitis due to *Flavobacterium odoratum* in a 6-week-old infant. Initial treatment with cefotaxime 50 mg per kg body-weight administered intravenously 4 times a day for 4 days produced no significant reduction in the number of organisms in the ventricular fluid.— D. E. Macfarlane *et al.*, *J. Infect.*, 1985, *11*, 233.

Preparations

Cefotaxime Sodium Injection *(U.S.P.)*. Maintain in the frozen state and thaw just prior to use.

Sterile Cefotaxime Sodium *(U.S.P.)*

Proprietary Preparations

Claforan *(Roussel, UK)*. *Injection*, powder for reconstitution, cefotaxime 0.5, 1, and 2 g (as sodium salt).

Proprietary Names and Manufacturers

Cefacron *(Faes, Spain)*; Claforan *(Roussel, Austral.; Roussel, Canad.; Hoechst, Denm.; Eire; Roussel, Fr.; Hoechst, Ger.; Hong Kong; Roussel Maestretti, Ital.; Hoechst, Norw.; Roussel, S.Afr.; Roussel, Spain; Hoechst, Swed.; Roussel, Switz.; Roussel, UK; Hoechst, USA)*; Primafen *(Hoechst, Spain)*; Zariviz *(Hoechst, Ital.)*.

15313-a

Cefotetan Disodium *(BANM, USAN, rINNM)*.

ICI-156834; YM-09330 (both cefotetan or disodium salt). (7*S*)-7-[(4-Carbamoylcarboxymethylene-1,3-dithietan-2-yl)carboxamido]-7-methoxy-3-[(1-methyl-1*H*-tetrazol-5-yl)thiomethyl]-3-cephem-4-carboxylic acid, disodium salt.

$C_{17}H_{15}N_7Na_2O_8S_4$=619.6.

CAS — 69712-56-7 (cefotetan); 74356-00-6 (disodium salt).

1.08 g of monograph substance is approximately equivalent to 1 g of cefotetan. Each g of monograph substance represents about 3.2 mmol of sodium.

Aqueous solutions of cefotetan disodium are reported to be **stable** for 24 hours at 25° and for 96 hours at 5°.

Adverse Effects and Precautions

As for Cephalothin Sodium, p.176.

ADMINISTRATION IN RENAL FAILURE. For reference to the precautions to be observed in renal failure, see under Administration in Renal Failure in Uses, below.

EFFECTS ON THE BLOOD. From a prospective evaluation of coagulation profiles of patients treated with cefotetan or latamoxef, it was suggested that underlying disease or infection may contribute towards coagulopathies reported to be associated with these agents.— M. L. Berman *et al.*, *Curr. ther. Res.*, 1984, *36*, 893.

From a study of 11 patients with normal or impaired renal function given cefotetan, it was concluded that when given in recommended doses it has no effect on platelet function. Bleeding time, however, was increased in one malnourished patient on haemodialysis given high doses of cefotetan. Thus cefotetan may interfere with vitamin K-dependent clotting factors in patients at risk; in these patients prothrombin time should be monitored and prophylactic vitamin K administered.— K. Andrassy *et al.*, in *Cefotetan— a long-acting antibiotic for polymicrobial infections*, H. Lode *et al.* (Ed.), London, Churchill Livingstone, 1985, p.131.

See also under Cephamandole Sodium, p.179.

EFFECTS ON THE GASTRO-INTESTINAL TRACT. *Clostridium difficile* was isolated in 4 of 6 healthy subjects within 14 days of being given a single 2-g intravenous dose of cefotetan; toxin was also detected in two subjects.— N. S. Ambrose *et al.*, *J. antimicrob. Chemother.*, 1985, *15*, 319.

EFFECTS ON THE KIDNEY. Administration of intravenous cefotetan 2 g twice daily for 3 days to 15 healthy subjects did not appear to affect creatinine clearance or urinary excretion of alanine aminopeptidase (a brush-border enzyme of the proximal renal tubule considered to be a sensitive indicator of renal damage). Mean urinary excretion of total protein did increase and there was also a slight increase in urinary excretion of albumin, but these changes were not considered to indicate a potential nephrotoxic effect.— A. W. Mondorf *et al.*, in *Cefotetan— a long-acting antibiotic for polymicrobial infections*, H. Lode *et al.* (Ed.), London, Churchill Livingstone, 1985, p.117.

INTERACTIONS. *Alcohol*. Since cefotetan disodium contains a methylthiotetrazole group the manufacturers state that a disulfiram-like reaction with alcohol may occur and that patients receiving the drug should therefore avoid alcohol during and for at least several days after treatment. In a review of cefotetan disodium, Ward and Richards (*Drugs*, 1985, *30*, 382) stated that to date no reports of such a reaction had been published. In a placebo-controlled study in 8 healthy subjects, facial flushing occurred in 5 subjects and was accompanied by a significant increase in heart-rate in 4 when alcohol was administered one hour after the last of 3 intravenous 2-g doses of cefotetan given at 12-hourly intervals. However, none reported nausea, vomiting, or clinical evidence of a severe disulfiram-type reaction (S. S. Kline *et al.*, *Antimicrob. Ag. Chemother.*, 1987, *31*, 1328).

See also under Cephamandole Sodium, p.180.

INTERFERENCE WITH DIAGNOSTIC TESTS. The manufacturers state that high concentrations of cefotetan may produce falsely elevated urine and serum creatinine concentrations when measured by the Jaffé method.

PREGNANCY AND THE NEONATE. For reference to the precautions to be taken in pregnancy with agents possessing a methylthiotetrazole side-chain, see under Cephamandole Sodium, p.180.

Antimicrobial Action and Resistance

Cefotetan is a cephamycin antibiotic, which like the other beta-lactam antibiotics is bactericidal and is considered to act through the inhibition of bacterial cell wall synthesis. It has a similar spectrum of activity to cefotaxime (see p.152) although it is generally less active against Gram-positive bacteria and some Gram-negative bacteria, including *Enterobacter* and *Citrobacter* spp., *Haemophilus influenzae*, and *Neisseria gonorrheae*; it has little activity against *Pseudomonas aeruginosa*. Cefotetan is more active than cefotaxime against *Bacteroides fragilis*.

Cefotetan is a cephamycin antibiotic with a 7α-methoxy substitution on the cephalosporin nucleus and is therefore structurally similar to cefoxitin and latamoxef. The commercially-available product exists as 2 epimers (*R* and *S*) although in weakly alkaline solutions a third tautomeric form is present; all 3 tautomers have equal antibacterial activity. Cefotetan is generally classified as a third-generation cephalosporin. Organisms with an MIC of 16 μg or less per mL may be considered susceptible to cefotetan, and those with an MIC of 64 μg or more per mL, resistant. The activity of cefotetan against Gram-positive organisms is similar to that of latamoxef. Cefotetan is active against a wide range of

Gram-negative bacteria. The MIC of 90% of strains of *Escherichia coli*, *Klebsiella* spp., *Proteus mirabilis*, and *Pr. vulgaris* is usually 1 µg or less per mL, that of 90% of strains of *Salmonella* and *Shigella* spp. and of *Yersinia enterolitica* 2 µg or less per mL, and that of 90% of isolates of *Providencia* spp., other indole-positive and indole-negative *Proteus* spp., *Morganella morganii*, *Neisseria* spp., and *Haemophilus influenzae* between 2 and 4 µg per mL. Many strains of *Enterobacter* and *Citrobacter* spp. are resistant, and resistant isolates of *Serratia* spp. do occur. Although cefotetan shows very little *in vitro* activity against *Pseudomonas aeruginosa*, it has shown some activity against other *Pseudomonas* spp. The activity *in vitro* of cefotetan against anaerobic bacteria shows wide variability between laboratories, and therefore local testing of isolates should be undertaken. In general, cefotetan, cefoxitin, and latamoxef are more active than the [true] cephalosporins against most clinically important *Bacteroides* spp., but less active than clindamycin, metronidazole, and imipenem. Cefotetan appears to be more active than cefoxitin and many third-generation cephalosporins against *Clostridium difficile*.

The incidence of synergistic interactions between cefotetan and aminoglycosides or other beta-lactam antibiotics appears to be relatively low. Antagonism between such combinations has been reported rarely.

Cefotetan has marked stability *in vitro* against a variety of beta-lactamases produced by Gram-negative bacteria. It shows some degree of hydrolysis by beta-lactamases produced by *Ps. aeruginosa* and occasional strains of *Enterobacter cloacae*. Cefotetan also possesses direct beta-lactamase inhibitory properties.— A. Ward and D. M. Richards, *Drugs*, 1985, *30*, 382.

Cefotetan has been shown to inhibit growth of *Mycobacterium fortuitum in vitro* at concentrations of 100 µg per mL and below. When given to *mice* in relatively large doses it was observed to have a therapeutic effect.— H. Saito *et al.*, *Antimicrob. Ag. Chemother.*, 1984, *26*, 270.

ACTIVITY WITH OTHER ANTIMICROBIAL AGENTS. There was little interaction *in vitro* between cefotetan and cefsulodin against aerobic organisms, and no antagonism was observed. However, synergy was observed against a large proportion of *Bacteroides fragilis* strains and against a few strains of other anaerobes; antagonism of cefotetan by cefsulodin was observed against two strains of *Clostridium perfringens* and *B. vulgatus*. Although cefotetan is reported to be a good inducer of Type I beta-lactamases, the combination did not show any antagonism against *Pseudomonas aeruginosa*.— B. Watt and F.V. Brown (letter), *J. antimicrob. Chemother.*, 1986, *18*, 766.

Absorption and Fate

Cefotetan is administered parenterally as the disodium salt. After intramuscular injection of the equivalent of 1 or 2 g of cefotetan, peak plasma concentrations of about 65 and 90 µg per mL respectively have been reported approximately 1.5 to 3.0 hours after a dose. The half-life of cefotetan is usually in the range of 3.0 to 4.6 hours and is slightly prolonged in patients with renal impairment. The amount of cefotetan in the circulation bound to plasma proteins is reported to vary between 78 and 91%.

Cefotetan is widely distributed in body tissues and fluids. It diffuses across the placenta and is excreted in breast-milk in low concentrations.

Cefotetan is excreted chiefly in the urine as unchanged drug; up to 81% of a dose is recovered in the urine in 24 hours and high concentrations are achieved.

About 12% of a dose is reported to be excreted in the bile.

A review of the absorption and fate of cefotetan disodium.— A. Ward and D. M. Richards, *Drugs*, 1985, *30*, 382.

The pharmacokinetics of cefotetan disodium in 8 healthy subjects given an intravenous infusion of the drug with or without a preceding bolus injection. The tautomeric form of cefotetan was detected in almost all plasma and urine samples.— H. K. Adam *et al.*, *J. antimicrob. Chemother.*, 1983, *11*, *Suppl.* A, 193.

A study of the pharmacokinetics of cefotetan disodium in 10 healthy subjects. The mean peak plasma concentrations after intravenous injection of doses equivalent to cefotetan 0.25, 0.5, 1.0, and 2.0 g were 42, 79, 142, and 237 µg per mL respectively. After the 1-g dose mean concentrations in the urine of 2.0 and 0.1 mg per mL were achieved 0 to 1 and 8 to 10 hours after the injection respectively. The corresponding figures for the 2-g dose were 4.1 and 0.3 mg per mL.— R. A. Yates *et al.*, *J. antimicrob. Chemother.*, 1983, *11*, *Suppl.* A, 185.

ADMINISTRATION IN RENAL FAILURE. For reference to the pharmacokinetics of cefotetan in renal failure, see under Administration in Renal Failure in Uses, below.

DIFFUSION INTO BODY TISSUES AND FLUIDS. The penetration of cefotetan into peritoneal fluid after administration of 1 g by intravenous injection was considered adequate for the prophylaxis or treatment of abdominal sepsis.— R. Wise *et al.*, *Antimicrob. Ag. Chemother.*, 1983, *24*, 279.

DRUG EXCRETION. Seventeen patients undergoing biliary-tract or pancreatic surgery were given cefotetan 1 g (as the disodium salt) by intravenous injection. Cefotetan was detected in bile from the common bile duct in concentrations greater than 250 µg per mL in all patients with unobstructed ducts who were sampled up to 8 hours after administration. Concentrations in bile from the gall-bladder were greater than in that from the common bile duct, except in patients with poor or no gall-bladder function.— A. W. M. C. Owen *et al.*, *J. antimicrob. Chemother.*, 1983, *11*, *Suppl.* A, 217.

After administration of cefotetan 0.5 g twice daily by intramuscular injection to 10 elderly patients with urinary-tract infections, mean concentrations in the urine were 0.7 and 1.1 mg per mL after one and five days of treatment respectively. Concentrations of 0.09 and 0.20 mg per mL were measured in urine from 2 patients 48 hours after the last dose had been administered.— R. J. Whale *et al.*, *in Cefotetan—a long-acting antibiotic for polymicrobial infections*, H. Lode *et al.* (Ed.), London, Churchill Livingstone, 1985, p.102.

Uses and Administration

Cefotetan is a cephamycin antibiotic which is given as the disodium salt for the treatment or prophylaxis of susceptible infections. Because of its activity against *Bacteroides fragilis* and other anaerobic organisms it may be useful for infections of mixed aerobic and anaerobic origin such as intra-abdominal or gynaecological infections.

It is administered by deep intramuscular injection or intravenously by slow injection over 3 to 5 minutes or by infusion. To decrease pain on intramuscular injection it may be administered in a 0.5 or 1% solution of lignocaine hydrochloride. Doses are expressed in terms of the equivalent amount of cefotetan. The usual dose for adults is 1 to 2 g twice daily. For the treatment of life-threatening infections, 3 g twice daily may be given intravenously. If cefotetan disodium is administered in association with an aminoglycoside, the drugs should be given separately.

For infection prophylaxis during surgical procedures an intravenous dose of 1 to 2 g is administered 30 to 60 minutes prior to surgery.

A detailed review of the actions and uses of cefotetan disodium. Cefotetan disodium has been investigated in both open and comparative studies in a wide range of bacterial infections. Particularly high success rates have been obtained in infections which may involve anaerobic and/or Gram-negative bacteria, such as intra-abdominal, soft-tissue, and obstetric and gynaecological infections, or the prophylaxis of postoperative wound sepsis. It has also been used successfully in large numbers of patients with chronic complicated urinary-tract infections and lower respiratory-tract infections. Studies of its use in immunocompromised patients with infections, patients with septicaemia, otorhinolaryngological infections, gonorrhoea, or infections of the bones and joints have involved only small numbers. Cefotetan disodium is not indicated for suspected or proven pseudomonal infections, nor for bacterial meningitis.

Although cefotetan disodium is usually administered twice daily, many studies have used single daily doses. There has been a limited number of studies of the use of cefotetan disodium in paediatric patients, and the equivalent of cefotetan 40 to 60 mg per kg body-weight daily in two divided doses has been suggested for children.— A. Ward and D. M. Richards, *Drugs*, 1985, *30*, 382. A brief review of cefotetan disodium. It has similar activity to cefoxitin (*in vitro*), but controlled studies comparing these agents for surgical prophylaxis or treatment of intra-abdominal and pelvic infections have not been adequate to establish comparable efficacy. When used alone, cefotetan disodium appears to be inadequate for the treatment of suspected sepsis in granulocytopenic patients.— *Med. Lett.*, 1986, *28*, 70.

For proceedings of symposia on cefotetan disodium, see *J. antimicrob. Chemother.*, 1983, *11*, *Suppl.* A, 1—236; *Cefotetan—a long-acting antibiotic for polymicrobial infections*, H. Lode *et al.*, (Ed.), London, Churchill Livingstone, 1985, p.1—289.

ADMINISTRATION IN RENAL FAILURE. A study of the pharmacokinetics of cefotetan disodium in subjects with varying degrees of renal function. They were divided into 3 groups: those with a creatinine clearance (CC) greater than 80 mL per minute (group 1), those with a CC between 40 and 80 mL per minute (group 2), and those with a CC between 10 and 39 mL per minute (group 3). The mean half-life increased from 4.2 to 9.9 hours in subjects from groups 1 to 3 respectively; the urinary excretion over 24 hours decreased from 49 to 27%. The results suggested that cefotetan is excreted in the urine primarily by glomerular filtration, but also by tubular secretion. The mean percentage of the dose excreted in the urine as cefotetan tautomer (U-18864) was not significantly affected by the degree of renal impairment.

Dosage adjustments are probably only required in patients with a CC of 30 mL per minute or less; either the dosage interval could be increased or the dose reduced. The following modifications were proposed: patients with CC above 30 mL per minute, 1 to 2 g every 12 hours; those with CC between 10 and 30 mL per minute, 1 to 2 g every 24 hours, or 0.5 to 1 g every 12 hours; those with CC less than 10 mL per minute, 1 to 2 g every 48 hours, or 0.25 to 0.5 g every 12 hours. A loading dose of 1 to 2 g should be given if the reduced-dose regimen is used.— B. R. Smith *et al.*, *Antimicrob. Ag. Chemother.*, 1986, *29*, 887.

The mean half-life of cefotetan disodium was 20.4 hours in 6 patients with end-stage renal failure (ESRF) given the drug between haemodialysis sessions; in 6 patients given cefotetan disodium during dialysis the mean half-life was 7.5 hours. In 5 patients given cefotetan while undergoing continuous ambulatory peritoneal dialysis (CAPD), the mean half-life was 15.5 hours and 5 to 9% of a dose was recovered in the dialysate over the 24 hours following the dose. It was suggested that patients with ESRF on intermittent haemodialysis could be given one-quarter of the usual dose on days between dialyses, increasing to one-half the usual dose on the day of dialysis. In patients undergoing CAPD one-half of the usual dose could be given at a dosage interval of at least 24 hours.— M. J. Browning *et al.*, *J. antimicrob. Chemother.*, 1986, *18*, 103.

Further references: N. Wright *et al.*, *J. antimicrob. Chemother.*, 1983, *11*, *Suppl.* A, 213; M. Ohkawa *et al.*, *Antimicrob. Ag. Chemother.*, 1983, *23*, 31.

Proprietary Names and Manufacturers

Apacef *(I.C.I.-Pharma, Fr.)*; Apatef *(ICI, Denm.; ICI, Ger.)*; Cefotan *(Stuart Pharmaceuticals, USA)*; Manufacturers also include—*Yamanouchi, Jpn.*

12542-q

Cefotiam Hydrochloride *(BANM, USAN, rINNM)*. Abbott-48999; CGP-14221/E; SCE-963. 7-[2-(2-Aminothiazol-4-yl)acetamido]-3-[1-(2-dimethylaminoethyl)-1*H*-tetrazol-5-ylthiomethyl]-3-cephem-4-carboxylic acid dihydrochloride.

$C_{18}H_{23}N_9O_4S_3,2HCl = 598.6$.

CAS — 61622-34-2 (cefotiam); 66309-69-1 (hydrochloride).

1.13 g of monograph substance is approximately equivalent to 1 g of cefotiam.

Cefotiam hydrochloride is a cephalosporin antibiotic with actions and uses similar to cephamandole (see p.179). It is administered by the intravenous or intramuscular route usually in doses up to the equivalent of cefotiam 4 g daily in two to four divided doses.

ADVERSE EFFECTS AND PRECAUTIONS. *Interactions*. No pharmacokinetic interaction was observed when cefotiam and cefsulodin were administered concomitantly to patients with impaired renal function.— J. B. Lecaillon *et al.*, *Antimicrob. Ag. Chemother.*, 1984, *26*, 368.

ANTIMICROBIAL ACTION. Reports suggesting that cefotiam is more active than cefoxitin or cefuroxime against members of the Enterobacteriaceae: R. Wise *et al.*, *J. antimicrob. Chemother.*, 1981, *7*, 343; B. Watt and F. V. Brown, *ibid.*, 1982, *10*, 391.

Further references to the antimicrobial action of cefotiam: G. P. Bodey *et al.*, *Antimicrob. Ag. Chemother.*, 1981, *20*, 226; B. Wiedemann and A. H. Seeberg, *J. antimicrob. Chemother.*, 1984, *13*, 111.

Activity with other antimicrobial agents. Demonstration *in vitro* of synergism between cefotiam and mezlocillin against various Gram-negative bacteria.— J. R. Rodríguez *et al.*, *Curr. ther. Res.*, 1984, *36*, 902.

Cefotiam was a less potent inducer of the beta-lactamases of *Enterobacter cloacae* and *Serratia marcescens* than cefoxitin and cefmetazole. It diminished the activity of some third-generation cephalosporins against these organisms to a small extent.— K. Okonogi *et al., J. antimicrob. Chemother.*, 1985, *16*, 31.

ABSORPTION AND FATE. After intravenous infusion of cefotiam to healthy subjects, Daschner *et al.* (*Antimicrob. Ag. Chemother.*, 1982, *22*, 958) demonstrated dose-dependent pharmacokinetics. In a study in 16 healthy subjects, Brisson *et al.* (*ibid.*, 1984, *26*, 513) could not verify these results. After intramuscular injection of 0.5 or 1 g, mean peak concentrations of 7.7 and 14.3 µg per mL after about 0.75 hours were obtained respectively. Up to 51 or 59% of a dose was excreted in the urine within 12 hours after intramuscular and intravenous administration respectively. The half-life varied from 0.9 to 1.2 hours. Although Rouan *et al.*, (*ibid.*, 1985, *27*, 177) did demonstrate some dose-dependency in cefotiam pharmacokinetics, he considered the deviation from linearity to be small and of little clinical significance.

Further references to the absorption and fate of cefotiam: K. Satake *et al., J. antimicrob. Chemother.*, 1982, *10*, 141 (biliary excretion in patients with biliary disease); I. Miyakawa *et al., Antimicrob. Ag. Chemother.*, 1984, *25*, 147 (transplacental transfer); I. G. Alonso *et al., Int. J. Pharmaceut.*, 1984, *19*, 345 (pharmacokinetics in healthy subjects).

USES AND ADMINISTRATION. Reports of the use of cefotiam hydrochloride: G. De Rosa *et al., Curr. ther. Res.*, 1983, *34*, 117 (various infections); J. R. Lentino *et al., Antimicrob. Ag. Chemother.*, 1984, *25*, 778 (skin and soft-tissue infections); M. A. Polis and C. U. Tuazon, *ibid.*, 1985, *28*, 576 (respiratory-tract infections).

Administration in renal failure. There was a moderate increase in the half-life of cefotiam in patients with renal impairment, accompanied by a decrease in the urinary excretion. The dose may only need to be reduced in patients with severe renal failure and even then only when the dose has to be given at dose intervals of less than 12 hours.— M. C. Rouan *et al., J. antimicrob. Chemother.*, 1984, *13*, 611. For patients with a creatinine clearance of less than 15 mL per minute, a standard dose of cefotiam could be given every 24 to 36 hours. A dose supplement may be required at the end of haemodialysis.— K. Konishi and Y. Ozawa, *Antimicrob. Ag. Chemother.*, 1984, *26*, 647.

Proprietary Names and Manufacturers

Halospor *(Ciba-Geigy, Jpn; Ciba, Switz.)*; Pansporin *(Takeda, Jpn)*; Pansporine *(Takeda, Fr.)*; Spizef *(Takeda, Ger.)*; Sporidyn *(Cyanamid, Ital.)*.

33-d

Cefoxitin Sodium *(BANM, USAN, rINNM).*

L-620388; MK-306. Sodium 3-carbamoyloxymethyl-7-methoxy-7-(2-thienylacetamido)-3-cephem-4-carboxylate.

$C_{16}H_{16}N_3NaO_7S_2$=449.4.

CAS — 35607-66-0 (cefoxitin); 33564-30-6 (sodium salt).

Pharmacopoeias. In *Jpn* and *U.S.*

White to off-white, somewhat hygroscopic powder or granules with a slight characteristic odour. 1.05 g of the monograph substance is approximately equivalent to 1 g of cefoxitin. Each g of monograph substance represents about 2.2 mmol of sodium. Very **soluble** in water; slightly soluble in acetone; sparingly soluble in dimethylformamide; soluble in methyl alcohol; insoluble in chloroform and ether. A 10% solution in water has a pH of 4.2 to 7.0. The *U.S.P.* injection has a pH of 4.5 to 8.0.

Store in airtight containers. Injections containing 1 g in 10 mL are reported to be **stable** for 24 hours if stored at room temperature, for one week if stored below 5°, and for at least 30 weeks if stored at −20°. Cefoxitin sodium tends to darken on storage.

Incompatibility or loss of activity has been reported with metronidazole.

Adverse Effects

As for Cephalothin Sodium, p.176.

About 8% of 1924 patients from 108 studies experienced drug-related adverse effects after receiving cefoxitin. After intravenous infusion, thrombophlebitis was reported in 89 of 1678 patients (5.3%) and occurred more frequently when indwelling polyethylene catheters were used rather than butterfly needles. Skin rashes occurred in 2.2% of patients. Reported changes in laboratory estimations after intravenous cefoxitin included eosinophilia (2.9% of patients tested), positive direct Coombs' tests (2.4%, haemolysis was not reported), increased serum aminotransferases (about 3%), and increased serum creatinine (0.7%). Intramuscular injections prepared with 0.5 or 1% lignocaine solutions were well-tolerated by 159 of 175 patients.— C. van Winzum, *J. antimicrob. Chemother.*, 1978, *4, Suppl.* B, 91.

ALLERGY. For a report of hypotension with or without bronchospasm following the rapid infusion of cefoxitin, see Cephalothin Sodium, p.177.

EFFECTS ON THE BLOOD. Reports of adverse effects on the blood associated with the administration of cefoxitin sodium: M. Shansky and C. W. Greenlaw (letter), *Ann. intern. Med.*, 1980, *92*, 874 (leucopenia); O. H. DeTorres, *Drug Intell. & clin. Pharm.*, 1983, *17*, 816 (haemolytic anaemia and pancytopenia).

EFFECTS ON THE GASTRO-INTESTINAL TRACT. Mulligan *et al.* (*Antimicrob. Ag. Chemother.*, 1984, *26*, 343) observed changes in the anaerobic, facultative, and aerobic faecal flora of 6 patients treated with cefoxitin. Five acquired *Clostridium difficile* during or after therapy, 2 of whom developed colitis requiring discontinuation of the drug. Ambrose *et al.* (*J. antimicrob. Chemother.*, 1985, *15*, 319) isolated *Cl. difficile* in the faeces of 2 of 6 healthy subjects within 7 days of being given a single intravenous dose of cefoxitin 2 g.

EFFECTS ON THE SKIN. Exfoliative dermatitis in an 84-year-old man during intramuscular therapy with cefoxitin sodium.— D. W. Kannangara *et al., Archs intern. Med.*, 1982, *142*, 1031. See also K. J. Tietze and J. A. Gaska, *Clin. Pharm.*, 1983, *2*, 582.

Precautions

As for Cephalothin Sodium, p.177.

There is some evidence of cross-allergenicity between cephamycins and other beta-lactam antibiotics. Cefoxitin should not be given to patients who are known to be allergic to cephalosporins and should be given with great care to those who are allergic to penicillin or have known histories of allergy.

Report of an increased incidence of *Pseudomonas aeruginosa* infections in an intensive care unit in association with increased use of cefoxitin. *Ps. aeruginosa* is naturally resistant to cefoxitin.— J. M. Martinez-Forde *et al.* (letter), *Lancet*, 1982, *2*, 719.

INTERACTIONS. The serum half-life of cefoxitin is not affected to a measurable extent by concomitant administration with moderate doses of frusemide by mouth.— B. Trollfors and R. Norrby (letter), *J. antimicrob. Chemother.*, 1980, *6*, 405.

INTERFERENCE WITH DIAGNOSTIC TESTS. Urine- and serum-creatinine concentrations measured by the Jaffé method were falsely elevated after the administration of cefoxitin sodium to healthy subjects. Serum-creatinine estimations should be delayed until at least 2 and preferably 4 hours after cefoxitin administration. Even then, estimations of creatinine clearance should not be relied on clinically.— S. R. Durham *et al., J. clin. Path.*, 1979, *32*, 1148. The extent of interference of cefoxitin sodium with measurements of serum-creatinine varied widely according to the version of the Jaffé method used. In patients with mild to moderate renal failure, measurement should be delayed until 6 to 8 hours after a dose of cefoxitin sodium; in patients with severe renal failure the assay is unreliable.— A. J. Saah *et al., J. Am. med. Ass.*, 1982, *247*, 205. See also D. R. P. Guay *et al., Am. J. Hosp. Pharm.*, 1983, *40*, 435.

Cefoxitin may interfere with the measurement of urinary 17-hydroxycorticosteroids using the Porter-Silber reaction.— F. H. Faas *et al.* (letter), *Clin. Chem.*, 1983, *29*, 1311.

Antimicrobial Action

Cefoxitin is a cephamycin antibiotic, which like the other beta-lactam antibiotics, is bactericidal and is considered to act through the inhibition of bacterial cell wall synthesis.

Cefoxitin has a similar spectrum of activity to cephamandole (see p.180) but is resistant to a wider range of beta-lactamases. It is generally more active than cephamandole against *Serratia marcescens*, but less active against some Gram-positive bacteria and against *Enterobacter* spp. Unlike cephamandole, many strains of *Bacteroides fragilis* are susceptible to cefoxitin.

Cefoxitin can induce the production of beta-lactamases by some bacteria, and therefore combinations of cefoxitin with other beta-lactam antibiotics have been shown to be antagonistic *in vitro*.

Reports indicating cefoxitin to be active against various organisms: C. A. M. McNulty *et al., Antimicrob. Ag. Chemother.*, 1985, *28*, 837 (*Campylobacter pyloridis*); E. J. C. Goldstein *et al., ibid.*, 1980, *18*, 832 (*Eikenella corrodens*); M. J. Sanson-Le Pors *et al., J. antimicrob. Chemother.*, 1983, *11*, 271 (*Haemophilus ducreyi*); A. W. Pasculle *et al., Antimicrob. Ag. Chemother.*, 1981, *20*, 793 (*Legionella* spp.); M. Casal and F. Rodriguez, *Tubercle*, 1982, *63*, 125. and J. M. Swenson *et al., Antimicrob. Ag. Chemother.*, 1985, *28*, 807 (*Mycobacterium fortuitum* and *M. chelonae*).

ACTIVITY AGAINST ANAEROBES. A study of the antimicrobial susceptibilities of anaerobic bacteria including *Bacteroides* spp. isolated from women with genital-tract infections. Susceptibilities were often unpredictable, particularly with latamoxef, cefoperazone, cefotaxime, and cefoxitin, although cefoxitin was most often more active than the third-generation cephalosporins tested. These agents, however, generally lacked the high degree of activity and/or breadth of spectrum associated with clindamycin, chloramphenicol, metronidazole, and imipenem.— G. B. Hill and O. M. Ayers, *Antimicrob. Ag. Chemother.*, 1985, *27*, 324.

ACTIVITY AGAINST GONOCOCCI. A study of the *in vitro* antimicrobial susceptibility of isolates of *Neisseria gonorrhoeae* obtained from patients in Bangkok. Isolates which did not produce penicillinase had significantly higher cefoxitin MICs than did the penicillinase-producing strains.— S. Brown *et al., Lancet*, 1982, *2*, 1366.

Further references to the activity of cefoxitin against *N. gonorrhoeae*: S. B. Kerbs *et al., Antimicrob. Ag. Chemother.*, 1983, *23*, 541; J. Y. Riou *et al., J. antimicrob. Chemother.*, 1985, *16, Suppl.* A, 209.

ACTIVITY WITH OTHER ANTIMICROBIAL AGENTS. A study assessing the extent and mechanisms of *in-vitro* antagonism between cefoxitin and other beta-lactam antibiotics against Gram-negative bacteria. For the penicillins, azlocillin was most frequently antagonised, followed by piperacillin, mezlocillin, and carbenicillin. Cefoxitin did not antagonise mecillinam or imipenem. For the cephalosporins tested, cefotaxime was most frequently antagonised, followed by cephamandole and latamoxef. No antagonism of cephalexin was observed. The frequency of antagonism was highest in strains possessing inducible cephalosporinases. Two mechanisms of antagonism were postulated. Firstly, cefoxitin may induce beta-lactamases capable of inactivating the second drug. Secondly, enzymes may be induced which cannot inactivate the drug but serve as a barrier against access to penicillin-binding proteins (PBPs). This mechanism is most efficient for drugs that bind to PBPs 1 and 3.— C. C. Sanders *et al., Antimicrob. Ag. Chemother.*, 1982, *21*, 968. The barrier effect of induced beta-lactamases has been questioned. After induction of large quantities of beta-lactamases even enzyme-stable drugs may be inactivated.— D. M. Livermore, *J. antimicrob. Chemother.*, 1985, *15*, 511.

For further discussion of induction of beta-lactamases by cefoxitin and their effect on the activity of other beta-lactam agents, see under Antimicrobial Action and Resistance in Imipenem, p.248.

Resistance

As for Cephalothin Sodium, p.178.

Cefoxitin has good stability to beta-lactamases produced by many bacteria including *Bacteroides fragilis*.

RESISTANCE OF BACTEROIDES FRAGILIS. Report of a study carried out in 8 centres in the *USA* of the susceptibility of clinical isolates of the *Bacteroides fragilis* group to 12 antibiotics. Taking a breakpoint for resistance of 16 µg per mL, the incidence of strains resistant to cefoxitin increased over the 3 years from 1981 to 1983, with rates of 8, 10, and 16%, respectively. Taking a breakpoint of 32 µg per mL, however, the resistance rate showed little change, being 2, 3, and 3% in the 3 years respectively. There were wide variations, however, in the resistance rates between laboratories which may be due to the different test methods used.— F. P. Tally *et al., Antimicrob. Ag. Chemother.*, 1985, *28*, 675. In the 2-year report of this study, cefoxitin resistance was associated with a high incidence of cross-resistance to other beta-lactam antibiotics.— G. J. Cuchural *et al.*, *ibid.*, 1984, *26*, 145.

The mechanism of resistance to cefoxitin reported in *Bacteroides fragilis* is unclear. Possible mechanisms that have been suggested include hydrolysis of cefoxitin by beta-lactamases (G.J. Cuchural *et al.*, *Antimicrob. Ag. Chemother.*, 1983, *24*, 936) or alterations in penicillin-binding proteins or in outer membrane porin proteins (L.J.V. Piddock and R. Wise, *J. antimicrob. Chemother.*, 1987, *19*, 161). Cuchural *et al.* (*Antimicrob. Ag. Chemother.*, 1986, *29*, 918) demonstrated that beta-lactamase-mediated cefoxitin resistance in *B. fragilis* is transferable by conjugation.

Absorption and Fate

Cefoxitin is not absorbed from the gastro-intestinal tract; it is given parenterally as the sodium salt. After 1 g by intramuscular injection a peak plasma concentration of up to 30 µg per mL at 20 to 30 minutes has been reported whereas concentrations of 125, 72, and 25 µg per mL have been achieved after the intravenous injection of 1 g over 3, 30, and 120 minutes respectively. Cefoxitin is about 70% bound to plasma proteins. It has a half-life of 45 to 60 minutes which is prolonged in renal impairment. Cefoxitin is widely distributed in the body but there is normally little penetration into the cerebrospinal fluid. It diffuses across the placenta and has been detected in the milk of nursing mothers.

The majority of a dose is excreted unchanged by the kidneys, about 2% being metabolised to descarbamylcefoxitin which is virtually inactive. Cefoxitin is excreted in the urine by glomerular filtration and tubular secretion and about 85% of a dose is recovered within 6 hours; probenecid slows this excretion. After an intramuscular dose of 1 g, peak concentrations in the urine are usually greater than 3 mg per mL. Small amounts of cefoxitin appear in bile.

For reviews of the absorption and fate of cefoxitin, see J. J. Schrogie *et al.*, *J. antimicrob. Chemother.*, 1978, *4, Suppl.* B, 69; R. N. Brogden *et al.*, *Drugs*, 1979, *17*, 1.

Use of lignocaine hydrochloride 0.5 or 1% solution as a solvent for cefoxitin sodium reduced the pain of intramuscular injection without apparently affecting the pharmacokinetics of cefoxitin.— P. F. Sonneville *et al.*, *Eur. J. clin. Pharmac.*, 1977, *12*, 273.

Further references to the pharmacokinetics of cefoxitin: N. Buchanan *et al.* (letter), *Br. J. clin. Pharmac.*, 1980, *9*, 623 (children with kwashiorkor); W. E. Feldman *et al.*, *Antimicrob. Ag. Chemother.*, 1980, *17*, 669 (children).

ADMINISTRATION IN RENAL FAILURE. The pharmacokinetics of cefoxitin during haemofiltration in patients with terminal renal impairment. The mean half-life fell from 11.9 hours in 7 patients in the interfiltration period to 3.4 hours in 7 patients during a session. For patients undergoing haemofiltration every 48 hours, a dose of 15 to 30 mg per kg body-weight at the start and end of each session was recommended.— M. J. Garcia *et al.*, *Eur. J. clin. Pharmac.*, 1983, *25*, 395.

The pharmacokinetics of intraperitoneal cefoxitin in 9 patients on continuous ambulatory peritoneal dialysis (CAPD). Non-renal clearance appeared to be the major route of elimination in such patients. The clearance of cefoxitin by CAPD from plasma was low at a mean of 4.1 mL per minute. An intraperitoneal dose of 100 mg per litre of dialysate was recommended for patients with peritonitis. For those with accompanying systemic infection the drug should also be administered intravenously.— A. Arvidsson *et al.*, *Eur. J. clin. Pharmac.*, 1985, *28*, 333. See also W. L. Greaves *et al.*, *Antimicrob. Ag. Chemother.*, 1981, *19*, 253.

References to the pharmacokinetics of cefoxitin in patients with renal impairment: J. P. Fillastre *et al.*, *J. antimicrob. Chemother.*, 1978, *4, Suppl.* B, 79; M. J. Garcia *et al.*, *Eur. J. clin. Pharmac.*, 1979, *16*, 119; D. Kampf *et al.*, *Antimicrob. Ag. Chemother.*, 1981, *20*, 741.

See also under Administration in Renal Failure in Uses, below.

DIFFUSION INTO BODY TISSUES AND FLUIDS. Concentrations of cefoxitin in the cerebrospinal fluid (CSF) were measured in 23 infants and children with bacterial meningitis after 3 consecutive doses of intravenous cefoxitin 75 mg per kg body-weight every 6 hours were given, beginning on days 4 and 9 of treatment. Concentrations of 2.5 µg per mL or higher, considered able to kill 90% of isolated causative organisms *in vitro*, were achieved in only 11 patients, and therefore the dosage was considered to be inadequate. No significant difference was observed in penetration of cefoxitin into the CSF on the 2 days.— W. E. Feldman *et al.*, *Antimicrob. Ag. Chemother.*, 1982, *21*, 468. Further studies on cefoxitin concentrations in the cerebrospinal fluid of patients with meningitis.— P. A. A. Galvao *et al.*, *Antimicrob. Ag. Chemother.*, 1980, *17*, 526; G. Humbert *et al.*, *ibid.*, 675.

Further references to the diffusion of cefoxitin: R. E. Bawdon *et al.*, *Antimicrob. Ag. Chemother.*, 1982, *22*, 999 (pelvic tissues); E. J. Perea *et al.*, *ibid.*, 1983, *23*, 323 (lung tissue); G. Tyden and A. S. Malmborg (letter), *Lancet*, 1985, *1*, 1046 (pancreatic juice).

DRUG EXCRETION. An intravenous infusion of cefoxitin 2 g was administered over 30 minutes prior to cholecystectomy in 17 patients. Bile-cefoxitin concentrations were greater than 16 µg per mL in 10 of 11 patients in whom bile was sampled within 3 hours of drug administration and who did not have biliary obstruction. Cefoxitin could be detected in the bile of 3 patients with obstruction of the bile duct or cystic duct.— J. F. Hansbrough and J. E. Clark, *Antimicrob. Ag. Chemother.*, 1982, *22*, 709.

PREGNANCY AND THE NEONATE. In studies involving 51 women given a single intramuscular dose of cefoxitin 1 g, the drug was detectable in the foetal serum and amniotic fluid of pregnant women, but not in the breast milk of nursing mothers.— M. Dubois *et al.*, *J. clin. Pharmac.*, 1981, *21*, 477. After an intramuscular dose of cefoxitin 2 g to 5 women, cefoxitin could be detected in breast milk in concentrations of up to 0.65 µg per mL. A. Dresse *et al.*, *ibid.*, 1983, *23*, 438.

Cefoxitin was administered to 15 neonates under 2 months of age, as an intravenous injection over 15 minutes every 8 hours in a total daily dose of 90 mg per kg body-weight. The mean half-life was 1.4 hours and was inversely related to postnatal age.— M. B. Regazzi *et al.*, *Eur. J. clin. Pharmac.*, 1983, *25*, 507.

Uses and Administration

Cefoxitin is a cephamycin antibiotic which differs structurally from the cephalosporins by the addition of a 7-α-methoxy group to the 7-β-aminocephalosporanic acid nucleus. It is given as the sodium salt for the treatment of susceptible infections similarly to cephamandole (see p.181). Because of its activity against *Bacteroides fragilis* and other anaerobic organisms it may also be used in the treatment of intra-abdominal infections, pelvic inflammatory disease, and infections of the female genital tract, or of infections of mixed aerobic and anaerobic origin.

Cefoxitin sodium is administered by deep intramuscular injection, by slow intravenous injection over 3 to 5 minutes, or by intermittent or continuous intravenous infusion. Intramuscular injections are painful but may be prepared using a 0.5 or 1% solution of lignocaine hydrochloride.

Doses are expressed in terms of the equivalent amount of cefoxitin. The usual dose is 1 or 2 g every 8 hours although it may be given more frequently (every 4 or 6 hours). In severe infections up to 12 g daily has been recommended. Children and neonates may be given 20 to 40 mg per kg body-weight every 12 hours for neonates up to 1 week old, every 8 hours for those aged 1 to 4 weeks, and every 6 to 8 hours for infants and children; in severe infections, up to 200 mg per kg daily may be given.

In renal insufficiency, dosage should be reduced according to the creatinine-clearance rate, after an initial loading dose of 1 to 2 g. Suggested maintenance doses are: 1 to 2 g every 8 to 12 hours with a clearance of 30 to 50 mL per minute, 1 to 2 g every 12 to 24 hours with a clearance of 10 to 29 mL per minute, 0.5 to 1 g every 12 to 24 hours with a clearance of 5 to 9 mL per minute, and 0.5 to 1 g every 24 to 48 hours when the clearance is below 5 mL per minute.

Cefoxitin sodium has been administered intramuscularly in a dose equivalent to cefoxitin 1 g twice daily for the treatment of urinary-tract infections, and as a single dose of 2 g, in association with probenecid 1 g by mouth, for the treatment of penicillin-resistant gonorrhoea.

Cefoxitin is used for surgical infection prophylaxis particularly for procedures which may be contaminated with anaerobic organisms. The usual dose, given by the intramuscular or intravenous route, is cefoxitin 2 g prior to the procedure and then every 6 hours, not usually for more than 24 hours. Infants and children are given doses of 30 to 40 mg per kg body-weight, at the same time intervals as adults; neonates are also given 30 to 40 mg per kg, but at intervals of 8 to 12 hours.

A review of the actions and uses of cefoxitin sodium. Cefoxitin can be used as a single agent in the treatment of most mixed aerobic/anaerobic skin and soft-tissue infections, pelvic infections, and community-acquired intra-abdominal sepsis. For nosocomial intra-abdominal sepsis, an aminoglycoside should be added to the regimen to expand the coverage for aerobic Gram-negative bacilli. Cefoxitin should not be used to treat bacterial meningitis or infections caused by enterococci or methicillin-resistant *Staphylococcus aureus*.— C. V. Sanders *et al.*, *Ann. intern. Med.*, 1985, *103*, 70.

Guidelines on the choice of drugs for treating anaerobic infections. Useful drugs include benzylpenicillin, metronidazole, clindamycin, chloramphenicol, and cefoxitin, but the best antimicrobial regimen varies according to the site of infection. Intra-abdominal infections and infections of the female genital tract are often of mixed bacterial origin; an aminoglycoside may be required in addition to the anti-anaerobic agent to cover coliforms, and a penicillin may be required to cover enterococci.— *Med. Lett.*, 1984, *26*, 87. See also J. G. Bartlett, *Lancet*, 1982, *2*, 478.

For reference to the use of cefoxitin in the treatment of atypical mycobacterial infections, see Amikacin Sulphate, p.111.

Beneficial effect of cefoxitin in the treatment of empyema due to *Legionella bozemanii* in a patient with an underlying lymphoma.— L. R. Brettman *et al.* (letter), *Ann. intern. Med.*, 1986, *105*, 146.

ADMINISTRATION IN RENAL FAILURE. The normal half-life for cefoxitin of 0.7 hour was increased to 13 to 22 hours in patients with end-stage renal failure. The normal dose interval of 8 hours should be increased to 8 to 12 hours in patients with a glomerular filtration-rate (GFR) of 10 to 50 mL per minute and to 24 to 48 hours in those with a GFR of less than 10 mL per minute. A dose supplement should be given to patients undergoing haemodialysis.— W. M. Bennett *et al.*, *Am. J. Kidney Dis.*, 1983, *3*, 155.

See also under Absorption and Fate, above, and Peritonitis, below.

ARTHRITIS, BACTERIAL. For reference to the use of cefoxitin in the treatment of bacterial arthritis, see Osteomyelitis, below.

BILIARY-TRACT INFECTIONS. Intravenous cefoxitin 1 g every 4 to 6 hours could be used in the treatment of biliary-tract infections such as acute cholecystitis and acute or recurrent cholangitis.— R. Munro and T. C. Sorrell, *Drugs*, 1986, *31*, 449.

ENDOCARDITIS. Intravenous cefoxitin 8 g daily in four divided doses was successful in 11 of 14 patients with endocarditis due mainly to *Staphylococcus* and *Streptococcus* spp. Treatment failed in the one patient whose endocarditis was due to a mixture of *Staph. aureus* and anaerobes.— D. Webb and H. Thadepalli, *Curr. ther. Res.*, 1983, *34*, 311.

GONORRHOEA. For the use of cefoxitin in the treatment of gonorrhoea, see under Ceftriaxone Sodium, p.170.

MOUTH INFECTIONS. For the use of cefoxitin sodium in the treatment of infections of the mouth, see under Benzylpenicillin Sodium, p.137.

OSTEOMYELITIS. Cefoxitin could be used in a dose of 2 g administered intravenously every 8 hours for the treatment of osteomyelitis or bacterial arthritis caused by anaerobes.— A. S. Dickie, *Drugs*, 1986, *32*, 458.

PELVIC INFLAMMATORY DISEASE. For the treatment of pelvic inflammatory disease in out-patients a single intramuscular dose of cefoxitin 2 g or ceftriaxone 250 mg, followed by doxycycline 100 mg twice daily by mouth for 10 days is recommended; cefoxitin is given with probenecid 1 g by mouth. For hospitalised patients, the recommended regimen is intravenous treatment with cefoxitin 2 g four times daily in association with doxycycline 100 mg twice daily until improvement occurs followed by oral doxycycline 100 mg twice daily to complete a total of 10 days of treatment. Alternative therapy for hospitalised patients is intravenous treatment with clindamycin 600 mg four times daily in association with gentamicin in an initial dose of 2 mg per kg body-weight followed by 1.5 mg per kg three times daily. Once improvement occurs, clindamycin 450 mg four times daily by mouth is given to complete 10 to 14 days of treatment.— *Med. Lett.*, 1988, *30*, 5.

PERITONITIS. Cefoxitin has been administered to patients with peritonitis undergoing continuous ambulatory dialysis intraperitoneally, in a dose of 100 mg added to each litre of dialysis fluid, or intravenously in a dose of 1 g every 12 to 24 hours.— D. K. Scott and D. E. Roberts, *Pharm. J.*, 1985, *1*, 621.

See also under Administration in Renal Failure, above.

RESPIRATORY-TRACT INFECTIONS. Cefoxitin may be a more appropriate choice than penicillin for the treatment of aspiration pneumonia since penicillin may be inadequate cover for many mixed aerobic/anaerobic infections. In the initial treatment of aspiration pneumonia, parenteral cefoxitin should be given in association with an aminoglycoside because of the possibility of infection with *Pseudomonas aeruginosa* or *Enterobacter* spp.— R. V. McCloskey, *Curr. ther. Res.*, 1983, *33*, 740.

Cefoxitin was effective treatment, as assessed by resolution of systemic and local signs of infection, in 32 of 36 patients with community-acquired pneumonia. The causative organism in over half the patients was *Haemophilus influenzae*.— C. Salzman *et al.*, *Curr. ther. Res.*, 1987, *41*, 785.

SURGICAL INFECTION PROPHYLAXIS. Cefoxitin sodium has been recommended in preference to first-generation cephalosporins such as cephazolin, for surgical infection prophylaxis in colorectal surgery and appendectomy because of its greater activity against bowel anaerobes including *Bacteroides fragilis* (*Med. Lett.*, 1987, *29*, 91). However, it is usually reserved for situations in which the use of oral antibiotics (neomycin and erythromycin) is impossible, such as bowel obstructions or emergencies, or is inadequate, as in delayed closure (A.B. Kaiser, *New Engl. J. Med.*, 1986, *315*, 1129). For other abdominal and pelvic operations, including many gynaecological and obstetric procedures, and for other clean and clean-contaminated surgical procedures, cephazolin appears to be as effective as cefoxitin.

Specific procedures for which cefoxitin has been recommended (A.B. Kaiser, 1986) include: caesarean section when irrigating antibiotics are used (cefoxitin 2 g in 1 litre of sodium chloride 0.9% has been shown to be effective), amputation of a lower limb, in colonic surgery when neomycin and erythromycin cannot be used, appendectomy, and surgery for penetrating abdominal trauma. In the management of emergency abdominal surgery when perforation of a hollow viscus is suspected, cefoxitin with or without an aminoglycoside may be used although it has been suggested that antibiotic combinations involving metronidazole may be preferable to cefoxitin sodium alone.

See also under Prophylactic Use of Antibiotics, p.103.

Preparations

Cefoxitin Sodium Injection *(U.S.P.)*

Sterile Cefoxitin Sodium *(U.S.P.)*

Proprietary Preparations

Mefoxin *(Merck Sharp & Dohme, UK). Injection,* powder for reconstitution, cefoxitin 1 or 2 g (as sodium salt).

Proprietary Names and Manufacturers

Betacef *(FIRMA, Ital.)*; Cefociclin *(Panthox & Burck, Ital.)*; Cefoxinol *(Magis, Ital.)*; Farmoxin *(Carlo Erba, Ital.)*; Mefoxin *(Merck Sharp & Dohme, Austral.; Frosst, Canad.; Merck Sharp & Dohme-Chibret, Fr.; Merck Sharp & Dohme, Ital.; Lux.; Neth.; NZ; Merck Sharp & Dohme, S.Afr.; Merck Sharp & Dohme, UK; Merck Sharp & Dohme, USA)*; Mefoxitin *(Merck Sharp & Dohme, Denm.; Merck Sharp & Dohme, Ger.; Merck Sharp & Dohme, Norw.; Merck Sharp & Dohme, Spain; MSD, Swed.; Chibret, Switz.)*; Siglen *(Neopharmed, Ital.)*; Stovaren *(Lifepharma, Ital.)*; Tifox *(Aandersen, Ital.)*.

16567-h

Cefpimizole Sodium *(USAN, rINNM).*

AC-1370 *(cefpimizole)*; U-63196 *(cefpimizole)*; U-63196E. The sodium salt of (1-4-carboxy-7-[(*R*)-2-(5-carboxyimidazol-4-ylcarboxamido)-2-phenylacetamido]-3-cephem-3-ylmethyl}-4-pyridinio)ethylsulphate.

$C_{28}H_{25}N_6NaO_{10}S_2$=692.7.

CAS — 84880-03-5 (cefpimizole); 85287-61-2 (sodium salt).

1.03 g of monograph substance is approximately equivalent to 1 g of cefpimizole. Each g of monograph substance represents about 1.4 mmol of sodium.

Cefpimizole sodium is a cephalosporin antibiotic which is administered by the parenteral route.

ANTIMICROBIAL ACTION. Studies *in vitro* have generally shown cefpimizole to have a similar spectrum of activity to other third-generation cephalosporins but to be less active against staphylococci, Enterobacteriaceae, *Haemophilus influenzae*, and *Neisseria gonorrhoeae* (H.C. Neu and P. Labthavikul, *Antimicrob. Ag. Chemother.*, 1983, *24*, 375; R.N. Jones *et al.*, *ibid.*, 1985, *27*, 982; J.L. LeFrock *et al.*, *ibid.*, *28*, 133). Although it has some activity against *Pseudomonas aeruginosa*, it is less than that of cefsulodin and ceftazidime (B. Gordts *et al.*, *J. antimicrob. Chemother.*, 1984, *14*, 25). Synergy against *Ps. aeruginosa* has been demonstrated between cefpimizole and tobramycin (G.M. Eliopoulos *et al.*, *Antimicrob. Ag. Chemother.*, 1984, *25*, 401); it has also been shown between cefpimizole and clindamycin against a few strains of *Klebsiella pneumoniae* and *Escherichia coli*, although antagonism occurred against all enterococci and methicillin-resistant *Staphylococcus aureus* strains tested and some Gram-negative bacteria (W.D. Welch *et al.*, *J. antimicrob. Chemother.*, 1984, *14*, 553).

Studies *in vitro* with human neutrophils demonstrating augmentation of phagocytosis by cefpimizole.— H. Ohnishi *et al.*, *Antimicrob. Ag. Chemother.*, 1983, *23*, 874.

ABSORPTION AND FATE. A study of the pharmacokinetics of cefpimizole sodium. Six healthy subjects all received single intravenous infusions equivalent to cefpimizole 1, 2, and 4 g on separate occasions. The mean half-life was 1.9 hours, and 75% of a dose was excreted in the urine within 6 hours.— D. B. Lakings *et al.*, *Antimicrob. Ag. Chemother.*, 1984, *26*, 802. After intramuscular injection of 0.5 and 1 g to 12 and 6 healthy subjects respectively, mean peak plasma concentrations of 15.5 and 38.6 μg per mL were obtained after approximately 1 hour.— D. B. Lakings *et al.*, *ibid.*, 1986, *29*, 271.

Further references to the absorption and fate of cefpimizole sodium: E. Novak *et al.*, *Antimicrob. Ag. Chemother.*, 1987, *31*, 1706 (pharmacokinetics after intramuscular administration).

USES AND ADMINISTRATION. *Gonorrhoea.* A study indicating that an intramuscular dose of cefpimizole sodium equivalent to cefpimizole 1 g, administered as two injections at separate sites, would be necessary for acceptable efficacy in gonococcal urethritis. However, because of a relatively high incidence of mild leucopenia, mild elevation in hepatic enzymes, and pain on injection cefpimizole appears to offer no advantage over currently available antibiotics for the treatment of uncomplicated gonorrhoea.— E. T. Sandberg *et al.*, *Antimicrob. Ag. Chemother.*, 1986, *29*, 849.

Proprietary Names and Manufacturers

Ajicef *(Ajinomoto, Jpn)*; Renilan *(Mochida, Jpn)*.
Manufacturers also include—*Upjohn, USA.*

16569-b

Cefpiramide Sodium *(USAN, rINNM).*

SM-1652; WY-44635 *(cefpiramide)*. Sodium 7-[(*R*)-2-(4-hydroxy-6-methylnicotinamido)-2-(4-hydroxyphenyl)acetamido]-3-(1-methyl-1*H*-tetrazol-5-ylthiomethyl)-3-cephem-4-carboxylate.

$C_{25}H_{23}N_8NaO_7S_2$=634.6.

CAS — 70797-11-4 (cefpiramide); 74849-93-7 (sodium salt).

1.04 g of monograph substance is approximately equivalent to 1 g of cefpiramide. Each g of monograph substance represents about 1.6 mmol of sodium.

Cefpiramide is a cephalosporin antibiotic which is structurally related to cefoperazone, p.148.

ADVERSE EFFECTS. Two children were given cefpiramide 20 mg per kg body-weight three times daily as an intravenous injection over 5 minutes for 5 or 7 days. Both experienced diarrhoea during and after therapy, and all micro-organisms except yeasts were absent from faecal specimens during treatment. This was attributed to the high biliary excretion of cefpiramide.— K. Fujita *et al.* (letter), *Lancet*, 1983, *1*, 423.

ANTIMICROBIAL ACTION. Studies *in vitro* have generally indicated that cefpiramide has a similar range of antimicrobial action to other third-generation cephalosporins such as cefotaxime. Against Gram-positive bacteria it has a similar potency; against Enterobacteriaceae, however, it is less active and some resistant strains have been observed (M. Kato *et al.*, *Antimicrob. Ag. Chemother.*, 1982, *22*, 721; H. Wexler *et al.*, *ibid.*, 1984, *25*, 162; M.A. Pfaller *et al.*, *ibid.*, 368; A.L. Barry *et al.*, *J. antimicrob. Chemother.*, 1985, *16*, 315). Its activity against *Pseudomonas aeruginosa* has been reported to be comparable to that of cefsulodin (M. Fukasawa *et al.*, *Antimicrob. Ag. Chemother.*, 1983, *23*, 195). Although Khan *et al.* (*ibid.*, 1984, *26*, 585) failed to confirm the good antipseudomonal activity of cefpiramide, they used isolates with moderate resistance to gentamicin and tobramycin.

A synergistic interaction between cefpiramide and gentamicin has been reported against half or more of strains of *Ps. aeruginosa*, *Enterobacter cloacae*, or *Klebsiella pneumoniae*. Cefoxitin, however, antagonised the activity of cefpiramide against all strains of *E. cloacae* and the majority of *Ps. aeruginosa* (J.D. Allan *et al.*, *ibid.*, 1985, *27*, 782). Hooton *et al.*, (*ibid.*, 1984, *26*, 535) observed synergy between cefpiramide and a range of aminoglycosides against only a small proportion of Gram-negative bacteria tested.

ABSORPTION AND FATE. The pharmacokinetics of cefpiramide after single or multiple intravenous doses. The overall mean half-life in 15 subjects who received a single dose of 0.5 or 1 g was 4.44 hours.— K. Nakagawa *et al.*, *Antimicrob. Ag. Chemother.*, 1984, *25*, 221.

Renal impairment had little effect on the total clearance of cefpiramide from the plasma, thus no change in dosage would be required for patients with renal insufficiency providing hepatic function is normal. Cefpiramide is highly bound to plasma proteins, although the degree of binding is decreased in patients on haemodialysis.— J. E. Conte, *Antimicrob. Ag. Chemother.*, 1987, *31*, 1585.

See also Adverse Effects, above.

Proprietary Names and Manufacturers

Sepatren *(Sumitomo, Jpn)*; Suncefal *(Yamanouchi, Jpn)*.

Manufacturers also include—*Wyeth, USA.*

18924-d

Cefpirome *(rINN).*

HR-810. (*Z*)-7-[2-(2-Aminothiazol-4-yl)-2-methoxyiminoacetamido]-3-(1-pyrindiniomethyl)-3-cephem-4-carboxylate.

$C_{22}H_{22}N_6O_5S_2$=514.6.

CAS — 84957-29-9.

Cefpirome is a cephalosporin antibiotic.

References to the antibacterial activity *in vitro* of cefpirome: R. N. Jones *et al.*, *Antimicrob. Ag. Chemother.*, 1984, *25*, 710. and *ibid.*, *26*, 949 (correction); M. A. Bertram *et al.*, *ibid.*, 277; H. Goossens *et al.*, *ibid.*, 1985, *27*, 388; R. N. Jones and E. H. Gerlach, *ibid.*, 413; P. Van der Auwera and B. Scorneaux, *ibid.*, *28*, 37; E. J. C. Goldstein and D. M. Citron, *ibid.*, 160; A. M. Clarke *et al.*, *J. antimicrob. Chemother.*, 1985, *15*, 305; R. Wise *et al.*, *ibid.*, 449; P. H. Chandrasekar *et al.*, *ibid.*, *16*, 179; K. V. I. Rolston *et al.*, *ibid.*, 1986, *17*, 453; P. C. Appelbaum *et al.*, *ibid.*, *18*, 675; K. E. Aldridge and C. V. Sanders, *Curr. ther. Res.*, 1986, *40*, 1069; A. Pascual *et al.* (letter), *J. antimicrob. Chemother.*, 1987, *19*, 701.

Proprietary Names and Manufacturers

Hoechst, Ger.

12543-p

Cefroxadine *(USAN, rINN).*

CGP-9000. (7*R*)-[D-2-Amino-2-(cyclohexa-1,4-dienyl)acetamido]-3-methoxy-3-cephem-4-carboxylic acid.

$C_{16}H_{19}N_3O_5S$=365.4.

CAS — 51762-05-1.

Cefroxadine is a cephalosporin antibiotic which is administered by mouth.

Cefroxadine had similar activity *in vitro* to cephalexin against Gram-positive organisms; cefroxadine was more active against cephalexin-susceptible Gram-negative organisms.— K. Yasuda *et al.*, *Antimicrob. Ag. Chemother.*, 1980, *18*, 105.

Studies indicating similar pharmacokinetics of cefroxadine and cephalexin after oral administration.— J. Lecaillon *et al.*, *Antimicrob. Ag. Chemother.*, 1980, *18*, 656. See also H. Lode *et al.*, *ibid.*, 1979, *16*, 1; A. Gerardin *et al.*, *J. Pharmacokinet. Biopharm.*, 1982, *10*, 15.

The half-life of cefroxadine of 0.8 to 1 hours was increased to 40 hours in end-stage renal disease. In patients with a glomerular filtration-rate (GFR) of over 50 mL per minute 65 to 100% of the normal dose could be given. In those with a GFR of 10 to 50 mL per minute, the dose should be reduced to 15 to 65%, and in those with a GFR of less than 10 mL per minute it should be reduced to 10 to 15%.— W. M. Bennett *et al.*, *Am. J. Kidney Dis.*, 1983, *3*, 155. In 17 patients with terminal renal impairment undergoing haemodialysis, the mean half-life of cefroxadine was 23.55 hours between dialysis sessions, and 3.40 hours during dialysis.— M. J. Nieto *et al.*, *Eur. J. clin. Pharmac.*, 1983, *24*, 109.

In a study of 44 patients with urinary-tract infections, treatment by mouth for 10 days with cefroxadine 250 mg four times daily was as effective as that with cephalexin 500 mg four times daily as assessed both clinically and bacteriologically. Several reinfections were noted, however, at follow-up in both treatment groups.— J. Hess *et al.*, *Infection*, 1984, *12*, 270. See also T. Ahrens and K. G. Naber, *ibid.*, 1983, *11*, 25.

Proprietary Names and Manufacturers

Oraspor *(Ciba, Ital.)*.

12544-s

Cefsulodin Sodium *(BANM, USAN, rINNM).*

Abbott-46811; CGP-7174E; SCE-129; Sulcephalosporin Sodium. The monosodium salt of 3-(4-carbamoylpyridiniomethyl)-7-[(2*R*)-2-phenyl-2-sulphoacetamido]-3-cephem-4-carboxylate.
$C_{22}H_{19}N_4NaO_8S_2$=554.5.

CAS — 62587-73-9 (cefsulodin); 52152-93-9 (sodium salt).

1.04 g of monograph substance is approximately equivalent to 1 g of cefsulodin. Each g of monograph substance represents about 1.8 mmol of sodium.

Aqueous solutions of cefsulodin sodium are reported to be **stable** for 12 hours at 23° and for 24 hours at 5°. They are most stable at pH 4 to 7. Solutions with a pH above 7 should be used immediately after preparation. Solutions may become yellow on storage, but slight discoloration does not affect potency.

Adverse Effects and Precautions

As for Cephalothin Sodium, p.176.

For reference to nausea and vomiting on intravenous infusion of cefsulodin sodium, see under Respiratory-tract Infections, Cystic Fibrosis, in Uses, below.

ADMINISTRATION IN RENAL FAILURE. For reference to the precautions to be observed in renal failure, see under Administration in Renal Failure in Uses, below.

INTERACTIONS. No pharmacokinetic interaction was observed when cefotiam and cefsulodin were administered concomitantly to patients with impaired renal function.— J. B. Lecaillon *et al.*, *Antimicrob. Ag. Chemother.*, 1984, *26*, 368.

Antimicrobial Action and Resistance

Cefsulodin is a bactericidal antibiotic with activity against *Pseudomonas aeruginosa* equal to or slightly less than that of ceftazidime, and greater than that of cefoperazone. It has no significant activity against other Gram-negative organisms. It has similar activity to ceftazidime (see p.162) against Gram-positive organisms and anaerobes.

Cefsulodin is stable to hydrolysis by many beta-lactamases. Emergence of resistant *Ps. aeruginosa* has been reported during treatment with cefsulodin.

A study of the antibacterial activity of cefsulodin.— A. L. Barry *et al.*, *Antimicrob. Ag. Chemother.*, 1981, *20*, 525.

ACTIVITY AGAINST ANAEROBES. In a study *in vitro* cefsulodin had only moderate activity against 115 strains of Gram-negative anaerobic bacteria. Its activity against organisms of the *Bacteroides fragilis* group was poor, less than half of the strains being inhibited by a concentration of 128 µg per mL. Activity was slightly better against Gram-positive anaerobes. A significant inoculum effect was observed, particularly in *B. fragilis*. A synergistic interaction between cefsulodin and cefoxitin was observed in 58% of *Bacteroides* spp. and 22% of anaerobic cocci tested.— B. Watt and F. V. Brown, *J. antimicrob. Chemother.*, 1981, *7*, 269.

ACTIVITY AGAINST BRANHAMELLA. A concentration of 4 µg per mL of cefsulodin was required to inhibit 90% of 17 beta-lactamase-negative strains of *Branhamella catarrhalis*. The corresponding figure for 11 beta-lactamase-producing strains was 64 µg per mL.— E. E. Stobberingh *et al.*, *J. antimicrob. Chemother.*, 1984, *13*, 55.

ACTIVITY AGAINST PSEUDOMONAS. The *in-vitro* activity of cefsulodin was similar against 43 isolates of *Pseudomonas aeruginosa* from patients with cystic fibrosis, and against 55 strains from other chronically infected patients; concentrations of 8.2 and 10.0 µg per mL were required to inhibit 90% of strains from the 2 groups respectively. Tobramycin was the most active agent in cystic fibrosis patients, but apart from this ceftazidime and cefsulodin were the most active of several antipseudomonal agents tested, including the antipseudomonal penicillins and aztreonam.— B. Gordts *et al.*, *J. antimicrob. Chemother.*, 1984, *14*, 25. The inhibitory activity of cefsulodin against 37 isolates of *Ps. aeruginosa* responsible for causing endocarditis was similar to that of aztreonam, less than that of tobramycin and imipenem, and greater than that of ticarcillin. MIC values for cefsulodin were in the range of 4 to 32 µg per mL. Taking a breakpoint for susceptibility of 16 µg per mL, 92% of strains were inhibited, but only 19% killed by cefsulodin at this concentration. Inhibitory and bactericidal synergy was observed between cefsulodin and tobramycin in 22 and 89% of strains respectively.— F. A. Zar and R. J. Kany, *Antimicrob. Ag. Chemother.*, 1985, *27*, 1.

Most of 131 isolates of *Pseudomonas aeruginosa* had MICs of cefsulodin of 1 to 4 µg per mL, but concentrations of 8 to 64 µg per mL were required to inhibit highly carbenicillin-resistant strains. A significant inoculum effect was only observed with these latter isolates. Cefsulodin was also active against *Ps. maltophilia*.— A. King *et al.*, *Antimicrob. Ag. Chemother.*, 1980, *17*, 165. A comparison of the *in-vitro* activity of cefsulodin, cefoperazone, ceftazidime, cefotaxime, latamoxef, and ceftriaxone against *Ps. aeruginosa*. Strains which were susceptible to carbenicillin were also sensitive to the cephalosporins. Carbenicillin-resistant strains could, however, be divided into two groups. Those with moderate to high carbenicillin resistance also had decreased susceptibility to all of the cephalosporins. Five strains with extremely high resistance to carbenicillin showed enhanced resistance to only cefoperazone and cefsulodin whilst remaining sensitive to the other agents. This resistance to cefoperazone and cefsulodin appeared to be due to the presence of a constitutive beta-lactamase.— D. M. Livermore *et al.*, *J. antimicrob. Chemother.*, 1981, *8*, 323. Unlike ceftazidime the antibacterial activity of cefsulodin decreased in strains of *Ps. aeruginosa* which produced certain beta-lactamases, particularly the highly ticarcillin-resistant isolates producing a carbenicillinase.— A. Philippon *et al.*, *ibid.*, *Suppl.* B, 119. Studies supporting the view that the constitutive production of beta-lactamase is not an adequate explanation for resistance of *Ps. aeruginosa* to cefsulodin.— L. E. Bryan *et al.*, *Antimicrob. Ag. Chemother.*, 1984, *25*, 382.

A study of the *in vitro* activities of cefsulodin and gentamicin against isolates of *Pseudomonas aeruginosa* from five hospitals in Japan. In 1982 and 1983 the sensitivity to both drugs was decreased compared with that in 1980 and 1981, largely because of the isolation of numbers of cefsulodin-gentamicin cross-resistant bacteria from 3 of the 5 hospitals.— T. Furusawa *et al.*, *J. antimicrob. Chemother.*, 1986, *17*, 755.

See also under Respiratory-tract Infections, Cystic Fibrosis in Uses, below.

ACTIVITY WITH OTHER ANTIMICROBIAL AGENTS. Both synergy and antagonism were observed *in vitro* against *Pseudomonas aeruginosa* between cefsulodin and either tobramycin or amikacin. The incidence of these interactions, however, depended on whether a chequerboard method or a 6- or 24-hour time-kill study was used. The 24-hour time-kill method was the best predictor of therapeutic outcome in 14 patients. Resistant pseudomonas emerged in 4 patients.— P. H. Chandrasekar *et al.*, *J. antimicrob. Chemother.*, 1987, *19*, 321. See also above under Activity against Pseudomonas.

A combination of cefsulodin and fosfomycin was synergistic against 83% of strains of *Pseudomonas aeruginosa* tested. This was increased to 100% by addition of tobramycin.— K. Takahashi and H. Kanno, *Antimicrob. Ag. Chemother.*, 1984, *26*, 789.

Synergy *in vitro* between cefsulodin and mezlocillin was demonstrated in a small proportion of gentamicin-sensitive strains of *Pseudomonas aeruginosa*, but in none of the gentamicin-resistant strains tested. A low incidence of synergy was also shown between these antibiotics against some organisms of the Enterobacteriaceae.— J. R. Rodriguez *et al.*, *Curr. ther. Res.*, 1984, *36*, 902.

The beta-lactamase inhibitor, clavulanic acid reduced the mode MIC of cefsulodin against 20 strains of *Bacteroides fragilis* from 512 to 4 µg per mL. This effect was less marked with non-*fragilis* strains.— J. P. Maskell *et al.*, *J. antimicrob. Chemother.*, 1984, *13*, 23. A similar effect was produced by cefsulodin in association with sulbactam or cefoxitin against *Bacteroides* spp.— K. P. Fu *et al.*, *ibid.*, 257. See also above under Activity against Anaerobes.

For a report of antimicrobial interaction between cefsulodin and cefotetan, see Cefotetan Disodium, p.157.

Absorption and Fate

Cefsulodin is administered parenterally as the sodium salt. It has a half-life of approximately 1.6 hours and up to 30% of cefsulodin in the circulation is bound to plasma proteins. Therapeutic concentrations have been reported in a wide range of body tissues and fluids. The major route of excretion of cefsulodin is via the urine, mainly by glomerular filtration.

Six groups of 4 or 5 healthy subjects were given cefsulodin sodium in varying doses intramuscularly or intravenously. The mean peak plasma concentrations after intramuscular administration of the equivalent of 0.25, 0.5 or 1 g of cefsulodin were 5.6, 12.7, and 20.1 µg per mL respectively, and were obtained approximately 1.5 hours after the dose. The mean urinary excretion within 24 hours varied between 50 and 55% of the dose. After intravenous administration of 0.5, 1, or 2 g between 52 and 60% of a dose was excreted in the urine within 24 hours.— G. R. Granneman *et al.*, *Clin. Pharmac. Ther.*, 1982, *31*, 95.

Pharmacokinetics of cefsulodin sodium in 12 patients with cystic fibrosis.— M. D. Reed *et al.*, *Antimicrob. Ag. Chemother.*, 1984, *25*, 579.

Further references to the absorption and fate of cefsulodin sodium: C. D. Findlay *et al.*, *J. antimicrob. Chemother.*, 1981, *7*, 637.

ADMINISTRATION IN RENAL FAILURE. The pharmacokinetics of cefsulodin sodium in 19 patients with varying degrees of renal function. Group I (6 patients) had a creatinine clearance (CC) of greater than 100 mL per minute; group II (7 patients) had a CC of 12 to 42 mL per minute; and group III (5 patients) had a CC of less than 10 mL per minute. Mean 24-hour cumulative urinary excretion of cefsulodin was 61.5, 33.5, and 7% in the three groups respectively, and mean half-lives were 1.8, 6.4, and 10.1 hours.— G. R. Matzke and W. F. Keane, *Antimicrob. Ag. Chemother.*, 1983, *23*, 369. Similar results. In 5 patients undergoing haemodialysis, the mean half-life of cefsulodin during dialysis was 2.1 hours. Studies both on and off dialysis in 3 of these patients indicated that haemodialysis resulted in a 57% decrease in plasma-cefsulodin concentrations.— T. P. Gibson *et al.*, *Clin. Pharmac. Ther.*, 1982, *31*, 602.

See also under Administration in Renal Failure in Uses, below.

DIFFUSION INTO BODY TISSUES AND FLUIDS. For reference to the penetration of cefsulodin sodium into sputum, see under Respiratory-tract Infections, Cystic Fibrosis in Uses, below.

Uses and Administration

Cefsulodin sodium is a cephalosporin antibiotic used for the treatment of infections of the urinary and respiratory tracts, and also of the soft tissue and bone, caused by susceptible strains of *Pseudomonas aeruginosa*. It is administered by intramuscular injection, usually dissolved in 0.5% lignocaine hydrochloride solution to decrease pain, or intravenously by slow injection or by infusion. Doses are expressed in terms of the equivalent amount of cefsulodin. The usual dose for adults is 1 to 4 g daily in two to four divided doses; in severe infections daily doses of 6 g or more may be required. Children may be given doses of 20 to 50 mg per kg body-weight daily.

Patients with renal impairment should be given cefsulodin sodium in a usual loading dose; subsequent doses should be reduced or the dosage interval prolonged.

Reviews of the actions and uses of cefsulodin sodium. Apart from pseudomonal infections of the urinary and respiratory tracts, skin and bone, it has also been investigated in a few patients with septicaemia, often in association with an aminoglycoside, or in patients with meningitis.— B. R. Smith, *Clin. Pharm.*, 1984, *3*, 373; D. B. Wright, *Drug Intell. & clin. Pharm.*, 1986, *20*, 845.

Forty-eight patients with 51 *Pseudomonas aeruginosa* infections were treated with cefsulodin 0.5 to 2 g every 6 hours administered as a 30-minute intravenous infusion. Sixteen patients had osteomyelitis, some of whom received additional antibiotics due to concurrent infection with Enterobacteriaceae or Gram-positive organisms. In 10 patients *Ps. aeruginosa* was eradicated during therapy, and 12 were considered to have a satisfactory clinical response. On follow-up for up to 2 years, recurrence of *Ps. aeruginosa* infection occurred in 4 patients who had bacteriological cure or a satisfactory clinical response during treatment. Thus no conclusions could be drawn about the long-term efficacy of cefsulodin therapy in these patients. Although a satisfactory clinical response was obtained in 2 patients with infected knee prostheses, both were bacteriological failures.
Bacteriological eradication and satisfactory clinical response, however, occurred in all 23 patients with superficial infections such as wound infections and skin ulcers, although two patients developed superinfections, one each with *Enterobacter cloacae* and *Staphylococcus aureus*.
Bacteriological eradication was also obtained in 4 of 7 patients with *Ps. aeruginosa* infections of the urinary tract, and 2 of 3 with infections of the respiratory tract.
Adverse effects occurred in 3 of the 48 patients. One patient had a mild increase in liver enzyme values on the final day of cefsulodin therapy, and 2 experienced nausea and vomiting.
It was concluded that although single-agent therapy with cefsulodin appeared to be satisfactory in many of these patients with serious *Ps. aeruginosa* infections, studies are required with control groups treated with another antipseudomonal beta-lactam antibiotic, or with cefsulodin in association with an aminoglycoside.— A. Routman *et al.*, *J. int. med. Res.*, 1986, *14*, 242.

ADMINISTRATION IN RENAL FAILURE. The half-life of cefsulodin of 1.7 to 2 hours was increased to 13 hours in end-stage renal disease. In patients with a glomerular filtration-rate (GFR) of over 50 mL per minute 50 to 100% of the normal dose could be given. In those with a GFR of 10 to 50 mL per minute the dose should be reduced to 15 to 50%, and in those with a GFR of less than 10 mL per minute it should be reduced to 10 to 15%. A dose supplement should be given to patients undergoing haemodialysis.— W. M. Bennett *et al.*, *Am. J. Kidney Dis.*, 1983, *3*, 155.

For further reference to the pharmacokinetics of cefsulodin sodium in patients with renal impairment, see under Absorption and Fate, above.

BONE AND SKIN INFECTIONS. For reference to the use of cefsulodin for the treatment of infections of the skin and bones, see above.

RESPIRATORY-TRACT INFECTIONS. *Cystic fibrosis.* A satisfactory clinical response was achieved with cefsulodin in 9 of 10 patients with cystic fibrosis and acute exacerbations of lower respiratory-tract infections, with *Pseudomonas aeruginosa* isolated from their sputum. Patients received 0.5, 1, or 1.5 g of cefsulodin by intravenous infusion over 30 minutes every 6 hours for 10 to 22 days. Concentrations of cefsulodin in sputum ranged from 2 to 5 μg per mL in 19 samples from 8 patients and were less than 2 μg per mL in 18 samples from 7 patients. Typical of patients with cystic fibrosis, colonisation of lower respiratory secretions persisted after therapy. MICs for 13 isolates from 6 patients were 32 μg or more per mL after therapy and 3 patients had isolates which appeared to have developed resistance only after therapy.— I. Cabezudo *et al.*, *Antimicrob. Ag. Chemother.*, 1984, *25*, 4. A comparative study of 7 new antipseudomonal penicillins and cephalosporins in the treatment of pseudomonal lung infections in patients with cystic fibrosis. Cefsulodin may be a useful agent for infections caused by organisms resistant to traditional antipseudomonal antibiotics. Nausea and vomiting occurring in patients treated with cefsulodin appeared to be related to the rate of infusion.— G. Mastella *et al.*, *J. antimicrob. Chemother.*, 1983, *12*, *Suppl.* A, 297.

URINARY-TRACT INFECTIONS. Beneficial effect of intravenous treatment with cefmenoxime in association with cefsulodin for complicated urinary-tract infections caused by *Pseudomonas aeruginosa* alone or with other organisms.— T. Doi *et al.*, *Chemotherapy, Basle*, 1986, *32*, 299.

Proprietary Preparations

Monaspor *(Ciba, UK)*. *Injection*, powder for reconstitution, cefsulodin 0.5 and 1 g (as sodium salt).

Proprietary Names and Manufacturers

Cefomonil *(Tap, Canad.)*; Monaspor *(Ciba, Denm.*; *Ciba, Switz.*; *Ciba, UK)*; Pseudocef *(Takeda, Ger.)*; Pyocefal *(Takeda, Fr.)*; Takesulin *(Jpn)*; Tilmapor *(Jpn)*; Ulfaret *(Abello, Spain)*.

12545-w

Ceftazidime *(BAN, USAN, rINN)*.

GR-20263; LY-139381. (*Z*)-(7*R*)-7-[2-(2-Aminothiazol-4-yl)-2-(1-carboxy-1-methylethoxyimino)acetamido]-3-(1-pyridiniomethyl)-3-cephem-4-carboxylate pentahydrate. $C_{22}H_{22}N_6O_7S_2,5H_2O=636.7$.

CAS — 72558-82-8 (anhydrous); 78439-06-2 (pentahydrate).

Ceftazidime pentahydrate 1.16 g is approximately equivalent to 1 g of anhydrous ceftazidime.

INCOMPATIBILITY. It has been reported that ceftazidime does not cause decreased activity when incubated in solution with gentamicin or tobramycin at 37° (T.S.J. Elliott *et al.*, *J. antimicrob. Chemother.*, 1984, *14*, 668; *idem*, 1986, *17*, 680). However the manufacturers recommend that ceftazidime, like most other beta-lactam antibiotics, should not be mixed with an aminoglycoside in the same giving set or syringe because of potential interaction.
A report of physical incompatibility between ceftazidime and vancomycin.— C. J. Cairns and J. Robertson (letter), *Pharm. J.*, 1987, *1*, 577.

STABILITY. Ceftazidime for injection is essentially stable in the dry state and may be stored at room temperature, but should be protected from light. When reconstituted with Water for Injections loss of potency occurs slowly and it is recommended that it should be used within 6 hours if stored at room temperature or 24 hours if stored in a refrigerator. The stability of ceftazidime for injection in lignocaine hydrochloride injection 1% is of a similar order to that obtained after reconstitution with water. Storage of ceftazidime for injection in 5 commonly used intravenous fluids showed very small potency losses after 48 hours at 4°. Losses of between 5 and 7% occurred after 24 hours at 25° for solutions in sodium chloride injection 0.9%, glucose injection 5%, sodium chloride and glucose injection, and Compound Sodium Lactate Injection, but solutions in Sodium Bicarbonate Injection decomposed at a slightly faster rate. The maximum recommended storage times for solutions of ceftazidime for injection in the different intravenous fluids are 48 hours at 4° for all solutions tested and 24 hours at room temperature for all the solutions except sodium bicarbonate, which should not be stored for longer than 6 hours at room temperature.— B. L. Richardson *et al.*, *Glaxo, UK*, *J. antimicrob. Chemother.*, 1981, *8*, *Suppl.* B, 233.
Reconstituted 1-g vials of ceftazidime for injection added to 50-mL minibags of sodium chloride injection 0.9% were found to be stable for 97 days when stored at −20°. A frozen shelf-life of 42 days was suggested to allow for a refrigeration life of 4 days followed by 24 hours at room temperature.— A. F. Brown *et al.*, *Br. J. parent. Ther.*, 1985, *6*, 43.

Adverse Effects and Precautions

As for Cephalothin Sodium, p.176.

In an analysis by the manufacturers of data from clinical studies of ceftazidime involving 2607 patients, 232 (8.9%) experienced adverse events, 15% of which were considered to be unrelated to the drug and 33% were of unknown relationship; the drug was discontinued in 2.4% of patients because of side-effects. The most common adverse effects were local intolerance, hypersensitivity, and gastro-intestinal effects, which each occurred in over 2% of patients receiving the drug; other effects involved the CNS, genito-urinary, and cardiovascular systems. Reported changes in laboratory tests thought to be due to ceftazidime included positive Coombs' test (in 4.7% of patients tested), eosinophilia (3.7%), blood disorders (1.4%), thrombocytosis (0.4%), abnormal liver enzyme values (7.0%), and abnormal renal function tests (1.2%). Of 1614 patients studied with 1906 infected sites superinfections were reported in 2.5% of sites. The incidence of adverse effects was not significantly different to that experienced by 466 patients who received one or more comparative antibiotics.— R. D. Foord, *J. antimicrob. Chemother.*, 1983, *12*, *Suppl.* A, 399. A low incidence of adverse effects was reported in a study of patients in Japan who received ceftazidime mainly in doses of 1 to 2 g daily. Only 32 of 1529 (2.1%) patients experienced adverse effects and these were mainly skin rashes, diarrhoea, and nausea and vomiting; fever and dizziness were also reported, each in 2 patients. None of the abnormalities in laboratory findings were judged to be severe. They were mainly slight elevations of serum glutamic-oxaloacetic transaminase (SGOT), glutamic pyruvic transaminase (SGPT), alkaline phosphatase, and eosinophil counts, occurring with an incidence of 2.8, 3.2, 0.8, and 1.6%, respectively, in those patients examined. Leucopenia was present in only 6 of 1333 patients (0.5%).— K. Ishibiki, *ibid.*, 123.
In a study involving 30 patients with serious bacterial infections there were 19 instances of laboratory or clinical reactions attributable to ceftazidime, most of which were considered clinically insignificant. The side-effects consisted of minimal eosinophilia (6 patients), minor liver function abnormalities (4), thrombocytosis (2), leucopenia (2), abnormal creatinine (2), diarrhoea (2), and rash (1); the drug was discontinued in 4 of these patients because of leucopenia, *Clostridium difficile* toxin-induced diarrhoea, rash, or mild azotaemia.— L. J. Eron *et al.*, *Antimicrob. Ag. Chemother.*, 1983, *23*, 236.

EFFECTS ON THE GASTRO-INTESTINAL TRACT. In a study of 8 healthy subjects given ceftazidime 2 g by intravenous infusion over 20 minutes every 12 hours for 8 days, gastro-intestinal side-effects were reported in 3 subjects; 2 had loose stools or moderate self-limiting diarrhoea, and one complained of slight nausea. After 8 days of therapy the main change in the intestinal flora was a suppression in numbers of *Escherichia coli*; anaerobic bacteria were not significantly affected. Two weeks after discontinuation of ceftazidime the antibiotic's influence on the intestinal flora was still apparent and ampicillin- and cephazolin-resistant *E. coli* and other Enterobacteriaceae were isolated.— B. Kemmerich *et al.*, *Antimicrob. Ag. Chemother.*, 1983, *24*, 333.
Clostridium difficile or its exotoxin were detected in 2 of 7 patients who experienced diarrhoea with ceftazidime therapy.— K. Ishibiki, *J. antimicrob. Chemother.*, 1983, *12*, *Suppl.* A, 123. See also P. Francioli *et al.*, *ibid.*, 139.
Three of 27 patients who received ceftazidime reported a metallic taste immediately following injection.— H. Schoengut and R. Jelinek, *J. antimicrob. Chemother.*, 1983, *12*, *Suppl.* A, 219.

EFFECTS ON THE LIVER. Reversible elevation of liver enzyme values particularly serum glutamic oxaloacetic transaminase (SGOT) and serum glutamic pyruvic transaminase (SGPT) has occurred with ceftazidime therapy (G. De Sandre *et al.*, *J. antimicrob. Chemother.*, 1981, *8*, *Suppl.* B, 307; N. Clumeck *et al.*, *Antimicrob. Ag. Chemother.*, 1983, *24*, 176). The reported incidence has ranged from about 2 to 20% (G.K. Daikos *et al.*, *J. antimicrob. Chemother.*, 1981, *8*, *Suppl.* B, 331; D.I. Gozzard *et al.*, *Lancet*, 1982, *1*, 1152). Transient elevation of liver enzyme values has been reported with many beta-lactam antibiotics and is often considered to be of no clinical significance, however, some workers feel that it is indicative of minor liver damage (F. Rusconi *et al.*, *Antimicrob. Ag. Chemother.*, 1984, *25*, 395).

LOCAL IRRITANT EFFECTS. Of 50 patients who received ceftazidime 1 or 2 g three times daily intramuscularly 10 complained on questioning of pain at the injection site; the pain was severe in 2 cases and these patients refused further injections.— T. Pettersson *et al.*, *J. antimicrob. Chemother.*, 1983, *12*, *Suppl.* A, 31.
None of 50 patients with recurrent chest infections given ceftazidime arginine 1 or 2 g intramuscularly 3 times daily for 10 days had local pain necessitating lignocaine administration, compared with 5 of 49 similar patients given similar intramuscular doses of ceftazidime sodium. No difference in clinical efficacy was noted between the 2 formulations although small differences were noted in pharmacokinetic parameters. The lack of pain after intramuscular ceftazidime arginine may confer an advantage over ceftazidime sodium.— B. I. Davies *et al.*, *J. antimicrob. Chemother.*, 1987, *20*, 133.

Antimicrobial Action

Ceftazidime has a bactericidal action and broad spectrum of activity similar to cefotaxime sodium (see p.152), but increased activity against *Pseudomonas* spp. Ceftazidime is highly stable to hydrolysis by most beta-lactamases produced by Gram-negative and Gram-positive bacteria.

Ceftazidime is active *in vitro* against many Gram-negative bacteria including many *Pseudomonas* spp. and Enterobacteriaceae including *Citrobacter* and *Enterobacter* spp., *Escherichia coli*, *Klebsiella* spp., both indole-positive and indole-negative *Proteus*, *Providencia*, *Salmonella*, *Serratia*, and *Shigella* spp., and *Yersinia enterocolitica*. Other susceptible Gram-negative organisms include *Haemophilus* and *Neisseria* spp. Among Gram-positive organisms it is active against some staphylococci and streptococci, but methicillin-resistant staphylococci, enterococci, and *Listeria monocytogenes* are generally resistant. Ceftazidime is active against some anaerobes but most strains of *Bacteroides fragilis* and *Clostridium difficile* are resistant. Minimum inhibitory concentrations for susceptible organisms range from about 0.03 to 16 µg per mL.

The activity of ceftazidime against *Pseudomonas aeruginosa* and some Enterobacteriaceae may be enhanced by aminoglycosides.

For the proceedings of a symposium on ceftazidime, see *J. antimicrob. Chemother.*, 1981, *8, Suppl.* B, 1–358.

A study of the activity of ceftazidime *in vitro* compared with other beta-lactams, aminoglycosides, and chloramphenicol. From testing nearly 13 000 consecutive clinical isolates ceftazidime was found to be superior to cephamandole and comparable in spectrum and activity to gentamicin against Enterobacteriaceae. Of 8038 Enterobacteriaceae tested over 98% were inhibited by ceftazidime 8 µg or less per mL; the most resistant isolates were *Citrobacter freundii* and *Enterobacter aerogenes* which required 32 µg per mL to inhibit 90% of the organisms. More than 90% of *Pseudomonas aeruginosa* isolates were inhibited by ceftazidime at concentrations of 4 µg per mL. Staphylococci strains were less susceptible to ceftazidime than to cephamandole or gentamicin, but beta-haemolytic streptococci and pneumococci were more susceptible to ceftazidime; enterococci and *Listeria monocytogenes* isolates were resistant to ceftazidime. When compared with other cephalosporins, ceftazidime had a similar spectrum of activity to cefotaxime, cefoperazone, and latamoxef against Enterobacteriaceae, staphylococci, and streptococci. Of the cephalosporins tested only ceftazidime, cefsulodin, and cefoperazone showed significant activity against *Ps. aeruginosa*; ceftazidime generally showed the best activity against *Ps. aeruginosa* and the other pseudomonads, although *Ps. maltophilia* was fairly resistant. Ceftazidime was also active against *Neisseria gonorrhoeae*, *N. meningitidis*, and *Haemophilus influenzae*. It was considered that ceftazidime had an antimicrobial spectrum comparable to that of broad-spectrum aminoglycosides.— R. N. Jones *et al.*, *J. antimicrob. Chemother.*, 1981, *8, Suppl.* B, 187. See also H. C. Neu, *ibid.*, 131.

Further studies comparing the activity of ceftazidime with other antibiotics: G. P. Bodey *et al.*, *Antimicrob. Ag. Chemother.*, 1981, *20*, 226; W. Brumfitt and J. M. T. Hamilton-Miller, *J. antimicrob. Chemother.*, 1981, *8, Suppl.* B, 15; H. Knothe and G. A. Dette, *ibid.*, 33; A. J. Bint *et al.*, *ibid.*, 47; A. M. Clarke and S. J. V. Zemcov, *ibid.*, 57; R. Vanhoof *et al.*, *ibid.*, 63; A. M. Emmerson *et al.*, *Curr. med. Res. Opinion*, 1985, *9*, 480.

Ceftazidime was highly active against most aerobic Gram-negative bacteria and was found to be stable to hydrolysis by nearly all beta-lactamases studied including plasmid-mediated beta-lactamases produced by *Escherichia coli* and *Pseudomonas aeruginosa* and chromosomally-determined beta-lactamases produced by *Citrobacter freundii*, *Enterobacter cloacae*, *E. coli*, *Klebsiella*, *Proteus*, *Providencia*, and *Serratia* spp., *Pseudomonas aeruginosa*, and *Bacteroides fragilis*; hydrolysis was only detectable with the enzyme produced by one strain of *Ent. cloacae* and one strain of *B. fragilis*.— I. Phillips *et al.*, *J. antimicrob. Chemother.*, 1981, *8, Suppl.* B, 23. See also R. P. Mouton *et al.*, *ibid.*, 147; H. C. Neu and P. Labthavikul, *Antimicrob. Ag. Chemother.*, 1982, *21*, 11.

ACTIVITY AGAINST ANAEROBES. In a study *in vitro* of 586 clinical isolates of anaerobic bacteria, ceftazidime, at a concentration of 16 µg per mL, inhibited only 60% of the isolates compared with 79% by cefuroxime, 81% by latamoxef, and 80% by cefoxitin. Ceftazidime was relatively inactive against *Bacteroides fragilis* group, *Lactobacillus*, and *Clostridium* spp. other than *Cl. perfringens*. *Peptococcus*, *Peptostreptococcus*, *Cl. perfringens*, microaerophilic streptococci, and *Propionibacterium* were readily inhibited.— A. W. Chow and K. H. Bartlett, *J. antimicrob. Chemother.*, 1981, *8, Suppl.* B, 91.

ACTIVITY AGAINST ENTEROBACTERIACEAE. The activity *in vitro* of ceftazidime against some Enterobacteriaceae and non-fermentative Gram-negative bacilli was compared with cefotaxime, latamoxef, cefoperazone, and gentamicin. For most strains tested ceftazidime was very active and the minimum bactericidal concentrations were very similar to minimum inhibitory concentrations. Ceftadizime was more active than gentamicin against most Enterobacteriaceae tested. Ceftazidime, cefotaxime, and latamoxef showed approximately the same activity for *Escherichia coli*. Ceftazidime was particularly active against *Proteus mirabilis* and *Pr. vulgaris* with all strains inhibited by 0.125 µg per mL, and also against *Serratia marcescens* strains which were inhibited by 0.25 µg per mL. Only latamoxef showed comparable activity against *Pr. vulgaris*, but on average ceftazidime was 10 times more active than latamoxef against *Serratia*.— H. H. Schassan and J. Fedder, *J. antimicrob. Chemother.*, 1981, *8, Suppl.* B, 79.

Salmonellae. Ceftazidime showed excellent activity *in vitro* against multiresistant strains of *Salmonella newport* and *S. typhi* isolated in Peru; minimum inhibitory concentrations ranged from less than 0.097 to 1.56 µg per mL.— H. Goossens *et al.* (letter), *Lancet*, 1982, *2*, 769. See also H. Goossens *et al.*, *J. antimicrob. Chemother.*, 1984, *13*, 559.

ACTIVITY AGAINST HAEMOPHILUS. Ceftazidime was highly active against 169 blood and cerebrospinal fluid isolates of *Haemophilus influenzae*, inhibiting both beta-lactamase-positive and -negative strains with concentrations ranging from 0.0156 to 0.25 µg per mL.— R. M. Bannatyne *et al.*, *J. antimicrob. Chemother.*, 1985, *15*, 187.

ACTIVITY AGAINST PSEUDOMONAS. Ceftazidime has been shown to have good activity *in vitro* against carbenicillin-susceptible and carbenicillin-resistant strains of *Pseudomonas aeruginosa* (N. Kelly *et al.*, *J. antimicrob. Chemother.*, 1981, *8, Suppl.* B, 175; D. Greenwood and A. Eley, *Antimicrob. Ag. Chemother.*, 1982, *21*, 204; M.O.S. Ferreira *et al.*, *J. int. med. Res.*, 1984, *12*, 356). Minimum inhibitory concentrations for 90% of organisms of 5.0 and 2.8 µg per mL have been reported for isolates from cystic fibrosis patients and other chronically infected patients, respectively (B. Gordts *et al.*, *J. antimicrob. Chemother.*, 1984, *14*, 25). In a more recent study minimum inhibitory concentrations of ceftazidime against *Ps. aeruginosa* ranged from 0.25 to 64 µg per mL and isolates of *Ps. fluorescens* were inhibited by 16 µg per mL, but poor activity against *Ps. maltophilia* was demonstrated. In general, the organisms tended to be less susceptible *in vitro* to agents such as ceftazidime which are in clinical use than to newer agents such as the 4-quinolones which had not been used clinically (K.V.I. Rolston *et al.*, *J. antimicrob. Chemother.*, 1987, *19*, 193). It has been demonstrated that sublethal concentrations of ceftazidime reduce adherence of mucoid strains to epithelial cells, which may partly explain its efficacy in patients with cystic fibrosis (S. Vishwanath *et al.*, *J. antimicrob. Chemother.*, 1987, *19*, 579). The activity of ceftazidime against *Pseudomonas aeruginosa* may be enhanced by an aminoglycoside, see below.

The stability of ceftazidime to pseudomonal beta-lactamases.— D. M. Livermore *et al.*, *J. antimicrob. Chemother.*, 1981, *8, Suppl.* B, 163.

In a study *in vitro* of 9 strains of *Pseudomonas pseudomallei*, ceftazidime showed promising activity with a mean minimum inhibitory concentration of 1.5 µg per mL. Ceftazidime was essentially stable to the beta-lactamase produced by the organism.— D. M. Livermore *et al.*, *J. antimicrob. Chemother.*, 1987, *20*, 313.

For reference to a study comparing the bactericidal activity of ceftazidime and cefoperazone against *Pseudomonas aeruginosa*, see under Cefoperazone Sodium, p.149. See also under Cefsulodin Sodium, p.161.

ACTIVITY WITH OTHER ANTIMICROBIAL AGENTS. Enhanced activity against *Pseudomonas aeruginosa* and some other Gram-negative bacteria has been demonstrated *in vitro* between ceftazidime and aminoglycosides including amikacin, gentamicin, netilmicin, and tobramycin; the combination of ceftazidime with an aminoglycoside may help to prevent emergence of resistance against either drug (R.K. Scribner *et al.*, *Antimicrob. Ag. Chemother.*, 1982, *21*, 939; R.N. Jones and R.R. Packer, *ibid.*, *22*, 985; A.S. Bayer *et al.*, *ibid.*, 1984, *25*, 725; J. Blaser *et al.*, *ibid.*, 1985, *28*, 64; F.M. Gordin *et al.*, *ibid.*, 1987, *31*, 398). The combined activity of ceftazidime with another beta-lactam antibiotic such as piperacillin appears to have no advantage over single-agent activity and is inferior to beta-lactam-aminoglycoside combinations (D.E. Johnson *et al.*, *Antimicrob. Ag. Chemother.*, 1985, *27*, 735). Some workers have, however, suggested that the combination of piperacillin plus latamoxef or ceftazidime may be advantageous if aminoglycoside toxicity is a concern (D.J. Winston *et al.*, *J. antimicrob. Chemother.*, 1986, *17*, *Suppl.* A, 55). The development of resistance to beta-lactam agents during treatment of *Ps. aeruginosa* infections is a continuing problem. Theoretically the best approach is therapy with a combination of antimicrobial agents which is minimally susceptible to changes in permeability and beta-lactamase production, such as an aminoglycoside, which may increase the permeability of the outer membrane, in combination with a beta-lactamase-resistant beta-lactam antibiotic. Clinical experience supports this view, while single or double beta-lactam therapy should be considered with caution (C.W. Stratton and F. Tausk, *J. antimicrob. Chemother.*, 1987, *19*, 413). The combinations of ciprofloxacin or pefloxacin and ceftazidime have tended to exhibit mixed or additive effects against *Ps. aeruginosa* although some synergy has been observed (N.N. Farrag *et al.*, *J. antimicrob. Chemother.*, 1986, *18*, 770; H.B. Drugeon *et al.*, *ibid.*, 1987, *19*, 197).

Clavulanic acid has been reported to enhance the activity of ceftazidime against beta-lactamase-producing isolates of the *Bacteroides fragilis* group, however, the effect appears much less marked against non-*fragilis* strains (J.P. Maskell *et al.*, *J. antimicrob. Chemother.*, 1984, *13*, 23). Some synergy has also been demonstrated between ceftazidime and clindamycin against mainly anaerobic bacteria (W.L. George, *Antimicrob. Ag. Chemother.*, 1984, *25*, 657).

Antagonism has been demonstrated between ceftazidime and chloramphenicol against Gram-negative organisms *in vitro* and also *in vivo* during treatment of Gram-negative meningitis (G.L. French *et al.*, *Br. med. J.*, 1985, *291*, 636). Antagonism has also been demonstrated between ceftazidime and ampicillin against group B streptococci and *Listeria monocytogenes* (J.-E. Brorson *et al.*, *J. antimicrob. Chemother.*, 1985, *16*, 406).

Resistance

As for Cefotaxime Sodium, p.153.

In a study of 30 patients with serious bacterial infections treated with ceftazidime, clinical failure occurred in one patient because of superinfection with a strain of *Enterobacter agglomerans*; the organism became resistant to ceftazidime during therapy. Superinfection with a resistant *E. agglomerans* strain also occurred in another patient. Development of resistance to ceftazidime during therapy was also noted in *E. cloacae* and *Pseudomonas aeruginosa*. Mucocutaneous candidiasis was a minor inconvenience in 4 instances, and 3 cases of *Enterococcus faecalis* (*Streptococcus faecalis*) colonisation were noted during therapy. *Clostridium difficile* toxin-induced diarrhoea occurred in one patient.— L. J. Eron *et al.*, *Antimicrob. Ag. Chemother.*, 1983, *23*, 236.

The development of multiple beta-lactam resistance in *Enterobacter cloacae* following therapy with ceftazidime in a 12-year-old neutropenic patient.— A. S. Black and J. Cohen (letter), *Lancet*, 1985, *2*, 331. A similar report of the emergence of resistance to ceftazidime and other beta-lactams in a *Pseudomonas aeruginosa* strain after therapy with ceftazidime in a patient with 40% burns. Multiple beta-lactam resistance has been shown to arise in certain groups of organisms, *Enterobacter* spp., *Ps. aeruginosa*, *Citrobacter* spp., *Serratia* spp., and indole-positive *Proteus*, which share the potential to produce class 1 beta-lactamases. The genes responsible for chromosomally-mediated, inducible enzymes are usually repressed and very little beta-lactamase is produced. However, the newer cephalosporins can induce these beta-lactamases by derepression, and this may result in resistance in clinical practice.— M. J. Weinbren and R. M. Perinpanayagam (letter), *ibid.*, 673.

For a similar report of the selection of strains of *Enterobacter cloacae* resistant to third-generation cephalosporins, see under Cefuroxime Sodium, Uses, Pregnancy and the Neonate, p.173.

Isolation of *Klebsiella pneumoniae* strains resistant to ceftazidime but which remained more or less sensitive to cefotaxime, ceftriaxone, and latamoxef.— J. Sirot *et al.* (letter), *J. antimicrob. Chemother.*, 1987, *20*, 611.

RESISTANCE OF PSEUDOMONAS. From a national survey in 24 British hospitals of antibiotic resistance in *Pseudomonas aeruginosa*, the incidence of resistance to ceftazidime was low (0.3% of 1866 isolates) at a breakpoint of 16 µg per mL (R.J. Williams *et al.*, *J. antimicrob. Chemother.*, 1984, *14*, 9); an incidence of 0.6% has been reported in the Netherlands (A.J. De Neeling *et al.*, *ibid.*, 1987, *19*, 703). However, resistance to ceftazidime may be expected to increase among strains of *Ps. aeruginosa* with increase in clinical use (H. Knothe *et al.*, *ibid.*, 136). Resistance has developed during treatment with ceftazidime and may be due to excessive production of chromosomally mediated beta-lactamases (S.J.

Hudson and H.R. Ingham, *Lancet*, 1985, *1*, 464). Induction or derepression of these beta-lactamases may produce simultaneous resistance to the broad-spectrum penicillins, monobactams, most of the second- and third-generation cephalosporins, and the cephamycins (C.C. Sanders, *J. antimicrob. Chemother.*, 1981, *13*, 1). Cross-resistance has been demonstrated between beta-lactam antibiotics (R.H.K. Eng *et al.*, *ibid.*, 1986, *17*, 717).

Resistance in *Ps. aeruginosa* seems to depend on the interaction between the penetration-rate of the drug and the rate of removal by hydrolysis and/or trapping by beta-lactamase; *Ps. aeruginosa* utilises a number of different mechanisms simultaneously to become resistant to antibacterial agents of virtually every class (C.W. Stratton and F. Tausk, *J. antimicrob. Chemother.*, 1987, *19*, 413). Aminoglycoside resistance has been associated with significant beta-lactam resistance in *Ps. aeruginosa* isolated from the sputum of patients with cystic fibrosis (S.C. Aronoff and J.D. Klinger, *J. antimicrob. Chemother.*, 1985, *15*, 545); the use of ceftazidime or cefsulodin monotherapy in cystic fibrosis patients may have been partly responsible for increasing the prevalence of multiresistant *Ps. aeruginosa*, including resistance to aminoglycosides, in a cystic fibrosis centre (S.S. Pedersen *et al.*, *ibid.*, 1986, *17*, 505). However, in a survey using clinical isolates of *Ps. aeruginosa* subjected to beta-lactamase induction using imipenem, emergence of cross-resistance to aminoglycosides was very rare (C.W. Stratton *et al.*, *J. antimicrob. Chemother.*, 1987, *19*, 21).

Absorption and Fate

Ceftazidime is administered by injection as the sodium salt. Mean peak serum concentrations of 17 and 39 µg per mL have been reported approximately one hour after intramuscular administration of the equivalent of 0.5 and 1 g of ceftazidime, respectively. Five minutes after intravenous bolus injections of the equiv. of 0.5, 1, and 2 g of ceftazidime, mean serum concentrations of 45, 90, and 170 µg per mL, respectively, have been reported. The plasma elimination half-life of ceftazidime is about 1.8 to 2.2 hours, but this is prolonged in patients with severe renal failure and in neonates. It is about 10 to 17% bound to plasma proteins.

Ceftazidime is widely distributed in body tissues and fluids including bone, synovial fluid, heart, bile, sputum, and aqueous humour; therapeutic concentrations have been achieved in the cerebrospinal fluid when the meninges are inflamed. It diffuses across the placenta and is excreted in breast milk.

Ceftazidime is excreted by the kidneys almost exclusively by glomerular filtration; probenecid has little effect on the excretion of ceftazidime. About 80 to 90% of a dose is recovered unchanged in the urine within 24 hours. It is removed by haemodialysis to some extent.

Studies of the pharmacokinetics of ceftazidime in healthy subjects: R. Wise *et al.*, *J. antimicrob. Chemother.*, 1981, *8*, *Suppl.* B, 277; R. Lüthy *et al.*, *Antimicrob. Ag. Chemother.*, 1981, *20*, 567; D. K. Sommers *et al.*, *ibid.*, 1983, *23*, 892; G. L. Drusano *et al.*, *ibid.*, 1984, *26*, 388.

A study of the pharmacokinetics of ceftazidime administered either alone or in combination with piperacillin or tobramycin to 21 febrile cancer patients. The observed elimination half-life was longer, the serum clearance smaller, and the volume of distribution larger than previously reported in studies of healthy subjects, probably due to the lower creatinine clearances in the cancer patients. The addition of either piperacillin or tobramycin did not influence the pharmacokinetic behaviour of ceftazidime.— G. L. Drusano *et al.*, *Antimicrob. Ag. Chemother.*, 1985, *27*, 605. See also I. Garcia *et al.*, *ibid.*, 1983, *24*, 141.

ADMINISTRATION IN CYSTIC FIBROSIS. The total body clearance of ceftazidime appears to be increased in patients with cystic fibrosis compared with healthy subjects (N. Martini *et al.*, *J. clin. Hosp. Pharm.*, 1984, *9*, 303; S. Leeder *et al.*, *Clin. Pharmac. Ther.*, 1984, *35*, 254). Some workers have reported that the elimination half-life does not appear to be altered in cystic fibrosis, but the distribution half-life appears to be prolonged, although large interindividual variations in pharmacokinetic parameters make results inconclusive (C.M. Kercsmar *et al.*, *J. antimicrob. Chemother.*, 1983, *12*, *Suppl.* A, 289; A. Turner *et al.*, *ibid.*, 1984, *14*, 521). Following an intravenous bolus dose of ceftazidime 50 mg per kg body-weight, Kercsmar *et al.* reported peak serum concentrations of 200 to 300 µg per mL and following the same dose for various lengths of treatment, concentrations of ceftazidime in the sputum of patients with cystic fibrosis have been reported to range from 1.4 to 12.1 µg per mL (H. Permin *et al.*, *J. antimicrob. Chemother.*, 1983, *12*, *Suppl.* A, 313).

ADMINISTRATION IN THE ELDERLY. In a study of the pharmacokinetics of ceftazidime after a 1-g intravenous bolus dose in 6 healthy elderly subjects (mean age 63 years) and 12 young subjects (mean age 23 years), the mean renal clearance of ceftazidime was 66.0 and 96.6 mL per minute, respectively; the reduced renal clearance reflected the normal ageing of the kidneys. The volume of distribution was also decreased in the elderly group, probably because of a reduction in total body water and lean mass. However, there was no significant difference in the elimination half-life between the 2 groups. Dosage adjustment is considered unnecessary in otherwise healthy elderly patients requiring ceftazidime.— M. LeBel *et al.*, *Antimicrob. Ag. Chemother.*, 1985, *28*, 713.

ADMINISTRATION IN RENAL FAILURE. A study of the pharmacokinetics of ceftazidime in 5 patients with normal renal function and 19 patients with various degrees of impaired renal function. The apparent elimination half-life increased with renal impairment from a mean of 1.57 hours in patients with normal renal function, to 3.74 hours in patients with a creatinine clearance (CC) of 39 to 73 mL per minute, 9.25 hours in those with a CC of 14 to 27 mL per minute, 15.33 hours in patients with a CC of 2 to 12 mL per minute, and about 25 hours in anuric patients. During a 6- to 8-hour haemodialysis procedure concentrations of ceftazidime in the plasma rapidly decreased and the mean elimination half-life was 2.8 hours. Patients should be given an additional dose at the end of haemodialysis. There was no evidence of accumulation of ceftazidime in 4 patients with severe and chronic renal impairment who received doses of 0.5 to 1 g intravenously every 24 hours for 10 days.— A. Leroy *et al.*, *Antimicrob. Ag. Chemother.*, 1984, *25*, 638. See also L. S. Welage *et al.*, *ibid.*, 201; B. H. Ackerman *et al.*, *ibid.*, 785.

Pharmacokinetics of ceftazidime during continuous ambulatory peritoneal dialysis and intermittent peritoneal dialysis. Ceftazidime readily penetrates the non-inflamed peritoneal membrane whether given by the intravenous or intraperitoneal route.— T. J. Comstock *et al.*, *Drug Intell. & clin. Pharm.*, 1983, *17*, 453. See also A. Tourkantonis and P. Nicolaidis, *J. antimicrob. Chemother.*, 1983, *12*, *Suppl.* A, 263.

DIFFUSION INTO BODY TISSUES AND FLUIDS. The penetration of ceftazidime into the cerebrospinal fluid (CSF) of 11 patients with bacterial meningitis undergoing concurrent treatment with other antibiotics was evaluated. CSF concentrations obtained 120 or 180 minutes after the fourth dose of ceftazidime 2 g infused intravenously over 30 minutes every 8 hours, ranged from 2 to 30 µg per mL. The mean concentrations found between days 2 and 4 of antibiotic treatment, when the meninges were the most inflamed, were somewhat higher than those found when the same dose regimen of ceftazidime was administered between days 11 and 20, when the meninges were supposedly healed, however, the difference was not significant.— J. Modai *et al.*, *Antimicrob. Ag. Chemother.*, 1983, *24*, 126. See also I. W. Fong and K. B. Tomkins, *ibid.*, 1984, *26*, 115; K. Alestig *et al.* (letter), *Lancet*, 1985, *1*, 161.

In a study of 73 surgical patients ceftazidime 2 g was administered intravenously before the operation and the total concentrations of bound and unbound ceftazidime in the tissues removed during the operation were determined. Mean tissue:serum ratios of ceftazidime calculated on the basis of the serum concentration at the time of removal of the tissue were found to be: for the myometrium, 0.632; skeletal muscle, 0.600; prostate, 0.579; skin, 0.441; gall-bladder wall, 0.413; breast, 0.368; peritoneal tissue, 0.305; and fatty tissue 0.244. These ratios were generally higher than had been previously reported by Daschner *et al.* (*J. antimicrob. Chemother.*, 1983, *12*, *Suppl.* A, 247) and Adam *et al.* (*ibid.*, 269), but this was because both bound and unbound drug was measured rather than only the extractable component.— L. H. Loebis, *J. antimicrob. Chemother.*, 1985, *16*, 757. See also R. M. Smith *et al.*, *Br. J. clin. Pract.*, 1985, *39*, 94.

Further references to the diffusion of ceftazidime into various body tissues and fluids: D. M. Ryan *et al.*, *J. antimicrob. Chemother.*, 1981, *8*, *Suppl.* B, 283 (subcutaneous fluid); D. H. Wittmann *et al.*, *ibid.*, 293 (bone, bile, tissue fluid, and peritoneal fluid); E. Bouza *et al.*, *Antimicrob. Ag. Chemother.*, 1983, *24*, 104 (bile); G. Benoni *et al.*, *ibid.*, 1984, *25*, 760 (ascitic fluid); A. M. A. Abbas *et al.*, *J. antimicrob. Chemother.*, 1985, *15*, 119 (prostate gland); C. R. R. Corbett *et al.*, *ibid.*, *16*, 261 (peritoneal fluid); D. A. Leigh *et al.*, *ibid.*, 637 (bone); R. A. Walstad *et al.*, *Eur. J. clin. Pharmac.*, 1986, *31*, 327 (gall bladder and bile); U. Frank *et al.*, *Antimicrob. Ag. Chemother.*, 1987, *31*, 813 (heart valves, and subcutaneous and muscle tissue); D. B. Clements and V. Tailor, *Br. J. Ophthal.*, 1987, *71*, 433 (aqueous humour and serum concentrations following subconjunctival administration).

PREGNANCY AND THE NEONATE. Ceftazidime 2 g intravenously every 8 hours for 5 days was administered to 11 puerperal women. The mean concentrations of ceftazidime in the milk collected 30 minutes before the next dose, 1 hour after a dose, and 3 hours after a dose were 3.8, 5.2, and 4.5 µg per mL, respectively. Ceftazidime was excreted in breast milk at relatively constant concentrations between days 2 and 4 of therapy.— J. D. Blanco *et al.*, *Antimicrob. Ag. Chemother.*, 1983, *23*, 479.

A study of the pharmacokinetics of ceftazidime in 16 preterm or term neonates. Peak serum concentrations ranging from 54 to 102 µg per mL were reached 30 to 60 minutes after an intramuscular injection of ceftazidime 50 mg per kg body-weight. Mean elimination half-lives of 4.7 and 3.8 hours were calculated following intravenous and intramuscular administration of a single dose of 50 mg per kg, respectively; the difference was not significant.— A. Boccazzi *et al.*, *Antimicrob. Ag. Chemother.*, 1983, *24*, 955. During multiple-dose therapy in 29 neonates given ceftazidime 50 mg per kg body-weight by intravenous infusion every 12 hours in the first week of life and every 8 hours thereafter, for 3 to 5 days, mean peak plasma concentrations ranged from 102 to 124 µg per mL. Mean elimination half-lives after one or two doses ranged from 4.2 to 6.7 hours and varied inversely with gestational age; after multiple doses the mean half-lives were from 2.9 to 3.7 hours.— G. H. McCracken *et al.*, *ibid.*, 1984, *26*, 583. See also J. G. Prinsloo *et al.*, *J. antimicrob. Chemother.*, 1983, *12*, *Suppl.* A, 361.

Uses and Administration

Ceftazidime is a third-generation cephalosporin antibiotic with enhanced activity against *Pseudomonas aeruginosa.* It is used in the treatment of susceptible infections including respiratory-tract infections such as pneumonia and lung infections in patients with cystic fibrosis, urinary-tract infections, skin and soft tissue infections, bone and joint infections, peritonitis and other abdominal infections, septicaemia, and meningitis. It is often used alone, but can be used in association with an aminoglycoside or vancomycin in patients with severe neutropenia, or, if infection with *Bacteroides fragilis* is suspected, it may be used in association with an antibiotic active against anaerobes such as clindamycin or metronidazole. The drugs should generally be administered separately.

Ceftazidime is available as the pentahydrate but it is formulated with sodium carbonate to form the sodium salt in solution. Doses are expressed in terms of anhydrous ceftazidime. It is administered by deep intramuscular injection, slow intravenous injection, or intravenous infusion in doses of 1 to 6 g daily in divided doses every 8 or 12 hours. The higher doses are used in severe infections especially in immunocompromised patients. In patients with cystic fibrosis who have pseudomonal lung infections, high doses of 100 to 150 mg per kg body-weight daily in 3 divided doses are used; up to 9 g daily has been given to adults with normal renal function. If pain is considered a problem with intramuscular use, ceftazidime may be reconstituted with lignocaine hydrochloride 0.5% or 1% injection.

Children are usually given ceftazidime 30 to 100 mg per kg daily in 2 or 3 divided doses, but in severely ill children up to 150 mg per kg daily to a maximum of 6 g daily may be given in 3 divided doses. Neonates and infants up to 2 months old have been given 25 to 60 mg per kg daily in 2 divided doses.

In patients with impaired renal function the dosage of ceftazidime may need to be reduced to compensate for slower excretion of the drug. For patients with creatinine clearances of 31 to 50, 16 to 30, 6 to 15, and 5 or less mL per minute, doses of 1 g every 12 hours, 1 g every 24 hours,

0.5 g every 24 hours, and 0.5 g every 48 hours, respectively, have been recommended. In severe infections these doses may need to be increased by 50%. In patients undergoing peritoneal dialysis a loading dose of 1 g may be given followed by 500 mg every 24 hours; ceftazidime may also be added to the dialysis fluid, usually 125 to 250 mg for 2 litres of dialysis fluid. In patients on haemodialysis the appropriate maintenance dose of ceftazidime should be repeated after each dialysis period.

Reviews of the actions and uses of ceftazidime: B. R. Smith, *Clin. Pharm.*, 1984, *3*, 373; J. Burnie and R. Matthews, *Drugs Today*, 1984, *20*, 555; D. M. Richards and R. N. Brogden, *Drugs*, 1985, *29*, 105; R. L. Yost and R. Ramphal, *Drug Intell. & clin. Pharm.*, 1985, *19*, 509; *Med. Lett.*, 1985, *27*, 85.

ADMINISTRATION IN LIVER DISORDERS. From a study of the pharmacokinetics of ceftazidime in 12 patients with chronic hepatic dysfunction it appeared that dose modification based on hepatic dysfunction is unnecessary in patients who have relatively normal renal function.— M. T. Pasko *et al.*, *J. antimicrob. Chemother.*, 1985, *15*, 365.

GYNAECOLOGICAL INFECTIONS. In a study of 77 patients with obstetric and gynaecological infections, ceftazidime 2 g intravenously every 8 hours produced similar results to clindamycin 600 mg in association with tobramycin 1.5 mg per kg body-weight, both given intravenously every 8 hours; 89.5 and 87.2% of patients, respectively, responded to treatment.— J. D. Blanco *et al.*, *Antimicrob. Ag. Chemother.*, 1983, *24*, 500.

Further references: Z. Takase, *J. antimicrob. Chemother.*, 1983, *12*, *Suppl.* A, 383.

IMMUNOCOMPROMISED PATIENTS. For the use of ceftazidime in the treatment of febrile episodes in immunocompromised patients, see under Septicaemia, below.

MENINGITIS. Including the patient reported by Alestig *et al.* (*Lancet*, 1985, *1*, 161), clinical success has been reported with ceftazidime in 32 of 35 patients with *Pseudomonas* meningitis; 16 patients received ceftazidime alone. Adults were usually given ceftazidime 2 g every 8 hours and infants usually 100 to 150 mg per kg body-weight daily. All patients received ceftazidime intravenously, but three also had intraventricular administration in doses of 50 mg every 48 hours, 25 mg every 72 hours, or 250 mg every 48 hours; the 250-mg dose was probably excessive but was well tolerated.— K. J. Williams and R. D. Foord, *Glaxo, UK* (letter), *Lancet*, 1985, *1*, 464. See also K. J. Williams (letter), *ibid.*, 634.

Beneficial results in 4 neonates with Gram-negative bacillary meningitis given ceftazidime 90 to 150 mg per kg body-weight daily in 3 divided doses, in association with gentamicin. Doses of both antibiotics were adjusted to maintain the recommended serum concentrations.— T. S. J. Elliott *et al.*, *J. antimicrob. Chemother.*, 1986, *17*, 245.

For comments on the problems associated with the empirical use of cephalosporins in the treatment of meningitis, see under Cefotaxime Sodium, p.155.

OSTEOMYELITIS. Of 21 patients with acute or chronic osteomyelitis due to both Gram-negative and Gram-positive organisms who received ceftazidime 1 or 2 g three times daily by intravenous infusion, 18 patients were cured, a further patient improved, and 2 failed to respond to therapy. Adequate drainage and debridement was also important.— J. P. Dutoy and G. Wauters, *J. antimicrob. Chemother.*, 1983, *12*, *Suppl.* A, 229. Seven of 9 patients with pseudomonal osteomyelitis improved or were cured following intravenous therapy with ceftazidime usually in doses of 3 to 6 g daily; some of the patients had polymicrobial infections.— L. J. Eron *et al.*, *ibid.*, 161.

In a study of 18 patients with Gram-negative osteomyelitis 9 patients received ceftazidime 2 g every 12 hours intravenously and 9 patients received both ticarcillin 3 g every 4 hours and tobramycin 100 to 360 mg daily in divided doses; treatment was given for 26 to 63 days. The osteomyelitis was considered to be arrested in all 9 patients receiving ticarcillin and tobramycin, but there were 3 treatment failures in the ceftazidime group, however, 2 of these were considered to be surgical failures.— T. G. Sheftel and J. T. Mader, *Antimicrob. Ag. Chemother.*, 1986, *29*, 112.

Further references: M. C. Bach and D. M. Cocchetto, *Antimicrob. Ag. Chemother.*, 1987, *31*, 1605.

For mention of the use of ceftazidime in the treatment of osteomyelitis due to *Salmonella typhimurium*, see under Salmonellosis, below.

OTITIS. All 4 patients with severe purulent *Pseudomonas aeruginosa* otitis with chondritis and abscesses responded to treatment with ceftazidime, but 2 relapsed after 15 and 90 days despite ceftazidime therapy for 3 and 6 weeks, respectively. In both cases the *Ps. aeruginosa* were still sensitive to ceftazidime.— P. Francioli *et al.*, *J. antimicrob. Chemother.*, 1983, *12*, *Suppl.* A, 139.

Otitis media. In a study of 17 children aged 5 months to 3 years with recurrent or chronic otitis media complicated by *Pseudomonas aeruginosa* infection, pseudomonas was eradicated from the middle-ear effusion in 11 patients given ceftazidime 50 mg per kg body-weight intramuscularly every 12 hours for a median duration of 10 days. In 3 additional cases clinical improvement occurred but pseudomonas continued to grow in the discharge from the ear, and in 3 cases the clinical response was poor.— P. Lautala *et al.*, *J. antimicrob. Chemother.*, 1983, *12*, *Suppl.* A, 365.

PERITONITIS. Ceftazidime has been used in peritonitis associated with continuous ambulatory peritoneal dialysis (CAPD). The British Society for Antimicrobial Chemotherapy has recommended that a loading dose of 1 g may be administered intravenously or intraperitoneally in the severely ill patient, and a maintenance dose of 125 mg per litre of dialysis fluid should be given intraperitoneally.— *Lancet*, 1987, *1*, 845.

Ceftazidime has been used in association with vancomycin to treat CAPD-associated peritonitis.— H. H. Gray and S. J. Eykyn (letter), *Lancet*, 1983, *1*, 349; I. Muscat *et al.* (letter), *ibid.*, 1987, *1*, 1142.

For comparison of the antimicrobial activities of various cephalosporins and the problems associated with the use of a cephalosporin as first-line therapy for peritonitis, see under Cefuroxime Sodium, p.172. See also under Choice of Antibiotic, p.99.

PREGNANCY AND THE NEONATE. Ceftazidime 100 mg per kg body-weight daily, in 2 divided doses by intravenous bolus injection, has been used successfully in febrile neonates with clinical signs of persisting infection or positive blood culture and it has been suggested that ceftazidime is a suitable broad-spectrum antibiotic for the initial treatment of infections in neonates (S. Snelling *et al.*, *J. antimicrob. Chemother.*, 1983, *12*, *Suppl.* A, 353; J. de Louvois and A.B. Mulhall, *Archs Dis. Childh.*, 1985, *60*, 891). However, some treatment failures and colonisation with *Enterococcus faecalis* (*Streptococcus faecalis*) have been reported following treatment with ceftazidime 25 mg per kg every 12 hours and some workers feel that ceftazidime should not be recommended as a single agent in bacteriologically unproven infections (D.C. Low *et al.*, *Archs Dis. Childh.*, 1985, *60*, 360), especially as it is considered inappropriate therapy for confirmed cases of group B streptococcal and *Staphylococcus aureus* infection, 2 of the commonest neonatal pathogens (*idem*, 892). More experience with ceftazidime was considered necessary before the situation could be resolved (I. Blumenthal, *ibid.*, 785; D.C. Low and J.G. Bissenden, *ibid.*).

More recently, ceftazidime 50 mg per kg every 12 hours during the first 7 days of life and every 8 hours thereafter, given by intravenous infusion over 10 to 15 minutes for a minimum of 10 days, was found to be more effective than therapy with amikacin in association with carbenicillin in treating neonatal sepsis (C.M. Odio *et al.*, *Pediat. infect. Dis. J.*, 1987, *6*, 371); this difference was principally due to the superiority of ceftazidime in treating *Pseudomonas* infections. Odio *et al.* did not believe that ceftazidime or any other cephalosporin should be used singly or in combination with ampicillin as routine initial empirical therapy of suspected sepsis in neonates. However, they suggested that ceftazidime either alone or with an aminoglycoside should be considered when, as in their nursery, neonatal septicaemia or meningitis is frequently caused by Gram-negative enteric bacilli or by *Ps. aeruginosa* that are resistant to the penicillins and one or more of the aminoglycosides, but susceptible to ceftazidime.

RESPIRATORY-TRACT INFECTIONS. Ceftazidime has been used in the treatment of serious infections of the lower respiratory tract particularly in patients with severe underlying lung disease where pulmonary defence mechanisms are seriously impaired (T.H. Peirce *et al.*, *J. antimicrob. Chemother.*, 1983, *12*, *Suppl.* A, 21). Ceftazidime, usually in doses of 1 to 2 g three times daily intravenously or intramuscularly for about 10 to 14 days, has produced satisfactory clinical responses in approximately 85 to 95% of patients with either community- or hospital-acquired pneumonia; there have, however, been some reports of the development of colonisation with resistant isolates or superinfection during ceftazidime therapy (T. Pettersson *et al.*, *J. antimicrob. Chemother.*, 1983, *12*, *Suppl.* A, 31; J.C. Engle *et al.*, *Antimicrob. Ag. Chemother.*, 1985, *28*, 146; B.G. Yangco *et al.*, *J. antimicrob. Chemother.*, 1986, *18*, 521). It appears to be as efficacious as cephazolin plus tobramycin for the treatment of acute exacerbations of chronic bronchitis (N. Vetter *et al.*, *J. antimicrob. Chemother.*, 1983, *12*, *Suppl.* A, 35) and pneumonia caused by Gram-negative organisms such as *Klebsiella* spp., *Serratia marcescens*, and *Pseudomonas aeruginosa* (L.A. Mandell *et al.*, *ibid.*, 9; J.C. Pottage *et al.*, *ibid.*, 223; L.A. Mandell *et al.*, *ibid.*, 1987, *20*, 95).

For further mention of the use of ceftazidime in pneumonia, see under Septicaemia, below.

Cystic fibrosis. Clinical improvement with marked reduction in cough and amount of sputum has been reported with ceftazidime therapy administered, alone or in association with tobramycin, in the treatment of acute pulmonary exacerbations in patients with cystic fibrosis (B. Strandvik *et al.*, *J. antimicrob. Chemother.*, 1983, *12*, *Suppl.* A, 283; J. Dodge *et al.*, *ibid.*, 325). Ceftazidime has been found to be at least as good as therapy with carbenicillin and tobramycin and is considered a good alternative to traditional antibiotics (G. Mastella *et al.*, *ibid.*, 297; T.J. David *et al.*, *ibid.*, 337). Ceftazidime is often given in doses of 50 mg per kg body-weight intravenously every 8 hours for about 14 days and this dosage appears to produce the maximal clinical response (M.D. Reed *et al.*, *Antimicrob. Ag. Chemother.*, 1987, *31*, 698). However, in common with other antipseudomonal antibiotics, therapy rarely eradicates the organism and the first course of ceftazidime is usually the most successful, with subsequent courses being less effective (R.T. Cullen *et al.*, *J. antimicrob. Chemother.*, 1983, *12*, *Suppl.* A, 369). Resistance to ceftazidime may also develop during treatment and the possibility that more widespread use of the agent may favour the development of resistant strains is a matter of concern (H. Permin *et al.*, *ibid.*, 313).

Ceftazidime has been reported to suppress both mucoid and non-mucoid strains of *Ps. aeruginosa*, but appears to have little effect on sputum colony counts of *Ps. cepacia* (R. Gold *et al.*, *ibid.*, 331).

Melioidosis. Beneficial results with ceftazidime in the treatment of pulmonary melioidosis caused by a multiresistant strain of *Pseudomonas pseudomallei* in an immunocompromised patient.— S. Y. So *et al.*, *Am. Rev. resp. Dis.*, 1983, *127*, 650.

SALMONELLOSIS. Ceftazidime showed excellent activity *in vitro* against multiresistant strains of *Salmonella newport* and *S. typhi* isolated in Peru (H. Goossens *et al.*, *Lancet*, 1982, *2*, 769). There has, however, been a report of treatment failure with ceftazidime 1 g three times daily by intravenous injection for 6 days in a patient with salmonellosis due to *S. newport*, despite an MIC of 0.25 µg per mL (D.I. Gozzard *et al.*, *ibid.*, *1*, 1152). The dose may have been rather low; ceftazidime 2 or 3 g twice daily has been used successfully in the treatment of a patient with osteomyelitis due to *S. typhimurium* with an MIC of 0.25 µg per mL (P.M. Shah and W. Stille, *ibid.*, 1419).

SEPTICAEMIA. Beneficial results have been obtained with ceftazidime in the treatment of septicaemia and other serious infections due to susceptible Gram-negative organisms including *Pseudomonas aeruginosa* (N. Clumeck *et al.*, *Antimicrob. Ag. Chemother.*, 1983, *24*, 176; P. Lundbergh *et al.*, *J. antimicrob. Chemother.*, 1983, *12*, *Suppl.* A, 199; M.J. Maslow *et al.*, *ibid.*, 213; M. Joshi *et al.*, *Antimicrob. Ag. Chemother.*, 1986, *30*, 90). Ceftazidime appears to be as effective as ticarcillin with tobramycin for serious infections including septicaemia and pneumonia in non-neutropenic patients, although superinfection with organisms such as *Pseudomonas maltophilia* or *Enterococcus faecalis* (*Streptococcus faecalis*) has been reported (L.A. Cone *et al.* , *Antimicrob. Ag. Chemother.*, 1985, *28*, 33). Ceftazidime monotherapy has also been used successfully for childhood infections (M.D. Reed, *et al.* , *Antimicrob. Ag. Chemother*, 1984, *26*, 318) and in elderly patients with multiple underlying chronic diseases (T.A. Taft *et al.*, *Curr. ther. Res.*, 1986, *40*, 830).

For the use of ceftazidime in the treatment of febrile neonates with septicaemia, see Pregnancy and the Neonate, above.

For a comparison of ceftazidime with aztreonam in the treatment of Gram-negative septicaemia in patients with severe underlying diseases, see Aztreonam, p.127.

Immunocompromised patients. Ceftazidime has been used with beneficial results in the treatment of febrile episodes in immunosuppressed patients (J.T. Reilly *et al.*, *J. antimicrob. Chemother.*, 1983, *12*, *Suppl.* A, 89; B.E. de Pauw *et al.*, *ibid.*, 93; J.J. Gomes d'Oliveira *et al.*, *J. int. med. Res.*, 1986, *14*, 30), including infections due to *Pseudomonas aeruginosa* (C. Verhagen *et al.*, *J. infect.*, 1986, *13*, 125). It has been shown by some workers to be of similar efficacy to combination therapies with azlocillin and tobramycin (G. Morgan *et al.*, *J. antimicrob. Chemother.*, 1983, *12*, *Suppl.* A, 347), piperacillin, netilmicin, and cefotaxime (J.P. Donnelly *et al.*, *J. infect.*, 1985, *11*, 205), or tobramycin and cefuroxime (S. Rödjer *et al.*, *J. antimicrob. Chemother.*, 1987, *20*, 109). However, although ceftazidime is useful in treating Gram-negative infections there are gaps in its spectrum including enterococci, methicillin-resistant *Staphylococcus aureus*, *Staph. epidermidis*, non-aeruginosa pseudomonas such as *Ps. maltophilia*, and, to some extent, anaerobes (J.W. Hathorn and P.A. Pizzo, *J. antimicrob. Chemother.*, 1986, *17*, *Suppl.* A, 41) and superinfection may occur during therapy; the emergence of resistance to ceftazidime by *Ps. aeruginosa* during therapy is also of concern (R. Ramphal *et al.*, *J. antimicrob. Chemother.*, 1983, *12*, *Suppl.* A, 81; J.A.A. Hoogkamp-Korstanje *et al.*, *ibid.*, 1985, *15*, 743).

Some workers therefore feel that ceftazidime cannot be recommended as a single agent for initial empirical therapy of febrile immunosuppressed patients and that an agent to cover Gram-positive infection such as vancomycin or an aminoglycoside should be added to the treatment until the infecting organism is identified (R. Ramphal *et al.*, *J. antimicrob. Chemother.*, 1983, *12*, *Suppl.* A, 81; V. Fainstein *et al.*, *ibid.*, 101; P.J. Darbyshire *et al.*, *ibid.*, 357; J.A.A. Hoogkamp-Korstanje *et al.*, *ibid.*, 1985, *15*, 743; B.S. Kramer *et al.*, *Antimicrob. Ag. Chemother.*, 1986, *30*, 64). Other workers, however, feel that monotherapy is reasonable, but may need to be modified if resistant Gram-positive organisms or mycotic infections are encountered (C.S. Verhagen *et al.*, *Antimicrob. Ag. Chemother.*, 1987, *31*, 191). In a study of over 600 episodes of fever in neutropenic cancer patients, undertaken by the USA National Cancer Institute, ceftazidime was found to be as successful as standard combination therapy during the initial 72 hours of management. Overall 13% of patient-episodes treated with ceftazidime also needed to receive an aminoglycoside during their treatment course, which means that over 85% of patients presenting with fever and neutropenia might be successfully treated without an aminoglycoside. Antibiotic modifications may be required in patients with prolonged neutropenia or once the organism causing the fever is identified (J.W. Hathorn and P.A. Pizzo, *J. antimicrob. Chemother.*, 1986, *17*, *Suppl.* A, 41).

SKIN INFECTIONS. In a study involving 197 patients, ceftazidime 0.5 or 1 g administered by intravenous infusion every 8 hours was found to be effective and well tolerated in the treatment of skin and skin structure infections including cellulitis, abscesses, skin ulcers, and wound infections. The higher dosage regimen tended to be more effective, especially against *Staphylococcus aureus* infections.— L. C. Parish *et al.*, *Int. J. Derm.*, 1986, *25*, 258.

Further references: W. M. Gooch and E. Swenson, *Curr. ther. Res.*, 1985, *37*, 3.

SURGICAL INFECTION PROPHYLAXIS. Favourable results with ceftazidime 2 g twice daily for 8 to 15 days, beginning during the operation, in 27 patients undergoing cholecystectomy.— H. Schoengut and R. Jelinek, *J. antimicrob. Chemother.*, 1983, *12*, *Suppl.* A, 219.

URINARY-TRACT INFECTIONS. Ceftazidime 1 g intramuscularly twice daily for 7 days resulted in clinical improvement or cure in 29 predominantly geriatric patients with urinary-tract infection. A positive bacteriological response to treatment was obtained in 21 (72.9%) of all patients or in 18 of 20 (90%) if those with indwelling catheters were excluded. *Enterococcus faecalis* (*Streptococcus faecalis*) was cultured in all 8 unsuccessful cases.— A. Kasanen *et al.*, *Curr. med. Res. Opinion*, 1982, *8*, 266.

Ceftazidime 0.5 g every 12 hours intramuscularly appeared to be at least as effective as tobramycin 3 mg per kg body-weight daily in 3 divided doses intramuscularly, in the treatment of 62 patients with complicated urinary-tract infections; the antibiotics were given for 5 to 17 days. Thirty-one of 33 ceftazidime-treated patients and 26 of 29 tobramycin-treated patients were considered clinically cured and, at follow-up 5 to 9 days after the end of treatment, 30 and 25 patients were cured, respectively.— C. E. Cox *et al.*, *J. antimicrob. Chemother.*, 1983, *12*, *Suppl.* A, 47. See also P. O. Madsen and P. C. Frimodt-Møller, *ibid.*, 77.

Beneficial results in paediatric patients with severe urinary-tract infections due to *Pseudomonas* spp. Fourteen patients were given ceftazidime 87.4 to 111.1 mg per kg body-weight daily by intramuscular injection in 2 divided doses for 10 to 18.5 days. A further patient with chronic renal failure (glomerular filtration-rate, 18 mL per minute per 1.73 m^2) received a single daily dose of 33 mg per kg for 13 days.— F. Rusconi *et al.*, *Antimicrob. Ag. Chemother.*, 1984, *25*, 395.

Proprietary Preparations

Fortum *(Glaxo, UK)*. *Injection*, powder for reconstitution, ceftazidime 0.25, 0.5, 1, and 2 g (as pentahydrate) with sodium carbonate 118 mg per g of ceftazidime.

Proprietary Names and Manufacturers

Ceftim *(Bonomelli, Ital.)*; Fortam *(Glaxo, Spain; Glaxo, Switz.)*; Fortaz *(Glaxo, Canad.; Glaxo, USA)*; Fortum *(Glaxo, Denm.; Glaxo, Fr.; Cascan, Ger.; Glaxo, Norw.; Glaxo, S.Afr.; Glaxo, Swed.; Glaxo, UK)*; Glazidim *(Glaxo, Ital.)*; Kefamin *(Lilly, Spain)*; Magnacef *(Ayerst, Canad.)*; Panzid *(Duncan, Ital.)*; Potendal *(Liade, Spain)*; Spectrum *(Sigmatau, Ital.)*; Starcef *(FIRMA, Ital.)*; Tazicef *(Smith Kline & French, USA)*; Tazidime *(Lilly, USA)*.

2899-x

Cefteram *(rINN)*.

T-2525. (*Z*)-7-[2-(2-Aminothiazol-4-yl)-2-methoxyiminoacetamido]-3-(5-methyl-2*H*-tetrazol-2-ylmethyl)-3-cephem-4-carboxylic acid.

$C_{16}H_{17}N_9O_5S_2$=479.5.

CAS — 82547-58-8.

Cefteram is a cephalosporin antibiotic. It may be administered by mouth as the pivaloyloxymethyl ester, cefteram pivoxil (T-2588).

Studies of antibacterial activity *in vitro*: S. Okamoto *et al.*, *Antimicrob. Ag. Chemother.*, 1987, *31*, 1111.

Proprietary Names and Manufacturers

Toyama, Jpn.

34-n

Ceftezole Sodium *(rINNM)*.

Sodium 7*R*-7-[2-(1 *H*-tetrazol-1-yl)acetamido]-3-(1,3,4-thiadiazol-2-ylthiomethyl)-3-cephem-4-carboxylate.

$C_{13}H_{11}N_8NaO_4S_3$=462.5.

CAS — 26973-24-0 (ceftezole); 41136-22-5 (sodium salt).

Ceftezole sodium is a cephalosporin antibiotic with similar properties to those of cephalothin sodium, (see p.176). It may be administered by the intramuscular or intravenous route.

For studies of the actions and uses of ceftezole, see *Chemotherapy, Tokyo*, 1976, *24*, 573-1252.

Absorption and fate.— M. Nishida *et al.*, *Antimicrob. Ag. Chemother.*, 1976, *10*, 1.

Proprietary Names and Manufacturers

Alomen *(Schering, Ital.)*; Celoslin *(Fujisawa, Jpn)*; Falomesin *(Chugai, Jpn)*.

12546-e

Ceftizoxime Sodium *(BANM, USAN, rINNM)*.

FK-749; FR-13749; SKF-88373-Z. Sodium (*Z*)-7-[2-(2-aminothiazol-4-yl)-2-methoxyiminoacetamido]-3-cephem-4-carboxylate.

$C_{13}H_{12}N_5NaO_5S_2$=405.4.

CAS — 68401-81-0 (ceftizoxime); 68401-82-1 (sodium salt).

Pharmacopoeias. In *U.S.*

1.06 g of monograph substance is approximately equivalent to 1 g of ceftizoxime. Each g of monograph substance represents about 2.5 mmol of sodium.

A 10% solution in water has a pH of 6 to 8. The *U.S.P.* injection has a pH of 5.5 to 8.0. **Store** in airtight containers.

Aqueous solutions of ceftizoxime are reported to be stable for at least 8 hours at room temperature. Solutions of ceftizoxime may become yellow on storage, but slight discoloration does not affect potency.

Adverse Effects and Precautions

As for Cephalothin Sodium, p.176.

ADMINISTRATION IN RENAL FAILURE. For reference to the precautions to be observed in renal failure, see under Administration in Renal Failure in Uses, below.

INTERFERENCE WITH ASSAY PROCEDURES. Ceftizoxime sodium did not appear to interfere with theophylline assay by high-performance liquid chromatography.— R. H. Gannon and R. M. Levy, *Am. J. Hosp. Pharm.*, 1984, *41*, 1185.

INTERFERENCE WITH DIAGNOSTIC TESTS. Although high concentrations of ceftizoxime produced false elevations of serum and urine creatinine concentrations using the Jaffé reaction, these were considered to be above the serum-ceftizoxime concentrations achieved clinically (D.R.P. Guay *et al.*, *Am. J. Hosp. Pharm.*, 1983, *40*, 435). Peterson *et al.* (*Antimicrob. Ag. Chemother.*, 1982, *22*, 878) and LeBel *et al.*, (*Drug Intell. & clin. Pharm.*, 1983, *17*, 908) also concluded that ceftizoxime is not likely to have a significant effect on such measurements.

Antimicrobial Action and Resistance

As for Cefotaxime Sodium, p.152.

A review of the antimicrobial action of ceftizoxime. Its range and potency of activity is generally similar to that of cefotaxime. In general its activity against *Staphylococcus* spp., however, appears to be slightly less than that of cefotaxime, ceftriaxone, or cefoperazone, and slightly greater than that of ceftazidime or latamoxef. In most studies, a concentration of more than 32 μg per mL was required to inhibit 90% of clinical isolates of *Pseudomonas aeruginosa*. Many beta-lactamase-positive strains and strains resistant to carbenicillin or gentamicin were also resistant to ceftizoxime. Aminoglycosides, and also piperacillin appear to be more active than ceftizoxime against this organism.

MICs for 90% of strains of *Listeria monocytogenes* of 25 and 64 μg per mL have been reported. Other organisms against which ceftizoxime is reported to have some activity include *Yersinia enterocolitica, Vibrio cholerae*, and *Branhamella* spp.

Ceftizoxime appears to have only a low or intermediate propensity to derepress (induce) the production of inducible beta-lactamases.— D. M. Richards and R. C. Heel, *Drugs*, 1985, *29*, 281.

General studies of the antimicrobial activity of ceftizoxime: A. L. Barry *et al.*, *J. antimicrob. Chemother.*, 1982, *10*, *Suppl.* C, 25; M. F. Parry *et al.*, *Curr. ther. Res.*, 1983, *34*, 807.

Studies indicating *in-vitro* activity of ceftizoxime against various organisms: D. L. Smalley *et al.*, *Antimicrob. Ag. Chemother.*, 1983, *23*, 161 (*Pseudomonas paucimobilis*); S. Oie *et al.*, *ibid.*, *24*, 905 (*Leptospira* spp.); R. T. Nozawa *et al.*, *ibid.*, 1985, *27*, 132 (*Mycobacterium avium-intracellulare*); E. Palenque *et al.*, *ibid.*, 1986, *29*, 182 (*Brucella melitensis*).

For reference to studies comparing the bactericidal activity of some third-generation cephalosporins, see under Cefoperazone Sodium, p.148.

ACTIVITY WITH OTHER ANTIMICROBIAL AGENTS. The results of tests *in vitro* for synergism between ceftizoxime and other antibiotics have been variable and dependent on differences in strains and techniques. Synergy has been reported between ceftizoxime and aminoglycosides (including amikacin, gentamicin, and netilmicin) against a variable percentage of strains of Enterobacteriaceae and *Pseudomonas aeruginosa*. Synergy appears to have occurred less often between ceftizoxime and the anti-pseudomonal penicillins (azlocillin, mezlocillin, piperacillin, ticarcillin, and carbenicillin) against these organisms. Antagonism between ceftizoxime and another antibiotic was uncommon, except for the combination with cefoxitin against several Gram-negative species. Clavulanic acid and ceftizoxime were antagonistic against some strains of *Ps. aeruginosa*.— D. M. Richards and R. C. Heel, *Drugs*, 1985, *29*, 281.

Further references to the activity of ceftizoxime with other antimicrobial agents: C. Kim *et al.*, *J. antimicrob. Chemother.*, 1982, *10*, *Suppl.* C, 57; A. S. Bayer *et al.*, *Antimicrob. Ag. Chemother.*, 1984, *25*, 725; J. W. King and R. L. Penn, *ibid.*, 770.

Absorption and Fate

Ceftizoxime is administered parenterally as the sodium salt. After intramuscular injection of the equivalent of 0.5 and 1 g of ceftizoxime, mean peak serum concentrations of about 14 and 39 μg per mL respectively have been reported after about 1 hour. The half-life of ceftizoxime is about 1.5 hours and is prolonged in renal impairment. At least 30% of ceftizoxime in the circulation is bound to plasma proteins.

Ceftizoxime is widely distributed in body tissues and fluids; therapeutic concentrations have been achieved in the cerebrospinal fluid when the meninges are inflamed. It diffuses across the placenta and is excreted in breast milk in low concentrations.

Up to 100% of a dose is excreted unchanged in the urine within 24 hours of administration, thus achieving high urine concentrations. The concomitant administration of probenecid results in higher and more prolonged plasma concentrations of ceftizoxime.

A review of the absorption and fate of ceftizoxime.— D. M. Richards and R. C. Heel, *Drugs*, 1985, *29*, 281.

A comparison of the pharmacokinetics of ceftizoxime and cefotaxime in 6 healthy subjects given a single intravenous dose of each drug. Since ceftizoxime lacks the acetoxy group of cefotaxime it is not metabolised; it therefore achieves a higher peak serum concentration, has a longer half-life, and produces more prolonged and higher urine concentrations than cefotaxime. However, the contribution of the microbiologically active desacetyl metabolite of cefotaxime to the action of cefotaxime must be taken into account when comparing these two drugs.— N. S. Jordan *et al.*, *Curr. ther. Res.*, 1986, *40*, 133.

Further studies of the pharmacokinetics of ceftizoxime: N. Nakashima *et al.*, *J. clin. Pharmac.*, 1981, *21*, 388; *idem*, 1982, *22*, 28; L. R. Peterson *et al.*, *Antimicrob. Ag. Chemother.*, 1982, *22*, 878; J. Dubb *et al.*, *Clin. Pharmac. Ther.*, 1982, *31*, 516.

ADMINISTRATION IN LIVER DISORDERS. The elimination of ceftizoxime in the immediate postoperative period appeared normal in paediatric liver transplant patients who had no impairment of renal function.— G. J. Burckart *et al.*, *Drug Intell. & clin. Pharm.*, 1985, *19*, 450.

ADMINISTRATION IN RENAL FAILURE. For reference to the pharmacokinetics of ceftizoxime in renal failure, see under Administration in Renal Failure in Uses, below.

DRUG EXCRETION. From a study of 5 healthy subjects it was concluded that ceftizoxime is excreted in the kidney by renal tubular secretion and reabsorption as well as by glomerular filtration. Biliary excretion accounted for only 0.2 to 7.8% of the dose.— U. Gundert-Remy *et al.*, *Eur. J. clin. Pharmac.*, 1985, *28*, 463.

Uses and Administration

Ceftizoxime sodium is a cephalosporin antibiotic which is used similarly to cefotaxime sodium (see p.154) for the treatment of susceptible infections. It is administered by deep intramuscular injection, or intravenously as a slow injection over 3 to 5 minutes or as a continuous or intermittent infusion. If pain following intramuscular injection is a problem, ceftizoxime may be administered in a 0.5% solution of lignocaine hydrochloride. If 2 g of ceftizoxime is injected intramuscularly the dose should be divided between sites.

Doses are expressed in terms of the equivalent amount of ceftizoxime. It is usually given in a dose of 1 to 2 g every 8 to 12 hours. In severe or life-threatening infections 2 to 3 g every 8 hours may be given, although doses of up to 12 g daily have been used. Children over 3 months of age may be given 30 to 60 mg per kg body-weight daily in 2 to 4 divided doses; this may be increased to 100 to 150 mg per kg daily in severe infections, although higher doses have sometimes been given.

For the treatment of urinary-tract infections, a dose of 0.5 to 1 g every 12 hours has been used. A single intramuscular dose of 1 g has been given in gonorrhoea.

Doses should be modified in patients with impaired renal function.

A detailed review of the actions and uses of ceftizoxime sodium. Ceftizoxime has been shown to be clinically and bacteriologically effective in a wide variety of infections caused by Gram-negative and Gram-positive bacteria. Comparative studies have been small, but it appears to be similar in efficacy to several standard antibiotics. Infections in which ceftizoxime has been investigated include those of the genito-urinary and respiratory tracts, the skin, bones, and joints, intra-abdominal, obstetric, and gynaecological infections, bacteraemia, meningitis and gonorrhoea. It has also been investigated for the prophylaxis of surgical infections, particularly for intra-abdominal, obstetric, or gynaecological procedures. During treatment with ceftizoxime, the emergence of resistant strains of *Pseudomonas aeruginosa*, *Staphylococcus aureus*, *Klebsiella oxytoca*, and *Enterobacter cloacae* has been reported. As with several other third-generation cephalosporins, ceftizoxime cannot be considered a drug of choice for infections caused by Gram-positive cocci, or of known or suspected pseudomonal infections. Its relatively low *in-vitro* activity against *Bacteroides fragilis* and enterococci may restrict its use in intra-abdominal, and obstetric and gynaecological infections.— D. M. Richards and R. C. Heel, *Drugs*, 1985, *29*, 281.

Further brief reviews of the actions and uses of ceftizoxime sodium: *Med. Lett.*, 1983, *25*, 109; *Lancet*, 1984, *1*, 260.

For proceedings of a symposium on ceftizoxime sodium, see *J. antimicrob. Chemother.*, 1982, *10*, *Suppl.* C, 1–350.

For reference to the use of ceftizoxime in association with ticarcillin for febrile episodes in non-neutropenic patients with cancer, see Ticarcillin Sodium, p.325.

ADMINISTRATION IN RENAL FAILURE. The manufacturers recommend that the dosage regimen of ceftizoxime sodium be modified in patients with renal impairment according to the creatinine clearance (CC), after an initial loading dose of 0.5 to 1 g. For patients with a CC of 50 to 79 mL per minute the equivalent of ceftizoxime 0.5 to 1.5 g may be given every 8 hours according to the severity of the infection. For those with a CC of 5 to 49 mL per minute, 0.25 to 1 g every 12 hours may be given, and for a CC of less than 5 mL per minute ceftizoxime may be administered in a dose of 0.25 to 0.5 g every 24 hours, or 0.5 to 1 g every 48 hours. A dose supplement is not required following haemodialysis, however the dose should be given at the end of the dialysis session.

The half-life for ceftizoxime of 1.4 hours was increased to 30 hours in end-stage renal failure. In patients with a glomerular filtration-rate (GFR) of greater than 50 mL per minute 45 to 100% of the normal dose could be given; in those with a GFR of 10 to 50 mL per minute the dose should be reduced to 10 to 45%; and in those with a GFR of less than 10 mL per minute it should be reduced to 5 to 10%.— W. M. Bennett *et al.*, *Am. J. Kidney Dis.*, 1983, *3*, 155.

Intravenous ceftizoxime 3 g was administered to 12 patients undergoing continuous ambulatory peritoneal dialysis (CAPD). The overall serum clearance of ceftizoxime was 17.1 mL per minute. This was composed of the renal clearance of 0.8 mL per minute, the peritoneal clearance of 2.8 mL per minute, and the nonrenal clearance. A dose of 3 g every 48 hours would achieve adequate concentrations of ceftizoxime in peritoneal dialysate for most susceptible organisms in such patients, however administration every 12 hours may be required for those organisms which are less susceptible.— E. D. Burgess and A. D. Blair, *Antimicrob. Ag. Chemother.*, 1983, *24*, 237. After intravenous administration of ceftizoxime in patients on CAPD, approximately 4 to 5% of the dose was eliminated through the peritoneal membrane in 6 hours. After intraperitoneal administration, ceftizoxime was rapidly absorbed into the central vascular compartment, and effective concentrations were achieved in serum and in peritoneal dialysate.— M. L. Gross *et al.*, *Clin. Pharmac. Ther.*, 1983, *34*, 673.

Further studies of the pharmacokinetics of ceftizoxime in patients with renal failure: R. E. Cutler *et al.*, *J. antimicrob. Chemother.*, 1982, *10*, *Suppl.* C, 91; M. Ohkawa *et al.*, *Antimicrob. Ag. Chemother.*, 1982, *22*, 308; S. F. Kowalsky *et al.*, *ibid.*, 1983, *24*, 151.

See also under Peritonitis, below.

GONORRHOEA. In a study involving 219 patients with gonorrhoea caused by non-penicillinase-producing *Neisseria gonorrhoeae*, a single intramuscular dose of ceftizoxime 0.5 or 1 g was considered to be as effective as intramuscular procaine penicillin 4.8 g in association with probenecid 1 g by mouth.— B. Lutz *et al.*, *J. antimicrob. Chemother.*, 1982, *10*, *Suppl.* C, 229.

MENINGITIS. Twelve infants and children and 6 adults with proven bacterial meningitis were treated with intravenous ceftizoxime 200 mg per kg body-weight daily in 6 divided doses, up to a maximum of 12 g daily. Ceftizoxime was administered until the patient had been afebrile for 5 days, or for a minimum of 10 days for meningitis caused by *Neisseria meningitidis* or *Streptococcus pneumoniae*, or 14 days for that caused by *Haemophilus influenzae*. All patients had a satisfactory clinical response to treatment, becoming afebrile after 1 to 14 days of therapy, and having negative CSF cultures after 24 to 48 hours. The MBC of ceftizoxime against all recovered bacterial isolates, which included *Escherichia coli*, *H. influenzae*, *Str. pneumoniae*, *N. meningitidis*, and an α-streptococcus were well below the measured concentrations of antibiotic in the spinal fluid.— G. D. Overturf *et al.*, *Antimicrob. Ag. Chemother.*, 1984, *25*, 258.

PERITONITIS. Ceftizoxime has been administered intravenously in a dose of 500 mg every 12 to 24 hours for the treatment of bacterial peritonitis in patients on continuous ambulatory peritoneal dialysis.— D. K. Scott and D. E. Roberts, *Pharm. J.*, 1985, *1*, 621.

PNEUMONIA. Report of a double-blind study involving 135 patients with bacterial pneumonia who had at least one of several risk factors including alcoholism, chronic obstructive pulmonary disease, corticosteroid therapy, diabetes mellitus, age over 70 years, or presence of a solid tumour. They received intravenous or intramuscular therapy with either ceftizoxime 2 to 4 g every 8 hours, latamoxef 2 to 4 g every 8 hours, or cefotaxime 1 to 2 g every 4 hours. Of the 84 patients who were evaluable, clinical cure was achieved in 20 of 22 (91%), 31 of 35 (89%), and 23 of 27 (85%), and bacteriological cure in 20 (91%), 31 (89%), and 26 (96%) of patients in the three groups, respectively. It was concluded that the three drugs were similarly effective in such patients, but that there was a higher incidence of adverse effects associated with latamoxef administration.— B. G. Yangco *et al.*, *J. antimicrob. Chemother.*, 1987, *19*, 239.

Further references to the use of ceftizoxime sodium in the treatment of pneumonia: J. R. Ebright *et al.*, *Curr. ther. Res.*, 1983, *33*, 39 (comparison with cephamandole).

PREGNANCY AND THE NEONATE. Twenty neonates and infants aged 1 to 53 days were treated for suspected bacterial infections with intramuscular or intravenous ceftizoxime 140 to 300 mg per kg body-weight daily in 3 divided doses. Clinical response was considered satisfactory in 13 of 15 evaluable cases. In one patient, *Serratia marcescens* sensitive to ceftizoxime *in vitro* persisted despite treatment.— T. Yamauchi *et al.*, *J. antimicrob. Chemother.*, 1982, *10*, *Suppl.* C, 297.

SEPTICAEMIA. For reference to the use of ceftizoxime sodium in the treatment of septicaemia, see under Cefotaxime Sodium, p.155.

SURGICAL INFECTION PROPHYLAXIS. Report of a small study failing to show any advantage for the prophylactic use of ceftizoxime in major gynaecological surgery.— A. Hitchcock *et al.*, *Br. J. clin. Pract.*, 1987, *41*, 879.

Preparations

Ceftizoxime Sodium Injection *(U.S.P.)*. Store in the frozen state.

Sterile Ceftizoxime Sodium *(U.S.P.)*

Proprietary Preparations

Cefizox *(Wellcome, UK)*. *Injection*, powder for reconstitution, ceftizoxime 0.5, 1, and 2 g (as sodium salt).

Proprietary Names and Manufacturers

Cefizox *(Pharmuka, Fr.; Smith Kline & French, Spain; Wellcome, UK; Smith Kline & French, USA)*; Ceftix *(Boehringer Mannheim, Ger.)*; Epocelin *(CEPA, Spain)*;Eposerin *(Farmitalia, Ital.)*.

12547-l

Ceftriaxone Sodium *(BANM, USAN, rINNM)*.

Ro-13-9904. (*Z*)-7-[2-(2-Aminothiazol-4-yl)-2-methoxyiminoacetamido]-3-[(2,5-dihydro-6-hydroxy-2-methyl-5-oxo-1,2,4-triazin-3-yl)thiomethyl]-3-cephem-4-carboxylic acid, disodium salt.

$C_{18}H_{16}N_8Na_2O_7S_3$=598.6.

CAS — 73384-59-5 (ceftriaxone); 74578-69-1 (disodium salt).

Pharmacopoeias. U.S. includes Sterile Ceftriaxone Sodium.

1.08 g of monograph substance is approximately equivalent to 1 g of ceftriaxone. Each g of monograph substance represents about 3.3 mmol of sodium.

A 10% solution in water has a pH of 6 to 8.

Solutions of ceftriaxone sodium of up to 100 mg per mL in water, sodium chloride 0.9% injection, or glucose 5 or 10% injection, are reported to be **stable** for 3 days at 25° and for 10 days at 4°. Solutions of 250 mg per mL in water, sodium chloride 0.9% injection, or glucose 5% injection, are stable for 24 hours at 25° and 3 days at 4°. Solutions of ceftriaxone sodium may darken on storage.

Adverse Effects

As for Cephalothin Sodium, p.176.

A report of the clinical adverse reactions to ceftriaxone from studies of its safety and efficacy. Of 2640 patients treated with the drug, 215 (8.1%) experienced adverse effects considered to be possibly or probably related to treatment. These were: local reactions including phlebitis in 49 (1.86%); hypersensitivity reactions such as rash, pruritus, fever or chills, bronchospasm and serum sickness in 73 (2.77%); headache or dizziness in 7 (0.27%); gastro-intestinal reactions including diarrhoea, nausea or vomiting, abdominal pain, colitis, jaundice, dysgeusia, flatulence and dyspepsia in 91 (3.45%); and candidal overgrowth in 6 (0.23%). Other reactions included diaphoresis (5 patients), flushing (3), a disulfiram reaction to alcohol (1), palpitations (1), and epistaxis (1).— B. L. Moskovitz, *Am. J. Med.*, 1984, *77, Suppl.* 4C, 84. In the same group of patients, 479 of 2526 patients (19%) evaluated had one or more abnormal laboratory test values considered to be possibly or probably related to administration of ceftriaxone. Haematological abnormalities occurred in 14.14% including eosinophilia, thrombocytosis, leucopenia, and thrombocytopenia. Abnormal values for tests of hepatic function occurred in 5% of patients; abnormalities for renal function tests were reported in 1.4% and included increases in blood-urea nitrogen and creatinine, and abnormalities in urinalysis.— M. Oakes *et al.*, *ibid.*, 89.

EFFECTS ON THE BLOOD. Hypoprothrombinaemia associated with clinically significant bleeding has been observed in a patient on chronic haemodialysis given ceftriaxone; the defect was rapidly corrected by administration of vitamin K (A. Haubenstock *et al.*, *Lancet*, 1983, *1*, 1215). In a study of 10 patients given ceftriaxone 1 g daily (G. Agnelli, *et al.*, *Antimicrob. Ag. Chemother.*, 1986, *29*, 1108) prolongation of the bleeding time and a reduction in factor VII activity was observed, although the degree of the effect was considered unlikely to be of clinical significance. Ceftriaxone contains a triazine ring instead of a methylthiotetrazole side-chain. The presence of a sulphydryl group in ceftriaxone and also in cephalosporins with a methylthiotetrazole side-chain, such as cephamandole, was considered responsible for the effect of these agents on blood.

EFFECTS ON THE GASTRO-INTESTINAL TRACT. In reviewing the adverse effects of ceftriaxone, Richards *et al.*, (*Drugs*, 1984, *27*, 469) noted that effects on the gastro-intestinal tract, such as soft stools, diarrhoea, stomatitis, nausea, and vomiting have generally been the most frequently reported, occurring in about 2 to 3% of patients, although in some individual studies the incidence of diarrhoea had been higher. In a study of 6 healthy subjects given a single 2-g dose of ceftriaxone, Ambrose, *et al.*, (*J. antimicrob. Chemother.*, 1985, *15*, 319) isolated *Clostridium difficile* from the faeces of 2; toxin was also detected in one. Arvidsson *et al.*, (*ibid.*, 1982, *10*, 207) considered that suppression of aerobic and anaerobic colonic flora, and colonisation by potentially pathogenic bacteria and yeasts in subjects given ceftriaxone could be attributed to the relatively high biliary excretion of this drug.

EFFECTS ON THE KIDNEY. In a review of ceftriaxone, it was noted that the administration of ceftriaxone 3 g daily for 3 days to 10 healthy subjects caused no rise in urinary brush border-bound alanine aminopeptidase activity, considered to be a useful parameter for determining the presence of tubular lesions. A literature survey of 3961 patients treated with ceftriaxone in therapeutic trials had only found 6 instances of elevated serum creatinine or blood urea nitrogen concentrations.— D. M. Richards *et al.*, *Drugs*, 1984, *27*, 469.

Precautions

As for Cephalothin Sodium, p.177.

ADMINISTRATION IN LIVER DISORDERS AND RENAL FAILURE. For reference to the precautions to be observed in liver disorders and renal failure, see under Administration in Liver Disorders and Administration in Renal Failure in Uses, below.

INTERACTIONS. For mention of a disulfiram reaction to alcohol during therapy with ceftriaxone, see Adverse Effects, above.

For the effects of other drugs on the antimicrobial activity of ceftriaxone, see below under Antimicrobial Action.

INTERFERENCE WITH ASSAY PROCEDURES. Ceftriaxone sodium did not appear to interfere with theophylline assay by high-performance liquid chromatography.— R. H. Gannon and R. M. Levy, *Am. J. Hosp. Pharm.*, 1984, *41*, 1185.

INTERFERENCE WITH DIAGNOSTIC TESTS. In concentrations of up to 1.5 mg per mL ceftriaxone did not interfere with the measurement of serum creatinine using the Jaffé reaction.— M. LeBel *et al.*, *Drug Intell. & clin. Pharm.*, 1983, *17*, 908. See also D. R. P. Guay *et al.*, *Am. J. Hosp. Pharm.*, 1983, *40*, 435.

PREGNANCY AND THE NEONATE. A study performed on blood samples from icteric neonates suggesting that ceftriaxone displaces bilirubin from albumin binding sites. This effect was significant at concentrations obtained during therapeutic use, and therefore caution was considered necessary in administering the drug to high-risk jaundiced neonates.— J.-M. Gulian *et al.*, *J. antimicrob. Chemother.*, 1987, *19*, 823.

Antimicrobial Action and Resistance

As for Cefotaxime Sodium, p.152.

A review of the antimicrobial action of ceftriaxone; the spectrum and potency of its activity is generally very similar to that of cefotaxime. Results of its activity against *Pseudomonas aeruginosa* are very variable, although at least 32 µg per mL was generally required to inhibit 90% of isolates. It was usually less active than aminoglycosides; it also tended to be less active than piperacillin, similar in activity to ticarcillin, and more active than carbenicillin, although many studies specifically tested carbenicillin-resistant or beta-lactamase-producing strains of *Ps. aeruginosa*. Ceftriaxone was one of the most active of all beta-lactam antibiotics yet studied against *Neisseria gonorrhoeae*, with 90% of isolates being inhibited by 0.025 µg or less per mL. Less commonly encountered organisms against which ceftriaxone has been reported to have some activity *in vitro* include some *Aeromonas, Branhamella*, and *Yersinia* spp. and *Nocardia asteroides*.

In general the beta-lactamase stability pattern of ceftriaxone was similar in rate and percentage of inactivation to that of cefotaxime and cefuroxime. There has generally been little difference observed between the MIC and MBC values for ceftriaxone, and little inoculum effect against most Gram-positive and Gram-negative organisms.— D. M. Richards *et al.*, *Drugs*, 1984, *27*, 469.

General studies of the antimicrobial activity of ceftriaxone *in vitro*: M. F. Parry *et al.*, *Curr. ther. Res.*, 1984, *36*, 86; A. M. Emmerson *et al.*, *Curr. med. Res. Opinion*, 1985, *9*, 480.

Studies indicating *in-vitro* activity of ceftriaxone against various organisms: R. Yogev *et al.*, *Antimicrob. Ag. Chemother.*, 1986, *29*, 179 (*Actinobacillus actinomycetemcomitans*); E. E. Stobberingh *et al.*, *J. antimicrob. Chemother.*, 1984, *13*, 55 (*Branhamella catarrhalis*); J. Bosch *et al.*, *J. antimicrob. Chemother.*, 1986, *17*, 459; E. Palenque *et al.*, *Antimicrob. Ag. Chemother.*, 1986, *29*, 182 (both *Brucella melitensis*).

ACTIVITY WITH OTHER ANTIMICROBIAL AGENTS. In reviewing *in-vitro* studies of combinations of ceftriaxone with other antimicrobial agents, ceftriaxone was generally synergistic with various aminoglycoside antibiotics against 20 to 80% of *Pseudomonas aeruginosa* strains tested; synergism had also been observed against some aminoglycoside-resistant strains. It had been reported, however, not to be synergistic with tobramycin in any of 18 multidrug-resistant strains of *Ps. aeruginosa*. Some instances of antagonism between ceftriaxone and aminoglycosides have been reported against this organism. Combinations of ceftriaxone and aminoglycosides have in addition been shown to be synergistic against members of the Enterobacteriaceae.

Synergy with antipseudomonal penicillins, such as carbenicillin, piperacillin, and mezlocillin, has been reported against *Ps. aeruginosa* and against various of the Enterobacteriaceae. Synergism has also been demonstrated with dicloxacillin against *Ps. aeruginosa*, and with ampicillin against *Neisseria meningitidis*; antagonism has been reported with cefoxitin, a strong inducer of beta-lactamases, against some bacteria.— D. M. Richards *et al.*, *Drugs*, 1984, *27*, 469.

A study of the activity of combinations of beta-lactam antibiotics against neonatal meningitis pathogens. When ceftriaxone was combined with benzylpenicillin, ampicillin, or piperacillin in chequerboard studies, synergism was observed for a low percentage of strains of *Escherichia coli*, a higher percentage of Group B streptococci, and for the majority of strains of *Listeria monocytogenes*, although ceftriaxone was not active against the latter organism when tested alone. However, killing curve studies did not generally correlate with these results.— J. A. A. Hoogkamp-Korstanje, *J. antimicrob. Chemother.*, 1985, *16*, 327.

A combination of ceftriaxone and fosfomycin was synergistic *in vitro* against some methicillin-susceptible and methicillin-resistant strains of *Staphylococcus aureus* and *Staph. epidermidis*. There was, however, poor correlation between chequerboard and timed killing curve methods.— R. J. Courcol and G. R. Martin (letter), *J. antimicrob. Chemother.*, 1987, *19*, 276.

RESISTANCE. Resistant mutants of *Pseudomonas aeruginosa* were produced *in vitro* after incubation with ceftriaxone. These mutants showed cross-resistance to a range of other beta-lactam antibiotics, and although they produced a cephalosporinase, the significance of this in the mechanism of resistance is unknown.— R. H. K. Eng *et al.*, *J. antimicrob. Chemother.*, 1986, *17*, 717.

Development of resistant strains of *Pseudomonas aeruginosa* in 2 of 5 cystic fibrosis patients treated for chest infections with intravenous ceftriaxone alone, and in 3 of 4 who were also given tobramycin. The majority of the resistant strains exhibited non-reversible derepression of a chromosomally-mediated beta-lactamase. Thus the value of ceftriaxone in cystic fibrosis chest infections, and its potentially-synergistic combination with tobramycin, may be limited.— A. Paull and J. R. Morgan, *J. antimicrob. Chemother.*, 1986, *18*, 635.

Absorption and Fate

Ceftriaxone is administered by injection as the sodium salt. After intramuscular injection mean peak plasma concentrations of about 43 and 80 µg per mL have been reported about 2 hours after the equivalent of 0.5 and 1 g of ceftriaxone respectively. Ceftriaxone demonstrates non-linear, dose-dependent pharmacokinetics. This is due to binding to plasma proteins which varies from 85 to 95% in a dose-dependent manner. The elimination half-life of ceftriaxone is not dependent on the dose and varies between 6 and 9 hours; it is prolonged in neonates.

Ceftriaxone is widely distributed in body tissues and fluids; therapeutic concentrations have been achieved in the cerebrospinal fluid when the meninges are inflamed. It diffuses across the placenta and is excreted in breast milk in low concentrations.

About 40 to 65% of a dose of ceftriaxone is excreted unchanged in the urine, principally by glomerular filtration; the remainder is excreted in the bile and is ultimately found in the faeces as microbiologically inactive compounds.

A review of the absorption and fate of ceftriaxone.— D. M. Richards *et al.*, *Drugs*, 1984, *27*, 469.

From a computer-simulated pharmacokinetic study it was considered that for a drug like ceftriaxone, which demonstrates concentration-dependent protein binding, the time course of the unbound drug concentration is more relevant than that of total drug.— P. J. McNamara *et al.*, *Eur. J. clin. Pharmac.*, 1983, *25*, 399. An extension of these principles to the pharmacokinetics of ceftriaxone in uraemic patients.— *idem*, 407.

A review of age-associated changes in the pharmacokinetics of ceftriaxone. The half-life was longest and showed the greatest interindividual variability in newborns. It fell rapidly with increasing age up to 6 years and then increased steadily with age throughout the remainder of the life-span. The kidneys eliminated about 70% of a dose of ceftriaxone in newborns, and this fraction declined as age increased up to 6 years. In adults, the kidneys eliminated about 40 to 50% of a dose and this fraction remained relatively constant with age. Plasma binding affinity and capacity for ceftriaxone were reduced in neonates, infants, and young children compared with adult values.— W. L. Hayton and K. Stoeckel, *Clin. Pharmacokinet.*, 1986, *11*, 76. In a study of the effects of age on ceftriaxone kinetics, it was concluded that dosage adjustment in ceftriaxone therapy is probably not necessary for elderly subjects unless they are debilitated, malnourished, or have marked impairment in renal function.— J. R. Luderer *et al.*, *Clin. Pharmac. Ther.*, 1984, *35*, 19.

Further references to the absorption and fate of ceftriaxone: P. Salvador *et al.*, *Antimicrob. Ag. Chemother.*, 1983, *23*, 583 (pharmacokinetics in patients with neoplastic disease).

ADMINISTRATION IN LIVER DISORDERS. For reference to the pharmacokinetics of ceftriaxone in liver disorders, see under Administration in Liver Disorders in Uses, below.

ADMINISTRATION IN RENAL FAILURE. For reference to the pharmacokinetics of ceftriaxone in renal failure, see under Administration in Renal Failure in Uses, below.

DIFFUSION INTO BODY TISSUES AND FLUIDS. Mean concentrations of ceftriaxone in the CSF after the administration of a single dose of ceftriaxone 50 mg per kg body-weight (as the sodium salt), by intravenous infusion over 10 to 15 minutes to 19 infants and children with bacterial meningitis, were 2.1, 2.2, 3.2, 2.5, and 4.2 μg per mL, 0.5, 1, 2, 4, and 6 hours after the dose respectively. When ceftriaxone was administered as an initial dose of 75 mg per kg followed by 50 mg per kg every 8 hours, CSF concentrations ranged from 1.8 μg per mL at 0.5 hour to 7.2 μg per mL at 6 hours after the first dose, and from 5.2 μg per mL at 0.5 hour to 4.8 μg per mL at 6 hours after multiple doses. When ceftriaxone was administered in the same dosage regimen, but at 12-hourly intervals, the mean CSF concentration 12 hours after the first dose was 2.8 μg per mL, and 1.6 μg per mL after multiple doses.— M. Del Rio *et al.*, *Antimicrob. Ag. Chemother.*, 1982, *22*, 622. See also R. Latif and A. S. Dajani, *ibid.*, 1983, *23*, 46; R. W. Steele *et al.*, *ibid.*, 191; M. D. Reed *et al.*, *Clin. Pharm.*, 1983, *2*, 558.

Ceftriaxone was administered intravenously over 30 minutes to 14 adult patients either as a single 2-g dose or as three 2-g doses at 12-hourly intervals. The mean concentration of ceftriaxone in the CSF was 2.12 μg per mL in 11 patients with uninflamed meninges, and 2.03 μg per mL in 3 who were recovering from meningitis.— P. H. Chandrasekar *et al.*, *J. antimicrob. Chemother.*, 1984, *14*, 427.

Further studies of the diffusion of ceftriaxone into various body tissues and fluids: C. S. Bryan *et al.*, *Antimicrob. Ag. Chemother.*, 1984, *25*, 37 (sternal bone and atrial appendage); G. Benoni *et al.*, *J. antimicrob. Chemother.*, 1985, *16*, 267 (ascitic fluid); J. R. Morgan *et al.*, *ibid.*, 367 (synovial fluid); G. Benoni *et al.*, *Antimicrob. Ag. Chemother.*, 1986, *29*, 906 (pleural fluid); F. Lucht *et al.* (letter), *J. antimicrob. Chemother.*, 1986, *17*, 545 (liver).

DRUG EXCRETION. A study of the biliary excretion of ceftriaxone in 19 patients undergoing cholecystectomy and given varying dosage regimens of the drug. The ratio of bile to plasma ceftriaxone concentrations after single and multiple doses exceeded 1 in most subjects but showed considerable inter-subject variation, as well as day-to-day variability in some subjects. Concentrations of ceftriaxone in the bile were considered to be adequate for the treatment of biliary-tract infections caused by most susceptible organisms.— W. L. Hayton *et al.*, *Eur. J. clin. Pharmac.*, 1986, *30*, 445. See also W. Hayton and K. Stoeckel (letter), *ibid.*, *31*, 123; D. P. Maudgal *et al.*, *Br. J. clin. Pharmac.*, 1982, *14*, 213.

PREGNANCY AND THE NEONATE. A study of the distribution of ceftriaxone to the foetus, and its penetration into breast milk.— D. A. Kafetzis *et al.*, *Antimicrob. Ag. Chemother.*, 1983, *23*, 870.

Uses and Administration

Ceftriaxone sodium is a cephalosporin antibiotic which is used similarly to cefotaxime sodium (see p.154) for the treatment of susceptible infections. It is administered by intermittent intravenous infusion or by deep intramuscular injection. If pain following intramuscular injection is a problem, ceftriaxone sodium may be administered in a 1.0% solution of lignocaine hydrochloride. Doses are expressed in terms of the equivalent amount of ceftriaxone. It is usually given in a dose of 1 to 2 g daily as a single dose or in 2 divided doses. In severe infections up to 4 g daily may be given. Children may be given 50 to 75 mg per kg body-weight daily in 2 divided doses.

For the treatment of meningitis in adults and children, ceftriaxone is given in a dose of 100 mg per kg daily in two divided doses, sometimes with a loading dose of 75 mg per kg. A single intramuscular dose of 250 mg is recommended for the treatment of gonorrhoea in adults.

Ceftriaxone is also used for surgical infection prophylaxis; a single dose of 1 g is administered 0.5 to 2 hours prior to surgery.

A review of the actions and uses of ceftriaxone sodium. It was considered worthy of consideration in the initial treatment of seriously ill patients having infections of undetermined aetiology when Gram-negative aerobes (other than *Pseudomonas* spp.) are the suspected pathogens and in patients with infections due to Gram-negative organisms with suspected or demonstrated resistance to other antibiotics. The unusually long half-life of ceftriaxone, allowing once or twice daily administrations could have significant cost and convenience benefits in some clinical situations.

Results from a small number of patients with infections caused by *Pseudomonas aeruginosa* and other *Pseudomonas* spp. suggest that ceftriaxone may not be suitable as sole therapy for such infections, although the doses used may have been insufficient. Many of the treatment failures that have occurred have been due to the emergence of resistant organisms. Ceftriaxone does, however, appear more promising in urinary-tract infections due to *Pseudomonas* spp; this may be because of the extensive excretion of unchanged drug in the urine. However, there have been recurrences in many patients with complicated infections.— D. M. Richards *et al.*, *Drugs*, 1984, *27*, 469.

Further reviews: *Med. Lett.*, 1985, *27*, 37.

Reports of the use of ceftriaxone sodium in the treatment of serious bacterial infections: in children.— A. L. Kovatch *et al.*, *Curr. ther. Res.*, 1983, *34*, 946; S. C. Aronoff *et al.*, *Antimicrob. Ag. Chemother.*, 1983, *24*, 663; T. Chonmaitree *et al.*, *J. antimicrob. Chemother.*, 1984, *13*, 511; B. L. Congeni *et al.*, *Antimicrob. Ag. Chemother.*, 1985, *27*, 181.

In adults.— J. S. Epstein *et al.*, *Antimicrob. Ag. Chemother.*, 1982, *21*, 402; R. W. Bradsher, *ibid.*, *22*, 36; M. J. Maslow *et al.*, *ibid.*, 103; M. J. Bittner *et al.*, *ibid.*, 1983, *23*, 261; L. J. Eron *et al.*, *J. antimicrob. Chemother.*, 1983, *12*, 65; I. M. Hoepelman *et al.*, *Lancet*, 1988, *1*, 1305.

ADMINISTRATION. Ceftriaxone has been administered into the eye by intravitreal injection.— T. S. Lesar and R. G. Fiscella, *Drug Intell. & clin. Pharm.*, 1985, *19*, 642.

ADMINISTRATION IN THE ELDERLY. For reference to possible dosage adjustments in elderly patients, see Absorption and Fate, above.

ADMINISTRATION IN LIVER DISORDERS. A study of the pharmacokinetics of ceftriaxone in patients with various liver disorders. Dosage adjustments should not be required in patients with chronic liver disease because of the relative safety of cephalosporins, including ceftriaxone, over a wide range of concentrations. However, on the basis of plasma concentrations of unbound drug, the dose could be decreased by half in patients with severe cirrhosis with or without ascites. Dosage adjustment will be required in patients who have serious impairment of both hepatic and renal function.— K. Stoeckel *et al.*, *Clin. Pharmac. Ther.*, 1984, *36*, 500. See also F. Lucht *et al.* (letter), *J. antimicrob. Chemother.*, 1986, *17*, 545.

ADMINISTRATION IN RENAL FAILURE. A study of the pharmacokinetics of ceftriaxone in patients with varying degrees of renal impairment. In patients with a creatinine clearance greater than 5 mL per minute the elimination of ceftriaxone is only moderately reduced and therefore dosage adjustment should not be necessary if the dose does not exceed 2 g daily. Since a substantially prolonged half-life has been observed in a small number of patients maintained on haemodialysis, plasma-ceftriaxone concentrations should be monitored in such patients. Ceftriaxone is not significantly removed during haemodialysis, therefore a supplemental dose should not be necessary. I. H. Patel *et al.*, *Antimicrob. Ag. Chemother.*, 1984, *25*, 438.

The pharmacokinetics of ceftriaxone in patients undergoing continuous ambulatory peritoneal dialysis (CAPD). After administration by the intravenous route only 4.5% of a dose was eliminated by the peritoneal route. After intraperitoneal administration, ceftriaxone was rapidly absorbed into the vascular compartment, however only about 40% was absorbed from the peritoneal space. A dose of 1 g intraperitoneally every 24 hours was suggested for the treatment of bacterial peritonitis in patients on CAPD.— H. Albin *et al.*, *Eur. J. clin. Pharmac.*, 1986, *31*, 479.

Further studies of the pharmacokinetics of ceftriaxone in patients with renal impairment: D. Cohen *et al.*, *Antimicrob. Ag. Chemother.*, 1983, *24*, 529; K. Stoeckel *et al.*, *Clin. Pharmac. Ther.*, 1983, *33*, 633; T. -Y. Ti *et al.*, *Antimicrob. Ag. Chemother.*, 1984, *25*, 83; S. F. Kowalsky *et al.*, *Clin. Pharm.*, 1985, *4*, 177.

ENTERIC INFECTIONS. *Shigellosis.* Patients with stool cultures positive for *Shigella* spp. were randomised to treatment with either a single intravenous injection of ceftriaxone 1 g (34 patients), or ampicillin 4 g (30), or to placebo (30). Ceftriaxone and ampicillin were no more effective than placebo in resolving diarrhoea, abdominal pain, or tenesmus, although they did reduce the mean duration of fever and stool frequencies on certain days. The mean duration of positive stool cultures for *Shigella* spp. was reduced significantly by ampicillin treatment, but not by ceftriaxone. Ceftriaxone was, however, considered to be potentially useful for achieving a clinical cure of shigellosis in areas where resistance to ampicillin and co-trimoxazole occurs, although no patients with ampicillin-resistant organisms were treated with ceftriaxone in this study.— I. Kabir *et al.*, *Antimicrob. Ag. Chemother.*, 1986, *29*, 645.

Typhoid fever. Fourteen patients with bacteraemic typhoid fever were treated with intravenous ceftriaxone 50 to 60 mg per kg body-weight daily given in 2 divided doses for 7 days. In 10 patients defervescence occurred after 6 or less days of treatment. Failure to defervesce in 3 patients was due either to associated medical conditions or to thrombophlebitis or drug fever associated with ceftriaxone therapy; in the other patient it was due to treatment failure. Thirteen patients were considered cured although one was a convalescent carrier of *Salmonella typhi*. No relapse was observed in the 11 patients who were followed up for a period of 1 to 8 months.— T. -Y. Ti *et al.*, *Antimicrob. Ag. Chemother.*, 1985, *28*, 540.

LYME DISEASE. In a study of 23 patients with late Lyme disease ceftriaxone 2 g intravenously every 12 hours for 14 days was found to be more effective than penicillin 4 million units intravenously every 4 hours for 10 days, as primary therapy for late Lyme borreliosis; after treatment only 1 of 13 patients given ceftriaxone, but 5 of 10 given penicillin were considered to be treatment failures. In an additional 31 patients given ceftriaxone 2 or 4 g daily, 4 patients were considered to be treatment failures; the rates of response to the 2 doses of ceftriaxone were similar. Three of the 5 patients unresponsive to ceftriaxone had been treated with corticosteroids, and an association between previous steroid treatment and lack of response to ceftriaxone was considered to be significant.— R. J. Dattwyler *et al.*, *Lancet*, 1988, *1*, 1191.

MENINGITIS. Ceftriaxone sodium has been suggested as an alternative to conventional treatment for meningitis due to both Gram-positive and Gram-negative organisms. Comparative studies have shown twice-daily treatment with ceftriaxone sodium to be as effective as conventional treatment with ampicillin and chloramphenicol (M. del Rio *et al.*, *Lancet*, 1983, *1*, 1241; S.C. Aronoff *et al.*, *J. antimicrob. Chemother.*, 1984, *13*, 143), or with ampicillin and either chloramphenicol or gentamicin (B.L. Congeni, *Antimicrob. Ag. Chemother.*, 1984, *25*, 40) in a wide age range of patients, particularly infants and children with infections due to *Haemophilus influenzae*. Although del Rio *et al.* showed ceftriaxone to have a greater mean bactericidal activity in CSF than conventional treatment, they could only observe a trend towards more rapid sterilisation. In most studies ceftriaxone sodium caused a higher incidence of diarrhoea than conventional therapy.

In the above studies ceftriaxone sodium was administered intravenously in a dose equivalent to ceftriaxone 50 mg per kg body-weight twice daily, with or without a loading dose of 75 mg per kg. It has been suggested, however, (E. Martin, *Lancet*, 1983, *2*, 43) that a dose of 100 mg per kg once daily may produce a higher amount of unbound drug available to cross the blood-brain barrier and hence a more rapid sterilisation of the CSF. Ceftriaxone sodium is usually given for at least 10 days, except for the treatment of meningitis caused by *Neisseria meningitidis*, when 7 days may be sufficient. Although Lin *et al.* (*J. Am. med. Ass.*, 1985, *253*, 3559) demonstrated treatment for 7 or 10 days to be equally effective for bacterial meningitis due to various organisms, they could not recommend that the shorter regimen be given routinely to all patients.

See also under Cefotaxime Sodium, p.155.

For the use of ceftriaxone in gonococcal meningitis, see under Sexually Transmitted Diseases, below.

Prophylaxis. A single dose of intramuscular ceftriaxone 125 mg was effective in eradicating pharyngeal carriage of *Neisseria meningitidis* in 29 patients who were being treated for anogenital gonorrhoea. Of 9 patients treated with intramuscular spectinomycin 2 g, only one was cured of meningococcal carriage.— F. N. Judson and J. M. Ehret (letter), *Lancet*, 1984, *2*, 1462.

In a study of 347 contacts of patients with meningococcal disease, a single intramuscular dose of ceftriaxone 250 mg for adults or 125 mg for children under 15 years old, was significantly more effective, in eradicating pharyngeal carriage of meningococci, than rifampicin 600 mg for adults or 10 mg per kg body-weight per dose for children given twice daily for 2 days; six days after treatment ceftriaxone had eradicated carriage in 66 of 68 (97%) persons compared with 27 of 36 (75%) in the rifampicin group. Ceftriaxone was considered to be an attractive alternative to rifampicin for prophylaxis of meningococcal disease in contacts.— B. Schwartz *et al.*, *Lancet*, 1988, *1*, 1239.

PELVIC INFLAMMATORY DISEASE. For the use of ceftriaxone in the treatment of pelvic inflammatory disease, see under Cefoxitin Sodium, p.159.

PERITONITIS. For reference to the use of intraperitoneal ceftriaxone sodium for the treatment of peritonitis, see

Administration in Renal Failure, above.

PREGNANCY AND THE NEONATE. Ceftriaxone 50 mg per kg body-weight as a single intravenous or intramuscular injection daily for up to 5 days was found to be safe and effective in a study involving 104 neonates with suspected or proven infections. Colonisation with resistant organisms was potentially the most serious complication.— J. James *et al.*, *J. Infect.*, 1985, *11*, 25.

Ophthalmia neonatorum. One-hundred and twenty-two neonates in Nairobi, Kenya with positive ocular cultures for *Neisseria gonorrhoeae* were treated with one of the following three regimens: a single intramuscular dose of ceftriaxone 125 mg plus ocular washes with cooled boiled water 3 to 4 times daily until the ocular discharge resolved (61 patients), a single intramuscular dose of kanamycin 75 mg plus gentamicin 1% eye ointment four times daily for 7 days (32 patients), or the same dose of kanamycin plus tetracycline 1% eye ointment four times daily for 7 days (29 patients). Of 105 infants who returned for at least one follow-up, 3 who received either of the kanamycin regimens had persistent or recurrent gonococcal conjunctivitis, as compared with none of 61 who received ceftriaxone. There was no difference between the 3 groups in the rapidity with which the signs of conjunctivitis resolved. Ceftriaxone was also extremely effective in eradicating extraocular gonococcal infections. It was concluded that a single dose of ceftriaxone should be considered as a first-line treatment for gonococcal ophthalmia neonatorum in areas with greater than 10% incidence of penicillin-resistant gonococci. Kanamycin combined with either topical gentamicin or tetracycline ointment are acceptable alternatives.— M. Laga *et al.*, *New Engl. J. Med.*, 1986, *315*, 1382.

RESPIRATORY-TRACT INFECTIONS. *Bronchitis.* In a study of the value of ceftriaxone in patients with acute purulent exacerbations of chronic bronchitis clinical results immediately after ceftriaxone 1 or 2 g given daily as a single intramuscular injection for 10 days were considered excellent in 13 of 19 patients given the higher and in 15 of 17 patients given the lower dose. One week after the course of therapy these results had fallen to 6 and 9 respectively, the main problem being recurrence of *Branhamella catarrhalis* in the sputum. Of the respiratory pathogens found in patients' sputum *Haemophilus influenzae* and *Streptococcus pneumoniae* were both found to be exquisitely sensitive to ceftriaxone *in vitro* but *Bran. catarrhalis* was only moderately sensitive and most *Pseudomonas aeruginosa* strains were resistant. In 4 patients pharmacokinetic studies found no ceftriaxone in the sputum in the first 24 hours of treatment and in a further 4 sputum concentrations were lower than expected; 7 of these patients had infections with beta-lactamase-producing strains of *Bran. catarrhalis*. Ceftriaxone yields excellent results at the end of the main treatment course in patients with acute purulent exacerbations but follow-up results are inferior to those which have been reported after cefotaxime or ceftazidime.— F. P. V. Maesen *et al.*, *J. antimicrob. Chemother.*, 1984, *14*, 653.

Cystic fibrosis. For reference to the development of resistant strains of *Pseudomonas aeruginosa* in cystic fibrosis patients treated with ceftriaxone alone or in association with tobramycin, see Antimicrobial Action and Resistance, above.

Pneumonia. A comparative study of intravenous ceftriaxone or cephamandole in the treatment of respiratory-tract infections, mainly pneumonia, in 30 predominantly elderly patients all but one of whom had underlying diseases. Clinical cure or improvement was reported in 15 of 16 treated with ceftriaxone, and in 11 of 14 treated with cephamandole. Of 2 patients treated with ceftriaxone who improved clinically, one developed a resistant strain of *Serratia marcescens* in their sputum, and the other had a superinfection with resistant *Pseudomonas aeruginosa*. The one patient in whom therapy with ceftriaxone failed also developed a superinfection with a resistant strain of *Ps. aeruginosa*.— M. J. Bittner *et al.*, *J. antimicrob. Chemother.*, 1986, *18*, 621.

SEPTICAEMIA. For reference to the use of ceftriaxone sodium in the treatment of septicaemia, see under Cefotaxime Sodium, p.155.

SEXUALLY TRANSMITTED DISEASES. *Chancroid.* An oral course of erythromycin 500 mg by mouth four times daily for 7 days, or of co-trimoxazole 960 mg (or other comparable trimethoprim-sulphonamide combination) twice daily for 5 days, is recommended for the treatment of chancroid. Limited data suggest that adequate cure-rates can also be obtained with thiamphenicol 2 to 5 g by mouth for 2 days, single intramuscular doses of ceftriaxone 250 mg or spectinomycin 2 g, or a single dose of co-trimoxazole 3.84 g by mouth (WHO Expert Committee on Venereal Diseases and Treponematoses, *Tech. Rep. Ser. Wld Hlth Org. No. 736*, 1986, p. 130). There have, however, been recent reports of treatment failures with co-trimoxazole regimens in some areas, and some authorities now recommend intramuscular ceftriaxone or oral erythromycin as drugs of choice, with a 7-day course of co-trimoxazole as an alternative (*Med. Lett.*, 1986, *28*, 23).

Further references to the use of ceftriaxone in the treatment of chancroid: M. I. Bowmer *et al.*, *Antimicrob. Ag. Chemother.*, 1987, *31*, 67.

Gonorrhoea. For the treatment of uncomplicated urogenital and rectal gonococcal infections, in areas where chromosomal gonococcal resistance has reduced the efficacy of antimicrobial agents such as benzylpenicillin, tetracycline, and co-trimoxazole to below 95%, and in areas where the prevalence of beta-lactamase-producing gonococci exceeds 5%, the WHO recommends the use of ceftriaxone 250 mg intramuscularly, cefotaxime 1 g intramuscularly, cefoxitin 2 g intramuscularly with probenecid 1 g by mouth, or spectinomycin 2 g intramuscularly. In pharyngeal infections ceftriaxone 250 mg intramuscularly may be used. For disseminated infection, cefotaxime 500 mg or cefoxitin 1 g may be given intravenously 4 times daily for 7 days, ceftriaxone 250 mg may be given intravenously or intramuscularly twice daily for 7 days, or spectinomycin 2 g may be given intramuscularly twice daily for 5 days. For adult conjunctivitis, cefoxitin 1 g intravenously 4 times daily for 5 days, or spectinomycin 2 g intramuscularly twice daily for 3 days have been recommended; irrigation of the eyes with saline or buffered ophthalmic solutions and application of a topical antibiotic preparation is also required (WHO Expert Committee on Venereal Diseases and Treponematoses, *Tech. Rep. Ser. Wld Hlth Org. No. 736*, 1986, p. 118). Other cephalosporins such as cefuroxime have also been used (A.E. Washington, *Drugs*, 1984, *28*, 355).

In the treatment of severe gonococcal infections such as meningitis, higher doses of cephalosporins such as cefotaxime 2 g every 4 hours or ceftriaxone 2 g daily, both administered intravenously for at least 10 days have been used as an alternative to benzylpenicillin (*Med. Lett.*, 1986, *28*, 23).

Recommendations have also been made for the treatment of gonococcal infections in children. Urogenital, anal, or pharyngeal gonorrhoea in children has been treated with intramuscular ceftriaxone 125 mg or with amoxycillin plus probenecid by mouth. Gonococcal arthritis or meningitis in children may be treated with intravenous cephalosporins as alternatives to benzylpenicillin. For arthritis, ceftriaxone 50 mg per kg body-weight daily, cefotaxime 50 mg per kg daily in divided doses, or cefoxitin 100 mg per kg daily in divided doses, may all be given for 7 days. For meningitis, ceftriaxone 100 mg per kg daily for 7 days, or cefotaxime 200 mg per kg daily for at least 10 days may be given (*Med. Lett.*, 1986, *28*, 23).

Further references to the use of ceftriaxone sodium in the treatment of gonorrhoea: F. N. Judson *et al.*, *Antimicrob. Ag. Chemother.*, 1983, *23*, 218 (comparison with procaine penicillin); H. H. Handsfield and V. L. Murphy, *Lancet*, 1983, *2*, 67 (comparison with spectinomycin); F. N. Judson *et al.*, *J. Am. med. Ass.*, 1985, *253*, 1417 (comparison with spectinomycin in pharyngeal and ano-rectal gonorrhoea); F. N. Judson, *Sex. transm. Dis.*, 1986, *13, Suppl.*, 199 (review of the use of ceftriaxone in uncomplicated gonorrhoea).

For reference to the use of ceftriaxone in neonatal gonococcal conjunctivitis, see Pregnancy and the Neonate, above.

Syphilis. Beneficial effect of intramuscular ceftriaxone in a study involving 20 men with primary syphilis.— T. T. Moorthy *et al.*, *Sex. transm. Dis.*, 1987, *14*, 116.

SKIN AND BONE DISORDERS. Reports of the use of ceftriaxone sodium in the treatment of infections of the skin and bones: L. J. Eron *et al.*, *Antimicrob. Ag. Chemother.*, 1983, *23*, 731 (use in infections of the bones and soft tissues caused by Gram-positive and Gram-negative bacteria); N. H. Goldstein *et al.*, *Curr. ther. Res.*, 1984, *36*, 653 (comparison with cephazolin in cellulitis due mainly to staphylococci and streptococci); F. M. Gordin *et al.*, *Antimicrob. Ag. Chemother.*, 1985, *27*, 648 (comparison with cephazolin in skin and soft-tissue infections due to Gram-positive and Gram-negative bacteria).

SURGICAL INFECTION PROPHYLAXIS. A review of the perioperative prevention of infection in cardiac surgery. Although no difference in the rate of infection had been observed after prophylaxis with ceftriaxone or cephazolin, it was considered that ceftriaxone may be more effective in protecting against infections caused by Gram-negative organisms. It was also noted that the half-life of ceftriaxone was prolonged in patients on cardiopulmonary bypass.— T. R. Beam, *Antibiotics Chemother.*, 1985, *33*, 114.

Further references to the use of ceftriaxone for surgical infection prophylaxis: D. L. Hemsell *et al.*, *Surgery Gynec. Obstet.*, 1985, *161*, 197 (vaginal or abdominal hysterectomy).

URINARY-TRACT INFECTIONS. A study in 54 women with acute urinary-tract infections concluding that a single intramuscular dose of ceftriaxone 500 mg is as effective as a 7-day course of co-trimoxazole 960 mg twice daily.— A. Iravani and G. A. Richard, *Antimicrob. Ag. Chemother.*, 1985, *27*, 158.

Preparations

Sterile Ceftriaxone Sodium *(U.S.P.)*

Proprietary Names and Manufacturers

Rocefacin *(Roche, Spain)*; Rocefin *(Roche, Ital.)*; Rocephin *(Roche, Austral.*; *Roche, Ger.*; *Roche, S.Afr.*; *Roche, USA)*; Rocephine *(Roche, Belg.*; *Roche, Fr.*; *Roche, Switz.)*.

16570-x

Cefuroxime Axetil *(BANM, USAN)*.

CCI-15641. The 1-(acetyloxy)ethyl ester of (*Z*)-3-carbamoyloxymethyl-7-[2-(2-furyl)-2-methoxyiminoacetamido]-3-cephem-4-carboxylic acid.

$C_{20}H_{22}N_4O_{10}S$=510.5.

CAS — 64544-07-6.

1.20 g of the monograph substance is approximately equivalent to 1 g of cefuroxime.

Adverse Effects and Precautions

As for Cefuroxime Sodium, p.171.

Gastro-intestinal disturbances, including diarrhoea, nausea, and vomiting have occurred in a small proportion of patients receiving cefuroxime axetil.

Absorption and Fate

Cefuroxime axetil is absorbed from the gastro-intestinal tract and is rapidly hydrolysed in the intestinal mucosa and blood to cefuroxime. The absorption of cefuroxime axetil is enhanced in the presence of food.

Single doses of cefuroxime axetil 1 g by mouth were given after fasting and after food to 23 healthy subjects and were compared with intravenous doses of cefuroxime 1 g, as the sodium salt. Serum concentrations of cefuroxime with cefuroxime axetil given after food were above those after intravenous doses from 2.5 hours after administration onwards. Mean concentrations after oral and intravenous doses were 8.8 and 5.5 µg per mL at 4 hours, respectively, and 1.2 and 0.8 µg per mL at 8 hours. The kinetics of cefuroxime elimination were very similar after oral and intravenous doses. Absolute bioavailability of cefuroxime after cefuroxime axetil was similar in male and female subjects. Absorption ranged from 21% to 44% in the fasting state but rose by about one third after food. It was recommended that cefuroxime axetil should be taken shortly after food.— P. E. O. Williams and S. M. Harding, *J. antimicrob. Chemother.*, 1984, *13*, 191.

Further studies of the absorption and fate of cefuroxime axetil: S. M. Harding *et al.*, *Antimicrob. Ag. Chemother.*, 1984, *25*, 78; D. K. Sommers *et al.*, *ibid.*, 344; D. K. Sommers *et al.*, *Br. J. clin. Pharmac.*, 1984, *18*, 535; R. Wise *et al.*, *J. antimicrob. Chemother.*, 1984, *13*, 603; C. M. Ginsburg *et al.*, *Antimicrob. Ag. Chemother.*, 1985, *28*, 504.

For reference to inconsistencies in the absorption of cefuroxime axetil, see Respiratory-tract Infections and Urinary-tract Infections under Uses, below.

Uses and Administration

Cefuroxime axetil is the acetoxyethyl ester of cefuroxime (see p.172) to which it is hydrolysed after administration. It is given by mouth in doses of 125 to 500 mg twice daily; a single dose of 1 g may be given for the treatment of gonorrhoea. A dose of 125 to 250 mg twice daily is recommended for children. Since the absorption of cefuroxime axetil is enhanced by food, it should be administered after meals.

For parenteral administration, cefuroxime sodium (see below) is used.

GONORRHOEA. Cefuroxime axetil 1 g by mouth with probenecid 1 g was effective in 29 of 30 urethral and 6 of 6 rectal gonococcal infections in men; given alone, 22 of 23 urethral and 4 of 6 rectal infections were considered to be cured.— A. Gottlieb and J. Mills, *Antimicrob. Ag. Chemother.*, 1986, *30*, 333.

Further references I. W. Fong *et al.*, *Antimicrob. Ag. Chemother.*, 1986, *30*, 321 (comparison with amoxycillin).

RESPIRATORY-TRACT INFECTIONS. In a double-blind, comparative study in 40 patients with acute bacterial lower respiratory-tract infections, the response rate for patients given cefuroxime axetil 500 mg two or three times daily by mouth compared favourably with that of those given amoxycillin 500 mg three times daily by mouth. Treatment was considered to be satisfactory if sputum became mucoid and no additional antibiotic therapy was required. The infecting organisms were mainly *Haemophilus influenzae* and *Streptococcus pneumoniae*.— T. J. Cooper *et al.*, *J. antimicrob. Chemother.*, 1985, *16*, 373.

Twelve children with a total of 14 episodes of lower respiratory-tract infections were given cefuroxime axetil 15 to 32 mg per kg body-weight daily as tablets given in 2 divided doses after meals for 10 days. Clearance of *Haemophilus influenzae* occurred in only 2 of 4 episodes caused by this organism; in another 2 cases *H. influenzae* appeared in the sputum after the onset of treatment. The poor clinical and bacteriological responses in this study may be attributed to the variable serum-cefuroxime concentrations which were recorded.— J. W. K. Carson *et al.*, *J. antimicrob. Chemother.*, 1987, *19*, 109.

SKIN DISORDERS. The use of cefuroxime axetil in bacterial infections of the skin and soft tissue.— A. C. Gudgeon *et al.*, *Br. J. clin. Pract.*, 1987, *41*, 954.

URINARY-TRACT INFECTIONS. Cefuroxime axetil by mouth was given after meals in a dose of 500 mg two or three times daily for 5 or 7 days, to 31 predominantly elderly patients with symptomatic bacteriuria. Twenty-eight were assessed as clinically cured or improved. When assessed bacteriologically, the causative organism was eradicated during and at the end of therapy in 27. At 1-week and 3- to 6-week follow-ups, 17 and 13 patients respectively remained free of bacteriuria. Transient haematological, biochemical, or urinary abnormalities were observed in 13 patients. Diarrhoea occurred in 6, three of whom had severe pseudomembranous colitis. This resulted in termination of the study in one of the 2 centres. It was considered that anomalies in the bioavailability of cefuroxime axetil may be responsible; pharmacokinetic studies in healthy subjects had produced inconsistent results attributed to problems in the dissolution of the film-coated tablets.— D. H. Adams *et al.*, *J. antimicrob. Chemother.*, 1985, *16*, 359.

Poor results in studies of cefuroxime axetil for the treatment of recurrent urinary-tract infections could be explained by variable bioavailability. The manufacturers have changed the formulation to achieve an improved and more consistent bioavailability.— W. Brumfitt *et al.*, *Antimicrob. Ag. Chemother.*, 1987, *31*, 1442.

Treatment of acute urinary-tract infections with cefuroxime axetil 125 mg every 12 hours was compared in 2 separate studies with cefaclor 250 mg every 8 hours and cephalexin 250 mg every 6 hours. All agents were administered by mouth for 10 days. There was little difference in the clinical or bacteriological efficacy between the 3 antibiotics in patients with uncomplicated infections, however, more patients with complicated infections were reported to be clinically cured after treatment with cefuroxime axetil.— C. E. Cox *et al.*, *Curr. ther. Res.*, 1987, *42*, 124.

Proprietary Preparations

Zinnat *(Glaxo, UK). Tablets,* cefuroxime 125 and 250 mg (as cefuroxime axetil).

35-h

Cefuroxime Sodium *(BANM, rINNM).*

640/359 *(cefuroxime).* Sodium (*Z*)-3-carbamoyloxymethyl-7-[2-(2-furyl)-2-methoxyiminoacetamido]-3-cephem-4-carboxylate.

$C_{16}H_{15}N_4NaO_8S=446.4$.

CAS — 55268-75-2 (cefuroxime); 56238-63-2 (sodium salt).

NOTE. Cefuroxime is *USAN*.

Pharmacopoeias. In *It. U.S.* includes Sterile Cefuroxime Sodium.

1.05 g of monograph substance is approximately equivalent to 1 g of cefuroxime. Each g of monograph substance represents about 2.2 mmol of sodium. A 10% solution in water has a pH of 6.0 to 8.5.

Suspensions of cefuroxime sodium for intramuscular injection and solutions for direct intravenous injection should be used within 5 hours of preparation if stored below 25° or within 48 hours if stored in a refrigerator. Solutions for intravenous infusion in sodium chloride injection 0.9%, glucose injection 5%, combined injections of sodium chloride and glucose, or of compound sodium lactate may be expected to retain their potency for up to 24 hours at 25°. Darkening of the solution may occur on storage. Cefuroxime sodium may be **incompatible** with aminoglycosides.

Adverse Effects and Precautions

As for Cephalothin Sodium, p.176.

Cefuroxime may cause false-negative reactions in the ferricyanide test for blood glucose.

ADMINISTRATION IN RENAL FAILURE. There were no signs of nephrotoxicity in 19 of 20 patients with pre-existing renal impairment when they were treated with cefuroxime, with or without frusemide, for 2 weeks. Decreased renal function occurred in one patient who had received an overdose of cefuroxime.— B. Trollfors *et al.*, *J. antimicrob. Chemother.*, 1980, *6*, 665.

See also under Administration in Renal Failure in Uses, below.

EFFECTS ON THE GASTRO-INTESTINAL TRACT. Of 6 healthy subjects given a single intravenous dose of cefuroxime 1.5 g, *Clostridium difficile* and its toxin were isolated from the faeces of one, 4 days later.— N. S. Ambrose *et al.*, *J. antimicrob. Chemother.*, 1985, *15*, 319.

EFFECTS ON THE NERVOUS SYSTEM. Intravenous cefuroxime was considered to have induced a psychotic reaction in a 69-year-old man with underlying renal failure.— W. Vincken (letter), *Lancet*, 1984, *1*, 965.

INTERACTIONS. From a study involving 21 immunocompromised patients, cefuroxime was not considered to potentiate the nephrotoxicity of tobramycin when both drugs are administered in moderate doses.— B. Trollfors *et al.*, *J. antimicrob. Chemother.*, 1983, *12*, 641.

INTERFERENCE WITH ASSAY PROCEDURES. Cefuroxime sodium did not appear to interfere with theophylline assay by high-performance liquid chromatography.— R. H. Gannon and R. M. Levy, *Am. J. Hosp. Pharm.*, 1984, *41*, 1185.

PORPHYRIA. Cefuroxime was considered to be unsafe in patients with acute porphyria although there is conflicting experimental evidence on porphyrinogenicity.— M. R. Moore and K.E.L. McColl, *Porphyrias, Drug Lists*, Glasgow, Porphyria Research Unit, University of Glasgow, 1987.

Antimicrobial Action and Resistance

Cefuroxime is bactericidal and has a similar spectrum of antimicrobial action and pattern of resistance to cephamandole (see p.180). It is more resistant to hydrolysis by beta-lactamases than cephamandole, and is therefore more active against some beta-lactamase-producing strains.

ACTIVITY AGAINST BRANHAMELLA. A study of the sensitivity of 28 strains of *Branhamella catarrhalis* to a range of antibiotics. For 17 non-beta-lactamase-producing strains 90% were inhibited by 2 µg per mL of cefuroxime; the corresponding concentration for 11 beta-lactamase-producing strains was 8 µg per mL.— E. E. Stobberingh *et al.*, *J. antimicrob. Chemother.*, 1984, *13*, 55. In a similar study of 35 strains of *B. catarrhalis*, the MIC of 90% of strains was 0.25 µg or less per mL for 26 non-beta-lactamase-producing strains, and 2 µg or less per mL for 35 beta-lactamase-producing strains.— F. Ahmad *et al.*, *Antimicrob. Ag. Chemother.*, 1984, *26*, 424.

ACTIVITY AGAINST ENTEROBACTER. For reference to the selection of resistant strains of *Enterobacter cloacae* by cefuroxime, see under Pregnancy and the Neonate in Uses, below.

ACTIVITY AGAINST GONOCOCCI. A study of the *in-vitro* antimicrobial susceptibility of isolates of *Neisseria gonorrhoeae* obtained from patients in Bangkok. Isolates which did not produce penicillinase (non-PPNG) had significantly higher cefuroxime MICs than did the penicillinase-producing strains (PPNG).— S. Brown *et al.*, *Lancet*, 1982, *2*, 1366. Contrary results in a similar study of *N. gonorrhoeae* isolated from a London hospital; the MICs of cefuroxime were significantly higher for PPNG than for non-PPNG. It was suggested that the relative resistance of non-PPNG in the Bangkok study could be chromosomally-mediated.— C. Herzog *et al.* (letter), *ibid.*, 1983, *1*, 304.

The MIC of cefuroxime against 41 penicillinase-negative isolates of *Neisseria gonorrhoeae* ranged from 0.016 to 0.25 µg per mL. The range was 0.016 to 0.5 µg per mL for 33 penicillinase-positive strains. Cefuroxime was the most active of the second-generation cephalosporins tested (cefuroxime, cefoxitin, and cephamandole), and was as active as several third-generation agents.— D. A. Strandberg *et al.*, *Curr. ther. Res.*, 1983, *34*, 955.

ACTIVITY AGAINST HAEMOPHILUS. The MICs of cefuroxime for 30 strains of *Haemophilus ducreyi*, (including 27 beta-lactamase-producing strains) ranged between 0.12 and 1 µg per mL.— M. J. Sanson-Le Pors *et al.*, *J. antimicrob. Chemother.*, 1983, *11*, 271.

The MIC of cefuroxime against 169 clinical isolates of *Haemophilus influenzae*, including beta-lactamase- and non-beta-lactamase-producing strains, ranged from 0.125 to 1 µg per mL. Of the antibiotics tested, cefuroxime was considered to have intermediate, but useful activity.— R. M. Bannatyne *et al.*, *J. antimicrob. Chemother.*, 1985, *15*, 187.

ACTIVITY AGAINST NOCARDIA. The MIC of cefuroxime against 12 clinical isolates of *Nocardia asteroides* ranged between 1 and 16 µg per mL. Cefuroxime had the best activity of the cephalosporins tested.— L. Gutmann *et al.*, *Antimicrob. Ag. Chemother.*, 1983, *23*, 248.

ACTIVITY AGAINST STAPHYLOCOCCI. A study comparing the activity *in vitro* of 8 antimicrobial agents against coagulase-negative staphylococci from patients with peritonitis associated with continuous ambulatory peritoneal dialysis. The MICs for cefuroxime were distributed over a relatively wide range (0.125 to greater than 32 µg per mL), with 4 strains having an MIC of 16 µg per mL or above.— M. A. Wilcox *et al.*, *J. antimicrob. Chemother.*, 1985, *15*, 297.

ACTIVITY WITH OTHER ANTIMICROBIAL AGENTS. Synergy or an additive effect against *E. coli, Klebsiella, Proteus,* and *Serratia* spp. was demonstrated *in vitro* between aminoglycosides, especially amikacin, and cefuroxime.— H. Gaya *et al.*, *Proc. R. Soc. Med.*, 1977, *70, Suppl.* 9, 51.

Absorption and Fate

Cefuroxime is poorly absorbed from the gastro-intestinal tract and is given by intramuscular or intravenous injection as the sodium salt. Peak plasma concentrations of 26 to 34 µg per mL have been achieved about 45 minutes after an intramuscular dose of 750 mg with measurable amounts present 8 hours after a dose; after a dose of 1 g peak concentrations are 32 to 40 µg per mL. About 33% of cefuroxime in the circulation is bound to plasma proteins. The plasma half-life is about 70 minutes and is prolonged in patients with renal impairment and in neonates.

Cefuroxime is widely distributed in the body including pleural fluid, sputum, bone, synovial fluid, and aqueous humour. It diffuses across the placenta and has been detected in breast milk, but only achieves therapeutic concentrations in the CSF when the meninges are inflamed.

Most of a dose of cefuroxime is excreted unchanged, by glomerular filtration and renal tubular secretion, within 24 hours, and the majority within 6 hours; high concentrations are achieved in the urine. Probenecid competes for renal tubular secretion with cefuroxime resulting in higher and more prolonged plasma concentrations of cefuroxime. Small amounts of cefuroxime are excreted in bile.

The mean serum concentrations of cefuroxime in 7 healthy subjects reached a peak of 37.8 µg per mL at the end of a 30 minute intravenous infusion of cefuroxime 500 mg given in 90 mL of sodium chloride 0.9% injection, and remained above 10 µg per mL for at least 1.5 hours after the start of the infusion; after a similar 750-mg dose the mean serum concentration in 8 healthy subjects reached a peak of 51 µg per mL and remained above 10 µg per mL for at least 2.0 hours.— C. S. Goodwin *et al.*, *J. antimicrob. Chemother.*, 1977, *3*, 253.

ADMINISTRATION IN THE ELDERLY. A study of the pharmacokinetics of cefuroxime in 18 elderly patients. Since the creatinine clearance decreases with age, the dose should be adjusted appropriately in such patients.— J. Broekhuysen *et al.*, *Br. J. clin. Pharmac.*, 1981, *12*, 801.

ADMINISTRATION IN LIVER DISORDERS. The absorption and fate of cefuroxime sodium in 11 patients with hepatic cirrhosis without ascites, was not significantly different from that in 11 healthy subjects.— L. Okolicsanyi *et al.*, *Arzneimittel-Forsch.*, 1982, *32*, 777.

ADMINISTRATION IN RENAL FAILURE. Studies of the pharmacokinetics of cefuroxime in patients with renal insufficiency.— R. van Dalen *et al.*, *J. antimicrob. Chemother.*, 1979, *5*, 281; R. W. Bundtzen *et al.*, *Antimicrob. Ag. Chemother.*, 1981, *19*, 443; R. A. Walstad *et al.*, *Eur. J. clin. Pharmac.*, 1983, *24*, 391.

See also under Administration in Renal Failure in Uses, below.

DIFFUSION INTO BODY TISSUES AND FLUIDS. The permeability of the peritoneal membrane to cefuroxime after intravenous or intraperitoneal administration was increased in patients with peritonitis.— M. E. McIntosh *et al.*, *Eur. J. clin. Pharmac.*, 1985, *28*, 187.

Further studies of the diffusion of cefuroxime into body tissues and fluids: N. Martini *et al.* (letter), *J. antimicrob. Chemother.*, 1981, *7*, 107 (pericardial fluid); B. R. Bullen *et al.*, *ibid.*, 163 (tissues and wound exudates from ischaemic limbs); A. Martini and L. Xerri, *ibid.*, 1982, *10*, 197 (middle ear effusions); M. A. del Rio *et al.*, *Antimicrob. Ag. Chemother.*, 1982, *22*, 990 (CSF concentrations in infants and children with meningitis); A. J. Davies *et al.*, *J. antimicrob. Chemother.*, 1986, *17*, 637 (bone concentrations in patients undergoing total hip replacement); D. A. Leigh, *ibid.*, *18*, 609 (bone concentrations in patients undergoing knee arthroplasty).

DRUG EXCRETION. A study on concentrations of cefuroxime in the bile, gall-bladder wall, liver, muscle, and skin after intravenous administration in patients undergoing cholecystectomy.— M. Severn and S. J. A. Powis, *J. antimicrob. Chemother.*, 1979, *5*, 183.

PREGNANCY AND THE NEONATE. In a study of 7 women given single intravenous doses of cefuroxime 750 mg, plasma-cefuroxime concentrations were lower during pregnancy than after, when the menstrual cycle had been re-established and breast feeding discontinued. Concentrations at the time of delivery were intermediate between these values. Transplacental transfer of cefuroxime was also demonstrated.— A. Philipson and G. Stiernstedt, *Am. J. Obstet. Gynec.*, 1982, *142*, 823.

A study of the transplacental transfer of cefuroxime in 15 pregnant women.— G. Coppi *et al.*, *Curr. ther. Res.*, 1982, *32*, 712.

For reference to the pharmacokinetics of cefuroxime in neonates, see under Pregnancy and the Neonate in Uses, below.

Uses and Administration

Cefuroxime sodium is a cephalosporin antibiotic which is used similarly to cephamandole (see p.181), in the treatment of susceptible infections. It is administered by deep intramuscular injection, by slow intravenous injection over 3 to 5 minutes, or by intravenous infusion. A usual dose is the equivalent of 750 mg of cefuroxime every 8 hours but in more severe infections up to 1.5 g may be given 6-hourly. Infants and children can be given 30 to 60 mg per kg body-weight daily, increased to 100 mg per kg daily if necessary, given in 3 or 4 divided doses. Neonates may be given similar total daily doses but administered in 2 or 3 divided doses.

For the treatment of meningitis due to sensitive strains of bacteria, cefuroxime sodium may be administered intravenously in doses equivalent to cefuroxime 3 g every 8 hours. Infants and children are given 200 to 240 mg per kg daily in 3 or 4 divided doses, which may be decreased to 100 mg per kg daily after 3 days. For neonates, a dose of 100 mg per kg daily, decreased to 50 mg per kg daily when indicated, has been recommended.

In the treatment of penicillin-resistant gonorrhoea a single dose of 1.5 g by intramuscular injection has been suggested. The dose may be divided between 2 injection sites, and may be given in conjunction with probenecid by mouth.

Cefuroxime sodium is used for surgical infection prophylaxis, usually in a dose equivalent to 1.5 g of cefuroxime intravenously prior to the procedure followed by 750 mg intravenously or intramuscularly every 8 hours for up to 24 to 48 hours. For total joint replacement 1.5 g of cefuroxime powder may be mixed with the methylmethacrylate cement.

Cefuroxime is also administered by mouth as the ester, cefuroxime axetil (see p.170).

Reviews of the actions and uses of cefuroxime sodium: B. R. Smith and J. L. LeFrock, *Ther. Drug Monit.*, 1983, *5*, 149; *Med. Lett.*, 1984, *26*, 15; T. A. Tartaglione and R. E. Polk, *Drug Intell. & clin. Pharm.*, 1985, *19*, 188.

A mention that cefuroxime, in association with amikacin, has been successfully used in the treatment of 6 patients infected with *Nocardia asteroides*.— L. Gutmann *et al.*, *Antimicrob. Ag. Chemother.*, 1983, *23*, 248.

ADMINISTRATION IN RENAL FAILURE. The manufacturers of cefuroxime sodium consider that dosage adjustment in renal insufficiency is only necessary if the creatinine clearance is less than 20 mL per minute. They recommend that the equivalent of cefuroxime 750 mg be given twice daily for patients whose creatinine clearance is between 10 and 20 mL per minute, and once daily for those with a creatinine clearance of less than 10 mL per minute. Patients undergoing haemodialysis should receive a further 750 mg at the end of each dialysis session, and those on continuous ambulatory peritoneal dialysis 750 mg twice daily.

The half-life for cefuroxime of 1.6 to 2.2 hours was increased to 17 hours in end-stage renal failure. Cefuroxime could be administered to patients with renal failure by adjusting the dosage interval. A dosage interval of 8 to 12 hours is suitable for patients whose glomerular filtration-rate exceeds 50 mL per minute; an interval of 24 to 48 hours between doses is advisable for rates of between 10 and 50 mL per minute. Where the rate is less than 10 mL per minute, the dosage interval should be 48 to 72 hours. A dose supplement should be given to patients undergoing haemodialysis or peritoneal dialysis.— W. M. Bennett *et al.*, *Am. J. Kidney Dis.*, 1983, *3*, 155.

See also under Peritonitis, below.

ARTHRITIS, BACTERIAL. For reference to the use of cefuroxime in the treatment of bacterial arthritis, see Osteomyelitis, below.

GONORRHOEA. Cefuroxime sodium has been suggested for the treatment of gonorrhoea in patients infected with penicillinase-producing *Neisseria gonorrhoeae* (PPNG) which are resistant to spectinomycin, or in whom spectinomycin is contra-indicated (*Med. Lett.*, 1984, *26*, 5). In a study of 358 patients with uncomplicated gonorrhoea, Lossick *et al.* (*Antimicrob. Ag. Chemother.*, 1982, *22*, 409, and 1090—minor corrections) demonstrated single intramuscular doses of cefuroxime 1.5 g and procaine penicillin 4.8 g to be equally efficacious; both drugs were given with probenecid 1 g by mouth, and the cure-rates were 96 and 95% respectively. Tupasi *et al.* (*Br. J. vener. Dis.*, 1983, *59*, 172), in a study of 428 women with 562 gonococcal infections, showed cefuroxime with probenecid to be as effective as a single dose of intramuscular spectinomycin or of thiamphenicol by mouth in infections caused by PPNG; in infections caused by non-PPNG it was more effective than both intramuscular procaine penicillin given with oral probenecid, or thiamphenicol by mouth. Graudal *et al.* (*Sex. transm. Dis.*, 1985, *12*, 49), however, did not consider cefuroxime to be effective for treatment of gonococcal infections of the pharynx.

See also under Antimicrobial Action (above), and Pregnancy and the Neonate (below).

MENINGITIS. Pfenninger *et al.* (*Archs Dis. Childh.*, 1982, *57*, 539) obtained favourable results with intravenous cefuroxime sodium in a series of 30 children over 3 months of age with suspected or proven bacterial meningitis, caused in most cases by *Haemophilus influenzae*, *Neisseria meningitidis*, or *Streptococcus pneumoniae*. Sirinavin *et al.* (*Antimicrob. Ag. Chemother.*, 1984, *25*, 273) used cefuroxime successfully to treat 5 children with *H. influenzae* and 2 with *Salmonella* meningitis. In an open multicentre study (Swedish Study Group, *Lancet*, 1982, *1*, 295), adults and children over 3 months of age with suspected, acute bacterial meningitis were treated with cefuroxime sodium alone or a combination of ampicillin and chloramphenicol. Cefuroxime sodium was given to adults in a dose equivalent to cefuroxime 3 g every 8 hours and to children in a dose of 60 to 75 mg per kg body-weight every 8 hours. Excellent clinical results with complete resolution of symptoms were recorded in 18 of 21 evaluable patients treated with cefuroxime, and 14 of 19 treated with ampicillin and chloramphenicol. Meningitis was caused by *H. influenzae* in 20 patients, by meningococci in 11, by pneumococci in 5, and by other bacterial species in 4. One patient in each group was infected with beta-lactamase-producing *H. influenzae*, and both were considered cured. Concentrations of cefuroxime in the CSF were high, and in most cases therapeutic concentrations were maintained throughout the intervals between doses. They concluded that cefuroxime sodium is at least as effective as a combination of ampicillin and chloramphenicol for the treatment of acute bacterial meningitis caused by susceptible pathogens.

In a review of the treatment of bacterial meningitis, Lambert (*Br. med. J.*, 1983, *286*, 741) considered that several of the newer cephalosporins, including cefuroxime sodium, may be suitable for the treatment of *Haemophilus* meningitis if resistance to chloramphenicol and ampicillin becomes more common. Whitby and Finch (*Drugs*, 1986, *31*, 266), gave cefuroxime as one of the standard regimens for the treatment of meningitis caused by *H. influenzae* and as an alternative for that caused by *Str. pneumoniae* or *N. meningitidis*. For empirical therapy, it was considered an alternative treatment for infants and children (but not neonates), and for adults, excluding immunosuppressed patients and those who have undergone neurosurgery. For all age ranges a dose of 150 mg per kg daily, given in divided doses every 8 hours was suggested.

See also under Choice of Antibiotic, p.98.

MOUTH INFECTIONS. A satisfactory response was obtained in 50 of 55 patients with odontogenic or maxillofacial infections after treatment with parenteral cefuroxime in association with surgical drainage. A large range of aerobic and anaerobic organisms were recovered from infection-site specimens.— M. F. Zide *et al.*, *Curr. ther. Res.*, 1986, *40*, 278.

OSTEOMYELITIS. Cefuroxime could be used in a dose of 750 mg to 1.5 g administered intravenously every 6 to 8 hours for the treatment of osteomyelitis or bacterial arthritis caused by *Haemophilus influenzae* or members of the Enterobacteriaceae.— A. S. Dickie, *Drugs*, 1986, *32*, 458.

Further references: H. Z. Herold *et al.*, *Curr. ther. Res.*, 1983, *33*, 892 (osteomyelitis and septic arthritis).

PERITONITIS. Cefuroxime, cephalothin, cephamandole, cefotaxime, and ceftazidime have been used successfully in peritonitis associated with continuous ambulatory peritoneal dialysis, and have the advantage of lower toxicity than the aminoglycosides. These cephalosporins are active against many Gram-negative and Gram-positive bacteria, but not *Enterococcus faecalis*. Cefotaxime and ceftazidime are less active than the other agents against Gram-positive cocci but are more active against Gram-negative bacilli; ceftazidime also has activity against *Pseudomonas aeruginosa*. Problems with the use of a cephalosporin as first-line therapy have included *Clostridium difficile*-associated colitis, failures with resistant *Staphylococcus epidermidis*, and fungal superinfection. Cefuroxime has been widely used in the UK and is the agent recommended by the British Society for Antimicrobial Chemotherapy (BSAC), (*Lancet*, 1987, *1*, 845), although some workers have reported low cure-rates (I. Muscat *et al.*, *ibid.*, 1142). The BSAC recommend that a loading dose of 750 mg be administered either intravenously or intraperitoneally in the severely ill patient, and a maintenance dose of 125 mg per litre of dialysis fluid be given intraperitoneally. Some units have used slightly different dosage regimens, for example a loading dose of 250 mg intravenously and a maintenance dose of 125 to 250 mg per litre intraperitoneally, or, in rapid exchange peritoneal dialysis a maintenance dose of 50 to 250 mg per litre intraperitoneally has been used (D.K. Scott and D.E. Roberts, *Pharm. J.*, 1985, *1*, 621).

For the initial empirical treatment of peritonitis, see under Choice of Antibiotic, Peritonitis, p.99.

PREGNANCY AND THE NEONATE. Twenty-eight neonates (23 preterm), who were considered to be at risk of infection were treated with intramuscular or intravenous cefuroxime 50 mg per kg body-weight daily in 2 divided doses for 5 days. Specimens from 7 patients revealed pathogenic or potentially pathogenic organisms; these were *Listeria monocytogenes* (1 patient), *Klebsiella pneumoniae* (1), *Escherichia coli* (3), *Haemophilus influenzae* (1), and *Staphylococcus epidermidis* (1), and were all sensitive to cefuroxime. The only cefuroxime-resistant organisms occasionally encountered in the special care baby unit before or during the study were pseudomonads from environmental swabs. Twenty-six babies were clinically improved after 5 days of treatment with cefuroxime. The condition of one neonate deteriorated after 24 hours, and treatment was changed to gentamicin and penicillin; another patient who was still unwell after the course of cefuroxime was also changed to this treatment.

In 17 neonates given intramuscular cefuroxime, peak serum concentrations were reached in a median time of 0.8 hours; median serum concentrations at 0.5 and 12 hours were 45 and 10.5 μg per mL respectively, and the half-lives ranged from 2.1 to 10.8 hours. There was no evidence of accumulation of cefuroxime, and steady-state was reached by 24 hours.— J. de Louvois *et al.*, *Archs Dis. Childh.*, 1982, *57*, 59.

The increasing use of cefuroxime sodium in a neonatal unit for the treatment of *Staphylococcus epidermidis* infections resistant to gentamicin, appeared to be responsible for the selection of strains of *Enterobacter cloacae* resistant to cefuroxime. This led to an increase in the number of infants colonised with this organism. The cefuroxime-resistant strains of *E. cloacae* were initially sensitive to cefotaxime and ceftazidime, but as more infants were colonised organisms resistant to these third-generation cephalosporins occurred.— N. Modi *et al.*, *Archs Dis. Childh.*, 1987, *62*, 148.

Ophthalmia neonatorum. Ophthalmia neonatorum caused by beta-lactamase-producing gonococci in premature identical twins was successfully treated with sulphacetamide 30% eye-drops every 6 hours and erythromycin by drip feed replaced after 24 hours by cefuroxime 100 mg per kg body-weight daily intramuscularly in 3 divided doses for 7 days. Recovery of gonococci from sites other than the eye pointed to the need for systemic antigonococcal treatment in such babies.— E. M. C. Dunlop *et al.*, *Br. med. J.*, 1980, *281*, 483. See also E. M. C. Dunlop, *Br. J. Hosp. Med.*, 1983, *29*, 6.

RESPIRATORY-TRACT INFECTIONS. A comparative study of cefuroxime sodium and co-trimoxazole in the treatment of respiratory-tract infections. Cefuroxime was considered to be a useful drug in such infections, although the dose of 750 mg every 8 hours used in this study should be increased to 1.5 g every 8 hours in severe chest infections.— S. Mehtar *et al.*, *J. antimicrob. Chemother.*, 1982, *9*, 479.

Beneficial effect of cefuroxime sodium in 2 patients with pneumonia caused by *Acinetobacter calcoaceticus*.— P. Guérisse (letter), *Lancet*, 1981, *2*, 96.

SURGICAL INFECTION PROPHYLAXIS. Cefuroxime sodium has been studied as prophylaxis against infection during surgery for a large variety of procedures. It may be used in combination with metronidazole in gynaecological and colorectal surgery where anaerobic organisms may be present. References: Cardiac surgery.— M. Abbate *et al.*, *Clin. Trials J.*, 1984, *21*, 348; T. G. Slama *et al.*, *Antimicrob. Ag. Chemother.*, 1986, *29*, 744; C. D. Peterson *et al.*, *Drug Intell. & clin. Pharm.*, 1987, *21*, 728. Intestinal surgery.— N. J. Mitchell *et al.*, *J. antimicrob. Chemother.*, 1980, *6*, 393; B. E. B. Claesson *et al.*, *Br. J. Surg.*, 1986, *73*, 953.

For comments on the use of cefuroxime for surgical infection prophylaxis, see under Ceforanide, p.151.

URINARY-TRACT INFECTIONS. Of 20 patients with bacterial cystitis given a single dose of cefuroxime 1.5 g intramuscularly, 14 were considered to be cured, compared with 19 of 20 patients given a 5-day course of co-trimoxazole 960 mg twice daily by mouth.— R. R. Bailey *et al.*, *N.Z. med. J.*, 1982, *95*, 699.

Preparations

Sterile Cefuroxime Sodium *(U.S.P.)*

Proprietary Preparations

Zinacef *(Glaxo, UK)*. *Injection*, powder for reconstitution, cefuroxime 250 mg, 750 mg, or 1.5 g (as sodium salt).

Proprietary Names and Manufacturers

Biociclin *(Del Saz & Filippini, Ital.)*; Biofurex *(Janus, Ital.)*; Bioxima *(Ital Suisse, Ital.)*; Cefamar *(FIRMA, Ital.)*; Cefoprim *(Esseti, Ital.)*; Cefumax *(Locatelli, Ital.)*; Cefur *(Tiber, Ital.)*; Cefurex *(Salus, Ital.)*; Cefurin *(Magis, Ital.)*; Colifossim *(Coli, Ital.)*; Curoxim *(Glaxo, Ital.)*; Curoxima *(Glaxo, Spain)*; Curoxime *(Glaxo, Fr.)*; Deltacef *(Pulitzer, Ital.)*; Duxima *(Dukron, Ital.)*; Gibicef *(Gibipharma, Ital.)*; Ipacef *(IPA, Ital.)*; Itorex *(Ausonia, Ital.)*; Kefox *(CT, Ital.)*; Kefurox *(Lilly, USA)*; Kesint *(Proter, Ital.)*; Lafurex *(Lafare, Ital.)*; Lamposporin *(Von Boch, Ital.)*; Medoxim *(Medici, Ital.)*; Polixima *(Herdel, Ital.)*; Supero *(Lifepharma, Ital.)*; Ultroxim *(Duncan, Ital.)*; Zinacef *(Glaxo, Canad.; Glaxo, Denm.; Hoechst, Ger.; Neth.; Glaxo, Norw.; Glaxo, S.Afr.; Glaxo, Swed.; Glaxo, UK; Glaxo, USA)*.

2900-x

Cefuzonam *(rINN)*.

(*Z*)-7-[2-(2-Aminothiazol-4-yl)-2-methoxyiminoacetamido]-3-(1,2,3-thiadiazol-5-ylthiomethyl)-3-cephem-4-carboxylic acid.

$C_{16}H_{15}N_7O_5S_4$=513.6.

CAS — 82219-78-1.

Cefuzonam is a cephalosporin antibiotic; it may be administered as the sodium salt.

Proprietary Names and Manufacturers of Cefuzonam or its Sodium Salt

Lederle, USA.

36-m

Cephacetrile Sodium *(USAN)*.

BA-36278A; Cefacetrile Sodium *(pINNM)*. Sodium (7*R*)-7-(2-cyanoacetamido)cephalosporanate; Sodium (7*R*)-3-acetoxymethyl-7-(2-cyanoacetamido)-3-cephem-4-carboxylate.

$C_{13}H_{12}N_3NaO_6S$=361.3.

CAS — 10206-21-0 (cephacetrile); 23239-41-0 (sodium salt).

1.06 g of monograph substance is approximately equivalent to 1 g of cephacetrile. Each g of monograph substance represents about 2.8 mmol of sodium.

Adverse Effects and Precautions

As for Cephalothin Sodium, p.176.

After an infusion of cephacetrile 8 g over 30 minutes, 9 of 15 healthy subjects had temporary proximal renal tubule damage, shown by increased excretion of alanine-aminopeptidase (a brush-border enzyme).— A. W. Mondorf *et al.*, *Eur. J. clin. Pharmac.*, 1978, *13*, 357.

INTERFERENCE WITH ASSAY PROCEDURES. For precautions to be observed when assaying cephacetrile in whole blood, see Cephalothin Sodium, p.177.

Antimicrobial Action and Resistance

As for Cephalothin Sodium, p.177.

Studies *in vitro* of the antibacterial activity of cephacetrile: F. Knüsel *et al.*, *Antimicrob. Ag. Chemother.*, 1970, 140; H. C. Neu and E. B. Winshell, *J. Antibiot., Tokyo*, 1972, *25*, 400.

Absorption and Fate

Cephacetrile is poorly absorbed from the gastro-intestinal tract and is given by intramuscular or intravenous injection. Following a dose of 1 g given intramuscularly peak plasma concentrations of up to 23 μg per mL have been achieved within one hour. From 20 to 40% of cephacetrile may be bound to plasma proteins and reported values for plasma half-lives range from 0.5 to 1.5 hours. Cephacetrile diffuses into many body tissues and fluids including bone, pleural and pericardial fluids, and the cerebrospinal fluid, especially when the meninges are inflamed. It also crosses the placenta into the foetal circulation.

It is excreted in the urine mainly by glomerular filtration but with some renal tubular secretion; up to 25% may appear as the desacetyl metabolite. Biliary excretion is low in patients with normal renal function.

A review of the absorption and fate of cephacetrile.— C. H. Nightingale *et al.*, *J. pharm. Sci.*, 1975, *64*, 1899.

In a study of 23 patients with varying degrees of renal function about 97% of a dose of cephacetrile was excreted in the urine of those with normal kidney function; the biological half-life was about 1 hour. In anuric patients the half-life was about 30 hours.— P. Spring *et al.*, *Schweiz. med. Wschr.*, 1973, *103*, 783.

A study of the pharmacokinetics of cephacetrile in patients on haemodialysis.— A. Dominguez-Gil *et al.*, *Eur. J. clin. Pharmac.*, 1979, *16*, 49.

DIFFUSION INTO BODY TISSUES AND FLUIDS. Into *bone*: H. Stuflesser *et al.* (letter), *J. antimicrob. Chemother.*, 1978, *4*, 188; *cerebrospinal fluid*: L. Dettli (letter), *Br. med. J.*, 1976, *2*, 110; A. Windorfer and U. Gasteiger, *Infection*, 1977, *5*, 242.

Uses and Administration

Cephacetrile sodium is a cephalosporin antibiotic with the actions and uses of cephalothin sodium (see p.178).

The usual dose is the equivalent of cephacetrile 2 to 6 g daily in divided doses given by intramuscular injection or intravenously by slow injection or by infusion; in severe infections up to 12 g daily may be given. A suggested dose for children is 50 to 100 mg per kg body-weight daily.

Reduced doses should be used in patients with impaired renal function.

MENINGITIS. Suggested doses of cephacetrile for the treatment of neonatal meningitis, based on concentrations achieved in the serum and CSF.— A. Windorfer and U. Gasteiger, *Infection*, 1977, *5*, 242.

A report of the use of cephacetrile in the treatment of 30 cases of pneumococcal meningitis.— H. Gallais *et al.*, *Med. trop. Marseille*, 1983, *43*, 163.

Proprietary Names and Manufacturers

Celospor *(Ciba, Fr.; Ciba, Ger.; Grünenthal, Ger.; Chinoin, Hung.; Ciba, Ital.; Jpn; Ciba, Spain; Ciba, Switz.)*; Celtol *(Jpn)*; Cristacef *(Istituto Wassermann, Ital.)*.

37-b

Cephalexin *(BAN, USAN)*.

66873; Cefalexin *(pINN)*. (7*R*)-3-Methyl-7-(α-D-phenylglycylamino)-3-cephem-4-carboxylic acid monohydrate.

$C_{16}H_{17}N_3O_4S,H_2O$=365.4.

CAS — 15686-71-2 (anhydrous); 23325-78-2 (monohydrate).

Pharmacopoeias. In *Br.*, *Braz.*, *Chin.*, *Cz.*, *Egypt.*, *Ind.*, *It.*, *Jpn*, *Jug.*, and *U.S.*

A white to cream-coloured, crystalline powder with a characteristic odour. Slightly **soluble** in water; practically insoluble in alcohol, chloroform, and ether. The *B.P.* specifies that a 0.5% solution in water has a pH of 3.5 to 5.5. The *U.S.P.* specifies that a 5% suspension in water has a pH of 3.0 to 5.5. **Store** at a temperature not exceeding 30° in airtight containers. Protect from light.

Adverse Effects

Side-effects of cephalexin include nausea, vomiting, diarrhoea, and abdominal discomfort. Allergic reactions, such as skin rashes, urticaria, eosinophilia, angioedema, and anaphylaxis may occur, and rises in liver enzyme values have been noted. Neutropenia has been reported. Supra-infection with resistant micro-organisms, particularly *Candida*, may follow treatment. There is the possibility of development of pseudomembranous colitis.

Of 12 917 patients treated with cephalexin in controlled clinical trials, 771 (6%) reported adverse effects, leading to withdrawal of the drug in 156 (1.2%). There was a probable or definite relationship of the reported reaction to cephalexin therapy in 385 patients (3%), and only an uncertain relationship in 386 (3%). Adverse effects involving the gastro-intestinal system were reported by 379 (3.1%) patients, and included nausea, vomiting, diarrhoea, gastro-intestinal upset or pain, anorexia, glossitis or stomatitis, oral candidiasis, and pruritus ani. Hypersensitivity reactions including skin reactions, angioedema, or positive direct Coombs' test occurred in 36 patients (0.3%). Only 21 of 462 patients with known penicillin sensitivity developed sensitivity to cephalexin. Other adverse effects reported included effects on the central nervous system such as headache and dizziness, and genito-urinary effects such as genital candidiasis, vaginitis, and pruritus vulvae. Abnormal laboratory results were observed in 170 patients (1.3%); these included abnormalities in urinalysis and other indices of renal function, liver enzymes, and haematological measurements.— R. A. P. Burt, *Postgrad. med. J.*, 1983, *59*, *Suppl.* 5, 47.

ALLERGY. A clinical picture of a hypersensitivity reaction producing a peripheral eosinophilia with pulmonary infiltration and a bullous rash, was described in a 44-year-old man after administration of cephalexin by mouth for 7 days. The condition resolved after treatment with prednisolone for one month.— J. H. Smith and V. F. Weinstein (letter), *Br. med. J.*, 1987, *294*, 776.

EFFECTS ON THE BLOOD. Reports of adverse effects on the blood associated with cephalexin administration: C. D. Forbes *et al.*, *Postgrad. med. J.*, 1972, *48*, 186 (acute intravascular haemolysis in a haemophiliac); M. Le Porrier *et al.*, *Ann. Méd. interne*, 1976, *127*, 461 (agranulocytosis).

EFFECTS ON THE EAR. Ototoxicity associated with cephalexin in 2 patients with renal failure. Both patients developed dizziness and vertigo, without tinnitus or hearing loss; the dizziness persisted for about one month after discontinuation of cephalexin in both cases.— J. Sennesael *et al.* (letter), *Lancet*, 1982, *2*, 1154.

EFFECTS ON ELECTROLYTE HOMOEOSTASIS. Hypokalaemia occurred in 9 of 11 patients with leukaemia after being given courses of gentamicin 80 mg intravenously every 8 hours with cephalexin 1 g every 6 hours by mouth. Most of the patients were also receiving antineoplastic therapy.— G. P. Young *et al.* (letter), *Lancet*, 1973, *2*, 855.

EFFECTS ON THE KIDNEY. Isolated reports of nephrotoxicity associated with cephalexin.— C. G. Fung-Herrera and W. P. Mulvaney, *J. Am. med. Ass.*, 1974, *229*, 318; S. Verma and E. Kieff, *ibid.*, 1975, *234*, 618; A. L. Linton *et al.*, *Ann. intern. Med.*, 1980, *93*, 735.

EFFECTS ON THE LIVER. Of 95 cases of granulomatous hepatitis diagnosed from 1500 liver biopsies, one was probably related to cephalexin administration.— K. R. McMaster and G. R. Hennigar, *Lab. Invest.*, 1981, *44*, 61. See also C. G. Fung-Herrera and W. P. Mulvaney, *J. Am. med. Ass.*, 1974, *229*, 318.

EFFECTS ON THE NERVOUS SYSTEM. A 46-year-old woman with uraemia who was treated with cephalexin developed convulsions and a toxic psychosis which were attributed to raised serum levels of cephalexin, as high as 120 µg per mL. The patient returned to normal 11 days after cessation of treatment with cephalexin.— B. M. Saker *et al.*, *Med. J. Aust.*, 1973, *1*, 497.

Precautions

Patients who are known or suspected to be allergic to other cephalosporins should not be treated with cephalexin. About 10% of penicillin-sensitive patients will also be allergic to cephalosporins and therefore great care should be taken if cephalexin is given to patients known to be hypersensitive to penicillins. Care is also necessary in patients with known histories of allergy. Reduced dosage is recommended in patients with severe renal impairment.

The urine of patients taking cephalexin may give a false positive reaction for glucose with copper-reduction reagents. Positive results to the Coombs' test have been reported with cephalexin and these can interfere with blood cross matching.

For reference to the possible alteration in the disposition of cephalexin in various disease states, see Absorption and Fate, below.

ADMINISTRATION IN RENAL FAILURE. For reference to the precautions to be observed in renal failure, see under Administration in Renal Failure in Uses, below.

INTERACTIONS. Mean peak plasma concentrations of cephalexin were reduced in healthy subjects when they also took cholestyramine.— R. L. Parsons and G. M. Paddock, *J. antimicrob. Chemother.*, 1975, *1*, *Suppl.* (Sept.), 59.

Pregnancy occurred in a woman taking an oral contraceptive after she had been given a course of cephalexin by mouth for urinary-tract infection.— M. Friedman *et al.*, *J. Obstet. Gynaecol.*, 1982, *2*, 195.

INTERFERENCE WITH DIAGNOSTIC TESTS. The manufacturers state that cephalexin can give falsely-high readings with the alkaline picrate assay for creatinine (Jaffé method), although this is unlikely to be of clinical importance.

PORPHYRIA. Cephalexin was considered to be unsafe in patients with acute porphyria although there is conflicting experimental evidence on porphyrinogenicity.— M. R. Moore and K.E.L. McColl, *Porphyrias, Drug Lists*, Glasgow, Porphyria Research Unit, University of Glasgow, 1987.

Antimicrobial Action and Resistance

As for Cephalothin Sodium, p.177, although cephalexin is generally less potent. Some strains of Gram-negative organisms may be inhibited only by concentrations that can usually be achieved only in the urinary tract. *Haemophilus influenzae* shows varying sensitivity to cephalexin.

A review of the antimicrobial activity of cephalexin comparing current data with previously published results, and examining its *in vitro* activity against more recently isolated pathogens. In general, members of the Enterobacteriaceae and Gram-positive cocci are less susceptible to cephalexin than to the first-generation parenteral cephalosporins. However, this did not appear to compromise the clinical effect of cephalexin; urinary-tract infections caused by *Escherichia coli, Klebsiella* spp., and *Proteus mirabilis* were given as examples. It was noted that data from recent studies have shown a decrease in MICs of cephalexin against the Enterobacteriaceae; this may be accounted for by improvements and standardisation in dilution procedures. *Branhamella catarrhalis* appears to be very susceptible to cephalexin, with MICs ranging from 2 to 4 µg per mL for non-beta-lactamase-producing strains, and from 1 to 16 µg per mL for beta-lactamase-producing strains. Studies have indicated that cephalexin enters bacterial cells as readily as cephalothin and has a high affinity for penicillin-binding proteins. It was considered to be one of the most stable first-generation cephalosporins to beta-lactamases, and therefore to be active against some beta-lactamase-producing strains of *Branhamella, Haemophilus* and *Neisseria* spp. The wide range of MICs reported against the Enterobacteriaceae emphasises the variable incidence of endemic resistance to cephalexin throughout the world. Rates of resistance might range from less than 10% to 50% for *E. coli*, but the lowest rates of less than 10% are usually found for other enteric bacilli.— R. N. Jones; D. A. Preston, *Postgrad. med. J.*, 1983, *59*, *Suppl.* 5, 9.

Of 2753 strains of *Shigella dysenteriae, Sh. flexneri*, and *Sh. boydii* examined at the Central Public Health Laboratory from 1979 to mid 1983 0.8% were resistant to cephalexin at a concentration of 4 µg per mL.— R. J. Gross *et al.*, *Br. med. J.*, 1984, *288*, 784.

Results of a study of the antibiotic susceptibility of organisms isolated from 293 consecutive urine specimens collected from May to July 1983 from general practice patients. The number, and percentage of isolates fully sensitive to cephalexin were 195 (93.7%) for *Escherichia coli*, 25 (80.6%) for *Proteus* spp., 21 (100%) for staphylococci or micrococci, 0 (0%) for faecal streptococci, and 10 (100%) for *Klebsiella* spp. These results appeared to be essentially the same as those in previous similar reports.— S. R. Marper and P. Noone (letter), *J. antimicrob. Chemother.*, 1985, *15*, 251.

ACTIVITY WITH OTHER ANTIMICROBIAL AGENTS. Studies *in vitro* indicating a synergistic interaction between cephalexin and fosfomycin.— N. A. Carlone *et al.*, *Drugs exp. & clin. Res.*, 1984, *10*, 47.

A consideration of the clinical importance of minor synergistic and antagonistic interactions between antimicrobial agents. It was noted that Atherton *et al.* (*Antimicrob. Ag. Chemother.*, 1981, *20*, 470) had reported synergy between cephalexin and alafosfalin *in vivo*, although the interaction *in vitro* would not be regarded as synergistic by most microbiologists.— M. C. Berenbaum (letter), *J. antimicrob. Chemother.*, 1987, *19*, 271.

Absorption and Fate

Cephalexin is almost completely absorbed from the gastro-intestinal tract and produces peak plasma concentrations about 1 hour after administration. A dose of 500 mg produces a peak plasma concentration of about 18 µg per mL; doubling the dose doubles the peak concentration. If cephalexin is taken with food, absorption may be delayed, but the total amount absorbed is not appreciably altered. Up to 15% of a dose is bound to plasma proteins. The half-life has been reported to range from 0.5 to 2.0 hours and this increases with reduced renal function.

Cephalexin is widely distributed in the body but does not enter the cerebrospinal fluid in significant quantities. It diffuses across the placenta and small quantities are found in the milk of nursing mothers. About 80% or more of a dose is excreted unchanged in the urine in the first 6 hours by glomerular filtration and tubular secretion; urinary concentrations greater than 1 mg per mL have been achieved after a dose of 500 mg. Probenecid delays urinary excretion and has been reported to increase biliary excretion. Therapeutically effective concentrations may be found in the bile.

Reviews of the absorption and fate of cephalexin: C. H. Nightingale *et al.*, *J. pharm. Sci.*, 1975, *64*, 1899; R. S. Griffith, *Postgrad. med. J.*, 1983, *59*, *Suppl.* 5, 16.

ABSORPTION AND FATE IN DISEASE STATES. The absorption and urinary excretion of cephalexin were increased in patients with coeliac disease or small bowel diverticulosis but absorption was reduced and delayed in patients with Crohn's disease or fibrocystic disease.— R. L. Parsons and G. M. Paddock, *J. antimicrob. Chemother.*, 1975, *1*, *Suppl.* (Sept.), 59.

There was little impairment in absorption of cephalexin in 18 patients with obstructive jaundice, 14 with gastric achlorhydria, 22 with partial gastrectomy and 6 patients with congestive cardiac failure compared with 21 healthy subjects. Although absorption was not impaired in 9 elderly subjects (mean age 78 years) serum concentrations of cephalexin were sustained compared with those in 12 younger subjects (mean age 29 years).— J. A. Davies and J. M. Holt, *J. antimicrob. Chemother.*, 1975, *1*, *Suppl.* (Sept.), 69.

PREGNANCY AND THE NEONATE. A mean peak serum concentration of about 4.5 µg per mL was obtained in 13 neonates 6 hours after administration of cephalexin 15 mg per kg body-weight 2 hours after a feed; the half-life for cephalexin was 63 hours.— J. A. Raeburn *et al.*, *J. antimicrob. Chemother.*, 1975, *1*, *Suppl.* (Sept.), 53.

A study of the pharmacokinetics of cephalexin in pregnant women.— G. Creatsas *et al.*, *Curr. med. Res. Opinion*, 1980, *7*, 43.

Uses and Administration

Cephalexin is a first-generation cephalosporin antibiotic. It is administered by mouth for the treatment of infections of the respiratory and urinary tracts and of the skin, for otitis media, and other infections due to sensitive organisms. For severe infections treatment with parenteral cephalosporins is to be preferred.

The usual dose for adults is 1 to 2 g daily given in divided doses at 6-, 8-, or 12-hourly intervals; in severe or deep-seated infections the dose can be increased to up to 6 g daily but when high doses are required the use of a parenteral cephalosporin should be considered. A single dose of 2 to 3 g has been given in association with probenecid 0.5 to 1 g for the treatment of gonorrhoea. Infants and children may be given 25 to 100 mg per kg body-weight daily in divided doses to a maximum of 4 g daily. A common dosage regimen is: children aged 5 to 12 years, 250 mg three times daily; 1 to 5 years, 125 mg three times daily; under 1 year, 125 mg twice daily.

Cephalexin sodium or cephalexin lysinate are available in some countries for parenteral use.

For the proceedings of a conference on cephalexin, see *Postgrad. med. J.*, 1983, *59*, *Suppl.* 5, 1–56.

Studies of the use of a combination of cephalexin and fosfomycin (cephemic cofosfolactamine): T. Barreca *et al.*, *Drugs exp. & clin. Res.*, 1984, *10*, 55; P. Mangini *et al.*, *Chemioterapia*, 1985, *4*, 222.

ADMINISTRATION IN RENAL FAILURE. The half-life of cephalexin in healthy subjects of 0.9 hours was increased to 20 to 40 hours in patients with end-stage renal disease. Cephalexin could be administered to patients with renal failure by adjusting the dosage interval. A dosage interval of 6 hours is suitable for patients whose glomerular filtration-rate (GFR) exceeds 50 mL per minute and an interval of 6 to 8 hours between doses is advisable for rates of between 10 and 50 mL per minute. Where the GFR is less than 10 mL per minute, the dosage interval should be 12 hours. A dose supplement should be given to patients undergoing haemodialysis.— W. M. Bennett *et al.*, *Am. J. Kidney Dis.*, 1983, *3*, 155.

Significant reduction in the removal of cephalexin from the body does not occur until there is marked reduction in renal function. All patients can be given a usual initial dose of cephalexin and subsequent doses reduced in proportion to the degree of renal impairment. Various nomograms have been devised for adjusting the dosage regimen which utilise an increase in the dosage interval and/or a decrease in the dose. The dosage interval may be increased according to the creatinine clearance (J.A. Linquist *et al.*, *New Engl. J. Med.*, 1970, *283*, 720): for creatinine clearance values in the range, greater than 30 mL per minute, 15 to 30 mL per minute, 4 to 15 mL per minute, or 1 to 4 mL per minute, cephalexin could be administered at a dosage interval of 4 to 6 hours, 8 to 12 hours, 24 hours, or 40 to 60 hours respectively. Cephalexin appears to be removed by haemodialysis at a rate comparable to the removal of creatinine.— R. S. Griffith, *Postgrad. med. J.*, 1983, *59*, *Suppl.* 5, 16.

Studies investigating the relationship between renal insufficiency and transport of cephalexin in the kidney. Dosage adjustment based on creatinine clearance alone may not be appropriate for drugs which are actively secreted by the kidney tubule.— R. Hori *et al.*, *Clin. Pharmac. Ther.*, 1983, *34*, 792. A nomogram for adjusting the dosage regimen in renal insufficiency, taking into account both the glomerular filtration and the tubular secretion of cephalexin.— R. Hori *et al.*, *ibid.*, 1985, *38*, 290.

In a study of 5 patients undergoing continuous ambulatory peritoneal dialysis given cephalexin by mouth the peritoneal clearance was calculated to be 2.29 mL per minute; thus the dosage regimen for patients with renal failure need not be altered in such patients. Cephalexin, by mouth, may not however be useful for treating intraperitoneal infection since consistently adequate concentrations of cephalexin in the peritoneal fluid may not be obtained.— C. M. Bunke *et al.*, *Clin. Pharmac. Ther.*, 1983, *33*, 66.

BILIARY-TRACT INFECTIONS. Of the orally-active cephalosporins, the biliary recovery of cephalexin is the greatest. It may therefore be of value in the treatment of biliary-tract infections, such as recurrent cholangitis or uncomplicated acute cholecystitis, in a dose of 250 to 500 mg every 6 hours. References: J. S. Dooley *et al.*, *Gut.* 1984, *25*, 988; R. Munro; T. C. Sorrell, *Drugs*, 1986, *31*, 449.

ENDOCARDITIS, PROPHYLAXIS. For reference to the use of cephalexin in the prophylaxis of endocarditis, see Cephazolin Sodium, p.184.

INFECTIOUS MONONUCLEOSIS. An impression that cephalexin may be of benefit in confirmed or suspected glandular fever.— J. Lakic, *Br. med. J.*, 1983, *286*, 1617. Criticism of the methodology and statistical analysis.— P. J. Williamson and P. M. Hawkey (letter), *ibid.*, 1974. Reply.— J. Lakic (letter), *ibid.*, 1975.

OTITIS MEDIA. See under Respiratory-tract Infections, below.

PERITONITIS. Cephalexin concentrations in dialysates and the clinical response achieved in a study of 13 patients with uncomplicated peritonitis associated with continuous ambulatory peritoneal dialysis suggested that treatment with oral cephalexin was satisfactory when sensitive organisms were involved. Thus, intra-peritoneal antibiotic administration appeared to be unnecessary in many such patients but cephalexin was not considered the agent of choice because of the high incidence of resistant strains.— P. J. T. Drew *et al.*, *J. antimicrob. Chemother.*, 1984, *13*, 153.

See also Administration in Renal Failure, above.

PREGNANCY AND THE NEONATE. See under Urinary-tract Infections, below.

RESPIRATORY-TRACT INFECTIONS. A review of cephalexin in the treatment of infections of the upper respiratory tract. Early studies assessing the use of cephalexin in pharyngitis and tonsillitis caused by beta-haemolytic streptococci have generally found it similar in efficacy to the penicillins and cephalosporins with which it has been compared. Studies have also found it to be satisfactory in the treatment of otitis media, except that caused by *Haemophilus influenzae*. Children with otitis media may require a dose of 75 to 100 mg per kg body-weight daily.— F. A. Disney, *Postgrad. med. J.*, 1983, *59*, *Suppl.* 5, 28. Cefaclor was considered to be the only oral cephalosporin with sufficient activity against *Haemophilus* to be of value in the treatment of otitis media.— *Drug & Ther. Bull.*, 1984, *22*, 53.

Cephalexin has been used with success in various infections of the lower respiratory tract, and may be useful for continuation of therapy in patients no longer requiring parenteral antibiotics. Its use is limited, however, by the resistance of some strains of *Haemophilus influenzae* to cephalexin; this is particularly important in infections in children, and in acute exacerbations of chronic bronchitis.— M. J. Raff, *Postgrad. med. J.*, 1983, *59*, *Suppl.* 5, 32.

For reference to the use of cephalexin in association with bromhexine hydrochloride in the treatment of respiratory-tract infections, see Bromhexine Hydrochloride, p.906.

SURGICAL INFECTION PROPHYLAXIS. A comparative study of the use of intravenous cephalexin or cefuroxime for the prophylaxis of infection during cardiac surgery.— M. Abbate *et al.*, *Clin. Trials J.*, 1984, *21*, 348.

URINARY-TRACT INFECTIONS. A review of the use of cephalexin for infections of the urinary tract. The concentrations of cephalexin achieved in the urine are high and prolonged; significant concentrations are obtained even after relatively low doses and after modification of the dose for renal impairment, but not if the patient is anuric. The concentrations obtained are often sufficient to inhibit relatively resistant strains of likely urinary pathogens. Extensive experience, indicating a good response rate, has been obtained with cephalexin in acute, uncomplicated urinary-tract infections, particularly those caused by *Escherichia coli*, *Klebsiella* spp., and *Proteus mirabilis*. Chronic infections, however, are often due to organisms not susceptible to cephalexin. Cephalexin has been effective in chronic infections caused by susceptible bacteria but reinfection or relapse are common. Penetration of cephalexin into prostatic tissue appears variable.— A. J. Weinstein, *Postgrad. med. J.*, 1983, *59*, *Suppl.* 5, 40.

Results of a study in 35 patients with long-term urethral catheters indicating that routine treatment of asymptomatic bacteriuria with cephalexin is not warranted. There was no difference between the control and treatment groups in prevalence of bacteriuria, incidence of bacteriuria, the number of bacterial strains present, the number of febrile days, or catheter obstructions. However, more resistant organisms were isolated from the patients treated with cephalexin.— J. W. Warren *et al.*, *J. Am. med. Ass.*, 1982, *248*, 454.

Of 59 episodes of bacteriuria in 58 pregnant women, 28 were treated with cephalexin 250 mg, and 31 with a combination of amoxycillin 250 mg and clavulanic acid 125 mg, both therapies being administered three times daily by mouth for 7 days. Of those treated with cephalexin there were 5 treatment failures 2 weeks after starting therapy and a further 5 after 6 weeks. In the group treated with amoxycillin and clavulanic acid there were 7 treatment failures after 2 weeks, but no additional failures after 6 weeks.— S. J. Pedler and A. J. Bint, *Antimicrob. Ag. Chemother.*, 1985, *27*, 508.

There is little information available on the use of the oral cephalosporins such as cephalexin, cefaclor, and cephradine in pregnancy. However, there appeared to be no significant risk to the foetus although there was the possibility of sensitising the foetus during the second and third trimesters. Cephalexin was considered to be a suitable choice for the treatment of asymptomatic bacteriuria or cystitis in pregnant women.— R. Wise, *Br. med. J.*, 1987, *294*, 42.

For reference to a comparative study of cephalexin, cefaclor, and cefuroxime axetil for the treatment of urinary-tract infections, see Cefuroxime Axetil p.171.

Prophylaxis. Although cephalexin 125 mg by mouth at night has been recommended for the prophylaxis of urinary-tract infections (P.E. Gower, *J. antimicrob. Chemother.*, 1975, *1*, *Suppl.* (Sept.), 93), in a review of the management of infections of the urinary tract in childhood, White (*Archs Dis. Childh.*, 1987, *62*, 421) considered it unsuitable due to the ready development of bacterial resistance.

Single-dose therapy. A single dose of cephalexin 3 g by mouth produced a successful response in 61 of 91 (67%) of women with acute, uncomplicated urinary-tract infections, and in 27 of 28 patients with acute urethral syndrome.— J. Cardenas *et al.*, *Antimicrob. Ag. Chemother.*, 1986, *29*, 383.

Preparations

Cephalexin Capsules *(B.P.)*

Cephalexin Capsules *(U.S.P.)*

Cephalexin Oral Suspension *(B.P.)*. Cephalexin Mixture

Cephalexin for Oral Suspension *(U.S.P.)*

Cephalexin Tablets *(B.P.)*

Cephalexin Tablets *(U.S.P.)*

Proprietary Preparations

Ceporex *(Glaxo, UK)*. *Capsules*, cephalexin 250 and 500 mg.
Tablets, cephalexin 250 and 500 mg.
Paediatric drops, granules for reconstitution, cephalexin 125 mg/1.25 mL when reconstituted with water.
Suspension, cephalexin 125 and 250 mg/5 mL.
Syrup, granules for reconstitution, cephalexin 125, 250, and 500 mg/5 mL when reconstituted with water.

Keflex *(Lilly, UK)*. *Capsules*, cephalexin 250 and 500 mg.
Tablets, cephalexin 250 mg.
Tablets, scored, cephalexin 500 mg.
Suspension, granules for reconstitution, cephalexin 125 and 250 mg/5 mL when reconstituted with water.

Keflex-C *(Lilly, UK)*. *Tablets*, chewable, cephalexin 250 mg.

Proprietary Names and Manufacturers of Cephalexin and its Salts

Abiocef *(Nuovo, Ital.)*; Acaxina *(Spain)*; Acinipan *(Spain)*; Adcadina *(Pentafarm, Spain)*; Alfaspoven *(Ital.)*; Ambal *(Medical, Spain)*; Amplicefal *(Spain)*; Basporin *(Spain)*; Bilatox *(Spain)*; Bioporina *(Cheminova, Spain)*; Bioscefal *(Graino, Spain*; *Unibios, Spain)*; Bor-Cef *(Borromeo, Ital.)*; Brisoral *(Spain)*; Céporexine *(Glaxo, Fr.)*; Cefabiot *(Spain)*; Cefadina *(Antibioticos, Spain)*; Cefadros *(Proter, Ital.)*; Cefa-Iskia *(Spain)*; Cefaleh Ina *(Oftalmiso, Spain)*; Cefalekey *(Inkey, Spain)*; Cefalepir *(Spain)*; Cefalescord *(Spain)*; Cefalexgobens *(Normon, Spain)*; Cefalival *(Valles Mestre, Spain)*; Cefalogobens *(Spain)*; Cefalorex *(Dibios, Spain)*; Cefaloticum *(Kairon, Spain)*; Cefaloto *(Spain)*; Cefamiso *(Oftalmiso, Spain)*; Cefa-Reder *(Reder, Spain)*; Cefaxin *(Bristol Italiana Sud, Ital.)*; Ceferran *(Ferran, Spain)*; Cefexin *(Spain)*; Cefibacter *(Rubio, Spain)*; Cefipan *(Spain)*; Ceflor *(Ital.)*; Cepexin *(Aust.)*; Cephalomax *(Jpn)*; Cephazal *(Jpn)*; Cepo *(Glaxo, Ital.)*; Cepol *(Jpn)*; Ceporex *(Glaxo, Austral.*; *Belg.*; *Glaxo, Canad.*; *Glaxo, Ital.*; *Neth.*; *Glaxo, S.Afr.*; *Glaxo, Spain*; *Glaxo, Switz.*; *Glaxo, UK)*; Ceporexin *(Arg.*; *Hoechst, Ger.)*; Ceporexina *(Fin.)*; Ceporexine *(Glaxo, Fr.)*; CEX *(Jpn)*; Chemosporal *(Ital.)*; Cilicef *(Hortel, Spain)*; Cipomin *(Jpn)*; Coliceflor *(Coli, Ital.)*; Cusisporina *(Cusi, Spain)*; Defaxina *(Smaller, Spain)*; Derantel *(Jpn)*; Derantel-D *(Jpn)*; Domucef *(Medici Domus, Ital.)*; Doriman *(Vir, Spain)*; Efalexin *(Spain)*; Efemida *(Llorens, Spain)*; Erifalecin *(Dreikehl, Spain)*; Falecina *(Spain)*; Farexin *(Ital.)*; Fergon *(Carol, Spain)*; Garasin *(Jpn)*; Grafalex *(Spain)*; Henina *(Spain)*; Huberlexina *(Spain)*; Ibilex *(Ibi, Ital.)*; Iwalexin *(Jpn)*; Janocilin *(Spain)*; Keflet *(Dista, USA)*; Keflex *(Lilly, Austral.*; *Lilly, Canad.*; *Lilly, Denm.*; *Jpn*; *Lilly, Norw.*; *Lilly, S.Afr.*; *Lilly, Swed.*; *Lilly, Switz.*; *Lilly, UK*; *Dista, USA)*; Keflex-C *(Lilly, UK)*; Kefloridina *(Lilly, Spain)*; Keforal *(Arg.*; *Belg.*; *Lilly, Fr.*; *Lilly, Ital.*; *Neth.)*; Kelfison *(Spain)*; Lafarin *(Lafare, Ital.)*; Laquisporin *(Spain)*; Larixin *(Jpn)*; Latoral *(Dukron, Ital.)*; Lefosporina *(Bicther, Spain)*; Lensafrend *(Lensa, Spain)*; Lerporina *(Lersa, Spain)*; Lexibiotico *(Llano, Spain)*; Lexicef *(Edmond Pharma, Ital.)*; Lexincef *(Serra Pamies, Spain)*; Libesporal *(Liberman, Spain)*; Llenas Biotic *(Spain)*; Llonexina *(Spain)*; Lorexina *(Crosara, Ital.)*; Madlexin *(Jpn)*; Mecilex *(Spain)*; Mepilacin-DS *(Jpn)*; Neolexina *(Spain)*; Nessaxina *(Nessa, Spain)*; Nilexina *(Spain)*; Novolexin *(Novopharm, Canad.)*; Ohlexin *(Jpn)*; Oracef *(Thomae, Ger.)*; Oracocin *(Jpn)*; Oralexine *(Swed.)*; Oroxin *(Jpn)*; Ortisporina *(IBE, Spain)*; Palitrex *(Switz.)*; Porinabis *(Spain)*; Pracefal *(Spain)*; Prindex *(Hosbon, Spain)*; Pyassan *(Hung.)*; Rinesal *(Jpn)*; Rogeridina *(Spain)*; Sartosona *(Spain)*; Sasperos *(Istituto Wassermann, Ital.)*; Sayra *(Spain)*; Segoramin *(Jpn)*; Sencephalin *(Jpn)*; Septilisin *(Arg.)*; Septosporina *(Spain)*; Seromicina *(Valles Mestre, Spain)*; Sintolexyn *(ISF, Ital.)*; Sporol *(Cantabria, Spain)*; Sulquipen *(Bohm, Spain)*; Syncel *(Jpn)*; Taicelexin *(Jpn)*; Talinsul *(Cheminova, Spain)*; Testaxina *(Spain)*; Tokiolexin *(Jpn)*; Tokiolexin-DS *(Jpn)*; Torlasporin *(Torlan, Spain)*; Ultralexin *(Almirall, Spain)*; Valesporin *(Valles Mestre, Spain)*; Vapocilin *(Wassermann, Spain)*; Xahl *(Jpn)*.

38-v

Cephaloglycin *(BAN, USAN)*.

39435; Cefaloglycin *(pINN)*. (7*R*)-7-(α-D-Phenylglycylamino)cephalosporanic acid dihydrate; (7*R*)-3-Acetoxymethyl-7-(α-D-phenylglycylamino)-3-cephem-4-carboxylic acid dihydrate.

$C_{18}H_{19}N_3O_6S,2H_2O = 441.5$.

CAS — 3577-01-3 (anhydrous); 22202-75-1 (dihydrate).

Cephaloglycin is a cephalosporin antibiotic with properties similar to those of cephalexin (p.173). It has been given by mouth in the treatment of infections of the urinary tract. It is, however, poorly absorbed and does not produce sufficiently high plasma concentrations to be useful in the treatment of systemic infections.

A brief review of the absorption and fate of cephaloglycin.— C. H. Nightingale *et al.*, *J. pharm. Sci.*, 1975, *64*, 1899.

Proprietary Names and Manufacturers

Kafocin *(Lilly, USA)*.

39-g

Cephalonium *(BAN).*
41071; Carbamoylcefaloridine; Cefalonium *(pINN).*
(7*R*)-3-(4-Carbamoyl-1-pyridiniomethyl)-7-[2-(2-thienyl)acetamido]-3-cephem-4-carboxylate.
$C_{20}H_{18}N_4O_5S_2$=458.5.

CAS — 5575-21-3.

Cephalonium is a cephalosporin antibiotic used in veterinary practice.

Proprietary Veterinary Names and Manufacturers
Cepravin *(Glaxovet, UK).*

40-f

Cephaloridine *(BAN, USAN).*
40602; Cefaloridine *(pINN)*; Cefaloridinum. (7*R*)-3-(1-Pyridiniomethyl)-7-[(2-thienyl)acetamido]-3-cephem-4-carboxylate.
$C_{19}H_{17}N_3O_4S_2$=415.5.

CAS — 50-59-9.

Pharmacopoeias. In *Aust., Br., Eur., Fr., Ger., Ind., It., Jpn, Neth.*, and *Swiss.*

It is derived from cephalosporin C produced by the growth of certain strains of various *Cephalosporium* spp. or obtained by other means.
A white or almost white crystalline powder. The α-form contains not more than 0.5% of water and the δ-form not more than 3%.
Soluble in water; slightly soluble in alcohol; practically insoluble in chloroform and ether. A 10% solution in water has a pH of 4 to 6. **Store** in airtight containers at a temperature of 8° to 15°. Protect from light.

Adverse Effects and Precautions
As for Cephalothin Sodium, below, although it causes less pain on intramuscular injection. Cephaloridine is considered to be the most nephrotoxic of the cephalosporins, and for this reason is seldom used. Acute and potentially fatal renal failure may occur, which is probably due to proximal tubular necrosis. It appears to be dose-related as it occurs more frequently when the total daily dose exceeds 4 to 6 g.

References to adverse effects associated with cephaloridine: J. B. Eastwood *et al., Br. J. Derm.*, 1969, *81*, 750 (shedding of nails in 2 anephric patients on haemodialysis given large doses of cephaloridine and cloxacillin); U. Mintz *et al.* (letter), *J. Am. med. Ass.*, 1971, *216*, 1200 (extrapyramidal syndrome after intravenous administration); H. Yoshioka *et al., Infection*, 1975, *3*, 123 (convulsions in an infant following intrathecal administration); R. Taylor *et al., Br. med. J.*, 1981, *283*, 409 (encephalopathy after intravenous administration in a patient with renal failure); N. P. Bown, *Adverse Drug React. Bull.*, 1984, (Apr.), 388 (chromosomal damage *in vitro*).

Antimicrobial Action and Resistance
As for Cephalothin Sodium, p.177, although it is reported to be more active against Gram-positive organisms. Cephaloridine appears to be inhibited by staphylococcal beta-lactamases more than most other cephalosporins.
The minimum inhibitory concentrations of cephaloridine for susceptible Gram-positive organisms range from about 0.01 to 1 µg per mL; for most susceptible Gram-negative organisms concentrations of at least 1 µg per mL are required for inhibition.

Of 2753 strains of *Shigella dysenteriae, Sh. flexneri*, and *Sh. boydii* examined at the Central Public Health Laboratory from 1979 to mid 1983 6.2% were resistant to cephaloridine at a concentration of 4 µg per mL.— R. J. Gross *et al., Br. med. J.*, 1984, *288*, 784.

ACTIVITY WITH OTHER ANTIMICROBIAL AGENTS. The activity of cephaloridine *in vitro* against some strains of *Bacteroides fragilis* was enhanced by clavulanic acid.— J. P. Maskell *et al., J. antimicrob. Chemother.*, 1984, *13*, 23.

Absorption and Fate
Cephaloridine is poorly absorbed from the gastro-intestinal tract and must be given by injection. Peak plasma concentrations of 15 to 20 µg per mL are achieved ½ to 1 hour after the intramuscular injection of 500 mg and 30 to 35 µg per mL after a 1-g dose.
Cephaloridine is widely distributed in body tissues and fluids except the brain and cerebrospinal fluid although it diffuses into the CSF when the meninges are inflamed. Cephaloridine diffuses across the placenta into the foetal circulation and it is excreted in the milk of nursing mothers. Only about 20% of a dose is bound to plasma proteins. The half-life of cephaloridine has been reported to be about 1 to 1.5 hours.
Cephaloridine is rapidly excreted unchanged in urine mainly by glomerular filtration and about 80% is eliminated within 24 hours. High urine concentrations have been reported following normal dosage. A small amount is excreted in bile.

A review of the absorption and fate of cephaloridine.— C. H. Nightingale *et al., J. pharm. Sci.*, 1975, *64*, 1899.

DIFFUSION INTO BODY TISSUES AND FLUIDS. References to the penetration of cephaloridine into various body tissues and fluids after parenteral administration: A. B. Richards *et al., Br. J. Ophthal.*, 1972, *56*, 531 (aqueous humour); A. H. Chignell, *Br. J. Ophthal.*, 1973, *57*, 421 (subretinal fluid); T. R. Tetzlaff *et al., J. Pediat.*, 1978, *92*, 135 (pus and bone of children with osteomyelitis).

Uses and Administration
Cephaloridine is a cephalosporin antibiotic with similar uses to Cephalothin Sodium, p.178. Its use, however, has been limited by nephrotoxicity. It is administered intramuscularly or intravenously in doses of 0.5 to 1 g two to four times daily. Children may be given up to 50 mg per kg body-weight daily in divided doses. A daily dosage of 6 g for adults should not normally be exceeded.
Cephaloridine should preferably not be given to patients with impaired renal function because of its nephrotoxicity.

SURGICAL INFECTION PROPHYLAXIS. The use of a topical solution of cephaloridine 1 g in 2 mL instilled into surgical wounds has been shown to reduce the rate of infection of contaminated wounds (C. Evans *et al., Br. J. Surg.*, 1974, *61*, 133), and to be as effective as a single intravenous injection of 1 g (M. J. Greenall *et al., J. antimicrob. Chemother.*, 1981, *7*, 223). Topical cephaloridine has been compared with various other topical antibiotics; Lindsey *et al.* (*ibid.*, 1984, *14*, 196) could demonstrate no difference between 5% solutions of cephaloridine and benzylpenicillin instilled intra-incisionally for the prophylaxis of traumatic wound infection.

Preparations
Cephaloridine Injection *(B.P.)*

Proprietary Names and Manufacturers
Acaporina *(Spain)*; Aliporina *(Spain)*; Amplicerina *(Spain)*; Ampligram *(Organon, Spain)*; Bioporina *(Spain)*; Céporine *(Glaxo, Fr.)*; Cefabena *(Spain)*; Cefabiot *(Galepharma, Spain)*; Cefalisan *(Spain)*; Cefalobiotic *(Kairon, Spain)*; Cefalogobens *(Spain)*; Cefalomiso *(Oftalmiso, Spain)*; Cefamusel *(Cruz, Spain)*; Cefa-Resan *(Alacan, Spain)*; Cefipan *(Spain)*; Ceflorin *(Arg.)*; Cepaloridin *(Ger.)*; Cepalorin *(Belg.; Neth.)*; Ceporan *(Austral.; Glaxo, Canad.; Denm.; Glaxo, S.Afr.; Glaxo, Spain; Swed.)*; Ceporin *(Glaxo, Ital.; Switz.; Glaxo, UK)*; CER *(Jpn)*; Cidan Cef *(Cidan, Spain)*; Cilicef *(Hortel, Spain)*; Cilifor *(Spain)*; Cobalcina *(Spain)*; Cusisporina *(Cusi, Spain)*; Dinasint *(Proter, Ital.)*; Eldia *(Spain)*; Endosporol *(Cantabria, Spain)*; Enebiotico *(Spain)*; Etrocefal *(Albofarma, Spain)*; Faredina *(Lafare, Ital.)*; Filoklin *(Sabater, Spain)*; Floridin *(Coli, Ital.)*; Gencefal *(Morgens, Spain)*; Glaxoridin *(Aust.)*; Henina *(Spain)*; Huberlexina *(Spain)*; Inex *(Inexfa, Spain)*; Intrasporin *(Torlan, Spain)*; Janosina *(Spain)*; Keflodin *(Belg.; Fr.; Lilly, Ital.; Neth.; Norw.; Lilly, Spain)*; Kelfison *(Davur, Spain)*; Latorex *(Dukron, Ital.)*; Lauridin *(Locatelli, Ital.)*; Lersina *(Lersa, Spain)*; Libesporina *(Liberman, Spain)*; Liexina *(Spain)*; Llenas Biotic *(Spain)*; Lloncefal *(Spain)*; Loridine *(Austral.; USA)*; Pantotiber *(Valles Mestre, Spain)*; Poricefal *(Spain)*; Prinderin *(Hosbon, Spain)*; Rogeridina *(Spain)*; Sasperin *(Istituto Wassermann, Ital.)*; Sintoridyn *(Ital.)*; Sporanicum *(Spain)*; Talinsul *(Cheminova, Spain)*; Tapiola *(Tafir, Spain)*; Testadina *(Spain)*; Thompen *(Llano, Spain)*; Totalmicina *(Valles Mestre, Spain)*.

41-d

Cephalothin Sodium *(BANM, USAN).*
Cefalotin Sodium *(pINNM)*; Sodium Cephalothin. Sodium (7*R*)-7-[2-(2-thienyl)acetamido)cephalosporanate; Sodium (7*R*)-3-acetoxymethyl-7-[2-(2-thienyl)acetamido]-3-cephem-4-carboxylate.
$C_{16}H_{15}N_2NaO_6S_2$=418.4.

CAS — 153-61-7 (cephalothin); 58-71-9 (sodium salt).

Pharmacopoeias. In *Br., Braz., Chin., Egypt., It., Jpn*, and *U.S.*

A white to off-white, almost odourless, crystalline powder. 1.06 g of monograph substance is approximately equivalent to 1 g of cephalothin. Each g of monograph substance represents 2.39 mmol of sodium.
Soluble 1 in 3.5 of water; slightly soluble in alcohol; freely soluble in 0.9% sodium chloride solution and in glucose solutions; practically insoluble in chloroform, ether, and most other organic solvents. A 10 or 25% solution in water has a pH of 4.5 to 7.0. **Store** at a temperature not exceeding 25° in airtight containers.
Aqueous solutions of cephalothin sodium are reported to be **stable** for 12 hours at 25° and for 48 hours at 5°. Solutions of cephalothin sodium in water, 0.9% sodium chloride, or 5% glucose which have been frozen immediately after reconstitution in their original containers are reported to be stable for 12 weeks at −20°.
Solutions of cephalothin sodium may darken on storage, especially at room temperature, but slight discoloration does not affect potency.
Precipitation may occur in solutions with a pH of less than 5. A precipitate may also form in refrigerated solutions; this can be dissolved by gently warming to room temperature.
Cephalothin sodium should not be mixed with blood products or other proteinaceous fluids such as protein hydrolysates.
Cephalothin sodium has been reported to be **incompatible** with aminoglycosides, tetracyclines, and other antimicrobial agents including benzylpenicillin, erythromycin, nitrofurantoin, polymyxin B sulphate, and sulphafurazole diethanolamine. Incompatibility or loss of activity has also been reported with aminophylline, soluble barbiturates, bleomycin sulphate, calcium salts, colistin sulphomethate sodium, diphenhydramine hydrochloride, dopamine hydrochloride, doxorubicin hydrochloride, methylprednisolone sodium succinate, noradrenaline acid tartrate, prochlorperazine edisylate, and certain fluids for parenteral nutrition including fat emulsions.

Units
One unit of cephalothin is contained in 0.0010661 mg of the first International Reference Preparation (1965) of cephalothin sodium which contains 938 units per mg.

Adverse Effects
Allergic reactions, including skin rashes, urticaria, eosinophilia, fever, reactions resembling serum sickness, and anaphylaxis may occur in patients receiving cephalothin sodium, especially if they are hypersensitive to penicillins or other cephalosporins. Neutropenia, leucopenia, thrombocytopenia, and haemolytic anaemia have occasionally been reported.
Nephrotoxicity has occurred particularly in patients with existing renal impairment or in patients receiving concomitant nephrotoxic drugs. Transient increases in liver enzyme values, including serum aspartate aminotransferase and alkaline phosphatase, have been reported. Neurological disturbances including encephalopathy have occurred occasionally.
There may be pain at the injection site following intramuscular administration and thrombophlebitis has occurred following intravenous infusion, usually of more than 6 g daily for more than 3 days.
Gastro-intestinal adverse effects have been reported rarely. Prolonged use may result in overgrowth of non-susceptible organisms and, as with other broad-spectrum antibiotics, pseudomembranous colitis may develop.

ALLERGY. A report of 2 cases in which administration of cephalothin sodium during surgery resulted in anaphylaxis and death. One patient had a history of allergy to penicillin.— F. G. Spruill *et al.*, *J. Am. med. Ass.*, 1974, *229*, 440.

The Boston Collaborative Drug Surveillance Program monitored consecutively 32 812 medical in-patients. Drug-induced anaphylaxis occurred in 1 of 1273 patients given cephalothin sodium.— J. Porter and H. Jick, *Lancet*, 1977, *1*, 587.

In a study involving 253 patients suspected of being allergic to penicillin 29 (11.5%) had positive skin tests to benzylpenicillin or a pencillin derivative and 6 of 178 patients (3.4%) demonstrated significant skin reactivity when tested with a minor determinant mixture of cephalothin; none had a positive skin-test reaction to cephalothin alone. Of the patents with positive skin tests to penicillin derivatives 29.1% of those tested also responded to the cephalothin derivative.— R. J. Warrington *et al.*, *Can. med. Ass. J.*, 1978, *118*, 787. See also under Allergy in Precautions, below.

Antibodies to cephalothin were present in the serum of 2 patients who had received whole blood from donor blood which was found to have plasma-cephalothin antibodies. One of the patients experienced a mild allergic reaction while receiving cephalothin therapy.— D. R. Branch and H. Gifford, *J. Am. med. Ass.*, 1979, *241*, 495.

Hypotension with or without bronchospasm occurred in 3 patients following rapid intravenous administration of large doses of cephalothin or cefoxitin, but no reaction was observed with smaller doses given slowly. These cases are not typical of true anaphylaxis and some patients' responses to small test doses of cephalosporins may not accurately predict the hypotension and bronchospasm that may accompany the rapid administration of large doses. It is therefore recommended that intravenous cephalosporins should be administered slowly.— C. H. L'Hommedieu and J. Erickson, *Anesthesiol. Rev.*, 1983, *10*, 10.

From an analysis of 148 reported episodes of drug fever 46 were caused by antimicrobial agents and of these 7 were due to cephalothin.— P. A. Mackowiak and C. F. LeMaistre, *Ann. intern. Med.*, 1987, *106*, 728.

EFFECTS ON THE BLOOD. Neutropenia has been associated with each generation of cephalosporins. Evaluable case reports of cephalothin-induced neutropenia outnumber those of other cephalosporins, but this is probably because of the widespread use of cephalothin. In most reports the course of neutropenia has closely followed the characteristic pattern of an immunological reaction (C.F. Kirkwood *et al.*, *Clin. Pharm.*, 1983, *2*, 569). The incidence of cephalothin-induced granulocytopenia in one hospital was reported in 1974 to be 4 out of about 3800 patients (M.-A. DiCato and L. Ellman, *Ann. intern. Med.*, 1975, *83*, 671).

For a discussion on beta-lactam-induced neutropenia, see under Benzylpenicillin Sodium p.132.

A positive direct antiglobulin test (Coombs' test) may occur in patients receiving cephalothin, but haemolysis does not usually occur; the responsible mechanism is frequently non-immune adsorption of serum proteins to cephalothin-exposed erythrocytes. However, haemolysis associated with specific anti-cephalothin antibodies has occasionally been reported with cephalothin therapy indicating that cephalothin can also induce an immune haemolysis similar to pencillin.— R. N. Rubin and E. R. Burka (letter), *Ann. intern. Med.*, 1977, *86*, 64.

Further references to blood disorders associated with cephalothin therapy: H. R. Gralnick *et al.*, *J. Am. med. Ass.*, 1971, *217*, 1193 (haemolytic anaemia and a positive direct Coombs' test); H. R. Gralnick *et al.*, *Ann. intern. Med.*, 1972, *77*, 401 (thrombocytopenia); D. MacCulloch *et al.* (letter), *Br. med. J.*, 1974, *4*, 163 (red cell aplasia); N. E. Tartas *et al.*, *J. Am. med. Ass.*, 1981, *245*, 1148 (reversible pancytopenia).

EFFECTS ON THE CARDIOVASCULAR SYSTEM. Reports of tachycardia associated with cephalothin administration: G. M. Lemole *et al.*, *J. Am. med. Ass.*, 1972, *221*, 593; R. A. Kaslow (letter), *J. Am. med. Ass.*, 1972, *222*, 833.

EFFECTS ON THE GASTRO-INTESTINAL TRACT. *Colitis.* A report of pseudomembranous colitis due to *Clostridium difficile* in 17 patients in whom the only antimicrobial agent administered was a cephalosporin; cephalothin was involved in 5 patients.— J. G. Bartlett *et al.*, *J. Am. med. Ass.*, 1979, *242*, 2683.

The intraperitoneal administration of cephalothin appeared to be the cause of diarrhoea, mediated by *Clostridium difficile* toxin, in a 62-year-old man. He was treated successfully with vancomycin.— D. L. Coleman *et al.* (letter), *Lancet*, 1981, *1*, 1004.

EFFECTS ON THE KIDNEY. Acute renal failure has occurred during therapy with cephalothin sodium (J.R. Burton *et al.*, *J. Am. med. Ass.*, 1974, *229*, 679). Some instances of cephalothin nephropathy appear to be toxic in nature with the appearance of acute tubular necrosis, whereas others exhibit signs of hypersensitivity with the development of rash and eosinophilia as well as impairment of renal function indicating the possibility of acute interstitial nephritis (G.B. Appel and H.C. Neu, *New Engl. J. Med.*, 1977, *296*, 663; M. Barza, *J. infect. Dis.*, 1978, *137*, *Suppl.* (May), S60). It has been suggested that factors associated with the nephrotoxicity include excessive dosage usually greater than 12 g daily, impaired renal function, an age of over 50 years, reduction in renal clearance due to factors such as surgical operation, dehydration, or shock, hypersensitivity reactions to pencillin or cephalosporins, or concomitant use of other potentially nephrotoxic antibiotics or diuretics (R.D. Foord, *J. antimicrob. Chemother.*, 1975, *1*, *Suppl.* (Sept.), 119). Some controversy has existed over whether the use of cephalothin with an aminoglycoside results in increased nephrotoxicity. Review of data from the Boston Collaborative Drug Surveillance Program revealed no appreciable enhanced renal toxicity arising from the use of gentamicin with cephalothin (W.L. Fanning *et al.*, *Antimicrob. Ag. Chemother.*, 1976, *10*, 80). However, there have been reports of significant increases in nephrotoxicity in patients receiving both aminoglycosides and cephalothin (S.L. Barriere, *Clin. Pharm.*, 1986, *5*, 24). In a study of cancer patients receiving aminoglycosides and cephalothin nephrotoxicity occurred in about 18%, but the incidence appeared to be higher in patients over 50 years of age (J.C. Wade *et al.*, *Archs intern. Med.*, 1981, *141*, 1789); other workers have reported a lower incidence, especially in children (A.E. Brown *et al.*, *Antimicrob. Ag. Chemother.*, 1982, *21*, 592).

EFFECTS ON THE LIVER. Hepatic dysfunction during cephalothin therapy occurred in a patient who had previously developed hepatitis due to oxacillin administration and hepatic dysfunction during nafcillin therapy.— W. I. Miller *et al.*, *Clin. Pharm.*, 1983, *2*, 465.

EFFECTS ON THE NERVOUS SYSTEM. A report of severe encephalopathy occurring in a man with renal failure who received a total of 22 g of cephalothin over 5 days. Very high cephalothin concentrations in the CSF (9.6 μg per mL) and serum (170 μg per mL) were recorded.— M. -J. Wu *et al.* (letter), *Ann. intern. Med.*, 1978, *89*, 429.

Neuropsychiatric sequelae in a uraemic patient given cephalothin and benzylpenicillin.— G. Tollefson (letter), *J. clin. Psychiat.*, 1984, *45*, 96.

Precautions

Cephalothin sodium should not be given to patients who are hypersensitive to it or to other cephalosporins. About 10% of penicillin-sensitive patients will also be allergic to cephalosporins and therefore great care should be taken if cephalothin is to be given to patients who are known to be allergic to penicillins. Care is also necessary in patients with known histories of allergy.

Cephalothin sodium should be given with caution to patients with renal impairment; a dosage reduction may be necessary. The concomitant use of diuretics such as frusemide and nephrotoxic antibiotics such as gentamicin may increase the risk of kidney damage. Renal and haematological status should be monitored especially during prolonged and high-dose therapy.

Interactions. Positive results to the direct Coombs' test have been found during treatment with cephalothin and these can interfere with blood cross-matching. The urine of patients being treated with cephalothin may give false-positive reactions for glucose using copper-reduction reactions.

ADMINISTRATION IN RENAL FAILURE. For the precautions to be observed in renal failure, see under Uses and Administration, below.

ALLERGY. A review of immunological cross-reactivity between penicillins and cephalosporins.— L. D. Petz, *J. infect. Dis.*, 1978, *137*, *Suppl.* (May), S74.

Allergic reactions have been reported to occur in 2 to 5% of all persons receiving cephalosporins and in 5 to 16% of patients with a history of penicillin allergy (B.E. Murray and R.C. Moellering, *Clin. Ther.*, 1979, *2*, 155). Most authorities avoid giving any of the cephalosporins or cephamycins to patients with a history of anaphylaxis or immediate-type hypersensitivity reaction to the penicillins. However, it is not unreasonable to consider their cautious use when indicated in patients with a history of less severe reactions to the penicillins, such as eosinophilia, morbilliform rash, or drug fever.— R. C. Moellering, *J. Am. med. Ass.*, 1980, *244*, 2562.

INTERFERENCE WITH ASSAY PROCEDURES. Cephalosporins with a 3-acetoxymethyl group, including cephalothin, cephaloglycin, cephacetrile, cefapirin, and cefotaxime, are deacetylated by lysed whole blood and this should be taken into account when assays must be run in whole blood or on tissues containing whole blood.— W. E. Wright and J. A. Frogge, *Antimicrob. Ag. Chemother.*, 1980, *17*, 99.

INTERFERENCE WITH DIAGNOSTIC TESTS. When urine of patients treated with cephalothin was tested for protein with 20% sulphosalicylic acid, a heavy white precipitate developed if cephalothin concentrations were 10 mg per mL or more. This precipitate was indistinguishable from that seen in proteinuria due to renal damage and awareness of this false positive reaction is important in the treatment of the patients.— M. Levy and M. Eliakim (letter), *J. Am. med. Ass.*, 1972, *219*, 908.

Cephalothin interfered with the determination of creatinine concentrations in plasma and urine using the Jaffé method and might produce falsely high values. This effect should be borne in mind when monitoring renal function.— L. I. Rankin *et al.*, *Antimicrob. Ag. Chemother.*, 1979, *15*, 666.

Cephalothin could interfere with urinary 17-hydroxycorticosteroid determination using the Porter-Silber reaction.— F. H. Faas *et al.* (letter), *Clin. Chem.*, 1983, *29*, 1311.

PORPHYRIA. Cephalosporins were considered to be unsafe in patients with acute porphyria although there is conflicting experimental evidence on porphyrinogenicity.— M.R. Moore and K.E.L. McColl, *Porphyrias, Drug Lists*, Glasgow, Porphyria Research Unit, University of Glasgow, 1987.

Antimicrobial Action

Cephalothin is bactericidal and acts similarly to the penicillins by inhibiting synthesis of the bacterial cell wall. It is active against a wide range of bacteria including many Gram-positive organisms and some Gram-negative organisms. Most Gram-positive cocci are sensitive including both penicillinase- and non-penicillinase-producing staphylococci, although methicillin-resistant *Staphylococcus aureus* are usually resistant; most streptococci are also sensitive, but enterococci are usually resistant. Some Gram-positive anaerobes are also sensitive. Among the Gram-negative organisms cephalothin has activity against some Enterobacteriaceae including strains of *Escherichia coli*, *Klebsiella pneumoniae*, *Proteus mirabilis*, and *Salmonella* and *Shigella* spp.; it is also active against *Haemophilus influenzae* and *Neisseria* spp.

Cephalothin is usually inactive against *Listeria monocytogenes*, *Bacteroides fragilis*, *Enterobacter* and *Pseudomonas* spp., indole-positive *Proteus*, *Serratia* spp., mycobacteria, mycoplasma, and fungi.

The minimum inhibitory concentrations of cephalothin for susceptible Gram-positive organisms range from about 0.1 to 1 μg per mL; for most susceptible Gram-negative organisms concentrations of 1 to 16 μg or more per mL are usually required.

Only cefoxitin and cephalothin appeared resistant to inactivation by beta-lactamase-producing *Staph. aureus* in a study of 8 cephalosporins. It was considered that cephalothin was generally the best cephalosporin to use in severe staphylococcal infections.— I. W. Fong *et al.*, *Antimicrob. Ag. Chemother.*, 1976, *9*, 939.

Cephalothin, cefapirin, and cefotaxime are all converted to desacetyl derivatives *in vivo*. The metabolites retain some antibacterial activity but are approximately 4 to 16 times less potent than the parent compounds. Several studies have demonstrated that the metabolites can act synergistically with the parent compound *in vitro*. Cephalothin and cefapirin have been shown to be synergistic with their respective metabolites against a wide variety of Enterobacteriaceae and *Staphylococcus aureus*. Synergy has been demonstrated for cefotaxime and its metabolite against an even wider range of bacteria, including *Bacteroides fragilis*, although antagonism was seen against *Morganella morganii* and *Proteus vulgaris*; *Pseudomonas aeruginosa* and enterococci were not affected by the combination. The cephalosporins that are transformed to desacetyl derivatives may, therefore, perform better *in vivo* than would be predicted from susceptibility tests *in vitro*.— S. L. Barriere, *Clin. Pharm.*, 1986, *5*, 24.

ACTIVITY WITH OTHER ANTIMICROBIAL AGENTS. Reports of enhanced activity: J. Klastersky, *Antimicrob. Ag. Chemother.*, 1972, *1*, 441 (with gentamicin against oxacillin-resistant strains of *Staphylococcus aureus*); R. S. Baltimore *et al*, *ibid.*, 1976, *9*, 701 (with mecillinam against *Klebsiella pneumoniae* and some *Proteus* spp.); R. M. D'Alessandri *et al.*, *ibid.*, *10*, 889 (with gentamicin against *Klebsiella* spp.); J. Wüst and T. D. Wilkins, *ibid.*, 1978, *13*, 130 (with clavulanic acid against penicillin-resistant strains of the *Bacteroides* spp.); R. T. Jackson *et al.*, *ibid.*, *14*, 118 (with clavulanic acid against cephalothin-resistant *Klebsiella pneumoniae*); M. E. Ein *et al.*, *ibid.*, 1979, *16*, 655 (with rifampicin or vancomycin against methicillin-resistant *Staphylococcus epidermidis*); R. H. Glew and R. A. Pavuk, *ibid.*, 1984, *26*, 378 (with amikacin against multiple-resistant Enterobacteriaceae).

Reports of diminished activity: F. D. Lowy *et al.*, *Antimicrob. Ag. Chemother.*, 1979, *16*, 314 (with gentamicin or vancomycin against methicillin-resistant *Staphylococcus epidermidis* infections in *mice*).

MICROBE SENSITIVITY TESTS. A study of the accuracy of diffusion susceptibility tests with disks containing 30 µg of cephamandole or cephalothin indicated that although the same interpretive zone standards could be applied to tests with either disk the two drugs could not be tested interchangeably.— A. L. Barry *et al.*, *Antimicrob. Ag. Chemother.*, 1979, *15*, 140.

Resistance

Resistance of bacteria to cephalothin may be due to several mechanisms: the drug may be prevented from reaching its site of action, for example in some Gram-negative organisms the cell wall may be a potential barrier; the target penicillin-binding proteins may be altered so that cephalothin cannot bind with these proteins; or, most importantly, the organism may produce beta-lactamases (cephalosporinases). Cephalothin is relatively resistant to hydrolysis by staphylococcal penicillinase but is inactivated by a variety of beta-lactamases produced by Gram-negative organisms; resistance of Gram-negative organisms often depends on more than one factor. Resistance can be chromosomally or plasmid-mediated and may sometimes be inducible by cephalosporins.

Certain strains of bacteria may be inhibited but not killed by cephalosporins or penicillins and in such cases the minimum bactericidal concentration (MBC) is much greater than the minimum inhibitory concentration (MIC); this is known as tolerance.

As well as with other cephalosporins, some cross-resistance may occur between cephalothin and the penicillinase-resistant penicillins.

Strains of *Streptococcus pneumoniae* isolated from 5 children were partially resistant to cephalothin.— P. C. Appelbaum *et al.*, *Lancet*, 1977, *2*, 995.

Methicillin-resistant coagulase-negative staphylococci showed nearly total cross-resistance to 8 cephalosporins tested *in vitro*, including cephalothin. Beta-lactamases produced by the staphylococci had little hydrolytic effect on the 5 cephalosporins tested and there was no correlation between anti-staphylococcal activity and resistance to beta-lactamases.— J. F. John and W. F. McNeill, *Antimicrob. Ag. Chemother.*, 1980, *17*, 179. See also N. Frimodt-Møller *et al.*, *J. antimicrob. Chemother.*, 1986, *18*, 27.

Cephalothin and cephaloridine have some activity against the common Enterobacteriaceae, however, with their increasing use, resistant strains, often klebsiellae or *Serratia* spp., are being reported. Such strains usually produce beta-lactamases capable of hydrolysing these otherwise fairly beta-lactamase-stable compounds.— R. Wise, *Lancet*, 1982, *2*, 140.

TOLERANCE. Of 7 strains of *Staph. aureus* which displayed tolerance to penicillins, 5 were cross-tolerant to the bactericidal effect of cephalothin.— L. D. Sabath *et al.*, *Lancet*, 1977, *1*, 443.

Further reports of tolerance to cephalothin: J. J. Bradley *et al.*, *Antimicrob. Ag. Chemother.*, 1978, *13*, 1052 (*Staph. aureus*); A. S. Bayer *et al.*, *ibid.*, *14*, 720 (lactobacilli); J. T. Noble *et al.* (letter), *Lancet*, 1980, *2*, 982 (Lancefield group G streptococci); C. G. Mayhall and E. Apollo, *Antimicrob. Ag. Chemother.*, 1980, *18*, 784 (*Staph. aureus*); K. V. I. Rolston *et al.*, *J. antimicrob. Chemother.*, 1984, *13*, 389 (group G streptococci).

Absorption and Fate

Cephalothin is poorly absorbed from the gastro-intestinal tract. After intramuscular injection peak plasma concentrations of about 10 and 20 µg per mL are achieved within 30 minutes of doses of 0.5 and 1 g, respectively. Concentrations of 30 to 60 µg per mL have been reported 15 minutes after the intravenous injection of a 1-g dose; a range of 14 to 20 µg per mL has been achieved by the continuous intravenous infusion of 500 mg per hour.

Cephalothin is widely distributed in body tissues and fluids except the brain and cerebrospinal fluid where the concentrations achieved are low and unpredictable. It readily diffuses across the placenta into the foetal circulation and low concentrations have been detected in breast milk. The biological half-life varies from about 30 to 50 minutes, and is shorter than that of many other cephalosporins. About 70% of cephalothin in the circulation is bound to plasma proteins.

Approximately 20 to 30% of cephalothin is rapidly deacetylated in the liver and about 60 to 70% of a dose is excreted in the urine by the renal tubules within 6 hours as cephalothin and the relatively inactive metabolite, desacetylcephalothin. High urine concentrations of 0.8 and 2.5 mg per mL have been observed following intramuscular doses of 0.5 and 1 g, respectively. Probenecid blocks the renal excretion of cephalothin. A very small amount is excreted in bile.

A review of the pharmacokinetics and clinical use of cephalosporin antibiotics including cephalothin.— C. H. Nightingale *et al.*, *J. pharm. Sci.*, 1975, *64*, 1899.

ADMINISTRATION IN THE ELDERLY. A study of the pharmacokinetics of cephalothin 1 g administered by intravenous bolus injection in 4 bedridden elderly patients compared with 7 healthy young subjects. The mean serum concentration of cephalothin was 7 µg per mL after 4 hours in the elderly patients while in the healthy subjects it was not detectable after 2.5 hours; the mean half-life was found to be 56.4 and 19.7 minutes, respectively, and the mean volume of distribution was 0.283 and 0.176 litres per kg, respectively. In the elderly patients about 32% of the administered dose was excreted in the first 2 hours and about 42% in 24 hours. In healthy subjects about 53% was excreted in the first 2 hours and then excretion was slight totalling only 57% after 24 hours. In bedridden elderly patients decreased renal excretion of cephalothin appears to be related to decreased renal function and an increased volume of distribution which may be due to slower peripheral circulation and a decrease in serum albumin concentration.— H. Yasuhara *et al.*, *J. clin. Pharmac.*, 1982, *22*, 403.

ADMINISTRATION IN LIVER DISORDERS. A study of the pharmacokinetics and protein binding of cephalothin in 20 patients with cirrhosis or hepatitis, but with normal renal function, compared with 12 healthy subjects. Protein binding was not significantly reduced, but systemic clearance of cephalothin was decreased by cirrhosis, probably reflecting the diminished hepatic metabolism. However, no dosage reduction appears to be necessary, even in severe hepatic impairment, unless the patient also has renal dysfunction.— K. Ohashi *et al.*, *J. antimicrob. Chemother.*, 1986, *17*, 347.

ADMINISTRATION IN RENAL FAILURE. After intravenous administration of cephalothin 2 g every 8 hours or 1 g every 6 hours to 7 patients with normal renal function, the mean serum half-life of cephalothin, calculated after the first dose, was 28 minutes and the deacetyl metabolite was eliminated fairly rapidly from the circulatory system. However, in 5 patients with severely impaired renal function given cephalothin 1 g every 12 or 24 hours, the half-life of cephalothin was 221 minutes and there was a continuous accumulation of deacetylcephalothin during the 5-day treatment period. For satisfactory monitoring of antibiotic concentrations in uraemic patients, individual quantitation of cephalothin and its deacetyl metabolite are required since a relatively low level of antibacterial activity may conceal a high concentration of the metabolite.— I. Nilsson-Ehle and P. Nilsson-Ehle, *J. infect. Dis.*, 1979, *139*, 712.

The normal half-life of cephalothin of 0.5 to 0.9 hours is increased in end-stage renal disease to 3 to 18 hours. A dialysis half-life of 3.3 hours has been reported in patients undergoing haemodialysis.— C. -s. C. Lee and T. C. Marbury, *Clin. Pharmacokinet.*, 1984, *9*, 42. See also under Administration in Renal Failure in Uses, below.

DIFFUSION INTO BODY TISSUES AND FLUIDS. Reports on the diffusion of cephalothin into body tissues and fluids: J. S. Tan and S. J. Salstrom, *Antimicrob. Ag. Chemother.*, 1977, *11*, 698 (interstitial fluid); R. H. Fitzgerald *et al.*, *ibid.*, 1978, *14*, 723 (bone and synovial tissues); W. J. Cady *et al.*, *Drug Intell. & clin. Pharm.*, 1983, *17*, 645 (bone and synovial fluid).

Uses and Administration

Cephalothin sodium is a first-generation cephalosporin antibiotic which is used in the treatment of infections due to susceptible organisms including skin and soft tissue infections, bone and joint infections, and infections of the respiratory and urinary tracts. It is less susceptible to penicillinase than many other cephalosporins and may be more effective in infections caused by penicillin-resistant staphylococci.

Cephalothin sodium is given by slow intravenous injection over 3 to 5 minutes or by intermittent or continuous infusion. It may be given intramuscularly but this route is painful. Doses are expressed in terms of the equivalent amount of cephalothin. The usual dose is 0.5 to 1 g of cephalothin every 4 to 6 hours; doses of 12 g daily may be given in severe infections. Children may be given 80 to 160 mg per kg body-weight daily in divided doses.

Reduced doses are recommended if cephalothin has to be given to patients with impaired renal function; patients with anuria may be given maintenance doses of 1 to 1.5 g or occasionally 3 g daily in divided doses. With creatinine clearances below 10, 25, 50, or 80 mL per minute doses of 0.5, 1, 1.5, or 2 g respectively may be given every 6 hours. Alternatively, the interval between doses has been increased (see under Administration in Renal Failure, below).

Cephalothin sodium is also used perioperatively for contaminated surgical procedures or when postoperative infection could be especially serious. Cephalothin 1 to 2 g may be administered approximately half an hour before surgical incision and again during surgery depending on the length of operation. A dose of 1 g every 6 hours should be given postoperatively for 24 hours.

The cephalosporins have been used as alternatives to penicillins in patients allergic to penicillins, but such patients may also have allergic reactions to cephalosporins. For parenteral treatment of staphylococcal or non-enterococcal streptococcal infections, a 'first-generation' cephalosporin such as cephalothin, cefapirin, cephradine, or cephazolin can be used; for staphylococcal endocarditis, some workers prefer cephalothin or cefapirin. Methicillin-resistant strains of staphylococci are also resistant to cephalosporins. The second- and third-generation cephalosporins have greater activity against enteric Gram-negative bacilli.— *Med. Lett.*, 1986, *28*, 33.

ADMINISTRATION. Some manufacturers have recommended that if intravenous infusions of cephalothin are given in doses larger than 6 g daily for periods longer than 3 days, the veins may have to be alternated. The addition of 10 to 25 mg of hydrocortisone to intravenous solutions containing 4 to 6 g of cephalothin may reduce the incidence of thrombophlebitis and the use of small intravenous needles in the larger available veins may be preferred.

ADMINISTRATION IN INFANTS AND CHILDREN. For severe infections in children cephalothin has been given intravenously in doses of 100 to 160 mg per kg body-weight daily in 4 to 6 divided doses. However, the first- and second-generation cephalosporins have limited application in the treatment of severe infections in infants and children because they do not penetrate sufficiently into the cerebrospinal fluid to be effective in treating or preventing meningitis.— K. H. Rhodes and C. M. Johnson, *Mayo Clin. Proc.*, 1983, *58*, 158.

ADMINISTRATION IN LIVER DISORDERS. For comment on dosage adjustment in patients with hepatic impairment, see Absorption and Fate, above.

ADMINISTRATION IN RENAL FAILURE. The dosage interval should be increased from 6 to 8 hours in patients with moderate renal failure, and to 12 to 24 hours in those with severe renal failure.— P. Sharpstone, *Br. med. J.*, 1977, *2*, 36.

After a loading dose of 1 to 3 g cephalothin could be given in a dose of 1 to 2 g every 4 to 6 hours to patients with a creatinine clearance (CC) of 40 to 80 mL per minute, every 6 to 8 hours to those with a CC of 10 to 40 mL per minute, and every 8 to 12 hours to those with a CC of less than 10 mL per minute. In haemodialysis 1 to 2 g could be given every 8 to 12 hours and 1 to 2 g after dialysis.— J. S. Cheigh, *Am. J. Med.*, 1977, *62*, 555.

Cephalothin could be administered to patients with renal failure by adjusting the dosage interval. A dosage interval of 6 hours is suitable for patients whose glomerular filtration-rates are 10 mL or more per minute; an interval of 8 to 12 hours between doses is advisable for rates of less than 10 mL per minute. A dose supplement should be given to patients undergoing haemodialysis or peritoneal dialysis.— W. M. Bennett *et al.*, *Am. J. Kidney Dis.*, 1983, *3*, 155.

For the intraperitoneal administration of cephalothin in patients undergoing continuous ambulatory peritoneal dialysis, see Peritonitis, below.

ARTHRITIS, BACTERIAL. For reference to the use of cephalothin in bacterial arthritis, see Flucloxacillin Sodium, p.232.

ENDOCARDITIS. Endocarditis due to *Streptococcus sanguis* was successfully treated in 2 women with cephalothin alone or cephalothin plus gentamicin. Cephalothin could be used for the initial treatment of streptococcal endocarditis in patients allergic to penicillin instead of the more toxic regimen of vancomycin plus gentamicin which has been recommended by the British Society for Antimicrobial Chemotherapy (BSAC) (R.C. Spencer and K.G. Kristinsson, *Lancet*, 1985, *2*, 1250). In reply, the BSAC felt that they could not recommend cephalothin or any other cephalosporin for use in patients allergic to penicillins because about 10% of penicillin-sensitive patients will also be allergic to the cephalosporins (N.A. Simmons, *ibid.*).

NEUTROPENIA. For mention of the use of cephalothin in association with gentamicin, carbenicillin, or ticarcillin in the management of febrile episodes in neutropenic patients, see under Piperacillin Sodium, p.287.

OSTEOMYELITIS. For reference to the use of cephalothin in osteomyelitis, see Flucloxacillin Sodium, p.232.

PERITONITIS. Cephalothin has been used in patients with peritonitis undergoing continuous ambulatory peritoneal dialysis. The British Society for Antimicrobial Chemotherapy has recommended that a loading dose of 1 g may be administered intravenously or intraperitoneally in the severely ill patient, and a maintenance dose of 250 mg per litre of dialysis fluid should be given intraperitoneally.— *Lancet*, 1987, *1*, 845. See also.— D. K. Scott and D. E. Roberts, *Pharm. J.*, 1985, *1*, 621. For comparison of the antimicrobial activities of various cephalosporins and the problems associated with the use of a cephalosporin as first-line therapy for peritonitis, see under Cefuroxime Sodium, p.172. See also under Choice of Antibiotic, p.99.

SURGICAL INFECTION PROPHYLAXIS. A report indicating that, unlike cephaloridine and cephazolin, cephalothin may not be effective in the prophylaxis of surgical wound infection. Cephalothin sodium attained, but did not maintain, wound concentrations consistent with effective antimicrobial activity even with 2-g doses given intravenously. There did not appear to be a reasonable likelihood of protection in any operation lasting more than one hour.— H. C. Polk *et al.*, *J. Am. med. Ass.*, 1980, *244*, 1353.

In a study of chemoprophylaxis in 48 patients undergoing orthopaedic surgery, bone concentrations of cephalothin showed a rather rapid decay, compared with concentrations of cefoxitin which were maintained for at least 2 hours, following a single 1-g dose of antibiotic given by intravenous bolus injection. No significant difference in morbidity was observed in either treatment group.— M. B. Rosenfeld *et al.*, *Antimicrob. Ag. Chemother.*, 1981, *19*, 826.

For comparison of the prophylactic use of cephalothin with cephamandole in cardiac surgery, see under Cephamandole Sodium, p.182.

Preparations

Cephalothin Injection *(B.P.)*. Contains cephalothin sodium; to be reconstituted before use.

Cephalothin Sodium Injection *(U.S.P.)*. Store in the frozen state. pH 6.0 to 8.5.

Cephalothin Sodium for Injection *(U.S.P.)*

Sterile Cephalothin Sodium *(U.S.P.)*

Proprietary Preparations

Keflin *(Lilly, UK)*. *Injection*, powder for reconstitution, cephalothin 1 g (as sodium salt).

Proprietary Names and Manufacturers

Averon *(Spain)*; Cephation *(Jpn)*; Ceporacin *(Glaxo, Austral.; Belg.; Glaxo, Canad.; Neth.; Glaxo, Spain)*; Cepovenin *(Hoechst, Ger.)*; CET *(Jpn)*; Coaxin *(Jpn)*; Keflin *(Arg.; Lilly, Austral.; Belg.; Lilly, Canad.; Lilly, Denm.; Lilly, Fr.; Lilly, Ital.; Neth.; Lilly, Norw.; Lilly, S.Afr.; Lilly, Spain; Lilly, Swed.; Lilly, UK; Lilly, USA)*; Keflin N *(Lilly, Switz.)*; Seffin *(Arg.; Glaxo, USA)*; Synclotin *(Jpn)*; Toricelocin *(Jpn)*.

42-n

Cephamandole *(BAN)*.

83405; Cefamandole *(USAN, rINN)*. (7*R*)-7-D-Mandelamido-3-(1-methyl-1*H*-tetrazol-5-ylthiomethyl)-3-cephem-4-carboxylic acid.

$C_{18}H_{18}N_6O_5S_2$=462.5.

CAS — 34444-01-4.

18358-s

Cephamandole Nafate *(BAN)*.

106223; Cefamandole Nafate *(USAN, rINNM)*. Sodium (7*R*)-7-[(2*R*)-2-formyloxy-2-phenylacetamido]-3-(1-methyl-1*H*-tetrazol-5-ylthiomethyl)-3-cephem-4-carboxylate.

$C_{19}H_{17}N_6NaO_6S_2$=512.5.

CAS — 42540-40-9.

Pharmacopoeias. U.S. includes Sterile Cefamandole Nafate.

1.11 g of monograph substance is approximately equivalent to 1 g of cephamandole activity and represents 2.2 mmol of sodium. Proprietary preparations (Kefadol and Mandol) contain sodium carbonate and the total sodium content of these preparations is approximately 3.3 mmol per g of cephamandole activity.

Freely **soluble** in water; practically insoluble in most organic solvents. A 10% solution has a pH of 3.5 to 7.0; a 10% solution of Cefamandole Nafate for Injection *(U.S.P.)* has a pH of between 6 and 8.

Cephamandole nafate has been reported to be **incompatible** with aminoglycosides and cimetidine hydrochloride. Formulations of cephamandole nafate available for injection contain sodium carbonate and are incompatible with solutions containing calcium or magnesium salts. When reconstituted with water the sodium carbonate rapidly hydrolyses about 30% of the ester to cephamandole sodium; during storage of the reconstituted solution at room temperature carbon dioxide is produced. Solutions for injection should be used within 96 hours if stored at 5° or within 24 hours if kept at 25°.

A study of the stability of cephamandole nafate injection with parenteral solutions and additives. Greater than 90% potency was retained in all intramuscular and intravenous solutions for at least 2 days when stored at 25° and 10 days at 5°. Conservative limits of 24 hours for cephamandole nafate solutions stored at 25° or 96 hours at 5° are, however, recommended because of the potential for contamination and subsequent microbial growth in extemporaneously prepared solutions. Visual incompatibility in the form of a haze was noted in several solutions including those containing Ringer's injection, Isolyte M with dextrose 5% injection *(McGraw, USA)*, and Plasma-Lyte injection *(Travenol, USA)*. Cephamandole nafate was incompatible with tobramycin sulphate, gentamicin sulphate, calcium gluceptate, and calcium gluconate. Lignocaine hydrochloride 0.5, 1.0, and 2.0% intramuscular solutions were compatible with cephamandole nafate at a concentration greater than 100 mg per mL, and lignocaine hydrochloride 0.1 and 0.2% intravenous solutions were compatible with cephamandole nafate concentrations less than 100 mg per mL; admixtures at concentrations other than these produced turbidity or precipitation immediately or during storage.— R. A. Frable *et al.*, *Am. J. Hosp. Pharm.*, 1982, *39*, 622 and 1479 (correction). See also V. Das Gupta and K. R. Stewart, *ibid.*, 1981, *38*, 875.

STORAGE. Comment from the manufacturers *(Lilly, USA)* that reconstituted solutions of cephamandole nafate do not need to be protected from light. The powder will, however, discolour upon prolonged exposure to light.— A. L. Fites (letter), *Am. J. Hosp. Pharm.*, 1980, *37*, 334.

Frozen solutions of cephamandole nafate in Water for Injection, sodium chloride injection 0.9%, or glucose injection 5% were found to be stable for at least 26 weeks when stored at −20° in the original glass vials or in polyvinyl chloride plastic containers.— M. Bornstein *et al.*, *Am. J. Hosp. Pharm.*, 1980, *37*, 98. See also C. J. Holmes *et al.*, *Drug Intell. & clin. Pharm.*, 1980, *14*, 353.

43-h

Cephamandole Sodium *(BANM)*.

Cefamandole Sodium *(USAN, rINNM)*. The monosodium salt of cephamandole.

$C_{18}H_{17}N_6NaO_5S_2$=484.5.

CAS — 30034-03-8.

Pharmacopoeias. U.S. includes Sterile Cefamandole Sodium.

1.05 g of monograph substance is approximately equivalent to 1 g of cephamandole and represents 2.2 mmol of sodium. A 10% solution has a pH of 3.5 to 7.0; a 10% solution of Cefamandole Sodium for Injection *(U.S.P.)* has a pH of between 6.0 and 8.5.

Adverse Effects and Precautions

As for Cephalothin Sodium, p.176.

Cephamandole may cause hypoprothrombinaemia which is usually reversible with administration of vitamin K; care should be taken in patients receiving anticoagulants. A disulfiram-like interaction with alcohol may occur and patients receiving cephamandole should therefore avoid alcohol during, and for at least several days after treatment.

In a study of cephamandole 6 to 12 g daily for the treatment of soft tissue and skeletal infections, 12 of 38 patients experienced adverse drug reactions: maculopapular rash, 1; maculopapular rash and eosinophilia, 2; eosinophilia without rash, 1; blood urea nitrogen (BUN) and creatinine elevation, 2; proteinuria, 1; serum glutamic-oxaloacetic transaminase (SGOT) and alkaline phosphatase elevation, 3; pancytopenia, 1; and leucopenia, 1.— J. L. LeFrock *et al.*, *Drug Intell. & clin. Pharm.*, 1981, *15*, 951.

From an analysis of 148 reported episodes of drug fever 46 were caused by antimicrobial agents and of these 1 was due to cephamandole.— P. A. Mackowiak and C. F. LeMaistre, *Ann. intern. Med.*, 1987, *106*, 728.

ADMINISTRATION IN RENAL FAILURE. For the precautions to be observed in renal failure, see under Uses and Administration, below.

EFFECTS ON THE BLOOD. *Hypoprothrombinaemia.* Cephamandole has been associated with hypoprothrombinaemia particularly in patients with a poor dietary intake, such as seriously ill patients receiving parenteral nutrition, and in patients with renal failure; severe bleeding has occurred in some patients and a fatality has been reported. An antibiotic-associated deficit in vitamin K has been proposed as a cause of the hypoprothrombinaemia and the prolongation of prothrombin time has responded to administration of vitamin K. Some workers have suggested that the combination of low vitamin K intake and limited synthesis of the vitamin, due to suppression of intestinal bacterial flora by antibiotic secreted in the bile, may produce a prothrombin deficiency (C.A. Hooper *et al.*, *Lancet*, 1980, *1*, 39; W. Rymer and C.W. Greenlaw, *Drug Intell. & clin. Pharm.*, 1980, *14*, 780). However, some cases of hypoprothrombinaemia have occurred in patients who were not severely compromised nutritionally and the nutritional significance of vitamin K derived from intestinal flora has been questioned (C.M. Clancy and R.H. Glew, *Lancet*, 1983, *1*, 250; K. Bruch, *ibid.*, 535). Also, many antibiotics are secreted in bile but are not associated with an increased incidence of hypoprothrombinaemia. Therefore, other workers have reasoned that cephamandole causes inhibition of the vitamin-K-dependent aspects of synthesis of prothrombin in the liver. The *N*-methylthiotetrazole side chain which is present in cephamandole and several other cephalosporins including cefmetazole, cefmenoxime, cefoperazone, and latamoxef, appears to be associated with hypoprothrombinaemia (H.C. Neu, *Ann. intern. Med.*, 1983, *98*, 415). It has been proposed that the methylthiotetrazole group inhibits the gamma carboxylation of glutamic acid which is a necessary reaction in the synthesis of prothrombin; vitamin K is a cofactor for this reaction (J.J. Lipsky,

Lancet, 1983, *2*, 192; F. R. Sattler, *Ann. intern. Med.*, 1986, *105*, 924). More recently the sulphydryl group in the side chain has been related to hypoprothrombinaemia, although additional factors are thought to be necessary to cause clinically significant haemorrhagic complications (G. Agnelli *et al.*, *Antimicrob. Ag. Chemother.*, 1986, *29*, 1108).

Neutropenia. Neutropenia has been reported in 3 patients who received large doses of cephamandole; 2 patients received more than 150 mg per kg body-weight daily. Onset of symptoms occurred after 18 to 21 days and recovery within 4 days.— C. F. Kirkwood *et al.*, *Clin. Pharm.*, 1983, *2*, 569.

EFFECTS ON THE SKIN. A report of toxic epidermal necrolysis associated with the administration of cephamandole.— R. N. Greenberg *et al.*, *Antimicrob. Ag. Chemother.*, 1979, *15*, 337.

INTERACTIONS. *Alcohol.* There have been several reports of a disulfiram-like reaction to alcohol in patients receiving cephamandole or some other cephalosporins (H. Portier *et al.*, *Lancet*, 1980, *2*, 263; S. Drummer *et al.*, *New Engl. J. Med.*, 1980, *303*, 1417). This reaction is attributed to the methylthiotetrazole side chain which has a molecular similarity to disulfiram (H.C. Neu, *Ann. intern. Med.*, 1983, *98*, 415). It has been suggested that this side chain is liberated *in vivo* and oxidised to 5,5′-dithiobis(1-methyltetrazole) which, like disulfiram, is a rapid inactivator of cytoplasmic aldehyde dehydrogenase so that acetaldehyde accumulates during alcohol metabolism (T.M. Kitson, *Lancet*, 1984, *2*, 1338). Interactions are also possible with preparations which contain significant amounts of alcohol such as cyclosporin preparations (L.E. Kerr, *Clin. Pharm.*, 1984, *3*, 346) or theophylline elixir (K.R. Brown *et al.*, *Ann. intern. Med.*, 1982, *97*, 621).

Warfarin. Since cephamandole may cause hypoprothrombinaemia its effects on the response to warfarin were studied retrospectively in patients who had undergone cardiac valve replacement surgery. Fourteen of 44 patients (32%) receiving prophylactic cephamandole therapy compared with 1 of 16 patients (6%) receiving vancomycin were considered to have an enhanced response to postoperative warfarin; 3 of the 14 given cephamandole and the one given vancomycin had received additional drugs that may have interacted with warfarin. Excessively high prothrombin times within 2 days of an initial warfarin dose were observed in patients with apparently adequate nutrition and normal prothrombin times before surgery; older cardiac valve replacement patients were considered to be at a high risk for profound cephamandole-induced warfarin sensitivity early in the postoperative period of anticoagulant therapy.— D. M. Angaran *et al.*, *Ann. Surg.*, 1984, *199*, 107.

PREGNANCY AND THE NEONATE. The view that cephamandole and other cephalosporins containing an *N*-methyltetrazole side chain should be avoided in pregnancy on theoretical grounds of interference with vitamin K metabolism.— R. Wise, *Br. med. J.*, 1987, *294*, 42.

THROMBOPHLEBITIS. A comparison of the incidence of phlebitis due to cephamandole, cefapirin, or buffered cephalothin in 12 healthy men given a total of 530 doses of antibiotics through 56 intravenous sites. Approximately 50% of intravenous sites developed mild phlebitis and 25% developed moderate phlebitis. The frequency of mild phlebitis did not differ significantly among the 3 cephalosporins, however, moderate phlebitis occurred most frequently with cephamandole and least often with buffered cephalothin.— S. Berger *et al.*, *Antimicrob. Ag. Chemother.*, 1976, *9*, 575.

Of 46 patients with infusion phlebitis, cephamandole was implicated as the causative agent in 10 patients. The incidence of cephamandole-induced phlebitis was reduced when the drug was administered in 100-mL volumes of solution rather than 50-mL. It was recommended that a dose of 1 to 2 g should be administered with at least 150 mL of intravenous fluid over 30 to 60 minutes.— C. A. Harrigan, *NITA*, 1984, *7*, 478.

Antimicrobial Action

Cephamandole is bactericidal and acts similarly to cephalothin, but has a broader spectrum of activity than the older cephalosporins. It generally has similar or less activity against Gram-positive cocci but is resistant to some beta-lactamases produced by Gram-negative bacteria and is more active against many of the Enterobacteriaceae including some strains of *Enterobacter, Escherichia coli, Klebsiella* and *Salmonella* spp. and indole-positive *Proteus* spp. Cephamandole is very active *in vitro* against *Haemophilus influenzae* although an inoculum effect has been reported. Cephamandole is active against many anaerobes although most strains of *Bacteroides fragilis* are usually resistant. *Pseudomonas* spp. are also resistant.

The minimum inhibitory concentrations of cephamandole for susceptible Gram-positive organisms have been reported to range from about 0.1 to 2.0 µg per mL; for most susceptible Gram-negative organisms concentrations of 0.5 to 8.0 µg per mL are usually required.

The activities of cephamandole, cefoxitin, cephalexin, and cephalothin were compared *in vitro* in broth and agar dilutions against 645 strains of bacteria from clinical sources. Cephamandole and cephalothin were the most effective against Gram-positive organisms while cephamandole and cefoxitin were most effective against Gram-negative organisms. Cephamandole was more active than cefoxitin against *Proteus mirabilis, Pr. rettgeri,* and *Enterobacter* spp. as well as *Neisseria meningitidis, N. gonorrhoeae*, and *Haemophilus influenzae.* An inoculum effect was demonstrated for cephamandole when testing *H. influenzae.*— T. C. Eickhoff and J. M. Ehret, *Antimicrob. Ag. Chemother.*, 1976, *9*, 994. Another study of the activity *in vitro* of cefoxitin and cephamandole showed diminished activity of cephamandole in broth compared with agar medium; this was not the case with cefoxitin. The main advantage of cephamandole over cefoxitin was in its action against some strains of *Enterobacter.*— H. G. Adams *et al.*, *ibid.*, 1019. Discrepancies in the sensitivity of *Enterobacter* spp. to cephamandole measured by agar and broth dilutions appeared to be due to a relatively high mutation-rate to resistance.— C. M. Findell and J. C. Sherris, *ibid.*, 970.

Depending on the test used, cephamandole nafate had about one-tenth the antibacterial activity *in vitro* of cephamandole but since cephamandole nafate was rapidly hydrolysed to cephamandole the activities *in vivo* were virtually identical.— J. R. Turner *et al.*, *Antimicrob. Ag. Chemother.*, 1977, *12*, 67. Since cephamandole nafate did not have the equivalent antibacterial activity of cephamandole *in vitro*, it was recommended that before microbiological assay the nafate should be hydrolysed. It might be advisable to use either the sodium or lithium salts of cephamandole in microbiological studies.— C. L. Winely *et al.*, *Antimicrob. Ag. Chemother.*, 1979, *16*, 424.

The *in vitro* activity of cephamandole against Gram-negative organisms did not correlate well with its stability to beta-lactamases.— K. P. Fu and H. C. Neu, *J. infect. Dis.*, 1978, *137*, *Suppl.* (May), S38.

A study of the accuracy of diffusion susceptibility tests with disks containing 30 µg of cephamandole or cephalothin indicated that although the same interpretive zone standards could be applied to tests with either disk the two drugs could not be tested interchangeably.— A. L. Barry *et al.*, *Antimicrob. Ag. Chemother.*, 1979, *15*, 140.

ACTIVITY AGAINST ENTEROBACTERIACEAE. *Escherichia.* Cephamandole was the most active of 7 cephalosporins against *E. coli* but it was not resistant to all 4 of the beta-lactamases tested. Cefoxitin and to a lesser extent cefuroxime were resistant to the beta-lactamases and only slightly less active than cephamandole against *E. coli.*— M. H. Richmond and S. Wotton, *Antimicrob. Ag. Chemother.*, 1976, *10*, 219.

Sub-inhibitory concentrations of cephamandole and gentamicin enhanced phagocytosis and killing of *E. coli* by hepatic macrophages *in vitro.* At one-fifth of the minimum inhibitory concentration for *E. coli* cephamandole induced elongation of bacteria due to its effect on cell wall synthesis.— A. Andreana *et al.*, *Antimicrob. Ag. Chemother.*, 1984, *25*, 182.

Salmonellae. Cephamandole had a similar activity to cefaclor, and was more active than cephazolin, cephalothin or cephalexin *in vitro* against 67 strains of *Salmonella typhi* and 54 strains of *S. paratyphi* A.— L. J. Strausbaugh *et al.*, *Antimicrob. Ag. Chemother.*, 1978, *13*, 134.

ACTIVITY AGAINST HAEMOPHILUS. Cephamandole has activity against both ampicillin-susceptible and ampicillin-resistant strains of *Haemophilus influenzae* (J.H. Jorgensen and G.A. Alexander, *Antimicrob. Ag. Chemother.*, 1978, *13*, 342), although limited bactericidal activity has been demonstrated particularly for ampicillin-resistant strains (E. Yourassowsky *et al.*, *ibid.*, 1979, *15*, 325; M.G. Bergeron *et al.*, *ibid.*, 1981, *19*, 101). An inoculum effect for beta-lactamase-producing organisms has been observed and cephamandole could not therefore be recommended for the treatment of ampicillin-resistant *H. influenzae* meningitis (V.P. Syriopoulou *et al.*, *Antimicrob. Ag. Chemother.*, 1979, *16*, 510; M.C. Thirumoorthi *et al.*, *ibid.*, 1981, *20*, 208).

ACTIVITY AGAINST STAPHYLOCOCCI. Cephamandole has been reported to have comparable activity to cephalothin or cephazolin against *Staphylococcus aureus in vitro.* However, 4 patients with *Staph. aureus* bacteraemia failed to respond to treatment with cephamandole. Cephamandole and cephazolin are more readily destroyed by staphylococcal beta-lactamase than cephalothin or the penicillinase-resistant penicillins such as methicillin and, in addition, cephamandole and cephazolin may be more susceptible to the effects of inoculum size. It has been reported that small differences detected in the beta-lactamase stability may be important and could explain the observed clinical failures with certain cephalosporins (R.H.K. Eng *et al.*, *J. antimicrob. Chemother.*, 1985, *16*, 663).

The cross-resistance reported between methicillin and cephalosporins for both coagulase-positive and coagulase-negative staphylococcal strains does not appear to occur with cephamandole *in vitro* (R.F. Frongillo *et al.*, *Antimicrob. Ag. Chemother.*, 1984, *25*, 666; K.V.I. Rolston *et al.*, *J. antimicrob. Chemother.*, 1985, *16*, 659). However, cephamandole given to *mice* with methicillin-resistant *Staph. aureus* infection required a dosage of approximately 20 times that needed for infection due to methicillin-sensitive strains, despite the fact that the minimum inhibitory concentrations *in vitro* were similar. Therefore conventional sensitivity testing of *Staph. aureus* to cephamandole does not appear suitable for predicting its efficiency *in vivo* (A. Hirschl *et al.*, *J. antimicrob. Chemother.*, 1984, *13*, 429).

See also under Uses, Septicaemia, below.

ACTIVITY WITH OTHER ANTIMICROBIAL AGENTS. Synergy has been reported *in vitro* between cephamandole and gentamicin or amikacin against Enterobacteriaceae (K.P. Fu and H.C. Neu, *J. infect. Dis.*, 1978, *137*, *Suppl.* (May), S38; R.H. Glew and R.A. Pavuk, *Antimicrob. Ag. Chemother.*, 1984, *26*, 378), cephamandole and fosfomycin against methicillin-resistant *Staphylococcus aureus* (S. Alvarez *et al.*, *ibid.*, 1985, *28*, 689), and between cephamandole and erythromycin against *Bacteroides fragilis* (R.S. Griffith *et al.*, *ibid.*, 1977, *11*, 813). However, antagonism has also been reported with cephamandole and erythromycin against *Staph. aureus* and *Escherichia coli* (J.R. Cohn *et al.*, *ibid.*, 1980, *18*, 872). Antagonism has been demonstrated with cephamandole and cefoxitin against *Enterobacter cloacae* infections *in mice* and it appeared to be due to a reversible induction of beta-lactamases by cefoxitin (R.V. Goering *et al.*, *Antimicrob. Ag. Chemother.*, 1982, *21*, 963).

Resistance

As for Cephalothin Sodium, p.178.

Cephamandole is slightly less susceptible than cephalothin to inhibition by some Gram-negative beta-lactamases.

Strains of *Streptococcus pneumoniae* isolated from 5 children were partially resistant to cephamandole.— P. C. Appelbaum *et al.*, *Lancet*, 1977, *2*, 995.

There was little correlation between beta-lactamase production and decreased susceptibility of strains of Enterobacteriaceae to cephamandole or cefoxitin. It was suggested that other characteristics such as decreased cell permeability and increased intrinsic resistance might be responsible for resistance.— J. L. Ott *et al.*, *Antimicrob. Ag. Chemother.*, 1979, *15*, 14. Studies *in vitro* indicated the presence of cefoxitin-inducible beta-lactamases among many strains of cephalothin-resistant, cephamandole-susceptible Enterobacteriaceae. The enzymes were highly active against cephamandole but less so against cefoxitin.— C. C. Sanders and W. E. Sanders, *ibid.*, 792.

Since discrepancies between susceptibility tests *in vitro* and results *in vivo* have been noted with cephamandole, resistance and the presence of inducible beta-lactamases was studied in 5 seriously ill patients in whom problems with cephamandole therapy were encountered. Resistance to cephamandole emerged during therapy with the drug in 3 patients, two of whom were infected with *Enterobacter* spp. and one with *E. coli*; resistance was associated with enhanced enzyme concentrations and/or with changes in the substrate specificities of the beta-lactamases. Concurrent development of resistance to beta-lactam antibiotics other than cephamandole also occurred and was not always associated with enhanced beta-lactamase activity. In the fourth patient routine disk diffusion tests failed to detect resistance to cephamandole in *E. cloacae*; this resistance would have been detected had a broth dilution test been used. The fifth patient developed postoperative wound infection with a cephamandole-resistant strain of *Enterobacter* during prophylaxis with the drug. All of the isolates from these patients, except the *E. coli* strain, possessed inducible beta-lactamases that were active against cephamandole.

The observations from this study and studies *in vitro* suggest that certain micro-organisms may be especially prone to becoming resistant to cephamandole during therapy or prophylaxis.— C. C. Sanders *et al.*, *J. infect. Dis.*, 1982, *145*, 118.

In a comparison of the activity of cephamandole *in vitro* and *in vivo* 20 patients received cephamandole 8 to 12 g daily by intermittent intravenous infusion for a variety of cephalothin-resistant Gram-negative bacillary infections. All infecting organisms were susceptible *in vitro* using the disk diffusion test, but 3 were resistant on determination of MIC by tube-dilution technique; of these 3, one was from a patient who exhibited delayed bacteriological clearing, and one was from 1 of 3 patients who subsequently relapsed. The 3 patients who relapsed all had closed-space infections and were treated for at least 28 days. Cephamandole should not be used alone for serious infections due to *Enterobacter, Serratia* or indole-positive *Proteus* spp., especially if a prolonged course of antibiotic therapy is anticipated; for less severe infections it may be used alone provided the organisms are susceptible by the tube dilution technique.— P. E. Kopp *et al.*, *Curr. ther. Res.*, 1984, *35*, 627.

The bactericidal effect of beta-lactam drugs was found to be considerably weaker against organisms in colonies than would be expected from tests on isolated bacteria. When an *E. coli* strain producing high concentrations of TEM-1 beta-lactamase constituted 6% or more of the population it enabled survival of all the non-beta-lactamase-producing strains at much higher concentrations of cephamandole than conventional minimum inhibitory concentrations. A limited selection of the resistant subpopulation can lead to an important protection of the whole population. This could probably explain, at least partially, the presence of sensitive isolates in infections that fail to respond to apparently appropriate antibiotic treatment.— F. Baquero *et al.*, *J. antimicrob. Chemother.*, 1985, *15*, 151.

Absorption and Fate

Cephamandole is poorly absorbed from the gastro-intestinal tract. It is given intramuscularly or intravenously, usually as the nafate which is rapidly hydrolysed to release cephamandole *in vivo*. Peak plasma concentrations for cephamandole of about 13 and 25 µg per mL have been achieved 0.5 to 2 hours after intramuscular doses of 0.5 and 1 g respectively; concentrations are very low after 6 hours. Immediately after the intravenous infusion of 1 g over 30 minutes a plasma concentration of about 85 µg per mL has been reported. About 70% is bound to plasma proteins. Plasma half-lives vary from about 0.5 to 1.2 hours depending on the route of injection.

Cephamandole is widely distributed in body tissues and fluids including bone, joint fluid, and pleural fluid; it diffuses into the CSF when the meninges are inflamed, but concentrations are unpredictable. Cephamandole has also been detected in breast milk. It is rapidly excreted unchanged by glomerular filtration and renal tubular secretion; about 80% of a dose is excreted within 6 hours and high urinary concentrations are achieved. Probenecid competes for renal tubular secretion with cephamandole resulting in higher and prolonged plasma concentrations of cephamandole. Cephamandole is excreted in bile.

A comparison of the pharmacokinetics of cephamandole and other cephalosporins.— H. C. Neu, *J. infect. Dis.*, 1978, *137, Suppl.* (May), S80.

In a study of 10 healthy subjects serum concentrations of cephamandole were about 5 times higher than those of cephalothin 0.5 to 1 hour after an intravenous injection of 1 g of cephamandole or cephalothin. The mean serum concentration of cephamandole 3 hours after administration was 2.2 µg per mL compared with less than 0.1 µg per mL for cephalothin.— V. C. Simon *et al.*, *J. antimicrob. Chemother.*, 1978, *4*, 85.

The pharmacokinetics of cephamandole in morbidly obese surgical patients, including penetration into adipose tissue and postoperative wound drainage.— H. J. Mann and H. Buchwald, *Drug Intell. & clin. Pharm.*, 1986, *20*, 869.

ADMINISTRATION IN BILIARY DISORDERS. A study of the bile concentrations of cephamandole achieved in 16 patients with hepatobiliary disease, but normal renal function. Administration of 1 g by intravenous infusion over 15 to 20 minutes every 4 or 6 hours for 4 to 24 doses before surgery resulted in therapeutic bile concentrations in all 13 common bile duct samples studied; in 11 they were 350 µg or more per mL. Similarly, and in the absence of cystic duct obstruction, gall-bladder bile concentrations exceeded serum concentrations many fold; the antibiotic was undetectable in 2 patients with aseptic cystic duct obstruction, but detectable concentrations occurred when duct obstruction was associated with infection. The results suggest that the high biliary concentrations of cephamandole are not appreciably affected by nonobstructing calculi, and therapeutically effective gall-bladder bile concentrations may be attained in the presence of cystic duct obstruction if there is also an acute inflammatory reaction.— M. Uwaydah *et al.*, *Antimicrob. Ag. Chemother.*, 1982, *22*, 1087. Maximum biliary concentrations of cephamandole in 6 patients with previous total biliary obstruction did not exceed 50 µg per mL even when a 2-g dose was administered as late as 7 days after biliary decompression. This compares with reported mean peak concentrations of cephamandole in unobstructed bile of approximately 125 to 150 µg per mL per 1-g dose given intravenously. In patients with total biliary obstruction the hepatocytes do not appear to recover full secretory capacity for this drug, and possibly for other cephalosporins as well, for up to several days after restoration of the biliary flow.— J. U. Levi *et al.*, *ibid.*, 1984, *26*, 944.

ADMINISTRATION IN INFANTS AND CHILDREN. Blood concentrations and urinary excretion of cephamandole in 30 children and infants (3 months to 13 years) were similar to those previously reported by Meyers *et al.* (*Antimicrob. Ag. Chemother.*, 1976, *9*, 140) in healthy adults. The half-life for cephamandole following intramuscular administration was about 66 minutes in children under 1 year and 88 minutes in children 1 year or over; half-lives following intravenous injection were about 46 and 48 minutes respectively.— C. T. Chang *et al.*, *Antimicrob. Ag. Chemother.*, 1978, *14*, 838.

Cephamandole 37 mg per kg body-weight given intravenously every 6 hours was used successfully to treat 62 children with various infections. The serum half-life of cephamandole in children older than 1 year was between 1.0 and 1.5 hours, but in patients younger than 3 months the half-life appeared to be prolonged and was approximately 2 hours. Concentrations in the cerebrospinal fluid of 11 children ranged from 0.25 to 2.4 µg per mL; serum concentrations ranged from 0.86 to 30.2 µg per mL. The average CSF concentration was 4% of the mean serum concentration in children without active meningitis and 23% of the mean serum concentration in children with active meningitis.— S. H. Walker and V. P. Gahol, *Antimicrob. Ag. Chemother.*, 1978, *14*, 315.

A study of the pharmacokinetics and safety of cephamandole in the newborn.— M. M. Agbayani *et al.*, *Antimicrob. Ag. Chemother.*, 1979, *15*, 674.

In a study involving 34 children aged over 6 months, the mean serum half-life for cephamandole was 34 minutes following doses of 25 mg per kg body-weight intravenously or intramuscularly. Mean serum concentrations of 26.2 and 1.8 µg per mL occurred 1 hour and 3 hours, respectively, after the end of intravenous infusion of 25 mg per kg administered over 30 minutes at 4-hourly intervals, for one or more doses. However, when cephamandole 37.5 mg per kg was given as a 30-minute intravenous infusion every 6 hours, the mean serum concentration was 0.9 µg per mL at 4 hours and this was extrapolated to fall to 0.1 µg per mL at 6 hours. Cephamandole half-lives were shorter than previously reported and it appeared that cephamandole should be administered every 4 hours in the treatment of serious infections.— M. C. Thirumoorthi *et al.*, *Antimicrob. Ag. Chemother.*, 1981, *20*, 21.

ADMINISTRATION IN RENAL FAILURE. A half-life for cephamandole of 12.3 to 18 hours occurred in 4 patients with stable renal failure.— B. R. Meyers and S. Z. Hirschman, *Antimicrob. Ag. Chemother.*, 1977, *11*, 248.

Cephamandole nafate 1 g was administered intramuscularly to 22 patients with varying degrees of renal function. Mean peak plasma concentrations occurred 1 to 2 hours after administration; at 2 hours, plasma concentrations ranged from 17 µg per mL in patients with normal renal function to 42 µg per mL in anephric patients. Mean plasma half-lives were 1.49 hours in patients with normal renal function, 2.42 hours in patients with a creatinine clearance (CC) of 39 to 50 mL per minute, 6.03 hours in patients with a CC of 7 to 20 mL per minute, and 11.48 hours in anephric patients. Haemodialysis resulted in increased elimination of cephamandole. Whereas patients with a CC of 39 mL or more per minute excreted about 48% of a dose in the urine within 8 hours, patients with a CC of less than 20 mL per minute excreted only about 17%. There was significant variance in calculated plasma half-lives in patients with a CC of less than 20 mL per minute and it was recommended that in these patients doses should be adjusted according to serum-cephamandole concentrations.— A. W. Czerwinski and J. A. Pederson, *Antimicrob. Ag. Chemother.*, 1979, *15*, 161.

A study on the pharmacokinetics of cephamandole in uraemic patients undergoing haemodialysis. The half-life of cephamandole in 6 patients on haemodialysis ranged from 3.6 to 4.4 hours; in 3 patients who were off dialysis the half-life ranged from 9.3 to 17.3 hours. In this study dialysis reduced the half-life of cephamandole by 50 to 70%, but using the data from this and other studies, haemodialysis appears to reduce the half-life by approximately 15 to 35%.— J. G. Gambertoglio *et al.*, *Clin. Pharmac. Ther.*, 1979, *26*, 592.

A study of the disposition kinetics of cephamandole during continuous ambulatory peritoneal dialysis (CAPD). Half-lives of 4.6 to 9.7 hours were reported in 6 patients on CAPD following cephamandole 1 g given by intravenous infusion over 30 minutes; the terminal elimination-rate constant was linearly correlated with creatinine clearance which varied between 0.7 to 10.9 mL per minute. Renal clearance accounted for approximately 54% of systemic clearance and a non-renal mechanism, possibly hepatobiliary clearance, accounted for the additional clearance. An average of 5% of the dose was dialysed. CAPD did not affect the distribution or contribute significantly to the elimination of cephamandole in patients with end-stage renal disease. Dosing of cephamandole in such patients should therefore be based upon the degree of renal dysfunction, as indicated by creatinine clearance, in addition to the site and severity of infection.— M. Bliss *et al.*, *Antimicrob. Ag. Chemother.*, 1986, *29*, 649.

Further studies of the pharmacokinetics of cephamandole during continuous ambulatory peritoneal dialysis: D. M. Janicke *et al.*, *Clin. Pharmac. Ther.*, 1986, *40*, 209.

DIFFUSION INTO BODY TISSUES AND FLUIDS. Cephamandole diffused into interstitial fluid. This diffusion was related to the amount of protein binding.— J. S. Tan and S. J. Salstrom, *Antimicrob. Ag. Chemother.*, 1977, *11*, 698.

In a study involving 27 patients given cephamandole 2 g intravenously over 5 minutes, mean concentrations of 105.8 µg per mL, 41.6 µg per g, and 20.8 µg per g were obtained in serum, pulmonary tissue, and subcutaneous tissue, respectively, within one hour of administration. Concentrations fell to 4.4 µg per mL, 2.3 µg per g, and 1.1 µg per g, respectively, within 4 hours.— F. Daschner *et al.* (letter), *J. antimicrob. Chemother.*, 1979, *5*, 474.

Cephamandole has been detected in the aqueous humour in peak concentrations of 0.6 and 1.6 µg per mL following intravenous administration of 1 and 2 g, respectively. However, it could not be detected following a dose of 1 g intramuscularly.— T. S. Lesar and R. G. Fiscella, *Drug Intell. & clin. Pharm.*, 1985, *19*, 642.

Further references to the diffusion of cephamandole into various body tissues and fluids: L. D. Mullany *et al.*, *Antimicrob. Ag. Chemother.*, 1982, *21*, 416 (heart tissue and pericardial fluid); M. G. Bergeron *et al.*, *ibid.*, 1985, *27*, 928 (heart tissue); A. J. Davies *et al.*, *J. antimicrob. Chemother.*, 1986, *17*, 637 (hip bone and surrounding tissue).

For mention of concentrations of cephamandole achieved in the CSF, see Administration in Infants and Children, above.

DRUG EXCRETION. The mean peak concentrations of cephamandole, cephazolin, and cephalothin in bile were 352, 46, and 12 µg per mL respectively in 8 patients 30 minutes after receiving 1 g of each antibiotic intravenously on separate occasions; the mean peak serum concentrations were 55.0, 92.8, and 32.4 µg per mL. The amount of cephamandole, cephazolin, and cephalothin excreted in the bile up to 6 hours after administration was 4.12, 1.2, and 0.25 mg respectively.— K. R. Ratzan *et al.*, *Antimicrob. Ag. Chemother.*, 1978, *13*, 985. See also Administration in Biliary Disorders, above.

Uses and Administration

Cephamandole is a second-generation cephalosporin antibiotic which is used in the treatment of infections due to susceptible organisms including infections of the respiratory, genito-urinary, and biliary tracts, bones and joints, skin and soft tissue, and in septicaemia.

Cephamandole is given as the nafate and sodium salts and doses are expressed in terms of the equivalent amount of cephamandole. It is administered by deep intramuscular injection, by slow intravenous injection over 3 to 5 minutes, or by intermittent or continuous infusion in doses of

0.5 to 2 g every 4 to 8 hours depending on the severity of the infection. Children may be given 50 to 100 mg per kg body-weight daily in divided doses; 150 mg per kg daily may be given in severe infections, but this dose should not be exceeded.

Doses should be reduced for patients with impaired renal function. After an initial dose of 1 to 2 g the following maintenance doses have been recommended: 0.75 to 2 g every 6 hours for patients with a creatinine clearance (CC) of 50 to 80 mL per minute; 0.75 to 2 g every 8 hours for a CC of 25 to 50 mL per minute; 0.5 to 1.25 g every 8 hours for a CC of 10 to 25 mL per minute; 0.5 to 1 g every 12 hours for a CC of 2 to 10 mL per minute; and 0.25 to 0.75 g every 12 hours for a CC of less than 2 mL per minute.

If the addition of an aminoglycoside to cephamandole therapy is necessary, then both drugs should be administered separately.

Cephamandole is also used for surgical infection prophylaxis and a dose of 1 to 2 g intravenously or intramuscularly one-half to one hour prior to surgical incision, followed by 1 or 2 g every 6 hours for 24 hours, is recommended. For patients undergoing procedures involving implantation of prosthetic devices, cephamandole should be continued for up to 72 hours.

Cephamandole lithium is available for use in sensitivity tests *in vitro*.

Proceedings of a symposium on cephamandole.— *J. infect. Dis.*, 1978, *137, Suppl.* (May), S1-S194.

A critical review of the current status of cephamandole in the treatment and prophylaxis of infections. Although it has been recommended in empiric therapy for patients undergoing abdominal, pelvic, or cardiovascular surgery, other regimens are less expensive or provide better coverage or both. Cephamandole should not be used to treat infections caused by *Enterobacter*, ampicillin-resistant *Haemophilus influenzae*, enterococci, or methicillin-resistant *Staphylococcus aureus*, nor to treat bacterial meningitis. Cephamandole has poor activity against *Bacteroides fragilis* and should not be used to treat intra-abdominal anaerobic infections.— C. V. Sanders *et al.*, *Ann. intern. Med.*, 1985, *103*, 70.

ADMINISTRATION. For comment on the volume of intravenous fluid necessary to reduce infusion phlebitis associated with cephamandole, see under Thrombophlebitis in Adverse Effects and Precautions, above.

ADMINISTRATION IN INFANTS AND CHILDREN. For severe infections in children cephamandole could be given intravenously in a dose of 150 mg per kg body-weight daily in 4 to 6 divided doses. However, the first- and second-generation cephalosporins have limitations in the treatment of serious bacterial infections in children because they do not penetrate sufficiently into the cerebrospinal fluid to be effective in treating or preventing meningitis.— K. H. Rhodes and C. M. Johnson, *Mayo Clin. Proc.*, 1983, *58*, 158.

ADMINISTRATION IN RENAL FAILURE. Cephamandole could be administered to patients with renal failure by adjusting the dosage interval. A dosage interval of 6 hours is suitable for patients whose glomerular filtration-rates exceed 50 mL per minute; an interval of 6 to 8 hours between doses is advisable for rates of between 10 and 50 mL per minute. Where the rate is less than 10 mL per minute, the dosage interval should be 8 hours. A dose supplement should be given to patients undergoing haemodialysis.— W. M. Bennett *et al.*, *Am. J. Kidney Dis.*, 1983, *3*, 155.

See also under Absorption and Fate (above).

PERITONITIS. Cephamandole has been administered intraperitoneally in patients undergoing continuous ambulatory peritoneal dialysis. A maintenance dose of 500 mg per litre has been used in some units.— D. K. Scott and D. E. Roberts, *Pharm. J.*, 1985, *1*, 621.

Cephamandole has been used as first-line therapy for peritonitis associated with continuous ambulatory peritoneal dialysis, with gentamicin or tobramycin added to cover Gram-negative organisms. However, due to increasing resistance of staphylococci to cephamandole, vancomycin is now considered the drug of choice administered in association with netilmicin.— T. A. McAllister *et al.*, *J. antimicrob. Chemother.*, 1987, *19*, 95.

For comment on the use of cephamandole in the management of peritonitis associated wih continuous ambulatory peritoneal dialysis, see under Cefuroxime Sodium, p.172.

RESPIRATORY-TRACT INFECTIONS. References to the use of cephamandole in the treatment of lower respiratory-tract infections: B. G. Petty *et al.*, *Antimicrob. Ag. Chemother.*, 1978, *14*, 13 (pneumonia); J. C. Engle *et al.*, *ibid.*, 1985, *28*, 146 (pneumonia); M. J. Bittner *et al.*, *J. antimicrob. Chemother.*, 1986, *18*, 621 (pneumonia or bronchitis in the elderly); L. Dall *et al.*, *Curr. ther. Res.*, 1986, *39*, 946 (pneumonia).

For a comparison of cephamandole with ampicillin in the initial treatment of community-acquired pneumonia, see under Ampicillin Trihydrate, p.121.

SEPTICAEMIA. The view that cephamandole should not be used for the treatment of serious, invasive *Haemophilus* infections. *H. influenzae* meningitis has been reported to occur during therapy and cephamandole has been found relatively inefficient in the treatment of such meningitis.— M. I. Marks, *J. Pediat.*, 1981, *98*, 910.

Results of a study of 80 patients with staphylococcal bacteraemia, bronchopneumonia, or severe staphylococcal infection treated with cephamandole alone, cephamandole and tobramycin, or vancomycin alone, indicated that cephamandole or another beta-lactamase-resistant cephalosporin is suitable initial therapy for suspected staphylococcal infection and that there is no need for a combination with an aminoglycoside. Vancomycin should probably be substituted when methicillin or cephalosporin resistance occurs, although the combination of a cephalosporin and an aminoglycoside might be effective as well.— L. Coppens *et al.*, *Antimicrob. Ag. Chemother.*, 1983, *23*, 36. Cephamandole showed good clinical activity in the treatment of 80 patients with many kinds of staphylococcal infections caused by both methicillin-susceptible and methicillin-resistant *Staph. aureus* and methicillin-susceptible and methicillin-resistant coagulase-negative staphylococci, particularly in the less severe, non-deep-seated infections. The clinical and bacteriological outcome of the patients with septicaemia was considered satisfactory, however, a poor response to cephamandole, even when used in combination with other antistaphylococcal agents, was observed in 4 patients with endocarditis. Cephamandole was considered a useful drug for the treatment of many staphylococcal infections, however, there were limits to its activity in deep-seated infections.— F. Frongillo *et al.*, *ibid.*, 1986, *29*, 789. A study of the sensitivity patterns of 97 coagulase-negative staphylococci, including *Staphylococcus epidermidis* and *Staph. haemolyticus*, isolated from neonates. Of 18 antibiotics tested cephamandole was the most active cephalosporin and netilmicin the most active aminoglycoside. However, as cephalosporins have been shown to have unpredictable clinical activity against coagulase-negative staphylococci despite activity *in vitro*, they should probably not be used in 'blind' therapy of serious infections.— A. J. Davies *et al.*, *J. antimicrob. Chemother.*, 1986, *17*, 155. See also Activity against Staphylococci, in Antimicrobial Action, above.

SURGICAL INFECTION PROPHYLAXIS. Cephamandole has been given parenterally for prophylaxis in open-heart surgery (G.L. Archer *et al.*, *Antimicrob. Ag. Chemother.*, 1978, *13*, 924; R.E. Polk *et al.*, *Clin. Pharmac. Ther.*, 1978, *23*, 473; T.G. Slama *et al.*, *Antimicrob. Ag. Chemother.*, 1986, *29*, 744), and also for total hip replacement. Although the pharmacokinetic properties of cephamandole have been demonstrated to be superior to those of cephalothin, some workers have found that the overall postoperative infection-rates do not appear to be lower than with first-generation cephalosporins (J.T. DiPiro *et al.*, *Clin. Pharm.*, 1982, *1*, 135; J. T. DiPiro *et al.*, *J. Am. med. Ass.*, 1984, *252*, 3277). Other workers have found cephamandole nafate to be superior to cephalothin sodium for prophylaxis during open-heart surgery (R. Mészáros *et al.*, *Cor Vasa*, 1986, *28*, 61) and for high-risk patients undergoing cholecystectomy (C.A. Crenshaw *et al.*, *Surgery Gynec. Obstet.*, 1981, *153*, 546). Cephamandole has, however, been shown to have no pharmacokinetic advantage over cephazolin in open-heart surgery prophylaxis (M. Toscani *et al.*, *J. clin. Pharmac.*, 1985, *25*, 455).

Irrigation with a solution containing cephamandole nafate 2 g has been found to significantly decrease post-caesarean endometritis and other forms of infection-related morbidity compared with irrigation with 800 mL saline (E.E. Dashow *et al.*, *Obstet. Gynec.*, 1986, *68*, 473).

See also under Choice of Antibiotic, p.103.

For a comparison of cephamandole and doxycycline prophylaxis in women undergoing vaginal hysterectomy, see under Doxycycline Hydrochloride, p.220.

TYPHOID FEVER. Cephamandole 2 g intravenously every 6 hours for 14 days was successfully used in one patient with *Salmonella typhi* bacteraemia (S.Z. Hirschman *et al.*, *Antimicrob. Ag. Chemother.*, 1977, *11*, 369). However, therapeutic failures were reported in 7 of 19 patients with salmonella bacteraemia given cephamandole 60 to 240 mg per kg body-weight daily although all the salmonella strains isolated were susceptible *in vitro* (E.M. De Carvalho *et al.*, *ibid.*, 1982, *21*, 334). In a study of 9 patients with typhoid fever, all 5 patients who received cephamandole 8 g daily by continuous intravenous drip responded satisfactorily to treatment whereas the infection was not controlled in 3 of 4 patients who received the antibiotic intermittently by short intravenous infusions in doses of 1 g every 3 or 4 hours. It appeared that successful treatment in enteric fever correlated with a dosage schedule which allowed maintenance of serum-drug concentrations high above the minimum inhibitory concentrations for the longest time intervals possible (M. Uwaydah *et al.*, *ibid.*, 1984, *26*, 426).

URINARY-TRACT INFECTIONS. Eleven of 26 patients with pyelonephritis and 3 of 5 with cystitis were re-infected with the same or different organisms within 10 days of completing at least 5 days of therapy with cephamandole 1.5 to 8 g given daily intravenously or intramuscularly in divided doses. Many patients had serious underlying medical problems which were frequently responsible for therapeutic failures, however, the number of re-infections produced by *Pseudomonas aeruginosa* suggested that the use of cephamandole could lead to secondary infections by such resistant organisms.— H. D. Short *et al.*, *J. antimicrob. Chemother.*, 1976, *2*, 345.

Cephamandole 1 g every 8 hours for 5 to 8 days administered intramuscularly to 20 patients with urinary-tract infections caused by susceptible organisms resulted in elimination of the original infecting organism in 15 patients. All 5 treatment failures were in patients with abnormal pyelograms; 4 of the 15 patients who were successfully treated also had abnormal pyelograms. Local pain despite the addition of lignocaine 2% was sufficiently prolonged and severe to make multiple-dose intramuscular administration unacceptable; the intravenous route might be preferable for prolonged treatment.— A. Nankervis *et al.*, *Med. J. Aust.*, 1980, *1*, 427.

A single intramuscular injection of cephamandole 1 g was effective in 37 of 53 episodes (70%) of infection in a group of 46 patients with recurrent urinary-tract infections caused by cephamandole-susceptible organisms.— P. G. Shaw *et al.*, *Med. J. Aust.*, 1980, *1*, 489.

Preparations

Cefamandole Nafate for Injection *(U.S.P.)*

Sterile Cefamandole Nafate *(U.S.P.)*

Cefamandole Sodium for Injection *(U.S.P.)*

Sterile Cefamandole Sodium *(U.S.P.)*

Proprietary Preparations

Kefadol *(Dista, UK)*. *Injection*, powder for reconstitution, cephamandole 0.5, 1, or 2 g (as nafate) with sodium carbonate. The total sodium content is approximately 77 mg per g of cephamandole activity.

Continued production of carbon dioxide after the repackaging of reconstituted solutions of Mandol (cephamandole nafate) into syringes led to an explosive-like reaction in which the rubber closure was forced out of the syringe body.— M. A. Palmer and C. C. Fraterrigo (letter), *Am. J. Hosp. Pharm.*, 1979, *36*, 596; *idem*, 1025. When intended for intramuscular or direct intravenous injection Mandol solution should be left in the original containers and withdrawn into syringes immediately before use.— P. R. Klink and C. W. McKeehan, *Lilly, USA* (letter), *ibid.*, 597.

Proprietary Names and Manufacturers of Cephamandole Salts

Bergacef *(Bergamon, Ital.)*; Cedol *(Tiber, Ital.)*; Cefam *(Magis, Ital.)*; Cefaseptolo *(Miba, Ital.)*; Cefiran *(Pierrel, Ital.)*; Cemado *(Lifepharma, Ital.)*; Fado *(Caber, Ital.)*; Forcef *(Chiesi, Ital.)*; Kefadol *(Dista, UK)*; Kefandol *(Lilly, Fr.)*; Lampomandol *(AGIPS, Ital.)*; Mancef *(Dukron, Ital.)*; Mandokef *(Lilly, Denm.*; *Lilly, Ger.*; *Lilly, Ital.*; *Lilly, S.Afr.*; *Lilly, Spain*; *Lilly, Switz.)*; Mandol *(Lilly, Austral.*; *Lilly, Canad.*; *Neth.*; *NZ)*; Mandolsan *(San Carlo, Ital.)*; Neocefal *(Gibipharma, Ital.)*; Pavecef *(IBP, Ital.)*.

18366-s

Cephazolin *(BAN)*.

Cefazolin *(USAN, pINN)*. 3-[(5-Methyl-1,3,4-thiadiazol-2-yl)thiomethyl]-7-(tetrazol-1-ylacetamido)-3-cephem-4-carboxylic acid.

$C_{14}H_{14}N_8O_4S_3$=454.5.

CAS — 25953-19-9.

Pharmacopoeias. In *U.S.*

Store in airtight containers.

44-m

Cephazolin Sodium *(BANM)*.

46083; Cefazolin Sodium *(USAN, pINNM)*; SKF-41558.

$C_{14}H_{13}N_8NaO_4S_3$=476.5.

CAS — 27164-46-1.

Pharmacopoeias. In *It.* and *Jpn. U.S.* includes Sterile Cefazolin Sodium.

A white to off-white almost odourless crystalline powder. 1.05 g of monograph substance is approximately equivalent to 1 g of cephazolin. Each g of monograph substance represents about 2.1 mmol of sodium.

Freely **soluble** in water, 0.9% sodium chloride solution, and glucose solutions; very slightly soluble in alcohol; practically insoluble in ether and chloroform. A 10% solution in water has a pH of 4.5 to 6.0. **Protect** from light.

Solutions of cephazolin sodium are reported to be **stable** for 24 hours at 25° and for 96 hours at 5°. Solutions of cephazolin sodium in water, 5% glucose, or 0.9% sodium chloride which have been frozen immediately after reconstitution in their original containers are reported to be stable for 12 weeks at −20°.

A precipitate may form in refrigerated solutions; this can be dissolved by warming to room temperature.

Cephazolin sodium should not be mixed with blood products or other proteinaceous fluids such as protein hydrolysates.

Cephazolin sodium has been reported to be **incompatible** with aminoglycosides, tetracyclines, and other antimicrobial agents including erythromycin gluceptate and polymyxin B sulphate. Incompatibility or loss of activity has also been reported with amylobarbitone sodium, ascorbic acid, bleomycin sulphate, calcium gluceptate, calcium gluconate, cimetidine hydrochloride, colistin sulphomethate sodium, lignocaine hydrochloride, pentobarbitone sodium, and vitamin B complex with vitamin C.

Cephazolin sodium when added to either sodium chloride 0.9% or glucose 5% in water to give concentrations of 10 mg per mL for intermittent infusion, may be filtered through a Millipore membrane filter without adversely affecting the concentration of active drug.— D. J. Stennett *et al.*, *Am. J. Hosp. Pharm.*, 1979, *36*, 657.

A report of crystal formation occurring at room temperature in 1-g vials of cephazolin sodium which had been reconstituted with 2.5 mL of 0.9% sodium chloride injection. There was no crystal formation during the 24 hours after reconstitution with sterile water for injection.— C. S. Senholzi and M. P. Kerns, *Am. J. Hosp. Pharm.*, 1985, *42*, 129. Comment from a manufacturer (*Lilly, USA*). Although the crystals formed can be redissolved by warming, 0.9% sodium chloride injection is no longer recommended as a diluent for 1-g vials of cephazolin sodium.— M. Bornstein and R. J. Templeton (letter), *ibid.*, 2436.

Adverse Effects

Side-effects are similar to those of cephalothin sodium (p.176) but phlebitis after the intravenous administration of cephazolin sodium and pain after intramuscular injection appear to be less frequent.

A report of crystalluria in a 37-year-old man receiving cephazolin sodium.— A. A. Nanji (letter), *Clin. Pharm.*, 1984, *3*, 19.

EFFECTS ON THE BLOOD. Kurz *et al.*, (*J. antimicrob. Chemother.*, 1986, *18*, 772) reported clinical bleeding associated with abnormal coagulation tests in one patient after administration of cephazolin; this resolved on administration of vitamin K. Lerner and Lubin (*New Engl. J. Med.*, 1974, *290*, 1324) have also reported hypoprothrombinaemia in one patient. From a study in rats, Lipsky *et al.*, (*J. antimicrob. Chemother.*, 1986, *18*, 131) suggested that the effect of cephazolin on coagulation could be attributed to the 2-methyl-1,3,4-thiadiazole-5-thiol group.

EFFECTS ON THE GASTRO-INTESTINAL TRACT. Of 6 healthy subjects given a single intravenous injection of cephazolin 1 g, one had *Clostridium difficile* isolated from the stools after 14 days. Cephazolin appeared to have no demonstrable effect on other aerobic and anaerobic flora.— N. S. Ambrose *et al.*, *J. antimicrob. Chemother.*, 1985, *15*, 319.

EFFECTS ON THE LIVER. Report of a 36-year-old woman given intramuscular cephazolin sodium 1 g daily and cefadroxil 1 g twice daily by mouth for treatment of acute febrile salpingitis. On the sixth day of treatment, the patient noted alcoholic stools and dark urine followed by increasing jaundice associated with severe itching. Laboratory tests indicated severe cholestatic jaundice. The condition resolved after treatment with prednisone for 5 weeks followed by cholestyramine and phenobarbitone for 4 weeks. A hypersensitivity reaction to cephalosporins was supposed.— R. Ammann *et al.* (letter), *Lancet*, 1982, *2*, 336.

EFFECTS ON THE NERVOUS SYSTEM. Convulsions in a 52-year-old man with renal failure were associated with treatment with cephazolin 12 g daily later reduced to 2 g daily.— M. E. Gardner *et al.*, *Drug Intell. & clin. Pharm.*, 1978, *12*, 268.

Tonic-clonic seizures developed in 3 patients after intravenous therapy with cephazolin sodium, and were associated with high concentrations of cephazolin in the CSF.— T. P. Bechtel *et al.*, *Am. J. Hosp. Pharm.*, 1980, *37*, 271.

Precautions

As for Cephalothin Sodium, p.177.

ADMINISTRATION IN RENAL FAILURE. For reference to the precautions to be observed in renal failure, see under Administration in Renal Failure in Uses, below.

INTERACTIONS. A study in 6 healthy subjects to investigate the mechanisms whereby frusemide and piretanide affect the urinary excretion of cephazolin. Both diuretics appeared capable of enhancing the excretion of cephazolin, but were unlikely to affect antibiotic activity *in vivo*.— C. Morgant *et al.*, *Antimicrob. Ag. Chemother.*, 1984, *25*, 618.

For the effects of other drugs on the antimicrobial activity of cephazolin, see below under Antimicrobial Action.

Antimicrobial Action

As for Cephalothin Sodium, p.177. The minimum inhibitory concentrations of cephazolin for susceptible Gram-positive organisms range from about 0.1 to 1 µg per mL; for most susceptible Gram-negative organisms concentrations of greater than 1 µg per mL are required.

For reference to the action of cephazolin against staphylococci, see Cephamandole Sodium, p.180.

ACTIVITY WITH OTHER ANTIMICROBIAL AGENTS. Studies *in vitro* have shown both synergy and antagonism when cephazolin is combined with other beta-lactam antibiotics. Studies have investigated combinations with azlocillin or mezlocillin (H.C. Neu and K.P. Fu, *Antimicrob. Ag. Chemother.*, 1978, *13*, 813) and with temocillin (K. Jules and H.C. Neu, *ibid.*, 1982, *22*, 453; L. Verbist and J. Verhaegen, *ibid.*, 1984, *25*, 142) against a range of Gram-negative bacteria. Synergy has been reported between cephazolin and mecillinam against *Proteus* and *Klebsiella* spp. (R.S. Baltimore *et al.*, *Antimicrob. Ag. Chemother.*, 1976, *9*, 701). An *in vitro* study (K. Okonogi *et al.*, *J. antimicrob. Chemother.*, 1985, *16*, 31), indicated that cephazolin could induce beta-lactamases, though to a lesser extent than cefoxitin and cefmetazole. When added to cefmenoxime, ceftizoxime, latamoxef, or cefoperazone the activity of these drugs against a strain of *Enterobacter cloacae* was diminished.

Synergy has been demonstrated *in vitro* with gentamicin against enterococci (M. Bourque *et al.*, *Antimicrob. Ag. Chemother.*, 1976, *10*, 157), and with amikacin against most oxacillin-resistant strains of *Staphylococcus aureus* (J. Levy and J. Klastersky, *J. antimicrob. Chemother.*, 1979, *5*, 365).

In a study of the effect of combinations of beta-lactam antibiotics with antineoplastic agents (Y. Ueda *et al.*, *Antimicrob. Ag. Chemother.*, 1983, *23*, 374) the only effect of cephazolin was antagonism with carboquone against *Klebsiella pneumoniae.*

Resistance

As for Cephalothin Sodium, p.178. Cephazolin is considered to be more susceptible to staphylococcal beta-lactamase than other cephalosporins, except cephaloridine.

Absorption and Fate

Cephazolin sodium is poorly absorbed from the gastro-intestinal tract and is given by intramuscular or intravenous injection. Following a dose of 500 mg given intramuscularly, peak plasma concentrations of 30 µg or more per mL are obtained after 1 to 2 hours. Up to 90% of cephazolin in the circulation may be bound to plasma proteins. The plasma half-life of cephazolin is about 1.8 hours, and is increased in patients with renal impairment. Cephazolin diffuses into bone and ascitic, pleural, and synovial fluid but not appreciably into the cerebrospinal fluid. It diffuses across the placenta into the foetal circulation and low concentrations are excreted in the milk of nursing mothers.

Cephazolin is excreted unchanged in the urine, mainly by glomerular filtration with some renal tubular secretion, at least 80% of a dose given intramuscularly being excreted within 24 hours. Peak urine concentrations of more than 1 and 4 mg per mL have been reported after intramuscular doses of 0.5 and 1 g respectively. Probenecid delays excretion.

High biliary concentrations have been reported.

A review of the absorption and fate of cephazolin.— C. H. Nightingale *et al.*, *J. pharm. Sci.*, 1975, *64*, 1899.

A study in 5 women suggesting a decrease in the total body clearance of cephazolin in the hypothyroid state.— P. Chanson *et al.*, *Antimicrob. Ag. Chemother.*, 1987, *31*, 635.

Further references to the pharmacokinetics of cephazolin: K. W. Miller *et al.*, *Clin. Pharmac. Ther.*, 1980, *27*, 550 (effect of cardiopulmonary bypass).

ADMINISTRATION IN RENAL FAILURE. For reference to the pharmacokinetics of cephazolin in renal failure, see under Administration in Renal Failure in Uses, below.

Dialysis. The serum-protein binding of cephazolin fell from an average of 72.5 down to an average of 22.4% in 12 uraemic patients who underwent haemodialysis.— D. S. Greene and A. D. Tice, *J. pharm. Sci.*, 1977, *66*, 1508.

A study of the pharmacokinetics of intravenous or intraperitoneal cephazolin in patients undergoing continuous ambulatory peritoneal dialysis (CAPD). Cephazolin appeared to diffuse from peritoneal fluid to plasma easily, peak plasma concentrations being obtained 4 to 5 hours after intraperitoneal administration. The movement from plasma to peritoneal fluid, however, was slow and hence cephazolin could be administered parenterally to patients on CAPD in the conventional doses for patients with renal failure.— C. M. Bunke *et al.*, *Clin. Pharmac. Ther.*, 1983, *33*, 66. See also T. W. Paton *et al.*, *Clin. Pharmacokinet.*, 1985, *10*, 404.

ADMINISTRATION IN LIVER DISORDERS. In a study of the disposition of cephazolin in patients with liver disorders the half-life was 2.57 hours in patients with normal liver function, 1.82 hours in those with severe cirrhosis and oesophageal varices or ascites, and 2.45 hours in those with chronic active hepatitis or fatty liver. The decrease in half-life could possibly be related to the concurrent decrease in protein binding observed in the patients with liver disorders. However, no dosage modification of cephazolin was considered necessary in patients with hepatic impairment.— K. Ohashi *et al.*, *J. antimicrob. Chemother.*, 1986, *17*, 347.

DIFFUSION INTO BODY TISSUES AND FLUIDS. Studies of the diffusion of cephazolin into body tissues and fluids after intramuscular or intravenous administration: D. R. Cole and J. Pung, *Antimicrob. Ag. Chemother.*, 1977, *11*, 1033 (pleural fluid); T. R. Tetzlaff *et al.*, *J. Pediat.*, 1978, *92*, 135 (pus and bone of children with osteomyelitis); R. L. Parsons *et al.*, *Br. J. clin. Pharmac.*, 1978, *5*, 331 (bone and hip capsule); M. N. Dudley *et al.*, *Antimicrob. Ag. Chemother.*, 1984, *26*, 347 (atrial appendage and pericardial fluids).

PREGNANCY AND THE NEONATE. Studies in 6 pregnant women indicating lower plasma-cephazolin concentrations and shorter half-life during pregnancy.— A. Philipson *et al.*, *Clin. Pharmacokinet.*, 1987, *12*, 136.

Uses and Administration

Cephazolin sodium is a cephalosporin antibiotic

with the actions and uses of Cephalothin Sodium, p.178.

The usual adult dose is the equivalent of 500 mg of cephazolin every 12 hours by intramuscular or slow intravenous injection over 3 to 5 minutes or by infusion, increased if necessary to 0.5 to 1.5 g every 6 hours. The usual maximum daily dose is 6 g, although up to 12 g has been used in severe life-threatening infections. Children over 1 month may be given 25 to 50 mg per kg body-weight daily in divided doses increased in severe infections to a maximum of 100 mg per kg daily. For the prophylaxis of infection during surgery, cephazolin sodium is administered parenterally in a dose equivalent to 1 g half to one hour prior to the operation, followed by 0.5 to 1 g during surgery for lengthy procedures. A dose of 0.5 to 1 g is given every 6 to 8 hours postoperatively for 24 hours, or up to 5 days in certain cases.

Various dosage modifications are recommended for patients with renal impairment; usually the dosage interval is increased and often this is accompanied by a decrease in the dose. After a loading dose of 500 mg patients with anuria may be given up to 200 mg every 24 hours; with a creatinine clearance below 20 mL per minute maintenance doses of 75 to 400 mg may be given every 24 hours and with clearances below 40 and 70 mL per minute doses of 125 to 600 mg and 0.25 to 1.25 g respectively may be given every 12 hours.

ADMINISTRATION. Cephazolin has been administered intraperitoneally in patients undergoing continuous ambulatory peritoneal dialysis. A loading dose of 500 mg per litre of dialysis fluid followed by a maintenance dose of 125 to 250 mg per litre has been used.— D. K. Scott and D. E. Roberts, *Pharm. J.*, 1985, *1*, 621. See also D. Kaye *et al.*, *Antimicrob. Ag. Chemother.*, 1978, *14*, 318.

Cephazolin could be administered into the eye by subconjunctival or intravitreal injection, or by the use of topical eye-drops.— T. S. Lesar and R. G. Fiscella, *Drug Intell. & clin. Pharm.*, 1985, *19*, 642.

ADMINISTRATION IN RENAL FAILURE. The normal half-life for cephazolin of 1.4 to 2.2 hours was increased to 18 to 36 hours in end-stage renal failure. The interval between doses should be extended from 8 hours to 12 hours in those with a glomerular filtration-rate (GFR) of 10 to 50 mL per minute, and to 24 to 48 hours in those with a GFR of less than 10 mL per minute. A dose supplement should be given to patients undergoing haemodialysis.— W. M. Bennett *et al.*, *Am. J. Kidney Dis.*, 1983, *3*, 155.

Dialysis. Haemodialysis over 4 hours removed about 46% of cephazolin and patients undergoing haemodialysis should receive a further half dose after haemodialysis. Peritoneal dialysis did not affect the half-life of cephazolin.— T. Madhavan *et al.*, *Antimicrob. Ag. Chemother.*, 1975, *8*, 63. See also C. P. Craig and S. I. Rifkin, *Clin. Pharmac. Ther.*, 1976, *19*, 825.

ARTHRITIS, BACTERIAL. For reference to the use of cephazolin in bacterial arthritis, see Flucloxacillin Sodium, p.232.

ENDOCARDITIS. Both patients with endocarditis caused by group A beta-haemolytic streptococci, and 18 of 22 with endocarditis caused by *Staphylococus aureus* were considered cured after therapy with cephazolin in doses of 4 to 8 g daily.— D. Webb and H. Thadepalli, *Curr. ther. Res.*, 1983, *34*, 311.

Prophylaxis. Cephazolin 1 g by intramuscular injection 30 minutes before the incision, followed by cephalexin 500 mg by mouth 6 hours later could be used as prophylaxis against staphylococcal endocarditis during drainage of abscesses in intravenous drug abusers. Alternatively, cephalexin 1 g one hour before the incision followed by 500 mg after 4 and 8 hours may be used. For areas where methicillin-resistant coagulase-positive staphylococci have been isolated vancomycin or co-trimoxazole could be used.— D. Kaye (letter), *Ann. intern. Med.*, 1986, *105*, 299.

ENTERIC FEVER. Nine patients with acute enteric fever due in 7 to *Salmonella typhi* and in 2 to *S. paratyphi* B were effectively treated with cephazolin 3 to 6 g by intravenous or intramuscular injection daily in divided doses for 11 to 16 days. One patient relapsed during a follow-up period of 5 to 8 weeks.— M. Uwaydah, *Antimicrob. Ag. Chemother.*, 1976, *10*, 52.

OSTEOMYELITIS. For reference to the use of cephazolin in osteomyelitis, see Flucloxacillin Sodium, p.232.

PROSTATITIS. Mention that local injections of cephazolin sodium into the prostate gland have been studied in the treatment of chronic bacterial prostatitis, although there have been treatment failures.— P. M. Hanus and L. H. Danziger, *Clin. Pharm.*, 1984, *3*, 49.

SURGICAL INFECTION PROPHYLAXIS. Cephazolin is the most studied of the first-generation cephalosporins in the prophylaxis of infections during surgery. In clean and clean-contaminated procedures in which the most likely pathogens are usually susceptible to first-generation agents, the second- or third-generation cephalosporins provide no better prophylaxis than cephazolin. Procedures for which cephazolin has been recommended, often as the drug of choice, include caesarean section, abortion, abdominal or vaginal hysterectomy, joint repair or replacement, reduction of fractures, cholecystectomy, gastric resection, head and neck surgery, and cardiothoracic and vascular surgery.— A. B. Kaiser, *New Engl. J. Med.*, 1986, *315*, 1129. See also *Med. Lett.*, 1987, *29*, 91. A view that second- and third-generation cephalosporins are normally used for the prophylaxis of wound infection in surgical procedures except in biliary surgery when cephazolin is used. Anaerobic organisms are rarely involved in biliary sepsis, therefore the use of broader-spectrum agents, or their combination with metronidazole, is unnecessary.— A. P. Ball, *Pharm. J.*, 1984, *2*, 77.

Reports and discussions of the use of cephazolin in surgical infection prophylaxis:. Biliary-tract surgery.— J. S. Dooley *et al.*, *Gut*, 1984, *25*, 988; R. Munro and T. C. Sorrell, *Drugs*, 1986, *31*, 449. Caesarean section; comparison of intrauterine irrigation and intravenous administration.— A. E. Donnenfeld *et al.*, *J. reprod. Med.*, 1986, *31*, 15. Cardiac surgery.— T. G. Slama *et al.*, *Antimicrob. Ag. Chemother.*, 1986, *29*, 744. Head and neck surgery.— J. T. Johnson *et al.*, *Arch. Otolaryngol. Head Neck Surg.*, 1986, *112*, 151. Hip replacement, total.— C. Hill *et al.*, *Lancet*, 1981, *1*, 795; F. Doyon *et al.* (letter), *ibid.*, 1987, *1*, 860. Hysterectomy, abdominal or vaginal.— B. F. Polk *et al.*, *Lancet*, 1980, *1*, 437; M. Shapiro *et al.*, *New Engl. J. Med.*, 1982, *307*, 1661. Intestinal surgery; use with metronidazole.— S. Smith *et al.*, *Br. J. clin. Pract.*, 1985, *39*, 12; W. E. G. Thomas *et al.*, *J. antimicrob. Chemother.*, 1985, *16*, 121.

See also under Prophylactic Use of Antibiotics, p.103.

Preparations

Cefazolin Sodium Injection *(U.S.P.)*. A sterile solution of cephazolin and sodium bicarbonate. Store in the frozen state.

Sterile Cefazolin Sodium *(U.S.P.)*. Cephazolin sodium suitable for parenteral use.

Proprietary Preparations

Kefzol *(Lilly, UK)*. *Injection*, powder for reconstitution, cephazolin 0.5 and 1 g (as sodium salt).

Proprietary Names and Manufacturers

Acef *(Tiber, Ital.)*; Ancef *(Smith Kline & French, Canad.; Smith Kline & French, USA)*; Areuzolin *(Areu, Spain)*; Atirin *(Fisons, Ital.)*; Biazolina *(Panthox & Burck, Ital.)*; Bor-Cefazol *(Proter, Ital.)*; Brizolina *(Bristol-Myers, Spain)*; Caricef *(Antibioticos, Spain)*; Cefacene *(Centrum, Spain)*; Cefacidal *(Belg.; Denm.; Alland, Fr.; Neth.)*; Cefadrex *(Vir, Spain)*; Cefakes *(Albofarma, Spain)*; Cefalomicina *(Arg.)*; Cefamezin *(Carlo Erba, Ital.; Knoll-Made, Spain)*; Cefazil *(Giustini, Ital.)*; Cefazina *(Chemil, Ital.)*; Cef-Llorens *(Llorens, Spain)*; Cefralay *(Ralay, Spain)*; Celmetin *(Swed.)*; Cromezin *(Crosara, Ital.)*; Dacovo *(Tafir, Spain)*; Elzogram *(Lilly, Ger.)*; Fazoplex *(Bicther, Spain)*; Fidesporin *(Fides, Spain)*; Firmacef *(FIRMA, Ital.)*; Gramaxin *(Boehringer Mannheim, Ger.)*; Intercefal *(Interpharma, Spain)*; Kefol *(Lilly, Spain)*; Kefzol *(Lilly, Austral.; Belg.; Lilly, Canad.; Denm.; Lilly, Fr.; Neth.; Lilly, S.Afr.; Lilly, Switz.; Lilly, UK; Lilly, USA)*; Kezolin *(Lilly, Ital.)*; Kurgan *(Normon, Spain)*; Lampocef *(Lampugnani, Ital.)*; Lifezolina *(Spain)*; Neofazol *(Rubio, Spain)*; Novaporin *(Spain)*; Recef *(Aandersen, Ital.)*; Sicef *(Ital Suisse, Ital.)*; Tasep *(Septa, Spain)*; Tecfazolina *(Bohm, Spain)*; Totacef *(Bristol Italiana Sud, Ital.)*; Zolicef *(Ger.)*; Zolin *(Locatelli, Ital.)*; Zolisint *(Locatelli, Ital.)*; Zolival *(Valles Mestre, Spain)*.

180-e

Cephoxazole Sodium *(BANM)*.

291/1 *(acid)*; Cefoxazole Sodium *(rINNM)*. Sodium (7*R*)-7-[3-(2-chlorophenyl)-5-methylisoxazole-4-carboxamido]cephalosporanate; Sodium (7*R*)-3-acetoxymethyl-7-[3-(2-chlorophenyl)-5-methylisoxazole-4-carboxamido]ceph-3-em-4-carboxylate.

$C_{21}H_{17}ClN_3NaO_7S$=513.9.

CAS — 36920-48-6 (cephoxazole).

Cephoxazole sodium is a cephalosporin antibiotic used in veterinary practice.

Proprietary Veterinary Names and Manufacturers
Glaxovet, UK.

45-b

Cephradine *(BAN, USAN)*.

Cefradine *(rINN)*; SKF-D-39304; SQ-11436. (7*R*)-7-(α-D-Cyclohexa-1,4-dienylglycylamino)-3-methyl-3-cephem-4-carboxylic acid.

$C_{16}H_{19}N_3O_4S$=349.4.

CAS — 38821-53-3 (anhydrous); 58456-86-3 (dihydrate).

Pharmacopoeias. In *Br.*, *It.*, *Jpn*, and *U.S.* which allows either the anhydrous form or the dihydrate.

A white to cream-coloured crystalline powder. *B.P.* **solubilities** are: slightly soluble in water; soluble 1 in 70 of methyl alcohol; freely soluble in propylene glycol; insoluble in alcohol, chloroform, and ether. *U.S.P.* solubilities are: sparingly soluble in water; very slightly soluble in alcohol and chloroform; practically insoluble in ether. A 1% solution in water has a pH of 3.5 to 6.0. Solutions for injection are prepared with the aid of sodium carbonate or arginine to enhance stability. **Store** at a temperature not exceeding 30° in airtight containers. Protect from light.

Solutions containing up to 25% cephradine are reported to be **stable** for 2 hours at 25° and 24 hours at 5°. Solutions of 5% cephradine for intravenous infusion are reported to be stable for 10 hours at 25° and for 48 hours at 5°; solutions containing 5% cephradine which have been frozen immediately after reconstitution in their original containers with Water for Injections are reported to be stable for 6 weeks at −20°.

Cephradine solutions may vary in colour from light to straw yellow but this does not affect the potency.

Cephradine should not be mixed with blood products or other proteinaceous fluids such as protein hydrolysates.

Some injections contain sodium carbonate and are **incompatible** with solutions such as compound sodium lactate injection which contain calcium salts.

STABILITY IN SOLUTION. Solutions containing 1% cephradine in various diluents and maintained at 25°, were found to be more stable when neutralised with arginine than with sodium carbonate. No significant difference in stability was observed at concentrations of 5 and 25%.— Y.-C. J. Wang and D. C. Monkhouse, *Am. J. Hosp. Pharm.*, 1983, *40*, 432.

Adverse Effects and Precautions

As for Cephalexin, p.173. Intramuscular injections of cephradine can be painful and thrombophlebitis has occurred following intravenous injection.

ADMINISTRATION IN RENAL FAILURE. For reference to the precautions to be observed in renal failure, see under Administration in Renal Failure in Uses, below.

EFFECTS ON THE GASTRO-INTESTINAL TRACT. Reports of pseudomembranous colitis, sometimes fatal, associated with the administration of cephradine.— R. J. Newman and C. M. McCollum, *Br. J. clin. Pract.*, 1979, *33*, 32; M. Sankarankutty *et al.*, *Postgrad. med. J.*, 1982, *58*, 726.

In a study of neonates and children treated with cephradine or ampicillin by mouth for 5 days, ampicillin appeared to select for ampicillin-resistant *Escherichia coli* in the faeces to a greater extent than cephradine.

No cephradine-resistant organisms were isolated after treatment with either drug. The effect of ampicillin appeared greater in the older children than the neonates. In the neonatal group, both antibiotics selected Gram-negative bacteria (other than *E. coli*), resistant to one or both antibiotics; these were mainly *Klebsiella* and *Proteus* spp., and *Pseudomonas aeruginosa*. Alterations in salivary flora were small in the older children; in neonates both ampicillin and cephradine selected some resistant Gram-negative bacteria which generally correlated with the organisms selected in the faeces.— J. Asquith and R. W. Lacey, in *Cephradine 12 years on — a routine antibiotic for therapy and prophylaxis, International Congress and Symposium Series No. 85*, A. Percival and P. Woods (Ed.), London, The Royal Society of Medicine, 1985, p.1.

For a similar study in elderly patients, see under Urinary-tract Infection in Amoxycillin Trihydrate, p.114.

PORPHYRIA. Cephradine was considered to be unsafe in patients with acute porphyria although there is conflicting experimental evidence on porphyrinogenicity.— M. R. Moore and K.E.L. McColl, *Porphyrias, Drug Lists*, Glasgow, Porphyria Research Unit, University of Glasgow, 1987.

Antimicrobial Action and Resistance

As for Cephalexin, p.174.

Reports of the antimicrobial activity of cephradine: W. Brumfitt *et al., Lancet*, 1982, *1*, 394 (anaerobic bacteria); E. J. C. Goldstein *et al., Antimicrob. Ag. Chemother.*, 1983, *24*, 418 (*Gardnerella vaginalis*); E. E. Stobberingh *et al., J. antimicrob. Chemother.*, 1984, *13*, 55 (*Branhamella catarrhalis*).

ACTIVITY WITH OTHER ANTIMICROBIAL AGENTS. A report of enhanced activity *in vitro* with cephradine and mecillinam against 16 of 36 multi-resistant strains of Gram-negative bacilli.— B. Chattopadhyay and I. Hall, *J. antimicrob. Chemother.*, 1979, *5*, 549.

Absorption and Fate

Cephradine is rapidly absorbed from the gastro-intestinal tract. Doses of 250 and 500 mg given by mouth produce peak plasma concentrations of about 9 and 17 µg per mL respectively at 1 hour and are similar to those achieved with cephalexin. A more rapid absorption with a higher peak plasma concentration may be achieved if the same dose is given as a syrup. Absorption is delayed by the presence of food although the total amount absorbed is not appreciably altered. Following intramuscular injection peak plasma concentrations of about 6 and 10 µg per mL are obtained within 1 to 2 hours of doses of 500 mg and 1 g respectively.

About 6 to 20% is reported to be bound to plasma proteins. A plasma half-life of about 50 minutes has been reported; this is prolonged in renal failure. Cephradine is widely distributed to body tissues and fluids. Cephradine does not enter the cerebrospinal fluid in significant quantities. Therapeutic concentrations may be found in the bile. It diffuses across the placenta into the foetal circulation and is excreted in small amounts in the milk of nursing mothers.

Cephradine is excreted unchanged in the urine by glomerular filtration and tubular secretion, up to 90% of a dose being recovered within 6 hours. Peak urinary concentrations greater than 1 mg per mL have been achieved after a 500-mg dose by mouth.

Probenecid delays excretion.

A review of the absorption and fate of cephradine.— C. H. Nightingale *et al., J. pharm. Sci.*, 1975, *64*, 1899.

Absorption of cephradine after intramuscular injection was lower in 6 healthy women than in 6 healthy men, especially after injection into the gluteus maximus.— R. A. Vukovich *et al., Clin. Pharmac. Ther.*, 1975, *18*, 215.

ADMINISTRATION IN RENAL FAILURE. After the administration of intravenous cephradine, therapeutic concentrations were achieved in the dialysate of patients on continuous ambulatory peritoneal dialysis for up to 20 to 24 hours; peritonitis resulted in higher dialysate concentrations.— E. G. Anastassiades and J. R. Curtis, in *Cephradine 12 years on — a routine antibiotic for therapy and prophylaxis, International Congress and Symposium Series No. 85*, A. Percival and P. Woods (Ed.), London, The Royal Society of Medicine, 1985, p.55.

For reference to the pharmacokinetics of cephradine in renal failure, see under Administration in Renal Failure in Uses, below.

DIFFUSION INTO BODY TISSUES AND FLUIDS. Studies of the diffusion of cephradine into body tissues and fluids: I. J. Kiss *et al., Br. J. clin. Pharmac.*, 1976, *3*, 891 (Lung tissues); J. R. T. Monson *et al.*, in *Cephradine 12 years on — a routine antibiotic for therapy and prophylaxis, International Congress and Symposium Series No. 85*, A. Percival and P. Woods (Ed.), London, The Royal Society of Medicine, 1985, p.89 (tissue concentrations in patients with ischaemic limbs); A. J. Davies *et al., J. antimicrob. Chemother.*, 1986, *17*, 637 (bone).

PREGNANCY AND THE NEONATE. Studies in 12 pregnant women indicating lower plasma-cephradine concentrations and shorter half-life during pregnancy.— A. Philipson *et al., Clin. Pharmacokinet.*, 1987, *12*, 136.

Uses and Administration

Cephradine, a cephalosporin antibiotic, is administered by mouth similarly to cephalexin (see p.174) and by the parenteral route similarly to cephalothin sodium (see p.178) in the treatment of susceptible infections and in the prophylaxis of infections during surgical procedures.

Cephradine is given by mouth in doses of 1 to 2 g daily in two to four divided doses; up to 4 g daily may be given by this route. In severe infections it should be given parenterally, by intramuscular injection or intravenously by slow injection over 3 to 5 minutes or by infusion, in doses of 2 to 4 g daily in four divided doses; up to 8 g daily may be given by the parenteral route. The usual daily dose by mouth for children is 25 to 50 mg per kg body-weight; by injection 50 to 100 mg per kg increasing to 300 mg per kg daily in severe infections.

For surgical infection prophylaxis, 1 to 2 g is given pre-operatively by the intramuscular or intravenous route; subsequent parenteral or oral doses are given as appropriate.

For the proceedings of a symposium on cephradine, see *Cephradine 12 years on — a routine antibiotic for therapy and prophylaxis, International Congress and Symposium Series No. 85*, A. Percival and P. Woods (Ed.), London, The Royal Society of Medicine, 1985, 1–121.

ADMINISTRATION IN RENAL FAILURE. A dosage schedule for cephradine in patients with varying degrees of renal impairment: those with creatinine clearances of up to 5, from 5 to 20, and above 20 mL per minute could be given 250 mg every 12 hours, 250 mg every 6 hours, and 500 mg every 6 hours respectively. Patients on long-term intermittent haemodialysis could be given 250 mg at the beginning of dialysis, 250 mg after 12 hours, and 250 mg 42 hours after the beginning of dialysis. A dose of 250 mg could be given at the beginning of the next dialysis procedure provided this was 30 hours or more after the previous dose.— A. E. Solomon *et al., Br. J. clin. Pharmac.*, 1975, *2*, 443.

The normal half-life for cephradine of 1.3 hours was increased to 8 to 15 hours in end-stage renal failure. Doses should be reduced to 50% in patients with a glomerular filtration-rate (GFR) of 10 to 50 mL per minute, and to 25% in those with a GFR of less than 10 mL per minute. A dose supplement should be given to patients undergoing haemodialysis or peritoneal dialysis.— W. M. Bennett *et al., Am. J. Kidney Dis.*, 1983, *3*, 155.

The *UK* manufacturers have recommended that in patients with renal impairment a loading dose of 750 mg of cephradine be given followed by maintenance doses of 500 mg. For patients with creatinine clearances of greater than 20, 15 to 19, 10 to 14, 5 to 9, and less than 5 mL per minute, the dosage interval should be 6 to 12, 12 to 24, 24 to 40, 40 to 50, and 50 to 70 hours respectively.

ENDOCARDITIS. Twelve of 13 patients with endocarditis caused by *Staphylococcus aureus* or streptococci had a favourable response to treatment with cephradine.— D. Webb and H. Thadepalli, *Curr. ther. Res.*, 1983, *34*, 311.

PERITONITIS. Treatment of peritonitis associated with continuous ambulatory peritoneal dialysis (CAPD) was considered to be as effective with oral as with intraperitoneal administration of cephradine. Oral cephradine could be used as a first-line antibiotic for peritonitis. Although infections caused by methicillin-resistant *Staphylococcus epidermidis* responded well initially, change to another antibiotic was required for complete recovery.— E. W. Boeschoten *et al., J. antimicrob. Chemother.*, 1985, *16*, 789. A series of studies to assess the efficacy of a single intramuscular injection of cephradine followed by treatment by mouth for one week in the treatment of CAPD-associated peritonitis. The primary resolution rates were 81, 66, and 50% in a pilot study, a comparison with intraperitoneal cefuroxime during one year, and during routine use in the following year, respectively. This decrease in response was considered to reflect the increase in infection by coliforms, and the emergence of resistant strains of *Staph. albus*. These authors, however, use oral cephradine as first-line treatment with gentamicin, vancomycin, and cefuroxime as alternatives.— G. V. Raman, in *Cephradine 12 years on — a routine antibiotic for therapy and prophylaxis, International Congress and Symposium Series No. 85*, A. Percival and P. Woods (Ed.), London, The Royal Society of Medicine, 1985, p.47.

See also Absorption and Fate, above.

PREGNANCY AND THE NEONATE. For reference to the use of cephradine during pregnancy, see under Urinary-tract Infections in Cephalexin, p.175.

SEXUALLY TRANSMITTED DISEASES. Reports of the use of cephradine by intramuscular injection in sexually transmitted diseases: A. Theodoridis *et al., Curr. ther. Res.*, 1976, *19*, 20 (gonorrhoea); A. Theodoridis *et al., ibid.*, *20*, 254. and A. Theodoridis *et al., ibid.*, 1984, *35*, 184 (syphilis).

SURGICAL INFECTION PROPHYLAXIS. Cephradine is used for surgical infection prophylaxis for a wide range of surgical procedures. In abdominal or gynaecological surgery where anaerobic organisms may be present it may be used in combination with metronidazole.

References to prophylactic use of cephradine in various surgical procedures: B. R. Bullen *et al., Curr. med. Res. Opinion*, 1982, *8*, 5 (Cholecystectomy); A. R. L. Penketh *et al.* (letter), *Lancet*, 1985, *1*, 1500 (coronary artery bypass); D. F. Hawkins and J. A. Giles, in *Cephradine 12 years on — a routine antibiotic for therapy and prophylaxis, International Congress and Symposium Series No. 85*, A. Percival and P. Woods (Ed.), London, The Royal Society of Medicine, 1985, p.23 (gynaecological surgery; in combination with metronidazole).

URINARY-TRACT INFECTIONS. Experience with cephradine by mouth for the treatment of urinary-tract infections in patients with a history of recurrent infections, and for long-term prophylaxis in such patients. The susceptibility of urinary pathogens to cephradine was considered not to have changed significantly over the past 12 years.— W. Brumfitt and J. M. T. Hamilton-Miller, in *Cephradine 12 years on — a routine antibiotic for therapy and prophylaxis, International Congress and Symposium Series No. 85*, A. Percival and P. Woods (Ed.), London, The Royal Society of Medicine, 1985, p.61.

For reference to a comparative study of cephradine and amoxycillin in the treatment of urinary-tract infections, see Amoxycillin Trihydrate p.114.

Preparations

Cephradine Capsules *(B.P.)*

Cephradine Capsules *(U.S.P.)*

Cephradine for Injection *(U.S.P.)*. pH of a 1% solution 8.0 to 9.6.

Sterile Cephradine *(U.S.P.)*

Cephradine for Oral Suspension *(U.S.P.)*

Cephradine Tablets *(U.S.P.)*

Proprietary Preparations

Velosef *(Squibb, UK)*. *Capsules*, cephradine 250 and 500 mg.
Syrup, powder for reconstitution, cephradine 250 mg/5 mL when reconstituted with water.
Injection, powder for reconstitution, cephradine 0.5 and 1 g.

Proprietary Names and Manufacturers

Anspor *(Smith Kline & French, USA)*; Cefamid *(Gibipharma, Ital.)*; Cefrabiotic *(Von Boch, Ital.)*; Cefradex *(Ausonia, Ital.)*; Cefradina *(Spain)*; Cefrag *(Magis, Ital.)*; Cefraian *(ISOM, Ital.)*; Cefral *(Unibios, Spain)*; Cefrasol *(Radiumfarma, Ital.)*; Cefril *(Squibb, S.Afr.)*; Cefro *(Jpn)*; Cefrum *(San Carlo, Ital.)*; Celex *(Lagap, Ital.)*; Cesporan *(Caber, Ital.)*; Citicef *(CT, Ital.)*; Dicefalin *(Jpn)*; Dimacef *(Fisons, Ital.)*; Ecosporina *(Ecobi, Ital.)*; Eskacef *(Austral.; Belg.; Smith Kline & French, Fr.; Ger.; Smith Kline & French, Ital.; Spain; Smith Kline & French, UK)*; Eskefrin *(Arg.)*; Lenzacef *(Lenza, Ital.)*; Lisacef *(Lisapharma, Ital.)*; Maxisporin *(Belg.; Neth.)*; Medicef *(Ital.)*; Megacef *(Fr.)*; Noblitina *(Spain)*; Protocef *(Ripari-Gero, Ital.)*; Samedrin *(Savoma, Ital.)*; Sefril *(Heyden, Ger.; Spain; Squibb, Switz.)*; Septacef *(Septa, Spain)*; Velocef *(Arg.; Squibb, Ital.; Squibb, Spain)*; Velosef *(Austral.; Belg.; Squibb, Canad.;*

Squibb, Denm.; Squibb, Fr.; Neth.; Squibb, Swed.; Squibb, UK; Squibb, USA).

49-p

Chloramphenicol *(BAN, USAN, rINN).*

Chloramphenicolum; Chloranfenicol; Cloranfenicol; Kloramfenikol; Laevomycetinum. 2,2-Dichloro-*N*-[(αR,βR)-β-hydroxy-α-hydroxymethyl-4-nitrophenethyl]acetamide.

$C_{11}H_{12}Cl_2N_2O_5$=323.1.

CAS — 56-75-7.

Pharmacopoeias. In *Arg., Aust., Belg., Br., Chin., Cz., Egypt., Eur., Fr., Ger., Hung., Ind., Int., It., Jpn, Jug., Mex., Neth., Nord., Pol., Port., Roum., Rus., Span., Swiss, Turk.,* and *U.S.* Also in *B.P. Vet.*

Rus. also includes chloramphenicol stearate.

An antimicrobial substance produced by the growth of certain strains of *Streptomyces venezuelae*, but now mainly prepared synthetically.

A white to greyish-white or yellowish-white, fine crystalline powder or fine crystals, needles, or elongated plates. M.p. 149° to 153°. *U.S.P.* specifies not less than 900 μg per mg.

Soluble 1 in 400 of water, 1 in 2.5 of alcohol, and 1 in 7 of propylene glycol; freely soluble in acetone and ethyl acetate; slightly soluble in ether. A 2.5% suspension in water has a pH of 4.5 to 7.5. **Store** in airtight containers. Protect from light.

A study on the 3 polymorphic forms of chloramphenicol stearate.— R. Cameroni *et al., Farmaco, Edn prat.,* 1978, *33,* 141.

Bilirubin could interfere with the colorimetric assay of chloramphenicol. A method using activated charcoal was devised to overcome the problem.— E. O. Mason *et al., Antimicrob. Ag. Chemother.,* 1979, *15,* 544.

SOLUBILITY. Urea increased the solubility of chloramphenicol in water. A solid solution of chloramphenicol in urea had a dissolution-rate up to 4 times that of chloramphenicol alone.— A. H. Goldberg *et al., J. pharm. Sci.,* 1966, *55,* 581.

The solubility of chloramphenicol in water was increased by the addition of benzalkonium chloride. The 2 substances had a synergistic action *in vitro* against *Pseudomonas aeruginosa.*— R. T. Yousef and A. A. Ghobashy, *Acta pharm. suec.,* 1968, *5,* 385.

STABILTY. In a study of the stability of chloramphenicol in some ophthalmic ointment bases, degradation followed first-order kinetic behaviour during storage for 12 months at 25° and 35°. Chloramphenicol was more stable in an absorption basis containing wool fat than one containing cetyl alcohol during storage for 12 months. Sodium metabisulphite and disodium edetate improved the stability of chloramphenicol in both absorption bases at 35°. Chloramphenicol was more stable in oil-in-water emulsion bases than in water-in-oil emulsion bases.— M. A. Attia *et al., Pharmazie,* 1985, *40,* 629.

STABILITY IN SOLUTION. Chloramphenicol in aqueous solution was very stable over a wide pH range. Hydrolysis did not occur at ordinary temperatures at pH 2 to 7. Decomposition was catalysed by mono-hydrogen phosphate and mono- and di-hydrogen citrate ions and undissociated acetic acid, and it was recommended that only weakly buffered solutions should be dispensed.— T. Higuchi *et al., J. Am. pharm. Ass., scient. Edn,* 1954, *43,* 129.

Aqueous solutions lost about half their chloramphenicol content by hydrolysis on storage for 290 days at 20° to 22°; under the same conditions, solutions buffered (with borax) at pH 7.4 lost about 14%. The loss on heating the solutions at 100° for 15 minutes was about 3%.— A. Brunzell, *Svensk farm. Tidskr.,* 1957, *6,* 129.

Chloramphenicol was degraded by light in 0.25% aqueous solution and the solution became yellow and acid. The major degradation products were formed by oxidation, reduction, and subsequent condensation.— I. K. Shih, *J. pharm. Sci.,* 1971, *60,* 1889.

Photochemical decomposition of chloramphenicol in eye-drops containing 0.25% and in a therapeutic intraocular concentration.— H. de Vries *et al., Int. J. Pharmaceut.,* 1984, *20,* 265.

STERILISATION OF SOLUTIONS. Chloramphenicol in aqueous solution could be heated at 100° for 30 minutes, with a predicted loss of only 3.66% potency. A loss of 10% potency would occur in 29 minutes at 115°. Heating at 98° to 100° for 30 minutes would be an acceptable method of sterilisation for chloramphenicol eye-drops and the drops would not lose more than 10% potency in 4 months' storage at 20° or 2 years at 4°.— M. Heward *et al., Pharm. J.,* 1970, *1,* 386. Comments.— K. C. James and R. H. Leach, *ibid.,* 477.

48-q

Chloramphenicol Palmitate *(BANM, USAN, rINNM).*

Chloramphenicol α-Palmitate; Chloramphenicoli Palmitas; Palmitylchloramphenicol. (2*R*,3*R*)-2-(2,2-Dichloroacetamido)-3-hydroxy-3-(4-nitrophenyl)propyl palmitate.

$C_{27}H_{42}Cl_2N_2O_6$=561.5.

CAS — 530-43-8.

Pharmacopoeias. In *Br., Braz., Chin., Cz., Egypt., Eur., Fr., Ger., Hung., Ind., It., Jug., Nord., Swiss, Turk.,* and *U.S.*

A fine, white or almost white, unctuous, crystalline powder. M.p. 87° to 95°. 1.7 g of monograph substance is approximately equivalent to 1 g of chloramphenicol. The *U.S.P.* specifies a potency equivalent to not less than 555 μg and not more than 595 μg of chloramphenicol per mg.

Practically **insoluble** in water; soluble 1 in 45 of alcohol, 1 in 6 of chloroform, and 1 in 14 of ether; freely soluble in acetone; very slightly soluble in hexane. **Store** in airtight containers. Protect from light.

Chloramphenicol palmitate occurs in several polymorphic forms and the thermodynamically stable form has low bioavailability following oral administration. The *B.P.* specifies a limit for the biologically inactive polymorph A in Chloramphenicol Oral Suspension.

Three polymorphic forms of the palmitate were demonstrated, of which polymorph B was the best absorbed. Peak blood concentrations were up to 8 times higher for polymorph B than polymorph A, both of about 5 μm particle size. Increasing the mean diameter of form B to 25 μm did not reduce blood concentrations.— A. J. Aguiar *et al., J. pharm. Sci.,* 1967, *56,* 847.

Suspensions containing the equivalent of 250 mg of chloramphenicol as the polymorph A or amorphous forms of chloramphenicol palmitate with 2% of polysorbate 80 were administered to up to 10 children aged 5 to 7 years. Serum concentrations of chloramphenicol after 2 and 4 hours were less after administration of suspensions containing polymorph A compared with the amorphous form. After 6 hours, the blood concentration was higher with the polymorph A suspension and at 8 hours there was little difference between the two.— S. Banerjee *et al., J. pharm. Sci.,* 1971, *60,* 153.

STABILITY. The polymorph B (α-form) of chloramphenicol palmitate was stable at room and higher temperatures; aqueous suspensions were also stable, with and without wetting agents. Polymorph C was less stable and rapidly converted to polymorph A (β-form) at elevated temperatures.— L. Borka, *Acta pharm. suec.,* 1971, *8,* 365.

Chloramphenicol palmitate suspension in a syrup basis became curdled and discoloured after storage in a rigid amber polyvinyl chloride bottle for 2 years, but kept well when stored in amber glass bottles for the same period.— R. C. Shah *et al., Pharm. J.,* 1978, *2,* 58.

46-v

Chloramphenicol Sodium Succinate *(BANM, USAN, rINNM).*

Chloramphenicol α-Sodium Succinate. Sodium (2*R*,3*R*)-2-(2,2-dichloroacetamido)-3-hydroxy-3-(4-nitrophenyl)propyl succinate.

$C_{15}H_{15}Cl_2N_2NaO_8$=445.2.

CAS — 982-57-0.

Pharmacopoeias. In *Br., Chin., Cz., Egypt., Ind.,* and *It. U.S.* includes Sterile Chloramphenicol Sodium Succinate. Also in *B.P. Vet.*

A white or yellowish-white hygroscopic powder. 1.4 g of monograph substance is approximately equivalent to 1 g of chloramphenicol. Each g of monograph substance represents about 2.2 mmol of sodium. The *U.S.P.* specifies that Sterile Chloramphenicol Sodium Succinate has a potency equivalent to not less than 650 μg and not more than 765 μg of chloramphenicol per mg.

Soluble 1 in less than 1 of water, 1 in 1 of alcohol; practically insoluble in chloroform and ether. A 25% solution in water has a pH of 6 to 7. **Store** in airtight containers. Protect from light. Sterile solutions are stable for 30 days at room temperature. A slight change of colour is not indicative of loss of potency, but cloudy solutions should not be employed.

Incompatibility or loss of activity has been reported between chloramphenicol sodium succinate and aminophylline, ampicillin, ascorbic acid, calcium chloride, carbenicillin sodium, chlorpromazine hydrochloride, erythromycin salts, gentamicin sulphate, hydrocortisone sodium succinate, hydroxyzine hydrochloride, methicillin sodium, methylprednisolone sodium succinate, nitrofurantoin sodium, oxytetracycline hydrochloride, phenytoin sodium, polymyxin B sulphate, prochlorperazine salts, promazine hydrochloride, promethazine hydrochloride, sulphafurazole diethanolamine, tetracycline hydrochloride, tripelennamine hydrochloride, vancomycin hydrochloride, and vitamin B complex.

Despite discrepancies in the literature, diluents containing benzyl alcohol should be satisfactory for the preparation of chloramphenicol sodium succinate solutions.— E. A. Parker, *Abbott* (letter), *Am. J. Hosp. Pharm.,* 1969, *26,* 197.

Adverse Effects

Chloramphenicol may cause serious and sometimes fatal adverse effects and it should be discontinued immediately on the appearance of toxic symptoms. The most serious adverse effect of chloramphenicol is its depression of the bone marrow, which can take 2 different forms. The first is a fairly common dose-related reversible depression occurring usually when plasma-chloramphenicol concentrations exceed 25 μg per mL and is characterised by morphological changes in the bone marrow, decreased iron utilisation, reticulocytopenia, anaemia, leucopenia, and thrombocytopenia. This effect may be due to inhibition of protein synthesis in the mitochondria of bone marrow cells.

The second and apparently unrelated form of bone-marrow toxicity is severe irreversible aplastic anaemia which is fairly rare, although the incidence varies throughout the world; it is not considered to be dose-related. The aplasia usually develops after a latent period of weeks or even months and it is considered that victims may have some biochemical predisposition. Unfortunately there is no way of identifying susceptible patients and many may die. Survival is most likely in those with early onset aplasia but they may subsequently develop myeloblastic leukaemia.

Haemolytic anaemia has occurred in some persons with a genetic deficiency of glucose-6-phosphate dehydrogenase activity.

A toxic manifestation— 'the grey syndrome'— which is characterised by abdominal distension, vomiting, ashen colour, hypothermia, progressive pallid cyanosis, irregular respiration, and circulatory collapse followed by death in a few hours or days, has occurred in premature and other newborn infants receiving large doses of chloramphenicol. In most cases, the dose of chloramphenicol has been more than 25 mg per kg body-weight daily. A similar syndrome has been reported in adults and older children given very high doses.

Prolonged oral administration of chloramphenicol may induce bleeding, either by bone-marrow depression or by reducing the intestinal flora with consequent inhibition of vitamin K synthesis and greatly increased prothrombin time.

Peripheral as well as optic neuritis has been reported in patients receiving chloramphenicol, usually over prolonged periods. Although ocular symptoms are often reversible if treatment is withdrawn early, optic atrophy with blindness has occurred.

Hypersensitivity reactions may occur especially after topical use. Jarisch-Herxheimer-like reactions may also occur. Gastro-intestinal symptoms including nausea, vomiting, and diarrhoea can follow oral administration. Disturbances of the oral and intestinal flora may cause stomatitis, glossitis, and rectal irritation. Patients may experience an intensely bitter taste following rapid intravenous administration of chloramphenicol sodium succinate.

ALLERGY. Of 620 persons with dermatitis or eczema submitted to patch testing with chloramphenicol 50% in yellow soft paraffin, 1.7% gave a positive reaction.— E. Rudzki and D. Kleniewska, *Br. J. Derm.*, 1970, *83*, 543.

A report of anaphylaxis following intravenous chloramphenicol sodium succinate in a 46-year-old man with a history of alcoholism, hepatic cirrhosis, and penicillin allergy. Anaphylaxis is rare following chloramphenicol administration, but physicians should be aware of this complication, especially in patients with prior exposure to the drug.— B. A. Palchick *et al.*, *Am. J. med. Sci.*, 1984, *288*, 43.

Urticaria and angioedema in a 30-year-old woman and urticaria in a 54-year-old woman following the use of topically applied chloramphenicol 3% ointment.— M. Schewach-Millet and D. Shpiro (letter), *Archs Derm.*, 1985, *121*, 587.

EFFECTS ON THE BLOOD. In a study of 76 infants and children aged 2 months to 15 years who received chloramphenicol in doses of 31 to 133 mg per kg bodyweight daily for 10 to 76 days for infections, hyperferraemia occurred in 36 and haemopoietic toxicity in 21. Hyperferraemia was more common in children above 6 years and at dosage levels above 75 mg per kg bodyweight daily. In 15 patients with haemopoietic toxicity chloramphenicol was continued and 10 received additional phenylalanine or riboflavine; recovery was variable. However therapy should be discontinued if neutropenia or thrombocytopenia develop.— D. W. O'G. Hughes, *Med. J. Aust.*, 1973, *2*, 1142.

Aplastic anaemia. An analysis of blood dyscrasias reported to the Swedish Adverse Drug Reactions Committee during a 10-year period, 1966–75, showed that aplastic anaemia attributable to chloramphenicol had been reported on 5 occasions (4 fatal); no case of chloramphenicol-induced aplasia was, however, reported during the last 5 years of the study period (L.E. Böttiger *et al.*, *Acta med. scand.*, 1979, *205*, 457). Other sources have reported the risk of developing pancytopenia or aplastic anaemia after oral chloramphenicol treatment to be about 13 times greater than the risk of idiopathic aplastic anaemia in the general population (F.T. Fraunfelder and S.M. Meyer, *Med. Toxicol.*, 1987, *2*, 287); and others have estimated the frequency of this reaction to be in the range of 1 in 10 000 to 1 in 40 000 (P.C. Vincent, *Drugs*, 1986, *31*, 52). However, the frequency varies; chloramphenicol sales in Hong Kong are unusually high, but the incidence of aplastic anaemia in the community does not appear to be unusual (C.R. Kumana *et al.*, *Lancet*, 1987, *2*, 449).

It was originally thought that aplastic anaemia occurred less frequently when the drug was given exclusively by the parenteral route, but analysis of chloramphenicol-associated blood dyscrasias reported to the American Medical Association Registry revealed that among 149 cases, the route was oral in 83%, parenteral in 14%, and rectal in 3%, although it could not be determined whether any of the patients treated parenterally also received the drug by mouth (M.E. Plaut and W.R. Best, *New Engl. J. Med.*, 1982, *306*, 1486). It must, therefore, be assumed that this adverse effect can occur when chloramphenicol is administered by any route. Blood dyscrasias or aplastic anaemia have also been reported following topical ocular chloramphenicol as ointment or eye-drops (G. Carpenter, *Lancet*, 1975, *2*, 326; S.M. Abrams *et al.*, *Archs intern. Med.*, 1980, *140*, 576; F.T. Fraunfelder and G.C. Bagby, *New Engl. J. Med.*, 1983, *308*, 1536; R. McGuinness, *Med. J. Aust.*, 1984, *140*, 383). There has also been a report of fatal bone-marrow hypoplasia in a shepherd using a spray containing chloramphenicol on his sheep; he would probably have inhaled the product and significant cutaneous contact was also likely. (G.S. Del Giacco *et al.*, *Lancet*, 1981, *1*, 945).

The majority of these haematological reactions have occurred within 4 months of initiation of chloramphenicol therapy and the dyscrasias have been fatal in approximately half of the patients (F.T. Fraunfelder and S.M. Meyer, *Med. Toxicol.*, 1987, *2*, 287).

The analogue thiamphenicol differs from chloramphenicol by substitution of the *p*-nitro group with the methylsulphonyl moiety. The observation that thiamphenicol does not appear to be associated with an increased incidence of aplastic anaemia has opened the question of a structure-toxicity relationship. It has been proposed that the *p*-nitro group of chloramphenicol is the structural feature underlying aplastic anaemia caused by this drug. In the predisposed host, chloramphenicol and/or its nitroso or hydroxylamine derivatives may cause DNA changes and mutation, ultimately leading to aplastic anaemia and/or leukaemia (A.A. Yunis, *Sex. transm. Dis.*, 1985, *11, Suppl.*, 340). Other workers have proposed that the molecular basis of this chloramphenicol toxicity is probably due to the one-electron nitro radical anion derivative of chloramphenicol (I.M. Skolimowski *et al.*, *J. antimicrob. Chemother.*, 1983, *12*, 535).

For further reference to fatal aplastic anaemia following chloramphenicol administration, see under Effects on the Liver, below.

Haemolytic anaemia. Chloramphenicol 1 to 2 g daily had been reported to cause haemolytic anaemia in certain individuals with a deficiency of glucose-6-phosphate dehydrogenase in conjunction with factors such as infection.— E. Beutler, *Pharmac. Rev.*, 1969, *21*, 73.

Chloramphenicol did not cause haemolysis in Chinese patients with glucose-6-phosphate dehydrogenase deficiency.— T. K. Chan *et al.*, *Br. med. J.*, 1976, *2*, 1227.

Leukaemia. Three women treated with chloramphenicol developed pancytopenia leading to myeloblastic leukaemia. The continued widespread administration of chloramphenicol, often for trivial complaints, was considered to be a possible cause of some forms of leukaemia, particularly those of the relatively indolent hypoplastic type.— M. J. Brauer and W. Dameshek, *New Engl. J. Med.*, 1967, *277*, 1003.

Three further cases of acute leukaemia had occurred in patients previously treated with chloramphenicol. This took the total reported in the literature up to 27.— P. Lechat *et al.*, *Thérapie*, 1976, *31*, 129.

A study of chloramphenicol use and childhood leukaemia. More than 30 cases of chloramphenicol-related leukaemia have been reported in the literature, with acute non-lymphocytic leukaemia (ANLL) predominating; the period from initial drug use to onset of leukaemia has ranged from 2 months to 8 years. A large population-based case-control study conducted in the Shanghai area during 1985 and 1986 revealed a dose-response relation with the use of chloramphenicol and the risk of both acute lymphocytic leukaemia (ALL) and ANLL; treatment for more than 10 days was associated with relative risks of 11.0 and 12.0, respectively compared with a risk of 1.0 for no exposure. The use of syntomycin, a racemic mixture of chloramphenicol, was also associated with a risk of 12.6 for ANLL. Although the association may have non-causal explanations, the results warrant cautious prescribing of chloramphenicol in children. Since the risk of leukaemia increases sharply with increasing days of use, there should be rapid screening of cultures so that treatment can be quickly changed if organisms prove to be sensitive to other antibiotics.— X. O. Shu *et al.*, *Lancet*, 1987, *2*, 934. Criticism.— C. R. Kumana *et al.* (letter), *ibid.*, 1988, *1*, 476. Reply.— X. O. Shu *et al.* (letter), *ibid.*

EFFECTS ON THE EAR. Chloramphenicol sodium succinate 5% in Ringer's solution and propylene glycol 10% both caused irreversible deafness when instilled into the middle ear cavity in *guinea-pigs*. It was recommended that propylene glycol should not be used as a solvent for chloramphenicol ear drops, and that higher concentrations of chloramphenicol should not be used in the middle-ear cavity.— T. Morizono and B. M. Johnstone, *Med. J. Aust.*, 1975, *2*, 634.

Of 47 children treated for *Haemophilus influenzae* meningitis, 3 showed some loss of hearing. They included 1 of 27 given ampicillin only, 1 of 12 given chloramphenicol only, and 1 of 8 given both antibiotics.— F. E. Jones and D. R. Hanson, *Develop. Med. Child Neurol.*, 1977, *19*, 593.

A report of progressive bilateral profound sensorineural hearing loss in a 20-year-old woman after systemic administration of chloramphenicol for typhoid fever on two occasions.— S. M. Iqbal and C. B. P. Srivatsav, *J. Lar. Otol.*, 1984, *98*, 523.

EFFECTS ON THE EYE. For reports of chloramphenicol causing optic neuritis, see under Effects on the Nervous System, below.

EFFECTS ON THE GASTRO-INTESTINAL TRACT. Not one of 437 hospital in-patients in a Boston Collaborative Drug Surveillance Program who received chloramphenicol developed colitis.— R. R. Miller and H. Jick, *Clin. Pharmac. Ther.*, 1977, *22*, 1. Chloramphenicol has been associated with pseudomembranous colitis.— M. H. Gross, *Clin. Pharm.*, 1985, *4*, 304.

EFFECTS ON THE LIVER. Five patients developed hepatitis then fatal aplastic anaemia following the administration of chloramphenicol.— R. Hodgkinson, *Med. J. Aust.*, 1973, *1*, 939.

EFFECTS ON THE NERVOUS SYSTEM. Reversible symptoms of encephalopathy, namely acute delirium, developed in 3 patients treated with chloramphenicol.— P. H. Levine *et al.*, *Clin. Pharmac. Ther.*, 1970, *11*, 194.

Optic neuritis. Reports of optic neuritis associated with chloramphenicol.— N. N. Huang *et al.*, *J. Pediat.*, 1966, *68*, 32; S. Charache *et al.*, *Johns Hopkins med. J.*, 1977, *140*, 121; L. Rothkoff *et al.*, *Ann. Ophthal.*, 1979, *11*, 105; V. Godel *et al.*, *Archs Ophthal., N.Y.*, 1980, *98*, 1417.

OVERDOSAGE. Charcoal haemoperfusion was found to be far superior to exchange transfusion in the removal of chloramphenicol from blood, although it did not prevent death in a 7-week-old infant with the grey baby syndrome following a dosage error.— M. Freundlich *et al.*, *J. Pediat.*, 1983, *103*, 485.

Further reports on the treatment of accidental chloramphenicol overdosage in infants: S. M. Mauer *et al.*, *J. Pediat.*, 1980, *96*, 136 (charcoal haemoperfusion); D. L. Kessler *et al.*, *ibid.*, 140 (exchange transfusion).

See also under Administration in Infants and Children in Uses, below.

Precautions

Chloramphenicol is contra-indicated in patients with a history of hypersensitivity or toxic reaction to the drug. It should never be given for minor infections or for prophylaxis. Repeated courses and prolonged treatment should be avoided. Routine periodic blood examinations are advisable in all patients, but will not warn of aplastic anaemia.

Reduced doses should be given to patients with impaired liver function. Excessive blood concentrations may also occur following administration of usual doses to patients with severe renal failure and in premature and full-term neonates who have immature metabolic processes.

Because of the risk of the 'grey syndrome' newborn infants should never be given chloramphenicol, unless it may be life-saving and there is no alternative treatment. The use of chloramphenicol is probably best avoided during pregnancy, and in nursing mothers since chloramphenicol given to the mother is excreted in the milk.

Concomitant administration of chloramphenicol with other drugs liable to depress bone-marrow function should be avoided.

Chloramphenicol may interfere with the development of immunity and it should not be given during active immunisation.

Chloramphenicol is inactivated in the liver and may, therefore, interact with drugs which are metabolised by hepatic microsomal enzymes. Chloramphenicol enhances the effects of coumarin anticoagulants such as dicoumarol and warfarin sodium, some hypoglycaemic agents such as chlorpropamide and tolbutamide, and antiepileptics such as phenytoin. The half-life or plasma concentrations of chloramphenicol may be affected by paracetamol, phenobarbitone, phenytoin, or rifampicin.

INTERACTIONS. *Alcohol.* Mention of a potential disulfiram-like reaction with alcohol and chloramphenicol.— *FDA Drug Bull.*, 1979, *9*, 10. See also *Med. Lett.*, 1981, *23*, 33.

Anticoagulants. For reference to the effect of chloramphenicol on anticoagulants, see under Warfarin Sodium, p.345.

Antiepileptics. In a newborn infant with *Escherichia coli* meningitis unresponsive to ampicillin and gentamicin, chloramphenicol was given intravenously for 3 weeks and blood concentrations measured after each injection. The dose had to be increased gradually from 20 to 95 mg per kg body-weight daily in order to maintain the blood concentration in the therapeutic range of 10 to 20 μg per mL. The concomitant use of phenobarbitone and phenytoin might have stimulated the metabolism of chloramphenicol.— S. B. Black *et al.*, *J. Pediat.*, 1978, *92*, 235.

Phenobarbitone reduced the blood-chloramphenicol concentration in 2 children being treated with the antibiotic for meningitis due to *H. influenzae*.— R. A. Bloxham *et al.*, *Archs Dis. Childh.*, 1979, *54*, 76.

In a study involving 34 infants and children receiving chloramphenicol succinate 25 mg per kg body-weight every 6 hours by intravenous infusion, concurrent administration of phenobarbitone resulted in decreased serum concentrations of chloramphenicol compared with patients who received chloramphenicol succinate alone. Concurrent administration of phenytoin and chloramphenicol succinate, with or without phenobarbitone, resulted in elevated serum concentrations of chloramphenicol into the potentially toxic range. While phenytoin may, like phenobarbitone, cause induction of hepatic microsomal enzymes, its major interaction with chloramphenicol appears to be competition for binding sites. This interaction most probably explains the elevated serum-chloramphenicol concentration and also the previously described occurrence of increased serum phenytoin and phenytoin toxicity when the 2 drugs were given concurrently.— K. Krasinski *et al.*, *Pediatr. infect. Dis.*, 1982, *1*, 232.

For the effect of chloramphenicol on serum concentrations of phenobarbitone, see Phenobarbitone, p.405.

Antimicrobial agents. Eight of 11 children treated for *Haemophilus influenzae* meningitis with ampicillin and chloramphenicol had long-term sequelae compared with 4 of 32 given ampicillin alone and 4 of 22 given chloramphenicol alone. An increased risk was suggested for this combination.— J. Lindberg *et al.*, *Pediatrics*, 1977, *60*, 1. See also T. Matthews (letter), *Lancet*, 1978, *2*, 376.

A report of a reduction in serum concentrations of chloramphenicol to below the therapeutic range in 2 children with *Haemophilus influenzae* type b meningitis, following concomitant administration of rifampicin. Rifampicin, like phenobarbitone, which has also been shown to reduce serum-chloramphenicol concentrations, is an inducer of hepatic enzymes. If patients are treated with chloramphenicol for serious *H. influenzae* infections and, as recommended by the American Academy of Pediatrics, rifampicin is given in an attempt to eradicate *H. influenzae* from the nasopharynx before discharge, there is a risk that serum concentrations of chloramphenicol will be reduced to subtherapeutic levels resulting in treatment failure.— C. G. Prober *et al.* (letter), *New Engl. J. Med.*, 1985, *312*, 788.

For reports of the effects of chloramphenicol and other antibiotics on each other's antimicrobial activity, see below under Antimicrobial Action.

Cimetidine. Fatal aplastic anaemia in a patient who received intravenous chloramphenicol and cimetidine concomitantly. As there is usually a latent period of 2 weeks to 12 months before aplastic anaemia develops following chloramphenicol therapy and in this case there was evidence of bone-marrow depression after less than 1 week of chloramphenicol administration, it is plausible that an additive or synergistic effect may have occurred between the 2 drugs to cause bone-marrow toxicity. Avoidance of this combination is perhaps warranted until further studies can be carried out.— B. F. Farber and J. P. Brody, *Sth. med. J.*, 1981, *74*, 1257.

Cyclophosphamide. For the effect of chloramphenicol on cyclophosphamide, see under Cyclophosphamide, p.612.

Diuretics. The urinary excretion of chloramphenicol in healthy subjects was decreased by frusemide but the excretion of its metabolites as aryl amines and total nitro compounds was increased.— O. Schück *et al.*, *Experientia*, 1975, *31*, 1434. The urinary excretion of chloramphenicol and its metabolites was increased in healthy subjects when ethacrynic acid, hydrochlorothiazide, or clopamide were taken with a 1-g dose of chloramphenicol. There were no significant changes in serum concentrations of chloramphenicol and its metabolites.— O. Schück *et al.*, *Int. J. clin. Pharmac. Biopharm.*, 1978, *16*, 217.

Oral contraceptives. There have been isolated reports of unintended pregnancies in women taking oral contraceptives following the use of antimicrobial agents including chloramphenicol.— *Drug Interact. News.*, 1985, *5*, 7.

Paracetamol. Paracetamol has been reported to alter the pharmacokinetics of chloramphenicol. Buchanan and Moodley (*Br. med. J.*, 1979, *2*, 307) reported an increase in chloramphenicol half-life from 3.25 to 15 hours in 6 patients given paracetamol 100 mg intravenously 2 hours after receiving chloramphenicol 1 g intravenously. However, Kearns *et al.* (*J. Pediat.*, 1985, *107*, 134) found no pharmacokinetic interaction between chloramphenicol sodium succinate given intravenously and the prior or concomitant adminstration of paracetamol by mouth. In contrast, a further study in children by Spika *et al.* (*Archs Dis. Childh.*, 1986, *61*, 1121) demonstrated increased clearance of chloramphenicol during therapy with oral paracetamol and a decreased half-life from 3 to 1.2 hours. Therapeutic drug monitoring is therefore required when the 2 drugs are administered together.

PORPHYRIA. Chloramphenicol was considered to be unsafe in patients with acute porphyria as it has been associated with acute attacks.— M.R. Moore and K.E.L. McColl, *Porphyrias, Drug Lists*, Glasgow, Porphyria Research Unit, University of Glasgow, 1987.

PREGNANCY AND THE NEONATE. Chloramphenicol should not be administered after the 28th week of pregnancy. A serious adverse effect of chloramphenicol, the 'grey syndrome', has been seen not only when the antibiotic has been administered to premature or full-term babies, but also in newborns borne to women who had taken chloramphenicol during the final stage of pregnancy. Chloramphenicol penetrates well into the foetal circulation; the levels reach 30 to 80% of the concentrations in maternal blood.— H. Knothe and G. A. Dette, *Infection*, 1985, *13*, 49.

Chloramphenicol should be avoided in pregnancy because of the risk of grey baby syndrome during the second and third trimesters. There is little evidence of ill effects to the foetus in early pregnancy, but there is still the possibility of maternal blood dyscrasias. Usually a safer choice can be made. During breast feeding, the grey baby syndrome is most unlikely, as concentrations are too low, but the possibility of infant marrow toxicity necessitates either avoiding this agent or stopping breast feeding.— R. Wise, *Br. med. J.*, 1987, *294*, 42.

Chloramphenicol has the potential to cause bone-marrow depression. Some publications advise that its use is contra-indicated in breast feeding, while the American Academy of Pediatrics notes no reported symptoms in breast-fed infants. Several adverse effects have been reported including refusal to feed, falling asleep during feeding, intestinal gas, and heavy vomiting after feeding. Other antibiotics should be preferred for nursing mothers.— R. L. Nation and N. Hotham, *Med. J. Aust.*, 1987, *146*, 308.

For comment on the absorption and fate of chloramphenicol in pregnancy and in the neonate, see under Absorption and Fate, below.

Antimicrobial Action

Chloramphenicol is a broad-spectrum antibiotic which acts by interfering with bacterial protein synthesis. It is usually bacteriostatic and is effective against a wide range of Gram-negative and Gram-positive organisms including *Salmonella typhi, Haemophilus influenzae, Neisseria meningitidis, Streptococcus pneumoniae,* and *Bacteroides fragilis.* It has antirickettsial activity, and is also active against chlamydias of the psittacosis-lymphogranuloma group, mycoplasmas, and *Vibrio* spp. *Pseudomonas aeruginosa* is usually resistant.

Minimum inhibitory concentrations for susceptible organisms have been reported to range from 0.1 to 16 µg per mL.

Chloramphenicol was bactericidal *in vitro* against most isolates of meningeal pathogens such as *Haemophilus influenzae, Streptococcus pneumoniae,* and *Neisseria meningitidis* at clinically achievable concentrations but was only bacteriostatic against the Enterobacteriaceae and *Staphylococcus aureus.*— J. J. Rahal and M. S. Simberkoff, *Antimicrob. Ag. Chemother.*, 1979, *16*, 13. Chloramphenicol demonstrated a wide spectrum of activity against 96 clinical isolates from patients with meningitis; 88% of the strains were susceptible.— R. N. Jones and A. L. Barry (letter), *J. antimicrob. Chemother.*, 1987, *19*, 843.

Reports of the activity *in vitro* of chloramphenicol against: *Aeromonas* spp.— M. R. Motyl *et al.*, *Antimicrob. Ag. Chemother.*, 1985, *28*, 151. *Branhamella catarrhalis.*— F. Ahmad *et al.*, *ibid.*, 1984, *26*, 424. *Campylobacter* spp.— J. Michel *et al.*, *ibid.*, 1983, *23*, 796; H. Sagara *et al.*, *ibid.*, 1987, *31*, 713. *Haemophilus* spp.— E. O. Mason *et al.*, *ibid.*, 1980, *17*, 470; V. Schauf *et al.*, *ibid.*, 1983, *23*, 364; R. M. Bannatyne *et al.*, *J. antimicrob. Chemother.*, 1985, *15*, 187. *Legionella* spp.— C. Thornsberry *et al.*, *Antimicrob. Ag. Chemother.*, 1978, *13*, 78; A. W. Pasculle *et al.*, *ibid.*, 1981, *20*, 793. *Listeria monocytogenes.*— G. L. Wiggins *et al.*, *ibid.*, 1978, *13*, 854. *Neisseria gonorrhoeae.*— P. D. Duck *et al.*, *ibid.*, *14*, 788. *Pseudomonas paucimobilis.*— D. L. Smalley *et al.*, *ibid.*, 1983, *23*, 161. *Rochalimaea quintana.*— W. F. Myers *et al.*, *ibid.*, 1984, *25*, 690. *Salmonella* spp.— S. R. Preblud *et al.*, *ibid.*, 327. *Streptococcus pneumoniae.*— J. Michel *et al.*, *ibid.*, 1983, *23*, 397; Y. Glupczynski *et al.* (letter), *J. antimicrob. Chemother.*, 1983, *11*, 488. *Vibrio* spp.— F. O'Grady *et al.*, *Bull. Wld Hlth Org.*, 1976, *54*, 181; S. W. Joseph *et al.*, *Antimicrob. Ag. Chemother.*, 1978, *13*, 244. *Yersinia enterocolitica.*— M. Raevuori *et al.*, *ibid.*, 888; J. A. A. Hoogkamp-Korstanje, *J. antimicrob. Chemother.*, 1987, *20*, 123.

ACTIVITY AGAINST ANAEROBIC BACTERIA. A study *in vitro* of the activity of 10 antimicrobial agents against 124 strains of *Bacteroides fragilis* and 57 strains of other anaerobic bacteria indicated that clindamycin, metronidazole, and chloramphenicol were the most effective agents against *B. fragilis.*— J. Dubois *et al.*, *J. antimicrob. Chemother.*, 1978, *4*, 329.

In a study *in vitro* of the antimicrobial susceptibilities of 230 anaerobic bacteria isolated from female genital tract infections, the isolates were, in general, very susceptible to chloramphenicol; minimum inhibitory concentrations ranged from less than 0.25 to 8.0 µg per mL.— G. B. Hill and O. M. Ayers, *Antimicrob. Ag. Chemother.*, 1985, *27*, 324.

Further references: F. P. Tally *et al.*, *Antimicrob. Ag. Chemother.*, 1985, *28*, 675 (*Bacteroides fragilis* group).

ACTIVITY WITH OTHER AGENTS. *Diminished activity.* Gentamicin did not affect the activity of chloramphenicol against *Bacteroides fragilis.* However, chloramphenicol inhibited the bactericidal activity of gentamicin against *E. coli.*— J. Klastersky and M. Husson, *Antimicrob. Ag. Chemother.*, 1977, *12*, 135. Antagonism between chloramphenicol and aminoglycoside antibiotics has been reported *in vitro* and has been confirmed *in vivo* in *animals.*— P. J. Sanderson (letter), *Lancet*, 1978, *2*, 210.

Antagonism occurred against some strains of *Staph. aureus* when the activity of chloramphenicol was tested *in vitro* with bleomycin.— J. Y. Jacobs *et al.*, *Antimicrob. Ag. Chemother.*, 1979, *15*, 580.

Chloramphenicol and other antibacterial agents considered to be bacteriostatic, have been shown to antagonise the activity *in vitro* of some beta-lactam antibiotics which are usually bactericidal. Chloramphenicol has antagonised the activity of ampicillin against group B streptococci (J.L. Weeks *et al.*, *Antimicrob. Ag. Chemother.*, 1981, *20*, 281), ampicillin or benzylpenicillin against *Listeria monocytogenes* (D.L. Winslow *et al.*, *ibid.*, 1983, *23*, 555), and ampicillin against *Haemophilus influenzae* (V. Rocco and G. Overturf, *ibid.*, 1982, *21*, 349; A.M.R. Mackenzie and F.T.H. Chan, *ibid.*, 1986, *29*, 565; J.-R. Lapointe *et al.*, *ibid.*, 1986, *29*, 594). Antagonism has also been demonstrated between chloramphenicol and cephalosporins against *Klebsiella pneumoniae* (T.H. Brown and R.H. Alford, *ibid.*, 1984, *25*, 405) and against *Salmonella enteritidis* both *in vitro* and *in vivo* (G.L. French *et al.*, *Br. med. J.*, 1985, *291*, 636).

For comments on the antagonism of ampicillin by chloramphenicol and the clinical problems in treating meningitis with the 2 drugs, see under Ampicillin Trihydrate, p.117.

For mention of antagonism between chloramphenicol and benzylpenicillin, see under Benzylpenicillin Sodium, p.133.

Enhanced activity. Synergism usually occurred when chloramphenicol was tested *in vitro* with actinomycin D or mitomycin against *Staph. aureus.* The effect of mitomycin was obtained at concentrations below those usually obtainable in serum.— J. Y. Jacobs *et al.*, *Antimicrob. Ag. Chemother.*, 1979, *15*, 580.

For reference to enhanced activity between chloramphenicol and fosfomycin, see Fosfomycin, p.233.

For a report of enhanced activity with chloramphenicol and benzalkonium chloride, see above under Solubility.

Resistance

The incidence of resistance to chloramphenicol has increased slowly and resistant strains of the majority of sensitive species have been reported. Resistance is often due to production of an enzyme, acetyltransferase, that acetylates the drug to the inactive derivative, or due to alteration in the permeability of the cell wall to chloramphenicol. Resistance is usually plasmid-mediated and may be transferable. A single plasmid may confer resistance to several antibiotics, as has occurred in salmonellae resistant to chloramphenicol, tetracycline, streptomycin, and sulphonamides. Cross-resistance with thiamphenicol also occurs.

A review of bacterial resistance to chloramphenicol.— W. V. Shaw, *Br. med. Bull.*, 1984, *40*, 36.

RESISTANCE OF BACTEROIDES. Severe anaerobic infections, mainly due to *Bacteroides fragilis*, in 10 patients who failed to respond to chloramphenicol but were later successfully treated with clindamycin.— H. Thadepalli *et al.*, *Curr. ther. Res.*, 1977, *22*, 421.

A report of strains of *B. fragilis* moderately resistant (MIC 12.5 µg per mL) to chloramphenicol due to production of chloramphenicol acetyltransferase.— M. L. Britz and R. G. Wilkinson, *Antimicrob. Ag. Chemother.*, 1978, *14*, 105.

The identification in a strain of *Bacteroides ochraceus* of a conjugative plasmid which specifies resistance to chloramphenicol, tetracycline, kanamycin, and streptomycin and which could be transferred by conjugation to *E. coli*.— D. G. Guiney and C. E. Davis, *Nature*, 1978, *274*, 181. See also J. R. Saunders, *ibid.*, 113.

A study *in vitro* of the susceptibility of 228 strains of the *Bacteroides fragilis* group isolated from 40 subjects who had had no antimicrobial therapy for at least 1 month before the sampling, and 20 patients who had received antimicrobial agents during the period of sampling and 1 week before. Only 2% of strains showed resistance to chloramphenicol at a breakpoint of 16 µg per mL.— A. E. C. C. de Almeida and M. de Uzeda, *Antimicrob. Ag. Chemother.*, 1987, *31*, 617.

RESISTANCE OF ESCHERICHIA. Of 232 strains of enteropathogenic *Escherichia coli* 29 were resistant to chloramphenicol at a concentration of 8 µg per mL; 28 were resistant at 256 µg per mL.— R. J. Gross *et al.*, *Br. med. J.*, 1982, *285*, 472.

See also under Resistance of Salmonellae, and Resistance of Shigellae, below.

RESISTANCE OF GONOCOCCI. For mention of chromosomal mutations in *Neisseria gonorrhoeae* causing increased resistance to benzylpenicillin, chloramphenicol, and other antibacterial agents, see under Benzylpenicillin Sodium, p.134.

RESISTANCE OF HAEMOPHILUS. Meningitis due to chloramphenicol-resistant *Haemophilus influenzae* type b.— A. -L. Kinmonth *et al.*, *Br. med. J.*, 1978, *1*, 694. See also R. J. P. Garvey and G. P. McMullin, *ibid.*, 1983, *287*, 1183.

Of 9 chloramphenicol-resistant isolates of *Haemophilus influenzae* with a minimum inhibitory concentration of chloramphenicol of 15 µg or more per mL, all contained conjugative plasmids encoding resistance to chloramphenicol and tetracycline, or chloramphenicol, tetracycline, and ampicillin, and produced chloramphenicol acetyltransferase.— M. C. Roberts *et al.*, *Antimicrob. Ag. Chemother.*, 1980, *18*, 610.

A report of a permeability barrier as a mechanism of chloramphenicol resistance in *Haemophilus influenzae*.— J. L. Burns *et al.*, *Antimicrob. Ag. Chemother.*, 1985, *27*, 46.

In a multicentre study of the resistance of clinical isolates of *Haemophilus influenzae* in the *UK* during the first 3 months of 1986, 1.7% of strains were considered to be resistant to chloramphenicol; the prevalence of resistance to chloramphenicol had not increased significantly when compared with a similar study in 1981. Of the resistant strains, 40 had minimum inhibitory concentrations (MICs) for chloramphenicol greater than 4 µg per mL and 2 strains had a MIC of 2 µg per mL. All 42 strains were shown to produce chloramphenicol acetyltransferase and were resistant to tetracycline, 13 produced beta-lactamase, and 11 were resistant to trimethoprim and sulphamethoxazole. Two strains were resistant to ampicillin, tetracycline, trimethoprim, sulphamethoxazole, and chloramphenicol.— M. Powell *et al.*, *Br. med. J.*, 1987, *295*, 176. See also A. J. Howard *et al.* (letter), *Lancet*, 1986, *2*, 745; A. J. Howard (letter), *Br. med. J.*, 1987, *295*, 608.

References to *Haemophilus influenzae* strains resistant to chloramphenicol and ampicillin: J. Philpott-Howard, *J. antimicrob. Chemother.*, 1984, *13*, 199; J. N. Walterspiel *et al.*, *J. Am. med. Ass.*, 1984, *251*, 884; A. P. Fraise *et al.*, *Archs Dis. Childh.*, 1986, *61*, 1134; Y. M. Coovadia *et al.*, *J. Infect.*, 1986, *12*, 247.

For further reference to *Haemophilus influenzae* type b resistant to both chloramphenicol and ampicillin, see under Ampicillin Trihydrate, p.118.

RESISTANCE OF PSEUDOMONAS. A report of transposon-mediated resistance to chloramphenicol in *Pseudomonas aeruginosa* due to decreased antibiotic penetration.— J. L. Burns *et al.*, *Antimicrob. Ag. Chemother.*, 1986, *29*, 445.

RESISTANCE OF SALMONELLAE. A study of multiple-drug resistance in isolates of *Salmonella* in India over the period 1972–8 indicated that since 1975 appreciable numbers of serotypes from human and non-human sources had emerged with multiple resistance to between 2 to 6 antimicrobial agents. Isolates of *S. typhi* uniformly resistant to chloramphenicol, streptomycin, sulphafurazole and tetracycline had been obtained. All the isolates studied were sensitive *in vitro* to co-trimoxazole.— K. B. Sharma *et al.*, *J. antimicrob. Chemother.*, 1979, *5*, 15.

S. typhi, in a patient with enteric fever, acquired resistance to both chloramphenicol and co-trimoxazole during treatment.— N. Datta *et al.*, *Lancet*, 1981, *1*, 1181.

A study *in vitro* of the susceptibility of salmonellae isolated in 3 different continents of the world to antimicrobial agents. The percentages of organisms resistant to chloramphenicol with minimum inhibitory concentrations of 25 µg or more per mL were: in Belgium, 13% for non-typhi salmonellae and 5% for *Salmonella typhi*; in Peru, 70% for *S. typhimurium* and 23% for *S. typhi*; and in 2 central Africa countries, 67% for non-typhi salmonellae and 4% for S. typhi.— H. Goossens *et al.*, *J. antimicrob. Chemother.*, 1984, *13*, 559.

During a study of an outbreak of enteritis caused by contaminated raw milk, isolates of *Salmonella typhimurium* were found resistant to chloramphenicol, ampicillin, carbenicillin, kanamycin sulphate, streptomycin, tetracycline, and sulphafurazole. Single isolates of *Escherichia coli* and of *Citrobacter freundii* resistant to chloramphenicol were also found.— C. O. Tacket *et al.*, *J. Am. med. Ass.*, 1985, *253*, 2058.

A report of chloramphenicol-resistant *Salmonella newport* isolated from hamburgers and traced back to the dairy farms of origin.— J. S. Spika *et al.*, *New Engl. J. Med.*, 1987, *316*, 565.

RESISTANCE OF SHIGELLAE. Of 2753 strains of *Shigella dysenteriae, Sh. flexneri*, and *Sh. boydii* examined at the Central Public Health Laboratory from 1979 to mid 1983 41.4% were resistant to chloramphenicol at a concentration of 8 µg per mL. The incidence of resistance to chloramphenicol had increased from 2.6% in 1974 to 52.1% in the first half of 1983.— R. J. Gross *et al.*, *Br. med. J.*, 1984, *288*, 784.

An account of a large-scale epidemic in West Bengal of severe bacillary dysentery, predominantly due to *Shigella dysenteriae* 1. The organisms were considered to be resistant to chloramphenicol, streptomycin, and tetracycline.— S. C. Pal (letter), *Lancet*, 1984, *1*, 1462. During the West Bengal outbreak, 27 of 45 (60%) enteroinvasive *Escherichia coli* and 18 of 32 (56.2%) *Shigella* spp. tested were resistant to chloramphenicol.— B. D. Chatterjee and S. N. Sanyal (letter), *ibid.*, *2*, 574.

RESISTANCE OF STREPTOCOCCI. Of 1176 strains of group A streptococci isolated in Japan in the period 1972 to 1974, 241 were resistant to tetracycline, 234 to tetracycline and chloramphenicol, 427 to tetracycline, chloramphenicol, erythromycin, oleandomycin, josamycin, midecamycin, and lincomycin, and 19 to chloramphenicol alone. Seven of 83 strains of group B streptococci were resistant to tetracycline and chloramphenicol and 26 to tetracycline alone.— Y. Miyamoto *et al.*, *Antimicrob. Ag. Chemother.*, 1978, *13*, 399.

Chloramphenicol-resistant pneumococci in West Africa.— D. Hansman (letter), *Lancet*, 1978, *1*, 1102.

Three of 866 strains of *Str. pneumoniae* were resistant to chloramphenicol.— A. J. Howard *et al.*, *Br. med. J.*, 1978, *1*, 1657. See also J. Garau *et al.* (letter), *Lancet*, 1981, *2*, 147.

In a study of antibiotic resistance of *Streptococcus pneumoniae* in healthy childhood carriers, 68 of 159 strains (42.8%) were resistant to chloramphenicol at a concentration of 16 µg or more per mL.— J. L. Pérez *et al.* (letter), *J. antimicrob. Chemother.*, 1987, *19*, 278.

Absorption and Fate

Chloramphenicol is readily absorbed when given by mouth. Blood concentrations of about 10 µg per mL may be reached 2 hours after a single dose of 1 g by mouth; a dose of 500 mg every 6 hours usually maintains blood concentrations above 4 µg per mL. Chloramphenicol palmitate in hydrolysed to chloramphenicol in the gastro-intestinal tract prior to absorption, and the sodium succinate, which is given parenterally, is hydrolysed to free drug in the liver, lungs, and kidneys. Chloramphenicol sodium succinate is, however, only partially hydrolysed so that blood concentrations of chloramphenicol obtained after parenteral administration of the sodium succinate are often lower than those obtained after administration of chloramphenicol by mouth.

Chloramphenicol is widely distributed in body tissues and fluids; it enters the cerebrospinal fluid, even in the absence of meningitis, giving concentrations of about 50% of those existing in the blood; it diffuses across the placenta into the foetal circulation, into breast milk, and into the aqueous and vitreous humours of the eye. Up to about 60% in the circulation is bound to plasma protein. The half-life of chloramphenicol has been reported to range from 1.5 to 5 hours; the half-life is prolonged in patients with severe liver impairment.

Chloramphenicol is excreted mainly in the urine but only 5 to 10% of an oral dose appears unchanged; the remainder is inactivated in the liver, mostly by conjugation with glucuronic acid; reduction to aryl amines has also been reported. About 3% is excreted in the bile. However, most is reabsorbed and only about 1%, mainly in the inactive form, is excreted in the faeces. After intravenous administration of chloramphenicol sodium succinate approximately 30% is excreted unchanged in the urine, although the amount is very variable.

A detailed review of the clinical pharmacokinetics of chloramphenicol and chloramphenicol succinate.— P. J. Ambrose, *Clin. Pharmacokinet.*, 1984, *9*, 222.

Pharmacokinetics of chloramphenicol sodium succinate in critically ill patients.— R. L. Slaughter *et al.*, *Clin. Pharmac. Ther.*, 1980, *28*, 69.

A study of serum concentrations of chloramphenicol during treatment of 10 paediatric patients aged 0.38 to 17.15 years given chloramphenicol succinate 19 to 26 mg per kg body-weight every 6 hours intravenously over 0.5 to 1 hour. The steady-state peak serum concentrations of chloramphenicol succinate decreased from a range of 22.9 to 181.6 µg per mL (mean 77.1 µg per mL), when measured between days 3 to 8 of illness, to a range of 24.7 to 75.4 µg per mL (mean 42.2 µg per mL), when measured between days 8 to 23. The steady-state peak serum concentrations of chloramphenicol also fell from a mean of 27.7 µg per mL to 24.9 µg per mL. The mean elimination half-life of chloramphenicol ranged from 1.5 to 5.4 hours (mean 3.0 hours) on the first occasion and from 1.2 to 3.8 hours (mean 2.3 hours) on the second. The decrease in serum concentrations of chloramphenicol during repeated chloramphenicol succinate dosing may be clinically important in patients with serious infections and, therefore, serum concentrations should be monitored frequently.— M. C. Nahata and D. A. Powell, *Clin. Pharmac. Ther.*, 1983, *33*, 308.

ABSORPTION AND FATE IN MALNUTRITION. In a study of the metabolism of chloramphenicol in malnourished children only 35 to 55% of an oral dose, given as the palmitate, appeared in the conjugated form compared with 75 to 80% in normal children.— S. Mehta *et al.*, *Am. J. clin. Nutr.*, 1975, *28*, 977.

A study involving 39 Ethiopian children with different nutritional states demonstrated that the pathophysiological changes which occur in malnourished children may offset one another; plasma concentrations within the therapeutic range were obtained in children with kwashiorkor given standard intravenous doses of chloramphenicol, despite decreased plasma clearance and increased half-life compared with children with normal nutritional status. The absorption of chloramphenicol was, however, erratic in severely malnourished children after oral administration of chloramphenicol palmitate which suggests that this route should be avoided in such patients.— M. Eriksson *et al.*, *Eur. J. clin. Pharmac.*, 1983, *24*, 819.

ADMINISTRATION IN INFANTS AND CHILDREN. Studies of the pharmacokinetics of chloramphenicol in infants and children demonstrating wide variations in serum concentrations and clearance of the drug. Serum concentrations should, therefore, be monitored, especially in neonates: G. J. Burckart *et al.*, *J. clin. Pharmac.*, 1982, *22*, 49; G. J. Burckart *et al.*, *ibid.*, 1983, *23*, 106; A. Mulhall *et al.*, *J. antimicrob. Chemother.*, 1983, *12*, 629; H. Ekblad *et al.*, *ibid.*, 1985, *15*, 489.

For comments on reduced hydrolysis of chloramphenicol palmitate and chloramphenicol sodium succinate to active chloramphenicol in neonates, see under Administration in Infants and Children in Uses and Administration, below.

ADMINISTRATION IN LIVER DISORDERS. In a study of 21 patients there was a significant correlation between serum trough concentrations of chloramphenicol and dose in patients with normal liver function but no such correlation in patients with impaired liver function. Mean serum protein binding of chloramphenicol was 53% in 10 patients with normal liver function, 42% in 15 patients with cirrhosis, and 32% in 20 premature infants. Reduced binding in neonates suggests that a lower therapeutic range of total chloramphenicol concentration of 3.5 to 13.9 µg per mL might be required compared with the usual adult range of 5 to 20 µg per mL.

Half of the patients with impaired liver function had serum concentrations of above 25 μg per mL after usual doses of chloramphenicol. The degree of intrapatient variation suggests that frequent monitoring of serum concentrations is necessary with empirical adjustment of dosage when indicated.— J. R. Koup *et al.*, *Antimicrob. Ag. Chemother.*, 1979, *15*, 651.

ADMINISTRATION IN RENAL FAILURE. For reference to the slightly increased half-life of chloramphenicol in patients with end-stage renal failure, see under Uses and Administration, below.

BIOAVAILABILITY. In a study of 18 children aged 2 months to 14 years, the bioavailability of active chloramphenicol following administration of chloramphenicol palmitate by mouth was greater than that following intravenous administration of chloramphenicol succinate; the relative bioavailability of chloramphenicol succinate was calculated to be 70% compared with chloramphenicol palmitate. Urinary excretion of chloramphenicol succinate was highly variable with a mean value of 36% (range 6 to 73%). This amount is virtually identical to and may account for the 30% reduction in bioavailability of the intravenous dosage form relative to that of the oral preparation.— R. E. Kauffman *et al.*, *J. Pediat.*, 1981, *99*, 963.

A comparison of the bioavailability of chloramphenicol in 12 adult patients following the administration of chloramphenicol succinate intravenously, and chloramphenicol palmitate and chloramphenicol base by mouth. Doses used were equivalent to chloramphenicol base 1 g every 6 hours and a minimum of 7 doses was given before blood samples were obtained for analysis; initial therapy was always by intravenous infusion. Mean peak plasma-chloramphenicol concentrations of 16.6, 22.3, and 22.8 μg per mL occurred at a mean of 1.18, 1.53, and 2.12 hours after administration of the succinate, base, and palmitate respectively. From 3 to 6 hours after administration, plasma-chloramphenicol concentrations following the use of the palmitate were significantly higher and peaked significantly later compared to the other two preparations; this was probably because of the necessity for the palmitate ester to be hydrolysed prior to absorption of the active chloramphenicol. The bioavailability of active chloramphenicol was generally less from the succinate intravenously than from the two oral forms. The urinary excretion of 10% to 44% of chloramphenicol succinate as unchanged drug might be responsible for this lower availability; there was excellent correlation for the succinate between the percentage of dose excreted unchanged and the availability of active chloramphenicol. The wide interpatient variability of urinary excretion of the succinate supports the need for monitoring of plasma-chloramphenicol concentrations.— W. G. Kramer *et al.*, *J. clin. Pharmac.*, 1984, *24*, 181.

Although it is widely believed that chloramphenicol sodium succinate is poorly absorbed after intramuscular administration, a prospective study in children indicated that adequate serum concentrations of chloramphenicol could be achieved by this route.— F. Shann *et al.*, *New Engl. J. Med.*, 1985, *313*, 410.

Local hydrolysis of chloramphenicol sodium succinate occurred after topical administration of the drug to 16 patients with superficial or deep soft-tissue infections, and microbiologically active concentrations of chloramphenicol were achieved. Chloramphenicol sodium succinate was administered with dextran gel in concentrations of 2 to 5% w/v and applied twice daily; the amount of drug administered varied between 50 mg and 1 g on each occasion. Seven patients had measurable but low chloramphenicol concentrations in the serum, with peak values ranging from 0.3 to 2.4 μg per mL; two further subjects had peak serum concentrations of 19.7 and 47.9 μg per mL, but these patients were also treated with systemic co-trimoxazole which interfered with the assay for chloramphenicol.— I. Nilsson-Ehle and S. Å. Hedström (letter), *J. antimicrob. Chemother.*, 1987, *19*, 138.

DIFFUSION INTO BODY TISSUES AND FLUIDS. The penetration of chloramphenicol from eye-drops or ointment was assessed in 183 patients. The concentration of chloramphenicol in tears fell below 1 μg per mL within about 5 minutes of a single application of a 0.5% solution to the eye and repeated instillation during several hours was necessary to achieve a concentration in aqueous humour of 1 μg per mL. A single application of chloramphenicol 1% ointment produced concentrations in aqueous humour of about 2 μg per mL at 2 hours, falling to 1 μg per mL at 4 hours; repeated applications of the ointment every 15 minutes gave a concentration of up to 77 μg per mL.— C. Hanna *et al.*, *Archs Ophthal., N.Y.*, 1978, *96*, 1258.

Peak serum concentrations of chloramphenicol and concentrations in cerebrospinal fluid ranged from 14.1 to 54.4 μg per mL and from 13.0 to 36.6 μg per mL respectively in 3 premature infants with intracranial sepsis who received chloramphenicol 25 to 35 mg per kg body-weight daily in 2 divided intravenous infusions of one hour each.— L. M. Dunkle, *Antimicrob. Ag. Chemother.*, 1978, *13*, 427. Following intravenous doses of chloramphenicol succinate of 20 to 30 mg per kg body-weight given every 6 hours to 2 infants with hydrocephalus and ventriculitis peak serum and peak ventricular fluid concentrations occurred after 30 minutes and 3 hours respectively. Ventricular fluid concentrations of chloramphenicol could not be predicted from serum concentrations; the peak ventricular fluid concentration was 57.5% of the peak serum concentration in one patient and only 22.5% in the other.— R. Yogev and T. Williams, *Antimicrob. Ag. Chemother.*, 1979, *16*, 7. Sequential measurement of CSF-chloramphenicol concentrations over a 6-hour dosage interval in a patient with an indwelling lumbar subarachnoid catheter. Therapeutic concentrations (5 μg or more per mL) were achieved during the entire dosage interval after oral administration of chloramphenicol palmitate suspension 12.5 mg per kg body-weight every 6 hours.— E. R. Rensimer *et al.* (letter), *Lancet*, 1981, *1*, 165.

References to the diffusion of chloramphenicol into various body tissues and fluids: D. N. Gerding *et al.*, *Ann. intern. Med.*, 1977, *86*, 708 (ascitic fluid); F. J. George and C. Hanna, *Archs Ophthal., N.Y.*, 1977, *95*, 879 (eye); J. R. Koup *et al.*, *Antimicrob. Ag. Chemother.*, 1979, *15*, 658 (saliva).

PREGNANCY AND THE NEONATE. In a study involving 21 healthy lactating women beginning on the fourth postpartum day, a single dose of chloramphenicol 500 mg or thiamphenicol 500 mg produced mean peak plasma concentrations of 5.5 and 3.7 μg per mL after a mean of 1.4 and 1.6 hours, respectively; mean peak milk concentrations of 2.9 and 2.2 μg per mL for chloramphenicol and thiamphenicol were reached after a mean of 1.4 and 2.6 hours, respectively. Following repeated oral doses of 500 mg three times daily for 2 days, mean plasma and milk concentrations at 24 hours were 3.7 and 1.7 μg per mL, respectively, for chloramphenicol, and 2.9 and 1.9 μg per mL for thiamphenicol; at 48 hours the respective concentrations were 1.1 and 0.6 μg per mL for chloramphenicol and 1.2 and 1.6 μg per mL for thiamphenicol.— T. A. Plomp *et al.*, *Vet. hum. Toxicol.*, 1983, *25*, 167.

There is a high degree of placental transfer of chloramphenicol, with a foetal to maternal serum concentration ratio of 0.7 to 1.0. In the neonate decreased hepatic conjugation may result in toxic accumulation of chloramphenicol, particularly in the preterm infant, who lacks both the enzyme responsible for glucuronyl conjugation and the functionally mature renal system required for effective tubular excretion of the free drug. The serum half-life of chloramphenicol is markedly prolonged in these neonates. Chloramphenicol is excreted in breast milk and concentrations of 1 to 3.5 μg per mL have been detected.— A. W. Chow and P. J. Jewesson, *Rev. infect. Dis.*, 1985, *7*, 287.

See also under Administration in Infants and Children, and Administration in Liver Disorders, above.

Uses and Administration

The liability of chloramphenicol to provoke life-threatening adverse effects, particularly bone-marrow aplasia, has severely limited its clinical usefulness, although it is still widely used in some countries. It should never be given for minor infections and regular blood estimations should be made during treatment of all patients. Typhoid fever and other severe salmonellal infections are the prime indications for the use of chloramphenicol, though it will not eliminate the carrier state.

It is used in serious infections due to *Haemophilus influenzae*, including meningitis attributed to ampicillin-resistant strains, but if children are to be treated the 'grey syndrome' (see Adverse Effects, above) should be taken into consideration; it has also been used in severe respiratory-tract infections including epiglottitis and pneumonia. Chloramphenicol has been used to treat severe anaerobic infections due to *Bacteroides fragilis* especially those involving the central nervous system, and rickettsial infections such as typhus and Rocky Mountain spotted fever when tetracyclines are not indicated. Chloramphenicol is applied topically for a variety of eye infections due to sensitive organisms and has also been used in skin infections.

Chloramphenicol is usually administered by mouth in capsules or as a suspension of chloramphenicol palmitate. When oral administration is not feasible water-soluble chloramphenicol sodium succinate may be given intravenously, but oral therapy should be substituted as soon as possible; an intravenous dose should be injected over at least one minute. Administration by intramuscular injection is controversial because of doubts whether absorption is adequate (but see under Administration in Infants and Children, below). In some countries it is given rectally as suppositories.

Doses are expressed in terms of chloramphenicol base and are similar whether administered by mouth or intravenously. For adults and children the usual dose is 50 mg per kg body-weight daily in divided doses every 6 hours; up to 100 mg per kg daily may be given in severe infections due to moderately resistant organisms, although these higher doses should be reduced as soon as possible. To minimise the risk of relapse it has been recommended that treatment should be continued for 4 days after the patient's temperature has returned to normal in rickettsial diseases and for 8 to 10 days in typhoid fever.

In cases of severe infection, premature and full-term neonates may be given daily doses of 25 mg per kg body-weight and full-term infants over the age of 2 weeks may be given up to 50 mg per kg daily, in 4 divided doses. However, chloramphenicol should only be used when there is no other suitable treatment for the severe infection and when blood concentrations can be monitored.

In patients with impaired hepatic function or severe renal failure the dose of chloramphenicol may need to be reduced because of decreased metabolism or excretion of chloramphenicol.

Reviews of the actions and uses of chloramphenicol: A. Kucers, *Lancet*, 1982, *2*, 425; I. Shalit and M. I. Marks, *Drugs*, 1984, *28*, 281; W. R. Wilson and F. R. Cockerill, *Mayo Clin. Proc.*, 1987, *62*, 906.

References to the use of chloramphenicol in anaerobic infections: J. G. Bartlett, *Lancet*, 1982, *2*, 478; R. E. Van Scoy *et al.*, *Mayo Clin. Proc.*, 1984, *59*, 842; *Med. Lett.*, 1984, *26*, 87.

Chloramphenicol reduced the white cell and blast count in a patient with chronic myeloid leukaemia.— M. A. Schwarz and B. G. Firkin, *Med. J. Aust.*, 1976, *1*, 687. See also B. Klein *et al.*, *Acta haemat.*, 1980, *64*, 246.

A report of beneficial effects with chloramphenicol in a 13-year-old boy with severe chronic neutropenia. His absolute neutrophil count rose from below 250 per mm^3 to 6000 per mm^3 2 weeks after starting chloramphenicol therapy, and remained normal for 5 months while taking chloramphenicol 1.75 g daily by mouth. There was no response to thiamphenicol.— G. R. Adams and H. A. Pearson, *New Engl. J. Med.*, 1983, *309*, 1039. Subtherapeutic concentrations of chloramphenicol stimulate granulocyte/monocyte colony-forming units *in vitro* and this may represent a mechanism for the increase in neutrophils.— B. Bostrom *et al.* (letter), *ibid.*, 1984, *310*, 723.

ADMINISTRATION. In general, peak serum-chloramphenicol concentrations of 10 to 20 μg per mL and trough concentrations of 5 to 10 μg per mL are desirable to ensure efficacy and avoid toxicity; factors such as the sensitivity of the specific organism and the severity of illness must also be considered. Concentration-dependent bone-marrow suppression has been associated with sustained peak serum-chloramphenicol concentrations of 25 μg or more per mL and trough concentrations in excess of 10 μg per mL; treatment duration is also an important factor for toxicity. The 'grey syndrome' has been associated with serum-chloramphenicol concentrations greater than 40 μg per mL.— P. J. Ambrose, *Clin. Pharmacokinet.*, 1984, *9*, 222.

ADMINISTRATION IN INFANTS AND CHILDREN. A review of the clinical pharmacology of chloramphenicol in paediatrics.— A. M. Ristuccia, *Ther. Drug Monit.*, 1985, *7*, 159.

A suggested parenteral dose of chloramphenicol for children is 50 to 100 mg per kg body-weight daily in 4 divided doses. For neonates a suggested dose is 25 mg per kg in a single daily dose for babies aged 0 to 1 week, 25 to 50 mg per kg daily in 1 or 2 divided doses for those aged 1 to 4 weeks, and 25 to 50 mg per kg daily in 2 or 3 divided doses for those aged over 4 weeks. Because of considerable individual variations in the serum concentrations achieved and the high potential for serious toxicity, appropriate doses must be determined by frequent monitoring of serum concentrations.— K. H. Rhodes and C. M. Johnson, *Mayo Clin. Proc.*, 1983, *58*, 158.

Chloramphenicol was given to 64 neonates for life-threatening infections and 10 showed signs of chloramphenicol toxicity, mainly due to overprescription or overdosage of chloramphenicol; peak serum concentrations were reported to range from 28 to 180 μg per mL in these patients.Three of the 64 received a 10-fold overdose and one was given the drug intraventricularly instead of intravenously. Though many babies tolerated serum-chloramphenicol concentrations in excess of 25 μg per mL, it is recommended that the concentration be maintained in the range 15 to 25 μg per mL. Arithmetic errors must be avoided.— A. Mulhall *et al.*, *Br. med. J.*, 1983, *287*, 1424.

There is some controversy over the route of administration of chloramphenicol and the dose to be given in seriously ill children. Some workers feel that although treatment with chloramphenicol may be given initially as the succinate by the intravenous route, there are good reasons, in may cases, for giving the antibiotic by mouth as soon as the child is well enough to take oral medication: chloramphenicol is usually given to children as the palmitate, which is rapidly and completely hydrolysed by pancreatic lipases followed by almost complete absorption; peak serum concentrations are reached some 2 hours after an oral dose, but exceed those after intravenous and intramuscular injection. In older children there seems to be little reason for using parenteral chloramphenicol after the first few doses as long as the oral drug is tolerated; some workers have observed, however, that marrow toxicity is more likely after oral than parenteral chloramphenicol, although there is probably insufficient evidence to support this view. The oral route should probably be avoided in neonates in whom there may be delayed and incomplete absorption as a result of deficient lipase activity (J. Symonds, *Archs Dis. Childh.*, 1984, *59*, 501). Neonates also hydrolyse chloramphenicol succinate to active chloramphenicol more slowly than older infants and children do, and the apparent half-life of cloramphenicol may vary from 3 to 12 hours. In pre-term babies especially, the ability to hydrolyse chloramphenicol succinate may be very variable, and chloramphenicol cannot be relied upon to give a good therapeutic result (K.J. Christiansen *et al.*, *Lancet*, 1983, *1*, 651).

Care must be taken when changing from chloramphenicol succinate to chloramphenicol palmitate as the bioavailability of the palmitate is higher and therefore the dose may need to be reduced (J.N. Walterspiel, *Lancet*, 1985, *2*, 1069). A reduction in dosage may not be appropriate in malnourished children who may have impaired absorption of chloramphenicol palmitate because of an inability to hydrolyse the drug (F. Shann and A. Mackenzie, *New Engl. J. Med.*, 1986, *314*, 451). Shann and others, working in Papua New Guinea, have advocated the intramuscular administration of chloramphenicol rather than the intravenous route. They reported adequate serum concentrations after intramuscular injection, contrary to the widely held belief that chloramphenicol sodium succinate is poorly absorbed by this route, and claimed that pain on injection was minimal (F. Shann *et al.*, *New Engl. J. Med.*, 1985, *313*, 410). Following a study in children with bacterial meningitis they suggested treatment with intramuscular chloramphenicol for 2 or 3 days, followed by oral therapy (F. Shann *et al.*, *Lancet*, 1985, *2*, 681). However, Coulthard and Lamb (*ibid.*, 1015) have found that children describe intramuscular chloramphenicol as amongst the worst treatments they ever receive, and certainly much worse than the insertion of intravenous cannulae. They suggest the use of venous cannula in developed countries, or, in developing countries, the use of a long-acting oil-based preparation of chloramphenicol (Tifomycin) given intramuscularly every 2 to 3 days. The serum concentrations achieved with the long-acting preparation may, however, be rather low (F. Shann, *ibid.*, 1986, *1*, 507).

Several workers feel that a daily dose of chloramphenicol greater than 75 mg per kg body-weight should be used with caution, and, if possible, serum concentrations should be monitored; serum concentrations greater than 50 μg per mL have been found in about 10% of patients receiving a dosage of 100 mg per kg daily (F. Shann *et al.*, *New Engl. J. Med.*, 1985, *313*, 410; M. Schreiner *et al.*, *ibid.*, 1986, *314*, 451).

For further comments on the doses of chloramphenicol used to treat serious infections in infants and children, see under Meningitis, below.

For reference to the reduced protein binding of chloramphenicol in premature infants, see above under Absorption and Fate, Administration in Liver Disorders.

ADMINISTRATION IN LIVER DISORDERS. For a report of reduced protein binding and elevated serum concentrations of chloramphenicol in patients with impaired liver function, see above under Absorption and Fate.

ADMINISTRATION IN RENAL FAILURE. The normal half-life of 2 to 4 hours was increased to 3 to 7 hours in end-stage renal failure; the half-life might be markedly prolonged in the joint presence of renal and hepatic impairment. No dosage adjustment was considered necessary for patients with renal failure. Chloramphenicol was ineffective for urinary-tract infections when the glomerular filtration-rate was less than 40 mL per minute. A dose supplement should be given to patients undergoing haemodialysis, but is not necessary for patients undergoing peritoneal dialysis.— W. M. Bennett *et al.*, *Am. J. Kidney Dis.*, 1983, *3*, 155 (the manufacturers have stated that doses of chloramphenicol may need to be adjusted in patients with renal impairment).

BRAZILIAN PURPURIC FEVER. Brazilian purpuric fever (BPF), first recognised in 1984 in Brazil, presents in children aged 1 to 10 years with the acute onset of fever, commonly associated with vomiting and abdominal pain; there is also an association with a preceding purulent conjunctivitis, and *Haemophilus aegyptius* has been isolated from conjunctivae, oropharynx, and blood of patients with BPF. Without treatment death usually occurs 24 to 48 hours after the onset of symptoms. Topical therapy of *H. aegyptius* conjunctivitis does not appear effective in preventing systemic disease, but early intravenous antimicrobial therapy improves survival. In affected areas, children with otherwise unexplained fever who have a history of conjunctivitis should receive high-dose intravenous antimicrobials that have proven activity against *H. aegyptius*, such as ampicillin and chloramphenicol.— Brazilian Purpuric Fever Study Group, *Lancet*, 1987, *2*, 761.

ENTERIC INFECTIONS. In patients with typhoid or paratyphoid infections, severe salmonella gastro-enteritis, or those with salmonella septicaemia treatment with an appropriate drug such as chloramphenicol, co-trimoxazole, or amoxycillin is essential; the choice of drug depends on the sensitivity of the patient's organism as drug resistance is common (*Drug & Ther. Bull.*, 1983, *21*, 101). Chloramphenicol should be given in a dose of 750 mg four times daily in adults until the fever falls and then 500 mg four times daily to complete treatment for 14 days. Relapses occur in about 5% of patients, but this can be reduced if a 4-week course of amoxycillin is given after the primary antibiotic (A.P. Hall *Br. J. Hosp. Med.*, 1986, *35*, 420).

Chloramphenicol by mouth or intramuscular injection was compared with ampicillin and co-trimoxazole in the treatment of 89 patients with bacteriologically confirmed typhoid fever. Chloramphenicol 50 mg per kg body-weight given by mouth daily in divided doses for 12 days provided the best treatment. Chloramphenicol given by mouth produced higher blood concentrations than the same dose given intramuscularly. However, in a second smaller study just involving these 2 routes of administration of chloramphenicol the response from the oral route was no better than that from the intramuscular route.— M. J. Snyder *et al.*, *Lancet*, 1976, *2*, 1155.

In a comparative study of chloramphenicol and co-trimoxazole in patients with typhoid and paratyphoid fever, treatment with chloramphenicol was more successful initially but gave rise to a greater number of carriers.— S. Ramachandran *et al.*, *J. trop. Med. Hyg.*, 1978, *81*, 36. See also under Co-trimoxazole, p.211.

A favourable report of surgery with peritoneal irrigation, using a solution of dextran in which chloramphenicol 4 g per litre together with aprotinin 1 million units had been dissolved, in the treatment of typhoid perforation.— O. A. Badejo and A. O. Arigbabu, *Gut*, 1980, *21*, 141.

During a period of 12 years, 109 children with enteric fever due to *Salmonella typhi* or *S. paratyphi A* were treated with chloramphenicol in doses of either 50 mg per kg body-weight daily until 10 days after the temperature fell to normal, or 100 mg per kg daily, to a maximum of 2 g, until the fever subsided, followed by 50 mg per kg daily for 10 days; 65 children received the lower dose during the period 1970–78 and 44 received the higher dose during 1978–81. Treatment failed in 41 (63%) children treated with the lower dose and in 10 (24%) treated with the higher dose. In the children who received chloramphenicol alone, the higher dose produced a clinical response in a mean of 5.4 days compared with 7 days with the lower dose. It was recommended that children with typhoid or paratyphoid fever be given chloramphenicol in an initial dose of 100 mg per kg daily until the fever subsided and then half that dose for a further 10 days.— P. Raghupathy *et al.*, *Ann. trop. Paediatr.*, 1984, *4*, 201.

See also under Resistance, p.189, and under Choice of Antibiotic, p.97.

For the use of chloramphenicol in the treatment of cholera and yersiniosis, and for mention of resistance to chloramphenicol in *Shigella* infections, see under Tetracycline Hydrochloride, p.318.

EYE INFECTIONS. In a study of the aetiology and treatment of acute bacterial infections of the external eye, chloramphenicol remained the most effective of 5 antibiotics tested for topical treatment of infection; overall resistance was least for chloramphenicol with 6% of organisms showing resistance. Chloramphenicol was less effective against coliform bacilli, for which gentamicin was preferred.— D. V. Seal *et al.*, *Br. J. Ophthal.*, 1982, *66*, 357. Ophthalmologists in the *UK* frequently use topical chloramphenicol in the treatment of external ocular disease and for prophylaxis in routine surgical cases. It is likely that systemic absorption occurs after ocular administration as there have been reports of bone-marrow depression. Concern has also been expressed about chloramphenicol and childhood leukaemia. Further studies into the systemic absorption of this drug after topical use are indicated, and the drug's application, especially in children for relatively minor conditions and prophylaxis, should be reviewed.— J. D. Stevens and G. P. Mission (letter), *Lancet*, 1987, *2*, 1456.

The treatment of traumatic corneal abrasion involves instillation of antibiotic drops or ointment such as chloramphenicol, and perhaps a mydriatic drop such as homatropine, followed by padding of the eye. It used to be claimed that ointment should not be used because globules could become trapped beneath the epithelium and therby be incorporated in the cornea, but this notion has been comprehensively disproved. Ointment is in fact preferable to drops, since it provides a longer contact time with the antibiotic and lubrication between the epithelial break and the lids.— *Lancet*, 1987, *2*, 1250.

For mention of the topical use of chloramphenicol to treat neonatal conjunctivitis, see Pregnancy and the Neonate, below.

LISTERIOSIS. For comments on the use of chloramphenicol in the treatment of listeriosis, see under Listeriosis and Meningitis in Ampicillin Trihydrate, p.120.

MELIOIDOSIS. For mention of the use of chloramphenicol in association with tetracycline for the treatment of melioidosis, see under Tetracycline Hydrochloride, p.319.

MENINGITIS. Chloramphenicol has been used either alone or in association with other drugs such as ampicillin in the treatment of meningitis due to *Haemophilus influenzae*, and it has also been given in the treatment of meningococcal meningitis in penicillin-allergic patients. Doses of chloramphenicol have varied from 75 to 100 mg per kg body-weight daily in divided doses for meningitis due to *H. influenzae*; the higher dose may, however, produce undesirably high blood concentrations (H.P. Lambert, *Br. J. Hosp. Med.*, 1983, *29*, 128; M. Schreiner *et al.*, *New. Engl. J. Med.*, 1986, *314*, 451). Neonatal doses have also varied, but therapeutic concentrations of chloramphenicol may be achieved in the serum and the cerebrospinal fluid with daily doses of 25 mg per kg body-weight in preterm and term infants during the first week of life, and 50 mg per kg for older term babies, administered in 2 or 3 divided doses (A. Mulhall *et al.*, *Lancet*, 1983, *1*, 284). The duration of treatment has ranged from 7 to 14 days. Because of the toxicity of chloramphenicol, peak serum concentrations should be monitored where possible regardless of the dose and route of administration. If therapy is changed from the parenteral route using chloramphenicol sodium succinate to the oral route using chloramphenicol palmitate, care should be taken with the dose as the bioavailability of the palmitate is higher than the succinate, and children may be unnecessarily exposed to the risks of toxic chloramphenicol concentrations (J.N. Walterspiel, *Lancet*, 1985, *2*, 1069); children with malnutrition may, however, have impaired absorption of the palmitate due to an inability to hydrolyse the drug (F. Shann, *ibid.*, 1986, *1*, 507).

Several workers advocate the use of chloramphenicol alone in the treatment of bacterial meningitis in children, especially if caused by *H. influenzae*. Shann *et al.* (*Lancet*, 1985, *2*, 681) studied 367 children with cerebrospinal-fluid findings suggestive of bacterial meningitis. They found chloramphenicol sodium succinate given alone intramuscularly to be as effective as chloramphenicol sodium succinate plus benzylpenicillin both given intravenously. Shann *et al.* concluded that intramuscular administration of chloramphenicol alone for 2 or 3 days followed by oral administration of chloramphenicol palmitate had several advantages over intravenous therapy with both chloramphenicol and benzylpenicillin, especially in developing countries. The single-drug therapy was considered to be cheaper, less staff intensive, and without the risks of sepsis and overhydration of intravenous therapy. However, other workers are concerned about the development of resistance to chloramphenicol (C.G. Prober *et al.*, *Lancet*, 1983, *2*, 158) and also to ampicillin, and so prefer the use of a third-generation cephalosporin such as cefotaxime or ceftriaxone (S.J. Eykyn, *Prescribers' J.*, 1983, *23*, 58; D. Hansman, *Med. J. Aust.*, 1987, *146*, 111). For further comments on the use of chloramphenicol with or without ampicillin in the treatment of meningitis, see under Ampicillin Trihydrate, p.120.

For comments on the route of administration and dosage of chloramphenicol to treat infants and children with severe bacterial infections, see Administration in Infants and Children, above.

Further references to the treatment of *Haemophilus influenzae* meningitis in children: P. C. Y. Chan and P. J. Sanderson (letter), *Lancet*, 1984, *1*, 1478 (use with rifampicin; no apparent antagonism); V. A. Nottidge, *J. Infect.*, 1985, *11*, 109 (use with penicillin).

Meningococcal meningitis was cured in 35 of 49 children over 1-year-old by a single injection of chloramphenicol given intramuscularly as an oily suspension. Only 4 of 17 children with pneumococcal meningitis were cured. The dose ranged from 1 to 3 g according to age.— P. Saliou *et al.*, *Med. trop. Marseille*, 1977, *37*, 189. See also J. B. Puddicombe *et al.*, *Trans. R. Soc. trop. Med. Hyg.*, 1984, *78*, 399.

Meningitis caused by *Campylobacter fetus* subspp. *jejuni* in a 34-year-old man was successfully treated with chloramphenicol. The organism was resistant to ampicillin but was sensitive also to metronidazole.— R. Norrby *et al.*, *Br. med. J.*, 1980, *280*, 1164.

For reference to the use of chloramphenicol to treat gonococcal meningitis, see under Sexually Transmitted Diseases, below.

MOUTH INFECTIONS. For mention of the use of chloramphenicol to treat serious or refractory oral infections, see under Benzylpenicillin Sodium, p.137.

PERICARDITIS. For a report of the use of chloramphenicol, ampicillin, and gentamicin in the treatment of pericarditis due to *Haemophilus influenzae* type b, see under Ampicillin Trihydrate, p.121.

PLAGUE. For mention of the use of chloramphenicol in the treatment of plague, see under Tetracycline Hydrochloride, p.320.

PREGNANCY AND THE NEONATE. For comments on the dose and route of administration of chloramphenicol in neonates, see Administration in Infants and Children, above.

Neonatal conjunctivitis. Chloramphenicol 0.5% and neomycin 0.5% ointments are widely used and effective in most acute bacterial infections of the eye in neonates although neomycin is inactive against streptococci. Chloramphenicol should be avoided if possible when chlamydial infection is a possibilty, since it may suppress but not eradicate chlamydia.— *Lancet*, 1984, *2*, 1375. See also J. M. Pierce *et al.*, *Br. J. Ophthal.*, 1982, *66*, 728.

For concern over the topical use of chloramphenicol for relatively minor eye conditions, see Eye Infections, above.

RELAPSING FEVER, LOUSE-BORNE. For a study comparing chloramphenicol, tetracycline, doxycycline, erythromycin, and penicillin in the treatment of louse-borne relapsing fever, see under Tetracycline Hydrochloride, p.320.

RESPIRATORY-TRACT INFECTIONS. *Epiglottitis.* Mention of the use of parenteral chloramphenicol to treat acute epiglottitis caused by *Haemophilus influenzae* type b.— T. J. Coleman (letter), *Lancet*, 1982, *2*, 613.

See also under Ampicillin Trihydrate, p.121.

Pneumonia. In a study involving 748 children with severe pneumonia, treatment with chloramphenicol alone was found to be as effective as chloramphenicol plus benzylpenicillin. The study took place in Papua New Guinea, where most cases of pneumonia are caused by *Haemophilus influenzae* or *Streptococcus pneumoniae*.— F. Shann *et al.*, *Lancet*, 1985, *2*, 684.

RICKETTSIAL INFECTIONS. For mention of the use of chloramphenicol and tetracyclines in the treatment of rickettsioses, see under Doxycycline Hydrochloride, p.220.

SEPTICAEMIA. Comment that an antibiotic such as chloramphenicol or gentamicin should initially be given to patients with septicaemia or other serious infections caused by *Campylobacter* spp. until the results of sensitivity tests are known.— C. A. M. McNulty, *J. antimicrob. Chemother.*, 1987, *19*, 281.

SEXUALLY TRANSMITTED DISEASES. Mention of the use of chloramphenicol as an alternative treatment to cephalosporins for gonococcal meningitis in adults and children.— *Med. Lett.*, 1988, *30*, 5.

SKIN DISORDERS. Chloramphenicol has been used topically in the treatment of acne vulgaris but is considered to be less effective than benzoyl peroxide. Resistant strains may rarely develop in the skin flora as a result of its use, and sensitisation uncommonly occurs.— W. J. Cunliffe, *Prescribers' J.*, 1987, *27*, 23.

WHIPPLE'S DISEASE. For mention of the use of chloramphenicol to treat Whipple's disease, see under Benzylpenicillin Sodium, p.138.

Preparations of Chloramphenicol and its Salts

Chloramphenicol Capsules *(B.P., U.S.P.)*

Chloramphenicol Cream *(U.S.P.)*

Chloramphenicol Ear Drops *(B.P.)*. Chloramphenicol in propylene glycol. Small amounts of water reduce the solubility of chloramphenicol in propylene glycol.

Chloramphenicol Otic Solution *(U.S.P.)*. A sterile solution of chloramphenicol in a suitable solvent. pH 4 to 8, when diluted with an equal volume of water.

Chloramphenicol Eye Drops *(B.P.)*. CPL

Chloramphenicol Eye Drops *(A.P.F.)*. Chloramphenicol 500 mg, boric acid 1.5 g, borax 300 mg, phenylmercuric nitrate 2 mg, and Water for Injections to 100 mL.

Chloramphenicol for Ophthalmic Solution *(U.S.P.)*. A sterile dry mixture of chloramphenicol. To be reconstituted.

Chloramphenicol Ophthalmic Solution *(U.S.P.)*

Chloramphenicol and Hydrocortisone Acetate for Ophthalmic Suspension *(U.S.P.)*. A sterile dry mixture of chloramphenicol and hydrocortisone acetate. To be reconstituted.

Chloramphenicol Eye Ointment *(B.P., A.P.F.)*

Chloramphenicol Ophthalmic Ointment *(U.S.P.)*

Chloramphenicol and Polymyxin B Sulfate Ophthalmic Ointment *(U.S.P.)*

Chloramphenicol, Polymyxin B Sulfate, and Hydrocortisone Acetate Ophthalmic Ointment *(U.S.P.)*

Chloramphenicol and Prednisolone Ophthalmic Ointment *(U.S.P.)*

Chloramphenicol Sodium Succinate Injection *(B.P.)*

Sterile Chloramphenicol *(U.S.P.)*

Sterile Chloramphenicol Sodium Succinate *(U.S.P.)*

Chloramphenicol Oral Suspension *(B.P.)*. Chloramphenicol Palmitate Mixture; Chloramphenicol Suspension. A suspension of chloramphenicol palmitate.

Chloramphenicol Palmitate Oral Suspension *(U.S.P.)*. pH 4.5 to 7.0.

Proprietary Preparations of Chloramphenicol and its Salts

Actinac *(Roussel, UK)*. *Lotion*, powder for reconstitution, chloramphenicol 40 mg, hydrocortisone acetate 40 mg, butoxyethyl nicotinate ($C_{12}H_{17}NO_3$ = 223.3) 24 mg, allantoin 24 mg, precipitated sulphur 320 mg/g, supplied with diluent.

Alcon Opulets Chloramphenicol 0.5% *(Alcon, UK)*. *Eye-drops*, chloramphenicol 0.5%, in single-use disposable applicators.

Chloromycetin *(Parke, Davis, UK)*. *Capsules*, chloramphenicol 250 mg.
Suspension, chloramphenicol 125 mg (as palmitate)/5 mL.
Injection, powder for reconstitution, chloramphenicol (as sodium succinate) in vials of 300 mg and 1.2 g.
Eye-drops (Redidrops), chloramphenicol 0.5%.
Eye ointment, chloramphenicol 1%.

Chloromycetin Hydrocortisone *(Parke, Davis, UK)*. *Eye ointment*, chloramphenicol 1%, hydrocortisone acetate 0.5%.

Kemicetine *(Farmitalia Carlo Erba, UK)*. *Injection*, powder for reconstitution, chloramphenicol (as sodium succinate), in vials of 1 g.

Minims Chloramphenicol *(Smith & Nephew Pharmaceuticals, UK)*. *Eye-drops*, chloramphenicol 0.5% in single-use disposable applicators.

Sno Phenicol *(Smith & Nephew Pharmaceuticals, UK)*. *Eye-drops*, chloramphenicol 0.5%.

Proprietary Names and Manufacturers of Chloramphenicol or its Salts

Ak-Chlor *(Akorn, Canad.; Akorn, USA)*; Alcon Opulets Chloramphenicol *(Alcon, UK)*; Amphicol *(USA)*; Antibiopto *(Prof. Pharmacal, USA)*; Aquamycetin *(Winzer, Ger.)*; Arcomicetina *(Clarben, Spain)*; Biomicin *(Tosi, Ital.)*; Bioticaps *(Arg.)*; Cafenolo *(Dessy, Ital.)*; Cébénicol *(Chauvin-Blache, Fr.; Novopharma, Switz.)*; Chemicetina *(Carlo Erba, Ital.; Ifesa, Spain)*; Chemyzin *(Ital.)*; Chlomin *(USV, Austral.)*; Chloramex *(Dumex, Denm.; MPS Lab., S.Afr.)*; Chloramol *(Austral.)*; Chlorates *(Pharmadrug, Ger.)*; Chlorcol *(Propan, S.Afr.)*; Chlorofair *(Pharmafair, USA)*; Chloromycetin *(Arg.; Parke, Davis, Austral.; Belg.; Parke, Davis, Canad.; Parke, Davis, Denm.; Parke, Davis, Ital.; Parke, Davis, Norw.; Parke, Davis, S.Afr.; Parke, Davis, Spain; Parke, Davis, Swed.; Parke, Davis, Switz.; Parke, Davis, UK; Parke, Davis, USA)*; Chloroptic *(Allergan, Austral.; Allergan, Canad.; Allergan, Ger.; Allergan, S.Afr.; Allergan, USA)*; Chlorsig *(Sigma, Austral.)*; Cloramfen *(Sclavo, Ital.)*; Cloramplast *(Llorens, Spain)*; Clorbiotina *(Spain)*; Clorfenicol Wolner *(Kairon, Spain)*; Clorofenicina *(Antibioticos, Spain)*; Cloromicetin *(Spain)*; Cloromisol *(Spain)*; Cloromoin *(Spain)*; Cloroptic *(Arg.)*; Cutispray No. 4 *(Switz.)*; Doctamicina *(Switz.)*; Econochlor *(Alcon Laboratories, USA)*; Espectro Medical *(Medical, Spain)*; Farmicetina *(Montedison, Arg.)*; Fenicol *(Belg.; Alcon, Canad.)*; Globenicol *(Belg.; Neth.)*; Hortfenicol *(Hortel, Spain)*; I-Chlor *(Americal, USA)*; Iprobiot *(Arg.)*; Isopto Fenicol *(Alcon, Canad.; Alcon, Spain; Alcon, Swed.; Switz.)*; Kamaver *(Ger.)*; Kemicetina *(Belg.)*; Kemicetine *(S.Afr.; Farmitalia Carlo Erba, UK)*; Kloramfenikol Minims *(Smith & Nephew, Denm.; Smith & Nephew, Norw.)*; Labamicol *(Switz.)*; Lennacol *(Lennon, S.Afr.)*; Leukomycin *(Bayer, Ger.)*; Levomicetina *(Ital.)*; Lomecitina *(Ital.)*; Micoclorina *(Ital.)*; Micodry *(Zambon, Ital.)*; Minims Chloramphenicol *(Smith & Nephew, Austral.; Smith & Nephew, S.Afr.; Smith & Nephew Pharmaceuticals, UK)*; Mycetin *(Farmigea, Ital.)*; Mychel *(Rachelle, USA)*;
Nevimycin *(Ger.)*; Normofenicol *(Normon, Spain)*; Novochlorocap *(Novopharm, Canad.)*; Ocu-Chlor *(Ocumed, USA)*; Oftalent *(Weiders, Norw.)*; Oleomycetin *(Winzer, Ger.)*; Opclor *(Austral.)*; Ophtaphénicol *(Faure, Fr.)*; Ophthochlor *(Parke, Davis, USA)*; Paidomicetina *(Ital.)*; Pantofenicol *(Arg.; Promesa, Spain)*; Pantovernil *(Ger.)*; Paraxin *(Boehringer Mannheim, Ger.)*; Paraxin Succinat A *(Jpn)*; Pentamycetin *(Berlex, Canad.)*; Plastodermo *(Labaz, Spain)*; Quemicetina *(Arg.)*; Ranphenicol *(Ind.)*; Rivomycine *(Switz.)*; Septicol *(Switz.)*; Sificetina *(SIFI, Ital.)*; Sintomicetina *(Arg.)*; Sno Phenicol *(Smith & Nephew Pharmaceuticals, UK)*; Solnicol Ercé *(Fr.)*; Solu-Paraxin *(Switz.)*; Sopamycetin *(Canad.)*; Spersanicol *(Dispersa, Switz.)*; Succicaf *(Farber-Ref, Ital.)*; Synthomycetine *(Belg.)*; Thilocanfol C *(Thilo, Ger.)*; Tifomycine *(Roussel, Fr.)*; Tramina *(Faes, Spain)*; Troymycetin *(SCS, S.Afr.)*; Vernacetin *(Vernleigh, S.Afr.)*.

The following names have been used for multi-ingredient preparations containing chloramphenicol or its salts— Acne-sol *(Fawns & McAllan, Austral.)*; Actinac *(Roussel, Canad.; Roussel, UK)*; Chlorocort *(Parke, Davis, Austral.)*; Chloromycetin Hydrocortisone *(Parke, Davis, UK; Parke, Davis, USA)*; Chloromyxin *(Parke, Davis, Austral.)*; Elase-Chloromycetin *(Parke, Davis, Canad.; Parke, Davis, USA)*; Ginetris *(Farmitalia Carlo Erba, UK)*; Ophthocort *(Parke, Davis, Canad.; Parke, Davis, USA)*; Otopred *(Loveridge, UK)*; Pentamycetin-HC *(Berlex, Canad.)*; Tanderil Chloramphenicol *(Zyma, UK)*.

51-h

Chlortetracycline Calcium *(BANM, rINNM)*.

The calcium salt of 7-chlorotetracycline.

CAS — 57-62-5 (chlortetracycline); 5892-31-9 (calcium).

52-m

Chlortetracycline Hydrochloride *(BANM, USAN, rINNM)*.

Biomycin Hydrochloride.

$C_{22}H_{23}ClN_2O_8$,HCl=515.3.

CAS — 64-72-2.

NOTE. Aureomycin and aureomycin hydrochloride were used as nonproprietary names for chlortetracycline hydrochloride; these names are now used in some countries as proprietary names.

Pharmacopoeias. In *Arg., Aust., Belg., Br., Braz., Chin., Cz., Egypt., Eur., Fr., Ger., Int., It., Jug., Neth., Rus., Span., Swiss,* and *U.S.* Also in *B.P. Vet. U.S.* includes Chlortetracycline Bisulfate for veterinary use.

An antimicrobial substance produced by the growth of certain strains of *Streptomyces aureo-*

faciens or by any other means.

Yellow odourless crystals. The *B.P.* specifies that chlortetracycline hydrochloride contains not less than 950 units per mg calculated with reference to the dried substance. The *U.S.P.* specifies not less than 900 µg per mg. Slightly **soluble** in water and in alcohol; soluble in solutions of alkali hydroxides and carbonates; practically insoluble in acetone, chloroform, dioxan, and ether. A 1% solution in water has a pH of 2.3 to 3.3. **Store** in airtight containers. Protect from light.

Chlortetracycline hydrochloride has been reported to be **incompatible** with amikacin sulphate, ammonium chloride, calcium chloride, calcium gluconate, cefapirin sodium, cephalothin sodium, cephazolin sodium, colistin sulphomethate sodium, dextrans, fructose, lactated Ringer's injection, polymyxin B sulphate, promazine hydrochloride, protein hydrolysate, and Ringer's injection.

In a study of the stability of chlortetracycline hydrochloride in some ophthalmic ointment bases, loss of activity during storage for 12 months at 25° and 35° displayed first-order kinetic behaviour. Chlortetracycline hydrochloride was more stable in absorption bases containing wool fat than in those containing cetyl alcohol. It was also more stable in water-in-oil emulsion bases than in oil-in-water emulsion ointment bases stored at 25° for 12 months, but the stability of the drug was approximately the same in the two bases stored at 35° for 12 months.— M. A. Attia *et al.*, *Pharmazie*, 1985, *40*, 629.

Units

One unit of chlortetracycline is contained in 0.001 mg of the second International Standard Preparation (1969) of chlortetracycline hydrochloride which contains 1000 units per mg.

Adverse Effects and Precautions

As for Tetracycline Hydrochloride, p.314.

Absorption and Fate

As for Tetracycline Hydrochloride, p.317.

Chlortetracycline is poorly absorbed from the gastro-intestinal tract compared with other tetracyclines. It is reported to be rapidly inactivated in the body and is largely eliminated by biliary excretion. Only a small amount is excreted in the urine and although it is not recommended in patients with renal impairment accumulation would not be likely.

Some 47% of chlortetracycline was bound in the body to serum proteins. The half-life in serum was 5.6 hours and 18% was excreted in urine.— C. M. Kunin, *Ann. intern. Med.*, 1967, *67*, 151.

The biological half-life of chlortetracycline was variously reported as 2.3 to 5.6 hours; in renal failure this might be increased to 7 to 11 hours.— W. A. Ritschel, *Drug Intell. & clin. Pharm.*, 1970, *4*, 332.

Uses and Administration

Chlortetracycline hydrochloride has the antimicrobial activity and uses described under tetracycline hydrochloride (see p.315).

The usual dose is 250 to 500 mg four times daily by mouth, preferably one hour before, or 2 hours after, meals. It is also used as a 1% ophthalmic ointment and as a 3% cream or ointment for application to the skin.

Chlortetracycline 1% eye ointment has been used for local treatment of ophthalmia neonatorum including chlamydial infection (J.M. Pierce *et al.*, *Br. J. Ophthal.*, 1982, *66*, 728; E.M.C. Dunlop, *Br. J. Hosp. Med.*, 1983, *29*, 6). However, even if the baby appears to have responded satisfactorily, organisms may sometimes be re-isolated from the eyes or pharynx (E. Rees *et al.*, *Archs Dis. Childh.*, 1981, *56*, 193) and confirmed chlamydial ophthalmia must be treated with systemic antibiotics such as erythromycin (*Lancet*, 1984, *2*, 1375). For further comment on the use of topical tetracyclines in the treatment of ophthalmia neonatorum (neonatal conjunctivitis), see under Tetracycline Hydrochloride, Pregnancy and the Neonate, p.320.

Persistent ulceration following too deep an injection of BCG vaccine could be treated with chlortetracycline 3% ointment or cream; the ointment could also be used for discharging abscesses if aspiration was unsuccessful.— J. Verbov, *Practitioner*, 1984, *228*, 1069.

A double-blind placebo-controlled study involving 57 patients with recurrent aphthous ulcers. Chlortetracycline 250 mg in 10 mL of water used as a mouth rinse for one minute 4 times daily for 4 consecutive days and repeated if necessary after a rinse-free period of one week, was found to be an effective local treatment.— V. Henricsson and T. Axéll, *Acta odontol. scand.*, 1985, *43*, 47.

For the use of chlortetracycline hydrochloride in the treatment of trachoma, see under Tetracycline Hydrochloride, Trachoma, p.322.

Preparations

Chlortetracycline Capsules *(B.P.)*. Capsules containing chlortetracycline hydrochloride.

Chlortetracycline Hydrochloride Capsules *(U.S.P.)*

Sterile Chlortetracycline Hydrochloride *(U.S.P.)*

Chlortetracycline Eye Ointment *(A.P.F.)*. Contains chlortetracycline hydrochloride.

Chlortetracycline Eye Ointment *(B.P.)*. Chlortetracycline Hydrochloride Eye Ointment

Chlortetracycline Hydrochloride Ophthalmic Ointment *(U.S.P.)*

Chlortetracycline Hydrochloride Ointment *(U.S.P.)*

Chlortetracycline Ointment *(A.P.F.)*. Contains chlortetracycline hydrochloride.

Chlortetracycline Ointment *(B.P.C. 1973)*. Contains chlortetracycline hydrochloride.

Proprietary Preparations

Aureomycin *(Lederle, UK)*. *Capsules*, chlortetracycline hydrochloride 250 mg.
Cream, chlortetracycline equivalent to chlortetracycline hydrochloride 3%.
Ointment, chlortetracycline hydrochloride 3%.
Eye ointment, chlortetracycline hydrochloride 1%.

Proprietary Names and Manufacturers of Chlortetracycline and Chlortetracycline Hydrochloride

Auréomycine *(Fr.; Lederle, Switz.)*; Aureomicina *(Cyanamid, Ital.; Cyanamid, Spain)*; Aureomycin *(Lederle, Austral.; Belg.; Lederle, Canad.; Lederle, Denm.; Cyanamid-Lederle, Ger.; Neth.; Lederle, Norw.; S.Afr.; Lederle, Swed.; Switz.; Lederle, UK; Lederle, USA)*; Aureum *(Ital.)*; Chlortet *(Austral.)*; Clorciclina *(Ital.)*.

The following names have been used for multi-ingredient preparations containing chlortetracycline and chlortetracycline hydrochloride—Aureocort *(Lederle, Canad.; Lederle, UK)*; Betnovate-A *(Glaxo, Austral.; Glaxo, UK)*; Deteclo *(Lederle, UK)*; Propaderm-A *(Allen & Hanburys, UK)*; Trimovate Ointment *(Glaxo, UK)*.

63-g

Ciclacillin *(BAN, rINN)*.

Cyclacillin *(USAN)*; Wy-4508. (6*R*)-6-(1-Aminocyclohexanecarboxamido)penicillanic acid.

$C_{15}H_{23}N_3O_4S = 341.4$.

CAS — 3485-14-1.

Pharmacopoeias. In *Jpn* and *U.S.*

A 1% solution has a pH of 4.0 to 6.5. **Store** in airtight containers.

Ciclacillin is an aminopenicillin with similar actions and uses to ampicillin (see p.116), although it is generally less active *in vitro*. Ciclacillin is given in usual doses of 250 to 500 mg four times daily by mouth. Children may be given half the adult dose.

Ciclacillin is well-absorbed from the gastro-intestinal tract and peak serum concentrations of about 12 µg per mL have been reported about ½ to 1 hour after a single 500 mg dose. It is rapidly excreted, about 80% of a dose being excreted in the urine within 6 hours, mainly as ciclacillin.

Ciclacillin has been reported to cause a lower incidence of diarrhoea than ampicillin.

Brief reviews of ciclacillin.— *Med. Lett.*, 1980, *22*, 13; *Drug & Ther. Bull.*, 1981, *19*, 78.

For comparative reviews and reports of aminopenicillins, see Ampicillin Trihydrate p.119.

ABSORPTION AND FATE. Investigation in *rats* demonstrated that ciclacillin caused sex-related nephropathy. The nephrotoxic effect was noted only in male *rats* and in correlation with this a metabolite of ciclacillin, 1-aminocyclohexanecarboxylic acid accumulated to a greater extent in the male. Nephrotoxicity was not noted in *dogs, rhesus monkeys*, or man. The principal excretion product in man was unchanged ciclacillin (60 to 70% of the dose), about 15 to 20% was penicilloic acid, and about 1 to 2% was 1-aminocyclohexanecarboxylic acid, this amount being independent of the sex of the subjects.— W. E. Tucker *et al.*, *Toxic. appl. Pharmac.*, 1974, *29*, 1.

Results of a study involving 27 infants indicating that the absorption of ciclacillin from the gastro-intestinal tract is not affected by administration with milk or milk formula.— C. M. Ginsburg *et al.*, *Antimicrob. Ag. Chemother.*, 1981, *19*, 1086.

ADMINISTRATION IN RENAL FAILURE. Ciclacillin is 20 to 25% bound to plasma proteins and has a normal half-life of 0.5 hours which is increased to 8 to 10 hours in end-stage renal failure. The interval between doses should be extended from 6 hours to up to 12 hours in patients with a glomerular filtration-rate (GFR) of 10 to 50 mL per minute, and to up to 24 hours in those with a GFR of less than 10 mL per minute. Supplements should be given to patients undergoing haemodialysis.— W. M. Bennett *et al.*, *Am. J. Kidney Dis.*, 1983, *3*, 155.

INTERFERENCE WITH DIAGNOSTIC TESTS. In a study *in vitro* of the effects of various antibiotics on tests for glycosuria, ciclacillin in the urine could give falsely elevated readings with a test using a copper-reduction method (Clinitest). It had no effect however on glucose oxidase methods (Diastix and Tes-Tape) of estimating glycosuria.— W. A. Parker and M. E. MacCara, *Am. J. Hosp. Pharm.*, 1984, *41*, 125.

URINARY-TRACT INFECTIONS. Single doses of co-trimoxazole 1.92 g, or amoxycillin 3 g, or ciclacillin 3 g, each given by mouth, were compared in a single-blind study of the treatment of 38 women with acute cystitis. After 2 weeks the overall cure-rates were: co-trimoxazole group, 85%, amoxycillin group, 50%, ciclacillin group, 30%. Relapses from initial cure had occurred in all groups. The study was prematurely stopped when it appeared that the cure-rate was unusually low.— T. M. Hooton *et al.*, *J. Am. med. Ass.*, 1985, *253*, 387.

Preparations

Cyclacillin for Oral Suspension *(U.S.P.)*. A dry mixture of ciclacillin for reconstitution.

Cyclacillin Tablets *(U.S.P.)*. Tablets containing ciclacillin.

Proprietary Preparations

Calthor *(Ayerst, UK)*. *Tablets*, scored, ciclacillin 250 and 500 mg.
Suspension, granules for reconstitution, ciclacillin 125 and 250 mg/5 mL when reconstituted with water.

Proprietary Names and Manufacturers

Calthor *(Ayerst, UK)*; Citocilina *(Spain)*; Citocillin *(S.Afr.)*; Citosarin *(Jpn)*; Cyclapen-W *(Wyeth, USA)*; Orfilina *(Spain)*; Ultracillin *(Ger.; Switz.)*; Vastcillin *(Jpn)*; Vatracin *(Jpn)*; Vipicil *(Arg.)*; Wyvital *(Jpn)*.

16578-v

Cilastatin Sodium *(BANM, USAN, rINNM)*.

MK-791. (*Z*)-(*S*)-6-Carboxy-6-[(*S*)-2,2-dimethylcyclopropanecarboxamido]-hex-5-enyl-L-cysteine, monosodium salt.

$C_{16}H_{25}N_2NaO_5S = 380.4$.

CAS — 81129-83-1; 82009-34-5 (cilastatin).

Cilastatin sodium is an inhibitor of dehydropeptidase I, an enzyme found in the brush border of the renal tubules. It is administered concurrently with the antibiotic imipenem (see p.247) to prevent its renal metabolism and thereby increase the concentrations of imipenem achieved in the urine.

A review of the development of the combination of imipenem and cilastatin, including the action and disposition of cilastatin.— F. M. Kahan *et al.*, *J. antimicrob. Chemother.*, 1983, *12*, *Suppl.* D, 1.

Cilastatin is a highly selective reversible competitive inhibitor of dehydropeptidase-I. Studies in *animals* have provided no evidence that inhibition of this enzyme produces any adverse effects during short periods of therapy, and cilastatin has been well tolerated when administered at high doses for long periods. High doses of imipenem have caused acute proximal tubular necrosis in *rabbits* and *monkeys* similar to that described for cephaloridine. Co-administration of cilastatin has produced a dose-dependent amelioration of this damage in *rabbits*, an imipenem to cilastatin ratio of 1 to 1 affording total protection.

Cilastatin is devoid of antibacterial activity and inhibitory effects on beta-lactamases, and neither potentiates nor antagonises the effects of imipenem.— S. P. Clissold *et al.*, *Drugs*, 1987, *33*, 183.

Cilastatin did not inhibit superoxide dismutase *in vitro*.— R. A. Proctor and J. A. Textor, *Antimicrob.*

Ag. Chemother., 1985, 28, 691.

For reference to studies of the absorption and fate of cilastatin, see Imipenem p.249.

Proprietary Names and Manufacturers

The following names have been used for multi-ingredient preparations containing cilastatin sodium— Primaxin *(Merck Sharp & Dohme, UK; Merck Sharp & Dohme, USA)*; Tienam *(Merck Sharp & Dohme, Swed.; Chibret, Switz.)*; Zienam *(Merck Sharp & Dohme, Ger.)*.

5655-n

Cinoxacin *(BAN, USAN, rINN)*.

Azolinic Acid; Compound 64716. 1-Ethyl-1,4-dihydro-4-oxo-1,3-dioxolo[4,5-*g*]cinnoline-3-carboxylic acid.

$C_{12}H_{10}N_2O_5$=262.2.

CAS — 28657-80-9.

Pharmacopoeias. In *U.S.*

White to yellowish-white, odourless crystalline solid. Practically **insoluble** in water and in most common organic solvents; soluble in alkaline solution. **Store** in airtight containers.

The manufacturer has stated that decomposition occurs in aqueous solutions with an alkalinity of pH 10 or more.

Adverse Effects

Adverse effects of cinoxacin are similar to those for nalidixic acid (see p.266) but the overall incidence appears to be lower.

The most common adverse effects for cinoxacin are nausea, vomiting, abdominal cramps, dizziness, headache, and hypersensitivity reactions including rash, pruritus, oedema, and urticaria.

Other adverse reactions reported less frequently include anorexia, diarrhoea, insomnia, tingling sensations, perineal burning, photophobia, and tinnitus. Transient changes in liver function tests have also occurred.

EFFECTS ON THE SKIN. Report of a bullous eruption attributed to cinoxacin in a patient also using a domestic UVA sunlamp.— A. Highet, *Br. med. J.*, 1986, *292*, 732.

Precautions

As for Nalidixic Acid, p.267.

ADMINISTRATION IN RENAL FAILURE. For reference to the precautions to be observed in renal failure, see under Uses, Administration in renal failure.

INTERACTIONS. For reference to studies indicating that concurrent administration of probenecid increases the serum half-life and peak plasma concentrations of cinoxacin, see under Absorption and Fate.

Antimicrobial Action and Resistance

Cinoxacin is bactericidal and has a similar antibacterial spectrum to nalidixic acid (see p.267). Most sensitive organisms are inhibited at minimum inhibitory concentrations of 8 to 16 μg or less per mL. Bacterial resistance may develop rapidly and cross-resistance with nalidixic acid and oxolinic acid occurs. As for nalidixic acid, bacterial resistance does not appear to be transferable or R-plasmid mediated.

References indicating that the antibacterial spectrum of cinoxacin is similar to that of nalidixic acid.— R. M. Lumish and C. W. Norden, *Antimicrob. Ag. Chemother.*, 1975, *7*, 159; H. Giamarellou and G. G. Jackson, *ibid.*, 688; R. N. Jones and P. C. Fuchs, *ibid.*, 1976, *10*, 146; R. C. Gordon *et al.*, *ibid.*, 918; P. A. Mårdh *et al.*, *J. antimicrob. Chemother.*, 1977, *3*, 411.

Cinoxacin was more active than ampicillin or chloramphenicol *in vitro* against various nontyphoid strains of *Salmonella* and against *Shigella sonnei*. Cinoxacin and chloramphenicol were equally effective against strains of *Sh. flexneri* and *Sh. boydii*; ampicillin was less effective.— E. Rubinstein and B. Shainberg, *Antimicrob. Ag. Chemother.*, 1977, *11*, 577.

Absorption and Fate

Cinoxacin is rapidly and almost completely absorbed following administration by mouth. Peak serum concentrations of about 15 μg per mL have been obtained 1 to 3 hours after a 500-mg dose. The plasma half-life is about 1 to 1.5 hours. Cinoxacin has been reported to be more than 60% bound to plasma proteins.

Cinoxacin appears to be metabolised in the liver and is excreted via the kidney. Over 95% of a dose appears in the urine within 24 hours, over half as unaltered drug and the remainder as inactive metabolites. Mean urinary concentrations of about 300 μg per mL have been achieved during the first 4 hours after administration of a 500-mg dose by mouth.

The degree of plasma protein binding for cinoxacin has varied according to the method of determination. While Wick *et al.* (*Antimicrob. Ag. Chemother.*, 1973, *4*, 415) found cinoxacin to be 16% bound other workers have reported values ranging from 68 to 83% (R. C. Gordon *et al.*, *Antimicrob. Ag. Chemother.*, 1976, *10*, 918; H.R. Black *et al.*, *ibid.*, 1979, *15*, 165).

There was considerable variation in the peak serum concentration of cinoxacin (mean 16.9 μg per mL; range 2.4 to 28 μg per mL) obtained in 13 patients following administration of a 500-mg dose twice daily. Peak concentrations were usually reached within 3 hours. Mean concentrations of cinoxacin in bladder tissue and prostatic tissue were 71% and 63% respectively of those simultaneously found in serum. There was no clear relation between concentrations in renal tissues and serum.— S. Colleen *et al.*, *J. antimicrob. Chemother.*, 1977, *3*, 579. See also R. A. P. Burt *et al.*, *Br. J. Urol.*, 1977, *49*, 147.

Studies indicating that concurrent use of probenecid decreases the renal clearance, prolongs the serum half-life, increases peak plasma concentrations and reduces urinary concentrations of cinoxacin.— K. S. Israel *et al.*, *J. clin. Pharmac.*, 1978, *18*, 491; N. Rodriguez *et al.*, *Antimicrob. Ag. Chemother.*, 1979, *15*, 465.

Pharmacokinetic studies involving 55 healthy male subjects indicated that cinoxacin was rapidly and almost completely absorbed after oral administration. Mean peak serum concentrations of 7.1, 15.5, and 20.9 μg per mL occurred 1 hour after administration of single doses of 0.25, 0.5, and 1 g respectively, falling to 2.3, 4.2, and 10.5 μg per mL 4 hours after administration. Serum concentrations were still detectable at 12 hours. Mean urine concentrations of 432 and 390 μg per mL were obtained during the first 2 hours after administration of the single doses of 0.25 and 0.5 g respectively and 450 μg per mL was obtained during the first 6 hours after the 1-g dose; concentrations remained above the MIC for most common Gram-negative urinary pathogens for at least 12 hours. About 48 to 54% of a single dose was excreted unaltered in the urine within 24 hours. The presence of food delayed the absorption and reduced the mean peak serum concentration of cinoxacin but did not significantly reduce the overall recovery in the urine in 24 hours.— H. R. Black *et al.*, *Antimicrob. Ag. Chemother.*, 1979, *15*, 165.

Acidification of the urine with ammonium chloride in 9 healthy subjects administered a 500-mg dose of cinoxacin resulted in an increase of the plasma half-life of cinoxacin from 1.1 to 2 hours and a decrease in renal clearance; alkalinisation with sodium bicarbonate produced a decrease in the half-life to 0.6 hour and an increase in renal clearance. Urinary concentrations and the amount of cinoxacin recovered in the urine were significantly increased by alkalinisation but the corresponding reductions associated with acidification were generally not significant. The change in urinary pH had no effect on the absorption or the volume of distribution of cinoxacin. Increasing the pH was associated with a reduction of antibacterial activity *in vitro*, although it was considered that this was unlikely to diminish the clinical effect.— R. H. Barbhaiya *et al.*, *Antimicrob. Ag. Chemother.*, 1982, *21*, 472.

Further references: R. L. Wolen *et al.*, *Clin. Pharmac. Ther.*, 1976, *19*, 119; J. M. Brogard *et al.*, *Eur. J. Drug Metab. Pharmacokinet.*, 1983, *8*, 251.

Uses and Administration

Cinoxacin is a 4-quinolone antimicrobial agent with actions and uses similar to those of nalidixic acid (see p.267). In the treatment of urinary-tract infections the usual dose is 250 mg given four times daily or 500 mg given twice daily for 7 to 14 days; for prophylaxis a single dose of 500 mg daily at bedtime may be given. Dosage should be reduced in renal impairment.

Reviews and discussions on cinoxacin.— J. M. Scavone *et al.*, *Pharmacotherapy*, 1982, *2*, 266; T. S. Sisca *et al.*, *Drugs*, 1983, *25*, 544.

For a series of papers on cinoxacin, see *Chemotherapy, Tokyo*, 1980, *28*, *Suppl.* 4, 1-576.

ADMINISTRATION IN RENAL FAILURE. A study suggesting that for patients with a creatinine clearance rate of less than 30 mL per minute, one-half to one-quarter of the normal dose of cinoxacin should be given.— J. J. Szwed *et al.*, *J. antimicrob. Chemother.*, 1978, *4*, 451. See also.— M. Ohkawa *et al.*, *ibid.*, 1981, *8*, 447.

The following maintenance dosage regimen has been recommended for cinoxacin in patients with renal impairment: for patients with a creatinine clearance (CC) of 50 to 80 mL per minute, 250 mg three times daily, for those with a CC of 20 up to 50 mL per minute, 250 mg twice daily, and for those with a CC of less than 20 mL per minute, 250 mg once daily. Administration to anuric patients is not recommended.— T. S. Sisca *et al.*, *Drugs*, 1983, *25*, 544.

URINARY-TRACT INFECTIONS. Cinoxacin 1 g given daily in divided doses has been used effectively in the treatment of uncomplicated urinary-tract infections caused by Entcrobacteriaceae (J.S. Welles *et al.*, *Curr. Chemother.*, 1978, *2*, 1041) although in one study in patients with recurrent urinary-tract infections Brumfitt *et al.* (*J. antimicrob. Chemother.*, 1985, *16*, 781) found that the dosage could be reduced to 250 mg given twice daily without loss of efficacy. Several other studies have shown cinoxacin to have similar efficacy to that of amoxycillin (R.R. Landes, *Urology*, 1981, *17*, 505), co-trimoxazole (J. Klastersky and L. Kahan-Coppens, *Curr. Chemother.*, 1978, *1*, 702; P. de Jersey and H.O. Wooller, *Med. J. Aust.*, 1982, *1*, 267), and nitrofurantoin (R. Lindan, *Urology*, 1981, *17*, 502; R.E. Schneider, *Clin. Ther.*, 1982, *4*, 390). Emergence of resistant strains in follow-up cultures has been reported in up to 12% of patients treated with cinoxacin (T.S. Sisca, *Drugs*, 1983, *25*, 544).

For a comparison of the efficacy of cinoxacin and other 4-quinolone antimicrobial agents in the treatment or prophylaxis of urinary-tract infections, see Norfloxacin, p.275.

Prophylaxis. In a double-blind study 70 patients with a history of recurrent urinary-tract infections received either cinoxacin 500 mg or placebo at night for up to 6 months. No infections occurred during treatment in the 38 patients receiving cinoxacin but there were 15 recurrences in the 32 patients receiving placebo. After the end of treatment with cinoxacin, re-infection had occurred within 3 months in 5 patients and within 12 months in 12. No resistant urinary pathogens emerged during treatment with cinoxacin and all recurrences were due to organisms still susceptible to cinoxacin or by organisms usually resistant. Adverse effects were considered to be mild and infrequent.— R. R. Landes, *J. Urol., Baltimore*, 1980, *123*, 47. Cinoxacin 500 mg given at night for 6 months was not significantly more effective than placebo in the prophylaxis of recurrent urinary-tract infection in a study involving 30 women.— A. J. Schaeffer *et al.*, *J. Urol., Baltimore*, 1982, *127*, 1128.

Preparations

Cinoxacin Capsules *(U.S.P.)*

Proprietary Preparations

Cinobac *(Lilly, UK)*. *Capsules*, cinoxacin 500 mg.

Proprietary Names and Manufacturers

Cinobac *(Lilly, Ital.; Lilly, Switz.; Lilly, UK; Dista, USA)*; Cinobactin *(Lilly, Ger.; Dista, S.Afr.; Lilly, Swed.)*; Nofrin *(Dista, Spain)*; Nossacin *(Corvi, Ital.)*; Uronorm *(Alfa Farmaceutici, Ital.)*; Uroxacin *(Malesci, Ital.)*.

16850-v

Ciprofloxacin *(BAN, USAN, rINN)*.

Bay-o-9867 (hydrochloride); Bay-o-9867/0163; Bay-q-3939. 1-Cyclopropyl-6-fluoro-1,4-dihydro-4-oxo-7-piperazin-1-ylquinoline-3-carboxylic acid.

$C_{17}H_{18}FN_3O_3$=331.3.

CAS — 85721-33-1 (ciprofloxacin); 86483-48-9 (hydrochloride); 86393-32-0 (hydrochloride, monohydrate); 97867-33-9 (lactate).

Ciprofloxacin lactate 127 mg is approximately equivalent to 100 mg of ciprofloxacin. Ciprofloxacin hydrochloride monohydrate 291.1 mg is approximately equivalent to 250 mg of ciprofloxacin.

Admixture of equal parts of solutions of ciprofloxacin lactate 2 mg per mL and heparin sodium 10 units per mL produced a white precipitate. The reaction was not pH dependent.— D. Lyall and J. Blythe (letter), *Pharm. J.*, 1987, *1*, 290.

Adverse Effects

As for Norfloxacin, p.274. Pain and local irritation may occur at the site of injection accompanied rarely by phlebitis or thrombophlebitis.

A review of the adverse effects of ciprofloxacin.— P. Ball, *J. antimicrob. Chemother.*, 1986, *18, Suppl.* D, 187.

Treatment with ciprofloxacin for a pulmonary infection due to *Pseudomonas aeruginosa* was associated with the development of asymptomatic haematuria on 3 separate occasions in a 24-year-old patient with cystic fibrosis.— F. Garlando *et al.*, *Infection*, 1985, *13*, 177.

A 16-year-old girl with cystic fibrosis developed arthropathy of both knees after 3 weeks of treatment with ciprofloxacin 750 mg given twice daily. All symptoms resolved completely within 2 weeks of the withdrawal of ciprofloxacin.— M. Alfaham *et al.*, *Br. med. J.*, 1987, *295*, 699.

Precautions

As for Nalidixic Acid, p.267.

Caution is advised during concomitant administration of ciprofloxacin and theophylline as ciprofloxacin and other 4-quinolone antimicrobials have been reported to inhibit the metabolism of theophylline.

Patients should maintain an adequate fluid intake during treatment with ciprofloxacin as there may be a risk of crystalluria.

ADMINISTRATION IN RENAL FAILURE. For reference to the precautions to be observed in renal failure, see under Uses, Administration in renal failure.

INTERACTIONS. *Antacids.* Peak serum concentrations and urinary excretion of ciprofloxacin have been reduced by over 90% when ciprofloxacin was administered with antacids containing magnesium hydroxide and aluminium hydroxide (G. Höffken *et al.*, *Eur. J. clin. Microbiol.*, 1985, *4*, 345). However, serum concentrations of ciprofloxacin appeared to be unaffected by antacids containing calcium carbonate (L. W. Fleming *et al.*, *Lancet*, 1986, *2*, 294).

Xanthines. For the interaction of 4-quinolone antimicrobial agents with caffeine and theophylline, see p.1523 and p.1529.

INTERFERENCE WITH DIAGNOSTIC TESTS. Ciprofloxacin did not interfere with determination of urinary glucose concentrations carried out with Clinitest, Diastix, or Tes-Tape.— T. A. Tartaglione and N. B. Flint, *Am. J. Hosp. Pharm.*, 1985, *42*, 602.

MYASTHENIA GRAVIS. A report of repeated exacerbation of myasthenia gravis in a patient receiving ciprofloxacin.— B. Moore *et al.* (letter), *Lancet*, 1988, *1*, 882.

Antimicrobial Action and Resistance

Ciprofloxacin has a similar spectrum of activity to norfloxacin (p.274), but is more active. MICs for susceptible Gram-negative aerobic organisms range from 0.004 to 2 µg per mL and for Gram-positive organisms from 0.12 to 4 µg per mL (R. Wise *et al.*, *Antimicrob. Ag. Chemother.*, 1983, *23*, 559; N.-X. Chin and H.C. Neu, *ibid.*, 1984, *25*, 319; A. King *et al.*, *J. antimicrob. Chemother.*, 1984, *13*, 325). There are many other studies of its comparative activity *in vitro* against a range of organisms. (Some references: R.J. Fass, *Antimicrob. Ag. Chemother.*, 1983, *24*, 568; L.J. Goodman *et al.*, *ibid.*, 1984, *25*, 504; P.M. Hawkey and C.A. Hawkey, *J. antimicrob. Chemother.*, 1984, *14*, 485).

Susceptible organisms in addition to those mentioned under norfloxacin include: *Chlamydia trachomatis* (F.W.A. Heessen and H.L. Muytjens, *Antimicrob. Ag. Chemother.*, 1984, *25*, 123), *Gardnerella vaginalis* (K. Machka, *Eur. J. clin. Microbiol.*, 1984, *3*, 374), *Mycoplasma hominis* (A. Escalante *et al.*, *Eur. J. sex. transm. Dis.*, 1985, *2*, 85), and some *Mycobacterium* spp. (J.D. Gay *et al.*, *Antimicrob. Ag. Chemother.*, 1984, *26*, 94). Activity against *Ureaplasma urealyticum* is variable (J. Aznar *et al.*, *Antimicrob Ag. Chemother.*, 1985, *27*, 76; G.L. Ridgway *et al.*, *Eur. J. clin. Microbiol.*, 1984, *3*, 344).

The anaerobic organisms *Bacteroides* and *Clostridium* spp. may be susceptible (M.V. Borobio and E.J. Perea, *Antimicrob. Ag. Chemother.*, 1984, *25*, 342) or they may not (V.L. Sutter *et al.*, *ibid.*, 1985, *27*, 427). Some Gram-positive aerobic organisms are susceptible to ciprofloxacin. Methicillin-resistant staphylococci are reported to be sensitive (E.C. Moorhouse *et al.*, *J. antimicrob. Chemother.*, 1985, *15*, 291; S.M. Smith and R.H.K. Eng, *Antimicrob. Ag. Chemother.*, 1985, *27*, 688); *Streptococcus pneumoniae* resistant to other antibiotics have also been inhibited by ciprofloxacin (M.E. Gombert and T.M. Aulicino, *Antimicrob. Ag. Chemother.*, 1984, *26*, 933). Studies *in vitro* and in *animals* indicate that ciprofloxacin may be active against intracellular organisms (C. S. F. Easmon *et al.*, *J. antimicrob. Chemother.*, 1986, *18*, *Suppl.* D, 43). There have been some reports of enhanced activity *in vitro* when ciprofloxacin has been used with other antimicrobial agents such as azlocillin against *Staphylococcus aureus* and *Pseudomonas aeruginosa* (J.A. Moody *et al.*, *Antimicrob. Ag. Chemother.*, 1985, *28*, 849), imipenem against *Ps. aeruginosa* (H. Giamarellou and G. Petrikkos, *Antimicrob. Ag. Chemother.*, 1987, *31*, 959) and cefotaxime or clindamycin against anaerobic bacteria (J.L. Whiting *et al.*, *Antimicrob. Ag. Chemother.*, 1987, *31*, 1379).

Organisms resistant to ciprofloxacin are usually cross-resistant to other 4-quinolone antimicrobial agents. There have been reports of resistant organisms being isolated from patients who had been given ciprofloxacin. The affected organisms include *Ps. aeruginosa* (S.M. Crook *et al.*, *Lancet*, 1985, *1*, 1275; C.M. Roberts *et al.*, *ibid.*, 1442), *Enterobacter cloacae and Kleb. pneumoniae* (S. T. Chapman *et al.*, *ibid.*, *2*, 39), *Staphylococcus* (H. Humphreys and E. Mulvihill, *ibid.*, 383; G. M. Smith *et al.*, *ibid.*, 949), and *Corynebacterium jeikeium* (P.G. Murphy and W.P. Ferguson, *J. antimicrob. Chemother.*, 1987, *20*, 922). Furthermore, there have also been reports of resistance to ciprofloxacin developing in *Ps. aeruginosa* and *Serratia marcescens* during combination therapy with other antimicrobial agents (C. C. Sanders and C. Watanakunakorn, *J. infect. Dis.*, 1986, *153*, 617; B.S. Azadian *et al.*, *J. antimicrob. Chemother.*, 1986, *18*, 771). Like norfloxacin, the antimicrobial activity of ciprofloxacin is reduced in acid media (H. Giamarellou *et al.*, *Arzneimittel-Forsch.*, 1984, *34*, 1775).

Inhibitory concentrations can be achieved in urine and may be achieved in other body fluids and tissues.

Absorption and Fate

A 500-mg dose of ciprofloxacin given by mouth produces a peak plasma concentration of about 2.5 µg per mL after 1 to 2 hours. The half-life of ciprofloxacin is about 3.5 to 4.5 hours and there is evidence of modest accumulation. Figures for protein binding vary but range upwards from about 20%.

About 30 to 50% of an oral dose of ciprofloxacin is excreted in the urine within 24 hours as unchanged drug and biologically active metabolites. Peak urinary concentrations ranging from about 300 to 500 µg per mL have been achieved after a 500-mg dose given by mouth. Significant amounts of an oral dose appear in the faeces. Ciprofloxacin penetrates into many body fluids and tissues in therapeutic concentrations.

A comparative study of the pharmacokinetics of five 4-quinolone antimicrobials including ciprofloxacin.— R. Wise *et al.*, *J. antimicrob. Chemother.*, 1986, *18*, *Suppl.* D, 71.

Ciprofloxacin 500 mg given by mouth was rapidly absorbed in 6 healthy subjects producing mean peak serum concentrations of about 2.3 µg per mL about 1.25 hours after administration. The mean terminal serum half-life was 3.9 hours. Concentrations in blister fluid reached a mean peak of 1.4 µg per mL about 2.6 hours after administration, exceeded serum concentrations after 3 hours, and remained above 0.1 µg per mL 12 hours after administration. The mean terminal half-life in blister fluid was 5.6 hours. Concentrations of ciprofloxacin in urine showed great interindividual variation but exceeded 2 µg per mL in all subjects in the sample taken over 12 to 24 hours after administration. A mean of 30.6% of a dose was recovered as microbiologically active drug in the urine during the first 24 hours.— B. Crump *et al.*, *Antimicrob. Ag. Chemother.*, 1983, *24*, 784.

Multiple-dose pharmacokinetics for ciprofloxacin were determined in 8 healthy subjects receiving ciprofloxacin 250 mg by mouth every 12 hours for 13 doses. The mean elimination half-life increased from 3.6 hours after the first dose to 6.1 hours after the last dose while the mean peak plasma concentration increased from 1.1 to 1.6 µg per mL. A steady state for peak plasma concentrations was obtained between 3 and 4 days after the start of administration. Plasma clearance decreased during administration while the volume of distribution was unchanged. It was considered that modest drug accumulation occurred with ciprofloxacin.— C. H. Kenner *et al.*, *Clin. Pharmac. Ther.*, 1984, *35*, 250.

The multiple-dose pharmacokinetics of ciprofloxacin were studied in 12 healthy subjects given ciprofloxacin 500 mg every 12 hours for 7 days. There was a significant increase in mean serum concentrations of ciprofloxacin during the study, mean peak serum concentrations increasing from about 1.9 to 2.8 µg per mL from day one to day 7. The mean half-life also increased from 3.3 to 4 hours over the same period. About 40% of an administered dose was excreted in the urine during the first 12-hour period after dosing and mean trough concentrations of ciprofloxacin in urine were 105 µg per mL on day one and 174 µg per mL on day 7. Concentrations of ciprofloxacin in the faeces on day 7 ranged from 185 to 2220 µg per g (mean 891 µg per g) and were considered to be due to poor absorption rather than recycling via the bile, since biliary excretion, although clinically significant is not sufficient to account for the amounts of drug recovered.— W. Brumfitt *et al.*, *Antimicrob. Ag. Chemother.*, 1984, *26*, 757. See also.— M. A. Gonzalez *et al.*, *ibid.*, 741.

The pharmacokinetics of ciprofloxacin were determined in 12 healthy subjects given on separate occasions ciprofloxacin 50, 100, or 750 mg by mouth or ciprofloxacin 50 or 100 mg by intravenous infusion. For intravenous administration ciprofloxacin was dissolved in 50 mL of a 0.9% solution of sodium chloride and infused over 15 minutes. Following intravenous administration mean serum concentrations of ciprofloxacin declined from 1.23 to 0.07 µg per mL after 4 hours with the 50-mg dose and from 2.8 to 0.18 µg per mL after 4 hours and then to 0.03 µg per mL after 12 hours with the 100-mg dose. There was considerable interindividual variation in serum concentrations. The mean terminal elimination half-life was about 180 minutes after the 50-mg dose and 185 minutes after the 100-mg dose. Ciprofloxacin had a high volume of distribution suggesting effective diffusion into the extravascular space. Urinary concentrations ranged from 172 to 741 µg per mL in the first 3 hours after administration and from 15 to 187 µg per mL between 3 to 6 hours after administration. Ciprofloxacin was rapidly absorbed after administration by mouth with mean peak serum concentrations of 0.28 µg per mL with the 50-mg dose, 0.49 µg per mL with the 100-mg dose, and 2.65 µg per mL with the 750-mg dose occurring about 35, 50, and 69 minutes after administration respectively. The mean terminal elimination half-life was about 206 minutes for the 50-mg dose, 246 minutes for the 100-mg dose, and 285 minutes for the 750-mg dose. The calculated bioavailability varied between 63 and 77%. About 62% of each dose was excreted in the urine as biologically active drug during the first 24 hours after intravenous administration and about 33 to 36% after oral administration; concentrations of ciprofloxacin measured using high-pressure liquid chromatography were lower, which may indicate the presence of biologically active metabolites. The proportion of the relative amounts of metabolites to the total amount of drug excreted in urine increased from 29.7% after intravenous administration to 42.7% after oral administration indicating a first-pass effect.— G. Höffken *et al.*, *Antimicrob. Ag. Chemother.*, 1985, *27*, 375.

Although food intake delayed absorption of ciprofloxacin, it did not appear to induce other changes in its pharmacokinetics.— B. Ledergerber *et al.*, *Antimicrob. Ag. Chemother.*, 1985, *27*, 350 and 992.

Further references to the pharmacokinetics of ciprofloxacin: R. Wise *et al.*, *Antimicrob. Ag. Chemother.*, 1984, *26*, 208 (intravenous administration); W. Wingender *et al.*, *Eur. J. clin. Microbiol.*, 1984, *3*, 355 (oral and intravenous administration); D. Höffler *et al.*, *ibid.*, 363 (oral administration); R. L. Davis *et al.*, *Antimicrob. Ag. Chemother.*, 1985, *28*, 74 (oral administration); D. C. Brittain *et al.*, *J. clin. Pharmac.*, 1985, *25*, 82 (oral administration); M. A. Gonzalez *et al.*, *Clin. Pharmac. Ther.*, 1985, *37*, 633 (intravenous administration); T. A. Tartaglione *et al.*, *Antimicrob. Ag. Chemother.*, 1986, *29*, 62 (oral administration); K. I. Plaisance *et al.*, *Antimicrob. Ag. Chemother.*, 1987, *31*, 956 (bioavailability).

DIFFUSION. Concentrations of ciprofloxacin that could be considered to be clinically useful were detected in: Aqueous humour.— A. I. Fern *et al.*, *Trans. ophthal. Soc. U.K.*, 1986, *105*, 650. Bone and muscle.— I. W. Fong *et al.*, *Antimicrob. Ag. Chemother.*, 1986, *29*, 405. Bronchial mucosa.— D. Honeybourne *et al.* (letter), *Lancet*, 1987, *1*, 1040. Cerebrospinal fluid.— M. Wolff *et al.*, *Antimicrob. Ag. Chemother.*, 1987, *31*, 899. Neutrophils.— C. S. F. Easmon and J. P. Crane, *J. antimicrob. Chemother.*, 1985, *16*, 67. Peritoneal fluid.— L. W. Fleming *et al.*, *J. antimicrob. Chemother.*, 1987, *19*, 493. Prostatic tissue and fluid.— J. B. J. Boerema *et al.*, *Chemotherapy, Basle*, 1985, *31*, 13. Saliva.— M. A. Gonzalez *et al.*, *Antimicrob. Ag. Chemother.*, 1984, *26*, 741. Sputum (indicating possible value in cystic fibrosis).— J. Goldfarb *et al.*, *J. clin. Pharmac.*, 1986, *26*, 222. Tonsils.— N. Falser *et al.*, *Infection*, 1984, *12*, 355.

PROTEIN BINDING. Ciprofloxacin has been reported to be between 19 and 43% bound to serum proteins (R. Wise *et al.*, *Antimicrob. Ag. Chemother.*, 1983, *23*, 559; D.S. Reeves *et al.*, *J. antimicrob. Chemother.*, 1984, *13*, 333; G. Höffken *et al.*, *Antimicrob. Ag. Chemother.*, 1985, *27*, 375).

Uses and Administration

Ciprofloxacin is a fluorinated 4-quinolone antimicrobial agent with a similar antibacterial spectrum to norfloxacin (p.274) but greater activity. As antibacterial concentrations of ciprofloxacin are obtained in serum and body tissues as well as in the urine following administration by mouth, ciprofloxacin has been suggested for use in the treatment of a wide range of infections caused by susceptible organisms including infections of the urinary, respiratory, and gastro-intestinal tracts, gonorrhoea, and septicaemia. Ciprofloxacin may also be administered by intravenous infusion for the treatment of severe infections.

Ciprofloxacin is administered by mouth as the hydrochloride in doses equivalent to 250 to 750 mg of ciprofloxacin twice daily depending on the severity and nature of the infection. A single oral dose of 250 mg has been suggested for the treatment of gonorrhoea. Ciprofloxacin is also administered as the lactate by intravenous infusion over a period of 30 to 60 minutes in doses ranging from the equivalent of 100 to 200 mg of ciprofloxacin twice daily. A single dose of 100 mg given intravenously has also been suggested for the treatment of gonorrhoea.

Reviews on the actions and uses of ciprofloxacin.— D. E. Nix and J. M. DeVito, *Clin. Pharm.*, 1987, *6*, 105; D. K. Terp and M. J. Rybak, *Drug Intell. & clin. Pharm.*, 1987, *21*, 568; *Drug & Ther. Bull.*, 1987, *25*, 69; *Med. Lett.*, 1988, *30*, 11; D. M. Campoli-Richards *et al.*, *Drugs*, 1988, *35*, 373.

Series of papers on ciprofloxacin.— D. S. Reeves (Ed.), *Eur. J. clin. Microbiol.*, 1984, *3*, 325-375; *Drugs exp. & clin. Res.*, 1985, *11*, 317-356.

Bactericidal activity of ciprofloxacin in serum of 10 healthy subjects was satisfactory only against *Escherichia coli* and *Klebsiella pneumoniae* following administration of 500-mg doses by mouth every 12 hours for 3 doses; activity was inadequate against *Pseudomonas aeruginosa*, *Staphylococcus aureus*, and *Enterococcus faecalis*. However bactericidal activity in urine was high against all strains tested even 8 to 12 hours after administration.— H. Lagast *et al.*, *J. antimicrob. Chemother.*, 1985, *16*, 341. Encouraging results in an open study of 100 patients treated with ciprofloxacin 500 mg by mouth every 12 hours for 2 to 107 days (mean 15.1 days). Infections treated included bacteraemia (41 patients), skin and soft tissue (17), gastro-intestinal (6), bone and joint (11), respiratory (21), and urinary-tract (4). Overall 88 patients obtained a clinical resolution with the infecting organism being eradicated in 87. Adverse effects developed in 4 patients, discontinuation of therapy being required in only one patient. The organisms involved in the systemic infections and eradicated by ciprofloxacin included: *Salmonella*, *Shigella*, *Klebsiella*, *Proteus*, *Staphylococcus*, and *Streptococcus* spp., *Escherichia coli*, and *Pseudomonas aeruginosa*.— C. A. Ramirez *et al.*, *Antimicrob. Ag. Chemother.*, 1985, *28*, 128.

Ciprofloxacin was given in a daily dosage ranging from 0.75 to 2.25 g by mouth in the treatment of 96 infections due to *Pseudomonas aeruginosa* involving 71 patients. Many of the isolates were resistant to carbenicillin and aminoglycoside antibiotics. Overall the clinical improvement-rate was 77% while the bacteriological cure-rate was 34%. Infections treated were exacerbations of cystic fibrosis respiratory disease (35), other respiratory-tract infections (21), urinary-tract infections (19), osteomyelitis (6), and soft-tissue infections (15). There was concern over the incidence of resistance to ciprofloxacin which developed in 25 of the infections though no resistance developed in urinary-tract infections.— B. E. Scully *et al.*, *Lancet*, 1986, *1*, 819. Similar treatment was also evaluated in 34 patients with infections caused by multiple resistant bacteria other than *Pseudomonas aeruginosa* although some patients had concomitant infections with this organism. The overall clinical response rate was 88% and the bacteriological response was 65%, or 76% if the pseudomonal infections were excluded. Resistance to ciprofloxacin developed in *Serratia marcescens* in one patient.— B. E. Scully and H. C. Neu, *J. antimicrob. Chemother.*, 1986, *18*, *Suppl.* D, 179.

The efficacy of ciprofloxacin in the treatment of 17 patients with life threatening infections caused by *Staphylococcus aureus* was poor. Ciprofloxacin had initially been given intravenously in a dose of 200 mg twice daily until defervescence, followed by 750 mg twice daily by mouth to a total of 2 weeks therapy. Clinical failure occurred in 5 patients but bacteriological failure occurred in 12. The poor outcome was not due to emergence of bacterial resistance or tolerance.— J. Righter, *J. antimicrob. Chemother.*, 1987, *20*, 595. Ciprofloxacin 750 mg was given twice daily by mouth for 7 to 28 days to 20 patients with infections caused by methicillin-resistant *Staphylococcus aureus*. Therapy was considered to be successful in 11 of 14 completed courses but recolonisation with *Staph. aureus* had occurred within 1 month in 4 patients and after 10 months in another patient. Bacteria isolated after the 3 unsuccessful courses showed resistance to ciprofloxacin.— M. E. Mulligan *et al.*, *Am. J. Med.*, 1987, *82*, *Suppl.* 4A 215. Further references.— H. Giamarellou *et al.*, *Eur. J. clin. Microbiol.*, 1986, *5*, 232.

ADMINISTRATION IN CYSTIC FIBROSIS. Results indicating that when ciprofloxacin is given by mouth to patients with cystic fibrosis it may need to be administered every 8 or 6 hours.— M. Le Bel *et al.*, *Antimicrob. Ag. Chemother.*, 1986, *30*, 260. Evidence that dosage regimens do not need to be altered for patients with cystic fibrosis.— R. L. Davis *et al.*, *ibid.*, 1987, *31*, 915.

ADMINISTRATION IN THE ELDERLY. Although the rate of absorption and total urinary recovery following oral administration of ciprofloxacin were similar in elderly and young adults both renal and non-renal clearance were significantly reduced in the elderly. The dosage interval should be not less than every 12 hours in the elderly.— M. Le Bel *et al.*, *Pharmacotherapy*, 1986, *6*, 87. Results indicating that ciprofloxacin 100 mg given twice daily by mouth produces adequate therapeutic urinary concentrations for the treatment of urinary-tract infections in the elderly.— A. P. Ball *et al.*, *J. antimicrob. Chemother.*, 1986, *17*, 629.

ADMINISTRATION IN RENAL FAILURE. The mean plasma elimation half-life of ciprofloxacin was 8.7 hours in 6 patients with a creatinine clearance (CC) of less than 20 mL per minute compared with 4.4 hours in 6 patients with a CC of more than 60 mL per minute. The amounts of ciprofloxacin recovered in the urine within 24 hours were 5.3 and 37% respectively of the administered oral dose. To maintain plasma concentrations in the same range as in patients with normal renal function the oral maintenance dose of ciprofloxacin should be halved in patients with a CC of less than 20 mL per minute. Urinary concentrations would of course be lower but might still be useful to treat urinary-tract infections. Patients with a CC of more than 20 mL per minute could probably receive the usual dose. The influence of a 4-hour dialysis in 5 patients was considered to be only moderate and dose supplementation at the end of haemodialysis does not seem to be indicated.— J. Boelaert *et al.*, *J. antimicrob. Chemother.*, 1985, *16*, 87.

It is suggested that when ciprofloxacin is used in the treatment of urinary-tract infections the usual oral dosage of 250 mg given twice daily should be reduced to 100 mg given three times daily in patients with a creatinine clearance (CC) of less than 30 mL per minute and to 200 mg twice daily in patients with a CC of 30 to 50 mL per minute.— D. E. Roberts *et al.*, *J. Pharm. Pharmac.*, 1985, *37*, *Suppl.*, 159P.

Recommendation that the dosing interval for ciprofloxacin should be doubled in patients with chronic renal failure.— E. Singlas *et al.*, *Eur. J. clin. Pharmac.*, 1987, *31*, 589.

Because of the unpredictability of half-life of ciprofloxacin even for anephric patients it would be safer to alter the dose size and maintain the dosing interval in patients with renal failure. The maximum dosing interval for patients with serious infections should be 12 hours.— G. L. Drusano *et al.*, *Antimicrob. Ag. Chemother.*, 1987, *31*, 860.

The following dosage schedules have been suggested for the intravenous administration of ciprofloxacin. For the treatment of systemic infections the following doses can be given twice daily: 200 mg for patients with a creatinine clearance (CC) of more than 50 mL per minute, 150 mg for patients with a CC of 30 to 50 mL per minute, and 100 mg for patients with a CC of less than 30 mL per minute. For the treatment of urinary-tract infections ciprofloxacin 100 mg can be given twice daily to patients with a CC of 30 mL or more per minute and three times daily to patients with a CC of less than 30 mL per minute.— D. B. Webb *et al.*, *J. antimicrob. Chemother.*, 1986, *18*, *Suppl.* D, 83. Experience in one patient with a severe soft-tissue infection did not support the recommendation that the intravenous dose of ciprofloxacin needed to be halved in acute renal failure. A starting dose of 300 mg given intravenously twice daily (i.e. 6 to 7 mg per kg body-weight daily) appeared to be more appropriate, with subsequent doses being modified according to serum concentrations.— J. B. Dibble *et al.* (letter), *ibid.*, 1987, *20*, 454.

BILIARY-TRACT INFECTIONS. One group of workers using ciprofloxacin have obtained a cure in 83% of 12 patients with biliary-tract infections (C.J. Chrysanthopoulos *et al.*, *Am. J. Med.*, 1987, *82*, *Suppl.* 4A, 357). Ciprofloxacin was initially given in a dose of 200 mg twice daily by intravenous infusion for 2 to 10 days followed by 750 mg twice daily by mouth for 4 to 6 days. There have also been isolated reports on the successful use of relatively long-term treatment with ciprofloxacin for recurrent cholangitis and in neonates with cholangitis arising after hepatic portoenterostomy (R.H.J. Houwen *et al.*, *Lancet*, 1987, *1*, 1367; L. Lonka and R. Smith Pederson, *ibid.*, *2*, 212).

BONE AND JOINT INFECTIONS. For reference to the use of ciprofloxacin in osteomyelitis and joint infections, see under Skin and Soft-tissue Infections, below.

EAR INFECTIONS. The role of ciprofloxacin in the treatment of ear infections remains to be determined but some clinicians do not advocate its use in the treatment of otitis media (*Drug & Ther. Bull.*, 1987, *25*, 69). In one small pilot study favourable results have been obtained with oral treatment in chronic otitis media and otitis externa but response was poor in cases with cholesteatoma or mastoid cavity (P.H. Van De Heyning *et al.*, *Pharm. Weekbl. Ned.*, *scient. Edn.*, 1986, *8*, 63).

ENTERIC INFECTIONS. Ciprofloxacin has been reported to be effective in the treatment of acute salmonella gastroenteritis (H. Pichler *et al.*, *Eur. J. clin. Microbiol.*, 1986, *5*, 241) and ciprofloxacin 500 mg and co-trimoxazole 960 mg given twice daily for 5 days have been found to be equally effective in the treatment of travellers' diarrhoea (C.D. Ericsson *et al.*, *Ann. intern. Med.*, 1987, *106*, 216). Ciprofloxacin 500 mg given twice daily has also been reported to be effective in the treatment of typhoid fever (C.A. Ramirez *et al.*, *Antimicrob. Ag. Chemother.*, 1985, *28*, 128) and there have been individual reports of its use to cure immunocompromised patients with salmonella septicaemia unresponsive to other antimicrobial agents (W.N. Patton *et al.*, *J. antimicrob. Chemother.*, 1985, *16*, 667; M.J. Connolly *et al.*, *ibid.*, 1986, *18*, 647). Chronic carriage of *Salmonella typhi* and other salmonella has also been treated successfully using doses of 750 mg given once or twice daily for up to 4 weeks (S.J. Hudson *et al.*, *Lancet*, 1985, *1*, 1047; K. Sammalkorpi *et al.*, *ibid.*, 1987, *2*, 164).

GONORRHOEA. From a review of the use of ciprofloxacin in the treatment of gonorrhoea Oriel (*J. antimicrob. Chemother.*, 1986, *18*, *Suppl.* D, 129) concluded that ciprofloxacin given in single doses by mouth was effective against urogenital gonococcal infections and probably also against rectal and pharyngeal infections. Most workers have used 250-mg doses but 100- and 500-mg doses have also produced good results. Ciprofloxacin given alone has produced cure-rates similar to those obtained after treatment with ampicillin and probenecid (R.E. Roddy *et al.*, *Antimicrob. Ag. Chemother.*, 1986, *30*, 267; G. R. Scott *et al.*, *J. antimicrob. Chemother.*, 1987, *20*, 117) but ciprofloxacin is effective against penicillinase- and non-penicillinase-producing strains of *Neisseria gonorrhoeae*. However, it appears to be ineffective against concomitant infections with *Chlamydia trachomatis*; even 500 to 750 mg twice daily for 7 days has produced poor results in postgonococcal and non-specific urethritis (O.P. Arya *et al.*, *Genitourinary Med.*, 1986, *62*, 170; I. W. Fong *et al.*, *Am. J. Med.*, 1987, *82*, *Suppl.* 4A, 311) although longer courses have sometimes produced better results (E. Montereiro *et al.*, *Genitourinary Med.*, 1986, *62*, 403).

IMMUNOCOMPROMISED PATIENTS. Favourable results have been obtained in preliminary studies of the use of ciprofloxacin given intravenously in the treatment of infections in immunocompromised patients.— G. M. Smith *et al.*, *J. antimicrob. Chemother.*, 1986, *18*, *Suppl.* D, 165; M. E. Wood and A. C. Newland, *ibid.*, 175.

Prophylaxis. From a review of the effect of quinolone antimicrobial agents on gastro-intestinal flora Reeves (*J. antimicrob. Chemother.*, 1986, *18*, *Suppl.* D, 89) considered that newer agents, such as ciprofloxacin and norfloxacin, may be suitable for selective gut decontamination, treatment of intestinal infections, and the prevention of re-infection of the urinary tract. They appear to have a similar effect on faecal flora, producing a small or no reduction in the numbers of most anaerobic species and a marked reduction in aerobic enterobacteria; the number of aerobic streptococci may also be reduced. The emergence of resistant enterobacteria is uncommon and replacement by resistant organisms such as yeasts is not often a problem. Dekker *et al.* (*Ann. intern. Med.*, 1987, *106*, 7) found ciprofloxacin 500 mg twice daily to be more effective than co-trimoxazole and colistin as part of a prophylactic regimen given to patients with acute leukaemia.

MENINGITIS AND VENTRICULITIS. Ciprofloxacin given intravenously with an aminoglycoside antibiotic has been used successfully to treat a neonate with pseudomonas ventriculitis (D. Isaacs *et al.*, *J. antimicrob. Chemother.*, 1986, *17*, 535) and a 56-year-old patient with *Pseudomonas aeruginosa* meningitis (M.R. Millar *et al.*, *Lancet*, 1986, *1*, 1325).

Prophylaxis. In a double-blind study meningococcal carriage was eliminated in 54 of 56 patients given ciprofloxacin 250 mg twice daily for 2 days compared with 7 of 53 patients who received placebo.— O.-V. Renkonen *et al.*, *Antimicrob. Ag. Chemother.*, 1987, *31*, 962. Similar results using ciprofloxacin 500 mg twice daily for 5 days.— M. P. Pugsley *et al.*, *J. infect. Dis.*, 1987, *156*, 211.

RESPIRATORY-TRACT INFECTIONS. Apart from its use in pseudomonal infections in patients with cystic fibrosis (see below) the role of ciprofloxacin in respiratory-tract infections remains to be determined. Doses of 500 to 750 mg given twice daily have produced good results in respiratory-tract infections including acute exacerbations of chronic bronchitis (J. A. A. Hoogkamp-Korstanje and S. J. Klein, *J. antimicrob. Chemother.*, 1986, *18*, 407; S. Raoof *et al.*, *ibid.*, 1986, *18*, *Suppl.* D, 139) caused by Gram-negative bacteria including *Haemophilus influenzae* and *Branhamella catarrhalis*. Some studies have demonstrated similar activity to that of ampicillin or amoxycillin (I. C. Gleadhill *et al.*, *J. antimicrob. Chemother.*, 1986, *18*, *Suppl.* D, 133; C. M. Wollschlager *et al.*, *Am. J. Med.*, 1987, *82*, *Suppl.* 4A, 164). Results have been variable against pneumococcal infections (B. Davies *et al.*, *Eur. J. clin. Microbiol.*, 1986, *5*, 226) and some consider that because of its marginal activity against these organisms ciprofloxacin may be unsuitable for empirical treatment of respiratory infections (*Drug & Ther. Bull.*, 1987, *25*, 69).

Cystic fibrosis. The proceedings of some workshops and symposia on the use of ciprofloxacin in the treatment of patients with cystic fibrosis and pulmonary infections caused by *Pseudomonas aeruginosa* have recently been reported (J.A. Raeburn *et al.*, *J. antimicrob. Chemother.*, 1987, *20*, 295; H.R. Stutman, *Pediatr. infect. Dis.*, 1987, *6*, 932). Because of evidence that quinolone antimicrobials may cause arthropathy in the young few studies have been carried out in patients under 18 years of age and its role remains investigational in this group of patients. However, in adults, ciprofloxacin 1.5 g daily by mouth in divided doses appears to be of similar efficacy to standard parenteral therapy of azlocillin with gentamicin or tobramycin (M.E. Hodson *et al.*, *Lancet*, 1987, *1*, 235; J.A. Bosso *et al.*, *Am. J. Med.*, 1987, *82*, *Suppl.* 4A, 180) and the ability to treat these patients on an outpatient basis is considered to be a valuable advance (*Drug & Ther. Bull.*, 1987, *25*, 69). Concern has been expressed over resistance to ciprofloxacin emerging during therapy and although resistant organisms have usually reverted to being sensitive on discontinuation of therapy, isolated reports of resistance persisting for long periods (B. Salh and A.K. Webb, *Lancet*, 1987, *1*, 749) have cast doubt on the value of ciprofloxacin in the long-term management of cystic fibrosis. Although optimum dosage regimens remain to be determined it has been suggested that therapy should be limited to 2 to 4 weeks with repeated courses being given to patients with advanced disease. At present there is no data to evaluate the usefulness of ciprofloxacin as a prophylactic agent or in chronic suppressive therapy and there are no controlled studies of its use with aminoglycosides and other antipseudomonal agents.

SKIN AND SOFT-TISSUE INFECTIONS. Ciprofloxacin has been reported to produce beneficial results in the treatment of osteomyelitis, joint infections, and skin and soft-tissue infections (M.J. Wood and M.N. Logan, *J. antimicrob. Chemother.*, 1986, *18*, *Suppl.* D, 159; R.N. Greenberg *et al.*, *Antimicrob. Ag. Chemother.*, 1987, *31*, 151) but controlled studies of its efficacy are lacking. The majority of treatment failures appear to have been in infections caused by Gram-positive organisms. In one double-blind study (P.L. Self *et al.*, *Am. J. Med.*, 1987, *82*, *Suppl.* 4A, 239) ciprofloxacin 750 mg given by mouth twice daily and cefotaxime 2 g given every 8 hours intravenously were of similar efficacy when given for a minimum of 5 days in skin and soft-tissue infections. Some (*Drug & Ther. Bull.*, 1987, *25*, 69) consider that ciprofloxacin is unsuitable for empirical use in soft-tissue infections because infections caused by Gram-negative bacteria are rare and its activity against Gram-positive organisms is relatively poor and it has none against anaerobes.

SUPPRESSION OF INTESTINAL FLORA. For reference to the potential value of 4-quinolone antimicrobial agents for selective decontamination of the gastro-intestinal tract see under Immunocompromised Patients, above.

URINARY-TRACT INFECTIONS. Ciprofloxacin given by mouth has been used effectively in the treatment of both uncomplicated and complicated upper and lower urinary-tract infections caused by a wide range of organisms including *Pseudomonas aeruginosa* and multiple-resistant bacteria (H. Giamarellou *et al.*, *Arzneimittel-Forsch.*, 1984, *34*, 1775; *Drug Intell. & clin. Pharm.*, 1987, *21*, 568). Doses of 100 to 250 mg given twice daily for 5 or more days have produced results comparable to those of co-trimoxazole or trimethoprim (N.K. Henry *et al.*, *J. antimicrob. Chemother.*, 1986, *18*, *Suppl.* D, 103; A. H. Williams; R. N. Grüneberg, *ibid.*, 107; S. Newsom *et al.*, *ibid.*, 111). In one study single oral doses of ciprofloxacin 100 or 250 mg were equally effective in the treatment of uncomplicated urinary-tract infections in 38 women and produced a cure in more than 80% (F. Garlando *et al.*, *Antimicrob. Ag. Chemother.*, 1987, *31*, 354). Dosage regimens of 500 mg or more twice daily have also been used. Ciprofloxacin has also produced encouraging results in difficult infections such as those in patients with complicated or chronic urinary-tract infections caused by *Ps. aeruginosa* (D.A. Leigh *et al.*, *J. antimicrob. Chemother.*, 1986, *18*, *Suppl.* D, 117; E.M. Brown *et al.*, *ibid.*, 123) although some treatment failures have been associated with the development of resistance.

Proprietary Preparations

Ciproxin *(Bayer, UK)*. *Intravenous infusion*, ciprofloxacin 2 mg (as lactate)/mL in bottles of 50 and 100 mL. *Tablets*, ciprofloxacin 250 mg (as hydrochloride).

Proprietary Names and Manufacturers

Ciflox *(Bayer, Fr.)*; Cipro *(Miles Pharmaceuticals, USA)*; Ciprobay *(Bayer, Ger.)*; Ciproxin *(Bayer, UK)*.

18258-v

Clavulanic Acid *(BAN, rINN)*.

BRL-14151; MM-14151. (*Z*)-(2*R*,5*R*)-3-(2-Hydroxyethylidene)-7-oxo-4-oxa-1-azabicyclo-[3.2.0]heptane-2-carboxylic acid.
$C_8H_9NO_5 = 199.2$.

CAS — 58001-44-8 (clavulanic acid); 57943-81-4 (sodium salt).

153-p

Potassium Clavulanate *(BANM)*.

BRL-14151K; Clavulanate Potassium *(USAN)*.
$C_8H_8KNO_5 = 237.3$.

CAS — 61177-45-5.

Pharmacopoeias. In *U.S.*

A 1% solution has a pH of 5.5 to 8.0.
Store in airtight containers.

Studies on the combined stability and administration of amoxycillin sodium and potassium clavulanate in a range of intravenous vehicles. Potassium clavulanate is reported to be very moisture sensitive.— J. Ashwin *et al.*, *Pharm. J.*, 1987, *1*, 116.

Clavulanic acid is produced by cultures of *Streptomyces clavuligerus*. It has a beta-lactam structure resembling that of the penicillin nucleus except that the fused thiazolidine ring of the penicillins is replaced by an oxazolidine ring. In general, clavulanic acid has only weak antibacterial activity. It is a potent progressive inhibitor of beta-lactamases of the Richmond-Sykes types II, III, IV, and V produced by Gram-negative bacteria including *Haemophilus influenzae, Neisseria gonorrhoeae, Branhamella catarrhalis, Bacteroides fragilis*, and some *Enterobacteriaceae*. It is also an inhibitor of the beta-lactamases produced by *Staphylococcus aureus*. Clavulanic acid can permeate bacterial cell walls and can therefore inactivate both extracellular enzymes and those which are bound to the cell. Its mode of action depends on the particular enzyme inhibited, but it generally acts as a competitive, and often irreversible, inhibitor. Clavulanic acid consequently enhances the activity of penicillin and cephalosporin antibiotics against many resistant strains of bacteria. The activity of cefoxitin, which is thought to be resistant to most beta-lactamases, does not appear to be enhanced.

Clavulanic acid is given as potassium clavulanate by mouth and injection in combination with amoxycillin (see p.113), and by injection in combination with ticarcillin (see p.325). Doses are usually 125 to 250 mg three times daily by mouth and 100 to 200 mg every 6 to 8 hours intravenously.

Sodium clavulanate has also been used.

In 18 patients given 23 courses of ticarcillin with clavulanic acid in association with tobramycin, clavulanic acid was associated with the development of a positive direct antiglobulin test in 10 courses.— M. E. Williams *et al.*, *Antimicrob. Ag. Chemother.*, 1985, *27*, 125.

In a comment on the ratio of antibiotic to clavulanic acid in proprietary combination preparations it was emphasised that the aim of such formulations was to provide adequate doses of each of the two components in the body. The activity of the combination is governed not by the ratio of antibiotic to clavulanic acid, but by the concentration of clavulanic acid. Thus, combinations with proportionately less clavulanic acid may appear to be less active in sensitivity tests *in vitro*.— *G. N. Rolinson (letter), J. antimicrob. Chemother.*, 1985, *15*, 256.

A study *in vitro* indicating that potassium clavulanate may inactivate aminoglycoside antibiotics, although the effect was small at clinically-achievable concentrations, particularly with amikacin. Addition of potassium clavulanate to ticarcillin, however, did not significantly increase the inactivation of aminoglycosides by ticarcillin.— R. J. Courcol and G. R. Martin (letter), *J. antimicrob. Chemother.*, 1986, *17*, 682.

ANTIMICROBIAL ACTION. Reports of the ability of clavulanic acid to inhibit *in vitro* beta-lactamases produced by various organisms: R. Zemelman *et al., J. antimicrob. Chemother.*, 1984, *14*, 575 (*Aeromonas hydrophila*); T. Farmer and C. Reading, *Drugs*, 1986, *31*, *Suppl.* 3, 70 (*Branhamella catarrhalis*); M. H. Cynamon and G. S. Palmer, *Antimicrob. Ag. Chemother.*, 1983, *23*, 935 (*Mycobacterium fortuitum*); *idem*, *24*, 429 (*Mycobacterium tuberculosis*); M. D. Kitzis *et al., J. antimicrob. Chemother.*, 1985, *15*, 23 (*Nocardia asteroides*); S. B. Calderwood *et al., Antimicrob. Ag. Chemother.*, 1982, *22*, 266 (Pseudomonas aeruginosa); Y. Saino *et al., ibid.*, 1984, *25*, 362 (*Pseudomonas maltophilia*).

Reports of the ability of clavulanic acid to enhance the action of penicillins (other than amoxycillin and ticarcillin) and cephalosporins against various bacteria *in vitro*.— M. B. Bansal *et al., Antimicrob. Ag. Chemother.*, 1984, *26*, 606 (azlocillin); M. A. Crosby and D. W. Gump, *ibid.*, 1982, *22*, 398 (cefoperazone); H. C. Neu, *ibid.*, 518 (mecillinam); H. C. Neu and K. P. Fu, *ibid.*, 1980, *18*, 582 (piperacillin).

ABSORPTION AND FATE. Studies have shown the absorption and fate of clavulanic acid to be similar to that of amoxycillin and ticarcillin with which it is administered. Clavulanic acid does not appear to alter the pharmacokinetics of these drugs although Höffken *et al.*, (*J. antimicrob. Chemother.*, 1985, *16*, 763) observed it to cause a slight decrease in the renal elimination of ticarcillin in a study in 10 healthy subjects. These authors also noted that ticarcillin caused a slight decrease in the non-renal clearance of clavulanic acid. Adam *et al.* (*Antimicrob. Ag. Chemother.*, 1982, *22*, 353) reported an increase in the absorption of clavulanic acid when administered with amoxycillin by mouth, resulting in slightly higher serum concentrations, and also an increase in its urinary excretion. Administration of clavulanic acid as the sodium or potassium salt either alone (R. Münch *et al., J. antimicrob. Chemother.*, 1981, *8*, 29), in combination with amoxycillin (J.D. Nelson *et al., Antimicrob. Ag. Chemother.*, 1982, *21*, 681; U.B. Schaad *et al., ibid.*, 1983, *23*, 252; K.E. Forslew *et al., J. clin. Pharmac.*, 1984, *24*, 452; I. Nilsson-Ehle *et al., J. antimicrob. Chemother.*, 1985, *16*, 491; U.B. Schaad *et al., ibid.*, 1986, *17*, 341) or with ticarcillin (S. Bennett *et al., Antimicrob. Ag. Chemother.*, 1983, *23*, 831; G.P. Bodey *et al., Clin. Pharmac. Ther.*, 1985, *38*, 134; T. Bergan *et al., J. antimicrob. Chemother.*, 1986, *17*, 97) have shown it to have the following pharmacokinetic properties: peak concentrations of about 2 to 4 μg per mL obtained about 1 hour after administration of 125 mg by mouth; half-life of approximately 1 hour; variable urinary excretion of unchanged drug of up to 60% of the total dose within 6 hours of oral administration. The excretion of clavulanic acid is not significantly affected by the administration of probenecid, suggesting that it is cleared predominantly by glomerular filtration (D.H. Staniforth *et al., J. antimicrob. Chemother.*, 1983, *12*, 273). Up to 30% of clavulanic acid has been stated to be bound to plasma proteins, and it appears to be metabolised to some extent.

Clavulanic acid is reported to be well distributed into body fluids and tissues. Variable concentrations have been achieved in sputum (R.J. Wallace *et al., Antimicrob. Ag. Chemother.*, 1985, *27*, 912; F.P.V. Maesen *et al., J. antimicrob. Chemother.*, 1987, *19*, 372). Wise *et al.* (*ibid.*, 1983, *11*, 57) observed concentrations in peritoneal fluid 66% of those in serum after intravenous administration with amoxycillin. Similar results were observed after administration with ticarcillin (N. Manek *et al., ibid.*, 1987, *19*, 363). In a study of the administration of clavulanic acid with amoxycillin to patients with varying degrees of renal impairment or on haemodialysis (F.F. Horber *et al., Antimicrob. Ag. Chemother.*, 1986, *29*, 614), although the clearance of clavulanic acid decreased with decreasing renal function, this did not occur to the same extent as for amoxycillin. The pharmacokinetics of clavulanic acid in patients with renal impairment has also been studied after administration with ticarcillin (P. Koeppe *et al., Arzneimittel-Forsch.*, 1987, *37*, 203). Slaughter *et al.* (*Ther. Drug Monit.*, 1984, *6*, 424) observed removal of significant amounts of clavulanic acid when administered with amoxycillin to one patient on haemodialysis. Clavulanic acid has also been stated to be removed by peritoneal dialysis.

Preparations

Sterile Clavulanate Potassium (*U.S.P.*)

For further preparations containing potassium clavulanate, see Amoxycillin Trihydrate, p.115, and Ticarcillin Sodium, p.326.

Proprietary Names and Manufacturers

The following names have been used for multi-ingredient preparations containing potassium clavulanate— Augmentan (*Beecham-Wülfing, Ger.*); Augmentin (*Beecham, Austral.*; *Beecham-Sevigne, Fr.*; *Beecham, S.Afr.*; *Beecham, Switz.*; *Beecham Research, UK*; *Beecham Laboratories, USA*); Clavulin (*Beecham, Canad.*); Timenten (*Beecham, Switz.*); Timentin (*Beecham Research, UK*; *Beecham Laboratories, USA*).

53-b

Clemizole Penicillin (*BAN, rINN*).

Penicillinclemizole. 1-[1-(4-Chlorobenzyl)benzimidazol-2-ylmethyl]pyrrolidinium (6*R*)-6-(2-phenylacetamido)penicillanate.

$C_{16}H_{18}N_2O_4S,C_{19}H_{20}ClN_3$=660.2.

CAS — 6011-39-8.

Clemizole penicillin is a long-acting preparation of benzylpenicillin, with similar properties and uses (see p.131). It is given by deep intramuscular injection in doses of 1.1 g, which contains about 600 mg (1 million units) of benzylpenicillin.

Proprietary Names and Manufacturers

Megacillin (*Grünenthal, Ger.*); Megacilline (*Grünenthal, Switz.*); Prevecillin (*Grünenthal, S. Afr.*).

55-g

Clindamycin Hydrochloride (*BANM, USAN, rINNM*).

(7*S*)-Chloro-7-deoxylincomycin; Chlorodeoxylincomycin Hydrochloride; U-21251 (*clindamycin*). Methyl 6-amino-7-chloro-6,7,8-trideoxy-*N*-[(2*S*,4*R*)-1-methyl-4-propylprolyl]-1-thio-β-L-*threo*-D-*galacto*-octopyranoside hydrochloride monohydrate.

$C_{18}H_{33}ClN_2O_5S,HCl,H_2O$=479.5.

CAS — 18323-44-9 (clindamycin); 21462-39-5 (hydrochloride, anhydrous); 58207-19-5 (hydrochloride, monohydrate).

NOTE. The name Clinimycin was formerly used for Clindamycin. It has been used for a preparation of oxytetracycline.

Pharmacopoeias. In *Br.*, *Braz.*, *Chin.*, *It.*, and *U.S.*

A white or almost white crystalline powder, odourless or with a faint mercaptan-like odour. 1.13 g of monograph substance is approximately equivalent to 1 g of clindamycin. *B.P.* **solubilities** are: soluble 1 in 2 of water, and 1 in 4 of dimethylformamide; slightly soluble in alcohol; very slightly soluble in chloroform. *U.S.P.* solubilities are: freely soluble in water, dimethylformamide, and methyl alcohol; soluble in alcohol; practically insoluble in acetone. A 10% solution in water has a pH of 3.0 to 5.5. **Store** at a temperature not exceeding 30° in airtight containers.

54-v

Clindamycin Palmitate Hydrochloride (*BANM, USAN, rINNM*).

U-25179E. Clindamycin 2-palmitate hydrochloride.

$C_{34}H_{63}ClN_2O_6S,HCl$=699.9.

CAS — 36688-78-5 (clindamycin palmitate); 25507-04-4 (hydrochloride).

Pharmacopoeias. In *U.S.*

A white to off-white amorphous powder with a characteristic odour. The *U.S.P.* specifies not less than the equivalent of 540 μg of clindamycin per mg. 1.6 g of monograph substance is approximately equivalent to 1 g of clindamycin. **Soluble** 1 in 3 of alcohol and 1 in 9 of ethyl acetate; freely soluble in water, chloroform, and ether; very soluble in dimethylformamide. A 1% solution in water has a pH of 2.8 to 3.8. **Store** in airtight containers.

In buffered aqueous solution, clindamycin showed maximum stability at pH 3 to 5; after storage for 2 years at 25° not more than 10% degradation would occur in the pH range 1 to 6.5. At pH 0.4 to 4 hydrolysis of clindamycin to 1-dethiomethyl-1-hydroxyclindamycin and methyl mercaptan occurred; at pH 5 to 10 lincomycin was formed.— T. O. Oesterling, *J. pharm. Sci.*, 1970, *59*, 63.

Units

One unit of clindamycin is contained in 0.0011947 mg of the first International Reference Preparation (1971) of clindamycin hydrochloride which contains 837 units per mg.

Adverse Effects

Clindamycin may cause diarrhoea, which can be severe and persistent, nausea, vomiting, abdominal cramps, and abnormality of taste. Severe pseudomembranous colitis has occurred in some patients and has occasionally been fatal; this appears to be caused by a toxin produced by *Clostridia* spp. particularly *Cl. difficile*. Colitis and diarrhoea have been reported during treatment or up to several weeks after its completion. Hypersensitivity reactions, including skin rashes and urticaria, may occur and transient leucopenia and eosinophilia, abnormalities of liver function tests, and jaundice have been reported. Agranulocytosis, thrombocytopenia, and erythema multiforme have been observed.

Irritant reactions or contact dermatitis have been reported after topical application of clindamycin.

Few adverse reactions had occurred in about 22 000 casualty patients given lincomycin or clindamycin over 4 years. Three patients had a skin rash after clindamycin and an occasional patient complained of diarrhoea.— D. H. Wilson (letter), *Br. med. J.*, 1974, *4*, 288.

EFFECTS ON THE GASTRO-INTESTINAL TRACT. *Clostridium difficile* and its cytotoxin are closely associated with pseudomembranous colitis and with a spectrum of gastro-intestinal illness ranging from mild self-limiting diarrhoea to fulminant colitis. Pseudomembranous colitis is known to pre-date the antibiotic era, but is now most frequently seen as a complication of antibiotic administration. Many commonly used antimicrobials have been implicated and it is probable that most antibiotics have the potential to be associated with pseudomembranous colitis. The most extensively studied form has been that associated with clindamycin although the reported incidence has ranged from 0.01 to 10%. In 38 cases of histologically-confirmed pseudomembranous colitis, 18 were associated with clindamycin/lincomycin and 15 with ampicillin/amoxycillin. In 98 patients with *Cl. difficile* and/or toxin-positive stools, 22 were associated with clindamycin/lincomycin and 37 with ampicillin/amoxycillin. The incidence of pseudomembranous colitis appears to be increased in females and the elderly.— S. P. Borriello and H. E. Larson, *J. antimicrob. Chemother.*, 1981, *7*, *Suppl.* A, 53.

In a prospective study of 200 patients treated with clindamycin by mouth or injection 42 (21%) developed diarrhoea and 20 (10%) had proctoscopic evidence of pseudomembranous colitis. The colitis was not dose-dependent but it was more common following administration by mouth than injection.— F. J. Tedesco *et al., Ann. intern. Med.*, 1974, *81*, 429. The incidence of diarrhoea in a group of patients treated with lincomycin or clindamycin was closely comparable with a similar group receiving ampicillin. Of 96 receiving lincomycin, only 1 developed pseudomembranous colitis after 2 prolonged courses.— M. B. Robertson *et al., Med. J. Aust.*, 1977, *1*, 243. Severe diarrhoea occurred in 25 of 160 patients who received clindamycin or lincomycin for bacterial infections, but it could not be related to a change in faecal flora. Diarrhoea occurred more frequently when clindamycin was given prophylactically and the incidence was higher in women (19%) than in men (13%) and in patients over 60 years of age. Clindamycin should be used cautiously in elderly patients.— D. A. Leigh and K. Simmons, *J. clin. Path.*, 1978, *31*, 439. Between 1964 and 1978 the Committee on Safety of Medicines (according to Adverse Reaction Series No.17, 1979) had received 174 reports of colitis attributed to antibiotics; 116, including 27 deaths, were associated with clindamycin and 27, including 10 deaths, with lincomycin. All but 4 of the reports associated with clindamycin were received after 1974, when the condition known as pseudomembranous colitis was identified. Clindamycin and lincomycin should not be given for minor infections.— *Pharm. J.*, 1979, *1*, 518. Antibiotic-induced diarrhoea was seen in 43 (12%) of 368 patients given lincomycin or clindamycin but there were no cases of pseudomembranous colitis.— D. A. Leigh *et al.*, *J. antimicrob. Chemother.*, 1980, *6*, 639. Pseudomembranous colitis associated with the topical application of clindamycin phosphate.— M. F. Parry and C. -K. Rha, *Archs Derm.*, 1986, *122*, 583.

See also Hazards of Antibiotic Therapy, p.104.

After administration of clindamycin 150 mg every 6 hours by mouth for 7 days to 10 healthy subjects, there was a decrease in the numbers of oropharyngeal aerobic streptococci and anaerobic organisms. In the intestine, enterococci were increased and anaerobes decreased.— C. E. Nord and A. Heimdahl, *J. antimicrob. Chemother.*, 1986, *18*, *Suppl.* C, 159.

Oesophageal ulceration. A report of oesophageal ulceration due to the disintegration of a capsule of clindamycin in the oesophagus.— D. R. Sutton and J. K. Gosnold (letter), *Br. med. J.*, 1977, *1*, 1598.

EFFECTS ON THE LIVER. Liver enzyme abnormalities occurred in a patient receiving clindamycin phosphate intravenously. Biopsy demonstrated lobular disruption, pseudogranulomas, necrosis, eosinophilic bodies, and mononuclear cell infiltration. The liver enzymes returned to normal when clindamycin was withdrawn and biopsy taken 15 days later showed improvement.— M. Elmore *et al.*, *Am. J. Med.*, 1974, *57*, 627.

EFFECTS ON THE NEUROMUSCULAR SYSTEM. Mention that clindamycin and lincomycin, because of their neuromuscular blocking activity, may cause postoperative respiratory depression.— R. J. M. Lane and P. A. Routledge, *Drugs*, 1983, *26*, 124.

EFFECTS ON THE SKIN. A patient who had been taking clindamycin 150 mg four times daily for a dental infection developed erythema multiforme (the Stevens-Johnson syndrome) 14 days after the start of treatment. Her condition improved after she received prednisone 60 mg daily (decreasing after 6 days) for 3 weeks.— D. D. Fulghum and P. M. Catalano, *J. Am. med. Ass.*, 1973, *223*, 318.

Leucocytoclastic angiitis involving the skin, occurred in a 56-year-old diabetic man, and was associated with the intravenous administration of clindamycin.— W. C. Lambert *et al.*, *Cutis*, 1982, *30*, 615.

Treatment of Adverse Effects

Clindamycin should be withdrawn if significant diarrhoea or colitis occurs. Vancomycin in doses of 125 to 500 mg by mouth every 6 hours has been used successfully in the treatment of antibiotic-associated pseudomembranous colitis.

For reference to the treatment of antibiotic-induced colitis, including the use of vancomycin, metronidazole, other antibiotics, and anion-exchange resins, see Vancomycin Hydrochloride, p.335.

Precautions

Clindamycin should not be given to patients known to be hypersensitive or who have experienced reactions with lincomycin. It should not be used in patients with diarrhoeal states and it should be used with caution in patients with impaired liver and renal function.

Since clindamycin is reported to possess neuromuscular blocking activity it should be used cautiously with other drugs having similar activity.

ADMINISTRATION IN LIVER DISORDERS AND RENAL FAILURE. For reference to the precautions to be observed in liver disorders and in renal failure, see under Uses, below.

INTERACTIONS. In 16 healthy subjects given clindamycin alone and with a kaolin-pectin suspension it was found that the suspension had no effect on the extent of clindamycin absorption but did markedly reduce the absorption rate.— K. S. Albert *et al.*, *J. pharm. Sci.*, 1978, *67*, 1579.

For the effects of other drugs on the antimicrobial activity of clindamycin, see below under Antimicrobial Action.

Antimicrobial Action

Clindamycin is bacteriostatic or bactericidal depending on the concentration and has a range of antimicrobial activity and mode of action similar to that of erythromycin. It is active against most aerobic Gram-positive bacteria including streptococci, staphylococci, *Bacillus anthracis*, and *Corynebacterium diphtheriae*; enterococci, however, are generally resistant. Most Gram-negative aerobic bacteria, including the Enterobacteriaceae, are resistant to clindamycin; unlike erythromycin, *Neisseria gonorrhoeae*, *N. meningitidis*, and *Haemophilus influenzae* are generally resistant to clindamycin.

Clindamycin has good activity against a wide range of anaerobic bacteria. Susceptible Gram-positive anaerobes include *Eubacterium*, *Propionibacterium*, *Peptococcus*, *Peptostreptococcus*, and most strains of *Clostridium perfringens* and *Cl. tetani*. Among Gram-negative anaerobes susceptible to clindamycin are *Fusobacterium* spp. and *Bacteroides* spp. including the *B. fragilis* group.

Apart from *Mycoplasma hominis*, clindamycin is generally less active than erythromycin against *Mycoplasma* spp.

Minimum inhibitory concentrations for sensitive Gram-positive cocci have been reported to range from about 0.002 to 0.8 µg per mL. Most strains of *Bacteroides* spp. have been found to be inhibited by 2 µg or less per mL of clindamycin.

Proceedings of a symposium on the effects of clindamycin on bacterial virulence and host defences.— *J. antimicrob. Chemother.*, 1983, *12*, *Suppl.* C, 1–124.

A study *in vitro* indicating that subinhibitory concentrations of clindamycin reduce the ability of *Escherichia coli* to adhere to epithelial cells, a prerequisite for the colonisation and development of infection; phagocytosis and killing of *E. coli in vitro* by normal human polymorphonuclear leucocytes were promoted, indicating that clindamycin had not rendered the organisms resistant to phagocytosis.— H. P. Bassaris *et al.*, *J. antimicrob. Chemother.*, 1984, *13*, 361.

Further references to good uptake of clindamycin by phagocytes and of enhancement of the immune system by clindamycin: P. E. Lianou *et al.*, *J. antimicrob. Chemother.*, 1985, *15*, 481; H. Faden *et al.*, *ibid.*, *16*, 649; H. P. Bassaris *et al.*, *ibid.*, 1987, *19*, 467; T. H. Steinberg and W. L. Hand, *Antimicrob. Ag. Chemother.*, 1987, *31*, 660.

ACTIVITY AGAINST ANAEROBES. The MIC of clindamycin and lincomycin against two strains of *Propionibacterium* spp. was 0.02 and 0.08 µg per mL respectively. In subinhibitory concentrations, clindamycin inhibited the production of lipase by these organisms.— S. E. Unkles and C. G. Gemmell, *Antimicrob. Ag. Chemother.*, 1982, *21*, 39.

A study of the susceptibility of anaerobic bacteria from several hospitals in France to metronidazole, cefoxitin, and clindamycin. On comparing the MIC for 50% of strains, clindamycin had comparable activity to metronidazole against most anaerobes, but was more active than cefoxitin. There were however more anaerobes showing resistance to clindamycin and cefoxitin than to metronidazole. At a break-point of 4 µg per mL, 16% of all anaerobes tested were resistant to clindamycin. The respective resistance-rates for metronidazole and cefoxitin were 8 and 11% at break-points of 8 and 16 µg per mL. Rates of resistance to clindamycin ranging from 8 to 29% were reported for *Bacteroides* spp., *Clostridia* spp. including *Cl. perfringens*, *Fusobacterium*, *Eubacterium*, *Propionibacterium*, *Actinomyces*, *Bifidobacterium*, *Peptococcus*, *Peptostreptococcus*, and *Streptococcus* spp.— L. Dubreuil *et al.*, *Antimicrob. Ag. Chemother.*, 1984, *25*, 764.

A study of the antimicrobial susceptibilities of anaerobic bacteria isolated from women with genital-tract infections concluded that clindamycin, chloramphenicol, metronidazole, and imipenem had the greatest degree of activity and breadth of spectrum. The newer cephalosporins, including cefoxitin, were generally less active and displayed unpredictable activity.— G. B. Hill and O. M. Ayers, *Antimicrob. Ag. Chemother.*, 1985, *27*, 324.

Further references to the activity of clindamycin against anaerobic organisms: C. E. Nord and B. Olsson-Liljequist, *Scand. J. infect. Dis.*, 1984, *Suppl.* 43, 44.

See also under Resistance, below.

ACTIVITY AGAINST CAMPYLOBACTER. The MIC of clindamycin against 178 strains of *Campylobacter* spp. was in the range of 0.25 to greater than 32 µg per mL. Strains isolated from *swine* (mainly *C. coli*) were generally less susceptible than those isolated from humans.— W. -L. L. Wang *et al.*, *Antimicrob. Ag. Chemother.*, 1984, *26*, 351. See also R. Vanhoof *et al.*, *ibid.*, 1982, *21*, 990; J. Michel *et al.*, *ibid.*, 1983, *23*, 796.

For reference to the comparative activity of macrolides and related antibiotics, including clindamycin, against *Campylobacter* spp., see Erythromycin, p.224.

ACTIVITY AGAINST CHLAMYDIA. For reference to the reported MIC of clindamycin against *Chlamydia trachomatis*, see Pelvic Inflammatory Disease under Uses, below.

ACTIVITY AGAINST GARDNERELLA. Erythromycin and clindamycin were the most active of 21 antimicrobial agents tested *in vitro* against 56 strains of *Gardnerella vaginalis* (*Haemophilus vaginalis*); all strains were inhibited by 0.06 µg or less per mL [metronidazole was not tested].— L. R. McCarthy *et al.*, *Antimicrob. Ag. Chemother.*, 1979, *16*, 186.

ACTIVITY AGAINST LEGIONELLA. For reference to the activity of clindamycin and lincomycin against *Legionella* spp., see Erythromycin, p.223.

ACTIVITY AGAINST PROTOZOA. Clindamycin possessed marked antiplasmodial activity.— C. Lewis, *J. Parasit.*, 1968, *54*, 169.

Clindamycin has been shown to be effective for the treatment of toxoplasmosis in *animals* (F.G. Araujo and J.S. Remington, *Antimicrob. Ag. Chemother.*, 1974, *5*, 647). It had no effect *in vitro*, however, on extracellular or intracellular *Toxoplasma gondii* whether studied alone or with sulphadiazine or sulphadiazine plus pyrimethamine (D.G. Mack and R. McLeod, *ibid.*, 1984, *26*, 26).

ACTIVITY WITH OTHER ANTIMICROBIAL AGENTS. Clindamycin has been reported to diminish the activity *in vitro* of ampicillin or gentamicin against *Staphylococcus aureus* (P.D. Meers, *Lancet*, 1973, *2*, 573). Other workers, however, have observed variable degrees of synergy between clindamycin and gentamicin against some anaerobes (I. Brook and R.I. Walker, *J. antimicrob. Chemother.*, 1984, *15*, 31; I. Brook *et al.*, *Antimicrob. Ag. Chemother.*, 1984, *25*, 71). Clindamycin did not diminish the bactericidal activity of cephamandole against a strain of *Enterobacter cloacae*, or of latamoxef against a strain of *Pseudomonas aeruginosa* (C.C. Sanders *et al.*, *J. antimicrob. Chemother.*, 1983, *12*, *Suppl.* C, 97); there was some evidence of enhanced bactericidal activity which may be associated with the ability demonstrated by clindamycin to prevent derepression of beta-lactamase production. Synergy has been reported between clindamycin and ceftazidime (W.L. George, *Antimicrob. Ag. Chemother.*, 1984, *25*, 657), and between clindamycin and metronidazole (D.F. Busch *et al.*, *J. infect. Dis.*, 1976, *133*, 321) against some *Bacteroides fragilis* strains. Synergy has also been reported between clindamycin and ciprofloxacin against some anaerobic organisms (J.L. Whiting *et al.*, *Antimicrob. Ag. Chemother.*, 1987, *31*, 1379).

Antagonism occurred against some strains of *Staph. aureus* when the activity of clindamycin was tested *in vitro* with actinomycin D, daunorubicin, doxorubicin, bleomycin, or plicamycin and synergism usually occurred when clindamycin was tested with mitomycin. The effect of mitomycin was obtained at concentrations below those usually obtainable in serum (J.Y. Jacobs *et al. Antimicrob. Ag. Chemother.*, 1979, *15*, 580).

For reference to antagonism between erythromycin and lincosamides, see under Resistance in Erythromycin, p.223.

Resistance

The pattern and mechanism of bacterial resistance to clindamycin is similar to that of erythromycin (see p.223). Cross-resistance occurs between clindamycin and lincomycin and is often observed between the lincosamide, macrolide, and streptogramin groups of antibiotics. Some erythromycin-resistant organisms may be sensitive to clindamycin, but resistance may develop *in vivo*.

For reference to resistance to clindamycin and lincomycin associated with resistance to macrolide and streptogramin-B-type antibiotics, in *Bacteroides* and *Mycoplasma* spp., staphylococci, and streptococci, see Erythromycin, p.223.

RESISTANCE OF ANAEROBES. In a study in Spain about 11 to 12% of clinically isolated strains of the *Bacteroides fragilis* group were resistant to clindamycin, at a break-point of 4 µg per mL, over the years 1980 to 1983, with peaks of resistance of 22 to 23% on 2 occasions during this period. At a break-point of 8 µg per mL, a similar pattern was observed. The results suggested that clusters of resistant *Bacteroides* could occasionally be located in different areas or institutions. Resistance of the *B. fragilis* group to clindamycin was not, however, confined to hospital strains, but also occurred in out-patients, in healthy subjects, and in patients not treated with antibiotics of the macrolide-lincosamide-streptogramin group.— M. Reig *et al.*, *J. antimicrob. Chemother.*, 1984, *14*, 595. A study of the antimicrobial susceptibility of organisms of the *Bacteroides fragilis* group isolated from 8 centres in the *USA*. Taking a break-point of 4 µg per mL, 6, 3, and 7% of strains were resistant to clindamycin in the 3 years from 1981 to 1983. Taking a break-point of 8 µg per mL, the corresponding resistance-rates were 5, 2, and 7%.— F. P. Tally *et al.*, *Antimicrob. Ag. Chemother.*, 1985, *28*, 675.

Most clindamycin-resistant *Bacteroides* are also tetracycline-resistant, as well as showing resistance to erythromycin and streptogramins.— F. P. Tally *et al.*, *Scand. J. infect. Dis.*, 1984, *Suppl.* 43, 34.

Anaerobic bacteria resistant to clindamycin were isolated from patients who had been treated with clindamycin in association with an aminoglycoside or aztreonam for pelvic soft-tissue infections. The clinical significance of these findings was unknown as all patients recovered and remained well.— M. J. Ohm-Smith *et al.*, *Antimicrob. Ag. Chemother.*, 1986, *30*, 11.

In a study of the susceptibility *in vitro* of strains of the *Bacteroides fragilis* group isolated from patients in Brazil, 37% were resistant to clindamycin compared with rates of resistance for metronidazole, chloramphenicol, cefoxitin, and carbenicillin of 0, 2, 21, and 13% respectively. The high rate of resistance to clindamycin may be related to a high use of erythromycin in Brazil.— A. E. C. C. de Almeida and M. de Uzeda, *Antimicrob. Ag. Chemother.*, 1987, *31*, 617.

See also Antimicrobial Action, above.

Absorption and Fate

About 90% of a dose of clindamycin hydrochloride is absorbed from the gastro-intestinal tract and peak plasma concentrations are achieved more rapidly than with lincomycin; concentrations of about 2.5 µg per mL occur within 1 hour after a 150-mg dose of clindamycin, with average concentrations of about 0.7 µg per mL after 6 hours. After doses of 300 and 600 mg peak plasma concentrations of 4 and 8 µg per mL, respectively, have been reported. The biological half-life is about 2.5 hours. Absorption is not significantly diminished by food in the stomach but the rate of absorption may be reduced. Clindamycin palmitate hydrochloride is rapidly hydrolysed following oral administration to provide free clindamycin. Between 80 and 90% of clindamycin in the circulation is bound to plasma proteins.

Clindamycin is widely distributed in body fluids and tissues including bone but it does not reach the CSF in significant concentrations. It diffuses across the placenta into the foetal circulation and has been reported to appear in breast milk. High concentrations occur in bile.

Clindamycin undergoes metabolism, presumably in the liver, to the active *N*-demethyl and sulphoxide metabolites, and also some inactive metabolites. About 10% of a dose is excreted in the urine as active drug or metabolites and about 4% in the faeces. It is not effectively removed from the blood by dialysis.

For the pharmacokinetics of clindamycin administered parenterally, see clindamycin phosphate (p.201).

Studies of 52 children aged 6 months to 14 years indicated that the equivalent of clindamycin 8 to 16 mg per kg body-weight daily in divided doses gave effective serum concentrations during a 17-dose course of clindamycin palmitate hydrochloride in flavoured granules. Mean serum concentrations 1 hour after the 17th dose of a course of clindamycin 2 or 4 mg per kg body-weight every 6 hours in two groups of children were 2.46 and 3.79 µg per mL, respectively. Elimination half-lives of 1.51 (range 0.57 to 3.14) and 2.22 (range 0.87 to 3.49) hours were estimated for the 2 dosage regimens.— R. M. DeHaan and D. Schellenberg, *J. clin. Pharmac.*, 1972, *12*, 74.

ADMINISTRATION IN LIVER DISORDERS AND RENAL FAILURE. For reference to the pharmacokinetics of clindamycin in liver disorders and renal failure, see under Uses, below.

DRUG ABSORPTION. In a crossover study of the absorption of clindamycin 12 men received clindamycin 300 mg as a suspension prepared from the palmitate hydrochloride, while fasting, immediately before food, or 1 hour after food. Serum concentrations of clindamycin were higher at the peak time of 1 hour when the drug was given immediately before food than when it was given to fasting patients. Serum concentrations were lower at 0.5 and 1 hour but higher at 3 and 4 hours when patients received the drug 1 hour after food than when they were given it immediately before food. With all drug regimens clindamycin appeared in the blood within half an hour.— R. M. DeHaan *et al.*, *J. clin. Pharmac.*, 1972, *12*, 205.

In 18 patients with acne vulgaris who had applied an aqueous/alcoholic solution of clindamycin hydrochloride 1% twice to 4 times daily for 6 to 150 days there was no evidence of systemic absorption.— R. J. Algra *et al.*, *Archs Derm.*, 1977, *113*, 1390. Urinary concentrations of clindamycin of up to 0.7 µg per mL had been reported in 4 of 9 subjects who had received daily topical applications containing clindamycin 20 mg for 1 to 7 weeks.— D. A. Voron (letter), *Archs Derm.*, 1978, *114*, 798. After topical application of a 1% solution of clindamycin as the hydrochloride to 13 patients with acne vulgaris, on average 4 to 5% of a dose entered the circulation although there was wide interindividual variation. Clindamycin could be detected in urine, but not in the serum.— M. Barza *et al.*, *J. Am. Acad. Derm.*, 1982, *7*, 208.

The absorption of clindamycin was increased in patients with coeliac disease or Crohn's disease.— P. G. Welling and F. L. S. Tse, *J. clin. Hosp. Pharm.*, 1984, *9*, 163.

PREGNANCY AND THE NEONATE. Tests on aborted foetuses showed that both clindamycin and erythromycin given by mouth to the mothers crossed the placental barrier, although erythromycin was less predictable than clindamycin. Foetal tissues, especially liver, were able to concentrate the antibiotics.— A. Philipson *et al.*, *New Engl. J. Med.*, 1973, *288*, 1219.

Concentrations of clindamycin in breast milk after oral administration were generally small but very variable.— B. Stéen and A. Rane, *Br. J. clin. Pharmac.*, 1982, *13*, 661.

Uses and Administration

Clindamycin, a lincosamide antibiotic, is a chlorinated derivative of the antibiotic lincomycin, and is used in the treatment of serious anaerobic infections especially those caused by *Bacteroides fragilis*. It has been recommended as an alternative to penicillin in some severe staphylococcal and streptococcal infections, including staphylococcal osteomyelitis. It is unlikely to be effective in infections of the CNS because of poor penetration of the blood-brain barrier. Because of its potential toxicity (see Adverse Effects) clindamycin should only be used when there is no suitable alternative.

Clindamycin has also been used in the treatment of some protozoal infections.

Clindamycin is given by mouth as capsules containing the hydrochloride or as oral liquid preparations containing the palmitate hydrochloride. The capsules should be taken with a glass of water. Doses are expressed in terms of the equivalent amount of clindamycin. Adults are given 150 to 300 mg every 6 hours; in severe infections the dose may be increased to 450 mg every 6 hours. Children may be given 3 to 6 mg per kg body-weight every 6 hours; those under one-year-old or weighing 10 kg or less should receive at least 37.5 mg every 8 hours.

It may be given by injection as clindamycin phosphate (see below).

Topical preparations of clindamycin hydrochloride or phosphate may be used in the treatment of acne vulgaris.

Clindamycin has been widely used, often in association with an aminoglycoside, for the treatment or prophylaxis of infections in sites where anaerobic organisms may be present, particularly intra-abdominal and gynaecological infections. However, less toxic regimens are now being investigated involving the newer cephalosporins (see cefoxitin sodium, p.158, and latamoxef disodium, p.252), imipenem (see p.247), or the antipseudomonal penicillins (see piperacillin sodium, p.285). Metronidazole (see p.666) is also widely used.

Brief reviews of clindamycin: J. G. Bartlett, *Lancet*, 1982, *2*, 478; W. R. Wilson *et al.*, *Mayo Clin. Proc.*, 1987, *62*, 906.

Proceedings of symposia on clindamycin.— *J. antimicrob. Chemother.*, 1981, *7*, *Suppl.* A, 1–85; *Scand. J. infect. Dis.*, 1984, *Suppl.* 43, 1–90.

The choice of antibiotics for anaerobic infections.— *Med. Lett.*, 1984, *26*, 87.

Clindamycin phosphate was given intravenously in doses of 300 to 450 mg every 6 to 8 hours to 42 patients with severe anaerobic infection. The mean serum concentration was always well in excess of the MIC. The mortality-rate in the 19 patients with bacteraemia was 21% compared with 27% in 48 similar patients treated with chloramphenicol. The infected sites healed in 21 of 23 non-bacteraemic patients and of 32 of the total group on whom follow-up cultures were done, 31 were cured bacteriologically. Treatment was well tolerated.— A. W. Chow *et al.*, *Archs intern. Med.*, 1974, *134*, 78. Of 18 patients with *Bacteroides fragilis* infection 14 responded to treatment with clindamycin. The response-rate (78%) was little higher than 93 (65%) in 142 patients given no antibiotics or antibiotics to which the organism was not sensitive.— D. A. Leigh, *Br. med. J.*, 1974, *3*, 225. Excellent results were obtained following concurrent administration of clindamycin and gentamicin to 38 patients with life-threatening infections, 29 of whom had failed to respond to prior antibiotic therapy. The good results were mainly attributed to the activity of clindamycin against anaerobic bacteria, particularly *B. fragilis*. Of the patients treated 30 recovered, 2 improved but required alternative therapy owing to the development of rashes, and 6 relapsed or failed to respond.— R. J. Fass *et al.*, *Archs intern. Med.*, 1977, *137*, 28. In a study of 70 patients with proven anaerobic infections, parenteral treatment with clindamycin or chloramphenicol was of similar clinical efficacy.— R. E. Van Scoy *et al.*, *Mayo Clin. Proc.*, 1984, *59*, 842.

Further references to the use of clindamycin in various infections: R. J. Fass *et al.*, *Ann. intern. Med.*, 1973, *78*, 853; D. A. Leigh *et al.*, *J. antimicrob. Chemother.*, 1977, *3*, 493.

ABSCESS, LUNG. For reference to the use of clindamycin in the treatment of lung abscess, see Benzylpenicillin Sodium, p.135.

ADMINISTRATION, OCULAR. Clindamycin has been administered into the eye topically, or by subconjunctival or intravitreal injection.— T. S. Lesar and R. G. Fiscella, *Drug Intell. & clin. Pharm.*, 1985, *19*, 642.

ADMINISTRATION IN LIVER DISORDERS. Five hours after the administration of clindamycin 600 mg by intravenous injection the mean serum concentration in patients with moderate to severe hepatic dysfunction was 24.3 µg per mL whereas in patients with normal function it was 8.3 µg per mL. It was suggested that the dose of clindamycin should be modified in patients with liver disease.— D. N. Williams *et al.*, *Antimicrob. Ag. Chemother.*, 1975, *7*, 153. Clindamycin 300 mg was given intravenously every 12 hours for 2 days to patients with cirrhosis or acute or chronic hepatitis or to controls. There was no deterioration in the liver disorder. Although there was a slight but significant delay in excretion between controls and patients with cirrhosis the half-lives in all groups were considered to be in normal ranges.— D. R. Hinthorn *et al.*, *ibid.*, 1976, *9*, 498.

A study of the pharmacokinetics of clindamycin in patients with anaerobic infections suggesting that there is a direct correlation between serum concentrations of indirect bilirubin and the half-life of clindamycin. The dose of clindamycin could thus be calculated for patients with liver disease providing there are no factors contributing to increased bilirubin production or biliary obstruction.— R. H. K. Eng *et al.*, *J. antimicrob. Chemother.*, 1981, *8*, 277.

ADMINISTRATION IN RENAL FAILURE. Peritoneal dialysis did not affect serum concentrations of clindamycin, but peak concentrations were twice as high in anephric patients as in normal subjects and so the normal dose should be halved for such patients.— R. F. Malacoff *et al.*, *Antimicrob. Ag. Chemother.*, 1975, *8*, 574.

The half-life for clindamycin was 2 to 4 hours in healthy subjects and 3 to 5 hours in end-stage renal disease. Clindamycin could be given in usual doses to patients with impaired renal function, and a supplemental dose was not required in patients on haemodialysis or peritoneal dialysis.— W. M. Bennett *et al.*, *Am. J. Kidney Dis.*, 1983, *3*, 155.

BABESIOSIS. Clindamycin, 1.2 g twice daily by parenteral administration or 600 mg three times daily by mouth, in association with quinine, 650 mg three times daily by mouth, was recommended for the treatment of babesiosis. Children could be given clindamycin 20 to 40 mg per kg body-weight daily and quinine 25 mg per kg daily both in 3 divided doses. Treatment should be continued for 7 days.— *Med. Lett.*, 1986, *28*, 9.

CRYPTOSPORIDIOSIS. The Centers for Disease Control in the *USA* had received 6 reports of AIDS patients and one bone-marrow transplant patient with cryptosporidiosis who were treated with a combination of quinine and clindamycin both given by mouth. Three patients did not respond after 7 to 14 days of therapy, and in a further three the drugs were discontinued because of adverse effects; one developed a severe rash, another severe vomiting, and the third thrombocytopenia. Symptoms improved in 2 of these 3 patients during the first few days of therapy. In one patient with AIDS, diarrhoea resolved within 2 days of initiating therapy although stool examinations continued to show occasional *Cryptosporidium*.— *Morb. Mortal.*, 1984, *33*, 117.

For brief comment on cryptosporidiosis in immunocompromised patients and the view that of the drugs tried so far spiramycin has offered the greatest promise, see spiramycin (p.296).

ENDOCARDITIS PROPHYLAXIS. The European Society of Cardiology has suggested clindamycin 600 mg by mouth taken one hour before a dental procedure as a possible alternative to erythromycin for the prophylaxis of infective endocarditis in patients allergic to penicillin (J. Delaye *et al.*, *Eur. Heart J.*, 1985, *6*, 826). Clindamycin has been used in preference to erythromycin in Switzerland, since it has been considered to be better absorbed, better tolerated, and more effective in the experimental *animal* model of endocarditis. Patients at high risk of endocarditis may be given 7 doses of clindamycin 300 mg at intervals of 6 hours following the initial 600-mg dose (D.C. Shanson, *J. antimicrob. Chemother.*, 1987, *20*, *Suppl.* A, 119; M. Glauser, *ibid.*, 133).

The British Society for Antimicrobial Chemotherapy, however, could not recommend the use of clindamycin for endocarditis prophylaxis because of the risk, albeit small, of pseudomembranous colitis (N.A. Simmons *et al.*, *Lancet*, 1986, *1*, 1267).

EYE INFECTIONS. Two patients with keratitis caused by *Capnocytophaga* responded to treatment with clindamycin topically, one drop of a 5% solution every 15 minutes, and subconjunctivally 75 mg twice daily.— T. J. Roussel *et al.*, *Br. J. Ophthal.*, 1985, *69*, 187.

MALARIA. Clindamycin has been used in the treatment of falciparum malaria resistant to 4-aminoquinolines. If used alone it acts only slowly, but if it is given in association with quinine for rapid reduction of parasitaemia the incidence and intensity of gastro-intestinal effects are exacerbated. Thus its use is not recommended.— Advances in malaria chemotherapy, *Tech. Rep. Ser. Wld. Hlth. Org. No. 711*, 1984, p.60. See also A. P. Hall *et al.*, *Br. med. J.*, 1975, *2*, 12.

MOUTH INFECTIONS. For reference to the use of clindamycin for treatment of orodental infections likely to involve anaerobic organisms, see Benzylpenicillin Sodium, p.137.

OSTEOMYELITIS. In a retrospective study, 33 of 35 children aged 5 to 15 years with acute osteomyelitis were successfully treated with clindamycin 75 or 150 mg 4 times daily for 4 to 8 weeks. Therapy for 4 weeks was adequate.— M. R. Wharton and F. H. Beddow, *Postgrad. med. J.*, 1975, *51*, 166.

Clindamycin was used successfully in the treatment of acute and chronic osteomyelitis in 25 and 4 children respectively. The majority of patients were given the equivalent of 50 mg per kg body-weight daily by intravenous injection for 3 weeks followed by 25 mg per kg daily by mouth for 4 to 6 weeks. *Staphylococcus aureus* was isolated in 22 of the patients and nearly all isolates were penicillin-resistant.— W. Rodriguez *et al.*, *Am. J. Dis. Child.*, 1977, *131*, 1088.

The successful use of clindamycin in the treatment of bone and joint infections.— A. M. Geddes *et al.*, *J. antimicrob. Chemother.*, 1977, *3*, 501.

PELVIC INFLAMMATORY DISEASE. Thirty-six women with pelvic inflammatory disease were treated with a standard regimen of clindamycin and tobramycin. An adequate short-term clinical response was observed in 16 of 19 patients who were evaluated after treatment, but patients with severe salpingitis responded slowly. *Chlamydia trachomatis* was present in the initial cultures of all 3 patients classified as clinical failures, although cervical, urethral, and rectal cultures from all patients evaluated after treatment were clear of this organism. The MIC of clindamycin against *C. trachomatis* has been reported to be approximately 1 μg per mL; such concentrations may have been achieved after the high intravenous and oral doses used.— J. N. Wasserheit *et al.*, *Ann. intern. Med.*, 1986, *104*, 187.

For reference to standard regimens involving clindamycin for the treatment of pelvic inflammatory disease, see under Cefoxitin Sodium, p.159.

PERITONITIS. Clindamycin base has been used in the treatment of peritonitis in patients on continuous ambulatory peritoneal dialysis (CAPD). It has been administered intraperitoneally in a loading dose of 300 mg per litre of dialysis fluid, followed by a maintenance dose of 50 mg per litre or 1.2 g daily. It has also been administered intraperitoneally as the phospate.— D. K. Scott and D. E. Roberts, *Pharm. J.*, 1985, *1*, 621.

The first-line treatment of peritonitis in patients on CAPD was changed from clindamycin and gentamicin to vancomycin and netilmicin because of the emergence of strains of multiply-resistant *Staphylococcus epidermidis*.— L. Brauner *et al.*, *J. antimicrob. Chemother.*, 1985, *15*, 751.

PNEUMONIA. All of 28 children with aspiration pneumonia due to aerobic and anaerobic bacteria responded to therapy with clindamycin phosphate 25 to 40 mg per kg body-weight given daily in 3 divided doses. Gentamicin 3 to 6 mg per kg given daily in 3 divided doses was added to the regimen when aerobic Gram-negative bacilli were predominant. The average length of treatment was about 14 days.— I. Brook, *Antimicrob. Ag. Chemother.*, 1979, *15*, 342.

For reference to the use of clindamycin in association with aztreonam or tobramycin in the treatment of pneumonia, see Aztreonam, p.127.

SKIN DISORDERS. *Acne*. For a review of the treatment of acne including the oral and topical use of clindamycin, see Tetracycline Hydrochloride, p.321.

References to the topical use of clindamycin in the treatment of acne vulgaris: J. D. Guin, *Int. J. Derm.*, 1979, *18*, 164 (use of 1% solutions of clindamycin hydrochloride or clindamycin phosphate); M. G. Lee and S. Richards (letter), *Pharm. J.*, 1983, *1*, 448 (formulae for topical solutions of clindamycin hydrochloride and clindamycin phosphate); S. B. Tucker *et al.*, *Br. J. Derm.*, 1984, *110*, 487 (comparison of clindamycin phosphate 1% solution and benzoyl peroxide 5% gel); L. R. Braathen, *Scand. J. infect. Dis.*, 1984, *Suppl.* 43, 71 (comparison of clindamycin phosphate 1% solution and tetracycline by mouth); M. J. Petersen *et al.*, *Curr. ther. Res.*, 1986, *40*, 232 (comparison of a 1% lotion and solution of clindamycin phosphate); A. Katsambas *et al.*, *Br. J. Derm.*, 1987, *116*, 387 (comparison of clindamycin phosphate 1% solution and tetracycline by mouth).

For conflicting reports on the systemic absorption of clindamycin after its topical use, see under Absorption and Fate.

For reference to clindamycin inhibiting lipase production by *Propionibacterium* spp., see under Antimicrobial Action, above.

SURGICAL INFECTION PROPHYLAXIS. Clindamycin has been used for prophylaxis of infection during surgical procedures particularly if contamination with anaerobic organisms is possible. It has been given alone in craniotomy, and in association with an aminoglycoside in major surgery involving an incision through the oral or pharyngeal mucosa or in procedures involving a ruptured viscus. Clindamycin is usually given in a pre-operative intravenous dose of 300 or 600 mg followed by further doses at intervals of 4 to 8 hours (A.B. Kaiser, *New Engl. J. Med.*, 1986, *315*, 1129; *Med. Lett.*, 1987, *29*, 91).

Further references to the use of clindamycin in surgical infection prophylaxis: R. L. Nichols *et al.*, *New Engl. J. Med.*, 1984, *311*, 1065 (similar efficacy of prophylaxis with clindamycin in association with gentamicin, and cefoxitin after penetrating abdominal trauma).

TOXOPLASMOSIS. Beneficial results with pyrimethamine together with clindamycin in 5 AIDS patients with toxoplasmosis of the CNS.— B. A. Navia *et al.*, *Ann. Neurol.*, 1986, *19*, 224. Comment from a National Institutes of Health conference on AIDS that there is no clearly effective alternative to pyrimethamine with sulphadiazine in the treatment of toxoplasmosis of the CNS. Convincing clinical reports to support the use of other drugs including clindamycin have not been published.— D. T. DeVita *et al.*, *Ann. intern. Med.*, 1987, *106*, 568.

See also Antimicrobial Action, above.

WOUND INFECTIONS. The use of clindamycin, doxycycline, and an aminoglycoside in 3 patients with sternal wound infections and mediastinitis caused by *Mycoplasma hominis*. A cure was achieved in one patient with the above therapy and concomitant surgery. The other two achieved microbiological cure, but later died after complications developed.— D. O. Steffenson *et al.*, *Ann. intern. Med.*, 1987, *106*, 204.

Preparations

Clindamycin Capsules *(B.P.)*. Capsules containing clindamycin hydrochloride.

Clindamycin Hydrochloride Capsules *(U.S.P.)*

Clindamycin Palmitate Hydrochloride for Oral Solution *(U.S.P.)*. Reconstituted solution has a pH of 2.5 to 5.0.

Proprietary Preparations

Dalacin C *(Upjohn, UK)*. *Capsules*, clindamycin 75 and 150 mg (as hydrochloride).

Paediatric suspension, granules for reconstitution, clindamycin 75 mg (as palmitate hydrochloride)/5 mL when reconstituted with water.

Topical solution (Dalacin T), see under clindamycin phosphate (below).

Proprietary Names and Manufacturers of Clindamycin Hydrochloride and Clindamycin Palmitate Hydrochloride

Cleocin *(Upjohn, USA)*; Dalacin *(Denm.; Upjohn, Norw.; Upjohn, Spain)*; Dalacin C *(Arg.; Upjohn, Austral.; Belg.; Upjohn, Canad.; Upjohn, Ital.; Neth.; Upjohn, S.Afr.; Upjohn, Switz.; Upjohn, UK)*; Dalacina *(Upjohn, Swed.)*; Dalacine *(Upjohn, Fr.)*; Sobelin *(Upjohn, Ger.)*.

NOTE. Some of the above names have also been used to denote preparations of clindamycin phosphate.

56-q

Clindamycin Phosphate *(BANM, USAN, rINNM)*.

U-28508. Clindamycin 2-(dihydrogen phosphate).
$C_{18}H_{34}ClN_2O_8PS = 505.0$.

CAS — 24729-96-2.

Pharmacopoeias. In *U.S.*

A white to off-white, odourless or almost odourless, hygroscopic, crystalline powder. The *U.S.P.* specifies not less than the equivalent of 758 μg of clindamycin per mg. 1.2 g of monograph substance is approximately equivalent to 1 g of clindamycin. **Soluble** 1 in 2.5 of water; slightly soluble in dehydrated alcohol; very slightly soluble in acetone; practically insoluble in chloroform and ether. A 1% solution in water has a pH of 3.5 to 4.5 and the *U.S.P.* injection has a pH or 5.5 to 7.0. **Store** in airtight containers.

It is reported to be **incompatible** with aminophylline, ampicillin sodium, barbiturates, calcium gluconate, magnesium sulphate, and phenytoin sodium. Solutions with tobramycin sulphate in glucose injection are reported to be unstable.

Clindamycin phosphate was less bitter than clindamycin hydrochloride, and was most stable in solution at pH 3.5 to 6.5.— T. O. Oesterling and E. L. Rowe, *J. pharm. Sci.*, 1970, *59*, 175.

A study of the effect of freezing and thawing on the stability of intravenous infusions of clindamycin phosphate.— C. J. Holmes *et al.*, *Am. J. Hosp. Pharm.*, 1982, *39*, 104.

A study of the compatibility and stability of clindamycin phosphate with intravenous fluids.— W. R. Porter *et al.*, *Am. J. Hosp. Pharm.*, 1983, *40*, 91.

Stability of clindamycin phosphate with aztreonam, ceftazidime sodium, ceftriaxone sodium, or piperacillin sodium in glucose 5% or sodium chloride 0.9% intravenous solutions.— D. A. Marble *et al.*, *Am. J. Hosp. Pharm.*, 1986, *43*, 1732.

Adverse Effects, Treatment, and Precautions

As for clindamycin (p.198).

Thrombophlebitis may occur after intravenous administration of clindamycin phosphate.

A report of an anaphylactic reaction to intravenous infusion of clindamycin.— A. J. Pomerance *et al.* (letter), *Drug Intell. & clin. Pharm.*, 1979, *13*, 348.

Cardiac arrest occurred in a 50-year-old woman after rapid injection of 600 mg of undiluted clindamycin phosphate into a central intravenous line. Further injections were given over 30 minutes without cardiovascular complications.— P. Aucoin *et al.*, *Sth. med. J.*, 1982, *75*, 768.

Absorption and Fate

Clindamycin phosphate is biologically inactive but is rapidly hydrolysed in the blood to clindamycin. When the equivalent of 300 mg of clindamycin is injected intramuscularly every 8 hours a mean peak plasma concentration of 6 μg per mL is achieved within 3 hours; 600 mg every 12 hours gives a peak concentration of 9 μg per mL. In children, peak concentrations may be reached within one hour. When the same doses are infused intravenously every 8 hours peak concentrations of 7 and 10 μg per mL are achieved by the end of infusion.

About 8% and 28% of intramuscular and intravenous doses of clindamycin, respectively, have been recovered from the urine within 8 hours.

A dose of clindamycin phosphate equivalent to 150 mg of clindamycin per m^2 body-surface given to 4 children intramuscularly produced adequate serum activity of 2.4 μg per mL at 8 hours, the half-life of serum activity being 3.4 hours. A dose of 117 mg per m^2 in 8 children produced an inadequate mean serum concentration of 1 μg per mL at 8 hours where the half-life was 2.4 hours.— R. E. Kauffman *et al.*, *Clin. Pharmac. Ther.*, 1972, *13*, 704.

In a study of 19 patients treated with clindamycin phosphate given parenterally, the equivalent of 900 mg of base was the usual dose which was given intravenously every 8 hours. After 30-minute infusions serum concentrations ranged from 11.1 to 39 μg per mL with a mean of 23.6 μg per mL. At 2 to 4 hours concentrations were 3.4 to 15 μg per mL (mean 9.6 μg per mL) and by 8 hours 0.9 to 10.7 μg per mL (mean 5.4 μg per mL). Maximum concentrations at 1 to 4 and at 8 hours in the 5 patients given 900 mg intramuscularly were similar to those after intravenous injection.— R. J. Fass *et al.*, *Ann. intern. Med.*, 1973, *78*, 853.

Clindamycin phosphate given intravenously was rapidly hydrolysed to clindamycin which disappeared from serum within 2 hours. Activity in bile, due to a *N*-demethyl derivative, persisted for up to 18 hours. Following intramuscular injection a peak serum concentration of clindamycin was found within 2 to 3 hours, with some still present after 4 hours, and the salivary concentration reached a peak at about 90 to 120 minutes after administration. Activity in urine, due to metabolites, persisted for up to 4 days after a single dose of clindamycin phosphate. The minimum effective dose was considered to be 300 mg every 12 hours.— R. M. DeHaan *et al.*, *J. clin. Pharmac.*, 1973, *13*, 190.

The pharmacokinetics of clindamycin phosphate in 10 critically ill patients, all of whom were receiving other antibiotics concomitantly. Most appeared to have decreased hepatic clearance of clindamycin compared to that in 6 healthy subjects.— H. J. Mann *et al.*, *Clin. Pharm.*, 1987, *6*, 154.

A crossover, pharmacokinetic study in 6 healthy subjects suggesting that intravenous infusion over 30 minutes of clindamycin phosphate, in a dosage regimen equivalent to clindamycin 900 mg every 8 hours, may be an acceptable alternative to 600 mg every 6 hours. A regimen of 600 mg every 8 hours was considered to be pharmacokinetically inferior.— R. J. Townsend and R. P. Baker, *Drug Intell. & clin. Pharm.*, 1987, *21*, 279. Criticism of the methods used and the conclusions.— J. K. Walters (letter), *ibid.*, 661. Reply; clinical studies are required to assess clinical equality of different dosage regimens.— R. J. Townsend and R. P. Baker (letter), *ibid.*, 662.

DIFFUSION INTO BODY TISSUES AND FLUIDS. Studies of the distribution of clindamycin after parenteral administration of clindamycin phosphate: bones.— P. Nicholas *et al.*, *Antimicrob. Ag. Chemother.*, 1975, *8*, 220; K. Dornbusch *et al.*, *J. antimicrob. Chemother.*, 1977, *3*, 153. skin and bone taken from patients undergoing excision of decubitus ulcers.— S. A. Berger *et al.*, *Antimicrob. Ag. Chemother.*, 1978, *14*, 498. intestinal wall and faeces.— L. Kager *et al.*, *ibid.*, 1981, *20*, 736. peritoneal fluid, intestine, and muscle of neonates and infants.— M. J. Bell *et al.*, *Curr. ther. Res.*, 1983, *33*, 751.

DRUG EXCRETION. Clindamycin phosphate 600 mg was given intravenously to 14 patients about 1 hour before biliary tract surgery; 7 had total obstruction of the common bile duct and 7 had patent biliary tracts. Those with patent ducts had average serum concentrations of 19.2 and 14.5 μg per mL at 30 and 60 minutes respectively and achieved high concentrations of clindamycin in specimens of gall-bladder bile (33.9 μg per mL), common duct bile (41.7 μg per mL), gall-bladder wall (12.0 μg per g), and liver (33.9 μg per g) obtained during surgery. In those with obstructed ducts average serum concentrations were 15.4 and 11.3 μg per mL at 30 and 60 minutes respectively. They had no measurable drug in the common duct bile and a reduced concentration in the gall-bladder wall (4.6 μg per g). Concentrations in the liver were however slightly higher (41.5 μg per g) than in the other group and clindamycin could therefore be used for intrahepatic infections in patients with common bile duct obstruction.— R. E. Brown *et al.*, *Ann. intern. Med.*, 1976, *84*, 168.

Uses and Administration

Clindamycin phosphate has the actions and uses of clindamycin (see p.198). It is administered by intramuscular injection or slow intravenous infusion in doses equivalent to 0.6 to 2.7 g of clindamycin daily in divided doses. Not more than 1.2 g should be infused in one hour, and not more than 600 mg should be given in a single intramuscular injection. Up to 4.8 g daily has been given intravenously in very severe infections but again no more than 1.2 g should be infused in 1 hour. Clindamycin phosphate may be administered by continuous infusion following an initial intravenous dose. Children over the age of 1 month may be given the equivalent of 15 to 40 mg per kg body-weight daily in divided doses; in severe infections they should receive a total dose of not less than 300 mg of clindamycin daily. Neonates have been given 15 to 20 mg per kg daily.

A 1% solution or gel of clindamycin phosphate is used for the topical treatment of acne vulgaris.

For reference to a pharmacokinetic study comparing different dosage regimens of clindamycin phosphate, see Absorption and Fate, above.

Preparations

Clindamycin Phosphate Injection *(U.S.P.)*

Clindamycin Phosphate Topical Solution *(U.S.P.)*. pH 4 to 7.

Sterile Clindamycin Phosphate *(U.S.P.)*

Proprietary Preparations

Dalacin C Phosphate Sterile Solution *(Upjohn, UK)*. *Injection*, clindamycin 150 mg(as phosphate)/mL in ampoules of 2 and 4 mL.

Dalacin T *(Upjohn, UK)*. *Topical solution*, clindamycin 1% (as phosphate).

Proprietary Names and Manufacturers

Cleocin *(Upjohn, USA)*; Cleocin T *(Upjohn, USA)*; Dalacin *(Upjohn, Denm.; Upjohn, Norw.)*; Dalacin C *(Arg.; Upjohn, Austral.; Belg.; Upjohn, Canad.; Upjohn, Ital.; Neth.; Upjohn, S.Afr.; Upjohn, Switz.; Upjohn, UK)*; Dalacin T *(Upjohn, UK)*; Dalacina *(Upjohn, Swed.)*; Dalacine *(Upjohn, Fr.)*; Sobelin *(Basotherm, Ger.; Upjohn, Ger.)*.

NOTE. Some of the above names have also been used to denote preparations of clindamycin hydrochloride or clindamycin palmitate hydrochloride.

57-p

Clometocillin Potassium *(rINNM)*.

3,4-Dichloro-α-methoxybenzylpenicillin potassium; Penicillin 356 (clometocillin). Potassium (6*R*)-6-[2-(3,4-dichlorophenyl)-2-methoxyacetamido]penicillanate.
$C_{17}H_{17}Cl_2KN_2O_5S$=471.4.

CAS — 1926-49-4 (clometocillin); 15433-28-0 (potassium salt).

Clometocillin has properties and uses similar to those of benzylpenicillin (see p.131) but is acid-stable and well-absorbed from the gastro-intestinal tract. It is given by mouth in a dose of 500 mg as the potassium salt, two to three times daily.

Proprietary Names and Manufacturers

Rixapen *(RIT, Belg.; Smith Kline & French, Fr.)*.

59-w

Clomocycline Sodium *(BANM, rINNM)*.

Chlormethylenecycline Sodium; N^2-(Hydroxymethyl)chlortetracycline Sodium; Methylolchlortetracycline Sodium. The sodium salt of 7-chloro-N^2-(hydroxymethyl)tetracycline.
$C_{23}H_{24}ClN_2NaO_9$=530.9.

CAS — 1181-54-0 (clomocycline).

A yellow powder. Very **soluble** in water. A 2% solution in water has a pH of about 8.4. Solutions in water lose most of their activity after 24 hours. **Store** in airtight containers. Protect from light.

Adverse Effects and Precautions

As for Tetracycline Hydrochloride, p.314.

PREGNANCY AND THE NEONATE. A report of the birth of an infant with multiple abnormalities to a woman who had taken clomocycline for the first 8 weeks of pregnancy. A causal relationship was not established but it was considered that prolonged tetracycline treatment for acne should not be given to women having unprotected intercourse and that it should be withdrawn as soon as possible in an unplanned pregnancy.— R. Corcoran and J. M. Castles, *Br. med. J.*, 1977, *2*, 807.

Absorption and Fate

As for Tetracycline Hydrochloride, p.317.

Serum concentrations of about 1 μg per mL have been reported to follow 2 or 3 hours after a single 170-mg dose of clomocycline sodium by mouth and concentrations of about 2 μg per mL after repeated doses. Its biological half-life is about 5.8 hours. About 30% of the administered dose is excreted in the urine.

Uses and Administration

Clomocycline sodium has the antimicrobial activity and uses described under tetracycline hydrochloride (see p.315).

It is given by mouth in usual doses of 170 or 340 mg three or four times daily.

Clomocycline produced marked improvement in 10 of 24 patients with pustular or pustular and cystic acne and moderate improvement in a further 12. The patients had shown negligible improvement with previous local and antibiotic therapy. Dosage was usually 170 mg four times daily for 1 week, then 170 mg twice daily, and treatment lasted for 2 weeks to 11 months. One patient experienced heartburn and another an irritant erythematous macular rash.— J. L. Verbov, *Br. J. clin. Pract.*, 1968, *22*, 37.

In a double-blind crossover study completed by 40 of 60 patients with persistent palmoplantar pustulosis, 15 responded to treatment with clomocycline 170 mg three times daily for 2 weeks and then twice daily for 10 weeks, 1 responded to treatment and the placebo, and 2 patients responded only to the placebo. There was no response in 22 patients.— J. M. Ward *et al.*, *Br. J. Derm.*, 1976, *95*, 317.

Proprietary Preparations

Megaclor *(Pharmax, UK)*. *Capsules*, clomocycline sodium 170 mg.

12594-t

Cloxacillin Benzathine *(BANM, USAN)*.

The *NN'*-dibenzylethylenediamine salt of cloxacillin.
$C_{16}H_{20}N_2,(C_{19}H_{18}ClN_3O_5S)_2$=1112.1.

CAS — 23736-58-5; 32222-55-2.

Pharmacopoeias. In *U.S.* for veterinary use only. Also in *B.P. Vet.*

A white or almost white powder. Slightly **soluble** in water, alcohol, and isopropyl alcohol; soluble 1 in 18 of chloroform and 1 in 3 of methyl alcohol. The pH of a 1% suspension is 3.0 to 6.5. **Store** at a temperature not exceeding 25° in airtight containers.

Cloxacillin benzathine has the actions and uses of cloxacillin sodium (see below). It is used in veterinary medicine as an ophthalmic ointment, or as an intramammary injection in the treatment of bovine mastitis.

Proprietary Veterinary Names and Manufacturers

Embaclox Dry Cow *(RMB Animal Health, UK)*; Orbenin Dry Cow *(Beecham Animal Health, UK)*; Orbenin Ophthalmic Ointment *(Beecham Animal Health, UK)*.

60-m

Cloxacillin Sodium *(BANM, USAN, rINNM)*.

BRL-1621; Cloxacillinum Natricum; P-25; Sodium Cloxacillin. Sodium (6*R*)-6-[3-(2-chloro-

phenyl)-5-methylisoxazole-4-carboxamido]penicillanate monohydrate.
$C_{19}H_{17}ClN_3NaO_5S,H_2O=475.9$.

CAS — 61-72-3 (cloxacillin); 642-78-4 (sodium salt, anhydrous); 7081-44-9 (sodium salt, monohydrate).

Pharmacopoeias. In *Br., Chin., Egypt., Ind., Int., It., Jpn, Jug., Nord., Roum.*, and *U.S.* Also in *B.P. Vet.*

A white, odourless, hygroscopic, crystalline powder. 1.09 g of monograph substance is approximately equivalent to 1 g of anhydrous cloxacillin. Each g of monograph substance represents about 2.1 mmol of sodium.

Soluble 1 in 2.5 of water and 1 in 30 of alcohol; slightly soluble in chloroform. The *B.P.* specifies that a 10% solution in water has a pH of 5 to 7. The *U.S.P.* specifies that a 1% solution in water has a pH of 4.5 to 7.5.

Store at a temperature not exceeding 25° in airtight containers.

Aqueous solutions of cloxacillin sodium are reported to be **stable** for up to 24 hours at 25° and for up to 72 hours at 5°. However, it is recommended that reconstituted solutions of cloxacillin sodium for injection should be administered immediately after preparation. Cloxacillin sodium should not be mixed with blood products or other proteinaceous fluids such as protein hydrolysates.

Cloxacillin sodium has been reported to be **incompatible** with aminoglycosides, tetracyclines, and other antimicrobial agents including erythromycin and polymyxin B sulphate.

Adverse Effects

As for Benzylpenicillin Sodium, p.132.

Febrile reactions were noted in 9 patients after the intravenous infusion of cloxacillin. Shaking chills and fever lasting 20 to 30 minutes occurred, in some patients after each dose and in others only intermittently.— J. Portnoy *et al.* (letter), *Can. med. Ass. J.*, 1975, *112*, 280.

An analysis of 148 reported episodes of drug fever; 46 were caused by antimicrobial agents and of these 2 were due to cloxacillin.— P. A. Mackowiak and C. F. LeMaistre, *Ann. intern. Med.*, 1987, *106*, 728.

EFFECTS ON THE BLOOD. Agranulocytosis developed in a 42-year-old man about one month after starting treatment with cloxacillin 500 mg four times daily by mouth.— E. L. Westerman *et al.*, *Am. J. clin. Path.*, 1978, *69*, 559.

EFFECTS ON THE GASTRO-INTESTINAL TRACT. Non-pseudomembranous colitis, presenting with abdominal pain, bloody diarrhoea, and fever was associated with the administration of a combination of cloxacillin and ampicillin in one patient.— M. Iida *et al.*, *Endoscopy*, 1985, *17*, 64.

EFFECTS ON THE LIVER. Intrahepatic cholestatic jaundice which occurred in a woman receiving nitrofurantoin, ampicillin, and cloxacillin re-appeared when the patient was treated with cloxacillin 2 years later. A macrophage inhibition factor test confirmed that cloxacillin was the offending drug.— R. Enat *et al.*, *Br. med. J.*, 1980, *280*, 982.

LOCAL IRRITANT EFFECTS. For reference to the incidence of phlebitis after intravenous infusion of cloxacillin, see Flucloxacillin Sodium (p.230).

Precautions

As for Benzylpenicillin Sodium, p.133. Lens opacities have occurred after ocular use of cloxacillin sodium in *animals*.

For reference to a possible change in the disposition of cloxacillin in patients with cystic fibrosis, see under Absorption and Fate, below.

ADMINISTRATION IN RENAL FAILURE. For reference to the precautions to be observed in renal failure, see below under Uses, Administration in Renal Failure.

INTERFERENCE WITH DIAGNOSTIC TESTS. Cloxacillin affected the estimation of urinary 17-oxosteroids and 17-oxogenic steroids.— *Adverse Drug React. Bull.*, 1972, June, 104.

PREGNANCY AND THE NEONATE. In a study in neonates given ampicillin, cloxacillin, flucloxacillin, or sulphafurazole, all except ampicillin reduced bilirubin-binding capacity. Sulphafurazole was already known to have precipitated kernicterus in preterm infants and it was suggested that cloxacillin and flucloxacillin should be used with caution in jaundiced neonates.— L. A. Friedman and P. J. Lewis, *Br. J. clin. Pharmac.*, 1977, *4*, 395P. See also *idem*, 1980, *9*, 61.

Antimicrobial Action and Resistance

Cloxacillin sodium has an antibacterial activity similar to that of flucloxacillin sodium (see p.231).

Absorption and Fate

Cloxacillin sodium is incompletely absorbed from the gastro-intestinal tract after oral administration, and absorption is further reduced by the presence of food in the stomach. After an oral dose of 500 mg, a peak plasma concentration of 7 to 14 μg per mL is obtained in fasting subjects in 1 to 2 hours. Absorption is more complete when given by intramuscular injection and peak plasma concentrations of about 15 μg per mL have been observed 30 minutes after a dose of 500 mg. Doubling the dose can double the plasma concentration. About 94% of cloxacillin in the circulation is bound to plasma proteins. Cloxacillin has been reported to have a plasma half-life of approximately 0.5 hour in healthy subjects. The half-life is prolonged in neonates.

Cloxacillin diffuses across the placenta into the foetal circulation and is excreted in breast milk. There is little diffusion into the CSF except when the meninges are inflamed. Therapeutic concentrations can be achieved in pleural and synovial fluids and in bone.

Cloxacillin is metabolised to a limited extent, and the unchanged drug and metabolites are excreted in the urine by glomerular filtration and renal tubular secretion. About 35% of an oral dose is excreted in the urine and up to 10% in the bile. Serum concentrations are enhanced if probenecid is given concomitantly.

In a study involving 16 patients with cystic fibrosis and 12 healthy subjects, serum concentrations of cloxacillin were lower in patients with cystic fibrosis both after intravenous and oral administration. This appeared to be due mainly to an increase in non-renal clearance. The bioavailability of cloxacillin in patients with cystic fibrosis was very variable.— M. Spino *et al.*, *J. Pediat.*, 1984, *105*, 829.

ADMINISTRATION IN RENAL FAILURE. For reference to the pharmacokinetics of cloxacillin in renal failure, see below under Uses, Administration in Renal Failure.

DIFFUSION INTO BODY TISSUES AND FLUIDS. The penetration of cloxacillin into joint fluid after administration by mouth.— J. D. Nelson *et al.*, *J. Pediat.*, 1978, *92*, 131.

Thirty-four patients undergoing cardiac surgery were given cloxacillin 1 g by intravenous infusion over 5 minutes, at induction of anaesthesia then every 4 hours to a total of 6 injections. The mean serum concentrations 1, 2, and 4 hours after the infusion were 30.8, 19.4, and 12.4 μg per mL respectively. The mean half-life of cloxacillin in 27 patients was 1.73 hours. A total of 39 heart specimens (36 atrial appendages and 3 mitral valves) were taken 16 to 200 minutes after the injections. Concentrations of cloxacillin in these specimens were very variable: none could be detected in 5, and the highest detectable concentration was 60 μg per g. In 14 patients in whom the atrial appendage and serum concentrations were measured at approximately the same time, the mean heart to serum-cloxacillin concentration ratio was 0.73 after 1 hour.— M. G. Bergeron *et al.*, *Antimicrob. Ag. Chemother.*, 1985, *27*, 928.

Ten patients undergoing open-heart surgery for valvular diseases, were given antibiotic prophylaxis with cloxacillin 2 g and benzylpenicillin 6 g (both as the sodium salt), by intravenous infusion at induction of anaesthesia, and repeated after 4 hours. Concentrations of the drugs in the atrium and diseased valve were measured between 17 and 135 minutes after the initial dose and were very variable. The mean concentrations of cloxacillin in these tissues represented 22 and 28% of those in the serum respectively. The corresponding values for benzylpenicillin were 56 and 45%. These concentrations were considered adequate, the second dose being recommended for operations lasting longer than 4 hours.— R. Pieper *et al.*, *Scand. J. thorac. cardiovasc. Surg.*, 1985, *19*, 49.

After the intravenous administration of cloxacillin 4 g, in association with probenecid, the peak concentration of cloxacillin in aqueous humour was 1 μg per mL.— T. S. Lesar and R. G. Fiscella, *Drug Intell. & clin. Pharm.*, 1985, *19*, 642.

METABOLISM. About 22% of a 500-mg dose of cloxacillin was metabolised. Within 12 hours of the dose being taken by 6 healthy subjects about 49% was recovered in the urine, 11% as penicilloic acid.— M. Cole *et al.*, *Antimicrob. Ag. Chemother.*, 1973, *3*, 463.

The metabolite of cloxacillin had similar antibacterial properties to the parent compound.— H. H. W. Thijssen and H. Mattie, *Antimicrob. Ag. Chemother.*, 1976, *10*, 441.

Uses and Administration

Cloxacillin sodium is an isoxazolyl penicillin with similar uses to flucloxacillin (p.231). When administered by mouth it should be given about 1 hour before or at least 2 hours after meals as the presence of food in the stomach reduces absorption.

Cloxacillin sodium is administered in usual doses equivalent to cloxacillin 250 to 500 mg four times daily by mouth or 250 mg by intramuscular injection every 4 to 6 hours. The equivalent of cloxacillin 500 mg may be given by slow intravenous injection over 3 to 4 minutes every 4 to 6 hours or by intravenous infusion. All systemic doses may be doubled in severe infections.

Cloxacillin sodium has been administered by other routes in conjunction with systemic therapy. It has been given in a dose equivalent to cloxacillin 500 mg daily administered by intra-articular injection, dissolved if necessary in a 0.5% solution of lignocaine hydrochloride, or by intrapleural injection. Using powder for injection, 125 to 250 mg has been dissolved in 3 mL of sterile water and inhaled by nebuliser four times daily.

Children up to 2 years of age may be given one-quarter the adult dose and those aged 2 to 10 years, one-half the adult dose. Children have been given doses of 12.5 to 25 mg per kg body-weight four times daily.

Cloxacillin may be administered in combination with other antibiotics, particularly ampicillin, to produce a wider spectrum of antibacterial activity.

For reference to the use of cloxacillin for the treatment and prophylaxis of various staphylococcal infections, see under Neutropenia, Osteomyelitis, Peritonitis, and Surgical Infection Prophylaxis in Flucloxacillin Sodium p.231.

ADMINISTRATION IN RENAL FAILURE. The normal half-life for cloxacillin of 0.4 to 0.6 hour was increased to 0.8 hour in end-stage renal failure. It could be given in usual doses to patients with renal failure. A dosage supplement was not required for patients undergoing haemodialysis.— W. M. Bennett *et al.*, *Am. J. Kidney Dis.*, 1983, *3*, 155.

ANIMAL BITES. For reference to the use of cloxacillin in the treatment of animal bites, see Benzylpenicillin Sodium, p.136.

MENINGITIS. A retrospective survey of 20 patients with meningitis, ventricular shunt infection, or brain abscess caused by *Staphylococcus aureus* or *epidermidis* who were treated with cloxacillin; cure was reported in 15.— I. W. Fong, *J. antimicrob. Chemother.*, 1983, *12*, 607.

See also Flucloxacillin Sodium, p.231.

PREGNANCY AND THE NEONATE. There appeared to be no significant risk to the foetus from cloxacillin when administered during pregnancy, although there was the possibility of sensitising the foetus during the second and third trimesters.— R. Wise, *Br. med. J.*, 1987, *294*, 42.

Preparations

Cloxacillin Capsules *(B.P.)*. Capsules containing cloxacillin sodium.

Cloxacillin Sodium Capsules *(U.S.P.)*

Cloxacillin Oral Solution *(B.P.)*. Cloxacillin Elixir; Cloxacillin Syrup. A dry mixture of cloxacillin sodium to be reconstituted before use.

Cloxacillin Sodium for Oral Solution *(U.S.P.)*

Cloxacillin Injection *(B.P.)*. Cloxacillin sodium to be reconstituted before use.

Proprietary Preparations

Orbenin *(Beecham Research, UK)*. *Capsules*, cloxacillin 250 and 500 mg (as sodium salt).

Syrup, powder for reconstitution, cloxacillin 125 mg (as sodium salt)/5 mL when reconstituted with water.
Injection, powder for reconstitution, cloxacillin 0.25, 0.5, and 1 g (as sodium salt).

Proprietary Names and Manufacturers
Anaclosil *(Antibioticos, Spain)*; Apo-Cloxi *(Apotex, Canad.)*; Austrastaph *(Commonwealth Serum Laboratories, Austral.)*; Bactopen *(Beecham, Canad.)*; Clocillin *(Jpn)*; Cloxapen *(Canad.; Ital.; Beecham Laboratories, USA)*; Cloxilean *(Canad.)*; Cloxypen *(Allard, Fr.)*; Ekvacillin *(Astra, Denm.; Astra, Norw.; Astra, Swed.)*; Landerclox *(Landerlan, Spain)*; Novocloxin *(Novopharm, Canad.)*; Orbénine *(Beecham Products, Fr.)*; Orbenin *(Beecham, Austral.; Belg.; Ayerst, Canad.; Ital.; Neth.; Beecham, S.Afr.; Beecham, Spain; Beecham, Switz.; Beecham Research, UK)*; Penstapho N *(Belg.)*; Staphybiotic *(Fr.)*; Tegopen *(Bristol, Canad.; Bristol, USA)*.

The following names have been used for multi-ingredient preparations containing cloxacillin sodium— Ampiclox *(Beecham, S.Afr.; Beecham Research, UK)*.

61-b

Colistin Sulphate *(BANM, pINNM)*.

Colistin Sulfate *(USAN)*; Colistini Sulfas; Polymyxin E Sulphate.

CAS — 1066-17-7 (colistin); 1264-72-8 (sulphate).

Pharmacopoeias. In *Br., Eur., Fr., Jug., Neth., Swiss,* and *U.S.*

A mixture of the sulphates of polypeptides produced by certain strains of *Bacillus polymyxa* var. *colistinus* or obtained by any other means. A white to slightly yellow, odourless or almost odourless, hygroscopic powder. The *B.P.* specifies not less than 19 000 units per mg calculated on the dried substance; *U.S.P.* specifies not less than 500 μg of colistin per mg.

B.P. **solubilities** are: soluble 1 in less than 2 of water; slightly soluble in alcohol; practically insoluble in acetone, chloroform, and ether. *U.S.P.* solubilities are: freely soluble in water; slightly soluble in methyl alcohol; insoluble in acetone and ether. The *B.P.* states that a 1% solution in water has a pH of 4.0 to 6.0, and the *U.S.P.* that it has a pH of 4.0 to 7.0. **Store** in airtight containers. Protect from light.

The base is precipitated from aqueous solution above pH 7.5.

62-v

Colistin Sulphomethate Sodium *(BANM)*.

Colistimethate Sodium *(USAN, rINN)*; Colistimethatum Natrium; Colistineméthanesulfonate Sodique; Sodium Colistimethate; Sodium Colistinmethanesulphonate; W-1929.

CAS — 8068-28-8.

Pharmacopoeias. In *Br., Eur., Fr., Jpn, Neth.,* and *Swiss. U.S.* includes Sterile Colistimethate Sodium.

An antimicrobial substance prepared from colistin by the action of formaldehyde and sodium bisulphite, whereby amino groups are sulphomethylated. A white to slightly yellow, odourless or almost odourless, hygroscopic powder. The *B.P.* specifies not less than 11 500 units per mg calculated on the dried substance; *U.S.P.* specifies not less than 390 μg of colistin per mg.

B.P. **solubilities** are: soluble 1 in less than 2 of water; slightly soluble in alcohol; practically insoluble in acetone, chloroform, and ether. *U.S.P.* solubilities are: freely soluble in water; soluble in methyl alcohol; insoluble in acetone and ether. The *B.P.* states that a 1% solution in water has a pH of 6.2 to 7.7, and the *U.S.P.* that it has a pH of 6.5 to 8.5.

Store in airtight containers. Protect from light.

Incompatibility or loss of activity has been reported with carbenicillin sodium, cephalothin sodium, cephazolin sodium, erythromycin lactobionate, hydrocortisone sodium succinate, and kanamycin sulphate.

Units

One unit of colistin is contained in 0.00004878 mg of the first International Standard Preparation (1968) of colistin sulphate which contains 20 500 units per mg. One unit of colistin sulphomethate is contained in 0.00007874 mg of the first International Reference Preparation (1966) of colistin sulphomethate which contains 12 700 units per mg.

Based on the above, 50 mg of colistin sulphate is approximately equivalent to 1 million units of colistin, and 80 mg of colistin sulphomethate is approximately equivalent to 1 million units of colistin sulphomethate. In the *USA* the potency of the national standard is expressed in terms of μg per mg but it is accepted for comparative purposes that each 'μg' of colistin base is equivalent to 30 units.

Adverse Effects, Treatments, and Precautions

As for Polymyxin B Sulphate, p.290.

Colistin sulphate is poorly absorbed from the gastro-intestinal tract and adverse effects do not normally follow its administration in the usual oral doses. Overgrowth of non-susceptible organisms, particularly *Proteus* spp., may occur after prolonged administration.

Adverse effects developed in 72 of 288 patients (25.1%) given 317 courses of treatment with colistin sulphomethate intramuscularly; 205 patients were given a total dose of less than 1 g, 69 between 1 and 2 g, and 43 were given doses greater than 2 g. Nephrotoxicity occurred in 20.2% of courses; the incidence increased with the age of the patient and with the concomitant administration of cephalothin sodium. Neurotoxic reactions, mainly paraesthesias and respiratory depression with apnoea, were found in 7.3% and allergic reactions in 2.2% of courses. There was a higher reaction-rate for any given dose calculated on body-weight in heavy patients than in lighter patients.— J. Koch-Weser *et al., Ann. intern. Med.*, 1970, *72*, 857.

ADMINISTRATION IN RENAL FAILURE. For reference to the precautions to be observed in renal failure, see under Administration in Renal Failure in Uses, below.

EFFECTS ON THE EAR. A solution of colistin applied directly into the middle ear of *guinea pigs* caused substantial sensory cell damage in the cochlea.— H. Stupp *et al., Audiology*, 1973, *12*, 350.

EFFECTS ON THE KIDNEY. Colistin sulphomethate sodium 26 million units daily was given to 14 severely ill patients with refractory *Klebsiella* chest and/or urinary-tract infections. Acute renal failure, sometimes with acute tubular necrosis, was evident in all patients, and contributed to the final cause of death in some of the 8 patients who died.— D. J. E. Price and D. I. Graham, *Br. med. J.*, 1970, *4*, 525. Criticisms.— E. Sproston and M. P. McConnell (letter), *ibid.*, 748.

Acute renal failure occurred in 4 patients given colistin sulphomethate sodium. All the patients had reduced glomerular filtration-rates and had either received cephalothin before, or concomitantly with, colistin sulphomethate sodium. It was recommended that dosage should be calculated from a measure of the glomerular filtration-rate rather than from body-weight.— S. Adler and D. P. Segel, *Am. J. med. Sci.*, 1971, *261*, 109.

EFFECTS ON THE NERVOUS SYSTEM. A 26-year-old woman with diabetes and renal failure developed a severe polyneuropathy which coincided with high blood concentrations of colistin sulphomethate sodium following daily doses of 1 million units and which resolved when treatment was discontinued.— J. F. Bridgman and S. M. Rosen (letter), *Br. med. J.*, 1971, *2*, 527. See also G. Richet *et al., ibid.*, 1970, *2*, 394.

EFFECTS ON THE NEUROMUSCULAR SYSTEM. Respiratory arrest occurred in a man with myasthenia gravis 2½ hours after he received an intramuscular injection of colistin sulphomethate sodium. Recovery of respiratory function took 11 days but other affected muscles improved after the intramuscular injection of neostigmine methylsulphate 2 mg and an intravenous injection of edrophonium chloride 10 mg.— D. A. Decker and R. W. Fincham, *Archs Neurol., Chicago*, 1971, *25*, 141.

A report of prolonged respiratory depression due to interaction of pancuronium bromide with colistin in one patient. A normal pattern of breathing was reinstated after 20 mL of a 10% solution of calcium gluconate was given in 2 divided doses.— M. M. Giala and A. G. Paradelis (letter), *J. antimicrob. Chemother.*, 1979, *5*, 234.

OVERDOSAGE. A 10-month-old boy developed acute renal failure after the accidental administration of an overdose of colistin sulphomethate. Two exchange transfusions were used successfully to remove colistin after peritoneal dialysis had failed. Renal function appeared to return to normal and no neurotoxicity was seen.— J. M. Brown *et al., Med. J. Aust.*, 1970, *2*, 923.

PORPHYRIA. Colistin was considered to be unsafe in patients with acute porphyria because it has been shown to be porphyrinogenic in *animals* or *in vitro* systems.— M.R. Moore and K.E.L. McColl, *Porphyrias, Drug Lists*, Glasgow, Porphyria Research Unit, University of Glasgow, 1987.

Antimicrobial Action and Resistance

The antimicrobial spectrum and mode of action of colistin is similar to that of polymyxin B (see p.290) but it is slightly less active.

The mean MIC of colistin against 6 isolates of the Legionnaires' disease bacterium was 72 units per mL.— C. Thornsberry *et al., Antimicrob. Ag. Chemother.*, 1978, *13*, 78.

Studies of the mode of action of colistin using *Mycobacterium aurum*.— H. L. David and N. Rastogi, *Antimicrob. Ag. Chemother.*, 1985, *27*, 701.

ACTIVITY WITH OTHER ANTIMICROBIAL AGENTS. In 19 of 20 strains of *Pseudomonas aeruginosa*, sulphamethoxazole and sulphamethizole enhanced the bactericidal effects of colistin.— N. A. Simmons and D. J. McGillicuddy, *Br. med. J.*, 1969, *3*, 693. Colistin and sulphamethoxazole were antagonistic *in vitro* when tested against *Ps. aeruginosa.* There was also some indication that carbenicillin and colistin were antagonistic.— A. C. Dalton and M. E. Plaut, *Am. J. med. Sci.*, 1971, *261*, 335. For a report of enhanced activity of colistin sulphomethate and co-trimoxazole against *Serratia marcescens*, see Uses, below.

A report of colistin diminishing the activity *in vitro* of amikacin against gentamicin-resistant strains of *Ps. aeruginosa*.— Y. Kobayashi, *Keio J. Med.*, 1976, *25*, 151.

Absorption and Fate

Colistin sulphate and colistin sulphomethate sodium are poorly absorbed from the gastro-intestinal tract. Peak plasma concentrations of colistin usually occur 2 to 3 hours after an intramuscular injection of the sulphomethate sodium. Detectable concentrations persist for about 8 hours. Half-lives of 2 to 5 hours have been reported for colistin sulphomethate sodium.

Colistin is mainly excreted by glomerular filtration and up to 80% of a parenteral dose of the sulphomethate sodium may be excreted in the urine within 8 hours. Excretion is more rapid in children than in adults; it is diminished in patients with impaired kidney function. Colistin diffuses across the placenta but diffusion into the cerebrospinal fluid is negligible except occasionally in infants. It has been detected in bile and in breast milk.

ADMINISTRATION IN RENAL FAILURE. Colistin sulphomethate was administered intramuscularly in a dose of 75 mg to 10 healthy persons and 8 patients with renal failure. The biological half-life was 4.8 hours in normal persons and 18 hours in patients with renal failure. A substantial change in drug distribution occurred as indicated by the smaller volume of distribution in the patients with renal failure.— M. Gibaldi and D. Perrier, *J. clin. Pharmac.*, 1972, *12*, 201.

See also under Uses, below.

PREGNANCY AND THE NEONATE. The biological half-life of colistin sulphomethate sodium was variously reported as 9 hours in newborn infants falling to 2.6 hours 3 or 4 days later and 2.3 to 2.6 hours (according to age) in premature infants.— W. A. Ritschel, *Drug Intell. & clin. Pharm.*, 1970, *4*, 332.

Uses and Administration

Colistin is a polymyxin antibiotic given by mouth, as the sulphate, for the treatment of intestinal infections due to susceptible micro-organisms and, usually in association with other antibiotics, for the suppression of bowel flora. The usual adult dose is 1.5 to 3 million units three times daily, although higher doses have been given. Children weighing up to 15 kg body-weight may be given 250 000 to 500 000 units three times daily and those weighing from 15 to 30 kg may be given 0.75 to 1.5 million units three times daily.

Colistin sulphate may also be applied topically as an ointment, powder, or solution in a concentration of 1%.

Colistin sulphomethate sodium is the form of colistin used for parenteral administration and has similar uses to polymyxin B sulphate (see p.290). The normal dose for adults is 6 million units daily in divided doses by intramuscular injection or intravenously by slow injection over 3 to 5 minutes or infusion. Infusions should be completed within 6 hours. Children may be given 50 000 units per kg body-weight daily in 3 divided doses. Doses should be reduced in renal impairment. Colistin sulphomethate sodium has been given intrathecally.

Colistin sulphomethate sodium is also given as an aerosol for respiratory infections in doses similar to those given by injection, and supplemented by parenteral administration. A solution of one million units in 50 mL of water or saline may be instilled into the bladder twice daily. In the treatment of eye infections it has been given by subconjunctival injection.

Co-trimoxazole and colistin sulphomethate showed enhanced activity against multiple drug-resistant strains of *Serratia marcescens*. Four of 6 patients with serious *Serratia* infections responded to treatment with 1.92 g of co-trimoxazole and 2 to 5 mg per kg body-weight of colistin sulphomethate daily.— F. E. Thomas *et al.*, *Antimicrob. Ag. Chemother.*, 1976, *9*, 201.

ADMINISTRATION IN RENAL FAILURE. The *UK* manufacturers have recommended that the dose of colistin sulphomethate sodium be reduced in patients with renal impairment according to the creatinine clearance. Patients with a creatinine clearance (CC) of 20 to 72 mL per minute should be given 1 to 2 million units every 8 hours; those with a CC of 10 to 20 mL per minute, 1 million units every 12 to 18 hours; and those with a CC of less than 10 mL per minute, 1 million units every 18 to 24 hours. Additional guidance by monitoring of blood concentrations is recommended; a concentration in the range of 10 to 15 μg per mL should be adequate.

Further references: J. R. Curtis and J. B. Eastwood, *Br. med. J.*, 1968, *1*, 484; N. J. Goodwin and E. A. Friedman, *Ann. intern. Med.*, 1968, *68*, 984; P. Sharpstone, *Br. med. J.*, 1977, *2*, 36.

CYSTIC FIBROSIS. Seven young patients with cystic fibrosis were treated with nebulised colistin sulphomethate sodium 500 000 units twice daily soon after *Pseudomonas* was first isolated from routine respiratory cultures. The results suggested that such therapy may reduce both the number of organisms isolated and also the frequency of isolation.— J. M. Littlewood *et al.* (letter), *Lancet*, 1985, *1*, 865.

In a double-blind placebo-controlled study, 20 cystic fibrosis patients with chronic bronchopulmonary infections caused by *Pseudomonas aeruginosa* were treated twice daily for 90 days with nebulised colistin sulphomethate sodium one million units. All patients had previously received a course of parenteral antipseudomonal antibiotics. Colistin inhalation appeared to reduce the deterioration in well-being and pulmonary function, and also to reduce the inflammatory response that otherwise occurs after a course of parenteral therapy. Resistance to colistin, or other antipseudomonal agents, or superinfection with colistin-resistant organisms was not observed. Bronchospasm was not reported.— T. Jensen *et al.*, *J. antimicrob. Chemother.*, 1987, *19*, 831.

SUPPRESSION OF INTESTINAL FLORA. Selective decontamination is a technique for the prevention of colonisation and infection in high-risk patients. It is achieved by elimination of aerobic, potentially pathogenic, organisms from throat and intestines whilst preserving the indigenous, mostly anaerobic, flora. Of many regimens tried, 3 have some value for the suppression of intestinal flora: non-absorbable gentamicin, vancomycin, and nystatin (GVN); non-absorbable framycetin, colistin, and nystatin (FRACON); and absorbable co-trimoxazole in association with non-absorbable colistin and amphotericin (SXTPAM). Neomycin may be substituted for framycetin in the FRACON regimen [NEOCON]. Several studies have demonstrated that these oral regimens reduce the incidence of infections, but not of febrile episodes. From the microbiological point of view, however, intestinal colonisation rates have remained high indicating incomplete flora elimination. Antimicrobial agents used for selective decontamination should fulfil the following criteria: they should be active against all Enterobacteriaceae, Pseudomonadaceae, and *Acinetobacter* spp., but not against the indigenous intestinal flora; they should have low MBCs for potentially pathogenic aerobes; they should be non-absorbable hence achieving high intraluminal concentrations; and they should show minimal inactivation by food and faecal compounds and no degradation by faecal enzymes. Colistin, gentamicin, and neomycin are moderately inactivated by faeces. Assessed by these four criteria, the GVN regimen may be considered neither selective nor effective, whilst FRACON and SXTPAM may be considered selective but not effective. Failure of these regimens to prevent infection, particularly pneumonia, may be due to poor elimination of oral flora.

An oral non-absorbable regimen of colistin, tobramycin, and amphotericin (PTA) has been applied to the buccal mucosa as a paste in carboxymethylcellulose and administered as a suspension via a nasogastric tube, both four times daily, in long-term ventilated patients. The regimen has been successful in virtually preventing pneumonia and septicaemia and its routine use over 5 years has resulted in only rare emergence of resistant organisms. A PTA regimen is also being studied for prevention of infection in bone-marrow transplantation patients.— H. K. F. Van Saene and C. P. Stoutenbeek, *J. antimicrob. Chemother.*, 1987, *20*, 462.

Report of a prospective study of 324 consecutive patients admitted over 16 months to an intensive therapy unit. Antibiotic prophylaxis was not given to the first 161 patients; the following 163 patients received a selective parenteral and enteral anti-sepsis regimen (SPEAR). This consisted of selective decontamination of the gastro-intestinal tract with colistin, tobramycin, and amphotericin [PTA] applied topically as a sticky ointment to the oropharynx and as a suspension via a nasogastric tube, and also systemic administration of cefotaxime 50 mg per kg body-weight daily. The group of patients given the SPEAR regimen showed a consistent reduction in colonisation of the gastro-intestinal tract with aerobic Gram-negative bacilli, and a substantial reduction in the incidence of acquired infection. Mortality in certain categories of patients such as those suffering from acute trauma was also reduced. It was emphasised that detailed and continuous microbiological surveillance designed to allow early detection of resistant strains must be an essential component of such a SPEAR regimen.— I. M. Ledingham *et al.*, *Lancet*, 1988, *1*, 785. In a discussion of SPEAR regimens it was considered that there is now good evidence that they can prevent infection and reduce mortality in selected groups of intensive care patients. The role of cefotaxime still needs proper analysis and the relevance of SPEAR to all intensive care patients and its impact on microbiology services needs to be assessed.— *ibid.*, 803.

Crohn's disease. In a study of 32 patients with active Crohn's disease, a regimen of an elemental diet and non-absorbable framycetin, colistin, and nystatin [FRACON], appeared to be as effective as conventional treatment with prednisolone by mouth as assessed by subjective and objective parameters of disease activity. However, five patients receiving the former regimen were not evaluated because of intolerance; this was mainly nausea and vomiting induced by the antibiotics.— S. Saverymuttu *et al.*, *Gut*, 1985, *26*, 994.

Preparations

Colistin Sulphomethate Injection *(B.P.)*. A sterile solution of colistin sulphomethate sodium, reconstituted in Sodium Chloride Intravenous Infusion.

Sterile Colistimethate Sodium *(U.S.P.)*. Colistin sulphomethate sodium suitable for parenteral use.

Colistin Tablets *(B.P.)*. Tablets containing colistin sulphate.

Colistin Sulfate for Oral Suspension *(U.S.P.)*. Reconstituted suspension has a pH of 5 to 6.

Colistin and Neomycin Sulfates and Hydrocortisone Acetate Otic Suspension *(U.S.P.)*. Sterile suspension of colistin sulphate, neomycin sulphate, and hydrocortisone acetate. pH 4.8 to 5.2.

Proprietary Preparations

Colomycin *(Pharmax, UK)*. *Tablets*, scored, colistin sulphate 1.5 million units.
Syrup, powder for reconstitution, colistin sulphate 250 000 units/5 mL when reconstituted with water.
Injection, powder for reconstitution, colistin sulphomethate sodium 0.5 and 1 million units.
Topical powder, sterile, colistin sulphate in vials of 1 g.

Proprietary Names and Manufacturers of Colistin Salts

Belcomycine *(Neth.)*; Colimicina *(UCB, Ital.; Syntex-Latino, Spain)*; Colimycin *(Lundbeck, Denm.; Lundbeck, Norw.)*; Colimycine *(Belg.; Bellon, Fr.; Neth.; Rhone-Poulenc, Switz.)*; Colomycin *(Pharmax, UK)*; Coly-Mycin M *(Warner, Austral.; Parke, Davis, Canad.; Parke, Davis, USA)*; Coly-Mycin S *(Parke, Davis, USA)*.

The following names have been used for multi-ingredient preparations containing colistin salts— Coly-Mycin Otic *(Warner, Austral.; Parke, Davis, Canad.)*; Coly-Mycin S Otic *(Parke, Davis, USA)*.

12612-v

Co-tetroxazine *(BAN)*.

A mixture of tetroxoprim and sulphadiazine in the proportion of 1:2.5.

CAS — 73173-12-3.

Co-tetroxazine has the general properties of co-trimoxazole (see p.206) and is used in the treatment of infections of the respiratory and urinary tracts. It is given by mouth in an initial dose of 700 mg (tetroxoprim 200 mg and sulphadiazine 500 mg), followed by 350 mg twice daily.

Studies of the absorption and fate of co-tetroxazine: H. Vergin *et al.*, *Int. J. clin. Pharmac. Ther. Toxic.*, 1981, *19*, 350 (pharmacokinetics in patients with chronic obstructive airway disease; comparison with co-trimoxazole); H. J. Peters *et al.*, *Int. J. clin. Pharmacol. Res.*, 1982, *2*, 259 (tissue diffusion in patients with benign prostatic hyperplasia).

Proprietary Names and Manufacturers

Sterinor *(Heumann, Ger.; ABC, Ital.)*; Tibirox *(Roche, Ger.; Roche, Switz.)*.

4902-z

Co-trifamole *(BAN)*.

CN-3123. A mixture of 5 parts of sulphamoxole and 1 part of trimethoprim.

Co-trifamole has similar actions and uses to co-trimoxazole (p.206). It is given by mouth in an initial dose of 960 mg (trimethoprim 160 mg and sulphamoxole 800 mg) followed by 480 mg every 12 hours. Lower doses may be necessary in patients with impaired renal function.

Proceedings of a symposium on co-trifamole.— Current Concepts in Antibacterial Chemotherapy Sulfamoxole/Trimethoprim (Co-trifamole), H. Knothe (Ed.), *International Congress and Symposium Series, No. 15*, London, The Royal Society of Medicine, 1980. See also: *Arzneimittel-Forsch.*, 1976, *26*, 596–683.

An unfavourable review of the use of co-trifamole for urinary-tract and respiratory-tract infections.— *Drug & Ther. Bull.*, 1983, *21*, 19.

Studies of the pharmacokinetics of sulphamoxole and trimethoprim after their administration together: J. Kuhne *et al.*, *Arzneimittel-Forsch.*, 1976, *26*, 651; J. K. Seydel and E. Wempe, *ibid.*, 1977, *27*, 1521; I. D. Watson *et al.*, *Br. J. clin. Pharmac.*, 1982, *14*, 437.

Studies of the antimicrobial activity of sulphamoxole-trimethoprim combinations: F. W. Kohlmann and H. Sous, *Arzneimittel-Forsch.*, 1976, *26*, 613; *idem*, 618; F. Legler, *ibid.*, 658; V. Hingst and H. -G. Sonntag, *Medsche Welt, Stuttg.*, 1979, *30*, 1199; R. N. Grüneberg, *Curr. med. Res. Opinion*, 1982, *8*, 128.

Proprietary Names and Manufacturers

Co-Fram *(Abbott, UK)*; Nevin *(Ger.)*; Supristol *(Gallier, Fr.; Ger.; Switz.)*; Sulmen *(Menarini, Ital.)*.

4903-c

Co-trimazine *(BAN)*.

A mixture of about 5 parts of sulphadiazine and 1 part of trimethoprim.

CAS — 39474-58-3.

Co-trimazine has similar actions and uses to co-trimoxazole (p.206). It has been given by mouth in a dose of 500 mg (trimethoprim 90 mg and sulphadiazine 410 mg) every 12 hours. Suggested doses of co-trimazine to be given to children twice daily are: 3 months to 5 years of age, 125 to 250 mg; 5 to 12 years, 250 to 500 mg. Lower doses may be necessary in patients with impaired renal function.

Proceedings of a symposium on trimethoprim-sulphonamide preparations including co-trimazine.— *Infection*, 1979, *7, Suppl.* 4, S309–S420.

A review of the clinical pharmacokinetics of co-trimazine, and comparison with co-trimoxazole.— T. Bergan *et al., Clin. Pharmacokinet.*, 1986, *11*, 372.

Clinical studies of the use of co-trimazine in the treatment of infections: P. Federspil and P. Bamberg, *J. int. med. Res.*, 1981, *9*, 478 (maxillary sinusitis); J. Aarbakke *et al., Eur. J. clin. Pharmac.*, 1983, *24*, 267 (acute urinary-tract infections in children); G. Leone *et al., J. int. med. Res.*, 1984, *12*, 1 (acute exacerbations of chronic bronchitis); J. Wallin *et al., Eur. J. sex. transm. Dis.*, 1984, *1*, 141 (gonorrhoea).

Proprietary Names and Manufacturers of Sulphadiazine/Trimethoprim Preparations

Adiprim *(Fin.)*; Antrima *(Théraplix, Fr.)*; Coptin *(Jouveinal, Canad.; Pfizer, UK)*; Kombinax *(Bracco, Ital.)*; Syntrizin *(Denm.)*; Triglobe *(Fr.; Astra, Ger.; Switz.)*; Trimin *(Astra, Swed.)*; Trobacter *(Spain)*.

4904-k

Co-trimoxazole *(BAN)*.

A mixture of 5 parts of sulphamethoxazole and 1 part of trimethoprim.

CAS — 8064-90-2.

The *B.P.* concentrate for intravenous infusion has a pH of 9.5 to 11.0 and is **sterilised** by autoclaving; the *U.S.P.* concentrate for infusion has a pH of 9.5 to 10.5. Preparations of co-trimoxazole should be **protected** from light.

A study indicating that co-trimoxazole injection (480 mg in 5 mL) may be diluted 1 ampoule to 125 mL (to give a concentration of co-trimoxazole 3.84 mg per mL) with either glucose 5% or sodium chloride 0.9% injections resulting in clear, colourless, and stable admixtures for up to 4 hours. If smaller dilutions are desired, such as 1 ampoule diluted to 50 mL (to give a concentration of 9.6 mg per mL), the preferred vehicle is glucose 5%, but the stability of this admixture is no longer than 2 hours. Dilutions of 1 ampoule to 25 mL (to give a concentration of 19.2 mg per mL) in either diluent result in obvious precipitation within 30 minutes. The solutions were stored in a volume-control set made of cellulose propionate and polyvinyl chloride at an ambient temperature of 21 to 23°.— L. J. Lesko *et al., Am. J. Hosp. Pharm.*, 1981, *38*, 1004. After storage in glass containers at ambient temperatures of 23 to 25°, co-trimoxazole injection was stable for at least 12 hours at dilutions of 3.84, 4.8, 6.4, and 9.6 mg per mL in all 5 intravenous fluids tested (glucose 5%, sodium chloride 0.45% and 0.9%, glucose 5% and sodium chloride 0.45%, and lactated Ringer's injection).— K. W. Deans *et al., ibid.*, 1982, *39*, 1681.

INCOMPATIBILITY. A transient precipitate was noted when verapamil hydrochloride and co-trimoxazole were added to infusions of sodium chloride 0.9% or glucose 5%. This may have been the result of a temporary, localised pH change at the point of mixing.— M. R. Cutie, *Am. J. Hosp. Pharm.*, 1983, *40*, 1205.

Adverse Effects and Treatment

As for Sulphamethoxazole, p.306, and Trimethoprim, p.328.

Hypersensitivity reactions particularly involving the skin are among the most common adverse effects caused by co-trimoxazole and are usually due to the sulphonamide component. The Stevens-Johnson and Lyell's syndromes have been reported in patients receiving co-trimoxazole. Adverse effects on the gastro-intestinal tract may also occur fairly frequently. The possiblity of blood dyscrasias like those associated with sulphonamides should be borne in mind.

A high incidence of adverse effects occurs in AIDS patients treated with high doses of co-trimoxazole. The adverse effects include skin rash, recurrent fever, neutropenia, thrombocytopenia, and raised liver enzyme values.

Analysis of reports of the early use of co-trimoxazole in 9909 patients showed gastro-intestinal side-effects in 3.3%, skin reactions in 1.5%, blood disorders in 0.8%, and other side-effects in 0.6%. Analysis of reports to the end of 1972 covered 37 914 patients estimated to cover 0.1% of the total use of co-trimoxazole. Excluding side-effects where it was not possible to assess the incidence, analysis showed gastro-intestinal side-effects in 2.9%, skin reactions in 1.32% (including exanthema, rash, erythema, urticaria, pruritus, allergic dermatitis, epidermal necrolysis—Lyell's syndrome, and erythema multiforme), blood disorders in 0.35% (including anaemia, leucopenia, neutropenia, granulocytopenia, thrombocytopenia, agranulocytosis, pancytopenia, and eosinophilia), and other side-effects in 0.48% (including headache, vertigo, renal complications, hepatic complications, sweating, weakness, insomnia, and allergic reactions). Severe side-effects were: megaloblastic anaemia (3 patients), haemolytic anaemia (1), agranulocytosis (5), pancytopenia (2), and Lyell's syndrome (2, one fatal).— L. Havas *et al., Roche, Clin. Trials J.*, 1973, *10* (3), 81.

Of the 29 524 medical in-patients monitored by the Boston Collaborative Drug Surveillance Program since 1966, 649 had received co-trimoxazole. Of these, 52 patients (8%) experienced adverse effects none of which was severe and all of which were reversible. The commonest side-effects were skin rashes in 23 patients (3.5%) and upper gastro-intestinal effects in 22 (3.4%); half occurred within 3 days of starting treatment. Adverse effects were more common in female patients (10.6%) than in males (4.8%). In no patient was a deterioration in renal function attributed to co-trimoxazole.— D. H. Lawson and H. Jick, *Am. J. med. Sci.*, 1978, *275*, 53.

In a follow-up study of 4828 children below 10 years of age who had received 1 or more prescriptions for oral co-trimoxazole between January 1979 and December 1981, none was subsequently admitted to hospital for any blood disorder or leukaemia. Among a subset of 2622 unselected children who received co-trimoxazole 66 (2.5%) had an adverse event which was attributed to the drug. Of these events 46 (70%) were rashes, 3 of which were described as erythema multiforme, and 15 (23%) were episodes of vomiting and/or diarrhoea. The remaining reactions were 1 each of the following: dizziness, headache, swollen lips, blue lips and hands, and constipation. In no case was the child admitted to hospital because of the adverse reaction, and in all cases there was rapid recovery after the drug was stopped. There were no reports of lowered white blood cell counts, nor of any other type of blood disorder.— S. S. Jick *et al.* (letter), *Lancet*, 1984, *2*, 631.

During the period 1973–81 there were 379 non-fatal adverse reactions to co-trimoxazole, mostly dermatological, reported to the New Zealand Committee on Adverse Drug Reactions. Other non-fatal reactions reported were anaphylaxis (4 cases), jaundice (4), and rash with blood-count depression (25). There were 11 fatal drug-associated cases, all in adults, including 4 severe skin reactions and 5 with an element of bone-marrow suppression. Co-trimoxazole was prescribed at a rate of approximately 600 000 prescriptions per year from 1978 to 1984 and the data suggested a rate of 1 fatal drug reaction per 600 000 prescriptions.— D. Lennon (letter), *Lancet*, 1984, *2*, 1152.

The Committee on Safety of Medicines (CSM) reported in 1985 on deaths associated with the use of co-trimoxazole and also with trimethoprim alone (*Current Problems Series No.15*). The 85 deaths associated with co-trimoxazole were predominantly due to blood dyscrasias (50 reports) and skin reactions (14 reports) and the 3 deaths attributed to trimethoprim were all due to blood dyscrasias. Further analysis of the fatal reports associated with co-trimoxazole showed a marked increase with age: below 40 years, there were 0.25 reported deaths per million prescriptions, but for patients over 65 years of age the number of reported deaths per million prescriptions was more than 15-fold greater. Experience with trimethoprim alone was considered to be too limited to enable firm conclusions to be drawn about its relative safety compared with that of co-trimoxazole. The CSM felt that it would be unwise to assume that trimethoprim is substantially less liable to cause fatal adverse reactions. However, Lacey *et al.* (*Br. med. J.*, 1985, *291*, 481) have commented that most of the deaths associated with the use of co-trimoxazole are typical of sulphonamide toxicity. They suggested that the indications for the use of co-trimoxazole should be reduced and that, from the data presented by the CSM, withdrawal of co-trimoxazole in the elderly seemed warranted. The CSM (A. Goldberg, *Br. med. J.*, 1985, *291*, 673) state that their main message is that the risks of treatment of co-trimoxazole are more apparent in the elderly, but that at present there is no significant difference between the numbers of reports received for serious adverse reactions to trimethoprim and co-trimoxazole when corrected for prescription volumes.

ALLERGY. Anaphylactic shock occurred in a 53-year-old woman 2 hours after taking co-trimoxazole 960 mg; she had taken co-trimoxazole 2 months previously which had been discontinued owing to development of a rash.— J. Dry *et al., Thérapie*, 1975, *30*, 705.

A patient developed fatal wide-spread reactions associated with co-trimoxazole and affecting skin, lungs, kidneys, liver, pancreas, and central nervous system with probable loss of central neural control of the heart.— J. Brøckner and E. Boisen (letter), *Lancet*, 1978, *1*, 831. A similar patient recovered after intensive treatment.— W. B. Finlayson and G. Johnson (letter), *ibid.*, 1978, *2*, 682.

A generalised allergic reaction followed by acute interstitial nephritis developed in a 16-month-old child after administration of co-trimoxazole.— M. J. Kraemer *et al., Ann. Allergy*, 1982, *49*, 323.

See also under Effects on the Kidney and Effects on the Skin, below.

EFFECTS ON THE BLOOD. Thrombocytopenia occurred in an 86-year-old woman who had been treated with allopurinol, dipyridamole 600 mg daily, and a 6-day course of co-trimoxazole. The thrombocytopenia was attributed to the combination of allopurinol and co-trimoxazole.— E. Raik and P. C. Vincent (letter), *Med. J. Aust.*, 1973, *2*, 468. Over 7 years the Australian Adverse Drug Reactions Registry received 31 reports of thrombocytopenia related to co-trimoxazole therapy. Of these 2 patients died, 26 recovered, and the outcome was unknown in 3.— H. G. Dickson, *ibid.*, 1978, *2*, 5. A further report of severe thrombocytopenia in 2 patients while taking co-trimoxazole; one patient died.— M. D. Hagen and R. D. White, *Sth. med. J.*, 1983, *76*, 503.

A 53-year-old woman developed red-cell hypoplasia after taking co-trimoxazole 960 mg twice daily for about 16 months.— M. E. M. Stephens, *Postgrad. med. J.*, 1974, *50*, 235.

A 4-year-old boy developed transient mild leucopenia 5 days after finishing a 14-day course of co-trimoxazole. Over the following 3 years he received another 4 courses of co-trimoxazole without adverse reactions but during the sixth course agranulocytosis developed after 8 days of therapy.— U. Lasson, *Dt. med. Wschr.*, 1977, *102*, 1287.

Acute pancytopenia due to megaloblastic arrest developed in 3 elderly patients during treatment with co-trimoxazole. Two of these patients died, one was also taking allopurinol, the other was taking digoxin, frusemide, and indomethacin in addition to co-trimoxazole and had previously received allopurinol, spironolactone, and lanatoside C.— E. A. Blackwell *et al., Med. J. Aust.*, 1978, *2*, 38. Comment.— I. S. Collins (letter), *ibid.*, 26. A further report of pancytopenia associated with co-trimoxazole therapy in an elderly patient.— C. E. Corallo and R. Martyres, *Aust. J. Hosp. Pharm.*, 1984, *14*, 12.

Haematological abnormalities occurred in 24 of 50 children (48%) treated with co-trimoxazole by mouth for 10 days in the management of acute otitis media or uncomplicated urinary-tract infections, compared with only 2 of 20 (10%) given amoxycillin. Neutropenia developed in 17 patients treated with co-trimoxazole; it was noted during the first week of treatment in 13 patients and at the end of treatment in the other 4. Thrombocytopenia, eosinophilia, and anaemia developed in 6, 7, and 3 of the children treated with co-trimoxazole, respectively.— B. I. Asmar *et al., Am. J. Dis. Child.*, 1981, *135*, 1100.

In 1985 the Committee on Safety of Medicines (CSM) received 19 reports of aplastic anaemia and 42 reports of depressed peripheral white cell counts associated with antimicrobial agents. Co-trimoxazole was suspected of causing blood dyscrasias in 9 cases and was one of the most commonly reported individual drugs causing these reactions.— *Br. med. J.*, 1986, *293*, 688.

See also under Immunocompromised Patients, below.

Haemolysis. A patient with glucose-6-phosphate dehydrogenase deficiency developed haemolysis during treatment with co-trimoxazole.— S. K. Owusu (letter), *Lancet*, 1972, *2*, 819.

No haemolysis was observed in 10 infants with glucose-6-phosphate dehydrogenase deficiency given co-trimoxazole. However, since haemolysis had been reported in similar patients, co-trimoxazole should be administered to such infants and children with care.— M. C. K. Chan and H. B. Wong (letter), *Lancet*, 1975, *1*, 410.

Megaloblastic anaemia. Co-trimoxazole was considered to be the main cause of megaloblastic anaemia in 4 of 112 patients studied over 2 years.— S. El Tamtamy (letter), *Lancet*, 1974, *1*, 929.

A report of megaloblastic anaemia in a patient taking co-trimoxazole daily and pyrimethamine 50 mg weekly.— A. F. Fleming *et al.* (letter), *Lancet*, 1974, *2*, 284. See also V. E. Ansdell *et al.* (letter), *ibid.*, 1976, *2*, 1257.

EFFECTS ON FERTILITY. After receiving co-trimoxazole for suspected seminal infections, reductions in sperm count of up to 88% were noted in 14 of 40 men attending a fertility clinic.— A. Murdia *et al.* (letter), *Lancet*, 1978, *2*, 375. The effect did not appear to be due to co-trimoxazole.— J. Guillebaud (letter), *ibid.*, 523.

EFFECTS ON THE GASTRO-INTESTINAL TRACT. Fatal pseudomembranous colitis occurred in an 80-year-old woman treated with co-trimoxazole for a urinary-tract infection after surgery for a fractured femur.— A. Cameron and M. Thomas, *Br. med. J.*, 1977, *1*, 1321.

Pseudomembranous colitis developed in 4 patients after they had received co-trimoxazole.— C. R. Pennington (letter), *New Engl. J. Med.*, 1980, *303*, 1533. Comment.— R. H. Rubin and M. N. Swartz (letter), *ibid.*, 1534.

A report of prolonged hiccups in a 14-year-old boy probably due to co-trimoxazole-induced oesophageal ulceration.— D. Seibert and F. Al-Kawas (letter), *Ann. intern. Med.*, 1986, *105*, 976.

EFFECTS ON THE KIDNEY. Deterioration in kidney function seen in 16 patients, most of whom had some pre-existing renal abnormality, was associated with the use of co-trimoxazole. Microscopic examination of tissue samples indicated acute tubular necrosis. Kidney damage in 3 of the patients was permanent and in 1 of these given a second course of treatment further irreversible damage occurred. It was recommended that co-trimoxazole should not be given to patients with a serum-creatinine concentration of more than 20 µg per mL.— S. Kalowski *et al.*, *Lancet*, 1973, *1*, 394.

Acute renal failure occurred in 2 patients given co-trimoxazole parenterally; one died. Both patients had hypoalbuminaemia reducing binding of sulphamethoxazole to plasma protein; competitive binding by penicillin and metronidazole, previously given, might also have contributed.— N. Buchanan, *Br. med. J.*, 1978, *2*, 172.

Reversible rise in plasma creatinine concentrations and reduction in creatinine clearance in 6 subjects with normal kidney function given co-trimoxazole 960 mg three times daily by mouth for 6 to 8 days.— D. Shouval *et al.*, *Lancet*, 1978, *1*, 244. Criticisms.— P. R. W. Tasker and H. E. de Wardener (letter), *ibid.*, 711; A. Bye and A. S. E. Fowle (letter), *ibid;* J. P. Guignard *et al.* (letter), *ibid.*, 712. Co-trimoxazole administered for 3 to 6 months to 16 children with normal renal function but with urinary-tract infection and/or vesico-ureteric reflux did not alter kidney function or interfere with renal function maturation.— J. -P. Guignard *et al.*, *Curr. ther. Res.*, 1983, *34*, 801.

A hypersensitivity rash and acute renal failure occurred together in 4 patients who received co-trimoxazole, 2 of whom were elderly and died. The dosage was inappropriately high in relation to the patients' renal function hence accumulation of sulphonamide could have been a contributing factor. Possibly co-trimoxazole should be avoided in the elderly. Trimethoprim alone might be adequate and preferable therapy for urinary-tract infections.— J. M. Richmond *et al.* (letter), *Lancet*, 1979, *1*, 493.

A report of interstitial nephritis attributed to co-trimoxazole.— D. Saltissi *et al.*, *Br. med. J.*, 1979, *1*, 1182.

Interstitial nephritis associated with co-trimoxazole in renal transplant recipients.— E. J. Smith *et al.*, *J. Am. med. Ass.*, 1980, *244*, 360.

See also Allergy, above.

EFFECTS ON THE LIVER. A patient accidentally given co-trimoxazole 7.68 g daily for 2.5 days (4 times the usual twice-daily dose) developed jaundice which persisted for 2.5 weeks; liver-function tests were normal 3 months later.— A. C. B. Wicks and T. J. Stamps (letter), *Br. med. J.*, 1970, *4*, 52.

A report of hepatic necrosis which resulted in the death of a patient who had been given co-trimoxazole.— C. F. Colucci and M. L. Cicero (letter), *J. Am. med. Ass.*, 1975, *233*, 952.

Jaundice occurred in a 54-year-old man after receiving co-trimoxazole for 7 days. Two months later he was inadvertently rechallenged with co-trimoxazole and developed cholestasis with jaundice and mild cytotoxic hepatic changes within 72 hours.— P. W. Thies and W. L. Dull, *Archs intern. Med.*, 1984, *144*, 1691.

Further references: S. S. Nair *et al.*, *Ann. intern. Med.*, 1980, *92*, 511; A. L. Ogilvie and P. J. Toghill, *Postgrad. med. J.*, 1980, *56*, 202; R. M. Oliver *et al.*, *Br. J. clin. Pract.*, 1987, *41*, 975.

EFFECTS ON MENTAL FUNCTION.

A report of psychosis manifesting as mutism and bizarre mannerisms in a 55-year-old man after receiving 6 doses of co-trimoxazole 1.44 g by intravenous infusion every 8 hours. The symptoms resolved within 24 hours of discontinuation of the drug.— L. A. Mermel *et al.*, *J. clin. Psychiat.*, 1986, *47*, 269.

EFFECTS ON THE NERVOUS SYSTEM. Aseptic meningitis occurred in a 30-year-old woman after treatment with co-trimoxazole had been started for a suspected urinary-tract infection. The symptoms cleared spontaneously and completely within 2 days of withdrawal of the drug, but reappeared on rechallenge with co-trimoxazole.— I. Kremer *et al.* (letter), *New Engl. J. Med.*, 1983, *308*, 1481. A similar report.— E. J. Haas (letter), *J. Am. med. Ass.*, 1984, *252*, 346.

A report of 2 cases of severe reversible ataxia that developed during intravenous co-trimoxazole therapy for *Pneumocystis carinii* pneumonia.— L. X. Liu *et al.* (letter), *Ann. intern. Med.*, 1986, *104*, 448.

EFFECTS ON THE PANCREAS. A report of acute pancreatitis with the occurrence of abdominal symptoms in a 33-year-old man during treatment with co-trimoxazole for a brain abscess. The symptoms recurred on rechallenge.— D. R. Antonow, *Ann. intern. Med.*, 1986, *104*, 363.

EFFECTS ON THE SKIN. A report of 2 patients with fixed drug eruptions of the genitals associated with the use of co-trimoxazole.— M. D. Talbot, *Practitioner*, 1980, *224*, 823. See also J. Amir *et al.*, *Drug Intell. & clin. Pharm.*, 1987, *21*, 41.

Drug-induced toxic epidermal necrolysis associated with co-trimoxazole in 3 patients.— J. -C. Roujeau *et al.*, *Lancet*, 1985, *1*, 609.

Co-trimoxazole was one of the drugs most commonly reported to the Australian Drug Reactions Advisory Committee as causing photosensitivity reactions. During the period from November 1972 to March 1984 there were 39 such reports.— K. Stone, *Aust. J. Pharm.*, 1985, *66*, 415.

A generalised pustular dermatosis occurred in 4 patients during treatment with co-trimoxazole by mouth and resolved spontaneously when the drug was stopped.— K. J. S. MacDonald *et al.*, *Br. med. J.*, 1986, *293*, 1279.

Analysis, by the Boston Collaborative Drug Surveillance Program, of data on 15 438 patients hospitalised between 1975 and 1982 detected 36 allergic skin reactions attributed to co-trimoxazole among 1066 recipients of the drug. For the purposes of the study, reactions were defined as being generalised morbilliform exanthems, urticaria, or generalised pruritus only.— M. Bigby *et al.*, *J. Am. med. Ass.*, 1986, *256*, 3358.

Stevens-Johnson syndrome. Twenty-eight cases of Stevens-Johnson syndrome have been reported in patients who had taken co-trimoxazole and 11 cases of erythema multiforme have been reported. The aetiological role of viral, bacterial and mycoplasmal infections and of sulphonamides and other antibacterial drugs made it difficult to establish the precise causative factor in any individual case.— L. S. Berstein and J. Cooper (letter), *Lancet*, 1978, *1*, 988.

A clear case of Stevens-Johnson syndrome in a 44-year-old woman after receiving co-trimoxazole for a urinary infection.— S. Kikuchi and T. Okazaki (letter), *Lancet*, 1978, *2*, 580.

Further reports of the Stevens-Johnson syndrome following treatment with co-trimoxazole.— J. A. C. Thorpe and A. Nysenbaum (letter), *Lancet*, 1978, *1*, 276.

IMMUNOCOMPROMISED PATIENTS. An extraordinarily high frequency of adverse reactions to co-trimoxazole has been reported in patients with AIDS being treated for *Pneumocystis carinii* pneumonia. Masur (*Ann. intern. Med.*, 1984, *100*, 92) commented that, when therapeutic doses of co-trimoxazole are used, hypersensitivity rashes and leucopenia each develop in 30% of patients compared to less than 5% for each complication in patients without AIDS. Higher incidences have been reported for skin rashes which may develop 1 to 9 days after initiation of therapy with co-trimoxazole. Adverse reactions also appear to be unusually frequent when prophylactic doses are used (R. Mitsuyasu *et al.*, *New Engl. J. Med.*, 1983, *308*, 1535). Other adverse effects include recurrent fevers and increasing malaise, nausea, and headache (H.S. Jaffe *et al.*, *Lancet*, 1983, *2*, 1109).

The occurrence of high serum concentrations of sulphamethoxazole in AIDS patients has been proposed as a contributing factor to the high incidence of adverse effects. However, McLean *et al.* (*Lancet*, 1987, *2*, 857) demonstrated no difference in the frequency of side-effects when the sulphamethoxazole dose was modified.

A lower frequency of cutaneous reactions has been reported among African, Haitian, and American black AIDS patients compared with white AIDS patients suggesting a genetic susceptibility for such reactions (R. Colebunders *et al.*, *Ann. intern. Med.*, 1987, *107*, 599).

Some workers have used diphenhydramine alone or with adrenaline to manage hypersensitivity reactions associated with co-trimoxazole therapy thus allowing continuation of treatment (R.B. Gibbons and J.A. Lindauer, *J. Am. med. Ass.*, 1985, *253*, 1259) and other workers have tried desensitisation to co-trimoxazole in a patient with AIDS (R.M. Smith *et al.*, *Ann. intern. Med.*, 1987, *106*, 335).

For comparison of the toxicity associated with co-trimoxazole and pentamidine in the treatment of *Pneumocystis carinii* pneumonia in AIDS patients, see under pentamidine (p.675).

In a double-blind placebo-controlled crossover study of 37 children with acute lymphocytic leukaemia, co-trimoxazole 900 mg per m^2 body-surface daily by mouth administered prophylactically for about 6 months was found to be an effective prophylactic antibacterial agent. However, there were significant reductions in the mean white blood cell count, absolute neutrophil count, absolute lymphocyte count, and platelet count during the 6 months of co-trimoxazole administration compared with the 6-month placebo period. It was considered that the myelosuppression associated with co-trimoxazole prophylaxis could potentially hamper the administration of maintenance cancer chemotherapy.— W. G. Woods *et al.*, *J. Pediat.*, 1984, *105*, 639.

Reports of aplasia associated with co-trimoxazole administration in children with acute leukaemia: H. C. Drysdale and L. F. Jones (letter), *Lancet*, 1982, *1*, 448; C. E. M. Unter and G. D. Abbott, *Archs Dis. Childh.*, 1987, *62*, 85.

Precautions

As for Sulphamethoxazole, p.307 and Trimethoprim, p.328.

Co-trimoxazole should not be given to patients with a history of sensitivity to it or to the sulphonamides or trimethoprim. Because of possible interference with human folate metabolism by trimethoprim, co-trimoxazole should be given with caution to patients with actual or possible folate deficiency. Its use should be avoided during pregnancy. Co-trimoxazole should also be used with caution in patients receiving pyrimethamine. Care should be taken in immunocompromised patients such as those suffering from AIDS or patients receiving immunosuppressive therapy. Adverse effects on the blood may be more severe in malnourished or elderly patients; there also appears to be an increased risk of thrombocytopenia in elderly patients concurrently receiving diuretics, mainly thiazides. All patients receiving prolonged treatment with co-trimoxazole should be given regular blood examinations.

Co-trimoxazole should be used cautiously and in reduced dosage in patients with impaired renal function. Because of the risk of crystalluria, an adequate fluid intake should be maintained and the administration of alkalis may be necessary if very large doses are used.

The absorptions of trimethoprim and sulphamethoxazole (taken as co-trimoxazole) were increased in patients with coeliac disease, small bowel diverticulosis, or Crohn's disease. There was a disproportionate increase in the plasma concentrations of trimethoprim in patients with coeliac disease or diverticulosis and peak plasma concentrations of sulphamethoxazole in patients with Crohn's disease were increased about threefold. Mean peak plasma concentrations of co-trimoxazole were reduced in healthy subjects when they also took cholestyramine.— R. L. Parsons and G. M. Paddock, *J. antimicrob. Chemother.*, 1975, *1*, *Suppl.* (Sept.), 59.

Two patients had reduced survival of transfused platelets while taking co-trimoxazole; a third patient developed thrombocytopenia. Serum from the 3 patients contained antibodies against donor platelets incubated with co-trimoxazole; the effect was against the trimethoprim component. Since co-trimoxazole is used for treatment and prophylaxis of infections in leukaemia its effect on platelets is of great importance.— F. H. J. Claas *et al.*, *Br. med. J.*, 1979, *2*, 898.

The incidences and duration of neutropenia and thrombocytopenia in 6 renal allograft recipients who received azathioprine and long-term prophylaxis (22 days or more) with co-trimoxazole were greater than in 25 similar patients who received azathioprine alone. In a further 9 patients who received azathioprine and treatment with co-trimoxazole (6 to 16 days) the incidences were not different to those in patients receiving azathioprine alone.— P. P. Bradley *et al.*, *Ann. intern. Med.*, 1980, *93*, 560.

In healthy subjects co-trimoxazole 960 mg twice daily for 10 days caused a significant reduction in free thyroxine index and in serum concentrations of thyroxine and tri-iodothyronine but did not significantly affect concentrations of thyroid-stimulating hormone. Although it could not be concluded that co-trimoxazole causes hypothyroidism it was suggested that tests of thyroid function should be interpreted with caution in patients on such treatment and that those on long-term therapy should have their thyroid function regularly assessed.— H. N. Cohen *et al.*, *Br. med. J.*, 1980, *281*, 646. Findings suggesting that trimethoprim does not have significant antithyroid activity, supporting the view that the sulphonamide component is responsible for the lowering of the thyroid hormone concentrations observed previously.— *idem* (letter), *Lancet*, 1981, *1*, 676.

For comments on an increased incidence of adverse effects associated with co-trimoxazole administration in patients with AIDS, and the problems associated with myelosuppression due to co-trimoxazole prophylaxis in children with acute leukaemia, see under Immunocompromised Patients in Adverse Effects, above.

INTERACTIONS. Co-trimoxazole has been reported to interact with several drugs often by inhibiting their metabolism: drugs which may have enhanced activity when administered with co-trimoxazole include anticoagulants (see Warfarin Sodium, p.345), antiepileptics (see Phenytoin Sodium, p.409), and sulphonylurea antidiabetic agents (see Chlorpropamide, p.388). Co-trimoxazole has also been reported to interact with some antineoplastic agents causing increased toxicity (see Methotrexate, pp.637-8). Intravenous co-trimoxazole formulated with alcohol may cause a disulfiram-like reaction with drugs such as metronidazole (see p.667).

For reports of interactions between trimethoprim and various drugs, see under Trimethoprim, p.329.

INTERFERENCE WITH DIAGNOSTIC TESTS. Co-trimoxazole administered by mouth interfered with measurements of plasma-urea concentrations using a reagent strip method based on the reaction of amides with *o*-phthalaldehyde. It was considered that the sulphamethoxazole component of co-trimoxazole was responsible for the interaction.— J. Gregory and E. Lester (letter), *Lancet*, 1982, *2*, 443.

Antimicrobial Action

The two components of co-trimoxazole interfere with the bacterial synthesis of tetrahydrofolic acid, an essential stage in the production of thymidine, purines, and subsequently nucleic acids. Enhanced antibacterial activity has been reported when sulphamethoxazole and trimethoprim are used together *in vitro* although there is doubt as to whether sequential blockade of the bacterial synthetic pathway is responsible. The clinical relevance of this enhanced activity is uncertain especially in urinary-tract infections where inhibitory concentrations of trimethoprim appear to be dominant.

Co-trimoxazole has a wide spectrum of activity similar to that of sulphamethoxazole (p.307) and trimethoprim (p.329). It is also active against *Pneumocystis carinii*.

When testing for the antimicrobial activity of co-trimoxazole *in vitro*, the culture media should be free of thymine and thymidine, specific antagonists for trimethoprim.

Observations that sulphonamides can be moderately potent inhibitors of bacterial dihydrofolate reductase led to the hypothesis that multiple simultaneous inhibition of the enzyme might be responsible for the enhanced activity seen *in vitro* with sulphonamides and trimethoprim rather than sequential inhibition.— M. Poe, *Science*, 1976, *194*, 533. The suggestion that sulphonamides and trimethoprim bind simultaneously to dihydrofolate reductase is not an adequate explanation of the synergistic inhibition of growth of *Escherichia coli* organisms observed.— J. J. Burchall, *Wellcome*, *ibid.*, 1977, *197*, 1300. Further criticism.— R. Then, *Roche, Switz.*, *ibid.*, 1301. Reply.— M. Poe, *ibid.* Agreement with the hypothesis of Poe. Although there may be enhanced activity with sulphamethoxazole and trimethoprim under defined conditions *in vitro*, synergy *in vivo* is only likely to occur where the local concentration of trimethoprim is sub-inhibitory.— R. W. Lacey, *J. antimicrob. Chemother.*, 1979, *5*, *Suppl.* B, 75.

Using an *in vitro* model of an infected urinary bladder and concentrations of sulphamethoxazole and trimethoprim well within those achievable therapeutically in urine, the presence of sulphonamide had no influence on the inhibitory activity of trimethoprim against *Escherichia coli*.— D. Greenwood, *J. antimicrob. Chemother.*, 1979, *5*, *Suppl.* B, 85. Similar findings.— J. D. Anderson *et al.*, *J. clin. Path.*, 1974, *27*, 619.

Further references on the rationale for combining sulphonamides with trimethoprim: R. N. Grüneberg, *J. antimicrob. Chemother.*, 1979, *5*, *Suppl.* B, 27.

References to the activity of co-trimoxazole against various micro-organisms: C. U. Tuazon *et al.*, *Antimicrob. Ag. Chemother.*, 1982, *21*, 525 (*Listeria monocytogenes*); A. C. Rodloff, *J. antimicrob. Chemother.*, 1982, *9*, 195 (nontuberculous mycobacteria); T. J. Walsh *et al.*, *ibid.*, 1985, *15*, 435 (methicillin-resistant *Staphylococcus aureus*; see also under Resistance); J. Bosch *et al.*, *ibid.*, 1986, *17*, 459 (*Brucella melitensis*).

ACTIVITY AGAINST ANAEROBIC ORGANISMS. There is some disagreement regarding the efficacy of co-trimoxazole *in vitro* against bacteria of the *Bacteroides fragilis* group. Some workers have demonstrated that co-trimoxazole is relatively inactive against this group of bacteria as well as other anaerobes (J.E. Rosenblatt and P.R. Stewart, *Antimicrob. Ag. Chemother.*, 1974, *6*, 93) whereas others have demonstrated promising activity *in vitro* against *B. fragilis* isolates and some other anaerobes (J. Wüst and T.D. Wilkins, *ibid.*, 1978, *14*, 384). The disparity in results probably reflects variations in the choice of media, inoculum size, and time of incubation (T.V. Riley, *ibid.*, 1981, *20*, 731; G.L. Jackson-York *et al. J. antimicrob. Chemother.*, 1983, *12*, 515). The ratio of the trimethoprim and sulphamethoxazole also affects activity; synergy has been shown to be more marked when the ratio of the 2 components is nearer 1:1 (R.L. Then and P. Angehrn, *Antimicrob. Ag. Chemother.*, 1979, *15*, 1).

ACTIVITY AGAINST BRANHAMELLA. All of 54 clinical isolates of *Branhamella catarrhalis* were resistant to trimethoprim, but were susceptible to co-trimoxazole. For trimethoprim, the minimum inhibitory concentration for 90% of the organisms, both beta-lactamase positive and negative strains, was 32 μg per mL, whereas for co-trimoxazole it was 8.0 and 4.0 μg per mL, respectively.— F. Ahmad *et al.*, *Antimicrob. Ag. Chemother.*, 1984, *26*, 424. See also K. G. Sweeney *et al.*, *ibid.*, 1985, *27*, 499.

ACTIVITY AGAINST CHLAMYDIA. Synergy was demonstrated *in vitro* between trimethoprim and sulphamethoxazole against *Chlamydia trachomatis*. The lowest inhibitory combinations were achieved with trimethoprim present at 2 μg per mL and sulphamethoxazole at 0.5 μg per mL (a ratio of 4:1), or trimethoprim 8 μg per mL and sulphamethoxazole 0.125 μg per mL (64:1). It is possible that previous investigators have not detected antichlamydial synergy between these 2 agents because sulphamethoxazole, which has the lower minimum inhibitory concentration, has predominated over trimethoprim and masked its effect.— S. J. How *et al.*, *J. antimicrob. Chemother.*, 1985, *15*, 533. See also M. R. Hammerschlag and J. C. Vuletin, *ibid.*, 209.

ACTIVITY AGAINST ENTEROPATHOGENS. A study of the activities *in vitro* of 10 antimicrobial agents against 243 bacterial enteropathogens including *Salmonella* and *Shigella* spp., enterotoxigenic *Escherichia coli, Yersinia enterocolitica, Aeromonas hydrophila, Plesiomonas shigelloides, Vibrio parahaemolyticus*, and *Campylobacter jejuni*. Trimethoprim and co-trimoxazole were inhibitory against all test strains except *C. jejuni* isolates. Minimum inhibitory concentrations for 90% of the susceptible organisms ranged from 0.5 μg or less per mL to 2 μg per mL for trimethoprim and 1 to 8 μg per mL for co-trimoxazole, although 32 μg of co-trimoxazole per mL was required to inhibit 90% of *Y. enterocolitica* strains. For *C. jejuni* concentrations of both antibiotics of 128 μg per mL were required to inhibit 50% of organisms.— J. R. Carlson *et al.*, *Antimicrob. Ag. Chemother.*, 1983, *24*, 509. See also P. L. Turgeon *et al.*, *Curr. ther. Res.*, 1987, *41*, 584.

Further references to the activity of co-trimoxazole against Enterobacteriaceae and other enteropathogens: S. Hammerberg *et al.*, *Antimicrob. Ag. Chemother.*, 1977, *11*, 566 (*Yersinia enterocolitica*); J. W. Paisley and J. A. Washington, *ibid.*, 1978, *14*, 656 (activity with gentamicin against *Escherichia coli* and *Klebsiella pneumoniae*); A. P. Panwalker *et al.*, *ibid.*, 1980, *18*, 877 (*Klebsiella* spp.); J. F. Reinhardt and W. L. George, *ibid.*, 1985, *27*, 643 (*Aeromonas* spp. and *Plesiomonas shigelloides*); M. R. Motyl *et al.*, *ibid.*, *28*, 151 (*Aeromonas* spp.).

Enterococci. Although Crider and Colby (*Antimicrob. Ag. Chemother.*, 1985, *27*, 71) reported that, in certain media, co-trimoxazole was bactericidal at low concentrations against enterococci, other reports have raised questions about the clinical application of this observation (M.J. Zervos and D.R. Schaberg, *ibid.*, *28*, 446). Investigation of the activity of co-trimoxazole *in vitro* against 20 strains of *Streptococcus faecalis* [*Enterococcus faecalis*] failed to demonstrate a consistent bactericidal effect. Minimum inhibitory concentrations for all strains were 0.5 μg or less per mL, but although some bactericidal activity was seen, the majority of tests showed minimum bactericidal concentrations of greater than 32 μg per mL; results were affected by varying the inoculum size and the length of incubation after subculturing.— A. Najjar and B. E. Murray, *Antimicrob. Ag. Chemother.*, 1987, *31*, 808.

ACTIVITY AGAINST GONOCOCCI. Trimethoprim or sulphamethoxazole lacked antibacterial activity against 10 isolates of penicillin-resistant *Neisseria gonorrhoeae* when either was used alone but inhibitory concentrations as low as 0.31 μg per mL for trimethoprim and 5.9 μg per mL for sulphamethoxazole were achieved when they were used in combination.— T. T. Yoshikawa and S. A. Shibata (letter), *J. antimicrob. Chemother.*, 1979, *5*, 618.

In a study using 168 strains of *Neisseria gonorrhoeae*, enhanced activity for sulphamethoxazole and trimethoprim was greatest when the 2 agents were used in the ratio 1:1. Enhanced activity was minimal and antagonism sometimes occurred when they were used together in the ratio usually achievable in serum after administration by mouth (19:1).— M. F. Rein *et al.*, *Antimicrob. Ag. Chemother.*, 1980, *17*, 247.

Further references: R. Widy-Wirski *et al.*, *Bull. Wld Hlth Org.*, 1982, *60*, 959.

ACTIVITY AGAINST HAEMOPHILUS. A report of enhanced activity *in vitro* with trimethoprim and sulphamethoxazole (ratio 1:20) against *Haemophilus influenzae*, including ampicillin-resistant strains.— S. Pelton *et al.*, *Antimicrob. Ag. Chemother.*, 1977, *12*, 649.

During an outbreak of chancroid in California 37 of 41 isolates of *Haemophilus ducreyi* showed resistance to both sulphamethoxazole and tetracycline, but susceptibility to erythromycin and co-trimoxazole.— C. A. Blackmore *et al.*, *J. infect. Dis.*, 1985, *151*, 840.

Further references to the activity of co-trimoxazole against *Haemophilus* spp.: R. Sinai *et al.*, *Antimicrob. Ag. Chemother.*, 1978, *13*, 861 (*Haemophilus influenzae*).

ACTIVITY AGAINST LEGIONELLA. Sulphamethoxazole-trimethoprim had an MIC of 4.8-0.25 μg per mL against 6 isolates of the legionnaires' disease bacterium.— C. Thornsberry *et al.*, *Antimicrob. Ag. Chemother.*, 1978, *13*, 78.

Activity of co-trimoxazole against *Legionella micdadei* pneumonia in *guinea-pigs*.— A. W. Pasculle *et al.*, *Antimicrob. Ag. Chemother.*, 1985, *28*, 730.

ACTIVITY AGAINST NOCARDIA. A study *in vitro* suggested that fixed-dose commercial combinations of trimethoprim and sulphamethoxazole contained too little trimethoprim for optimum activity against isolates of *Nocardia*.— J. E. Bennett and A. E. Jennings, *Antimicrob. Ag. Chemother.*, 1978, *13*, 624.

Twenty-six clinical isolates of *Nocardia asteroides* showed moderate resistance to co-trimoxazole; the minimum inhibitory concentration for 90% of the organisms was 8 to 160 μg per mL.— M. E. Gombert, *Antimicrob. Ag. Chemother.*, 1982, *21*, 1011.

ACTIVITY AGAINST PSEUDOMONAS. All of 82 strains of *Pseudomonas aeruginosa* were resistant to trimethoprim and sulphamethoxazole when tested alone and together using a disk containing trimethoprim and sulphamethoxazole in the conventional ratio of 1:19. However, marked enhanced activity was demonstrated with trimethoprim and sulphamethoxazole against 22 strains of moderately-resistant *Ps. aeruginosa* in agar-plate dilution tests. Mean MICs were: trimethoprim 108 μg per mL, sulphamethoxazole 227 μg per mL, and trimethoprim with sulphamethoxazole 11.4-16.4 μg per mL. The MICs for the combination are well within concentrations achieved in urine and are also in a similar ratio. A disk containing trimethoprim and sulphamethoxazole in the ratio of 1:2 should be used for sensitivity testing of urinary isolates.— D. Grey and J. M. T. Hamilton-Miller, *J. med. Microbiol.*, 1977, *10*, 273.

All of 14 isolates of *Pseudomonas maltophilia* were susceptible *in vitro* to trimethoprim 0.09 μg per mL-sulphamethoxazole 1.78 μg per mL with a median MIC of 0.5-0.89 μg per mL. Enhanced activity was obtained against 12 of the strains when trimethoprim-sulphamethoxazole were used with carbenicillin.— T. P. Felegie *et al.*, *Antimicrob. Ag. Chemother.*, 1979, *16*, 833.

All of 20 clinical isolates of *Pseudomonas paucimobilis* were sensitive to co-trimoxazole; minimum inhibitory concentrations ranged from 0.5 to 9.5 μg per mL.— D.

L. Smalley *et al.*, *Antimicrob. Ag. Chemother.*, 1983, *23*, 161.

Of 104 nosocomial strains of *Pseudomonas cepacia* 96 (92.3%) were inhibited by 16 μg per mL.— M. O. S. Ferreira *et al.*, *J. int. med. Res.*, 1985, *13*, 270.

SENSITIVITY TESTING. A recommendation that disks for sensitivity testing of urinary isolates should contain trimethoprim and sulphamethoxazole in the ratio of 1:2.— D. Grey and J. M. T. Hamilton-Miller, *J. med. Microbiol.*, 1977, *10*, 273.

A study *in vitro* indicated that the use of thymine-free and thymidine-free agar might not give a realistic assessment of the activity *in vivo* of sulphamethoxazole and trimethoprim since thymidine may possibly be present in the urine of patients.— A. Stokes and R. W. Lacey, *J. clin. Path.*, 1978, *31*, 165. A comment that sensitivity testing using thymidine-free media is an adequate guide to treatment.— R. Maskell and O. A. Okubadejo (letter), *ibid.*, 808.

A discussion on sources of error in the determination of sensitivity to co-trimoxazole and its components.— J. M. T. Hamilton-Miller, *J. antimicrob. Chemother.*, 1979, *5*, *Suppl.* B, 61.

Resistance

Resistance of bacteria to sulphonamides, including sulphamethoxazole (see p.307), is common. Resistance has also been reported with trimethoprim (see p.329).

A report of thymine-requiring bacteria occurring in the urine or sputum of patients who had received co-trimoxazole for several months. Thymine-like compounds were present in the urine from which the mutant strains were isolated.— R. Maskell *et al.*, *Lancet*, 1976, *1*, 834. A further report of the isolation of thymine-requiring mutant bacteria resistant to trimethoprim.— O. A. Okubadejo and R. Maskell (letter), *ibid.*, 1977, *2*, 926. See also J. J. Plorde and T. Bailey (letter), *Ann. intern. Med.*, 1979, *91*, 134. See also under Sensitivity Testing in Antimicrobial Action, above.

Emergence of resistance to trimethoprim was monitored in 30 patients with chronic urinary-tract infections who received long-term low dosage treatment with co-trimoxazole over a period of up to 5 years. About 5% of the isolates examined were found to carry plasmids conferring transferable resistance to trimethoprim and about 17% had a resistance to trimethoprim of a non-transferable type.— K. J. Towner *et al.*, *J. antimicrob. Chemother.*, 1979, *5*, 45.

An outbreak of plasmid-mediated trimethoprim resistance in coliform bacilli was related to prior exposure to co-trimoxazole, sulphonamides, and ampicillin.— R. N. Grüneberg and M. J. Bendall, *Br. med. J.*, 1979, *2*, 7.

In a study of 41 children with acute lymphoblastic leukaemia who received infection prophylaxis with co-trimoxazole, 25 (61%) were found to be excreting trimethoprim-resistant bacteria in their faeces. In contrast only 79 of 568 (14%) control children who were not receiving co-trimoxazole were excreting resistant bacteria. *Escherichia coli* was the predominant resistant isolate in both groups. Co-trimoxazole also apparently coselected for resistance to sulphonamides as 24 (96%) of the trimethoprim-resistant bacteria isolated from the study group were also resistant to sulphamethoxazole, whereas 65 (82%) of those obtained from the control group were similarly resistant.— H. P. McDowell *et al.*, *Archs Dis. Childh.*, 1987, *62*, 573.

For discussion of the selection of resistance to trimethoprim with the use of co-trimoxazole or trimethoprim, see under Trimethoprim, p.329.

RESISTANCE OF ENTEROBACTERIACEAE. Reports of the development of resistance to co-trimoxazole in Enterobacteriaceae, during oral prophylactic therapy with co-trimoxazole, in patients with acute leukaemia.— J. M. Wilson and D. G. Guiney, *New Engl. J. Med.*, 1982, *306*, 16; O. -P. Lehtonen and T. -T. Pelliniemi (letter), *ibid.*, *307*, 60. A similar report of the emergence of high-level trimethoprim resistance in faecal *Escherichia coli* during oral administration of trimethoprim or co-trimoxazole given to healthy subjects for the prevention of diarrhoea.— B. E. Murray *et al.*, *ibid.*, *306*, 130.

For further reports of the development of resistance to trimethoprim in Enterobacteriaceae in patients treated with co-trimoxazole, see under Trimethoprim, p.330. See also above.

A report of high levels of co-trimoxazole resistance in Enterobacteriaceae isolates from Jamaica. Similar high levels of co-trimoxazole resistance have been reported in *Escherichia coli* isolates from Chile, Thailand, Brazil, Honduras, and Costa Rica (B.E. Murray *et al.*, *J. infect. Dis.*, 1985, *152*, 1107). It has been suggested that free availability of co-trimoxazole and the high incidence of diarrhoeal disease in developing countries may be to blame for increased resistance to co-trimoxazole. In Jamaica, this antimicrobial cannot be obtained without a doctor's prescription, however, profligate use of co-trimoxazole for respiratory, urinary, and gastro-intestinal tract infections together with poor sanitation allowing frequent faecal-oral transmission of coliforms with transferable resistance determinants may explain the high levels of resistance in Jamaica.— D. E. MacFarlane (letter), *Lancet*, 1986, *1*, 923.

Salmonellae. *Salmonella typhi* in the bowel of a patient with enteric fever treated with chloramphenicol and co-trimoxazole acquired resistance to these drugs.— N. Datta *et al.*, *Lancet*, 1981, *1*, 1181.

Plasmid-mediated resistance to co-trimoxazole in *Salmonella krefeld* strains isolated in the United States.— J. J. Mathewson and B. E. Murray, *Antimicrob. Ag. Chemother.*, 1983, *23*, 495.

Shigellae. A report of the rapid acquisition of trimethoprim resistance in an epidemic strain of *Shigella dysenteriae* type 1 in Zaire. The causative strain was resistant to ampicillin, chloramphenicol, tetracyclines, streptomycin, and sulphonamides and so during the summer of 1981 co-trimoxazole was introduced for treatment. However, by September strains resistant to trimethoprim were being isolated with increasing regularity. It appeared that the original strain acquired a plasmid, possibly from a non-pathogenic organism resistant to trimethoprim which was already present in the population.— J. A. Frost *et al.* (letter), *Lancet*, 1982, *1*, 963.

Of 80 clinical strains of *Shigella sonnei* isolated in a hospital in Spain, 71 (89%) were resistant to trimethoprim and 80 (100%) to sulphamethoxazole. Co-trimoxazole is so widely used in Spain that it would seem reasonable to assume that this high consumption would play a role in the high incidence reported.— E. Palenque *et al.* (letter), *J. antimicrob. Chemother.*, 1983, *11*, 196.

Further reports of co-trimoxazole-resistant *Shigella* spp. isolated in various parts of the world: R. M. Bannatyne *et al.* (letter), *Lancet*, 1980, *1*, 425 (Canada); M. Finlayson (letter), *Can. med. Ass. J.*, 1980, *123*, 718 (Canada); K. M. Tiemens *et al.*, *Antimicrob. Ag. Chemother.*, 1984, *25*, 653 (Brazil); M. J. Albert (letter), *Lancet*, 1985, *2*, 948 (India).

RESISTANCE OF GONOCOCCI. Of all chromosomally mediated beta-lactamase negative resistant *Neisseria gonorrhoeae* isolates submitted to the Centers for Disease Control (CDC) in the *US* for agar dilution susceptibility testing during 1983-84, only 47.0% were susceptible to less than 0.5 μg of trimethoprim per mL and 9.5 μg of sulphamethoxazole per mL.— *Morb. Mortal.*, 1984, *33*, 408.

RESISTANCE OF HAEMOPHILUS. Of 874 strains of *Haemophilus influenzae* 69 had an MIC for sulphamethoxazole of 32 μg or more per mL; the apparent incidence of resistance was reduced when the inoculum was reduced. Only 2 strains had an MIC for trimethoprim of 32 μg or more per mL.— A. J. Howard *et al.*, *Br. med. J.*, 1978, *1*, 1657.

In a study in 1986 of the resistance of 2434 clinical isolates of *Haemophilus influenzae* collected in the *UK*, 102 strains (4.2%) were resistant to trimethoprim with a minimum inhibitory concentration of 2 or more μg per mL. Of these, 47 strains were also resistant to sulphamethoxazole and 12 produced beta-lactamase. Determining the minimum inhibitory concentrations of sulphamethoxazole by the agar dilution method produced a larger range of values compared with results of tube dilution assays. Of the 193 strains with a reduced zone diameter, 85 (3.5% of the total number of strains tested) required a minimum inhibitory concentration of sulphamethoxazole of 32 or more μg per mL. The resistance to trimethoprim and sulphamethoxazole had increased from 1.4 and 1.5%, respectively, in 1981.— M. Powell *et al.*, *Br. med. J.*, 1987, *295*, 176. See also J. Campos and S. Garcia-Tornel, *J. antimicrob. Chemother.*, 1987, *19*, 297.

RESISTANCE OF STAPHYLOCOCCI. Resistance to co-trimoxazole was found in nearly all of 40 isolates of methicillin-resistant coagulase-negative staphylococci.— R. A. Proctor, *J. antimicrob. Chemother.*, 1987, *20*, 223.

RESISTANCE OF STREPTOCOCCI. In a study of 10 neutropenic leukaemic patients with septicaemia caused by viridans streptococci, 7 of 8 strains tested were resistant to co-trimoxazole. It was considered possible that resistance had been induced by selection during long-term prophylaxis with this drug, although co-trimoxazole resistance may be inherent in viridans streptococci.— J. Cohen *et al.*, *Lancet*, 1983, *2*, 1452.

Further references to the resistance of streptococci: J. Michel *et al.*, *Antimicrob. Ag. Chemother.*, 1983, *23*, 397 (pneumococci).

RESISTANCE OF VIBRIO. Development of plasmid-mediated resistance in *Vibrio cholerae* during treatment with co-trimoxazole.— M. -J. Dupont *et al.*, *Antimicrob. Ag. Chemother.*, 1985, *27*, 280.

Absorption and Fate

See sulphamethoxazole (p.307) and trimethoprim (p.330). When co-trimoxazole is administered by mouth, plasma concentrations of trimethoprim and sulphamethoxazole are generally in the ratio of 1:20; in urine this ratio may vary from 1:1 to 1:5 depending on the pH. About 50% of administered trimethoprim and 50% of sulphamethoxazole is excreted in the urine in 24 hours; a larger proportion of sulphamethoxazole appears as inactive metabolite.

A review of the pharmacokinetics of trimethoprim and trimethoprim-sulphonamide preparations.— D. S. Reeves and P. J. Wilkinson, *Infection*, 1979, *7*, *Suppl.* 4, S330.

A review of the clinical pharmacokinetics of co-trimoxazole.— R. B. Patel and P. G. Welling, *Clin. Pharmacokinet.*, 1980, *5*, 405.

The apparent volume of distribution of trimethoprim was 5 to 6 times greater than that of sulphamethoxazole; this explained why the ratio of trimethoprim to sulphamethoxazole used clinically was higher than the optimum ratio of 1:20 *in vitro*. The half-lives of trimethoprim and sulphamethoxazole were 10.1 and 11.4 hours respectively. Peak plasma concentrations of trimethoprim in 6 healthy men after a single dose of 960 mg of co-trimoxazole were 2.7 μg per mL and 3.5 μg per mL after 15 twelve-hourly doses. Peak concentrations of unconjugated sulphamethoxazole were 40 and 90 μg per mL respectively. Suggested dose regimens in renal impairment included: the standard regimen of 960 mg of co-trimoxazole every 12 hours if the creatinine clearance exceeded 25 mL per minute; for clearances of 15 to 25 mL per minute the standard dose was used for 3 days then 960 mg daily, provided the total sulphamethoxazole concentration did not exceed 200 μg per mL.— A. S. E. Fowle, *Med. J. Aust.*, 1973, *1*, *Suppl.* (June 30), 26.

Peak-serum-nonacetylated sulphamethoxazole concentrations of between 27.9 and 45.2 μg per mL were obtained in healthy subjects 2 and 4 hours after sulphamethoxazole 800 mg in conjunction with trimethoprim 160 mg. In uraemic patients peak sulphamethoxazole concentrations were achieved at 4 or 6 hours and ranged from 18.8 to 35 μg per mL. Peak serum-trimethoprim concentrations ranging from 0.9 to 1.5 μg per mL were achieved in healthy subjects at 1 and 2 hours and similar values were obtained in uraemic patients. The serum half-lives for nonacetylated sulphamethoxazole and trimethoprim were 9.3 and 10.6 hours respectively in the healthy subjects and there was little difference when each compound was administered singly. As renal function deteriorated, the half-lives became more prolonged but both compounds were removed by haemodialysis at rates similar to the excretion in subjects with healthy kidneys. The serum-binding of unchanged sulphamethoxazole was reduced in uraemic patients and was further reduced in uraemic patients with low serum-protein concentrations; no changes were detected in the binding of trimethoprim to serum proteins. In the first 48 hours about 30% of nonacetylated sulphamethoxazole and 53% of trimethoprim were excreted in the urine. It was found that acidification of the urine increased the excretion of trimethoprim, alkalinisation decreased its excretion and increased that of free sulphamethoxazole, and renal impairment reduced the excretion of both compounds.— W. A. Craig and C. M. Kunin, *Ann. intern. Med.*, 1973, *78*, 491.

Following single doses of co-trimoxazole 60 mg per kg body-weight administered to children aged 2 to 6 years maximum plasma concentrations were much lower than those observed in adults who had received comparable doses. The average plasma half-life for both drugs in children was generally about half of that for adults.— P. Kremers *et al.*, *Thérapie*, 1973, *28*, 1177.

Administration of 960 mg of co-trimoxazole twice daily to 5 healthy subjects for 9 days gave steady-state plasma concentrations of the constituents after 3 days; for active sulphamethoxazole this was between 52.5 and 63.1 μg per mL, and for trimethoprim 1.61 and 1.91 μg per mL.— P. Kremers *et al.*, *J. clin. Pharmac.*, 1974, *14*, 112.

Seven healthy subjects who took 9 tablets of co-trimoxazole, a dose of 4.32 g, achieved in the first 8 hours mean serum concentrations of 6.12 to 8.32 μg per mL for trimethoprim and 98 to 128 μg per mL for sulphamethoxazole; at 24 hours the respective average concentrations were 2.16 and 31.70 μg per mL. This high dose could be useful in the treatment of uncomplicated gonorrhoea.— T. T. Yoshikawa and L. B. Guze, *Antimicrob. Ag. Chemother.*, 1976, *10*, 462.

In healthy subjects given 12 tablets of co-trimoxazole, elimination half-lives for trimethoprim and sulphamethoxazole were longer than those for smaller doses. Ratios of serum concentrations of trimethoprim to free sulphamethoxazole ranged from about 1:16 to 1:30 during the first 24 hours; urinary concentrations were much higher and the ratios ranged from about 1:2 to 1:4. Side-effects were severe.— R. J. Fass *et al.*, *Antimicrob. Ag. Chemother.*, 1977, *12*, 102.

Peak serum concentrations of trimethoprim and sulphamethoxazole in 6 healthy subjects occurred about 40 minutes and 2 hours respectively after an intramuscular injection of trimethoprim 4 mg per kg body-weight as the pantothenate and sulphamethoxazole 20 mg per kg.— A. Lázaro *et al.* (letter), *J. antimicrob. Chemother.*, 1978, *4*, 287.

Co-trimoxazole 960 mg was given every 8 hours by intravenous infusion over one hour to 11 cancer patients. At the end of the first infusion mean plasma concentrations for trimethoprim and free sulphamethoxazole were 3.4 and 46.3 μg per mL respectively and had fallen to 1.8 and 23.8 μg per mL at 8 hours. On the fourth day mean plasma concentrations immediately after an infusion were 8.8 μg per mL for trimethoprim and 105.6 μg per mL for sulphamethoxazole and had fallen to 5.8 and 69 μg per mL at 8 hours. The estimated half-life of 7.7 hours for trimethoprim on day 1 increased to 11.3 hours on day 4 and likewise increased for sulphamethoxazole from 8.5 to 12.8 hours. About 22% of the dose of trimethoprim appeared in the urine within 8 hours and during the same time 22% of the dose of sulphamethoxazole appeared as free sulphamethoxazole and about 10% as metabolites.— W. E. Grose *et al.*, *Antimicrob. Ag. Chemother.*, 1979, *15*, 447. See also D. J. Morgan and K. Raymond, *ibid.*, 1980, *17*, 132.

Steady-state pharmacokinetics of co-trimoxazole in healthy subjects after rectal administration.— R. Liedtke and W. Haase, *Arzneimittel-Forsch.*, 1979, *29*, 345.

The pharmacokinetics of co-trimoxazole during peritoneal dialysis and haemodialysis.— R. L. Slaughter *et al.*, *Drug Intell. & clin. Pharm.*, 1983, *17*, 440.

Pharmacokinetics of co-trimoxazole in the elderly.— O. Varoquaux *et al.*, *Br. J. clin. Pharmac.*, 1985, *20*, 575.

DIFFUSION INTO BODY TISSUES AND FLUIDS. A review of tissue penetration of trimethoprim and sulphonamides. Trimethoprim is widely distributed in the body with some sequestration inside cells whereas sulphonamides are more confined to the blood and extracellular fluid. After the administration of co-trimoxazole the concentration ratios of trimethoprim to sulphonamide in body fluids other than blood are usually in the range 1:2 to 1:5, with wide individual variations.— P. J. Wilkinson and D. S. Reeves, *J. antimicrob. Chemother.*, 1979, *5*, *Suppl.* B, 159.

Co-trimoxazole 960 mg given to 6 patients with cataracts gave therapeutically effective concentrations in the aqueous humour.— P. E. J. Pohjanpelto *et al.*, *Br. J. Ophthal.*, 1974, *58*, 606. See also J. D. Salmon *et al.*, *J. antimicrob. Chemother.*, 1975, *1*, 205.

Concentrations of sulphamethoxazole and trimethoprim in middle ear fluid.— J. J. Klimek *et al.*, *J. Pediat.*, 1980, *96*, 1087.

Penetration of co-trimoxazole into skin blister fluid.— A. Nowak *et al.*, *Eur. J. clin. Pharmac.*, 1983, *25*, 825.

Penetration of sulphamethoxazole and trimethoprim into synovial fluid.— M. A. Sattar *et al.*, *J. antimicrob. Chemother.*, 1983, *12*, 229.

Ventricular cerebrospinal fluid concentrations of trimethoprim and sulphamethoxazole after intravenous infusion of co-trimoxazole in patients undergoing ventriculoperitoneal shunt surgery.— E. E. L. Wang and C. G. Prober, *J. antimicrob. Chemother.*, 1983, *11*, 385.

Pharmacokinetics of trimethoprim and sulphamethoxazole in serum and cerebrospinal fluid of adult patients with normal meninges.— M. N. Dudley *et al.*, *Antimicrob. Ag. Chemother.*, 1984, *26*, 811.

Results in 2 patients with Gram-negative bacillary meningitis suggesting that co-trimoxazole given by intravenous infusion achieves adequate CSF concentrations and may be useful in the therapy of uncommon types of meningitis, particularly those resistant or only moderately susceptible to beta-lactam antibiotics.— R. E. Levitz *et al.* (letter), *J. antimicrob. Chemother.*, 1984, *13*, 400.

EFFECT OF DISEASES STATES. The absorption of sulphamethoxazole from co-trimoxazole was increased in patients with coeliac disease.— R. L. Parsons *et al.*, *J. antimicrob. Chemother.*, 1975, *1*, 39.

Rapid elimination of trimethoprim-sulphamethoxazole in patients with cystic fibrosis.— M. D. Reed *et al.*, *J. Pediat.*, 1984, *104*, 303.

The pharmacokinetics of high-dose co-trimoxazole in 7 patients with *Pneumocystis carinii* pneumonia associated with AIDS. Patients were given daily doses of trimethoprim 20 mg per kg body-weight and sulphamethoxazole 100 mg per kg either by mouth or intravenously and serum was collected 1.5 hours after an oral dose or 1.5 hours after completion of the intravenous infusion. On days 2 to 4 of treatment, mean trimethoprim serum-concentrations were 8.7 (range 7.0 to 11.0) μg per mL and mean sulphamethoxazole concentrations were 274.2 (range 241 to 317) μg per mL; on days 8 to 10, mean blood concentrations were 9.4 (range 4.7 to 11.9) μg per mL and 342.5 (range 277 to 536) μg per mL, respectively. Absolute sulphamethoxazole concentrations were higher and trimethoprim:sulphamethoxazole ratios were lower than those cited in other similar studies. Although Gordin *et al.* (*Ann. intern. Med.*, 1984, *100*, 495) have discounted high serum concentrations of sulphamethoxazole as a contributing factor to the high frequency of side-effects of co-trimoxazole in AIDS patients, these results suggest that high serum-sulphamethoxazole concentrations may be partly responsible, and, in such patients, it may be necessary to administer trimethoprim and sulphamethoxazole separately in a lower dosage and in a different ratio to that in co-trimoxazole.— F. J. Bowden *et al.* (letter), *Lancet*, 1986, *1*, 853.

PREGNANCY AND THE NEONATE. A brief discussion on the pharmacokinetics of co-trimoxazole in pregnancy and labour.— A. Philipson, *Clin. Pharmacokinet.*, 1979, *4*, 297.

Uses and Administration

Co-trimoxazole is used similarly to the sulphonamides (see Sulphamethoxazole, p.307) but in a wider variety of infections. Its indications for use include genito-urinary-tract infections, respiratory-tract infections such as bronchitis and *Pneumocystis carinii* pneumonia, and enteric infections. Trimethoprim (p.330) alone may be preferred to co-trimoxazole in urinary-tract infections (see also under Antimicrobial Action, above).

Co-trimoxazole is usually given by mouth in a dose of 960 mg (trimethoprim 160 mg and sulphamethoxazole 800 mg) twice daily for at least 5 days; in severe infections 2.88 g daily in 2 divided doses may be given. Lower doses are given for long-term treatment and in patients with renal impairment; co-trimoxazole is generally not recommended when the creatinine clearance is less than 15 mL per minute unless facilities for haemodialysis are available.

Suggested doses of co-trimoxazole to be given twice daily to children are: from 6 weeks to 5 months of age, 120 mg; 6 months to 5 years, 240 mg; 6 to 12 years, 480 mg.

Higher doses of co-trimoxazole of 120 mg per kg body-weight daily given in 2 to 4 divided doses for 14 days are used in the treatment of *Pneumocystis carinii* pneumonia; blood concentrations of sulphamethoxazole should be monitored.

Co-trimoxazole is available for parenteral use when treatment by mouth is not possible. A solution of co-trimoxazole 960 mg in 3 mL is given by deep intramuscular injection in similar doses to the oral regimen. The intramuscular route should not be used for longer than 5 successive days, or 3 days if the maximum dose is given, and should not be used in children under 6 years of age. For serious infections co-trimoxazole may be given initially by intravenous infusion as a solution diluted immediately before use in the usual glucose or electrolyte solutions; a suggested dose is 960 mg in 250 mL twice daily, up to a maximum of 1.44 g in 500 mL twice daily, each dose infused over about 60 to 90 minutes (but see under Administration, below). The maximum dose should not be given for more than 3 days. A dose of 18 mg per kg body-weight twice daily has been suggested in children.

Reviews on the actions and uses of co-trimoxazole: *Med. Lett.*, 1981, *23*, 102; G. P. Wormser *et al.*, *Drugs*, 1982, *24*, 459; F. R. Cockerill and R. S. Edson, *Mayo Clin. Proc.*, 1987, *62*, 921.

A review of the significance of the sulphonamide component for the clinical efficacy of trimethoprim-sulphonamide combinations.— L. G. Burman, *Scand. J. infect. Dis.*, 1986, *18*, 89. See also P. Ball, *J. antimicrob. Chemother.*, 1986, *17*, 694.

Reviews comparing co-trimoxazole and trimethoprim: W. Brumfitt and J. M. T. Hamilton-Miller, *Drugs*, 1982, *24*, 453; *Drug & Ther. Bull.*, 1986, *24*, 17.

Criticism of the unnecessarily large amount of sulphamethoxazole in co-trimoxazole.— J. K. Seydel and E. Wempe, *Arzneimittel-Forsch.*, 1977, *27*, 1521.

For reports and comments on trimethoprim as an antibacterial agent in its own right, see Trimethoprim, p.330.

ADMINISTRATION. Comment that hyponatraemia may be associated with the large volumes of fluid required for high-dose intravenous treatment with co-trimoxazole. Because co-trimoxazole is unstable in solution, the manufacturers [*US*] recommend that each ampoule of 480 mg be dissolved in 125 mL of glucose 5% in water; if fluid restriction is required, 75 mL of this diluent can be used. A typical patient weighing 70 kg given co-trimoxazole 120 mg per kg body-weight daily will require 1.35 to 2.25 litres of glucose 5% in water daily and such large volumes of salt-free solution could result in hyponatraemia. As a partial solution to this problem Deans *et al.* (*Am. J. Hosp. Pharm.*, 1982, *39*, 1681) showed that normal saline in a smaller volume of 50 mL could be used. However, this regimen would still require 900 mL daily in a 70-kg person. Caution is advised in the use of intravenous high-dose co-trimoxazole and serum-sodium concentrations should be monitored.— Y.-H. Ahn and J. M. Goldman (letter), *Ann. intern. Med.*, 1985, *103*, 161. *UK* manufacturers have recommended a range of diluents for co-trimoxazole by intravenous infusion including solutions of glucose, fructose, or sodium chloride. One suggests that, when fluid restriction is necessary, co-trimoxazole may be given in a higher concentration such as 480 mg in 50 mL or 75 mL of glucose 5% in water.

Co-trimoxazole may cause oesophagitis or oesophageal ulceration and tablets should therefore be given with at least 100 mL of water while the patient is in an upright sitting position.— S. K. Vong and R. K. Parekh (letter), *Pharm. J.*, 1987, *1*, 5.

ADMINISTRATION IN RENAL FAILURE. Co-trimoxazole was given to 20 patients with varying degrees of renal impairment to treat respiratory or urinary-tract infections. There was no deterioration in renal function in 17 and in the other 3 factors other than co-trimoxazole might have been responsible. The dose of co-trimoxazole was based on plasma-creatinine concentrations; for a creatinine clearance above 25 mL per minute and a plasma-creatinine concentration of less than 20 μg per mL for women or 30 μg per mL for men the dose was 960 mg twice daily. With a creatinine clearance of 25 to 15 mL per minute and a plasma concentration of 20 to 45 μg per mL for women and 30 to 70 μg per mL for men the dose was 960 mg twice daily for 3 days then once daily. Where the creatinine clearance was below 15 mL per minute and the plasma concentrations were greater than 45 or 70 μg per mL respectively for women and men, the dose was 960 mg daily.— P. R. W. Tasker *et al.*, *Lancet*, 1975, *1*, 1216.

Accumulation of conjugated sulphamethoxazole was reported in 9 uraemic patients with creatinine clearances of less than 20 mL per minute.— L. Gotloib (letter), *Lancet*, 1975, *2*, 365.

See also under Sulphamethoxazole, p.308 and Trimethoprim, p.330.

Dialysis. Co-trimoxazole has been given to patients undergoing continuous ambulatory peritoneal dialysis in a loading dose of 480 mg per litre intraperitoneally followed by a maintenance dose of 30 mg per litre of dialysate fluid intraperitoneally or 960 mg by mouth daily.— D. K. Scott and D. E. Roberts, *Pharm. J.*, 1985, *1*, 621.

Comment on the administration of high-dose co-trimoxazole for treating *Pneumocystis carinii* pneumonia in patients receiving acute haemodialysis. A patient with severe renal failure, receiving haemodialysis for 4 hours daily with a blood flow of 200 mL per minute, was given co-trimoxazole 480 mg twice daily intravenously after dialysis, and his plasma concentrations of trimethoprim and sulphamethoxazole before the next dialysis were 7.61 and 19.5

μg per mL, respectively; when given co-trimoxazole 1.44 g twice daily the plasma concentrations were 13.6 and 67.9 μg per mL, respectively. For maximum efficacy in treating *Pn. carinii* infection, the steady-state serum concentration of trimethoprim should be maintained above 5 μg per mL. It seems that with the haemodialysis schedule used in this patient, the fairly small intravenous dose of 480 mg twice daily is appropriate for treating *Pn. carinii* pneumonia, although it is advisable to monitor drug concentrations.— G. G. Wathen *et al., Br. med. J.*, 1987, *295*, 333.

ANIMAL BITES. The use of co-trimoxazole in an attempt to reduce wound infection rates in dog-bite wounds.— D. A. Jones and T. N. Stanbridge, *Postgrad. med. J.*, 1985, *61*, 593.

ATYPICAL MYCOBACTERIAL INFECTIONS. There have been 2 main approaches to the therapy of atypical mycobacterial infections, the first uses various combinations of antituberculous agents and the second uses other antimicrobial agents including sulphamethoxazole with or without trimethoprim, erythromycin, doxycycline, or amikacin. There is limited evidence that co-trimoxazole may be of benefit in mycobacterial infections due to *Mycobacterium chelonei, M. xenopi, M. marinum*, and perhaps *M. avium* when used with other drugs.— J. M. Grange, *J. antimicrob. Chemother.*, 1984, *13*, 308.

Skin lesions due to *Mycobacterium marinum* from infected tropical fish tanks occurred in 3 patients and were successfully controlled with co-trimoxazole given by mouth. Complete resolution took up to 3 months.— M. M. Black and S. J. Eykyn, *Br. J. Derm.*, 1977, *97*, 689. See also R. Kelly, *Med. J. Aust.*, 1976, *2*, 681; C. Maloney *et al., Br. J. Derm.*, 1986, *115, Suppl.* 30, 32.

BILIARY-TRACT INFECTIONS. A review of the treatment of biliary infection including the use of co-trimoxazole or trimethoprim.— J. S. Dooley *et al., Gut*, 1984, *25*, 988.

BRUCELLOSIS. Twenty patients with chronic brucellosis were treated with co-trimoxazole 1.44 g twice daily till afebrile then 960 mg twice daily for 2 months. Fever subsided in 2 to 7 days. Two patients relapsed; in the other serum agglutination titres fell or became negative in a 2-year follow-up.— P. A. Kontoyannis *et al., Br. med. J.*, 1975, *2*, 480.

A good therapeutic response was seen in 12 children aged 3 to 14 years old with brucellar arthritis treated with high-dose co-trimoxazole by mouth. The children were given the following daily dosage regimen: 90 to 100 mg of sulphamethoxazole per kg body-weight [co-trimoxazole 108 to 120 mg per kg] for the first week; 50 to 60 mg of sulphamethoxazole per kg [co-trimoxazole 60 to 72 mg per kg] during weeks 2 to 4; and 25 to 30 mg of sulphamethoxazole per kg [co-trimoxazole 30 to 36 mg per kg] during weeks 5 to 12. The arthritis subsided within 2 to 3 months in all the patients, although 2 patients with hip involvement still had functional limitation of the joint.— F. J. Gómez-Reino *et al., Ann. rheum. Dis.*, 1986, *45*, 256.

Further references: A. M. Kambal *et al., Trans. R. Soc. trop. Med. Hyg.*, 1983, *77*, 820 (co-trimoxazole in association with streptomycin to treat children); I. O. Al-Orainey *et al., J. Infect.*, 1987, *14*, 141 (co-trimoxazole with doxycycline or rifampicin to treat brucella meningitis).

For comment on the use of co-trimoxazole in the treatment of brucellosis, see under Doxycycline Hydrochloride, p.218.

DIARRHOEA. Travellers' diarrhoea usually starts within 14 days of arrival and the disease usually resolves untreated in 48 to 72 hours. Many different pathogens can be responsible for the symptoms, but the major causative agents are usually *Escherichia coli* and *Shigella*. Avoidance of infected food and water is the ideal means of prevention, but many antibiotics have been used for attempted prophylaxis. A study carried out in Mexico demonstrated a beneficial effect with co-trimoxazole (H.L. DuPont *et al., Gastroenterology*, 1983, *84*, 75); doxycycline has also been demonstrated to be effective. However, the successful prophylactic use of an antibiotic must be weighed against the undesirable side-effects of antibiotics. Antibiotics also increase the risk of superinfection by other pathogens and the development of resistance is a major problem. There are certain groups in whom prophylaxis with co-trimoxazole or doxycycline is advisable including patients with achlorhydria, inflammatory bowel disease, and those in whom electrolyte disturbance may have dangerous consequences, including patients taking diuretics. In addition, it may be justifiable to give antibiotic prophylaxis to people on important business trips and to military populations (G.C. Cook, *Gut*, 1983, *24*, 1105). Co-trimoxazole has been used prophylactically in a single dose of 960 mg daily; trimethoprim 200 mg once daily may also prevent travellers' diarrhoea (*Med. Lett.*, 1987, *29*, 53). Priority chemoprophylaxis should be given to those at risk for the shortest periods of time (2 to 5 days), and should be avoided when the period of risk exceeds 2 weeks. Prophylaxis should be commenced on the first day of travel, and probably continued for 2 days after returning home, although this point has not been well studied (H.L. DuPont *et al., Ann. intern. Med.*, 1985, *102*, 260).

In the treatment of mild travellers' diarrhoea, antidiarrhoeal drugs may be used, but co-trimoxazole may be appropriate for more severe illness (S.L. Gorbach, *New Engl. J. Med.*, 1982, *307*, 881; S. Hughes, *Drugs*, 1983, *26*, 80). Early treatment with antibiotics is considered by some workers to be a reasonable alternative to prophylaxis. DuPont *et al.* (*New Engl. J. Med.*, 1982, *307*, 841) demonstrated beneficial effects with twice daily administration of co-trimoxazole 960 mg or trimethoprim 200 mg given for 5 days in travellers from the United States to Mexico.

ENDOCARDITIS. For mention of the use of co-trimoxazole to treat Q fever endocarditis, see under Q fever, below.

ENTERIC INFECTIONS. A prolonged dysentery-like syndrome associated with repeated recovery of *Aeromonas hydrophilia* from stool cultures in a patient was relieved by the administration of co-trimoxazole 960 mg twice daily.— A. F. M. S. Rahman and J. M. T. Willoughby, *Br. med. J.*, 1980, *281*, 976.

Cholera. For mention of co-trimoxazole in the prophylaxis and treatment of cholera, see under Tetracycline Hydrochloride, p.318.

Salmonellosis. Comparable results with co-trimoxazole or amoxycillin in the treatment of chloramphenicol-sensitive and chloramphenicol-resistant typhoid fever. Both regimens were effective but co-trimoxazole resulted in more rapid lysis of fever in infections due to chloramphenicol-sensitive strains.— R. H. Gilman *et al., J. infect. Dis.*, 1975, *132*, 630.

A report recommending ampicillin or co-trimoxazole in the treatment of typhoid fever due to *S. typhi* resistant to chloramphenicol, streptomycin, sulphonamide, and tetracycline.— T. Butler *et al., Antimicrob. Ag. Chemother.*, 1977, *11*, 645.

In a study in Indonesia of patients with typhoid fever treated with co-trimoxazole or chloramphenicol, co-trimoxazole was more effective in sterilising the blood, but in other respects the results of treatment were the same for both drugs. From a review of the literature of 31 reports involving 1184 patients with typhoid fever treated with co-trimoxazole, there were 38 relapses (3.2%) and 13 deaths (1.1%). The time for defervescence was 3 to 9 days (median 5.1 days). In 17 of the 31 reports, treatment with co-trimoxazole was compared with chloramphenicol: co-trimoxazole resulted in a more favourable outcome in 7 reports, the 2 drugs were equally effective in 4 reports, but more prolonged fever occurred with co-trimoxazole in 5 reports, and there was a higher relapse rate and more prolonged bacteraemia with co-trimoxazole in one report. Co-trimoxazole was considered to be an effective alternative to chloramphenicol for the treatment of typhoid fever.— T. Butler *et al., Rev. infect. Dis.*, 1982, *4*, 551.

See also under Chloramphenicol, p.191.

Shigellosis. Co-trimoxazole was as effective as ampicillin in a study of 28 children with acute shigellosis and was also active against ampicillin-resistant strains of *Shigella*.— J. D. Nelson *et al., J. Am. med. Ass.*, 1976, *235*, 1239.

Infections with strains of *Shigella dysenteriae* type 1 that are resistant to several drugs continue to wreak havoc in developing countries. Resistance to co-trimoxazole, nalidixic acid, and ampicillin has varied and their use should be based on susceptibility tests *in vitro*. Drugs offer only short-term solutions. The organism very quickly becomes resistant and there is the risk of normal gut flora acquiring resistance.— M. J. Albert (letter), *Lancet*, 1985, *2*, 948.

Further references: F. A. Barada and R. L. Guerrant, *Antimicrob. Ag. Chemother.*, 1980, *17*, 961.

For comparison of co-trimoxazole and trimethoprim in the treatment of severe bacillary dysentery, see under Trimethoprim, p.331.

Yersiniosis. Treatment of *Yersinia enterocolitica* infection in 4 children with co-trimoxazole. The role of antibiotic agents in the management of this enteritis is controversial.— D. J. E. Marriott *et al., Med. J. Aust.*, 1985, *143*, 489.

For further mention of the use of co-trimoxazole in the treatment of yersiniosis, see under Tetracycline Hydrochloride, p.319.

For a recommendation to use co-trimoxazole for prophylaxis against systemic yersiniosis in patients with homozygous β-thalassaemia who become febrile, see under Precautions in Desferrioxamine, p.837.

GRANULOMATOUS DISEASES. A review and discussion on chronic granulomatous disease. Chronic granulomatous disease is a rare inherited disease of abnormal phagocyte oxidative metabolism, characterised by recurrent, life-threatening infections with catalase-positive micro-organisms and excessive inflammatory reactions that lead to granuloma formation. Retrospective studies have indicated that prophylactic antibiotic therapy, particularly with co-trimoxazole, prolongs the disease-free intervals to greater than 40 months. For patients who have allergic reactions to co-trimoxazole, trimethoprim alone or dicloxacillin may be tried, but the efficacy of this approach has not been evaluated.— J. I. Gallin *et al., Ann. intern. Med.*, 1983, *99*, 657.

Wegener's granulomatosis is a systemic disease that is characterised pathologically by necrotising granulomas and vasculitis involving both arteries and veins; it affects the upper and lower respiratory tract, often in association with focal necrotising glomerulitis. Some published reports have implicated bacterial or viral infections in relapses of Wegener's granulomatosis and the disease has been controlled or ameliorated with the use of antimicrobial treatment alone or added to a regimen of cyclophosphamide and prednisone. The clinical course improved in 11 of 12 patients who received this treatment chiefly with co-trimoxazole.— R. A. DeRemee *et al., Mayo Clin. Proc.*, 1985, *60*, 27. A further report of sustained and complete remission in a patient with Wegener's granulomatosis given co-trimoxazole 960 mg twice daily initially followed by 960 mg daily.— B. C. West *et al., Ann. intern. Med.*, 1987, *106*, 840.

IMMUNOCOMPROMISED PATIENTS. *Prophylaxis*. Periods of neutropenia and damaged membranes of the oropharynx, gut, and lung due to chemotherapy and radiotherapy permit predominantly Gram-negative organisms to enter the systemic circulation or the lung parenchyma more readily and patients with leukaemia are particularly susceptible to severe infections, many of which are due to endogenous gastro-intestinal organisms. Non-absorbable antibiotics have been used in an attempt to reduce the level of microbial flora in the gut, but because the presence of anaerobic organisms may protect against colonisation with exogenous Gram-negative pathogens, selective aerobic decontamination with co-trimoxazole has been adopted (R.E. Marcus and J.M. Goldman, *Br. med. J.*, 1986, *293*, 406).

Co-trimoxazole has been shown to be effective in both reducing the incidence of pneumonia due to *Pneumocystis carinii* in children with leukaemia in remission (see *Pneumocystis carinii* Infections, below) and lowering their risk for relatively mild bacterial infections of skin and soft tissue (L.S. Young, *Ann. intern. Med.*, 1987, *106*, 144). In the *UK* the Medical Research Council (MRC) has recommended prophylactic co-trimoxazole for children with acute lymphoblastic leukaemia (ALL) and although its use has not been advocated in adults, some workers feel that its routine use should be considered in adults with ALL (D.W. Milligan *et al., Lancet*, 1987, *1*, 867). However, studies in adults with haematological malignancies in relapse are more controversial. Concern has been raised about the use of co-trimoxazole because of its inhibitory effect on myelopoiesis, the high incidence of adverse effects, and the selection of resistant Gram-negative bacilli and superinfecting fungi. When co-trimoxazole has been used extensively as prophylaxis in compromised hosts, almost 40% of the gut flora and most of the organisms causing extra-intestinal bacterial infections have become resistant to this compound (L.S. Young, *Ann. intern. Med.*, 1987, *106*, 144). Because of this, when used for selective aerobic decontamination of the bowel, agents such as colistin, a non-absorbed antibiotic, may have to be added to the regimen. The risk of fungal colonisation may be reduced by the concomitant use of amphotericin and nystatin, or by ketoconazole (E. Estey *et al., Archs intern. Med.*, 1984, *144*, 1562; R.E. Marcus and J.M. Goldman, *Br. med. J.*, 1986, *293*, 406). Newer agents such as the 4-fluoroquinolones appear to offer a promising alternative to prophylaxis with co-trimoxazole (A.W. Dekker *et al., Ann. intern. Med.*, 1987, *106*, 7; L.S. Young, *ibid.*, 144).

Further references to the prophylactic use of co-trimoxazole in granulocytopenic patients: EORTC International Antimicrobial Therapy Project Group, *J. infect. Dis.*, 1984, *150*, 372; E. J. Bow *et al., Am. J. Med.*, 1984, *76*, 223.

For reference to regimens used to prevent colonisation and infection by the selective decontamination of the gastro-intestinal tract, see Colistin Sulphomethate Sodium, p.205.

A study of the efficacy of co-trimoxazole 480 mg daily by mouth for prophylaxis against urinary-tract infection following renal transplantation. It was considered that co-trimoxazole prophylaxis should be initiated soon after transplantation regardless of renal function, as delaying prophylaxis increased the risk of urinary-tract infections.— M. S. Maddux *et al.*, *Drug Intell. & clin. Pharm.*, 1985, *19*, 452.

For the use of co-trimoxazole in the *treatment* of immunocompromised patients infected with various organisms, see Isosporiasis, *Pneumocystis carinii* Infections, and Toxoplasmosis, below.

ISOSPORIASIS. A patient with chronic coccidiosis caused by *Isospora belli* was successfully treated with co-trimoxazole 960 mg every 6 hours for 10 days followed by 960 mg twice daily for 3 weeks.— E. L. Westerman and R. P. Christensen, *Ann. intern. Med.*, 1979, *91*, 413.

Comment on infection with *Isospora belli* (isosporiasis) and the difficulty of treatment; nitrofurantoin, pyrimethamine and sulphonamide, and co-trimoxazole have all been tried with limited success.—WHO Scientific Working Group, *Bull. Wld Hlth Org.*, 1980, *58*, 819.

Co-trimoxazole was considered the drug of choice for parasitic infections due to *Isospora belli*; a dosage of 960 mg four times daily for 10 days, then twice daily for 3 weeks was recommended.— *Med. Lett.*, 1988, *30*, 15.

Isospora belli was an opportunistic pathogen in 20 of 131 (15%) patients with AIDS who were treated in Haiti during 1983 to 1984. Fifteen patients initially had isosporiasis as their sole coccidial infection and had a weight loss of at least 10% during the 2 months before diagnosis of the disorder. Treatment of these 15 patients with co-trimoxazole 960 mg administered by mouth 4 times daily for 10 days and then twice daily for 3 weeks resulted in a dramatic clinical response, with cessation of diarrhoea within 2 days. However, in contrast to this favourable initial outcome, there was a high rate of recurrence of isosporiasis (47%) with most patients becoming symptomatic within 8 weeks of completing therapy. The initial 4½-week course of therapy may have been excessive, and an initial shorter course of co-trimoxazole for 1 to 2 weeks, followed by prophylaxis for an indefinite period with either daily doses of co-trimoxazole or weekly doses of pyrimethamine-sulfadoxine may be more appropriate.— J. A. DeHovitz *et al.*, *New Engl. J. Med.*, 1986, *315*, 87.

LEISHMANIASIS. A favourable response was obtained in a patient with systemic leishmaniasis (kala-azar) after treatment with co-trimoxazole and metronidazole. Enhanced activity might have been obtained when these 2 agents were used together.— K. J. Murphy and A. C. W. Bong (letter), *Lancet*, 1981, *1*, 323. Doubt as to the diagnosis of kala-azar, and a report of a patient who did not respond to co-trimoxazole.— J. Guardia (letter), *ibid.*, 501. Doubt as to the role of co-trimoxazole. A rapid response had been obtained in a patient treated with metronidazole alone.— J. Masramon *et al.* (letter), *ibid.*, 669.

MALAKOPLAKIA. The successful medical management of an 11-year-old child with bilateral renal malakoplakia. She became afebrile several days after starting treatment with co-trimoxazole. Maintenance consisted of co-trimoxazole with intermittent bladder catheterisation.— E. B. Charney *et al.*, *Archs Dis. Childh.*, 1985, *60*, 254.

MALARIA. Co-trimoxazole has been evaluated in the treatment of *Plasmodium falciparum* malaria (C.F. Hansford and J. Hoyland, *S. Afr. med. J.*, 1982, *61*, 512). However, co-trimoxazole and the pyrimethamine-compound antimalarials work by inhibiting the enzymes dihydrofolic acid synthetase and dihydrofolic acid reductase and, therefore, widespread use of co-trimoxazole in malarial areas might be expected to select for malarial parasites resistant to sulfadoxine-pyrimethamine or dapsone-pyrimethamine (F. Shann, *Lancet*, 1984, *2*, 1477 and *ibid.*, 1985, *1*, 358).

MELIOIDOSIS. The successful use of co-trimoxazole in the treatment of chronic prostatic melioidosis.— R. E. Morrison *et al.*, *J. Am. med. Ass.*, 1979, *241*, 500.

MENINGITIS. A review of the use of co-trimoxazole in the treatment of bacterial meningitis.— R. E. Levitz and R. Quintiliani, *Ann. intern. Med.*, 1984, *100*, 881.

Successful treatment of *Klebsiella pneumoniae* meningitis with intravenous co-trimoxazole in one patient.— D. D. Hickstein and J. T. Dillon, *J. Am. med. Ass.*, 1982, *248*, 1212. Comment.— R. H. Gates and C. E. McCall, *ibid.*, 1217.

Further references: G. Jacquette and P. H. Dennehy, *Ann. intern. Med.*, 1985, *102*, 866 (*Listeria monocytogenes* meningitis).

MYCETOMA. In a study of the medical treatment of 144 patients with actinomycetoma, initially 12 received sulfadoxine, 12 received dapsone, and 12 received co-trimoxazole, for an average of 3 months. On statistical analysis the latter 2 were superior to sulfadoxine which was therefore dropped from the study. The 36 patients were then incorporated into second- and third-stage studies together with an additional 108 patients; each patient served as his own control. The following drug regimens were given: co-trimoxazole, dapsone, co-trimoxazole with streptomycin, dapsone with streptomycin, sulfadoxine with pyrimethamine and streptomycin, and rifampicin with streptomycin. Of the 144 patients, 91 (63.2%) were cured and 31 (21.5%) obtained great improvement; all infections caused by *Actinomadura pelletieri* (14), *A. madurae* (13) and *Nocardia brasiliensis* (4) were easily cured; the few cases that did not respond to treatment were among the 133 caused by *Streptomyces somaliensis*. Cures were obtained within 4 to 24 months (average about 9 months), treatment being successful even when bone involvement was advanced. Dapsone with streptomycin and co-trimoxazole with streptomycin were the most effective treatments, neither drug association being clearly superior, although certain strains appeared to respond better to one or other regimen. Good results were also obtained in the few patients treated with the other 2 regimens, making them a useful second line of therapy. Side-effects to all the drugs included moderate to severe leucopenia and/or anaemia, and reversible streptomycin-associated tinnitus developed in 3 patients. Although only 2 of 20 patients with maduromycetoma caused by *Madurella mycetomatis* were cured by griseofulvin (7 mg per kg body-weight daily in a single dose after a fatty lunch) together with penicillin, this association was considered to have an indication as an adjunct to surgery. Despite being effective *in vitro* clotrimazole was ineffective by mouth or by infiltration of the lesions with a 1% solution, and was toxic. Usual doses of the drugs given were as follows: clotrimazole 20 mg per kg body-weight three times daily; sulfadoxine 14 mg per kg on 3 days a week; dapsone 1.5 mg per kg morning and evening; co-trimoxazole 13.8 mg per kg twice daily; streptomycin sulphate 14 mg per kg daily for a month then reduced to alternate days; rifampicin 4.3 mg per kg morning and evening; and tablets containing sulfadoxine 500 mg and pyrimethamine 25 mg at a dose of 7.5 mg per kg once or twice a week.— E. S. Mahgoub, *Bull. Wld Hlth Org.*, 1976, *54*, 303.

NOCARDIOSIS. A report and discussion of 3 patients with haematological malignancies who developed *Nocardia asteroides* infections after splenectomy. The infections responded to treatment with co-trimoxazole 3.84 g daily by mouth in divided doses. Sulphonamides have been the mainstay of treatment for nocardiosis. Addition of trimethoprim to sulphamethoxazole reduces the mean inhibitory concentration of the latter, although the synergism of this combination depends on the strain of *Nocardia*, the duration of incubation, and the ratio of the 2 drugs. If used alone, the suggested therapeutic dose of sulphonamide is 4 to 8 g daily. If co-trimoxazole or sulphonamides cannot be used due to allergy to sulphonamides or other cause, a combination of ampicillin/amoxycillin and erythromycin has been suggested. To prevent relapses antibiotics should be continued for at least 3 months and up to one year. Treatment is further aided by the proper drainage of any localised abscess.— E. A. Abdi *et al.*, *Postgrad. med. J.*, 1987, *63*, 455.

Comment that co-trimoxazole may have an advantage over sulphonamides alone for subsets of patients with disseminated disease or central nervous system (CNS) involvement. Both trimethoprim and sulphamethoxazole penetrate well into most body fluids and tissues, including the cerebrospinal fluid and brain parenchyma, and reach concentrations at these sites in ratios that achieve synergistic *in-vitro* killing of *Nocardia*. Due to the lack of availability of parenteral sulphonamides in the *USA*, co-trimoxazole is often the drug of choice as serious pulmonary, CNS, and disseminated nocardiosis preclude confident reliance on oral sulphonamide therapy alone.— R. A. Smego *et al.* (letter), *Lancet*, 1987, *1*, 456. Disagreement as to the superiority of co-trimoxazole; when used appropriately, sulphonamides alone have proved very effective in immunosuppressed patients with moderate to severe nocardiosis. Some data *in vitro* suggest that the combination is superior, but others suggest that there may be antagonism, and also susceptibility tests of *Nocardia* spp. have not been shown to predict clinical outcome. One cannot conclude that the combination is better or worse than a sulphonamide alone. There is no rationale or empirical support for the recommendation that intravenous therapy must be used to treat mildly or moderately ill patients. Intravenous therapy is indicated for patients who are critically ill or who cannot ingest or absorb antinocardial drugs normally.— G. A. Filice (letter), *ibid.*, 1261.

Further references: M. Roman and E. Reiss-Levy (letter), *Med. J. Aust.*, 1984, *140*, 447 (*Nocardia asteroides* infection in 2 patients); J. De Luca *et al.*, *Postgrad. med. J.*, 1986, *62*, 673 (*N. asteroides* osteomyelitis in 1 patient); Y. Girouard *et al.*, *Can. med. Ass. J.*, 1987, *136*, 844 (cutaneous nocardiosis due to *N. caviae* in 1 patient).

OTITIS MEDIA. Reviews and discussions of the treatment of otitis media including the use of co-trimoxazole: J. Fry and J. W. Stephenson, *Prescribers' J.*, 1984, *24*, 15; *Drug & Ther. Bull.*, 1986, *24*, 22.

A study of 223 children comparing co-trimoxazole with cefaclor in the treatment of acute otitis media; both drugs were found to be effective and with few side-effects.— W. Feldman *et al.*, *Archs Dis. Childh.*, 1982, *57*, 594.

Beneficial effects with co-trimoxazole for prophylaxis of recurrent otitis media.— J. D. Gaskins *et al.*, *Drug Intell. & clin. Pharm.*, 1982, *16*, 387.

A discussion of antibiotic treatment of acute otitis media. Co-trimoxazole may be considered a reasonable alternative to amoxycillin, although the clinician must be aware of the potential for serious side-effects and provide appropriate parent education to monitor for the appearance of a rash, indicating the initial signs of adverse effect.— B. L. True and D. K. Helling, *Drug Intell. & clin. Pharm.*, 1986, *20*, 666.

PEDICULOSIS CAPITIS. A study in 20 patients with lice infestation showed that co-trimoxazole in doses of 480 mg twice daily for 3 days caused the lice to leave infested areas during the first day, and die after leaving the body. Neither sulphamethoxazole nor trimethoprim alone had any effect and co-trimoxazole had no effect on eggs present. A second course of treatment 10 days after the first was given to free the patients from lice.— C. H. Shashindran *et al.*, *Br. J. Derm.*, 1978, *98*, 699.

PLAGUE. All of 50 strains of *Yersinia pestis* were sensitive to co-trimoxazole, which had been successfully used in the treatment of 12 patients.— Nguyen-Van-Ai *et al.* (letter), *Br. med. J.*, 1973, *4*, 108.

For a report of streptomycin being more successful than co-trimoxazole in the treatment of plague, see Streptomycin, p.298.

PNEUMOCYSTIS CARINII INFECTIONS. Overt pneumonitis due to *Pneumocystis carinii* occurs almost exclusively in severely immunocompromised patients, whereas subclinical asymptomatic infection occurs in the majority of healthy people early in life. The rapidly escalating prevalence of this pneumonitis is mainly due to the epidemic of acquired immunodeficiency syndrome (AIDS) and also due to advances in medical practice causing the population of other susceptible immunosuppressed patients to increase. Differences in the disease have been observed between patients with AIDS and those without AIDS; the course may be more subtle and chronic in patients with AIDS than in other immunocompromised hosts. Also the response to treatment is slower and relapse occurs more frequently in patients with AIDS than in most other groups of immunocompromised hosts. Once *Pn. carinii* pneumonitis becomes discernible on chest radiography in immunocompromised hosts without AIDS, the mortality rate approximates 100% if the disease is not treated. However, patients with AIDS may, at times, survive without treatment for relatively long periods with chronic low-grade pneumonitis (W.T. Hughes, *New Engl. J. Med.*, 1987, *317*, 1021).

Initially, pentamidine was the standard treatment for *Pn. carinii* pneumonia. However, pentamidine is toxic, and in a comparative study in children with acute leukaemia or other malignancies, co-trimoxazole was found to be as effective as pentamidine in the treatment of *Pn. carinii* pneumonia, but to be less toxic (see also under pentamidine, p.676). Therefore, co-trimoxazole is usually preferred in the treatment of *Pn. carinii* pneumonia in immunosuppressed patients because it is less toxic and is available in oral as well as parenteral forms for administration. Unfortunately, a much higher incidence of adverse reactions to co-trimoxazole has been noted in patients with AIDS than in other immunosuppressed patients, and also more prolonged therapy is often necessary (J. A. Kovacs *et al.*, *Ann. intern. Med.*, 1984, *100*, 663; H. W. Haverkos, *Am. J. Med.*, 1984, *76*, 501).

For the initial treatment of *Pn. carinii* pneumonia, many workers recommend co-trimoxazole 120 mg per kg body-weight daily in 3 or 4 divided doses for 2 to 3 weeks in patients with AIDS and for 2 weeks in other immunocompromised patients; doses are usually given by the intravenous route initially and then by mouth. Pentamidine is used for patients with a history of severe allergy to a sulphonamide or those unable to tolerate, or failing to respond to, co-trimoxazole within 4 to 7 days of therapy. However, pentamidine is often ineffective if the patient has not responded to initial treatment with co-trimoxazole. Many patients with AIDS treated for second episodes of *Pn. carinii* pneumonia do not respond to co-trimoxazole and in these circumstances the more frequent use of pentamidine may be justified. There is no advantage in using both drugs together, and the drug toxicities could be additive (J. F. Murray *et al.*, *New Engl. J. Med.*, 1984, *310*, 1682; A. Millar, *Br. med. J.*, 1987, *294*, 1334; *Med. Lett.*, 1987, *29*, 103). The 2 drugs have been reported to be equally effective in treating *Pn. carinii* pneumonia in patients with AIDS with a 60 to 80% response rate but with a 50 to 60% incidence of adverse reactions (J.M. Wharton *et al.*, *Ann. intern. Med.*, 1986, *105*, 37; V. T. DeVita *et al.*, *ibid.*, 1987, *106*, 568). However, some workers have reported co-trimoxazole to be more toxic than pentamidine in AIDS patients (F.M. Gordin *et al.*, *Ann. intern. Med.*, 1984, *100*, 495). Although many workers continue to recommend co-trimoxazole, some feel that pentamidine might be the drug of choice for the initial treatment of *Pn. carinii* pneumonia in AIDS patients, with co-trimoxazole more appropriate in patients without AIDS (K.L. Goa and D.M. Campoli-Richards, *Drugs*, 1987, *33*, 242). Additional compounds are needed because of the failure rate and the high incidence of adverse reactions in patients with AIDS: drugs currently under study include dapsone alone or in combination with trimethoprim, pyrimethamine and sulfadoxine, eflornithine hydrochloride, and trimetrexate.

Prophylaxis against *Pn. carinii* pneumonia has been tried in patients at risk. Co-trimoxazole 900 mg per m^2 body-surface daily in 2 divided doses by mouth or as an intermittent regimen given in the same daily dose but only on 3 consecutive days a week has been used successfully in the prevention of *Pn. carinii* pneumonia in children with acute lymphoblastic leukaemia (W.T. Hughes *et al.*, *New Engl. J. Med.*, 1977, *297*, 1419; W. T. Hughes *et al.*, *ibid.*, 1987, *316*, 1627). However, other workers have found no benefit with co-trimoxazole prophylaxis (L.J. Wolff and R.L. Baehner, *Am. J. Dis. Child.*, 1978, *132*, 525). Co-trimoxazole 24 to 48 mg per kg body-weight daily given in 2 divided doses has been recommended by some for prophylaxis in AIDS patients, although an increased incidence of disseminated candidiasis has been reported with such prophylaxis (N. Dozier *et al.*, *Drug Intell. & clin. Pharm.*, 1983, *17*, 798; see also Immunocompromised Patients, above).

A report of cutaneous pneumocystosis in a 42-year-old man with the acquired immunodeficiency syndrome which responded to treatment with intravenous co-trimoxazole 120 mg per kg body-weight daily for 7 days followed by oral co-trimoxazole for 3 weeks.— C. U. Coulman *et al.*, *Ann. intern. Med.*, 1987, *106*, 396.

PROSTATITIS. Chronic bacterial prostatitis is difficult both to diagnose and to treat. Initial response to antimicrobial therapy is usually satisfactory and patients remain free of symptoms as long as bladder urine is sterile. Nevertheless, after withdrawal of short-course antimicrobial therapy, bacteria persisting in the prostate usually reinfect the bladder, and symptoms recur after days or months. Three approaches to therapy have been pursued, the most important being administration of an antibiotic capable of crossing prostatic epithelium into prostatic fluid. Transurethral prostatectomy has also been tried, and a third approach has been to maintain patients on long-term low-dose antimicrobial therapy, although this is seldom curative and drug withdrawal leads to return of symptomatic urinary infection. Only lipid-soluble antibiotics are able to cross the epithelial membranes, and only the uncharged fraction of a drug is able to pass into prostatic fluid since the ionised or charged fraction is lipid-insoluble: sulphonamides are acids and therefore undergo ion-trapping in the plasma, so that prostatic fluid concentrations are usually much lower than those in serum, however, trimethoprim fulfils the theoretical criteria for diffusion into prostatic fluid. Despite this, co-trimoxazole has proved disappointing in treating bacterial prostatitis. This may, in some cases, be due to the pH of prostatic fluid being unsuitable in patients with chronic prostatitis, thus reducing antimicrobial penetration, or other factors such as prostatic calculi may contribute to the persistence of infection. Alternative drugs are, therefore, being studied.— *Lancet*, 1983, *1*, 393. See also P. M. Hanus and L. H. Danziger, *Clin. Pharm.*, 1984, *3*, 49.

See also under Urinary-tract Infections, below.

Q FEVER. Successful treatment of Q fever endocarditis with co-trimoxazole.— R. Freeman and M. E. Hodson, *Br. med. J.*, 1972, *1*, 419. Failure of co-trimoxazole in Q fever endocarditis in one patient.— N. I. Subramanya *et al.*, *ibid.*, 1982, *285*, 343.

RESPIRATORY INFECTIONS. A review of the use of co-trimoxazole and other combinations of trimethoprim with sulphonamides in the treatment of respiratory-tract infections.— D. T. D. Hughes, *J. antimicrob. Chemother.*, 1983, *12*, 423. See also D. Reeves, *Lancet*, 1982, *2*, 370.

For comparison of co-trimoxazole with trimethoprim in the treatment of respiratory-tract infections, see Trimethoprim, p.331.

Bronchitis. A recommendation to use ampicillin or co-trimoxazole to treat acute exacerbations of bronchitis. Prophylaxis in chronic bronchitis is controversial but if considered necessary, tetracycline or co-trimoxazole may be used.— D. T. D. Hughes and D. W. Empey, *Practitioner*, 1979, *223*, 771. There was a significant benefit with antibiotic therapy using co-trimoxazole, amoxycillin, or doxycycline for 10 days, compared with placebo, for the treatment of exacerbations of chronic obstructive pulmonary disease.— N. R. Anthonisen *et al.*, *Ann. intern. Med.*, 1987, *106*, 196. Comment that the question of the need for antibiotic treatment in exacerbations of chronic bronchitis remains unanswered. Whilst it seems appropriate to use antibiotics in an acute exacerbation, since up to 50% of exacerbations respond to placebo some restraint should be exercised in less severe episodes.— *Lancet*, 1987, *2*, 23.

Pertussis. There were no cases of pertussis in 24 children at risk who had received co-trimoxazole prophylactically.— A. S. Cullen and H. B. Cullen (letter), *Lancet*, 1978, *1*, 556.

For mention of the use of co-trimoxazole as an alternative agent to erythromycin in the treatment of pertussis, see under Erythromycin, p.226.

Pneumonia. Co-trimoxazole or erythromycin are usually recommended for the treatment of atypical pneumonia due to *Branhamella catarrhalis*, although the organisms are invariably resistant to trimethoprim *in vitro*. Co-trimoxazole is effective against pneumococcus and haemophilus, but is considered one of the less satisfactory alternatives to penicillins for treating community-acquired pneumonia. It is highly effective against enterobacter and serratia, causative pathogens of nosocomial pneumonia.— J. T. Macfarlane, *Lancet*, 1987, *2*, 1446.

SEXUALLY TRANSMITTED DISEASES. Beneficial results with co-trimoxazole in the treatment of men and women with gonorrhoea and simultaneous infection with *Chlamydia trachomatis*.— W. E. Stamm *et al.*, *New Engl. J. Med.*, 1984, *310*, 545. See also P. A. Csángó *et al.*, *Br. J. vener. Dis.*, 1984, *60*, 95.

Chancroid. Co-trimoxazole 960 mg twice daily by mouth for 5 days, or trimethoprim with a sulphonamide component comparable to sulphamethoxazole, is one of the 2 regimens recommended by the World Health Organization for the treatment of chancroid due to *Haemophilus ducreyi*; erythromycin given for 7 days is the other regimen. Limited data suggest that adequate cure-rates can also be obtained with thiamphenicol given for 2 days, or with single-dose regimens of co-trimoxazole 3.84 g, or trimethoprim with a comparable sulphonamide component, ceftriaxone, or spectinomycin. However, treatment failures with co-trimoxazole have been observed in some areas (WHO Expert Committee on Venereal Diseases and Treponematoses, Sixth Report, *Tech. Rep. Ser. Wld Hlth Org. No. 736*, 1986, p.130). Treatment with co-trimoxazole has also been given for longer periods ranging from 7 to 14 days, although some workers prefer the single-dose regimen. Resistance of *H. ducreyi* to sulphonamides has been reported and the continuing spread of plasmid-mediated resistance among *H. ducreyi* has curtailed the usefulness of sulphonamides for the treatment of chancroid; resistance has also been reported to trimethoprim (*Lancet*, 1982, *2*, 747; A. R. Ronald and F. A. Plummer, *Ann. intern. Med.*, 1985, *102*, 705). Significant geographical variation in the susceptibility of *H. ducreyi* to sulphamethoxazole and trimethoprim suggests that this combination may become increasingly less effective (G. P. Schmid, *J. Am. med. Ass.*, 1986, *255*, 1757).

Gonorrhoea. Co-trimoxazole 1.92 g by mouth twice daily for 2 days has been suggested as one of the alternative regimens for gonococcal urethritis in patients who are allergic to penicillin. Co-trimoxazole is not as effective as penicillin, but since co-trimoxazole is not treponemicidal it may be given to those patients being investigated for suspected syphilis. The regimen is suggested for use only in the *UK* and regimens in other countries will depend on the sensitivities of the gonococcus and the availability of antibiotics.— M. W. Adler, *Br. med. J.*, 1983, *287*, 1452.

One of the suggested regimens for the treatment of uncomplicated gonorrhoea or rectal infections is co-trimoxazole 4.8 g daily by mouth for 3 days, or trimethoprim with a sulphonamide component comparable to sulphamethoxazole. Unfortunately this regimen is often ineffective in localities where it has been used regularly for the treatment of gonorrhoea. Co-trimoxazole has also been given in the same dosage for 5 days to treat pharyngeal infections.— WHO Expert Committee on Venereal Diseases and Treponematoses, Sixth Report, *Tech. Rep. Ser. Wld Hlth Org. No. 736*, 1986, p.118. In the *USA*, a dosage of co-trimoxazole 4.32 g daily as a single dose by mouth for 5 days has been suggested as an alternative regimen for the treatment of pharyngeal infections due to *Neisseria gonorrhoeae*.— *Med. Lett.*, 1988, *30*, 5.

Granuloma inguinale. Ulcers were healed and Donovan bodies eradicated within 14 days in 10 patients with granuloma inguinale who were treated with co-trimoxazole 960 mg twice daily.— B. R. Garg *et al.*, *Br. J. vener. Dis.*, 1978, *54*, 348.

Co-trimoxazole 960 mg twice daily by mouth for 14 days, or trimethoprim with a sulphonamide component comparable to sulphamethoxazole, was considered to be the regimen of choice for the treatment of granuloma inguinale (donovanosis). Alternative agents included chloramphenicol or thiamphenicol with gentamicin, or tetracycline hydrochloride.— WHO Expert Committee on Venereal Diseases and Treponematoses, Sixth Report, *Tech. Rep. Ser. Wld Hlth Org. No. 736*, 1986, p.133.

SKIN DISORDERS. Treatment with co-trimoxazole, in doses reduced at weekly intervals from 1.92 g daily to 480 mg daily and continued for a total of 7 weeks, was effective in reducing pustular lesions and in preventing scaling and atrophy for at least the following 6 months in 23 of 24 Nigerian patients with dermatitis cruris pustulosa et atrophicans.— W. K. Jacyk, *Br. J. Derm.*, 1976, *95*, 71.

For the treatment of skin lesions due to *Mycobacterium marinum*, see Atypical Mycobacterial Infections, above.

Acne. Similar therapeutic results with co-trimoxazole and oxytetracycline in the treatment of children over the age of 12 years with acne vulgaris.— J. W. Harcup and J. Cooper, *Practitioner*, 1980, *224*, 747.

For mention of the use of co-trimoxazole or trimethoprim in the treatment of acne vulgaris, see under Tetracycline Hydrochloride, p.321.

SURGICAL INFECTION PROPHYLAXIS. In a double-blind study co-trimoxazole 960 mg given intravenously one hour before surgery reduced wound sepsis and postoperative pulmonary complications compared with a placebo; in groups of 48 and 47 patients respectively the incidence of wound sepsis was 21 and 4% and that of pulmonary complications 49 and 19%. Trimethoprim, but not sulphamethoxazole, was concentrated in the bile.— C. Morran *et al.*, *Br. med. J.*, 1978, *2*, 462.

Beneficial results in patients undergoing appendicectomy given routine antibiotic prophylaxis with metronidazole pre-operatively and, in patients with gangrenous or perforated appendix, or appendiceal abscess, given co-trimoxazole and metronidazole postoperatively.— E. Arnbjörnsson and C. Mikaelsson (letter), *Lancet*, 1984, *2*, 1279.

Mention of the use of co-trimoxazole for prophylaxis in transurethral prostatectomy and neurosurgery. Results of a study by Blomstedt (*J. Neurosurg.*, 1985, *62*, 694) indicated that prophylaxis with co-trimoxazole in patients undergoing cerebrospinal-fluid shunt implantation may decrease the incidence of infection after this procedure. However, other studies have shown no benefit with antimicrobial prophylaxis for this procedure.— *Med. Lett.*, 1985, *27*, 105. Further comment.— R. Yogev (letter), *New Engl. J. Med.*, 1987, *316*, 1089.

TOXOPLASMOSIS. In 7 patients with toxoplasmosis good therapeutic results were observed with co-trimoxazole in 5 with lymphoglandular toxoplasmosis and a significant reduction in dye test titres in 6. Treatment was discontinued in 1 patient because of an allergic reaction, and 1 patient relapsed 6.5 months after the end of treatment.— R. Norrby *et al.*, *Scand. J. infect. Dis.*, 1975, *7*, 72.

Dramatic recovery in an 11½-year-old girl with generalised toxoplasmosis after she was given co-trimoxazole 480 mg twice daily for one month.— M. Williams and D. C. L. Savage (letter), *Archs Dis. Childh.*, 1978, *53*, 829.

Although clinical experience with co-trimoxazole in toxoplasmosis is very limited it could be useful, especially in toxoplasmic meningitis.— F. J. Nye, *J. antimicrob. Chemother.*, 1979, *5*, 244.

Five patients with the acquired immune deficiency syndrome (AIDS) suffering from cerebral toxoplasmosis were successfully treated with co-trimoxazole given for 3 weeks at the dosage recommended for *Pneumocystis carinii* pneumonia. Although pyrimethamine with a sulphonamide is the treatment of choice for cerebral toxoplasmosis in patients with AIDS, co-trimoxazole should be considered in patients who cannot tolerate pyrimethamine plus sulphonamide.— R. Esposito *et al.* (letter), *Br. med. J.*, 1987, *295*, 668.

URINARY-TRACT INFECTIONS. A review of the management of urinary-tract infections in children including the use of co-trimoxazole and trimethoprim.— A. W. Asscher, *Prescribers' J.*, 1982, *22*, 19. A similar review. Nowadays, even first urinary-tract infections in children are often at least partially resistant to sulphonamides, and co-trimoxazole has no advantage over trimethoprim alone.— R. H. R. White, *Archs Dis. Childh.*, 1987, *62*, 421.

A study of bacteriuria in elderly institutionalised men. Therapy with co-trimoxazole or tobramycin for asymptomatic bacteriuria was considered to be neither necessary nor effective.— L. E. Nicolle *et al.*, *New Engl. J. Med.*, 1983, *309*, 1420.

A review of the treatment of uncomplicated urinary-tract infections in women including the use of co-trimoxazole or trimethoprim. Women with uncomplicated urinary-tract infections require only short (3-day) courses of treatment or even single large doses: co-trimoxazole 960 mg twice daily or trimethoprim 200 mg twice daily may be used. A single dose of co-trimoxazole 1.92 g has been shown to be effective in women with no recent history of urinary-tract infection, who present within 2 days of onset of symptoms. Longer courses of treatment are required for recurrent infections.— W. R. Cattell, *Prescribers' J.*, 1983, *23*, 81. See also A. L. Komaroff, *New Engl. J. Med.*, 1984, *310*, 368.

In a study of 60 women with acute renal infection, including 39 women with acute pyelonephritis, patients were treated with co-trimoxazole 960 mg twice daily or ampicillin 500 mg every 6 hours given for 2 or 6 weeks. Of the patients treated for 2 weeks, 19 of 21 (90%) and 11 of 17 (65%) receiving co-trimoxazole and ampicillin, respectively, were cured; of those treated for 6 weeks, 10 of 12 (83%) and 4 of 10 (40%), respectively, were cured. The 2-week regimen of co-trimoxazole was considered suitable for the treatment of acute pyelonephritis in outpatients, longer periods of therapy having no additional benefit.— W. E. Stamm *et al.*, *Ann. intern. Med.*, 1987, *106*, 341. Comment.— A. R. Ronald, *ibid.*, 467.

Comparative studies. Comparative efficacy and safety of co-trimoxazole and nalidixic acid in the treatment of acute urinary-tract infections in women.— A. Iravani *et al.*, *Antimicrob. Ag. Chemother.*, 1981, *19*, 598.

Comparison of co-trimoxazole twice daily and co-trimazine once daily in the treatment of urinary-tract infections in children.— D. Adam *et al.*, *J. antimicrob. Chemother.*, 1982, *10*, 453.

Co-trimoxazole and trimethoprim were found to be equally effective in the treatment of patients with acute urinary-tract infections. There was also no significant difference in the incidence of adverse effects.— A. J. Martin and R. W. Lacey, *Practitioner*, 1984, *228*, 545.

Further references: M. Gringras and J. Cooper, *Practitioner*, 1979, *223*, 357 (comparison with nitrofurantoin).

Prophylaxis. In a prospective double-blind study completed by 74 patients co-trimoxazole prophylaxis produced a highly significant reduction in the incidence of bacteriuria after prostatectomy.— N. H. Hills *et al.*, *Br. med. J.*, 1976, *2*, 498.

A study of 28 women with persistent urinary-tract infections who received 6-month courses of low-dose co-trimoxazole (240 mg daily), or nitrofurantoin 100 mg daily. Although nitrofurantoin prophylaxis is adequate for the simpler problems of re-infection, where bacteriuria persisted co-trimoxazole is indicated.— T. A. Stamey *et al.*, *New Engl. J. Med.*, 1977, *296*, 780. Comment.— S. B. Levy, *ibid.*, 813.

A study in 32 women who suffered from recurrent urinary-tract infections indicated that thrice weekly treatment with co-trimoxazole 240 mg was effective for prophylaxis and did not predispose to colonisation or infection with trimethoprim-resistant Enterobacteriaceae.— G. K. M. Harding *et al.*, *J. Am. med. Ass.*, 1979, *242*, 1975.

Both co-trimoxazole and trimethoprim are used for long-term prophylaxis in patients with recurrent urinary-tract infections. However, R-factors conferring high-level resistance to trimethoprim are becoming widespread, and it appears that co-trimoxazole and trimethoprim may only have a limited time span of continued efficacy for long-term therapy.— W. Brumfitt *et al.*, *Br. J. Hosp. Med.*, 1983, *30*, 381. See also W. Brumfitt and J. M. T. Hamilton-Miller (letter), *Br. med. J.*, 1987, *295*, 390.

In a study on the prophylaxis of recurrent urinary-tract infections in children, co-trimoxazole 12 mg per kg body-weight given daily as a single dose and co-trimoxazole 12 mg per kg given three times a week were both effective. There was a slightly higher incidence of infection in children treated three times a week but fewer side-effects were noted in this group.— J. Labbé, *Can. med. Ass. J.*, 1984, *131*, 1229.

Comment on the management of recurrent urinary-tract infection including the use of co-trimoxazole and trimethoprim, and the role of self-medication.— *Lancet*, 1985, *1*, 1199.

Single-dose regimen. A single dose of co-trimoxazole 2.88 g given to adults and 0.72, 0.96, or 1.44 g to children aged 1 to 2 years, 2 to 5 years, and 5 to 12 years respectively, was as effective in the treatment of uncomplicated urinary-tract infections as conventional 5- to 7-day courses of co-trimoxazole given every 12 hours.— R. R. Bailey and G. D. Abbott, *Can. med. Ass. J.*, 1978, *118*, 551.

Single-dose treatment with co-trimoxazole is satisfactory only for lower urinary-tract infection; recurrent infections always require further investigations.— J. Z. Shainhouse (letter), *Can. med. Ass. J.*, 1978, *119*, 308.

Further references: W. R. Pitt *et al.*, *Archs Dis. Childh.*, 1982, *57*, 229; H. J. Schultz *et al.*, *Mayo Clin. Proc.*, 1984, *59*, 391; K. J. Carlson and A. G. Mulley, *Ann. intern. Med.*, 1985, *102*, 244; E. S. Wong *et al.*, *ibid.*, 302.

WHIPPLE'S DISEASE. For mention of the use of co-trimoxazole in the treatment of Whipple's disease, see under Benzylpenicillin Sodium, p.138.

Preparations

Co-trimoxazole Intravenous Infusion *(B.P.).* Co-trimoxazole Injection. A sterile solution prepared immediately before use by diluting Strong Sterile Co-trimoxazole Solution with 25 to 35 volumes of Glucose Intravenous Infusion or Sodium Chloride Intravenous Infusion.

Strong Sterile Co-trimoxazole Solution *(B.P.).* Strong Sterile Co-trimoxazole Solution for the preparation of Co-trimoxazole Intravenous Infusion. A sterile solution of sulphamethoxazole sodium (prepared by the interaction of sulphamethoxazole and sodium hydroxide) and trimethoprim in the proportion 5:1, in Water for Injections containing propylene glycol 40% v/v. Dilute before use.

Sulfamethoxazole and Trimethoprim Concentrate for Injection *(U.S.P.).* A sterile solution of sulphamethoxazole and trimethoprim in Water for Injections. Suitable for intravenous infusion after dilution with glucose 5% injection.

Co-trimoxazole Oral Suspension *(B.P.).* Co-trimoxazole Mixture; Sulphamethoxazole and Trimethoprim Mixture; Sulphamethoxazole and Trimethoprim Oral Suspension. A suspension containing sulphamethoxazole 8% and trimethoprim 1.6%. pH 5.0 to 6.5. Store at a temperature not exceeding 30°.

Paediatric Co-trimoxazole Oral Suspension *(B.P.).* Paediatric Co-trimoxazole Mixture; Paediatric Sulphamethoxazole and Trimethoprim Mixture; Paediatric Sulphamethoxazole and Trimethoprim Oral Suspension. A suspension containing sulphamethoxazole 4% and trimethoprim 0.8%. pH 5.0 to 6.5. Store at a temperature not exceeding 30°.

Sulfamethoxazole and Trimethoprim Oral Suspension *(U.S.P.).* pH 5.0 to 6.5.

Co-trimoxazole Tablets *(B.P.).* Sulphamethoxazole and Trimethoprim Tablets

Dispersible Co-trimoxazole Tablets *(B.P.).* Dispersible Sulphamethoxazole and Trimethoprim Tablets

Paediatric Co-trimoxazole Tablets *(B.P.).* Paediatric Sulphamethoxazole and Trimethoprim Tablets. Tablets each containing co-trimoxazole 120 mg.

Sulfamethoxazole and Trimethoprim Tablets *(U.S.P.)*

Proprietary Preparations

Bactrim *(Roche, UK). Drapsules*, film-coated tablets, co-trimoxazole 480 mg.
Paediatric tablets, co-trimoxazole 120 mg.
Tablets, dispersible, scored, co-trimoxazole 480 mg.
Tablets, scored, co-trimoxazole 960 mg.
Paediatric syrup, suspension, co-trimoxazole 240 mg/5 mL.
Suspension, co-trimoxazole 480 mg/5 mL.
Intramuscular injection, co-trimoxazole 320 mg/mL, in a vehicle containing glycofurol 52%, in ampoules of 3 mL.
Concentrate for intravenous infusion, co-trimoxazole 96 mg/mL, in a vehicle containing propylene glycol 40%, in ampoules of 5 mL. Dilute before use.

Chemotrim *(R.P. Drugs, UK). Paediatric suspension*, co-trimoxazole 240 mg/5 mL.

Comox *(Norton, UK). Tablets*, scored, co-trimoxazole 480 mg.
Tablets, dispersible, co-trimoxazole 480 mg.
Tablets, (Comox Forte), scored, co-trimoxazole 960 mg.
Paediatric suspension, co-trimoxazole 240 mg/5 mL.

Fectrim *(DDSA Pharmaceuticals, UK). Paediatric tablets*, co-trimoxazole 120 mg.
Tablets, dispersible, co-trimoxazole 480 mg.
Tablets (Fectrim Forte), dispersible, co-trimoxazole 960 mg.

Laratrim *(Lagap, UK). Tablets*, co-trimoxazole 480 mg.
Tablets (Laratrim Forte), co-trimoxazole 960 mg.
Paediatric suspension, co-trimoxazole 240 mg/5 mL.
Suspension, co-trimoxazole 480 mg/5 mL.

Septrin *(Wellcome, UK). Paediatric tablets*, scored, dispersible, co-trimoxazole 120 mg.
Tablets, co-trimoxazole 480 mg.
Tablets, dispersible, co-trimoxazole 480 mg.
Tablets (Septrin Forte), scored, co-trimoxazole 960 mg.
Paediatric suspension, co-trimoxazole 240 mg/5 mL.
Suspension, co-trimoxazole 480 mg/5 mL.
Intramuscular injection, co-trimoxazole 320 mg/mL, in a vehicle containing glycofurol 52%, in ampoules of 3 mL.
Concentrate for intravenous infusion, co-trimoxazole 96 mg/mL, in a vehicle containing propylene glycol 40%, in ampoules of 5 mL. Dilute before use.

Proprietary Names and Manufacturers

Abacin *(Gentili, Ital.)*; Abactrim *(Spain)*; Ampliespectrum *(Spain)*; Apo-Sulfatrim *(Apotex, Canad.)*; Bactekod *(Biogalenique, Fr.)*; Bacterial *(CT, Ital.)*; Bacticel *(Arg.)*; Bactifor *(Spain)*; Bactoreduct *(Azuchemie, Ger.)*; Bactramin *(Jpn)*; Bactrim *(Arg.; Roche, Austral.; Belg.; Roche, Canad.; Denm.; Roche, Fr.; Roche, Ger.; Roche, Ital.; Roche, Norw.; Roche, S.Afr.; Roche, Swed.; Roche, Switz.; Roche, UK; Roche, USA)*; Bactrimel *(Neth.)*; Baktar *(Jpn)*; Biosulten *(Spain)*; Brogenit *(Spain)*; Chemitrim *(Biomedica Foscama, Ital.)*; Chemotrim *(R.P. Drugs, UK)*; Comox *(Norton, UK)*; Comoxol *(Squibb, USA)*; Co-Trim *(Beiersdorf, Ger.; S.Afr.)*; Cotrim *(Engelhard, Ger.; Kettelhack Riker, Ger.; Klinge-Nattermann, Ger.; Ratiopharm, Ger.; Spirig, Switz.; Lemmon, USA)*; Cotrimox *(Unimed, UK)*; Cotrimstada *(Stadapharm, Ger.)*; Cozole *(Be-Tabs, S.Afr.)*; Dhas *(Spain)*; Drylin *(Merckle, Ger.)*; Duobiocin *(Dorsch, Ger.)*; Duratrimet *(Durachemie, Ger.)*; Durobac *(Supramed, S.Afr.)*; Escoprime *(Streuli, Switz.)*; Espectrin *(Braz.; Hong Kong; Malaysia; Philipp.; Singapore)*; Eusaprim *(Aust.; Belg.; Fin.; Wellcome, Fr.; Wellcome, Ger.; Wellcome, Ital.; Neth.; Wellcome, Norw.; Wellcome, Swed.; Wellcome, Switz.)*; Fectrim *(DDSA Pharmaceuticals, UK)*; Gantaprim *(Ausonia, Ital.)*; Gantrim *(Geymonat, Ital.)*; Groprim *(Grossmann, Switz.)*; Helveprim *(Switz.)*; Hulin *(Spain)*; Imexim *(Cimex, Switz.)*; Isotrim *(Ghimas, Ital.)*; Ixazolina *(Spain)*; Kepinol *(Pfleger, Ger.)*; Kitaprim *(Spain)*; Lagatrim *(Lagamed, S.Afr.; Lagap, Switz.)*; Laratrim *(Lagap, UK)*; Lescot *(Arg.)*; Linaris *(RAN, Ger.)*;
Magisprim *(Magis, Ital.)*; Medixin *(Pierrel, Ital.)*; Metoprin *(Spain)*; Mezenol *(Pharmador, S.Afr.)*; Microtrim *(Chephasaar, Ger.)*; Missile *(Arg.)*; Moxotrim *(Wilson, Pakistan)*; Nodilon *(Berk Pharmaceuticals, UK)*; Nopil *(Mepha, Switz.)*; Omsat *(Galenus Mannheim, Ger.)*; Oxaprim *(Otifarma, Ital.)*; Paitrin *(Ital.)*; Protrin *(Pro Doc, Canad.)*; Purbac *(Lennon, S.Afr.)*; Resprim *(Alphapharm, Austral.)*; Roubac *(Rougier, Canad.)*; Septocid *(Ital.)*; Septra *(Braz.; Wellcome, Canad.; Wellcome, USA)*; Septran *(Ind.; Pakistan; Wellcome, S.Afr.; Urug.)*; Septrin *(Arg.; Wellcome, Austral.; Spain; Wellcome, UK)*; Sigaprim *(Siegfried, Ger.; Sigamed, Switz.)*; Sinerbactin *(Spain)*; Soifasul *(Spain)*; Strepto-plus *(Molteni, Ital.)*; Sulfacet *(Winthrop, Ger.)*; Sulfatrim *(Schein, USA)*; Sulfotrim *(Denm.; Neth.; Switz.)*; Sulfotrimin *(Combustin, Ger.)*; Supracombin *(Grünenthal, Ger.)*; Suprin *(Valeas, Ital.)*; Syntran *(Ind.)*; System *(Chiesi, Ital.)*; Tacumil *(Spain)*; Teleprim *(Ital.)*; Thiocuran *(Sagitta, Ger.)*; Thoxaprim *(S.Afr.)*; TMS *(TAD, Ger.; TAD, Switz.)*; Trib *(Protea, Austral.)*; Trigonyl *(Hoyer, Ger.)*; Trim *(Giustini, Ital.)*; Trimesulf *(LPB, Ital.)*; Trimethoprim comp.-ratiopharm *(Ger.)*; Trimetoprim-Sulfa *(KabiVitrum, Norw.; Swed.)*; Trisazol *(Spain)*; Trisural *(Denm.)*; Ultrasept *(Sundrychem, S.Afr.)*; Ultrazole *(Rolab, S.Afr.)*; Uro-Septra *(Braz.)*; Uro-Sigaprim *(Siegfried, Ger.)*.

65-p

Demeclocycline *(BAN, USAN, rINN).*

Demethylchlortetracycline. 7-Chloro-6-demethyltetracycline.
$C_{21}H_{21}ClN_2O_8$=464.9.

CAS — 127-33-3; 13215-10-6 (sesquihydrate).

Pharmacopoeias. In *U.S.*

A yellow odourless crystalline powder. The *U.S.P.* specifies that it contains not less than the equivalent of 970 µg of demeclocycline hydrochloride per mg, calculated on the anhydrous basis. Sparingly **soluble** in water; soluble 1 in 200 of alcohol and 1 in 40 of methyl alcohol; soluble in 3N hydrochloric acid and in alkaline solutions. A 1% solution in water has a pH of 4 to 5.5. **Store** in airtight containers. Protect from light.

66-s

Demeclocycline Hydrochloride *(BANM, USAN, rINNM).*

Demethylchlortetracycline Hydrochloride.
$C_{21}H_{21}ClN_2O_8$,HCl=501.3.

CAS — 64-73-3.

Pharmacopoeias. In *Aust., Br., Eur., Fr., Ger., Ind., It., Neth., Nord., Swiss,* and *U.S.*

An antimicrobial substance produced by the growth of certain strains of *Streptomyces aureofaciens* or by any other means. It occurs as a yellow, odourless, crystalline powder. The *B.P.* specifies not less than 950 units per mg and *U.S.P.* specifies not less than 900 µg per mg, both calculated on the anhydrous basis.

Soluble 1 in 30 to 60 of water and 1 in 50 of methyl alcohol; slightly soluble in alcohol; practically insoluble in acetone, chloroform, and ether; soluble in aqueous solutions of alkali hydroxides and carbonates. A 1% solution in water has a pH of 2 to 3. **Store** in airtight containers. Protect from light.

The sulphates of copper, nickel, ferrous iron, and magnesium all destroyed or reduced the activity of demeclocycline when added to a solution of the antibiotic. Tests *in vitro* showed enhancement of antibiotic activity in the presence of zinc sulphate.— M. E. Hamner, *Antibiotics Chemother.*, 1961, *11*, 498.

Units

One unit of demeclocycline is contained in 0.001 mg of the first International Reference Preparation (1962) which contains 1000 units per mg.

Adverse Effects and Precautions

As for Tetracycline Hydrochloride, p.314.

Phototoxic reactions occur more frequently with demeclocycline than with other tetracyclines and patients should avoid exposure to direct sunlight. Reversible nephrogenic diabetes insipidus with polyuria, polydipsia, and weakness may occur in patients treated with demeclocycline.

EFFECTS ON THE KIDNEY. Nonoliguric acute renal failure occurred in a patient with cirrhosis given demeclocycline 300 mg three times daily. Demeclocycline should be used with great caution in correcting impaired renal diluting ability especially in cirrhotic patients.— J. R. Oster and M. Epstein (letter), *Lancet*, 1977, *1*, 52. See also F. Carrilho *et al.*, *Ann. intern. Med.*, 1977, *87*, 195.

Hypophosphataemia with an inappropriate phosphaturia occurred in a 62-year-old woman during therapy with demeclocycline 300 mg twice daily for inappropriate secretion of antidiuretic hormone.— G. Decaux *et al.* (letter), *New Engl. J. Med.*, 1985, *313*, 1480.

Further references: P. L. Padfield *et al.*, *Postgrad. med. J.*, 1978, *54*, 623.

EFFECTS ON THE SKIN. A 64-year-old woman who developed photodermatitis one day after treatment with demeclocycline developed photo-onycholysis 5 weeks later.— H. J. N. Bethell, *Br. med. J.*, 1977, *2*, 96.

Of the tetracyclines, demeclocycline is the most potent phototoxic agent. It causes both immediate and delayed reactions in most individuals, according to dose. Studies have demonstrated that the action spectrum for demeclocycline phototoxicity is above 320 nm and that complement and polymorphonuclear leucocytes are required as amplifiers or effectors of the phototoxicity. Therapy of acute phototoxic responses includes the use of topical cool wet dressings, soothing lotions, topical corticosteroids, and systemic antipruritic agents; if the process is severe enough, systemic corticosteroids may be indicated.— J. H. Epstein and B. U. Wintroub, *Drugs*, 1985, *30*, 42.

INTERACTIONS. Diuresis induced by amiloride and metolazone was enhanced in a patient when demeclocycline was given concomitantly.— R. R. Ghose and R. Bonser (letter), *Br. med. J.*, 1978, *1*, 1282.

Absorption and Fate

As for Tetracycline Hydrochloride, p.317.

Peak plasma concentrations of about 2.4 µg per mL have been reported 3 to 6 hours after an oral dose of 500 mg of demeclocycline hydrochloride and persist for longer than after a similar dose of tetracycline, only falling to about 1 µg per mL after 24 hours. Its biological half-life is about 12 hours. The renal clearance of demeclocycline is about half that of tetracycline.

Uses and Administration

Demeclocycline hydrochloride has the antimicrobial activity and uses described for tetracycline hydrochloride (see p.315). It is excreted more slowly and effective blood concentrations are maintained for a longer period.

The usual adult dosage is 600 mg of demeclocycline hydrochloride daily by mouth in 2 or 4 divided doses preferably one hour before or 2 hours after meals; 900 mg daily in divided doses may be given for mycoplasmal pneumonia. Children have been given 6 to 12 mg per kg body-weight daily in divided doses, but the effect of tetracyclines on teeth should be considered.

Demeclocycline may be given to adults in the treatment of chronic hyponatraemia associated with the inappropriate secretion of antidiuretic hormone, when water restriction has proved ineffective. Initially demeclocycline hydrochloride 0.9 to 1.2 g is given daily in divided doses, reduced to maintenance doses of 0.6 to 0.9 g daily.

HYPONATRAEMIA. Water excess or water intoxication due to increased intake or inability to excrete water normally results in hypo-osmolality, a small increase in extracellular fluid, and progressive hyponatraemia (S.M. Willatts, *Br. J. Hosp. Med.*, 1984, *32*, 8). Causes of impaired ability to excrete water include the syndrome of inappropriate secretion of antidiuretic hormone (SIADH). Possible treatment in patients with chronic or persistent SIADH, in whom water restriction has failed, includes demeclocycline, lithium, urea and sodium supplements, or frusemide. Lithium and demeclocycline interfere with the cellular action of antidiuretic hormone to produce nephrogenic diabetes insipidus. Since the report that demeclocycline was superior to lithium (J.N. Forrest *et al.*, *New Engl. J. Med.*, 1978, *298*, 173), demeclocycline has become the preferred treatment for chronic SIADH if water restriction is unsuccessful (R.W. Schrier, *New Engl. J. Med.*, 1985, *312*, 1121), although fluid restriction is still the treatment of choice. However, it has been noted that since demeclocycline caused nephrogenic diabetes insipidus (delayed onset of 5 to 8 days) and nephrotoxicity in patients with cardiac or hepatic disease, its usefulness in the treatment of hyponatraemic states might be limited; this view was supported by studies in patients with cardiac failure (D. Zegers de Beyl *et al.*, *Br. med. J.*, 1978, *1*, 760) and cirrhosis (P.D. Miller *et al.*, *J. Am. med. Ass.*, 1980, *243*, 2513). (See also under Effects on the Kidney in Adverse Effects, above). More recently the use of vasopressin antagonists has shown promise.

RESPIRATORY-TRACT INFECTIONS. For the use of demeclocycline in the treatment of bronchitis, see under Tetracycline Hydrochloride, p.320.

Preparations

Demeclocycline Capsules *(B.P.).* Capsules containing demeclocycline hydrochloride.

Demeclocycline Hydrochloride Capsules *(U.S.P.)*

Demeclocycline Hydrochloride Tablets *(U.S.P.)*

Demeclocycline Oral Suspension *(U.S.P.).* Potency is expressed in terms of demeclocycline hydrochloride. pH 4.0 to 5.8.

Demeclocycline Hydrochloride and Nystatin Capsules *(U.S.P.)*

Demeclocycline Hydrochloride and Nystatin Tablets *(U.S.P.)*

Proprietary Preparations

Ledermycin *(Lederle, UK). Capsules,* demeclocycline hydrochloride 150 mg.
Tablets, demeclocycline hydrochloride 300 mg.

Proprietary Names and Manufacturers of Demeclocycline and its Salts

Actaciclina *(Ital.)*; Benaciclin *(Spain)*; Bioterciclin *(Ital.)*; Clortetrin *(Medosan, Ital.)*; Compleciclin *(Spain)*; Declomycin *(Lederle, Canad.; Lederle, USA)*; Demeplus *(Boniscontro & Gazzone, Ital.)*; Deme-Proter *(Proter, Ital.)*; Demetetra *(Ital.)*; Demetraciclina *(Ital.)*; Demetraclin *(Ital.)*; Detracin *(Ital.)*; Detravis *(Vis, Ital.)*; Dimeral *(Ital.)*; Diuciclin *(Benvegna, Ital.)*; Elkamicina *(Ital.)*; Fidocin *(Ital.)*; Isodemetil *(Ital.)*; Latomicina *(Ital.)*; Ledermicina *(Arg.; Cyanamid, Ital.; Spain)*; Ledermycin *(Lederle, Austral.; Belg.; Lederle, Denm.; Cyanamid-Lederle, Ger.; Neth.; Norw.; Lederle, S.Afr.; Lederle, Swed.; Lederle, Switz.; Lederle, UK)*; Ledermycine *(Fr.)*; Magis-Ciclina *(Ital.)*; Mirciclina *(Ital.)*; Neo Cromaciclin *(Ital.)*; Provimicina *(Sabater, Spain)*; Rynabron *(Landerlan, Spain)*; Tetradek *(Ital.)*; Tollerclin *(Ital.)*; Veraciclina *(Ital.)*; Wolnerciclina *(Kairon, Spain)*.

The following names have been used for multi-ingredient preparations containing demeclocycline and its salts—

Deteclo *(Lederle, UK)*; Ledermix *(Lederle, UK)*; Lederstatin *(Lederle, UK)*.

67-w

Dibekacin Sulphate *(BANM, rINNM).*

3′,4′-Dideoxykanamycin B. 6-*O*-(3-Amino-3-deoxy-α-D-glucopyranosyl)-2-deoxy-4-*O*-(2,6-diamino-2,3,4,6-tetradeoxy-α-D-glucopyranosyl)-D-streptamine sulphate.
$C_{18}H_{37}N_5O_8$,xH_2SO_4=451.5 (dibekacin).

CAS — 34493-98-6 (dibekacin); 58580-55-5 (sulphate).

Pharmacopoeias. In *Jpn.*

Dibekacin sulphate is **incompatible** with beta-lactam antibiotics (see Gentamicin Sulphate, p.236).

Dibekacin is an aminoglycoside antibiotic derived from kanamycin with actions and uses similar to those of gentamicin (see p.236). It has been given as the sulphate, intramuscularly or intravenously in various dosage regimens (see below).

A review of the actions and uses of dibekacin. Dibekacin has been used in relatively low doses in the Far East; 1 mg per kg body-weight twice daily or 2 mg per kg once daily intravenously or intramuscularly has been a standard regimen in many reported studies. Dosage regimens in Europe have generally been 3 mg per kg daily in 2 or 3 divided doses although one large study used 3 mg per kg every 12 hours. The lack of controlled clinical studies makes it difficult to evaluate the true role of this aminoglycoside.— P. Noone, *Drugs*, 1984, *27*, 548.

See also Gentamicin Sulphate, p.242, for further reviews of aminoglycoside antibiotics.

For reference to a comparative study of the antimicrobial activity of 11 aminoglycosides including dibekacin, see Gentamicin Sulphate, p.239, and for reference to its activity against atypical *Mycobacterium* spp., see Amikacin Sulphate, p.110.

Proprietary Names and Manufacturers

Debekacyl *(Bellon, Fr.)*;
Decabicin *(Faes, Spain)*; Icacine *(Bristol, Fr.)*; Kappabi *(Carlo Erba, Ital.)*; Klobamicina *(Almirall, Spain)*; Orbicin *(Mack, Illert., Ger.; Pfizer, Ger.)*; Panimycin *(Jpn)*.

68-e

Dicloxacillin Sodium *(BANM, USAN, rINNM).*

P-1011; Sodium Dicloxacillin. Sodium (6*R*)-6-[3-(2,6-dichlorophenyl)-5-methylisoxazole-4-carboxamido]penicillanate monohydrate.
$C_{19}H_{16}Cl_2N_3NaO_5S$,$H_2O$=510.3.

CAS — 3116-76-5 (dicloxacillin); 343-55-5 (sodium salt, anhydrous); 13412-64-1 (sodium salt, monohydrate).

Pharmacopoeias. In *Braz., It., Jpn,* and *U.S.*

A white to off-white crystalline powder. 1.09 g of monograph substance is approximately equivalent to 1 g of anhydrous dicloxacillin. Each g of monograph substance represents approximately 2 mmol of sodium. Freely **soluble** in water. A 1% solution in water has a pH of 4.5 to 7.5. **Store** in airtight containers.

Adverse Effects

As for Benzylpenicillin Sodium, p.132.

EFFECTS ON THE GASTRO-INTESTINAL TRACT. The isolation of toxin-producing *Clostridium difficile* from 2 children with dicloxacillin- and oxacillin-associated diarrhoea, respectively.— I. Brook, *Pediatrics*, 1980, *65*, 1154.

Non-pseudomembranous colitis, presenting with abdominal pain and bloody diarrhoea, was associated with the administration of a combination of dicloxacillin and ampicillin in 3 patients.— M. Iida *et al.*, *Endoscopy*, 1985, *17*, 64.

LOCAL IRRITANT EFFECTS. Ischaemia followed by gangrene requiring amputation occurred in the hand and lower arm of 2 patients each given dicloxacillin accidentally by intra-arterial injection.— H. Ehringer *et al.*, *Wien. med. Wschr.*, 1971, *121*, 710.

Precautions

As for Benzylpenicillin Sodium, p.133.

For reference to a possible change in the disposition of dicloxacillin in patients with cystic fibrosis, see below under Absorption and Fate.

ADMINISTRATION IN RENAL FAILURE. For reference to the precautions to be observed in renal failure, see below under Uses, Administration in Renal Failure.

INTERACTIONS. For reference to the effect of mezlocillin on the pharmacokinetics of dicloxacillin, see Oxacillin Sodium p.277.

For the effects of other drugs on the antimicrobial activity of dicloxacillin sodium, see below under Antimicrobial Action.

Antimicrobial Action

Dicloxacillin sodium has a range of antibacterial activity similar to that of flucloxacillin (see p.231), but is generally reported to be more active.

ENHANCED ACTIVITY. No synergy was shown *in vitro* between combinations of dicloxacillin and fusidic acid, or dicloxacillin and rifampicin when tested against 10 clinical isolates of *Staphylococcus epidermidis* implicated in endocarditis. A combination of all 3 drugs, however, was synergistic against 5 of the isolates.— V. L. Yu *et al.*, *J. antimicrob. Chemother.*, 1984, *14*, 359.

For reference to reported synergism between dicloxacillin and amoxycillin, see Amoxycillin Trihydrate p.112.

Resistance

As for Methicillin Sodium, p.259.

Absorption and Fate

Dicloxacillin sodium, like flucloxacillin sodium, is about twice as well absorbed from the gastro-intestinal tract as cloxacillin sodium but absorption is also reduced by the presence of food in the stomach. After an oral dose of 500 mg, peak plasma concentrations of 10 to 18 μg per mL are obtained in about 1 hour in fasting subjects. Doubling the dose can double the plasma concentration. About 97% of dicloxacillin in the circulation is bound to plasma proteins. Dicloxacillin has been reported to have a plasma half-life of about 0.5 hour in healthy subjects. The half-life is prolonged in neonates.

The distribution of dicloxacillin in body tissues and fluids is similar to that of cloxacillin sodium, p.203.

Dicloxacillin is metabolised to a limited extent and the unchanged drug and metabolites are excreted in the urine by glomerular filtration and renal tubular secretion. About 60% of a dose given by mouth is excreted in the urine. Only small amounts are excreted in the bile.

Serum concentrations are enhanced if probenecid is given concomitantly.

Serum concentrations of dicloxacillin after the administration of a single dose by mouth were lower in patients with cystic fibrosis than in healthy subjects. This appeared to be due to an increase in renal clearance although pharmacokinetic parameters varied greatly between patients.— W. J. Jusko *et al.*, *Pediatrics*, 1975, *56*, 1038.

ADMINISTRATION IN RENAL FAILURE. For reference to the pharmacokinetics of dicloxacillin in renal failure, see below under Uses, Administration in Renal Failure.

DIFFUSION INTO BODY TISSUES AND FLUIDS. Studies of the penetration of dicloxacillin into bone and joint fluid after systemic administration: J. D. Nelson *et al.*, *J. Pediat.*, 1978, *92*, 131; T. R. Tetzlaff *et al.*, *J. Pediat.*, 1978, *92*, 135.

METABOLISM. About 10% of a 500-mg dose of dicloxacillin was metabolised. Within 12 hours of the dose being taken by 6 healthy subjects about 37% was recovered in the urine, 4% as penicilloic acid.— M. Cole *et al.*, *Antimicrob. Ag. Chemother.*, 1973, *3*, 463.

Dicloxacillin was metabolised to a slightly less potent antibacterial compound.— H. H. W. Thijssen and H. Mattie, *Antimicrob. Ag. Chemother.*, 1976, *10*, 441.

Uses and Administration

Dicloxacillin sodium is an isoxazolyl penicillin with similar uses to flucloxacillin, p.231.

Dicloxacillin sodium is administered by mouth about 1 hour before, or at least 2 hours after meals since the presence of food in the stomach reduces absorption. The usual dose is the equivalent of 125 to 500 mg of dicloxacillin four times daily. Children may be given the equivalent of 12.5 to 25 mg of dicloxacillin per kg body-weight daily in divided doses. Dicloxacillin sodium has also been given parenterally in doses equivalent to 500 mg of dicloxacillin every 6 hours. Doses may be increased in severe infections.

ADMINISTRATION. Dicloxacillin sodium was given as an example of a drug with a high specific gravity whose administration may be unpredictable when given by slow intravenous infusion.— S. C. Smith and R. E. Crass (letter), *Drug Intell. & clin. Pharm.*, 1984, *18*, 530.

ADMINISTRATION IN RENAL FAILURE. The normal half-life for dicloxacillin of 0.5 to 0.9 hour was increased to 1 to 1.6 hours in end-stage renal failure. It could be given in usual doses to patients with renal failure. A dosage supplement was not required for patients undergoing haemodialysis.— W. M. Bennett *et al.*, *Am. J. Kidney Dis.*, 1983, *3*, 155.

Preparations

Dicloxacillin Sodium Capsules *(U.S.P.)*

Sterile Dicloxacillin Sodium *(U.S.P.)*

Dicloxacillin Sodium for Oral Suspension *(U.S.P.)*

Proprietary Names and Manufacturers

Dichlor-Stapenor *(Bayer, Ger.)*; Diclo *(FIRMA, Ital.)*; Diclocil *(Bristol, Belg.; Bristol-Myers, Denm.; Bristol, Fr.; Bristol Italiana Sud, Ital.; Bristol, Neth.; Bristol, Norw.; Antibioticos, Spain; Bristol, Swed.; Bristol, Switz.)*; Diclocillin *(Lagap, Ital.)*; Diclomax *(Pulitzer, Ital.)*; Dicloxapen *(Magis, Ital.)*; Diflor *(Coli, Ital.)*; Dycill *(Beecham Laboratories, USA)*; Dynapen *(Bristol, Canad.; Bristol, USA)*; Maclicine *(Christiaens, Belg.)*; Novapen *(IBP, Ital.)*; Pathocil *(Wyeth, USA)*; Stafopenin *(Astra, Swed.)*; Veracillin *(Ayerst, USA)*.

71-g

Dihydrostreptomycin Sulphate *(BAN, rINNM)*.

Dihydrostreptomycin Sulfate *(USAN)*; Dihydrostreptomycini Sulfas. 4-*O*-[2-*O*-(2-Deoxy-2-methylamino-α-L-glucopyranosyl)-5-deoxy-3-*C*-hydroxymethyl-α-L-lyxofuranosyl]-*NN'*-diamidino-D-streptamine sulphate.

$(C_{21}H_{41}N_7O_{12})_2,3H_2SO_4$=1461.4.

CAS — 128-46-1 (dihydrostreptomycin); 5490-27-7 (sulphate).

Pharmacopoeias. In *Arg., Aust., Belg., Eur., Fr., It., Mex., Nord., Port.,* and *Swiss.* Also in *B.P. Vet.* and in *U.S.P.* for veterinary use only.

Dihydrostreptomycin *(Span. P.)* is the hydrochloride or the sulphate.

A white or almost white powder; it may be hygroscopic. The *B.P. Vet.* specifies not less than 730 units per mg with reference to the dried substance. The *U.S.P.* specifies a potency equivalent to not less than 650 μg of dihydrostreptomycin per mg, or not less than 725 μg per mg if it is crystalline, and not less than 450 μg per mg if it is for oral use only. 1.25 g of monograph substance is approximately equivalent to 1 g of dihydrostreptomycin.

Freely **soluble** in water; practically insoluble in alcohol, acetone, chloroform, and methyl alcohol. A 25% solution in water has a pH of 5 to 7.

Store at a temperature not exceeding 30° in airtight containers. Protect from light.

Units

One unit of dihydrostreptomycin is contained in 0.001219 mg of the second International Standard Preparation (1966) of dihydrostreptomycin sulphate which contains 820 units per mg.

Dihydrostreptomycin sulphate is an aminoglycoside antibiotic with actions and uses similar to those of Streptomycin Sulphate, p.297. It has been given intramuscularly in doses equivalent to 0.5 to 1 g of dihydrostreptomycin. However, since it is more likely than streptomycin to cause partial or complete loss of hearing it is rarely used. Dihydrostreptomycin sulphate is widely used in veterinary medicine.

Proprietary Names and Manufacturers

Abiocine *(Lepetit, Fr.)*; Coliriocilina DHD Estrepto *(Medical, Spain)*; Diestreptopab *(Spain)*; Dihidro-Cidan Sulfato *(Cidan, Spain)*; Entera-strept *(Heyl, Ger.)*; Estreptoluy *(Spain)*; Sanestrepto *(Santos, Spain)*; Solvo-Strept *(Heyl, Ger.)*.

The following names have been used for multi-ingredient preparations containing dihydrostreptomycin sulphate— Diarstop *(Schering, Ital.)*; Guanimycin *(Allen & Hanburys, UK)*; Streptomagma *(Wyeth, Austral.)*.

5656-h

Dihydroxymethylfuratrizine

N-[6-(5-Nitrofurfurylidenemethyl)-1,2,4-triazin-3-yl]-iminodimethanol.

$C_{11}H_{11}N_5O_5$=293.2.

CAS — 794-93-4.

Dihydroxymethylfuratrizine is a nitrofuran antibacterial agent which was formerly used in the treatment of urinary-tract infections.

Proprietary Names and Manufacturers

Panfuran-S *(Toyama, Jpn)*.

72-q

Doxycycline *(BAN, USAN, rINN)*.

Doxycycline Monohydrate. 6-Deoxy-5β-hydroxytetracycline monohydrate.

$C_{22}H_{24}N_2O_8,H_2O$=462.5.

CAS — 564-25-0 (anhydrous); 17086-28-1 (monohydrate).

Pharmacopoeias. In *U.S.*

A yellow crystalline powder containing 880 to 980 μg of anhydrous doxycycline per mg. Very slightly **soluble** in water; sparingly soluble in alcohol; practically insoluble in chloroform and ether; freely soluble in dilute acids and alkali hydroxides. A 1% aqueous suspension has a pH of 5.0 to 6.5. **Store** in airtight containers. Protect from light.

73-p

Doxycycline Calcium *(BANM, USAN, rINNM).*

A complex prepared from doxycycline hydrochloride and calcium chloride.

18633-l

Doxycycline Fosfatex *(BAN, USAN).*

AB08. 6-Deoxy-5β-hydroxytetracycline—metaphosphoric acid—sodium metaphosphate in the ratio 3:3:1.

$(C_{22}H_{24}N_2O_8)_3(HPO_3)_3NaPO_3$=1675.2.

CAS — 83038-87-3.

74-s

Doxycycline Hydrochloride *(BANM).*

6-Deoxy-5β-hydroxytetracycline Hydrochloride; Dossiciclina Iclato; Doxycycline Hyclate *(USAN)*; Doxycyclini Hyclas. Doxycycline hydrochloride hemiethanolate hemihydrate.

$C_{22}H_{24}N_2O_8$,HCl,½C_2H_5OH,½H_2O=512.9.

CAS — 10592-13-9 ($C_{22}H_{24}N_2O_8$,HCl); 24390-14-5 ($C_{22}H_{24}N_2O_8$,HCl,½C_2H_5OH,½H_2O).

Pharmacopoeias. In *Br., Braz., Chin., Cz., Eur., Fr., Ind., It., Jpn, Neth., Nord., Swiss,* and *U.S.*

A yellow hygroscopic crystalline powder. The *B.P.* specifies that it contains not less than 880 units per mg calculated with reference to the anhydrous and alcohol-free substance. The *U.S.P.* specifies that it contains 800 to 920 µg of doxycycline per mg. Doxycycline hydrochloride 115 mg is approximately equivalent to 100 mg of doxycycline. **Soluble** 1 in 3 of water and 1 in 4 of methyl alcohol; sparingly soluble in alcohol; practically insoluble in chloroform and ether; soluble in solutions of alkali hydroxides and carbonates. A 1% solution in water has a pH of 2 to 3. The *U.S.P.* injection has a pH of 1.8 to 3.3. **Store** in airtight containers. Protect from light.

Solutions in sodium chloride injection or glucose injection should be used within 48 hours of preparation and protected from direct sunlight; they may be stored for up to 72 hours at a temperature between 2° and 8°, but infusion must then be completed within 12 hours.

LOSS OF ACTIVITY. Riboflavine reduced the antimicrobial activity *in vitro* of doxycycline hydrochloride by 56.5%.— M. A. El-Nakeeb *et al., Can. J. pharm. Sci.*, 1976, *11*, 85.

Units

One unit of doxycycline is contained in 0.0011494 mg of the first International Reference Preparation (1973) of doxycycline hydrochloride which contains 870 units per mg.

Adverse Effects

As for Tetracycline Hydrochloride, p.314.

Doxycycline has a lower affinity for binding with calcium and it may cause less tooth discoloration than other tetracyclines.

Tetracyclines, especially doxycycline, have been reported to interfere with host defence mechanisms including depression of chemotaxis, phagocytosis, and intracellular metabolism of polymorphonuclear leucocytes. However, the literature is limited and often contradictory (J.M. Oleske, *J. antimicrob. Chemother.*, 1984, *13*, 413). The significance of the effect of tetracyclines on polymorphonuclear leucocyte migration *in vitro* has been challenged and a single oral dose of doxycycline 200 mg given to healthy subjects was shown to have no inhibitory effect on the subsequent migration of polymorphonuclear leucocytes *in vitro* (O. Bäck and B. Norberg, *Eur. J. clin. Pharmac.*, 1985, *28*, 193).

ALLERGY. A report of an anaphylactoid reaction in a 71-year-old woman who received intravenous doxycycline during general anaesthesia and beta-blockade treatment. The manufacturer had received 5 other reports of anaphylactoid reactions due to doxycycline.— J. C. Raeder, *Drug Intell. & clin. Pharm.*, 1984, *18*, 481. Comment that the antibiotic may have been administered too rapidly.— R. L. Barkin and Z. L. G. Stein (letter), *ibid.*, 999. Reply.— J. C. Raeder (letter), *ibid.*

Analysis, by the Boston Collaborative Drug Surveillance Program, of data on 15 438 patients hospitalised between 1975 and 1982 detected 2 allergic skin reactions attributed to doxycycline among 425 recipients of the drug.— M. Bigby *et al., J. Am. med. Ass.*, 1986, *256*, 3358.

DEPOSITION IN BONES AND TEETH. Of 25 children who had been born prematurely and who had received doxycycline in total doses of from 9 to 37 mg soon after birth, only 1 was found to have a discoloration of the milk teeth. The upper incisors had a slight spotted discoloration.— G. Forti and C. Benincori (letter), *Lancet*, 1969, *1*, 782.

EFFECTS ON THE GASTRO-INTESTINAL TRACT. There have been a number of reports of oesophagitis or oesophageal ulceration associated with administration of doxycycline tablets or capsules (G.J. Hatheway, *Drug Intell. & clin. Pharm.*, 1982, *16*, 879; A. Geschwind, *Med. J. Aust.*, 1984, *140*, 223; B. Bissonnette and P. Biron, *Can. med. Ass. J.*, 1984, *131*, 1186; M.A. Amendola and T.D. Spera, *J. Am. med. Ass.*, 1985, *253*, 1009; S. Adib-Bagheri, *Gut*, 1986, *27*, A1269). Other tetracyclines including tetracycline, oxytetracycline, and minocycline have also been reported to cause oesophagitis (M. Atkinson, *Prescribers' J.*, 1982, *22*, 129; T.D. Spera and M.A. Amendola, *J. Am. med. Ass.*, 1985, *254*, 508). Most patients have taken too little fluid with the drug and have often gone to bed almost immediately, thus delaying passage through the oesophagus (*Drug & Ther. Bull.*, 1985, *23*, 73; A.D. Shiff, *J. Am. med. Ass.*, 1986, *256*, 1893). The acidity of tetracycline and doxycycline and the rate of dissolution and release of the drug have been linked to the toxic effects (O. Brors, *Med. Toxicol.*, 1987, *2*, 105); the doxycycline monohydrate free base formulation has been found to be less toxic to the *cat* oesophageal mucosa than the hydrochloride (B. Carlborg and J.C. Farmer, *Curr. ther. Res.*, 1983, *34*, 110) and dispersible tablets are less likely than capsules to stick to oesophageal mucosa (*Drug & Ther. Bull.*, 1982, *20*, 76). Symptoms usually resolve within about 1 week without stricture formation, however, oesophagitis may persist considerably longer than this (*Drug & Ther. Bull.*, 1981, *19*, 33; P.M. Jost, *J. Am. med. Ass.*, 1985, *254*, 508).

A report of the impact of orally administered antimicrobial agents on human oropharyngeal and colonic microflora. Doxycycline 100 mg daily for 7 days given to 10 subjects resulted in only moderate changes in the microflora with a decrease in the number of enterococci and streptococci in 8 subjects, enterobacteria in 5, and fusobacteria in 3. There was, however, a marked emergence of doxycycline resistance among both aerobic and anaerobic bacteria.— C. E. Nord and A. Heimdahl, *J. antimicrob. Chemother.*, 1986, *18*, *Suppl.* C, 159.

EFFECTS ON MEMORY. In a double-blind placebo-controlled study of 32 healthy subjects doxycycline 200 mg given by mouth at bedtime impaired memory of material learned during the night.— C. Idzikowski and I. Oswald, *Psychopharmacology*, 1983, *79*, 108.

EFFECTS ON THE SKIN. Doxycycline, methacycline, minocycline, oxytetracycline, and tetracycline have been reported to cause photosensitivity reactions; demeclocycline is a frequent cause. Drugs such as doxycycline that only cause reactions occasionally are used so frequently that they may be common causes of photosensitivity.— *Med. Lett.*, 1986, *28*, 51.

See also Allergy, above.

THROMBOPHLEBITIS. Of 46 patients with infusion phlebitis, doxycycline hydrochloride was implicated as the causative agent in 11 patients. The incidence of doxycycline-induced phlebitis was reduced when the drug was administered in 100-mL rather than 50-mL solutions. It was recommended that a dose of 100 mg should be administered with at least 200 to 250 mL of intravenous fluid over 1 to 2 hours.— C. A. Harrigan, *NITA*, 1984, *7*, 478.

Precautions

As for Tetracycline Hydrochloride, p.315.

Absorption of doxycycline appears to be less affected by milk or food than the other tetracyclines. Doxycycline may also be less likely to aggravate renal disease.

Renal function deteriorated acutely but reversibly in a patient with chronic renal failure given doxycycline for 14 days.— L. H. Orr *et al., Archs intern. Med.*, 1978, *138*, 793.

INTERACTIONS. In 5 subjects the mean half-life of doxycycline after a 100-mg intravenous dose was significantly reduced from a mean of 15.3 hours to a mean of 11.1 hours after the administration for 10 days of phenobarbitone 50 mg three times daily. In 5 further patients on long-term barbiturates the mean half-life was 7.7 hours. Phenytoin similarly reduced the half-life of doxycycline.— P. J. Neuvonen and O. Penttilä, *Br. med. J.*, 1974, *1*, 535.

The mean half-life of doxycycline after intravenous injection of 100 mg was 15.1 hours in 9 controls, but was 7.2 hours in 7 patients who had taken phenytoin for from 4 months to 10 years, 8.4 hours in 5 patients who had taken carbamazepine for from 4 months to 4 years, and 7.4 hours in 4 patients taking phenytoin and carbamazepine.— O. Penttilä *et al., Br. med. J.*, 1974, *2*, 470.

Concurrent oral ferrous sulphate administration lowered the serum concentration of doxycycline administered by mouth, and shortened the serum half-life after a single intravenous injection. The interaction could not be avoided completely by leaving a 3-hour interval between doses of the two drugs.— P. J. Neuvonen and O. Penttilä, *Eur. J. clin. Pharmac.*, 1974, *7*, 361. The therapeutic effect of doxycycline was not considered to be at risk provided doxycycline and iron were given several hours apart.— V. M. K. Venho *et al., Eur. J. clin. Pharmac.*, 1978, *14*, 277.

Doxycycline is more lipid soluble than tetracycline and also undergoes more extensive hepatic metabolism. Doxycycline kinetics are therefore more likely to be altered by agents which inhibit or induce hepatic metabolism. Short-term administration of alcohol has been shown to increase the elimination half-life of doxycycline, and the half-life of doxycycline has been reported to be reduced in recently abstinent alcoholic patients compared with healthy controls.— E. A. Lane *et al., Clin. Pharmacokinet.*, 1985, *10*, 228.

PORPHYRIA. Doxycycline was considered to be unsafe in patients with acute porphyria because it has been shown to be porphyrinogenic in *animals* or *in vitro* systems.— M.R. Moore and K.E.L. McColl, *Porphyrias, Drug Lists*, Glasgow, Porphyria Research Unit, University of Glasgow, 1987.

Antimicrobial Action and Resistance

Doxycycline hydrochloride has a range of antimicrobial activity and mode of action similar to that of tetracycline hydrochloride (see p.315). It is more effective than tetracycline against many species.

A study of the activity *in vitro* of doxycycline, minocycline, and oxytetracycline against anaerobic bacteria; both doxycycline and minocycline showed enhanced antibacterial activity compared with oxytetracycline. At least 90% of the *Bacteroides fragilis* group, *B. melaninogenicus, Fusobacterium* spp., *Clostridium perfringens, Cl. difficile*, and *Propionibacterium acnes* isolates were inhibited by an achievable serum concentration of 4 µg per mL of doxycycline or minocycline. Oxytetracycline is considered no longer useful in the treatment of possible anaerobic infection, but doxycycline and minocycline could be used when the infecting organisms are known to be sensitive.— M. Robbins *et al., J. antimicrob. Chemother.*, 1987, *20*, 379. See also under Minocycline Hydrochloride, p.263.

References to the activity of doxycycline against various organisms: J. R. Carlson *et al., Antimicrob. Ag. Chemother.*, 1983, *24*, 509 (bacterial enteropathogens); W. F. Myers *et al., ibid.*, 1984, *25*, 690 (*Rochalimaea quintana*); S. Larsson *et al., ibid.*, 1985, *28*, 12 (*Listeria monocytogenes*); A. W. Pasculle *et al., ibid.*, 730 (*Legionella micdadei*); J. M. Swenson *et al., ibid.*, 807 (*Mycobacterium fortuitum* and *M. chelonae*); J. Bosch *et al., J. antimicrob. Chemother.*, 1986, *17*, 459 (*Brucella melitensis*); A. A. Crouch *et al., Trans. R. Soc. trop. Med. Hyg.*, 1986, *80*, 893 (*Giardia lamblia*); M. R. Scavizzi *et al., Antimicrob. Ag. Chemother.*, 1987, *31*, 523 (*Yersinia enterocolitica*); J. A. A. Hoogkamp-Korstanje, *J. antimicrob. Chemother.*, 1987, *20*, 123 (*Y. enterocolitica*).

ACTIVITY WITH OTHER ANTIMICROBIAL AGENTS. Doxycycline antagonised the bactericidal action of ampicillin and benzylpenicillin against *Listeria monocytogenes in vitro*.— D. L. Winslow *et al., Antimicrob. Ag. Chemother.*, 1983, *23*, 555.

Absorption and Fate

As for Tetracycline Hydrochloride, p.317.

Doxycycline hydrochloride is readily absorbed from the gastro-intestinal tract and absorption is not significantly affected by the presence of food in the stomach or duodenum. Mean peak plasma concentrations of 2.6 µg per mL have been reported 2 hours after a 200-mg dose by mouth, falling to 1.45 µg per mL at 24 hours. Following repeated doses of 100 mg daily, concentrations of about 2 µg per mL are maintained. Similar values are reported after intravenous infusions.

From 80 to 95% of doxycycline in the circulation is reported to be bound to plasma proteins. Its biological half-life varies from about 15 to 22 hours. Doxycycline is more lipid-soluble than tetracycline. It is widely distributed in body tissues and fluids but only low concentrations are achieved in cerebrospinal fluid. Doxycycline is slowly excreted in the urine and it is also excreted in the faeces following chelation in the intestines. There is also some inactivation in the liver. It is stated not to accumulate significantly in patients with renal impairment although excretion in the urine is reduced; increased amounts of doxycycline are excreted in the faeces in these patients. Nevertheless there have been reports of some accumulation in renal failure. Removal of doxycycline by haemodialysis is insignificant.

In 6 healthy subjects urinary excretion of doxycycline after a single 200-mg dose by mouth was 60.8% when urine pH was 7.4 to 8.0 and 37.1% at pH 5.3 to 6.3. The mean half-life in each case was 9 and 13.2 hours respectively. During a multiple dose regimen urinary excretion of doxycycline was 65% at pH 7.7 to 8.4 and 52.8% at pH 5.6 to 6.7. The mean half-lives under these conditions were 11.8 and 17 hours respectively.— J. M. Jaffe *et al.*, *J. pharm. Sci.*, 1974, *63*, 1256.

A study of the pharmacokinetics of doxycycline polyphosphate after ingestion of milk. The absorption of doxycycline polyphosphate, administered by mouth as a single dose equivalent to 200 mg of doxycycline to 6 healthy subjects, was not significantly impaired by simultaneous administration of milk, although there was a moderate increase in the lag time. The clearance of doxycycline was, however, increased due to an apparent reduction in enterohepatic recycling; the mean terminal half-life was decreased from 28.1 to 15.8 hours.— M. -C. Saux *et al.*, *Eur. J. Drug Metab. Pharmacokinet.*, 1983, *8*, 43.

For the effect of phenobarbitone, phenytoin, and alcohol on the pharmacokinetics of doxycycline, see Precautions, Interactions, above.

ADMINISTRATION IN RENAL FAILURE. Doxycycline in a dose of 200 mg produced peak serum concentrations after 4 hours of 9 µg per mL in patients with impaired kidney function and 4.2 µg per mL in other patients. The urine concentration, 24 hours after administration, was 20.9 µg per mL in patients with normal kidney function, a value much greater than the MIC for most sensitive organisms. Urine measurements of patients with renal failure showed low doxycycline concentrations.— W. A. Mahon *et al.*, *Can. med. Ass. J.*, 1970, *103*, 1031.

Doxycycline appears to accumulate to some extent in impaired renal function. After a 200-mg intravenous dose, the serum half-life was significantly prolonged from 13.8 to 20.6 hours in 8 patients with chronic stable renal failure (creatinine clearance less than 5 mL per minute) compared with 8 subjects with normal renal function. In those with renal failure only 2% of the dose was recovered in the urine over 72 hours compared with 57% in normal subjects.— D. Heaney and G. Eknoyan, *Clin. Pharmac. Ther.*, 1978, *24*, 233.

The half-life of doxycycline was 15 to 36 hours in patients with end-stage renal disease compared with 14 to 25 hours in those with normal renal function.— W. M. Bennett *et al.*, *Am. J. Kidney Dis.*, 1983, *3*, 155.

A study of the effects of chronic renal insufficiency on the pharmacokinetics of doxycycline. It appeared that the renal capacity of doxycycline elimination decreases when renal failure worsens, but that the free fraction of the drug is increased in parallel, which favours hepatic elimination, leading to an unchanged overall total clearance.— G. Houin *et al.*, *Br. J. clin. Pharmac.*, 1983, *16*, 245.

METABOLISM. Doxycycline was considered, by some workers, to be metabolically inert because metabolites could not be detected (H.J.C.F. Nelis and A.P. De Leenheer, *J. pharm. Sci.*, 1981, *70*, 226). More recently, however, a metabolite of doxycycline has been detected in organs of laboratory *animals* and in human urine (R. Böcker *et al.*, *Lancet*, 1982, *2*, 1155).

Uses and Administration

Doxycycline hydrochloride is used for the same purposes as tetracycline hydrochloride (see p.318). It is readily absorbed and excreted more slowly than most other tetracyclines and effective blood concentrations are maintained for longer periods so that dosage once daily is usually adequate.

It may be given, with care, to patients with renal impairment but its low renal clearance could make it unsuitable for the treatment of urinary-tract infections.

Doxycycline is normally administered by mouth in capsules or tablets as the hydrochloride or in syrup or suspension as the calcium chelate or monohydrate. The hydrochloride may also be given by slow intravenous infusion. Doses are expressed in terms of doxycycline. The usual dose by either route is 200 mg of doxycycline on the first day (as a single dose or 100 mg repeated after 12 hours), followed by 100 mg daily. Children weighing 50 kg or less may be given 4 mg per kg body-weight initially and thereafter 2 mg per kg daily but the effect of tetracyclines on teeth should be considered. In severe infections the initial dosage is maintained throughout the course of treatment.

The equivalent of 300 or 600 mg has been given over one day in the treatment of gonorrhoea.

ADMINISTRATION. Doxycycline hydrochloride must be diluted before intravenous administration. It may be given by intermittent infusion when it should be diluted to at least 1 mg per 2.5 mL and infused over at least 2 hours; piggyback volume must be at least 250 mL to minimise postinfusion phlebitis. For continuous intravenous infusion a concentration of 0.1 to 0.4 mg per mL should be used and infused over 2 to 12 hours.— R. P. Rapp *et al.*, *Drug Intell. & clin. Pharm.*, 1984, *18*, 218. The manufacturer recommends a minimum infusion time of one hour for 100 mg of a 0.5 mg per mL solution. Concentrations lower than 0.1 mg per mL or higher than 1.0 mg per mL are not recommended, and the infusion should be completed within 12 hours after reconstitution to ensure adequate stability.

Doxycycline may cause oesophagitis or oesophageal ulceration and tablets or capsules should therefore be given with at least 100 mL of water while the patient is in an upright sitting position.— S. K. Vong and R. K. Parekh (letter), *Pharm. J.*, 1987, *1*, 5.

ADMINISTRATION IN RENAL FAILURE. The manufacturers have stated that no dosage adjustment is necessary in patients with renal impairment and that usual doses of doxycycline do not lead to excessive accumulation.

Bennett *et al.* (*Am. J. Kidney Dis.*, 1983, *3*, 155) suggested that the dosage interval should be adjusted in patients with renal failure according to their glomerular filtration-rate as follows: glomerular filtration-rate greater than 50 mL per minute, a dosage interval of 12 hours; 10 to 50 mL per minute, 12 to 18 hours; less than 10 mL per minute, 18 to 24 hours. However, maintenance doses of doxycycline in patients with normal renal function are usually given only every 24 hours, so their recommendations may be academic.

For the pharmacokinetics of doxycycline in patients with renal failure, see Absorption and Fate (above).

ANTHRAX. There was rapid systemic improvement in 33 patients with cutaneous anthrax given a single dose of doxycycline 7 to 32 mg per kg body-weight by mouth. All lesions were free of infection within 4 days.— S. N. Saggar *et al.*, *E. Afr. med. J.*, 1974, *51*, 889.

ATYPICAL MYCOBACTERIAL INFECTIONS. For reference to the use of doxycycline in the treatment of atypical myobacterial infections, see Amikacin Sulphate, p.111.

BRUCELLOSIS. For the treatment of brucellosis the WHO currently recommends doxycycline 200 mg in association with rifampicin 600 to 900 mg both given daily in the morning as a single dose, for at least 6 weeks. This has superseded the previous regimen of tetracycline 500 mg every 6 hours by mouth for 6 weeks in association with streptomycin 1 g daily intramuscularly for the first 3 weeks. Patients are considered more likely to comply with one daily doxycycline dose than with tetracycline given 4 times daily. Co-trimoxazole is also effective but relapse is common when co-trimoxazole is prescribed alone. A Herxheimer reaction at the start of antibiotic treatment may warrant intravenous hydrocortisone. Certain complications such as spondylitis or endocarditis may require urgent surgical intervention and several courses of antibiotic treatment may be necessary in chronic brucellosis. Following accidental contamination with *Brucella* organisms, including live vaccines, antibiotic treatment should be started immediately, its duration depending on the degree of exposure and the results of serial antibody tests (Sixth Report of the Joint FAO/WHO Expert Committee on Brucellosis, *Tech. Rep. Ser. Wld Hlth Org. No. 740*, 1986, p.56). For recommendations for the treatment of brucellosis in pregnancy see under Rifampicin, p.575.

Some workers have reported a higher relapse rate with doxycycline and rifampicin compared with tetracycline and streptomycin when given for a period of 30 days or less, although when doxycycline and rifampicin are given for longer periods such as 45 days the relapse rate is reduced (J. Ariza *et al.*, *Antimicrob. Ag. Chemother.*, 1985, *28*, 548); others have reported doxycycline and rifampicin to be better than tetracycline and streptomycin (W. Brumfitt and J.M.T. Hamilton-Miller, *Br. med. J.*, 1984, *289*, 496). However, treatment failure and development of rifampicin resistance have been reported in a patient who received treatment with doxycycline and rifampicin for 6 weeks (Y.M. De Rautlin De La Roy *et al.*, *J. antimicrob. Chemother.*, 1986, *18*, 648). The use of variable doses and duration of therapy depending on whether non-focal or mono- or multi-focal localised forms of brucellosis are being treated, has been suggested, with therapy continuing for 9 months for multifocal forms (J. De Mello Vieira, *Curr. ther. Res.*, 1984, *35*, 944).

Tetracycline, streptomycin, co-trimoxazole, and rifampicin have all been used in the treatment of neurobrucellosis. The length of therapy is important; recurrences may occur after short courses of treatment lasting only 2 to 3 weeks. A regimen of tetracycline 2 g daily and rifampicin 600 to 900 mg daily for 8 to 12 weeks with streptomycin 1 g daily for 6 weeks has been recommended (R. A. Shakir, *Postgrad. med. J.*, 1986, *62* 1077), although regimens using combinations of doxycycline, rifampicin, or co-trimoxazole have also been effective (I.O. Al-Orainey *et al.*, *J. infect.*, 1987, *14*, 141). Tetracycline with streptomycin and rifampicin have been used successfully in the treatment of *Brucella melitensis* endocarditis (D.S. Pratt *et al.*, *Am. J. Med.*, 1978, *64*, 897; Z. Farid and B. Trabolsi, *Br. med. J.*, 1985, *291*, 110) and tetracycline 10 mg per kg body-weight every 6 hours by mouth for 3 weeks with streptomycin 15 mg per kg every 12 hours intramuscularly for 2 weeks has been used with beneficial results in children with cardiac involvement due to infections with *B. melitensis* (M. Lubani *et al.*, *Archs Dis. Childh.*, 1986, *61*, 569).

Further references to the use of tetracyclines in brucellosis: *Br. med. J.*, 1981, *282*, 1180; A. M. Kambal *et al.*, *Trans. R. Soc. trop. Med. Hyg.*, 1983, *77*, 820.

DIARRHOEA. *Prophylaxis.* Travellers' diarrhoea is often due to enterotoxigenic *Escherichia coli* and *Shigella* spp. Care with food and drink is the most practical means of reducing the likelihood of developing diarrhoea while in areas of high risk, but chemoprophylactic measures may be useful for some patients. Both doxycycline 100 mg daily and co-trimoxazole have been shown to be useful in minimising illness during travel to endemic areas; Sack (*Scand. J. Gastroenterol.*, 1983, *84*, (*Suppl.*), 111) reported the 2 drugs to be 70% and 95% effective, respectively. However, not all travellers can be advised to take such drugs because of the occurrence of side-effects, such as photosensitivity with doxycycline, and because of resistance among enteric bacterial pathogens in certain areas. There is also the possibility of developing resistance in the intestinal flora during prophylactic therapy, which may cause problems in treating patients who develop diarrhoea after prophylaxis is discontinued, or in treating patients prone to develop other infections such as urinary-tract infections. It is generally recommended that the prophylactic use of doxycycline or co-trimoxazole should be restricted to persons visiting high-risk areas on important business trips for short periods of time such as 2 to 5 days, and persons with underlying health problems that might increase susceptibility to diarrhoea or the likelihood of complications from dehydration; chemoprophylaxis should be avoided when the period of risk exceeds 2 weeks. For most travellers early treatment of diarrhoea is considered sufficient.— H. L. DuPont *et al.*, *Ann. intern. Med.*, 1985, *102*, 260. See also G. C. Cook, *Gut*, 1983, *24*, 1105; *Med. Lett.*, 1987, *29*, 53.

ENTERIC INFECTIONS. *Cholera.* Doxycycline 2 mg per kg body-weight initially, again at 12 hours, then daily for a total of 5 doses given to 17 patients with actively purging cholera was as effective as tetracycline 20 mg per kg daily given to 15 patients in divided 6-hourly doses for 4 days and more effective than placebo. However, vibrios were eradicated more rapidly with tetracycline (1.8 days) than with doxycycline (2.6 days). In spite of this and of a risk of incomplete absorption due to reduced transit time in cholera, the reduced number of doses of doxycycline and its safety in renal impairment offered advantages over tetracycline.— M. M. Rahaman *et al.*, *Antimicrob. Ag. Chemother.*, 1976, *10*, 610.

In a comparative study in cholera patients, doxycycline 300 mg as a single dose was almost as effective as tetracycline 500 mg every 6 hours for 48 hours.— S. De *et al.*, *Bull. Wld Hlth Org.*, 1976, *54*, 177.

In cholera patients, a single 200-mg dose of doxycycline was as effective as 100 mg, repeated after 12 hours and then given daily for 3 days. Tetracycline remained the treatment of choice.— D. A. Sack *et al.*, *Antimicrob. Ag. Chemother.*, 1978, *14*, 462.

From a study in 276 contacts of cholera patients, 137 of whom were given doxycycline, a single dose of doxycycline was considered an effective prophylactic agent. The dose was 300 mg for persons over 15 years of age and 6 mg per kg body-weight for younger persons.— P. G. Sen Gupta *et al.*, *Bull. Wld Hlth Org.*, 1978, *56*, 323.

For further comment on the use of doxycycline in the treatment of cholera, see under Tetracycline Hydrochloride, p.318.

EPERYTHROZOONOSIS. Doxycycline 100 mg every 12 hours for 18 days resulted in clinical cure in a 28-year-old woman infected with *Eperythrozoon* spp. (in the order Rickettsiales). Tetracycline has been reported as the drug of choice for eperythrozoonosis.— V. Puntaric *et al.* (letter), *Lancet*, 1986, *2*, 868.

EYE INFECTIONS. For the use of doxycycline in the treatment of trachoma and paratrachoma, see under Trachoma, below.

INFERTILITY. Results suggesting that T-mycoplasma (*Ureaplasma urealyticum*) infection in the genital tract may have an important role in infertility. Doxycycline 100 mg twice daily was given for 4 weeks to 161 men with T-mycoplasma infection in their seminal fluid and to their wives. Among the 129 couples in which infection had been eradicated in the men, the 3-year rate of successful pregnancy was 60% compared with only 5% in 32 couples where infection had not been eradicated.— A. Toth *et al.*, *New Engl. J. Med.*, 1983, *308*, 505. See also J. Friberg and H. Gnarpe, *Am. J. Obstet. Gynec.*, 1973, *116*, 23; G. H. Cassell *et al.*, *New Engl. J. Med.*, 1983, *308*, 502. Studies which do not support any role for genital mycoplasmas in the pathogenesis of infertility.— D. W. Gump *et al.*, *ibid.*, 1984, *310*, 937. Comment.— H. W. Horne (letter), *ibid.*, *311*, 407. Reply.— D. W. Gump and M. Gibson (letter), *ibid.* See also J. de Louvois *et al.*, *Lancet*, 1974, *1*, 1073; R. F. Harrison *et al.*, *ibid.*, 1975, *1*, 605.

ISRAELI SPOTTED FEVER. Doxycycline 2.2 mg per kg body-weight twice daily for the first day and 1.1 mg per kg twice daily on subsequent days was given by mouth to a 2-year-old boy with Israeli spotted fever. His temperature returned to normal after 5 doses of doxycycline, but treatment was continued for an additional 24 hours. However, following cessation of treatment for 1 day he relapsed becoming febrile and lethargic. Doxycycline therapy was restarted and continued for 1 week after the fever had resolved. Recovery was uneventful.— P. Yagupsky and E. M. Gross (letter), *Trans. R. Soc. trop. Med. Hyg.*, 1985, *79*, 139.

See also Rickettsial Infections, below.

LEGIONNAIRES' DISEASE. Experience suggesting that doxycycline is clinically effective in legionnaires' disease. Erythromycin remains the drug of choice, but if the diagnosis is uncertain and legionnaires' disease is only one of a number of diagnostic possibilities, empirical therapy with doxycycline is preferred.— B. A. Cunha and M. Jonas (letter), *Lancet*, 1981, *1*, 1107.

Successful treatment of a 54-year-old woman with empyema due to *Legionella bozemanii* given doxycycline 100 mg every 12 hours, intravenously and orally, after erythromycin treatment had failed. Because patients may not respond or may have a relapse on erythromycin therapy, doxycycline should be considered an alternative therapeutic agent for *L. bozemanii* infection as well as for *L. pneumophila* and *L. micdadei* infections.— M. J. Strampfer *et al.* (letter), *Ann. intern. Med.*, 1986, *105*, 626.

LEPTOSPIROSIS. In a double-blind randomised study of 29 patients with leptospirosis, doxycycline administered early in the course of the illness produced beneficial results. In 14 patients who received doxycycline hydrochloride 100 mg twice daily by mouth for 7 days, the duration of illness was reduced by 2 days and also the number of days of fever, malaise, headache, and myalgias were reduced compared with 15 patients given placebo. Doxycycline also prevented leptospiruria which was found in only 1 patient receiving doxycycline, but in 13 patients given placebo.— J. B. L. McClain *et al.*, *Ann. intern. Med.*, 1984, *100*, 696.

Prophylaxis. A double-blind study of prophylaxis with doxycycline against leptospirosis in *US* soldiers deployed in Panama for about 3 weeks. Only one leptospirosis infection occurred in the 469 soldiers given doxycycline 200 mg weekly by mouth compared with 20 infections in the 471 given placebo. The feasibility of chemoprophylaxis on a more prolonged basis needs to be evaluated.— E. T. Takafuji *et al.*, *New Engl. J. Med.*, 1984, *310*, 497. Comments on the possible development of resistant organisms if doxycycline is used prophylactically against leptospirosis; widespread use of doxycycline prophylaxis is not indicated.— W. K. Krick (letter), *ibid.*, *311*, 54; E. T. Takafuji *et al.* (letter), *ibid.*

LYME DISEASE. Doxycycline 200 mg daily for 3 weeks resulted in rapid recovery in a 48-year-old man with meningoradiculitis associated with infection by *Borrelia burgdorferi*, the aetiological agent of Lyme disease.— O. Weill *et al.* (letter), *Lancet*, 1985, *1*, 1400.

Successful treatment of a patient with early Lyme disease given doxycycline 100 mg twice daily for 30 days.— I. McCrossin, *Med. J. Aust.*, 1986, *144*, 724.

Further references: G. Stanek *et al.* (letter), *Lancet*, 1987, *1*, 1490.

MALARIA. Doxycycline 100 mg daily has been suggested for malaria chemoprophylaxis in areas such as Southeast Asia, notably Thailand, the Amazon region of Brazil, and East Africa, where malaria due to *Plasmodium falciparum* resistant to both chloroquine and pyrimethamine with sulfadoxine has been reported.— *Med. Lett.*, 1987, *29*, 53.

For further comment on the use of doxycycline in the prophylaxis and treatment of malaria, see under Tetracycline Hydrochloride, p.319.

MALIGNANT EFFUSIONS. Beneficial results with doxycycline hydrochloride 200 to 300 mg instilled at a concentration of 20 mg per mL into the pericardial cavity of 7 patients with carcinomatous pericarditis and pericardial effusion secondary to lung or breast cancer.— S. Kitamura *et al.*, *Curr. ther. Res.*, 1981, *30*, 589.

MEDITERRANEAN SPOTTED FEVER. Successful treatment of 3 patients with Mediterranean spotted fever due to *Rickettsia conori* with doxycycline 200 mg daily; a 7-year-old boy also responded to treatment with doxycycline.— S. Staszewski *et al.* (letter), *Lancet*, 1984, *2*, 1466.

See also Rickettsial Infections, below.

MELIOIDOSIS. For the use of doxycycline in the treatment of melioidosis, see under Tetracycline Hydrochloride, p.319.

MOUTH INFECTIONS. *Periodontal disease.* For the use of tetracyclines including doxycycline hydrochloride in the treatment of periodontal disease, see under Tetracycline Hydrochloride, p.320.

MYCETOMA. Mycetoma due to *Nocardia brasiliensis* in the lower leg of a 41-year-old man was completely cured following treatment with doxycycline 200 mg daily in association with ketoconazole 400 mg daily for one year.— R. G. M. Lecluse and B. E. W. L. van Huystee, *Br. J. Derm.*, 1985, *112*, 229.

PELVIC INFLAMMATORY DISEASE. The Centers for Disease Control (CDC) recommends that hospitalised patients with pelvic inflammatory disease (PID) should be treated with doxycycline 100 mg intravenously twice daily plus cefoxitin 2 g intravenously 4 times daily, both for at least 4 days, followed by doxycycline given by mouth for 10 or more days. For ambulatory patients the CDC recommends single-dose therapy for *Neisseria gonorrhoeae* with cefoxitin, ceftriaxone, procaine penicillin, amoxycillin, or ampicillin, the latter 3 being given with probenecid, followed by doxycycline 100 mg twice daily by mouth for 10 to 14 days. Many other treatment regimens such as clindamycin plus gentamicin or tobramycin, or doxycycline plus metronidazole might be effective and practical, and perhaps PID in ambulatory patients should be treated with drugs more effective against anaerobes than those recommended by the CDC.— T. A. Bell and J. T. Grayston, *Ann. intern. Med.*, 1986, *104*, 524.

Until more data are available, the treatment of acute pelvic inflammatory disease should be with doxycycline and an appropriate beta-lactam antibiotic such as cefoxitin sodium which together offer activity against both *Neisseria gonorrhoeae* and *Chlamydia trachomatis*.— P. Wølner-Hanssen *et al.*, *J. Am. med. Ass.*, 1986, *256*, 3262.

For the management of severe to moderate acute pelvic inflammatory disease, a suggested treatment was benzylpenicillin 1.2 g intravenously every 4 hours until symptoms and signs improve, in association with doxycycline 200 mg daily by mouth for 2 to 4 weeks. Mild symptoms could be treated with doxycycline in the regimen described above.— G. L. Gilbert, *Med. J. Aust.*, 1987, *146*, 205.

For further reference to the use of doxycycline in the treatment of pelvic inflammatory disease, see under Cefoxitin Sodium, p.159.

For the prophylactic use of doxycyline, before gynaecological surgery, to prevent pelvic infection, see under Surgical Infection Prophylaxis, below.

Salpingitis. Mild forms of acute salpingitis may be treated with doxycycline 100 mg daily for 14 days in association with rectal metronidazole 500 mg twice daily for 7 to 14 days; if the patient is pregnant, erythromycin should be substituted for doxycycline. In severe cases where the patient requires hospitalisation, a suitable regimen would be spectinomycin 4 to 6 g every 6 hours for 24 hours in association with doxycycline 100 mg twice daily for 7 days and daily for a further 14 days, and rectal metronidazole 500 mg twice daily for 10 days. An alternative regimen would be penicillin 7.2 to 12 g daily in divided doses, switching after 72 hours to a tetracycline, such as doxycycline 100 mg twice daily, or erythromycin 500 mg four times daily for 7 to 10 days; gentamicin 2 to 5 mg per kg body-weight daily is also given in divided doses, together with rectal metronidazole 500 mg twice daily for 10 days.— S. L. Stanton, *Br. med. J.*, 1987, *295*, 621.

PERITONEAL INFECTIONS. Diffuse peritonitis, chronic ascites, and vaginal discharge due to infection with *Chlamydia trachomatis* in 2 women without liver disease, responded quickly to doxycycline 200 mg daily.— U. A. Marbet *et al.*, *Br. med. J.*, 1986, *293*, 5.

Q FEVER. Acute Q fever infections usually respond to a course of one of the tetracyclines, of which doxycycline is possibly the most active against *Coxiella burnetii*. The treatment of chronic infections, especially if associated with endocarditis, may be difficult, and a regimen of a tetracycline plus clindamycin has been recommended; these antibiotics are bacteriostatic and treatment has to be continued for many months, sometimes for as long as a year. Rifampicin has been suggested as an alternative antibiotic for refractory Q fever endocarditis, as it is more active *in vitro* than the tetracyclines. Patients being prepared for heart valve replacement who live, or have lived, in rural areas and patients who work in abattoirs or who visit the countryside could be screened for antibodies and if positive they could be given a pre-operative course of a tetracycline to eradicate any latent focus of infection.— A. M. Geddes, *Br. med. J.*, 1983, *287*, 927.

See also Rickettsial Infections, below.

RELAPSING FEVER, LOUSE-BORNE. Doxycycline in a single dose of 100 mg by mouth was effective in the treatment of 26 patients with confirmed louse-borne relapsing fever due to *Borrelia recurrentis* spirochaetes. Each patient experienced a Jarisch-Herxheimer reaction and in 5 the cardiac failure with hypotension required treatment with digoxin 500 μg intravenously. Also 10 patients with serologically confirmed typhus were given doxycycline 100 mg and between 38 and 128 hours they became afebrile and symptom-free.— P. L. Perine *et al.*, *Lancet*, 1974, *2*, 742.

See also under Tetracycline Hydrochloride, p.320.

RESPIRATORY-TRACT INFECTIONS. A study using doxycycline and placebo indicating that in otherwise healthy patients with cough and purulent sputum the symptoms would usually get better without antibiotic treatment.— N. C. H. Stott and R. R. West, *Br. med. J.*, 1976, *2*, 556. Comment.— *ibid.*, 550. There was a significant benefit with antibiotic therapy using doxycycline, co-trimoxazole, or amoxycillin for 10 days, compared with placebo, for the treatment of exacerbations of chronic obstructive pulmonary disease.— N. R. Anthonisen *et al.*, *Ann. intern. Med.*, 1987, *106*, 196.

Bronchitis. A study of 40 patients with acute purulent exacerbations of chronic bronchitis to assess the effectiveness of doxycycline therapy. The patients received doxycycline 100 mg twice daily for 10 days by mouth before food, and the sputum was examined microbiologically before and after treatment. *Branhamella catarrhalis* and *Streptococcus pneumoniae* organisms were eradicated from the sputum except in one patient who developed *Str. pneumoniae* septicaemia with a resistant pneumococcus while receiving doxycycline treatment. Only *Haemophilus influenzae* seemed to present difficulties in eradication, but 4 patients developed superinfections with *Pseudomonas aeruginosa*. Of 39 evaluable patients clinical results were excellent or good in 29 (74%) of the patients on day 10 and 25 (64%) on day 17; sputum examination was completely negative on day 17 in 24 (61%) of patients. Despite a reported resistance of about 7% of *Str. pneumoniae* and 5% of *H. influenzae* strains, doxycycline is still considered a valuable antibiotic for patients with exacerbations of chronic bronchitis especially for *B. catarrhalis* infections. One advantage of tetracyclines is that they are also active against *Mycoplasma pneumoniae*.— F. P. V. Maesen *et al., J. antimicrob. Chemother.*, 1986, *18*, 531.

See also under Tetracycline Hydrochloride, p.320.

Legionnaires' disease. For comment on the use of doxycycline hydrochloride in Legionnaires' disease, see above.

RICKETTSIAL INFECTIONS. Tetracyclines and chloramphenicol are used for the treatment of rickettsioses and doxycycline has the advantage of reduced frequency of administration and prolonged action. Doxycycline 100 to 200 mg as a single dose may be given for the treatment of louse-borne typhus, and perhaps scrub typhus; in the case of louse-borne typhus doxycycline 50 mg may be given to children. Other rickettsioses such as murine typhus, Rocky Mountain spotted fever, and perhaps infections with other tick-borne rickettsioses (spotted fever group), and Q fever require antibiotic therapy over a period of several days and doxycycline 200 mg daily is suitable; chronic Q fever infections and endocarditis will require more prolonged therapy, which in the case of endocarditis may be for many months.— WHO Working Group on Rickettsial Diseases, *Bull. Wld Hlth Org.*, 1982, *60*, 157.

For further mention of the use of doxycycline in the treatment of rickettsial infections, see under Israeli Spotted Fever, Mediterranean Spotted Fever, and Q Fever, above, and Typhus, below. See also under Eperythrozoonosis, above.

SEXUALLY TRANSMITTED DISEASES. Doxycycline 100 mg twice daily for 28 days, repeated every 3 to 4 months, was effective and well tolerated in 51 patients with syphilis at various stages.— Y. Onoda, *Br. J. vener. Dis.*, 1979, *55*, 110.

For mention of the use of doxycycline hydrochloride and other tetracyclines in the treatment of gonococcal infections, lymphogranuloma venereum, and nongonococcal urethritis, see under Tetracycline Hydrochloride, p.321. See also under Trachoma, below.

SKIN DISORDERS. *Acne.* For mention of the use of doxycycline in the treatment of acne see Tetracycline Hydrochloride, p.321.

SURGICAL INFECTION PROPHYLAXIS. Experience involving 2950 women undergoing induced abortion indicated that a single prophylactic dose of doxycycline 500 mg by mouth considerably reduced the incidence of pelvic infection after abortion, compared with placebo.— C. Brewer, *Br. med. J.*, 1980, *281*, 780. In a study involving 557 women of whom 70 had *Chlamydia trachomatis* isolated from the cervix, a single intravenous dose of doxycycline hydrochloride 200 mg given before and during the operation appeared to have no protective effect against the development of chlamydia-associated pelvic inflammatory disease (PID) after therapeutic abortion.— E. Qvigstad *et al., Br. J. vener. Dis.*, 1983, *59*, 189.

In a study of 51 premenopausal women undergoing vaginal hysterectomy, a single pre-operative dose of doxycycline 200 mg intravenously over a period of 2 hours before the operation was as effective at preventing post-hysterectomy pelvic infection as was cephamandole 2 g pre-operatively followed by 1 g at 3 successive intervals of 6 hours. The incidence of postoperative pelvic infection was 19.2% for 26 women given doxycycline and 16% for women given cephamandole.— D. L. Hemsell *et al., Surgery Gynec. Obstet.*, 1985, *161*, 462.

In a double-blind study of single-dose chemoprophylaxis in elective colorectal surgery, doxycycline 400 mg in association with metronidazole 1.5 g or doxycycline 400 mg plus saline were given by intravenous infusion pre-operatively. The total rate of septic complications related to the surgical procedures was 4 of 135 patients (3.0%) in the doxycycline plus metronidazole group and 20 of 126 (15.9%) in the doxycycline group. The single-dose administration of doxycycline and metronidazole reduced the postoperative septic complications in elective colorectal surgery to almost the same as in "clean" surgery.— L. Bergman and J. H. Solhaug, *Ann. Surg.*, 1987, *205*, 77.

For comment on the use of doxycycline prophylaxis in patients being prepared for heart valve replacement, see Q fever, above.

TRACHOMA. A double-blind controlled study of topical oxytetracycline twice daily for 7 days each month or doxycycline 5 mg per kg body-weight once a month by mouth in hyperendemic trachoma. There was no marked difference between the two treatments.— S. Darougar *et al., Br. J. Ophthal.*, 1980, *64*, 291.

A study of various oral dosage regimens of doxycycline for the treatment of adult chlamydial ophthalmia (paratrachoma). A single dose of doxycycline 300 mg (5 mg per kg body-weight) reduced the severity of clinical signs and stopped the shedding of *Chlamydia trachomatis* in about half of the patients. Treatment with doxycycline 300 mg weekly for 3 weeks or 100 mg daily for one week was equally effective in producing clinical and microbiological cure in all the patients. The best results, however, were obtained with doxycycline 100 mg daily for 2 weeks, when a rapid resolution of clinical signs was achieved.— N. D. Viswalingam *et al., Br. J. Ophthal.*, 1986, *70*, 301.

For further reference to the use of doxycycline in the treatment of trachoma, see under Tetracycline Hydrochloride, p.322.

TYPHUS. A single dose of doxycycline 200 mg was as effective as a 7-day course of treatment with tetracycline for patients with scrub typhus.— G. W. Brown *et al., Trans. R. Soc. trop. Med. Hyg.*, 1978, *72*, 412.

A double-blind placebo-controlled study of doxycycline prophylaxis for scrub typhus. Nine of 10 healthy subjects given doxycycline 200 mg weekly by mouth for 7 doses, who were exposed to *Leptotrombidium fletcheri* chiggers infected with *Rickettsia tsutsugamushi* 2 days after prophylaxis started, remained well during prophylaxis although some symptoms such as malaise were experienced; 8 of the 9 developed significant levels of antibody to strains of *R. tsutsugamushi*. However, 9 of 10 similar subjects given placebo required treatment for scrub typhus. Doxycycline in weekly 200-mg doses appears to provide effective prophylaxis of scrub typhus if prophylaxis is started before exposure to infection and continued for 6 weeks after exposure. A single dose of doxycycline 200 mg given on the third day of illness to the 10 subjects who developed scrub typhus was initially effective but was frequently followed by relapse and cannot be recommended.— J. C. Twartz *et al., J. infect. Dis.*, 1982, *146*, 811.

For further reference to the use of doxycycline in the treatment of typhus, see Relapsing Fever, Louse-borne, above. See also Rickettsial Infections, above.

URINARY-TRACT INFECTIONS. In a study of 62 women with acute urethral syndrome, doxycycline was significantly more effective than placebo in eradicating urinary symptoms, pyuria, and the infecting micro-organisms, including coliforms, staphylococci, or *Chlamydia trachomatis*. Women without pyuria did not benefit from treatment with doxycycline.— W. E. Stamm *et al., New Engl. J. Med.*, 1981, *304*, 956. The urethral syndrome is a self-limiting illness. In a double-blind study treatment with doxycycline was of no benefit.— T. C. O'Dowd *et al., Br. med. J.*, 1984, *288*, 1349.

Doxycycline 300 mg given by mouth with food as a single dose resulted in clinical cure in 38 of 45 women with bacterial cystitis compared with 44 of 45 women given co-trimoxazole 960 mg every 12 hours for 5 days.— R. R. Bailey *et al., N.Z. med. J.*, 1982, *95*, 699.

Purulent urethritis in a 26-year-old man responded to treatment with a single dose of ampicillin and probenecid, followed by a 7-day course of doxycycline by mouth, for presumed gonococcal urethritis. The infection was found to be due to *Branhamella catarrhalis* organisms which were positive for beta-lactamase and resistant to ampicillin but sensitive to tetracycline, however, since both ampicillin and tetracycline were used, the patient was adequately treated before culture results were available.— G. L. Smith (letter), *New Engl. J. Med.*, 1987, *316*, 1277.

For the use of doxycycline in the treatment of nongonococcal urethritis, see under Tetracycline Hydrochloride, Sexually Transmitted Diseases, p.321.

WOUND INFECTIONS. The use of doxycycline, clindamycin, and an aminoglycoside in the treatment of sternal wound infections due to *Mycoplasma hominis* in 3 patients.— D. O. Steffenson *et al., Ann. intern. Med.*, 1987, *106*, 204.

For the use of doxycycline with benzylpenicillin in the treatment of penetrating intestinal injuries, see under Benzylpenicillin Sodium, p.138.

Preparations

Doxycycline Capsules *(B.P.)*. Capsules containing doxycycline hydrochloride.

Doxycycline Hyclate Capsules *(U.S.P.)*. Capsules containing doxycycline hydrochloride.

Doxycycline Hyclate Delayed-release Capsules *(U.S.P.)*. Capsules containing doxycycline hydrochloride.

Doxycycline Hyclate for Injection *(U.S.P.)*. A sterile dry mixture or a sterile-filtered and lyophilised mixture of doxycycline hydrochloride and a suitable buffer. To be reconstituted before use.

Sterile Doxycycline Hyclate *(U.S.P.)*. Doxycycline hydrochloride suitable for parenteral use.

Doxycycline Calcium Oral Suspension *(U.S.P.)*. Prepared from doxycycline hydrochloride. pH 6.5 to 8.0.

Doxycycline for Oral Suspension *(U.S.P.)*. pH 5.0 to 6.5 when reconstituted.

Doxycycline Hyclate Tablets *(U.S.P.)*. Tablets containing doxycycline hydrochloride.

Proprietary Preparations

Nordox *(Panpharma, UK)*. *Capsules*, doxycycline 100 mg (as hydrochloride).

Vibramycin *(Pfizer, UK)*. *Capsules*, doxycycline 50 and 100 mg (as hydrochloride).
Syrup, doxycycline 50 mg (as calcium chelate)/5 mL.

Vibramycin-D *(Pfizer, UK)*. *Tablets*, dispersible, doxycycline 100 mg (as monohydrate).

Proprietary Names and Manufacturers of Doxycycline and its Salts

Abadox *(Lafar, Ital.)*; Amplidox *(Ital.)*; Azudoxat *(Azuchemie, Ger.)*; Bassado *(Poli, Ital.)*; Biostar *(Ausonia, Ital.)*; Cirenyl *(Edmond Pharma, Ital.)*; Clisemina *(Unibios, Spain)*; Cyclidox *(Protea, Austral.; Triomed, S.Afr.)*; Diocimex *(Cimex, Switz.)*; Docostyl *(Pentafarm, Spain)*; Doryx *(Faulding, Austral.; Parke, Davis, USA)*; Dosil *(Llorens, Spain)*; Dossil *(Ital.)*; Doxacin *(Ital.)*; Doxaclen *(Hortel, Spain)*; Doxatet *(Cox, UK)*; Doxi *(Isola-Ibi, Ital.)*; Doxibiotic *(Ital.)*; Doxicento *(Recordati, Ital.)*; Doxiclat *(Inkey, Spain)*; Doxiclin *(Maipe, Spain)*; Doxi-Crisol *(Crisol, Spain)*; Doxidima *(Fisons, Ital.)*; Doxifin *(IFI, Ital.)*; Doxigram *(Ital.)*; Doxilen *(Lenza, Ital.)*; Doxileo *(ISF, Ital.)*; Doxin *(G.P. Laboratories, Austral.)*; Doxina *(IBP, Ital.)*; Doxinate *(Torlan, Spain)*; Doxitard *(Ger.)*; Doxitenbio *(Frumtost, Spain)*; Doxitrecina *(Spain)*; Doxivis *(Vis, Ital.)*; Dox-Life *(Spain)*; Doxoral *(IBIS, Ital.)*; Doxy-100 *(Elerte, Fr.)*; Doxy-basan *(Schönenberger, Switz.)*; Doxybiocin *(Dorsch, Ger.)*; Doxy-Caps *(Edwards, USA)*; Doxychel *(Rachelle, USA)*; Doxyclin *(Pharmador, S.Afr.)*; Doxycline *(Spirig, Switz.)*; Doxygram *(Negma, Fr.)*; Doxylag *(Lagap, Switz.)*; Doxylar *(Lagap, UK)*; Doxy-Lemmon *(Lemmon, USA)*; Doxylin *(Alphapharm, Austral.; Apothekernes Laboratorium, Norw.)*; Doxymycin *(Neth.; Continental Ethicals, S.Afr.)*; Doxysept *(Chassot, Switz.)*; Dumoxin *(Dumex, Denm.; Neth.; Dumex, Norw.; MPS Lab., S.Afr.)*; Duradoxal *(Durachemie, Ger.)*; Ecodox *(Ital.)*; Ekaciclina *(Ital.)*; Emidox *(Ital.)*; Esaciclina *(Ital.)*; Esadoxi *(Benvegna, Ital.)*; Falorciclina *(Ital.)*; Farmacina *(Spain)*; Farmodoxi *(Lifepharma, Ital.)*; Fenoseptil *(Spain)*; Fortaciclina *(Spain)*; Furdox *(Ital.)*; Geobiotico Depot *(Spain)*; Germiciclin *(Mendelejeff, Ital.)*; Ghimadox *(Ghimas, Ital.)*; Gibidox *(Ital.)*; Gram-Val *(Polifarma, Ital.)*; Granudoxy *(Leurquin, Fr.)*; Grodoxin *(Grossmann, Switz.)*; Hiclamicina *(Spain)*; Hovione *(Port.)*; Hydramycin *(Jpn)*; Icidox *(Ital.)*; Iclados *(Panthox & Burck, Ital.)*; Idocyklin *(Norw.; Leo, Swed.)*; Isodox *(Ital.)*; Lampodox *(Ital.)*; Libeciclina *(Spain)*; Liomycin *(Jpn)*; Liviatin *(Juste, Spain)*; Mespafin *(Merckle, Ger.)*; Microciclina *(Ital.)*; Minidox *(CT, Ital.)*; Miraclin *(Farmacologico Milanese, Ital.)*; Monocline *(Doms, Fr.)*; Monodoxin *(Crosara, Ital.)*; Mundicyl *(Mundipharma, Ger.)*; Neociclina *(Ital.)*; Nivocilin *(Spain)*; Nordox *(Panpharma, UK)*; Novaciclin *(Ital.)*; Novelciclina *(Sabater, Spain)*; Peraseptum *(Spain)*; Philcociclina *(Biotrading, Ital.)*; Plenomicin *(Spain)*; Plumbiot *(Bicther, Spain)*; Pocaciclina *(Ital.)*; Puramicina *(Wasserman, Spain)*; Radox *(Radiumfarma, Ital.)*; Relociclina *(Cheminova, Spain)*; Retens *(Wasserman, Spain)*; Rodomicina *(Antibioticos, Spain)*; Roximycin *(Jpn)*; Samecin *(Savoma, Ital.)*; Saramicina *(Ital.)*; Semelciclina *(Proter, Ital.)*; Semelin *(Fargal-Pharmasint, Ital.)*; Severciclina *(Ital.)*; Sferamicina *(Ital.)*; Sigadoxin *(Siegfried, Ger.)*; Sigadoxine *(Sigamed, Switz.)*; Sincromicyn *(Ital.)*; SK-Doxycycline Hyclate *(Smith Kline & French, USA)*; Solupen *(Aristegui, Spain)*; Spanor *(Pharmascience, Fr.)*; Stamicina *(Torre, Ital.)*; Supracyclin *(Grünenthal, Ger.)*; Tecacin *(Ital.)*; Tecnomicina *(Ital.)*; Tetradox *(Ind.)*; Tetrasan *(Federico Bonet, Spain)*; Thedox *(Vesta, S.Afr.)*; Unacil *(FIRMA, Ital.)*; Uniciclina *(Ital.)*; Unidox *(Ital.)*; Unidoxi *(Jorba, Spain)*; Vibracina *(Pfizer, Spain)*; Vibradoxil *(Ital.)*; Vibralex *(Neopharmed, Ital.)*; Vibramicina *(Arg.; Ital.)*; Vibramycin *(Pfizer, Austral.; Pfizer, Canad.; Pfizer, Denm.; Pfizer, Ger.; Jpn; Neth.; Pfizer, Norw.; Pfizer, S.Afr.; Pfizer, Swed.; Pfizer, UK; Pfizer, USA; Roerig, USA)*; Vibramycin-D *(Pfizer, UK)*; Vibramycine *(Belg.; Pfizer, Fr.; Pfizer, Switz.)*; Vibra-Tabs *(Pfizer, Austral.; Pfizer, USA)*; Vibraveineuse *(Pfizer, Fr.; Pfizer, Switz.)*; Vibravenös *(Pfizer, Ger.)*; Vibravenosa *(Pfizer, Spain)*; Vip-Ciclina *(Ital.)*; Vivox *(Squibb, USA)*; Ximicina *(Rottapharm, Ital.)*; Zadorine *(Mepha, Switz.)*.

16623-k

Enoxacin *(BAN, USAN, rINN).*

AT-2266; CI-919; PD-107779. 1-Ethyl-6-fluoro-1,4-dihydro-4-oxo-7-(1-piperazinyl)-1,8-naphthyridine-3-carboxylic acid.

$C_{15}H_{17}F_4O_3$=320.3.

CAS — 74011-58-8.

Adverse Effects

As for Norfloxacin, p.274.

Adverse effects were reported by 17 of 18 healthy subjects after receiving enoxacin 400 to 800 mg twice daily for 14 days in a double-blind manner compared with 3 of 6 who received placebo. Rashes were observed in 7 subjects receiving enoxacin and in several the rash was most prominent over sun-exposed areas. Other adverse effects reported after enoxacin were: fatigue (10), headache (8), dizziness (4), nausea (7), and lack of appetite (5).— R. Wolf *et al., J. antimicrob. Chemother.*, 1984, *14, Suppl.* C, 63.

A report of an 18-year-old man who had a generalised tonic-clonic seizure 3 hours after receiving his third dose of enoxacin 400 mg which was being given twice daily for a soft-tissue infection. There was no history of head injury but the patient had had a convulsion at the age of 14 months. Caution is required when administering enoxacin to patients with a history of convulsions or active epilepsy.— K. J. Simpson and M. J. Brodie (letter), *Lancet*, 1985, *2*, 161.

Precautions

As for Nalidixic Acid, p.267. Enoxacin has been reported to interact with theophylline by inhibiting its metabolism.

INTERACTIONS. *Warfarin.* Enoxacin was found not to affect the hypoprothombinaemic response produced by warfarin but did reduce the clearance of the least pharmacologically active enantiomer (*R*)-warfarin.— S. Toon *et al., Clin. Pharmac. Ther.*, 1987, *42*, 33.

Xanthines. For the interaction of 4-quinolone antimicrobial agents with caffeine and theophylline, see p.1523 and p.1529.

Antimicrobial Action and Resistance

As for Norfloxacin, p.274.

Some references to the antibacterial activity of enoxacin that demonstrate its similarity to norfloxacin: N. -X. Chin and H. C. Neu, *Antimicrob. Ag. Chemother.*, 1983, *24*, 754; R. Wise *et al., J. antimicrob. Chemother.*, 1984, *13*, 237; C. Siporin and G. Towse, *ibid.*, *14, Suppl.* C, 47; R. M. Bannatyne *et al.* (letter), *Lancet*, 1984, *2*, 172 and 362; J. T. Rudrick *et al., Antimicrob. Ag. Chemother.*, 1984, *26*, 97; C. M. Bassey *et al., ibid.*, 417; C. H. Teoh-Chan *et al., J. antimicrob. Chemother.*, 1985, *15*, 45; A. King *et al., ibid.*, 551; P. Van der Auwera, *ibid.*, *16*, 581.

References to enoxacin resistance or cross-resistance: J. H. T. Wagenvoort *et al.* (letter), *J. antimicrob. Chemother.*, 1986, *18*, 429; D. I. Limb *et al., ibid.*, 1987, *19*, 65; L. J. V. Piddock *et al.* (letter), *Lancet*, 1987, *2*, 907.

Absorption and Fate

Enoxacin given by mouth in doses of 200 to 600 mg has produced peak plasma concentrations ranging from about 1 to 4 µg per mL after 1 to 2 hours. Serum half-lives ranging from 3.4 to 6.7 hours have been reported.

Enoxacin is mainly excreted by the kidneys and about 60% of a dose may appear in the urine within 24 hours. Enoxacin appears to penetrate into body fluids and tissues in therapeutic concentrations.

A comparative study of the pharmacokinetics of enoxacin and four other 4-quinolone antimicrobial agents.— R. Wise *et al., J. antimicrob. Chemother.*, 1986, *18, Suppl.* D, 71.

Details of a method using high-performance liquid chromatography for the determination of enoxacin and its 5 metabolites in plasma and/or urine. Enoxacin 400 mg given by mouth to one subject produced a peak plasma concentration of enoxacin of 2.86 µg per mL one hour after administration. Plasma concentrations of enoxacin's major metabolite were about one-tenth of those of enoxacin. Enoxacin had an apparent terminal elimination half-life of 5.3 hours. About 54% of the dose was excreted in the urine within 24 hours as unchanged drug with about 8% being excreted as the major metabolite and about 2% as minor metabolites.— R. Nakamura *et al., J. Chromatogr. biomed. Appl.*, 1983, *278*, 321.

Enoxacin was given in single doses ranging from 200 to 1600 mg to 12 healthy subjects in a capsule formulation and later as an oral suspension. Peak plasma concentrations of 1.19 to 8.29 µg per mL were observed 0.75 to 2.25 hours after administration of the suspension and 0.5 to 2.75 hours after the capsules. The apparent elimination half-life ranged from about 3.4 to 6.4 hours. About 23 to 54% of the administered dose was excreted unchanged in the urine within 72 hours. Plasma concentrations of enoxacin following administration of 400 to 800 mg twice daily for 14 days to 18 similar subjects were greater than after the corresponding single doses, and had reached steady-state levels by the third day. In the group receiving enoxacin 400 mg twice daily, trough plasma concentrations were in the range of 1 to 1.5 µg per mL and average urinary concentrations exceeded 100 µg per mL for 8 hours or more following each dose at steady-state. The increase in plasma concentrations of enoxacin after 14 days of administration was greater than would have been predicted by simple addition; there was also a 15 to 26% increase in the mean half-life of enoxacin and a 21 to 49% reduction in the mean total body clearance of enoxacin after 14 days of administration.— R. Wolf *et al., J. antimicrob. Chemother.*, 1984, *14, Suppl.* C, 63.

Steady-state plasma concentrations of enoxacin were obtained in 18 healthy subjects about 4 days after starting enoxacin 400 mg given twice daily for 14 days. At steady-state the mean plasma concentration 1.5 hours after administration was 3.53 µg per mL compared with 2.38 µg per mL after the first dose and the mean plasma trough concentration was 1.25 µg per mL.— S. E. Tsuei *et al., J. antimicrob. Chemother.*, 1984, *14, Suppl.* C, 71.

DIFFUSION. Diffusion of enoxacin into blister fluid.— R. Wise *et al., J. antimicrob. Chemother.*, 1984, *14, Suppl.* C, 75. Prostatic tissue.— S. Rannikko and A. -S. Malmborg (letter), *ibid.*, 1986, *17*, 123. Sputum.— B. I. Davies *et al., ibid.*, 1984, *14, Suppl.* C, 83.

PROTEIN BINDING. The plasma protein binding of enoxacin was 18% at a concentration of 5 µg per mL.— R. Wise *et al., J. antimicrob. Chemother.*, 1984, *13*, 237.

Uses and Administration

Enoxacin is a fluorinated 4-quinolone antimicrobial agent with actions similar to those of norfloxacin (see p.275). It has been suggested for use in the treatment of a range of infections due to Gram-negative and Gram-positive organisms, including those of the urinary tract.

Proceedings of a symposium on enoxacin.— I. Phillips *et al.* (Ed.), *J. antimicrob. Chemother.*, 1984, *14, Suppl.* C, 1-96. See also D. Speller and R. Wise (Ed.), *ibid.*, 1988, *21, Suppl.* B 1-137.

ADMINISTRATION IN THE ELDERLY. Findings of a pharmacokinetic study suggesting that there is no need for alteration in enoxacin dosage in elderly patients.— R. Wise *et al., J. antimicrob. Chemother.*, 1987, *19*, 343.

CHANCROID. Enoxacin 400 mg given twice daily was effective within 7 to 12 days in the treatment of 7 patients with chancroid. All patients were bacteriologically negative after 3 to 7 days and ulcerations were healed in 5 to 8 days. However, one of the patients with severely enlarged inguinal lymph nodes required an increase in dosage to 600 mg twice daily for a further 5 days after receiving 7 days of treatment.— H. Mensing, *Acta derm.-vener., Stockh.*, 1985, *65*, 455.

CYSTIC FIBROSIS. A 12-year-old boy hospitalised with cystic fibrosis and a persistent respiratory infection due to *Ps. aeruginosa* was given enoxacin 200 mg twice daily for 7 days by mouth after he failed to respond satisfactorily to high-dose intravenous antibiotic therapy. Enoxacin 400 mg was then given twice daily at home for 14-day periods, 9, 16, 20, and 26 weeks after the first course. Improvement obtained after the second course of treatment was sustained during other courses but at no time was his sputum free of *Pseudomonas* organisms. A strain resistant to enoxacin was isolated at the start of the third course of treatment but no resistance was detected at the end of the course. Mild nausea lasting 2 days was the only adverse effect reported and no accumulation of enoxacin in serum was detected.— M. G. Miller *et al.* (letter), *Lancet*, 1985, *1*, 646.

GONORRHOEA. In a double-blind pilot study a cure was obtained in all of 11 patients with uncomplicated urogenital gonorrhoea who received enoxacin 600 mg as a single dose and in all of 11 patients who received enoxacin 400 mg repeated after 4 hours. No adverse effects were noted.— A. Notowicz *et al., J. antimicrob. Chemother.*, 1984, *14, Suppl.* C, 91.

A single dose of 200 mg or 400 mg of enoxacin produced a 90% or 92% cure rate in a study involving 155 men with uncomplicated urethral gonorrhoea. Postgonococcal urethritis occurred in 42% of those given 200 mg and 26% of those given 400 mg.— A. H. van der Willigen *et al., Antimicrob. Ag. Chemother.*, 1987, *31*, 535.

OSTEOMYELITIS. Enoxacin 400 mg given by mouth every 12 hours produced a cure in a patient with osteomyelitis of the spine caused by 2 strains of *Pseudomonas aeruginosa* both of which were resistant to aminoglycoside, cephalosporin, and semi-synthetic penicillin antibiotics. Fluid and tissue cultures were negative after 15 days and all clinical signs resolved during 128 days of treatment.— R. R. Bailey and E. Newman (letter), *N.Z. med. J.*, 1985, *98*, 508.

RESPIRATORY-TRACT INFECTIONS. Of 20 patients with severe bronchopulmonary infection 17 were cured or improved after receiving enoxacin 400 mg given by mouth every 12 hours for 7 to 10 days. Infecting organisms included Gram-positive and Gram-negative bacteria; those identified in treatment failures were *Streptococcus pneumoniae* and *Legionella pneumophila.*— F. P. Joet (letter), *Eur. J. clin. Microbiol.*, 1985, *4*, 512.

Further references: W. J. A. Wijnands *et al., J. antimicrob. Chemother.*, 1986, *18*, 719.

See also under Cystic fibrosis.

SHIGELLOSIS. Comparable clinical and bacteriological improvement with enoxacin and nalidixic acid in shigellosis.— P. De Mol *et al., J. antimicrob. Chemother.*, 1987, *19*, 695.

URINARY-TRACT INFECTIONS. Enoxacin was given in a dosage of 400 mg twice daily with food for up to 7 days to the first 11 of 25 patients being treated for moderate or severe urinary-tract infections but this was reduced to 200 mg given twice daily for the remaining patients due to the number of side-effects being reported. Seven days after treatment 18 patients were cured, 5 had had a relapse, infection being due to organisms sensitive to enoxacin, and 2 had become re-infected with a resistant strain of *Enterococcus faecalis.* Most side-effects reported were either neurological or involved the gastro-intestinal tract, the most common being: nausea, unpleasant taste, strange sensation, vertigo, and visual disturbances. One patient developed a widespread reversible arthralgia which lasted for 6 weeks and another an Achilles tendinitis for 8 weeks.— R. R. Bailey and B. A. Peddie, *N.Z. med. J.*, 1985, *98*, 286.

A cure was obtained in 16 of 20 patients with urinary-tract infection following treatment with enoxacin 200 mg or 400 mg given twice daily with food for 7 or 14 days. Of the 4 treatment failures 3 had pyelonephritis and the other had an infection due to *Enterococcus faecalis*. Nine patients reported mild side-effects including: depression (5), nausea (4), taste disturbance (3), headache (2), vomiting (1). Adverse effects were no more common in those receiving the higher dosage regimen or the longer course.— M. G. Thomas and R. B. Ellis-Pegler, *J. antimicrob. Chemother.*, 1985, *15*, 759.

Further references: K. G. Naber *et al., Infection*, 1985, *13*, 219.

WOUND INFECTION. A report of the successful use of enoxacin in the treatment of a 69-year-old man whose surgical wound became infected with a strain of *Pseudomonas aeruginosa* resistant to a wide range of antimicrobial agents.— J. M. Hubrechts *et al.* (letter), *Lancet*, 1984, *1*, 860.

Proprietary Names and Manufacturers

Flumark *(Dainippon, Jpn)*; Gyramid *(Parke, Davis, Ger.).*

75-w

Enramycin *(rINN).*

Enduracidin.

CAS — 11115-82-5.

Enramycin is a polypeptide antibiotic derived from cultures of *Streptomyces fungicidicus* B5477 and active against Gram-positive bacteria. It was formerly given by intramuscular injection and has been used as an animal feed additive.

Proprietary Names and Manufacturers

Takeda, Jpn.

76-e

Epicillin *(BAN, USAN, rINN).*
SQ-11302. (6*R*)-6-(α-D-Cyclohexa-1,4-dienylglycylamino)penicillanic acid.
$C_{16}H_{21}N_3O_4S$=351.4.

CAS — 26774-90-3.

Epicillin is an aminopenicillin with actions and uses similar to those of ampicillin (see p.116), although it has been reported to have greater *in vitro* activity against *Pseudomonas aeruginosa.* It is administered by mouth in doses of 250 to 1000 mg every 6 hours. Children weighing less than 20 kg may be given 25 to 100 mg per kg body-weight daily in divided doses. It has also been administered by mouth as the hydrochloride. Epicillin may be administered by intramuscular or intravenous injection as the sodium salt; doses of up to 16 g daily have been given.

Proprietary Names and Manufacturers of Epicillin and its Salts
Dexacilina *(Byk Liprandi, Arg.)*; Dexacillin *(Squibb, Austral.; Squibb, Belg.; Squibb, Ital.)*; Dexacilline *(Squibb, Fr.)*; Dex-Cillin *(Squibb, S.Afr.)*; Florispec *(Squibb, Neth.)*; Omnisan *(Spain)*; Spectacillin *(Sandoz, Ger.)*; Spectacilline *(Sandoz, Switz.)*.

77-l

Erythromycin *(BAN, USAN, rINN).*

Eritromicina; Erythromycinum. Erythromycin A is (2*R*,3*S*,4*S*,5*R*,6*R*,8*R*,10*R*,11*R*,12*S*,13*R*)-5-(3-amino-3,4,6-trideoxy-*N*,*N*-dimethyl-β-D-*xylo*-hexopyranosyloxy)-3-(2,6-dideoxy-3-*C*,3-*O*-dimethyl-α-L-*ribo*-hexopyranosyloxy)-13-ethyl-6,11,12-trihydroxy-2,4,6,8,10,12-hexamethyl-9-oxotridecan-13-olide.
$C_{37}H_{67}NO_{13}$=733.9.

CAS — 114-07-8 (erythromycin A).

Pharmacopoeias. In *Aust., Belg., Br., Braz., Chin., Cz., Egypt., Eur., Fr., Ger., Ind., Int., It., Jpn, Jug., Neth., Rus., Swiss, Turk.,* and *U.S.* Also in *B.P. Vet.*

Erythromycin is produced by the growth of a strain of *Streptomyces erythreus* and is a mixture of macrolide antibiotics consisting largely of erythromycin A.

It occurs as white or slightly yellow, odourless or almost odourless, slightly hygroscopic crystals or powder. The *B.P.* specifies not less than 920 units per mg and the *U.S.P.* not less than 850 μg per mg, both calculated on the anhydrous basis.

B.P. **solubilities** are: slightly soluble in water; less soluble at higher temperatures; soluble 1 in 5 of alcohol; soluble in chloroform, methyl alcohol, and 2M hydrochloric acid. *U.S.P.* solubilities are: soluble 1 in 1000 of water; soluble in alcohol, chloroform, and ether. A 0.067% solution in water has a pH of 8.0 to 10.5. **Store** in airtight containers. The *B.P.* recommends storage at a temperature not exceeding 30°. Protect from light.

The water solubility and bitterness of the salts of erythromycin were related to the size of the alkyl group attached to the acid used to prepare the salt. In addition, the bitterness was related to the stability of the salt. The stearyl sulphate salt was the least bitter.— P. H. Jones *et al., J. pharm. Sci.,* 1969, *58,* 337.

Units

One unit of erythromycin is contained in 0.001087 mg of the second International Standard Preparation (1978) of erythromycin A base which contains 920 units per mg.

Collaborative assay of the material proposed as the second International Standard for erythromycin.— J. W. Lightbown and M. V. Mussett, *J. biol. Stand.,* 1981, *9,* 209.

The Committee had noted in its thirty-third report that a discrepancy of about 4 to 8% had been demonstrated between the International Unit as defined by the second International Standard and the microgram of erythromycin activity as defined by the *US* Master Standard for Erythromycin used in the collaborative assay of the first International Standard for Erythromycin. Following investigation it was agreed that the first and second International Standards for Erythromycin had been shown to be stable and that there was no evidence that the activity defined by the International Unit had changed. The possibility of establishing an authentic chemical reference substance would be investigated.— Thirty-fourth Report of WHO Expert Committee on Biological Standardization, *Tech. Rep. Ser. Wld Hlth Org. No. 700,* 1984.

Adverse Effects

Gastro-intestinal disturbances are fairly common with erythromycin, especially with large doses, but serious side-effects are rare. Supra-infection following the oral administration of erythromycin is also rare, as is sensitisation to erythromycin; skin reactions have been reported, but only isolated cases of anaphylaxis.

Reversible deafness has occurred after high doses of erythromycin.

Hepatotoxicity has been reported after administration of erythromycin, most commonly as the estolate (see p.227).

Irritation or sensitivity reactions may occur after the topical administration of erythromycin.

EFFECTS ON THE EAR. Partial deafness developed in a woman after 4 days' therapy with erythromycin 4 g daily. When the dose was reduced to 2 g daily 3 days later her hearing returned to normal.— M. R. Eckman *et al.* (letter), *New Engl. J. Med.,* 1975, *292,* 649.

Reversible loss of hearing occurred in 2 patients, with uraemia and liver disease, given erythromycin 4 g daily by intravenous injection of the lactobionate; it was associated with very high blood concentrations of erythromycin.— G. V. Quinnan and W. R. McCabe (letter), *Lancet,* 1978, *1,* 1160.

Administration of erythromycin stearate 500 mg four times daily to 2 patients on chronic intermittent dialysis caused reversible ototoxicity.— W. F. van Marion *et al.* (letter), *Lancet,* 1978, *2,* 214.

An acute psychotic reaction was associated temporarily with ototoxicity in 2 patients given intravenous erythromycin lactobionate. Both patients had some degree of hepatic dysfunction, moderate renal impairment, and were receiving other ototoxic drugs.— G. S. Umstead and K. H. Neumann, *Archs intern. Med.,* 1986, *146,* 897.

Further references to ototoxicity associated with erythromycin administration: V. G. Schweitzer and N. R. Olson, *Archs Otolar.,* 1984, *110,* 258; K. Yoong *et al., Can. J. Hosp. Pharm.,* 1987, *40,* 97.

EFFECTS ON THE GASTRO-INTESTINAL TRACT. A report of pseudomembranous colitis associated with the administration of erythromycin ethyl succinate.— N. M. Gantz *et al., Ann. intern. Med.,* 1979, *91,* 866.

After administration of erythromycin 500 mg twice daily by mouth for 7 days to 10 healthy subjects, there was a suppression of oropharyngeal aerobic streptococci but no effect on the anaerobic flora. In the intestine erythromycin decreased the numbers of most anaerobic bacteria, and also of enterococci and streptococci in some subjects.— C. E. Nord and A. Heimdahl, *J. antimicrob. Chemother.,* 1986, *18, Suppl.* C, 159.

Erythromycin 500 mg twice daily by mouth was given 30 minutes before food for at least 6 months to 607 patients with acne. The most common adverse effect was diarrhoea (44 patients, 7.2%). Other side-effects were abdominal colic (39, 6.4%), nausea (10, 1.6%), indigestion or dyspepsia (4, 0.7%), increased flatus (1, 0.2%), constipation (1, 0.2%), thrush (14, 2.3%), headache (1, 0.2%), and dizziness (1, 0.2%). Ninety-seven patients (16%) had one or more adverse effects, although in most they were mild and self-limiting.— B. R. Hughes and W. J. Cunliffe (letter), *Lancet,* 1987, *2,* 1340.

The simultaneous intake of BA yoghurt (yoghurt containing viable *Bifidobacterium longum*) with erythromycin reduced the frequency of gastro-intestinal disorders seen in healthy subjects taking erythromycin and placebo yoghurt. The sharp fall in clostridial spore count suggests that BA yoghurt may reduce antibiotic-induced alterations of the intestinal flora.— J. F. Colombel *et al.* (letter), *Lancet,* 1987, *2,* 43.

For reference to the effect of erythromycin on gastro-intestinal motility, see Erythromycin Lactobionate, p.229.

EFFECTS ON THE KIDNEY. Interstitial nephritis and acute renal failure associated with erythromycin therapy in a 39-year-old woman.— J. Rosenfeld *et al., Br. med. J.,* 1983, *286,* 938.

EFFECTS ON THE LIVER. A 57-year-old man developed acute liver failure after treatment with erythromycin base. Transient selective factor X deficiency was also observed. J. P. Hosker and D. P. Jewell, *Postgrad. med. J.,* 1983, *59,* 514.

For further reports of hepatotoxicity associated with erythromycin, see Erythromycin Estolate (p.227), Erythromycin Ethyl Succinate (p.228), Erythromycin Propionate (p.229), and Erythromycin Stearate (p.230).

EFFECTS ON THE NERVOUS SYSTEM. For reference to an acute psychotic reaction associated with ototoxicity after administration of erythromycin lactobionate, see under Effects on the Ear, above.

EFFECTS ON THE SKIN. Analysis, by the Boston Collaborative Drug Surveillance Program, of data on 15 438 patients hospitalised between 1975 and 1982 detected 3 allergic skin reactions attributed to erythromycin among 147 recipients of the drug.— M. Bigby *et al., J. Am. med. Ass.,* 1986, *256,* 3358.

Precautions

Erythromycin should not be used in patients with a known history of allergy to it and should be given with caution to patients with impaired liver function.

Erythromycin may potentiate the action of some drugs, including carbamazepine, cyclosporin, theophylline, and warfarin, probably by inhibition of their hepatic metabolism.

Erythromycin may interfere with some diagnostic tests including measurements of urinary catecholamines, 17-hydroxycorticosteroids, and 17-ketosteroids, and with the microbiological measurements of blood folate.

To avoid the ototoxicity of erythromycin in patients with renal failure it is suggested that the daily dosage should not exceed 1.5 g in patients with serum creatinine above 180 μmol per litre; hearing acuity should be tested before and during treatment, especially in the elderly; and erythromycin should not be given with other potentially ototoxic drugs.— J. -P. Méry and A. Kanfer (letter), *New Engl. J. Med.,* 1979, *301,* 944.

For reference to the precautions to be observed in renal failure, see under Administration in Renal Failure in Uses, below.

INTERACTIONS. There have been a number of reports indicating that macrolide antibiotics may be involved in clinically significant interactions with several drugs. Triacetyloleandomycin has been the most commonly implicated, followed by erythromycin; josamycin has been involved on a few occasions, while there appear to be no reports with midecamycin and spiramycin. Biochemical and *animal* studies have suggested that some of these interactions may be due to inhibition of hepatic metabolism by the macrolide. From case reports and pharmacokinetic studies triacetyloleandomycin appears to inhibit the hepatic metabolism and therefore potentiate the effect of carbamazepine, methylprednisolone, and theophylline. It has also been reported to increase the risk of jaundice in patients taking oral contraceptives, and of acute ergotism in patients being treated with ergot alkaloids, but the mechanism of these reactions has not been elucidated. Studies have suggested that erythromycin may inhibit the hepatic metabolism of carbamazepine, methylprednisolone, theophylline, and also warfarin.— J. Descotes *et al., J. antimicrob. Chemother.,* 1985, *15,* 659. In *rats* and humans, triacetyloleandomycin, and erythromycin and some of its derivatives, induce microsomal enzymes; the nitrosoalkane metabolites so formed produce stable inactive complexes with the iron of cytochrome P-450. Eventually the oxidative metabolism of other drugs may be decreased. These effects are marked after administration of triacetyloleandomycin, moderate after erythromycin, small after oleandomycin, and absent or negligible after josamycin, midecamycin, or spiramycin.— D. Pessayre *et al., ibid., 16, Suppl.* A, 181. A further review of pharmacokinetic interactions of macrolide antibiotics. Erythromycin has been reported to increase serum-digoxin concentrations; this may be due to an inhibiting effect of the antibiotic on the formation of digoxin reduction products in the gut.— T. M. Ludden, *Clin. Pharmacokinet.,* 1985, *10,* 63. A discussion of the interaction between erythromycin and cyclosporin.— *Drug Interact. News.,* 1987, *7,* 23.

For the effect of macrolide antibiotics on plasma-theophylline concentrations, see Theophylline Hydrate, p.1528.

For the effects of other drugs on the antimicrobial activity of erythromycin, see below under Antimicrobial Action.

PORPHYRIA. Erythromycin was considered to be unsafe in patients with acute porphyria because it has been shown to be porphyrinogenic in *animals* or *in vitro* systems.— M.R. Moore and K.E.L. McColl, *Porphyrias, Drug Lists,* Glasgow, Porphyria Research Unit, University of Glasgow, 1987.

Antimicrobial Action

Erythromycin is a macrolide antibiotic. It interferes with bacterial protein synthesis by binding to the 50S subunit of ribosomes. It is bacteriostatic or bactericidal depending on its concentration and the type of organism. Activity increases with increases in pH up to about pH 8.5. Its range of antimicrobial action is similar to that of penicillin. It is active against most Gram-positive bacteria including staphylococci, streptococci, *Corynebacterium diphtheriae*, and *Listeria monocytogenes*. Susceptible Gram-negative bacteria include *Bordetella pertussis*, *Branhamella catarrhalis*, *Campylobacter* and *Neisseria* spp., *Legionella* spp. including *L. pneumophila*, and *Haemophilus* spp., although *H. influenzae* may be only moderately susceptible. Although *Pseudomonas aeruginosa* and the Enterobacteriaceae are generally resistant to erythromycin, some strains of *Escherichia coli* and *Klebsiella* spp. have been reported to be sensitive at an alkaline pH. Other susceptible organisms include *Chlamydia* spp., *Mycoplasma pneumoniae* but not *M. hominis*, some non-tuberculous mycobacteria, *Ureaplasma urealytica*, *Treponema pallidum*, *Entamoeba histolytica*, and some rickettsiae. Many Gram-positive anaerobes are susceptible to erythromycin, but its activity against Gram-negative anaerobes is variable; some strains of *Bacteroides fragilis* and *Fusobacterium* spp. are resistant. Fungi, yeasts, and viruses are resistant to erythromycin.

The minimum inhibitory concentrations of erythromycin for sensitive micro-organisms have been reported to range from less than 0.1 to about 2 µg per mL.

Antibacterial activities of erythromycins A, B, C, and D and some of their derivatives.— I. O. Kibwage *et al.*, *Antimicrob. Ag. Chemother.*, 1985, *28*, 630.

In tissue culture studies, erythromycin penetrated into human cells in high concentrations.— J. R. Martin *et al.*, *Antimicrob. Ag. Chemother.*, 1985, *27*, 314. Erythromycin was also concentrated by human lymphocytes and polymorphonuclear leucocytes *in vitro*.— G. A. Dette and H. Knothe, *J. antimicrob. Chemother.*, 1986, *18*, 73.

The MIC of erythromycin against 2 strains of *Rochalimaea quintana*, the aetiological agent of trench fever, ranged between 0.04 and 0.07 µg per mL.— W. F. Myers *et al.*, *Antimicrob. Ag. Chemother.*, 1984, *25*, 690.

ACTIVITY AGAINST BORDETELLA. The MIC of erythromycin against 50 clinical isolates of *Bordetella pertussis* ranged between 0.012 and 0.1 µg per mL. Susceptibility had not changed from isolates tested about 10 years previously. Erythromycin was the most active of a range of antibiotics tested.— R. M. Bannatyne and R. Cheung, *Antimicrob. Ag. Chemother.*, 1982, *21*, 666.

ACTIVITY AGAINST BRANHAMELLA. The geometric mean MIC of erythromycin against 28 strains of *Branhamella catarrhalis* was 0.07 µg per mL.— E. E. Stobberingh *et al.*, *J. antimicrob. Chemother.*, 1984, *13*, 55. See also F. Ahmad *et al.*, *Antimicrob. Ag. Chemother.*, 1984, *26*, 424; N. J. Slevin *et al.*, *Lancet*, 1984, *1*, 782; J. -E. Brorson and P. Larsson (letter), *J. antimicrob. Chemother.*, 1985, *15*, 644.

ACTIVITY AGAINST CAMPYLOBACTER. All of 70 isolates of *Campylobacter pyloridis* were susceptible to erythromycin *in vitro*; the MIC was in the range 0.015 to 0.5 µg per mL.— C. A. M. McNulty *et al.*, *Antimicrob. Ag. Chemother.*, 1985, *28*, 837.

For the action of erythromycin against *Campylobacter coli* and *C. jejuni*, see below under Resistance.

ACTIVITY AGAINST GONOCOCCI. Erythromycin inhibited about 92, 98, and 100% of 517 of non-beta-lactamase-producing isolates of *Neisseria gonorrhoeae in vitro* at an MIC of 0.5, 1, and 2 µg per mL respectively. It inhibited about 39, 92, and 100% of 13 beta-lactamase-producing isolates at MICs of 0.5, 1, and 2 µg per mL.— J. R. Dillon *et al.* (letter), *J. antimicrob. Chemother.*, 1978, *4*, 477. See also R. Widy-Wirski *et al.*, *Bull. Wld Hlth Org.*, 1982, *60*, 959.

All 100 strains of *Neisseria gonorrhoeae* isolated from men with acute urethritis, had good or intermediate sensitivity *in vitro* to erythromycin, spiramycin, josamycin, and pristinamycin; 12% of strains were resistant to oleandomycin, and 75% resistant to lincomycin.— A. Thabaut *et al.*, *J. antimicrob. Chemother.*, 1985, *16*, *Suppl.* A, 213.

ACTIVITY AGAINST HAEMOPHILUS. Of 68 strains of *Haemophilus influenzae*, 34 were inhibited by erythromycin at a concentration of 0.06 µg per mL, 17 at 0.12 µg per mL, 13 at 0.25 µg per mL, and 4 at 0.5 µg per mL.— J. D. Williams and J. Andrews, *Br. med. J.*, 1974, *1*, 134. The MIC of erythromycin against 83 isolates of *H. influenzae* resistant to both ampicillin and chloramphenicol ranged from 0.5 to 16 µg per mL. It was one of the least active of a range of antibiotics tested.— J. Campos and S. Garcia-Tornel, *J. antimicrob. Chemother.*, 1987, *19*, 297.

All of 30 strains of *Haemophilus ducreyi* were susceptible *in vitro* to erythromycin; the MIC ranged from 0.002 to 0.032 µg per mL.— M. J. Sanson-Le Pors *et al.*, *J. antimicrob. Chemother.*, 1983, *11*, 271. See also Y. R. Bilgeri *et al.*, *Antimicrob. Ag. Chemother.*, 1982, *22*, 686.

ACTIVITY AGAINST LEGIONELLA. Demonstration that *Legionella* multiplying within human polymorphonuclear leucocytes are destroyed by erythromycin A base.— M. F. Miller *et al.* (letter), *Lancet*, 1984, *1*, 348. The fact that it accumulates in macrophages points to erythromycin as the drug of choice in the treatment of legionellosis; however, it probably acts by bacteriostatic rather than bactericidal activity, allowing the cell-mediated immune system time to eradicate the bacterium.— F. G. Rodgers and T. S. J. Elliott (letter), *ibid.*, 683.

A study of the susceptibility of 36 strains of *Legionella* spp. to a range of macrolides and related antibiotics. The most active were josamycin (MIC ranging from 0.06 to 0.25 µg per mL), pristinamycin (0.06 to 0.5 µg per mL), and erythromycin (0.12 to 0.5 µg per mL). Midecamycin (0.12 to 1 µg per mL) and spiramycin (0.5 to 4 µg per mL) also had useful activity. The MIC ranges for other antibiotics tested were 0.5 to 8 µg per mL for oleandomycin, 0.5 to 16 µg per mL for clindamycin, and 16 to 128 µg per mL for lincomycin. The MIC for some of the agents depended on the media used for testing.— N. Bornstein *et al.*, *J. antimicrob. Chemother.*, 1985, *15*, 17.

ACTIVITY AGAINST LISTERIA. There was no evidence of change in the susceptibility of *Listeria monocytogenes* to erythromycin in Sweden over the years 1958 to 1982. The MIC of 90% of strains was between 0.125 and 0.25 µg per mL.— S. Larsson *et al.*, *Antimicrob. Ag. Chemother.*, 1985, *28*, 12.

ACTIVITY AGAINST MYCOBACTERIA. A study *in vitro* of the antimicrobial susceptibility of 258 clinical isolates of *Mycobacterium fortuitum* and *M. chelonae*. In general, all *M. fortuitum* biovariants should be considered resistant to erythromycin. Some strains of both subspecies of *M. chelonae* tested were susceptible.— J. M. Swenson *et al.*, *Antimicrob. Ag. Chemother.*, 1985, *28*, 807.

ACTIVITY AGAINST SHIGELLAE. The MIC of erythromycin against 22 strains of *Shigella* spp. ranged from 2 to 62 µg per mL, concentrations attainable in faeces.— R. N. Greenberg *et al.*, *Antimicrob. Ag. Chemother.*, 1982, *21*, 347.

ACTIVITY AGAINST STREPTOCOCCI. A study *in vitro* of the antibiotic susceptibilities of 68 strains of *Streptococcus milleri* indicating that the most appropriate antibiotic for the treatment of *Str. milleri* infections is benzylpenicillin. In penicillin-allergic patients erythromycin is a suitable alternative.— G. S. Tillotson and L. A. Ganguli (letter), *J. antimicrob. Chemother.*, 1984, *14*, 557.

ACTIVITY WITH OTHER ANTIMICROBIAL AGENTS. Since erythromycin may exhibit bacteriostatic activity, antagonism of bactericidal agents is possible. Erythromycin has been shown to antagonise the bactericidal activity *in vitro* of benzylpenicillin, ampicillin, or gentamicin against *Listeria monocytogenes* (R.L. Penn *et al.*, *Antimicrob. Ag. Chemother.*, 1982, *22*, 289; D.L. Winslow *et al.*, *ibid.*, 1983, *23*, 555). Cohn *et al.* (*ibid.*, 1980, *18*, 872) demonstrated both antagonism and synergism between erythromycin and either ampicillin, cephamandole, or gentamicin depending on the organism; antagonism occurred particularly in *Staphylococcus aureus*.

A synergistic interaction has been reported between erythromycin and sulphamethoxazole against some strains of *Haemophilus influenzae* (M.I. Marks, *Can. med. Ass. J.*, 1975, *112*, 170), and erythromycin has been shown to accelerate the killing of a meningococcal culture by rifampicin without emergence of rifampicin resistance (R.A. Wall and R.N. Grüneberg, *Lancet*, 1982, *2*, 1346).

Depending on the assay method used, chloroquine and erythromycin have demonstrated synergy against chloroquine-resistant *Plasmodium falciparum* (P. Gershon and R.E. Howells, *Trans. R. Soc. trop. Med. Hyg.*, 1986, *80*, 753).

Synergy against some strains of *Staph. aureus* has also been observed when erythromycin was tested *in vitro* with daunorubicin, mitomycin, or doxorubicin (J.Y. Jacobs *et al.*, *Antimicrob. Ag. Chemother.*, 1979, *15*, 580).

For reference to antagonism between erythromycin and either lincosamides or spiramycin, see under Resistance, below.

Resistance

Resistance of bacteria to erythromycin may be due to a decreased affinity of the antibiotic for its site of action. This results from alterations in the 50S subunit of the bacterial ribosome, and may be plasmid-mediated or by chromosomal mutation.

Such resistance to erythromycin is most commonly found in staphylococci and streptococci and is often associated with cross-resistance to other macrolide, lincosamide, or streptogramin antibiotics.

Resistance to erythromycin may also be due to enzymatic inactivation. Intrinsic resistance in Gram-negative bacteria may in part be due to poor penetration of the bacterial cell wall by erythromycin.

Development of bacterial strains resistant to erythromycin is not usually a serious clinical problem during successful short courses of treatment; it is more common during prolonged treatment of infections more difficult to eradicate.

A discussion of the mechanisms of bacterial resistance to macrolide, lincosamide, and streptogramin-B-type antibiotics, known collectively as MLS_B antibiotics. Resistance may be associated with alteration in the target site; specifically N^6-dimethylation of adenine in the 23S ribosomal RNA results in a markedly reduced affinity between MLS_B antibiotics and the ribosome. In certain strains, this resistance is inducible by subinhibitory concentrations of MLS_B antibiotics and in others is expressed constitutively or zonally. This resistance phenotype is widely spread among clinical isolates: it was first reported for *Staphylococcus* spp., and since then has been detected in *Streptococcus* spp., *Corynebacterium diphtheriae*, *Bacteroides fragilis*, *Clostridium perfringens*, *Lactobacillus casei*, and *Streptomyces erythreus*. Many of the genes mediating resistance to MLS_B antibiotics are borne by plasmids which are capable of self-transfer by congugation or can be mobilised by conjugative plasmids.

Resistance of some bacterial species, for example *Lactobacillus* spp., *Clostridium perfringens*, *Streptomyces* spp., and *Escherichia coli* may be mediated by the enzymic inactivation of macrolides. Such strains may also be resistant to lincosamides and streptogramins, but this may be due to the synthesis of several different enzymes by the organism. This resistance may be related to the use of some of these antibiotics as growth-promoting agents in animal feeds.

Intrinsic low-level MLS_B resistance of Gram-negative bacteria may be due both to alteration of the ribosomal binding site and to cellular impermeability.— P. Courvalin *et al.*, *J. antimicrob. Chemother.*, 1985, *16*, *Suppl.* A, 91.

A review of the evolution and epidemiology of resistance to macrolide, lincosamide, and streptogramin-B-type (MLS_B) antibiotics. MLS_B resistance in *Staphylococcus aureus* is characterised in general by a fairly moderate speed of emergence of resistant strains; the incidence of resistance is about 30 to 40% in hospitals and 5 to 10% in general practice and has been fairly stable for the past 20 years. Local variations are mainly linked to usage and epidemics. Acquired MLS_B resistance in streptococci is governed by the same biochemical mechanisms as resistance in *Staph. aureus*, and the genes governing this mechanism are also homologous in many ways. MLS_B resistance in both these species can also cause antagonism between erythromycin and the lincosamides or between erythromycin and spiramycin. MLS_B resistance in streptococci and staphylococci is rarely isolated, but is often associated with other types of resistance, especially to tetracycline and/or chloramphenicol. Under the same selection pressures, MLS_B resistance affected streptococci a few years after it affected staphylococci. The incidence of resistance in streptococci is usually lower than that of staphylococci, usually reaching levels noted for *Staph. aureus* in general practice. Results from Japan, however, show that resistance in streptococci can reach high frequencies under the influence of intensive use of macrolides and epidemic spread of resistant strains.

MLS_B resistance has also been found in the *Bacteroides*

fragilis group, but the genetic determinants implicated appear to be different from those in staphylococci and streptococci.— J. Duval, *J. antimicrob. Chemother.*, 1985, *16, Suppl.* A, 137.

A report of the resistance of *Staphylococcus aureus* to macrolide, lincosamide, and streptogramin (MLS) antibiotics in hospitals. The phenotypes of resistance to macrolides and related compounds can be classified into 3 types: Type A, constitutive resistance to all macrolides and lincosamides; Type B, resistance to erythromycin and oleandomycin, and sensitivity to spiramycin and the lincosamides, although resistance to these latter two antibiotics can be induced by brief contact with subinhibitory concentrations of erythromycin and oleandomycin; Type C, resistance to erythromycin, the only antibiotic able to induce resistance to other antibiotics. Among macrolide-resistant strains of *Staph. aureus* there is a marked predominance of strains showing resistance of Type A; there is a low incidence of Type C resistance, whereas Type B resistance has generally been increasing since 1978. Over recent years, there has been a marked increase to 12% of strains of *Staph. aureus* showing resistance to a wide range of antibiotics including methicillin, macrolides, and aminoglycosides.— A. Thabaut *et al.*, *J. antimicrob. Chemother.*, 1985, *16, Suppl.* A, 205.

Further references to the mechanisms of resistance to macrolides, lincosamides, and streptogramins: B. Weisblum, *J. antimicrob. Chemother.*, 1985, *16, Suppl.* A, 63; R. P. Novick and E. Murphy, *ibid.*, 101; T. Horaud *et al.*, *ibid.*, 111; M. Arthur *et al.*, *ibid.*, 1987, *20*, 783.

RESISTANCE OF BACTEROIDES. A study *in vitro* indicating that erythromycin resistance in *Bacteroides* spp. is linked to diminished clindamycin susceptibility.— M. Reig *et al.*, *Antimicrob. Ag. Chemother.*, 1987, *31*, 665.

RESISTANCE OF CAMPYLOBACTER. Along with rifabutin, the quinolones and cefpirome, erythromycin has been reported to be one of the most active of 27 antibiotics tested *in vitro* against 200 strains of *Campylobacter jejuni* (P. Van der Auwera and B. Scorneaux, *Antimicrob. Ag. Chemother.*, 1985, *28*, 37); the MIC of erythromycin was in the range of 0.62 to 20 μg per mL, 8% of strains being considered resistant. Most studies have demonstrated only a few *C. jejuni* resistant to erythromycin, but a higher rate of resistance has been shown among *C. coli* (D.A Secker, *J. antimicrob. Chemother.*, 1983, *12*, 414; R.D. Burridge and I. Phillips, *ibid.*, 1984, *14*, 307). Some *C. coli* resistant to erythromycin have also shown resistance to tetracycline and kanamycin, and in one case to chloramphenicol also (H. Sagara *et al.*, *Antimicrob. Ag. Chemother.*, 1987, *31*, 713). Resistance has been shown to be more common among *Campylobacter* spp. isolated from *hogs* (mainly *C. coli*) rather than from humans (mainly *C. jejuni*) (W.-L.L. Wang *et al.*, *ibid.*, 1984, *26*, 351). In comparing the susceptibility of *Campylobacter* spp. to a range of macrolides and related antibiotics, erythromycin, josamycin, clindamycin, and ASE-136-BS (a new erythromycin derivative) were the most active against human strains of *C. jejuni*; oleandomycin, spiramycin, lincomycin, and pristinamycin were less active. Most human *C. coli* had a similar pattern of susceptibility to *C. jejuni*, but *C. coli* isolated from *swine* were highly resistant to all the agents tested except pristinamycin (Z. Elharrif *et al.*, *ibid.*, 1985, *28*, 695).

RESISTANCE OF ENTEROBACTERIACEAE. The incidence of intestinal carriage of highly erythromycin-resistant strains of Enterobacteriaceae in a haematological oncology unit was strongly associated with individual exposure to erythromycin.— A. Andremont *et al.*, *Antimicrob. Ag. Chemother.*, 1986, *29*, 1104.

RESISTANCE OF LEGIONELLA. Variants of *Legionella* spp. demonstrating resistance to erythromycin were produced *in vitro*. Various patterns of cross-resistance to macrolide, lincosamide, and streptogramin B antibiotics were observed.— J. N. Dowling *et al.*, *Antimicrob. Ag. Chemother.*, 1985, *27*, 272.

RESISTANCE OF MYCOPLASMA. A few strains of *Mycoplasma pneumoniae* resistant to erythromycin have been isolated from patients treated with the drug, particularly for prolonged periods. Some such strains studied *in vitro* also showed resistance to other macrolide, lincosamide, and streptogramin B antibiotics. Induction of resistance was observed, but the mechanism responsible appeared to be different from that seen in *Staphylococcus aureus*.— T. Stopler and D. Branski, *J. antimicrob. Chemother.*, 1986, *18*, 359.

RESISTANCE OF STAPHYLOCOCCI. Isolation of strains of staphylococci from *cows*, suggesting naturally occurring resistance to macrolide, lincosamide, and streptogramin B (MLS) antibiotics. Previous reports of MLS resistance in staphylococci have been of acquired resistance in clinical cases.— P. K. Saikia *et al.* (letter), *J. antimicrob. Chemother.*, 1986, *17*, 685.

RESISTANCE OF STREPTOCOCCI. Antibiotic resistance of *Streptococcus pneumoniae* in childhood carriers; a few strains showed multiple resistance including resistance to benzylpenicillin, tetracycline, chloramphenicol, erythromycin, clindamycin, and co-trimoxazole.— J. L. Pérez *et al.* (letter), *J. antimicrob. Chemother.*, 1987, *19*, 278.

Localised incidences of increased resistance of *Streptococcus pyogenes* in Sweden may not be related to clinical usage, but to the use of macrolides such as tylosin in animal feeds.— P. B. Fernandes and D. Garmaise (letter), *J. antimicrob. Chemother.*, 1987, *20*, 449.

See also under Pharyngitis in Uses, Respiratory-tract Infections.

Absorption and Fate

Erythromycin is destroyed by gastric acid, and is usually administered either as base in enteric-coated formulations or as the more stable salts or esters. Depending on the formulation, food can interfere with the absorption of erythromycin so administration may be best 30 minutes or more before food. Peak plasma-erythromycin concentrations of about 0.5 and 1.0 μg per mL are achieved within 4 hours of doses of 250 and 500 mg of the base respectively. However, higher peak plasma concentrations have been reported after administration of erythromycin every 6 hours for a few days. Plasma half-lives from 1.2 to 4 hours have been reported.

Erythromycin is widely distributed throughout body tissues and fluids with some retention in the liver and spleen. Diffusion into the aqueous, but not the vitreous humour of the eye has been reported to be good. Only low concentrations appear in cerebrospinal fluid. Up to 20% of the maternal plasma concentration of erythromycin has been measured in the blood of the foetus; it appears in breast milk. Erythromycin is excreted in high concentrations in the bile and up to 5% of an oral dose appears in the urine; considerable amounts may also be inactivated in the body.

Intravenous administration results in higher but less sustained plasma concentrations and a greater degree of urinary excretion.

ADMINISTRATION IN LIVER DISORDERS. In 8 patients with alcoholic liver disease given enteric-coated erythromycin base tablets by mouth, the lag time for absorption and the time to peak serum concentrations was shorter than in 6 healthy subjects. Although the half-life was decreased in these patients, the rate of elimination of erythromycin appeared to be slower than in the healthy subjects.— P. D. Kroboth *et al.*, *Antimicrob. Ag. Chemother.*, 1982, *21*, 135.

The mean half-life of erythromycin after administration by mouth was 2.0 hours in 6 healthy subjects and 3.2 hours in 6 patients with alcoholic liver disease. This increase was not considered to be clinically significant.— K. W. Hall *et al.*, *J. clin. Pharmac.*, 1982, *22*, 321.

Erythromycin has been reported to be bound mainly to α_1-acid glycoprotein in plasma and to a minor extent to albumin. In a study *in vitro*, a marked elevation of free fraction of erythromycin was associated with lowered concentrations of α_1-acid glycoprotein in serum from patients with cirrhosis of the liver.— J. Barre *et al.* (letter), *Br. J. clin. Pharmac.*, 1984, *18*, 652. See also J. Barre *et al.*, *ibid.*, 1987, *23*, 753.

ADMINISTRATION IN RENAL FAILURE. For reference to the pharmacokinetics of erthromycin in renal failure, see under Administration in Renal Failure in Uses, below.

DIFFUSION INTO BODY TISSUES AND FLUIDS. Therapeutic sputum concentrations of erythromycin after rectal administration in adult patients with bronchitis.— E. Pozzi *et al.*, *Curr. ther. Res.*, 1983, *33*, 681.

Penetration of erythromycin into bronchial secretions after oral administration of propionyl erythromycin mercaptosuccinate (RV-11).— E. Concia *et al.*, *J. int. med. Res.*, 1986, *14*, 137.

DRUG ABSORPTION. A brief comparative review of oral erythromycin preparations. Claims for superior bioavailability of different formulations of oral erythromycins are difficult to evaluate, partly because similar studies have in some instances yielded opposite results. In general, however, the pathogens for which oral erythromycin is recommended are susceptible to low concentrations of the drug, and all of the different preparations are usually absorbed well enough to reach serum concentrations higher than those needed to inhibit the growth of these organisms.— *Med. Lett.*, 1985, *27*, 1. For reference to reports suggesting greater efficacy of erythromycin estolate compared with other erythromycin salts, see under the respiratory-tract infections Pertussis and Pharyngitis in Uses, below.

The absorption of erythromycin was reported to be accelerated in patients with coeliac disease. In those with Crohn's disease the absorption of the stearate ester was reported to be reduced, and that of the ethyl succinate unchanged.— P. G. Welling and F. L. S. Tse, *J. clin. Hosp. Pharm.*, 1984, *9*, 163.

Influence of bariatric surgery (surgical treatment of obesity) on erythromycin absorption.— R. A. Prince *et al.*, *J. clin. Pharmac.*, 1984, *24*, 523.

Studies demonstrating improved absorption of erythromycin from capsules containing enteric-coated pellets of the base when compared with other formulations including enteric-coated erthromycin tablets, film-coated erythromycin stearate tablets, and erythromycin ethyl succinate tablets: K. Josefsson *et al.*, *Br. J. clin. Pharmac.*, 1982, *13*, 685; T. Hovi *et al.*, *Eur. J. clin. Pharmac.*, 1983, *25*, 271; A. Digranes *et al.*, *Curr. ther. Res.*, 1984, *35*, 313; T. Hovi and M. Heikinheimo, *Eur. J. clin. Pharmac.*, 1985, *28*, 231; G. J. Yakatan *et al.*, *J. clin. Pharmac.*, 1985, *25*, 36; K. Josefsson *et al.*, *Curr. ther. Res.*, 1986, *39*, 131.

PROTEIN BINDING. There have been varying reports of the amount of erythromycin bound to plasma proteins: Some 18% of erythromycin in the circulation was bound to serum proteins. The half-life in serum was 1.4 hours and 15% was excreted in urine.— C. M. Kunin, *Ann. intern. Med.*, 1967, *67*, 151. About 81% of erythromycin was bound to serum proteins when measured by ultrafiltration and about 84% when equilibrium dialysis was used.— R. G. Wiegand and A. H. C. Chun, *J. pharm. Sci.*, 1972, *61*, 425. About 73% of erythromycin and 92.6% of erythromycin propionate was bound to serum proteins as measured by ultrafiltration with 100% serum and tube dilution. The low degree of protein-binding previously reported could have been due to measurements based only on tube dilution and not using whole serum.— R. C. Gordon *et al.*, *J. pharm. Sci.*, 1973, *62*, 1074. Erythromycin was 64.5% bound to plasma proteins as measured by equilibrium dialysis. It was mainly bound to α_1-acid glycoprotein, with some binding also to albumin.— J. Prandota *et al.*, *J. int. med. Res.*, 1980, *8, Suppl.* 2, 1.

Uses and Administration

Erythromycin is used in the treatment of infections due to susceptible organisms; it is often used as an alternative to penicillin in infections due to Gram-positive cocci, especially streptococci, and *Listeria monocytogenes*. In penicillin-sensitive patients it is given in place of penicillin in the prophylaxis of endocarditis and in the treatment of syphilis. For the treatment of otitis media caused by *Haemophilus influenzae* it may be given in combination with a sulphonamide.

Erythromycin may be given as an adjunct to antitoxin in the treatment of diphtheria or used alone to eradicate the carrier state. In the management of pertussis, it may be used to render the patient non-infectious or be given prophylactically to contacts. It is used in infections due to *Mycoplasma pneumoniae* and *Chlamydia trachomatis*, in legionnaires' disease, in enteritis due to *Campylobacter* spp., chancroid, and, similarly to tetracycline, in the treatment of severe acne vulgaris.

An effective blood concentration for moderately severe infections in adults may be maintained by a dose by mouth of 1 g daily in 2 to 4 divided doses; for severe infections 2 to 4 g may be given daily. For children the dose is usually about 30 to 50 mg per kg body-weight daily although it may be doubled in severe infections; a recommended dose for children aged 2 to 8 years is 1 g daily in divided doses, and for infants and children up to 2 years of age, 500 mg daily in divided doses. To avoid destruction by gastric juice, erythromycin is usually given as enteric-coated formulations. It may be preferable to administer erythromycin on an empty stomach, as its absorption from some formulations is delayed by the presence of food. It is also given by mouth as the estolate, ethyl succinate, propionate, or stearate. The ethyl carbonate was formerly used.

In the patient who is unable to take erythromycin by mouth and in severely ill patients in whom it is necessary to attain an immediate high blood concentration, erythromycin may be given intravenously in the form of one of its more soluble salts such as the gluceptate or the lactobionate.

Erythromycin may occasionally be given intramuscularly as a solution of erythromycin ethyl succinate.

Erythromycin is used as a 0.5% ophthalmic ointment for the treatment and prophylaxis of infections of the eye, particularly of neonatal conjunctivitis. It may also be applied topically, usually as a 2% solution for the treatment of acne vulgaris.

Erythromycin thiocyanate is used in veterinary medicine.

Reviews and discussions of the actions and uses of erythromycin: J. A. Washington and W. R. Wilson, *Mayo Clin. Proc.*, 1985, *60*, 189; *idem*, 271; A. -S. Malmborg, *J. antimicrob. Chemother.*, 1986, *18*, 293; W. R. Wilson *et al.*, *Mayo Clin. Proc.*, 1987, *62*, 906.

A review of antibacterial agents used in anaerobic infections. The usefulness of erythromycins appears to be limited by the resistance *in vitro* of some strains, especially *Bacteroides fragilis* and fusobacteria, by the low serum concentrations achieved with oral administration, by the difficulties of intravenous administration, and most importantly by the scarcity of data indicating clinical efficacy.— J. G. Bartlett, *Lancet*, 1982, *2*, 478.

For reference to the use of erythromycin in the treatment of atypical mycobacterial infections, see Amikacin Sulphate, p.111.

ADMINISTRATION, OCULAR. Erythromycin has been administered to the eye topically, or by subconjunctival or intravitreal injection.— T. S. Lesar and R. G. Fiscella, *Drug Intell. & clin. Pharm.*, 1985, *19*, 642.

ADMINISTRATION, RECTAL. A report of the successful use of erythromycin suppositories in a patient who had undergone an almost total small bowel resection. Suppositories of erythromycin base in Witepsol H15 were prepared; a displacement value of 3.7 was calculated for erythromycin. Adequate serum concentrations were achieved by the insertion four times daily of two 4-g suppositories, each containing 1 g of erythromycin.— S. Hall and S. Potter (letter), *Pharm. J.*, 1981, *2*, 115.

ADMINISTRATION IN RENAL FAILURE. The normal half-life for erythromycin of 1.2 to 2.6 hours was increased to 4 to 6 hours in end-stage renal failure. It could be given in usual doses to patients with renal failure.— W. M. Bennett *et al.*, *Am. J. Kidney Dis.*, 1983, *3*, 155.

Serum concentrations of erythromycin do increase in patients with moderate to severe renal insufficiency and the dose of erythromycin should probably be adjusted because of the risk of deafness.— R. E. Van Scoy and W. R. Wilson, *Mayo Clin. Proc.*, 1983, *58*, 246.

A study indicating insignificant removal of erythromycin by haemodialysis.— A. Iliopoulou and K. Downey, *Br. J. clin. Pharmac.*, 1982, *13*, 611P.

See also under Peritonitis, below.

DIPHTHERIA. In a comparison in 294 subjects between a single injection of benzathine penicillin and a 7-day course of clindamycin or erythromycin by mouth, erythromycin was recommended as the drug of choice for the treatment of diphtheria carriers.— R. V. McCloskey *et al.*, *Ann. intern. Med.*, 1974, *81*, 788. Bacteriological follow-up should be carried out 2 weeks after completing treatment with erythromycin or penicillin.— L. W. Miller *et al.*, *Antimicrob. Ag. Chemother.*, 1974, *6*, 166.

The successful use of erythromycin with diphtheria antitoxin to treat a 10-week-old child with a toxigenic strain of *Corynebacterium diphtheriae mitis*. Carriers were also treated with erythromycin.— L. E. Simmons *et al.*, *Lancet*, 1980, *1*, 304.

ENDOCARDITIS. In patients with streptococcal endocarditis who are allergic to penicillins, oral treatment with erythromycin may be substituted after 2 weeks of intravenous therapy with vancomycin and gentamicin according to *in-vitro* susceptibility studies and the clinical response of the patient (British Society for Antimicrobial Chemotherapy, *Lancet*, 1985, *2*, 815). Its use [by the intravenous route] in association with fusidic acid or vancomycin has also been suggested for the treatment of endocarditis caused by *Staphylococcus aureus*, including methicillin-resistant strains (S.J. Eykyn, *J. antimicrob. Chemother.*, 1987, *20*, *Suppl.* A, 161; C.M. Oakley, *ibid.*, 181).

Prophylaxis. When administered by mouth, erythromycin has been shown to be effective in reducing the prevalence of streptococcal bacteraemia after dental extraction (D.C. Shanson *et al.*, *J. antimicrob. Chemother.*, 1985, *15*, 83). It is therefore widely recommended for oral prophylaxis against infective endocarditis in at-risk patients who are allergic to penicillins. For patients undergoing dental procedures, the British Society for Antimicrobial Chemotherapy (BSAC) (*Lancet*, 1982, *2*, 1323 and *ibid.*, 1986, *1*, 1267) recommend a single dose of amoxycillin 3 g by mouth, but since erythromycin is less predictably bactericidal *in vitro* against many oral streptococci and is less reliably absorbed from the gastro-intestinal tract, two doses of erythromycin are necessary. They therefore recommend that penicillin-allergic patients should be given erythromycin stearate 1.5 g by mouth 1 to 2 hours before the procedure followed by 0.5 g six hours later. Children under 10 years of age should be given half the adult dose, and children under 5, one-quarter. A 2-g dose of erythromycin stearate may produce more reliable bactericidal plasma concentrations, but it has been associated with a higher incidence of adverse gastro-intestinal effects (D.C. Shanson *et al.*, *ibid.*, 1983, *1*, 299). The BSAC used to recommend that patients who had received penicillins in the previous month be given prophylaxis with erythromycin stearate because of the possibility of carriage of oral streptococci with a reduced sensitivity to amoxycillin. However, Harrison *et al.* (*J. antimicrob. Chemother.*, 1985, *15*, 471 and 501), demonstrated that this may also occur after repeated doses of erythromycin stearate and possibly to a greater extent. Therefore the BSAC now state that amoxycillin may be given twice in a month if necessary.

The recommendations of the European Society of Cardiology for prophylaxis during dental procedures are very similar to those of the BSAC (J. Delaye *et al.*, *Eur. Heart J.*, 1985, *6*, 826).

Although the American Heart Association (AHA) recommend phenoxymethylpenicillin for oral prophylaxis in patients undergoing dental procedures and surgery of the upper respiratory tract, they also advocate the use of erythromycin in penicillin-allergic patients (S.T. Shulman *et al.*, *Circulation*, 1984, *70*, 1123A). They recommend a dose of 1 g of erythromycin given one hour prior to the procedure followed by 500 mg six hours later. Children may be given 20 mg per kg body-weight followed by 10 mg per kg.

The choice of erythromycin salt administered by mouth should be determined by the plasma concentrations achieved at the expected time of bacteraemia. In a study in 11 healthy subjects, Shanson *et al.* (*J. antimicrob. Chemother.*, 1984, *14*, 157) considered that erythromycin stearate was more likely to produce adequate serum bactericidal concentrations against viridans streptococci during the 6-hour period following bacteraemia than erythromycin ethyl succinate although more subjects preferred taking the ethyl succinate.

Although the BSAC and AHA recommend that vancomycin be used instead of a penicillin in penicillin-allergic patients requiring parenteral therapy, Gammage *et al.* (*Br. med. J.*, 1984, *289*, 1516) have suggested the use of erythromycin lactobionate 500 mg in association with gentamicin 1.5 mg per kg for women at risk of endocarditis attending for insertion of an intra-uterine contraceptive device. Both agents should be administered intravenously 30 minutes before the procedure and repeated twice at 8-hour intervals.

See also under Phenoxymethylpenicillin Potassium, p.283, and Prophylactic Use of Antibiotics, p.102.

ENTERIC INFECTIONS. *Campylobacter enteritis.* Erythromycin has been used for the treatment of enteritis caused by *Campylobacter* spp., particularly *C. jejuni*. A study involving 29 patients, however, demonstrated that a 5-day course of erythromycin by mouth promptly eradicated the organisms from the faeces but had no effect on the clinical course of the infection (B.J. Anders *et al.*, *Lancet*, 1982, *1*, 131). Treatment was not commenced until about 5 to 6 days after onset of the illness. Mandal *et al.* (*J. antimicrob. Chemother.*, 1984, *13*, 619) reached similar conclusions, but Taylor *et al.* (*Antimicrob. Ag. Chemother.*, 1987, *31*, 438) could find no effect of erythromycin on the duration of excretion of *Campylobacter* spp. This latter study involved 100 infants in Bangkok with diarrhoea caused by *Campylobacter* spp., *Shigella* spp., or other organisms, and treatment was commenced within 24 hours of the onset of symptoms. A high incidence of resistance among *Campylobacter* strains was reported, however, particularly among institutionalised children; in some cases this resistance occurred independently of tetracycline resistance. Most authors reviewing the management of *Campylobacter* enteritis have considered it to be a self-limiting condition usually requiring only symptomatic treatment as for diarrhoea of any other cause (J. Symonds, *Br. med. J.*, 1983, *286*, 243; C.A.M. McNulty, *J. antimicrob. Chemother.*, 1987, *19*, 281). Administration of erythromycin may be advisable if symptoms have been prolonged, bloody diarrhoea is severe, or relapses occur. Human faecal-oral transmission appears to play only a very minor role in the epidemiology of *Campylobacter* enteritis, but may become more important in children in residential or day-care centres and in food-handlers. Asymptomatic food handlers excreting *C. jejuni* seem to constitute little risk.

GASTRITIS. Rapid healing of acute purulent gastritis associated with campylobacter-like organisms has been reported in a 28-year-old woman after administration of erythromycin (M. Salmeron *et al.*, *Lancet*, 1986, *2*, 975). In a study of 50 patients with gastritis associated with *Campylobacter pyloridis*, however, erythromycin ethyl succinate by mouth was little different from placebo and less effective than bismuth salicylate in clearing *Campylobacter* and improving gastritis; symptomatic response was difficult to assess (C.A.M. McNulty *et al.*, *Br. med. J.*, 1986, *293*, 645).

LEGIONNAIRES' DISEASE. Erythromycin is usually considered to be the drug of choice for infections caused by *Legionella pneumophila* (*Med. Lett.*, 1986, *28*, 33) including legionnaires' disease. It is given in a dose of 2 to 4 g daily, administered initially by the intravenous route in the seriously ill followed by oral maintenance treatment. Rifampicin may be added if there is no response to erythromycin alone. Treatment should be continued for 3 weeks as relapse has been noted after shorter courses (D.C. Flenley, *Br. med. J.*, 1983, *286*, 955; K. Rashed *et al.*, *Lancet*, 1986, *1*, 197). There have been reports of the failure of therapy with erythromycin and rifampicin, mainly in immunocompromised patients (A. Mercatello *et al.*, *J. Infect.*, 1985, *10*, 282), thus higher doses may be required (J.A. Washington and W.R. Wilson, *Mayo Clin. Proc.*, 1985, *60*, 271). Aerosol administration has been investigated in *animals* as a possible adjunct to parenteral therapy (R.B. Fitzgeorge *et al.*, *Lancet*, 1986, *1*, 502). Erythromycin has also been used to treat pneumonia caused by other *Legionella* spp. such as *L. micdadei* (P.N. Gobbo *et al.*, *ibid.*, *2*, 969), *L. wadsworthii* (P. H. Edelstein *et al.*, *Ann. intern. Med.*, 1982, *97*, 809), and *L. bozemanii* (C.R. Swinburn *et al.*, *Lancet*, 1988, *1*, 472).

LISTERIOSIS. For reference to the use of erythromycin in listeria infections, see Ampicillin Trihydrate, p.120.

LYME DISEASE. For reference to the use of erythromycin in the treatment of Lyme disease, see Tetracycline Hydrochloride, p.319.

MALARIA. Studies in *animals* have suggested that erythromycin may potentiate the action of chloroquine against chloroquine-resistant *Plasmodium* spp. Studies in Eastern Thailand in patients with chloroquine-resistant falciparum malaria, however, have shown unsatisfactory results when erythromycin was added to treatment with chloroquine (R.E. Phillips *et al.*, *Lancet*, 1984, *1*, 300), amodiaquine (S. Looareesuwan *et al.*, *ibid.*, 1985, *2*, 805), or quinine (L.W. Pang *et al.*, *Bull. Wld Hlth Org.*, 1985, *63*, 739).

MEDITERRANEAN SPOTTED FEVER. For a comparative study of erythromycin in the treatment of Mediterranean spotted fever in children, see Tetracycline Hydrochloride, p.319.

MENINGITIS. For reference to the precautions to be observed in using erythromycin and ampicillin in the treatment of listeria meningitis, see Ampicillin Trihydrate, p.120.

OTITIS MEDIA. In a study of 81 children with otitis media due to *Haemophilus influenzae*, erythromycin ethyl succinate equivalent to erythromycin 50 mg per kg body-weight daily combined with trisulphapyrimidines [sulphadiazine, sulphamerazine, and sulphadimidine in equal parts] 150 mg per kg daily was significantly more effective than erythromycin used alone. However, there was no significant difference in the results obtained with ampicillin 50 to 60 mg per kg daily and those achieved with either the combined regimen or erythromycin alone.— S. H. Sell *et al.*, *Sth. med. J.*, 1978, *71*, 1493.

Studies of the use of a combination preparation of erythromycin and sulphafurazole in the treatment of otitis media in children: W. J. Rodriguez *et al.*, *Am. J. Dis. Child.*, 1985, *139*, 766; M. J. Corwin *et al.*, *Int. J. pediatr. Otorhinolaryngol.*, 1986, *11*, 109.

See also under Choice of Antibiotic, p.98.

PELVIC INFLAMMATORY DISEASE. For reference to the use of erythromycin in the treatment of acute salpingitis, see Choice of Antibiotic, p.99.

PERITONITIS. Erythromycin has been administered intra-peritoneally to patients with peritonitis associated with continuous ambulatory peritoneal dialysis. A loading dose of 150 mg per litre of dialysis fluid followed by a maintenance dose of 75 mg per litre has been given.

Transient deafness has occurred after the administration of a maintenance dose of 250 mg per exchange.— D. K. Scott and D. E. Roberts, *Pharm. J.*, 1985, *1*, 621.

Use of a single dose of rifampicin 10 mg per kg body-weight by mouth in association with erythromycin 2 g daily in divided doses, or flucloxacillin in patients intolerant to erythromycin, for the management of exit-site infections during continuous ambulatory peritoneal dialysis.— A. R. Morton *et al.* (letter), *Lancet*, 1987, *1*, 1258.

Further references to the use of erythromycin in peritonitis: R. Wens *et al.*, *J. Infect.*, 1985, *10*, 249 (*Campylobacter fetus* infection).

PREGNANCY AND THE NEONATE. For the use of erythromycin in the treatment of chlamydial infections in pregnant women and neonates, see Chlamydial Infections under Sexually Transmitted Diseases, below.

For WHO recommendations for the use of erythromycin in the prophylaxis and treatment of neonatal conjunctivitis, see under Tetracycline Hydrochloride, p.320.

PSITTACOSIS. For reference to the use of erythromycin in psittacosis, see Psittacosis under Respiratory-tract Infections in Tetracycline Hydrochloride, p.320.

Q FEVER. Five patients with Q fever pneumonia (diagnosed retrospectively) have been reported to respond promptly to treatment with intravenous erythromycin lactobionate (L.J. D'Angelo and R. Hetherington, *Br. med. J.*, 1979, *2*, 305). Marrie *et al.* (*Lancet*, 1986, *1*, 427) have also found it to be adequate for mild cases of the disease, but considered that a controlled trial is needed to confirm its superiority over placebo. Tetracyclines are usually regarded as the treatment of choice for Q fever.

RELAPSING FEVER, LOUSE-BORNE. For a study concluding that the treatment of choice was a single 500-mg dose of tetracycline or erythromycin by mouth, see Tetracycline Hydrochloride, p.320.

RESPIRATORY-TRACT INFECTIONS. *Bronchitis.* References to the use of erythromycin in the treatment of bronchitis: acute bronchitis.— P. -S. Pekkanen and K. Josefsson, *J. int. med. Res.*, 1983, *11*, 285 (use of capsules containing enteric-coated pellets of erythromycin base). chronic bronchitis.— E. T. Peel and G. Anderson, *Postgrad. med. J.*, 1983, *59*, *Suppl.* 3, 190 (use of erythromycin stearate as prophylaxis against acute exacerbations); P. B. Ryan *et al.*, *Curr. ther. Res.*, 1986, *39*, 93 (comparison with cephalexin in treatment of acute exacerbations).

Pertussis. Erythromycin, tetracycline, and chloramphenicol have been shown to be effective in achieving an early bacteriological cure in patients with pertussis providing the drug diffuses sufficiently into respiratory-tract secretions. These agents do not alter the subsequent clinical course of the illness if given in the paroxysmal stage of the disease when the diagnosis is most often first suspected. Administration to patients at any stage of pertussis may however render them non-infectious, hence the rationale for antimicrobial treatment of this infection (J.W. Bass, *Pediatr. infect. Dis.*, 1985, *4*, 614). Erythromycin is most often considered the drug of choice for *Bordetella pertussis* infections, with co-trimoxazole or ampicillin as alternatives (*Med. Lett.*, 1986, *28*, 33). Bass considered that reports of the failure of erythromycin to eradicate pertussis organisms are associated with inadequate concentrations of the drug in the serum or respiratory secretions and that this most often occurs after administration of the ethyl succinate or stearate esters. He recommended the use of the estolate ester in a dosage of 50 mg [expressed as the base] per kg body-weight daily (or a maximum of 1 to 2 g daily) for 14 days to treat patients with pertussis at any stage of the infection. An alternative treatment regimen must reliably produce comparable blood-erythromycin concentrations. Although pertussis organisms are eliminated from the nasopharynx of patients on this regimen after 4 days, courses of 10 days or less are associated with a 10% incidence of bacteriological relapse. He considered that the above factors also explain reports of the failure of erythromycin to protect contacts from infection when administered prophylactically (P.R. Grob, *Lancet*, 1981, *1*, 772; M. Spencely and H.P. Lambert, *ibid.*). Treatment for 14 days was considered to be adequate to protect exposed unvaccinated individuals and to control outbreaks of infections; it should be administered in the same dose as for treatment.

Pharyngitis. In a study involving 102 children with Group A streptococcal pharyngitis the failure-rates were 4.3 and 17.5% in groups of 5 patients treated with erythromycin as the estolate or ethyl succinate esters respectively. The estolate was administered in a dose equivalent to erythromycin 15 mg per kg body-weight twice daily and the ethyl succinate in a dose equivalent to 25 mg per kg twice daily, both given by mouth for 10 days. There was a higher incidence of gastro-intestinal effects in patients treated with the ethyl succinate, which may, in part, have contributed to the higher failure rate.— C. M. Ginsburg *et al.*, *Am. J. Dis. Child.*, 1984, *138*, 536.

Penicillin remains the standard treatment for Group A streptococcal pharyngitis; erythromycin is recommended for penicillin-allergic patients, except in Japan where significant resistance is emerging. However, the use of erythromycin may increase with the growing importance of *Corynebacterium haemolyticum* as a cause of pharyngitis, since erythromycin appears to be more effective than penicillin in eradicating this organism.— *Lancet*, 1987, *1*, 1241.

For a report of the use of erythromycin in the treatment of pharyngitis caused by *Corynebacterium haemolyticum*, see Benzathine Penicillin, p.130.

Pneumonia. Erythromycin has been shown to have similar efficacy to ampicillin followed by amoxycillin (J.T. Macfarlane *et al.*, *J. Infect.*, 1983, *7*, 111) and to ampicillin in association with flucloxacillin (D.C. Shanson *et al.*, *J. antimicrob. Chemother.*, 1984, *14*, 75) in the treatment of community-acquired pneumonia; intravenous treatment may be required initially. Some workers have recommended that pneumonia in previously fit individuals be treated immediately with a penicillin effective against *Streptococcus pneumoniae* and erythromycin to cover mycoplasma and legionella. When influenza A is prevalent in the community an anti-staphylococcal antibiotic such as flucloxacillin should be added (C.K. Connolly and B. Harrison, *Br. med. J.*, 1985, *290*, 1586; M.A. Woodhead and J.T. Macfarlane, *ibid.*, 1745).

In 17 children with pneumonia caused by *Mycoplasma pneumoniae*, treatment with erythromycin 40 mg per kg body-weight daily for 7 to 10 days reduced the duration of fever but had no effect on duration of hospitalisation, duration of cough, or duration of radiological changes, and had no significant effect on long-term impaired pulmonary function.— A. R. Sabato *et al.*, *Archs Dis. Childh.*, 1984, *59*, 1034.

For reference to the use of erythromycin in other atypical pneumonias, see Chlamydial Infections under Sexually Transmitted Diseases, Legionnaires' Disease, Psittacosis, and Q Fever.

RHEUMATIC FEVER PROPHYLAXIS. In patients allergic to both penicillin and sulphonamides, erythromycin may be used for the prevention of recurrent attacks of rheumatic fever. Appropriate doses have not been definitely established, but 250 mg twice daily by mouth has been suggested.— S. T. Shulman *et al.*, *Circulation*, 1984, *70*, 1118A.

SEPTICAEMIA. Beneficial effect of erythromycin in the treatment of a patient with septicaemia caused by *Bacillus cereus*.— P. Casella and N. Monzani (letter), *Eur. J. clin. Microbiol.*, 1984, *3*, 35.

As a few strains of *Campylobacter* spp. are resistant to erythromycin, sensitivity testing is advised for patients with septicaemia or other serious infections caused by these organisms. An antibiotic with more certain activity, such as chloramphenicol or gentamicin, should be given initially.— C. A. M. McNulty, *J. antimicrob. Chemother.*, 1987, *19*, 281.

Toxic-shock syndrome. Use of erythromycin in a patient with diarrhoea and bacteraemia caused by *Campylobacter intestinalis* and indistinguishable from classical toxic-shock syndrome.— J. C. van der Zwan (letter), *Lancet*, 1984, *1*, 449.

SEXUALLY TRANSMITTED DISEASES. *Chancroid.* Erythromycin 500 mg four times daily by mouth for 7 days is one of the recommended agents for the treatment of chancroid (WHO Expert Committee on Venereal Diseases and Treponematoses, *Tech. Rep. Ser. Wld Hlth Org. No. 736*, 1986; *Med. Lett.*, 1986, *28*, 23). The most common alternative agents are co-trimoxazole and ceftriaxone.

Further references to the treatment of chancroid with erythromycin: G. P. Schmid, *J. Am. med. Ass.*, 1986, *255*, 1757.

Chlamydial infections. The WHO recommends the use of erythromycin for the treatment of uncomplicated urethral, endocervical, or rectal infections caused by *Chlamydia trachomatis* in patients who cannot tolerate tetracyclines or in whom they are contra-indicated (WHO Expert Committee on Venereal Diseases and Treponematoses, *Tech. Rep. Ser. Wld Hlth Org. No. 736*, 1986). It should be administered in a dose of 500 mg four times daily for 7 days. In men with nongonococcal urethritis this dose should reliably eradicate *C. trachomatis* and *Ureaplasma urealyticum*; it is not, however, reliable against *Neisseria gonorrhoeae* (W.R. Bowie, *Drugs*, 1984, *27*, 459).

The WHO recommends the use of erythromycin for the treatment of pregnant women who have *C. trachomatis* infections and of pregnant women whose sexual partners have nongonococcal urethritis. It should be given in the above dose, or, for women who cannot tolerate this, in a dose of 250 mg four times daily for 14 days. The optimal dose and duration of antibiotic therapy for pregnant women have not, however, been established. In women with proven treatment failure, a second course of erythromycin in either of the above dosage regimens should be administered. Concurrent treatment of the male partner with a tetracycline is an important part of therapy. A study involving 184 pregnant women concluded that erythromycin ethyl succinate 400 mg four times daily by mouth for 7 days during the 36th week of pregnancy was a reasonably effective, but not ideal, therapy for eradicating chlamydial infection in pregnant women and for preventing perinatal transmission to their infants (J. Schachter *et al.*, *New Engl. J. Med.*, 1986, *314*, 276).

The most common neonatal complications of perinatally acquired *C. trachomatis* infection are conjunctivitis and pneumonia. The WHO recommends that erythromycin syrup 50 mg per kg body-weight daily by mouth in 4 divided doses be given for 2 weeks for conjunctivitis and for 3 weeks for pneumonia, although they state that the optimal duration of treatment for pneumonia has not been established. If inclusion conjunctivitis recurs after therapy has been completed, erythromycin treatment should be repeated for a further 2 weeks. For further reference to the treatment and prevention of neonatal conjunctivitis, see Tetracycline Hydrochloride, p.320.

Erythromycin, 500 mg by mouth four times daily for 2 weeks, is also one of several alternatives to tetracycline recommended by the WHO for the treatment of chlamydial lymphogranuloma.

See also under Trachoma, below.

Gonorrhoea. For reference to the use of erythromycin in association with rifampicin for the treatment of gonorrhoea, see Rifampicin, p.575.

Syphilis. For WHO recommendations for the use of erythromycin in the treatment of syphilis in penicillin-allergic patients, see Tetracycline Hydrochloride, p.321.

SKIN DISORDERS. In a review of erythromycin, it was considered to be an effective alternative to benzylpenicillin for the treatment of streptococcal skin infections such as erysipelas, cellulitis, lymphangitis, and impetigo. Although it may also be useful for the treatment of minor cutaneous infections caused by penicillin-resistant *Staphylococcus aureus*, the emergence of an appreciable number of resistant strains restricts its use for the treatment of serious staphylococcal infections.— J. A. Washington and W. R. Wilson, *Mayo Clin. Proc.*, 1985, *60*, 271.

Further references to the use of erythromycin by mouth in the treatment of various skin disorders: B. L. Connor, *Br. J. Derm.*, 1972, *87*, *Suppl.* 8, 48 (impetigo); S. Bitnun (letter), *Lancet*, 1985, *1*, 345 (prophylactic use in a patient with erysipelas).

Abscess. Resolution of a cutaneous abscess caused by *Legionella micdadei* in an immunosuppressed patient after 6 weeks' therapy with erythromycin.— N. M. Ampel *et al.*, *Ann. intern. Med.*, 1985, *102*, 630.

Acne. For a review of the treatment of acne including the oral and topical use of erythromycin, see Tetracycline Hydrochloride, p.321.

References to the use of erythromycin in the treatment of acne vulgaris: Oral use.— R. Greenwood and W. J. Cunliffe, *Br. J. Derm.*, 1982, *107*, *Suppl.* 22, 24 (treatment of patients with a very greasy skin); J. Bleeker, *J. int. med. Res.*, 1983, *11*, 38 (comparison of erythromycin stearate tablets and capsules containing enteric-coated pellets of erythromycin base); R. Greenwood *et al.*, *Br. J. Derm.*, 1986, *114*, 353 (evaluation of optimum dosage regimen); B. R. Hughes and W. J. Cunliffe, *ibid.*, 1987, *117*, *Suppl.* 32, 27 (duration of treatment). Topical use:— R. A. Prince *et al.*, *Drug Intell. & clin. Pharm.*, 1981, *15*, 372 (use in inflammatory acne); M. A. Llorca *et al.*, *Curr. ther. Res.*, 1983, *33*, 14 (use of erythromycin lauryl sulphate); J. H. Exner *et al.*, *ibid.*, 1983, *34*, 762 (use of a preparation containing erythromycin and zinc acetate); B. Burke *et al.*, *Br. J. Derm.*, 1983, *108*, 199 (comparison of erythromycin and benzoyl peroxide).

BCG vaccination, local reactions. A 2- to 4-week course of erythromycin by mouth has been reported to accelerate the healing of abscesses or ulcers complicating BCG vaccination (J.T. Power *et al.*, *Br. J. Dis. Chest*, 1984, *78*, 192; G. Singh and M. Singh, *Lancet*, 1984, *2*, 979). Power *et al.*, however, found the *in-vitro* MIC of erythromycin for the BCG organism to be over 64 μg per mL. Hanley *et al.* (*Br. med. J.*, 1985, *290*, 970) found no difference in the response of children with post-BCG abscess or ulcers to a one-month course of isoniazid or erythromycin, and considered that possibly neither drug had any effect on the natural resolution of the lesions. Erythromycin may be of benefit if secondary bacterial infection of the injection site contributes to the adverse local reaction.

Pemphigoid. For mention of the use of erythromycin or tetracycline in association with nicotinamide for the treatment of bullous pemphigoid, see under Tetracycline Hydrochloride, p.321.

SURGICAL INFECTION PROPHYLAXIS. In the *USA*, the oral administration of 1 g each of neomycin and erythromycin base at 1, 2, and 11p.m. on the day before surgery is the treatment of choice for infection prophylaxis during colonic surgery, except for emergency surgery, or situations precluding oral prophylaxis (*Med. Lett.*, 1987, *29*, 91; A.B. Kaiser, *New Engl. J. Med.*, 1986, *315*, 1129). In the *UK*, however, oral, parenteral, or rectal administration of metronidazole, together with an antibiotic active against aerobic Gram-negative rods is more widely used. There has been controversy over the most effective regimen: the following studies have suggested that regimens containing metronidazole are more effective than those containing erythromycin (C. Brass *et al.*, *Am. J. Surg.*, 1978, *135*, 91; A.V. Pollock and M. Evans, *New Engl. J. Med.*, 1980, *303*, 1066).

TRACHOMA. Erythromycin and related macrolides administered by mouth or topically to the eye have been shown to have a beneficial effect on trachoma, but they have not been widely used. A few strains of *Chlamydia trachomatis* are resistant to erythromycin.— C. R. Dawson *et al.*, *Guide to Trachoma Control*, Wld Hlth Org., Geneva, 1981, p.40.

Further references to the use of erythromycin in the treatment of trachoma: C. R. Dawson *et al.*, *Bull. Wld Hlth Org.*, 1981, *59*, 91 (eye ointment); C. R. Dawson *et al.*, *ibid.*, 1982, *60*, 347 (oral).

See also Chlamydial Infections under Sexually Transmitted Diseases, above.

TYPHUS. A study concluding that although erythromycin appears to be less effective than tetracycline in the treatment of tick bite fever, it may be a useful alternative when tetracycline is contra-indicated.— G. B. Miller and J. H. S. Gear, *S. Afr. med. J.*, 1984, *66*, 694.

URINARY-TRACT INFECTIONS. Treatment with erythromycin estolate 500 mg or 1 g three times daily for 14 days in conjunction with sodium bicarbonate 18 g daily to render the urine alkaline eliminated the infecting Gram-negative bacteria from the urine of 27 of the 37 patients with chronic bacteriuria.— S. H. Zinner *et al.*, *Lancet*, 1971, *1*, 1267.

Reviews of chronic bacterial prostatitis with conflicting conclusions as to the usefulness of erythromycin in this condition: *Lancet*, 1983, *1*, 393; P. M. Hanus and L. H. Danziger, *Clin. Pharm.*, 1984, *3*, 49.

For reference to the use of erythromycin in the treatment of nongonococcal urethritis, see Chlamydial Infections under Sexually Transmitted Diseases, above.

Preparations

Erythromycin Tablets (*B.P.*). They are enteric-coated.

Erythromycin Tablets (*U.S.P.*)

Erythromycin Delayed-release Tablets (*U.S.P.*). They are enteric-coated.

Erythromycin Delayed-release Capsules (*U.S.P.*). Erythromycin Capsules

Erythromycin Ointment (*U.S.P.*)

Erythromycin Ophthalmic Ointment (*U.S.P.*)

Erythromycin Pledgets (*U.S.P.*). Absorbent pads impregnated with Erythromycin Topical Solution (*U.S.P.*).

Erythromycin Topical Solution (*U.S.P.*)

Erythromycin and Benzoyl Peroxide Topical Gel (*U.S.P.*)

Proprietary Preparations

Erycen (*Berk Pharmaceuticals, UK*). *Tablets*, enteric-coated, erythromycin 250 and 500 mg.

Erymax (*Parke, Davis, UK*). *Capsules*, containing enteric-coated pellets, erythromycin 250 mg. *Sprinkle capsules* (paediatric), containing enteric-coated pellets, erythromycin 125 mg. The pellets can be sprinkled on to food.

Erythromid (*Abbott, UK*). *Tablets*, enteric-coated, erythromycin 250 mg.
Tablets (Erythromid DS), enteric-coated, erythromycin 500 mg.

Retcin (*DDSA Pharmaceuticals, UK*). *Tablets*, enteric-coated, erythromycin 250 mg.

Stiemycin (*Stiefel, UK*). *Topical solution*, erythromycin 2% in an alcoholic basis.

Proprietary Names and Manufacturers

Abboticin (*Abbott, Denm.*; *Abbott, Swed.*); Abboticine (*Fr.*); Aknefug-EL (*Wolff, Ger.*); Akne-Mycin (*Hermal, Ger.*; *Hermal, Switz.*; *Hermal, USA*); Aknin (*Schwarzhaupt, Ger.*); Apo-Erythro Base (*Apotex, Canad.*); A/T/S (*Hoechst, USA*); Biorythrin (*S.Afr.*); Bram-mycin (*Austral.*); Cimetrin (*Cimex, Switz.*); Emu-V (*Upjohn, Austral.*; *Belg.*; *Upjohn, S.Afr.*); Emu-Ve (*Arg.*); E-Mycin (*Upjohn, Canad.*; *Upjohn, USA*); Endoeritrin (*Wasserman, Spain*); Eratrex (*Austral.*); Ermysin (*Britannia Health, UK*); ERYC (*Faulding, Austral.*; *Parke, Davis, Canad.*; *Parke, Davis, USA*); Erycen (*Berk Pharmaceuticals, UK*); Erycette (*Ortho Dermatological, USA*); Erycinum (*Schering, Ger.*); Eryderm (*Abbott, S.Afr.*; *Abbott, Switz.*; *Abbott, USA*); Eryfluid (*Pierre Fabre, Fr.*); Ery-Max (*Astra, Norw.*); Erymax (*Warner, S.Afr.*; *Parke, Davis, UK*; *Herbert, USA*); Ery-maxin (*Astra, Denm.*); Ery-Tab (*Abbott, USA*); Erythrogel (*Biorga, Fr.*); Erythromid (*Abbott, Canad.*; *Abbott, S.Afr.*; *Abbott, UK*); ETS (*Paddock, USA*); Ilocap (*Lilly, Austral.*); Iloticina (*Ital.*; *Derly, Spain*); Ilotycin (*Lilly, Canad.*; *Neth.*; *Switz.*; *Lilly, UK*; *Dista, USA*); Ilotycin TS (*Dista, S.Afr.*); Oftalmolets (*Arg.*); Orizina (*Perga, Spain*); Paediathrocin (*Abbott, Ger.*); Pantomicina (*Arg.*); PCE (*Abbott, USA*); Pharyngocin (*Upjohn, Ger.*); Polarmycina (*Medipolar, Swed.*); Proterytrin (*Proter, Ital.*); Retcin (*DDSA Pharmaceuticals, UK*); Robimycin Robitabs (*Robins, USA*); Staticin (*Westwood, Canad.*; *Westwood, USA*); Stiemycin (*Stiefel, Ger.*; *Stiefel, UK*); T-Stat (*Westwood, USA*).

The following names have been used for multi-ingredient preparations containing erythromycin— Benzamycin (*Dermik, USA*).

NOTE. Some of the above names have also been used to denote preparations of erythromycin esters.

78-y

Erythromycin Estolate *(BAN, USAN, rINNM).*

Erythromycin Propionate Lauryl Sulfate; Erythromycin Propionate Lauryl Sulphate; Erythromycini Estolas; Propionyl Erythromycin Lauryl Sulphate. Erythromycin 2′-propionate dodecyl sulphate.

$C_{40}H_{71}NO_{14},C_{12}H_{26}O_4S = 1056.4$.

CAS — 3521-62-8.

Pharmacopoeias. In *Br.*, *Chin.*, *Eur.*, *Ind.*, *It.*, *Jug.*, and *U.S.*

A white, odourless or almost odourless, crystalline powder. The *B.P.* specifies not less than 610 units per mg and the *U.S.P.* specifies a potency equivalent to not less than 600 μg of erythromycin per mg, both calculated on the anhydrous basis. 1.44 g of monograph substance is approximately equivalent to 1 g of erythromycin.

B.P. **solubilities** are: practically insoluble in water; soluble 1 in 2 of alcohol; freely soluble in chloroform; practically insoluble in 2M hydrochloric acid. *U.S.P.* solubilities are: practically insoluble in water; soluble 1 in 20 of alcohol, 1 in 10 of chloroform, and 1 in 15 of acetone. A saturated solution in water has a pH of 4.5 to 7.0. **Store** in airtight containers.

Adverse Effects

As for Erythromycin, p.222.

Signs of liver damage consisting of upper abdominal pain, fever, liver enlargement, eosinophilia, raised serum bilirubin, and changes in other liver-function tests indicative of cholestasis, and jaundice (reversible on discontinuing treatment) have been reported in patients receiving erythromycin estolate for more than 10 days or immediately on starting a second course. These hepatotoxic effects appear to be limited almost entirely to adult patients.

In one year there were 6 cases of infantile hypertrophic pyloric stenosis out of an infant population of 963; 5 of these cases were attributed to erythromycin estolate given in a daily dose of 40 mg per kg body-weight. Vomiting began within 48 hours of starting erythromycin estolate in all 5 children and their condition deteriorated despite subsequent withdrawal of the antibiotic. Surgical treatment was required and a pyloric mass was confirmed in each of the 5 infants.— J. A. Sanfilippo, *J. pediat. Surg.*, 1976, *11*, 177.

EFFECTS ON THE LIVER. A review of the hepatotoxic potential of macrolide antibiotics. Hepatitis has occurred most often with triacetyloleandomycin or erythromycin, but only rarely, if at all, with josamycin, midecamycin, or spiramycin. It was long considered that only the estolate ester of erythromycin was hepatotoxic. It is now recognised, however, that other erythromycin derivatives may also produce hepatitis, although their hepatotoxic potential is probably less than that of the estolate. It may be postulated that hepatotoxicity is associated with nitrosoalkanes formed by complexation of triacetyloleandomycin or erythromycin with cytochrome P-450 after induction of this enzyme by the macrolide. There is evidence that both allergic and toxic mechanisms may be involved in the hepatotoxicity of macrolides.— D. Pessayre *et al.*, *J. antimicrob. Chemother.*, 1985, *16*, *Suppl.* A, 181.

The Committee on Safety of Medicines reported in Adverse Reaction Leaflet No. 10 that it had received 41 reports of jaundice associated with erythromycin, 40 of which related to erythromycin estolate. The jaundice usually lasted for 1 or 2 weeks and was reversible after the antibiotic was withdrawn. There were no fatalities. The Committee was not able to advise whether the risk of jaundice with erythromycin estolate was offset by greater efficacy.— *Pharm. J.*, 1973, *2*, 59. Up to May 1973 the Australian Drug Evaluation Committee had received 113 reports of jaundice or cholestasis associated with erythromycin estolate; only 2 of these dealt with children under the age of 6 years. Since the Committee did not consider that the estolate was more effective than other forms of erythromycin, its use, apart from the low-dose paediatric formulations, should be restricted.— *Med. J. Aust.*, 1973, *2*, 192. Data obtained by prescription monitoring and follow-up questionnaire, on some 8600 patients who had received either erythromycin estolate, erythromycin stearate, or tetracycline, cast grave doubts on the previously reported high incidence of jaundice seen with the estolate. Of about 3000 patients who had received the estolate, none had developed drug-related jaundice; the 3 possible cases detected by the survey were all amongst patients who had received erythromycin stearate.— W. H. W. Inman and N. S. B. Rawson, *Br. med. J.*, 1983, *286*, 1954.

A report of hepatotoxicity in a 7-year-old boy given erythromycin estolate.— J. D. Lloyd-Still *et al.*, *Am. J. Dis. Child.*, 1978, *132*, 320. A report of complete biliary obstruction in a 6-week-old infant associated with the administration of erythromycin estolate.— D. Krowchuk and J. H. Seashore, *Pediatrics*, 1979, *64*, 956.

Precautions

As for Erythromycin, p.222.

Erythromycin estolate should not be given to patients with impaired liver function or to patients who have developed jaundice or other symptoms of liver toxicity during previous treatment with erythromycin estolate. A second course of treatment with this ester should be given with caution.

INTERFERENCE WITH DIAGNOSTIC TESTS. Seven young men without evidence of jaundice or oedema were each given 1 g of erythromycin estolate 8-hourly for 4 doses, in each of 2 cycles of treatment 6 days apart. During 1 cycle they also took either sodium bicarbonate 18 g or acetazolamide 500 mg daily. All subjects apparently showed transient and sometimes marked elevations of serum aspartate aminotransferase (SGOT) values. The results were found to be due to a false positive colorimetric reaction, attributed to an unidentified trypsin-stable substance in the blood, possibly a metabolite of the antibiotic. Despite this finding, the authors stressed, any apparent rise in SGOT should not be disregarded during erythromycin estolate therapy, where real elevations of SGOT values had been demonstrated.— L. D. Sabath *et al.*, *New Engl. J. Med.*, 1968, *279*, 1137.

PREGNANCY AND THE NEONATE. Of 298 pregnant women who took erythromycin estolate, clindamycin, or placebo for 3 weeks or longer, about 14, 4, and 3% respectively had abnormally high serum aspartate aminotransferase (SGOT) values. Erythromycin estolate should probably not be given to pregnant women.— W. M. McCormack *et al.*, *Antimicrob. Ag. Chemother.*, 1977, *12*, 630.

Absorption and Fate

As for Erythromycin, p.224.

Erythromycin estolate is more stable than the free base to the acid of gastric juice; following administration by mouth, it is rapidly absorbed, whether given in the fasting state or with food, and appears in the blood as erythromycin base or as erythromycin propionate which hydrolyses to erythromycin. It is not clear whether the circulating concentrations of active base produced by erythromycin estolate are higher than those from other preparations though it appears that this may be so.

A detailed study *in vitro* of the antibacterial activity of 2'-esters of erythromycin suggested that they were only active when hydrolysed to erythromycin.— P. L. Tardrew *et al.*, *Appl. Microbiol.*, 1969, *18*, 159.

In 28 children given single and multiple doses of erythromycin estolate or ethyl succinate, higher concentrations of erythromycin were achieved in both serum and tonsils after the estolate.— C. M. Ginsburg *et al.*, *J. Pediat.*, 1976, *89*, 1011. Further studies indicating higher serum-erythromycin concentrations after administration of the estolate than after the ethyl succinate: L. D. Bechtol *et al.*, *Curr. ther. Res.*, 1976, *20*, 610; *idem*, 1981, *29*, 52; P. Patamasucon *et al.*, *Antimicrob. Ag. Chemother.*, 1981, *19*, 736.

DRUG ABSORPTION. In 10 healthy subjects higher plasma concentrations of total antibiotic were achieved with erythromycin estolate than with equivalent doses of the stearate but concentrations of free base were lower although more consistent. Increased absorption occurred with the estolate in the presence of food whereas the absorption of stearate was reduced.— P. G. Welling *et al.*, *J. pharm. Sci.*, 1979, *68*, 150. Single-dose studies in healthy subjects indicated that absorption of erythromycin estolate (as capsules) was enhanced after food compared to that after a 12-hour fast. Food had little effect on the bioavailability of erythromycin ethyl succinate suspension or enteric-coated erythromycin tablets.— L. D. Bechtol *et al.*, *Curr. ther. Res.*, 1979, *25*, 618.

Further references to comparative bioavailability studies of erythromycin estolate and other erythromycin preparations: A. R. DiSanto *et al.*, *J. clin. Pharmac.*, 1980, *20*, 437 (estolate and erythromycin base); J. Henry *et al.*, *Postgrad. med. J.*, 1980, *55*, 707 (estolate, propionate, and stearate); G. J. Yakatan *et al.*, *J. clin. Pharmac.*, 1980, *20*, 625 (estolate, stearate, and erythromycin base).

For further reference to the comparative bioavailability of different erythromycin preparations, see Erythromycin, above.

Uses and Administration

Erythromycin estolate has the actions and uses of erythromycin (see p.222) and is administered by mouth in similar doses.

PREGNANCY AND THE NEONATE. See under Precautions, above.

Preparations

Erythromycin Estolate Capsules *(B.P.)*

Erythromycin Estolate Capsules *(U.S.P.)*

Erythromycin Estolate for Oral Suspension *(U.S.P.)*. Reconstituted suspension has a pH of 5 to 7 or (pediatric drops) 5.0 to 5.5.

Erythromycin Estolate Oral Suspension *(U.S.P.)*. Store at a temperature not exceeding 8°. pH 3.5 to 6.5.

Erythromycin Estolate Tablets *(U.S.P.)*. They may be chewable.

Proprietary Preparations

Ilosone *(Dista, UK)*. *Capsules*, erythromycin 250 mg (as estolate).

Tablets, erythromycin 500 mg (as estolate).

Suspension, erythromycin 125 mg (as estolate)/5 mL.

Suspension forte, erythromycin 250 mg (as estolate)/5 mL.

Proprietary Names and Manufacturers

Dreimicina *(Dreikehl, Spain)*; Erimec *(Isola-Ibi, Ital.)*; Eritrobios *(Nuovo, Ital.)*; Eritrobiotic *(Ital.)*; Eritrocin *(Maipe, Spain)*; Eritroveinte *(Madariaga, Spain)*; Eritro-Wolf *(Spain)*; Eromycin *(Austral.)*; Espimina *(Spyfarma, Spain)*; Estomicina *(Bergamon, Ital.)*; Estomycin *(Columbia, S.Afr.)*; Ilosone *(Lilly, Austral.; Belg.; Lilly, Canad.; Lilly, Ital.; Dista, S.Afr.; Dista, Switz.; Dista, UK; Dista, USA)*; Liferitrin *(IBYS, Spain)*; Loderm *(Vinas, Spain)*; Manilina *(Ital.)*; Marocid *(Lifepharma, Ital.)*; Mistral *(Ital.)*; Neo-Erycinum *(Ger.)*; Neo-Iloticina *(Dista, Spain)*; Novorythro *(Canad.)*; Propiocine Enfant *(Fr.)*; Proterytrin *(Proter, Ital.)*; Purmycin *(Lennon, S.Afr.)*; Roxochemil *(Chemil, Ital.)*; Spectrasone *(Schwulst, S.Afr.)*; Stellamicina *(Pierrel, Ital.)*; Taimoxin *(Jpn)*; Togiren *(Lilly, Ger.)*.

NOTE. Some of the above names have also been used to denote preparations of other erythromycin esters.

80-q

Erythromycin Ethyl Succinate *(BANM)*.

Erythromycin Ethylsuccinate *(USAN)*; Erythromycini Ethylsuccinas. Erythromycin 2'-(ethylsuccinate).

$C_{43}H_{75}NO_{16}$=862.1.

CAS — 1264-62-6; 41342-53-4.

Pharmacopoeias. In *Br., Cz., Eur., Fr., Ger., It., Jpn, Neth., Swiss,* and *U.S.*

A white or slightly yellow, odourless or almost odourless, hygroscopic crystalline powder. The *B.P.* specifies not less than 780 units per mg and the *U.S.P.* specifies a potency equivalent to not less than 765 μg of erythromycin per mg, both calculated on the anhydrous basis. 1.17 g of monograph substance is approximately equivalent to 1 g of erythromycin.

B.P. **solubilities** are: practically insoluble in water; freely soluble in dehydrated alcohol, acetone, chloroform, and methyl alcohol. *U.S.P.* solubilities are: very slightly **soluble** in water; freely soluble in alcohol, chloroform, and macrogol 400. A 1% suspension in water has a pH of 6.0 to 8.5. **Store** in airtight containers. The *B.P.* recommends storage at a temperature not exceeding 30°. Protect from light.

Adverse Effects and Precautions

As for Erythromycin, p.222.

Pain may occur on intramuscular injection of erythromycin ethyl succinate.

EFFECTS ON THE GASTRO-INTESTINAL TRACT. See Erythromycin, p.222.

EFFECTS ON THE LIVER. A 9-year-old boy developed nausea, abdominal pain, and raised liver enzymes on the seventh day of a course of erythromycin ethyl succinate; symptoms resolved after withdrawal of the drug.— K. G. Phillips (letter), *Can. med. Ass. J.*, 1983, *129*, 411. See also D. Sullivan *et al.*, *J. Am. med. Ass.*, 1980, *243*, 1074.

Absorption and Fate

As for Erythromycin, p.224.

Erythromycin ethyl succinate is more stable than the free base to the acid of gastric juice; following administration by mouth it is well absorbed, and appears in the blood as both ester and erythromycin base.

DIFFUSION INTO BODY TISSUES AND FLUIDS. Good penetration of erythromycin into tonsillar tissue after administration of the ethyl succinate by mouth to children undergoing tonsillectomy.— M. Falchi *et al.*, *Curr. med. Res. Opinion*, 1985, *9*, 611. See also under Erythromycin Estolate.

For reference to the penetration of erythromycin ethyl succinate into lung tissue, see Erythromycin Lactobionate.

DRUG ABSORPTION. In 18 children aged 6 to 23 months given erythromycin ethyl succinate 40 to 50 mg per kg body-weight daily the mean serum concentration of total erythromycin was about 3.05 μg per mL after 1½ hours when given with food and 1.51 μg per mL after 1 hour when fasting. Thus, serum concentrations were significantly higher in the nonfasting state. Fasting serum concentrations were comparable to those found in adults receiving therapeutic doses.— T. C. Coyne *et al.*, *J. clin. Pharmac.*, 1978, *18*, 194. In a study of the influence of food on absorption of erythromycin ethyl succinate from film-coated tablets in adults, absorption was delayed by food, but was considered adequate whether taken before or after food. There was considerable inter- and intra-individual variation. For rapid absorption and high peak plasma concentrations, administration immediately before food was considered preferable.— P. J. Thompson *et al.*, *Antimicrob. Ag. Chemother.*, 1980, *18*, 829.

A bioavailability study of erythromycin ethyl succinate from tablet and mixture forms and a comparison with equivalent doses of erythromycin stearate.— A. -S. Malmborg, *Curr. ther. Res.*, 1980, *27*, 733.

For reference to the comparative bioavailability of different erythromycin preparations, including erythromycin ethyl succinate, see under Erythromycin and Erythromycin Estolate.

Uses and Administration

Erythromycin ethyl succinate has the actions and uses of erythromycin (see p.222) and is administered by mouth in similar doses. In the *USA* it is often administered in a dose equivalent to erythromycin 400 mg every 6 hours.

Erythromycin ethyl succinate may be given by intramuscular injection, but because of pain on injection this route is seldom used.

Preparations

Erythromycin Ethylsuccinate Tablets *(U.S.P.)*. May be chewable.

Erythromycin Ethylsuccinate for Oral Suspension *(U.S.P.)*. Reconstituted suspension has a pH of 7 to 9.

Erythromycin Ethylsuccinate Oral Suspension *(U.S.P.)*

Erythromycin Ethylsuccinate and Sulfisoxazole Acetyl for Oral Suspension *(U.S.P.)*. A dry mixture of erythromycin ethyl succinate and acetyl sulphafurazole. pH of the reconstituted suspension 5 to 7.

Erythromycin Ethylsuccinate Injection *(U.S.P.)*. A sterile solution of erythromycin ethyl succinate in macrogol 400 with butyl aminobenzoate 2% and a suitable preservative.

Sterile Erythromycin Ethylsuccinate *(U.S.P.)*

Proprietary Preparations

Arpimycin *(R.P. Drugs, UK)*. *Suspension*, granules for reconstitution, erythromycin 125, 250, and 500 mg (as ethyl succinate)/5 mL when reconstituted with water.

Erythrolar *(Lagap, UK)*. *Suspension*, erythromycin 250 mg (as ethyl succinate)/5 mL when reconstituted with water.

Erythroped *(Abbott, UK)*. *Oral granules* (Erythroped Sugar Free), erythromycin 250 mg (as ethyl succinate)/sachet. To be dispersed in water before administration.

Suspension (Erythroped PI), granules for reconstitution, erythromycin 125 mg (as ethyl succinate)/5 mL when reconstituted with water. Also available as single-dose sachets.

Suspension, granules for reconstitution, erythromycin 250 mg (as ethyl succinate)/5 mL when reconstituted with water. Also available as single-dose sachets.

Suspension (Erythroped Forte), granules for reconstitution, erythromycin 500 mg (as ethyl succinate)/5 mL when reconstituted with water. Also available as single-dose sachets.

Erythroped A *(Abbott, UK)*. *Tablets*, erythromycin 500 mg (as ethyl succinate).

Oral granules, erythromycin 1 g (as ethyl succinate)/sachet. To be dispersed in water before administration.

Proprietary Names and Manufacturers

Abboticin *(Denm.; Abbott, Norw.; Abbott, Swed.)*; Abboticine *(Belg.; Abbott, Fr.; Neth.)*; Ambamida *(Arg.)*; Anamycin *(Ger.)*; Apo-Erythro-ES *(Apotex, Canad.)*; Arpimycin *(R.P. Drugs, UK)*; Durapaediat *(Durachemie, Ger.)*; EES *(Abbott, Austral.; Abbott, Canad.; Abbott, USA)*; E-Mycin E *(Upjohn, USA)*; Eritrocina *(Abbott, Ital.)*; Eritroger *(Isnardi, Ital.)*; Eritrogobens *(Normon, Spain)*; Eromerzin *(Ger.)*; Ery *(Bouchara, Fr.; Distripharm, Switz.)*; Erycocci *(Leurquin, Fr.)*; Ery-Diolan *(Engelhard, Ger.)*; Eryliquid *(Karlspharma, Ger.)*; Ery-Max *(Astra, Swed.)*; Eryped *(Abbott, USA)*; Eryromycen *(Jpn)*; Erythrocin *(Abbott, Austral.; Abbott, Ger.; Abbott, UK)*; Erythrocine *(Belg.; Abbott, Fr.; Neth.; Abbott, Switz.)*; Erythro-ES *(Jpn)*; Erythroforte 500 *(Belg.)*; Erythrogram *(Negma, Fr.)*; Erythrolar *(Lagap, UK)*; Erythromycin-ES *(Jpn)*; Erythroped *(Abbott, S.Afr.; Abbott, UK)*; Erythroped A *(Abbott, UK)*; Esinol *(Jpn)*; Esmycin *(Jpn)*; Minotin *(Jpn)*; Monomycin *(Grünenthal, Ger.)*; Paediathrocin *(Abbott, Ger.)*; Pantomicina *(Arg.; Abbott, Spain)*; Pediamycin *(Ross, USA)*; Proterytrin *(Proter, Ital.)*; Refkas *(Jpn)*; Rossomicina *(Pierrel, Ital.)*; Servitrocine *(Servipharm, Switz.)*; Takasunon *(Jpn)*; Wyamycin E *(Wyeth, USA)*.

The following names have been used for multi-ingredient preparations containing erythromycin ethyl succinate— Pediazole *(Abbott, Canad.; Ross, USA)*.

NOTE. Some of the above names have also been used to denote preparations of erythromycin or other erythromycin esters.

81-p

Erythromycin Gluceptate *(BANM, USAN, rINNM)*.

Erythromycin glucoheptonate.

$C_{37}H_{67}NO_{13},C_7H_{14}O_8$=960.1.

CAS — 304-63-2; 23067-13-2.

Pharmacopoeias. U.S. includes Sterile Erythromycin Gluceptate.

A white, odourless or almost odourless, slightly hygroscopic powder. It has a potency equivalent to not less than 600 μg of erythromycin per mg calculated on the anhydrous basis. 1.3 g of monograph substance is approximately equivalent to 1 g of erythromycin.

Freely **soluble** in water, alcohol, and methyl alcohol; slightly soluble in acetone and chloroform; practically insoluble in ether. A 2.5% solution in water has a pH of 6 to 8.

Loss of activity or **incompatibility** may occur in solutions for intravenous infusion if erythromycin gluceptate is mixed with additives which result in a final pH of less than 5.5. Drugs which have been reported to be incompatible with erythromycin gluceptate include: amikacin sulphate, aminophylline, barbiturates, cephalothin sodium, cephazolin sodium, heparin sodium, phenytoin sodium, streptomycin sulphate, and tetracyclines.

Erythromycin gluceptate has the actions and uses of erythromycin (see p.222).

It is administered intravenously in similar doses to erythromycin lactobionate, below. To minimise venous irritation it is given by continous infusion or by intermittent infusion over 20 to 60 minutes.

For the preparation of solutions of erythromycin gluceptate for infusion, a primary solution containing not more than 5% of erythromycin should be prepared with Water for Injections. To avoid gel formation or slow and incomplete solution of the drug, sodium chloride injection should not be used in preparing the primary solution. It should be further diluted before intravenous administration with 0.9% sodium chloride or 5% glucose injection. If it is to be administered in glucose injection over a period of more than 4 hours, it should be buffered with sodium bicarbonate.

For reference to gastro-intestinal disturbances after intravenous administration of erythromycin, see Erythromycin Lactobionate, below.

Preparations

Sterile Erythromycin Gluceptate *(U.S.P.)*

Proprietary Names and Manufacturers

Erycinum *(Schering, Ger.)*; Ilotycin Gluceptate *(Lilly, Austral.; Dista, Switz.; Dista, USA).*

82-s

Erythromycin Lactobionate *(USAN).*

Erythromycin mono(4-*O*-*β*-D-galactopyranosyl-D-gluconate).

$C_{37}H_{67}NO_{13},C_{12}H_{22}O_{12}$=1092.2.

CAS — 3847-29-8.

Pharmacopoeias. In *Chin.* and *Roum. U.S.* includes Sterile Erythromycin Lactobionate.

White or slightly yellow crystals or powder with a faint odour. 1.5 g of monograph substance is approximately equivalent to 1 g of erythromycin.

Freely **soluble** in water, alcohol, and methyl alcohol; slightly soluble in acetone and chloroform; practically insoluble in ether. A 5% solution in water has a pH of 6.5 to 7.5. In acidic solutions, erythromycin lactobionate is unstable and rapidly loses potency below pH 5.5.

Loss of activity or *incompatibility* may occur in solutions for intravenous infusion if erythromycin lactobionate is mixed with sodium salts of biologically derived macromolecules such as antibiotics, or with additives which result in a final pH of less than 5.5. It should not be diluted in glucose injection unless buffered with sodium bicarbonate. Drugs which have been reported to be incompatible with erythromycin lactobionate include: ampicillin sodium, cephalothin sodium, colistin sulphomethate sodium, gentamicin sulphate, heparin sodium, metaraminol tartrate, and tetracyclines.

Adverse Effects and Precautions

As for Erythromycin, p.222.

Because of the risk of venous irritation associated with the intravenous administration of erythromycin lactobionate, bolus injection is not recommended.

EFFECTS ON THE EAR. For reports on the use of erythromycin lactobionate being associated with reversible loss of hearing, see Erythromycin, p.222.

EFFECTS ON THE GASTRO-INTESTINAL TRACT. In a study in 10 healthy subjects, the severity of gastro-intestinal disturbances after intravenous infusion of erythromycin lactobionate was correlated with the rate of infusion and with plasma-erythromycin concentrations.— K. M. Downey and D. M. Chaput de Saintonge, *Br. J. clin. Pharmac.*, 1986, *21*, 295.

A study in *dogs* suggesting that the gastro-intestinal disturbances observed after intravenous administration of erythromycin may be due to an effect on motility of the gastro-intestinal tract.— G. P. Zara *et al., J. antimicrob. Chemother.*, 1985, *16, Suppl.* A, 175. Studies in human subjects had shown that intravenous and oral erythromycin caused massive contractions in the stomach, but an inhibition of motility in the duodenum and jejunum.— G. P. Zara *et al.* (letter), *Lancet*, 1987, *2*, 1036.

See also under Local Irritant Effects, below.

EFFECTS ON THE HEART. Ventricular arrhythmias occurred in a 65-year-old woman on several occasions after intravenous administration of erythromycin lactobionate is association with cloxacillin sodium; erythromycin lactobionate was implicated.— J. M. McComb *et al., Am. J. Cardiol.*, 1984, *54*, 922.

LOCAL IRRITANT EFFECTS. Venous irritation occurred in 12 of 16 patients given intravenous infusions of erythromycin lactobionate over 30 or 60 minutes. The use of an inline filter set reduced the severity but not the incidence of the effect. Gastro-intestinal disturbances, including severe abdominal pain and nausea occurred in 8 patients.— G. E. Marlin *et al., Hum. Toxicol.*, 1983, *2*, 593.

Absorption and Fate

As for Erythromycin, p.224.

In 6 healthy subjects given erythromycin 2 g by infusion of the lactobionate over 12 hours, the mean peak plasma concentration of erythromycin at about 1 hour was 6.1 μg per mL with a second peak of 7.2 μg per mL at 4 hours. Effective concentrations were maintained at least 8 hours after the end of infusion.— R. L. Parsons *et al., Postgrad. med. J.*, 1978, *54*, 68. See also M. A. Neaverson, *Curr. med. Res. Opinion*, 1976, *4*, 359; G. E. Marlin *et al., Hum. Toxicol.*, 1983, *2*, 593.

DIFFUSION INTO BODY TISSUES AND FLUIDS. Between 0.5 and 1 g of erythromycin lactobionate was administered by continuous infusion to 8 patients before undergoing hip surgery. Concentrations in cancellous bone ranged from 0.6 to 11.5 μg per g with a mean value about 30% of the corresponding serum concentrations.— V. T. Rosdahl *et al., J. antimicrob. Chemother.*, 1979, *5*, 275.

Erythromycin, administered as the ethyl succinate or lactobionate, showed good penetration of both healthy and tumorous lung tissue, and compared favourably with amoxycillin.— Y. Brun *et al., J. antimicrob. Chemother.*, 1981, *8*, 459. A study, using positron tomography of pulmonary-erythromycin concentrations after the intravenous administration of erythromycin lactobionate to patients with lobar pneumonia. Concentrations considered to be effective for most sensitive organisms were reached in both the pneumonic and unaffected lung within 10 minutes of administration. Blood and lung concentrations reached equilibrium after approximately 45 minutes, and thereafter the concentrations in the extravascular compartment of the lung began to fall. Concentrations of erythromycin in the extravascular compartment of the pneumonic and unaffected lung were not significantly different.— P. Wollmer *et al., Lancet*, 1982, *2*, 1361.

DRUG EXCRETION. Biliary excretion of erythromycin after parenteral administration of the lactobionate.— P. Chelvan *et al., Br. J. clin. Pharmac.*, 1979, *8*, 233.

Uses and Administration

Erythromycin lactobionate has the actions and uses of erythromycin (see p.222). It is suitable for the preparation of solutions for intravenous administration to patients who are unable to tolerate oral medication or when it is necessary to produce a high blood concentration of erythromycin to control severe infections. Oral administration of erythromycin should replace parenteral administration as soon as practicable.

Doses are expressed in terms of the equivalent amount of erythromycin. The usual dose for adults is erythromycin 1 to 2 g daily increased to 4 g daily for severe infections. Children may be given 15 to 50 mg per kg body-weight daily. To reduce the risk of venous irritation it should be administered only by continuous or intermittent intravenous infusion of a solution containing not more than 0.5% of erythromycin. Intermittent infusions should be given every 6 hours over 20 to 60 minutes.

For the preparation of solutions of erythromycin lactobionate for infusion, a primary solution containing not more than 5% of erythromycin should be prepared with Water for Injections. To avoid precipitation of the drug, sodium chloride injection or other inorganic salt solution should not be used in preparing the primary solution. It should be further diluted before intravenous administration with 0.9% sodium chloride injection or other suitable intravenous fluid. Acidic solutions, such as glucose injection, should only be used if buffered with sodium bicarbonate.

Preparations

Erythromycin Lactobionate for Injection *(U.S.P.)*

Sterile Erythromycin Lactobionate *(U.S.P.)*

Proprietary Preparations

Erythrocin I.V. Lactobionate *(Abbott, UK). Intravenous infusion,* powder for reconstitution, erythromycin 1 g (as lactobionate). May be supplied with diluent.

Proprietary Names and Manufacturers

Abboticin *(Denm.; Abbott, Norw.; Abbott, Swed.)*; Erythrocin *(Abbott, Austral.; Abbott, Canad.; Abbott, Ger.; Abbott, S.Afr.; Abbott, UK; Abbott, USA)*; Erythrocine *(Neth.; Abbott, Switz.)*; Pantomicina *(Abbott, Spain)*; Stellamicina *(Pierrel, Ital.).*

NOTE. Some of the above names have also been used to denote preparations of erythromycin or other erythromycin esters.

83-w

Erythromycin Propionate *(USAN).*

Erythromycin 2′-propionate.

$C_{40}H_{71}NO_{14}$=790.0.

CAS — 134-36-1.

Pharmacopoeias. In *Fr.* and *Roum.*

1.08 g of monograph substance is approximately equivalent to 1 g of erythromycin.

Erythromycin propionate has the actions of erythromycin (see p.222) and is used similarly to the estolate, the lauryl sulphate salt of erythromycin propionate, in a dose equivalent to 1 to 2 g of erythromycin daily by mouth.

ABSORPTION AND FATE. A study comparing concentrations of erythromycin in plasma and saliva after administration of the propionate, estolate, and stearate esters.— J. Henry *et al., Postgrad. med. J.*, 1980, *56*, 707.

EFFECTS ON THE LIVER. Severe abdominal pains, cholestatic jaundice, and eosinophilia occurred in a patient after erythromycin propionate was given.— D. Pessayre and J. P. Benhamou (letter), *Br. med. J.*, 1979, *1*, 1357.

Proprietary Names and Manufacturers

Bio Exazol *(Andreu, Spain)*; Éry *(Bouchara, Fr.)*; Propiocine *(Roussel, Fr.; Roussel, Spain; Roussel, Switz.).*

84-e

Erythromycin Stearate *(BANM, USAN, rINNM)*.

Erythromycini Stearas.

$C_{37}H_{67}NO_{13}, C_{18}H_{36}O_2$=1018.4.

CAS — 643-22-1.

Pharmacopoeias. In *Br., Cz., Egypt., Eur., Fr., Ger., Ind., It., Jpn, Swiss,* and *U.S.*

The stearate of erythromycin with some uncombined stearic acid and sodium stearate.

Colourless or slightly yellow crystals or a white or slightly yellow powder, odourless or with a slight earthy odour. The *B.P.* specifies not less than 600 units per mg, and the *U.S.P.* specifies a potency equivalent to not less than 550 μg of erythromycin per mg calculated on the anhydrous basis. 1.39 g of monograph substance is approximately equivalent to 1 g of erythromycin.

B. P. **solubilities** are: practically insoluble in water; soluble in acetone, dehydrated alcohol, chloroform, and methyl alcohol. Solutions in acetone, dehydrated alcohol, chloroform, and methyl alcohol may be opalescent. *U.S.P.* solubilities are: practically insoluble in water; soluble in alcohol, chloroform, ether, and methyl alcohol. The *B.P.* states that a 1% aqueous suspension has a pH of 7.0 to 10.5 and *U.S.P.* that it has a pH of 6 to 11. **Store** in airtight containers. Protect from light. The *B.P.* recommends storage at a temperature below 30°.

Adverse Effects and Precautions

As for Erythromycin, p.222.

EFFECTS ON THE LIVER. Asymptomatic increase in liver enzyme values associated with administration of erythromycin stearate in a 73-year-old woman.— J. Alcalay *et al., Drug Intell. & clin. Pharm.*, 1986, *20*, 601.

See also under Erythromycin Estolate.

Absorption and Fate

As for Erythromycin, p.224.

Erythromycin stearate is relatively stable in gastric acid and when given by mouth it releases active erythromycin in the duodenum.

DRUG ABSORPTION. A mean peak serum-erythromycin concentration of 2.65 μg per mL occurred 2 hours after administration of erythromycin stearate equivalent to erythromycin 500 mg by mouth, with 250 mL of water, to 6 healthy subjects in the fasting state. In the same subjects following a standard meal high in carbohydrate, fat, or protein, or in a fasting state with only 20 mL of water, peak serum concentrations were reduced by about 50%. It was suggested that erythromycin stearate should be administered on an empty stomach with an adequate amount of water.— P. G. Welling *et al., J. pharm. Sci.*, 1978, *67*, 764.

Erythromycin was better absorbed when 15 healthy subjects took erythromycin stearate immediately before food rather than on an empty stomach. A mean peak plasma concentration of 2.8 μg per mL occurred one hour after a 500-mg dose was taken just before a standardised breakfast compared with only 1.3 μg per mL two hours after a similar dose was taken in the fasting state. Tablets of erythromycin stearate should be taken just before a meal and not as previously recommended.— A.-S. Malmborg, *Curr. med. Res. Opinion*, 1978, *5, Suppl.* 2, 15. See also *idem, J. antimicrob. Chemother.*, 1979, *5*, 591. Confirmation that preparations of erythromycin stearate should be given immediately before food for consistent and rapid absorption. In this study food did not affect the bioavailability of a preparation of erythromycin base.— J. Rutland *et al., Br. J. clin. Pharmac.*, 1979, *8*, 343.

In single-dose studies in healthy subjects, the bioavailability of a film-coated tablet of erythromycin stearate was enhanced when taken just before food, whereas that of an enteric-coated formulation was impaired.— J. Posti and M. Salonen, *Int. J. Pharmaceut.*, 1983, *17*, 225.

For reference to the comparative bioavailability of different erythromycin preparations, including erythromycin stearate, see under Erythromycin and Erythromycin Estolate.

Uses and Administration

Erythromycin stearate has the actions and uses of erythromycin (see p.222) and is administered by mouth in similar doses.

Preparations

Erythromycin Mixture *(B.P.C. 1973)*. Erythromycin Suspension. A suspension of erythromycin stearate containing the equivalent of 2% of erythromycin in a suitable coloured flavoured vehicle.

Erythromycin Stearate for Oral Suspension *(U.S.P.)*. Reconstituted suspension has a pH of 6 to 9.

Erythromycin Stearate Tablets *(B.P.)*

Erythromycin Stearate Tablets *(U.S.P.)*

Proprietary Preparations

Erythrocin *(Abbott, UK). Tablets*, erythromycin 250 and 500 mg (as stearate).

Erythrolar *(Lagap, UK). Tablets*, erythromycin 250 and 500 mg (as stearate).

Proprietary Names and Manufacturers

Abboticin *(Denm.; Abbott, Norw.; Abbott, Swed.)*; Abboticine *(Fr.)*; Apo-Erythro-S *(Apotex, Canad.)*; Bristamycin *(Swed.; Bristol, USA)*; Celtiacina *(Arg.)*; Cimetrin 500 Stearate *(Cimex, Switz.)*; Doranol *(Antibioticos, Spain)*; Dowmycin-E *(USA)*; DuraErythromycin *(Ger.)*; Emestid *(Abbott, Fr.)*; E-Mycin *(Protea, Austral.)*; Erios *(Mepha, Switz.)*; Eritrocina *(Abbott, Ital.)*; Eritroger *(Isnardi, Ital.)*; Eritrogobens *(Normon, Spain)*; Eritrolag *(Lagap, Switz.)*; Eromel *(Lagamed, S.Afr.)*; Erostin *(Medex, Austral.)*; Ery-Diolan *(Engelhard, Ger.)*; Erymycin *(Triomed, S.Afr.)*; Erypar *(Parke, Davis, USA)*; Erythrocin *(Abbott, Austral.; Abbott, Canad.; Abbott, Ger.; Abbott, S.Afr.; Abbott, UK; Abbott, USA)*; Erythrocine *(Belg.; Neth.; Abbott, Switz.)*; Erythrolar *(Lagap, UK)*; Erythro-S *(Jpn)*; Erytran *(Spirig, Switz.)*; Erytrocilin *(Lisapharma, Ital.)*; Ethimycin *(SCS, S.Afr.)*; Ethril *(Squibb, USA)*; Ethryn *(Faulding, Austral.)*; Infectocin *(Pharmador, S.Afr.)*; Lauromicina *(Dukron, Ital.)*; Novorythro *(Novopharm, Canad.)*; Pantomicina *(Abbott, Spain)*; Pfizer-E *(Pfipharmecs, USA)*; Rubimycin *(Lennon, S.Afr.)*; Rythrocaps *(S.Afr.)*; Servitrocine *(Servipharm, Switz.)*; SK-Erythromycin *(Smith Kline & French, USA)*; Takasunon *(Jpn)*; Tolerabiotico *(Iquinosa, Spain)*; Torlamicina *(Spain)*.

NOTE. Some of the above names have also been used to denote preparations of erythromycin or other erythromycin esters.

12750-z

Fibracillin *(rINN)*.

AL-70-35; Amidacilina. (6*R*)-6-{D-2-[2-(4-Chlorophenoxy)-2-methylpropionamido]-2-phenylacetamido}penicillanic acid.

$C_{26}H_{28}ClN_3O_6S$=546.0.

CAS — 51154-48-4.

Fibracillin is a penicillin given by mouth or by intramuscular injection in the treatment of susceptible bacterial infections. The sodium salt has also been used.

Proprietary Names and Manufacturers

Alongapen *(Lafarquim, Spain)*.

1792-n

Flomoxef *(rINN)*.

6315-S. 7*R*-7-[2-(difluoromethylthio)acetamido]-3-[1-(2-hydroxyethyl)-1*H*-tetrazol-5-ylthiomethyl]-7-methoxy-1-oxa-3-cephem-4-carboxylic acid.

$C_{15}H_{18}F_2N_6O_7S_2$=496.5.

CAS — 99665-00-6.

Flomoxef is an oxacephalosporin antibiotic.

References to the antibacterial activity of flomoxef *in vitro*: H. C. Neu and N. -X. Chin, *Antimicrob. Ag. Chemother.*, 1986, *30*, 638.

Proprietary Names and Manufacturers

Shionogi, Jpn.

3868-r

Flucloxacillin Magnesium *(BANM, rINNM)*.

Floxacillin Magnesium *(USAN)*. Magnesium (6*R*)-6-[3-(2-chloro-6-fluorophenyl)-5-methylisoxazole-4-carboxamido]penicillanate octahydrate.

$(C_{19}H_{16}ClFN_3O_5S)_2Mg,8H_2O$=1074.2.

CAS — 5250-39-5 (flucloxacillin); 58486-36-5 (magnesium salt).

Pharmacopoeias. In *Br.*

A white or almost white powder. 2.4 g of monograph substance is approximately equivalent to 1 g of anhydrous flucloxacillin. Each g of monograph substance represents about 0.9 mmol of magnesium.

Slightly **soluble** in water and in chloroform; soluble 1 in 1 of methyl alcohol. A 0.5% solution in water has a pH of 4.5 to 6.5. **Store** at a temperature not exceeding 25° in well-closed containers. Protect from moisture.

85-l

Flucloxacillin Sodium *(BANM, rINNM)*.

Floxacillin Sodium.

$C_{19}H_{16}ClFN_3NaO_5S,H_2O$=493.9.

CAS — 1847-24-1 (sodium salt, anhydrous); 34214-51-2 (sodium salt, monohydrate).

Pharmacopoeias. In *Br.*

A white or almost white hygroscopic powder. 1.09 g of monograph substance is approximately equivalent to 1 g of anhydrous flucloxacillin. Each g of monograph substance represents about 2 mmol of sodium.

Soluble 1 in 1 of water, 1 in 8 of alcohol, 1 in 8 of acetone, and 1 in 2 of methyl alcohol. A 10% solution in water has a pH of 5 to 7. **Store** at a temperature not exceeding 25° in well-closed containers. Protect from moisture.

Aqueous solutions of flucloxacillin sodium are reported to be **stable** for up to 24 hours at 25° and for up to 72 hours at 5°. However, it is recommended that reconstituted solutions of flucloxacillin sodium for injection should be administered immediately after preparation. Flucloxacillin sodium should not be mixed with blood products or other proteinaceous fluids such as protein hydrolysates.

Flucloxacillin sodium has been reported to be **incompatible** with aminoglycosides.

For reference to the degradation of flucloxacillin sodium in solution, see under Benzylpenicillin Sodium, p.132.

Adverse Effects

As for Benzylpenicillin Sodium, p.132.

Gangrene, requiring amputation of thumb and fingers occurred in a woman after inadvertent intra-arterial injection of flucloxacillin.— D. A. Zideman and M. Morgan, *Anaesthesia*, 1981, *36*, 296.

EFFECTS ON THE LIVER. Intrahepatic cholestasis developed in 2 women after administration of flucloxacillin by mouth for 4 and 7 weeks respectively. Raised bilirubin concentrations and jaundice resolved slowly after cessation of therapy.— F. Bengtsson *et al., Scand. J. infect. Dis.*, 1985, *17*, 125.

LOCAL IRRITANT EFFECTS. In a study involving 22 patients, the incidence of phlebitis on administration of an intravenous infusion of flucloxacillin was independent of the solvent, water or sodium chloride, used. In a further double-blind study involving 32 patients, the incidence of phlebitis after administration of an infusion of flucloxacillin for 2, 3, and 4 days was 18, 47, and 79% respectively. The equivalent figures for an infusion of cloxacillin were 13, 21, and 50%.— Å. Svedhem *et al., Antimicrob. Ag. Chemother.*, 1980, *18*, 349. Correction.— *ibid.*, 1981, *19*, 940.

Precautions

As for Benzylpenicillin Sodium, p.133. Lens opacities have occurred after ocular use of flucloxacillin in *animals*.

ADMINISTRATION IN RENAL FAILURE. For reference to the precautions to be observed in renal failure, see below under Uses, Administration in Renal Failure.

PORPHYRIAS. Flucloxacillin was considered to be unsafe in patients with acute porphyria because it has been shown to be porphyrinogenic in *animals* or *in vitro* systems.— M.R. Moore and K.E.L. McColl, *Porphyrias, Drug Lists*, Glasgow, Porphyria Research Unit, University of Glasgow, 1987.

PREGNANCY AND THE NEONATE. For precautions to be observed on administration of flucloxacillin to jaundiced neonates, see Cloxacillin Sodium, p.203.

Antimicrobial Action

Flucloxacillin sodium is bactericidal with a mode of action similar to that of benzylpenicillin, but is resistant to staphylococcal penicillinase. It has an antibacterial spectrum similar to that of methicillin (see p.259). It is generally more active than methicillin sodium. Minimum inhibitory concentrations against most strains of staphylococci are in the range of 0.25 to 0.5 µg per mL. Its activity against streptococci is less than that of benzylpenicillin but sufficient to be useful when these organisms are present with penicillin-resistant staphylococci.

ACTIVITY WITH OTHER ANTIMICROBIAL AGENTS. A combination of flucloxacillin and temocillin *in vitro* was partially synergistic against the majority of methicillin-susceptible strains of *Staphylococcus aureus* tested. In a few cases synergism or indifference were demonstrated.— L. Verbist and J. Verhaegen, *Antimicrob. Ag. Chemother.*, 1984, *25*, 142.

For a report of antagonism *in vitro* between flucloxacillin and fusidic acid, see under Uses, Osteomyelitis.

Resistance

As for Methicillin Sodium, p.259.

Absorption and Fate

Flucloxacillin sodium, like dicloxacillin sodium, is about twice as well absorbed from the gastro-intestinal tract as cloxacillin sodium, but absorption is also reduced by the presence of food in the stomach. After an oral dose of 250 mg to 1 g, in fasting subjects, peak plasma concentrations in about 1 hour are usually in the range of 5 to 15 µg per mL. Serum concentrations following the intramuscular injection of flucloxacillin sodium are similar, but peak concentrations are achieved in about 30 minutes. Doubling the dose can double the plasma concentration. About 95% of flucloxacillin in the circulation is bound to plasma proteins. Flucloxacillin has been reported to have a plasma half-life of approximately 1 hour in healthy subjects. The half-life is prolonged in neonates.

The distribution of flucloxacillin into body tissues and fluids is similar to that of cloxacillin (p.203).

Flucloxacillin is metabolised to a limited extent, and the unchanged drug and metabolites are excreted in the urine by glomerular filtration and renal tubular secretion. About 50% of a dose by mouth and up to 90% of an intramuscular dose is excreted in the urine within 6 hours. Only small amounts are excreted in the bile.

Serum concentrations are enhanced if probenecid is given concomitantly.

DIFFUSION INTO BODY TISSUES AND FLUIDS. A study of the pharmacokinetics of flucloxacillin in 19 patients, aged between 40 and 88 years, undergoing pacemaker surgery. The mean half-life of flucloxacillin calculated after a single intravenous infusion of 1 g was 1.5 hours, which is longer than that reported in healthy subjects. From *in vitro* studies, 91% flucloxacillin was bound to plasma proteins, and 14% distributed to blood cells. The volume of distribution suggested possible intracellular distribution and substantial tissue binding. After a further 3 intravenous doses of flucloxacillin 1 g every 8 hours, the average ratio of flucloxacillin concentrations in pacemaker pocket fluid to plasma was 0.57. Thus, despite the high degree of plasma protein binding of flucloxacillin, these results suggest that it is rapidly distributed to extravascular compartments such as a pacemaker pocket.— P. Anderson *et al.*, *Eur. J. clin. Pharmac.*, 1985, *27*, 713.

In a study of 12 patients undergoing open-heart surgery, all received flucloxacillin 500 mg by intravenous injection after induction of anaesthesia and 6 received a further 500 mg at the end of the procedure. Post-operatively, all patients were given 500 mg intravenously every 6 hours for 2 days. In those receiving one dose initially the mean serum concentration fell from 69 to 9 µg per mL during surgery and was considered adequate. However, the concentration of flucloxacillin in wound fluid at the time of closure ranged from less than 2 to 7.8 µg per mL and was considered to be too low for adequate prophylaxis. In those receiving the 2 doses of flucloxacillin, mean serum concentrations were 16.9 µg per mL at the end of surgery, and wound fluid concentrations ranged from 8.6 to 23 µg per mL. This was considered more satisfactory, and thus the 2-dose regimen was recommended.— M. Farrington *et al.*, *J. antimicrob. Chemother.*, 1985, *16*, 253.

Studies of the penetration of flucloxacillin into the bone and joint capsule in patients receiving flucloxacillin alone or in combination with ampicillin for the prophylaxis of infection during hip replacement surgery: P. F. Unsworth *et al.*, *J. clin. Path.*, 1978, *31*, 705; R. L. Parsons *et al.*, *Br. J. clin. Pharmac.*, 1978, *6*, 135; J. P. Pollard *et al.*, *J. antimicrob. Chemother.*, 1979, *5*, 721; S. Brooks and A. R. Dent, *Pharmatherapeutica*, 1984, *3*, 649.

METABOLISM. About 10% of a 500-mg dose of flucloxacillin was metabolised. Within 12 hours of the dose being taken by 6 healthy subjects about 44% was recovered in the urine, 4% as penicilloic acid.— M. Cole *et al.*, *Antimicrob. Ag. Chemother.*, 1973, *3*, 463.

The metabolite of flucloxacillin had similar antibacterial properties to the parent compound.— H. H. W. Thijssen and H. Mattie, *Antimicrob. Ag. Chemother.*, 1976, *10*, 441. The pharmacokinetics of flucloxacillin and its 5-hydroxymethyl metabolite, hydroxyflucloxacillin, in patients with normal and impaired renal function. In renal disease relatively high plasma concentrations of the metabolite are reached which persist for longer than the parent compound.— H. H. W. Thijssen and J. Wolters, *Eur. J. clin. Pharmac.*, 1982, *22*, 429.

PREGNANCY AND THE NEONATE. Pharmacokinetics of flucloxacillin in neonates after administration of intravenous or oral doses of 50 mg per kg body-weight. The mean half-life was approximately 4.6 hours and was inversely proportional to gestational age. After intravenous administration, renal clearance constituted about 24% of total body clearance and was lower than values of 64 to 72% reported in adults.— L. Herngren *et al.*, *Eur. J. clin. Pharmac.*, 1987, *32*, 403.

Uses and Administration

Flucloxacillin is an isoxazolyl penicillin used primarily for the treatment of infections due to staphylococci resistant to benzylpenicillin, including infections of the skin and soft tissues, bones and joints, respiratory tract and urinary tract; otitis media, endocarditis, septicaemia, and meningitis. It is also used for mixed streptococcal and staphylococcal infections when the staphylococci are penicillin-resistant. Flucloxacillin is used for the prophylaxis of staphylococcal infections during major surgical procedures, particularly in cardiothoracic and orthopaedic surgery.

Flucloxacillin is administered by mouth as the sodium salt, in the form of capsules, or as the magnesium salt, in the form of a syrup or suspension. It should be given about 1 hour before meals as the presence of food in the stomach reduces absorption. It is administered parenterally as the sodium salt. All doses are expressed as flucloxacillin.

Flucloxacillin sodium is administered by mouth or by intramuscular injection in a usual dose of 250 mg four times daily. It is administered intravenously in a dose of 250 mg to 1 g four times daily by slow injection over 3 to 4 minutes or by intravenous infusion. All systemic doses may be doubled in severe infections.

Flucloxacillin has been administered by other routes in conjunction with systemic therapy. It has been administered in a dose of 250 to 500 mg daily by intra-articular injection, dissolved if necessary in a 0.5% solution of lignocaine hydrochloride, and by intrapleural injection in a dose of 250 mg daily. Using powder for injection, 125 to 250 mg has been dissolved in 3 mL of sterile water and inhaled by nebuliser 4 times daily.

Children up to 2 years of age may be given one-quarter the adult dose and those aged 2 to 10 years, one-half the adult dose. Children have been given doses of 12.5 to 25 mg per kg body-weight four times daily.

In staphylococcal meningitis parenteral treatment has been supplemented with intrathecal injections of flucloxacillin. Flucloxacillin specifically prepared for this purpose should be obtained from the manufacturer. The usual intrathecal dose is the equivalent of 5 mg for infants from birth up to 2 years of age, 10 mg for children up to 12 years of age, and 20 mg for adults, given as a single injection once daily. The dose should be dissolved in sodium chloride injection 0.9% immediately before use to give a solution containing 10 mg per mL. If two penicillins are given concurrently by the intrathecal route, the dose of each should be reduced so that the total daily penicillin dose does not exceed that given above.

Flucloxacillin may be administered in combination with other antibiotics, particularly ampicillin, to produce a wider spectrum of antibacterial activity. If used concurrently with an aminoglycoside the two antibiotics should not be mixed.

Flucloxacillin and related penicillinase-resistant antibiotics are used in a wide variety of staphylococcal infections. For further information see under Respiratory-tract Infections, Septicaemia, and Skin Disorders in Choice of an Antibiotic, p.99.

ADMINISTRATION IN RENAL FAILURE. Flucloxacillin can usually be given in normal doses to patients with renal failure. If, however, the creatinine clearance is less than 10 mL per minute, a reduction in dose or an increase in the dosage interval should be considered. A dosage supplement is not required for patients undergoing haemodialysis.

For reference to the administration of flucloxacillin by the intraperitoneal route in patients undergoing continuous ambulatory peritoneal dialysis, see under Peritonitis, below.

ANIMAL BITES. For reference to the use of penicillinase-resistant penicillins in the treatment of animal bites, see Benzylpenicillin Sodium, p.136.

ARTHRITIS, BACTERIAL. For reference to the use of flucloxacillin in bacterial arthritis, see under Osteomyelitis, below.

ENDOCARDITIS. Flucloxacillin should be added to therapy with a penicillin and aminoglycoside in the initial treatment of endocarditis before results of cultures are obtained if there is a strong possibility of staphylococcal infection, such as in drug addicts or patients with skin sepsis. For proven *Staphylococcus aureus* endocarditis the recommended regimen is flucloxacillin 12 g daily in 6 divided doses by intravenous injection, fusidic acid 500 mg every 8 hours by mouth, and intravenous gentamicin in an initial dose of 120 mg followed by 80 to 120 mg every 8 hours. Netilmicin may be used as an alternative to gentamicin in the elderly and in patients with impaired renal function. Treatment should continue for at least 4 weeks, although the gentamicin is seldom given for more than 14 days. Back titrations of serum bactericidal activity against the infecting organism should be used to monitor therapy. If the organism is resistant to flucloxacillin, or if the patient is allergic to penicillins, vancomycin alone is the recommended treatment. Endocarditis caused by *Staph. epidermidis* can be treated by the same regimen if the organisms are sensitive to the antibiotics, although even in such cases eradication of the infection is often impossible and valve replacement is necessary.— British Society for Antimicrobial Chemotherapy, *Lancet*, 1985, *2*, 815.

See also under Pregnancy and the Neonate, below.

FURUNCULOSIS. For reference to the use of isoxazolyl penicillins in the treatment of recurrent furunculosis, see Sodium Fusidate, p.236.

MENINGITIS. The isoxazolyl penicillins, flucloxacillin, cloxacillin, and oxacillin, or nafcillin were considered to be the treatment of choice for meningitis caused by *Staphylococcus aureus*. They should be given intravenously in high doses, such as 12 to 18 g daily in 4 to 6 divided doses for an adult. Intravenous rifampicin 10 mg per kg body-weight twice daily may be added, and vancomycin may be substituted for the penicillin.— M. Whitby and R. Finch, *Drugs*, 1986, *31*, 266.

For the treatment of meningitis due to other organisms, see under Choice of Antibiotic, p.98.

NEUTROPENIA. For reference to the use of antistaphylococcal penicillins for febrile episodes in neutropenic patients, see Piperacillin Sodium, p.287.

OSTEOMYELITIS. The isoxazolyl penicillins, for example flucloxacillin or cloxacillin 1 to 2 g every four hours, or benzylpenicillin 1.2 g every 4 hours (if the organism is sensitive), may be considered the antibiotics of choice for acute and chronic osteomyelitis or bacterial arthritis. Alternatives are first-generation cephalosporins, erythromycin, clindamycin, fusidic acid, rifampicin, or vancomycin. *Staphylococcus aureus* is a likely causative pathogen in all age groups; other likely pathogens depend on the age and condition of the patient and include streptococci, Enterobacteriaceae, *Haemophilus influenzae*, *Pseudomonas aeruginosa*, *Neisseria gonorrhoeae*, and other Gram-negative bacilli. Hence the recommended empirical regimens always include an antistaphylococcal agent but the need for additional agents varies.

In most adults, an isoxazolyl penicillin may be given alone, but in those with a major underlying illness an aminoglycoside, and either ticarcillin or piperacillin should be given in addition. In bacterial arthritis where infection with *N. gonorrhoeae* is a possibility, benzylpenicillin should be added. In neonates the isoxazolyl penicillin should be given in association with an aminoglycoside, in children aged one month to 3 years it is given in association with ampicillin.

In all the above regimens for empirical treatment, the isoxazolyl penicillin may be replaced by a first-generation cephalosporin such as cephalothin or cephazolin.

Neonates may be given flucloxacillin or cloxacillin in a dose of 75 mg per kg body-weight daily in divided doses every 6 to 8 hours; infants and children over one month of age may be given 150 mg per kg daily in divided doses every 4 hours.

In all cases of acute osteomyelitis, antibiotics should be given parenterally for a minimum of 3 weeks, except in certain uncomplicated cases where oral therapy may be substituted after 5 to 7 days. In all cases, a total of 6 weeks' therapy is recommended.

Surgical intervention may be required if there is no response to antibiotics within 48 hours.

Treatment of chronic osteomyelitis is primarily surgical; however, antibiotics should be given parenterally for 1 to 2 months over the period of surgical intervention followed by oral antibiotics for several more months. Bacterial arthritis caused by *Staph. aureus* or Gram-negative bacilli should be treated with parenteral antibiotics for at least 2 weeks; the total duration of treatment should be 4 to 6 weeks. Drainage of the joint is essential.— A. S. Dickie, *Drugs*, 1986, *32*, 458.

Unsuccessful treatment of a severe *Staphylococcus aureus* infection of the tibia with flucloxacillin and fusidic acid. Antagonism between the 2 drugs was demonstrated *in vitro* and the patient recovered after drainage of the tibial abscess and treatment with flucloxacillin alone.— S. J. Hudson (letter), *Lancet*, 1985, *2*, 1249. Comment.— N. A. Simmons (letter), *ibid.*, 1250.

PERITONITIS. Flucloxacillin or vancomycin are the recommended antibiotics for the treatment of continuous ambulatory peritoneal dialysis-associated peritonitis caused by *Staphylococcus aureus*. Cloxacillin could also be administered in a loading dose of 1 g given by the intravenous or intraperitoneal route, followed by a maintainance dose of 125 mg added to 1 litre of dialysis fluid.— British Society for Antimicrobial Chemotherapy, *Lancet*, 1987, *1*, 845. Flucloxacillin could be given by intravenous or intraperitoneal administration to patients undergoing continuous ambulatory peritoneal dialysis as a loading dose of 0.5 to 1 g, followed by a maintenance dose of 100 to 250 mg per litre intraperitoneally.— D. K. Scott and D. E. Roberts, *Pharm. J.*, 1985, *1*, 621.

PREGNANCY AND THE NEONATE. There appeared to be no significant risk to the foetus from flucloxacillin when administered during pregnancy although there was the possibility of sensitising the foetus during the second and third trimesters. If an antimicrobial agent had to be used during pregnancy, flucloxacillin, in association with fusidic acid, was recommended for the treatment of staphylococcal endocarditis.— R. Wise, *Br. med. J.*, 1987, *294*, 42.

RESPIRATORY-TRACT INFECTIONS. Amoxycillin and flucloxacillin both at a dose of 1 g per 20 kg body-weight twice daily by mouth produced a beneficial effect in patients with bronchiectasis associated with cystic fibrosis.— R. K. Knight (letter), *Lancet*, 1983, *2*, 970.

Pneumonia. For reference to the use of flucloxacillin in patients with pneumonia, see Ampicillin Trihydrate p.121.

SURGICAL INFECTION PROPHYLAXIS. *Cardiac surgery*. Flucloxacillin, and other beta-lactamase-stable penicillins such as cloxacillin, oxacillin, and nafcillin, are used alone or in combination with other antibiotics as intravenous prophylaxis in cardiothoracic surgery. An aminoglycoside is often added, partly due to its reported synergistic action with beta-lactam antibiotics. Cephalosporins are sometimes used in preference to a penicillin particularly in the *U.S.A.* (*Med. Lett.*, 1985, *27*, 105; *Lancet*, 1985, *2*, 701; *ibid.*, 1986, *1*, 537; A.B. Kaiser, *New Engl. J. Med.*, 1986, *315*, 1129; A.P.R. Wilson *et al.*, *Thorax*, 1986, *41*, 396), and vancomycin and rifampicin have been used in patients allergic to penicillins or who are infected with methicillin-resistant staphylococci.

In heart-valve and pacemaker operations antibiotic cover has been given to cover staphylococci, particularly *Staph. aureus* and *Staph. epidermidis*, and corynebacteria associated with prosthetic valve endocarditis; staphylococci may also be associated with infections of the wound. In coronary artery bypass surgery however, the main infection risk is of deep sternal wound infection and infections may also be caused by Gram-negative bacteria such as *Enterobacter* and *Acinetobacter* spp. Some workers (F.C. Wells *et al.*, *Lancet*, 1983, *1*, 1209; M. Farrington *et al.*, *ibid.*, *2*, 395; *idem*, *Br. J. Surg.*, 1985, *72*, 759) have suggested that such bacteria may be transferred from the leg to the heart with the saphenous vein graft possibly causing a higher rate of wound infection than with other heart procedures. Other workers, however, (R. Freeman and F.K. Gould, *Lancet*, 1986, *1*, 103) have found no difference in the rates of wound infection between cases of valve surgery and coronary artery bypass. In heart transplant surgery the main early infective complication is chest infection with Gram-negative bacilli.

Dosage regimens of antibiotics for prophylaxis in cardiothoracic surgery have been very variable. On the basis of pharmacokinetic studies of flucloxacillin (see Absorption and Fate, above) or cloxacillin (see p.203), a large antibiotic dose both before induction of anaesthesia and at the end of a long procedure has been recommended. This may be followed by intravenous antibiotics for a few days postoperatively.

In reviewing the use of prophylactic antibiotics in coronary artery bypass surgery, Farrington (*J. antimicrob. Chemother.*, 1986, *18*, 656) concluded that the emphasis should be on good surgical technique and intensive pre-operative skin disinfection rather than on broad-spectrum antibiotics; the value of pre-operative depilation was also emphasised. He considered that high-dose, narrow-spectrum, peri-operative prophylaxis may further decrease infection with sensitive organisms, although studies had not yet proved this. Prophylaxis with agents such as flucloxacillin has little effect on normal bacterial flora; broader spectrum cover with cephalosporins, or the addition of amoxycillin to flucloxacillin may encourage colonisation with Gram-negative organisms. Other workers (R. Freeman and F.K. Gould, *Lancet*, 1986, *1*, 103) agree with the choice of flucloxacillin for prophylaxis in coronary artery bypass and also in valve surgery.

Orthopaedic surgery. Prophylactic antibiotics were considered to be a cost-effective measure to reduce the incidence of infections after joint surgery, although special ventilation systems appear to be equally effective. Up to 3 doses of antibiotic at the time of the operation is sufficient to maintain high tissue concentrations during the critical period. Flucloxacillin or a cephalosporin alone may not be adequate due to the possibility of methicillin-resistant *Staphylococcus aureus* and *Staph. epidermidis*; up to 3 doses of flucloxacillin and gentamicin was suggested, although the effectiveness of this prophylaxis has not been proved.— *Lancet*, 1985, *1*, 378. Caution concerning the routine use of prophylactic gentamicin.— R. Freeman and F. K. Gould (letter), *ibid.*, 694. Risk of resistance to flucloxacillin or gentamicin, particularly in *Staph. epidermidis*.— A. J. Davies and M. El-Safty (letter), *ibid.*

For reference to the penetration of flucloxacillin into the bone and joint capsule after administration for prophylaxis of infection in hip replacement surgery, see Absorption and Fate, above.

Preparations

Flucloxacillin Capsules *(B.P.)*. Capsules containing flucloxacillin sodium.

Flucloxacillin Injection *(B.P.)*. Flucloxacillin sodium to be reconstituted before use.

Flucloxacillin Oral Solution *(B.P.)*. Flucloxacillin Elixir; Flucloxacillin Syrup. A dry mixture of flucloxacillin sodium for reconstitution.

Flucloxacillin Oral Suspension *(B.P.)*. Flucloxacillin Mixture. A dry mixture of flucloxacillin magnesium for reconstitution.

Proprietary Preparations

Abboflox *(Abbott, UK)*. *Capsules*, flucloxacillin 250 mg (as sodium salt).

Floxapen *(Beecham Research, UK)*. *Capsules*, flucloxacillin 250 and 500 mg (as sodium salt).
Syrup, powder for reconstitution, flucloxacillin 125 mg (as magnesium salt)/5 mL when reconstituted with water.
Syrup forte, powder for reconstitution, flucloxacillin 250 mg (as magnesium salt)/5 mL when reconstituted with water.
Oral powder (Unidose sachets), flucloxacillin 125 mg (as magnesium salt)/sachet. To be dispersed in water before administration.
Injection, powder for reconstitution, flucloxacillin 0.25, 0.5, and 1 g (as sodium salt).

Ladropen *(Berk Pharmaceuticals, UK)*. *Capsules*, flucloxacillin 250 and 500 mg (as sodium salt).

Stafoxil *(Brocades, UK)*. *Capsules*, flucloxacillin 250 and 500 mg (as sodium salt).

Staphlipen (formerly known as Staphcil) *(Lederle, UK)*. *Capsules*, flucloxacillin 250 and 500 mg (as sodium salt).
Injection, powder for reconstitution, flucloxacillin 0.25, 0.5, and 1 g (as sodium salt).

Proprietary Names and Manufacturers of Flucloxacillin Salts

Abboflox *(Abbott, UK)*; Dumpikal *(Spain)*; Flopen *(Commonwealth Serum Laboratories, Austral.)*; Floxapen *(Beecham, Austral.; Belg.; Ital.; Neth.; NZ; Bencard, S.Afr.; Beecham, Spain; Beecham, Switz.; Beecham Research, UK)*; Flupen *(Ital.)*; Heracillin *(Astra, Denm.; Astra, Swed.)*; Ladropen *(Berk Pharmaceuticals, UK)*; Lifecilina *(IBYS, Spain)*; Penplus *(Ital.)*; Stafoxil *(Brocades, UK)*; Staphcil *(Lederle, UK)*; Staphlipen *(Lederle, UK)*; Staphylex *(Beecham-Wülfing, Ger.)*.

The following names have been used for multi-ingredient preparations containing flucloxacillin salts— Flu-Amp *(Generics, UK)*; Magnapen *(Beecham Research, UK)*; Suprapen *(Bencard, S. Afr.)*.

12757-f

Flumequine *(BAN, USAN, rINN)*.

R-802. 9-Fluoro-6,7-dihydro-5-methyl-1-oxo-1*H*,5*H*-pyrido[3,2,1-*ij*]quinoline-2-carboxylic acid.
$C_{14}H_{12}FNO_3$=261.3.

CAS — *42835-25-6.*

Adverse Effects and Precautions

As for Nalidixic Acid, p.266.

Antimicrobial Action and Resistance

Flumequine is bactericidal and has a similar antibacterial spectrum to nalidixic acid (see p.267) though it is reported also to have activity against some Gram-positive organisms.

Cross-resistance with nalidixic acid and oxolinic acid occurs. Antagonism has been reported to occur between flumequine and nitrofurantoin or tetracycline.

Some references to the antibacterial activity of flumequine: G. Stilwell *et al.*, *Antimicrob. Ag. Chemother.*, 1975, *7*, 483; S. R. Rohlfing *et al.*, *ibid.*, 1976, *10*, 20; *idem*, *J. antimicrob. Chemother.*, 1977, *3*, 615; D. Greenwood, *Antimicrob. Ag. Chemother.*, 1978, *13*, 479.

Absorption and Fate

Flumequine is rapidly absorbed from the gastro-intestinal tract and metabolised in the liver before being excreted in the urine as inactive glucuronides and the active hydroxy metabolite; very little of a dose is excreted as unchanged drug.

Two hours after administration of single doses of flumequine 400, 800, or 1200 mg by mouth, to 10 healthy subjects, average plasma concentrations of flumequine were 13.5, 23.8, and 31.9 µg per mL respectively with corresponding peak urinary concentrations of 50, 105, and 131 µg per mL respectively being obtained 6 to 8 hours after administration. In 18 further healthy subjects who received flumequine 800 mg four times daily, the mean peak plasma concentrations were 27 µg per mL 2.5 to 3.5 hours after a single dose and 41 µg per mL at steady-state; trough plasma concentrations ranged from 21 to 23 µg per mL. The mean plasma elimination half-life increased from 7.1 to 8.5 hours with multiple dosing but this difference was not significant. Urinary concentrations of the active metabolite 7-hydroxyflumequine were usually higher than those of flumequine with overnight concentrations always exceeding 80 and 50 µg per mL respectively. Following a single 800-mg dose about 63% of the administered dose was recovered in the urine within 24 hours, 2.5% as unchanged flumequine, 5.6% as the hydroxy metabolite, and the rest as inactive urinary conjugates.— D. Schuppan *et al.*, *J. antimicrob. Chemother.*, 1985, *15*, 337.

Further references: D. Schuppan *et al.*, *Pharmacologist*, 1974, *16*, 262 (excretion); L. I. Harrison *et al.*, *Antimicrob. Ag. Chemother.*, 1984, *25*, 301 (urinary excretion of metabolite); J. Aubert and J. B. Fourtillan, *J. Urol., Paris*, 1985, *91*, 159 (renal and prostatic tissue concentrations).

Uses and Administration

Flumequine is a 4-quinolone antimicrobial agent used similarly to nalidixic acid (see p.267) in the treatment of urinary-tract infections. Doses of 400 mg have been given three times daily by mouth.

GONORRHOEA. The efficacy of short-term treatment with flumequine was evaluated in 239 patients with uncomplicated gonorrhoea. Three dosage regimens were studied: regimen (A): flumequine 1.2 g by mouth followed by 800 mg every 6 hours for 2 doses; regimen (B): flumequine 1.2 g followed by 800 mg after 6 hours; regimen (C): a single dose of flumequine 1.2 g. Treatment with regimen C was discontinued after being given to 23 patients when a failure-rate of 26% was noted. Treatment with regimens A or B, evaluated in 97 and 119 patients respectively, appeared to be equally effective with a cure-rate of 100% being obtained in female patients and a cure-rate of over 90% in male patients. Six of the 10 treatment failures had originally been infected with strains of gonococci with an MIC of 3.2 µg or more per mL while resistance to flumequine had developed during treatment in 2 patients. All patients infected with beta-lactamase producing strains were cured. Adverse efects reported included dizziness, confusion, and minor neurological disturbances.— H. B. Svindland *et al.*, *Br. J. vener. Dis.*, 1982, *58*, 317.

URINARY-TRACT INFECTIONS. The original infecting organism was eradicated in 22 of 26 female patients with significant bacteriuria after receiving flumequine 400 mg every 6 hours for 14 days. However, only 7 of 15 of the patients were free of infection at follow-up 6 months later. Resistance to flumequine developed during treatment in 3 of the 4 treatment failures. One patient stopped treatment after developing a rash on the face and hands. Other adverse effects reported were considered to be minor and included tiredness (2), transient rash (2), heartburn (1), giddiness (1), and transient diarrhoea (1).— C. R. Steer *et al.*, *J. antimicrob. Chemother.*, 1981, *7*, 643.

Proprietary Names and Manufacturers

Apurone *(Riker, Fr.)*; Flumural *(SPA, Ital.)*.

4905-a

Formosulphathiazole

Formosulfathiazole; Methylenesulfathiazole. A condensation product of sulphathiazole with formaldehyde.

CAS — 12041-72-4.

Formosulphathiazole is a sulphonamide with properties similar to sulphamethoxazole, p.306, which is used for the treatment of local intestinal infections. It is also used topically, with other antibacterial agents, in veterinary practice.

Proprietary Names and Manufacturers

Formilae *(Spain)*; Formo-Cibazol *(Ciba, Ger.)*; Ormidal *(Estedi, Spain)*; Sunfintestin *(Hosbon, Spain)*.

179-a

Fosfomycin *(BAN, USAN, pINN)*.

MK-955; Phosphomycin; Phosphonomycin. (−)-(1*R*,2*S*)-(1,2-Epoxypropyl)phosphonic acid.
$C_3H_7O_4P$=138.1.

CAS — 23155-02-4.

An antibiotic isolated from *Streptomyces fradiae*.

Adverse Effects

Gastro-intestinal disturbances, transient increases in serum concentrations of aminotransferases, and skin rashes have been reported following the use of fosfomycin. Eosinophilia has also occurred.

ADMINISTRATION IN RENAL FAILURE. For reference to the precautions to be observed in renal failure, see under Administration in Renal Failure in Uses, below.

Antimicrobial Action and Resistance

Fosfomycin is a bactericidal antibiotic and is reported to interfere with the first step in the synthesis of bacterial cell walls. It is active *in vitro* against a range of Gram-positive and Gram-negative bacteria including *Staphylococcus aureus*, some streptococci, most Enterobacteriaceae, *Haemophilus influenzae*, *Neisseria* spp., and some strains of *Pseudomonas aeruginosa*. *Bacteroides* spp. are not sensitive. MICs are very variable and depend on the type of test media used as well as inoculum size. Bacterial resistance to fosfomycin has been reported.

International collaborative study on standardisation of bacterial sensitivity to fosfomycin.— J. M. Andrews *et al.*, *J. antimicrob. Chemother.*, 1983, *12*, 357.

The MICs for fosfomycin against 50 clinical isolates of methicillin-resistant *Staphylococcus aureus* ranged from 0.25 to 32 µg per mL.— S. H. Guenthner and R. P. Wenzel, *Antimicrob. Ag. Chemother.*, 1984, *26*, 268.

A study on the inability of gentamicin and fosfomycin to kill intracellular Enterobacteriaceae.— E. Kihlström and L. Andåker, *J. antimicrob. Chemother.*, 1985, *15*, 723.

Further studies of the antimicrobial activity of fosfomycin: A. Forsgren and M. Walder, *J. antimicrob. Chemother.*, 1983, *11*, 467; G. A. Dette *et al.*, *ibid.*, 517.

RESISTANCE. Plasmid-mediated fosfomycin resistance appeared to be due to enzymatic modification of the antibiotic.— J. Llaneza *et al.*, *Antimicrob. Ag. Chemother.*, 1985, *28*, 163. See also C. J. Villar *et al.*, *ibid.*, 1986, *29*, 309.

ACTIVITY WITH OTHER ANTIMICROBIAL AGENTS. A synergistic interaction between fosfomycin and many antibiotics has been demonstrated *in vitro* against a wide range of bacteria. Studies in *animals* have also reported increased activity of such combinations over the individual agents in bacterial infections. Antibiotics with which synergy has been reported include penicillins, cephalosporins, aminoglycosides, chloramphenicol, tetracycline, erythromycin, rifamycin, and lincomycin. References: T. Olay *et al.*, *J. antimicrob. Chemother.*, 1978, *4*, 569 (a range of antibiotics); E. J. Perea *et al.*, *Antimicrob. Ag. Chemother.*, 1978, *13*, 705 (ampicillin and chloramphenicol); M. V. Vicente *et al.*, *ibid.*, 1981, *20*, 10 (benzylpenicillin and cefoxitin); N. A. Carlone *et al.*, *Drugs exp. & clin. Res.*, 1984, *10*, 47 (amoxycillin and cephalexin); K. Takahashi and H. Kanno, *Antimicrob. Ag. Chemother.*, 1984, *26*, 789 (cefoperazone, cefsulodin, and piperacillin); S. Alvarez *et al.*, *ibid.*, 1985, *28*, 689 (methicillin); A. Carvajal (letter), *J. antimicrob. Chemother.*, 1985, *16*, 677 (cefotaxime); R. J. Courcol and G. R. Martin (letter), *ibid.*, 1987, *19*, 276 (ceftriaxone).

Absorption and Fate

Fosfomycin calcium is poorly absorbed from the gastro-intestinal tract; absorption of the trometamol salt is reported to be better. Fosfomycin disodium is administered by the intramuscular or intravenous routes. The plasma half-life varies from 1.5 to 2 hours. Fosfomycin does not appear to be bound to plasma proteins. It diffuses across the placenta and is widely distributed in body fluids including the cerebrospinal fluid; small amounts have been found in breast milk and bile. The majority of a parenteral dose is excreted unchanged in the urine, by glomerular filtration, within 24 hours.

A study of the pharmacokinetics of fosfomycin in 7 healthy subjects. After the intravenous administration over 5 minutes of 20 or 40 mg per kg body-weight (as the disodium salt), peak serum concentrations of 132.1 and 259.3 µg per mL respectively were obtained; these concentrations fell to 4.4 and 6.8 µg per mL after 8 hours. The half-life of fosfomycin was about 2 hours and 80% of a dose was excreted in the urine in 24 hours. After administration by mouth (as the calcium salt) peak serum concentrations of 4.4 to 8.6 µg per mL and 6.9 to 13.4 µg per mL were reported about 2 to 3 hours after 20 or 40 mg per kg of fosfomycin respectively. The bioavailability of the oral preparation was calculated to be 0.28. The mean half-life was 3 hours after the lower oral dose and 5 hours after the higher dose; about 25% was excreted in the urine in 24 hours.— M. Goto *et al.*, *Antimicrob. Ag. Chemother.*, 1981, *20*, 393.

Further references to the pharmacokinetics of fosfomycin: K. C. Kwan *et al.*, *J. pharm. Sci.*, 1971, *60*, 678 (after intravenous administration); C. Fernandez Lastra *et al.*, *Antimicrob. Ag. Chemother.*, 1984, *25*, 458 (disposition in patients with pleural effusion).

ADMINISTRATION IN RENAL FAILURE. For reference to the pharmacokinetics of fosfomycin in renal failure, see under Administration in Renal Failure in Uses, below.

Uses and Administration

Fosfomycin is a phosphonic acid antibiotic which has been given by mouth as the calcium salt and by intramuscular or intravenous injection as the disodium salt in the treatment of a variety of infections. Usual adult doses have ranged from 2 to 4 g daily in divided doses, although up to 16 g daily has been administered intravenously in severe infections.

Fosfomycin has also been administered by mouth as the trometamol salt.

Proceedings of a symposium on the actions and uses of fosfomycin.— A. Gallego and J. M. Rubio (Ed.), *Chemotherapy, Basle*, 1977, *23*, *Suppl.* 1, 1-447.

A brief review of phosphonic acid antibiotics. Since the trometamol salt of fosfomycin is absorbed from the gastro-intestinal tract to a greater extent than the calcium or lysine salts and therefore produces higher concentrations of fosfomycin in the urine, it has been studied in single doses or in short courses for the treatment of uncomplicated urinary-tract infections. It has been suggested that fosfomycin may decrease the nephrotoxicity of aminoglycosides.— M. Neuman, *J. antimicrob. Chemother.*, 1984, *14*, 309.

Treatment of systemic infections with a combination of cephalexin and fosfomycin, described as cephemic cofosfolactamine.— P. Mangini *et al.*, *Chemioterapia*, 1985, *4*, 222.

ADMINISTRATION IN RENAL FAILURE. A study of the diffusion of fosfomycin into the interstitial fluid of subjects with normal renal function and patients with varying degrees of renal impairment. Elimination rates from interstitial fluid and serum were similar. The serum half-life of fosfomycin increased from 1.73 to 28.15 hours as the creatinine clearance decreased from 120 to less than 5 mL per minute. The dosage interval should be increased from 6 to 24 hours as the creatinine clearance decreases, and the maintenance dose could be decreased also in those with the most severe impairment.— C. Fernandez Lastra *et al.*, *Eur. J. clin. Pharmac.*, 1983, *25*, 333.

More than 60% of a single dose of fosfomycin 30 mg per kg body-weight given intravenously, to 10 patients with terminal renal impairment, immediately before a 4-hour haemofiltration session was eliminated during the session. Since patients subjected to haemofiltration showed 2 differentiated kinetic processes, one during the sessions and the other in the interfiltration periods, it was recommended that a dose of 30 mg per kg should be administered intravenously at the beginning and at the end of each haemofiltration session when the interfiltration periods are prolonged to 48 hours.— C. Fernandez Lastra *et al.*, *Br. J. clin. Pharmac.*, 1984, *17*, 477.

DIARRHOEA. Fosfomycin calcium (a suspension containing 50 mg per mL fosfomycin) 100 to 200 mg per kg body-weight daily in divided doses was given for about 7 days to 42 premature infants and children, including 3 carriers, with gastro-enteritis due to *Escherichia coli*. After a second course of treatment in 11 cases (6 re-infections, 5 relapses) a 92% cure was achieved. Fosfomycin was partly absorbed, a mean blood concentration of 2.8 (100 mg per kg) to 4.6 µg per mL (200 mg per kg) being detected in 23 patients 1 hour after the first dose. The remainder was eliminated in the faeces. In 11 patients (200 mg per kg) a mean of 3.7 µg per g of faeces was measured on day 3 to 4 of treatment. Fosfomycin was well tolerated.— F. Baquero *et al.*, *Archs Dis. Childh.*, 1975, *50*, 367.

ENDOCARDITIS. Successful use of fosfomycin and gentamicin in the treatment of a patient with endocarditis caused by *Haemophilus aphrophilus*.— S. Moreno *et al.* (letter), *J. antimicrob. Chemother.*, 1986, *18*, 771.

Proprietary Names and Manufacturers of Fosfomycin Salts

Afos *(Tiber, Ital.)*; Biocin *(Ibirn, Ital.)*; Biofos *(Von Boch, Ital.)*; Endociclina *(Del Saz & Filippini, Ital.)*; Faremicin *(Lafare, Ital.)*; Fonofos *(Pulitzer, Ital.)*; Fosfobiotic *(Bergamon, Ital.)*; Fosfocin *(Crinos, Ital.)*; Fosfocina *(CEPA, Spain)*; Fosfocine *(Midy, Fr.*; *Boehringer Mannheim, Switz.)*; Fosfogram *(FIRMA, Ital.)*; Fosforal *(Sis-Ter, Ital.)*; Fosfotricina *(Italfarmaco, Ital.)*; Foximin *(Caber, Ital.)*; Francital *(Francia Farm., Ital.)*; Gram-micina *(Lagap, Ital.)*; Ipamicina *(IPA, Ital.)*; Lancetina *(Aandersen, Ital.)*; Lofoxin *(Locatelli, Ital.)*; Neofocin *(Medici, Ital.)*; Palmofen *(Zambon, Ital.)*; Priomicina *(San Carlo, Ital.)*; Selemicina *(Ital.)*; Solufos *(Federico Bonet, Spain)*; Ultramicina *(Lisapharma, Ital.)*; Valemicina *(Lifepharma, Ital.)*; Vastocin *(Coli, Ital.)*; Veramina *(Roux-Ocefa, Arg.)*.

19200-a

Fosmidomycin *(rINN).*
FR-31564. [3-(*N*-Hydroxyformamido)propyl]phosphonic acid.
$C_4H_{10}NO_5P=183.1$.
CAS — 66508-53-0.

An antimicrobial substance produced by *Streptomyces lavendulae.*

Fosmidomycin is a phosphonic acid antibiotic.

A brief review of phosphonic acid antibiotics. Unlike fosfomycin, fosmidomycin has a narrow antibacterial spectrum limited to Gram-negative bacilli. It is active against enterobacteria and some *Pseudomonas* spp., but indole-positive *Proteus* spp. and *Serratia* spp. are resistant. The MIC for most enterobacteria is below 1 μg per mL, and synergy may occur with beta-lactams or aminoglycosides. Fosmidomycin has been administered by the intravenous, intramuscular, and oral routes. Its binding to plasma proteins is low and high concentrations are achieved in the urine, although bioavailability is limited after oral administration.— M. Neuman, *J. antimicrob. Chemother.*, 1984, *14*, 309.

Further references to fosmidomycin: H. C. Neu and T. Kamimura, *Antimicrob. Ag. Chemother.*, 1981, *19*, 1013; T. Murakawa *et al.*, *ibid.*, 1982, *21*, 224; H. C. Neu and T. Kamimura, *ibid.*, *22*, 560; H. P. Kuemmerle *et al.*, *Int. J. clin. Pharmac. Ther. Toxic.*, 1985, *23*, 515; H. P. Kuemmerle *et al.*, *ibid.*, 521.

Proprietary Names and Manufacturers
Fujisawa, Jpn.

86-y

Framycetin Sulphate *(BANM, rINNM).*

Framycetini Sulfas. The sulphate of neomycin B.
$C_{23}H_{46}N_6O_{13},3H_2SO_4=908.9$.

CAS — 119-04-0 (framycetin); 4146-30-9; 28002-70-2 (both sulphate).

Pharmacopoeias. In *Br. Eur., Fr., Neth.,* and *Swiss* specify xH_2SO_4.
Also in *B.P.Vet.*

Framycetin is an antimicrobial substance produced by certain strains of *Streptomyces fradiae* or *Streptomyces decaris* or by any other means. It contains not more than 3% of neomycin C (see p.268) and loses not more than 8% of its weight on drying. A white or yellowish-white, odourless or almost odourless, hygroscopic powder containing not less than 630 units of neomycin B per mg after drying.

Soluble 1 in 1 of water; very slightly soluble in alcohol; practically insoluble in acetone, chloroform, and ether. A 1% solution in water has a pH of 6 to 7. **Store** at a temperature not exceeding 30° in well-closed containers. Protect from light.

Units

One unit of framycetin is contained in 0.001492 mg of the first International Reference Preparation (1970) of framycetin sulphate which contains 670 units per mg.

Framycetin sulphate is an aminoglycoside antibiotic with actions and uses similar to those of neomycin sulphate (p.268) and is administered topically in the treatment of infections of the skin, eye, and ear. Adults have been given doses of up to 2 or sometimes 4 g daily by mouth for enteric infections.

Framycetin has been given prophylactically with colistin and nystatin (FRACON) to reduce the intestinal flora in patients with leukaemia.

ANTIMICROBIAL ACTION. Studies of the antimicrobial activity of framycetin sulphate: M. Laverdiere *et al.*, *Curr. ther. Res.*, 1983, *33*, 905 (comparison of the activity *in vitro* of framycetin sulphate and chlorhexidine acetate tulle dressings); B. D. Rawal, *J. antimicrob. Chemother.*, 1987, *20*, 537 (comparison of MIC and ET (extinction time) data for the activity of framycetin sulphate against *Pseudomonas aeruginosa*).

USES AND ADMINISTRATION. *Administration.* References to the subconjunctival injection of framycetin.— A. J. Bron *et al.*, *Br. J. Ophthal.*, 1970, *54*, 615; N. E. Christy and P. Lall, *Archs Ophthal., N.Y.*, 1973, *90*, 361.

Skin disorders. For reference to the use of topical antibiotics, including framycetin sulphate, in the treatment of infections of the skin, see Neomycin Undecenoate, p.269.

Suppression of intestinal flora. For reference to the use of framycetin in regimens to prevent colonisation and infection by the selective decontamination of the gastro-intestinal tract, and in the treatment of Crohn's disease, see Colistin Sulphomethate Sodium, p.205.

Preparations

Framycetin Gauze Dressing *(B.P.).* Framycetin Sulphate Gauze Dressing. Gauze impregnated with ointment containing framycetin sulphate 1% in a basis of white soft paraffin that contains 10% w/w of wool fat. The amount of wool fat may be adjusted for use in tropical countries. Supplied as sterile single pieces.

Proprietary Preparations

Framycort *(Fisons, UK). Drops,* for eye or ear, framycetin sulphate 0.5%, hydrocortisone acetate 0.5%.
Eye ointment, framycetin sulphate 0.5%, hydrocortisone acetate 0.5%.
Ointment, framycetin sulphate 0.5%, hydrocortisone acetate 0.5%.

Framygen *(Fisons, UK). Cream,* framycetin sulphate 0.5%.
Drops, for eye or ear, framycetin sulphate 0.5%.
Eye ointment, framycetin sulphate 0.5%.

Sofradex *(Roussel, UK). Ear drops,* framycetin sulphate 0.5%, dexamethasone sodium *m*-sulphobenzoate 0.05%, gramicidin 0.005%.
Ointment, for eye or ear, framycetin sulphate 0.5%, dexamethasone 0.05%, gramicidin 0.005%.

Soframycin *(Roussel, UK). Tablets,* scored, framycetin sulphate 250 mg.
Cream, framycetin sulphate 1.5%, gramicidin 0.005%.
Ointment, framycetin sulphate 1.5%, gramicidin 0.005%.
Eye-drops, framycetin sulphate 0.5%.
Eye ointment, framycetin sulphate 0.5%.

Sofra-Tulle *(Roussel, UK). Dressing,* paraffin gauze, impregnated, framycetin sulphate 1%.

Proprietary Names and Manufacturers

Framygen *(Austral.; Fisons, UK)*; Isofra *(Bouchara, Fr.)*; Isoframicol *(Fr.)*; Perframyl *(Arg.)*; Soframycin *(Roussel, Austral.; Roussel, Canad.; Roussel, Denm.; Neth.; Roussel, S.Afr.; Roussel, Switz.; Roussel, UK)*; Soframycine *(Belg.; Roussel, Fr.)*; Sofra-Tull *(Albert-Roussel, Ger.)*; Sofra-Tulle *(Roussel, Austral.; Roussel, Canad.; Neth.; Roussel, Norw.; Roussel, S.Afr.; Roussel, Swed.; Roussel, Switz.; Roussel, UK)*; Tuttomycin *(Mago, Ger.)*.

The following names have been used for multi-ingredient preparations containing framycetin sulphate—

Diprosone-F *(Essex, Austral.)*; Enterfram *(Fisons, UK)*; Framycort *(Fisons, UK)*; Proctosedyl *(Roussel, Canad.; Roussel, UK)*; Sofracort *(Roussel, Canad.)*; Sofradex *(Roussel, Austral.; Roussel, UK)*; Soframycin Cream *(Roussel, Austral.; Roussel, UK)*; Soframycin Nebuliser *(Roussel, Austral.)*; Soframycin Ointment *(Roussel, Austral.; Roussel, UK)*.

87-j

Fusafungine *(BAN, rINN).*
A depsipeptide antibiotic of *Fusarium lateritium 437.*
CAS — 1393-87-9.

Fusafungine is active against some Gram-positive and Gram-negative organisms and *Candida albicans.* It has also been stated to possess anti-inflammatory activity.
It is used in the form of an aerosol spray as an 0.25% solution in the treatment of infections of the upper respiratory tract.

References: D. Haler, *J. int. med. Res.*, 1977, *5*, 61; J. C. Vallé-Jones, *ibid.*, 65; M. F. Osman, *ibid.*, 139.

Proprietary Preparations

Locabiotal *(Servier, UK). Spray,* aerosol, fusafungine 125 μg/metered dose. Supplied with attachments for nasal or oral use. *Dose.* Nasal, 3 metered doses in each nostril 5 times daily; oral, 5 doses 5 times daily. Children: nasal, 1 to 3 doses in each nostril 5 times daily; oral, 2 to 4 doses three times daily.

Proprietary Names and Manufacturers

Fusaloyos *(Servier, Spain)*; Locabiosol *(Itherapia, Ger.)*; Locabiotal *(Arg.; Belg.; Servier, Fr.; Stroder, Ital.; Servier, S.Afr.; Switz.; Servier, UK)*.

88-z

Fusidic Acid *(BAN, USAN, rINN).*

SQ-16603. *ent*-16α-Acetoxy-3β,11β-dihydroxy-4β,8β,14α-trimethyl-18-nor-5β,10α-cholesta-(17*Z*)-17(20),24-dien-21-oic acid hemihydrate.
$C_{31}H_{48}O_6,\frac{1}{2}H_2O=525.7$.

CAS — 6990-06-3 (anhydrous).

Pharmacopoeias. In *Br.*

An antimicrobial substance produced by the growth of certain strains of *Fusidium coccineum* (K. Tubaki).

A white crystalline powder. Practically **insoluble** in water; soluble 1 in 5 of alcohol, 1 in 4 of chloroform, and 1 in 60 of ether. **Store** in well-closed containers. Protect from light.

69-l

Diethanolamine Fusidate

The diethanolamine salt of fusidic acid.
$C_{35}H_{59}NO_8=621.9$.

CAS — 16391-75-6.

1.15 g of monograph substance is approximately equivalent to 1 g of sodium fusidate.

The manufacturers recommend that diethanolamine fusidate should not be infused with amino acid solutions or in whole blood. Opalescence may occur with more acidic samples of glucose; such solutions should be discarded.

154-s

Sodium Fusidate *(BANM, rINNM).*

Fusidate Sodium *(USAN)*; SQ-16360. The sodium salt of fusidic acid.
$C_{31}H_{47}NaO_6=538.7$.

CAS — 751-94-0.

Pharmacopoeias. In *Br.*

A white or almost white, slightly hygroscopic, crystalline powder.

Soluble 1 in 1 of water, 1 in 1 of alcohol; slightly soluble in chloroform; practically insoluble in acetone and ether. A 1.25% solution in water has a pH of 7.5 to 9.0. **Store** in well-closed containers. Protect from light.

Adverse Effects and Precautions

Apart from mild gastro-intestinal upsets sodium fusidate appears to be well tolerated when given by mouth. Skin rashes have been reported. Treatment with fusidates, by mouth or by the intravenous route, has been associated with jaundice and changes in liver function; normal liver function is usually restored when treatment is discontinued. They should be given with caution to patients with impaired liver function.

Venospasm, thrombophlebitis, and haemolysis have occurred in patients given diethanolamine fusidate intravenously. To reduce this it is recommended that solutions be buffered and that the solution should be given as a slow infusion into a large vein where there is a good blood-flow. Hypocalcaemia has occurred after intravenous administration of doses above those recommended, and has been attributed to the phosphate-citrate buffer in the preparation.

Hypersensitivity reactions may occur after the topical administration of fusidates.

EFFECTS ON THE EYE. Treatment with sodium fusidate and erythromycin was associated with the development of tunnel vision in a patient with diphtheroid endocarditis. The visual impairment resolved when sodium fusidate was withdrawn.— G. Jackson and K. Saunders, *Br. Heart J.*, 1973, *35*, 931.

EFFECTS ON THE LIVER. In a retrospective study of patients with staphylococcal bacteraemia, jaundice developed during treatment in 38 of 112 patients given fusidic acid (in 32 of 66 given the intravenous preparation with or without oral treatment and in 6 of 46 given only the oral preparation) compared with 2 of 101 patients given other antimicrobial agents. It was suggested that since the jaundice was reversible the continuing use of this drug would seem to be justified but that the intravenous preparation should be diluted to a volume of 500 mL or the maximum volume compatible with the clinical condition of the patient and infused slowly over at least 6 to 8 hours, that liver function should be monitored regularly in any patient receiving the drug by this route, and that oral medication be given as soon as possible but stopped if the bilirubin concentration continues to rise.— M. W. Humble *et al., Br. med. J.*, 1980, *280*, 1495.

By September 1985 the Committee on Safety of Medicines in the *UK* had received 87 reports of hepatotoxicity occurring in both young and old patients who had been treated with sodium fusidate administered either intravenously or by mouth at conventional doses.— Committee on Safety of Medicines, *Current Problems Series No. 16*, 1986.

INTERACTIONS. For a report of hydrocortisone diminishing the activity of fusidic acid, see under Antimicrobial Action.

INTERFERENCE WITH DIAGNOSTIC TESTS. Fusidic acid might interfere with fluorimetric estimations of plasma hydrocortisone.— J. Millhouse, *Adverse Drug React. Bull.*, 1974, Dec., 164.

PREGNANCY AND THE NEONATE. *In vitro* studies indicating that fusidic acid competes with bilirubin for binding to serum albumin. Caution is therefore advised in neonates, especially if premature, icteric, acidotic, or in respiratory distress, because of the possibility of bilirubin displacement and consequent risk of kernicterus.— R. Brodersen, *Acta paediat. scand.*, 1985, *74*, 874.

Antimicrobial Action

Fusidic acid inhibits bacterial protein synthesis and it may be bacteriostatic or bactericidal. It is highly active against staphylococci, including some strains that are resistant to methicillin and to other antibiotics. It is also active, but less so, against streptococci, enterococci, *Corynebacterium diphtheriae*, and *Clostridium* spp. Among the Gram-negative bacteria the *Neisseria* spp. are sensitive; *Bacteroides fragilis* is less sensitive. It has some activity against *Mycobacterium tuberculosis*.

Fusidic acid has been reported to inhibit the growth of susceptible *Staph. aureus* in concentrations of 0.03 to 0.16 μg per mL and of streptococci in concentrations of up to 16 μg per mL.

ACTIVITY AGAINST ANAEROBES. Fusidic acid inhibited 12 of 14 strains of *Bacteroides fragilis in vitro* at a concentration of 2 μg per mL and all 14 at 8 μg per mL; the addition of serum to the medium raised the MIC considerably for most strains.— J. Stirling and S. Goodwin (letter), *J. antimicrob. Chemother.*, 1977, *3*, 523.

Sodium fusidate had an MIC of up to 1 μg per mL against 114 strains of *Clostridia* spp. and an MIC of up to 2 μg per mL against 41 isolates of other species of anaerobic Gram-positive rods. All of 156 strains of *Bacteroides* were inhibited over a range of concentrations of 0.06 to 8 μg per mL, but up to 16 μg per mL was required to inhibit strains of *B. fragilis* and up to 32 μg per mL to inhibit strains of *B. thetaiotaomicron* and *Fusobacterium necrophorum*. Sodium fusidate inhibited all of 130 anaerobic cocci at a concentration of up to 8 μg per mL.— G. E. Steinkraus and L. R. McCarthy, *Antimicrob. Ag. Chemother.*, 1979, *16*, 120.

ACTIVITY AGAINST BORDETELLA. The *in-vitro* susceptibility of *Bordetella pertussis* to fusidic acid had not changed in the two decades from 1960 to 1981. Values for the MIC ranged from 0.03 to 0.5 μg per mL.— R. M. Bannatyne and R. Cheung, *Antimicrob. Ag. Chemother.*, 1982, *21*, 666.

ACTIVITY AGAINST PROTOZOA. Fusidic acid was active *in vitro* against 4 strains of *Plasmodium falciparum* at concentrations well within the range achievable by oral administration of 500 mg three times daily.— F. T. Black *et al.* (letter), *Lancet*, 1985, *1*, 578.

Sodium fusidate had moderate activity *in vitro* against *Giardia lamblia*; it was less than that of metronidazole.— M. J. G. Farthing and P. M. G. Inge, *J. antimicrob. Chemother.*, 1986, *17*, 165.

ACTIVITY AGAINST STAPHYLOCOCCI. Fusidic acid had the greatest inhibitory activity against 50 isolates of methicillin-resistant *Staphylacoccus aureus* (MRSA) of a range of antistaphylococcal agents tested. It was considered, however, that more information on its bactericidal action was needed to define its clinical efficacy.— S. H. Guenthner and R. P. Wenzel, *Antimicrob. Ag. Chemother.*, 1984, *26*, 268. Only 3 of 100 strains of MRSA were sensitive to fusidic acid with MICs of 0.06 μg per mL. The remainder had MICs of above 32 μg per mL. Fusidic acid should be administered with a second antibiotic to prevent development of resistance.— E. C. Moorhouse *et al., J. antimicrob. Chemother.*, 1985, *15*, 291.

For reference to the inhibitory and bactericidal activity of fusidic acid against coagulase-negative staphyloccoci, see Vancomycin Hydrochloride, p.333.

ACTIVITY AGAINST VIRUSES. For reference to the action *in vitro* of fusidic acid against HIV, see AIDS under Uses, below.

ACTIVITY WITH OTHER AGENTS. In studies *in vitro* 2-way antagonism has been demonstrated between fusidic acid and each of several penicillins against the majority of staphylococci tested (F. O'Grady and D. Greenwood, *J. med. Microbiol.*, 1973, *6*, 441). This antagonism was considered unlikely to be of clinical significance for 2 reasons: firstly the combinations remained bactericidal; secondly the effects were unlikely to be so marked *in vivo* because of pharmacokinetic differences between the drugs, and under these circumstances the penicillins still appeared to control the emergence of fusidic acid-resistant mutants. Although Farber *et al.* (*Antimicrob. Ag. Chemother.*, 1986, *30*, 174) demonstrated synergy between fusidic acid and rifampicin against coagulase-positive and -negative staphylococci, the incidence depended very much on the method used. Foldes *et al.* (*J. antimicrob. Chemother.*, 1983, *11*, 21), however, could show no enhancement or inhibition of growth of *Staph. aureus* resistant to methicillin, and in most cases also to gentamicin, with combinations of fusidic acid and either rifampicin or vancomycin. Yu *et al.* (*ibid.*, 1984, *14*, 359) also found no synergistic interaction between 2-drug combinations of fusidic acid, dicloxacillin, and rifampicin against *Staph. epidermidis* isolates from patients with endocarditis; he did, however, observe synergy in 5 of 10 isolates when all 3 drugs were tested together.

The antibacterial activity *in vitro* of fusidic acid against *Staph. aureus* was markedly decreased in the presence of hydrocortisone.— W. P. Raab, *Br. J. Derm.*, 1971, *84*, 582.

Resistance

Bacterial resistance to fusidic acid is readily acquired in the laboratory and has been reported to occur during treatment, especially when topical preparations have been used in hospital skin wards. There have been increasing reports of strains of methicillin-resistant *Staphylococcus aureus* resistant to fusidic acid. To prevent the emergence of resistant organisms it is usually recommended that fusidates be used in conjunction with other antibiotics.

RESISTANCE OF STAPHYLOCOCCI. In a study in Birmingham between 1967 and 1975 strains of *Staph. aureus* resistant to fusidic acid emerged during 1967 in dermatology wards and increased despite restrictions on the topical use of the antibiotic. In contrast, resistance to fusidic acid was low in burns wards.— G. A. J. Ayliffe *et al., J. clin. Path.*, 1977, *30*, 40.

For further reference to resistance of staphylococci to fusidic acid, see under Antimicrobial Action, above.

Absorption and Fate

Sodium fusidate is absorbed from the gastro-intestinal tract. A single 500-mg dose produces plasma concentrations of about 30 μg per mL after 2 to 3 hours in fasting subjects. Food has been reported to delay absorption. Higher concentrations may occur with repeated doses; concentrations of 50 to 100 μg per mL have been reported after treatment with 500 mg every 8 hours for 4 days. Concentrations of fusidic acid in the blood are higher after administration of solid oral dosage forms of sodium fusidate than after fusidic acid suspension. About 95% of sodium fusidate in the circulation is bound to plasma proteins. Although the plasma half-life of fusidic acid is usually 5 to 6 hours, some studies have suggested that it may increase during repeated dosing. It is widely distributed in body tissues and fluids but it does not diffuse into the cerebrospinal fluid when the meninges are not inflamed. Concentrations have been detected in the foetal circulation and in the milk of nursing mothers.

Sodium fusidate is excreted in the bile and about 2% appears unchanged in the faeces; metabolites, some with weak antimicrobial activity, have been detected in the bile. Little is excreted in the urine or removed by haemodialysis.

A review of the absorption and fate of fusidic acid and its salts.— D. S. Reeves, *J. antimicrob. Chemother.*, 1987, *20*, 467.

The absorption of sodium fusidate was increased in patients with coeliac disease.— R. L. Parsons *et al., J. antimicrob. Chemother.*, 1975, *1*, 39.

The pharmacokinetics of suspension, capsule, and intravenous forms of fusidic acid.— R. Wise *et al., Br. J. clin. Pharmac.*, 1977, *4*, 615.

DIFFUSION INTO BODY TISSUES AND FLUIDS. *Bone and connective tissue.* References: G. Hierholzer *et al., Arzneimittel-Forsch.*, 1966, *16*, 1549.

Brain. Fusidic acid seemed to penetrate well into intracranial pus.— J. de Louvois *et al., Br. med. J.*, 1977, *2*, 985.

Burn crusts. In patients given fusidic acid as tablets or solution by mouth in the prophylactic treatment of burns, the antibiotic was found in the burn crusts in a concentration considerably higher than that in the serum.— B. Sørensen *et al., Acta chir. scand.*, 1966, *131*, 423.

Eye. Study of 18 patients having cataract extractions showed that sodium fusidate was present in therapeutic concentrations in the aqueous humour after doses of 500 mg thrice daily for 3 days. As sodium fusidate binds with protein, a higher concentration might be expected in the inflamed eye.— A. J. Chadwick and B. Jackson, *Br. J. Ophthal.*, 1969, *53*, 26. See also J. Williamson *et al., ibid.*, 1970, *54*, 126.

Skin. Tests *in vitro* showed that sodium fusidate and fusidic acid penetrated human skin when applied locally and that absorption was increased by the addition of dimethyl sulphoxide or salicylic acid.— C. F. H. Vickers, *Br. J. Derm.*, 1969, *81*, 902.

Uses and Administration

Fusidic acid and its salts are used in the treatment of infections due to staphylococci, especially strains resistant to other antibiotics. To prevent emergence of resistant strains it is usually given in conjunction with other agents. Fusidic acid is used particularly for infections of the skin, bones, and joints, and for the treatment of bacterial endocarditis.

Sodium fusidate is administered as tablets or capsules in a dose of 500 mg by mouth every 8 hours. In severe infections the dose may be doubled. Fusidic acid is used for the preparation of aqueous suspensions for administration by mouth and the following doses of fusidic acid have been recommended for children: up to 1 year, 50 mg per kg body-weight daily in 3 divided doses; 1 to 5 years, 250 mg three times daily; and 5 to 12 years, 500 mg three times daily (250 mg of fusidic acid is stated to be therapeutically equivalent to 175 mg of sodium fusidate). To reduce gastro-intestinal disturbances, doses may be taken with meals.

In severe infections diethanolamine fusidate 580 mg, equivalent to 500 mg of sodium fusidate, is given three times daily by slow intravenous infusion over not less than 6 hours. Each 500-mg dose is administered as a buffered solution (pH 7.5) diluted to 500 mL with sodium chloride injection or other suitable intravenous solution. For children and adults weighing less than 50 kg a dose of 6 to 7 mg per kg body-weight of diethanolamine fusidate three times daily is recommended.

Sodium fusidate as an ointment (2%), or fusidic acid as a cream or gel (2%), are used in the local treatment of skin infections. A sterile gel of fusidic acid (2%) is used for the treatment of abscesses. Topical use may lead to problems of resistance.

For reference to the treatment of serious infections due to methicillin-resistant staphylococci including the use of fusidic acid, see Vancomycin Hydrochloride, p.334.

ABSCESS. Sterile fusidic acid gel was introduced into the abscess cavity (after incision and curetting) on a single occasion in 87 patients and sodium fusidate ointment dressings were applied daily after similar pretreatment in a further 71 patients. Mean healing times were 4.8 and 9.9 days respectively. A similar significant reduction of healing times occurred in each subgroup of patients analysed according to the size and site of abscess. *Staphylococcus aureus* was responsible for 82% of the infections and was resistant to penicillin and ampicillin in 49%.— I. C. Ritchie, *Br. med. J.*, 1972, *2*, 381.

There was more rapid healing of 23 abscesses all packed with 5 g of a preparation of fusidic acid 2% gel (Fucidin Caviject) compared to the healing of 20 packed with fusidic acid-impregnated wick.— A. Franklin and R. F. Calver (letter), *Lancet*, 1973, *2*, 573. See also *idem, Practitioner*, 1974, *212*, 388.

There was no significant difference between the mean time to healing in 17 patients who had a 2% fusidic acid gel introduced into abscess cavities compared with 22 similar patients who also received flucloxacillin 250 mg four times daily by mouth.— J. Kotowski, *Practitioner*, 1979, *222*, 269.

ADMINISTRATION IN RENAL FAILURE. The dosage interval of sodium fusidate was not affected in renal failure.— P. Sharpstone, *Br. med. J.*, 1977, *2*, 36.

AIDS. Striking clinical improvement occurred in a patient with AIDS after fusidic acid was added to his previously unsuccessful treatment regimen for *Mycobacterium tuberculosis* infection. It was considered that fusidic acid might have a direct effect against human immunodeficiency virus (HIV) and subsequent studies *in vitro* demonstrated an anti-HIV effect at concentrations readily attainable *in vivo*. It does not appear to inhibit reverse transcriptase and further studies into its mode of action are underway.— V. Faber *et al.*, *Lancet*, 1987, *2*, 827. Studies *in vitro* indicating that the antiviral effects of fusidic acid can all be attributed to toxicity to host cells.— D. D. Richman *et al.* (letter), *ibid.*, 1988, *1*, 1051.

ANTIBIOTIC-ASSOCIATED COLITIS. For reference to the treatment of antibiotic-associated colitis, including the possible use of fusidic acid, see Vancomycin Hydrochloride, p.335.

ENDOCARDITIS. For recommendations regarding the use of fusidic acid in the treatment of endocarditis, see Flucloxacillin Sodium, p.231.

EYE INFECTIONS. Fusidic acid eye-drops appeared effective for the treatment of bacterial conjunctivitis in 114 Egyptian children.— O. P. van Bijsterveld *et al.*, *Infection*, 1987, *15*, 16.

OSTEOMYELITIS. A report of a method for eradicating staphylococcal bone or joint infections by fusidic acid irrigation.— A. C. Mackechnie-Jarvis (letter), *Lancet*, 1985, *1*, 1035.

For the unsuccessful treatment of osteomyelitis with fusidic acid and flucloxacillin, and antagonism between the 2 agents *in vitro*, see Flucloxacillin Sodium, p.232.

SKIN DISORDERS. *Acne vulgaris*. Application of fusidic acid cream for 8 weeks by 36 patients with mild to moderate acne vulgaris resulted in a significantly greater fall in the average number of papules and pustules compared with 34 patients applying placebo in a double-blind randomised study.— B. Hansted *et al.*, *Curr. ther. Res.*, 1985, *37*, 249.

Furunculosis. Following a study involving 80 patients with recurrent staphylococcal furunculosis the following management strategy was recommended: treatment with an isoxazolyl penicillin [such as flucloxacillin] 0.5 to 1 g twice daily for 10 to 14 days, possibly in conjunction with probenecid, followed immediately by prophylactic fusidic acid ointment applied to the nares twice daily for every fourth week in the patient and all family carriers of the lesion strain.— S. A. Hedstrom, *Scand. J. infect. Dis.*, 1985, *17*, 55.

Preparations

Fusidic Acid Oral Suspension *(B.P.)*. Fusidic Acid Mixture. pH 4.8 to 5.2. Store at a temperature not exceeding 25°.

When the strength is not specified, a mixture containing the equivalent of anhydrous fusidic acid 250 mg/5mL should be dispensed or supplied.

Sodium Fusidate Capsules *(B.P.)*

Sodium Fusidate Gauze Dressing *(B.P.)*. Cotton fabric of leno weave impregnated with Sodium Fusidate Ointment. Sterile.

Sodium Fusidate Ointment *(B.P.)*

Proprietary Preparations

Fucidin *(Leo, UK)*. *Tablets*, film-coated, sodium fusidate 250 mg.

Suspension, fusidic acid 250 mg (therapeutically equivalent to sodium fusidate 175 mg)/5 mL.

Intravenous infusion, powder for reconstitution, diethanolamine fusidate 580 mg (equivalent to sodium fusidate 500 mg), supplied with diluent.

Cream and *Gel*, fusidic acid 2%.

Caviject gel, sterile, fusidic acid 2%, in single-dose applicators of 7 g.

Ointment, sodium fusidate 2%.

Intertulle, impregnated dressing, sodium fusidate 2% (as ointment).

Fucidin H *(Leo, UK)*. *Cream* and *Gel*, fusidic acid 2%, hydrocortisone acetate 1%.

Ointment, sodium fusidate 2%, hydrocortisone acetate 1%.

Fucithalmic *(Leo, UK)*. *Eye-drops*, fusidic acid 1%, in an aqueous sustained-release formulation.

Proprietary Names and Manufacturers of Fusidic Acid and its Salts

Fucidin *(Smith Kline & French, Austral.; Leo, Canad.; Leo, Denm.; Sigmatau, Ital.; Neth.; Leo, Norw.; Leo, S.Afr.; Lövens, Swed.; Switz.; Leo, UK)*; Fucidine *(Belg.; Leo, Fr.; Thomae, Ger.; Alter, Spain; Leo, Switz.)*; Fucithalmic *(Leo, Denm.; Leo, UK)*; Stafusid *(Italfarmaco, Ital.)*.

The following names have been used for multi-ingredient preparations containing fusidic acid and its salts— Fucibet *(Leo, UK)*; Fucidin H *(Leo, UK)*.

89-c

Gentamicin Sulphate *(BANM, pINNM)*.

Gentamicin Sulfate *(USAN)*; NSC-82261; Sch-9724. The sulphates of a mixture of antimicrobial substances produced by *Micromonospora purpurea*.

CAS — 1403-66-3 (gentamicin); 1405-41-0 (sulphate).

Pharmacopoeias. In *Br., Braz., Chin., Cz., Egypt., Eur., Fr., Ind., It., Jug., Neth., Swiss,* and *U.S.*

Gentamicin sulphate is a complex mixture of the sulphates of gentamicin C_1, gentamicin C_{1A}, and gentamicin C_2. Some commercial samples may contain significant quantities of the minor components gentamicin C_{2A} and gentamicin C_{2B}. It contains when dried not less than 590 units of gentamicin per mg.

A white to almost white powder.

B.P. **solubilities** are: freely soluble in water; practically insoluble in alcohol, chloroform, and ether. *U.S.P.* solubilities are: soluble in water, insoluble in alcohol and acetone. A 4% solution in water has a pH of 3.5 to 5.5. The *B.P.* injection has a pH of 3.0 to 4.5; the *U.S.P.* injection has a pH of 3.0 to 5.5. Solutions are **sterilised** by filtration. The powder has been sterilised by irradiation. **Store** in airtight containers.

Incompatibilities, see below.

Potency of gentamicin sulphate was lost in plastic disposable syringes and a brown precipitate formed. Storage in glass disposable syringes should not exceed 30 days.— B. Weiner *et al.*, *Am. J. Hosp. Pharm.*, 1976, *33*, 1254.

Report of potency loss of gentamicin in serum samples stored for up to 63 days at −60°.— L. G. Carlson *et al.*, *Antimicrob. Ag. Chemother.*, 1982, *21*, 192.

INCOMPATIBILITY. The aminoglycosides are inactivated by various beta-lactam antibiotics *in vitro* by interaction with the beta-lactam ring. The extent of inactivation is dependent upon temperature, duration of contact, and the concentration of beta-lactam antibiotic and also varies according to the aminoglycoside and beta-lactam combination (P. Noone and J.R. Pattison, *Lancet*, 1971, *2*, 575; J.L. Henderson *et al.*, *Am. J. Hosp. Pharm.*, 1981, *38*, 1167). Several studies have indicated that amikacin is the most resistant of the aminoglycosides to inactivation *in vitro* and tobramycin the most susceptible; gentamicin, dibekacin, sissomicin, and netilmicin appear to be of intermediate stability (H.A. Holt *et al.*, *Infection*, 1976, *4*, 107; R.H. Glew and R.A. Pavuk, *Antimicrob. Ag. Chemother.*, 1983, *24*, 474; A.S. Navarro *et al.*, *J. antimicrob. Chemother.*, 1986, *17*, 83). Several workers have also studied the relative degree of inactivation produced by various beta-lactam antibiotics especially the antipseudomonal penicillins (L.K. Pickering and P. Gearhart, *Antimicrob. Ag. Chemother.*, 1979, *15*, 592; J.L. Henderson *et al.*, *Am. J. Hosp. Pharm.*, 1981, *38*, 1167; H. Konishi *et al.*, *Antimicrob. Ag. Chemother.*, 1983, *23*, 653; D.N. Wright *et al.*, *Antimicrob. Ag. Chemother.*, 1986, *29*, 353). Tindula *et al.* (*Drug Intell. & clin. Pharm.*, 1983, *17*, 906) found that ampicillin, benzylpenicillin, carbenicillin, and ticarcillin produced marked inactivation while cephazolin and cephamandole produced little inactivation; nafcillin, cephapirin, and cefoxitin produced moderate inactivation. Other beta-lactams reported to produce little or no inactivation have included ceftazidime, imipenem, aztreonam, latamoxef, and cefotaxime (R.H. Glew and R.A. Pavuk, *Antimicrob Ag. Chemother.*, 1983, *24*, 474; T.S.J. Elliott *et al.*, *J. antimicrob. Chemother.*, 1986, *17*, 680). Inactivation has also been reported to occur with the beta-lactamase inhibitor clavulanic acid which also has a beta-lactam structure (R.J. Courcol and G.R. Martin, *J. antimicrob. Chemother.*, 1986, *17*, 682).

It is generally recommended that when these antibiotics need to be used together they should be administered at different sites and not mixed in infusion solutions or given through the same intravenous lines. Care should also be taken to limit the amount of aminoglycoside inactivated *in vitro* in blood samples taken for analysis (see under Precautions, Interference with Assay Procedures, p.238). For other clinical implications of the incompatibility of aminoglycosides and beta-lactam antibiotics see under Precautions, Interactions (p.238).

Other antimicrobial agents reported to be incompatible *in vitro* with gentamicin include erythromycin, chloramphenicol, and sulphadiazine sodium (B.B. Riley, *J. Hosp. Pharm.*, 1970, *28*, 228; *Med. Lett.*, 1972, *14*, (Jan.), *Suppl.*, 32).

Gentamicin is also incompatible with heparin and sodium bicarbonate and there have been reports of incompatibility with frusemide (D.F. Thompson *et al.*, *Am. J. Hosp. Pharm.*, 1985, *42*, 116).

For the effect of dopamine hydrochloride on gentamicin, see Dopamine Hydrochloride, p.1460.

Units

One unit of gentamicin is contained in 0.00156 mg of the first International Reference Preparation (1968) of gentamicin sulphate which contains 641 units per mg.

80 000 units of gentamicin is approximately equivalent to 80 mg of gentamicin.

Adverse Effects

All aminoglycoside antibiotics can produce irreversible ototoxicity following systemic treatment. Vestibular damage is more common with gentamicin than hearing loss which, when it occurs, is greatest in the high-tone range. Ototoxicity has also occurred following the topical application of aminoglycosides, especially neomycin, to mucous membranes, large areas of denuded skin, or burns. Previous exposure to other ototoxic drugs may be a contributory factor.

Reversible nephrotoxicity may occur and acute renal failure has been reported, often in association with the concurrent administration of other nephrotoxic agents.

Many risk factors have been suggested for ototoxicity and nephrotoxicity in patients receiving aminoglycosides. Patients especially at risk are those whose condition may lead to raised plasma concentrations such as in patients with renal failure. Peak plasma concentrations of gentamicin above 10 to 12 μg per mL and trough plasma concentrations, that is those immediately before the next dose, of more than 2 μg per mL may be associated with a greater risk of toxicity.

Aminoglycosides possess a neuromuscular blocking action and respiratory depression and muscular paralysis have been reported, usually after intrapleural or intraperitoneal instillation. Neomycin has the most potent action and several deaths have been associated with its use. Hypersensitivity reactions have occurred, especially after local use, and cross-sensitivity between aminoglycosides may occur. Hypomagnesaemia, hypocalcaemia, and hypokalaemia have also occurred when aminoglycosides have been given for prolonged periods, especially in association with antineoplastic agents. Although pseudomembranous colitis has occurred in patients treated with aminoglycosides as part of multiple antibiotic therapy their causal role, if any, is unclear. Infrequent effects reported for gentamicin include

anaemia, purpura, convulsions, visual disturbances, increased serum aminotransferase values, and increased serum-bilirubin concentrations.

A review of the toxicity of gentamicin.— W. L. Hewitt, *Postgrad. med. J.*, 1974, *50*, (Nov.), *Suppl.* 7, 55.

ALLERGY. An anaphylactic reaction to gentamicin in one patient. Collapse with tachycardia, hypotension, and apnoea occurred within a minute of starting to inject 80 mg intravenously.— F. J. Hall (letter), *Lancet*, 1977, *2*, 455. A large or concentrated dose of an antibiotic could produce adverse effects due to the release of endotoxin in patients whose bloodstreams contained a heavy infection of Gram-negative bacteria. This should be considered as a cause of anaphylaxis. One patient had died in endotoxic shock 20 minutes after receiving gentamicin intravenously for a suspected heavy bacteraemia following surgical disturbance of a large pelvic abscess.— D. A. B. Hopkin (letter), *ibid.*, 603.

Of 15 438 hospital inpatients monitored by the Boston Collaborative Drug Surveillance Program between 1975 and 1982 allergic skin reactions were detected in 3 of 670 patients given gentamicin.— M. Bigby *et al.*, *J. Am. med. Ass.*, 1986, *256*, 3358.

EFFECTS ON THE BLOOD. There have been isolated reports of gentamicin producing adverse effects on the blood including granulocytopenia (R. Bussien, *Nouv. Presse méd.*, 1974, *3*, 1236), reversible agranulocytosis (J.C. Chang and B. Reyes, *J. Am. med. Ass.*, 1975, *232*, 1154), and thrombocytopenia (J.-H. Chen *et al.*, *N.Y. St. J. Med.*, 1980, *80*, 1134).

See also under Effects on Immune Function, below.

EFFECTS ON THE EAR. Although all aminoglycosides are potentially ototoxic they vary in the degree of impairment they produce in cochlear and vestibular function. Ototoxicity appears to be related to accumulation of aminoglycosides in the perilymph and endolymph and as subsequent elimination is slow it can occur even after discontinuation of therapy. Because destroyed or damaged cochlear hair cells are unable to regenerate, ototoxicity is often irreversible and is cumulative in nature being related to the dose and duration of therapy.

As aminoglycosides may be absorbed from serous surfaces and mucous membranes ototoxicity has occurred not only after parenteral administration but also following topical application to burns and wounds and after irrigation of body cavities especially with agents such as neomycin. It has been suggested that ototoxicity occurs more frequently with gentamicin when peak serum concentrations exceed 10 to 12 µg per mL, but evidence from clinical studies is conflicting (M. Wenk *et al.*, *Clin. Pharmacokinet.*, 1984, *9*, 475). Others consider that ototoxicity is more commonly associated with sustained rather than peak concentrations (J.M. Symonds, *J. antimicrob. Chemother.*, 1978, *4*, 199; I. Phillips, *Lancet*, 1982, *2*, 311). However, despite monitoring of aminoglycoside concentrations, ototoxicity may still occur. Ototoxicity does not correlate well with development of symptoms; many patients found to have measurable ototoxicity are asymptomatic (L. Koegel, *Am. J. Otol.*, 1985, *6*, 190).

Other risk factors for ototoxicity may be similar to those suggested for nephrotoxicity (see under Effects on the Kidney) (A. Whelton, *J. clin. Pharmac.*, 1985, *25*, 67) but may also include noise and increased susceptibility in the neonate and the elderly. However, the clinical value of many of these factors for predicting toxicity remains to be confirmed in clinical studies. A retrospective study by Moore *et al.* (*J. infect. Dis.*, 1984, *149*, 23) indicated that duration of therapy, total aminoglycoside dosage, elevated body temperature, bacteraemia, liver dysfunction, and the initial ratio of serum concentrations of urea nitrogen and creatinine were associated with increased risk of ototoxicity.

Whether aminoglycoside therapy contributes significantly to deafness in preterm infants requiring intensive care may be difficult to ascertain because of the multiple insults to which they are exposed, however, it has been suggested that there is little evidence to support the belief that it does (*Lancet*, 1985, *1*, 1373). Finitzo-Hieber *et al.* (*J. Pediat.*, 1985, *106*, 129) found no significant difference in the incidence of hearing impairment in neonates given amikacin or netilmicin compared with matched controls but the number of patients involved may have been too small to detect an increased incidence (P. Davey, *Lancet*, 1985, *2*, 612). Although concurrent use of ethacrynic acid is considered to potentiate the auditory toxicity of the aminoglycosides the use of frusemide does not appear to be an important factor (see under Precautions, below).

Retrospective reviews (L.A. Cone, *Clin. Ther.*, 1982, *5*, 155; G. Kahlmeter and J.I. Dahlager, *J. antimicrob. Chemother.*, 1984, *Suppl. A.*, 9) indicate that netilmicin is less cochleotoxic than gentamicin and tobramycin which are each less toxic than amikacin; netilmicin also exhibited the least vestibular toxicity while gentamicin, tobramycin, and amikacin were of similar toxicity.

A report of vestibular toxicity associated with gentamicin and presenting as severe rombergism.— R. Duncan and I. D. Melville (letter), *Br. med. J.*, 1987, *295*, 1141.

EFFECTS ON ELECTROLYTE HOMOEOSTASIS. Hypomagnesaemia, hypocalcaemia, and hypokalaemia have been reported when aminoglycoside antibiotics have been administered for prolonged periods (G.L. Goodhart and S. Handelsman, *Ann. intern. Med.*, 1985, *103*, 645; R. Wilkinson *et al.*, *Br. med. J.*, 1986, *292*, 818) especially in patients with leukaemia or other malignant diseases also receiving antineoplastic agents (M.J. Keating *et al.*, *Cancer*, 1977, *39*, 1410; P. Davey *et al.*, *J. antimicrob. Chemother.*, 1985, *15*, 623— see also under Antineoplastic Agents, p.581). Renal tubular leakage of magnesium may persist for several months after the end of treatment. Electrolyte status should be monitored when aminoglycoside antibiotics are given for prolonged periods or with antineoplastic agents.

EFFECTS ON THE EYE. For a report of severe retinal ischaemia associated with intra-ocular injection of gentamicin, see under Local Irritant Effects, below.

EFFECTS ON IMMUNE FUNCTION. Although aminoglycoside antibiotics have been reported to interfere with human polymorphonuclear leucocyte function *in vitro* (M.M. Seklecki *et al.*, *Antimicrob. Ag. Chemother.*, 1978, *13*, 552; J.M. Oleske, *J. antimicrob. Chemother.*, 1984, *13*, 413) Venezio and DiVincenzo (*Antimicrob. Ag. Chemother.*, 1985, *27*, 712) found that function was unimpaired *in vivo*.

EFFECTS ON THE KIDNEY. The nephrotoxicity of gentamicin and the other aminoglycosides has been reviewed by Luft (*J. antimicrob. Chemother.*, 1984, *13*, *Suppl.* A, 23) and Whelton (*J. clin. Pharmac.*, 1985, *25*, 67). Aminoglycoside antibiotics accumulate in the renal cortex and produce morphological changes in the proximal tubular cells. Impairment of renal function is usually mild and non-oliguric but acute tubular necrosis and interstitial nephritis have occurred (O. Kourilsky *et al.*, *Medicine, Baltimore*, 1982, *61*, 258). The first clinical signs of nephrotoxicity may include an increase in the excretion of renal tubular enzymes in the urine, proteinuria, and the appearance of urinary casts and although these signs have been used by some clinicians as an early indicator of renal toxicity their clinical usefulness remains to be determined. A decrease in glomerular filtration-rate is usually seen only after several days of therapy and may even occur after therapy has been discontinued. Impairment of renal function is usually reversible on discontinuation of therapy. Associated electrolyte disturbances (see under Effects on Electrolyte Homoeostasis, above) may occur rarely. A Fanconi syndrome has also been reported in one patient (J.C. Russo and R.D. Adelman, *J. Pediat.*, 1980, *96*, 151). Although nephrotoxicity has been associated with plasma trough concentrations of gentamicin greater than 2 µg per mL (M.E. Burton *et al.*, *Clin. Pharmacokinet.*, 1985, *10*, 1) evidence from clinical studies is conflicting (M. Wenk *et al.*, *Clin. Pharmacokinet.*, 1984, *9*, 475) and nephrotoxicity may still occur despite monitoring to ensure that trough concentrations are maintained below this value (J.J. Schentag *et al.*, *Antimicrob. Ag. Chemother.*, 1982, *21*, 721). A number of other risk factors for developing aminoglycoside nephrotoxicity have been suggested by findings from *animal* studies including duration of therapy, dehydration, hypokalaemia, age, sex, pre-existing renal dysfunction, liver disease, and recent prior therapy with aminoglycosides or other nephrotoxic agents. Although there is some confirmatory evidence from studies in humans for a number of these factors (R.D. Moore *et al.*, *Ann. intern. Med.*, 1984, *100*, 352; A. Whelton, *J. clin. Pharmac.*, 1985, *25*, 67; C.L. Sawyers *et al.*, *J. infect. Dis.*, 1986, *153*, 1062) some still consider they have limited value in predicting toxicity (F.C. Luft, *J. antimicrob. Chemother.*, 1984, *13*, *Suppl.* A, 23; Y.W.F. Lam *et al.*, *J. Am. med. Ass.*, 1986, *255*, 639).

While *animal* studies have indicated differences in nephrotoxicity between the aminoglycosides (G.A. Porter *et al.*, *J. clin. Pharmac.*, 1983, *23*, 445) there is little clinical evidence to support these findings in humans. Although many studies have been conducted to determine the relative incidence of nephrotoxicity for the aminoglycosides it is often difficult to evaluate the results due to the use of different criteria to denote nephrotoxicity. Furthermore, few of the studies have adopted a rigorous trial methodology. Several retrospective reviews have failed to reveal any major difference between the nephrotoxicity of gentamicin, tobramycin, amikacin, and netilmicin, although there is some evidence to suggest that netilmicin may be less nephrotoxic than these other aminoglycosides and tobramycin may be slightly less nephrotoxic than gentamicin (L.A. Cone, *Clin. Ther.*, 1982, *5*, 155; G. Kahlmeter and J.I. Dahlager, *J. antimicrob. Chemother.*, 1984, *13*, *Suppl.* A, 9; W.S. Burkle, *Clin. Pharm.*, 1986, *5*, 514). However, since renal impairment is usually mild any difference may have little clinical significance and other factors may be more important in selecting which aminoglycoside to use (F.C. Luft, *J. antimicrob. Chemother.*, 1984, *13*, *Suppl.* A, 23). It has also been suggested that differences in incidence may be related to the severity of the infection itself as nephrotoxicity may be potentiated by the release of bacterial endotoxin (M.G. Bergeron and Y. Bergeron, *Antimicrob. Ag. Chemother.*, 1986, *29*, 7).

Aminoglycoside-induced auditory toxicity (see under Effects on the Ear, above) and nephrotoxicity appear to be independent events (C.R. Smith *et al.*, *Antimicrob. Ag. Chemother.*, 1979, *15*, 780).

Some controversy exists over whether an aminoglycoside used in association with a cephalosporin antibiotic results in increased nephrotoxicity. Evidence for cephalothin has been conflicting (see p.177) and few studies have been conducted on the relative effect of other cephalosporins.

Following results suggesting that neonates may be less susceptible than adults to gentamicin-induced nephrotoxicity (D.B. Haughey, *et al.*, *J. Pediat.*, 1980, *96*, 325) Tessin *et al.* (*Archs Dis. Childh.*, 1982, *57*, 758) found that despite increased concentrations of urinary enzymes indicating damage to proximal tubule cells no other signs of nephrotoxicity could be detected in neonates during treatment with gentamicin.

EFFECTS ON MENTAL STATE. Visual hallucinations were reported in 3 patients who had each received a total of 880 mg, 780 mg, and 1200 mg of gentamicin respectively by intramuscular injection; normal mental states were recovered within 72 hours of withdrawal of gentamicin.— G. J. Byrd (letter), *Drug Ther.*, 1976, *6*, 11. See also G. J. Byrd, *J. Am. med. Ass.*, 1977, *238*, 53.

EFFECTS ON THE NERVOUS SYSTEM. Review of the literature reveals that in *animal* studies administration of aminoglycosides such as gentamicin by the intracisternal or intraventricular route has been associated with various types of neurotoxicity including ventriculitis and ataxia (S.R. Snavely and G.R. Hodges, *Ann. intern. Med.*, 1984, *101*, 92). There have also been rare isolated clinical reports of meningeal irritation and arachnoiditis with polyradiculitis in patients given gentamicin and tobramycin intrathecally (I. Watanabe *et al.*, *Ann. Neurol.*, 1978, *4*, 564; J. W. Hollifield *et al.*, *J. Am. med. Ass.*, 1976, *236*, 1264); meningeal irritation has also been associated with streptomycin administered by this route. Although one study group (G.H. McCracken *et al.*, *Lancet*, 1980, *1*, 787) found that the death-rate was unexpectedly high in infants with meningitis given intraventricular gentamicin in addition to parenteral antibiotics when compared to infants receiving parenteral therapy only, the contribution of gentamicin-neurotoxicity if any to the outcome remains unclear.

There has also been a report of polyneuropathy and, in part, encephalopathy following [parenteral] administration of gentamicin (A. Bischoff *et al.*, *Schweiz. med. Wschr.*, 1977, *107*, 3).

Benign intracranial hypertension in a 26-year-old man with cystic fibrosis was attributed to gentamicin which had been given, 80 mg intramuscularly twice daily, for 5 days prior to his admission to hospital with headaches and transient blurring of vision. Gentamicin was discontinued on the second day in hospital and the headaches subsided.— R. Boe and C. S. Conner (letter), *J. Am. med. Ass.*, 1973, *226*, 567.

A patient experienced convulsions following the use of gentamicin to irrigate the needle-puncture site of a lumbar laminectomy. The convulsions may have been due to leakage of gentamicin into the subdural space through the puncture.— R. C. Marcove and M. R. Rask, *J. neurol. orthop. Med. & Surg.*, 1985, *6*, 123.

EFFECTS ON THE NEUROMUSCULAR SYSTEM. Aminoglycoside antibiotics have produced a curare-like neuromuscular blockade leading to muscular paralysis and respiratory depression. Most cases have been associated with the use of aminoglycosides in patients undergoing general anaesthesia and those receiving other drugs with neuromuscular blocking activity. Other patients at risk include those with renal failure, myasthenia gravis and other diseases affecting neuromuscular transmission. Potentiation of neuromuscular weakness has also been reported in a neonate with hypermagnesaemia (C.S. L'Hommedieu *et al.*, *J. Pediat.*, 1983, *102*, 629) and in neonates with botulism (J.I. Santos *et al.*, *Pediatrics*, 1981, *68*, 50). Blockade has usually been associated with intraperitoneal or intrapleural instillation of large doses but there have been reports following parenteral or oral administration especially in patients at risk (J.L. Holtzmann, *Ann. intern. Med.*, 1976, *84*, 55). Although all aminoglycosides may produce neuromuscular blockade neomycin appears to have the most potent action and several deaths have been associated with its use (C.B. Pittinger *et al.*, *Anaesth. Analg.*, 1970, *49*, 487). The exact mechanism for the neuromuscular blockade remains to be determined but appears to be due to both pre- and postsynaptic action on acetylcholine release and uptake (F.L. Mastaglia, *Drugs*, 1982, *24*, 304); it may be reversed by the administration of calcium salts; the use of neostigmine has been less successful (A.G. Paradelis, *J. antimicrob. Chemother.*, 1979, *5*, 737).

EFFECTS ON THE SKIN. See also under Allergy, above.

Alopecia. A 15-year-old boy complained of dizziness, tinnitus, and blurred vision during treatment with gentamicin, and there was progressive loss of hair and eyebrows. The blood concentration of gentamicin was 14 µg per mL. Hair began to grow again when treatment was discontinued.— H. Yoshioka and I. Matsuda (letter), *J. Am. med. Ass.*, 1970, *211*, 123.

LOCAL IRRITANT EFFECTS. There have been several reports of cutaneous necrosis following subcutaneous administration of gentamicin in patients also receiving anticoagulant therapy (J. Taillandier *et al.*, *Presse méd.*, 1984, *13*, 1574; D. Penso *et al.*, *ibid.*, 1575; M.S. Doutre *et al.*, *Thérapie*, 1985, *40*, 266).

A report of 5 patients with severe retinal ischaemia associated with intra-ocular injection of gentamicin. Three of the patients had erroneously received large doses of gentamicin in mistake for other ophthalmic solutions. The cause of toxicity in the other 2 patients was unclear but may have been related to the technique of administration. It was recommended that all intravitreal injections should be performed slowly, in the anterior vitreous, with the needle bevel upwards.— H. R. McDonald *et al.*, *Ophthalmology*, 1986, *93*, 871.

Following examination of nearly 200 sites of administration there was no evidence to confirm a previous report by Blakey *et al.* (*Pharm. J.*, 1987, *2*, 541) that intravenous infusion of gentamicin over short periods increased the incidence of thrombophlebitis.— A. Willson and J. F. Hecker (letter), *Pharm. J.*, 1987, *2*, 572.

OVERDOSAGE. An accidental overdose of 160 mg of gentamicin (2 mg per kg body-weight) instead of 2 mg was given intrathecally on two occasions to a patient; the only signs of toxicity were transient calf pain and weakness.— J. Smilack and R. V. McCloskey (letter), *Ann. intern. Med.*, 1972, *77*, 1002.

Treatment of Adverse Effects

Aminoglycoside antibiotics may be removed by haemodialysis or to a lesser extent by peritoneal dialysis. Calcium salts given intravenously have been used to counter neuromuscular blockade; the effectiveness of neostigmine has been variable.

Haemoperfusion through acrylic resin-coated charcoal together with haemodialysis removed about 70% of the gentamicin given, in excessive dosage, to an anuric patient.— N. Wright and A. Bhamjee, *Postgrad. med. J.*, 1980, *56*, 140.

Complexation of gentamicin or tobramycin with ticarcillin was considered to be as effective as haemodialysis for reduction of excessive serum-aminoglycoside concentrations and appeared to have a lower risk of adverse effects. Patients with elevated amikacin concentrations may obtain less benefit as amikacin does not readily form complexes with ticarcillin.— J. J. Schentag *et al.*, *Pharmacotherapy*, 1984, *4*, 374.

For reference to studies indicating that gentamicin is removed from serum during arteriovenous haemofiltration, see under Uses, Administration in Renal Failure, p.243.

Precautions

Gentamicin is contra-indicated in patients with a known history of allergy to it and probably to other aminoglycosides. If symptoms of ototoxicity occur gentamicin should be withdrawn immediately.

Although gentamicin should be given with care and in reduced dosage to patients with impaired renal function the pharmacokinetics of gentamicin and other aminoglycosides are affected by many other factors and disease states and dosage requirements in all patients are best determined by individual monitoring. The dosage should be adjusted if the plasma concentration of gentamicin approaches 10 to 12 µg per mL or if the concentration immediately before the next dose exceeds 2 µg per mL.

Aminoglycosides should be avoided in patients with myasthenia gravis and care should be exerted when they are given to patients receiving other drugs with a neuromuscular blocking activity or which are ototoxic or nephrotoxic. Antiemetics may mask ototoxic symptoms.

Since aminoglycosides have been shown to be incompatible with beta-lactam antibiotics such as carbenicillin sodium *in vitro* (see Incompatibility, above), these antibiotics should be administered separately when both are required. No antagonism has been shown *in vivo* except when these two antibiotics have been used together in patients with severe renal impairment, when the activity of the aminoglycoside has been diminished.

Many workers consider that aminoglycosides such as gentamicin that are given systemically should not be used topically because of the serious risk of developing bacterial resistance.

Neomycin and netilmicin, but not tobramycin, were found to have antithyroid activity. Whereas netilmicin produced a significant decrease in serum concentrations of tri-iodothyronine, neomycin significantly reduced serum concentrations of both tri-iodothyronine and thyroglobulin. Although the antithyroid activity of aminoglycosides may not be of clinical significance in patients with an intact hypothalamic-thyroid axis it might be of importance in patients with low concentrations of tri-iodothyronine or in those receiving thyroxine.— P. du Souich *et al.*, *Clin. Pharmac. Ther.*, 1985, *38*, 686.

INTERACTIONS. *Antimicrobial agents.* Aminoglycoside antibiotics are inactivated if mixed *in vitro* with ticarcillin or carbenicillin or some other beta-lactam antibiotics. Although there have been occasional reports of reduced concentrations of aminoglycoside (J.E. McLaughlin and D.S. Reeves, *Lancet*, 1971, *1*, 261; J. Murillo *et al.*, *J. Am. Med. Ass.*, 1979, *241*, 2401) in patients with normal renal function this effect does not usually appear to be of clinical significance (S. Eykyn *et al.*, *Lancet*, 1971, *1*, 545) if these agents are administered at separate sites because the relative time of contact *in vivo* is minimal. However in patients with renal failure contact time is longer and the degree of inactivation may be sufficient to reduce antimicrobial efficacy. For *in vitro* reports of the relative inactivating potential of some of the beta-lactam antibiotics and the relative resistance of the aminoglycosides to inactivation, see Incompatibility, p.236. *In vivo* ticarcillin has been variously reported to inactivate gentamicin to a greater or lesser degree than carbenicillin (F.R. Ervin *et al.*, *Antimicrob. Ag. Chemother.*, 1976, *9*, 1004; H. Konishi *et al.*, *ibid.*, 1983, *23*, 653); piperacillin and mezlocillin appear to produce less inactivation than ticarcillin or carbenicillin (M.I.B. Thompson *et al.*, *Antimicrob. Ag. Chemother.*, 1982, *21*, 268; H. Konishi *et al.*, *ibid.*, 1983, *23*, 653; A.-F. Viollier *et al.*, *J. antimicrob. Chemother.*, 1985, *15*, 597). Studies and reports indicate that amikacin may be less susceptible to inactivation than gentamicin (D.C. Blair *et al.*, *Antimicrob. Ag. Chemother.*, 1982, *22*, 376) and that gentamicin may be less susceptible than tobramycin (G.R. Matzke *et al.*, *Pharmacotherapy*, 1984, *4*, 158). However, these differences may not necessarily be reflected in relative clinical efficacy because of differences in the initial activity of these combinations.

In a retrospective study, the incidence of aminoglycoside-related toxicity, including ototoxicity, nephrotoxicity, and drug rashes, appeared to be significantly increased when mezlocillin rather than ticarcillin was used with gentamicin in the treatment of pyrexia in 25 patients with leukaemia (E.M. Rankin *et al.*, *J. antimicrob. Chemother.*, 1984, *14*, 411). However, many aspects of this study have been criticised and Noone *et al.* (*J. antimicrob. Chemother.*, 1985, *15*, 785) have reported that in a properly controlled randomised study involving many more patients there was no evidence of excessive toxicity associated with the use of mezlocillin with an aminoglycoside.

High concentrations (18.75 mg per mL) of sulphacetamide increased the mean bactericidal concentration of gentamicin *in vitro* against 37 strains of *Pseudomonas aeruginosa*. As such concentrations are often reached the use of sulphacetamide with gentamicin in the treatment of eye infections was not recommended.— L. M. Burger *et al.*, *Am. J. Ophthal.*, 1973, *75*, 314.

Serum concentrations of gentamicin were higher than expected in 2 renal transplant patients also receiving flucytosine.— P. Noone *et al.*, *Br. med. J.*, 1978, *2*, 470.

Results indicating that concurrent administration of amphotericin significantly increases the serum half-life of gentamicin and tobramycin in children.— C. F. Stewart *et al.*, *Clin. Pharmac. Ther.*, 1984, *35*, 277.

For reports and discussions on the incidence of nephrotoxicity when aminoglycosides are administered with other antimicrobial agents see under Cephalothin Sodium, p.177 and under Vancomycin Hydrochloride, p.333.

For reports on the effects of other drugs on the antimicrobial activity of gentamicin, see p.239.

Cisplatin. Apart from the risk of additive nephrotoxicity and increased renal wasting of magnesium when cisplatin and aminoglycosides are used together cisplatin has been shown to significantly reduce gentamicin elimination. Both renal function and magnesium status should be monitored when these agents are used together.— *Drug Interact. News.*, 1985, *5*, 49.

Diuretics. Concomitant administration of frusemide has been shown to increase the nephrotoxicity and the ototoxicity of the aminoglycosides in *animal* studies (I. Ohtani *et al.*, *Chemotherapy, Tokyo*, 1977, *25*, 2348). Studies of the effect of frusemide on the pharmacokinetics of aminoglycosides have produced differing results. While some workers (W.J. Tilstone *et al.*, *Clin. Pharmac. Ther.*, 1977, *22*, 389; D.H. Lawson *et al.*, *J. clin. Pharmac.*, 1982, *22*, 254) found that frusemide reduced the renal and plasma clearance of gentamicin with resultant increases in plasma concentrations. Whiting *et al.* (*Br. J. clin. Pharmac.*, 1981, *12*, 795) found that frusemide and piretanide both increased the renal clearance of gentamicin. From an evaluation of data obtained from randomised double-blind controlled studies Smith and Lietman (*Antimicrob. Ag. Chemother.*, 1983, *23*, 133) concluded that frusemide administration should not be considered a major risk factor for the development of nephrotoxicity or ototoxicity with aminoglycosides; they noted, however, that the use of ethacrynic acid with an aminoglycoside may cause severe auditory toxicity.

Indomethacin. Peak and trough serum concentrations of gentamicin or amikacin were significantly increased in 20 preterm infants with patent ductus arteriosus when indomethacin was added to treatment. A significant increase in mean serum creatinine concentrations and decreases in serum concentrations of sodium and chloride also occurred; 6 of the infants developed hyponatraemia. It appears advisable to reduce aminoglycoside dosage prior to starting therapy with indomethacin.— Y. Zarfin *et al.*, *J. Pediat.*, 1985, *106*, 511.

INTERFERENCE WITH ASSAY PROCEDURES. The implications of drug interference with assays for aminoglycoside antibiotics have been reviewed by Yosselson-Superstine (*Clin. Pharmacokinet.*, 1984, *9*, 67). A number of other antimicrobial agents and antineoplastic antibiotics may alter the results of microbiological assays but this might be overcome by selection of an appropriate assay organism. Microbiological assays for aminoglycosides in samples also containing imipenem could be accomplished by using cysteine hydrochloride to inactivate imipenem since it is stable to most beta-lactamases and resistant strains are extremely rare (K.M. McLeod *et al.*, *J. antimicrob. Chemother.*, 1986, *17*, 828). Because aminoglycoside antibiotics may be inactivated by penicillins and cephalosporins it has been recommended that aminoglycoside sampling times should be chosen to coincide with a trough plasma concentration for the beta-lactam antibiotic. Samples should also be frozen if there is to be a delay before they are assayed (R.J. Tindula *et al.*, *Drug Intell. & clin. Pharm.*, 1983, *17*, 906) or a penicillinase added. However, one group of workers have reported loss of gentamicin activity after storage at −60° before assay (L.G. Carlson *et al.*, *Antimicrob. Ag. Chemother.*, 1982, *21*, 192). Furthermore, there have been reports that concentrations of aminoglycosides in patients also receiving beta-lactam antibiotics are overestimated using a homogenous enzyme immunoassay, probably because of an inability to differentiate between active drug and inactivated products (S.C. Ebart and W.A. Clementi, *Drug Intell. & clin. Pharm.*, 1983, *17*, 451; C. Dalmady-Israel *et al.*, *Ann. intern. Med.*, 1984, *100*, 460). The radionuclide gallium-67 interferes with radio-enzymatic assays and it has been suggested that an agar diffusion method should be used in patients who have received a gallium scan (I. Bhattacharya *et al.*, *Antimicrob. Ag. Chemother.*, 1978, *14*, 448; K. Shannon *et al.*, *J. antimicrob. Chemother.*, 1980, *6*, 285). Heparin has been shown to produce underestimation of aminoglycoside concentrations when using microbiological, enzymatic, or immunoassays (L. Nilsson, *Antimicrob. Ag. Chemother.*, 1980, *17*, 918 and 1980, *18*, 839; L. Nilsson *et al.*, *ibid.*, 1981, *20*, 155; M.B.

O'Connell *et al.*, *Drug Intell. & clin. Pharm.*, 1984, *18*, 503). It has been recommended that either serum should be used or that blood samples should not be collected in heparinised tubes or from indwelling catheter lines. Some consider that concentrations of heparin reached in the blood of patients receiving heparin are too low to affect gentamicin (C. Regamey *et al.*, *Antimicrob. Ag. Chemother.*, 1972, *1*, 329). Falsely low concentrations have also been reported in microbiological assays in the presence of zinc salts (R.H. George and D.E. Healing, *J. antimicrob. Chemother.*, 1978, *4*, 186).

Heat treatment of whole blood to inactivate human immunodeficiency virus leads to an increase in the concentration of gentamicin subsequently found on assay, apparently due to lysis of red blood cells. The clinical significance of this effect is unclear.— A. Eley *et al.* (letter), *Lancet*, 1987, *2*, 335.

INTERFERENCE WITH DIAGNOSTIC TESTS. Aminoglycoside antibiotics did not interfere with determination of urinary glucose concentrations carried out with either copper-reduction (Clinitest) or glucose oxidase (Diastix or TesTape) methods (M.E. MacCara and W.A. Parker, *Am. J. Hosp. Pharm.*, 1981, *38*, 1340; W.A. Parker and M.E. MacCara, *ibid.*, 1984, *41*, 125).

PREGNANCY AND THE NEONATE. If given during pregnancy aminoglycosides, including gentamicin sulphate, might cause damage to the eighth cranial nerve of the foetus.— *Med. Lett.*, 1987, *29*, 61.

Antimicrobial Action

Gentamicin and other aminoglycoside antibiotics interfere with bacterial protein synthesis by binding primarily to the 30S subunit of bacterial ribosomes. Other mechanisms of action may contribute to the bactericidal effect of gentamicin. It is effective against many strains of Gram-negative bacteria including species of *Campylobacter, Citrobacter, Escherichia, Enterobacter, Klebsiella, Proteus, Providencia, Pseudomonas,* and *Serratia.* Minimum inhibitory concentrations have been reported to range from 0.06 to 8 μg per mL.

Among the Gram-positive organisms most strains of *Staphylococcus aureus* are highly sensitive to gentamicin with minimum inhibitory concentrations being reported within the range of 0.12 to 1 μg per mL. *Listeria monocytogenes* and some strains of *Staph. epidermidis* may also be sensitive to gentamicin. Although gentamicin has only low or no activity against enterococci and streptococci, enhanced activity may occur *in vitro* when ampicillin or benzylpenicillin are added. Enhanced activity may also occur against *Ps. aeruginosa* between gentamicin and antipseudomonal penicillins such as carbenicillin. Some mycoplasmas have been reported to be sensitive to gentamicin; anaerobic organisms, yeasts, and fungi are resistant.

It is more active in an alkaline medium.

For a comprehensive review of the antimicrobial mode of action of the aminoglycoside antibiotics, see R. E. W. Hancock, *J. antimicrob. Chemother.*, 1981, *8*, 249 and 429.

Apart from the three main components, gentamicin C_1, gentamicin C_{1A}, and gentamicin C_2, gentamicin contains several minor components including gentamicin C_{2A} (the 6'-*C* epimer of gentamicin C_2) and C_{2B} (micronomicin). Recently the C_{2A} component has been found to be present in commercial samples of gentamicin in higher proportions than previously thought, but as it has a similar activity *in vitro* to the C_2 component this increase will not change the activity of gentamicin.— L. Verbist *et al.* (letter), *J. antimicrob. Chemother.*, 1985, *15*, 250.

The activity of 11 aminoglycoside antibiotics was tested *in vitro* against nearly 800 clinical isolates of Gram-negative aerobic bacteria and staphylococci obtained mainly from immunocompromised patients who had received multiple antibiotic therapy. Between 20 and 30% of the strains of *Pseudomonas aeruginosa, Proteus mirabilis,* and indole-positive *Proteus* and 82% of coagulase-negative staphylococci were resistant to gentamicin. However, resistance to amikacin and netilmicin was less common and there were only slight differences between the activities of these two aminoglycosides. Although netilmicin was active against fewer isolates than amikacin, it was generally more active on a weight for weight basis. Gentamicin, tobramycin, and sissomicin had similar activity to each other except that sissomicin was the most active against *Proteus mirabilis* and gentamicin was the most active against *Serratia* spp. While tobramycin was the most active against *Ps. aeruginosa* it was also the least active against *Escherichia coli.* Dibekacin had a similar spectrum of activity to these agents but was marginally more active against *Ps. aeruginosa.* Of all the aminoglycosides tested the newer aminoglycoside pentisomicin (5-epi-sissomicin) had the best all round activity. It inhibited over 92% of the strains tested and was also the most active aminoglycoside against *Ps. aeruginosa.* Another new aminoglycoside, isepamicin, also had good activity and was the most active against staphylococci and indole-positive *Proteus* spp.— M. A. Guimaraes *et al.*, *J. antimicrob. Chemother.*, 1985, *16*, 555. See also T. O. Kurtz *et al.*, *Antimicrob. Ag. Chemother.*, 1980, *18*, 645.

ACTIVITY AGAINST GRAM-NEGATIVE BACTERIA. *Activity against Acinetobacter.* Report of a study showing good activity of aminoglycosides against *Acinetobacter calcoaceticus in vitro* and in urinary-tract infections in *mice.*— Y. Obana *et al.*, *J. antimicrob. Chemother.*, 1985, *15*, 441. Discussion of decreasing susceptibility of *A. calcoaceticus* to aminoglycosides, and mechanisms of resistance.— M. L. Joly-Guillou *et al.*, *J. antimicrob. Chemother.*, 1987, *20*, 773.

Activity against Aeromonas. An *in-vitro* study of the activity of 22 antimicrobial agents against 60 strains of *Aeromonas* spp. including *A. hydrophila* indicated that 90% of the isolates were inhibited by 1 μg per mL of gentamicin and 2 μg per mL of amikacin; tobramycin was generally less active. Cefotaxime and tetracycline were the most active of all the agents tested.— M. R. Motyl *et al.*, *Antimicrob. Ag. Chemother.*, 1985, *28*, 151.

Activity against Branhamella. Studies indicating that beta-lactamase-producing and non-beta-lactamase-producing strains of *Branhamella catarrhalis* were inhibited by gentamicin and other aminoglycosides *in vitro* at clinically achievable concentrations.— E. E. Stobberingh *et al.*, *J. antimicrob. Chemother.*, 1984, *13*, 55; K. G. Sweeney *et al.*, *Antimicrob. Ag. Chemother.*, 1985, *27*, 499.

Activity against Campylobacter. Gentamicin has been found to be one of the most active of antimicrobial agents *in vitro* against various species of *Campylobacter* (C.J. Gebhart *et al.*, *Antimicrob. Ag. Chemother.*, 1985, *27*, 55) including erythromycin-resistant strains of *Campylobacter jejuni* (R. Vanhoof *et al.*, *Antimicrob. Ag. Chemother.*, 1978, *14*, 553; M. Walder, *ibid.*, 1979, *16*, 37; J. Michel *et al.*, *ibid.*, 1983, *23*, 796). Although gentamicin is also very active against *C. pyloridis*, this species, unlike other *Campylobacter*, is more susceptible to benzylpenicillin and erythromycin (C.A.M. McNulty *et al.*, *Antimicrob. Ag. Chemother.*, 1985, *28*, 837).

Activity against Citrobacter. A study of the *in-vitro* antimicrobial susceptibility of 27 strains of *Citrobacter freundii* and 14 of *C. diversus.* Amikacin and imipenem were among the most active of the 16 agents tested. For *C. freundii*, MICs were in the following ranges: amikacin 0.25 to 4 μg per mL, gentamicin less than 0.06 to 16 μg per mL, and netilmicin less than 0.06 to 32 μg per mL. For *C. diversus*, MICs were: amikacin 0.3 to 2 μg per mL, gentamicin 0.25 to 64 μg per mL, and netilmicin 0.25 to 2 μg per mL.— G. Samonis *et al.*, *Antimicrob. Ag. Chemother.*, 1987, *31*, 829.

Activity against Legionella. Gentamicin was shown to be bactericidal *in vitro* against *Legionella micdadei* at readily achievable concentrations. Poor clinical outcome in patients with pneumonia due to *L. micdadei* treated with aminoglycosides cannot therefore be ascribed to lack of bactericidal action.— J. N. Dowling *et al.*, *Antimicrob. Ag. Chemother.*, 1982, *22*, 272.

Activity against Pseudomonas. A study of the antibacterial activity of aminoglycoside antibiotics against *Pseudomonas aeruginosa* in peritoneal dialysis fluid.— I. Shalit *et al.*, *Antimicrob. Ag. Chemother.*, 1985, *27*, 908.

Activity against Yersinia. Studies *in vitro* have indicated that most strains of *Yersinia* spp. are inhibited by 1 μg per mL of gentamicin, tobramycin, or netilmicin, 2 μg per mL of neomycin, or 8 μg per mL of amikacin or kanamycin (M. Raevuori *et al.*, *Antimicrob. Ag. Chemother.*, 1978, *13*, 888; A.M. Lewis and B. Chattopadhyay, *J. antimicrob. Chemother.*, 1987, *3*, 406). However, Lewis and Chattopadhyay questioned the clinical significance of these results as most *Yersinia* infections were usually self-limiting. Furthermore, they had found ciprofloxacin to be the most active agent against *UK* strains with all isolates being inhibited by 0.03 μg per mL.

ACTIVITY AGAINST MYCOBACTERIA. For reference to the activity of gentamicin against atypical *Mycobacterium* spp., see Amikacin Sulphate, p.110.

While very large doses of amikacin, streptomycin, and kanamycin had significant activity against *Mycobacterium leprae* in *mice*, gentamicin and tobramycin were relatively inactive. Further *animal* studies of the aminoglycosides for use against *M. leprae* alone or in combination with rifampicin are in progress.— R. H. Gelber *et al.*, *Lepr. Rev.*, 1984, *55*, 341.

ACTIVITY AGAINST STAPHYLOCOCCI. See under Resistance, below.

ACTIVITY WITH OTHER ANTIMICROBIAL AGENTS. The activity of the aminoglycosides has been evaluated *in vitro* with a variety of antimicrobial agents against a wide range of organisms. Addition of agents such as beta lactams which disrupt the bacterial cell wall may enhance the penetration of aminoglycosides into the organism and thus increase their activity. Enhanced activity has sometimes been demonstrated for certain combinations, particularly against *Pseudomonas aeruginosa, Staphylococcus aureus*, and the enterococci. The activity of the various combinations may vary greatly according to the aminoglycoside and other antimicrobial agent used (T.M. Hooton *et al.*, *Antimicrob. Ag. Chemother.*, 1984, *26*, 535).

The activity of aminoglycosides with other antimicrobial agents against *Ps. aeruginosa* has been discussed by Baltch and Smith (*Am. J. Med.*, 1985, *79*, *Suppl.* 1A, 8); enhanced activity has been obtained for the aminoglycosides when used with the antipseudomonal penicillins including carbenicillin, ticarcillin, piperacillin, azlocillin, and mezlocillin, several of the cephalosporins, and with some other beta-lactam antibiotics such as latamoxef and aztreonam (R. Skalova *et al.*, *J. antimicrob. Chemother.*, 1982, *9*, 103; R.K. Scribner *et al.*, *Antimicrob. Ag. Chemother.*, 1982, *21*, 939; H.O. Hallander *et al.*, *ibid.*, *22*, 743; H. Giamarellou *et al.*, *ibid.*, 1984, *25*, 534; M.A. Buseing and J.H. Jorgenson, *ibid.*, 283; M.D. Lyon *et al.*, *ibid.*, 1986, *30*, 25; J.A. Bosso *et al.*, *ibid.*, 1987, *31*, 1403). However, results may be unpredictable, the effect on activity sometimes depending on the test method or the strain used (P.K.W. Yu *et al.*, *Antimicrob. Ag. Chemother.*, 1983, *23*, 179; J.W. King and R.L. Penn, *ibid.*, 1984, *25*, 770). The activity of gentamicin against *Ps. aeruginosa* has been reported to be antagonised to some degree by several agents including: calcium and magnesium ions (D.N. Gilbert *et al.*, *J. infect. Dis.*, 1971, *124*, *Suppl.*, S37), colistin (S.D. Davis and A. Iannetta, *Appl. Microbiol.*, 1972, *23*, 775), sulphacetamide, sulphafurazole (L.M. Burger *et al.*, *Am. J. Ophthal.*, 1973, *75*, 314), acetylcysteine (M.F. Parry and H.C. Neu, *J. clin. Microbiol.*, 1977, *5*, 58).

Although some other antimicrobial agents such as cefotaxime and cephazolin (M. Bourque *et al.*, *Antimicrob. Ag. Chemother.*, 1976, *10*, 157; A.M. Elliott *et al.*, *ibid.*, 1983, *24*, 847) have been reported to enhance the activity of the aminoglycosides to some degree against the enterococci, activity *in vitro* is usually greatest when combined with a penicillin (M.J. Basker and R. Sutherland, *J. antimicrob. Chemother.*, 1977, *3*, 273; S.A. Calderwood *et al.*, *Antimicrob. Ag. Chemother.*, 1977, *12*, 401; J.J. Rahal and M.S. Simberkoff, *J. antimicrob. Chemother.*, 1986, *17*, 585). High-level resistance of enterococci to gentamicin, however, has been reported to prevent synergy with penicillin (P.J. Sanderson, *Br. med. J.*, 1984, *289*, 638). See also Resistance of Enterococci under Resistance p.240, and Endocarditis under Uses, p.243.

Antimicrobial agents reported to enhance the activity of gentamicin against staphylococci include some penicillins (C.U. Tuazon *et al.*, *Curr. ther. Res.*, 1978, *23*, 760; R.J.P. Hemmer *et al.*, *Antimicrob. Ag. Chemother.*, 1979, *15*, 34; C. Watanakunakorn and C. Glotzbecker, *J. antimicrob. Chemother.*, 1979, *5*, 151) and some cephalosporins (J. Klastersky, *Antimicrob. Ag. Chemother.*, 1972, *1*, 441; R.L. Marier *et al.*, *ibid.*, 1975, *8*, 571). Lowy *et al.*, (*Antimicrob. Ag. Chemother.*, 1979, *16*, 314) found that although the use of cephalothin, vancomycin, or rifampicin with gentamicin did not improve the bactericidal activity of gentamicin against methicillin-resistant strains of *Staphlococcus epidermidis in vitro* the emergence of gentamicin-resistant strains was suppressed. Lowy *et al.* also found that in *mice* the most effective regimen was vancomycin with gentamicin; however, there was an increased death-rate when cephalothin or nafcillin were used with gentamicin but this was not due to drug-drug inactivation. Yu *et al.* (*J. antimicrob. Chemother.*, 1984, *14*, 359) have also demonstrated enhanced activity *in vitro* for the triple combination of gentamicin, vancomycin, and rifampicin. The actions of gentamicin and coumermycin have been reported to be antagonistic *in vitro* against *Staph. aureus* (B.R. Meyers *et al.*, *Antimicrob. Ag. Chemother.*, 1985, *28*, 706).

Although enhanced activity has been obtained against *Listeria monocytogenes* by using gentamicin and ampicillin together (G.L. Wiggins *et al.*, *Antimicrob. Ag. Chemother.*, 1978, *13*, 854) the use of gentamicin with erythromycin for penicillin-allergic patients may offer no advantage as antagonism has occurred when these two agents have been tested together *in vitro* (R.L. Penn *et al.*, *Antimicrob. Ag. Chemother.*, 1982, *22*, 289).

The activity of the aminoglycosides is poor against anaerobic bacteria or other bacteria under anaerobic conditions (A.V. Reynolds *et al.*, *Lancet*, 1976, *1*, 447) and the effect of gentamicin on the activity of metronidazole or clindamycin against anaerobic bacteria including *Bacteroides fragilis* has been varied (I. Brook *et al.*, *Antimicrob. Ag. Chemother.*, 1984, *25*, 71; I. Brook and R.I. Walker, *J. antimicrob. Chemother.*, 1984, *15*, 31; B.A.C. Dijkmans *et al.*, *ibid.*, 77). There have been reports of clindamycin antagonising the activity of gentamicin against aerobic bacteria (P.D. Meers, *Lancet*, 1973, *2*, 573; R.J. Snyder *et al.*, *Antimicrob. Ag. Chemother.*, 1975, *7*, 333) although some workers have failed to confirm these findings (E. Ekwo and G. Peter, *Antimicrob. Ag. Chemother.*, 1976, *10*, 893; J. Klastersky and M. Husson, *ibid.*, 1977, *12*, 135).

Diminished activity has also been reported for gentamicin against some species of bacteria in the presence of the antineoplastic agents actinomycin D, cytarabine, daunorubicin, or doxorubicin but activity has been reported to be enhanced in the presence of mitomycin (M.R. Moody *et al.*, *Antimicrob. Ag. Chemother.*, 1978, *14*, 737; J.Y. Jacobs *et al.*, *ibid.*, 1979, *15*, 580). Chloramphenicol and gentamicin may also be antagonistic *in vitro* (P.J. Sanderson, *Lancet*, 1978, *2*, 210; A.P. Panwalker *et al.*, *Antimicrob. Ag. Chemother.*, 1980, *18*, 877).

Further reports of enhanced activity for the aminoglycosides with other antimicrobial agents *in vitro* include:

Enterobacteriaceae—Fass *et al.*, *Antimicrob. Ag. Chemother.*, 1976, *10*, 34 (minocycline); Neu and Fu, *ibid.*, 1978, *13*, 813 (azlocillin); Paisley and Washington, *ibid.*, *14*, 656 (co-trimoxazole); Bayer *et al.*, *ibid.*, 1984, *25*, 725 (cephalosporins); *Klebsiella* spp.—Klastersky *et al.*, *Am. J. med. Sci.*, 1971, *262*, 283 (cephalothin); D'Alessandri *et al.*, *Antimicrob. Ag. Chemother.*, 1976, *10*, 889 (cephalothin); Panwalker *et al.*, *ibid.*, 1980, *18*, 877 (beta-lactam antibiotics); *Serratia marcescens*—Markowitz and Sibilla, *ibid.*, 1980, *18*, 651 (cephalosporins).

Streptococci—Cooper *et al.*, *Animicrob. Ag. Chemother.*, 1979, *15*, 484 (ampicillin); Lam and Bayer, *ibid.*, 1984, *26*, 260 (benzylpenicillin, vancomycin, or cefotaxime).

Lactobacilli—Bayer *et al.*, *ibid.*, 1980, *17*, 359 (ampicillin or benzylpenicillin).

MICROBIOLOGICAL TEST METHODS. There have been problems associated with the accuracy of some microbiological assays and susceptibility tests for the aminoglycosides and the reliability of some agar diffusion tests has been evaluated against *E. coli* and *Staph. aureus* (G. Kahlmeter, *J. antimicrob. Chemother.*, 1980, *6*, 43). Error-rates associated with newly proposed breakpoints for disk agar diffusion tests against *Ps. aeruginosa* suggest this method may have limitations and dilution tests have been recommended instead (B.F. Woolfrey *et al.*, *Antimicrob. Ag. Chemother.*, 1983, *24*, 764). False readings of susceptibility to aminoglycosides may also be obtained for *Ps. aeruginosa* or methicillin-resistant staphylococci using a semi-automated testing system (Autobac I) (J.B. Mayo, *Antimicrob. Ag. Chemother*, 1982, *21*, 412). Addition of sodium chloride to growth media has been reported to interfere with susceptibility testing of staphylococci and some *Vibrio* spp. (S.W. Joseph *et al.*, *Antimicrob. Ag. Chemother.*, 1978, *13*, 244; J.M. Campos *et al.*, *ibid.*, 1986, *29*, 152). Calcium and magnesium ions have also been reported to antagonise the antimicrobial action of the aminoglycosides (see under Activity with other Antimicrobial Agents, above). Since enterococci highly resistant to aminoglycosides are unlikely to be inhibited even by the usually synergistic combination of penicillin and aminoglycoside antibiotics a disk sensitivity test has been developed to distinguish between these organisms and enterococci with the usual degree of susceptibility to the aminoglycosides (S.L. Rosenthal and L.F. Freundlich, *J. antimicrob. Chemother.*, 1982, *10*, 459).

Resistance

Widespread use of aminoglycoside antibiotics has led to an increase in the incidence of resistance found in staphylococci, enterococci, *Pseudomonas aeruginosa*, the Enterobacteriaceae, and other Gram-negative organisms.

The incidence of resistance to aminoglycosides appears generally to be higher in the *US* than in Europe.

Resistance to the aminoglycoside antibiotics occurs by three main mechanisms. The first is by mutation leading to reduced affinity for binding to ribosomal target sites; this type of resistance is generally only relevant for streptomycin and then it appears to be rare in Gram-negative bacteria. Secondly, penetration of aminoglycosides into bacterial cells is by an oxygen-dependent active transport process and resistance may also occur because of elimination or reduction of this uptake; this mechanism not infrequently affects all aminoglycosides and leads to some degree of cross-resistance. However, by far the most important cause of resistance to the aminoglycosides is inactivation by enzymatic modification. Enzyme production is plasmid-determined and resistance can be acquired by conjugation or transfer of these resistance factors between bacteria, even between organisms of different species. Multiple-resistance to unrelated antibacterials may also be transferred at the same time. Although numerous individual enzymes have been found they usually belong to one of three main classes: *O*-phosphotransferases, *O*-nucleotidyltransferases or adenyltransferases, and *N*-acetyltransferases. Each enzyme produces a characteristic pattern of resistance among the aminoglycosides depending on the presence or absence of the specific chemical group within the aminoglycoside. The overlapping substrate profiles of individual enzymes can result in a wide range of permutations for cross-resistance within the aminoglycoside antibiotics. Some organisms have also been found to possess the ability to produce more than one inactivating enzyme. While some of these enzymes are widely distributed among bacteria the occurrence of others may be more limited. The prevalence of individual enzymes varies according to geographical location and time but there appears to be no clear relationship to usage of individual aminoglycosides. Amikacin and, to a lesser degree, netilmicin are both susceptible to fewer inactivating enzymes than the other aminoglycosides.

It was considered that gentamicin 240 mg daily would be effective only against very susceptible bacteria with an MIC of up to 1 µg per mL.— R. Bickenbach *et al.*, *Arzneimittel-Forsch.*, 1977, *27*, 2023.

A discussion of resistance to antibiotics related to topical use.— *Br. med. J.*, 1978, *2*, 649.

Despite reports of simultaneous resistance to aminoglycosides and beta-lactam antibiotics emerging in *Pseudomonas aeruginosa* and *Serratia marcescens* during therapy (L.C. Preheim *et al.*, *Antimicrob. Ag. Chemother.*, 1982, *22*, 1037; C.C. Sanders and C. Watanakunakorn, *J. infect. Dis.*, 1986, *153*, 617) findings of an *in vitro* study by Stratton *et al.* (*J. antimicrob. Chemother.*, 1987, *19*, 21) suggest that this is a rare phenomenon.

For reference to the change in the incidence of gentamicin resistance in Gram-negative bacteria after replacement of gentamicin by amikacin as the aminoglycoside of routine use, see Amikacin Sulphate, p.110.

RESISTANCE OF ACINETOBACTER. See under Antimicrobial Action, above.

RESISTANCE OF ENTEROBACTERIACEAE. Of 232 strains of enteropathogenic *Escherichia coli* none was resistant to gentamicin at a concentration of 4 µg per mL.— R. J. Gross *et al.*, *Br. med. J.*, 1982, *285*, 472.

Studies indicating that development of resistance to nitrofurantoin and associated resistance to aminoglycoside antibiotics in *E. coli* may be R-plasmid mediated or due to impaired bacterial uptake of these agents.— E. E. Obaseiki-Ebor and A. S. Breeze, *J. antimicrob. Chemother.*, 1984, *13*, 567; A. S. Breeze and E. E. Obaseiki-Ebor, *ibid.*, *14*, 477.

Of 2753 strains of *Shigella dysenteriae*, *Sh. flexneri*, and *Sh. boydii* examined at the Central Public Health Laboratory from 1979 to mid 1983, 0.5% were resistant to gentamicin at a concentration of 4 µg per mL.— R. J. Gross *et al.*, *Br. med. J.*, 1984, *288*, 784.

A survey of resistance to gentamicin among *Salmonella* spp. in India between 1973 and 1982. Of the isolates tested in 1982 2.1% were resistant to 10 µg or more per mL of gentamicin but a peak of nearly 19% had been found for isolates tested in 1979.— S. Ahuja *et al.*, *Antonie van Leeuwenhoek*, 1984, *50*, 161.

Reports from the *UK* and France indicate that the intensive use of apramycin in *animal* husbandry has led to the emergence of apramycin- and gentamicin-resistant strains of *Salmonella typhimurium* in both cattle and humans (E. J. Threlfall *et al.*, *J. antimicrob. Chemother.*, 1986, *18*, *Suppl.* C, 175; E. Chaslus-Dancla *et al.*, *Antimicrob. Ag. Chemother.*, 1986, *29*, 239).

RESISTANCE OF ENTEROCOCCI. A discussion on enterococci with special reference to the emergence of high-level resistance to gentamicin. Unlike most other streptococci, enterococci are resistant to the majority of antibiotics, including most beta lactams. Even antibiotics, such as penicillin, ampicillin, and vancomycin, that do have intrinsic activity against enterococci are not bactericidal against most strains; however, combinations of these agents with aminoglycosides do achieve bactericidal synergy even though the MICs of the aminoglycosides typically range from 6 to 64 µg per mL. Enterococci have become progressively more resistant to antimicrobial agents such as erythromycin and the tetracyclines, but the evolution of aminoglycoside resistance has been of greatest clinical significance. For many years enterococci have been known to have differing rates of high-level resistance to streptomycin, kanamycin, and amikacin, but as recently as 1977 a study of clinical isolates found no high-level resistance to gentamicin. However, in 1979, Horodniceanu *et al.* (*Antimicrob. Ag. Chemother.*, 1979, *16*, 686) reported isolates of *Enterococcus faecalis* (*Streptococcus faecalis*) resistant to gentamicin concentrations of more than 16 000 µg per mL. Other reports followed and high-level resistance to gentamicin has now been shown to be endemic in many parts of the *US* and to be present in other countries including the *UK*. It is mediated by plasmids which are usually transferable and organisms are generally resistant to all other aminoglycosides, except occasionally streptomycin. High-level resistance to gentamicin invariably entails the loss of bactericidal synergy between gentamicin and a penicillin or vancomycin.— S. A. Hoffmann and R. C. Moellering, *Ann. intern. Med.*, 1987, *106*, 757.

RESISTANCE OF PSEUDOMONAS. Of 1866 isolates of *Pseudomonas aeruginosa* from British hospitals studied in a 3-month survey during 1982, 5.5% were resistant to gentamicin (MIC greater than 2 µg per mL) and 9.6% to carbenicillin (MIC greater than 128 µg per mL). In contrast to findings in the *US*, there was little evidence of increased resistance of *Ps. aeruginosa* to gentamicin in the *UK* and both these antipseudomonal agents appeared to have largely retained their activity.— R. J. Williams *et al.*, *J. antimicrob. Chemother.*, 1984, *14*, 9.

Further references: T. Furusawa *et al.*, *J. antimicrob. Chemother.*, 1986, *17*, 755 (resistance to gentamicin and cefsulodin in Japan); A. J. De Neeling *et al.* (letter), *ibid.*, 1987, *19*, 703 (resistance to aminoglycosides and beta-lactam antibiotics in the Netherlands).

RESISTANCE OF STAPHYLOCOCCI. An outbreak of gentamicin-resistant strains of *Staphylococcus aureus* involving 23 patients and 3 members of staff in the Dermatological Unit of a hospital appeared to be associated with the increased topical use of gentamicin.— T. D. Wyatt *et al.*, *J. antimicrob. Chemother.*, 1977, *3*, 213. More than 10% of isolates of coagulase-negative staphylococci survived despite exposure *in vitro* for 4 hours to concentrations of gentamicin or streptomycin greater than those used for topical prophylaxis in neurosurgical procedures.— P. R. Fischer *et al.*, *Antimicrob. Ag. Chemother.*, 1984, *25*, 502.

Evidence suggesting a new mechanism of resistance to gentamicin in *Staphylococcus aureus*.— R. R. Cutler, *J. antimicrob. Chemother.*, 1983, *11*, 263.

A report of probable chromosomal mutation in *Staph. aureus* conferring resistance to all aminoglycosides following the therapeutic use of gentamicin.— J. Heritage *et al.*, *J. antimicrob. Chemother.*, 1986, *17*, 571.

For a discussion on gentamicin resistance in methicillin-resistant strains of *Staphylococcus aureus*, including the appearance of simultaneous resistance to antiseptic agents, see under Resistance in Methicillin Sodium, p.259.

All infants admitted to a special-care baby unit during a 3-month study subsequently became colonised with strains of coagulase-negative staphylococci resistant to gentamicin and benzylpenicillin, and often to other antibiotics. Similar strains were found in the environment and nasal carriage was detected in up to 60% of the staff of the unit.— R. A. Simpson *et al.*, *J. Hosp. Infect.*, 1986, *7*, 108. Isolates of coagulase-negative staphylococci from two special-care baby units demonstrated resistance to gentamicin if there had been considerable previous exposure to an aminoglycoside. Netilmicin was reported to be the most active aminoglycoside against these organisms.— A. J. Davies *et al.*, *J. antimicrob. Chemother.*, 1986, *17*, 155.

Absorption and Fate

Gentamicin and other aminoglycosides are poorly absorbed from the gastro-intestinal tract but are rapidly absorbed after intramuscular injection. Average peak plasma concentrations of about 4 µg per mL have been obtained 30 to 60 minutes after intramuscular administration of a dose equivalent to 1 mg of gentamicin per kg body-weight although there may be considerable individual variation and higher concentrations in patients with renal failure. Similar concentrations are obtained after intravenous administration. Several doses are required before equilibrium concentrations are obtained in the plasma and this may represent the saturation of binding sites in body tissues such as the kidney. Binding of gentamicin to plasma proteins is usually low.

Following parenteral administration gentamicin and other aminoglycosides diffuse mainly into extracellular fluids and factors which affect the volume of distribution will also affect plasma concentrations. However, there is little diffusion into the cerebrospinal fluid and even when the meninges are inflamed effective concentrations may not be achieved; diffusion into the eye is also poor. Aminoglycosides diffuse readily into the perilymph of the inner ear. Gentamicin crosses the placenta but only small amounts have been reported in breast milk.

Systemic absorption of gentamicin and other aminoglycosides has been reported after topical use on denuded skin and burns and following instillation into and irrigation of wounds, body-cavities, and joints.

The plasma elimination half-life for gentamicin has been reported to be 2 to 3 hours though it may be considerably longer in neonates and patients with renal impairment. Gentamicin and other aminoglycosides do not appear to be metabolised and are excreted virtually unchanged in the urine by glomerular filtration. At steady-state at least 70% of a dose may be recovered in the urine in 24 hours and urine concentrations in excess of 100 µg per mL may be obtained. However, gentamicin and the other aminoglycosides appear to accumulate in body tissues to some extent, mainly in the kidney, although the relative degree to which this occurs may vary with different aminoglycosides. Release from these sites is slow and aminoglycosides may be detected in the urine for up to 20 days or more after administration ceases. Small amounts of gentamicin appear in the bile.

A review of the clinical pharmacokinetics of aminoglycoside antibiotics.— J. -C. Pechere and R. Dugal, *Clin. Pharmacokinet.*, 1979, *4*, 170.

The pharmacokinetics of gentamicin have been found to be altered by many disease states and other factors, especially those that affect the volume of distribution and the rate of glomerular filtration including:

age (L.A. Bauer and R.A. Blouin, *Eur. J. clin. Pharmac.*, 1983, *24*, 639);

blood disorders and neoplastic disease (R.P. Manny and P.R. Hutson, *Clin. Pharm.*, 1986, *5*, 629);

body-weight and obesity (I. Sketris *et al.*, *J. clin. Pharmac.*, 1981, *21*, 288; L.A. Bauer *et al.*, *Eur. J. clin. Pharmac.*, 1983, *24*, 643; M.M. Tointon *et al.*, *Clin. Pharm.*, 1987, *6*, 160);

burns (R.J. Sawchuk and T.S. Rector, *Clin. Pharmacokinet.*, 1980, *5*, 548);

cystic fibrosis (G.L. Kearns *et al.*, *J. Pediat.*, 1982, *100*, 312; N.E. McDonald *et al.*, *ibid.*, 1983, *103*, 985; L.A. Bauer *et al.*, *Clin. Pharm.*, 1983, *2*, 262; J.A. Bosso *et al.*, *ibid.*, 1987, *6*, 54);

intravenous drug abuse (C.H. King *et al.*, *Antimicrob. Ag. Chemother.*, 1985, *27*, 285);

kwashiorkor and protein intake (N. Buchanan *et al.*, *Br. J. clin. Pharmac.*, 1979, *8*, 451; C.J. Dickson *et al.*, *Clin. Pharmac. Ther.*, 1986, *39*, 325);

pregnancy (see under Pregnancy and the Neonate, below);

sepsis (H.J. Mann *et al.*, *Clin. Pharm.*, 1987, *6*, 148);

spinal cord injury (J.L. Segal *et al.*, *Clin. Pharm.*, 1984, *3*, 418 and *Curr. ther. Res.*, 1986, *39*, 961);

surgery (D.D. Kloth *et al.*, *Clin. Pharm.*, 1985, *4*, 182).

While some workers (J.F. Giudicelli and J.P. Tillement, *Clin. Pharmacokinet.*, 1977, *2*, 157) have found that there are sex-linked differences in gentamicin pharmacokinetics they did not consider dosage modification to be warranted.

Renal clearance of gentamicin was not significantly affected by changes of urine pH.— C. Mariel *et al.* (letter), *Br. med. J.*, 1972, *2*, 406.

Intrathecal injections of gentamicin 4 mg given to 12 patients produced CSF concentrations of up to 45 µg per mL which were eliminated within 2 to 24 hours to residual concentrations of 0.3 µg per mL. At 14 hours the concentrations in all samples were 7.8 µg or less.— J. J. Rahal (letter), *Ann. intern. Med.*, 1972, *77*, 1003.

The disposition of gentamicin C_1, C_{1a} and C_2.— R. L. Nation *et al.*, *Eur. J. clin. Pharmac.*, 1978, *13*, 459.

Comparison of methods for estimating gentamicin clearance.— P. G. Davey *et al.*, *Br. J. clin. Pharmac.*, 1984, *17*, 147.

Further references to the pharmacokinetics of gentamicin: C. Thuillier *et al.* (letter), *J. antimicrob. Chemother.*, 1977, *3*, 527; J. J. Schentag and W. J. Jusko (letter), *Lancet*, 1977, *1*, 486; G. Kahlmeter *et al.*, *J. antimicrob. Chemother.*, 1978, *4*, 143; O. L. Laskin *et al.*, *Clin. Pharmac. Ther.*, 1983, *34*, 644.

ABSORPTION. Absorption of gentamicin from wounds.— H. H. Stone *et al.*, *Am. Surg.*, 1968, *34*, 639.

Systemic absorption ranged from 1.5 to 34% in patients with pneumonia who were given gentamicin (1 patient) or tobramycin (9 patients) by endotracheal instillation; all had a creatinine clearance of 40 or more mL per minute. Although some patients absorbed significant amounts of aminoglycosides, serum concentrations above 1 µg per mL did not occur.— S. S. Crosby *et al.*, *Antimicrob. Ag. Chemother.*, 1987, *31*, 850.

ADMINISTRATION. For reference to the modification of gentamicin doses according to plasma-gentamicin concentrations in all patients, including those with renal impairment, see under Uses, Administration and Administration in Renal Failure, p.242.

ADMINISTRATION IN INFANTS AND CHILDREN. The pharmacokinetics of gentamicin in neonates have been briefly reviewed by Morselli *et al.* (*Clin. Pharmacokinet.*, 1980, *5*, 485) and Edwards (*Pharm. J.*, 1986, *2*, 518). The volume of distribution of gentamicin in neonates and children is greater than that in adults and therefore neonates require larger doses to achieve similar serum concentrations (see under Administration in Infants and Children in Uses). As gentamicin and other aminoglycoside antibiotics are eliminated primarily unchanged by glomerular filtration through the kidney the rate of clearance is low in neonates, especially the premature, who have relatively immature renal function. The elimination half-life for gentamicin therefore decreases as renal function matures and some studies have found clearance to be related to postconceptional age; reported values have ranged from 9.5 hours in neonates of less than 28 weeks' gestation to about 5 hours at 39 weeks (S.J. Szefler *et al.*, *J. Pediat.*, 1980, *97*, 312; J.W. Kasik *et al.*, *ibid.*, 1985, *106*, 502; C. Edwards, *Pharm. J.*, 1986, *2*, 518).

Some further references to the pharmacokinetics of gentamicin in infants and children: D. B. Haughey *et al.*, *J. Pediat.*, 1980, *96*, 325 (premature neonates); K. W. Hindmarsh *et al.*, *Eur. J. clin. Pharmac.*, 1983, *24*, 649 (low birth-weight preterm infants); K. E. Zenk *et al.*, *Clin. Pharm.*, 1984, *3*, 170 (effect of body-weight on neonatal pharmacokinetics); A. W. Kelman *et al.*, *Br. J. clin. Pharmac.*, 1984, *18*, 685 (clearance and volume of distribution in neonates and children); G. Koren *et al.*, *Pediat. Pharmacol.*, 1985, *5*, 79 (low birth-weight preterm infants).

ADMINISTRATION, INTRANASAL. A mean serum concentration of 2.48 µg per mL was obtained in 7 healthy subjects 30 minutes after intranasal administration of gentamicin 2 mg per kg body-weight in a solution with sodium glycocholate 1%. Concentrations were similar to those obtained after an intramuscular dose of 0.3 mg per kg. Gentamicin was undetectable in the serum when sodium glycocholate was omitted from the solution. There was slight nasal irritation after a single dose.— A. Rubinstein, *Antimicrob. Ag. Chemother.*, 1983, *23*, 778.

DIALYSIS. Gentamicin was rapidly absorbed from the peritoneal cavity in patients undergoing continuous ambulatory peritoneal dialysis with about 49% of the dose added to the dialysate being absorbed over a 6-hour period. However, it was estimated that it may take as long as 48 hours for equilibrium to be achieved between serum and peritoneal fluid. Dialysis clearance was low and 48 hours of dialysis would be necessary to remove 50% of the amount of gentamicin absorbed.— S. Pancorbo and C. Comty, *Antimicrob. Ag. Chemother.*, 1981, *19*, 605. See also M. de Paepe *et al.*, *Clin. Nephrol.*, 1983, *19*, 107.

DIFFUSION INTO BODY TISSUES AND FLUIDS. Gentamicin is widely distributed in body tissues and fluids following intramuscular or intravenous administration but concentrations are usually lower than those in serum.

Although biliary concentrations of gentamicin are usually 30 to 40% of those in serum (H.A. Pitt *et al.*, *J. infect. Dis.*, 1973, *127*, 299; J. Mendelson *et al.*, *Antimicrob. Ag. Chemother.*, 1973, *4*, 538) concentrations 2 to 4 times higher than those in serum have been obtained in gall-bladder tissue in patients with acute cholecystitis which may explain the effectiveness of gentamicin in hepatobiliary infections (B.A. Cunha *et al.*, *Curr. ther. Res.*, 1981, *30*, 522).

Diffusion into bronchial secretions is poor and endotracheal administration has been used to obtain therapeutic concentrations (W. Odio *et al.*, *J. clin. Pharmac.*, 1975, *15*, 518).

Antibacterial concentrations are not achieved in the vitreous humour and are variable in the aqueous humour following parenteral administration or topical application of gentamicin and intravitreal and subconjunctival injection respectively are required to treat infections at these sites (M.B.R. Mathalone and A. Harden, *Br. J. Ophthal.*, 1972, *56*, 609; J.S. Hillman *ibid.*, 1979, *63*, 794).

Richey and Schleupner (*Antimicrob. Ag. Chemother.*, 1981, *19*, 312) considered diffusion of gentamicin into peritoneal fluid to be therapeutically adequate in cirrhotic patients with spontaneous peritonitis when serum concentrations were also maintained in the therapeutic range. However, Lapalus *et al.* (*Thérapie*, 1983, *38*, 247) found that intraperitoneal administration was necessary to achieve therapeutic concentrations in ascitic fluid in similar patients with ascites. Creatsas *et al.* (*Int. J. clin. Pharmac. Biopharm.*, 1979, *17*, 225) considered that concentrations of gentamicin obtained in cervical fluid, mucus, and menses would be sufficient for the treatment of certain genital infections.

Therapeutic concentrations have been obtained in synovial fluid after intramuscular injection of gentamicin (D.C. Marsh *et al.*, *J. Am. med. Ass.*, 1974, *228*, 607) and some consider that intra-articular injections may not be necessary in the treatment of infectious arthritis (T.H. Dee and F. Kozin, *Antimicrob. Ag. Chemother.*, 1977, *12*, 548).

Aminoglycosides have been reported to penetrate into burn eschar in therapeutic concentrations (R.E. Polk *et al.*, *Archs Surg.*, 1983, *118*, 295).

Studies in humans and *animals* have shown that gentamicin accumulates in the kidney with most drug being concentrated in the renal cortex (C.Q. Edwards *et al.*, *Antimicrob. Ag. Chemother.*, 1976, *9*, 925).

Schentag and Jusko (*Lancet*, 1977, *1*, 486) reported that 40% of the total amount of gentamicin in the body was present in the kidney. Accumulation appears to be due to tubular reabsorption followed by active transport of gentamicin into the renal cortex (C.H. Hsu, *Antimicrob. Ag. Chemother.*, 1977, *12*, 192); tissue concentrations in patients with renal failure have been low or undetectable (W.M. Bennett *et al.*, *J. Lab. clin. Med.*, 1977, *90*, 389). Whether high concentrations are of benefit in the therapy of pyelonephritis appears to be a matter of controversy (M.G. Bergeron, *J. antimicrob. Chemother.*, 1985, *15*, 4). The relative amount of reabsorption and accumulation varies between the aminoglycosides.

PREGNANCY AND THE NEONATE. Gentamicin 40 mg given by intramuscular injection to 37 pregnant women just before delivery produced a mean peak serum concentration of 3.65 µg per mL within 30 minutes and a peak of 1.25 µg per mL in the cord serum within 1 to 2 hours.— H. Yoshioka *et al.*, *J. Pediat.*, 1972, *80*, 121.

The rate of elimination of gentamicin has been reported to be increased during pregnancy and immediately postpartum probably due to increases in renal blood flow and glomerular filtration (D.E. Zaske *et al.*, *Obstet. Gynec.*, 1980, *56*, 559; D.K. Gardner and P.J. Schneider, *Clin. Pharm.*, 1984, *3*, 416). However, compared to other postpartum patients McNeeley *et al.* (*Am. J. Obstet. Gynec.*, 1985, *153*, 793) found that elimination was significantly longer in those with severe pre-eclampsia.

See also under Administration in Infants and Children, above.

PROTEIN BINDING. Results of studies on the protein binding of gentamicin have been conflicting and reported values have ranged from 0 to 30%. While Ramirez-Ronda *et al.* (*Antimicrob. Ag. Chemother.*, 1975, *7*, 239) found no significant binding to serum proteins under physiological conditions, in studies by Myers *et al.* (*Clin. Pharmac. Ther.*, 1978, *23*, 356) gentamicin was about 20% protein bound under the same conditions. However, both groups of workers agreed that gentamicin binding was enhanced in the absence of calcium and magnesium ions. Ramirez-Ronda suggested that although under normal conditions binding did not appear to be of clinical significance it might be in certain pathological states. Myers *et al.* were unable to demonstrate a significant difference between the binding capacity of serum from healthy subjects and that from uraemic patients receiving chronic haemodialysis but did find that protein binding appeared to be increased in the presence of heparin due to direct binding of gentamicin to heparin.

Uses and Administration

Gentamicin sulphate is an aminoglycoside antibiotic and is used to treat septicaemia, including neonatal sepsis, and other severe systemic infections due to sensitive Gram-negative organisms. It is also used in the treatment and prophylaxis of endocarditis due to streptococci, enterococci, and sometimes staphylococci. It has been used for surgical infection prophylaxis. Gentamicin is often given in association with other antibiotics either to delay the development of resistance or because of reported synergy *in vitro*. It may be given with an antipseudomonal penicillin or cephalosporin for the treatment of pseudomonal infections, with ampicillin or benzylpenicillin for enterococcal and streptococcal infections, or with metronidazole or clindamycin for mixed aerobic-anaerobic infections. Gentamicin and other antibiotics should be administered separately (see Incompatibility, p.236).

Doses of gentamicin sulphate are expressed in terms of gentamicin base. It is usually given intramuscularly every 8 hours; the total daily dose is 3 to 5 mg of gentamicin per kg body-weight. Infants and children may be given 5 to 7.5 mg of gentamicin per kg daily in divided doses (see also under Administration in Infants and Children, below). The course of treatment should generally be limited to 7 to 10 days. As gentamicin is poorly distributed into fatty tissue some authorities suggest that dosage calculations should be based on an estimate of lean body-weight. Dosage should be reduced in renal insufficiency, but in all patients doses should be adjusted according to plasma-gentamicin concentrations. In general, peak plasma concentrations (measured about one hour after intramuscular or intravenous injection) should not exceed 10 µg per mL and trough concentrations (measured just before the next dose) should be less than 2 µg per mL, but see under Administration (below) for further details.

Gentamicin is also given intravenously; however, there is controversy over the optimum method of administration (see Administration, Intravenous Route, below). Doses for intravenous administration are the same as those used intramuscularly. It has sometimes been given by mouth for enteric infections and to suppress intestinal flora. In meningitis it has been administered intrathecally or intraventricularly usually in doses of 1 to 5 mg daily in conjunction with intramuscular therapy. Doses of 10 to 40 mg have been given by subconjunctival injection.

A bone cement impregnated with gentamicin is used in orthopaedic surgery. Acrylic beads containing gentamicin and threaded on to surgical wire are implanted in the management of bone infections.

Gentamicin is also used topically in concentrations of 0.1 to 0.3%, but as topical use may lead to the emergence of resistance it is considered inadvisable.

Reviews of the actions and uses of gentamicin and other aminoglycosides: I. Phillips, *Lancet*, 1982, *2*, 311; R. S. Edson and C. L. Terrell, *Mayo Clin. Proc.*, 1987, *62*, 916.

A review of research into new aminoglycoside antibiotics.— K. E. Price, *Antimicrob. Ag. Chemother.*, 1986, *29*, 543.

Reviews of the treatment of pseudomonal infections, including the use of aminoglycosides: S. J. Eykyn, *Br. J. Hosp. Med.*, 1984, *31*, 136; J. C. Rotschafer and L. R. Shikuma, *Drug Intell. & clin. Pharm.*, 1986, *20*, 575.

ADMINISTRATION. Clinical outcome has been shown to correlate well with plasma concentrations of gentamicin and other aminoglycoside antibiotics (R.D. Moore *et al.*, *Am. J. Med.*, 1984, *77*, 657 and *J. infect. Dis.*, 1984, *149*, 443). Depending on the nature of the infection, it is generally recommended that doses should be adjusted to achieve minimum peak concentrations of 4 to 5 µg per mL for gentamicin and tobramycin and 15 and 8 µg per mL for amikacin and netilmicin respectively (A. Richens, *Prescribers' J.*, 1983, *23*, 1; M. Wenk *et al.*, *Clin. Pharmacokinet.*, 1984, *9*, 475). However, it is still not known for how long concentrations must exceed the MIC to eradicate infection and for how long concentrations may be sub-inhibitory without allowing recrudescence (see also under Antimicrobial Action, above and under Administration, Intravenous Route, below). Although adverse effects such as ototoxicity and nephrotoxicity have been associated with peak plasma concentrations of gentamicin exceeding 10 to 12 µg per mL and trough concentrations above 2 µg per mL (see under Adverse Effects) some consider that neither concentration has proved to be a reliable indicator for toxicity (M. Wenk *et al.*, *Clin. Pharmacokinet.*, 1984, 9, 475) and there is some evidence to suggest that transiently high concentrations produced by once daily dosing may be less toxic and more effective than those following continuous administration (see under Intravenous Route, below). To complicate matters, many studies have indicated that plasma concentrations correlate poorly with dosage for gentamicin and administration of standard doses cannot be expected to produce predictable concentrations in individual patients. There appear to be many factors affecting the relationship between dose and plasma concentration for gentamicin including renal function, lean body-weight, age, fever, degree of hydration, concurrent therapy with penicillin, burns, surgical procedures, and the degree and nature of the infection and other concomitant conditions such as pregnancy and cystic fibrosis. Correlation of serum creatinine or creatinine clearance to gentamicin clearance is sometimes poor and the use of renal function alone may not be sufficient for accurate dosage calculation. Consequently it is advised that plamsa concentrations of aminoglycosides should be determined regularly; it has been suggested that patients with unstable renal function should be monitored at least 3 times a week and other patients twice weekly (R.Wise, *Lancet*, 1987, *2*, 1251).

Much controversy still exists over the best method for calculating dosage requirements for the aminoglycosides and the problem has been addressed in a review by Burton (*Clin. Pharmacokinet.*, 1985, *10*, 1). Many workers have suggested dosage regimens for individual patient groups and several predictive nomograms have been devised to aid dosage calculations including those of Hull and Sarubbi (*Ann. intern. Med.*, 1976, *85*, 183 and *ibid.*, 1978, *89*, 612). However, although they are better than the use of standard regimens many predictive algorithms assume a constant volume of distribution for aminoglycosides derived from population averages and may therefore be inappropriate in patients with atypical or changing volumes of distribution such as neonates (see under Administration in Infants and Children, below) and those with ascites or oedema. Studies (T.S. Lesar, *J. Am. med. Ass.*, 1982, *248*, 1190; D.R. Platt *et al.*, *Clin. Pharm.*, 1982, *1*, 361) have shown than nomograms predict peak and trough concentrations less reliably than methods which are based on the use of individualised pharmacokinetic parameters such as the Sawchuk-Zaske method (R.J. Sawchuk *et al.*, *Clin. Pharmac. Ther.*, 1977, *21*, 362). This method has adequately controlled gentamicin concentrations in a range of different patient groups (D.E. Zaske *et al.*, *Antimicrob. Ag. Chemother.*, 1982, *21*, 407) and survival of patients with burns was increased when gentamicin dosage was individualised for each patient compared with the use of standard dose regimens (D.E. Zaske *et al.*, *Surgery*, 1982, *91*, 142). However, some consider the Sawchuk-Zaske method impractical for routine use. Another method which uses fewer measured serum-aminoglycoside concentrations is a computerised statistical method based on Baye's theorem. It has been shown to be of similar efficacy to the Sawchuk-Zaske method (M.E. Burton *et al.*, *Clin. Pharmac. Ther.*, 1984, *35*, 230 and *Clin. Pharm.*, 1986, *5*, 143). A number of other computer programs have also been devised for dose adjustment.

Although sex-linked differences in pharmacokinetics exist for gentamicin, dosage modification does not appear to be warranted.— J. F. Giudicelli and J. P. Tillement, *Clin. Pharmacokinet.*, 1977, *2*, 157.

Intravenous route. Opinions vary on the optimum method for the intravenous administration of gentamicin. In the *USA* the manufacturers have recommended infusing a dose in 50 to 200 mL of saline or glucose solution over a period of 30 minutes to 2 hours. In the *UK* some manufacturers recommend direct intravenous injection of a 2-mL dose over 2 to 3 minutes while others recommend infusion with smaller volumes than in the *USA* and shorter infusion times or recommend that gentamicin should not be given as a slow infusion at all. Furthermore, there has been some variance in the time at which peak plasma concentrations have been measured following intravenous administration and reported peak concentrations may therefore be difficult to interpret or compare. In the *UK*, it has been suggested that peak plasma concentrations should be measured 1 hour after the start of administration as this allows for distribution and equilibration of gentamicin in extravascular tissue and as this is also the usual time for monitoring peak concentrations following intramuscular injection it would eliminate any potential source of confusion and error in aminoglycoside dosage monitoring arising from differences in the mode of administration (D.S. Reeves, *Lancet*, 1985, *2*, 1420). Stratford *et al.* (*Lancet*, 1974, *1*, 378) reported that concentrations of about 10 µg per mL were obtained 5 minutes after administration of 80 mg or 1 mg per kg body-weight of gentamicin given by intravenous injection over 2½ to 3 minutes. However, Bailey and Lynn (*Lancet*, 1974, *1*, 730) warned that toxic concentrations might be achieved as they had found that a similar rapid bolus injection had produced a peak serum concentration of 18.3 µg per mL after 2.5 minutes falling to 9.3 µg per mL at 10 minutes and 5.1 µg per mL at 1 hour. Subtherapeutic concentrations have been reported after the use of large-volume infusions of gentamicin (S. Kaumeier and P. Lücker, *Arzneimittel-Forsch.*, 1977, *27*, 1212) and some consider (T.S.J. Elliott, *Lancet*, 1985, *2*, 1184) that the use of infusions should be discouraged as they may also produce prolonged serum trough concentrations above 2 µg per mL. However, Meunier *et al.* (*J. antimicrob. Chemother.*, 1987, *19*, 225) calculated that the pharmacokinetics and the peak serum concentration of gentamicin at equilibrium were similar after a slow bolus injection or an infusion over 15 minutes. They considered that infusion over 15 minutes would avoid the large variations in peak serum concentrations obtained with longer infusion times. While some clinicians (H. Colding *et al.*, *Archs Dis. Childh.*, 1982, *57*, 602) have found that, for neonates also requiring parenteral nutrition, continuous infusion of gentamicin in the parenteral nutrition solution was as effective as, and more convenient than, intermittent intramuscular or intravenous administration others consider that the use of continuous infusion for neonates is not warranted until the nephrotoxicity and long-term hazards of this mode of administration are more clearly established (G.P. Giacoia and J.J. Schentag, *J. Pediat.*, 1986, *109*, 715). Furthermore, *animal* studies have indicated that the transiently high concentrations produced by once or twice daily administration of aminoglycosides may be more effective and less toxic than prolonged exposure to the concentrations following continuous infusions (*Lancet*, 1986, 2, 670; W.A. Craig and B. Vogelman, *Ann. intern. Med.*, 1987, *106*, 900). Feld *et al.* (*Am. J. med. Sci.*, 1977, *274*, 179) found that continuous infusion of sissomicin was not significantly more effective than intermittent infusion in the treatment of febrile episodes in cancer patients. Some favourable results have been reported after the use of once-daily administration of aminoglycosides (S.H. Powell *et al.*, *J. infect. Dis.*, 1983, *147*, 918) but experience is limited and controlled clinical studies are required.

Problems associated with the slow intravenous administration of aminoglycoside antibiotics to paediatric patients have been discussed by Smith and Crass (*Drug Intell. & clin. Pharm.*, 1984, *18*, 530). Some studies have suggested that less than 10% of a dose would be lost due to adsorption to the giving equipment and filter during in-line filtration (D.R. Nazeravich and N.H.H. Otten, *Am. J. Hosp. Pharm.*, 1983, *40*, 1961; D.F. Thompson *et al.*, *Infusion*, 1984, *8*, 31).

ADMINISTRATION IN INFANTS AND CHILDREN. Gentamicin toxicity in neonates appears to be rare and there is little evidence to suggest that the use of adult limits for peak and trough plasma concentrations of gentamicin (see above under Administration) are appropriate for neonates, infants, and children. Rylance (*Archs Dis. Childh.*, 1983, *58*, 900) suggested that manipulation of dosing intervals to conform with these concentrations could even compromise efficacy but considered that it was reasonable to use these guidelines until more definitive data is available. Dosage requirements for gentamicin in relation to its pharmacokinetics in neonates have been briefly reviewed by Edwards (*Pharm. J.*, 1986, *2*, 518). Since neonates have a higher volume of distribution for the aminoglycosides than adults higher doses are generally required to achieve comparable serum concentrations. A commonly recommended dose is 2.5 mg per kg body-weight but recommended dosage intervals vary according to age and weight. Kasik *et al.* (*J. Pediat.*, 1985, *106*, 502) have shown that postconceptional age (gestational age plus postnatal age) is more important than postnatal age for the prediction of optimal dosage for aminoglycosides and this supports findings that the renal function of neonates matures at a steady rate rather than suddenly in 2 stages at 34 to 36 weeks and one week after birth. However, most dosage recommendations still reflect the concept of an increase in renal function one week after birth. A dosage interval of 12 hours has been used for neonates of 36 or more weeks' gestation during the first week of life, followed by administration every 8 hours thereafter. Studies have indicated that for low birth-weight infants and infants of less than 35 weeks' gestation the dosage interval should be increased to 18 hours during the first week of life (S.J. Szefler *et al.*, *J. Pediat.*, 1980, *97*, 312; A.Mulhall *et al.*, *Archs Dis. Childh.*, 1983, *58*, 897; G. Koren *et al.*, *Pediat. Pharmacol.*, 1985, *5*, 79). However, Hindmarsh *et al.* (*Eur. J. clin. Pharmac.*, 1983, *24*, 649) also found that 3 mg per kg given every 24 hours was as effective and more convenient. Edwards *et al.* (*Lancet*, 1986, *1*, 508) have extended these recommendations by suggesting a dose of 2.5 mg per kg given every 24 hours to neonates of 28 weeks or less. For full-term neonates Zenk *et al.* (*Clin. Pharm.*, 1984, *3*, 170) considered that dosage did not need to be altered if they were large-for-age. For older children Rhodes and Johnson (*Mayo Clin. Proc.*, 1983, *58*, 158) have suggested the following doses given three times daily: 6 months to 5 years of age, 2.5 mg per kg; 5 to 10 years of age, 2 mg per kg; older than 10 years, 1.5 mg per kg. While Siber *et al.* (*J. Pediat.*, 1979, *94*, 135) obtained predictable peak concentrations in patients ranging from 8 months to 73 years of age when the dosage of gentamicin was based on body-surface area rather than body-weight, Evans *et al.* (*ibid.*, 139) found that the use of either method produced equally unpredictable concentrations in children. Although several nomograms have been devised for dosage prediction in neonates and young children, ideally, dosage adjustments during treatment should be determined, as for adults, by monitoring peak and trough plasma concentrations.

As plasma-gentamicin concentrations were decreased following exchange transfusion in neonates it was recommended that an attempt should be made to co-ordinate the time of exchange transfusion to precede the next scheduled dose of gentamicin.— R. M. Kliegman *et al.*, *J. Pediat.*, 1980, *96*, 927.

ADMINISTRATION IN RENAL FAILURE. Although a number of nomograms, schedules, and rules have been devised for the calculation of aminoglycoside dosage in renal failure, where possible dosage modification should be based on the monitoring of individual pharmacokinetic parameters (see under Administration, above). Standard dosage calculation methods should not be used for patients undergoing dialysis as they may require supplementary post-dialysis doses.

Methods and data for predicting removal of gentamicin by conventional haemodialysis: T. P. Gibson and H. A. Nelson, *Clin. Pharmacokinet.*, 1977, *2*, 403; D. R. Goetz, *Am. J. Hosp. Pharm.*, 1980, *37*, 1077; G. R. Matzke *et al.*, *Antimicrob. Ag. Chemother.*, 1984, *25*, 128.

Rebound of serum concentrations of aminoglycosides has been reported to occur following haemodialysis (L.A. Bauer, *Ther. Drug Monit.*, 1982, *4*, 99; C.E. Halstenson *et al.*, *Drug Intell. & clin. Pharm.*, 1984, *18*, 493), but Catolico *et al.*, (*Drug Intell. & clin. Pharm.*, 1987, *21*, 46) considered that the small increase they found might not be of clinical significance with regard to the time of determination of postdialysis concentrations.

Gentamicin has been reported to be removed from serum in patients undergoing continuous arteriovenous haemofiltration and dosage adjustments and monitoring would therefore be required in patients receiving this treatment (B.J.M. Zarowitz *et al.*, *Drug Intell. & clin. Pharm.*, 1985, *19*, 459; M.E. Lehman and K.W. Kolb, *Clin. Pharm.*, 1985, *4*, 327). An accurate knowledge of the ultrafiltration-rate is considered to be necessary for precise dosage calculation and the effect on the first dose and after any filter change of drug binding to the membrane must also be accounted for. A method for calculating the effect of ultrafiltration on aminoglycoside clearance has been outlined by Cairns (*Pharm. J.*, 1987, *2*, 222).

For recommendations on the amount of gentamicin to be added to dialysate to achieve therapeutic serum concentrations in patients undergoing continuous ambulatory peritoneal dialysis, see S. Pancorbo and C. Comty, *Antimicrob. Ag. Chemother.*, 1981, *19*, 605.

A study indicating that loss of gentamicin from dialysate may occur due to binding to the administration set during continuous ambulatory peritoneal dialysis.— M. Kane *et al.*, *Am. J. Hosp. Pharm.*, 1986, *43*, 81.

For reference to the intraperitoneal administration of aminoglycosides for the treatment of peritonitis in patients on continuous ambulatory peritoneal dialysis, see Peritonitis, below.

ANIMAL BITES. For reference to the use of aminoglycosides for the prevention or treatment of infection in animal bites, see Benzylpenicillin Sodium, p.136.

ARTHRITIS, BACTERIAL. For reference to the use of aminoglycosides in the treatment of bacterial arthritis, see Osteomyelitis, below.

BILIARY-TRACT INFECTIONS. Although biliary concentrations of aminoglycosides are less than those in serum, these agents, particularly gentamicin, may be used in antibiotic regimens for the treatment of acute cholecystitis in severely ill or septicaemic patients and of acute cholangitis. Usually an aminoglycoside, a ureidopenicillin such such as mezlocillin, or a cephalosporin such as cefotaxime are given in association with metronidazole or clindamycin to provide anaerobic cover. However various three-drug combinations of the above agents have also been used (J.S. Dooley *et al.*, *Gut*, 1984, *25*, 988; R. Munro and T.C. Sorrell, *Drugs*, 1986, *31*, 449).

ENDOCARDITIS. The British Society for Antimicrobial Chemotherapy (BSAC) has recommended the use of an aminoglycoside and a penicillin for the treatment of endocarditis, before the results of cultures are available, when there is a firm clinical diagnosis of endocarditis or if the patient is very ill (*Lancet*, 1985, *2*, 815). This combination is aimed primarily at streptococci since two-thirds of cases are caused by these organisms, although it has some activity against staphylococci. Flucloxacillin should be added if there is a strong possibility of staphylococcal infection, for example in drug addicts or in patients with skin sepsis. The penicillin is usually benzylpenicillin and the aminoglycoside, gentamicin.

In the treatment of streptococcal endocarditis when the MBC for benzylpenicillin is 1 µg or less per mL, benzylpenicillin 7.2 g daily by intravenous injection in 6 divided doses should be given with gentamicin in initial doses of 80 mg twice daily by intravenous injection; subsequent doses of gentamicin will depend upon blood concentrations. After 14 days the gentamicin should be discontinued and the benzylpenicillin replaced by amoxycillin 0.5 to 1 g three times daily by mouth for another 14 days. Probenecid may be administered concurrently. Back-titrations of serum bactericidal activity against the infecting organism should be used to monitor treatment. In the *USA* it has been recommended that endocarditis caused by viridans streptococci, *Str. bovis*, or *Str. pneumoniae* which are fully sensitive to penicillin be treated with benzylpenicillin alone for a minimum of 4 weeks especially if there are contra-indications to the use of an aminoglycoside (W.R. Wilson, *J. antimicrob. Chemother.*, 1987, *20*, *Suppl.* A, 147). The BSAC, however, recommend the addition of gentamicin to a penicillin in order to achieve the maximum bactericidal effect since this combination is usually synergistic against streptococci. If the MBC for benzylpenicillin is greater than 1 µg per mL the BSAC recommend that gentamicin should be given with penicillin for at least 4 weeks, although some workers consider that a minimum of 6 weeks' therapy is required for enterococcal endocarditis (W.R. Wilson, 1987). In patients who are allergic to penicillins, vancomycin may be substituted for benzylpenicillin.

A combination of flucloxacillin and either gentamicin or fusidic acid is recommended by the BSAC for the treatment of endocarditis caused by *Staphylococcus aureus* whether the infected valve is natural or prosthetic. The initial dose of gentamicin should be 120 mg; subsequent doses will vary from about 80 to 120 mg intravenously every 8 hours depending on the weight of the patient and blood concentrations. Flucloxacillin is given in a dose of 12 g daily in 6 divided doses by intravenous injection. The total duration of antibiotic treatment should be at least 4 weeks; however because of the relatively high blood concentrations of gentamicin required (greater than in the treatment of streptococcal endocarditis) gentamicin should seldom be continued for more than 14 days. In patients allergic to penicillins, or if the organism is resistant to methicillin or flucloxacillin, treatment should be with vancomycin alone. If endocarditis is caused by *Staph. epidermidis*, treatment may be as for *Staph. aureus* if the organisms are shown to be sensitive to these agents.

In the *USA*, streptomycin is often used in preference to gentamicin (W.R. Wilson, 1987). Although studies *in vitro* and *in animals* have suggested an equivalent response with gentamicin- and streptomycin-containing regimens, data from humans is limited (W.M. Scheld, *J. antimicrob. Chemother.*, 1987, *20*, *Suppl.* A, 71). The choice between these 2 aminoglycosides is particularly controversial in the treatment of enterococcal endocarditis since synergism has not been observed between streptomycin and penicillin *in vitro* or *in vivo* against enterococci, which are resistant to streptomycin, whereas gentamicin does appear to act synergistically with ampicillin or benzylpenicillin against most streptomycin-resistant strains. Streptomycin may be given intramuscularly in a dose of 7.5 mg per kg body-weight, up to a maximum of 500 mg every 12 hours.

The BSAC have recommended gentamicin as the aminoglycoside of choice since they consider that most physicians have experience in the administration of gentamicin and that most laboratories have experience in monitoring the blood concentrations. They do, however, state that netilmicin could be considered as an alternative to gentamicin in elderly patients or when there is impaired renal function since it is claimed to be less nephrotoxic than gentamicin.

References to the treatment of endocarditis caused by various organisms with antimicrobial regimens which include gentamicin sulphate: S. Moreno *et al.* (letter), *J. antimicrob. Chemother.*, 1986, *18*, 771 (*Haemophilus aphrophilus*); A. J. Davies *et al.*, *J. Infect.*, 1986, *12*, 169 (*Lactobacillus* spp).

Prophylaxis. The British Society for Antimicrobial Chemotherapy (BSAC) recommend the use of gentamicin in regimens for the prophylaxis of endocarditis during dental or surgical procedures in patients referred to hospital for a general anaesthetic or because they are at high risk of endocarditis (*Lancet*, 1982, *2*, 1323; *ibid.*, 1986, *1*, 1267). Although gentamicin alone is not very active against streptococci the combination of gentamicin and amoxycillin is synergistic, therefore the following regimen is recommended for patients undergoing dental procedures: amoxycillin 1 g intramuscularly in 2.5 mL of lignocaine 1% and gentamicin 120 mg intramuscularly given immediately before induction if a general anaesthetic is to be given, or if not, 15 minutes before the procedure. A further 0.5 g of amoxycillin is given by mouth 6 hours later. In children under 10 years of age the dose of amoxycillin should be halved, and the dose of gentamicin should be 2 mg per kg body-weight. Adults who are allergic to penicillins should be given vancomycin 1 g by slow intravenous infusion over 60 minutes followed by gentamicin 120 mg intravenously immediately before induction of anaesthesia. Children under 10 years may be given vancomycin 20 mg per kg followed by gentamicin 2 mg per kg. The above regimens may also be given to patients undergoing genito-urinary surgery or instrumentation and in those with prosthetic valves undergoing obstetric and gynaecological procedures, gastro-intestinal procedures, or surgery or instrumentation of the upper respiratory tract. The Council on Cardiovascular Disease in the Young (CCD) in the *USA* (S.T. Shulman, *Circulation*, 1984, *70*, 1123A) recommend similar prophylactic regimens to the BSAC but use parenteral ampicillin followed by oral phenoxymethylpenicillin instead of amoxycillin. Doses are as follows: ampicillin 1 to 2 g and gentamicin 1.5 mg per kg body-weight both administered intramuscularly or intravenously half-an-hour prior to the procedures, followed by phenoxymethylpenicillin 1 g six hours later. Alternatively the parenteral regimen may be repeated once 8 hours later. Children may be given ampicillin 50 mg per kg and gentamicin 2 mg per kg. For penicillin-allergic patients vancomycin may be used alone for dental procedures and other surgery except for that of the gastro-intestinal or genito-urinary tracts when gentamicin should be added. The BSAC considers that although vancomycin has been successfully used in the treatment of streptococcal, including enterococcal, endocarditis the combination of vancomycin and gentamicin is more reliably bactericidal.

ENTERIC INFECTIONS. *Cholera.* For the use of an aminoglycoside in association with tetracycline or chloramphenicol for the treatment of *Vibrio vulnificus* septicaemia, see Enteric Infections, Cholera, in Tetracycline Hydrochloride, p.318.

Yersiniosis. For reference to the treatment of yersiniosis including mention of the use of gentamicin for severe disease, see Tetracycline Hydrochloride, p.319.

EYE INFECTIONS. References to the use of gentamicin sulphate in infections of the eye: G. A. Peyman *et al.*, *Br. J. Ophthal.*, 1977, *61*, 260 (reduction of the incidence of endophthalmitis by a single injection of gentamicin into the anterior chamber of the eye after cataract extraction); D. V. Seal *et al.*, *ibid.*, 1982, *66*, 357 (aetiology and treatment with topical antibiotics of acute bacterial infection of the external eye); D. D. Bodé *et al.*, *ibid.*, 1985, *69*, 915 (intra-ocular use in endophthalmitis due to coagulase-negative staphylococci); D. J. Coster and P. R. Badenoch, *ibid.*, 1987, *71*, 96 (a review of 87 cases of microbial keratitis supporting the choice of gentamicin and a cephalosporin as initial topical therapy).

For the use of gentamicin eye ointment in association with intramuscular kanamycin for the treatment of gonococcal neonatal conjunctivitis, see Ceftriaxone Sodium, p.170.

GONORRHOEA. References to the use of gentamicin in the treatment of gonorrhoea: G. D. Morrison and D. S. Reeves, *Br. J. vener. Dis.*, 1973, *49*, 513; W. Bowie *et al.*, *ibid.*, 1974, *50*, 208; S. K. Hira *et al.*, *Sex. transm. Dis.*, 1985, *12*, 52.

For the use of gentamicin eye ointment in association with intramuscular kanamycin for the treatment of gonococcal neonatal conjunctivitis, see Ceftriaxone Sodium, p.170.

INTRA-ABDOMINAL INFECTIONS. A review of the role of aminoglycoside antibiotics in the treatment of intra-abdominal infections. Several published studies have compared combinations of an aminoglycoside (usually gentamicin or tobramycin) in association with clindamycin with the newer beta-lactam agents such as cefoxitin, imipenem, or latamoxef which have good activity against *Bacteroides fragilis* and facultative Gram-negative bacilli. Tobramycin has also been used in association with cefoxitin. In general no difference in efficacy has been demonstrated between regimens which do or do not contain an aminoglycoside, even in studies of seriously ill patients and those whose initial cultures contained beta-lactam-resistant bacteria. There also appeared to be no difference in the incidence of superinfections. However, most studies involved only small numbers of patients, insufficient to assess whether an aminoglycoside may be of benefit in patients with infections caused by *Pseudomonas aeruginosa* or *Enterobacter* spp. Apart from these patients, there appears to be no benefit in continuing treatment with an aminoglycoside if cultures fail to yield beta-lactam-resistant bacteria.— J. L. Ho and M. Barza, *Antimicrob. Ag. Chemother.*, 1987, *31*, 485.

See also Peritonitis, below.

LISTERIOSIS. For the use of gentamicin in association with ampicillin in the treatment of listeriosis, see Ampicillin Trihydrate, p.120.

MENINGITIS. Aminoglycosides are used in the treatment of meningitis and are particularly important in the therapy of infections caused by Gram-negative organisms. They have a broad spectrum of antimicrobial activity and are rapidly bactericidal although their ototoxicity and nephrotoxicity restrict the doses that can be used. Gentamicin has been given in association with ampicillin for meningitis caused by *Escherichia coli* or *Listeria monocytogenes*, and with ampicillin or benzylpenicillin for that caused by Group B streptococci; tobramycin has been given with an antipseudomonal penicillin such as azlocillin or ticarcillin in the treatment of meningitis caused by *Pseudomonas aeruginosa*. Ampicillin in association with gentamicin is commonly used for the empirical treatment of neonatal meningitis. (For further discussion of the regimens used for the treatment of meningitis and of the benefit in adding an aminoglycoside to treatment with ampicillin or benzylpenicillin, see Ampicillin Trihydrate, p.120).
Gentamicin or tobramycin may be administered intravenously in a dose of 5 to 7 mg per kg body-weight daily in divided doses. All aminoglycosides, however, have poor penetration into the CSF and therefore concomitant intravenous and either intrathecal or intraventricular administration has been investigated. Studies of the intrathecal administration of gentamicin to neonates, however, have not demonstrated a decrease in mortality or neurological sequelae of meningitis. Although one study of intraventricular gentamicin has shown a higher mortality than in patients given systemic antibiotics alone, a study with amikacin administered via a percutaneously implanted reservoir demonstrated an increase in survival rate. Further controlled clinical studies are required to resolve this conflicting evidence. There have been reports of neurotoxicity associated with the intrathecal or intraventricular administration of aminoglycosides (see Adverse Effects, Effects on the Nervous System, p.237).— M. Whitby and R. Finch, *Drugs*, 1986, *31*, 266.

Further references to the use of gentamicin sulphate in the treatment of meningitis: T. S. J. Elliott *et al.*, *J. antimicrob. Chemother.*, 1986, *17*, 245 (use of gentamicin and ceftazidime in Gram-negative bacillary meningitis in neonates); H. Goossens *et al.*, *Lancet*, 1986, *2*, 146 (use of gentamicin and ampicillin in an outbreak of *Campylobacter jejuni* meningitis in neonates).

NEUTROPENIA. For reference to the use of gentamicin sulphate in the treatment of febrile episodes in neutropenic patients, see Septicaemia, below.

OSTEOMYELITIS. Aminoglycosides may be used in the treatment of osteomyelitis and bacterial arthritis. They are often used with ampicillin or vancomycin for infections caused by enterococci, with an antipseudomonal penicillin such as ticarcillin or piperacillin for those caused by *Pseudomonas aeruginosa*, or alone for those caused by Enterobacteriaceae. An aminoglycoside may also be used in association with flucloxacillin or a first-generation cephalosporin such as cephalothin for the empirical therapy of these infections in neonates; ticarcillin or piperacillin may be added in the empirical treatment of infections in adults with a major underlying illness. However, due to the relatively poor penetration of aminoglycosides into joint fluid and their poor activity at the low pH found in septic joints a beta-lactam antibiotic may be preferred in the treatment of bacterial arthritis.— A. S. Dickie, *Drugs*, 1986, *32*, 458.
For further reference to the treatment of osteomyelitis and bacterial arthritis, see Flucloxacillin Sodium, p.232.

A brief discussion of the use of gentamicin-polymethylmethacrylate beads in the treatment of osteomyelitis. Such a drug delivery system should provide high antibiotic concentrations at the site of implantation for several weeks whilst avoiding high systemic concentrations. Studies have shown the gentamicin beads to give comparative or superior results in the treatment of infections to conventional therapy such as irrigation suction drainage.— H. Wahlig (letter), *J. antimicrob. Chemother.*, 1982, *10*, 463.

PELVIC INFLAMMATORY DISEASE. For the use of gentamicin in association with clindamycin in the treatment of pelvic inflammatory disease, see under Cefoxitin Sodium, p.159.

For reference to the use of gentamicin in the treatment of acute salpingitis, see Choice of Antibiotic, p.99.

PERITONITIS. Aminoglycosides are used with vancomycin in the empirical treatment of peritonitis associated with continuous ambulatory peritoneal dialysis (CAPD), and with an antipseudomonal penicillin or ceftazidime for infections caused by *Pseudomonas aeruginosa* (British Society for Antimicrobial Chemotherapy (BSAC), *Lancet*, 1987, *1*, 845). For recommendations of the BSAC on duration of treatment and mode of administration, and comments on the possible additive toxicity of aminoglycosides and vancomycin, see Vancomycin Hydrochloride, p.336. The BSAC consider that in the absence of bacterial resistance there is no evidence of superior activity for any of the aminoglycosides. Some workers, however, have changed from gentamicin to netilmicin for routine use because of the greater *in-vitro* activity of netilmicin against *Staphylococcus epidermidis* including strains demonstrating multiple antibiotic resistance (L. Brauner *et al.*, *J. antimicrob. Chemother.*, 1985, *15*, 751; T.A. McAllister *et al.*, *ibid.*, 1987, *19*, 95). Other considerations as to choice of aminoglycosides are the possible lower toxicity of some agents such as netilmicin and tobramycin. The BSAC recommend the following doses. An intravenous or intraperitoneal loading dose is only required in severely ill patients; this should be given in the following doses, gentamicin and tobramycin, 1.7 mg per kg body-weight, netilmicin 2.5 mg per kg, and amikacin 7.5 mg per kg. For most patients gentamicin, tobramycin, or netilmicin should be administered intraperitoneally in a dose of 8 mg per litre of dialysis fluid added to each bag for 48 hours. Since this dose results in high serum concentrations it should then be decreased to 4 mg per litre added to each bag or 8 mg per litre to every other bag. Amikacin is added to the dialysis fluid in a dose of 25 mg per litre. Blood-aminoglycoside concentrations should be monitored.

PREGNANCY AND THE NEONATE. Gentamicin may be used in various neonatal infections including conjunctivitis (see Ceftriaxone Sodium, p.170), listeriosis (see Ampicillin Trihydrate, p.120), meningitis (see above), and sepsis (see Neonate under Pregnancy and the Neonate in Choice of Antibiotic, p.99).

Neonatal necrotising enterocolitis. Reference to the prophylaxis of neonatal necrotising enterocolitis with gentamicin given by mouth.— L. Grylack and J. W. Scanlon (letter), *Lancet*, 1977, *2*, 506.

For reference to a change in intravenous treatment of neonatal necrotising enterocolitis from gentamicin and ampicillin to vancomycin and cefotaxime, see Vancomycin Hydrochloride, p.336.

RESPIRATORY TRACT INFECTIONS. *Cystic fibrosis.* Aminoglycosides, such as gentamicin, netilmicin, or tobramycin are administered parenterally in the treatment of *Pseudomonas aeruginosa* infections of the respiratory tract in patients with cystic fibrosis. They are commonly given in association with an antipseudomonal penicillin or cephalosporin. Gentamicin and tobramycin have also been administered by nebuliser. For discussion of treatment regimens in these patients, see Carbenicillin Sodium, p.141.

Pneumonia. For reference to the poor response of patients with *Legionella micdadei* pneumonia to aminoglycosides, see Antimicrobial Action, above.

SEPTICAEMIA. Aminoglycosides are widely used, usually in association with other antibiotics, in regimens for the treatment of septicaemia (*Drug & Ther. Bull.*, 1986, *24*, 33; *Med. Lett.*, 1986, *28*, 33), septic shock (R.A. Eskridge, *Drug Intell. & clin. Pharm.*, 1983, *17*, 92), and febrile episodes in neutropenic patients (S.H. Zinner, *Am. J. Med.*, 1985, *79*, *Suppl.* 1A, 17; L.S. Young, *ibid.*, 21). Amikacin may be of use where there is a high incidence of Gram-negative bacteria resistant to gentamicin, tobramycin, or netilmicin. For a detailed discussion of the regimens used in the treatment of febrile episodes in neutropenic patients, see Piperacillin Sodium, p.287.

For reference to the use of gentamicin in the treatment of septicaemia or other serious infections caused by *Campylobacter* spp., see Erythromycin, p.226.

See also under Choice of Antibiotic, p.100.

SKIN DISORDERS. For discussion on the topical use of antibiotics, see Neomycin Sulphate, p.269.

SUPPRESSION OF INTESTINAL FLORA. For reference to regimens used to prevent colonisation and infection by the selective decontamination of the gastro-intestinal tract, see Colistin Sulphomethate Sodium, p.205.

SURGICAL INFECTION PROPHYLAXIS. Although parenteral aminoglycosides have been used in combination with a number of beta-lactam antibiotics, there are limited indications for the routine use of this class of antibiotic in surgical infection prophylaxis. When appropriately controlled studies have demonstrated its usefulness, or when the risk of infection by an organism resistant to cephalosporins is high, a loading dose of gentamicin 1.5 to 2.0 mg per kg body-weight should be given. There are insufficient data for determination of the timing of or the need for subsequent doses.
Intravenous gentamicin and clindamycin given pre-operatively then at 8-hourly intervals for 2 further doses has been recommended as prophylaxis during major surgical procedures involving incision through the oral or pharyngeal mucosa. A single dose of this combination may be an effective alternative in patients undergoing gastric resection who are allergic to beta-lactams but data are limited. Gentamicin in association with metronidazole, or gentamicin alone have been shown to be effective when given pre-operatively and for a further 3 doses at 8-hourly intervals in patients allergic to beta-lactams undergoing colonic surgery or cholecystectomy respectively. Single doses of intramuscular gentamicin and intravenous vancomycin may be given as prophylaxis during craniotomy. Gentamicin has also been used with other antibiotics in patients undergoing abdominal surgery when perforation of a hollow viscus is suspected.— A. B. Kaiser, *New Engl. J. Med.*, 1986, *315*, 1129.

In a study of the use of gentamicin-polymethylmethacrylate chains for infection prophylaxis in colorectal surgery 5 patients received the beads transperitoneally and 7 acted as controls; a further patient had the beads inserted in a perineal wound. Two of the 5 patients with transperitoneal beads developed a purulent discharge and one developed a serous ooze; some difficulty was experienced in removing the beads in all these patients. In view of the problems associated with this route the study was discontinued. No difficulty was experienced in removing the beads from the perineal wound. A further 5 patients had the beads placed subcutaneously in the abdominal wounds and 2 of these developed wound infections; little difficulty was experienced in the removal of the beads in these 5 patients. The use of gentamicin-polymethylmethacrylate beads in colorectal surgery in those situations where beads are placed intraperitoneally could not be recommended and there seems little benefit in using the beads in abdominal wounds. The beads could have a role in perineal wounds and this deserves further study.— R. A. J. Spence *et al.*, *Br. J. clin. Pract.*, 1984, *38*, 252.

References to the use of aminoglycosides in regimens for surgical infection prophylaxis: M. T. Cafferkey *et al.*, *J. antimicrob. Chemother.*, 1982, *9*, 471 (urological procedures); R. L. Nichols *et al.*, *New Engl. J. Med.*, 1984, *311*, 1065 (penetrating abdominal trauma).

For reference to the use of gentamicin sulphate for prophylaxis of infection in cardiac and orthopaedic surgery, see Flucloxacillin Sodium (p.232).

See also Prophylactic Use of Antibiotics, p.103.

URINARY-TRACT INFECTIONS. Gentamicin is generally only indicated for the treatment of infections of the urinary tract when they are severe or unresponsive to other antimicrobial agents. A 5-day course may be used for the treatment of recurrent uncomplicated infections in women (W.R. Cattell, *Prescribers' J.*, 1983, *23*, 81). When there is evidence of bacteraemia or pyelonephritis, gentamicin may be useful when added to therapy with ampicillin or parenteral cephalosporins if it is necessary to start treatment before susceptibility tests are available (*Med. Lett.*, 1981, *23*, 69; W.A. Gillespie, *J. antimicrob. Chemother.*, 1986, *18*, 149). Gentamicin and other aminoglycosides accumulate within the kidneys but whether the high concentrations achieved are actually of benefit in the treatment of pyelonephritis is still a matter of controversy. Although the aminoglycosides are commonly used for the treatment of severe urinary-tract infections there appears to be no data comparing their long-term efficacy with that of standard therapy. However, in *animal* studies, addition of gentamicin for the first 3 days of a 2-week course of ampicillin, cephalothin, or trimethoprim, was more effective than any of the agents used alone (M.G. Bergeron, *J. antimicrob. Chemother.*, 1985, *15*, 4). Controlled studies are required to establish whether such short-duration therapy will reduce the nephrotoxic potential of the aminoglycosides. Administration of gentamicin in a once-daily dose of up to 160 mg for 8 to 15 days may be suitable for the treatment of recurrent infections of the lower urinary-tract in adults (E. Labovitz *et al.*, *Antimicrob. Ag. Chemother.*, 1974, *6*, 465; V. Prát *et al.*, *Infection*, 1978, *6*, 29; S.D. Sharma, *Curr. ther. Res.*, 1984, *35*, 937). Although once-daily administration has also been used in children (N. Principi *et al.*, *Helv. paediat. Acta.*, 1977, *32*, 343; A. Shankar and S.D. Sharma, *Curr. ther. Res.*, 1987, *41*, 599) some consider that because urinary-tract infections are often serious in infants and may be accompanied by septicaemia, children should receive a combination such as amoxycillin and gentamicin in full dosage. Gentamicin and other aminoglycosides have also been given in single-dose therapy of urinary-tract infections (J.A. Whitworth, *Med. J. Aust.*, 1986, *144*, 136).

Although gentamicin is more active in alkaline media *in vitro* no evidence was found to indicate that alkalinisation of urine increased the efficacy of gentamicin in urinary-tract infections in *animals*. Manipulation of urinary flow also appeared to have no effect.— T. Miller and S. Phillips, *Antimicrob. Ag. Chemother.*, 1983, *23*, 422.

Prophylaxis. For reference to a comparison between gentamicin and nitrofurantoin for the prophylaxis of urinary-tract infections during trans-urethral resection, see Nitrofurantoin Sodium, p.274.

Preparations

Gentamicin Injection *(B.P.).* Contains gentamicin sulphate.

Gentamicin Sulfate Injection *(U.S.P.).* It may contain suitable buffers, preservatives, and sequestering agents unless intended for intrathecal use, when it contains only suitable agents to adjust tonicity.

Gentamicin Cream *(B.P.).* A viscous oil-in-water emulsion containing gentamicin sulphate in solution in the aqueous phase.

Gentamicin Sulfate Cream *(U.S.P.)*

Gentamicin Ointment *(B.P.).* A dispersion of gentamicin sulphate in microfine powder in white soft paraffin or other anhydrous greasy basis.

Gentamicin Sulfate Ointment *(U.S.P.)*

Gentamicin Eye Drops *(B.P.).* GNT. Contain gentamicin sulphate.

Gentamicin Sulfate Ophthalmic Solution *(U.S.P.).* A sterile buffered solution of gentamicin sulphate with preservatives. pH 6.5 to 7.5.

Gentamicin Sulfate Ophthalmic Ointment *(U.S.P.)*

Proprietary Preparations

Cidomycin *(Roussel, UK). Injection*, gentamicin 40 mg (as sulphate)/mL in ampoules or vials of 2 mL, and 80 mg (as sulphate)/mL in ampoules of 2 mL.
Paediatric injection, gentamicin 10 mg (as sulphate)/mL in vials of 2 mL.
Intrathecal injection, gentamicin 5 mg (as sulphate)/mL in ampoules of 1 mL.
Powder, for the preparation of sub-conjunctival injections, gentamicin (as sulphate) in bottles of 1 g.
Cream, gentamicin 0.3% (as sulphate).
Ointment, gentamicin 0.3% (as sulphate).
Drops, for eye or ear, gentamicin 0.3% (as sulphate).
Eye ointment, gentamicin 0.3% (as sulphate).

Garamycin *(Kirby-Warrick, UK). Drops*, for eye or ear, gentamicin 0.3% (as sulphate).
Chains, gentamicin sulphate 7.5 mg (equivalent to gentamicin base 4.5 mg), zirconium dioxide 20 mg/polymethylmethacrylate-methylacrylate copolymer bead, in chains of 30 beads.

Genticin *(Nicholas, UK). Injection*, gentamicin 40 mg (as sulphate)/mL in ampoules or vials of 2 mL.
Paediatric injection, gentamicin 10 mg (as sulphate)/mL in vials of 2 mL.
Intrathecal injection, gentamicin 1 mg (as sulphate)/mL in ampoules of 2 mL.
Powder, for the preparation of injections, gentamicin (as sulphate) in vials of 0.5 and 1 g.
Cream, gentamicin 0.3% (as sulphate).
Ointment, gentamicin 0.3% (as sulphate).
Drops, for eye or ear, gentamicin 0.3% (as sulphate).
Eye ointment, gentamicin 0.3% (as sulphate).

Genticin HC *(Nicholas, UK). Cream*, gentamicin 0.3% (as sulphate), hydrocortisone acetate 1%.
Ointment, gentamicin 0.3% (as sulphate), hydrocortisone acetate 1%.

Gentisone HC *(Nicholas, UK). Ear drops*, gentamicin 0.3% (as sulphate), hydrocortisone acetate 1%.

Lugacin *(Lagap, UK). Injection*, gentamicin 40 mg (as sulphate)/mL in ampoules of 2 mL.

Minims Gentamicin Sulfate *(Smith & Nephew Pharmaceuticals, UK). Eye-drops*, gentamicin 0.3% (as sulphate), in single-dose disposable applicators.

Septopal *(E. Merck, UK). Chains*, gentamicin sulphate 7.5 mg (equivalent to gentamicin 4.5 mg), zirconium dioxide 20 mg/polymethylmethacrylate-methylmethacrylate copolymer bead, in chains of 10 or 30 beads.

Proprietary Names and Manufacturers

Alcomicin *(Alcon, Canad.; Alcon, Spain)*; BayGent *(Bay, USA)*; Biogen *(Cusi, Spain)*; Biomargen *(Cheminova, Spain)*; Cidomycin *(Roussel, Austral.; Roussel, Canad.; Roussel, S.Afr.; Roussel, Switz.; Roussel, UK)*; Dianfarma *(Andalucia, Spain)*; Duragentam *(Durachemie, Ger.)*; Espectrocina *(Centrum, Spain)*; Garamycin *(Essex, Austral.; Schering, Canad.; Schering, Denm.; Neth.; Schering, Norw.; Scherag, S.Afr.; Essex, Switz.; Kirby-Warrick, UK; Schering, USA)*; Garamycina *(Schering, Swed.)*; Genalfa *(Ital.)*; Genoptic *(Allergan, Austral.; Allergan, USA)*; Gensumycin *(Roussel, Denm.; Roussel, Norw.; Roussel, Swed.)*; Gentacidin *(Coopervision, USA)*; Gentacin *(Jpn)*; Gentadavur *(Davur, Spain)*; Gentafair *(Pharmafair, USA)*; Genta-Gobens *(Normon, Spain)*; Gentak *(Akorn, USA)*; Gentallenas *(Spain)*; Gentalline *(Unicet, Fr.)*; Gentalyn *(Essex, Ital.)*; Gentamedical *(Medical, Spain)*; Gentamen *(Pierrel, Ital.)*; Gentamicin BDH *(E. Merck, UK)*; Gentamicin L-BDH *(E. Merck, UK)*; Gentamin *(Medix, Spain)*; Gentamina *(Arg.)*; Gentamival *(Valles Mestre, Spain)*; Gentamix *(Baxter, Ger.)*; Gentamorgens *(Morgens, Spain)*; Gentamytrex *(Mann, Ger.)*; Gentibioptal *(Farmila, Ital.)*; Genticin *(Nicholas, UK)*; Genticina *(Antibioticos, Spain)*; Genticol *(SIFI, Ital.)*; Gentigan *(E. Merck, UK)*; Gentisum *(Hortel, Spain)*; Gento *(Spain)*; Gentofarma *(Unibios, Spain)*; Gentogram *(Merck-Clévenot, Fr.)*; Gentollorens *(Llorens, Spain)*; Gentoma *(Spain)*; Gent-Ophtal *(Winzer, Ger.)*; Gentopine *(Dulcis, Mon.)*; Gentralay *(Ralay, Spain)*; Geomycine *(Belg.)*; Gevramycin *(Essex, Spain)*; Glevomicina *(Arg.)*; G-Myticin *(Pedinol, USA)*;
Hosbogen *(Hosbon, Spain)*; Lugacin *(Lagap, UK)*; Martigenta *(Martinet, Fr.)*; Metrorrigen *(Inexfa, Spain)*; Minims Gentamicin Sulfate *(Smith & Nephew Pharmaceuticals, UK)*; Nichogencin *(Nicholas, Ger.)*; Nuclogen *(Vir, Spain)*; Ocu-Mycin *(Ocumed, USA)*; Ophtagram *(Chauvin-Blache, Fr.)*; Palacos LV with Gentamicin *(Kirby-Warrick, UK)*; Palacos R with Gentamicin *(Kirby-Warrick, UK)*; Palacos-R with Garamycin *(Essex, Austral.)*; Quintamicina *(Albofarma, Spain)*; Refobacin *(Aust.; E. Merck, Ger.; E. Merck, Swed.)*; Rexgenta *(Areu, Spain)*; Ribomicin *(Farmigea, Ital.)*; Rovixida *(Arg.)*; Septopal *(Ciba, Austral.; E. Merck, Denm.; E. Merck, Ger.; E. Merck, Norw.; E. Merck, Swed.; E. Merck, Switz.; E. Merck, UK)*; Sintepul *(Arg.)*; Sulgemicin *(Spain)*; Sulmycin *(Essex, Ger.)*; Supragenta *(Spain)*; Tamadit *(Esteve, Spain)*.

The following names have been used for multi-ingredient preparations containing gentamicin sulphate— Celestone-VG *(Essex, Austral.)*; Diprogen *(Schering, Canad.)*; Garasone *(Schering, Canad.)*; Genticin HC *(Nicholas, UK)*; Gentisone HC *(Nicholas, UK)*; Valisone-G *(Schering, Canad.)*.

90-s

Gramicidin *(USAN, rINN).*

Gramicidin D; Gramicidin (Dubos).

CAS — 1405-97-6 (gramicidin); 113-73-5 (gramicidin S).

NOTE. The name gramicidin was formerly applied to tyrothricin.

Pharmacopoeias. In *U.S.*

An antimicrobial cyclic polypeptide produced by the growth of *Bacillus brevis* Dubos; it may be obtained from tyrothricin (see p.331), of which it is one of the principal components.

It occurs as a white or almost white, odourless, crystalline powder containing not less than 900 µg of gramicidin per mg calculated on the dried basis. **Insoluble** in water; soluble in alcohol. **Store** in airtight containers.

Units

One unit of gramicidin is contained in 0.001 mg of the first International Reference Preparation (1966) which contains 1000 units per mg.

Adverse Effects and Precautions

As for Tyrothricin, p.331.

Gramicidin was considered to be unsafe in patients with acute porphyria because it has been shown to be porphyrinogenic in *animals* or *in vitro* systems.— M.R. Moore and K.E.L. McColl, *Porphyrias, Drug Lists*, Glasgow, Porphyria Research Unit, University of Glasgow, 1987.

Uses and Administration

Gramicidin has actions similar to those of tyrothricin (see p.331) and is too toxic to be administered systemically. It has been used for the local treatment of susceptible infections.

Gramicidin S or 'Soviet gramicidin' ($C_{60}H_{92}N_{12}O_{10}$ = 1141.5) has been used in the *USSR.*

Preparations

Some official preparations containing gramicidin are described under neomycin sulphate.

Some proprietary preparations containing gramicidin are described under framycetin sulphate, neomycin sulphate, and triamcinolone.

Proprietary Names and Manufacturers

Bafucin *(Ferrosan, Swed.).*

The following names have been used for multi-ingredient preparations containing gramicidin— Adcortyl with Graneodin *(Squibb, UK)*; Ak-Spore Ophthalmic Solution *(Akorn, USA)*; Biomydrin *(Warner, UK)*; Graneodin *(Squibb, Austral.; Squibb, UK)*; Kenacomb *(Squibb, Austral.; Squibb, Canad.)*; Kenalog-S *(USA)*; Lidecomb *(Syncare, Canad.)*; Mycolog *(Squibb, USA)*; Myco-Triacet *(Lemmon, USA)*; Mytrex *(Savage, USA)*; Neosporin Cream *(Wellcome, Canad.)*; Neosporin Ophthalmic Solution *(Wellcome, Austral.; Wellcome, Canad.; Wellcome, UK; Wellcome, USA)*; Neosporin-G *(Wellcome, USA)*; Nyst-olone *(Schein, USA)*; Ocu-Spor-G *(Ocumed, USA)*; Ocutricin Solution *(Pharmafair, USA)*; Polysporin *(Wellcome, Canad.)*; Sofracort *(Roussel, Canad.)*; Sofradex *(Roussel, Austral.; Roussel, UK)*; Soframycin Cream *(Roussel, Austral.; Roussel, UK)*; Soframycin Nebuliser *(Roussel, Austral.; Roussel, UK)*; Soframycin Ointment *(Roussel, Austral.; Roussel, UK)*; Spectrocin *(Squibb, Canad.)*; Tri-Adcortyl *(Squibb, UK)*; Tri-Thalmic *(Schein, USA)*; Viaderm-KC *(Taro, Canad.)*.

12804-y

Guamecycline Dihydrochloride *(BANM, rINNM).*

Tetrabiguanide. N^2-(4-Guanidinoformimidoylpiperazin-1-ylmethyl)tetracycline dihydrochloride.

$C_{29}H_{38}N_8O_8,2HCl = 699.6.$

CAS — 16545-11-2 (guamecycline); 13040-98-7 (dihydrochloride); 19115-46-9 (xHCl).

An antibiotic with the general properties of tetracycline.

Proprietary Names and Manufacturers

Bronco-Was *(Spain)*; Guanamycine *(Prospa, Belg.)*; Xantociclina *(SPA, Ital.)*.

183-j

Hetacillin *(BAN, USAN, pINN).*

BL-P-804; BRL-804; Hetacillinum; Isopropylidene-aminobenzylpenicillin; Phenazacillin. (6*R*)-6-(2,2-Dimethyl-

5-oxo-4-phenylimidazolidin-1-yl)penicillanic acid.
$C_{19}H_{23}N_3O_4S$=389.5.

CAS — 3511-16-8.

Pharmacopoeias. In *Fr.* and *U.S.*

A white or off-white crystalline powder. Practically **insoluble** in water and most organic solvents; soluble in methyl alcohol and in dilute solutions of sodium hydroxide. A 1% solution in water has a pH of 2.5 to 5.5. **Store** in airtight containers.

92-e

Hetacillin Potassium *(BANM, USAN, pINNM).*

Hetacillinum Kalicum; Isopropylideneaminobenzylpenicillin Potassium. The potassium salt of hetacillin.
$C_{19}H_{22}KN_3O_4S$=427.6.

CAS — 5321-32-4.

Pharmacopoeias. In *Jpn* and *U.S.*

A white to light buff crystalline powder. 1.1 g of monograph substance is approximately equivalent to 1 g of hetacillin and 900 mg of ampicillin. Each g of monograph substance represents about 2.3 mmol of potassium. Freely **soluble** in water; soluble in alcohol. A 1% solution in water has a pH of 7 to 9. **Store** in airtight containers.

Hetacillin has actions and uses similar to those of ampicillin (see p.116), to which it is rapidly converted after administration by mouth or by injection. It is given as the acid or potassium salt in doses equivalent to 250 to 500 mg of hetacillin four times daily by mouth; the potassium salt may be given by injection. Hetacillin is also administered as the hydrochloride.

A study indicating that usual therapeutic doses of hetacillin strongly interfere with colour vision.— J. Laroche and C. Laroche, *Annls pharm. fr.*, 1977, *35*, 173.

Preparations

Hetacillin Potassium Capsules *(U.S.P.)*

Sterile Hetacillin Potassium *(U.S.P.)*

Hetacillin for Oral Suspension *(U.S.P.)*

Hetacillin Tablets *(U.S.P.).* Chewable tablets containing hetacillin.

Proprietary Names and Manufacturers of Hetacillin and its Salts

Etaciland *(Landerlan, Spain)*; Etasepti *(Spain)*; Hetancinato *(Spain)*; Hystra *(Cidan, Spain)*; Versapen *(Allard, Fr.; Bristol Italiana Sud, Ital.; Bristol-Myers, Spain; Bristol, USA)*; Versapen-K *(Bristol, USA)*; Viderbiotic *(Spain).*

5657-m

Hexamine

Aminoform; E239; Esametilentetrammina; Esammina; Formine; Hexamethylenamine; Metenammina; Methenamine *(USAN, rINN)*; Urotropine. Hexamethylenetetramine; 1,3,5,7-Tetraazatricyclo[3.3.1.1^{3,7}]decane.
$C_6H_{12}N_4$=140.2.

CAS — 100-97-0.

Pharmacopoeias. In *Arg., Aust., Belg., Braz., Chin., Cz., Fr., Ger., Hung., Jug., Mex., Neth., Pol., Port., Roum., Rus., Span., Swiss,* and *U.S.*

Almost odourless, colourless, lustrous crystals or white crystalline powder with a bitter-sweet taste. It sublimes at about 260° without melting.

Soluble 1 in 1.5 of water, 1 in 12.5 of alcohol, 1 in 10 of chloroform, and 1 in 320 of ether. Solutions in water are alkaline to litmus.

Adverse Effects

Hexamine and its salts are generally well tolerated but may cause gastro-intestinal disturbances such as nausea, vomiting, and diarrhoea. Comparatively large amounts of formaldehyde are formed during prolonged administration or when large doses are used, and may give rise to irritation and inflammation of the urinary tract especially the bladder, painful and frequent micturition, haematuria, and proteinuria. The effect of the formaldehyde may be diluted by administering alkalinising agents such as sodium bicarbonate or large quantities of water but it is then less effective. Skin rashes have occasionally been reported.

Precautions

Hexamine and its salts are contra-indicated in patients with hepatic insufficiency because of the liberation of ammonia in the gastro-intestinal tract. Hexamine salts should be avoided in patients with moderate or severe renal failure, severe dehydration, metabolic acidosis, or gout. Hexamine compounds should not be given concomitantly with sulphonamides such as sulphamethizole because crystalluria may occur at urinary pH values necessary for hexamine to be effective. Agents that alkalinise the urine such as acetazolamide or potassium citrate should not be used.

Interference with laboratory estimations for catecholamines, 17-hydroxycorticosteroids, and oestrogens in the urine has been reported.

Antimicrobial Action

The antimicrobial action of hexamine is due to formaldehyde which is liberated during acid hydrolysis; most micro-organisms are susceptible to formaldehyde. Hexamine and its salts are effective *in vitro* against a range of Gram-negative and Gram-positive bacteria. Activity for hexamine hippurate and hexamine mandelate has been reported *in vitro* against *Escherichia coli, Pseudomonas aeruginosa,* and some *Klebsiella, Staphylococcus,* and *Streptococcus* spp. However, urea-splitting micro-organisms such as *Proteus* and some *Pseudomonas* spp. tend to increase urinary pH and therefore inhibit the release of formaldehyde.

Antimicrobial resistance to formaldehyde or to hexamine and its salts does not appear to occur.

Absorption and Fate

Hexamine is readily absorbed from the gastro-intestinal tract and is rapidly eliminated in the urine. In acid urine, hexamine is slowly hydrolysed to formaldehyde and ammonia and peak concentrations of formaldehyde are attained in about 2 hours. The same reaction occurs in the acid gastric secretion and may account for a loss of 10 to 30% of the administered dose.

Urinary formaldehyde concentrations in patients on intermittent catheterisation treated with hexamine mandelate.— M. C. Nahata *et al., J. fam. Pract.*, 1983, *16*, 398.

Uses and Administration

Hexamine is used, usually as the hippurate or mandelate (see below), in the prophylaxis and treatment of recurrent urinary-tract infections. It has also been administered as the anhydromethylenecitrate, camphorate, ethyliodide, and the orthophosphate salts.

Topically, hexamine has been used in deodorant preparations, since in the presence of acid sweat it liberates formaldehyde.

Hexamine is a permitted preservative for use in Provolone cheese and marinated herring and mackerel.

Estimated acceptable daily intake of hexamine: up to 150 µg per kg body-weight. The toxic effects are due to liberated formaldehyde and formic acid. Because of possible nitrosamine formation it should not be used with nitrites.— Seventeenth Report of FAO/WHO Expert Committee on Food Additives, *Tech. Rep. Ser. Wld Hlth Org. No. 539*, 1974.

A favourable report of the use of hexamine topically in hyperhidrosis.— S. I. Cullen, *Archs Derm.*, 1975, *111*, 1158.

Preparations

Methenamine and Monobasic Sodium Phosphate Tablets *(U.S.P.).* Tablets containing hexamine and sodium acid phosphate. Store in airtight containers.

Methenamine Elixir *(U.S.P.).* An elixir containing hexamine, with 19 to 21% of alcohol. Store in airtight containers.

Methenamine Tablets *(U.S.P.).* Tablets containing hexamine.

Proprietary Names and Manufacturers of Hexamine and some of its Salts

Aci-steril *(Heyl, Ger.)*; Antihydral *(Robugen, Ger.; Medipharm, Switz.)*; Dehydral *(Trans Canaderm, Canad.)*; Elmitolo *(Bayer, Ital.)*; Jodoibs *(Benvegna, Ital.)*; Urasal *(Horner, Canad.)*; Uromandelin *(Lazar, Arg.)*; Urotropina *(Schering, Arg.; Schering, Ital.).*

The following names have been used for multi-ingredient preparations containing hexamine and some of its salts— Trac Tabs *(Hyrex, USA)*; Urised *(Webcon, USA)*; Uroblue *(Geneva, USA)*; Uro-phosphate *(Poythress, USA).*

5660-r

Hexamine Hippurate *(BAN).*

Methenamine Hippurate *(USAN, rINNM).*
Hexamethylenetetramine hippurate.
$C_6H_{12}N_4,C_9H_9NO_3$=319.4.

CAS — 5714-73-8.

Pharmacopoeias. In *U.S.*

Adverse Effects and Precautions

As for Hexamine, above.

ADMINISTRATION IN RENAL FAILURE. For reference to the precautions to be observed in renal failure, see under Uses, Administration in Renal Failure.

INTERFERENCE WITH DIAGNOSTIC TESTS. In 5 pregnant women given hexamine hippurate, urine concentrations of oestriol, an assessment of foetoplacental function and foetal well-being, promptly fell to below normal values. Oestriol concentrations in the plasma and foetal well-being were not affected by the drug.— S. Kivinen and R. Tuimala, *Br. med. J.*, 1977, *2*, 682.

Antimicrobial Action

Hexamine hippurate has the antimicrobial action of hexamine (see above); hippuric acid, a bacteriostat, may also contribute to its action.

Absorption and Fate

As for Hexamine, above.

Hippuric acid is rapidly excreted unchanged in the urine, by both glomerular filtration and tubular secretion.

Uses and Administration

Hexamine hippurate is used similarly to hexamine mandelate (see below) in the prophylaxis and treatment of chronic or recurrent infections of the urinary tract.

The usual adult dose is 1 g twice daily by mouth; children aged 6 to 12 years may be given 0.5 to 1 g twice daily.

ADMINISTRATION IN RENAL FAILURE. Hexamine hippurate is not recommended for urinary-tract infections if the creatinine clearance is less than 20 mL per minute.— J. S. Cheigh, *Am. J. Med.*, 1977, *62*, 555.

URINARY-TRACT INFECTIONS. Some authorities consider that hexamine should no longer be used in urinary-tract infections because it is only bacteriostatic, requires acidification of the urine, and frequently causes adverse-effects.— A. Morley *et al., Pharm. J.*, 1986, *2*, 662.

A comparative crossover study of hexamine hippurate 1 g twice daily and hexamine mandelate 1 g four times daily in 73 patients demonstrated that while both treatments were satisfactory for the prevention of lower urinary-tract infection, the incidence of side-effects, particularly gastro-intestinal, was significantly lower with hexamine hippurate.— J. G. Gow, *Practitioner*, 1974, *213*, 97.

A double-blind study indicating that hexamine hippurate was effective in the long-term prophylaxis of recurrent acute cystitis in women.— S. Cronberg *et al., Br. med. J.*, 1987, *294*, 1507. Hexamine hippurate, while still useful, has been superseded by more effective agents for the control of recurrent urinary-tract infections.— W. Brumfitt and J. M. T. Hamilton-Miller, *ibid.*, *295*, 390.

For the use of hexamine in patients undergoing catheterisation, see Hexamine Mandelate, p.247.

Preparations

Methenamine Hippurate Tablets *(U.S.P.).* Tablets containing hexamine hippurate.

Proprietary Preparations

Hiprex *(Riker, UK). Tablets,* scored, hexamine hippurate 1 g.

Proprietary Names and Manufacturers

Haiprex *(Riker, Denm.)*; Hipeksal *(Norw.)*; Hippramine *(Riker, S.Afr.)*; Hippuran *(Orion, Swed.)*; Hiprex *(Riker, Austral.; Belg.; Riker, Canad.; Riker, Norw.; Riker, Swed.; Riker 3M, Switz.; Riker, UK; Merrell Dow, USA)*; Urex *(Riker, USA)*; Urotractan *(Klinge, Ger.).*

5661-f

Hexamine Mandelate

Mandelato de Metenamina; Methenamine Mandelate *(USAN, rINNM)*. Hexamethylenetetramine mandelate.

$C_6H_{12}N_4,C_8H_8O_3$=292.3.

CAS — 587-23-5.

Pharmacopoeias. In *Braz.* and *U.S.*

A white crystalline almost odourless powder. M.p. about 127° with decomposition.

Very **soluble** in water; soluble 1 in 10 of alcohol, 1 in 20 of chloroform, and 1 in 350 of ether. Solutions in water have a pH of about 4.

Adverse Effects and Precautions

As for Hexamine, p.246.

A 2½-year-old child who accidentally ingested at least 8 g of hexamine mandelate developed haemorrhagic cystitis, mild transient uraemia, and acidosis. He recovered without specific treatment.— R. P. Ross and G. F. Conway, *Am. J. Dis. Child.*, 1970, *119*, 86.

ADMINISTRATION IN RENAL FAILURE. For reference to the precautions to be observed in renal failure, see under Uses, Administration in Renal Failure.

INTERFERENCE WITH DIAGNOSTIC TESTS. Patients taking hexamine mandelate might show an apparent elevation of urinary excretion of 17-hydroxycorticosteroids if a colorimetric method using phenylhydrazine was performed.— L. E. Braverman *et al.*, *Clin. Chem.*, 1968, *14*, 374.

Antimicrobial Action

Hexamine mandelate has the antimicrobial actions of both hexamine and mandelic acid.

Absorption and Fate

As for Hexamine, p.246.

Uses and Administration

Hexamine mandelate is used in the treatment of infections of the urinary tract. It is only active in acid urine (pH below 5.5), when formaldehyde is released, and although mandelic acid helps to acidify the urine, administration of ammonium chloride or ascorbic acid may be necessary. If urea-splitting bacteria such as *Proteus* or some *Pseudomonas* spp. are present they may produce so much ammonia that the urine cannot be acidified.

Hexamine mandelate should not be used in upper urinary-tract infections because it is eliminated too rapidly to exert an effect, or in acute urinary infections. It may be used in the treatment of chronic or recurrent, uncomplicated, lower urinary-tract infections and asymptomatic bacteriuria. It is suitable for long-term use because acquired resistance does not appear to develop.

The usual dose in adults is 1 g four times daily by mouth, after meals and at bedtime. A suggested dose for children is 50 mg per kg bodyweight daily in 4 divided doses.

ADMINISTRATION IN RENAL FAILURE. Hexamine mandelate is not recommended for urinary-tract infections if the creatinine clearance is less than 20 mL per minute.— J. S. Cheigh, *Am. J. Med.*, 1977, *62*, 555.

Hexamine mandelate could be administered in usual doses to patients with a glomerular filtration-rate greater than 50 mL per minute, but should be avoided in those with a glomerular filtration-rate less than this.— W. M. Bennett *et al.*, *Am. J. Kidney Dis.*, 1983, *3*, 155.

URINARY-TRACT INFECTIONS. Some authorities consider that hexamine should no longer be used in urinary-tract infections because it is only bacteriostatic, requires acidification of the urine, and frequently causes adverse-effects.— A. Morley *et al.*, *Pharm. J.*, 1986, *2*, 662.

Hexamine with acidification of the urine has been used in patients requiring catheterisation in an attempt to prevent urinary-tract infections. Although Norberg *et al.* (*Eur. J. clin. Pharmac.*, 1980, *18*, 497) found that administration of hexamine hippurate 1 g three times daily prolonged catheter life in patients with indwelling catheters. Vainrub and Musher (*Antimicrob. Ag. Chemother.*, 1977, *12*, 625) considered hexamine mandelate to be ineffective for the suppression or prophylaxis of urinary-tract infections in para- and quadraplegic patients with indwelling catheters or in those undergoing intermittent catheterisation. Furthermore, Kostiala *et al.* (*J. Hosp. Infect.*, 1982, *3*, 357) found that prophylaxis with hexamine hippurate or nitrofurantoin did not prevent bacteriuria in elderly patients undergoing long-term catheterisation but only delayed its emergence. However, they considered that these agents could be of use for a short time after catheterisation and other workers have obtained beneficial results using hexamine mandelate or hexamine hippurate in patients requiring intermittent catheterisation for the management of neurogenic bladder dysfunction (C.G. Kevorkian *et al.*, *Mayo Clin. Proc.*, 1984, *59*, 523) and in those requiring short-term catheterisation after uterovaginal surgery (N.-O. Tyreman *et al.*, *Acta obstet. gynec. scand.*, 1986, *65*, 731).

For a comparative study of hexamine hippurate and hexamine mandelate in the prevention of lower urinary-tract infection, see Hexamine Hippurate, above.

Preparations

Methenamine Mandelate for Oral Solution *(U.S.P.)*. Hexamine mandelate as granules for reconstitution.

Methenamine Mandelate Oral Suspension *(U.S.P.)*. A suspension of hexamine mandelate in a vegetable oil. Store in airtight containers.

Methenamine Mandelate Tablets *(U.S.P.)*. Tablets containing hexamine mandelate.

Proprietary Names and Manufacturers

Cedulamin *(Switz.)*; Hexydal *(Norw.)*; Lemandine *(Spain)*; Mandaze *(Austral.)*; Mandelamine *(Warner, Austral.*; *Belg.*; *Parke, Davis, Canad.*; *Gödecke, Ger.*; *Warner, S.Afr.*; *Warner-Lambert, Switz.*; *Warner, UK*; *Parke, Davis, USA)*; Metenamin *(Denm.)*; Methandine *(Canad.)*; Reflux *(Neth.)*; Renelate *(USA)*; Sterine *(Canad.)*; Urocedulamin *(Neth.)*.

The following names have been used for multi-ingredient preparations containing hexamine mandelate— G500 *(Cox, UK)*; Thiacide *(Beach, USA)*; Uroqid-Acid *(Beach, USA)*.

93-l

Hydrabamine Phenoxymethylpenicillin

Penicillin V Hydrabamine *(USAN)*. *NN'*-Bis-[(1,2,3,4,4a,9,10,10a-octahydro-7-isopropyl-1,4a-dimethylphenanthr-1-yl)methyl]ethylenediamine bis[(6*R*)-6-(2-phenoxyacetamido)penicillanate].

$(C_{16}H_{18}N_2O_5S)_2,C_{42}H_{64}N_2$=1299.8.

CAS — 6591-72-6.

Hydrabamine phenoxymethylpenicillin has properties and uses similar to benzylpenicillin (see p.131). It is given by mouth in doses of 250 to 500 mg every 6 hours in the treatment of mild to moderate infections caused by susceptible Gram-positive organisms. The hydrabamine portion of the molecule is not absorbed to any significant extent after oral administration.

Hydrabamine phenoxymethylpenicillin 1.85 g is approximately equivalent to 1 g of phenoxymethylpenicillin.

Proprietary Names and Manufacturers

Abbocillin-V *(Abbott, Austral.)*; Compocillin *(Abbott, Austral.)*; Compocillin-V *(Abbott, Austral.*; *Abbott, NZ*; *Abbott, S.Afr.*; *Ross, USA)*; Flavopen *(G.P. Laboratories, Austral.)*; Pfipen V *(Pfizer, Austral.)*.

16849-l

Imipenem *(BAN, USAN, rINN)*.

Imipemide; *N*-Formimidoyl Thienamycin; MK-0787; MK-787. (5*R*,6*S*)-6-[(*R*)-1-Hydroxyethyl]-3-(2-iminomethylaminoethylthio)-7-oxo-1-azabicyclo[3.2.0]hept-2-ene-2-carboxylic acid monohydrate.

$C_{12}H_{17}N_3O_4S,H_2O$=317.4.

CAS — 64221-86-9 (anhydrous); 74431-23-5 (monohydrate).

The *N*-formimidoyl derivative of thienamycin an antibiotic produced by Streptomyces cattleya.

On incubation *in vitro* of imipenem for 24 hours at 37°, there was a decrease in activity of 17% both with and without addition of gentamicin. Imipenem did not, however, decrease the activity of gentamicin.— T. S. J. Elliott *et al.* (letter), *J. antimicrob. Chemother.*, 1984, *14*, 668. Similar results on incubation of imipenem with tobramycin.— *idem* (letter), 1986, *17*, 680.

Studies *in vitro* indicating first-order hydrolysis of imipenem in sodium chloride 0.9% and human serum.— D. J. Swanson *et al.*, *Antimicrob. Ag. Chemother.*, 1986, *29*, 936.

Studies of the stability of a combination of imipenem and cilastatin in intravenous fluids.— F. P. Bigley *et al.*, *Am. J. Hosp. Pharm.*, 1986, *43*, 2803.

Adverse Effects

Imipenem is only given in association with the enzyme inhibitor cilastatin and thus clinical experience relates to the combination. However, adverse effects appear to be similar to those with other beta-lactam antibiotics. Allergic reactions, including skin rashes, urticaria, eosinophilia, and fever may occur in patients receiving imipenem. Nausea and vomiting may occur, and sometimes have been related to rapid intravenous infusion of imipenem; diarrhoea has also been reported. Administration of imipenem may result in the overgrowth of non-susceptible organisms, and there is the possibility that pseudomembranous colitis may develop.

Local reactions such as pain or thrombophlebitis have been reported following the intravenous administration of imipenem.

Other adverse effects reported include seizures, increases in liver enzymes, and abnormalities in haematological parameters.

An analysis from the manufacturers of the safety of a combination of imipenem and cilastatin in 3470 patients entered into studies in all countries except Japan. The most common group of clinical adverse effects were those related to the gastro-intestinal system: nausea, vomiting, and diarrhoea probably or definitely related to drug administration occurred in 1.4, 0.9, and 0.9% of patients respectively. Hypertrophy of tongue papillae and pseudomembranous colitis also occurred in a few patients. Problems at the site of intravenous injection probably or definitely related to the combination occurred in 1.7%, and included phlebitis, thrombophlebitis, and pain. Drug-associated rash, pruritus, or urticaria occurred in 1.4% of patients; some, but not all, patients who had experienced rashes while on therapy with other beta-lactam antibiotics developed a rash during treatment with imipenem and cilastatin. Patients who had anaphylactic reactions to other beta-lactams were excluded from the studies in this analysis. No anaphylactic reactions were reported to imipenem and cilastatin.

Seizures or myoclonus were considered to be probably or definitely related to drug therapy in 7 patients, most of whom had renal insufficiency, and/or background history of CNS lesions. Seizures occurred most commonly 2 to 6 days after starting therapy. Adverse effects reported in a few patients only, included hypotension, tachycardia, hyperhidrosis, and taste alteration. Renal insufficiency and bleeding occurred only in patients with risk factors for these conditions.

The most common abnormalities in laboratory values reported after administration of imipenem and cilastatin were increases in liver enzyme values. Abnormalities in haematological parameters included eosinophilia, leucopenia, granulocytopenia, and a positive Coombs' test, and were transient. Drug-related changes in platelets and abnormal prothrombin times were rare. Increase blood-urea-nitrogen (BUN) in one patient, and increased creatinine in 3 patients were considered probably or definitely related to drug therapy.— G. B. Calandra *et al.*, *J. antimicrob. Chemother.*, 1986, *18*, *Suppl.* E, 193.

EFFECTS ON THE GASTRO-INTESTINAL TRACT. Since imipenem has a broad spectrum of antimicrobial activity it may be expected to have a profound effect on the faecal flora. Most studies with the combination of imipenem and cilastatin, however, have demonstrated only minor alterations, and this has been attributed to the low faecal concentrations of imipenem. Results from a study of 21 infants and children given the combination for 3 to 15 days suggested that organisms which are relatively less susceptible to imipenem, such as *Entero-*

coccus spp. and some Enterobacteriaceae, or that are resistant to imipenem, such as *Candida* spp. increase in faecal flora early in the course of therapy (C.J. Welkon *et al.*, *Antimicrob. Ag. Chemother.*, 1986, *29*, 741). In a similar study imipenem again only had a small impact on the faecal flora, except in patients who had previously been treated with another antibiotic known to alter the gastro-intestinal flora; in which case the effect was prolonged by the administration of imipenem (J.C. Borderon *et al.*, *J. antimicrob. Chemother.*, 1986, *18*, *Suppl.* E, 121).

EFFECTS ON THE KIDNEY. For reference to nephrotoxicity of imipenem in *animals*, and the protective effect of cilastatin, see Cilastatin Sodium, p.193.

EFFECTS ON THE NERVOUS SYSTEM. Reports of seizures associated with the administration of a combination of imipenem and cilastatin: T. J. Brotherton and R. L. Kelber, *Clin. Pharm.*, 1984, *3*, 536; C. S. T. Tse *et al.* (letter), *Drug Intell. & clin. Pharm.*, 1987, *21*, 659.

Precautions

Imipenem should not be given to patients known to be hypersensitive to it and should be administered with caution to patients known to be hypersensitive to other beta-lactam antibiotics because of the possibility of cross-sensitivity. Care is also necessary in patients with a history of allergy.
Imipenem should be given with caution in patients with renal impairment; a dosage reduction may be required. Care has been advised in patients with CNS disorders such as epilepsy.

ADMINISTRATION IN RENAL FAILURE. For reference to the precautions to be observed in renal failure, see under Administration in Renal Failure in Uses, below.

INTERFERENCE WITH DIAGNOSTIC TESTS. Interference with a copper-reduction method for determination of urinary glucose (Clinitest), occurred only at very low concentrations of a combination of imipenem and cilastatin. Falsely low glucose concentrations were obtained, but the interaction was not considered of great clinical importance.— T. A. Tartaglione and N. B. Flint, *Am. J. Hosp. Pharm.*, 1985, *42*, 602.

Antimicrobial Action

Imipenem is bactericidal and acts similarly to the penicillins by inhibiting synthesis of the bacterial cell wall. It has a very broad spectrum of activity *in vitro* including activity against Gram-positive and Gram-negative aerobic and anaerobic organisms. Most Gram-positive cocci are sensitive including both penicillinase- and non-penicillinase-producing staphylococci, although its activity against methicillin-resistant *Staphylococcus aureus* is variable. Most streptococci are also sensitive; imipenem has good to moderate activity against *Enterococcus faecalis* (*Streptococcus faecalis*), but most *E. faecium* are resistant. Among Gram-negative organisms, imipenem is active against many of the Enterobacteriaceae including *Citrobacter* and *Enterobacter* spp., *Escherichia coli, Klebsiella, Proteus, Providencia, Salmonella, Serratia, Shigella,* and *Yersinia* spp. Its activity against *Pseudomonas aeruginosa* is similar to that of ceftazidime. Imipenem is also reported to be active against *Acinetobacter* spp., *Campylobacter jejuni*, *Haemophilus influenzae*, and *Neisseria* spp. Many anaerobic organisms, including *Bacteroides* spp., are sensitive to imipenem, but *Clostridium difficile* is only moderately susceptible. Imipenem is inactive against *Chlamydia* and *Mycoplasma* spp., and against fungi and viruses.
Imipenem is a potent inducer of beta-lactamases of some Gram-negative bacteria; there have been reports of antagonism between imipenem and other beta-lactam antibiotics *in vitro*.

Imipenem has been found to have an extremely broad spectrum of antibacterial activity *in vitro*. Overall it appears to bind preferably to penicillin-binding protein (PBP) 2, although as the concentration is increased it binds to other PBPs. Organisms with an MIC of 4 µg or less per mL may be regarded as susceptible to imipenem, and those with an MIC of 16 µg or more per mL as resistant; those with intermediate MICs may be considered as moderately susceptible.
The MIC of imipenem against most staphylococci and streptococci is in the range 0.08 to 4 µg per mL. Although there have been encouraging results from studies against methicillin-resistant and rifampicin-resistant *Staphylococcus aureus*, other studies have demonstrated tolerant strains and decreased activity on prolonged incubation, and have suggested that imipenem may not be useful against these organisms. Most strains of enterococci including *Enterococcus faecalis* have been found to be susceptible or moderately susceptible to imipenem, but *E. faecium* is generally resistant. *Listeria monocytogenes* is also reported to be susceptible to imipenem.
Imipenem has excellent antibacterial activity against a wide range of Enterobacteriaceae; MIC values are generally 0.1 µg or more per mL. It is also active against organisms resistant to many penicillins and cephalosporins. Imipenem has good activity against *Pseudomonas* spp. except for *Ps. maltophilia* and *Ps. cepacia*. The concentration of imipenem which inhibited 90% of strains ranged between 2 and 8 µg per mL in 4 studies evaluating a large number of clinical isolates of *Ps. aeruginosa* including some multiresistant strains. The inhibitory concentration of imipenem was lower than for most other agents tested including penicillins, cephalosporins, and aminoglycosides.
Imipenem appears to be less potent than some broad-spectrum cephalosporins against *Haemophilus influenzae, Neisseria gonorrhoeae*, and *N. meningitidis*.
Imipenem has good activity against many Gram-positive and Gram-negative anaerobes; its activity has been reported to be comparable to or greater than that of clindamycin, and comparable to that of metronidazole against some anaerobes including *Bacteroides* spp.
Other organisms that have been reported to be susceptible to imipenem include *Achromobacter xylosoxidans, Aeromonas, Alcaligenes,* and *Bordetella* spp., *Eikenella corrodens, Gardnerella vaginalis, Legionella* spp. including *L. pneumophila, Mycobacterium fortuitum*, and *Nocardia* spp.
The MBC of imipenem has been reported to be more than 8 times greater than the MIC for some strains of *Ps. aeruginosa, Enterococcus faecalis*, methicillin-resistant *Staph. aureus*, and some Enterobacteriaceae. Imipenem has been demonstrated to exert a postantibiotic effect [persistent suppression of bacterial growth after short exposure of a micro-organism to an antimicrobial agent] *in vitro* against some organisms.— S. P. Clissold *et al.*, *Drugs*, 1987, *33*, 183. In reviewing imipenem, it was concluded that *in vitro* it is as active as benzylpenicillin against streptococci and more active than cephalosporins against staphylococci, including penicillinase-producing strains. Its activity against Gram-negative aerobic bacilli, except for *Proteus* spp., is similar to the most potent third-generation cephalosporins, and its activity against *Pseudomonas aeruginosa* is similar to that of ceftazidime. It is also more active than the broad-spectrum penicillins such as piperacillin and the aminoglycosides against Gram-negative bacteria.— M. Barza, *Ann. intern. Med.*, 1985, *103*, 552.

Studies of the serum bactericidal activity of imipenem: H. C. Standiford *et al.*, *Antimicrob. Ag. Chemother.*, 1986, *29*, 412 (comparison with latamoxef); P. Van der Auwera *et al.*, *ibid.*, *30*, 122 (comparison between imipenem, imipenem plus amikacin, and ceftazidime plus amikacin); P. Van der Auwera *et al.*, *J. antimicrob. Chemother.*, 1987, *19*, 205 (comparison with clindamycin, latamoxef, and metronidazole against anaerobes).

For the action of imipenem against organisms which are inducible producers of beta-lactamases, see below under Resistance.

ACTIVITY WITH OTHER ANTIMICROBIAL AGENTS. Imipenem has been reported to antagonise the antibacterial effects of a number of beta-lactam antibiotics, including aztreonam (N.M. Ampel *et al.*, *J. antimicrob. Chemother.*, 1984, *13*, 398), piperacillin (M.A. Bertram and L.S. Young, *Antimicrob. Ag. Chemother.*, 1984, *26*, 272), and ticarcillin, mezlocillin, latamoxef, cefotaxime, and cefoperazone (F. Tausk *et al.*, *ibid.*, 1985, *28*, 41). This has been attributed to the induction of beta-lactamases by imipenem. Shannon and Phillips (*J. antimicrob. Chemother.*, 1986, *18*, *Suppl.* E, 15) concluded, however, from studies *in vitro* that continued induction of beta-lactamase by imipenem or cefoxitin is necessary for susceptibility to other compounds to be decreased, the temporary phenomenon of induction does not have a detectable effect on subsequently determined susceptibility to other beta-lactams, in contrast to the permanent phenomenon in which an antibiotic selects variants with genetically derepressed beta-lactamase synthesis. Concern over possible antagonism had led some workers to recommend that combinations of imipenem and other beta-lactams be avoided although there have been a few reports of synergistic combinations (S.P. Clissold *et al.*, *Drugs*, 1987, *33*, 183), and Brorson and Larsson (*J. antimicrob. Chemother.*, 1984, *14*, 667) considered antagonism of aztreonam by imipenem to be unusual and possibly of low clinical importance.
When combined with aminoglycosides *in vitro* various incidences of synergy have been reported against enterococci (C. Watanakunakorn and J.C. Tisone, *Antimicrob. Ag. Chemother.*, 1982, *22*, 1082; M.E. Gombert *et al.*, *ibid.*, 1983, *23*, 245; J.A. Indrelie *et al.*, *ibid.*, 1984, *26*, 909) and *Listeria monocytogenes* (S.K. Kim, *ibid.*, 1986, *29*, 289); Aznar *et al.* (*J. antimicrob. Chemother.*, 1984, *13*, 129) also reported some antagonism against enterococci, particularly with amikacin.
In reviewing imipenem, Clissold *et al.* (*Drugs*, 1987) cited reports of synergistic interactions between imipenem and norfloxacin against some multiresistant strains of *Pseudomonas aeruginosa*, and between imipenem, ethambutol, and rifampicin against multiresistant *Mycobacterium avium-intracellulare*.
Some degree of antagonism of the antibacterial activity of imipenem against *Klebsiella pneumoniae* by chloramphenicol has also been observed *in vitro* (T.H. Brown and R.H. Alford, *Antimicrob. Ag. Chemother.*, 1984, *25*, 405).

Resistance

Imipenem is stable to hydrolysis by beta-lactamases produced by most bacterial species. Emergence of resistant *Pseudomonas aeruginosa* has occurred during treatment with imipenem.

Imipenem had a moderate affinity for a range of plasmid- and chromosome-mediated penicillinases, and chromosome-mediated cephalosporinases studied, but hydrolysis of imipenem was not detected. Resistance to hydrolysis was attributed to its uncommon chemical structure (R. Labia *et al.*, *J. antimicrob. Chemother.*, 1986, *18*, *Suppl.* E, 1). A few organisms, including *Pseudomonas maltophilia, Aeromonas hydrophila,* and *Bacteroides fragilis*, have been reported to produce beta-lactamases which hydrolyse imipenem. Imipenem is a very potent inducer of chromosomal beta-lactamases; it is moreover stable to these induced enzymes and has been shown to inhibit some of them. Imipenem therefore retains a high degree of activity against organisms which are inducible producers of beta-lactamases (R.J. Williams *et al.*, *ibid.*, 9). In an *in-vitro* study, Ashby *et al.* (*ibid.*, 1987, *20*, 15) demonstrated that although both cefoxitin and imipenem induced beta-lactamases of Enterobacteriaceae, only cefoxitin selected stably derepressed mutants. These mutants showed a substantial increase in beta-lactamase activity and exhibited decreased susceptibility to all antibiotics tested except imipenem. Williams *et al.* considered that other factors by which imipenem may circumvent resistance in Gram-negative rods were its high affinity for penicillin-binding protein (PBP) 2 and its ability to penetrate efficiently to its target site.

RESISTANCE OF BACTEROIDES. Isolation of a strain of *Bacteroides fragilis* resistant to imipenem, metronidazole, and other beta-lactam antibiotics in a patient who had received neither imipenem nor metronidazole previously.— F. Lamothe *et al.* (letter), *J. antimicrob. Chemother.*, 1986, *18*, 642.

RESISTANCE OF PSEUDOMONAS. Knothe *et al.* (*J. antimicrob. Chemother.*, 1987, *19*, 136) have isolated several strains of *Pseudomonas aeruginosa* and one of *Klebsiella pneumoniae* resistant to imipenem, ceftazidime, or both, from patients who had received neither drug. They have shown this resistance to be chromosomal in origin and non-transferable. Slow hydrolysis of imipenem was demonstrated *in vitro* but may not be the sole mechanism responsible for resistance. Emergence of resistant strains of *Ps. aeruginosa* has occurred during treatment with imipenem. This appears to be independent of beta-lactamase production, but may be attributed to a change in the outer membrane proteins. Cross-resistance between imipenem and other beta-lactams is considered unlikely (G. Calandra *et al.*, *Lancet*, 1986, *2*, 340; R.H.K. Eng *et al.*, *J. antimicrob. Chemother.*, 1986, *17*, 717; K.-H. Büscher *et al.*, *Antimicrob. Ag. Chemother.*, 1987, *31*, 703; M.J. Lynch *et al.*, *ibid.*, 1892).

RESISTANCE OF STAPHYLOCOCCI. Eight of 25 clinical isolates of coagulase-negative staphylococci showed some pattern of resistance to imipenem; only 2 of the patients were being treated with the drug. All imipenem-resistant strains were also resistant to a range of other antibiotics.— R. M. Blumenthal *et al.*, *Antimicrob. Ag. Chemother.*, 1983, *24*, 61. Demonstration of inducible resistance of methicillin-resistant *Staphylococcus aureus* to imipenem by subinhibitory concentrations of the drug *in vitro*.— B. A. Forbes *et al.*, *ibid.*, 1984, *25*, 491.

Absorption and Fate

Imipenem is not appreciably absorbed from the gastro-intestinal tract and is therefore administered parenterally. It has a half-life of approximately one hour, and up to 20% of imipenem in the circulation is bound to plasma proteins. It is widely distributed in body tissues and fluids. Imipenem is excreted primarily in the urine by glomerular filtration and tubular secretion. However, it undergoes partial metabolism in the kidneys by dehydropeptidase I to an inactive metabolite, and only 5 to 45% of a dose is excreted in the urine as unchanged drug. Therefore, imipenem is administered in conjunction with cilastatin sodium (see p.193), an inhibitor of the enzyme, resulting in increased urinary-imipenem concentrations.

Up to 1% of imipenem is excreted in the faeces.

A review of the absorption and fate of imipenem and cilastatin. Imipenem is hydrolysed in the kidneys to an open lactam metabolite by dehydropeptidase I, a zinc metallo-enzyme in the brush border of the renal tubules. When administered alone, urinary recovery of imipenem ranged from 6 to 34%; a bimodal distribution of urinary recovery was noted, implying the existence of low and high post-excretion metabolisers of the drug. Co-administration of increasing amounts of cilastatin altered the total urinary recovery of unchanged imipenem with a maximum of about 70% being achieved at a ratio of imipenem to cilastatin of 4 to 1. In order to provide clinically appropriate concentrations of imipenem in the urine for 8 to 10 hours, however, a ratio of 1 to 1 was chosen for introduction into clinical practice. Cilastatin causes a slight increase in the area under the concentration-time curve of imipenem, but this is not accompanied by a change in half-life.

Cilastatin is also metabolised in the kidneys. In a study using radiolabelled imipenem and cilastatin, about 12% of the radiolabel of cilastatin was accounted for as *N*-acetyl cilastatin.

The effect of probenecid on the disposition of imipenem and cilastatin has been studied. Probenecid blocked virtually all the active tubular secretion of imipenem, decreasing the renal clearance by approximately 30%. Total plasma clearance, however, fell by only 14% suggesting the increasing importance of an extra-renal cilastatin-insensitive metabolic pathway for imipenem. In contrast, probenecid decreased both the plasma and renal clearance of cilastatin by 60%; total urinary recovery of unchanged cilastatin was delayed but not altered. These results can predict the handling of the combination in patients with renal impairment. The half-life of imipenem increased from 1 hour in healthy subjects to about 4 hours in functionally anephric patients in one study. The half-life of cilastatin increased from 0.8 to over 16 hours.

Both imipenem and cilastatin are removed by haemodialysis.— G. L. Drusano, *J. antimicrob. Chemother.*, 1986, *18, Suppl.* E, 79.

Imipenem 1 g in combination with cilastatin 1 g was administered by intravenous infusion over 30 minutes every 6 hours for 40 doses to 6 healthy subjects. The mean plasma-imipenem concentration at the end of the infusion was 52.1, 57.4, and 66.9 μg per mL after doses 1, 17, and 37 respectively, and the mean half-life was 0.93 hour. The mean concentration of imipenem in the urine during the time intervals 0 to 2, 2 to 4, and 4 to 6 hours was 886.8, 562.8, and 175.8 μg per mL respectively. The mean total amount of imipenem excreted within 6 hours after the dose was 540.3 mg.

The mean plasma-cilastatin concentrations measured at the same times were 65.04, 65.18, and 64.37 μg per mL respectively, and the half-life was 0.84 hour. The mean cumulative excretion of cilastatin in 6 hours was 698.6 mg.— G. L. Drusano *et al., Antimicrob. Ag. Chemother.*, 1984, *26*, 715.

A study in 15 patients with cystic fibrosis suggesting similar disposition of imipenem with cilastatin to that reported in healthy subjects.— M. D. Reed *et al., Antimicrob. Ag. Chemother.*, 1985, *27*, 583.

Further references to the pharmacokinetics of imipenem in combination with cilastatin: G. L. Drusano *et al., Antimicrob. Ag. Chemother.*, 1987, *31*, 1420 (febrile neutropenic cancer patients).

ADMINISTRATION IN THE ELDERLY. A study of the pharmacokinetics of imipenem in combination with cilastatin in 6 elderly patients. No effects of age, apart from those dependent on decreased renal function, were detected.— R. G. Finch *et al., J. antimicrob. Chemother.*, 1986, *18, Suppl.* E, 103. See also S. Toon *et al., Br. J. clin. Pharmac.*, 1987, *23*, 143.

ADMINISTRATION IN RENAL FAILURE. References to the pharmacokinetics of a combination of imipenem and cilastatin in patients with renal impairment: G. A. Verpooten *et al., Br. J. clin. Pharmac.*, 1984, *18*, 183; L. Verbist *et al., J. antimicrob. Chemother.*, 1986, *18, Suppl.* E, 115.

DIFFUSION INTO BODY TISSUES AND FLUIDS. A study of the penetration of imipenem and cilastatin into the CSF after the intravenous administration of a combination of the 2 drugs to 20 infants and children with bacterial infections of the CNS. From concentrations measured 1.5 to 2.5 hours after administration, the ratio of CSF to serum concentrations of imipenem was in the range of 0.15 to 0.27, after either a single dose or 3 doses given in the early or late stage of infection. For cilastatin, however, the ratio of CSF to serum concentrations was 0.16 and 0.66 in the early and late stages after a single dose respectively, and 0.29 and 0.21 in the early and late stages after multiple doses.— R. F. Jacobs *et al., Antimicrob. Ag. Chemother.*, 1986, *29*, 670.

Further studies of the penetration of imipenem into body tissues and fluids after the administration of imipenem with cilastatin: R. R. MacGregor *et al., Antimicrob. Ag. Chemother.*, 1986, *29*, 188 (inflammatory exudates in seriously ill patients); R. Wise *et al., J. antimicrob. Chemother.*, 1986, *18, Suppl.* E, 93 (cantharides-induced inflammatory exudate and peritoneal fluid); P. C. Gartell *et al., ibid.*, 109 (plasma and tissue concentrations in patients undergoing colorectal surgery); C. Muller-Serieys *et al.* (letter), *ibid.*, 1987, *20*, 618 (bronchial secretions); G. Benoni *et al., ibid.*, 725 (lung tissue and pericardial fluid in patients undergoing thoracotomy).

DRUG EXCRETION. Studies of the biliary excretion of a combination of imipenem and cilastatin in 12 patients undergoing cholecystectomy and 12 with constant drainage of the biliary system. Less than 0.3% of each drug was recovered in the bile.— A. L. Graziani *et al., Antimicrob. Ag. Chemother.*, 1987, *31*, 1718.

PREGNANCY AND THE NEONATE. The mean half-life of imipenem in 30 neonates given varying doses of imipenem with cilastatin as a single intravenous dose or multiple doses ranged from 1.7 to 2.4 hours. The half-life of cilastatin ranged from 3.9 to 6.4 hours. These half-lives were greater than the values of about 1 hour reported for both substances in adults. Half-lives were particularly prolonged in premature infants.— B. J. Freij *et al., Antimicrob. Ag. Chemother.*, 1985, *27*, 431. See also W. C. Gruber *et al., ibid.*, 511.

Uses and Administration

Imipenem is a carbapenem antibiotic. Carbapenems are beta-lactam antibiotics which differ from the penicillins in that the 5-membered ring is unsaturated and contains a carbon rather than a sulphur atom. Since imipenem is metabolised in the kidney by the enzyme dehydropeptidase I it is administered in combination with cilastatin sodium (see p.193), an inhibitor of the enzyme, to enhance urinary concentrations of active drug. Commercial preparations contain imipenem and cilastatin sodium in a ratio of 1 to 1. Doses of the combination are expressed in terms of the amount of anhydrous imipenem. Imipenem is used for the treatment of infections caused by susceptible organisms; it appears to be particularly useful for the empirical treatment of polymicrobial infections. It may be given in conjunction with an aminoglycoside, especially for infections caused by *Pseudomonas aeruginosa*, in order to prevent the emergence of resistant organisms; the drugs should not, however, be mixed in the same container.

Imipenem is administered by intravenous infusion; doses of 250 to 500 mg are infused over 20 to 30 minutes, and doses of 1 g over 40 to 60 minutes. It is given in doses ranging between 250 mg and 1 g every 6 hours or between 500 mg and 1 g every 8 hours depending on the severity of the infection. A maximum daily dose of 4 g or 50 mg per kg body-weight is recommended.

A review of the actions and uses of imipenem with cilastatin. It has been shown to be effective in many small comparative and non-comparative studies for a wide range of infections including those of the respiratory and urinary tracts, the skin, soft tissues, bones, and joints, septicaemia, intra-abdominal and obstetric and gynaecological infections, and a few cases of endocarditis. There have been few studies of its use in infections of the CNS. It appears to be comparable to treatment with clindamycin and an aminoglycoside in intra-abdominal and pelvic infections involving mixed aerobic and anaerobic pathogens. Although it has been investigated for use in prophylaxis of infections during surgery, the need for such a broad-spectrum agent is questionable.

Imipenem with cilastatin has been investigated for the treatment of some paediatric infections; it has been administered in doses of 15 to 25 mg per kg body-weight every 6 hours.

It was concluded that the use of imipenem with cilastatin is difficult to justify in simple community-acquired, mild to moderate, and/or monomicrobial infections, particularly when the pathogen has been isolated and is susceptible to one or more standard antimicrobial agents. It is most likely to be of value in intra-abdominal and pelvic infections, difficult to treat monomicrobial infections, and as empiric monotherapy of serious hospital-acquired infections such as septicaemia and respiratory-tract infections. In pseudomonal infections the addition of an aminoglycoside may be necessary.— S. P. Clissold *et al., Drugs*, 1987, *33*, 183.

Further reviews of the actions and uses of imipenem with cilastatin: M. Barza, *Ann. intern. Med.*, 1985, *103*, 552; *Med. Lett.*, 1986, *28*, 29; D. A. Pastel, *Clin. Pharm.*, 1986, *5*, 719; R. J. Williams, *Postgrad. med. J.*, 1986, *62, Suppl.* 2, 75; *Lancet*, 1988, *2*, 376.

For proceedings of symposia on imipenem, see *J. antimicrob. Chemother.*, 1983, *12, Suppl.* D, 1–156; *ibid.*, 1986, *18, Suppl.* E, 1–214.

Imipenem with cilastatin has been investigated and shown to be effective in many open studies for the empirical treatment of serious, often polymicrobial, infections in patients with underlying disorders such as trauma, or malignant neoplasms (often including patients with neutropenia). Many of the patients studied had been treated unsuccessfully with other antibiotics either singly or in combinations of up to 3 agents, and/or were infected with organisms resistant to a wide range of agents including the newer cephalosporins and quinolones. Infections that have been successfully treated, usually with imipenem and cilastatin alone, cover a wide range of body systems, particularly the respiratory and urinary tracts, bones and soft tissues, and also septicaemia, and intra-abdominal infections such as peritonitis (D.J. Winston *et al., Antimicrob. Ag. Chemother.*, 1984, *26*, 673; B.A. Zajac *et al., ibid.*, 1985, *27*, 745; E.H. Freimer *et al., J. antimicrob. Chemother.*, 1985, *16*, 499; J. Garau *et al., ibid.*, 1986, *18, Suppl.* E, 131; F.W. Reutter, *ibid.*, 141; M.S.C. Dirksen *et al., ibid.*, 145; G.P. Bodey *et al., ibid.*, 161; H. Giamarellou *et al., ibid.*, 175; C. Wang *et al., ibid.*, 185). A few cases of endocarditis have also been treated with imipenem. Not many patients given imipenem with cilastatin have had infections of the CNS, but one study (E. Rouveix *et al., ibid.*, 153) included 8 patients with *Acinetobacter calcoaceticus* meningo-ventriculitis, 6 of whom also received intravenous and/or local aminoglycosides. A group of neutropenic children with malignancies who were treated with imipenem with cilastatin in association with an aminoglycoside have also been studied (A. Baruchel *et al., ibid.*, 167).

Infections have been caused by a wide range of Gram-positive cocci, Gram-negative bacilli, and anaerobic organisms. There have been encouraging results in the treatment of infections caused by *Staphylococcus aureus*, including some methicillin-resistant strains (W. Fan *et al., Antimicrob. Ag. Chemother.*, 1986, *29*, 26). Although a wide range of infections caused by various organisms has been successfully treated by imipenem with cilastatin as monotherapy, pseudomonal infections have been particularly difficult to treat; the MIC of imipenem for *Pseudomonas aeruginosa* has often been reported to increase during treatment, organisms have often persisted, and most studies have noted emergence of a few resistant organisms. In some studies there have been infections caused by *Ps. maltophilia* which is not usually susceptible to imipenem. Authors have therefore emphasised the need for careful monitoring of the susceptibility of organisms during and at the end of treatment, particularly for *Ps. aeruginosa*, and it has generally been recommended that an aminoglycoside be added for the treatment of pseudomonal infections (these are particularly likely to occur in immunocompromised patients). Emergence of resistant *Ps. aeruginosa* has, however, been reported during treatment with imipenem and an aminoglycoside (E. Rouveix *et al., ibid.*, 153).

Only a few studies have compared imipenem with cilastatin against alternative agents for the empirical treatment of serious infections. Two small studies have compared the combination with latamoxef (L.J. Eron *et al., Antimicrob. Ag. Chemother.*, 1983, *24*, 841; M.S. Topiel *et al., Curr. ther. Res.*, 1986, *40*, 7), one showing a tendency towards the superior efficacy of imipenem; another small study (J.D. Baumgartner and M.P. Glauser, *J. antimicrob. Chemother.*, 1983, *12, Suppl.* D, 141) showed it to have similar efficacy to cefotaxime. A Scandinavian Study Group (*Lancet*, 1984, *1*, 868) compared treatment with imipenem and cilastatin with a combination of gentamicin and clindamycin; again there was a trend in favour of imipenem, but this may have been due to a higher frequency of abdominal infections or septicaemia in the gentamicin and clindamycin group. A study involving 66 patients concluded that both imipenem and ciprofloxacin were good to excellent in the treatment of severe bacterial infections (H. Lode *et al.*, *Antimicrob. Ag. Chemother.*, 1987, *31*, 1491).

Thus these initial studies suggest that imipenem with cilastatin may be effective monotherapy for the empirical treatment of severe bacterial infections, particularly polymicrobial infections in seriously ill patients, although the addition of an aminoglycoside may be prudent for pseudomonal infections in order to prevent the development of resistance. The adverse effects of imipenem and cilastatin, including superinfection and colonisation, appear to be comparable with other treatments. Advantages of imipenem over other beta-lactam agents originate from its antimicrobial action; they include its broad spectrum of action encompassing some enterococci, the apparent absence of cross resistance to other agents if resistance to imipenem should occur, and its activity against organisms which are inducible producers of chromosomal beta-lactamases and against derived mutants which are constitutive in their enzyme production (R.J. Williams *et al.*, *J. antimicrob. Chemother.*, 1986, *18*, *Suppl.* E, 9).

ADMINISTRATION IN RENAL FAILURE. The manufacturers have recommended that the dosage of imipenem with cilastatin (expressed in terms of the dose of imipenem) should be adjusted in patients whose creatinine clearance (CC) is 70 mL per minute or less as follows: for a CC of 30 to 70 mL per minute, 500 mg every 6 to 8 hours; for a CC of 20 to 30 mL per minute, 500 mg every 8 to 12 hours; and for a CC of less than 20 mL per minute, 250 to 500 mg every 12 hours. A dose supplement should be given to patients on haemodialysis.

See also under Absorption and Fate, above.

LEGIONNAIRES' DISEASE. Successful treatment with imipenem of 2 patients with pneumonia caused by *Legionella pneumophila*.— I. D. Farrell *et al.*, *J. antimicrob. Chemother.*, 1985, *16*, 61.

RESPIRATORY-TRACT INFECTIONS. *Cystic fibrosis*. Ten cystic fibrosis patients (aged 11 to 30 years) with chronic *Pseudomonas aeruginosa* lung infections were treated with imipenem 45 mg per kg body-weight daily with cilastatin for 14 days, administered as 30-minute intravenous infusions four times daily. A clinical response was obtained in all patients particularly during the first week, but in none of the patients was the organism eradicated. The mean MIC of imipenem increased during treatment; in 3 patients resistance to imipenem developed in the initial isolated strain, and in the other 7 a new resistant strain was selected.— S. S. Pedersen *et al.*, *J. antimicrob. Chemother.*, 1985, *16*, 629. A further 10 patients (aged 8 to 33 years) were treated with imipenem 100 mg per kg daily with cilastatin, in association with tobramycin 15 mg per kg daily; both were given intravenously four times daily. High-dose imipenem and cilastatin was however poorly tolerated leading to discontinuation in 3 patients, and similar problems of imipenem resistance occurred. Thus imipenem and cilastatin could not be recommended for routine treatment of cystic fibrosis patients with *Ps. aeruginosa* infection.— S. S. Pedersen *et al.*, *ibid.*, 1987, *19*, 101.

Pneumonia. Beneficial results with imipenem plus cilastatin in acute bacterial pneumonia.— R. J. Gebhart *et al.*, *J. antimicrob, Chemother.*, 1985, *15*, 233.

One patient with a severe pneumonitis and blood cultures positive for *Acinetobacter baumanii* recovered after administration of imipenem in association with pefloxacin, the only bactericidal combination found *in vitro*.— J. -F. Ygout *et al.* (letter), *Lancet*, 1987, *1*, 802.

For reference to the use of imipenem in pneumonia caused by *Legionella pneumophila*, see above under Legionnaires' Disease.

Proprietary Preparations

Primaxin *(Merck Sharp & Dohme, UK)*. *Intravenous infusion*, powder for reconstitution, imipenem 250 mg (as monohydrate) with cilastatin 250 mg (as sodium salt), and imipenem 500 mg with cilastatin 500 mg.

Proprietary Names and Manufacturers

The following names have been used for multi-ingredient preparations containing imipenem—

Primaxin *(Merck Sharp & Dohme, Austral.; Merck Sharp & Dohme, UK; Merck Sharp & Dohme, USA)*; Tienam *(Merck Sharp & Dohme, Swed.; Chibret, Switz.)*; Zienam *(Merck Sharp & Dohme, Ger.)*.

2173-v

Isepamicin *(BAN, USAN, rINN)*.

HAPA-B; HAPA-gentamicin B; Sch-21420. 4-*O*-(6-Amino-6-deoxy-α-D-glucopyranosyl)-1-*N*-(3-amino-L-lactoyl)-2-deoxy-6-*O*-(3-deoxy-4-*C*-methyl-3-methylamino-β-L-arabinopyranosyl)streptamine; 1*N*-(*S*-3-Amino-2-hydroxypropionyl)-gentamicin B.

$C_{22}H_{43}N_5O_{12}$=569.6.

CAS — 58152-03-7.

Isepamicin is an aminoglycoside antibiotic.

References to the antimicrobial activity of isepamicin *in vitro*: P. K. W. Yu and J. A. Washington, *Antimicrob. Ag. Chemother.*, 1978, *13*, 891; C. C. Sanders *et al.*, *ibid.*, *14*, 178; S. A. Kabins and C. Nathan, *ibid.*, 786; M. A. Guimaraes *et al.*, *J. antimicrob. Chemother.*, 1985, *16*, 555.

For reference to a comparative study of the antimicrobial activity of 11 aminoglycosides including isepamicin, see Gentamicin Sulphate, p.239.

Proprietary Names and Manufacturers

Essex, Jpn; Schering, USA.

94-y

Josamycin *(USAN, rINN)*.

EN-141. 3-Acetoxy-5-[3,6-dideoxy-4-*O*-(2,6-dideoxy-4-*O*-isovaleryl-3-*C*-methyl-α-L-*ribo*-hexopyranosyl)-3-dimethylamino-β-D-glucopyranosyloxy]-6-formylmethyl-9-hydroxy-4-methoxy-8-methylhexadecan-10,12-dien-15-olide.

$C_{42}H_{69}NO_{15}$=828.0.

CAS — 16846-24-5; 56689-45-3.

Pharmacopoeias. In *Jpn* which also includes Josamycin Propionate.

Josamycin is a macrolide antibiotic with actions and uses similar to those of erythromycin (see p.222) although it may be more active *in vitro* against some anaerobic bacteria. It has been given by mouth in doses of up to 2 g daily in divided doses in the treatment of susceptible infections. Josamycin propionate is used in oral suspensions.

ADVERSE EFFECTS AND PRECAUTIONS. For reference to the hepatotoxic potential of macrolide antibiotics, see under Effects on the Liver in Erythromycin Estolate, p.227.

Interactions. Administration of josamycin caused a slight decrease in the clearance of carbamazepine in 8 epileptic patients, but none showed clinical signs of an interaction.— G. Vinçon *et al.*, *Eur. J. clin. Pharmac.*, 1987, *32*, 321.

For reference to possible interactions with macrolide antibiotics, and their effect on hepatic metabolism, see Erythromycin, p.222.

ANTIMICROBIAL ACTION. In a comparative study *in vitro* josamycin showed similar activity to erythromycin and clindamycin against Gram-positive aerobic cocci. It was more active than erythromycin and ampicillin against anaerobes, 90% of isolates of *Bacteroides fragilis* being inhibited by 0.78 µg per mL, and comparable with clindamycin.— E. L. Westerman *et al.*, *Antimicrob. Ag. Chemother.*, 1976, *9*, 988. Against *Bacteroides fragilis*, josamycin had similar inhibitory activity but less bactericidal activity than metronidazole, rosaramicin, or clindamycin.— J. Santoro *et al.*, *ibid.*, *10*, 188.

Josamycin was as or more active than erythromycin *in vitro* against anaerobic Gram-positive organisms and against *Bacteroides* spp.; it was inactive against *Fusobacterium* spp. About 75% of anaerobic organisms tested were inhibited by 1.56 µg per mL of josamycin. At 3.12 µg per mL all strains of *Bacteroides fragilis* were inhibited and at this concentration josamycin was as active as clindamycin. Such a serum concentration, however, was not achieved with oral therapy.— R. E. Reese *et al.*, *Antimicrob. Ag. Chemother.*, 1976, *10*, 253.

Further references to the antimicrobial activity of josamycin: S. Shadomy *et al.*, *Antimicrob. Ag. Chemother.*, 1976, *10*, 773.

For reference to the activity of josamycin against *Campylobacter* and *Legionella* spp., and *Neisseria gonorrhoeae*, and for reference to bacterial resistance to macrolide antibiotics, see Erythromycin, p.223.

ABSORPTION AND FATE. The pharmacokinetics of josamycin following administration by mouth were similar to those of erythromycin stearate in a study of 21 healthy subjects. Josamycin tended to accumulate over the first 48 hours of administration and the plasma half-life varied from 1.34 to 1.56 hours. The urinary excretion over 24 hours ranged from 4.4 to 17.5% as treatment progressed. Josamycin was also present in saliva, sweat, and tears and mean concentrations of 1.03, 0.95, and 2.62 µg per mL respectively were measured in 4 subjects given 1.5 g as a loading dose then 0.5 g every six hours for 10 days.— L. J. Strausbaugh *et al.*, *Antimicrob. Ag. Chemother.*, 1976, *10*, 450.

USES AND ADMINISTRATION. Josamycin 1.5 g daily was as effective as erythromycin stearate 1 g daily, both in divided doses, in reducing the nasal carriage of *Staphylococcus aureus* in a controlled study of 75 subjects.— S. Z. Wilson *et al.*, *Antimicrob. Ag. Chemother.*, 1977, *11*, 407.

An oral suspension of josamycin propionate was given to 1908 children with infections, mainly of the respiratory tract; the usual dose was 50 mg per kg body-weight daily in 2 to 4 divided doses. Treatment was considered successful in 97% of 1880 evaluable children. Adverse effects, mainly gastro-intestinal disturbances and hypersensitivity reactions such as skin rashes, were observed in 98 patients (about 5%) although the majority were also receiving other drugs. Adverse effects were generally mild, necessitating interruption of treatment in 28 (about 1.5%).— G. Privitera *et al.*, *Int. J. clin. Pharmacol. Res.*, 1984, *4*, 201.

Proprietary Names and Manufacturers of Josamycin or Josamycin Propionate

Iosalide *(Schering, Ital.)*; Jomybel *(Belg.)*; Josacine *(Spret-Mauchant, Fr.; Mack, Switz.)*; Josamina *(Novag, Spain)*; Josamy *(Yamanouchi, Jpn; Endo, USA)*; Josaxin *(UCB, Ital.; Liade, Spain)*; Wilprafen *(Mack, Illert., Ger.)*.

95-j

Kanamycin Acid Sulphate *(BANM)*.

Kanamycini Sulfas Acidus. A form of kanamycin sulphate prepared by adding sulphuric acid to a solution of kanamycin sulphate and drying by a suitable method.

$C_{18}H_{36}N_4O_{11},1.7H_2SO_4$=651.2.

Pharmacopoeias. In *Belg., Br., Chin., Eur., Fr., Ind., It., Neth.*, and *Swiss*.

A white or almost white, odourless or almost odourless, hygroscopic powder containing not less than 670 units per mg and 23 to 26% of sulphate, calculated on the dried material. 1.34 g of monograph substance is approximately equivalent to 1 g of kanamycin.

Soluble 1 in 1 of water; practically insoluble in alcohol, acetone, chloroform, and ether. A 1% solution in water has a pH of 5.5 to 7.5. **Store** in well-closed containers.

96-z

Kanamycin Sulphate *(BANM, rINNM)*.

Kanamycin A Sulphate; Kanamycin Monosulphate; Kanamycin Sulfate *(USAN)*; Kanamycini Monosulfas. 6-*O*-(3-Amino-3-deoxy-α-D-glucopyranosyl)-4-*O*-(6-amino-6-deoxy-α-D-glucopyranosyl)-2-deoxy-D-streptamine monosulphate.

$C_{18}H_{36}N_4O_{11},H_2SO_4,H_2O$=600.6.

CAS — 59-01-8 (kanamycin); 25389-94-0 (sulphate, anhydrous).

Pharmacopoeias. In *Belg., Br., Chin., Egypt., Eur., Fr., Ind., It., Jpn, Neth., Roum., Rus., Swiss*, and *U.S.*

Br. and *Eur.* specify the monohydrate; *Jpn* has xH_2SO_4.

The sulphate of an antimicrobial substance produced by the growth of *Streptomyces kanamyceticus*.

A white or almost white, odourless or almost odourless, crystalline powder. The *B.P.* specifies not less than 750 units per mg and 15.0 to 17.0% of sulphate, calculated on the dried material; *U.S.P.* specifies not less than 750 µg per mg. 1.2 g of monograph substance is approximately equivalent to 1 g of kanamycin.

Soluble 1 in 8 of water; practically insoluble in alcohol, acetone, chloroform, ether, and ethyl acetate. A 1% solution in water has a pH of 6.5 to 8.5. **Store** in airtight containers.

Incompatibility or loss of activity has been reported between kanamycin and some cephalosporins or penicillins (see Gentamicin Sulphate, p.236), and also with amphotericin, barbiturates, chlorpromazine, colistin sulphomethate sodium, heparin, hydrocortisone sodium succinate, nitrofurantoin sodium, phenytoin sodium, prochlorperazine edisylate, sulphafurazole diethanolamine, and some electrolytes such as calcium, magnesium, citrate, or phosphate ions.

There was no significant loss of potency when kanamycin injection was added to 3 commercially available 0.5% hypromellose solutions in plastic squeezy bottles (Lacril, pH 5.9; Tearisol, pH 7.3; Isoptotears, pH 7.4) and the resulting solutions of kanamycin 30 mg per mL kept at 25° for 7 days.— E. Osborn *et al.*, *Am. J. Ophthal.*, 1976, *82*, 775.

Units

10 345 units of kanamycin are contained in approximately 12.7 mg of kanamycin sulphate in one ampoule of the second International Standard Preparation (1985).

Adverse Effects, Treatment, and Precautions

As for Gentamicin Sulphate, p.236.

Like neomycin, kanamycin is more likely to cause auditory than vestibular toxicity.

The occurrence of neurotoxic reactions is greatly reduced if the dose is adjusted so that the concentration of kanamycin in the plasma does not exceed 30 µg per mL. Minor side-effects such as headache and paraesthesia sometimes occur. Gastro-intestinal disorders may occur after administration of kanamycin by mouth (see Neomycin Sulphate, p.268).

Calcium ions inhibited the antimicrobial activity *in vitro* of kanamycin against some organisms, so that prophylactic administration of calcium salts with kanamycin in an attempt to reduce antibiotic-induced neuromuscular blockade could be unwise.— K. Sakurai *et al.*, *Am. Surg.*, 1965, *31*, 165.

EFFECTS ON THE LIVER. Kanamycin was the cause of hepatitis in 1 patient.— S. Imoto *et al.* (letter), *Ann. intern. Med.*, 1979, *91*, 129.

PREGNANCY AND THE NEONATE. It was estimated that a breast-fed infant of a mother receiving kanamycin sulphate would ingest about 0.95% of the usual therapeutic dose for an infant.— D. E. Snider and K. E. Powell, *Archs intern. Med.*, 1984, *144*, 589.

Antimicrobial Action

Kanamycin sulphate is bactericidal; it has a mode of action and antimicrobial spectrum similar to that of gentamicin (see p.239), although it is not active against *Pseudomonas aeruginosa*. Some strains of *Mycobacterium tuberculosis* are sensitive.

The minimum inhibitory concentration of kanamycin for susceptible organisms ranges from 0.12 to 8 µg per mL.

For reports of the antimicrobial activity of kanamycin, see Amikacin Sulphate, p.110 (atypical *Mycobacterium* spp.); Gentamicin Sulphate, p.239 (*Yersinia* spp.; *Mycobacterium leprae*; activity with other antimicrobial agents).

For the effect of calcium on kanamycin, see under Adverse Effects, Treatment, and Precautions, above.

Resistance

Resistance has been observed in strains of most of the organisms reported to be sensitive to kanamycin. There is cross-resistance between kanamycin, neomycin, framycetin, and paromomycin and partial cross-resistance between kanamycin and streptomycin.

For the mechanisms of resistance of bacteria to aminoglycosides, see Gentamicin Sulphate, p.240.

Absorption and Fate

As for Gentamicin Sulphate, p.241.

After intramuscular injection peak plasma concentrations of kanamycin of about 20 and 30 µg per mL are attained in about 1 hour following doses of 0.5 and 1 g respectively but amounts are negligible after 12 hours. A plasma half-life of about 3 hours has been reported.

Kanamycin is rapidly excreted by glomerular filtration and most of a parenteral dose appears in the urine within 6 hours, during which time concentrations in excess of 100 µg per mL may be produced. Kanamycin does not diffuse into the cerebrospinal fluid if the meninges are not inflamed. It has been detected in cord blood and in breast milk.

The pharmacokinetics of kanamycin by intravenous infusion and intramuscular injection.— J. T. Clarke *et al.*, *Clin. Pharmac. Ther.*, 1974, *15*, 610. See also J. -C. Pechere and R. Dugal, *Clin. Pharmacokinet.*, 1979, *4*, 170.

ADMINISTRATION IN INFANTS AND CHILDREN. In 65 neonates treated with kanamycin 7.5 or 10 mg per kg body-weight by intramuscular injection every 12 hours, mean peak serum concentrations varied with dose, birth-weight, and postnatal age and were lower in infants weighing 2 kg or more at birth. Half-lives were correlated inversely with gestational and chronological age. In 21 infants with meningitis given kanamycin 7.5 mg per kg intramuscularly every 12 hours, peak concentrations detected in the CSF 3 to 4 hours after administration ranged from 2.4 to 12 µg per mL (mean of 5.6 µg per mL) compared with a mean peak serum concentration of 13 µg per mL. Penetration into the CSF roughly correlated with the degree of meningeal inflammation.— J. B. Howard and G. H. McCracken, *J. Pediat.*, 1975, *86*, 949.

DIFFUSION INTO BODY TISSUES AND FLUIDS. Studies of the penetration of kanamycin into body tissues and fluids: E. A. Baciocco and R. L. Iles, *Clin. Pharmac. Ther.*, 1971, *12*, 858 (synovial fluid); J. F. Hansbrough *et al.*, *Antimicrob. Ag. Chemother.*, 1981, *20*, 515 (gall-bladder bile and wall).

Uses and Administration

Kanamycin is an aminoglycoside antibiotic with actions and uses similar to gentamicin sulphate (p.242). It has also been used as a secondary antituberculous agent, but other safer agents are usually preferred.

The sulphate or acid sulphate salts are used. Doses are expressed in terms of kanamycin base. It is usually given by intramuscular injection and in acute infections adults may be given 15 mg per kg body-weight daily, to a maximum of 1.5 g daily given in 2 to 4 divided doses for 6 days. Children can receive the same daily dose of 15 mg per kg. For the treatment of chronic infections adults may be given 3 to 4 g of kanamycin weekly in doses of 1 g on alternate days or 1 g every 12 hours twice a week; the total amount of kanamycin given should not exceed 50 g.

In overwhelming infections, kanamycin may be given as a slow intravenous infusion of a 0.25% solution in sodium chloride 0.9% or glucose 5% injection at the rate of 3 to 4 mL per minute to a total of 15 mg per kg body-weight daily in 2 or 3 divided doses; daily doses of up to 30 mg per kg have also been recommended. As an adjunct to systemic therapy kanamycin has been administered intrathecally. Doses should be reduced in patients with impaired renal function. In all patients, dosage should be adjusted according to plasma-kanamycin concentrations; recommended peak plasma concentrations of 15 to 30 µg per mL, and trough concentrations of 5 to 10 µg per mL should not generally be exceeded (see also under Uses, Administration, in Gentamicin Sulphate, p.242).

Kanamycin has been used by mouth similarly to neomycin (see p.269), for the suppression of intestinal flora. For pre-operative use, the equivalent of 1 g of kanamycin may be given every hour for 4 hours, then 1 g every 6 hours for 36 to 72 hours. In the management of hepatic encephalopathy (hepatic coma) 8 to 12 g daily in divided doses may be given.

For the inhalation treatment of respiratory infections kanamycin has been administered 2 to 4 times daily as an aerosol containing 250 mg in 1 mL of water diluted with 3 mL of saline. Solutions of kanamycin 0.25% have been used for the irrigation of body cavities.

Kanamycin, given as a single intramuscular dose of 2 g, has been used in the treatment of penicillin-resistant gonorrhoea.

See Gentamicin Sulphate, p.242 for general reviews of the aminoglycoside antibiotics.

ADMINISTRATION IN INFANTS AND CHILDREN. Intramuscular doses of kanamycin for infants weighing less than 2 kg at birth were: 12-hourly doses of 7.5 mg per kg body-weight for those aged 7 days or less or 10 mg per kg for those over 7 days. For infants over 2 kg at birth body-weight: 10 mg per kg every 12 hours for those aged 7 days or less or every 8 hours for those over 7 days. If necessary, doses could be given by constant intravenous infusion over 20 minutes. Kanamycin was considered safe when given in these doses for not more than 12 days.— H. F. Eichenwald and G. H. McCracken, *J. Pediat.*, 1978, *93*, 337.

Results indicating that in older children kanamycin in a dose of 30 mg per kg body-weight daily intramuscularly or intravenously produced optimal peak serum concentrations without drug accumulation or toxicity. This dose, given in 3 divided doses, is recommended for children over 2 months of age, but must be reconsidered if therapy beyond 14 days is necessary.— J. P. Hieber *et al.*, *J. Pediat.*, 1980, *96*, 1089.

GONORRHOEA. A single intramuscular injection of kanamycin 2 g may be used for the treatment of uncomplicated urogenital and rectal gonococcal infections. Although it is active against beta-lactamase-producing gonococci, kanamycin shows considerable geographical variation in its efficacy, sometimes curing less that 95% of infections. It is not recommended for use in pregnant women.— WHO Expert Committee on Venereal Diseases and Treponematoses, *Tech. Rep. Ser. Wld Hlth Org. No. 736*, 1986.

For reference to the use of kanamycin in the treatment of neonatal gonococcal conjunctivitis, see under Pregnancy and the Neonate, below.

HEPATIC ENCEPHALOPATHY. Kanamycin given by mouth and then intramuscularly to 14 patients with cirrhosis of the liver reduced blood and urine ammonia and urine amino acid concentrations but had no effect on plasma amino acids. Ten of the patients had chronic hepatic encephalopathy and 6 improved when kanamycin was given intramuscularly.— F. Nealon *et al.*, *Clin. Pharmac. Ther.*, 1971, *12*, 298.

LISTERIOSIS. For the use of kanamycin in association with ampicillin in the treatment of listeriosis, see Ampicillin Trihydrate, p.120.

MELIOIDOSIS. For reference to the use of kanamycin in association with tetracycline and chloramphenicol for the treatment of melioidosis, see Tetracycline Hydrochloride, p.319.

PREGNANCY AND THE NEONATE. *Neonatal conjunctivitis.* Although kanamycin 25 mg per kg body-weight daily by intramuscular injection in 4 divided doses for 3 days has been recommended for the treatment of neonates with gonococcal conjunctivitis, concern has been expressed regarding the possible ototoxic effects of a 3-day course. Systemic therapy should be accompanied by hourly conjunctival irrigation with saline or buffered ophthalmic solutions, and application of a topical antibiotic preparation until the discharge is eliminated. If hospitalisation of the patient is not possible a single intramuscular injection of kanamycin 25 mg per kg in association with topical treatment with tetracycline hydrochloride 1% or erythromycin 0.5% eye ointment for 10 days may be given in areas where the prevalence of penicillin-resistant gonococci is more than 1% or is unknown. Suitable prophylactic regimens have not been determined for infants exposed to gonorrhoea at birth in areas with a high prevalence of chromosomally resistant gonococci or penicillinase-producing *Neisseria gonorrhoeae*. A single intramuscular injection of kanamycin in a dose of 15 mg per kg for infants of less than 2 kg or 25 mg per kg for those over 2 kg may be considered.— WHO Expert Committee on Venereal Diseases and Treponematoses, *Tech. Rep. Ser. Wld Hlth Org. No. 736*, 1986.

A study involving 117 infants demonstrating that a single intramuscular dose of kanamycin of 75 or 150 mg in association with gentamicin 1% eye ointment for 3 days is an effective treatment for ophthalmia neonatorum due to penicillin-sensitive and penicillinase-producing *Neisseria gonorrhoeae*. One of 15 neonates given kanamycin 150 mg with chloramphenicol eye-drops did not repond to treatment.— L. Fransen *et al.*, *Lancet*, 1984, *2*, 1234.

For comparison of the treatment of neonatal gonococcal conjunctivitis with intramuscular kanamycin in association with topical gentamicin or tetracycline ointment, or with intramuscular ceftriaxone, see Ceftriaxone Sodium, p.170.

Neonatal necrotising enterocolitis. Kanamycin given prophylactically prevented necrotising enterocolitis in infants under 1.5 kg body-weight at birth.— E. A. Egan *et al.*, *J. Pediat.*, 1976, *89*, 467. See also E. A. Egan *et al.* (letter), *ibid.*, 1977, *90*, 331. Two of 9 infants under 2 kg body-weight given kanamycin 15 mg per kg daily for at least 6 days to prevent necrotising enterocolitis developed the condition.— M. M. Conroy *et al.* (letter), *Lancet*, 1978, *1*, 613.

Preparations

Kanamycin Injection *(B.P.)*. A sterile solution of kanamycin sulphate containing sulphuric acid (pH 4.0 to 6.0), or a solution prepared with kanamycin acid sulphate immediately before use (pH 5.5 to 7.5). Protect from light.

Kanamycin Sulfate Capsules *(U.S.P.)*

Kanamycin Sulfate Injection *(U.S.P.)*. pH 3.5 to 5.0.

Sterile Kanamycin Sulfate *(U.S.P.)*

Proprietary Preparations

Kannasyn *(Winthrop, UK)*. *Injection*, kanamycin 250 mg (as sulphate)/mL in vials of 4 mL.
Injection, powder for reconstitution, kanamycin 1 g (as acid sulphate).

Proprietary Names and Manufacturers of Kanamycin Salts

Anamid *(Beecham, Canad.)*; Cristalomicina *(Arg.)*; Enterokanacin *(Salus, Ital.)*; Kamycine *(Bristol, Fr.)*; Kamynex *(Belg.; Neth.)*; Kanabiot *(Galepharma, Spain)*; Kanacet *(Ital.)*; Kanacetic *(Ital.)*; Kanacolirio *(Medical, Spain)*; Kanacyn *(Belg.; Neth.)*; Kanafluid *(Bicther, Spain)*; Kanahidro *(Medical, Spain)*; Kanamytrex *(Belg.; Basotherm, Ger.)*; Kanapiam *(Piam, Ital.)*; Kanaplus *(Roger, Spain)*; Kanaqua *(Spain)*; Kanasig *(Sigma, Austral.)*; Kanatrol *(Lusofarmaco, Ital.)*; Kanescin *(Torlan, Spain)*; Kannasyn *(Winthrop, UK)*; Kantrex *(Arg.; Bristol-Myers, Austral.; Canad.; Denm.; Bristol Italiana Sud, Ital.; Norw.; S.Afr.; Bristol-Myers, Spain; Switz.; Bristol, USA)*; Keimicina *(Boehringer Biochemia, Ital.)*; Klebcil *(USA)*; Tannamicina *(Panthox & Burck, Ital.)*.

The following names have been used for multi-ingredient preparations containing kanamycin salts— Kanfotrex *(Bristol-Myers Pharmaceuticals, UK)*; Kantrexil *(Bristol-Myers Pharmaceuticals, UK)*.

12876-g

Kasugamycin

$C_{14}H_{25}N_3O_9$=379.4.

CAS — 6980-18-3.

An antimicrobial substance produced by the growth of *Streptomyces kasugaensis*.

Kasugamycin is an aminoglycoside antibiotic with antifungal activity and generally weak antibacterial properties.

97-c

Kitasamycin *(USAN, rINN)*.

CAS — 1392-21-8.

Pharmacopoeias. In *Jpn* which also includes Acetylkitasamycin.

An antimicrobial substance produced by *Streptomyces kitasatoensis*.

Kitasamycin is a macrolide antibiotic with similar actions and uses to erythromycin (p.222), but weaker antimicrobial activity. It has been administered by mouth as kitasamycin base or intravenously as the tartrate. Acetylkitasamycin has also been administered by mouth.

In 81 patients with acute respiratory infections, including 56 with mixed bacterial infections, kitasamycin 1.6 g daily for 5 days, resulted in bacteriological and clinical cure in 34 and clinical cure only in 25. In 10 patients with wound infections, all were considered cured clinically, but 1 was a bacteriological failure.— B. C. Stratford and S. Dixson, *Med. J. Aust.*, 1974, *1*, 1029.

Proprietary Names and Manufacturers of Kitasamycin, its Salts and Derivatives
Acetyl Leucomycin *(Toyo Jozo, Jpn)*; Ayermicina *(Ayerst, Ital.)*; Leucomycin *(Toyo Jozo, Jpn)*.

186-k

Latamoxef Disodium *(BANM, rINNM)*.

6059-S; LY-127935; Moxalactam Disodium *(USAN)*. (7*R*)-7-[2-Carboxy-2-(4-hydroxyphenyl)acetamido]-7-methoxy-3-(1-methyl-1*H*-tetrazol-5-ylthiomethyl)-1-oxa-3-cephem-4-carboxylic acid, disodium salt.
$C_{20}H_{18}N_6Na_2O_9S$=564.4.

CAS — 64952-97-2 (latamoxef); 64953-12-4 (disodium salt).

1.08 g of monograph substance is approximately equivalent to 1 g of latamoxef. Each g of monograph substance represents about 3.5 mmol of sodium.

A 10% solution in water of the *U.S.P.* substance for injection has a pH of 4.5 to 7.0.

Incompatibility or loss of activity has been reported between latamoxef disodium and some aminoglycosides.

Adverse Effects

As for Cephalothin Sodium, p.176.

Latamoxef disodium may interfere with haemostasis; thus abnormalities in haematological tests may be observed and these may be associated with bleeding episodes. If bleeding occurs and the prothrombin time is prolonged vitamin K should be administered. Administration of fresh frozen plasma, packed red cells, and platelet concentrates may also be necessary. If bleeding is due to platelet dysfunction, latamoxef should be discontinued. Latamoxef should also be discontinued if bleeding times are unduly prolonged.

EFFECTS ON THE BLOOD. Latamoxef disodium has been reported to interfere with haemostasis by three mechanisms: hypoprothrombinaemia, inhibition of platelet function, and, very rarely, immune-mediated thrombocytopenia. Coagulopathies, including prolonged prothrombin time, depletion of vitamin K-dependent clotting factors, prolonged bleeding time, and decreased platelet count have been attributed to the administration of the drug (F.M. MacLennan *et al.*, *Lancet*, 1983, *1*, 1215; S. Lee *et al.*, *J. Am. med. Ass.*, 1983, *249*, 2019; J.P. Au and G.S. Geiger, *Drug Intell. & clin. Pharm.*, 1984, *18*, 140). In some cases these have been associated with bleeding episodes (R.L. Pakter *et al.*, *J. Am. med. Ass.*, 1982, *248*, 1100; M.R. Weitekamp and R.C. Aber, *ibid.*, 1983, *249*, 69; C.E. Slonaker and W.E. Luper, *ibid.*, *250*, 729; S.R. Jones and R.C. Kimbrough, *Ann. intern. Med.*, 1983, *99*, 126; L. Beeley and F. Beadle, *Br. med. J.*, 1983, *287*, 1028; S. Meisel, *Drug Intell. & clin. Pharm.*, 1984, *18*, 721), including some fatalities (M.A.R. Al-Fallouji and N.K.S. Al-Quisi, *Br. J. clin. Pract.*, 1985, *39*, 249). Such reports have occurred most often in patients who are debilitated or malnourished or who have impaired renal function. The effect of latamoxef on platelet function appears to be dose- and time-dependent (M. R. Weitekamp *et al.*, *J. antimicrob. Chemother.*, 1985, *16*, 95), therefore the manufacturers recommend limitation of the dose to 4 g daily. They also recommend administration of vitamin K 10 mg weekly to all patients as prophylaxis against hypoprothrombinaemia. There has, however, been a report of serious bleeding in 4, and prolonged prothrombin time in 2, of 23 surgical patients with colorectal disease given two doses of latamoxef 2 g for infection prophylaxis together with intravenous vitamin K 10 mg (P.J. Fabricius *et al.*, *Gut*, 1984, *25*, A553). As a result of a prospective evaluation of coagulation profiles of patients treated with cefotetan or latamoxef, Berman *et al.* (*Curr. ther. Res.*, 1984, *36*, 893) suggested that underlying disease or infection may contribute towards coagulopathies reported to be associated with these agents. A study in children has suggested that platelet function, as assessed by bleeding time, may be impaired by latamoxef, but not to the same degree as in adults (S.L. Kaplan *et al.*, *Antimicrob. Ag. Chemother.*, 1987, *31*, 467).

For a discussion on the possible mechanisms of latamoxef-induced hypoprothrombinaemia, including the role of vitamin K deficiency, and of the *N*-methylthiotetrazole side-chain of latamoxef, see Cephamandole Sodium, p.179.

EFFECTS ON THE GASTRO-INTESTINAL TRACT. As with many antibiotics, therapy with latamoxef disodium has been reported to result in changes in the faecal microflora. After administration of intravenous latamoxef to 5 healthy subjects for 7 days, Benno *et al.* (*Antimicrob. Ag. Chemother.*, 1986, *29*, 175) reported a marked suppression in faecal counts of anaerobic bacteria and Enterobacteriaceae, but an increase in counts of *Streptococcus* and *Lactobacillus* spp. The faecal flora had not recovered to pretreatment levels 7 days after discontinuation of the drug. Although these authors did not detect *Clostridium difficile*, Ambrose *et al.* (*J. antimicrob. Chemother.*, 1985, *15*, 319) did isolate this organism from the faeces of 3 of 6 healthy subjects given a single intravenous dose of latamoxef 2 g. Deery *et al.* (*ibid.*, 1984, *13*, 521) reported stool cultures positive for *Cl. difficile* in 7 of 27 patients following therapy with latamoxef for a variety of bacterial infections. One of the colonised patients experienced profuse diarrhoea, but although the stools were positive for cytotoxin, no pseudomembranes were seen, and colitis was not proven. Because of the high rate of colonisation with *Cl. difficile* observed in these patients, these authors suggested that patients who have received latamoxef should be followed closely for symptoms of antibiotic-associated colitis, especially after the antibiotic has been discontinued.

There have been several reports of superinfection with enterococci after treatment with latamoxef disodium; Yu (*Ann. intern. Med.*, 1981, *94*, 784) observed four cases of superinfection and 5 of colonisation by enterococcus in a study involving 41 patients, and Thomas (*Archs. intern. Med.*, 1983, *143*, 1780) reported the development of an enterococcal liver abscess in a 62-year-old man treated with the drug. Moellering (*Rev. infect. Dis.*, 1982, *4*, *Suppl.*, S708) reported enterococcal superinfections in 45 of 2107 patients (2.1%) treated with latamoxef; the incidence in patients with urinary-tract infections however, was 6.6%.

Precautions

As for Cephalothin Sodium, p.177.

All patients treated with latamoxef disodium should be given vitamin K 10 mg weekly as prophylaxis against hypoprothrombinaemia. Inhibition of platelet function caused by latamoxef is dose-dependent and can usually be avoided by limiting the dose to 4 g daily. Bleeding time should be monitored in patients receiving more than 4 g daily for longer than 3 days, and in patients with significantly impaired renal function. Latamoxef disodium should not be administered to patients receiving concomitant therapy with high-dose heparin or with oral anticoagulants. Aspirin or other non-steroidal anti-inflammatory drugs which can affect haemostasis may increase the risk of bleeding.

A disulfiram-like interaction with alcohol may occur, and patients receiving latamoxef disodium should therefore avoid alcohol during, and for at least several days after treatment.

ADMINISTRATION IN RENAL FAILURE. For reference to the precautions to be observed in renal failure, see under Administration in Renal Failure in Uses, below.

INTERACTIONS. *Alcohol.* A study in 10 healthy subjects of the disulfiram-like reaction of latamoxef with alcohol. The reaction occurred on 2 occasions when subjects were given latamoxef for four doses before taking alcohol. No reactions were observed when they received alcohol one hour before a single dose of latamoxef.— R. M. Elenbaas *et al.*, *Clin. Pharmac. Ther.*, 1982, *32*, 347.

References to reports of a disulfiram-like reaction in patients ingesting alcohol or alcohol-containing preparations during or after therapy with latamoxef disodium: H. C. Neu and A. S. Prince (letter), *Lancet*, 1980, *1*, 1422; K. R. Brown *et al.*, *Ann. intern. Med.*, 1982, *97*, 621.

For a discussion on the possible mechanism of the disulfiram-like reaction to alcohol in patients receiving latamoxef or some other cephalosporins, see Cephamandole Sodium, p.180.

Piperacillin. Piperacillin appeared to decrease the clearance of latamoxef when the drugs were administered concomitantly to 8 healthy subjects, but the need for an alteration in the dose of latamoxef was considered unlikely.— J. E. Kapusnik *et al.*, *Clin. Pharmac. Ther.*, 1984, *35*, 250.

Tobramycin. For reference to pharmacokinetic interaction between latamoxef and tobramycin, see Tobramycin Sulphate, p.326.

INTERFERENCE WITH ASSAY PROCEDURES. Latamoxef disodium did not appear to interfere with theophylline assay by high-performance liquid chromatography.— R. H. Gannon and R. M. Levy, *Am. J. Hosp. Pharm.*, 1984, *41*, 1185.

INTERFERENCE WITH DIAGNOSTIC TESTS. Although high

concentrations of latamoxef interfered with determinations of urine and serum creatinine using the Jaffé method, this was not observed at clinically achievable concentrations.— D. R. P. Guay *et al.*, *Am. J. Hosp. Pharm.*, 1983, *40*, 435.

PREGNANCY AND THE NEONATE. Latamoxef and other cephalosporins containing an *N*-methylthiotetrazole side-chain should be avoided in pregnancy on theoretical grounds of interference with vitamin K metabolism.— R. Wise, *Br. med. J.*, 1987, *294*, 42.

A review of drug-induced bilirubin displacement. Some studies *in vitro* have demonstrated displacement of bilirubin by latamoxef, but a study in neonates given latamoxef 100 mg per kg body-weight daily (J. de Louvois *et al.*, *Archs. Dis. Childh.*, 1984, *59*, 346) could not confirm these results.— P. C. Walker, *Clin. Pharmacokinet.*, 1987, *13*, 26.

Antimicrobial Action

Latamoxef is an oxacephalosporin antibiotic which, like the other beta-lactam antibiotics, is bactericidal and is considered to act through the inhibition of bacterial cell wall synthesis. It has a similar spectrum of activity to cefotaxime (see p.152) although it is generally slightly less active against Gram-positive bacteria. It is more active than cefotaxime against *Bacteroides fragilis*.

Although latamoxef is structurally an oxalactam, in terms of its antimicrobial activity it is classified as a third-generation cephalosporin. Its spectrum and potency of activity is very similar to that of cefotaxime. Latamoxef exists as 2 epimers (*R* and *S*). The *R* form is twice as active *in vitro* as the *S* form, however the clinical significance of this is unknown. Bacterial isolates are generally considered to be susceptible to latamoxef at MICs of 16 µg or less per mL and resistant at MICs of 64 µg or more per mL, although different breakpoints have been used.

A concentration of 8 to 32 µg per mL inhibits 50% of *Pseudomonas aeruginosa* isolates. However, as with cefotaxime, a proportion are resistant and therefore concentrations of 64 µg or more per mL are often required to inhibit 90% of strains tested. Only a small proportion of *Ps. aeruginosa* resistant to gentamicin or carbenicillin are sensitive to latamoxef. In general, latamoxef is less active *in vitro* against *Ps. aeruginosa* than cefoperazone, cefsulodin, ceftazidime, amikacin, gentamicin, tobramycin, piperacillin, and azlocillin, comparable to ticarcillin and cefotaxime, and more active than carbenicillin and mezlocillin.

The activity of latamoxef against *Haemophilus influenzae* is similar to cefotaxime, and is not affected by the presence of beta-lactamase or by resistance to ampicillin and chloramphenicol. Both beta-lactamase-producing, and non-beta-lactamase-producing strains of *Neisseria gonorrhoeae* are highly susceptible to latamoxef. Although the activity of latamoxef against *Enterobacter* spp. is comparable to cefotaxime, latamoxef is more active against gentamicin- and mezlocillin-resistant strains.

Most isolates of *Acinetobacter calcoaceticus* are resistant to latamoxef, but latamoxef is reported to be very active *in vitro* against *Yersinia enterocolitica*.

There is wide variation in susceptibility to latamoxef of anaerobes of the same genera or even the same species. Hence, sensitivity testing of local isolates is advisable. In general, latamoxef appears to be more active than cefoxitin against *Bacteroides fragilis* and has similar or less activity against the other species of the *B. fragilis* group. Cefotaxime and cefoperazone are usually less active than latamoxef against *B. fragilis*, and clindamycin and chloramphenicol are more active. Most isolates of *Clostridium difficile* are resistant to latamoxef.

Certain strains of some bacterial species have demonstrated tolerance to latamoxef, and a marked inoculum effect has been observed with many of the Enterobacteriaceae and some *Ps. aeruginosa*.

Latamoxef has marked stability *in vitro* against a variety of beta-lactamases, and resists hydrolysis by *B. fragilis* beta-lactamase to a greater degree than cefotaxime. Two types of beta-lactamase produced by *Ps. aeruginosa* can hydrolyse latamoxef; resistance of this organism to latamoxef may not, however, be related to beta-lactamase production, but to alterations in cell permeability. Like cefotaxime, latamoxef also possesses some beta-lactamase inhibitory properties.— A. A. Carmine *et al.*, *Drugs*, 1983, *26*, 279.

Studies indicating *in-vitro* activity of latamoxef against various organisms: E. J. C. Goldstein *et al.*, *Antimicrob. Ag. Chemother.*, 1980, *18*, 832 (*Eikenella corrodens*); A. W. Pasculle *et al.*, *ibid.*, 1981, *20*, 793 (*Legionella* spp.); M. J. Sanson-Le Pors *et al.*, *J. antimicrob. Chemother.*, 1983, *11*, 271 (*Haemophilus ducreyi*); E. Palenque *et al.*, *Antimicrob. Ag. Chemother.*, 1986, *29*, 182 (*Brucella melitensis*).

Some studies of the antimicrobial activity *in vitro* of latamoxef compared with other antibiotics: N. T. Sutphen *et al.*, *J. antimicrob. Chemother.*, 1982, *10*, 11; A. Digranes *et al.*, *Curr. ther. Res.*, 1984, *35*, 610.

For reference to studies comparing the bactericidal activity of some third-generation cephalosporins, see under Cefoperazone Sodium, p.148.

ACTIVITY AGAINST ANAEROBES. For a study of the susceptibilities of anaerobic bacteria isolated from women with genital-tract infections to a range of antimicrobial agents, including latamoxef, see Cefoxitin Sodium, p.158.

ACTIVITY AGAINST BRANHAMELLA. On a weight-for-weight basis, latamoxef was the most active of a range of beta-lactam antibiotics tested *in vitro* against *Branhamella catarrhalis*. It was similarly active against both beta-lactamase- and non-beta-lactamase-producing strains of disease-producing and colonising isolates of the organism.— K. G. Sweeney *et al.*, *Antimicrob. Ag. Chemother.*, 1985, *27*, 499. See also E. E. Stobberingh *et al.*, *J. antimicrob. Chemother.*, 1984, *13*, 55.

ACTIVITY WITH OTHER ANTIMICROBIAL AGENTS. Results of synergism testing between latamoxef and other antimicrobial agents has been variable depending on differences in technique and definitions of synergism used. Several studies have demonstrated a synergistic interaction between latamoxef and aminoglycosides against *Pseudomonas aeruginosa*, Enterobacteriaceae, and *Staphylococcus aureus* including some gentamicin-resistant strains. Aminoglycosides tested include amikacin (T.O. Kurtz *et al.*, *Antimicrob. Ag. Chemother.*, 1981, *20*, 239; R.H. Glew and R.A. Pavuk, *ibid.*, 1984, *26*, 378), gentamicin (A.P. Panwalker *et al.*, *ibid.*, 1980, *18*, 877; R. Skalova *et al.*, *J. antimicrob. Chemother.*, 1982, *9*, 103; P.K.W. Yu *et al.*, *Antimicrob. Ag. Chemother.*, 1983, *23*, 179) and tobramycin (R.J. Fass, *ibid.*, 1982, *21*, 1003). Hallander *et al.* (*ibid.*, 1982, *22*, 743) demonstrated synergy between latamoxef and gentamicin or netilmicin, but the effect was reduced if the drugs were not added to the inocula simultaneously.

There have also been studies of combinations of latamoxef with antipseudomonal penicillins such as azlocillin, mezlocillin, and piperacillin against Gram-positive and Gram-negative bacteria. The rate of occurrence of synergism has been variable (C.H. Ramírez-Ronda *et al.*, *Curr. ther. Res.*, 1984, *35*, 64; J.R. Rodríguez *et al.*, *ibid.*, *36*, 902) and antagonism against *Pseudomonas aeruginosa* has been reported on a few occasions (J.A. Moody *et al.*, *Antimicrob. Ag. Chemother.*, 1984, *26*, 256). Barriere *et al.* (*J. antimicrob. Chemother.*, 1985, *16*, 49) demonstrated an increased bactericidal effect of latamoxef and piperacillin against *Ps. aeruginosa* when administered concurrently at high concentrations to healthy subjects.

Antagonism against *Klebsiella pneumoniae* has been reported between a combination of latamoxef and chloramphenicol (T.H. Brown and R.H. Alford, *Antimicrob. Ag. Chemother.*, 1984, *25*, 405), but no significant interactions have been observed between latamoxef and mecillinam (R.J. Fass, *Antimicrob. Ag. Chemother.*, 1982, *21*, 188) or benzylpenicillin (P.H. Azimi and M.G. Dunphy, *ibid.*, 521) against Gram-negative bacteria.

Resistance

As for Cefotaxime Sodium, p.153.

Latamoxef has a high degree of stability to beta-lactamases produced by many bacteria, including *Bacteroides fragilis*.

Latamoxef induced the production of beta-lactamases in strains of *Enterobacter cloacae*, *Morganella morganii*, and *Pseudomonas aeruginosa* to a low to moderate extent.— T. H. Farmer and C. Reading (letter), *J. antimicrob. Chemother.*, 1987, *19*, 401.

For reference to the susceptibility of latamoxef to various beta-lactamases, see Antimicrobial Action, above.

RESISTANCE OF BACTEROIDES FRAGILIS. A study of the susceptibility to a range of antibiotics of clinical isolates of the *Bacteroides fragilis* group from 8 centres in the USA. Taking a breakpoint for resistance of 16 µg per mL, the rates of resistance for latamoxef in the 3 years from 1981 to 1983 were 22, 12, and 12% respectively. Taking a breakpoint of 32 µg per mL, the resistance-rates were 12, 7, and 7%.— F. P. Tally *et al.*, *Antimicrob. Ag. Chemother.*, 1985, *28*, 675. In the 2-year report of this study it was noted that isolates resistant to latamoxef were also likely to be resistant to other beta-lactam agents.— G. J. Cuchural *et al.*, *ibid.*, 1984, *26*, 145. See also H. M. Wexler and S. M. Finegold, *J. antimicrob. Chemother.*, 1987, *19*, 143.

RESISTANCE OF PSEUDOMONAS AERUGINOSA. The emergence of resistant strains of *Pseudomonas aeruginosa* during or after treatment with latamoxef, alone or in combination with tobramycin, in 4 patients. In 2 patients this was associated with decreased susceptibility to aminoglycosides. It was considered that latamoxef should not be used as single-agent therapy in infections caused by *Ps. aeruginosa*.— L. C. Preheim *et al.*, *Antimicrob. Ag. Chemother.*, 1982, *22*, 1037.

RESISTANCE OF SERRATIA MARCESCENS. Different mechanisms of resistance to latamoxef in *Serratia marcescens*.— L. Gutmann and Y. A. Chabbert, *J. antimicrob. Chemother.*, 1984, *13*, 15.

Absorption and Fate

Latamoxef is administered parenterally as the disodium salt. Plasma concentrations after intramuscular administration have been very variable; peak concentrations ranging from 15 to 24 µg per mL after 0.5 g and from 23 to 52 µg per mL after 1 g have been reported 0.5 to 2 hours after a dose. The plasma elimination half-life of latamoxef is approximately 2 hours and is prolonged in renal impairment and in neonates. About 50% of latamoxef in the circulation is bound to plasma proteins.

Latamoxef is widely distributed in body tissues and fluids. It diffuses into the cerebrospinal fluid particularly when the meninges are inflamed. It diffuses across the placenta and is excreted in breast milk in low concentrations.

Latamoxef is excreted principally by glomerular filtration; up to 90% of a dose appears unchanged in the urine within 24 hours and thus high urinary concentrations are achieved.

A small proportion of a dose of latamoxef is excreted in the faeces via the bile.

A review of the absorption and fate of latamoxef disodium. In plasma, the ratio of the *R* to *S* epimers varies with time after drug administration in patients with normal renal function because of an apparent preferential excretion of the *R* epimer. Since the *S* epimer is less active than the *R* form, the antimicrobial activity of the mixture of epimers two hours or more after drug administration may be decreased relative to that at the end of injection. Thus plasma concentrations measured at this time by microbiological assay may be lower than those obtained by HPLC.— A. A. Carmine *et al.*, *Drugs*, 1983, *26*, 279.

References to the pharmacokinetics of latamoxef disodium:. general pharmacokinetics studies.— K. S. Israel *et al.*, *Antimicrob. Ag. Chemother.*, 1982, *22*, 94; A. M. Shepherd *et al.*, *J. antimicrob. Chemother.*, 1983, *12*, 377.

comparisons with cephazolin.— S. Srinivasan *et al.*, *Antimicrob. Ag. Chemother.*, 1981, *19*, 302; W. M. Scheld *et al.*, *ibid.*, 613; R. E. Polk *et al.*, *ibid.*, *20*, 576.

comparisons with cefoxitin.— B. G. Charles *et al.*, *Aust. J. Hosp. Pharm.*, 1986, *16*, 238.

comparisons with ceftazidime.— T. B. Tjandramaga *et al.*, *Antimicrob. Ag. Chemother.*, 1982, *22*, 237; G. L. Drusano *et al.*, *ibid.*, 1984, *26*, 388.

comparisons with other agents.— R. Lüthy *et al.*, *ibid.*, 1981, *20*, 567 (with cefotaxime and ceftazidime); B. Kemmerich *et al.*, *ibid.*, 1983, *23*, 429 (with cefoperazone and cefotaxime); H. C. Standiford *et al.*, *ibid.*, 1986, *29*, 412 (with imipenem in association with cilastatin).

further pharmacokinetic studies.— E. H. Estey *et al.*, *ibid.*, 1981, *19*, 639 (in patients with malignancies); M. C. Nahata *et al.*, *Clin. Pharmac. Ther.*, 1982, *31*, 528 (epimer kinetics in children); M. D. Reed *et al.*, *Antimicrob. Ag. Chemother.*, 1983, *24*, 383 (in infants and children); M. H. Andritz *et al.*, *ibid.*, 1984, *25*, 33 (in elderly subjects).

ADMINISTRATION IN RENAL FAILURE. A study of the pharmacokinetics of intravenous latamoxef in patients on continuous ambulatory peritoneal dialysis (CAPD). The peritoneal excretion was low, only 17% of the dose being extracted over 24 hours. Concentrations of latamoxef in the dialysate were, however, above the MIC for many organisms susceptible to latamoxef.— E. Singlas *et al.*, *Clin. Pharmac. Ther.*, 1983, *34*, 403. See also G. Morse *et al.*, *ibid.*, 1985, *38*, 150.

Studies of the pharmacokinetics of latamoxef disodium in patients with renal impairment: W. K. Bolton *et al.*, *Antimicrob. Ag. Chemother.*, 1980, *18*, 933; E. J. Jacobsen *et al.*, *Clin. Pharmac. Ther.*, 1981, *30*, 487; N. Wright *et al.*, *J. antimicrob. Chemother.*, 1981, *8*, 395; M. Lam *et al.*, *Antimicrob. Ag. Chemother.*, 1981, *19*, 461; G. R. Aronoff *et al.*, *ibid.*, 575; A. Leroy *et al.*, *ibid.*, 965; L. R. Peterson *et al.*, *ibid.*, *20*, 378; S. Srinivasan and H. C. Neu, *ibid.*, 398; D. Hoffler *et al.*, *Arzneimittel-Forsch.*, 1984, *34*, 317.

For dosage recommendations in renal failure, see under Administration in Renal Failure in Uses, below.

DIFFUSION INTO BODY TISSUES AND FLUIDS. Eleven adults with bacterial meningitis were given 3 intravenous infusions of latamoxef 20 mg per kg body-weight at 8-hourly intervals, once between days 2 and 4 and again between days 11 and 20 of treatment with other antibiotics. Concentrations of latamoxef in the CSF ranged from 2.0 to 11.0 µg per mL and from 1.5 to 6.0 µg per mL on the two occasions, respectively, indicating that latamoxef has good penetrability when the meninges are inflamed.— J. Modai *et al.*, *Antimicrob. Ag. Chemother.*, 1982, *21*, 551. Report of a study in 3 neurosurgical patients with ventricular catheters being treated with intravenous latamoxef 2 g every four hours for presumed or culture-positive meningitis. The mean ratios of CSF to serum latamoxef concentrations were 7.8, 11.2, 14.2, and 15.0, at one, 2, 3, and 4 hours after a dose respectively.— R. J. Creger *et al.*, *ibid.*, 1985, *28*, 839.

A study in healthy subjects indicating that latamoxef does not readily penetrate saliva. Since salivary penetration was considered to be an indicator of ability to eradicate *Haemophilus influenzae* type b from the nasopharynx, patients with *H. influenzae* meningitis treated with latamoxef should receive rifampicin afterwards to reduce the likelihood of persistent colonisation.— D. T. Casto *et al.*, *Clin. Pharm.*, 1985, *4*, 67.

Further studies of the distribution of latamoxef into body tissues and fluids: R. E. Polk *et al.*, *Antimicrob. Ag. Chemother.*, 1982, *22*, 201 (atrial appendage); R. P. Smith *et al.*, *ibid.*, 1983, *24*, 15 (prostatic tissue); J. Stewart *et al.*, *J. antimicrob. Chemother.*, 1984, *13*, 377 (tissues of patients undergoing amputation of ischaemic limbs); H. M. Faris and D. W. Potts (letter), *Ann. intern. Med.*, 1984, *101*, 144. and H. Yamada *et al.*, *Antimicrob. Ag. Chemother.*, 1985, *27*, 93 (both pleural fluid).

DRUG EXCRETION. In a study involving 6 healthy subjects, probenecid did not affect the pharmacokinetics of latamoxef. Thus latamoxef appears to be eliminated via the kidney primarily by glomerular filtration, with no involvement of tubular secretion.— K. A. DeSante *et al.*, *Antimicrob. Ag. Chemother.*, 1982, *21*, 58.

A comparison of latamoxef concentrations in bile and gall-bladder wall in 34 patients undergoing cholecystectomy who received latamoxef, either 1 g intramuscularly 1 hour prior to surgery or 0.5 g intravenously with anaesthetic induction. Concentrations in the serum, gall-bladder wall, and bile were generally comparable in both groups and were above the MIC of many pathogens. However, concentrations within the groups were variable. Concentrations of latamoxef in the common-duct bile were higher than in gall-bladder bile or wall, being more than double the serum concentrations. The intravenous dose of latamoxef was favoured for infection prophylaxis in biliary surgery.— P. Vowden *et al.*, *J. antimicrob. Chemother.*, 1986, *18*, 227. See also O. V. Martinez *et al.*, *Antimicrob. Ag. Chemother.*, 1981, *20*, 231.

PREGNANCY AND THE NEONATE. Latamoxef 100 mg per kg body-weight daily in 2 divided doses was given to 31 neonates for 2 to 10 days. Peak serum concentrations of 105 µg per mL and 128 µg per mL were achieved respectively after single and multiple injections, with half-lives of 8.9 and 5.8 hours. Apart from the time to peak concentrations there was no significant difference between intravenous and intramuscular injection.— J. de Louvois *et al.*, *Archs Dis. Childh.*, 1984, *59*, 346.

In a study involving 12 pregnant women, serum-latamoxef concentrations were lower immediately postpartum than 4 months later. The total body clearance of latamoxef was almost doubled early in the puerperium. Doses may need to be adjusted accordingly.— D. Charles and B. Larsen, *Antimicrob. Ag. Chemother.*, 1986, *29*, 873.

A novel pharmacokinetic method for analysis of placental transfer of latamoxef in pregnant women.— T. Yamamoto *et al.*, *Clin. Pharmacokinet.*, 1986, *11*, 154.

Uses and Administration

Latamoxef disodium is an oxacephalosporin antibiotic; it differs from the cephalosporins in that the sulphur atom of the beta-lactam nucleus is replaced by oxygen. It is used similarly to the third-generation cephalosporin cefotaxime sodium for the treatment of susceptible infections (see p.154). It is administered by deep intramuscular injection or intravenously by slow injection over 3 to 5 minutes or by continuous or intermittent infusion. Intramuscular doses of 2 g or more should not be administered at one injection site. If pain following intramuscular injection is a problem latamoxef disodium may be administered in a 0.5 or 1% solution of lignocaine hydrochloride. Doses are expressed in terms of the equivalent amount of latamoxef. The usual dose for adults is 0.5 to 4 g daily in two divided doses. For the treatment of serious or life-threatening infections up to 4 g every 8 hours may be given; however, to avoid the risk of bleeding disorders that have been associated with the use of latamoxef disodium, the manufacturers generally recommend limitation of the dose to 4 g daily and the prophylactic administration of vitamin K 10 mg weekly (see above under Adverse Effects and Precautions).

Infants and children may be given latamoxef in doses of 50 mg per kg body-weight every 12 hours; neonates up to one week of age may be given 25 mg per kg every 12 hours, and those aged 1 to 4 weeks, 25 mg per kg every 8 hours. These doses may be doubled in serious infections. In the treatment of meningitis, a loading dose of 100 mg per kg may be given.

Doses may need to be modified in patients with renal impairment.

If latamoxef disodium is administered in association with an aminoglycoside, the drugs should be administered separately.

Reviews of the actions and uses of latamoxef disodium: *Lancet*, 1981, *2*, 23; *Med. Lett.*, 1982, *24*, 13; A. A. Carmine *et al.*, *Drugs*, 1983, *26*, 279.

ADMINISTRATION. Latamoxef has been administered into the eye topically, or by subconjunctival or intravitreal injection.— T. S. Lesar and R. G. Fiscella, *Drug Intell. & clin. Pharm.*, 1985, *19*, 642.

ADMINISTRATION IN INFANTS AND CHILDREN. Infants and children could be given latamoxef intravenously in a dose of 200 to 300 mg per kg body-weight daily in 4 to 6 divided doses for the treatment of severe infections.— K. H. Rhodes and C. M. Johnson, *Mayo Clin. Proc.*, 1983, *58*, 158.

ADMINISTRATION IN RENAL FAILURE. The manufacturers of latamoxef have recommended that patients with impaired renal function be given an initial dose of 1 to 2 g followed by a maintenance dose adjusted according to the creatinine clearance (CC).

For a CC of more than 80 mL per minute (normal renal function), 0.25 to 2 g every 8 to 12 hours (maximum, 4 g every 8 hours);
between 50 and 80 mL per minute, 0.25 to 1 g every 8 hours (maximum, 3 g every 8 hours);
between 25 and 50 mL per minute, 0.25 to 1 g every 12 hours (maximum, 2 g every 8 hours or 3 g every 12 hours);
between 2 and 25 mL per minute, 0.25 to 0.5 g every 8 hours (maximum, 1 g every 8 hours or 1.25 g every 12 hours);
less than 2 mL per minute, 0.25 to 0.5 g every 12 hours (maximum, 1 g every 24 hours). Maintenance doses should be repeated following regular haemodialysis.

The half-life of latamoxef was increased from 2.3 to between 18 and 23 hours in end-stage renal failure. Latamoxef could be administered to patients with renal failure by adjusting the dosage interval. A dosage interval of 8 hours is suitable for patients whose glomerular filtration-rates exceed 50 mL per minute; an interval of 12 hours between doses is advisable for rates of between 10 and 50 mL per minute. Where the rate is less than 10 mL per minute, the dosage interval should be 12 to 24 hours. A dose supplement should be given to patients undergoing haemodialysis.— W. M. Bennett *et al.*, *Am. J. Kidney Dis.*, 1983, *3*, 155.

Latamoxef has been administered intraperitoneally in a dose of 200 mg per litre of dialysis fluid to patients on continuous ambulatory peritoneal dialysis who develop peritonitis.— D. K. Scott and D. E. Roberts, *Pharm. J.*, 1985, *1*, 621.

For reference to pharmacokinetic studies in patients with renal impairment, see Absorption and Fate, above.

GONORRHOEA. Treatment with a single intramuscular dose of latamoxef 1 g was effective in eradicating *Neisseria gonorrhoeae* at follow-up after 3 to 7 days, from 120 evaluable patients with acute gonorrhoea. They included 2 patients with penicillin-resistant isolates and 5 women with rectal infection.— B. Lutz *et al.*, *Clin. Ther.*, 1983, *5*, 509.

MENINGITIS. Latamoxef has been investigated in the treatment of meningitis due to a broad range of bacteria. In a study involving 63 neonates and infants less than one year of age presenting with meningitis due to Gram-negative enteric bacilli (G.H. McCracken *et al.*, *J. Am. med. Ass.*, 1984, *252*, 1427), parenteral therapy with latamoxef together with ampicillin sodium appeared to be comparable to ampicillin sodium with amikacin sulphate; the number of patients was too small to detect a difference. Other authors have reported success with latamoxef as sole therapy for Gram-negative meningitis in a few patients, (D.A. Olson *et al.*, *Ann. intern. Med.*, 1981, *95*, 302; M. Uwaydah *et al.*, *Antimicrob. Ag. Chemother.*, 1983, *23*, 289), including one report of meningitis caused by a *Vibrio* spp. (R.B. Bode *et al.*, *Ann intern. Med.*, 1986, *104*, 55). Latamoxef has also been reported to be as effective as ampicillin or chloramphenicol in the treatment of *Haemophilus influenzae* type b meningitis in a study in 91 children (S.L. Kaplan *et al.*, *J. Pediat.*, 1984, *104*, 447).

A combination of latamoxef and ampicillin has therefore been suggested as an alternative to ampicillin and gentamicin for empirical therapy of neonatal meningitis. Latamoxef should not, however, be used alone because of poor activity against pneumococci, group B streptococci, and *Listeria monocytogenes* (M. Whitby and R. Finch, *Drugs*, 1986, *31*, 266).

See also Absorption and Fate, above.

NEUTROPENIA. For reference to the use of latamoxef in febrile episodes in neutropenic patients, see below under Septicaemia.

PNEUMONIA. A report of the treatment of 78 patients with community- or hospital-acquired pneumonia treated with intravenous latamoxef disodium. There was a high mortality rate, but this was attributed to the poor general medical condition of the patients and to the presence of serious Gram-negative bacterial infections. It was concluded that latamoxef disodium was effective single-agent therapy against a wide range of susceptible organisms although precautions must be observed when administering high doses.— D. K. Payne *et al.* (letter), *Drug Intell. & clin. Pharm.*, 1987, *21*, 293.

For reference to a comparative report of cefotaxime, ceftizoxime, and latamoxef in the treatment of pneumonia, see Ceftizoxime Sodium, p.167.

SEPTICAEMIA. Because of its broad spectrum of antimicrobial action, latamoxef disodium has been investigated for the treatment of suspected or confirmed serious infections in various groups of patients including neonates (J. de Louvois *et al.*, *Archs Dis. Childh.*, 1984, *59*, 346), non-neutropenic patients with suspected bacteraemia (W.R. Wilson *et al.*, *Mayo Clin. Proc.*, 1984, *59*, 318), neutropenic patients with febrile episodes (W.R. Bezwoda *et al.*, *J. antimicrob. Chemother.*, 1985, *15*, 239), patients with life-threatening Gram-negative infections (M. Joshi *et al.*, *Antimicrob. Ag. Chemother.*, 1986, *30*, 90), and other hospitalised patients (T.F. Murphy and M. Barza, *ibid.*, 1982, *21*, 568; R. L. Marier *et al.*, *ibid.*, 650; G. E. Mathisen *et al.*, *ibid.*, 780; W. Salzer *et al.*, *ibid.*, 1983, *23*, 565). Because of the activity of latamoxef against *Bacteroides* spp. (*Med. Lett.*, 1984, *26*, 87) it may be more appropriate than other third-generation cephalosporins for the treatment of anaerobic infections, such as localised abscesses (H. Lagast *et al.*, *Antimicrob. Ag. Chemother.*, 1982, *22*, 604; *Drug & Ther. Bull.*, 1986, *24*, 33), or mixed aerobic/anaerobic infections such as intra-abdominal or necrotising soft-tissue surgical sepsis (F.P. Tally *et al.*, *Antimicrob. Ag. Chemother.*, 1986, *29*, 244). Some workers (P. Davey, *J. antimicrob. Chemother.*, 1984, *13*, 204), however, have suggested that in neutropenic patients such anti-anaerobic activity may impair colonisation-resistance of the gastro-intestinal tract resulting in superinfections. Studies of the use of latamoxef disodium in serious infections have in general indicated that it is not appropriate sole therapy for infections caused by Gram-positive organisms or *Pseudomonas aeruginosa*, and that there may be a danger of the emergence of resistant organisms during treatment. To overcome some of these deficits, latamoxef has been used in association with an aminoglycoside or another beta-lactam antibiotic, particularly the penicillins with antipseudomonal activity. Several studies have compared these regimens, for example latamoxef with either piperacillin or amikacin (D. J. Winston *et al.*, *Am. J. Med.*, 1984, *77*, 442), or latamoxef with ticarcillin or tobramycin (V. Fainstein *et al.*, *Archs intern. Med.*, 1984, *144*, 1766). Although these studies found no significant difference in overall efficacy between their two regimens, Young (*J. antimicrob. Chemother.*, 1985, *16*, 4), considered that therapy with two beta-lactam antibiotics should not be used routinely in immunocompromised patients, particularly in those with proven or suspected pseudomonal infections. Another potential problem of such a combination is the induction of beta-lactamases by some beta-lactams

such as cefoxitin and imipenem.
More recently the empirical use of latamoxef for the treatment of bacteraemia (*Med. Lett.*, 1986, *28*, 33) or for febrile episodes in neutropenic patients (L.S. Young, *J. antimicrob. Chemother.*, 1985, *16*, 4) has been advised against because of its association with coagulopathies and serious, sometimes fatal, bleeding disorders. Alternative cephalosporins or related compounds are available, and it would appear especially prudent not to use latamoxef in thrombocytopenic patients.

SURGICAL INFECTION PROPHYLAXIS. Because of its broad antimicrobial spectrum, latamoxef has been investigated for the prophylaxis of infection during surgical procedures. It has been reported to be as effective as cephazolin for caesarean section (W. Rayburn *et al.*, *Antimicrob. Ag. Chemother.*, 1985, *27*, 337), as effective as a combination of cephazolin and metronidazole for colorectal surgery (W.E.G. Thomas *et al.*, *J. antimicrob. Chemother.*, 1985, *16*, 121), and as effective as cefoxitin for vaginal hysterectomy (R.P. Rapp *et al.*, *Clin. Pharm.*, 1986, *5*, 988). Latamoxef, cefotaxime, and cefoperazone were equally effective in preventing sepsis in patients undergoing surgery for early appendicitis, but latamoxef was more effective in late cases, including those with gangrenous or perforated appendicitis (W.-Y. Lau *et al.*, *Antimicrob. Ag. Chemother.*, 1985, *28*, 639). This was assumed to be due to its greater activity against *Bacteroides fragilis*. Crots *et al.* (*Clin. Pharm.*, 1985, *4*, 316) showed latamoxef to be as effective as a combination of gentamicin and clindamycin in preventing infection after penetrating abdominal trauma; antibiotics were given for between 3 and 18 days.
However, serious bleeding in 4 patients and prolonged prothrombin time in 2, has been observed in a group of 23 surgical patients with colorectal diseases given infection prophylaxis with two doses of latamoxef 2 g in association with intravenous vitamin K 10 mg (P.J. Fabricius *et al.*, *Gut*, 1984, *25*, A553). From a study in 20 patients also undergoing colorectal surgery, Kager *et al.* (*J. antimicrob. Chemother.*, 1984, *14*, 171) concluded that a single dose may be sufficient for prophylaxis and may avoid the risk of adverse effects on the microbial flora. It should also be remembered that some workers consider that the first-generation cephalosporins and cefoxitin are the preferred cephalosporins for surgical infection prophylaxis in most procedures and that there is no reason to use a third-generation agent (*Med. Lett.*, 1985, *27*, 105).

TYPHOID FEVER. An evaluation of different dosage regimens of latamoxef in the treatment of 25 patients with typhoid fever. Although latamoxef appears to be effective therapy especially when given for 10 to 11 days, it should probably be reserved for use only when conventional therapy is ineffective or contra-indicated.— M. Uwaydah *et al.*, *Antimicrob. Ag. Chemother.*, 1986, *30*, 338.

URINARY-TRACT INFECTIONS. In a study of 49 patients with complicated urinary-tract infections, parenteral treatment with latamoxef or gentamicin was considered to be equally efficacious. An additional 10 patients with gentamicin-resistant organisms were treated with latamoxef; 4 of these had complete bacteriological cure. Resistance to latamoxef developed in 3 *Pseudomonas aeruginosa* isolates during therapy with the drug, and 2 of these isolates demonstrated a concurrent decrease in susceptibility to aminoglycosides. These findings suggest that latamoxef should not be used as sole therapy for severe infections caused by this organism.— P. G. Penn *et al.*, *Antimicrob. Ag. Chemother.*, 1983, *24*, 494. See also A. S. Lea *et al.*, *ibid.*, 1982, *22*, 32 (comparison with cephazolin).

Preparations

Moxalactam Disodium for Injection (*U.S.P.*). Contains latamoxef disodium.

Proprietary Preparations

Moxalactam (*Lilly, UK*). *Injection*, powder for reconstitution, latamoxef 0.5, 1, and 2 g (as disodium salt).

Proprietary Names and Manufacturers

Baxal (*Ital Suisse, Ital.*); Betalactam (*Bergamon, Ital.*); Latoxacef (*Magis, Ital.*); Mactam (*Coli, Ital.*); Moxatres (*Radiumfarma, Ital.*); Moxacef (*Pulitzer, Ital.*); Moxalactam (*Lilly, Austral.*; *Lilly, Fr.*; *Lilly, Ger.*; *Lilly, S.Afr.*; *Lilly, Spain*; *Lilly, Switz.*; *Lilly, UK*); Moxam (*Lilly, Canad.*; *Lilly, USA*); Oxacef (*Gibipharma, Ital.*); Priolatt (*San Carlo, Ital.*); Sectam (*Locatelli, Ital.*).

16873-l

Lenampicillin (*rINN*).

KBT-1585. 2,3-Dihydroxy-2-butenyl(2*S*,5*R*,6*R*)-6-[(*R*)-2-amino-2-phenylacetamido]-3,3-dimethyl-7-oxo-4-thia-1-azabicyclo[3.2.0]heptane-2-carboxylate, cyclic carbonate.
$C_{21}H_{23}N_3O_7S$=461.5.
CAS — 86273-18-9.

Lenampicillin is an ester of ampicillin and is administered by mouth.

References to lenampicillin: A. Saito and M. Nakashima, *Antimicrob. Ag. Chemother.*, 1986, *29*, 948 (pharmacokinetics).

Proprietary Names and Manufacturers
Kanebo, Jpn.

98-k

Lincomycin Hydrochloride (*BANM, USAN, rINNM*).

NSC-70731; U-10149 (*lincomycin*). Methyl 6-amino-6,8-dideoxy-*N*-[(2*S*,4*R*)-1-methyl-4-propylprolyl]-1-thio-α-D-*erythro*-D-*galacto*-octopyranoside hydrochloride monohydrate.
$C_{18}H_{34}N_2O_6S,HCl,H_2O$=461.0.
CAS — 154-21-2 (lincomycin); 859-18-7 (hydrochloride, anhydrous); 7179-49-9 (hydrochloride, monohydrate).

Pharmacopoeias. In *Br.*, *Chin.*, *Egypt.*, *Ind.*, *It.*, *Jpn*, and *U.S.* Also in *B.P. Vet.*

An antimicrobial substance produced by the growth of *Streptomyces lincolnensis* var. *lincolnensis* or by any other means.
A white or almost white crystalline powder, odourless or with a slight characteristic odour. The *B.P.* specifies that not more than 5% is lincomycin B. The *U.S.P.* specifies not less than 790 μg of lincomycin per mg. 1.13 g of monograph substance is approximately equivalent to 1 g of lincomycin.
Soluble 1 in 2 of water, 1 in 40 of alcohol, and 1 in 20 of dimethylformamide; very slightly soluble in acetone; practically insoluble in chloroform and ether. A 10% solution of lincomycin hydrochloride in water has a pH of 3.0 to 5.5. Solutions are **sterilised** by filtration. **Store** at a temperature not exceeding 30° in airtight containers. The *B.P.* injection should be protected from light.

Lincomycin hydrochloride is stated to be **incompatible** with kanamycin sulphate and novobiocin sodium.

Units

One unit of lincomycin is contained in 0.0011351 mg of the first International Reference Preparation (1965) of lincomycin hydrochloride which contains 881 units per mg.

Adverse Effects

As for Clindamycin Hydrochloride, p.198.
Phlebitis may occur when large doses of lincomycin hydrochloride are given intravenously. Hypotension and on rare occasions cardiac arrest have followed too rapid intravenous injections.

A patient given lincomycin 4 to 6 g daily by rapid intermittent intravenous infusion developed reversible glucose intolerance, hyperlipidaemia, and hypertriglyceridaemia.— C. J. O'Connell and M. E. Plaut, *Curr. ther. Res.*, 1969, *11*, 478.

EFFECTS ON THE BLOOD. A report of a 58-year-old woman who developed sideroblastic anaemia and pseudomembranous enterocolitis after lincomycin therapy. After withdrawal of the lincomycin and administration of pyridoxine and blood transfusions, the anaemia resolved.— G. Kokkini *et al.*, *Postgrad. med. J.*, 1983, *59*, 796.

EFFECTS ON THE GASTRO-INTESTINAL TRACT. For reports of diarrhoea and pseudomembranous colitis associated with the administration of lincomycin hydrochloride, see Clindamycin Hydrochloride, p.198.

EFFECTS ON THE NEUROMUSCULAR SYSTEM. See under Clindamycin Hydrochloride, p.199.

OVERDOSAGE. Chest compliance decreased within 15 minutes of the inadvertent administration of a 12-g bolus intravenous injection of lincomycin instead of 1.2 g. Cardiac arrest immediately followed intubation. It was considered that cardiac arrest was not due to reflex bradycardia or hypoxia after intubation but to a cardiac depressant action.— J. L. Daubeck *et al.*, *Anesth. Analg. curr. Res.*, 1974, *53*, 563.
A 10-year-old girl with osteomyelitis erroneously received lincomycin 6 g intravenously on 2 occasions within 10 hours without signs of toxicity, apart from fatigue and unpleasant taste sensation.— K. Widhalm and G. Salzman, *Arzneimittel-Forsch.*, 1978, *28*, 1428.

Treatment of Adverse Effects

As for Clindamycin Hydrochloride, p.199.

Precautions

As for Clindamycin Hydrochloride, p.199.
Lincomycin should not be given to patients who are known to be hypersensitive to it or who have experienced reactions with clindamycin. Kaolin and cyclamates reduce the absorption of lincomycin from the gastro-intestinal tract.

ADMINISTRATION IN LIVER DISORDERS AND RENAL FAILURE. For reference to the precautions to be observed in liver disorders and in renal failure, see under Uses, below.

PREGNANCY AND THE NEONATE. A study over 7 years of the children of mothers who received lincomycin in the 3 trimesters of pregnancy indicated that the incidence of abnormalities was no greater than in a normal population.— A. Mickal and J. D. Panzer, *Am. J. Obstet. Gynec.*, 1975, *121*, 1071.

Antimicrobial Action and Resistance

Lincomycin has an antimicrobial spectrum similar to that of clindamycin (see p.199) but it is less potent. The minimum inhibitory concentrations of lincomycin have been reported to range from 0.02 to 3.1 μg per mL for many strains of sensitive Gram-positive cocci. Most strains of *Bacteroides* spp. have been reported to be inhibited by about 6 μg or less per mL of lincomycin.
Bacterial resistance to lincomycin is similar to that to clindamycin.

Absorption and Fate

About 20 to 35% of a dose of lincomycin given by mouth is absorbed from the gastro-intestinal tract and following a 500-mg dose, peak plasma concentrations of 1 to 6 μg per mL are reached within 2 to 4 hours. Food markedly reduces the rate and extent of absorption. The intramuscular injection of 600 mg produces peak plasma concentrations of 8 to 12 μg per mL within 1 to 2 hours; peak plasma concentrations within 30 minutes have been reported.
The biological half-life of lincomycin is about 5 hours. Lincomycin is widely distributed in the tissues including bone and body fluids but diffusion into the cerebrospinal fluid is poor unless the meninges are inflamed. It diffuses across the placenta and is excreted in the milk of nursing mothers. About 5 to 10% of a 500-mg dose given by mouth is excreted in the urine within 24 hours but 30% or more of a dose given parenterally may be excreted in the urine, most of it within 4 hours. It is not effectively removed from the blood by dialysis. High concentrations are achieved in the bile and about 40% of a dose given by mouth and up to 14% of a dose given by injection can be excreted in the faeces. It is considered that lincomycin not accounted for by urinary and faecal excretion is inactivated, probably in the liver.

Pharmacokinetic studies of lincomycin: intravenous infusion.— E. Novak *et al.*, *Clin. Pharmac. Ther.*, 1971, *12*, 793; P. R. Gwilt and R. B. Smith, *J. clin. Pharmac.*, 1986, *26*, 87; intramuscular injection.— R. B. Smith *et al.*, *ibid.*, 1981, *21*, 411.

ADMINISTRATION IN LIVER DISORDERS AND RENAL FAILURE. For references to the pharmacokinetics of lincomycin in liver disorders and renal failure, see under Uses, below.

DRUG ABSORPTION. The absorption of lincomycin may

be reduced in patients with Crohn's disease.— P. G. Welling and F. L. S. Tse, *J. clin. Hosp. Pharm.*, 1984, *9*, 163.

DIFFUSION INTO BODY TISSUES AND FLUIDS. Reports of the distribution of lincomycin hydrochloride: P. A. Thomas and P. C. Jolly, *Am. Rev. resp. Dis.*, 1967, *96*, 1044 (pleural fluid); P. I. Lerner, *Am. J. med. Sci.*, 1969, *257*, 125 (CSF); R. L. Parsons *et al.*, *Br. J. clin. Pharmac.*, 1977, *4*, 433 (bone and synovial fluid); J. Gabka and W. Platz, *Arzneimittel-Forsch.*, 1978, *28*, 87 (tonsils).

PREGNANCY AND THE NEONATE. Diffusion of lincomycin into the foetal circulation, cord blood, and amniotic fluid after intramuscular administration to 60 pregnant women shortly before delivery.— N. M. Duignan *et al.*, *Br. med. J.*, 1973, *3*, 75.

PROTEIN BINDING. Using an ultrafiltration method, protein binding of lincomycin varied between 28 and 86% depending on the concentration of drug in the serum.— P. R. Gwilt and R. B. Smith, *J. clin. Pharmac.*, 1986, *26*, 87.

Uses and Administration

Lincomycin is a lincosamide antibiotic with actions and uses similar to its chlorinated derivative, clindamycin (see p.198). Clindamycin is usually preferred now to lincomycin because of its greater activity and better absorption.

Lincomycin hydrochloride is administered by mouth in doses equivalent to 500 mg of lincomycin 3 or 4 times daily taken at least 1 hour before food; by intramuscular injection, 600 mg once or twice daily; by slow intravenous infusion over not less than one hour, 600 mg two or three times daily in at least 250 mL of sodium chloride 0.9% infusion or glucose 5% infusion. Higher doses have been given in very severe infections. Children over the age of 1 month may be given 30 to 60 mg per kg body-weight daily in divided doses by mouth or 10 to 20 mg per kg daily in divided doses by intramuscular injection or intravenous infusion.

Lincomycin hydrochloride may be administered into the eye by subconjunctival injection in a dose equivalent to 75 mg of lincomycin.

A brief review of lincomycin.— J. G. Bartlett, *Lancet*, 1982, *2*, 478.

ADMINISTRATION IN LIVER DISORDERS. The mean serum half-life for lincomycin was 8.96 hours (range 6.11-11.8 hours) in 9 patients with hepatic insufficiency, but normal renal function, given 600 mg intramuscularly compared with 4.85 hours (range 4.45 to 5.67 hours) in 6 controls with normal hepatic and renal functions. Doses may need to be reduced in patients with liver disease.— H. M. Bellamy *et al.*, *Antimicrob. Ag. Chemother.*, 1966, 36.

ADMINISTRATION IN RENAL FAILURE. The *US* manufacturers have recommended that patients with severe renal impairment be given lincomycin in a dose 25 to 30% of that used in patients with normal renal function. The normal half-life for lincomcyin of 4 to 5 hours was increased to 10 to 20 hours in end-stage renal disease. The interval between doses should be extended from 6 hours to 12 hours in those with a glomerular filtration-rate (GFR) of 10 to 50 mL per minute, and to 24 hours in those with a GFR of less than 10 mL per minute. A supplemental dose of lincomycin was not required for patients on haemodialysis or peritoneal dialysis.— W. M. Bennett *et al.*, *Am. J. Kidney Dis.*, 1983, *3*, 155.

Preparations

Lincomycin Capsules *(B.P.)*. Capsules containing lincomycin hydrochloride.

Lincomycin Hydrochloride Capsules *(U.S.P.)*

Lincomycin Hydrochloride Syrup *(U.S.P.)*

Lincomycin Injection *(B.P.)*. A sterile solution of lincomycin hydrochloride in Water for Injections. *U.S.P.* (Lincomycin Hydrochloride Injection) contains benzyl alcohol as a preservative.

Sterile Lincomycin Hydrochloride *(U.S.P.)*

Proprietary Preparations

Lincocin *(Upjohn, UK)*. *Capsules*, lincomycin 500 mg (as hydrochloride). *Syrup*, lincomycin 250 mg (as hydrochloride)/5 mL. *Injection*, lincomycin 300 mg (as hydrochloride)/mL in ampoules of 2 mL.

Proprietary Names and Manufacturers

Albiotic *(Upjohn, Ger.; Ind.)*; Cillimicina *(Hoechst, Ital.; Normon, Spain)*; Cillimycin *(Hoechst, Ger.; Norw.)*; Frademicina *(Arg.)*; Lincocin *(Upjohn, Austral.; Belg.; Upjohn, Canad.; Denm.; Upjohn, Ital.; Neth.; Upjohn, Norw.; Upjohn, S.Afr.; Upjohn, Spain; Upjohn, Swed.; Upjohn, Switz.; Upjohn, UK; Upjohn, USA)*; Lincocine *(Upjohn, Fr.)*; Mycivin *(Boots, UK)*.

99-a

Lividomycin *(rINN)*.

Lividomycin A. 4-*O*-(2-Amino-2,3-dideoxy-α-D-*ribo*-hexopyranosyl)-2-deoxy-5-*O*-[3-*O*-(4-*O*-α-D-mannopyranosyl-2,6-diamino-2,6-dideoxy-β-L-idopyranosyl)-β-D-ribofuranosyl]-D-streptamine.

$C_{29}H_{55}N_5O_{18}$=761.8.

CAS — 36441-41-5.

An antimicrobial substance produced by the growth of *Streptomyces lividus*.

Lividomycin is an aminoglycoside antibiotic.

Proprietary Names and Manufacturers

Livaline *(Bellon, Fr.)*.

100-a

Lymecycline *(BAN, rINN)*.

Lumecycline; Tetracycline-L-methylenelysine. A water-soluble combination of tetracycline, lysine, and formaldehyde with a molecular weight of approximately 603.

CAS — 992-21-2.

Pharmacopoeias. In *Br.*

A yellow very hygroscopic powder. The *B.P.* specifies that it contains not less than 900 units per mg of anhydrous lymecycline. Lymecycline 408 mg is approximately equivalent to 300 mg of tetracycline and to 324 mg of tetracycline hydrochloride. **Soluble** 1 in less than 1 of water; slightly soluble in alcohol; practically insoluble in acetone, chloroform, and ether. A 1% solution in water has a pH of 7.8 to 8.1. **Store** at a temperature not exceeding 25° in well-closed containers. Protect from light.

Accelerated degradation studies showed that the loss of potency of lymecycline powder stored in ampoules at −20° would be less than 1% over 10 years.— J. W. Lightbown *et al.*, *Bull. Wld Hlth Org.*, 1972, *47*, 343.

Units

One unit of lymecycline is contained in 0.0010548 mg of the second International Reference Preparation (1971) which contains 948 units per mg.

Adverse Effects and Precautions

As for Tetracycline Hydrochloride, p.314.

Absorption and Fate

As for Tetracycline Hydrochloride, p.317.

A mean concentration of 1.4 µg of lymecycline per mL was achieved in sinus secretions 3 to 5 hours after 300 mg was taken by mouth by 15 patients on twice-daily dosage.— K. Lundin and J. -E. Brorson (letter), *J. antimicrob. Chemother.*, 1978, *4*, 187.

In a study of the bioavailability of lymecycline and tetracycline hydrochloride given by mouth to 12 healthy subjects in doses equivalent to 300 mg tetracycline base every 12 hours for 7 doses, the relative bioavailability of lymecycline was only 70% compared with tetracycline hydrochloride.— G. Sjölin-Forsberg and J. Hermansson, *Br. J. clin. Pharmac.*, 1984, *18*, 529.

Uses and Administration

Lymecycline has antimicrobial activity and uses similar to those of tetracycline hydrochloride (see p.315).

Doses are expressed in terms of the equivalent amount of tetracycline base. The usual adult dose is the equivalent of 300 mg of tetracycline administered twice daily by mouth; in severe infections doses of up to 1.2 g may be given over 24 hours.

For the use of lymecycline in the treatment of bronchitis, see under Tetracycline Hydrochloride, Respiratory-tract Infections, p.320.

Preparations

Lymecycline Capsules *(B.P.)*

Proprietary Preparations

Tetralysal *(Farmitalia Carlo Erba, UK)*. *Capsules*, lymecycline 408 mg equivalent to tetracycline base 300 mg.

Proprietary Names and Manufacturers

Ciclisin *(Ital.)*; Ciclolysal *(Arg.)*; Lisinbiotic *(Ital.)*; Lisinciclina *(Ital.)*; Tancilina *(Arg.)*; Tetralysal *(Belg.; Farmitalia, Denm.; Fr.; Carlo Erba, Ital.; Farmitalia, Norw.; Farmitalia Carlo Erba, S.Afr.; Ifesa, Spain; Farmitalia Carlo Erba, Swed.; Farmitalia Carlo Erba, UK)*; Tralisin *(FIRMA, Ital.)*.

101-t

Lysostaphin *(USAN)*.

An antibiotic derived from the growth of *Staphylococcus staphylolyticus*.

CAS — 9011-93-2.

Lysostaphin is an antibacterial enzyme highly active *in vitro* against staphylococci and causes rapid lysis of the cell wall of the organism.

Proprietary Names and Manufacturers

Mead Johnson Laboratories, USA.

4908-r

Mafenide Acetate *(BANM, USAN, rINNM)*.

NSC-34632 *(mafenide)*. α-Aminotoluene-*p*-sulphonamide acetate.

$C_7H_{10}N_2O_2S,C_2H_4O_2$=246.3.

CAS — 138-37-4 (hydrochloride); 138-39-6 (mafenide); 13009-99-9 (acetate).

Pharmacopoeias. In *Braz.*, *Chin.*, and *U.S.*

A white crystalline powder. 11.2 g of monograph substance is approximately equivalent to 8.5 g of mafenide. Freely **soluble** in water. A 10% solution in water has a pH of 6.4 to 6.8. **Store** in airtight containers. Protect from light.

Adverse Effects, Treatment, and Precautions

As for Sulphamethoxazole, p.306 since mafenide is absorbed by the skin. Its action is not, however, antagonised by *p*-aminobenzoic acid or related compounds.

Mafenide acetate cream may cause pain or a burning sensation on application to the burnt area, particularly on burns of partial skin thickness. Allergic reactions associated with a maculopapular rash, urticaria, an eczematoid reaction, contact dermatitis, and erythema multiforme have occurred. The separation of the eschar may be delayed and fungal invasion of the wound has been reported. By its action in inhibiting carbonic anhydrase mafenide may cause metabolic acidosis and hyperventilation; acid-base balance should therefore be monitored, particularly in patients with extensive burns, and treatment should be temporarily suspended and continuous fluid therapy given if persistent acidosis occurs.

Absorption and Fate

Mafenide is absorbed from wounds into the circulation and is metabolised to *p*-carboxybenzenesulphonamide which is excreted in the urine. The metabolite has no antibacterial action but retains the ability to inhibit carbonic anhydrase.

Uses and Administration

Mafenide is a sulphonamide which is not inactivated by *p*-aminobenzoic acid or by pus and serum. The acetate is used as a cream, in conjunction with debridement, for the prevention and treatment of infection, particularly by *Pseudomonas aeruginosa*, in second- and third-degree burns. It is applied to a thickness of 1 to 2 mm once or twice daily by a sterile gloved hand and, although not usually necessary, may be covered by a thin gauze dressing. Treatment is continued until healing is progressing satisfactorily or the burn site is ready for skin grafting. Mafenide hydrochloride and mafenide propionate have also been used.

Preparations

Mafenide Acetate Cream *(U.S.P.)*. Store at a temperature not exceeding 40°.

Proprietary Preparations

Sulfamylon *(Sterling Research, UK)*. *Cream*, mafenide 8.5% (as acetate).

Proprietary Names and Manufacturers of Mafenide Salts

Mafylon *(S.Afr.)*; Napaltan *(Ger.; Switz.)*; Sulfamylon *(Arg.; Austral.; Winthrop, Canad.; Denm.; Fr.; Swed.; Sterling Research, UK; Winthrop-Breon, USA)*; Sulfomyl *(Winthrop, UK)*.

5662-d

Mandelic Acid

Amygdalic Acid; Racemic Mandelic Acid; Phenylglycollic Acid. 2-Hydroxy-2-phenylacetic acid.
$C_8H_8O_3$=152.1.

CAS — 90-64-2; 17199-29-0 (+); 611-72-3 (±); 611-71-2 (−).

Pharmacopoeias. In *Arg.*, *Aust.*, and *Neth. Arg.*, *Nord.*, and *Span.*, include calcium mandelate.

Adverse Effects and Precautions

Mandelic acid has occasionally caused side-effects such as giddiness, tinnitus, gastric disturbances, dysuria, haematuria and, rarely, an urticarial rash.

It should be avoided in patients with impaired renal function.

Uses and Administration

Mandelic acid has bacteriostatic properties and has been used in the treatment of urinary-tract infections, usually as the ammonium or calcium salt.

It is excreted unchanged in the urine and has been effective against infections due to *Escherichia coli* and *Enterococcus faecalis (Streptococcus faecalis)* provided that the pH is maintained below 5.5. Mandelic acid is also used as a 1% flushing solution for the maintenance of indwelling urinary catheters.

See also Hexamine Mandelate, p.247.

Proprietary Preparations

Uro-Tainer Mandelic Acid *(Vifor, Switz.: CliniMed, UK)*. *Irrigation solution*, sterile, mandelic acid 1%. For flushing of indwelling urinary catheters.

102-x

Mecillinam *(BAN, rINN)*.

Amdinocillin *(USAN)*; FL-1060; Ro-10-9070.
(6*R*)-6-(Perhydroazepin-1-ylmethyleneamino)penicillanic acid.
$C_{15}H_{23}N_3O_3S$=325.4.

CAS — 32887-01-7.

Pharmacopoeias. U.S. includes Sterile Amdinocillin.

A 10% solution in water has a pH of 4.0 to 6.2.
A 10% aqueous solution is reported to be **stable** for 24 hours at 25° and for 3 days at 5°. A 20% aqueous solution is reported to be stable for 16 hours at 25° and for 24 hours at 5°. It is recommended that reconstituted solutions of mecillinam for injection should be administered immediately after preparation.

Adverse Effects and Precautions

As for Benzylpenicillin Sodium, p.132.

ADMINISTRATION IN RENAL FAILURE. For reference to the precautions to be observed in renal failure, see under Uses, Administration in Renal Failure, below.

INTERFERENCE WITH DIAGNOSTIC TESTS. In a study *in vitro* mecillinam, unlike the other penicillins tested, had no effect on urinary glucose estimations using Clinitest Reagent Tablets.— W. A. Parker and M. E. MacCara, *Am. J. Hosp. Pharm.*, 1984, *41*, 125.

Antimicrobial Action

Mecillinam is a derivative of amidinopenicillanic acid which, unlike benzylpenicillin and related antibiotics, is very active against a wide range of Gram-negative bacteria including most of the Enterobacteriaceae. *Pseudomonas aeruginosa, Haemophilus influenzae, Bacteroides* spp., and indole-positive *Proteus* spp. are considered to be resistant. It is much less active against Gram-positive bacteria; enterococci including *Enterococcus faecalis* are resistant.

Mecillinam interferes with the synthesis of the bacterial cell wall by binding with a different penicillin-binding protein from benzylpenicillin. This difference in the mode of action may explain the synergism against many Gram-negative organisms that has been reported *in vitro* between mecillinam and various penicillins or cephalosporins.

Mecillinam is more stable against beta-lactamases than ampicillin.

Mecillinam inhibited 5, 33, 44, 53, 74, 89, and all of 92 strains of *Neisseria gonorrhoeae in vitro* at an MIC of 0.25, 0.5, 1, 2, 4, 8, and 16 µg per mL respectively.— B. A. Watts *et al.*, *J. antimicrob. Chemother.*, 1977, *3*, 331.

In a study *in vitro*, the MIC_{90} values (minimum concentration at which 90% of strains tested are inhibited) of mecillinam against beta-lactamase-producing and non-beta-lactamase-producing strains of *Branhamella catarrhalis* were 64 and 8 µg per mL respectively.— E. E. Stobberingh *et al.*, *J. antimicrob. Chemother.*, 1984, *13*, 55.

Of 2753 strains of *Shigella dysenteriae*, *S. flexneri*, and *S. boydii* isolated from the faeces of patients and examined at the Central Public Health Laboratory from 1979 to mid 1983, 7.1% were resistant to mecillinam at a concentration of 2 µg per mL.— R. J. Gross *et al.*, *Br. med. J.*, 1984, *288*, 784.

A study of the sensitivity to a range of antibiotics of 293 organisms isolated from urine specimens collected between May and July 1983. A total of 156 (53%) of isolates were fully sensitive to mecillinam, including 64% of *Escherichia coli*, 55% of *Proteus* spp. and 40% of *Klebsiella* spp.— S. R. Marper and P. Noone (letter), *J. antimicrob. Chemother.*, 1985, *15*, 251.

ACTION. A study of the mechanism of action of mecillinam. Although it binds to penicillin-binding protein, PBP-2 in Gram-negative bacteria, its mode of action in most Gram-positive bacteria is probably no different from that of other beta-lactam antibiotics.— B. G. Spratt, *J. antimicrob. Chemother.*, 1977, *3*, *Suppl.* B, 13.

ENHANCED ACTIVITY. Mecillinam binds avidly and virtually exclusively, to a minor penicillin-binding protein, PBP-2, a transpeptidase which appears to be essential for the determination of normal bacterial cell shape. *Escherichia coli* exposed to low or high concentrations of mecillinam are converted to osmotically stable round forms, which lyse slowly after a number of hours. On combination with any of several beta-lactam antibiotics which bind preferentially to PBP-3 extensive and rapid lysis of bacteria may be observed. However, a synergistic interaction has been shown only against about half of the strains of enteric Gram-negative bacteria tested, and there is no way of predicting which strains will respond.— W. E. Farrar, *Ann. intern. Med.*, 1984, *101*, 389. Mecillinam is most often synergistic *in vitro* with older beta-lactam antibiotics such as ampicillin, cephazolin, cephamandole, cefoxitin, and carbenicillin, which are less active against Enterobacteriaceae than newer compounds. Synergy is less frequently seen with more potent, broad-spectrum agents such as piperacillin and latamoxef. The role of mecillinam may be limited, however, since many of the newer cephalosporins may be more active than combinations of mecillinam with the above beta-lactam agents.— S. L. Barriere, *Clin. Pharm.*, 1986, *5*, 24.

Clavulanic acid and mecillinam or sulbactam and mecillinam demonstrated synergy *in vitro* against the majority of isolates of *Escherichia coli*, *Klebsiella*, *Citrobacter*, *Salmonella*, and *Serratia* spp. resistant to mecillinam alone. Neither beta-lactamase inhibitor however, increased the activity of mecillinam against a significant number of mecillinam-susceptible strains.— H. C. Neu, *Antimicrob. Ag. Chemother.*, 1982, *22*, 518.

Absorption and Fate

Mecillinam is poorly absorbed from the gastro-intestinal tract. Peak plasma concentrations of about 6 and 12 µg per mL have been achieved half an hour after intramuscular doses of 200 and 400 mg, respectively. A plasma half-life of 1 hour has been reported. Between 5 and 15% of mecillinam is reported to be bound to plasma proteins. Mecillinam is widely distributed into body tissues and fluids; little passes into the CSF unless the meninges are inflamed. It diffuses across the placenta and has been detected in amniotic fluid; little appears to be excreted in breast milk. Mecillinam is metabolised to only a limited extent. From 50 to 70% of a parenteral dose may be excreted in the urine within 6 hours by glomerular filtration and tubular secretion. Renal tubular secretion can be reduced by the concomitant use of probenecid. High concentrations are achieved in bile.

Studies of the pharmacokinetics of mecillinam after intravenous or intramuscular administration to healthy subjects: K. Roholt, *J. antimicrob. Chemother.*, 1977, *3*, *Suppl.* B, 71; M. Mitchard *et al.*, *ibid.*, 83; J. G. Gambertoglio *et al.*, *Antimicrob. Ag. Chemother.*, 1980, *18*, 952; S. L. Barriere *et al.*, *ibid.*, 1982, *21*, 54; B. R. Meyers *et al.*, *ibid.*, 1983, *23*, 827.

ADMINISTRATION IN RENAL FAILURE. For reference to the absorption and fate of mecillinam in patients with impaired renal function, see under Uses, Administration in Renal Failure, below.

DIFFUSION INTO BODY TISSUES AND FLUIDS. A study of 53 patients undergoing surgery for acute or chronic cholecystitis or for obstructive jaundice given mecillinam 800 mg intramuscularly 1 hour before the operation. In non-jaundiced patients, there was a mean mecillinam-concentration of 12 µg per mL in the serum and 49 µg per mL in the common bile duct. In the 26 patients with normal gall-bladder function the mean concentration in the gall-bladder bile was 40 µg per mL. The equivalent figure for the 16 patients with a non-functioning gall-bladder was 12 µg per mL. In the 11 jaundiced patients the mean concentrations of mecillinam in common duct bile and gall-bladder bile were 8 and 12 µg per mL respectively. The 7 patients with severe jaundice, however, had a mean gall-bladder bile concentration of less than 1 µg per mL. The poor concentration of mecillinam in the biliary tree in jaundiced patients was associated with a slight elevation of the serum-mecillinam concentration to 17 µg per mL, as compared with 12 µg per mL in the non-jaundiced group.— M. M. Hares *et al.*, *J. antimicrob. Chemother.*, 1982, *9*, 217.

Combination with ampicillin. Ten patients undergoing prostatectomy were given a single intravenous dose of mecillinam 5 mg per kg body-weight and ampicillin 12 mg per kg, one to six hours prior to surgery. Drug concentrations in the prostate gland up to 6 hours after administration were 32 to 100% of those in the serum for mecillinam, and 35 to 85% for ampicillin.— N. Jeppesen and C. Frimodt-Møller, *Curr. med. Res. Opinion*, 1984, *9*, 213.

Mecillinam 400 mg with ampicillin 1000 mg were administered as a single intravenous injection to 13 patients 1 to 4 hours before partial or total nephrectomy. The mean kidney-to-serum ratios at biopsy were 1.4 and 2.4 for mecillinam and ampicillin respectively.— P. Ostri and C. Frimodt-Møller, *Curr. med. Res. Opinion*, 1986, *10*, 117.

Uses and Administration

Mecillinam has the same penicillanic acid nucleus as the penicillins and a substituted amidino group has been introduced at the 6-position. It is given by intravenous injection over 3 to 4 minutes, by intravenous infusion over 15 to 30 minutes usually in glucose (5%) or sodium chloride (0.9%) injection, or intramuscularly in the treatment of severe Gram-negative infections. For urinary-tract infections a dose of 5 mg per kg body-weight may be given every 6 to 8 hours. In severe infections 10 mg per kg may be given 4- to 6-hourly. A suggested dose in the treatment of enteric fever is 12.5 to 15 mg per kg every 6 hours; probenecid may be taken concomitantly to delay the excretion of mecillinam.

Mecillinam has been administered in combination with other beta-lactam antibiotics, particularly ampicillin (p.116), to increase its spectrum of

antimicrobial activity to Gram-positive organisms and because of reported synergism against Gram-negative bacteria *in vitro* (see Antimicrobial Action, above).
For the oral use of mecillinam as its pivaloyloxymethyl ester, see Pivmecillinam p.289.

Reviews of the actions and uses of mecillinam: W. E. Farrar, *Ann. intern. Med.*, 1984, *101*, 389; *Med. Lett.*, 1985, *27*, 30; H. C. Neu, *Pharmacotherapy*, 1985, *5*, 1.

ADMINISTRATION IN RENAL FAILURE. The mean elimination half-life of mecillinam was 1.1 hours in 5 healthy subjects, and 1.3, 2.4, and 4.0 hours in patients with creatinine clearances of 51 to 100 mL per minute (5 patients), 16 to 50 mL per minute (9), and 5 to 15 mL per minute (9), respectively, after they were given a 15-minute intravenous infusion of mecillinam 10 mg per kg body-weight. Although the concentrations of mecillinam in the urine of the patients with the most severe renal impairment were generally lower than those found for the other groups, they were still considered to exceed the MIC values for pathogens likely to be responsible for urinary-tract infections. It was recommended that in patients with severe renal impairment the usual dose of mecillinam could be administered, but the dosage interval should be increased from 4 hours to between 6 and 8 hours.
In 5 patients who received haemodialysis for 4 hours immediately after the drug infusion, 32 to 72% of the administered dose was recovered in the dialysate. Concentrations were considered to have remained in the therapeutic range, and therefore supplemental doses of mecillinam either during or at the end of the dialysis procedure should not be required. In 2 patients who underwent peritoneal dialysis, less than 4% of the administered dose was lost into the dialysate.— I. H. Patel *et al.*, *Antimicrob. Ag. Chemother.*, 1985, *28*, 46. See also: K. Bailey *et al.* (letter), *Br. J. clin. Pharmac.*, 1980, *10*, 177; P. L. Svarva and T. Wessel-Aas, *Scand. J. infect. Dis.*, 1980, *12*, 303; A. Schapira, *Clin. Pharmacokinet.*, 1984, *9*, 364.

ENTERIC INFECTIONS. For reference to the use of mecillinam in enteric fever and *Salmonella* carrier states, see Pivmecillinam p.289.

Preparations

Sterile Amdinocillin *(U.S.P.)*. Mecillinam suitable for parenteral use.

Proprietary Preparations

Selexidin *(Burgess, UK)*. *Injection*, powder for reconstitution, mecillinam 200 and 400 mg.

Proprietary Names and Manufacturers

Coactin *(Roche, USA)*; Selecidin *(Alter, Spain)*; Selexid *(Hässle, Denm.; Neth.; Leo, Norw.)*; Selexidin *(Lövens, Swed.; Burgess, UK)*.

103-r

Meclocycline Sulfosalicylate *(USAN)*.

GS-2989 (meclocycline); Meclocycline Sulphosalicylate; NSC-78502 (meclocycline). 7-Chloro-6-demethyl-6-deoxy-5β-hydroxy-6-methylenetetracycline 5-sulphosalicylate.
$C_{22}H_{21}ClN_2O_8,C_7H_6O_6S$=695.0.

CAS — 2013-58-3 (meclocycline); 73816-42-9 (sulfosalicylate).

NOTE. Meclocycline is *BAN*, *USAN*, and *rINN*.

Pharmacopoeias. In *U.S.*

The *U.S.P.* specifies that meclocycline sulfosalicylate contains not less than 620 μg of meclocycline per mg. A 1% solution in water has a pH of 2.5 to 3.5. **Store** in airtight containers. Protect from light.

Meclocycline sulfosalicylate is a tetracycline antibiotic which is applied topically for the treatment of acne vulgaris and superficial skin infections. Potency is expressed in terms of meclocycline.

Preparations

Meclocycline Sulfosalicylate Cream *(U.S.P.)*

Proprietary Names and Manufacturers

Meclan *(Ortho Dermatological, USA)*; Meclocil *(Esseti, Ital.)*; Mecloderm *(Schwarz, Ital.)*; Meclosorb *(Basotherm, Ger.)*; Meclutin Semplice *(ABC, Ital.)*; Quoderm *(Isdin, Spain)*; Traumatociclina *(Biomedica Foscama, Ital.)*.

185-c

Metampicillin *(rINN)*.

(6*R*)-6-(D-2-Methyleneamino-2-phenylacetamido)penicillanic acid.
$C_{17}H_{19}N_3O_4S$=361.4.

CAS — 6489-97-0.

Metampicillin has actions and uses similar to ampicillin (see p.116).
After oral administration it is almost completely hydrolysed to ampicillin. When given parenterally however, a proportion of the administered dose exists in the circulation as unchanged metampicillin which has some antibacterial activity of its own and is excreted in high concentrations in the bile.
Metampicillin is given by mouth in doses of 2 g daily in 2 to 4 divided doses. It may also be given intramuscularly or intravenously. Metampicillin is often administered as the sodium salt.

In a study involving 35 cholecystectomised patients and 10 healthy subjects, total biliary excretion of metampicillin in the cholecystectomised patients was 8.3% of a 500-mg intravenous dose compared with 0.19% of a dose of carbenicillin 1 g intramuscularly and 0.1% of a dose of ampicillin 500 mg given by mouth or intravenously. When metampicillin was given by mouth only 0.16% of a 500-mg dose was excreted in the bile. In the healthy subjects 5.8% of the dose of metampicillin given intravenously was recovered in the duodenal juice compared with 0.04% and 0.11% after intravenous doses of ampicillin and carbenicillin respectively. Antibiotic activity in patients given metampicillin was assayed in terms of ampicillin because of its partial hydrolysis to ampicillin.— M. Pinget *et al.*, *J. antimicrob. Chemother.*, 1976, *2*, 195. See also J. M. Brogard *et al.*, *ibid.*, 363.

Proprietary Names and Manufacturers of Metampicillin and Metampicillin Sodium

Actuapen *(Spain)*; Ampilprats *(Prats, Spain)*; Ampimetacil *(Spain)*; Ampliopenil *(Spain)*; Baldacilina *(Spain)*; Cetinmicina *(Carol, Spain)*; Co-Metampicil *(Spain)*; Daniven *(Spain)*; Darkepen *(Tilfarma, Spain)*; Demetilina *(Spain)*; Doctamicina *(Spain)*; Dompil *(Spyfarma, Spain)*; Durmetan *(Spain)*; Fedacilina *(Spain)*; Italcina *(Spain)*; Janopen *(Spain)*; Lermetan *(Spain)*; Madecilina *(Spain)*; Magnipen *(Clin Midy, Fr.; Midy, Ital.)*; Maipen *(Maipe, Spain)*; Marcomycina *(Spain)*; Mempil *(Spain)*; Meta-Alvar *(Oftalmiso, Spain)*; Metabacter *(Rubio, Spain)*; Metabiot *(Spain)*; Metacidan *(Cidan, Spain)*; Metaclarben *(Clarben, Spain)*; Metacostyl *(Pentafarm, Spain)*;
Meta-Espectral *(Spain)*; Meta-Ferran *(Ferran, Spain)*; Meta-Framan *(Oftalmiso, Spain)*; Metainexfa *(Inexfa, Spain)*; Metakes *(Albofarma, Spain)*; Metalcor *(Alcor, Spain)*; Metamas *(Tafir, Spain)*; Metambac *(Kairon, Spain)*; Metamico *(Kairon, Spain)*; Metampen *(Almirall, Spain)*; Metampicef *(Llorens, Spain)*; Metampikel *(Spain)*; Metampilene *(Hortel, Spain)*; Metam-Piror *(Spain)*; Metamplimedix *(Medix, Spain)*; Metanova *(Cheminova, Spain)*; Metapenyl *(Spain)*; Metaval *(Valles Mestre, Spain)*; Metiskia *(Spain)*; Micinovo *(Andreu, Spain)*; Neo-Togram *(Morgens, Spain)*; Ocelina *(Roux-Ocefa, Arg.)*; Pemet *(Graino, Spain)*; Penapli *(Spain)*; Pirobiotic *(Clariana, Spain)*; Pluriespec *(Spain)*; Pramet *(Spain)*; Serfabiotic *(Serra Pamies, Spain)*; Soifamet *(Spain)*; Suvipen *(Spedrog-Caillon, Arg.; Sarbach, Fr.; Spain)*; Tablebiotin *(Santos, Spain)*; Tampilen *(Sabater, Spain)*; Tisquibron *(Maipe, Spain)*; Totalbiotico *(Llano, Spain)*; Venzoquimpe *(Quimpe, Spain)*; Viderpen *(Seid, Spain)*; Vigocina *(Spain)*.

105-d

Methacycline Hydrochloride *(BANM, USAN)*.

6-Methyleneoxytetracycline Hydrochloride; GS-2876 (methacycline); Méthylènecycline Hydrochloride; Metacycline Hydrochloride *(pINNM)*; Metacyclini Chloridum. 6-Demethyl-6-deoxy-5β-hydroxy-6-methylenetetracycline hydrochloride.
$C_{22}H_{22}N_2O_8$,HCl=478.9.

CAS — 914-00-1 (methacycline); 3963-95-9 (hydrochloride).

Pharmacopoeias. In *Jug.*, *Nord.*, and *U.S.*

A yellow crystalline powder. The *U.S.P.* specifies that it contains not less than 832 μg of methacycline per mg. Methacycline 92 mg is approximately equivalent to 100 mg of methacycline hydrochloride. **Soluble** 1 in 100 of water and 1 in 300 of alcohol; practically insoluble in chloroform and ether; soluble in dilute solutions of sodium hydroxide. A 1% solution in water has a pH of 2 to 3. **Store** in airtight containers. Protect from light.

Units

One unit of methacycline is contained in 0.001082 mg of the first International Reference Preparation (1969) of methacycline hydrochloride which contains 924 units per mg.

Adverse Effects and Precautions

As for Tetracycline Hydrochloride, p.314.

A report of pigment deposits in the eyes and skin exposed to the light in 6 patients during prolonged treatment with methacycline; a further patient experienced conjunctival pigmentation only.— K. Dyster-Aas *et al.*, *Acta derm.-vener., Stockh.*, 1974, *54*, 209.

For mention of methacycline causing photosensitivity reactions, see under Doxycycline Hydrochloride, p.217.

Absorption and Fate

As for Tetracycline Hydrochloride, p.317.
About 80 to 90% of methacycline in the circulation is bound to plasma proteins. Plasma concentrations of up to 2.6 μg per mL have been reported 4 hours after a 300-mg dose of methacycline hydrochloride. Its biological half-life is about 15 hours. About 50% of a dose is slowly excreted unchanged in the urine.

The average concentration of methacycline in lung tissue in 5 patients 8 hours after taking methacycline 300 mg was 0.83 μg per g compared with an average serum concentration of 0.64 μg per mL. In another group of 10 patients given 2 doses of 300 mg twenty and eight hours before the assay, the average lung tissue concentration was 0.98 μg per g and the average serum concentration was 1.28 μg per mL.— J. J. Timmes *et al.*, *Clin. Pharmac. Ther.*, 1971, *12*, 920.

Uses and Administration

Methacycline hydrochloride has the antimicrobial activity and uses described for tetracycline hydrochloride (see p.315). Like demeclocycline it is excreted more slowly than tetracycline and effective blood concentrations are maintained for longer periods.
It is administered by mouth in a usual dose of 600 mg daily in 2 or 4 divided doses, preferably one hour before or 2 hours after meals. Children have been given 6.5 to 13 mg per kg body-weight daily but the effect of tetracyclines on teeth should be considered.

For mention of the use of methacycline hydrochloride in the treatment of bronchitis, see under Tetracycline Hydrochloride, Respiratory-tract Infections, p.320.

Preparations

Methacycline Hydrochloride Capsules *(U.S.P.)*

Methacycline Hydrochloride Oral Suspension *(U.S.P.)*. pH 6.5 to 8.0. Potency is expressed in terms of methacycline.

Proprietary Names and Manufacturers

Apriclina *(Aandersen, Ital.)*; Benciclina *(Benvegna, Ital.)*; Bialatan *(Spain)*; Boscillina *(Ital.)*; Brevicillina *(Ital.)*; Ciclobiotic *(Beta, Ital.)*; Ciclum *(Ital.)*; Duecap *(Ital.)*; Duplaciclina *(Locatelli, Ital.)*; Duramicina *(Bergamon, Ital.)*; Dynamicin *(Ital.)*; Esarondil *(Terapeutico M.R., Ital.)*; Esquilin *(Edmond Pharma, Ital.)*; Fitociclina *(Ital.)*; Franciclina *(Francia Farm., Ital.)*; Francomicina *(Nuovo, Ital.)*; Gammaciclina *(Ital.)*; Globociclina *(Ital.)*; Idrossimicina *(Ital.)*; Isometa *(Ital.)*; Largomicina *(Ital.)*; Medomycin *(Medosan, Ital.)*; Metabiotic *(Ital.)*; Metabioticon B.G. *(Boniscontro & Gazzone, Ital.)*; Metac *(Ital.)*; Metacil *(Ibirn, Ital.)*; Metaclin *(Ital.)*; Metaclor *(Ital.)*; Metadomus *(Medici Domus, Ital.)*; Metagram *(Biochimica Zanardi, Ital.)*; Metamicina *(Rottapharm, Ital.)*; Metilenbiotic *(Ital.)*; Micociclina *(Ital.)*; Mit-Ciclina *(Ital.)*; Molciclina *(Ital.)*;
Optimycine *(Sandoz, Switz.)*; Ossirondil *(Ital.)*; Paveciclina *(IBP, Ital.)*; Physiomycine *(Millot-Solac, Fr.)*; Piziacina *(Lifepharma, Ital.)*; Pluramycine *(Belg.)*; Plurigram *(Lafare, Ital.)*; Prontomicina *(Tosi-Novara, Ital.)*; Quickmicina *(Panthox & Burck, Ital.)*; Radiomicina *(Ital.)*; Rindex *(Salus, Ital.)*; Rondomicina *(Ital.)*; Rondomycin *(Warner, Austral.; Roerig, Swed.; Pfizer, UK; Wallace, USA)*; Rondomycine *(Belg.; Fr.; Pfizer, Switz.)*; Rotilen *(Terapeutico M.R., Ital.)*; Sernamicina

(Ital.); Stafilon *(AGIPS, Ital.)*; Tachiciclina *(Ital.)*; Tetrabios *(Ausonia, Ital.)*; Tiberciclina *(Ital.)*; Ticomicina *(Ital.)*; Treis-Ciclina *(Ecobi, Ital.)*; Valcin *(Ital.)*; Wassermicina *(IFI, Ital.)*; Yatrociclina *(Ital.)*; Zermicina *(Ital.)*.

106-n

Methicillin Sodium *(BANM, USAN)*.

Dimethoxyphenecillin Sodium; Dimethoxyphenyl Penicillin Sodium; Meticillin Sodium *(pINNM)*; Meticillinum Natricum; Sodium Methicillin.
Sodium (6*R*)-6-(2,6-dimethoxybenzamido)penicillanate monohydrate.
$C_{17}H_{19}N_2NaO_6S,H_2O=420.4$.

CAS — 61-32-5 (methicillin); 132-92-3 (sodium salt, anhydrous); 7246-14-2 (sodium salt, monohydrate).

Pharmacopoeias. In *Cz., Int., It., Jug., Nord., Roum., Rus.,* and *Turk. U.S.* includes Sterile Methicillin Sodium.

A fine white crystalline powder, odourless or with a slight odour. 1.11 g of monograph substance is approximately equivalent to 1 g of anhydrous methicillin. Each g of monograph substance represents about 2.4 mmol of sodium.

Freely **soluble** in water and methyl alcohol; slightly soluble in amyl alcohol, chloroform, and propyl alcohol; practically insoluble in ether and acetone. A 1% solution in water has a pH of 5.0 to 7.5.

Solutions of methicillin sodium are reported to be **stable** for 24 hours at 25° and for 4 days at 5°. A 10% solution is reported to be stable for 7 days at 5°; a 50% solution is reported to be stable for 4 weeks at −20°. However, it is recommended that reconstituted solutions of methicillin sodium for injection should be administered immediately after preparation. Methicillin sodium should not be mixed with blood products or other proteinaceous fluids such as protein hydrolysates.

Methicillin sodium has been reported to be **incompatible** with aminoglycosides, tetracyclines, and other antimicrobial agents including erythromycin ethylsuccinate, lincomycin hydrochloride, sulphafurazole diethanolamine, sulphadiazine sodium, and vancomycin hydrochloride. It has been reported to be incompatible with acidic drugs such as ascorbic acid, atropine sulphate, metaraminol tartrate, and vitamins of the B group, and alkaline drugs such as aminophylline, methohexitone sodium, and sodium bicarbonate. Incompatibility or loss of activity has also been reported with salts of opioid analgesics, canrenoate potassium, chlorpromazine hydrochloride, coliston sulphomethate sodium, fat emulsions, hydrocortisone sodium succinate, prochlorperazine edisylate, and promethazine hydrochloride.

For reference to the degradation of methicillin sodium in solution, see under Benzylpenicillin Sodium, p.132.

Adverse Effects and Precautions

As for Benzylpenicillin Sodium, p.132.

Interstitial nephritis has occurred in patients given methicillin sodium. Blood disorders have occasionally been reported.

An analysis of 148 reported episodes of drug fever; 46 were caused by antimicrobial agents and of these 6 were due to methicillin.— P. A. Mackowiak and C. F. LeMaistre, *Ann. intern. Med.*, 1987, *106*, 728.

EFFECTS ON THE BLOOD. Methicillin sodium may cause bone-marrow depression and both leucopenia and agranulocytosis have been reported. There appears to be a high incidence of methicillin-associated neutropenia; the incidence of neutropenia caused by penicillinase-resistant penicillins has been reported to approach 5% (C.F. Kirkwood *et al.*, *Clin. Pharm.*, 1983, *2*, 569). In some cases anaemia has also been reported and there has been a report of thrombocytopenia in one patient (C.A. Schiffer *et al.*, *Ann. intern. Med.*, 1976, *85*, 338).

EFFECTS ON THE GASTRO-INTESTINAL TRACT. Methicillin 150 to 200 mg per kg body-weight daily administered intravenously to 8 children caused alteration of the faecal flora with suppression of *Bifidobacterium*, *Streptococcus*, and *Lactobacillus* spp.— H. Sakata *et al.*, *Antimicrob. Ag. Chemother.*, 1986, *29*, 225.

EFFECTS ON THE KIDNEYS AND URINARY BLADDER. Methicillin sodium has been reported to cause acute interstitial nephritis which has an immunological mechanism and is usually reversible on withdrawal of the drug (S.A. Sanjad *et al.*, *J. Pediat.*, 1974, *84*, 873; K. Solex *et al.*, *J. clin. Pharmac.*, 1983, *23*, 484). Haemorrhagic cystitis has also been reported usually following administration of high doses of methicillin for 8 to 21 days (R. Bracis *et al.*, *Antimicrob. Ag. Chemother.*, 1977, *12*, 438). The cause of methicillin-induced haemorrhagic cystitis is unclear and both direct bladder toxicity and hypersensitivity reactions have been suggested. One patient developed haemorrhagic cystitis, acute interstitial nephritis, and agranulocytosis during methicillin therapy, and the coincident occurrence of complications of immunological origin suggested an immunological mechanism might be involved for the bladder lesions and bone-marrow depression (M. Godin *et al.*, *J. antimicrob. Chemother.*, 1980, *6*, 296).

INTERACTIONS. Sequential administration of intravenous bolus doses of streptomycin 500 mg and methicillin 1 g, over a period of 5 minutes through a subclavian-vein catheter, had caused rigors in postoperative coronary-artery bypass patients, within 30 minutes of administration. Administration of the 2 drugs separated by an interval of 4 hours appeared to avoid this.— P. C. Robinson *et al.* (letter), *Lancet*, 1978, *2*, 1056.

Antimicrobial Action

Methicillin sodium has a similar mode of action to that of benzylpenicillin but is resistant to staphylococal penicillinase. It is active against both penicillinase-producing and non-penicillinase-producing staphylococci, and also against group A beta-haemolytic streptococci, *Streptococcus pneumoniae*, and some viridans streptococci. It is virtually ineffective against *Entercoccus faecalis*.

The minimum inhibitory concentration against susceptible penicillinase-producing and non-penicillinase-producing staphylococci, is usually within the range of 1 to 4 µg per mL. However, its activity against penicillin-sensitive staphylococci and streptococci is less than that of benzylpenicillin.

In a study of the susceptibility of the penicillinase-resistant penicillins to penicillinase of *Staphylococcus aureus*, methicillin, cloxacillin, and nafcillin were relatively resistant to penicillinase but flucloxacillin was much less resistant.— R. W. Lacey and A. Stokes, *J. clin. Path.*, 1977, *30*, 35. In another study methicillin was found to be the most stable, followed in descending order of stability by cloxacillin, dicloxacillin, and flucloxacillin (equal stabilities); oxacillin, cephalothin, cephradine, and cephalexin (equal); and cephazolin and cephaloridine (equal).— M. J. Basker *et al.*, *J. antimicrob. Chemother.*, 1980, *6*, 333. Similar results showing methicillin to be the most stable against *Staph. aureus* penicillinase followed by dicloxacillin, cloxacillin, flucloxacillin, and oxacillin.— N. Frimodt-Møller *et al.*, *J. antimicrob. Chemother.*, 1986, *18*, 27.

ACTIVITY WITH OTHER ANTIMICROBIAL AGENTS. Synergy has been demonstrated *in vitro* between methicillin and fosfomycin against methicillin-resistant *Staphylococcus aureus*.— S. Alvarez *et al.*, *Antimicrob. Ag. Chemother.*, 1985, *28*, 689.

Resistance

Resistance of staphylococci to methicillin is intrinsic and does not depend directly upon penicillinase production. Cross-resistance to other penicillins, including the penicillinase-resistant penicillins, such as cloxacillin, dicloxacillin, flucloxacillin, nafcillin, and oxacillin, and to the cephalosporins usually occurs. Methicillin-resistant staphylococci are also frequently resistant to other antibiotics including chloramphenicol, erythromycin, and tetracycline, and some strains may also be resistant to clindamycin, lincomycin, and gentamicin or other aminoglycosides.

Outbreaks of hospital infection with methicillin-resistant *Staphylococcus aureus* (MRSA) first occurred in the 1960s; this resistance also affected flucloxacillin and other isoxazolyl penicillins. The incidence of hospital infections with MRSA appeared to decline, but in 1976 a strain resistant to both methicillin and gentamicin was described in London, and a few years later in Australia there began a nationwide outbreak of hospital infection with *Staph. aureus* resistant to penicillin, methicillin, gentamicin, cephalosporins, erythromycin, and tetracyclines. Since then outbreaks have occurred in Europe, the *USA*, South Africa, and the Middle East (P.J. Sanderson, *Br. med. J.*, 1986, *293*, 573).

Resistance to methicillin appears to be an intrinsic characteristic of the bacterial cell wall; MRSA synthesise a penicillin-binding protein that impedes the action of beta-lactam antibiotics on the final stages of cell wall synthesis. The genes coding for methicillin resistance are chromosomal. Strains from hospitals in Australia and London seem to be closely related and may have a common origin. They differ from Dublin isolates in that genes coding for resistance to gentamicin, tobramycin, and kanamycin, are commonly located in plasmids and linked to determinants for resistance to propamidine and quaternary ammonium compounds, some of which are commonly used as antiseptics; resistance to chlorhexidine has also been reported. The clinical implications are uncertain but it is possible that the use of such disinfectants, particularly at suboptimal concentrations, may favour survival of antibiotic-resistant strains (*Lancet*, 1985, *2*, 189).

About one-third of *UK* hospital groups have been reported to have some methicillin-resistant strains of *Staph. aureus* which are also resistant to gentamicin, and such strains comprise over 5% of the total number of staphylococcal isolates in some hospitals; in large Australian hospitals about 20 to 40% of total staphylococcal isolations are resistant to methicillin and gentamicin. MRSA now seem to be endemic in many large hospitals in eastern Australia and in America. Community-acquired infection has also occurred in Australia and the *USA* (K. King and K. Harvey, *Med. J. Aust.*, 1985, *142*, 88).

Resistance to methicillin *in vitro* implies resistance to all beta-lactams including the cephalosporins. Vancomycin has become the mainstay for treatment of serious infections due to multiple-antibiotic-resistant MRSA strains. Occasionally another antibiotic such as gentamicin or rifampicin may be used in association with vancomycin. Other agents including teicoplanin and quinolones, such as ciprofloxacin, also show promise *in vitro*, but their clinical efficacy remains to be established.

One of the most important means of spread of MRSA is by interhospital transmission, usually by the introduction of a colonised or infected patient from another hospital, or by staff who work in more than one hospital. An epidemic strain is mainly spread between patients via the hands or contaminated clothing of staff, and if an outbreak is not controlled quickly then the strain is likely to become endemic (D.C. Shanson, *Br. J. Hosp. Med.*, 1986, *35*, 312). Guidelines for the control of epidemic methicillin-resistant *Staph. aureus* have been published by a combined working party of the Hospital Infection Society and the British Society for Antimicrobial Chemotherapy. The guidelines include: prompt isolation of infected or colonised patients, bacteriological screening of patients and staff in contact with such patients, the use of protective clothing and handwashing with a suitable antiseptic detergent or an alcoholic rub, and the use of topical antiseptics to treat carriage sites (*J. Hosp. Infect.*, 1986, *7*, 193).

Difficulty in controlling epidemic MRSA may occur because of problems in detecting methicillin resistance. MRSA strains usually show a heterogeneous resistance which is poorly expressed at temperatures of 37° or above, at pH 5, or under conditions of low tonicity; resistance is fully expressed at neutral pH, low temperatures, or in hypertonic media (R.W. Lacey, *J. antimicrob. Chemother.*, 1986, *18*, 435). Detection of MRSA, especially in patients with low levels of colonisation or in patients with lesions which are heavily colonised with a wide range of Gram-positive and Gram-negative organisms may prove difficult and modifications to the growth media have been suggested (P.A. Wilson and D.N. Petts, *Lancet*, 1987, *1*, 558).

The antibiotic sensitivity of *Staph. epidermidis* (a coagulase-negative staphylococcus) is less predictable than that of *Staph. aureus*. Coagulase-negative staphylococci resistant to a wide range of antibiotics have been reported and methicillin or gentamicin resistance is frequently observed. In *Staph. aureus* resistance to cephalosporins normally parallels resistance to flucloxacillin, but in coagulase-negative staphylococci there is a differing sensitivity pattern for flucloxacillin and cephalosporins. Many coagulase-negative staphylococci are now multiresistant but may be sensitive *in vitro* to cephalosporins such as cephamandole or cefuroxime. Transfer of resistance from coagulase-negative staphylococci to *Staph. aureus* seems rare, although it has been shown both *in vitro* and *in vivo* (A.J. Davies, *Br. med. J.*, 1985, *290*, 1230).

Absorption and Fate

Methicillin is inactivated by gastric acid and must be given by injection. Peak plasma concentrations are attained within ½ to 1 hour of an intramuscular injection; concentrations of 10 µg or more per mL have been reported 1 hour after a dose of 1 g. A half-life of 0.5 to 1 hour has been reported, although this may be increased to 3 to 6 hours in renal failure. About 40% of the methicillin in the circulation is bound to plasma proteins. It diffuses into ascitic, pleural, pericardial, and synovial fluids; high concentrations are achieved in the bile and in bone tissue. There is little diffusion into the cerebrospinal fluid unless the meninges are inflamed. Methicillin also diffuses across the placenta. It is rapidly excreted by tubular secretion and glomerular filtration; up to 80% of an injected dose has been detected unchanged in the urine. Excretion can be delayed by probenecid.

In a study of 7 patients with cystic fibrosis and 6 healthy subjects, higher renal clearance-rates appeared to be responsible for lower serum concentrations of methicillin after a single intravenous dose in those with cystic fibrosis. Dosage might have to be increased in such patients.— S. J. Yaffe *et al.*, *J. infect. Dis.*, 1977, *135*, 828.

A study of the pharmacokinetics of methicillin in neonatal infants. The average serum half-life values ranged from 1 to 3 hours and were inversely correlated with birth weight, gestational age, and chronological age.— L. D. Sarff *et al.*, *J. Pediat.*, 1977, *90*, 1005.

There is a high degree of placental transfer of methicillin and a foetal-to-maternal serum concentration ratio of 0.8 to 1.4 has been reported. Trace amounts of methicillin are excreted in breast milk.— A. W. Chow and P. J. Jewesson, *Rev. infect. Dis.*, 1985, *7*, 287.

DIFFUSION INTO BODY TISSUES AND FLUIDS. Penetration of methicillin into bone and synovial tissues.— R. H. Fitzgerald *et al.*, *Antimicrob. Ag. Chemother.*, 1978, *14*, 723.

METABOLISM. Within 12 hours of the intramuscular administration of a 500-mg dose of methicillin to 6 healthy subjects, 75% was recovered unchanged in the urine with a further 7% recovered as penicilloic acid.— M. Cole *et al.*, *Antimicrob. Ag. Chemother.*, 1973, *3*, 463.

Uses and Administration

Methicillin sodium is used only in the treatment of infections due to penicillinase-producing staphylococci. The usual dosage of methicillin sodium is 1 g intramuscularly every 4 to 6 hours; it may be given intravenously, 1 g being dissolved in 20 to 50 mL of Water for Injections and injected slowly over 3 to 5 minutes. In more severe infections up to 12 g daily can be given intravenously in divided doses by slow injection or by intermittent infusion. Higher doses have been given in staphylococcal endocarditis. A usual children's dose is 100 mg per kg body-weight daily in divided doses by intramuscular or intravenous injection. If pain is a problem, intramuscular injections may be prepared using a 0.5% lignocaine hydrochloride solution.

Doses of 0.5 to 1 g have been given daily by intra-articular injection, dissolved if necessary in a 0.5% solution of lignocaine hydrochloride, and by intrapleural injection. Doses of up to 500 mg have been given daily by subconjunctival injection.

In staphylococcal infections of the lung methicillin sodium has been administered by nebuliser, a dose of 500 mg being dissolved in 5 mL of sterile water and inhaled 4 times daily.

ADMINISTRATION IN INFANTS AND CHILDREN. The suggested dose of methicillin for infants of more than 37 weeks' gestation was 25 mg per kg body-weight given intramuscularly or intravenously, by very slow bolus injection, every 12 hours for the first 48 hours of life, every 8 hours from the 3rd day to 2 weeks, then every 6 hours. For immature infants (those of less than 37 weeks' gestation) this dose should be given every 12 hours for the 1st week of life, every 8 hours from then to 4 weeks of age, and every 6 hours thereafter.— P. A. Davies, *Br. med. J.*, 1978, *2*, 676. For severe infections in neonates a suggested daily dose of methicillin administered intravenously was: 0 to 1 week, 75 to 100 mg per kg body-weight in 2 to 3 divided doses; 1 to 4 weeks, 100 to 150 mg per kg in 3 to 4 divided doses; over 4 weeks, 150 to 200 mg per kg in 3 to 4 divided doses. For severe infections in children a suggested intravenous dose was 200 to 300 mg per kg in 4 to 6 divided doses.— K. H. Rhodes and C. M. Johnson, *Mayo Clin. Proc.*, 1983, *58*, 158. Neonates requiring intensive care often have immature organs and multiple problems and therefore the dose of antibiotic should be adjusted according to serum concentrations.

ADMINISTRATION IN RENAL FAILURE. No dose change was required in patients with mild renal failure; 1 to 2 g every 8 hours was recommended in uraemia and this was also suitable during peritoneal dialysis. A dose of 1 g every 6 hours was recommended for patients undergoing haemodialysis.— G. B. Appel and H. C. Neu, *New Engl. J. Med.*, 1977, *296*, 663.

Methicillin could be administered to patients with renal failure by adjusting the dosage interval. A dosage interval of 4 hours is suitable for patients whose glomerular filtration-rates exceed 50 mL per minute; an interval of 4 to 8 hours between doses is advisable for rates of between 10 and 50 mL per minute. Where the rate is less than 10 mL per minute, the dosage interval should be 8 to 12 hours. No dose supplement is necessary for patients undergoing haemodialysis or peritoneal dialysis.— W. M. Bennett *et al.*, *Am. J. Kidney Dis.*, 1983, *3*, 155.

SURGICAL INFECTION PROPHYLAXIS. In a double-blind study of patients undergoing vascular reconstructive surgery, 79 patients received a prophylactic regimen of methicillin 2 g and netilmicin 200 mg administered intravenously in 2 separate injections at the start of general anaesthesia and again at 8 and 16 hours after the initial dose, and 72 patients received placebo. Antimicrobial prophylaxis was effective in reducing the wound infection rate compared with placebo; postoperative wound infections occurred in 4 patients (5.8%) in the treatment group and 12 patients (16.7%) in the placebo group. In addition prophylaxis tended to reduce the frequency of septicaemia and urinary-tract infections. However, in 3 of the 4 cases where prophylaxis failed the pathogens were fully sensitive to both drugs, which illustrated that antimicrobial coverage is no absolute safeguard against complications.— A. M. Worning *et al.*, *J. antimicrob. Chemother.*, 1986, *17*, 105.

For the use of penicillinase-resistant penicillins in cardiac surgery infection prophylaxis, see under Flucloxacillin Sodium, p.232.

Preparations

Methicillin Sodium for Injection *(U.S.P.)*. pH of a 1% solution 6.0 to 8.5.

Sterile Methicillin Sodium *(U.S.P.)*

Proprietary Preparations

Celbenin *(Beecham Research, UK)*. *Injection*, powder for reconstitution, methicillin sodium 1 g.

Proprietary Names and Manufacturers

Azapen *(USA)*; Baclyn *(Sifarma, Ital.)*; Celbenin *(Austral.; Belg.; Neth.; Switz.; Beecham Research, UK; Beecham Laboratories, USA)*; Celpillina *(Ital.)*; Ellecillina *(Ital.)*; Esapenil BG *(Boniscontro & Gazzone, Ital.)*; Flabelline *(Fr.)*; Lucopenin *(Astra, Denm.)*; Metin *(Commonwealth Serum Laboratories, Austral.)*; Pénistaph *(Bristol, Fr.)*; Penaureus *(Arg.)*; Penysol *(Edmond Pharma, Ital.)*; Sintespen *(Ital.)*; Staficyn *(FIRMA, Ital.)*; Staphcillin *(Canad.; Norw.; Bristol, USA)*.

12942-d

Methocidin *(rINN)*.

Hydroxymethyl Gramicidin.

CAS — 1407-05-2.

Methocidin is an antimicrobial agent with the actions and uses of gramicidin (see p.245) from which it is derived. It is used in association with cetylpyridinium chloride as nasal drops for respiratory infections.

Proprietary Names and Manufacturers
Argicilline *(Aron, Fr.)*.

12954-b

Metioprim *(BAN, USAN, rINN)*.

5-(3,5-Dimethoxy-4-methylthiobenzyl)pyrimidine-2,4-diyldiamine.
$C_{14}H_{18}N_4O_2S = 306.4$.

CAS — 68902-57-8.

Metioprim is closely related structurally to trimethoprim (see p.328), and has antibacterial activity.

The trimethoprim analogues, brodimoprim and metioprim, were 2 to 4 times more active than trimethoprim against anaerobic bacteria *in vitro*. The combinations, brodimoprim plus sulfamerazine, and metioprim plus sulphadiazine were, however, slightly less active than trimethoprim plus sulphamethoxazole.— J. Wüst and J. Schwarzenbach, *Antimicrob. Ag. Chemother.*, 1983, *23*, 490.

Pharmacokinetics of metioprim in healthy subjects and in patients with impaired renal function.— H. Vergin *et al.*, *Antimicrob. Ag. Chemother.*, 1983, *24*, 190.

Proprietary Names and Manufacturers
Heumann, Ger.

107-h

Mezlocillin Sodium *(BANM, USAN, rINNM)*.

BAY-f-1353. Sodium (6*R*)-6-[D-2-(3-mesyl-2-oxoimidazolidine-1-carboxamido)-2-phenylacetamido]penicillanate monohydrate.
$C_{21}H_{24}N_5NaO_8S_2,H_2O = 579.6$.

CAS — 51481-65-3 (mezlocillin); 42057-22-7; 59798-30-0 (both sodium salt, anhydrous).

Pharmacopoeias. *U.S.* includes Sterile Mezlocillin Sodium.

1.07 g of monograph substance is approximately equivalent to 1 g of anhydrous mezlocillin. Each g of monograph substance represents about 1.7 mmol of sodium. A 10% solution in water has a pH of 4.5 to 8.0.

A 10% solution of mezlocillin sodium in water, sodium chloride 0.9%, or glucose 5% is reported to be **stable** for up to 48 hours at 25°, up to 7 days at 5°, and up to 28 days at −12°; a 25% solution in water, sodium chloride 0.9%, or lignocaine hydrochloride 0.5 or 1% is reported to be stable for up to 24 hours at 25°. However, it is recommended that reconstituted solutions of mezlocillin sodium for injection should be administered immediately after preparation.

Incompatibility or loss of activity has been reported with aminoglycosides.

Adverse Effects

As for Carbenicillin Sodium, p.139. As mezlocillin sodium has a lower sodium content than carbenicillin sodium, hypernatraemia and hypokalaemia are less likely to occur.

An evaluation of the incidence of adverse effects of mezlocillin given in multiple doses to 1148 patients over 2 years of age for the treatment of systemic or urinary-tract infections. Adverse reactions probably or possibly caused by mezlocillin occurred in 10.5% of patients. Local reactions were reported in 34 patients (3%) and included thrombophlebitis, erythema, cellulitis, and vein irritation. Cutaneous reactions occurred in 22 (1.9%) and included maculopapular rashes, urticaria, pruritus, and one case of exfoliative dermatitis. Fever or chills occurred in 5 (0.4%). Fifteen patients (1.3%) experienced nausea or diarrhoea; there were no cases of pseudomembranous colitis. Adverse effects on the blood included a positive Coomb's test (2 patients), thrombocytosis (2), thrombocytopenia (1), leucopenia (2), and eosinophilia (25). Reversible hepatotoxicity, as indicated by elevated liver enzyme values, was observed in 10 (0.9%) instances; an additional 11 patients developed hyperbilirubinaemia but its relationship to mezlocillin administration was unclear. Other adverse effects included hypokalaemia in 8 patients (0.7%), and 2 reports of azotaemia.— M. F. Parry and H. C. Neu, *J. antimicrob. Chemother.*, 1982, *9*, *Suppl.* A, 273.

EFFECTS ON THE BLOOD. In studies in healthy subjects, mezlocillin appeared less likely than ticarcillin (P. Somani *et al.*, *J. antimicrob. Chemother.*, 1983, *11*, *Suppl.* C, 33) or carbenicillin (E.A. Copelan *et al.*, *ibid.*, 43; J.O. Ballard *et al.*, *Antimicrob. Ag. Chemother.*, 1984, *25*, 153) to cause abnormalities in haemostasis. Some patients had a minor increase in bleeding time, and Copelan *et al.* also reported abnormal platelet aggregation.

Precautions

As for Carbenicillin Sodium, p.139.

INTERACTIONS. *Aminoglycosides.* For reference to the *in vitro* and *in vivo* inactivation of aminoglycosides by mezlocillin see Gentamicin Sulphate p.236 and p.238.

Cephalosporins. For the effect of mezlocillin on the clearance of cefotaxime, see Cefotaxime Sodium, p.152.

Penicillins. For reference to the effect of mezlocillin on the pharmacokinetics of dicloxacillin and oxacillin, see Oxacillin Sodium p.277.

INTERFERENCE WITH DIAGNOSTIC TESTS. In a study *in vitro* of the effect of various antibiotics on tests for glycosuria, mezlocillin in the urine could give falsely elevated readings with a test using a copper-reduction method (Clinitest). It had no effect however on glucose oxidase methods (Diastix and Tes-Tape) of estimating glycosuria.— W. A. Parker and M. E. MacCara, *Am. J. Hosp. Pharm.*, 1984, *41*, 125.

See also.— M. LeBel *et al.*, *Drug Intell. & clin. Pharm.*, 1984, *18*, 617.

Antimicrobial Action and Resistance

Mezlocillin has a similar antimicrobial action to carbenicillin (p.139), although it is active against a wider range of Gram-negative organisms including *Klebsiella pneumoniae*. It is generally more active *in vitro*, especially against *Pseudomonas aeruginosa* and the Enterobacteriaceae, although its activity against *Ps. aeruginosa* is less than that of azlocillin or piperacillin.

Mezlocillin has a similar pattern of resistance to carbenicillin.

Studies of the antibacterial activity of mezlocillin *in vitro*: K. P. Fu and H. C. Neu, *Antimicrob. Ag. Chemother.*, 1978, *13*, 930; G. W. White *et al.*, *Antimicrob. Ag. Chemother.*, 1979, *15*, 540; H. Thadepalli *et al.*, *Antimicrob. Ag. Chemother.*, 1979, *15*, 487; R. Wise and J. M. Andrews, *J. antimicrob. Chemother.*, 1982, *9*, *Suppl.* A, 1; C. C. Sanders, *ibid.*, 15; M. F. Parry and D. Folta, *ibid.*, 1983, *11*, *Suppl.* C, 97.

ACTIVITY WITH OTHER ANTIMICROBIAL AGENTS. See under Azlocillin Sodium, p.124.

Absorption and Fate

Mezlocillin sodium is not absorbed from the gastro-intestinal tract to any significant extent. It is well absorbed after intramuscular administration, peak plasma concentrations of up to 45 μg per mL being observed 45 to 90 minutes after a dose of 1 g. Doubling the intramuscular or intravenous dose of mezlocillin sodium more than doubles the plasma concentrations. Between 16 and 42% of mezlocillin in the circulation is bound to plasma proteins. Mezlocillin is reported to have a dose-dependent plasma half-life which is usually about one hour. The half-life is slightly prolonged in neonates and in patients with renal failure.

Mezlocillin is widely distributed in body tissues and fluids. It diffuses across the placenta into the foetal circulation and is excreted in small amounts in breast milk. There is little diffusion into CSF except when the meninges are inflamed.

Mezlocillin is reported to be metabolised to a limited extent. About 55% of a dose is excreted unchanged in the urine by glomerular filtration and tubular secretion within 6 hours of administration, hence achieving high urinary concentrations. High concentrations are also found in the bile; up to 30% of a dose has been reported to be excreted by this route.

Serum concentrations are enhanced if probenecid is administered concomitantly.

Mezlocillin is removed by haemodialysis, and to a smaller extent by peritoneal dialysis.

A review of the pharmacokinetics of mezlocillin.— T. Bergan, *J. antimicrob. Chemother.*, 1983, *11*, *Suppl.* C, 1.

References to the pharmacokinetics of mezlocillin after intravenous administration: T. Bergan, *Antimicrob. Ag. Chemother.*, 1978, *14*, 801.

A study of the pharmacokinetics of mezlocillin in children with malignancies.— W. G. Kramer *et al.*, *Antimicrob. Ag. Chemother.*, 1984, *25*, 62.

ADMINISTRATION IN LIVER DISORDERS AND RENAL FAILURE. For reference to the pharmacokinetics of mezlocillin sodium in renal and hepatic failure, see below under Uses, Administration in Renal Failure, and Administration in Liver Disorders.

DIFFUSION INTO BODY TISSUES AND FLUIDS. References to the diffusion of mezlocillin into body tissues and fluids: K. G. Naber and D. Adam, *J. antimicrob. Chemother.*, 1983, *11*, *Suppl.* C, 17 (comparison of prostate tissue concentrations after intravenous administration by bolus injection or by infusion); P. Pederzoli *et al.* (letter), *J. antimicrob. Chemother.*, 1986, *17*, 397 (pancreatic juice); F. Pirali *et al.* (letter), *Lancet*, 1987, *1*, 505 (bronchial aspirates and mucosa).

DRUG EXCRETION. A study of the biliary excretion of mezlocillin in 14 patients some of whom had varying degrees of hepatic and renal impairment. Biliary excretion was very variable, 0.05 to 26.6% of the dose being excreted by this route; the lower values tended to be found in those with hepatic impairment.— U. Gundert-Remy *et al.*, *J. antimicrob. Chemother.*, 1982, *9*, *Suppl.* A, 65.

PREGNANCY AND THE NEONATE. Studies of the pharmacokinetics of mezlocillin sodium in neonates. The half-life of mezlocillin was about 4.5 hours in neonates aged 7 days or less, and 1.6 to 2.5 hours in those older than 7 days: T. Rubio *et al.*, *J. antimicrob. Chemother.*, 1982, *9*, *Suppl.* A, 241; C. Odio *et al.*, *Antimicrob. Ag. Chemother.*, 1984, *25*, 556.

Uses and Administration

Mezlocillin sodium is a ureido-penicillin with uses similar to Piperacillin Sodium, p.286. It may be used for prophylaxis of infection during abdominal surgery. Mezlocillin sodium is commonly administered in association with an aminoglycoside; however they should not be administered in the same infusion as they have been shown to be incompatible. It has also been given in association with other beta-lactam agents.

The usual dosage of mezlocillin sodium is the equivalent of 2 to 4 g of mezlocillin intravenously or 0.5 to 2 g intramuscularly given every 4 to 8 hours. For the treatment of life-threatening infections or those due to unidentified organisms or to *Pseudomonas* spp. the equivalent of 5 g every 6 to 8 hours or 4 g every 4 hours should be given intravenously. The usual maximum daily dose is 24 g. Uncomplicated gonorrhoea may be treated by a single intramuscular or intravenous dose equivalent to mezlocillin 1 to 2 g.

For the prophylaxis of infection during surgery an intravenous pre-operative dose of the equivalent of mezlocillin 2 g, followed by 2 postoperative doses at 8-hourly intervals may be given. Alternatively, a single pre-operative 5-g dose may be given.

When the intravenous route is employed, a 10% solution in a suitable diluent is infused over 15 to 20 minutes for 5-g doses; lower doses may be injected over 2 to 4 minutes. Intramuscular injections may be painful so mezlocillin sodium may be administered in a 0.5 to 1.0% solution of lignocaine hydrochloride. Single intramuscular doses should not exceed 2 g. Probenecid 1 g by mouth may be given half-an-hour before the injection.

Suggested intravenous doses of mezlocillin for children are 75 mg per kg body-weight twice daily by prolonged infusion for premature infants and neonates, and 75 mg per kg three times daily by injection or infusion for infants and older children.

Reviews of the actions and uses of mezlocillin: J. Russo and M. E. Russo, *Clin. Pharm.*, 1982, *1*, 207; G. M. Eliopoulos and R. C. Moellering, *Ann. intern. Med.*, 1982, *97*, 755.

Proceedings of symposia on mezlocillin sodium: *J. antimicrob. Chemother.*, 1982, *9*, *Suppl.* A, 1 to 291; *ibid.*, 1983, *11*, *Suppl.* C, 1 to 105.

ADMINISTRATION IN INFANTS AND CHILDREN. A dose equivalent to mezlocillin 300 mg per kg body-weight daily given in divided doses every 4 to 6 hours could be administered intravenously to children for the treatment of severe infection.— K. H. Rhodes and C. M. Johnson, *Mayo Clin. Proc.*, 1983, *58*, 158.

ADMINISTRATION IN LIVER DISORDERS. Mezlocillin 3 g was administered by intravenous infusion to 8 healthy subjects and to 4 patients with hepatic insufficiency secondary to cirrhosis. In those with hepatic impairment the half-life was increased from 0.96 to 2.6 hours and the fraction excreted in the urine from 36 to 86% as compared with those with normal hepatic function. The results were considered to indicate a decrease in non-renal clearance. For these patients a dose reduction of 50% was suggested.— C. M. Bunke *et al.*, *Clin. Pharmac. Ther.*, 1983, *33*, 73. See also B. R. Meyers *et al.*, *J. antimicrob. Chemother.*, 1986, *18*, 709; B. E. Cooper *et al.*, *Clin. Pharm.*, 1986, *5*, 764.

ADMINISTRATION IN RENAL FAILURE. Most authorities recommend that the dosage of mezlocillin sodium need only be adjusted in patients with severe renal impairment, usually considered as a glomerular filtration-rate (GFR) of less than 30 mL per minute. Bennett *et al.* (*Am. J. Kidney Dis.*, 1983, *3*, 155) stated that the half-life in patients with normal renal function ranged from 0.6 to 1.2 hours and was increased to 2.6 to 5.4 hours in end-stage renal disease. They have therefore suggested that in patients with a GFR between 10 and 50 mL per minute the dosage interval be increased from 4 to 6 hours to 6 to 8 hours, and in those with a GFR of less than 10 mL per minute, mezlocillin sodium be administered every 8 hours. The *US* manufacturers recommend similar dosage adjustments but suggest a dosage interval of 6 hours in the treatment of life-threatening infections even in the most severe renal impairment. The *UK* manufacturers recommend a dosage interval of 12 hours in patients with renal insufficiency, accompanied by monitoring of serum concentrations to ensure that adequate and constant concentrations are maintained. The *US* manufacturers recommend that patients on haemodialysis should be given mezlocillin sodium twice daily with an additional dose after each dialysis.

Further references to the pharmacokinetics of mezlocillin in patients with renal impairment and on haemodialysis: D. M. Janicke *et al.*, *Antimicrob. Ag. Chemother.*, 1981, *20*, 590; G. R. Aronoff, *J. antimicrob. Chemother.*, 1982, *9*, *Suppl.* A, 77; A. Mangione *et al.*, *ibid.*, 81; G. L. Drusano *et al.*, *Antimicrob. Ag. Chemother.*, 1984, *26*, 686.

For reference to the administration of mezlocillin sodium by the intraperitoneal route in patients undergoing continuous ambulatory peritoneal dialysis, see under Peritonitis in Azlocillin Sodium, p.125.

BILIARY-TRACT INFECTIONS. The acylaminopenicillins mezlocillin, azlocillin, and piperacillin produce high biliary concentrations. These drugs have therefore been suggested for the treatment and prophylaxis of infections of the biliary tract. They have a broad spectrum of activity and are effective against *Pseudomonas aeruginosa* and some pathogenic anaerobes. Dooley *et al.* (*Gut*, 1984, *25*, 988) suggested the use of an intravenous infusion of mezlocillin 2 to 5 g or cefotaxime 1 g given as a single dose 0.5 hour before the procedure. Munro and Sorrell (*Drugs*, 1986, *31*, 449), however, considered that the acylaminopenicillins and the newer cephalosporins are generally no more effective than the older agents, and are more expensive. Dooley *et al.* also suggested the use of mezlocilllin 5 g every 8 hours or cefotaxime 1 g every 6 hours in association with gentamicin and metronidazole for the intravenous treatment of acute cholecystisis in septicaemic patients, or of acute cholangitis. Again, Munro and Sorrell considered that the acylaminopenicillins offer few practical advantages over older agents.

GONORRHOEA. Studies of the use of mezlocillin sodium for the treatment of gonorrhoea: W. Fowler and M. H. Khan, *Curr. med. Res. Opinion*, 1979, *5*, 790; A. Lassus and O. -V. Renkonen, *Br. J. vener. Dis.*, 1979, *55*, 191; M. H. Khan and J. G. Tomkyns, *Curr. med. Res. Opinion*, 1982, *8*, 247.

MENINGITIS. The successful use of intravenous mezlocillin sodium for the treatment of meningitis in 30 children.— J. Llorens-Terol *et al.*, *Arzneimittel-Forsch.*, 1979, *29*, 2001.

NEUTROPENIA. For reference to the use of mezlocillin sodium in empiric antibiotic regimens in neutropenic patients with febrile episodes, see Piperacillin Sodium, p.287.

PERITONITIS. For reference to the use of mezlocillin sodium in the treatment of peritonitis, see Azlocillin Sodium, p.125.

PREGNANCY AND THE NEONATE. For reference to the use of mezlocillin sodium in pregnancy, see Piperacillin Sodium, p.287.

SURGICAL INFECTION PROPHYLAXIS. *Appendectomy*. In a double-blind randomised study in 94 patients undergoing emergency appendectomy, 4 of 46 given metronidazole 500 mg by intravenous infusion during surgery developed postoperative wound infection which was not significantly different from the 3 cases in the remaining 48, who received mezlocillin 5 g by intravenous infusion. Dosage was halved in children under 10 years of age. Although mezlocillin has been shown to be very effective in dealing with the anaerobic organisms encountered at appendectomy, the study does not demonstrate any advantage over metronidazole alone.— G. S. McIntosh et al., *J. antimicrob. Chemother.*, 1984, *14*, 537.

Biliary-tract surgery. See Biliary-tract Infections, above.

URINARY-TRACT INFECTIONS. A review of the treatment with mezlocillin sodium of urinary-tract infections in 149 patients from 7 different medical centres. The drug was administered intravenously in doses of 1.5 to 4 g every 6 to 8 hours, and the infections treated were classified as acute (82 patients), chronic (33), recurrent (30), or unspecified (4). The clinical response to mezlocillin was assessed as resolution in 120 patients, improvement in 17, failure in 11, or indeterminate in 1. Bacteriologically 105 infections were considered to be eliminated by treatment, 42 to be persistent, and 2 indeterminate; mezlocillin was successful in eliminating a wide range of bacteria. A total daily dosage of 6 g was considered to be satisfactory for the treatment of uncomplicated urinary-tract infections, particularly those confined to the bladder. Doses of 12 to 16 g daily, however, should be used for patients with complicated infections, those involving the upper tract, or those associated with bacteraemia.— C. E. Cox, *J. antimicrob. Chemother.*, 1982, *9*, *Suppl.* A, 173.

Further references: P. O. Madsen and O. S. Nielsen, *J. antimicrob. Chemother.*, 1982, *9*, *Suppl.* A, 179.

Preparations

Sterile Mezlocillin Sodium *(U.S.P.)*

Proprietary Preparations

Baypen *(Bayer, UK). Injection*, powder for reconstitution, mezlocillin 0.5, 1, and 2 g (as sodium salt). *Intravenous infusion*, powder for reconstitution, mezlocillin 5 g (as sodium salt).

Proprietary Names and Manufacturers

Baypen *(Bayer, Austral.*; *Bayer, Fr.*; *Bayer, Ger.*; *Bayer, Ital.*; *Bayer, Spain*; *Bayer, Swed.*; *Bayer, Switz.*; *Bayer, UK)*; Mezlin *(Miles Pharmaceuticals, USA)*.

736-p

Micronomicin Sulphate *(pINNM)*.

6′*N*-Methylgentamicin C_{1A} Sulphate; Gentamicin C_{2B} Sulphate; KW-1062 *(micronomicin)*; Sagamicin Sulphate. *O*-2-Amino-2,3,4,6-tetradeoxy-6-(methylamino)-α-D-*erythro*-hexopyranosyl-(1→4)-*O*-[3-deoxy-4-*C*-methyl-3-(methylamino)-β-L-arabinopyranosyl-(1→6)]-2-deoxy-D-streptamine hemipentasulphate.
$(C_{20}H_{41}N_5O_7)_2,5H_2SO_4$=1417.5.

CAS — 52093-21-7 (micronomicin).

Micronomicin sulphate is an aminoglycoside antibiotic.

Proprietary Names and Manufacturers
Sagamicin *(Kyowa, Jpn)*; Santemycin *(Santen, Jpn)*.

108-m

Midecamycin *(rINN)*.

Mydecamycin. 5-[3,6-Dideoxy-4-*O*-(2,6-dideoxy-3-*C*-methyl-4-*O*-propionyl-α-L-*ribo*-hexopyranosyl)-3-dimethylamino-β-D-glucopyranosyloxy]-6-formylmethyl-9-hydroxy-4-methoxy-8-methyl-3-propionyloxyhexadecan-10,12-dien-15-olide.
$C_{41}H_{67}NO_{15}$=814.0.

CAS — 35457-80-8.

Pharmacopoeias. In *Jpn*.

Midecamycin is a macrolide antibiotic produced by the growth of *Streptomyces mycarofaciens* and with actions and uses similar to those of erythromycin (see p.222). It has been given by mouth in a dose of 0.8 to 1.6 g daily in divided doses; children have been given 20 to 50 mg per kg body-weight daily.

A study of the antimicrobial activity *in vitro* of midecamycin.— H. C. Neu, *Antimicrob. Ag. Chemother.*, 1983, *24*, 443.

For reference to the hepatotoxic potential of macrolide antibiotics, see under Effects on the Liver in Erythromycin Estolate, p.227.

For reference to possible interactions with macrolide antibiotics, and their effect on hepatic metabolism, see Erythromycin, p.222.

Proprietary Names and Manufacturers
Medemycin *(Jpn)*; Midécacine *(Midy, Fr.)*; Midecin *(Farmaka, Ital.)*; Rubimycin *(Nikken, Jpn)*.

12960-h

Mikamycin *(BAN, rINN)*.

Antimicrobial substances produced by *Streptomyces mitakaensis*.

CAS — 11006-76-1.

Mikamycin is a streptogramin antibiotic with actions and uses similar to virginiamycin (p.337). It is applied topically.

For discussion on the streptogramin group of antibiotics, see Virginiamycin, p.337.

Proprietary Names and Manufacturers
Banyu, Jpn.

12962-b

Miloxacin *(rINN)*.

AB-206. 1,4-Dihydro-6,7-methylenedioxy-1-methoxy-4-oxoquinoline-3-carboxylic acid.
$C_{12}H_9NO_6$=263.2.

CAS — 37065-29-5.

Miloxacin is a 4-quinolone antimicrobial agent with actions similar to those of norfloxacin (p.274). It has been tried in the treatment of urinary-tract and respiratory-tract infections.

For a series of papers on miloxacin, including clinical studies in urinary-tract and respiratory-tract infections, see *Chemotherapy, Tokyo*, 1978, *26*, *Suppl.* 4, 1-388.

Further references.— A. Izawa *et al.*, *Antimicrob. Ag. Chemother.*, 1980, *18*, 37 (antimicrobial activity); A. Yoshitake *et al.*, *ibid.*, 45 (pharmacokinetics).

Proprietary Names and Manufacturers
Sumitomo, Jpn.

109-b

Minocycline Hydrochloride *(BANM, USAN, rINNM)*.

6-Demethyl-6-deoxy-7-dimethylaminotetracycline hydrochloride.
$C_{23}H_{27}N_3O_7$,HCl=493.9.

CAS — 10118-90-8 (minocycline); 13614-98-7 (hydrochloride).

Pharmacopoeias. In *Br.*, *Braz.*, *Jpn*, and *U.S. Br.* specifies the monohydrate.

A yellow crystalline powder. The *U.S.P.* specifies that it contains the equivalent of 875 to 950 μg of minocycline per mg calculated on the anhydrous basis. Minocycline hydrochloride 108 mg is approximately equivalent to 100 mg of minocycline. **Soluble** in water and solutions of alkali hydroxides and carbonates; slightly soluble in alcohol; practically insoluble in chloroform and ether. A solution equivalent to 1% of minocycline has a pH of 3.5 to 4.5; the *U.S.P.* specifies that a similar solution of sterile Minocycline Hydrochloride has a pH of 2.0 to 3.5. **Store** in airtight containers. Protect from light.

For a report of visual incompatibility between minocycline or tetracycline and several opioid analgesics, see under Tetracycline Hydrochloride, p.314.

Units

One unit of minocycline is contained in 0.0011587 mg of the first International Reference Preparation (1975) of minocycline hydrochloride which contains 863 units per mg.

Adverse Effects and Precautions

As for Tetracycline Hydrochloride, p.314.

Vestibular side-effects including dizziness or vertigo occur with minocycline and patients should be advised not to drive or operate machinery if affected. Minocycline has also been associated with pigmentation of the skin and other tissues.

ALLERGY. A patient who had developed contact sensitivity to minocycline after 3 months' treatment presented the same widespread immunological response when he inadvertently received minocycline by mouth for the treatment of a urinary-tract infection 2 months later.— W. B. Shelley and C. L. Heaton, *J. Am. med. Ass.*, 1973, *224*, 125.

Pulmonary infiltrates and eosinophilia were associated with minocycline administration in a 55-year-old woman. She experienced fever, chills, night sweats, and fatigue, and chest x-ray showed diffuse bilateral fine reticulonodular infiltrates involving all lobes but most prominent in the lung bases. A hypersensitivity reaction to minocycline was thought to be the cause.— M. Otero and H. C. Goodpasture (letter), *J. Am. med. Ass.*, 1983, *250*, 2602.

EFFECTS ON THE EYE. For a report of conjunctival pigmentation in a patient who had received long-term treatment with minocycline and tetracycline, see under Tetracycline Hydrochloride, p.314. See also Effects on the Skin, below.

EFFECTS ON THE GASTRO-INTESTINAL TRACT. For mention of oesophagitis caused by minocycline and other tetracyclines, see under Doxycycline Hydrochloride, p.217.

EFFECTS ON THE KIDNEY. A report of interstitial nephritis attributed to minocycline given in a dose of 250 mg four times daily for 5 days.— R. G. Walker *et al.*, *Br. med. J.*, 1979, *1*, 524. The dose was 5 times that recommended in the UK and a causal relationship was not established.— G. W. R. Hill and M. Roach, *Lederle* (letter), *ibid.*, 820.

EFFECTS ON THE LIVER. Acute hepatic injury associated with intravenous minocycline in one patient.— A. Burette *et al.*, *Archs intern. Med.*, 1984, *144*, 1491.

EFFECTS ON THE NERVOUS SYSTEM. *Vestibular disturbances*. Vestibular side-effects including dizziness or vertigo, ataxia, weakness, nausea, and vomiting have been reported with minocycline therapy; these effects are often acute and may be severe, but are reversible on withdrawal of the drug (D.N. Williams *et al.*, *Lancet*, 1974, *2*, 744). The incidence of these adverse effects has been reported to vary from about 5% to 90% (A. Yeadon, *Lancet*, 1975, *1*, 109; W.L. Fanning and D.W. Gump, *Archs intern. Med.*, 1976, *136*, 761) and is higher in women than in men (C.S. Nicol and J.D. Oriel, *Lancet*, 1974, *2*, 1260). It has been suggested that this higher incidence in women could be attributed to higher serum-minocycline concentrations which might be a reflection of their smaller size (W.L. Fanning *et al.*, *Antimicrob. Ag. Chemother.*, 1977, *11*, 712). However, further study showed that women taking minocycline 150 mg daily had approximately the same serum concentrations as men taking minocycline 200 mg daily, but the women still had a considerably higher incidence of side-effects than the men (D.W. Gump *et al.*, *ibid.*, *12*, 642). Alteration of the dosage schedule from 100 mg twice daily to 50 mg four times daily may possibly reduce adverse effects (T.P. Greco *et al.*, *Curr. ther. Res.*, 1979, *25*, 193).

EFFECTS ON THE SKIN. Minocycline-related pigmentation of the skin has been described in a variety of forms. One type is characterised by dark blue-black macules localised to areas of depressed acne scarring or at sites of cutaneous inflammation. The source of the pigment appears to be an iron-containing compound, possibly haemosiderin or an iron chelate of minocycline, within dermal macrophages. It has been proposed that the pigment remains in the skin because of minocycline affecting the formation of intact lysosomal membranes to surround toxic iron derivatives within the macrophage. A second type is characterised by hyperpigmented macules or a more diffuse hyperpigmentation occurring distant from the site of inflammation or infection, often in the lower legs as well as areas commonly exposed to sunlight. A third form is the "muddy skin syndrome" which is characterised by a diffuse dark brown-grey discoloration suggesting an off-colour suntan and is generalised over most of the body with less darkening of nonexposed areas. It has been proposed that minocycline causes stimulation of melanin production by epidermal melanocytes which could explain both the photodistributed and muddy skin types of presentation. Cutaneous pigmentation will resolve spontaneously on cessation of minocycline therapy; those with the most profound colour changes can be expected to take the longest to clear completely. Tissue staining in various organs other than the skin has also been described in patients receiving long-term minocycline; the thyroid gland, bone, teeth, sclerae, and breast milk have been affected.— R. S. W. Basler, *Archs Derm.*, 1985, *121*, 606.

A report of cutaneous blue-black pigmentation with generalised pruritus and areas of erythema in an 83-year-old man who had been taking minocycline 200 mg daily for chronic pulmonary disease. The erythema cleared on discontinuing minocycline. The patient subsequently died of cardiac disease and on post-mortem examination the major findings were diffusely darkened areas of aorta, endocardium, and ribs; thyroid and prostate were black on gross examination.— A. M. Zijdenbos and K. J. Balmus, *Br. J. Derm.*, 1984, *110*, 117.

For mention of minocycline causing photosensitivity reactions, see under Doxycycline Hydrochloride, p.217.

EFFECTS ON THE THYROID. A black thyroid was found post mortem in a 69-year-old man who had taken minocycline for a year up to 4 months before death. Similar effects had been seen in some *animals*.— H. D. Attwood and X. Dennett, *Br. med. J.*, 1976, *2*, 1109.

Further reports: R. A. Billano *et al.*, *J. Am. med. Ass.*, 1983, *249*, 1887.

See also Effects on the Skin, above.

INTERACTIONS. For the effect of iron salts, antacids containing calcium, magnesium, or aluminium salts, milk, or food on the absorption of minocycline, see under Absorption and Fate, below.

Antimicrobial Action and Resistance

Minocycline has a spectrum of activity and mode of action similar to that of tetracycline hydrochloride (see p.315) but it is more active against many species. In addition it is reported to be effective *in vitro* against some tetracycline-resistant staphylococci, streptococci and certain strains of tetracycline-resistant *Escherichia coli* and *Haemophilus* spp.

Minocycline was generally more active *in vitro* than tetracycline against both tetracycline-sensitive and -resistant strains of *Haemophilus influenzae* and *Streptococcus pneumoniae* and inhibited all of the 51 strains of *H. influenzae* at a concentration of 2 µg per mL. Although minocycline was more active than tetracycline *in vitro* against strains of group A streptococci, MICs were still greater than 4 µg per mL.— M. J. Wood *et al.*, *J. antimicrob. Chemother.*, 1975, *1*, 323.

Minocycline showed greater activity than tetracycline against 50 strains of *Bacteroides fragilis*, 48% of strains being inhibited by 0.1 µg per mL of minocycline but 14% by 0.1 µg per mL of tetracycline. With an average blood concentration of 2 to 3 µg per mL for minocycline 78% of strains would be inhibited compared with an inhibition of 60% by tetracycline in an average blood concentration of 2 to 4 µg per mL.— D. A. Leigh and K. Simmons, *Lancet*, 1975, *1*, 51. Minocycline was more active than tetracycline or doxycycline against 624 strains of anaerobic bacteria *in vitro*. At 5 µg per mL minocycline, doxycycline, and tetracycline inhibited 84, 74, and 66% respectively of 241 strains of *Bacteroides* spp.— V. Bach *et al.*, *Curr. ther. Res.*, 1978, *23*, 206. See also under Doxycycline Hydrochloride, p.217.

Of 152 tetracycline-resistant strains of *Staph. aureus* tested by disk diffusion only 33 (22%) were considered to be sensitive to minocycline.— B. Chattopadhyay and E. Harding (letter), *Lancet*, 1975, *1*, 405.

Of 169 strains of penicillin-resistant *Staph. aureus* 84.5% were sensitive to tetracycline and minocycline. However 13.5% were resistant to tetracycline but sensitive to minocycline. Also 48 of 311 isolates of Enterobacteriaceae were sensitive to minocycline but resistant to tetracycline.— C. Candanoza and P. D. Ellner, *Antimicrob. Ag. Chemother.*, 1975, *7*, 227.

Amongst 7 tetracyclines minocycline then doxycycline were the most active against strains of *Staph. aureus* and *Staph. epidermidis*; oxytetracycline was the least active.— L. D. Sabath *et al.*, *Antimicrob. Ag. Chemother.*, 1976, *9*, 962.

Plasmids bearing tetracycline resistance determinants mediate considerably less resistance to the lipophilic analogue minocycline than to tetracycline. Minocycline has been found to cross the outer membrane of *Escherichia coli* 10 to 20 times faster than tetracycline. It is possible that lipophilicity for the tetracyclines increases the rate of uptake and at the same time decreases the ability of the efflux system in resistant cells to handle the drug.— L. M. McMurry *et al.*, *Antimicrob. Ag. Chemother.*, 1982, *22*, 791.

Further references to the antimicrobial activity of minocycline: E. G. Maderazo *et al.*, *Antimicrob. Ag. Chemother.*, 1975, *8*, 54 (*Acinetotobacter calcoaceticus; Serratia marcescens*); J. Z. Montgomerie *et al.*, *ibid.*, 1976, *10*, 102 (*Acinetobacter anitratus*); W. Brown and R. J. Fallon, *J. antimicrob. Chemother.*, 1980, *6*, 91 (*Neisseria meningitidis*); M. Tsukamura, *Tubercle*, 1980, *61*, 37 (*Mycobacterium* spp.); M. E. Gombert *et al.*, *Antimicrob. Ag. Chemother.*, 1987, *31*, 2013 (*Nocardia asteroides*).

ACTIVITY WITH OTHER ANTIMICROBIAL AGENTS. Demonstration *in vitro* of enhanced antimicrobial activity with a combination of gentamicin and minocycline against the Enterobacteriaceae, especially *E. coli*.— R. J. Fass *et al.*, *Antimicrob. Ag. Chemother.*, 1976, *10*, 34. In a study *in vitro* of 30 strains of Enterobacteriaceae and 10 strains of *Pseudomonas aeruginosa* the combination of minocycline and an aminoglycoside was usually additive with some synergy, but partial antagonism occurred in about 10 to 40% of the strains depending on the aminoglycoside.— P. Van der Auwera, *J. antimicrob. Chemother.*, 1985, *16*, 581.

Minocycline enhanced the activity of amphotericin *in vitro* against 30 strains of *Candida albicans, Cryptococcus neoformans, Torulopsis glabrata*, and strains of *Candida* other than *albicans*. Minocycline alone had no activity against any of the strains.— M. A. Lew *et al.*, *Antimicrob. Ag. Chemother.*, 1978, *14*, 465.

Absorption and Fate

Minocycline is readily absorbed from the gastro-intestinal tract and is not significantly affected by the presence of food or moderate amounts of milk, although absorption is impaired by the concomitant administration of iron salts or antacids containing calcium, magnesium or aluminium salts. Normal doses of 200 mg followed by 100 mg every 12 hours produced plasma concentrations within the range of 1 to 4 µg per mL. It is more lipid-soluble than doxycycline and the other tetracyclines and is widely distributed in body tissues and fluids, including the cerebrospinal fluid. A higher ratio of CSF to blood concentrations has been reported with minocycline than with doxycycline. It crosses the placenta and diffuses into milk of nursing mothers. About 75% of minocycline in the circulation is bound to plasma proteins. It has a lower renal clearance than doxycycline and its plasma half-life ranges from 11 to 23 hours. Only about 11% of a dose is excreted in the urine in 96 hours and up to about 34% is excreted in the faeces. Little minocycline is removed by dialysis. The plasma half-life tends to be prolonged in patients with severe renal impairment.

The plasma half-life of minocycline determined in 20 healthy adults was 13.7 hours, and was not dependent on the dose administered or time of administration. Plasma half-life was prolonged in patients with renal dysfunction but was not affected by hepatic dysfunction.— B. Bernard *et al.*, *J. clin. Pharmac.*, 1971, *11*, 332. The urinary excretion of minocycline was not slowed significantly in a study of 12 patients with renal impairment.— M. C. McHenry *et al.*, *Clin. Pharmac. Ther.*, 1972, *13*, 146. After a 200-mg intravenous dose of minocycline the serum half-life was prolonged from 14.6 to 17.3 hours in 8 patients with chronic stable renal failure (creatinine clearance less than 5 mL per minute) compared with 8 subjects with normal renal function. However, excretion appeared to be almost independent of renal function since only 0.7% of the dose was recovered over 72 hours from the urine of those with renal failure compared with 11% in the normal subjects.— D. Heaney and G. Eknoyan, *Clin. Pharmac. Ther.*, 1978, *24*, 233.

In healthy subjects absorption of minocycline was rapid and complete and the serum half-life was about 16 hours after a single oral dose of 150 mg. An average of 76% binding to serum protein was found and urinary excretion tests demonstrated that minocycline was partly metabolised. Following multiple oral doses (200 mg initially then 100 mg twice daily) steady-state serum concentrations of 2.3 to 3.5 µg per mL were reached. Administration of minocycline to patients prior to surgery revealed favourable tissue penetration, the highest concentrations being reached in the intestinal tract, liver, gall-bladder, and bile, suggesting a hepatic role in excretion. After a dosage of 100 mg twice daily in healthy subjects antibiotic concentrations were found in skin, scalp, sebum, and sweat. Minocycline was also shown to pass more effectively into the CSF than doxycycline.— H. Macdonald *et al.*, *Clin. Pharmac. Ther.*, 1973, *14*, 852.

ABSORPTION. A study in 10 healthy subjects confirmed that minocycline absorption is not significantly affected by food.— C. Smith *et al.* (letter), *J. antimicrob. Chemother.*, 1984, *13*, 93. The absorption of minocycline in 8 healthy subjects was decreased by concomitant administration of iron, milk, or food; absorption was reduced by 77%, 27%, and 13%, respectively. However, the inhibitory effect on absorption with food and milk was significantly greater for tetracycline than for minocycline.— J. J. Leyden, *J. Am. Acad. Derm.*, 1985, *12*, 308.

DIFFUSION INTO BODY TISSUES AND FLUIDS. Minocycline concentrations in serum, saliva, sputum, pleural exudate, and lung extracts in patients with respiratory-tract infections.— D. Sommerwerck *et al.*, *Dt. med. Wschr.*, 1978, *103*, 822.

Minocycline is more lipophilic than doxycycline, oxytetracycline, or tetracycline. Concentrations in saliva and tears known to be inhibitory to meningococci, were attained in 5 healthy subjects given minocycline 100 mg every 12 hours for 5 days. With doxycycline 100 mg every 12 hours the mean MIC for *Neisseria meningitidis* was only just reached.— P. D. Hoeprich and D. M. Warshauer, *Antimicrob. Ag. Chemother.*, 1974, *5*, 330.

Further references: D. Worgan and R. J. E. Daniel, *Scott. med. J.*, 1976, *21*, 197 (sinus secretions); D. MacCulloch *et al.*, *N.Z. med. J.*, 1974, *80*, 300 (sputum); T. D. Brogan *et al.*, *J. antimicrob. Chemother.*, 1977, *3*, 247 (sputum).

METABOLISM. Isolation of 6 minocycline metabolites from human urine.— H. J. C. F. Nelis and A. P. de Leenheer (letter), *Lancet*, 1981, *2*, 938.

Uses and Administration

Minocycline hydrochloride has actions and uses similar to those of tetracycline hydrochloride (see p.318). It has been used in the elimination of the meningococcal carrier state although the risk of vestibular disturbances may make such a use unwise.

There is controversy about the safe use of minocycline in patients with renal impairment; if used the dosage should be reduced.

Minocycline hydrochloride is normally given by mouth but may be given by slow intravenous infusion; doses are expressed in terms of minocycline base. The usual dose by either route is 200 mg of minocycline daily in divided doses, usually every 12 hours. A dose of 50 mg twice daily by mouth is used for the treatment of acne.

Children have been given 4 mg per kg bodyweight initially followed by 2 mg per kg every 12 hours but the effect of tetracyclines on teeth should be considered.

Report of a 39-year-old woman with hypogammaglobulinaemia who had chronic joint infection with *Mycoplasma salivarium*. Following synovectomy the knee remained hot and slightly tender despite treatment with erythromycin 250 mg four times daily by mouth. However, when minocycline 100 mg twice daily was substituted her symptoms resolved rapidly.— A. K. L. So *et al.*, *Br. med. J.*, 1983, *286*, 762.

ADMINISTRATION. Minocycline hydrochloride must be diluted before intravenous administration. It is given by continuous intravenous infusion because of the volume of fluid required; a dose of 100 mg should be reconstituted in 500 to 1000 mL of intravenous fluid.— R. P. Rapp *et al.*, *Drug Intell. & clin. Pharm.*, 1984, *18*, 218.

ADMINISTRATION IN RENAL FAILURE. There appeared to be no reduction in drug clearance in a study of single and repeated doses of minocycline given to patients with various degrees of renal function.— P. G. Welling *et al.*, *Antimicrob. Ag. Chemother.*, 1975, *8*, 532. The view that minocycline should be avoided in patients with renal failure; doxycycline should be used if a tetracycline is needed.— G. B. Appel and H. C. Neu, *New Engl. J. Med.*, 1977, *296*, 663. Minocycline could be administered to patients with renal failure; no dosage adjustment is necessary and no supplement is required for patients undergoing haemodialysis or peritoneal dialysis.— W. M. Bennett *et al.*, *Am. J. Kidney Dis.*, 1983, *3*, 155.

See also under Absorption and Fate.

GRANULOMA. Considerable improvement was achieved with minocycline 100 mg twice daily for 2 months given to a 26-year-old man with swimming pool granuloma (a slowly enlarging lump in the skin of the wrist due to *Mycobacterium marinum*).— H. H. J. Teunissen, *Br. J. Derm.*, 1985, *112*, 229. For reference to the use of minocycline in the treatment of atypical mycobacterial infections, see Atypical Mycobacterial Infections in Amikacin Sulphate, p.111.

MALARIA. For comment on the use of tetracyclines, including minocycline, in the prophylaxis and treatment of malaria, see under Tetracycline Hydrochloride, p.319.

MENINGOCOCCAL MENINGITIS PROPHYLAXIS. Minocycline has been found effective in the prevention of meningococcal disease in military recruits. It has been shown to be slightly less effective than rifampicin in reducing meningococcal carriage rates, but when used either with rifampicin or followed by rifampicin the 2 drugs have been shown to be effective in reducing carriage in both military populations and in family studies. However, the use of minocycline for chemoprophylaxis has been complicated by the high frequency of vestibular reactions and also the risk of dental staining in young household contacts, and therefore rifampicin is the drug recommended for prophylaxis in contacts of patients with meningococcal meningitis.— C. V. Broome, *J. antimicrob. Chemother.*, 1986, *18, Suppl.* A, 25.

See also under Rifampicin, p.576.

MOUTH INFECTIONS. *Periodontal disease.* For the use of tetracyclines including minocycline hydrochloride in the treatment of periodontal disease, see under Tetracycline Hydrochloride, p.320.

NOCARDIOSIS. For mention of the use of minocycline in the treatment of nocardiosis, see under Respiratory-tract Infections, below.

PROSTATITIS. Minocycline has been evaluated in the treatment of bacterial prostatitis: its lipid solubility is greater than that of older tetracyclines and it yields concentrations in prostatic fluid similar to those in serum. However, side-effects such as vertigo and gastro-intestinal disturbance will often make it unsuitable for long-term use.— *Lancet*, 1983, *1*, 393.

Reports of the use of minocycline in the treatment of bacterial prostatitis.— D. F. Paulson and R. D. White, *J. Urol., Baltimore*, 1978, *120*, 184; S. K. P. Kan and R. W. W. Kay, *Trans. R. Soc. trop. Med. Hyg.*, 1978, *72*, 522.

RESPIRATORY-TRACT INFECTIONS. Beneficial results in 5 severely immunocompromised cardiac transplant patients with pulmonary nocardiosis treated with minocycline hydrochloride usually in a dose of 300 mg twice daily by mouth for 6 months to 1 year. Optimal dosage or duration of treatment was not established.— E. A. Petersen *et al.*, *J. Am. med. Ass.*, 1983, *250*, 930.

For the use of tetracyclines including minocycline in the treatment of bronchitis, see under Tetracycline Hydrochloride, p.320.

SEXUALLY TRANSMITTED DISEASES. *Gonorrhoea.* Single doses of 300 or 400 mg of minocycline were given to 349 men with uncomplicated gonococcal urethritis. Of the 328 who returned 13 were treatment failures and 16 had or developed non-specific urethritis by day 29. Side-effects included dizziness in 2 patients and nausea in 3.— G. Masterton and C. B. S. Schofield, *Br. J. vener. Dis.*, 1976, *52*, 43.

Single oral doses of minocycline 300 mg were more effective than talampicillin 1.5 g in the treatment of uncomplicated gonococcal urethritis in 230 men. Failure-rates were 3.2% and 8.7% respectively.— A. Saeed and R. B. Roy, *Br. J. clin. Pract.*, 1979, *33*, 199.

In the treatment of uncomplicated gonococcal infections minocycline hydrochloride 100 mg twice daily by mouth for 5 days was as effective as procaine penicillin 4.8 g by intramuscular injection in association with probenecid 1 g by mouth. Minocycline eliminated the infection from 143 of 146 men and all of 70 women, compared with 133 of 137 men and 68 or 70 women given procaine penicillin.— B. Lutz *et al.*, *Curr. ther. Res.*, 1985, *37*, 165.

Gonorrhoea prophylaxis. In a prospective study in the Far East of 1080 men exposed to the risk of gonococcal infection, postexposure prophylaxis with a single dose of minocycline 200 mg completely prevented infection by gonococci susceptible to 0.75 µg per mL of tetracycline hydrochloride, reduced the risk of infection or prolonged the incubation period in those exposed to gonococci with MICs of 1 to 2 µg per mL, did not reduce infection or prolong incubation in those exposed to gonococci resistant to 2 µg per mL, and did not increase the risk of asymptomatic infection. However, the widespread prophylactic use of minocycline for the control of gonorrhoea is probably of limited value because of the tendency of this regimen to select gonococci that are relatively resistant to tetracycline. Of 27 men with symptomatic gonorrhoea given minocycline 900 mg over 4 days, only 11 were cured.— W. O. Harrison *et al.*, *New Engl. J. Med.*, 1979, *300*, 1074.

Nongonococcal urethritis. Treatment with minocycline 100 mg twice daily was compared with oxytetracycline 250 mg twice daily or tetracycline (sustained-release) 250 mg twice daily, all given for 7 days, in 505 patients with nonspecific urethritis. Of those available for assessment after 3 months, 29 of 102 given minocycline had relapsed compared with 42 of 109 given oxytetracycline and 43 of 103 who received tetracycline.— B. A. Evans, *Br. J. vener. Dis.*, 1978, *54*, 107.

In a placebo-controlled study of 244 men with nongonococcal urethritis, mainly due to chlamydiae ureaplasmas, or *Mycoplasma hominis*, a single dose of minocycline 300 mg by mouth was compared with treatment for 2 and 10 days given as a loading dose of 200 mg of minocycline followed by 100 mg twice daily by mouth. Irrespective of the micro-organisms isolated and the number of previous attacks, the clinical response was not significantly different between patients receiving single-dose treatment or treatment for 2 days, with failure rates of 26% (20 of 76 patients) and 28% (25 of 89 patients), respectively. However, failure was significantly less for patients who received treatment for 10 days compared with 1 or 2 days, and occurred in only 8 of 79 patients (10%). More than half the men who were experiencing at least their third attack and from whom micro-organisms were not isolated failed to respond to the short regimens. However, for men suffering first attacks and from whom only ureaplasmas, with or without *M. hominis*, had been isolated only 1 of 24 (4%) failed to respond to short treatment.— D. Taylor-Robinson *et al.*, *Genitourinary Med.*, 1986, *62*, 19.

See also under Tetracycline Hydrochloride, p.321, and under Prostatitis, above.

SKIN DISORDERS. *Acne.* In a double-blind study of 16 patients with severe acne vulgaris, minocycline was as effective as doxycycline when 100 mg of either was given daily for 3 months.— F. Smit, *Dermatologica*, 1978, *157*, 186. Of 25 patients with acne vulgaris who had not responded to treatment with tetracycline 1 g daily for 6 to 8 weeks, 22 responded to minocycline 50 mg twice daily given for a similar period. No vestibular side-effects were noted.— S. I. Cullen, *Cutis*, 1978, *21*, 101.

A study of minocycline treatment for therapy-resistant and recurrent forms of severe acne vulgaris. Of 28 evaluable patients, 20 reacted favourably to minocycline 100 mg daily by mouth for 1 month reduced to 100 mg every other day during the second and third month of treatment; topical benzoyl peroxide 5 or 10% was also used. Improvement occurred within 2 to 4 weeks of starting treatment.— H. Degreef, *Curr. ther. Res.*, 1983, *33*, 8.

All of 22 patients with nodulocystic acne vulgaris resistant to previous dermatological therapy, including an antecedent 3-month course of minocycline 50 mg three times daily by mouth, responded within one month of ibuprofen 400 mg three times daily being added to their minocycline treatment. Improvement, demonstrated by a decreased number of nodulocystic lesions, varied between 75% and 90%.— L. S. Funt (letter), *J. Am. Acad. Derm.*, 1985, *13*, 524.

Further references: P. M. Cohen, *J. int. med. Res.*, 1985, *13*, 214; E. D. Millar *et al.*, *Br. J. clin. Pract.*, 1987, *41*, 882.

For further comment on the use of tetracyclines in the treatment of acne vulgaris, see under Tetracycline Hydrochloride, p.321.

Granuloma. For the treatment of granulomatous lesions with minocycline, see Granuloma, above.

URINARY-TRACT INFECTIONS. Minocycline 50 mg four times a day for 10 days was given to 124 women with symptomatic urinary-tract infection. Of 65 women with bacteriuria who completed treatment 52 were cured. Adverse effects occurred in 24 women and necessitated discontinuation of therapy in 16. Vestibular toxicity occurred in 14 women while other side-effects reported included headache, nausea, and vomiting.— T. P. Greco *et al.*, *Curr. ther. Res.*, 1979, *25*, 193.

See also Prostatitis and Sexually Transmitted Diseases, above.

Preparations

Minocycline Hydrochloride Capsules *(U.S.P.)*

Minocycline Hydrochloride Oral Suspension *(U.S.P.)*

Minocycline Hydrochloride Tablets *(U.S.P.)*

Minocycline Tablets *(B.P.)*. Tablets containing minocycline hydrochloride.

Sterile Minocycline Hydrochloride *(U.S.P.)*

Proprietary Preparations

Minocin *(Lederle, UK)*. *Tablets*, minocycline 50 and 100 mg (as hydrochloride).

Proprietary Names and Manufacturers

Klinomycin *(Cyanamid-Lederle, Ger.)*; Minocin *(Belg.; Lederle, Canad.; Cyanamid, Ital.; Neth.; Cyanamid, Spain; Lederle, Switz.; Lederle, UK; Lederle, USA)*; Minomycin *(Lederle, Austral.; Jpn; Lederle, S.Afr.)*; Mynocine *(Lederle, Fr.)*; Ultramycin *(Canad.)*; Vectrin *(USA)*.

16897-x

Miocamycin

Miokamycin; MOM. 9,3″-Diacetylmidecamycin.

$C_{45}H_{71}NO_{17}$=898.1.

CAS — 55881-07-7.

Miocamycin is a macrolide antibiotic administered by mouth.

Studies *in vitro* of the antibacterial activity of miocamycin: G. L. Ridgway *et al.*, *J. antimicrob. Chemother.*, 1983, *12*, 511; R. W. Lacey *et al.*, *ibid.*, 1984, *13*, 5.

Good clinical and bacteriological results were achieved in 86 patients with respiratory-tract infections given miocamycin 900 mg daily by mouth in 3 divided doses for 5 to 20 days. Penetration of the drug into bronchial secretions was considered good.— R. Rimoldi *et al.*, *Drugs exp. & clin. Res.*, 1985, *11*, 263.

Proprietary Names and Manufacturers

Macroral *(Zambeletti, Ital.)*; Miocamen *(Menarini, Ital.)*; Miokacin *(Hammer Pharma. Ital.)*.

12970-b

Mocimycin *(rINN)*.

MYC-8003. An antibiotic obtained from *Streptomyces ramocissimus* or by any other means.

$C_{43}H_{60}N_2O_{12}$=797.0.

CAS — 50935-71-2; 52212-85-8.

Mocimycin has been added to animal feeding stuffs for promoting growth.

16906-v

Mupirocin *(BAN, USAN, rINN)*.

BRL-4910A; Pseudomonic Acid. 9-[(2*E*)-4-[(2*S*,3*R*,4*R*,5*S*)-5-[(2*S*,3*S*,4*S*,5*S*)-2,3-Epoxy-5-hydroxy-4-methylhexyl]tetrahydro-3,4-dihydroxy-pyran-2-yl]-3-methylbut-2-enoyloxy]nonanoic acid.

$C_{26}H_{44}O_9$=500.6.

CAS — 12650-69-0.

An antibiotic produced by *Pseudomonas fluorescens*.

Adverse Effects and Precautions

Local reactions such as burning, stinging, and itching may occur after the application of mupirocin to the skin.

Antimicrobial Action and Resistance

Mupirocin is an antibiotic which inhibits bacterial protein synthesis by binding to iso-leucyl transfer RNA synthetase. Most strains of staphylococci and streptococci are very susceptible to mupirocin and it is also active against some Gram-negative bacteria. It is primarily bacteriostatic, although it may be bactericidal in the high concentrations achieved on the skin. At these concentrations it may have some activity against organisms reported to be relatively resistant to mupirocin *in vitro*.

Studies of the antimicrobial activity of mupirocin. Mupirocin inhibited staphylococci and most streptococci at low concentrations *in vitro*. All 310 clinical isolates of *Staphylococcus aureus* were susceptible with MICs in the range of 0.06 to 0.25 µg per mL. Penicillin-susceptible, penicillin-resistant, and methicillin-resistant strains were equally susceptible. Mupirocin was also active against multiply-resistant strains and there was no evidence of cross-resistance between mupirocin and any of the major groups of antibiotics. Similar results were observed with 71 isolates of *Staph. aureus* and coagulase-negative staphylococci. Three clinical strains of staphylococci with reduced susceptibility to mupirocin were also tested. Most streptococci tested had MICs of between 0.12 and 0.5 µg per mL. *Enterococcus faecalis* (*Streptococcus faecalis*), *E. faecium*, and *Str. bovis*, however, were only inhibited by concentrations of 32 to 64 µg per mL. The test strains of *Erysipelothrix rhusiopathiae* and *Listeria monocytogenes* were relatively susceptible to the antibiotic (MIC 8.0 µg per mL).

Other aerobic bacteria, including *Corynebacterium* spp. and *Micrococcus luteus* were less susceptible, as were the anaerobic Gram-positive bacteria tested, *Peptostreptococcus anaerobius, Peptococcus prevotii, Clostridium* spp., and *Propionibacterium acnes*.
Test strains of the following Gram-negative bacteria had MICs in the range of 0.02 to 0.25 µg per mL: *Haemophilus influenzae, Neisseria gonorrhoeae, N. meningitidis, Branhamella catarrhalis, Bordetella pertussis*, and *Pasteurella multocida*. *Pseudomonas aeruginosa* and members of the Enterobacteriaceae, however, had MICs ranging between 64 and 6400 µg per mL. *Bacteroides fragilis* was resistant to mupirocin.
Mupirocin was ineffective in inhibiting the growth of *Chlamydia trachomatis* in tissue culture and had only low activity against a variety of fungi tested.
Staphylococci resistant to mupirocin emerged only slowly *in vitro*, and these variants showed no cross-resistance with other antibiotics. Mupirocin was more active in acid than neutral or alkaline media; its activity was reduced in the presence of human serum due to high binding. In general, the MBCs of mupirocin against *Staph. aureus* were 8- to 32-fold higher than the corresponding MICs.— R. Sutherland *et al., Antimicrob. Ag. Chemother.*, 1985, *27*, 495. A similar study. The MICs for a range of clinical isolates of *Staph. aureus* were between 0.015 and 0.06 µg per mL.— M. W. Casewell and R. L. R. Hill, *J. antimicrob. Chemother.*, 1985, *15*, 523.

RESISTANCE. Two distinct strains of *Staphylococcus aureus* with high-level resistance (MICs above 700 µg per mL) had been isolated from 14 patients. One strain was resistant to penicillin, erythromycin, and mupirocin, and the other also to tetracycline. Some coagulase-negative staphylococci had also become resistant. The *Staph. aureus* strains were considered to have become resistant, probably by acquisition of a plasmid, during therapy with mupirocin; long-term use of the drug should be avoided.— M. Rahman *et al.* (letter), *Lancet*, 1987, *2*, 387. Isolation of strains of *Staph. aureus* with MICs of 32 to 64 µg per mL, considered resistant to mupirocin. These resistant strains had been slowly spreading in the dermatology wards of a hospital during the past 6 months. Some coagulase-negative staphylococci had also become resistant.— D. Baird and J. Coia (letter), *ibid.* The incidence of mupirocin resistance in clinical isolates of *Staph. aureus* (MIC of 8 µg or more per mL) rose from 3% in 1986 to 6% in 1987; the modal MIC resistant isolates in these 2 years was 8 and 64 µg per mL respectively. There was no association between mupirocin and methicillin resistance and the isolates did not share a common antibiotic resistance profile or phage type. These isolates were considered to demonstrate low-level resistance which may develop *in vivo* on exposure to mupirocin and is unlikely to be plasmid-mediated. High-level resistance is uncommon, unstable, and plasmid-mediated and hence transferable, as found by Rahman *et al.*— J. Kavi *et al.* (letter), *ibid.*, 1472. Emergence of low-level mupirocin-resistance in methicillin-resistant *Staph. aureus* after use of mupirocin for about 3 weeks.— M. D. Smith *et al.* (letter), *ibid.*

Absorption and Fate

Only very small amounts of topically applied mupirocin are absorbed into the systemic circulation where it is rapidly metabolised to monic acid.

Uses and Administration

Mupirocin is an antibiotic which is applied topically as a 2% ointment in a macrogol basis in the treatment of various bacterial skin infections. It should be applied up to three times a day for up to 10 days. This ointment is not suitable for application to mucous membranes and mupirocin in a paraffin basis is used for eradication of the nasal carriage of epidemic methicillin-resistant *Staphylococcus aureus*.

Reviews of the actions and uses of mupirocin: A. Ward and D. M. Campoli-Richards, *Drugs*, 1986, *32*, 425; J. Rumsfield *et al., Drug Intell. & clin. Pharm.*, 1986, *20*, 943; K. A. Pappa (letter), *ibid.*, 1987, *21*, 466; M. W. Casewell and R. L. R. Hill, *J. antimicrob. Chemother.*, 1987, *19*, 1; *Drug & Ther. Bull.*, 1987, *25*, 7.

For proceedings of a symposium on mupirocin, see *Mupirocin, a novel topical antibiotic International Congress and Symposium Series No. 80*, D.S. Wilkinson and J.D. Price (Ed.), London, The Royal Society of Medicine, 1984, 1 to 181.

CONTROL OF EPIDEMIC MRSA. Guidelines for the control of epidemic methicillin-resistant *Staphylococcus aureus* (MRSA). The application of mupirocin in a paraffin basis to the anterior nares three times daily for at least 5 days was considered to be the most effective treatment for nasal carriage. Other topical agents such as chlorhexidine 1% cream or a cream containing chlorhexidine 0.1% and neomycin 0.5% had generally been less effective at eradicating epidemic MRSA although they may reduce the number of organisms in the nose. Antiseptics were recommended for reduction of staphylococci on the skin; mupirocin, however, may be particularly effective in lesions such as eczema or pressure sores.— *J. Hosp. Infect.*, 1986, *7*, 193.
Studies of the use of mupirocin in the elimination of nasal carriage of *Staphylococcus aureus*: J. E. Dacre *et al.* (letter), *Lancet*, 1983, *2*, 1036; M. W. Casewell and R. L. R. Hill, *J. antimicrob. Chemother.*, 1986, *17*, 365.

SKIN DISORDERS. Mupirocin has been investigated for the topical treatment of both primary skin infections, including impetigo, and secondary infections, including infected eczema, atopic dermatitis, or psoriasis, and infected wounds, burns, and ulcers. Clinical success rates of 80 to 100% in primary infections and 75 to 100% in secondary infections have been reported. However, in some studies the success rates with the macrogol vehicle have also been high and little different from those with mupirocin ointment. Bacteriologically, mupirocin has been shown to be superior to vehicle in most studies. Comparative studies of mupirocin with other antibacterial agents have been few and generally in small groups of patients.— A. Ward and D. M. Campoli-Richards, *Drugs*, 1986, *32*, 425.
Comparative studies of topical mupirocin and systemic antibiotics in the treatment of skin infections: J. W. Villiger *et al., Curr. med. Res. Opinion*, 1986, *10*, 339 (erythromycin or flucloxacillin); P. H. Dux *et al., Curr. ther. Res.*, 1986, *40*, 933 (cloxacillin or erythromycin); O. Welsh and C. Saenz, *ibid.*, 1987, *41*, 114 (ampicillin); J. L. Arredondo, *ibid.*, 121 (dicloxacillin).

Proprietary Preparations

Bactroban *(Beecham Research, UK). Ointment*, mupirocin 2% in a macrogol basis.
Nasal Ointment (Bactroban Nasal), mupirocin 2% in a basis of white soft paraffin.

Proprietary Names and Manufacturers

Bactroban *(Beecham, Canad.; Beecham Research, UK).*

110-x

Nafcillin Sodium *(BANM, USAN, rINNM).*

Nafcillinum Natricum; Sodium Nafcillin. Sodium (6*R*)-6-(2-ethoxy-1-naphthamido)penicillanate monohydrate.
$C_{21}H_{21}N_2NaO_5S,H_2O$=454.5.

CAS — 147-52-4 (nafcillin); 985-16-0 (sodium salt, anhydrous); 7177-50-6 (sodium salt, monohydrate).

Pharmacopoeias. In *Braz., Int.*, and *U.S.*

A white to yellowish-white powder with not more than a slight characteristic odour. 1.1 g of monograph substance is approximately equivalent to 1 g of anhydrous nafcillin. Each g of monograph substance represents 2.2 mmol of sodium.
Freely **soluble** in water and chloroform; soluble in alcohol. A 3% solution in water has a pH of 5 to 7. **Store** in airtight containers.
Solutions of nafcillin sodium are reported to be **stable** for 3 months at −20°. Solutions containing up to 20% are reported to be stable for 24 hours at 25° and for 4 days at 5°; a 25% solution is reported to be stable for 3 days at 25°, and for 7 days at 5°. However, it is recommended that reconstituted solutions of nafcillin sodium should be administered immediately after preparation.
Nafcillin sodium has been reported to be **incompatible** with aminoglycosides, aztreonam, tetracyclines, and polymyxin B. It has been reported to be incompatible with acidic drugs such as ascorbic acid, metaraminol tartrate, suxamethonium, and vitamins of the B group, and alkaline drugs such as aminophylline. Incompatibility or loss of activity has also been reported with salts of opioid analgesics, droperidol, hydrocortisone sodium succinate, methylprednisolone sodium succinate, promazine hydrochloride, and verapamil hydrochloride.

Adverse Effects

As for Benzylpenicillin Sodium, p.132.

Thrombophlebitis may occur when nafcillin sodium is given by intravenous injection, and tissue damage has been reported on extravasation.

EFFECTS ON THE BLOOD. Various adverse effects on the blood have been reported after the administration of nafcillin sodium, including neutropenia (M. Sandberg *et al., J. Am. med. Ass.*, 1975, *232*, 1152; C. Wilson *et al., Lancet*, 1979, *1*, 1150; M.P. Dutro *et al., Am. J. Hosp. Pharm.*, 1981, *38*, 889) and agranulocytosis (S.M. Markowitz *et al., J. Am. med. Ass.*, 1975, *232*, 1150). These effects have most often occurred after administration of high, intravenous doses over a prolonged period, and have resolved after withdrawal of the drug. Prolongation of the bleeding time has been reported in 2 patients (D.P. Alexander *et al., Antimicrob. Ag. Chemother*, 1983, *23*, 59), also given high-dose, intravenous nafcillin sodium; one of the patients also had a bleeding episode. In the other patient abnormal platelet aggregation was demonstrated.

EFFECTS ON ELECTROLYTE HOMOEOSTASIS. Hypokalaemia with excessive urinary potassium loss in one patient given intravenous nafcillin sodium 8 g daily. The serum-potassium concentration was not corrected by intravenous administration of potassium chloride, but did return to normal after decreasing the dose of nafcillin sodium to 4 g daily.— J. A. Mohr *et al., J. Am. med. Ass.*, 1979, *242*, 544.

EFFECTS ON THE KIDNEYS. Nephritis which had developed in a 6-year-old boy who received methicillin recurred when he was given nafcillin 150 mg per kg body-weight daily.— M. F. Parry *et al.* (letter), *J. Am. med. Ass.*, 1973, *225*, 178. The nephropathy was also exacerbated by cephalothin.— S. N. Cohen and J. E. Conte (letter), *ibid.*, 1974, *227*, 325.
Further references to interstitial nephritis associated with nafcillin: T. W. Bodendorfer (letter), *J. Am. med. Ass.*, 1980, *244*, 2609.

LOCAL IRRITANT EFFECTS. A report of cutaneous necrosis in 4 infants associated with the extravasation of nafcillin sodium on intravenous administration.— S. J. Tilden *et al., Am. J. Dis. Child.*, 1980, *134*, 1046.

Precautions

As for Benzylpenicillin Sodium, p.133.

ADMINISTRATION IN LIVER DISORDERS. For reference to the precautions to be observed in liver disorders, see below under Uses, Administration in Liver Disorders.

ADMINISTRATION IN RENAL FAILURE. For reference to the precautions to be observed in renal failure, see below under Uses, Administration in Renal Failure.

INTERACTIONS. For the effect of nafcillin on warfarin, see Warfarin Sodium p.345.
For the effect of other drugs on the antimicrobial activity of nafcillin sodium, see below under Antimicrobial Action.

INTERFERENCE WITH DIAGNOSTIC TESTS. False-positive results for proteinuria occurred in 2 patients; very high doses of nafcillin caused a heavy urinary sediment.— D. E. Line *et al., J. Am. med. Ass.*, 1976, *235*, 1259.

Antimicrobial Action

Nafcillin sodium has an antibacterial activity similar to that of Methicillin Sodium, p.259, although it is generally more active.

Studies *in vitro* indicating that in the presence of polyvinylchloride catheters coagulase-negative staphylococci, especially slime-producing strains, are able to survive exposure to concentrations of nafcillin exceeding the expected minimum bactericidal concentrations.— N. K. Sheth *et al., Lancet*, 1985, *2*, 1266. Comment suggesting that the degree of adherence, whether associated with slime production or not, is the more important factor in the survival of coagulase-negative staphylococcal strains exposed to nafcillin.— R. Edwards *et al.* (letter), *ibid.*, 1986, *1*, 330.

ACTIVITY WITH OTHER ANTIMICROBIAL AGENTS. *Aminoglycosides.* Studies *in vitro* have demonstrated enhanced activity of nafcillin against clinical isolates of *Staphylococcus aureus* when combined with netilmicin or sissomicin (C. Watanakunakorn and C. Glotzbecker, *Antimicrob. Ag. Chemother.*, 1977, *12*, 346), or with gentamicin sulphate (C.U. Tuazon *et al., Curr. ther. Res.*, 1978, *23*, 760). Enhanced activity of nafcillin in combination with gentamicin or netilmicin has also been shown against enterococci (J.J. Rahal and M.S. Simberkoff, *J. antimicrob. Chemother.*, 1986, *17*, 585).

Ampicillin. Synergy between nafcillin and ampicillin was demonstrated *in vitro* against ampicillin-resistant strains of *Haemophilus influenzae*.— R. Yogev *et al.*,

Antimicrob. Ag. Chemother., 1980, *17*, 461.

Rifampicin. Variable antimicrobial interactions against *Staphylococcus aureus* have been demonstrated *in vitro* with a combination of nafcillin and rifampicin. In one study (C.U. Tuazon *et al.*, *Antimicrob. Ag. Chemother.*, 1978, *13*, 759) the 2 drugs enhanced each other's activity against 12 strains; however their activities were additive or antagonistic against 2 and 6 strains respectively. In another study, however (C. Watanakunakorn and J.C. Tisone, *ibid.*, 1982, *22*, 920), rifampicin diminished the activity of nafcillin against all 20 strains tested. Nafcillin has also been shown to reduce the emergence of rifampicin resistance when methicillin-sensitive *Staph. aureus* were incubated with rifampicin and nafcillin (R.H.K. Eng *et al.*, *J. antimicrob. Chemother.*, 1985, *15*, 201).

Resistance

As for Methicillin Sodium, p.259.

Absorption and Fate

Nafcillin sodium is incompletely and irregularly absorbed from the gastro-intestinal tract, especially when administered after a meal. Peak plasma concentrations of 1.5 to 8 µg per mL have been reported 1 hour after a dose of 0.5 to 1 g given by mouth to fasting subjects. After intramuscular injection it is absorbed more reliably, an injection of 0.5 to 1 g producing peak plasma concentrations of 5 to 8 µg per mL within about 0.5 to 2 hours. Up to 90% of nafcillin in the circulation is bound to plasma proteins. Nafcillin has been reported to have a plasma half-life of about 0.5 to 1 hour. The half-life is prolonged in neonates.

Nafcillin diffuses across the placenta into the foetal circulation and is excreted in breast milk. There is little diffusion into the CSF except when the meninges are inflamed. Therapeutic concentrations can be achieved in pleural and synovial fluids and in bone.

Nafcillin differs from most other penicillins in that it is largely inactivated by hepatic metabolism. It is excreted via the bile though some reabsorption takes place in the small intestine. Only about 10% of a dose given by mouth before food and about 30% of a dose given intramuscularly is excreted in the urine.

Serum concentrations are enhanced if probenecid is given concomitantly.

Reports of the pharmacokinetics of nafcillin given intravenously.— W. E. Feldman *et al.*, *J. Pediat.*, 1978, *93*, 1029 (infants and children); W. Banner *et al.*, *Antimicrob. Ag. Chemother.*, 1980, *17*, 691 (premature infants).

ADMINISTRATION IN LIVER DISORDERS. For reference to the pharmacokinetics of nafcillin in liver disorders, see below under Uses, Administration in Liver Disorders.

ADMINISTRATION IN RENAL FAILURE. For reference to the pharmacokinetics of nafcillin in renal failure, see below under Uses, Administration in Renal Failure.

DIFFUSION INTO BODY TISSUES AND FLUIDS. In a study of 9 patients with either staphylococcal sepsis or meningitis who received nafcillin intravenously in varying dosage regimens, cerebrospinal fluid concentrations of nafcillin ranged from 0.13 to 88 µg per mL, while serum concentrations ranged from 5.8 to 615 µg per mL. Although there was considerable individual variation, nafcillin concentrations in the CSF usually exceeded the minimum bactericidal concentrations for *Staph. aureus* but a dose of at least 100 to 200 mg per kg body-weight daily was recommended for the treatment of meningitis caused by *Staph. aureus*.— J. G. Kane *et al.*, *Ann. intern. Med.*, 1977, *87*, 309. See also W. J. Sanders (letter), *ibid.*, 1978, *88*, 271.

Nafcillin sodium diffused into the CSF in 16 patients with non-inflamed meninges given a dose of 40 mg per kg body-weight by intravenous infusion. At 1 hour the mean CSF concentration was 0.05 µg of nafcillin per mL compared with a serum concentration of 34.4 µg per mL; at 2 hours the figures were 0.12 and 12.7 µg per mL; at 3 hours 0.09 and 4.9 µg per mL. At 4 hours detectable CSF concentrations were present in 3 of 4 patients. Large doses of nafcillin were considered to be appropriate for the prophylaxis and treatment of staphylococcal meningitis.— B. E. Fossieck *et al.*, *Antimicrob. Ag. Chemother.*, 1977, *11*, 965.

Concentrations of nafcillin in aqueous humour ranged between 0.4 and 2.0 µg per mL after the intravenous administration of nafcillin 2 g.— T. S. Lesar and R. G. Fiscella, *Drug Intell. & clin. Pharm.*, 1985, *19*, 642.

Uses and Administration

Nafcillin sodium has similar indications for use to flucloxacillin (p.231).

Nafcillin sodium is administered by intramuscular injection in a usual dose equivalent to 0.5 to 1 g of nafcillin every 4 to 6 hours. Children may be given 25 mg per kg body-weight twice daily, and neonates 10 mg per kg twice daily. Nafcillin sodium may also be given intravenously by slow injection over 5 to 10 minutes or by slow infusion; adult doses are 0.5 to 1 g of nafcillin every 4 hours, although it is usually recommended that it be used for not more than 24 to 48 hours because of the risk of thrombophlebitis.

Nafcillin sodium may be given by mouth. The dose by mouth for adults is the equivalent of 0.25 to 1 g of nafcillin every 4 to 6 hours, for children 6.25 to 12.5 mg per kg four times daily, and for neonates 10 mg per kg three or four times daily, given about one hour before or at least 2 hours after meals.

All these doses may be increased in serious infections.

A study concluding that cefotaxime is probably safer and more effective than nafcillin in association with tobramycin for the initial empirical treatment of patients with serious infections.— C. R. Smith *et al.*, *Ann. intern. Med.*, 1984, *101*, 469.

For reference to the use of nafcillin for the treatment and prophylaxis of various staphylococcal infections, see under Meningitis, Neutropenia, and Surgical Infection Prophylaxis in Flucloxacillin Sodium, p.231.

ADMINISTRATION IN INFANTS AND CHILDREN. Nafcillin could be administered by the intravenous route to children with severe infections in a dose of 150 to 200 mg per kg body-weight daily given in divided doses every 4 to 6 hours.— K. H. Rhodes and C. M. Johnson, *Mayo Clin. Proc.*, 1983, *58*, 158.

ADMINISTRATION IN LIVER DISORDERS. Plasma clearance of nafcillin was reduced in patients with biliary obstruction or cirrhosis and lower doses might be necessary in such patients.— J. P. Marshall *et al.*, *Gastroenterology*, 1977, *73*, 1388.

ADMINISTRATION IN RENAL FAILURE. The normal half-life for nafcillin of 0.5 hours was increased to 1.2 hours in end-stage renal failure. It could be given in usual doses to patients with renal failure. Doses should be reduced, however, in combined hepatic and renal failure. A dosage supplement was not required for patients undergoing haemodialysis.— W. M. Bennett *et al.*, *Am. J. Kidney Dis.*, 1983, *3*, 155.

ENDOCARDITIS. A study involving 48 drug addicts and 30 non-addicts comparing parenteral nafcillin alone for 6 weeks, or with gentamicin for the first 2 weeks for the treatment of endocarditis caused by *Staphylococcus aureus*. There were some advantages to the mixture, especially in the addicts; in the non-addicts the increased clearance of bacteraemia was associated with an increase in azotaemia.— O. Korzeniowski *et al.*, *Ann. intern. Med.*, 1982, *97*, 496.

Preparations

Nafcillin Sodium Capsules *(U.S.P.)*

Nafcillin Sodium for Injection *(U.S.P.)*. pH 6.0 to 8.5.

Sterile Nafcillin Sodium *(U.S.P.)*

Nafcillin Sodium for Oral Solution *(U.S.P.)*

Nafcillin Sodium Tablets *(U.S.P.)*. Protect from light.

Proprietary Names and Manufacturers

Nafcil *(Bristol, USA)*; Unipen *(Wyeth, Canad.; Wyeth, USA)*.

5663-n

Nalidixic Acid *(BAN, USAN, rINN)*.

Nalidixinic Acid; Win-18320. 1-Ethyl-1,4-dihydro-7-methyl-4-oxo-1,8-naphthyridine-3-carboxylic acid.

$C_{12}H_{12}N_2O_3$=232.2.

CAS — 389-08-2.

Pharmacopoeias. In *Br., Braz., Chin., Cz., Egypt., Ind., It., Jpn,* and *U.S.*

White to very pale yellow odourless or almost odourless crystalline powder.

B.P. **solubilities** are: practically insoluble in water; slightly soluble in alcohol and solutions of alkali hydroxides; soluble 1 in 35 of chloroform. *U.S.P.* solubilities are: very slightly soluble to practically insoluble in water; soluble 1 in 910 of alcohol and 1 in 29 of chloroform; very slightly soluble in ether; soluble in solutions of fixed alkali hydroxides and carbonates.

Store in airtight containers. Protect from light.

Adverse Effects

About 8% of patients are considered to experience adverse effects with nalidixic acid. The most frequent adverse reactions involve the gastro-intestinal tract, skin, or the central nervous system. Common side-effects on the gastro-intestinal tract include nausea and vomiting. Diarrhoea and abdominal pain have also occurred.

Neurological side-effects include visual disturbances, headache, dizziness or vertigo, and drowsiness. Confusion, mental depression, excitement, hallucinations, and psychoses have also occurred as have peripheral neuropathies, muscular weakness, and myalgia. Convulsions have occurred after large doses or in patients with predisposing factors such as cerebrovascular insufficiency, parkinsonism, and epilepsy. There have been reports of intracranial hypertension especially in infants and young children.

Adverse effects on the skin include photosensitivity reactions with erythema and bullous eruptions, allergic rashes, urticaria, and pruritus. Eosinophilia, fever, angioedema, and arthralgia occur occasionally.

Cholestatic jaundice, thrombocytopenia, and leucopenia have occurred rarely, as has haemolytic anaemia in patients who may or may not be deficient in glucose-6-phosphate dehydrogenase.

EFFECTS ON THE BLOOD. *Haemolytic anaemia.* Haemolytic anaemia has occurred in patients deficient in glucose-6-phosphate dehydrogenase and given nalidixic acid (L.P. Vargas and C.S. González, *Lancet*, 1967, *2*, 97; B.K. Mandal and J. Stevenson, *ibid.*, 1970, *1*, 614; L. Alessio and G. Morselli, *Br. med. J.*, 1972, *4*, 110) as well as in an infant without any evidence of deficiency (E.M. Belton and R.V. Jones, *Lancet*, 1965, *2*, 691). Fatal auto-immune haemolytic anaemia has occurred in elderly patients (C. Gilbertson and D.R. Jones, *Br. med. J.*, 1972, *4*, 493; O. Tafani *et al.*, *ibid.*, 1982, *285*, 936).

Thrombocytopenia. A report, from the Netherlands Centre for Monitoring of Adverse Reactions to Drugs, of 6 patients who had developed profound but transient thrombocytopenia probably induced by nalidixic acid. All recovered after withdrawal of the drug. It was noted that 5 of the patients were over 65 years-of-age and that 2 of them had impaired renal function.— R. H. B. Meyboom, *Br. med. J.*, 1984, *289*, 962.

EFFECTS ON THE EAR. A report suggesting a possible adverse effect of nalidixic acid on hearing. A newly-born infant who accidentally received 10 times the normal dose of nalidixic acid developed tachypnoea and transient acidosis but subsequently recovered and appeared in good health. Approximately 2½ years later the child was discovered to have severe bilateral hearing impairment. A second child who received nalidixic acid in normal doses for 4 to 5 days at the age of 3 months showed some signs of hypotonia and was subsequently found, at the age of 2, to suffer from profound deafness. Neither child had any indications suggesting a hereditary cause for the handicap.— J. -P. de Reynier, *Rev. méd. Suisse romande*, 1977, *97*, 437.

EFFECTS ON THE JOINTS. For reference to studies indicating that nalidixic acid and related compounds can induce arthropathy in juvenile *animals*, see under Precautions.

EFFECTS ON METABOLISM. Severe metabolic acidosis with serum concentrations of nalidixic acid 297 µg per mL was reported in a previously healthy 18-year-old man who had taken an overdose of nalidixic acid together with probenecid and other drugs. The mean serum concentration of nalidixic acid 8 hours after dosage was increased 3-fold when the dose followed probenecid 500 mg in 2 subjects.— H. Dash and J. Mills (letter), *Ann. intern. Med.*, 1976, *84*, 570.

A report of coma and metabolic acidosis in a 17-

month-old child following administration of a single dose of about 100 mg of nalidixic acid.— C. Corsini *et al.*, *Anest. Rianim.*, 1982, *23*, 31.

Hyperglycaemia. Reports of hyperglycaemia and convulsions associated with usual doses or overdosage of nalidixic acid: M. A. Islam and T. Sreedharan, *J. Am. med. Ass.*, 1965, *192*, 1100; A. G. Fraser and A. D. B. Harrower, *Br. med. J.*, 1977, *2*, 1518; P. J. A. Leslie *et al.*, *Hum. Toxicol.*, 1984, *3*, 239.

EFFECTS ON THE NERVOUS SYSTEM. Reports of intracranial hypertension in infants and children given nalidixic acid: T. Deonna and J. P. Guignard, *Archs Dis. Childh.*, 1974, *49*, 743; C. Kilpatrick and P. Ebeling (letter), *Med. J. Aust.*, 1982, *1*, 252; W. Gedroyc and S. D. Shorvon, *Neurology*, 1982, *32*, 212. Increased intracranial pressure in a 20-year-old woman given nalidixic acid 2 g.— G. Granström and B. Santesson, *Acta med. scand.*, 1984, *216*, 237.

Precautions

Nalidixic acid and related 4-quinolone antimicrobial agents should be given with care to patients with damage of the central nervous system, to patients subject to convulsions, and to those with impaired renal or hepatic function.

Their use should be avoided in babies less than 3 months old. Since nalidixic acid and related antimicrobial agents have been shown to cause degenerative changes in weight-bearing joints of young *animals*, it has been suggested that these compounds should not be used in prepubertal children, pregnant women, or during lactation.

Exposure to strong sunlight should be avoided during treatment with nalidixic acid.

Nitrofurantoin and nalidixic acid are antagonistic *in vitro* and should not be used together. Nalidixic acid can displace oral anticoagulants from their plasma binding sites. Because the anticoagulant is rapidly redistributed, this displacement may not result in an enhanced anticoagulant effect. However, in the event of any enhancement, the dose of the anticoagulant should be reduced.

Nalidixic acid may cause false-positive reactions in urine tests for glucose using copper reduction methods.

Studies indicating that nalidixic acid and related compounds can induce degenerative changes in weight-bearing joints in juvenile *animals*.— B. Ingham *et al.*, *Toxicol. Lett.*, 1977, *1*, 21 (nalidixic acid, oxolinic acid, pipemidic acid); L. C. Howard *et al.*, *Toxic. appl. Pharmac.*, 1979, *48*, A145 (cinoxacin); A. Gough *et al.*, *ibid.*, *51*, 177 (oxolinic acid, pipemidic acid); M. Nomura *et al.*, *Chemotherapy, Tokyo*, 1984, *32*, *Suppl.*1, 1105 (ofloxacin).

ADMINISTRATION IN RENAL FAILURE. See under Uses.

INTERACTIONS. Nalidixic acid was highly bound to albumin and displaced warfarin from its binding sites *in vitro*.— E. M. Sellers and J. Koch-Weser, *Clin. Pharmac. Ther.*, 1970, *11*, 524. See also.— *idem*, *Ann. N.Y. Acad. Sci.*, 1971, *179*, 213.

For reports of antagonistic effects on activity when nalidixic acid is used with other antimicrobial agents, see under Antimocrobial Action. For a report of probenecid increasing serum concentrations of nalidixic acid, see under Effects on Metabolism in Adverse Effects. For the interaction of 4-quinolone antimicrobial agents with xanthines such as caffeine and theophylline, see p.1523 and p.1529.

INTERFERENCE WITH DIAGNOSTIC TESTS. Reports of nalidixic acid interfering with various laboratory tests: O. Llerena and O. H. Pearson, *New Engl. J. Med.*, 1968, *279*, 983 (urinary steroids); *Adverse Drug React. Bull.*, 1972, June, 104 (plasma steroids); *Drug & Ther. Bull.*, 1972, *10*, 69 (urinary vanilmandelic acid); J. Millhouse, *Adverse Drug React. Bull.*, 1974, Dec., 164 (glucose).

PORPHYRIA. Nalidixic acid was considered to be unsafe in patients with acute porphyria because it has been shown to be porphyrinogenic in *animals* or *in-vitro* systems.— M. R. Moore and K. E. L. McColl, *Porphyrias, Drug Lists*, Glasgow, Porphyria Research Unit, University of Glasgow, 1987.

PREGNANCY AND THE NEONATE. From the results of a retrospective study of 63 women who received nalidixic acid during pregnancy (6 during the first trimester, 26 during the second, 30 during the third, and one at term) Murray (*Br. med. J.*, 1981, *282*, 224) concluded that nalidixic acid did not appear to cause congenital deformity or intracranial hypertension in the foetus. Asscher (*ibid.*, 1977, *1*, 1332) had previously recommended that nalidixic acid should be avoided in the late stages of pregnancy since it might produce hydrocephalus in the foetus even in low dosage.

Antimicrobial Action and Resistance

Nalidixic acid is active against Gram-negative bacteria including *Escherichia coli, Klebsiella* spp., *Proteus* spp., *Enterobacter* spp., *Salmonella* spp., and *Shigella* spp. It is usually bactericidal. Most susceptible organisms are inhibited by 16 µg or less per mL. *Pseudomonas aeruginosa* is usually resistant. Bacterial resistance may develop rapidly, sometimes within a few days, but it does not appear to be transferable or R-plasmid mediated. Cross-resistance with oxolinic acid and cinoxacin occurs.

Unlike nitrofurantoin, Gram-positive urinary-tract pathogens are relatively resistant, also the antibacterial activity of nalidixic acid is not significantly affected by differences in urinary pH. Antagonism between nitrofurantoin and nalidixic acid has been demonstrated *in vitro*.

Nalidixic acid is considered to act by inhibiting the replication of bacterial DNA probably by interfering with DNA gyrase (topoisomerase) activity.

For a report that oxolinic acid was more effective *in vitro* than nalidixic acid or cinoxacin against *Shigella sonnei* and *Sh. flexneri*, see Oxolinic Acid, p.278.

ACTIVITY WITH OTHER ANTIMICROBIAL AGENTS. Results of a study of the activity of nalidixic acid with various antibiotics on 95 strains of Enterobacteriaceae indicated that most other antimicrobial agents quite frequently produce an antagonistic effect when used with nalidixic acid. Potential combinations should be tested *in vitro* before being used clinically.— J. Michel *et al.*, *Antimicrob. Ag. Chemother.*, 1973, *4*, 201.

Ampicillin and chloramphenicol. Evidence of some degree of antagonism between nalidixic acid and ampicillin or chloramphenicol *in vitro*.— J. Brisou and F. Denis, *Path. Biol., Paris*, 1971, *19*, 655.

Metronidazole. Synergism of nalidixic acid and metronidazole *in vitro* against *Bacteroides fragilis*.— A. R. Salem *et al.*, *J. antimicrob. Chemother.*, 1975, *1*, 387. See also E. D. Ralph and Y. E. Amatnieks, *Antimicrob. Ag. Chemother.*, 1980, *17*, 379.

Nitrofurantoin. Reports of nitrofurantoin inhibiting the antimicrobial activity of nalidixic acid *in vitro*.— W. Stille and K. H. Ostner, *Klin. Wschr.*, 1966, *44*, 155; J. D. Piguet, *Annls Inst. Pasteur, Paris*, 1969, *116*, 43.

Rifampicin. A report of antagonism between nalidixic acid and rifampicin *in vitro*.— J. -G. Baudens and Y. -A. Chabbert, *Path. Biol., Paris*, 1969, *17*, 391. Rifampicin and nalidixic acid enhanced the activity of each other when used together *in vitro* against various Gram-negative bacteria and suppressed the emergence of resistant bacteria that occurred when each drug was used alone.— D. Greenwood and J. Andrew, *J. antimicrob. Chemother.*, 1978, *4*, 533.

BACTERIAL RESISTANCE. Apparent absence of transferable resistance to nalidixic acid in pathogenic Gram-negative bacteria.— L. G. Burman, *J. antimicrob. Chemother.*, 1977, *3*, 509.

Of 232 strains of enteropathogenic *Escherichia coli* none was resistant to nalidixic acid at a concentration of 20 µg per mL.— R. J. Gross *et al.*, *Br. med. J.*, 1982, *285*, 472.

Of 2753 strains of *Shigella dysenteriae, Sh. flexneri*, and *Sh. boydii* examined at the Central Public Health Laboratory from 1979 to mid 1983 0.1% were resistant to nalidixic acid at a concentration of 20 µg per mL.— R. J. Gross *et al.*, *Br. med. J.*, 1984, *288*, 784. See also H. B. Hansson *et al.*, *Antimicrob. Ag. Chemother.*, 1981, *19*, 271.

A report of plasmid-mediated resistance to nalidixic acid in *Shigella dysenteriae* type 1 isolated during an epidemic of shigellosis in Bangladesh.— M. H. Munshi *et al.*, *Lancet*, 1987, *2*, 419. Confirmation is required; this report should not be taken as indicating that plasmid-mediated resistance to the newer 4-quinolones is imminent.— G. C. Crumplin (letter), *ibid.*, 854.

Absorption and Fate

Nalidixic acid is rapidly and almost completely absorbed from the gastro-intestinal tract and peak plasma concentrations of 20 to 50 µg per mL have been reported 2 hours after the administration of 1 g by mouth. Plasma half-lives of about 1 to 2.5 hours have been reported.

Nalidixic acid is partially metabolised to hydroxynalidixic acid, which also has antibacterial activity and accounts for about 30% of active drug in the blood. About 93% of nalidixic acid and 63% of hydroxynalidixic acid are bound to plasma proteins. Both nalidixic acid and hydroxynalidixic acid are rapidly metabolised to inactive glucuronide and dicarboxylic acid derivatives. Nalidixic acid and its metabolites are excreted rapidly in the urine, nearly all of a dose being eliminated within 24 hours. About 80 to 90% of the drug excreted in the urine is as inactive metabolites but urinary concentrations of unchanged drug and active metabolite ranging from 25 to 250 µg per mL are achieved after a single 1-g dose. Hydroxynalidixic acid accounts for about 80 to 85% of activity in the urine.

Only traces of nalidixic acid appear in breast-milk and cerebrospinal fluid; traces also appear to cross the placenta. About 4% of a dose is excreted in the faeces.

In a multiple-dose study of the pharmacokinetics of nalidixic acid the apparent mean elimination half-life for nalidixic acid and hydroxynalidixic acid was found to be about 6 to 7 hours after using more specific and sensitive assay techniques and longer sampling periods than previously used.— N. Ferry *et al.*, *Clin. Pharmac. Ther.*, 1981, *29*, 695.

From the results of a study in 23 patients with varying renal function it appears that the elimination-rate of nalidixic acid is not markedly altered by renal insufficiency. However, the elimination of hydroxynalidixic acid is significantly reduced and therefore hydroxynalidixic acid accumulates in patients with renal insufficiency. 7-Carboxynalidixic acid which could not be detected in the plasma of patients with normal renal function, also appeared in the plasma of patients with renal insufficiency.— G. Cuisinaud *et al.*, *Br. J. clin. Pharmac.*, 1982, *14*, 489.

There were significant variations between the pharmacokinetic parameters of nalidixic acid in 8 young subjects (mean age 25.4 years) and those in 6 elderly subjects (mean age 77.3 years). Plasma concentrations were generally higher in the elderly and the mean half-life of active drug was 2.7 hours in the young group and 11.5 hours in the elderly. Diminished renal function may explain the slower elimination in the elderly subjects. It may be wise to reduce the dosage of nalidixic acid when treating elderly patients.— G. Barbeau and P. -M. Belanger, *J. clin. Pharmac.*, 1982, *22*, 490.

The pharmacokinetics of nalidixic acid in healthy subjects following intravenous infusion.— R. Cadórniga *et al.*, *An. R. Acad. Farm., Madr.*, 1983, *49*, 411.

Uses and Administration

Nalidixic acid is a 4-quinolone antimicrobial agent used in the treatment of uncomplicated lower urinary-tract infections due to Gram-negative bacteria other than *Pseudomonas* spp. It may be effective in urinary infections which have not responded to treatment with other agents. Its antibacterial activity does not appear to be influenced by urinary pH although the concomitant administration of sodium bicarbonate or sodium citrate does increase the concentration of active drug in the urine. It has also been used in the treatment of shigellosis resistant to treatment with other antimicrobial agents, although there is concern that if used routinely resistance to nalidixic acid may also develop.

The usual adult dose is 4 g daily in 4 divided doses for at least 7 days in acute infections. Since bacterial resistance may develop rapidly it has been suggested that if treatment with nalidixic acid has not resulted in a negative urine culture within 48 to 72 hours another antimicrobial agent should be used. If therapy continues for longer than 2 weeks the dose should usually be halved. Children may be given 50 to 55 mg per kg body-weight daily in 4 divided doses reduced to 30 to 33 mg per kg daily for prolonged treatment.

A suggested dose of nalidixic acid, in conjunction with sodium citrate, is 660 mg three times daily for 3 days.

The sodium salt of nalidixic acid has been given by intravenous infusion.

ADMINISTRATION IN THE ELDERLY. See under Absorption and Fate (above).

ADMINISTRATION IN RENAL FAILURE. Nalidixic acid is not recommended for urinary-tract infections if the creatinine clearance is less than 20 mL per minute.— J. S. Cheigh, *Am. J. Med.*, 1977, *62*, 555.

Nalidixic acid could be given in usual doses if the glomerular filtration-rate was more than 50 mL per minute but should be avoided at glomerular filtration-rates less than this because metabolites accumulated.— W. M. Bennett *et al.*, *Am. J. Kidney Dis.*, 1983, *3*, 155.

SHIGELLOSIS. There have been several reports of nalidixic acid being effective in the treatment of *Shigella* infections (J.G. McCormack, *Lancet*, 1983, *2*, 1091; H.E. Parry, *ibid.*, 1206; M. Malengreau, *ibid.*, 1984, *2*, 172) without there being any problems of emerging resistance. However, concern about the dangers of resistance developing in gut flora has been voiced (B.R. Panhotra and B. Desai, *Lancet*, 1983, *2*, 1420) as well as resistance in *Shigella* (R. Bose *et al.*, *Lancet*, 1984, *2*, 1160; B.R. Panhotra *et al.*, *ibid.*, 1985, *1*, 763).

URINARY-TRACT INFECTIONS. A review of the actions and uses of nalidixic acid. It was considered that only a few studies could pass current standards. Those that were interpretable indicated amongst other things that nalidixic acid is effective for acute symptomatic urinary-tract infections due to *Escherichia coli*, *Proteus* spp., and *Enterobacter* spp. although it is no better than other standard therapy. It is also considered to be suitable for patients sensitive to penicillins or sulphonamides.— R. Gleckman *et al.*, *Am. J. Hosp. Pharm.*, 1979, *36*, 1071.

Some references to nalidixic acid being assessed in urinary-tract infections: A. Iravani *et al.*, *Antimicrob. Ag. Chemother.*, 1981, *19*, 598; R. B. Light *et al.*, *Scand. J. infect. Dis.*, 1981, *13*, 195; J. K. Preiksaitis *et al.*, *J. infect. Dis.*, 1981, *143*, 603.

Use with sodium citrate. Studies have not shown the use of nalidixic acid with sodium citrate (Mictral) to be more effective than ampicillin, co-trimoxazole, or nitrofurantoin in the treatment of acute lower urinary-tract infection. However, its use may be considered in patients who have not responded to standard therapy and a 3-day course may prove to be more effective and less toxic than nalidixic acid given alone.— *Drug & Ther. Bull.*, 1981, *19*, 72.

Preparations

Nalidixic Acid Oral Suspension *(B.P.).* Nalidixic Acid Mixture

Nalidixic Acid Oral Suspension *(U.S.P.)*

Nalidixic Acid Tablets *(B.P.)*

Nalidixic Acid Tablets *(U.S.P.)*

Proprietary Preparations

Mictral *(Winthrop, UK). Granules*, effervescent, nalidixic acid 660 mg, sodium citrate 3.75 g, citric acid 250 mg, sodium bicarbonate 250 mg/sachet. *Dose.* The contents of one sachet to be taken in water three times daily for 3 days.

Negram *(Sterling Research, UK). Tablets*, nalidixic acid 500 mg.

Suspension, nalidixic acid 300 mg/5 mL.

Uriben *(R.P. Drugs, UK). Suspension*, nalidixic acid 300 mg/5 mL.

Proprietary Names and Manufacturers

Betaxina *(Terapeutico M.R., Ital.)*; Chemiurin *(Ital.)*; Dixiben *(Ital.)*; Dixilina *(Ital.)*; Dixinal *(Biochimica Zanardi, Ital.)*; Dixurol *(ABC, Ital.)*; Enexina *(SIT, Ital.)*; Entolon *(Jpn)*; Eucistin *(San Carlo, Ital.)*; Faril *(Edmond Pharma, Ital.)*; Gramoneg *(Ind.)*; Innoxalon *(Jpn)*; Jicsron *(Jpn)*; Kusnarin *(Jpn)*; Mictral *(Winthrop, UK)*; Nalicidin *(Rhone-Poulenc, Ital.)*; Nalidicron *(Jpn)*; Nalidixin *(Nuovo, Ital.; Spain)*; Nalidixol *(Spain)*; Naligen *(Savio, Ital.)*; Naligram *(Geymonat, Ital.)*; Nalissina *(Rorer, Ital.)*; Nalitucson *(Jpn)*; Nalix *(Ital.)*; Naluran *(Ital.)*; Narigix *(Jpn)*; Naxivalene *(Valles Mestre, Spain)*; Naxuril *(Esterfarm, Ital.)*; Negabatt *(Dessy, Ital.)*; NegGram *(Winthrop, Canad.; Maggioni-Winthrop, Ital.; Winthrop-Breon, USA)*; Negram *(Aust.; Winthrop, Austral.; Belg.; Winthrop, Denm.; Fin.; Winthrop, Fr.; Iceland; Neth.; Winthrop, Norw.; Sterling-Winthrop, Swed.; Winthrop, Switz.; Sterling Research, UK)*; Nicelate *(Jpn)*; Nogacit *(Winthrop, Ger.)*; Nogermin *(Spain)*; Nogram *(Winthrop, Ger.)*; Notricel *(Hortel, Spain)*; Oxoranil *(Jpn)*; Pielos *(Ital.)*; Poleon *(Jpn)*; Puromylon *(Lennon, S.Afr.)*; Sicmylon *(Jpn)*; Specifin *(Bergamon, Ital.)*; Unaserus *(Jpn)*; Uralgin *(Ceccarelli, Ital.)*; Uretrene *(Ital.)*; Uriben *(R.P. Drugs, UK)*; Uriclar *(Ital.)*; Uri-Flor *(AGIPS, Ital.)*; Urisco *(Schwarz, Ital.)*; Uristeril *(Ital.)*; Urodixin *(Ital.)*; Urogram *(FIRMA, Ital.)*; Urolex *(Ital.)*; Uroman *(Jpn)*; Uromina *(Ausonia, Ital.)*; Uronax *(Damor, Ital.)*; Uroneg *(Ibirn, Ital.)*; Uropan *(Tiber, Ital.)*; Valuren *(Ital.)*; Wintomylon *(Arg.; Jpn; Winthrop, S.Afr.; Sterwin, Spain)*; Wintron *(Jpn)*.

111-r

Neomycin *(BAN, rINN).*

A mixture of 2 isomers, neomycins B and C, and neomycin A (neamine), an inactive component and degradation product of neomycins B and C. Neomycin B is 2-deoxy-4-*O*-(2,6-diamino-2,6-dideoxy-α-D-glucopyranosyl)-5-*O*-[3-*O*-(2,6-diamino-2,6-dideoxy-β-L-idopyranosyl)-β-D-ribofuranosyl]-D-streptamine.

$C_{23}H_{46}N_6O_{13}$=614.7.

CAS — 1404-04-2 (neomycin); 3947-65-7 (neomycin A); 119-04-0 (neomycin B); 66-86-4 (neomycin C).

Framycetin (see p.234) consists mainly of neomycin B with not more than 3% of neomycin C.

The *B.P.* states that when Neomycin is prescribed or demanded, Neomycin Sulphate must be dispensed or supplied.

112-f

Neomycin Sulphate *(BANM, rINNM).*

Fradiomycin Sulphate; Neomycin Sulfate *(USAN)*; Neomycini Sulfas.

CAS — 1405-10-3.

Pharmacopoeias. In *Arg., Aust., Belg., Br., Braz., Chin., Cz., Egypt., Eur., Fr., Ger., Hung., Ind., Int., It., Jpn, Jug., Neth., Nord., Pol., Port., Roum., Rus., Swiss, Turk.*, and *U.S.*
Also in *B.P. Vet.*

Neomycin sulphate is a mixture of the sulphates of the antimicrobial substances produced by the growth of certain selected strains of *Streptomyces fradiae*. The *B.P.* specifies not less than 680 units per mg, and the *U.S.P.* not less than the equivalent of 600 µg of neomycin per mg, both calculated on the dried substance.

Neomycin sulphate occurs as a white or yellowish-white, odourless or almost odourless, hygroscopic powder.

B.P. **solubilities** are: slowly soluble 1 in 1 of water and readily soluble 1 in 3 of water; very slightly soluble in alcohol; practically insoluble in acetone, chloroform, and ether. *U.S.P.* solubilities are: soluble 1 in 1 of water; very slightly soluble in alcohol; insoluble in acetone, chloroform, and ether. A 1% solution in water has a pH of 5.0 to 7.5. **Store** at a temperature not exceeding 30° in airtight containers. Protect from light.

113-d

Neomycin Undecenoate *(BANM, rINNM).*

Neomycin Undecylenate *(USAN)*. The 10-undecenoate salt of neomycin.

CAS — 1406-04-8.

Units

One unit of neomycin is contained in 0.0012903 mg of the second International Reference Preparation (1974) of neomycin sulphate which contains 775 units per mg.

Collaborative assay by 11 laboratories of the material now established as the Second International Reference Preparation of Neomycin. Chemical examination in 4 or 5 laboratories showed a mean of 91.05% of neomycin B, 8.62% of neomycin C, and less than 1% of neamine.— J. W. Lightbown *et al.*, *J. biol. Stand.*, 1979, *7*, 227.

Adverse Effects and Treatment

As for Gentamicin Sulphate, p.236.

Neomycin may cause irreversible partial or total deafness when given by injection, by mouth, by enema or by instillation into cavities, or when applied as solutions or aerosols to open wounds or damaged skin. The effect is dose-related and is enhanced by renal or hepatic impairment. The risk of nephrotoxicity is not great when neomycin is given by mouth in recommended doses, as neomycin is poorly absorbed.

When given by mouth neomycin in large doses causes nausea, vomiting, and diarrhoea. Prolonged oral therapy may cause a malabsorption syndrome with steatorrhoea and diarrhoea which can be very severe. Supra-infection may occur, especially with prolonged oral treatment.

Neomycin has a neuromuscular blocking action similar to but stronger than that of gentamicin and respiratory depression and arrest has followed the intraperitoneal instillation of neomycin.

Hypersensitivity reactions, usually of the delayed type, occur frequently during local treatment with neomycin but may be masked by the combined use of a corticosteroid. Cross-sensitivity with other aminoglycoside antibiotics may occur.

ALLERGY. Of 2175 subjects who were patch-tested with a preparation containing neomycin sulphate 20%, only 2 out of 22 who had reactions were judged to have clear-cut contact allergy. All the other reactions were described as being of a non-allergic irritant type.— J. J. Leyden and A. M. Kligman, *J. Am. med. Ass.*, 1979, *242*, 1276.

EFFECTS ON THE EAR. Profound deafness was diagnosed 11 months after birth in a preterm infant who had been treated neonatally, around the umbilical stump, with a topical antibiotic spray containing bacitracin, polymyxin, and neomycin. Gentamicin had also been given intravenously. Serum concentrations in a premature baby whose umbilical stump was treated with an antibiotic spray for 1 second on 6 occasions over the first 36 hours of life indicated significant aminoglycoside absorption.— P. Morrell *et al.* (letter), *Lancet*, 1985, *1*, 1167.

See also Gentamicin Sulphate, p.237.

EFFECTS ON THE GASTRO-INTESTINAL TRACT. Lactose malabsorption and reduction in disaccharidases in the small bowel was induced after 3 days' therapy with neomycin sulphate, 8 g daily. Histological study of the bowel mucosa suggested that neomycin had a direct toxic action.— G. D. Cain *et al.*, *Archs intern. Med.*, 1968, *122*, 311.

Clostridium difficile-associated colitis in a patient treated with neomycin responded to treatment with metronidazole.— R. P. Bolton, *Br. med. J.*, 1979, *2*, 1479.

Salmonella meningitis, attributed to *Salmonella oranienburg*, developed in a 17-year-old boy after the successful treatment of salmonella enteritis with neomycin by mouth. There was also evidence of concurrent pericarditis. It was suggested that neomycin-induced damage of the gastro-intestinal mucosa might have aided the invasion of *S. oranienburg* into the blood stream.— C. Hardy *et al.*, *Postgrad. med. J.*, 1984, *60*, 284.

EFFECTS ON THE NEUROMUSCULAR SYSTEM. For reference to the neuromuscular blocking effect of neomycin, see Gentamicin Sulphate, p.237.

OVERDOSAGE. A patient who was inadvertently given 6 g of neomycin by intramuscular injection for hepatic coma developed anuria but was managed successfully by haemodialysis.— F. A. Krumlovsky *et al.*, *Ann. intern. Med.*, 1972, *76*, 443.

A fatality preceded by deafness in a patient inadvertently given 8 g of neomycin intramuscularly instead of by mouth.— L. D. Lowry *et al.*, *Ann. Otol. Rhinol. Lar.*, 1973, *82*, 876.

Precautions

As for Gentamicin Sulphate, p.238.

Neomycin is contra-indicated for intestinal disinfection when an obstruction is present and in patients with a known history of allergy to neomycin. It should be used with great care in patients with kidney or liver disease and in those with impaired hearing. The topical use of neomycin in patients with extensive skin damage or perforated tympanic membranes may result in deafness. Neomycin sulphate should not be applied topically or for urological purposes in doses greater than 1 g daily; it should not be used urologically for longer than 10 days. The parenteral use of neomycin is no longer recommended.

Prolonged local use should be avoided as it may lead to skin sensitisation. Neomycin by mouth and possibly the parenteral administration of other aminoglycosides such as gentamicin, might cause immediate skin sensitivity reactions in patients previously sensitised by the topical use of neomycin.

Neomycin, taken by mouth, has been reported to impair the absorption of other drugs including phenoxymethylpenicillin, digoxin, methotrexate, and some vitamins; the efficacy of oral contraceptives might be reduced.

For reference to the antithyroid activity of neomycin, see Gentamicin Sulphate, p.238.

INTERACTIONS. For the effect of neomycin sulphate on warfarin, see Warfarin Sodium, p.345.

PREGNANCY AND THE NEONATE. Deafness in the infant of a mother given neomycin during pregnancy has been reported.— J. M. Forrest, *Med. J. Aust.*, 1976, *2*, 138.

Antimicrobial Action

Neomycin has a mode of action and spectrum of activity similar to that of gentamicin sulphate (p.239). It is not, however, active against *Pseudomonas aeruginosa*, and resistant strains of Gram-negative bacteria are more common than with gentamicin.

For reference to the activity of neomycin against *Yersinia* spp., see Gentamicin Sulphate, p.239.

Resistance

Frequent and long-term topical or oral use of neomycin has led to the emergence of resistant bacteria. There is almost complete cross-resistance between neomycin, kanamycin, paromomycin, and framycetin.

For the mechanisms of resistance of bacteria to aminoglycosides, see Gentamicin Sulphate, p.240.

In 11 of 14 patients who had taken neomycin for at least 3 months for hypercholesterolaemia, coliform bacteria from the gut were resistant to several antimicrobial agents and the resistance was transferable to *Escherichia coli*.— M. V. Valtonen *et al.*, *Br. med. J.*, 1977, *1*, 683.

Of 232 strains of enteropathogenic *Escherichia coli* 21 were resistant to neomycin at a concentration of 8 µg per mL.— R. J. Gross *et al.*, *Br. med. J.*, 1982, *285*, 472.

Of 2753 strains of *Shigella dysenteriae*, *Sh. flexneri*, and *Sh. boydii* examined at the Central Public Health Laboratory from 1979 to mid 1983 1.9% were resistant to neomycin at a concentration of 8 µg per mL.— R. J. Gross *et al.*, *Br. med. J.*, 1984, *288*, 784.

Absorption and Fate

Neomycin is poorly absorbed from the alimentary tract, about 97% of an orally administered dose being excreted unchanged in the faeces. Doses of 3 to 4 g by mouth produce peak plasma concentrations of up to 4 µg per mL and absorption is similar after administration by enema. It is, however, rapidly absorbed after intramuscular injection, a dose of 0.5 g producing a plasma concentration of about 20 µg per mL. Absorption has also been reported to occur from the peritoneum, respiratory tract, bladder, wounds, and inflamed skin.

Once neomycin is absorbed it is rapidly excreted by the kidneys in active form. It has been reported to have a half-life of 2 to 3 hours.

Uses and Administration

Neomycin sulphate is an aminoglycoside antibiotic administered topically in the treatment of infections of the skin and eye due to susceptible staphylococci and other organisms. Neomycin undecenoate or sulphate is used in ear-drops.

To prevent the development of resistant strains, another antibacterial agent such as bacitracin or polymyxin B is sometimes used in conjunction with neomycin.

A cream containing neomycin sulphate and chlorhexidine hydrochloride has been used for application to the nostrils in the treatment of staphylococcal nasal carriers but resistant organisms have developed.

Because neomycin sulphate is poorly absorbed from the gastro-intestinal tract, it has been given by mouth for the suppression of bacterial growth in the intestine before abdominal surgery although the development of resistant organisms may be encouraged and supra-infection may occur; in the *USA* it is administered with erythromycin prior to colonic surgery. It is also used similarly, with other antibacterial agents, to prevent infection in neutropenic patients. Neomycin is given to patients with hepatic encephalopathy (hepatic coma) to suppress ammonia-forming bacteria in the gastro-intestinal tract. It is no longer recommended for use in the treatment of gastro-intestinal infections.

For pre-operative use, 1 g of neomycin sulphate has been given hourly for 4 hours and then every 4 hours for up to 3 days; children over 12 years of age may be given 1 g of neomycin sulphate every 4 hours for no longer than 3 days.

As an adjunct in the management of hepatic encephalopathy, 4 to 12 g may be given daily in divided doses; prolonged administration may cause malabsorption.

For general reviews of aminoglycoside antibiotics, see Gentamicin Sulphate, p.242.

Successful use of neomycin in the treatment of D-lactic acidosis developing after jejuno-ileal bypass.— M. Traube *et al.*, *Ann. intern. Med.*, 1983, *98*, 171.

CONTROL OF EPIDEMIC MRSA. For the use of a cream containing neomycin and chlorhexidine in the eradication of nasal carriage of epidemic methicillin-resistant *Staphylococcus aureus* (MRSA), see Mupirocin, p.265.

EYE DISORDERS. A report of the successful topical treatment of acanthamoeba keratitis with dibromopropamidine and propamidine isethionates, and neomycin.— P. Wright *et al.*, *Br. J. Ophthal.*, 1985, *69*, 778.

For reference to the use of neomycin eye ointment in the treatment of neonatal conjunctivitis, see under Pregnancy and the Neonate, below.

HEPATIC ENCEPHALOPATHY. Neomycin is used in the treatment of hepatic encephalopathy. It appears to reduce the concentration of urease-containing bacteria in the intestinal flora thereby decreasing the production of ammonia from proteins and amino acids. It may be given by mouth or by enema. About 1 to 3% of the dose is absorbed when administered by these routes, and although this may give rise to ototoxicity and nephrotoxicity, both are rare. Treatment failures have occurred with neomycin and may be due to neomycin-resistant strains of *Klebsiella* or *Proteus*. Alternative antibiotics to neomycin include ampicillin, kanamycin, tetracycline, or sulphonamides (C.L. Fraser and A.I. Arieff, *New Engl. J. Med.*, 1985, *313*, 865). In theory, neomycin may suppress the activity of the bacteria necessary for the hydrolysis of lactulose, but studies have indicated that when administered together these agents may result in a greater decrease in intestinal ammonia production and in blood-ammonia concentrations than when given alone. This suggests that the effects of each drug are mediated by different bacterial populations. No studies to date, however, have demonstrated an enhanced clinical efficacy of the combination in the treatment of hepatic encephalopathy (I.R. Crossley and R. Williams, *Gut*, 1984, *25*, 85).

HYPERCHOLESTEROLAEMIA. A review of drugs used in the treatment of hyperlipoproteinaemia. Neomycin should be regarded as a second-line agent for use in patients with primary hypercholesterolaemia who are unable to take bile acid sequestrants such as colestipol and cholestyramine. The hypocholesterolaemic effect of neomycin appears to be mediated by a reduction in the absorption of exogenous and endogenous cholesterol from the gastro-intestinal tract, mainly due to its action on the intestinal flora. Neomycin has been reported to reduce plasma-low-density lipoprotein cholesterol concentrations by 15 to 20% in patients with hypercholesterolaemia but to have no effect on the concentrations of high-density-lipoproteins or triglyceride; its cholesterol-lowering effect can be potentiated by bile acid sequestrants or nicotinic acid. The clinical use of neomycin in the treatment of hypercholesterolaemia was, however, considered to be limited by its adverse effects. It should not be used in patients with impaired renal function or in those with gastro-intestinal disorders in which the absorption of neomycin may be increased. Patients maintained on neomycin should have periodic hearing tests and assessments of renal function, even though the frequency of changes in these parameters appears to be low. The usual dose of neomycin for the treatment of hypercholesterolaemia is 1 g twice daily by mouth.— D. R. Illingworth, *Drugs*, 1987, *33*, 259.

For a discussion of the adverse effects of neomycin when given by mouth for the treatment of hypercholesterolaemia, see L. C. Knodel and R. L. Talbert, *Med. Toxicol.*, 1987, *2*, 10.

PREGNANCY AND THE NEONATE. Both neomycin (0.5%) and chloramphenicol (0.5%) eye ointments are widely used in the treatment of neonatal conjunctivitis and are effective in most acute bacterial infections. Neomycin has the disadvantage of being inactive against streptococci, and chloramphenicol may suppress but not eradicate infections caused by *Chlamydia* spp. Failure to respond clinically to treatment with neomycin or chloramphenicol within 48 hours should suggest the need for chlamydia investigation.— *Lancet*, 1984, *2*, 1375. In 152 babies from whom pathogens were isolated from eye swabs, gonococcal infection was much less frequent than conjunctivitis due to other acquired pyogenic bacteria, notably *Staphylococcus aureus*, lactose-fermenting coliforms, and *Haemophilus* spp. Topical neomycin would rapidly cure most of these non-gonococcal infections.— H. Mallinson *et al.* (letter), *ibid.*, 1985, *1*, 380.

REYE'S SYNDROME. Lactulose and neomycin given by nasogastric tube had been used in the treatment of Reye's syndrome to reduce the production of toxic nitrogenous metabolites in the colon, however, this use needed to be evaluated.— J. F. T. Glasgow, *Archs Dis. Childh.*, 1984, *59*, 230.

SKIN DISORDERS. A review of the use of topical antibiotics and antiseptics for the treatment of infections of the skin. Neomycin is the treatment of choice for impetigo, especially in children. Contact sensitisation is unlikely when it is applied for only a week or two. However, bacterial resistance to neomycin and framycetin spreads easily, particularly among hospital inpatients. Combinations of a corticosteroid with an antibiotic or antiseptic have been advocated for secondarily infected eczema; most studies of such combinations containing neomycin have suggested the combination to be clinically and microbiologically more effective than the steroid alone. Oral flucloxacillin should be given to patients with impetigo or infected eczema who are systemically ill. Leg ulcers should not in general be treated with topical antibiotics; they do not reduce the bacterial population but encourage colonisation by more resistant organisms and are liable to sensitise the patient.— *Drug & Ther. Bull.*, 1987, *25*, 97.

References to the use of neomycin in various skin disorders: R. S. Dillon (letter), *New Engl. J. Med.*, 1984, *311*, 540 (foot infections; use of a neomycin sulphate 0.5% soak in saline); *Lancet*, 1985, *2*, 81 (recurrent furunculosis; use of a cream containing neomycin sulphate and chlorhexidine to eliminate nasal carriage of *Staphylococcus aureus*); *ibid* (tinea pedis).

For reference to the treatment of acne including the use of topical antibiotics such as neomycin, see Tetracycline Hydrochloride, p.321.

SUPPRESSION OF INTESTINAL FLORA. For reference to regimens used to prevent colonisation and infection by the selective decontamination of the gastro-intestinal tract, see Colistin Sulphomethate Sodium, p.205.

The effects of neomycin in several other disorders have been attributed to its action on the intestinal flora. See under: Hepatic Encephalopathy, Hypercholesterolaemia, and Reye's Syndrome (above), and Surgical Infection Prophylaxis (below).

SURGICAL INFECTION PROPHYLAXIS. For reference to the use of neomycin and erythromycin by mouth for infection prophylaxis during colonic surgery, see Erythromycin, p.227.

References to the use of a topical spray containing neomycin, bacitracin, and polymyxin B for the prophylaxis of wound infections: S. J. Hildred and C. J. Henderson, *Br. med. J.*, 1977, *2*, 869; V. C. Wright *et al.*, *Can. med. Ass. J.*, 1978, *118*, 1395. See also Effects on the Ear under Adverse Effects, above.

Preparations

Aerosols

Neomycin and Polymyxin B Sulfates and Bacitracin Zinc Topical Aerosol *(U.S.P.)*

Creams

Neomycin Cream *(B.P.C. 1973).* Neomycin sulphate 500 mg, chlorocresol 100 mg, disodium edetate 10 mg, cetomacrogol emulsifying ointment 30 g, and freshly boiled and cooled water 69.39 g. A phosphate buffer may be included.

Neomycin Sulfate Cream *(U.S.P.)*

Hydrocortisone and Neomycin Cream *(B.P.)*. Contains neomycin sulphate and hydrocortisone.

Neomycin Sulfate and Dexamethasone Sodium Phosphate Cream *(U.S.P.)*

Neomycin Sulfate and Fluocinolone Acetonide Cream *(U.S.P.)*

Neomycin Sulfate and Flurandrenolide Cream *(U.S.P.)*. Contains neomycin sulphate and flurandrenolone.

Neomycin Sulfate and Hydrocortisone Cream *(U.S.P.)*

Neomycin Sulfate and Hydrocortisone Acetate Cream *(U.S.P.)*

Neomycin Sulfate and Methylprednisolone Acetate Cream *(U.S.P.)*

Neomycin and Polymyxin B Sulfates Cream *(U.S.P.)*

Neomycin and Polymyxin B Sulfates and Gramicidin Cream *(U.S.P.)*

Neomycin and Polymyxin B Sulfates, Gramicidin, and Hydrocortisone Acetate Cream *(U.S.P.)*

Neomycin and Polymyxin B Sulfates and Hydrocortisone Acetate Cream *(U.S.P.)*

Neomycin Sulfate and Triamcinolone Acetonide Cream *(U.S.P.)*

Ear-drops

Bacitracin, Neomycin and Polymyxin Ear Drops *(A.P.F.)*. Contain neomycin sulphate, bacitracin, and polymyxin B sulphate. These ear-drops should be freshly prepared, stored at a temperature not exceeding 8°, and used within 1 week.

Hydrocortisone and Neomycin Ear Drops *(B.P.)*. A suspension of hydrocortisone acetate in a solution of neomycin sulphate. pH 6.5 to 8.0.

Neomycin Sulfate and Hydrocortisone Otic Suspension *(U.S.P.)*. When no strength is specified a suspension containing in each mL the equivalent of 3.5 mg of neomycin and the equivalent of 10 mg of hydrocortisone is supplied. pH 4.5 to 6.0.

Neomycin and Polymyxin B Sulfates and Hydrocortisone Otic Solution *(U.S.P.)*. When no strength is specified a solution containing in each mL the equivalent of 3.5 mg of neomycin, the equivalent of 10 000 units of polymyxin B, and hydrocortisone 10 mg is supplied. pH 2.0 to 4.5.

Neomycin and Polymyxin B Sulfates and Hydrocortisone Otic Suspension *(U.S.P.)*. When no strength is specified a suspension containing in each mL the equivalent of 3.5 mg of neomycin, the equivalent of 10 000 units of polymyxin B, and hydrocortisone 10 mg is supplied. pH 3.0 to 5.5.

Eye-drops

Neomycin Eye Drops *(B.P.)*. Neomycin Sulphate Eye Drops; NEO

Neomycin Eye Drops *(A.P.F.)*. Contain neomycin sulphate 0.5%. Sterilised by maintaining at 98° to 100° for 30 minutes. Store at a temperature below 25°.

Bacitracin, Neomycin and Polymyxin Eye Drops *(A.P.F.)*. Contain neomycin sulphate, bacitracin, and polymyxin B sulphate. Prepared aseptically or sterilised by filtration. These eye-drops should be freshly prepared, stored below 8°, and used within 1 week.

Hydrocortisone and Neomycin Eye Drops *(B.P.)*. A sterile suspension of hydrocortisone acetate in a solution of neomycin sulphate.

Neomycin Sulfate and Dexamethasone Sodium Phosphate Ophthalmic Solution *(U.S.P.)*. When no strength is specified a solution containing in each mL the equivalent of 3.5 mg of neomycin and the equivalent of 1 mg of dexamethasone phosphate is supplied. pH 6 to 8.

Neomycin Sulfate and Hydrocortisone Acetate Ophthalmic Suspension *(U.S.P.)*. pH 5.5 to 7.5.

Neomycin and Polymyxin B Sulfates Ophthalmic Solution *(U.S.P.)*. pH 5 to 7.

Neomycin and Polymyxin B Sulfates and Dexamethasone Ophthalmic Suspension *(U.S.P.)*. pH 3.5 to 6.0.

Neomycin and Polymyxin B Sulfates and Gramicidin Ophthalmic Solution *(U.S.P.)*. pH 4.7 to 6.0.

Neomycin and Polymyxin B Sulfates and Hydrocortisone Ophthalmic Suspension *(U.S.P.)*. pH 4.1 to 7.0.

Neomycin and Polymyxin B Sulfates and Hydrocortisone Acetate Ophthalmic Suspension *(U.S.P.)*. pH 5 to 7.

Neomycin and Polymyxin B Sulfates and Prednisolone Acetate Ophthalmic Suspension *(U.S.P.)*. pH 5 to 7.

Neomycin Sulfate and Prednisolone Acetate Ophthalmic Suspension *(U.S.P.)*. pH 5.5 to 7.5.

Eye Ointments

Neomycin Eye Ointment *(B.P.)*. Neomycin Sulphate Eye Ointment

Neomycin Sulfate Ophthalmic Ointment *(U.S.P.)*

Hydrocortisone and Neomycin Eye Ointment *(B.P.)*. Contains neomycin sulphate and hydrocortisone acetate.

Neomycin Sulfate and Dexamethasone Sodium Phosphate Ophthalmic Ointment *(U.S.P.)*. When no strength is specified an ointment containing in each g the equivalent of 3.5 mg of neomycin and the equivalent of 500 µg of dexamethasone phosphate is supplied.

Neomycin Sulfate and Hydrocortisone Acetate Ophthalmic Ointment *(U.S.P.)*

Neomycin and Polymyxin B Sulfates Ophthalmic Ointment *(U.S.P.)*

Neomycin and Polymyxin B Sulfates and Bacitracin Ophthalmic Ointment *(U.S.P.)*

Neomycin and Polymyxin B Sulfates and Bacitracin Zinc Ophthalmic Ointment *(U.S.P.)*

Neomycin and Polymyxin B Sulfates, Bacitracin, and Hydrocortisone Acetate Ophthalmic Ointment *(U.S.P.)*

Neomycin and Polymyxin B Sulfates, Bacitracin Zinc, and Hydrocortisone Ophthalmic Ointment *(U.S.P.)*

Neomycin and Polymyxin B Sulfates, Bacitracin Zinc, and Hydrocortisone Acetate Ophthalmic Ointment *(U.S.P.)*

Neomycin and Polymyxin B Sulfates and Dexamethasone Ophthalmic Ointment *(U.S.P.)*

Neomycin Sulfate and Prednisolone Acetate Ophthalmic Ointment *(U.S.P.)*

Neomycin Sulfate and Prednisolone Sodium Phosphate Ophthalmic Ointment *(U.S.P.)*. When no strength is specified an ointment containing in each g the equivalent of 3.5 mg of neomycin and the equivalent of 2.5 mg of prednisolone phosphate is supplied.

Neomycin Sulfate, Sulfacetamide Sodium, and Prednisolone Acetate Ophthalmic Ointment *(U.S.P.)*

Neomycin Sulfate and Triamcinolone Acetonide Ophthalmic Ointment *(U.S.P.)*

Injections

Sterile Neomycin Sulfate *(U.S.P.)*

Insufflations

Bacitracin, Neomycin and Polymyxin Insufflation *(A.P.F.)*. Contains neomycin sulphate, bacitracin zinc, and polymyxin B sulphate. Prepared aseptically. Store below 25°.

Irrigations

Neomycin and Polymyxin B Sulfates Solution for Irrigation *(U.S.P.)*. pH 4.5 to 6.0. For use, after dilution, for bladder irrigation.

Lotions

Neomycin Sulfate and Flurandrenolide Lotion *(U.S.P.)*. Contains neomycin sulphate and flurandrenolone.

Neomycin Sulfate and Hydrocortisone Acetate Lotion *(U.S.P.)*

Ointments

Neomycin Sulfate Ointment *(U.S.P.)*

Hydrocortisone Acetate and Neomycin Ointment *(B.P.)*. Contains neomycin sulphate and hydrocortisone acetate.

Neomycin and Bacitracin Ointment *(B.P.C. 1973)*. Neomycin sulphate 500 mg, bacitracin zinc 50 000 units, liquid paraffin 10 g, white soft paraffin to 100 g. The ointment may be expected to retain its potency for 2 years provided that the moisture content does not exceed 0.2%.

Neomycin Sulfate and Bacitracin Ointment *(U.S.P.)*

Neomycin Sulfate and Bacitracin Zinc Ointment *(U.S.P.)*

Neomycin Sulfate and Fluorometholone Ointment *(U.S.P.)*

Neomycin Sulfate and Flurandrenolide Ointment *(U.S.P.)*. Contains neomycin sulphate and flurandrenolone.

Neomycin Sulfate and Gramicidin Ointment *(U.S.P.)*

Neomycin Sulfate and Hydrocortisone Ointment *(U.S.P.)*

Neomycin Sulfate and Hydrocortisone Acetate Ointment *(U.S.P.)*

Neomycin and Polymyxin B Sulfates and Bacitracin Ointment *(U.S.P.)*

Neomycin and Polymyxin B Sulfates and Bacitracin Zinc Ointment *(U.S.P.)*

Neomycin and Polymyxin B Sulfates, Bacitracin, and Hydrocortisone Acetate Ointment *(U.S.P.)*

Neomycin and Polymyxin B Sulfates, Bacitracin Zinc, and Hydrocortisone Ointment *(U.S.P.)*

Neomycin and Polymyxin B Sulfates, Bacitracin Zinc, and Lidocaine Ointment *(U.S.P.)*. Contains neomycin sulphate, polymyxin B sulphate, bacitracin zinc, and lignocaine.

Neomycin Sulfate and Prednisolone Acetate Ointment *(U.S.P.)*

Oral Solutions

Neomycin Oral Solution *(B.P.)*. Neomycin Mixture; Neomycin Sulphate Elixir. pH of 4 to 5. Store at a temperature not exceeding 15°.

Neomycin Sulfate Oral Solution *(U.S.P.)*. pH 5.0 to 7.5.

Powders

Neomycin and Polymyxin B Sulfates and Bacitracin Zinc Topical Powder *(U.S.P.)*

Tablets

Neomycin Tablets *(B.P.)*. Contain neomycin sulphate.

Neomycin Sulfate Tablets *(U.S.P.)*

Proprietary Preparations

NOTE. Proprietary preparations containing a corticosteroid and neomycin sulphate which are used mainly for their anti-inflammatory effects are described in the section on Corticosteroids, p.872.

Audicort *(Lederle, UK)*. *Ear drops*, neomycin undecenoate equivalent to neomycin 3.5 mg and undecenoic acid 7 mg, triamcinolone acetonide 1 mg, benzocaine 50 mg.

Cicatrin *(Calmic, UK)*. *Cream*, neomycin sulphate 3300 units, bacitracin zinc 250 units, glycine 10 mg, L-cysteine 2 mg, DL-threonine 1 mg/g.
Topical powder, ingredients as for cream.
Topical powder spray, aerosol, neomycin sulphate 16 500 units, bacitracin zinc 1250 units, glycine 60 mg, L-cysteine 12 mg/g.

Graneodin *(Squibb, UK)*. *Ointment*, neomycin 0.25% (as sulphate), gramicidin 0.025%.
Eye ointment, ingredients as for ointment.

Gregoderm *(Unigreg, UK)*. *Ointment*, neomycin sulphate 4 mg, polymyxin B sulphate 7250 units, hydrocortisone 10 mg, nystatin 100 000 units/g.

Maxitrol *(Alcon, UK)*. *Eye-drops*, neomycin 3.5 mg (as sulphate)/mL, polymyxin B sulphate 6000 units/mL, dexamethasone 0.1%, in a vehicle containing hypromellose 0.5%.
Eye ointment, neomycin 3.5 mg (as sulphate)/g, polymyxin B sulphate 6000 units/g, dexamethasone 0.1%.

Minims Neomycin Sulphate *(Smith & Nephew Pharmaceuticals, UK)*. *Eye-drops*, neomycin sulphate 0.5%, in single-dose disposable applicators.

Mycifradin *(Upjohn, UK)*. *Powder*, neomycin sulphate 500 mg. For the preparation of irrigations and topical solutions.

Myciguent *(Upjohn, UK)*. *Ointment*, neomycin sulphate 0.5%.
Eye ointment, neomycin sulphate 0.5%.

Neo-Cortef *(Upjohn, UK)*. *Drops*, for eye or ear, neomycin sulphate 0.5%, hydrocortisone acetate 1.5%.
Ointment, for eye or ear, neomycin sulphate 0.5%, hydrocortisone acetate 1.5%.

Neosporin *(Calmic, UK)*. *Eye-drops*, neomycin sulphate 1700 units, gramicidin 25 units, polymyxin B sulphate 5000 units/mL.

Nivemycin *(Boots, UK)*. *Tablets*, neomycin sulphate 350 000 units (approximately equivalent to 500 mg).
Elixir, neomycin sulphate 62 500 units (approximately equivalent to 100 mg)/5mL.

Otosporin *(Calmic, UK)*. *Ear drops*, neomycin sulphate 3400 units, polymyxin B sulphate 10 000 units, hydrocortisone 10 mg/mL.

Polybactrin *(Calmic, UK)*. *Bladder irrigation* (Soluble GU), powder for reconstitution, neomycin sulphate 20 000 units, bacitracin 1000 units, polymyxin B sulphate 75 000 units.
Topical powder spray, aerosol, neomycin sulphate 495 000 units, bacitracin zinc 37 500 units, polymyxin B sulphate 150 000 units/115 mL.

Tribiotic *(Riker, UK)*. *Topical spray*, aerosol, neomycin sulphate 500 000 units, bacitracin zinc 10 000 units, polymyxin B sulphate 150 000 units/110 g.

Proprietary Names and Manufacturers of Neomycin Salts

Biofradin *(Spain)*; Burn-Gel *(Organon, Spain)*; Bykomycin *(Byk Gulden, Ger.)*; Dermonalef *(Spain)*; Emelmycin *(S.Afr.)*; Endomixin *(Lusofarmaco, Ital.)*; Filmaseptic *(Switz.)*; Fradyl *(Belg.)*; Herisan Antibiotic *(Canad.)*; Larmicin *(Spain)*; Minims Neomycin *(Smith & Nephew, Austral.)*; Minims Neomycin Sulphate *(Smith & Nephew, S.Afr.; Smith & Nephew Pharmaceuticals, UK)*; Myacyne *(Schur, Ger.)*; Mycifradin *(Upjohn, Austral.; Upjohn, Canad.; Upjohn, S.Afr.; Upjohn, UK; Upjohn, USA)*; Myciguent *(Upjohn, Austral.; Upjohn, Canad.; Upjohn, S.Afr.; Upjohn, UK; Upjohn, USA)*; Néomycine Médial *(Syntex, Switz.)*; Neobiotic *(Pfipharmecs, USA)*; Neocin *(Canad.)*; Neo-Gelicil *(S.Afr.)*; Neointestin *(Hosbon, Spain)*; Neomas Bowers *(Arg.)*; Neomate *(Austral.)*; Neomin *(Glaxo, UK)*; Neopan *(S.Afr.)*; Neopt *(Sigma, Austral.)*; Neosulf *(Protea, Austral.)*; Nivemycin *(Boots, UK)*; Otobiotic *(Schering,*

USA); Quintress-N *(Austral.)*; Siguent Neomycin *(Sigma, Austral.)*; Tampovagan N *(Norgine, Austral.; S.Afr.; Norgine, UK)*.

The following names have been used for multi-ingredient preparations containing neomycin salts— Adcortyl with Graneodin *(Squibb, UK)*; Aerocortin *(Wellcome, Austral.)*; Ak-Spore Ophthalmic Ointment *(Akorn, USA)*; Ak-Spore Ophthalmic Solution *(Akorn, USA)*; Ak-Trol *(Akorn, USA)*; Aminoderm *(Desbergers, Canad.)*; Audicort *(Lederle, UK)*; Bacticort *(Rugby, USA)*; BaySporin *(Bay, USA)*; Betnesol-N *(Glaxo, UK)*; Betnovate-N *(Glaxo, Austral.; Glaxo, Canad.; Glaxo, UK)*; Biomydrin *(Warner, UK)*; Biotren *(Carlton Laboratories, UK)*; Carmycin *(Carlton Laboratories, UK)*; Cicatrene; Cicatrex; Cicatrin *(Wellcome, Austral.; Wellcome, Canad.; Calmic, UK)*; Cicatrinsone GA Dental Paste *(Biorex, UK)*; Coly-Mycin Otic *(Warner, Austral.; Parke, Davis, Canad.)*; Coly-Mycin S Otic *(Parke, Davis, USA)*; Cordran-N *(Dista, USA)*; Cortisporin Cream *(Wellcome, Canad.; Wellcome, USA)*; Cortisporin Ointment *(Wellcome, Canad.; Wellcome, USA)*; Decaspray *(Merck Sharp & Dohme, UK)*; Dermamed Ointment *(Medo, UK)*; Dermovate-NN *(Glaxo, UK)*; Dexacidin *(Coopervision, USA)*; Dexa-Rhinaspray *(Boehringer Ingelheim, UK)*; Dexasporin *(Pharmafair, USA)*; Di-Hydrotic *(Legere, USA)*; Dispray Antibiotic Powder Spray *(Stuart, UK)*; Donnagel with Neomycin *(Robins, Canad.; Robins, UK)*; Drotic *(Ascher, USA)*; Duobac *(Stuart, UK)*; Eumovate-N *(Glaxo, UK)*; FML-Neo *(Allergan, Canad.; Allergan, UK)*; Framyspray *(Fisons, UK)*; Graneodin *(Squibb, Austral.; Squibb, UK)*; Gregoderm *(Unigreg, UK)*;
Halcicomb *(Squibb, Canad.; FAIR Laboratories, UK)*; Hydroderm *(Merck Sharp & Dohme, UK)*; Hydromycin-D *(Boots, UK)*; Ivax *(Boots, UK)*; Kaomycin *(Upjohn, Austral.; Upjohn, Canad.; Upjohn, UK)*; Kenacomb *(Squibb, Austral.; Squibb, Canad.)*; Kenalog-S *(USA)*; LazerSporin-C *(Pedinol, USA)*; Lidecomb *(Syncare, Canad.)*; Lomotil with Neomycin *(Searle, UK)*; Maxitrol *(Alcon, Canad.; Alcon, UK; Alcon Laboratories, USA)*; Mycitracin *(Upjohn, Austral.)*; Mycolog *(Squibb, USA)*; Myco-Triacet *(Lemmon, USA)*; Mytrex *(Savage, USA)*; Naseptin *(ICI, Austral.; ICI Pharmaceuticals, UK)*; Nemdyn *(Hamilton, Austral.)*; Neo Hycor *(Sigma, Austral.)*; Neobacrin *(Glaxo, UK)*; Neo-Cortef *(Upjohn, Austral.; Upjohn, Canad.; Upjohn, UK)*; NeoDecadron *(Merck Sharp & Dohme, Canad.)*; Neodecadron *(Merck Sharp & Dohme, USA)*; Neo-Medrol *(Upjohn, Austral.; Upjohn, Canad.)*; Neo-Medrone Acne Lotion *(Upjohn, UK)*; Neo-Medrone Cream *(Upjohn, UK)*; Neo-Polycin *(Merrell Dow, USA)*; Neosporin Aerosol *(Wellcome, Canad.)*; Neosporin Cream *(Wellcome, Canad.; Wellcome, USA)*; Neosporin Irrigation Solution *(Wellcome, Canad.; Wellcome, USA)*; Neosporin Ointment *(Wellcome, Austral.; Wellcome, Canad.; Wellcome, USA)*; Neosporin Ophthalmic Ointment *(Wellcome, Austral.; Wellcome, Canad.; Wellcome, USA)*; Neosporin Ophthalmic Solution *(Wellcome, Austral.; Wellcome, Canad.; Calmic, UK; Wellcome, USA)*; Neosporin Powder *(Wellcome, Canad.)*; Neosporin-G *(Wellcome, USA)*; Neo-Synalar *(Syntex, USA)*; Neotracin *(Cilag, Austral.)*; Neotulle *(Fisons, UK)*; Neovax *(Norton, UK)*; Nyst-olone *(Schein, USA)*;
Octicair *(Pharmafair, USA)*; Ocu-Cort *(Ocumed, USA)*; Ocu-Spor-B *(Ocumed, USA)*; Ocu-Spor-G *(Ocumed, USA)*; Ocutricin HC Ointment *(Pharmafair, USA)*; Ocutricin Ointment *(Pharmafair, USA)*; Ocutricin Solution *(Pharmafair, USA)*; Ocu-Trol *(Ocumed, USA)*; Otizol-HC *(Nadeau, Canad.)*; Otocort *(Lemmon, USA)*; Otoseptil *(Napp, UK)*; Otosporin *(Calmic, UK)*; Pimafucort *(Astra, Austral.)*; Plegettes *(Hamilton, Austral.)*; Polybactrin *(Wellcome, Austral.; Calmic, UK)*; Polynorm Ointment *(Norma, UK)*; Poly-Pred *(Allergan, USA)*; Predsol-N *(Glaxo, UK)*; Proctosone *(Technilab, Canad.)*; Propaderm-N *(Allen & Hanburys, UK)*; Retrografin *(Squibb, Canad.)*; Rikospray Antibiotic *(Riker, UK)*; Silderm *(Lederle, UK)*; Spectrocin *(Squibb, Canad.)*; Spersin *(Sigma, Austral.)*; Stiedex LPN *(Stiefel, UK)*; Synalar Biotic *(Syncare, Canad.)*; Synalar-N *(ICI Pharmaceuticals, UK)*; Topisporin *(Pharmafair, USA)*; Tri-Adcortyl *(Squibb, UK)*; Tribactric Dusting Powder *(Stuart, UK)*; Tribiotic *(Riker, UK)*; Trisep *(Stuart, UK)*; Tri-Thalmic *(Schein, USA)*; Unidiarea *(Unigreg, UK)*; Uniroid *(Unigreg, UK)*; Viaderm-KC *(Taro, Canad.)*; Vibrocil *(Zyma, UK)*; Vista-Methasone N *(Richard Daniel, UK)*.

114-n

Netilmicin Sulphate *(BANM, rINNM)*.

N-Ethyl Sissomicin; Netilmicin Sulfate *(USAN)*; Sch-20569. 4-*O*-[(2*S*,3*S*)-3-Amino-6-aminomethyl-3,4-dihydro-2*H*-pyran-2-yl]-2-deoxy-6-*O*-[3-deoxy-4-*C*-methyl-3-methylamino-β-L-arabinopyranosyl]-1-*N*-ethyl-D-streptamine sulphate. $(C_{21}H_{41}N_5O_7)_2,5H_2SO_4=1441.6$.

CAS — 56391-56-1 (netilmicin); 56391-57-2 (sulphate).

Pharmacopoeias. In *U.S.*

A semi-synthetic derivative of sissomicin. It has a potency equivalent to not less than 595 μg of netilmicin per mg, calculated with reference to the dried substance. 1.5 g of monograph substance is approximately equivalent to 1 g of netilmicin. A 4% solution in water has a pH between 3.5 and 5.5. The *U.S.P.* injection has a pH of 3.5 to 6.0. **Store** in airtight containers.

Incompatibility or loss of activity has been reported between netilmicin sulphate and many cephalosporins or penicillins (see Gentamicin Sulphate, p.236), and also with frusemide (D.F. Thompson *et al., Am. J. Hosp. Pharm.*, 1985, *42*, 116).

Studies of the stability of netilmicin sulphate in a range of commonly used intravenous fluids, and of its compatibility with a range of other drugs.— I. A. Chaudry *et al., Am. J. Hosp. Pharm.*, 1981, *38*, 1737.

Adverse Effects, Treatment, and Precautions

See Gentamicin Sulphate, p.236.

Peak plasma concentrations of netilmicin greater than 16 μg per mL, and trough concentrations greater than 4 μg per mL should be avoided.

A survey of the efficacy and toxicity of netilmicin in adult and paediatric patients involved in over 150 clinical studies. Netilmicin was administered either intravenously or intramuscularly in doses ranging from 3 to 8 mg per kg body-weight daily. Of 3376 patients assessed for the safety of netilmicin, nephrotoxicity was probably associated with administration of the drug in 57 (1.7%). In general, these declines in renal function were mild and transient. Definitive decreases in auditory acuity probably associated with netilmicin were observed in 22 (1.6%) of patients. The audiometric abnormalities usually occurred in the higher frequencies and were not generally associated with subjective hearing losses. Abnormalities of vestibular function, including vertigo, dizziness, or nystagmus were probably related to netilmicin administration in 12 (0.36%) of patients. Other adverse effects which were reported included transient elevations in liver enzymes, itching, rash, nausea, vomiting, and headache.— A. Z. Lane, *J. antimicrob. Chemother.*, 1984, *13, Suppl.* A, 67.

For reference to the antithyroid activity of netilmicin, see Gentamicin Sulphate, p.238.

EFFECTS ON THE EAR. For reference to studies indicating that netilmicin may be less ototoxic than gentamicin, see Gentamicin Sulphate, p.237.

EFFECTS ON THE KIDNEY. For reference to studies suggesting that the nephrotoxic potential of netilmicin may be less than that of gentamicin, see Gentamicin Sulphate, p.237.

Antimicrobial Action and Resistance

Netilmicin has an antimicrobial action and spectrum of activity similar to that of gentamicin (see p.239), although it is reported to be slightly less active against *Pseudomonas aeruginosa*. Netilmicin appears to be resistant to some of the bacterial enzymes which inactivate gentamicin and it is active against some gentamicin-resistant isolates. It is considered to be active against fewer gentamicin-resistant Gram-negative organisms than amikacin, but because of different enzyme susceptibilities netilmicin may be effective where amikacin is not.

For the mechanisms of resistance of bacteria to aminoglycosides, see Gentamicin Sulphate, p.240.

For reference to a comparative study of the antimicrobial activity of 11 aminoglycosides including netilmicin, and for studies of the activity of netilmicin against *Citrobacter* and *Yersinia* spp. and coagulase-negative staphylococci, see under Antimicrobial Action and Uses, Peritonitis, in Gentamicin Sulphate, p.239 and p.244.

Further references to the antimicrobial activity of netilmicin: E. Yourassowsky *et al., Curr. ther. Res.*, 1987, *41*, 823 (comparison of bactericidal activity with piperacillin).

ACTIVITY WITH OTHER ANTIMICROBIAL AGENTS. For reference to the effect of other agents on the *in-vitro* antimicrobial activity of aminoglycosides, see Gentamicin Sulphate, p.239.

References to studies of the antibacterial activity of netilmicin in association with other antimicrobial agents: J. Blaser *et al., Antimicrob. Ag. Chemother.*, 1985, *28*, 64 (with ceftazidime); J. J. Rahal and M. S. Simberkoff, *J. antimicrob. Chemother.*, 1986, *17*, 585 (with penicillins); D. C. Shanson *et al., ibid.*, *18*, 479 (with penicillins).

RESISTANCE. A report of *Serratia marcescens* resistant to netilmicin in a special-care baby unit where netilmicin had been used as a 'blind' treatment.— D. A. Lewis *et al., Br. med. J.*, 1983, *287*, 1701.

Absorption and Fate

The absorption and fate of netilmicin is similar to that of gentamicin (see p.241).

The half-life of netilmicin is usually 2.0 to 2.5 hours. About 80% of a dose is excreted in the urine within 24 hours.

In a comparative study 13 healthy subjects were given netilmicin or gentamicin 1 mg per kg body-weight intramuscularly and intravenously. After intramuscular injection, mean peak serum concentrations were 3.76 μg per mL for each antibiotic; there was less individual variation with netilmicin but the peak concentration was achieved more slowly. After intravenous administration over 3 to 5 minutes netilmicin disappeared from serum more rapidly than gentamicin, had a greater volume of distribution, less variability in elimination half-life, and less was recovered in the urine.— L. J. Riff and G. Moreschi, *Antimicrob. Ag. Chemother.*, 1977, *11*, 609. See also O. L. Laskin *et al., Clin. Pharmac. Ther.*, 1983, *34*, 644 (multidose pharmacokinetics).

A mean peak serum concentration of 16.56 μg per mL was achieved 3 minutes after the intravenous infusion of netilmicin 2 mg per kg body-weight over 30 minutes in 10 healthy subjects. Of the dose infused, 39% was excreted in the urine during the first 8 hours.— B. R. Meyers *et al., Antimicrob. Ag. Chemother.*, 1977, *12*, 122.

In 8 infants and children with cystic fibrosis and in 8 age-matched patients without cystic fibrosis the half-life was the only pharmacokinetic parameter of netilmicin to be significantly different between the 2 groups. The mean values were 1.4 and 2.3 hours respectively; this difference was not considered sufficient to warrant dosage modification in patients with cystic fibrosis.— H. Michalsen and T. Bergan, *Antimicrob. Ag. Chemother.*, 1981, *19*, 1029. A pharmacokinetic study in 10 patients with cystic fibrosis suggesting that higher doses may be required to achieve therapeutic peak serum concentrations of netilmicin.— J. A. Bosso *et al., ibid.*, 1985, *28*, 829.

The pharmacokinetics of netilmicin after once- or twice-daily administration by subcutaneous injection.— R. J. Courcol *et al.* (letter), *J. antimicrob. Chemother.*, 1986, *18*, 646.

A comparative study of the pharmacokinetics of netilmicin and tobramycin after single intravenous doses.— N. E. Winslade *et al., Antimicrob. Ag. Chemother.*, 1987, *31*, 605.

Further pharmacokinetic studies of netilmicin: D. J. Edwards *et al., Antimicrob. Ag. Chemother.*, 1981, *20*, 714; J. Blaser *et al., Eur. J. clin. Pharmac.*, 1983, *24*, 399.

DIFFUSION INTO BODY TISSUES AND FLUIDS. Studies of the penetration of netilmicin into body tissues and fluids: O. Brückner *et al., J. antimicrob. Chemother.*, 1983, *11*, 565 (cerebrospinal fluid); G. Tyden and A. S. Malmborg (letter), *Lancet*, 1985, *1*, 1046 (pancreatic juice).

PREGNANCY AND THE NEONATE. The pharmacokinetics of netilmicin were studied in 101 neonates. Mean peak serum concentrations which occurred 30 minutes after intramuscular administration were directly related to birth-weight and gestational age and ranged from 5.6 to 6.9 μg per mL after 3 mg per kg body-weight and from 7.8 to 8.4 μg per mL after 4 mg per kg. Six hours after administration mean serum concentrations had fallen to 2.3 to 3.5 μg per mL with the higher concentrations after the 4-mg per kg dose. Serum half-lives of netilmicin ranged from 3.4 to 4.7 hours. The pharmacokinetics of netilmicin were similar after intravenous and intramuscular administration. Average concentrations in urine after intramuscular administration of 3 and 4 mg per kg were 46 and 69 μg per mL respectively during the first 3 hours after administration and 29 and 103 μg per mL during the next 3 hours.— J. D. Siegel *et al.*, *Antimicrob. Ag. Chemother.*, 1979, *15*, 246.

See also under Administration in Infants and Children in Uses, below.

Uses and Administration

Netilmicin sulphate is a semisynthetic aminoglycoside antibiotic which has been used similarly to gentamicin (see p.242). It may be used as an alternative to amikacin sulphate, p.111, in the treatment of infections caused by susceptible bacteria which are resistant to gentamicin and tobramycin. As with gentamicin, netilmicin may be used with penicillins and with cephalosporins; the injections should be given separately.

Doses are expressed in terms of the equivalent amount of netilmicin. It may be given intramuscularly or intravenously in doses of 4 to 6 mg per kg body-weight daily in two or three divided doses in the treatment of Gram-negative infections; up to 7.5 mg per kg may be given daily in divided doses every 8 hours in severe infections. Children may be given 6.0 to 7.5 mg per kg body-weight daily in 3 divided doses. A dose of 2.5 to 3.0 mg per kg three times daily has been recommended for infants and neonates over one week of age and of 3 mg per kg twice daily for premature or full-term neonates one week old or less (but see also under Administration in Infants and Children, below).

When administered intravenously netilmicin may be injected slowly over 3 to 5 minutes or infused over 0.5 to 2 hours in 50 to 200 mL of infusion fluid, usually sodium chloride 0.9% or glucose 5% injection.

Treatment with netilmicin is usually given for 7 to 14 days. Peak plasma concentrations greater than 16 μg per mL and trough plasma concentrations greater than 4 μg per mL should be avoided. Dosage should be reduced in patients with renal impairment. In all patients, dosage should be adjusted according to plasma-netilmicin concentrations (see under Uses, Administration in Gentamicin Sulphate, p.242).

Reviews of the actions and uses of netilmicin: *Drug & Ther. Bull.*, 1982, *20*, 61; *Med. Lett.*, 1983, *25*, 65; D. R. P. Guay, *Drug Intell. & clin. Pharm.*, 1983, *17*, 83; P. Noone, *Drugs*, 1984, *27*, 548.

For the proceedings of a symposium on netilmicin, see *J. antimicrob. Chemother.*, 1984, *13*, *Suppl.* A, 1–83.

See also under Gentamicin Sulphate, p.242, for general reviews of the aminoglycoside antibiotics.

ADMINISTRATION. A study examining the *in-vitro* pharmacokinetics and bactericidal activity of netilmicin. The concept of administering high doses of aminoglycosides once daily was upheld.— J. Blaser *et al.*, *Antimicrob. Ag. Chemother.*, 1985, *27*, 343.

ADMINISTRATION IN INFANTS AND CHILDREN. In a study involving 80 neonates a dosage regimen for netilmicin of 3 mg per kg body-weight followed by 2 mg per kg every 12 hours given by intravenous injection over 3 minutes was considered suitable for preterm and term infants younger than one week. This generally produced plasma-netilmicin concentrations within the desired range (peak concentrations not exceeding 12 μg per mL; trough concentrations not exceeding 3 μg per mL). Although dosage regimens of 2.5 or 3.0 mg per kg every 12 hours were satisfactory for the term neonates, trough concentrations were too high in the preterm infants.— A. M. R. Phillips and R. D. G. Milner, *Archs Dis. Childh.*, 1983, *58*, 451.

CYSTIC FIBROSIS. Aminoglycosides, such as gentamicin, netilmicin, or tobramycin are administered parenterally in the treatment of *Pseudomonas aeruginosa* infections of the respiratory tract in patients with cystic fibrosis. They are commonly given in association with an antipseudomonal penicillin or cephalosporin. Gentamicin and tobramycin have also been administered by nebuliser. For discussion of treatment regimens in these patients, see Carbenicillin Sodium, p.141.

ENDOCARDITIS. For reference to the use of netilmicin sulphate in the treatment of infective endocarditis, see Gentamicin Sulphate, p.243.

GONORRHOEA. A single intramuscular injection of netilmicin 300 mg achieved a cure in all of 1200 patients with uncomplicated gonorrhoea (excluding pharyngeal infections).— J. Söltz-Szöts *et al.*, *Genitourinary Med.*, 1987, *63*, 95.

MEDITERRANEAN SPOTTED FEVER. The use of netilmicin in the treatment of mediterranean spotted fever.— G. Di Lascio and R. Elisei, *G. Mal. infett. parassit.*, 1985, *37*, 1140.

NEUTROPENIA. For reference to the use of netilmicin sulphate in the treatment of febrile episodes in neutropenic patients, see under Septicaemia in Gentamicin Sulphate, p.244.

References to the use of netilmicin in the treatment of immunocompromised patients: P. Noone, *J. antimicrob. Chemother.*, 1984, *13*, *Suppl.* A, 51.

PERITONITIS. For reference to the use of netilmicin sulphate in the treatment of peritonitis associated with continuous ambulatory peritoneal dialysis, see Gentamicin Sulphate, p.244.

SEPTICAEMIA. For reference to the use of netilmicin sulphate in the treatment of septicaemia and septic shock, see Gentamicin Sulphate, p.244.

SURGICAL INFECTION PROPHYLAXIS. References to the use of netilmicin sulphate for the prophylaxis of infection during surgical procedures: T. N. Stanbridge and D. J. B. Greenall, *J. antimicrob. Chemother.*, 1984, *13*, *Suppl.* A, 59 (open-heart surgery); A. M. Worning *et al.*, *ibid.*, 1986, *17*, 105 (with methicillin in vascular reconstructive surgery).

See also under Gentamicin Sulphate, p.244.

URINARY-TRACT INFECTIONS. Bacteriological cure was evident in 32 of 37 patients with urinary-tract infection, at follow-up 7 or 8 days after a single intramuscular injection of netilmicin sulphate 150 mg. *Escherichia coli* was the predominant causative pathogen.— B. F. Murphy and K. F. Fairley (letter), *Med. J. Aust.*, 1984, *140*, 311.

Preparations

Netilmicin Sulfate Injection *(U.S.P.)*

Proprietary Preparations

Netillin *(Kirby-Warrick, UK)*. *Injection*, netilmicin 10 mg (as sulphate)/mL in ampoules of 1.5 mL, 50 mg (as sulphate)/mL in ampoules of 1 mL, and 100 mg (as sulphate)/mL in ampoules of 1, 1.5, or 2 mL.

Proprietary Names and Manufacturers

Certomycin *(Essex, Ger.)*; Netillin *(Kirby-Warrick, UK)*; Netilyn *(Schering Corp., Denm.*; *Schering, Norw.*; *Schering, Swed.)*; Netrocin *(Essex, Spain)*; Netromicine *(Unicet, Fr.)*; Netromycin *(Essex, Austral.*; *Schering, Canad.*; *Scherag, S.Afr.*; *Schering, USA)*; Netromycine *(Essex, Switz.)*; Nettacin *(Essex, Ital.)*; Zetamicin *(Menarini, Ital.)*.

13016-c

Nifurtoinol *(rINN)*.

Hydroxymethylnitrofurantoin. 3-Hydroxymethyl-1-(5-nitrofurfurylideneamino)hydantoin.

$C_9H_8N_4O_6$=268.2.

CAS — 1088-92-2.

Nifurtoinol is a nitrofuran antibacterial agent used similarly to nitrofurantoin (below) in the treatment of urinary-tract infections. It has been given by mouth in divided doses of 160 mg daily.

A study comparing the incidence of vomiting with nifurtoinol and nitrofurantoin.— A. J. Beysens and H. C. L. V. Kock, *Pharm. Weekbl. Ned.*, 1973, *108*, 149.

Pharmacokinetic study indicating that *in vivo* nifurtoinol acts as a pro-drug of nitrofurantoin.— R. H. A. Sorel and H. Roseboom, *Int. J. Pharmaceut.*, 1979, *3*, 93.

Proprietary Names and Manufacturers

Urfadyn *(Inpharzam, Belg.*; *Arsac, Fr.*; *Zambon, Ital.*; *Inpharzam, Neth.)*; Urfadyne *(Inpharzam, Ger.*; *Inpharzam, Switz.)*.

13021-y

Nisin

234. An antimicrobial substance produced by the growth of *Streptococcus lactis*.

CAS — 1414-45-5.

Units

One unit of nisin is contained in 0.001 mg of the first International Reference Preparation (1969) of nisin which contains 1000 units per mg.

Uses.

Nisin is a polypeptide antibiotic used as a preservative for cheese and canned foods.

A study of the mode of action of nisin suggesting that its primary target is the cytoplasmic membrane and that membrane disruption accounts for its bactericidal action.— E. Ruhr and H. -G. Sahl, *Antimicrob. Ag. Chemother.*, 1985, *27*, 841.

5651-x

Nitrofurantoin *(BAN, USAN, rINN)*.

Furadoninum; Nitrofurantoinum. 1-(5-Nitrofurfurylideneamino)hydantoin; 1-(5-Nitrofurfurylideneamino)imidazolidine-2,4-dione.

$C_8H_6N_4O_5$=238.2.

CAS — 67-20-9 (anhydrous); 17140-81-7 (monohydrate).

Pharmacopoeias. In *Belg.*, *Br.*, *Chin.*, *Cz.*, *Eur.*, *Fr.*, *Int.*, *It.*, *Jug.*, *Neth.*, *Nord.*, *Pol.*, *Roum.*, *Swiss*, and *Turk*. *Rus.* specifies the monohydrate; *Braz.*, *Egypt.*, *Ind.*, and *U.S.* specify anhydrous or monohydrate.

Yellow odourless or almost odourless crystals or fine powder with a bitter after-taste. It is discoloured by alkalis and by exposure to light.

Very slightly **soluble** in water and alcohol; soluble 1 in 16 of dimethylformamide. **Store** at a temperature not exceeding 25° in airtight containers and avoid contact with metals other than stainless steel or aluminium. Protect from light.

The crystal size affects the absorption of nitrofurantoin.

5652-r

Nitrofurantoin Sodium *(BANM, rINNM)*.

$C_8H_5N_4NaO_5$=260.1.

CAS — 54-87-5.

INCOMPATIBILITY. Nitrofurantoin was incompatible in intravenous solutions with amphotericin, kanamycin, oxacillin, polymyxin b, and tetracycline.— *Med. Lett.*, 1972, *14*, (Jan.), *Suppl.*, 32.

Nitrofurantoin sodium was incompatible with amikacin sulphate in a variety of diluents.— B. C. Nunning and A. P. Granatek, *Curr. ther. Res.*, 1976, *20*, 417.

Oral suspensions of nitrofurantoin were found to contain an impurity, identified as 3-(5-nitrofurfurylideneamino)hydantoic acid, in concentrations ranging from 20 to 300 μg per mL. Presence of the impurity was attributed to a reaction between nitrofurantoin and the citrate buffer.— E. C. Juenge *et al.*, *J. pharm. Sci.*, 1985, *74*, 100.

Adverse Effects

The most common adverse effects encountered with nitrofurantoin involve the gastro-intestinal tract. They are dose-related and generally include nausea, vomiting, and anorexia; abdominal pain and diarrhoea occur less frequently. It has been reported that adverse effects on the gastro-intestinal tract are less common when nitrofurantoin is administered in a macrocrystalline form or with food.

Neurological adverse effects include headache, drowsiness, vertigo, dizziness, nystagmus, and myalgia. Peripheral neuropathy, usually related to high blood concentrations, has occurred in patients with impaired renal function or after prolonged administration or the administration of large doses.

Allergic reactions such as skin rashes, urticaria, pruritus, fever, and angioedema may occur. Anaphylaxis and arthralgia have also been reported. Acute pulmonary sensitivity reactions characterised by sudden onset of fever, chills, cough, chest pain, dyspnoea, pulmonary infiltration, and pleural effusion associated with eosinophilia may occur within hours to a few days of beginning therapy, but they usually resolve on discontinuation. Patients with a history of asthma may experience acute asthmatic attacks.

Chronic pulmonary symptoms including interstitial pneumonitis and pulmonary fibrosis may develop insidiously in patients on long-term therapy and these are not always reversible.

Hepatotoxicity including cholestatic jaundice and hepatitis may develop rarely. Other adverse effects include megaloblastic anaemia, agranulocytosis, and haemolytic anaemia in persons with a genetic deficiency of glucose-6-phosphate dehydrogenase. Transient alopecia has been reported.

While Koch-Weser *et al.* (*Archs intern. Med.*, 1971, *128*, 399) found an incidence of 9.2% for severe reactions in patients treated with nitrofurantoin between April 1967 and July 1968, D'Arcy (*Drug Intell. & clin. Pharm.*, 1985, *19*, 540) in a review of worldwide data obtained from the manufacturer (*Norwich-Eaton, USA*) for the period 1953-1984 calculated, that at worst, the incidence was 0.003%. The Swedish Adverse Drug Reaction Committee (L. Holmberg *et al.*, *Am. J. Med.*, 1980, *69*, 733) found an increase in the incidence of reactions as the use of nitrofurantoin increased. During the period 1966-1976 they had received reports of 921 adverse reactions of which 651 were severe enough to require hospitalisation and 11 were fatal. These reports from Sweden were compared by Penn and Griffin (*Br. med. J.*, 1982, *284*, 1440) with those reported to the Committee on Safety of Medicines in the UK for the period 1964-1980 and also with those reported to the Netherlands Drug Registration Authority for 1975-1980. Overall 455 reports were made in the UK and 88 in Holland. Because of the differing incidences they found for the various types of adverse reactions, Penn and Griffin considered that it would be unwise to make comparisons of the ranges of adverse reactions between countries. However, bearing this in mind, the most common reactions were: allergic reactions (182 reports in the UK, 384 in Sweden, and 37 in Holland); acute pulmonary reactions (64 reports in the UK, 398 in Sweden, and 11 in Holland; D'Arcy calculated an incidence of 0.0009% based on 1138 reports from the manufacturer); liver damage and gastro-intestinal disturbances (73 reports in the UK, 50 in Sweden, 12 in Holland, and 312 reports (0.0003%) of hepatic reactions from the manufacturer); peripheral neuropathy (64 reports in the UK, 20 in Sweden, 8 in Holland, and 847 reports (0.0007%) from the manufacturer); chronic pulmonary reactions (9 reports in the UK, 49 in Sweden, 3 in Holland, and 281 reports (0.0002%) from the manufacturer); haematological reactions (11 reports in the UK, 20 in Sweden, 6 in Holland, and 500 reports (0.0004%) from the manufacturer). Data from the manufacturer reviewed by D'Arcy also included 22 reports of subacute pulmonary reactions (calculated incidence: 0.00002%) and a further 283 reports of miscellaneous pulmonary reactions (calculated incidence: 0.0002%). Reports of miscellaneous reactions in the UK had included: headache (4); dizziness, giddiness, and vertigo (7); depression (4); confusion (3); hallucinations (1); schizophrenic reaction (1); slurred speech (2); drowsiness (2); abnormal vision (2); deafness (1); shaking (1); salivary gland enlargement (3).

Precautions

Nitrofurantoin should not be given to patients with impaired renal function since antibacterial concentrations in the urine may not be attained and toxic concentrations in the plasma can occur. Concomitant administration of probenecid should be avoided since it may reduce the excretion of nitrofurantoin. Nitrofurantoin is also contra-indicated in patients known to be hypersensitive, in those with a deficiency of glucose-6-phosphate dehydrogenase, and in infants less than one month old. It has been suggested that nitrofurantoin should not be used in pregnant patients at term because of the possibility of producing haemolytic anaemia in the neonate. Since nitrofurantoin has been detected in breast milk its use should also be avoided in nursing mothers of infants with a deficiency of glucose-6-phosphate dehydrogenase.

Patients should be warned to report early signs of peripheral neuropathy such as paraesthesia. Patients undergoing prolonged therapy should be monitored for changes in pulmonary function.

Nitrofurantoin and nalidixic acid are antagonistic *in vitro* and should not be used together. Nitrofurantoin has also been reported to antagonise the effects of oxolinic acid *in vitro* against some organisms. Nitrofurantoin may cause false positive reactions in urine tests for glucose using copper reduction methods.

INTERACTIONS. Although agents which reduce gastric emptying, such as atropine, propantheline, or diphenoxylate have been reported to delay the absorption and excretion of nitrofurantoin, its overall bioavailability is usually increased (J.M. Jaffe, *J. Pharm. Sci.*, 1975, *64*, 1730; M. Callahan *et al.*, *Fedn Proc.*, 1974, *33*, 513; P. Männistö, *Int. J. clin. Pharmac.*, 1978, *16*, 223). A similar effect has also been reported when nitrofurantoin was taken with food or pyridoxine (I. Amon *et al.*, *Dte GesundhWes.*, 1973, *28*, 1157). Likewise, agents such as metoclopramide, which increase gastric emptying decrease the bioavailability of nitrofurantoin. Männistö also found that the bioavailability of nitrofurantoin was reduced by administration with an antacid preparation of magnesium hydroxide, aluminium hydroxide, and magnesium carbonate but the mechanism of action was unclear. From a review of the literature D'Arcy and McElnay (*Drug Intell. & clin. Pharm.*, 1987, *21*, 607) considered that it was unlikely that nitrofurantoin interacted with common antacid preparations although some adsorption onto magnesium trisilicate may occur. Findings by Naggar and Khalil (*Clin. Pharmac. Ther.*, 1979, *25*, 857) that the rate and extent of absorption were reduced following administration with magnesium trisilicate appear to have been extrapolated in review literature to general interaction between antacids and nitrofurantoin, although there is no substantive clinical evidence for this.

PORPHYRIA. Nitrofurantoin was considered to be unsafe in patients with acute porphyria although there is conflicting experimental evidence on porphyrinogenicity.— M.R. Moore and K.E.L. McColl, *Porphyrias, Drug Lists*, Glasgow, Porphyria Research Unit, University of Glasgow, 1987.

The *US* manufacturers are not aware of any clinical reports of a disulfiram-like reaction with alcohol and nitrofurantoin although the latter has been used in a great number of patients over many years.— B. Rowles and D. B. Worthen (letter), *New Engl. J. Med.*, 1982, *306*, 113.

PREGNANCY AND THE NEONATE. A retrospective analysis of 91 pregnancies in 81 women treated with nitrofurantoin for urinary-tract infection during pregnancy indicated that the incidence of death, malformation, prematurity and low birth-weight in neonates born to these women was not significantly different from that in the United States population, nor was there a difference observed which could be attributed to duration of therapy. Thirty-six of the urinary-tract infections had been treated during the first trimester, 48% in the second, and 16% in the third.— F. J. Hailey *et al.*, *J. int. med. Res.*, 1983, *11*, 364. Printer's correction.— *ibid.*, 1984, *12* (No.1).

Nitrofurantoin is usually well tolerated but it can cause serious adverse effects. Although these reactions are not particularly related to pregnancy the availability of safer alternatives makes the use of nitrofurantoin inadvisable.— *Med. Lett.*, 1986, *28*, 32.

Antimicrobial Action

Nitrofurantoin is bactericidal *in vitro* to most Gram-positive and Gram-negative urinary-tract pathogens and minimum inhibitory concentrations have been reported to range from 4 to 100 µg per mL. Most strains of *Escherichia coli* are particularly sensitive to nitrofurantoin but *Enterobacter* and *Klebsiella* spp. are less susceptible and some may be resistant. *Pseudomonas aeruginosa* is usually resistant and most strains of *Proteus* spp. are moderately resistant. It is most active in acid urine, and if the pH exceeds 8 most of the antibacterial activity is lost. Resistance rarely develops during nitrofurantoin treatment.

Antagonism between nitrofurantoin and nalidixic acid and nitrofurantoin and oxolinic acid has been demonstrated *in vitro*.

The precise mode of action of nitrofurantoin is unknown but it does appear to interfere with a number of bacterial enzymes.

Nitrofuran antimicrobial agents may exert an antimicrobial effect against some bacteria by damaging their DNA.— D. R. McCalla (letter), *J. antimicrob. Chemother.*, 1977, *3*, 517.

BACTERIAL RESISTANCE. Isolation of aminoglycoside-antibiotic-resistant mutants of *Escherichia coli* cross-resistant to high concentrations of nitrofurazone or nitrofurantoin under aerobic and anaerobic conditions *in vitro*.— E. E. Obaseiki-Ebor and A. S. Breeze, *J. antimicrob. Chemother.*, 1984, *13*, 567. See also.— A. S. Breeze and E. E. Obaseiki-Ebor, *ibid.*, *14*, 477.

Absorption and Fate

Nitrofurantoin is readily absorbed from the gastro-intestinal tract and up to about 60% is bound to plasma proteins. Plasma half-lives of 0.3 to 1 hour have been reported. Nitrofurantoin diffuses across the placenta and low concentrations appear in the foetal circulation. It has also been detected in milk. It is metabolised in the liver and most body tissues and about 30 to 50% of a dose is excreted rapidly in the urine as nitrofurantoin. Average doses give a concentration of 50 to 200 µg per mL in the urine in patients with normal renal function.

The absorption of nitrofurantoin is dependent on crystal size. The macrocrystalline form has slower dissolution and absorption rates, produces lower serum concentrations than the microcrystalline form, and takes longer to achieve peak concentrations in the urine. The presence of food in the gastro-intestinal tract may increase the bioavailability of nitrofurantoin and prolong the duration of therapeutic urinary concentrations.

A mean terminal half-life of 58.1 minutes was obtained in 6 healthy subjects after intravenous infusion of about 50 mg of nitrofurantoin. Plasma protein binding was about 60%. In contrast to the findings of other workers, the increase in the absolute bioavailability of nitrofurantoin obtained in the same subjects when nitrofurantoin was given with food as compared with administration after fasting was not significant. A mean of 1.2% of an oral dose was excreted in the urine as aminofurantoin. Although nitrofurantoin appeared to be nearly completely absorbed after doses by mouth the absorption rate-profile was erratic. This could lead to inadequate urinary concentrations; urinary concentrations in 2 subjects failed to reach 32 µg per mL.— B. Hoener and S. E. Patterson, *Clin. Pharmac. Ther.*, 1981, *29*, 808.

BIOAVAILABILITY. A review of the bioavailability of nitrofurantoin.— D. E. Cadwallader *et al.*, *J. Am. pharm. Ass.*, 1975, *NS15*, 409.

Studies of the bioavailability of nitrofurantoin.— M. C. Meyer *et al.*, *J. pharm. Sci.*, 1974, *63*, 1693; J. Bron *et al.*, *Arzneimittel-Forsch.*, 1979, *29*, 1614; H. Maier-Lenz *et al.*, *ibid.*, 1898.

Uses and Administration

Nitrofurantoin is a nitrofuran derivative which is used in the treatment of uncomplicated lower urinary-tract infections although sulphonamides or antibiotics are generally the agents of choice. Antimicrobial concentrations are not reached in the blood but nitrofurantoin is concentrated in the urine and bactericidal concentrations are achieved. It is used prophylactically and for long-term suppressive therapy.

It is given by mouth usually in a dose of 50 to 100 mg four times daily, during or immediately after meals, and at bedtime with food or milk. Treatment is usually continued for up to 14 days. A usual prophylactic dose is 50 to 100 mg at bedtime. Preparations of the macrocrystalline form of nitrofurantoin are available for patients who have suffered nausea with the microcrystalline form.

Infants over 1 month of age and older children may be given 1.25 to 1.75 mg per kg bodyweight 4 times daily by mouth. The dosage should be reduced if continued beyond 10 to 14 days or if used for prophylaxis.

Nitrofurantoin sodium has been given intravenously to patients unable to take the drug by mouth; the usual dose is the equivalent of

180 mg of nitrofurantoin twice daily given by intravenous infusion.

URINARY-TRACT INFECTIONS. Due to the frequency and potential severity of adverse reactions to nitrofurantoin and its inability to achieve therapeutic blood concentrations, nitrofurantoin was considered to be an agent of secondary importance. However, indications for use could include the treatment of acute symptomatic bacterial cystitis or recurrent urinary-tract infections in patients with hypersensitivity to penicillins or cephalosporins and it may be of use in chronic prophylactic treatment for adults or children who experience recurrent urinary-tract infections. It should not be used to treat patients with bacteraemia or acute bacterial pyelonephritis. Furthermore it should not be used to treat recurrent urinary-tract infections in men as these were often caused by chronic prostatitis or infection stones.— R. Gleckman *et al.*, *Am. J. Hosp. Pharm.*, 1979, *36*, 342.

Studies in children indicating that a 3-day course of nitrofurantoin may be as effective as a 10-day course.— J. A. Lohr *et al.*, *J. Pediat.*, 1981, *99*, 980; U. Roberto *et al.* (letter), *ibid.*, 1984, *104*, 483.

Prophylaxis. There was no significant difference between the clinical efficacy of single-day treatment with nitrofurantoin or gentamicin in the prophylaxis of urinary-tract infections in 39 patients who underwent trans-urethral resection. Nitrofurantoin 180 mg or gentamicin 80 mg was given by intravenous infusion during surgery followed by a second dose after 12 or 8 hours respectively. Infection rates were considered to be similar to those after prophylactic treatment given for 5 days.— A. V. Bono *et al.*, *Curr. ther. Res.*, 1983, *33*, 450.

In a 12-month study nitrofurantoin 100 mg at night was more effective but less well tolerated than trimethoprim 100 mg at night in the long-term prophylaxis of recurrent urinary-tract infections. Of the evaluable patients, 88% of 34 who received nitrofurantoin and 58% of 38 who received trimethoprim were abacteriuric during treatment while 62 and 34% of the patients respectively remained asymptomatic. While the 5 breakthrough infections in patients receiving nitrofurantoin were due to nitrofurantoin-sensitive organisms, 28 infections in patients who received trimethoprim were predominantly caused by trimethoprim-resistant organisms; faecal isolates also became resistant to trimethoprim. However, of 40 patients who received nitrofurantoin 6 had to stop treatment because of side-effects and overall 16 reported some form of adverse effect.— W. Brumfitt *et al.*, *J. antimicrob. Chemother.*, 1985, *16*, 111.

Pivmecillinam 100 or 200 mg or nitrofurantoin 1.5 mg per kg body-weight given at night by mouth were equally effective in the long-term prophylaxis of recurrent urinary-tract infections in a crossover study involving 35 children aged between 1 and 13 years but, pivmecillinam was significantly better tolerated.— N. L. T. Carlsen *et al.*, *J. antimicrob. Chemother.*, 1985, *16*, 509.

Single-dose therapy. In an evaluation of the treatment of 151 women with uncomplicated lower urinary-tract infection, nitrofurantoin 200 mg given as a single dose was found to be as effective as nitrofurantoin 50 mg given four times daily for 10 days. Of 218 women originally involved in the study adverse reactions occurred in 4% treated with a single dose and in 13% of those treated with a 10-day regimen.— G. Gossius, *Curr. ther. Res.*, 1984, *35*, 925.

Preparations

Nitrofurantoin Capsules *(U.S.P.)*

Nitrofurantoin Oral Suspension *(B.P.)*. Nitrofurantoin Suspension; Nitrofurantoin Mixture. The preparation should not be diluted.

Nitrofurantoin Oral Suspension *(U.S.P.)*. A suspension of nitrofurantoin 0.46 to 0.54% w/v in a suitable aqueous basis. pH 4.5 to 6.5.

Nitrofurantoin Tablets *(B.P.)*

Nitrofurantoin Tablets *(U.S.P.)*. Potency is expressed in terms of anhydrous nitrofurantoin.

Proprietary Preparations

Furadantin *(Norwich-Eaton, UK)*. *Tablets*, scored, nitrofurantoin 50 and 100 mg.
Suspension, nitrofurantoin 25 mg/5 mL.

Macrodantin *(Norwich-Eaton, UK)*. *Capsules*, nitrofurantoin 50 and 100 mg (as macrocrystals).

Urantoin *(DDSA Pharmaceuticals, UK)*. *Tablets*, scored, nitrofurantoin 50 and 100 mg.

Proprietary Names and Manufacturers of Nitrofurantoin and Nitrofurantoin Sodium

Berkfurin *(Berk Pharmaceuticals, UK)*; Chemiofuran *(Ital.)*; Chemiofurin *(Torlan, Spain)*; Cistofuran *(Crosara, Ital.)*; Cyantin *(USA)*; Cystit *(Heyden, Ger.)*; Fua-Med *(Ger.)*; Furadantin *(Norwich-Eaton, Austral.; Röhm, Ger.; Formenti, Ital.; Pharmacia, Norw.; Eaton, S.Afr.; Pharmacia, Swed.; Norwich-Eaton, UK; Norwich Eaton, USA)*; Furadantina *(Arg.)*; Furadantine *(Belg.; Oberval, Fr.; Neth.; Boehringer Mannheim, Switz.)*; Furadöine *(Fr.)*; Furan *(Chelsea Drug & Chemical, UK)*; Furantoina *(Uriach, Spain)*; Furatine *(Canad.)*; Furedan *(Scharper, Ital.)*; Furil *(OFF, Ital.)*; Furobactina *(Esteve, Spain)*; Furophen *(Krewel, Ger.)*; Ituran *(Belg.; Promonta, Ger.)*; Ivadantin *(Norwich Eaton, USA)*; Macrodantin *(Norwich-Eaton, Austral.; Norwich-Eaton, Canad.; Eaton, S.Afr.; Norwich-Eaton, UK; Norwich Eaton, USA)*; Microdoine *(Gomenol, Fr.)*; Micturol Simple *(Liade, Spain)*; Nephronex *(Cortunon, Canad.)*; Nierofu *(Hoyer, Ger.)*; Nifuran *(Canad.)*; Nitrex *(Star, USA)*; Nitrofurin G.W. *(Panthox & Burck, Ital.)*; Novofuran *(Novopharm, Canad.)*; Phenurin *(Merckle, Ger.)*; Trantoin *(USA)*; Trocurine *(Labatec-Pharma, Switz.)*; Urantoin *(DDSA Pharmaceuticals, UK)*; Urefuran *(Jpn)*; Uretoin *(Jpn)*; Uriston *(Wilson, Pakistan)*; Urodin *(Switz.)*; Urolisa *(Lisapharma, Ital.)*; Urolong *(Thiemann, Ger.; Sodip, Switz.)*; Urosagen *(Jpn)*; Uro-Tablinen *(Beiersdorf, Ger.)*; Uvamin retard *(Switz.)*; Uvamine *(Mepha, Switz.)*.

The following names have been used for multi-ingredient preparations containing nitrofurantoin— Ceduran *(Tillotts, UK)*.

5664-h

Nitroxoline *(BAN, pINN)*.

5-Nitroquinolin-8-ol.
$C_9H_6N_2O_3$=190.2.

CAS — 4008-48-4.

Nitroxoline is an antimicrobial agent used in the treatment of urinary-tract infections in usual doses of 300 to 600 mg daily by mouth.

Studies of the use of a preparation containing nitroxoline with sulphamethizole (Nicene) for the treatment of urinary-tract infections.— M. R. Bednarek *et al.*, *Curr. ther. Res.*, 1986, *39*, 505; A. J. N. Du Raan, *ibid.*, 1987, *42*, 77.

Proprietary Names and Manufacturers

Nibiol *(Belg.; Debat, Fr.; Debat, Neth.; Inofarma, Spain; Debat, Switz.)*; Uro-Coli *(Roussel Maestretti, Ital.)*.

The following names have been used for multi-ingredient preparations containing nitroxoline— Nicene *(Chephasaar, Ger.; Adcock Ingram, S.Afr.)*.

12349-g

Norfloxacin *(BAN, USAN, rINN)*.

AM-715; MK-0366; MK-366. 1-Ethyl-6-fluoro-1,4-dihydro-4-oxo-7-(piperazin-1-yl)quinoline-3-carboxylic acid.
$C_{16}H_{18}FN_3O_3$=319.3.

CAS — 70458-96-7.

Adverse Effects

Adverse effects reported after the use of norfloxacin include nausea and other gastro-intestinal disturbances, drowsiness, headache, dizziness, and skin rashes. Crystalluria has occurred with high doses.

A brief discussion of the adverse effects of fluoroquinolones.— C. R. Smith, *J. antimicrob. Chemother.*, 1987, *19*, 709.

A 22-year-old woman developed a systemic reaction with dry mouth, extreme anxiety, glassy eyes, disorientation, tachycardia, a swollen tongue, and a fine erythematous rash, 100 minutes after receiving her first dose of norfloxacin 400 mg for urinary-tract infection. The reaction gradually settled over 3 hours.— R. R. Bailey *et al.* (letter), *N.Z. med. J.*, 1983, *96*, 446.

Tendinitis developed in 2 immunosuppressed patients with poorly functioning renal transplants, during long-term treatment with norfloxacin given in doses of 800 reducing to 200 mg daily. Symptoms settled on withdrawal of norfloxacin or on reduction of the dosage. One patient had a recurrence of tendinitis when norfloxacin was again administered at a dosage of 400 mg twice daily.— R. R. Bailey *et al.* (letter), *N.Z. med. J.*, 1983, *96*, 590.

See also under Urinary-tract Infections in Uses.

The quinolones were capable of releasing substantial quantities of endotoxin from a culture of *Escherichia coli*. Their use in serious sepsis might be associated with endotoxaemia.— J. S. McConnell and J. Cohen (letter), *J. antimicrob. Chemother.*, 1986, *18*, 765.

CRYSTALLURIA. For a report of crystalluria following administration of large doses of norfloxacin, see under Absorption and Fate.

Precautions

As for Nalidixic Acid, p.267.

Because of the risk of crystalluria, patients should maintain an adequate fluid intake during treatment with norfloxacin.

For reference to the precautions to be observed in renal failure, see under Uses, Administration in Renal Failure.

Antimicrobial Action and Resistance

There are many studies on the antimicrobial activity *in vitro* of norfloxacin and some have been the subject of detailed reviews (S.W.B. Newsom, *J. antimicrob. Chemother.*, 1984, *13*, *Suppl.* B, 25; B. Holmes *et al.*, *Drugs*, 1985, *30*, 482).

It has been shown to be bactericidal, with the MIC being close to the MBC, (H.C. Neu and P. Labthavikul, *Antimicrob. Ag. Chemother.*, 1982, *22*, 23; S.R. Norrby and M. Jonsson, *ibid.*, 1983, *23*, 15) and to act by inhibiting the A subunit of DNA gyrase (topoisomerase) which is essential in the reproduction of bacterial DNA (G.C. Crumplin *et al.*, *J. antimicrob. Chemother.*, 1984, *13*, *Suppl.* B, 9).

Resistance can be induced (J.H. Tenney *et al.*, *Antimicrob. Ag. Chemother.*, 1983, *23*, 188) as can cross-resistance between the 4-quinolones—although it has been considered unlikely that such resistance would diminish any clinical effect since the increased MICs are still within achievable concentrations *in vitro* (J.T. Smith, *Eur. J. clin. Microbiol.*, 1984, *3*, 347). The activity of norfloxacin also appears to be influenced by pH with its activity being diminished in acid media (D. Greenwood *et al.*, *J. antimicrob. Chemother.*, 1984, *13*, 315; R.W. Lacey *et al.*, *ibid.*, *Suppl.* B, 49).

Sensitive Gram-negative organisms include *Escherichia coli*, *Citrobacter*, *Enterobacter*, *Klebsiella*, *Proteus*, *Salmonella*, *Shigella*, and *Yersinia* spp. (A. King *et al.*, *Antimicrob. Ag. Chemother.*, 1982, *21*, 604; S.R. Norrby and M. Jonsson, 1983; D.L. Shungu *et al.*, *Antimicrob. Ag. Chemother.*, 1983, *23*, 86). *Pseudomonas aeruginosa* is susceptible as are other *Pseudomonas* spp., but to a lesser degree (H.C. Neu and P. Labthavikul, 1982). *Haemophilus*, *Neisseria*, and *Acinetobacter* spp. are sensitive as are *Campylobacter*, *Providencia*, *Serratia*, (A. King *et al.*, 1982; H.C. Neu and P. Labthavikul, 1982) and *Legionella* spp. (D. Greenwood and A. Laverick, *Lancet*, 1983, *2*, 279). Gram-positive organisms are less sensitive (A. King *et al.*, 1982; H.C. Neu and P. Labthavikul, 1982) although staphylococci, streptococci, and *Listeria* spp. can be inhibited.

The reported minimum inhibitory concentrations for susceptible bacteria range from about 0.006 to 16 μg per mL.

Norfloxacin has little antifungal activity but it has enhanced the activity of amphotericin against *Candida albicans* (M. Vangdal and T. Bergan, *Drugs exp. & clin. Res.*, 1984, *10*, 443).

Many studies have compared norfloxacin with other 4-quinolones as well as established antimicrobial agents. Clinical studies (see below) have shown norfloxacin to be as effective as amoxycillin, as or more effective than co-trimoxazole, and more effective than nalidixic acid in the treatment of urinary-tract infections.

Absorption and Fate

Maximum plasma concentrations of about 1.5 μg of norfloxacin per mL have been achieved 1 to 2 hours after the administration of a 400-mg dose by mouth. Norfloxacin has been reported to be

14% bound to plasma proteins. The plasma half-life is about 4 hours. About 30% of a dose is excreted unchanged in the urine within 24 hours thus producing high urinary concentrations. Some metabolism occurs, possibly in the liver, and several metabolites have been identified, some of which have antibacterial activity.

Norfloxacin has been detected in bile, prostatic fluid, umbilical cord blood, and amniotic fluid.

Reviews of the absorption and fate of norfloxacin.— S. R. Norrby, *Eur. J. Chemother. Antibiot.*, 1983, *3*, 19; R. Wise, *J. antimicrob. Chemother.*, 1984, *13, Suppl.* B, 59.

A study of 5 healthy subjects administered norfloxacin 200 mg by mouth indicated that renal clearance of norfloxacin is due to renal tubular secretion in addition to glomerular filtration. The mean percentage dose recovered in the urine after 12 hours was reduced from 28% to 13.9% by prior administration of probenecid 1 g.— J. Shimada *et al.*, *Antimicrob. Ag. Chemother.*, 1983, *23*, 1.

Single doses of norfloxacin 0.2, 0.4, 0.8, 1.2, and 1.6 g were given to 14 healthy subjects at weekly intervals. Mean peak serum and urine concentrations were usually obtained 1 to 2 hours after each dose; mean peak concentrations for increasing doses were 0.75, 1.58, 2.41, 3.15, and 3.87 µg per mL respectively in serum and 200, 478, 697, 992, and 1045 µg per mL respectively in urine. The apparent serum elimination half-life was about 7 hours. Approximately 30% of each dose was excreted in the urine as unmetabolised norfloxacin in the first 48 hours after administration. The urinary solubility of norfloxacin was dependent on pH and temperature, with norfloxacin being least soluble at pH 7.5 when maximal solubility was about 450 µg per mL at 25° and 1200 µg per mL at 37°. Norfloxacin also had solubilities greater than 40 mg per mL at 37° for urinary pH values of 5.5 or less. Crystals were occasionally observed during microscopic examination of urine following doses of norfloxacin 1.2 or 1.6 g.— B. N. Swanson *et al.*, *Antimicrob. Ag. Chemother.*, 1983, *23*, 284.

A mean intraprostatic concentration of norfloxacin of 0.98 µg per g was obtained in 10 patients who had received norfloxacin 400 mg by mouth, repeated 11 hours later, before undergoing prostatectomy. The mean serum concentration was 1.09 µg per mL. Blood and prostate-tissue samples were obtained 14 to 15 hours after the first dose.— M. Bologna *et al.*, *Lancet*, 1983, *2*, 280.

Differences between the pharmacokinetic parameters of norfloxacin in 3 patients with hepatic damage, 3 patients with moderate renal failure, and 6 healthy subjects were slight and not statistically significant. Administration of norfloxacin 400 mg by mouth produced maximum plasma concentrations of 1.30 µg per mL in patients with hepatic damage, 1.47 µg per mL in patients with renal impairment, and 1.35 µg per mL in healthy subjects in about 1 to 1.5 hours; mean half-lives were 5.47, 6.50, and 4.28 hours respectively. About 30% of a dose was excreted unmetabolised in the urine within 24 hours of administration and mean urinary concentrations of norfloxacin were much higher than the MIC and MBC of most urinary-tract pathogens.— M. Eandi *et al.*, *Eur. J. clin. Microbiol.*, 1983, *2*, 253. See also.— G. Arrigo *et al.*, *Int. J. clin. Pharmac. Biopharm.*, 1985, *23*, 491 (renal failure). See also under Administration in renal failure in Uses.

Norfloxacin was rapidly absorbed in 6 healthy subjects following administration of a single 400-mg dose by mouth, with serum concentrations of about 0.4 µg per mL occurring within 30 minutes. A mean peak serum concentration of 1.45 µg per mL was obtained after about 1.5 hours and concentrations in excess of 0.2 µg per mL were detected up to 8 hours after administration. The mean terminal elimination half-life was 3.25 hours. After 24 hours a mean of 27% of the administered dose was recovered in the urine as microbiologically active compound. Norfloxacin also penetrated blister fluid rapidly with a peak concentration of 1.01 µg per mL occurring after 2 to 3 hours. Thereafter, blister fluid concentrations of norfloxacin paralleled but exceeded serum concentrations.— Z. N. Adhami *et al.*, *J. antimicrob. Chemother.*, 1984, *13*, 87.

Following administration of norfloxacin 400 mg by mouth to 12 healthy male subjects, recovery of norfloxacin in the faeces during the following 48 hours ranged from 8.3 to 53.3% (mean 29%) of the administered dose. Peak faecal concentrations were usually greater than 200 µg per g. Most subjects had faecal drug concentrations greater than 50 µg per g for at least 24 hours.— R. D. Cofsky *et al.*, *Antimicrob. Ag. Chemother.*, 1984, *26*, 110.

Further references: R. Wise *et al.*, *J. antimicrob. Chemother.*, 1986, *18*, *Suppl.* D, 71.

Uses and Administration

Norfloxacin is a fluorinated 4-quinolone antimicrobial agent structurally related to nalidixic acid but with a wider antibacterial spectrum and greater activity.

Administration of norfloxacin by mouth readily produces urinary concentrations that are bactericidal to most urinary-tract pathogens, including *Pseudomonas aeruginosa*. It is therefore used in the treatment of urinary-tract infections in usual doses of 400 mg given twice daily by mouth for 7 to 10 days. The treatment period may be extended to up to 21 days in some patients. It has also been tried in gonococcal urethritis as well as bacterial gastroenteritis.

Review of norfloxacin.— B. Holmes *et al.*, *Drugs*, 1985, *30*, 482.

Series of papers on the action and use of norfloxacin.— J. F. Acar and R. Norrby (Ed.), *Eur. J. clin. Microbiol.*, 1983, *2*, 225-276; *J. antimicrob. Chemother.*, 1984, *13*, *Suppl.* B, 1-142. See also *Chemotherapy, Tokyo*, 1981, *29*, *Suppl.* 4, 1-1000.

A decrease in morbidity and Gram-negative infections in patients with acute leukaemia given norfloxacin 400 mg by mouth every 12 hours throughout periods of granulocytopenia.— J. E. Karp *et al.*, *Ann. intern. Med.*, 1987, *106*, 1.

ADMINISTRATION IN RENAL FAILURE. From results of a study of the pharmacokinetics of norfloxacin in 5 healthy subjects and 11 patients with impaired renal function it was recommended that the usual dosage of norfloxacin should be halved in patients with a glomerular filtration-rate of less than 30 mL per minute. Even in patients with the most severe renal impairment the urinary concentration of norfloxacin exceeded 4 µg per mL after a 400-mg dose.— P. J. Hughes *et al.*, *J. antimicrob. Chemother.*, 1984, *13*, *Suppl.* B, 55.

The mean elimination half-life of norfloxacin in 18 uraemic patients following norfloxacin 400 mg by mouth ranged from 4.4 to 7.6 hours, increasing with increasing renal impairment, compared with 2.3 hours in 5 healthy subjects. The mean half-life of norfloxacin was 7.99 hours between dialysis sessions in 5 of the patients who required haemodialysis and was not influenced by haemodialysis. It appeared that norfloxacin 400 mg given every 12 hours by mouth would be an appropriate dosage for patients with a creatinine clearance of 20 mL or more per minute but for patients with a creatinine clearance of 2 to 10 mL per minute, it is recommended that the dosage interval should be doubled or the dose halved.— J. P. Fillastre *et al.* (letter), *J. antimicrob. Chemother.*, 1984, *14*, 439.

See also under Absorption and Fate.

ENTERIC INFECTIONS. As the results of an open study involving 30 patients indicated that 5-day courses of norfloxacin 400 mg given twice daily and nalidixic acid 1 g given three times daily were of similar efficacy in the treatment of shigellosis it has been suggested that norfloxacin may be useful in areas where nalidixic acid resistant strains of *Shigella* occur (F. Rogerie *et al.*, *Antimicrob. Ag. Chemother.*, 1986, *29*, 883). Encouraging results have also been obtained with norfloxacin given in daily doses of 400 mg for prophylaxis of traveller's diarrhoea (P.C. Johnson *et al.*, *Antimicrob. Ag. Chemother.*, 1986, *30*, 671; J. Wiström *et al.*, *J. antimicrob. Chemother.*, 1987, *20*, 563).

GONORRHOEA. Open studies suggest that a single 800-mg dose of norfloxacin given by mouth may be effective in the treatment of men and women with uncomplicated urethral and anorectal gonorrhoea due to penicillinase and non-penicillinase producing organisms (B. Romanowski *et al.*, *Antimicrob. Ag. Chemother.*, 1986, *30*, 514; J. Bogaerts *et al.*, *ibid.*, 1987, *31*, 434). Crider *et al.* (*New Engl. J. Med.*, 1984, *311*, 137) found that norfloxacin 600 mg given by mouth and repeated after 4 hours and spectinomycin 2 g given intramuscularly were equally effective in the treatment of uncomplicated gonococcal urethritis in men infected with penicillinase or non-penicillinase producing organisms. However, norfloxacin is reported to be ineffective in the treatment of nongonococcal urethritis caused by *Chlamydia trachomatis* (W.R. Bowie *et al.*, *Antimicrob. Ag. Chemother.*, 1986, *30*, 594).

URINARY-TRACT INFECTIONS. Analysis of the results of 4 multicentre studies indicated that norfloxacin 400 mg given twice daily is as effective in eradicating bacteriuria as amoxycillin 250 mg given three times a day or co-trimoxazole 960 mg given twice daily in a 7-day course of treatment and is more effective than nalidixic acid with sodium citrate in a 3-day course of treatment. A 3-day course of norfloxacin appeared to be as effective as a 7-day course. All organisms encountered were sensitive to norfloxacin except some strains of *Enterococcus faecalis*. The incidence of resistance for norfloxacin was 0.2% compared with 5.2% for trimethoprim, 22.2% for amoxycillin, and 15.2% for nalidixic acid. Of a total of 758 patients who received norfloxacin 71 (9%) experienced adverse effects considered to be due to norfloxacin, with 5 (0.7%) discontinuing therapy as a result. Adverse effects reported included: lightheadedness (7), depression (3), drowsiness (6), headache (4), insomnia (2), confusion (1), nausea (20), vomiting (4), constipation (1), abdominal pain (2), diarrhoea (2), 'swollen stomach' (2), vaginal discharge (10), swollen finger joint (1), sore mouth (4), and rash (4).— R. Vogel *et al.*, *J. antimicrob. Chemother.*, 1984, *13*, *Suppl.*, B, 113.

[Some of the individual studies appear to be: N.B. Deaney *et al.*, *Practitioner*, 1984, *228*, 111; B. Watt *et al.*, *J. antimicrob. Chemother.*, 1984, *13*, *Suppl.* B, 89; D. S. Reeves *et al. ibid.*, 99]

Studies indicating that norfloxacin is of similar or greater efficacy than co-trimoxazole in the treatment of urinary-tract infections.— J. G. Guerra *et al.*, *Eur. J. clin. Microbiol.*, 1983, *2*, 260; H. Giamarellou *et al.*, *ibid.*, 266; G. Panichi *et al.*, *J. antimicrob. Chemother.*, 1983, *11*, 589; D. A. Haase *et al.*, *Antimicrob. Ag. Chemother.*, 1984, *26*, 481; A. J. Schaeffer and G. A. Sisney, *J. Urol., Baltimore*, 1985, *133*, 628; J. Sabbaj *et al.*, *Antimicrob. Ag. Chemother.*, 1985, *27*, 297; E. J. C. Goldstein *et al.*, *ibid.*, 422.

The efficacy of norfloxacin, oxolinic acid, cinoxacin, or nalidixic acid was evaluated in 125 patients with urinary-tract infections due to *Escherichia coli*, *Klebsiella* spp., or *Proteus* spp. Dosage regimens were oxolinic acid 1.5 g or nalidixic acid 4 g given daily for 14 days, cinoxacin 500 mg given twice daily for 10 days, or norfloxacin 400 mg given every 12 hours for 10 days. There were no significant differences in the overall success-rates of the different agents, treatment being considered to be successful in 14 of 20 patients (70%) for nalidixic acid, 16 of 20 patients (80%) for oxolinic acid, 58 of 70 patients (83%) for cinoxacin, and 14 of 15 patients (93%) for norfloxacin. Epigastric discomfort was reported by patients receiving nalidixic acid, oxolinic acid, or cinoxacin. Nalidixic acid, oxolinic acid, or cinoxacin, given in the doses above for 6 weeks, were also evaluated in the prophylaxis of urinary-tract infections in a further 30 similar patients. At follow-up 9 months after the end of therapy, recurrence of infection had been prevented in 7 of 10 patients given nalidixic acid, in 8 of 10 given oxolinic acid, and in 9 of 10 given cinoxacin.— M. S. Sabbour *et al.*, *Infection*, 1984, *12*, 377.

Norfloxacin 400 mg given twice daily for 5 to 10 days (or norfloxacin 800 mg given twice daily for 10 days in one patient) eradicated the infection in 16 (84%) of 19 courses of treatment in 17 patients with urinary-tract infection caused by *Pseudomonas aeruginosa* or *Ps. fluorescens*. Two treatment failures in one patient were attributed to underlying urinary-tract disease; the other failure was due to a resistant strain of *Ps. aeruginosa*.— D. A. Leigh and F. X. S. Emmanuel, *J. antimicrob. Chemother.*, 1984, *13*, *Suppl.* B, 85.

Further references.— L. A. Ganguli *et al.*, *Drugs exp. & clin. Res.*, 1985, *11*, 177; S. Hill *et al.* (letter), *J. antimicrob. Chemother.*, 1985, *15*, 505.

Proprietary Names and Manufacturers

Amicrobin *(Hosbon, Spain)*; Baccidal *(Kyorin, Jpn; Liade, Spain)*; Barazan *(Merck Sharp & Dohme, Ger.)*; Buccidal; Esclebin *(Boizot, Spain)*; Espeden *(Vita, Spain)*; Fulgram *(ABC, Ital.)*; Lexinor *(Astra, Swed.)*; Nalion *(Lesvi, Spain)*; Noroxin *(Merck Sharp & Dohme, Austral.; Merck Sharp & Dohme, Canad.; Merck Sharp & Dohme, Ital.; Merck Sharp & Dohme, Spain; Chibret, Switz.; Merck Sharp & Dohme, USA)*; Noroxine *(Merck Sharp & Dohme-Chibret, Fr.)*; Primoxin; Sebercim *(ISF, Ital.)*; Senro *(Madaus Cerafarm, Spain)*; Uroctal *(Funk, Spain)*; Zoroxin *(Merck Sharp & Dohme, Denm.)*.

13034-a

Nosiheptide *(BAN, USAN, rINN).*
RP-9671. A peptide antibiotic obtained from cultures of *Streptomyces actuosus* or by any other means.
$C_{51}H_{43}N_{13}O_{12}S_6$=1222.4.

CAS — 56377-79-8.

Nosiheptide is used as a food additive in veterinary practice to promote growth.

115-h

Novobiocin *(BAN, rINN).*

Streptonivicin. 4-Hydroxy-3-[4-hydroxy-3-(3-methylbut-2-enyl)benzamido]-8-methylcoumarin-7-yl 3-*O*-carbamoyl-5,5-di-*C*-methyl-4-*O*-methyl-α-L-*lyxo*-hexopyranoside.
$C_{31}H_{36}N_2O_{11}$=612.6.

CAS — 303-81-1.

An antimicrobial substance produced by the growth of *Streptomyces niveus* and *S. spheroides* or related organisms.

116-m

Novobiocin Calcium *(BANM, USAN, rINNM).*

Calcium Novobiocin; Novobiocinum Calcium.
The calcium salt of novobiocin.
$(C_{31}H_{35}N_2O_{11})_2Ca$=1263.3.

CAS — 4309-70-0.

Pharmacopoeias. In *Int.* and *U.S.*

It contains not less then 840 µg per mg of the dried substance. 1.03 g of monograph substance is approximately equivalent to 1 g of novobiocin. A 2.5% suspension in water has a pH of 6.5 to 8.5. **Store** in airtight containers.

117-b

Novobiocin Sodium *(BANM, USAN, rINNM).*

Novobiocinum Natricum; Sodium Novobiocin.
The monosodium salt of novobiocin.
$C_{31}H_{35}N_2NaO_{11}$=634.6.

CAS — 1476-53-5.

Pharmacopoeias. In *Fr., Ind., Int., Rus.,* and *U.S.*

It contains not less than 850 µg per mg of the dried substance. 1.04 g of monograph substance is approximately equivalent to 1 g of novobiocin. Each g of monograph substance represents about 1.6 mmol of sodium. A 2.5% solution in water has a pH of 6.5 to 8.5. **Store** in airtight containers.

INCOMPATIBILITY. *For reference to incompatibilities with novobiocin in intravenous infusions, see Martindale 28th Edn, p. 1193.*

Units

One unit of novobiocin is contained in 0.001031 mg of the first International Standard Preparation (1965) of novobiocin acid which contains 970 units per mg.

Adverse Effects and Precautions

Novobiocin produces many side-effects. Nausea, colic, vomiting, and diarrhoea frequently occur but are usually not sufficiently severe to necessitate stopping treatment. Sensitisation reactions are common with courses lasting more than 1 week and symptoms include urticarial and maculopapular skin eruptions, often with fever. Erythema multiforme has been reported. Eosinophilia, leucopenia, thrombocytopenia, and occasionally haemolytic anaemia have occurred. Total and differential blood counts should be made routinely during treatment.

A yellow pigment which may appear in the plasma of patients treated with novobiocin is a metabolite of the drug; it may be deposited in the skin or sclerae and may interfere with the determination of serum bilirubin. In a few cases, novobiocin appears to have produced some degree of liver dysfunction with raised serum-bilirubin concentration; this is a special risk in neonates.

INTERACTIONS. In a study in 10 healthy subjects, rifampicin decreased the mean serum concentrations of novobiocin after multiple oral doses of both drugs. The degree of change was, however, unlikely to be of clinical significance.— G. L. Drusano *et al., Antimicrob. Ag. Chemother.,* 1986, *30,* 42.

PORPHYRIA. Novobiocin was considered to be unsafe in patients with acute porphyria because it has been shown to be porphyrinogenic in *animals* or *in vitro* systems.— M.R. Moore and K.E.L. McColl, *Porphyrias, Drug Lists,* Glasgow, Porphyria Research Unit, University of Glasgow, 1987.

Antimicrobial Action

Novobiocin appears to act in several ways; it interferes with the synthesis of bacterial cell walls, and also with protein and nucleic acid synthesis, by inhibition of the enzyme DNA gyrase (topoisomerase). In high concentrations it is bactericidal against highly susceptible species.

It is active against Gram-positive micro-organisms such as *Staphylococcus aureus, Clostridia, Corynebacterium diphtheriae,* and *Streptococcus pneumoniae.* Activity against other streptococci is variable; *Enterococcus faecalis,* (*Streptococcus faecalis*) is usually resistant. Of the Gram-negative bacteria, *Haemophilus influenzae, Neisseria gonorrhoeae,* and *N. meningitidis* are sensitive. *Proteus vulgaris* is variable in its reaction to novobiocin. *Pseudomonas pseudomallei* may be sensitive at high concentrations. *Escherichia coli, Ps. aeruginosa, Klebsiella, Salmonella,* and *Shigella* spp. are resistant to novobiocin.

The usual minimum inhibitory concentration of novobiocin for sensitive strains of Gram-positive bacteria has been reported to range from 0.1 to 4 µg per mL.

The antimicrobial activity of novobiocin was enhanced in alkaline urine.— S. A. Kabins, *J. Am. med. Ass.,* 1972, *219,* 206.

Novobiocin, an inhibitor of DNA gyrase, could be used to eliminate (cure) plasmids from bacterial hosts. References: D. C. Hooper *et al., Antimicrob. Ag. Chemother.,* 1984, *25,* 586; Y. Michel-Briand *et al., J. antimicrob. Chemother.,* 1986, *18,* 667.

ACTIVITY AGAINST BACTERIA. Novobiocin inhibited all 10 multiply-resistant strains of *Streptococcus pneumoniae* tested at a concentration of 1 to 2 µg per mL.— M. E. Gombert and T. M. Aulicino, *Antimicrob. Ag. Chemother.,* 1984, *26,* 933.

Novobiocin had variable, but possibly useful activity against 30 clinical strains of *Corynebacterium* Group D2. The MIC ranged from less than 0.25 to 32 µg per mL at pH 7.4, and was substantially higher at pH 8.5.— M. Santamaria *et al., Antimicrob. Ag. Chemother.,* 1985, *28,* 845.

Novobiocin had good activity *in vitro* against *Pseudomonas cepacia*; MICs were in the range of 0.5 to 8 µg per mL.— M. O. S. Ferreira *et al., J. int. med. Res.,* 1985, *13,* 270.

All 103 isolates of methicillin-resistant *Staphylococcus aureus* tested were susceptible to novobiocin at concentrations of 0.25 µg or less per mL. The MICs and MBCs were very similar.— T. J. Walsh *et al., J. antimicrob. Chemother.,* 1985, *15,* 435.

ACTIVITY AGAINST PROTOZOA. Novobiocin and its structural analogue clorobiocin antagonised the growth of *Trypanosoma cruzi* amastigotes in cell-free medium. The concentration of novobiocin required, however, was at the limits of achievable, nontoxic drug concentrations in the sera of patients.— P. G. Pate *et al., Antimicrob. Ag. Chemother.,* 1986, *29,* 426.

ACTIVITY AGAINST VIRUSES. Novobiocin suppressed the multiplication of herpes virus *in vitro* and was found to have greater activity at an acid pH. Novobiocin enhanced the activity of idoxuridine against herpes virus and vaccinia virus and the emergence of resistant herpes virus appeared to be delayed.— T. Chang and L. Weinstein, *Antimicrob. Ag. Chemother.,* 1970, 165.

Novobiocin showed a dose-dependent inhibition of human cytomegalovirus replication in cell cultures. It had no effect, however, on replication of adenovirus type 37.— M. P. Landini and B. Baldassarri, *J. antimicrob. Chemother.,* 1982, *10,* 533. Activity of novobiocin against cytomegalovirus infection in *mice.*— G. Furlini *et al., ibid.,* 1983, *12,* 503.

ACTIVITY WITH OTHER ANTIMICROBIAL AGENTS. Novobiocin and rifampicin enhanced the activity of each other *in vitro* against 17 of 18 strains of *Salmonella typhi.*— D. C. Shanson and T. Leung, *J. antimicrob. Chemother.,* 1976, *2,* 81.

Synergy was observed *in vitro* between novobiocin and rifampicin or vancomycin against some strains of methicillin-resistant *Staphylococcus aureus.* However, the frequency of synergy depended on the method used.— T. J. Walsh *et al., J. antimicrob. Chemother.,* 1986, *17,* 75. See also R. A. Proctor *et al., ibid.,* 1987, *20,* 223.

Resistance

Many species of bacteria are capable of developing resistance to novobiocin. *Staphylococcus aureus* readily develops resistance both *in vitro* and *in vivo.*

Absorption and Fate

Novobiocin given as the calcium or sodium salt is absorbed from the gastro-intestinal tract, giving maximum plasma concentrations of about 10 µg per mL within 1 to 4 hours of a dose equivalent to about 250 mg. Over 90% of novobiocin in the circulation is bound to plasma proteins.

Novobiocin is excreted mainly in the bile from which it is repeatedly reabsorbed and eventually excreted in the faeces. No more than 3% is excreted in the urine. It diffuses into the pleural and ascitic fluids but not into the cerebrospinal fluid unless the meninges are inflamed.

It is excreted in milk.

Some 95.5% of novobiocin in the body was bound to serum proteins. The half-life in serum was 2.3 hours and 1.5 to 3.3% was excreted in urine.— C. M. Kunin, *Ann. intern. Med.,* 1967, *67,* 151. See also J. G. Wagner and R. E. Damiano, *J. clin. Pharmac.,* 1968, *8,* 102.

Uses and Administration

There appears to be little reason for the continued use of novobiocin as alternative therapy for susceptible infections is usually safer. Apart from being used in staphylococcal infections, it has formed part of the treatment of melioidosis due to *Pseudomonas pseudomallei.*

Novobiocin is given by mouth as the sodium or calcium salt in doses of 250 mg (of base) every 6 hours, although higher doses have been used in severe infections. Children have been given 30 mg per kg body-weight daily. Novobiocin sodium has also been given by the parenteral route.

Preparations

Novobiocin Calcium Oral Suspension *(U.S.P.).* Prepared from novobiocin calcium or novobiocin sodium reacted with a suitable calcium salt. pH 6.0 to 7.5. Protect from light.

Novobiocin Sodium Capsules *(U.S.P.).* Protect from light.

Proprietary Names and Manufacturers of Novobiocin Salts

Albamycin *(Belg.; Upjohn, UK; Upjohn, USA)*; Cathomycine *(Fr.)*; Catomicina *(Spain)*; Novobioplast *(Spain)*; Robiocina *(Ital.; Spain).*

The following names have been used for multi-ingredient preparations containing novobiocin salts— Albamycin GU *(Upjohn, UK)*; Albamycin T *(Upjohn, UK).*

16935-w

Ofloxacin *(BAN, USAN, rINN).*
DL-8280; HOE-280; RU-43280. (±)-9-Fluoro-2,3-dihydro-3-methyl-10-(4-methyl-1-piperazinyl)-7-oxo-7*H*-pyrido[1,2,3-*de*]-1,4-benzoxazine-6-carboxylic acid.
$C_{18}H_{20}FN_3O_4$=361.4.

CAS — 82419-36-1; 83380-47-6.

Ofloxacin is a fluorinated 4-quinolone antimicrobial agent with actions similar to those of norfloxacin (see p.274). It is being studied in both systemic and urinary-tract infections.

For a series of papers on ofloxacin, including clinical studies in urinary-tract infections, respiratory-tract infections, skin infections, and ENT infections and in the fields of obstetrics and gynaecology and surgery, see *Chemotherapy, Tokyo*, 1984, *32, Suppl.* 1, 1-1210. For another series, see *Drugs*, 1987, *34, Suppl.* 1, 1-187.

A review of the antibacterial activity, pharmacokinetics, and therapeutic use of ofloxacin.— J. P. Monk and D. M. Campoli-Richards, *Drugs*, 1987, *33*, 346.

ABSORPTION AND FATE. A mean peak serum concentration of 10.7 µg per mL was obtained in 6 healthy subjects about 1.2 hours after administration of ofloxacin 600 mg by mouth. Serum concentrations of ofloxacin exceeded 1 µg per mL in all subjects 12 hours after administration. The mean serum elimination half-life was 7 hours with 72.9% of a dose being recovered in the urine within 24 hours and 80.3% being recovered within 48 hours. Ofloxacin penetrated into blister fluid reaching a mean peak concentration of 5.2 µg per mL after about 5.3 hours. Concentrations in blister fluid exceeded 1.8 µg per mL after 12 hours.— M. R. Lockley *et al.*, *J. antimicrob. Chemother.*, 1984, *14*, 647.

Ofloxacin 200 mg given by mouth produced a mean peak serum concentration of 2.3 µg per mL in 6 healthy subjects 0.7 hours after administration. The terminal elimination half-life was 5.9 hours with 77% of the dose being recovered in the urine within 48 hours of administration. Results indicated considerable tubular secretion in addition to glomerular filtration.— D. Beermann *et al.*, *J. clin. Pharmac.*, 1984, *24*, 403.

Further references to the pharmacokinetics of ofloxacin R. Wise *et al.*, *J. antimicrob. Chemother.*, 1986, *18, Suppl.* D, 71 (comparative pharmacokinetics of 5 quinolones); H. Lode *et al.*, *Antimicrob. Ag. Chemother.*, 1987, *31*, 1338 (oral and parenteral administration); A. Fisch *et al.* (letter), *J. antimicrob. Chemother.*, 1987, *20*, 453 (distribution into aqueous humour and lens).

ANTIMICROBIAL ACTION. As for Norfloxacin, p.274. Some references: K. Sato *et al.*, *Antimicrob. Ag. Chemother.*, 1982, *22*, 548; Y. Osada and H. Ogawa, *ibid.*, 1983, *23*, 509; R. Wise *et al.*, *J. antimicrob. Chemother.*, 1984, *13*, 237; J. M. G. Bailey *et al.*, *Antimicrob. Ag. Chemother.*, 1984, *26*, 13; A. King *et al.*, *J. antimicrob. Chemother.*, 1985, *15*, 551; C. Heppleston *et al.*, *ibid.*, 645; J. F. Chantot and A. Bryskier, *ibid.*, *16*, 475; T. Kumada and H. C. Neu, *ibid.*, 563; H. Goossens *et al.*, *Antimicrob. Ag. Chemother.*, 1985, *27*, 388; A. Saito *et al.*, *ibid.*, *28*, 15; M. Tsukamura, *Am. Rev. resp. Dis.*, 1985, *131*, 348; P. B. Fernandes *et al.*, *ibid.*, 693; J. Weisser and B. Wiedemann, *J. antimicrob. Chemother.*, 1986, *18*, 575; D. I. Limb, *ibid.*, 1987, *19*, 65.

Isomers. (−)-Ofloxacin was 8 to 128 times more active than (+)-ofloxacin *in vitro* against Gram-negative and Gram-positive bacteria and about twice as active as the racemate (±)-ofloxacin.— I. Hayakawa *et al.*, *Antimicrob. Ag. Chemother.*, 1986, *29*, 163.

CAMPYLOBACTER INFECTIONS. Treatment failure with ofloxacin and the development of resistance in *Campylobacter pylori* infection.— Y. Glupczynski *et al.* (letter), *Lancet*, 1987, *1*, 1096. See also E. Bayerdörffer *et al.*, *ibid.*, *2*, 1467.

RESPIRATORY INFECTIONS. Some references to ofloxacin in respiratory infections: F. P. V. Maesen *et al.*, *J. antimicrob. Chemother.*, 1986, *18*, 629 (acute purulent exacerbations of chronic respiratory disease); B. Kemmerich *et al.*, *Antimicrob. Ag. Chemother.*, 1987, *31*, 417 (experimental *Haemophilus influenzae* pneumonia); N. M. Jitta and Ch. A. Sumajow, *Curr. ther. Res.*, 1987, *42*, 39 (acute exacerbations of chronic bronchitis).

Pulmonary tuberculosis. A pilot study of the clinical effect of ofloxacin on pulmonary tuberculosis was carried out in 19 patients with chronic cavitary lung tuberculosis who were considered to be 'treatment failures'. The patients had received various regimens of antituberculous agents without negative conversion of sputum cultures and were excreting tubercle bacilli resistant to various antituberculous agents. The regimens were continued in most patients together with ofloxacin 300 mg given daily as a single dose for 6 or 8 months. A decrease in the number of tubercle bacilli in the sputum was observed in almost all patients and negative conversion was obtained in 5. Tubercle bacilli resistant to ofloxacin appeared in the 3rd to 4th month of treatment in most patients who did not show negative conversion.— M. Tsukamura *et al.*, *Am. Rev. resp. Dis.*, 1985, *131*, 352. See also.— R. J. O'Brien and D. E. Snider, *ibid.*, 309.

SALMONELLAL INFECTIONS. The successful treatment of a chronic salmonella excretor with ofloxacin 400 mg daily for 7 days.— A. Löffler and H. Graf von Westphalen (letter), *Lancet*, 1986, *1*, 1206.

Proprietary Names and Manufacturers
Tarivid *(Hoechst, Ger.; Daiichi, Jpn).*

118-v

Oleandomycin Phosphate *(BANM, rINNM).*
3-(2,6-Dideoxy-3-*O*-methyl-α-L-*arabino*-hexopyranosyloxy)-8,8-epoxymethano-11-hydroxy-2,4,6,10,12-pentamethyl-9-oxo-5-(3,4,6-trideoxy-3-dimethylamino-β-D-*xylo*-hexopyranosyloxy)tetradecan-13-olide phosphate.
$C_{35}H_{61}NO_{12},H_3PO_4$=785.9.

CAS — 3922-90-5 (oleandomycin); 7060-74-4 (phosphate).

The phosphate of an antimicrobial substance produced by the growth of certain strains of *Streptomyces antibioticus*.

Units
One unit of oleandomycin is contained in 0.001176 mg of the first International Standard Preparation (1964) of oleandomycin chloroform adduct which contains 850 units per mg.

Oleandomycin is a macrolide antibiotic with actions and uses similar to those of erythromycin (see p.222). It has antimicrobial activity weaker than that of erythromycin; cross-resistance occurs between oleandomycin and the other macrolides.

Oleandomycin phosphate has been used in the treatment of susceptible infections but more effective antibiotics are generally preferred. It has been given by mouth or intravenously in a dose of 1 to 2 g daily in divided doses. The intramuscular route has been used only rarely since such injections are painful.

Oleandomycin has also been given by mouth as the triacetyl ester, triacetyloleandomycin (see p.328).

References: E. Semenitz, *J. antimicrob. Chemother.*, 1978, *4*, 455 (antibacterial activity).

For reference to possible interactions with macrolide antibiotics, and their effect on hepatic metabolism, see Erythromycin, p.222.

Proprietary Names and Manufacturers of Oleandomycin or Oleandomycin Phosphate
Matromycin *(Pfizer Taito, Jpn)*; Mittamycin *(Jpn)*; Oleandocyn *(Pfizer, Ger.)*; Taocin-P *(Jpn)*; Triolmicina *(Ripari-Gero, Ital.).*

119-g

Oxacillin Sodium *(BANM, USAN, rINNM).*

(5-Methyl-3-phenyl-4-isoxazolyl)penicillin Sodium; Oxacillinum Natricum; Oxacillinum Natrium; Sodium Oxacillin. Sodium (6*R*)-6-(5-methyl-3-phenylisoxazole-4-carboxamido)penicillanate monohydrate.
$C_{19}H_{18}N_3NaO_5S,H_2O$=441.4.

CAS — 66-79-5 (oxacillin); 1173-88-2 (sodium salt, anhydrous); 7240-38-2 (sodium salt, monohydrate).

Pharmacopoeias. In *Braz.*, *Chin.*, *Cz.*, *Int.*, *Roum.*, *Rus.*, *Turk.*, and *U.S.*

A fine white crystalline powder, odourless or with a slight odour. 1.1 g of monograph substance is approximately equivalent to 1 g of anhydrous oxacillin. Each g of monograph substance represents about 2.3 mmol of sodium.

Freely **soluble** in water and in methyl alcohol; slightly soluble in dehydrated alcohol and chloroform; practically insoluble in ether. A 3% solution in water has a pH of 4.5 to 7.5. **Store** in airtight containers.

Aqueous solutions containing 17% are reported to be stable for 3 days at room temperature and for 7 days when stored in a refrigerator. Oxacillin Sodium has been reported to be **incompatible** with aminoglycosides and tetracyclines.

Adverse Effects
As for Benzylpenicillin Sodium, p.132.

EFFECTS ON THE BLOOD. Neutropenia associated with oxacillin sodium: J. M. Leventhal and A. B. Silken, *J. Pediat.*, 1976, *89*, 769.

Agranulocytosis attributed to oxacillin sodium: J. B. Kahn (letter), *J. Am. med. Ass.*, 1978, *240*, 2632; R. D. Scalley and R. D. Roark, *Drug Intell. & clin. Pharm.*, 1977, *11*, 420.

EFFECTS ON THE GASTRO-INTESTINAL TRACT. Pseudomembranous colitis after the administration of oxacillin: E. Thomas and J. B. Mehta, *Sth. med. J.*, 1984, *77*, 532. See also under Dicloxacillin Sodium, p.216.

EFFECTS ON THE KIDNEYS. Renal failure with acute interstitial nephritis associated with the administration of oxacillin by mouth.— J. R. Burton *et al.*, *Johns Hopkins med. J.*, 1974, *134*, 58.

Further references: D. B. Tillman *et al.*, *Archs intern. Med.*, 1980, *140*, 1552.

EFFECTS ON THE LIVER. There have been several reports of hepatotoxicity after the intravenous administration of oxacillin sodium (W.E. Dismukes, *J. Am. med. Ass.*, 1973, *226*, 861; R.N. Olans and L.B. Weiner, *J. Pediat.*, 1976, *89*, 835; I. Klein and H. Tobias, *Am. J. Gastroent. N.Y.*, 1976, *65*, 546; A. Denny *et al.*, *Ann. intern. Med.*, 1979, *90*, 277; C. Taylor *et al.*, *ibid.*, 857; P.A. Michelson, *Can. J. Hosp. Pharm.*, 1981, *34*, 83). Most of these reactions were characterised by raised liver enzyme values, particularly serum aspartate and alanine aminotransferases (SGOT and SGPT), accompanied in some cases by fever, nausea, vomiting, eosinophilia, rash, or liver enlargement or tenderness. Onorato and Axelrod (*Ann. intern. Med.*, 1978, *89*, 497) carried out a retrospective study of the records of 54 patients who had received oxacillin by intravenous injection at a daily dosage greater than 6 g. Eight had developed hepatitis during treatment, the symptoms occurring 2 to 21 days after its commencement and after a total dose of 16 to 300 g.

The authors of most of the above reports concluded that the adverse effects of oxacillin on the liver were probably due to a hypersensitivity reaction, and in most patients liver function returned to normal after withdrawal of the drug. In a few patients, nafcillin or benzylpenicillin was substituted for oxacillin without ill-effect. Several authors recommended evaluation of liver function tests in patients receiving therapy with intravenous oxacillin, particularly if given in high doses or for long periods.

Although most of the hepatic reactions to oxacillin that have been reported appear to be anicteric, Ten Pas and Quinn (*J. Am. med. Ass.*, 1965, *191*, 674) reported cholestatic jaundice in a 65-year-old woman after she had received oxacillin sodium by mouth.

EFFECTS ON THE NERVOUS SYSTEM. For a report of convulsions associated with oxacillin therapy in one patient, see Benzylpenicillin Sodium, p.133.

Precautions
As for Benzylpenicillin Sodium, p.133.

ADMINISTRATION IN RENAL FAILURE. For reference to the precautions to be observed in renal failure, see below under Uses, Administration in Renal Failure.

INTERACTIONS. *Antimicrobials.* Concurrent administration of mezlocillin and oxacillin to 16 patients caused an increase in plasma-oxacillin concentrations as a result of a reduction in both its renal and non-renal elimination. The decrease in renal clearance was probably largely due to competitive inhibition of a saturable tubular transport system. In contrast, mezlocillin caused no relevant change in the pharmacokinetics of dicloxacillin; the only statistically significant change was a decrease in the cumulative urinary recovery of dicloxacillin over 36 hours. The difference between the effect of mezlocillin on these 2 isoxazolyl penicillins may be attributable to the greater non-renal clearance of oxacillin.— D. Kampf, *J. antimicrob. Chemother.*, 1983, *11*, *Suppl.* C, 25.

Anti-epileptics. For the effect of oxacillin on phenytoin, see under Phenytoin Sodium, p.408.

Oral contraceptives. Report of a pregnancy occurring after administration of oxacillin sodium by mouth for 6 weeks to a woman regularly taking an oral contraceptive.— T. J. Silber, *J. adolesc. Health Care*, 1983, *4*, 287.

For the effects of other drugs on the antimicrobial activity of oxacillin sodium, see below under Antimicrobial Action.

Antimicrobial Action
Oxacillin sodium has a range of antibacterial activity similar to that of flucloxacillin sodium (see p.231).

A concentration of oxacillin of 1 mg per mL was required *in vitro* to kill 90% of 48 clinical isolates of coagulase-negative staphylococci after one hour of exposure to the drug. This concentration may be useful for short-term topical application to shunts and tissues during neurological surgery.— P. R. Fischer *et al.*, *Antimicrob. Ag. Chemother.*, 1984, *25*, 502.

ACTIVITY WITH OTHER ANTIMICROBIAL AGENTS. *Aminoglycosides.* Studies *in vitro* have shown synergistic activity between oxacillin and various aminoglycosides. Watanakunakorn and Glotzbecker (*Antimicrob. Ag. Chemother.*, 1977, *12*, 346) demonstrated enhancement of the activity of oxacillin against *Staphylococcus aureus* when used in conjunction with netilmicin or sissomicin. In an earlier study (*idem.*, 1974, *6*, 802), however, its activity was enhanced by a range of aminoglycosides against fewer strains of *Staph. aureus* than for most of the other antibiotics tested. Enhanced oxacillin activity by gentamicin or netilmicin has also been reported against some enterococci (J.J. Rahal and M.S. Simberkoff, *J. antimicrob. Chemother.*, 1986, *17*, 585).

AMPICILLIN. Ampicillin and oxacillin enhanced the activity of each other *in vitro* against 7 strains of enterococci.— J. Garau and S. A. Kabins, *J. antimicrob. Chemother.*, 1979, *5*, 31.

Rifampicin. Watanakunakorn and Tisone (*Antimicrob. Ag. Chemother.*, 1982, *22*, 920) have demonstrated antagonism between rifampicin and oxacillin *in vitro* against strains of *Staphylococcus aureus*. Traczewski *et al.* (*ibid.*, 1983, *23*, 571), however, observed either a synergistic, additive or indifferent, or antagonistic effect of the combination depending on the method used and the concentration of the 2 drugs.

Resistance

As for Methicillin Sodium, p.259.

Absorption and Fate

Oxacillin sodium is incompletely absorbed from the gastro-intestinal tract. Absorption is reduced by the presence of food in the stomach and is less than with cloxacillin. Peak plasma concentrations of 3 to 6 µg per mL are achieved 1 hour after a dose of 500 mg given by mouth to fasting subjects. Following the intramuscular injection of 500 mg peak plasma concentrations of up to 15 µg per mL are achieved after 30 minutes. Doubling the dose can double the plasma concentration. About 93% of the oxacillin in the circulation is bound to plasma proteins. Oxacillin has been reported to have a plasma half-life of approximately 0.5 hour in healthy subjects. The half-life is prolonged in neonates.

The distribution of oxacillin into body tissues and fluids is similar to that of cloxacillin (p.203).

Oxacillin undergoes some metabolism, and the unchanged drug and metabolites are excreted in the urine by glomerular filtration and renal tubular secretion.

About 20% to 30% of an oral dose and more than 40% of an intramuscular dose is rapidly excreted in the urine. Oxacillin is also excreted in the bile.

Serum concentrations are enhanced if probenecid is given.

ADMINISTRATION IN RENAL FAILURE. For reference to the pharmacokinetics of oxacillin in renal failure, see below under Uses, Administration in Renal Failure.

DIFFUSION INTO BODY TISSUES AND FLUIDS. A study of the penetration of oxacillin into bone and synovial tissue in patients receiving prophylactic intravenous oxacillin for hip replacement surgery.— R. H. Fitzgerald *et al.*, *Antimicrob. Ag. Chemother.*, 1978, *14*, 723.

No oxacillin could be detected in the aqueous humour after the intramuscular administration of 4 doses of oxacillin 500 mg every 6 hours, in association with probenecid.— T. S. Lesar and R. G. Fiscella, *Drug Intell. & clin. Pharm.*, 1985, *19*, 642.

METABOLISM. About 49% of a 500-mg dose of oxacillin was metabolised. Within 12 hours of the dose being taken by 6 healthy subjects 33% was recovered in the urine, 16% as penicilloic acid.— M. Cole *et al.*, *Antimicrob. Ag. Chemother.*, 1973, *3*, 463.

Oxacillin was metabolised to a slightly less potent antibacterial compound.— H. H. W. Thijssen and H. Mattie, *Antimicrob. Ag. Chemother.*, 1976, *10*, 441.

Uses and Administration

Oxacillin sodium is an isoxazolyl penicillin with similar uses to flucloxacillin, p.231.

Oxacillin sodium is administered by mouth preferably 1 or 2 hours before, or at least 2 hours after meals as the presence of food in the stomach reduces absorption. It is given in usual doses equivalent to 500 mg to 1 g of oxacillin four times daily. It may also be given by intramuscular injection in doses of 250 mg to 1 g every 4 to 6 hours. The same dose is given by slow intravenous injection over about 10 minutes, or by intravenous infusion.

Children weighing less than 40 kg should be given the equivalent of 12.5 to 25 mg per kg body-weight every 4 to 6 hours by mouth or parenterally.

A dose of 25 mg per kg body-weight daily in divided doses by injection has been suggested for newborn and premature infants.

All doses may be increased in severe infections.

Oxacillin in association with rifampicin in the treatment of staphylococcal infections.— P. Van der Auwera *et al.*, *Antimicrob. Ag. Chemother.*, 1985, *28*, 467.

For reference to the use of oxacillin for the treatment and prophylaxis of various staphylococcal infections, see under Meningitis, Neutropenia, and Surgical Infection Prophylaxis in flucloxacillin sodium (p.231).

ADMINISTRATION IN INFANTS AND CHILDREN. Doses of intravenous oxacillin sodium for the treatment of severe infections in children and neonates. Suggested doses for neonates were: up to 1 week of age, the equivalent of 75 to 100 mg per kg body-weight of oxacillin daily in 2 to 3 divided doses; from 1 to 4 weeks of age, 100 to 150 mg per kg daily in 3 to 4 divided doses; and above 4 weeks of age, 150 to 200 mg per kg in 3 to 4 divided doses. A suggested dose for children was the equivalent of oxacillin 200 to 300 mg per kg daily given in 4 to 6 divided doses.— K. H. Rhodes and C. M. Johnson, *Mayo Clin. Proc.*, 1983, *58*, 158.

ADMINISTRATION IN RENAL FAILURE. The normal half-life for oxacillin of 0.4 hour was increased to 1 hour in end-stage renal failure. It could be given in usual doses to patients with renal failure. A dosage supplement was not required for patients undergoing haemodialysis or peritoneal dialysis.— W. M. Bennett *et al.*, *Am. J. Kidney Dis.*, 1983, *3*, 155.

ANIMAL BITES. Of 5 patients with cat-bite wounds given prophylaxis with oxacillin 500 mg four times daily by mouth for 5 days, none developed infection. There were 4 infections, however, in the 6 patients given placebo, 3 of which were caused by *Pasteurella multocida*. All infections occurred in patients with puncture wounds, which were considered to be more prone to infection than laceration injuries as are often found after dog bites.— R. M. Elenbaas *et al.*, *Ann. emerg. Med.*, 1984, *13*, 155.

SURGICAL INFECTION PROPHYLAXIS. *Cardiac surgery.* For reference to the use of oxacillin sodium for prophylaxis of infection in cardiac surgery, see flucloxacillin sodium (p.232).

Neurosurgery. A study of the use of oxacillin for prophylaxis of meningitis in patients undergoing neurosurgery for implantation of a CSF shunt. In the group of 30 patients given intravenous oxacillin 200 mg per kg daily in divided doses every 4 hours for a period of 24 hours covering the operation, meningitis caused by *Acinetobacter* occurred in one. In the control group, meningitis developed in 6 of 30 patients; cultures were positive in only 3, and yielded methicillin-susceptible staphylococci in all cases.— M. Djindjian *et al.*, *Surg. Neurol.*, 1986, *25*, 178.

For reference to the possible topical use of oxacillin in neurosurgery, see Antimicrobial Action, above.

Preparations

Oxacillin Sodium Capsules *(U.S.P.)*

Oxacillin Sodium for Injection *(U.S.P.)*. pH of a 3% solution 6.0 to 8.5.

Sterile Oxacillin Sodium *(U.S.P.)*

Oxacillin Sodium for Oral Solution *(U.S.P.)*

Proprietary Names and Manufacturers

Bactocill *(Beecham Laboratories, USA)*; Bristopen *(Bristol, Fr.)*; Cryptocillin *(Hoechst, Ger.)*; Penistafil *(Antibioticos, Spain)*; Penstapho *(Bristol, Belg.*; *Bristol Italiana Sud, Ital.)*; Pro-Staphlin *(Lundbeck, Denm.)*; Prostaphlin *(Bristol, Canad.*; *Bristol, USA)*; Stapenor *(Bayer, Ger.)*.

5665-m

Oxolinic Acid *(BAN, USAN, rINN).*

W-4565. 5-Ethyl-5,8-dihydro-8-oxo-1,3-dioxolo[4,5-*g*]-quinoline-7-carboxylic acid.

$C_{13}H_{11}NO_5$=261.2.

CAS — 14698-29-4.

Pharmacopoeias. In *Cz.*

Adverse Effects and Precautions

As for nalidixic acid (p.266). The incidence of adverse effects on the CNS is greater with oxolinic acid.

Nitrofurantoin has been reported to antagonise the activity of oxolinic acid *in vitro*.

Antimicrobial Action

Oxolinic acid is bactericidal and has a similar antibacterial spectrum and mode of action to nalidixic acid (see p.267) but is reported to be more active *in vitro*; in addition activity against *Staphylococcus aureus* has been demonstrated. Minimum inhibitory concentrations below 5 µg per mL have been reported for Gram-negative urinary pathogens.

Bacterial resistance may develop rapidly and cross-resistance with nalidixic acid and cinoxacin occurs. Nitrofurantoin may antagonise the activity of oxolinic acid against some organisms.

Oxolinic acid was more active *in vitro* than nalidixic acid or cinoxacin against 138 strains of *Shigella sonnei* and *Sh. flexneri* with an MIC of 1.56 µg per mL compared with 6.25 µg per mL for the other two.— R. C. Gordon *et al.*, *Antimicrob. Ag. Chemother.*, 1976, *10*, 918.

Absorption and Fate

Oxolinic acid is poorly but rapidly absorbed from the gastro-intestinal tract. It is extensively metabolised and conjugated, and then excreted in the urine. Some metabolites are active.

Excretion in milk and faeces is also stated to occur.

A mean peak serum concentration of 0.8 µg per mL was obtained 2 to 6 hours after a dose of oxolinic acid in a study involving 15 healthy subjects who received oxolinic acid 750 mg every 12 hours for one or more doses. The mean peak urinary concentration of 9.1 µg per mL achieved after one dose increased to 19.7 µg per mL after 5 doses, with a wide range of individual urinary concentrations being obtained. About 1% of a dose was excreted in the urine as active drug within 8 hours.— M. J. Kershaw and D. A. Leigh, *J. antimicrob. Chemother.*, 1975, *1*, 311.

Between 80 and 85% of oxolinic acid was bound to serum protein.— R. C. Gordon *et al.*, *Antimicrob. Ag. Chemother.*, 1976, *10*, 918.

On the first day of administration of oxolinic acid 750 mg twice daily for 7 days, mean peak serum concentrations of 1.4 µg per mL (total drug) and 0.7 µg per mL (unconjugated drug) were obtained after 3 hours in 10 healthy subjects; these concentrations had risen to 6.4 and 3.6 µg per mL respectively by the third day and were similar on the seventh day. The apparent half-life was about 4 hours for the first 3 days but on the seventh day a two-process elimination was seen with half-lives of 1½ and 15 hours. Steady-state urinary concentrations of 570 µg per mL (total drug) and 35 µg per mL (unconjugated drug) were obtained during the study. Oxolinic acid was about 77 to 81% bound to plasma proteins.— P. T. Männistö, *Clin. Pharmac. Ther.*, 1976, *19*, 37.

Uses and Administration

Oxolinic acid is a 4-quinolone antimicrobial agent and has been used similarly to nalidixic acid (see p.267) in the treatment of urinary-tract infections. It has been given in a usual dose of 750 mg every 12 hours for 7 to 14 days, preferably after food.

URINARY-TRACT INFECTIONS. Although review of the literature suggests that oxolinic acid is effective in the treatment of acute and recurrent urinary-tract infections it appears to offer little advantage over other agents (R. Gleckman *et al.*, *Am. J. Hosp. Pharm.*, 1979, *36*, 1077) and some workers consider that because of the high incidence of adverse effects oxolinic acid is not suitable for routine use (S. Kalowski and P. Kincaid-Smith, *Clin. exp. Pharmac. Physiol.*, 1978, *5*, 244). However, it may be of some use as an alternative form of therapy in the treatment of recurrent urinary-tract infections uncomplicated by bacteraemia in patients hypersensitive to penicillins, cephalosporins, or sulphonamides or for the treatment of infections highly resistant to other therapy (S. Kalowski *et al.*, *Med. J. Aust.*, 1979, *1*, 345).

For a comparison of the efficacy of oxolinic acid and other 4-quinolone antimicrobial agents in the treatment/prophylaxis of urinary-tract infections, see Norfloxacin, p.275.

Proprietary Names and Manufacturers
Decme *(Poli, Ital.)*; Emyrenil *(Valles Mestre, Spain)*; Gramurin *(Chinoin, Hung.)*; Nefroclar *(Hosbon, Spain)*; Nidantin *(Sasse, Ger.)*; Oribiox *(Bohm, Spain)*; Ossian *(Bioindustria, Ital.)*; Oxalin *(Prodes, Spain)*; Oxobid *(Warner, NZ)*; Oxoboi *(Boi, Spain)*; Oxoinex *(Inexfa, Spain)*; Oxol *(Spain)*; Oxolin *(Prodes, Spain)*; Oxolina *(Rorer, Ital.)*; Pelvis *(Coli, Ital.)*; Pietil *(Argentia, Arg.)*; Prodoxol *(Warner, S.Afr.*; *Warner, UK)*; Tilvis *(Scharper, Ital.)*; Tiurasin *(Bouty, Ital.)*; Tropodil *(Elea, Arg.)*; Urinox *(Parke, Davis, Arg.)*; Uristatic *(Frumtost, Spain)*; Uritrate *(Parke, Davis, Ital.*; *Parke, Davis, Spain)*; Uro-Alvar *(Oftalmiso, Spain)*; Uropax *(Spain)*; Urotrate *(Substantia, Fr.)*; Uroxin *(Von Boch, Ital.)*; Uroxol *(Ausonia, Ital.)*; Utibid *(Warner, Austral.*; *Parke, Davis, USA)*.

121-d

Oxytetracycline *(BAN, USAN, rINN)*.

5-Hydroxytetracycline; Oxytetracycline Dihydrate; Oxytetracyclinum; Terrafungine. 5β-Hydroxytetracycline.
$C_{22}H_{24}N_2O_9$=460.4.

CAS — 79-57-2 (anhydrous); 6153-64-6 (dihydrate).

Pharmacopoeias. In *Arg., Aust., Br., Cz., Eur., Fr., Ger., Hung., Ind., It., Jug., Neth., Nord., Pol., Rus., Swiss,* and *U.S.*. Also in *B.P. Vet. Swiss* specifies the anhydrous form.

An antimicrobial substance produced by the growth of certain strains of *Streptomyces rimosus*, or by any other means. It contains a variable quantity of water. It occurs as an odourless yellow to tan-coloured crystalline powder. The *B.P.* specifies that it contains not less than 930 units per mg, calculated with reference to the anhydrous substance. The *U.S.P.* specifies not less than 832 µg of oxytetracycline per mg. Stable in air but darkens on exposure to strong sunlight. Oxytetracycline dihydrate 1.08 g is approximately equivalent to 1 g of oxytetracycline.

Very slightly **soluble** in water; soluble 1 in 66 of dehydrated alcohol and 1 in 6250 of ether; sparingly soluble in alcohol; practically insoluble in chloroform; soluble in dilute acids and alkalis. A 1% suspension in water has a pH of 4.5 to 7.5; the *U.S.P.* injection has a pH of 8.0 to 9.0. It deteriorates in solutions having a pH of less than 2 and is rapidly destroyed by alkali hydroxide solutions. **Store** in airtight containers. Protect from light.

120-f

Oxytetracycline Calcium *(BANM, USAN, rINNM)*.

The calcium salt of 5β-hydroxytetracycline.
$C_{44}H_{46}CaN_4O_{18}$=958.9.

CAS — 15251-48-6 (xCa).

Pharmacopoeias. In *Br.* and *U.S.*

A pale yellow to greenish-fawn or light brown crystalline powder. The *U.S.P.* specifies that it contains not less than 865 µg of oxytetracycline per mg calculated on the anhydrous basis. Oxytetracycline calcium 1.04 g is approximately equivalent to 1 g of oxytetracycline.

Practically **insoluble** in water; soluble in dilute acids and in dilute solutions of sodium hydroxide. A 2.5% suspension in water has a pH of about 6 to 8. **Store** in a cool place in airtight containers. Protect from light.

122-n

Oxytetracycline Hydrochloride *(BANM, USAN, rINNM)*.

Chlorhydrate de Terrafungine. 5β-Hydroxytetracycline hydrochloride.
$C_{22}H_{24}N_2O_9$,HCl=496.9.

CAS — 2058-46-0.

Pharmacopoeias. In *Arg., Aust., Belg., Br., Chin., Cz., Egypt., Eur., Fr., Ger., Hung., Ind., Int., It., Jpn, Jug., Neth., Nord., Rus., Swiss, Turk.,* and *U.S.* Also in *B.P. Vet.*

A yellow, odourless, hygroscopic, crystalline powder. The *B.P.* specifies that it contains not less than 860 units per mg of anhydrous oxytetracycline hydrochloride. The *U.S.P.* specifies that it contains not less than 835 µg of oxytetracycline per mg calculated on the dried basis. Oxytetracycline hydrochloride 1.08 g is approximately equivalent to 1 g of oxytetracycline. It decomposes above 180°. It darkens on exposure to sunlight or to moist air above 90°, but there is little loss of potency.

Soluble 1 in 2 of water and 1 in 45 of alcohol; less soluble in dehydrated alcohol; practically insoluble in chloroform and ether. The *B.P.* specifies that a 1% solution in water has a pH of 2.3 to 2.9; the *U.S.P.* specifies that a 1% solution has a pH of 2.0 to 3.0 and a 2.5% solution of the injection has a pH of 1.8 to 2.8.

Solutions in water become turbid on standing owing to hydrolysis and precipitation of oxytetracycline base. Oxytetracycline hydrochloride deteriorates in solutions having a pH of less than 2 and is rapidly destroyed by alkali hydroxide solutions. **Store** in airtight containers. Protect from light.

Incompatibility has been reported with alkalis, aminophylline, amphotericin, ampicillin sodium, soluble barbiturates, benzylpenicillin, carbenicillin sodium, cefapirin sodium, cephalothin sodium, cephazolin sodium, cloxacillin sodium, erythromycin salts, iron dextran injection, methicillin sodium, oxacillin sodium, phenytoin sodium, sodium bicarbonate, sulphadiazine sodium, and sulphafurazole diethanolamine. Incompatibility has also been reported, generally less consistently, with calcium chloride, calcium gluconate, chloramphenicol sodium succinate, heparin sodium, hydrocortisone sodium succinate, lactated Ringer's injection, protein hydrolysate, and sodium lactate, and, depending on the diluent, with amikacin sulphate.

STABILITY IN SOLUTION. Oxytetracycline in glucose injection 5% at pH 3.22 lost 17% activity in 12 hours, increasing to 25% after 24 hours.— J. N. Bair and D. P. Carew, *Bull. parent. Drug Ass.*, 1965, *19*, 153.

A study of the effects of pH and temperature on the degradation of oxytetracycline in aqueous solutions. Maximum stability occurred at pH 2.— B. Vej-Hansen *et al.*, *Arch. Pharm. Chemi, scient. Edn*, 1978, *6*, 151.

Units

One unit of oxytetracycline is contained in 0.0011364 mg of the second International Standard Preparation (1966) of oxytetracycline base dihydrate which contains 880 units per mg.

Adverse Effects and Precautions

As for Tetracycline Hydrochloride, p.314.

Oxytetracycline may produce less tooth discoloration than most other tetracyclines.

In a study involving 7 geriatric patients given parenteral nutrition with an amino acid solution and glucose, infusions of oxytetracycline 1 g daily produced a negative nitrogen balance within 1 or 2 days and very high peak blood concentrations. A dose of 500 mg had a similar effect on nitrogen balance. Folic acid supplements for those with folate deficiency prevented this effect. Doxycycline 100 mg by infusion daily had only slight if any effect on nitrogen balance.— J. Korkeila, *Ann. clin. Res.*, 1974, *6*, 25.

Oxytetracycline tablets may cause oesophagitis in the normal oesophagus.— D. A. W. Edwards, *Postgrad. med. J.*, 1984, *60*, 737. See also under Effects on the Gastro-intestinal Tract in Doxycycline Hydrochloride, p.217.

A report of pseudomembranous colitis in a 51-year-old woman who received oral oxytetracycline for perioral dermatitis. The Committee on Safety of Medicines had had no reports of pseudomembranous colitis in association with tetracycline and the association between tetracyclines and pseudomembranous colitis is presumably rare, but recognition that it may occur with this group of antibiotics is important.— A. J. Treloar and A. N. Hamlyn (letter), *Br. med. J.*, 1987, *295*, 1001.

For mention of oxytetracycline causing photosensitivity reactions, see under Doxycycline Hydrochloride, p.217.

PREGNANCY AND THE NEONATE. Oxytetracycline and hydrocortisone ointment has been used to control hypergranulation in burns and open wounds. Although oxytetracycline produces less severe tooth discoloration than tetracycline, chlortetracycline, demeclocycline, or methacycline, it would seem sensible to avoid applying this ointment to excessive raw areas during the last 2 trimesters of pregnancy and in children under 7 years of age.— L. Beeley, *Br. med. J.*, 1983, *286*, 1206.

Absorption and Fate

As for Tetracycline Hydrochloride, p.317.

Some 20 to 35% of oxytetracycline was bound in the body to serum proteins. The half-life in serum was 9.6 hours and 70% was excreted in urine.— C. M. Kunin, *Ann. intern. Med.*, 1967, *67*, 151.

Studies in 36 subjects with normal or impaired renal function demonstrated that in normal subjects the half-life in serum was 9.3 hours and that the urinary clearance was 82% of the glomerular filtration. In those subjects with impaired kidney function urinary excretion decreased in proportion to the decrease in glomerular filtration and so lengthened the half-life in serum. In 3 patients with a creatinine clearance rate between 0 and 2 mL per minute, the mean serum half-life of oxytetracycline was reduced from 54 to 12 hours by haemodialysis.— G. Mérier *et al.*, *Schweiz. med. Wschr.*, 1970, *100*, 1442.

DIFFUSION INTO BODY TISSUES AND FLUIDS. A study of tissue concentrations of oxytetracycline following intravenous administration.— F. Legler and K. Schwemmle, *Arzneimittel-Forsch.*, 1974, *24*, 185.

Sputum. The average sputum concentration of oxytetracycline in 9 patients with acute exacerbations of chronic chest disease was 1 µg per mL after receiving oxytetracycline 500 mg 4 times daily for 4 days; the corresponding serum concentration was 3.7 µg per mL.— T. D. Brogan *et al.*, *J. antimicrob. Chemother.*, 1977, *3*, 247.

PREGNANCY AND THE NEONATE. The concentration of oxytetracycline in foetal blood was one-quarter that of the maternal blood.— P. Demers *et al.*, *Can. med. Ass. J.*, 1968, *99*, 849.

Uses and Administration

Oxytetracycline has the antimicrobial activity and uses described for tetracycline hydrochloride (see p.315).

Oxytetracycline is usually used in tablets, the calcium salt in aqueous oral suspensions, and the hydrochloride in capsules and intravenous injections; the calcium and hydrochloride salts are also used in topical preparations. Doses are expressed confusingly as oxytetracycline, the dihydrate, or the hydrochloride; in practice this appears to make little difference.

Oxytetracycline is usually given in doses of 250 to 500 mg four times daily by mouth, usually one hour before food or 2 hours after food; up to 2 g daily may be given by intravenous infusion in divided doses. Children have been given 25 to 50 mg per kg body-weight daily by mouth, in 4 divided doses, and up to 20 mg per kg daily by intravenous infusion, but the effect of tetracyclines on teeth should be considered.

Oxytetracycline is sometimes given intramuscularly, but this route may be painful and produces lower blood concentrations than oral administration in the recommended doses.

ADMINISTRATION. Oxytetracycline may cause oesophagitis or oesophageal ulceration and tablets or capsules should therefore be given with at least 100 mL of water while the patient is in an upright sitting position.— S. K. Vong and R. K. Parekh (letter), *Pharm. J.*, 1987, *1*, 5.

ADMINISTRATION IN RENAL FAILURE. The use of oxytetracycline should be avoided in patients with even mild renal failure; doxycycline may be used if necessary.— G. B. Appel and H. C. Neu, *New Engl. J. Med.*, 1977, *296*, 663.

EYE INFECTIONS. Ocular rosacea responded to treatment with oxytetracycline 250 mg twice daily by mouth for 6 weeks in 11 of 35 patients, and with repeated or continuous treatment 19 of 35 patients achieved a sustained remission for 8 months. Most patients showed a delay of 2 weeks in response to oxytetracycline, and relapses generally occurred 2 to 3 weeks after drug withdrawal.— R. S. Bartholomew *et al.*, *Br. J. Ophthal.*, 1982, *66*, 386.

For reference to the use of oxytetracycline in the treatment of trachoma, see under Trachoma, below. See also under Tetracycline Hydrochloride, p.322.

LEGIONNAIRES' DISEASE. For mention of the use of oxytetracycline in association with rifampicin in the treatment of legionnaires' disease, see under Rifampicin, p.576.

MEDITERRANEAN SPOTTED FEVER. Oxytetracycline 50 mg per kg body-weight daily by mouth for 7 days was effective in the treatment of 60 children with boutonneuse fever, also known as Mediterranean fever, which is prevalent in Mediterranean areas and is caused by *Rickettsia conorii*.— F. A. Moraga *et al.*, *Archs Dis. Childh.*, 1982, *57*, 149.

PREGNANCY AND THE NEONATE. A report of chlamydial pneumonia in 5 neonates who did not respond to treatment with either erythromycin or sulphonamides. Three patients improved, however, when treated with oxytetracycline given intravenously. Neonates with pneumonia associated with isolation of *Chlamydia trachomatis* in their tracheal secretions should initially be treated with erythromycin or a sulphonamide for 2 weeks. If no improvement occurs, however, treatment with oxytetracycline for 2 weeks may be justifiable.— A. A. Attenburrow and C. M. Barker, *Archs Dis. Childh.*, 1985, *60*, 1169.

RESPIRATORY-TRACT INFECTIONS. For comment on the use of tetracyclines in the treatment of bronchitis, see under Tetracycline Hydrochloride, p.320.

SEXUALLY TRANSMITTED DISEASES. Tetracyclines have been the standard treatment for nongonococcal urethritis for many years. The dosage of oxytetracycline has varied considerably, ranging from the smallest effective dose of 250 mg twice daily for 7 days, to 500 mg four times daily for 7 or 10 days. Where oxytetracycline is specifically contra-indicated, as in patients with renal failure, then doxycycline should be considered; where tetracyclines are contra-indicated, then erythromycin should be used.— *Drug & Ther. Bull.*, 1983, *21*, 25.

Oxytetracycline 500 mg four times daily by mouth for 14 days, or 21 days if there are complications, is effective treatment for chlamydial genital infections in adults. Tetracyclines should not, of course, be given to pregnant or lactating women.— E. M. C. Dunlop, *Br. J. Hosp. Med.*, 1983, *29*, 6.

In a study of 138 male patients with their first attack of non-specific urethritis oxytetracycline 250 mg four times daily or rifampicin 600 mg daily, both given by mouth for 10 days, were equally effective with a cure rate of 97%, although rifampicin was not considered suitable for routine treatment. Co-trimoxazole or trimethoprim were less effective with cure rates of 75 and 57.5%, respectively.— K. C. Mohanty and R. B. Roy, *Br. J. clin. Pract.*, 1986, *40*, 78.

For further reference to the use of oxytetracycline in the treatment of nongonococcal urethritis, see under Tetracycline Hydrochloride, p.321.

SEPTICAEMIA. Septicaemia due to *Kingella kingae* (*Moraxella kingae*) in a 21-year-old woman with a clinical presentation resembling disseminated gonococcal infection, responded to oxytetracycline 500 mg every 6 hours by mouth.— D. C. Shanson and B. G. Gazzard, *Br. med. J.*, 1984, *289*, 730.

SKIN DISORDERS. *Acne.* Oxytetracycline 500 mg twice daily before meals for at least 6 months is considered the drug of choice for systemic antibacterial treatment of acne vulgaris. If patients are intolerant of oxytetracycline or show no improvement after 3 months, erythromycin 500 mg twice daily before meals may be substituted. Trimethoprim, minocycline, or doxycycline are other possible alternatives.— W. J. Cunliffe, *Prescribers' J.*, 1987, *27*, (4), 23.

See also under Tetracycline Hydrochloride, p.321.

Further references: J. R. Gibson *et al.*, *Br. J. Derm.*, 1982, *107*, 221.

Perioral dermatitis. For the use of oxytetracycline in the treatment of perioral dermatitis, see under Tetracycline Hydrochloride, p.321.

Rosacea. For comparison of oxytetracycline and metronidazole in the treatment of rosacea, see under Metronidazole, p.672.

TRACHOMA. References to the use of oxytetracycline in the treatment of trachoma: S. Darougar *et al.*, *Br. J. Ophthal.*, 1980, *64*, 37; S. Darougar *et al.*, *ibid.*, 291.

See also under Tetracycline Hydrochloride, p.322.

URINARY-TRACT INFECTIONS. For the use of oxytetracycline in the treatment of nongonococcal urethritis, see Sexually Transmitted Diseases, above.

Preparations

Oxytetracycline Capsules *(B.P.)*. Capsules containing oxytetracycline hydrochloride.

Oxytetracycline Hydrochloride Capsules *(U.S.P.)*

Oxytetracycline and Nystatin Capsules *(U.S.P.)*

Oxytetracycline and Phenazopyridine Hydrochlorides and Sulfamethizole Capsules *(U.S.P.)*

Oxytetracycline Hydrochloride for Injection *(U.S.P.)*

Sterile Oxytetracycline Hydrochloride *(U.S.P.)*

Oxytetracycline Injection *(U.S.P.)*

Sterile Oxytetracycline *(U.S.P.)*

Oxytetracycline Hydrochloride and Hydrocortisone Ointment *(U.S.P.)*

Oxytetracycline Hydrochloride and Polymyxin B Sulfate Ointment *(U.S.P.)*

Oxytetracycline Hydrochloride and Polymyxin B Sulfate Ophthalmic Ointment *(U.S.P.)*

Oxytetracycline Hydrochloride and Hydrocortisone Acetate Ophthalmic Suspension *(U.S.P.)*

Oxytetracycline and Nystatin for Oral Suspension *(U.S.P.)*

Oxytetracycline Calcium Oral Suspension *(U.S.P.)*. It may contain *N*-acetylglucosamine. pH 5 to 8.

Oxytetracycline Tablets *(B.P.)*

Oxytetracycline Tablets *(U.S.P.)*

Oxytetracycline Hydrochloride and Polymyxin B Sulfate Topical Powder *(U.S.P.)*

Oxytetracycline Hydrochloride and Polymyxin B Sulfate Vaginal Tablets *(U.S.P.)*

Proprietary Preparations containing Oxytetracycline or its Salts

Berkmycen *(Berk Pharmaceuticals, UK)*. *Tablets*, oxytetracycline 250 mg.

Imperacin *(ICI Pharmaceuticals, UK)*. *Tablets*, oxytetracycline 250 mg.

Oxymycin *(DDSA Pharmaceuticals, UK)*. *Tablets*, oxytetracycline 250 mg.

Terra-Cortril *(Pfizer, UK)*. *Ear-drops*, oxytetracycline 5 mg (as hydrochloride), polymyxin B sulphate 10 000 units, hydrocortisone acetate 15 mg/mL.
Ointment, oxytetracycline 3% (as hydrochloride), hydrocortisone 1%.
Topical spray, aerosol, oxytetracycline 0.5% (as hydrochloride), hydrocortisone 0.17%.

Terra-Cortril Nystatin *(Pfizer, UK)*. *Cream*, oxytetracycline 3% (as calcium salt), nystatin 100 000 units/g, hydrocortisone 1%.

Terramycin *(Pfizer, UK)*. *Capsules*, oxytetracycline 250 mg (as hydrochloride).
Tablets, oxytetracycline 250 mg.

Unimycin *(Unigreg, UK)*. *Capsules*, oxytetracycline hydrochloride 250 mg.

Proprietary Names and Manufacturers of Oxytetracycline or its Salts

Abbocin *(Abbott, UK)*; Berkmycen *(Berk Pharmaceuticals, UK)*; Betacycline *(Restan, S.Afr.)*; Bramcycline *(Austral.)*; Chemocycline *(Consolidated Chemicals, UK)*; Clinimycin *(Glaxo, UK)*; Clinmycin; Crisamicin *(Spain)*; Duratetracyclin *(Durachemie, Ger.)*; Elaciclina *(Spain)*; E.P. Mycin *(Edwards, USA)*; Galenomycin *(Galen, UK)*; Geobiotico *(Spain)*; Gynamousse *(Fr.)*; Huberbiotic *(Spain)*; Humusmycin *(Spain)*; Imperacin *(ICI Pharmaceuticals, UK)*; Inoxtet *(S.Afr.)*; Lenocyclin *(S.Afr.)*; Macocyn *(Mack, Illert., Ger.)*; O-4 Cycline *(GS, S.Afr.)*; Oppamycin *(LRC Products, UK)*; Oxim *(S.Afr.)*; Oxycyclin *(Dumex, Denm.)*; Oxycycline *(Austral.)*; Oxydon *(R.P. Drugs, UK)*; Oxy-Dumocyclin *(Dumex, Norw.; Dumex, Swed.)*; Oxylag *(Switz.)*; Oxymed *(Unimed, UK)*; Oxymycin *(Lennon, S.Afr.; DDSA Pharmaceuticals, UK; Forest Pharmaceuticals, USA)*; Oxypan *(Propan, S.Afr.)*; Oxy-Rivo *(Switz.)*; Oxytetral *(A.L., Denm.; Apothekernes Laboratorium, Norw.; A. L., Swed.)*; Posicycline *(P.O.S., Fr.)*; Proteroxyna *(Proter, Ital.)*; Roxy *(Rio, S.Afr.)*; Stecsolin *(Squibb, UK)*; Terraject *(Belg.)*; Terramicina *(Ital.; Pfizer, Spain)*; Terramycin *(Pfizer, Austral.; Canad.; Pfizer, Ger.; Neth.; Pfizer, S.Afr.; Switz.; Pfizer, UK; Pfizer, USA)*; Terramycin Intramuscular *(Roerig, USA)*; Terramycine *(Belg.; Pfizer, Fr.; Pfizer, Switz.)*; Terramyfar *(Spain)*; Terraveineuse *(Pfizer, Switz.)*; Terraven *(Arg.; Belg.)*; Terravenös *(Pfizer, Ger.; Switz.)*; Tetramel *(MPS Lab., S.Afr.)*; Tetra-Tablinen *(Beiersdorf, Ger.)*; Unimycin *(Unigreg, UK)*; Uri-Tet *(American Urologicals, USA)*; Vendarcin *(Belg.; Neth.; Switz.)*; Vernacycline *(Vernleigh, S.Afr.)*.

The following names have been used for multi-ingredient preparations containing oxytetracycline or its salts—
Bisolvomycin *(Boehringer Ingelheim, UK)*; Terra-Bron *(Pfizer, UK)*; Terra-Cortril *(Roerig, USA)*; Terra-Cortril Ear Suspension *(Pfizer, UK)*; Terra-Cortril Nystatin *(Pfizer, UK)*; Terra-Cortril Spray *(Pfizer, UK)*; Terra-Cortril Topical Ointment *(Pfizer, UK)*; Terramycin Ointment *(Pfipharmecs, USA)*; Terramycin Ophthalmic Ointment with Polymyxin B Sulphate *(Pfizer, Austral.; Pfizer, UK; Roerig, USA)*; Terramycin SF *(Pfizer, UK)*; Trimovate Cream *(Glaxo, UK)*; Urobiotic *(Roerig, USA)*.

123-h

Paromomycin Sulphate *(BANM, rINNM)*.

Aminosidinum Sulfuricum; Amminosidina Solfato; Catenulin; Paromomycin Sulfate *(USAN)*.

4-*O*-(2-Amino-2-deoxy-α-D-glucopyranosyl)-2-deoxy-5-*O*-[3-*O*-(2,6-diamino-2,6-dideoxy-β-L-idopyranosyl)-β-D-ribofuranosyl]-D-streptamine sulphate.

$C_{23}H_{45}N_5O_{14},xH_2SO_4$=615.6 (paromomycin).

CAS — 7542-37-2 (paromomycin); 1263-89-4 (sulphate).

NOTE. Aminosidin Sulphate (Crestomycin Sulphate) produced by the growth of *Streptomyces chrestomyceticus* was shown by R.T. Schillings and C.P. Schaffner (*Antimicrob. Ag. Chemother.*, 1961, 274) to be identical with paromomycin sulphate.

Monomycin, an antibiotic, isolated from *Streptomyces circulatus* var. *monomycini* (see *Martindale 26th Edn.*, p.1386) is considered to be identical with paromomycin.

Pharmacopoeias. In *Chin.*, *It.*, and *U.S.*

A mixture of the sulphates of the antimicrobial substances produced by the growth of certain strains of *Streptomyces rimosus* forma *paromomycinus*.

A creamy-white to light yellow, odourless or almost odourless, hygroscopic powder containing not less than 675 μg per mg, calculated on the dried material.

Very **soluble** in water; practically insoluble in alcohol, chloroform, and ether. A 3% solution in water has a pH of 5.0 to 7.5. **Store** in airtight containers.

Units

One unit of paromomycin is contained in 0.001333 mg of the first International Reference Preparation (1965) of paromomycin sulphate which contains 750 units per mg.

Adverse Effects, Treatment, and Precautions

As for Neomycin Sulphate, p.268.

Antimicrobial Action

Paromomycin sulphate has an antimicrobial spectrum similar to that of neomycin sulphate (p.269). *Entamoeba histolytica* has also been reported to be sensitive to paromomycin.

Good activity *in vitro* of paromomycin sulphate against *Leishmania major* in mouse peritoneal macrophages.—

J. El-On and C. L. Greenblatt, *Curr. ther. Res.*, 1983, *33*, 660.

Resistance

There is cross-resistance between paromomycin, kanamycin, framycetin, and neomycin.

Absorption and Fate

Paromomycin is poorly absorbed from the gastro-intestinal tract and most of the dose is eliminated in the faeces.

Uses and Administration

Paromomycin sulphate is an aminoglycoside antibiotic which has been administered by mouth in the treatment of intestinal amoebiasis. A recommended dose for both adults and children is the equivalent of 25 to 35 mg of paromomycin per kg body-weight daily in 3 divided doses for 5 to 10 days. Paromomycin has also been effective in the treatment of tapeworm infection.

It has also been used similarly to neomycin (see p.269) in the suppression of intestinal flora both pre-operatively and in the management of hepatic coma.

AMOEBIASIS. Treatment of amoebiasis in 114 homosexual men with paromomycin sulphate.— P. M. Sullam (letter), *New Engl. J. Med.*, 1987, *316*, 690.

BALANTIDIASIS. For a description of balantidiasis and mention of the use of paromomycin sulphate in its treatment, see under Antiprotozoal Agents, p.659.

LEISHMANIASIS. In a preliminary study, 2 patients with recurrent cutaneous leishmaniasis caused by *Leishmania tropica* were treated with an ointment containing paromomycin sulphate 15% and methylbenzethonium chloride 1% twice daily for 80 to 85 days. Healing was complete after treatment in one patient and within 3 to 4 weeks of the end of treatment in the other.— J. El-On *et al.*, *Br. med. J.*, 1985, *291*, 704. Encouraging results in 67 patients with acute cutaneous leishmaniasis caused by *L. major* treated twice daily for 10 days with a similar ointment. Pigmentation and inflammation occurred in some treated lesions.— J. El-On *et al.* (letter), *ibid.*, 1280.

TAPEWORM INFECTIONS. Paromomycin may be used as an alternative to the anthelmintics niclosamide and praziquantel in the treatment of tapeworm infections. The usual dose is 1 g for adults, or 11 mg per kg body-weight for children, given every 15 minutes for 4 doses. For *Hymenolepis nana* infections adults and children may be given a dose of 45 mg per kg once daily for 5 to 7 days.— *Med. Lett.*, 1986, *28*, 9.

Preparations

Paromomycin Sulfate Capsules *(U.S.P.)*
Paromomycin Sulfate Syrup *(U.S.P.)*

Proprietary Names and Manufacturers

Aminoxidin *(Ital.)*; Gabbromicina *(Montedison, Arg.)*; Gabbromycin *(Farmitalia, Ger.)*; Gabbroral *(Montedison, Arg.*; *Farmitalia Carlo Erba, Belg.*; *Carlo Erba, Ital.)*; Gabromicina *(Farmitalia, Spain)*; Gabroral *(Farmitalia, Spain)*; Humagel *(Substantia, Fr.)*; Humatin *(Belg.*; *Substantia, Fr.*; *Parke, Davis, Ger.*; *Parke, Davis, Ital.*; *Substantia, Neth.*; *Parke, Davis, Spain*; *Parke, Davis, Swed.*; *Parke, Davis, Switz.*; *Parke, Davis, UK*; *Parke, Davis, USA)*; Paramicina *(Ragionieri, Ital.)*; Sinosid *(SIFI, Ital.)*.

16941-p

Pefloxacin *(BAN, USAN)*.

1589-RB; EU-5306; Pefloxacine *(rINN)*; Perfloxacin; RB-1589. 1-Ethyl-6-fluoro-1,4-dihydro-7-(4-methyl-1-piperazinyl)-4-oxo-3-quinolinecarboxylic acid.
$C_{17}H_{20}FN_3O_3$=333.4.

CAS — 70458-92-3.

Pefloxacin is a fluorinated 4-quinolone antimicrobial agent with actions similar to those of norfloxacin (see p.274). It is administered as the mesylate for the treatment of both systemic and urinary-tract infections. One of its metabolites is norfloxacin.

The usual dose is 400 mg twice daily by mouth. It has also been given by intravenous infusion in similar doses.

ABSORPTION AND FATE. Three healthy subjects were given on separate occasions pefloxacin in doses of 200, 400, 600, or 800 mg by mouth or by intravenous infusion over one hour. After intravenous infusion plasma concentrations showed a biphasic decline with mean half-lives of about 9 minutes and 11.5 hours respectively. Pharmacokinetic parameters were similar after intravenous and oral administration and remained constant in the dose range used. The bioavailability of the oral form was close to 100%. About 13.5 to 14.5% of the orally administered dose was excreted unchanged in the urine.— J. Barre *et al.*, *J. pharm. Sci.*, 1984, *73*, 1379.

Administration of pefloxacin 400 mg by mouth as the dihydrate mesylate to 6 healthy subjects produced mean peak plasma concentrations of 3.77 µg per mL as determined by bioassay or 3.84 µg per mL as determined using high pressure liquid chromatography; the mean apparent elimination half-lives were 10.1 hours and 8.6 hours respectively. Pefloxacin was about 20 to 30% bound to plasma proteins. The *N*-desmethyl metabolite of pefloxacin (norfloxacin) and pefloxacin *N*-oxide were detected in plasma. Following administration of pefloxacin 800 mg by mouth to 5 healthy subjects mean urinary concentrations of pefloxacin and norfloxacin during the first 24 hours were 42 and 80 µg per mL respectively. About 8.7% of a dose was recovered in the urine within 72 hours as pefloxacin and 20.2% as norfloxacin. Other metabolites detected in urine were pefloxacin *N*-oxide, oxonorfloxacin, oxopefloxacin, and pefloxacin glucuronide. The *N*-oxide and glucuronide metabolites were the only metabolites which showed little antimicrobial activity *in vitro*. Total recovery in urine of pefloxacin and its identified metabolites was about 59% of the dose. Microbiologically active concentrations between 5 and 30 µg per mL were found in the bile of 3 subjects between 2 and 24 hours after receiving pefloxacin 800 mg, the activity mainly being due to unchanged pefloxacin; the most common metabolites in bile were norfloxacin, the *N*-oxide, and the glucuronide. Biliary concentrations of pefloxacin 2 to 12 hours after dosing were 2 to 5 times greater than plasma concentrations. The mean ratio of conjugated to free pefloxacin in bile was 0.9.— G. Montay *et al.*, *Antimicrob. Ag. Chemother.*, 1984, *25*, 463.

Administration of pefloxacin 800 mg as the mesylate by mouth to 20 patients with respiratory infections produced mean concentrations of pefloxacin in bronchial mucus of 9, 11, 8.1, and 14.1 µg per mL after 1, 2, 3, and 4 hours respectively. The mean percentage ratio of the concentrations of pefloxacin in bronchial mucus to those in serum ranged from about 75% to 116%. Concentrations obtained after 3 days of administration of pefloxacin 400 mg twice daily were similar to those obtained on the first day. Similar results were obtained in a further 15 patients.— C. Morel *et al.*, *Path. Biol., Paris*, 1984, *32*, 516.

The diffusion of pefloxacin into cerebrospinal fluid (CSF) was evaluated in 15 patients receiving treatment with other antibiotics for purulent meningitis and/or ventriculitis. Pefloxacin was administered at 12-hourly intervals in doses of 7.5 mg per kg body-weight or 15 mg per kg given either by mouth (4 patients) or as an intravenous infusion over one hour (11 patients). A mean peak plasma concentration of 10.28 µg per mL and a mean trough concentration of 3.54 µg per mL was obtained in 6 patients who received the low dose intravenously, the corresponding mean concentration in CSF being 4.8 µg per mL. In 5 patients who received the high dose intravenously the mean peak plasma concentration was 20.15 µg per mL, the mean trough concentration 8.21 µg per mL, and the mean concentration in the CSF 8.3 µg per mL. The ratio for pefloxacin in CSF to that in plasma was 58% after the low dose and 52% after the high dose. When pefloxacin was administered by mouth, peak plasma concentrations of 8.2 and 10.0 µg per mL were obtained in one patient who received the low dose. Corresponding trough concentrations were 6.8 and 3.5 µg per mL respectively and concentrations of 3.8 and 3.0 µg per mL were obtained in the CSF. In 3 patients who received the high dose by mouth the mean peak plasma concentration was 21.24 µg per mL and the mean concentration in CSF was 10.17 µg per mL.— M. Wolff *et al.*, *Antimicrob. Ag. Chemother.*, 1984, *26*, 289.

Pefloxacin 400 mg was given by mouth every 12 hours for 7 days to 10 healthy subjects. Concentrations of pefloxacin in saliva were similar to those in serum and were higher on day 7 than day 1. Mean concentrations in the faeces ranged from 122 µg per g on day 2 to 645 µg per g on day 8. On day 10 the mean value was 395 µg per g. There was no effect on buccal flora. With regard to faecal flora, there was a decrease in enterobacteria and *Enterococcus faecalis*.— N. Janin *et al.*, *Antimicrob. Ag. Chemother.*, 1987, *31*, 1665.

Further references to the pharmacokinetics of pefloxacin: A. Salvanet *et al.*, *J. antimicrob. Chemother.*, 1986, *18*, 199 (concentrations in aqueous humour and lens); R. Wise *et al.*, *ibid.*, *Suppl.* D, 71 (comparative pharmacokinetics with 4 other quinolones).

ADMINISTRATION IN HEPATIC FAILURE. The plasma clearance of pefloxacin in 16 patients with cirrhosis was about 30% of that in 12 healthy subjects. It was proposed that this reduction may be due to a reduced rate of hepatic metabolism in patients with cirrhosis. It appears that a single daily dose of 8 mg per kg body-weight given intravenously might be sufficient in these patients.— G. Danan *et al.*, *Clin. Pharmac. Ther.*, 1985, *38*, 439.

ADMINISTRATION IN RENAL FAILURE. Preliminary findings in 15 patients with various degrees of renal failure suggest that modification of the dosage regimen of pefloxacin is not required in renal impairment since its pharmacokinetics are barely affected. This may be due to the importance of metabolism in elimination of the drug. No accumulation of the active *N*-desmethyl metabolite was observed but further study of accumulation of this and the *N*-oxide metabolite after repeated administration is required. Removal of pefloxacin was poor following 4 hours of haemodialysis in 6 further patients with anuria.— G. Montay *et al.*, *Eur. J. clin. Pharmac.*, 1985, *29*, 345.

ANTIMICROBIAL ACTION. As for Norfloxacin, p.274. Some references: A. M. Clarke *et al.*, *J. antimicrob. Chemother.*, 1985, *15*, 39; E. E. J. Ligtvoet and T. Wickerhoff-Minoggio, *ibid.*, *16*, 485.

BRONCHITIS. Forty-three patients with acute purulent exacerbations of chronic bronchitis were treated with pefloxacin 400 mg given twice daily by mouth as the mesylate for 10 days, the first 20 patients receiving the first dose as an intravenous infusion. Although all strains of *Haemophilus influenzae* and *Branhamella catarrhalis* had been eradicated from the sputum of the 42 patients evaluated the day after treatment *Streptococcus pneumoniae* remained in the sputum of 8 of 13 patients originally infected and *Pseudomonas aeruginosa* in 4 of 6 patients. The mean peak sputum concentration of pefloxacin had been about 4.6 µg per mL but it appeared that both *Ps. aeruginosa* and *Str. pneumoniae* frequently became more resistant during treatment, the mean MICs required rising from 2.97 to 16 µg per mL and from 3.8 to 8.3 µg per mL respectively during treatment. The sputum should be examined in order to exclude the presence of *Str. pneumoniae* and *Ps. aeruginosa* before 4-quinolone antimicrobial agents are used to treat lower respiratory-tract infections.— F. P. V. Maesen *et al.*, *J. antimicrob. Chemother.*, 1985, *16*, 379.

BURNS. *Animal* studies of topical burn wound therapy indicated that the silver derivative of pefloxacin was effective against strains of *Pseudomonas aeruginosa* resistant to silver sulphadiazine and also possessed antifungal activity *in vitro*. Pefloxacin mesylate alone lacked significant antifungal activity. There was little systemic absorption of pefloxacin or silver following topical treatment.— S. Modak *et al.*, *Burns*, 1984, *10*, 170.

INTERACTIONS. For the interaction of 4-quinolone antimicrobial agents with xanthines such as caffeine and theophylline, see p.1523 and p.1529.

Proprietary Names and Manufacturers

Peflacine *(Bellon, Fr.)*.

127-g

Penimepicycline *(rINN)*.

N^2-[4-(2-Hydroxyethyl)piperazin-1-ylmethyl]tetracycline (6*R*)-6-(2-phenoxyacetamido)penicillanate.
$C_{45}H_{56}N_6O_{14}S$=937.0.

CAS — 4599-60-4.

Penimepicycline is the phenoxymethylpenicillin salt of a tetracycline compound with the expected actions of these antibiotics.

Proprietary Names and Manufacturers

Cilipenuve *(Hortel, Spain)*; Criseosil *(Montedison, Arg.)*; Mucosiris *(Osiris, Arg.)*; Pénétracyne *(Midy, Fr.)*; Penetracyn *(Midy, Ital.)*; Peniltetra 500 *(Ital.)*; Prestociclina *(Chemil, Ital.)*; Pulmobiotic *(Spain)*; Tetrabiomar *(Cheminova, Spain)*; Ultrabiotic *(Spain)*.

129-p

Phenethicillin Potassium *(BANM)*.

Penicillin B; Pheneticillin Potassium *(rINNM)*; Pheneticillinum Kalicum; Potassium α-Phenoxyethylpenicillin. A mixture of the D(+)- and L(−)-isomers of potassium (6*R*)-6-(2-phenoxypropionamido)penicillanate.
$C_{17}H_{19}KN_2O_5S$=402.5.

CAS — 147-55-7 (phenethicillin); 132-93-4 (potassium salt).

Pharmacopoeias. In *Br., Int.,* and *Jpn.*

A white or almost white powder. 1.1 g of monograph substance is approximately equivalent to 1 g of phenethicillin. Each g of monograph substance represents about 2.5 mmol of potassium. **Soluble** 1 in 1.5 of water, 1 in 85 of alcohol; slightly soluble in dehydrated alcohol and chloroform; practically insoluble in ether. A 10% solution in water has a pH of 5.5 to 7.5. **Store** in well-closed containers.

Adverse Effects and Precautions

These are similar to those of benzylpenicillin (see p.132).

Antimicrobial Action

Phenethicillin potassium has a range of antimicrobial activity similar to that of benzylpenicillin (see p.133) and a similar mode of action. However, it is generally less active than benzylpenicillin or phenoxymethylpenicillin against many susceptible organisms particularly Gram-negative micro-organisms. Phenethicillin is slightly less susceptible to penicillinase than benzylpenicillin and phenoxymethylpenicillin.

Absorption and Fate

Phenethicillin is more resistant to inactivation by the acid of gastric secretions and is more completely absorbed than benzylpenicillin from the gastro-intestinal tract following administration by mouth. Absorption is generally rapid, although variable and is decreased by the presence of food. It is stated to produce higher blood concentrations than phenoxymethylpenicillin. About 75% is bound to plasma protein. The distribution and elimination of phenethicillin is similar to that of benzylpenicillin (see p.135).

A comparison of the pharmacokinetics of phenethicillin potassium and phenoxymethylpenicillin in 10 patients.— D. Overbosch *et al., Br. J. clin. Pharmac.,* 1985, *19,* 657.

METABOLISM. About 31% of a 500-mg dose of phenethicillin was metabolised. Within 12 hours of the dose being taken by 6 healthy subjects, 72% was recovered in the urine, about 22% as penicilloic acid.— M. Cole *et al., Antimicrob. Ag. Chemother.,* 1973, *3,* 463.

Uses and Administration

Phenethicillin potassium is a phenoxypenicillin used similarly to benzylpenicillin (see p.135) in the treatment of mild to moderate infections caused by susceptible Gram-positive organisms.

The usual dosage is the equivalent of 250 to 500 mg of phenethicillin by mouth every 6 hours. Children under 2 years of age may be given one quarter the adult dose and from 2 to 10 years, one half the adult dose. Doses should preferably be taken ½ to 1 hour before food.

The sodium and iodide salts of phenethicillin have also been used.

Preparations

Phenethicillin Capsules *(B.P.).* Capsules containing phenethicillin potassium.

Phenethicillin Oral Solution *(B.P.).* Phenethicillin Elixir; Phenethicillin Syrup. A dry mixture of phenethicillin potassium for reconstitution. pH 4 to 7.

Phenethicillin Tablets *(B.P.).* Tablets containing phenethicillin potassium.

Proprietary Preparations

Broxil *(Beecham Research, UK). Capsules,* phenethicillin 250 mg (as potassium salt). *Syrup,* powder for reconstitution, phenethicillin 125 mg (as potassium salt)/5 mL when reconstituted with water.

Proprietary Names and Manufacturers of Phenethicillin Salts

Altocillin *(Ital.)*; Bendralan *(Antibioticos, Spain)*; Broxil *(Neth.; S.Afr.; Beecham Research, UK)*; Drastina *(Landerlan, Spain)*; Esterloven *(Spain)*; Metilpen *(Ital.)*; Optipen *(Commonwealth Serum Laboratories, Austral.)*; Penicilloral *(Terapeutico M.R., Ital.)*; Penorale *(Lusofarmaco, Ital.)*; Pensig *(Sigma, Austral.)*; Syncillin *(USA)*.

130-n

Phenoxymethylpenicillin *(BAN, rINN)*.

Penicillin V *(USAN)*; Phénomycilline; Phenoxymethyl Penicillin; Phenoxymethylpenicillinum. (6*R*)-6-(2-Phenoxyacetamido)penicillanic acid.
$C_{16}H_{18}N_2O_5S$=350.4.

CAS — 87-08-1.

Pharmacopoeias. In *Arg., Aust., Br., Egypt., Eur., Fr., Ger., Int., It., Jug., Neth., Pol., Roum., Rus., Swiss, Turk.,* and *U.S.* Also in *B.P. Vet.*

Phenoxymethylpenicillin is an antimicrobial acid produced by the growth of certain strains of *Penicillium notatum* or related organisms on a culture medium containing an appropriate precursor, or obtained by any other means.

It is a white crystalline powder; odourless or with a slight characteristic odour.

Very slightly **soluble** in water; soluble 1 in 7 of alcohol; freely soluble in acetone; practically insoluble in fixed oils and liquid paraffin. The *B.P.* specifies that a 0.5% solution in water has a pH of 2.4 to 4.0. The *U.S.P.* specifies that a 3% suspension in water has a pH of 2.5 to 4.0. **Store** in airtight containers.

131-h

Phenoxymethylpenicillin Calcium *(BANM, rINNM)*.

Penicillin V Calcium; Phenoxymethylpenicillinum Calcicum. The dihydrate of the calcium salt of phenoxymethylpenicillin.
$(C_{16}H_{17}N_2O_5S)_2Ca,2H_2O$=774.9.

CAS — 147-48-8 (anhydrous).

Pharmacopoeias. In *Br.* and *Int.* Also in *B.P. Vet.*

A white crystalline powder. 2.2 g of monograph substance is approximately equivalent to 1 g of phenoxymethylpenicillin. Each g of monograph substance represents about 1.3 mmol of calcium. Slowly **soluble** 1 in 120 of water; practically insoluble in fixed oils and liquid paraffin. A 0.5% solution in water has a pH of 5.0 to 7.5. **Store** in well-closed containers.

132-m

Phenoxymethylpenicillin Potassium *(BANM, rINNM)*.

Penicillin V Potassium *(USAN)*; Phenoxymethylpenicillinum Kalicum. The potassium salt of phenoxymethylpenicillin.
$C_{16}H_{17}KN_2O_5S$=388.5.

CAS — 132-98-9.

Pharmacopoeias. In *Br., Braz., Cz., Eur., Fr., Ind., Int., It., Jpn, Neth., Nord., Pol., Swiss,* and *U.S.* Also in *B.P. Vet.*

A white crystalline powder; odourless or with a slight characteristic odour. 1.1 g of monograph substance is approximately equivalent to 1 g of phenoxymethylpenicillin. Each g of monograph substance represents about 2.6 mmol of potassium.

Soluble 1 in 1.5 of water and 1 in 150 of alcohol; practically insoluble in acetone, chloroform, ether, fixed oils, and liquid paraffin. The *B.P.* specifies that a 0.5% solution in water has a pH of 5.5 to 7.5. The *U.S.P.* specifies that a 3% solution in water has a pH of 4.0 to 7.5. **Store** in airtight containers.

STABILITY IN SOLUTION. Results from a study into the penicillin content and stability of diluted antibiotic syrups indicated that these parameters were dependent upon the techniques used to reconstitute the syrups from dry mixtures. Phenoxymethylpenicillin syrups became less stable as the sucrose content of the diluent increased, and separation of dry granules into portions before reconstitution resulted in wide dosage variations. The effect of sucrose content on the stability of ampicillin preparations was found to be more complex, due to the system being a suspension rather than a solution.— J. M. Hempenstall *et al., Int. J. Pharmaceut.,* 1985, *23,* 131.

For a report of a study on the formation of N-formylpenicillamine and penicillamine as degradation products of various penicillins in solution, including phenoxymethylpenicillin, see Benzylpenicillin Sodium, p.132.

Units

One unit of phenoxymethylpenicillin was contained in 0.00059 mg of the first International Standard Preparation (1957) which contained 1695 units per mg. The International Standard was discontinued in 1968.

Adverse Effects

These are similar to those of benzylpenicillin (see p.132).

Phenoxymethylpenicillin is usually well tolerated but may occasionally cause transient nausea and diarrhoea.

EFFECTS ON THE GASTRO-INTESTINAL TRACT. In a study in 10 healthy subjects, Nord and Heimdahl (*J. antimicrob. Chemother.,* 1986, *18, Suppl.* C, 159) observed only minor changes in the oropharyngeal microflora after administration of phenoxymethylpenicillin 800 mg by mouth every 12 hours for 7 days. There was a slight decrease in the numbers of *Streptococcus salivarius* and fusobacteria in most subjects, but no increase in the numbers of resistant bacterial strains. This may have been explained by the absence of detectable concentrations of the drug in saliva. Phenoxymethylpenicillin could not be detected in the faeces, and produced no significant changes in the numbers of aerobic or anaerobic organisms in the intestinal microflora or in the numbers of resistant bacterial strains. Sakata *et al.* (*Antimicrob. Ag. Chemother.,* 1986, *29,* 225), however, noted a considerable suppression in the numbers of bifidobacteria and streptococci, a small decrease in the numbers of lactobacilli, and a small increase in the numbers of yeasts of the intestinal flora of 5 children given phenoxymethylpenicillin 30 mg per kg body-weight daily by mouth in divided doses for 5 to 14 days. There was no notable change in the numbers of enterobacteriaceae, clostridia, bacteroidaceae, or staphylococci, and the disturbed flora returned to normal within 3 to 6 days of cessation of therapy.

Larson *et al.* (*Br. med. J.,* 1977, *1,* 1246) reported the development of pseudomembranous colitis in a 12-year-old girl after a short course of phenoxymethylpenicillin by mouth. There have also been reports of non-pseudomembranous colitis after the administration of oral phenoxymethylpenicillin (R.B. Toffler *et al., Lancet,* 1978, *2,* 707; I.G. Barrison and S.P. Kane, *ibid.,* 843).

EFFECTS ON THE LIVER. A severe systemic reaction with liver impairment occurred in a patient given phenoxymethylpenicillin.— L. Beeley *et al.* (letter), *Lancet,* 1976, *2,* 1297. See also L. I. Goldstein and K. G. Ishak, *Archs Path.,* 1974, *98,* 114.

Precautions

As for Benzylpenicillin, p.133.

For a reference to impaired absorption of phenoxymethylpenicillin in patients with coeliac disease, see under Absorption and Fate, below.

INTERACTIONS. The average serum concentration of penicillin in 5 healthy subjects given a 250-mg dose of phenoxymethylpenicillin was reduced by more than 50% after 7 days' dosage with neomycin 12 g daily. The average 24-hour recovery of penicillin in the subjects' urine was reduced by a similar amount. Phenoxymethylpenicillin administered to the same subjects 6 days after withdrawal of neomycin produced the expected serum concentrations.— S. H. Cheng and A. White, *New Engl. J. Med.,* 1962, *267,* 1296.

Of 38 cases of failure of oral contraceptive steroids in

women receiving antibiotics reported to the Committee on the Safety of Medicines, 2 patients had taken phenoxymethylpenicillin (one in association with oxytetracycline).— D. J. Back *et al.*, *Drugs*, 1981, *21*, 46.

A report of fatal anaphylactic reactions in 2 patients who received a course of phenoxymethylpenicillin by mouth in association with beta-blocker therapy (nadolol or propranolol) for hypertension. Beta-adrenergic blockade may potentiate anaphylactic reactions.— R. L. Berkelman *et al.* (letter), *Ann. intern. Med.*, 1986, *104*, 134.

Since guar gum may slow the speed of absorption of phenoxymethylpenicillin, patients should take the antibiotic 30 minutes before food and guar to ensure maximum peak blood concentrations.— R. Levin (letter), *Pharm. J.*, 1987, *2*, 422.

For a report of chloroquine diminishing the antibacterial action of phenoxymethylpenicillin, see below under Antimicrobial Action.

Antimicrobial Action and Resistance

Phenoxymethylpenicillin has a range of antimicrobial activity similar to that of benzylpenicillin (see p.133) and a similar mode of action. However, it is slightly less active against many susceptible organisms particularly Gram-negative micro-organisms. It is inactivated by penicillinase.

The mechanisms and patterns of resistance to phenoxymethylpenicillin are similar to those of benzylpenicillin.

DIMINISHED ACTIVITY. Chloroquine phosphate decreased the antibacterial effect *in vitro* of benzylpenicillin and phenoxymethylpenicillin against *Staphylococcus aureus*.— M. A. Toama *et al.*, *J. pharm. Sci.*, 1978, *67*, 23.

Absorption and Fate

Phenoxymethylpenicillin is more resistant to inactivation by the acid of gastric secretions and is more completely absorbed than benzylpenicillin from the gastro-intestinal tract following administration by mouth. Absorption is usually rapid, although variable, up to 60% of a dose by mouth being absorbed. The calcium and potassium salts are better absorbed than the free acid. Peak serum concentrations of 3 to 6 µg per mL have been observed following a dose of 250 to 500 mg. The effect of food on absorption appears to be slight and variable. The plasma half-life of phenoxymethylpenicillin is about 30 minutes which may be increased to about 4 hours in renal failure, and about 80% is reported to be protein bound. The distribution and elimination of phenoxymethylpenicillin is similar to that of benzylpenicillin (see p.135). It is metabolised in the liver to a greater extent than benzylpenicillin; several metabolites have been identified including penicilloic acid. The unchanged drug and metabolites are excreted rapidly in the urine. Only small concentrations are excreted in the bile.

In a study of 13 infants coeliac disease, but not diarrhoea, impaired the absorption of phenoxymethylpenicillin.— P. Bolme *et al.*, *Acta paediat. scand.*, 1977, *66*, 573. See also A. E. Davis and R. C. Pirola, *Australas. Ann. Med.*, 1968, *17*, 63.

A comparison of the pharmacokinetics of phenoxymethylpenicillin and phenethicillin potassium in 10 patients.— D. Overbosch *et al.*, *Br. J. clin. Pharmac.*, 1985, *19*, 657.

For reference to the distribution of phenoxymethylpenicillin into the saliva, see under Adverse Effects, above.

Uses and Administration

Phenoxymethylpenicillin is used similarly to benzylpenicillin (see p.135) in the treatment or prophylaxis of infections caused by susceptible Gram-positive organisms. It is used only for the treatment of mild to moderate infections, and should not be used for chronic, severe, or deep-seated infections such as subacute bacterial endocarditis, meningitis, or syphilis. Patients treated initially with parenteral benzylpenicillin may continue treatment with phenoxymethylpenicillin by mouth once a satisfactory clinical response has been obtained.

For the treatment of infections, phenoxymethylpenicillin is administered in a dose of 125 to 500 mg usually given every 4 to 6 hours. Dosage may need to be modified in severe renal impairment. Children may be given the following doses every 6 hours: up to 1 year, 62.5 mg; 1 to 5 years, 125 mg; and 6 to 12 years, 250 mg.

For doses of phenoxymethylpenicillin recommended for the prophylaxis of infective endocarditis or rheumatic fever, see below.

Phenoxymethylpenicillin is administered by mouth, either as the free acid or as its potassium or calcium salt, preferably 30 minutes before or at least 2 hours after food.

ADMINISTRATION. A view that if phenoxymethylpenicillin by mouth is used it should be given in a dose of 500 mg every 4 hours.— R. Wise, *Lancet*, 1982, *2*, 140.

A recommendation that penicillin administered by mouth should be given with at least 100 mL of water while the patient is in an upright sitting position to avoid oesophagitis or oesophageal ulceration.— S. K. Vong and R. K. Parekh (letter), *Pharm. J.*, 1987, *1*, 5.

ANTHRAX. For reference to the use of phenoxymethylpenicillin potassium in the treatment of anthrax, see Benzylpenicillin Sodium, p.136.

ENDOCARDITIS. *Prophylaxis.* In patients at risk of endocarditis undergoing dental procedures or surgery of the upper respiratory tract the American Heart Association has recommended a standard regimen of phenoxymethylpenicillin 2 g administered by mouth one hour prior to the procedure and then 1 g six hours later; children less than 27 kg should receive one-half the adult dose. For patients in whom maximal protection is desired, for example those with prosthetic heart valves, parenteral ampicillin and gentamicin could be substituted for the first and possibly also the second dose of phenoxymethylpenicillin; these drugs should be given half-an-hour before and 8 hours after the procedure (S.T. Shulman *et al.*, *Circulation*, 1984, *70*, 1123A). However, the Working Party of the British Society for Antimicrobial Chemotherapy has recommended the use of a single dose of amoxycillin 3 g by mouth (*Lancet*, 1982, *2*, 1323) which is considered to be better absorbed than phenoxymethylpenicillin (*Drug & Ther. Bull.*, 1985, *23*, 53).

Results of a study to assess the prophylactic effect of phenoxymethylpenicillin or erythromycin by mouth on the incidence and type of bacteraemia subsequent to dental surgery. Fifty-one patients underwent 60 dental extractions; prophylaxis with either phenoxymethylpenicillin 2 g (as the potassium salt), one to 1.5 hours pre-operatively (20 procedures), erythromycin 500 mg, 1.5 to 2.5 hours pre-operatively (20), or no antibiotic treatment (20) was given. Although the total numbers of bacteria isolated from the blood during the operation were lower in the antibiotic-treated patients than those not treated, the incidence of bacteraemia was similar (50, 55, and 55% in the 3 groups respectively). The incidences of bacteraemia 10 minutes after the operation, however, were 15, 20, and 30%. One aerobic and 17 anaerobic isolates were recovered from patients given phenoxymethylpenicillin. The corresponding numbers were 6 and 30 for erythromycin-treated and 12 and 37 for untreated patients. The most commonly detected anaerobes were of the genera *Streptococcus*, *Peptococcus*, *Veillonella*, *Actinomyces*, and *Bacteroides*. Among the aerobes detected, staphylococci and viridans streptococci predominated. The efficacy of phenoxymethylpenicillin in reducing the number of anaerobic bacteria was further supported by the low MICs and MBCs obtained for most isolates. Only 2 anaerobic strains, identified as *Veillonella parvula* and *Bacteroides* spp., were resistant. Two aerobic strains, *Enterococcus faecium* and a beta-lactamase-producing strain of *Staph. epidermidis*, were also resistant. In contrast, erythromycin was less effective in reducing the number of anaerobic bacteria, and high MBCs were obtained for 16 anaerobic strains including *Veillonella parvula*, *Peptococcus*, *Eubacterium*, and *Bacteroides* spp., and *Fusobacterium nucleatum*. Three aerobic strains were resistant to erythromycin, including the 2 resistant to phenoxymethylpenicillin.— K. Josefsson *et al.*, *J. antimicrob. Chemother.*, 1985, *16*, 243.

See also under Prophylactic Use of Antibiotics, p.102.

INFECTION PROPHYLAXIS, HYPOSPLENISM. In a multicentre double-blind study of 215 children with sickle-cell anaemia, prophylaxis with phenoxymethylpenicillin potassium 125 mg given twice daily by mouth resulted in a significant reduction in the incidence of severe pneumococcal infection compared with placebo. Pneumococcal infection occurred in 2 of 105 children receiving phenoxymethylpenicillin compared with 13 of 110 receiving placebo, and no deaths occurred from pneumococcal septicaemia in the penicillin group whereas 3 deaths occurred in the placebo group. Pneumococcal vaccine had been administered to 93.2% and 95.2% of the children over one year of age in the placebo and penicillin groups, respectively. It was recommended that infants with sickle-cell anaemia should receive prophylactic penicillin not later than 4 months after birth and that prophylaxis should probably be continued beyond the third birthday.— M. H. Gaston *et al.*, *New Engl. J. Med.*, 1986, *314*, 1593.

See also under Prophylactic Use of Antibiotics, p.102.

LYME DISEASE. Phenoxymethylpenicillin potassium 250 mg by mouth administered 4 times daily for 10 days had been used successfully in the treatment of Lyme disease (J.L. Benach *et al.*, *New Engl. J. Med.*, 1983, *308*, 740) and phenoxymethylpenicillin potassium 500 mg given by mouth 4 times daily for 10 days had also been used to treat simultaneous occurrence of babesiosis and Lyme disease (E. Grunwaldt *et al.*, *ibid.*, 1166). However, although erythema chronicum migrans and its associated symptoms resolved with either phenoxymethylpenicillin 250 mg or tetracycline 250 mg given 4 times daily for 10 days, and minor late complications occurred after either drug, major late complications had occurred in 3 of 40 patients treated with penicillin, but in none of 39 patients given tetracycline. Treatment with tetracycline was therefore recommended for adults with early manifestations of Lyme disease, although a higher dose of phenoxymethylpenicillin might be as effective as the tetracycline regimen; it was also recommended that children should receive phenoxymethylpenicillin 50 mg per kg body-weight daily (not less than 1 g or more than 2 g daily) for at least 10 days (A. C. Steere *et al.*, *Ann. intern. Med.*, 1983, *99*, 22).

See also under Benzylpenicillin Sodium, p.136.

MOUTH INFECTIONS. For reference to a comparative study of phenoxymethylpenicillin and amoxycillin in the treatment of acute dento-alveolar abscess, see p.114.

PREGNANCY AND THE NEONATE. For reference to the use of phenoxymethylpenicillin during pregnancy, see under Benzylpenicillin Sodium, p.137.

RESPIRATORY-TRACT INFECTIONS. *Pharyngitis.* Of 44 children with suspected streptococcal pharyngitis 26 (59%) had an initial throat culture which was positive for group A beta-haemolytic streptococci. In 11 of these culture-positive children early treatment with phenoxymethylpenicillin 250 mg by mouth administered 3 times daily for 3 days, beginning at the initial consultation, resulted in a significant clinical improvement compared with 15 children who received placebo. Some workers favoured delay in treatment of streptococcal pharyngitis pending throat culture results as a delay of up to several days did not appear to place the patient at risk of developing rheumatic fever, however, the clinical benefits of early treatment should be taken into consideration.— M. S. Krober *et al.*, *J. Am. med. Ass.*, 1985, *253*, 1271.

A study involving 99 children indicating that phenoxymethylpenicillin 250 mg by mouth was equally effective in the treatment of streptococcal pharyngitis whether given 2 or 3 times daily.— M. A. Gerber *et al.*, *Am. J. Dis. Child.*, 1985, *139*, 1145.

For reference to the use of a combination of phenoxymethylpenicillin potassium and rifampicin in the treatment of group A streptococcal pharyngitis, see Rifampicin, p.576.

Tonsillitis. A study of the minimum amount of penicillin prophylaxis required to control an epidemic of acute tonsillitis associated with *Streptococcus pyogenes* infection in a closed community of boys aged 14 to 17 years old. Phenoxymethylpenicillin 500 mg administered daily as a single dose by mouth for 10 days after entry into the community was found to be effective.— A. Colling *et al.*, *Br. med. J.*, 1982, *285*, 95.

Phenoxymethylpenicillin remains the drug of choice for oral treatment of tonsillitis caused by *Streptococcus pyogenes*. While studies indicate that treatment for 10 days is more effective than shorter courses, in practice a 7 day course is often given.— R. H. George, *Br. med. J.*, 1986, *293*, 682.

RHEUMATIC FEVER PROPHYLAXIS. For the use of phenoxymethylpenicillin in the prevention of initial or recurrent attacks of rheumatic fever, see under Benzathine Penicillin, p.130. See also Respiratory-tract Infections, above.

WHIPPLE'S DISEASE. For the use of phenoxymethylpenicillin in the treatment of Whipple's disease, see Benzylpenicillin Sodium, p.138.

Preparations

Phenoxymethylpenicillin Capsules *(B.P.)*. Penicillin VK Capsules ; Phenoxymethylpenicillin Potassium Capsules

Penicillin V for Oral Suspension *(U.S.P.)*

Penicillin V Potassium for Oral Solution *(U.S.P.)*

Phenoxymethylpenicillin Oral Solution *(B.P.)*. Phenoxymethylpenicillin Elixir; Phenoxymethylpenicillin Syrup. A dry mixture of phenoxymethylpenicillin potassium for reconstitution.

Phenoxymethylpenicillin Oral Suspension *(B.P.)*. Phenoxymethylpenicillin Mixture. A suspension of phenoxymethylpenicillin calcium or phenoxymethylpenicillin potassium.

Penicillin V Tablets *(U.S.P.)*

Penicillin V Potassium Tablets *(U.S.P.)*

Phenoxymethylpenicillin Tablets *(B.P.)*. Penicillin VK Tablets. Tablets containing phenoxymethylpenicillin potassium.

Proprietary Preparations

Apsin VK *(Approved Prescription Services, UK)*. *Tablets*, scored, phenoxymethylpenicillin 250 mg (as potassium salt).
Syrup, granules for reconstitution, phenoxymethylpenicillin 125 and 250 mg (as potassium salt)/5 mL when reconstituted with water.

Distaquaine V-K *(Dista, UK)*. *Tablets*, scored, phenoxymethylpenicillin 125 and 250 mg (as potassium salt).
Elixir, granules for reconstitution, phenoxymethylpenicillin 62.5 mg (as potassium salt)/5 mL when reconstituted with water.
Syrup, granules for reconstitution, phenoxymethylpenicillin 125 and 250 mg (as potassium salt)/5 mL when reconstituted with water.

Econocil VK *(DDSA Pharmaceuticals, UK)*. *Capsules*, phenoxymethylpenicillin 250 mg (as potassium salt).
Tablets, phenoxymethylpenicillin 125 and 250 mg (as potassium salt).

Stabillin V-K *(Boots, UK)*. *Tablets*, phenoxymethylpenicillin 250 mg (as potassium salt).
Elixir, granules for reconstitution, phenoxymethylpenicillin 62.5, 125, and 250 mg (as potassium salt)/5 mL when reconstituted with water.

V-Cil-K *(Lilly, UK)*. *Capsules*, phenoxymethylpenicillin 250 mg (as potassium salt).
Tablets, phenoxymethylpenicillin 125 and 250 mg (as potassium salt).
Paediatric syrup, granules for reconstitution, phenoxymethylpenicillin 62.5 and 125 mg (as potassium salt)/5 mL when reconstituted with water.
Syrup, granules for reconstitution, phenoxymethylpenicillin 250 mg (as potassium salt)/5 mL when reconstituted with water.

Proprietary Names and Manufacturers of Phenoxymethylpenicillin and its Salts

Abbocillin-VK *(Abbott, Austral.; Ger.)*; Acipen-V *(Neth.)*; Antibiocin *(Dorsch, Ger.)*; Apocillin *(Apothekernes Laboratorium, Norw.)*; Apopen *(Swed.)*; Apo-Pen-VK *(Apotex, Canad.)*; Apsin VK *(Approved Prescription Services, UK)*; Arcasin *(Engelhard, Ger.; Cimex, Switz.)*; Beepen-VK *(Beecham Laboratories, USA)*; Beromycin *(Boehringer Ingelheim, Ger.)*; Betapen-VK *(Bristol, USA)*; Bramcillin *(Austral.)*; Brunocilline *(Mepha, Switz.)*; Calciopen *(Leo, Swed.)*; Calcipen *(Leo, Denm.; Leo, Norw.; Alter, Spain; Switz.)*; Cilicaine VK *(Sigma, Austral.)*; Cliacil *(Arg.; Hoechst, Switz.)*; Co-Caps Penicillin V-K *(Co-Caps, UK)*; Compocillin VK *(Austral.; NZ)*; Copen *(Covan, S.Afr.)*; Crystapen V *(Glaxo, UK)*; Crystapen VK *(Austral.; NZ)*; CVK *(Abbott, UK)*; Darocillin *(SCS, S.Afr.)*; Deltacillin *(MPS Lab., S.Afr.)*; Distaquaine V-K *(Austral.; S.Afr.; Dista, UK)*; Dowpen VK *(USA)*; DQVK *(NZ)*; Durapenicillin *(Durachemie, Ger.)*; Econocil VK *(DDSA Pharmaceuticals, UK)*; Falcopen VK *(Faulding, Austral.)*; Femepen *(NAF, Norw.)*; Fenospen *(Carlo Erba, Ital.)*; Fenoxcillin *(Novo, Denm.)*; Fenoxypen *(Novo, Norw.; S.Afr.; Novo, Swed.; Novo, Switz.)*; GPV *(Galen, UK)*; Icipen *(ICI Pharmaceuticals, UK)*; Incil-VK *(S.Afr.)*; Isocillin *(Hoechst, Ger.)*; Ispenoral *(Chephasaar, Ger.)*; Jatcillin *(S.Afr.)*; Kavepenin *(Astra, Swed.)*; Ledercillin *(Lederle, UK)*; Ledercillin VK *(Lederle, Canad.; Lederle, USA)*; Len VK *(Lennon, S.Afr.)*; LPV *(Commonwealth Serum Laboratories, Austral.)*; Megacillin *(Grünenthal, Ger.)*; Monocillin *(Chassot, Switz.)*; Nadopen-V *(Nadeau, Canad.)*; Norcillin *(R.P. Drugs, UK)*; Novopen-VK *(Novopharm, Canad.)*; Novo-VK *(Novo, S.Afr.)*; Nutracillin *(Propan, S.Afr.)*; Oracillin VK *(SCS, S.Afr.)*; Oracilline *(Belg.; Théraplix, Fr.)*; Orpenic *(Belg.)*; Ospen *(Sandoz, Fr.; Sandoz, Ger.; Sandoz, Switz.)*; Paclin VK *(USA)*; Penadur VK *(Wyeth, Switz.)*; Penapar VK *(Parke, Davis, USA)*; Penbec-V *(Canad.)*; Pencompren *(E. Merck, Ger.)*; Pengrocill *(Grossmann, Switz.)*; Penicals *(Lövens, Swed.)*; Penicillat *(Azuchemie, Ger.)*; Peni-oral *(Belg.)*; Pen-Oral *(Arg.)*; Penoral *(S.Afr.)*; Pentabs *(Belg.)*; Pentid *(Arg.)*; Pen-Vee *(Wyeth, Canad.)*; Pen-Vee-K *(Wyeth, USA)*; Pfipen V *(Austral.)*; Pfizerpen VK *(Pfipharmecs, USA)*; Phenocilline *(Streuli, Switz.)*; P-Mega *(Beiersdorf, Ger.)*; Primcillin *(Astra, Denm.)*; Propen VK *(Austral.)*; PVF K *(Frosst, Canad.)*; PVK *(Lilly, Austral.)*; PVO *(Fawns & McAllan, Austral.)*; Robicillin VK *(Robins, USA)*; Rocilin *(Austral.; Rosco, Denm.; Rosco, Norw.)*; Ro-Cillin VK *(USA)*; Roscopenin *(Rosco, Swed.)*; Servipen-V *(Servipharm, Switz.)*; SK-Penicillin VK *(Smith Kline & French, USA)*; Stabicilline *(Vifor, Switz.)*; Stabillin V-K *(Boots, UK)*; Ticillin V-K *(Ticen, Eire)*; Tripapenicillina *(Ital.)*; Uticillin VK *(Upjohn, USA)*; V-Cil-K *(NZ; Dista, S.Afr.; Lilly, UK)*; V-Cillin K *(Lilly, Canad.; Lilly, USA)*; VC-K 500 *(Lilly, Canad.)*; Veekay *(S.Afr.)*; Veetids *(Squibb, USA)*; Vepen *(Swed.)*; Vepicombin *(DAK, Denm.)*; Viraxacillin-V *(Austral.)*; Weifapenin *(Weiders, Norw.)*; Widocilline *(Wiedenmann, Switz.)*.

The following names have been used for multi-ingredient preparations containing phenoxymethylpenicillin and its salts— Tonsillin *(Winthrop, UK)*; V-Cil-K Sulpha *(Lilly, UK)*.

4912-k

Phthalylsulphathiazole *(BAN)*.

Ftalilsulfatiazol; Phthalazolum; Phthalylsulfathiazole *(rINN)*; Phthalylsulfathiazolum; Sulfaphtalylthiazol. 4′-(Thiazol-2-ylsulphamoyl)phthalanilic acid.
$C_{17}H_{13}N_3O_5S_2$=403.4.

CAS — 85-73-4.

Pharmacopoeias. In *Arg., Br., Braz., Chin., Cz., Eur., Fr., Ind., Int., It., Jug., Neth., Nord., Port., Roum., Rus., Span., Swiss,* and *Turk.* Also in *B.P. Vet.*

White or yellowish-white, odourless crystalline powder. Practically **insoluble** in water, chloroform, and ether; slightly soluble in alcohol and in acetone; freely soluble in dimethyl formamide. **Protect** from light.

Phthalylsulphathiazole is a sulphonamide with properties similar to Sulphamethoxazole, p.306. It is slowly hydrolysed to sulphathiazole in the large intestine and only about 5% is absorbed.

Phthalylsulphathiazole has been used in the treatment of bacillary dysentery but most strains of *Shigella* are now resistant to sulphonamides. A suggested adult dose in acute bacillary dysentery is 5 g or more daily in divided doses; for short-term prophylaxis 1 g twice daily has been given.

Phthalylsulphathiazole has also been used to reduce the bacterial count in the large bowel in patients undergoing surgery but many doubt its value. A suggested dose is 250 mg per kg body-weight initially, followed by 12 g daily in divided doses every 3 hours, with treatment beginning 4 days before surgery and continuing for 4 days postoperatively.

Proprietary Names and Manufacturers of Phthalylsulphathiazole or its Derivatives

Colicitina *(Panthox & Burck, Ital.)*; Crematalil *(Spain)*; Enterosteril *(Ital.)*; Ilentazol *(Belg.; Switz.)*; Novosulfina *(Ital.)*; Phthazol *(USV, Austral.)*; Sulfathalidin *(Andreu, Spain)*; Sulfathalidine *(Canad.)*; Sulftalyl *(Pharmacia, Swed.)*; Sulmatren *(Ralay, Spain)*; Talidine *(Fr.)*; Thalazole *(May & Baker, Austral.; May & Baker, S.Afr.; May & Baker, UK)*.

The following names have been used for multi-ingredient preparations containing phthalylsulphathiazole or its derivatives— Neo-Sulfazon *(Wallace Mfg Chem., UK)*; Sulphamagna *(Wyeth, UK)*.

5666-b

Pipemidic Acid *(rINN)*.

1489-RB; Piperamic Acid. 8-Ethyl-5,8-dihydro-5-oxo-2-(piperazin-1-yl)pyrido[2,3-*d*]pyrimidine-6-carboxylic acid.
$C_{14}H_{17}N_5O_3$=303.3.

CAS — 51940-44-4.

Adverse Effects and Precautions

As for nalidixic acid (see p.266). The most frequently reported adverse effects are gastro-intestinal symptoms and allergic reactions.

EFFECTS ON THE SKIN. A 25-year-old woman developed toxic epidermal necrolysis (Lyell's syndrome) about 2 weeks after she had started treatment with pipemidic acid 800 mg daily.— F. Vachon *et al., Nouv. Presse méd.*, 1977, *6*, 1239.

Antimicrobial Action

As for Norfloxacin, p.274.

Some references to the antibacterial activity of pipemidic acid: M. Shimizu *et al., Antimicrob. Ag. Chemother.*, 1975, *8*, 132; S. Nakamura *et al., ibid.*, 1976, *10*, 779; S. Inoue *et al., ibid.*, 1978, *14*, 240; G. Peters *et al., Dt. med. Wschr.*, 1979, *104*, 946; H. L. Muytjens *et al., Antimicrob. Ag. Chemother.*, 1983, *24*, 302.

Absorption and Fate

Peak plasma concentrations of 3.5 to 4.5 µg per mL of pipemidic acid have been achieved 1 to 2 hours after oral doses of 400 or 500 mg.

Pipemidic acid is excreted by the kidney and about 50 to 85% of a dose appears in the urine within 24 hours. Urinary concentrations usually exceed 100 µg per mL for up to 12 hours following doses of 400 or 500 mg. Traces have been detected in breast milk.

The amount of pipemidic acid diffusing across the placenta was very small.— M. Kanao *et al., Chemotherapy, Tokyo*, 1975, *23*, 2939.

Therapeutic concentrations of pipemidic acid could be achieved in prostatic tissue.— J. P. Archimbaud and A. Leriche, *J. Urol. Néphrol.*, 1979, *85*, 191.

Following administration by mouth pipemidic acid was excreted largely unchanged in the urine with the metabolites acetylpipemidic acid, formylpipemidic acid, and oxopipemidic acid each representing less than 2% of unchanged pipemidic acid excreted. It was considered that these metabolites contributed little to overall activity in urine as they were about 3 to 10 times less active than pipemidic acid.— N. Kurobe *et al., Xenobiotica*, 1980, *10*, 37.

A calculated mean peak plasma concentration of 4.48 µg per mL was obtained in 10 healthy subjects 1.3 hours after administration of a single 400-mg dose of pipemidic acid. The biological half-life was 2.15 hours. Mean urinary concentrations were about 510 µg per mL over the first 6 hours and 131 µg per mL between 9 and 12 hours after administration. About 83% of a dose was recovered in the urine within 12 hours.— J. M. Brogard *et al., Eur. J. Drug Metab. Pharmacokinet.*, 1983, *8*, 251.

At steady-state the mean peak serum concentration of pipemidic acid in 10 healthy subjects receiving pipemidic acid 500 mg twice daily was 4.27 µg per mL and occurred 1.2 hours after administration. The serum elimination half-life was 3.4 hours. Minimum urinary concentrations exceeded 100 µg per mL with 57% of a dose being excreted in the urine within 12 hours and about 61% within 24 hours. Plasma protein binding ranged from about 13 to 39% depending on the plasma concentration.— E. Klinge *et al., Antimicrob. Ag. Chemother.*, 1984, *26*, 69.

Further references.— M. Shimizu *et al., Antimicrob. Ag. Chemother.*, 1975, *7*, 441.

Uses and Administration

Pipemidic acid is a 4-quinolone antimicrobial agent used similarly to nalidixic acid (see p.267).

Doses of 400 mg administered as the trihydrate morning and night are used in the treatment of urinary-tract infections.

SUPPRESSION OF INTESTINAL FLORA. Pipemidic acid, in combination with antifungal prophylaxis, may be useful for selective decontamination of the gastro-intestinal tract for infection prophylaxis in neutropenic patients.— H. L. Muytjens *et al., Antimicrob. Ag. Chemother.*, 1983, *24*, 902.

URINARY-TRACT INFECTIONS. Pipemidic acid 400 mg twice daily by mouth was as effective as nalidixic acid 1 g four times daily when both were given for 7 days in the treatment of urinary-tract infections. An excellent or good response was obtained in 11 of 16 patients given pipemidic acid and in 13 of 16 given nalidixic acid. Adverse effects were more frequent with nalidixic acid.— A. Manganelli *et al.*, *Drugs exp. & clin. Res.*, 1979, *5*, 321.

In a double-blind study involving 123 patients pipemidic acid 500 mg or sulphadiazine 500 mg both given twice daily for 10 days were equally effective in the treatment of acute lower urinary-tract infections and produced a cure in over 90% of the patients at evaluation 4 to 5 days after treatment. The majority of patients infected with *Staphylococcus saprophyticus* were cured by their respective treatments despite resistance *in vitro* to pipemidic acid. Of 49 patients followed up from each treatment group for 3 to 4 weeks recurrence of infection occurred in 8% of the patients treated with pipemidic acid and in 6% of those treated with sulphadiazine.— P. Mäkelä *et al.*, *Curr. ther. Res.*, 1983, *34*, 757.

Pipemidic acid 1 g twice daily was more effective than nalidixic acid 1 g four times daily when administered for 2 weeks in a double-blind study of 82 elderly patients with recurrent lower urinary-tract infections but was associated with more side-effects. Urine was examined after treatment and of the 44 given pipemidic acid, 26 (59%) had sterile urine, 1 (2%) was a treatment failure, and 15 (34%) were re-infected with a new bacterial strain; 2 patients in whom treatment was discontinued were not followed up. Of the 38 given nalidixic acid, 10 (26%) had sterile urine, 16 (42%) were treatment failures, and 12 (32%) were re-infected. The majority of treatment failures were due to bacterial resistance. The high incidence of adverse effects with pipemidic acid was probably due to the age of the patients and the high dose used. Side-effects were reported in 12 patients given pipemidic acid and included: rash (2 patients), itching (2), nausea (3), gastro-intestinal symptoms (1), dizziness and weakness (2). Two patients who experienced grand mal convulsions were both about 90 years of age and had advanced cerebral arteriosclerosis. Treatment was discontinued by 8 patients because of adverse effects.— L. Niinistö *et al.*, *Curr. ther. Res.*, 1984, *35*, 57.

Proprietary Names and Manufacturers

Acipem *(Caber, Ital.)*; Biopim *(Ital Suisse, Ital.)*; Cistomid *(Crosara, Ital.)*; Deblaston *(Madaus, Ger.*; *Madaus, S.Afr.*; *Madaus, Switz.)*; Diperpen *(Francia Farm., Ital.)*; Filtrax *(Biomedica Foscama, Ital.)*; Galusan *(Almirall, Spain)*; Nuril *(High Noon, Pakistan*; *Prodes, Spain)*; Pipeacid *(Del Saz & Filippini, Ital.)*; Pipedac *(Mediolanum, Ital.)*; Pipedase *(Logifarm, Ital.)*; Pipefort *(Lampugnani, Ital.)*; Pipemid *(Gentili, Ital.)*; Pipram *(Bellon, Fr.*; *Rhone-Poulenc, Ital.)*; Pipurin *(Brocchieri, Ital.)*; Septidron *(Ethimed, S.Afr.)*; Solupemid *(Recordati, Ital.)*; Tractur *(Damor, Ital.)*; Urisan *(Zambeletti, Spain)*; Urodene *(OFF, Ital.)*; Uropimid *(CT, Ital.)*; Uropipedil *(Inofarma, Spain)*; Urosan *(AGIPS, Ital.)*; Urosetic *(Von Boch, Ital.)*; Urosten *(Bonomelli, Ital.)*; Urotractin *(Zambeletti, Ital.)*; Uroval *(FIRMA, Ital.)*; Uticid *(Erco, Denm.)*; Utivec *(Orion, Fin.)*.

133-b

Piperacillin Sodium *(BANM, USAN, rINNM)*.

CL-227193; T-1220. Sodium (6*R*)-6-[D-2-(4-Ethyl-2,3-dioxopiperazine-1-carboxamido)-2-phenylacetamido]penicillanate.

$C_{23}H_{26}N_5NaO_7S$=539.5.

CAS — 61477-96-1 (piperacillin); 59703-84-3 (sodium salt).

Pharmacopoeias. In *Jpn. U.S.* includes Sterile Piperacillin Sodium.

1.04 g of monograph substance is approximately equivalent to 1 g of piperacillin. Each g of monograph substance represents 1.85 mmol of sodium. A 40% solution in water has a pH of 5.5 to 7.5.

It is recommended that reconstituted solutions of piperacillin sodium for injection should be administered immediately after preparation. Piperacillin sodium should not be mixed with blood products or other proteinaceous fluids such as protein hydrolysates.

Incompatibility or loss of activity has been reported with aminoglycosides and sodium bicarbonate.

Adverse Effects

As for Carbenicillin Sodium, p.139. As piperacillin sodium has a lower sodium content than carbenicillin sodium, hypernatraemia and hypokalaemia are less likely to occur.

Adverse reactions which could possibly, probably, or definitely be related to therapy with piperacillin were observed in 105 of 758 patients (13%), treated with the drug in initial studies to assess its safety and efficacy. Allergic reactions, including rash and pruritus, occurred with an incidence of 4%, and gastro-intestinal disturbances, including diarrhoea, bloody diarrhoea, nausea, or vomiting, with an incidence of about 4%. Thrombophlebitis was observed in 4% of instances, and pain at the injection site, induration, or erythema in 1.3%. Reversible leucopenia and a frequently associated neutropenia occurred in 4% of courses of piperacillin treatment; they were most common after treatment for 3 or more weeks. Eosinophilia occurred with an incidence of 6%. Transient elevations in liver enzyme values (3% of courses), bilirubin concentrations (3%), and a direct positive Coombs test (2%) were also reported. One patient developed cholestatic hepatitis which reappeared with increased severity on rechallenge. Hypokalaemia occurred primarily in severely ill immunocompromised patients, or those receiving potent diuretics.— P. G. Gooding *et al.*, *J. antimicrob. Chemother.*, 1982, *9*, *Suppl.* B, 93. Leucopenia and/or neutropenia was only definitely associated with piperacillin in 4 of the 38 reported cases; there was a probable association in a further 7.— P. G. Gooding (letter), *ibid.*, *10*, 560.

ALLERGY. There have been several reports of adverse reactions after administration of piperacillin sodium to patients with cystic fibrosis. Stead *et al.* (*Thorax*, 1985, *40*, 184) reported the development of swinging fever, requiring discontinuation of treatment, in 9 of 38 patients given intravenous therapy with piperacillin in association with an aminoglycoside. Two patients also developed a rash. The reactions occurred after 5 to 28 days of treatment, and usually resolved within 24 hours of withdrawal; fever recurred in 2 patients in whom piperacillin was re-introduced. Strandvik *et al.* (*Lancet*, 1984, *1*, 1362) observed adverse reactions in 13 of 18 patients with cystic fibrosis, also treated with piperacillin and an aminoglycoside. Reactions included fever (11 patients), rash (3), pruritus (2), tender lymphadenitis (2), eosinophilia (2), and respiratory symptoms (1). Eight patients reacted during their first course of treatment after 9 to 22 days, and 5 after up to 15 days of their second course. Eight of these patients had previously been treated with azlocillin; 2 had experienced a similar reaction to this drug. Two patients who reacted to piperacillin had tolerated azlocillin, but had reacted seriously to carbenicillin.

Stead *et al.* observed fevers and/or urticaria in 4 of 36 patients given azlocillin and in 2 of 35 given carbenicillin. Strandvik *et al.* reported reactions in 4 of 28 patients given azlocillin. Brock and Roach, however, (*ibid.*, 1071) considered that patients with cystic fibrosis were particularly prone to allergy and cited earlier reports in which 16 of 84 patients given carbenicillin had similar reactions, and 5 of 18 patients who received azlocillin had symptoms of serum sickness. McDonnell and FitzGerald (*ibid.*, 1301) reported penicillin-hypersensitivity reactions in 10 of 63 patients with cystic fibrosis; 4 of these had received carbenicillin, 3 ticarcillin, 1 ampicillin, and 2 ampicillin in association with cloxacillin. They considered that this unusually high incidence of hypersensitivity might be related to exposure to complex antipseudomonal penicillins in the presence of a hyperimmune state. In spite of this, Stead *et al.*, Strandvik *et al.*, and others (M.E. Hodson, *Postgrad. med. J.*, 1984, *60*, 225) considered piperacillin to cause a higher incidence of adverse reactions than other related agents in patients with cystic fibrosis, and that it should be best avoided in such patients.

Mead and Smith (*Lancet*, 1985, *2*, 499) observed allergic skin reactions in 9 of 22 leukaemia patients with neutropenic fever after the administration of antibiotic regimens which included piperacillin. Since all 9 patients had acute myeloid leukaemia (AML), they concluded that piperacillin might be associated with a higher incidence of allergic reactions in such patients. Anderson *et al.* (*ibid.*, 723) reported the development of skin rashes in 15 of 156 cancer patients treated with piperacillin and netilmicin, all 15 of whom had AML. Schimpff *et al.* (*ibid.*), however, could not confirm these observations in a review of 5 prospective studies of the use of empirical antibiotic regimens in chemotherapy-associated neutropenia. In each study the frequency of skin rash was low (10% or less), and there was no difference in the incidence of reactions associated with piperacillin or other antibiotics, or in patients with AML or other malignancies.

EFFECTS ON THE BLOOD. Piperacillin was administered in a dose of 100, 200, or 300 mg per kg body-weight daily for 7 days by intravenous infusion to 15 healthy subjects. One subject receiving the lowest dose, and 2 receiving the highest had prolonged bleeding times at the end of the study, and some abnormality in platelet aggregation was observed in 13.— L. O. Gentry *et al.*, *Antimicrob. Ag. Chemother.*, 1981, *19*, 532.

Neutropenia. Reports of neutropenic reactions to piperacillin in patients who had previously shown a similar reaction to another penicillin: C. Wilson *et al.* (letter), *Lancet*, 1979, *1*, 1150 (cross-reaction with nafcillin); C. F. Kirkwood and G. M. Lasezkay, *Drug Intell. & clin. Pharm.*, 1985, *19*, 112 (cross-reaction with mezlocillin). See also above.

EFFECTS ON THE SKIN. See Allergy, above.

Precautions

As for Carbenicillin Sodium, p.139.

For reference to precautions to be observed in patients with cystic fibrosis, see under Adverse Effects, Allergy, above.

ADMINISTRATION IN LIVER DISORDERS AND RENAL FAILURE. For reference to the precautions to be observed in renal and liver failure, see under Uses, Administration in Renal Failure, below.

INTERACTIONS. For reference to the *in vitro* and *in vivo* inactivation of aminoglycosides by piperacillin, see Gentamicin Sulphate, p.236 and p.238.

For the effect of piperacillin sodium on latamoxef, see Latamoxef Disodium, p.252.

For the effects of other drugs on the antimicrobial activity of piperacillin, see below under Antimicrobial Action.

INTERFERENCE WITH DIAGNOSTIC TESTS. In a study *in vitro* of the effects of various antibiotics on tests for glycosuria, piperacillin in the urine could give falsely elevated readings with a test using a copper-reduction method (Clinitest). It had no effect however on glucose oxidase methods (Diastix and Tes-Tape) of estimating glycosuria.— W. A. Parker and M. E. MacCara, *Am. J. Hosp. Pharm.*, 1984, *41*, 125.

See also.— M. LeBel *et al.*, *Drug Intell. & clin. Pharm.*, 1984, *18*, 617.

Antimicrobial Action

Piperacillin has a similar antimicrobial action to carbenicillin, p.139, although it is active against a wider range of Gram-negative organisms including *Klebsiella pneumoniae*. It is generally more active *in vitro*, especially against *Pseudomonas aeruginosa* and the *Enterobacteriaceae*.

A review of the antimicrobial activity of piperacillin, including comparisons with other extended-spectrum penicillins, and with some aminoglycosides and cephalosporins. Piperacillin has been reported to demonstrate an inoculum effect *in vitro*, the MIC for a wide range of organisms increasing as the size of the inoculum is increased.— B. Holmes *et al.*, *Drugs*, 1984, *28*, 375.

A comparison *in vitro* of the activities of piperacillin and metronidazole against anaerobic bacilli. Two distinct populations of *Bacteroides fragilis* were demonstrated as regards susceptibility to piperacillin, 48% of strains being inhibited by 0.125 μg per mL or less, and the remainder by a wide range of MICs from 2 to over 32 μg per mL. The MICs of metronidazole for the majority of strains, however, were in a narrow range between 0.5 and 8 μg per mL. A similar pattern of 2 populations for piperacillin and one for metronidazole was also shown with *Clostridium* spp. Therefore, although piperacillin has marked *in vitro* activity against anaerobic bacilli, it is no more active than metronidazole, and strains with relative resistance to piperacillin occasionally occur.— D. A. Leigh (letter), *J. antimicrob. Chemother.*, 1984, *13*, 525. Similar results. Resistance rates of piperacillin for anaerobic bacteria, using a breakpoint of 128 μg per mL were no more than 6%. With the spread of resistance to clindamycin and cefoxitin in some areas, piperacillin could be of use in the treatment of infections caused by such organisms, but extreme caution is needed to reduce the spread of resistance.— M. Mandelli *et al.* (letter), *ibid.*, 1985, *15*, 252.

A report of the results after 3 years of a survey carried out in 8 centres throughout the *USA* of the susceptibility of clinical isolates of the *Bacteroides fragilis* group to a range of antimicrobials. Piperacillin was the most active of the 5 beta-lactams tested: cefoperazone, cefotaxime, cefoxitin, latamoxef, and piperacillin. Taking an MIC of 64 μg per mL as the breakpoint for susceptibility, the resistance rates were 12, 7, and 8% of strains tested in the 3 years from 1981 to 1983 respectively. Taking a breakpoint of 128 μg per mL, the equivalent figures were 8, 5, and 4%.— F. P. Tally *et al.*, *Antimicrob. Ag. Chemother.*, 1985, *28*, 675.

ACTIVITY WITH OTHER ANTIMICROBIAL AGENTS. *Aminoglycosides.* Studies *in vitro* of the activity of combinations of piperacillin and aminoglycosides have been unpredictable, depending on the definitions of combined action used and also on the method of the test. Many studies have shown synergy (P. Chanbusarakum and P.R. Murray, *Antimicrob. Ag. Chemother.*, 1978, *14*, 505; R.J. Fass, *ibid.*, 1982, *21*, 1003; A. Proietti *et al.*, *Curr. ther. Res.*, 1983, *34*, 297; R.H. Glew and R.A. Pavuk, *Antimicrob. Ag. Chemother.*, 1983, *23*, 902; *idem.*, 1984, *26*, 378; S.C. Aronoff and J.D. Klinger, *ibid.*, *25*, 279; M.D. Lyon *et al.*, *ibid.*, 1986, *30*, 25), but against a variable proportion of the strains studied, and the combinations have often shown indifference. The aminoglycosides studied include amikacin, gentamicin, netilmicin, and tobramycin, and their effect with piperacillin has been investigated against *Pseudomonas aeruginosa* and the *Enterobacteriaceae*, including strains resistant to the agents studied. Synergy between these antibiotics has been attributed to enhanced penetration of the aminoglycoside into the organism, via the action of piperacillin on the cell wall. Takahashi and Kanno (*ibid.*, 1984, *26*, 789) have demonstrated a synergistic interaction between piperacillin, fosfomycin, and tobramycin, 3 agents considered to act at different stages of bacterial growth.

Antineoplastics. A study *in vitro* of the interactions between piperacillin and some antineoplastic agents against *Pseudomonas aeruginosa* and various *Enterobacteriaceae*. Synergism was demonstrated with bleomycin, mitomycin, and fluorouracil against some organisms, and antagonism with carboquone. Combinations with doxorubicin were neither synergistic nor antagonistic.— Y. Ueda *et al.*, *Antimicrob. Ag. Chemother.*, 1983, *23*, 374.

Beta-lactams. Combinations of piperacillin with other beta-lactam agents have been investigated *in vitro* with a view that they would be less toxic *in vivo* than combinations including an aminoglycoside. Results have been unpredictable, depending on the method used, on the concentrations of the drugs, and on the definitions of combined effects. Studies using a checkerboard technique (N.A. Kuck *et al.*, *Antimicrob. Ag. Chemother.*, 1981, *19*, 634; T.O. Kurtz *et al.*, *ibid.*, *20*, 239; M.B. Bansal and H. Thadepalli, *ibid.*, 1983, *23*, 166; D.H. Wu *et al.*, *ibid.*, 1984, *26*, 519; C.H. Ramirez-Ronda *et al.*, *Curr. ther. Res.*, 1984, *35*, 64; J.A.A. Hoogkamp-Korstanje, *J. Antimicrob. Chemother.*, 1985, *16*, 327) have demonstrated mainly synergistic or additive/indifferent effects, but some antagonism has been shown. The beta-lactams with which piperacillin was combined included: aztreonam, cefoperazone, cefotaxime, cefoxitin, ceftizoxime, ceftriaxone, cephalothin, cephamandole, and latamoxef. They were tested against a wide range of organisms including *Pseudomonas aeruginosa, Bacteroides fragilis, Escherichia coli, Klebsiella pneumoniae, Serratia marcescens*, and *Listeria monocytogenes*, some strains of which were resistant to aminoglycosides. Hoogkamp-Korstanje could not back up the synergistic effects observed, by demonstration of increased bactericidal rates in killing-curve studies. Although Barriere *et al.* (*ibid.*, 49) found no synergy between piperacillin and latamoxef against *Ps. aeruginosa* by the chequerboard method, after administration of the drugs to 4 healthy subjects they observed an area under the bactericidal-activity-curve (AUBC) for the drugs administered together which was 2.5 times the sum of the AUBCs when they were given alone. This method takes into account both the antibacterial activity of the drugs and their pharmacokinetics. In an *in vitro* study (M.A. Bertram and L.S. Young, *Antimicrob. Ag. Chemother.*, 1984, *26*, 272), imipenem antagonised the activity of piperacillin against 28 of 35 strains of *Ps. aeruginosa*; this was associated with the induction of beta-lactamases by imipenem. Cefoxitin has also been reported to induce beta-lactamases. Antagonistic effects between beta-lactams may also be due to competition for, or an alteration of, target protein sites.

Clavulanic acid. Clavulanic acid has been shown *in vitro* to decrease the MIC of piperacillin against some strains of bacteria resistant to piperacillin by virtue of beta-lactamase production (H.C. Neu and K.P. Fu, *Antimicrob. Ag. Chemother.*, 1980, *18*, 582; C.N. Simpson *et al.*, *J. antimicrob. Chemother.*, 1984, *14*, 133).

Resistance

As for Carbenicillin Sodium, p.140.

In a review of case reports of all patients treated with piperacillin sodium which were submitted to the manufacturer from January 1978 to July 1981, Marier *et al.* (*J. antimicrob. Chemother.*, 1982, *9*, *Suppl.* B, 85) concluded that emergence of resistance to piperacillin was uncommon, and relatively unimportant. The overall rates of emergence of resistant organisms were 1.3% for piperacillin as compared with 2.3% during therapy with carbenicillin. Emergence of resistance was associated with infections caused by aerobic Gram-negative bacteria and with prolonged therapy. There may also have been an association with underdosing, with relatively lower initial susceptibility of organisms, and with cystic fibrosis. There have, however, been reports of the emergence of *Pseudomonas aeruginosa* resistant to piperacillin, some of which have been associated with superinfection or treatment failure. These have occurred most often during treatment with piperacillin alone (G.L. Simon *et al.*, *Antimicrob. Ag. Chemother.*, 1980, *18*, 167; M.J. Gribble *et al.*, *ibid.*, 1983, *24*, 388), although it has also been reported when piperacillin is administered with an aminoglycoside (A.J. Godfrey *et al.*, *ibid.*, 1981, *19*, 705) or another beta-lactam (M. Placzek *et al.*, *Archs. Dis. Childh.*, 1983, *58*, 1006). Godfrey demonstrated that the *Ps. aeruginosa* strains resistant to piperacillin were also resistant to carbenicillin, ticarcillin, cefsulodin, and cefotaxime, and that the resistance was probably due to an alteration in the target proteins of the bacteria. In some of the above studies, other organisms, including enterococci and other Gram-negative bacilli, also acquired resistance. Such reports of resistance have led to recommendations that piperacillin sodium should be used in conjunction with other antibacterials, particularly for infections caused by *Ps. aeruginosa*.

Absorption and Fate

Piperacillin sodium is not absorbed from the gastro-intestinal tract after oral administration. It is well absorbed after intramuscular administration, peak plasma concentrations of 30 to 40 μg per mL being observed 30 to 50 minutes after a dose of 2 g. The pharmacokinetics of piperacillin sodium have been reported to be dose-dependent. About 20% of piperacillin in the circulation is bound to plasma proteins. Piperacillin is reported to have a dose-dependent plasma half-life which is usually about one hour. The half-life is prolonged in neonates and in patients with renal failure.

Piperacillin is widely distributed in body tissues and fluids. It diffuses across the placenta into the foetal circulation and is excreted in small amounts in breast milk. There is little diffusion into the CSF except when the meninges are inflamed.

About 60 to 80% of a dose is excreted unchanged in the urine by glomerular filtration and tubular secretion within 24 hours, achieving high concentrations. High concentrations are also found in the bile; up to 25% of a dose has been reported to be excreted by this route.

Serum concentrations are enhanced if probenecid is administered concomitantly.

Piperacillin is removed by haemodialysis to some extent.

A review including the absorption and fate of piperacillin sodium.— B. Holmes *et al.*, *Drugs*, 1984, *28*, 375.

Studies of the pharmacokinetics of piperacillin sodium after intravenous administration: M. A. L. Evans *et al.*, *J. antimicrob. Chemother.*, 1978, *4*, 255; T. B. Tjandramaga *et al.*, *Antimicrob. Ag. Chemother.*, 1978, *14*, 829.

In a study of 12 women, serum-piperacillin concentrations were lower 2 or 3 days postpartum compared with those measured after administration of the same dose 6 months later.— D. Charles and B. Larsen, *Gynec. Obstet. Invest.*, 1985, *20*, 194.

ADMINISTRATION IN LIVER DISORDERS AND RENAL FAILURE. For reference to the pharmacokinetics of piperacillin in renal and liver failure, see under Uses, Administration in Renal Failure, below.

DIFFUSION INTO BODY TISSUES AND FLUIDS. Concentrations of piperacillin in cardiac valvular tissue, subcutaneous tissue, and muscle in patients given a dose of 4 g intravenously before undergoing open-heart surgery.— F. D. Daschner *et al.*, *J. antimicrob. Chemother.*, 1982, *9*, 489.

DRUG EXCRETION. Although the mean recovery of piperacillin in urine was reduced from about 70% in patients with normal renal function to about 20% in patients with severe renal impairment, the antibiotic concentration in urine was high in all individuals capable of producing urine. The concentrations achieved in the urine after an intravenous dose of 1 or 4 g were considered to be adequate for the treatment of infections caused by most urinary-tract pathogens.— P. G. Welling *et al.*, *Antimicrob. Ag. Chemother.*, 1983, *23*, 881.

Uses and Administration

Piperacillin sodium is a piperazine derivative of ampicillin which is used for the treatment of infections known or suspected to be caused by susceptible organisms, particularly *Pseudomonas aeruginosa*. It has been used to treat infections of the bones, joints, skin and soft tissues, respiratory tract, and urinary tract, and also gynaecological and intra-abdominal infections, septicaemia, endocarditis, and gonorrhoea. It may also be used for prophylaxis of infections during surgery, particularly abdominal surgery, vaginal hysterectomy, and caesarean section. It is often recommended that piperacillin sodium be administered in association with another antimicrobial agent for the treatment of serious infections. It is commonly given with an aminoglycoside with which synergism has been demonstrated *in vitro*; however they should not be administered in the same infusion as they have been shown to be incompatible. Piperacillin sodium may also be given in association with other beta-lactams or with metronidazole.

For the treatment of serious or complicated infections, piperacillin sodium is given in doses equivalent to 3 to 4 g of piperacillin every 4 to 8 hours intravenously. In life-threatening infections, particularly those caused by *Pseudomonas* or *Klebsiella* spp., it should be given in a dose of not less than 16 g daily. The usual maximum daily dose is 24 g, although this has been exceeded. For mild or uncomplicated infections, the equivalent of 2 g of piperacillin every 6 to 8 hours, or 4 g every 12 hours by intravenous administration, or 2 g every 8 to 12 hours by intramuscular injection may be given. Uncomplicated gonorrhoea may be treated by a single intramuscular dose equivalent to piperacillin 2 g. Probenecid 1 g by mouth may be given half an hour before the injection.

For serious infections, piperacillin sodium is administered by slow intravenous injection over 3 to 5 minutes, or by intravenous infusion over 20 to 40 minutes. For less severe infections, or for maintenance therapy after a response has been obtained to intravenous therapy, it may be given by deep intramuscular injection. Single doses of more than 2 g for adults or 0.5 g for children should not be given by the intramuscular route. To avoid pain on intramuscular injection it may be administered in a 0.5 to 1.0% solution of lignocaine hydrochloride.

For the prophylaxis of infection during surgery, the equivalent of 2 g piperacillin just before the procedure, or when the umbilical cord is clamped in caesarean section, followed by at least 2 doses of 2 g at 4- to 6-hourly intervals may be given.

Children aged 2 months to 12 years may be given piperacillin sodium equivalent to piperacillin 100 to 300 mg per kg body-weight daily in 3 or 4 divided doses. Neonates and infants may be given 100 to 300 mg per kg in 2 divided doses.

Doses of piperacillin sodium may need to be reduced in renal failure.

Reviews of the action and uses of piperacillin sodium.— J. Russo and M. E. Russo, *Clin. Pharm.*, 1982, *1*, 207; G. M. Eliopoulos and R. C. Moellering, *Ann. intern. Med.*, 1982, *97*, 755; *Med. Lett.*, 1982, *24*, 48; *Drug & Ther. Bull.*, 1983, *21*, 71; P. Sesin *et al.*, *Hosp. Formul.*, 1984, *19*, 380; B. Holmes *et al.*, *Drugs*, 1984, *28*, 375.

Guidelines on the choice of drugs for treating anaerobic infections. The antipseudomonal penicillins, carbenicillin, ticarcillin, piperacillin, mezlocillin, and azlocillin, in high dosages may be useful for some *Bacteroides fragilis* infections caused by strains that are relatively resistant to penicillin.— *Med. Lett.*, 1984, *26*, 87.

A suggestion that piperacillin, azlocillin, or mezlocillin in association with an aminoglycoside be used for the treatment of infections with strains of *Pseudomonas aeruginosa* and *Enterobacteriaceae* shown to be inducible for class I beta-lactamases by a disc induction technique. Therapeutic failures due to the emergence of stably derepressed mutants producing significant amounts of these beta-latamases were considered less likely to occur with these penicillins than with the third generation cephalosporins.— M. J. Weinbren and R. M. Perinpanayagam (letter), *Lancet*, 1985, *2*, 673; *idem* (letter), 1986, *1*, 102.

ADMINISTRATION. Piperacillin could be administered into the eye as a 5% topical solution, or by subconjunctival injection in a dose of 100 mg in 0.5 mL.— T. S. Lesar and R. G. Fiscella, *Drug Intell. & clin. Pharm.*, 1985, *19*, 642.

ADMINISTRATION IN LIVER DISORDERS. See below under Administration in Renal Failure.

ADMINISTRATION IN RENAL FAILURE. The normal half-life for piperacillin of 0.8 to 1.5 hours was increased to 3.3 to 5.1 hours in end-stage renal disease (W.M. Bennett *et al.*, *Am. J. Kidney Dis.*, 1983, *3*, 155). Bennett *et al.* have therefore suggested that piperacillin can be given in usual doses to patients with a glomerular filtration-rate (GFR) greater than 50 mL per minute, the dosage interval being 4 to 6 hours. The dosage interval should be increased to 6 to 8 hours in patients with a GFR between 10 and 50 mL per minute, and to 8 hours in those with a GFR less than 10 mL per minute. The manufacturer's recommendations are similar, but they suggest a dosage interval of 12 hours for those patients with the most severe renal impairment. For patients on haemodialysis, they recommend a dosage of 2 g every 8 hours, supplemented by 1 g after each dialysis period.

The half-life of piperacillin in a patient who developed renal and liver failure was estimated to be 32 hours. Careful monitoring of serum concentrations will be necessary in such patients.— L. Green *et al.*, *Drug Intell. & clin. Pharm.*, 1985, *19*, 427.

Further references: P. J. De Schepper *et al.*, *J. antimicrob. Chemother.*, 1982, *9*, *Suppl.* B, 49; G. R. Aronoff *et al.*, *Eur. J. clin. Pharmac.*, 1983, *24*, 543; B. Holmes *et al.*, *Drugs*, 1984, *28*, 375.

For reference to the administration of piperacillin sodium by the intraperitoneal route in patients undergoing continuous ambulatory peritoneal dialysis, see under Peritonitis in Azlocillin Sodium, p.125.

ARTHRITIS, BACTERIAL. For reference to the use of piperacillin sodium in the treatment of bacterial arthritis, see under Osteomyelitis in Flucloxacillin Sodium, p.232.

BILIARY-TRACT INFECTIONS. For reference to the use of piperacillin sodium for the prophylaxis of infection during surgical procedures of the biliary tract, see Mezlocillin Sodium p.261.

GONORRHOEA. In a study involving 142 men with uncomplicated gonococcal urethritis caused by non-beta-lactamase-producing strains of *Neisseria gonorrhoeae*, half were treated with piperacillin 2 g and half with procaine penicillin 4.8 g. Both agents were administered by intramuscular injection into 2 sites, and all patients were given probenecid 1 g by mouth before the injection. All evaluable patients in both groups had a bacteriological and clinical cure.— S. J. Landis *et al.*, *Antimicrob. Ag. Chemother.*, 1981, *20*, 693. In a similar study, all patients with urethritis were cured. All patients with rectal or pharyngeal gonorrhoea were cured except one patient with pharyngeal infection who received piperacillin. After therapy, 4 men in the piperacillin group returned with positive pharyngeal cultures which had been sterile on the initial visit.— M. L. Simpson *et al.*, *ibid.*, 1982, *21*, 727.

MENINGITIS. Reports of intravenous piperacillin sodium in the treatment of meningitis: J. Karpuch *et al.* (letter), *J. Infect.*, 1985, *11*, 272.

NEUTROPENIA. The extended-spectrum penicillins showing high activity against *Pseudomonas aeruginosa*, such as piperacillin, are widely used as part of empirical antibiotic regimens for febrile episodes in neutropenic patients. They have been used alone, but studies with mezlocillin have indicated that their spectrum of activity may be inadequate particularly against *Ps. aeruginosa* and *Staphylococcus aureus* (B.F. Issell and G.P. Bodey, *Antimicrob. Ag. Chemother.*, 1980, *17*, 1008), and that emergence of resistant organisms may occur (J.C. Wade *et al.*, *ibid.*, *18*, 299). Standard regimens in many centres involve an aminoglycoside in association with either an antipseudomonal penicillin, an antistaphylococcal penicillin, or a cephalosporin (R.E. Marcus and J.M. Goldman, *Br. med. J.*, 1986, *293*, 406; J.W. Hathorn and P.A. Pizzo, *J. antimicrob. Chemother.*, 1986, *17*, *Suppl.* A, 41). Such combinations provide a broad spectrum of activity against the majority of likely pathogens, as well as demonstrating a synergistic action *in vitro* in many cases. Vancomycin should be added if *Staph. epidermidis* or other Gram-positive organisms have been isolated on admission. In an early study the European Organization for Research on Treatment of Cancer (EORTC) International Antimicrobial Therapy Project Group (*J. infect. Dis.*, 1978, *137*, 14) compared the following regimens (therapeutic trial I): gentamicin and carbenicillin or ticarcillin; gentamicin and cephalothin; and cephalothin and carbenicillin or ticarcillin. Although the efficacy of these regimens was comparable, the combination of gentamicin and carbenicillin or ticarcillin was preferred because of both its wide antibacterial spectrum and the low frequency of renal dysfunction associated with its use. The EORTC therapeutic trial III (J. Klastersky *et al.*, *Antimicrob. Ag. Chemother.*, 1986, *29*, 263) compared 2-drug therapy involving amikacin in association with azlocillin, ticarcillin, or cefotaxime; the response rates were 66, 47, or 37% respectively in patients with bacteraemia due to Gram-negative bacilli. The lower activity of ticarcillin as compared with azlocillin could be partly ascribed to a high degree of resistance of *Escherichia coli* isolates to ticarcillin. The reason for the poor response to amikacin and cefotaxime was not clear, but there appeared to be a low activity of the combination against infections caused by *Ps. aeruginosa* and *E. coli* in spite of their susceptibility *in vitro*. When selecting an antipseudomonal penicillin for use in association with an aminoglycoside piperacillin, azlocillin, or mezlocillin may be preferred to carbenicillin or ticarcillin in institutions where there is a relatively high prevalence of *Ps. aeruginosa* infections and of carbenicillin- or ticarcillin-resistant organisms (D.J. Winston *et al.*, *J. antimicrob. Chemother.*, 1986, *17*, *Suppl.* A, 55). Also these agents have a lower sodium content than carbenicillin or ticarcillin, hence less effect on electrolyte balance. Ticarcillin has the advantage over carbenicillin that it can be used in lower doses because of its greater antipseudomonal activity and hence has less effect on electrolyte balance and platelet function (K.H. Mayer and O.H. DeTorres, *Drugs*, 1985, *29*, 262).

Due to the toxicity of aminoglycosides, there have been many studies comparing combinations including an aminoglycoside with those of 2 beta-lactam antibiotics, such as latamoxef with either piperacillin or amikacin (D.J. Winston *et al.*, *Am. J. Med.*, 1984, *77*, 442), or latamoxef with ticarcillin or tobramycin (V. Fainstein *et al.*, *Archs intern. Med.*, 1984, *144*, 1766). Neither of these studies observed a significant difference in overall efficacy between the 2 regimens investigated. On assessing these 2 studies Young (*J. antimicrob. Chemother.*, 1985, *16*, 4) considered that there were sufficient problems with double-beta-lactam therapy to warrant caution in the use of such regimens routinely in the immunocompromised host. Some beta-lactams, such as cefoxitin and imipenem, are inducers of beta-lactamases and have shown antagonism with such agents as piperacillin *in vitro*. Young therefore advised that such combinations might be used in immunocompromised patients above the age of 60 years who have borderline or impaired renal and/or auditory nerve function, and could also be justified in patients receiving nephrotoxic agents such as cyclosporin and amphotericin in whom *Ps. aeruginosa*, *Enterobacter*, and *Serratia* spp. have not been isolated. He considered a combination of an antipseudomonal penicillin and an aminoglycoside best for patients with likely or proven *Ps. aeruginosa* infection.

Many centres use 3-drug empirical antibiotic regimens consisting of an aminoglycosde, an antipseudomonal penicillin, and either a first-generation cephalosporin or an antistaphylococcal penicillin (J.W. Hathorn and P.A. Pizzo, *J. antimicrob. Chemother.*, 1986, *17*, *Suppl.* A, 41). The EORTC therapeutic trial II (*J. clin. Oncol.*, 1983, *1*, 597) compared a regimen of carbenicillin or ticarcillin and amikacin with one which also included cephazolin, but could demonstrate no advantage from addition of the cephalosporin.

With the advent of newer beta-lactams, such as ceftizoxime, ceftazidime, cefoperazone, and latamoxef, with broad-spectrum antibacterial activity that includes *Ps. aeruginosa*, and with a bactericidal activity greater than many traditional synergistic combinations, single-agent therapy has again been studied (M. Piccart *et al.*, *Antimicrob. Ag. Chemother.*, 1984, *26*, 870; P.A. Pizzo *et al.*, *New Engl. J. Med.*, 1986, *315*, 552; B.S. Kramer *et al.*, *Antimicrob. Ag. Chemother.*, 1986, *30*, 64). The efficacy of such therapy appears similar to that with regimens using 2 or more agents, and the incidence of adverse effects may be lower, however Hathorn and Pizzo advised caution because of the risk of resistance developing and because of the relatively low activity of these agents against anaerobic organisms and Gram-positive bacteria.

Davey (*J. antimicrob. Chemother.*, 1984, *13*, 204) commented on the design of comparative clinical studies of antibiotic regimens for febrile episodes in neutropenic patients, and considered that the results of many could be predicted from sensitivity tests of recent isolates.

It thus appears that while the newer broad spectrum beta-lactams offer promise, treatment with an antipseudomonal penicillin and an aminoglycoside is for the time being the best option for febrile episodes in neutropenic patients.

For references to studies of a combination of ticarcillin sodium and potassium clavulanate in the treatment of febrile episodes in neutropenic patients, see Ticarcillin Sodium p.325.

OSTEOMYELITIS. For reference to the use of piperacillin sodium in the treatment of osteomyelitis, see Flucloxacillin Sodium, p.232.

PERITONITIS. For reference to the use of piperacillin sodium in the treatment of peritonitis, see Azlocillin Sodium, p.125.

PREGNANCY AND THE NEONATE. Seventy neonates who were suspected of having a bacterial infection in the first 48 hours of life, were treated with either piperacillin and flucloxacillin (study group), or penicillin and gentamicin (control group). Doses of piperacillin (100 mg per kg body-weight) and flucloxacillin (25 mg per kg), or gentamicin (2.5 mg per kg) and penicillin (36 mg per kg) were given intravenously every 12 hours. Antibiotics were continued for 5 to 16 days when infection was confirmed, but discontinued after 3 to 4 days in the absence of clinical and bacteriological evidence of infection. In the group receiving piperacillin and flucloxacillin, infection was eradicated in all patients in whom it was confirmed, including one with a positive blood culture. Four neonates in the control group had a confirmed infection; one deteriorated and therapy was changed to piperacillin and amikacin. Two of the 70 patients developed septicaemia with associated meningitis, one due to *Escherichia coli* and one to *Pseudomonas*; the CSF was rendered sterile after treatment with piperacillin 200 mg per kg every 12 hours, in association with amikacin in one patient. CSF concentrations were considered adequate for the majority of likely pathogens in patients both with and without meningeal inflammation. Although all the bacteria responsible for early infections were fully sensitive to piperacillin, 4 neonates treated with piperacillin and flucloxacillin, and 7 treated with penicillin and gentamicin developed colonisation by Gram-negative organisms moderately or completely resistant to piperacillin. It was therefore recommended that if piperacillin is used for the treatment of early infections, an alternative antibiotic should be used for later infections. Because of the absence of staphylococci in early neonatal infection in this hospital, flucloxacillin was no longer considered essential. It was recommended, however, that piperacillin be used in conjunction with an aminoglycoside or third generation cephalosporin in critically ill neonates with severe neutropenia, and in neonatal meningitis, due to the possibility of resistance of Gram-negative bacteria to piperacillin.— M. Placzek *et al.*, *Archs Dis. Childh.*, 1983, *58*, 1006.

There is little information available on the use of antipseudomonal penicillins, such as azlocillin, carbenicillin, mezlocillin, piperacillin, and ticarcilllin, in pregnancy. It was considered that these agents should be reserved for the treatment of serious infections such as sepsis.— R. Wise, *Br. med. J.*, 1987, *294*, 42.

RESPIRATORY-TRACT INFECTIONS. *Cystic fibrosis*. For reference to a recommendation that piperacillin sodium may best be avoided in patients with cystic fibrosis, see under Allergy in Adverse Effects.

SURGICAL INFECTION PROPHYLAXIS. *Biliary-tract surgery*. For reference to the use of piperacillin sodium for the treatment of infections of the biliary-tract, see Mezlocillin Sodium, p.261.

Caesarean section. Report of a double-blind, multicentre study indicating piperacillin to be as effective as cefoxitin for the prophylaxis of infection during caesarean section. Both drugs were administered by intravenous infusion in 3 doses of 2 g, given immediately after clamping the umbilical cord, and then 4 and 8 hours later. A satisfactory response, defined as no clinical or bacteriological evidence of infection within the 3 to 10 week follow-up period, was observed in 121 of 136 (89%) evaluable patients given piperacillin, and in 136 of 147 (93%) evaluable patients given cefoxitin.— B. B. Benigno *et al.*, *Surgery Gynec. Obstet.*, 1986, *162*, 1.

Intestinal surgery. Report of a double-blind, multicentre study indicating piperacillin to be as effective as cephalothin or cefoxitin for the prophylaxis of infection during intra-abdominal surgery. All drugs were administered intravenously to a total of 8 to 12 g. Of 112 evaluable patients given piperacillin, 106 (95%) had a satisfactory response as defined by no clinical or bacteriological evidence of infection within the 3 to 10 week follow-up period. The corresponding figures for cephalothin and cefoxitin were 63 of 71 patients (89%), and 32 of 36 patients (89%) respectively.— R. J. Baker *et al.*, *Surgery Gynec. Obstet.*, 1985, *161*, 409.

Prostatectomy. In a study of 40 patients undergoing transurethral prostatectomy, 20 received prophylaxis with intravenous piperacillin 2 g every 6 hours for 48 hours. One and 6 patients had a urinary-tract infection 3 and 21 days after the procedure, respectively. The corresponding figures for those patients who received no antibiotic prophylaxis were 8 and 4. Piperacillin appeared to have no effects on the composition of the faecal flora.— J. A. A. Hoogkamp-Korstanje *et al.*, *J. antimicrob. Chemother.*, 1985, *16*, 773.

Preparations

Sterile Piperacillin Sodium *(U.S.P.)*. Suitable for parenteral use.

Proprietary Preparations

Pipril *(Lederle, UK)*. *Injection*, powder for reconstitution, piperacillin 1 and 2 g (as sodium salt).
Intravenous infusion, powder for reconstitution, piperacillin 4 g (as sodium salt), supplied with diluent.

Proprietary Names and Manufacturers

Avocin *(Cyanamid, Ital.)*; Ivacin *(Lederle, Denm.; Lederle, Swed.)*; Pentcillin *(Jpn)*; Piperilline *(Lederle, Fr.)*; Pipracil *(Lederle, Canad.; Lederle, USA)*; Pipril *(Lederle, Austral.; Cyanamid-Lederle, Ger.; Lederle, S.Afr.; Cyanamid, Spain; Lederle, Switz.; Lederle, UK)*.

147-w

Pirlimycin Hydrochloride *(USAN, rINNM)*.

U-57930E. Methyl 7-chloro-6,7,8-trideoxy-6-(*cis*-4-ethyl-L-pipecolamido)-1-thio-L-*threo*-α-D-*galacto*-octopyranoside monohydrochloride monohydrate.
$C_{17}H_{31}ClN_2O_5S,HCl,H_2O$=465.4.

CAS — 79548-73-5 (pirlimycin); 77495-92-2 (hydrochloride).

Pirlimycin hydrochloride is a lincosamide antibiotic.

Studies *in vitro* and in *animals* of the antimicrobial activity of pirlimycin: M. E. Evans *et al.*, *Antimicrob. Ag. Chemother.*, 1982, *22*, 334 (comparison with clindamycin of activity against *Staphylococcus aureus*); J. A. Garcia-Rodriguez *et al.*, *ibid.*, 893 (activity against organisms of the *Bacteroides fragilis* group); G. A. Denys *et al.*, *ibid.*, 1983, *23*, 335 (activity against *Propionibacterium acnes*); A. A. Divo *et al.*, *ibid.*, 1985, *27*, 21 (activity against *Plasmodium falciparum*); R. J. Yancey *et al.*, *J. antimicrob. Chemother.*, 1985, *15*, 219 (activity in *murine* staphylococcal mastitis).

Proprietary Names and Manufacturers

Upjohn, USA.

5667-v

Piromidic Acid *(rINN)*.

PD-93. 8-Ethyl-5,8-dihydro-5-oxo-2-(pyrrolidin-1-yl)pyrido[2,3-*d*]pyrimidine-6-carboxylic acid.
$C_{14}H_{16}N_4O_3$=288.3.

CAS — 19562-30-2.

Piromidic acid is a 4-quinolone antimicrobial agent with similar actions and uses to those of nalidixic acid (see p.267). It is less active than nalidixic acid against Gram-negative organisms but activity against some staphylococci has been reported. Cross-resistance with nalidixic acid occurs. It has been used in the treatment of urinary-tract infections in a dose of 2 g daily in divided doses.

Antimicrobial activity.— M. Shimizu *et al.*, *Antimicrob. Ag. Chemother.*, 1970, 117.

Metabolism.— M. Shimizu *et al.*, *Antimicrob. Ag. Chemother.*, 1970, 123; Y. Sekine *et al.*, *Xenobiotica*, 1976, *6*, 185.

Renal failure in 2 patients possibly associated with the administration of piromidic acid.— *Jpn med. Gaz.*, 1978, *15* (Apr. 20), 10.

Proprietary Names and Manufacturers

Actrun C *(Jpn)*; Bactamyl *(Carrion, Fr.)*; Coltix *(Gramon, Arg.)*; Panacid *(Jpn)*; Panerco *(Erco, Denm.)*; Pirodal *(SIT, Ital.)*; Purim *(Laphal, Fr.)*; Septural *(Grünenthal, Ger.)*; Uriclor *(Almirall, Spain)*; Urol *(Janus, Ital.)*; Uropir *(Salus, Ital.)*.

188-t

Pivampicillin *(BAN, rINN)*.

MK-191. Pivaloyloxymethyl (6*R*)-6-(α-D-phenylglycylamino)penicillanate.
$C_{22}H_{29}N_3O_6S$=463.6.

CAS — 33817-20-8.

1.3 g of monograph substance is approximately equivalent to 1 g of ampicillin.

135-g

Pivampicillin Hydrochloride *(BANM, USAN, rINNM)*.

The hydrochloride of pivampicillin.
$C_{22}H_{29}N_3O_6S,HCl$=500.0.

CAS — 26309-95-5.

Pharmacopoeias. In *Nord.*

1.43 g of monograph substance is approximately equivalent to 1 g of ampicillin.

Adverse Effects and Precautions

As for ampicillin (p.116). Pivampicillin is reported to cause a lower incidence of diarrhoea than ampicillin, although upper gastro-intestinal discomfort may be more frequent. These effects appear to be more common when pivampicillin is taken on an empty stomach.

Ampicillin concentrations in serum, urine, and urogenital tissue were determined in 64 patients given pivampicillin 700 mg by mouth pre-operatively. Absorption of pivampicillin was significantly reduced after 1 hour in patients who received pre-operative medication with atropine and pethidine.— O. Alfthan and O. V. Renkonen, *Arzneimittel-Forsch.*, 1975, *25*, 1831.

For the possibility of pivampicillin causing oesophageal ulceration, see below under Uses, Administration.

For reduced absorption in coeliac disease, see below under Absorption and Fate.

PORPHYRIA. Pivampicillin was considered to be unsafe in patients with acute porphyria as it has been associated with acute attacks.— M.R. Moore and K.E.L. McColl, *Porphyria, Drug Lists*, Glasgow, Porphyria Research Unit, University of Glasgow, 1987.

Antimicrobial Action

Pivampicillin has the antimicrobial activity of ampicillin *in vivo* (see p.117).

Absorption and Fate

Pivampicillin is acid-stable and is readily absorbed from the gastro-intestinal tract. It is rapidly and almost completely hydrolysed to ampicillin by esterases in tissues and blood to produce plasma-ampicillin concentrations 1 hour after administration that are approximately 2 to 3 times higher than those obtained after an equivalent dose of ampicillin. The absorption of pivampicillin is generally not significantly affected by food, although reports have been variable. About 70% of a dose is excreted in the urine as ampicillin within 6 hours.

The absorption of pivampicillin was impaired after administration by mouth to patients with coeliac disease.— R. L. Parsons *et al.*, *J. antimicrob. Chemother.*, 1975, *1*, 39.

See also under Ampicillin Trihydrate, p.119.

Uses and Administration

Pivampicillin has the actions and uses of ampicillin (see p.119) and may be given in doses of 0.5 to 1 g twice daily with food. In gonorrhoea a single dose of 1.5 to 2 g has been given, often in association with probenecid 1 g.

Pivampicillin may also be administered in association with pivmecillinam hydrochloride, see p.289.

A brief review of the actions and uses of pivampicillin.— *Drug & Ther. Bull.*, 1981, *19*, 78.

For comparative reviews and reports of aminopenicillins, see Ampicillin Trihydrate p.119.

ADMINISTRATION. A recommendation that pivampicillin administered by mouth should be given with at least 100 mL of water while the patient is in an upright sitting position to avoid oesophagitis or oesophageal ulceration.— S. K. Vong (letter), *Pharm. J.*, 1987, *1*, 5.

ENDOCARDITIS. Pivampicillin has been used instead of amoxycillin for the oral treatment of streptococcal endocarditis following standard intravenous therapy. Satisfactory trough serum bactericidal titres were obtained after a dose of 2 g given three times daily.— E. G. Smyth and A. P. Pallet (letter), *Lancet*, 1987, *2*, 110.

RESPIRATORY-TRACT INFECTIONS. A study involving 463 patients indicating no overall difference between pivampicillin and amoxycillin administered by mouth in the treatment of respiratory-tract infections.— D. G. Moran, *J. int. med. Res.*, 1983, *11*, 370.

SURGICAL INFECTION PROPHYLAXIS. For reference to the use of pivampicillin in infection prophylaxis for patients undergoing first-trimester abortion, see Benzylpenicillin Sodium, p.138.

ULCERS. *Peptic ulcer.* A suggestion that pivampicillin might be a suitable systemically-active antimicrobial to be used with a locally-active bismuth salt to achieve eradication of *Campylobacter pyloridis*, an organism strongly associated with gastritis, duodenitis, and duodenal ulceration.— C. A. M. McNulty, *Practitioner*, 1987, *231*, 176.

URINARY-TRACT INFECTIONS. Report of a study of 158 women with acute uncomplicated urinary-tract infections treated with pivampicillin 500 mg twice daily by mouth for 5 days. Ninety-five (60%), were symptom-free after treatment, and of 41 with significant bacteriuria the original organism was eradicated in 38.— J. B. Sutton, *J. int. med. Res.*, 1983, *11*, 375.

Proprietary Preparations

Pondocillin *(Burgess, UK)*. *Tablets*, pivampicillin 500 mg.
Oral granules, pivampicillin 175 mg/sachet. To be dispersed in water before administration.
Suspension, powder for reconstitution, pivampicillin 175 mg/5 mL when reconstituted with water.

For preparations of pivampicillin in combination with pivmecillinam hydrochloride, see Pivmecillinam Hydrochloride, p.290.

Proprietary Names and Manufacturers of Pivampicillin and Pivampicillin Hydrochloride

Acerum *(Spain)*; Bensamin *(Spain)*; Berocillin *(Ger.)*; Brotalcilina *(Spain)*; Centurina *(Arg.; Spain)*; Co-Pivam *(Smaller, Spain)*; Crisbiotic *(Crisol, Spain)*; Devonian *(Spain)*; Fasis-pen *(Spain)*; Inacilin *(Inibsa, Spain)*; Isvitrol *(Spain)*; Kesmicina *(Albofarma, Spain)*; Lanzabiotic *(Lanzas, Spain)*; Lervipan *(Lersa, Spain)*; Maxifen *(Ger.)*; Oxidina *(Arg.)*; Penimenal *(Spain)*; Pibena *(Spain)*; Piva Efesal *(IBE, Spain)*; Pivabiot *(Spain)*; Pivacid *(Bicther, Spain)*; Pivacilin-Base *(Boehringer Ingelheim, Spain)*; Pivacostyl *(Pentafarm, Spain)*; Pivadilon *(Cruz, Spain)*; Pivamag *(Spain)*; Pivamboi *(Spain)*; Pivaminol *(Spain)*; Pivamiser *(Serra Pamies, Spain)*; Pivamkey *(Spain)*; Pivam-Piror *(Spain)*; Pivapen *(Spain)*; Pivascel *(Ital.)*; Pivastol *(Spain)*; Pivatil *(Belg.)*; Piviotic *(Spain)*; Pondocil *(Leo, Fr.)*; Pondocillin *(Belg.; Leo, Canad.; Leo, Denm.; Neth.; Leo, Norw.; Leo, S.Afr.; Lövens, Swed.; Burgess, UK)*; Pondocillina *(Ital.)*; Pondocilline *(Leo Suede, Switz.)*; Proampi *(Pharmeurop, Fr.)*; Tam-Cilin *(Spain)*; Tryco *(Spain)*; Vampi-Framan *(Oftalmiso, Spain)*.

The following names have been used for multi-ingredient preparations containing pivampicillin and pivampicillin hydrochloride— Miraxid *(Fisons, UK)*; Pondocillin Plus *(Leo, UK)*.

13138-m

Pivcephalexin Hydrochloride

Pivcefalexin Hydrochloride; ST-21. Pivaloyloxymethyl (7*R*)-3-methyl-7-(α-D-phenylglycylamino)-3-cephem-4-carboxylate hydrochloride.
$C_{22}H_{27}N_3O_6S,HCl$=498.0.

CAS — 27726-31-4.

Pivcephalexin is the pivaloyloxymethyl ester of cephalexin (see p.173). It is administered by mouth as the hydrochloride.

Proprietary Names and Manufacturers

Pivacef *(FIRMA, Ital.)*; Sigmacef *(Sigmatau, Ital.)*.

136-q

Pivmecillinam *(BAN, rINN).*
Amdinocillin Pivoxil *(USAN)*; FL-1039; Ro-10-9071. Pivaloyloxymethyl (6*R*)-6-(perhydroazepin-1-ylmethyleneamino)penicillanate.
$C_{21}H_{33}N_3O_5S$=439.6.
CAS — 32886-97-8.

137-p

Pivmecillinam Hydrochloride *(BANM, rINNM).*

$C_{21}H_{33}N_3O_5S,HCl$=476.0.
CAS — 32887-03-9.

Pivmecillinam 1.35 g and pivmecillinam hydrochloride 1.46 g are each approximately equivalent to 1 g of mecillinam.

Adverse Effects and Precautions
As for Benzylpenicillin Sodium, p.132. Gastro-intestinal adverse effects such as nausea and vomiting may be more common after administration of pivmecillinam on an empty stomach.

EFFECTS ON THE GASTRO-INTESTINAL TRACT. Pivmecillinam 1.2 to 2.4 g administered daily by mouth to healthy subjects greatly reduced *E. coli* and other Enterobacteriaceae of gut flora.— H. Knothe, *Arzneimittel-Forsch.*, 1976, *26*, 427.

Symptoms of oesophageal injury after taking pivmecillinam by mouth had been reported to the Swedish adverse drug reaction advisory committee (20 patients) and to the Committee on Safety of Medicines (5 patients). Pivmecillinam should therefore be taken during a meal while sitting or standing, and washed down with at least half a glass of water.— *Pharm. J.*, 1987, *1*, 443.

Antimicrobial Action
Pivmecillinam has the antimicrobial activity of mecillinam to which it is hydrolysed *in vivo* (see p.257).

Absorption and Fate
Pivmecillinam is well absorbed from the gastro-intestinal tract and is rapidly hydrolysed by esterases in tissues and blood to the active drug mecillinam (see p.257). The presence of food in the stomach does not appear to have a significant effect on absorption. Peak plasma concentrations of mecillinam of up to 5 μg per mL have been achieved 1 to 2 hours after a 400-mg dose of pivmecillinam.
About 45% of a dose may be excreted in the urine as mecillinam, mainly within the first 6 hours of a dose.

Mean serum-mecillinam concentrations of 3.93, 3.48, 1.3, and 0.74 μg per mL were achieved 1, 2, 4, and 6 hours respectively after pivmecillinam 400 mg was given to 22 patients with urinary-tract infections. Urine concentrations of mecillinam at 6 hours ranged from 37 to 787 μg per mL (mean 187 μg per mL) in 33 patients.— R. Wise *et al.*, *Chemotherapy, Basle*, 1976, *22*, 335.

The absorption of pivmecillinam from the gastro-intestinal tract was not altered in patients with coeliac disease.— R. L. Parsons *et al.*, *Br. J. clin. Pharmac.*, 1977, *4*, 267.

Pharmacokinetic studies of bacmecillinam and pivmecillinam, esters of mecillinam.— K. Josefsson *et al.*, *Eur. J. clin. Pharmac.*, 1982, *23*, 249.

COMBINATION WITH PIVAMPICILLIN. Ten patients with urinary-tract infections were given a combination preparation containing pivmecillinam 200 mg and pivampicillin 250 mg three times daily by mouth for 7 to 14 days. The pharmacokinetics of the 2 drugs were similar, and a constant ratio in serum of 2 parts mecillinam to 5 parts ampicillin was maintained.— N. Jeppesen and C. Frimodt-Møller, *Curr. med. Res. Opinion*, 1984, *9*, 213.

Uses and Administration
Pivmecillinam is the pivaloyloxymethyl ester of mecillinam (see p.257), to which it is hydrolysed on administration, and is used in the treatment of Gram-negative infections. Doses of pivmecillinam are expressed in a confusing manner since no differentiation is made between the hydrochloride, used in tablets, and the base, used in suspensions for oral use. In urinary-tract infections the usual dose is 200 to 400 mg of the base or hydrochloride taken three to four times daily, although twice daily regimens have been investigated; children may be given about 20 to 40 mg per kg body-weight daily. Up to 2.4 g daily for 14 days has been recommended for salmonellal infections; carriers may receive the same dose for 2 to 4 weeks.
Pivmecillinam should preferably be taken with food.
Pivmecillinam has been administered in combination with other beta-lactam antibiotics, particularly pivampicillin (p.288), to increase its spectrum of antimicrobial activity to Gram-positive organisms and because of reported synergism against Gram-negative bacteria *in vitro* (see Mecillinam, p.257).
For parenteral administration mecillinam (see p.257) is used.

ENTERIC INFECTIONS. A study in 44 patients suggesting that oral pivmecillinam may be as effective as ampicillin in the treatment of shigellosis. Two strains of *Shigella* spp. were resistant to both ampicillin and pivmecillinam, and a further 4 were resistant to ampicillin alone.— I. Kabir *et al.*, *Antimicrob. Ag. Chemother.*, 1984, *25*, 643.

Mecillinam by mouth [pivmecillinam] 200 mg each morning appeared to be effective prophylaxis against traveller's diarrhoea in 32 students visiting Mexico. The enteric pathogens responsible for the diarrhoea were not detected. Changes in the intestinal flora and its resistance to a range of antibiotics were noted.— K. Gaarslev and J. Stenderup, *Curr. med. Res. Opinion*, 1985, *9*, 384.

Enteric fever. Pivmecillinam by mouth, often preceded by parenteral mecillinam, has been investigated for use in enteric fever. In a retrospective study (A.P. Ball and A.M. Geddes, *Am. J. Med.*, 1983, *75*, *Suppl.*, 130), the response rates to treatment with pivmecillinam or co-trimoxazole were similar, 23 of 26 and 18 of 21 responding satisfactorily in the two groups respectively. The mean times to temperature defervescence were 6.4 and 5.2 days. The overall incidence of complications to treatment or to the disease, and of relapse were similar. The major difference between the 2 treatments was a higher incidence of faecal excretion of the causative organism immediately after treatment in the group receiving pivmecillinam; this resulted in a longer hospital stay. Only one patient in each group became a chronic carrier (positive stools after 3 months).
Because of this defect in pivmecillinam therapy, and also unsatisfactory results reported by Mandal *et al.* (*Br. med. J.*, 1979, *1*, 586), it has been investigated in combination with pivampicillin with encouraging results (D. Tanphaichitra *et al.*, *J. antimicrob. Chemother.*, 1981, *8*, 23). Limson *et al.* (*ibid.*, 1982, *9*, 405) treated 40 patients with enteric fever with pivmecillinam 400 mg four times daily by mouth (12 patients), pivmecillinam 200 mg in association with pivampicillin 250 mg both given four times daily by mouth (15), or chloramphenicol 500 mg four times daily by mouth (13). In some cases treatment during the first 3 to 5 days was given by the parenteral form of the drugs; the total treatment period was 14 days. *Salmonella typhi* or *S. paratyphi A, B,* or *C* was isolated from pre-treatment blood cultures from 24 patients. Several isolates were resistant to chloramphenicol and/or ampicillin; all were sensitive to mecillinam and mecillinam with ampicillin. Patients infected with chloramphenicol-resistant pathogens were not randomised to treatment with chloramphenicol. A satisfactory clinical response, accompanied by negative blood and stool cultures on completion of therapy, was achieved in 35 patients, including 12 of those treated with chloramphenicol and all 15 treated with pivmecillinam and pivampicillin. Only 8 patients given pivmecillinam alone, however, responded clinically. The 4 in whom treatment failed subsequently responded to chloramphenicol or co-trimoxazole. The incidence of relapses or persistent faecal excretion were not monitored.
Pivmecillinam has also been investigated in the eradication of chronic carriage of *Salmonella* spp. Jonsson (*ibid.*, 1977, *3*, *Suppl.* B, 103) treated 12 chronic carriers with pivmecillinam 300 mg four times daily by mouth for 28 days followed when necessary after 5 weeks by 1.2 g four times daily for a further week. Of 8 patients who appeared to have been cured one year after treatment, one had been cured after cholecystectomy during treatment and 2 had been cured only after receiving both courses of treatment and undergoing cholecystectomy. Nye and Roberts (*Br. med. J.*, 1978, *2*, 1502), however, were not so successful in eradicating organisms from the stools of faecal excreters of *Salmonella* using pivmecillinam or mecillinam by mouth, although they used a shorter course of treatment initially and did not follow it by high-dose treatment.

PREGNANCY AND THE NEONATE. See under Urinary-tract Infections, below.

RESPIRATORY-TRACT INFECTIONS. *Combination with pivampicillin.* In a comparative study of 49 patients with acute exacerbations of chronic bronchitis, 25 were given pivmecillinam 300 mg in association with pivampicillin 375 mg twice daily by mouth while 24 were given co-trimoxazole 480 mg twice daily by mouth, both for 10 days. Both treatments were equally effective clinically; one patient in the co-trimoxazole group withdrew from the study after 4 days due to side-effects.— S. Lal *et al.*, *J. antimicrob. Chemother.*, 1984, *14*, 179. See also M. J. Atkins and D. J. Talbot, *J. int. med. Res.*, 1987, *15*, 115.

Further studies of the use of a combination of pivmecillinam and pivampicillin in the treatment of respiratory-tract infections: K. Shenderey *et al.*, *Pharmatherapeutica*, 1985, *4*, 300 (comparison with amoxycillin); R. B. Wallace *et al.*, *Curr. med. Res. Opinion*, 1985, *9*, 659 (comparison with co-trimoxazole); D. McGhie *et al.*, *J. int. med. Res.*, 1986, *14*, 254 (comparison with a combination of amoxycillin and clavulanic acid).

SURGICAL INFECTION PROPHYLAXIS. *Prostatectomy. Combination with pivampicillin.* Report of a study concluding that a short course of pivmecillinam in association with pivampicillin by mouth could be used as an alternative to a parenteral antibiotic such as cefotaxime for the prophylaxis of bacteriuria in patients undergoing transurethral prostatic resection.— M. Grabe *et al.*, *Scand. J. infect. Dis.*, 1986, *18*, 567.

URINARY-TRACT INFECTIONS. Pivmecillinam has been used in various dosage regimens in the "blind" treatment of urinary symptoms such as frequency and dysuria in non-hospitalised patients. Such symptoms are not always associated with a significant bacteriuria. Pettersson *et al.* (*Curr. ther. Res.*, 1984, *35*, 618) considered a dosage of 200 or 400 mg three times daily by mouth for 7 days to be equally effective, while Marsh and Menday (*J. int. Med. Res.*, 1980, *8*, 105) found no difference between 200 mg three times daily for 3 or 7 days. Twice daily regimens have also been investigated, Sutlieff (*Curr. med. Res. Opinion*, 1982, *7*, 563) obtaining a similar response after a dosage regimen of 400 mg initially followed by 200 mg three times daily for 3 days as after 200 mg twice daily for 5 days. Richards (*ibid.*, 1984, *9*, 197) concluded treatment with pivmecillinam 400 mg twice daily for 3 or 7 days to be equally effective. All these studies assessed both the symptomatic and bacteriological response to treatment.

Twenty children, aged 5 months to 14 years, with acute pyelonephritis were treated with pivmecillinam 25 to 40 mg per kg body-weight daily given by mouth in 2 to 3 divided doses for 10 days. Bacteriuria was eradicated 4 to 7 days after commencing treatment in 16 patients with *Escherichia coli* and 2 patients with *Klebsiella pneumoniae* infection; and also in one patient with infection due to *Staphylococcus saprophyticus* although this showed resistance to mecillinam *in vitro*. In the one patient with infection due to a mixed Gram-positive flora, treatment was changed to ampicillin. During a follow-up period of at least one month after the end of treatment, recurrent infection occurred in only one patient who had a congenital abnormality of the urinary tract.— I. Helin, *J. int. med. Res.*, 1983, *11*, 113.

Pivmecillinam was an effective treatment for bacteriuria in 33 of 38 pregnant women given 200 mg three times daily by mouth for a week. A further 6 women could not be evaluated, 2 of whom ceased treatment due to side-effects. Ten of the successfully treated women went on to receive pivmecillinam 100 mg by mouth on alternate days for 2 to 3 months, in an unsuccessful attempt to determine whether subsequent low-dose prophylactic therapy would prevent further episodes of bacteriuria. Thirty-nine of the 41 women followed to term delivered normal infants; there was one still-birth and another child was born with a cleft palate, but it was unlikely that the drug was implicated. Pivmecillinam was considered a safe agent for use in pregnancy: further prospective studies of its potential value for low-dose prophylaxis of bacteriuria are needed.— P. Sanderson and P. Menday, *J. antimicrob. Chemother.*, 1984, *13*, 383.

Combination with pivampicillin. A study of 58 patients with symptoms of urinary frequency, dysuria, or loin pain, treated for 5 days by mouth with a combination of pivmecillinam 200 mg and pivampicillin 250 mg given twice daily, or of amoxycillin 250 mg and clavulanic acid 125 mg given three times daily. Of those patients who had significant bacteriuria, 19 of 23 and 12 of 18 were bacteriologically cured one month after commencing treatment in the 2 groups respectively. Symptomatic response, however, was less satisfactory, 10 and 5 patients respectively still presenting with symptoms after one week.— T. C. O'Dowd *et al.*, *Curr. med. Res. Opinion*, 1984, *9*, 310.

Further studies of the use of a combination of pivmecillinam and pivampicillin in the treatment of urinary-tract infections: H. Gippert *et al.*, *J. antimicrob. Chemother.*, 1981, *7*, 185 (comparison with pivmecillinam); C. Frimodt-Møller and R. Vejlsgaard, *J. int. med. Res.*, 1981, *9*, 283 (comparison with pivmecillinam); C. S. Iosif *et al.*, *Acta obstet. gynec. scand.*, 1983, *62*, 515 (comparison with co-trimoxazole).

For reference to a comparative study of pivmecillinam and nitrofurantoin in the prophylaxis of recurrent urinary-tract infections in children, see Nitrofurantoin, p.274.

Proprietary Preparations

Miraxid *(Fisons, UK)*. *Tablets*, pivmecillinam hydrochloride 100 mg, pivampicillin 125 mg.
Tablets, (Miraxid 450), pivmecillinam hydrochloride 200 mg, pivampicillin 250 mg.
Paediatric suspension, pivmecillinam 46.2 mg, pivampicillin 62.5 mg/sachet. To be dispersed in water before administration.

Pondocillin Plus *(Leo, UK)*. *Tablets*, pivmecillinam hydrochloride 200 mg, pivampicillin 250 mg.

Selexid *(Burgess, UK)*. *Tablets*, pivmecillinam hydrochloride 200 mg.
Oral granules, pivmecillinam 100 mg/sachet. To be dispersed in water before administration.

Proprietary Names and Manufacturers of Pivmecillinam and Pivmecillinam Hydrochloride

Maxibiol *(Berenguer-Beneyto, Spain)*; Melicin *(Jpn)*; Selecid *(Alter, Spain)*; Selexid *(Leo, Canad.*; *Hässle, Denm.*; *Leo, Fr.*; *Neth.*; *Leo, Norw.*; *Burgess, UK)*; Selexidin *(Lövens, Swed.)*; Tindacilin *(Hosbon, Spain)*.

The following names have been used for multi-ingredient preparations containing pivmecillinam and pivmecillinam hydrochloride— Miraxid *(Fisons, UK)*; Pondocillin Plus *(Leo, UK)*.

139-w

Polymyxin B Sulphate *(BANM, rINNM)*.

Polymyxin B Sulfate *(USAN)*; Polymyxini B Sulfas.

CAS — 1404-26-8 (polymyxin B); 1405-20-5 (sulphate).

Pharmacopoeias. In *Arg.*, *Aust.*, *Belg.*, *Br.*, *Braz.*, *Egypt.*, *Eur.*, *Fr.*, *Ger.*, *Int.*, *It.*, *Jpn*, *Jug.*, *Neth.*, *Nord.*, *Swiss*, *Turk.*, and *U.S.*

A mixture of the sulphates of polypeptides produced by the growth of certain strains of *Bacillus polymyxa* or obtained by other means. A white or buff-coloured, hygroscopic powder, odourless or with a slight odour. The *B.P.* specifies that it contains not less than 6500 units per mg and the *U.S.P.* specifies not less than 6000 units of polymyxin B per mg both calculated on the dried substance.

The *B.P.* states **soluble**, and the *U.S.P.* freely soluble in water; both state slightly soluble in alcohol. The *B.P.* states that a 2% solution in water has a pH of 5 to 7, and the *U.S.P.* that a 0.5% solution has a pH of 5.0 to 7.5.

Store in a cool place in airtight containers. Protect from light.

Incompatibility or loss of activity has been reported with many other antimicrobial agents including amphotericin, ampicillin sodium, cephalothin sodium, cephazolin sodium, chloramphenicol sodium succinate, nitrofurantoin sodium, and tetracycline hydrochloride; and also with calcium and magnesium salts, heparin sodium, and prednisolone sodium phosphate. Polymyxin B sulphate is rapidly inactivated by strong acids and alkalis.

Units

One unit of polymyxin B is contained in 0.000119 mg of the second International Standard Preparation (1969) of polymyxin B sulphate which contains 8403 units per mg.

NOTE. The available forms of polymyxin B sulphate are generally less pure than the International Standard Preparation and doses are sometimes stated in terms of pure polymyxin base; 100 mg of pure polymyxin B is considered to be equivalent to 1 million units (1 mega unit).

Adverse Effects

Neurotoxic reactions including dizziness, ataxia, and sensory disturbances of the face and extremities are fairly common following the parenteral administration of polymyxin B sulphate and appear to be dose-related. Reversible neuromuscular blockade resulting in respiratory paralysis has occurred especially in patients with impaired renal function. Serious dose-related nephrotoxicity can develop and produce haematuria, proteinuria, and tubular necrosis. Meningeal irritation may follow the intrathecal administration of polymyxin B when given in doses of 50 000 to 100 000 units. Other side-effects include fever and skin rashes; pain following intramuscular injection can be severe. Bronchial irritation may occur on inhalation of polymyxin B sulphate.

ALLERGY. A study in 26 patients with atopic asthma suggesting that bronchospasm after inhalation of polymyxin B sulphate is due to mast-cell degranulation.— P. Górski *et al.*, *Allergy*, 1985, *40*, 70.

EFFECTS ON THE EAR. Intratympanic application of a 0.1% solution of polymyxin B sulphate appeared to be harmless in *guinea pigs*, but concentrations of 0.2 to 2.5% produced sensory cell degeneration in the cochlea, ranging from loss of a few hair cells to complete destruction of the organ of Corti. Other less toxic drugs might be safer where prolonged local therapy for chronic otitis media is required.— A. Kohonen and J. Tarkkanen, *Acta oto-lar.*, 1969, *68*, 90.

A reminder of the increased risk of drug-induced deafness in patients with perforation of the tympanic membrane when otitis externa is treated topically with preparations containing polymyxins. It is important to ensure that there is no perforation before such preparations are prescribed.— Committee on Safety of Medicines, Current Problems Series No. 5, February 1981.

EFFECTS ON ELECTROLYTE HOMOEOSTASIS. Severe hypochloraemia, hypokalaemia, hyponatraemia, and nitrogen retention developed in 57 adults with acute leukaemia given 107 courses of treatment with polymyxin B. Hypocalcaemia was evident in most patients whose serum calcium was determined. These electrolyte abnormalities were considered to be early indications of polymyxin B toxicity. The toxicity was related to the duration of treatment.— V. Rodriguez *et al.*, *Clin. Pharmac. Ther.*, 1970, *11*, 106.

Treatment of Adverse Effects

Most of the adverse effects of polymyxin B are reversible although recovery may be slow. Patients with respiratory paralysis can be treated with artificial respiration; the administration of calcium salts may be of some benefit. Neostigmine has been used with conflicting results and probably has no place in the treatment of such patients.

There have been conflicting reports of the value of peritoneal dialysis or haemodialysis in the removal of polymyxins from the blood.

For a report of the successful use of exchange transfusion in the treatment of colistin overdosage, see Colistin Sulphomethate Sodium, p.204.

Precautions

Polymyxin B sulphate should not be given to patients with a history of hypersensitivity to the polymyxins. Reduced dosage should be employed in patients with impaired renal function. Because polymyxin may give rise to muscular weakness and respiratory depression, patients should be constantly supervised during parenteral therapy; special care is required for patients with myasthenia gravis and those who have received neuromuscular blocking agents, general anaesthetics, or drugs such as colistin or gentamicin and the other aminoglycosides which are neurotoxic. It should be used cautiously if other potentially nephrotoxic drugs are used.

Ear-drops containing polymyxin B or colistin should not be used in patients with perforated ear-drums.

Antimicrobial Action

Polymyxin B and the other polymyxin antibiotics act primarily by binding to and changing the permeability of the bacterial cytoplasmic membrane. Polymyxin B has a bactericidal action on most Gram-negative bacilli except *Proteus* spp. It is particularly effective against *Pseudomonas aeruginosa*, *Escherichia coli*, *Enterobacter*, and *Klebsiella* spp. Of the other Gram-negative organisms, *Haemophilus influenzae*, *Bordetella pertussis*, *Salmonella*, and *Shigella* spp. are sensitive. Classical *Vibrio cholerae* is sensitive but the *eltor* biotype is resistant. *Serratia marcescens* and *Bacteroides fragilis* are usually resistant. It is not active against *Neisseria gonorrhoeae*, *N. meningitidis*, fungi, and Gram-positive bacteria.

In the presence of large amounts of serum, polymyxin B is reported to lose about 50% of its activity *in vitro*. Most sensitive organisms are inhibited by 0.1 to 0.2 units (0.01 to 0.02 μg) per mL.

Polymyxin B inhibited all of 12 strains of *Coccidioides immitis in vitro* at a concentration of 10 μg per mL. Fungistatic activity was demonstrated in *mice* infected with the organism.— M. S. Collins and D. Pappagianis, *Antimicrob. Ag. Chemother.*, 1976, *10*, 318.

Polymyxin B showed slight activity *in vitro* against *Acanthamoeba* spp.— R. J. Duma and R. Finley, *Antimicrob. Ag. Chemother.*, 1976, *10*, 370.

There was no evidence of any change in the susceptibility of strains of *Bordetella pertussis* over the 2 decades between 1960 and 1981. All isolates had MICs of polymyxin B in the range 0.03 to 0.12 μg per mL.— R. M. Bannatyne and R. Cheung, *Antimicrob. Ag. Chemother.*, 1982, *21*, 666.

An *in-vitro* study in *Escherichia coli* to investigate the mechanism of action of polymyxin B.— R. A. Dixon and I. Chopra, *J. antimicrob. Chemother.*, 1986, *18*, 557.

ACTIVITY WITH OTHER ANTIMICROBIAL AGENTS. The activities of polymyxin B and rifampicin were enhanced when used together *in vitro* against 52 isolates of *Serratia marcescens*.— R. C. Ostenson *et al.*, *Antimicrob. Ag. Chemother.*, 1977, *12*, 655.

Polymyxin B protected *Pr. mirabilis in vitro* against usually bactericidal concentrations of benzylpenicillin.— I. J. Sud and D. S. Feingold, *Antimicrob. Ag. Chemother.*, 1978, *14*, 916.

Resistance

Bacteria do not readily acquire resistance to polymyxins, but when resistance does occur *in vitro* there is complete cross-resistance between polymyxin B and colistin. Resistant strains of *Pseudomonas aeruginosa* have occasionally been reported.

Evidence for 2 distinct mechanisms of resistance to polymyxin B in *Pseudomonas aeruginosa*.— R. A. Moore *et al.*, *Antimicrob. Ag. Chemother.*, 1984, *26*, 539.

Absorption and Fate

Polymyxin B sulphate is not absorbed from the gastro-intestinal tract, except in the newborn. It is not absorbed through the intact skin.

Peak plasma concentrations after intramuscular administration are usually obtained within 2 hours, but are variable. Accumulation may occur after repeated doses. Polymyxin B is reported to have a half-life of about 6 hours. There is no diffusion into the CSF.

Polymyxin B sulphate is excreted mainly by the kidneys, up to 60% being recovered in the urine, but there is a considerable time lag before an effective concentration is built up in the urine.

Faecal binding of polymyxin B.— M. P. Hazenberg *et al.*, *J. antimicrob. Chemother.*, 1986, *17*, 333.

Uses and Administration

Polymyxin B as the sulphate is used by intravenous or sometimes by intramuscular injection in the treatment of systemic and urinary-tract infections due to susceptible organisms which are resistant to other less toxic antibiotics, particularly *Pseudomonas aeruginosa*. Meningitis has been treated by intrathecal injections. Polymyxin B sulphate, often in association with neomycin (see p.269) and bacitracin (see p.129), is applied topically in the treatment of skin, ear, and eye infections and solutions are used for inhalation and/or bladder irrigation.

It has been given orally in association with other oral antibiotics for the suppression of intestinal flora.

In systemic infections the usual dose is 15 000 to 25 000 units per kg body-weight daily administered, diluted in glucose 5%, by continuous intravenous infusion or as 2 infusions administered over 1 to 2 hours and given 12 hours apart. Infants have been given up to 40 000 units per kg daily. Intramuscular administration is not recommended routinely because of severe pain at injection sites but doses of 15 000 to 30 000 units per kg have been given daily in divided doses every 4 to 6 hours. Neonates have been given up to 45 000 units per kg daily. Pain may be reduced by administration in procaine hydrochloride solution 1%. Parenteral doses of polymyxin B sulphate should be reduced in patients with impaired renal function. In meningeal infections a dose of 50 000 units in 1 mL of 0.9% sodium chloride injection may be given daily by intrathecal injection to adults and 20 000 units daily to children under 2 years of age; it may be administered on alternate days once the CSF is sterile. Concurrent parenteral therapy is required if a systemic infection is present. In eye infections doses of up to 100 000 units daily have been injected subconjunctivally and 0.1 to 0.25% solutions have been administered as drops. A 0.01 to 0.1% solution of polymyxin B sulphate may be used for inhalation, and a 0.1 to 1% solution, cream, or ointment for topical administration.

Eight of 12 patients with nosocomial infections due to multiple-resistant strains of *Serratia marcescens* had a favourable response to treatment with polymyxin B given intravenously and rifampicin taken by mouth 2 hours before each infusion of polymyxin B. Three patients died and one of the deaths was associated with supra-infection with *Proteus mirabilis*. Another patient developed jaundice which regressed when the antibiotics were withdrawn.— R. C. Ostenson *et al.*, *Antimicrob. Ag. Chemother.*, 1977, *12*, 655.

ADMINISTRATION IN RENAL FAILURE. The manufacturer has recommended that patients with renal impairment be given a dose of polymyxin B sulphate 25 000 units per kg body-weight on the first day. Subsequent doses should be as follows: for a creatinine clearance 30 to 80% of normal, 10 000 to 15 000 units per kg daily; for a creatinine clearance 25% of normal, 10 000 to 15 000 units per kg every 2 to 3 days; for anuric patients 10 000 units per kg every 5 to 7 days. Additional guidance should be obtained by regular monitoring of serum-polymyxin B concentrations which should be kept below 10 μg per mL.

EYE INFECTIONS. Use of an ophthalmic solution containing polymyxin B and trimethoprim in the treatment of bacterial conjunctivitis.— J. R. Gibson, *J. antimicrob. Chemother.*, 1983, *11*, 217.

Preparations

Polymyxin Injection *(B.P.C. 1973)*. Polymyxin B Sulphate Injection

Sterile Polymyxin B Sulfate *(U.S.P.)*

Polymyxin Ear Drops *(A.P.F.)*. Contain polymyxin B sulphate.

Polymyxin Eye Drops *(A.P.F.)*. Contain polymyxin B sulphate.

Polymyxin and Bacitracin Eye Ointment *(B.P.)*. Polymyxin B Sulphate and Bacitracin Zinc Eye Ointment

Polymyxin B Sulfate and Bacitracin Zinc Topical Aerosol *(U.S.P.)*

Polymyxin B Sulfate and Bacitracin Zinc Topical Powder *(U.S.P.)*

Polymyxin B Sulfate and Hydrocortisone Otic Solution *(U.S.P.)*. pH 3 to 5.

For other preparations containing polymyxin B sulphate, see under bacitracin zinc, chloramphenicol, neomycin, and oxytetracycline hydrochloride.

Proprietary Preparations

Aerosporin *(Calmic, UK)*. *Injection*, powder for reconstitution, polymyxin B sulphate 500 000 units.

Polyfax *(Calmic, UK)*. *Eye ointment*, polymyxin B sulphate 10 000 units, bacitracin zinc 500 units/g. *Ointment*, ingredients as for eye ointment.

For other proprietary preparations containing polymyxin B sulphate, see under Neomycin Sulphate, p.270, and Trimethoprim, p.331.

Proprietary Names and Manufacturers

Aerosporin *(Wellcome, Canad.; Switz.; Calmic, UK; Wellcome, USA)*.

The following names have been used for multi-ingredient preparations containing polymyxin b sulphate—

Aerocortin *(Wellcome, Austral.)*; Aerosporin *(Wellcome, Austral.)*; Ak-Spore Ophthalmic Ointment *(Akorn, USA)*; Ak-Spore Ophthalmic Solution *(Akorn, USA)*; Ak-Trol *(Akorn, USA)*; Bacticort *(Rugby, USA)*; BaySporin *(Bay, USA)*; Chloromyxin *(Parke, Davis, Austral.)*; Cortisporin Cream *(Wellcome, Canad.; Wellcome, USA)*; Cortisporin Ointment *(Wellcome, Canad.; Wellcome, USA)*; Dexacidin *(Coopervision, USA)*; Dexasporin *(Pharmafair, USA)*; Di-Hydrotic *(Legere, USA)*; Dispray Antibiotic Powder Spray *(Stuart, UK)*; Drotic *(Ascher, USA)*; Gregoderm *(Unigreg, UK)*; LazerSporin-C *(Pedinol, USA)*; Lidosporin *(Wellcome, Canad.)*; Maxitrol *(Alcon, Canad.; Alcon, UK; Alcon Laboratories, USA)*; Mycitracin *(Upjohn, Austral.)*; Neo-Polycin *(Merrell Dow, USA)*; Neosporin Aerosol *(Wellcome, Canad.)*; Neosporin Cream *(Wellcome, Canad.; Wellcome, USA)*; Neosporin Cream-G *(Wellcome, USA)*; Neosporin Irrigation Solution *(Wellcome, Canad.; Wellcome, USA)*; Neosporin Ointment *(Wellcome, Austral.; Wellcome, Canad.; Wellcome, USA)*; Neosporin Ophthalmic Ointment *(Wellcome, Austral.; Wellcome, Canad.; Wellcome, USA)*; Neosporin Ophthalmic Solution *(Wellcome, Austral.; Wellcome, Canad.; Calmic, UK; Wellcome, USA)*; Neosporin Powder *(Wellcome, Canad.)*; Neotracin *(Cilag, Austral.)*; Octicair *(Pharmafair, USA)*; Ocu-Cort *(Ocumed, USA)*; Ocumycin *(Pharmafair, USA)*; Ocu-Spor-B *(Ocumed, USA)*; Ocu-Spor-G *(Ocumed, USA)*; Ocutricin HC Ointment *(Pharmafair, USA)*; Ocutricin Ointment *(Pharmafair, USA)*; Ocutricin Solution *(Pharmafair, USA)*; Ocu-Trol *(Ocumed, USA)*; Ophthocort *(Parke, Davis, Canad.; Parke, Davis, USA)*; Otobiotic *(Schering, USA)*; Otocort *(Lemmon, USA)*; Otosporin *(Calmic, UK)*; Ototrips *(Consolidated Chemicals, UK)*; Polybactrin *(Wellcome, Austral.; Calmic, UK)*; Polyfax *(Calmic, UK)*; Poly-Pred *(Allergan, USA)*; Polysporin *(Wellcome, Canad.; Wellcome, USA)*; Polytrim *(Wellcome, UK)*; Pyocidin-Otic *(Forest Pharmaceuticals, USA)*; Rikospray Antibiotic *(Riker, UK)*; Spersin *(Sigma, Austral.)*; Synalar Bi-otic *(Syncare, Canad.)*; Terra-Cortril Ear Suspension *(Pfizer, UK)*; Terramycin Ointment *(Pfipharmecs, USA)*; Terramycin Ophthalmic Ointment with Polymyxin B Sulphate *(Pfizer, Austral.; Pfizer, UK; Roerig, USA)*; Topisporin *(Pharmafair, USA)*; Tribiotic *(Riker, UK)*; Tri-Thalmic *(Schein, USA)*; Uniroid *(Unigreg, UK)*.

140-m

Pristinamycin *(BAN, rINN)*.

RP-7293.

CAS — 11006-76-1.

Antimicrobial substances produced by the growth of *Streptomyces pristina spiralis*.

Pristinamycin is a streptogramin antibiotic with actions and uses similar to virginiamycin (p.337). It is administered by mouth in the treatment of susceptible infections in a dose of 2 to 4 g daily in divided doses. Children have been given 50 to 100 mg per kg body-weight daily.

A study of the activity *in vitro* of pristinamycin against oral streptococci, compared with that of amoxycillin, vancomycin, and erythromycin.— J. P. Maskell and J. D. Williams, *J. antimicrob. Chemother.*, 1987, *19*, 585.

See also Erythromycin, p.223.

Proprietary Names and Manufacturers

Pyostacine *(Rhone-Poulenc, Belg.; Specia, Fr.)*.

141-b

Procaine Penicillin *(BAN)*.

Benzylpenicillin Novocaine; Benzylpenicillinum Procainum; Penicillin G Procaine *(USAN)*; Procaine Benzylpenicillin; Procaine Penicillin G; Procaini Benzylpenicillinum. 2-(4-Aminobenzoyloxy)ethyldiethylammonium (6*R*)-6-(2-phenylacetamido)penicillanate monohydrate.

$C_{13}H_{20}N_2O_2,C_{16}H_{18}N_2O_4S,H_2O=588.7$.

CAS — 54-35-3 (anhydrous); 6130-64-9 (monohydrate).

Pharmacopoeias. In *Arg., Aust., Belg., Br., Braz., Chin., Cz., Egypt., Eur., Fr., Ger., Hung., Ind., Int., Jpn, Jug., Mex., Neth., Nord., Pol., Port., Roum., Rus., Span., Swiss,* and *Turk. U.S.* includes Sterile Penicillin G Procaine. Also in *B.P. Vet.*

A white, crystalline powder with a faint characteristic odour. Procaine penicillin 600 mg is approximately equivalent to 360 mg of benzylpenicillin (600 000 units).

The *B.P.* **solubilities** are: slightly soluble in water; freely soluble in alcohol. *U.S.P.* solubilities are: soluble 1 in 250 of water, 1 in 30 of alcohol, and 1 in 60 of chloroform. A 0.33% solution in water has a pH of 5.0 to 7.5. It is rapidly inactivated by acids, alkali hydroxides, and oxidising agents.

Store at a temperature not exceeding 30° in airtight containers. Protect from moisture.

Adverse Effects and Precautions

As for Benzylpenicillin Sodium, p.132.

Severe, usually transient, reactions with symptoms of severe anxiety and agitation, psychotic reactions, including visual and auditory disturbances, seizures, tachycardia and hypertension, cyanosis, and a sensation of impending death have occasionally been reported with procaine penicillin and may be due to accidental intravascular injection. Procaine has been implicated as a cause of these reactions, especially after injection of high doses. This reaction has been termed non-allergic, pseudoallergic, pseudoanaphylactic, or Hoigné's syndrome.

Procaine penicillin should not be injected intravascularly since ischaemic reactions may occur.

Procaine penicillin should not be given to patients known to be hypersensitive to procaine.

Reports of non-allergic reactions to procaine penicillin: J. E. Galpin *et al.*, *Ann. intern. Med.*, 1974, *81*, 358; T. F. Downham and D. P. Ramos, *Mich. Med.*, 1973, *72*, 223; H. E. Menke and L. Pepplinkhuizen (letter), *Lancet*, 1974, *2*, 723; R. L. Green *et al.*, *New Engl. J. Med.*, 1974, *291*, 223; T. J. Silber and L. D'Angelo, *Am. J. Dis. Child.*, 1985, *139*, 335.

Absorption and Fate

When procaine penicillin is given by intramuscular injection, it forms a depot from which it is slowly released and hydrolysed to benzylpenicillin (see p.135). Peak plasma concentrations are produced in 1 to 4 hours, and effective concentrations of benzylpenicillin are usually maintained for 12 to 24 hours. However, plasma concentrations are lower than those following an equivalent dose of benzylpenicillin.

Results of a study to investigate the CSF concentrations of penicillin achieved after varying dosage schedules of procaine penicillin in patients with late or congenital syphilis. Treponemicidal concentrations (considered to be 18 ng of benzylpenicillin per mL) were achieved in none of 4 patients given intramuscular procaine penicillin 600 mg for 10 days and 2 of 3 given the same dose of procaine penicillin in association with probenecid 500 mg every 6 hours by mouth; and also in 4 of 5 patients given procaine penicillin 1.2 g with probenecid, and 9 of 9 given 2.4 g with probenecid.— E. M. C. Dunlop *et al.*, *J. Am. med. Ass.*, 1979, *241*, 2538.

For reference to the serum concentrations of procaine penicillin after its intramuscular administration in association with benzathine penicillin, see p.130.

Uses and Administration

Procaine penicillin is administered by deep intramuscular injection to create a depot from which benzylpenicillin is slowly liberated. It has the same antimicrobial action as benzylpenicillin (see p.133) and is used for similar purposes in doses of 600 mg to 1.2 g daily in one or two doses, often divided between 2 injection sites. However, because of the relatively low blood concentrations produced, its use should be restricted to infections caused by micro-organisms that are highly sensitive to penicillin. Procaine penicillin should not be used as the sole treatment for severe acute infections, and when bacteraemia is present.

In the treatment of gonorrhoea 4.8 g is given as a single dose with probenecid, usually 1 g by mouth, taken about 30 minutes before the injection. Children may be given procaine penicillin 100 mg per kg body-weight intramuscularly with probenecid 25 mg per kg by mouth. Patients with early syphilis are given procaine penicillin 600 mg daily for 8 to 10 days, or for longer in late syphilis. Children with congenital syphilis have been given 50 to 100 mg per kg body-weight daily for 10 days.

For a report of the use of procaine penicillin in the treatment of louse-borne relapsing fever, see Tetracycline Hydrochloride, p.320.

ANTHRAX. For reference to the use of procaine penicillin in the treatment of anthrax, see Benzylpenicillin Sodium, p.136.

ENDOCARDITIS. Intramuscular procaine penicillin could be used as an alternative to intravenous benzylpenicillin for selected patients in the treatment of penicillin-sensitive streptococcal infective endocarditis. A dose of 1.2 g every 6 hours could be given for 2 or 4 weeks in association with intramuscular streptomycin 7.5 mg per kg body-weight every 12 hours for 2 weeks. Patients with suspected intracranial mycotic aneurysm or cerebritis, and those with decreased peripheral perfusion were not treated with procaine penicillin because of presumed decreased absorption from the intramuscular site.— W. R. Wilson *et al.*, *Mayo Clin. Proc.*, 1982, *57*, 95.

Prophylaxis. Postextraction bacteraemia occurred in 17 of 82 children with cardiac disease given procaine penicillin 900 mg and benzylpenicillin 180 mg both by intramuscular injection for prophylactic cover 45 minutes before dental extraction; none developed endocarditis. Children under 6 years of age were given half this dose. Viridans streptococci were cultured from 10 children, other aerobes from 8 and anaerobes from 5. The mean serum-penicillin concentration did not differ between those with positive and negative blood cultures.— J. Hess *et al.*, *Pediatrics*, 1983, *71*, 554.

PREGNANCY AND THE NEONATE. For reference to the use of procaine penicillin in the neonate and during pregnancy see under Sexually Transmitted Diseases, below, and in Benzylpenicillin Sodium, p.137.

SEXUALLY TRANSMITTED DISEASES. *Gonorrhoea.* In areas where gonococci are known to have maintained chromosomal sensitivity to penicillin and where beta-lactamase-producing gonococci comprise less than 1% of isolates, procaine penicillin 4.8 g intramuscularly administered in association with probenecid 1 g by mouth is considered useful for the treatment of rectal or pharyngeal gonococcal infections (WHO Expert Committee on Venereal Diseases and Treponematoses, *Tech. Rep. Ser. Wld Hlth Org. No. 736*, 1986). This regimen may also be used for treatment of gonococcal infections in pregnant women (*Conjunctivitis of the newborn: prevention and treatment at the primary health care level*, World Health Organization, Geneva, 1986, p.12). Some workers, however, have recommended ceftriaxone as the drug of choice for gonorrhoea, because it is effective against penicillin-resistant strains (*Med. Lett.*, 1986, *28*, 23). Other workers have felt that the risk of postgonococcal chlamydial infections is unacceptably high using penicillin plus probenecid or ceftriaxone and that another drug such as tetracycline should be given in addition to the beta-lactam antibiotic (W.E. Stamm *et al.*, *New Engl. J. Med.*, 1984, *310*, 545; *Med Lett.*, 1986, *28*, 23).

See also Choice of Antibiotic, p.101.

Syphilis. For the use of procaine penicillin in the treatment of syphilis, see Benzathine Penicillin, p.130.

WHIPPLE'S DISEASE. For the use of procaine penicillin in the treatment of Whipple's disease, see Benzylpenicillin Sodium, p.138.

Preparations

Procaine Penicillin Injection *(B.P.)*. Procaine Benzylpenicillin Injection. Store in a cool place. Protect from light.

Fortified Procaine Penicillin Injection *(B.P.)*. A sterile suspension of procaine penicillin and benzylpenicillin potassium or benzylpenicillin sodium to be diluted before use. Store in a cool place.

Sterile Penicillin G Procaine *(U.S.P.)*

Sterile Penicillin G Procaine Suspension *(U.S.P.)*. It may contain procaine hydrochloride up to 2%. Store at 2° to 8°.

Sterile Penicillin G Procaine for Suspension *(U.S.P.)*

Sterile Penicillin G Procaine with Aluminum Stearate Suspension *(U.S.P.)*. PAM

Proprietary Preparations

Bicillin *(Brocades, UK)*. *Injection*, powder for reconstitution, procaine penicillin 3 g, benzylpenicillin sodium 600 mg. *Dose.* 400 000 units (equivalent to procaine penicillin 300 mg with benzylpenicillin sodium 60 mg) every 12 or 24 hours.

Depocillin *(Brocades, UK)*. *Injection*, powder for reconstitution, procaine penicillin 3 g.

Proprietary Names and Manufacturers

Aquacaine G *(Austral.)*; Aquacillin *(Faulding, Austral.)*; Aquicilina *(Antibioticos, Spain)*; Ayercillin *(Ayerst, Canad.)*; Cilicaine Syringe *(Sigma, Austral.; NZ)*; Crysticillin AS *(Squibb, USA)*; Depocillin *(Brocades, UK)*; Depocilline Vloeibaar *(Neth.)*; Duracillin AS *(Lilly, USA)*; Farmaproina *(CEPA, Spain)*; Fradicilina *(Galepharma, Spain)*; Hostacillin *(Hoechst, S.Afr.)*; Klaricina *(Spain)*; Megacillin *(Faulding, Austral.)*; Novocillin *(Novo, S.Afr.)*; Penicil Dermol *(Arg.)*; Peniern *(Ern, Spain)*; Penifasa '900' *(Spain)*; Pfizerpen-AS *(Roerig, USA)*; Provipen Procaina *(Sabater, Spain)*; Sanciline Procaina '300' *(Spain)*; Wycillin *(Wyeth, Canad.; Wyeth, USA)*.

The following names have been used for multi-ingredient preparations containing procaine penicillin— Bicillin *(Brocades, UK)*; Bicillin All Purpose *(Wyeth, Austral.)*; Bicillin A-P *(Wyeth, Canad.)*; Bicillin C-R *(Wyeth, USA)*; Tampovagan PSS *(Norgine, UK)*; Triplopen *(Glaxo, UK)*; Wycillin and Probenecid *(Wyeth, USA)*.

142-v

Propicillin Potassium *(BANM, pINNM)*.

Potassium α-Phenoxypropylpenicillin; Propicillinum Kalicum. A mixture of the D(+)- and L(−)-isomers of potassium (6*R*)-6-(2-phenoxybutyramido)penicillanate.

$C_{18}H_{21}KN_2O_5S$=416.5.

CAS — 551-27-9 (propicillin); 1245-44-9 (potassium salt).

Pharmacopoeias. In *Int.*

Each g of monograph substance represents about 2.4 mmol of potassium. 1.1 g of monograph substance is approximately equivalent to 1 g of propicillin.

Propicillin is a phenoxypenicillin with properties similar to benzylpenicillin (see p.131). It is generally less active than benzylpenicillin or phenoxymethylpenicillin against many susceptible organisms, particularly Gram-negative micro-organisms. It is slightly less susceptible to penicillinase than benzylpenicillin and phenoxymethylpenicillin.

Propicillin is relatively stable in acid gastric secretion and its absorption is generally rapid but can be variable. Up to 90% is bound to plasma proteins.

Propicillin is given by mouth, as the potassium salt, for the treatment of mild to moderate infections caused by susceptible Gram-positive organisms.

METABOLISM. About 32% of a 500-mg dose of propicillin was metabolised within 12 hours of the dose being taken by 6 healthy subjects; 66% was recovered in the urine, 21% as penicilloic acid.— M. Cole, *Antimicrob. Ag. Chemother.*, 1973, *3*, 463.

Proprietary Names and Manufacturers

Baycillin *(Bayer, Ger.)*; Bayercillin *(Bayer, Ital.)*; Bayercilline *(Bayer, Belg.)*; Delprosyn *(Gist-Brocades, Neth.)*; Oricillin *(Grünenthal, Ger.; Grünenthal, Switz.)*; Ultrapen *(Pfizer, UK)*.

143-g

Puromycin *(BAN, USAN, pINN)*.

CL-13900; L-3123; P-638. 3′-[2-Amino-3-(4-methoxyphenyl)propionamido]-3′-deoxy-*NN*-dimethyladenosine.

$C_{22}H_{29}N_7O_5$=471.5.

CAS — 53-79-2.

NOTE. Puromycin was at first called achromycin in the scientific literature but in 1953 this name became a trade-name for tetracycline hydrochloride.

An antibiotic produced by the growth of *Streptomyces albo-niger*. It has generally been used as the hydrochloride (CL-16536, $C_{22}H_{29}N_7O_5$,2HCl=544.4).

Puromycin has been used experimentally because of its ability to inhibit protein synthesis.

144-q

Ribostamycin Sulphate *(BANM, rINNM)*.

SF-733 *(ribostamycin)*. 2-Deoxy-4-*O*-(2,6-diamino-2,6-dideoxy-α-D-glucopyranosyl)-5-*O*-β-D-ribofuranosyl-streptamine sulphate.

$C_{17}H_{34}N_4O_{10}$,xH_2SO_4=454.5 (ribostamycin).

CAS — 25546-65-0 (ribostamycin); 53797-35-6 (sulphate).

Pharmacopoeias. In *Jpn.*

An aminoglycoside antibiotic derived from *Streptomyces ribosidificus* or prepared synthetically.

Ribostamycin sulphate is an aminoglycoside antibiotic with actions and uses similar to those of gentamicin sulphate (see p.236). It has been given by mouth or by intramuscular injection.

The antibacterial spectrum of ribostamycin against 161 strains of Gram-negative bacilli was identical with that of kanamycin. It was slightly less active than kanamycin against sensitive strains.— E. Yourassowsky and M. P. B. Linden, *Arzneimittel-Forsch.*, 1976, *26*, 184.

Proprietary Names and Manufacturers

Ibistacin *(Ibi, Ital.)*; Ribastamin *(Morrith, Spain)*; Ribomed *(Maggioni-Winthrop, Ital.)*; Ribomycine *(Delalande, Fr.)*; Ribostamin *(Delalande, Ital.)*; Ribostat *(Farmaka, Ital.)*; Vistamycin *(Meiji, Jpn)*.

145-p

Rifamide *(BAN, USAN, pINN)*.

Rifamycin B *NN*-diethylamide.

$C_{43}H_{58}N_2O_{13}$=810.9.

CAS — 2750-76-7.

Rifamide is a rifamycin antibiotic with activity against *Mycobacterium tuberculosis* and various other bacteria. It was formerly used in the treatment of susceptible infections of the respiratory and biliary tracts. It was given by intramuscular injection, as the sodium salt.

Proprietary Names and Manufacturers

Rifocin M *(Austral.; Lepetit, UK)*.

146-s

Rifamycin Sodium *(BANM, rINNM)*.

M-14 *(rifamycin)*; Rifamicina; Rifamycin SV Sodium; Rifamycinum Natricum. Sodium (12*Z*,14*E*,24*E*)-(2*S*,16*S*,17*S*,18*R*,19*R*,20*R*,21*S*,22*R*,23*S*)-21-acetoxy-1,2-dihydro-6,9,17,19-tetrahydroxy-23-methoxy-2,4,12,16,18,20,22-heptamethyl-1,11-dioxo-2,7-(epoxypentadeca-1,11,13-trienimino)-naphtho[2,1-*b*]furan-5-olate.

$C_{37}H_{46}NNaO_{12}$=719.8.

CAS — 6998-60-3 (rifamycin); 14897-39-3; 15105-92-7 (both sodium salt).

Pharmacopoeias. In *Aust., Br., Eur., Fr., Ger., Neth.*, and *Swiss.*

The monosodium salt of rifamycin SV, a substance obtained by chemical transformation of rifamycin B which is produced during growth of certain strains of *Streptomyces mediterranei*. Rifamycin SV may also be obtained directly from certain mutants of *Streptomyces mediterranei*. Rifamycin sodium contains not less than 900 units per mg calculated on the anhydrous substance.

A red, fine or slightly granular powder. **Soluble** in water; freely soluble in dehydrated alcohol and methyl alcohol; practically insoluble in chloroform and ether. A 5% solution has a pH of 6.5 to 7.5. **Store** in airtight containers. Protect from light.

Units

One unit of rifamycin is contained in 0.001127 mg of the first International Reference Preparation (1967) of rifamycin sodium which contains 887 units per mg.

Adverse Effects and Precautions

Some gastro-intestinal side-effects have occurred following injections of rifamycin sodium. High doses may produce alterations in liver function. Skin reactions have rarely been reported. Transient orange coloration of the tissues may occur after the infusion of high doses of rifamycin sodium.

Antimicrobial Action

Rifamycin sodium is active against Gram-positive and some Gram-negative bacteria, and also against *Mycobacterium tuberculosis*.

Rifamycin was effective *in vitro* against the amoeba *Naegleria fowleri*.— Y. H. Thong *et al.* (letter), *Lancet*, 1977, *2*, 876.

Absorption and Fate

Rifamycin sodium is not effectively absorbed from the gastro-intestinal tract. Plasma concentrations of 2 µg per mL have been achieved 2 hours after a dose of 250 mg by intramuscular injection.

It is excreted mainly in the bile and only small amounts appear in the urine.

Uses and Administration

Rifamycin sodium has been used in the treatment of infections caused by susceptible organisms. It has been given by intramuscular injection in doses of up to 1 g daily, and by slow intravenous infusion in doses of up to 2 g daily. Rifamycin sodium has also been administered by local instillation, and into the eye as a 1% ointment or drops.

Reference to the use of rifamycin in the treatment of herpes zoster.— L. Bruni *et al.*, *J. int. med. Res.*, 1980, *8*, 1. See also L. Bruni *et al.*, *ibid.*, 1984, *12*, 255.

MENINGITIS. Three neonates with meningitis due to *Flavobacterium meningosepticum* were given effective treatment with rifamycin 20 mg per kg body-weight every 12 hours by intramuscular or slow intravenous injection; rifamycin 2 to 5 mg daily in sodium chloride injection 2 mL was also instilled into the ventricles to treat ventriculitis. Treatment was continued although jaundice lasting for from 4 to 8 weeks occurred in 2 patients. Hydrocephalus occurred in all 3 patients and in 1 patient development was delayed by neurological defect.— E. L. Lee *et al.*, *Archs Dis. Childh.*, 1976, *51*, 209. See also I. Rios *et al.*, *Antimicrob. Ag. Chemother.*, 1978, *14*, 444.

Proprietary Names and Manufacturers

Otofa *(Bouchara, Fr.)*; Rifobac *(Liade, Spain)*; Rifocin *(Lepetit, Ital.)*; Rifocina *(Lepetit, Spain)*; Rifocine *(Merrell Dow, Belg.*; *Lepetit, Fr.*; *Neth.*; *Merrell Dow, Switz.)*.

503-j

Rifaximin *(rINN)*.

L-105; Rifaximine.

(2S,16Z,18E,20S,21S,22R,23R,24R,25S,26S,27S,28E)-5,6,21,23,25-Pentahydroxy-27-methoxy-2,4,11,16,20,22,24,26-octamethyl-2,7-(epoxypentadeca-[1,11,13]trienimino)benzofuro[4,5-*e*]pyrido[1,2-*a*]benzimidazole-1,15(2*H*)-dione, 25-acetate.

$C_{43}H_{51}N_3O_{11}$=785.9.

CAS — 80621-81-4.

NOTE. The code L-105 has also been applied to a cephalosporin antibiotic under investigation.

Rifaximin is a rifamycin antibiotic which is poorly absorbed from the gastro-intestinal tract. Its antimicrobial spectrum is reported to include both Gram-positive and Gram-negative organisms. It has been given by mouth in the treatment of gastro-intestinal infections.

References to the use of rifaximin: gastro-intestinal infections.— V. Alvisi *et al.*, *Clin. Trials J.*, 1984, *21*, 215; M. Vinci *et al.*, *Curr. ther. Res.*, 1984, *36*, 92; S. Lombardo and G. Santangelo, *Farmaco, Edn prat.*, 1984, *39*, 170; V. Alvisi *et al.*, *J. int. med. Res.*, 1987, *15*, 49. hepatic encephalopathy.— F. De Marco *et al.*, *Curr. ther. Res.*, 1984, *36*, 668.

Proprietary Names and Manufacturers

Normix *(Alfa Farmaceutici, Ital.)*.

148-e

Ristocetin *(BAN, rINN)*.

A mixture of 2 antimicrobial substances produced by the growth of *Nocardia lurida* (Actinomycetaceae).

CAS — 1404-55-3.

Ristocetin was formerly used in the treatment of severe staphylococcal infections unresponsive to other antibiotics but has been superseded by less toxic antibiotics.

A specific test for diagnosis of von Willebrand's disease using ristocetin.— H. Gralnick, *J. Am. med. Ass.*, 1977, *238*, 1625.

Ristocetin sulphate when added to plasma samples from 22 patients accelerated the thrombin clotting time in 20.— A. Aronstam *et al.*, *J. clin. Path.*, 1978, *31*, 1106.

2827-b

Rokitamycin *(rINN)*.

3″-*O*-Propionyl-leucomycin A_5; TMS-19-Q.

[(4R,5S,6S,7R,9R,10R,11E,13E,16R)-7-(formylmethyl)-4,10-dihydroxy-5-methoxy-9,16-dimethyl-2-oxooxacyclohexadeca-11,13-dien-6-yl]-3,6-dideoxy-4-*O*-(2,6-dideoxy-3-*C*-methyl-α-L-*ribo*-hexopyranosyl)-3-(dimethylamino)-β-D-glucopyranoside 4″-butyrate 3″-propionate.

$C_{42}H_{69}NO_{15}$=828.0.

CAS — 74014-51-0.

Rokitamycin is a macrolide antibiotic administered by mouth.

The administration of rokitamycin had no significant effect on the serum concentrations of theophylline or digoxin in studies of 11 and 10 patients respectively.— T. Ishioka, *Acta ther.*, 1987, *13*, 17.

Activity *in vitro* of rokitamycin against *Mycoplasma pneumoniae*.— T. Misu *et al.*, *Antimicrob. Ag. Chemother.*, 1987, *31*, 1843.

Proprietary Names and Manufacturers

Ricamycin *(Toyo Jozo, Jpn)*.

149-l

Rolitetracycline *(BAN, USAN, rINN)*.

PMT; Pyrrolidinomethyltetracycline. N^2-(Pyrrolidin-1-ylmethyl)tetracycline.

$C_{27}H_{33}N_3O_8$=527.6.

CAS — 751-97-3.

Pharmacopoeias. In *It. U.S.* includes Sterile Rolitetracycline.

A light yellow crystalline powder with a characteristic musty amine-like odour, containing not less than 900 µg per mg, calculated on the anhydrous basis. Rolitetracycline 275 mg is approximately equivalent to 250 mg of tetracycline hydrochloride.

Soluble 1 in 1.1 of water and 1 in 200 of alcohol; slightly soluble in dehydrated alcohol; soluble in acetone; very slightly soluble in ether. A 1% solution has a pH of 7 to 9; the *U.S.P.* injection has a pH of 3.0 to 4.5. **Store** in airtight containers. Protect from light.

Rolitetracycline may be physically or chemically **incompatible** with substances that alter the pH. It should not be mixed with other antibiotics, aminophylline, calcium salts, heparin sodium, or hydrocortisone.

150-v

Rolitetracycline Nitrate *(BANM, USAN, rINNM)*.

Pyrrolidinomethyltetracycline Nitrate Sesquihydrate.

$C_{27}H_{33}N_3O_8,HNO_3,1\frac{1}{2}H_2O$=617.6.

CAS — 20685-78-3 (anhydrous); 26657-13-6 (sesquihydrate).

Pharmacopoeias. In *Cz.*

LOSS OF ACTIVITY. Storage for 30 days at 37° and 100% relative humidity resulted in the almost complete loss of activity of rolitetracycline.— V. C. Walton *et al.*, *J. pharm. Sci.*, 1970, *59*, 1160.

STABILITY IN SOLUTION. Solutions in water of both rolitetracycline nitrate and base were more than 50% hydrolysed to tetracycline in 3 hours at 25°.— D. W. Hughes *et al.* (letter), *J. Pharm. Pharmac.*, 1974, *26*, 79.

Reconstituted injections of rolitetracycline base lost 15% of their original antibiotic content in 21 to 25 hours when stored at 5° (the manufacturers' recommendation was 2° to 10°). Injections of the nitrate lost 15% of their content 1.5 to 3.5 hours after reconstitution and more than 60% in 8 to 20 hours when stored at 25° (the manufacturers' recommended storage at 21°). The major decomposition product was tetracycline.— W. L. Wilson *et al.*, *Can. J. pharm. Sci.*, 1976, *11*, 126.

Units

One unit of rolitetracycline is contained in 0.001004 mg of the first International Standard Preparation (1968) which contains 996 units per mg.

Adverse Effects and Precautions

As for Tetracycline Hydrochloride, p.314.

Shivering and more rarely rigor may be associated with the first few injections of rolitetracycline in infections due to organisms highly sensitive to tetracyclines. Injections may be followed by a peculiar taste sensation, often similar to ether. Rapid intravenous injection may cause transient giddiness, hot flushes, reddening of the face and, occasionally, peripheral circulatory failure. Symptoms of myasthenia gravis have been exacerbated by the intravenous administration of rolitetracycline.

A report of the accidental intra-arterial injection of rolitetracycline in one infant causing arteriolar obstruction followed by gangrene of the affected limb.— J. M. Wynne, *Archs Dis. Childh.*, 1978, *53*, 396.

JARISCH-HERXHEIMER REACTION. A study of the Jarisch-Herxheimer-like reaction in louse-borne relapsing fever. All of the 12 patients who received rolitetracycline 275 mg by slow intravenous injection or procaine penicillin with aluminium monostearate (PAM) 600 000 units intramuscularly developed a Jarisch-Herxheimer-like reaction. Compared with the tetracycline, slow-release penicillin induced a reaction that peaked later, was less often associated with rigors, and caused a smaller increase in temperature and decrease in peripheral leucocyte count; however, the fever was protracted and the spirochaetes were cleared from the blood more slowly. A tetracycline was considered to be the agent of choice especially in severely ill patients because of the rapid clearance of spirochaetes from the blood. Also the circulatory abnormalities, which are the probable cause of most fatalities during the Jarisch-Herxheimer-like reaction, although a little more severe, were of significantly shorter duration than in patients treated with the penicillin.— D. A. Warrell *et al.*, *J. infect. Dis.*, 1983, *147*, 898.

Absorption and Fate

As for Tetracycline Hydrochloride, p.317.

Rolitetracycline is not absorbed from the gastro-intestinal tract. When administered by injection about 50% of rolitetracycline in the circulation is bound to plasma proteins. Peak plasma concentrations of about 4 to 6 µg per mL have been reported about 0.5 to 1 hour after a dose of 350 mg given intramuscularly and therapeutic concentrations may still be detected 24 hours after the injection. The half-life has been reported to range from about 5 to 8 hours. About 50% of a dose is excreted in the urine.

Uses and Administration

Rolitetracycline has antimicrobial activity and uses similar to those of tetracycline hydrochloride (see p.315). It has been given by deep intramuscular injection, usually with a local anaesthetic, or by slow intravenous injection or infusion. Treatment with an oral tetracycline should be substituted as soon as possible.

Adults may be given up to 350 mg once daily intramuscularly, or 275 mg once daily by slow intravenous injection; in severe infections the intravenous dose may be given up to 3 times daily. Extravasation into subcutaneous tissues should be avoided.

Children have been given 10 mg per kg body-weight daily in one or 2 doses by either route but the effect of tetracyclines on teeth should be considered.

Preparations

Rolitetracycline for Injection *(U.S.P.)*

Sterile Rolitetracycline *(U.S.P.)*

Proprietary Names and Manufacturers

Bristacin *(Bristol, Neth.)*; Farmaciclina *(Selvi, Ital.)*; Reverin *(Hoechst, Arg.*; *Hoechst, Austral.*; *Hoechst, Belg.*; *Hoechst, Canad.*; *Hoechst, Denm.*; *Hoechst, Ger.*; *Hoechst, Ital.*; *Hoechst, Neth.*; *Hoechst, S.Afr.)*; Reverine *(Hoechst, Switz.)*; Tetralidina *(Ital Suisse, Ital.)*; Tetrex-

PMT *(Bristol-Myers Pharmaceuticals, UK)*; Transcycline *(Hoechst, Fr.)*.

151-g

Rosaramicin *(BAN, USAN, rINN)*.
Rosamicin; Sch-14947. 12,13-Epoxy-6-formylmethyl-3-hydroxy-4,8,12,14-tetramethyl-9-oxo-5-(3,4,6-trideoxy-3-dimethylamino-β-D-*xylo*-hexopyranosyloxy)heptadec-10-en-15-olide.
$C_{31}H_{51}NO_9$=581.7.

CAS — 35834-26-5.

Rosaramicin is a macrolide antibiotic derived from *Micromonospora rosaria*. It has an antimicrobial spectrum similar to that of erythromycin (see p.223) but is generally more active than erythromycin against Gram-negative bacteria. Several salts and esters of rosaramicin have also been studied.

ANTIMICROBIAL ACTION. General studies of the antimicrobial activity of rosaramicin *in vitro*: S. Shadomy *et al.*, *Antimicrob. Ag. Chemother.*, 1976, *10*, 773; C. C. Sanders and W. E. Sanders, *ibid.*, 1977, *12*, 293; R. W. Lacey, *J. antimicrob. Chemother.*, 1981, *7*, 293; J. A. Smith *et al.*, *ibid.*, 505.

Activity of rosaramicin against specific organisms: anaerobic bacteria.— J. Santoro *et al.*, *Antimicrob. Ag. Chemother.*, 1976, *10*, 188; Y. -Y. Kwok *et al.*, *J. antimicrob. Chemother.*, 1979, *5*, 61.
Campylobacter jejuni.— V. I. Ahonkhai *et al.*, *Antimicrob. Ag. Chemother.*, 1981, *20*, 850.
Chlamydia trachomatis.— C. -C. Kuo *et al.*, *ibid.*, 1977, *12*, 80; T. F. Smith and H. E. Washton, *ibid.*, 1978, *14*, 493; W. R. Bowie, *ibid.*, 1980, *18*, 978.
Neisseria gonorrhoeae.— J. W. Biddle and C. Thornsberry, *ibid.*, 1979, *15*, 243.

ABSORPTION AND FATE. References to the absorption and fate of rosaramicin: A. Baumueller *et al.*, *Antimicrob. Ag. Chemother.*, 1977, *12*, 240 (concentrations in the prostate); C. -C. Lin *et al.*, *ibid.*, 1984, *26*, 522 (pharmacokinetics and metabolism in healthy subjects).

Proprietary Names and Manufacturers
Schering, USA.

680-p

Roxithromycin *(USAN, rINN)*.
RU-28965; RU-965. Erythromycin 9-{*O*-[(2-methoxyethoxy)methyl]oxime}.
$C_{41}H_{76}N_2O_{15}$=837.1.

CAS — 80214-83-1.

Roxithromycin is a macrolide antibiotic with actions and uses similar to those of erythromycin (see p.222). It is given by mouth in a dose of 150 mg twice daily in the treatment of susceptible infections.

For proceedings of symposia on the actions and uses of roxithromycin, see *J. antimicrob. Chemother.*, 1987, *20*, *Suppl.* B, 1–187; *Br. J. clin. Pract.*, 1988, *42*, *Suppl.* 55, 1–119.

ANTIMICROBIAL ACTION. General studies of the antimicrobial activity of roxithromycin *in vitro*: R. N. Jones *et al.*, *Antimicrob. Ag. Chemother.*, 1983, *24*, 209; T. Barlam and H. C. Neu, *ibid.*, 1984, *25*, 529; H. Goossens *et al.*, *ibid.*, 1985, *27*, 388; E. J. C. Goldstein *et al.*, *ibid.*, 1986, *29*, 556; K. V. I. Rolston *et al.*, *J. antimicrob. Chemother.*, 1986, *17*, 161; S. C. Aronoff *et al.* (letter), *ibid.*, 1987, *19*, 275.

Activity of roxithromycin against specific organisms: J. H. Jorgensen *et al.*, *Antimicrob. Ag. Chemother.*, 1986, *29*, 921 (*Haemophilus influenzae*); S. Czinn *et al.*, *ibid.*, *30*, 328 (*Campylobacter pyloridis*); M. -J. Sanson-Le Pors *et al.*, *ibid.*, 512 (*Haemophilus ducreyi*); W. E. Stamm and R. Suchland, *ibid.*, 806 (*Chlamydia trachomatis*); W. R. Bowie *et al.*, *ibid.*, 1987, *31*, 470 (*Chlamydia trachomatis* and *Neisseria gonorrhoeae*); M. Casal *et al.*, *Tubercle*, 1987, *68*, 141 (*Mycobacterium tuberculosis*); A. Pascual *et al.* (letter), *J. antimicrob. Chemother.*, 1987, *19*, 701 (anaerobic bacteria); R. N. Jones and A. L. Barry (letter), *ibid.*, 841 (*Legionella* spp).

ABSORPTION AND FATE. A review of the pharmacokinetics of roxithromycin. Roxithromycin is rapidly absorbed from the gastro-intestinal tract and its bioavailability is not markedly affected by milk or food. It has a half-life of approximately 10 hours. After oral doses, high concentrations of roxithromycin are achieved in pulmonary, prostatic, and tonsillar tissues, and in tear and pleural fluids. It is not, however, detected in the CSF of subjects with non-inflamed meninges or in saliva. Less than 0.05% of a dose is excreted in the breast milk of lactating women. About 53% of the drug is excreted in the faeces, approximately 13% in expired air, and 8% in the urine as unchanged compound. Although only the parent drug is detected in plasma, 3 metabolites have been identified in the urine, and 5 in the faeces. The half-life is increased in patients with severe renal insufficiency or liver cirrhosis, but dosage adjustment is not considered necessary. It was concluded that a dose of 150 mg twice daily or 300 mg once daily would provide plasma concentrations well above the MICs required for antibacterial activity.— S. K. Puri and H. B. Lassman, *J. antimicrob. Chemother.*, 1987, *20*, *Suppl.* B, 89. See also O. G. Nilsen, *ibid.*, 81; R. Wise *et al.*, *Antimicrob. Ag. Chemother.*, 1987, *31*, 1051.

Penetration of roxithromycin into the lungs.— J. Chastre *et al.*, *Antimicrob. Ag. Chemother.*, 1987, *31*, 1312.

USES AND ADMINISTRATION. A study involving 225 patients with throat infections caused by *Streptococcus pyogenes* treated by mouth for 10 days with roxithromycin, either 150 mg twice daily or 300 mg once daily, or erythromycin ethylsuccinate 400 mg four times daily. Clinical response-rates with either dose of roxithromycin compared favourably with erythromycin; bactericidal eradication was however less satisfactory with the once-daily regimen of roxithromycin. There were fewer side-effects associated with roxithromycin than erythromycin therapy.— J. M. Herron, *J. antimicrob. Chemother.*, 1987, *20*, *Suppl.* B, 139.

A summary of 5 comparative and non-comparative studies of the use of roxithromycin in the treatment of nongonococcal urethritis. Of a total of 637 patients treated with a dose of 150 mg twice daily by mouth, 91 and 90% were considered to be clinical and bacteriological successes respectively. Roxithromycin was effective in eradicating 97% of isolates of *Chlamydia trachomatis*, 88% of *Ureaplasma urealyticum*, 73% of *Mycoplasma hominis*, and 57% of *Gardnerella vaginalis*. Roxithromycin compared well with lymecycline and doxycycline; a higher dose of 450 mg daily did not appear to offer any significant advantage.— A. Lassus and A. Seppala, *J. antimicrob. Chemother.*, 1987, *20*, *Suppl.* B, 157.

Further studies of the use of roxithromycin: L. O. Gentry, *J. antimicrob. Chemother.*, 1987, *20*, *Suppl.* B, 145 (lower respiratory-tract infections); D. A. Kafetzis and F. Blanc, *ibid.*, 171 (paediatric infections).

Proprietary Names and Manufacturers
Rulid *(Roussel, Fr.)*.

4913-a

Silver Sulphadiazine

Silver Sulfadiazine *(USAN)*. The silver salt of N^1-(pyrimidin-2-yl)sulphanilamide.
$C_{10}H_9AgN_4O_2S$=357.1.

CAS — 22199-08-2.

Pharmacopoeias. In *Chin.*

Adverse Effects, Treatment, and Precautions

As for Sulphamethoxazole, p.306, as absorption of sulphadiazine may occur. Its action is not antagonised by *p*-aminobenzoic acid or related compounds.

Local reactions have been reported in patients treated with silver sulphadiazine; the separation of the eschar may be delayed and fungal invasion of the wound may occur.

Transient leucopenia has occurred although its association with application of silver sulphadiazine has not been consistently confirmed.

Some adverse effects occurring after application of silver sulphadiazine preparations have been attributed to additional constituents present in some formulations: C. L. Fligner *et al.*, *J. Am. med. Ass.*, 1985, *253*, 1606 (hyperosmolality following cardiorespiratory arrest in an 8-month-old infant, attributed to propylene glycol); M. C. Cantarell *et al.*, *Ann. intern. Med.*, 1987, *106*, 478 (acute oliguric renal failure in 5 patients associated with diethylene glycol).

Antimicrobial Action and Resistance

Silver sulphadiazine has broad antimicrobial activity against Gram-positive and Gram-negative bacteria including *Pseudomonas aeruginosa*, yeasts, and fungi. It has also been reported to be active *in vitro* against herpes virus and *Treponema pallidum*. Silver sulphadiazine has a bactericidal action; in contrast to sulphadiazine, the silver salt acts primarily on the cell membrane and cell wall and its action is not antagonised by *p*-aminobenzoic acid. Resistance to silver sulphadiazine has been reported.

Absorption and Fate

Silver sulphadiazine is slowly metabolised in contact with wound exudates. Up to about 10% of the sulphadiazine may be absorbed; concentrations in blood of 10 to 20 µg per mL have been reported although higher concentrations may be achieved when extensive areas of the body are treated. Probably not more than 1% of the silver content is absorbed.

Following daily cleansing and application of 1% silver sulphadiazine cream to 12 patients with burns covering 7 to 63% of the body-surface, plasma concentrations of total sulphonamide were less than 6 µg per mL.— P. Delaveau and P. Friedrich-Noue, *Thérapie*, 1977, *32*, 563.

Uses and Administration

Silver sulphadiazine is a sulphonamide which is used, in conjunction with debridement, for the prevention and treatment of infection, particularly by *Pseudomonas aeruginosa*, in severe burns. A 1% cream is usually applied daily to a thickness of 3 to 5 mm by a sterile spatula or gloved hand. Treatment is continued until healing is progressing satisfactorily or the burn site is ready for skin grafting.

Silver sulphadiazine has also been used in other skin conditions, such as leg ulcers, where infection may prevent healing.

Nine of 10 strains of varicella zoster virus were completely inactivated *in vitro* by silver sulphadiazine in a concentration of 10 µg per mL. All of 42 patients treated for herpes zoster with a 1% silver sulphadiazine cream showed a definite clinical response.— L. F. Montes *et al.*, *Cutis*, 1986, *38*, 363.

Proprietary Preparations

Flamazine *(Smith & Nephew Pharmaceuticals, UK)*. *Cream*, silver sulphadiazine 1%.

Proprietary Names and Manufacturers

Argent-Eze *(Lennon, S.Afr.)*; Flamazine *(Smith & Nephew, Canad.; Smith & Nephew, Denm.; Smith & Nephew, Norw.; Smith & Nephew, S.Afr.; Smith & Nephew Pharmaceuticals, UK)*; Flammazine *(Belg.; Duphar, Fr.; Duphar, Ger.; Neth.; Kali-Farma, Spain; Duphar, Switz.)*; Flint SSD *(Flint, USA)*; Silvadene *(Max Ritter, Switz.; Marion Laboratories, USA)*; Silvazine *(Smith & Nephew, Austral.)*; Silvederma *(Aldo, Spain)*; Sofargen *(Sofar, Ital.)*; Ustionil *(Schwarz, Ital.)*.

152-q

Sissomicin Sulphate *(BANM)*.
Antibiotic 6640; Sch-13475 *(sissomicin)*; Sisomicin Sulfate *(USAN)*; Sisomicin Sulphate *(rINNM)*. 4-*O*-[(2*S*,3*S*)-3-Amino-6-aminomethyl-3,4-dihydro-2*H*-pyran-2-yl]-2-deoxy-6-*O*-(3-deoxy-4-*C*-methyl-3-methylamino-β-L-arabinopyranosyl)-D-streptamine sulphate.
$(C_{19}H_{37}N_5O_7)_2,5H_2SO_4$=1385.5.

CAS — 32385-11-8 (sissomicin); 53179-09-2 (sulphate).

Pharmacopoeias. In *U.S.*

Sissomicin is an antibiotic produced by *Micromonospora inyoensis* and closely related to gentamicin C_{1A}.
It contains not less than 580 µg of sissomicin per mg, calculated with reference to the dried substance. 1.5 g of monograph substance is approximately equivalent to 1 g of sissomicin. A 4% solution has a pH of 3.5 to 5.5. The

U.S.P. injection has a pH of 2.5 to 5.5. **Store** in airtight containers.
Sissomicin is **incompatible** with beta-lactam antibiotics (see Gentamicin Sulphate, p.236).

Units
35 200 units of sissomicin are contained in approximately 56.5 mg of sissomicin sulphate in one ampoule of the first International Standard Preparation (1984).

Adverse Effects, Treatment, and Precautions
See Gentamicin Sulphate, p.236.
Peak plasma concentrations of sissomicin greater than 12 μg per mL and trough concentrations greater than 2 μg per mL should be avoided.

Antimicrobial Action and Resistance
Sissomicin has a mode of action and spectrum of antimicrobial activity similar to that of gentamicin (see p.239), although it appears to be slightly more active against *Pseudomonas aeruginosa*. There is almost complete cross-resistance between the two antibiotics.

Studies *in vitro* suggested that tobramycin was more active than gentamicin, kanamycin, or sissomicin against *Pseudomonas* spp., whilst sissomicin and gentamicin were most active against *Serratia* spp. Against other species differences were slight. *In vivo* sissomicin was the most active of the 4 antibiotics.— J. A. Waitz *et al., Antimicrob. Ag. Chemother.*, 1972, *2,* 431. See also C. C. Crowe and E. Sanders, *ibid.*, 1973, *3,* 24.

For reference to a comparative study of the antimicrobial activity of 11 aminoglycosides including sissomicin, see Gentamicin Sulphate, p.239.

ACTIVITY WITH OTHER ANTIMICROBIAL AGENTS. For reference to the effect of other agents on the *in-vitro* antimicrobial activity of aminoglycosides, see Gentamicin Sulphate, p.239.

Absorption and Fate
The absorption and fate of sissomicin is similar to that of gentamicin (see p.241).

After intramuscular doses of sissomicin 20 and 40 mg per m^2 body-surface mean peak serum concentrations achieved after 1 hour were 2.5 and 4 μg per mL respectively; within 6 hours the urinary excretion was 49 and 61%. After an intravenous injection of 30 mg per m^2, mean peak serum concentrations of 5.1 μg per mL were achieved after ½ hour.— V. Rodriguez *et al., Antimicrob. Ag. Chemother.*, 1975, *7,* 38.

In a comparative study of the pharmacokinetics of gentamicin, sissomicin, and tobramycin in doses of 1 mg per kg body-weight sissomicin gave the highest serum concentration of 4.66 μg per mL and the serum-concentration curve exceeded that of the other 2 antibiotics.— H. Lode *et al., Antimicrob. Ag. Chemother.*, 1975, *8,* 396.

The pharmacokinetics of sissomicin were studied in 10 healthy subjects given doses of 1 mg per kg body-weight intramuscularly or intravenously as an infusion in 250 mL of glucose injection over 30 minutes. Peak serum-sissomicin concentrations of 3.08 μg per mL at 1 hour after intramuscular injection and 7.12 μg per mL 30 minutes after infusion were obtained. No serum concentration was detectable at 24 hours following either route. About 34% of the intramuscular dose was excreted in the urine during the first 8 hours and about 6% during the next 16; comparable figures for the intravenous dose were about 30 and 4%. The half-life for the beta phase was 2.63 hours following intramuscular administration and 2.55 hours following intravenous administration.— B. R. Meyers *et al., Antimicrob. Ag. Chemother.*, 1976, *10,* 25.

Uses and Administration
Sissomicin is an aminoglycoside antibiotic which has been used, as the sulphate, similarly to gentamicin (see p.242). The usual dose for adults is the equivalent of 3 mg of sissomicin per kg body-weight daily given intramuscularly or intravenously in 3 divided doses. A dose of 2 mg per kg daily in 2 divided doses may be given for the treatment of urinary-tract infections. Dosage should be reduced in patients with renal impairment.

A review of the actions and uses of sissomicin.— P. Noone, *Drugs*, 1984, *27,* 548.

See also Gentamicin Sulphate, p.242, for further reviews of aminoglycoside antibiotics.

ADMINISTRATION. For a discussion on the adjustment of aminoglycoside dosage see under Uses, Administration in Gentamicin Sulphate (p.242).
It has been suggested that nomograms for determining the dosage of gentamicin may also be used for sissomicin; trough concentrations should be kept below 2 μg per mL (P. Noone, *Drugs*, 1984, *27,* 548).

RESPIRATORY-TRACT INFECTIONS. A study of 20 tracheotomised or intubated patients with Gram-negative bronchopulmonary infections. The addition of systemic sissomicin to treatment with sissomicin 25 mg by rapid endotracheal injection three times daily in association with intravenous mezlocillin did not appear to be necessary in the absence of bacteraemia. Care should be taken during endotracheal administration since it was associated with a high rate of selection of bacteria resistant to sissomicin.— J. P. Sculier *et al., J. antimicrob. Chemother.*, 1982, *9,* 63.
The use of sissomicin in association with mezlocillin or ticarcillin in the treatment of bacteraemia or bronchopneumonia.— B. Hanson *et al., J. antimicrob. Chemother.*, 1982, *10,* 335.

Preparations
Sisomicin Sulfate Injection *(U.S.P.)*

Proprietary Names and Manufacturers
Baymicin *(Bayer, Ital.; Bayer, S.Afr.)*; Baymicina *(Bayer, Spain)*; Baymicine *(Bayer, Belg.; Bayer, Fr.)*; Extramycin *(Bayer, Ger.; Bayer, Switz.)*; Mensiso *(Menarini, Ital.)*; Pathomycin *(Byk Essex, Ger.)*; Siseptin *(Scherag, S.Afr.)*; Sismine *(Schering, Belg.)*; Sisobiotic *(Von Boch, Ital.)*; Sisolline *(Unicet, Fr.)*; Sisomin *(Essex, Ital.; Schering, Switz.)*; Sisomina *(Essex, Arg.; Essex, Spain)*.

155-w

Spectinomycin *(BAN, rINN).*

Actinospectacin. Decahydro-4a,7,9-trihydroxy-2-methyl-6,8-bis(methylamino)-4*H*-pyrano[2,3-*b*]-[1,4]benzodioxin-4-one.
$C_{14}H_{24}N_2O_7$=332.4.

CAS — 1695-77-8.

An antimicrobial substance produced by the growth of *Streptomyces spectabilis* or by any other means.

157-l

Spectinomycin Hydrochloride *(BANM, USAN, rINNM).*

M-141; U-18409AE. Spectinomycin dihydrochloride pentahydrate.
$C_{14}H_{24}N_2O_7,2HCl,5H_2O$=495.4.

CAS — 21736-83-4 (anhydrous); 22189-32-8 (pentahydrate).

Pharmacopoeias. In *Br., Braz.,* and *It. U.S.* includes Sterile Spectinomycin Hydrochloride. Also in *B.P. Vet.*

A white or almost white crystalline powder. The *B.P.* specifies a potency of not less than 780 units per mg calculated on the anhydrous substance, and the *U.S.P.* a potency of not less than 603 μg of spectinomycin per mg. 1.5 g of monograph substance is approximately equivalent to 1 g of spectinomycin. **Soluble** 1 in 10 of water; practically insoluble in alcohol, chloroform, and ether. The *B.P.* states that a 10% and the *U.S.P.* that a 1% solution in water has a pH of 3.8 to 5.6. The *B.P.* injection has a pH of 4 to 7. **Store** in well-closed containers at a temperature not exceeding 30°.

STABILITY. The stability of spectinomycin was a function of pH and temperature. No significant degradation occurred in 0.1M hydrochloric acid and at pH 4.65 for over 43 days at 30°, but degradation was significant in alkaline solution. Spectinomycin should be stable enough for practical purposes below pH 5.— E. R. Garrett and G. R. Umbreit, *J. pharm. Sci.*, 1962, *51,* 436.

Units
One unit of spectinomycin is contained in 0.00149 mg of the first International Reference Preparation (1975) which contains 671 units per mg.

Adverse Effects and Precautions
Nausea, headache, dizziness, fever, and urticaria have occasionally occurred with single doses of spectinomycin hydrochloride. Mild to moderate pain has been reported in a few patients following intramuscular injections. Alterations in kidney and liver function and a decrease in haemoglobin and blood count have occasionally been observed with repeated doses. Spectinomycin should not be used to treat syphilis.

Healthy subjects given up to 8 g of spectinomycin hydrochloride daily for 5 days showed no evidence of ototoxicity, hepatotoxicity, or nephrotoxicity.— E. Novak *et al., J. clin. Pharmac.*, 1974, *14,* 442. See also *idem, J. infect. Dis.*, 1974, *130,* 50.

ALLERGY. A report of anaphylaxis after the intramuscular administration of spectinomycin.— B. S. Bender *et al., Sth. med. J.*, 1983, *76,* 1456.

EFFECTS ON THE LIVER. Cholestatic jaundice occurred in a 20-year-old man and was considered to be associated with a single intramuscular injection of spectinomycin.— D. R. Skillman and M. K. Taormina (letter), *Ann. intern. Med.*, 1985, *103,* 805.

INTERACTIONS. For the effect of spectinomycin on lithium, see Lithium Carbonate, p.367.

Antimicrobial Action
Spectinomycin shows activity against a wide range of Gram-positive and Gram-negative organisms but its main effect is against *Neisseria gonorrhoeae*, most strains of which are inhibited by less than 7.5 to 20 μg per mL. It acts by inhibiting bacterial protein synthesis.

The majority of 100 strains of *Bacteroides fragilis* were inhibited *in vitro* by spectinomycin at a concentration of 16 μg per mL. Although the MIC was not significantly affected by the inoculum size, type of medium, or presence of serum it was markedly increased at low pH and diminished at high pH. Studies *in vitro* suggested that *Bacteroides fragilis* slowly acquired resistance to spectinomycin.— I. Phillips and C. Warren, *J. antimicrob. Chemother.*, 1975, *1,* 91. The addition of clindamycin or metronidazole had little effect.— R. Wise *et al.* (letter), *ibid.*, 439. Spectinomycin was not a potent inhibitor of *Bacteroides fragilis* or other clinically significant anaerobes and would probably not be effective in the treatment of anaerobic infection.— J. E. Rosenblatt and A. M. Gerdts, *Antimicrob. Ag. Chemother.*, 1977, *12,* 37.

The activity of 9 aminoglycosides and spectinomycin was tested *in vitro* against 351 strains of Enterobacteriaceae, 34 of *Pseudomonas aeruginosa*, 38 gentamicin-sensitive and 42 gentamicin-resistant strains of the *Pseudomonas* spp., 20 of the *Acinetobacter* spp., 17 of *Haemophilus influenzae* and 41 strains of *Neisseria gonorrhoeae*; spectinomycin inhibited 63, 0, 32, 0, 55, 100, and 100% of the strains respectively at a concentration of 16 μg per mL.— I. Phillips *et al., J. antimicrob. Chemother.*, 1977, *3,* 403.

Resistance
Resistant gonococci have been reported. Resistance to spectinomycin has also developed amongst other bacteria.

For reports of resistance to spectinomycin in both penicillinase- and non-penicillinase-producing *Neisseria gonorrhoeae*, see under Uses, below.

Absorption and Fate
Spectinomycin is rapidly absorbed following the intramuscular injection of the hydrochloride. A 2-g dose produces peak plasma concentrations of about 100 μg per mL at 1 hour while a 4-g dose produces peak concentrations of about 160 μg per mL at 2 hours. Therapeutic plasma concentrations are maintained for up to 8 hours. Spectinomycin is excreted in an active form in the urine and up to 100% of a dose has been recovered within 48 hours. Mean half-lives of about 2.5 hours have been reported.

Uses and Administration
Spectinomycin is used as the hydrochloride in the treatment of gonorrhoea when penicillin, tetracycline, or co-trimoxazole treatment is ineffective or inadvisable. It is usually administered by deep intramuscular injection as a single dose equivalent to 2 g of spectinomycin, although a dose of 4 g may sometimes be required. Multiple-dose courses have been used for the treatment of disseminated infections and conjunctivitis. Although spectinomycin may be effective in infections caused by *Ureaplasma urealyticum*, it is not effective in those caused by *Chlamydia trachomatis*. Since co-existing infections with these organisms frequently occur in patients with

gonorrhoea, a suitable antibiotic such as a tetracycline may be required following spectinomycin therapy.

Doses equivalent to spectinomycin 40 mg per kg body-weight have been administered to children.

Spectinomycin sulphate is used for veterinary purposes.

PELVIC INFLAMMATORY DISEASE. For reference to the use of spectinomycin in the treatment of acute salpingitis, see Choice of Antibiotic, p.99.

SEXUALLY TRANSMITTED DISEASES. *Chancroid.* Limited data suggest that in the treatment of chancroid (*Haemophilus ducreyi* infection), adequate cure-rates can be obtained with a single intramuscular injection of spectinomycin 2 g.— WHO Expert Committee on Venereal Diseases and Treponematoses, *Tech. Rep. Ser. Wld Hlth Org. No. 736*, 1986, p. 130.

Patients with chancroid were treated with either a single intramuscular injection of spectinomycin 2 g (32 patients) or a 5-day course of co-trimoxazole 960 mg twice daily by mouth (20 patients). The 2 treatments were considered equally effective. By day fourteen, 29 and 19 patients in the two groups respectively were considered to be improved or cured. The MIC of spectinomycin was 8, 16, and 32 µg per mL for 12, 14, and 27 isolates of *Haemophilus ducreyi*, respectively.— L. Fransen *et al.*, *Sex. transm. Dis.*, 1987, *14*, 98.

Gonorrhoea. Spectinomycin, or cefotaxime, cefoxitin, or ceftriaxone, may be used for the treatment of gonococcal infections in areas where chromosomal gonococcal resistance has reduced the efficacy of penicillins, tetracycline, or co-trimoxazole to below 95%, and in areas where the prevalence of beta-lactamase-producing gonococci exceeds 5%. A single intramuscular injection of spectinomycin 2 g may be effective in uncomplicated urogenital infections and in rectal infections, but not in infections of the pharynx. A dosage regimen of 2 g twice daily intramuscularly for 5 days is used in the treatment of disseminated infection. Spectinomycin may be used to treat pregnant women. In a dose of 2 g twice daily by intramuscular injection for 3 days, spectinomycin is one of the recommended treatment regimens for adults with gonococcal conjunctivitis; this should be accompanied by regular irrigation of the eyes with saline or buffered ophthalmic solutions.— WHO Expert Committee on Venereal Diseases and Treponematoses, *Tech. Rep. Ser. Wld Hlth Org. No. 736*, 1986.

Emergence of resistance after spectinomycin treatment of gonorrhoea due to a beta-lactamase-producing strain of *Neisseria gonorrhoeae*.— C. S. F. Easmon *et al.*, *Br. med. J.*, 1982, *284*, 1604. See also W. A. Ashford *et al.*, *Lancet*, 1981, *2*, 1035.

The prevalence of penicillinase-producing *Neisseria gonorrhoeae* (PPNG) at a London clinic rose from less than 0.5% to 6.5% between 1978 and 1982. Thus, from January 1983 spectinomycin was used as first-line treatment for uncomplicated, heterosexual, anogenital gonorrhoea and cured 95% of such patients. However, its use failed to influence the prevalence of PPNG to any degree; this may in part have been due to spectinomycin resistance in both penicillinase-producing and non-penicillinase-producing *N. gonorrhoeae*. To date, spectinomycin resistance was not considered a major problem, although once resistance has occurred it could build up to serious levels very rapidly.— C. S. F. Easmon *et al.*, *Br. med. J.*, 1984, *289*, 1032. See also C. A. Ison *et al.*, *ibid.*, 1983, *287*, 1827.

Of 97 *US* servicemen in Korea with uncomplicated gonococcal urethritis who were treated with a single intramuscular injection of spectinomycin 2 g, 8 (8.2%) were considered to be treatment failures. A further dose of 4 g given to 5 at follow-up was unsuccessful. Six of 7 isolates of *Neisseria gonorrhoeae* from these patients had MICs of spectinomycin of 100 µg or more per mL. Spectinomycin-resistant isolates were generally susceptible to other antibiotics, including penicillin, although several were relatively resistant to tetracycline. Most experimental evidence suggests that high-level resistance to spectinomycin in gonococci results from a single-step chromosomal mutation affecting ribosome structure. Ceftriaxone was subsequently used for the primary treatment of gonorrhoea because of the high prevalence of resistance to spectinomycin.— J. W. Boslego *et al.*, *New Engl. J. Med.*, 1987, *317*, 272.

Preparations

Spectinomycin Injection *(B.P.)*. Spectinomycin Hydrochloride Injection

Sterile Spectinomycin Hydrochloride *(U.S.P.)*

Proprietary Preparations

Trobicin *(Upjohn, UK)*. *Injection*, powder for reconstitution, spectinomycin 2 g (as hydrochloride), supplied with diluent.

Proprietary Names and Manufacturers

Delspectin *(Neth.)*; Kempi *(Upjohn, Spain)*; Stanilo *(Ger.)*; Togamycin *(Arg.)*; Trobicin *(Upjohn, Austral.; Belg.; Upjohn, Canad.; Upjohn, Denm.; Upjohn, Ital.; Jpn; Upjohn, Norw.; Upjohn, S.Afr.; Upjohn, Swed.; Upjohn, Switz.; Upjohn, UK; Upjohn, USA)*; Trobicine *(Upjohn, Fr.)*.

158-y

Spiramycin *(BAN, USAN, rINN)*.

IL-5902; NSC-55926; NSC-64393 (hydrochloride); Spiramycinum.

(4*R*,5*S*,6*S*,7*R*,9*R*,10*R*,16*R*)-(11*E*,13*E*)-6-[(*O*-2,6-dideoxy-3-*C*-methyl-α-L-*ribo*-hexapyranosyl-(1→4)-(3,6-dideoxy-3-dimethylamino-β-D-glucopyranosyl)-oxy]-7-formylmethyl-4-hydroxy-5-methoxy-9,16-dimethyl-10-[(2,3,4,6-tetradeoxy-4-dimethylamino-D-*erythro*-hexopyranosyl)oxy]-oxacyclohexadeca-11,13-dien-2-one.

$C_{43}H_{74}N_2O_{14}$=843.1.

CAS — 8025-81-8.

Pharmacopoeias. In *Eur., Fr., Ger., It., Neth.,* and *Swiss.* Also in *B.P. Vet. Jpn* includes Acetylspiramycin.

A macrolide antibiotic produced by the growth of certain strains of *Streptomyces ambofaciens* or obtained by any other means. The main component is described above.

A white or slightly yellowish slightly hygroscopic powder with a slight odour. It contains not less than 3900 units per mg, calculated with reference to the dried substance.

Slightly **soluble** in water; freely soluble in alcohol, acetone, and methyl alcohol; sparingly soluble in ether. **Store** in airtight containers.

Units

One unit of spiramycin is contained in 0.0003125 mg of the first International Reference Preparation (1962) which contains 3200 units per mg.

Adverse Effects and Precautions

As for Erythromycin, p.222.

There have been only a few reports of untoward reactions following the use of spiramycin; these include nausea, vomiting, diarrhoea, epigastric pain, and skin sensitisation.

ALLERGY. Bronchial asthma occurred in 2 patients after occupational inhalation of spiramycin powder.— G. Moscato *et al*, *Clin. Allergy*, 1984, *14*, 355.

EFFECTS ON THE GASTRO-INTESTINAL TRACT. A 27-year-old man developed acute colitis on the fifth day of taking spiramycin 500 mg four times daily for 5 days for a tooth infection. A barium enema showed marked spasm, nodularity, and micro-ulcerations in the descending colon. All complaints disappeared within 24 hours of stopping the antibiotic.— G. M. Decaux and C. Devroede (letter), *Lancet*, 1978, *2*, 993.

EFFECTS ON THE LIVER. For reference to the hepatotoxic potential of macrolide antibiotics, see Erythromycin Estolate, p.227.

INTERACTIONS. For reference to possible interactions with macrolide antibiotics, and their effect on hepatic metabolism, see Erythromycin, p.222.

Antimicrobial Action and Resistance

Spiramycin has antimicrobial activity and pattern of resistance similar to that of erythromycin (see p.223), although it is less potent against *Haemophilus influenzae*.

A study of the antimicrobial activity *in vitro* of a combination of spiramycin and metronidazole. Synergy was observed against some organisms.— T. C. Quee *et al.*, *Antimicrob. Ag. Chemother.*, 1983, *24*, 445.

An evaluation of spiramycin derivatives including structure activity relationships. Spiramycin itself is a complex of macrolide antibiotics with 3 major components, Spiramycin I, II, and III.— S. Omura *et al.*, *J. antimicrob. Chemother.*, 1985, *16*, *Suppl.* A, 1.

For reference to the activity of spiramycin against *Campylobacter* and *Legionella* spp., and *Neisseria gonorrhoeae*, see Erythromycin, p.223.

Absorption and Fate

Spiramycin is irregularly absorbed from the gastro-intestinal tract and is widely distributed in the tissues. A dose of 1 g produces blood concentrations of approximately 1 µg per mL after 2 to 3 hours; high blood concentrations are maintained for 4 to 6 hours after a single dose. High tissue concentrations are achieved and persist long after the plasma concentration has fallen to low levels. From 12 to 16% of the maternal blood concentration has been reported in the amniotic fluid; it does not diffuse into the cerebrospinal fluid to an appreciable extent.

Spiramycin is slowly eliminated; substantial amounts are excreted in the bile and about 10% in the urine. High concentrations appear in the milk of nursing mothers.

Uses and Administration

Spiramycin is a macrolide antibiotic which is given by mouth and has been used similarly to erythromycin (see p.224) in the treatment of susceptible infections. It has also been used to treat the protozoal infections cryptosporidiosis and toxoplasmosis. The adult dose is 2 to 4 g daily, usually in 2 divided doses. Spiramycin has also been administered locally in the treatment of eye infections.

Acetylspiramycin and spiramycin adipate are also used.

Spiramycin is used in some countries as an additive for animal feeding stuffs. Spiramycin and its embonate salt are used in veterinary practice.

CRYPTOSPORIDIOSIS. *Cryptosporidium muris* is a coccidian parasite that infects the gastro-intestinal tract. In immunocompetent adults cryptosporidiosis presents as a mild 'flu-like' illness with diarrhoea but in immunocompromised individuals, including those with AIDS or receiving immunosuppressive therapy for transplants or tumours, the disease is often severe and life-threatening. There is thus an urgent need for a safe and effective agent to treat cryptosporidiosis. Of the antimicrobial agents tried spiramycin offers the greatest promise so far.— A. Hart and D. Baxby, *J. antimicrob. Chemother.*, 1985, *15*, 3.

After treatment with spiramycin, 5 of 10 immunosuppressed patients (9 with AIDS) with intestinal cryptosporidiosis had complete resolution of diarrhoea within the first week of treatment, one had resolution within one month, and the remaining patients had some symptomatic improvement. The 9 adults received spiramycin 3 g daily in divided doses and a 2-year-old child received 1 g daily; treatment was continued for 1 to 16 weeks. It was considered that spiramycin may produce a significant clinical improvement even if the parasite is not eradicated from the stool.— D. Portnoy *et al.*, *Ann. intern. Med.*, 1984, *101*, 202. See also A. C. Collier *et al.*, *ibid.*, 205; *Morb. Mortal.*, 1984, *33*, 117.

RESPIRATORY-TRACT INFECTIONS. Comparative reports of spiramycin and erythromycin in the treatment of acute tonsillo-pharyngitis: Zulkifli *et al.*, *Curr. med. Res. Opinion*, 1984, *8*, 708; Suprihati *et al.*, *ibid.*, *9*, 192; T. Soekrawinata *et al.*, *ibid.*, 296.

TOXOPLASMOSIS. Spiramycin may be used as an alternative to pyrimethamine in association with trisulphapyrimidines for the treatment of toxoplasmosis (infection due to *Toxoplasma gondii*). Adults may be given 2 to 4 g daily and children 50 to 100 mg per kg body-weight daily; treatment should be continued for 3 to 4 weeks. In ocular toxoplasmosis, corticosteroids should also be used for their anti-inflammatory action on the eyes.— *Med. Lett.*, 1986, *28*, 9.

Congenital toxoplasmosis. Spiramycin 2 to 3 g daily in divided doses for 3 weeks, repeated at 2-weekly intervals, was given to pregnant women with toxoplasmosis and reduced the overall incidence of foetal infections when compared with an untreated group of mothers but did not influence significantly the course of established foetal toxoplasmosis.— G. Desmonts and J. Couvreur, *New Engl. J. Med.*, 1974, *290*, 1110. Comment on the problem of congenital toxoplasmosis. Spiramycin therapy has been suggested for pregnant women found to convert serologically from negative to positive, but the detection and avoidance of a single case would be very costly.— *Lancet*, 1980, *1*, 578. See also D. G. Fleck, *Archs Dis. Childh.*, 1981, *56*, 494; A. O. Carter and J. W. Frank, *Can. med. Ass. J.*, 1986, *135*, 618.

Immunocompromised patients. Successful use of spiramycin in addition to conventional treatment with pyrimethamine and sulphonamides for the management of disseminated toxoplasmosis in patients undergoing cardiac transplantation. These patients were on immunosuppressive therapy.— M. Hakim *et al.*, *Br. med. J.*, 1986, *292*, 1108.

From experience in 4 patients, 3 of them with AIDS, it was concluded that spiramycin 2 g daily by mouth does not prevent the occurrence of neurotoxoplasmosis in immunosuppressed patients. This may be due to poor diffusion of spiramycin into the CNS.— C. Leport *et al.* (letter), *J. Am. med. Ass.*, 1986, *255*, 2290. Brief comment from a National Institutes of Health conference on AIDS that pyrimethamine plus sulphadiazine was the only regimen clearly effective in treating encephalitis caused by the protozoan *Toxoplasma gondii* in patients with AIDS. No convincing clinical reports to support the use of other drugs, including spiramycin had been published.— V. T. DeVita *et al.*, *Ann. intern. Med.*, 1987, *106*, 568.

Proprietary Names and Manufacturers

Dicorvin *(Hubber, Spain)*; Rovamicina *(Carlo Erba, Ital.)*; Rovamycin *(Rhone-Poulenc, Denm.*; *Rhône-Poulenc, Norw.*; *Leo Rhodia, Swed.*; *May & Baker, UK)*; Rovamycine *(Rhodia, Arg.*; *Rhone-Poulenc, Belg.*; *Rhône-Poulenc, Canad.*; *Specia, Fr.*; *Rhône-Poulenc, Ger.*; *Specia, Neth.*; *Rhone, Spain*; *Rhone-Poulenc, Switz.)*; Selectomycin *(Grünenthal, Ger.)*.

160-q

Streptomycin *(BAN, rINN)*.

Estreptomicina. 4-*O*-[2-*O*-(2-Deoxy-2-methylamino-α-L-glucopyranosyl)-5-deoxy-3-*C*-formyl-α-L-lyxofuranosyl]-*NN'*-diamidino-D-streptamine.

$C_{21}H_{39}N_7O_{12}$=581.6.

CAS — 57-92-1.

NOTE. Under the name Streptomycin, *Mex. P.* and *Span. P.* include the calcium chloride complex, the hydrochloride, the phosphate, and the sulphate.

An antimicrobial organic base produced by the growth of certain strains of *Streptomyces griseus*, or by any other means.

NOTE. The *B.P.* directs that when Streptomycin is prescribed or demanded, Streptomycin Sulphate (see below) be dispensed or supplied. The quantity of streptomycin specified is interpreted as referring to streptomycin base.

161-p

Streptomycin Calcium Chloride

$(C_{21}H_{39}N_7O_{12},3HCl)_2,CaCl_2$=911.3.

Pharmacopoeias. In *Mex.* and *Span.* See also above under Streptomycin.

162-s

Streptomycin Hydrochloride

$C_{21}H_{39}N_7O_{12},3HCl$=691.0.

CAS — 6160-32-3.

Pharmacopoeias. In *Mex.* and *Span.* See also above under Streptomycin.

1.19 g of monograph substance is approximately equivalent to 1 g of streptomycin.

163-w

Streptomycin Sulphate *(BANM, rINNM)*.

Sulfato de Estreptomicina; Streptomycin Sulfate *(USAN)*; Streptomycini Sulfas.

$(C_{21}H_{39}N_7O_{12})_2,3H_2SO_4$=1457.4.

CAS — 3810-74-0.

Pharmacopoeias. In *Arg.*, *Aust.*, *Belg.*, *Br.*, *Braz.*, *Chin.*, *Cz.*, *Egypt.*, *Fr.*, *Ger.*, *Hung.*, *Ind.*, *Int.*, *It.*, *Jpn*, *Jug.*, *Mex.*, *Neth.*, *Nord.*, *Pol.*, *Roum.*, *Rus.*, *Span.*, *Swiss*, and *Turk.* Also in *B.P. Vet.*
U.S. includes Sterile Streptomycin Sulfate.

A white or almost white hygroscopic powder, odourless or almost odourless. The *B.P.* specifies not less than 720 units per mg calculated on the dried substance; the *U.S.P.* specifies not less than 650 μg and not more than 850 μg of streptomycin per mg. 1.25 g of monograph substance is approximately equivalent to 1 g of streptomycin. *B.P.* **solubilities** are: very soluble in water; practically insoluble in alcohol, chloroform, and ether. *U.S.P.* solubilities are: freely soluble in water; very slightly soluble in alcohol; practically insoluble in chloroform. A 25% solution in water has a pH of 4.5 to 7.0. The *B.P.* injection has a pH of 5.0 to 6.5; the *U.S.P.* injection has a pH of 5.0 to 8.0. **Incompatible** with acids and alkalis. **Store** in airtight containers and protect from moisture.

CAUTION. *Streptomycin may cause severe dermatitis in sensitised persons, and pharmacists, nurses, and others who handle the drug frequently should wear masks and rubber gloves.*

INCOMPATIBILITY. The increase in colour of a solution of streptomycin sulphate in the presence of *procaine hydrochloride* was due to a reaction between the carbonyl group of the streptomycin and the *p*-amino group of the procaine.— A. V. Puccini and A. J. Spiegel, *J. pharm. Sci.*, 1962, *51*, 496.

For reference to the inactivation of aminoglycosides by beta-lactam antibiotics, see Gentamicin Sulphate, p.236.

Units

78 500 units of streptomycin are contained in 100 mg of streptomycin sulphate in one ampoule of the third International Standard Preparation (1980).

Adverse Effects and Treatment

As for Gentamicin Sulphate, p.236.

Paraesthesia in and around the mouth has been reported following the intramuscular injection of streptomycin sulphate. Hypersensitivity reactions may occur and sensitisation is common among those who handle streptomycin occupationally. It should not therefore be administered topically or by inhalation. Ototoxicity has been observed in infants whose mothers had been given streptomycin during pregnancy.

Meningeal irritation has occurred after intrathecal injections of streptomycin, and some authorities do not recommend administration by this route.

Desensitisation may be attempted following hypersensitivity reactions if the use of streptomycin is considered essential for the provision of adequate antituberculous chemotherapy (see p.546).

EFFECTS ON THE BLOOD. Spontaneous transient inhibition of blood-clotting factor V occurred in a patient. Streptomycin might have been implicated in this effect, as it might have been in 5 of 7 other patients who were known to have had the same inhibition.— D. I. Feinstein *et al.*, *Ann. intern. Med.*, 1973, *78*, 385.

Acute haemolytic anaemia and renal failure developed in a 45-year-old man shortly after he injected himself with streptomycin and ampicillin. Antibodies to streptomycin were demonstrated. He had used streptomycin repeatedly over the previous 15 years.— J. M. -L. Letona *et al.*, *Br. J. Haemat.*, 1977, *35*, 561.

EFFECTS ON THE EAR. A report of 3 families supporting the view that there may be a familial susceptibility to streptomycin ototoxicity.— X. Chan and Y. Xie, *Br. med. J.*, 1986, *293*, 1158.

EFFECTS ON THE EYE. Streptomycin might cause optic neuritis, optic atrophy, toxic amblyopia, loss of vision, and scotoma.— H. I. Silverman, *Am. J. Optom.*, 1972, *49*, 335.

EFFECTS ON THE SKIN. Seven cases of toxic epidermal necrolysis had been reported associated with the use of streptomycin.— E. D. Lowney *et al.*, *Archs Derm.*, 1967, *95*, 359.

A report of Stevens-Johnson syndrome associated with the administration of streptomycin.— S. K. Sarkar *et al.*, *Tubercle*, 1982, *63*, 137.

Precautions

As for Gentamicin Sulphate, p.238.

Peak plasma concentrations greater than 40 μg per mL, and trough concentrations greater than 5 μg per mL should be avoided.

INTERACTIONS. Sequential administration of intravenous bolus doses of streptomycin 500 mg and methicillin 1 g, over a period of 5 minutes through a subclavian vein catheter, had caused rigors in postoperative coronary bypass patients, within 30 minutes of administration. Administration of the 2 drugs separated by an interval of 4 hours appeared to avoid this.— P. C. Robinson *et al.* (letter), *Lancet*, 1978, *2*, 1056.

INTERFERENCE WITH DIAGNOSTIC TESTS. Streptomycin could interfere technically with chemical estimations for urea in the blood to produce erroneous lowered results.— *Drug & Ther. Bull.*, 1972, *10*, 69.

PREGNANCY AND THE NEONATE. It was estimated that a breast-fed infant of a mother receiving streptomycin sulphate would ingest about 9.5% of the usual therapeutic dose for an infant.— D. E. Snider and K. E. Powell, *Archs intern. Med.*, 1984, *144*, 589.

Antimicrobial Action

Streptomycin has a mode of action and antimicrobial spectrum similar to that of gentamicin (see p.239), although most strains of *Pseudomonas aeruginosa* are resistant. It is effective against *Yersinia pestis*, *Francisella tularensis*, and *Brucella* spp. Some strains of staphylococci are sensitive but it is ineffective against most other Gram-positive cocci and bacilli; *Enterococcus faecalis* (*Streptococcus faecalis*) is invariably resistant but may be inhibited by streptomycin in conjunction with penicillin. Streptomycin has particular activity against *Mycobacterium tuberculosis*; for the role of this activity in the treatment of tuberculosis see the section on Antimycobacterial Agents, p.546.

The minimum inhibitory concentration of streptomycin for most susceptible organisms is in the range of 1 to 8 μg per mL.

The MIC of streptomycin for 95 strains of *Brucella melitensis* ranged from 0.12 to 1 μg per mL. Doxycycline and tetracycline were the most active of the agents tested.— J. Bosch *et al.*, *J. antimicrob. Chemother.*, 1986, *17*, 459.

ACTIVITY AGAINST MYCOBACTERIA. For reference to the activity of streptomycin against *Mycobacterium tuberculosis*, see the section on Antimycobacterial Agents, p.546; against *Mycobacterium leprae*, see Gentamicin Sulphate, p.239; and against atypical *Mycobacterium* spp., see Amikacin Sulphate, p.110.

ACTIVITY WITH OTHER ANTIMICROBIAL AGENTS. For reference to the effect of other agents on the *in-vitro* antimicrobial activity of aminoglycosides, see Gentamicin Sulphate, p.239. For the particular effect of streptomycin and benzylpenicillin against enterococci, see Uses, Endocarditis, in Gentamicin Sulphate, p.243.

Resistance

Resistance has been observed in strains of most of the organisms reported to be sensitive to streptomycin and many strains of bacteria initially sensitive to streptomycin become resistant during therapy. For reference to primary and secondary resistance of *Mycobacterium tuberculosis* to streptomycin, see the section on Antimycobacterial Agents, p.546. The emergence of resistant strains may be delayed by combining the streptomycin therapy with the administration of other antibiotics or other chemotherapeutic agents.

There is complete cross-resistance between streptomycin and dihydrostreptomycin, and partial cross-resistance between streptomycin, neomycin, framycetin, kanamycin, and paromomycin.

For the mechanisms of resistance of bacteria to aminoglycosides, see Gentamicin Sulphate, p.240.

Although streptomycin has been used for the management of chancroid, treatment failures have been observed since 1980. These appear to be associated with an increase in the incidence of strains of *Haemophilus ducreyi* showing resistance to streptomycin and kanamycin *in vitro*.— V. S. Rajan and E. H. Sng (letter), *Lancet*, 1982, *2*, 1043.

Of 232 strains of enteropathogenic *Escherichia coli* 106 were resistant to streptomycin at a concentration of 16 μg per mL.— R. J. Gross *et al.*, *Br. med. J.*, 1982,

285, 472.

Of 2753 strains of *Shigella dysenteriae, Sh. flexneri*, and *Sh. boydii* examined at the Central Public Health Laboratory from 1979 to mid 1983 72.0% were resistant to streptomycin at a concentration of 16 µg per mL.— R. J. Gross *et al., Br. med. J.*, 1984, *288*, 784.

For reports of resistance to streptomycin in the treatment of tuberculosis, see Antimycobacterial Agents, p.546.

Absorption and Fate

As for Gentamicin Sulphate, p.241. After intramuscular injection of streptomycin, maximum concentration in the blood is reached in 0.5 to 2 hours but the time taken and the concentration attained, which may be as high as 40 or 50 µg per mL after a dose of 1 g, vary considerably. Following intramuscular injection of 1 g of streptomycin detectable amounts may still be present after 24 hours. The half-life of streptomycin is about 2½ hours. About one-third of streptomycin in the circulation is bound to plasma proteins. The rate of urinary excretion varies in different individuals and the concentration of streptomycin in the urine is often very high with about 30 to 90% of a dose usually being excreted within 24 hours.

Uses and Administration

Streptomycin is an aminoglycoside antibiotic mainly used in the treatment of tuberculosis, in conjunction with other antituberculous agents (see p.547) and may be classified as a first-line or primary antituberculous agent.

Streptomycin and penicillin have a synergistic action against some bacteria and are used together in the treatment of bacterial endocarditis.

Streptomycin is effective in the treatment of plague, tularaemia, and, in conjunction with tetracycline, in brucellosis. It was formerly used by mouth in the treatment of infections of the intestine and prior to abdominal surgery.

Streptomycin is used as the sulphate and is given by intramuscular injection as a solution in Water for Injections or sodium chloride 0.9% injection. Intravenous administration is not advisable because it produces high and potentially toxic blood concentrations.

Doses should be reduced in patients with impaired renal function. In all patients dosage should be adjusted according to plasma-streptomycin concentrations; peak plasma concentrations should be less than 40 µg per mL and trough concentrations not more than 5 µg per mL (see also Administration under Gentamicin Sulphate, Uses, p.242).

In tuberculosis, streptomycin is given with other antituberculous agents; administration of streptomycin is generally restricted to the first 2 months of treatment regimens. In intermittent regimens streptomycin has been given 2 or 3 times a week rather than daily. The usual dose of streptomycin is 1 g daily by intramuscular injection, although in general, for patients over 40 years of age the dose of streptomycin should not exceed 750 mg daily and for those over 60 years of age it should not exceed 500 mg because of the greater risk of vestibular disturbance. Children have been given up to 40 mg per kg body-weight daily in divided doses although for long-term treatment a daily dose of 20 mg per kg body-weight is usually recommended.

In tuberculous meningitis, intramuscular administration has sometimes been supplemented by intrathecal injections of streptomycin; adults may be given 50 mg daily, dissolved in at least 10 mL of sodium chloride 0.9% injection. Children have been given 1 mg per kg body-weight. However, streptomycin has caused meningeal irritation and some authorities do not recommend administration by this route.

For the treatment of non-tuberculous infections, the usual dose is 1 g daily for not more than 5 to 10 days because of the possibility of inducing drug resistance; higher doses are recommended in the treatment of plague and tularaemia.

For reviews of the actions and uses of streptomycin and other aminoglycoside antibiotics, see Gentamicin Sulphate, p.242.

For reference to the treatment of atypical mycobacterial infections including the use of streptomycin, see Antimycobacterial Agents, p.553.

BRUCELLOSIS. For reference to the use of streptomycin and tetracycline in the treatment of brucellosis, see Doxycycline Hydrochloride, p.218.

CHANCROID. For reference to the use of streptomycin in the treatment of chancroid, see under Resistance, above.

ENDOCARDITIS. For reference to the use of streptomycin in the treatment of infective endocarditis, see Gentamicin Sulphate, p.243.

LEPTOSPIROSIS. For reference to the use of streptomycin in leptospirosis, see Benzylpenicillin Sodium, p.136.

MÉNIÈRE'S DISEASE. The neurotoxic effect of streptomycin was used therapeutically in Ménière's disease. The usual dose was 1 g thrice daily for 3 to 4 weeks or until the caloric response disappeared in the more seriously affected labyrinth. Ataxia often occurred and could be more disabling than the original disease. The treatment should not be given to patients over 50 years of age or to those with unilateral disease.— *Br. med. J.*, 1970, *1*, 614.

An improvement in vestibular symptoms without hearing loss was achieved in 8 patients with bilateral Ménière's disease treated with intramuscular injections of streptomycin sulphate. In all but one patient streptomycin was given in the following dosage regimen: 1 g twice daily for 5 days a week for 2 weeks and then titration of the dose until a response was obtained or until adverse effects, such as hearing loss or oscillopsia, occurred. Total doses of 30 to 60 g were required.— M. D. Graham *et al., Otolaryngol. Head Neck Surg.*, 1984, *92*, 440.

MYCETOMA. For reference to the successful antibacterial therapy of actinomycetoma using regimens incorporating streptomycin, see Co-trimoxazole, p.212.

PLAGUE. In a study of 10 patients with *Yersinia pestis* infection (plague) who were randomly assigned to treatment with streptomycin or co-trimoxazole for 10 days, all patients survived. Streptomycin was given in a dose of 1 g twice daily by intramuscular injection (patients weighing less than 25 kg received half this dose). Co-trimoxazole was given intravenously for 3 to 5 days and then by mouth. Those treated with streptomycin had a shorter duration of fever and fewer complications and it was considered that streptomycin should remain the drug of choice.— T. Butler *et al., J. infect. Dis.*, 1976, *133*, 493. See also *idem*, 1977, *136*, 317.

For further references to the use of streptomycin in plague, see Tetracycline Hydrochloride, p.320.

TUBERCULOSIS. For the use of streptomycin in the treatment of tuberculosis, see Treatment of Tuberculosis in Antimycobacterial Agents, p.547.

TULARAEMIA. A report of 2 small outbreaks of tularaemia. One was successfully treated with tetracycline and the other with intramuscular streptomycin. Streptomycin was considered the drug of choice for severe tularaemia as relapses were less common than with tetracycline or chloramphenicol.— L. Ford-Jones *et al., Can. med. Ass. J.*, 1982, *127*, 298.

WHIPPLE'S DISEASE. For reference to the use of streptomycin in Whipple's disease, see Benzylpenicillin Sodium, p.138.

Preparations

Streptomycin Injection *(B.P.)*. Streptomycin Sulphate Injection. Protect from light and store at a temperature not exceeding 20°.

Streptomycin Sulfate Injection *(U.S.P.)*

Sterile Streptomycin Sulfate *(U.S.P.)*

Proprietary Preparations

Streptomycin Sulphate *(Evans Medical, UK)*. *Injection*, powder for reconstitution, streptomycin 1 g (as sulphate).

Proprietary Names and Manufacturers

Cidan Est *(Cidan, Spain)*; Darostrep *(S.Afr.)*; Dif-Estrepto E *(Spain)*; Estrepto E *(Spain)*; Estreptomade *(Spain)*; Estrepto-Wolner *(Kairon, Spain)*; Neodiestreptobap *(Spain)*; Novostrep *(Novo, S.Afr.)*; Novo-Strep *(Novo, Denm.)*; Orastrep *(Dista, UK)*; Servistrep *(Servipharm, Switz.)*; Solvo-strept S *(Ger.)*; Streptocidan *(Cidan, Spain)*; Streptocol *(Molteni, Ital.)*; Strycin *(Squibb, Ital.)*.

The following names have been used for multi-ingredient preparations containing streptomycin sulphate— Crystamycin *(Glaxo, UK)*; Streptotriad *(May & Baker, UK)*; Sulphamagna *(Wyeth, UK)*.

4914-t

Succinylsulphathiazole *(BAN)*.

Succinilsolfatiazolo; Succinylsulfathiazole *(rINN)*; Succinylsulfathiazolum. 4′-(Thiazol-2-ylsulphamoyl)succinanilic acid monohydrate.

$C_{13}H_{13}N_3O_5S_2,H_2O=373.4$.

CAS — 116-43-8 (anhydrous).

Pharmacopoeias. In *Arg., Aust., Br., Braz., Eur., Fr., Ger., Ind., Int., It., Mex., Neth., Span., Swiss,* and *Turk.*

White or yellowish-white, odourless crystalline powder. M.p. about 190° with decomposition. It darkens on exposure to light.

Very slightly **soluble** in water; slightly soluble in alcohol; practically insoluble in ether; dissolves in aqueous solutions of alkali hydroxides and carbonates. **Protect** from light.

Succinylsulphathiazole is a sulphonamide with properties similar to those of sulphamethoxazole, p.306. It is hydrolysed to sulphathiazole in the large intestine and only about 5% is absorbed.

Succinylsulphathiazole has been given by mouth in the treatment of gastro-intestinal infections. Usual adult doses of succinylsulphathiazole are in the range of 10 to 20 g daily in divided doses.

Preparations

Paediatric Succinylsulphathiazole Mixture *(B.P.C. 1973)*. Mist. Succinylsulphathiaz. pro Inf. Contains succinylsulphathiazole 0.5 g per 5 mL. *Dose.* Children 1 to 2 years, 10 mL four times daily; 3 to 5 years, 20 mL four times daily.

Proprietary Names and Manufacturers

SS Thiazole *(Austral.)*; Sulfasuxidine *(Canad.; Merck Sharp & Dohme, UK)*; Thiacyl *(Fr.)*.

The following names have been used for multi-ingredient preparations containing succinylsulphathiazole— Cremomycin *(Merck Sharp & Dohme, UK)*; Cremostrep *(Merck Sharp & Dohme, UK)*; Cremosuxidine *(Merck Sharp & Dohme, UK)*; Kaovax *(Norton, UK)*.

13275-l

Sulbactam *(BAN, rINN)*.

CP-45889-2 *(sodium salt)*; CP-45899; CP-47904 *(pivsulbactam; pivaloyloxymethyl penicillanate 1,1-dioxide; sulbactam pivoxil)*. Penicillanic acid 1,1-dioxide; (2*S*,5*R*)-3,3-Dimethyl-7-oxo-4-thia-1-azabicyclo[3.2.0]heptane-2-carboxylic acid 4,4-dioxide.

$C_8H_{11}NO_5S=233.2$.

CAS — 68373-14-8 (sulbactam); 69388-84-7 (sodium salt); 69388-79-0 (pivsulbactam).

NOTE. Sulbactam Sodium is *USAN*.

Sulbactam is a penicillanic acid sulphone with beta-lactamase inhibitory properties. It generally has only weak antibacterial activity, except against *Neisseria gonorrhoeae* and *N. meningitidis*, but it is an irreversible inhibitor of several beta-lactamases including Richmond-Sykes types II, III, IV, and V. Sulbactam may therefore enhance the activity of many beta-lactam antibiotics against bacteria that are normally resistant because of the production of beta-lactamases, including staphylococci, *Bacteroides fragilis* and other *Bacteroides* spp., *Haemophilus influenzae, Neisseria gonorrhoeae*, and some Enterobacteriaceae.

Sulbactam is poorly absorbed after oral administration and is therefore administered parenterally. The basic pharmacokinetic characteristics of sulbactam are similar to those of ampicillin after parenteral administration. Sulbactam may be given in association with ampicillin (see p.119) or with cefoperazone in the treatment of various infections where beta-lactamase production is suspected. Sulbactam is usually given with ampicillin in a ratio of 1:2, respectively. An adult dosage of sulbactam 0.25 to 1 g plus ampicillin 0.5 to 2 g given intravenously or intramuscularly every 6 hours has been used.

Sulbactam is available as the sodium salt and also as pivsulbactam (sulbactam pivoxil). A preparation of sulbactam combined via ester linkages with ampicillin is also under study (see Sultamicillin, p.310).

Reviews of the antibacterial activity, pharmacokinetic properties, and therapeutic use of sulbactam in association with ampicillin: D. M. Campoli-Richards and R. N. Brogden, *Drugs*, 1987, *33*, 577–609; *Med. Lett.*, 1987, *29*, 79.

Proceedings of a symposium on sulbactam/ampicillin.— *Drugs*, 1988, *35*, *Suppl.* 7, 1-94.

ADVERSE EFFECTS. Data collected by the manufacturer involving 1764 patients who received sulbactam in association with ampicillin showed that less than 10% of patients reported side-effects and only 0.7% discontinued therapy because of adverse effects. The most frequent adverse effects were pain at the injection site, usually associated with intramuscular administration (3.6%), diarrhoea (1.9%), and phlebitis (1.2%) (D.M. Campoli-Richards and R.N. Brogden, *Drugs*, 1987, *33*, 577). In this and other studies adverse effects reported in patients receiving both drugs have also included other gastro-intestinal disorders such as flatulence or vomiting, skin reactions including itching and rashes, and CNS disorders such as headache and dizziness (J. Gunning, *Drugs*, 1986, *31*, *Suppl.* 2, 14; D.L. Hemsell, *ibid.*, 22).

ANTIMICROBIAL ACTION. Several studies have demonstrated synergy *in vitro* between sulbactam and ampicillin (R. Wise *et al.*, *J. antimicrob. Chemother.*, 1980, *6*, 197; J.A. Retsema *et al.*, *Antimicrob. Ag. Chemother.*, 1980, *17*, 615); a concentration ratio of 1 part sulbactam to 2 parts ampicillin has been reported to be optimal, although other ratios have also been used (D.M. Campoli-Richards and R.N. Brogden, *Drugs*, 1987, *33*, 577). Synergy between sulbactam and ampicillin has been demonstrated against beta-lactamase-producing strains of *Staphylococcus aureus*, *Bacteroides* spp., *Haemophilus influenzae*, and *H. ducreyi*, and some beta-lactamase-producing Enterobacteriaceae (R.J. Fass, *Antimicrob. Ag. Chemother.*, 1981, *19*, 361; M.R. Jacobs *et al.*, *ibid.*, 1986, *29*, 980; B.M. Jones *et al.*, *ibid.*, 1110; R. Auckenthaler *et al.*, *Curr. ther. Res.*, 1986, *40*, 1078). Sulbactam and clavulanic acid have been reported to have no effect on the activity of various beta-lactams, including ampicillin, against *Campylobacter jejuni* (P. Van der Auwera and B. Scorneaux, *Antimicrob. Ag. Chemother.*, 1985, *28*, 37).

Synergy against beta-lactamase-producing organisms has also been reported between sulbactam and other beta-lactam antibiotics that are hydrolysed by beta-lactamases: the activity of cefsulodin or cefoperazone has been enhanced against *B. fragilis* organisms (K.P. Fu *et al.*, *J. antimicrob. Chemother.*, 1984, *13*, 257; M.B.S. Dias *et al.*, *ibid.*, 1986, *18*, 467); the activity of cefoperazone enhanced against *H. influenzae* (P.K.W. Yu and J.A. Washington, *Antimicrob. Ag. Chemother.*, 1981, *20*, 63); the activity of mecillinam enhanced against *Escherichia coli*, *Enterobacter* spp., and some other Enterobacteriaceae (H.C. Neu, *ibid.*, 1982, *22*, 518); and the activity of azlocillin enhanced against *Ps. aeruginosa* (S.E. Calderwood *et al.*, *ibid.*, 266). Other workers have found no synergy with other extended spectrum penicillins including ticarcillin and piperacillin against *Ps. aeruginosa*, but some synergy with ticarcillin against *Ps. maltophilia* (M.R. Jacobs *et al.*, *J. antimicrob. Chemother.*, 1986, *18*, 177).

Sulbactam generally appears to be a less potent inhibitor of most types of beta-lactamases than clavulanic acid, on a weight-for-weight basis, however, the relative effectiveness will depend on the organism being challenged (M.R. Jacobs *et al.*, *Antimicrob Ag. Chemother.*, 1986, *29*, 980). The effect of increasing the inoculum size has been reported to increase the resistance level of multi-resistant *E. coli*, *H. influenzae*, *Ps. aeruginosa*, and methicillin-resistant staphylococci to sulbactam plus ampicillin or clavulanic acid plus ampicillin (K. E. Aldridge *et al.*, *J. antimicrob. Chemother.*, 1986, *17*, 463).

ABSORPTION AND FATE. Sulbactam is poorly absorbed from the gastro-intestinal tract. It is administered parenterally often in association with ampicillin, both drugs having similar half-lives of about one hour. Serum concentrations of sulbactam have been reported to be about 1.5 times those of ampicillin when both drugs are administered intravenously in a dose of 0.5 g (R.M. Brown *et al.*, *Antimicrob. Ag. Chemother.*, 1982, *21*, 565). Peak serum concentrations of 20 and 43 µg per mL have been reported following administration of single intravenous doses of sulbactam 0.5 and 1.0 g respectively, infused over 30 minutes. Mean peak serum concentrations of 13 and 28 µg per mL have been reported approximately 30 minutes following intramuscular administration of sulbactam 0.5 and 1.0 g, respectively. Co-administration of sulbactam and ampicillin resulted in only minor changes in serum concentrations compared with those reported with administration of either drug alone (G. Foulds *et al.*, *ibid.*, 1983, *23*, 692).

Following intravenous administration, sulbactam has been detected in various body tissues and fluids including intestinal mucosa, peritoneal fluid, myometrium, fallopian tube, ovary, and breast milk (L. Kager *et al.*, *Antimicrob. Ag. Chemother.*, 1982, *22*, 208; E.T. Houang *et al.*, *ibid.*, 1985, *28*, 165; G. Foulds *et al.*, *Clin. Pharmac. Ther.*, 1985, *38*, 692; U. Schwiersch *et al.*, *Drugs*, 1986, *31*, *Suppl.* 2, 26). Sulbactam penetrates into the CSF of patients with bacterial meningitis to a similar extent to that of ampicillin after intravenous administration (J.-P. Stahl *et al.*, *Rev. infect. Dis.*, 1986, *8*, *Suppl.* 5, S612).

Sulbactam is mainly excreted in the urine; about 70% of a parenteral dose of sulbactam is excreted unchanged in the urine in the first 6 hours after a dose and about 85% within 24 hours (R.M. Brown *et al.*, *Antimicrob. Ag. Chemother.*, 1982, *21*, 565; G. Foulds *et al.*, *ibid*, 1983, *23*, 692). The half-life of sulbactam is increased in patients with renal failure (N. Wright and R. Wise, *J. antimicrob. Chemother.*, 1983, *11*, 583).

USES AND ADMINISTRATION. *Administration in liver disorders.* A study of the clinical efficacy and safety of sulbactam administered in association with ampicillin to 41 patients suffering from chronic liver disease. The drugs were administered in doses ranging from ampicillin 1 g with sulbactam 0.5 g given intramuscularly twice daily to ampicillin 2 g with sulbactam 1 g given 2 or 3 times daily by intravenous infusion, for 5 to 21 days depending on the site and severity of infection. A favourable clinical response was achieved in about 85% of the patients and no significant change in liver function tests and/or blood chemistry parameters were observed in any of the patients.— D. Galante *et al.*, *J. antimicrob. Chemother.*, 1987, *19*, 527.

Administration in renal failure. The mean half-life of sulbactam 0.5 g administered as a single intravenous dose to 12 patients with various degrees of renal dysfunction increased with diminishing renal function from 1.1 hours in patients with a glomerular filtration-rate (GFR) of 30 to 100 mL per minute to 21.3 hours in patients with terminal renal failure. In 5 similar patients given the same dose of sulbactam intravenously and also ampicillin 0.5 g intravenously, the pharmacokinetic properties of the 2 drugs were found to be similar. Thus the ratio of the 2 drugs present in the plasma remained the same whatever the extent of renal dysfunction. If drug-accumulation is to be avoided in patients with renal failure, a dose of sulbactam 0.5 g in association with ampicillin 0.5 g, both given 6 hourly to patients with normal renal function, should be reduced to twice daily in patients with GFRs between 15 and 30 mL per minute, once daily for GFRs between 5 and 14 mL per minute, and every second day for rates of less than this.— N. Wright and R. Wise, *J. antimicrob. Chemother.*, 1983, *11*, 583.

Administration with ampicillin. Eleven patients with non-life-threatening infections due to ampicillin-resistant organisms, including infections of the urinary tract and skin and soft tissue, were successfully treated with ampicillin 500 mg in association with sulbactam 500 mg both given intravenously every 6 hours for 5 to 10 days.— J. F. Plouffe, *Antimicrob. Ag. Chemother.*, 1982, *21*, 519.

In a study involving 54 patients with severe respiratory-tract or abdominal infections, sulbactam 500 mg was administered in conjunction with ampicillin 500 mg or 1 g given parenterally every 6 hours. The combinations of sulbactam with ampicillin in either a 1:1 or 1:2 ratio were found to be equally effective.— S. Mehtar *et al.*, *J. antimicrob. Chemother.*, 1986, *17*, 389.

A symposium on beta-lactamase inhibitors in obstetrics and gynaecology, covering mainly the use of sulbactam in association with ampicillin.— D. L. Hemsell and H. H. Werner, *Drugs*, 1986, *31*, *Suppl.* 2, pp.1-28.

Further references to the use of sulbactam in association with ampicillin to treat various bacterial infections: V. O. Oviasu and A. O. Obasohan, *Curr. ther. Res.*, 1987, *41*, 99 (lobar pneumonia); A. T. Dutse *et al.*, *ibid.*, 128 (meningococcal meningitis); T. Odugbemi, *ibid.*, 542 (gonorrhoea); N. A. Rotowa *et al.*, *ibid.*, *42*, 351 (gonorrhoea).

For references to the use of sulbactam in association with ampicillin in the treatment of meningitis, pelvic inflammatory disease, gonorrhoea, respiratory-tract infections, and surgical infection prophylaxis, see under Ampicillin Sodium, Uses, p.120.

Gonorrhoea. Although sulbactam has activity *in vitro* against *Neisseria gonorrhoeae*, its clinical efficacy was poor in the treatment of patients with acute uncomplicated gonorrhoea due to beta-lactamase-negative *N. gonorrhoeae*. Sulbactam 2 g given as 2 simultaneous intramuscular injections with probenecid 1 g by mouth, or sulbactam given alone as 2 intramuscular doses of 0.5 g administered 4 hours apart, resulted in cure in only 5 of 10 and 6 of 10 patients, respectively. In the regimens studied sulbactam alone is not suitable for the treatment of gonorrhoea.— V. A. Caine *et al.*, *Antimicrob. Ag. Chemother.*, 1984, *26*, 683.

Proprietary Names and Manufacturers

Pfizer, UK.

The following names have been used for multi-ingredient preparations containing sulbactam— Unasyn *(Roerig, USA)*.

164-e

Sulbenicillin Sodium *(rINNM)*.

α-Sulfobenzylpenicillin Sodium; Sulfocillin Sodium. The disodium salt of (6*R*)-6-(2-phenyl-2-sulphoacetamido)penicillanic acid.

$C_{16}H_{16}N_2Na_2O_7S_2$=458.4.

CAS — 34779-28-7; 41744-40-5 (both sulbenicillin).

Pharmacopoeias. In *Jpn.*

1.1 g of monograph substance is approximately equivalent to 1 g of sulbenicillin. Each g of monograph substance represents about 4.4 mmol of sodium.

Sulbenicillin sodium has actions and uses similar to those of Carbenicillin Sodium, p.139. It is given by intramuscular or intravenous injection usually in doses equivalent to sulbenicillin 2 to 4 g daily. It has also been administered as eye-drops.

Sulbenicillin or its major metabolite α-sulphobenzylpenicilloic acid interfered with platelet aggregation *in vitro*, the metabolite producing a greater effect.— Y. Ikeda *et al.*, *Antimicrob. Ag. Chemother.*, 1978, *13*, 881.

Further references to sulbenicillin sodium: I. Hansen *et al.*, *Clin. Pharmac. Ther.*, 1975, *17*, 339 (pharmacokinetic studies); B. A. Watts *et al.*, *J. antimicrob. Chemother.*, 1977, *3*, 331 (*in vitro* activity against *Neisseria gonorrhoeae*); K. Tsuchiya and M. Kondo, *Antimicrob. Ag. Chemother.*, 1978, *13*, 536 (*in vitro* activity against *Pseudomonas* spp.); I. Miyakawa *et al.*, *ibid.*, 1982, *21*, 838 (transplacental transfer); F. Ginesu *et al.*, *Drugs exp. & clin. Res.*, 1985, *11*, 885 (use in treatment of respiratory-tract infections).

Proprietary Names and Manufacturers

Kedacillina *(Bracco, Ital.)*; Lilacillin *(Takeda, Jpn)*; Sulbenil *(Gist-Brocades, Neth.)*; Sulpelin *(Senju, Jpn)*.

4915-x

Sulfabenzamide *(USAN, rINN)*.

N-Sulphanilylbenzamide.

$C_{13}H_{12}N_2O_3S$=276.3.

CAS — 127-71-9.

Pharmacopoeias. In *U.S.*

A white, practically odourless, fine powder. **Insoluble** in water and in ether; soluble in acetone, alcohol, and sodium hydroxide 4% solution. **Store** in well-closed containers. Protect from light.

Sulfabenzamide is a sulphonamide with properties similar to those of sulphamethoxazole (see p.306). It is used with sulphacetamide and sulphathiazole in pessaries or a vaginal cream for the treatment of vaginitis.

For a study of the action of sulfabenzamide (an ingredient in Sultrin vaginal tablets) against *Gardnerella vaginalis*, see Sulphacetamide Sodium, p.302.

Proprietary Names and Manufacturers

The following names have been used for multi-ingredient preparations containing sulfabenzamide— Gyne-Sulf *(G & W, USA)*; Sultrin *(Cilag, Austral.*; *Ortho, Canad.*; *Ortho-Cilag, UK*; *Ortho Pharmaceutical, USA)*; Trysul *(Savage, USA)*.

4916-r

Sulfacytine *(BAN, USAN).*
CI-636; Sulfacitine *(pINN).* 1-Ethyl-N^4-sulphanilylcytosine; N^1-(1-Ethyl-1,2-dihydro-2-oxopyrimidin-4-yl)sulphanilamide.
$C_{12}H_{14}N_4O_3S$=294.3.
CAS — 17784-12-2.

Sulfacytine is a short-acting sulphonamide with actions and uses similar to those of sulphamethoxazole, p.306. It has been used only in the treatment of urinary-tract infections because of its rapid excretion by the kidneys; after a loading dose of 500 mg, sulfacytine 250 mg has been given four times daily for 10 days.

Proprietary Names and Manufacturers
Renoquid *(Glenwood, USA).*

13277-j

Sulfadicramide *(rINN).*
3-Methyl-*N*-sulphanilylcrotonamide.
$C_{11}H_{14}N_2O_3S$=254.3.
CAS — 115-68-4.

Sulfadicramide is a sulphonamide with properties similar to those of sulphamethoxazole (see p.306). It is used as a 15% ointment for topical application to the eye.

Proprietary Names and Manufacturers
Irgamid *(Zyma-Galen, Belg.; Dispersa, Denm.; Dispersa, Ger.; Zyma, Neth.; Dispersa, Switz.).*

4917-f

Sulfadoxine *(BAN, USAN, rINN).*

Ro-4-4393; Sulformethoxine; Sulforthomidine; Sulphormethoxine; Sulphorthodimethoxine. N^1-(5,6-Dimethoxypyrimidin-4-yl)sulphanilamide.
$C_{12}H_{14}N_4O_4S$=310.3.
CAS — 2447-57-6.

Pharmacopoeias. In *Br., Fr., Ind.,* and *U.S.* Also in *B.P. Vet.*

A white or creamy-white odourless or almost odourless crystalline powder. Very slightly **soluble** in water; slightly soluble in alcohol and in methyl alcohol; practically insoluble in ether. **Store** in well-closed containers and protect from light.

Adverse Effects, Treatment, and Precautions
As for sulphamethoxazole, p.306. For reference to the adverse effects, including the Stevens-Johnson syndrome, of a combination of sulfadoxine and pyrimethamine, see Pyrimethamine, p.516.

If side-effects occur, sulfadoxine has the disadvantage that several days are required for elimination from the body.

Stevens-Johnson syndrome occurred in 22 people after mass prophylaxis of 149 000 inhabitants of Beira, Mozambique with sulfadoxine to control an outbreak of cholera. Sulfadoxine was given to adults in a single 2-g dose; the dose in children was reduced according to age. The interval between administration of sulfadoxine and onset of symptoms of the reaction ranged from 3 to 46 days. Treatment of the more serious cases was mainly by supportive care and systemic corticosteroids and antibiotics. Three patients died, 7, 10, and 16 days after admission.— A. Hernborg (letter), *Lancet,* 1985, *2,* 1072.

Antimicrobial Action and Resistance
As for sulphamethoxazole, p.307.

Absorption and Fate
Sulfadoxine is readily absorbed from the gastro-intestinal tract. High concentrations in the blood are reached in about 4 hours; the half-life in the blood is about 4 to 8 days. About 90 to 95% is reported to be bound to plasma proteins.

Sulfadoxine is widely distributed to body tissues and fluids; it passes into the foetal circulation and has been detected in low concentrations in breast milk.

About 5% of sulfadoxine in the blood is present as the acetyl derivative, and 2% as the glucuronide. Sulfadoxine is very slowly excreted, only about 8% being recovered from the urine in 24 hours and about 30% in 7 days, up to 60% being excreted as the acetyl derivative and about 10% as the glucuronide.

Uses and Administration
Sulfadoxine is a long-acting sulphonamide which has been used in the treatment of various infections including leprosy. It is now rarely used alone, but has been given in an initial dose of 2 g by mouth, followed by 1 to 1.5 g weekly.

It is given with pyrimethamine in the treatment and prophylaxis of falciparum malaria resistant to other therapies. Its prophylactic use has, however, declined due to reports of the Stevens-Johnson syndrome (sometimes fatal) associated with the sulfadoxine component. In the treatment of malaria, the usual dose is 1 to 1.5 g of sulfadoxine with 50 to 75 mg of pyrimethamine; this should not be repeated for at least 7 days. For prophylaxis a dose of 500 mg of sulfadoxine with 25 mg of pyrimethamine should be repeated every 7 days. For further information on the uses and administration of a combination of sulfadoxine and pyrimethamine, see Pyrimethamine, p.517.

A mixture of 5 parts of sulfadoxine with 1 part trimethoprim is used in veterinary medicine.

MALARIA. For reference to recommendations for the use of a combination of sulfadoxine and pyrimethamine in the treatment and prophylaxis of malaria, see p.505.

RESPIRATORY-TRACT INFECTIONS. For reference to reports of the use of a combination of sulfadoxine and pyrimethamine for the prophylaxis of *Pneumocystis carinii* pneumonia, see Pyrimethamine, p.517.

Proprietary Preparations
For description of a combination preparation of sulfadoxine and pyrimethamine (Fansidar), see Pyrimethamine, p.518.

Proprietary Names and Manufacturers
Fanaril; Fanasil *(Roche, Ital.; Roche, UK);* Fanasulf; Fanzil; Fontasul.

The following names have been used for multi-ingredient preparations containing sulfadoxine— Fansidar *(Roche, Austral.; Roche, Fr.; Roche, UK; Roche, USA);* Fansimef *(Roche, Switz.).*

4918-d

Sulfamerazine *(BAN, USAN, rINN).*
Solfamerazina; Sulfamerazinum; Sulfamethyldiazine; Sulfamethylpyrimidine; Sulphamerazine. N^1-(4-Methylpyrimidin-2-yl)sulphanilamide.
$C_{11}H_{12}N_4O_2S$=264.3.
CAS — 127-79-7.

Pharmacopoeias. In *Arg., Aust., Braz., Eur., Fr., Ger., Int., It., Jug., Neth., Nord., Span., Swiss,* and *U.S.* Also in *B.P. Vet.*

A white or faintly pinkish- or yellowish-white, odourless or almost odourless, crystalline powder; it slowly darkens on exposure to light.

Soluble 1 in 6250 of water at 20°, 1 in 3300 of water at 37°; sparingly soluble in acetone; slightly soluble in alcohol; very slightly soluble in chloroform and in ether; dissolves in dilute mineral acids and in solutions of alkali hydroxides. **Store** in well-closed containers. Protect from light.

4919-n

Sulfamerazine Sodium *(BANM, rINN).*
Soluble Sulphamerazine; Sulfamerazinum Natricum; Sulphamerazine Sodium.
$C_{11}H_{11}N_4NaO_2S$=286.3.
CAS — 127-58-2.

Pharmacopoeias. In *Aust., Braz.* and *Int.*

1.08 g of monograph substance is approximately equivalent to 1 g of sulfamerazine.

Sulfamerazine is a short-acting sulphonamide with actions and uses similar to those of sulphamethoxazole, p.306. It is usually administered in conjunction with other sulphonamides.

Sulfamerazine is used in veterinary medicine.

For a study of the renal elimination of sulfamerazine, see Sulphadimidine Sodium, p.304.

For reference to the use of sulfamerazine in the determination of acetylator status, see Sulphadimidine Sodium, p.304.

Preparations
Sulfamerazine Tablets *(U.S.P.)*

Proprietary Names and Manufacturers of Sulfamerazine
The following names have been used for multi-ingredient preparations containing sulfamerazine— Dosulfin *(Geigy, Ger.; Geigy, UK);* Dosulfine *(Gomenol, Fr.);* Neotrizine *(Lilly, USA);* Sulphatriad *(May & Baker, UK);* Terfonyl *(Squibb, USA);* Trisulfaminic *(Ancalab, Canad.).*

13278-z

Sulfametomidine *(rINN).*
N^1-(6-Methoxy-2-methylpyrimidin-4-yl)sulphanilamide.
$C_{12}H_{14}N_4O_3S$=294.3.
CAS — 3772-76-7.

Sulfametomidine is a sulphonamide with actions and uses similar to those of sulphamethoxazole (see p.306).

For a study of the renal elimination of sulfametomidine, see Sulphasomidine, p.309.

Proprietary Names and Manufacturers
Télémid *(Nativelle, Fr.).*

4920-k

Sulfametopyrazine *(BAN).*

AS-18908; NSC-110433; Solfametopirazina; Solfametossipirazina; Sulfalene *(USAN, pINN);* Sulfamethoxypyrazine; Sulfapirazinmetossina; Sulfapyrazin Methoxyne; Sulphalene. N^1-(3-Methoxypyrazin-2-yl)sulphanilamide.
$C_{11}H_{12}N_4O_3S$=280.3.
CAS — 152-47-6.

Pharmacopoeias. In *Ind.* and *It.*

Adverse Effects, Treatment, and Precautions
As for Sulphamethoxazole, p.306.

If side-effects occur, sulfametopyrazine has the disadvantage that several days are required for its elimination from the body.

ADMINISTRATION IN RENAL FAILURE. For reference to the precautions to be observed on administration of a combination of sulfametopyrazine and trimethoprim, see Absorption and Fate, below.

Antimicrobial Action and Resistance
As for Sulphamethoxazole, p.307.

Absorption and Fate
Sulfametopyrazine is readily absorbed from the gastro-intestinal tract; 60 to 80% is bound to plasma proteins. About 5 to 10% of sulfametopyrazine in the blood is in the form of the acetyl derivative. It is slowly excreted, about 70% as the acetyl derivative. The biological half-life has been reported to be about 65 hours.

Sulfametopyrazine was bound to plasma protein to the extent of 72 to 81%. Concentrations of sulfametopyrazine in cerebrospinal fluid in 2 patients were about one-third of concentrations in the blood. An initial dose of 1.25 g, followed by daily doses of 250 mg, could be expected to produce a blood concentration of 70 μg per mL.— R. L. Herting *et al., Antimicrob. Ag. Chemother.,* 1964, 554.

Sulfametopyrazine and trimethoprim given together in doses of 600 and 750 mg respectively for the first day then 200 and 250 mg daily for 9 days produced blood concentrations in the ratio of 10 or 20 to 1 after 10 days. Antibacterial concentrations were maintained throughout treatment.— V. de Pascale *et al., Farmaco, Edn prat.,* 1977, *32,* 228.

The pharmacokinetics of sulfametopyrazine and trimethoprim in healthy subjects following administration of a preparation containing sulfametopyrazine and trimethoprim in the ratio 4:5 (Kelfiprim).— D. S. Reeves *et al., J. antimicrob. Chemother.*, 1980, *6*, 647.

ADMINISTRATION IN RENAL FAILURE. A study of the pharmacokinetics of sulfametopyrazine and trimethoprim in patients with renal insufficiency following administration of a single dose by mouth of trimethoprim 250 mg in association with sulfametopyrazine 200 mg. Results suggested that dosage modification was not required in patients with mild renal impairment (creatinine clearance greater than 40 mL per minute).— A. Cantaluppi *et al., Eur. J. clin. Pharmac.*, 1984, *27*, 345.

DIFFUSION INTO BODY TISSUES AND FLUIDS. Concentrations of sulfametopyrazine and trimethoprim in female reproductive tissues after administration of a combination of the 2 drugs (Kelfiprim).— P. C. Preza *et al., J. int. med. Res.*, 1986, *14*, 101.

Uses and Administration

Sulfametopyrazine is a long-acting sulphonamide with actions and uses similar to those of sulphamethoxazole, p.306. It is usually given by mouth in a single dose of 2 g once a week.

Sulfametopyrazine is also used with trimethoprim, in the ratio 4 parts sulfametopyrazine to 5 parts trimethoprim, similarly to co-trimoxazole (p.210).

A study of the clinical efficacy and tolerance of a combination of sulfametopyrazine and trimethoprim (Kelfiprim) in 5885 patients.— F. Celotti *et al., J. int. med. Res.*, 1986, *14*, 236.

ADMINISTRATION IN RENAL FAILURE. For reference to the administration of a combination of sulfametopyrazine and trimethoprim in patients with renal impairment, see Absorption and Fate, above.

MALARIA. Report of a Tanzanian study involving 336 asymptomatic carriers of *Plasmodium falciparum* to ascertain resistance to chloroquine and to a combination of sulfametopyrazine and pyrimethamine.— C. M. Kihamia *et al., Curr. ther. Res.*, 1986, *40*, 141.

URINARY-TRACT INFECTIONS. References to the use of a combination of sulfametopyrazine and trimethoprim (Kelfiprim) in urinary-tract infections: H. Bröll *et al., Curr. med. Res. Opinion*, 1983, *8*, 338 (comparison with ampicillin); F. Calais da Silva *et al., Curr. ther. Res.*, 1984, *36*, 646 (comparison with co-trimoxazole).

Proprietary Preparations

Kelfizine W *(Farmitalia Carlo Erba, UK). Tablets*, dispersible, sulfametopyrazine 2 g.

Proprietary Names and Manufacturers

Dalysep *(Syntex, UK)*; Kelfizina *(Arg.; Belg.; Farmitalia, Ital.; Neth.)*; Kelfizine W *(Farmitalia Carlo Erba, UK)*; Longum *(Arg.; Belg.; Farmitalia, Ger.; Farmitalia, Spain; Neth.)*; Policydal *(Jpn)*.

The following names have been used for multi-ingredient preparations containing sulfametopyrazine— Kelfiprim; Kelfiprin; Trimed *(Armour, Ital.)*.

4921-a

Sulfametrole *(BAN, rINN).*

N^1-(4-Methoxy-1,2,5-thiadiazol-3-yl)sulphanilamide.
$C_9H_{10}N_4O_3S_2$=286.3.

CAS — 32909-92-5.

Sulfametrole is a sulphonamide with actions and uses similar to sulphamethoxazole, p.306. It is used with trimethoprim in the ratio of 5 parts sulfametrole to 1 part trimethoprim, similarly to co-trimoxazole (p.210).

A combination of sulfametrole 20 parts with trimethoprim 1 part *in vitro* had a similar antibacterial activity to co-trimoxazole.— G. Nabert-Bock and H. Grims, *Arzneimittel-Forsch.*, 1977, *27*, 1109. Of 100 coliforms tested *in vitro*, 63% were sensitive to a combination of sulfametrole and trimethoprim (Lidaprim), and 52% were sensitive to co-trimoxazole.— E. F. Abdel-Messih *et al., J. int. med. Res.*, 1984, *12*, 219.

A study of the pharmacokinetics of sulfametrole, alone or in combination with trimethoprim, in 8 healthy subjects. Sulfametrole had a half-life of 10 hours, which is of the same order of magnitude as trimethoprim. The N_4-acetyl metabolite accounts for about 40% of the total plasma-sulphonamide concentration. The renal clearance of sulfametrole, but not of its metabolite increased with increasing urinary pH.— Y. A. Hekster *et al., J. antimicrob. Chemother.*, 1981, *8*, 133.

Report of a double-blind study of 78 men with chancroid comparing a single dose of sulfametrole 3200 mg in combination with trimethoprim 640 mg, with 5-day regimens of either sulfametrole 800 mg with trimethoprim 160 mg, or trimethoprim 200 mg each given twice daily. Rates of ulcer and bubo resolution, mean healing times, microbiological response, the number of treatment failures, and the number of recurrent ulcers were similar in all 3 treatment groups.— F. A. Plummer *et al., New Engl. J. Med.*, 1983, *309*, 67. Comment that from pharmacokinetic and solubility considerations the risk of crystalluria after a large single dose of sulfametrole with trimethoprim may be reduced by encouraging adequate fluid intake and by alkalinisation of the urine.— D. R. Webster and D. M. Paton (letter), *ibid.*, 1652. Reply that until the theoretical risk of crystalluria has been quantified by clinical studies, advising patients to drink additional fluids would seem sufficient.— F. A. Plummer *et al.* (letter), *ibid.*

Proprietary Names and Manufacturers

The following names have been used for multi-ingredient preparations containing sulfametrole— Lidaprim *(Chemie-Linz, Aust.)*; Lidatrim *(Warrick, Neth.)*; Maderan *(Ciba, Switz.)*; Pharbil *(Belg.; Hormonchemie, Ger.)*; Trimetrol *(Essex, Belg.)*.

4922-t

Sulfamonomethoxine *(USAN, rINN).*

DJ-1550; DS-36; ICI-32525; Ro-4-3476. N^1-(6-Methoxypyrimidin-4-yl)sulphanilamide monohydrate.
$C_{11}H_{12}N_4O_3S,H_2O$=298.3.

CAS — 1220-83-3 (anhydrous).

Pharmacopoeias. In *Chin.* and *Jpn.*

Sulfamonomethoxine is a sulphonamide with actions and uses similar to those of sulphamethoxazole, p.306.

The biological half-life of sulfamonomethoxine was 30 hours.— W. A. Ritschel, *Drug Intell. & clin. Pharm.*, 1970, *4*, 332.

Proprietary Names and Manufacturers

Daimeton *(Daiichi, Jpn)*.

13280-s

Sulfaperin *(rINN).*

BT-325. N^1-(5-Methylpyrimidin-2-yl)sulphanilamide.
$C_{11}H_{12}N_4O_2S$=264.3.

CAS — 599-88-2.

Sulfaperin is a sulphonamide with actions and uses similar to those of sulphamethoxazole (see p.306). It has been given by mouth or rectally.

Proprietary Names and Manufacturers

Grosulan *(Grossmann, Switz.)*; Ipersulfidin *(Francia Farm., Ital.)*; Palidin *(Ital.)*; Pallidin *(E. Merck, Ger.)*; Retardon *(Chassot, Switz.)*; Retardsulf *(Ital.)*; Rexulfa *(Ital.)*; Sintosulfa *(Ital.)*; Sulfalast *(Ital.)*; Sulfapenta *(Ital.)*; Sulfatreis *(Ital.)*; Sulfixone *(Ital.)*; Sulfopiran *(Ital.)*; Sulfopirimidina *(Ital.)*; Ultrasulfon *(Streuli, Switz.)*.

4923-x

Sulfapyrazole *(BAN, rINN).*

Ba-18605; Sulfamethylphenazole; Sulfazamet *(USAN)*. N^1-(3-Methyl-1-phenylpyrazol-5-yl)sulphanilamide.
$C_{16}H_{16}N_4O_2S$=328.4.

CAS — 852-19-7.

Pharmacopoeias. In *B.P. Vet.*

A white or creamy-white, odourless or almost odourless, crystalline powder. Practically **insoluble** in water; soluble in alcohol; slightly soluble in chloroform; freely soluble in methyl alcohol. **Protect** from light.

Sulfapyrazole is a sulphonamide with properties similar to those of sulphamethoxazole, p.306. It is used in veterinary medicine.

Proprietary Veterinary Names and Manufacturers

Vesulong *(Ciba-Geigy Agrochemicals, UK)*.

4924-r

Sulfaquinoxaline *(BAN, rINN).*

Sulfabenzpyrazine; Sulphaquinoxalina; Sulphaquinoxaline. N^1-(Quinoxalin-2-yl)sulphanilamide.
$C_{14}H_{12}N_4O_2S$=300.3.

CAS — 59-40-5; 967-80-6 (sodium).

Pharmacopoeias. In *Fr.* and *Nord.* Also in *B.P. Vet. Fr.* also includes Sulfaquinoxaline Sodium, $C_{14}H_{11}N_4NaO_2S$ = 322.3.

A yellow, odourless powder. Practically **insoluble** in water; very slightly soluble in alcohol; practically insoluble in ether; freely soluble in aqueous solutions of alkalis. **Store** in well-closed containers. Protect from light.

Sulfaquinoxaline is a sulphonamide with properties similar to those of sulphamethoxazole, p.306, used in the treatment of coccidiosis in poultry. It has been used as an additive to veterinary feedstuffs.

For a study of the *in-vitro* activity of sulfaquinoxaline against *Leishmania major*, see Sulphamoxole, p.309.

4927-n

Sulphacetamide *(BAN).*

Acetosulfaminum; Sulfacetamide *(USAN, rINN)*. *N*-Sulphanilylacetamide.
$C_8H_{10}N_2O_3S$=214.2.

CAS — 144-80-9.

Pharmacopoeias. In *Arg., Aust., Neth., Pol.,* and *U.S.*

A white, odourless, crystalline powder.

Slightly **soluble** in water and in ether; soluble in alcohol; very slightly soluble in chloroform; freely soluble in dilute mineral acids and solutions of alkali hydroxides. Solutions in water are acid to litmus and sensitive to light; they are unstable when acidic or strongly alkaline. **Store** in well-closed containers. Protect from light.

4928-h

Sulphacetamide Sodium *(BANM).*

Soluble Sulphacetamide; Sulfacetamide Sodium *(USAN, rINNM)*; Sulfacetamidum Natricum; Sulfacylum; Sulphacetamidum Sodium.
$C_8H_9N_2NaO_3S,H_2O$=254.2.

CAS — 127-56-0 (anhydrous); 6209-17-2 (monohydrate).

Pharmacopoeias. In *Arg., Belg., Br., Braz., Chin., Cz., Egypt., Eur., Fr., Ger., Hung., Ind., Int., It., Jug., Neth., Pol., Rus., Swiss, Turk.,* and *U.S.*

White or yellowish-white, odourless crystals or crystalline powder. It slowly darkens on exposure to light. 1.19 g of monograph substance is approximately equivalent to 1 g of sulphacetamide.

B.P. **solubilities** are: soluble 1 in 1.5 of water; slightly soluble in alcohol; practically insoluble in chloroform and ether. *U.S.P.* solubilities are: soluble 1 in 2.5 of water; sparingly soluble in alcohol; practically insoluble in chloroform and ether. A 5% solution in water has a pH of 8.0 to 9.5. When solutions are sterilised by heat, hydrolysis occurs forming sulphanilamide which may be deposited as crystals, especially from concentrated solutions and under cold storage conditions. **Store** in airtight containers. Protect from light.

Solutions of sulphacetamide sodium were incompatible with benzalkonium chloride. Solutions of sulphacetamide sodium 10 or 30% containing sodium metabisulphite 0.1% and infected with *Ps. aeruginosa* were not resterilised within 1 hour in the presence of phenylmercuric nitrate 0.002%, thiomersal 0.01%, chlorhexidine acetate 0.01%, or chlorocresol 0.05%. Solutions were resterilised within 1 hour in the presence of phenylmercuric nitrate 0.002% plus disodium edetate 0.05% and phenethyl alcohol 0.4%. The effect of thiomersal was less improved. Solutions were sterilised within 1 hour in the presence of chlorhexidine acetate 0.01% or chlorocresol 0.05% plus in each case either disodium edetate 0.05% or phenethyl alcohol 0.4% or both disodium edetate and phenethyl alcohol. Chlorocresol was considered the preservative of choice because it was least affected by the presence or absence of sodium metabisulphite. Resterilisation times were prolonged after storage for 7 days in the presence of phenylmercuric nitrate, thiomersal, or chlorhexidine, probably due to the formation of a complex between the preservative and sodium metabisulphite. Chlorocresol did not appear to be so affected. There was no evidence of degradation of sulphacetamide to sulphanilamide in solutions stored in the dark for 7 days.— R. M. E. Richards and R. J. McBride, *Pharm. J.*, 1973, *1*, 118.

STABILITY OF SOLUTIONS. The development of a yellowish-brown to deep reddish-brown coloration which occurred in sulphacetamide sodium solutions on keeping was thought to be due to oxidation, and was preceded by the formation of sulphanilamide by hydrolysis. Oxidation products included azobenzene-4,4′-disulphonamide and/or azoxybenzene-4,4′-disulphonamide.— P. A. Clarke, *Pharm. J.*, 1965, *1*, 375.

The rate of hydrolysis of sulphacetamide was independent of pH in the range 7.15 to 8.9, and a more acid pH caused increased discoloration. The hydrolysis reaction-rate was first order and a 0.2M to 1.0M solution had a half-life of 22 hours. Heating in an autoclave at 120° for 20 minutes or at 115° for 30 minutes resulted in a 1% loss of potency. Heating with a bactericide at 98° to 100° for 30 minutes gave a loss of less than 0.5%. Autoclaving was the method of choice.— R. A. Anderson, *Australas. J. Pharm.*, 1966, *47*, S26.

STORAGE OF SOLUTIONS. Avoid contact with metals, particularly copper, which causes darkening of the solutions.— A. J. Cobcroft, *Australas. J. Pharm.*, 1954, *35*, 361.

Low-density polyethylene containers were unsuitable for sulphacetamide eye-drops, which were discoloured within 1 week at 32°.— B. T. O'Boyle (letter), *Pharm. J.*, 1973, *1*, 201.

Adverse Effects, Treatment, and Precautions

As for Sulphamethoxazole, p.306.

Local application of sulphacetamide sodium to the eye may cause burning or stinging but this is rarely severe enough to necessitate discontinuance of treatment. Sulphacetamide sodium ointment should not be applied to penetrating wounds of the cornea.

A 73-year-old man who had been taking sulphamethoxazole developed the Stevens-Johnson syndrome shortly after starting treatment with sulphacetamide sodium 30% eye-drops.— Z. Rubin (letter), *Archs Derm.*, 1977, *113*, 235.

A report of fatal systemic lupus erythematosus associated with the use of an ophthalmic preparation containing sulphacetamide sodium.— J. D. Adams, *Aust. J. Derm.*, 1978, *19*, 31.

For a study suggesting that sulphacetamide and gentamicin should not be used together in the treatment of eye infections, see Gentamicin Sulphate, p.238.

Antimicrobial Action and Resistance

As for Sulphamethoxazole, p.307.

Gardnerella vaginalis, often concomitant with *Bacteroides* spp., was isolated from women with nonspecific vaginitis. These organisms were inhibited by very high concentrations of the sulphonamides present in Sultrin vaginal tablets (sulphacetamide, sulfabenzamide, and sulphathiazole); such concentrations could be achieved locally after the use of this preparation.— B. M. Jones *et al.*, *Antimicrob. Ag. Chemother.*, 1982, *21*, 870.

Absorption and Fate

Sulphacetamide is readily absorbed from the gastro-intestinal tract. It is rapidly excreted in the urine, largely unchanged.

When sulphacetamide sodium is applied to the eye high concentrations are achieved in ocular tissues and fluids; sulphonamide may be absorbed into the blood when the conjunctiva is inflamed.

The biological half-life of sulphacetamide is variously reported as 7 to 12.8 hours.— W. A. Ritschel, *Drug Intell. & clin. Pharm.*, 1970, *4*, 332.

Uses and Administration

Sulphacetamide is a short-acting sulphonamide which was formerly used in the treatment of bacterial infections of the urinary tract.

Sulphacetamide is used with sulfabenzamide and sulphathiazole in preparations for vaginal use.

Sulphacetamide sodium is used mainly by local application in infections or injuries of the eyes although its efficacy appears doubtful. Eye-drops containing sulphacetamide sodium 10% to 30% are instilled every 2 to 6 hours; eye-ointments containing 2.5, 6, or 10% are applied 2 to 4 times daily or at night. In the *UK* the use of sulphacetamide and its salts in cosmetics is prohibited.

Preparations

Sulfacetamide Sodium Ophthalmic Ointment *(U.S.P.)*

Sulfacetamide Sodium Ophthalmic Solution *(U.S.P.)*

Sulphacetamide Eye Drops *(A.P.F.)*. Gutt. Sulphacetam. Contain sulphacetamide sodium 10%. Sterilise by autoclaving.

Sulphacetamide Eye Drops Strong *(A.P.F.)*. Gutt. Sulphacetam. Fort. Contain sulphacetamide sodium 30%.

Sulphacetamide Eye Drops *(B.P.)*. Sulphacetamide Sodium Eye Drops; SULF. Contain sulphacetamide sodium. pH 6.6 to 8.6.

The *B.P.C. 1973* specified that when the strength is not specified or when Weak Sulphacetamide Eye-drops are ordered or prescribed, a solution containing 10% of sulphacetamide sodium is supplied. When Strong Sulphacetamide Eye-drops are ordered or prescribed, a solution containing 30% of sulphacetamide sodium is supplied. Store at a temperature not exceeding 25°.

Sulphacetamide Eye Ointment *(B.P.)*. Sulphacetamide Sodium Eye Ointment. Contains sulphacetamide sodium.

Sulfacetamide Sodium and Prednisolone Acetate Ophthalmic Ointment *(U.S.P.)*

Proprietary Preparations

Albucid *(Nicholas, UK)*. *Eye-drops*, sulphacetamide sodium 10, 20, and 30%.

Eye ointment, sulphacetamide sodium 2.5, 6, and 10%.

Cortucid *(Nicholas, UK)*. *Eye drop cream*, sulphacetamide sodium 10%, hydrocortisone acetate 0.5%.

Minims Sulphacetamide Sodium *(Smith & Nephew Pharmaceuticals, UK)*. *Eye-drops*, sulphacetamide sodium 10%, in single-use disposable applicators.

Ocusol *(Boots, UK)*. *Eye-drops*, sulphacetamide sodium 5%, zinc sulphate 0.1%.

Sultrin *(Ortho-Cilag, UK)*. *Pessaries*, sulphacetamide 143.75 mg, sulfabenzamide 184.0 mg, sulphathiazole 172.5 mg.

Vaginal cream (Triple Sulfa), sulphacetamide 2.86%, sulfabenzamide 3.7%, sulphathiazole 3.42%.

Proprietary Names and Manufacturers of Sulphacetamide or Sulphacetamide Sodium

Acetopt *(Sigma, Austral.)*; Ak-Sulf *(Akorn, Canad.; Akorn, USA)*; Albucid *(Arg.; Austral.; Scherag, S.Afr.; Nicholas, UK)*; Antebor *(Belg.; Laboratoires Biologiques de l'Île-de-France, Fr.; Switz.)*; Blef *(Arg.)*; Bleph-10 *(Allergan, Austral.; Allergan, Canad.; S.Afr.; Allergan, UK; Allergan, USA)*; Buco-Albucid *(Spain)*; Cetamide *(Alcon, Canad.; Alcon Laboratories, USA)*; Covosulf *(Covan, S.Afr.)*; Drugtets *(Pharmadrug, Ger.)*; Isopto Cetamida *(Arg.)*; Isopto Cetamide *(Alcon, Austral.; Alcon, Canad.; Neth.; Alcon, UK; Alcon Laboratories, USA)*; Minims Sulfacetamid *(Smith & Nephew, Denm.)*; Minims Sulphacetamide Sodium *(Smith & Nephew, Austral.; Smith & Nephew, S.Afr.; Smith & Nephew Pharmaceuticals, UK)*; Ocu-Sul *(Ocumed, USA)*; Optamide *(McGloin, Austral.)*; Optosulfex *(Canad.)*; Opulets Sulphacetamide *(Pharmax, UK)*; Prontamid *(SIT, Ital.)*; Sebizon *(Schering, USA)*; Sodium Sulamyd *(Schering, Canad.; Schering, USA)*; Spersacet *(Dispersa, Switz.)*; Sulf-10 *(Canad.; Coopervision, USA)*; Sulf-30 *(Canad.)*; Sulfableph *(Allergan, Ger.)*; Sulfair *(Pharmafair, USA)*; Sulfex *(Charton, Canad.)*; Sulphacalyre *(Wallace Mfg Chem., UK)*; Sulten-10 *(Bausch & Lomb, USA)*; Vasosulf *(S.Afr.; Knox, UK: CooperVision, UK)*.

The following names have been used for multi-ingredient preparations containing sulphacetamide or sulphacetamide sodium— Ak-Cide *(Akorn, Canad.; Akorn, USA)*; Blephamide *(Allergan, Austral.; Allergan, Canad.; Allergan, USA)*; Celestone-S *(Schering, Canad.)*; Cetapred *(Alcon, Canad.; Alcon Laboratories, USA)*; Cortucid *(Nicholas, UK)*; Gyne-Sulf *(G & W, USA)*; Isopto Cetapred *(Alcon, Canad.; Alcon Laboratories, USA)*; Metimyd *(Schering, Canad.; Schering, USA)*; Ocu-Lone-C *(Ocumed, USA)*; Ocusol *(Boots, UK)*; Optimyd *(Schering, USA)*; Predsulfair *(Pharmafair, USA)*; Sulfacet-R *(Rorer, Canad.; Dermik, USA)*; Sulfacort *(Rugby, USA)*; Sulfapred *(Wallace Mfg Chem., UK)*; Sulphrin *(Bausch & Lomb, USA)*; Sulpred *(Pharmafair, USA)*; Sultrin *(Cilag, Austral.; Ortho, Canad.; Ortho-Cilag, UK; Ortho Pharmaceutical, USA)*; Trysul *(Savage, USA)*; Vasocidin *(Coopervision, Canad.; Coopervision, USA)*; Vasosulf *(Coopervision, Canad.; Coopervision, USA)*.

4930-t

Sulphadiazine *(BAN)*.

Solfadiazina; Solfapirimidina; Sulfadiazine *(USAN, rINN)*; Sulfadiazinum. N^1-(Pyrimidin-2-yl)sulphanilamide.

$C_{10}H_{10}N_4O_2S$=250.3.

CAS — 68-35-9.

Pharmacopoeias. In *Arg., Aust., Belg., Br., Chin., Egypt., Eur., Fr., Ger., Ind., Int., It., Jug., Mex., Neth., Nord., Port., Roum., Span., Swiss, Turk.*, and *U.S.* Also in *B.P. Vet.*

White, yellowish-white, or pinkish-white, odourless or almost odourless, crystals or powder, slowly darkening on exposure to light.

Soluble 1 in 13 000 of water; slightly to sparingly soluble in acetone; very slightly to sparingly soluble in alcohol; practically insoluble in chloroform; freely soluble in dilute mineral acids and in solutions of alkali hydroxides. **Store** in well-closed containers. Protect from light.

4931-x

Sulphadiazine Sodium *(BANM)*.

Sodium Sulfadiazine; Soluble Sulphadiazine; Sulfadiazine Sodium *(USAN, rINN)*; Sulfadiazinum Natricum.

$C_{10}H_9N_4NaO_2S$=272.3.

CAS — 547-32-0.

Pharmacopoeias. In *Aust., Belg., Egypt., Int., Jug., Mex., Turk.*, and *U.S.*

A white powder. On prolonged exposure to humid air it absorbs carbon dioxide with the liberation of sulphadiazine and becomes incompletely soluble in water. 1.09 g of monograph substance is approximately equivalent to 1 g of sulphadiazine.

Soluble 1 in 2 of water; slightly soluble in alcohol. The *B.P.* injection has a pH of 10 to 11, and the *U.S.P.* injection a pH of 8.5 to 10.5. The *B.P.* injection is **sterilised** by heating in an autoclave. **Store** in airtight containers. Protect from light.

Incompatibility may occur in solutions for intravenous infusion if sulphadiazine sodium is mixed with acidic drugs, or with fructose, iron salts, or salts of heavy metals.

Adverse Effects, Treatment, and Precautions

As for Sulphamethoxazole, p.306.

Because of the low solubilities of sulphadiazine and its acetyl derivative in urine, crystalluria is more likely after administration of sulphadiazine than after sulphamethoxazole.

Renal complications occur more frequently with intravenous than with oral administration. Sulphadiazine sodium solution is strongly alkaline; it should therefore be administered intravenously in a strength not exceeding 5% to reduce the risk of thrombosis of the vein; extravasation may cause sloughing and necrosis. For the same reason, intramuscular injections are painful and sulphadiazine sodium should not be given by intrathecal or subcutaneous injection.

ALLERGY. A report of successful desensitisation to sulphadiazine in 3 patients with the acquired immunodeficiency syndrome and cerebral toxoplasmosis who had had severe sulphonamide reactions.— E. T. Bell *et al.* (letter), *Lancet*, 1985, *1*, 163.

EFFECTS ON THE EYE. Numerous white stone-like concretions of sulphadiazine occurred in the conjunctiva of a woman who had used sulphadiazine eye-drops for about one year.— E. A. Boettner *et al.*, *Archs Ophthal., N.Y.*, 1974, *92*, 446.

INTERACTIONS. For the effect of sulphadiazine in inhibiting the metabolism of phenytoin, see Phenytoin Sodium, p.409.

OVERDOSAGE. A 3-year-old girl weighing 13 kg developed crystalluria and hypoglycaemia after excessive doses of sulphadiazine—300 to 450 mg per kg body-weight per 24 hours.— A. W. Craft *et al.*, *Postgrad. med. J.*, 1977, *53*, 103.

PREGNANCY AND THE NEONATE. For reference to the ability of sulphonamides, including sulphadiazine to displace bilirubin and hence the risk of causing kernicterus in neonates, see sulphamethoxazole, p.307.

Antimicrobial Action and Resistance

As for Sulphamethoxazole, p.307.

Absorption and Fate

Sulphadiazine is readily absorbed from the gastro-intestinal tract, peak blood concentrations being reached 3 to 6 hours after a single dose; 20 to 55% has been reported to be bound to plasma proteins. It penetrates into the cerebrospinal fluid to produce therapeutic concentrations, which may be more than half of those in the blood, within 4 hours of administration by mouth. Up to 40% of sulphadiazine in the blood is present as the acetyl derivative.

About 50% of a single dose of sulphadiazine given by mouth is excreted in the urine in 24 hours; 15 to 40% is excreted as the acetyl derivative.

The biological half-life of sulphadiazine is variously reported as 8 to 16.8 hours.— W. A. Ritschel, *Drug Intell. & clin. Pharm.*, 1970, *4*, 332. The half-life of sulphadiazine ranges from 7 to 12 hours and that of its metabolite from 8 to 18 hours.— T. B. Vree *et al.*, *Clin. Pharmacokinet.*, 1980, *5*, 274.

DRUG EXCRETION. The urinary excretion of sulphadiazine and the acetyl derivative is dependent on pH. About 30% is excreted unchanged in both fast and slow acetylators when the urine is acidic whereas about 75% is excreted unchanged by slow acetylators when the urine is alkaline.— T. B. Vree *et al.*, *Clin. Pharmacokinet.*, 1980, *5*, 274.

For a study of the renal elimination of sulphadiazine, see Sulphadimidine Sodium, p.304.

Uses and Administration

Sulphadiazine is a short-acting sulphonamide with similar uses to sulphamethoxazole, p.307. In the treatment of susceptible infections it may be given by mouth in an initial dose of 2 to 4 g followed by up to 4 g daily in divided doses; a suggested dose in children is 75 mg per kg body-weight initially then 150 mg per kg daily in divided doses to a maximum of 6 g daily. A concentration in the blood of 100 to 150 µg per mL is desirable. Nocardiosis has been treated successfully with sulphadiazine. In toxoplasmosis, sulphadiazine is given with pyrimethamine (p.517).

In severe meningococcal meningitis sulphadiazine is given intravenously although meningococci resistant to sulphonamides are common. Sulphadiazine sodium in an initial dose of 2 to 3 g followed by 1 g four times daily is given intravenously for 2 days; sulphadiazine is then given by mouth; children may be given the equivalent of 50 mg per kg body-weight initially and then 100 mg per kg daily in 4 divided doses. In cases where susceptibility to sulphonamides has been demonstrated sulphadiazine may be given for 2 days by mouth in the following doses as prophylaxis against meningococcal disease in contacts: for adults, 1 g twice daily; for children aged 1 to 12 years, 500 mg twice daily, and for infants aged 2 months to 1 year, 500 mg once daily.

Intravenous doses of sulphadiazine sodium are given by infusion or by slow intravenous injection of a solution containing up to 5%. It may be diluted with sodium chloride 0.9% injection. Sulphadiazine sodium has been given by deep intramuscular injection but great care must be exercised to prevent damage to subcutaneous tissues and the intravenous route is preferred. It must not be given intrathecally or subcutaneously. Oral administration should begin as soon as possible.

For the use of sulphadiazine with trimethoprim, see Co-trimazine, p.205. Sulphadiazine has also been given in association with other sulphonamides, particularly sulfamerazine and sulphadimidine.

For reference to the use of sulphadiazine in the determination of acetylator status, see Sulphadimidine Sodium, p.304.

MALARIA. Quinine sulphate with pyrimethamine, both for 3 days, and sulphadiazine 500 mg four times daily for 5 days is the treatment of choice in uncomplicated attacks of malaria due to chloroquine-resistant strains of *Plasmodium falciparum*. Pyrimethamine and sulphadiazine are considered to lower the rate of recurrence.— *Med. Lett.*, 1988, *30*, 15.

MENINGITIS. Although sulphonamides such as sulphadiazine and sulphadimidine penetrate the CSF well even in the absence of inflammation, these drugs are less widely used in the treatment of meningitis than in the past due to toxicity and drug resistance, particularly among meningococci (M. Whitby and R. Finch, *Drugs*, 1986, *31*, 266). Sulphonamides should not be used for initial treatment of meningococcal meningitis although oral sulphadiazine, sulphadimidine, or sulphafurazole may be substituted for parenteral penicillin once susceptibility to sulphonamides has been established (H.P. Lambert, *Br. J. Hosp. Med.*, 1983, *29*, 128).

Prophylaxis. Rifampicin has replaced sulphonamides as treatment of choice for chemoprophylaxis in contacts of patients with meningococcal meningitis (see p.576) due to an increased incidence of *Neisseria meningitidis* resistant to sulphonamides. Sulphadiazine or sulphadimidine may be given where sensitivity has been demonstrated (C.V. Broome, *J. antimicrob. Chemother.*, 1986, *18*, *Suppl.* A, 25; H. Smith, *Archs Dis. Childh.*, 1986, *61*, 4). Smith suggested a dosage regimen of 0.5 to 1 g every 8 hours for 3 days for sulphadiazine or sulphadimidine (but see under Uses and Administration, above).

RHEUMATIC FEVER PROPHYLAXIS. Sulphadiazine 1 g once daily may be given for the continuous prophylaxis of rheumatic fever in patients at low risk of recurrences; those weighing less than 27 kg are given 500 mg daily. Sulphonamides should not be used to treat streptococcal infections since they will not eradicate the streptococcus.—Report of the Committee on Rheumatic Fever and Infective Endocarditis of the American Heart Association, S. T. Shulman *et al.*, *Circulation*, 1984, *70*, 1118A.

TOXOPLASMOSIS. For the use of sulphadiazine with pyrimethamine in the treatment of toxoplasmosis, see Pyrimethamine, p.517.

URINARY-TRACT INFECTIONS. Findings from pharmacokinetic and clinical studies of sulphadiazine that a dose of 250 mg or 500 mg twice daily for adults or 4 mg per kg body-weight twice daily for children is adequate in the treatment of acute urinary-tract infections.— J. Seppänen, *Ann. clin. Res.*, 1980, *12*, *Suppl.* 25, 1–51.

Preparations

Sulfadiazine Sodium Injection *(U.S.P.)*. A sterile solution of sulphadiazine sodium in Water for Injections.

Sulfadiazine Tablets *(U.S.P.)*

Sulphadiazine Injection *(B.P.)*. A sterile solution of sulphadiazine sodium in Water for Injections free from dissolved air.

Trisulfapyrimidines Oral Suspension *(U.S.P.)*. A suspension containing equal parts of sulphadiazine, sulphadimidine, and sulfamerazine. Store in airtight containers at a temperature above freezing.

Trisulfapyrimidines Tablets *(U.S.P.)*. Tablets containing equal parts of sulphadiazine, sulphadimidine, and sulfamerazine.

Proprietary Preparations

Sulphadiazine Sodium *(May & Baker, UK)*. *Injection*, sulphadiazine 250 mg (as sodium salt)/mL in ampoules of 4 mL.

Proprietary Names and Manufacturers of Sulphadiazine or Sulphadiazine Sodium

Adiazine *(Belg.; Théraplix, Fr.)*; Diazyl Dulcet *(Austral.)*; S-Diazine *(Austral.)*.

The following names have been used for multi-ingredient preparations containing sulphadiazine or sulphadiazine sodium— Neotrizine *(Lilly, USA)*; Streptotriad *(May & Baker, UK)*; Sulphamagna *(Wyeth, UK)*; Sulphatriad *(May & Baker, UK)*; Terfonyl *(Squibb, USA)*; Trisulfaminic *(Ancalab, Canad.)*.

4932-r

Sulphadimethoxine *(BAN)*.

Solfadimetossina; Solfadimetossipirimidina; Sulfadimethoxine *(rINN)*. N^1-(2,6-Dimethoxypyrimidin-4-yl)sulphanilamide.

$C_{12}H_{14}N_4O_4S$=310.3.

CAS — 122-11-2.

Pharmacopoeias. In *Br.*, *Fr.*, *Ind.*, *It.*, *Jug.*, and *Nord.*

A white, or creamy white, odourless or almost odourless, crystalline powder.

Very slightly **soluble** in water; slightly soluble in alcohol; dissolves in dilute mineral acids and in solutions of alkali hydroxides and carbonates. **Protect** from light.

Sulphadimethoxine is a long-acting sulphonamide with actions and uses similar to those of Sulphamethoxazole, p.306. It is readily absorbed from the gastro-intestinal tract, and about 90% is bound to plasma proteins. Half-lives of up to 41 hours have been reported.

The initial dose is 1 or 2 g, according to the severity of the infection, followed by a dose of 0.5 to 1 g daily.

For the effect of sulphadimethoxine in inhibiting the metabolism of phenytoin, see Phenytoin Sodium, p.409.

For a study of the renal elimination of sulphadimethoxine, see Sulphasomidine, p.309.

Preparations

Sulphadimethoxine Tablets *(B.P.)*

Proprietary Names and Manufacturers

Bensulfa *(Ital.)*; Chemiosalfa *(Salfa, Ital.)*; Crozinal *(Ital.)*; Deltin *(IFI, Ital.)*; Diasulfa *(Ital.)*; Diazinol *(Ital.)*; Dimetossilina *(Ital.)*; Dimetoxan *(Nessa, Spain)*; Emerazina *(Croce Bianca, Ital.)*; Fultamid *(Ital.)*; Ipersulfa *(Ital.)*; Jatsulph *(S.Afr.)*; Lensulpha *(S.Afr.)*; Lenterap *(Arg.)*; Levisul *(Ital.)*; Madribon *(Austral.; Belg.; Canad.; Roche, Denm.; Fr.; Ger.; Roche, Ital.; Roche, S.Afr.; Spain; Swed.; Roche, Switz.; Roche, UK)*; Madroxine *(Pol.)*; Micromega *(Ital.)*; Neosulfamyd *(Ital.)*; Oxazina *(Spain)*; Pansulph *(S.Afr.)*; Redifal *(Ital.)*; Risulpir *(Lisapharma, Ital.)*; Ritarsulfa *(Benvegna, Ital.)*; Sulfabon *(Ital.)*; Sulfadomus *(Ital.)*; Sulfadren *(Biotrading, Ital.)*; Sulfaduran *(Ital.)*; Sulfastop *(Vis, Ital.)*; Sulfathox *(SCS, S.Afr.)*; Sulfomikron *(Ital.)*; Sulfoplan *(Denm.)*; Sulfreten *(Spain)*; Tempodiazina *(Ital.)*; Unisulph *(Vernleigh, S.Afr.)*.

4933-f

Sulphadimidine *(BAN)*.

Solfametazina; Sulfadimerazine; Sulfadimezinum; Sulfadimidine *(rINN)*; Sulfadimidinum; Sulfamethazine *(USAN)*; Sulphadimethylpyrimidine; Sulphamethazine. N^1-(4,6-Dimethylpyrimidin-2-yl)sulphanilamide.

$C_{12}H_{14}N_4O_2S$=278.3.

CAS — 57-68-1.

NOTE. Sulfadimethylpyrimidine has been used as a synonym for sulphasomidine (p.309). Care should be taken to avoid confusion between the two compounds, which are isomeric.

Pharmacopoeias. In *Arg.*, *Aust.*, *Br.*, *Chin.*, *Cz.*, *Egypt.*, *Eur.*, *Fr.*, *Ger.*, *Hung.*, *Ind.*, *Int.*, *It.*, *Jug.*, *Neth.*, *Nord.*, *Pol.*, *Roum.*, *Rus.*, *Swiss*, *Turk.*, and *U.S.* Also in *B.P. Vet.*

White or yellowish-white, almost odourless, crystals or powder. It darkens on exposure to light.

Very slightly **soluble** in water; soluble in acetone; slightly soluble in alcohol; very slightly soluble to practically insoluble in ether; soluble in dilute mineral acids and in aqueous solutions of alkali hydroxides and carbonates. **Store** in well-closed containers. Protect from light.

4934-d

Sulphadimidine Sodium *(BANM)*.

Soluble Sulphadimethylpyrimidine; Soluble Sulphadimidine; Soluble Sulphamethazine; Sulfadimidine Sodium; Sulfamethazine Sodium.

$C_{12}H_{13}N_4NaO_2S$=300.3.

CAS — 1981-58-4.

Pharmacopoeias. In *Aust.*, *Br.*, *Cz.*, *Egypt.*, *Ind.*, *Pol.*, and *Turk.* Also in *B.P. Vet.*

White or creamy-white, odourless or almost odourless, hygroscopic crystals or powder. 1.08 g of monograph substance is approximately equivalent to 1 g of sulphadimidine.

Soluble 1 in 2.5 of water and 1 in 60 of alcohol. A 10% solution has a pH of 10 to 11. Solutions are most stable at pH 10 to 11; precipitation of sulphadimidine occurs below pH 10. The *B.P.* injection has a pH of 10 to 11 and is **sterilised** by heating in an autoclave. **Incompatible** with acids, iron salts, and salts of heavy metals. Protect from light.

INCOMPATIBILITY. A haze developed over 3 hours when sulphadimidine sodium was mixed with amiphenazole hydrochloride in sodium chloride injection. An immediate precipitate occurred with chlorpromazine hydrochloride, promazine hydrochloride, promethazine hydrochloride, and a yellow colour with a precipitate developing over 3 hours occurred with hydralazine hydrochloride in glucose injection or sodium chloride injection. An immediate precipitate occurred when sulphadimidine sodium was mixed with prochlorperazine mesylate in sodium chloride injection, but when they were mixed in glucose injection a haze developed over 3 hours.— B. B. Riley, *J. Hosp. Pharm.*, 1970, *28*, 228.

Adverse Effects, Treatment, and Precautions

As for Sulphamethoxazole, p.306.

Sulphadimidine and its acetyl derivative are relatively soluble in urine; the risk of crystalluria is therefore slight, but adequate fluid intake is recommended.

Sulphadimidine sodium should not be given intrathecally or subcutaneously; intramuscular injections are painful.

For reference to the detection of sulphadimidine residues in meat after its use in veterinary medicine, see Antibiotics in Food, p.104.

INTERACTIONS. Short-term alcohol administration may decrease the half-life of sulphadimidine and lead to misclassification of slow acetylators as rapid acetylators.— E. A. Lane *et al.*, *Clin. Pharmacokinet.*, 1985, *10*, 228.

Decreased serum-cyclosporin concentrations in 5 patients, leading to rejection episodes in 2, were attributed to sulphadimidine therapy. Intravenous sulphadimidine and trimethoprim were used for treatment of *Pneumocystis carinii* pneumonia.— D. K. Jones *et al.*, *Br. med. J.*, 1986, *292*, 728.

Antimicrobial Action and Resistance

As for Sulphamethoxazole, p.307, although it may be less active.

Absorption and Fate

Sulphadimidine is readily absorbed from the gastro-intestinal tract and over half is bound to plasma proteins. It penetrates into the cerebrospinal fluid, but less readily than sulphadiazine; concentrations of sulphadimidine in body fluids may be more than half those in the blood.

About 40% of sulphadimidine in the blood is present as the acetyl derivative. About 50% of a dose may be excreted in the urine in 2 days, 70% being in the form of the acetyl derivative.

Sulphadimidine tablets, 50% of which dissolved in 1 to 5 minutes *in vitro*, were given to 9 subjects in a 3-g dose, and gave average serum concentrations of free plus acetylated sulphadimidine at 0.5, 1, 4, 10, and 24 hours of 19, 43.7, 82, 59.5, and 17.5 µg per mL respectively. Average serum concentrations of free sulphadimidine at the same times were 17.2, 37, and about 57, 32, and 8 µg per mL respectively.— M. J. Taraszka and R. A. Delor, *J. pharm. Sci.*, 1969, *58*, 207.

In 20 healthy men the biological half-life of sulphadimidine was 4 and 8.8 hours for rapid and slow acetylators respectively.— M. C. B. van Oudtshoorn and F. J. Potgieter, *J. Pharm. Pharmac.*, 1972, *24*, 357.

The half-life of sulphadimidine is about 1.5 hours in fast acetylators compared with 5.5 hours in slow acetylators; half-lives for the N^4-acetyl metabolite are 5 and 7 hours respectively. The average renal clearance of the metabolite is about 7 to 20 times greater than that of the parent compound. In a fast acetylator there was no significant difference between plasma half-lives or urinary excretion when the urine was acidic compared with when it was alkaline.— T. B. Vree *et al.*, *Clin. Pharmacokinet.*, 1980, *5*, 274.

For reference to the use of sulphadimidine in determination of acetylator phenotype, see under Uses, below.

ADMINISTRATION IN RENAL FAILURE. In healthy adults, urinary clearance of sulphadimidine sodium was directly related to urinary pH; in 1 person, clearances were 4.2 and 12.7 mL per minute at pH 5.4 and 7.2 respectively. Urinary clearance was significantly greater in 10 patients with uraemia. Urine concentrations in 8 of the uraemic patients exceeded 60 mg per litre after a 1-g dose intravenously and were considered satisfactory for the treatment of infections due to sensitive pathogens.— D. M. Williams *et al.*, *Lancet*, 1968, *2*, 1058.

The mean renal clearance of sulphadimidine was 2.4 mL per minute in 10 uraemic patients given 1 g intravenously compared with 8.5 mL per minute in 10 healthy subjects given the same dose, and the excretion-rates were 86.9 µg per minute and 356.7 µg per minute respectively. There was less protein-bound sulphadimidine in the plasma of the uraemic patients whereas these patients had a higher concentration of acetylated sulphadimidine than did the control subjects. After 24 hours no sulphadimidine could be detected in the control subjects' plasma but 7 to 23 µg per mL was found in that of the uraemic patients.— E. Fischer, *Lancet*, 1972, *2*, 210.

In 9 healthy subjects given sulphadimidine 1 g four times daily for 3 days mean plasma concentrations of unconjugated sulphadimidine on the third day were 139 µg per mL, with total sulphadimidine 205 µg per mL, and unconjugated sulphadimidine in urine 574 µg per mL. In 3 patients with renal failure and plasma-creatinine concentrations of 25 to 109 µg per mL mean plasma concentrations of unconjugated sulphadimidine on the third day were 149 µg per mL, while in 7 patients with plasma-creatinine concentrations in excess of 50 µg per mL mean urine concentrations of unconjugated sulphadimidine were 45 µg per mL, probably less than the MIC for *Escherichia coli*. In 3 patients undergoing peritoneal dialysis, for whom sulphadimidine 100 or 200 µg per mL was added to the dialysate, concentrations of unconjugated sulphonamide in plasma reached these levels in 4 or 5 days.— W. R. Adam *et al.*, *Med. J. Aust.*, 1973, *1*, 936.

DRUG EXCRETION. The effects of the molecular structure of closely related N^1-substituents of sulphonamides on the pathways of elimination; the acetylation-deacetylation equilibrium and renal clearance of sulfamerazine, sulphadiazine, and sulphadimidine. These 3 sulphonamides are excreted by glomerular filtration followed by passive tubular reabsorption of the parent drug and predominantly active tubular secretion of the N^4-acetyl metabolite.— T. B. Vree *et al.*, *Pharm. Weekbl. Ned., scient. Edn*, 1983, *5*, 49.

Uses and Administration

Sulphadimidine is a short-acting sulphonamide used similarly to sulphamethoxazole, p.307.

In the treatment of susceptible infections sulphadimidine may be given by deep intramuscular or slow intravenous injection in an initial dose of 3 g, with a subsequent dosage of 1.0 to 1.5 g every 6 hours. Children have been given the following dosage regimens: from 12 to 16 years, 2.5 g initially followed by 1.0 to 1.25 g every 6 hours; from 8 to 12 years, 2 g initially followed by 0.75 g to 1.0 g every 6 hours; from 4 to 8 years, 1.5 g initially followed by 0.75 g every 6 hours; from 6 months to 4 years, 1 g initially followed by 0.5 g every 6 hours; and for infants under 6 months of age, 0.5 g initially followed by 0.25 g every 6 hours. The initial and maintenance doses for adults and children may be increased by one-third in very severe infections.

Sulphadimidine may also be given by mouth in doses similar to those given by injection.

Sulphadimidine has also been used with trimethoprim similarly to co-trimoxazole (p.210) and in association with other sulphonamides, particularly sulfamerazine and sulphadiazine.

A review of *N*-acetylation pharmacogenetics. Several sulphonamides, including sulphadiazine, sulphadimidine, sulfamerazine, sulphapyridine, and sulphasalazine have been used to determine acetylator status. Until recently, when sulphadimidine approved for human use has become difficult to obtain, determinations of acetylator status in the *US* were frequently carried out with sulphadimidine in preference to isoniazid. Rapid and slow acetylators may be differentiated by determination of the ratio of acetylsulphadimidine to sulphadimidine in urine, or preferably, venous blood. A dose of sulphadimidine 10 mg per kg body-weight produces a more accurate determination of acetylator status than a dose of 40 mg per kg as the pharmacokinetics of sulphadimidine become non-linear at the higher dosage.— W. W. Weber and D. W. Hein, *Pharmac. Rev.*, 1985, *37*, 25. See also D. W. J. Clark, *Drugs*, 1985, *29*, 342.

MENINGITIS. For reference to the use and a suggested dosage regimen of sulphadimidine in the treatment and prophylaxis of meningococcal meningitis, see sulphadiazine, p.303.

URINARY-TRACT INFECTIONS. Recommended doses for sulphadimidine may be too large; 500 mg every 6 hours should be adequate for simple urinary-tract infections.— D. S. Reeves *et al.*, *Br. med. J.*, 1978, *2*, 410.

Preparations

Paediatric Sulphadimidine Oral Suspension *(B.P.)*. Paediatric Sulphadimidine Mixture. Contains sulphadimidine 500 mg/5 mL.

Sulphadimidine Injection *(B.P.)*. Sulphadimidine Sodium Injection; Sulfadimidine Injection. A sterile solution of sulphadimidine sodium in Water for Injections free from dissolved air, prepared either from sulphadimidine sodium or by the interaction of sulphadimidine and sodium hydroxide.

Sulphadimidine Tablets *(B.P.)*

Proprietary Preparations

Sulphamezathine *(ICI Pharmaceuticals, UK)*. *Injection*, sulphadimidine sodium 1 g/3 mL in ampoules of 3 mL.

Proprietary Names and Manufacturers of Sulphadimidine or Sulphadimidine Sodium

Col Lersa *(Lersa, Spain)*; Deladine *(S.Afr.)*; Diazil *(Ital.)*; Nutradimidine *(S.Afr.)*; S-Dimidine *(Protea, Austral.)*; Sulfa-D *(Vernleigh, S.Afr.)*; Sulphamezathine *(Austral.; ICI Pharmaceuticals, UK)*.

The following names have been used for multi-ingredient preparations containing sulphadimidine or sulphadimidine sodium—

Neotrizine *(Lilly, USA)*; Penbritin KS *(Beecham Research, UK)*; Poteseptyl *(Alkaloida Chemical Factory, Hung.)*; Streptotriad *(May & Baker, UK)*; Terfonyl *(Squibb, USA)*; Trisulfaminic *(Ancalab, Canad.)*; V-Cil-K Sulpha *(Lilly, UK)*.

4936-h

Sulphafurazole *(BAN)*.

Sulfafurazole *(pINN)*; Sulfafurazolum; Sulfisoxazole *(USAN)*; Sulphafuraz. N^1-(3,4-Dimethylisoxazol-5-yl)sulphanilamide.

$C_{11}H_{13}N_3O_3S = 267.3$.

CAS — 127-69-5.

Pharmacopoeias. In *Arg.*, *Br.*, *Braz.*, *Cz.*, *Egypt.*, *Fr.*, *Ind.*, *Int.*, *It.*, *Jpn*, *Jug.*, *Nord.*, *Roum.*, *Turk.*, and *U.S.*

A white or yellowish-white, odourless or almost odourless, crystalline powder.

Soluble 1 in 7700 of water, 1 in 50 of alcohol, 1 in 10 of boiling alcohol, and 1 in 30 of a solution of sodium bicarbonate; slightly soluble in chloroform and ether and soluble in 3N hydrochloric acid. **Store** in airtight containers. Protect from light.

4937-m

Acetyl Sulphafurazole

Sulfisoxazole Acetyl *(USAN)*. N^1-Acetyl Sulphafurazole; *N*-(3,4-Dimethylisoxazol-5-yl)-*N*-sulphanilylacetamide.

$C_{13}H_{15}N_3O_4S = 309.3$.

CAS — 80-74-0.

NOTE. Acetyl sulphafurazole is to be distinguished from the N^4-acetyl derivative formed from sulphafurazole by conjugation in the body.

Pharmacopoeias. In *U.S.*

A white to slightly yellow, tasteless, crystalline

powder. 1.16 g of monograph substance is approximately equivalent to 1 g of sulphafurazole.
Practically **insoluble** in water; soluble 1 in about 180 of alcohol, 1 in 35 of chloroform, 1 in about 200 of methyl alcohol, and 1 in about 1100 of ether. **Store** in airtight containers. Protect from light.

4938-b

Sulphafurazole Diethanolamine

Sulfafurazole Diolamine *(pINNM)*; Sulfisoxazole Diolamine *(USAN)*; Sulphafurazole Diolamine.
The 2,2′-iminobisethanol salt of sulphafurazole.
$C_{11}H_{13}N_3O_3S,C_4H_{11}NO_2$=372.4.

CAS — 4299-60-9.

Pharmacopoeias. In *U.S.*

An odourless, white to off-white, fine, crystalline powder. 1.39 g of monograph substance is approximately equivalent to 1 g of sulphafurazole.
Soluble 1 in 2 of water, 1 in 16 of alcohol, 1 in 1000 of chloroform, 1 in 4 of methyl alcohol, and 1 in 250 of isopropyl alcohol; practically insoluble in ether. **Store** in airtight containers. Protect from light.

Sulphafurazole diethanolamine is **incompatible** with *aminophylline, ascorbic acid injection, cephalothin sodium, promazine hydrochloride,* and *thiopentone sodium.* It is also reported to be incompatible with *ammonium chloride, hydroxyzine hydrochloride, insulin, opioid analgesics, oxytetracycline hydrochloride, phenytoin sodium, procaine hydrochloride, prochlorperazine edisylate, promethazine hydrochloride, streptomycin sulphate, tetracycline hydrochloride, vancomycin hydrochloride,* and *vitamin B complex with vitamin C*; and less consistently reported to be incompatible with *amikacin sulphate, chloramphenicol sodium succinate, heparin, kanamycin sulphate,* and *methicillin sodium.*
Solutions for intravenous administration should be diluted only in Water for Injections because of the risk of crystallisation in other parenteral fluids, depending on their composition and initial pH.

Adverse Effects, Treatment, and Precautions

As for sulphamethoxazole, p.306.
Sulphafurazole and its acetyl derivative are relatively soluble in urine and the risk of crystalluria is generally slight, nevertheless adequate fluid intake is recommended.
Sulphafurazole has been reported to increase the anaesthetic effect of thiopentone sodium.
Eye preparations of sulphafurazole diethanolamine should not be applied concomitantly with preparations of silver salts.

ADMINISTRATION IN LIVER DISORDERS. A study of the pharmacokinetics of sulphafurazole in 6 patients with alcoholic cirrhosis and 6 healthy subjects. Except in the most severe cases, cirrhosis appeared to have no effect on clearance of the unbound drug.— J. P. Cello and S. Øie, *J. Pharmacokinet. Biopharm.*, 1985, *13*, 1.

ADMINISTRATION IN RENAL FAILURE. For precautions to be observed in patients with impaired renal function, see under Absorption and Fate, and Uses, below.

INTERACTIONS. For a report of sulphafurazole enhancing the anticoagulant effect of warfarin, see Warfarin Sodium, p.345.

Antimicrobial Action and Resistance

As for sulphamethoxazole, p.307.

Absorption and Fate

Sulphafurazole is readily absorbed from the gastro-intestinal tract; about 85% is bound to plasma proteins. Sulphafurazole readily diffuses into extracellular fluid, but very little diffuses into cells. Concentrations in the cerebrospinal fluid are about one-third of those in the blood. It crosses the placenta into the foetal circulation and is excreted in breast milk. About 30% of sulphafurazole in the blood and in the urine is in the form of the N^4-acetyl derivative.
It is excreted rapidly, up to 95% of a single dose being eliminated in 24 hours. Both sulphafurazole and its acetyl derivative are more soluble than sulphadiazine and many other sulphonamides in urine.
It is believed that acetyl sulphafurazole (the N^1-acetyl derivative) is broken down in the gastro-intestinal tract releasing sulphafurazole, with a consequent delay in absorption.

The elimination half-life of sulphafurazole was reduced from 6.3 hours under normal urine conditions to 4.4 hours under alkaline urine conditions.— A. P. Goossens and M. C. B. van Oudtshoorn (letter), *J. Pharm. Pharmac.*, 1970, *22*, 224.

The half-life of sulphafurazole after oral administration was 4.6 to 7.8 hours; after intramuscular administration, 5.0 to 7.6 hours; and after intravenous administration, 4.6 to 6.9 hours.— S. A. Kaplan *et al.*, *J. pharm. Sci.*, 1972, *61*, 773.

References to the pharmacokinetics and protein binding of sulphafurazole: R. L. Suber *et al.*, *J. pharm. Sci.*, 1981, *70*, 981; S. Øie *et al.*, *J. Pharmacokinet. Biopharm.*, 1982, *10*, 157; R. A. Shastri (letter), *Br. J. clin. Pharmac.*, 1982, *13*, 249.

ADMINISTRATION IN RENAL FAILURE. The elimination of unbound sulphafurazole in 8 renal transplant patients was similar to that in 6 healthy subjects when differences in renal function were taken into consideration. There were, however, notable changes in the elimination of total sulphafurazole, due mainly to a lower binding to plasma proteins in the transplant patients; this may be related to a lower albumin concentration and to an accumulation of the metabolite N^4-acetyl sulphafurazole which is a displacer of the parent drug. It was considered that sulphafurazole may be used as prophylaxis against urinary-tract infections in this group of patients if the creatinine clearance is not less than 20 mL per minute. If this precaution and maintenance of adequate fluid intake is observed, the risk of crystalluria should be minimised. If renal function deteriorates, the acetyl metabolite, which is less soluble and more difficult to remove by haemodialysis than the parent drug, will accumulate.— M. Shermantine *et al.*, *Antimicrob. Ag. Chemother.*, 1985, *28*, 535.

See also under Uses, below.

Uses and Administration

Sulphafurazole is a short-acting sulphonamide which is used similarly to sulphamethoxazole (see p.307).
It is usually administered by mouth. In the treatment of susceptible infections sulphafurazole is given in an initial dose of 2 to 4 g followed by 4 to 8 g daily in divided doses every 4 to 6 hours. For children, the dose is 75 mg per kg bodyweight initially, followed by 150 mg per kg daily in divided doses to a maximum of 6 g daily. Acetyl sulphafurazole is tasteless and is used in liquid oral preparations of the drug; doses are expressed in terms of sulphafurazole.
Sulphafurazole has also been given by subcutaneous injection or slow intravenous injection or infusion as a 5% solution prepared by diluting a 40% solution of sulphafurazole in the form of the diethanolamine salt with Water for Injections. It has also been given intramuscularly. Doses are expressed in terms of the equivalent amount of sulphafurazole. A suggested parenteral dose for children and adults is 50 mg per kg body-weight initially, followed by 100 mg per kg daily in divided doses. Oral administration should commence as soon as possible.
Sulphafurazole diethanolamine has been used, as an ophthalmic ointment or solution containing the equivalent of 4% of sulphafurazole, in the topical treatment of susceptible eye infections.
In the *UK* the use of sulphafurazole and its salts in cosmetics is prohibited.

Sulphonamide therapy appeared to provide a considerable protective effect in 4 of 5 patients with chronic granulomatous disease. Studies *in vitro* showed that white blood-cells from the 5 patients gained increased bactericidal activity in the presence of sulphafurazole.— R. B. Johnston *et al.*, *Lancet*, 1975, *1*, 824.

ADMINISTRATION IN RENAL FAILURE. The normal half-life for sulphafurazole of 3 to 7 hours was increased to 6 to 12 hours in end-stage renal failure. The interval between doses should be extended from 6 hours to 8 to 12 hours in patients with a glomerular filtration-rate (GFR) of 10 to 50 mL per minute, and to 18 to 24 hours in those with a GFR of less than 10 mL per minute. A dosage supplement should be given to patients undergoing haemodialysis or peritoneal dialysis.— W. M. Bennett *et al.*, *Am. J. Kidney Dis.*, 1983, *3*, 155.

See also under Absorption and Fate, above.

MENINGITIS. For reference to the use of sulphafurazole in the treatment of meningitis, see Sulphadiazine, p.303.

OTITIS MEDIA. For references to the use of a combination preparation of erythromycin and sulphafurazole in the treatment of otitis media in children, see Erythromycin p.225.

PREGNANCY AND THE NEONATE. Sulphafurazole has been suggested as an alternative to erythromycin in the treatment of neonatal pneumonia caused by *Chlamydia trachomatis* in infants over 4 weeks of age.— *Med. Lett.*, 1986, *28*, 23.

Reports of the use of sulphafurazole in the treatment of infants with chlamydial pneumonia.— J. A. Embil *et al.*, *Can. med. Ass. J.*, 1978, *119*, 1199; M. O. Beem *et al.*, *Pediatrics*, 1979, *63*, 198.

SEXUALLY TRANSMITTED DISEASES. Sulphafurazole 500 mg four times daily by mouth for 10 days may be used as an alternative to tetracycline or erythromycin in the treatment of urethritis or cervicitis caused by *Chlamydia trachomatis.*— *Med. Lett.*, 1986, *28*, 23.

Sulphafurazole 500 mg four times daily for 10 days was effective in the treatment of all 13 men with urethritis due to *Chlamydia trachomatis.* It was considered ineffective in urethritis due to *Ureaplasma urealyticum.*— W. R. Bowie *et al.*, *Lancet*, 1976, *2*, 1276.

URINARY-TRACT INFECTIONS. Urinary-tract infection in 29 girls was considered cured in 27 (possibly in 29) after single doses of sulphafurazole 200 mg per kg body-weight.— G. Källenius and J. Winberg, *Br. med. J.*, 1979, *1*, 1175.

See also under Sexually Transmitted Diseases, above.

Prophylaxis. For the use of sulphafurazole for the prophylaxis of urinary-tract infections in renal transplant patients, see Administration in Renal Failure, under Absorption and Fate, above.

Preparations

Sulfisoxazole Acetyl Oral Suspension *(U.S.P.).* A suspension containing acetyl sulphafurazole. pH 5.0 to 5.5.

Sulfisoxazole Diolamine Injection *(U.S.P.).* A sterile solution of sulphafurazole diethanolamine in Water for Injections. pH 7.0 to 8.5.

Sulfisoxazole Diolamine Ophthalmic Ointment *(U.S.P.).* A sterile eye ointment containing sulphafurazole diethanolamine.

Sulfisoxazole Diolamine Ophthalmic Solution *(U.S.P.).* A sterile solution of sulphafurazole diethanolamine. pH 7.2 to 8.2.

Sulfisoxazole Tablets *(U.S.P.).* Tablets containing sulphafurazole.

Sulphafurazole Tablets *(B.P.)*

Proprietary Names and Manufacturers of Sulphafurazole or its Derivatives

Chemovag *(USA)*; Gantrisin *(Roche, Austral.; Belg.; Roche, Canad.; Roche, Denm.; Ger.; Neth.; S.Afr.; Swed.; Switz.; Roche, UK; Roche, USA)*; Gantrisine *(Fr.)*; Gantrisona *(Spain)*; Koro-Sulf *(Youngs, USA)*; Lipo Gantrisin *(Roche, USA)*; Novosoxazole *(Novopharm, Canad.)*; Pancid *(Ital.)*; SK-Soxazole *(Smith Kline & French, USA)*; Sosol *(USA)*; Soxa *(USA)*; Soxomide *(USA)*; Sulfagan *(USA)*; Sulfalar *(USA)*; Sulfazole *(Protea, Austral.)*; Sulfizin *(Reid-Provident, USA)*; Sulfizole *(Canad.)*; Urazole *(S.Afr.)*; Urizole *(USA)*; Urogan *(Austral.)*; Velmatrol *(USA)*.

The following names have been used for multi-ingredient preparations containing sulphafurazole or its derivatives— Azo Gantrisin *(Roche, Canad.; Roche, USA)*; Azo-Sulfisoxazole *(Schein, USA)*; Pediazole *(Abbott, Canad.; Ross, USA)*.

4939-v

Sulphaguanidine *(BAN).*

Solfaguanidina; Sulfaguanidine *(rINN)*; Sulfaguanidinum; Sulfamidinum; Sulginum. 1-Sulphanilylguanidine; N'-Amidinosulphanilamide monohydrate.
$C_7H_{10}N_4O_2S,H_2O$=232.3.

CAS — 57-67-0 (anhydrous); 6190-55-2 (monohydrate).

Pharmacopoeias. In *Arg., Aust., Egypt., Fr., Ger., Hung., Int., It., Jug., Mex., Pol., Rus., Span., Swiss,* and *Turk.* Also in *B.P.C. 1973.*

Adverse Effects, Treatment, and Precautions
As for Sulphamethoxazole, below.

Antimicrobial Action and Resistance
As for Sulphamethoxazole, p.307.

Absorption and Fate
Sulphaguanidine is absorbed to a varying degree from the gastro-intestinal tract; blood concentrations of 15 to 40 μg per mL after single doses of 1 to 7 g have been reported. It is rapidly excreted in the urine, about one-third being in the form of the acetyl derivative.

Uses and Administration
Sulphaguanidine is a sulphonamide which has been employed for the treatment of local intestinal infections, particularly bacillary dysentery, but phthalylsulphathiazole and succinylsulphathiazole are less toxic. It has been given in doses of up to 3 g four times daily.

Preparations
Sulphaguanidine Tablets *(B.P.C. 1973)*

Proprietary Names and Manufacturers
Ganidan *(Fr.)*; Resulfon *(Ger.)*; S-Guanidine *(Austral.)*.

The following names have been used for multi-ingredient preparations containing sulphaguanidine— Guanimycin *(Allen & Hanburys, UK)*; Pomalin *(Winthrop, Canad.)*.

4940-r

Sulphaguanole

Sulfaguanole *(rINN)*. N^1-[(4,5-Dimethyloxazol-2-yl)amidino]sulphanilamide.
$C_{12}H_{15}N_5O_3S$=309.3.

CAS — 27031-08-9.

Sulphaguanole is a sulphonamide with properties similar to sulphamethoxazole, below. It has been given by mouth in a dose of 800 mg three times daily on the first day, then 400 mg three times daily in the treatment of gastro-intestinal infections.

Maximum plasma concentrations were reached 3.5 hours after a dose of sulphaguanole. The plasma half-life was 7 hours.— R. Denk *et al., Arzneimittel-Forsch.*, 1973, *23*, 187.

After administration by mouth to 14 children, 8% of a dose of sulphaguanole was absorbed and excreted within 30 hours.— E. Gladtke, *Arzneimittel-Forsch.*, 1973, *23*, 191.

Proprietary Names and Manufacturers
Asorec *(Radiumfarma, Ital.)*; Enterocura *(Nordmark, Ger.; De Angeli, Ital.)*.

4941-f

Sulphamethizole *(BAN)*.

Sulfamethizole *(USAN, rINN)*. N^1-(5-Methyl-1,3,4-thiadiazol-2-yl)sulphanilamide.
$C_9H_{10}N_4O_2S_2$=270.3.

CAS — 144-82-1.

Pharmacopoeias. In *Br., Fr., Ind., Jpn, Neth., Nord., Swiss,* and *U.S.*

Odourless or almost odourless, colourless crystals or white or creamy-white crystalline powder. **Soluble** 1 in 2000 of water, 1 in 60 of boiling water, 1 in 25 to 38 of alcohol, 1 in 13 to 15 of acetone, and 1 in 1900 of chloroform and ether; freely soluble in solutions of alkali hydroxides and in dilute mineral acids. **Store** in well-closed containers. Protect from light.

Adverse Effects, Treatment, and Precautions
As for Sulphamethoxazole, below.
Crystalluria occurs very rarely but an adequate fluid intake should generally be maintained.

INTERACTIONS. For the effect of sulphamethizole in inhibiting the metabolism of phenytoin, see Phenytoin Sodium, p.409.

Antimicrobial Action and Resistance
As for Sulphamethoxazole, p.307.

Absorption and Fate
Sulphamethizole is readily absorbed from the gastro-intestinal tract; about 90% has been reported to be bound to plasma proteins. It is only slightly acetylated in the body and is rapidly excreted, about 60% of a dose being eliminated in the urine in 5 hours. Sulphamethizole and its acetyl derivative are readily soluble in urine over a wide pH range.

The biological half-life of sulphamethizole is 1.5 to 1.6 hours.— W. A. Ritschel, *Drug Intell. & clin. Pharm.*, 1970, *4*, 332.

Following administration of sulphamethizole 14.3 mg per kg body-weight to 7 healthy geriatric subjects, the mean half-life was 181 minutes and the mean blood concentration after 6 hours was 14.2 μg per mL; in 6 young subjects given the same dose, the mean values were 105 minutes and 5 μg per mL respectively.— E. J. Triggs *et al., Eur. J. clin. Pharmac.*, 1975, *8*, 55.

Uses and Administration
Sulphamethizole is a short-acting sulphonamide which is given by mouth in the treatment of infections of the urinary tract.
It is given in adult doses of 1.5 to 4 g daily in 3 to 4 divided doses. A suggested dose for children is 30 to 45 mg per kg body-weight daily in 4 divided doses.

URINARY-TRACT INFECTIONS. Sensitivity of bacteria cultured from the urine of spinal-cord injury patients to sulphamethizole in combination with nitroxoline (Nicene).— R. D. Shrosbree and P. Engel, *Curr. ther. Res.*, 1984, *35*, 321. Studies of the use of a combination of sulphamethizole and nitroxoline in the treatment of urinary-tract infections: M. R. Bednarek *et al., ibid.*, 1986, *39*, 505; A. J. N. Du Raan, *ibid.*, 1987, *42*, 77.

Preparations
Sulfamethizole Oral Suspension *(U.S.P.)*
Sulfamethizole Tablets *(U.S.P.)*
Sulphamethizole Tablets *(B.P.)*

Proprietary Names and Manufacturers
Lucosil *(Belg.; Lundbeck, Denm.; Neth.; Lundbeck, Norw.; Lundbeck, Switz.)*; Methisul *(R.P. Drugs, UK)*; Microsul *(Star, USA)*; Proklar-M *(USA)*; Rufol *(Debat, Fr.; Roussel Maestretti, Ital.)*; Salimol *(Jpn)*; S-Methizole *(Protea, Austral.)*; Sulfametin *(Swed.)*; Sulfapyelon *(Belg.)*; Thiosulfil *(Austral.; Canad.; Ayerst, Ital.; Ayerst, USA)*; Tiosulfan *(Inibsa, Spain)*; Urocydal *(Jpn)*; Urolex *(Austral.)*; Urolucosil *(Warner, Austral.; Belg.; Neth.; Lundbeck, Switz.; Parke, Davis, UK)*; Uroz *(Austral.)*.

The following names have been used for multi-ingredient preparations containing sulphamethizole— Azotrex *(Bristol, USA)*; Nicene *(Adcock Ingram, S.Afr.)*; Thiosulfil-A *(Ayerst, USA)*; Urobiotic *(Roerig, USA)*.

4942-d

Sulphamethoxazole *(BAN)*.

Ro-4-2130; Sulfamethoxazole *(USAN, rINN)*; Sulfamethoxazolum; Sulfisomezole. N^1-(5-Methylisoxazol-3-yl)sulphanilamide.
$C_{10}H_{11}N_3O_3S$=253.3.

CAS — 723-46-6.

Pharmacopoeias. In *Belg., Br., Braz., Chin., Cz., Egypt., Eur., Fr., Ger., Ind., Int., It., Jpn, Jug., Neth., Swiss,* and *U.S.*

A white or off-white, odourless or almost odourless, crystalline powder.
Soluble 1 in 3400 of water; soluble 1 in 50 of alcohol and 1 in 3 of acetone; slowly and usually incompletely soluble 1 in 2 of carbon disulphide; soluble 1 in 1000 of chloroform and ether; soluble in solutions of alkali hydroxides. The filtrate of a 5% solution in carbon dioxide-free water has a pH of 4 to 5. **Store** in well-closed containers; the *U.S.P.* suspension should be stored in airtight containers. Protect from light.

Adverse Effects
Nausea, vomiting, and diarrhoea are relatively common following the administration of sulphamethoxazole and other sulphonamides.
Hypersensitivity reactions may occur; those involving the skin include rashes, photosensitivity reactions, exfoliative dermatitis, toxic epidermal necrolysis (Lyell's syndrome), and erythema nodosum. A severe, potentially fatal, form of erythema multiforme, associated with widespread lesions of the skin and mucous membranes, termed the Stevens-Johnson syndrome, has occurred in patients treated with sulphonamides. Dermatitis may occur on contact of sulphonamides with the skin. Systemic lupus erythematosus, particularly exacerbations of pre-existing disease, has also been reported.
Nephrotoxic reactions, which may result in renal failure, have been attributed to hypersensitivity to sulphamethoxazole. Lumbar pain, haematuria, oliguria, and anuria may also occur due to crystallisation in the urine of sulphamethoxazole or its less soluble acetylated metabolite.
Blood disorders have occasionally occurred during treatment with the sulphonamides including sulphamethoxazole, and include agranulocytosis, aplastic anaemia, thrombocytopenia, leucopenia, hypoprothrombinaemia, and eosinophilia. Acute haemolytic anaemia is a rare complication which may be associated with glucose-6-phosphate dehydrogenase deficiency. Many of these effects on the blood may result from hypersensitivity reactions.
Other adverse effects which may be manifestations of a generalised hypersensitivity reaction to sulphonamides include a syndrome resembling serum sickness, hepatotoxic reactions, myocarditis, pancreatitis, pulmonary eosinophilia, and vasculitis including polyarteritis nodosa. Anaphylaxis has been reported only very rarely.
Sulphonamides may rarely cause cyanosis due to methaemoglobinaemia or sulphaemoglobinaemia.
Other adverse reactions that have been reported after the administration of sulphamethoxazole or other sulphonamides include effects on the eyes such as optic neuropathy or transient myopia, fever, hypothyroidism, and neurological reactions including ataxia, dizziness, fatigue, headache, insomnia, peripheral neuritis, and vertigo.
As with other antimicrobial agents, sulphamethoxazole may cause alterations of the bacterial flora in the gastro-intestinal tract. There is, therefore, the possibility, although it appears to be small, that pseudomembranous colitis may occur.
Slow acetylators of sulphamethoxazole may be at greater risk of adverse reactions than fast acetylators.

Reports dealing with the adverse effects of sulphamethoxazole given with trimethoprim are provided under Co-trimoxazole, p.206.
Two patients aged 4½ years and 14 months respectively developed benign intracranial hypertension after completing courses of treatment with sulphamethoxazole.— L. T. Ch'ien (letter), *New Engl. J. Med.*, 1970, *283*, 47.
During the years 1964 to 1985 the Committee on Safety of Drugs and the Committee on Safety of Medicines received 322 reports of adverse reactions to the sulphonamides (11 fatal); this was considered to demonstrate under-reporting. Ninety-two reports described rashes, 15 the Stevens-Johnson syndrome (2 fatal), and 44 blood dyscrasias (4 fatal).— *Br. med. J.*, 1986, *293*, 1163.

ALLERGY. Discussion on the hypersensitivity reactions observed with sulphonamides with reference to a study by Shear *et al.* (*Ann. intern. Med.*, 1986, *105*, 179) of 6 children who had severe reactions to a triple sulphonamide preparation (sulphadiazine, sulphadimidine, and sulfamerazine). Susceptibility to such reactions may be due to a combination of increased production of a reactive metabolite under control of the gene regulating *N*-acetylation together with a relative inability of the tissues to detoxify it; a secondary immunological response produces the symptoms of a multisystem hypersensitivity disorder.— *Lancet*, 1986, *2*, 958.

EFFECTS ON THE BLOOD. Comment that most sulphonamides do not produce haemolysis in glucose-6-phosphate dehydrogenase-deficient patients.— E. Beutler, *J. Am. med. Ass.*, 1985, *254*, 1234. The following sulphonamides may cause clinically significant haemolytic anaemia in patients with glucose-6-phosphate dehydrogenase deficiency: sulphamethoxazole, sulphacetamide, sulphanilamide, and sulphapyridine.— *Ann. intern. Med.*, 1985, *103*, 245.

Treatment of Adverse Effects

Treatment of overdosage with sulphamethoxazole is primarily symptomatic. Fluids should be administered to maintain a high urine output and thus assist elimination of the drug in the urine. The risk of crystalluria may also be minimised by administration of sodium bicarbonate. Severe crystalluria may require ureteric catheterisation and irrigation with warm sodium bicarbonate 2.5% solution.

Sulphamethoxazole is removed moderately well by haemodialysis but not by peritoneal dialysis.

Precautions

In patients receiving sulphamethoxazole, adequate fluid intake is necessary to reduce the risk of crystalluria; the daily urine output should be 1500 mL or more. The administration of compounds which render the urine acid may increase the risk of crystalluria; the risk may be reduced with alkaline urine.

Treatment with sulphamethoxazole should be discontinued immediately a rash appears because of the danger of severe allergic reactions such as the Stevens-Johnson syndrome.

Sulphamethoxazole is contra-indicated in patients with severe renal or hepatic failure or with blood disorders; it should not be given to patients with acute porphyria as it may cause exacerbations of the disease. Complete blood counts and urinalyses with microscopic examination should be carried out particularly during prolonged therapy with sulphamethoxazole. Sulphamethoxazole should not be given to patients with a history of hypersensitivity to sulphonamides as cross-sensitivity may occur between agents of this group; cross-sensitivity has also been observed between sulphonamides and chemically related drugs such as some diuretics, particularly acetazolamide and thiazides, and the sulphonylurea hypoglycaemic agents.

Sulphamethoxazole and other sulphonamides are not usually given to infants within 1 to 2 months of birth because of the risk of producing kernicterus; for the same reason, they are generally contra-indicated in women prior to delivery or in nursing mothers.

Reduction of dosage may be required in patients with renal impairment.

Sulphamethoxazole and other sulphonamides may potentiate the effects of some drugs, such as oral anticoagulants (see p.345), methotrexate, and phenytoin; this may be due to displacement of the drug from plasma protein binding sites or to inhibition of metabolism. However, the clinical significance of these interactions appears to depend on the particular sulphonamide involved.

High doses of sulphonamides have been reported to have a hypoglycaemic effect; the antidiabetic effect of the sulphonylurea compounds may be enhanced by the concomitant administration of sulphonamides.

The action of sulphonamides may be antagonised by *p*-aminobenzoic acid and compounds derived from it, particularly the procaine group of local anaesthetics.

Paraldehyde has been reported to increase the acetylation of sulphonamides with subsequent increased risk of crystalluria.

Sulphonamides have been reported to interfere with some diagnostic tests including those for urea, creatinine, and urinary glucose and urobilinogen.

Reports dealing with the precautions to be observed with sulphamethoxazole given with trimethoprim are provided under Co-trimoxazole, p.207.

Warnings that sulphonamides may cause discoloration of the urine.— J. Karlstrand, *J. Am. pharm. Ass.*, 1977, *NS17*, 735 (rust yellow to brown); D. K. Watkins, *Pharm. J.*, 1987, *1*, 68 (greenish blue).

ADMINISTRATION IN RENAL FAILURE. For reference to the precautions to be observed in renal failure, see Administration in Renal Failure in Uses, below.

INTERFERENCE WITH ASSAY PROCEDURES. For the interference of some sulphonamides with theophylline assays, see Theophylline Hydrate, p.1530.

PREGNANCY AND THE NEONATE. Some sulphonamides have been shown to cause foetal abnormalities including cleft palate in *animals*, but fears of teratogenic effects in humans do not appear to be substantiated. Sulphonamides are probably safe in the first trimester of pregnancy although throughout pregnancy they should be used only in the absence of a suitable alternative drug; they should be avoided within 2 days of delivery, because of the risk of kernicterus (R. Wise, *Br. med. J.*, 1987, *294*, 42; *Med. Lett.*, 1987, *29*, 61).

A review of drug-induced bilirubin displacement. The initial evidence suggesting a kernicterus-promoting effect of drugs in neonates was reported for sulphafurazole and this drug now serves as a standard displacing agent against which other drugs are evaluated. Although all sulphonamides are highly protein bound, each has a different capacity to displace bilirubin. Sulphadiazine and sulphanilamide have been found to be the least displacing of the sulphonamides and the effects of sulphadiazine on bilirubin may not be clinically significant; an increased incidence of hyperbilirubinaemia and kernicterus has not been demonstrated following its use for prophylaxis of rheumatic fever during pregnancy. Sulphasalazine should theoretically cause significant bilirubin displacement, but studies suggest that the drug may be given to pregnant and lactating patients with Crohn's disease. Metabolites of sulphonamides have also been evaluated for kernicterus-promoting effects; glucuronide metabolites are expected to compete for binding sites less effectively than the parent compound, whereas acetylated metabolites of some sulphonamides appear to be more potent bilirubin displacers.— P. C. Walker, *Clin. Pharmacokinet.*, 1987, *13*, 26.

Antimicrobial Action

Sulphamethoxazole and other sulphonamides have a similar structure to *p*-aminobenzoic acid and interfere with the synthesis of nucleic acids in sensitive micro-organisms by blocking the conversion of *p*-aminobenzoic acid to the co-enzyme dihydrofolic acid, a reduced form of folic acid; in man, dihydrofolic acid is obtained from dietary folic acid so sulphonamides do not affect human cells.

The broad spectrum of bacteriostatic antimicrobial activity of sulphonamides has been decreased by an increase in resistance of many organisms (see below). Among Gram-negative bacteria the following organisms may be susceptible: Enterobacteriaceae including *Escherichia coli*; *Haemophilus ducreyi* and *H. influenzae*; *Neisseria gonorrhoeae* and *N. meningitidis*; and *Vibrio cholerae*. Among Gram-positive organisms, some staphylococci and streptococci, and *Clostridium perfringens* and *Cl. tetani* may be susceptible. Other sensitive organisms include *Actinomyces* and *Nocardia* spp., *Chlamydia trachomatis*, and the protozoa *Plasmodium falciparum* and *Toxoplasma gondii*.

Sulphamethoxazole and other sulphonamides demonstrate synergy with the dihydrofolate reductase inhibitors pyrimethamine and trimethoprim which inhibit a later stage in folic acid synthesis. For reports of the antimicrobial activity of sulphamethoxazole with trimethoprim, see Co-trimoxazole, p.208.

The *in vitro* antimicrobial activity of sulphamethoxazole is very dependent on both the culture medium and size of inoculum used.

Resistance

Acquired resistance to sulphamethoxazole and other sulphonamides is common and has been reported in the majority of pathogenic micro-organisms sensitive to sulphonamides. It has particularly limited the usefulness of these agents in infections caused by *Neisseria gonorrhoeae* and *N. meningitidis*, shigellae, staphylococci, and streptococci. Resistance to sulphamethoxazole may develop during therapy, particularly if prolonged.

Most strains of *Enterococcus faecalis* (*Streptococcus faecalis*) are resistant to sulphamethoxazole.

Resistance to sulphamethoxazole may be plasmid-mediated, as in many Gram-negative bacteria, or chromosomally mediated.

Cross resistance generally occurs between sulphonamides.

Of 232 strains of enteropathogenic *Escherichia coli* 106 were resistant to sulphonamides at a concentration of 100 µg per mL.— R. J. Gross *et al.*, *Br. med. J.*, 1982, *285*, 472.

Of 2753 strains of *Shigella dysenteriae*, *Sh. flexneri*, and *Sh. boydii* examined at the Central Public Health Laboratory from 1979 to mid 1983, 75.8% were resistant to sulphonamides at a concentration of 100 µg per mL.— R. J. Gross *et al.*, *Br. med. J.*, 1984, *288*, 784.

Bacterial resistance to antifolate antimicrobial agents mediated by plasmids.— J. T. Smith and S. G. B. Amyes, *Br. med. Bull.*, 1984, *40*, 42.

Absorption and Fate

Sulphamethoxazole is readily absorbed from the gastro-intestinal tract and peak plasma concentrations are reached after about 2 hours. Doses of 1 g twice daily should produce blood concentrations of unconjugated sulphamethoxazole in excess of 50 µg per mL. About 65% is bound to plasma proteins and the plasma half-life is about 10 hours.

Sulphamethoxazole, like most sulphonamides, diffuses freely throughout the body tissues and may be detected in the urine, saliva, sweat, and bile, in the cerebrospinal, peritoneal, ocular, and synovial fluids, and in pleural and other effusions. It crosses the placenta into the foetal circulation, and is excreted in low concentrations in breast milk.

Sulphamethoxazole undergoes conjugation mainly in the liver, chiefly to the inactive N^4-acetyl derivative; this metabolite represents about 15% of the total amount of sulphamethoxazole in the blood. Elimination in the urine is dependent on pH. About 25% of a single 2-g dose of sulphamethoxazole has been reported to be excreted in the urine within 8 hours, about 60% being in the form of the acetyl derivative.

Reports dealing with the absorption and fate of sulphamethoxazole given with trimethoprim are provided under Co-trimoxazole, p.209.

A study in 10 healthy subjects indicated that urine flow and urine pH are the 2 main variables influencing the excretion and metabolism of sulphamethoxazole. When urine was maintained between pH 7 and 8, 22 to 43% of a dose was excreted unchanged in the urine over 60 hours and 31 to 72% was excreted as N^4-acetylsulphamethoxazole. With urine maintained between pH 5 and 6.5, 3.4 to 26% was excreted unchanged and 24 to 52% appeared as acetylated derivative. Although fast and slow acetylators of procainamide took part in the study, a similar classification could not be made in terms of sulphamethoxazole acetylation.— T. B. Vree *et al.*, *Clin. Pharmacokinet.*, 1978, *3*, 319.

The pharmacokinetics of N^1-acetyl- and N^4-acetylsulphamethoxazole in healthy subjects.— T. B. Vree *et al.*, *Clin. Pharmacokinet.*, 1979, *4*, 310.

A review of the determination of the acetylator phenotype and pharmacokinetics of sulphonamides.— T. B. Vree *et al.*, *Clin. Pharmacokinet.*, 1980, *5*, 274.

Circulating concentrations of sulphamethoxazole might be increased in coeliac disease and Crohn's disease.— P. G. Welling and F. L. S. Tse, *J. clin. Hosp. Pharm.*, 1984, *9*, 163.

ADMINISTRATION IN RENAL FAILURE. For reference to the pharmacokinetics of sulphamethoxazole, see Administration in Renal Failure in Uses, below.

PROTEIN BINDING. For reference to the protein binding of sulphonamides and their capacity to displace bilirubin, see Pregnancy and the Neonate under Precautions, above.

Uses and Administration

The use of sulphamethoxazole and other sulphonamides has been limited by the increasing incidence of resistant organisms. Their main use is in the treatment of acute, uncomplicated urinary-tract infections, particularly those caused by *Escherichia coli*. They are not generally recommended for the treatment of pyelonephritis.

Sulphamethoxazole is an intermediate-acting sulphonamide given in a usual dose of 2 g initially, followed by 1 g twice daily. A total daily dose of 3 g should not be exceeded.

A suggested dose for children is 50 to 60 mg per kg body-weight initially, followed by 25 to 30 mg per kg twice daily. A total daily dose of 75 mg per kg should not be exceeded.

Reduction of dosage may be required in patients with renal impairment.

Sulphamethoxazole is used with trimethoprim in Co-trimoxazole, p.210.

A review of sulphonamides and trimethoprim. There are only minor differences in antimicrobial activity between sulphonamide derivatives and the choice of sulphonamide depends principally on pharmacokinetic properties. Sulphonamides, as single antibacterial agents, are of declining use, being replaced by other synthetic agents and by antibiotics which often have less toxic potential and are becoming cheaper relative to their previous cost.— D. Reeves, *Lancet*, 1982, *2*, 370. A brief historical perspective of the sulphonamides and their current clinical status. Today, the general indications for sulphonamides are restricted to the treatment of cystitis and to the eradication of meningococci from pharyngeal carriers, although in both these cases bacterial resistance has undermined their usefulness. Specific uses for sulphonamides include silver sulphadiazine for burns and sulphasalazine for ulcerative colitis. Sulphonamides demonstrate synergy with diaminopyrimidines such as trimethoprim and pyrimethamine, and numerous clinical indications for the co-trimoxazole combination have been proposed. The combination of pyrimethamine with sulphonamides is widely used for antimalarial prophylaxis and for the treatment of toxoplasmosis.— *Lancet*, 1985, *1*, 378.

A sulphonamide was considered to be an alternative to amphotericin or ketoconazole in the treatment of infections caused by *Paracoccidioides brasiliensis*.— *Med. Lett.*, 1986, *28*, 41.

For reference to the use of sulphonamides in the treatment of atypical mycobacterial infections, see Amikacin Sulphate, p.111.

ADMINISTRATION. The *U.S.* manufacturers of sulphamethoxazole have recommended that blood concentrations be measured in patients receiving sulphonamides for serious infections. The following concentrations of free sulphonamide in the blood were considered to be therapeutically effective; for most infections, 50 to 150 μg per mL, and for serious infections, 120 to 150 μg per mL. Concentrations of 200 μg per mL should not be exceeded since the incidence of adverse reactions may be increased.

ADMINISTRATION IN RENAL FAILURE. The normal half-life for sulphamethoxazole of 9 to 11 hours was increased to 20 to 50 hours in end-stage renal failure. Protein binding might be decreased in end-stage renal failure. The usual dosage interval of 12 hours could be increased to 18 hours in patients with a glomerular filtration-rate (GFR) of 10 to 50 mL per minute, and to 24 hours in those with a GFR of less than 10 mL per minute. A dosage supplement should be given to patients undergoing haemodialysis but not to those undergoing peritoneal dialysis.— W. M. Bennett *et al.*, *Am. J. Kidney Dis.*, 1983, *3*, 155.

NOCARDIOSIS. For reference to the use of sulphonamides in the treatment of infections caused by *Nocardia asteroides*, see Co-trimoxazole, p.212.

OTITIS MEDIA. A single bedtime dose of sulphamethoxazole daily appeared to be effective prophylaxis for preventing ear infections in young children prone to otitis media.— R. H. Schwartz *et al.*, *Archs Dis. Childh.*, 1982, *57*, 590.

PREGNANCY AND THE NEONATE. For reference to the use of sulphonamides during pregnancy, see Precautions, above.

RHEUMATOID ARTHRITIS. Evidence of a second-line effect of sulphamethoxazole 2 g daily by mouth for 3 months in 12 patients with rheumatoid arthritis. Eleven further patients, however, withdrew from the study because of adverse effects; these were mainly nausea and vomiting, but abnormal liver function tests occurred in one patient.— G. Ash *et al.*, *Br. J. Rheumatol.*, 1986, *25*, 285.

SEXUALLY TRANSMITTED DISEASES. *Chancroid*. For the use of sulphonamides in the treatment of chancroid, see Co-trimoxazole, p.213.

Gonorrhoea. For the use of sulphonamides in the treatment of gonorrhoea, see Co-trimoxazole, p.213.

Granuloma inguinale. For the use of sulphonamides in the treatment of granuloma inguinale, see Co-trimoxazole, p.213.

Lymphogranuloma venereum. Sulphamethoxazole 1 g twice daily by mouth for 2 weeks, or equivalent doses of other sulphonamides, may be used as an alternative to tetracycline in the treatment of infections with lymphogranuloma venereum (LGV) biovars of *Chlamydia trachomatis*. Sulphonamides are active against LGV serotypes *in vitro* but have not been extensively evaluated in culture-confirmed cases of this infection.— WHO Expert Committee on Venereal Diseases and Treponematoses, Sixth Report, *Tech. Rep. Ser. Wld Hlth Org. No. 736*, 1986, p.125.

TRACHOMA. Topical therapy of trachoma with sulphonamides appears only partially effective; adequate treatment with oral sulphonamides requires full therapeutic doses for approximately 2 to 3 weeks and may be associated with adverse reactions. Topical and oral tetracyclines are generally used for the treatment of this condition.— C. R. Dawson *et al.*, *Guide to Trachoma Control*, Geneva, World Health Organization, 1981, p.40.

Preparations

Sulfamethoxazole Oral Suspension *(U.S.P.)*
Sulfamethoxazole Tablets *(U.S.P.)*

Proprietary Names and Manufacturers

Gantanol *(Roche, Austral.; Roche, Canad.; Roche, Norw.; Roche, Spain; Roche, Switz.; Roche, UK; Roche, USA)*.

The following names have been used for multi-ingredient preparations containing sulphamethoxazole— Azo Gantanol *(Roche, USA)*; Uro Gantanol *(Roche, Canad.)*.

4943-n

Sulphamethoxydiazine *(BAN)*.

AHR-857; Sulfameter *(USAN)*; Sulfamethoxydiazine; Sulfametin; Sulfametorinum; Sulfametoxydiazine *(rINN)*; Sulphamethoxydin. N^1-(5-Methoxypyrimidin-2-yl)sulphanilamide.
$C_{11}H_{12}N_4O_3S$=280.3.

CAS — 651-06-9.

Pharmacopoeias. In *Chin.*, *Cz.*, and *Roum.*

Sulphamethoxydiazine is a long-acting sulphonamide with actions and uses similar to those of sulphamethoxazole (see p.306). It has been given to adults in an initial dose of 1 g followed by 500 mg daily.

Proprietary Names and Manufacturers

Bayrena *(Bayer, Arg.; Bayer, Austral.; Bayer, Belg.; Bayer, Denm.; Bayer, Fr.; Bayer, Neth.; Bayer, S.Afr.; Bayer, Spain; Bayer, Swed.; Bayer, Switz.)*; Durenat *(Bayer, Ger.)*; Durenate *(Bayer, UK)*; Kinecid *(Schering, Spain)*; Kirocid *(Schering, Austral.)*; Kiron *(Schering, Belg.; Schering, Ital.)*; Panafil *(Arg.)*; Sulla *(Robins, Canad.; Robins, USA)*.

4944-h

Sulphamethoxypyridazine *(BAN)*.

Solfametossipiridazina; Sulfamethoxypyridazine *(rINN)*; Sulfamethoxypyridazinum. N^1-(6-Methoxypyridazin-3-yl)sulphanilamide.
$C_{11}H_{12}N_4O_3S$=280.3.

CAS — 80-35-3.

Pharmacopoeias. In *Br.*, *Braz.*, *Fr.*, *Hung.*, *Int.*, *It.*, *Jug.*, *Nord.*, and *Turk.* Also in *B.P. Vet.*

A white or yellowish-white, odourless or almost odourless, crystalline powder.

Very slightly **soluble** in water; sparingly soluble in alcohol; soluble 1 in 25 of acetone; dissolves in dilute mineral acids and solutions of alkali hydroxides. **Protect** from light.

4945-m

Acetyl Sulphamethoxypyridazine

N-(6-Methoxypyridazin-3-yl)-*N*-sulphanilylacetamide.
$C_{13}H_{14}N_4O_4S$=322.3.

CAS — 3568-43-2.

NOTE. Acetyl sulphamethoxypyridazine is to be distinguished from the N^4-acetyl derivative formed from sulphamethoxypyridazine by conjugation in the body.

1.15 g of monograph substance is approximately equivalent to 1 g of sulphamethoxypyridazine.

Adverse Effects, Treatment, and Precautions

As for Sulphamethoxazole, p.306.

If side-effects occur, sulphamethoxypyridazine has the disadvantage that several days are required for its elimination from the body.

Sulphamethoxypyridazine is readily soluble in urine, but the acetyl derivative is much less soluble. Adequate fluid intake should be maintained during therapy and for 2 or 3 days thereafter.

EFFECTS ON THE SKIN. Between 1958 and 1965, a total of 71 cases of erythema multiforme, the Stevens-Johnson syndrome, and epidermal necrolysis, Lyell's syndrome, associated with the use of sulphamethoxypyridazine were reported in the world medical literature.— H. Seneca, *J. Am. med. Ass.*, 1966, *198*, 975.

Antimicrobial Action and Resistance

As for Sulphamethoxazole, p.307.

Absorption and Fate

Sulphamethoxypyridazine is readily absorbed from the gastro-intestinal tract. After a single dose peak blood concentrations are reached within 5 hours; about 85% is bound to plasma proteins. Concentrations of sulphamethoxypyridazine in the cerebrospinal fluid of 5 to 10% of those in the blood have been reported. About 10 to 15% of sulphamethoxypyridazine in the blood is present as the N^4-acetyl derivative.

Sulphamethoxypyridazine is excreted slowly and may be detected in the blood for up to 7 days after stopping treatment; about 25% is excreted in the urine in 24 hours, and a further 20% in the next 24 hours; 40 to 70% is excreted as the acetyl derivative and a smaller amount as glucuronide conjugate.

The biological half-life of sulphamethoxypyridazine is variously reported as 34.6 to 63 hours.— W. A. Ritschel, *Drug Intell. & clin. Pharm.*, 1970, *4*, 332.

Uses and Administration

Sulphamethoxypyridazine is a long-acting sulphonamide with uses similar to those of sulphamethoxazole (see p.307). It has been given by mouth in doses of up to 500 mg daily.

Acetyl sulphamethoxypyridazine is hydrolysed in the gastro-intestinal tract forming sulphamethoxypyridazine; it is tasteless and has been used in liquid oral preparations.

The sodium derivative of sulphamethoxypyridazine is also used.

Sulphamethoxypyridazine has also been used with trimethoprim similarly to co-trimoxazole.

DERMATITIS HERPETIFORMIS. Mention that sulphamethoxypyridazine was being used to control the rash of dermatitis herpetiformis.— C. E. M. Griffiths *et al.*, *Br. J. Derm.*, 1985, *112*, 443.

Preparations

Sulphamethoxypyridazine Tablets *(B.P.)*

Proprietary Names and Manufacturers of Sulphamethoxypyridazine, its Salts, or Derivatives

Aseptilex *(Spain)*; Asey-Sulfa *(Spain)*; Durasul *(Spain)*; Eusulfa *(Ital.)*; Exazol *(Andreu, Spain)*; Ketiak *(Edmond Pharma, Ital.)*; Lederkyn *(Austral.; Belg.; Denm.; Ger.; Cyanamid, Ital.; Neth.; Switz.; Lederle, UK)*; Longisul *(Landerlan, Spain)*; Metazina *(Piam, Ital.)*; Microcid *(Ital.)*; Midicel *(Austral.; Parke, Davis, UK)*; Midikel *(Spain)*; Minikel *(Belg.)*; Sulfadepot *(Spain)*; Sulfadin *(Ital.)*; Sulfaintensa *(Spain)*; Sulfalex *(Ital.)*; Sulfamizina *(Ital.)*; Sulfamyd *(Ital.)*; Sulfatar *(Arnaldi, Ital.)*; Sulfa-Ulta *(Spain)*; Sulfocidan *(Cidan, Spain)*; Sulforetent *(Ital.)*; Sulfo-Rit *(Ital.)*; Sultirène *(Fr.)*; Unisulfa *(Angelini, Ital.)*.

The following names have been used for multi-ingredient preparations containing sulphamethoxypyridazine, its salts, or derivatives.— Velaten *(Corvi, Ital.)*.

4946-b

Sulphamoxole *(BAN).*
Sulfamoxole *(USAN, rINN)*; Sulphadimethyloxazole. N^1-(4,5-Dimethyloxazol-2-yl)sulphanilamide.
$C_{11}H_{13}N_3O_3S$=267.3.

CAS — 729-99-7.

Pharmacopoeias. In *Fr.*

Sulphamoxole is a sulphonamide with actions and uses similar to those of sulphamethoxazole (see p.306). It has been given by mouth in a dose of 500 mg twice daily.
For the use of sulphamoxole with trimethoprim, see Co-trifamole, p.205.

The biological half-life of sulphamoxole is variously reported as 4.4 to 10.6 hours.— W. A. Ritschel, *Drug Intell. & clin. Pharm.*, 1970, *4*, 332.

Sulphamoxole and sulfaquinoxaline, but not 11 other sulphonamides tested, inhibited the *in vitro* growth of promastigotes of *Leishmania major*. In contrast to the action of sulphonamides in bacteria and malaria parasites, the mode of action in *L. major* did not appear to be at the level of *de novo* synthesis of folate.— M. P. Peixoto and S. B. Beverley, *Antimicrob. Ag. Chemother.*, 1987, *31*, 1575.

Proprietary Names and Manufacturers
Justamil *(Anphar-Rolland, Fr.)*; Sulfmidil *(Astra, Swed.)*; Sulfuno *(Belg.; Ferrosan, Denm.; Nordmark, Ger.; Noristan, S.Afr.; Ferrosan, Swed.)*.

4947-v

Sulphanilamide *(BAN).*
Solfammide; Streptocidum; Sulfaminum; Sulfanilamide *(rINN)*; Sulfanilamidum. 4-Aminobenzenesulphonamide.
$C_6H_8N_2O_2S$=172.2.

CAS — 63-74-1.

Pharmacopoeias. In *Arg., Aust., Belg., Fr., Int., Mex., Nord., Pol., Port., Rus., Span.,* and *Turk.* Also in *B.P. Vet.*
Rus. P. also includes Streptocidum Solubile, sodium *p*-sulphamoylanilinomethanesulphonate,
$C_7H_9N_2NaO_5S_2$ = 288.3.

A white, or almost white, odourless crystalline powder. Slightly **soluble** in water and in alcohol; practically insoluble in chloroform and in ether; freely soluble in solutions of alkali hydroxides. **Store** in well-closed containers. Protect from light.

Sulphanilamide is a short-acting sulphonamide with properties similar to those of sulphamethoxazole (see p.306). It has been used topically, including as pessaries or as a vaginal cream.
Sulphanilamide is used in veterinary medicine.

A woman experienced acute transient myopia after applying a vaginal cream containing sulphanilamide.— M. A. Maddalena, *Archs Ophthal., N.Y.*, 1968, *80*, 186.

There was no evidence that sulphanilamide or sulphafurazole in vaginal creams were effective in most common forms of vaginitis.— *FDA Drug Bull.*, 1980, *10*, 6.

Proprietary Names and Manufacturers
Astreptine *(Belg.)*; Azol *(Andreu, Spain)*; Buco-Pental *(Pental, Spain)*; Exoseptoplix *(Belg.; Théraplix, Fr.)*; Oxidermiol Sulfamida *(Spain)*; Pental Micronizado *(Spain)*; Pulvi-bacteramide *(Bailly, Fr.)*; Streptamin *(Switz.)*; Streptosil *(Ital.)*; Sulfamida *(Spain)*; Sulfonamid-Spuman *(Ger.)*; Tablamide *(Fr.)*; Vagitrol *(Lemmon, USA)*.

The following names have been used for multi-ingredient preparations containing sulphanilamide— AVC *(Merrell Dow, Canad.)*; Rhinamid *(Bailly, Fr.: Bengué, UK)*; Tampovagan PSS *(Norgine, UK)*; Vagimide *(Legere, USA)*.

4948-g

Sulphaphenazole *(BAN).*
Sulfaphenazole *(rINN)*; Sulphaphenylpyrazol. N^1-(1-Phenylpyrazol-5-yl)sulphanilamide.
$C_{15}H_{14}N_4O_2S$=314.4.

CAS — 526-08-9.

Pharmacopoeias. In *Ind., Jug.,* and *Roum.*

Sulphaphenazole is a sulphonamide with actions and uses similar to those of sulphamethoxazole (see p.306). It has been administered by mouth.

INTERACTIONS. For the effect of sulphaphenazole on other drugs, see Cyclophosphamide p.612, and Phenytoin Sodium, p.409.

Proprietary Names and Manufacturers
Fenazolo *(Ital.)*; Orisul *(Ciba, Austral.; Ciba, Belg.; Ciba, Ger.; Ciba, Neth.; Ciba-Geigy, Switz.)*; Orisulf *(Ciba, NZ; Ciba, UK)*; Sulfapadil *(Padil, Ital.)*; Sulforal *(Farber-Ref, Ital.)*.

13286-z

Sulphaproxyline *(BAN).*
Sulfaproxyline *(rINN)*. N^1-(4-Isopropoxybenzoyl)sulphanilamide; *p*-Isopropoxy-*N*-sulphanilylbenzamide.
$C_{16}H_{18}N_2O_4S$=334.4.

CAS — 116-42-7.

Sulphaproxyline is a sulphonamide with actions and uses similar to those of sulphamethoxazole, p.306. It is used, usually with sulfamerazine, in the treatment of susceptible infections.

Proprietary Names and Manufacturers
The following names have been used for multi-ingredient preparations containing sulphaproxyline— Dosulfin *(Geigy, Ger.; Geigy, UK)*; Dosulfine *(Gomenol, Fr.)*.

4949-q

Sulphapyridine *(BAN).*
Sulfapyridine *(USAN, rINN)*. N^1-(2-Pyridyl)sulphanilamide.
$C_{11}H_{11}N_3O_2S$=249.3.

CAS — 144-83-2.

Pharmacopoeias. In *Arg., Br., Fr., Port., Span.,* and *U.S.*

A white or yellowish-white, odourless or almost odourless, crystalline powder or granules. It slowly darkens on exposure to light.
Soluble 1 in 3500 of water, 1 in 440 of alcohol, 1 in 65 of acetone; freely soluble in dilute mineral acids and aqueous solutions of alkali hydroxides. **Store** in well-closed containers. Protect from light.

4950-d

Sulphapyridine Sodium *(BANM).*
Soluble Sulphapyridine; Sulfapyridine Sodium *(rINNM)*.
$C_{11}H_{10}N_3NaO_2S$=271.3 (or with $1H_2O$ = 289.3).

CAS — 127-57-1 (anhydrous); 6101-41-3 (monohydrate).

Pharmacopoeias. In *Arg.*

Adverse Effects, Treatment, and Precautions
As for Sulphamethoxazole, p.306.
Adverse effects are common with sulphapyridine, and nausea and vomiting may render continued therapy difficult. Sulphapyridine and its acetyl derivative have low solubilities in urine and crystalluria may occur; solubilities are not greatly increased with increased pH.

Antimicrobial Action and Resistance
As for Sulphamethoxazole, p.307.

Absorption and Fate
Sulphapyridine is irregularly absorbed from the gastro-intestinal tract, and is bound to plasma proteins to the extent of 10 to 45%. It penetrates into the cerebrospinal fluid. Up to about 75% of sulphapyridine in the blood is present as the acetyl derivative. The rate of excretion appears to be irregular.

The biological half-life of sulphapyridine is 6.5 to 9.4 hours.— W. A. Ritschel, *Drug Intell. & clin. Pharm.*, 1970, *4*, 332.

Uses and Administration
Sulphapyridine is a short-acting sulphonamide, whose main use, because of its toxicity, is in the treatment of dermatitis herpetiformis when patients do not respond to dapsone and in certain other dermatoses. It is given by mouth in an initial dose of 2 to 4 g daily which may be reduced to the minimum effective maintenance dose when improvement occurs.
Sulphapyridine is a component of sulphasalazine. For discussion of the role of the sulphapyridine moiety when sulphasalazine is used to treat inflammatory bowel diseases and rheumatoid arthritis, see Action under Uses and Administration in Sulphasalazine, p.1110.
For reference to the use of sulphapyridine in the determination of acetylator status, see Sulphadimidine, p.304.

SKIN DISORDERS. A review on the use of sulphapyridine and dapsone in dermatology.— P. G. Lang, *J. Am. Acad. Derm.*, 1979, *1*, 479.

The favourable response of 2 young children with chronic bullous dermatosis to treatment with sulphapyridine.— N. B. Esterly *et al.*, *Archs Derm.*, 1977, *113*, 42.

Dermatitis herpetiformis. A review of dermatitis herpetiformis and its treatment, including the use of sulphapyridine.— S. I. Katz *et al.*, *Ann. intern. Med.*, 1980, *93*, 857.

Pemphigus. A retrospective review of patients with pemphigus seen between 1968 and 1975 showed that in 6 of 41 patients with bullous pemphigoid there was significant response to treatment with sulphapyridine or dapsone; in 5 of these patients the condition was completely controlled. Three other patients responded to treatment given together with corticosteroids and in 3 further patients response to treatment with sulphapyridine or dapsone was transient.— J. R. Person and R. S. Rogers, *Mayo Clin. Proc.*, 1977, *52*, 54.

Pyoderma gangrenosum. Sulphapyridine, 1 or 2 g three or four times daily, was effective, if given early in the course of the disease, in controlling the chronic indolent ulcers of pyoderma gangrenosum.— *J. Am. med. Ass.*, 1968, *206*, 2229.

Preparations
Sulfapyridine Tablets *(U.S.P.)*
Sulphapyridine Tablets *(B.P.)*

Proprietary Names and Manufacturers of Sulphapyridine
Dagenan *(Rhône-Poulenc, Canad.)*; M & B 693 *(May & Baker, Austral.; S.Afr.; May & Baker, UK)*.

4952-h

Sulphasomidine *(BAN).*
Sulfa-isodimérazine; Sulfaisodimidine; Sulfasomidine; Sulfisomidine *(rINN)*. N^1-(2,6-Dimethylpyrimidin-4-yl)sulphanilamide.
$C_{12}H_{14}N_4O_2S$=278.3.

CAS — 515-64-0.

NOTE. Sulfadimethylpyrimidine has been used as a synonym for sulphasomidine, and sulphadimethylpyrimidine is sometimes used as a synonym for sulphadimidine (p.303). Care should be taken to avoid confusion between the two compounds, which are isomeric.

Pharmacopoeias. In *Fr.* and *Ger.*

Sulphasomidine is a short-acting sulphonamide with actions and uses similar to those of sulphamethoxazole (see p.306). It has been applied topically and administered by mouth. The sodium salt has also been used.

The biological half-life of sulphasomidine was 6 to 8 hours.— W. A. Ritschel, *Drug Intell. & clin. Pharm.*, 1970, *4*, 332.

The effects of methoxy groups in the N^1-substituent of sulphonamides on the pathways of elimination; the acetylation-deacetylation equilibrium and mechanisms of renal excretion of sulfametomidine, sulphadimethoxine, and sulphasomidine. No acetylator phenotype was observed for these agents.— T. B. Vree *et al.*, *Pharm. Weekbl. Ned., scient. Edn*, 1984, *6*, 150.

Proprietary Names and Manufacturers
Aristamid *(Nordmark, Ger.)*; Elcosine *(Ciba, Fr.)*; Elkosin *(Ciba, Denm.; Ciba, Ger.; Ciba, Norw.; Ciba, Swed.)*; Elkosina *(Ciba, Spain)*; Elkosine *(Ciba, Belg.; Ciba, Neth.; Ciba, Switz.)*; Isosulf *(Apothekernes Laboratorium, Norw.)*; Pepsilphen *(Cambridge Laboratories, Austral.)*.

4953-m

Sulphathiazole *(BAN).*
M & B 760; Norsulfazolum; Solfatiazolo; Sulfanilamidothiazolum; Sulfathiazole *(USAN, rINN)*; Sulfathiazolum; Sulfonazolum. N^1-(Thiazol-2-yl)sulphanilamide.
$C_9H_9N_3O_2S_2$=255.3.

CAS — 72-14-0.

Pharmacopoeias. In *Arg., Aust., Belg., Br., Cz., Fr., Hung., Int., It., Mex., Pol., Port., Roum., Rus., Span., Swiss,* and *U.S.*

A white or yellowish-white, odourless or almost odourless, crystalline powder.
Very slightly **soluble** in water; slightly soluble in alcohol; soluble in acetone; dissolves in dilute mineral acids and solutions of alkali hydroxides and carbonates. **Store** in well-closed containers. Protect from light.

4954-b

Sulphathiazole Sodium *(BANM).*
Soluble Sulphathiazole; Sulfathiazole Sodium *(rINNM)*; Sulfathiazolum Natricum.
$C_9H_8N_3NaO_2S_2,5H_2O$=367.4.

CAS — 144-74-1 (anhydrous); 6791-71-5 (pentahydrate).

Pharmacopoeias. In *Arg., Aust.,* and *Mex.* (all $1\frac{1}{2}H_2O$); in *Int.* and *Pol.* ($1\frac{1}{2}H_2O$ or $5H_2O$); and in *Rus.* ($6H_2O$). Also in *B.P. Vet.* ($1\frac{1}{2}H_2O$ or $5H_2O$).

A white or yellowish-white crystalline powder or granules with a slight odour. 1.44 g of monograph substance is approximately equivalent to 1 g of sulphathiazole.
Freely **soluble** in water; soluble in alcohol. A solution in water containing the equivalent of 1% of the anhydrous substance has a pH of about 9 to 10. **Store** in well-closed containers. Protect from light.

Sulphathiazole is a short-acting sulphonamide with actions and uses similar to those of sulphamethoxazole (see p.306). It is now rarely used systemically due to its toxicity which includes a high incidence of crystalluria.
Sulphathiazole is used with other sulphonamides, usually sulfabenzamide and sulphacetamide, in preparations for the topical treatment of vaginal infections.
Sulphathiazole sodium was formerly given by intravenous injection.

For a study of the action of sulphathiazole (an ingredient in Sultrin vaginal tablets) against *Gardnerella vaginalis*, see Sulphacetamide Sodium, p.302.

Preparations

Sulphathiazole Tablets *(B.P.)*

Proprietary Names and Manufacturers
Cibazol *(Ger.; Switz.)*; Edifeno *(Faes, Spain)*; Formotablin Antidiarreico *(Wasserman, Spain)*; Septozol *(Switz.)*; Sulfamul *(Canad.)*; Sulfavitina *(CT, Ital.)*; Sulfintestin *(Hosbon, Spain)*; Thiazamide *(S.Afr.; May & Baker, UK)*.

The following names have been used for multi-ingredient preparations containing sulphathiazole— Gyne-Sulf *(G & W, USA)*; Septex Cream No. 2 *(Norton, UK)*; Streptotriad *(May & Baker, UK)*; Sulfex *(Smith Kline & French, UK)*; Sulphatriad *(May & Baker, UK)*; Sultrin *(Cilag, Austral.; Ortho, Canad.; Ortho-Cilag, UK; Ortho Pharmaceutical, USA)*; Tampovagan PSS *(Norgine, UK)*; Trysul *(Savage, USA)*.

13288-k

Sulphatolamide *(BAN).*
Sulfatolamide *(rINN)*. The *N*-sulphanilylthiourea salt of α-amino-*p*-toluenesulphonamide.
$C_{14}H_{19}N_5O_4S_3$=417.5.

CAS — 1161-88-2.

Sulphatolamide is a sulphonamide with properties similar to those of sulphamethoxazole (see p.306). It has been used topically in local infections.

Proprietary Names and Manufacturers
Marbadal *(Hartmann, Ger.)*; Marbaletten *(Bayer, Switz.)*.

4956-g

Sulphaurea *(BAN).*
Sulfacarbamide *(rINN)*; Sulfanilcarbamide; Sulphacarbamide; Sulphanilylurea; Urosulphanum. Sulphanilylurea monohydrate.
$C_7H_9N_3O_3S,H_2O$=233.2.

CAS — 547-44-4 (anhydrous); 6101-35-5 (monohydrate).

Pharmacopoeias. In *Rus.*

Adverse Effects, Treatment, and Precautions
As for Sulphamethoxazole, p.306.

Antimicrobial Action and Resistance
As for Sulphamethoxazole, p.307.

Absorption and Fate
Sulphaurea is readily absorbed from the gastro-intestinal tract and most of a single dose is removed from the blood in 12 hours. It is rapidly excreted; 10 to 15% of sulphaurea in the urine is in the form of the acetyl derivative. Sulphaurea and its acetyl derivative are relatively highly soluble in urine.

Uses and Administration
Sulphaurea is a sulphonamide which is used in the treatment of urinary-tract infections, usually in conjunction with a urinary analgesic such as phenazopyridine. The adult dose of sulphaurea is 1 g three times daily; children may be given one-half the adult dose.

Proprietary Preparations
Uromide *(Consolidated Chemicals, UK). Tablets,* sulphaurea 500 mg, phenazopyridine hydrochloride 50 mg.

Proprietary Names and Manufacturers
Euvernil *(Heyden, Ger.; Squibb, Switz.)*.

165-l

Sulphomyxin Sodium *(BAN).*
Sulfomyxin *(USAN)*; Sulfomyxin Sodium *(rINNM)*. A mixture of sulphomethylated polymyxin B and sodium bisulphite.

CAS — 1405-52-3.

Sulphomyxin sodium has actions and antimicrobial activity resembling those of polymyxin B (see p.290) and has been given by intramuscular injection.

Proprietary Names and Manufacturers
Thiosporin *(Wellcome, UK)*.

17000-k

Sultamicillin *(BAN, USAN, rINN).*
CP-49952. Penicillanoyloxymethyl (6*R*)-6-(D-2-phenylglycylamino)penicillanate *S'*,*S'*-dioxide.
$C_{25}H_{30}N_4O_9S_2$=594.7.

CAS — 76497-13-7.

Sultamicillin is a prodrug of ampicillin (p.116) and the beta-lactamase inhibitor sulbactam (p.298); it consists of the two compounds linked chemically as a double ester and formulated as the tosylate salt. During absorption the ester is hydrolysed, releasing equimolar quantities of ampicillin and sulbactam.
Sultamicillin has been tried in the treatment of infections where beta-lactamase-producing organisms might occur, including uncomplicated gonorrhoea, otitis media, and respiratory-tract infections. It has been administered by mouth or by injection, however, a high incidence of adverse gastro-intestinal effects has limited its use by mouth.

A cross-over study of the pharmacokinetics and acceptability of sultamicillin administered by mouth compared with ampicillin. Six healthy subjects received sultamicillin 250 mg (containing 147 mg of available ampicillin and 98 mg of sulbactam), sultamicillin 500 mg, and ampicillin 250 mg each given 8 hourly for one week. Mean peak serum concentrations of ampicillin of 2.1, 3.2, and 5.6 μg per mL were achieved 2 hours, 40 minutes, and 1 hour after ampicillin 250 mg, sultamicillin 250 and 500 mg, respectively. The serum half-lives of ampicillin after the administration of sultamicillin were estimated to be 1.2 and 1.0 hours following the 250- and 500-mg doses, respectively. Mean peak serum concentrations of sulbactam 2.2 and 4.0 μg per mL were achieved about 1 hour after administration of sultamicillin 250 and 500 mg, respectively; the serum half-lives were estimated to be 1.1 and 1.2 hours, respectively. Following ampicillin 250 mg, 35% of the dose was excreted in the urine; the 250- and 500-mg doses of sultamicillin (equivalent to 147 and 294 mg of ampicillin) produced ampicillin recovery rates of 62% and 80%, respectively. Thus the bioavailability of ampicillin was greater as sultamicillin. However, diarrhoea or loose stools occurred in all subjects given sultamicillin compared with only 1 subject given ampicillin, and therefore, intravenous or intramuscular injection may be the preferred mode of administration for sultamicillin.— S. Hartley and R. Wise, *J. antimicrob. Chemother.*, 1982, *10,* 49.

Pharmacokinetics and bioavailability of sultamicillin estimated by high performance liquid chromatography.— H. J. Rogers *et al., J. antimicrob. Chemother.*, 1983, *11,* 435.

Pharmacokinetics of sultamicillin in infants and children.— C. M. Ginsburg *et al., J. antimicrob. Chemother.*, 1985, *15,* 345.

Beneficial results in a study of 30 patients with acute exacerbations of chronic bronchitis who received sultamicillin 0.75 or 1 g twice daily for 10 days by mouth. Mean peak sputum concentrations of ampicillin of 0.7 and 1.2 μg per mL were found about 2 to 4 hours after administration of sultamicillin 0.75 or 1 g, respectively. Two of the 30 patients discontinued therapy due to severe diarrhoea and a further 7 patients noted loose stools.— B. I. Davies *et al., J. antimicrob. Chemother.*, 1984, *13,* 161.

Further references to the use of sultamicillin: S. C. Aronoff *et al., J. antimicrob. Chemother.*, 1984, *14,* 261 (childhood streptococcal pharyngitis); A. P. Ball *et al., ibid.*, 395 (urinary-tract infections); S. Jones *et al., Antimicrob. Ag. Chemother.*, 1985, *28,* 832 (acute sinusitis); J. Goldfarb *et al., ibid.*, 1987, *31,* 663 (superficial skin and soft tissue infections in children).

Proprietary Names and Manufacturers
Pfizer, UK.

166-y

Talampicillin Hydrochloride *(BANM, USAN, rINNM).*
BRL-8988. Phthalidyl (6*R*)-6-(α-D-phenylglycylamino)penicillanate hydrochloride.
$C_{24}H_{23}N_3O_6S,HCl$=518.0.

CAS — 47747-56-8 (talampicillin); 39878-70-1 (hydrochloride).

A white to off-white hygroscopic powder with a slight characteristic odour. 1.48 g of monograph substance is approximately equivalent to 1 g of ampicillin. **Soluble** 1 in 4 of water, 1 in 2 of chloroform, and 1 in 2 of methyl alcohol; practically insoluble in ether. A 1% solution in water has a pH of 3.0 to 4.5.

167-j

Talampicillin Napsylate *(BANM).*
Talampicillin Napsilate *(rINNM)*. Phthalidyl (6*R*)-6-(α-D-phenylglycylamino)penicillanate naphthalene-2-sulphonate.
$C_{24}H_{23}N_3O_6S,C_{10}H_8O_3S$=689.8.

CAS — 71953-01-0.

A white to pale yellow hygroscopic powder with a slight characteristic odour. 1.33 g of monograph substance is approximately equivalent to 1 g of talampicillin hydrochloride and 674 mg of ampicillin. Practically **insoluble** in water and ether; soluble 1 in 3 of chloroform, and 1 in 2 of methyl alcohol.

Adverse Effects and Precautions
As for ampicillin, (p.116).
Diarrhoea has been reported to occur less frequently with talampicillin.

EFFECTS ON THE GASTRO-INTESTINAL TRACT. Non-pseudomembranous colitis, presenting with abdominal pain and bloody diarrhoea, was associated with the administration of talampicillin by mouth in 2 patients.— M. Iida *et al., Endoscopy*, 1985, *17,* 64.

Antimicrobial Action
Talampicillin has the antimicrobial action of

ampicillin *in vivo* (see p.117). It possesses no intrinsic activity and requires to be hydrolysed to ampicillin.

Absorption and Fate

Talampicillin is more rapidly and completely absorbed from the gastro-intestinal tract than ampicillin, to which it is hydrolysed after administration. Peak plasma-ampicillin concentrations are obtained about 40 to 60 minutes after administration, and are approximately twice those obtained after an equivalent dose of ampicillin. The presence of food in the stomach does not appear to affect the total amount of talampicillin absorbed. About 50% of a dose is excreted in the urine as ampicillin within 6 hours.

Hydrolysis also releases the phthalidyl moiety of talampicillin and this is metabolised to 2-hydroxymethylbenzoic acid which is excreted in the urine.

Uses and Administration

Talampicillin is the phthalidyl ester of ampicillin and has the actions and uses of ampicillin (see p.119). It is given by mouth as the hydrochloride or napsylate and doses of the napsylate are expressed in terms of the hydrochloride. The usual dose is 250 to 500 mg of the hydrochloride three times daily; children may be given half the adult dose. Under 2 years, 3 to 7 mg per kg body-weight may be given three times daily. A single dose of 1.5 to 2 g may be used in the treatment of gonorrhoea often in association with probenecid 1 g by mouth.

For reference to comparative reviews and reports of aminopenicillins, see Ampicillin p.119.

GONORRHOEA. Of 460 women treated for uncomplicated gonorrhoea with a single dose of talampicillin 1.5 g by mouth and who returned for follow-up, treatment had failed in only 4 by the second week after treatment. All the strains of *Neisseria gonorrhoeae* isolated were sensitive to talampicillin.— K. C. Mohanty and R. B. Roy, *Br. J. vener. Dis.*, 1982, *58*, 180. Further favourable studies: R. R. Wilcox, *ibid.*, 1976, *52*, 184; J. D. Price *et al.*, *ibid.*, 1977, *53*, 113; S. Al-Egaily *et al.*, *ibid.*, 1978, *54*, 243.

Proprietary Preparations

Talpen *(Beecham Research, UK). Tablets*, talampicillin hydrochloride 250 mg.
Syrup, powder for reconstitution, talampicillin napsylate equivalent to talampicillin hydrochloride 125 mg/5 mL when reconstituted with water.

Proprietary Names and Manufacturers of Talampicillin Hydrochloride and Talampicillin Napsylate

Ausotal *(Ausonia, Ital.)*; Diampen *(Boizot, Spain)*; Fisiopen *(Hosbon, Spain)*; Penbritin-T *(Beecham, S.Afr.)*; Pre-cillin *(Edmond Pharma, Ital.)*; Talacilin *(Ferrer, Spain)*; Talat *(Polifarma, Ital.)*; Talmen *(Ferrer, Spain)*; Talpen *(Beecham Research, UK)*; Yamacillin *(Jpn)*.

18689-v

Teicoplanin *(BAN, USAN, rINN)*.

A-8327; DL-507-IT; L-12507; MDL-507; Teichomycin A_2.

CAS — 61036-62-2 (teichomycin); 61036-64-4 (teichomycin A_2).

An antibiotic obtained from cultures of Actinoplanes teichomyceticus or the same substance obtained by any other means.

Adverse Effects and Precautions

For reference to adverse effects reported in clinical studies of teicoplanin, see under Uses, below.

ADMINISTRATION IN RENAL FAILURE. For reference to the precautions to be observed in renal failure, see under Uses, Administration in Renal Failure, below.

ALLERGY. Allergic cross-reactivity of teicoplanin and vancomycin in one patient.— M. J. McElrath *et al.* (letter), *Lancet*, 1986, *1*, 47.

EFFECTS ON THE BLOOD. Clinical bleeding, associated with a circulating inhibitor of factor VIII occurred in a 57-year-old man and was possibly related to administration of teicoplanin and rifampicin.— J. C. Legrand *et al.* (letter), *J. antimicrob. Chemother.*, 1987, *19*, 850.

Studies in 8 healthy subjects concluding that in therapeutic concentrations teicoplanin has no effect on platelet function and blood coagulation. *In vitro*, platelet function was only affected by concentrations far higher than those achievable clinically.— G. Agnelli *et al.*, *Antimicrob. Ag. Chemother.*, 1987, *31*, 1609.

EFFECTS ON THE EAR. A report of ototoxicity associated with teicoplanin in a patient with Down's syndrome.— E. R. Maher *et al.* (letter), *Lancet*, 1986, *1*, 613.

INTERACTIONS. For reference to the binding *in vitro* of teicoplanin by cholestyramine, and to the effect of other agents on its antimicrobial activity, see under Antimicrobial Action, below.

Antimicrobial Action and Resistance

Teicoplanin has a similar mode of action and spectrum of antimicrobial activity to vancomycin (see p.333).

Studies *in vitro* have shown teicoplanin to have a similar range of antimicrobial activity to vancomycin. Among Gram-positive aerobic organisms it has good activity against *Staphylococcus aureus* including methicillin-resistant strains, *Staph. epidermidis*, streptococci, enterococci, *Listeria monocytogenes* and Group JK corynebacteria. The MIC of teicoplanin against these organisms has generally been reported to be similar to or slightly less than that of vancomycin. References: V. Fainstein *et al.*, *Antimicrob. Ag. Chemother.*, 1983, *23*, 497; H. C. Neu and P. Labthavikul, *ibid.*, *24*, 425; L. Verbist *et al.*, *ibid.*, 1984, *26*, 881.

A study of the mechanism of action of teicoplanin. Similarly to the other glycopeptides, vancomycin and ristocetin, teicoplanin interferes with bacterial cell wall synthesis by binding to the D-Ala-D-Ala termini of peptidoglycan or peptidoglycan precursors.— S. Somma *et al.*, *Antimicrob. Ag. Chemother.*, 1984, *26*, 917.

ACTIVITY AGAINST ANAEROBIC ORGANISMS. Teicoplanin is active against many Gram-positive anaerobes including *Clostridium* spp., *Propionibacterium acnes*, and *Peptostreptococcus* and *Peptococcus* spp. Of 57 Gram-positive anaerobic isolates tested *in vitro*, none had MIC values greater than 1.56 µg per mL for teicoplanin as compared with 3.12 µg per mL for vancomycin (Y. Glupczynski *et al.*, *Eur. J. clin. Microbiol.*, 1984, *3*, 50). In general teicoplanin was more active than vancomycin, particularly against *Clostridium difficile*. Newsom *et al.* (*J. antimicrob. Chemother.*, 1985, *15*, 648) reported MICs of less than 0.007 to 0.125 µg per mL for teicoplanin, and of 0.06 to 0.5 for vancomycin against 23 strains of *Cl. difficile*, and both drugs were more active than imipenem or a range of quinolones tested. Pantosti *et al.* (*Antimicrob. Ag. Chemother.*, 1985, *28*, 847) reported MICs of 0.12 to 0.5 µg per mL for teicoplanin and 0.25 to 1 µg per mL for vancomycin against 75 strains isolated from stool samples of patients with pseudomembranous colitis or antibiotic-associated diarrhoea. They also demonstrated teicoplanin to be almost entirely bound by cholestyramine *in vitro* whereas vancomycin was 80% bound.

ACTIVITY AGAINST ENTEROCOCCI. Teicoplanin had marked activity against 56 isolates of *Enterococcus faecalis* (*Streptococcus faecalis*) or *E. faecium* (*Str. faecium*), and was more active than vancomycin, ampicillin, piperacillin, gentamicin, or cefpirome. The MIC and MBC values against 90% of strains were both 1.6 µg per mL, whereas for vancomycin they were 4 and 16 µg per mL respectively.— P. H. Chandrasekar *et al.*, *J. antimicrob. Chemother.*, 1985, *16*, 179.

ACTIVITY AGAINST STAPHYLOCOCCI. Studies of the activity of teicoplanin against methicillin-resistant *Staphylococcus aureus*. MICs have been in the range of 0.06 to 1 µg per mL and have been similar to or slightly less than those of vancomycin: S. H. Guenthner and R. P. Wenzel, *Antimicrob. Ag. Chemother.*, 1984, *26*, 268; K. E. Aldridge *et al.*, *ibid.*, 1985, *28*, 634; E. C. Moorhouse *et al.*, *J. antimicrob. Chemother.*, 1985, *15*, 291.

See also under Resistance of Staphylococci, below.

ACTIVITY WITH OTHER ANTIMICROBIAL AGENTS. Variable interactions have been reported *in vitro* between teicoplanin and rifampicin. Varaldo *et al.* (*Antimicrob. Ag. Chemother.*, 1983, *23*, 402) reported mainly indifference against a range of Gram-positive bacteria and observed similar results with a combination of vancomycin and rifampicin. Van der Auwera and Joly (*J. antimicrob. Chemother.*, 1987, *19*, 313) demonstrated antagonism or synergy against *Staphylococcus aureus* depending on the relative concentrations of teicoplanin and rifampicin used, and Tuazon and Miller (*Antimicrob. Ag. Chemother.*, 1984, *25*, 411) observed a fairly high incidence of synergy against staphylococci; both groups of workers demonstrated higher rates of synergy between teicoplanin and rifampicin than between vancomycin and rifampicin.

Effects have also varied with combinations of teicoplanin and aminoglycosides. Watanakunakorn (*J. antimicrob. Chemother.*, 1987, *19*, 439) reported synergy with teicoplanin and rifampicin against just over half of the coagulase-negative staphylococci tested, whereas there was synergy or antagonism between teicoplanin and gentamicin or tobramycin against only a few strains. Tuazon and Miller observed a higher incidence of synergy against enterococci when an aminoglycoside was added to teicoplanin than to vancomycin. Van der Auwera and Klastersky (*ibid.*, 623) found an increase in serum bactericidal activity against most staphylococci when amikacin was added to teicoplanin or vancomycin administration in healthy subjects.

RESISTANCE OF STAPHYLOCOCCI. Reports of coagulase-negative staphylococci resistant to teicoplanin.

A strain of *Staphylococcus haemolyticus* was isolated from a patient 8 days after administration of teicoplanin for prophylaxis during cardiac surgery with an MIC and MBC to teicoplanin of 16 and 32 µg per mL respectively. The corresponding figures for vancomycin were both 2 µg per mL. No clinical infection was associated with the culture.— A. P. R. Wilson *et al.* (letter), *Lancet*, 1986, *2*, 973. Isolation of a strain of *Staph. epidermidis* with an MIC to teicoplanin of 12.8 µg per mL from a patient on continuous ambulatory peritoneal dialysis (CAPD) with peritonitis. In a study of 6 patients who had received vancomycin and/or gentamicin but not teicoplanin, 4 had significant numbers of commensal coagulase-negative staphylococci with reduced sensitivity to teicoplanin. All such isolates studied so far have been susceptible to vancomycin but resistant to gentamicin.— A. C. Grant *et al.* (letter), *ibid.*, 1166. Eleven of 29 isolates of *Staph. haemolyticus* had MIC values for teicoplanin of 16 to 32 µg per mL and should be considered resistant.— A. Arioli and R. Pallanza (letter), *ibid.*, 1987, *1*, 39.

For reference to resistance to teicoplanin in isolates of *Staphylococcus haemolyticus* with reduced susceptibility to vancomycin, see Vancomycin Hydrochloride, p.333.

Absorption and Fate

Pharmacokinetics of teicoplanin after administration of single doses of 2 or 3 mg per kg body-weight by 30-minute intravenous infusion to groups of 5 healthy subjects. Peak serum-teicoplanin concentrations ranged from 12.7 to 19.5 µg per mL for the lower dose and from 20.3 to 23.5 µg per mL for the higher dose. The half-life of teicoplanin was between 20 and 77 hours, and a mean of 52% of a dose was excreted unchanged in the urine within 96 hours.— G. L. Traina and M. Bonati, *J. Pharmacokinet. Biopharm.*, 1984, *12*, 119.

After the intramuscular administration of teicoplanin 3 mg per kg body-weight to 6 healthy subjects a mean peak plasma concentration of 7.1 µg per mL was obtained after approximately 2 hours. Bioavailability was 90% as compared with intravenous administration. The mean half-life after either intramuscular or intravenous administration of doses of 3 or 6 mg per kg ranged from 44 to 47 hours, and total urinary recovery from 46 to 54%.— L. Verbist *et al.*, *Antimicrob. Ag. Chemother.*, 1984, *26*, 881.

Six healthy subjects were administered teicoplanin 440 mg by intravenous injection over 2 to 4 minutes. The mean serum-teicoplanin concentration remained above 3.5 µg per mL throughout the study period of 49 hours. Penetration of teicoplanin into blister fluid was 77.4% and maximum concentrations were obtained after 2 to 3 hours. The mean elimination half-life was 34.5 hours and ranged from 28.7 to 38.2 hours. Elimination of teicoplanin in the urine was slow; 25% of the dose was excreted within 24 hours and 48% within 96 hours. Teicoplanin was reported to be 90% bound to plasma proteins.— C. A. M. McNulty *et al.*, *J. antimicrob. Chemother.*, 1985, *16*, 743.

A comparison of the pharmacokinetics and bactericidal activity of teicoplanin and vancomycin. After intravenous infusion over 3 minutes of teicoplanin sodium 200 mg to 6 healthy subjects, mean serum concentrations of 22.2, 6.9, 4.9, and 1.9 µg per mL occurred 1, 12, 24 and 96 hours after the infusion respectively. The mean half-life of teicoplanin was 33.2 hours as compared with 5.8 hours for vancomycin, and 62 and 92% of the administered dose of the 2 drugs was excreted in the urine. The serum bactericidal activities of both drugs at one hour against *Staphylococcus aureus* and *Staph. epidermidis* were comparable. Serum killing-rate studies showed similar killing-rates for *Staph. epidermidis*, but a slower rate of killing of *Staph. aureus* with teicoplanin than with vancomycin. No useful serum bactericidal activity or killing was observed for either drug against *Enterococcus faecalis*.— H. Lagast *et al.*, *J. antimicrob. Chemother.*, 1986, *18*, 513.

For further reference to serum concentrations of teicoplanin, see under Endocarditis Prophylaxis in Uses, below.

ADMINISTRATION IN RENAL FAILURE. For reference to the pharmacokinetics of teicoplanin in renal failure, see under Administration in Renal Failure in Uses, below.

DIFFUSION INTO BODY TISSUES AND FLUIDS. Seven patients, aged 1 to 74 years, with bacterial meningitis were given an intravenous dose of teicoplanin 400 mg by infusion over 15 minutes on two occasions 3 days apart. In one patient concentrations of 0.8 and 1.3 µg per mL were achieved in the CSF 2 hours after the infusions, otherwise no patient showed a concentration above 0.3 µg per mL as measured 2 to 8 hours after the infusion.— J. P. Stahl *et al.* (letter), *J. antimicrob. Chemother.*, 1987, *20*, 141.

Uses and Administration

Teicoplanin is a glycopeptide antibiotic with similar properties to vancomycin hydrochloride (see p.334). It may be administered by the intravenous or intramuscular route.

A review of teicoplanin.— A. H. Williams and R. N. Grüneberg, *J. antimicrob. Chemother.*, 1984, *14*, 441.

Evaluation of teicoplanin in the treatment of severe infections caused by Gram-positive bacteria. Forty-seven patients with infections in a variety of body sites were given a loading dose of 400 mg followed by 200 mg once daily given by the intravenous or intramuscular route. Overall, the clinical response-rate was 63.8% and eradication of the causative organisms after a minimum follow-up of 4 weeks was 53.2%. Cure or improvement occurred more often in non-bacteraemic than in bacteraemic patients. Failure of teicoplanin therapy did not appear to be related to inadequate serum concentrations. The following adverse effects were reported: superinfections due to Gram-negative bacteria (6 patients), mild thrombophlebitis (2), pain at the site of intramuscular injection (1), moderate pruritus (1), allergic maculopapular rash requiring discontinuation (1), and mild and transient eosinophilia (2).— Y. Glupczynski *et al.*, *Antimicrob. Ag. Chemother.*, 1986, *29*, 52. In a similar study, 69 patients received an intravenous bolus dose of teicoplanin 400 mg, followed by a single daily intramuscular or intravenous dose of 200 to 400 mg (3 to 6 mg per kg body-weight). In the most severe illnesses or in mixed infections, another antibiotic was also given, including rifampicin, an aminoglycoside, ceftazidime, or piperacillin. Another agent was also added if therapy with teicoplanin alone was not successful. The overall clinical response was 86%, and the microbiological response 73%. Side-effects were: superinfections (6 patients), drug fever (2), pain at the site of the injection (3), nausea and vomiting (2), neutropenia (1). Two patients had an anaphylactoid reaction with bronchospasm after the first injection of teicoplanin and the administration of the drug was interrupted. Treatment had to be discontinued in 5 cases.— S. Pauluzzi *et al.*, *J. antimicrob. Chemother.*, 1987, *20*, 431.

ADMINISTRATION IN RENAL FAILURE. The half-life of teicoplanin was increased from 41 hours in healthy subjects to 157 hours in anuric patients. Only 6.8% of an intravenous dose was recovered in the peritoneal fluid of patients on continuous ambulatory peritoneal dialysis (CAPD), and only traces of the drug were detected in the dialysate of patients on haemodialysis. In patients with renal insufficiency, either the dose could be decreased or the dosage interval increased; alterations by a factor of 2 in mild to moderate renal impairment and a factor of 3 in severe impairment were suggested.— M. Bonati *et al.*, *Clin. Pharmacokinet.*, 1987, *12*, 292. See also G. L. Traina *et al.*, *Eur. J. clin. Pharmac.*, 1986, *31*, 501.

Further references to the pharmacokinetics of teicoplanin in patients with renal impairment: C. Falcoz *et al.*, *Antimicrob. Ag. Chemother.*, 1987, *31*, 1255; Y. Domart *et al.*, *ibid.*, 1600.

ENDOCARDITIS. The use of teicoplanin in 12 patients with bacterial endocarditis; the drug was administered as a loading dose of 400 mg followed by a once daily injection of 200 mg by intramuscular or intravenous injection.— A. Webster *et al.*, *Postgrad. med. J.*, 1987, *63*, 621.

Prophylaxis. Three groups of 10 patients undergoing dental extraction were given either intramuscular teicoplanin 200 mg, amoxycillin 3 g by mouth, or no prophylaxis. The antibiotics were administered one hour prior to the procedure. Detectable bacteraemia due to oral streptococci and anaerobes occurred in 6, 4, and 10 patients in the 3 groups respectively although the degree of bacteraemia was less in those given antibiotics. Substantially fewer anaerobic organisms were isolated from patients given amoxycillin compared with teicoplanin. The mean serum-teicoplanin concentration at the time of extraction was 1 µg per mL. When tested *in vitro* against isolates of oral streptococci both teicoplanin and amoxycillin showed only minimal bactericidal activity during the first few hours of incubation.— J. P. Maskell *et al.*, *J. antimicrob. Chemother.*, 1986, *17*, 651. In a similar study, 3 groups of 40 patients were given either a rapid intravenous injection of teicoplanin 400 mg after induction of anaesthesia, an intramuscular injection of amoxycillin 1 g shortly before anaesthesia, or no antibiotic. Teicoplanin was more effective than amoxycillin in reducing the prevalence of streptococcal bacteraemia immediately following the extraction, although after 4 and 24 hours of exposure to amoxycillin there was a clear reduction in streptococcal isolations compared with the control group. The mean serum concentration of teicoplanin at the time of the extraction and 4 hours later was 36.8 and 9.7 µg per mL respectively.— D. C. Shanson *et al.*, *ibid.*, 1987, *20*, 85.

NEUTROPENIA. Febrile episodes in granulocytopenic patients with acute leukaemia were treated with amikacin and ceftazidime, with or without the addition of teicoplanin. Teicoplanin was administered intravenously in an initial dose of 8 mg per kg body-weight (maximum of 600 mg) followed by 5 mg per kg (maximum of 400 mg) once daily. An improvement occurred in 14 of 25 (56%) of episodes treated with the 2-drug regimen, and in 18 of 22 (82%) treated with the 3 drugs. The higher response-rate with the teicoplanin regimen was most evident in infections caused by Gram-positive organisms and in patients with profound and persistent neutropenia. These good results were confirmed by treatment with the 3 drugs of 20 febrile episodes in 14 patients undergoing allogenic bone-marrow transplantation; 7 of 8 Gram-positive bacteraemias related to central venous catheters were cleared, and only one required catheter removal.— A. Del Favero *et al.*, *Antimicrob. Ag. Chemother.*, 1987, *31*, 1126.

PERITONITIS. In a pilot study, 11 patients on continuous ambulatory peritoneal dialysis with 12 episodes of proven Gram-positive peritonitis were treated with teicoplanin; 20 mg was added to each litre of dialysis fluid, and a single intravenous dose of 400 mg given if the patient was febrile. The dosage regimen was modified in the second and third week of treatment to maintain serum concentrations of below 10 µg per mL. Cure was achieved in 10 patients. Teicoplanin was well tolerated; there was no evidence of ototoxicity as determined by serial audiometry, or of further decline in residual renal function. All 10 patients remained well at follow-up after 4 weeks to 11 months. Emergence of teicoplanin-resistant strains of coagulase-negative staphylococci did not occur. In future studies aztreonam was to be added to treatment with teicoplanin to provide cover for Gram-negative infection.— L. O. Neville *et al.* (letter), *Lancet*, 1987, *1*, 1320.

Proprietary Names and Manufacturers

Targocid *(Merrell, Fr.)*.

17002-t

Temocillin Sodium *(BANM, rINNM)*.

BRL-17421; Temocillin Disodium. The disodium salt of (6*S*)-6-[2-carboxy-2-(3-thienyl)acetamido]-6-methoxypenicillanic acid.

$C_{16}H_{16}N_2Na_2O_7S_2$=458.4.

CAS — 66148-78-5 (temocillin); 61545-06-0 (disodium salt).

NOTE. Temocillin is *USAN*.

Adverse Effects and Precautions

As for Benzylpenicillin Sodium, p.132.

A rise in serum-alkaline phosphatase concentration was observed in one patient during treatment with temocillin. The alkaline phosphatase was shown to originate from bone.— G. Lindsay *et al.*, *Drugs*, 1985, *29*, *Suppl.* 5, 191.

EFFECTS ON THE BLOOD. In a study of 8 healthy subjects, the administration of intravenous temocillin 4 g every 12 hours for 7 days had no significant effect on bleeding time, although bleeding stopped less abruptly in 4 subjects, and appeared to have little, if any effect on platelet responsiveness.— B. Nunn *et al.*, *Antimicrob. Ag. Chemother.*, 1985, *27*, 858.

EFFECTS ON THE GASTRO-INTESTINAL TRACT. Studies in *hamsters* (R.J. Boon and A.S. Beale, *Drugs*, 1985, *29*, *Suppl.* 5, 57) and *mice* (H.G. De Vries-Hospers *et al.*, *ibid.*, 227) have suggested that temocillin might not have a significant effect on the resistance of the gastro-intestinal tract to colonisation. Mittermayer (*ibid.*, 43) administered intravenous temocillin 1 g twice daily for 6 to 7 days to 6 healthy subjects; the only significant change in the intestinal flora was a decrease in the number of *Enterobacteriaceae* during and immediately after treatment, although there was a slight increase in the number of enterococci. De Vries-Hospers suggested that for this reason, temocillin might be suitable for the selective decontamination of the gastro-intestinal tract. Temocillin, administered in various intramuscular doses, was quite effective for this purpose in 7 of 10 healthy subjects. Veringa and van der Waaij (*J. antimicrob. Chemother.*, 1984, *14*, 605) demonstrated in 6 healthy subjects that temocillin was resistant to inactivation by faecal suspensions *in vitro*; it was, however, completely inactivated in one patient.

EFFECTS ON THE LIVER. Plasma-alanine aminotransferase concentrations were increased in 2 patients without recorded liver function impairment after treatment with temocillin.— B. Schulze and H. -D. Heilmann, *Drugs*, 1985, *29*, *Suppl.* 5, 207.

Antimicrobial Action

Temocillin is a bactericidal antibiotic active *in vitro* against the majority of Gram-negative aerobic bacteria, including many of the *Enterobacteriaceae, Haemophilus influenzae, Branhamella catarrhalis*, and *Neissera gonorrhoeae*. It exhibits no significant activity against *Pseudomonas aeruginosa* and *Acinetobacter* spp., Gram-negative anaerobes such as *Bacteroides fragilis*, and Gram-positive organisms. Temocillin is highly resistant to a wide range of beta-lactamases produced by Gram-negative bacteria.

The MIC values for susceptible *Enterobacteriaceae* are generally in the range of 1 to 16 µg per mL. Other susceptible organisms often have MIC values lower than this.

Studies investigating the *in vitro* activity of temocillin have shown sensitive *Enterobacteriaceae* to include *Citrobacter* and *Enterobacter* spp., *Escherichia coli, Klebsiella, Proteus, Providencia, Salmonella, Serratia, Shigella*, and *Yersinia* spp. (D. Greenwood *et al.*, *Antimicrob. Ag. Chemother.*, 1982, *22*, 198; K. Jules and H.C. Neu, *ibid.*, 453; I. Phillips *et al.*, *J. antimicrob. Chemother.*, 1982, *10*, 271; A.M. Clark and S.J.V. Zemcov, *ibid.*, 1983, *11*, 319; H.W. Van Landuyt *et al.*, *Drugs*, 1985, *29*, *Suppl.* 5, 1).

There have been many studies comparing the activity of temocillin with other penicillins, particularly carbenicillin, mezlocillin, piperacillin, and ticarcillin, as well as with cephalosporins (H.W. Van Landuyt *et al.*, *Drugs*, 1985, *29*, *Suppl.* 5, 1; A. Bauernfeind, *ibid.*, 9; M. Gobernado and E. Canton, *ibid.*, 24; H.Y. Chen and J.D. Williams, *ibid.*, 85; J. Martinez-Beltran *et al.*, *ibid.*, 91). In general the intrinsic activity of temocillin against susceptible organisms is similar to the broad-spectrum penicillins and first and second generation cephalosporins, but less than that of the third generation cephalosporins. Due to its high stability against a wide range of beta-lactamases produced by Gram-negative bacteria, however, (R.A. Edmondson and C. Reading, *ibid.*, 64) it is also active against many beta-lactamase-producing strains of bacteria including *Haemophilus influenzae* (H.Y. Chen and J.D. Williams, *ibid.*, 85) and *Neisseria gonorrhoeae* (A.E. Jephcott and S.I. Egglestone, *ibid.*, 18). Although the newer cephalosporins are generally resistant to beta-lactamases, there have been reports of these cephalosporins being inactivated. Temocillin has been shown to be active against such strains (B. Slocombe *et al.*, *ibid.*, 49; R. Malottke and J. Potel, *ibid.*, 67), and also against strains showing multiple resistance to beta-lactam agents (J. Focht *et al.*, *ibid.*, 78). Thus temocillin demonstrates a uniform activity, with MIC values within a narrow range against a wide variety of Gram-negative organisms.

Like other penicillins, temocillin is considered to exert its antibacterial action through binding to penicillin-binding proteins (R. Labia *et al.*, *Antimicrob. Ag. Chemother.*, 1984, *26*, 335; *Drugs*, 1985, *29*, *Suppl.* 5, 98).

There has been a report (K.H. Tjian *et al.*, *Eur. J. clin. Microbiol.*, 1984, *3*, 39) suggesting that temocillin may have useful activity against *Chlamydia trachomatis*, the MIC values being in the range of 5 to 10 µg per mL.

ACTIVITY WITH OTHER ANTIMICROBIAL AGENTS. Some beta-lactam antibiotics which are stable to beta-lactamases have been reported to induce the production of beta-lactamases and hence to antagonise the action of non-beta-lactamase-stable beta-lactams when combined *in vitro*. Jules and Neu (*Antimicrob. Ag. Chemother.*, 1982, *22*, 453) have demonstrated antagonism between temocillin and ticarcillin or cephazolin against some bacteria. Verbist and Verhaegen (*Drugs*, 1985, *29*, *Suppl.* 5, 32) and Slocombe *et al.* (*ibid.*, 49) showed a moderate degree of synergy and only occasional antagonism when temocillin was combined with these and other beta-lactam antibiotics and tested against strains of *Enterobacteriaceae, Pseudomonas aeruginosa*, or Gram-positive organisms. Combinations of temocillin with aminoglycosides against a similar range of organisms (B. Slocombe *et al., ibid.*, 49; H.-M. Just *et al., ibid.*, 74) have shown synergy against a small proportion of strains and indifference against the majority.

Chen and Williams (*ibid.*, 85) could demonstrate no synergy between temocillin and clavulanic acid *in vitro*; this is probably due to the stability of temocillin to beta-lactamases.

RESISTANCE. Resistance to temocillin has been observed *in vitro* in some strains of bacteria usually susceptible to temocillin, particularly in strains of *Serratia marcescens* (J. Martinez-Beltran *et al., Drugs*, 1985, *29, Suppl.* 5, 91); this resistance does not appear to be related to hydrolysis by beta-lactamases.

Resistance of temocillin to Gram-negative bacilli such as *Pseudomonas aeruginosa* appears to be due to a failure of the drug to pass through the cell wall of the organism, whereas resistance to Gram-positive bacteria is probably due to poor binding to penicillin-binding proteins (K. Jules and H.C. Neu, *Antimicrob. Ag. Chemother.*, 1982, *22*, 453; *Drugs*, 1985, *29, Suppl.* 5, 98).

Absorption and Fate

Temocillin is not absorbed from the gastro-intestinal tract. After intramuscular and intravenous administration, high and prolonged plasma concentrations are obtained. It has a plasma half-life of about 4.5 hours, which is longer than for most penicillins. About 85% of temocillin in the circulation is bound to plasma proteins. A small proportion of temocillin is metabolised and excreted in the faeces via the bile; 70 to 80% is excreted in the urine mainly by glomerular filtration.

The mean peak serum concentration of temocillin after the intramuscular administration of 0.25, 0.5, or 1 g to groups of 6 healthy subjects was 25, 48, and 70 µg per mL respectively, achieved after about 2 hours. After the 0.5-g dose drug concentrations were maintained above 20 µg per mL for 8 hours, and after the 1-g dose concentrations were above 18 µg per mL for 12 hours. After administration of a single intravenous dose of 1 g to 6 subjects, serum concentrations were in excess of 25 µg per mL for up to 6 hours, and of 12 µg per mL after 12 hours. Temocillin could not be detected in the serum after 24 hours.— B. Slocombe *et al., Antimicrob. Ag. Chemother.*, 1981, *20*, 38. See also.— B. Hampel *et al., Drugs*, 1985, *29, Suppl.* 5, 99.

Concentrations of temocillin in serum and urine were measured after administration of the pro-drug, BRL-20330 to 12 healthy subjects.— M. J. Basker *et al., J. antimicrob. Chemother.*, 1986, *18*, 399.

DIFFUSION INTO BODY TISSUES AND FLUIDS. Several studies have investigated the excretion of temocillin in the bile with a view to its use in the treatment and prophylaxis of infections of the gall bladder and biliary tract. Maudgal *et al.* (*Drugs*, 1985, *29, Suppl.* 5, 146) reported that 2% of a dose of temocillin given by intravenous injection was excreted in the bile, using duodenal perfusion studies in 6 healthy subjects. This study, and other studies in patients with a variety of biliary-tract or gall-bladder diseases (F. Spelsberg *et al., ibid.*, 122; G.J. Poston *et al., ibid.*, 140; M. Uwaydah *et al., ibid.*, 186) have all found concentrations of temocillin in the bile to be widely variable after intramuscular or intravenous administration. They have all concluded, however, that in most cases they would be above the MIC for the majority of common biliary-tract pathogens. Concentrations in the bile were generally higher than in serum, and were higher in common bile-duct bile than in gall-bladder bile. Poston *et al.* could detect no temocillin in the gall-bladder bile of 3 patients with non-functioning gall bladders. Uwaydah *et al.* found lower concentrations in bile from patients with bile-duct obstruction than without, and even lower concentrations in those with biliary sepsis. Concentrations in gall-bladder tissue have been found to be lower than in the bile, but again were considered to be sufficiently high to inhibit most likely organisms.

Ten patients with severe respiratory-tract infections who were producing copious purulent sputum, were given intravenous temocillin 1 g twice daily for 6 to 15 days. Sputum concentrations were usually poor on the first day, but by the final day of treatment reached concentrations ranging between 1.5 and 2.8 µg per mL. In two patients given 2 g twice daily, temocillin was detected in the sputum one hour after the first dose and rose to about 2 µg per mL after 12 hours.— J. S. Legge *et al., Drugs*, 1985, *29, Suppl.* 5, 118.

A study of the penetration of temocillin into the CSF after intravenous administration to 8 patients with some degree of impairment of the blood-brain barrier. Like other penicillins, temocillin does not appear to enter the CSF readily and would not be expected to accumulate in patients with normal renal function.— O. Brückner *et al., Drugs*, 1985, *29, Suppl.* 5, 162.

Temocillin was widely distributed in the body as demonstrated by concentrations measured in various tissue samples.— J. G. Gould *et al., Drugs*, 1985, *29, Suppl.* 5, 167. See also.— R. R. Wittke *et al., ibid.*, 221.

Further studies measuring the concentration of temocillin in various body tissues and fluids: R. Wise *et al., J. antimicrob. Chemother.*, 1983, *12*, 93 (peritoneal fluid); T. Bergan *et al., Drugs*, 1985, *29, Suppl.* 5, 114 (peripheral lymph); W. Cowan *et al., ibid.*, 151 (lung tissue); E. R. Weissenbacher *et al., ibid.*, 178 (gynaecological tissues).

DRUG EXCRETION. The increase in the renal clearance of temocillin with increasing plasma concentrations could be accounted for by a decrease in protein binding. Concomitant administration of probenecid resulted in a decrease in renal clearance of temocillin, but not an increase in serum concentrations. Tubular excretion is probably less important for temocillin than for other penicillins.— D. Overbosch *et al., Drugs*, 1985, *29, Suppl.* 5, 128.

Uses and Administration

Temocillin sodium is the 6-α-methoxy derivative of ticarcillin, and is used for the treatment of infections caused by susceptible bacteria. It is administered by the intramuscular or intravenous route in doses equivalent to 0.5 to 2 g of temocillin twice daily. Temocillin sodium may be administered in a 0.5 to 1% solution of lignocaine hydrochloride to avoid pain on intramuscular injection.

BRL-20330, an ester of temocillin which is converted to temocillin after absorption from the gastro-intestinal tract, is under investigation.

Proceedings of a symposium on temocillin.— *Drugs*, 1985, *29, Suppl.* 5, 1-243.

Temocillin has been investigated in a wide variety of infections considered to be caused by susceptible Gram-negative bacteria. These include the treatment of biliary-tract infections (M. Uwaydah *et al., Drugs*, 1985, *29, Suppl.* 5, 186; D. Tanphaichitra *et al., ibid.*, 201) or their prophylaxis during surgery (R.R. Wittke *et al., ibid.*, 221), enteric infections (D. Tanphaichitra *et al., ibid.*, 201), gonorrhoea (G. Reimer *et al., ibid.*, 210), gynaecological infections (E.R. Weissenbacher *et al., ibid.*, 178), peritonitis (M. Pfeiffer and R.R.E. Fock, *ibid.*, 194), respiratory-tract infections (J.M.B. Gray *et al., ibid.*, 197), septicaemia (H.W. Van Landuyt *et al., ibid.*, 182; G. Offenstadt *et al., ibid.*, 213), and uncomplicated and complicated infections of the urinary tract (M. Libert and C.C. Schulman, *Curr. ther. Res.*, 1983, *33*, 887; J. Kosmidis, *Drugs*, 1985, *29, Suppl.* 5, 172; H.W. Asbach *et al., ibid.*, 175). It has also been investigated for selective decontamination of the gastro-intestinal tract (see Adverse Effects and Precautions, above).

ADMINISTRATION IN RENAL FAILURE. Temocillin sodium, equivalent to temocillin 15 mg per kg body-weight was administered by intravenous injection to 28 patients with varying degrees of renal impairment. The half-life increased to 3.5, 12.7, and 17.5 hours as the creatinine clearance decreased from greater than 70, between 20 and 70, and less than 20 mL per minute respectively. Thus it was recommended that patients with a creatinine clearance of greater than 20 mL per minute could be given temocillin 1 to 2 g every 24 hours, and those with a creatinine clearance of less than 20 mL per minute, 1 g every 48 hours.

In the 7 patients receiving haemodialysis, the half-life was 15.7 and 7.3 hours off and on dialysis respectively, and the haemodialysis extraction ratio was reported to be 6%. A dose of 1 g every 48 hours, preferably at the end of dialysis, or 0.5 g daily if dialysis is carried out every day, could be given to such patients. Continuous ambulatory peritoneal dialysis in 5 patients resulted in little change in the pharmacokinetics of temocillin, and only 8% of the dose was recovered from the dialysate over 24 hours. These patients could be given 1 g every 48 hours.— J. Boelaert *et al., Drugs*, 1985, *29, Suppl.* 5, 109.

A study of the pharmacokinetics of temocillin in renal failure, and the use of dose-reduction factors to calculate a suitable dose.— D. Höffler and P. Koeppe, *Drugs*, 1985, *29, Suppl.* 5, 135.

Further references: N. Wright *et al., J. antimicrob. Chemother.*, 1983, *11*, 481; A. Leroy *et al., ibid.*, *12*, 47.

Proprietary Names and Manufacturers

Negaban *(Beecham, Belg.)*; Temopen *(Beecham-Wülfing, Ger.)*;

Manufacturers also include—*Beecham Research, UK.*

168-z

Tetracycline *(BAN, USAN, rINN).*

Tetraciclina; Tetracyclinum. A hydrated form of (4*S*,4a*S*,5a*S*,6*S*,12a*S*)-4-Dimethylamino-1,4,4a,5,5a,6,11,12a-octahydro-3,6,10,12,12a-pentahydroxy-6-methyl-1,11-dioxonaphthacene-2-carboxamide.

$C_{22}H_{24}N_2O_8$=444.4.

CAS — 60-54-8 (anhydrous); 6416-04-2 (trihydrate).

Pharmacopoeias. In *Br., Eur., Fr., Ind., It., Jpn, Neth., Roum., Rus., Swiss,* and *U.S.*

A yellow, odourless, crystalline powder. It darkens in strong sunlight in a moist atmosphere. The *B.P.* specifies not less than 1000 units per mg calculated with reference to the dried substance; *U.S.P.* specifies a potency of not less than 975 µg of tetracycline hydrochloride calculated on the anhydrous basis. Tetracycline (anhydrous) 1 g is approximately equivalent to 1.08 g of tetracycline hydrochloride.

Soluble 1 in 2500 of water and 1 in 50 of alcohol; soluble in methyl alcohol; sparingly soluble in acetone; freely soluble in dilute acids and, with decomposition, in solutions of alkali hydroxides; practically insoluble in chloroform and ether. The *B.P.* specifies that a 1% suspension in water has a pH of 3.5 to 6.0; the *U.S.P.* specifies a pH of 3 to 7. The potency of tetracycline is reduced in solutions having a pH below 2. **Store** in airtight containers. Protect from light.

169-c

Tetracycline Hydrochloride *(BANM, USAN, rINNM).*

$C_{22}H_{24}N_2O_8$,HCl=480.9.

CAS — 64-75-5.

Pharmacopoeias. In *Aust., Belg., Br., Braz., Chin., Cz., Egypt., Eur., Fr., Ger., Hung., Ind., Int., It., Jpn, Jug., Neth., Nord., Pol., Port., Roum., Rus., Swiss, Turk.,* and *U.S. U.S.* also includes Epitetracycline Hydrochloride.

A yellow, odourless, hygroscopic, crystalline, amphoteric powder. Tetracycline hydrochloride darkens in moist air when exposed to strong sunlight. The *B.P.* specifies not less than 950 units per mg calculated with reference to the dried substance; *U.S.P.* specifies not less than 900 µg per mg.

Soluble 1 in 10 of water and 1 in 100 of alcohol; soluble in aqueous solutions of alkali hydroxides and carbonates, although it is rapidly destroyed by alkali hydroxide solutions; practically insoluble in acetone, chloroform, and ether. A 1% solution in water has a pH of 1.8 to 2.8. The *B.P.* and *U.S.P.* specify a pH of 2 to 3 for the injection. Solutions in water become turbid on standing owing to hydrolysis and precipitation of tetracycline. The potency of tetracycline hydrochloride is reduced in solutions having a pH below 2.

Store in airtight containers. Protect from light.

Incompatibility has been reported with alkalis, amikacin sulphate, aminophylline, amphotericin, ampicillin sodium, soluble barbiturates, benzylpenicillin, carbenicillin sodium, cefapirin sodium, cephalothin sodium, cephazolin sodium, chloramphenicol sodium succinate, chlorothiazide sodium, chlorpromazine, cloxacillin sodium, cyanocobalamin, dimenhydrinate, erythromycin salts, heparin sodium, hydrocortisone sodium succinate, methicillin sodium, methyldopa, nitrofurantoin sodium, novobiocin sodium, oxacillin sodium, phenytoin sodium, polymyxin B sulphate, prochlorperazine, riboflavine, sodium bicarbonate, sulphadiazine sodium, sulphafurazole diethanolamine, vitamin B complex, and warfarin sodium. Incompatibility has also been reported, generally less consistently, with methyldopate hydrochloride, metoclopramide hydrochloride, various inorganic ions including calcium, magnesium, aluminium, manganese, and iron, and also with blood.

The effect of vehicle on tetracycline applied to the eye.— J. Y. Massey *et al.*, *Am. J. Ophthal.*, 1976, *81*, 151.

EFFECT OF GAMMA-IRRADIATION. Sterilisation of tetracycline ophthalmic ointments by gamma-irradiation.— R. A. Nash, *Bull. parent. Drug Ass.*, 1974, *28*, 181.

The sterilisation of tetracycline hydrochloride by gamma-irradiation.— G. P. Jacobs, *Pharm. Acta Helv.*, 1977, *52*, 302.

EPIMERISATION. Epimerisation at carbon atom 4 of tetracycline occurred at pH 2 to 6, producing a ratio of epimer to tetracycline of 0.6:1 in 24 hours. The epi-isomers were less active therapeutically. Alkaline degradation occurred but tetracyclines were fairly stable to oxidation.— H. S. Carlin and A. J. Perkins, *Am. J. Hosp. Pharm.*, 1968, *25*, 270.

INCOMPATIBILITY. Aqueous tetracycline solutions showed maximum degradation, by air and light, in the presence of *riboflavine* 0.01 to 0.1%. Maximum degradation at 37° and pH 4.5, in the absence of light, occurred with riboflavine 1%. Ascorbic acid suppressed the degradation of tetracycline by riboflavine.— L. J. Leeson and J. F. Weidenheimer, *J. pharm. Sci.*, 1969, *58*, 355.

When reconstituted with bacteriostatic water for injection and mixed with 500 mL of Ringer's injection or lactated Ringer's injection, each with 40 mmol of potassium chloride added, tetracycline hydrochloride 500 mg, as Achromycin Intravenous (*Lederle*), maintained at least 90% of its stated potency for 24 hours at ambient conditions and for 48 hours when refrigerated. Under these conditions chelation with calcium salts was not a problem, confirming that tetracycline can be given in compound sodium lactate injection.— M. Roach, *Lederle* (letter), *Pharm. J.*, 1978, *1*, 143.

Tetracyline hydrochloride was incompatible with a total nutrient admixture, resulting in signs of creaming, oiling out, and phase separation. The disruptive effect of tetracycline hydrochloride on the lipid emulsion was attributed to the highly acid pH of the ascorbic acid present in the tetracycline product.— R. J. Baptista and R. W. Lawrence, *Am. J. Hosp. Pharm.*, 1985, *42*, 362.

Visual incompatibilities were reported when 1 mL of a solution containing tetracycline hydrochloride 2.5 mg per mL or minocycline hydrochloride 0.2 mg per mL was mixed with 1 mL of a solution of morphine sulphate 1 mg per mL, hydromorphone hydrochloride 0.2 mg per mL, or pethidine hydrochloride 10 mg per mL; all solutions were prepared in 5% glucose injections. The colour of the admixtures changed from pale yellow to light green within the first hour.— A. L. Nieves-Cordero *et al.*, *Am. J. Hosp. Pharm.*, 1985, *42*, 1108.

LOSS OF ACTIVITY. A study of the effect of the antibiotic and preservative on each other's binding to pharmaceutical adjuvants in mixtures containing benzalkonium chloride or chlorocresol and tetracycline hydrochloride.— M. A. El-Nakeeb and M. H. Ali, *Mfg Chem.*, 1976, *47*, (Mar.), 37.

STABILITY. Tetracycline hydrochloride lost 10% potency when stored for 2 months at 37° and 66% relative humidity. The presence of citric acid increased the degradation of tetracycline hydrochloride to anhydrotetracycline and epianhydrotetracycline when stored under the same conditions.— V. C. Walton *et al.*, *J. pharm. Sci.*, 1970, *59*, 1160.

STABILITY IN SOLUTION. Tetracycline hydrochloride in intravenous solutions of pH 3 to 5 was chemically stable for 6 hours, but had lost 8 to 12% potency in 24 hours at room temperature.— E. A. Parker, *Am. J. Hosp. Pharm.*, 1967, *24*, 434.

Tetracycline hydrochloride 1 g per 100 mL lost 50% activity in glucose injection after 14 days at 25°.— J. F. Gallelli *et al.*, *Am. J. Hosp. Pharm.*, 1969, *26*, 630.

Tetracycline hydrochloride 970 mg per litre was stable in sodium chloride injection for 24 hours. The pH of the mixture was 3.1.— R. L. Nedich, *Bull. parent. Drug Ass.*, 1973, *27*, 228.

A study on the effects of pH on the degradation of tetracycline in aqueous solution at 60°. Maximum stability occurred at about pH 3.— B. Vej-Hansen and H. Bundgaard, *Arch. Pharm. Chemi, scient. Edn*, 1978, *6*, 201.

The stability of alcoholic solutions for topical use containing tetracycline hydrochloride and 4-epitetracycline hydrochloride.— R. Vancaillie *et al.*, *J. Pharm. Belg.*, 1985, *40*, 168.

See also above under Incompatibility.

STABILITY IN SUSPENSION. A study of the stability of tetracycline suspensions demonstrated that slightly acid pH values between 4 and 7 produced good stability. The solubility of tetracycline is about constant over pH 4 to 7, but below this pH solubility increases rapidly. Tetracycline in solution at pH 2 to 6 undergoes epimerisation with the formation of 4-epitetracycline. The equilibrium ratio is affected by the pH and is in favour of tetracycline at higher pH values. At lower pH values anhydrotetracycline and 4-epianhydrotetracycline are also formed. Epitetracycline is about five times more soluble than tetracycline at pH 5.5. The stability of aqueous tetracycline suspensions at pH 4 to 7 is due to the poor solubility of tetracycline and the relatively better solubility of epitetracycline, so that formation of epitetracycline stops when equilibrium between epimers is reached in the liquid phase of the suspension.— A. Grobben-Verpoorten *et al.*, *Pharm. Weekbl. Ned., scient. Edn*, 1985, *7*, 104.

Units

One unit of tetracycline is contained in 0.00101833 mg of the second International Standard Preparation (1970) of tetracycline hydrochloride which contains 982 units per mg.

Adverse Effects

The side-effects of tetracycline hydrochloride are common to all tetracyclines. Gastro-intestinal effects including nausea, vomiting, and diarrhoea are common especially with high doses and most are attributed to irritation of the mucosa. Oesophageal ulceration has also been reported, particularly after ingestion of capsules or tablets with insufficient water, at bedtime. Oral candidiasis, vulvovaginitis, and pruritus ani occur mainly due to overgrowth with *Candida albicans* and there may be overgrowth of resistant coliform organisms, such as *Pseudomonas* spp. and *Proteus* spp., causing diarrhoea. More serious superinfection with resistant staphylococci causing enterocolitis, and also pseudomembranous colitis due to *Clostridium difficile* have occasionally been reported.

Usual therapeutic doses given to patients with renal disease increase the severity of uraemia with increased excretion of nitrogen and losses of sodium, accompanied by acidosis and hyperphosphataemia. These effects are related to the dose and the severity of renal impairment and are probably due to the anti-anabolic effects of the tetracycline.

Severe and sometimes fatal hepatotoxicity associated with fatty changes in the liver and pancreatitis has been reported in pregnant women given tetracycline intravenously for pyelonephritis, and in patients with renal impairment or those given high doses.

Tetracyclines are deposited in deciduous and permanent teeth causing discoloration and enamel hypoplasia. They are also deposited in calcifying areas in bone and the nails and when given in therapeutic doses to young infants or women during the late stages of pregnancy tetracyclines interfere with bone growth. An increase in intracranial pressure, which may be associated with a bulging fontanelle in infants, has been reported in patients given tetracyclines.

Allergic reactions to tetracycline and its analogues have been reported, usually as skin reactions; cross-sensitisation between tetracyclines is common. Photosensitivity of the skin and nails has occurred, especially after demeclocycline, and onycholysis may be associated with nail discoloration. Local irritation can occur when tetracyclines are given parenterally and thrombophlebitis may follow intravenous injections. A Jarisch-Herxheimer-like reaction has been reported in patients with relapsing fever treated with tetracycline.

Haemolytic anaemia, eosinophilia, neutropenia, and thrombocytopenia have been reported rarely. The use of out-of-date or deteriorated tetracyclines has been associated with the development of a reversible Fanconi-type syndrome characterised by polyuria and polydipsia with nausea, proteinuria, glycosuria, acidosis, aminoaciduria, hypophosphataemia, and hypokalaemia; these effects have been attributed to the presence of degradation products.

Increased urinary excretion of ascorbic acid during tetracycline therapy.— A. C. M. Windsor *et al.*, *Br. med. J.*, 1972, *1*, 214. Folate deficiency with megaloblastic anaemia was associated with tetracycline 250 mg which had been given twice daily for 3 years.— C. C. Jones, *Ann. intern. Med.*, 1973, *78*, 910. Tetracyclines reduce serum vitamin B_{12}, B_6, and pantothenic acid concentrations, and long-term treatment might possibly cause vitamin deficiencies particularly in the elderly. There is no evidence that the use of vitamin B complex is beneficial in patients who are taking short- or long-term antibiotics.— C. W. H. Havard, *Br. med. J.*, 1984, *289*, 741.

Myospherulotic lesions, which appeared to be composed of shrunken distorted erythrocytes, were associated with the packing of cavities, following ENT surgery, with soft paraffin-based ointments containing tetracycline.— *Lancet*, 1978, *2*, 358.

A report of irregular menses or amenorrhoea in 5 patients associated with the administration of tetracycline in the treatment of acne.— S. P. Stone (letter), *J. Am. Acad. Derm.*, 1979, *1*, 151.

For comment on the effect of tetracyclines on host defence mechanisms, see under Doxycycline Hydrochloride, p.217.

ALLERGY. Although allergic reactions to tetracyclines are considerably less common than with beta-lactam antibiotics, various allergic reactions, usually affecting the skin, have been reported. In a retrospective study of 86 patients with fixed eruptions during the period 1971–1980, tetracyclines were the agents responsible in 5 cases (K. Kauppinen and S. Stubb, *Br. J. Derm.*, 1985, *112*, 575). Tetracycline has also been associated with drug fever in 2 patients (P.A. Mackowiak and C.F. LeMaistre, *Ann. intern. Med.*, 1987, *106*, 728). A fatal anaphylactic reaction to tetracycline has been reported (C.V. Singh *et al.*, *Anaesthesia*, 1977, *32*, 268), and tetracyclines have been incriminated in hypersensitivity myocarditis (*Lancet*, 1985, *2*, 1165).

See also under Effects on the Skin, below.

DEPOSITION IN BONES AND TEETH. Treatment with tetracyclines can permanently stain children's teeth a greyish-brown or yellow colour; children are at risk from the fourteenth week *in utero*, when calcification of deciduous teeth begins, to their seventh year when calcification of the permanent teeth is complete (*Drug & Ther. Bull.*, 1984, *22*, 55). In a survey carried out in Belfast in 1982 (M.J. Kinirons, *Br. med. J.*, 1983, *287*, 1515), the proportion of children with tetracycline deposits in their teeth was about 15% compared with 70% in a similar survey in 1973, indicating that exposure of young children to tetracyclines had decreased considerably. However, this level of exposure was still unacceptably high (C. Gilks, *ibid.*, 1984, *288*, 151); although the number of paediatric preparations in the UK has declined, continued availability encourages their general use. Many workers feel that tetracycline syrups should be withdrawn completely. The lower age limit at which tetracyclines may be used in children has not been agreed, but their use in children under 8 years has been strongly condemned (*Drug & Ther. Bull.*, 1984, *22*, 55) and some prefer to avoid administration of tetracyclines in children up to the age of 12 years. However, in a very few clinical situations tetracyclines have been used in paediatric patients where no alternative, less toxic drug is available (K.H. Rhodes and C.M. Johnson, *Mayo Clin. Proc.*, 1983, *58*, 158). Little has been done about the cosmetic problem of children exposed to tetracyclines, although some workers have bleached stained teeth (K.D. Hay and P.C. Reade, *Drugs*, 1983, *26*, 268).

EFFECTS ON THE BLOOD. Prothrombin activity was modestly or markedly reduced in 14 patients given tetracycline intravenously.— R. L. Searcy *et al.*, *Clin. Res.*, 1964, *12*, 230.

A report of haemolytic anaemia associated wtih tetracycline therapy in a 43-year-old patient.— M. B. Simpson *et al.*, *New Engl. J. Med.*, 1985, *312*, 840.

EFFECTS ON THE EYE. Acute transient myopia has been reported rarely in some patients taking tetracyclines. It is possible that transient hydration of the lens leads to its greater thickening and so the eye becomes myopic.— S. I. Davidson, *Br. J. Hosp. Med.*, 1980, *24*, 24.

A report of conjunctival pigmentation in a 26-year-old man associated with long-term oral administration of tetracycline and minocycline for the treatment of acne vulgaris. He had been taking tetracycline for more than 12 years and minocycline for over 6 years.— D. M. Brothers and A. A. Hidayat, *Ophthalmology*, 1981, *88*, 1212. Tetracycline fluorescence was detected in the conjunctiva of 5 patients who were receiving long-term tetracycline by mouth.— P. N. Dilly and I. A. Mackie, *Br. J. Ophthal.*, 1985, *69*, 25.

Permanent yellow discoloration of the foetal corneas and lenses was detected following administration of tetracycline in a total dose of 6 to 8 g by mouth to 8 pregnant women during the first 8 to 12 weeks of pregnancy.— L. Krejčí and I. Brettschneider, *Ophthalmic Paediatr. Genet.*, 1983, *3*, 59.

For a report of ocular irritation after concurrent treatment with tetracyclines in patients using a contact lens solution containing thiomersal, see under Thiomersal, p.970.

EFFECT ON THE GASTRO-INTESTINAL TRACT. Oesophageal ulceration was associated with the ingestion of tetracycline or doxycycline capsules in 3 patients. Capsules taken at night were believed to have lodged in the oesophagus.— T. D. Crowson *et al.*, *J. Am. med. Ass.*, 1976, *235*, 2747. See also K. S. Channer and D. Hollanders, *Br. med. J.*, 1981, *282*, 1359.

Of 1517 hospital in-patients in a Boston Collaborative Drug Surveillance Program who received tetracycline none developed colitis.— R. R. Miller and H. Jick, *Clin. Pharmac. Ther.*, 1977, *22*, 1. For a report of pseudomembranous colitis associated with a tetracycline, see under Oxytetracycline Hydrochloride, p.279.

Steatorrhoea occurred in 6 of 27 patients given tetracycline or demeclocycline for labelling bone prior to bone biopsy.— T. H. Mitchell *et al.*, *Br. med. J.*, 1982, *285*, 780. These modest rises in faecal fat should not be regarded as evidence of tetracycline toxicity unless confirmed by more precise methods of measurement of faecal fat output.— F. G. Simpson (letter), *ibid.*, 1423.

A report of metallic taste associated with oral tetracycline therapy in one patient.— L. D. Magnasco and A. J. Magnasco, *Clin. Pharm.*, 1985, *4*, 455.

EFFECTS ON THE KIDNEY. Tetracycline could produce 3 types of renal disease: acute renal failure without oliguria in patients with fatty liver or pancreatitis, a Fanconi-like syndrome, and uraemia in patients with impaired renal function.— H. T. Lew and S. W. French, *Archs intern. Med.*, 1966, *118*, 123. See also *Lancet*, 1978, *2*, 558.

Simultaneous lactic acidosis and Fanconi syndrome developed in a 41-year-old woman following ingestion of tetracycline tablets which had accidentally become wet, been dried, and stored for over a year.— J. Montoliu *et al.*, *Br. med. J.*, 1981, *283*, 1576.

EFFECTS ON MENTAL STATE. Reports of lassitude by patients receiving therapeutic doses of antibiotics including tetracycline.— J. H. Scotson, *Practitioner*, 1984, *228*, 669.

EFFECTS ON THE NERVOUS SYSTEM. Tetracyclines have been associated with benign intracranial hypertension. The patients tend to be young, often 22 years old or less, and predominantly female. Patients have usually been receiving tetracyline for acne, but the time to the development of symptoms has been variable, ranging from 24 hours to several months. Symptoms regress rapidly on stopping the drug. Several mechanisms by which tetracyclines cause benign intracranial hypertension have been proposed including interference with the action of antidiuretic hormone, interference with cerebrospinal fluid reabsorption, or potentiation of vitamin A to cause benign intracranial hypertension. However, the mechanism involved remains obscure.— D. Chadwick, *J. antimicrob. Chemother.*, 1982, *9*, 88.

Concern at the increasing number of reports of benign intracranial hypertension associated with long-term oral therapy of acne with a tetracycline. Reports received were: minocycline (9), tetracycline (5), demeclocycline (2), and oxytetracycline (1); almost all had received normal dosage regimens.— *UK* Committee on Safety of Medicines, *Current Problems*, No. 23, 1988.

EFFECTS ON THE NEUROMUSCULAR SYSTEM. Myopathy apparently due to tetracycline treatment for acne vulgaris has been reported in a 15-year-old girl (D. Sinclair and C. Phillips, *New Engl. J. Med.*, 1982, *307*, 821). There have also been reports of respiratory paralysis after administration of tetracyclines to unanaesthetised myasthenic patients (C.B. Pittinger *et al.*, *Anesth. Analg. Curr. Res.*, 1970, *49*, 487). The neuromuscular blockade seems to involve primarily the post-synaptic receptor to which tetracycline reversibly binds causing decreased sensitivity to acetylcholine (R.J.M. Lane and P.A. Routledge, *Drugs*, 1983, *26*, 124; J.M. Hunter, *Br. J. Anaesth.*, 1987, *59*, 46).

EFFECTS ON THE SKIN. Tetracycline had been implicated in the Stevens-Johnson syndrome.— D. B. Coursin, *J. Am. med. Ass.*, 1966, *198*, 113.

In 3 patients fixed drug reactions occurred 2 to 4 days after starting tetracycline therapy.— S. T. Brown (letter), *J. Am. med. Ass.*, 1974, *227*, 801.

Tetracycline was implicated as the causative agent in 2 patients with toxic epidermal necrolysis.— H. L. Chan, *J. Am. Acad. Derm.*, 1984, *10*, 973. Toxic epidermal necrolysis and markedly elevated serum amylase in a 59-year-old woman following tetracycline treatment.— F. M. Tatnall *et al.* (letter), *Br. J. Derm.*, 1985, *113*, 629.

See also under Allergy, above.

Photosensitivity. Photosensitivity accounted for 35% of the 235 adverse reactions to tetracyclines recorded by the Australian Registry. It was more frequent with the longer acting forms such as demeclocycline, doxycycline, and methacycline.— *Med. J. Aust.*, 1972, *1*, 435.

Porphyria-like skin changes in 5 patients taking tetracycline and exposed to the sun.— J. H. Epstein *et al.*, *Archs Derm.*, 1976, *112*, 661.

Photo-onycholysis in 2 patients receiving low-dose tetracycline therapy for acne.— H. Baker (letter), *Br. med. J.*, 1977, *2*, 519.

JARISCH-HERXHEIMER REACTION. For comparison of the severity of the Jarisch-Herxheimer-like reaction in patients with louse-borne relapsing fever treated with a tetracycline or a penicillin, see under Rolitetracycline Nitrate, p.293.

LUPUS ERYTHEMATOSUS. Tetracycline had been implicated in the provocation of lupus erythematosus in 3 patients.— C. A. Domz *et al.*, *Ann. intern. Med.*, 1959, *50*, 1217.

PREGNANCY AND THE NEONATE. For adverse effects on the foetus following administration of tetracycline to the mother, see Deposition in Bones and Teeth, and Effects on the Eye, above.

Precautions

The tetracyclines with the exception of doxycycline and possibly minocycline are generally contra-indicated in patients with renal impairment. Care must be taken when liver function is impaired. Potentially hepatotoxic drugs should not be given with tetracyclines nor should compounds such as methoxyflurane that can be nephrotoxic.

The use of tetracyclines in pregnancy should be avoided. When administered to women during the latter half of pregnancy, to nursing mothers, or during childhood up to the age of 12 years, permanent discoloration of the child's teeth may occur.

Tetracyclines should not be given to patients with known hypersensitivity to any of this group of antibiotics. They should be avoided in patients with systemic lupus erythematosus. Symptoms of myasthenia gravis may be exacerbated by tetracyclines.

Absorption of tetracyclines is diminished by milk, alkalis, aluminium hydroxide, and the salts of other trivalent and divalent cations including calcium, iron, and magnesium, when these are taken concomitantly.

Because of possible antagonism of the action of the penicillins by predominantly bacteriostatic tetracyclines it has been recommended that the two types of antibiotic should not be given concomitantly, especially when a rapid bactericidal action is necessary.

Tetracycline may interfere with some diagnostic tests including determination of urine catecholamines or glucose.

INTERACTIONS. The absorption of tetracycline is reduced by certain drugs and foods including milk and milk products because of chelation with calcium ions (K.R. Hunter, *Prescribers' J.*, 1981, *21*, 177), drugs which release calcium such as calcium polystyrene sulphonate or polycarbophil calcium, and other metal ions including iron salts (P.J. Neuvonen *et al.*, *Br. J. clin. Pharmac.*, 1975, *2*, 94), zinc salts (K.-E. Andersson *et al.*, *Eur. J. clin- Pharmac.*, 1976, *10*, 59), magnesium- and aluminium-containing preparations such as antacids or sucralfate (M.J.S. Langman and C.J. Hawkey, *Prescribers' J.*, 1984, *24*, 106). It has been suggested that binding of tetracyclines to organic macromolecules within the gut is increased by calcium and probably also by other di- and trivalent metal ions resulting in impaired permeation across the absorbing epithelium (P. F. D'Arcy and J. C. McElnay, *Drug Intell. & clin. Pharm.*, 1987, *21*, 607). Other drugs which affect the absorption of tetracycline include other antacid preparations such as sodium bicarbonate, probably due at least in part to the limited dissolution of tetracycline at pH 5 to 6 compared with pH 1 to 3 (W.H. Barr *et al.*, *Clin. Pharmac. Ther.*, 1971, *12*, 779), and antidiarrhoeal agents such as bismuth salicylate or kaolin-pectin which have an adsorptive mechanism of action (K.S. Albert *et al.*, *J. pharm. Sci.*, 1979, *68*, 586). Serum-tetracycline concentrations also appear to be reduced by test meals compared with the fasting state (P.G. Welling and F.L.S. Tse, *J. antimicrob. Chemother.*, 1982, *9*, 7). Other drugs which affect the pH or motility of the gastro-intestinal tract may also affect the absorption of tetracycline: there have been variable reports with cimetidine (J.J. Cole *et al.*, *Lancet*, 1980, *2*, 536; H.J. Rogers *et al.*, *ibid.*, 694; M. Garty and A. Hurwitz, *Clin. Pharmac. Ther.*, 1980, *28*, 203), whilst metoclopramide has been reported to increase the absorption of tetracycline (*Med. Lett.*, 1985, *27*, 21).

Tetracyclines may affect other drugs taken concomitantly. They may enhance the effects of oral anticoagulants and methotrexate, and diminish the effectiveness of oral contraceptives (see p.1391). For reports of the effect of tetracycline on lithium carbonate, see p.367, and on theophylline, see p.1529.

Tetracyclines should not be administered concurrently with other potentially hepatotoxic drugs. These included erythromycin estolate, triacetyloleandomycin, chloramphenicol, sulphonamides, aminosalicylic acid, isoniazid, chlorpromazine and other phenothiazine derivatives, phenytoin and other anti-epileptics, cinchophen, phenylbutazone, chlorpropamide, methyltestosterone, phenindione, and chlorothiazide.— H. F. Dowling and M. H. Lepper, *J. Am. med. Ass.*, 1964, *188*, 307.

When 1957 patients were screened for increases in blood-urea-nitrogen concentrations, rises were confined to those patients receiving diuretics in addition to tetracycline therapy. Patients on diuretic therapy should be given alternative antibiotics.—A report from the Boston Collaborative Drug Surveillance Program, *J. Am. med. Ass.*, 1972, *220*, 377.

PORPHYRIA. Tetracyclines were considered to be unsafe in patients with acute porphyria although there is conflicting experimental evidence on porphyrinogenicity.— M. R. Moore and K. E. L. McColl, *Porphyrias, Drug Lists*, Glasgow, Porphyria Research Unit, University of Glasgow, 1987.

PREGNANCY AND THE NEONATE. Tetracyclines should be avoided in pregnant women. Severe adverse effects such as lethal fatty liver degeneration have been reported in pregnant women undergoing tetracycline therapy, often at high dosage; the danger of adverse effects to the woman is probably greatest during the last trimester of pregnancy. The concentration of tetracyclines in umbilical cord blood amounts to about 50% of the concentration in the maternal blood and adverse effects typical of tetracyclines have been seen in the foetus following intra-uterine exposure. Tetracyclines given during the period of calcification of the teeth are deposited as a calcium complex in the mineralisation zones and cause greyish-brown or yellow discoloration of the teeth as well as hypoplasia and enamel defects. Similarly tetracyclines are deposited in growing bones with possible disturbances of longitudinal growth. Congenital limb malformations due to tetracyclines have also been discussed.— H. Knothe and G. A. Dette, *Infection*, 1985, *13*, 49. See also *Med. Lett.*, 1987, *29*, 61. See also under Adverse Effects, Deposition in Bones and Teeth, and Effects on the Eye, above.

Tetracyclines should be avoided during breast feeding because of a theoretical, rather than real, risk to the infant of teeth discoloration. Chelation of tetracycline by the calcium ions in milk probably overcomes this problem.— R. Wise, *Br. med. J.*, 1987, *294*, 42. The risk may be greater with doxycycline and minocycline, whose gastro-intestinal absorption is not affected markedly by milk.— R. L. Nation and N. Hotham, *Med. J. Aust.*, 1987, *146*, 308.

For a report of congenital abnormalities associated with the use of a tetracycline during pregnancy, see Clomocycline, p.202.

Antimicrobial Action

The group of tetracycline antibiotics are mainly bacteriostatic, with a broad spectrum of antimicrobial activity. They interfere with bacterial protein synthesis by reversibly binding to bacterial 30S ribosomal subunit, thus preventing the binding of aminoacyl transfer RNA to the messenger RNA ribosome complex. They are usually active against mycoplasmas, rickettsias, and spirochaetes, and also against many aerobic and anaerobic Gram-positive and Gram-negative pathogenic bacteria, and some protozoa.

Organisms usually sensitive to tetracyclines include *Actinomyces*, *Chlamydia*, and *Mycoplasma* spp., *Ureaplasma urealyticum*, rickettsias including *Coxiella burnettii*, and spirochaetes including *Borrelia*, *Leptospira*, and *Treponema* spp. Sensitive Gram-negative aerobic bacteria include *Bordetella pertussis*, *Brucella* spp., *Calymmatobacterium granulomatis*, *Campylobacter* spp., some Enterobacteriaceae including *Yersinia pestis* (*Serratia marcescens* and most *Proteus* spp. are usually resistant), *Francisella tularensis*, *Haemophilus*, *Neisseria*, and *Pasteurella* spp., *Pseudomonas mallei* and *Ps. pseudomallei* (*Ps. aeruginosa* is usually resistant), and *Vibrio* spp. Sensitive Gram-positive aerobic bacteria include *Bacillus anthracis*, *Listeria monocytogenes*, and some staphylococci and streptococci. Some anaerobic organisms are sensitive including some *Bacteroides*, *Fusobacterium*, and *Clostridium* spp., although resistance occurs frequently. Some protozoa including *Plasmodium falciparum* may also be sensitive.

Fungi, yeasts, and true viruses are resistant.

Susceptible organisms are usually inhibited by tetracycline 4 µg per mL.

Comment on how low concentrations of antibiotics including tetracyclines can interfere with bacterial adhesion, resulting, in some cases, in effective treatment with antibiotic concentrations below the minimum inhibitory concentration.— I. Chopra, *J. antimicrob. Chemother.*, 1986, *18*, 553. See also under Activity against Propionibacterium, below.

For comparison of the activities of tetracycline, minocycline, and other tetracyclines against various organisms, see under Minocycline Hydrochloride, p.263.

References to the activity of tetracycline against various microorganisms: D. L. Stevens *et al.*, *Antimicrob. Ag. Chemother.*, 1979, *16*, 322 (*Pasteurella multocida*); V. L. Sutter *et al.*, *ibid.*, 1981, *20*, 270 (*Capnocytophaga* strains); R. M. Bannatyne and R. Cheung, *ibid.*, 1982, *21*, 666 (*Bordetella pertussis*); R. Vanhoof *et al.*, *ibid.*, 990 (*Campylobacter jejuni*); D. L. Smalley *et al.*, *ibid.*, 1983, *23*, 161 (*Pseudomonas paucimobilis*); W. F. Myers *et al.*, *ibid.*, 1984, *25*, 690 (*Rochalimaea quintana*); J. F. Reinhardt and W. L. George, *ibid.*, 1985, *27*, 643 (*Aeromonas* spp. and *Plesiomonas shigelloides*); M. R. Motyl *et al.*, *ibid.*, *28*, 151 (*Aeromonas* spp.); J. Bosch *et al.*, *J. antimicrob. Chemother.*, 1986, *17*, 459 (*Brucella melitensis*).

ACTIVITY AGAINST ENTEROBACTERIACEA. *Escherichia.* The activity of tetracycline *in vitro* against *E. coli* was enhanced when used with human serum.— B. S. Dutcher *et al.*, *Antimicrob. Ag. Chemother.*, 1978, *13*, 820.

Escherichia coli sensitivity to tetracycline involves transport and accumulation of the antibiotic within the cell. Transport of tetracycline into susceptible *E. coli* cells has 2 components, an initial rapid uptake system which does not require energy and a second slow energy-dependent uptake system.— L. McMurry and S. B. Levy, *Antimicrob. Ag. Chemother.*, 1978, *14*, 201. Depending on the medium, *E. coli* cells can actively excrete tetracyclines.— L. M. McMurray *et al.*, *ibid.*, 1983, *24*, 544. See also L. M. McMurray *et al.*, *ibid.*, 1981, *20*, 307; M. C. M. Smith and I. Chopra, *ibid.*, 1984, *25*, 446.

Tetracycline penetrated well into epithelial cells and inhibited, but did not kill, enteroinvasive *Escherichia coli*.— P. R. Chadwick and A. R. Mellersh, *J. antimicrob. Chemother.*, 1987, *19*, 211.

Klebsiella. Iron and to some extent copper neutralised the effects of tetracyclines on klebsiellae.— A. A. Miles and J. P. Maskell, *J. antimicrob. Chemother.*, 1986, *17*, 481.

ACTIVITY AGAINST GONOCOCCI. All of 70 isolates of non-beta-lactamase-producing *Neisseria gonorrhoeae* from the Central African Republic were inhibited by tetracycline 4 µg or less per mL.— R. Widy-Wirski *et al.*, *Bull. Wld Hlth Org.*, 1982, *60*, 959. The susceptibility of 83 penicillinase-producing *Neisseria gonorrhoeae* strains to tetracycline varied with the culture media. At a concentration of 4 µg per mL all organisms were inhibited on a medium from the Institut Pasteur Production whereas only 61.7% of the organisms were inhibited on a medium based on Oxoid diagnostic sensitivity test agar.— J. Y. Riou *et al.*, *J. antimicrob. Chemother.*, 1985, *16*, *Suppl.* A, 209.

ACTIVITY AGAINST PROPIONIBACTERIUM. Tetracycline in concentrations which do not inhibit growth of *Propionibacterium acnes* can suppress the production of bacterial extracellular lipases. These are thought to be of importance in the appearance and development of inflammatory skin lesions, due to the release of irritating and comedogenic free fatty acids from sebum triglycerides (G.F. Webster *et al.*, *Br. J. Derm.*, 1981, *104*, 453; S.E. Unkles and C.G. Gemmell, *Antimicrob. Ag. Chemother.*, 1982, *21*, 39). Subminimal inhibitory concentrations of tetracyclines have also been shown to produce a significant suppression of chemotactic factor production in susceptible strains of *P. acnes* (G.F. Webster *et al.*, *ibid.*, 770).

ACTIVITY WITH OTHER AGENTS. Some synergy occurred against some strains of *Staphylococcus aureus* when the activity of tetracycline was tested *in vitro* with actinomycin D or mitomycin.— J. Y. Jacobs *et al.*, *Antimicrob. Ag. Chemother.*, 1979, *15*, 580.

Synergy *in vitro* between amphotericin and tetracycline or minocycline against a strain of *Naegleria fowleri*.— K. K. Lee *et al.*, *Antimicrob. Ag. Chemother.*, 1979, *16*, 217.

Tetracycline and other ribosome inhibitors induced lysis in non-growing *Escherichia coli* cultures treated with ampicillin which usually only acts during active cell growth.— W. Kusser and E. E. Ishiguro, *Antimicrob. Ag. Chemother.*, 1986, *29*, 451.

Resistance

Resistance to the tetracyclines is usually plasmid-mediated and transferable. It is often inducible and appears to be associated with the ability to prevent accumulation of the antibiotic within the bacterial cell. It generally develops relatively slowly in susceptible organisms but the incidence of resistance to these antibiotics has risen with their continued use so that resistant strains of the majority of sensitive species have now been reported. Resistance has increased particularly among Enterobacteriaceae such as *Escherichia coli* and *Shigella* spp., many staphylococci and streptococci, and some gonococci. An organism resistant to one of the tetracyclines is usually resistant to all other members of the group although some tetracycline-resistant staphylococci may be sensitive to minocycline and some resistant strains of *Bacteroides fragilis* may be sensitive to doxycycline.

Administration of tetracycline-containing feeds to farm *animals* led within 3 to 5 months to an increase in tetracycline-resistant intestinal bacteria in the farm workers. Antibiotic-supplemented feeds contributed to the selection of human resistant strains of bacteria; this form of animal treatment should be re-evaluated.— S. B. Levy *et al.*, *New Engl. J. Med.*, 1976, *295*, 583. See also Resistance of Enterobacteriaceae, below.

A survey of the use of tetracycline in the community and its possible relation to the excretion of tetracycline-resistant bacteria.— M. H. Richmond and K. B. Linton, *J. antimicrob. Chemother.*, 1980, *6*, 33.

Plasmid-mediated tetracycline resistance has been studied in many aerobic and anaerobic bacterial species carrying different plasmids, and the full expression of the resistance is generally inducible by subinhibitory concentrations of the antibiotic. In a study of 63 strains of the *Bacteroides fragilis* group, tetracycline resistance was frequently transferable, and both expression of tetracycline resistance and its transferability was generally inducible by tetracycline although some constitutive resistant mutants could also be selected. Resistance to erythromycin and clindamycin could be cotransferred with tetracycline resistance and was transferred independently of tetracycline resistance in only one strain.— G. Privitera *et al.*, *Antimicrob. Ag. Chemother.*, 1981, *20*, 314.

Discussion of plasmid-mediated tetracycline resistance resulting from decreased drug accumulation. Membrane-located resistance proteins are considered to promote energy-dependent tetracycline efflux. The synthesis of these proteins is inducible and involves classical genetic regulatory systems. The high prevalence of plasmid-determined tetracycline resistance has undoubtedly reduced the value of tetracycline for human and veterinary medicine.— I. Chopra, *Br. med. Bull.*, 1984, *40*, 11. See also *idem*, *J. antimicrob. Chemother.*, 1986, *18*, *Suppl.* C, 51.

In a study of 11 families comprising 26 people, long-term tetracycline therapy for acne vulgaris in 5 patients selected for multiple antibiotic-resistant aerobic bowel flora in both patients and their immediate relatives. In contrast, the administration of erythromycin to 6 patients did not appear to affect antibiotic resistance levels in patients or their relatives.— S. J. Adams *et al.*, *J. invest. Derm.*, 1985, *85*, 35. See also M. V. Valtonen *et al.*, *Br. J. Derm.*, 1976, *95*, 311.

RESISTANCE OF ANAEROBES. Of 705 isolates of the *Bacteroides fragilis* group, 63% were resistant to tetracycline at a break point of 4 µg per mL. This confirms the widespread resistance to tetracycline in *Bacteroides* spp. that was first recognised in the 1960s. Tetracycline resistance has also been encountered in anaerobic cocci and clostridia and these observations relegate tetracycline to a drug of primarily historical interest in the treatment of anaerobic infections.— F. P. Tally *et al.*, *Antimicrob. Ag. Chemother.*, 1983, *23*, 536. See also A. R. Fox and I. Phillips, *J. antimicrob. Chemother.*, 1987, *20*, 477.

For comment on the transferability of tetracycline resistance in *B. fragilis*, see above.

RESISTANCE OF CAMPYLOBACTER. Resistance to high concentrations of tetracycline (64 µg or more per mL) in strains of *Campylobacter jejuni* and *C. coli* is plasmid-mediated and appears to have evolved quite separately from that observed in the Enterobacteriaceae. The tetracycline-resistant plasmids can be transferred within the *Campylobacter* genus, but transfer has not been achieved between *Campylobacter* spp. and Enterobacteriaceae.— D. E. Taylor *et al.*, *Antimicrob. Ag. Chemother.*, 1983, *24*, 930.

Further references: H. Sagara *et al.*, *Antimicrob. Ag. Chemother.*, 1987, *31*, 713.

For a report of resistance of *Campylobacter* spp. and other enteropathogens, see under Resistance of Enterobacteriaceae, below.

RESISTANCE OF CORYNEBACTERIUM. Only 19 of 133 (14%) clinical isolates of *Corynebacterium diphtheriae* from patients in Jakarta, Indonesia, were sensitive to tetracycline with a minimum inhibitory concentration of 0.5 µg per mL; the remaining isolates required 32 µg or more per mL. This high level of resistance was in contrast to that reported in other countries.— R. C. Rockhill *et al.*, *Antimicrob. Ag. Chemother.*, 1982, *21*, 842.

RESISTANCE OF ENTEROBACTERIACEAE. The decrease in tetracycline resistance in *Salmonella* of human and porcine origin that has occurred in the Netherlands since 1974, appears to coincide with the legislative ban by the EEC on incorporation of tetracycline in animal feeds.— W. J. van Leeuwen *et al.*, *Antimicrob. Ag. Chemother.*, 1979, *16*, 237. Resistance to tetracycline increased significantly among *Salmonella* spp. isolated from humans in the *USA* in 1984-1985 compared with that observed during 1979-1980; of 485 isolates collected during 1984-1985, 13% were resistant compared with 8.6% of 511 isolates collected during the earlier years. The increase in resistance was compatible with the use of subtherapeutic concentrations of tetracycline in cattle; a recent national survey indicated that 61% of cattle raisers used low-dose tetracycline in animal feed.— K. L. MacDonald *et al.*, *J. Am. med. Ass.*, 1987, *258*, 1496.

For a report of multiple-antibiotic resistance, including resistance to tetracycline, in *Salmonella typhimurium* isolated from contaminated raw milk, see Resistance of Salmonellae in Chloramphenicol Sodium Succinate, p.189.

Of 232 strains of enteropathogenic *Escherichia coli* isolated from faeces of infants under 3 years old 67 were resistant to tetracycline at a concentration of 16 µg per mL. R. J. Gross *et al.*, *Br. med. J.*, 1982, *285*, 472.

Of 2753 strains of *Shigella dysenteriae*, *S. flexneri*, and *S. boydii* examined at the Central Public Health Laboratory from 1979 to mid 1983 60.8% were resistant to tetracycline at a concentration of 16 µg per mL. The incidence of resistance to tetracycline had increased from 15% in 1974 to 69.2% in the first half of 1983.— R. J. Gross *et al.*, *Br. med. J.*, 1984, *288*, 784. See also S. C. Pal (letter), *Lancet*, 1984, *1*, 1462.

In a study of the activity of tetracycline *in vitro* against 108 enteropathogens resistant organisms occurred in *Campylobacter*, *Salmonella*, and *Shigella* spp. At a breakpoint of 4 µg per mL, 16.1, 8.9, 73.3, and 0% of strains of *Campylobacter*, *Salmonella*, *Shigella*, and *Yersinia* spp., respectively, were resistant to tetracycline.— P. L. Turgeon *et al.*, *Curr. ther. Res.*, 1987, *41*, 584. Most of 75 strains of *Yersinia* spp. were resistant to tetracycline; only 50% of the strains were inhibited by 8 µg per mL.— A. M. Lewis and B. Chattopadhyay (letter), *J. antimicrob. Chemother.*, 1987, *19*, 406.

RESISTANCE OF GONOCOCCI. The Centers for Disease Control has confirmed 79 cases of plasmid-mediated tetracycline-resistant *Neisseria gonorrhoeae* infection (TRNG) between February 1985 when it was first identified and March 1986. Three of the cases have also been confirmed as combined tetracycline-resistant penicillinase-producing *N. gonorrhoeae*.— *J. Am. med. Ass.*, 1986, *256*, 25. Eight of 1500 gonococcal isolates from patients attending a London clinic since September 1986 were resistant to tetracycline. All 8 resistant strains were isolated in 1988 and had MICs of above 16 µg per mL for tetracycline, 0.25 µg per mL for penicillin, and 16 to 32 µg per mL for spectinomycin.— C. A. Ison *et al.* (letter), *Lancet*, 1988, *1*, 651.

RESISTANCE OF HAEMOPHILUS. In a study of 2434 clinical isolates of *Haemophilus influenzae* collected from 23 laboratories in the United Kingdom in 1986, 66 (2.7%) strains were resistant to tetracycline with a minimum inhibitory concentration of 4 µg or more per mL; 23 strains also produced beta-lactamase. The prevalence of strains resistant to tetracycline had not increased significantly since 1981.— M. Powell *et al.*, *Br. med. J.*, 1987, *295*, 176. See also A. J. Howard (letter), *ibid.*, 608.

From a comparison of the susceptibility of ampicillin- and chloramphenicol-resistant *Haemophilus influenzae* to 15 antibiotics, tetracycline was one of the least active drugs. Of the 83 strains studied 55.5% were simultaneously resistant to ampicillin, chloramphenicol, tetracycline, sulphamethoxazole, trimethoprim, and co-trimoxazole.— J. Campos and S. Garcia-Tornel, *J. antimicrob. Chemother.*, 1987, *19*, 297.

An increase in beta-lactamase-producing strains of *Haemophilus ducreyi* combined with resistance to tetracycline was observed in Amsterdam from 1978 to 1985; the resistance appeared to be due to a plasmid-mediated mechanism. Only 11 (19%) of 57 *H. ducreyi* strains did not produce beta-lactamase and showed minimum inhibitory concentrations for tetracycline of 2 µg or less per mL, and 10 of these strains were isolated in the first 4 years of the study.— A. W. Sturm, *J. antimicrob. Chemother.*, 1987, *19*, 187. See also Y. R. Bilgeri *et al.*, *Antimicrob. Ag. Chemother.*, 1982, *22*, 686; W. L. Albritton *et al.*, *ibid.*, 1984, *25*, 187.

RESISTANCE OF MYCOPLASMA. Clinical isolates of *Mycoplasma hominis* resistant to tetracycline contained DNA sequences similar to those found in tetracycline-resistant streptococcal strains. This suggested the direct spread of resistance from streptococcal spp. to *M. hominis*, but independent acquired resistance could not be ruled out.— M. C. Roberts *et al.*, *Antimicrob. Ag. Chemother.*, 1985, *28*, 141.

RESISTANCE OF STAPHYLOCOCCI. Periodic surveys in a general hospital indicated a decline in the proportions of patients with strains of *Staph. aureus* in their noses resistant to tetracycline, erythromycin, kanamycin, methicillin, and novobiocin. This was associated with a large reduction in the use of tetracycline, but no overall reduction in the use of antibiotics. Replies from microbiologists in 20 British hospitals also confirmed published reports of a reduced incidence of resistant hospital strains of *Staph. aureus*. No similar reduction was noted in a hospital for diseases of the skin where tetracyclines are commonly used. A dramatic fall in tetracycline-resistant and multiresistant *Staph. aureus* was noted in a burns unit (where tetracycline was rarely used) associated with unusually low numbers of patients and little antibiotic use; this was reversed when both increased, the increase in novobiocin- and tetracycline-resistant strains probably being due to selection by treatment with erythromycin.— G. A. J. Ayliffe *et al.*, *Lancet*, 1979, *1*, 538.

Of 102 endocervical isolates of staphylococci, comprising 4 *Staphylococcus aureus* and 98 coagulase-negative staphylococci, only 41% were susceptible to tetracycline. Of 60 isolates resistant to at least 8 µg of tetracycline per mL, 43 contained a plasmid similar in mass to a tetracycline resistance plasmid previously reported in staphylococci.— R. C. Cooksey and J. N. Baldwin, *Antimicrob. Ag. Chemother.*, 1985, *27*, 234.

RESISTANCE OF STREPTOCOCCI. Of 1176 strains of group A streptococci isolated in Japan in the period 1972 to 1974, 241 were resistant to tetracycline, 234 to tetracycline and chloramphenicol, 427 to tetracycline, chloramphenicol, erythromycin, oleandomycin, josamycin, midecamycin, and lincomycin, and 19 to chloramphenicol alone. Seven of 83 strains of group B streptococci were resistant to tetracycline and chloramphenicol and 26 to tetracycline alone. It was considered that because resistance to a single macrolide antibiotic was rare and that acquisition of resistance to tetracycline and/or chloramphenicol appeared to be a prerequisite for resistance to macrolide antibiotics, restriction of the use of tetracycline and chloramphenicol would lead to a decline in the frequency of macrolide-antibiotic resistance.— Y. Miyamoto *et al.*, *Antimicrob. Ag. Chemother.*, 1978, *13*, 399.

Of 433 clinical isolates of group B streptococci 92.4% were resistant to tetracycline, and in the majority of cases tetracycline resistance plasmids could not be identified; of 30 strains examined in detail only 3 were found to contain tetracycline resistance plasmids. This is in contrast to the findings with Gram-negative bacteria, whose tetracycline resistance is almost always plasmid-associated.— V. Burdett, *Antimicrob. Ag. Chemother.*, 1980, *18*, 753.

Pneumococci. Of 159 strains of *Streptococcus pneumoniae* isolated from the nasopharynx of unselected children aged 4 to 5 years old, 104 (65.4%) were resistant to tetracycline with a minimum inhibitory concentration of 8 µg or more per mL. Thirty-one strains showed multiple resistance, with penicillin, tetracycline, chloramphenicol, and co-trimoxazole being the most frequent pattern of resistance.— J. L. Pérez *et al.* (letter), *J. antimicrob. Chemother.*, 1987, *19*, 278.

RESISTANCE OF VIBRIO CHOLERAE. During the first 6 months of the fourth cholera epidemic in Tanzania, determination of the MICs of 110 isolates of *Vibrio cholerae* taken from 102 patients, revealed rapid emergence of resistance to tetracycline, which was used extensively for both prophylaxis and treatment. Whereas all isolates were fully sensitive to tetracycline during the first month 76% were resistant (MIC greater than 100 µg per mL) after 5 months of extensive use. Tetracycline resistance, however, was not the only factor which led to continued excretion of *V. cholerae* since the concentration of tetracycline in the faeces may reach considerably more than 100 µg per mL and although some patients with isolates with MICs above 100 µg per mL continued to excrete *V. cholerae* after tetracycline treatment, several did not. The MICs of isolates taken from 8 resistant patients measured both before and after tetracycline therapy did not change indicating that resistance did not develop *in vivo*. The results reaffirmed the view that resistance of *V. cholerae* to chemotherapeutic agents is complex and that further studies are needed before resistance to chemotherapeutic agents *per se* can be blamed for failure of chemotherapy. Resistance to chloramphenicol, which was used less than tetracycline, developed more slowly. Resistance to nitrofurantoin, neomycin, ampicillin, and sulphadimidine (which were not used in the outbreak) also developed more slowly.— F. S. Mhalu *et al.*, *Lancet*, 1979, *1*, 345. This is one of the first examples of a widespread outbreak of R plasmid-carrying strains of *V. cholerae*. The appearance of resistance to tetracycline demonstrates the way in which plasmid-mediated resistance can emerge and rapidly spread under the heavy selection pressure of mass prophylaxis.— K. J. Towner *et al.* (letter), *ibid.*, *2*, 147. See also K. J. Towner *et al.*, *Bull. Wld Hlth Org.*, 1980, *58*, 747.

Absorption and Fate

Most tetracyclines are incompletely absorbed from the gastro-intestinal tract. The degree of absorption is diminished by the presence of divalent and trivalent metal ions with which tetracyclines form stable complexes and to a variable degree by milk or food. It has been recommended that tetracyclines should be given before food; however, doxycycline and minocycline are more completely absorbed compared with the other tetracyclines, and they are little affected by food. Formulation with phosphate may enhance the absorption of tetracycline.

Doses of 250 to 500 mg by mouth every 6 hours produce plasma concentrations of tetracycline ranging from about 1 to 5 µg per mL. Intravenous injections of 250 to 500 mg produce plasma concentrations of about 15 to 20 µg per mL at 0.5 hours falling to 4 to 10 µg per mL at 1 to 2 hours, though at 12 hours 1 to 3 µg per mL may still be present. Intramuscular doses of 100 mg yield plasma concentrations of up to 2 µg per mL and 250-mg doses up to 3.6 µg per mL at 3 to 4 hours.

In the circulation, tetracyclines are bound to plasma proteins in varying degrees, and the following figures have been reported: from 20 to 40% for oxytetracycline, from 24 to 65% for tetracycline, about 47% for chlortetracycline, from 41 to 90% for demeclocycline, about 75% for minocycline, and about 80% to 95% for methacycline and doxycycline. They are widely distributed throughout the body tissues and fluids. Concentrations in cerebrospinal fluid are relatively low, but may be raised if the meninges are inflamed. Small amounts appear in saliva, tears, and intra-ocular fluids; higher concentrations are achieved with minocycline and doxycycline. Tetracyclines appear in the milk of nursing mothers where concentrations may be 60% or more of those in the plasma. They diffuse across the placenta and appear in the foetal circulation in concentrations of about 25 to 75% of those in the maternal blood. Tetracyclines are retained at sites of new bone formation and recent calcification and in developing teeth.

The biological half-life of tetracycline has been reported to be about 8 to 10 hours; comparable figures reported for other tetracyclines are chlortetracycline 5.5 hours, clomocycline 5.8 hours, demeclocycline 12 hours, doxycycline 15 to 22 hours, methacycline 15 hours, minocycline 11 to 23 hours, and oxytetracycline 9.5 hours.

The tetracyclines are excreted in the urine and in the faeces. Renal clearance is by glomerular filtration and concentrations in the urine of up to 300 µg per mL of tetracycline may be reached 2 hours after a usual dose is taken and be maintained for about 6 to 12 hours. Up to 60% of an intravenous dose of tetracycline and rather less of a dose by mouth is eliminated unchanged in the urine; for most tetracyclines about 40 to 70% of a dose is excreted in the urine, but for chlortetracycline, doxycycline, and minocycline rather less is eliminated by this route.

The tetracyclines are excreted in the bile where concentrations 5 to 20 times those in plasma can occur. Since there is some reabsorption complete elimination is slow. Considerable quantities occur in the faeces after administration by mouth and lesser amounts after administration by injection.

In a study of 170 men and 142 women given various antibiotics, blood concentrations following tetracycline 370 mg were 19% higher in the females at 2 hours and 21.5% higher at 6 hours.— R. Scotti, *Chemotherapy, Basle*, 1973, *18*, 205.

The renal excretion of tetracycline and doxycycline was enhanced by rendering the urine alkaline and was probably the result of altered tubular reabsorption.— J. M. Jaffe *et al.*, *J. Pharmacokinet. Biopharm.*, 1973, *1*, 267.

ABSORPTION. A discussion of factors affecting the absorption of tetracyclines.— P. J. Neuvonen, *Drugs*, 1976, *11*, 45.

No difference in either rate or extent of tetracycline absorption after administration by mouth was found between 5 elderly patients with achlorhydria and 5 controls. It was suggested that previous reports of reduced absorption in patients with elevated gastric pH may have resulted from using poorly formulated preparations.— P. A. Kramer *et al.*, *Clin. Pharmac. Ther.*, 1978, *23*, 467.

See also under Precautions (above).

BIOAVAILABILITY. A review of the bioavailability of tetracycline.— T. D. Sokoloski *et al.*, *J. Am. pharm. Ass.*, 1975, *NS15*, 709.

Bioavailability tests *in vivo* of tetracycline should cover a period of 96 hours. Absorption from a capsule and 2 film-coated tablets did not show any significant differences until after 6 hours.— C. M. Davis *et al.*, *Am. J. med. Sci.*, 1973, *265*, 69.

The bioavailability of tetracycline from tablets and suspension was found to be similar.— P. Fisher *et al.*, *Br. J. clin. Pharmac.*, 1980, *9*, 153.

DIFFUSION INTO BODY TISSUES AND FLUIDS. Mean sputum concentrations of tetracycline after a 500-mg dose were 200 and 100 ng per mL 4 to 6 and 24 hours, respectively, after oral administration to 23 patients with chronic bronchitis.— C. G. C. MacArthur *et al.*, *J. antimicrob. Chemother.*, 1978, *4*, 509.

A study indicating that tetracycline rapidly enters red blood cells *in vitro*.— H. W. Jun and B. H. Lee, *J. pharm. Sci.*, 1980, *69*, 455.

Ocular tetracycline concentrations of 3 to 7, 1 to 2, and 0 to 2 µg per mL have been reported following intravenous administration of tetracycline 500 mg, topical administration of a 0.5% preparation every 4 minutes for 6 applications, and subconjunctival administration of 1.2 mg, respectively.— T. S. Lesar and R. G. Fiscella, *Drug Intell. & clin. Pharm.*, 1985, *19*, 642.

MALNUTRITION. A report that the protein binding of tetracycline was significantly reduced in malnutrition and probably accounted for its more rapid elimination by the kidneys in such patients.— A. K. Shastri and K. Krishnaswamy, *Clinica chim. Acta*, 1976, *66*, 157.

In patients with severe protein-energy malnutrition (nutritional oedema), systemic availability of tetracycline was higher than in healthy subjects and total body clearance and renal clearance were significantly decreased. These results were different to those obtained in patients with mild and moderate degrees of malnutrition, mainly due to the decreased clearance of the drug; glomerular filtration is reported to be reduced in severe protein-energy malnutrition. Therefore suitable alterations in dosage regimens of tetracycline should be based on the severity of malnutrition.— T. C. Raghuram and K. Krishnaswamy, *Chemotherapy, Basle*, 1982, *28*, 428.

PREGNANCY AND THE NEONATE. A high degree of placental transfer has been reported for tetracyclines with a foetal to maternal serum concentration ratio of 0.5 to 0.7. Although tetracyclines are excreted in breast milk the bioavailability is considered to be low because of chelation with milk calcium.— A. W. Chow and P. J. Jewesson, *Rev. infect. Dis.*, 1985, *7*, 287.

Uses and Administration

The tetracyclines have a wide spectrum of activity and have been used in the treatment of a large number of infections caused by susceptible organisms. With the emergence of bacterial resistance and the development of other antibacterial agents their use may be restricted increasingly to the treatment of rickettsial infections, including typhus, Rocky Mountain spotted fever, and Q fever; chlamydial infections, including psittacosis, lymphogranuloma venereum, trachoma, and inclusion conjunctivitis; and mycoplasmal infections, especially those caused by *Mycoplasma pneumoniae*.

Tetracyclines are used, often in association with streptomycin, in the treatment of brucellosis and plague, and as an alternative to streptomycin in the treatment of tularaemia. Tetracyclines are also used in the treatment of chronic bronchitis, chancroid, granuloma inguinale, and urinary-tract infections, especially non-specific urethritis, and are given in low doses in the long-term treatment of acne. The tetracyclines are used in the treatment of malabsorption syndromes such as tropical sprue and Whipple's disease, and also in the treatment of cholera in conjunction with fluid and electrolyte replacements. Relapsing fever responds to treatment with tetracycline but a Jarisch-Herxheimer-like reaction appears to be a frequent complication. Tetracycline is also used in the treatment of leptospirosis, and in the early stages of Lyme disease. It has been given in conjunction with quinine in the management of malaria especially when resistant to chloroquine. Tetracyclines have also been used in the treatment of balantidiasis and they have been used in association with an amoebicide in the treatment of amoebic dysentery.

In penicillin-hypersensitive patients tetracyclines have been used in the treatment of certain stages of syphilis, and in yaws, gonorrhoea, actinomycosis, anthrax, rat-bite fever, and acute necrotising ulcerative gingivitis (Vincent's infection).

Tetracycline has been used topically in the treatment of chlamydial infections of the eye, but systemic treatment is also necessary.

In the treatment of systemic infections the tetracyclines are usually administered by mouth. In severe acute infections they may be given by slow intravenous infusion or, occasionally, by intramuscular injection; parenteral therapy should be substituted by oral administration as soon as practicable. Doses of tetracycline base and tetracycline hydrochloride are expressed in terms of tetracycline hydrochloride.

The usual adult dosage of tetracycline hydrochloride is 250 or 500 mg every 6 hours by mouth, preferably one hour before or 2 hours after meals. In severe infections, tetracycline hydrochloride may be administered by slow intravenous infusion every 12 hours as a solution containing not more than 0.5%. The usual dose is 1 g daily but up to 2 g daily has been given to patients with normal renal function. If the intramuscular route is to be used, a solution containing not more than 5% tetracycline hydrochloride is usually given in a dosage of 200 to 300 mg in divided doses with a maximum of 600 mg daily. As intramuscular injections are painful, procaine hydrochloride is usually included in the solution.

In children, the effects on teeth should be considered and tetracyclines only used when absolutely essential. Tetracycline hydrochloride has been given to older children in doses of 25 to 50 mg per kg body-weight daily by mouth in divided doses and in doses of 10 to 20 mg per kg daily by intravenous infusion. If the intramuscular route is used, the dose should not exceed 250 mg daily.

Tetracyclines, apart from doxycycline and possibly minocycline, should generally be avoided in patients with renal impairment and care should be taken in elderly patients.

Reviews of the actions and uses of the tetracyclines: I. Chopra *et al.*, *J. antimicrob. Chemother.*, 1981, *8*, 5; A. Kucers, *Lancet*, 1982, *2*, 425; W. R. Wilson and F. R. Cockerill, *Mayo Clin. Proc.*, 1987, *62*, 906.

'Seal finger' infection due to an unidentified organism and contracted by hunters handling seals and polar bears could be controlled within 7 days by tetracycline given by mouth; erythromycin, penicillin, and sulphonamide were ineffective.— B. Beck and T. G. Smith (letter), *Can. med. Ass. J.*, 1976, *115*, 105. See also E. Sargent (letter), *J. Am. med. Ass.*, 1980, *244*, 437.

Tetracycline was considered the treatment of choice in cat scratch fever but it should not be given prophylactically.— *Br. med. J.*, 1978, *1*, 427.

Beneficial results were achieved with tetracycline in 2 patients in the early stages of immunoproliferative small intestine disease (IPSID) (C. Matuchansky *et al.*, *New Engl. J. Med.*, 1983, *309*, 1126). The response rate, however, has appeared to decline with increased dystrophic changes of mucosal lymphoplasmacytic infiltrate (A. Khojasteh *et al.*, *ibid.*, *308*, 1401); the use of tetracycline and prednisone, with or without cyclophosphamide, is under investigation. For the general treatment of lymphomas including IPSID-associated lymphoma, see under Choice of Antineoplastic Agent, Hodgkin's Disease and other Lymphomas, p.586.

ADMINISTRATION. Tetracycline may cause oesophagitis or oesophageal ulceration and tablets or capsules should therefore be given with at least 100 mL of water while the patient is in an upright sitting position.— S. K. Vong and R. K. Parekh (letter), *Pharm. J.*, 1987, *1*, 5.

ADMINISTRATION IN RENAL FAILURE. Tetracycline hydrochloride should be avoided in patients with even mild renal failure; doxycycline may be used if necessary.— G. B. Appel and H. C. Neu, *New Engl. J. Med.*, 1977, *296*, 663. See also R. E. Van Scoy and W. R. Wilson, *Mayo Clin. Proc.*, 1983, *58*, 246.

Haemodialysis has been reported to clear tetracycline from blood to a lesser extent than creatinine and urea. Peritoneal dialysis does not appear to remove significant amounts either.— A. S. Watanabe, *Drug Intell. & clin. Pharm.*, 1977, *11*, 407.

ANTHRAX. Tetracycline 3.75 mg per kg body-weight administered by mouth every 6 hours for 5 to 7 days is recommended for the treatment of cutaneous anthrax in patients who cannot take penicillin. Tetracyline 1 g intravenously every 24 hours has been reported effective in treating some cases of intestinal anthrax.— G. B. Knudson, *Milit. Med.*, 1986, *151*, 71.

BRUCELLOSIS. For the use of tetracyclines in the treatment of brucellosis, see under Doxycycline Hydrochloride, p.218.

CYSTS. *Thyroid cyst.* A study of the treatment of thyroid cysts in 35 euthyroid patients. Most of the cystic nodules were simple cysts without any other definite disease and could be treated successfully by aspiration alone or, if recurrence occurred, by a second aspiration and instillation of tetracycline solution as a sclerosant. One mL of tetracycline hydrochloride 100 mg per mL in sodium chloride 0.9% solution was injected into small cysts and 2 mL was injected if the volume aspirated exceeded 15 mL.— C. J. Edmonds and M. Tellez, *Br. med. J.*, 1987, *295*, 529.

Hydrocele. A study of 24 patients with hydrocele treated by sclerotherapy using tetracycline 2.5, 5, or 10% solutions. Pain immediately after the injection was the only side-effect noted and one patient discontinued treatment because of severe pain after sclerotherapy with a 10% solution of tetracycline; there was, however, no significant difference in the degree of pain between the different concentrations of tetracycline used. In the remaining 23 patients fluid did not reaccumulate in the hydrocele during the follow-up period of 6 to 18 months. The number of treatments required ranged from 1 to 5 and appeared to be related to the size of the hydrocele and not the concentration of tetracycline used.— K. -N. Hu *et al.*, *Urology*, 1984, *24*, 572.

For further reference to tetracycline used as a sclerosant, see under Malignant Effusions and Pneumothorax, below.

DIARRHOEA. Comment that the administration of a broad-spectrum antibiotic such as tetracycline, given intermittently one week in four, often relieves symptoms of diarrhoea in diabetic autonomic neuropathy, but improvement may coincide with natural remission. However, it was considered that such treatment should only be given if metoclopramide is not effective.— D. J. Ewing and B. F. Clarke, *Br. med. J.*, 1982, *285*, 916. It seems prudent to administer a 2-week course of antibiotics such as tetracycline 0.5 to 1 g daily to any diabetic patient with unexplained chronic diarrhoea, especially if steatorrhoea is also present. Some patients may need intermittent or chronic antibiotic therapy, although often only a temporary remission is achieved.— M. Feldman and L. R. Schiller, *Ann. intern. Med.*, 1983, *98*, 378.

For comment on the use of a long-acting tetracycline for prophylaxis against travellers' diarrhoea, see under Doxycycline Hydrochloride, Diarrhoea, p.218.

ENTERIC INFECTIONS. *Balantidiasis.* The incidence of balantidiasis is low in man, but many mammals including *pigs* are naturally infected with *Balantidium coli*. Balantidiasis in humans is often self-limiting and asymptomatic, but in some individuals, especially malnourished children, *B. coli* causes deep penetrating ulcerations of the colon resulting in a dysenteric syndrome. Tetracyclines are usually considered the drug of choice (WHO Scientific Working Group, *Bull Wld Hlth Org.*, 1980, *58*, 819) with 5-nitroimidazole derivatives such as metronidazole, di-iodohydroxyquinoline, or paromomycin as alternative drugs. In adults tetracycline is given in doses of 500 mg four times daily for 10 days. For children a dose of 10 mg per kg body-weight four times daily, to a maximum of 2 g daily, for 10 days has been suggested (*Med. Lett.*, 1986, *28*, 9), but the effects on teeth should be borne in mind.

Campylobacter enteritis. Tetracyclines may be considered as an alternative to erythromycin in the treatment of uncomplicated campylobacter enteritis. However, they have the disadvantage of a broad spectrum of activity and they are contra-indicated in children; resistance rates of up to 20% have also been reported.— C. A. M. McNulty, *J. antimicrob. Chemother.*, 1987, *19*, 281.

Cholera. Correction of dehydration is the single most important measure in the treatment of cholera, but chemotherapy with tetracycline, doxycycline, chloramphenicol, or co-trimoxazole can accelerate the disappearance of vibrios from the stools and diminish the volume and duration of diarrhoea (J. Lindenbaum *et al.*, *Bull Wld Hlth Org.*, 1967, *36*, 871; *Drug & Ther. Bull.*, 1983, *21*, 101). The World Health Organization recommended tetracycline or chloramphenicol intravenously or by mouth in doses of 250 or 500 mg every 6 hours for the treatment of cholera (WHO Expert Committee on Cholera, Second Report, *Tech. Rep. Ser. Wld Hlth Org. No. 352*, 1967). Multiple-dose tetracycline therapy remains the best choice; a single dose of tetracycline 1 or 2 g appears to be a reasonable alternative to multiple doses, although clinical relapses are more likely to occur (M.R. Islam, *Gut*, 1987, *28*, 1029). Tetracycline probably reduces the duration of other *Vibrio* diarrhoeas, although these are often mild and may only require oral rehydration. For extra-intestinal *Vibrio* infections, the use of antimicrobial agents is advisable and for *V. vulnificus* septicaemia treatment should probably include tetracycline or chloramphenicol, plus an aminoglycoside (P.A. Blake, *Ann. intern. Med.*, 1983, *99*, 558; J.G. Morris and R.E. Black, *New Engl. J. Med.*, 1985, *312*, 343).

It has been suggested that, because the protection afforded by cholera vaccination is poor, when travelling into an area where there is an epidemic of cholera, tetracycline 250 mg four times daily should be given prophylactically and continued for 2 days after leaving the area (A.G. Higginson, *Practitioner*, 1979, *223*, 529). However, chemotherapy is considered by some workers to be of limited value in high-cholera-endemic areas (B.C. Deb *et al.*, *Bull. Wld Hlth Org.*, 1976, *54*, 171). Tetracycline administered to cholera carriers for 3 days has been shown to decrease the number of vibrio excretors, but on withdrawal of the drug the number of excretors rose again (Report of a Joint ICMR-GWB-WHO Cholera Study Group, Calcutta, India, *Bull. Wld*

Hlth Org., 1971, *45*, 451). Three hospital outbreaks of cholera in Tanzania have, however, been controlled by isolation of infective patients and administration of antibacterial chemoprophylaxis of tetracycline or co-trimoxazole to all at-risk patients and their accompanying relatives (F.S. Mhalu *et al.*, *Lancet*, 1984, *2*, 82).

Dysentery. Comment that *Shigella dysenteriae* 1 strains isolated recently from various geographical locations have been resistant to older antimicrobials such as tetracycline, chloramphenicol, streptomycin, and sulpha drugs, and these drugs should no longer be used for treating dysentery due to *Sh. dysenteriae* 1.— M. J. Albert (letter), *Lancet*, 1985, *2*, 948.

Yersiniosis. Yersiniosis usually manifests itself as enteritis and is a self-limiting disease requiring only symptomatic treatment without antibiotics. However, antibiotics are indicated in patients with septicaemia, intra-abdominal sepsis, or severe terminal ileitis. Most strains of *Yersinia pseudotuberculosis* and *Y. enterocolitica* are susceptible to antibiotics active against Gram-negative rods. Tetracycline is the drug of choice in adults, but should not be used in children. Chloramphenicol, streptomycin, and gentamicin should be reserved for severe disease. Co-trimoxazole is also effective (WHO Working Group Report on Yersiniosis, *Euro Reports and Studies 60, World Health Organization, Copenhagen*, 1983, p.24; *Lancet*, 1986, *2*, 761). Some workers have suggested co-trimoxazole as the drug of choice in children and adults (M. Mäki *et al.*, *Archs Dis. Childh.*, 1980, *55*, 861).

EPERYTHROZOONOSIS. For mention of the use of tetracyclines in the treatment of eperythrozoonosis, see under Doxycycline Hydrochloride, p.219.

EYE INFECTIONS. Comments on the use of tetracycline for topical treatment of acute bacterial infection of the external eye.— D. V. Seal *et al.*, *Br. J. Ophthal.*, 1982, *66*, 357.

See also under Trachoma, below.

INFERTILITY. For the treatment of male infertility due to inflammatory reactions, both antimicrobial and anti-inflammatory agents are employed. The choice of antibiotic depends on the organism, however, in most cases tetracyclines are considered suitable.— W. -B. Schill and M. Michalopoulos, *Drugs*, 1984, *28*, 263.

Mention of the use of tetracyclines in treating *Chlamydia* and *Mycoplasma* infections in patients with habitual abortion.— A. DeCherney and M. L. Polan, *Br. J. Hosp. Med.*, 1984, *31*, 261.

Further references: *Ann. intern. Med.*, 1985, *103*, 906.

For further mention of tetracyclines to treat infertility, see under Doxycycline Hydrochloride, p.219.

LEPTOSPIROSIS. For mention of tetracycline in the treatment of leptospirosis, see under Benzylpenicillin Sodium, p.136. For the use of a tetracycline in the prophylaxis and treatment of leptospirosis, see under Doxycycline Hydrochloride, p.219.

LYME DISEASE. Lyme disease is a seasonal infectious disease caused by the spirochaete *Borrelia burgdorferi* which is transmitted primarily by ixodes ticks. Tetracycline 250 mg four times daily for 10 days has been recommended for the early treatment of Lyme disease in adults; children should receive phenoxymethylpenicillin (A. Parke, *Br. med. J.*, 1987, *294*, 525). Erythema chronicum migrans and its associated symptoms have been reported to resolve faster in tetracycline- or phenoxymethylpenicillin-treated patients than in those given erythromycin, and major late complications of meningoencephalitis, myocarditis, or recurrent attacks of arthritis, appear to be less likely to occur after tetracycline than with phenoxymethylpenicillin or erythromycin treatment (A.C. Steere *et al.*, *Ann. intern. Med.*, 1983, *99*, 22). However, late neurological complications of Lyme disease have been reported in 5 patients who received tetracycline therapy for early Lyme disease given at or above the recommended dosage of 250 mg 4 times daily for 10 days. It has been suggested that tetracycline may not effectively penetrate into some tissues and that this dosage may not be adequate to inhibit some strains of *B. burgdorferi*. Further studies are necessary to determine the optimal therapy for early Lyme disease (R.J. Dattwyler and J.J. Halperin, *Arthritis Rheum.*, 1987, *30*, 448).

For severe complications of Lyme disease treatment with intravenous benzylpenicillin is usually preferred, but if the patient is allergic to penicillin, tetracycline 500 mg four times daily by mouth for 30 days may be a suitable alternative (A.C. Steere *et al.*, *Ann. intern. med.*, 1983, *99*, 767); successful treatment of Lyme meningitis has been reported with this tetracycline regimen (A. Ackley and M. Lupovici, *ibid.*, 1986, *105*, 630).

MALARIA. Tetracyclines given for 7 or more consecutive days may be used in the treatment of infections due to *Plasmodium falciparum*. Tetracycline hydrochloride 1 or 2 g daily in 4 equal doses, doxycycline 200 mg daily, or minocycline 100 to 400 mg daily are equally effective, but because the infection does not usually respond for 3 or 4 days it is essential to administer a rapidly acting blood schizontocide, such as quinine or amodiaquine, at the beginning of the course of treatment. In areas where both 4-aminoquinolines and antifolate-sulphonamide combinations are considered ineffective, the World Health Organization recommends the use of mefloquine, or alternatively quinine alone or in association with tetracycline 1 to 2 g daily given for at least 7 days; other tetracyclines such as doxycycline or minocycline may be acceptable alternatives. Tetracycline is not, however, recommended for use in pregnancy or in children (Advances in Malaria Chemotherapy, *Tech. Rep. Ser. Wld Hlth Org. No. 711*, 1984; WHO Expert Committee on Malaria, 18th Report, *Tech. Rep. Ser. Wld Hlth Org. No. 735*, 1986).

Tetracycline is active against both pre-erythrocytic and blood stages of malaria and it has been suggested for prophylactic use in travellers. However, it has not been used in large studies and its efficacy and safety for travellers has not been assessed (T.E.A. Peto and C.F. Gilks, *Lancet*, 1986, *1*, 1256). If doxycycline is to be used patients should at least be advised to limit direct exposure to the sun to minimise the possibility of a photosensitivity reaction (*Med. Lett.*, 1986, *28*, 9). One study involving healthy children aged 10 to 15 years living in Thailand, demonstrated that doxycycline 100 mg daily for those over 40 kg or 50 mg daily for those less than 40 kg, gave substantial, but not complete, suppressive or causal protection against falciparum malaria in an area of high multidrug resistance; the study population had some malaria immunity and therefore the results should not be applied to non-immune populations (L.W. Pang *et al.*, *Lancet*, 1987, *1*, 1161). In view of the probable development of doxycycline resistance in *P. falciparum* and the possibility of side-effects, it has been suggested that prophylactic doxycycline is not justified as a method of malaria control (L.J. Bruce-Chwatt, *ibid.*, 1487). Some workers feel, however, that tetracyclines can be used for chemoprophylaxis against falciparum malaria but their use should be limited to non-immune individuals visiting or working temporarily in areas with a high transmission of multidrug resistant strains, and that tetracyclines should not be used extensively by people living in endemic areas. However, in many malarious countries there is indiscriminate exposure of many human and animal populations to tetracyclines and therefore the deployment of tetracyclines as antimalarial agents would probably not contribute significantly to the emergence of tetracycline-resistant organisms. A further problem with tetracycline prophylaxis is that it cannot be taken by young children and pregnant women, the segment of a community most vulnerable to malaria in many endemic areas (K.H. Rieckmann, *Lancet*, 1987, *2*, 507). Some workers have suggested that doxycycline should be started one week before and continued for 6 weeks after exposure in the endemic area (*Med. Lett.*, 1986, *28*, 44). However, Rieckmann (1987) considered that protection against malaria should be possible if a tetracycline is started just before arrival in a malarious area and discontinued shortly after leaving the area; further prophylaxis for several weeks, as recommended for chloroquine, should not be necessary since tetracyclines inhibit completely the development of pre-erythrocytic stages of *P. falciparum* and are therefore not needed to act against parasites that may pass from the liver to the bloodstream after departure from an endemic area. For *P. vivax* infection, the pre-erythrocytic stages are only partly affected by the tetracyclines and administration of primaquine may also be necessary. Rieckmann concluded that precise recommendations for the optimum use of tetracyclines in malaria prophylaxis will only be possible after the evaluation of different drug regimens.

For overall recommendations for the prophylaxis and treatment of malaria, see under Antimalarial Agents, p.505.

Further references: S. Pinichpongse *et al.*, *Bull. Wld Hlth Org.*, 1982, *60*, 907; S. Noeypatimanond *et al.*, *Trans. R. Soc. trop. Med. Hyg.*, 1983, *77*, 338.

MALIGNANT EFFUSIONS. Comment on the instillation of tetracycline for the management of malignant effusions.— *Lancet*, 1981, *1*, 198.

Tetracycline was successfully used in the management of cardiac tamponade secondary to malignant pericardial effusion in 6 patients. A solution of 0.5 to 1 g of tetracycline hydrochloride dissolved in 20 mL of sterile saline was instilled intrapericardially, the cannula flushed with a further 30 mL of saline, and the whole procedure repeated every 48 to 96 hours until total sclerosis occurred or no more fluid could be drained.— S. Davis *et al.*, *New Engl. J. Med.*, 1978, *299*, 1113. Further studies have demonstrated that symptomatic pericardial effusions can be effectively controlled with intrapericardial instillation of tetracycline in 81 to 91% of cases.— O. W. Press and R. Livingston, *J. Am. med. Ass.*, 1987, *257*, 1088. See also J. H. Horgan, *Br. med. J.*, 1987, *295*, 563.

Tetracycline 0.5 to 1 g as a single dose has been administered intrapleurally for treatment of malignant pleural effusions, and is considered, by some, to be the agent of choice. It is easily administered, has few side-effects, is effective and cheap (G.N. Fox, *J. Am. med. Ass.*, 1979, *242*, 1362; D.P. Dhillon and S.G. Spiro, *Br. J. Hosp. Med.*, 1983, *29*, 506). However, variable results have been reported, with control of effusion achieved in 48 to 87% of patients, and some workers prefer the use of other agents such as talc. Instillation of tetracycline produces severe pain and therefore lignocaine hydrochloride should be added to the solution (I.S. Fentiman, *Br. J. Hosp. Med.*, 1987, *37*, 421). A precipitate of tetracycline has been reported to occur 4 to 12 hours after preparation of solutions of tetracycline hydrochloride with lignocaine hydrochloride at pH 2.2 to 2.4. When buffered to pH 1.75, however, no precipitation occurred after storage for 3 days at room temperature (T. Meo *et al.*, *Aust. J. Hosp. Pharm.*, 1984, *14*, 134).

For further reference to tetracycline used as a sclerosant, see under Cysts, above, and Pneumothorax, below.

MALIGNANT NEOPLASMS. The results of a retrospective study of 218 patients with tumours of the larynx or nasopharynx, who had subsequently died, suggested that the addition of tetracyclines to their treatment had prolonged the survival of some patients. Inhibition of mitochondrial protein synthesis by the tetracyclines was proposed as a possible mechanism of this effect.— J. A. Leezenberg *et al.*, *Eur. J. clin. Pharmac.*, 1979, *16*, 237.

Diagnosis. Bladder tumours were diagnosed in patients given tetracycline when epithelial cells radiated a bright yellow fluorescence.— M. Kafkas, *J. Urol., Baltimore*, 1977, *117*, 581.

Tetracycline labelling was used to detect an increased rate of bone calcification in a patient with acute leukaemia and fibrosis.— D. P. Schenkein *et al.*, *Ann. intern. Med.*, 1986, *105*, 375.

MEDITERRANEAN SPOTTED FEVER. Mediterranean spotted fever is an acute infectious disease caused by *Rickettsia conorii* which is generally benign but usually has severe clinical manifestations with intense malaise. In a randomised study of 81 children aged between 1 and 13 years with Mediterranean spotted fever, tetracycline 40 mg per kg body-weight daily was superior to erythromycin 50 mg per kg daily, as the stearate, both given by mouth in 4 divided doses for 10 days. Although both regimens proved effective, symptoms disappeared significantly more rapidly in the group treated with tetracycline. One patient who had persistence of fever, headache, myalgias, and prostration on the eighth day of treatment with erythromycin responded to tetracycline therapy after 2 days of treatment. However, tetracyclines are not usually recommended for children, and erythromycin could constitute an acceptable therapeutic alternative to tetracycline for children under 8 years with Mediterranean spotted fever, except those with severe symptoms or serious illness.— T. Muñoz-Espin *et al.*, *Archs Dis. Childh.*, 1986, *61*, 1027.

MELIOIDOSIS. A review of 20 cases of melioidosis due to *Pseudomonas pseudomallei* in far north Queensland. In the acute fulminating form of the disease the overall mortality rate for septicaemic patients was 75% and many of these patients died before receiving effective antibiotic treatment. As *Ps. pseudomallei* is resistant to most antibiotics commonly used in the initial treatment of undiagnosed septicaemic illnesses, a high index of clinical suspicion is required. Treatment with tetracycline in high dosage in association with chloramphenicol and possibly kanamycin has been used, although little appears to be gained by the addition of kanamycin. All of 7 patients with positive blood cultures but clinically not septicaemic responded well to initial therapy with tetracycline or doxycycline (in 2 cases combined with other agents) and there were no deaths. Patients with the pulmonary form of the disease, the most common form encountered in Australia, responded well to doxycycline 200 mg daily for 3 to 6 months. Treatment of the chronic or subacute nonbacteraemic form of the disease is usually with tetracycline, although co-trimoxazole has also been shown to be effective. Treatment should be continued for a prolonged period such as 3 to 6 months, although longer periods may be necessary; the optimal length of treatment has not been determined.— R. W. Guard *et al.*, *Am. J. trop. Med. Hyg.*, 1984, *33*, 467.

MOUTH INFECTIONS. In patients undergoing cytotoxic or

immunosuppressive chemotherapy a mouth-wash of tetracycline and nystatin is useful in reducing both secondary infection and the likelihood of candidiasis; tetracycline used topically as a mouth-wash can cause acute oral candidiasis and must therefore be administered with an antifungal agent. An example of a tetracycline/nystatin mouth-rinse is tetracycline 1.25 g, nystatin 1 250 000 units, compound tragacanth powder 2 g, chloroform water double strength 50 mL, glycerol to 1000 mL; the mixture should be strained through gauze and dispensed in amber glass bottles. Five to 10 mL of the mouth-wash should be held in the mouth for 5 minutes, as required.— K. D. Hay and P. C. Reade, *Drugs,* 1983, *26,* 268. Tetracycline and amphotericin syrup (Mysteclin) may be used in the same way.— R. A. Cawson, *Prescribers' J.,* 1984, *24,* 124.

Periodontal disease. Tetracycline has been used both systemically and topically in the management of periodontal disease. In the absence of scaling, systemic tetracycline therapy appears to have a beneficial but transient effect, lasting about 6 to 16 weeks, and the possibility of introducing tetracycline-resistant strains must be borne in the mind. In the majority of cases, the use of systemic tetracycline as an adjunct to scaling does not appear to enhance treatment when compared with debridement alone. Tetracycline may be of some benefit, however, in particular refractory, active, or surgical cases that do not respond to mechanical debridement. Encouraging results have been found using topical tetracycline released from cellulose fibres filled with the antibiotic and tied around involved teeth. Local delivery of tetracycline combined with conventional scaling probably offers very little advantage over scaling alone, but in situations where tetracycline may be useful, local delivery may be a viable alternative to systemic antibiotic.

Systemic minocycline may be used as an alternative to tetracycline and has the advantages of longer serum half-life and lower urinary excretion-rate allowing lower doses to be used. Minocycline 200 mg daily for 7 days as well as scaling has produced favourable results in terms of gingival health and bacterial counts compared with scaling alone (M. Marder and P. Milgrom, *Drug Intell. & clin. Pharm.*, 1984, *18*, 466).

The tetracyclines, tetracycline, minocycline, and doxycycline, have been shown to inhibit polymorphonuclear leucocyte collagenase activity *in vitro*. This anti-collagenase activity may explain, at least in part, their effectiveness in treating periodontal disorders in which the destruction of collagen fibres during the inflammatory disease is attributed partially to the activity of leucocyte collagenase (*J. Am. med. Ass.*, 1984, *252*, 1989).

Perioral dermatitis. For the use of tetracyclines in the treatment of perioral dermatitis, see under Skin Disorders, below.

Ulcers, aphthous. For the use of tetracycline and amphotericin in the treatment of aphthous ulcers, see Ulcers, Aphthous, below.

PELVIC INFLAMMATORY DISEASE. For the use of tetracyclines in the treatment of pelvic inflammatory disease, see under Cefoxitin Sodium, p.159. See also under Doxycycline Hydrochloride, p.219.

PLAGUE. Prompt treatment was essential in human plague especially in the pneumonic type where it was necessary to start specific treatment within 15 hours of overt illness if it was to have a favourable effect on the outcome of the disease. Tetracycline was the recommended treatment for bubonic and pneumonic plague. It should be given in a dosage of 4 to 6 g daily during the first 48 hours. Intravenous therapy, in conjunction with treatment by mouth if tolerated, was essential for the treatment of severely ill patients. Streptomycin, though effective, caused severe intoxication and should be given with other antibiotics, in doses of 500 mg intramuscularly 4-hourly for 2 days, followed by 500 mg six-hourly until clinical improvement had occurred. Chloramphenicol given in a dose of 50 to 75 mg per kg body-weight had also been given by mouth up to a total dose of 20 to 25 g. Sulphadiazine 12 g daily for 4 to 7 days had reduced mortality in bubonic plague but not in the pneumonic disease. Less severe infections had been treated with a 4-g initial dose, 2 g four-hourly until the temperature was normal, and 500 mg four-hourly to complete a course of 7 to 10 days.— *Tech. Rep. Ser. Wld Hlth Org. No. 447,* 1970.

In a report prepared by the Public Health Laboratory Service Communicable Disease Surveillance Centre, treatment of plague with streptomycin, tetracycline, or chloramphenicol was considered to be highly effective in all forms of human disease if recognised early.— *Br. med. J.*, 1983, *287,* 118.

PNEUMOTHORAX. A report of the successful management of pneumothorax in 2 patients with the intrapleural instillation of 500 mg of tetracycline dissolved in 50 mL of sodium chloride injection.— R. C. Goldszer *et al., J. Am. med. Ass.*, 1979, *241,* 724.

Tetracycline 2 g in 50 mL of saline solution for adult patients has been found to be effective in causing pleurodesis in patients with pneumothorax and active pulmonary-pleural air leak provided the lung is expanded; the procedure is usually carried out for 3 days in a row. If tetracycline is used alone it frequently causes a quite severe scalding chest pain which does not appear to be alleviated by prior administration of analgesics, sedatives, or lignocaine or bupivacaine hydrochloride. However, ketamine 0.2 to 0.75 mg per kg body-weight administered intravenously before the tetracycline is instilled appears to effectively control the pain.— L. W. Stephenson, *Chest,* 1985, *88,* 803.

For further reference to tetracycline used as a sclerosant, see under Cysts and Malignant Effusions, above.

PREGNANCY AND THE NEONATE. In most developing countries the risk of neonatal gonococcal or chlamydial conjunctivitis (ophthalmia neonatorum) is high and eye prophylaxis is essential. The World Health Organisation (WHO) recommends careful cleaning of the eyes immediately after birth followed by application to the conjunctivae of silver nitrate 1% eye-drops, tetracycline hydrochloride 1% eye ointment, or erythromycin 0.5% eye ointment. All 3 preparations are considered to be effective in preventing gonococcal infection in the newborn, but erythromycin eye ointment is not widely available and silver nitrate has no proven effect against chlamydial conjunctivitis. In industrialised countries gonococcal conjunctivitis of the newborn is less of a problem but the incidence of chlamydial infection of the newborn is increasing.

For the treatment of neonatal conjunctivitis due to *Neisseria gonorrhoeae* the WHO recommends that systemic therapy with cefotaxime, kanamycin, or benzylpenicillin should be accompanied by hourly conjunctival irrigation with saline or buffered ophthalmic solutions, and application of a topical antibiotic preparation until the discharge is eliminated. The topical antibiotic can be either tetracycline hydrochloride 1% or erythromycin 0.5% eye ointment which should be administered hourly for the first 24 hours, every 3 hours for the second 24 hours, and then every 6 hours for a further 8 days (WHO Expert Committee on Venereal Diseases and Treponematoses, *Tech. Rep. Ser. Wld Hlth Org. No. 736*, 1986; *Conjunctivitis of the Newborn: prevention and treatment at the primary health care level*, Geneva, World Health Organization, 1986). Some workers feel that, if adequate systemic treatment is given, there is no evidence that topical antibiotics are necessary, although in practice many clinicians continue to use both (J.D. Oriel, *J. antimicrob. Chemother*., 1984, *14*, 209).

For the treatment of nongonococcal conjunctivitis of the newborn, with onset of infection after 7 days and minimal discharge, topical tetracycline hydrochloride 1% or erythromycin 0.5% ointment may be used 4 times daily for 14 days. However, for infants with chlamydial infection erythromycin should be given by mouth (*Conjunctivitis of the Newborn; prevention and treatment at the primary health care level*, Geneva, World Health Organization, 1986). Topical antimicrobial therapy, even with agents which are active *in vitro* such as tetracycline or erythromycin often fails in neonatal chlamydial conjunctivitis because about one-third of affected babies have concurrent nasopharyngeal colonisation. Confirmed chlamydial ophthalmia must be treated with systemic antibiotics (E. Rees *et al., Archs Dis. Childh.*, 1981, *56*, 193; *Lancet*, 1984, *2*, 1375). For neonatal conjunctivitis caused by other organisms such as streptococci, chloramphenicol is recommended for topical therapy (J.M. Pierce *et al., Br. J. Ophthal.*, 1982, *66*, 728).

Studies comparing topical tetracycline hydrochloride with erythromycin or silver nitrate for prophylaxis against neonatal conjunctivitis: E. M. Zola, *Drug Intell. & clin. Pharm.*, 1984, *18*, 692; V. N. Jarvis *et al., Br. J. Ophthal.*, 1987, *71*, 295; R. C. Brunham *et al.* (letter), *New Engl. J. Med.*, 1987, *316*, 1549.

Q FEVER. For comment on the use of tetracyclines to treat Q fever, see under Doxycycline Hydrochloride, p.219.

RELAPSING FEVER, LOUSE-BORNE. In an evaluation of single-dose antibiotic regimens in patients with louse-borne relapsing fever due to *Borrelia recurrentis*, 21 patients were given either tetracycline or erythromycin by mouth and 30 received either tetracycline 250 mg intravenously or procaine penicillin 600 mg intramuscularly. Although tetracycline given intravenously was superior to procaine penicillin, the treatment of choice was considered to be a single 500-mg dose of tetracycline or erythromycin by mouth. In 15 similar patients given paracetamol 650 mg, hydrocortisone sodium succinate 500 mg intravenously, or no drug 2 hours before and 2 hours after a dose of erythromycin, rigor was not prevented although defervescence occurred earlier in those given hydrocortisone. The best management of a possible Jarisch-Herxheimer reaction was considered to be the prophylactic infusion of sodium chloride injection to prevent hypotension.— T. Butler *et al., J. infect. Dis.*, 1978, *137*, 573.

In a study of 377 patients with louse-borne relapsing fever, a single oral dose of tetracycline 500 mg, doxycycline 100 mg, erythromycin 500 mg, or chloramphenicol 500 mg, or a single intramuscular injection of penicillin with aluminium monostearate were all considered to be equally effective. All patients who received antibiotic treatment for their first attack of louse-borne relapsing fever experienced a Jarisch-Herxheimer reaction. Of the 253 patients treated with a non-penicillin drug 64 (25%) had another episode of fever 4 to 6 days after the resolution of the Jarisch-Herxheimer reaction, and it was therefore considered prudent to treat louse-borne relapsing fever patients with multiple doses of an effective antibiotic for 2 days whenever possible.— P. L. Perine and B. Teklu, *Am. J. trop. Med. Hyg.*, 1983, *32,* 1096.

A tetracycline such as tetracycline hydrochloride is considered the drug of choice for relapsing fever due to *Borrelia recurrentis*, although tetracyclines should generally be avoided in pregnant women, infants, and children aged 8 years or younger; doxycycline is recommended for uraemic patients. Benzylpenicillin may be used as an alternative drug.— *Med. Lett.*, 1986, *28,* 33.

RESPIRATORY-TRACT INFECTIONS. *Bronchitis.* Tetracycline hydrochloride 1 g daily is of moderate clinical efficacy for the treatment of clinically mild cases of purulent exacerbations of chronic bronchitis; it is relatively inexpensive and causes few side-effects. Equivalent daily dosages of other tetracyclines such as doxycycline 100 mg, demeclocycline 600 mg, lymecycline 600 mg, methacycline hydrochloride 600 mg, minocycline hydrochloride 200 mg, or the preparation of chlortetracycline, tetracycline, and demeclocycline (Deteclo) produce similar results; higher doses may be required for more severe illness. Tetracyclines may retain their usefulness in areas where the incidence of resistant pneumococci and *Haemophilus influenzae* remains low. In addition, mild cases of aspiration pneumonia may be due to mycoplasma which are sensitive to tetracyclines, but not to ampicillin or co-trimoxazole. However, long-term treatment of chronic bronchitis with tetracycline is largely ineffective and bactericidal antibiotics such as ampicillin, amoxycillin, and cefuroxime are to be preferred (A. Pines, *J. antimicrob. Chemother.*, 1982, *9*, 333). Conflicting data on the value of antibiotic administration in the therapy of acute exacerbation of chronic bronchitis have been obtained. Some workers have found no substantial benefit using tetracycline therapy compared with placebo (M.B. Nicotra *et al., Ann. intern. Med.*, 1982, *97*, 18), whereas others have reported a greater overall failure rate (no resolution of symptoms or deterioration) in patients receiving placebo compared to patients receiving antibiotic treatment, particularly when the severity of symptoms increased (N.R. Anthonisen *et al., Ann. intern. Med.*, 1987, *106*, 196).

Pertussis. For comment on the use of tetracycline in patients with pertussis, see under Erythromycin, p.226.

Pneumonia. Tetracyclines were ineffective in preventing or treating bacterial pneumonia complicating viral pneumonia in 35 patients.— C. Ellenbogen *et al., Am. J. Med.*, 1974, *56*, 169.

Community-acquired pneumonia due to *Legionella bozemanii* in an immunocompetent patient was unresponsive to erythromycin but addition of intravenous tetracycline to the regimen resulted in a favourable response.— S. Ruiz-Santana *et al.* (letter), *Ann. intern. Med.*, 1986, *105,* 969.

Psittacosis. Psittacosis due to *Chlamydia psittaci* is one of the more common causes of atypical pneumonia and pyrexia of unknown origin seen in general practice. It may be transmitted by both ill and well birds, but may also be spread from person to person. Three patients who presented with the signs and symptoms of a localised chest infection, but failed to improve when treated with broad-spectrum antibiotics, expectorants, and bronchodilators, were found to have chlamydial infection and made gradual but full recoveries when given courses of tetracycline antibiotics (J. C. Jemmett and S. R. Palmer, *J. R. Coll. gen. Pract.*, 1985, *35*, 413). A new *C. psittaci* strain, TWAR, has been isolated, and in a study of 386 students with acute respiratory-tract infections, the TWAR strain occurred most often in patients with pneumonia (12%), but also in patients with bronchitis (5%) or pharyngitis (1%); it appeared to spread from human to human. Erythromycin 1 g daily for 5 to 10 days was found to be inadequate as many of the patients had continuing or recurring symptoms. Therefore until it is possible to study various treatments for TWAR infections it would seem reasonable to use treatment schedules recommended for chlamydia, that is tetracycline 2 g daily for 7 to 10 days or 1 g daily for 21 days (J. T. Grayson *et al.*, *New Engl. J. Med.*, 1986, *315*, 161.

RICKETTSIAL INFECTIONS. For the use of tetracycline in rickettsial infections, see under Mediterranean Spotted Fever, above, and Typhus, below. See also under Doxycycline Hydrochloride, Q Fever, p.219 and Rickettsial Infections, p.220.

SEXUALLY TRANSMITTED DISEASES. *Gonorrhoea.* Tetracycline has been recommended by the World Health Organization as one of the treatments for uncomplicated gonococcal infections, although it is not recommended for rectal or pharyngeal infections. A dose of tetracycline hydrochloride 500 mg 4 times daily by mouth for 7 days or doxycycline hydrochloride 100 mg twice daily by mouth for 7 days has been suggested (WHO Expert Committee on Venereal Diseases and Treponematoses, *Tech. Rep. Ser. Wld Hlth Org. No. 736*, 1986, p.118). However, because of tetracycline-resistance some workers no longer recommend the use of tetracycline alone (F. Brewer *et al.*, *New Engl. J. Med.*, 1986, *315*, 1548) and current treatment recommendations for gonorrhoea such as amoxycillin plus probenecid or ceftriaxone tend to reflect the emergence of tetracycline-resistant *Neisseria gonorrhoeae* and the increasing prevalence of penicillinase-producing strains (*Med. Lett.*, 1986, *28*, 23). However, these regimens are not reliably effective against *Chlamydia trachomatis* infection which has been reported to be present in up to about 45% of patients with gonorrhoea (A.E. Washington, *Drugs*, 1984, *28*, 355; E.W. Hook and K.K. Holmes, *Ann. intern. Med.*, 1985, *102*, 229). Many clinicians, therefore, recommend that all patients with gonorrhoea be treated with a suitable agent against gonococci and in addition a 7-day course of tetracycline or doxycycline to cover chlamydial infection (W.R. Bowie, *Drugs*, 1984, *27*, 459; W.E. Stamm *et al.*, *New Engl. J. Med.*, 1984, *310*, 545; A.E. Washington *et al.*, *J. Am. med. Ass.*, 1987, *257*, 2056; H.H. Handsfield, *ibid.*, 2073).

For the use of tetracycline hydrochloride eye ointment in the prophylaxis and treatment of neonatal conjunctivitis, see Pregnancy and the Neonate, above.

Granuloma inguinale. Some workers consider a tetracycline to be the drug of choice in the treatment of granuloma inguinale due to *Calymmatobacterium granulomatis* (P.J.B. Smith and A.V. Kaisary, *Practitioner*, 1984, *228*, 733; *Med. Lett.*, 1986, *28*, 33). However, the World Health Organization recommends the use of co-trimoxazole as the drug of choice, and tetracycline hydrochloride 500 mg four times daily by mouth for 14 days, or chloramphenicol or thiamphenicol in association with gentamicin, as alternative regimens depending on regional variations in the efficacy of these regimens. The causal organism is difficult to isolate and culture, and there have been few clinical studies (WHO Expert Committee on Venereal Diseases and Treponematoses, *Tech. Rep. Ser. Wld Hlth Org. No. 736*, 1986, p.133).

Lymphogranuloma venereum. The World Health Organization recommends that infections with lymphogranuloma venereum (LGV) biovars of *Chlamydia trachomatis* should be treated with tetracycline hydrochloride 500 mg four times daily by mouth for 2 weeks. Alternative regimens include doxycycline 100 mg twice daily, erythromycin 500 mg four times daily, or sulphamethoxazole 1 g twice daily, all given by mouth for 2 weeks (WHO Expert Committee on Venereal Diseases and Treponematoses, *Tech. Rep. Ser. Wld Hlth Org. No. 736*, 1986, p.125). However, some workers recommend that treatment is continued for 21 days (*Med. Lett.*, 1986, *28*, 23; T.A. Bell and J.T. Grayston, *Ann. intern. Med.*, 1986, *104*, 524).

Nongonococcal urethritis and cervicitis. Nongonococcal urethritis or nonspecific urethritis is usually caused by infection with *Chlamydia trachomatis* or *Ureaplasma urealyticum*. Tetracycline 500 mg four times daily by mouth for 7 days, or other tetracyclines such as doxycycline 100 mg twice daily, minocycline 100 mg twice daily, or oxytetracycline 500 mg four times daily, all given for 7 days, or alternatively erythromycin 500 mg four times daily by mouth for 7 days, are usually effective against both organisms, although tetracycline-resistant strains of *U. urealyticum* have been reported (A.E. Washington, *Drugs*, 1984, *28*, 355; J.D. Oriel, *J. antimicrob. Chemother.*, 1986, *18*, *Suppl.* A, 67; *Med. Lett.*, 1986, *28*, 23). For uncomplicated urethral, endocervical, or rectal infections with *C. trachomatis* the World Health Organization recommends treatment with doxycycline or tetracycline, and erythromycin as an alternative regimen for patients in whom tetracyclines are contra-indicated as in pregnancy (WHO Expert Committee on Venereal Diseases and Treponematoses, *Tech. Rep. Ser. Wld Hlth Org. No. 736*, 1986, p.124). There has been a report of therapeutic failue with tetracycline or doxycycline in 3 patients with *C. trachomatis* infection which was successfully treated with rifampicin (M. Midulla *et al.*, *Br. med. J.*, 1987, *294*, 742). However, it is possible that the diagnosis of chlamydial infection was mistaken and, as yet, there have been no confirmed reports of resistance of *C. trachomatis* to tetracycline either *in vitro* or *in vivo*. Erythromycin is considered to be a more appropriate alternative than rifampicin in cases of apparent tetracycline failure (D. Taylor-Robinson, *ibid.*, 1161; M. Viswalingam *et al.*, *ibid.*, 1352).

For mention of the use of tetracycline in the management of other chlamydial infections, see Pregnancy and the Neonate and Respiratory-tract Infections, Psittacosis, above, and Trachoma, below.

Reiter's disease. Aseptic arthritis may complicate sexually transmitted genital-tract infection and certain bacterial gut infections. When sexually transmitted infection is the trigger, both the patient and the regular sex partner should be treated with an antibiotic until signs of urethritis or cervicitis have disappeared. A one- to three-week course of tetracycline 1 to 2 g daily by mouth is usually sufficient, although recurrence of genital-tract inflammation is common. However, there have been no adequate studies to determine whether antibiotic therapy can either prevent the development of arthritis or influence its severity, extent, or duration.— *Lancet*, 1987, *2*, 1125.

Syphilis. Tetracycline hydrochloride 500 mg four times daily by mouth for 15 days, or erythromycin given in the same dose, are recommended by the World Health Organization as alternative regimens to benzathine or procaine penicillins for penicillin-allergic patients with early syphilis; the treatment should be given for 30 days in patients with late syphilis. Tetracyclines are not recommended for pregnant patients and pregnant women with syphilis who are allergic to penicillins should be treated with erythromycin (WHO Expert Committee on Venereal Diseases and Treponematoses, *Tech. Rep. Ser. Wld Hlth Org. No. 736*, 1986, p.126). Since erythromycin is considered to be less effective than penicillins or tetracycline, compliance and follow-up must be assured before prescribing, especially in pregnant women (A.E. Washington, *Drugs*, 1984, *28*, 355). If erythromycin is used, the neonate should be fully treated with a penicillin at birth, because of the unpredictable placental transfer of erythromycin (G. Buttigieg, *Br. J. Hosp. Med.*, 1985, *33*, 28; C. I. Ewing *et al.*, *Archs Dis. Childh.*, 1985, *60*, 1128).

SKIN DISORDERS. *Acne.* Oral antibiotics such as tetracycline, oxytetracycline, or erythromycin are used, usually in association with topical preparations such as benzoyl peroxide, in the treatment of moderate to severe acne vulgaris. Doses of the antibiotic may vary from 250 mg twice daily to 1 g or even 2 g daily, depending on the severity of the disease. Treatment is recommended for at least 6 months, during which time the dosage may be reduced (W.J. Cunliffe, *Br. med. J.*, 1980, *280*, 1394; *idem.*, 1982, *285*, 912; *Lancet*, 1982, *2*, 1138). One cause of treatment failure is non-compliance, and therefore patients should be told to expect little improvement in the first month of treatment, but gradual improvement over 6 months. If tetracycline or oxytetracycline are prescribed, patients should also be told that their medication should not be taken with milk, antacids, or oral iron preparations (W. J. Cunliffe, *Prescribers. J.*, 1987, *27*(4), 23).

Systemic treatment with tetracycline hydrochloride in doses greater than 1 g daily reduces the number of *Propionibacterium acnes*, but low doses of 500 mg or less daily tend to have less effect on the bacterial numbers. However, apart from antibacterial activity tetracycline has been reported to have other effects including anti-inflammatory activity, reduction of keratin in pilosebaceous ducts, and inhibition of complement activation, chemotaxis, phagocytosis, cell-mediated immunity, and lipase activity (E. A. Eady *et al.*, *J. antimicrob. Chemother.*, 1982, *10*, 89). Tetracycline has also been shown to be an effective superoxide scavenger and oxidation products of unsaturated skin lipids are believed to be comedogenic (H.M.J. van Baar *et al.*, *Br. J. Derm.*, 1987, *117*, 131). One problem associated with long-term therapy is the increase in gastro-intestinal tract bacterial flora with resistance to tetracycline and other antibiotics (M.V. Valtonen *et al.*, *Br. J. Derm.*, 1976, *95*, 311). Concern has also been expressed over increased resistance of *P. acnes* to antibiotics used in the treatment of acne (J.M. Brown and S.M. Poston, *J. med. Microbiol.*, 1983, *16*, 271).

Other antibiotics which have been tried systemically as alternative treatments for acne include other tetracyclines such as doxycycline or minocycline; co-trimoxazole or trimethoprim, although some workers feel that their use should be restricted because of their wide use in urinary-tract and respiratory-tract infections; and clindamycin which although effective in acne, when taken orally may cause antibiotic-associated colitis and its use is therefore restricted (E.A. Eady *et al.*, *J. antimicrob. Chemother.*, 1982, *10*, 89; *Lancet*, 1982, *2*, 1138; W.J. Cunliffe, *Prescribers' J.*, 1987, *27*(4), 23). In refractory cases of acne in women, hormonal treatments with high-oestrogen-containing oral contraceptives, combinations of oestrogen and anti-androgen, or spironolactone reduce sebum excretion and can be of value (W.J. Cunliffe, *Prescribers' J.*, 1987, *27*(4), 23). Treatment with oestrogen-cyproterone has been shown to be at least as effective as tetracycline and may be tried in women whose oral contraception is jeopardised by antibiotic-induced diarrhoea, or in patients whose acne has improved with conventional treatment, but show no sign of further improvement after 3 to 6 months. Little benefit has been demonstrated using both tetracycline and oestrogen-cyproterone (R. Greenwood *et al.*, *Br. med. J.*, 1985, *291*, 1231). In the treatment of severe acne, isotretinoin may also be of benefit (A.R. Shalita, *Cosmet. Toilet.*, 1983, *98* (July), 57).

Patients with mild acne should be treated with topical preparations such as benzoyl peroxide or tretinoin (W.J. Cunliffe, *Prescribers' J.*, 1987, *27*(4), 23). Topical preparations of antibiotics such as clindamycin, erythromycin, neomycin, or tetracycline have been used, but many dermatologists believe that topical antibiotics are generally less effective than conventional oral treatment. Also many workers feel that no antibiotic which is used systemically or which is related to a systemic drug should be applied topically because of the risks of promoting allergy or resistance to other useful systemic antibiotics. Although tetracycline, erythromycin, and clindamycin have a very low topical sensitising potential, they all readily select for resistance, particularly in staphylococci. Changing from oral to topical antibiotic treatment means that instead of a predominantly antibiotic-resistant Gram-negative gut flora the patient acquires an antibiotic-resistant Gram-positive skin flora. There is also a risk that resistant strains of *P. acnes* could be selected. However, another view is that sensitisation is rare and although resistant bacterial strains undoubtedly arise with topical antibiotics, more side-effects such as gastro-intestinal intolerance and candidiasis are associated with systemic antibiotic therapy (*Lancet*, 1982, *2*, 1138). With topical tetracycline treatment there is, however, a problem of yellow discoloration of the skin and glowing in ultraviolet light. The colouring can be minimised by the use of a low pH wash. A topical preparation of meclocycline sulfosalicylate has also been shown to be clinically effective. There appears to be little point in withholding either topical or oral preparations of tetracyclines because their use in general medicine is declining. However, the beneficial effect of topical benzoyl peroxide or retinoic acid should not be ignored (E.A. Eady *et al.*, *J. antimicrob. Chemother.*, 1982, *10*, 89; *idem*, *Br. J. Derm.*, 1982, *107*, 235). Alternative topical agents include older drugs such as salicylic acid, resorcinol, and sulphur (A. R. Shalita, *Cosmet. Toilet.*, 1983, *98* (July), 57).

Pemphigoid. A preliminary report of clinical improvement in 4 patients with bullous pemphigoid given oral tetracycline or erythromycin in association with nicotinamide. A regimen of tetracycline hydrochloride or erythromycin in doses of 1 to 2.5 g daily in association with nicotinamide 1.5 to 2.5 g daily was suggested to avoid the adverse effects of corticosteroid treatment for bullous pemphigoid. If this regimen alone is insufficient, other drugs such as dapsone or steroids may be added to the regimen. After 6 months of therapy, if complete remission occurs while the patient is undergoing treatment with the antibiotic and nicotinamide, a trial of gradual drug withdrawal would be appropriate.— M. A. Berk and A. L. Lorincz, *Archs Derm.*, 1986, *122*, 670.

Perioral dermatitis. Perioral dermatitis resulting from the use of potent topical corticosteroids may be cured in most patients by a 6- to 8-week course of systemic tetracyclines.— *Lancet*, 1980, *1*, 75. A suggested course of treatment is oxytetracycline 250 mg twice daily for 4 weeks, followed by a further month's treatment with one tablet daily, and the withdrawal of all topical corticosteroids as soon as possible.— *Br. med. J.*, 1980, *280*, 136.

Rosacea. A dose of tetracycline of 250 mg once daily is usually adequate in the treatment of rosacea; it might have to be taken permanently.— *Br. med. J.*, 1978, *2*, 750.

SURGICAL INFECTION PROPHYLAXIS. Irrigation of appendicectomy wounds with tetracycline 250 mg in sodium chloride injection 50 mL reduced the incidence of infection from 7 of 30 control patients to 3 of 41 treated patients.— E. A. Benson *et al.* (letter), *Lancet*, 1973, *2*, 322.

In 1504 consecutive abdominal operations, surgical techniques to minimise contamination were supplemented, when there was potential or actual contamination, by tetracycline lavage (1 g per litre of 0.9% sodium chloride) of the wound and peritoneal cavity together with a single prophylactic pre-operative dose of tetracycline 500 mg given intravenously. The overall incidence of wound and peritoneal cavity infection was 2.8% and 0.8% respectively, which compared favourably with the results achieved in studies of the conventional prophylactic use of antibiotics. Tetracycline lavage was considered to be an important component of the regimen.— Z. H. Krukowski *et al.*, *Br. med. J.*, 1984, *288*, 278.

For comment on the topical application of antibiotics for surgical infection prophylaxis, see Prophylactic Use of Antibiotics, p.103.

TRACHOMA. The tetracyclines (tetracycline, chlortetracycline, and oxytetracycline) have been widely used for the treatment of trachoma (due to *Chlamydia trachomatis*), usually by topical application of a 1% ophthalmic ointment; higher concentrations up to 3% have been prepared but are less well tolerated. Oily suspensions of tetracyclines have also been used at a concentration of 1%, and although they are more expensive they have the advantage that they are easier to apply, involve less wastage than ointments, and cause less inconvenience to the recipients. Topical chemotherapy for trachoma must be intensive and prolonged, 6 weeks being the minimum recommended duration for continuous intensive treatment with tetracycline. With less frequent applications, the duration of treatment must be prolonged and may need to be extended to months or even years. The recommended intermittent treatment schedule consists of applications of tetracycline twice daily for 5 consecutive days or once daily for 10 days, each month and for 6 months each year, to be repeated as necessary. Short courses with tetracyclines can be used for the control of bacterial infections during seasonal epidemics of conjunctivitis and may have to be repeated annually.

Oral therapy with tetracycline given 4 times daily or doxycycline given once daily for 3 to 4 weeks have been effective for selective treatment in well monitored programmes, but cannot be recommended for community-wide use to replace topical chemotherapy. Oral tetracyclines should not be administered to pregnant women because of the possible adverse effects on the foetus.— C. R. Dawson *et al.*, *Guide to Trachoma Control*, World Health Organization, Geneva, 1981, p.40.

Further references: C. R. Dawson *et al.*, *Bull. Wld Hlth Org.*, 1981, *59*, 91; C. R. Dawson *et al.*, *ibid.*, 1982, *60*, 347.

See also under Sexually Transmitted Diseases, above.

TULARAEMIA. For comment on the use of tetracycline in the treatment of tularaemia, see under Streptomycin Sulphate, p.298.

TYPHUS. A report of 3 patients with severe tick-bite fever, the diagnosis of which was delayed. One patient died, but the other 2 responded to treatment with tetracycline 500 mg every 6 hours. Tick-bite fever, the variety of tick typhus or spotted fever occurring in southern Africa, is caused by *Rickettsia conori* var. *pijperi* and is usually a relatively mild illness; however, in middle-aged and elderly individuals the disease tends to be more severe. If there is doubt about the diagnosis but tick-bite fever is suspected, then treatment with tetracycline should be prescribed in addition to other antibiotics which may be indicated.— J. H. S. Gear *et al.*, *S. Afr. med. J.*, 1983, *63*, 807.

ULCERS, APHTHOUS. In a double-blind study in 20 patients with recurrent aphthous ulcers 5 mL of syrup containing tetracycline hydrochloride 125 mg and amphotericin 25 mg, used as a mouthwash three times daily, was significantly more effective than placebo in relieving pain and reducing the incidence of new ulcers.— A. M. Denman and A. A. Schiff, *Br. med. J.*, 1979, *1*, 1248.

URINARY-TRACT INFECTIONS. A study in 62 nonpregnant women with signs and symptoms of uncomplicated urinary-tract infections to compare single-dose tetracycline hydrochloride with conventional therapy. Twelve of 16 women (75%) with positive urine cultures were cured with a single dose of tetracycline 2 g by mouth compared with 15 of 16 (94%) who received tetracycline 500 mg four times daily by mouth for 10 days, and 7 of 13 (54%) who received a single dose of amoxycillin 3 g by mouth. Mild nausea occurred in 3 of 20 patients (15%) who received single-dose tetracycline therapy whereas 8 of 25 patients in the multi-dose tetracycline group experienced severe nausea requiring the drug to be stopped. Although the study only involved small numbers of patients, the potential advantage of single-dose tetracycline for uncomplicated urinary-tract infections warrants further investigation.— J. Rosenstock *et al.*, *Antimicrob. Ag. Chemother.*, 1985, *27*, 652.

See also under Sexually Transmitted Diseases, Nongonococcal Urethritis, above.

Preparations

Tetracycline Capsules *(B.P.)*. Capsules containing tetracycline hydrochloride.

Tetracycline Hydrochloride Capsules *(U.S.P.)*

Tetracycline and Amphotericin B Capsules *(U.S.P.)*

Tetracycline Hydrochloride and Nystatin Capsules *(U.S.P.)*

Tetracycline and Procaine Injection *(B.P.C. 1973)*. A sterile solution of tetracycline hydrochloride and procaine hydrochloride. The injection deteriorates on storage and should be used within 24 hours of preparation.

Tetracycline Hydrochloride for Injection *(U.S.P.)*. If it contains an anaesthetic agent it is intended for intramuscular use only.

Tetracycline Intravenous Infusion *(B.P.)*. Tetracycline Injection. A sterile solution of tetracycline hydrochloride. The injection should be stored at a temperature not exceeding 4° and used within 72 hours of preparation. For intravenous use only in a well-diluted solution.

Sterile Tetracycline Hydrochloride *(U.S.P.)*

Tetracycline Hydrochloride Ointment *(U.S.P.)*

Tetracycline Hydrochloride Ophthalmic Ointment *(U.S.P.)*

Tetracycline Hydrochloride Ophthalmic Suspension *(U.S.P.)*. A sterile suspension of tetracycline hydrochloride in a suitable oil.

Tetracycline Oral Suspension *(B.P.)*. Tetracycline Mixture. pH 3.5 to 6.0.

Tetracycline Oral Suspension *(U.S.P.)*. pH 3.5 to 6.0.

Tetracycline and Amphotericin B Oral Suspension *(U.S.P.)*

Tetracycline Hydrochloride Tablets *(U.S.P.)*

Tetracycline Tablets *(B.P.)*. Tablets containing tetracycline hydrochloride.

Tetracycline Hydrochloride for Topical Solution *(U.S.P.)*. A dry mixture of tetracycline hydrochloride with epitetracycline hydrochloride and sodium metabisulphite, with a suitable aqueous vehicle. pH of reconstituted solution 1.9 to 3.5.

Proprietary Preparations

Achromycin *(Lederle, UK)*. *Capsules*, tetracycline hydrochloride 250 mg.
Tablets, tetracycline hydrochloride 250 mg.
Syrup, tetracycline 125 mg (as hydrochloride)/5 mL.
Intramuscular injection, powder for reconstitution, tetracycline hydrochloride 100 mg, procaine hydrochloride 40 mg.
Intravenous injection, powder for reconstitution, tetracycline hydrochloride 250 and 500 mg.
Eye-drops, tetracycline hydrochloride 1%.
Ointment, for ear or eye, tetracycline hydrochloride 1%.
Ointment, tetracycline hydrochloride 3%.

Achromycin V *(Lederle, UK)*. *Capsules*, tetracycline equivalent to tetracycline hydrochloride 250 mg.

Chymocyclar *(Rorer, UK)*. *Capsules*, tetracycline hydrochloride 250 mg, proteolytic activity (provided by a concentrate of trypsin and chymotrypsin) 50 000 Armour units.

Deteclo *(Lederle, UK)*. *Tablets 300 mg*, tetracycline hydrochloride 115.4 mg, chlortetracycline hydrochloride 115.4 mg, demeclocycline hydrochloride 69.2 mg. *Dose*. 1 tablet every 12 hours; may be increased to 3 or 4 tablets daily for short periods.

Economycin *(DDSA Pharmaceuticals, UK)*. *Capsules*, tetracycline hydrochloride 250 mg.
Tablets, tetracycline hydrochloride 250 mg.

Mysteclin *(Squibb, UK)*. *Tablets*, tetracycline hydrochloride 250 mg, nystatin 250 000 units.
Syrup, tetracycline equivalent to tetracycline hydrochloride 125 mg, amphotericin 25 mg/5 mL. For bacterial infections in patients liable to candidiasis.

Sustamycin *(MCP Pharmaceuticals, UK)*. *Capsules*, sustained-release, tetracycline hydrochloride 250 mg. *Dose*. 2 capsules initially, then 1 every 12 hours.

Tetrabid-Organon *(Organon, UK)*. *Capsules*, sustained-release, tetracycline hydrochloride 250 mg. *Dose*. 2 capsules initially, then 1 capsule every 12 hours; in acne, 1 capsule daily.

Tetrachel *(Berk Pharmaceuticals, UK)*. *Capsules*, tetracycline hydrochloride 250 mg.
Tablets, tetracycline hydrochloride 250 mg.

Topicycline *(Norwich-Eaton, UK)*. *Topical solution*, powder for reconstitution, tetracycline hydrochloride, 4-epitetracycline hydrochloride, providing tetracycline hydrochloride 2.2 mg per mL when reconstituted with solvent containing *n*-decyl methyl sulphoxide and citric acid in 40% alcohol.

Proprietary Names and Manufacturers of Tetracycline and Tetracycline Hydrochloride

Achromycin *(Lederle, Austral.; Lederle, Canad.; Lederle, Denm.; Cyanamid-Novalis, Ger.; Neth.; Norw.; S.Afr.; Lederle, Swed.; Switz.; Lederle, UK; Lederle, USA)*; Achromycin V *(Lederle, Austral.; Lederle, Canad.; Switz.; Lederle, UK; Lederle, USA)*; Achromycine *(Lederle, Switz.)*; Acromicina *(Arg.; Cyanamid, Ital.; Spain)*; Akne-Pyodron *(Artesan, Ger.)*; Ambramicina *(Ital.; Merrell Dow, Spain)*; Apo-Tetra *(Apotex, Canad.)*; Archiciclina *(Ital.)*; Austramycin *(Commonwealth Serum Laboratories, Austral.)*; Austramycin V *(Commonwealth Serum Laboratories, Austral.)*; Binicap *(Ital.)*; Bio-Tetra *(Canad.)*; Bristaciclina *(Antibioticos, Spain)*; Bristacycline *(USA)*; Calociclina *(ISI, Ital.)*; Cefracycline *(Canad.)*; Centet *(USA)*; Chemiciclina *(Ifesa, Spain)*; Ciclotetryl *(Arg.)*; Co-Caps Tetracycline *(Co-Caps, UK)*; Cyclabid *(Script Intal, S.Afr.)*; Cyclopar *(Parke, Davis, USA)*; Diocyclin *(Cimex, Switz.)*; Dumocyclin *(Dumex, Denm.; Norw.)*; Economycin *(DDSA Pharmaceuticals, UK)*; Fermentmycin *(Spain)*; Florocycline *(Fr.)*; Friciclin *(Spain)*;

Gammatet *(S.Afr.)*; Grocyclin *(Switz.)*; Grocycline *(Grossmann, Switz.)*; Guayaciclina *(Novag, Spain)*; Hexacycline *(Diamant, Fr.)*; Hortetracin *(Hortel, Spain)*; Hostaciclina *(Spain)*; Hostacyclin *(Hoechst, Ger.)*; Hostacycline *(Austral.; Belg.; S.Afr.; Hoechst, Switz.)*; Hydracycline *(Fawns & McAllan, Austral.)*; Ibicyn *(Ibi, Ital.)*; Itaglucina *(ITA, Ital.)*; Kinciclina *(Kin, Spain)*; Lauroanginol *(Spain)*; Medicycline *(Canad.)*; Mephacycline *(Mepha, Switz.)*; NC *(Jpn)*; Neo-Tetrine *(Neolab, Canad.)*; Novotetra *(Novopharm, Canad.)*; Omnaze *(Arg.)*; Oppacyn *(LRC Products, UK)*; Panmycin *(Upjohn, USA)*; Panmycin-P *(Upjohn, Austral.)*; Pervasol *(Arg.)*; Piracaps *(Reid-Provident, USA)*; Polycycline *(Austral.)*; Quadcin *(Austral.)*; Quatrax *(Austral.)*; Quimpe Antibiotico *(Quimpe, Spain)*; Reacton *(Nezel, Spain)*; Remicyclin *(Schaper & Brümmer, Ger.)*; Retet *(Reid-Provident, USA)*; Retet-S *(Reid-Provident, USA)*; Riocyclin *(Adcock Ingram, S.Afr.)*; Robitet *(Robins, USA)*; Roviciclina *(Rovi, Spain)*; Rubibacter *(Rubio, Spain)*; Sanbiotetra *(Santos, Spain)*; Sifacycline *(Fr.)*; SK-Tetracycline *(Smith Kline & French, USA)*; Spaciclina *(SPA, Ital.)*; Steclin *(Arg.; Heyden, Ger.; Squibb, UK)*; Steclin-V *(Squibb, Austral.; Squibb, S.Afr.)*; Sumycin *(Squibb, USA)*; Supramycin *(Grünenthal, Ger.)*; Sustamycin *(MCP Pharmaceuticals, UK)*;

T-Caps *(Canad.)*; Teciclina *(Spain)*; Teclinazets *(Spain)*; Tefilin *(Hermal, Ger.)*; Tetra Hubber *(Hubber, Spain)*; Tetra-B *(Spain)*; Tetrabakat *(Dorsch, Ger.)*; Tetrabid-Organon *(Organon, UK)*; Tetrabioptal *(Farmila, Ital.)*; Tetrablet *(Makara, Ger.; Makapharm, Switz.)*; Tetracap *(Austral.; S.Afr.)*; Tetrachel *(Neth.; Berk Pharmaceuticals, UK; Rachelle, USA)*; Tetraciclene *(Spain)*; Tetracitro *(Chephasaar, Ger.)*; Tetracrine *(Canad.)*; Tetracyn *(Austral.; Pfizer, Canad.; Pfizer, UK; Pfipharmecs, USA)*; Tetracyn-V *(Austral.)*; Tetralean *(Canad.)*; Tetralen *(CEPA, Spain)*; Tetra-Liser *(Spain)*; Tetralution *(Merckle, Ger.)*; Tetramavan *(Switz.)*; Tetramig *(Biogalenique, Fr.)*; Tetramykoin *(Boucher & Muir, Austral.)*; Tetranovin *(Denm.)*; Tetraplus *(Ital.)*; Tetra-Proter *(Proter, Ital.)*; Tetrarco *(Neth.)*; Tetrarco LA *(Switz.)*; Tetrarco Simple *(Clarben, Spain)*; Tetraseptin *(Switz.)*; Tetrasuiss *(Switz.)*; Tetratets *(Pharmadrug, Ger.)*; Tetrivo Bicaps *(Switz.)*; Topicycline *(Stockhausen, Ger.; Procter & Gamble, Switz.; Norwich-Eaton, UK; Norwich Eaton, USA)*; Totomycin *(Boots, UK)*; Triacycline *(Canad.)*; Triphacyclin *(Switz.)*; Ultraciclina *(Ital.)*; Unitetra *(Ausonia, Ital.)*; U-Tet *(USA)*; Zyler *(Spain)*.

The following names have been used for multi-ingredient preparations containing tetracycline and tetracycline hydrochloride—

Achrocidin *(Lederle, Canad.)*; Achrostatin *(Lederle, Austral.)*; Albamycin T *(Upjohn, UK)*; Chymocyclar *(Rorer, UK)*; Comycin *(Upjohn, Austral.)*; Deteclo

(Lederle, UK); Mysteclin Syrup *(Squibb, UK)*; Mysteclin Tablets *(Squibb, UK)*; Mysteclin-F *(Squibb, USA)*; Mysteclin-V *(Squibb, Austral.)*; Tetracyn SF *(Pfizer, UK)*; Tetrex-F *(Astra, Austral.)*.

170-s

Tetracycline Phosphate Complex *(BAN, USAN)*.
A complex of sodium metaphosphate and tetracycline.

CAS — 1336-20-5.

Pharmacopoeias. In *U.S.*
Jpn includes Tetracycline Metaphosphate ($C_{22}H_{24}N_2O_8,HPO_3,1/5NaPO_3$=544.8).

A yellow crystalline powder with a faint characteristic odour and a potency of not less than 750 µg per mg, as tetracycline hydrochloride, calculated on the anhydrous basis. A 1% aqueous suspension has a pH of 2 to 4; the *U.S.P.* injection has a pH of 2 to 3. **Soluble** 1 in 31 of water, 1 in 130 of alcohol; slightly soluble in methyl alcohol; very slightly soluble in acetone. **Store** in airtight containers. Protect from light.

Small amounts of anhydrotetracycline and epianhydrotetracycline were found in newly manufactured tetracycline phosphate preparations. Storage in warm humid conditions increased the percentage of these degradation products.— V. C. Walton *et al.*, *J. pharm. Sci.*, 1970, *59*, 1160.

Tetracycline phosphate complex has the same actions and uses as tetracycline hydrochloride (see p.313) but has been claimed to be more readily absorbed. Potency is expressed in terms of tetracycline or tetracycline hydrochloride. It is usually given by mouth in a dose equivalent to 1 g of tetracycline daily in 2 to 4 divided doses. The parenteral route has also been used.

The administration of tetracycline phosphate complex, 500 mg every 12 hours to 10 healthy subjects resulted in mean serum concentrations of about 1.5 µg per mL after 2 hours, falling to 0.64 µg after 12 hours, rising and maintained between 2 and 4 µg after the first 24 hours' treatment. About 95 mg of the drug was recovered from the urine during the first 24 hours.— L. P. Olon and D. N. Holvey, *Clin. Med.*, 1968, *75*, (Jan.), 33.

Tissue concentrations of tetracycline following the administration of tetracycline complex by mouth.— G. Racz, *Curr. ther. Res.*, 1971, *13*, 553.

Preparations

Tetracycline Phosphate Complex Capsules *(U.S.P.)*

Tetracycline Phosphate Complex for Injection *(U.S.P.)*. A sterile dry mixture of tetracycline phosphate complex and magnesium chloride or magnesium ascorbate to be reconstituted before use.

Sterile Tetracycline Phosphate Complex *(U.S.P.)*

Proprietary Preparations

Tetrex *(Bristol-Myers Pharmaceuticals, UK)*. *Capsules*, tetracycline 250 mg (as phosphate complex).

Proprietary Names and Manufacturers

Binicap *(Ital.)*; Biocheclina *(Kairon, Spain)*; Bristaciclina Retard *(Spain)*; Ciclindif Infantil *(Spain)*; Conciclina *(Lusofarmaco, Ital.)*; Hostacycline-P *(Hoechst, Austral.; Hoechst, S.Afr.)*; Tetradecin Novum *(Swed.)*; Tetrafosammina *(FIRMA, Ital.)*; Tetramin *(Spain)*; Tetrazetas Retard *(Spain)*; Tetrex *(Astra, Austral.; Belg.; Canad.; Bristol Europe, Ital.; S.Afr.; Switz.; Bristol-Myers Pharmaceuticals, UK; Bristol, USA)*.

The following names have been used for multi-ingredient preparations containing tetracycline phosphate complex— Azotrex *(Bristol, USA)*; Resteclin *(Squibb, Canad.)*.

13315-b

Tetroxoprim *(BAN, USAN, rINN)*.
5-[3,5-Dimethoxy-4-(2-methoxyethoxy)benzyl]pyrimidine-2,4-diyldiamine.
$C_{16}H_{22}N_4O_4$=334.4.

CAS — 53808-87-0.

Tetroxoprim is closely related chemically to trimethoprim (see p.328). It is a dihydrofolate reductase inhibitor. It is used as co-tetroxazine (see p.205) in conjunction with sulphadiazine.
Tetroxoprim embonate has also been used.

Proprietary Names and Manufacturers
Heumann, Ger.

171-w

Thiamphenicol *(BAN, USAN, rINN)*.

CB-8053; Dextrosulphenidol; Thiamfenicol; Thiamphenicolum; Thiophenicol; Tiamfenicolo; Win-5063-2. 2,2-Dichloro-*N*-[($\alpha R,\beta R$)-β-hydroxy-α-hydroxymethyl-4-mesylphenethyl]acetamide.
$C_{12}H_{15}Cl_2NO_5S$=356.2.

CAS — 15318-45-3; 847-25-6 (racephenicol).

NOTE. Racephenicol is the racemic form of thiamphenicol.

Pharmacopoeias. In *Belg., Br., Eur., Fr., It., Neth.*, and *Swiss.*

A fine white to yellowish-white odourless crystalline powder or crystals. M.p. 163° to 167°. Slightly **soluble** in water, ether, and ethyl acetate; soluble in methyl alcohol; sparingly soluble in dehydrated alcohol and acetone; freely soluble in dimethylformamide and acetonitrile; very soluble in dimethylacetamide. **Store** in well-closed containers. Protect from light and moisture.

172-e

Thiamphenicol Glycinate Hydrochloride

Thiamphenicol Aminoacetate Hydrochloride; Tiamfenicolo Glicinato Cloridrato. (2*R*,3*R*)-2-(2,2-Dichloroacetamido)-3-hydroxy-3-(4-mesylphenyl)propyl glycinate hydrochloride.
$C_{14}H_{18}Cl_2N_2O_6S,HCl$=449.7.

CAS — 2393-92-2 (thiamphenicol glycinate); 2611-61-2 (hydrochloride).

Pharmacopoeias. In *It.*

1.26 g of monograph substance is approximately equivalent to 1 g of thiamphenicol.

Adverse Effects and Precautions

As for chloramphenicol (p.186).

Thiamphenicol is probably more liable to cause dose-dependent reversible depression of the bone marrow than chloramphenicol but it is not usually associated with aplasia. Thiamphenicol also appears to be less likely to cause the 'grey syndrome' in neonates.

Doses of thiamphenicol should be reduced in patients with renal impairment. It is probably not necessary to reduce doses in patients with impaired liver function.

EFFECTS ON THE BLOOD. References to the haematological side-effects of thiamphenicol: J. P. Kaltwasser *et al.*, *Arzneimittel-Forsch.*, 1974, *24*, 190; *idem*, 343 and 561; R. Franceschinis, *Arzneimittel-Forsch.*, 1974, *24*, 944; A. Cornet *et al.*, *Sem. Hôp. Paris*, 1974, *50*, 1567.

For comment on the structural differences between thiamphenicol and chloramphenicol and a proposed structure-toxicity relationship associated with chloramphenicol-induced aplastic anaemia, see under Chloramphenicol Sodium Succinate, p.187.

EFFECTS ON THE NERVOUS SYSTEM. Reports of peripheral neuritis due to thiamphenicol.— *Jpn med. Gaz.*, 1977, *14*, (Dec. 20), 12; Y. Shinohara *et al.*, *Eur. Neurol.*, 1977, *16*, 161.

Antimicrobial Action

Thiamphenicol has a broad spectrum of activity resembling that of chloramphenicol (see p.188) although in general it is less active.

Cross-resistance has been reported between thiamphenicol and chloramphenicol.

Thiamphenicol inhibited 97.5, 99.6, and 100% of 517 strains of *Neisseria gonorrhoeae* at concentrations of 2, 4, and 8 µg per mL respectively and inhibited 76.9 and 100% of 13 beta-lactamase-producing strains of *N. gonorrhoeae* at concentrations of 2 and 4 µg per mL respectively.— P. D. Duck *et al.*, *Antimicrob. Ag. Chemother.*, 1978, *14*, 788. See also J. Y. Riou *et al.*, *J. antimicrob. Chemother.*, 1985, *16*, *Suppl.* A, 209.

A study *in vitro* comparing the antimicrobial activities of thiamphenicol and chloramphenicol. Although thiamphenicol was generally 2 to 4 times less active than chloramphenicol against most species, minimum inhibitory concentrations (MICs) were similar for the 2 drugs against *Streptococcus pyogenes* and *Strep. pneumoniae.* Thiamphenicol also had similar or enhanced activity compared with chloramphenicol against *Haemophilus influenzae* and *Neisseria meningitidis* when both MICs and minimum bactericidal concentrations (MBCs) were measured.— F. O'Grady *et al.*, *Chemotherapy, Basle*, 1980, *26*, 116.

Minimum inhibitory concentrations (MICs) of 196 clinical isolates of *Streptococcus pneumoniae* showed important variations in their sensitivity to thiamphenicol and chloramphenicol; MICs ranged from 0.4 to greater than 100 µg per mL and less than 0.1 to 12.5 µg per mL, respectively.— Y. Glupczynski *et al.* (letter), *J. antimicrob. Chemother.*, 1983, *11*, 488.

Absorption and Fate

Thiamphenicol is absorbed from the gastro-intestinal tract following oral administration and peak serum concentrations of 3 to 6 µg per mL have been achieved about 2 hours after a 500-mg dose. Concentrations from about 7 to 13 µg per mL have been reported one hour after 500 mg administered intramuscularly as the glycinate.

Thiamphenicol has been reported to diffuse into the cerebrospinal fluid, across the placenta, into breast milk, and to penetrate well into purulent and mucous sputum. The half-life of thiamphenicol is similar to that of chloramphenicol (see p.189), but unlike chloramphenicol most of the administered dose of thiamphenicol is excreted unchanged in the urine; the half-life is increased in patients with renal failure. Only 5 to 10% is conjugated with glucuronic acid in the liver. A small amount is excreted in the bile.

Plasma concentrations, half-life, and urinary excretion of thiamphenicol were studied in 13 healthy subjects, 19 patients with cirrhosis of the liver, and 16 with acute viral hepatitis. Disturbed liver function did not influence the metabolism or excretion of the drug. High doses of heparin seemed to decrease the activity of thiamphenicol.— H. P. Menz *et al.*, *Arzneimittel-Forsch.*, 1974, *24*, 99.

In patients with renal failure the half-life of thiamphenicol was prolonged to 13.5 hours during the interval between dialysis treatment. During haemodialysis the half-life was still 2 to 3 times longer than in patients with normal renal function.— H. P. Menz *et al.*, *Arzneimittel-Forsch.*, 1974, *24*, 102.

The absorption and excretion of thiamphenicol palmitate in *rats* and humans.— D. D. Bella *et al.*, *Arzneimittel-Forsch.*, 1974, *24*, 836.

The pharmacokinetics of thiamphenicol were unaltered by peritoneal dialysis in anephric patients.— K. I. Furman *et al.*, *Antimicrob. Ag. Chemother.*, 1976, *9*, 557.

PREGNANCY AND THE NEONATE. The placental transfer of thiamphenicol.— T. A. Plomp *et al.*, *Eur. J. Obstet. Gynec. reprod. Biol.*, 1977, *7*, 383.

For the excretion of thiamphenicol and chloramphenicol in breast milk, see under Chloramphenicol, p.190.

Uses and Administration

Thiamphenicol has been used similarly to chloramphenicol (see p.190) in the treatment of susceptible infections. The usual adult dose is 1.5 g daily by mouth in divided doses; up to 3 g daily has been given initially in severe infections. Equivalent doses may be administered by intramuscular or intravenous injection as the more water-soluble glycinate.

Thiamphenicol has also been used as thiamphenicol glycinate acetylcysteinate, and thiamphenicol palmitate.

Beneficial results with thiamphenicol in patients with non-sporing anaerobic infections.— B. M. Limson *et al.*, *Curr. ther. Res.*, 1981, *29*, 438.

PROSTATITIS. Of 10 patients with chronic bacterial prostatitis who received thiamphenicol 500 mg every 8 hours for 6 weeks, 8 had a good or excellent response to treatment. Mean concentrations of thiamphenicol in blood and ejaculate were 5.3 and 2.3 µg per mL respectively 2 hours after the start of therapy and 7.3 and 13.9 µg per mL respectively after 24 hours.— T. A. Plomp *et al.*, *J. antimicrob. Chemother.*, 1978, *4*, 65. See also T. A. Plomp *et al.*, *Chemotherapy, Basle*, 1979, *25*, 254.

Treatment of recurrent chronic bacterial prostatitis in 29 patients by local injection of thiamphenicol. A 20-mL physiological saline solution containing thiamphenicol glycinate 2 g and lignocaine hydrochloride 20 mg injected using a long fine needle via the perineal route directly into the prostate lobes was curative in 19

(66%) of the patients; eleven patients were cured after one injection, 5 required 2 injections, and 3 obtained sterile cultures after 3 injections.— T. A. Plomp *et al.*, *Urology*, 1980, *15*, 542.

SEXUALLY TRANSMITTED DISEASES. In a study of 120 patients with urethritis caused by *Neisseria gonorrhoeae*, *Chlamydia trachomatis*, *Mycoplasma hominis*, or *Ureaplasma urealyticum*, 111 patients were subjectively free of symptoms after treatment with thiamphenicol 2.5 g by mouth as a single dose on the first day followed by 0.5 g three times daily for the next 3 days. All of 51 patients infected with *N. gonorrhoeae* were cured; treatment was successful in 31 of 32 (97%) infected with *C. trachomatis*, 11 of 12 (90%) infected with mycoplasma or ureaplasma, 9 of 26 (29%) infected with Gram-positive bacilli, and 4 of 23 (7%) infected with Gram-negative bacilli.— H. Mensing *et al.*, *Eur. J. sex. transm. Dis.*, 1985, *3*, 47.

Chancroid. Beneficial response in Zimbabwe to single-dose thiamphenicol therapy for chancroid. Patients were given thiamphenicol 2.5 g by mouth followed by a second dose of 1.5 g if the ulcer remained tender a week later. If the treatment was judged ineffective after two weeks patients were given co-trimoxazole 960 mg three times daily for 10 days. Of 341 patients who completed the full observation period, 206 had healed ulcers after the first dose and 122 after the second; only 13 did not respond.— A. S. Latif *et al.* (letter), *Lancet*, 1982, *2*, 1225.

For further mention of the use of thiamphenicol in the treatment of chancroid, see under Choice of Antibiotic, p.101.

Gonorrhoea. Thiamphenicol, 2.5 g by mouth, has been recommended as one of the drugs which may be used to treat uncomplicated urogenital gonococcal infections. It is active against beta-lactamase-producing gonococci, but may show considerable geographical variation in its efficacy, sometimes curing less than 95% of infections. It is not recommended for pregnant women.— WHO Expert Committee on Venereal Diseases and Treponematoses, Sixth Report, *Tech. Rep. Ser. Wld Hlth Org. No. 736*, 1986, p.118.

A report of a high failure rate of single-dose thiamphenicol to treat uncomplicated gonorrhoea in Rwanda. Of 46 evaluable patients only 35 (76%) were cured with thiamphenicol 2.5 g given by mouth. This corresponded with low susceptibility *in vitro* of the infecting strain.— J. Bogaerts *et al.*, *Antimicrob. Ag. Chemother.*, 1987, *31*, 434.

For comparison of thiamphenicol with cefuroxime sodium in the treatment of penicillinase- and non-penicillinase-producing *Neisseria gonorrhoeae* infections, see under Cefuroxime Sodium, p.172.

Proprietary Names and Manufacturers

Flogotisol *(Zambon, Ital.)*; Glitisol *(Zambon, Ital.)*; Hyrazin *(Jpn)*; Neomyson *(Jpn)*; Rincrol *(Jpn)*; Thiamcol *(Jpn)*; Urfamycin *(Montpellier, Arg.; Rio, S.Afr.; Zambon, Spain)*; Urfamycine *(Inpharzam, Belg.; Inpharzam, Ger.; Inpharzam, Neth.; Inpharzam, Switz.)*.

173-l

Ticarcillin Sodium *(BANM, pINNM)*.

BRL-2288; Ticarcillin Disodium *(USAN)*. The disodium salt of (6*R*)-6-[2-carboxy-2-(3-thienyl)acetamido]penicillanic acid.

$C_{15}H_{14}N_2Na_2O_6S_2$=428.4.

CAS — 34787-01-4; 3973-04-4 (both ticarcillin); 4697-14-7; 29457-07-6 (both disodium salt).

Pharmacopoeias. In *Jpn. U.S.* includes Sterile Ticarcillin Disodium.

A white to pale yellow powder. 1.1 g of monograph substance is approximately equivalent to 1 g of ticarcillin. Each g of monograph substance represents about 4.7 mmol of sodium.

Freely **soluble** in water. A solution in water containing about 1% has a pH of 6 to 8.

Aqueous solutions retain their potency for up to 24 hours at 25° and for up to 3 days at 5°. It is recommended that reconstituted solutions of ticarcillin sodium for injection should be administered immediately after preparation. Ticarcillin sodium should not be mixed with blood products or other proteinaceous fluids such as protein hydrolysates. **Incompatibility** or loss of activity has been reported with aminoglycosides and fat emulsions.

Adverse Effects

As for Carbenicillin Sodium, p.139.

Combination with clavulanic acid. An evaluation of the safety and tolerance of 4 formulations of ticarcillin sodium with potassium clavulanate in 1659 patients included in clinical studies in Europe and the *USA*. A total of 161 adverse effects were reported in 151 patients (9.1%), 36 of whom (2.2%) discontinued treatment. The spectrum and intensity of the reactions observed were similar to those associated with ticarcillin therapy.— E. A. P. Croydon and C. Hermoso, *J. antimicrob. Chemother.*, 1986, *17*, *Suppl.* C, 233.

ALLERGY. For comparison of the incidence of allergic reactions to antipseudomonal penicillins in patients with cystic fibrosis, see Piperacillin Sodium, p.285.

EFFECTS ON THE BLOOD. A dose-related prolongation of bleeding time was observed in 17 healthy subjects given ticarcillin 100 to 300 mg per kg body-weight intravenously (C.H. Brown *et al.*, *Antimicrob. Ag. Chemother.*, 1975, *7*, 652). Platelet aggregation was also abnormal in all subjects. These observations were supported by a study by Somani *et al.* (*J. antimicrob. Chemother.*, 1983, *11*, *Suppl.* C, 33) in 6 healthy subjects. Andrassy *et al.* (*New Engl. J. Med.*, 1975, *292*, 109) noted that a haemorrhagic diathesis had been observed after ticarcillin administration.

Other adverse effects on the blood associated with ticarcillin administration include neutropenia (D. Gastineau *et al.*, *Ann. intern. Med.*, 1981, *94*, 711; C.F. Kirkwood *et al.*, *Clin. Pharm.*, 1983, *2*, 569) and a case of thrombocytosis when ticarcillin was administered with clavulanic acid (S.B. Moody and K.S. Pawlicki, *Drug Intell. & clin. Pharm.*, 1987, *21*, 292).

See also Effects on the Kidney and Urinary Bladder, below.

EFFECTS ON ELECTROLYTE HOMOEOSTASIS. Thrombocytosis and hyperkalaemia occurred in one patient after administration of ticarcillin in association with clavulanic acid (as the potassium salt). The potassium content of potassium clavulanate was considered insufficient to be responsible for the hyperkalaemia which was supposed to be secondary to the thrombocytosis.— S. B. Moody and K. S. Pawlicki (letter), *Drug Intell. & clin. Pharm.*, 1987, *21*, 292.

EFFECTS ON THE KIDNEYS AND URINARY BLADDER. Haemorrhagic cystitis occurred in a 12-year-old boy with cystic fibrosis after receiving treatment with intravenous ticarcillin and netilmicin. This recurred 3 months later when he was treated with ticarcillin and tobramycin. On this occasion the condition resolved on substitution of cefoxitin for ticarcillin.— M. V. Relling and J. E. Schunk, *Clin. Pharm.*, 1986, *5*, 590.

Precautions

As for Carbenicillin Sodium, p.139.

INTERACTIONS. For reference to the *in vitro* and *in vivo* inactivation of aminoglycosides by ticarcillin, see Gentamicin Sulphate p.236 and p.238.

See also under Antimicrobial Action (below).

INTERFERENCE WITH DIAGNOSTIC TESTS. In a study *in vitro* of the effects of various antibiotics on tests for glycosuria, ticarcillin in the urine could give falsely elevated readings with a test using a copper-reduction method (Clinitest). It had no effect however on glucose oxidase methods (Diastix and Tes-Tape) of estimating glycosuria.— M. LeBel *et al.*, *Drug Intell. & clin. Pharm.*, 1984, *18*, 617.

Antimicrobial Action

Ticarcillin is bactericidal and has a mode of action and range of activity similar to that of carbenicillin (see p.139) but is reported to be 2 to 4 times more active against *Pseudomonas aeruginosa*.

Combinations of ticarcillin and aminoglycosides have been shown to be synergistic *in vitro*. The activity of ticarcillin against organisms usually resistant due to the production of certain beta-lactamases is enhanced by clavulanic acid, p.197.

ACTIVITY WITH OTHER ANTIMICROBIAL AGENTS. Ticarcillin has been shown to be synergistic *in vitro* against *Pseudomonas aeruginosa* with amikacin (T.T. Yoshikawa and S. A. Shibata, *Antimicrob. Ag. Chemother.*, 1978, *13*, 997; S.C. Aronoff and J.D. Klinger, *ibid.*, 1984, *25*, 279), gentamicin (P. Acred *et al.*, *ibid.*, 1970, 396), and tobramycin (K.R. Comber *et al.*, *ibid.*, 1977, *11*, 956; F.A. Zar and R.J. Kany, *ibid.*, 1985, *27*, 1); these studies have shown synergy against some strains resistant to ticarcillin and/or the aminoglycoside. Synergy has also been shown with amikacin or gentamicin against bacteria of the *Enterobacteriaceae* (R.H. Glew and R.A. Pavuk, *ibid.*, 1983, *23*, 902) and with amikacin against a range of Gram-negative aerobic organisms (S.H. Guenthner *et al.*, *J. antimicrob. Chemother.*, 1986, *18*, 550).

There have been many studies showing the beta-lactamase inhibitor clavulanic acid to extend the spectrum of activity of ticarcillin to organisms which produce certain beta-lactamases (J.W. Paisley and J.A. Washington, *Antimicrob. Ag. Chemother.*, 1978, *14*, 224; P.C. Fuchs *et al.*, *ibid.*, 1984, *25*, 392; A.M. Clarke and S.J.V. Zemcov, *J. antimicrob. Chemother.*, 1984, *13*, 121; B. Chattopadhyay and I. Hall, *Curr. med. Res. Opinion*, 1984, *9*, 157; I.M. Gould *et al.*, *J. antimicrob Chemother.*, 1987, *19*, 307). Clavulanic acid potentiated the action of ticarcillin *in vitro* against *Staphylococcus aureus*, coagulase-negative staphylococci, *Bacteroides* spp. and some *Enterobacteriaceae* including *Klebsiella* spp., *Proteus mirabilis* and most of the *Escherichia* and *Acinetobacter* strains. Activity against *Enterobacter cloacae*, *Serratia marcescens*, and *Pseudomonas aeruginosa* was not potentiated (G. Pulverer *et al.*, *J. antimicrob. Chemother.*, 1986, *17*, *Suppl.* C, 1).

A combination of ticarcillin and temocillin *in vitro* (L. Verbist and J. Verhaegen, *Antimicrob. Ag. Chemother.*, 1984, *25*, 142) showed some antagonism and synergism, but mainly indifference against a range of Gram-negative aerobes.

Resistance

As for Carbenicillin Sodium, p.140. Cross-resistance between carbenicillin and ticarcillin is usual.

Report of the isolation of resistant strains of *Pseudomonas aeruginosa* after treatment with a combination of ticarcillin and clavulanic acid. The resistant isolates demonstrated elevated production of beta-lactamase and had a stable multiresistant phenotype.— R. G. Masterton *et al.* (letter), *Lancet*, 1987, *2*, 975.

Absorption and Fate

Ticarcillin sodium is not absorbed from the gastro-intestinal tract. After the intramuscular injection of the equivalent of ticarcillin 1 g approximate peak plasma concentrations in the range of 20 to 30 μg per mL are achieved after 0.5 to 1 hour. About 45% of ticarcillin in the circulation is bound to plasma proteins. A plasma half-life of 70 minutes has been reported. The half-life is prolonged in neonates and in patients with renal failure.

Distribution of ticarcillin in the body is similar to that of carbenicillin and concentrations have been detected in interstitial, cerebrospinal, pleural, and peritoneal fluids and also in sputum and bile.

Ticarcillin is reported to be metabolised to a limited extent. Ticarcillin is excreted by glomerular filtration and tubular secretion. Concentrations of 2 to 4 mg per mL are achieved in the urine after the intramuscular injection of the equivalent of 1 or 2 g; up to 90% of a dose is excreted unchanged in the urine mostly within 6 hours after administration. The concomitant administration of probenecid produces higher plasma-ticarcillin concentrations.

Ticarcillin is partly removed by haemodialysis.

Studies of the pharmacokinetics of ticarcillin sodium after intravenous administration: R. Sutherland and P. J. Wise, *Antimicrob. Ag. Chemother.*, 1970, 402; J. Klastersky *et al.*, *J. clin. Pharmac.*, 1974, *14*, 172; A. Dalhoff and D. Höffler, *J. int. med. Res.*, 1977, *5*, 308.

For further reference to the pharmacokinetics of a combination of ticarcillin sodium and potassium clavulanate, see under Uses, Administration in Renal Failure, below, and in Clavulanic Acid, p.198.

ADMINISTRATION IN RENAL FAILURE. For reference to the pharmacokinetics of ticarcillin sodium in renal failure, see under Uses, Administration in Renal Failure.

DIFFUSION INTO BODY TISSUES AND FLUIDS. A study in 20 patients given an intravenous injection of either 1 g or 3 g of ticarcillin at anaesthetic induction before cholecystectomy. Bile was aspirated during surgery and venous blood sampled at the same time; a sample of gall-bladder wall was taken immediately after the operation. Mean ticarcillin concentrations for the groups given 1 and 3 g were: in serum, 64 and 271 μg per mL respectively; in gall-bladder bile, 10 and 53 μg per mL respectively; in gall-bladder wall, 23 and 104 μg per mL respectively; and in common bile-duct bile, 60 and 77 μg per mL respectively. There were, however, large interindividual variations in all these concentrations, and those in the gall-bladder bile were reduced in the presence of cystic duct obstruction. The 3-g dose was considered to provide adequate bactericidal concentrations if ticarcillin is used as indicated by sensitivity testing.— D. W. Forrester *et al.*, *Br. J. clin. Pract.*, 1984, *38*, 350.

Combination with clavulanic acid. In a study involving 38 patients given intravenous ticarcillin with clavulanic acid, both drugs penetrated well into the peritoneal fluid, and to a similar extent. The concentrations in peritoneal fluid declined in parallel to serum concentrations, and the ratio of ticarcillin to clavulanic acid in serum and peritoneal fluid did not vary significantly with time.— N. Manek *et al.*, *J. antimicrob. Chemother.*, 1987, *19*, 363.

DRUG EXCRETION. *Combination with clavulanic acid.* Biliary pharmacokinetics of a combination of ticarcillin and clavulanic acid in 26 patients who required biliary surgery.— A. W. M. C. Owen and E. B. Faragher, *J. antimicrob. Chemother.*, 1986, *17*, *Suppl.* C, 65.

METABOLISM. About 15% of a 1-g dose of ticarcillin, given intramuscularly to 6 healthy subjects, was metabolised to penicilloic acid and recovered in the urine within 12 hours. The remainder of the dose was excreted unchanged.— M. Cole *et al.*, *Antimicrob. Ag. Chemother.*, 1973, *3*, 463.

PREGNANCY AND THE NEONATE. *Combination with clavulanic acid.* Ticarcillin 75 mg per kg body-weight (as sodium salt) in combination with clavulanic acid 5 mg per kg (as potassium salt) were given prophylactically every 12 hours by slow intra-arterial injection to 24 neonates at risk of infection, 22 of whom were preterm. The mean peak concentrations 15 minutes after the first dose were 183 μg per mL for ticarcillin and 2.4 μg per mL for clavulanic acid; the half-lives of the drugs were 4.5 and 2.0 hours respectively. High urinary concentrations of both drugs were maintained throughout the 0 to 6 and 6 to 12 hour collection periods. The mean peak urinary concentrations were 1169 μg per mL for ticarcillin and 112 μg per mL for clavulanic acid. Twenty-two organisms were isolated from 12 infants; 15 of these were sensitive to the combination.— S. B. Fayed *et al.*, *J. antimicrob. Chemother.*, 1987, *19*, 113.

Uses and Administration

Ticarcillin sodium is a carboxypenicillin with actions and uses similar to those of carbenicillin sodium (see p.140) and is indicated in the treatment of severe Gram-negative infections, especially those due to *Pseudomonas aeruginosa*. The usual adult dose is the equivalent of 15 to 20 g of ticarcillin daily in divided doses every 4 to 8 hours although 3 g has been given every 3 hours in very severe infection. It is administered by slow intravenous injection over 3 to 4 minutes or by infusion over 30 to 40 minutes. Children may be given 200 to 300 mg per kg body-weight daily in divided doses.

The concomitant administration of probenecid 1 g three times daily by mouth may achieve higher and more prolonged serum concentrations of ticarcillin but caution is recommended in patients with impaired renal function. Doses of ticarcillin may need to be reduced in renal failure.

In the treatment of uncomplicated urinary-tract infections the usual dose is the equivalent of 3 to 4 g in divided doses daily intramuscularly or by slow intravenous injection. Children have been given 50 to 100 mg per kg body-weight daily in divided doses. If intramuscular injections prove painful they may be prepared using a 0.5% to 1.0% solution of lignocaine hydrochloride. Not more than 2 g of ticarcillin should be injected intramuscularly into one site.

As an adjunct to systemic use, ticarcillin may be given by intra-articular injection in doses of 500 mg to 1 g, by intrapleural injection in doses of 1 g daily, and by local irrigation as a 0.2% solution. The equivalent of ticarcillin 500 mg dissolved in 3 to 5 mL of water may be nebulised and inhaled 3 to 4 times daily.

As with carbenicillin, ticarcillin may be used with an aminoglycoside but the injections must be administered separately because of possible incompatibility.

Ticarcillin sodium may also be administered in a combination preparation with clavulanic acid (see p.197), a beta-lactamase inhibitor, to widen its antibacterial spectrum to organisms usually resistant to ticarcillin due to the production of beta-lactamases. This combination is administered by intravenous infusion in a ratio of 15 or 30 parts of ticarcillin (as the sodium salt) to 1 part of clavulanic acid (as the potassium salt). It is given in doses according to the content of ticarcillin, as specified above.

Reviews of the actions and uses of ticarcillin: R. N. Brogden *et al.*, *Drugs*, 1980, *20*, 325.

Report of a symposium on ticarcillin in association with clavulanic acid.— *J. antimicrob. Chemother.*, 1986, *17*, *Suppl.* C, 1 to 240.

Reviews of the actions and uses of a combination of ticarcillin sodium with potassium clavulanate: *Med. Lett.*, 1985, *27*, 69 and 84.

A study of the use of ticarcillin in association with ceftizoxime in the treatment of infections in non-neutropenic cancer patients. A favourable response was observed in 16 of 21 patients with bacteraemia, 19 of 31 with pneumonia, 8 of 9 with urinary-tract infections, 10 of 11 with skin and soft-tissue infections, and 8 of 9 with miscellaneous infections. One strain of *Escherichia coli* developed resistance to ticarcillin during therapy. There were no serious adverse effects to therapy. Three patients developed phlebitis towards the end of therapy, one patient developed a rash, and 3 had laboratory evidence of coagulation abnormalities but no clinical bleeding. There was a 5% incidence of superinfections.— K. V. I. Rolston *et al.*, *J. antimicrob. Chemother.*, 1987, *19*, 367.

Clinical studies of the use of ticarcillin sodium in association with potassium clavulanate: T. M. File *et al.*, *Antimicrob. Ag. Chemother.*, 1984, *26*, 310 (comparison with piperacillin for urinary-tract and respiratory-tract infections, and with latamoxef for soft-tissue infections); G. A. Roselle *et al.*, *ibid.*, 1985, *27*, 291 (use in a range of bacterial infections).

For the possible use of ticarcillin to reduce excessively high plasma-aminoglycoside concentrations, see Gentamicin Sulphate, p.238.

ADMINISTRATION. Ticarcillin could be administered into the eye as a 5% topical solution, or by subconjunctival injection in a dose of 100 mg in 0.5 mL.— T. S. Lesar and R. G. Fiscella, *Drug Intell. & clin. Pharm.*, 1985, *19*, 642.

ADMINISTRATION IN INFANTS AND CHILDREN. The following doses of ticarcillin were suggested for intravenous administration in the treatment of severe infections in neonates: up to 1 week old, 150 to 200 mg per kg body-weight daily in 2 or 3 divided doses; 1 to 4 weeks old, 200 to 300 mg per kg daily in 3 or 4 divided doses; greater than 4 weeks old, 300 to 400 mg per kg in 4 to 6 divided doses. Older children could be given 200 to 300 mg per kg daily in 4 to 6 divided doses.— K. H. Rhodes and C. M. Johnson, *Mayo Clin. Proc.*, 1983, *58*, 158.

ADMINISTRATION IN RENAL FAILURE. The normal half-life for ticarcillin of 1.0 to 1.5 hours was increased to 16 hours in end-stage renal disease (W.M. Bennett *et al.*, *Am. J. Kidney Dis.*, 1983, *3*, 155). Bennett *et al.* have therefore suggested that ticarcillin be administered every 8 to 12 hours to patients with a glomerular filtration-rate (GFR) greater than 50 mL per minute, every 12 to 24 hours to those with a GFR of 10 to 50 mL per minute, and every 24 to 48 hours to those with a GFR of less than 10 mL per minute. Alternatively, the *US* manufacturers, expressing renal function in terms of creatinine clearance values, suggest that ticarcillin be given intravenously in the following doses: 3 g every 4 hours for creatinine clearances greater than 60 mL per minute; 2 g every 4 hours for creatinine clearances of 30 to 60 mL per minute; 2 g every 8 hours for creatinine clearances of 10 to 30 mL per minute; 2 g every 12 hours for creatinine clearances less than 10 mL per minute. In this last group of patients ticarcillin may be given intramuscularly in a dose of 1 g every 6 hours. The *UK* manufacturers recommended adjustment of dosage according to serum-ticarcillin concentrations. Since ticarcillin is removed during haemodialysis the manufacturers recommend a supplement of 2 to 3 g during or at the end of haemodialysis. For patients on peritoneal dialysis, the *UK* manufacturers recommend a dosage of 2 g every 8 hours, and the *US* manufacturers a dosage of 3 g every 12 hours.

For reference to the administration of ticarcillin sodium by the intraperitoneal route in patients undergoing continuous ambulatory peritoneal dialysis, see under Peritonitis in Azlocillin Sodium, p.125.

Combination with clavulanic acid. A study of the pharmacokinetics of ticarcillin administered in association with clavulanic acid in healthy subjects and in patients with renal impairment. The half-life of both components was increased in patients with renal insufficiency, and therefore an increase in the dosage interval was recommended.— P. Koeppe *et al.*, *Arzneimittel-Forsch.*, 1987, *37*, 203. See also F. Dalet *et al.*, *J. antimicrob. Chemother.*, 1986, *17*, *Suppl.* C, 57.

BURNS. *Combination with clavulanic acid.* Twenty-one patients with infected burns were treated with a combination of ticarcillin and clavulanic acid; ten cases of septicaemia with *Staphylococcus aureus* were cured, but treatment failed in 3 patients with septicaemia caused by *Pseudomonas aeruginosa* and infections with methicillin-resistant *Staph. aureus*.— E. Diem and W. Graninger, *J. antimicrob. Chemother.*, 1986, *17*, *Suppl.* C, 123.

MENINGITIS. The optimal treatment for meningitis caused by *Pseudomonas aeruginosa* has still to be established. At present the following regimens were recommended: either ticarcillin 300 mg per kg body-weight daily or azlocillin 200 mg per kg daily, both given intravenously 4 times a day in association with an aminoglycoside, such as tobramycin 5 to 7 mg per kg daily in 3 divided doses. Alternatively ceftazidime in association with tobramycin could be used.— M. Whitby and R. Finch, *Drugs*, 1986, *31*, 266.

NEUTROPENIA. For reference to the use of ticarcillin sodium for febrile episodes in neutropenic patients, see Piperacillin Sodium, p.287.

Combination with clavulanic acid. Ticarcillin sodium in combination with clavulanic acid has been investigated for the empirical treatment of febrile episodes in neutropenic patients, including some patients with septicaemia. The mixture has been used alone (J.P. Bru *et al.*, *J. antimicrob. Chemother.*, 1986, *17*, *Suppl.* C, 203), or most commonly in association with an aminoglycoside such as amikacin (F. Meunier *et al.*, *ibid.*, 195), netilmicin (G. Schaison *et al.*, *ibid.*, 177), or tobramycin (O. Krieger *et al.*, *ibid.*, 211). In association with tobramycin, the mixture has been shown to be as effective as piperacillin used with tobramycin (M.J. Mackie *et al.*, *ibid.*, 219). However, in the study by Meunier *et al.*, the regimen used was considered to be suboptimal for the treatment of Gram-positive septicaemia, and the emergence of Gram-positive cocci during therapy to be a possible additional problem.

OSTEOMYELITIS. For reference to the use of ticarcillin sodium in the treatment of osteomyelitis and bacterial arthritis, see Flucloxacillin Sodium, p.232.

PERITONITIS. For reference to the use of ticarcillin sodium in the treatment of peritonitis, see Azlocillin Sodium, p.125.

PREGNANCY AND THE NEONATE. For reference to the use of ticarcillin sodium in pregnancy, see Piperacillin Sodium, p.287.

RESPIRATORY-TRACT INFECTIONS. *Cystic fibrosis.* For reference to the use of ticarcillin sodium in the treatment of pseudomonal chest infections in patients with cystic fibrosis, see Carbenicillin Sodium, p.141.

SURGICAL INFECTION PROPHYLAXIS. *Combination with clavulanic acid.* Infection prophylaxis with 3 injections of either a combination of ticarcillin and clavulanic acid or cephamandole, was given to 484 patients undergoing vascular or thoracic surgery. Postoperative infections occurred in 6 and 9 patients in the 2 groups respectively. In addition, 10 and 6 patients developed infections of the urinary or respiratory tract. Cephamandole resistance was detected in 56% of isolates, and resistance to ticarcillin and clavulanic acid in 24%.— M. Kitzis *et al.*, *J. antimicrob. Chemother.*, 1986, *17*, *Suppl.* C, 183.

URINARY-TRACT INFECTIONS. *Combination with clavulanic acid.* A study of 16 patients with urinary-tract infections and underlying or complicating urological conditions. In the group of 37 patients treated with a combination of ticarcillin and clavulanic acid, 39 of 43 causative pathogens were eradicated, including all 6 responsible for septicaemia. One isolate of *Klebsiella pneumoniae* failed to respond and there were 3 relapses; four reinfections or superinfections were also reported. Of 39 patients treated with piperacillin, 33 of 43 pathogens were eliminated including 3 of 4 organisms isolated from the blood. Four isolates of *Escherichia coli*, 2 of *Pseudomonas aeruginosa* and 1 of *Kleb. pneumoniae* did not respond. There were 3 relapses, and 5 reinfections or superinfections. Only one patient in each group was classified as a clinical failure.— C. E. Cox, *J. antimicrob. Chemother.*, 1986, *17, Suppl.* C, 93. See also M. Westenfelder *et al.*, *ibid.*, 97.

Preparations

Sterile Ticarcillin Disodium *(U.S.P.)*

Sterile Ticarcillin Disodium and Clavulanate Potassium *(U.S.P.)*. pH of a 10% solution 5.5 to 7.5.

Proprietary Preparations

Ticar *(Beecham Research, UK)*. *Injection*, powder for reconstitution, ticarcillin 1 and 5 g (as sodium salt). *Intravenous infusion*, powder for reconstitution, ticarcillin 5 g (as sodium salt), supplied with diluent.

Timentin *(Beecham Research, UK)*. *Intravenous infusion* (Timentin 800 mg), powder for reconstitution, ticarcillin 750 mg (as sodium salt), clavulanic acid 50 mg (as potassium salt).
Intravenous infusion (Timentin 1.6 g), powder for reconstitution, ticarcillin 1.5 g (as sodium salt), clavulanic acid 100 mg (as potassium salt).
Intravenous infusion (Timentin 3.2 g), powder for reconstitution, ticarcillin 3 g (as sodium salt), clavulanic acid 200 mg (as potassium salt).

Proprietary Names and Manufacturers

Aerugipen *(Beecham-Wülfing, Ger.)*; Tarcil *(Beecham, Austral.)*; Ticar *(Beecham, Canad.; Beecham Research, UK; Beecham Laboratories, USA)*; Ticarpen *(Beecham-Sevigne, Fr.; Neth.; Beecham, Spain; Switz.)*; Ticillin *(Commonwealth Serum Laboratories, Austral.)*.

The following names have been used for multi-ingredient preparations containing ticarcillin sodium—Timenten *(Beecham, Switz.)*; Timentin *(Beecham Research, UK; Beecham Laboratories, USA)*.

18310-c

Tobramycin *(BAN, USAN, rINN)*.

47663; Nebramycin Factor 6. 6-*O*-(3-Amino-3-deoxy-α-D-glucopyranosyl)-2-deoxy-4-*O*-(2,6-diamino-2,3,6-trideoxy-α-D-*ribo*-hexopyranosyl)-D-streptamine.

$C_{18}H_{37}N_5O_9$=467.5.

CAS — 32986-56-4.

Pharmacopoeias. In *Br.* and *U.S.*

An antibiotic substance produced by the growth of *Streptomyces tenebrarius* or by any other means. The *B.P.* specifies not less than 930 units of tobramycin per mg and the *U.S.P.* specifies not less than 900 μg per mg, both calculated on the anhydrous basis.

A white or almost white hygroscopic powder. **Soluble** 1 in 1.5 of water; very slightly soluble in alcohol; practically insoluble in chloroform and ether. A 10% solution in water has a pH of 9.0 to 11.0. **Store** at a temperature not exceeding 25° in airtight containers.

174-y

Tobramycin Sulphate *(BANM, rINNM)*.

Tobramycin Sulfate *(USAN)*.

$(C_{18}H_{37}N_5O_9)_2,5H_2SO_4$=1425.4.

CAS — 49842-07-1; 79645-27-5.

Pharmacopoeias. U.S. includes Sterile Tobramycin Sulfate.

It has a potency of not less than 634 μg and not more than 739 μg of tobramycin per mg. 1.5 g of monograph substance is approximately equivalent to 1 g of tobramycin. A 4% solution in water has a pH of 6.0 to 8.0. The *B.P.* injection has a pH of 3.5 to 6.0; the *U.S.P.* injection has a pH of 3.0 to 6.5. Solutions are **sterilised** by filtration.

Incompatibility or loss of activity has been reported between tobramycin sulphate and some cephalosporins or penicillins (see Gentamicin Sulphate, p.236), and also with heparin sodium. Solutions with clindamycin phosphate in glucose injection are reported to be unstable.

A study of the effect of freezing and thawing on the stability of tobramycin added to intravenous fluids in plastic bags.— C. J. Holmes *et al.*, *Am. J. Hosp. Pharm.*, 1982, *39*, 104.

Units

9800 units of tobramycin are contained in approximately 10.2 mg of tobramycin in one ampoule of the second International Standard Preparation (1985).

Adverse Effects, Treatment, and Precautions

As for Gentamicin Sulphate, p.236.

Peak plasma-tobramycin concentrations greater than 12 μg per mL and trough concentrations greater than 2 μg per mL should be avoided.

EFFECTS ON THE EAR. For reference to the ototoxicity of tobramycin, see Gentamicin Sulphate, p.237.

EFFECTS ON THE KIDNEY. For reference to studies suggesting the nephrotoxic potential of tobramycin may be less than that of gentamicin, see Gentamicin Sulphate, p.237.

EFFECTS ON MENTAL STATE. A report on delirium possibly associated with the intravenous administration of tobramycin sulphate.— C. F. McCartney *et al.*, *J. Am. med. Ass.*, 1982, *247*, 1319.

INTERACTIONS. Single doses of tobramycin and latamoxef were administered by intravenous injection alone, or concomitantly at separate sites, to 6 healthy subjects and also to 5 anuric patients on dialysis. Latamoxef increased the elimination rate of tobramycin in both groups; this appeared to be related to an increase in the nonrenal clearance of tobramycin. Tobramycin, however, had the effect of decreasing the elimination of latamoxef in the healthy subjects only; this appeared to be related to a decrease in the renal clearance of latamoxef. It was considered that the magnitude of these changes may be of clinical significance. No interaction occurred when the drugs were mixed *in vitro*.— G. R. Aronoff *et al.*, *J. infect. Dis.*, 1984, *149*, 9.

Eight of 9 patients had a significant decrease in the peak serum-tobramycin concentration when they also received therapy with intravenous miconazole.— S. M. Hatfield *et al.*, *Clin. Pharm.*, 1986, *5*, 415.

For reference to the inactivation of tobramycin by antipseudomonal penicillins *in vivo*, see Gentamicin Sulphate, p.238.

For reference to the effect of amphotericin on the half-life of tobramycin, see Gentamicin Sulphate, p.238.

OVERDOSAGE. For reference to the reduction of excessive plasma-tobramycin concentrations by complexation with ticarcillin, see Gentamicin Sulphate, p.238.

Antimicrobial Action

Tobramycin is bactericidal and has a mode of action, antimicrobial spectrum, and minimum inhibitory concentrations similar to those of gentamicin (see p.239), but is reported to be 2 to 4 times more active against *Pseudomonas aeruginosa* and less active against *Serratia marcescens*. It may also be active against some strains of *Ps. aeruginosa* demonstrating low-level resistance to gentamicin.

For reference to a comparative study of the antimicrobial activity of 11 aminoglycosides including tobramycin, and for studies of the activity of tobramycin against *Aeromonas* and *Yersinia* spp., see Gentamicin Sulphate, p.239.

ACTIVITY AGAINST MYCOBACTERIA. For reference to the activity of tobramycin against atypical *Mycobacterium* spp., see Amikacin Sulphate, p.110.

For reference to the activity of tobramycin against *Mycobacterium leprae* infection in *mice*, see Gentamicin Sulphate, p.239.

ACTIVITY WITH OTHER ANTIMICROBIAL AGENTS. For reference to the effect of other agents on the *in-vitro* antimicrobial activity of aminoglycosides, see Gentamicin Sulphate, p.239.

Studies showing synergy *in vitro* between tobramycin and other antimicrobial agents: R. J. Fass, *Antimicrob. Ag. Chemother.*, 1982, *21*, 1003 (ceftriaxone, latamoxef, or piperacillin; against *Pseudomonas aeruginosa* and multidrug-resistant Enterobacteriaceae); A. Proietti *et al.*, *Curr. ther. Res.*, 1983, *34*, 297 (piperacillin; against *Ps. aeruginosa*); K. Takahashi and H. Kanno, *Antimicrob. Ag. Chemother.*, 1984, *26*, 789 (addition of tobramycin to combinations of fosfomycin and a penicillin or cephalosporin; against *Ps. aeruginosa*).

For reference to the ability of different tests for synergy or antagonism between tobramycin and cefsulodin to predict for therapeutic outcome, see Cefsulodin, p.161.

Resistance

Mechanisms of resistance of bacteria to aminoglycosides are described under Gentamicin Sulphate (p.240). Cross-resistance occurs between gentamicin and tobramycin but it may not be complete for *Pseudomonas aeruginosa*.

For reference to the change in the incidence of tobramycin resistance in Gram-negative bacteria after replacement of gentamicin by amikacin as the aminoglycoside of routine use, see Amikacin Sulphate, p.110.

RESISTANCE OF PSEUDOMONAS. Strains of *Pseudomonas aeruginosa* isolated from patients without cystic fibrosis were significantly more resistant to tobramycin than strains from patients with the disease. Tobramycin was, however, the most active of a range of antimicrobial agents tested *in vitro* against the strains from the cystic fibrosis group.— B. Gordts *et al.*, *J. antimicrob. Chemother.*, 1984, *14*, 25.

A study *in vitro* suggesting that growth of *Pseudomonas aeruginosa* in a thick biofilm adherent to a urinary catheter may confer resistance of the bacteria to tobramycin.— J. C. Nickel *et al.*, *Antimicrob. Ag. Chemother.*, 1985, *27*, 619.

Absorption and Fate

As for Gentamicin Sulphate, p.241.

Following intramuscular administration of tobramycin peak plasma concentrations are achieved within half to 1 hour and concentrations of about 4 μg per mL have been reported following doses of 80 to 100 mg. After injection tobramycin has been detected in body fluids but concentrations in the cerebrospinal fluid are low even when there is meningeal inflammation. It crosses the placenta and small amounts have been detected in breast milk. A plasma half-life of 2 hours has been reported. Most of a dose is excreted by glomerular filtration in the urine within 24 hours.

Intramuscular injections of tobramycin produced average peak serum concentrations of 1.14, 2.09, and 2.71 μg per mL in 1 hour after doses of 25, 50, and 75 mg respectively, and the corresponding urine concentrations were 12.28, 21, and 54 μg per mL, mostly during the 12 hours after injection.— H. R. Black and R. S. Griffith, *Antimicrob. Ag. Chemother.*, 1970, 314.

When tobramycin 100 mg was administered intramuscularly to 10 fasting volunteers serum concentrations reached a peak of 3.77 and 3.75 μg per mL at 30 minutes and 1 hour respectively. Following intravenous injections peak serum concentrations of 5.5 and 6.02 μg per mL were achieved at 30 minutes following doses of 1 mg and 1.5 mg per kg body-weight respectively. The half-life after an intramuscular injection was 2 hours and after an intravenous injection 1.3 hours. Serum concentrations of gentamicin after similar doses were generally higher.— B. R. Meyers and S. Z. Hirschman, *J. clin. Pharmac.*, 1972, *12*, 321.

Similar serum concentrations were achieved following intravenous infusions and intramuscular injections of tobramycin and gentamicin.— C. Regamey *et al.*, *Clin. Pharmac. Ther.*, 1973, *14*, 396.

Tobramycin given as a slow bolus intravenous injection over 2.5 to 3 minutes to 5 healthy subjects in a standard dose of 80 mg produced a peak serum concentration of about 11 μg per mL within 5 minutes. A dose of 1 mg per kg body-weight produced a slightly lower peak of about 10 μg per mL. The regression curves for both doses were similar.— B. C. Stratford *et al.*, *Lancet*, 1974, *1*, 378.

A study of 20 patients with burns and 8 healthy subjects demonstrated that glomerular filtration-rate was increased in those with burns, especially the younger patients, and that the plasma half-life of tobramycin was consequently reduced.— P. Loirat *et al.*, *New Engl. J. Med.*, 1978, *299*, 915.

The mean half-life for tobramycin of 67.3 minutes, after intramuscular injection in 4 children with kwashiorkor, was shorter than that in normal subjects and was reduced to only 50.2 minutes on recovery.— N. Buchanan and C. Eyberg (letter), *S. Afr. med. J.*, 1978, *53*, 273.

The pharmacokinetics of tobramycin in obese patients.— R. A. Blouin *et al.*, *Clin. Pharmac. Ther.*, 1979, *26*, 508. See also L. A. Bauer *et al.*, *Eur. J. clin. Pharmac.*, 1983, *24*, 643.

The total clearance of tobramycin was increased by 20% in 12 patients with cystic fibrosis compared with 6 controls with other diseases. There was no change in renal clearance.— J. Levy *et al.*, *J. Pediat.*, 1984, *105*, 117. In patients with mild to moderate cystic fibrosis, results suggested no effect of the disease on renal clearance, total clearance, or volume of distribution of tobramycin.— C. W. Kildoo *et al.*, *Drug Intell. & clin. Pharm.*, 1987, *21*, 639. See also L. A. Bauer *et al.*, *Clin.*

Pharm., 1983, *2*, 262; G. W. Horner and D. A. Stempel, *Drug Intell. & clin. Pharm.*, 1987, *21*, 276.

The effect of plasmaphaeresis on the pharmacokinetics of drugs. Studies involving a total of 3 subjects had found plasmaphaeresis procedures to remove between 4 and 10% of the total body stores of tobramycin.— J. V. Jones *et al.*, *Dialysis Transplant.*, 1985, *14*, 225.

For reference to the systemic absorption of tobramycin after endotracheal instillation, see Gentamicin Sulphate, p.241.

Further references to the pharmacokinetics of tobramycin: C. H. King *et al.*, *Antimicrob. Ag. Chemother.*, 1985, *27*, 285 (in intravenous drug abusers); N. E. Winslade *et al.*, *ibid.*, 1987, *31*, 605 (comparison with netilmicin); H. J. Mann *et al.*, *Clin. Pharm.*, 1987, *6*, 148 (in critically ill patients with sepsis).

ADMINISTRATION IN THE ELDERLY. Increased age had no effect on the pharmacokinetics of tobramycin in patients with normal renal function.— L. A. Bauer and R. A. Blouin, *Antimicrob. Ag. Chemother.*, 1981, *20*, 587.

Pharmacokinetics of tobramycin after intramuscular administration to elderly patients.— P. R. Mayer *et al.*, *Drug Intell. & clin. Pharm.*, 1986, *20*, 611.

ADMINISTRATION IN INFANTS AND CHILDREN. In 40 children given tobramycin 5 mg per kg body-weight daily in 3 divided doses by intramuscular injection, the mean serum concentration was 2.77 µg per mL one hour after injection, falling to 0.4 µg per mL after 8 hours. The serum half-life was about 4.5 hours.— F. J. Da Nobrega *et al.*, *Curr. ther. Res.*, 1977, *21*, 741.

See also under Uses, below.

DIFFUSION INTO BODY TISSUES AND FLUIDS. The concentration of tobramycin in *synovial fluid* ranged from 60 to 105% that of simultaneous serum concentrations in 6 patients with non-traumatic joint effusions 90 or 120 minutes after they received tobramycin 1 to 1.5 mg per kg body-weight intramuscularly.— T. H. Dee and F. Kozin, *Antimicrob. Ag. Chemother.*, 1977, *12*, 548.

Following a single dose of tobramycin 10 mg by subconjunctival injection, therapeutically effective concentrations were achieved in *aqueous humour* whilst negligible concentrations were reached after intramuscular injection of tobramycin 80 or 100 mg.— A. Petounis *et al.*, *Br. J. Ophthal.*, 1978, *62*, 660. Tobramycin concentrations of 3 to 4 µg per mL were achieved in the aqueous humour of patients with cataract 1 hour after the intravenous infusion of 1 mg per kg body-weight, compared with peak serum concentrations of 2.93 to 3.70 µg per mL half an hour after administration. After the intramuscular injection of a similar dose peak concentrations in the aqueous humour were only 0.22 to 0.32 µg per mL four hours after injection. Variable concentrations occurred in the aqueous humour of 4 patients after the subconjunctival injection of tobramycin 10 or 20 mg.— F. P. Furgiuele *et al.*, *Am. J. Ophthal.*, 1978, *85*, 121.

Antipseudomonal activity of tobramycin in *bronchial secretions*.— G. Mombelli *et al.*, *Antimicrob. Ag. Chemother.*, 1981, *19*, 72. Correction.— *ibid.*, *20*, 279.

A study of the influence of ascites on tobramycin pharmacokinetics in 8 men with marked ascites and clinical alcoholic cirrhosis of the liver; 5 of the men subsequently had a resolution of the ascites and acted as their own controls. The presence of ascites had no significant effect on the plasma half-life of tobramycin but the disappearance of tobramycin from *ascitic fluid* was considerably slower than from plasma. Uptake of tobramycin into ascitic fluid was also quite slow with maximum ascitic fluid concentrations being reached an average of 4.4 hours after intravenous administration. The volume of distribution of tobramycin was significantly greater in the presence of ascites suggesting that a larger loading dose might be needed, but since the clearance did not change there would be no need to alter the total daily dose.— R. Sampliner *et al.*, *J. clin. Pharmac.*, 1984, *24*, 43. Intraperitoneal administration of tobramycin was required to achieve adequate concentrations of tobramycin in ascitic fluid of cirrhotic patients.— P. Lapalus *et al.*, *Thérapie*, 1983, *38*, 247. See also T. Hodgman *et al.*, *Clin. Pharm.*, 1984, *3*, 203.

Tobramycin could not be detected in 32 of 34 *saliva* specimens from patients given the drug intravenously. Thus saliva cannot be used as an indirect method of measuring serum-tobramycin concentrations.— L. Hendeles *et al.*, *Drug Intell. & clin. Pharm.*, 1985, *19*, 378.

PREGNANCY AND THE NEONATE. Concentrations of tobramycin in the breast milk of one patient were 0.6 and 0.58 µg per mL one and 8 hours respectively after the intramuscular injection of 80 mg, with corresponding serum concentrations of 4.2 and 0.8 µg per mL.— M. Uwaydah *et al.*, *J. antimicrob. Chemother.*, 1975, *1*, 429.

Tobramycin 2 mg per kg body-weight was given intramuscularly to 35 pregnant women before abortion. Foetal assay showed transplacental diffusion, tobramycin being detected in foetal serum, kidney, urine, and amniotic fluid. Low concentrations were detected in the cerebrospinal fluid of 9 of 15 foetuses of less than 17 weeks gestation; none was found in the CSF of older foetuses. The placental mean concentration of 1.4 µg per g for at least 24 hours was considered to be sufficiently high to suggest tobramycin for the treatment of placental infections.— B. Bernard *et al.*, *Antimicrob. Ag. Chemother.*, 1977, *11*, 688.

For reference to the pharmacokinetics of tobramycin in neonates, see Administration in Infants and Children under Uses, below.

PROTEIN BINDING. Tobramycin did not exhibit any protein binding in studies *in vitro* of human serum under controlled physiological conditions using an ultra-filtration technique.— R. C. Gordon *et al.*, *Antimicrob. Ag. Chemother.*, 1972, *2*, 214. See also U. Ullmann (letter), *J. antimicrob. Chemother.*, 1976, *2*, 213.

Uses and Administration

Tobramycin is an aminoglycoside antibiotic with actions and uses similar to those of gentamicin (see p.242). It is used as the sulphate, mainly in the treatment of pseudomonal infections.

As with gentamicin, tobramycin may be used with penicillins or cephalosporins; the injections should be administered separately.

Doses are expressed in terms of the equivalent amount of tobramycin. The usual dose for adults is 3 mg of tobramycin per kg body-weight daily in divided doses every 8 hours; up to 5 mg per kg daily in divided doses every 6 to 8 hours may be given in serious infections. Children may be given 6 to 7.5 mg per kg daily in divided doses although higher doses may sometimes be required. A dose of 2 mg per kg every 12 hours has been suggested for premature or full-term neonates aged up to 1 week (but see also under Administration in Infants and Children, below). It is given by intramuscular injection, or by intravenous infusion over 20 to 60 minutes in 50 to 100 mL of sodium chloride 0.9% or glucose 5% injection; proportionately less fluid should be given to children. It has also been given by direct intravenous injection. Treatment should generally continue for not longer than 7 to 10 days, and peak plasma concentrations greater than 12 µg per mL or trough concentrations greater than 2 µg per mL should be avoided. Doses are reduced for patients with impaired renal function. In all patients, dosage should be adjusted according to plasma-tobramycin concentrations (see under Uses, Administration, in Gentamicin Sulphate, p.242).

Tobramycin may be administered into the eye as a 0.3% ointment or drops.

A brief comparative review of tobramycin and gentamicin.— *Drug & Ther. Bull.*, 1982, *20*, 11.

See also under Gentamicin Sulphate (p.242) for general reviews of the aminoglycoside antibiotics.

ADMINISTRATION. A study in 17 patients aged 2 to 27 years with normal renal function to compare 5 strategies used for monitoring serum-tobramycin concentrations. It was concluded that desired serum concentrations could be as reliably achieved by determining individual dosage regimens from population pharmacokinetic parameters as from individual values. This could be attributed to the large intra-individual variation but small interindividual variation observed in pharmacokinetic parameters. The study failed to demonstrate a superior prediction of concentrations when doses were calculated on body-surface as opposed to body-weight.— T. P. Green *et al.*, *Clin. Pharmacokinet.*, 1984, *9*, 457. See also Gentamicin Sulphate, p.242.

A description of the preparation of tobramycin-impregnated polymethylmethacrylate beads, a study of their *in-vitro* release characteristics, and a report of their use in a patient with infection of the bones.— J. A. Goodell *et al.*, *Am. J. Hosp. Pharm.*, 1986, *43*, 1454.

ADMINISTRATION IN INFANTS AND CHILDREN. In a study of the effects of birth-weight and gestational age on the pharmacokinetics of tobramycin, 26 neonates with birth-weights between 1.0 and 3.5 kg and gestational ages from 28 to 40 weeks were given tobramycin 2.5 mg per kg body-weight by intravenous infusion every 12 hours for at least 48 hours. When neonates were divided by birth-weight there were 7 between 1.0 and 1.25 kg, 6 between 1.26 and 1.5 kg, 7 from 1.51 to 2.0 kg, and 6 from 2.1 to 3.5 kg and these four groups had mean elimination half-lives of tobramycin of 11.3, 8.2, 7.5, and 5.6 hours respectively. There were also significant differences when the infants were divided by gestational age; mean elimination half-life was 9.3 hours in the 9 neonates with gestational ages from 28 to 30 weeks, compared with 8.9 hours in 11 neonates over 30 and less than 34 weeks, and 5.6 hours in the remaining 6, with gestational ages from 34 to 40 weeks. A suggested preliminary dosage regimen in newborns might be: in infants greater than 34 weeks gestational age, 2.5 mg per kg every 12 hours; in those of 34 weeks gestational age or less but more than 1.25 kg birth-weight, 2.5 mg per kg every 18 hours; and in neonates with gestational age of 34 weeks or less and birth-weight less than 1.25 kg, tobramycin 3.0 mg per kg every 24 hours.— M. C. Nahata *et al.*, *J. antimicrob. Chemother.*, 1984, *14*, 59. The half-life of tobramycin in 8 infants of gestational age 24 to 30 weeks and birth-weight of 0.60 to 0.97 kg ranged from 7.7 to 12.6 hours. Intravenous administration of tobramycin by infusion pump in doses ranging from 2.5 mg per kg every 18 hours to 3 mg per kg every 24 hours produced satisfactory peak and trough serum-tobramycin concentrations.— M. C. Nahata *et al.*, *Br. J. clin. Pharmac.*, 1986, *21*, 325.

EAR INFECTIONS. References to the successful use of parenteral tobramycin and an antipseudomonal penicillin for the treatment of malignant (or invasive) external otitis, a pseudomonal ear infection often occurring in elderly diabetic patients: I. E. Salit *et al.*, *Can. med. Ass. J.*, 1985, *132*, 381; H. A. Lovitt and R. G. Kimpton, *Aust. J. Hosp. Pharm.*, 1986, *16*, 123.

EYE INFECTIONS. For reports of the penetration of tobramycin into the aqueous humour after intramuscular or intravenous injection and the concentrations achieved after subconjunctival injections, see Absorption and Fate (above).

INTRA-ABDOMINAL INFECTIONS. For reference to the use of tobramycin in the treatment of intra-abdominal infections, see Gentamicin Sulphate, p.244. See also Peritonitis, below.

MENINGITIS. For reference to the use of tobramycin sulphate in the treatment of meningitis, see Gentamicin Sulphate, p.244.

NEUTROPENIA. For reference to the use of tobramycin sulphate in the treatment of febrile episodes in neutropenic patients, see under Septicaemia in Gentamicin Sulphate, p.244.

OSTEOMYELITIS. For reference to a comparison of tobramycin in association with ticarcillin, and ceftazidime in the treatment of osteomyelitis, see Ceftazidime, p.165.

PELVIC INFLAMMATORY DISEASE. For use of tobramycin in association with clindamycin in the treatment of pelvic inflammatory disease, see Clindamycin, p.201.

PERITONITIS. For reference to the use of tobramycin sulphate in the treatment of peritonitis associated with continuous ambulatory peritoneal dialysis, see Gentamicin Sulphate, p.244.

Recurrence of peritonitis due to *Campylobacter fetus* occurred six weeks after apparently effective treatment with tobramycin, 8 mg per litre, and cephazolin, 150 mg per litre, added to dialysis fluid in a patient undergoing continuous ambulatory peritoneal dialysis. Subsequent intraperitoneal tobramycin, 8 mg per litre, for 3 weeks followed by erythromycin, 3 g daily by mouth for one month achieved a cure.— R. Wens *et al.*, *J. Infect.*, 1985, *10*, 249.

RESPIRATORY-TRACT INFECTIONS. *Cystic fibrosis*. Aminoglycosides, such as gentamicin, netilmicin, or tobramycin are administered parenterally in the treatment of *Pseudomonas aeruginosa* infections of the respiratory tract in patients with cystic fibrosis. They are commonly given in association with an antipseudomonal penicillin or cephalosporin. Gentamicin and tobramycin have also been administered by nebuliser. For discussion of treatment regimens in these patients, see Carbenicillin Sodium, p.141.

Further references to the use of tobramycin in the treatment of pseudomonal pulmonary infections in patients with cystic fibrosis: G. L. Fraser *et al.*, *Drug Intell. & clin. Pharm.*, 1985, *19*, 757 (evaluation of high-dose tobramycin and carbenicillin parenteral therapy); S. S. Pedersen *et al.*, *Antimicrob. Ag. Chemother.*, 1987, *31*, 594 (cumulative and acute toxicity of repeated high-dose treatment with parenteral tobramycin).

SEPTICAEMIA. For reference to the use of tobramycin sulphate in the treatment of septicaemia and septic shock, see Gentamicin Sulphate, p.244.

SUPPRESSION OF INTESTINAL FLORA. For reference to regimens used to prevent colonisation and infection by the selective decontamination of the gastro-intestinal tract, see Colistin Sulphomethate Sodium, p.205.

Preparations

Tobramycin Injection *(B.P.)*. A sterile solution of tobramycin containing sufficient sulphuric acid to adjust the pH to 3.5 to 6.0.

Tobramycin Sulfate Injection *(U.S.P.)*. Prepared using tobramycin and sulphuric acid.

Tobramycin Ophthalmic Ointment *(U.S.P.)*

Tobramycin Ophthalmic Solution *(U.S.P.)*. pH 7.0 to 8.0.

Sterile Tobramycin Sulfate *(U.S.P.)*

Proprietary Preparations

Nebcin *(Lilly, UK)*. *Injection*, tobramycin 10 mg(as sulphate)/mL in vials of 2 mL, and 40 mg(as sulphate)/mL in vials of 1 and 2 mL.

Tobralex *(Alcon, UK)*. *Eye-drops*, tobramycin 0.3%.

Proprietary Names and Manufacturers of Tobramycin and Tobramycin Sulphate

Brulamycin *(Hung.)*; Gernebcin *(Lilly, Ger.)*; Nebcin *(Lilly, Austral.; Lilly, Canad.; Lilly, S.Afr.; Lilly, UK; Lilly, USA)*; Nebcina *(Lilly, Denm.; Lilly, Norw.; Lilly, Swed.)*; Nebcine *(Lilly, Fr.)*; Nebicina *(Lilly, Ital.)*; Obracin *(Belg.; Neth.; Lilly, Switz.; Lilly, UK)*; Tobra *(Arg.)*; Tobracin *(Jpn)*; Tobradistin *(Dista, Spain)*; Tobra-Gobens *(Normon, Spain)*; Tobral *(Alcon, Ital.)*; Tobra-Laf *(Andalucia, Spain)*; Tobralex *(Alcon, UK)*; Tobramaxin *(Alcon, Ger.)*; Tobrex *(Alcon, Austral.; Alcon, Canad.; FIRMA, Ital.; Alcon, S.Afr.; Alcon, Switz.; Alcon Laboratories, USA)*.

175-j

Triacetyloleandomycin *(BAN)*.

Troleandomycin *(USAN, rINN)*. The triacetyl ester of oleandomycin.

$C_{41}H_{67}NO_{15}$=814.0.

CAS — 2751-09-9.

Pharmacopoeias. In *Fr.* and *U.S.*

Contains the equivalent of not less than 750 µg of oleandomycin per mg. 1.18 g of monograph substance is approximately equivalent to 1 g of oleandomycin. A 10% solution in alcohol (50%) has a pH of 7.0 to 8.5. **Store** in airtight containers.

Units

One unit of triacetyloleandomycin is contained in 0.0012 mg of the first International Reference Preparation (1962) which contains 833 units per mg.

Adverse Effects

Reported side-effects include hypersensitivity reactions and gastro-intestinal disturbances. After administration of triacetyloleandomycin for 2 weeks or more, or in repeated courses, hepatotoxicity with transient disturbances of liver function and jaundice, as described for erythromycin estolate (see p.227), have occurred.

EFFECTS ON THE LIVER. For reference to the hepatotoxic potential of macrolide antibiotics including triacetyloleandomycin, see Erythromycin Estolate, p.227.

Precautions

Triacetyloleandomycin should not generally be administered for longer than 14 days or in repeated courses unless tests of liver function are made frequently. It should not be given to patients with impaired liver function or to patients who have developed jaundice or other symptoms of liver toxicity during previous treatment with triacetyloleandomycin.

Similarly to erythromycin, triacetyloleandomycin may potentiate the action of some drugs, probably by inhibition of their hepatic metabolism.

INTERACTIONS. An investigation of the interaction between triacetyloleandomycin and methylprednisolone. Triacetyloleandomycin inhibits the elimination of methylprednisolone, and hence has a steroid-sparing effect.— S. J. Szefler *et al.*, *Clin. Pharmac. Ther.*, 1982, *32*, 166.

Pharmacokinetic interaction between triacetyloleandomycin and triazolam in healthy subjects.— D. Warot *et al.*, *Eur. J. clin. Pharmac.*, 1987, *32*, 389.

For reference to possible interactions with macrolide antibiotics including triacetyloleandomycin, and their effect on hepatic metabolism, see Erythromycin, p.222.

Antimicrobial Action and Resistance

Triacetyloleandomycin is hydrolysed *in vivo* to oleandomycin (see p.277) which has a range of activity similar to but, in general, less effective than that of erythromycin (see p.223). It has a similar pattern of resistance to erythromycin.

Absorption and Fate

Triacetyloleandomycin is more rapidly and completely absorbed from the gastro-intestinal tract than is oleandomycin, to which it is hydrolysed *in vivo*. Peak plasma-oleandomycin concentrations of about 2 µg per mL are attained 2 hours after a single dose of 500 mg, and detectable amounts are present in plasma after 12 hours. It is excreted in the urine and bile; about 20% of the dose can be recovered in active form from the urine.

The mean ratio of antibiotic concentration in tonsillar tissue to the concentration in serum was significantly higher in 6 patients given triacetyloleandomycin for 2 days pre-operatively than in 6 further patients given similar doses of erythromycin.— S. Georgiew *et al.* (letter), *J. antimicrob. Chemother.*, 1978, *4*, 472.

Uses and Administration

Triacetyloleandomycin is a macrolide antibiotic and has been given by mouth in the treatment of susceptible infections but more effective antibiotics are generally preferred. The usual adult dose is the equivalent of 1 to 2 g daily of oleandomycin in divided doses. Children have been given the equivalent of 30 to 50 mg per kg body-weight daily.

ASTHMA. The successful use of triacetyloleandomycin together with methylprednisolone in 11 steroid-dependent children with poorly controlled, severe, chronic asthma.— R. W. Eitches *et al.*, *Am. J. Dis. Child.*, 1985, *139*, 264.

Preparations

Troleandomycin Capsules *(U.S.P.)*. Capsules containing triacetyloleandomycin. Potency is expressed in terms of the equivalent amount of oleandomycin.

Troleandomycin Oral Suspension *(U.S.P.)*. A suspension of triacetyloleandomycin. pH 5 to 8. Store between 8° and 15°.

Proprietary Names and Manufacturers

Aovine *(Wyeth, Belg.)*; Cetilmin *(Lafare, Ital.)*; Evramycin *(Wyeth, UK)*; Isotriacin *(ISOM, Ital.)*; Micotil *(Magis, Ital.)*; Oleandocyn *(Pfizer, Ger.)*; Oleandom *(Coli, Ital.)*; TAO *(Pfizer, Austral.; Roerig, Belg.; Jouveinal, Fr.; Pfizer, Ital.; Pfizer, S.Afr.; Pfizer, Spain; Roerig, USA)*; Treis-Micina *(Ecobi, Ital.)*; Treolmicina *(Ital.)*; Triacet *(Ausonia, Ital.)*; Triocetin *(OFF, Ital.)*; Triolan *(Ital Suisse, Ital.)*; Viamicina *(Benvegna, Ital.)*; Wytrion *(Wyeth, Switz.)*.

1401-c

Trimethoprim *(BAN, USAN, rINN)*.

BW-56-72; NSC-106568; Trimethoprimum; Trimethoxyprim. 5-(3,4,5-Trimethoxybenzyl)pyrimidine-2,4-diamine.

$C_{14}H_{18}N_4O_3$=290.3.

CAS — 738-70-5.

Pharmacopoeias. In *Br., Belg., Chin., Cz., Egypt., Eur., Fr., Ind., Int., It., Jug., Neth., Swiss,* and *U.S.* Also in *B.P. Vet.*

White or yellowish-white, odourless or almost odourless crystals or crystalline powder. Very slightly **soluble** in water; slightly soluble in alcohol and acetone; soluble 1 in 55 of chloroform; soluble in benzyl alcohol; sparingly soluble in methyl alcohol; practically insoluble in ether and carbon tetrachloride. **Store** in airtight containers. Protect from light.

Trimethoprim (Syraprim) was considered to be compatible with glucose 5%, but Syraprim should not be added to any chloride-containing infusion.— *Pharm. J.*, 1984, *1*, 335. The manufacturer also states that Syraprim (trimethoprim lactate) should not be mixed with solutions of sulphonamides because of incompatibility.

Adverse Effects and Treatment

Side-effects include pruritus, skin rash, fever, nausea, vomiting, and sore mouth. Trimethoprim given over a prolonged period, or in high doses, may cause a depression of haemopoiesis due to interference of the drug in the metabolism of folic acid. Calcium folinate 3 to 6 mg daily by mouth or intramuscularly for 5 to 7 days may be given to counter this effect.

For reports of adverse effects of trimethoprim when used with sulphamethoxazole, see Co-trimoxazole, p.206.

For a report of fatalities associated with co-trimoxazole or trimethoprim alone, see under Co-trimoxazole, p.206.

EFFECTS ON THE BLOOD. Trimethoprim-associated marrow toxicity in one patient.— J. Sheehan (letter), *Lancet*, 1981, *2*, 692.

Trimethoprim inhibition of dihydrofolate reductase in human bone marrow has been shown to result in megaloblastic changes at trimethoprim concentrations achievable with usual doses. The prophylactic use of folinic acid has therefore been recommended for patients at risk of developing trimethoprim-induced haematotoxicity such as patients with pre-existing or borderline folate deficiency and patients receiving high doses of trimethoprim. The optimal dosing regimen for folinic acid for this purpose needs to be determined, but 15 mg daily has been suggested as prophylaxis during trimethoprim treatment. Existing trimethoprim-induced toxicity, however, may require higher doses of folinic acid.— B. J. Kinzie and J. W. Taylor (letter), *Ann. intern. Med.*, 1984, *101*, 565. Reservations about the routine use of folinic acid.— C. Stock (letter), *ibid.*, 1985, *102*, 277.

EFFECTS ON THE GASTRO-INTESTINAL TRACT. A report of pseudomembranous colitis in an 82-year-old man believed to be associated with trimethoprim given by mouth; the man had also received cefuroxime.— J. De Courcy and J. Mackinnon, *Br. med. J.*, 1985, *290*, 1112.

EFFECTS ON THE LIVER. A report of hepatic cholestasis in one patient induced by co-trimoxazole and during subsequent re-exposure to trimethoprim. The manufacturers of trimethoprim (*Duphar*) had received 4 reports of hepatic reactions: hepatitis (2), jaundice (1), and cholestatic jaundice (1).— A. R. Tanner, *Br. med. J.*, 1986, *293*, 1072.

EFFECTS ON THE NERVOUS SYSTEM. A report of a patient with Sjögren's syndrome who had 4 episodes of aseptic meningitis temporally related to the use of co-trimoxazole, and a single episode of aseptic meningitis following the use of trimethoprim alone.— S. J. Derbes, *J. Am. med. Ass.*, 1984, *252*, 2865.

EFFECTS ON THE SKIN. In a study of 135 women with acute dysuria-frequency syndrome there was quite a high frequency of side-effects, in particular rash, when treatment with trimethoprim 200 mg twice daily by mouth was prolonged beyond 5 to 6 days; 7 of 64 patients given a 10-day course discontinued treatment because of a rash.— G. Gossius and L. Vorland, *Curr. ther. Res.*, 1985, *37*, 34.

Erythema multiforme. A report of erythema multiforme associated with trimethoprim in a patient known to be allergic to co-trimoxazole. In the *UK* 11 cases of erythema multiforme associated only with trimethoprim have been reported to the Committee on Safety of Medicines; other skin reactions are mainly exanthematous eruptions.— M. Penmetcha (letter), *Br. med. J.*, 1987, *295*, 556.

Fixed drug eruptions. In a retrospective study of fixed eruptions in 86 patients, confirmed by a positive challenge test in 84, trimethoprim was the agent responsible in 2 cases.— K. Kauppinen and S. Stubb, *Br. J. Derm.*, 1985, *112*, 575.

Further reports of trimethoprim-associated fixed drug eruptions: J. R. Gibson, *Br. med. J.*, 1982, *284*, 1529; B. R. Hughes *et al.*, *Br. J. Derm.*, 1987, *116*, 241.

OVERDOSAGE. Six hours after ingesting 80 tablets of trimethoprim 100 mg in a suicide attempt, a 28-year-old man vomited. Fourteen hours after ingestion he was admitted to hospital complaining of headache, swollen face, and weakness. Activated charcoal was given after gastric lavage. He was given intravenous fluids to ensure good diuresis, and during the 48 hours of observation his only complaint was mild epigastric pain after the lavage. Physically he remained normal throughout. He was estimated to have absorbed 3.2 g of trimethoprim, and the elimination of the drug followed first-order kinetics with a half-life of 11.9 hours.— K. Hoppu *et al.* (letter), *Lancet*, 1980, *1*, 778.

For comment on the effect of activated charcoal dose on the absorption of trimethoprim, see P. J. Neuvonen and K. T. Olkkola, *Eur. J. clin. Pharmac.*, 1984, *26*, 761.

Precautions

Trimethoprim should not be given to patients

with a history of hypersensitivity to the drug, and it should be discontinued if a skin rash appears. Care is necessary in administering trimethoprim to patients with impaired renal function. It should be used with caution in patients with severe hepatic damage as changes may occur in the absorption and metabolism of trimethoprim.

It is suggested that regular haematological examination should be made during prolonged courses of treatment; trimethoprim should not usually be given to patients with serious haematological disorders. Caution should be taken in patients with actual or possible folate deficiency and administration of folinic acid should be considered. Its use should be avoided during pregnancy. Elderly patients may be more susceptible to adverse effects and a lower dosage may be advisable.

For reports dealing with precautions for trimethoprim given with sulphamethoxazole, see Co-trimoxazole, p.207.

Interactions. Trimethoprim may potentiate the anticoagulant effect of warfarin. It also prolongs the half-life of phenytoin. Trimethoprim has been reported to interact with a number of drugs by interfering with their clearance; such drugs include digoxin, procainamide, and tolbutamide. Reversible deterioration in renal function has been reported in patients given trimethoprim and cyclosporin following renal transplantation. It is possible that patients receiving pyrimethamine may develop megaloblastic anaemia if trimethoprim is given concurrently.

Trimethoprim may interfere with some diagnostic tests including serum methotrexate assay where dihydrofolate reductase is used, and the Jaffé reaction for creatinine.

Four patients with megaloblastic anaemia who were given co-trimoxazole for concurrent infections failed to respond to haematinic therapy. Reticulocytosis was suppressed in 3 patients and the fourth failed to respond clinically until the antibacterial therapy was discontinued. Thrombocytopenia and neutropenia were prominent in 2 of the patients. Trimethoprim was suspected as the agent responsible.— I. Chanarin and J. M. England, *Br. med. J.*, 1972, *1*, 651.

A warning that trimethoprim and other folate antagonists should be avoided in children with the fragile X chromosome which is associated with mental retardation and is folate sensitive. Trimethoprim should also be avoided in pregnant women who are at risk of having a child with fragile X chromosome, until more is known about the expression of this chromosome.— F. Hecht and T. W. Glover (letter), *New Engl. J. Med.*, 1983, *308*, 285.

Blood concentrations of trimethoprim are increased in coeliac disease and in Crohn's disease.— P. G. Welling and F. L. S. Tse, *J. clin. Hosp. Pharm.*, 1984, *9*, 163.

INTERACTIONS. *Antineoplastic agents and immunosuppressants.* Trimethoprim caused serum-creatinine concentrations to rise in 4 renal transplant patients on cyclosporin treatment and 7 on azathioprine. Alternative drugs to trimethoprim should be given when possible in patients whose renal function has to be assessed, such as renal transplant patients.— G. Nyberg *et al.*, *Lancet*, 1984, *1*, 394. See also under Interference with Diagnostic Tests (below).

An 80-year-old woman with psoriasis developed necrotic skin ulceration and pancytopenia after concurrent administration of methotrexate, trimethoprim, and naproxen. Methotrexate toxicity was probably precipitated by concurrent treatment with trimethoprim; both drugs are folate antagonists which, given together, may produce a synergistic effect on folate metabolism.— H. W. K. Ng *et al.*, *Br. med. J.*, 1987, *295*, 752.

For a report of decreased cyclosporin serum-concentrations in a patient given sulphadimidine and trimethoprim, see under Cyclosporin, p.616.

Diuretics. A report of hyponatraemia in a 75-year-old woman associated with concurrent treatment with trimethoprim and amiloride with hydrochlorothiazide. Several other patients had also developed hyponatraemia while taking trimethoprim or co-trimoxazole; all of these patients were elderly and taking several drugs, including diuretics in all but one case.— R. Eastell and C. J. Edmonds, *Br. med. J.*, 1984, *289*, 1658.

INTERFERENCE WITH DIAGNOSTIC TESTS. Trimethoprim may be responsible for a reversible increase in serum-creatinine concentration which is probably caused by competitive inhibition of tubular secretion of creatinine. This must not be misinterpreted as deterioration in renal function.— T. Sandberg and B. Trollfors (letter), *J. antimicrob. Chemother.*, 1986, *17*, 123.

PORPHYRIA. Trimethoprim was considered to be unsafe in patients with acute porphyria because it has been shown to be porphyrinogenic in *animals* or *in vitro* systems.— M.R. Moore and K.E.L. McColl, *Porphyrias, Drug Lists*, Glasgow, Porphyria Research Unit, University of Glasgow, 1987.

Antimicrobial Action

Trimethoprim is a dihydrofolate reductase inhibitor. It inhibits the conversion of bacterial dihydrofolic acid to tetrahydrofolic acid which is necessary for the synthesis of certain amino acids, purines, thymidine, and ultimately DNA synthesis. It acts in the same metabolic pathway as the sulphonamides. Trimethoprim may be bacteriostatic or bactericidal depending on growth conditions; pus, for example, may inhibit the action of trimethoprim because of the presence of thymine and thymidine.

Trimethoprim is active against a wide range of aerobic Gram-negative and Gram-positive organisms including strains of most Enterobacteriaceae such as *Escherichia coli*, *Enterobacter*, *Klebsiella*, *Proteus*, and *Salmonella* spp., some staphylococci and streptococci, and *Listeria monocytogenes*. It is also active against certain protozoa including *Plasmodium* spp.

For testing the antimicrobial activity of trimethoprim, the media should contain minimal amounts of thymine or thymidine. Minimium inhibitory concentrations for most susceptible organisms have been reported to range from 0.1 to 5.0 μg per mL.

Synergy between trimethoprim and sulphonamides occurs against a wide spectrum of organisms, see under Co-trimoxazole (p.208). Enhanced activity has also been reported *in vitro* between trimethoprim and polymyxins, aminoglycosides, and rifampicin.

Trimethoprim was found to be markedly concentrated within human polymorphonuclear leucocytes. Entry into phagocytes is a necessary, but certainly not the only, determinant of the intracellular activity of an antibiotic and these results may help explain the success of trimethoprim, in combination with sulphamethoxazole, against intracellular pathogens such as *Pneumocystis carinii*.— W. L. Hand *et al.*, *Antimicrob. Ag. Chemother.*, 1987, *31*, 1553.

Trimethoprim-induced structural alterations in *Staphylococcus aureus* and the recovery of bacteria in drug-free medium.— T. Nishino *et al.*, *J. antimicrob. Chemother.*, 1987, *19*, 147.

References to the activity of trimethoprim against various organisms: J. R. Carlson *et al.*, *Antimicrob. Ag. Chemother.*, 1983, *24*, 509 (bacterial enteropathogens including *Salmonella* and *Shigella* spp., and enterotoxigenic *Escherichia coli*); S. Larsson *et al.*, *ibid.*, 1985, *28*, 12 (*Listeria monocytogenes*); S. R. Marper and P. Noone (letter), *J. antimicrob. Chemother.*, 1985, *15*, 251 (urinary-tract pathogens including *Escherichia coli*, *Proteus* spp., staphylococci, faecal streptococci, and *Klebsiella* spp.); E. Petersen, *Trans. R. Soc. trop. Med. Hyg.*, 1987, *81*, 238 (*Plasmodium falciparum*); A. M. Lewis and B. Chattopadhyay (letter), *J. antimicrob. Chemother.*, 1987, *19*, 406 (*Yersinia* spp.); J. A. A. Hoogkamp-Korstanje, *ibid.*, *20*, 123 (*Yersinia enterocolitica*).

ACTIVITY WITH OTHER ANTIMICROBIAL AGENTS. Reports of enhanced activity between trimethoprim and other antimicrobial agents: S. H. Zinner *et al.*, *Eur. J. clin. Microbiol.*, 1982, *1*, 144 (with aminoglycosides against Gram-negative bacilli); L. K. McDougal and C. Thornsberry, *J. antimicrob. Chemother.*, 1982, *9*, 369 (with rifampicin against *Haemophilus influenzae*).

Resistance

Resistance to trimethoprim may be due to several mechanisms. Clinical resistance is often due to plasmid-mediated dihydrofolate reductases that are resistant to trimethoprim. Resistance may also be due to overproduction of dihydrofolate reductase, changes in cell permeability, or bacterial mutants which are intrinsically resistant to trimethoprim because they depend on exogenous thymine and thymidine for growth.

It was previously considered that resistance would develop rapidly when trimethoprim was used alone; these fears are now considered to have been largely unjustified, although, as with all antimicrobial agents, resistance to trimethoprim has generally increased.

Trimethoprim-resistant variants have occurred in many bacterial species including staphylococci, streptococci, and some enterobacteria. Trimethoprim resistance in Enterobacteriaceae can be mediated by R-plasmids, by chromosomal mutation, and by transposons which are segments of DNA that can be transposed between plasmids and chromosomes; multiple drug resistance has been reported in *Escherichia coli*, *Salmonella*, and *Shigella* spp.

Resistance to trimethoprim with a sulphonamide is discussed under Co-trimoxazole, p.209.

Reviews of the selection and mechanisms of resistance to trimethoprim: R. W. Lacey, *J. med. Microbiol.*, 1982, *15*, 403; J. T. Smith and S. G. B. Amyes, *Br. med. Bull.*, 1984, *40*, 42; S. G. B. Amyes, *J. antimicrob. Chemother.*, 1986, *18*, *Suppl.* C, 215.

When co-trimoxazole was introduced in 1969 it was thought that use of the combination might delay the emergence of resistant bacteria and early experience in Finland, where trimethoprim was used first as a single agent, suggested that some resistance was associated with use of trimethoprim alone. However, more recent experience in Finland and in other countries suggests that trimethoprim alone is not particularly likely to select resistance. The typical incidence of acquired resistance to trimethoprim in the Enterobacteriaceae, notably *Escherichia coli*, in Europe and North America is now between 4 and 15%, which in general is still much less than resistance to ampicillin. However, a high incidence of resistance to trimethoprim in *E. coli* has been found in many developing countries and resistance in 40% or more of isolates has been reported from Santiago, Chile, and Bangkok, Thailand. The great majority of these isolates were highly resistant to trimethoprim and were also resistant to sulphonamides; most were also resistant to streptomycin, ampicillin, tetracycline, and chloramphenicol. The free availability of co-trimoxazole and the high incidence in these countries of diarrhoeal illness may be responsible for the prevalence of resistance to trimethoprim. It appears that the high incidence of multiresistant bacteria is not necessarily prevented by antibiotic combinations.— *Lancet*, 1986, *1*, 364. It may be the overall level of trimethoprim usage, irrespective of whether it is used alone or in combination with a sulphonamide, which will have the greatest influence in the future on the incidence of trimethoprim resistance.— *ibid.*, *2*, 791.

By the spring of 1987, nine different trimethoprim-resistant plasmid-encoded bacterial dihydrofolate reductase enzymes or their genes had been characterised; the mechanism of resistance of all these enzymes appears to be an alteration in the active site. Some of these enzymes are mediated by transposons such as the transposon Tn7. Although Tn7 was first identified in plasmids it has subsequently been found integrated into bacterial chromosomes. Some plasmid-encoded enzymes cause high-level resistance to trimethoprim with minimum inhibitory concentrations (MICs) of trimethoprim greater than 1 mg per mL, whereas other strains are only moderately resistant to trimethoprim, with MICs of 10 to 64 μg per mL; in the future, it will be important to monitor for intermediate-level transferable trimethoprim resistance. Plasmid-mediated trimethoprim resistance is a significant problem in developing countries, owing to the widespread use of trimethoprim, mostly in combination with sulphonamides. In industrialised countries, such as the *UK* and Finland, trimethoprim resistance tends to be a problem in hospitals, particularly geriatric units. In outpatients, recent findings have shown different trends in the development of trimethoprim resistance. Some studies indicate that resistance is falling or has reached a plateau level (R. Maskell, *Br. med. J.*, 1985, *290*, 156; P. Huovinen and P. Toivanen, *Lancet*, 1986, *2*, 1285), however, there are also areas where trimethoprim resistance is still increasing: Hamilton-Miller and Purves (*J. antimicrob. Chemother.* 1986, *18*, 643) described an increase from 6 to 19% in trimethoprim resistance among *E. coli* urinary-tract isolates from outpatients at the Royal Free Hospital, UK, from 1981 to 1985; and in the Helsinki area in Finland an increase from 3% in 1980 to 15% in 1986 occurred (P. Huovinen and P. Toivanen, *Lancet*, 1986, *2*, 1285). Several investigators have suggested that trimethoprim-resistant strains are spread from animals to humans, however, the use of trimethoprim for the treatment of human infections may be more significant. Whether trimethoprim alone promotes the development of resistance more than a trimethoprim-sulphonamide combination in clinical settings is not clear, although trimethoprim-resistant strains which are susceptible to sulphonamides have been reported since the introduction of trimethoprim monotherapy. Combination with a second agent has not, however, prevented the development of trimethoprim resistance and the best method for preventing the spread of resistance is the controlled use of trimethoprim and other antimicrobial agents.— P. Huovinen, *Antimicrob. Ag. Chemother.*, 1987, *31,* 1451.

For further mention of the development of resistance to trimethoprim in patients treated with co-trimoxazole, see under Co-trimoxazole, p.209.

RESISTANCE OF ENTEROBACTERIACEAE. Isolation of trimethoprim-resistant, sulphonamide-susceptible Enterobacteriaceae from patients with urinary-tract infections.— K. J. Towner *et al., Antimicrob. Ag. Chemother.*, 1983, *23,* 617.

Although firm national data are not available, it is reasonably certain that resistance of Enterobacteriaceae to trimethoprim has increased in the *UK* over the last few years; a recent national survey indicated that about 15% of isolates of *Escherichia coli* are now resistant to trimethoprim. In a study of 151 patients with urinary-tract infections, trimethoprim and co-trimoxazole, given by mouth, were found to select a similar incidence of resistance to trimethoprim in the intestinal flora.— R. Menon *et al., J. antimicrob. Chemother.*, 1986, *18,* 415.

Escherichia. Of 232 strains of enteropathogenic *Escherichia coli* 14 were resistant to trimethoprim at a concentration of 0.5 µg per mL.— R. J. Gross *et al., Br. med. J.*, 1982, *285,* 472.

Salmonellae. The incidence of trimethoprim-resistant strains of salmonellae was monitored in Britain over 12 years from January 1970 to December 1981. Strains of trimethoprim-resistant *Salmonella typhimurium* had increased and in 1981, 6.7% of strains isolated from man were resistant to trimethoprim; the use of antibiotics in animal husbandry was considered to have contributed to the resistance. In *S. typhi* trimethoprim resistance was rare, occurring in only 3 of 2870 strains received since 1970; in 2 patients resistance was acquired *in vivo* whilst the patients were receiving treatment with trimethoprim. Trimethoprim-resistance in man of salmonellae other than *S. typhi* and *S. typhimurium* also increased from 1980.— L. R. Ward *et al., Lancet*, 1982, *2,* 705.

A report of transferable resistance in *Salmonella saint-paul* from Tunis. A total of 18 multiple-resistant salmonella strains were isolated during a 6-month period in a single hospital, from patients on admission. In all the strains resistance was to ampicillin/carbenicillin, first generation cephalosporins, chloramphenicol, streptomycin, tetracycline, and trimethoprim.— J. Ďurkovský *et al.* (letter), *J. antimicrob. Chemother.*, 1987, *20,* 768.

Shigellae. Acquisition of trimethoprim resistance in an epidemic strain of *Shigella dysenteriae* type 1 from Zaire following use of co-trimoxazole.— J. A. Frost *et al.* (letter), *Lancet*, 1982, *1,* 963.

Of 2753 strains of *Shigella dysenteriae*, *S. flexneri*, and *S. boydii* examined at the Central Public Health Laboratory from 1979 to mid 1983, 5.8% were resistant to trimethoprim at a concentration of 0.5 µg per mL. The incidence of resistance to trimethoprim had increased from 0.3% in 1974 to 16.8% in the first half of 1983.— R. J. Gross *et al., Br. med. J.*, 1984, *288,* 784.

RESISTANCE OF HAEMOPHILUS. Of 2434 strains of *Haemophilus influenzae* collected in 1986 from 23 laboratories in the *UK*, 102 strains (4.2%) were resistant to trimethoprim with a minimum inhibitory concentration of 2 µg or more per mL. Of these 47 were also resistant to sulphamethoxazole and 12 produced beta-lactamase.— M. Powell *et al., Br. med. J.*, 1987, *295,* 176. See also J. Campos and S. Garcia-Tornel, *J. antimicrob. Chemother.*, 1987, *19,* 297.

In a study of the susceptibility of 57 strains of *Haemophilus ducreyi* isolated in Amsterdam from 1978 to 1985, an increase in the minimum inhibitory concentration of trimethoprim occurred: during 1978–81 all of 28 isolates were inhibited by 0.125 µg per mL, whereas in 1982–85 only 69% of 29 isolates were inhibited by this concentration and a concentration of 8 µg per mL was required to inhibit all strains.— A. W. Sturm, *J. antimicrob. Chemother.*, 1987, *19,* 187.

RESISTANCE OF STAPHYLOCOCCI. Of 386 strains of *Staphylococcus epidermidis* tested for susceptibility to trimethoprim 27.3% of clinical strains, but only 12.6% of strains from normal flora, were resistant to trimethoprim. All of 63 strains of *Staph. saprophyticus* were sensitive to trimethoprim being inhibited by 0.5 µg or less per mL.— J. F. Richardson, *J. antimicrob. Chemother.*, 1983, *11,* 163.

A report of plasmid-encoded trimethoprim resistance in *Staphylococcus aureus* and *Staph. epidermidis* isolates.— G. L. Archer *et al., Antimicrob. Ag. Chemother.*, 1986, *29,* 733.

RESISTANCE OF VIBRIO. Transposable resistance to trimethoprim in *Vibrio cholerae*.— F. Goldstein *et al., J. antimicrob. Chemother.*, 1986, *17,* 559.

Plasmid-mediated trimethoprim resistance in *Vibrio cholerae*.— H. -K. Young and S. G. B. Amyes, *J. antimicrob. Chemother.*, 1986, *17,* 697.

Absorption and Fate

Trimethoprim is rapidly and almost completely absorbed from the gastro-intestinal tract and peak concentrations in the circulation occur about 1 to 4 hours after an oral dose; peak plasma concentrations of about 1 µg per mL have been reported after a single dose of 100 mg. About 40 to 70% is bound to plasma proteins. Trimethoprim is widely distributed to various tissues and fluids including kidneys, liver, bronchial secretions, saliva, prostatic tissue and fluid, and vaginal secretions; tissue concentrations in the kidneys and lungs are reported to be higher than serum concentrations, but concentrations in the cerebrospinal fluid are about one-half of those in the blood. Trimethoprim readily crosses the placenta and it appears in breast milk. The half-life is about 8 to 10 hours, but is prolonged in severe renal failure. Trimethoprim is excreted primarily by the kidneys through glomerular filtration and tubular secretion. About 40 to 60% of a dose is excreted in the urine within 24 hours, predominantly as unchanged drug. About 10 to 20% of trimethoprim is metabolised primarily in the liver and small amounts are excreted in the faeces. Trimethoprim is removed from the blood by haemodialysis to some extent.

Pharmacokinetics of trimethoprim given to healthy subjects in a dose of 200 mg twice daily or 300 mg daily by mouth.— I. D. Watson *et al., J. int. med. Res.*, 1983, *11,* 137.

Bioavailability of trimethoprim combined with folic acid.— K. Soininen and T. Kleimola, *J. int. med. Res.*, 1983, *11,* 294.

Trimethoprim was reported to be 30 to 70% bound to plasma proteins. The normal half-life of 8 to 15 hours was increased to 24 hours in end-stage renal failure.— W. M. Bennett *et al., Am. J. Kidney Dis.*, 1983, *3,* 155.

ABSORPTION. Food decreased the amount of trimethoprim absorbed, but had no effect on the rate of absorption in 12 healthy subjects given trimethoprim 3 mg per kg body-weight as a suspension by mouth. These results suggest that trimethoprim given as a suspension should be administered between meals.— K. Hoppu *et al., Eur. J. clin. Pharmac.*, 1987, *32,* 427.

ADMINISTRATION IN INFANTS AND CHILDREN. In 18 children aged 3 months to 13 years given trimethoprim 10 mg per kg body-weight as a single dose by mouth the mean time to maximum concentration in plasma was 2.2 hours with wide individual variation. The mean elimination half-life calculated from plasma data (6.8 hours) or from urine data (7.9 hours) was considerably shorter than values of 7 to 17 hours reported for adults. Concentrations in urine were usually sustained for at least 16 hours above the MIC for common urinary pathogens. Recovery of only 34% of the dose in the urine in 24 hours suggested extrarenal elimination.— G. W. Rylance *et al., Archs Dis. Childh.*, 1985, *60,* 29. See also.— P. Kremers *et al., Thérapie*, 1973, *28,* 1177.

The pharmacokinetics of trimethoprim in children with renal insufficiency.— K. Hoppu *et al., Clin. Pharmac. Ther.*, 1987, *42,* 181.

DIFFUSION INTO BODY TISSUES AND FLUIDS. In 4 patients given trimethoprim 160 mg (as co-trimoxazole) concentrations in the CSF 0.5 to 1.5 hours after infusion were 20 to 44% of those in serum; in 5 patients treated by mouth concentrations in the CSF 2 to 4 hours after the dose were 13 to 34% of those in serum.— Å. Svedhem and S. Inwarson, *J. antimicrob. Chemother.*, 1979, *5,* 717.

Reports of the diffusion of trimethoprim into various body tissues and fluids: J. N. Bruun *et al., Antimicrob. Ag. Chemother.*, 1981, *19,* 82 (serum and skin blister fluid, combined with sulphonamides); S. J. McIntosh *et al.* (letter), *J. antimicrob. Chemother.*, 1983, *11,* 195 (sputum and saliva); A. M. Ristuccia *et al., Clin. Pharmac. Ther.*, 1984, *35,* 269 (prostate).

For further reference to the absorption and fate of trimethoprim with various sulphonamides, see under Co-trimazine, p.206, Co-trimoxazole, p.209, and Sulfametopyrazine, p.300.

Uses and Administration

Trimethoprim is an antibacterial agent used for the treatment of infections due to sensitive organisms particularly infections of the urinary and respiratory tracts.

In the treatment of acute urinary-tract infections the usual dose is 200 mg twice daily; doses of 200 mg daily in 1 or 2 divided doses or 300 mg daily as a single dose are also used. Children may be given 6 to 8 mg per kg body-weight daily in 2 divided doses: suggested regimens for children are, 6 to 12 years, 100 mg twice daily; 6 months to 5 years, 50 mg twice daily; 2 to 5 months, 25 mg twice daily. For long-term prophylaxis the usual dose is 100 mg at night, with 2 to 2.5 mg per kg for children. Trimethoprim is also used in the treatment of respiratory-tract infections, in doses similar to those used in acute urinary-tract infections. Trimethoprim is also administered intravenously by injection or infusion as the lactate in similar doses; total daily doses of up to 20 mg per kg in divided doses have been used in severely ill patients. Care should be taken in patients with renal failure; plasma concentrations should be monitored in patients with severe renal failure.

Trimethoprim is used in conjunction with sulphonamides in the treatment of bacterial infections. The most well known combination is co-trimoxazole (trimethoprim with sulphamethoxazole); other combinations are co-trimazine (with sulphadiazine) and co-trifamole (with sulphamoxole); trimethoprim is also used with sulfametopyrazine, sulfametrole, or sulphadimidine, and, in veterinary practice, with sulfadoxine.

Trimethoprim has been used in conjunction with sulphonamides in the treatment of chloroquine-resistant malaria but has not achieved wide acceptance.

For a review of the antibacterial activity, pharmacokinetics, and therapeutic use of trimethoprim in urinary-tract infections, see R. N. Brogden *et al., Drugs*, 1982, *23,* 405.

For an account of the antibacterial activity and uses of trimethoprim, see G. Rich and B. Mee, *Med. J. Aust.*, 1985, *142,* 350.

For comparative reviews of trimethoprim and co-trimoxazole, see Co-trimoxazole, p.210.

ADMINISTRATION IN INFANTS AND CHILDREN. In a study of 18 children, the elimination half-life of trimethoprim was reduced when compared with 12 healthy adults, because of the smaller volume of distribution and higher total clearance in children. The current dosage recommendations are based on adult data, and it appears that the dosage interval may need to be reduced in children.— K. Hoppu, *Clin. Pharmac. Ther.*, 1987, *41,* 336.

ADMINISTRATION IN RENAL FAILURE. Trimethoprim could be administered to patients with renal failure by adjusting the dosage interval. A dosage interval of 12 hours is suitable for patients whose glomerular filtration-rates exceed 50 mL per minute; an interval of 18 hours between doses is advisable for rates of between 10 and 50 mL per minute. Where the rate is less than 10 mL per minute, the dosage interval should be 24 hours. A dose supplement should be given to patients undergoing haemodialysis.— W. M. Bennett *et al., Am. J. Kidney Dis.*, 1983, *3,* 155.

DIARRHOEA. For comments on the use of trimethoprim in the prophylaxis and treatment of travellers' diarrhoea, see under Co-trimoxazole, p.211.

ENTERIC INFECTIONS. *Salmonellosis.* Of 71 patients with typhoid or paratyphoid fever, 63 were successfully treated with trimethoprim 300 mg every 12 hours, reducing to 200 mg every 12 hours after 48 to 72 hours; treatment was given for 14 days. Intravenous bolus injections were given initially followed by oral therapy in 42 patients, whilst the remaining patients received oral therapy throughout. Of the treatment failures, 4 suffering from typhoid fever remained febrile despite sterile blood cultures and so treatment was changed to chloramphenicol; in a further 3 patients trimethoprim therapy was discontinued because of the development of a rash, and one patient who had been ill for 2 weeks before admission to hospital died after developing disseminated intravascular coagulation and intestinal haemorrhage. Complete defervescence occurred in a mean of 4.9 days, but 3 patients relapsed clinically and bacteriologically after the end of trimethoprim therapy; 2 of these patients were successfully retreated with trimethoprim and one with chloramphenicol. Three patients continued to excrete *Salmonella typhi*. Trimethoprim was considered to be a satisfactory antimicrobial agent for the treatment of typhoid and paratyphoid fevers and also for other invasive salmonella infections.— P. Gargalianos *et al.*, *J. antimicrob. Chemother.*, 1986, *18*, 277.

Successful use of intravenous trimethoprim to treat neonatal typhoid fever.— K. C. Chin *et al.*, *Archs Dis. Childh.*, 1986, *61*, 1228.

Shigellosis. In a study of 20 patients with severe bacillary dysentery trimethoprim 300 mg twice daily was found to have activity comparable to co-trimoxazole 960 mg twice daily, both given by mouth for 5 days. With the exception of 4 patients harbouring trimethoprim-resistant strains, all responded clinically and bacteriologically within 48 hours of starting treatment.— J. Bogaerts *et al.*, *Trans. R. Soc. trop. Med. Hyg.*, 1985, *79*, 203.

IMMUNOCOMPROMISED PATIENTS. For reference to the use of trimethoprim with dapsone in the treatment of *Pneumocystis carinii* pneumonia in AIDS patients, see *Pneumocystis carinii* Infections, below.

MENINGITIS. Treatment of *Listeria* meningitis with cephalothin in association with trimethoprim in a penicillin-allergic patient.— P. H. J. van Keulen *et al.* (letter), *J. Infect.*, 1986, *13*, 303.

PNEUMOCYSTIS CARINII INFECTIONS. Patients with AIDS and a first episode of pneumonia due to *Pneumocystis carinii* were treated with dapsone 100 mg daily as a single dose and trimethoprim 20 mg per kg body-weight daily in 4 divided doses, both given by mouth for 21 days. All 15 patients improved clinically and radiographically usually within 3 to 10 days after starting treatment. Although side-effects occurred in 14 patients only 2 patients had to discontinue therapy after 10 days because of worsening skin rash.— G. S. Leoung *et al.*, *Ann. intern. Med.*, 1986, *105*, 45.

RESPIRATORY-TRACT INFECTIONS. In a prospective randomised double-blind study, 107 patients with chest infections were given trimethoprim 100 mg twice daily for 5 days and 109 similar patients were given co-trimoxazole 600 mg twice daily. The mean response of those who received trimethoprim alone was virtually identical to that of those who received co-trimoxazole. Twenty side-effects were noted in 16 patients who received trimethoprim compared with 46 in 25 patients treated with co-trimoxazole; bad taste, sore throat, and nausea were more common with co-trimoxazole than with trimethoprim. It was considered that in the treatment of acute respiratory-tract infections trimethoprim was as effective as co-trimoxazole and produced fewer side-effects, but since there were several types of respiratory infections, these results could mask differences for certain diagnoses.— R. W. Lacey *et al.*, *Lancet*, 1980, *1*, 1270.

Comment that although some workers have recommended the use of trimethoprim alone in respiratory-tract infections, caution should be taken where infections with *Branhamella (Moraxella) catarrhalis* are known to occur. These organisms have been found to be resistant to trimethoprim *in vitro*, but susceptible to co-trimoxazole.— T. G. Winstanley and R. C. Spencer (letter), *J. antimicrob. Chemother.*, 1986, *18*, 425.

Studies comparing trimethoprim with co-trimoxazole in the treatment of respiratory-tract infections: J. J. Ashford and L. J. Downey, *Br. J. clin. Pract.*, 1982, *36*, 152; M. Haataja *et al.*, *Curr. ther. Res.*, 1985, *37*, 191; M. Gonsalkorale, *Br. J. clin. Pract.*, 1987, *41*, 743.

A double-blind study of trimethoprim and amoxycillin in the treatment of upper respiratory-tract infections in general practice. There was no significant difference between the 2 drugs in efficacy and acceptability and trimethoprim was considered to be a suitable alternative treatment to amoxycillin. However, trimethoprim eradicated only 50% of group A streptococci and therefore penicillin is still the treatment of choice for such infections.— B. W. McGuinness *et al.*, *Practitioner*, 1986, *230*, 905. See also R. I. Gove and R. M. Cayton, *J. antimicrob. Chemother.*, 1985, *15*, 495.

SEXUALLY TRANSMITTED DISEASES. For the use of trimethoprim with a sulphonamide, in the treatment of chancroid, gonorrhoea, or granuloma inguinale, see under Co-trimoxazole, p.213.

For the use of trimethoprim alone or with sulfametrole in the treatment of chancroid, see under Sulfametrole, p.301.

SKIN DISORDERS. *Acne.* A single-blind comparative study, involving 53 patients, of trimethoprim or oxytetracycline by mouth in inflammatory acne vulgaris demonstrated no significant difference between the 2 treatments.— J. R. Gibson *et al.*, *Br. J. Derm.*, 1982, *107*, 221.

Comment that systemic trimethoprim can be considered as an alternative drug to treat acne vulgaris in patients intolerant of oxytetracycline therapy, but should not be used as first-line therapy.— W. J. Cunliffe, *Prescribers' J.*, 1987, *27* (4), 23.

URINARY-TRACT INFECTIONS. Several studies have demonstrated trimethoprim to be as effective as co-trimoxazole in the treatment of acute urinary-tract infections (Trimethoprim Study Group, *J. antimicrob. Chemother.*, 1981, *7*, 179; A.J. Martin and R.W. Lacey, *Practitioner*, 1984, *228*, 545; R. Menon *et al.*, *J. antimicrob. Chemother.*, 1986, *18*, 415). Various dosage regimens have been suggested for uncomplicated urinary-tract infections ranging from a single dose of trimethoprim 200 or 400 mg (R.B. Harbord and R.N. Grüneberg, *Br. med. J.*, 1981, *283*, 1301; J.A. Boscia *et al.*, *J. Am. med. Ass.*, 1987, *257*, 1067) to 10-day treatment regimens (G. Gossius and L. Vorland, *Curr. ther. Res.*, 1985, *37*, 34); shorter regimens improve patient compliance and reduce side-effects. The frequency of trimethoprim administration has also been discussed. A once-daily regimen of trimethoprim 300 mg was found to be as effective as 160 mg given twice daily for 7 days (A. Kasanen *et al.*, *Curr. ther. Res.*, 1984, *36*, 105).

In the long-term prophylaxis of urinary-tract infections, trimethoprim has been given in a dose of 100 mg at night, but as high-level resistance to trimethoprim becomes more widespread its use in long-term therapy may be limited (W. Brumfitt *et al.*, *Br. J. Hosp. Med.*, 1983, *30*, 381; W. Brumfitt *et al.*, *J. antimicrob. Chemother.*, 1985, *16*, 111). For the management of recurrent urinary-tract infections, treatment for 7 days with trimethoprim 300 mg at night has been found to be as effective as co-trimoxazole 960 mg given every 12 hours (W. Brumfitt *et al.*, *Infection*, 1982, *10*, 280).

Preparations

Trimethoprim Tablets *(B.P.)*

Proprietary Preparations

Ipral *(Squibb, UK)*. *Tablets*, trimethoprim 100 and 200 mg.
Paediatric suspension, trimethoprim 50 mg/5 mL.

Monotrim *(Duphar, UK)*. *Tablets*, scored, trimethoprim 100 and 200 mg.
Suspension, trimethoprim 50 mg/5 mL.
Injection, trimethoprim 20 mg (as lactate)/mL in ampoules of 5 mL.

Polytrim *(Wellcome, UK)*. *Eye-drops*, trimethoprim 0.1%, polymyxin B sulphate 10 000 units/mL.
Eye ointment, trimethoprim 0.5%, polymyxin B sulphate 10 000 units/g.

Syraprim *(Wellcome, UK)*. *Tablets*, scored, trimethoprim 100 and 300 mg.
Injection, trimethoprim 20 mg (as lactate)/mL in ampoules of 5 mL.

Tiempe *(DDSA Pharmaceuticals, UK)*. *Tablets*, trimethoprim 100 and 200 mg.

Trimogal *(Lagap, UK)*. *Tablets*, trimethoprim 100 and 200 mg.

Trimopan *(Berk Pharmaceuticals, UK)*. *Tablets*, scored, trimethoprim 100 and 200 mg.
Suspension, trimethoprim 50 mg/5 mL.

Proprietary Names and Manufacturers of Trimethoprim and Trimethoprim Lactate

Abaprim *(Gentili, Ital.)*; Alprim *(Alphapharm, Austral.)*; Delprim *(Delalande, Switz.)*; Idotrim *(Leo, Swed.)*; Ipral *(Squibb, UK)*; Methoprim *(Protea, Austral.)*; Monotrim *(GEA, Denm.*; *Biochimica, Switz.*; *Duphar, UK)*; Motrim *(Lannacher, Aust.)*; Primosept *(Chassot, Switz.)*; Proloprim *(Wellcome, Canad.*; *Wellcome, S.Afr.*; *Wellcome, USA)*; Syraprim *(Gayoso Wellcome, Spain*; *Wellcome, UK)*; Tediprima *(Estedi, Spain)*; Tiempe *(DDSA Pharmaceuticals, UK)*; Trentina *(Jorba, Spain)*; Trimanyl *(Tosse, Ger.)*; Trimogal *(Lagap, UK)*; Trimono *(Röhm, Ger.)*; Trimopan *(Farmos, Denm.*; *Fin.*; *Laakefarmos, Swed.*; *Berk Pharmaceuticals, UK)*; Trimpex *(Roche, USA)*; Triprim *(Wellcome, Austral.*; *Fisons, S.Afr.)*; Unitrim *(Unimed, UK)*; Uretrim *(Bastian, Ger.)*; Wellcoprim *(Wellcome, Fr.*; *Wellcome, Norw.*; *Wellcome, Swed.)*.

The following names have been used for multi-ingredient preparations containing trimethoprim and trimethoprim lactate—

Kelfiprim; Kelfiprin; Lidaprim *(Chemie-Linz, Aust.*; *Pharbil, Belg.)*; Lidatrim *(Warrick, Neth.)*; Maderan *(Ciba, Switz.)*; Polytrim *(Wellcome, UK)*; Poteseptyl *(Alkaloida Chemical Factory, Hung.)*; Rifaprim *(Lepetit, Arg.*; *Lepetit, Ital.)*; Trimed *(Armour, Ital.)*; Trimetrol *(Essex, Belg.)*; Velaten *(Corvi, Ital.)*.

13388-r

Tylosin *(BAN, rINN)*.

$C_{46}H_{77}NO_{17}$=916.1.

CAS — 1401-69-0.

Pharmacopoeias. In *B.P. Vet.*

A mixture of antimicrobial macrolides, produced by the growth of certain strains of *Streptomyces fradiae* or by any other means. It consists largely of tylosin A, but tylosin B (desmycosin), tylosin C (macrocin), and tylosin D (relomycin) may also be present.

An almost white to buff-coloured powder. Slightly **soluble** in water; soluble 1 in 15 of alcohol, 1 in 30 of chloroform, and 1 in 6 of methyl alcohol; soluble in dilute mineral acids. A 2.5% suspension in carbon-dioxide-free water has a pH of 8.5 to 10.5. **Store** in well-closed containers.

13389-f

Tylosin Tartrate *(BANM, rINNM)*.

$(C_{46}H_{77}NO_{17})_2,C_4H_6O_6$=1982.3.

CAS — 1405-54-5.

Pharmacopoeias. In *B.P. Vet.*

A white to buff-coloured powder. 1.1 g of monograph substance is approximately equivalent to 1 g of tylosin. **Soluble** 1 in 10 of water; slightly soluble in alcohol; freely soluble in chloroform; practically insoluble in ether. A 2.5% solution in water has a pH of 5.0 to 7.2. **Store** in well-closed containers.

Units

One unit of tylosin is contained in 0.001 mg of the first International Standard Preparation (1966) of tylosin base which contains 1000 units per mg.

Uses.

Tylosin is a macrolide antibiotic and has similar antimicrobial activity to erythromycin (p.222). Tylosin and its phosphate and tartrate salts are used in veterinary medicine in the prophylaxis and treatment of various infections caused by susceptible organisms.

Tylosin and tylosin phosphate are added to animal feeding stuffs as growth promoters for pigs.

A report of 2 cases of contact dermatitis due to tylosin contained in animal feed supplements. The second patient was also allergic to feed supplements containing nitrofurazone.— K. H. Neldner, *Archs Derm.*, 1972, *106*, 722.

A review of the use of tylosin in animal feeds and in veterinary medicine.— J. D. Mackinnon, in, *Ten Years on from Swann*, D.W. Jolly *et al.* (Ed.), London, The Association of Veterinarians in Industries, 1981, p.51.

Susceptibility of *Legionella* spp. to macrolide antibiotics including tylosin.— P. H. Edelstein *et al.*, *Antimicrob. Ag. Chemother.*, 1982, *22*, 90.

Proprietary Veterinary Names and Manufacturers of Tylosin and its Salts

Tylamix *(Elanco, UK)*; Tylan *(Elanco, UK)*.

176-z

Tyrothricin *(BAN, USAN, rINN)*.

Tirotricina.

CAS — 1404-88-2.

Pharmacopoeias. In *Arg.*, *Braz.*, *Fr.*, *Swiss*, and *U.S.*

An antimicrobial substance produced by the growth of *Bacillus brevis* Dubos. It is a mixture consisting chiefly of gramicidin and tyrocidine, the latter being usually present as the hydrochloride. Both components are mixtures of polypeptides.

Store in airtight containers.

Adverse Effects and Precautions

Tyrothricin is too toxic to be administered systemically; effects that have been reported include liver and kidney damage. It damages the sensory epithelium of the nose and instances of prolonged loss of smell have occurred after its use as a nasal spray or instillation. Tyrothricin should not be instilled into the nasal cavities or into closed body cavities.

EFFECTS ON THE SKIN. Tyrothricin had been implicated in the Stevens-Johnson syndrome.— D. B. Coursin, *J. Am. med. Ass.*, 1966, *198*, 113.

Uses and Administration

Tyrothricin is unsuitable for systemic treatment. It is active *in vitro* against many Gram-positive bacteria and has been used either alone or in conjunction with other antibacterial agents in the local treatment of infections of the skin and mouth.

Proprietary Preparations

Tyrozets *(Merck Sharp & Dohme, UK). Lozenges*, tyrothricin 1 mg, benzocaine 5 mg.

Proprietary Names and Manufacturers

Faringotricina *(SIT, Ital.)*; Ginotricina *(UCB, Ital.)*; Hydrotricine *(Belg.; Rhone-Poulenc, Ital.)*; Rinotricina *(SIT, Ital.)*; Solutricina *(UCB, Ital.)*; Solutricine *(Fr.)*; Soropon *(Purdue Frederick, Canad.)*; Tyrosur *(Engelhard, Ger.)*.

The following names have been used for multi-ingredient preparations containing tyrothricin—

Otoseptil *(Napp, UK)*; Tetrazets *(Merck Sharp & Dohme, UK)*; Tyrosolven *(Warner, UK)*; Tyrozets *(Merck Sharp & Dohme, UK)*.

177-c

Vancomycin Hydrochloride *(BANM, USAN, rINNM)*.

Vancomycini Hydrochloridum. (S_a)-(3*S*,6*R*,7*R*,22*R*,23*S*,26*S*,36*R*,38a*R*)-44-{[2-*O*-(3-Amino-2,3,6-trideoxy-3-*C*-methyl-α-L-*lyxo*-hexopyranosyl)-β-D-glucopyranosyl]oxy}-3-(carbamoylmethyl)-10,19-dichloro-2,3,4,5,6,7,23,24,25,26,36,37,38,38a-tetradecahydro-7,22,28,30,32-pentahydroxy-6-[(2*R*)-4-methyl-2-(methylamino)valeramido]-2,5,24,38,39-pentaoxo-22*H*-8,11:18,21-dietheno-23,36-(iminomethano)-13,16:31,35-dimetheno-1*H*,16*H*-[1,6,9]oxadiazacyclohexadecino[4,5-*m*]-[10,2,16]-benzoxadiazacyclotetracosine-26-carboxylic acid, monohydrochloride.

$C_{66}H_{75}Cl_2N_9O_{24}$,HCl=1485.7.

CAS — 1404-90-6 (vancomycin); 1404-93-9 (hydrochloride).

Pharmacopoeias. In *Br.*, *Int.*, and *U.S.*

A glycopeptide antimicrobial substance produced by the growth of certain strains of *Streptomyces orientalis*, or by any other means. A light brown, very hygroscopic, odourless powder. The *B.P.* specifies not less than 900 units per mg, and the *U.S.P.* not less than 900 µg of vancomycin per mg, both calculated on the anhydrous substance. One million units of vancomycin are approximately equivalent to 1 g of vancomycin. 1.03 g of monograph substance is approximately equivalent to 1 g of vancomycin.

B.P. **solubilities** are: soluble 1 in 10 of water; slightly soluble in alcohol and ether; practically insoluble in chloroform. *U.S.P.* solubilities are: freely soluble in water; insoluble in ether and chloroform. A 5% solution in water has a pH of 2.5 to 4.5.

Store in airtight containers. Solutions are most stable at pH 3 to 5; they should be stored in a refrigerator. Solutions of vancomycin hydrochloride equivalent to vancomycin 5% are stable for 96 hours if stored in a refrigerator.

Since vancomycin hydrochloride solutions have a low pH they may be physically **incompatible** with other drugs.

There was no significant loss of potency when vancomycin for injection was dissolved in water, added to each of 3 commercially available 0.5% hypromellose solutions in plastic squeezy bottles (Lacril, pH 5.9; Tearisol, pH 7.3; Isoptotears, pH 7.4), and the resulting solutions of vancomycin 31 mg per mL kept at 25° for 7 days. The relative potency of vancomycin varied according to the hypromellose solution used.— E. Osborn *et al.*, *Am. J. Ophthal.*, 1976, *82*, 775.

A poor therapeutic response to vancomycin was attributed to inactivation of the drug by heparin when they were administered through the same intravenous line.— N. L. Barg *et al.*, *Antimicrob. Ag. Chemother.*, 1986, *29*, 209.

Stability studies of vancomycin hydrochloride in sodium chloride 0.9% and glucose 5% injections at different temperatures.— V. Das Gupta *et al.*, *Am. J. Hosp. Pharm.*, 1986, *43*, 1729.

A study suggesting that vancomycin is insufficiently stable for use in an implantable drug pump delivery system.— R. N. Greenberg *et al.*, *Antimicrob. Ag. Chemother.*, 1987, *31*, 610.

Units

One unit of vancomycin is contained in 0.000993 mg of the first International Standard Preparation (1963) of vancomycin sulphate which contains 1007 units per mg.

Adverse Effects

Thrombophlebitis has been a common complication of vancomycin therapy; it may be minimised by slow intravenous injection of a dilute solution of the antibiotic, and by using different veins in rotation. Extravasation at the injection site may cause tissue necrosis.

A syndrome, characterised by a sudden fall in blood pressure, with or without a maculopapular rash over the face and upper body, and known as the 'red man' or 'red neck' syndrome has been associated with the intravenous administration of vancomycin; the hypotension appears to be related to a rapid rate of infusion.

Febrile reactions, chills, skin rashes, eosinophilia, and alterations in kidney function may occur, and anaphylaxis and neutropenia have been reported rarely. Hearing loss has been associated with the administration of vancomycin and may be irreversible; it is sometimes preceded by tinnitus which must be regarded as a sign to discontinue treatment. The use of vancomycin may be associated with the overgrowth of non-susceptible organisms. Some of the adverse effects of vancomycin may be related to high blood concentrations or prolonged treatment.

Few adverse effects have been reported after the oral administration of vancomycin.

A retrospective study of 98 patients given 100 courses of intravenous vancomycin between 1974 and 1981. Adverse effects reported included: rashes (3% of patients), phlebitis (13%), and neutropenia (2%). One patient developed transient fever associated with wheezing and chills after the first dose, another developed fever while receiving both vancomycin and rifampicin. There were no clinically apparent cases of ototoxicity, and no changes were observed in 5 patients who had serial audiograms. One patient developed vertigo. Ninety-four patients could be evaluated for nephrotoxicity. A significant increase in serum-creatinine concentrations occurred in 12 of 34 patients (35%) who received concomitant aminoglycosides. Increased serum creatinine occurred in 3 of the remaining patients (5%); all had trough serum-vancomycin concentrations between 30 and 65 µg per mL, and in 2 the creatinine concentration returned to baseline after dosage adjustment. The high incidence of nephrotoxicity in patients given vancomycin and aminoglycosides, although it may demonstrate an additive effect, may be as a result of bias in the method of identifying patients for the study.— B. F. Farber and R. C. Moellering, *Antimicrob. Ag. Chemother.*, 1983, *23*, 138. A prospective study of nephrotoxicity and ototoxicity in 34 patients given 39 courses of intravenous vancomycin often in association with other drugs including frusemide, antineoplastics, and aminoglycosides. Acute nephrotoxicity developed in 3 patients; only one had a steady reduction in renal function during vancomycin therapy. Increases in serum creatinine, observed on 3 occasions after completion of therapy may have been associated with the disease state. The authors could find no evidence of synergistic toxicity between vancomycin and aminoglycosides.

Tinnitus and dizziness were reported by 2 patients, one of whom was also receiving amikacin; symptoms resolved within 24 hours of discontinuing vancomycin. Acute hearing loss was noted during one of 23 courses of vancomycin analysed, and delayed onset hearing loss after one of 18 courses; this latter patient was also receiving gentamicin. Both patients were unaware of any change in their hearing.— J. A. Mellor *et al.*, *J. antimicrob. Chemother.*, 1985, *15*, 773. A further prospective study in 54 patients, the majority of whom were receiving other drugs including aminoglycosides. Thrombophlebitis occurred in all patients given vancomycin through peripheral venous cannulae, but in none in whom central venous cannulae or dialysis catheters were used. Maculopapular rashes could be attributed to vancomycin therapy in 3 patients, and subsided within 7 days of cessation of drug therapy. Hearing loss was not clinically demonstrable in any of the 34 patients in whom it could be tested, and no patient complained of vertigo or tinnitus. Of 11 patients who underwent audiometry, a right-sided hearing loss developed in one who was also receiving gentamicin. Serum-creatinine concentrations increased by more than 50% in 4 patients, all of whom were receiving concomitant therapy with aminoglycosides. The bilirubin concentration increased by more than 50% in one patient treated with vancomycin. There were no cases of haematological toxicity.— T. C. Sorrell and P. J. Collignon, *ibid.*, *16*, 235.

Low back pain after intravenous administration of vancomycin to 3 patients on continuous ambulatory peritoneal dialysis.— G. Gatterer, *Clin. Pharm.*, 1984, *3*, 87.

A report of profuse lachrymation on intravenous infusion of vancomycin.— D. Temperley *et al.* (letter), *Lancet*, 1987, *2*, 1337.

ALLERGY. A report of successful desensitisation to vancomycin after a severe systemic allergic reaction to the drug.— A. Lerner and J. M. Dwyer (letter), *Ann. intern. Med.*, 1984, *100*, 157.

EFFECTS ON THE BLOOD. Severe thrombocytopenia following the intravenous and intraperitoneal administration of vancomycin to a patient on continuous ambulatory peritoneal dialysis.— R. W. Walker and A. Heaton (letter), *Lancet*, 1985, *1*, 932.

Pancytopenia in a 42-year-old woman after rapid intravenous infusion of vancomycin.— A. J. Carmichael and M. F. Al-Zahawi (letter), *Br. med. J.*, 1986, *293*, 1103.

Reports of neutropenia associated with intravenous vancomycin therapy: C. D. R. Borland and W. E. Farrar (letter), *J. Am. med. Ass.*, 1979, *242*, 2392; H. H. Kesarwala *et al.* (letter), *Lancet*, 1981, *1*, 1423; R. L. Mackett and D. R. P. Guay, *Can. med. Ass. J.*, 1985, *132*, 39; K. B. Koo *et al.*, *Drug Intell. & clin. Pharm.*, 1986, *20*, 780.

EFFECTS ON THE EAR. For reports of the incidence of ototoxicity after administration of vancomycin, see above.

EFFECTS ON THE GASTRO-INTESTINAL TRACT. A 25-year-old woman developed *Clostridium difficile* colitis following a course of vancomycin and metronidazole, both by mouth, for pelvic inflammatory disease. The condition resolved after treatment with vancomycin given alone.— P. J. Bingley and G. M. Harding, *Postgrad. med. J.*, 1987, *63*, 993.

EFFECTS ON THE KIDNEY. For reports of the incidence of nephrotoxicity after administration of vancomycin alone or in association with an aminoglycoside, see above.

EFFECTS ON THE NERVOUS SYSTEM. Fever and encephalopathy occurred in a 14-year-old anephric girl on peritoneal dialysis given vancomycin 250 mg every 6 hours by mouth for pseudomembranous colitis. They were possibly associated with the unexpected accumulation of vancomycin to sustained serum concentrations of 34 µg per mL and a single CSF concentration of 4.2 µg per mL.— C. M. Thompson *et al.*, *Int. J. pediatr. Nephrol.*, 1983, *4*, 1.

EFFECTS ON THE SKIN. See under Hypotension, below.

HYPOTENSION. There have been several reports of the red man syndrome (characterised by sudden hypotension, with or without a maculopapular rash over the face and upper body) on rapid intravenous administration of vancomycin (J.C. Garrelts and J.D. Peterie, *New Engl. J. Med.*, 1985, *312*, 245; P.A. Southorn *et al.*, *Mayo Clin. Proc.*, 1986, *61*, 721); in one patient seizures also occurred (G.R. Bailie *et al.*, *Lancet*, 1985, *2*, 279). The reaction is probably caused by a histamine-release phenomenon and may be mistaken for an allergic reaction. It usually resolves on discontinuation of the infusion although administration of fluids, antihistamines, or corticosteroids may be beneficial. Most patients tolerate the drug on slow administration; a minimum infusion time of 60 minutes is recommended by the manufacturer. There have been reports of the characteristic rash, although not necessarily a fall in blood pressure, in one patient (A.K. Pau and R. Khakoo, *New Engl. J. Med.*, 1985, *313*, 756) and in 5 healthy subjects (R.L. Davis *et al.*, *Ann. intern. Med.*, 1986, *104*, 285) despite adherence to these recommendations. Cardiac arrest has also been reported after rapid intravenous administration of vancomycin (D. Glicklich and I. Figura, *ibid.*, 1984, *101*, 880).

Foetal bradycardia, secondary to maternal hypotension, occurred when a pregnant woman was given vancomycin intravenously over 3 minutes during labour (L.M. Hill, *Am. J. Obstet. Gynec.*, 1985, *153*, 74).

LOCAL IRRITANT EFFECTS. For reports of the incidence of thrombophlebitis after the intravenous administration of vancomycin, see above.

OVERDOSAGE. A patient with renal failure inadvertently received a total dose of 2.5 g of vancomycin (500 mg given intravenously every 6 hours). Haemoperfusion using an Amberlite resin, but not charcoal, was successful in decreasing serum-vancomycin concentrations.— R. Ahmad *et al.* (letter), *Br. med. J.*, 1982, *284*, 1953.

TREATMENT OF ADVERSE EFFECTS. A study concluding that multiple doses of activated charcoal by mouth do not enhance vancomycin clearance in subjects with normal renal function when serum concentrations are within the therapeutic range. Further study in patients with toxic vancomycin concentrations or prolonged elimination may be warranted.— R. L. Davis *et al.*, *Antimicrob. Ag. Chemother.*, 1987, *31*, 720.

For reference to the use of diphenhydramine in the treatment of adverse reactions to intravenous vancomycin, see Neurosurgery under Surgical Infection Prophylaxis in Uses, below.

Precautions

Vancomycin should not be given to patients who have experienced a hypersensitivity reaction to it. Vancomycin causes tissue necrosis and should not be injected intramuscularly. It is given parenterally by intravenous infusion; 500 mg of vancomycin should be given in at least 100 mL of fluid and infused over not less than 60 minutes to minimise thrombophlebitis and other adverse effects associated with rapid administration. It should be used with extreme caution in patients with renal insufficiency or who have a history of hearing loss. Adjustment of the parenteral dose, according to frequent determinations of serum-vancomycin concentrations, has been advised particularly in patients with renal impairment or in premature infants (see Administration under Uses). Monitoring of auditory function is advised, especially in elderly patients. Haematological status and kidney and liver function should be assessed periodically in all patients. Other ototoxic or nephrotoxic drugs should be used concurrently only with extreme caution.

Since vancomycin is poorly absorbed, toxicity is much less of a problem following oral administration than with the intravenous route.

ADMINISTRATION IN LIVER DISORDERS AND RENAL FAILURE. For reference to the precautions to be observed in liver disorders and in renal failure, see under Uses, below.

INTERACTIONS. For the effects of other agents on the antimicrobial activity of vancomycin, see under Antimicrobial Action, below.

Aminoglycosides. Nephrotoxicity, defined as a two-fold or greater increase in serum-creatinine concentrations, occurred in 4 children given vancomycin in association with an aminoglycoside. The elevated creatinine concentrations returned to pretreatment values within 3 to 6 days of stopping aminoglycoside therapy in 3 children.— C. Odio *et al.*, *J. Pediat.*, 1984, *105*, 491.

Patients receiving a combination of vancomycin and gentamicin appeared to excrete larger amounts of the proximal-tubule brush border enzyme alanine aminopeptidase in the urine than when given either agent alone. This may be an indication of additive nephrotoxicity.— M. J. Rybak *et al.*, *Antimicrob. Ag. Chemother.*, 1987, *31*, 1461.

For reference to conflicting reports on the increased incidence of nephrotoxicity in patients receiving vancomycin and aminoglycosides, see under Adverse Effects, above.

PREGNANCY AND THE NEONATE. Vancomycin should be given with caution during pregnancy as it may cause auditory or renal toxicity in the foetus.— *Med. Lett.*, 1987, *29*, 61.

For reference to foetal distress when a pregnant woman was given vancomycin rapidly during labour, see under Hypotension in Adverse Effects (above).

Antimicrobial Action

Vancomycin is a glycopeptide antibiotic which acts by interfering with bacterial cell wall synthesis. Most of the Gram-positive bacteria are sensitive to vancomycin but Gram-negative organisms, mycobacteria, and fungi are highly resistant.

Organisms are usually considered to be susceptible if the minimum inhibitory concentration of vancomycin is 5 µg or less per mL. In adequate concentrations it has bactericidal activity.

A review of the antimicrobial action of vancomycin. Vancomycin is a glycopeptide antibiotic; its primary action is the inhibition of cell wall synthesis of susceptible organisms but in a different manner from penicillins and cephalosporins. It prevents the synthesis of peptidoglycan by binding tightly to peptides containing D-alanyl-D-alanine at the free carboxyl end. Vancomycin has also been demonstrated to alter the permeability of the cell membrane and may selectively inhibit ribonucleic acid synthesis.

Organisms are considered to be susceptible to vancomycin if the MIC is 5 µg or less per mL. Vancomycin is active against almost all species of Gram-positive cocci and Gram-positive bacilli. With the exception of a few resistant strains tested in the 1950s, all *Staphylococcus aureus* strains tested since the 1960s had been susceptible to vancomycin. Methicillin-resistant strains, apart from a few in one study, have also been susceptible. Vancomycin is active against the majority of strains of *Staph. epidermidis, Staph. saprophyticus, Staph. haemolyticus, Staph. hominis, Staph. warneri*, and unspeciated coagulase-negative staphylococci. All strains of *Streptococcus pneumoniae* tested, including multi-resistant strains, have been susceptible to vancomycin; so also have all *Str. pyogenes* (group A), group C, and group G streptococci tested. Although vancomycin is active against the vast majority of *Str. agalactiae, Str. bovis*, enterococcal species, *Str. mutans*, and viridans streptococci, resistant strains have been detected. Other Gram-positive bacteria susceptible to vancomycin include all diphtheroids and *Listeria monocytogenes* tested, the majority of strains of *Clostridium difficile, Cl. perfringens, Cl. ramosum, Cl. botulinum, Cl. septicum*, and unspeciated clostridia, and some *Actinomyces* and *Lactobacillus* spp. Although vancomycin has been used to treat meningitis caused by *Flavobacterium meningosepticum*, a Gram-negative bacillus, all strains of *Flavobacterium* spp. tested have been resistant to vancomycin.— C. Watanakunakorn, *J. antimicrob. Chemother.*, 1984, *14*, *Suppl.* D, 7.

For reference to studies comparing the antimicrobial activity of vancomycin and teicoplanin, see Teicoplanin, p.311.

ACTIVITY AGAINST CORYNEBACTERIUM. Vancomycin and norfloxacin were the most active of a range of antimicrobial agents tested against 30 clinical strains of *Corynebacterium* group D2. The MIC of vancomycin ranged from less than 0.25 to 0.5 µg per mL at pH 7.4 and from 1 to 8 µg per mL at pH 8.5.— M. Santamaria *et al.*, *Antimicrob. Ag. Chemother.*, 1985, *28*, 845. See also R. Fernández-Roblas *et al.*, *ibid.*, 1987, *31*, 821.

ACTIVITY AGAINST LEUCONOSTOC. A report of 3 patients with infections due to *Leuconostoc* spp. which were initially identified as vancomycin-resistant *Streptococcus* spp. All 3 *Leuconostoc* strains were highly resistant to vancomycin.— H. W. Horowitz *et al.* (letter), *Lancet*, 1987, *2*, 1329. See also A. Buu-Hoï *et al.*, *Antimicrob. Ag. Chemother.*, 1985, *28*, 458.

ACTIVITY AGAINST STAPHYLOCOCCI. Exposure to vancomycin 100 µg per mL for one hour killed 90% of 48 clinical isolates of coagulase-negative staphylococci. Such bactericidal concentration may be useful for short-term topical prophylaxis in neurosurgical procedures.— P. R. Fischer *et al.*, *Antimicrob. Ag. Chemother.*, 1984, *25*, 502.

A study *in vitro* of antibiotic sensitivity in 43 strains of coagulase-negative staphylococci, isolated from patients with peritonitis complicating continuous ambulatory peritoneal dialysis (CAPD). Vancomycin appeared to have the most consistent activity of all the antibiotics tested; rifampicin, netilmicin, and cephamandole were also active against most of the strains.— L. D. Gruer *et al.*, *J. antimicrob. Chemother.*, 1984, *13*, 577. All of 23 strains of coagulase-negative staphylococci isolated from patients with CAPD-associated peritonitis were sensitive to vancomycin at concentrations between 2 and 8 µg per mL. Despite its relatively slow bactericidal activity, vancomycin achieved complete killing of all strains after 24 hours in broth and dialysate. Rifampicin had the lowest MIC values of the eight antistaphylococcal agents tested but its rate of bactericidal activity was variable. Both gentamicin and fusidic acid showed bimodal MIC distributions with approximately 40% of strains being resistant. Gentamicin was the most rapidly bactericidal agent; fusidic acid failed to achieve total killing of 4 strains in broth and dialysate. These *in-vitro* results suggested that fusidic acid would be unsuitable as the sole agent for the treatment of peritonitis caused by *Staphylococcus epidermidis*.— M. H. Wilcox *et al.*, *ibid.*, 1985, *15*, 297. Over a period of 6 years from October 1979 to June 1985, 64 episodes of bacterial peritonitis occurred in 26 children on continuous ambulatory peritoneal dialysis. Of the 74 bacterial isolates 59 were Gram-positive organisms including 27 *Staphylococcus epidermidis* and 24 *Staph. aureus*. Both species showed 100% sensitivity to vancomycin, rifampicin, or netilmicin, whereas only 52% of *Staph. epidermidis* and 96% of *Staph. aureus* were sensitive to cephamandole or methicillin.— T. A. McAllister *et al.*, *ibid.*, 1987, *19*, 95.

Although all of 90 isolates of coagulase-negative staphylococci were susceptible to vancomycin, the MBC was commonly 4 to 8 times greater than the MIC, and occasional tolerance was observed.— K. V. I. Rolston *et al.*, *J. antimicrob. Chemother.*, 1985, *16*, 659.

ACTIVITY AGAINST STREPTOCOCCI. Of 61 clinical isolates of group C and group G streptococci, tolerance to vancomycin, as defined by an MIC/MBC ratio of 32 or greater, was observed in one group G isolate.— K. V. I. Rolston *et al.*, *J. antimicrob. Chemother.*, 1984, *13*, 389. See also J. T. Noble *et al.* (letter), *Lancet*, 1980, *2*, 982.

ACTIVITY WITH OTHER AGENTS. *Aminoglycosides.* Vancomycin has been reported to be synergistic with streptomycin or gentamicin against enterococci (C. Watanakunakorn and C. Bakie, *Antimicrob. Ag. Chemother.*, 1973, *4*, 120), with gentamicin or tobramycin against the majority of tested isolates of methicillin-susceptible and -resistant *Staphylococcus aureus* (C. Watanakunakorn and J.C. Tisone, *ibid.*, 1982, *22*, 903), and with gentamicin against a large proportion of group G streptococci (K. Lam and A.S. Bayer, *ibid.*, 1984, *26*, 260).

Antineoplastics. Antagonism occurred against some strains of *Staphylococcus aureus* when the activity of vancomycin was tested *in vitro* with daunorubicin or doxorubicin.— J. Y. Jacobs *et al.*, *Antimicrob. Ag. Chemother.*, 1979, *15*, 580.

Cephalosporins. Enhanced activity against methicillin-resistant *Staphylococcus epidermidis* was demonstrated *in vitro* with vancomycin in association with cephamandole, cephalothin, or rifampicin.— M. E. Ein *et al.*, *Antimicrob. Ag. Chemother.*, 1979, *16*, 655. Although vancomycin decreased the activity of cephalothin against methicillin-resistant *Staph. epidermidis* in *animals*, this effect could not be demonstrated *in vitro*.— F. D. Lowy *et al.*, *ibid.*, 314.

Rifampicin. There have been conflicting studies on the antimicrobial interaction between vancomycin and rifampicin *in vitro*. Watanakunakorn and Tisone (*Antimicrob. Ag. Chemother.*, 1982, *22*, 915) observed antagonism in a few strains of enterococci but no synergy. For methicillin-susceptible and -resistant *Staphylococcus aureus*, Watanakunakorn and Guerriero (*ibid.*, 1981, *19*, 1089) reported mainly antagonism, Foldes *et al.* (*J. antimicrob. Chemother.*, 1983, *11*, 21) neither synergy nor antagonism, and Bayer and Morrison (*Antimicrob. Ag. Chemother.*, 1984, *26*, 220) either indifference, synergy, or antagonism depending on whether a checkerboard or timed-kill method was used. In *Staph. epidermidis.*, Yu *et al.* (*J. antimicrob. Chemother.*, 1984, *14*, 359) demonstrated no synergy between vancomycin and rifampicin, and some antagonism, although synergy occurred in most strains when gentamicin was added to the combination. Vancomycin does not appear to consistently prevent the development of rifampicin resistance in staphylococci (F.D. Lowy *et al.*, *Antimicrob. Ag. Chemother.*, 1983, *23*, 932; R.H.K Eng *et al.*, *J. antimicrob. Chemother.*, 1985, *15*, 201). The clinical significance of these results is, however, unclear. Although Morris and Tenney (*Ann. intern. Med.*, 1983, *99*, 283) demonstrated antagonism between vancomycin and rifampicin *in vitro*, the combination was clinically effective in a patient with an infection caused by a methicillin-resistant strain of *Staph. aureus* where vancomycin therapy had failed.

Resistance

Sensitive bacteria do not readily acquire resistance to vancomycin.

The MIC of vancomycin against *Staphylococcus haemolyticus*, a coagulase-negative staphylococcus, isolated from a patient with CAPD-related peritonitis increased from 2 to 8 µg per mL over a period of 88 days of vancomycin therapy. An isolate with such an MIC is usually considered to have intermediate sensitivity to vancomycin. However, vancomycin was ineffective in clearing the organism from the patient, and all peritoneal-fluid isolates contained stable subpopulations capable of growth *in vitro* at a vancomycin concentration of 8 μg per mL. Stepwise resistance was also documented *in vitro*. Thus, these studies suggest that coagulase-negative staphylococci have the ability to acquire resistance to vancomycin. Teicoplanin was ineffective against both the clinical isolates and the laboratory-selected resistant clones. Daptomycin (LY-146032), an investigational lipopeptide, was effective against all the organisms tested.— R. S. Schwalbe *et al.*, *New Engl. J. Med.*, 1987, *316*, 927.

Since November 1986, 55 strains of vancomycin-resistant enterococci derived from 22 patients with end-stage renal failure or multiple organ failure had been isolated. Faecal carriage of resistant organisms was present in some infected patients. All the strains were resistant to concentrations of vancomycin above 64 μg per mL, and 7 strains had MICs greater than 2000 μg per mL. Vancomycin resistance was associated with high level aminoglycoside resistance in 5 strains; most strains tested were also resistant to teicoplanin, penicillin, ampicillin, piperacillin, clindamycin, erythromycin, tetracycline, chloramphenicol, fusidic acid, rifampicin, sulphamethoxazole, and trimethoprim. Most were moderately susceptible to ciprofloxacin and all were very sensitive to daptomycin (LY-146032). Three months before the isolation of these resistant strains, vancomycin and ceftazidime were adopted for the management of acute sepsis. The use of vancomycin in this group of patients has been drastically reduced and the frequency of isolation of resistant strains has fallen.— A. H. C. Uttley *et al.* (letter), *Lancet*, 1988, *1*, 57.

For reference to reports of tolerance to vancomycin in staphylococci and streptococci, see under Antimicrobial Action, above.

Absorption and Fate

Vancomycin is only poorly absorbed from the gastro-intestinal tract. There is marked inter-individual variation in the pharmacokinetics of vancomycin after intravenous administration. Half-lives of between 3 and 13 hours have been reported, and are prolonged in patients with renal impairment.

The antibiotic diffuses into pleural, pericardial, ascitic, and synovial fluids, but does not readily penetrate the cerebrospinal fluid unless the meninges are inflamed. It has been reported to diffuse across the placenta and into breast milk in *animals*. Vancomycin is excreted by the kidneys, primarily by glomerular filtration; about 90% of the dose is excreted in urine within 24 hours.

A review of the pharmacokinetics of vancomycin. Values for the protein binding of vancomycin have varied between 10 and 82%, apparently due to methodological differences. Therapeutic concentrations of vancomycin (greater than 2.5 μg per mL) have been reported in ascitic, pericardial, pleural, and synovial fluids in patients with normal renal function after administration of single or multiple intravenous doses; only low concentrations are noted in aqueous humour and in bile. Therapeutic faecal concentrations have been detected after both oral and intravenous administration. Penetration of vancomycin, given intravenously, into the CSF in patients with and without meningitis has been quite variable; adequate concentrations may be obtained in some patients with inflamed meninges, although some authors have suggested intrathecal or intraventricular administration. Vancomycin is excreted mainly in the urine by glomerular filtration; there is no direct evidence of renal tubular secretion or reabsorption in humans. Some studies have suggested that a small proportion of non-renal clearance, possibly in the liver, may occur. Studies of the pharmacokinetics of vancomycin in neonates have been contradictory. The clearance of vancomycin in paediatric patients generally appears to be related primarily to the degree of renal function. However, since significant interpatient variability has been observed in the small numbers of premature infants studied, doses should be calculated for these patients with caution.— G. R. Matzke *et al.*, *Clin. Pharmacokinet.*, 1986, *11*, 257. See also R. C. Moellering, *J. antimicrob. Chemother.*, 1984, *14*, *Suppl.* D, 43.

Further studies of the pharmacokinetics of vancomycin: R. A. Blouin *et al.*, *Antimicrob. Ag. Chemother.*, 1982, *21*, 575 (morbidly obese subjects); J. -J. Garaud *et al.*, *J. antimicrob. Chemother.*, 1984, *14*, *Suppl.* D, 53 (critically ill patients); D. C. Brater *et al.*, *Clin. Pharmac. Ther.*, 1986, *39*, 631 (patients with burn injuries).

For reference to a comparative study of the pharmacokinetics and bactericidal activity of vancomycin and teicoplanin, see Teicoplanin, p.311.

ADMINISTRATION. For reference to the pharmacokinetics of vancomycin after various dosage regimens, and to the monitoring of serum-vancomycin concentrations, see under Administration and Administration in Renal Failure under Uses, below.

ADMINISTRATION IN THE ELDERLY. The mean half-lives of vancomycin in 2 groups each of 6 healthy subjects of average age 23 and 68 years were 7.2 and 12.1 hours respectively. The increased half-life in elderly subjects was related to an increase in the volume of distribution, attributed to enhanced tissue binding, and to a decrease in renal clearance.— N. R. Cutler *et al.*, *Clin. Pharmac. Ther.*, 1984, *36*, 803.

ADMINISTRATION IN LIVER DISORDERS AND IN RENAL FAILURE. For reference to the pharmacokinetics of vancomycin in liver disorders and in renal failure, see under Uses, below.

DIFFUSION INTO BODY TISSUES AND FLUIDS. A study of the penetration of vancomycin into heart tissues in patients undergoing open-heart surgery.— F. D. Daschner *et al.*, *J. antimicrob. Chemother.*, 1987, *19*, 359.

DRUG ABSORPTION. Although in general very little vancomycin is absorbed from the gastro-intestinal tract in healthy subjects following oral administration, absorption may be enhanced in patients with pseudomembranous colitis and renal impairment. References: C. S. Bryan and W. L. White, *Antimicrob. Ag. Chemother.*, 1978, *14*, 634 (low serum concentrations in 2 of 5 anephric subjects); C. M. Thompson *et al.*, *Int. J. pediatr. Nephrol.*, 1983, *4*, 1 (toxicity associated with high serum and CSF concentrations in an anephric patient with pseudomembranous colitis); P. G. Spitzer and G. M. Eliopoulos, *Ann. intern. Med.*, 1984, *100*, 533 (significant serum concentrations in a patient with pseudomembranous colitis and severe renal failure); M. N. Dudley *et al.* (letter), *ibid.*, *101*, 144 (detectable serum concentrations in 4 patients with pseudomembranous colitis and varying renal function); R. A. Lucas *et al.*, *J. clin. Pharm. Ther.*, 1987, *12*, 27 (none detected in the plasma of healthy subjects following oral administration in semi-solid matrix capsules or solution).

PREGNANCY AND THE NEONATE. For reference to the pharmacokinetics of vancomycin in neonates, see above.

Uses and Administration

Parenteral vancomycin hydrochloride is used in patients critically ill with infections caused by Gram-positive bacteria which are resistant to the commonly used antibiotics and for patients who are allergic to penicillin. It is particularly recommended for the treatment of infections caused by methicillin-resistant staphylococci; if a response is not obtained with vancomycin another agent may also be given. Vancomycin is recommended alone, or in association with gentamicin, as an alternative to penicillin in the treatment or prophylaxis of endocarditis; in association with an aminoglycoside for the treatment of peritonitis in patients on CAPD; or it may be added to regimens for the treatment of febrile episodes in neutropenic patients. It may also be used for the prophylaxis of infection in surgical procedures.

Vancomycin hydrochloride is administered intravenously, preferably by intermittent infusion, although continuous infusion has been used. For intermittent infusion, a concentrated solution containing the equivalent of 500 mg of vancomycin in 10 mL of Water for Injections is added to 100 to 200 mL of glucose 5% injection or of sodium chloride 0.9% injection and the diluted solution infused over at least 60 minutes. This method of administration should diminish the risk of both local reactions and of the 'red man' syndrome occurring (see Adverse Effects, above). For continuous intravenous infusion, the equivalent of 1 to 2 g is added to a sufficiently large volume of glucose or sodium chloride solution to permit the daily dose to be given over a period of 24 hours. The usual adult dose is the equivalent of 500 mg of vancomycin every 6 hours or 1 g every 12 hours. Children may be given 44 mg per kg body-weight daily in divided doses. Neonates may be given an initial dose of 15 mg per kg followed by 10 mg per kg every 12 hours in the first week of life, and every 8 hours up to the age of one month.

Since there is marked inter-individual variation in the pharmacokinetics of vancomycin it has been recommended that the dose be adjusted according to measurements of serum-vancomycin concentrations particularly in patients with renal impairment or in premature infants. Various recommendations have been made for peak and trough, or mean steady-state concentrations which are effective but not toxic (see under Administration and Administration in Renal Failure, below).

Vancomycin hydrochloride is administered by mouth in the treatment of staphylococcal enterocolitis and antibiotic-associated colitis including pseudomembranous colitis. It has also been investigated for the treatment of other syndromes of diarrhoea or colitis which may be associated with the overgrowth of *Clostridium difficile*. It is given in a dose of 125 to 500 mg four times daily; the 125-mg dose is often considered adequate. The dose for children should be adjusted according to their body-weight.

Reviews of the actions and uses of vancomycin: R. Brown and R. Wise, *Br. med. J.*, 1982, *284*, 1508; S. W. B. Newsom, *J. antimicrob. Chemother.*, 1982, *10*, 257; J. E. Geraci and P. E. Hermans, *Mayo Clin. Proc.*, 1983, *58*, 88; A. Kucers, *J. antimicrob. Chemother.*, 1984, *14*, 564; Lancet, 1985, *1*, 677; *Med. Lett.*, 1986, *28*, 121; P. E. Hermans and M. P. Wilhelm, *Mayo Clin. Proc.*, 1987, *62*, 901.

For proceedings of a symposium on vancomycin, see *J. antimicrob. Chemother.*, 1984, *14*, *Suppl.* D, 1–109.

Vancomycin is considered the mainstay for treatment of serious infections due to methicillin-resistant staphylococci (W.M.M. Kirby, *J. antimicrob. Chemother.*, 1984, *14*, *Suppl.* D, 73; D. Andrews, *Can. J. hosp. Pharm.*, 1986, *39*, 135; *J. hosp. Infect.*, 1986, *7*, 193; J. Klastersky and P. Van der Auwera, *J. antimicrob. Chemother.*, 1986, *17*, *Suppl.* A, 19). There is disagreement as to the value of adding rifampicin to treatment with vancomycin, due in part to conflicting *in vitro* data on the efficacy of such a combination and uncertainty as to the clinical significance of these findings (see Activity with other Agents under Antimicrobial Action, above). Vancomycin may also be used in association with an aminoglycoside since *in-vitro* and *animal* studies have indicated that aminoglycosides may increase the bactericidal effect of vancomycin. Most methicillin-resistant staphylococcal infections are treated initially with vancomycin alone, and a second agent, such as an aminoglycoside, rifampicin, or fusidic acid, added if the patient fails to respond. For reference to methicillin resistance in staphylococci and for guidelines on the control of epidemics caused by these organisms, see under Resistance in Methicillin Sodium, p.259. For further reference to the use of vancomycin in such infections see under individual headings, below.

Intravenous vancomycin was not effective in eradicating nasal carriage of *Staphylococcus aureus* in a haemodialysis unit.— V. L. Yu *et al.*, *New Engl. J. Med.*, 1986, *315*, 91.

ADMINISTRATION. A study in 11 healthy subjects of the pharmacokinetics of vancomycin after intravenous administration in 2 dosage regimens. After administration of 500 mg every 6 hours, the mean steady-state serum concentrations were 40.3, 27.4, and 22.6 μg per mL immediately after completion of the infusion, and 15 minutes and 1 hour later respectively. The corresponding concentrations for a dose of 1 g every 12 hours were 65.7, 41.0, and 33.7 μg per mL. Due to the long half-life of vancomycin, accumulation was significant for both regimens.

On reviewing the monitoring of serum-vancomycin concentrations, the authors noted disagreement on when blood samples should be obtained and the desired therapeutic concentrations; such disagreement may reflect, in part, the lack of reliable data which relate serum concentrations to either efficacy or toxicity. Times of 15 minutes, 1 hour, and 3 or more hours after completion of a one-hour infusion have been recommended for obtaining peak concentrations. Therapeutic peak serum concentrations of less than 80, less than 50 to 80, 30 to 40, 15 to 50, and 20 to 40 μg per mL have been proposed, but these recommendations have been made without regard to the dosage regimen. On the basis of their pharmacokinetic study, these authors recommend that peak serum-vancomycin concentrations be measured 1 hour after completion of the infusion. For a dosage regimen of 500 mg every 6 hours the peak concentration should be 15 to 30 μg per mL, and for 1 g every 12 hours it should be 25 to 40 μg per mL. Trough serum-vancomycin concentrations of 5 to 10 μg per mL have been recommended, but this study suggests that this requirement may be too restrictive.— D. P. Healy *et al.*, *Antimicrob. Ag. Chemother.*, 1987, *31*, 393. See also M. J. Rybak and S. C. Boike, *Drug Intell. & clin. Pharm.*, 1986, *20*, 757. For further reference to nomograms and guidelines for the calculation of vancomycin doses and their relation to serum-vancomycin concentrations, see under Administration in Renal Failure, below.

Discussion on the possible use of vancomycin in bone cement.— T. McGuire, *Aust. J. Hosp. Pharm.*, 1987, *17*, 151.

ADMINISTRATION IN INFANTS AND CHILDREN. Intravenous vancomycin could be administered to neonates for the treatment of severe infections in the following daily doses: up to one week of age, 30 mg per kg body-weight in 2 divided doses; one to 4 weeks, 40 mg per kg in 3 divided doses; over 4 weeks, 40 mg per kg in 3 to 4 divided doses.— K. H. Rhodes and C. M. Johnson, *Mayo Clin. Proc.*, 1983, *58*, 158.

See also under Absorption and Fate, above.

ADMINISTRATION, INTRATHECAL. For reference to local administration of vancomycin into the CNS, see Central Nervous System Infections, and Neurosurgery under Surgical Infection Prophylaxis, below.

ADMINISTRATION IN LIVER DISORDERS. The pharmacokinetics of vancomycin were altered in cancer patients with abnormal hepatic function. Liver function should be carefully monitored in such patients receiving vancomycin, and the dosage regimen adjusted accordingly.— N. Brown *et al.*, *Antimicrob. Ag. Chemother.*, 1983, *23*, 603.

ADMINISTRATION, OCULAR. Vancomycin has been administered into the eye, topically or by subconjunctival or intravitreal injection.— T. S. Lesar and R. G. Fiscella, *Drug Intell. & clin. Pharm.*, 1985, *19*, 642.

ADMINISTRATION IN RENAL FAILURE. The normal half-life for vancomycin of 6 to 8 hours was increased to 200 to 250 hours in end-stage renal failure. The interval between doses should be extended to 24 to 72 hours in patients with a glomerular filtration-rate (GFR) above 50 mL per minute (mild renal failure), to 72 to 240 hours in those with a GFR of 10 to 50 mL per minute, and to 240 hours in those with a GFR of less than 10 mL per minute. However, since elimination of vancomycin is variable in renal failure, serum concentrations are the best guide to therapy. A dosage supplement is not required for patients on haemodialysis or peritoneal dialysis.— W. M. Bennett *et al.*, *Am. J. Kidney Dis.*, 1983, *3*, 155.

Various methods have been proposed to ascertain the optimum dose of vancomycin according to renal function and serum concentrations.

A formula for calculating the maintenance dose of vancomycin based on the correlation observed between vancomycin clearance and glomerular filtration-rate.— H. E. Nielsen *et al.*, *Acta med. scand.*, 1975, *197*, 261. A nomogram for adjusting the dose of vancomycin according to the creatinine clearance of the patient, so as to produce a steady-state serum-vancomycin concentration of approximately 15 μg per mL. The nomogram gives the dose in mg per kg per 24 hours, however, since doses of 250 to 500 mg and not exceeding 1 g are optimal, patients with severe renal impairment may be given doses every several days. Such patients also require a loading dose of 15 mg per kg body-weight. The nomogram is not valid for functionally anephric patients on haemodialysis or peritoneal dialysis; these patients should be given vancomycin in a dose of 1.9 mg per kg every 24 hours.— R. C. Moellering *et al.*, *Ann. intern. Med.*, 1981, *94*, 343. Patients with normal renal function should be given initial intravenous doses of vancomycin 6.5 to 8 mg per kg body-weight every 6 to 12 hours. Subsequent doses should be modified to produce a peak serum concentration of 30 to 40 μg per mL and a trough concentration of 5 to 10 μg per mL. Longer dosage intervals may be required in older patients or in those with compromised renal function.— J. C. Rotschafer *et al.*, *Antimicrob. Ag. Chemother.*, 1982, *22*, 391. A further nomogram to adjust the dose of vancomycin according to creatinine clearance. A loading dose of 25 mg per kg body-weight is followed by a maintenance dose of 19 mg per kg given at a dosage interval estimated from the nomogram. This dosage regimen should maintain peak serum concentrations of 30 μg per mL and trough concentrations of 7.5 μg per mL. The nomogram is not valid for patients on peritoneal dialysis.— G. R. Matzke *et al.*, *ibid.*, 1984, *25*, 433. A comparison of the above 4 dosing methods for vancomycin. The method proposed by Matzke *et al.* was the most precise and showed the least bias, although that proposed by Moellering *et al.* would probably yield a clinically similar degree of accuracy. The method proposed by Nielsen *et al.* underpredicted and that proposed by Rotschafer *et al.* overpredicted the required maintenance dose.— G. R. Matzke *et al.*, *Clin. Pharm.*, 1985, *4*, 311. A method for calculating vancomycin dosage was proposed which uses measured serum-vancomycin concentrations to derive patient-specific pharmacokinetic data. This individualised method was compared with the above nomograms proposed by Moellering *et al.* and Matzke *et al.* Although all 3 methods tended to underpredict serum-vancomycin concentrations, the individualised method was more accurate in predicting steady-state serum concentrations. This may be because, unlike the nomograms, it does not assume a constant volume of distribution.— M. J. Rybak and S. C. Boike, *Drug Intell. & clin. Pharm.*, 1986, *20*, 64.

For further reference to the monitoring of serum-vancomycin concentrations, see under Administration, above.

Dialysis. A study in patients undergoing continuous ambulatory peritoneal dialysis (CAPD), indicating that vancomycin passes easily from the peritoneal fluid to the blood, but not in the reverse direction.— C. M. Bunke *et al.*, *Clin. Pharmac. Ther.*, 1983, *34*, 631. Similar results.— R. D. Blevins *et al.*, *Antimicrob. Ag. Chemother.*, 1984, *25*, 603. Vancomycin is efficiently and rapidly absorbed into the general circulation after intraperitoneal administration, however a loading dose is required to achieve rapid equilibriation of plasma and dialysate concentrations. An ideal loading dose would be approximately 38-times the maintenance dose. The intrinsic peritoneal clearance of vancomycin was considered to be much greater than previously reported values for apparent peritoneal clearance.— M. C. Rogge *et al.*, *ibid.*, 1985, *27*, 578. A pharmacokinetic study in patients with CAPD-associated peritonitis suggesting that a single intravenous dose of vancomycin 25 mg per kg body-weight may produce dialysate concentrations sufficient to inhibit the majority of *Staphylococcus epidermidis* strains for at least 4 days.— M. Whitby *et al.*, *J. antimicrob. Chemother.*, 1987, *19*, 351.

See also recommendations for dosage adjustment in renal impairment, above.

Haemofiltration. The effect of haemofiltration on the disposition of vancomycin. In 5 anuric patients given an intravenous infusion of vancomycin 18 mg per kg body-weight immediately after haemofiltration, the mean half-lives between and during haemofiltration procedures were 136 and 4.1 hours respectively, although there was large interpatient variability. Approximately 32% of a dose of vancomycin was removed by haemofiltration; thus doses may need to be increased to maintain therapeutic concentrations.— G. R. Matzke *et al.*, *Clin. Pharmac. Ther.*, 1986, *40*, 425. Comments on the disposition of drugs, including vancomycin, during continuous arteriovenous haemofiltration.— N. Barber *et al.* (letter), *Pharm. J.*, 1987, *2*, 114; C. J. Cairns (letter), *ibid.*, 222.

CENTRAL NERVOUS SYSTEM INFECTION. Vancomycin was administered locally, either directly into the shunt, intraventricularly, or by the lumbar intrathecal route, for the treatment of hydrocephalus shunt infections in 6 patients. All patients also received intravenous vancomycin or other antibiotics. Four patients responded well to therapy with eradication of staphylococcal meningitis, and 2 patients with malfunctioning shunts failed to respond. Apart from a suggestion of arachnoiditis in one patient no toxicity was observed.— J. H. Andrew and M. J. Waters (letter), *J. antimicrob. Chemother.*, 1986, *18*, 145.

A study of the use of intraventricular vancomycin for the treatment of 20 episodes of shunt-associated ventriculitis caused by staphylococci or streptococci in 15 patients. Intraventricular vancomycin was used alone in 4 episodes, together with intravenous vancomycin in 5 episodes, and in combination with other drugs in 11 episodes. It was administered in a daily intraventricular dose of 20 mg for adults and 10 mg for children, diluted to 2.5 mg per mL in distilled water, for 4 to 19 days. The infected shunts or drains were removed and replaced with an external drain. All patients responded to therapy and their CSF became sterile and free from pus; 8 patients have remained well for 5 months or more. It was considered that therapy with intraventricular vancomycin alone is probably sufficient unless the infection is complicated by cellulitis or wound infection requiring systemic therapy, or when vancomycin-tolerant strains are involved. In this latter case the addition of rifampicin may be useful.— R. Swayne *et al.*, *J. antimicrob. Chemother.*, 1987, *19*, 249.

ENDOCARDITIS. The British Society for Antimicrobial Chemotherapy (BSAC) have recommended that intravenous vancomycin be used in association with gentamicin for the treatment of streptococcal endocarditis in patients allergic to penicillins (*Lancet*, 1985, *2*, 815). The dose of vancomycin should initially be 1 g once or twice daily, and then adjusted according to daily blood concentrations to achieve a peak concentration of 30 μg per mL and a trough concentration of 5 to 10 μg per mL. The minimum inhibitory and bactericidal concentrations of vancomycin and other antibiotics should be determined and the patient's condition assessed each day. Depending on these investigations, consideration may be given to using vancomycin alone, substituting erythromycin for vancomycin and gentamicin, or stopping treatment after only 2 weeks.

They recommend vancomycin alone, in the same doses as for streptococcal endocarditis, for the treatment of endocarditis caused by *Staphylococcus aureus* in patients allergic to penicillins or when the organism is resistant to methicillin or flucloxacillin. Treatment should normally be continued for at least 4 weeks. *Staph. epidermidis* tends to infect prosthetic rather than natural valves and its sensitivity to antibiotics is much less predictable. When the organism is shown to be sensitive to the antibiotics recommended for the treatment of *Staph. aureus* endocarditis the same regimens can be used. However, eradication of this organism is frequently impossible and valve replacement is required.

One or two agents from rifampicin, erythromycin, or gentamicin have been added to therapy with vancomycin for the treatment of staphylococcal endocarditis, particularly infections of prosthetic valves with methicillin-resistant organisms (S.W.B. Newsom, *J. antimicrob. Chemother.*, 1984, *14*, *Suppl.* D, 79; S.J. Eykyn, *ibid.*, 1987, *20*, *Suppl.* A, 161; C.M. Oakley, *ibid.*, 181).

Prophylaxis. Vancomycin, alone or in combination with gentamicin, is used for the prophylaxis of endocarditis during dental or surgical procedures in patients at risk who are allergic to penicillins and cannot be given other antibiotics by mouth since they are undergoing general anaesthesia. The British Society for Antimicrobial Chemotherapy (BSAC) has recommended a dosage regimen of vancomycin 1 g by intravenous infusion over 60 minutes followed by gentamicin 120 mg intravenously before induction of anaesthesia for all procedures for which prophylaxis is indicated. Children under 10 years of age should be given vancomycin 20 mg per kg body-weight and gentamicin 2 mg per kg (*Lancet*, 1982, *2*, 1323; *ibid.*, 1986, *1*, 1267). The Council on Cardiovascular Disease in the Young (CCD) in the *USA*, however, have recommended the use of vancomycin 1 g alone, 1 hour prior to dental procedures or surgery of the upper respiratory tract; gentamicin 1.5 mg per kg by intramuscular or intravenous administration should be added during gastro-intestinal or genito-urinary procedures, and the administration of both drugs repeated once 8 to 12 hours later if required. (The BSAC considered that although vancomycin had been successful in the treatment of streptococcal, including enterococcal, endocarditis the combination of vancomycin and gentamicin was more reliably bactericidal.) During cardiac surgery, the use of vancomycin may be considered if there is a high prevalence of methicillin-resistant staphylococci (S.T. Shulman *et al.*, *Circulation*, 1984, *70*, 1123A). Similarly to the CCD, the European Society of Cardiology has recommended the use of vancomycin alone for prophylaxis of endocarditis during most procedures; gentamicin may be added and treatment continued for 72 hours in patients at high risk (J. Delaye *et al.*, *Eur. Heart J.*, 1985, *6*, 826).

See also under Prophylactic Use of Antibiotics, p.102.

GASTRO-INTESTINAL DISORDERS. Beneficial effect of oral vancomycin in 2 patients with metabolic acidosis associated with elevated plasma concentrations of D-lactic acid, presumed to be of intestinal origin.— L. Stolberg *et al.*, *New Engl. J. Med.*, 1982, *306*, 1344.

Successful use of oral vancomycin in the treatment of *Clostridium difficile*-related diarrhoea and colitis caused by the administration of antineoplastic drugs including methotrexate.— S. D. Miller and H. J. Koornhof, *Eur. J. clin. Microbiol.*, 1984, *3*, 10.

After a policy was introduced of treating all patients in a leukaemia unit carrying *Clostridium difficile* in their stools with vancomycin, the number of patients with stools positive for the organism and its cytotoxin decreased.— M. Delmee and J. -L. Michaux (letter), *Lancet*, 1986, *2*, 350. In a discussion of *Clostridium difficile* infections, it was recommended that hospital inpatients with diarrhoea whose stools are positive for the organism should be nursed in isolation and treated with metronidazole or oral vancomycin.— *ibid.*, 790.

Antibiotic-associated colitis. The oral administration of vancomycin is considered to be the treatment of choice for colitis associated with the administration of antibiotics (R. Fekety *et al., J. antimicrob. Chemother.*, 1984, *14, Suppl.* D, 97; D.W. Burdon, *ibid.*, 103). Antibiotic-associated colitis may present as pseudomembranous colitis or as a non-specific colitis without pseudomembranes, and may occur as late as 6 weeks after antibiotic therapy has been discontinued. The most important cause is an alteration of bowel flora and overgrowth of toxigenic *Clostridium difficile*. When antibiotics are discontinued and fluid and electrolyte losses replaced, diarrhoea usually resolves within 7 to 10 days. The use of diphenoxylate with atropine (Lomotil) or codeine to treat the diarrhoea is not usually advised (E. Novak *et al., J. Am. med. Ass.*, 1976, *235*, 1451). Early specific antibiotic therapy should be given to patients with severe illness characterised by high fever, marked abdominal pain, and marked leucocytosis and to elderly, toxic, or debilitated patients, or those unresponsive to supportive therapy.

The efficacy of oral vancomycin in the treatment of antibiotic-associated colitis is well documented; intravenous treatment is unreliable and should not be used. Absorption of vancomycin after administration by mouth is usually minimal, although significant serum concentrations have been detected in a few patients (see Drug Absorption in Absorption and Fate, above) and there has been a report of a possible toxic reaction after oral administration (C.M. Thompson *et al., Int. J. pediatr. Nephrol.*, 1983, *4*, 1). Thus concentrations of vancomycin are easily achieved in the colonic lumen to inhibit *Cl. difficile* and the production of its toxins. *Cl. difficile*, including organisms isolated from patients who have had recurrences of colitis after treatment with vancomycin, are generally highly susceptible to vancomycin. Vancomycin is administered by mouth in a dose of 125 to 500 mg four times daily; there does not appear to be a notable difference between these doses and the lower dose of 125 mg is being increasingly adopted. Response to vancomycin is usually good unless treatment has been delayed until the patient is moribund, or has ileus, toxic megacolon, or a colonic perforation. The severity of the diarrhoea often decreases within 48 to 72 hours, but cessation may take a week or more. Treatment should be continued for no more than 5 to 7 days if the response is prompt, but some patients require treatment for 14 to 21 days. Relapses have occurred after discontinuation of vancomycin and may be due to failure to eradicate *Cl. difficile* from the stools (B.A.J. Walters *et al., Gut*, 1983, *24*, 206). They usually respond to retreatment with vancomycin, or after administration of an alternative antibiotic.

Metronidazole by mouth has been used as an alternative to vancomycin in the treatment of antibiotic-associated colitis (see p.672). Some workers have considered it to be as effective as vancomycin (D.G. Teasley *et al., Lancet*, 1983, *2*, 1043), however, because of treatment failures in seriously ill patients, Fekety *et al.* have reserved it for use in mild cases. Burdon has also used metronidazole when the indications for therapy of colitis are less clear cut, and when long courses of therapy are given to patients who have relapsed.

Other antibiotics that appear to be effective in the treatment of antibiotic-associated colitis include fusidic acid (S. Cronberg *et al., Infection*, 1984, *12*, 276) and bacitracin (M.N. Dudley *et al., Archs intern. Med.*, 1986, *146*, 1101). Bacitracin 25 000 units or vancomycin hydrochloride, both given four times daily by mouth for 10 days, were equally effective in controlling diarrhoea in a study of 30 evaluable patients; bacitracin was not, however, as effective in eradicating *Cl. difficile* and its toxin from the faeces.

Rectal infusion of faeces successfully normalised bowel flora and function in a woman with recurrent *Cl. difficile*-associated colitis despite several courses of vancomycin therapy (A. Schwan *et al., Lancet*, 1983, *2*, 845). Oral administration of *Lactobacillus* GG has also been used with some success to terminate relapsing colitis due to *Cl. difficile* (S.L. Gorbach *et al., Lancet*, 1987, *2*, 1519).

The anion-exchange resins cholestyramine and colestipol hydrochloride have been shown to bind the *Cl. difficile* toxin *in vitro* (T.W. Chang *et al., Lancet*, 1978, *2*, 258), and cholestyramine has been used to treat pseudomembranous colitis (E.W. Kreutzer and F.D. Milligan, *Johns Hopkins med. J.*, 1978, *143*, 67). The use of vancomycin together with cholestyramine has been suggested and although vancomycin is bound by cholestyramine (R.H. George *et al., Lancet*, 1978, *2*, 624) a study *in vitro* (C.Y. King and S.L. Barriere, *Antimicrob. Ag. Chemother.*, 1981, *19*, 326) demonstrated that an immediate loss of antibacterial activity did not occur. King and Barriere suggested that the interaction was not important and that concomitant use of cholestyramine and vancomycin may enhance therapeutic response and prevent relapse of pseudomembranous colitis.

Inflammatory bowel diseases. Findings of *Clostridium difficile* toxin in the stools of 6 patients with chronic inflammatory bowel disease during symptomatic relapse. Five of the 6 patients obtained a beneficial response to vancomycin therapy, and the sixth was controlled with corticosteroids, sulphasalazine, and bowel rest. Stool toxin should be assayed in patients with symptomatic inflammatory bowel disease unresponsive to standard medical therapy, irrespective of previous antibiotic therapy. This will allow selection of a sub-group of patients who may benefit from vancomycin therapy.— J. T. LaMont and Y. M. Trnka, *Lancet*, 1980, *1*, 381. A study of the addition of oral vancomycin 500 mg every 6 hours or placebo for 7 days to routine medical therapy for exacerbations of ulcerative colitis or Crohn's disease. Although there was no significant overall difference in outcome between the 2 groups, there was a trend towards a reduction in the need for operative intervention in patients with ulcerative colitis treated with vancomycin compared with controls. The efficacy of vancomycin was not attributable to its action against *Cl. difficile* which was not isolated from any of the patients.— R. J. Dickinson *et al., Gut*, 1985, *26*, 1380.

Neonatal necrotising enterocolitis. The imposition of strict infection control measures and the use of oral vancomycin in all neonates admitted to a neonatal unit was considered responsible for controlling an outbreak of neonatal necrotising enterocolitis; *Clostridium difficile* appeared to have an aetiological role in the outbreak. They were initially given vancomycin 15 mg per kg body-weight daily for seven days.— V. K. M. Han *et al., Pediatrics*, 1983, *71*, 935.

In a Canadian hospital 46 infants with neonatal necrotising enterocolitis were treated with ampicillin 100 mg per kg body-weight daily and gentamicin 5 to 7.5 mg per kg daily in the years 1982 to 1983. Because of the isolation of cloxacillin-resistant coagulase-negative staphylococci, therapy was changed, and in the years 1984 to 1985, 44 neonates were treated with vancomycin 30 to 45 mg per kg daily and cefotaxime 150 mg per kg daily. All antibiotics were administered intravenously. Those over 2200 g birth-weight did well with either regimen; smaller neonates did better on vancomycin and cefotaxime. Clinically, the major difference in outcome between the treatment groups was the lower risk of culture-positive peritonitis in those given cefotaxime and vancomycin. This may be related to the marked suppression of aerobic faecal flora in patients given this regimen, as compared to those given ampicillin and gentamicin.— D. W. Scheifele *et al., J. antimicrob. Chemother.*, 1987, *20*, 421.

NEUTROPENIA. Parenteral vancomycin may be added to empiric antibiotic regimens for febrile episodes in neutropenic patients if Gram-positive organisms, particularly *Staphylococcus epidermidis* are likely to be present. For a discussion of such regimens, see Piperacillin Sodium, p.287.

PERITONITIS. Vancomycin is valuable in the treatment of peritonitis associated with continuous ambulatory peritoneal dialysis (CAPD), caused by staphylococci, streptococci, and diphtheroids. Its use has increased particularly because of activity against *Staphylococcus epidermidis* and other coagulase-negative staphylococci resistant to many other antibiotics (L. Brauner *et al., J. antimicrob. Chemother.*, 1985, *15*, 751; see also under Antimicrobial Action, above). For the initial empirical treatment of peritonitis, the British Society for Antimicrobial Chemotherapy (BSAC) recommend that vancomycin be used in association with an aminoglycoside, such as gentamicin, netilmicin, or tobramycin (*Lancet*, 1987, *1*, 845). This regimen covers most pathogens including *Staph. epidermidis* and Gram-negative bacilli including *Pseudomonas aeruginosa*. Once the pathogen and its sensitivity are known, either vancomycin or the aminoglycoside should be discontinued; in culture-negative episodes it is advisable to continue both agents provided the patients is responding. Cefuroxime or ceftazidime may be used as alternatives to the above regimen, although their activity against *Staph. epidermidis* should be confirmed. The optimum length of treatment is controversial, but the BSAC recommend continuation for at least 5 days after resolution of clinical signs and symptoms and clearing of the effluent; usually a total of 7 to 10 days is adequate. In severely ill patients, an intravenous or intraperitoneal loading dose of vancomycin 500 mg may be given to ensure prompt therapeutic concentrations. The recommended maintenance dose of vancomycin is 25 mg per litre of dialysate, and the BSAC state the maximum safe blood concentration of vancomycin to be 60 to 80 µg per mL. A single intraperitoneal dose of vancomycin 25 mg per litre may be used for prophylaxis of peritonitis during a known episode of contamination.

The BSAC recommend the use of intraperitoneal antibiotics for the treatment of CAPD-associated peritonitis, since precise therapeutic and non-toxic concentrations can be delivered directly to the site of infection. Some workers, however, have considered from pharmacokinetic studies that a single intravenous dose of 25 mg per kg body-weight would produce dialysate concentrations sufficient to inhibit the majority of *Staph. epidermidis* strains for at least 4 days (M. Whitby *et al., J. antimicrob. Chemother.*, 1987, *19*, 351).

Commenting on the BSAC recommendations, some workers considered that the combination of vancomycin and an aminoglycoside may have cumulative ototoxicity, and that the suggested maximum concentration of 60 µg per mL is too high (I. Muscat *et al., Lancet*, 1987, *1*, 1142). These authors had successfully used a combination of vancomycin and ceftazidime. For recurrent episodes of peritonitis caused by coagulase-negative staphylococci, after intraperitoneal treatment with vancomycin and netilmicin for 48 hours, rifampicin by mouth has been substituted for netilmicin (S.J. Pickering *et al., ibid.*, 1258).

For reference to a report of decreasing susceptibility to vancomycin of isolates of *Staphylococcus haemolyticus* in a patient with peritonitis, see under Resistance, above.

PREGNANCY AND THE NEONATE. For reference to the use of vancomycin in the neonate, see Administration in Infants and Children, and Neonatal Necrotising Enterocolitis under Gastro-intestinal Disorders, above.

SEPTICAEMIA. Successful use of intravenous vancomycin for the treatment of bacteraemia caused by a rapidly-growing *Mycobacterium* sp.— L. Jadeja *et al., Ann. intern. Med.*, 1983, *99*, 475.

A study recommending vancomycin as the agent of choice for the treatment of septicaemia caused by methicillin-resistant *Staphylococcus aureus*.— M. T. Cafferkey *et al., Antimicrob. Ag. Chemother.*, 1985, *28*, 819.

SUPPRESSION OF INTESTINAL FLORA. A study in 38 patients with leukaemia who received oral regimens of gentamicin, vancomycin, and nystatin (GVN) or gentamicin and nystatin for prophylactic suppression of intestinal flora, indicated that vancomycin could be safely omitted from the GVN regimen provided that microbiological monitoring was performed to detect the emergence of resistant organisms. Tolerance was improved when vancomycin was omitted.— J. F. Bender *et al., Antimicrob. Ag. Chemother.*, 1979, *15*, 455.

For further reference to the use of the GVN regimen to prevent colonisation and infection by the selective decontamination of the gastro-intestinal tract, see Colistin Sulphomethate Sodium, p.205.

SURGICAL INFECTION PROPHYLAXIS. Vancomycin may be useful for the prophylaxis of infection during clean surgical procedures in which both coagulase-positive and -negative staphylococci are important pathogens, such as orthopaedic, cardiac, and neurological surgery. It is, however, usually reserved for use in patients allergic to cephalosporins or where there is a high risk of methicillin-resistant staphylococcal infections. Vancomycin is usually administered in a single pre-operative intravenous dose of 1 g, although in coronary-artery bypass procedures 15 mg per kg body-weight has been given pre-operatively, 10 mg per kg after initiation of the bypass, followed by further doses every 8 hours for 48 hours. Vancomycin has also been given in association with gentamicin for infection prophylaxis prior to craniotomy (A.B. Kaiser, *New Engl. J. Med.*, 1986, *315*, 1129; *Med. Lett.*, 1987, *29*, 91).

Cardiac surgery. For reference to infection prophylaxis in cardiac surgery, including mention of the use of vancomycin, see Flucloxacillin Sodium, p.232.

Neurosurgery. In a study of 137 children receiving neurosurgical shunts, infection prophylaxis with vancomycin 15 or 20 mg per kg body-weight given intravenously before and 6 hours after operation, together with an intrathecal dose of vancomycin 10 mg during operation, did not significantly change the shunt-associated infection-rate. In children receiving the higher intravenous dosage, the first dose of which was given in the operating theatre, 22.7% became hypotensive; the lower dose, given on the ward to avoid possible potentiation of reactions by anaesthesia, did not provoke hypotension. Other reactions were flushing, urticaria, or pruritus; a slow rate of infusion and/or administration of diphenhydramine appeared to modify some but not all reactions.— P. H. Slight *et al.* (letter), *New Engl. J. Med.*, 1985, *312*, 921.

Preparations

Vancomycin Hydrochloride Capsules *(U.S.P.)*

Vancomycin Hydrochloride for Oral Solution *(U.S.P.)*. Reconstituted solution has a pH of 2.5 to 4.5.

Vancomycin Injection *(B.P.)*. Vancomycin hydrochloride to be reconstituted before use.

Sterile Vancomycin Hydrochloride *(U.S.P.)*

Proprietary Preparations

Vancocin *(Lilly, UK)*. *Capsules* (Vancocin Matrigel), vancomycin hydrochloride 125 and 250 mg.
Oral solution, powder for reconstitution, vancomycin 10 g (as hydrochloride). To be reconstituted with water to give a solution containing approximately 500 mg/6 mL.
Injection, powder for reconstitution, vancomycin 500 mg (as hydrochloride).
Injection (Vancocin CP), powder for reconstitution, chromatographically purified, vancomycin 500 mg (as hydrochloride).

Proprietary Names and Manufacturers

Diatracin *(Dista, Spain)*; Vancocin *(Lilly, Austral.; Belg.; Lilly, Canad.; Lilly, Denm.; Lilly, Norw.; Lilly, S.Afr.; Lilly, Swed.; Lilly, Switz.; Lilly, UK; Lilly, USA)*; Vancocina *(Lilly, Ital.)*; Vancoled *(Lederle, USA)*.

178-k

Virginiamycin *(BAN, USAN, rINN)*.

Antibiotic 899; SKF-7988; Virgimycin.

CAS — 11006-76-1; 21411-53-0 (virginiamycin M_1); 23152-29-6 (virginiamycin S_1).

A mixture consisting principally of 2 antimicrobial substances, virginiamycin M_1, and virginiamycin S_1, produced by the growth of *Streptomyces virginiae.*

Adverse Effects

Virginiamycin may cause gastro-intestinal irritation and vomiting. A few instances of hypersensitivity have been observed.

Antimicrobial Action and Resistance

Virginiamycin has a similar spectrum of antimicrobial activity to erythromycin. It is active against staphylococci and some streptococci; *Neisseria gonorrhoeae* and *Haemophilus influenzae* are reported to be sensitive. Cross-resistance is often observed between streptogramin, macrolide, and lincosamide antibiotics.

The streptogramin group of antibiotics includes the mikamycins, pristinamycins, oestreomycins, and virginiamycins, which are produced as secondary metabolites from a wide variety of *Streptomyces* spp. They are divided into 2 main groups: Group A or M which is composed of polyunsaturated cyclic peptidolides and Group B or S which is composed of cyclic hexadepsipeptides. Each component within these groups possesses good bacteriostatic activity on Gram-positive bacteria. However, the combination of one component from each group leads to an association which is strongly bactericidal and highly synergistic. For example, *Str. pristina spiralis* produces the 2 pristinamycins pristinamycin PI_A and pristinamycin PII_A.— F. Le Goffic, *J. antimicrob. Chemother.*, 1985, *16, Suppl.* A, 13. Streptogramins, or synergistins, comprise two factors which act with synergy. These factors are called I and II for pristinamycin, A and B for streptogramin, and S and M for virginiamycin. Thus, groups SBI and AMII may be used to describe the 2 factors, although current practice is to describe them using the A and B factors of streptogramin. Factor B has great structural similarity to the macrolides and is affected by macrolide-lincosamide-streptogramin-B-type (MLS_B) resistance but such resistant strains still appear to be sensitive to factor A and there is maintenance of A-B synergy.— J. Duval, *ibid.*, 137. A review of the molecular mechanism of action of virginiamycin-like antibiotics (synergimycins) on bacterial protein synthesis.— C. Cocito and G. Chinali, *ibid.*, 35.

For further reference to MLS_B resistance, see Erythromycin, p.223.

Absorption and Fate

Virginiamycin is rapidly absorbed from the gastro-intestinal tract, and is excreted in the urine and faeces.

In 2 volunteers given radioactive virginiamycin peak plasma and urinary concentrations were achieved about 4 hours after the dose; about 15 to 20% of the dose was excreted within 24 hours.— B. Boon *et al.*, *Thérapie*, 1973, *28*, 367.

Uses and Administration

Virginiamycin is a streptogramin antibiotic used for the treatment of infections due to sensitive organisms, particularly Gram-positive cocci. The usual dose by mouth is 2 to 4 g daily in divided doses. Children have been given 50 to 100 mg per kg body-weight daily. It has been applied locally in a dusting-powder (2%) or ointment (0.5%).

Virginiamycin is used as an additive for animal feeding stuffs.

Proprietary Names and Manufacturers

Stafilomicina *(Smith Kline & French, Ital.)*; Staphylomycine *(RIT, Belg.; Smith Kline & French, Fr.; Smith Kline & French, Neth.)*; Staxidin *(Smith Kline & French, Spain)*.

Proprietary Veterinary Names and Manufacturers

Eskalin *(Smith Kline Animal Health, UK)*.

Anticoagulants

4800-s

Anticoagulants may be divided into direct anticoagulants such as the heparins and indirect anticoagulants such as the coumarin and indanedione derivatives. Developments have led to low-molecular-weight heparins and heparinoids that are aimed at providing heparin's anticoagulant activity without its haemorrhagic hazards.

Other anticoagulants included in this section are ancrod, leech, and sodium pentosan polysulphate.

In general, anticoagulants are used in the management and prophylaxis of thrombo-embolic disorders; they are not thrombolytics or platelet aggregation inhibitors. As can be seen from the following reviews, their use in myocardial infarction and in strokes remains a subject of debate.

MYOCARDIAL INFARCTION. There have been a number of detailed studies showing that anticoagulant therapy could reduce the risk of reinfarction or of further emboli when given to patients after myocardial infarction. Recent studies have included daily subcutaneous low-dose heparin (G.G. Neri Serneri *et al.*, *Lancet*, 1987, *1*, 937) or the long-term use of oral coumarin anticoagulants in the Sixty Plus Reinfarction Study (*Lancet*, 1980, *2*, 989; *ibid.*, 1982, *1*, 64) or in the study by Weinreich *et al.* (*Ann. intern. Med.*, 1984, *100*, 789). There have been criticisms, of the Sixty Plus Reinfarction Study, for instance (*Drug & Ther. Bull.*, 1982, *20*, 49; E. Van der Does, *Br. med. J.*, 1982, *285*, 294), and there have been recent studies that have failed to show any benefits (R.J. Goldberg *et al.*, *Am. Heart J.*, 1985, *109*, 616; S. Arvan and K. Boscha, *ibid.*, 1987, *113*, 688).

Some centres that use thrombolytic therapy with streptokinase follow it up with several months' treatment with warfarin or an antiplatelet drug and there is evidence of some benefit in a scheme that employs heparin after thrombolytic therapy (K. Kaplan *et al.*, *Am. J. Cardiol.*, 1987, *59*, 241).

While the developments in thrombolytic therapy may alter the way anticoagulants might be used in patients with recent myocardial infarction, the developments in antiplatelet therapy (see under aspirin, p.6) confuse the role of anticoagulants. One study has shown no real difference in mortality and morbidity following myocardial infarction between patients given aspirin (1.5 g daily, rather than the lower doses used in some other studies) or those given an anticoagulant (The E.P.S.I.M. Research Group, *New Engl. J. Med.*, 1982, *307*, 701). The study did not investigate whether either treatment was better than no treatment.

STROKE AND TRANSIENT ISCHAEMIC ATTACKS. Anticoagulants are used following strokes to prevent further cerebrovascular incidents. However, their use is contra-indicated if the stroke was a result of haemorrhage. There have been reports of useful prophylaxis with heparin (J.D. Easton and D.G. Sherman, *Stroke*, 1980, *11*, 433; G.J. Martin and J. Biller, *Archs intern. Med.*, 1984, *144*, 1997; M.-G. Bousser *et al.*, *Stroke*, 1985, *16*, 199), but a more recent controlled study involving larger numbers of patients has shown no benefit with heparin in the prevention of further strokes (R.J. Duke *et al.*, *Ann. intern. Med.*, 1986, *105*, 825).

Anticoagulants are also recommended for the prophylaxis of cerebrovascular incidents in patients who have experienced transient ischaemic attacks and some studies have shown anticoagulants providing a better prophylactic effect than antiplatelet drugs (J.-E. Olsson *et al.*, *Stroke*, 1980, *11*, 4; S.-E. Eriksson, *Acta neurol. scand.*, 1985, *71*, 485) or a similar effect (A. Garde *et al.*, *Stroke*, 1983, *14*, 677). Yet again though, there are other studies that have shown no benefit (S.F. Putman and H.P. Adams, *Archs Neurol., Chicago*, 1985, *42*, 960; C. Warlow, *Drugs*, 1985, *29*, 474).

As with myocardial infarction, other reports on the value of antiplatelet drugs (see under aspirin, p.6) confuse the role of anticoagulants in the protection of patients from further cerebrovascular incidents.

4804-y

Ancrod *(BAN, USAN, rINN).*

An active enzymatic principle derived from the venom of the Malayan pit-viper (*Agkistrodon rhodostoma = Calloselasma rhodostoma*).

CAS — 9046-56-4.

Pharmacopoeias. The *B.P.* includes an injection.

The injection has a pH of 6.5 to 7.1. **Store** at 2 to 8°, do not freeze. Protect from light.

Units

55 units are contained in 16.90 mg with lactose and albumin in one ampoule of the first International Reference Preparation (1976).

Adverse Effects and Treatment

Haemorrhage may occur during treatment with ancrod and usually responds to its withdrawal. If severe it may be treated by an antiserum, each mL of which is sufficient to neutralise 70 units of ancrod. An initial dose of 0.2 mL is given subcutaneously, followed in the absence of untoward reaction after 30 minutes by 0.8 mL intramuscularly; in the absence of untoward reaction 1 mL is then given intravenously 30 minutes later. In emergency the intramuscular dose may be omitted in the absence of untoward reaction to the subcutaneous dose. In life-threatening haemorrhage it may be necessary to give antiserum intravenously without prior test doses but with adrenaline, antihistamines, and corticosteroids available against the possibility of anaphylactic shock. Fibrinogen 5 g or 1 litre of fresh blood or plasma should also be given to restore the fibrinogen concentration.

Precautions

As for Heparin, p.340.

Ancrod should not be given to patients with thrombocytopenia, coronary thrombosis, severe infections, septicaemia, or disseminated intravascular coagulation. It should be used cautiously in patients with cardiovascular disorders that may be complicated by defibrination and in stroke, uraemia, and renal colic. Dextran injections or aminocaproic acid should not be given concomitantly. It is important that when ancrod is given by intravenous infusion it should be given slowly over a period of not less than 4 hours to prevent the formation of large amounts of unstable fibrin.

Ancrod has caused foetal death in *animals* as a result of placental haemorrhage and is not recommended during pregnancy.

Uses and Administration

Ancrod reduces the blood-concentration of fibrinogen by the cleavage of microparticles of fibrin which are rapidly removed from the circulation by fibrinolysis or phagocytosis. It reduces blood viscosity but has no effect on established thrombi. Haemostatic concentrations of fibrinogen are normally restored in about 12 hours and normal concentrations in 10 to 20 days.

It is used in the treatment of thrombotic disorders including retinal vein occlusion and deep-vein thrombosis and to prevent thrombosis after surgery. It has also been given for priapism.

The usual initial dose is 2 to 3 units per kg body-weight in 50 to 500 mL of sodium chloride injection (0.9%) given over 4 to 12 hours (usually 6 to 8 hours). Maintenance doses of 2 units per kg are given every 12 hours by slow intravenous injection (over 5 minutes) or by infusion, usually for about 7 days. The blood-fibrinogen concentrations may be used to monitor treatment.

For the prevention of deep-vein thrombosis after hip surgery 280 units have been given by subcutaneous injection postoperatively, followed by 70 units daily for 8 days; a treatment period of 4 days has been used in some other surgical procedures. Resistance has developed to ancrod.

Twenty-three patients undergoing surgery for fracture of the neck of the femur, a procedure associated with a high incidence of deep-vein thrombosis, were treated with low-dose ancrod and the results compared with 24 similar patients. Ancrod, given for 72 hours after surgery, reduced the fibrinogen concentration of the blood and the effect persisted to the eighth day. Three patients in the control group died from pulmonary embolism and there were 3 more non-fatal cases; there was 1 non-fatal case of pulmonary embolism in the ancrod group. The incidence of deep-vein thrombosis was not significantly different. Initially the dose of ancrod was 0.5 unit per kg body-weight over 12 hours; after the first 10 patients this was increased to 1 unit per kg over the first 12 hours, then 0.5 unit per kg per 12 hours.— W. W. Barrier *et al.*, *Br. med. J.*, 1974, *4*, 130.

In a double-blind placebo-controlled study 55 patients received subcutaneous injections of ancrod (280 units initially followed by 70 units on the 4 subsequent days) after operation for fractured neck of femur; 55 similar patients received placebo injections. Bilateral ascending venography or necropsy carried out 6 to 16 days after surgery revealed no deep-vein thrombosis in 29 of 53 patients in the ancrod group and 14 of 52 in the placebo group. The incidence of total and bilateral deep-vein thrombosis was significantly lower in the ancrod group, the difference being even more marked if only major deep-vein thromboses were included. No complications were associated with ancrod therapy.— G. D. O. Lowe *et al.*, *Lancet*, 1978, *2*, 698.

The management of thrombosis with ancrod in a patient with systemic lupus erythematosus.— A. K. Dosekun *et al.*, *Archs intern. Med.*, 1984, *144*, 37.

A reduced loading dose of ancrod in 2 patients allowed a more gradual and controlled reduction in fibrinogen. Doses of 2.15 or 2.00 units per kg body-weight were excessive in 2 patients; doses of 0.86 or 1.27 units per kg were effective in producing a 74 or 77% depletion of fibrinogen in another 2 patients.— P. A. Taylor and P. W. Shaw, *Pharm. J.*, 1985, *2*, 21.

Preparations

Ancrod Injection *(B.P.)*

Arvin *(Armour, UK). Injection,* ancrod 70 units/mL in ampoules of 1 mL.

NOTE. 1-mL ampoules of antiserum specific against ancrod are available.

Proprietary Names and Manufacturers

Arvin *(Knoll, Canad.; Knoll-Made, Spain; Armour, UK).*

4805-j

Anisindione *(BAN, rINN).*

2-(4-Methoxyphenyl)indan-1,3-dione.

$C_{16}H_{12}O_3$=252.3.

CAS — 117-37-3.

Anisindione is an orally administered indanedione anticoagulant with actions and uses similar to those of warfarin sodium (see p.348), but like phenindione (p.343) it is more toxic than warfarin and this limits its use.

The usual initial dose is 300 mg on the first day, 200 mg on the second day, and 100 mg on the third. The maintenance dose may range from 25 to 250 mg daily.

During treatment with anisindione the urine may be coloured pink.

Proprietary Names and Manufacturers

Miradon *(Schering, USA)*; Unidone *(Unicet, Fr.).*

4806-z

Bromindione *(BAN, USAN, rINN).*

p-Bromindione. 2-(4-Bromophenyl)indan-1,3-dione.

$C_{15}H_9BrO_2$=301.1.

CAS — 1146-98-1.

Bromindione is an orally administered indanedione anticoagulant.

Proprietary Names and Manufacturers
Fluidane *(Fr.)*.

4807-c

Clorindione *(BAN, rINN)*.
Chlorphenindione; G-25-766. 2-(4-Chlorophenyl)indan-1,3-dione.
$C_{15}H_9ClO_2$=256.7.
CAS — 1146-99-2.

Clorindione is an orally administered indanedione anticoagulant.

Proprietary Names and Manufacturers
Indalitan *(Geigy, Switz.)*.

4808-k

Cumetharol *(BAN)*.
Coumetarol *(rINN)*. 3,3′-(2-Methoxyethylidene)bis(4-hydroxycoumarin).
$C_{21}H_{16}O_7$=380.4.
CAS — 4366-18-1.

Cumetharol is an orally administered coumarin anticoagulant with actions and uses similar to those of warfarin sodium (see p.344).

Proprietary Names and Manufacturers
Dicoumoxyl *(Labaz, Fr.)*.

4809-a

Cyclocoumarol *(BAN)*.
Cyclocumarol. 3,4-Dihydro-2-methoxy-2-methyl-4-phenylpyrano[3,2-*c*]chromen-5(2*H*)-one.
$C_{20}H_{18}O_4$=322.4.
CAS — 518-20-7.

Cyclocoumarol is an orally administered coumarin anticoagulant.

4811-l

Dicoumarol *(rINN)*.
Bishydroxycoumarin; Dicoumarolum; Dicumarinum; Dicumarol *(USAN)*; Melitoxin. 3,3′-Methylenebis(4-hydroxycoumarin).
$C_{19}H_{12}O_6$=336.3.
CAS — 66-76-2.

Pharmacopoeias. In *Braz., Int., Jug., Mex., Nord., Pol., Rus., Turk.,* and *U.S.*

A white or creamy-white crystalline powder with a faint pleasant odour.
Practically **insoluble** in water, alcohol, and ether; slightly soluble in chloroform; readily soluble in solutions of alkali hydroxides. **Store** in well-closed containers. Protect from light.

Adverse Effects, Treatment, and Precautions
As for warfarin sodium (p.344).
The absorption of dicoumarol is affected by food.
The interactions associated with oral anticoagulants are discussed in detail under warfarin. Specific references to interactions involving dicoumarol can be found under the headings for the following drug groups: analgesics; anti-arrhythmics; antibacterial agents; antidepressants; antidiabetic agents; anti-epileptics; corticosteroids and corticotrophin; gastro-intestinal agents; lipid regulating agents; sedatives and neuroleptics; sex hormones; thyroid and antithyroid agents; uricosuric agents; vasodilators; and vitamins.

EFFECTS ON THE LIVER. The cause of the rise in serum-aminotransferase concentrations which might occur during treatment with dicoumarol was obscure. The rise in serum-lactic dehydrogenase concentrations in some patients given dicoumarol might be as great as that produced by an acute myocardial infarction.— F. Clark, *Adverse Drug React. Bull.*, 1977, Oct., 232.

See also under warfarin sodium (p.344).

Absorption and Fate
Dicoumarol is irregularly absorbed from the gastro-intestinal tract and is extensively bound to plasma protein. It is metabolised in the liver and is excreted in the urine, mainly as metabolites.

Uses and Administration
Dicoumarol is an orally administered coumarin anticoagulant with actions and uses similar to those of warfarin sodium (p.348). The initial dose of dicoumarol is usually 200 to 300 mg with a daily maintenance dose according to coagulation tests of 25 to 200 mg.
Because of its slow onset and long duration of action and the unpredictability of response, dicoumarol has been largely replaced by warfarin sodium.

Preparations

Dicumarol Capsules *(U.S.P.)*. Capsules containing dicoumarol.

Dicumarol Tablets *(U.S.P.)*. Tablets containing dicoumarol.

Proprietary Names and Manufacturers
Apekumarol *(Ferrosan, Swed.)*; Dicumol *(ACF, Neth.)*; Dufalone *(Frosst, Canad.)*.

4812-y

Diphenadione *(BAN, pINN)*.
Diphacinone. 2-(Diphenylacetyl)indan-1,3-dione.
$C_{23}H_{16}O_3$=340.4.
CAS — 82-66-6.

Diphenadione is an orally administered indanedione anticoagulant with actions and uses similar to those of warfarin sodium (see p.348), but like phenindione (p.343) its use has declined in favour of the coumarins. During treatment with diphenadione the urine may be coloured pink.
Diphenadione is also used as a rodenticide.

4813-j

Ethyl Biscoumacetate *(BAN, rINN)*.
Aethylis Biscoumacetas; Ethyl Biscoumac.; Ethyldicoumarol; Ethylis Biscoumacetas; Neodicumarinum. Ethyl bis(4-hydroxycoumarin-3-yl)acetate.
$C_{22}H_{16}O_8$=408.4.
CAS — 548-00-5.

Pharmacopoeias. In *Arg., Egypt., Fr., Int., It., Jug., Rus.,* and *Turk.*

Adverse Effects, Treatment, and Precautions
As for warfarin sodium (p.344).
The interactions associated with oral anticoagulants are discussed in detail under warfarin. Specific references to interactions involving ethyl biscoumacetate can be found under the headings for the following drug groups: analgesics; antifungal agents; central stimulants; corticosteroids and corticotrophin; diuretics; sedatives and neuroleptics; and vasodilators.

Absorption and Fate
Ethyl biscoumacetate is readily absorbed from the gastro-intestinal tract and is extensively bound to plasma proteins. It is metabolised in the liver. Reported plasma half-life ranges from 2 to 3.5 hours.
Ethyl biscoumacetate has been reported to appear in only small amounts in breast milk.

Uses and Administration
Ethyl biscoumacetate is an orally administered coumarin anticoagulant with actions and uses similar to those of warfarin sodium (p.348).
It has been given in a dose of up to 1.2 g daily in divided doses for the first 2 or 3 days and subsequently 300 to 600 mg daily according to coagulation tests. It exists in 2 polymorphic forms.

Proprietary Names and Manufacturers
Stabilène *(Auclair, Fr.)*; Tromexan *(Geigy, Arg.; Geigy, Belg.; Geigy, Switz.; Geigy, UK)*; Tromexane *(Geigy, Fr.)*; Tromexano *(Padro, Spain)*.

4814-z

Ethylidene Dicoumarin
Ethylidene Dicoumarol. 3,3′-Ethylidenebis(4-hydroxycoumarin).
$C_{20}H_{14}O_6$=350.3.
CAS — 1821-16-5.

Ethylidene dicoumarin is an orally administered coumarin anticoagulant.

Proprietary Names and Manufacturers
Pertrombon *(Gerot, Belg.)*.

4815-c

Fluindione *(rINN)*.
Fluorindione; LM-123. 2-(4-Fluorophenyl)indan-1,3-dione.
$C_{15}H_9FO_2$=240.2.
CAS — 957-56-2.

Fluindione is an orally administered indanedione anticoagulant.

An 80-mg loading dose of fluindione reduced the prothrombin level to 37% in 24 hours; the effect lasted for 48 hours. The mean elimination half-life of fluindione was 31 hours; about 94% was bound to plasma proteins.— J.-P. Tillement *et al.*, *Eur. J. clin. Pharmac.*, 1975, *8*, 271.

Proprietary Names and Manufacturers
Préviscan *(Nativelle, Fr.)*.

4801-w

Heparin Calcium *(BAN, USAN)*.
Calcium Heparinate.

CAS — 9005-49-6 (heparin); 37270-89-6 (calcium salt).

Pharmacopoeias. In *Br., Eur., Fr., It., Neth., Swiss,* and *U.S.*

A preparation containing the calcium salt of a sulphated glucosaminoglycan present in mammalian tissues, and having the characteristic property of delaying the clotting of shed blood. It is prepared from the lungs of oxen or the intestinal mucosa of oxen, pigs, or sheep. The *B.P.* specifies that heparin calcium intended for use in the manufacture of a parenteral dosage form contains not less than 150 units per mg and heparin calcium not intended for use in the manufacture of a parenteral dosage form contains not less than 120 units per mg, both calculated with reference to the dried substance. The potency of Heparin Calcium (*U.S.P.*) calculated on the dried basis, is not less than 140 *U.S.P.* heparin units in each mg. The *B.P.* and *U.S.P.* require that the source of the material be stated on the label.
A white or almost white moderately hygroscopic powder. **Soluble** 1 in less than 5 of water. The *B.P.* specifies that a 1% solution in water has a pH of 5.5 to 8.0; the *U.S.P.* specifies a pH of 5.0 to 7.5. Solutions are **sterilised** by filtration. **Incompatibility.** See Heparin Sodium (below). **Store** in airtight containers.

4802-e

Heparin Sodium *(BAN, USAN, rINN)*.
Eparina; Heparin; Heparinum; Heparinum Natricum; Sodium Heparin; Soluble Heparin.

CAS — 9041-08-1.

Pharmacopoeias. In *Arg., Aust., Br., Braz., Chin., Cz., Egypt., Eur., Fr., Hung., Ind., Int., It., Jpn, Jug., Neth., Pol., Roum., Swiss, Turk.,* and *U.S.*

A preparation containing the sodium salt of a sulphated glucosaminoglycan present in mammalian tissues, and having the characteristic property of delaying the clotting of shed blood. It is prepared from the lungs of oxen or the intestinal mucosa of oxen, pigs, or sheep. The *B.P.* specifies that heparin sodium intended for use in the manufacture of a parenteral dosage form contains not less than 150 units per mg and heparin sodium not intended for use in the manufacture of a parenteral dosage form contains not less than 120 units per mg, both calculated with reference to the dried substance. The potency of Heparin Sodium (*U.S.P.*), calculated on the dried basis is not less than 140 *U.S.P.* units in each mg. The *B.P.* and *U.S.P.* require that the source of the material be stated on the label.

A white or almost white, odourless or almost odourless, moderately hygroscopic powder. *B.P.* solubilities are: **soluble** 1 in 2.5 of water and a 1% solution has a pH of 5.5 to 8.0. The *U.S.P.* solubilities are: soluble 1 in 20 of water and a 1% solution has a pH of 5.0 to 7.5. Solutions are **sterilised** by filtration. **Store** in airtight containers.

INCOMPATIBILITY. Incompatibility has been reported between heparin calcium or sodium and amikacin sulphate, amiodarone, ampicillin sodium, benzylpenicillin sodium, cephalothin sodium, ciprofloxacin lactate, daunorubicin hydrochloride, dobutamine hydrochloride, doxorubicin hydrochloride, erythromycin lactobionate, gentamicin sulphate, haloperidol lactate, hyaluronidase, hydrocortisone sodium succinate, kanamycin sulphate, methicillin sodium, opioid analgesics, oxytetracycline hydrochloride, polymyxin B sulphate, promazine hydrochloride, promethazine hydrochloride, streptomycin sulphate, sulphafurazole diethanolamine, tetracycline hydrochloride, tobramycin sulphate, and vancomycin hydrochloride. Glucose can have variable effects. Incompatibility has also been reported between heparin and fat emulsion.

Units

1780 units of heparin, porcine, are contained in one ampoule of the fourth International Standard Preparation (1983).

The *U.S.P.* states that the *U.S.P.* and international units are not equivalent.

Adverse Effects

Heparin can give rise to haemorrhage as a consequence of its action. It can also cause thrombocytopenia, either through a direct effect or through an immune effect producing a platelet-aggregating antibody. Consequent platelet aggregation and thrombosis may therefore exacerbate the condition being treated. The incidence of thrombocytopenia is reported to be greater with bovine than porcine heparin.

Allergic reactions may occur, as may local irritant effects, necrosis, alopecia, and spontaneous fractures.

Priapism in a 37-year-old man 7 hours after a heparin infusion. The patient demonstrated spontaneous platelet aggregation. There have been a number of reports of priapism with heparin; none were considered to have demonstrated altered platelet function.— B. J. Burke *et al.*, *Postgrad. med. J.*, 1983, *59*, 332.

EFFECTS ON THE ADRENAL GLANDS. Heparin inducing hypoaldosteronism.— D. Brohee and P. Neve, *Archs intern. Med.*, 1984, *144*, 1698. Suppression of aldosterone production by low-dose heparin.— R. A. Sherman, *Am. J. Nephrol.*, 1986, *6*, 165.

EFFECTS ON THE BLOOD. Haemorrhage is a recognised risk with heparin (A.M. Walker and H. Jick, *J. Am. med. Ass.*, 1980, *244*, 1209). The incidence of major bleeding in several studies has been summarised by Morabia (*Lancet*, 1986, *1*, 1278).

Thrombocytopenia has been reported with various doses of heparin including heparin flushes (P.S. Heeger and J.T. Backstrom, *Ann. intern. Med*, 1986, *105*, 143). The incidence appears to be higher with bovine heparin than other forms (W.R. Bell and R.M. Royall, *New Engl. J. Med.*, 1980, *303*, 902; D.J. King and J.G. Kelton, *Ann. intern. Med.*, 1984, *100*, 535). Two types of thrombocytopenia are recognised depending on whether there is an immunological basis or not. It is the immunological type that is associated with thrombo-embolic complications through a heparin-dependent antibody that can bind to platelets (B.H. Chong *et al.*, *Lancet*, 1982, *2*, 1246; H. Wolf and G. Wick, *ibid.*, 1986, *2*, 222) and other tissues (D.B. Cines *et al.*, *New Engl. J. Med.*, 1987, *316*, 581). Skin necrosis may be due to induced thromboses (see below) reported in some patients. The point has been made that thrombosis can occur with a reduced platelet count that might not be taken to represent 'full-blooded' thrombocytopenia (B.K. Phelan, *Ann. intern. Med.*, 1983, *99*, 637; D.P. Trono *et al.*, *ibid.*, 1984, *100*, 464; M. Ramirez-Lassepas and R.J. Cipolle, *ibid.*, 613).

There have been reports of low-molecular-weight fractions of heparin being used successfully in patients with heparin-induced thromboses (M. Goualt-Heilmann *et al.*, *Lancet*, 1983, *2*, 1374; J.H. Roussi *et al.*, *ibid.*, 1984, *1*, 1183).

EFFECTS ON BONE. See below under Pregnancy and the Neonate.

EFFECTS ON THE LIVER. Reversible increases in transaminase values in patients given heparin of bovine or porcine origin.— G. E. Dukes *et al.*, *Ann. intern. Med.*, 1984, *100*, 646. See also M. Sonnenblick *et al.*, *Br. med. J.*, 1975, *3*, 77.

EFFECTS ON SERUM LIPIDS. There have been a number of reports of heparin increasing concentrations of free fatty acids (M. Rubegni *et al.*, *Lancet*, 1974, *2*, 903; M. Wood and A.J.J. Wood, *Br. med. J.*, 1979, *2*, 611; S.J. Davies and J.H. Turney, *Lancet*, 1987, *2*, 1097). The point has been made by Riemersma *et al.* (*Lancet*, 1981, *2*, 471) that the true extent of plasma lipolysis induced by heparin may have been greatly overestimated.

EFFECTS ON THE SKIN. Heparin has been implicated in skin necrosis; this might be a complication of induced thrombosis (see under Effects on the Blood). References to some case reports: J. C. Hall *et al.*, *J. Am. med. Ass.*, 1980, *244*, 1831; A. M. Jackson and A. V. Pollock, *Br. med. J.*, 1981, *283*, 1087; P. Isaacs *et al.* (letter), *ibid.*, 1982, *284*, 201; L. E. Levine *et al.*, *Archs Derm.*, 1983, *119*, 400; G. R. Hasegawa, *Drug Intell. & clin. Pharm.*, 1984, *18*, 313; M. Monreal *et al.* (letter), *Lancet*, 1984, *2*, 820.

There have also been a few reports of skin reactions some of which are considered to be allergic; some also involve ecchymosis: P. J. Ulrick and A. Manoharan, *Med. J. Aust.*, 1984, *140*, 287; J. G. Barbaccia *et al.*, *Clin. Pharm.*, 1984, *3*, 184; M. Bigby *et al.*, *J. Am. med. Ass.*, 1986, *256*, 3358; C. A. Grodman-Gross and S. V. Sastri, *Drug Intell. & clin. Pharm.*, 1987, *21*, 180.

PREGNANCY AND THE NEONATE. Although heparin does not cross the placenta its use in pregnant women has resulted in an increased incidence of still-births and of premature births (R.M. Pauli and J.G. Hall, *Lancet*, 1979, *2*, 144; J.G. Hall *et al.*, *Am. J. Med.*, 1980, *68*, 122). Osteoporosis and compression fractures have also developed in pregnant women given heparin and appear to be associated with reduced concentrations of 1,25-dihydroxycholecalciferol (D. Aarskog *et al.*, *Lancet*, 1980, *2*, 650; P.H. Wise and A.J. Hull, *Br. med. J.*, 1980, *281*, 110; D. Aarskog *et al.*, *Am. J. Obstet. Gynec.*, 1984, *148*, 1141; H.T. Griffiths and D.T.Y. Liu, *Postgrad. med. J.*, 1984, *60*, 424).

Treatment of Adverse Effects

Slight haemorrhage due to overdosage can usually be treated by withdrawing heparin. Severe bleeding may be reduced by the slow intravenous administration of protamine sulphate (see p.852). 1 mg of protamine sulphate usually neutralises at least 80 or 100 international units of heparin derived from lung or mucosa respectively. If more than 15 minutes have elapsed since the injection of heparin, lower doses of protamine will be necessary.

Urokinase was effective in the treatment of thrombosis associated with heparin-induced thrombocytopenia.— S. K. Krueger *et al.* (letter), *Ann. intern. Med.*, 1985, *103*, 159. Another case.— G. D. Clifton and M. D. Smith, *Clin. Pharm.*, 1986, *5*, 597.

Precautions

Heparin is contra-indicated in patients with haemorrhagic diseases nor is it recommended in patients with thrombocytopenia. It should be withdrawn from patients who develop thrombosis associated with thrombocytopenia. Heparin is also contra-indicated in patients who are haemorrhaging or are at risk of haemorrhage and this includes those with haemophilia, subacute bacterial endocarditis, gastric or duodenal ulcer, or severe hypertension. Heparin is also contra-indicated in patients who have recently undergone surgery at sites where haemorrhage would be an especial risk. Patients with severely impaired liver or kidney function are at risk of haemorrhage from heparin. It is recommended that a test dose be given as a check for heparin sensitivity.

Heparin should be used with care in conjunction with oral anticoagulants or agents, such as aspirin and dipyridamole, which affect platelet function, with dextran injections, and thrombolytic enzymes such as streptokinase. Estimations of oral anticoagulant control may be modified by heparin's action on prothrombin.

Doses are reduced in old people; elderly women are especially susceptible to heparin toxicity.

Although heparin does not cross the placenta, there are risks associated with its use in pregnancy (see under Adverse Effects, above).

The preservatives used in heparin preparations have been implicated in unwanted effects. Benzyl alcohol has been suspected of contributing to heparin's toxicity in neonates; it has also inhibited the activation of lymphokine-activated killer cells in the laboratory (F.M. Marincola *et al.*, *Lancet*, 1987, *2*, 399). Chlorbutol present in another heparin preparation caused a sharp fall in blood pressure (G.M.R. Bowler *et al.*, *ibid.*, 1986, *1*, 848).

INTERACTIONS. *Aspirin.* Of 12 patients with fractures of the hip who received heparin 5000 units subcutaneously every 12 hours and aspirin 600 mg twice daily rectally before operation and by mouth after operation, 8 had serious bleeding complications.— H. S. Yett *et al.* (letter), *New Engl. J. Med.*, 1978, *298*, 1092.

Glipizide. Prolonged hypoglycaemia in one patient attributed to an interaction between heparin and glipizide.— G. McKillop *et al.*, *Br. med. J.*, 1986, *293*, 1073.

Glyceryl trinitrate. Glyceryl trinitrate given intravenously has reduced the activity of heparin also given intravenously: M. A. Habbab and J. I. Haft (letter), *Ann. intern. Med.*, 1986, *105*, 305; M. A. Habbab, *Archs intern. Med.*, 1987, *147*, 857.

Laboratory tests. Heparin which can be present in blood samples can interfere with a number of laboratory estimations. A number of reports have dealt with faulty aminoglycoside estimations, especially tobramycin. The activity of tobramycin may also be inhibited and affect microbiological estimations.

References to interference with laboratory estimations: L. Nilsson, *Antimicrob. Ag. Chemother.*, 1980, *17*, 918 (aminoglycoside assay); L. Nilsson *et al.*, *ibid.*, 1981, *20*, 155 (aminoglycoside assay); A. S. Hutchison *et al.*, *Br. med. J.*, 1983, *287*, 1131 (blood-gas analysis); J. Holliday (letter), *ibid.*, 1381 (blood-gas analysis); M. B. O'Connell *et al.*, *Drug Intell. & clin. Pharm.*, 1984, *18*, 503 (aminoglycoside assay); G. R. Matzke *et al.*, *ibid.*, 517 (aminoglycoside assay); J. S. McConnell and J. Cohen, *J. clin. Path.*, 1985, *38*, 430 (*Limulus* lysate assay for endotoxin).

Quinidine. For a report of decreased quinidine protein binding due to heparin, see p.86.

Tobacco smoking. Reduced half-life and increased elimination of heparin in smokers compared with non-smokers.— R. J. Cipolle *et al.*, *Clin. Pharmac. Ther.*, 1981, *29*, 387.

MALARIA. Bell has commented that heparin is contra-indicated in malaria (*Prescribers' J.*, 1983, *23*, 119). Gilbreath *et al.* (*Trans. R. Soc. trop. Med. Hyg.*, 1983, *77*, 546) found that heparin decreased the anti-lymphocyte activity in blood from patients with malaria.

Absorption and Fate

Heparin is not absorbed from the gastro-intestinal tract. Following intravenous or subcutaneous injection heparin is extensively bound to plasma proteins. It does not cross the placenta or appear in the milk of nursing mothers. Its half-life is affected by kidney or liver impairments; patients with pulmonary embolisms are reported to have a reduced heparin half-life. Heparin is taken up by the reticuloendothelial system.

A review of the clinical pharmacokinetics of heparin.— J. W. Estes, *Clin. Pharmacokinet.*, 1980, *5*, 204.

Apparent discrepancies in published values for the half-life of heparin are due to differing methods of dealing with the experimental data. The expression 'half-life' should be qualified in the case of heparin, so as to make clear precisely what has been measured.— T. J. McAvoy, *Clin. Pharmac. Ther.*, 1979, *25*, 372.

Uses and Administration

Heparin is an anticoagulant which inhibits clotting of blood *in vitro* and *in vivo* through its action on antithrombin III. Antithrombin III which is present in plasma inhibits the activity of thrombin and activated factor X (factor Xa); heparin increases the rate of this inhibition, but in a manner that is dependent on its dose. With normal therapeutic doses heparin has an inhibitory effect on both thrombin and factor Xa. Thus the conversion of fibrinogen to fibrin is blocked through the thrombin inhibition, while the conversion of prothrombin to thrombin is blocked by the inhibition of factor Xa. The low doses that are given subcutaneously for the prophylaxis of thrombo-embolisms have a selective effect on antithrombin III's inhibition of factor Xa. Very high doses are reported to reduce the activity of antithrombin III. Other effects of heparin include inhibition of the formation of a stable fibrin clot and an antilipaemic effect.

Heparin is used in the treatment and prophylaxis of deep-vein thrombosis and pulmonary embolism as well as peripheral arterial embolism. It is often used as a precursor to oral anticoagulation and is withdrawn once the oral anticoagulant is exerting its full effect. It is also used to prevent coagulation during dialysis and other extracorporeal circulatory procedures and as an adjunct to thrombolytic therapy. Other uses include the anticoagulation of blood samples and the flushing of catheters and cannulas to maintain patency.

Heparin may be given as the calcium or sodium salt and it is generally accepted that there is little difference in their effects. The dose should be adjusted according to the patient's response as measured by coagulation tests. Tests employed include the activated partial thromboplastin time as well as whole blood coagulation. A recommended range for the first is 1.5 to 2 times normal and for blood coagulation 2.5 to 3 times normal.

Doses normally used intravenously are 12 500 units as a loading dose followed by 5000 to 10 000 units every 4 hours or by a continuous infusion of 20 000 to 40 000 units over 24 hours. Subcutaneous doses used for prophylaxis are 5000 units 2 hours before surgery then every 8 to 12 hours usually until the patient is ambulant. Subcutaneous doses used in treatment are 10 000 to 20 000 units every 12 hours or 250 units per kg body-weight every 12 hours, adjusted daily according to coagulation tests.

Children have been given 50 units per kg body-weight by intravenous infusion increased to 100 units per kg every 4 hours.

Test doses are sometimes used in patients with a history of allergy.

Heparin is available in a variety of forms for administration by different routes. The two main salts are heparin sodium and heparin calcium and they are generally considered to be equally effective (but see below). The routes include intravenous injection, continuous intravenous infusion, and subcutaneous injection. Heparin flushes are intended to maintain the patency of catheters and are not for therapeutic use. The sodium salt is generally used for the intravenous route; either the sodium or the calcium salt is used for subcutaneous injection.

The importance of starting or continuing anticoagulant treatment on confirmation of a thrombo-embolism is emphasised in a *Lancet* editorial (*Lancet*, 1988, *1*, 275). This editorial considers that *US* workers have promoted heparin treatment periods of 7 to 14 days, although the recommendations of the American College of Chest Physicians and the National Heart, Lung, and Blood Institute are for a period of 7 to 10 days (J.E. Dalen and J. Hirsh, *Archs intern. Med.*, 1986, *146*, 462). The *UK* preference is reported to be for a period of 3 days' simultaneous treatment with heparin and an oral anticoagulant before withdrawing the heparin. It seems reasonable to start warfarin on the first day of heparin treatment and to stop heparin when warfarin has prolonged the International Normalised Ratio (INR) to its recommended range [2.0 to 3.0].

The intravenous and subcutaneous routes have been compared in the treatment of deep-vein thrombosis. Hull *et al.* (*New Engl. J. Med.*, 1986, *315*, 1109) found continuous intravenous infusion to be better than subcutaneous injection in the initial treatment of such thromboses. The greater incidence of recurrent thrombo-embolisms in the subcutaneous group was associated with inadequate initial anticoagulation. When the subcutaneous dose was adjusted after 12 and not 24 hours and when heparin calcium rather than heparin sodium was used for both the intravenous infusion and the subcutaneous injection, some of Hull's colleagues (D.J. Doyle *et al.*, *Ann. intern. Med.*, 1987, *107*, 441) found no difference between the 2 routes. They did however suggest that there might be a difference in response between the 2 salts. In another study, Walker *et al.* (*Br. med. J.*, 1987, *294*, 1189) found that subcutaneous heparin calcium was better than continuous intravenous heparin sodium in helping to lyse existing thrombi and in preventing their extension.

Heparin prophylaxis of thrombo-embolisms in patients at risk undergoing surgery has been the subject of many studies, some of them involving thousands of patients (*Lancet*, 1975, *2*, 45), and has been found to be effective. Colditz *et al.* (*Lancet*, 1986, *2*, 143) reviewed many of these studies and by amalgamating results considered that 27% of patients undergoing general surgery developed deep-vein thrombosis if they were in a control group or received no prophylaxis. The incidence when heparin prophylaxis was used was 9.6% or 6.3% when compression stockings were also used. A lower rate of 4.5% was achieved with stockings plus intermittent pneumatic compression and no heparin. However, Bounameaux and Krahenbuhl (*ibid.*, 456) commented that this rate of 4.5% was obtained from a summary of 3 studies involving a total of 137 patients that did not involve a placebo control.

Heparin is given intravenously during heart surgery. Lower doses are given subcutaneously for prophylaxis in other surgical procedures; these doses tend not to be adjusted according to laboratory coagulation tests apart from orthopaedic surgery where adjusted doses are recommended (*Lancet*, 1986, *1*, 1202; *J. Am. med. Ass.*, 1986, *256*, 744). Ultra-low doses of 1 unit per kg body-weight have been reported to provide effective prophylaxis (D. Negus *et al.*, *Lancet*, 1980, *1*, 891).

Heparin is sometimes given combined with dihydroergotamine, see p.1052.

Low-dose prophylaxis has been given for varying periods ranging from 6 days to 2 weeks or until the patient is mobile or discharged.

Low-molecular-weight heparins and heparinoids have been reported to provide efficient prophylaxis (A.G.G. Turpie *et al.*, *New Engl. J. Med.*, 1986, *315*, 925; *idem*, *Lancet*, 1987, *1*, 523) and as they are considered to carry less risk of haemorrhage their impact is awaited.

The use of heparin-agarose beads for the extracorporeal removal of low-density lipoprotein from the plasma.— P.-J. Lupien *et al.*, *Lancet*, 1976, *1*, 1261.

References to heparin being used to keep cannulas and catheters free of clots: J. R. Stradling, *Br. med. J.*, 1978, *2*, 1195; M. J. Bailey, *ibid.*, 1979, *1*, 1671; P. F. Hoar *et al.*, *New Engl. J. Med.*, 1981, *305*, 993; D. T. Mangano (letter), *ibid.*, 1982, *307*, 894; G. Alpam, *Pediatrics*, 1984, *74*, 375; R. Nelson (letter), *Am. J. Hosp. Pharm.*, 1984, *41*, 1992.

CONTROL. References to the control of heparin therapy: P. G. Hattersley *et al.*, *J. Am. med. Ass.*, 1983, *250*, 1413; H. E. Branson *et al.*, *J. clin. Path.*, 1985, *38*, 422; F. C. Chenella *et al.*, *Clin. Pharm.*, 1986, *5*, 510; A. G. Fennerty *et al.*, *Br. med. J.*, 1986, *292*, 579; A. Pollock (letter), *ibid.*, 1081; J. B. Groce *et al.*, *Clin. Pharm.*, 1987, *6*, 216. Circadian variations in anticoagulation should be taken into account in evaluating the dose of heparin.— H. A. Decousus *et al.*, *Br. med. J.*, 1985, *290*, 341.

DISSEMINATED INTRAVASCULAR COAGULATION. Heparin has been used with some success in disseminated intravascular coagulation associated with a variety of conditions (see *Martindale 28th Edition*, p.766). However, this use is considered by some to be controversial.

GALL-STONES. References to some responses to heparin given by local administration into the bile ducts for gall-stones: A. Iseil and D. L. Crosby (letter), *Lancet*, 1975, *1*, 583; B. Gardner *et al.*, *Am. J. Surg.*, 1975, *130*, 293; L. A. Christiansen *et al.*, *Scand. J. Gastroenterol.*, 1977, *12*, 337.

HAEMOLYTIC-URAEMIC SYNDROME. There have been some reports of heparin being of benefit in the haemolyticuraemic syndrome (G.S. Gilchrist *et al.*, *Lancet*, 1969, *1*, 1123; M.W. Moncrieff and E.F. Glasgow, *Br. med. J.*, 1970, *3*, 188; *Lancet*, 1976, *1*, 943). Other reports have shown no benefit (M. Vitacco *et al.*, *J. Pediat.*, 1973, *83*, 271; M.G. Coulthard, *Archs Dis. Childh.*, 1980, *55*, 393; B.T. Steele *et al.*, *Lancet*, 1984, *1*, 511).

MYOCARDIAL INFARCTION. For a discussion of anticoagulants in myocardial infarction, see p.338.

PREGNANCY AND THE NEONATE. Heparin calcium and dipyridamole might be useful in the prevention of placental insufficiency and its associated complications in mother and foetus as indicated by experience in treating 13 patients and comparing them with 21 untreated patients.— P. Capetta *et al.* (letter), *Lancet*, 1986, *1*, 919.

Some references to continuous heparin infusion in pregnant patients: Ch. P. Henny *et al.* (letter), *Lancet*, 1982, *1*, 615; A. W. Cohen *et al.*, *Am. J. Obstet. Gynec.*, 1983, *146*, 463; M. C. Brabeck, *J. Am. med. Ass.*, 1987, *257*, 1790.

Pulsatile infusion.— C. L. A. Hahn, *Am. J. Obstet. Gynec.*, 1986, *155*, 283.

See also under Adverse Effects, above.

STROKE AND TRANSIENT ISCHAEMIC ATTACKS. For a discussion of anticoagulants in strokes and transient ischaemic attacks, see p.338.

Preparations of Heparin Salts

Anticoagulant Heparin Solution *(U.S.P.)*. A sterile solution of heparin sodium in sodium chloride injection.

Heparin Calcium Injection *(U.S.P.)*

Heparin Injection *(B.P.)*. A sterile solution of heparin calcium or heparin sodium in Water for Injections.

Heparin Lock Flush Solution *(U.S.P.)*. A sterile solution of heparin sodium rendered isotonic with blood by the addition of not more than 1% of sodium chloride.

Heparin Sodium Injection *(U.S.P.)*

Proprietary Preparations of Heparin Salts

Calciparine *(Sanofi, UK)*. *Injection*, heparin calcium 25 000 units/mL, in ampoules of 0.5 and 0.8 mL.

Hep-Flush *(Leo, UK)*. *Solution*, heparin sodium 100 units/mL, in ampoules of 2 mL.

Heplok *(Leo, UK)*. *Solution*, heparin sodium 10 units/mL, in ampoules of 5 mL.

Hepsal *(CP Pharmaceuticals, UK)*. *Solution*, heparin sodium 10 units/mL, in ampoules of 5 mL.

Minihep *(Leo, UK)*. *Injection*, heparin sodium 25 000 units/mL, in 0.2 mL ampoules.

Minihep Calcium *(Leo, UK)*. *Injection*, heparin calcium 25 000 units/mL, in 0.2 mL ampoules.

Monoparin *(CP Pharmaceuticals, UK)*. *Injection*, heparin sodium 1000, 5000, and 25 000 units/mL, in ampoules of 1 mL; 1000 units/mL, in ampoules of 5 and 10 mL; 5000 units/mL, in ampoules of 0.2 mL.

Monoparin Calcium *(CP Pharmaceuticals, UK)*. *Injection*, heparin calcium 25 000 units/mL, in ampoules of 0.2 mL.

Multiparin *(CP Pharmaceuticals, UK)*. *Injection*, heparin sodium 1000, 5000, and 25 000 units/mL, in vials of 5 mL.

Pump-Hep *(Leo, UK)*. *Intravenous infusion*, heparin sodium 1000 units/mL, in ampoules of 5, 10, and 20 mL.

Unihep *(Leo, UK)*. *Injection*, heparin sodium 1000, 5000, 10 000, and 25 000 units/mL, in ampoules of 1 mL.

Uniparin *(CP Pharmaceuticals, UK)*. *Injection*, heparin sodium, 25 000 units/mL, in syringes of 0.2 mL.

Uniparin Calcium *(CP Pharmaceuticals, UK)*. *Injection*, heparin calcium 25 000 units/mL, in syringes of 0.2 mL.

Uniparin Forte *(CP Pharmaceuticals, UK)*. *Injection*, heparin sodium 25 000 units/mL, in ampoules of 0.4 mL.

Proprietary Names and Manufacturers of Heparin Salts

Alfa-Eparina *(Alfa Farmaceutici, Ital.)*; Ateroclar *(Mediolanum, Ital.)*; Calcihep *(Weddel, Austral.)*; Calcilean *(Organon Teknika, Canad.)*; Calciparin *(Labaz, Ger.)*; Calciparina *(Italfarmaco, Ital.*; *Labaz, Spain)*; Calciparine *(Bull, Austral.*; *Anglo-French Laboratories, Canad.*; *Choay, Fr.*; *Choay Lab, S.Afr.*; *Choay, Switz.*; *Sanofi, UK*; *American Critical Care, USA)*; Calparine *(Belg.*; *Neth.)*; Caprin *(Commonwealth Serum Laboratories, Austral.)*; Chemyparin *(SIT, Ital.)*; Clarisco *(Schwarz, Ital.)*; Clearane *(Ital.)*; Co-Lipase *(ABC, Ital.)*; Croneparina *(Mediolanum, Ital.)*; Cuthéparine *(Biosédra, Fr.*; *Switz.)*; Darkinal *(Spain)*; Disebrin *(Allergan, Ital.)*; Ecasolv *(Lepetit, Ital.)*; Eparical *(Nattermann, Ital.)*; Eparinoral *(Ital.)*; Eparinovis *(INTES, Ital.)*; Hämocura *(Ger.)*; HépaGel *(Spirig, Switz.)*; Héparine *(Fresenius, Switz.*; *KabiVitrum, Switz.*; *Novo, Switz.)*; Hepacarin *(Jpn)*; Hepalean *(Organon Teknika, Canad.)*; Heparinin *(Jpn)*; Hep-Flush *(Leo, UK)*; Hep-Lock *(Elkins-Sinn, USA)*; Heplok *(Leo, UK)*; Heprinar *(USA)*; Hep-Rinse *(Leo, UK)*; Hepsal *(CP Pharmaceuticals, UK)*; Lioton *(Menarini, Ital.)*; Lipo-Hepin *(Canad.*; *Riker, USA)*; Liquaemin *(Organon, USA)*; Liquémine *(Roche, Fr.*; *Roche, Switz.)*; Liquemin *(Roche, Ger.*; *Roche, Ital.*; *Neth.)*; Liquemine *(Arg.*; *Belg.*; *Roche, Spain)*; Minihep

(Leo, Canad.; Leo, UK); Minihep Calcium *(Leo, UK)*; Monoparin *(CP Pharmaceuticals, UK)*; Monoparin Calcium *(CP Pharmaceuticals, UK)*; Multiparin *(CP Pharmaceuticals, UK)*; Noparin *(Novo, Denm.; Novo, Swed.)*; Ox-Hep *(Leo, Denm.)*; Panheprin *(Jpn; USA)*; Percase *(Salac, Fr.)*; Praecivenin *(Pfleger, Ger.)*; Pularin *(Allen & Hanburys, S.Afr.; Evans Medical, UK)*; Pularin-Ca *(Evans Medical, UK)*; Pularine *(Belg.)*; Pump-Hep *(Leo, UK)*; Thrombareduct *(Azuchemie, Ger.)*; Thromboliquine *(Neth.; Organon, Swed.)*; Thrombophob *(Nordmark, Ger.; Nordmark, Swed.; Knoll, Switz.)*; Thrombo-Vetren *(Promonta, Ger.)*; Unihep *(Leo, UK)*; Uniparin *(Weddel, Austral.; CP Pharmaceuticals, UK)*; Uniparin Calcium *(CP Pharmaceuticals, UK)*; Uniparin Forte *(CP Pharmaceuticals, UK)*; Uniparin-Ca *(Weddel, Austral.)*; Vetren *(Promonta, Ger.; Wyeth, USA)*.

The following names have been used for multi-ingredient preparations containing heparin salts— Embolex *(Sandoz, USA)*; Hepacort Plus *(Lipha, UK)*; Lipactin *(Ciba-Geigy, Canad.)*; Reparil Gel *(Ibi Ital.)*.

18636-z

Low Molecular Weight Heparins

LMW Heparins.

NOTE. There are different forms of these heparin fractions. One fraction was formerly known as enoxaparin (PK-10169) and another as tedelparin.

Low molecular weight heparin fractions are used in the treatment and prophylaxis of thrombo-embolisms. They are not considered to have heparin's adverse effects on the platelets.

Low molecular weight heparin (enoxaparin) 30 mg was given subcutaneously twice daily in a placebo-controlled study of thrombo-embolism prophylaxis in 100 patients undergoing hip surgery. Treatment started 12 to 24 hours after surgery and continued for 14 days or until discharge. There was a significantly lower incidence of venous thrombosis in the group given low molecular weight heparin.— A. G. G. Turpie *et al., New Engl. J. Med.*, 1986, *315*, 925. Comment on the need for units for low-molecular-weight heparins as their specific activities may vary from batch to batch.— H. Bounameaux (letter), *ibid.*, *316*, 949.

References to the use of the low molecular weight heparin formerly known as tedelparin: M. Koller *et al., Thromb. Haemostasis*, 1986, *56*, 243 (surgery prophylaxis); B. Ljungberg *et al., Clin. Nephrol.*, 1987, *27*, 31 (use in haemodialysis).

Proprietary Names and Manufacturers

Fragmin *(Kabi, Ger.; Kabi, Swed.)*; Fragmine *(Kabivitrum, Fr.)*; Lovenox *(Pharmuka, Fr.)*.

3872-k

Heparinoids

A number of heparin derivatives, known as heparinoids, are in use or under investigation; these include A-73025 or SSHA-73025 and other glycosaminoglycan polysulphate compounds. Org-10172 and sodium apolate, though not heparin derivatives, are similar heparinoid substances. Preparations of these compounds are available with uses ranging from anticoagulation to the alleviation of inflammation.

There are also low molecular weight heparins, see above.

Proprietary Preparations

Anacal *(Panpharma, UK). Ointment* , a heparinoid 0.2%, prednisolone 0.15%, laureth 9 5%, hexachlorophane 0.5%.

Suppositories, a heparinoid 0.2%, prednisolone 0.05%, laureth 9 2.5%, hexachlorophane 0.25%. For haemorrhoids and ano-rectal disorders.

Hirudoid *(Panpharma, UK). Cream, Gel*, a heparinoid 300 mg (25 000 units)/100 g. For topical anticoagulant and anti-inflammatory therapy.

For reports of the use of Hirudoid, see B. S. S. Acharya, *Practitioner*, 1973, *211*, 371; H. Tronnier, *Clin. Trials J.*, 1973, *10*, 91; M. Fateh, *ibid.*, 122; P. P. Mehta *et al., Br. med. J.*, 1975, *3*, 614.

Movelat *(Panpharma, UK). Cream, Gel*, a heparinoid 200 mg, adrenal extract (total corticosteroid content 2%) 1 g, salicylic acid 2 g/ 100g. For inflammatory and arthritic conditions.

In a controlled study in 97 patients the application of Movelat three times daily over the cannula site reduced, by about half, the incidence of thrombophlebitis in patients receiving intravenous infusions expected to last 48 hours or longer.— C. R. J. Woodhouse, *Br. med. J.*, 1979, *1*, 454. Further references.— B. L. Bisley *et al., Br. J. clin. Pract.*, 1972, *26*, 477.

Proprietary Names and Manufacturers

Arteparon *(Luitpold, Ger.; Luitpold, Ital.; Luitpold, S.Afr.; Alfarma, Spain; Luitpold, Switz.)*; Fraxiparine *(Choay, Fr.)*; Hemeran *(Zyma, Ger.; Geigy, Switz.)*; Heparilene *(Clariana, Spain)*; Hirudoid *(Luitpold, Austral.; Luitpold, Denm.; Luitpold, Ger.; Luitpold, Ital.; Neth.; Luitpold, Norw.; Luitpold, S.Afr.; Alfarma, Spain; Luitpold, Switz.; Panpharma, UK)*; Lasoven *(Sigurtà, Ital.)*; Mesarin *(Spain)*.

The following names have been used for multi-ingredient preparations containing heparinoids— Anacal *(Panpharma, UK)*; Bayolin *(Bayer, UK)*; Feparil *(Madaus Cerafarm, Spain)*; Lasonil *(Bayer, Austral.; Bayer, UK)*; Mobilat; Movelat *(Luitpold, Austral.; Panpharma, UK)*; Reparil Gel *(Madaus, Ger.; Madaus, Switz.)*; Venostasin *(Madaus, Switz.)*.

4816-k

Leech

Blutegel; Hirudo; Sangsue; Sanguessugas; Sanguisuga.

Pharmacopoeias. In *Chin., Hung.*, and *Port.*

Leeches used in medicine are fresh-water annelids; the speckled or German leech and the green or Hungarian leech are varieties of *Hirudo medicinalis*, and the five-striped or Australian leech is *H. quinquestriata* (Hirudinidae).

Leeches should be stored in unglazed earthenware pans, half-filled with soft water, and having pebbles, turf, or moss and charcoal on the bottom; the pans should be securely covered with muslin and kept in a shady place at a temperature between 10° and 20°.

Leeches are used for withdrawing blood from inflamed and congested areas and have been found to be of value in plastic surgery. The buccal secretion of the leech contains the anticoagulant hirudin. The part to be bitten may be moistened with sugar solution before applying the leech. About 6 mL of blood is withdrawn by each leech. Once used a leech should not be applied to another patient.

There have been reports of wound infection from *Aeromonas hydrophila* transmitted by leeches.

Hirudin has been extracted from leeches and has more recently been prepared by recombinant technology.

A description of the leech, its care, and method of use.— P. S. Braidwood, *Pharm. J.*, 1987, *2*, 766.

Mention of enzymes from leeches, including hirudin which is an anticoagulant, hementin which is an antithrombin agent, and orgelase which degrades hyaluronic acid. These enzymes are prepared by *Biopharm, UK* which also supplies live leeches.— *Pharm. J.*, 1985, *2*, 48.

Dickson *et al.* (*Br. med. J.*, 1984, *289*, 1727) reported a case of wound infection due to *Aeromonas hydrophila* acquired from leeches used for decongestion in plastic surgery. Subsequently Mercer *et al.* (*ibid.*, 1987, *294*, 937) reported 6 cases of similar infection occurring over a period of 3 years when they would have used leeches on about 30 patients - an infection rate of 20%. All but one of the strains were resistant to penicillin and ampicillin; successful treatment was with amoxycillin, with or without clavulanic acid, or with cefuroxime.

4817-a

Nicoumalone *(BAN).*

Acenocoumarol *(rINN)*; Acenocumarin; G-23350. 4-Hydroxy-3-[1-(4-nitrophenyl)-3-oxobutyl]coumarin.

$C_{19}H_{15}NO_6$=353.3.

CAS — 152-72-7.

Pharmacopoeias. In *Br., Braz.*, and *Ind.*

An almost white to buff-coloured odourless or almost odourless powder.

Practically **insoluble** in water and ether; slightly soluble in alcohol and in chloroform; soluble in aqueous solutions of alkali hydroxides.

Adverse Effects, Treatment, and Precautions

As for warfarin sodium (p.344).

The interactions associated with oral anticoagulants are discussed in detail under warfarin. Specific references to interactions involving nicoumalone can be found there under the headings for the following drug groups: analgesics; anti-arrhythmics; antibacterial agents; antifungal agents; beta-blockers; diuretics; gastro-intestinal agents; sex hormones; uricosuric agents; vasodilators; and vitamins.

Deafness due to a haemorrhagic bulla in a patient taking nicoumalone. The bulla and the deafness resolved on withdrawing the nicoumalone.— R. Feinmesser *et al., Br. med. J.*, 1986, *292*, 992.

PREGNANCY AND THE NEONATE. For a report of nicoumalone embryopathy see Pregnancy and the Neonate in the Adverse Effects Section of warfarin sodium (p.344).

Absorption and Fate

Nicoumalone is readily absorbed from the gastro-intestinal tract and is excreted in the urine mainly as metabolites. Nicoumalone is extensively bound to plasma proteins. Reports show an elimination half-life ranging from 3 to 11 hours. Its stereo-isomers have different pharmacokinetics and actions.

References to the pharmacokinetics of nicoumalone: J. Godbillon *et al., Br. J. clin. Pharmac.*, 1981, *12*, 621; H. H. W. Thijssen and L. G. Baars, *ibid.*, 1983, *16*, 491; T. S. Gill *et al., J. Pharm. Pharmac.*, 1984, *36*, *Suppl.*, 12P.

Uses and Administration

Nicoumalone is an orally administered coumarin anticoagulant with actions and uses similar to those of warfarin sodium (p.348). The usual dose on the first day is 8 to 12 mg, on the second day 4 to 8 mg, and with a maintenance dose ranging from 1 to 8 mg depending on the response.

Whereas $R(+)$-nicoumalone produced an increase in the prothrombin time in 4 healthy subjects, $S(-)$-nicoumalone was ineffective in 3 subjects. The $R(+)$ enantiomer of nicoumalone was considered to be the pharmacologically active component of nicoumalone.— T. Meinertz *et al.* (letter), *Br. J. clin. Pharmac.*, 1978, *5*, 187.

Preparations

Nicoumalone Tablets *(B.P.)*

Proprietary Preparations

Sinthrome *(Geigy, UK). Tablets*, nicoumalone 1 mg and 4 mg (scored).

Proprietary Names and Manufacturers

Sinthrome *(Geigy, UK)*; Sintrom *(Arg.; Geigy, Austral.; Belg.; Geigy, Canad.; Geigy, Fr.; Ciba, Ger.; Geigy, Ital.; Neth.; Ciba, Spain; Geigy, Switz.)*.

3155-e

Org-10172

Org-10172 is a low-molecular-weight heparinoid isolated from porcine mucosa considered to carry a lower risk of haemorrhage than heparin but to have its anticoagulant activity.

The clinical pharmacology of Org-10172.— I. D. Bradbrook *et al., Br. J. clin. Pharmac.*, 1987, *23*, 667.

There was a significantly reduced incidence of venous thrombosis in 44 patients given Org-10172 following a stroke compared with 23 similar patients given placebo. The dose of Org-10172 consisted of a loading dose of 1000 anti-factor-Xa units intravenously followed by 750 units every 12 hours subcutaneously.— A. G. G. Turpie *et al., Lancet*, 1987, *1*, 523.

Further references to the use of Org-10172: Ch. P. Henny *et al., Lancet*, 1983, *1*, 890 (use in haemodialysis); J. Harenberg *et al.* (letter), *ibid.*, 986 (heparin-induced thrombocytopenia with thrombosis).

Proprietary Names and Manufacturers

Organon, Neth.

4818-t

Phenindione *(BAN, USAN, rINN).*
Fenindiona; Phenylindanedione; Phenylinium. 2-Phenylindan-1,3-dione.
$C_{15}H_{10}O_2$=222.2.

CAS — 83-12-5.

Pharmacopoeias. In *Arg., Br., Braz., Ind., Rus., Turk.,* and *U.S.*

Soft, odourless or almost odourless, white or creamy-white or pale yellow crystals or crystalline powder. *B.P.* **solubilities** are: very slightly soluble in water; slightly soluble in alcohol and in ether; freely soluble in chloroform. *U.S.P.* solubilities are: soluble 1 in 5000 of water, 1 in 100 of alcohol, 1 in 7 of chloroform, and 1 in 110 of ether, forming yellow to red solutions; soluble 1 in 100 of 0.1M sodium hydroxide solution. **Store** in well-closed containers.

Adverse Effects and Treatment
Like warfarin (p.344) phenindione and the other indanediones can cause haemorrhage and hypersensitivity reactions, but they are generally more toxic with the reactions involving many organs sometimes resulting in death. Some of the reactions include skin rashes, pyrexia, diarrhoea, vomiting, sore throat, liver and kidney damage, exfoliative dermatitis, myocarditis, agranulocytosis, leucopenia, eosinophilia, and a leukaemoid syndrome.
Phenindione may discolour the urine pink or orange and this is independent of any haematuria. Taste disturbances have been reported.
Treatment of adverse effects is as for warfarin (p.344).

EFFECTS ON THE GASTRO-INTESTINAL TRACT. There have been some early cases of paralytic ileus associated with phenindione, see: I. S. Menon (letter), *Lancet,* 1966, *1,* 1421; A. G. Nash (letter), *ibid.,* 1966, *2,* 51.

PREGNANCY AND THE NEONATE. Congenital malformations including hypoplasia of the nasal bones occurred in 3 infants whose mothers had received warfarin or phenindione during the first trimester of pregnancy. Other effects included stippling of epiphyses and bones.— J. M. Pettifor and R. Benson, *J. Pediat.,* 1975, *86,* 459.

Precautions
As for warfarin sodium (p.344).
Phenindione is not recommended in pregnancy. Unlike warfarin it is excreted in breast milk so should not be given to breast-feeding women.
The interactions associated with oral anticoagulants are described in detail under warfarin. Specific references to interactions involving phenindione can be found there under the headings for the following drug groups: analgesics; antibacterial agents; antifungal agents; corticosteroids and corticotrophin; gastro-intestinal agents; lipid regulating agents; sedatives and neuroleptics; sex hormones; and vasodilators.

Absorption and Fate
Phenindione is absorbed from the gastro-intestinal tract. It diffuses across the placenta and appears in breast milk. A metabolite of phenindione excreted in the urine is responsible for any discoloration.

Uses and Administration
Phenindione is an orally administered indanedione anticoagulant with actions and uses similar to those of warfarin sodium (see p.348), but because of its higher incidence of severe adverse effects it is now rarely employed.
The usual initial dose of phenindione is 200 mg on the first day, 100 mg on the second day, and then maintenance doses of 50 to 150 mg daily according to coagulation tests.

Preparations
Phenindione Tablets *(B.P.)*
Phenindione Tablets *(U.S.P.)*

Proprietary Preparations
Dindevan *(Duncan, Flockhart, UK). Tablets,* phenindione 10, 25, and 50 mg.

Proprietary Names and Manufacturers
Danilone *(Canad.)*; Dindevan *(Glaxo, Austral.; Nyco, Denm.; Allen & Hanburys, S.Afr.; Duncan, Flockhart, UK)*; Emandione *(Ital.)*; Hedulin *(USA)*; Pindione *(Belg.; Oberval, Fr.; Vaillant, Ital.; Switz.)*; Trombantin *(Norw.)*.

4819-x

Phenprocoumon *(BAN, USAN, rINN).*
Phenylpropylhydroxycoumarin. 4-Hydroxy-3-(1-phenylpropyl)coumarin.
$C_{18}H_{16}O_3$=280.3.

CAS — 435-97-2.

Pharmacopoeias. In *U.S.*

A fine white crystalline powder, odourless or with a slight odour. Practically **insoluble** in water; soluble in chloroform, methyl alcohol, and solutions of alkali hydroxides. **Store** in well-closed containers.

Adverse Effects and Treatment
As for warfarin sodium (p.344).

EFFECTS ON THE LIVER. A woman who had twice previously developed jaundice while taking phenprocoumon developed jaundice and parenchymal liver damage when, after some years, phenprocoumon was again given.— W. den Boer and E. A. Loeliger (letter), *Lancet,* 1976, *1,* 912. Two cases of phenprocoumon-associated hepatitis.— G. Slagboom and E. A. Loeliger, *Archs intern. Med.,* 1980, *140,* 1028.

Precautions
As for warfarin sodium (p.344).
The interactions associated with oral anticoagulants are discussed in detail under warfarin. Specific references to interactions involving phenprocoumon can be found there under the headings for the following drug groups: analgesics; anti-arrhythmics, antibacterial agents; antidepressants; antidiabetic agents; beta-blockers; gastro-intestinal agents; lipid regulating agents; sedatives and neuroleptics; sex hormones; uricosuric agents; and vasodilators.

Increased clearance of phenprocoumon in patients with liver cirrhosis. Possible mechanisms are altered enterohepatic circulation, decreased plasma protein binding, or a change in glucuronyl transferase activity.— N. R. Kitteringham *et al., Br. J. clin. Pharmac.,* 1983, *15,* 590P.

Absorption and Fate
Phenprocoumon is readily absorbed from the gastro-intestinal tract and is extensively bound to plasma proteins. It is excreted in the urine and faeces as conjugated hydroxy metabolites and parent compound.

The plasma half-life of phenprocoumon was 6.5 days.— R. A. O'Reilly and P. M. Aggeler, *Pharmac. Rev.,* 1970, *22,* 35. In 4 patients with acute myocardial infarction the half-life of phenprocoumon was 2.7 to 5.5 days, and 2.8 to 7.0 days in 5 patients with chronic cardiovascular disease.— S. Husted and F. Andreasen, *Eur. J. clin. Pharmac.,* 1977, *11,* 351.

Investigations *in vitro* into the binding of phenprocoumon to human serum albumin using fluorescence spectroscopy. Results indicated that the affinity for the *S*(−)-enantiomer of phenprocoumon is greater than the affinity for the *R*(+)-enantiomer for both the first and second binding site on crystalline human serum albumin and that the racemic form, the commercial form of phenprocoumon, had intermediate behaviour.— M. Otagiri *et al., J. Pharm. Pharmac.,* 1980, *32,* 478.

The metabolic fate of phenprocoumon in healthy subjects.— S. Toon *et al., J. pharm. Sci.,* 1985, *74,* 1037.

Uses and Administration
Phenprocoumon is an orally administered coumarin anticoagulant with actions and uses similar to those of warfarin sodium (p.348). Initial doses of up to 24 mg have been reported. Maintenance doses have ranged from 0.75 to 6 mg daily, depending on the response.

S(−)-phenprocoumon was a more potent anticoagulant than *R*(+)-phenprocoumon.— E. Jähnchen *et al., Clin. Pharmac. Ther.,* 1976, *20,* 342.

Preparations
Phenprocoumon Tablets *(U.S.P.)*

Proprietary Names and Manufacturers
Liquamar *(Organon, USA)*; Marcoumar *(Roche, Belg.; Roche, Denm.; Roche, Neth.; Roche, Switz.; Roche, UK)*; Marcumar *(Roche, Canad.; Roche, Ger.; Roche, Spain)*.

13240-n

Sodium Apolate *(BAN, rINN).*
Lyapolate Sodium *(USAN).* Poly(sodium ethylenesulphonate).
$(C_2H_3NaO_3S)_n$.

CAS — 25053-27-4.

Sodium apolate is a synthetic heparinoid anticoagulant. It has been tried in the topical treatment of haematomas and for the relief of sprains and contusions.

Proprietary Names and Manufacturers
Pergagel *(Albert-Roussel, Ger.)*.

The following names have been used for multi-ingredient preparations containing sodium apolate— Pergalen *(Hoechst, Austral.)*.

4820-y

Sodium Iodoheparinate
Iodohéparinate de Sodium.

Sodium iodoheparinate 1 mg is stated to be equivalent to 100 units of heparin.

Sodium iodoheparinate is a derivative of heparin (see p.339) that has been given or applied in a variety of inflammatory conditions.

Proprietary Names and Manufacturers
Dioparine *(Biosédra, Fr.; Faure, Fr.; Biosedra, Switz.)*.

4821-j

Sodium Pentosan Polysulphate
Sodium Xylanpolysulphate. A synthetic sulphated polyanion with heparin-like properties.

CAS — 37319-17-8.

Sodium pentosan polysulphate has anticoagulant and fibrinolytic properties; its anticoagulant effect is less than that of heparin. As well as being used in thrombo-embolic disorders it has been tried in a number of conditions including haemorrhagic cystitis following radiotherapy and in the inhibition of calcium oxalate stones.

References to the effect of sodium pentosan polysulphate on the blood: G. Frandoli *et al., Arzneimittel-Forsch.,* 1972, *22,* 759 (anticoagulant, fibrinolytic, and hypolipidaemic); S. Joffe, *Archs Surg.,* 1976, *111,* 37 (less effective than heparin); 1976, *235,* H. Greten *et al., Dt. med. Wschr.,* 1978, *103,* 204 (no lasting effect on serum lipids).

CYSTITIS. Successful management of radiation cystitis with sodium pentosan polysulphate.— C. L. Parsons, *J. Urol., Baltimore,* 1986, *136,* 813.

RENAL CALCULI. Inhibition of calcium oxalate crystallisation by sodium pentosan polysulphate.— R. W. Norman *et al., Br. J. Urol.,* 1984, *56,* 594.

Proprietary Names and Manufacturers
Fibrase *(Smith Kline & French, Ital.)*; Hémoclar *(Midy, Fr.)*; SP 54 *(Bene, Ger.)*; Tavan-SP 54 *(Ethimed, S.Afr.)*; Thrombocid *(Bene, Ger.; Smith Kline & French, Ital.; Lacer, Spain; Bene-Arzneimittel, Switz.)*.

13347-l

Tioclomarol *(rINN).*
LM-550. 3-[5-Chloro-α-(4-chloro-β-hydroxyphenethyl)-2-thenyl]-4-hydroxycoumarin.
$C_{22}H_{16}Cl_2O_4S$=447.3.

CAS — 22619-35-8.

Tioclomarol is an oral coumarin anticoagulant.

Proprietary Names and Manufacturers
Apegmone *(Oberval, Fr.)*.

4822-z

Warfarin Potassium *(BANM, USAN, rINNM).*

Potassium Warfarin; Warfarinum Kalicum.
$C_{19}H_{15}KO_4$=346.4.

CAS — 2610-86-8.

Pharmacopoeias. In *Jpn* and *U.S.*

A white odourless crystalline powder with a slightly bitter taste. **Soluble** 1 in 1.5 of water and 1 in 1.9 of alcohol; very slightly soluble in chloroform and in ether. A 1% solution in water has a pH of 7.2 to 8.3. **Store** in well-closed containers. Protect from light.

4823-c

Warfarin Sodium *(BANM, USAN, rINNM).*

Sodium Warfarin; Warfarin Sod.; Warfarinum Natricum. The sodium salt of 4-hydroxy-3-(3-oxo-1-phenylbutyl)coumarin.
$C_{19}H_{15}NaO_4$=330.3.

CAS — 81-81-2 (warfarin); 129-06-6 (sodium salt).

Pharmacopoeias. In *Br., Braz., Chin., Egypt., Int., Nord., Turk.,* and *U.S. B.P., Braz. P.,* and *U.S.P.* permit also the use of the crystalline clathrate with isopropyl alcohol.

A white odourless or almost odourless amorphous or crystalline powder; it is discoloured by light. **Soluble** 1 in less than 1 of water and alcohol; slightly or very slightly soluble in chloroform and ether. A 1% solution in water has a pH of 7.2 to 8.3. **Store** in well-closed containers. Protect from light.

Incompatibility has been reported with adrenaline hydrochloride, amikacin sulphate, metaraminol tartrate, oxytocin, promazine hydrochloride, tetracycline hydrochloride, and vancomycin hydrochloride.

NOTE. Commercial warfarin sodium is racemic.

Absorption of warfarin sodium increasing with time occurred when solutions in water were exposed to polyvinyl chloride infusion bags. Absorption was greater when glucose injection was the diluent.— P. Moorhatch and W. L. Chiou, *Am. J. Hosp. Pharm.*, 1974, *31*, 72.

Adverse Effects

The major risk from warfarin therapy is of haemorrhage from almost any organ of the body with the consequent effects of haematomas as well as anaemia. Skin necrosis is an occasional effect seen usually in obese elderly subjects. A purple discoloration of the toes has sometimes been observed. Other effects not necessarily associated with haemorrhage include alopecia, fever, nausea, vomiting, diarrhoea, hypersensitivity reactions, priapism, and skin reactions.

Warfarin is a recognised teratogen. Given in the first trimester of pregnancy it can cause a foetal warfarin syndrome with bone stippling (chondrodysplasia punctata) and facial and CNS abnormalities; the CNS abnormalities may develop following administration in the second or third trimester. Administration in the late stages of pregnancy is associated with foetal haemorrhage. In addition warfarin is associated with an increased abortion rate. The reported incidence of the foetal warfarin syndrome has ranged from about 5% up to about 30%.

In Great Britain the recommended exposure limits of wafarin are 0.1 mg per m^3 (long-term); 0.3 mg per m^3 (short-term).

Many of the adverse effects in the reports cited below can be attributed to the haemorrhage caused by the anticoagulant. Bleeding may arise through poor control, although Levine *et al.* (*Drugs*, 1985, *30*, 444) observed that haemorrhage often occurred when treatment appeared to be keeping the patient under control as specified by coagulation tests. There may be some improvement in this area with the increased use of the international normalised ratio (INR) for laboratory control. Levine *et al.* also pointed out that there was a risk of bleeding associated with the condition requiring anticoagulation and in addition that patients often had underlying risks, a point supported by Schuster *et al.* in their study of patients who developed haematuria (*J. Urol, Baltimore*, 1987, *137*, 923).

EFFECTS ON THE EYE. Retinal haemorrhage from warfarin leading to blindness.— K. Maddox (letter), *Med. J. Aust.*, 1977, *1*, 420.

EFFECTS ON THE KIDNEY. Spontaneous unilateral kidney rupture occurred in 2 patients who were treated with warfarin sodium. Nephrectomy was performed but only 1 patient survived.— I. Luna *et al.*, *J. Urol., Baltimore*, 1973, *109*, 788.

See also above for a reference to haematuria.

EFFECTS ON THE LIVER. Signs of liver cell necrosis in 2 patients regressed only when anticoagulants (warfarin and dicoumarol) were withdrawn.— N. Rehnquist, *Acta med. scand.*, 1978, *204*, 335.

Intrahepatic cholestasis following warfarin therapy; the patient recovered on withdrawal of warfarin.— D. B. Jones *et al.*, *Postgrad. med. J.*, 1980, *56*, 671.

Reports of hepatic rupture in patients taking warfarin: M. H. Roberts and F. R. Johnston, *Archs Surg.*, 1975, *110*, 1152; H. Dizadji *et al.*, *ibid.*, 1979, *114*, 734.

EFFECTS ON THE OVARY. Reports of haemorrhage from the corpus luteum in patients taking warfarin: J. R. Krause and R. Amores, *Sth. med. J.*, 1976, *69*, 1220; K. P. Wong and P. G. Gillett, *Can. med. Ass. J.*, 1977, *116*, 388; D. D. Tresch *et al.*, *Ann. intern. Med.*, 1978, *88*, 642.

EFFECTS ON THE SKIN. There have been a number of reports of necrosis of the skin and subcutaneous tissue in patients taking warfarin. Areas involved have included the breast and penis.— M. DiCato and L. Ellman (letter), *Ann. intern. Med.*, 1975, *83*, 233; J. P. Lacy and R. R. Goodin (letter), *ibid.*, *82*, 381; C. D. Haynes *et al.*, *Sth. med. J.*, 1983, *76*, 1091; W. G. McGehee *et al.*, *Ann. intern. Med.*, 1984, *101*, 59; G. Hermann *et al.*, *J. Am. med. Ass.*, 1986, *255*, 939.

Kirby and Brearley (*Br. J. Derm.*, 1978, *98*, 707) considered that the risk of necrosis should be reduced by following the usual practice of starting treatment with incremental doses of warfarin sodium rather than with a large loading dose. Protein C deficiency or depression might also play some part in the development of necrosis (W.G. McGehee *et al.*, 1984; A.W. Broekmans *et al.*, *Thromb. Haemostasis*, 1983, *49*, 251).

PREGNANCY AND THE NEONATE. Reviews of warfarin's effects on the foetus: R. M. Pauli and J. G. Hall (letter), *Lancet*, 1979, *2*, 144; J. G. Hall *et al.*, *Am. J. Med.*, 1980, *68*, 122; L. M. Hill and F. Kleinberg, *Mayo Clin. Proc.*, 1984, *59*, 755; *Drug & Ther. Bull.*, 1987, *25*, 1; M. De Swiet, *Br. med. J.*, 1987, *294*, 428; J. E. Dixon, *Br. J. Hosp. Med.*, 1987, *38*, 449.

Coumarin embryopathy occurred in 8 of 27 foetuses (29.6%) whose mothers continued nicoumalone throughout pregnancy; in 2 of 8 who had nicoumalone withdrawn between the 7th and 11th week and replaced by heparin; in 0 of 19 who had nicoumalone withdrawn before the 6th week and reinstated in the 13th week, heparin being used in the interim.— I. Iturbe-Alessio *et al.*, *New Engl. J. Med.*, 1986, *315*, 1390.

Treatment of Adverse Effects

Mild bleeding due to overdosage of warfarin sodium is usually adequately controlled by discontinuing the drug. Phytomenadione 2 to 10 or sometimes 20 mg by mouth is usually effective in treating the effects of overdosage. Severe hypoprothrombinaemia may be treated by the slow intravenous injection of 2.5 to 10 mg of phytomenadione. The dose of phytomenadione should be the smallest needed to control bleeding. Phytomenadione takes several hours to act and reduces the response to resumed therapy with anticoagulants for up to several weeks. A rapid response can be achieved by injecting fresh frozen plasma or concentrates of factors II, IX, and X.

The international normalised ratio (INR) should be used as a guide to the treatment or prevention of haemorrhage.

Cholestyramine was considered to have played a useful role in the elimination of warfarin in a patient being treated for warfarin overdose.— S. Renowden *et al.*, *Br. med. J.*, 1985, *291*, 513.

A suggestion that the administration of protein C to correct protein C deficiency at the beginning of treatment with warfarin could prevent warfarin-induced necrosis.— L. H. Clouse and P. C. Comp, *New Engl. J. Med.*, 1986, *314*, 1298.

Precautions

Warfarin should not be given to patients who are haemorrhaging. In general it should not be given to patients at serious risk of haemorrhage, although it has been used with very careful control; patients at risk include those with haemorrhagic blood disorders, peptic ulcers, severe wounds (including surgical wounds), and bacterial endocarditis. Severe kidney and liver impairment as well as severe hypertension are considered by some to be contra-indications. Pregnancy is also considered by some to be a contra-indication, but others have given warfarin to pregnant women during the periods of least risk.

The elderly and patients with vitamin-K deficiency require special care as do patients with hyperthyroidism.

Patients may display resistance to warfarin for any of the reasons apparent in this precautions section. However, a few patients have displayed a hereditary resistance.

Many compounds interact with warfarin and other oral anticoagulants. Details of these interactions are given below for all oral anticoagulants with different groups of drugs; if the anticoagulant is other than warfarin, then its identity is given after each reference. Readers should be aware that while interactions of a pharmacodynamic nature occurring with one anticoagulant may well apply to another, this is not necessarily the case with interactions of a pharmacokinetic nature.

An interaction may be due to increased or decreased anticoagulant metabolism; with warfarin some interacting drugs such as co-trimoxazole or phenylbutazone have a selective effect on its stereo-isomers. Altered absorption may sometimes play a part as with cholestyramine. Not all reports that have recorded an alteration in the pharmacokinetics of the anticoagulant have shown a corresponding change in clinical response.

There are drugs other than anticoagulants that are capable of altering the coagulation process and causing haemorrhage and this can play a part in their interactions with anticoagulants, as with thyroid hormones, and clofibrate; aspirin also has a complex action on coagulation. Even though interactions may not have been reported with anticoagulants and compounds with haematological effects, the potential for an increased risk of haemorrhage should be borne in mind. Some of the compounds that carry this risk and not covered in the details provided below include colaspase, some contrast media, epoprostenol, streptokinase, and urokinase.

Where there is a risk of serious haemorrhage from an interaction, then use of the 2 drugs is best avoided. In other instances the anticoagulant activity should be carefully monitored so as to increase or decrease the anticoagulant dose as required. Critical periods are when patients stabilised on an anticoagulant commence treatment with an interacting drug, or when patients stabilised on a regimen of an interacting drug and anticoagulant have the interacting drug withdrawn. Depending on the mechanism of the interaction, the clinical response to the interaction may be rapid or may take some days. Readers should also be aware that some interacting drugs do not produce predictable effects; there have for instance been reports of increased as well as decreased anticoagulant activity with allopurinol, with disopyramide, and with oral contraceptives. Another problem occurs with dipyridamole; it can cause bleeding when given to patients taking anticoagulants but without any changes in the measures used for anticoagulant control.

Drugs recognised or generally reported as enhancing oral anticoagulants are included in the following list. Further information on the interactions with these drugs and others where the interaction is not so well recognised is provided in

the referenced section below.
Alcohol (acute ingestion), allopurinol, amiodarone,
aspirin, azapropazone, bezafibrate,
cephamandole, chloral hydrate, chloramphenicol,
cimetidine, clofibrate, co-trimoxazole,
danazol, dextropropoxyphene, dipyridamole,
disulfiram, erythromycin, ethacrynic acid,
ethyloestrenol, glucagon, halofenate,
ketoconazole, latamoxef, meclofenamate sodium,
mefenamic acid, metronidazole, miconazole,
norethandrolone, oxymetholone, oxyphenbutazone,
paracetamol, phenylbutazone, piroxicam,
quinidine, quinine, stanozolol,
sulindac, sulphinpyrazone, sulphonamides,
tetracyclines, thyroid, tienilic acid,
vitamin E.

Drugs generally recognised as diminishing the effects of oral anticoagulants are included in the following list. Further information on the interactions with these drugs and others where the interaction is not so well recognised is provided in the referenced section below.
Acetomenaphthone, alcohol (chronic ingestion),
aminoglutethimide,
barbiturates, carbamazepine, dichloralphenazone,
ethchlorvynol, glutethimide, griseofulvin,
oral contraceptives, phytomenadione, primidone,
rifampicin, spironolactone.

ANTICOAGULANT RESISTANCE. Lefrere *et al.* (*J. clin. Path.*, 1987, *40*, 242) in proposing a classification of resistances to oral anticoagulants briefly listed the mechanisms of resistance as: noncompliance, excessive vitamin K intake, drug interactions, malabsorption, altered metabolism, and hereditary resistance. Some references to hereditary resistance: R. A. O'Reilly, *New Engl. J. Med.*, 1970, *282*, 1448; J. Zager *et al.*, *Ann. intern. Med.*, 1973, *78*, 775; D. B. Barnett and B. W. Hancock, *Br. med. J.*, 1975, *1*, 608; B. M. Alving *et al.*, *Archs intern. Med.*, 1985, *145*, 499.

Warfarin Interactions

Some reviews of drug interactions involving warfarin: *Drug Interact. News.*, 1982, *2*, 21; A. Scott and M. L'E. Orme, *Adverse Drug React. Bull.*, 1983, (Dec.), 380; M. J. Serlin and A. M. Breckenridge, *Drugs*, 1983, *25*, 610; P. A. Routledge, *Prescribers' J.*, 1986, *26*, 71.

ALCOHOL. Alcohol has a variable effect on warfarin. Heavy regular drinkers may experience a diminished effect, perhaps through enzyme induction; acute ingestion has enhanced the effect of warfarin. A moderate alcohol intake is not considered to cause problems.
Alcoholics taking disulfiram will experience an enhanced effect to warfarin (see below).
References: *J. Am. med. Ass.*, 1968, *206*, 1709; J. A. Udall, *Clin. Med.*, 1970, *77*, (Aug.), 20; A. Breckenridge and M. Orme, *Ann. N.Y. Acad. Sci.*, 1971, *179*, 421; J. Koch-Weser and E. M. Sellers, *New Engl. J. Med.*, 1971, *285*, 547; R. A. O'Reilly, *Am. J. med. Sci.*, 1979, *277*, 189.

ANALGESICS AND NON-STEROIDAL ANTI-INFLAMMATORY AGENTS. Compounds that affect platelet function such as aspirin can cause problems in patients taking warfarin. (Sulphinpyrazone is discussed below under Uricosuric Agents; Dipyridamole is discussed below under Vasodilators.) Also aspirin has an irritant effect on the gastro-intestinal tract so increasing the risks of haemorrhage. Furthermore, aspirin can increase the activity of warfarin. Patients requiring analgesics are therefore recommended to take paracetamol, for although there have been some reports of it enhancing warfarin's activity it does not generally cause problems. Nor do the opioid analgesics, with the possible exception of dextropropoxyphene which can enhance warfarin.
Phenylbutazone given to patients taking warfarin has led to serious haemorrhage. It affects the metabolism of warfarin's *R* and *S* isomers in complex and different ways, but with the net effect of enhancing its anti-coagulant activity. Azapropazone has also led to serious effects.
When considering other non-steroidal anti-inflammatory agents one should be aware that many can have some effect on platelets, although not so much as to lead to an embargo on their careful use in patients taking warfarin. Indeed not all studies have shown an alteration of warfarin's activity.
References:
Reviews T. Pullar and H. A. Capell, *Scott. med. J.*, 1983, *28*, 42; *Drug Interact. News.*, 1983, *3*, 49; J. W. O'Callaghan *et al.*, *Can. med. Ass. J.*, 1984, *131*, 857.
Aspirin and salicylates J. A. Udall, *Clin. Med.*, 1970, *77* (Aug.), 20; R. A. O'Reilly *et al.*, *Ann. N.Y. Acad. Sci.*, 1971, *179*, 173; K. J. Starr and J. C. Petrie, *Br. med. J.*, 1972, *4*, 133; P. Barth *et al.*, *Dt. med. Wschr.*, 1972, *97*, 1854 (phenprocoumon).
Azapropazone P. R. Powell-Jackson, *Br. med. J.*, 1977, *1*, 1193; A. E. Green *et al.* (letter), *ibid.*, 1532; J. C. McElnay and P. F. D'Arcy (letter), *ibid.*, *2*, 773; *idem*, *J. Pharm. Pharmac.*, 1980, *32*, 709.
Cinchophen S. Jarnum, *Scand. J. clin. Lab. Invest.*, 1974, *6*, 91.
Dextropropoxyphene M. Orme *et al.*, *Br. med. J.*, 1976, *1*, 200; R. V. Jones (letter), *ibid.*, 460; R. Smith *et al.* (letter), *Drug Intell. & clin. Pharm.*, 1984, *18*, 822; *Drug Interact. News.*, 1984, *4*, 43.
Diclofenac sodium F. Michot *et al.*, *J. int. med. Res.*, 1975, *3*, 153 (nicoumalone).
Diflunisal K. F. Tempero *et al.*, *Br. J. clin. Pharmac.*, 1977, *4*, 31S (nicoumalone); M. J. Serlin *et al.*, *ibid.*, 1980, *9*, 287P.
Fenbufen J. P. Savitsky *et al.*, *Clin. Pharmac. Ther.*, 1980, *27*, 284.
Fenoprofen M. Otagiri *et al.*, *J. Pharm. Pharmac.*, 1980, *32*, 478 (phenprocoumon).
Feprazone S. Chierichetti *et al.*, *Curr. ther. Res.*, 1975, *18*, 568.
Flurbiprofen G. A. Marbet *et al.*, *Curr. med. Res. Opinion*, 1977, *5*, 26 (phenprocoumon); B. H. C. Stricker and J. L. Delhez (letter), *Br. med. J.*, 1982, *285*, 812 (nicoumalone).
Glafenine J. K. Boeijinga and W. J. F. van der Vijgh, *Eur. J. clin. Pharmac.*, 1977, *12*, 291 (phenprocoumon); C. Raby, *Thérapie*, 1977, *32*, 293 (ethyl biscoumacetate and nicoumalone).
Ibuprofen L. Goncalves, *J. int. med. Res.*, 1973, *1*, 180; D. Thilo *et al.*, *J. int. med. Res.*, 1974, *2*, 276 (phenprocoumon); M. J. Boekhout-Mussert and E. A. Loeliger, *ibid.*, 279 (phenprocoumon); J. A. Penner and P. H. Abbrecht, *Curr. ther. Res.*, 1975, *18*, 862; J. T. Slattery and G. Levy (letter), *J. pharm. Sci.*, 1977, *66*, 1060; M. Otagiri *et al.*, *J. Pharm. Pharmac.*, 1980, *32*, 478 (phenprocoumon); J. C. McElnay and P. F. D'Arcy, *ibid.*, 709.
Indomethacin M. J. Rand, *Australas. J. Pharm.*, 1971, *52*, S17 (phenindione); J. Koch-Weser, *Clin. Pharmac. Ther.*, 1973, *14*, 139; T. H. Self *et al.* (letter), *Lancet*, 1975, *2*, 557; E. S. Vesell *et al.*, *J. clin. Pharmac.*, 1975, *15*, 486; J. C. McElnay and P. F. D'Arcy, *J. Pharm. Pharmac.*, 1980, *32*, 709.
Ketoprofen J. C. McElnay and P. F. D'Arcy, *J. Pharm. Pharmac.*, 1980, *32*, 709.
Meclofenamate sodium F. D. Baragar and T. C. Smith, *Curr. ther. Res.*, 1978, *23*, *Suppl.* 4S, S51.
Mefenamic acid E. L. Holmes, *Ann. phys. Med.*, 1966, *8*, *Suppl.*, 36; E. M. Sellers and J. Koch-Weser, *Clin. Pharmac. Ther.*, 1970, *11*, 524; J. C. McElnay and P. F. D'Arcy, *J. Pharm. Pharmac.*, 1980, *32*, 709.
Meptazinol hydrochloride E. Ryd-Kjellen and A. Alm, *Hum. Toxicol.*, 1986, *5*, 101.
Naproxen A. Jain *et al.*, *Clin. Pharmac. Ther.*, 1979, *25*, 61; J. T. Slattery *et al.*, *ibid.*, 51; J. C. McElnay and P. F. D'Arcy, *J. Pharm. Pharmac.*, 1980, *32*, 709.
Oxyphenbutazone N. Kaplinsky *et al.* (letter), *J. Am. med. Ass.*, 1980, *243*, 513.
Paracetamol A. M. Antlitz *et al.*, *Curr. ther. Res.*, 1968, *10*, 501 (warfarin; anisindione; dicoumarol; phenprocoumon); A. M. Antlitz and L. F. Awalt, *ibid.*, 1969, *11*, 360; J. A. Udall, *Clin. Med.*, 1970, *77*, (Aug.), 20; J. J. Boeijinga *et al.* (letter), *Lancet*, 1982, *1*, 506; *Drug Interact. News.*, 1983, *3*, 55.
Phenazone A. Breckenridge and M. Orme, *Ann. N.Y. Acad. Sci.*, 1971, *179*, 421; J. B. Whitfield *et al.*, *Br. med. J.*, 1973, *1*, 316.
Phenylbutazone M. J. Eisen, *J. Am. med. Ass.*, 1964, *189*, 64; B. I. Hoffbrand and D. A. Kininmonth (letter), *Br. med. J.*, 1967, *2*, 838; P. M. Aggeler *et al.*, *New Engl. J. Med.*, 1967, *276*, 496; J. A. Udall, *Clin. Med.*, 1970, *77*, (Aug.), 20; S. Chierichetti *et al.*, *Curr. ther. Res.*, 1975, *18*, 568; R. A. O'Reilly, *Archs intern. Med.*, 1982, *142*, 1634 (phenprocoumon); C. Banfield *et al.*, *Br. J. clin. Pharmac.*, 1983, *16*, 669.
Phenyramidol S. A. Carter, *New Engl. J. Med.*, 1965, *273*, 423 (warfarin; dicoumarol; phenindione).
Piroxicam R. S. Rhodes *et al.*, *Drug Intell. & clin. Pharm.*, 1985, *19*, 556.
Sulindac S. A. Carter (letter), *Lancet*, 1979, *2*, 698; J. R. Y. Ross and L. Beeley (letter), *ibid.*, 1075; J. P. Loftin and E. S. Vesell, *J. clin. Pharmac.*, 1979, *19*, 733.
Tiaprofenic acid S. J. Whittaker *et al.*, *Br. J. clin. Pract.*, 1986, *40*, 440 (nicoumalone).

ANTI-ARRHYTHMICS. Both disopyramide and quinidine have been reported to have variable effects on warfarin requiring increases or reductions in its dose. Also there is a report of quinidine necessitating a dose increase of dicoumarol. Amiodarone has been shown in several studies to increase the activity of warfarin and nicoumalone, probably through inhibition of metabolism. There is an early report of phenprocoumon not being affected by amiodarone. A more recent report indicates that propafenone can enhance warfarin.
References:
Amiodarone M. Verstraete et al., *Archs int. Pharmacodyn. Thér.*, 1968, *176*, 33 (phenprocoumon); U. Martinowitz *et al.* (letter), *New Engl. J. Med.*, 1981, *304*, 671; A. Rees *et al.*, *Br. med. J.*, 1981, *282*, 1756; M. J. Serlin *et al.* (letter), *ibid.*, *283*, 58; A. Hamer *et al.*, *Circulation*, 1982, *65*, 1025; M. Arboix *et al.*, *Br. J. clin. Pharmac.*, 1984, *18*, 355 (nicoumalone); A. H. Watt *et al.*, *ibid.*, 1985, *20*, 707; S. Almog *et al.*, *Eur. J. clin. Pharmac.*, 1985, *28*, 257; C. Richard *et al.*, *ibid.*, 625 (nicoumalone); R. A. O'Reilly *et al.*, *Clin. Pharmac. Ther.*, 1987, *42*, 290.
Disopyramide E. Haworth and A. K. Burroughs, *Br. med. J.*, 1977, *2*, 866; C. Sylvén and P. Anderson, *Br. med. J.*, 1983, *286*, 1181.
Propafenone R. E. Kates *et al.*, *Clin. Pharmac. Ther.*, 1987, *42*, 305.
Quinidine J. Koch-Weser, *Ann. intern. Med.*, 1968, *68*, 511; A. B. Gazzaniga and D. R. Stewart, *New Engl. J. Med.*, 1969, *280*, 711; J. A. Udall, *Clin. Med.*, 1970, *77*, (Aug.), 20; C. Sylvén and P. Anderson, *Br. med. J.*, 1983, *286*, 1181 (warfarin and dicoumarol).

ANTIBACTERIAL AGENTS. Several antibacterial agents have been involved in interactions with warfarin. Only a few reports are of serious effects and it is unlikely that any of the agents need to be contra-indicated with warfarin; careful control should suffice.
Most of the agents enhance the effects of warfarin. Erythromycin does so probably by inhibition of warfarin's metabolism. Co-trimoxazole may have a stereospecific inhibitory effect on warfarin's metabolism; co-trimoxazole has been reported not to influence the effect of phenindione. For the other compounds the mechanism of the enhancement is less clear. A diminished effect occurs with rifampicin due to an induction of warfarin's metabolism. There is a report of a similar effect with nafcillin. All the other reports cited below deal with an enhancement of warfarin's activity and most are but individual case reports.
Aztreonam and latamoxef are not included in the following references, but they could increase anti-coagulation if given with warfarin. Metronidazole is discussed below under Antiprotozoal Agents. Readers should also be aware that some other antibiotics such as chloramphenicol and tetracycline have been reported to possess anticoagulant properties of their own.
References:
Aminosalicylic acid T. H. Self (letter), *J. Am. med. Ass.*, 1973, *223*, 1285.
Benzylpenicillin M. A. Brown *et al.*, *Can. J. Hosp. Pharm.*, 1979, *32*, 18.
Cephamandole D. M. Angaran *et al.*, *Ann. Surg.*, 1984, *199*, 107.
Chloramphenicol L. K. Christensen and L. Skovsted, *Lancet*, 1969, *2*, 1397 (dicoumarol).
Co-trimoxazole C. Hassall *et al.* (letter), *Lancet*, 1975, *2*, 1155; J. de Swiet (letter), *Br. med. J.*, 1975, *3*, 491 (phenindione); W. J. Tilstone *et al.*, *Postgrad. med. J.*, 1977, *53*, 388; J. K. Errick and P. W. Keys, *Am. J. Hosp. Pharm.*, 1978, *35*, 1399; R. A. O'Reilly and C. H. Motley, *Ann. intern. Med.*, 1979, *91*, 34; R. A. O'Reilly, *New Engl. J. Med.*, 1980, *302*, 33.
Enoxacin S. Toon *et al.*, *Clin. Pharmac. Ther.*, 1987, *42*, 33.
Erythromycin W. R. Bartle (letter), *Archs intern. Med.*, 1980, *140*, 985; F. E. Husserl (letter), *ibid.*, 1983, *143*, 1831 and 1836; J. Schwartz *et al.*, *Sth. med. J.*, 1983, *76*, 91; K. Bachmann *et al.*, *Pharmacology*, 1984, *28*, 171; R. I. Sato *et al.*, *Archs intern. Med.*, 1984, *144*, 2413.
Isoniazid A. R. Rosenthal *et al.*, *J. Am. med. Ass.*, 1977, *238*, 2177.
Nafcillin G. D. Qureshi *et al.*, *Ann. intern. Med.*, 1984, *100*, 527.
Nalidixic acid E. M. Sellers and J. Koch-Weser, *Clin. Pharmac. Ther.*, 1970, *11*, 524; B. I. Hoffbrand (letter), *Br. med. J.*, 1974, *2*, 666; I. Potasman and H. Bassan (letter), *Ann. intern. Med.*, 1980, *92*, 571 (nicoumalone); J. Leor *et al.* (letter), *ibid.*, 1987, *107*, 601.
Neomycin J. A. Udall, *Clin. Med.*, 1970, *77*, (Aug.), 20.
Rifampicin F. Michot *et al.*, *Schweiz. med. Wschr.*, 1970, *100*, 583 (warfarin and nicoumalone); R. J. Boekhout-Mussert *et al.*, *J. Am. med. Ass.*, 1974, *229*, 1903 (phenprocoumon); R. A. O'Reilly, *Ann. intern. Med.*, 1974, *81*, 337; J. A. Romankiewicz and M. Ehrman, *ibid.*, 1975, *82*, 224; R. A. O'Reilly, *ibid.*, *83*, 506; H. Held, *Dt. med. Wschr.*, 1979, *104*, 1311 (phenprocoumon).
Sulphafurazole T. H. Self *et al.*, *Circulation*, 1975, *52*,

528; L. J. Sioris *et al.*, *Archs intern. Med.*, 1980, *140*, 546.
Sulphamethizole B. Lumholtz *et al.*, *Clin. Pharmac. Ther.*, 1975, *17*, 731.
Sulphaphenazole H. M. Solomon and J. J. Schrogie, *Biochem. Pharmac.*, 1967, *16*, 1219; D. R. Varma *et al.* (letter), *Br. J. clin. Pharmac.*, 1975, *2*, 467 (phenindione).
Tetracycline A. P. Klippel and B. Pitsinger, *Archs Surg.*, 1968, *96*, 266.

ANTIDEPRESSANTS. Nortriptyline has been reported to prolong the half-life of dicoumarol in healthy subjects. The few reports of investigations into the effect of tricyclic antidepressants on warfarin have not been conclusive of an interaction. Mianserin and phenprocoumon have been reported not to interact.
Some authorities consider that there is a theoretical risk of an interaction with monoamine oxidase inhibitors.
One patient required an increase in the dose of warfarin when taking trazodone. Fluvoxamine might increase warfarin concentrations.
References:
Amitriptyline or nortriptyline E. S. Vesell *et al.*, *Ann. N.Y. Acad. Sci.*, 1971, *179*, 752 (dicoumarol); J. Koch-Weser, *Clin. Pharmac. Ther.*, 1973, *14*, 139; S. M. Pond *et al.*, *ibid.*, 1975, *18*, 191 (warfarin and dicoumarol).
Mianserin H. Kopera *et al.*, *Eur. J. clin. Pharmac.*, 1978, *13*, 351 (phenprocoumon).
Trazodone J. -L. Hardy and A. Sirois, *Can. med. Ass. J.*, 1986, *135*, 1372.

ANTIDIABETIC AGENTS. There have been a few early instances of tolbutamide enhancing the activity of dicoumarol. However, this effect has not been observed in later studies involving dicoumarol, warfarin, and phenprocoumon, although one study did demonstrate altered dicoumarol pharmacokinetics. An absence of effect has been documented for phenprocoumon and insulin, glibenclamide, or glibornuride, while metformin has been reported to diminish phenprocoumon activity.
There has been one early isolated report of phenformin enhancing the anticoagulant activity of warfarin.
References:
Glibenclamide, glibornuride, and insulin P. Heine *et al.*, *Eur. J. clin. Pharmac.*, 1976, *10*, 31 (phenprocoumon).
Metformin E. E. Ohnhaus *et al.*, *Klin. Wschr.*, 1983, *61*, 851 (phenprocoumon).
Phenformin T. J. Hamblin (letter), *Lancet*, 1971, *2*, 1323.
Tolbutamide H. Chaplin and M. Cassell, *Am. J. med. Sci.*, 1958, *235*, 706 (dicoumarol); R. L. Poucher and T. J. Vecchio, *J. Am. med. Ass.*, 1966, *197*, 1069 (warfarin and dicoumarol); P. Heine *et al.*, *Eur. J. clin. Pharmac.*, 1976, *10*, 31 (phenprocoumon); E. Jähnchen *et al.*, *ibid.*, 349 (dicoumarol).

ANTI-EPILEPTICS. Phenobarbitone diminishes the activity of warfarin through increased metabolism. Carbamazepine is reported to have a similar effect while the anticoagulant may in turn affect the activity of carbamazepine. Reports of the effect of phenytoin on anticoagulants do not provide a clear picture; the effect of warfarin has been reported to be enhanced while that of dicoumarol diminished. Warfarin has also been reported to inhibit the metabolism of phenytoin.
References:
Carbamazepine J. M. Hansen *et al.*, *Clin. Pharmac. Ther.*, 1971, *12*, 539; J. R. Y. Ross and L. Beeley, *Br. med. J.*, 1980, *280*, 1415.
Phenytoin J. M. Hansen *et al.*, *Acta med. scand.*, 1971, *189*, 15 (dicoumarol); J. M. Nappi (letter), *Ann. intern. Med.*, 1979, *90*, 852.

ANTIFUNGAL AGENTS. Griseofulvin has been reported to diminish the activity of warfarin, whereas ketoconazole and miconazole have each been reported to enhance its activity, probably through altered metabolism. Miconazole has also enhanced the activity of several other anticoagulants.
References:
Griseofulvin S. I. Cullen and P. M. Catalano, *J. Am. med. Ass.*, 1967, *199*, 582; J. A. Udall, *Clin. Med.*, 1970, *77*, (Aug.), 20.
Ketoconazole A. G. Smith, *Br. med. J.*, 1984, *288*, 188 and 608.
Miconazole Proc. R. Soc. Med., 1977, *70*, *Suppl.* 1, 52 (nicoumalone); P. G. Watson *et al.*, *Br. med. J.*, 1982, *285*, 1045; E. Loupi *et al.*, *Thérapie*, 1982, *37*, 437 (ethyl biscoumacetate, nicoumalone, phenindione, and tioclomarol); M. C. Colquhoun *et al.* (letter), *Lancet*, 1987, *1*, 695.

ANTIHYPERTENSIVES. Diazoxide has been reported to displace warfarin from albumin *in vitro*, but there does not appear to have been any clinical interaction.
References:
Diazoxide E. M. Sellers and J. Koch-Weser, *Clin. Pharmac. Ther.*, 1970, *11*, 524; *idem*, *Ann. N.Y. Acad. Sci.*, 1971, *179*, 213.

ANTIMALARIALS. The ingestion of large amounts of tonic water by 2 patients necessitated a reduction in their warfarin dosage. The enhanced effect was attributed to the quinine content of the tonic water.
References:
Quinine D. J. Clark, *Br. med. J.*, 1983, *286*, 1258.

ANTINEOPLASTIC AGENTS. There have been several reports of interactions between warfarin and antineoplastic agents. No clear picture emerges from these reports which is not surprising considering that antineoplastic agents are often given in combination and that they can exert their own haematological effects. Cyclophosphamide for instance has been associated with an increase in warfarin's activity when given with methotrexate and fluorouracil but with a decrease when given with nonantineoplastic agents. Etoposide with vindesine has produced an increased anticoagulant effect as has tamoxifen. Aminoglutethimide and mitotane have each led to decreased warfarin activity, probably due to increased warfarin metabolism. Mercaptopurine has also decreased warfarin activity.
References:
Aminoglutethimide R. M. L. Murray *et al.*, *Med. J. Aust.*, 1981, *1*, 179; P. F. Bruning and J. G. M. Bonfrèr (letter), *Lancet*, 1983, *2*, 582; P. E. Lønning *et al.*, *Cancer Chemother. Pharmac.*, 1984, *12*, 10.
Cyclophosphamide C. K. Tashima, *Sth. med. J.*, 1979, *72*, 633; E. J. Seifter *et al.* (letter), *Cancer Treat. Rep.*, 1985, *69*, 244.
Etoposide with vindesine K. Ward and J. D. Bitran (letter), *ibid.*, 1984, *68*, 817.
Mercaptopurine A. S. D. Spiers and R. S. Mibashan (letter), *Lancet*, 1974, *2*, 221.
Mitotane P. G. Cuddy *et al.*, *Sth. med. J.*, 1986, *79*, 387.
Tamoxifen R. Lodwick *et al.* (letter), *Br. med. J.*, 1987, *295*, 1141.

ANTIPROTOZOAL AGENTS. Metronidazole enhances the activity of warfarin through selective inhibition of the metabolism of its *S*-isomer.
References:
Metronidazole R. A. O'Reilly, *New Engl. J. Med.*, 1976, *295*, 354; F. J. Kazmier, *Mayo Clin. Proc.*, 1976, *51*, 782; R. P. Dean and R. L. Talbert, *Drug Intell. & clin. Pharm.*, 1980, *14*, 864.

BETA BLOCKERS. Propranolol in normal doses has increased the area under the serum-warfarin concentration time curve without producing any change in anticoagulant response. Atenolol is reported to have no effect on the area under the curve. Metoprolol is reported to have no effect on warfarin or nicoumalone but has caused a transient increase in plasma-phenprocoumon concentrations, though without any increased anticoagulation. Atenolol is reported to have no effect on nicoumalone or phenprocoumon; similarly pindolol did not affect phenprocoumon.
One study has referred to the association of the lipid solubility of the beta blockers with the inhibition of liver enzymes and correlates this with the effect on warfarin kinetics.
References:
Atenolol and *metoprolol* F. Mantero *et al.*, *Br. J. clin. Pharmac.*, 1984, *17*, 94S (nicoumalone); H. Spahn *et al.*, *ibid.*, 97S (phenprocoumon).
Pindolol H. Vinazzer, *Int. J. clin. Pharmac. Biopharm.*, 1975, *12*, 458 (phenprocoumon).
Propranolol, metoprolol, and *atenolol* N. D. S. Bax *et al.*, *Br. J. clin. Pharmac.*, 1984, *17*, 553.
Propranolol A. K. Scott *et al.*, *ibid.*, 559.

CARDIAC INOTROPIC AGENTS. Digoxin has been reported not to interact with warfarin.
References:
Digoxin A. Breckenridge and M. Orme, *Ann. N.Y. Acad. Sci.*, 1971, *179*, 421.

CENTRAL STIMULANTS. While methylphenidate has been reported to increase the half-life of ethyl biscoumacetate, it has also been reported to have no effect on the half-life or on the anticoagulant activity of ethyl biscoumacetate.
References:
Methylphenidate L. K. Garrettson *et al.*, *J. Am. med. Ass.*, 1969, *207*, 2053; D. E. Hague *et al.*, *Clin. Pharmac. Ther.*, 1971, *12*, 259 (both ethyl biscoumacetate).

CORTICOSTEROIDS AND CORTICOTROPHIN. There are several early reports of corticosteroids or corticotrophin either enhancing or diminishing the effects of anticoagulants. Matters are further confused by corticosteroids being associated with increased coagulopathy.
References:
Corticotrophin and *cortisone* J. B. Chatterjea and L. Salomon, *Br. med. J.*, 1954, *2*, 790 (ethyl biscoumacetate).
Corticotrophin A. J. Hellem and J. H. Solem, *Acta med. scand.*, 1954, *150*, 389 (dicoumarol and phenindione); H. Van Cauwenberge and L. B. Jaques, *Can. med. Ass. J.*, 1958, *79*, 536 (ethyl biscoumacetate).
Prednisone J. Menczel and F. Dreyfuss, *J. Lab. clin. Med.*, 1960, *56*, 14 (dicoumarol); J. Sievers *et al.*, *Cardiologia*, 1964, *45*, 65 (dicoumarol).

DISULFIRAM. Disulfiram inhibits liver enzymes which probably accounts for its enhancement of warfarin activity. This interaction is complicated by the variable effects of alcohol on warfarin (see above). Special care is therefore called for when these drugs are used together.
References: E. Rothstein (letter), *J. Am. med. Ass.*, 1968, *206*, 1574; E. S. Vesell *et al.*, *Clin. Pharmac. Ther.*, 1971, *12*, 785; E. Rothstein (letter), *J. Am. med. Ass.*, 1972, *221*, 1052; R. A. O'Reilly, *Ann. intern. Med.*, 1973, *78*, 73; *idem*, *Clin. Pharmac. Ther.*, 1981, *29*, 332.

DIURETICS. There have been a number of studies on the effects of diuretics on anticoagulants. Tienilic acid produces the most serious interaction enhancing the activity of ethyl biscoumacetate, nicoumalone, and warfarin and has led to haemorrhage; the mechanism of this interaction is not clear, but considerable care is obviously required if tienilic acid is used with an anticoagulant. Ethacrynic acid has also been reported to enhance the activity of warfarin, but reports do not show as severe an effect as with tienilic acid.
Chlorthalidone and spironolactone have both been associated with a reduction in warfarin's activity and it has been suggested that this might be a consequence of the diuresis concentrating the circulating clotting factors. However, bumetanide, frusemide, and the thiazides are reported to have no effect on warfarin.
References:
Bumetanide C. M. Nilsson *et al.*, *J. clin. Pharmac.*, 1978, *18*, 91; H. Nipper *et al.*, *ibid.*, 1981, *21*, 654.
Chlorthalidone R. A. O'Reilly *et al.*, *Ann. N.Y. Acad. Sci.*, 1971, *179*, 173.
Ethacrynic acid E. M. Sellers and J. Koch-Weser, *Clin. Pharmac. Ther.*, 1970, *11*, 524; *idem*, *Ann. N.Y. Acad. Sci.*, 1971, *179*, 213; J. Koch-Weser, *Clin. Pharmac. Ther.*, 1973, *14*, 139; R. J. Petrick *et al.*, *J. Am. med. Ass.*, 1975, *231*, 843.
Frusemide C. M. Nilsson *et al.*, *J. clin. Pharmac.*, 1978, *18*, 91.
Spironolactone R. A. O'Reilly, *Clin. Pharmac. Ther.*, 1980, *27*, 198.
Thiazides D. S. Robinson and D. Sylwester, *Ann. intern. Med.*, 1970, *72*, 853; A. Breckenridge and M. Orme, *Ann. N.Y. Acad. Sci.*, 1971, *179*, 421.
Tienilic acid M. Detilleux *et al.*, *Nouv. Presse méd.*, 1976, *5*, 2395; H. Portier *et al.*, *ibid.*, 1977, *6*, 468 (both ethyl biscoumacetate); A. Grand *et al.*, *ibid.*, 2691 (nicoumalone); *Postgrad. med. J.*, 1979, *55*, *Suppl.* 3, 67; J. T. Slattery and G. Levy, *J. pharm. Sci.*, 1979, *68*, 393; D. A. McLain *et al.*, *J. Am. med. Ass.*, 1980, *243*, 763.

GASTRO-INTESTINAL AGENTS. Antacids may or may not interact with warfarin. Bismuth carbonate and magnesium trisilicate for example have been reported to reduce warfarin's absorption, but aluminium hydroxide has been observed to have no effect on warfarin or dicoumarol. Psyllium and magnesium hydroxide have also been reported to have no effect on warfarin, but the latter has increased the plasma concentrations of dicoumarol.
There has been one case report of sucralfate diminishing the effect of warfarin (Mungall *et al.*, 1983). However, this was not confirmed in subsequent studies.
Histamine H_2-antagonists have been much studied. A number of studies show that cimetidine can increase the plasma concentration and half-life of warfarin and that there is a selective inhibitory effect on the metabolism of its *R*-isomer. In some, but not all of these studies, there was an increase in prothrombin time. A similar interaction has also been observed with nicoumalone and cimetidine and with phenindione and cimetidine. There have also been reports of no effect of cimetidine on warfarin (Mills *et al.*, 1986) or on phenprocoumon (Harenberg *et al.*, 1982).
Studies of the effect of ranitidine on warfarin have usually shown that there is no interaction, although Desmond *et al.* (1984) did observe increased plasma concentration and reduced clearance of warfarin with both cimetidine and ranitidine.
The study that showed no interaction between cimetidine or ranitidine and warfarin (Mills *et al.*, 1986) observed that oxmetidine reduced the excretion of warfarin possibly by an inhibitory effect on the *S*-isomer rather than the *R*-isomer.
References:
Aluminium hydroxide J. J. Ambre and L. J. Fischer,

Clin. Pharmac. Ther., 1973, 14, 231 (warfarin and dicoumarol).
Bismuth carbonate J. C. McElnay *et al.* (letter), *Br. med. J.*, 1978, *2*, 1166.
Cimetidine A. C. Flind (letter), *Lancet*, 1978, *2*, 1054; M. J. Serlin *et al.*, *ibid.*, 1979, *2*, 317 (warfarin, nicoumalone, and phenindione); D. Hetzel *et al.* (letter), *ibid.*, 639; B. A. Silver and W. R. Bell, *Ann. intern. Med.*, 1979, *90*, 348; B. A. Wallin *et al.* (letter), *ibid.*, 993; J. Harenberg *et al.*, *Br. J. clin. Pharmac.*, 1982, *14*, 292 (phenprocoumon); B. Kerley and M. Ali (letter), *Can. med. Ass. J.*, 1982, *126*, 116; P. V. Desmond *et al.*, *Clin. Pharmac. Ther.*, 1984, *35*, 338; R. A. O'Reilly, *Archs intern. Med.*, 1984, *144*, 989; I. A. Choonara *et al.*, *Br. J. clin. Pharmac.*, 1986, *21*, 271; S. Toon *et al.* (letter), *ibid.*, 245; T. S. Gill *et al.*, *ibid.*, 564P (nicoumalone); S. Toon *et al.*, *ibid.*, 565P; J. G. Mills *et al.*, *ibid.*, 566P; W.R. Bell *et al.*, *Archs intern. Med.*, 1986, *146*, 2325.
Magnesium hydroxide J. J. Ambre and L. J. Fischer, *Clin. Pharmac. Ther.*, 1973, *14*, 231 (dicoumarol and warfarin).
Magnesium trisilicate J. C. McElnay *et al.* (letter), *Br. med. J.*, 1978, *2*, 1166.
Oxmetidine J. G. Mills *et al.*, *Br. J. clin. Pharmac.*, 1986, *21*, 566P.
Psyllium D. S. Robinson *et al.*, *Clin. Pharmac. Ther.*, 1971, *12*, 491.
Ranitidine M. J. Serlin *et al.*, *Br. J. clin. Pharmac.*, 1981, *12*, 791; P. V. Desmond *et al.*, *Clin. Pharmac. Ther.*, 1984, *35*, 338; R. A. O'Reilly, *Archs intern. Med.*, 1984, *144*, 989; S. Toon *et al.*, *Br. J. clin. Pharmac.*, 1986, *21*, 565P; J. G. Mills *et al.*, *ibid.*, 566P.
Sucralfate D. Mungall *et al.* (letter), *Ann. intern. Med.*, 1983, *98*, 557; R. L. Talbert *et al.*, *Drug Intell. & clin. Pharm.*, 1985, *19*, 456; P. J. Neuvonen *et al.* (letter), *Br. J. clin. Pharmac.*, 1985, *20*, 178.

GLUCAGON. A dose-dependent enhancement of warfarin's anticoagulant activity has been reported with glucagon.
References: J. Koch-Weser, *Ann. intern. Med.*, 1970, *72*, 331.

LIPID REGULATING AGENTS. Clofibrate can enhance the activity of warfarin, sometimes to the point of haemorrhage. The mechanism of this interaction is not clear, but it does not appear to be connected with any pharmacokinetic effect. Similar enhancement of activity has been reported when clofibrate is given to patients taking dicoumarol or phenindione. Bezafibrate is considered to enhance the effect of warfarin. Halofenate may exert the same effect.
An opposite effect may occur with cholestyramine which has reduced warfarin's serum concentration and half-life as well as its activity. The mechanisms of this interaction include binding of warfarin to cholestyramine and reduced absorption; the enterohepatic recycling of warfarin may have a part to play. However, cholestyramine can also reduce vitamin K absorption. Phenprocoumon's activity has also been reduced by cholestyramine.
Benfluorex and colestipol have been reported not to interact with phenprocoumon.
See also under Thyroid and Antithyroid Agents, below.
References:
Benfluorex P. De Witte and H. M. Brems, *Curr. med. Res. Opinion*, 1980, *6*, 478 (phenprocoumon).
Cholestyramine D. S. Robinson *et al.*, *Clin. Pharmac. Ther.*, 1971, *12*, 491; T. Meinertz *et al.*, *ibid.*, 1977, *21*, 731 (phenprocoumon); E. Jähnchen *et al.*, *Br. J. clin. Pharmac.*, 1978, *5*, 437.
Clofibrate M. F. Oliver *et al.*, *Lancet*, 1963, *1*, 143 (phenindione); J. J. Schrogie and H. M. Solomon, *Clin. Pharmac. Ther.*, 1967, *8*, 70 (dicoumarol); J. A. Udall, *Clin. Med.*, 1970, *77* (Aug.), 20; K. J. Starr and J. C. Petrie, *Br. med. J.*, 1972, *4*, 133; R. D. Eastham (letter), *Lancet*, 1973, *1*, 1450; S. M. Pond *et al.*, *Aust. N.Z. J. Med.*, 1975, *5*, 324; T. D. Bjornsson *et al.*, *J. Pharmacokinet. Biopharm.*, 1977, *5*, 495; T. D. Bjornsson *et al.*, *J. Pharmac. exp. Ther.*, 1979, *210*, 316.
Colestipol C. Harvengt and J. P. Desager, *Eur. J. clin. Pharmac.*, 1973, *6*, 19 (phenprocoumon).

PESTICIDES. Chlorinated insecticides have been reported to diminish the activity of warfarin in one patient.
References: W. H. Jeffery *et al.*, *J. Am. med. Ass.*, 1976, *236*, 2881.

PIRACETAM. Piracetam caused an increase in prothrombin time in one patient who had been stabilised on warfarin.
References: H. Y. M. Pan and R. P. Ng, *Eur. J. clin. Pharmac.*, 1983, *24*, 711.

SEDATIVES AND NEUROLEPTICS. The drugs in this group may enhance or more often diminish the activity of anticoagulants, but except in a few cases the interactions have not been considered to be a cause for great concern.
The barbiturates by inducing liver metabolism can reduce activity. The benzodiazepines on the other hand do not generally have any effect although there is the rare report of increased (Schunter *et al.*, 1978; Davis, 1984) or decreased activity (Breckenridge and Orme, 1971).
Chloral hydrate may increase the anticoagulant activity of warfarin, although here too there are exceptions and there has been a fall in warfarin concentrations (Breckenridge and Orme, 1971), in warfarin activity (Cucinell *et al.*, 1966), and in dicoumarol activity with a fatal outcome when chloral hydrate was withdrawn (Cucinell *et al.*, 1966). Triclofos has also increased warfarin's activity.
Reduced anticoagulant activity has been reported with dichloralphenazone, ethchlorvynol, and haloperidol. Reduction may generally occur with glutethimide. Compounds such as meprobamate and methaqualone have been reported to have no effect on anticoagulants.
References:
Chloral hydrate S. A. Cucinell *et al.*, *J. Am. med. Ass.*, 1966, *197*, 366 (warfarin and dicoumarol); E. M. Sellers and J. Koch-Weser, *New Engl. J. Med.*, 1970, *283*, 827; *idem, Ann. N.Y. Acad. Sci.*, 1971, *179*, 213; A. Breckenridge and M. Orme, *ibid.*, 421; Boston Collaborative Drug Surveillance Program, *New Engl. J. Med.*, 1972, *286*, 53; *Lancet*, 1972, *1*, 524; J. A. Udall, *Ann. intern. Med.*, 1974, *81*, 341; R. E. Galinsky *et al.* (letter), *ibid.*, 1975, *83*, 286.
Chloral hydrate or chloral betaine P. F. Griner *et al.*, *Ann. intern. Med.*, 1971, *74*, 540.
Chlordiazepoxide A. Breckenridge and M. Orme, *Ann. N.Y. Acad. Sci.*, 1971, *179*, 421; M. Orme *et al.*, *Br. med. J.*, 1972, *3*, 611; J. B. Whitfield *et al.*, *ibid.*, 1973, *1*, 316; P. P. deCarolis and M. L. Gelfand, *J. clin. Pharmac.*, 1975, *15*, 557.
Diazepam M. Orme *et al.*, *Br. med. J.*, 1972, *3*, 611; J. B. Whitfield *et al.*, *ibid.*, 1973, *1*, 316; P. P. deCarolis and M. L. Gelfand, *J. clin. Pharmac.*, 1975, *15*, 557; C. Schunter *et al.*, *Klin. Wschr.*, 1978, *56*, 305 (phenprocoumon); L. J. Davis *et al.*, *Drug Intell. & clin. Pharm.*, 1984, *18*, 509.
Dichloralphenazone A. Breckenridge and M. Orme, *Ann. N.Y. Acad. Sci.*, 1971, *179*, 421; J. B. Whitfield *et al.*, *Br. med. J.*, 1973, *1*, 316.
Ethchlorvynol S. I. Cullen and P. M. Catalano, *J. Am. med. Ass.*, 1967, *199*, 582; S. A. Johansson, *Acta med. scand.*, 1968, *184*, 297 (dicoumarol).
Flunitrazepam J. Dry *et al.* (letter), *Thérapie*, 1976, *31*, 805.
Glutethimide F. E. van Dam *et al.* (letter), *Lancet*, 1966, *2*, 1027 (ethyl biscoumacetate); M. G. MacDonald *et al.*, *Clin. Pharmac. Ther.*, 1969, *10*, 80; J. A. Udall, *Curr. ther. Res.*, 1975, *17*, 67.
Haloperidol D. P. Oakley and H. Lautch (letter), *Lancet*, 1963, *2*, 1231 (phenindione).
Lorazepam L. J. Davis *et al.*, *Drug Intell. & clin. Pharm.*, 1984, *18*, 509.
Meprobamate J. A. Udall, *Curr. ther. Res.*, 1970, *12*, 724; L. Gould *et al.*, *J. Am. med. Ass.*, 1972, *220*, 1460; P. P. deCarolis and M. L. Gelfand, *J. clin. Pharmac.*, 1975, *15*, 557.
Methaqualone J. B. Whitfield *et al.*, *Br. med. J.*, 1973, *1*, 316.
Nitrazepam A. Breckenridge and M. Orme, *Ann. N.Y. Acad. Sci.*, 1971, *179*, 421; R. Bieger *et al.*, *Clin. Pharmac. Ther.*, 1972, *13*, 361 (phenprocoumon); M. Orme *et al.*, *Br. med. J.*, 1972, *3*, 611; J. B. Whitfield *et al.*, *ibid.*, 1973, *1*, 316.
Triclofos E. M. Sellers *et al.*, *Clin. Pharmac. Ther.*, 1972, *13*, 911.

SEX HORMONES. There have been a number of reports of various anabolic steroids enhancing the activity of anticoagulant agents to the point of haemorrhage. Reports have covered oxymetholone enhancing warfarin and nicoumalone; stanozolol enhancing warfarin and dicoumarol; ethyloestrenol enhancing phenindione; and norethandrolone enhancing dicoumarol. The mechanism of this interaction is not clear although it is considered that it is not due to altered pharmacokinetics. Steroids with a 17-α-alkyl substituent appear to be most involved, but there has been a report of topically applied testosterone, which does not have such a substituent, enhancing warfarin. Another androgen involved in enhanced anticoagulation is methyltestosterone which has been reported to interact with phenprocoumon.
Oral contraceptives have also been implicated in interactions. However, while the effects of dicoumarol were diminished by an oestrogen progestogen mixture, those of nicoumalone were enhanced by other oestrogen and progestogen preparations.
An increase in prothrombin time with haematemesis has been associated with danazol given to a patient receiving warfarin and a range of other drugs.
References:
Danazol I. A. Goulbourne and D. A. D. Macleod, *Br. J. Obstet. Gynaec.*, 1981, *88*, 950.
Ethyloestrenol D. W. Vere and G. R. Fearnley (letter), *Lancet*, 1968, *2*, 281 (phenindione).
Methyltestosterone S. Husted *et al.*, *Eur. J. clin. Pharmac.*, 1976, *10*, 209 (phenprocoumon).
Norethandrolone J. J. Schrogie and H. M. Solomon, *Clin. Pharmac. Ther.*, 1967, *8*, 70 (dicoumarol).
Oral contraceptives J. J. Schrogie *et al.*, *Clin. Pharmac. Ther.*, 1967, *8*, 670 (dicoumarol); E. de Teresa *et al.*, *Br. med. J.*, 1979, *2*, 1260 (nicoumalone).
Oxymetholone B. H. B. Robinson (letter), *Lancet*, 1971, *1*, 1356; R. G. M. Longridge *et al.* (letter), *ibid.*, *2*, 90; M. S. Edwards and J. R. Curtis (letter), *ibid.*, 221; J. C. de Oya *et al.* (letter), *ibid.*, 259 (nicoumalone).
Stanozolol W. Howard *et al.* (letter), *Br. med. J.*, 1977, *1*, 1659 (dicoumarol); C. Acomb and P. W. Shaw, *Pharm. J.*, 1985, *1*, 73.
Testosterone S. McQ. Lorentz and R. T. Weibert, *Clin. Pharm.*, 1985, *4*, 332.

THYROID AND ANTITHYROID AGENTS. Since hyperthyroid patients are especially susceptible to anticoagulants it is not surprising that the activity of anticoagulants is enhanced by thyroid compounds, sometimes with serious consequences. It is considered that the thyroid compound has a direct effect on the clotting factors. Antithyroid compounds have not been reported to diminish the effect of anticoagulants but warfarin has been reported to increase the free fraction of propylthiouracil *in vitro* (p.687) and surprisingly propylthiouracil has been reported to have caused hypoprothrombinaemia (p.686).
References:
Dextrothyroxine J. C. Owens *et al.*, *New Engl. J. Med.*, 1962, *266*, 76; J. J. Schrogie and H. M. Solomon, *Clin. Pharmac. Ther.*, 1967, *8*, 70 (dicoumarol); H. M. Solomon and J. J. Schrogie, *ibid.*, 797.
Thyroxine D. C. Costigan *et al.*, *Clin. Pediat.*, 1984, *23*, 172.

TOBACCO. Tobacco smoking has been reported to have variable effects on warfarin.
References: P. F. D'Arcy, *Drug Intell. & clin. Pharm.*, 1984, *18*, 302.

URICOSURIC AGENTS. The two agents in this group that are implicated in interactions with anticoagulants are allopurinol and sulphinpyrazone.
With allopurinol there are conflicting reports of patients experiencing no interaction or an enhanced anticoagulant effect with dicoumarol, phenprocoumon, or warfarin.
Interactions with sulphinpyrazone have usually involved warfarin and, apart from 1 case of a mixed response, have involved increased anticoagulant activity, sometimes with haemorrhage, so calling for careful control. It is still not clear how sulphinpyrazone exerts its effect, but studies point to a stereoselective effect on warfarin metabolism where the *S*-isomer's metabolic clearance is inhibited but the *R*-isomer's is increased. Displacement of the *R*-isomer from plasma protein has also been reported to play a part. It should also be remembered that sulphinpyrazone affects platelets. The other anticoagulants involved with sulphinpyrazone in reports are nicoumalone, where its dose required reduction, and phenprocoumon, where there was a less significant interaction in healthy subjects.
References:
Allopurinol E. S. Vesell *et al.*, *Ann. N.Y. Acad. Sci.*, 1971, *179*, 752 (dicoumarol); M. D. Rawlins and S. E. Smith, *Br. J. Pharmac.*, 1973, *48*, 693; T. H. Self *et al.* (letter), *Lancet*, 1975, *2*, 557; S. M. Pond *et al.*, *Aust. N.Z. J. Med.*, 1975, *5*, 324; E. Jähnchen *et al.*, *Klin. Wschr.*, 1977, *55*, 759 (phenprocoumon).
Sulphinpyrazone D. Mattingly *et al.* (letter), *Br. med. J.*, 1978, *2*, 1786; J. W. Davis and L. E. Johns (letter), *New Engl. J. Med.*, 1978, *299*, 955; M. Weiss (letter), *Lancet*, 1979, *1*, 609; R. R. Bailey and J. Reddy (letter), *ibid.*, 1980, *1*, 254; A. Gallus and D. Birkett (letter), *ibid.*, 1980, *1*, 535; F. Michot *et al.*, *Schweiz. med. Wschr.*, 1981, *111*, 255 (nicoumalone); G. G. Nenci *et al.*, *Br. med. J.*, 1981, *282*, 1361; R. A. O'Reilly, *Circulation*, 1982, *65*, 202; F. G. Larsen *et al.*, *J. Pharm. Pharmac.*, 1984, *36*, 689; S. Toon and W. F. Trager (letter), *J. pharm. Sci.*, 1984, *73*, 1671; S. Toon *et al.*, *Clin. Pharmac. Ther.*, 1986, *39*, 15; L. D. Heimark *et al.*, *ibid.*, 1987, *42*, 312 (phenprocoumon).

VACCINES. Severe bleeding occurred in an elderly warfarin-stabilised patient following influenza vaccination (Sumner *et al.*, 1981) and stimulated a number of investigations into this possible interaction. Two of these studies have demonstrated some inconsistent increase in warfarin's activity following influenza vaccine (Kramer *et al.*, 1984; Weibert *et al.*, 1986). More commonly, other studies have shown no effect.

References:
Influenza vaccine H. W. Sumner *et al.*, *Geriatrics*, 1981, *36*, 83; P. Kramer and C. J. McClain, *New Engl. J. Med.*, 1981, *305*, 1262; P. A. Patriarca *et al.* (letter), *ibid.*, 1983, *308*, 1601; P. Kramer *et al.*, *Clin. Pharmac. Ther.*, 1984, *35*, 416; B. A. Lipsky *et al.*, *Ann. intern. Med.*, 1984, *100*, 835; A. K. Scott *et al.*, *Br. J. clin. Pharmac.*, 1985, *19*, 144P; I. H. Gomolin, *Can. med. Ass. J.*, 1986, *135*, 39; R. T. Weibert *et al.*, *Clin. Pharm.*, 1986, *5*, 499.

VASODILATORS. Dipyridamole and benziodarone have both been implicated in interactions with anticoagulants. Diltiazem has been investigated but found to have no effect on warfarin.

The interaction with dipyridamole is an oddity in that bleeding can occur without any alteration in prothrombin times; special care is therefore required as the usual method of monitoring the anticoagulant effect is of no value. This interaction has involved a small number of patients taking dipyridamole and warfarin or phenindione.

Twenty-five years ago Pyörälä *et al.* (1963) reported that the doses of warfarin, diphenadione, ethyl biscoumacetate, and nicoumalone needed to be reduced when benziodarone was given; the doses of clorindione, dicoumarol, phenindione, and phenprocoumon were not affected. Some years later Verstraete *et al.* (1968) observed the same effect with ethyl biscoumacetate and benziodarone, but found that the dose of phenprocoumon needed to be reduced if benziodarone was also given.

References:
Benziodarone K. Pyörälä *et al.*, *Acta med. scand.*, 1963, *173*, 385 (warfarin, clorindione, dicoumarol, diphenadione, ethyl biscoumacetate, nicoumalone, phenindione, and phenprocoumon); M. Verstraete *et al.*, *Archs int. Pharmacodyn. Ther.*, 1968, *176*, 33 (ethyl biscoumacetate and phenprocoumon).
Diltiazem D. R. Mungall *et al.*, *J. clin. Pharmac.*, 1984, *24*, 264.
Dipyridamole S. Kalowski and P. Kincaid-Smith, *Med. J. Aust.*, 1973, *2*, 164 (warfarin and phenindione).

VITAMINS. Since vitamin K reverses the effects of oral anticoagulants, it is not surprising that there have been reports of acetomenaphthone and phytomenadione reducing anticoagulant activity, or of foods or nutritional preparations containing phytomenadione doing the same.

Occasional reports of ascorbic acid reducing the activity of warfarin have not been confirmed in subsequent studies. There have also been isolated reports of vitamin E enhancing warfarin's activity.

References:
Acetomenaphthone G. E. Heald and L. Poller (letter), *Br. med. J.*, 1974, *1*, 455 (nicoumalone).
Ascorbic acid G. Rosenthal (letter), *J. Am. med. Ass.*, 1971, *215*, 1671; R. Hume *et al.* (letter), *ibid.*, 1972, *219*, 1479; E. C. Smith *et al.* (letter), *ibid.*, *221*, 1166; C. L. Feetam *et al.*, *Toxic. appl. Pharmac.*, 1975, *31*, 544.
Phytomenadione R. A. O'Reilly and D. A. Rytand (letter), *New Engl. J. Med.*, 1980, *303*, 160; M. Lee *et al.* (letter), *Ann. intern. Med.*, 1981, *94*, 140; S. J. Kempin (letter), *New Engl. J. Med.*, 1983, *308*, 1229; A. J. M. Watson *et al.*, *Br. med. J.*, 1984, *288*, 557.
Vitamin E J. J. Corrigan and F. I. Marcus, *J. Am. med. Ass.*, 1974, *230*, 1300; J. J. Schrogie (letter), *ibid.*, 1975, *232*, 19.

Absorption and Fate

Warfarin sodium is readily absorbed from the gastro-intestinal tract; it can also be absorbed through the skin. It is extensively bound to plasma proteins and its plasma half-life is about 37 hours. It crosses the placenta but does not occur in significant quantities in breast milk. Warfarin is administered as a racemic mixture. The *S*-isomer is reported to be more potent; the *R*- and *S*-isomers are both metabolised in the liver, though at different rates; the stereo-isomers may also be affected differently by other drugs (see Interactions, above). The inactive metabolites are excreted in the urine following reabsorption from the bile.

The pharmacokinetics of warfarin.— D. R. Mungall *et al*, *J. Pharmacokinet. Biopharm.*, 1985, *13*, 213; E. Chan *et al.*, *Br. J. clin. Pharmac.*, 1985, *19*, 571P; N. H. G. Holford, *Clin. Pharmacokinet.*, 1986, *11*, 483.

Uses and Administration

Warfarin is a coumarin anticoagulant which depresses the hepatic vitamin K-dependent synthesis of coagulation factors II (prothrombin), VII, IX, and X. It is equally effective either orally or intravenously. Since warfarin acts indirectly, it has no effect on existing clots. Also as the coagulation factors involved have half-lives ranging from 6 to 60 hours, several hours are required before an effect is observed. A therapeutic effect is usually apparent by 12 hours, but the peak effect may not be achieved until 2 or 3 days after a dose; the overall effect may last for 5 days.

Warfarin is used in the prevention and management of deep-vein thrombosis or pulmonary embolism. If an immediate effect on blood coagulation is required, heparin should be given intravenously or subcutaneously to cover the first 36 to 48 hours. Some clinicians give warfarin coincidentally or after the initial heparin treatment. Warfarin is also used for the prevention of thrombo-embolism in patients with atrial fibrillation or prosthetic heart valves; in the latter group it is sometimes used with antiplatelet drugs. Warfarin and other anticoagulants are used prophylactically in myocardial infarction, stroke, and transient ischaemic attacks, but their role in such conditions is not clear (see p.338).

Oral anticoagulants are sometimes used in peripheral venous thrombosis, but should not be used in peripheral arterial occlusion.

Some patients may show a hereditary resistance to warfarin.

Dosage must be determined as discussed below under Control. Initial doses of warfarin sodium are usually within the range of 10 to 15 mg daily for 3 days, but may be lower for patients at risk. Subsequent maintenance doses usually range from 2 to 30 mg daily.

Warfarin is also given as the potassium salt; warfarin-deanol has been tried.

Warfarin is a potent rodenticide although resistance has been reported in *rats*.

Control of Oral Anticoagulant Therapy.
Treatment with oral anticoagulants must be monitored to ensure that the dose is providing the required effect on the vitamin-K-dependent clotting factors; too small a dose provides inadequate anticoagulation, too large a dose puts the patient at risk of haemorrhage. This monitoring is commonly carried out by checking the clotting property of the patient's plasma against that of normal plasma using a suitable preparation of thromboplastin which contains a source of calcium. The time taken for the clot to form due to the effect of the thromboplastin preparation on prothrombin is known as the prothrombin time (PT). The prothrombin time ratio (PTR) is the prothrombin time of the patient's plasma divided by that for a standard plasma sample.

So that there is some consistency in prothrombin time ratios measured at different times or at different laboratories, it is now common practice for the manufacturer or control laboratory to calibrate their batches of thromboplastin against the international reference preparation. This calibration produces an international sensitivity index (ISI) appropriate to that thromboplastin. The laboratory measuring the clotting capacity of a sample of plasma is thus able to convert the prothrombin time ratio to an international normalised ratio (INR) using the sensitivity index through the formula

$$\mathrm{INR} = \mathrm{PTR}^{(\mathrm{ISI})}$$

Thus a prothrombin time ratio of 2.0 obtained with a thromboplastin with a declared international sensitivity index of 1.5 would be converted to an international normalised ratio of 2.8. An international normalised ratio is therefore equivalent to a prothrombin time ratio carried out using the primary international reference preparation of thromboplastin.

This method of standardisation has taken over from methods involving use of a standard reagent such as the British or Manchester comparative thromboplastin. Also preparations of thromboplastin derived from *rabbit* brain have superseded or are superseding those from human brain because of the dangers of viral transmission.

In the *UK* the following ranges of international normalised ratio recommended by the British Society for Haematology are considered desirable for patients given anticoagulant treatment or cover for the listed condition or procedures:

2.0 to 2.5 Prophylaxis of deep-vein thrombosis including high risk surgery.
2.0 to 3.0 Prophylaxis of deep-vein thrombosis for hip surgery and fractured femur; treatment of deep-vein thrombosis; pulmonary embolism; transient ischaemic attacks.
3.0 to 4.5 Recurrent deep-vein thrombosis and pulmonary embolism; arterial disease including myocardial infarction; arterial grafts; cardiac prosthetic valves and grafts.

In the *US* somewhat similar ranges have been recommended by the American College of Chest Physicians and the National Heart, Lung and Blood Institute:

2.0 to 3.0 Prophylaxis of venous thrombo-embolism in high-risk medical or surgical patients.
2.0 to 3.0 Treatment of proximal vein thrombosis and pulmonary embolism; warfarin should follow initial treatment with heparin.
2.0 to 3.0 Prophylaxis of embolism in patients with atrial fibrillation, valvular heart disease, bioprosthetic heart valves, or acute myocardial infarction.
3.0 to 4.5 Prophylaxis in patients with mechanical heart valves and in patients with recurrent systemic embolism.

Measurements should be carried out before treatment, on the 2nd and 3rd day of treatment, and then on alternate days. Once the dose has been established the measurement can be made at greater but regular intervals; allowances should be made for any events that might influence the activity of the anticoagulant.

In a review of warfarin Wessler and Gitel (*New Engl. J. Med.*, 1984, *311*, 645 and 1579) concisely discuss its actions. Before their release into the circulation, factors II, VII, IX, and X are altered by conversion of glutamic acid residues to γ-carboxyglutamic acid residues so that they can bind to phospholipids for activation. Warfarin by inhibiting vitamin K blocks the carboxylation system, so decreasing this binding to phospholipids. Warfarin can also influence the release of proteins deficient in γ-carboxyglutamic acid, although it is not clear how this affects its antithrombotic activity.

Wessler and Gitel comment that warfarin can increase the rate at which plasma inhibits clotting proteases as measured by the rate of factor Xa inhibition. One of the main plasma protease inhibitors is antithrombin III. However, while Winter and Douglas (*Postgrad. med. J.*, 1983, *59*, 677) cite studies showing an increase in antithrombin III, they cite other references as well as their own findings that show no such increase.

Warfarin also affects protein C and protein S, two other vitamin-K-dependent proteins in the coagulation sequence. Protein C inhibits coagulation factors V and VIII and is augmented by protein S. Warfarin is thus blocking an anticoagulant process, but this appears to be dwarfed by its inhibitory effect on other factors resulting in a net anticoagulation. Depression of protein C has however been linked to warfarin-induced skin necrosis (A.W. Broekmans *et al.*, *Thromb. Haemostasis*, 1983, *49*, 251). Patients deficient in protein C or S require artificial or exogenous anticoagulant control, and there are reports of them having been managed with warfarin or other oral anticoagulants (H.E. Branson *et al.*, *Lancet*, 1983, *2*, 1165; I. Garcia-Plaza *et al.*, *ibid.*, 1985, *1*, 634; N.P. Zauber and M.W. Stark, *Ann. intern. Med.*, 1986, *104*, 659; J.J. Michiels *et al.*, *Br. med. J.*, 1987, *295*, 641). Some of the effects of the deficiency in their reports included purpura and disseminated intravascular coagulation.

Guidelines on optimum anticoagulation are widely available and the *UK* and *US* recommended international normalised ratios (INRs) for different uses of oral anticoagulants are given above. The American recommendations were based mainly on a critical review of available publications (J.E. Dalen and J. Hirsh, *Archs intern. Med.*, 1986, *146*, 462).

A *Lancet* editorial in early 1988 (*Lancet*, 1988, *1*, 275) discussed various aspects of the management of venous thrombo-embolism. In this it is considered advisable to carry out objective tests, usually venography and/or radionuclide lung scanning, to establish that there is a thrombo-embolism. Ideally this should be done before anticoagulation is begun. Should such treatment have started before the test, then it should be discontinued if that test is negative. Should the test be positive and anticoagulation begun or continued, then the duration of that treatment is not clear. It is considered that *US* workers have promoted heparin treatment periods of 7 to 14 days, although the recommendations coordinated by Dalen and Hirsh (1986) give a period of 7 to 10 days while the *UK* preference is for a period of 3 days' simultaneous treatment with heparin and an oral anticoagulant before withdrawing the heparin. It seems reasonable to start warfarin on the first day of heparin treatment and to stop heparin when warfarin has prolonged the INR to its recommended range [2.0 to 3.0].

Oral anticoagulants are often continued for 3 to 6 months in the management of venous thrombo-embolisms, but there is a range of opinion for the duration of such treatment. Pragmatic advice provided in the *Lancet* editorial is to give oral anticoagulants for 6 weeks to 3 months for proven deep-vein thrombosis and for 3 to 6 months for proven pulmonary embolisms, although external factors can affect both these times.

Long-term warfarin treatment is recommended in Dalen and Hirsh's report (1986) for mitral valve disease, prosthetic heart valves, and atrial fibrillation.

A further commentary on the optimal intensity of oral anticoagulant therapy is provided by Hirsh and Levine (*J. Am. med. Ass.*, 1987, *258*, 2723) who highlight the problems that have arisen from the use of different thromboplastins.

Some references to the use of warfarin in thrombo-embolic disorders: C. I. Lagerstedt *et al.*, *Lancet*, 1985, *2*, 515 (prevention of recurrent calf-vein thrombosis); M. V. Huisman *et al.* (letter), *ibid.*, 1011 (criticism; the need for secondary prevention of calf-vein thrombosis was not demonstrated); C. K. Mok *et al.*, *Circulation*, 1985, *72*, 1059 (favourable comparison with anti-platelet therapy in the prophylaxis of prosthetic heart valve thrombo-embolism); A. Gallus *et al.*, *Lancet*, 1986, *2*, 1293 (the benefits of a short heparin treatment period with early warfarin substitution in venous thrombo-embolism); L. Poller *et al.*, *Br. med. J.*, 1987, *295*, 1309 (fixed minidose warfarin for prophylaxis of venous thrombosis following major surgery).

CONTROL. References to the control of oral anticoagulant therapy: The Thirty-third and Thirty-fourth Reports of the WHO Expert Committee on Biological Standardization. *Tech. Rep. Ser. Wld Hlth Org. No. 687* and *700*, 1983 and 1984; International Committee for Standardization in Haematology and International Committee on Thrombosis and Haemostasis, *J. clin. Path.*, 1985, *38*, 133; M. J. Allington and F. G. Bolton (letter), *Lancet*, 1986, *1*, 1088; M. Allardyce *et al.* (letter), *ibid.*, 1334; H. C. Wilkes *et al.* (letter), *ibid.*, 1987, *1*, 328; J. Hirsh, *Archs intern. Med.*, 1987, *147*, 769; L. Poller, *Br. med. J.*, 1987, *294*, 1184; R. V. Majer *et al.* (letter), *ibid.*, 1414.

Anticoagulant control using human brain thromboplastin allowed a less intensive warfarin regimen in patients who had received tissue heart valves compared with control using *rabbit* brain thromboplastin.— A. G. G. Turpie *et al.*, *Lancet*, 1988, *1*, 1242.

References to studies on warfarin dose predictions from laboratory values: G. M. Peterson *et al.* (letter), *Br. J. clin. Pharmac.*, 1985, *20*, 177; N. H. G. Holford, *Clin. Pharmacokinet.*, 1986, *11*, 483; B. L. Carter *et al.*, *Clin. Pharm.*, 1987, *6*, 37; C. Lee *et al.*, *ibid.*, 406.

See also S. Dobrzanski *et al.*, *J. clin. Hosp. Pharm.*, 1983, *8*, 75; D. M. Kirking *et al.*, *ibid.*, 1985, *10*, 101.

MYOCARDIAL INFARCTION. For a discussion of anticoagulants in myocardial infarction, see p.338.

STROKE AND TRANSIENT ISCHAEMIC ATTACKS. For a discussion of anticoagulants in strokes and transient ischaemic attacks, see p.338.

Preparations

Warfarin Potassium Tablets *(U.S.P.)*

Warfarin Sodium for Injection *(U.S.P.)*

Warfarin Sodium Tablets *(U.S.P.)*

Warfarin Tablets *(B.P.)*. Tablets containing warfarin sodium.

Proprietary Preparations

Marevan *(Duncan, Flockhart, UK)*. *Tablets*, warfarin sodium 1, 3, and 5 mg.

Warfarin *(Boehringer Ingelheim, UK)*. *Tablets*, scored, warfarin sodium 1, 3, and 5 mg.

Proprietary Names and Manufacturers of Warfarin Salts

Aldocumar *(Aldo, Spain)*; Athrombin-K *(Purdue Frederick, Canad.; Purdue Frederick, USA)*; Coumadan Sodico *(Arg.)*; Coumadin *(Du Pont, Austral.; Du Pont, Canad.; Merrell, Ger.; Crinos, Ital.; Boots, S.Afr.; Du Pont, USA)*; Coumadine *(Belg.; Merrell, Fr.)*; Marevan *(Glaxo, Austral.; Belg.; Nyco, Denm.; Nyco, Norw.; Allen & Hanburys, S.Afr.; Duncan, Flockhart, UK)*; Panwarfin *(Abbott, USA)*; Sofarin *(Lemmon, USA)*; Waran *(Nycomed, Swed.)*; Warfarin *(Boehringer Ingelheim, UK)*; Warfilone *(Frosst, Canad.)*; Warnerin *(Canad.)*.

NOTE. The name Sofarin has also been used to denote diclofenac sodium.

Antidepressants

2500-b

The main drugs used in the treatment of depression are classified into 2 groups according to whether they inhibit monoamine oxidase or whether they inhibit the re-uptake into, or potentiate the release of biogenic amines from nerve endings, but the mechanisms that account for their antidepressant activity are not clear.

Most of the *monoamine oxidase inhibitors* are hydrazine derivatives and include: phenelzine, p.377, iproniazid, p.364, isocarboxazid, p.365, mebanazine, p.372, and nialamide, p.374. Tranylcypromine (p.381) is a nonhydrazine monoamine oxidase inhibitor, as is pargyline which is used mainly in the treatment of hypertension and is described under Antihypertensive Agents (p.493). The selective monoamine oxidase inhibitor selegiline is described under Dopaminergic Antiparkinsonian Agents (p.1008).

The actions and uses of monoamine oxidase inhibiting antidepressants (MAOI) are described under Phenelzine Sulphate (p.377).

The second group of drugs described in this chapter causes changes in the electroencephalogram similar to those produced by the phenothiazines. Some of them have marked sedative actions. These drugs are mainly dibenzazepine or dibenzocycloheptene derivatives and because of their structures are commonly known as the *tricyclic antidepressants*, although it has been suggested that they might be more accurately classified according to their effect on biogenic amine re-uptake; they include: amineptine, p.350, amitriptyline, p.350, amoxapine, p.356, butriptyline, p.357, clomipramine, p.358, desipramine, p.359, dothiepin, p.360, doxepin, p.360, imipramine, p.362, lofepramine, p.371, nortriptyline, p.375, protriptyline, p.380, and trimipramine, p.383. Iprindole (p.364) has a different tricyclic structure; maprotiline (p.371) and mianserin (p.372) have a *tetracyclic* structure; trazodone (p.381), and viloxazine (p.384) have different structures; each has uses similar to those of the classical tricyclic antidepressants, but some have fewer side-effects.

The actions and uses of tricyclic antidepressants are described under Amitriptyline Hydrochloride (below).

The monoamine oxidase inhibitors are generally considered to be less effective than the tricyclic antidepressants in endogenous depression, but more effective in neurotic or 'atypical' depression.

Lithium salts are of value in the prophylaxis of bipolar illness (manic depression) and unipolar illness (recurrent depression) as well as in the prophylaxis and treatment of mania. The actions and uses of lithium are described under Lithium Carbonate (p.365).

Drugs formerly used in the treatment of depression include stimulants such as dexamphetamine, methylphenidate, and pipradrol which are described under Stimulants and Anorectics (p.1439) but these are no longer advocated. Tranquillisers such as diazepam (p.731) are often used in anxiety associated with depression; flupenthixol (p.738) is also used in depression.

ACTIONS AND USES. Reviews of the actions and uses of antidepressants: *Drugs in Psychiatric Practice*, P.J. Tyrer (Ed.), London, Butterworths, 1982, pp.177-249.; *Biomedical Aspects of Depression and its Treatment*, R.J. Baldessarini, Washington, American Psychiatry Press, 1983; *Drugs in Psychiatry*, Volume 1, Antidepressants, G.D. Burrows *et al.*, (Eds.), Oxford, Elsevier, 1983; *Handbook of Drug Therapy in Psychiatry*, J.G. Bernstein, Boston, John Wright PSG Inc., 1983, pp.73-113; B. R. Ballinger and J. Feely, *Br. med. J.*, 1983, *286*, 1885; J. W. Richardson, *Mayo Clin. Proc.*, 1984, *59*, 330; P. Blier and C. de Montigny, in *Pharmacotherapy of Affective Disorders: Theory and Practice*, W.G. Dewhurst and G.B. Baker (Eds.), London, Croom Helm, 1985, pp.338-381; E. F. Coccaro and L. J. Siever, *J. clin. Pharmac.*, 1985, *25*, 241; S. G. Bryant and C. S. Brown, *Clin. Pharm.*, 1986, *5*, 304; *Med. Lett.*, 1986, *28*, 99; J. A. Henry and A. J. Martin, *Med. Toxicol.*, 1987, *2*, 445.

ADVERSE EFFECTS. Adverse reactions to antidepressants and their incidence: *Br. med. J.*, 1985, *291*, 1638; B. E. Leonard (letter), *Lancet*, 1986, *2*, 1105; S. Cassidy and J. Henry, *Br. med. J.*, 1987, *295*, 1021 and 1382.

ANTIDEPRESSANT SELECTION. Reviews on the selection of an appropriate antidepressant: S. Brandon, *Br. med. J.*, 1982, *285*, 1594; P. Rowan (letter), *ibid.*, 1983, *286*, 225; A. J. Cooper and R. V. Magnus, *Can. med. Ass. J.*, 1984, *130*, 383; *Drug & Ther. Bull.*, 1984, *22*, 61; D. T. Nguyen, *Can. J. Hosp. Pharm.*, 1987, *40*, 57.

COMPARISON WITH ECT. In a retrospective study, the hospital records of 1495 patients with depression, consisting of 448 patients treated by electroconvulsive therapy (ECT), 246 patients treated with 'adequate' antidepressant therapy (4 or more weeks treatment with 2 or more weeks at specified doses), 478 patients treated with 'inadequate' antidepressant therapy, and 323 patients receiving neither antidepressants nor ECT, were studied. ECT caused marked improvement in 69.6% of patients, which was significantly higher than that seen in patients receiving 'adequate' (48.4%) or 'inadequate' (50.2%) antidepressant treatment, and in those receiving neither treatment (44.9%). When the groups were stratified according to sex, age, duration of illness, and subclasses of depression, ECT produced marked improvement more frequently than other treatments. It was concluded that, although the treatment groups were not comparable at baseline, ECT appeared to be significantly more effective than antidepressants in the treatment of acutely depressed hospitalised patients.— D. W. Black *et al.*, *Compreh. Psychiat.*, 1987, *28*, 169.

METABOLISM OF ANTIDEPRESSANTS. Metabolism of drugs used in affective disorders.— M.V. Rudorfer and W.Z. Potter, in *Pharmacotherapy of Affective Disorders: Theory and Practice*, W.G. Dewhurst and G.B. Baker (Eds.), London, Croom Helm, 1985, pp.382-448..

NEUROCHEMISTRY OF DEPRESSION. Reviews on neurotransmitters and depression, with mention of the monoamine theory of depression: H. M. Van Praag, *Lancet*, 1982, *2*, 1259; W. Z. Potter, *Drugs*, 1984, *28*, 127; G.B. Baker and W.G. Dewhurst, in *Pharmacotherapy of Affective Disorders: Theory and Practice*, W.G. Dewhurst and G.B. Baker (Eds.), London, Croom Helm, 1985, pp.1-59.

Some alternatives to the monoamine theory of depression: *Lancet*, 1982, *1*, 781 (altered α_2-adrenergic receptor sensitivity); K. Wood and A. Coppen (letter), *ibid.*, 1121 (altered α_2-adrenergic receptor sensitivity); S. A. Checkley *et al.* (letter), *ibid.*, 1359 (altered α_2-adrenergic receptor sensitivity); K. Wood *et al.* (letter), *ibid.*, 1983, *2*, 519 (altered histamine uptake by blood platelets); C. Thompson *et al.* (letter), *ibid.*, 1983, *1*, 1101 (β-adrenoceptor down regulation); J. Mendlewicz (letter), *ibid.*, *2*, 283 (β-adrenoceptor down regulation); W. Z. Potter *et al.*, *Clin. Pharmac. Ther.*, 1984, *35*, 267 (altered α_2-adrenergic receptor sensitivity); S. H. Snyder, *New Engl. J. Med.*, 1984, *311*, 254 (cholinergic mechanisms); D. P. Srinivasan, *Br. J. Hosp. Med.*, 1984, *32*, 77 (increased plasma vanadium concentration in manic depressives); J. A. Blair *et al.* (letter), *Lancet*, 1984, *2*, 163 (reduced CNS tetrahydrobiopterin synthesis); E. H. Reynolds *et al.*, *ibid.*, 196 (altered methylation in the nervous system); T. Bottiglieri *et al.* (letter), *ibid.*, 224 (altered methylation in the nervous system); J. J. Mann *et al.*, *New Engl. J. Med.*, 1985, *313*, 715 (reduced β-adrenergic receptor sensitivity).

12336-n

Alaproclate *(USAN, rINN).*
GEA-654. 4-Chloro-$\alpha\alpha$-dimethylphenethyl DL-alaninate; 2-(4-Chlorophenyl)-1,1-dimethylethyl ester of DL-alanine.
$C_{13}H_{18}ClNO_2$=255.7.

CAS — 60719-82-6.

Alaproclate is an antidepressant which selectively inhibits the re-uptake of serotonin. It has also been tried in senile dementia.

Proprietary Names and Manufacturers
Astra, USA.

12358-q

Amineptine Hydrochloride *(rINNM).*
S-1694. 7-(10,11-Dihydro-5*H*-dibenzo[*a,d*]cyclohepten-5-ylamino)heptanoic acid hydrochloride.
$C_{22}H_{27}NO_2$,HCl=373.9.

CAS — 57574-09-1 (amineptine); 30272-08-3 (hydrochloride).

Amineptine hydrochloride is a tricyclic antidepressant with actions and uses similar to those of amitriptyline (below). In the treatment of depression it has been given by mouth in doses of 100 to 200 mg daily. Hepatic adverse effects seem more common than with other tricyclic antidepressants.

Of 91 cases of hepatitis due to antidepressant therapy, 63 were associated with amineptine therapy. Most patients presented with abdominal pain and mixed liver damage with predominant cholestasis. One died after myocardial infarction, but all the others recovered. The mean amineptine dosage was 200 mg daily and no case was an overdose.— B. Lefebure *et al.*, *Thérapie*, 1984, *39*, 509.

For a further report of acute hepatitis associated with amineptine, and cross hepatotoxicity with clomipramine, see Clomipramine Hydrochloride, p.358.

A report of 5 cases of very severe acne-type lesions following the chronic administration of high doses of amineptine (200 to 1000 mg daily).— P. Vexiau *et al.* (letter), *Lancet*, 1988, *1*, 585.

Proprietary Names and Manufacturers
Maneon *(Poli, Ital.)*; Survector *(Eutherapie, Fr.; Stroder, Ital.; Servier, Spain).*

2501-v

Amitriptyline Embonate *(BANM, rINNM).*

$(C_{20}H_{23}N)_2,C_{23}H_{16}O_6$=943.2.

CAS — 50-48-6 (amitriptyline); 17086-03-2 (embonate).

Pharmacopoeias. In *Br.* and *Nord.*

A pale yellow to brownish-yellow odourless or almost odourless powder. Amitriptyline embonate 1.5 g is approximately equivalent to 1 g of amitriptyline hydrochloride and 0.88 g of amitriptyline. Practically **insoluble** in water; slightly soluble in alcohol; soluble 1 in 8 of chloroform. **Protect** from light.

2502-g

Amitriptyline Hydrochloride *(BANM, USAN, rINNM).*

Cloridrato de Amitriptilina. 3-(10,11-Dihydro-5*H*-dibenzo[*a,d*]cyclohepten-5-ylidene)propyldimethylamine hydrochloride.
$C_{20}H_{23}N$,HCl=313.9.

CAS — 549-18-8.

Pharmacopoeias. In *Br., Braz., Chin., Cz., Egypt., Eur., Ind., Int., It., Jpn, Jug., Nord., Swiss,* and *U.S.*

Odourless or almost odourless, colourless crystals or white or almost white powder.

Soluble 1 in 1 of water, 1 in 1.5 of alcohol, 1 in 1.2 of chloroform, and 1 in 1 of methyl alcohol; practically insoluble in ether. The *U.S.P.* specifies that a 1% solution in water has a pH between 5.0 and 6.0. The *U.S.P.* injection has a pH of between 4.0 and 6.0. **Store** in well-closed containers.

STABILITY. Decomposition occurred when solutions of amitriptyline hydrochloride in water or phosphate buffers were autoclaved at 115° to 116° for 30 minutes in the presence of excess oxygen.— R. P. Enever *et al.*, *J. pharm. Sci.*, 1975, *64*, 1497. The decomposition of amitriptyline as the hydrochloride in buffered aqueous solution was accelerated by metal ions particularly from amber glass ampoules. Disodium edetate 0.1% significantly reduced the decomposition rate of these amitriptyline solutions but propyl gallate and hydroquinone were less effective. Sodium metabisulphite produced an initial lowering of amitriptyline concentration and subsequently an acceleration of decomposition.— R. P. Enever *et al.*, *J. pharm. Sci.*, 1977, *66*, 1087.

Solutions of amitriptyline hydrochloride in water are stable for at least 8 weeks at room temperature if protected from light either by storage in a cupboard or in amber containers. Decomposition to ketone and, to a lesser extent, other unidentified products was found to occur on exposure to light.— J. Buckles and V. Walters, *J. clin. Pharm.*, 1976, *1*, 107.

The photochemical stability of *cis* and *trans* isomers of tricyclic neuroleptic drugs.— A. Li Wan Po and W. J. Irwin, *J. Pharm. Pharmac.*, 1980, *32*, 25.

Adverse Effects

Many side-effects of amitriptyline and the other tricyclic antidepressants are caused by their antimuscarinic actions. These include dry mouth, sour or metallic taste, constipation occasionally leading to paralytic ileus, urinary retention, blurred vision and disturbances in accommodation, palpitations, tachycardia, and impotence.

Other adverse effects of tricyclic antidepressants include drowsiness (but sometimes nervousness and insomnia may occur), headache, peripheral neuropathy, tremor, orthostatic hypotension, occasionally hypertension, dizziness, sweating, weakness and fatigue, ataxia, epileptiform seizures, occasional extrapyramidal symptoms including speech difficulties, tinnitus, stomatitis and gastric irritation with nausea and vomiting. Confusion or delirium may occur, particularly in the elderly. Anorexia with weight loss, or weight gain, sometimes with inappropriate appetite (carbohydrate craving) may occur. Allergic skin reactions and photosensitisation have been reported and, rarely, cholestatic jaundice and blood disorders, including eosinophilia, bone-marrow depression, thrombocytopenia, leucopenia, and agranulocytosis.

The tricyclic antidepressants have an adverse effect on the myocardium and can cause conduction defects and cardiac arrhythmias; an increased risk of sudden death has been suspected in cardiac patients receiving tricyclic antidepressants.

Endocrine effects associated with tricyclic antidepressant therapy include changes in libido, interference with sexual function, gynaecomastia and breast enlargement, and galactorrhoea. Changes in blood sugar concentrations may also occur, and, very occasionally, inappropriate secretion of antidiuretic hormone.

Symptoms of overdosage are excitement and restlessness with marked antimuscarinic effects, including dryness of the mouth, dilated pupils, tachycardia, urinary retention, and intestinal stasis. Severe symptoms include unconsciousness, convulsions and myoclonus, hyperreflexia, hypotension, and respiratory and cardiac depression, with life-threatening cardiac arrhythmias that may recur some days after apparent recovery.

ANTIMUSCARINIC EFFECTS. In an *in vitro* study, the relative antimuscarinic potency of various tricyclic and tetracyclic antidepressants was found to be, in descending order: amitriptyline, clomipramine, trimipramine, doxepin, imipramine, protriptyline, nortriptyline, desipramine, amoxapine, maprotiline, trazodone. The antimuscarinic property is not necessary for antidepressant efficacy, so this information would enable the clinician to choose an antidepressant for a patient who should not be given an antimuscarinic drug.— E. Richelson, *Mayo Clin. Proc.*, 1983, *58*, 40.

EFFECTS ON THE BLOOD. Agranulocytosis associated with tricyclic antidepressant use appeared to be a rare, idiosyncratic condition resulting from a direct toxic effect rather than an allergic mechanism, and particularly affecting the elderly from 4 to 8 weeks after beginning treatment.— R. S. Albertini and T. M. Penders, *J. clin. Psychiat.*, 1978, *39*, 483.

A report of a patient who developed neutropenia after separate exposure to 2 tricyclic antidepressants. It was suggested that cross-intolerance may occur.— B. M. Draper and A. Manoharan (letter), *Med. J. Aust.*, 1987, *146*, 452.

EFFECTS ON THE CARDIOVASCULAR SYSTEM. Reviews of the effects of tricyclic antidepressants on the cardiovascular system: A. H. Glassman, *Annu. Rev. Med.*, 1984, *35*, 503 (see also under nortriptyline hydrochloride, p.375); S. A. Mortensen, *Practitioner*, 1984, *228*, 1180.

Several reports have linked the therapeutic use of amitriptyline with sudden cardiac death, especially in patients with pre-existing cardiac disease (D.C. Coull *et al., Lancet*, 1970, *2*, 590; D.C. Moir, *et al., ibid.*, 1972, *2*, 561; D.C. Moir *et al., Eur. J. clin. Pharmac.*, 1973, *6*, 98), but the Boston Collaborative Drug Surveillance Program (*Lancet*, 1972, *1*, 529) could find no evidence of such an association.

The antimuscarinic activity of tricyclic antidepressants causes tachycardia and decreases conduction time through the atrioventricular node. The tricyclics also have a quinidine-like activity on the myocardium which may delay atrioventricular conduction. The net effect on the electrocardiogram in most studies is to prolong the PR and QT intervals. A further effect of the tricyclics is to decrease myocardial contractility though the clinical importance of this is not clear. Postural hypotension seen in some patients is probably due to a combination of these mechanisms rather than to peripheral α-adrenoceptor blockade, which is only seen with very high doses. Anecdotal reports have appeared of heart block, cardiac arrhythmias, and myocardial infarction in patients receiving tricyclics, but the general opinion seems to be that for most patients with mild disease these risks have been overemphasised.— M. L. Orme, *Br. med. J.*, 1984, *289*, 1.

A study of 7 female inpatients receiving combinations of tri- and tetracyclic antidepressants and 7 controls suggested that postural hypotension associated with antidepressant medication is caused in large part by a dose-related failure of reflex peripheral vasoconstriction.— H. C. Middleton *et al.,*, *Eur. J. clin. Pharmac.*, 1987, *31*, 647.

For a mention of the increased risk of cardiotoxicity from tricyclic antidepressants in patients with pre-existing cardiac disease, see under Cardiovascular Disease in Precautions, below.

Cardiomyopathy. A 50-year-old man was found to have congestive cardiomyopathy after taking tricyclic antidepressants for 4½ years (amitriptyline 6 months, imipramine 4 years). A cause-and-effect relationship could not be proved, but the patient's history was negative for all other known causes. Nine other cases of cardiomyopathy in patients taking tricyclic antidepressants had been reported. Physicians should discontinue such medication if cardiomyopathy develops and should use tricyclics with great caution in patients with cardiomyopathy because of the possible risk of ventricular fibrillation.— J. S. Howland *et al., Sth. med. J.*, 1983, *76*, 1455.

Malignant hypertension. A 66-year-old man with borderline hypertension developed malignant hypertension (blood pressure 210/120) after taking amitriptyline 50 mg daily for 3 weeks. Blood pressure was rapidly controlled on discontinuation of amitriptyline and the institution of metoprolol 50 mg twice daily.— F. G. Dunn, *Sth. med. J.*, 1982, *75*, 1124.

Myocarditis. Amitriptyline is one of the drugs that has been incriminated in the aetiology of hypersensitivity myocarditis.— *Lancet*, 1985, *2*, 1165.

EFFECTS ON THE ENDOCRINE SYSTEM. *Diabetogenic effect.* Occasional instances of diabetes mellitus, aggravation of existing diabetes, abnormal glucose tolerance, glycosuria, and hyperglycaemia have been reported after the use of antidepressants, such as amitriptyline.— *Br. med. J.*, 1980, *281*, 596.

Inappropriate ADH syndrome. Inappropriate secretion of antidiuretic hormone developed in 1 patient who had received amitriptyline hydrochloride 50 mg three times daily for 6 weeks.— D. Beckstrom *et al.* (letter), *J. Am. med. Ass.*, 1979, *241*, 133. See also W. A. Parker, *Drug Intell. & clin. Pharm.*, 1984, *18*, 890.

Hyperprolactinaemia. Drug-induced hyperprolactinaemia may result from the administration of tricyclic antidepressants.— P. H. Bayliss, *Adverse Drug React. Bull.*, 1986, (Feb.), 432.

EFFECTS ON THE GASTRO-INTESTINAL TRACT. During the past 13 years the Committee had received reports of ileus, probably resulting from the antimuscarinic effects of tricyclic antidepressants. Various tricyclics were taken by different patients, there being no suggestion that any one is especially liable to cause ileus. Fortunately the complication appears to be rare.— Committee on Safety of Medicines, *Current Problems No. 3*, Feb., 1978.

EFFECTS ON THE KIDNEY AND URINE. A 35-year-old woman taking carbamazepine 800 mg daily by mouth for temporal lobe epilepsy developed haematuria after about 5 days of treatment with amitriptyline 100 mg daily, which cleared over the 4 days following amitriptyline withdrawal. Re-challenge produced haematuria again.— M. A. Gillman and R. Sandyk (letter), *Am. J. Psychiat.*, 1984, *141*, 463.

Amitriptyline had been reported to colour urine blue-green, but this appeared to be rare.— L. Beeley, *Br. med. J.*, 1986, *293*, 750.

EFFECTS ON THE LIVER. Of 91 cases of hepatitis due to antidepressant therapy, 10 were due to tricyclic antidepressants.— B. Lefebure *et al.*, *Thérapie*, 1984, *39*, 509.

For a report of acute hepatitis following the administration of tricyclic antidepressants, see Clomipramine Hydrochloride, p.358. For reports of increased liver enzyme activity, abnormal liver function, hepatitis, jaundice, hepatocellular damage and hepatic failure with lofepramine, see under Lofepramine Hydrochloride, p.371.

EFFECTS ON THE NERVOUS SYSTEM. Amitriptyline and imipramine can cause a symmetrical polyneuropathy which is almost exclusively motor.— R. J. M. Lane and P. A. Routledge, *Drugs*, 1983, *26*, 124. See also J. Marley (letter), *Br. med. J.*, 1987, *294*, 1616 (peripheral neuritis with clomipramine).

For a report of amitriptyline causing the restless leg syndrome, see under Uses, p.356. For further effects on the nervous system, see under Epileptogenic Effect and Extrapyramidal Effects, below.

EFFECTS ON SEXUAL FUNCTION. Sedation due to tricyclic antidepressants may lead to loss of libido. Amitriptyline with its greater antimuscarinic activity is more likely than the others to cause erectile problems (*Med. Lett.*, 1980, *22*, 108), although most of the tricyclics have been reported to cause impotence (L. Beeley, *Adverse Drug React. Ac. Pois. Rev.*, 1984, *3*, 23). Amitriptyline, clomipramine, desipramine, doxepin, and trimipramine can all delay or inhibit ejaculation, and amoxapine and imipramine can also cause painful ejaculation. In women, anorgasmia or delayed orgasm has been reported with amitriptyline, amoxapine, clomipramine, and imipramine (L. Beeley, 1984; *Med. Lett.*, 1983, *25*, 73; W.W. Shen and L.S. Sata, *J. reprod. Med.*, 1983, *28*, 497). It should be remembered that loss of libido and impotence are common symptoms of depression, often making the role of drugs in producing sexual dysfunction difficult to assess. However, when due to depression, these symptoms usually improve with effective treatment (L. Beeley, 1984; *idem, Prescribers' J.*, 1982, *22*, 84).

EFFECTS ON THE SKIN. A review of cutaneous reactions with tricyclic antidepressants. Urticaria and angioneurotic oedema have occurred, the urticaria occasionally clearing without drug withdrawal. Pruritus is uncommon, but may be associated with transient erythema. Photosensitivity reactions are far less common than with phenothiazines, but have been reported. Rarely exfoliative dermatitis has developed, and purpura, pigmentation, and lichen planus have been noted in isolated reports.— J. Almeyda, *Br. J. Derm.*, 1971, *84*, 298.

Skin reactions to antidepressant drugs are rarely severe. Allergic reactions usually occur between 14 and 60 days after the start of medication.— F. Quitkin, *J. Am. med. Ass.*, 1979, *241*, 1625.

Severe persistent cutaneous photosensitivity in a 38-year-old woman after 2 daily doses of a tricyclic antidepressant (imipramine 75 mg by mouth).— W. G. Walter-Ryan *et al.*, (letter), *J. Am. med. Ass.*, 1985, *254*, 357.

EPILEPTOGENIC EFFECT. A study suggesting that the overall incidence of seizures during tricyclic treatment is approximately 1% and among non-epileptic patients is perhaps 0.5%.— M. R. Lowry and F. J. Dunner, *Am. J. Psychiat.*, 1980, *137*, 1461.

EXTRAPYRAMIDAL EFFECTS. *Akathisia.* Some patients with panic disorder are exquisitely sensitive to imipramine and respond with symptoms of insomnia, jitteriness, and irritability. Some of the frequently reported symptoms are "trouble sitting still" and "shakiness inside". These symptoms have also been observed in patients with panic disorder treated with low doses of desipramine. The symptoms usually subside when the dose of the tricyclic is gradually increased. V. K. Yeragani *et al.*, (letter), *Br. med. J.*, 1986, *292*, 1529.

Dysarthria. A 48-year-old woman developed dysarthria on the fourth day of treatment with amitriptyline 25 to 50 mg three times daily; the condition regressed when the drug was withdrawn.— S. E. Quader, *Br. med. J.*, 1977, *2*, 97. Dysarthria is not uncommon in patients taking tricyclic antidepressants in doses of 300 to 450 mg daily.— M. Saunders (letter), *ibid.*, 317.

Torsion dystonia. Acute torsion dystonias can occur

after treatment with tricyclic antidepressants, particularly among children and young adults.— R. J. M. Lane and P. A. Routledge, *Drugs*, 1983, *26*, 124.

Tremor. Tricyclic antidepressants can accentuate one or more frequencies of physiological postural tremor and increase the observed amplitude.— R. J. M. Lane and P. A. Routledge, *Drugs*, 1983, *26*, 124.

NEUROLEPTIC MALIGNANT SYNDROME. Of 16 cases of neuroleptic malignant syndrome reported to the *UK* Committee on Safety of Medicines by July 1986, 3 cases, one fatal, occurred in patients receiving a tricyclic antidepressant alone or in combination with perphenazine.— Committee on Safety of Medicines, *Current Problems No.18*, Sept., 1986.

OVERDOSAGE. A review of antidepressant overdosage. The most common clinical features of tricyclic antidepressant overdosage are sinus tachycardia, pyramidal neurological signs (increased tendon reflexes and extensor plantar responses), drowsiness and delirium, and antimuscarinic effects. Other effects include cardiovascular complications, coma, convulsions, respiratory complications, acid-base disturbances, temperature disturbances, and blisters. There was little evidence to suggest that the tricyclic antidepressants differ in their toxicity.— P. Crome, *Drugs*, 1982, *23*, 431.

Tricyclic antidepressants and monoamine oxidase inhibitors can precipitate hyperthermia both singly, and more commonly in combination, especially when taken in overdose.— P. G. Blain and M. D. Rawlins, *Prescribers' J.*, 1981, *21*, 204.

If a child has taken more than 10 mg per kg bodyweight of amitriptyline or imipramine, convulsions, coma, and respiratory depression occur rapidly. Hypotension and cardiac arrhythmias may occur and the child should be observed with a cardiac monitor.— H. B. Valman, *Br. med. J.*, 1982, *284*, 1178.

In a review of 20 cases of amitriptyline overdose, 12 initially had absent oculocephalic reflexes. In 3 patients tested, oculovestibular reflexes were also absent. Opthalmoplegia was not encountered in 10 cases of imipramine ingestion, but had been reported with doxepin.— M. F. Beal (letter), *Neurology*, 1982, *32*, 1409.

Evidence for an enhancing effect of benzodiazepines in fatal amitriptyline poisoning.— L. A. King (letter), *Lancet*, 1982, *2*, 982.

Ischaemic colitis developed in a 49-year-old woman who took 20 capsules of amitriptyline 50 mg in 48 hours. J. M. Gollock and J. P. S. Thomson, *Postgrad. med. J.*, 1984, *60*, 564.

In overdose, the membrane stabilising activity of the tricyclic antidepressants is widely accepted as being responsible for the profound hypotension, prolongation of the ECG QRS complex to over 100 milliseconds (a feature of severe overdose), and potentially fatal cardiac conduction abnormalities and arrhythmias.— J. A. Henry and S. L. Cassidy, *Lancet*, 1986, *1*, 1414.

A 53-year-old woman developed acute polyradiculoneuropathy after taking an overdose of 800 mg of amitriptyline.— D. Leys, *Br. med. J.*, 1987, *294*, 608.

WEIGHT CHANGES. Weight gain and a craving for carbohydrates were associated with amitriptyline in 51 female patients with depression.— E. S. Paykel *et al.*, *Br. J. Psychiat.*, 1973, *123*, 501. See also J. H. Brown and J. D. Brown (letter), *Can. med. Ass. J.*, 1967, *97*, 1361; *Br. med. J.*, 1974, *1*, 168.

Treatment of Adverse Effects

The stomach should be emptied by emesis or aspiration and lavage. The use of activated charcoal as an adjunct to gastric lavage has been recommended. Supportive therapy alone may then suffice for patients who are not severely poisoned.

In particular the patient should be monitored for cardiac arrhythmias and anti-arrhythmic measures instituted if cardiac output is jeopardised. Propranolol and phenytoin have been used in cardiac arrhythmias associated with tricyclic antidepressant poisoning, but digoxin is not recommended. Some of the cardiac effects respond to infusions of sodium bicarbonate or to the cautious administration of physostigmine salicylate (see p.1334) but the routine use of the latter is not recommended.

Convulsions can be managed by giving diazepam intravenously. Physostigmine may also be used to control convulsions but caution must be exercised, since among its other adverse effects it can also induce convulsions. Paraldehyde and inhalation anaesthetics with muscle relaxants have also been recommended for the management of convulsions. Forced diuresis, peritoneal dialysis, and haemodialysis are not of value in tricyclic antidepressant poisoning and charcoal haemoperfusion is of doubtful value.

A review of the clinical presentation and treatment of poisoning due to tricyclic antidepressant overdosage.— P. Crome, *Med. Toxicol.*, 1986, *1*, 261. See also A. T. Proudfoot, *Prescribers' J.*, 1986, *26*, 97; D. A. Frommer, *J. Am. med. Ass.*, 1987, *257*, 521. The management of arrhythmias in tricyclic antidepressant poisoning.— P. R. Pentel and N. L. Benowitz, *Med. Toxicol.*, 1986, *1*, 101.

A study of 18 fatal cases of tricyclic antidepressant overdosage led to the following guidelines for the management of tricyclic poisoning: after stomach emptying and the use of activated charcoal and laxatives in tricyclic antidepressant overdoses, the patient should then be observed for 6 hours. If at any time during this period he develops major signs of poisoning (decreased level of consciousness, respiratory depression, seizures, hypotension, arrhythmia, or conduction blocks), he should be hospitalised. If after 6 hours no major signs develop, the patient should receive a final dose of charcoal and may be discharged to psychiatric evaluation. Patients who after 6 hours demonstrate only minor signs (such as tachycardia with a heart rate less than 120 or slightly slurred speech) may be discharged if active bowel sounds are present and if signs of poisoning are decreasing rather than increasing. If bowel sounds are absent or markedly depressed, admission for further observation is prudent. Previous fears of unexpected late complications and fatalities have not been realised. Virtually all fatalities attributable to direct tricyclic antidepressant toxicity occur within the first 24 hours.— M. Callaham and D. Kassel, *Ann. emerg. Med.*, 1985, *14*, 1. See also R. J. Goldberg *et al.*, *J. Am. med. Ass.*, 1985, *254*, 1772.

In a study of 49 patients, it was concluded that prolongation of the maximal limb-lead QRS duration was of value in predicting the risk of seizures and ventricular arrhythmias in acute overdose with tricyclic antidepressants; serum drug concentrations were not of predictive value.— M. T. Boehnert and F. H. Lovejoy, *New Engl. J. Med.*, 1985, *313*, 474.

There have been several reports of the successful use of prolonged cardiac massage in tricyclic antidepressant poisoning where the patient had severe hypotension or asystole unresponsive to all the inotropic agents tried.— J. A. Henry, *Br. J. Anaesth.*, 1986, *58*, 223.

ACTIVATED CHARCOAL. The influence of the repeated administration of oral activated charcoal on the elimination of tricyclic antidepressants is not consistent; plasma half-lives of amitriptyline and doxepin, but not imipramine are reduced. It is unlikely that any useful reduction in elimination half-life of tricyclic antidepressants would be achieved because of their very large volume of distribution.— *Lancet*, 1987, *1*, 1013.

It was concluded that painful faecal impaction with spurious diarrhoea in a 32-year-old man after an unsuccessful suicide attempt was due to the combination of the antimuscarinic action of both amitriptyline and chlorpromazine taken in overdose, together with 350 g of high residue activated charcoal (Carbomix) given over the 36 hours following gastric lavage. Consideration should be given to using a preparation of activated charcoal reported to cause diarrhoea (Medicoal) and early and vigorous treatment of constipation.— I. M. Anderson and C. Ware (letter), *Br. med. J.*, 1987, *294*, 578.

DIALYSIS AND HAEMOPERFUSION. Tricyclic antidepressants, drugs with a large volume of distribution, are cleared poorly by haemoperfusion or haemodialysis.— P. R. Pentel *et al.*, *J. Toxicol. clin. Toxicol.*, 1982, *19*, 239.

Although at any one time only a very small part of a tricyclic antidepressant ingested is found in the plasma pool, major adverse effects correlate with the concentration of tricyclic antidepressant in plasma. If the plasma concentration can be kept beneath a critical value the prognosis may, therefore, be improved. A 56-year-old man who had ingested about 2 g of amitriptyline had a beneficial response to haemoperfusion through XAD-4 Amberlite resin.— R. S. Pedersen (letter), *Lancet*, 1980, *1*, 154. Mention of 4 patients with tricyclic antidepressant poisoning who responded to Amberlite haemoperfusion.— A. Heath *et al.* (letter), *ibid.*, 155. One indication for the use of resin (not charcoal) haemoperfusion is severe tricyclic intoxication.— A. Trafford *et al.* (letter), *ibid.*

DRY MOUTH. Bethanechol chloride 25 mg taken by mouth 3 times daily with food may restore salivation in patients with dry mouth due to tricyclic antidepressants.— H. C. Everett (letter), *New Engl. J. Med.*, 1984, *310*, 1122.

GASTRIC LAVAGE. Henry and Volans (*Br. med. J.*, 1984, *289*, 304) have recommended that gastric lavage or emesis should be performed if an adult has ingested over 750 mg or a child over 150 mg of a tricyclic antidepressant. They also advocated (*idem*, 1291) gastric lavage for up to 12 hours after tricyclic antidepressant overdose.

Bramble (*ibid.*, 1985, *290*, 467) felt that this procedure would only be of benefit up to 4 hours after the overdose, especially in view of the risk of cardiac arrest shortly after lavage. Volans and Henry (*ibid.*) however, upheld the view that gastric lavage was worthwhile up to 12 hours after overdose in patients who had taken large quantities of tricyclic antidepressant since these drugs inhibited gastric emptying.

PHYSOSTIGMINE. A 66-year-old woman who had ingested amitriptyline 500 mg and methotrimeprazine 250 mg developed delirium which was reversed by physostigmine 2 mg given intravenously; a total of 6 doses of physostigmine, the last 120 hours after ingestion of the tablets, was required to reverse recurring delirium. The patient had no prominent electrocardiographic or peripheral antimuscarinic signs.— I. H. Gomolin and C. A. Melmed, *Can. med. Ass. J.*, 1983, *129*, 1203.

For further comments on the use of physostigmine to reverse tricyclic antidepressant poisoning, see Physostigmine Sulphate, p.1334.

SODIUM BICARBONATE. Of 12 children with cardiac arrhythmias caused by tricyclic antidepressant poisoning, 9 promptly reverted to sinus rhythm after being given only sodium bicarbonate 0.5 to 2 mmol per kg bodyweight intravenously.— T. C. K. Brown, *Med. J. Aust.*, 1976, *2*, 382.

After ingestion of imipramine hydrochloride 5.35 g a 23-year-old woman developed ventricular tachycardia which persisted despite hyperventilation with 100% oxygen. Sodium bicarbonate 50 mmol immediately restored sinus rhythm despite the presence of respiratory alkalosis superimposed on metabolic acidosis. Although the patient had a blood pH greater than 7.35, sodium bicarbonate was successfully used on 2 further occasions to control arrhythmias that recurred despite continued hyperventilation and the administration of physostigmine. The use of sodium bicarbonate in the presence of combined metabolic and respiratory alkalosis is not without risk and should be reserved for life-threatening arrhythmias unresponsive to conventional therapy.— D. W. Molloy *et al.*, *Can. med. Ass. J.*, 1984, *130*, 1457. Comment on the mode of action of sodium bicarbonate in treating tricyclic antidepressant-induced arrhythmias.— B. G. Pollock and J. M. Perel (letter), *ibid.*, *131*, 717. Reply.— K. W. Hall and J. Rabson (letter), *ibid.*

A further report of the successful use of sodium bicarbonate intravenously, with hyperventilation, to control arrhythmias induced by tricyclic antidepressants.— D. Hodes, *Br. med. J.*, 1984, *288*, 1800. Comment supporting the conclusion that arterial pH and blood gas monitoring are mandatory in patients severely poisoned with tricyclic antidepressants.— B. M. Buckley *et al.* (letter), *ibid.*, *289*, 185.

TACRINE. Three patients who had taken an overdose of a tricyclic antidepressant in conjunction with other drugs were given the anticholinesterase tacrine intravenously in doses of 0.5 to 1.67 mg per kg body-weight over 10 to 90 minutes from 2 to 13 hours after overdose. One patient failed to respond, but in 2 there was improvement in the level of consciousness, respiration, pupil reaction, motor activity, and orientation; the duration of action of tacrine was longer than that of physostigmine.— W. K. Summers *et al.*, *Clin. Toxicol.*, 1980, *16*, 269.

Precautions

Amitriptyline and other tricyclic antidepressants should be used with caution in patients with cardiovascular disease and should be avoided in the immediate recovery phase after myocardial infarction and in patients with heart block. Tricyclic antidepressants should also be used with caution in patients with hyperthyroidism or with impaired liver function, and in those with a history of epilepsy, untreated narrow-angle glaucoma, urinary retention, prostatic hypertrophy, or constipation.

Psychosis may be activated in schizophrenic patients and manic-depressive patients may switch to a manic phase; use is not recommended in mania. Patients with suicidal tendencies should be carefully supervised during treatment. Blood-sugar concentrations may be altered in diabetic patients.

Although they have been used together under expert supervision (see p.355), tricyclic antidepressants should not generally be given to patients receiving monoamine oxidase inhibitors or for at least 14 days after their discontinuation; severe hypertensive reactions have been reported. Similarly, several days should elapse between withdrawing a tricyclic antidepressant and starting a monoamine oxidase inhibitor.

The effects of the direct-acting sympathomimetic agents adrenaline and noradrenaline are enhanced by tricyclic antidepressants and local anaesthetics containing these vasoconstrictors should be used with great caution. The interaction is liable to be considerably more hazardous if these agents are injected intravenously. It has been recommended that, where possible, tricyclic antidepressants should be stopped some days before elective surgery.

The effects of tricyclic antidepressants are influenced by drugs that affect their metabolism. Barbiturates and other enzyme inducers such as anti-epileptics increase their metabolism while neuroleptics, cimetidine, methylphenidate, and possibly oestrogens and oral contraceptives reduce it. CNS depressants including alcohol and antimuscarinic agents can have their effects increased by tricyclic antidepressants. Hyperthyroid patients or those taking thyroid preparations may show an enhanced response to tricyclic antidepressants. The effects of bethanidine, debrisoquine, guanethidine and possibly of clonidine are reduced by tricyclic antidepressants.

Elderly patients and children under 5 years of age can be especially sensitive to the side-effects of tricyclic antidepressants; reduced dosage should be used.

Drowsiness is often experienced at the start of tricyclic antidepressant therapy and patients if affected should not drive or operate machinery. Fur further details of the effects of antidepressant therapy on driving, see under Driving, below.

CARDIOVASCULAR DISEASE. Patients with mild heart disease, such as a history of myocardial infarction or mild angina, can probably be treated with any antidepressant. It would seem wise to be very careful about tricyclic antidepressant use in patients with severe heart disease, such as those suffering from heart failure, those with bundle branch block, or those with heart block in their electrocardiograms, and those who have recently had a myocardial infarction.— M. L. Orme, *Br. med. J.*, 1984, *289*, 1. Criticism. Overdosage with the older tricyclic antidepressants is likely to produce cardiotoxic effects, and some of these effects are also seen in therapeutic dosage. Depression occurs more often in older patients, who are more at risk of heart disease. Cardiotoxicity has been reported at low plasma concentrations, but the risk is substantially raised in those developing high concentrations, as can happen in many patients treated with standard doses. Patients with pre-existing heart disease seem to be at particular risk. Most studies suggest that certain antidepressants such as mianserin and nomifensine are less cardiotoxic than antidepressants such as amitriptyline. In patients with heart disease, whether mild or severe, those antidepressants thought to be safer should be prescribed.— R. Farmer and S. A. Montgomery (letter), *ibid.*, 559.

For details of the cardiotoxicity of tricyclic antidepressants, see under Effects on the Cardiovascular System in Adverse Effects, above. For the use of tricyclic antidepressants in depressed patients with cardiovascular disease, see Imipramine Hydrochloride, p.363 and Nortriptyline Hydrochloride, p.375.

CONTACT LENSES. The antimuscarinic action of tricyclic antidepressants may decrease tear flow enough to cause corneal drying and staining of contact lenses.— *Aust. J. Hosp. Pharm.*, 1987, *17*, 55.

DRIVING. While affective disorders probably adversely affect driving skill, treatment with antidepressant drugs may also be hazardous, although epidemiological studies are lacking. Impairment of performance is largely related to sedative and antimuscarinic effects both of which are more pronounced at the start of treatment. Sedative tricyclics, such as amitriptyline and doxepin, cause greater psychomotor impairment than less sedative drugs such as imipramine and nortriptyline. However, there are large individual differences between drugs, dosages, and duration of treatment; imipramine, nortriptyline, mianserin, and some monoamine oxidase inhibitors can all adversely affect psychomotor performance. Nomifensine and viloxazine, however, appear to be relatively safe. The effects on driving skills of some antidepressants, especially if sedative, are potentiated by alcohol.— H. Ashton, *Adverse Drug React. Bull.*, 1983, *98*, 360.

The Medical Commission on Accident Prevention recommended that patients on long-term psychotropic medication were unsuitable to be drivers of heavy goods or public service vehicles.— A. Cremona, *Br. J. Hosp. Med.*, 1986, *35*, 193.

ECT. It has been recommended that tricyclic antidepressants and monoamine oxidase inhibitors should be discontinued 2 weeks prior to an anaesthetic, but this may not be possible or advisable in most psychiatric patients, and concurrent therapy with tricyclics or monoamine oxidase inhibitors should not be a contra-indication to anaesthesia for ECT. However, tricyclic antidepressants and monoamine oxidase inhibitors augment the effects of barbiturates, increasing sleep time, duration of anaesthesia, and the incidence of fatality; lower barbiturate doses should be used in patients concomitantly taking tricyclic antidepressants or monoamine oxidase inhibitors.— G. Y. Gaines and D. I. Rees, *Anesth. Analg.*, 1986, *65*, 1345.

GLAUCOMA. The evidence for the antimuscarinic mydriatic and cycloplegic effects of tricyclic antidepressants and monoamine oxidase inhibitors triggering an acute attack of narrow-angle glaucoma in susceptible patients was very sparse indeed. There was virtually no evidence that an antimuscarinic reaction, such as could be induced by the tricyclics, had any harmful effect on intra-ocular pressure and if a patient was being treated for open-angle glaucoma, the standard treatment would easily counterbalance any possibility of aggravation of the condition by these drugs. These drugs were therefore not contra-indicated in primary glaucomatous conditions.— A. L. Crombie, *Prescribers' J.*, 1981, *21*, 222.

GRAFT-VERSUS-HOST DISEASE. For a report of failure to absorb amitriptyline after oral administration in a patient with graft-versus-host disease, and the suggestion that parenteral administration may be desirable, see under Absorption and Fate, below.

INTERACTIONS. *Alcohol.* As well as the recognised pharmacodynamic interaction with amitriptyline, alcohol decreases its hepatic first-pass extraction resulting in increased free plasma-amitriptyline concentrations, especially during the period of drug absorption.— P. Dorian *et al.*, *Eur. J. clin. Pharmac.*, 1983, *25*, 325.

Anticoagulants. For the effect of amitriptyline and other tricyclic antidepressants on anticoagulants, see Warfarin Sodium, p.346.

Antidepressants. A woman developed epileptic seizures on addition of lithium to her amitriptyline therapy.— J. G. Solomon, *Postgrad. Med.*, 1979, *66*, 145.

For a suggestion that antidepressants may cause hypomania or mania refractory to lithium, see Lithium Carbonate, p.367.

The combination of tricyclic antidepressants with monoamine oxidase inhibitors can result in agitation, delirium, hyperpyrexia, convulsions, and at times, hypertension, although it is usually safe for treating refractory depressions.— B. H. Guzé and L. R. Baxter, *New Engl. J. Med.*, 1985, *313*, 163. See also E. Marley and K. M. Wozniak, *Psychol. Med.*, 1983, *13*, 735.

Barbiturates. See under ECT, above.

Benzodiazepines. For evidence of an enhancing effect of benzodiazepines in fatal amitriptyline poisoning, see under Overdosage in Adverse Effects, above.

Clonidine. For the effect of tricyclic and related antidepressants on clonidine, see Clonidine Hydrochloride, p.473.

Dextropropoxyphene. The plasma-doxepin concentration in an 89-year-old man receiving doxepin 150 mg daily doubled 5 days after starting dextropropoxyphene 65 mg every 6 hours. The patient was lethargic whilst his plasma-doxepin concentration was raised, but improved when dextropropoxyphene was discontinued. Dextropropoxyphene inhibition of doxepin metabolism is consistent with the known properties of both drugs.— *Drug Interact. News.*, 1984, *4*, 43.

Disulfiram. Acute organic brain syndrome occurred in 2 patients receiving disulfiram when treatment with amitriptyline was started. Symptoms rapidly resolved on cessation of amitriptyline.— I. Maany *et al.* (letter), *Archs gen. Psychiat.*, 1982, *39*, 743.

Enflurane. For a report of amitriptyline enhancing enflurane-induced seizure activity, see Enflurane, p.1115.

Fenclonine. The antidepressant effect of imipramine was reversed by fenclonine.— B. Shopsin *et al.*, *Archs gen. Psychiat.*, 1976, *33*, 811.

Fenfluramine. In 3 subjects given amitriptyline 50 mg three times daily till a steady plasma-amitriptyline concentration had been reached, those concentrations rose when fenfluramine up to 60 mg daily was added to their treatment, and fell slowly over 1 to 2 weeks when fenfluramine was withdrawn.— L. Gunne *et al.*, *Postgrad. med. J.*, 1975, *51*, *Suppl.* 1, 117.

Furazolidone. A 49-year-old woman given amitriptyline 75 mg daily for depression developed a toxic psychosis 4 days after she started treatment with furazolidone, 300 mg daily. She developed blurred vision and profuse perspiration followed by alternating chills and hot flushes, restlessness, motor hyperactivity, persecutory delusions, auditory hallucinations, and visual illusions. These symptoms cleared 24 hours after stopping furazolidone. She was also taking conjugated oestrogens, diphenoxylate, and atropine. Furazolidone is a monoamine oxidase inhibitor.— R. M. Aderhold and C. E. Muniz (letter), *J. Am. med. Ass.*, 1970, *213*, 2080.

H_2 antagonist antihistamines. Available evidence indicates that cimetidine inhibits the elimination of doxepin, (D.R. Abernethy and E.L. Todd, *J. clin. Psychopharmacol.*, 1986, *6*, 8), imipramine, desipramine, and nortriptyline (*Drug Interact. News.*, 1984, *4*, 9). Adjustment of tricyclic antidepressant dosage may be required if cimetidine therapy is initiated or discontinued. Ranitidine does not affect imipramine (B.G. Wells *et al.*, *Eur. J. clin. Pharmac.*, 1986, *31*, 285) or doxepin pharmacokinetics, and may be the preferred H_2 antagonist antihistamine in patients requiring tricyclic antidepressants (D.L. Sutherland *et al.*, *ibid.*, 1987, *32*, 159).

Hexamethylmelamine. For a report of severe orthostatic hypotension in patients receiving concurrent hexamethylmelamine and tricyclic antidepressants, see Hexamethylmelamine, p.631.

Labetalol. The incidence of tremor with labetolol may be increased when it is given together with tricyclic antidepressants.— *Med. Lett.*, 1984, *26*, 83.

Levodopa. For the effect of tricyclic antidepressants on levodopa therapy, see p.1017.

Morphine. For a study suggesting that amitriptyline and clomipramine increase the bioavailability of morphine, see Morphine, p.1312.

Neuroleptics. Tricyclic antidepressants may increase neuroleptic concentration by competing for liver enzymes and it is anecdotally reported that this combination may be associated with an intensification of psychosis with confusional features (E.C. Johnstone, *Br. J. Hosp. Med.*, 1985, *34*, 198). Studies indicate that most neuroleptics inhibit the metabolism of imipramine and amitriptyline and, probably, their active metabolites, desipramine and nortriptyline. In patients receiving nortriptyline in combination with a neuroleptic, routine monitoring of plasma-nortriptyline concentrations may be helpful. Clinicians should also be alert for exaggerated side-effects from either antidepressants or neuroleptics when these drugs are given together (R.S. Lott, *Drug Interact. News.*, 1985, *5*, 31).

For further information on the effect of tricyclic antidepressants on neuroleptics, see Chlorpromazine, p.723 and Thioridazine, p.770.

Phenytoin. For the effect of tricyclic antidepressants on phenytoin see Phenytoin, p.408.

Sex hormones. Ethinyloestradiol given in doses of 50 µg together with imipramine 150 mg to 5 depressed patients, induced severe lethargy in all 5, hypotension in 4, coarse tremor in 2, and mild depersonalisation in 2. However, in a further trial in 30 women using doses of 25 µg and 50 µg of ethinyloestradiol with imipramine, patients on the lower dose of oestrogen and imipramine showed greater improvement than those taking the higher dose of oestrogen and imipramine or than those taking imipramine alone.— *J. Am. med. Ass.*, 1972, *219*, 143. See also R. C. Khurana (letter), *ibid.*, *222*, 702; S. M. Somani and R. C. Khurana (letter), *ibid.*, 1973, *223*, 560.

Of 5 men with depression given imipramine and methyltestosterone 15 mg daily, 4 showed a paranoid response which regressed when methyltestosterone was withdrawn.— I. C. Wilson *et al.*, *Am. J. Psychiat.*, 1974, *131*, 21.

Limited clinical information indicates that oral contraceptives reduce the first-pass metabolism of imipramine and may increase steady-state concentrations of clomipramine, although oral contraceptives have failed to alter clomipramine plasma concentrations. Until more is known about this interaction, one should be alert for evidence of altered response to tricyclic antidepressants if oral contraceptives are initiated or discontinued.— *Drug Interact. News.*, 1982, *2*, 41.

Smoking. Although no difference in the steady-state plasma concentrations of nortriptyline between tobacco smokers and non-smokers was observed in one study, two subsequent studies involving large numbers of patients demonstrated lower plasma concentrations of amitriptyline, desipramine, imipramine, and nortriptyline in smokers than non-smokers. The magnitude of the decreases in plasma drug concentrations associated with smoking appeared large enough to interfere with antidepressant efficacy in some patients.— *Drug Interact. News.*, 1982, *2*, 13.

Sympathomimetics. For the effect of amitriptyline and other tricyclic antidepressants on direct-acting sympathomimetics, see Noradrenaline, p.1471, and Phenylephrine, p.1474.

MANIA. For the risk of occurrence of mania in susceptible patients with tricyclic antidepressant therapy, see Phenelzine Sulphate, p.378.

PLASMA CONCENTRATIONS. Although spuriously low plasma concentrations of some tricyclic antidepressants and their metabolites previously resulted from the collection of blood samples in Vacutainer tubes (R.C. Veith and C. Perera, *New Engl. J. Med.*, 1979, *300*, 504), newer Vacutainer tubes no longer contained in the stopper the plasticiser that caused the leaching-displacement interaction although some Vacutainers with stoppers containing the plasticiser continued to be manufactured (V.P. Shah *et al.*, *Am. J. Hosp. Pharm.*, 1982, *39*, 1454).

PORPHYRIA. Imipramine was considered to be unsafe in patients with acute porphyria as it has been associated with acute attacks. Clomipramine was also considered to be unsafe as it has been shown to be porphyrinogenic in *animals* or *in vitro* systems. Amitriptyline and nortriptyline are considered to be unsafe, although there is conflicting experimental evidence of porphyrinogenicity.— M.R. Moore and K.E.L. McColl, *Porphyrias, Drug Lists*, Glasgow, Porphyria Research Unit, University of Glasgow, 1987.

PREGNANCY AND THE NEONATE. In a study in 836 infants with congenital malformations there was no significant difference in the maternal usage of tricyclic antidepressants during the first trimester of pregnancy compared with the use in 836 controls.— G. Greenberg *et al.*, *Br. med. J.*, 1977, *2*, 853. See also: D. L. Crombie *et al.* (letter), *Br. med. J.*, 1972, *1*, 745; M. Sim (letter), *ibid.*, *2*, 45; E. V. Kuenssberg and J. D. E. Knox (letter), *ibid.*, 292; G. S. Rachelefsky *et al.* (letter), *Lancet*, 1972, *1*, 838; P. Banister *et al.* (letter), *ibid;* J. Idänpään-Heikkilä and L. Saxén, *ibid.*, 1973, *2*, 282.

Case-control data from 11 mothers of children with birth defects, 5 treated antenatally with tri- and tetracyclic antidepressants and 6 untreated, did not show any association with infant central nervous system defects when tri- and tetracyclic antidepressants were given in the trimester before the last menstrual period and in the first trimester of pregnancy.— K. A. Winship *et al.*, *Archs Dis. Childh.*, 1984, *59*, 1052.

Individual reports and comments on congenital malformations in the infants of mothers given a tricyclic antidepressant during pregnancy: A. J. Barson (letter), *Br. med. J.*, 1972, *2*, 45; W. G. McBride (letter), *Med. J. Aust.*, 1972, *1*, 492; A. W. Morrow (letter), *ibid.*, 658.

Lactation. Although amitriptyline, amoxapine, desipramine, dothiepin, and imipramine are transferred into breast milk, there were no reported effects on lactation, or signs or symptoms in breast-fed infants.— *Pediatrics*, 1983, *72*, 375. See also L. Brixen-Rasmussen *et al.*, *Psychopharmacology*, 1982, *76*, 94.

REFLUX OESOPHAGITIS. The antimuscarinic action of tricyclic antidepressants causes relaxation of the lower oesophageal sphincter and could aggravate nocturnal symptoms of gastro-oesophageal reflux if given in the late evening.— M. Atkinson, *Prescribers' J.*, 1982, *22*, 129.

SURGERY. Tricyclic antidepressants increase the risk of ventricular arrhythmias and hypertension particularly when a directly-acting sympathomimetic is used during the operation. To reduce the risk of anaesthesia the drug has to be stopped for at least 2 weeks, which can be long enough to risk a relapse of depression. As this may outweigh the risk of anaesthesia, the patient is usually allowed to continue the drug and the anaesthetic is modified. If a vacoconstrictor is essential, felypressin is safer than adrenaline.— *Drug & Ther. Bull.*, 1984, *22*, 73.

TOLERANCE. Six patients with chronic or frequently recurrent non-bipolar major depression had full remission of symptoms with initial tricyclic antidepressant or monoamine oxidase inhibitor treatment, but relapsed within weeks or months of continued treatment. Remission was regained by serial increases in dose, unless or until side-effects intervened, or by changes of medication. Metabolic tolerance did not appear to account for the relapses.— B. M. Cohen and R. J. Baldessarini, *Am. J. Psychiat.*, 1985, *142*, 489.

WITHDRAWAL SYNDROMES. Antidepressant withdrawal syndromes seem to be characterised by 4 types of symptoms: a range of gastro-intestinal symptoms, sometimes with cardiac arrhythmias; insomnia followed by excessive, vivid dreams; extrapyramidal symptoms; and acute psychiatric disturbances. Withdrawal syndromes may occur after stopping a monoamine oxidase inhibitor and more rarely after a tricyclic. Antidepressants, particularly monoamine oxidase inhibitors, should be stopped gradually. Awareness of the possibility of withdrawal syndromes helps to avoid misinterpreting new symptoms after withdrawal as evidence of relapse.— *Drug & Ther. Bull.*, 1986, *24*, 29.

See also under Depression in Uses, below.

For reports of withdrawal syndromes in neonates whose mothers had received a tricyclic antidepressant during pregnancy, see Clomipramine Hydrochloride, p.358.

Absorption and Fate

Amitriptyline is readily absorbed from the gastro-intestinal tract, peak plasma concentrations occurring within about 6 hours of oral administration. Since amitriptyline slows gastro-intestinal transit time, absorption can, however, be delayed, particularly in overdosage.

Amitriptyline is extensively demethylated in the liver to its primary active metabolite, nortriptyline. Paths of metabolism of both amitriptyline and nortriptyline include hydroxylation (possibly to active metabolites) and *N*-oxidation. Amitriptyline is excreted in the urine, mainly in the form of its metabolites, either free or in conjugated form.

Amitriptyline and nortriptyline are widely distributed throughout the body and are extensively bound to plasma and tissue protein. Amitriptyline has been estimated to have a half-life ranging from 9 to 25 hours, which may be considerably extended in overdosage. Plasma concentrations of amitriptyline and nortriptyline vary very widely between individuals and no simple correlation with therapeutic response has been established.

Amitriptyline and nortriptyline cross the placental barrier and are excreted in breast milk (see under Precautions).

The pharmacokinetic properties of amitriptyline in psychiatric patients.— E. Mårtensson *et al.*, *Curr. ther. Res.*, 1984, *36*, 228.

A review of the discrepancies between pharmacokinetic studies of amitriptyline.— P. Schulz *et al.*, *Clin. Pharmacokinet.*, 1985, *10*, 257.

ABSORPTION. Amitriptyline given rectally relieved some symptoms of depression in a 56-year-old woman with colonic adenocarcinoma.— F. Adams (letter), *New Engl. J. Med.*, 1982, *306*, 996.

A 30-year-old woman with graft-versus-host disease of the gut failed to absorb amitriptyline after oral administration. In certain cases it may be desirable to give suitable antidepressants parenterally.— E. Freed *et al.* (letter), *Med. J. Aust.*, 1984, *140*, 509.

METABOLISM. Eight fasted subjects were given a single 50-mg dose of amitriptyline hydrochloride and urine was collected regularly for up to 180 hours. The approximate total excretion in the urine was amitriptyline 5%, 10-hydroxyamitriptyline 28%, nortriptyline and desmethylnortriptyline 6%, 10-hydroxynortriptyline 41%, and amitriptyline *N*-oxide 1%, 90% of the *N*-oxide being excreted during the first 12 hours.— G. Santagostino *et al.*, *J. pharm. Sci.*, 1974, *63*, 1690.

Amitriptyline, desipramine, imipramine, and nortriptyline share the debrisoquine/sparteine oxidation pathway, but as reports of possible associations between adverse reactions to tricyclics and poor metabolism of debrisoquine or sparteine have only been anecdotal, the clinical significance of this finding is not known.— D. W. J. Clark, *Drugs*, 1985, *29*, 342.

References to the influence of debrisoquine/sparteine oxidation phenotype on the metabolism of tricyclic antidepressants: K. Brøsen *et al.*, *Clin. Pharmac. Ther.*, 1986, *40*, 543; E. Spina *et al.*, *ibid.*, 1987, *41*, 314.

For a report suggesting a lack of correlation between hydroxylation phenotype and amitriptyline serum concentrations, see Nortriptyline Hydrochloride, p.375.

PLASMA CONCENTRATIONS. Controversy surrounds the relationship between plasma-amitriptyline concentration and clinical outcome. Three studies have shown a linear relationship like that found with imipramine. Three studies have revealed a curvilinear (window-like) relationship similar to that seen with nortriptyline, and 4 studies have found no relationship at all. From the available data on amitriptyline it is only possible to define certain plasma concentrations as extremely low and unlikely to be therapeutic.— American Psychiatric Association (APA) Task Force, *Am. J. Psychiat.*, 1985, *142*, 155.

For reports of spuriously low plasma concentrations of some tricyclic antidepressants and their metabolites resulting from the collection of blood samples in Vacutainer tubes, see under Precautions, above.

Uses and Administration

Amitriptyline is a tricyclic antidepressant. It has marked antimuscarinic and sedative properties, and prevents the re-uptake (and hence the inactivation) of noradrenaline and serotonin at nerve terminals. Its mode of action in depression is not fully understood.

Amitriptyline and other tricyclic antidepressants are used in the treatment of depression, particularly endogenous depression; they are less effective in reactive depression. Since up to a month may elapse before an antidepressant response is obtained, severely depressed or suicidal patients may require electroconvulsive therapy initially. The sedative action of tricyclics is not delayed.

Amitriptyline is usually given as the hydrochloride, by mouth, in a single or divided daily dose of 75 mg initially, gradually increased if necessary, to 150 mg daily, the additional doses being given in the late afternoon or evening. Therapy may also be initiated with a single dose of 50 to 100 mg at night increased by 25 or 50 mg as necessary to a total of 150 mg daily. Maintenance doses are usually 50 to 100 mg daily and therapy should be continued for at least 3 months before being gradually withdrawn. Hospital in-patients may be given amitriptyline hydrochloride in doses of up to 200 mg daily and, occasionally, up to 300 mg daily.

Adolescent or elderly patients often have reduced tolerance to tricyclic antidepressants and initial doses of amitriptyline hydrochloride 10 to 50 mg daily may be adequate, given either as divided doses or as a single dose, preferably at night. Half the usual maintenance dose will often be sufficient.

In the initial stages of treatment, if administration by mouth is impracticable or inadvisable, 20 to 30 mg of the hydrochloride may be given by intravenous or intramuscular injection 4 times daily, but oral administration should be substituted as soon as possible; in some countries only the intramuscular route is recommended. Amitriptyline may also be given as a syrup by mouth in the form of the embonate.

Amitriptyline is also given for the treatment of nocturnal enuresis in children. The use of tricyclic antidepressants for nocturnal enuresis in children is controversial, not least in view of the hazards of accidental overdosage. In particular, tricyclic antidepressant therapy is not suitable for younger children. Doses that have been suggested are 10 to 20 mg at bedtime for children aged 6 to 10 years, and 25 to 50 mg at bedtime for children over 11 years of age. Treatment should not continue for longer than 3 months.

The actions and uses of tricyclic antidepressants: R.H. Mindham, in *Drugs in Psychiatric Practice*, P.J. Tyrer (Ed.), London, Butterworths, 1982, p.177.; *Drugs in Psychiatry*, Volume 1, Antidepressants, G.D. Burrows *et al.*, (Eds.), Oxford, Elsevier, 1983, p.57; J.M. Baker and W.G. Dewhurst, in *Pharmacotherapy of Affective Disorders: Theory and Practice*, W.G. Dewhurst and G.B. Baker (Eds.), London, Croom Helm, 1985, p.262.

ADMINISTRATION. A review of dose response studies of antidepressants. Data suggested that patients without significant side-effects should be treated with imipramine 300 mg or its equivalent before concluding that the drug is ineffective.— F. M. Quitkin, *Br. J. Psychiat.*, 1985, *147*, 593.

ADMINISTRATION IN CARDIOVASCULAR DISEASE. For the successful use of tricyclic antidepressants in depressed patients with cardiovascular disease, see Imipramine Hydrochloride, p.363 and Nortriptyline Hydrochloride, p.375.

ADMINISTRATION IN THE ELDERLY. Owing to increased sensitivity to side-effects and, in some cases, impaired elimination, the elderly need smaller doses of antidepressants than the young, often a third to a half of the standard adult dose, although there is considerable variation in dose requirements.— *Drugs for the Elderly*, Geneva, Wld Hlth Org., 1985, p.124.

Amitriptyline dosage prediction in elderly patients from plasma concentration at 24 hours after a single 100-mg dose.— S. Dawling *et al.*, *Clin. Pharmacokinet.*, 1984, *9*, 261.

ADMINISTRATION IN RENAL FAILURE. Amitriptyline can be given in usual doses to patients with renal failure. Concentrations of amitriptyline are not affected by haemodialysis or peritoneal dialysis.— W. M. Bennett *et al.*, *Am. J. Kidney Dis.*, 1983, *3*, 155. Symptoms of encephalopathy developed in a patient on maintenance haemodialysis when given amitriptyline. Similar symptoms had occurred when he was taking flurazepam.— L. Taclob and M. Needle, *Lancet*, 1976, *2*, 704.

ADMINISTRATION, RECTAL. For the use of amitriptyline given rectally, see under Absorption in Absorption and Fate, above.

ANXIETY AND PHOBIAS. Amitriptyline, trimipramine, doxepin, and mianserin have useful secondary sedative properties and are the treatment of first choice in depressed patients with anxiety or agitation. They are not appropriate for patients with primary anxiety states.— M. Lader and H. Petursson, *Drugs*, 1983, *25*, 514.

Agoraphobia. For the use of a tricyclic antidepressant in agoraphobia and panic attacks, see Imipramine Hydrochloride, p.363.

Panic attacks. Tricyclic antidepressants and monoamine oxidase inhibitors are more effective than beta blockers for the treatment of recurrent panic attacks.— *Med. Lett.*, 1984, *26*, 61.

BEHAVIOUR DISORDERS. Eight of 12 patients with a syndrome of pathological laughing and weeping associated with multiple sclerosis showed clinical improvement within 48 hours of starting therapy with amitriptyline in a double-blind placebo-controlled crossover study; in 7 of these patients the improvement was dramatic. The dosage of amitriptyline used was lower than that usually required to affect mood and there was no evidence of a significant change in scores on depression-rating scales, suggesting that this effect of amitriptyline is not mediated by its antidepressant property.— R. B. Schiffer *et al.*, *New Engl. J. Med.*, 1985, *312*, 1480. Comment. Patients with emotional lability due to amyotrophic lateral sclerosis also showed dramatic improvement with the use of amitriptyline and imipramine in doses of 50 to 75 mg at bedtime.— J. T. Caroscio *et al.* (letter), *ibid.*, *313*, 1478.

CIGUATERA POISONING. Amitriptyline 25 mg twice daily by mouth resulted in resolution of dysaesthesias and pruritus and normalisation of electrocardiographic findings after one week in a 52-year-old man with ciguatera fish poisoning.— R. T. Davis and L. A. Villar (letter), *New Engl. J. Med.*, 1986, *315*, 65. See also P. B. Bowman (letter), *Med. J. Aust.*, 1984, *140*, 802.

DEPRESSION. Amitriptyline and imipramine are the 2 standard antidepressants by which others must be measured in the treatment of depression in general practice. The sedative properties of amitriptyline may be useful in agitated patients and those with broken sleep or early waking, when a single dose at night can be taken. In obese patients, trazodone may be used as it is often associated with loss of weight. Mianserin has found favour as having established efficacy, less antimuscarinic effects, probably less cardiotoxicity, and being safer in overdose. In patients with congestive heart failure, coronary artery disease, a conduction defect, or a recent myocardial infarction antidepressants are best avoided, but if they seem essential mianserin has a larger margin of safety than the tricyclics. Electroconvulsive therapy is safer and has a more rapid effect than drug therapy. Where epilepsy or a reduced threshold for fits is a problem, desipramine and trazodone or viloxazine are less likely to be associated with fits than other antidepressants, except the monoamine oxidase inhibitors. Monoamine oxidase inhibitors are still useful in some circumstances and may be used in combination with tricyclics. That combination is, however, sufficiently hazardous to be justified only in the hands of experts.

Compliance will be improved if the patient is warned both of the likely side-effects and of the delay of up to 2 or 3 weeks before maximum effects are likely to be achieved. The starting dose should be about one third of the standard adult dose and it may be increased in 2 stages after intervals of 3 or 4 days. Treatment should continue for one month before it can be regarded as having failed. The most common cause of failure is non-compliance and the second is inadequate dosage. If possible a single drug only should be prescribed. If an antidepressant in adequate dosage is not producing some improvement within 2 weeks, supplementary lithium, liothyronine, or oestrogens may increase response to the drug, or it may be advisable to change to a different drug. Once remission is achieved some continuing medication is required for 6 months if the risk of relapse is to be reduced. After 6 months' treatment withdrawal should be gradual, over 4 to 8 weeks.— S. Brandon, *Br. med. J.*, 1986, *292*, 287.

Results suggested that even with a fairly rapid increase in drug dose, a substantial minority of outpatient depressives unresponsive after 4 weeks of tricyclic antidepressant or monoamine oxidase inhibitor treatment achieve significant benefit if the drug trial is extended to 6 weeks. More data was needed.— F. M. Quitkin *et al.*, *Archs gen. Psychiat.*, 1984, *41*, 238.

For a report of studies examining the relationship between plasma-amitriptyline concentration and clinical outcome, see under Plasma Concentration in Absorption and Fate, above.

For the use of dexamphetamine as a predictive test for response to tricyclic antidepressants, see p.1441.

Combination therapy. As well as considering combinations of tricyclic antidepressants with liothyronine, with lithium, and with monoamine oxidase inhibitors (see below), this review considers the combination of tricyclic antidepressants with tryptophan. As tryptophan can boost the serotonin-potentiating effect of antidepressant drugs and is a relatively nontoxic drug, it is worth considering as an addition to the drug regimen of depressed patients where tricyclics or monoamine oxidase inhibitors, with or without lithium, have not proved beneficial.— C. L. E. Katona and T. R. E. Barnes, *Br. J. Hosp. Med.*, 1985, *34*, 168.

Combination therapy with liothyronine. For the use of liothyronine as a adjunct to tricyclic antidepressant therapy in depression, see Liothyronine, p.1487.

Combination therapy with lithium. For a report of clinical improvement following the addition of lithium therapy in patients with depression resistant to tricyclic antidepressants, see Lithium Carbonate, p.370.

Combination therapy with monoamine oxidase inhibitors. The risk of serious problems in combining tricyclic antidepressant and monoamine oxidase inhibitor antidepressant therapy is almost exclusively limited to sequential prescribing, in particular the addition of a tricyclic to established treatment with a monoamine oxidase inhibitor. The recommended procedure is to allow a drug-free interval of at least one week and then to start both drugs together at a low dosage. The dosage of both drugs is then gradually increased to around half that normally prescribed for the drugs when given on their own. The dietary restrictions for monoamine oxidase inhibitors alone apply equally to the combined antidepressant regimen. Amitriptyline and trimipramine seem to be the tricyclics least likely to produce side-effects in combination with monoamine oxidase inhibitors, while phenelzine and isocarboxazid are the safest monoamine oxidase inhibitors. There have been 3 recent studies comparing the combination of tricyclics and monoamine oxidase inhibitors with individual antidepressants (J.P.R. Young *et al.*, *Br. med. J.*, 1979, *2*, 1315; K. White *et al.*, *Am J. Psychiat.*, 1980, *137*, 1422; J. Razani *et al.*, *Archs gen. Psychiat.*, 1983, *40*, 657). In none of these was the combination demonstrably superior to individual antidepressants in the mild to moderately depressed patients studied. The effectiveness of the combination in refractory depression has not been systematically tested. Three open studies in refractory depression (D.R. Gander, *Lancet*, 1965, *2*, 107; F. Winston, *Br. J. Psychiat.*, 1971, *118*, 301; E.R. Sethna, *ibid.*, 1974, *124*, 265) claimed that the treatment was beneficial in a high proportion of patients, although it has been suggested that the improvement observed might be related to an anxiolytic rather than a specific antidepressant action. The only controlled study comparing combined tricyclic and monoamine oxidase inhibitor medication with ECT in refractory depression found ECT to be the superior treatment in both psychotic and neurotic depression (J. Davidson *et al.*, *Archs gen. Psychiat.*, 1978, *35*, 639).— C. L. E. Katona and T. R. E. Barnes, *Br. J. Hosp. Med.*, 1985, *34*, 168.

A retrospective study of combined tricyclic or tetracyclic and monoamine oxidase inhibitor antidepressant therapy in 94 patients refractory to alternative therapy concluded that combined treatment was effective and did not generally result in increased side-effects.— M. Schmauss *et al.*, *Pharmacopsychiatry*, 1986, *19*, 251.

For a description of the possible adverse reactions resulting from the combined administration of tricyclic antidepressants and monoamine oxidase inhibitors, see under Precautions, above. For reports suggesting that the combined administration of a monoamine oxidase inhibitor with amitriptyline may decrease the risk of a hypertensive reaction with oral tyramine, see Phenelzine Sulphate, p.379.

Combination therapy with monoamine oxidase inhibitors and central stimulants. In a retrospective study of 16 patients with treatment-resistant depression, a combination of tricyclic antidepressant and a monoamine oxidase inhibitor with a central stimulant (dexamphetamine or methylphenidate), or a monoamine oxidase inhibitor with a central stimulant produced fair to good improvement of depressive symptoms. Mean blood pressure was generally in the normal range with both these combinations and there were no hypertensive crises. The most frequent complication was orthostatic hypotension. It was suggested that therapy was initiated in the order: tricyclic antidepressant, monoamine oxidase inhibitor, central stimulant.— J. P. Feighner *et al.*, *J. clin. Psychiat.*, 1985, *46*, 206.

Delusional depression. In an open study 12 of 29 patients with delusional depression responded to treatment with amitriptyline, but it was noted that tricyclic antidepressants could exacerbate the psychosis of these patients, that the combination of a phenothiazine with a tricyclic was more efficacious than a tricyclic alone, and that other workers felt that ECT was the treatment of choice.— D. G. Spiker *et al.*, *J. clin. Psychiat.*, 1986, *47*, 243.

Depression in Alzheimer's disease. Antidepressants may be useful if depression accompanies the dementia. However, tricyclics may predispose to the development of delirium and make the patient worse. Monoamine oxidase inhibitors might be a better choice, but orthostatic hypotension limits their applicability.— L. E. Hollister, *Drugs*, 1985, *29*, 483.

Depression in cardiovascular disease. See under Administration in Cardiovascular Disease, above.

Depression in children. For the use of a tricyclic antidepressant in childhood depression, see Imipramine Hydrochloride, p.363.

Depression in the elderly. A review of the use of tricyclic antidepressants in the elderly.— T. L. Thompson *et al.*, *New Engl. J. Med.*, 1983, *308*, 194. Comment regarding adequacy of dosage.— B. S. Fogel (letter), *ibid.*, 1600. Reply.— T. L. Thompson *et al.*, *ibid.*, 1601. Further reference: J. C. A. Morrant, *Can. med. Ass. J.*, 1983, *129*, 245.

See also under Administration in the Elderly, above.

Depression in medical patients. The use of tricyclic and tetracyclic antidepressants in depressed medical patients.— *Lancet*, 1986, *1*, 949.

Depression in parkinsonism. Depression commonly accompanies Parkinson's disease and must be treated for the patient to benefit adequately from antiparkinsonian drugs. Tricyclic antidepressants may be useful (*Med. Lett.*, 1986, *28*, 62). Depression also occurs in half of all patients given levodopa and, again, is best controlled by tricyclics (J.M.S. Pearce, *Br. med. J.*, 1984, *288*, 1777).

For the effect of amitriptyline on levodopa therapy, see Levodopa, p.1016.

Depression in pregnancy. Endogenous depression may be treated in the normal way with tricyclic antidepressants if it occurs in pregnancy. The newer non-tricyclic antidepressants are best avoided in pregnancy.— J. B. Loudon, *Br. med. J.*, 1987, *294*, 167.

See also under Pregnancy and the Neonate, in Precautions, above.

Depression after stroke. A review of depression after stroke, including treatment with tricyclic antidepressants.— A. House, *Br. med. J.*, 1987, *294*, 76.

For the successful use of a tricyclic antidepressant for post-stroke depression, see Nortriptyline Hydrochloride, p.375.

Prophylaxis. For a study showing amitriptyline and lithium to have equal effectiveness in preventing recurrent depression, see Lithium Carbonate, p.370.

Withdrawal of therapy. In a study of 51 patients treated for depressive, anxiety, and phobic neuroses, the relatively small changes in symptoms following withdrawal from tricyclic antidepressants suggested that in most cases abrupt withdrawal from a low maintenance dose after less than 9 months' treatment would lead to no special clinical problems.— P. Tyrer, *J. Affect. Dis.*, 1984, *6*, 1. Results from a National Institute of Mental Health project indicated that withdrawal of tricyclic antidepressant therapy for major depressive episodes was safe only after the patient had been free of significant symptoms for 16 to 20 weeks. R. F. Prien and D. J. Kupfer, *Am. J. Psychiat.*, 1986, *143*, 18.

EATING DISORDERS. In the treatment of anorexia nervosa, no significant differences have been found between amitriptyline or clomipramine and placebo. However, imipramine and phenelzine have been shown to be significantly superior to placebo in reducing bulimic and depressive symptoms, although controlled studies of amitriptyline and mianserin did not yield similar findings.— D. B. Herzog and P. M. Copeland, *New Engl. J. Med.*, 1985, *313*, 295. See also H. G. Pope and J. I. Hudson, *J. clin. Psychiat.*, 1986, *47*, 339; W. S. Bond *et al.*, *Drug Intell. & clin. Pharm.*, 1986, *20*, 659.

For the beneficial use of other tricyclic antidepressants in bulimia, see Desipramine Hydrochloride, p.359 and Protriptyline Hydrochloride, p.380.

ENURESIS. For a review of the use of a tricyclic antidepressant in enuresis, see Imipramine Hydrochloride, p.364.

HEADACHE. Tricyclic antidepressants such as amitriptyline are effective in the prophylaxis of migraine and combined with propranolol are particularly helpful when common migraine and tension headaches occur together. The beneficial action of amitriptyline is independent of its antidepressant activity and may be due to its 5-HT receptor antagonism.— S. Nightingale, *J. clin. Hosp. Pharm.*, 1984, *9*, 271. Further references to amitriptyline in migraine: J. R. Couch *et al.*, *Neurology, Minneap.*, 1976, *26*, 121; J. R. Couch and R. S. Hassanein, *Archs Neurol., Chicago*, 1979, *36*, 695; N. T. Mathew, *Headache*, 1981, *21*, 105; V. Pfaffenrath *et al.*, *Cephalalgia*, 1986, *6*, *Suppl.* 5, 25.

HICCUP. Amitriptyline up to 30 mg daily by mouth in three divided doses resulted in the almost complete disappearance of intractable hiccups in a 17-year-old boy. No side-effects were observed. Gradual reduction of the dose to 10 mg daily after 5 months of treatment resulted in reappearance of the hiccups. Reinstating the 30-mg dose produced control and the patient had been free of hiccups for the last 6 months.— R. Stalnikowicz *et al.*, (letter), *New Engl. J. Med.*, 1986, *315*, 64.

MYOTONIA. For the use of amitriptyline in the symptomatic relief of myotonia, see Imipramine Hydrochloride, p.364.

PAIN. A review of the pharmacology, use, and effectiveness of tricyclic, tetracyclic, and monoamine oxidase inhibitor antidepressants in chronic pain. Antidepressants have a useful opiate-potentiating role in pain due to cancer, are valuable in the treatment of neuralgia when given with a phenothiazine and, in other conditions, may relieve depression-associated pain by their antidepressant action.— T. D. Walsh, *Clin. Neuropharmacol.*, 1983, *6*, 271.

Antidepressants are widely used in the treatment of chronic non-cancer pain, but have never been shown to be effective in the relief of acute pain. Certain chronic pain syndromes have been specifically regarded as being manifestations of an underlying depressive illness. Atypical facial pain, facial arthromyalgia, and low back pain with no identifiable cause are the conditions which have most often been described in these terms and do respond favourably to antidepressants.— G. W. Hanks, *Postgrad. med. J.*, 1984, *60*, 881.

Diabetic neuropathy. Initial reports suggested that amitriptyline and fluphenazine, separately or in combination, were effective in relieving the pain of diabetic neuropathy (J.L. Davis *et al.*, *J. Am. med. Ass.*, 1977, *238*, 2291; G.N. Gade *et al.*, *ibid.*, 1980, *243*, 1160), but a double-blind crossover study in non-depressed patients found the combination to be no more effective than placebo, although it was acknowledged that there is strong placebo response in this condition (C.M. Mendel *et al.*, *ibid.*, 1986, *255*, 637). However, a study comparing amitriptyline with a placebo which mimicked tricyclic antidepressant side-effects found amitriptyline to be more effective than placebo, and concluded that the analgesic effect is independent of mood change (M.B. Max *et al.*, *Neurology*, 1987, *37*, 589); in contrast, in depressed patients, the pain of diabetic neuropathy was felt to be a depressive symptom in many cases, and imipramine and amitriptyline produced both relief of depression and pain (R.W. Turkington, *J. Am. med. Ass.*, 1980, *243*, 1147). A crossover study also found imipramine to be more effective than placebo (B. Kvinesdal *et al.*, *ibid.*, 1984, *251*, 1727), but this study was criticised by Mendel *et al.*, (1986) on the grounds that the statistical analyses were incorrect and that the patients could distinguish imipramine from placebo by its side-effects.

Migraine. For the successful use of tricyclic anti-depressants in migraine, see under Headache, above.

Musculoskeletal and joint pain. In a double-blind study of 59 patients with fibrositis, amitriptyline 50 mg daily by mouth significantly improved morning stiffness, pain, sleep patterns, and physicians' global assessments compared with placebo (S. Carette *et al.*, *Arthritis Rheum.*, 1986, *29*, 655). Similar improvement was also seen in 62 fibrositic patients receiving amitriptyline 25 mg daily, and the concomitant administration of naproxen 500 mg twice daily did not produce any further improvement (D.L. Goldenberg *et al.*, *ibid.*, 1371). However, in 36 patients with definite or classical rheumatoid arthritis with pain not adequately controlled by non-steroidal anti-inflammatory drugs, the addition of amitriptyline therapy at daily doses of up to 75 mg did not improve joint pain and tenderness (E.M. Grace *et al.*, *Curr. med. Res. Opinion*, 1985, *9*, 426).

For a report of reduction of joint pain and tenderness after trimipramine administration in patients with rheumatoid arthritis, see Trimipramine Hydrochloride, p.383.

Pain of cortical origin. A 44-year-old woman with paroxysmal pain of cortical origin, resistant to opioid and other analgesics and non-steroidal anti-inflammatory drugs, experienced complete and prolonged relief of symptoms after taking amitriptyline 50 mg by mouth each night, although hyperalgesia remained.— R. Sandyk and M. A. Gillman, *Clin. Pharm.*, 1986, *5*, 108.

Postherpetic neuralgia. Amitriptyline at a median daily dose of 75 mg was superior to placebo in relieving postherpetic neuralgia, and produced analgesia in patients who were not depressed, suggesting an action other than an antidepressant effect (C.P. Watson *et al.*, *Neurology*, 1982, *32*, 671). Successful results have also been obtained using combinations of amitriptyline with perphenazine (O. Weis *et al.*, *S. Afr. med. J.*, 1982, *62*, 274), and with sodium valproate (H. Raftery, *J. Ir. med. Ass.*, 1979, *72*, 399). A tricyclic antidepressant, especially amitriptyline, seems a reasonable first choice for analgesia when therapy with traditional analgesics has failed (M. Thompson and M. Bones, *Clin. Pharm.*, 1985, *4*, 170; P.N. Robinson and N. Fletcher, *J. R. Coll. gen. Pract.*, 1986, *36*, 24). It has been suggested that a therapeutic window may exist for the analgesic action of amitriptyline in some patients, such that if the dose or blood concentrations are below or above this range, or window, the desired effect does not occur (C.P. Watson, *Can. med. Ass. J.*, 1984, *130*, 105).

PHOBIAS. For comments on the role of tricyclic antidepressants in the management of phobic states, see under Anxiety and Phobias, above.

RESTLESS LEG SYNDROME. Amitriptyline has not been shown to have any benefit over placebo in the treatment of the restless leg syndrome (C. Clough, *Br. med. J.*, 1987, *294*, 262); on the contrary amitriptyline 50 mg by mouth at night caused the syndrome in a 56-year-old woman, although when the drug was stopped the syndrome resolved (R. Sandyk and M.A. Gillman, *ibid.*, 1984, *289*, 162).

SLEEP DISORDERS. For a brief mention of the use of amitriptyline for night terrors and nightmares, see Imipramine Hydrochloride, p.364.

URINARY INCONTINENCE. In patients with urge incontinence due to detrusor instability, tricyclic antidepressants and antimuscarinic agents can be used either singly, or together as it appears that their site of action is not the same.— E. J. McGuire, *Br. J. Hosp. Med.*, 1984, *31*, 149.

Preparations

Amitriptyline Hydrochloride Injection *(U.S.P.)*

Amitriptyline Hydrochloride Tablets *(U.S.P.)*

Amitriptyline Oral Suspension *(B.P.)*. Amitriptyline Embonate Mixture; Amitriptyline Syrup. Potency is expressed in terms of the equivalent amount of amitriptyline. pH 5 to 7.

Amitriptyline Tablets *(B.P.)*. Tablets containing amitriptyline hydrochloride.

Chlordiazepoxide and Amitriptyline Hydrochloride Tablets *(U.S.P.)*. The potency of amitriptyline is expressed in terms of the equivalent amount of amitriptyline. Store in airtight containers. Protect from light.

Perphenazine and Amitriptyline Hydrochloride Tablets *(U.S.P.)*

Proprietary Preparations

Domical *(Berk Pharmaceuticals, UK)*. *Tablets*, amitriptyline hydrochloride, 10, 25, and 50 mg.

Elavil *(DDSA Pharmaceuticals, UK)*. *Tablets*, amitriptyline hydrochloride, 10 and 25 mg.

Lentizol *(Parke, Davis, UK)*. *Capsules*, sustained-release, amitriptyline hydrochloride 25 and 50 mg.

Limbitrol *(Roche, UK)*. *Capsules* (Limbitrol 5), amitriptyline 12.5 mg (as hydrochloride), chlordiazepoxide 5 mg.
Capsules (Limbitrol 10), amitriptyline 25 mg (as hydrochloride), chlordiazepoxide 10 mg.

Triptafen *(Allen & Hanburys, UK)*. *Tablets*, amitriptyline hydrochloride 25 mg, perphenazine 2 mg.
Tablets (Triptafen-M), amitriptyline hydrochloride 10 mg, perphenazine 2 mg.

Tryptizol *(Morson, UK)*. *Capsules* (Tryptizol 75), sustained-release, amitriptyline hydrochloride 75 mg.
Tablets, amitriptyline hydrochloride 10, 25, and 50 mg.
Syrup, amitriptyline 10 mg (as embonate)/5 mL.
Injection, amitriptyline hydrochloride 10 mg/mL, in vials of 10 mL.

Proprietary Names and Manufacturers of Amitriptyline or its Salts

Adepril *(Lepetit, Ital.)*; Amavil *(USA)*; Amilent *(Warner, S.Afr.)*; Amiline *(Canad.)*; Amilit *(IFI, Ital.)*; Amitid *(Squibb, USA)*; Amitril *(Parke, Davis, USA)*; Amitrip *(Protea, Austral.)*; Amitrip M *(Protea, Austral.)*; Amitriptol *(Ital.)*; Annolytin *(Jpn)*; Deprestat *(Propan, S.Afr.)*; Deprex *(Canad.)*; Domical *(Berk Pharmaceuticals, UK)*; Elavil *(Austral.; Merck Sharp & Dohme, Canad.; Merck Sharp & Dohme-Chibret, Fr.; DDSA Pharmaceuticals, UK; Merck Sharp & Dohme, USA)*; Endep *(Roche, USA)*; Equilibrin *(Natrapharm, Ger.)*; Laroxyl *(Roche, Austral.; Belg.; Roche, Fr.; Roche, Ger.; Roche, Ital.; Roche, Switz.)*; Larozyl *(Swed.)*; Lentizol *(Parke, Davis, UK)*; Levate *(ICN, Canad.)*; Meravil *(Canad.)*; Miketorin *(Jpn)*; Novotriptyn *(Novopharm, Canad.)*; Redomex *(Belg.)*; Saroten *(Nicholas, Austral.; Lundbeck, Denm.; Tropon, Ger.; Leo, S.Afr.; SCS, S.Afr.; Lundbeck, Swed.; Lundbeck, Switz.; Warner, UK)*; Sarotex *(Neth.; Lundbeck, Norw.)*; SK-Amitriptyline *(Smith Kline & French, USA)*; Teperin *(Hung.)*; Trepiline *(Lennon, S.Afr.)*; Triptizol *(Merck Sharp & Dohme, Ital.)*; Tryptanol *(Arg.; Frosst, Austral.; Merck Sharp & Dohme, S.Afr.)*; Tryptizol *(Belg.; Merck Sharp & Dohme, Denm.; Frosst, Ger.; Neth.; Merck Sharp & Dohme, Norw.; Merck Sharp & Dohme, Spain; MSD, Swed.; Merck Sharp & Dohme, Switz.; Morson, UK)*; Uxen *(Arg.)*.

The following names have been used for multi-ingredient preparations containing amitriptyline or its salts— Elavil Plus *(Merck Sharp & Dohme, Canad.)*; Etrafon *(Schering, Canad.; Schering, USA)*; Limbatril; Limbitrol *(Roche, UK; Roche, USA)*; Mutabon *(Essex, Austral.)*; Proavil *(Pro Doc, Canad.)*; Triamed *(Medic, Canad.)*; Triavil *(Merck Sharp & Dohme, Canad.; Merck Sharp & Dohme, USA)*; Triptafen *(Allen & Hanburys, UK)*; Triptafen-DA *(Allen & Hanburys, UK)*; Triptafen-Forte *(Allen & Hanburys, UK)*; Triptafen-M *(Allen & Hanburys, UK)*; Triptafen-Minor *(Allen & Hanburys, UK)*.

2503-q

Amoxapine *(BAN, USAN, rINN)*.

CL-67772. 2-Chloro-11-(piperazin-1-yl)dibenz-[*b,f*][1,4]oxazepine.

$C_{17}H_{16}ClN_3O$=313.8.

CAS — 14028-44-5.

Adverse Effects and Treatment

As for Amitriptyline Hydrochloride, p.351.

A brief review of adverse reactions to some antidepressants including amoxapine.— P. E. Hayes and C. A. Kristoff, *Clin. Pharm.*, 1986, *5*, 471.

ANTIDOPAMINERGIC EFFECTS. Amoxapine therapy has been associated with chorea (J.F. Patterson, *Sth. med. J.*, 1983, *76*, 1077), oculogyric crisis (A.K. Hunt-Fugate *et al.*, *Pharmacotherapy*, 1984, *4*, 35), akinesia, akathisia, withdrawal dyskinesia, reversible tardive dyskinesia, persistent dyskinesia, elevated serum concentration of prolactin, and galactorrhoea. All are symptoms of dopamine receptor blockade (G.K. Tao *et al.*, *Drug*

Intell. & clin. Pharm., 1985, *19*, 548).

EFFECTS ON THE ENDOCRINE SYSTEM. *Diabetogenic effect.* Reversible nonketotic hyperglycaemia developed in a 49-year-old woman with no history of diabetes mellitus within 5 days of therapy with amoxapine 50 mg three times daily by mouth. The patient had previously experienced nonketotic hyperglycaemic coma after loxapine 150 mg daily.— G. Tollefson and T. Lesar, *J. clin. Psychiat.*, 1983, *44*, 347.

Hyperprolactinaemia. For a report of galactorrhoea, due to elevated serum prolactin concentration, see under Antidopaminergic Effects, above.

EFFECTS ON THE SKIN. Toxic epidermal necrolysis developed in a 55-year-old woman 2 weeks after commencing therapy with amoxapine 50 mg three times daily. The patient was also receiving triamterene, hydrochlorothiazide, and conjugated oestrogens, but those were not considered to be the cause of the adverse reaction.— C. Camisa and C. Grines (letter), *Archs Derm.*, 1983, *119*, 709.

OVERDOSAGE. In overdosage, amoxapine is reported not to be cardiotoxic (K. Kulig *et al.*, *J. Am. med. Ass.*, 1982, *248*, 1092), but to cause acute renal failure (A.J. Pumariega *et al.*, *ibid.*, 3141; A.E. Jennings *et al.*, *Archs intern. Med.*, 1983, *143*, 1525), coma, and seizures (K. Kulig *et al.*, *J. Am. med. Ass.*, 1982, *248*, 1092; T.L. Litovitz and W.G. Troutman, *ibid.*, 1983, *250*, 1069; J.W. Jefferson, *ibid.*, 1984, *251*, 603). There is debate as to whether the incidence of seizures and death is higher with overdosage of amoxapine than other tricyclic antidepressants (H. Kiltie *et al.*, *ibid.*, 601; T.L. Litovitz and W.G. Troutman, *ibid.*, 602; K. Kulig and B.H. Rumack, *ibid.*; T.L. Litovitz and W.G. Troutman, *ibid.*, 603).

Clinical features and management of self-poisoning with amoxapine.— P. Crome and C. Ali, *Med. Toxicol.*, 1986, *1*, 411.

Precautions

As for Amitriptyline Hydrochloride, p.352.

PREGNANCY AND THE NEONATE. *Lactation.* For a report that although amoxapine is transferred into breast milk, there had been no reported effects on lactation, or signs or symptoms in breast-fed infants, see Amitriptyline Hydrochloride, p.354.

TOLERANCE. Eight patients treated with amoxapine in doses of 50 to 300 mg daily demonstrated rapid antidepressant response, often including mild euphoria, increased energy, and, in some cases, increased insomnia. All then experienced loss of antidepressant efficacy within 1 to 3 months and were refractory to upward or downward dosage adjustment, suggesting pharmacological tolerance to its antidepressant effect.— M. Zetin *et al.*, *Clin. Ther.*, 1983, *5*, 638.

For a further report of tolerance to antidepressants, see Amitriptyline Hydrochloride, p.354.

Absorption and Fate

Amoxapine is readily absorbed from the gastro-intestinal tract. Since amoxapine slows gastro-intestinal transit time, absorption can, however, be delayed, particularly in overdosage.

Amoxapine bears a close chemical relationship to loxapine and is similarly metabolised by hydroxylation. It is excreted in the urine, mainly as its metabolites in conjugated form as glucuronides.

Amoxapine has been reported to have a serum half-life of 8 hours and its major metabolites, 8-hydroxyamoxapine and 7-hydroxyamoxapine have been reported to have biological half-lives of 30 hours and 6.5 hours respectively. Both metabolites are pharmacologically active. Amoxapine is extensively bound to plasma proteins.

Uses and Administration

Amoxapine is a tricyclic antidepressant with actions and uses similar to those of amitriptyline (p.354). It is the *N*-desmethyl derivative of loxapine (p.749).

In the treatment of depression amoxapine is given in doses of 50 mg two or three times daily initially, gradually increased to 100 mg three times daily as necessary. Higher doses of up to 600 mg daily may be required in severely depressed hospital patients. A suggested dose for the elderly is 25 mg two or three times daily initially, increased gradually to a maximum of 300 mg daily as necessary.

Once-daily dosage regimens, usually given at night, are suitable for amoxapine up to 300 mg daily; divided-dosage regimens are recommended for doses above 300 mg daily.

Reviews of the actions and uses of amoxapine: *Med. Lett.*, 1981, *23*, 39; S. G. Jue *et al.*, *Drugs*, 1982, *24*, 1.

DEPRESSION. In the treatment of depression, amoxapine has been reported to be as effective as, but with a faster onset of action than, amitriptyline (D.M. McNair *et al.*, *Psychopharmacology*, 1984, *83*, 129), doxepin (L.J. Hekimian *et al.*, *J. clin. Psychiat.*, 1983, *44*, 248), and maprotiline (L.F. Fabre, *ibid.*, 1985, *46*, 521), although Gelenberg *et al.* (*ibid.*, 1984, *45*, 54) did not find an earlier onset of therapeutic effects than with imipramine.

For a general review of the role of antidepressants in depression, see Amitriptyline Hydrochloride, p.355.

Delusional depression. Four patients with delusional depression, which usually responds poorly to tricyclic antidepressants, had a favourable outcome after receiving amoxapine 200 to 400 mg daily. In 3 patients tested, the mean increase in serum prolactin was 147%, and it was suggested that this may reflect neuroleptic activity.— R. F. Anton and J. D. Sexauer, *Am. J. Psychiat.*, 1983, *140*, 1344.

Proprietary Names and Manufacturers

Asendin *(Lederle, Canad.; Lederle, USA)*; Demolox *(Lederle, Denm.; Lederle, S.Afr.; Cyanamid, Spain)*; Moxadil *(Lederle, Fr.)*; Omnipress *(Ger.)*.

12422-f

Befuraline Hydrochloride *(rINNM)*.

DIV-154. Benzofuran-2-yl 4-benzylpiperazin-1-yl ketone hydrochloride.

$C_{20}H_{20}N_2O_2$,HCl=356.9.

CAS — 41717-30-0 (befuraline); 41716-84-1 (hydrochloride).

Befuraline hydrochloride is reported to have antidepressant properties.

References: M. Gastpar *et al.*, *Pharmacopsychiatry*, 1985, *18*, 351.

Proprietary Names and Manufacturers

Hoechst, Ger.

12469-j

Bupropion Hydrochloride *(BANM, USAN)*.

Amfebutamone Hydrochloride *(rINNM)*; BW-323.

(±)-2-(*tert*-Butylamino)-3′-chloropropiophenone hydrochloride.

$C_{13}H_{18}ClNO$,HCl=276.2.

CAS — 34911-55-2 (bupropion); 31677-93-7 (hydrochloride).

Bupropion hydrochloride is a chlorpropiophenone antidepressant. The use of bupropion in bulimic patients was associated with a high incidence of seizures, which halted its release onto the market in 1986.

Proprietary Names and Manufacturers

Wellbutrin *(Wellcome, USA)*.

2505-s

Butriptyline Hydrochloride *(BANM, USAN, rINNM)*.

AY-62014. (±)-3-(10,11-Dihydro-5*H*-dibenzo-[*a,d*]cyclohepten-5-yl)-2-methylpropyldimethylamine hydrochloride.

$C_{21}H_{27}N$,HCl=329.9.

CAS — 35941-65-2 (butriptyline); 5585-73-9 (hydrochloride).

Adverse Effects, Treatment, and Precautions

As for Amitriptyline Hydrochloride, p.351.

Uses and Administration

Butriptyline hydrochloride is a tricyclic antidepressant with actions and uses similar to those of amitriptyline (p.354). In the treatment of depression it is given by mouth as the hydrochloride in doses equivalent to butriptyline 25 mg three times daily initially, gradually increased to a maximum of 100 to 150 mg daily as necessary.

Butriptyline was shown to differ from other tricyclic antidepressants in not inhibiting the pressor effect of tyramine.— K. Ghose *et al.* (letter), *Br. J. clin. Pharmac.*, 1977, *4*, 91.

Proprietary Preparations

Evadyne *(Ayerst, UK)*. *Tablets,* butriptyline hydrochloride, each containing the equivalent of 25 or 50 mg of butriptyline.

Proprietary Names and Manufacturers

Centrolyse *(Arg.)*; Evadene *(Ayerst, Ital.)*; Evadyne *(Belg.; Neth.; Ayerst, S.Afr.; Ayerst, UK)*.

2506-w

Caroxazone *(USAN, rINN)*.

FI-6654. 2-(3,4-Dihydro-2-oxo-2*H*-1,3-benzoxazin-3-yl)acetamide.

$C_{10}H_{10}N_2O_3$=206.2.

CAS — 18464-39-6.

Caroxazone has been used as an antidepressant.

18967-e

Cianopramine *(pINN)*.

Ro-11-2465. 5-[3-(Dimethylamino)propyl]-10,11-dihydro-5*H*-dibenz[*b,f*]azepine-3-carbonitrile.

$C_{20}H_{23}N_3$=305.4.

CAS — 66834-24-0.

Cianopramine is a tricyclic antidepressant which selectively inhibits the re-uptake of serotonin.

A study of the cardiovascular effects of cianopramine in healthy subjects indicated that it had positive inotropic effects.— S. Gasic *et al.*, *Eur. J. clin. Pharmac.*, 1982, *21*, 357.

DEPRESSION. In the treatment of depression, cianopramine has been shown to be as effective as amitriptyline (V.P. Avento *et al.*, *Drugs Exp. Clin. Res.*, 1984, *10*, 127; G.W. Mellsop *et al.*, *Clin. Ther.*, 1985, *7*, 699).

Proprietary Names and Manufacturers

Roche, Switz.

12564-y

Ciclazindol Hydrochloride *(BANM, rINNM)*.

Wy-23409. 10-(3-Chlorophenyl)-2,3,4,10-tetrahydropyrimido[1,2-*a*]indol-10-ol hydrochloride.

$C_{17}H_{15}ClN_2O$,HCl=335.2.

CAS — 37751-39-6 (ciclazindol); 37647-52-2 (hydrochloride).

Ciclazindol hydrochloride is a tetracyclic antidepressant with anorectic properties.

The use of ciclazindol in obesity: D. Wheatley, *Postgrad. med. J.*, 1982, *58*, 279; W. P. Leary *et al.*, *Curr. ther. Res.*, 1983, *34*, 728.

Anorectic and hypoglycaemic activity.—M. E. J. Lean and L. J. Borthwick, *Eur. J. clin. Pharmac.*, 1983, *25*, 41.

Proprietary Names and Manufacturers

Wyeth, UK.

12580-y

Cilobamine Mesylate *(USAN)*.

Cilobamine Mesilate *(rINNM)*; Clobamine Mesylate; MDL-81182EF; RMI-81182EF. *cis*-2-(3,4-Dichlorophenyl)-3-isopropylaminobicyclo[2.2.2]octan-2-ol methanesulphonate.

$C_{17}H_{23}Cl_2NO,CH_4O_3S$=424.4.

CAS — 69429-85-2; 69429-84-1 (cilobamine).

Cilobamine mesylate is reported to be an antidepressant.

Contrary to 3 earlier studies, a double-blind, placebo-controlled study in patients with major depression failed to demonstrate antidepressant activity for cilobamine.— J. D. Amsterdam *et al.*, *Curr. ther. Res.*, 1986, *39*, 87.

Proprietary Names and Manufacturers
Merrell Dow, USA.

12575-c

Citalopram Hydrobromide *(BANM, rINNM).*

Lu-10-171; Nitalapram Hydrobromide. 1-(3-Dimethylaminopropyl)-1-(4-fluorophenyl)-1,3-dihydroisobenzofuran-5-carbonitrile hydrobromide.
$C_{20}H_{21}FN_2O,HBr$=405.3.

CAS — 59729-33-8 (citalopram); 59729-32-7 (hydrobromide).

Citalopram hydrobromide is an antidepressant which selectively inhibits the re-uptake of serotonin.

References to the actions and uses of citalopram: N.F. Damlouji *et al.*, in *Pharmacotherapy of Affective Disorders: Theory and Practice*, W.G. Dewhurst and G.B. Baker (Eds), London, Croom Helm, 1985, p.286..

ALCOHOL ABUSE. In a double-blind crossover study of 39 non-depressed early-stage problem drinkers citalopram 40 mg daily, but not 20 mg daily, by mouth decreased the number of drinks consumed and increased the number of abstinent days.— C. A. Naranjo *et al.*, *Clin. Pharmac. Ther.*, 1987, *41*, 266.

DEPRESSION. In the treatment of depression, citalopram has been shown to be as effective as amitriptyline (D.M. Shaw *et al.*, *Br. J. Psychiat.*, 1986, *149*, 515; A. Gravem *et al.*, *Acta pychiat. scand.*, 1987, *75*, 478), less effective than clomipramine (J. Andersen *et al.*, *Psychopharmacology*, 1986, *90*, 131), and more effective than mianserin (J. de Wilde *et al.*, *Acta psychiat. scand.*, 1985, *72*, 89). Side-effects reported include dry mouth, drowsiness, sweating, headache, salivation, nausea, and sleep disturbance (J. de Wilde, 1985).

The relationship between clinical effects, serum-drug concentration, and serotonin uptake inhibition in depressed patients treated with citalopram.— L. Bjerkenstedt *et al.*, *Eur. J. clin. Pharmac.*, 1985, *28*, 553.

Proprietary Names and Manufacturers
Lundbeck, UK.

2507-e

Clomipramine Hydrochloride *(BANM, USAN, rINNM).*

Chlorimipramine Hydrochloride; G-34586; Monochlorimipramine Hydrochloride. 3-(3-Chloro-10,11-dihydro-5*H*-dibenz[*b,f*]azepin-5-yl)-propyldimethylamine hydrochloride.
$C_{19}H_{23}ClN_2,HCl$=351.3.

CAS — 303-49-1 (clomipramine); 17321-77-6 (hydrochloride).

Pharmacopoeias. In *Br.*, *Fr.*, *Jpn*, and *Nord.*

An odourless or almost odourless white or slightly yellow crystalline powder. Freely **soluble** in water, in alcohol, and in chloroform; slightly soluble in acetone, practically insoluble in ether. A 10% solution has a pH of 3.5 to 5.0.
Store in well-closed containers. Protect from light.

Adverse Effects and Treatment

As for Amitriptyline Hydrochloride, p.351.

EFFECTS ON THE EYE. For a report of concomitant trazodone and clomipramine causing excessive blinking, see Trazodone Hydrochloride, p.382.

EFFECTS ON THE LIVER. Acute hepatitis occurred in a 39-year-old woman 15 days after commencing amineptine therapy at a dose of 300 mg daily by mouth. She improved rapidly on withdrawal of the drug, but the hepatitis recurred 7 days after starting clomipramine 100 mg daily by mouth. This suggested that the tricyclic ring is involved in the mechanism of the deleterious effect on the liver. In patients in whom hepatitis had been induced by a tricyclic antidepressant, administration of another tricyclic should be avoided or carefully monitored by repeated liver function tests.— D. Larrey *et al.*, *Gut*, 1986, *27*, 726.

EFFECTS ON SEXUAL FUNCTION. A report of bizarre increases in sexual arousal associated with yawning in patients taking clomipramine. J. D. McLean *et al.*, *Can J. Psychiat.*, 1983, *28*, 569.
See also Amitriptyline Hydrochloride, p.351.

NEUROLEPTIC MALIGNANT SYNDROME. Of 16 cases of neuroleptic malignant syndrome reported to the *UK* Committee on Safety of Medicines by July 1986, one fatal case occurred in a patient receiving clomipramine.— Committee on Safety of Medicines, *Current Problems No. 18*, Sept., 1986.

Precautions

As for Amitriptyline Hydrochloride, p.352.

INTERACTIONS. Interactions involving tricyclic antidepressants are discussed under amitriptyline (p.353). References to interactions where clomipramine has been the tricyclic antidepressant affected can be found under the heading Sex Hormones.
Clomipramine has sometimes been the tricyclic antidepressant that has affected other drugs and information on these interactions can be found under miconazole nitrate (p.430) and morphine sulphate (p.1312). The combination of clomipramine and tranylcypromine is particularly hazardous, see phenelzine sulphate (p.378).

PORPHYRIA. For a report suggesting that clomipramine is unsafe in patients with acute porphyria, see under Amitriptyline Hydrochloride, p.354.

PREGNANCY AND THE NEONATE. For reports of neonatal clomipramine withdrawal, see under Withdrawal Syndromes, below.

WITHDRAWAL SYNDROMES. Withdrawal symptoms in a neonate whose mother received clomipramine throughout pregnancy. Phenobarbitone controlled the symptoms and may have also induced the hepatic conjugating enzymes needed to metabolise clomipramine.— A. Ben Musa and C. S. Smith (letter), *Archs Dis. Childh.*, 1979, *54*, 405.
Convulsions on the first day of life occurred in 2 neonates due to withdrawal from maternal clomipramine. Convulsions were controlled by parenteral phenobarbitone in the neonate whose mother had received clomipramine for the last 7 weeks of pregnancy, and by intravenous clomipramine in the neonate whose mother had received clomipramine throughout pregnancy.— L. Cowe *et al.*, *Br. med. J.*, 1982, *284*, 1837.

Absorption and Fate

Clomipramine is readily absorbed from the gastro-intestinal tract, and extensively demethylated by first-pass metabolism in the liver to its primary active metabolite, desmethylclomipramine. Since clomipramine slows gastro-intestinal transit time, absorption can, however, be delayed, particularly in overdosage.
Paths of metabolism of both clomipramine and desmethylclomipramine include hydroxylation and *N*-oxidation. Clomipramine is excreted in the urine, mainly in the form of its metabolites, either free or in conjugated form.
Clomipramine and desmethylclomipramine are widely distributed throughout the body and are extensively bound to plasma and tissue protein. Clomipramine has been estimated to have a plasma half-life ranging from 17 to 28 hours, which may be considerably extended in overdosage; that of desmethylclomipramine is longer.

Clomipramine was estimated to have a half-life ranging from 22 to 84 hours in 10 depressed subjects. The plasma concentration of desmethylclomipramine continued to increase after that of clomipramine had begun to fall, indicating that its half-life is longer than that of the parent compound.— S. Dawling *et al.*, *Postgrad. med. J.*, 1980, *56*, *Suppl.* 1, 115.

The pharmacokinetic properties of clomipramine in psychiatric patients.— E. Mårtensson *et al.*, *Curr. ther. Res.*, 1984, *36*, 228.

Uses and Administration

Clomipramine is a tricyclic antidepressant with actions and uses similar to those of amitriptyline (p.354). It is recommended in depression when sedation is required as well as in cataplexy associated with narcolepsy.
In the treatment of depression, clomipramine is given by mouth as the hydrochloride in doses of 10 mg daily initially, increasing gradually to 30 to 150 mg daily if required. Usual maintenance doses are 30 to 50 mg daily. Higher doses may be needed in some patients particularly those suffering from obsessional or phobic disorders. Where a higher dosage is required, the 75 mg sustained-release formulation may be preferable. A suggested initial dose for the elderly is 10 mg daily increasing to 30 to 75 mg daily if required. Half the normal maintenance dose may be sufficient. Clomipramine may be given in divided doses throughout the day, but since it has a prolonged half-life, once-daily dosage regimens are also suitable, usually given at night.
In the initial stages of treatment, if administration by mouth is impracticable or inadvisable, up to 150 mg of the hydrochloride may be given daily in divided doses by intramuscular injection, but oral administration should be substituted as soon as possible. Clomipramine hydrochloride may also be given by intravenous infusion in initial doses of 25 to 50 mg diluted to 200 to 500 mL with sodium chloride 0.9% injection or glucose 5% injection and infused over 2 hours to assess tolerance; the dose may then be increased by 25 mg daily until an optimum therapeutic dose is achieved; this is usually about 100 mg daily, although more may be required. As the initial dose is gradually increased the volume of infusion fluid may be decreased to a minimum of 125 mL, and the duration of infusion decreased to a minimum of 45 minutes. Infusions are usually given for 7 to 10 days. When a satisfactory response to intravenous infusion has been obtained it should be gradually decreased as oral therapy is substituted, initially giving double the maximum intravenous dose by mouth and subsequently adjusting to a satisfactory maintenance dose if necessary. Patients must be carefully supervised during intravenous infusion of clomipramine hydrochloride and the blood pressure carefully monitored owing to the risk of hypotension.

ANXIETY AND PHOBIAS. *Agoraphobia.* For a brief review of the management of agoraphobia, including the use of clomipramine, see Imipramine Hydrochloride, p.363.

DEPRESSION. A preliminary report of rapid remission of symptoms in 5 patients with moderately severe depression given clomipramine 75 mg by intravenous infusion, followed by 200 mg intravenously the following day. Sleep and depressive symptoms improved over the next 11 days despite the patients receiving no further medication. This response was significantly better than in matched control patients receiving intravenous saline.— B. G. Pollock *et al.* (letter), *New Engl. J. Med.*, 1985, *312*, 1130.

For a general review of the role of antidepressants in depression, see Amitriptyline Hydrochloride, p.355.

Combination therapy with oxitriptan. In a double-blind study 24 depressed patients were treated for 28 days with clomipramine 50 mg daily by mouth and either placebo or oxitriptan 300 mg daily. No tricyclic side-effects were noted in either group, but combination therapy was significantly more effective in relieving depressive symptoms than clomipramine alone.— M. Nardini *et al.*, *Int. J. clin. Pharmacol. Res.*, 1983, *3*, 239.

EATING DISORDERS. Clomipramine was no more effective than placebo in causing weight gain in a double-blind study in which 8 female anorectic patients were given clomipramine 50 mg at night and 8 similar patients were given placebo.— J. H. Lacey and A. H. Crisp, *Postgrad. med. J.*, 1980, *56*, *Suppl.* 1, 79.

OBSESSIVE COMPULSIVE DISORDER. A number of reports have suggested that clomipramine has a specific anti-compulsive effect; it should be considered as an adjunct to behaviour therapy.— P. T. Lelliott and W. O. Monteiro, *Drugs*, 1986, *31*, 75. Further references: T. R. Insel *et al.*, *Archs gen. Psychiat.*, 1983, *40*, 605 (comparison with clorgyline); I. M. Marks, *Br. J. Psychiat.*, 1983, *143*, 338 (review of antidepressants in phobic and obsessive compulsive disorders); M. F. Flament *et al.*, *Archs gen. Psychiat.*, 1985, *42*, 977 (use in children).

PREMATURE EJACULATION. Beneficial results with clomipramine in premature ejaculation.— H. Eaton, *J. int. med. Res.*, 1973, *1*, 432. See also B. Klug (letter), *Med. J. Aust.*, 1984, *141*, 71.

SLEEP DISORDERS. *Narcolepsy.* Seventy-five patients with cataplexy were treated with clomipramine 10 to 150 mg daily for 4 to 7 years. The frequency of cataplectic attacks fell within 24 to 48 hours of the start of treatment and there was total abolition or marked reduction of attacks in 66 patients; initially results were poor in 9 patients. Response to clomipramine was maintained for 4 to 7 years in 71 of the patients, but 4 had a progressive failure in response over 2 to 4 weeks after starting treatment. Clomipramine withdrawal was followed by an immediate increase in the severity and frequency of cataplexy lasting 2 to 4 days in 22 patients. Clomipramine alone did not alter the severity of narcolepsy, but usually abolished sleep paralysis.— J. D. Parkes and M. Schachter (letter), *Lancet*, 1979, *2*, 1085.

Sleep apnoea. Clomipramine has been tried in sleep apnoea as a respiratory stimulant, but there is little evidence for its efficacy.— M. C. P. Apps, *Br. J. Hosp. Med.*, 1983, *30*, 339.

Preparations

Clomipramine Capsules *(B.P.).* Clomipramine Hydrochloride Capsules

Proprietary Preparations

Anafranil *(Geigy, UK). Capsules*, clomipramine hydrochloride 10 mg, 25 mg, and 50 mg.
Tablets (Anafranil SR), sustained-release, clomipramine hydrochloride 75 mg.
Syrup, clomipramine hydrochloride 25 mg/5 mL.
Injection, clomipramine hydrochloride 12.5 mg/mL in ampoules of 2 mL.

Proprietary Names and Manufacturers

Anafranil *(Arg.; Geigy, Austral.; Belg.; Geigy, Canad.; Geigy, Denm.; Ciba, Fr.; Geigy, Ger.; Geigy, Ital.; Neth.; Geigy, Norw.; NZ; S.Afr.; Spain; Geigy, Swed.; Geigy, Switz.; Geigy, UK).*

2508-l

Clorgyline Hydrochloride *(BANM).*

Clorgiline Hydrochloride *(rINNM)*; M & B 9302. 3-(2,4-Dichlorophenoxy)propyl(methyl)prop-2-ynylamine hydrochloride.
$C_{13}H_{15}Cl_2NO,HCl=308.6$.

CAS — 17780-72-2 (clorgyline); 17780-75-5 (hydrochloride).

Clorgyline hydrochloride is a monoamine oxidase inhibitor which has been tried in the treatment of depression.

BEHAVIOUR DISORDERS. For a report suggesting clorgyline may be an alternative to dexamphetamine in the treatment of children with attention deficit disorder, see Tranylcypromine Sulphate, p.381.

MANIA AND MANIC DEPRESSION. Clorgyline given in doses of 5 to 30 mg daily by itself, or in combination with lithium carbonate prolonged the duration and lessened the severity of mood cycles in 4 of 5 patients with rapid-cycling manic depression.— W. Z. Potter *et al.*, *Archs gen. Psychiat.*, 1982, *39*, 505.

Proprietary Names and Manufacturers
May & Baker, UK.

12593-a

Clovoxamine *(rINN).*

DU-13811. 4′-Chloro-5-methoxyvalerophenone (*E*)-*O*-(2-aminoethyl)oxime.
$C_{14}H_{21}ClN_2O_2=284.8$.

CAS — 54739-19-4.

Clovoxamine is an antidepressant that is reported to inhibit serotonin and noradrenaline re-uptake.

References to the actions and uses of clovoxamine: N.F. Damlouji *et al.*, in *Pharmacotherapy of Affective Disorders: Theory and Practice*, W.G. Dewhurst and G.B. Baker (Eds.), London, Croom Helm, 1985, p.286..

Clovoxamine pharmacokinetics in depressed patients.— H. E. Hurst *et al.*, *Clin. Pharmac. Ther.*, 1983, *34*, 266.

DEPRESSION. In the treatment of depression, clovoxamine has been found to be as effective as amitriptyline (A.J. Gelenberg *et al.*, *J. clin. Psychopharmacol.*, 1985, 5, 30) and doxepin (G.J. Lodge and H.L. Freeman, *Br. J. Psychiat.*, 1986, *148*, 718). Adverse effects reported include nausea, vomiting, dry mouth, tremor, anorexia, insomnia, dizziness, constipation, somnolence, and headache (A.J. Gelenberg *et al.*, 1985).

Proprietary Names and Manufacturers
Duphar, Neth.

2509-y

Desipramine Hydrochloride *(BANM, USAN, rINNM).*

Desmethylimipramine Hydrochloride; DMI; EX-4355; G-35020; JB-8181; NSC-114901; RMI-9384A. 3-(10,11-Dihydro-5*H*-dibenz[*b*,*f*]-azepin-5-yl)-propyl(methyl)amine hydrochloride.
$C_{18}H_{22}N_2,HCl=302.8$.

CAS — 50-47-5 (desipramine); 58-28-6 (hydrochloride).

Pharmacopoeias. In *Aust., Br., Eur., Fr., Ger., It., Jug., Neth., Swiss,* and *U.S.*

A white or almost white, crystalline powder. **Soluble** 1 in 20 of water, 1 in 20 of alcohol, and 1 in 4 of chloroform; practically insoluble in ether; freely soluble in methyl alcohol. A 5% solution in water has a pH of 4.0 to 5.5. **Store** in airtight containers. Protect from light.

Adverse Effects, Treatment, and Precautions

As for Amitriptyline Hydrochloride, p.351.
The antimuscarinic and sedative actions of desipramine are reported to be less marked than those of amitriptyline.

EXTRAPYRAMIDAL EFFECTS. *Akathisia.* For a report of insomnia, jitteriness, and irritability in patients with panic disorder receiving low doses of desipramine, see Amitriptyline Hydrochloride, p.351.

INTERACTIONS. Interactions involving tricyclic antidepressants are discussed under amitriptyline (p.353). References to interactions where desipramine has been the tricyclic antidepressant affected can be found under the headings H_2 antagonist antihistamines, Neuroleptics, and Smoking.

PHAEOCHROMOCYTOMA. Phaeochromocytoma unmasked in one patient by desipramine therapy.— M. R. Achong and P. M. Keane, *Ann. intern. Med.*, 1981, *94*, 358.

PREGNANCY AND THE NEONATE. *Lactation.* For a report that although desipramine is transferred into breast milk, there had been no reported effects on lactation, or signs or symptoms in breast-fed infants, see Amitriptyline Hydrochloride, p.354.

Absorption and Fate

Desipramine is the principal active metabolite of imipramine. For an account of its metabolism, see Imipramine Hydrochloride, p.363.
Desipramine has been reported to have a longer plasma half-life than imipramine.

METABOLISM. For reference to possible associations between poor metabolism of debrisoquine or sparteine and adverse reactions to tricyclic antidepressants, see Amitriptyline Hydrochloride, p.354.

PLASMA CONCENTRATIONS. A linear relationship between plasma-desipramine concentration and clinical outcome has been described by 2 studies. Plasma concentrations above 125 ng/mL were significantly more effective than lower concentrations. However, the data available were not as extensive as with imipramine or nortriptyline and the therapeutic range should be considered tentative, pending confirmatory studies. Nevertheless plasma concentration measurements were unequivocally useful in problem patients who did not respond to usual oral doses or in high-risk patients who, because of age or medical illness, would be best treated with the lowest possible effective dose.— American Psychiatric Association (APA) Task Force, *Am. J. Psychiat.*, 1985, *142*, 155.

Uses and Administration

Desipramine is a tricyclic antidepressant with actions and uses similar to those of amitriptyline (p.354). It is the principal active metabolite of imipramine (p.362) and, like imipramine, has less marked sedative properties than amitriptyline. In the treatment of depression, desipramine is given by mouth as the hydrochloride in doses of 25 mg three times daily initially, gradually increased to 50 mg three or four times daily; higher doses of up to 300 mg daily may be required in severely depressed hospital patients. A suggested initial dose for adolescents and the elderly is 25 to 50 mg daily, gradually increased to 100 mg daily if necessary. Since desipramine has a prolonged half-life, once-daily dosage regimens are also suitable.

ADMINISTRATION IN RENAL FAILURE. Desipramine can be given in usual doses to patients with renal failure. Concentrations of desipramine were not affected by haemodialysis or peritoneal dialysis.— W. M. Bennett *et al.*, *Am. J. Kidney Dis.*, 1983, *3*, 155.

BEHAVIOUR DISORDERS. Desipramine 25 mg daily by mouth, increasing by 25 mg daily to 100 mg daily produced behavioural improvement by day 3 in 29 boys (mean age of 8.8 years) with attention deficit/hyperactivity. The improvement was sustained for the 14 days of the study. Behavioural improvement did not correlate with plasma concentrations of desipramine, hydroxydesipramine, or their sum at days 3 or 14.— M. Donnelly *et al.*, *Clin. Pharmac. Ther.*, 1986, *39*, 72.

DEPRESSION. A review of the use of desipramine in depression.— D. S. Janowsky *et al.*, *J. clin. Psychiat.*, 1984, *45*, (Oct.), 3.

For a report of studies describing a linear relationship between plasma-desipramine concentration and clinical outcome, see under plasma concentrations in Absorption and Fate, above.

For a general review of the role of antidepressants in depression, see Amitriptyline Hydrochloride, p.355.

EATING DISORDERS. In 22 patients with bulimia without major depression, desipramine 50 mg nightly increased by 50 mg every 3 days to reach 200 mg nightly was compared with placebo. After 6 weeks, patients taking desipramine had a mean 91% decrease in binge-eating frequency and patients taking placebo had a 19% increase.— P. L. Hughes *et al.*, *Archs gen. Psychiat.*, 1986, *43*, 182.

SLEEP DISORDERS. *Narcolepsy.* For a report suggesting that desipramine is effective in treating the auxiliary symptoms of cataplexy, see Imipramine Hydrochloride, p.364.

WITHDRAWAL SYNDROMES. In a study of 40 chronic cocaine or phencyclidine abusers who had discontinued their abuse, desipramine 150 mg daily was significantly more effective than placebo in alleviating withdrawal depression.— A. J. Giannini *et al.*, *J. clin. Pharmac.*, 1986, *26*, 211.

Preparations

Desipramine Hydrochloride Capsules *(U.S.P.)*

Desipramine Hydrochloride Tablets *(U.S.P.)*

Desipramine Tablets *(B.P.).* Tablets containing desipramine hydrochloride.

Proprietary Preparations

Pertofran *(Geigy, UK). Tablets*, desipramine hydrochloride 25 mg.

Proprietary Names and Manufacturers

Nebril *(Arg.)*; Norpramin *(Merrell Dow, Canad.; Merrell Dow, USA)*; Nortimil *(Chiesi, Ital.)*; Pertofran *(Geigy, Austral.; Geigy, Denm.; Geigy, Fr.; Geigy, Ger.; Neth.; Geigy, S.Afr.; Geigy, Switz.; Geigy, UK)*; Pertofrana *(Spain)*; Pertofrane *(Geigy, Canad.; USV Pharmaceutical Corp., USA)*; Pertofrin *(Geigy, Swed.)*; Sertofren *(Geigy, Norw.)*.

12636-y

Deximafen Hydrochloride *(rINNM).*

R-25540 (racemic); R-26333. (+)-2,3,5,6-Tetrahydro-5-(or 3-)-phenyl-1*H*-imidazo[1,2-*a*]imidazole hydrochloride.
$C_{11}H_{13}N_3,HCl=223.7$.

CAS — 42116-77-8 (deximafen).

NOTE. Deximafen is *USAN.*

Deximafen hydrochloride is reported to be an antidepressant.

Proprietary Names and Manufacturers
Janssen, Belg.

2510-g

Dibenzepin Hydrochloride *(BANM, USAN, rINNM).*
HF-1927. 10-(2-Dimethylaminoethyl)-5,10-dihydro-5-methyl-dibenzo[*b*,*e*][1,4]diazepin-11-one hydrochloride.
$C_{18}H_{21}N_3O,HCl$=331.8.

CAS — 4498-32-2 (dibenzepin); 315-80-0 (hydrochloride).

Dibenzepin hydrochloride is a tricyclic antidepressant with actions and uses similar to those of amitriptyline (p.350).

In the treatment of depression dibenzepin hydrochloride is given by mouth in doses of 240 mg to 480 mg daily; higher doses may be required.

Dibenzepin has also been given by intravenous infusion.

In 46 severely depressed patients, a 10-hour intravenous infusion of dibenzepin 720 mg daily on 2 or 3 successive days was as effective as an infusion of the same dose given continuously over 24 hours for 2 successive days. The shorter infusion was as effective as the longer, less demanding technically and in terms of nursing care, and did not result in a greater frequency or severity of general or cardiovascular side-effects.— M. Gastpar *et al.*, *Neuropsychobiology*, 1984, *11*, 44.

Proprietary Names and Manufacturers

Deprex *(Novo, Belg.; Novo, Denm.; Novo, Norw.)*; Écatril *(Sandoz, Fr.)*; Noveril *(Sandoz, Austral.; Wander, Belg.; Sandoz, Fr.; Wander, Ger.; Sandoz, Ital.; Wander, S.Afr.; Sandoz, Spain; Wander, Switz.; Wander, UK).*

12647-c

Diclofensine Hydrochloride *(rINNM).*
Moxifensine Hydrochloride; Ro-8-4650. (±)-4-(3,4-Dichlorophenyl)-1,2,3,4-tetrahydro-7-methoxy-2-methylisoquinoline hydrochloride.
$C_{17}H_{17}Cl_2NO,HCl$=358.7.

CAS — 67165-56-4 (diclofensine); 34041-84-4 (hydrochloride).

Diclofensine hydrochloride is an antidepressant which is reported to inhibit the re-uptake of dopamine, noradrenaline, and serotonin.

DEPRESSION. In the treatment of depression, diclofensine has been shown to be more effective and faster in onset of action than imipramine (R. Capponi *et al.*, *Neuropsychobiology*, 1985, *14*, 173) and as effective as maprotiline (C. Cherpillod and L.M.O. Omer, *J. int. med. Res.*, 1981, *9*, 324). Side-effects reported include tremor, fatigue, dizziness, agitation, insommia, dry mouth, constipation, tachycardia, and orthostatic hypotension (L.M.O. Omer, *Int. J. clin. Pharmac. Ther. Toxic.*, 1982, *20*, 320).

Proprietary Names and Manufacturers

Roche, Switz.

2511-q

Dimetacrine Tartrate *(rINNM).*
Dimetacrine Bitartrate; Dimetacrine Hydrogen Tartrate; Dimethacrine Tartrate; SD-709. 3-(9,9-Dimethylacridan-10-yl)-*NN*-dimethylpropylamine hydrogen tartrate.
$C_{20}H_{26}N_2,C_4H_6O_6$=444.5.

CAS — 4757-55-5(dimetacrine); 3759-07-7(tartrate).

Dimetacrine is a tricyclic antidepressant.

Proprietary Names and Manufacturers

Istonil *(Siegfried, Belg.; Siegfried, Ger.; Siegfried, Switz.)*; Linostil *(ACF, Neth.).*

2512-p

Dothiepin Hydrochloride *(BANM, USAN).*

Dosulepin Hydrochloride *(rINNM)*. 3-(Dibenzo-[*b*,*e*]thiepin-11-ylidene)propyldimethylamine hydrochloride.
$C_{19}H_{21}NS,HCl$=331.9.

CAS — 113-53-1 (dothiepin); 897-15-4 (monohydrate); 7081-53-0 (anhydrous).

Pharmacopoeias. In *Br.* and *Cz.*

A white to faintly yellow odourless or almost odourless crystalline powder. It consists chiefly of the *E*-isomer. **Soluble** 1 in 2 of water, 1 in 8 of alcohol, and 1 in 2 of chloroform; practically insoluble in ether. **Store** in well-closed containers. Protect from light.

Adverse Effects, Treatment, and Precautions

As for Amitriptyline Hydrochloride, p.351.

Dothiepin has been reported to have a lower incidence of antimuscarinic side-effects than amitriptyline.

NEUROLEPTIC MALIGNANT SYNDROME. Of 16 cases of neuroleptic malignant syndrome reported to the *UK* Committee on Safety of Medicines by July 1986, one case occurred in a patient receiving dothiepin.— Committee on Safety of Medicines, *Current Problems No.18*, Sept., 1986. See also R. Grant (letter), *Br. med. J.*, 1984, *288*, 1690.

PREGNANCY AND THE NEONATE. *Lactation.* For a report that although dothiepin is transferred into breast milk, there had been no reported effects on lactation, or signs or symptoms in breast-fed infants, see Amitriptyline Hydrochloride, p.354.

Absorption and Fate

Dothiepin is readily absorbed from the gastro-intestinal tract, and extensively demethylated by first-pass metabolism in the liver to its primary active metabolite, desmethyldothiepin (also termed northiaden). Since dothiepin slows gastro-intestinal transit time absorption can, however, be delayed, particularly in overdosage. Paths of metabolism also include *S*-oxidation. Dothiepin is excreted in the urine, mainly in the form of its metabolites; small amounts are also excreted in the faeces. A half-life of about 19 to 33 hours has been reported for dothiepin and its metabolites.

Dothiepin is excreted in breast milk.

Reviews of the pharmacokinetics of dothiepin: K. P. Maguire *et al.*, *Clin. Pharmacokinet.*, 1983, *8*, 179 (depressed patients); D. K. Yu *et al.*, *J. pharm. Sci.*, 1986, *75*, 582 (healthy subjects).

Uses and Administration

Dothiepin hydrochloride is a tricyclic antidepressant with actions and uses similar to those of amitriptyline (p.354). Like amitriptyline, it also has sedative properties.

In the treatment of depression, dothiepin hydrochloride is given by mouth in doses of 25 mg three times daily initially, gradually increased to 50 mg three times daily if necessary, or 75 or 150 mg as a single night-time dose; higher doses of up to 225 mg daily have been given in severely depressed hospital patients. The recommended initial dose for the elderly is 50 to 75 mg daily. Half the normal maintenance dose may be adequate.

DEPRESSION. An overview of 17 years experience with dothiepin in the treatment of depression in Europe.— B. J. Goldstein and J. L. Claghorn, *J. clin. Psychiat.*, 1980, *41*, 64.

For a general review of the role of antidepressants in depression, see Amitriptyline Hydrochloride, p.355.

PAIN. Dothiepin in a mean dose of 130 mg daily was shown to be superior to placebo in the relief of atypical facial pain. Pain relief appeared to be independent of antidepressant effects.— C. Feinmann *et al.*, *Br. med. J.*, 1984, *288*, 436.

Musculoskeletal and joint pain. Results of a preliminary study suggested that dothiepin was significantly more effective than placebo in improving the condition of patients with primary fibromyalgia syndrome.— I. Caruso *et al.*, *J. int. med. Res.*, 1987, *15*, 154.

Preparations

Dothiepin Capsules *(B.P.)*. Capsules containing dothiepin hydrochloride.

Prothiaden *(Boots, UK). Capsules*, dothiepin hydrochloride 25 mg.
Tablets, dothiepin hydrochloride 75 mg.

Proprietary Names and Manufacturers

Idom *(Kanoldt, Ger.)*; Prothiaden *(Boots, Austral.; Cz.; Boots, Denm.; Boots-Dacour, Fr.; Boots, S.Afr.; Boots, UK)*; Protiaden *(Boots-Formenti, Ital.).*

2513-s

Doxepin Hydrochloride *(BANM, USAN, rINNM).*

P-3693A. A mixture of the *Z* and *E* isomers of 3-(dibenz[*b*,*e*]oxepin-11-ylidene)propyl-dimethylamine hydrochloride.
$C_{19}H_{21}NO,HCl$=315.8.

CAS — 1668-19-5(doxepin); 1229-29-4(hydrochloride).

Pharmacopoeias. In *Br.*, *Nord.*, and *U.S.*

A white crystalline powder with a slight amine-like odour. Doxepin hydrochloride 113 mg is approximately equivalent to 100 mg of doxepin. **Soluble** 1 in 1.5 of water, 1 in 1 of alcohol, and 1 in 2 of chloroform. **Store** in well-closed containers. Protect from light.

Adverse Effects, Treatment, and Precautions

As for Amitriptyline Hydrochloride, p.351.

EFFECTS ON THE CARDIOVASCULAR SYSTEM. Initial studies with doxepin suggested that it was less cardiotoxic than the earlier tricyclic antidepressants (J. Vohra *et al.*, *Aust. N.Z. J. Med.*, 1975, *5*, 7), in spite of having similar antimuscarinic activity (J.B. Marshall and A.D. Forker, *Am. Heart J.*, 1982, *103*, 401), but more recent evidence has not confirmed this early finding (D.J. Luchins, *Am. J. Psychiat.*, 1983, *140*, 1006).— M. L. Orme, *Br. med. J.*, 1984, *289*, 1.

INTERACTIONS. Interactions involving tricyclic antidepressants are discussed under amitriptyline (p.353). References to interactions where doxepin has been the tricyclic antidepressant affected can be found under the headings Dextropropoxyphene and H_2 antagonist antihistamines.

PREGNANCY AND THE NEONATE. *Lactation.* An 8-week-old girl with persistent drowsiness and shallow respiration, whose mother was receiving doxepin 75 mg daily, returned to normal within 24 hours of breast feeding being stopped. On 2 occasions prior to stopping breast feeding, the infant's serum concentrations of desmethyldoxepin were similar to those found in the mother, although doxepin was almost undetectable. Doxepin should be given with great caution to women who are breast feeding because of the potential risk of sedating the infant, especially in the perinatal period.— I. Matheson *et al.* (letter), *Lancet*, 1985, *2*, 1124. See also J. Kemp *et al.*, *Br. J. clin. Pharmac.*, 1985, *20*, 497.

Absorption and Fate

Doxepin is readily absorbed from the gastro-intestinal tract, and extensively demethylated by first-pass metabolism in the liver, to its primary active metabolite, desmethyldoxepin. Since doxepin slows gastro-intestinal transit time absorption can, however, be delayed, particularly in overdosage.

Paths of metabolism of both doxepin and desmethyldoxepin include hydroxylation and *N*-oxidation. Doxepin is excreted in the urine, mainly in the form of its metabolites, either free or in conjugated form.

Doxepin and desmethyldoxepin are widely distributed throughout the body and are extensively bound to plasma and tissue protein. Doxepin has been estimated to have a plasma half-life ranging from 8 to 24 hours, which may be considerably extended in overdosage; that of desmethyldoxepin is longer.

Doxepin crosses the blood-brain barrier and the placental barrier. It is excreted in breast milk.

In 7 depressed patients receiving single daily doses of doxepin 150 mg by mouth for 1 to 3 weeks kinetics were in the normal range. Mean doxepin half-life after the first dose was 17.7 hours, rising to 21.8 hours after the last dose. Mean desmethyldoxepin half-life was not significantly affected by multiple dosing (34.2 hours after first dose, 37.1 hours after the last dose). Steady-state concentrations of doxepin and desmethyldoxepin were reached within 2 weeks of beginning doxepin dosing. There was strong correlation between total doxepin and desmethyldoxepin concentration and antidepressant effect.— R. D. Faulkner *et al.*, *Clin. Pharmac. Ther.*, 1983, *34*, 509.

Further reference to doxepin pharmacokinetics: P. R. Joyce and J. R. Sharman, *Clin. Pharmacokinet.*, 1985, *10*, 365.

Uses and Administration

Doxepin is a tricyclic antidepressant with actions and uses similar to those of amitriptyline (p.354). Like amitriptyline it has marked sedative properties.

In the treatment of depression doxepin is given by mouth as the hydrochloride in doses equivalent to doxepin 25 mg three times daily initially, gradually increased to 50 mg three times daily as necessary. Higher doses of up to 300 mg daily may be required, particularly in severely depressed hospital patients; mildly affected patients may respond to as little as 25 to 50 mg daily. A suggested starting dose in the elderly is 10 to 50 mg daily. A satisfactory response may be obtained in many elderly patients at a daily dose of 30 to 50 mg.

Since doxepin has a prolonged half-life, once-daily dosage regimens using doses up to 100 mg are also suitable; such doses are usually given at night.

ADMINISTRATION IN CARDIOVASCULAR DISEASE. For the successful use of doxepin in depressed patients with chronic heart disease, see Imipramine Hydrochloride, p.363.

See also under Adverse Effects, above.

ADMINISTRATION IN THE ELDERLY. In a study of 36 depressed patients aged 55 to 81 years, imipramine resulted in a significantly greater incidence of orthostatic hypotension than doxepin, although their mean daily doses of 83.3 and 76.1 mg did not differ significantly. The incidence of orthostatic hypotension with doxepin was not significantly different from that with placebo. The antidepressive efficacy of the 2 drugs was equal.— R. E. Neshkes *et al.*, *J. clin. Psychopharmacol.*, 1985, *5*, 102.

ADMINISTRATION IN RENAL FAILURE. Doxepin can be given in usual doses to patients with renal failure. Concentrations of doxepin were not affected by haemodialysis or peritoneal dialysis.— W. M. Bennett *et al.*, *Am. J. Kidney Dis.*, 1983, *3*, 155.

ANXIETY AND PHOBIAS. For a suggestion that antidepressants with secondary sedative properties, such as doxepin, are the treatment of first choice in depressed patients with anxiety or agitation, see Amitriptyline Hydrochloride, p.355.

DEPRESSION IN THE ELDERLY. In a double-blind study of 24 depressed patients aged 70 to 83 years, low-dose doxepin (10 to 20 mg daily) for 3 weeks produced a significantly greater decrease in depressive symptoms than placebo. There were no complaints of antimuscarinic side-effects or daytime drowsiness.— M. Lakshmanan *et al.*, *J. Am. Geriat. Soc.*, 1986, *34*, 421.

See also under Administration in the Elderly, above.

PEPTIC ULCERATION. Doxepin reduces gastric acid secretion (K.-E. Giercksky *et al.*, *Scand. J. Gastroenterol.*, 1984, *19*, 661) and, at doses of 50 to 100 mg daily, has been shown to be significantly more effective than placebo in healing duodenal ulcers (J. Bergsåker-Aspøy *et al.*, *ibid.*, 1983, *18*, *Suppl.* 86, 7; O.K. Andersen *et al.*, *ibid.*, 1984, *19*, 923), and as effective as cimetidine 1 to 1.2 g daily (G.S. Hoff *et al.*, *ibid.*, 1981, *16*, 1041; R.K. Shrivastava *et al.*, *Clin. Ther.*, 1985, *7*, 181). Doxepin has produced healing of duodenal ulcers where cimetidine has failed (J.C. Mangla and M. Pereira, *Archs intern. Med.*, 1982, *142*, 273) and may promote more rapid healing than cimetidine (R.K. Shrivastava *et al.*, *Clin. Ther.*, 1985, *7*, 319).

URTICARIA. Doxepin at doses of 10 to 75 mg daily has been shown to be an effective alternative to conventional H_1 antagonist antihistamines in the treatment of chronic urticaria (S.L. Greene *et al.*, *J. Am. Acad. Derm.*, 1985, *12*, 669; A. Harto *et al.*, *Dermatologica*, 1985, *170*, 90; A.B. Goldsobel *et al.*, *J. Allergy & clin. Immunol.*, 1986, *78*, 867).

Doxepin at doses of up to 75 mg daily also appeared to be an effective treatment for idiopathic cold urticaria (H. Neittaanmäki *et al.*, *J. Am. Acad. Derm.*, 1984, *11*, 483) although it was suggested that this was due to inhibition of platelet-activating factor-like lipid release (K.E. Grandel *et al.*, *New Engl. J. Med.*, 1985, *313*, 405).

WITHDRAWAL SYNDROMES. Doxepin at doses of 50 to 200 mg daily was found to be a useful adjunctive treatment in 46 depressed and/or anxious patients attending a methadone maintenance programme.— J. Titievsky *et al.*, *J. clin. Psychiat.*, 1982, *43*, 454.

Preparations

Doxepin Capsules *(B.P.)*. Capsules containing doxepin hydrochloride. Potency is expressed in terms of the equivalent amount of doxepin.

Doxepin Hydrochloride Capsules *(U.S.P.)*. Potency is expressed in terms of the equivalent amount of doxepin.

Doxepin Hydrochloride Oral Solution *(U.S.P.)*. Potency is expressed in terms of the equivalent amount of doxepin. pH 4 to 7. Store in airtight containers. To be diluted with water or other suitable fluid immediately before ingestion.

Proprietary Preparations

Sinequan *(Pfizer, UK)*. *Capsules*, doxepin 10, 25, 50, and 75 mg (as hydrochloride).

Proprietary Names and Manufacturers

Adapin *(Pennwalt, USA)*; Aponal *(Galenus Mannheim, Ger.)*; Co-Dox *(Smaller, Spain)*; Novoxapin *(Spain)*; Quitaxon *(Reckitt & Colman, Austral.; Belg.; Erco, Denm.; Pierre Fabre, Fr.; Neth.; S.Afr.)*; Sinequan *(Pfizer, Austral.; Belg.; Pfizer, Canad.; Pfizer, Fr.; Ital.; Neth.; Pfizer, Norw.; S.Afr.; Pfizer, Spain; Pfizer, UK; Roerig, USA)*; Sinquan *(Pfizer, Denm.; Pfizer, Ger.)*; Sinquane *(Pfizer, Switz.)*; Spectra *(Ind.)*; Toruan *(Spain)*; Triadapin *(Pennwalt, Canad.)*.

12721-w

Etoperidone Hydrochloride *(rINNM)*.

Clopradone Hydrochloride; ST-1191 *(etoperidone)*. 2-{3-[4-(3-Chlorophenyl)piperazin-1-yl]propyl}-4,5-diethyl-2,4-dihydro-1,2,4-triazol-3-one hydrochloride.
$C_{19}H_{28}ClN_5O,HCl=414.4$.

CAS — 52942-31-1 (etoperidone); 57775-22-1 (hydrochloride).

Etoperidone hydrochloride is reported to have antidepressant activity.

DEPRESSION. In 45 patients with severe depression, etoperidone and trazodone at daily doses of 200 to 600 mg by mouth, and maprotiline at a daily dose of 100 to 300 mg by mouth were found to be equally effective antidepressants; there were no significant differences in side-effects.— F. Aprile *et al.*, *Acta ther.*, 1983, *9*, 353.

Proprietary Names and Manufacturers

Centren *(Syntex-Latino, Spain)*; Depraser *(Farma-Lepori, Spain)*; Staff *(Sigmatau, Ital.)*.

16802-x

Femoxetine *(rINN)*.

FG-4963 (hydrochloride). (+)-*trans*-3-[(*p*-Methoxyphenoxy)methyl]-1-methyl-4-phenylpiperidine.
$C_{20}H_{25}NO_2=311.4$.

CAS — 59859-58-4.

Femoxetine is an antidepressant which selectively inhibits the re-uptake of serotonin.

DEPRESSION. In the treatment of depression, femoxetine has been shown to be as effective as, but with fewer side-effects than, amitriptyline (B.K. Skrumsager and K. Jeppesen, *Pharmacopsychiatry*, 1986, *19*, 368), and desipramine (L.-E. Dahl *et al.*, *Acta psychiat. scand.*, 1982, *66*, 9). Side-effects reported included nausea, dry mouth, and dizziness (B.K. Skrumsager and K. Jeppesen, 1986).

HEADACHE. In the treatment of migraine, femoxetine has been shown to be less effective than doxepin (O. Sjaastad, *Cephalalgia*, 1983, *3*, 53) and no more effective than placebo (I. Zeeberg, *Acta neurol. scand.*, 1981, *64*, 452; M. Orholm *et al.*, *Cephalalgia*, 1985, *5*, *Suppl.* 3, 516).

SLEEP DISORDERS. Beneficial effects of femoxetine in narcolepsy.— H. Schrader *et al.*, *Acta neurol. scand.*, 1986, *74*, 297.

Proprietary Names and Manufacturers

Malexil *(USA)*;

Manufacturers also include—*Ferrosan, Denm.*

12739-x

Fenmetozole Hydrochloride *(USAN, pINNM)*.

DH-524. 2-(3,4-Dichlorophenoxymethyl)-2-imidazoline hydrochloride.
$C_{10}H_{10}Cl_2N_2O,HCl=281.6$.

CAS — 41473-09-0 (fenmetozole); 23712-05-2 (hydrochloride).

Fenmetozole is reported to be an antidepressant.

Proprietary Names and Manufacturers

Merrell Dow, USA.

12742-z

Fenpentadiol *(rINN)*.

Rd-292. 2-(4-Chlorophenyl)-4-methylpentane-2,4-diol.
$C_{12}H_{17}ClO_2=228.7$.

CAS — 15687-18-0.

Fenpentadiol has been used as an antidepressant.

Proprietary Names and Manufacturers

Trédum *(Anphar-Rolland, Fr.)*.

12762-t

Fluotracen Hydrochloride *(USAN, rINNM)*.

SK&F-28175. (±)-*cis*-(9,10-Dihydro-*N,N*,10-trimethyl-2-(trifluoromethyl)-9-anthracenepropylamine hydrochloride.
$C_{21}H_{24}F_3N,HCl=383.9$.

CAS — 35764-73-9 (fluotracen); 57363-14-1 (hydrochloride).

Fluotracen hydrochloride is a tricyclic antidepressant.

DEPRESSION. In a double-blind study of 28 depressed patients, fluotracen was found to have significantly better antidepressant effects than amitriptyline.— T. M. Itil *et al.*, *Curr. ther. Res.*, 1984, *35*, 1014.

Proprietary Names and Manufacturers

Smith Kline & French, USA.

12763-x

Fluoxetine *(BAN, USAN, rINN)*.

Lilly-103472; Lilly-110140. (±)-*N*-Methyl-3-phenyl-3-(α,α,α-trifluoro-*p*-tolyloxy)propylamine.
$C_{17}H_{18}F_3NO=309.3$.

CAS — 54910-89-3.

Adverse Effects

Adverse effects reported with fluoxetine include nausea, nervousness, insomnia and anxiety, headache, tremor, drowsiness, dry mouth, sweating, and diarrhoea.

A report of side-effects noted in 1378 patients treated for up to 3 years with fluoxetine.— J. F. Wernicke, *J. clin. Psychiat.*, 1985, *46*, 59.

A 41-year-old woman developed hypersensitivity to zimeldine, characterised by joint pain, chills, headache, and raised serum liver enzyme levels. Zimeldine was discontinued, and when all symptoms had resolved, fluoxetine 20 mg daily increasing to 100 mg daily was given. The patient continued to receive fluoxetine for 4 months without symptoms of hypersensitivity or changes in liver enzyme levels. It was concluded that the potent and specific serotonergic re-uptake block common to the 2 drugs did not appear to be a factor in the development of hypersensitivity to zimeldine.— G. Chouinard and B. Jones (letter), *Can. med. Ass. J.*, 1984, *131*, 1190.

OVERDOSAGE. All of 21 patients who took overdoses of fluoxetine (between 80 and 3000 mg) either alone, or with other drugs, recovered. Some were treated with emetics or lavage, particularly those who took the highest doses. Others were left untreated or given antihistamines for urticaria. Signs and symptoms were generally mild.— P. Benfield *et al.*, *Drugs*, 1986, *32*, 481.

Absorption and Fate

Fluoxetine is readily absorbed from the gastro-intestinal tract and extensively metabolised in the liver to its primary active metabolite desmethylfluoxetine and other metabolites. Fluoxetine is excreted in the urine, mainly in the form of its metabolites, either free or in conjugated form; small amounts are also found in the faeces. Fluoxetine is widely distributed throughout the body and is extensively bound to plasma proteins. Fluoxetine has been estimated to have an elimination half-life ranging from 1 to 4 days after a single dose and 2 to 7 days after multiple doses.

Uses and Administration

Fluoxetine is an antidepressant which selectively inhibits the re-uptake of serotonin. It is reported to cause fewer antimuscarinic side-effects than tricyclic antidepressants. Its mode of action in depression is not fully understood. In the treatment of depression, fluoxetine is given by mouth in doses of 20 to 80 mg daily. The concomitant administration of a sedative may be required for anxiety and insomnia. Reduced doses are recommended for patients with hepatic failure. Fluoxetine has also been tried in obesity and alcohol abuse.

Reviews of the actions and uses of fluoxetine: *J. clin. Psychiat.*, 1985, *46*, 3-59; N.F. Damlouji *et al.*, in *Pharmacotherapy of Affective Disorders: Theory and Practice*, W.G. Dewhurst and G.B. Baker (Eds.), London, Croom Helm, 1985, p.286.; P. Benfield *et al., Drugs*, 1986, *32*, 481; R. W. Sommi *et al., Pharmacotherapy*, 1987, *7*, 1.

DEPRESSION. Fluoxetine has been shown to be superior to placebo in the treatment of major depression (L.F. Fabre and L. Crismon, *Curr. ther. Res.*, 1985, *37*, 115; K. Rickels *et al., ibid.*, 1986, *39*, 559; R.R. Fieve *et al., J. clin Psychiat.*, 1986, *47*, 560) and as, or more, effective than amitriptyline (G. Chouinard, *ibid.*, 1985, *46*, 32; J.P. Feighner, *ibid.*, 369), imipramine (F.W. Reimherr *et al., Psychopharmac. Bull.*, 1984, *20*, 70; J.D. Bremner, *J. clin. Psychiat.*, 1984, *45*, 414; J.B. Cohn and C. Wilcox, *ibid.*, 1985, *46*, 26; P. Stark and C.D. Hardison, *ibid.*, 53), and doxepin (J.P. Feighner and J.B. Cohn, *ibid.*, 20).

OBSESSIVE COMPULSIVE DISORDERS. Two small studies have found fluoxetine to be of benefit in the treatment of obsessive compulsive disorder (S.M. Turner *et al., J. clin. Psychopharmacol.*, 1985, *5*, 207; R. Fontaine and G. Chouinard, *ibid.*, 1986, *6*, 98).

SLEEP DISORDERS. Of 11 patients with narcolepsy and cataplexy treated with fluoxetine 60 mg daily or clomipramine 25 to 150 mg daily for 4 weeks, 4 found fluoxetine more effective, 2 found clomipramine more effective, and 5 found both treatments equally effective. The mean daily number of attacks was reduced from 2.1 before treatment to 0.5 and 0.6 following fluoxetine and clomipramine treatment respectively.— R. Sandyk and M. A. Gillman, *Sleep*, 1986, *9*, 371.

Proprietary Names and Manufacturers

Prozac *(Dista, S.Afr.; Lilly, USA)*.

12768-h

Fluvoxamine Maleate *(BANM, rINNM)*.

DU-23000. (*E*)-5-Methoxy-4′-trifluoromethylvalerophenone *O*-2-aminoethyloxime maleate.

$C_{15}H_{21}F_3N_2O_2,C_4H_4O_4$=434.4.

CAS — 54739-18-3 (fluvoxamine); 61718-82-9.

Adverse Effects

The most common side-effects of fluvoxamine maleate are nausea and vomiting, which are reported to diminish with continuing treatment. Convulsions have been reported. Drowsiness, agitation and insomnia, tremor, anorexia, constipation, reversible elevation of serum liver enzyme concentrations, and bradycardia with ECG changes have also been noted.

There had been 30 reports of overdosage with fluvoxamine. Three of these patients ingested between 600 and 1500 mg of fluvoxamine and were satisfactorily managed after evacuation of the stomach either by vomiting or lavage. Another patient ingested about 2500 mg of fluvoxamine, 100 brompheniramine sustained-release tablets, and about 6 flurazepam capsules. On admission to hospital, body temperature and pulse rate were elevated and the patient was in a mild hypomanic state. Recovery followed gastric lavage; a sedative was subsequently administered for restlessness and disturbed behaviour.— P. Benfield and A. Ward, *Drugs*, 1986, *32*, 313.

The *UK* Committee on Safety of Medicines reported in May 1988 (*Current Problems, No. 22*, 1988) that between 25 September 1986 and 23 March 1988 it had received 961 reports of adverse reactions to fluvoxamine and that these included 5 deaths. The most frequently reported reactions were nausea (183) and vomiting (101). Other reactions included dizziness, somnolence, agitation, headache, tremor, and, during the first few days, worsening of anxiety. There were 13 reports of convulsions. Reports of appetite stimulation and antimuscarinic reactions were rare. Some effects resolved with time or dose reduction.

Precautions

Fluvoxamine should be avoided in patients with a history of epilepsy. Treatment in patients with hepatic or renal impairment should commence with low doses of fluvoxamine. Plasma concentrations of propranolol and warfarin may be increased in patients receiving fluvoxamine, and the effects of alcohol enhanced. Fluvoxamine should not be given to patients receiving monoamine oxidase inhibitors or for at least 14 days after their discontinuation.

DRIVING. For a general comment on antidepressant therapy and driving, see Amitriptyline Hydrochloride, p.353.

Absorption and Fate

Fluvoxamine is readily absorbed from the gastro-intestinal tract and metabolised in the liver. It is excreted in the urine as inactive metabolites, and has an elimination half-life of about 15 hours.

References: H. De Bree *et al., Eur. J. Drug Metab. Pharmacokinet.*, 1983, *8*, 175; H. Overmars *et al., ibid.*, 269.

Uses and Administration

Fluvoxamine is an antidepressant. It selectively inhibits the re-uptake of serotonin but has relatively little effect on noradrenaline re-uptake. Its mode of action in depression is not fully understood. In the treatment of depression fluvoxamine is given by mouth as the maleate in doses of 100 to 200 mg daily; in some patients 300 mg daily may be required. It is recommended that daily dosages exceeding 100 mg should be given in divided doses.

Reviews and studies on the actions and uses of fluvoxamine: *Br. J. clin. Pharmac.*, 1983, *15, Suppl.* 3, 347S-449S; N.F. Damlouji *et al.*, in *Pharmacotherapy of Affective Disorders: Theory and Practice*, W.G. Dewhurst and G.B. Baker (Eds.), London, Croom Helm, 1985, p.286; P. Benfield and A. Ward, *Drugs*, 1986, *32*, 313., Correction.— *ibid.*, 1987, *33*, No.2 (correction on contents page); *Drug & Ther. Bull.*, 1988, *26*, 11.

ANXIETY AND PHOBIAS. In a double-blind study in 58 patients with phobic disorders or anxiety states, fluvoxamine 50 mg daily increasing over 2 weeks to 100 mg daily and clomipramine 25 mg daily increasing to 150 mg daily, both given for 6 weeks, were both effective, decreasing both anxiety and associated depressive symptoms equally.— J. A. den Boer *et al., Int. clin. Psychopharmacol.*, 1987, *2*, 21.

DEPRESSION. In the treatment of depression fluvoxamine has been shown to be as effective as clomipramine (P. Dick and E. Ferrero, *Br. J. clin. Pharmac.*, 1983, *15*, 419S; J.E. De Wilde *et al., ibid.*, 427S) and imipramine (J.D. Guelfi *et al., ibid.*, 411S; W. Guy *et al., Psychopharmac. Bull.*, 1984, *20*, 73; R.A. Dominguez *et al., J. clin. Psychiat.*, 1985, *46*, 84; Y.D. Lapierre *et al., ibid.*, 1987, *48*, 65).

In a double-blind study of 62 patients suffering from mild to moderate depression, fluvoxamine was given either as a single 100-mg daytime dose, a single night-time dose, or as 50 mg twice daily for 6 weeks. All 3 regimens produced significant improvement, and no significant difference was found in antidepressant activity between the groups. However, patients receiving a single night-time dose experienced fewer side-effects than in the other 2 groups.— U. A. Siddiqui *et al., Curr. med. Res. Opinion*, 1985, *9*, 681.

Depression in the elderly. In a multicentre double-blind study of 76 severely depressed patients over 60 years of age, it was concluded that fluvoxamine 100 to 300 mg daily was well tolerated, more effective than placebo, and more rapidly effective than imipramine.— J. S. Wakelin, *Int. clin. Psychopharmacol.*, 1986, *1*, 221.

EXTRAPYRAMIDAL DISORDERS. Improvement in a patient with a hypokinetic rigid syndrome following the use of fluvoxamine.— J. D. Meerwaldt (letter), *Lancet*, 1986, *1*, 977.

Proprietary Preparations

Faverin *(Duphar, UK). Tablets*, enteric-coated, fluvoxamine maleate 50 mg.

Proprietary Names and Manufacturers

Faverin *(Duphar, UK)*; Fevarin *(Ferrosan, Denm.; Duphar, Ger.)*; Floxyfral *(Duphar, Fr.; Duphar, Switz.)*;

2514-w

Imipramine *(BAN, rINN)*.

3-(10,11-Dihydro-5*H*-dibenz[*b,f*]azepin-5-yl)propyldimethylamine.

$C_{19}H_{24}N_2$=280.4.

CAS — 50-49-7.

Imipramine 0.88 g is approximately equivalent to 1 g of imipramine hydrochloride.

2515-e

Imipramine Embonate *(BANM, rINNM)*.

Imipramine Pamoate.

$(C_{19}H_{24}N_2)_2,C_{23}H_{16}O_6$=949.2.

CAS — 10075-24-8.

Imipramine embonate 1.5 g is approximately equivalent to 1 g of imipramine hydrochloride.

2516-l

Imipramine Hydrochloride *(BANM, USAN, rINNM)*.

Imipram. Hydrochlor.; Imipramini Chloridum; Imipramini Hydrochloridum; Imizine.

$C_{19}H_{24}N_2,HCl$=316.9.

CAS — 113-52-0.

Pharmacopoeias. In *Aust., Belg., Br., Braz., Cz., Egypt., Eur., Fr., Ger., Ind., It., Jpn, Jug., Neth., Nord., Roum., Rus., Swiss*, and *U.S.*

A white or slightly yellow, odourless or almost odourless, crystalline powder. **Soluble** 1 in 2 of water, 1 in 1.5 of alcohol; freely soluble in chloroform; soluble in acetone; practically insoluble in ether. A 10% solution in water has a pH of 3.6 to 5.0. **Store** in airtight containers. Protect from light.

Adverse Effects, Treatment, and Precautions

As for Amitriptyline Hydrochloride, p.351.

CARDIOVASCULAR DISEASE. The use of tricyclic antidepressants in patients with cardiovascular disease is discussed under the Precautions section of amitriptyline. There is also further information on the precautions in such patients under Administration in Cardiovascular Disease in Uses, below.

EFFECTS ON THE PERIPHERAL CIRCULATION. Within 10 days of starting treatment with imipramine 150 mg daily, a 37-year-old depressed woman noted that her hands and feet became cold and turned blue for 5 minutes to several hours several times daily, and radial pulses were diminished. These vasospastic episodes continued for 4 months after discontinuation of a 3-week course of imipramine.— P. S. Appelbaum and W. Kapoor, *Am. J. Psychiat.*, 1983, *140*, 913.

EFFECTS ON THE SKIN. For a report of severe persistent cutaneous photosensitivity after 2 daily doses of imipramine, see Amitriptyline Hydrochloride, p.351.

EXTRAPYRAMIDAL EFFECTS. *Akathisia.* For a report of insomnia, jitteriness, and irritability in patients with panic disorder receiving imipramine, see Amitriptyline Hydrochloride, p.351.

INTERACTIONS. Interactions involving tricyclic antidepressants are discussed under amitriptyline (p.353). References to interactions where imipramine has been the tricyclic antidepressant affected can be found under the headings Fenclonine, H_2 antagonist antihistamines, Neuroleptics, Sex hormones, and Smoking.

Imipramine has sometimes been the tricyclic antidepressant that has affected other drugs and information on these interactions can be found under levodopa (p.1017), phenytoin (p.408), phenylephrine hydrochloride (p.1474), and thyroxine sodium (p.1489). For a report of an adverse reaction to imipramine, but not trimipramine, in a patient receiving phenelzine, see phenelzine sulphate (p.379).

OVERDOSAGE. For a report of the use of sodium bicarbonate to restore sinus rhythm in a patient with ventricular tachycardia after an overdose of imipramine, see Amitriptyline Hydrochloride, p.352.

PHAEOCHROMOCYTOMA. A 36-year-old pregnant woman with an undetected phaeochromocytoma was given imipramine 25 mg every 8 hours for depression. About 6 hours after the fourth dose she experienced 3 grand mal seizures.— J. S. Kaufmann (letter), *J. Am. med. Ass.*, 1974, *229*, 1282.

In an 11-year-old girl imipramine 50 mg caused hypertension, tachycardia, and profuse sweating; the same dose 2 months earlier had had similar effects. She was later shown to have a phaeochromocytoma.— J. Mok and I. Swann, *Archs Dis. Childh.*, 1978, *53*, 676.

PORPHYRIA. For a report recommending that imipramine should not be used in porphyrics, see Amitriptyline Hydrochloride p.354.

PREGNANCY AND THE NEONATE. For studies finding no association between maternal tricyclic antidepressant usage and congenital malformation, see Amitriptyline Hydrochloride, p.354. For a report that although imipramine is transferred into breast milk, there had been no reported effects on lactation, or signs or symptoms in breast-fed infants, see Amitriptyline Hydrochloride, p.354.

WITHDRAWAL SYNDROMES. *Neonatal withdrawal.* Withdrawal symptoms were observed in 3 neonates whose mothers had taken imipramine during pregnancy.— E. Eggermont (letter), *Lancet*, 1973, *2*, 680. See also *idem* (letter), *Archs Dis. Childh.*, 1980, *55*, 81.

Absorption and Fate

Imipramine is readily absorbed from the gastro-intestinal tract, and extensively demethylated by first-pass metabolism in the liver, to its primary active metabolite, desipramine. Since imipramine slows gastro-intestinal transit time absorption can, however, be delayed, particularly in overdosage.

Paths of metabolism of both imipramine and desipramine include hydroxylation and *N*-oxidation. Imipramine is excreted in the urine, mainly in the form of its metabolites, either free or in conjugated form.

Imipramine and desipramine are widely distributed throughout the body and are extensively bound to plasma and tissue protein. Imipramine has been estimated to have a half-life ranging from 9 to 28 hours, which may be considerably extended in overdosage. Plasma concentrations of imipramine and desipramine vary very widely between individuals but some correlation with therapeutic response has been established.

Imipramine and desipramine cross the blood-brain barrier and placental barrier and are excreted in breast milk.

The pharmacokinetic properties of imipramine in psychiatric patients.— E. Mårtensson *et al.*, *Curr. ther. Res.*, 1984, *36*, 228.

METABOLISM. For reference to possible associations between poor metabolism of debrisoquine or sparteine and adverse reactions to tricyclic antidepressants, see Amitriptyline Hydrochloride, p.354.

PLASMA CONCENTRATIONS. Six studies of imipramine agreed that: interindividual metabolic differences do influence outcome; the percentage of patients responding favourably increases as blood levels of imipramine plus desmethyl metabolite are increased up to 200 to 250 ng/mL (although some patients may show favourable clinical response at lower blood levels); higher levels (more than 250 ng/mL) can produce more side-effects, but in five of the six studies, no change in antidepressant response was seen. Plasma level measurements were unequivocally useful in problem patients who did not respond to usual oral doses or in high-risk patients who, because of age or medical illness, would be best treated with the lowest possible effective dose of the drug.— American Psychiatric Association (A.P.A.) Task Force, *Am. J. Psychiat.*, 1985, *142*, 155.

Uses and Administration

Imipramine is a tricyclic antidepressant with actions and uses similar to those of amitriptyline (p.354). It has less marked sedative properties.

In the treatment of depression, imipramine is given by mouth as the hydrochloride in doses of 25 mg three times daily initially, gradually increased to 50 mg three or four times daily as necessary; higher doses of up to 300 mg daily may be required in severely depressed hospital patients. A suggested initial dose for adolescents and the elderly is 10 mg at night, increasing to 10 mg to 25 mg three times daily. Since imipramine has a prolonged half-life, once-daily dosage regimens are also suitable, usually given at night.

In the initial stages of treatment, if administration by mouth is impracticable or inadvisable, up to 100 mg of the hydrochloride may be given daily in divided doses by intramuscular injection, but oral administration should be substituted as soon as possible. In addition to the hydrochloride, imipramine is available as the embonate for oral administration, as capsules in strengths suitable for adults only.

Imipramine is also given for the treatment of nocturnal enuresis in children. Suggested doses are 25 mg for children aged 6 to 7 years, 25 to 50 mg for children aged 8 to 11 years, and 50 to 75 mg for children aged over 11 years. The dose should be taken just before bedtime and treatment should not continue for longer than 3 months. The use of tricyclic antidepressants for nocturnal enuresis in children is controversial, not least in view of the hazards of accidental overdosage. In particular, tricyclic antidepressant therapy is not suitable for younger children; for further comment, see below under Enuresis.

ADMINISTRATION. A possible means of predicting imipramine and desipramine dosage requirements following administration of a single dose.— D. J. Brunswick *et al.*, *Clin. Pharmac. Ther.*, 1979, *25*, 605. See also R. A. Braithwaite *et al.*, *Postgrad. med. J.*, 1980, *56*, *Suppl.* 1, 112.

Administration in cardiovascular disease. Twenty four depressed patients with chronic heart disease were treated with doxepin, imipramine, or placebo in a double-blind study. The starting dose of tricyclic antidepressant was 50 mg daily, increased every 3 days until side-effects supervened, or a daily dose of 150 mg was reached. After 4 weeks, the mean daily doses of doxepin and imipramine were 153 mg and 129 mg respectively. Depression was significantly improved in the doxepin and imipramine groups, but not in the placebo group. The tricyclic antidepressants had no effect on left ventricular ejection fraction at rest or during maximal exercise. Premature ventricular contractions were reduced by imipramine, but not consistently changed by doxepin or placebo, and there was no significant change in resting supine blood pressure in any treatment group. It was suggested that in the absence of severe impairment of myocardial performance, depressed patients with pre-existing heart disease could be effectively treated with tricyclic antidepressants without an adverse effect on ventricular rhythm or haemodynamic function.— R. C. Veith *et al.*, *New Engl. J. Med.*, 1982, *306*, 954. Comment. The imipramine dose used was low and the patients had minimal cardiac impairment. Higher doses had been used in patients with severely depressed left ventricular function without notable change in ejection fraction, but it was premature to imply that all tricyclic antidepressants could be given safely.— E. -G. V. Giardina (letter), *ibid.*, *307*, 821. Reply. The authors were aware of no evidence to suggest that comparable plasma concentrations of other tricyclic antidepressants should be expected to produce cardiovascular effects any greater than the observed effects of imipramine and doxepin.— R. C. Veith *et al.* (letter), *ibid.*,. Seven of 15 depressed patients with notable pre-existing left ventricular dysfunction experienced such severe orthostatic hypotension on administration of imipramine that the drug had to be discontinued. Plasma concentrations were essentially twice those usually seen. Although imipramine did not further impair resting left ventricular performance, it was not without risk.— A. H. Glassman *et al.*, *J. Am. med. Ass.*, 1983, *250*, 1997.

Cardiac arrhythmias. Imipramine and its metabolites have actions characteristic of class I antiarrhythmic drugs (M.E. Thase and J.M. Perel, *J. Am. med. Ass.*, 1982, *248*, 429). Imipramine and nortriptyline have been successfully used to control premature ventricular contractions (E.-G.V. Giardini and J.T. Bigger, *Am. J. Cardiol.*, 1982, *50*, 172), even in patients with moderate to severe left ventricular impairment (E.-G.V. Giardini *et al.*, *Am. Heart. J.*, 1985, *109*, 992), but imipramine was not shown to be more effective than other class I antiarrhythmics in treating ventricular tachycardia (S.J. Connolly *et al.*, *Am. J. Cardiol.*, 1984, *53*, 516).

The cardiotoxicity of tricyclic antidepressants and the cautions required when using them in patients with cardiovascular disease are discussed under the Adverse Effects and Precautions sections of amitriptyline (p.351).

ADMINISTRATION IN THE ELDERLY. For a study suggesting that imipramine resulted in a higher incidence of orthostatic hypotension in the elderly than doxepin, see Doxepin Hydrochloride, p.361.

ADMINISTRATION IN RENAL FAILURE. Imipramine can be given in usual doses to patients with renal failure. Concentrations of imipramine are affected by haemodialysis or peritoneal dialysis.— W. M. Bennett *et al.*, *Am. J. Kidney Dis.*, 1983, *3*, 155.

ANXIETY AND PHOBIAS. *Agoraphobia.* In a placebo-controlled study, phobic avoidance ratings were reduced more by imipramine or phenelzine than by placebo. Clomipramine has also been claimed to reduce phobic anxiety, but high doses may be needed and these have many side-effects in phobic patients, and there is a high risk of relapse when one of these drugs is discontinued. Controlled studies of monoamine oxidase inhibitors have shown a small but definite benefit. It is not clear whether improvement in agoraphobic patients following antidepressants is restricted to those with co-existing depression, and the additional benefit conferred by adding an antidepressant to behavioural treatments remains doubtful unless the patient is overtly depressed.— *Drug & Ther. Bull.*, 1983, *21*, 61.

Panic attacks. Most studies have confirmed the effectiveness of tricyclic antidepressants, notably imipramine, in the treatment of phobic disorders characterised by panic attacks. At the onset of treatment, the efficacy of imipramine may be enhanced by using benzodiazepines or behavioural therapy to decrease the anticipatory anxiety associated with such attacks. The duration of therapy is not well established.— J. T. Brown *et al.*, *Ann. intern. Med.*, 1984, *100*, 558. See also: D. V. Sheehan, *New Engl. J. Med.*, 1982, *307*, 156; P. H. Keefe and W. S. Agras (letter), *ibid.*, 1983, *308*, 341; I. Marks (letter), *ibid.*,; R. R. Neubig (letter), *ibid.*, 342; D. V. Sheehan (letter), *ibid.*

BEHAVIOUR DISORDERS. The efficacy of imipramine has been proved in the treatment of a variety of childhood behavioural disorders, including childhood depression, encopresis, episodic anxiety (particularly when manifested as school phobia), and attention deficit disorder (hyperkinesis or minimal brain dysfunction).— C. L. DeVane and K. M. Ahsanuddin, *Drug Intell. & clin. Pharm.*, 1983, *17*, 562. See also J. Biederman and M. S. Jellinek, *New Engl. J. Med.*, 1984, *310*, 968.

For further information on the use of imipramine in childhood depression, see under Depression, below.

For the beneficial use of imipramine in patients with emotional lability due to amyotrophic lateral sclerosis, see Amitriptyline Hydrochloride, p.355.

CARDIAC ARRHYTHMIAS. For references to the anti-arrhythmic activity of imipramine, see under Administration in Cardiovascular Disease, above.

DEPRESSION. For a general review of the role of antidepressants in depression, see Amitriptyline Hydrochloride, p.355.

For a report of studies examining the relationship between plasma-imipramine concentrations and clinical outcome, and with suggestions for patients who might benefit from plasma concentration measurements, see under Plasma Concentrations in Absorption and Fate, above.

Bipolar depression. See under Mania and Manic Depression, below.

Combination therapy with liothyronine. For the use of liothyronine as an adjunct to tricyclic antidepressant therapy in depression, see Liothyronine, p.1487.

Depression in children. In controlled studies of tricyclic antidepressants, particularly imipramine, in childhood depression, 60 to 75% of prepubertal children respond, whereas approximately one-third of adolescents benefit. Other investigators report that the positive effects do not differ from the improvement found in children receiving placebo. The efficacy of tricyclics may depend upon plasma levels. A recommended regimen consists of starting the drug at 1.5 mg per kg body-weight daily, then increasing to 3, 4, or a maximum of 5 mg per kg daily in 3 roughly equivalent doses every third or fourth day. Some clinicians prefer the administration of one evening dose to reduce the daytime sedative effect. A trial of at least 4 weeks is necessary and continuation for up to 3 or 4 months after initial recovery is suggested. A longer weaning time is recommended in adolescents.— G. P. Aylward, *J. Pediat.*, 1985, *107*, 1.

Prophylaxis. For studies showing imipramine to be as effective as, or more effective than lithium in preventing recurrent depression, see Lithium Carbonate, p.370.

EATING DISORDERS. For the beneficial use of imipramine in bulimia, see Amitriptyline Hydrochloride, p.356.

ENURESIS. Imipramine is the drug of choice in the pharmacological management of enuresis, but its use should be limited to older children and adolescents, and then only for very short-term special situations. Treatment is started with a dosage of 10 mg daily one or two hours before bedtime with gradual increases to a therapeutic level (25 to 75 mg daily depending on age and bodyweight). Although imipramine is very effective in reducing the frequency of enuretic events, some patients do not respond, and others develop tolerance. When treatment is withdrawn, the relapse rate is high. The exact mechanism of action of imipramine has not been identified, but may be related to the drug's antimuscarinic properties. Also, imipramine induces a significant increase in wakefulness during the night, which may allow the child more conscious control of micturition. This effect, coupled with a decrease in bladder excitability, which permits a greater bladder capacity, reduces enuretic events. Despite accumulated evidence for the effectiveness of this drug, a controlled comparison between the urine alarm method and drug therapy with imipramine showed a more effective outcome with the alarm (W. Wagner *et al.*, *J. Pediat.*, 1982, *101*, 302).— A. Kales *et al.*, *Ann. intern. Med.*, 1987, *106*, 582.

Imipramine was not superior to placebo in the treatment of diurnal enuresis in a double-blind trial in 27 children.— R. Meadow and I. Berg, *Archs Dis. Childh.*, 1982, *57*, 714.

MANIA AND MANIC DEPRESSION. Controlled studies suggest that imipramine has no place in the long-term prevention of manic depression and mania, because lithium is equally effective in preventing depressive recurrence and imipramine may even increase the risk of manic recurrences.— J. C. Cookson, *Br. J. Hosp. Med.*, 1985, *34*, 172.

MYOTONIA. A report of imipramine or amitriptyline in doses of 100 to 150 mg daily reducing symptomatic clinical myotonia, increasing testable muscle strength, reducing the frequency of or eliminating cardiac arrhythmias, and improving gastro-intestinal function in 35 patients with myotonic dystrophy.— R. A. Brumback and K. M. Carlson (letter), *Muscle Nerve*, 1983, *6*, 233.

OBSESSIVE COMPULSIVE DISORDERS. For a preliminary report of the successful use of imipramine in obsessive thoughts, see Phenelzine Sulphate, p.379.

PAIN. For conflicting results concerning the benefit of imipramine in relieving the pain of diabetic neuropathy, see Amitriptyline Hydrochloride, p.356.

PHOBIAS. For the use of imipramine in agoraphobia, see under Anxiety and Phobias, above.

SEXUAL DISORDERS. Administration of imipramine was associated with an ejaculate of normal volume and consistency, containing motile spermatozoa, in a man with aspermia following retroperitoneal lymph node dissection.— M. E. Kelly and M. A. Needle, *Urology*, 1979, *13*, 414.

In patients with retrograde ejaculation or failure of emission, anterograde ejaculation may be achieved by imipramine 25 to 50 mg daily.— W. -B. Schill and M. Michalopoulos, *Drugs*, 1984, *28*, 263.

SLEEP DISORDERS. *Narcolepsy.* Imipramine is the treatment of choice in cataplexy. It also alleviates sleep paralysis, but has little effect on narcoleptic sleep attacks. Imipramine acts more rapidly and requires a lower dose for cataplexy than when used as an antidepressant, generally 10 to 75 mg daily. Single or divided doses should be titrated to provide maximal protection for the time of day when symptoms usually occur; evening doses should be avoided to minimise nocturnal arousal. When a patient requires treatment for both sleep attacks and auxiliary symptoms including cataplexy, central stimulants and imipramine may be combined, but careful titration and monitoring are necessary because of the risk of serious side-effects such as hypertension. Clomipramine, desipramine, and protriptyline have also been found to be effective for treating auxiliary symptoms.— A. Kales *et al.*, *Ann. intern. Med.*, 1987, *106*, 434.

Parasomnias. Imipramine has been used for aggressive behaviour during sleep, and sometimes controls head banging during sleep, at least for a brief period. Imipramine and amitriptyline could be effective for night terrors and nightmares.— J. D. Parkes, *Lancet*, 1986, *2*, 1021.

URINARY INCONTINENCE. Imipramine has been used to control stress incontinence in women (I. Gilja *et al.*, *J. Urol., Baltimore*, 1984, *132*, 909), incontinence due to hyper-reflexic bladder in multiple sclerosis (B. Giesser, *Drugs*, 1985, *29*, 88), and urge incontinence in the elderly both on its own (B. Isaacs, *Prescribers' J.*, 1981, *21*, 285; J.C. Brocklehurst, *Practitioner*, 1984, *228*, 275; J.W. Rowe, *New Engl. J. Med.*, 1985, *312*, 827), and in combination with antimuscarinic agents (N.M. Resnick and S.V. Yalla, *ibid.*, *313*, 800; J.C. Gingell, *Br. med. J.*, 1986, *292*, 1180). Its site of action is thought to differ from that of the antimuscarinic agents (E.J. McGuire, *Br. J. Hosp. Med.*, 1984, *31*, 149).

Preparations

Imipramine Hydrochloride Injection *(U.S.P.)*

Imipramine Hydrochloride Tablets *(U.S.P.)*

Imipramine Tablets *(B.P.)*. Tablets containing imipramine hydrochloride.

Proprietary Preparations

Praminil *(DDSA Pharmaceuticals, UK). Tablets*, imipramine hydrochloride 10 and 25 mg.

Tofranil *(Geigy, UK). Tablets*, imipramine hydrochloride 10 and 25 mg.
Syrup, imipramine equivalent to imipramine hydrochloride 25 mg/5 mL.

Proprietary Names and Manufacturers

Antipress *(Lemmon, USA)*; Berkomine *(Berk Pharmaceuticals, UK)*; Chimoreptin *(Jpn)*; Deprinol *(Denm.)*; Dimipressin *(R.P. Drugs, UK)*; Dynaprin *(Ital.)*; Efuranol *(Jpn)*; Ethipramine *(SCS, S.Afr.)*; Imavate *(Robins, USA)*; Imidol *(Jpn)*; Imiprin *(Protea, Austral.)*; Impril *(ICN, Canad.)*; Iramil *(Austral.)*; Janimine *(Abbott, USA)*; Medipramine *(Vernleigh, S.Afr.)*; Melipramine *(Austral.)*; Norpramine *(Norton, UK)*; Novopramine *(Novopharm, Canad.)*; Oppanyl *(Oppenheimer, UK)*; Panpramine *(S.Afr.)*; Praminil *(DDSA Pharmaceuticals, UK)*; Presamine *(USV Pharmaceutical Corp., USA)*; Prodepress *(Austral.)*; SK-Pramine *(Smith Kline & French, USA)*; Somipra *(Austral.)*; Surplix *(Vis, Ital.)*; Tizipramine *(Ticen, Eire)*; Tofranil *(Arg.; Geigy, Austral.; Belg.; Geigy, Canad.; Geigy, Denm.; Geigy, Fr.; Geigy, Ger.; Geigy, Ital.; Neth.; Geigy, Norw.; Geigy, S.Afr.; Ciba, Spain; Geigy, Swed.; Geigy, Switz.; Geigy, UK; Geigy, USA)*; Tofranil-PM *(Geigy, USA)*; W.D.D. *(Tutag, USA)*.

2517-y

Imipramine Oxide Hydrochloride

Imipramine *N*-Oxide Hydrochloride; Imipraminoxide Hydrochloride; Imipraminoxidi Chloridum. 3-(10,11-Dihydro-5*H*-dibenz[*b,f*]azepin-5-yl)propyldimethylamine *N*-oxide hydrochloride.
$C_{19}H_{24}N_2O,HCl=332.9$.

CAS — 19864-71-2; 6829-98-7(imipramine oxide).

Pharmacopoeias. In *Nord.*

Imipramine oxide hydrochloride is an antidepressant with actions and uses similar to those of imipramine hydrochloride.

Proprietary Names and Manufacturers

Elepsin *(Andromaco, Arg.)*; Imiprex *(Dumex, Denm.; Dumex, Norw.; Lasa, Spain)*.

15324-r

Indeloxazine Hydrochloride *(USAN, rINNM)*.

CI-874. (±)-2-(Inden-7-yloxymethyl)morpholine hydrochloride.
$C_{14}H_{17}NO_2,HCl=267.8$.

CAS — 60929-23-9 (indeloxazine); 65043-22-3 (hydrochloride).

Indeloxazine hydrochloride is reported to be an antidepressant; it has also been tried in senile dementia.

Proprietary Names and Manufacturers

Elen *(Yamanouchi, Jpn)*;
Manufacturers also include—*Parke, Davis, USA*.

2518-j

Iprindole Hydrochloride *(BANM, rINNM)*.

Pramindole Hydrochloride; Wy-3263. 5-(3-Dimethylaminopropyl) -6,7,8,9,10,11- hexahydrocyclooct[*b*]indole hydrochloride.
$C_{19}H_{28}N_2,HCl=320.9$.

CAS — 5560-72-5 (iprindole); 68782-59-2 (hydrochloride).

NOTE. Iprindole is *USAN*.

Iprindole hydrochloride 16.9 mg is approximately equivalent to 15 mg of iprindole.

Adverse Effects, Treatment and Precautions

As for Amitriptyline Hydrochloride, p.351.

Antimuscarinic side-effects occur less frequently with iprindole than with imipramine, and are usually less severe.

Jaundice or bilirubinuria has been reported with iprindole, usually during the first 14 days of treatment; it should not be given to patients with impaired liver function or a history of liver disease.

Uses and Administration

Iprindole hydrochloride has actions and uses similar to those of the tricyclic antidepressants such as amitriptyline (p.354), but it only has weak antimuscarinic effects.

The initial dose in mild depression and in the elderly is the equivalent of 15 mg of iprindole three times daily. In moderate to severe depression, the initial dose is the equivalent of 30 mg of iprindole three times daily, which may be increased up to 60 mg three times daily. The usual maintenance dose is the equivalent of 30 mg of iprindole three times daily.

Proprietary Preparations

Prondol *(Wyeth, UK). Tablets*, iprindole 15 and 30 mg (as hydrochloride).

2519-z

Iproclozide *(BAN, rINN)*.

PC-603. 2-(4-Chlorophenoxy)-2′-isopropylacetohydrazide.
$C_{11}H_{15}ClN_2O_2=242.7$.

CAS — 3544-35-2.

Iproclozide is a monoamine oxidase inhibitor with actions and uses similar to those of phenelzine (p.377).

Proprietary Names and Manufacturers

Sursum *(Belg.; Ibsa, Switz.)*.

2520-p

Iproniazid Phosphate *(BANM, rINNM)*.

2′-Isopropylisonicotinohydrazide phosphate.
$C_9H_{13}N_3O,H_3PO_4=277.2$.

CAS — 54-92-2 (iproniazid); 305-33-9 (phosphate).

Iproniazid phosphate 155 mg is approximately equivalent to 100 mg of iproniazid.

Adverse Effects, Treatment, and Precautions

As for Phenelzine Sulphate, p.377.

EFFECTS ON THE LIVER. Of 91 cases of hepatitis due to antidepressant therapy, cytolytic reactions occurred in 11 treated with iproniazid. Five patients died, 3 of them after involuntary rechallenge. High levels of antimitochondrial antibody were found in 5 patients.— B. Lefebure *et al.*, *Thérapie*, 1984, *39*, 509.

PORPHYRIA. Iproniazid was considered to be unsafe in patients with acute porphyria because it has been shown to be porphyrinogenic in *animals* or *in vitro* systems.— M.R. Moore and K.E.L. McColl, *Porphyrias, Drug Lists*, Glasgow, Porphyria Research Unit, University Of Glasgow, 1987.

Uses and Administration

Iproniazid is a monoamine oxidase inhibitor with actions and uses similar to those of phenelzine (p.379).

In the treatment of depression iproniazid is given by mouth as the phosphate in doses equivalent to iproniazid

100 to 150 mg daily, usually in the morning. Once a response has been obtained the dosage may be gradually reduced for maintenance therapy; some patients may respond to 25 to 50 mg daily.
Iproniazid, which is the isopropyl derivative of isoniazid, was developed for use in tuberculosis but owing to its toxicity it is no longer used for this purpose.

Proprietary Names and Manufacturers
Marsilid *(Roche, Austral.; Belg.; Roche, Fr.; Spain; Roche, UK).*

2521-s

Isocarboxazid *(BAN, USAN, rINN).*
Ro-50831. 2′-Benzyl-5-methylisoxazole-3-carbohydrazide.
$C_{12}H_{13}N_3O_2$=231.3.

CAS — 59-63-2.

Pharmacopoeias. In *Ind.* and *U.S.*

A white or practically white, crystalline powder with a faint characteristic odour. **Soluble** 1 in 2000 of water, 1 in 83 of alcohol, 1 in 2 of chloroform, and 1 in 58 of ether. **Store** in well-closed containers.

Adverse Effects, Treatment, and Precautions
As for Phenelzine Sulphate, p.377.

EFFECTS ON THE SKIN. Isocarboxazid may cause photosensitivity reactions.— *Med. Lett.*, 1986, *28*, 51.

Absorption and Fate
Isocarboxazid is readily absorbed from the gastro-intestinal tract. It is metabolised by the liver, and excreted in the urine mainly in the form of metabolites.

Uses and Administration
Isocarboxazid is a monoamine oxidase inhibitor with actions and uses similar to those of phenelzine (p.379).
In the treatment of depression isocarboxazid is given in initial doses of 30 mg daily. If no improvement occurs after 4 weeks, doses up to 60 mg daily can be tried for 4 to 6 weeks. Once a response has been obtained the dosage may be gradually reduced to a maintenance of 10 to 20 mg daily, although doses up to 40 mg daily may be needed. Half the normal maintenance dose may be adequate in the elderly.

ADMINISTRATION. For a study suggesting that the doses of isocarboxazid formerly used were too low to be fully effective, see Phenelzine Sulphate, p.379.

DEPRESSION. For general comments on the role of monoamine oxidase inhibitors in depression, see Phenelzine Sulphate, p.379.

Combination therapy with tricyclic antidepressants. For a report suggesting that isocarboxazid and phenelzine are the monoamine oxidase inhibitors least likely to produce side-effects in combination with tricyclic antidepressants, see Amitriptyline Hydrochloride, p.355.

PREMATURE EJACULATION. Isocarboxazid 20 to 40 mg daily by mouth successfully treated premature ejaculation in a series of 6 patients.— D. Bennett (letter), *Lancet*, 1961, *2*, 1309.

Preparations

Isocarboxazid Tablets *(U.S.P.).* Protect from light.

Proprietary Preparations

Marplan *(Roche, UK). Tablets,* scored, isocarboxazid 10 mg.

Proprietary Names and Manufacturers
Marplan *(Roche, Austral.; Belg.; Roche, Canad.; Roche, Denm.; Fr.; Roche, Ital.; Roche, Switz.; Roche, UK; Roche, USA).*

5057-h

Lithium Carbonate *(BAN, USAN).*

CP-15467-61; Lithii Carbonas; Lithium Carb.
Li_2CO_3=73.89.

CAS — 554-13-2.

Pharmacopoeias. In *Aust., Br., Braz., Chin., Cz., Egypt., Eur., Fr., Ger., Ind., Int., It., Jpn, Jug., Neth., Nord., Port., Roum., Span., Swiss,* and *U.S. U.S.* also includes lithium citrate and lithium hydroxide.

A white, light odourless granular powder. Each g represents 27 mmol (27 mEq) of lithium.
B.P. **solubilities** are: slightly soluble in water; practically insoluble in alcohol. *U.S.P.* solubilities are: sparingly soluble in water, very slightly soluble in alcohol; dissolves, with effervescence, in dilute mineral acids. A saturated solution is alkaline to litmus. **Store** in well-closed containers.

Adverse Effects
The side-effects of lithium are dose-related and the margin between the therapeutic and toxic dose is narrow. Initial adverse effects of lithium therapy include nausea, vertigo, fine hand tremor, polyuria with thirst and polydipsia, muscle weakness, and a feeling of somnolence and lethargy. Some of these effects often abate with continued therapy. Besides these initial effects adverse effects occurring at therapeutic serum concentrations of lithium include diarrhoea, metallic taste, headache, vertigo, fine tremor, hyperparathyroidism with hypercalcaemia, leucocytosis, weight gain, oedema (which should not be treated with diuretics), hypermagnesaemia, cardiac arrhythmias with ECG changes, and exacerbation of skin conditions such as acne and psoriasis. Long-term adverse effects include hypothyroidism and/or goitre, rarely hyperthyroidism, kidney damage, impaired renal function, and nephrogenic diabetes insipidus, mild cognitive and memory impairment, and increased antinuclear antibody titres.
Toxic effects may be expected at serum-lithium concentrations of about 1.5 mmol per litre, although they can appear at lower concentrations. They call for immediate withdrawal of treatment and should always be considered very seriously.
Signs of toxicity include increasing diarrhoea, vomiting, anorexia, polyuria, muscle weakness, lethargy, ataxia, lack of co-ordination, tinnitus, blurred vision, coarse tremor of the extremities and lower jaw, muscle hyperirritability and twitching, hyperreflexia, choreoathetoid movements, dysarthria, disorientation, psychosis, drowsiness, and seizures. Coma and death may occur.

A review of the adverse effects of lithium and recommendations for the monitoring of lithium therapy.— R. B. Salem, *Drug Intell. & clin. Pharm.*, 1983, *17*, 346.

EFFECTS ON THE BLOOD. *Leucocytosis.* A reversible and apparently harmless leucocytosis was observed in patients treated with lithium.— B. Shopsin *et al., Clin. Pharmac. Ther.*, 1971, *12*, 923.

Leucopenia. For a report of severe leucopenia following lithium overdosage, see under Overdosage, below.

Leukaemia. Several reports have suggested a possible connection between lithium therapy and leukaemia (R.T.S. Jim, *Blood*, 1979, *53*, 1031; L.E. Orr and J.F. McKernan, *Lancet*, 1979, *1*, 449; W.P. Hammond and F. Appelbaum, *New Engl. J. Med.*, 1980, *302*, 808; J.L. Nielsen, *ibid.*, *303*, 283), but other workers, some retrospectively studying case notes, could find no association (D.L. Longo, *ibid.*; J. Lyskowski and H.A. Nasrallah, *Br. J. Psychiat.*, 1981, *139*, 256; G. Resek and S. Olivieri, *Lancet*, 1983, *1*, 940).

EFFECTS ON THE CARDIOVASCULAR SYSTEM. *Cardiac arrhythmias.* Lithium therapy has been associated with bradycardia due to sinus node dysfunction (G. Montalescot *et al., Int. J. Cardiol.*, 1984, *5*, 94), which has persisted after stopping lithium (E.V. Palileo *et al., Am. Heart J.*, 1983, *106*, 1443). Premature ventricular contractions (T.M. Tangedahl and G.T. Gau, *New Engl. J. Med.*, 1972, *287*, 867), atrioventricular block (C.M. Jaffe, *Am. J. Psychiat.*, 1977, *134*, 88; C.A. Martin and M.T. Piascik, *Can. J. Psychiat.*, 1985, *30*, 114), and T-wave depression (R.G. Demers and G.R. Heninger, *J. Am. med. Ass.*, 1971, *218*, 381) have also been reported. In general, lithium does not appear to be contra-indicated in patients with heart disease, but if used in patients with arrhythmias, electrocardiographic monitoring is essential to detect any possible, although unlikely, aggravation of the arrhythmia (A.G. Tilkian *et al., Am. J. Med.*, 1976, *61*, 665).

Malignant hypertension. For a report of severe hypertension occurring during acute lithium intoxication, see under Overdosage, below.

Myocarditis. Lithium can cause toxic myocarditis.— *Lancet*, 1985, *2*, 1165.

Thrombophlebitis. For a report of deep venous thrombophlebitis occurring in association with chronic lithium toxicity, see under Overdosage, below.

EFFECTS ON THE ENDOCRINE SYSTEM. A review of the endocrine and metabolic effects of lithium.— J. H. Lazarus, *Adverse Drug React. Ac. Pois. Rev.*, 1982, *1*, 181.

Diabetogenic effect. The occurrence of diabetes mellitus in patients taking lithium has been reported (B.B. Johnston, *Lancet*, 1977, *2*, 935; J. Craig *et al., ibid.*, 1028) and a worsening of the diabetic state was described in one patient taking lithium (R. Waziri and J. Nelson, *J. clin. Psychiat.*, 1978, *39*, 623), but administration of lithium in therapeutic doses to maturity-onset diabetics for one week has caused no deterioration in glucose and insulin response to a standard carbohydrate meal. No cases of acute diabetes mellitus in patients taking lithium have been reported since 1977 and it seems unlikely that lithium precipitates diabetes.— J. H. Lazarus, *Adverse Drug React. Ac. Pois. Rev.*, 1982, *1*, 181.

Hyperparathyroidism. A possible association between lithium, hypercalcaemia, and hyperparathyroidism in 6 patients.— T. A. T. Christensson (letter), *Lancet*, 1976, *2*, 144.
Another report of lithium producing a mild hyperparathyroidism in manic-depressive patients. This was considered to be a biochemical syndrome without clinical features, requiring neither withdrawal nor surgery.— C. Christiansen *et al.* (letter), *Lancet*, 1976, *2*, 969. See also G. A. MacGregor (letter), *Lancet*, 1977, *2*, 1129.
A report of hyperparathyroidism in 2 patients receiving lithium. In both patients improvement in plasma-calcium concentrations on discontinuation of lithium coincided with improvement in mental state.— A. Prasad, *Eur. J. clin. Pharmac.*, 1984, *27*, 499. See also L. E. Mallette and E. Eichhorn, *Archs intern. Med.*, 1986, *146*, 770.

Thyroid disorders. The prevalence of goitre in reported series has varied between 0 and 61.5%, but the examination methods in the series showing low prevalence were probably less than adequate. Goitre can appear early during lithium therapy and, for reasons still not understood, tend to regress during treatment. The most important effect of lithium on goitre formation is inhibition of thyroid hormone release, producing an increase in the pituitary secretion of thyroid-stimulating hormone. Some studies in humans have shown significantly lowered peripheral thyroid hormone concentrations, while others have found no depression. Other factors, such as the presence of thyroid autoantibodies and variable intra-thyroidal iodine concentrations, appear to contribute, as some patients develop goitre whilst others with similar exposure to lithium and similar serum-lithium concentrations do not. Most workers estimate the prevalence of lithium-induced hypothyroidism at about 3 to 5%, with an average duration of lithium therapy before diagnosis of about 18 months. Lithium-induced hypothyroidism is partly related to inhibition of thyroid secretion and possibly to antibody-mediated damage; 10 to 60% of patients with lithium induced hypothyroidism have thyroid antibodies. Hyperthyroidism and exophthalmos occurring during lithium therapy have been the subject of many reports, but there has been no proof of any pathogenic role of lithium; however, recent immunological data may stimulate enquiry into its role in the development of Graves' hyperthyroidism and exophthalmos.— J. H. Lazarus, *Adverse Drug React. Ac. Pois. Rev.*, 1982, *1*, 181.
A 47-year-old woman who had received lithium carbonate for 12 years developed marked clinical thyrotoxicosis and active ophthalmopathy 7 weeks after discontinuing the drug. During treatment she was considered to be clinically euthyroid but was noted to have bilateral exophthalmos and a smoothly enlarged thyroid gland. It was proposed that lithium might have initiated Graves' disease (autoimmune hyperthyroidism) by stimulating the production of thyroid autoantibodies, and that the antithyroid actions of lithium suppressed the symptoms.— C. J. Thompson and P. H. Baylis, *Postgrad. med. J.*, 1986, *62*, 295. Comment. Eleven more cases of this syndrome had previously been described (G.A. MacGregor, *Lancet*, 1977, *2*, 1129).— G. A. MacGregor (letter), *Postgrad. med. J.*, 1986, *62*, 1159. Reply. This patient differed from those described by MacGregor in that there was clear evidence of Graves' disease with high titres of circulating thyroid autoantibodies and marked ophthalmopathy.— C. J. Thompson and P. H. Baylis (letter), *ibid.*, 1160.

EFFECTS ON THE EYE. To date, there were 6 questionable cases of possible retinal changes associated with lithium use in the National Registry of Drug-Induced Side Effects, but in no case was there data to support a direct cause-and-effect relationship. So far, all lithium-related adverse ocular side-effects seemed to be reversible after withdrawal of therapy, such as decrease in vision, nystagmus, scotomas, conjunctival or lid oedema, exophthalmos, and myaesthenic neuromuscular blocking effects. Transitory blurred vision and even blindness can occur at toxic blood levels around 2 mmol per litre. These visual changes probably affect vision at a cortical level. Exophthalmos, unilateral or bilateral may occur at normal dosages, but may be due to the direct effect of lithium on the thyroid. One case of possible drug-related pseudotumour cerebri with papilloedema had been reported to the Registry.— F. T. Fraundfelder, *J. Am. med. Ass.*, 1983, *249*, 2389.

For a report of photophobia apparently associated with lithium intoxication, see under Overdosage, below.

EFFECTS ON THE GASTRO-INTESTINAL TRACT. Incomplete bowel obstruction with vomiting, abdominal pain, and distension, due to intestinal vasculitis with thrombosis and infarction of part of the ileal wall, occurred in a 57-year-old man who had been taking lithium carbonate for about 3 years. He had experienced severe episodic diarrhoea whilst taking lithium, but had no further diarrhoea after its discontinuation.— S. R. Cannon, *Postgrad. med. J.*, 1982, *58*, 445.

Nausea, vomiting, diarrhoea, anorexia, and epigastric bloating or pressure are common in the first few weeks of lithium therapy, but usually disappear with continued use. When these complaints occur later in therapy, lithium toxicity should be considered.— R. B. Salem, *Drug Intell. & clin. Pharm.*, 1983, *17*, 346.

EFFECTS ON THE KIDNEY. Polyuria (primarily associated with nephrogenic diabetes insipidus) and impaired renal concentrating ability are commonly associated with long-term lithium therapy (J.W. Jefferson, *J. Am. med. Ass.*, 1986, *255*, 3018), although it has been suggested that only a small subgroup of patients are affected (J.R. DePaulo *et al.*, *Am. J. Psychiat.*, 1986, *143*, 892). Interstitial fibrosis, tubular atrophy, and glomerular sclerosis have been associated with the long-term use of lithium (K. Solez *et al.*, *J. clin. Pharmac.*, 1983, *23*, 484) and some studies have reported a tendency towards a reduction in glomerular filtration-rate with time (J.W. Jefferson, 1986), although others have found no such reduction (C.A. Vaamonde *et al.*, *Am. J. Kidney Dis.*, 1986, *7*, 213). Nephrotic syndrome has also been associated with lithium therapy (K.M. Kalina and G.B. Burnett, *J. clin. Psychopharmacol.*, 1984, *4*, 148; R.A. Bear and M. Paul, *Can. med. Ass. J.*, 1985, *132*, 735). It has been suggested that a regimen involving a single daily dose may reduce both polyuria and morphological alterations (M. Schou *et al.*, *Psychopharmacology*, 1982, *77*, 387).

A review of the adverse effects of lithium on the kidney.— D. G. Waller and C. F. George, *Adverse Drug React. Ac. Pois. Rev.*, 1984, *3*, 65. See also H. E. Hansen, *Drugs*, 1981, *22*, 461.

For reference to the use of desmopressin to test renal function in patients receiving lithium therapy, see Desmopressin, p.1136.

EFFECTS ON THE MUSCULOSKELETAL SYSTEM. Lithium can cause acute myopathy and also muscle weakness (P.G. Blain, *Adverse Drug React. Bull.*, 1984, *Feb.*, 384), myalgia, and muscle cramps (F.L. Mastaglia, *Drugs*, 1982, *24*, 304).

For a report of transient polyarthritis following lithium intoxication, see under Overdosage, below.

EFFECTS ON THE NERVOUS AND NEUROMUSCULAR SYSTEMS. *Benign intracranial hypertension.* A report of benign intracranial hypertension in 3 patients taking lithium carbonate. Symptoms resolved in 2 who stopped treatment, but in the third, who continued to take lithium carbonate after a break, papilloedema and raised intracranial pressure persisted.— R. F. Saul *et al.*, *J. Am. med. Ass.*, 1985, *253*, 2869.

Extrapyramidal effects. Extrapyramidal symptoms in 2 patients receiving lithium carbonate which worsened following administration of orphenadrine.— P. Tyrer *et al.*, *Br. J. Psychiat.*, 1980, *136*, 191.

A 58-year-old woman experienced ataxia and confusion on 3 separate occasions a year or more apart following the administration of lithium. These symptoms abated several days after discontinuation of the drug on each occasion, but dysarthria and marked choreoathetoid movements of the extremities and trunk, which developed after lithium administration on the third occasion, persisted. Symptoms had, however, disappeared by 3 months.— C. F. Zorumski and G. L. Bakris, *Am. J. Psychiat.*, 1983, *140*, 1621.

There are 2 types of lithium-induced tremor. The first is a coarse tremor occurring with impending and actual lithium toxicity and appearing to have both cerebellar and parkinsonian components. It is often associated with inco-ordination, spasm of facial muscles, twitching of muscles and limbs, hyperactive reflexes, and more general systemic signs of toxicity. The second and more common type is a fine tremor, usually occurring within normal therapeutic concentrations, either transiently within a few days of starting treatment or later as a long-standing side-effect.— S. Johns and B. Harris (letter), *Br. med. J.*, 1984, *288*, 1309.

For a report of dysarthria and ataxia following lithium intoxication, see under Overdosage, below.

Impairment of memory. A study in 30 patients aged 21 to 62 years with bipolar affective disorder and with serum-lithium concentrations within the therapeutic range did not reveal any evidence of memory impairment.— A. M. Ghadirian *et al.*, *J. clin. Psychopharmacol.*, 1983, *3*, 313.

Impairment of taste perception. Of 450 patients treated with lithium about 5% complained of impaired taste of butter; celery and other foods were also involved.— J. M. Himmelhoch and I. Hanin (letter), *Br. med. J.*, 1974, *4*, 233. See also J. M. T. Willoughby, *Adverse Drug React. Bull.*, 1983, Jun., 368.

Myaesthenia. A myaesthenic syndrome of postoperative respiratory depression has been reported in patients taking lithium, and myaesthenic symptoms may be exacerbated or precipitated in patients with latent myaesthenia gravis.— R. J. M. Lane and P. A. Routledge, *Drugs*, 1983, *26*, 124.

Neurotoxicity. A report of 2 cases of neurotoxicity in patients whose serum-lithium concentrations were maintained at therapeutic levels. Neurotoxicity was characterised by confusion, disorientation, memory impairment, and ataxia, dysarthria, dysphasia, cognitive impairment, and hyperreflexia, or hallucinations and clouding of consciousness. Both patients showed improvement of symptoms on discontinuing lithium. It was recommended that lithium should be stopped promptly in all cases of a confusional state, whatever the serum-lithium concentration.— G. Hay and N. Simpson, *Lancet*, 1982, *2*, 160. Another report.— D. A. Lewis, *J. Am. med. Ass.*, 1983, *250*, 2029.

A report suggesting that acutely ill patients over 65 years of age are at increased risk of developing neurotoxicity with therapeutic serum-lithium concentrations and should be carefully and frequently monitored during treatment.— R. E. Smith and P. M. Helms, *J. clin. Psychiat.*, 1982, *43*, 94.

Further references to lithium-induced neurotoxicity: A. P. West and H. Y. Meltzer, *Am. J. Psychiat.*, 1979, *136*, 963; H. T. Pi and F. G. Surawicz, *Clin. Toxicol.*, 1978, *13*, 479.

Speech disturbance. A patient who had been taking lithium with amitriptyline for more than a year, and with a serum-lithium concentration within the therapeutic range, developed constructional dyspraxia with slight dysphasia. Lithium was stopped but the amitriptyline was continued. After one month there was marked improvement in the patient's condition.— E. P. Worrall and R. A. Gillham, *Br. med. J.*, 1983, *286*, 189.

Further reports of speech disturbance associated with lithium: K. Solomon and R. Vickers, *J. Am. med. Ass.*, 1975, *231*, 280; B. Johnels *et al.* (letter), *Br. med. J.*, 1976, *2*, 642; G. P. McGovern (letter), *ibid.*, 1983, *286*, 646.

EFFECTS ON POTASSIUM HOMOEOSTASIS. Hyperkalaemia in a woman given lithium.— F. C. Goggans, *Am. J. Psychiat.*, 1980, *137*, 860.

EFFECTS ON RESPIRATION. A patient with stable chronic airways obstruction and manic-depressive psychosis suffered an episode of reversible respiratory failure about 3 weeks after the start of lithium therapy. Recovery of consciousness and resolution of hypercapnia occurred within 24 to 36 hours of lithium discontinuation.— M. Weiner *et al.*, *New Engl. J. Med.*, 1983, *308*, 319.

See also Asthma under Uses, below.

EFFECTS ON THE SALIVARY GLANDS. A report of chronic submandibular sialadenitis in association with lithium therapy in a 25-year-old woman.— D. V. Forrest *et al.* (letter), *J. clin. Psychiat.*, 1983, *44*, 161.

EFFECTS ON SEXUAL FUNCTION. Lithium does not seem to interfere with sexual function in the majority of patients, but there have been isolated reports of impotence associated with loss of libido attributed to lithium therapy.— L. Beeley, *Adverse Drug React. Ac. Pois. Rev.*, 1984, *3*, 23.

EFFECTS ON THE SKIN AND HAIR. The administration of lithium has been associated with acneiform eruptions (Y. Kusumi, *Dis. nerv. Syst.*, 1971, *32*, 853; R. Ruiz-Maldonado *et al.*, *J. Am. med. Ass.*, 1973, *224*, 1534; F.W. Yoder, *Archs Derm.*, 1975, *111*, 396), cutaneous eruptions (C.L. Callaway *et al.*, *Am. J. Psychiat.*, 1968, *124*, 1124; R.E. Posey, *J. Am. med. Ass.*, 1972, *221*, 1517; S.B. Kurtin, *ibid.*, 1973, *223*, 802), exfoliative dermatitis (E.J. Kuhnley and A.L. Granoff, *Am. J. Psychiat.*, 1979, *136*, 1340), folliculitis (S.B. Kurtin, 1973; A. Rifkin *et al.*, *Am. J. Psychiat.*, 1973, *130*, 1018), precipitation or exacerbation of psoriasis (A. Skott *et al.*, *Br. J. Derm.*, 1977, *96*, 445; I. Skoven and J. Thormann, *Archs Derm.*, 1979, *115*, 1185), induction of the pustular phase of psoriasis (D.L. Evans and W. Martin, *Am. J. Psychiat.*, 1979, *136*, 1326; S.W. White, *J. Am. Acad. Derm.*, 1982, *7*, 660), and stomatitis (C.E. Muniz and D.H. Berghman, *J. Am. med. Ass.*, 1978, *239*, 2759). Hair loss or thinning has also been reported with lithium therapy (C.E. Muniz *et al.*, *Psychosomatics*, 1982, *23*, 312; R. Dawber and P. Mortimer, *Br. J. Derm.*, 1982, *107*, 124; A. Orwin, *ibid.*, 1983, *108*, 503).

References to the cutaneous side-effects of lithium: M. C. Y. Heng, *Br. J. Derm.*, 1982, *106*, 107; D. Sarantidis and B. Waters, *Br. J. Psychiat.*, 1983, *143*, 42.

EPILEPTOGENIC EFFECT. Lithium at therapeutic serum concentrations activated seizures with EEG changes in a 22-year-old patient. Clinical symptoms abated as serum concentrations fell.— E. W. Massey and W. N. Folger, *Sth. med. J.*, 1984, *77*, 1173.

Further references to seizures with lithium: R. Demers *et al.* (letter), *Lancet*, 1970, *2*, 315; D. Mayfield and R. G. Brown, *J. Psychiat. Res.*, 1966, *4*, 207; S. R. Platman and R. R. Fieve, *Br. J. Psychiat.*, 1969, *115*, 1185; C. C. Pfeiffer *et al.*, *J. clin. Pharmac.*, 1969, *9*, 298; R. A. Brumback *et al.*, *Pediatrics*, 1975, *56*, 831.

LUPUS. A controlled study of 50 patients who had been taking lithium carbonate for 2 months to 10 years indicated that antinuclear antibodies were more common in patients taking lithium carbonate than in controls. The absence of anti-DNA antibodies indicated that they did not have true systemic lupus erythematosus but patients ingesting lithium might be at risk.— A. P. Presley *et al.*, *Br. med. J.*, 1976, *2*, 280. See also: E. C. Johnstone and K. Whaley, *Br. med. J.*, 1975, *2*, 724; *idem*, *Br. J. clin. Pharmac.*, 1975, *2*, 377P; V. R. Shukla and R. L. Borison, *J. Am. med. Ass.*, 1982, *248*, 921.

MALIGNANT NEOPLASMS. See under Effects on the Blood, above.

NEUROLEPTIC MALIGNANT SYNDROME. For a report suggesting that the combined use of lithium and neuroleptics may increase the risk of an episode of neuroleptic malignant syndrome, see under Interactions, below.

OVERDOSAGE. Nausea, vomiting, and diarrhoea are common early features of lithium toxicity and are followed by coarse tremor, increased muscle tone, cogwheel rigidity, fasciculation, and myoclonus. Coma and convulsions may occur in the most serious cases and cardiac effects (first degree heart block and QRS and QT prolongation) have been described rarely. A patient may appear to be aware with open eyes but have an expressionless face and be unable to move or speak (coma vigil). Acute renal failure and nephrogenic diabetes insipidus may develop. Patients who develop features of lithium toxicity during long-term treatment usually have serum-lithium concentrations which are only modestly in excess of the upper limit of the recommended therapeutic range. Intoxication has been occasionally reported with concentrations within the accepted range. In contrast, acute massive overdosage may produce very high concentrations (occasionally as high as 7 mmol per litre) without immediate evidence of poisoning. If levels of this magnitude persist for some days, toxic features, even death, will occur.— A. T. Proudfoot, *Prescribers' J.*, 1986, *26*, 97.

Further reviews covering lithium overdosage and its clinical features: H. E. Hansen and A. Amdisen, *Q. J. Med.*, 1978, *47*, 123; P. Crome, *Drugs*, 1982, *23*, 431; J. Henry and G. Volans, *Br. med. J.*, 1984, *289*, 1291; E. H. Dyson *et al.*, *Hum. Toxicol.*, 1987, *6*, 325; A. Amdisen, *Med. Toxicol.*, 1988, *3*, 18.

ECG manifestations of lithium toxicity.— J. R. Mateer and M. R. Clark, *Ann. emerg. Med.*, 1982, *11*, 208.

A report of photophobia apparently associated with lithium intoxication.— R. P. Caplan and A. H. Fry, *Br. med. J.*, 1982, *285*, 1314.

Acute polyarthritis involving several large joints developed in a 33-year-old man concomitantly with toxic lithium levels. Symptoms resolved spontaneously on discontinuing lithium.— D. W. Black and R. Waziri, *J. clin. Psychiat.*, 1984, *45*, 135.

A report of severe hypertension in a 36-year-old woman during acute lithium intoxication.— J. Michaeli *et al.* (letter), *J. Am. med. Ass.*, 1984, *251*, 1680.

Deep venous thrombophlebitis, requiring acute anti-coagulant therapy, developed in a 59-year-old woman in association with chronic lithium toxicity.— M. R. Lyles, *J. natn. med. Ass.*, 1984, *76*, 633.

Neurotoxicity with persistent dysarthria, ataxia, and

muscle weakness following acute renal failure occurred in a 38-year-old woman with a serum-lithium concentration of 2.06 mmol per litre on a daily dosage of lithium carbonate 1.2 g.— J. B. Green, *Ann. Neurol.*, 1984, *15*, 111. See also M. Schou, *Acta psychiat. scand.*, 1984, *70*, 594.

At clinically toxic concentrations, lithium *in vitro* was found to have an antimuscarinic effect. This may explain such toxic symptoms of lithium as blurred vision, dry mouth, constipation, loss of memory, disorientation, confusion, ataxia, and in extreme cases, delirium and hallucinations.— S. Kanba and E. Richelson (letter), *New Engl. J. Med.*, 1984, *310*, 989.

From observations in one patient, it was suggested that reduction of the central temperature may be a prodrome of lithium poisoning.— J. -Y. Follézou and J. -M. Bleibel, *New Engl. J. Med.*, 1985, *313*, 1609.

Dystonia in a 3.5-year-old child associated with acute lithium poisoning.— M. G. Goetting, *Pediatrics*, 1985, *76*, 978.

A fatal case of self-poisoning with lithium carbonate in a 49-year-old man led to severe leucopenia before death. There were no appreciable changes in counts of circulating red cells and platelets.— S. T. Green and F. G. Dunn, *Br. med. J.*, 1985, *290*, 517.

PREGNANCY AND THE NEONATE. *Effects on the foetus.* By 1980, reports on 225 babies exposed to lithium *in utero* in the first trimester of pregnancy had been received by the Register of Lithium Babies. Of these, 25 had congenital malformations, including 18 with serious cardiovascular malformations, 6 of which were cases of Ebstein's anomaly. By March 1983, about 275 cases had been reported, and the findings had not changed substantially. On that basis, cardiovascular malformations are about 6 times as common in malformed 'lithium' babies as they are in other malformed babies and Ebstein's anomaly is about 150 times as common.— F. R. Frankenburg and J. F. Lipinski (letter), *New Engl. J. Med.*, 1983, *309*, 311.

Effects on the mother. In 4 healthy pregnant women given test doses of lithium carbonate, lithium clearances fell significantly after delivery. In 1 manic-depressive woman lithium clearance rose during pregnancy. Frequent assessments of serum-lithium concentrations were necessary during pregnancy and immediately after delivery so that the dose might be adjusted to avoid inadequate control during pregnancy or toxicity after delivery.— M. Schou *et al.*, *Br. med. J.*, 1973, *2*, 137. See also G. D. Wilbanks *et al.*, *J. Am. med. Ass.*, 1970, *213*, 865; M. Piton *et al.*, *Thérapie*, 1973, *28*, 1123; P. A. Sykes *et al.*, *Br. med. J.*, 1976, *2*, 1299.

Effects on the neonate. Hypotonia, poor sucking, and poor respiration in a newborn infant was attributed to lithium toxicity; the concentration of lithium in cord blood was 0.32 mmol per litre. The mother had been taking 800 mg of lithium carbonate daily, yielding serum-lithium concentrations of 0.06 to 0.2 mmol per litre.— J. K. Stothers *et al.* (letter), *Br. med. J.*, 1973, *3*, 233.

Atrial flutter (N. Wilson *et al.*, *Archs Dis. Childh.*, 1983, *58*, 538), polyuria, and hypotonia in the neonate, without any corresponding structural abnormalities, have also been reported in association with the maternal use of lithium throughout pregnancy (P. Morrell *et al.*, *ibid.*, 539). It was emphasised that such transplacental lithium poisoning could occur even if the maternal serum lithium concentration was maintained within the normal range (D. Stevens *et al.*, *ibid.*, 840).

See also under Precautions and Absorption and Fate.

WEIGHT CHANGES. A discussion of weight gain associated with lithium.— R. J. Kerry (letter), *Br. med. J.*, 1974, *2*, 441.

Evidence that patients gaining excessive amounts of weight during lithium therapy can lose weight by means of a calorie-controlled dietary regimen. Because electrolyte balance is important in the avoidance of lithium side-effects, it should be emphasised that weight loss can and should occur with a normal intake of sodium chloride.— G. M. Dempsey *et al.*, *Am. J. Psychiat.*, 1976, *133*, 1082.

Treatment of Adverse Effects

In the case of recent severe overdosage the stomach should be emptied by aspiration and lavage. As a result of the narrow margin between therapeutic and toxic serum concentrations, however, lithium poisoning may also develop during the course of therapeutic lithium administration.

Early lithium poisoning in patients with normal renal function may be treated by discontinuation of lithium and forced alkaline diuresis, but there is a danger of causing hypernatraemia. However, if the patient's condition deteriorates, or serum lithium concentration exceeds 4 mmol per litre, or the serum elimination half-life exceeds 30 hours, repeated haemodialysis should be initiated without delay; peritoneal dialysis is less effective and only appropriate if haemodialysis facilities are not available.

Maintenance of fluid and electrolyte balance is particularly important, due to the risk of hypernatraemia.

Reviews of the treatment of acute lithium overdosage: P. Crome, *Drugs*, 1982, *23*, 431; R. S. El-Mallakh, *Vet. hum. Toxicol.*, 1984, *26*, 31; J. Henry and G. Volans, *Br. med. J.*, 1984, *289*, 1291; A. T. Proudfoot, *Prescribers' J.*, 1986, *26*, 97; E. H. Dyson *et al.*, *Hum. Toxicol.*, 1987, *6*, 325.

The patients' clinical state will not improve dramatically with the fall in lithium concentration achieved by haemodialysis because toxicity is due to intracellular lithium which cannot be reduced speedily by any form of treatment.— A. T. Proudfoot, *Prescribers' J.*, 1986, *26*, 97. See also N. J. Clendeninn *et al.*, *J. Toxicol. clin. Toxicol.*, 1982, *19*, 341.

In a study in 9 patients with polyuria associated with long-term lithium therapy, amiloride in daily doses between 10 and 20 mg by mouth resulted in a significant reduction in urine volume and an increase in urine osmolality. Amiloride administration over several months had no significant effect on mean plasma potassium and lithium concentrations. That amiloride reduces urinary output without decreasing lithium clearance to any great extent, and that its use does not necessitate potassium supplementation, suggest that this agent may be the initial treatment of choice for lithium-induced polyuria.— D. C. Batlle *et al.*, *New Engl. J. Med.*, 1985, *312*, 408.

Precautions

The margin between the therapeutic and the toxic concentration of lithium is narrow, therefore it should be given under close medical supervision, and serum concentrations should be monitored regularly under controlled conditions, see Absorption and Fate (below). Unless deemed essential, lithium should be avoided in patients with any significant cardiovascular or renal impairment. It is contra-indicated in severe renal disease, in debilitated or dehydrated patients, and in those with sodium depletion; it is reported to be contra-indicated in Addison's disease.

Patients receiving lithium therapy should be taught to recognise the symptoms of early toxicity and, should these occur, to discontinue therapy and request medical aid at once. Among other factors, lithium requirements may change during fever, infection, and when mood swings occur. Patients should also be instructed to take their tablets at exactly the stipulated time, and not to compensate for an omitted dose by subsequently taking a double dose. Reduction in sodium intake increases the amount of lithium retained by the kidneys leading to a rise in serum-lithium concentrations; therefore, patients should avoid low-salt dietary regimens or other dietary changes which may reduce sodium intake, or circumstances which may cause excessive sodium loss such as those leading to excessive sweating, vomiting, or diarrhoea, with resultant dehydration. Conversely, increased sodium intake increases the amount of lithium excreted by the kidneys, leading to reduced serum-lithium concentrations; therefore, sodium-containing medicaments, such as sodium bicarbonate in indigestion mixtures or 'fruit salts', should not be given concomitantly with lithium salts. Concurrent administration of diuretics with lithium exerts a paradoxical antidiuretic effect in patients receiving lithium, and diuretics are normally contra-indicated in patients receiving lithium therapy.

Patients receiving lithium should be examined periodically for abnormal thyroid function, since goitre and hypothyroidism may develop. Cardiac and renal function should also be monitored regularly. Lithium should be used with particular care in the elderly. Impaired driving performance may occur in patients receiving lithium.

An increased incidence of cardiovascular abnormalities has been noted in the infants of women given lithium during the first 3 months of pregnancy. In pregnant women the dosage requirements of lithium can vary very abruptly, particularly immediately after delivery. The infants of women given lithium during late pregnancy may develop lithium intoxication. Lithium is excreted in breast milk and is contra-indicated in breast-feeding mothers.

BLOOD DONATION. It was considered that patients being treated with lithium would be acceptable as blood donors. The amount present in donor's blood at steady-state concentrations would have no biological significance when diluted in the recipient.— R. K. Gupta and S. Montgomery (letter), *Lancet*, 1975, *1*, 860.

CEREBROVASCULAR DISORDERS. The suggestion that, due to the possible trophic effect on serotoninergic nerve fibres, lithium may be contra-indicated in patients prone to cerebrovascular disorders.— K. Dhital *et al.* (letter), *Lancet*, 1985, *2*, 779.

DIURETIC THERAPY. When diuretic treatment is necessary for a patient taking lithium, the following procedure is suggested and plasma-lithium monitoring is essential. Ensure first that the plasma lithium concentration is in the therapeutic range. Reduce the dose of lithium by 50% when starting the diuretic, use the smallest dose of diuretic needed, and choose a loop diuretic such as frusemide, bumetanide, or ethacrynic acid. Monitor the plasma-lithium concentration twice weekly, and adjust the dose of lithium as necessary to regain the therapeutic range. During this period, the patient should be reminded of the gastro-intestinal and neurological symptoms of early lithium toxicity, and advised that should they occur, lithium must be stopped immediately until the plasma concentration has been checked at the earliest opportunity. If the diuretic treatment is stopped subsequently the dose of lithium will need to be increased and plasma levels monitored.— L. E. Ramsay, *Prescribers' J.*, 1984, *24*, 60.

DRIVING. Impaired driving performance in patients receiving lithium. The subjects usually felt that their performance had improved which might increase the driving risk.— T. Seppala *et al.*, *Drugs*, 1979, *17*, 389.

ECT. Although it is regarded as safe for patients receiving lithium to undergo ECT, when serum levels are outside the therapeutic range, even without overt signs of toxicity, interaction with barbiturate anaesthesia may lead to prolonged recovery times. Lithium may also interact with depolarising neuromuscular blockers, resulting in markedly prolonged action. The action of pancuronium is also prolonged; but no prolongation of neuromuscular blockade has been demonstrated following gallamine or tubocurarine.— G. Y. Gaines and D. I. Rees, *Anesth. Analg.*, 1986, *65*, 1345.

INTERACTIONS. Reviews of drug interactions with lithium: A. Amdisen, *Drugs*, 1982, *24*, 133; R. S. Lott, *Drug Interact. News.*, 1983, *3*, 17; L. Beeley, *Prescribers' J.*, 1986, *26*, 160.

Antibiotics. Two patients experienced lithium intoxication following the brief use of metronidazole. Persistent signs of renal damage later emerged.— M. H. Teicher *et al.* (letter), *J. Am. med. Ass.*, 1987, *257*, 3365.

Raised blood-lithium concentrations and signs of lithium toxicity developed in a woman receiving maintenance lithium therapy when she was treated with spectinomycin for gonorrhoea.— *Int. Drug Ther. Newslett.*, 1978, *13*, 15.

In a 30-year-old woman who had taken lithium carbonate for about 3 years with a stable serum-lithium concentration of 0.5 to 0.84 mmol per litre, that value rose to 1.7 mmol per litre and to 2.74 mmol per litre 2 and 4 days respectively after beginning a course of tetracycline.— A. J. McGennis, *Br. med. J.*, 1978, *1*, 1183. The toxicity might have been due to a low sodium intake possibly aggravated by tetracycline-induced diarrhoeal sodium loss.— U. Malt (letter), *ibid.*, 1978, *2*, 502. It had been the author's experience that lithium and tetracycline could be used together compatibly and that lower than usual doses need not be prescribed.— J. W. Jefferson (letter), *Br. J. Derm.*, 1982, *107*, 370.

Antidepressants. Antidepressants often cause or accentuate a switch from depression to hypomania or mania, with temporary refractoriness to lithium of the hypomania or mania.— D. Reginaldi *et al.*, *Int. Pharmacopsychiat.*, 1981, *16*, 124.

For the effect of lithium on amitriptyline, see Amitriptyline Hydrochloride, p.353.

Anti-epileptics. For reports of neurotoxicity in patients receiving carbamazepine and lithium, see Carbamazepine, p.401.

A report of severe CNS toxicity in a patient, possibly with minimal brain damage, taking phenytoin, phenobarbitone, and lithium carbonate 2 to 2.4 g daily; his serum-lithium concentration was 0.8 mmol per litre.— J. Speirs and S. R. Hirsch, *Br. med. J.*, 1978, *1*, 815.

Polydipsia, polyuria, and tremor in a patient taking lithium carbonate and phenytoin (each in doses to provide therapeutic concentrations) ceased when the phenytoin was replaced by carbamazepine.— W. A. G. MacCallum, *Br. med. J.*, 1980, *280*, 610. Comments.— E. Perucca and A. Richens (letter), *ibid.*, 863; K. Ghose (letter), *ibid.*, 1122.

Benzodiazepines. Hypothermia occurred on 4 occasions in a patient treated with lithium carbonate and diazepam, but not when either drug was given alone.— G. J. Naylor and A. McHarg, *Br. med. J.*, 1977, *2*, 22.

Calcium antagonists. There have been case reports of decreased serum-lithium concentrations in patients after the initiation of verapamil (L.A. Weinrauch *et al.*, *Am. Heart J.*, 1984, *108*, 1378), and of neurotoxicity when lithium is given concomitantly with verapamil or possibly diltiazem (*Drug Interact. News.*, 1987, *7*, 17).

Central stimulants. A woman who had been stabilised on lithium treatment for 15 months developed lithium toxicity within a few days of being given mazindol 2 mg daily.— M. S. Hendy *et al.*, *Br. med. J.*, 1980, *280*, 684.

For reports suggesting antagonism of the effects of amphetamines by lithium, see Dexamphetamine Sulphate, p.1441.

Cisplatin. Transient decreases in serum-lithium concentration occurred in a patient during intermittent administration of cisplatin. The relative contributions of cisplatin itself, or the fluid loading procedure involving intravenous fluids and mannitol, or their combined effects were unclear.— L. J. Pietruszka *et al.*, *Drug Intell. & clin. Pharm.*, 1985, *19*, 31.

Diuretics. Thiazide diuretics produce sodium depletion by inhibiting distal tubular sodium reabsorption. The consequent increase in proximal tubular reabsorption frequently results in an increase in plasma lithium concentrations (L. Beeley, *Prescribers' J.*, 1986, *26*, 160). Patients who are stabilised on lithium therapy and begin taking thiazide diuretics are at significant risk of developing lithium toxicity. Toxic plasma-lithium concentrations may be seen within 3 to 5 days of diuretic initiation. The development of toxicity depends upon prediuretic lithium concentrations, diuretic dose, and the degree of dietary sodium restriction. Loop diuretics (frusemide, bumetanide, and ethacrynic acid) seem less likely to cause lithium retention, although caution is warranted, especially with patients in whom dietary sodium is restricted (R.S. Lott, *Drug Interact. News.*, 1983, *3*, 17). Amiloride has no effect on lithium excretion, but acetazolamide increases lithium excretion. However, the diuretic action of acetazolamide is short-lived and the interaction may therefore be transient (L. Beeley, 1986).

For precautions to be taken when administering diuretics to patients receiving lithium, see under Precautions, above.

Enalapril. Plasma-lithium concentration rose to toxic levels when a patient stabilised on lithium carbonate was given concomitant enalapril. There was moderate alteration of renal function, which returned to normal 48 hours after discontinuation of both drugs, but it was felt that lithium retention was due to the increase in sodium excretion induced by enalapril.— P. Douste-Blazy *et al.*, *Lancet*, 1986, *1*, 1448.

Gastro-intestinal agents. Administration of sodium bicarbonate with lithium has led to reduced blood-lithium concentrations (C. McSwiggan, *Aust. J. Pharm.*, 1978, *59*, 6), but antacids containing combinations of aluminium and magnesium hydroxides and activated dimethicone had no effect on the dissolution and solubility of lithium carbonate *in vitro* (D.M. Schiessler *et al.*, *Am. J. Hosp. Pharm.*, 1983, *40*, 825), nor on its bioavailability *in vivo* (D.L. Goode *et al.*, *Clin. Pharm.*, 1984, *3*, 284).

Methyldopa. Concomitant administration of methyldopa appeared to induce signs of lithium toxicity in a patient stabilised on lithium carbonate.— G. J. Byrd (letter), *J. Am. med. Ass.*, 1975, *233*, 320. See also J. B. O'Regan (letter), *Can. med. Ass. J.*, 1976, *115*, 385.

Further references.— G. J. Byrd, *Clin. Toxicol.*, 1977, *11*, 1; E. Osanloo and J. H. Deglin (letter), *Ann. intern. Med.*, 1980, *92*, 433.

Muscle relaxants. For the effect of lithium on neuromuscular blockade, see Pancuronium Bromide, p.1236, and Suxamethonium Chloride, p.1239.

See also ECT under Precautions, above.

Neuroleptics. Lithium is excreted more rapidly during concurrent chlorpromazine treatment than when given alone (I. Sletten *et al.*, *Curr. ther. Res.*, 1966, *8*, 441), which can result in an abrupt rise in plasma-lithium concentration on withdrawing chlorpromazine (G.E. Pakes, *Lancet*, 1979, *2*, 701). Conversely, pre-treatment with lithium can reduce the plasma-chlorpromazine concentration following a dose of chlorpromazine compared with the concentration obtained before pre-treatment (L. Rivera-Calimlim *et al.*, *Clin. Pharmac. Ther.*, 1978, *23*, 451). There have been isolated reports of neurotoxicity or brain damage, characterised by delirium, seizures, encephalopathy, or an increased incidence of extrapyramidal symptoms in patients receiving lithium concomitantly with flupenthixol decanoate (A. West, *Br. med. J.*, 1977, *2*, 642), fluphenazine decanoate (S.V. Singh, *Lancet*, 1982, *2*, 278), high-dose haloperidol (W.J. Cohen and N.H. Cohen, *J. Am. med. Ass.*, 1974, *230*, 1283; J.B. Loudon and H. Waring, *Lancet*, 1976, *2*, 1088; C. Thomas *et al.*, *ibid.*, 1982, *1*, 626), or thioridazine (G.K. Spring, *J. clin. Psychiat.*, 1979, *40*, 135; H.M.A.S. Standish-Barry and M.A. Shelly, *Lancet*, 1983, *1*, 771; C.H. Cantor, *Med. J. Aust.*, 1986, *144*, 164). However, retrospective studies have failed to detect such adverse reactions in patients receiving lithium in combination with neuroleptics (P.C. Baastrup *et al.*, *J. Am. med. Ass.*, 1976, *236*, 2645; R. Prakash, *Lancet*, 1982, *1*, 1468), and in some cases the combination has been beneficial in reducing lithium-induced vomiting (R. Rosser and A. Herxheimer, *Lancet*, 1979, *2*, 97). It would be preferable to avoid the concurrent use of lithium with neuroleptics in patients with acute manic symptoms, and if lithium and haloperidol are used concomitantly careful attention should be paid to the dosage of both drugs, since large doses of one or both probably increases the likelihood of an adverse drug reaction (*Drug Interact. News.*, 1982, *2*, 17).

Although neuroleptic malignant syndrome classically follows the use of neuroleptics alone, a similar syndrome has been noted with the combined use of lithium and a neuroleptic. It is unclear whether these cases represent enhancement of the neurotoxicity of lithium, or a true neuroleptic malignant syndrome due to the use of high-potency dopamine-blocking neuroleptics such as haloperidol coincidently with lithium. Since lithium has been shown to enhance the extrapyramidal effects of neuroleptics, combined use in susceptible patients may increase the risk of an episode of neuroleptic malignant syndrome.— L. J. Birkhimer and C. L. DeVane, *Drug Intell. & clin. Pharm.*, 1984, *18*, 462.

Nonsteroidal anti-inflammatory drugs. Decreased clearance and increased serum concentrations of lithium, resulting in toxicity on some occasions, have been reported after the concomitant adminstration of lithium with ibuprofen (C.A. Kristoff *et al.*, *Clin. Pharm.*, 1986, *5*, 51; M. Ragheb, *J. clin. Psychiat.*, 1987, *48*, 161), indomethacin (I.W. Reimann *et al.*, *Archs gen. Psychiat.*, 1983, *40*, 283), naproxen (M. Ragheb and A. Powell, *J. clin. Psychopharmacol.*, 1986, *6*, 150), piroxicam (R.J. Kerry *et al.*, *Lancet*, 1983, *1*, 418; D.G. Walbridge *et al.*, *Br. J. Psychiat.*, 1985, *147*, 206), and may occur with diclofenac, mefenamic acid, and phenylbutazone (M.J. Kendall, *Prescribers' J.*, 1986, *26*, 135). However, serum-lithium concentration is not increased by the concomitant administration of sulindac (M.M. Furnell and J. Davies, *Drug Intell. & clin. Pharm.*, 1985, *19*, 374; M.A. Ragheb and A.L. Powell, *J. clin. Psychiat.*, 1986, *47*, 33), and possibly by aspirin (I.W. Reimann *et al.*, 1983), although serum lithium levels were increased in one patient (H. Bendz and M. Feinberg, *Archs gen. Psychiat.*, 1984, *41*, 310) but may have been due to variations in sodium intake (I. Reimann, *ibid.*, 311).

Sodium. Sodium salts increase lithium excretion, presumably by reducing sodium-linked lithium reabsorption from the proximal tubule. Some antacids and other medications with a high sodium content are best avoided. Sodium depletion stimulates proximal tubular reabsorption of both sodium and lithium with an increase in plasma-lithium concentration. Dietary sodium restriction in patients taking diuretics increases the risk of lithium toxicity (L. Beeley, *Prescribers' J.*, 1986, *26*, 160), and when patients commence very-low-energy diets, there is an initial, inevitable natriuresis (A.G. Wallace, *Med. J. Aust.*, 1984, *141*, 311).

See also under Diuretics and Gastro-intestinal agents, above.

Theophylline. Theophylline enhances the renal clearance of lithium, thus tending to reduce serum-lithium concentrations.— *Drug Interact. News.*, 1986, *6*, U-9.

PREGNANCY AND THE NEONATE. Since bradycardia and irregularity of the foetal heart may be caused by lithium toxicity, these signs do not necessarily mean foetal distress if the mother is receiving lithium.— D. Stevens *et al.*, *Archs Dis. Childh.*, 1983, *58*, 840.

The use of lithium during the first trimester may be related to an increased incidence of congenital defects, particularly of the cardiovascular system. Its use should be avoided during pregnancy if possible, especially during the first trimester. Use of the drug near term may produce severe toxicity in the neonate, which is usually reversible.— *Drugs in Pregnancy and Lactation*, 2nd Edn, G.G. Briggs *et al.* (Eds), Baltimore, Williams & Wilkins, 1986, 251/l.

See also I. F. Brockington, *Prescribers' J.*, 1979, *19*, 66.

See also under Adverse Effects, above, and Absorption and Fate, below.

Lactation. Although the American Academy of Pediatrics Committee on Drugs considered lithium to be a medication usually compatible with breast feeding (*Pediatrics*, 1983, *72*, 375), others consider lithium to be contra-indicated in women who are breast feeding (P.C. Rubin, *Br. med. J.*, 1986, *293*, 1415).

RENAL FUNCTION TESTING. The risk of renal complications from lithium therapy can be minimised by maintaining patients at the lowest effective serum level and scrupulously avoiding intoxication. Experts differ with regard to recommendations for both frequency and type of renal function monitoring. At the very least, serum creatinine level should be measured 2 or 3 times yearly together with a clinical estimate of urine volume. A more complete evaluation might also include yearly urinalysis and measurement of 24-hour urine volume and creatinine clearance. More elaborate testing is necessary only if dictated by clinical circumstances. Tests of renal concentrating ability are generally not considered routinely necessary.— J. W. Jefferson, *J. Am. med. Ass.*, 1986, *255*, 3018.

SURGERY. Lithium should be discontinued 2 to 3 days before major surgery, but need not be discontinued for minor surgery. Lithium treatment should be resumed as soon as possible after the operation, when kidney function and fluid-electrolyte balance have become normal. Patients with lithium-induced polyuria should be given fluids parenterally during the night before the operation, if they vomit copiously, or if they are unconscious for several hours.— M. Schou and H. Hippus (letter), *Br. J. Anaesth.*, 1987, *59*, 809.

TREMOR. With coarse tremor it is mandatory to decrease or stop lithium. With fine tremor, there is evidence to show that it is partly related to serum concentration, and a slight decrease in dose may be beneficial. Often, however, this may precipitate a relapse in the patient's condition, and in these cases propranolol has been shown to be effective, often without the need to reduce lithium concentrations (S. Johns and B. Harris, *Br. med. J.*, 1984, *288*, 1309). Oxprenolol, pindolol, and nadolol have also been reported to be beneficial, but other studies have found propranolol, practolol, and metoprolol ineffective (J.M. Kruse *et al.*, *Clin Pharm.*, 1984, *3*, 299). Alcohol and tricyclic antidepressants usually exacerbate lithium-induced tremor (J.B. Louden, *Br. J. Hosp. Med.*, 1977, *18*, 578; *idem*, 1978, *19*, 294).

WITHDRAWAL SYNDROMES. Relapses have been described after both abrupt withdrawal of lithium therapy (A. Margo and P. McMahon, *Br. J. Psychiat.*, 1982, *141*, 407) and after slower withdrawal over several weeks (D.G. Wilkinson, *Br. med. J.*, 1979, *1*, 235). It has been suggested that lithium does not improve the long-term prognosis if it is withdrawn (A.J. Mander, *Br. J. Psychiat.*, 1986, *149*, 498). However, in schizophrenics treated with lithium and concomitant tranquillisers, abrupt withdrawal of lithium is not always associated with relapse (N.J. Delva *et al.*, *ibid.*, 1982, *141*, 401).

Absorption and Fate

Lithium is readily and completely absorbed from the gastro-intestinal tract when taken in solution as one of its salts; when taken in the form of tablets small amounts are lost in the faeces. Peak plasma concentrations are obtained about 2 hours after ingestion from conventional tablets or capsules, and lithium is distributed throughout the body over a period of several hours, with higher concentrations occurring in the bones, the thyroid gland, and portions of the brain, than in the serum. Lithium is excreted in the kidneys and can be detected in sweat and saliva. It is not bound to plasma proteins. It crosses the placenta and is excreted in breast milk. It is reported to have a plasma half-life ranging from about 7 to 20 hours during the daytime; this value is considerably extended during the night and in those with impaired renal function.

Following administration of lithium salts there is wide intersubject variation between both the plasma concentrations obtained following a given dose, and between those required for therapeutic effect. Plasma concentrations also vary considerably according to factors such as the bioavailability of the lithium preparation taken, renal function, the dietary regimen of the patient, the patient's state of health, the time at which the blood sample is taken, and concomitant medication, such as sodium salts or diuretics. Moreover, there is only a narrow margin between the therapeutic and the toxic plasma concentration of lithium. Therefore, not only is individual titration of lithium dosage essential to ensure constant appropriate plasma concentrations for the patient involved, but the conditions under which the blood samples are taken for monitoring must be carefully controlled. In practice, the lithium ion concentration in the serum from a blood sample drawn 12 hours after the last dose of lithium in a patient who has been taking his daily lithium requirement at the scheduled hours during the past 48 hours is measured. Under such conditions the usual therapeutic plasma concentrations of lithium are 0.6 to 1.2 mmol per litre, with a reported effective range of 0.5 to 1.5 mmol per litre. At concentrations exceeding 1.5 mmol per litre, toxic effects may be expected.

A detailed account of the clinical pharmacokinetics of lithium and the special requirements for carefully monitoring serum-lithium concentrations during therapy.— A. Amdisen, *Clin. Pharmacokinet.*, 1977, *2*, 73. See also J. Gaillot *et al.*, *J. Pharmacokinet. Biopharm.*, 1979, *7*, 579; F. Nielsen-Kudsk and A. Amdisen, *Eur. J. clin. Pharmac.*, 1979, *16*, 271; A. Amdisen, *Ther. Drug Monit.*, 1980, *2*, 73.

ABSORPTION. From a study of slow-release lithium carbonate in 8 subjects, it was inferred that incomplete lithium absorption with some preparations was probably because some lithium is not released until the colon where it cannot be absorbed; the development of diarrhoea does not necessarily mean that lithium irritates the colon, but may represent the water required to keep the non-absorbed lithium and accompanying anion isotonic; and that an ideal slow-release preparation should spread lithium release over the small intestine, but leave no more lithium to be released after the ileum.— B. E. Ehrlich and J. M. Diamond, *Lancet*, 1983, *1*, 306.

Steady-state lithium blood level fluctuations following administration of a lithium carbonate conventional and controlled-release dosage form.— H. C. Caldwell *et al.*, *J. clin. Pharmac.*, 1981, *21*, 106.

Ordinary and sustained-release lithium carbonate tablets were administered in daily doses of 1.5 and 1.8 g respectively in a crossover fashion to 5 manic patients. Actual and theoretical steady-state serum levels of both preparations were determined. The sustained-release preparation gave observed serum levels that differed widely from predicted levels. It was suggested that this was a consequence of the combination of patient, diet, and sickness factors on drug absorption and it was recommended that morning blood sampling was the most appropriate, regardless of lithium formulation used.— D. P. Thornhill, *Int. J. clin. Pharmac. Ther. Toxic.*, 1986, *24*, 257.

DISTRIBUTION. *Erythrocyte concentrations.* Some correlation of the clinical effects of lithium with the ratio of erythrocyte to plasma lithium concentrations has been demonstrated (E. Sacchetti *et al.*, *Lancet*, 1977, *1*, 908; B.B. Johnston *et al.*, *Br. J. Psychiat.*, 1979, *134*, 482; T.A. Ramsey *et al.*, *Archs gen. Psychiat.*, 1979, *36*, 457).

Leucocyte concentrations. A strong correlation was obtained between white blood cell-lithium concentrations and the severity of observed side-effects in a group of 40 patients receiving prophylactic lithium therapy.— Y. L. Ong, *Br. J. Psychiat.*, 1983, *143*, 36.

Saliva and tear concentrations. Saliva lithium concentrations have been used to monitor therapy (C. Neu and A. Di Mascio, *Psychopharmac. Bull.*, 1977, *13*, 55; P. Ravenscroft *et al.*, *Archs gen. Psychiat.*, 1978, *35*, 1123; P.L. Man, *Psychosomatics*, 1979, *20*, 758; E. Othmer *et al.*, *J. clin. Psychiat.*, 1979, *40*, 525; R. Perry *et al.*, *J. clin. Psychopharmacol.*, 1984, *4*, 199), but the reliability of the method and correlation of saliva concentrations with plasma concentrations, especially at toxic levels, has been questioned (J.-L. Evrard *et al.*, *Acta psychiat. scand.*, 1978, *58*, 67; A. Sims *et al.*, *Br. J. Psychiat.*, 1978, *132*, 152; H. Vlaar *et al.*, *Acta psychiat. scand.*, 1979, *60*, 423; C.B. Khare *et al.*, *Int. J. clin. Pharmac. Ther. Toxic.*, 1983, *21*, 451; A. Sankaranarayanan *et al.*, *ibid.*, 1985, *23*, 365). Measurements in pure parotid saliva may be more reliable (D. Selinger *et al.*, *Biol. Psychiat.*, 1982, *17*, 99). Lithium concentrations in tears have been found to correlate closely with plasma concentrations (R. Brenner *et al.*, *Am. J. Psychiat.*, 1982, *139*, 678).

EXCRETION. In a study of 8 patients, there were no significant changes in either serum half-lives or renal lithium clearance when the total daily dosage of lithium carbonate was given as a single daily dose of conventional tablets, compared with a schedule of divided doses given twice daily. However, a significant decrease in the 24-hour urine output was noted on the single daily dose.— P. J. Perry *et al.*, *Acta psychiat. scand.*, 1981, *64*, 281.

The effect of age and renal function on lithium kinetics.— T. R. Norman *et al.*, *Clin. Pharmacokinet.*, 1984, *9*, 349.

Data suggesting that the clearance of lithium is not constant, but decreases with increasing serum level, within the therapeutic range of 0.6 to 1.2 mmol per litre. Caution was recommended when serum-lithium concentrations were over 1.0 mmol per litre since a small decrease in clearance could result in lithium intoxication.— S. R. Saklad *et al.*, *Drug Intell. & clin. Pharm.*, 1984, *18*, 507. See also P. J. Goodnick *et al.*, *Clin. Pharmac. Ther.*, 1981, *29*, 47.

PREGNANCY AND THE NEONATE. An analysis of figures from various sources showed that the breast milk of 8 mothers taking lithium had lithium concentrations of about one-half those of maternal serum. The lithium concentration of the infants' serum was one-half to one-third that of the maternal serum.— M. Schou and A. Amdisen, *Br. med. J.*, 1973, *2*, 138.

A healthy infant with normal neonatal blood concentrations of thyroxine and of thyrotrophin was born to a mother given lithium carbonate from the 11th week of pregnancy. There was no placental barrier to the diffusion of lithium ions, but the concentration of lithium in the amniotic fluid was higher than in the umbilical cord venous blood.— A. V. P. Mackay *et al.*, *Br. med. J.*, 1976, *1*, 878. See also H. Fries (letter), *Lancet*, 1970, *1*, 1233.

See also under Adverse Effects and Precautions.

Uses and Administration

Lithium carbonate is used as a source of lithium ions which may act by competing with sodium ions at various sites in the body. The mechanism by which it exerts its effect in affective disorders is not known. It is used in the prophylaxis and treatment of mania or hypomania, in the prophylaxis of manic depression (bipolar illness or bipolar depression) and recurrent depression (unipolar illness or unipolar depression), and to control aggressive or self-mutilating behaviour.

The usual dose of lithium carbonate for prophylactic therapy is 0.4 to 1.2 g daily, given in divided doses, or given once or twice daily in a sustained-release form. The initial dose given is adjusted after 2 to 7 days according to the results of serum-lithium estimations obtained under strictly controlled conditions. During the initial stages of lithium therapy, serum-lithium concentrations must then be checked at least once a week to ensure that they remain within the usual therapeutic range of 0.6 to 1.2 mmol per litre, 12 hours after the last dose (see under Absorption and Fate, above); when consistent concentrations have been achieved, estimations may be made monthly and, eventually, every 2 months.

In the acute treatment of mania and hypomania up to 1.5 to 2 g daily may be given for the first 5 to 7 days, together with close checks to maintain the serum-lithium concentration within the optimum range of 0.6 to 1.2 mmol per litre, 12 hours after the last dose. The dose may need to be reduced rapidly once the acute phase has passed.

The range between the toxic and the therapeutic concentration of lithium is narrow and efforts must be made to avoid toxic peaks in an otherwise therapeutic serum concentration. To this end the daily dosage, if not given in a sustained-release form should preferably be divided into at least 2 portions, which must always be taken at exactly the stipulated time of day, and the patient must be warned never to compensate for an omitted dose by subsequently taking a double dose. Sustained-release tablets are also useful in avoiding toxic peaks. Various formulations of lithium carbonate tablets are available which are not necessarily bioequivalent, and it is essential that patients should not be switched between these without special control of their serum-lithium concentrations.

Patients must also be taught to recognise the symptoms of early lithium intoxication (which may be expected at concentrations exceeding 1.5 mmol per litre) in order to omit further doses of lithium and seek medical care. Patients must similarly be warned that the following may affect lithium dosage requirements: intercurrent illnesses, including urinary-tract infections, manic or depressive phases, changes in dietary regimen, changes in temperature, pregnancy, and concomitant medication (in particular, sodium-containing preparations and diuretics). For further details see under Precautions (above).

The dosage of lithium should be reduced in elderly or light-weight patients. Other lithium salts have been used as a source of lithium ions and these include the acetate, aspartate, citrate, gluconate, orotate, and sulphate. Lithium hydroxide is used in the preparation of lithium citrate.

Reviews of the actions and uses of lithium: *Handbook of Lithium Therapy*, F.N. Johnson (Ed.), Lancaster, MTP, 1980; *Drug & Ther. Bull.*, 1981, *19*, 21; S. Tyrer and D.M. Shaw in *Drugs in Psychiatric Practice*, P.J. Tyrer (Ed.), London, Butterworths, 1982, p.280; M. T. Abou-Saleh and A. H. Ghodse, *Pharm. J.*, 1983, *2*, 618; *Lithium Encyclopedia for Clinical Practice*, J.W. Jefferson *et al.* (Ed.), Washington, American Psychiatric Press, 1983; G. Johnson, *Med. J. Aust.*, 1984, *141*, 595; S. P. Tyrer, *J. Affect. Dis.*, 1985, *8*, 251; *Med. Lett.*, 1986, *28*, 99; S. G. Bryant and C. S. Brown, *Clin. Pharm.*, 1986, *5*, 385.

ADMINISTRATION. Detailed recommendations for the management of lithium administration, with special reference to the monitoring of serum-lithium concentrations using the 12h-stSLi, which is the concentration of lithium ions in serum or plasma of a blood sample drawn in the morning, before the first lithium dose of the day, 12(±0.5) hours after the evening dose, from a patient complying completely with treatment in regard to dosage, dose regimen, and dose timing, taking the dosage in more than one dose per day (even for the controlled sustained-release tablets), and who is in steady-state equilibrium of dosage and excretion. Based on a study of the 12h-stSLi of 79 patients on successful long-term treatment, the therapeutic range of serum-lithium concentrations is 0.3 to 1.3 mmol per litre. The highest and lowest responders differ by a factor of about 3 in respect to the 12h-stSLi, while the corresponding factor for daily dose is about 7 (ranging from 8 to 54 mmol of lithium ions daily). Based on clinical experience, the therapeutic concentration at which intoxication may occur is 1.5 mmol per litre. With a patient commencing long-term treatment, whose concentration requirements are unknown, the adjustment should aim at 0.8 to 1.0 mmol per litre, because a majority of patients are seriously disturbed by adverse reactions at the upper end of the therapeutic range, before the adaptation period has elapsed; only patients suffering from relapse should subsequently be pushed to the upper concentrations. The 12h-stSLi should then be checked once a week over the following 6 months, monthly over the next 6 months, and every second month thereafter. In addition the patient should be trained to recognise the symptom association of poisoning of moderate intensity: speech difficulty, irregular tremor, myoclonic twitchings, muscular weakness, and ataxia which calls for immediate discontinuation of the treatment and referral to the physician for control of the 12h-stSLi.— A. Amdisen, Lithium, in *Therapeutic Relevance of Drug Assays*, F.A. de Wolff *et al.* (Ed.), Leiden University Press, 1979, p. 63.

The effectiveness of a pharmacokinetic method of predicting maintenance lithium dosage.— R. W. Fitzpatrick and R. B. Bye, *Pharm. J.*, 1986, *2*, 726.

Evaluation of 4 methods for predicting lithium dosage.— F. Lobeck *et al.*, *Clin. Pharm.*, 1987, *6*, 230. See also J. M. Patrias and F. H. Moore, *ibid.*, 1985, *4*, 77.

ADMINISTRATION IN CARDIOVASCULAR DISEASE. For a general comment that lithium does not appear to be contra-indicated in patients with heart disease, but that electrocardiographic monitoring is essential in patients with arrhythmias, see Effects on the Cardiovascular System under Adverse Effects, above.

ADMINISTRATION IN THE ELDERLY. In a study, 82 psychiatric out-patients were given lithium daily to give a plasma concentration of 1 mmol per litre. It was considered necessary to reduce the daily weight-related lithium dose by 50% over the age range of 20 to 79 years to compensate for an age-related decrease in lithium excretion and to reduce lithium side-effects to a level comparable to that acceptable in younger patients.— D. S. Hewick *et al., Br. J. clin. Pharmac.*, 1977, *4,* 201.

Further references.— J. R. Foster *et al., J. Geront.*, 1977, *32,* 299.

ADMINISTRATION IN RENAL FAILURE. Lithium carbonate could be administered to patients with renal failure by adjusting the dose. No dosage adjustment is necessary for patients whose glomerular filtration-rates exceed 50 mL per minute; 50 to 75% of the normal dose is advisable for rates of between 10 and 50 mL per minute. Where the rate is less than 10 mL per minute, 25 to 50% of the normal dose should be given. A dose supplement should be given to patients undergoing haemodialysis.— W. M. Bennett *et al., Am. J. Kidney Dis.*, 1983, *3,* 155. See also J. A. Koecheler *et al., Drug Intell. & clin. Pharm.*, 1986, *20,* 623.

During intermittent peritoneal dialysis, lithium has a peritoneal clearance of 14 mL per minute.— D. K. Scott and D. E. Roberts, *Pharm. J.*, 1985, *1,* 621.

ALCOHOLISM. A critical review of studies of the use of lithium in alcoholics concluded that lithium appeared to reduce the number of days incapacitated by alcohol in patients with affective disorders, to reduce depression in depressed alcoholics, particularly secondary alcoholics, and to increase abstinence (T.M. McMillan, *Br. J. Addict.*, 1981, *76,* 245). However, alcoholics without depression respond no better to lithium than to placebo (J.E. Peachey and C.A. Naranjo, *Drugs*, 1984, *27,* 171).

ASTHMA. There have been reports of patients with asthma and bipolar depression whose asthmatic as well as their affective symptoms have improved on receiving lithium (S.J. Nasr and R.W. Atkins, *Am. J. Psychiat.*, 1977, *134,* 1042). However, although asthmatic symptoms also respond in some patients without affective disorders, its toxicity argues against the use of lithium for asthma (E. Spitz *et al., Ann. Allergy*, 1982, *49,* 165).

See also Effects on Respiration under Adverse Effects, above.

BEHAVIOUR DISORDERS. Lithium has been shown to be more effective than placebo in controlling aggressive and self-mutilating behaviour in adults (A.F. Cooper and H.C. Fowlie, *Br. J. Psychiat.*, 1973, *122,* 370; M.H. Sheard *et al., Am. J. Psychiat.*, 1976, *133,* 1409; S.P. Tyrer *et al., Prog. Neuropsychopharmacol. biol. Psychiatry*, 1984, *8,* 751) and children (A. Vetró *et al., Neuropsychobiology*, 1985, *14,* 121). Lithium carbonate in doses of 500 to 2000 mg daily was similar to haloperidol 1 to 6 mg daily in controlling aggressive behaviour in children, but caused fewer side-effects (M. Campbell *et al., Archs gen. Psychiat.*, 1984, *41,* 650; J.E. Platt *et al., Psychopharmac. Bull.*, 1984, *20,* 93).

BLOOD DISORDERS. The therapeutic use of lithium salts is associated with neutrophilia, which reflects an expansion of the total blood granulocyte pool through increased production in the bone marrow. Lithium salts may also cause an increase in eosinophil and platelet counts, although this has not been a uniform finding (R.D. Barr and P.R. Galbraith, *Can. med. Ass. J.*, 1983, *128,* 123). In view of these effects, lithium has been used in aplastic anaemia (A.J. Barrett *et al., Lancet*, 1977, *1,* 202; S.F. Blum, *New Engl. J. Med.*, 1979, *300,* 677), drug-induced leucopenia (R. Yassa *et al., Am. J. Psychiat.*, 1978, *135,* 1423), Felty's syndrome (R.C. Gupta *et al., Am. J. Med.*, 1976, *61,* 29; R.A. Kaplan, *Ann. intern. Med.*, 1976, *84,* 342; M.J. Mant, *Archs intern. Med.*, 1986, *146,* 277), and hairy-cell leukaemia (S.F. Blum, *New Engl. J. Med.*, 1980, *303,* 464; J.R. Quesada *et al., Leukaemia Res.*, 1981, *5,* 463) with some success in isolated cases. Lithium has been used with greater success to ameliorate the granulocytopenia induced by cancer chemotherapy (D. Charron *et al., Lancet*, 1977, *1,* 1307; R.S. Stein *et al., New Engl. J. Med.*, 1977, *297,* 430; G.H. Lyman *et al., ibid.*, 1980, *302,* 257; N.J. Vogelzang and D.H. Frenning, *ibid.*, *303,* 525; G.H. Lyman *et al., Am. J. Med.*, 1981, *70,* 1222; P.G. Steinherz *et al., Am. J. ped. Hematol. Oncol.*, 1983, *5,* 39; C.M. Richman *et al., Am. J. Hematol.*, 1984, *16,* 313).

DEPRESSION. As an antidepressant, lithium is probably less effective than tricyclic antidepressants or monoamine oxidase inhibitors, but is an effective adjunct to these drugs in patients with resistant depressions. There is a trend for patients with bipolar depression to respond more favourably than patients with depression without such a history. Lithium salts, however, have been mainly used as a prophylactic treatment in the management of bipolar and unipolar illness. In unipolar patients, lithium is particularly effective in those with an endogenous profile of symptoms, a family history of depression, and who had shown less personality disturbance before the onset of their first episode of illness. Patients with unipolar illness with a non-endogenous symptom profile (neurotic depression) may benefit from lithium if it is combined with psychological treatment, particularly cognitive therapy.— M. T. Abou-Saleh, *Br. med. J.*, 1986, *293,* 251.

Bipolar depression. See under Mania and Manic Depression, below.

Combination therapy with monoamine oxidase inhibitors. Three patients with major depressive disorder unresponsive to a 3-week trial of adequate dosage of phenelzine (60 to 90 mg daily) responded within 5 days of receiving concomitant lithium therapy.— J. C. Nelson and R. Byck, *Br. J. Psychiat.*, 1982, *141,* 85.

Combination therapy with tricyclic antidepressants. De Montigny *et al. (Br. J. Psychiat.*, 1981, *138,* 252) reported dramatic clinical improvement within 48 hours of the addition of lithium in patients who had not responded to 3 weeks of tricyclic antidepressant treatment. The findings from this open study were confirmed by further studies involving the same investigators. Another group (G.R. Heninger *et al., Archs gen. Psychiat.*, 1983, *40,* 1335) carried out a double-blind study comparing the addition of lithium and placebo in patients failing to improve on tricyclics or mianserin. Although the addition of lithium was effective, improvement took between 6 and 12 days. The authors' experience was of a response similar to that reported by Heninger *et al.*, with clinically useful response occurring in the majority of cases in the second or third week after adding lithium. This drug strategy seemed to be a promising and worthwhile avenue in patients resistant to tricyclics alone.— C. L. E. Katona and T. R. E. Barnes, *Br. J. Hosp. Med.*, 1985, *34,* 168.

Delusional depression. In a retrospective study of 21 patients with delusional depression refractory to combined antipsychotic and antidepressant drug treatment, the addition of lithium was effective in 8 of 9 patients with bipolar depression, but only 3 of 12 with unipolar depression.— J. C. Nelson and C. M. Mazure, *Am. J. Psychiat.*, 1986, *143,* 363.

Prophylaxis. A recent MRC study showed that lithium and amitriptyline had equal effects in preventing recurrent depression, but more than two-thirds of the patients had at least one depressive episode during the 3 years of the study (*Psychol. Med.*, 1981, *11,* 409; *ibid.*, 1984, *14,* 37). A similar *US* study showed that imipramine was more effective than lithium in preventing depression, although a few patients developed mania (R.F. Prien *et al., Archs gen. Psychiat.*, 1984, *41,* 1096).— S. P. Tyrer, *Br. J. Hosp. Med.*, 1986, *35,* 145. See also: A. Coppen and M. T. Abou-Saleh, *J. R. Soc. Med.*, 1983, *76,* 297; C. P. Freeman, *Br. med. J.*, 1984, *289,* 512.

DIABETES INSIPIDUS, NEPHROGENIC. Findings that lithium carbonate was ineffective and had serious side-effects in the treatment of inappropriate secretion of antidiuretic hormone.— J. N. Forrest *et al., New Engl. J. Med.*, 1978, *298,* 173.

Further references.— M. G. White and C. D. Fetner, *New Engl. J. Med.*, 1975, *292,* 390; J. N. Forrest, *ibid.*, 423; N. Hendler *et al.* (letter), *ibid.*, 1976, *294,* 446; R. S. Baker *et al., J. Pediat.*, 1977, *90,* 480; E. Casado de Frias *et al., J. Pediat.*, 1980, *96,* 153.

EATING DISORDERS. Reports of weight gain in anorectic patients given lithium indicate that it was corporeal weight gain, rather than a weight gain secondary to fluid. However, in a double-blind study (H.A. Gross *et al., J. clin. Psychopharmacol.*, 1981, *1,* 376), lithium carbonate produced no significant change in pretreatment weight. The efficacy of lithium in anorexia is unproven and the risk of lithium-induced neurological and cardiac toxicity may be increased in a patient population already susceptible to electrolyte disturbances from abnormal eating behaviours (W.S. Bond *et al., Drug Intell. & clin. Pharm.*, 1986, *20,* 659).

In an uncontrolled study, 14 bulimic women were treated with lithium carbonate (L.K.G. Hsu, *Am. J. Psychiat.*, 1984, *141,* 1260) and 12 experienced a 75 to 100% reduction in their frequency of binge-eating episodes with a parallel reduction in depression. In most subjects improvement was maintained for 6 to 16 months follow-up, with 7 subjects able to discontinue lithium without relapse. In 7 patients who had shown an adequate response to their existing antidepressant regimens, one achieved remission, and 2 others had an improvement of about 50% in the frequency of their binge-eating after the addition of lithium. However, caution is indicated in administering lithium to bulimic patients with frequent vomiting and hypokalaemia (H.G. Pope and J.I. Hudson, *J. clin. Psychiat.*, 1986, *47,* 339).

EXTRAPYRAMIDAL DISORDERS. Lithium carbonate was given in increasing doses to 11 patients with torticollis, torsion dystonia, or choreoathetosis. Some improvement was observed in 3 patients with torticollis but 2 of these did not deteriorate when given placebo. Lithium was not considered effective in clinical dyskinesias.— J. A. McCaul and G. M. Stern (letter), *Lancet*, 1974, *1,* 1058.

See also under Extrapyramidal Effects in Adverse Effects, above.

Chorea. Although improvement has been observed in patients with Huntington's chorea after the addition of lithium to their neuroleptic therapy (P. Dalén, *Lancet*, 1973, *1,* 107; D.P. Leonard *et al., ibid.*, 1974, *2,* 1208), double-blind studies have failed to show any consistent benefit (M.J. Aminoff and J. Marshall, *ibid.*, *1,* 107; P. Vestergaard *et al., Acta psychiat. scand.*, 1977, *56,* 183).

Gilles de la Tourette's syndrome. Administration of lithium carbonate to 2 male patients with Gilles de la Tourette's syndrome. Complete remission of symptoms was obtained in one and the second was markedly improved.— F. S. Messiha *et al., Clin. Pharmac. Ther.*, 1977, *21,* 111.

Parkinsonism. Five of 6 patients with severe parkinsonism complicated by the 'on-off' phenomenon and treated with lithium carbonate in addition to regular antiparkinsonian medication had marked reductions in akinesia and improved one grade in Parkinson staging.— C. E. Coffey *et al., Ann. Neurol.*, 1982, *12,* 375. A similar study finding no significant improvement in symptoms.— A. Lieberman and G. Gopinathan, *ibid.*, 402.

In a double-blind placebo-controlled study in 7 patients with Parkinson's disease, lithium carbonate reduced or abolished painful 'off' period dystonias 1 to 16 days after starting therapy. The beneficial effect disappeared 1 to 14 days after stopping lithium.— N. Quinn and C. D. Marsden, *Lancet*, 1986, *1,* 1377.

Tardive dyskinesia. Although lithium has been reported to aggravate tardive dyskinesia (E.L. Crews and A.E. Carpenter, *Am. J. Psychiat.*, 1977, *134,* 933), other reports suggest certain patients may experience some alleviation of symptoms with lithium therapy (R.H. Ehrensing, *Lancet*, 1974, *2,* 1459; F.A. Reda *et al., Am. J. Psychiat.*, 1975, *132,* 560; R. Yassa and J. Ananth, *Int. Pharmacopsychiat.*, 1980, *15,* 301).

HEADACHE. Several open studies have found lithium to be a useful prophylactic agent in cluster headache (K. Ekbom, *Opusc. Med.*, 1974, *19,* 148; L. Kudrow in *Current Concepts in Migraine Research*, R. Green (Ed.), New York, Raven Press, 1978, p.159; G.M. Wyant and E.M. Ashenhurst, *Can. Anaesth. Soc. J.*, 1979, *26,* 38). The effective dose has ranged from 600 to 900 mg of lithium carbonate daily. Favourable responses occurred within the first week of therapy in the majority of patients, and the drug is often effective at plasma concentrations below those required for psychiatric purposes (R. Atkinson and O. Appenzeller, *Postgrad. med. J.*, 1984, *60,* 841). However, lithium may worsen migraine (R.C. Peatfield, *J.R. Soc. Med.*, 1981, *74,* 432).

HERPES SIMPLEX INFECTIONS. A double-blind placebo-controlled study in 73 patients with recurrent herpes genitalis indicated that an ointment containing lithium succinate 8% had a beneficial effect both for symptomatic relief and for lowering virus excretion.— G. R. B. Skinner (letter), *Lancet*, 1983, *2,* 288. Reports of remission of herpes labialis during systemic treatment with lithium carbonate: J. Lieb (letter), *New Engl. J. Med.*, 1979, *301,* 942; A. Gillis (letter), *Lancet*, 1983, *2,* 516 and 584.

HYPERTHYROIDISM. Lithium has been used to control the symptoms of hyperthyroidism in patients with Graves' disease (J.H. Lazarus *et al., Lancet*, 1974, *2,* 1160), and was as effective as methimazole in a study of thyrotoxic patients, although side-effects associated with lithium made treatment impracticable (O. Kristensen *et al., ibid.*, 1976, *1,* 603). Lithium has also been used as an adjunct to carbimazole (J.G. Turner and B.E.W. Brownlie, *ibid.*, *2,* 904). Pre- and post-treatment with lithium carbonate caused significant retention of iodine-131 by the thyroid, which might be useful where the total body radiation dose must be kept to a minimum (J.G. Turner *et al.*, *ibid.*, *1*, 614; K. Bakker *et al.*, *ibid.*, 1135).

See also Effects on the Endocrine System, under Adverse Effects, above.

MANIA AND MANIC DEPRESSION. *Acute mania.* Lithium is not sedative and its antimanic effect develops over 1 to 3 weeks. It is therefore the drug of first choice only in mild cases of mania. Lithium is often effective in patients who have shown only partial improvement on antipsychotic drugs, and is therefore frequently used in combination with these drugs for more extreme cases. About 20 to 30% of manic patients are refractory to lithium.— J. C. Cookson, *Br. J. Hosp. Med.*, 1985, *34*, 172.

Combination therapy. In patients with mania or manic depression (bipolar illness) poorly controlled by lithium therapy, small studies or anecdotal reports have suggested benefit from concomitant therapy with carbamazepine (J.F. Lipinski and H.G. Pope, *Am. J. Psychiat.*, 1982, *139*, 948; R. Keisling, *Archs gen. Psychiat.*, 1983, *40*, 223; J. Fawcett and H.M. Kravitz, *J. clin. Psychiat.*, 1985, *46*, 58), methylene blue (G.J. Naylor *et al.*, *Biol. Psychiat.*, 1986, *21*, 915), spironolactone (M.A. Gillman and F.J. Lichtigfeld, *Br. med. J.*, 1986, *292*, 661), L-tryptophan (T.D. Brewerton and V.I. Reus, *Am. J. Psychiat.*, 1983, *140*, 757), and sodium valproate (H.M. Emrich *et al.*, *Archs Psychiat. neurol. Sci.*, 1980, *229*, 1).

Prophylaxis. The use of long-term lithium is generally considered where a patient has had 3 or more definite affective episodes or 2 severe, socially disastrous episodes at intervals of less than 2 years.— M. H. Lader, *Prescribers' J.*, 1982, *22*, 112.

The value of lithium in the prophylaxis of bipolar illness (manic depression) was established in placebo-controlled studies. These involved bipolar patients with a history of at least 2 and usually 3 or more episodes in the previous 3 years. The patients were treated in the study for up to 2 years. The results showed that about 7 times as many patients on lithium went into continuous remission as did those on placebo. The frequency of manic episodes was reduced on average by a factor of 8, and depressive episodes by a factor of 3. The severity of episodes was also reduced. However, about 20% of these bipolar patients seemed to derive little benefit from receiving prophylactic lithium. There are, as yet, no reliable indicators of which bipolar or unipolar patients would benefit from lithium, although a family history of mania is suggested. Patients experiencing 4 or more episodes of mania or depression in a year ('rapid-cyclers') tend not to respond so well to lithium. A distinction between bipolar patients in whom mania precedes depression, and those in whom depression precedes mania may be useful, since lithium seems to be of more value in the former than the latter group. Low blood-folate concentrations were associated with greater affective morbidity over 2 years in patients on lithium. The prophylactic effect will usually occur with plasma-concentrations of lithium of 0.4 to 0.7 mmol per litre and there is not necessarily any advantage in maintaining higher levels.— J. C. Cookson, *Br. J. Hosp. Med.*, 1985, *34*, 172.

For studies demonstrating some correlation of the clinical effects of lithium with plasma, erythrocyte, leucocyte, saliva, or tear concentrations of lithium, see under Absorption and Fate, above.

MYOTONIA. A 37-year-old man experienced relief of myotonic symptoms with blood-lithium concentrations above 2.0 mmol per litre. There was no change in myotonic stiffness with blood concentrations of 1.5 mmol per litre.— J. W. Gerst *et al.*, (letter), *J. Neurol. Neurosurg. Psychiat.*, 1984, *47*, 1044.

PREMENSTRUAL SYNDROME. Studies have shown lithium to be no more effective than placebo for the relief of premenstrual symptoms (K. Singer *et al.*, *Br. J. Psychiat.*, 1974, *124*, 50; B. Mattsson and B.V. Schoultz, *Acta psychiat. scand.*, 1974, *Suppl.* 255, 75; M. Steiner *et al.*, *ibid.*, 1980, *61*, 96).

SCHIZOPHRENIA. In a review of the use of lithium for schizophrenia and schizoaffective disorders, lithium was found to be superior to placebo in all studies, with some improvement in psychotic as well as affective symptoms (N.J. Delva and F.J.J. Letemendia, *Br. J. Psychiat.*, 1982, *141*, 387). Lithium has been shown to be more effective than benzodiazepines in the treatment of psychotic disorders (G.W. Arana *et al.*, *Psychopharmac. Bull.*, 1986, *22*, 77) and as effective as carbamazepine (A. Lenzi *et al.*, *J. int. med. Res.*, 1986, *14*, 78).

Drug-induced psychosis. Lithium has been used successfully in the management of psychoses associated with the use of corticotrophin (W.E. Falk *et al.*, *J. Am. med. Ass.*, 1979, *241*, 1011), corticosteroids (F.P. Siegal, *New Engl. J. Med.*, 1978, *299*, 155), and levodopa (P. Dalén and G. Steg, *Lancet*, 1973, *1*, 936). Preliminary results suggested that lithium may also be of use in controlling psychotic symptoms associated with cocaine abuse (M.E. Scott and R.W. Mullaly, *Sth. med. J.*, 1981, *74*, 1475).

SEBORRHOEIC DERMATITIS. In a double-blind study, 17 patients with seborrhoeic dermatitis were treated twice daily with topical lithium succinate 8% ointment or inactive placebo ointment for 4 weeks, followed by the alternative treatment for 4 weeks. Fourteen showed improvement with lithium ointment, 2 had no response to either treatment and one responded to placebo. Lithium succinate did not inhibit the growth of pityrosporum yeasts and was presumed to act as an anti-inflammatory agent by some other mechanism.— J. Boyle *et al.*, *Br. med. J.*, 1986, *292*, 28.

Preparations

Lithium Carbonate Capsules *(U.S.P.)*

Lithium Carbonate Tablets *(B.P.)*

Lithium Carbonate Tablets *(U.S.P.)*

Lithium Citrate Syrup *(U.S.P.)*. Prepared from lithium citrate or from lithium hydroxide to which an excess of citric acid has been added. Potency is expressed in terms of the lithium content. pH 4 to 5.

Proprietary Preparations

Camcolit *(Norgine, UK)*. *Tablets*, scored, lithium carbonate 250 mg (6.8 mmol Li).
Tablets, scored, sustained-release, lithium carbonate 400 mg (10.8 mmol Li).

Liskonum *(Smith Kline & French, UK)*. *Tablets*, scored, sustained-release, lithium carbonate 450 mg (12.2 mmol Li).

Litarex *(CP Pharmaceuticals, UK)*. *Tablets*, sustained-release, lithium citrate 564 mg (6.0 mmol Li).

Phasal *(Lagap, UK)*. *Tablets*, sustained-release, lithium carbonate 300 mg (8.1 mmol Li).

Priadel *(Delandale, UK)*. *Tablets*, scored, sustained-release, lithium carbonate 200 and 400 mg (5.4 and 10.8 mmol Li).

Proprietary Names and Manufacturers of Lithium Salts

Arthri-Sel *(Fr.)*; Camcolit *(Norgine, Austral.*; *Camden, S.Afr.*; *Norgine, UK)*; Carbolith *(Drug Houses Austral., Austral.*; *ICN, Canad.)*; Carbolithium *(IFI, Ital.)*; Ceglution *(Arg.)*; Cibalith-S *(Ciba, USA)*; Duralith *(McNeil, Canad.)*; Eskalith *(Smith Kline & French, USA)*; Hypnorex *(Belg.*; *Delalande, Ger.*; *Delalande, Switz.)*; Lentolith *(Script Intal, S.Afr.)*; Liskonum *(Smith Kline & French, UK)*; Litarex *(Dumex, Denm.*; *Dumex, Norw.*; *Dumex, Swed.*; *Dumex, Switz.*; *CP Pharmaceuticals, UK)*; Lithane *(Pfizer, Canad.*; *Miles Pharmaceuticals, USA)*; Lithicarb *(Protea, Austral.)*; Lithiofor *(Vifor, Switz.)*; Lithionit *(Astra, Denm.*; *Astra, Norw.*; *Astra, Swed.)*; Lithium Oligosol *(Fr.)*; Lithium-Duriles *(Ger.)*; Lithiumorotat *(Ger.)*; Lithizine *(Paul Maney, Canad.)*; Lithobid *(Ciba, USA)*; Lithonate *(Rowell, USA)*; Lithonate-S *(USA)*; Lithotabs *(Rowell, USA)*; Lithuril *(Belg.)*; Litilent *(Arg.)*; Manialit *(ISF, Ital.)*; Manialith *(Muir & Neil, Austral.)*; Maniprex *(Belg.)*; Neurolithium *(Labcatal, Fr.)*; Oligosol Li *(Labcatal, Switz.)*; Phasal *(Lagap, UK)*; Plenur *(Lasa, Spain)*; Priadel *(Protea, Austral.*; *Neth.*; *Riker, S.Afr.*; *Delandale, UK)*; Quilonorm *(Smith Kline & French, Switz.)*; Quilonum *(Smith Kline Dauelsberg, Ger.*; *Dauelsberg, S.Afr.)*; Téralithe *(Théraplix, Fr.)*.

2522-w

Lofepramine Hydrochloride *(BANM, rINNM)*.

Leo-640; Lopramine Hydrochloride. 5-{3-[*N*-(Chlorophenacyl)-*N*-methylamino]propyl}10,11-5*H*-dihydrodibenz[*b,f*]azepine hydrochloride.

$C_{26}H_{27}ClN_2O,HCl = 455.4$.

CAS — 23047-25-8 (lofepramine); 26786-32-3 (hydrochloride).

Adverse Effects, Treatment, and Precautions

As for Amitriptyline Hydrochloride, p.351.

Antimuscarinic side-effects occur less frequently with lofepramine than with amitriptyline or imipramine, and lofepramine is reported to be less cardiotoxic than other tricyclic antidepressants.

EFFECTS ON THE LIVER. The *UK* Committee on Safety of Medicines had by the end of 1987 received 57 reports of abnormal liver function tests associated with lofepramine. They included hepatic failure (1), jaundice (9), and hepatitis (5). All reactions occurred within the first 8 weeks of treatment and all were reversible on discontinuation of the drug.— *Current Problems*, No. 23, 1988.

OVERDOSAGE. In a study of 13 cases of attempted suicide with lofepramine (A. Heath and B.-Å. Hultén, *Proceedings of VII World Congress of Psychiatry*, Vienna, 1983), the average age of the patients was 38.6 years and the amount of drug ingested ranged from 1.1 to 4.9 g. Other drugs were involved in 5 patients and alcohol was implicated in 3. One of the patients had a systolic blood pressure of 90 mmHg. No patient was in shock. Tachycardia was present in a single case, where ingestion of hyoscine had also occurred. No convulsions or arrhythmias were observed. Intraventricular conduction was slowed in the patient who had taken 4.9 g and he also required assisted ventilation due to an unrelated complication of bronchopneumonia. Only 2 patients displayed antimuscarinic symptoms whilst awaking, and 10 of the 13 had a coma grade score of 0 or 1.— T. Dorman, *J. int. med. Res.*, 1985, *13*, 77.

Clinical features and management of self-poisoning with lofepramine.— P. Crome and C. Ali, *Med. Toxicol.*, 1986, *1*, 411.

PORPHYRIA. Lofepramine was considered to be unsafe in patients with acute porphyria because it has been shown to be porphyrinogenic in *animals* or *in vitro* systems.— M.R. Moore and K.E.L. McColl, *Porphyrias, Drug Lists*, Glasgow, Porphyria Research Unit, University of Glasgow, 1987.

Absorption and Fate

Lofepramine is readily absorbed from the gastro-intestinal tract, and extensively demethylated by first-pass metabolism in the liver to its primary metabolite, desipramine. Since lofepramine slows gastro-intestinal transit time absorption can, however, be delayed, particularly in overdosage. Paths of metabolism also include *N*-oxidation and hydroxylation. Lofepramine is excreted in the urine, mainly in the form of its metabolites.

Uses and Administration

Lofepramine hydrochloride is a tricyclic antidepressant with actions and uses similar to those of amitriptyline (p.354). One of its metabolites is reported to be desipramine (p.359). Like imipramine and desipramine, it has less marked sedative properties than amitriptyline.

In the treatment of depression lofepramine is given by mouth in divided doses of 140 to 210 mg daily. Higher doses have been given in severe cases.

Reviews of the actions and uses of lofepramine: *Drug & Ther. Bull.*, 1983, *21*, 99; M. Peet, *Int. Med.*, 1987, *Suppl.* 11, 23.

DEPRESSION. The use of lofepramine in depression: P. F. Morse and T. G. C. Smith, *Br. J. clin. Pract.*, 1984, *38*, 301; J. M. C. Holden and P. F. Morse, *ibid.*, 1986, *40*, 59.

For a general review of the role of antidepressants in depression, see Amitriptyline Hydrochloride, p.355.

Proprietary Preparations

Gamanil *(E. Merck, UK)*. *Tablets*, scored, lofepramine 70 mg (as hydrochloride).

Proprietary Names and Manufacturers

Amplit *(Jpn)*; Deftan *(Igoda, Spain)*; Deprimil *(Port.)*; Emdalen-70 *(Merck, S.Afr.)*; Gamanil *(E. Merck, UK)*; Gamonil *(Arg.*; *Aust.*; *Egypt*; *E. Merck, Ger.*; *Greece*; *Switz.)*; Tymelyt *(Belg.*; *Pharmacia, Denm.*; *Leo, Swed.)*.

2524-l

Maprotiline Hydrochloride *(BANM, USAN, rINNM)*.

Ba-34276. 3-(9,10-Dihydro-9,10-ethanoanthracen-9-yl)(methyl)propylamine hydrochloride.

$C_{20}H_{23}N,HCl = 313.9$.

CAS — 10262-69-8 (maprotiline); 10347-81-6 (hydrochloride).

Pharmacopoeias. In *U.S.*

A fine white to off-white odourless crystalline powder. Freely **soluble** in methyl alcohol and in chloroform; slightly soluble in water.
Store in airtight containers.

Adverse Effects and Treatment

As for Amitriptyline Hydrochloride, p.351. Antimuscarinic effects may occur less frequently, but seizures seem more common.

Adverse reactions to maprotiline.— P. E. Hayes and C. A. Kristoff, *Clin. Pharm.*, 1986, *5*, 471.

By March 1985 the *UK* Committee on Safety of Medicines had received 124 reports of convulsions, 4 of hepatic reactions, and 8 of haematological reactions associated with maprotiline from a cumulative total of 2.5 million prescriptions. There had also been 454 reports of skin rashes.— Committee on Safety of Medicines, *Current Problems No. 15*, July, 1985..

EFFECTS ON THE CARDIOVASCULAR SYSTEM. Despite early reports of a lack of cardiotoxicity with maprotiline (K.-P. Bethge *et al.*, *J. cardiovasc. Pharmac.*, 1982, *4*, 142), atrial flutter has been reported in an 80-year-old woman (G. Tollefson *et al.*, *J. clin. Psychiat.*, 1984, *45*, 31).

EFFECTS ON MENTAL FUNCTION. A 59-year-old man lapsed into a catatonic stupor with electroencephalographic signs of epilepsy over a period of 72 hours after 12 days combined treatment with maprotiline 150 mg daily and thiothixene 5 mg daily.— P. B. Atri and D. A. Julius, *J. clin. Psychopharmacol.*, 1984, *4*, 207.

EFFECTS ON THE SKIN. An 83-year-old woman developed cutaneous vasculitis after therapy with maprotiline 25 mg daily increased to 125 mg daily over 3 weeks. The vasculitic skin eruptions resolved on discontinuation of the drug.— A. M. M. Oakley and L. Hodge, *Aust. N.Z. J. Med.*, 1985, *15*, 256.

EPILEPTOGENIC EFFECT. In a retrospective review of 186 psychiatric patients with no history of prior seizures, 5 of 32 patients receiving maprotiline developed generalised tonic-clonic seizures, compared with 1 of 45 receiving a tricyclic antidepressant. There were no seizures in the remaining patients who received other medications, or no drug treatment. Two of the 5 patients experiencing seizures with maprotiline were receiving daily doses of 75 to 150 mg daily, 2 were receiving daily doses of 200 to 300 mg, and one patient experienced partial complex seizures with a daily dose of 150 mg and generalised tonic-clonic seizures after increasing the daily dose to 300 mg.— B. Jabbari *et al.*, *Archs Neurol., Chicago*, 1985, *42*, 480.

Reports of seizures with maprotiline: B. F. Hoffman and R. Wachsmuth, *J. clin. Psychiat.*, 1982, *43*, 117; W. Holliday *et al.*, *Am. J. Psychiat.*, 1982, *139*, 673.

See also under Effects on Mental Function, above.

OVERDOSAGE. Experience with 41 cases of maprotiline overdosage has suggested that, unlike mianserin, the clinical features of maprotiline poisoning resemble those of the more conventional tricyclic antidepressants.— P. Crome and B. Newman (letter), *Br. med. J.*, 1977, *2*, 260.

A study of overdosage with maprotiline in 43 episodes in 41 patients; many had also taken other drugs, usually benzodiazepines and/or alcohol; the average ingested dose of maprotiline was 1.47 g. Coma was common and often prolonged; six patients required assisted ventilation; ECG abnormalities included first-degree atrioventricular block, and an increased QRS interval; hypotension occurred in 8 patients; 15 patients had seizures. Cardiotoxicity was at least equal to that with tricyclic antidepressants and seizures were more common. Physostigmine was given to 7 patients 6 of whom developed seizures; it should not therefore be used in maprotiline poisoning.— K. Knudsen and A. Heath, *Br. med. J.*, 1984, *288*, 601.

A fatal case of maprotiline overdosage associated with torsade de pointes.— R. A. Curtis *et al.*, *Drug Intell. & clin. Pharm.*, 1984, *18*, 716.

Clinical features and management of self-poisoning with maprotiline.— P. Crome and C. Ali, *Med. Toxicol.*, 1986, *1*, 411.

Precautions

As for Amitriptyline Hydrochloride, p.352. It should not be used in patients with a history of seizure disorders.

INTERACTIONS. *Anticoagulants.* Maprotiline did not appear to interact to any significant extent with coumarin anticoagulants.— *Drug Interact. News.*, 1982, *2*, 21.

Clonidine. Maprotiline did not affect the antihypertensive action of clonidine and was to be preferred to tricyclic antidepressants in patients taking clonidine for hypertension.— U. Gundert-Remy *et al.*, *Eur. J. clin. Pharmac.*, 1983, *25*, 595.

PREGNANCY AND THE NEONATE. For a report showing no association between infant central nervous system defects and the administration of tetracyclic antidepressants during the trimester before the last menstrual period, and in the first trimester of pregnancy, see Amitriptyline Hydrochloride, p.354.

Lactation. Significant amounts of maprotiline are present in breast milk and it was recommended that mothers receiving the drug should not breast-feed their infants.— *Drug & Ther. Bull.*, 1983, *21*, 48.

Absorption and Fate

Maprotiline is slowly but completely absorbed from the gastro-intestinal tract. Since maprotiline slows gastro-intestinal transit-time absorption may be further delayed in overdosage. Maprotiline is extensively demethylated to its principal active metabolite, desmethylmaprotiline; paths of metabolism of both maprotiline and desmethylmaprotiline include *N*-oxidation, aliphatic and aromatic hydroxylation, and the formation of aromatic methoxy derivatives. In addition to desmethylmaprotiline, maprotiline-*N*-oxide is also reported to be pharmacologically active. The elimination half-life of maprotiline is reported to be 51 hours. Maprotiline is excreted in the urine, mainly in the form of its metabolites, either in free or in conjugated form; appreciable amounts are also excreted in the faeces.

Maprotiline is widely distributed throughout the body and is extensively bound to plasma protein. It has been estimated to have a very prolonged plasma half-life of about 2 days. Maprotiline is excreted in breast milk.

The pharmacokinetics of maprotiline.— K. P. Maguire *et al.*, *Eur. J. clin. Pharmac.*, 1980, *18*, 249; D. Alkalay *et al.*, *Clin. Pharmac. Ther.*, 1980, *27*, 697.

Uses and Administration

Maprotiline is a *tetracyclic* antidepressant with structural similarities to the tricyclic antidepressants. It is used similarly to amitriptyline (p.354) in the treatment of depression. It has marked sedative properties, but can also cause convulsions.

In the treatment of depression maprotiline is given by mouth as the hydrochloride in doses of 25 mg to 75 mg daily in three divided doses, gradually increased to a maximum of 150 mg daily if necessary. The dosage should be adjusted after 1 or 2 weeks according to response. Because of the prolonged half-life of maprotiline the total daily dose may also be given as a single dose, usually at night. A suggested initial dose for elderly or other susceptible patients is 10 mg three times daily (or 30 mg at night).

A brief review of maprotiline.— *Med. Lett.*, 1981, *23*, 58.

CARDIAC ARRHYTHMIAS. In 9 patients with cardiac arrhythmias treatment with maprotiline reduced the incidence of ventricular premature beats, reduced the severity of arrhythmias, and reduced the incidence of exercise-induced ventricular premature beats.— E. A. Raeder *et al.*, *Br. med. J.*, 1979, *2*, 102.

DEPRESSION. For a general comment on the role of antidepressants in depression, see Amitriptyline Hydrochloride, p.355.

Depression in medical patients. The use of tricyclic and tetracyclic antidepressants in depressed medical patients.— *Lancet*, 1986, *1*, 949.

ENURESIS. Nocturnal enuresis in a 22-year-old woman only partially responsive to tricyclic antidepressants and not helped by physical devices abated within 6 days of starting treatment with maprotiline 25 mg at night. Enuresis was controlled for 4 months but recurred within 1 week of stopping maprotiline.— M. A. Gillman and R. Sandyk (letter), *J. clin. Psychiat.*, 1985, *46*, 546.

PAIN. A report of some patients experiencing pain relief with maprotiline.— P. G. Lindsay and R. B. Olsen, *J. clin. Psychiat.*, 1985, *46*, 226.

Preparations

Maprotiline Hydrochloride Tablets *(U.S.P.)*

Proprietary Preparations

Ludiomil *(Ciba, UK)*. *Tablets*, maprotiline hydrochloride 10, 25, 50, and 75 mg.

Proprietary Names and Manufacturers

Ludiomil *(Arg.; Belg.; Ciba, Canad.; Ciba, Denm.; Ciba, Fr.; Geigy, Ger.; Geigy, Ital.; Neth.; Ciba, S.Afr.; Ciba, Spain; Ciba, Swed.; Geigy, Switz.; Ciba, UK; Ciba, USA)*.

2525-y

Mebanazine *(BAN, rINN)*.

ICI-31397. α-Methylbenzylhydrazine.
$C_8H_{12}N_2$=136.2.

CAS — 65-64-5.

Mebanazine is a monoamine oxidase inhibitor which has been used in the treatment of depression.

Proprietary Names and Manufacturers
Actomol *(ICI Pharmaceuticals, UK)*.

12920-k

Medifoxamine Fumarate *(rINN)*.

NN-Dimethyl-2,2-diphenoxyethylamine fumarate.
$C_{16}H_{19}NO_2,C_4H_4O_4$=373.4.

CAS — 32359-34-5 (medifoxamine); 16604-45-8 (fumarate).

Medifoxamine fumarate is an antidepressant which has been given by mouth in a usual dose of 150 mg daily.

Proprietary Names and Manufacturers
Clédial *(Anphar-Rolland, Fr.)*; Gerdaxyl *(Sidus, Arg.; Gerda, Fr.; Promesa, Spain)*.

2526-j

Melitracen Hydrochloride *(USAN, rINNM)*.

N7001; U-24973A. 3-(9,10-Dihydro-10,10-dimethyl-9-anthrylidene)propyldimethylamine hydrochloride.
$C_{21}H_{25}N,HCl$=327.9.

CAS — 5118-29-6 (melitracen); 10563-70-9 (hydrochloride).

Melitracen hydrochloride 28.1 mg is approximately equivalent to 25 mg of melitracen.

Melitracen is a tricyclic antidepressant with actions and uses similar to those of amitriptyline (p.354). In the treatment of depression it is given as the hydrochloride in usual doses equivalent to melitracen 25 to 50 mg three times daily. It has also been given intramuscularly as the mesylate.

Proprietary Names and Manufacturers
Dixeran *(Lundbeck, Belg.; Lundbeck, Switz.)*; Melixeran *(Lusofarmaco, Ital.)*; Trausabun *(Promonta, Ger.; Byk, Neth.)*.

16892-z

Metralindole *(rINN)*.

2,4,5,6-Tetrahydro-9-methoxy-4-methyl-1-*H*-3,4,6a-triazafluoranthene.
$C_{15}H_{17}N_3O$=255.3.

CAS — 54188-38-4.

Metralindole is reported to possess antidepressant properties.

Proprietary Names and Manufacturers
Incazan *(USSR)*.

2527-z

Mianserin Hydrochloride *(BANM, USAN, pINNM)*.

Org-GB-94. 1,2,3,4,10,14b-Hexahydro-2-methyldibenzo[*c,f*]pyrazino[1,2-*a*]azepine hydrochloride.

$C_{18}H_{20}N_2,HCl=300.8$.

CAS — 24219-97-4 (mianserin); 21535-47-7 (hydrochloride).

Pharmacopoeias. In *Br.*

White or almost white odourless or almost odourless crystals or crystalline powder. **Soluble** 1 in 50 of water, 1 in 100 of alcohol, and 1 in 20 of chloroform. A 1% solution has a pH of 4.0 to 5.5. **Store** in well-closed containers. Protect from light.

Adverse Effects

The most common adverse effect associated with mianserin is drowsiness. Mianserin also causes bone-marrow depression with leucopenia, and agranulocytosis; aplastic anaemia has been reported. The elderly are considered to be especially sensitive. Other side-effects reported include convulsions, disturbances of liver function and jaundice, breast disorders (gynaecomastia, nipple tenderness, and non-puerperal lactation), dizziness, orthostatic hypotension, oedema, polyarthropathy, skin rash, sweating, and tremor. Antimuscarinic and cardiac side-effects are fewer and milder than with tricyclic antidepressants.

In overdosage mianserin is unlikely to cause severe cardiac arrhythmias, respiratory depression, convulsions, or coma; prolonged sedation is usual.

By March 1985 the *UK* Committee on Safety of Medicines had received 64 reports of convulsions, 57 of hepatic reactions, and 113 of haematological reactions (12 fatal) associated with mianserin from a cumulative total of 5 million prescriptions. The haematological reactions had predominantly been leucopenia or agranulocytosis, and the elderly appeared particularly susceptible. The hepatic reactions had included jaundice and other abnormalities of liver function, but no fatalities had been reported. Mianserin had also been suspected of causing malaise or an influenza-like syndrome, as well as arthralgia and arthritis.— Committee on Safety of Medicines, *Current Problems No. 15*, July 1985..

A prescription-event monitoring study indicating that both mianserin and amitriptyline are associated with a low risk of blood disorders, but that mianserin is safer in overdosage.—W. H. W. Inman, *Lancet*, 1988, *2*, 90. See also *idem*, 683.

EFFECTS ON THE BLOOD. Mianserin was the drug most commonly reported to the *UK* Committee on Safety of Medicines in 1985 as being suspected of causing aplastic anaemia or depressed peripheral white cell counts.— *Br. med. J.*, 1986, *293*, 688.

White cell depression usually occcurs early, typically between 4 and 6 weeks after the start of treatment with mianserin. The neutrophil count in most cases was severely reduced to 0.2×10^9 per litre or less but, typically, complete recovery occurred once the drug was withdrawn.— A. Wakeling, *Postgrad. med. J.*, 1983, *59*, 229.

Proposed mechanisms of mianserin haematotoxicity: J. L. O'Donnell *et al.*, *Br. med. J.*, 1985, *291*, 1375; B. H. C. Stricker *et al.*, *Br. J. clin. Pharmac.*, 1985, *19*, 102.

Reports of blood dyscrasias associated with mianserin therapy: C. E. Page, *Br. med. J.*, 1982, *284*, 1912 (agranulocytosis); K. N. Achar (letter), *ibid.*, *285*, 208 (agranulocytosis); S. Durrant and D. Read (letter), *ibid.*, 437 (aplastic anaemia); S. G. Braye *et al.* (letter), *ibid.*, 1117 (neutropenic enterocolitis during mianserin-induced agranulocytosis); P. C. Adams *et al.*, *Postgrad. med. J.*, 1983, *59*, 31 (leucopenia); J. Brume *et al.*, *Scott. med. J.*, 1983, *28*, 373 (agranulocytosis); J. Forgan-Smith and P. Leslie (letter), *Med. J. Aust.*, 1985, *143*, 398 (neutropenia); C. A. Morgan and M. D. Donaldson (letter), *ibid.*, 1986, *144*, 165 (agranulocytosis).

EFFECTS ON THE CARDIOVASCULAR SYSTEM. Two elderly patients receiving mianserin at doses of 30 to 70 mg daily developed signs of disturbed cardiac function (congestive cardiac failure, atrial and ventricular fibrillation, bradycardia, and frequent ventricular ectopic beats) which resolved after the drug was discontinued. One of the patients also developed hypokalaemia which was possibly caused by mianserin.— H. Whiteford *et al.*, *Med. J. Aust.*, 1984, *140*, 166.

EFFECTS ON THE LIVER. Mixed obstructive and hepatocellular liver damage, jaundice, and fevers occurred in a 65-year-old woman who had been taking mianserin 30 mg daily by mouth for 3 months, as well as prochlorperazine. The patient recovered when mianserin was stopped although prochlorperazine therapy continued (Adverse Drug Reactions Advisory Committee, *Med. J. Aust.*, 1980, *2*, 673). Cholestatic jaundice, accompanied by fever occurred in a 46-year-old woman after 11 days of treatment with mianserin 20 mg daily and resolved 7 days after discontinuing therapy (J.-P. Zarski *et al.*, *Gastroenterol. clin. biol.*, 1983, *7*, 220).

EFFECTS ON THE MUSCULOSKELETAL SYSTEM. A 36-year-old woman developed an acute polyarthritis affecting her hands and feet 6 days after commencing therapy with mianserin 30 mg each night. Arthritis resolved within 7 days of stopping mianserin. The *UK* Committee on Safety of Medicines had received 19 reports of arthritis and arthralgia associated with mianserin.— A. Hughes and J. Coote, *Br. med. J.*, 1986, *292*, 1050.

See also under Effects on the Skin, below.

EFFECTS ON THE SKIN. Toxic epidermal necrolysis in a 34-year-old woman might have been associated with mianserin.— P. Randell (letter), *Med. J. Aust.*, 1979, *2*, 653.

Widespread and severe lesions of erythema multiforme appeared on 2 occasions in a 38-year-old woman after 4 days of treatment with mianserin 30 mg daily (E. Quraishy, *Br. J. Derm.*, 1981, *104*, 481), and occurred with associated arthralgia in the hands in a 20-year-old woman who had been taking mianserin for 5 weeks (N.H. Cox, *Br. J. clin. Pract.*, 1985, *39*, 293).

EFFECTS ON THE TONGUE. Glossitis developed in 2 elderly patients within 4 to 14 days of starting mianserin at doses of 20 to 40 mg daily and disappeared within 3 to 7 days of stopping the drug.— J. R. de la Fuente and C. Berlanga (letter), *Lancet*, 1984, *1*, 233.

EFFECTS ON VITAMIN D METABOLISM. Low serum 1,25-dihydroxycholecalciferol concentration and hypophosphataemia was seen in a 51-year-old man who had been receiving short courses of mianserin 10 mg daily every 2 to 3 months for 6 years. It was suggested that mianserin may alter production and/or catabolism of 1,25-dihydroxycholecalciferol due to enzyme induction.— V. Lo Cascio *et al.* (letter), *Lancet*, 1984, *1*, 958.

EPILEPTOGENIC EFFECT. Of 40 patients reported to the *UK* Committee on Safety of Medicines because of convulsions occurring during mianserin treatment, a causal connection could be established only in a minority. It was suggested that mianserin is no more epileptogenic than tricyclic antidepressants.— J. G. Edwards and M. Glen-Bott, *Br. J. clin. Pharmac.*, 1983, *15*, 299S. See also A. Richens *et al.*, *ibid.*, 295S.

OVERDOSAGE. Experience with 44 patients confirmed that mianserin in overdosage did not cause the severe complications seen with tricyclic antidepressants.— P. Crome *et al.* (letter), *Br. med. J.*, 1978, *1*, 859.

Symptoms in 42 patients who had taken an overdose of mianserin alone included drowsiness (16), coma (2), hypertension (4), sinus tachycardia (3), bradycardia (2), vomiting (3), dizziness and ataxia (1), constricted pupils (1), dilated pupils (1), and hypotension (1).— W. L. Shaw, *Curr. med. Res. Opinion*, 1980, *6*, *Suppl.* 7, 44.

A further report of the lack of toxicity of mianserin in overdose.— S. Chand *et al.*,, *Pharmakopsychiatrie*, 1981, *14*, 15.

Pinpoint pupils unresponsive to naloxone were seen in a 33-year-old woman who had taken 750 to 1200 mg of mianserin and half a bottle of rum.— G. N. Fuller and J. Clarbour (letter), *Br. med. J.*, 1987, *294*, 1233.

WEIGHT CHANGES. Weight gain associated with unusual craving for bread and butter, chocolate, and bread respectively, was noted in 3 patients given mianserin for depression.— B. Harris and M. Harper (letter), *Lancet*, 1980, *1*, 590. Three women who, despite vigorous dieting efforts, had gained 6 to 20 kg above their normal weight on amitriptyline, regained their former weights on transfer to mianserin. Carbohydrate craving disappeared and weight loss began (in 2 cases associated with dieting) within one to two weeks.— W. Williams (letter), *Med. J. Aust.*, 1980, *1*, 132.

Treatment of Adverse Effects

The stomach should be emptied by emesis or aspiration and lavage. Supportive therapy alone may then suffice.

A review of the clinical features and management of self-poisoning with mianserin. In 54 patients who ingested mianserin alone, the following clinical features were noted: patient fully alert (41%), grade I to II coma (44%), hypotension (17%), sinus tachycardia (7%), sinus bradycardia (4%), hypertension (2%) (S. Chand *et al.*, *Pharmacopsychiat.*, 1981, *14*, 15). There had been isolated reports of heart block in patients who took mianserin and benzodiazepines (S.D.R. Green and P. Kendall-Taylor, *Br. med. J.*, 1977, *2*, 1190; N. Grabe, *Ugeskr. Laeg.*, 1983, *145*, 3413).— P. Crome and C. Ali, *Med. Toxicol.*, 1986, *1*, 411.

Precautions

Mianserin is contra-indicated in patients with severe liver disease and in patients with mania. Manic depressive patients may switch from a depressive to a manic phase during treatment with mianserin; whenever that occurs mianserin should be withdrawn.

Although mianserin does not have the cardiotoxicity of the tricyclic antidepressants, it should be used with caution in patients with cardiovascular disorders, such as heart block, or after recent myocardial infarction. It should be used with caution in patients with epilepsy, and hepatic or renal insufficiency. Patients with suicidal tendencies should be carefully supervised during treatment. Blood sugar concentrations may be altered in diabetic patients. Patients with narrow angle glaucoma or prostatic hypertrophy should be monitored even though antimuscarinic effects are rare. A full blood count is recommended every 4 weeks during the first 3 months of treatment, due to the risk of bone-marrow depression. Similarly, if a patient receiving mianserin develops fever, sore throat, stomatitis, or other signs of infection, treatment should be stopped and a full blood count obtained. The elderly are considered to be at special risk of blood disorders from mianserin.

It is recommended that mianserin should not be given to patients receiving monoamine oxidase inhibitors or for at least 14 days after their discontinuation. Mianserin does not diminish the effects of the antihypertensive agents guanethidine, hydralazine, propranolol, clonidine, or bethanidine. However, it is still recommended that blood pressure is monitored when mianserin is prescribed with antihypertensive therapy. Phenytoin plasma concentrations should be watched carefully in patients treated concurrently with mianserin. The sedative effects of mianserin may be enhanced by concurrent administration with alcohol.

Drowsiness is often experienced at the start of mianserin antidepressant therapy and patients if affected should not drive or operate machinery. For further details of the effects of antidepressant therapy on driving see amitriptyline hydrochloride (p.353).

Breast feeding should be discontinued during treatment with mianserin.

INTERACTIONS. *Anticoagulants.* Mianserin did not appear to interact with coumarin anticoagulants to any significant extent.— *Drug Interact. News.*, 1982, *2*, 21.

Anti-epileptics. Reduced plasma concentrations of mianserin and desmethylmianserin in 6 patients also receiving anti-epileptic therapy consisting of phenytoin with either carbamazepine or phenobarbitone.— S. Nawishy *et al.*, *Br. J. clin. Pharmac.*, 1982, *13*, 612P.

Clonidine. For a report stating that mianserin did not interfere with the antihypertensive action of clonidine, see Clonidine Hydrochloride, p.473.

Methyldopa. Mianserin did not interfere with the antihypertensive action of methyldopa.— H. L. Elliott *et al.*,, *Eur. J. clin. Pharmac.*, 1983, *24*, 15.

PREGNANCY AND THE NEONATE. For a report showing no association between infant central nervous system defects and the administration of tetracyclic antidepressants during the trimester before the last menstrual period, and in the first trimester of pregnancy, see Amitriptyline Hydrochloride, p.354.

Absorption and Fate

Mianserin is readily absorbed from the gastrointestinal tract, but its bioavailability is reduced to about 70% by extensive first-pass metabolism in the liver.

Paths of metabolism of mianserin include aromatic hydroxylation, *N*-oxidation, and *N*-demethylation. Desmethylmianserin and 8-hydroxymianserin are pharmacologically active.

Mianserin is excreted in the urine, almost entirely as its metabolites, either free or in conjugated form; some is also found in the faeces. Mianserin is widely distributed throughout the body and is extensively bound to plasma proteins. It has been found to have a biphasic plasma half-life with the duration of the terminal phase ranging from 6 to 39 hours.

Mianserin pharmacokinetics were studied in 8 depressed patients aged 25 to 42 years after a single 60-mg dose by mouth. Mean peak plasma concentrations were reached between 1 and 3 hours. The decline of mianserin plasma concentrations was biphasic with a mean elimination half-life of 21.6 hours (range 10.7 to 40.8 hours). The estimated mean first-pass loss was 37% (range 26 to 48%) and was lower than that reported for tertiary amine tricyclic antidepressants. The results indicated that mianserin kinetics are in most respects similar to those of tertiary amine tricyclics, such as imipramine, and the tetracyclic maprotiline.— P. D. Hrdina *et al.*, *Clin. Pharmac. Ther.*, 1983, *33*, 757.

Uses and Administration

Mianserin is a *tetracyclic* antidepressant. It does not appear to have significant antimuscarinic properties, but has a marked sedative action. Unlike amitriptyline, it does not prevent the peripheral re-uptake of noradrenaline; it blocks presynaptic alpha-adrenoceptors and increases the turnover of brain noradrenaline. It has little effect on central serotonin uptake but has been shown to increase peripheral serotonin uptake in depressed subjects. It has antihistamine properties. Although many of the effects of mianserin differ from those of amitriptyline, its activity in depression is similar. Like amitriptyline, its mode of action in depression is not fully understood. In the treatment of depression mianserin is given by mouth as the hydrochloride in doses of 30 to 40 mg daily for the first few days. The effective daily dosage is usually between 30 and 90 mg. The daily dosage may be divided throughout the day or given as a single dose at night. Divided daily dosages of up to 200 mg have been given. The recommended initial daily dose in the elderly is not more than 30 mg, which may be slowly increased if necessary.

The pharmacology of mianserin.— R. J. Marshall, *Br. J. clin. Pharmac.*, 1983, *15*, 263S.

Reviews of mianserin: M. L. Mashford, *Med. J. Aust.*, 1984, *141*, 308; *Drug & Ther. Bull.*, 1988, *26*, 17.

ADMINISTRATION. In a study of 17 depressed elderly patients, the relationship between plasma mianserin and desmethylmianserin concentrations at steady-state and at 16 and 24 hours after a single 30-mg test dose of mianserin was not sufficiently well-defined to allow a single test dose to be used for prediction of dosage requirements.— S. Dawling *et al.*, *Clin. Pharmacokinet.*, 1987, *12*, 73.

ANXIETY AND PHOBIAS. For a suggestion that antidepressants with secondary sedative properties, such as mianserin, are the treatment of first choice in depressed patients with anxiety or agitation, see Amitriptyline Hydrochloride, p.355.

DEPRESSION. In the treatment of depression, mianserin has been reported to be as effective as amitriptyline (M.C. Khan *et al.*, *Br. J. clin. Pract.*, 1982, *36*, 240; J.P. Feigher *et al.*, *Br. J. clin. Pharmac.*, 1983, *15*, 227S; W. Guy *et al.*, *Pharmacotherapy*, 1983, *3*, 45; J.G. Rabkin *et al.*, *Neuropsychobiology*, 1984, *12*, 224), dothiepin (M.J. Akhtar *et al.*, *Br. J. clin. Pract.*, 1984, *38*, 316; M.P. De Sousa and J.R. Tropa, *J. int. med. Res.*, 1986, *14*, 42), doxepin (M.C. Khan *et al.*, *Br. J. clin. Pharmac.*, 1983, *15*, 213S), imipramine (K. Eklund *et al.*, *Acta psychiat. scand.*, 1985, *72*, *Suppl.* 320, 54), indalpine (G.J. Naylor and B. Martin, *Br. J. Psychiat.*, 1985, *147*, 306), maprotiline (A.P. Palha *et al.*, *Clin. Ther.*, 1985, *7*, 584), nomifensine (R. Granier *et al.*, *Acta psychiat. scand.*, 1985, *72*, *Suppl.* 320, 67), nortriptyline (J. Hoc, *Curr. med. Res. Opinion*, 1982, *8*, 282), and trazodone (E.H. Bennie *et al.*, *ibid.*, 1984, *9*, 253).

For a general comment on the role of antidepressants in depression, see Amitriptyline Hydrochloride, p.355.

Depression in children. In an open study, mianserin at an average daily dose of 1 mg per kg body-weight was effective in treating depression in 80 depressed children and adolescents aged 8 to 19 years. Efficacy was noticeable by the end of the first week of treatment and was maintained throughout the 60-day study period. Side-effects were minimal leading to temporary withdrawal of treatment in only 7 cases. The profile of mianserin in children and adolescents was similar to that of adults.— M. Dugas *et al.*, *Acta psychiat. scand.*, 1985, *72*, *Suppl.* 320, 48.

Depression in medical patients. The use of tricyclic and tetracyclic antidepressants in depressed medical patients.— *Lancet*, 1986, *1*, 949.

DIAGNOSTIC USE. Mianserin could not be considered useful in the diagnosis of hyperprolactinaemic states.— E. Rolandi *et al.*, *Curr. ther. Res.*, 1983, *33*, 238.

EATING DISORDERS. For a report indicating a lack of benefit in bulimia with mianserin, see Amitriptyline Hydrochloride, p.356.

HEADACHE. Mianserin 30 to 60 mg daily produced a significantly greater reduction in migraine frequency and severity than placebo in a double-blind study in 38 patients.— P. Monro *et al.*, *Acta psychiat. scand.*, 1985, *72*, *Suppl.* 320, 98.

PAIN. In a double-blind study in 112 elderly patients suffering from chronic painful conditions, there was significant relief of pain and psychiatric morbidity with both mianserin and placebo, but no significant difference between the two.— D. Wheatley, *Practitioner*, 1986, *320*, 477.

Preparations

Mianserin Tablets *(B.P.)*. Mianserin Hydrochloride Tablets

Proprietary Preparations

Bolvidon *(Organon, UK)*. *Tablets*, mianserin hydrochloride 10, 20, and 30 mg.

Norval *(Bencard, UK)*. *Tablets*, mianserin hydrochloride 10, 20, and 30 mg.

Proprietary Names and Manufacturers

Athimil *(Chile; Organon, Peru)*; Athymil *(Organon, Fr.)*; Bolvidon *(Organon, UK)*; Lantanon *(Ravasini, Ital.; Organon, S.Afr.; Organon, Spain)*; Lerivon *(Belg.)*; Norval *(Bencard, UK)*; Tetramide *(Organon, Jpn)*; Tolvin *(Organon, Ger.)*; Tolvon *(Organon, Austral.; Organon, Denm.; Organon, Norw.; Organon, Switz.)*.

12963-v

Minaprine Hydrochloride *(BANM, USAN, rINNM)*.

Agr-1240; CB-30038. *N*-(4-Methyl-6-phenylpyridazin-3-yl)-2-morpholinoethylamine dihydrochloride.
$C_{17}H_{22}N_4O,2HCl=371.3$.

CAS — 25953-17-7; 25905-77-5 (minaprine).

Minaprine is an antidepressant with stimulant properties which has been given by mouth in doses of 100 to 300 mg daily. It has also been tried in senile dementia.

DEPRESSION. In the treatment of depression, minaprine has been reported to be as effective as imipramine (N. Bohacek *et al.*, *J. clin. Psychopharmacol.*, 1986, *6*, 320) and nomifensine (P. Mikus *et al.*, *Clin. Trials J.*, 1985, *22*, 477).

SENILE DEMENTIA. A placebo-controlled study of minaprine showed improvement in depressed mood and behaviour in senile dementia.— M. Passeri *et al.* (letter), *Lancet*, 1985, *1*, 824.

Proprietary Names and Manufacturers

Cantor *(Clin Midy, Fr.; Midy, Ital.)*; Isopulsan *(Labaz, Spain)*;
Manufacturers also include—*Taisho, Jpn.*

19529-x

Moclobemide *(rINN)*.

Ro-11-1163. *p*-Chloro-*N*-(2-morpholinoethyl)benzamide.
$C_{13}H_{17}ClN_2O_2=268.7$.

CAS — 71320-77-9.

Moclobemide is an antidepressant which reversibly inhibits type A monoamine oxidase.

Seven depressed patients received placebo and moclobemide 100 mg as single doses and five patients were also given chronic treatment with individually assessed optimal therapeutic doses (100 to 400 mg). No change in blood pressure, heart rate, ECG, or systolic time intervals was found.— S. Gasic *et al.*, *Eur. J. clin. Pharmac.*, 1983, *25*, 173.

No rise in blood pressure was noted in 6 healthy subjects who received cheddar cheese with a tyramine content of 65 to 70 mg before and after treatment with moclobemide. In 3 subjects treated with tranylcypromine the cheese caused a pronounced and sustained rise in blood pressure.— A. Korn *et al.*, *J. Pharm. Pharmac.*, 1984, *36*, *Suppl.*, 64W.

The pharmacokinetics of moclobemide.— F. -A. Wiesel *et al.*, *Eur. J. clin. Pharmac.*, 1985, *28*, 89.

DEPRESSION. Moclobemide was as effective as amitriptyline in a double-blind study involving 25 patients with depression. There was no difference in the onset of antidepressant effect.— T. R. Norman *et al.*, *J. Affect. Dis.*, 1985, *8*, 29.

Further references to moclobemide in depression.— J. U. Postma and D. Vranesic, *Acta ther.*, 1985, *11*, 249; K. Lensch *et al.*, *Int. clin. Psychopharmacol.*, 1987, *2*, 165.

Proprietary Names and Manufacturers

Auroxix *(Roche, Switz.)*.

12999-k

Napactadine Hydrochloride *(USAN, rINNM)*.

DL-588. *NN'*-Dimethylnaphthalene-2-acetamidine hydrochloride.
$C_{14}H_{16}N_2,HCl=248.8$.

CAS — 76631-45-3 (napactadine); 57166-13-9 (hydrochloride).

Napactadine hydrochloride is reported to have antidepressant activity.

Proprietary Names and Manufacturers

Merrell Dow, USA.

2528-c

Nialamide *(BAN, rINN)*.

N'-(2-Benzylcarbamoylethyl)isonicotinohydrazide.
$C_{16}H_{18}N_4O_2=298.3$.

CAS — 51-12-7.

Pharmacopoeias. In *Jug.*

Nialamide is a monoamine oxidase inhibitor which has been used in the treatment of depression.

Proprietary Names and Manufacturers

Niamid *(Roerig, Belg.; Pfizer, Denm.; Pfizer, Spain; Pfizer, UK)*; Niamide *(Pfizer, Fr.)*.

2529-k

Nomifensine Maleate *(BANM, USAN, rINNM)*.

36-984; Hoe-984. 1,2,3,4-Tetrahydro-2-methyl-4-phenylisoquinolin-8-ylamine maleate.
$C_{16}H_{18}N_2,C_4H_4O_4=354.4$.

CAS — 24526-64-5 (nomifensine); 32795-47-4 (maleate).

Nomifensine is a tetrahydroisoquinoline antidepressant. In the treatment of depression it was formerly given by mouth as the maleate in doses of 75 to 200 mg daily. It was also used in the diagnosis of pituitary adenomas. Nomifensine was withdrawn worldwide in January 1986 due to the risk of acute haemolytic anaemia, with intravascular haemolysis. In some cases, renal failure also developed.

Since 1977, up to half a million patients had been treated with nomifensine. The *UK* manufacturers had received a total of 296 adverse reaction reports including 43 of haemolytic anaemia. Of those 43, 26 were of the acute (immune) type and 16 of the 26 patients with that type of reaction had received a previous course of nomifensine. The remaining 17 cases comprised a chronic (auto-immune) form with a slow onset of haemolysis. Only 4 of the 17 patients with such a reaction had been previously exposed to the drug. In the *UK* 3 of the 8 deaths associated with nomifensine since its introduction in 1977 were associated with haemolytic anaemias.— *Pharm. J.*, 1986, *1*, 113.

Although haemolytic anaemia was the serious reaction with nomifensine most frequently reported to the CSM, other adverse effects also caused concern. Five reports described thrombocytopenia. Of the 51 reported cases of suspected hepatotoxicity with nomifensine (one fatal), 40 (including 28 women) were assessed as probably or possibly due to nomifensine, and 4 patients reacted positively on rechallenge. Two patients had both haemolytic anaemia and evidence of hepatotoxicity. Two reports described patients with a syndrome resembling acute allergic alveolitis after nomifensine; both patients recovered. The CSM had also received 48 reports describing febrile or influenza-like reactions. Many of these reports of suspected adverse reactions to nomifensine contained features that suggested an immunological mechanism. Recent studies have suggested that haemolysis is associated with the formation of immune complexes with nomifensine or its metabolites.— *Br. med. J.*, 1986, *293*, 41.

Proprietary Names and Manufacturers
Alival *(Belg.; Denm.; Fr.; Ger.; Neth.; Switz.)*; Anametrin *(Port.)*; Hostalival *(Arg.)*; Merital *(Hoechst, Austral.; S.Afr.; Hoechst, UK; Hoechst, USA)*; Merital AM *(Hoechst, UK)*; Merival *(Thai.)*; Psicronizer *(Ital.)*.

2530-w

Nortriptyline Hydrochloride *(BANM, USAN, rINNM)*.

3-(10,11-Dihydro-5*H*-dibenzo[*a,d*]cyclohepten-5-ylidene)propyl(methyl)amine hydrochloride.
$C_{19}H_{21}N,HCl = 299.8$.

CAS — 72-69-5 (nortriptyline); 894-71-3 (hydrochloride).

Pharmacopoeias. In *Br.*, *Cz.*, *Nord.*, and *U.S.*

A white or off-white powder with a slight characteristic odour. Nortriptyline hydrochloride 22.8 mg is approximately equivalent to 20 mg of nortriptyline.

B.P. **solubilities** are: soluble 1 in 50 of water and 1 in 10 of alcohol; freely soluble in chloroform; practically insoluble in ether. *U.S.P.* solubilities are: soluble 1 in 90 of water, 1 in 30 of alcohol, 1 in 20 of chloroform, and 1 in 10 of methyl alcohol; practically insoluble in most other organic solvents. A 1% solution in water has a pH of about 5. **Store** in airtight containers. Protect from light.

Adverse Effects, Treatment, and Precautions

As for Amitriptyline Hydrochloride, p.351. Nortriptyline is reported to be less sedating than amitriptyline but with a greater incidence of antimuscarinic effects.

EFFECTS ON THE CARDIOVASCULAR SYSTEM. In reviewing the cardiovascular effects of the tricyclic antidepressants, Glassman (*Annu. Rev. Med.*, 1984, *35*, 503) considered that nortriptyline had a negligible effect in inducing orthostatic hypotension. He cited a study by Freyschuss *et al.* (*Pharmacol. Clin.*, 1970, *2*, 68) and his own work (S.P. Roose, *et al.*, *J. clin. Psychopharmacol.* 1981, *1*, 316) to support this opinion.
The use of tricyclic antidepressants in patients with cardiovascular disease is discussed under the Precautions section of amitriptyline. There is also further information under Administration in Cardiovascular Disease in Uses, below.

EFFECTS ON VENTILATION. Severe hyperventilation developed in a 61-year-old man with end-stage renal disease after receiving nortriptyline 125 mg daily; mechanical ventilation was necessary to correct severe respiratory alkalosis.— S. Sunderrajan *et al.*, *Archs intern. Med.*, 1985, *145*, 746.

INTERACTIONS. Interactions involving tricyclic antidepressants are discussed under amitriptyline (p.353). References to interactions where nortriptyline has been the tricyclic antidepressant affected can be found under the headings H_2 Antagonist Antihistamines, Neuroleptics, and Smoking.
For a report indicating that nortriptyline does not affect the plasma protein binding of propylthiouracil, see propylthiouracil (p.687).

PORPHYRIA. Nortriptyline was considered to be unsafe in patients with acute porphyria, although there is conflicting experimental evidence of porphyrinogenicity; see Amitriptyline Hydrochloride, p.354.

PREGNANCY AND THE NEONATE. For studies finding no association between maternal tricyclic antidepressant usage and congenital malformation, see Amitriptyline Hydrochloride, p.354.

Absorption and Fate

Nortriptyline is the principal active metabolite of amitriptyline. For an account of its metabolism, see Amitriptyline Hydrochloride, p.354.

Nortriptyline has been reported to have a longer plasma half-life than that of amitriptyline. Nortriptyline is subject to extensive first-pass metabolism in the liver to 10-hydroxynortriptyline, which is active.

PLASMA CONCENTRATIONS. Nortriptyline appears to have a specific therapeutic window between 50 and 150 ng per mL within which favourable antidepressant responses occur. Above and below this specific plasma concentration range, there is a poor clinical response. Plasma concentration measurements were unequivocally useful in problem patients who did not respond to usual oral doses or in high-risk patients who, because of age or medical illness, would best be treated with the lowest possible effective dose of the drug.— American Psychiatric Association (APA) Task Force, *Am. J. Psychiat.*, 1985, *142*, 155.
In a study of 18 depressed patients with steady-state total nortriptyline plasma concentrations between 50 and 150 ng per mL, regression analyses predicted that the probability of antidepressant response would be 68% or more if the free nortriptyline concentration is between 7 and 10 ng per mL.— P. J. Perry *et al.*, *Drug Intell. & clin. Pharm.*, 1984, *18*, 510.

METABOLISM. There is evidence that individuals with a slow debrisoquine hydroxylation phenotype may be at greater risk of confusional states when taking nortriptyline (B.K. Park and N.R. Kitteringham, *Adverse Drug React. Bull.*, 1987, *122*, 456). This was thought to be because the polymorphic hydroxylation of debrisoquine and nortriptyline are mediated by similar enzymatic mechanisms, with slow oxidizers having higher plasma nortriptyline concentrations (C. Nordin *et al.*, *Br. J. clin. Pharmac.*, 1985, *19*, 832). There was no significant correlation between hydroxylation phenotype and amitriptyline serum concentrations, suggesting that demethylation is mediated by a different cytochrome P-450 isoenzyme to hydroxylation (L. Bertilsson *et al.*, *ibid.*, 1982, *14*, 602).
For further reference to possible associations between poor metabolism of debrisoquine or sparteine and adverse reactions to tricyclic antidepressants, see Amitriptyline Hydrochloride, p.354.

Uses and Administration

Nortriptyline is a tricyclic antidepressant with actions and uses similar to those of amitriptyline (p.354). It is the principal active metabolite of amitriptyline.

In the treatment of depression nortriptyline is given by mouth as the hydrochloride in doses equivalent to nortriptyline 20 to 40 mg daily in divided doses, increasing to 100 mg daily as necessary. The usual maintenance dose is 30 to 75 mg daily. A suggested initial dose for adolescents and the elderly is 10 mg three times daily. Since nortriptyline has a prolonged half-life, once-daily dosage regimens are also suitable, usually given at night.

Nortriptyline is also given for the treatment of nocturnal enuresis in children. Suggested doses are 10 mg for children aged 6 to 7 years (20 to 25 kg body-weight), 10 to 20 mg for children aged 8 to 11 years (25 to 35 kg), and 25 to 35 mg for children aged over 11 years (35 to 54 kg). The dose should be given 30 minutes before bedtime and treatment should not continue for longer than 3 months.

ADMINISTRATION. A means of predicting nortriptyline dosage requirements following administration of a single 100-mg dose.— S. A. Montgomery *et al.*, *Clin. Pharmacokinet.*, 1979, *14*, 129. See also: R. A. Braithwaite *et al.*, *Clin. Pharmac. Ther.*, 1978, *23*, 303; *idem*, *Postgrad. med. J.*, 1980, *56*, *Suppl.* 1, 112; S. Dawling *et al.*, *Eur. J. clin. Pharmac.*, 1980, *18*, 147; W. K. Fant *et al.*, *Clin. Pharmacokinet.*, 1984, *9*, 450; P. J. Perry *et al.*, *ibid.*, 555.

ADMINISTRATION IN CARDIOVASCULAR DISEASE. Only one of 21 depressed patients with left ventricular impairment and treated with nortriptyline developed orthostatic hypotension; ejection fraction was unchanged in all. It was concluded that nortriptyline is a relatively safe treatment for depression in patients with left ventricular impairment.— S. P. Roose *et al.*, *J. Am. med. Ass.*, 1986, *256*, 3253.

ADMINISTRATION IN RENAL FAILURE. Nortriptyline can be given in usual doses to patients with renal failure. Concentrations of nortriptyline were not affected by haemodialysis or peritoneal dialysis.— W. M. Bennett *et al.*, *Am. J. Kidney Dis.*, 1983, *3*, 155.

CARDIAC ARRHYTHMIAS. For the successful use of nortriptyline to control premature ventricular contractions, see Imipramine Hydrochloride, p.363.

DEPRESSION. For a general review of the role of antidepressants in depression, see Amitriptyline Hydrochloride, p.355.

Depression after stroke. In a double-blind study of 34 patients with post-stroke depression (17 with major depression), nortriptyline 20 mg daily by mouth increasing to 100 mg daily produced significantly greater improvement in depression than placebo. Three patients receiving active medication developed delirium with confusion, drowsiness, and sometimes agitation.— J. R. Lipsey *et al.*, *Lancet*, 1984, *1*, 297. Comments on the unacceptable incidence of delirium and the susceptibility of ageing and damaged brains to tricyclic complications: A. G. Fullerton (letter), *ibid.*, 519; M. Agerholm (letter), *ibid.* Reply. The delirium was reversible on withdrawal of nortriptyline and doses were only increased weekly, with careful monitoring, to try and avoid drug-induced delirium.— J. R. Lipsey and R. G. Robinson (letter), *ibid.*, 803.
For reports that nortriptyline appears to have a specific therapeutic window of plasma concentrations within which favourable antidepressant responses occur, see under Absorption and Fate, above.

NAUSEA AND VOMITING. The incidence, severity, and duration of nausea and vomiting was reduced in patients with breast cancer receiving antineoplastic agents when they were given fluphenazine 1.5 mg and nortriptyline 30 mg daily for 5 days. Fluphenazine alone, cyclizine, metoclopramide, or placebo were not effective.— C. Morran *et al.*, *Br. med. J.*, 1979, *1*, 1323.

URTICARIA. Nortriptyline 25 mg three times daily was given to 12 patients with urticarial wheals or dermographism for 4 weeks and a placebo was given for a further 4 weeks. Ten patients improved when taking nortriptyline, but not when taking the placebo. There was dramatic improvement in 3 of 4 with dermographism. Maintenance with nortriptyline was necessary for continued control of urticaria.— W. N. Morley, *Br. J. clin. Pract.*, 1969, *23*, 305.

Preparations

Nortriptyline Capsules *(B.P.)*. Capsules containing nortriptyline hydrochloride. Potency is expressed in terms of the equivalent amount of nortriptyline.

Nortriptyline Hydrochloride Capsules *(U.S.P.)*. Potency is expressed in terms of the equivalent amount of nortriptyline.

Nortriptyline Hydrochloride Oral Solution *(U.S.P.)*. The solution contains alcohol 3 to 5%. Potency is expressed in terms of the equivalent amount of nortriptyline. pH 2.5 to 4.

Nortriptyline Tablets *(B.P.)*. Tablets containing nortriptyline hydrochloride. Potency is expressed in terms of the equivalent amount of nortriptyline.

Proprietary Preparations

Allegron *(Dista, UK)*. *Tablets*, nortriptyline 10 mg (as hydrochloride).
Tablets, scored, nortriptyline 25 mg (as hydrochloride).

Aventyl *(Lilly, UK)*. *Capsules*, nortriptyline 10 and 25 mg (as hydrochloride).
Liquid, nortriptyline 10 mg/5mL (as hydrochloride).

Motipress *(Squibb, UK)*. *Tablets*, nortriptyline 30 mg (as hydrochloride), fluphenazine hydrochloride 1.5 mg.

Motival *(Squibb, UK)*. *Tablets*, nortriptyline 10 mg (as hydrochloride), fluphenazine hydrochloride 0.5 mg.

Proprietary Names and Manufacturers

Allegron *(Dista, Austral.; Belg.; Dista, UK)*; Altilev *(Fr.)*; Ateben *(Arg.)*; Aventyl *(Austral.; Lilly, Canad.; Lilly, S.Afr.; Lilly, UK; Lilly, USA)*; Kareon *(Arg.)*; Martimil *(Lafarquim, Spain)*; Noritren *(Lundbeck, Denm.; Recordati, Ital.; Lundbeck, Norw.; Lundbeck, Swed.)*; Nortab *(Squibb, Austral.)*; Nortrilen *(Belg.; Tropon, Ger.; Lundbeck, S.Afr.; Lundbeck, Switz.)*; Pamelor *(Sandoz, USA)*; Paxtibi *(Dista, Spain)*; Psychostyl *(Fr.)*; Sensaval *(Pharmacia, Swed.)*; Sensival *(Pharmacia, Denm.; Jpn; Switz.)*; Vividyl *(Lilly, Ital.)*.

2531-e

Noxiptyline Hydrochloride *(BANM).*
Bay-1521; Dibenzoxine Hydrochloride; Noxiptiline Hydrochloride *(rINNM).* 2-(10,11-Dihydro-5*H*-dibenzo-[*a,d*]cyclohepten-5-ylideneamino-oxy)ethyldimethylamine hydrochloride.
$C_{19}H_{22}N_2O,HCl=330.9$.

CAS — 3362-45-6 (noxiptyline); 4985-15-3 (hydrochloride).

Noxiptyline is a tricyclic antidepressant with actions and uses similar to those of amitriptyline (p.354).
In the treatment of depression noxiptyline has been given by mouth as the hydrochloride in doses of 10 to 150 mg daily; in hospital patients up to 200 mg daily has been given. It has also been given by intramuscular injection.
Nornoxiptyline has also been tried as an antidepressant.

Proprietary Names and Manufacturers
Agedal *(Dolorgiet, Ger.; Bayer, Ital.)*; Nogêdal *(Thér-aplix, Fr.).*

2532-l

Opipramol Hydrochloride *(BANM, USAN, rINNM).*
G-33040. 2-[4-(3-5*H*-Dibenz[*b,f*]azepin-5-ylpropyl)piper-azin-1-yl]ethanol dihydrochloride.
$C_{23}H_{29}N_3O,2HCl=436.4$.

CAS — 315-72-0 (opipramol); 909-39-7 (hydrochloride).

Opipramol is a tricyclic antidepressant with actions and uses similar to those of amitriptyline (p.354). Opipramol hydrochloride has been given in doses of 150 to 300 mg daily.

Proprietary Names and Manufacturers
Ensidon *(Geigy, Swed.)*; Insidon *(Geigy, Austral.; Geigy, Belg.; Geigy, Denm.; Geigy, Eire; Geigy, Fr.; Geigy, Ger.; Geigy, Ital.; Geigy, Neth.; Geigy, Norw.; Geigy, Switz.; Geigy, UK)*; Nisidana *(Padro, Spain).*

13054-f

Oxaprotiline Hydrochloride *(USAN, rINNM).*
C-49802B-Ba; CGP-12104. (±)-1-(9,10-Dihydro-9,10-ethanoanthracen-9-yl)-3-methylaminopropan-2-ol hydrochloride.
$C_{20}H_{23}NO,HCl=329.9$.

CAS — 56433-44-4 (oxaprotiline); 39022-39-4 (hydrochloride).

Oxaprotiline hydrochloride is a tetracyclic antidepressant. It is a hydroxylated derivative of maprotiline. Antimuscarinic side-effects have been reported.

The actions and uses of oxaprotiline: N.F. Damlouji *et al.*, in *Pharmacotherapy of Affective Disorders: Theory and Practice*, W.G. Dewhurst and G.B. Baker (Eds.), London, Croom Helm, 1985, p.286..

DEPRESSION. In the treatment of depression, oxaprotiline has been shown to be as effective as fluvoxamine (H.M. Emrich *et al., Pharmacopsychiatry*, 1987, *20*, 60) and maprotiline (M. Schmauss *et al., Curr. ther. Res.*, 1987, *41*, 342). Although one study found oxaprotiline to be as effective as amitriptyline (M. Roffman *et al., ibid.*, 1982, *32*, 247), a later study found it to be less effective (H. Geidke *et al., Eur. Arch. Psychiatry neurol. Sci.*, 1986, *235*, 329).

Proprietary Names and Manufacturers
Ciba-Geigy, USA.

12836-r

Oxitriptan *(rINN).*
5-HTP; Ro-0783/B; L-5-Hydroxytryptophan. L-2-Amino-3-(5-hydroxy-1*H*-indol-3-yl)propionic acid.
$C_{11}H_{12}N_2O_3=220.2$.

CAS — 4350-09-8; 56-69-9 (DL-5-Hydroxytryptophan).

5-Hydroxytryptophan is a precursor of serotonin (see p.1611). The L form as oxitriptan has been given in the treatment of depression sometimes with a peripheral decarboxylase inhibitor such as carbidopa. Adverse effects include gastro-intestinal effects and central stimulation. Neurotoxicity has also been reported. The concomitant use of a peripheral decarboxylase inhibitor is intended to reduce oxitriptan's peripheral adverse effects as well as increase the amount taken up by the brain.
Oxitriptan has also been tried in myoclonic disorders especially post-hypoxic myoclonus.
DL-5-Hydroxytryptophan has also been tried as an antidepressant.

Changes in mood, mostly elevation, were observed in 7 neurological patients without affective disorders and 1 healthy subject given oxitriptan 100 to 300 mg by intravenous infusion in sodium chloride injection. Carbidopa was also given to reduce the severity of vomiting which always occurred 30 to 90 minutes after infusion and to increase the amount of oxitriptan entering the brain. Neurotoxicity occurred with doses of 200 mg and above and included dilatation of the pupil, hyperreflexia, ataxia, and dysarthria. There was some similarity to the effects of alcohol.— M. Trimble *et al.* (letter), *Lancet*, 1975, *1*, 583. See also M. H. Greenwood *et al., Br. J. clin. Pharmac.*, 1975, *2*, 165.

ANXIETY AND PHOBIAS. In a double-blind study of 45 patients with phobic disorders treated for 8 weeks with oxitriptan, clomipramine (both in doses of 25 to 150 mg daily), or placebo by mouth, it was concluded that whilst clomipramine was highly effective in the treatment of anxiety disorders, oxitriptan showed moderate efficacy.— R. S. Kahn *et al., Int. clin. Psychopharmacol.*, 1987, *2*, 33.

BEHAVIOUR DISORDERS. The self-mutilation associated with the Lesch-Nyhan syndrome, an inborn error of purine metabolism, was abolished by oxitriptan in 4 patients.— T. -I. Mizuno and Y. Yugari (letter), *Lancet*, 1974, *1*, 761.

Administration of oxitriptan 1.6 g daily in divided doses with carbidopa 75 mg four times daily controlled the tics, vocalisations and self-mutilation in a 15-year-old boy with Gilles de la Tourette syndrome. Lip and buccal ulcers healed and it was possible to reduce major and minor tranquilliser therapy. Symptoms recurred during 3 periods of placebo therapy.— M. H. Van Woert *et al., New Engl. J. Med.*, 1977, *296*, 210.

Further references: C. D. Frith *et al., J. Neurol. Neurosurg. Psychiat.*, 1976, *39*, 656.

DEPRESSION. Oxitriptan has been shown to have equivocal beneficial effects in depression (N.S. Kline *et al., Am. J. Psychiat.*, 1964, *121*, 379; T. Persson and B.-E. Roos, *Lancet*, 1967, *2*, 987; I. Sano, *Münch. med. Wschr.*, 1972, *114*, 1713; G. d'Elia *et al., Acta psychiat. scand.*, 1978, *57*, 239; L.J. van Hiele, *Neuropsychobiology*, 1980, *6*, 230; W.F. Byerley *et al., J. clin. Psychopharmacol.*, 1987, *7*, 127). In one study of patients with depression unresponsive to oxaprotiline, fluvoxamine, and sleep deprivation, subsequent therapy with oxitriptan was significantly less effective than treatment with tranylcypromine (W.A. Nolen *et al., Br. J. Psychiat.*, 1985, *147*, 16).

Combination therapy with clomipramine. For a study showing combined therapy with oxitriptan and clomipramine to be more effective in relieving depressive symptoms than clomipramine alone, see under Clomipramine Hydrochloride, p.358.

EXTRAPYRAMIDAL DISORDERS. *Myoclonus.* Comment on the use of oxitriptan in the treatment of myoclonus and the view that in general its use should be discouraged. Oxitriptan is usually effective in posthypoxic intention myoclonus, a rare condition, but may exacerbate some other myoclonic syndromes. Significant adverse effects, especially gastro-intestinal disturbances, are almost universal, even when given with a peripheral decarboxylase inhibitor such as carbidopa.— R. R. Young, *J. Am. med. Ass.*, 1980, *243*, 1569.

Oxitriptan with carbidopa was administered to 23 patients with myoclonus and 16 patients with other neurological disorders. Following administration by mouth of maximum doses of 0.4 to 2 g daily with carbidopa 100 to 300 mg daily more than 50% improvement was obtained in 11 of 18 patients with intention myoclonus due to anoxia or other brain damage; only 1 patient obtained no improvement and in 3 it was 90% or more; some patients derived sustained benefit for more than 3 years. No benefit was obtained by 2 patients with athetotic cerebral palsy, 2 with multiple sclerosis, 2 with essential tremor, 4 with cerebellar intention tremor, 1 with infantile spasms, 2 with dystonia musculorum deformans, 2 with central pain syndromes, or 3 with idiopathic epilepsy; some benefit was obtained in 1 patient with myoclonus epilepsy and in 1 of 2 patients with familial essential myoclonus. Side-effects included anorexia, nausea, diarrhoea, and occasional vomiting. Prior administration of carbidopa for 1 or 2 days before therapy reduced the gastro-intestinal side-effects. During the first week of therapy 3 patients developed dyspnoea followed by hyperventilation and lightheadedness, with fainting in 1; pulmonary function tests remained normal. Varying degrees of mental stimulation occurred in 10 patients; these were reversible on dosage reduction and frequently disappeared or diminished after 4 to 6 weeks without reduction, but 2 patients required concurrent administration of perphenazine to maintain their antimyoclonic dosage. Other side-effects included mydriasis, blurring of vision, abdominal pain, and bradycardia.— M. H. Van Woert *et al., New Engl. J. Med.*, 1977, *296*, 70. Comment.— T. L. Munsat, *ibid.*, 101.

Studies suggesting that the treatment of intention myoclonus with oxitriptan and carbidopa in a 70-year-old man unmasked an abnormality in his ability to metabolise kynurenine and resulted in the development of a scleroderma-like illness.— E. M. Sternberg *et al., New Engl. J. Med.*, 1980, *303*, 782.

Further references: D. Chadwick *et al., Lancet*, 1975, *2*, 434; J. DeLéan and J. C. Richardson (letter), *ibid.*, 870; J. H. Growdon *et al., Neurology*, 1976, *26*, 1135; W. M. Carroll and P. J. Walsh, *Br. med. J.*, 1978, *2*, 1612.

Parkinsonism. Following administration of oxitriptan and a peripheral decarboxylase inhibitor to 7 parkinsonian patients significant increase in bradykinesia and rigidity occurred together with an exacerbation of functional disability.— T. N. Chase *et al., Neurology*, 1972, *22*, 479. See also T. N. Chase (letter), *Lancet*, 1970, *2*, 1029.

An antidepressant and tremor-decreasing effect was noted in the majority of 13 patients with Parkinson's disease after administration of oxitriptan by mouth. Any effect on muscle rigidity was difficult to evaluate.— I. Sano and K. Taniguchi, *Münch. med. Wschr.*, 1972, *114*, 1717.

MANGANESE POISONING. A beneficial response to DL-5-hydroxytryptophan, up to 3 g daily, was achieved in a patient in whom the symptoms of manganese poisoning failed to respond to levodopa.— I. Mena *et al., New Engl. J. Med.*, 1970, *282*, 5.

PHOBIA. See under Anxiety and Phobias, above.

PSYCHOSIS. After oral administration of oxitriptan with a peripheral decarboxylase inhibitor, mild to moderate improvement was obtained in 6 of 7 chronic undifferentiated schizophrenic patients who were resistant to phenothiazines. Of 4 chronic paranoid schizophrenic patients who were resistant to phenothiazines 2 became worse after treatment with oxitriptan and 1 improved. Some schizophrenic patients might have an abnormality in serotonin metabolism.— R. J. Wyatt *et al., Science*, 1972, *177*, 1124.

Further studies in schizophrenia: V. Zarcone *et al., Archs gen. Psychiat.*, 1973, *28*, 843; R. J. Wyatt *et al., ibid.*, *29*, 597.

SLEEP DISORDERS. Severe insomnia in a 33-year-old woman following a road accident responded to 4 consecutive nightly doses of oxitriptan totalling 3 g.— M. Webb and J. G. Kirker (letter), *Lancet*, 1981, *1*, 1365.

Proprietary Names and Manufacturers of Oxitriptan or Racemic 5-Hydroxytryptophan
Cincofarm *(Farma-Lepori, Spain)*; Dromia *(Knoll-Made, Spain)*; Lévotonine *(Pan Medica, Fr.)*; Levothym *(Karlspharma, Ger.)*; Natil *(Nativelle, Ital.)*; Oxyfan *(Coli, Ital.)*; Prétonine *(Synthelabo, Fr.)*; Quiétim *(Nativelle, Fr.)*; Serotonyl *(ICT-Lodi, Ital.)*; Telesol *(Lasa, Spain)*; Trimag *(Magis, Ital.)*; Triptene *(IRBI, Ital.)*; Tript-OH *(Sigmatau, Ital.).*

18670-k

Paroxetine Hydrochloride *(BANM, rINNM).*
BRL-29060; BRL-29060A (hydrochloride); FG-7051. (-)-*trans*-5-(4-*p*-Fluorophenyl-3-piperidylmethoxy)-1,3-benzodioxole hydrochloride.
$C_{19}H_{20}FNO_3,HCl=365.8$.

CAS — 61869-08-7 (paroxetine).

Paroxetine is an antidepressant which selectively inhibits the re-uptake of serotonin.

References to the actions and uses of paroxetine: N.F. Damlouji *et al.*, in *Pharmacotherapy of Affective Disorders: Theory and Practice*, W.G. Dewhurst and G.B. Baker (Eds.), London, Croom Helm, 1985, p.286..

In 12 subjects, paroxetine compared to placebo, caused more frequent awakening, reduced total sleep, and strongly suppressed REM sleep. When taken in the morning, paroxetine also delayed sleep onset and increased slow wave sleep.— I. Oswald and K. Adam,

Br. J. clin. Pharmac., 1986, *22*, 97.

DEPRESSION. In the treatment of depression, paroxetine has been shown to be as effective as amitriptyline. Side-effects reported included sweating, tiredness, difficulty in concentrating, dry mouth, and irritability.— R. Battegay *et al.*, *Neuropsychobiology*, 1985, *13*, 31.

MYOCLONUS. Mention of the unsuccessful use of paroxetine in severe resistant myoclonus.— K. Mondrup *et al.* (letter), *Lancet*, 1983, *2*, 1490.

Proprietary Names and Manufacturers
Aropax *(Beecham Laboratories, USA)*.

2533-y

Phenelzine Sulphate *(BANM, pINNM)*.

Phenelzine Sulfate *(USAN)*. Phenethylhydrazine hydrogen sulphate.
$C_8H_{12}N_2,H_2SO_4$=234.3.

CAS — 51-71-8 (phenelzine); 156-51-4 (sulphate).

Pharmacopoeias. In *Br.*, *Egypt.*, and *U.S.*

A white or yellowish-white powder or pearly platelets with a pungent odour. Phenelzine 15 mg is approximately equivalent to 25 mg of phenelzine sulphate. **Soluble** 1 in 7 of water; practically insoluble in alcohol, chloroform, and ether. A 1% solution has a pH of 1.4 to 1.9. **Store** in a cool place in airtight containers. Protect from light.

Adverse Effects

Adverse effects commonly associated with phenelzine and other monoamine oxidase inhibitors include orthostatic hypotension and attacks of dizziness. Other common side-effects include drowsiness, headache, weakness and fatigue, dryness of mouth, constipation and other gastro-intestinal disturbances (including nausea and vomiting), and oedema. Agitation and tremors, nervousness, insomnia and restless sleep, blurred vision, difficulty in micturition, hyperhidrosis, convulsions, skin rashes, leucopenia, sexual disturbances, delirium, and weight gain with inappropriate appetite may also occur. Psychotic episodes, with hypomanic behaviour, confusion, and hallucinations, may be induced in susceptible persons. Jaundice has been reported with hydrazine monoamine oxidase inhibitors and, on rare occasions, fatal progressive hepatocellular necrosis. Peripheral neuropathies associated with the hydrazine derivatives may be due to pyridoxine deficiency.

Symptoms of overdosage may not occur for some hours after ingestion. They include agitation with hyperactivity and hallucinations, tachycardia, hypertension sometimes with severe headache (hypotension may also develop), hyperreflexia and spasticity, profuse sweating and hyperthermia, dilated pupils, urinary retention, coma, convulsions, and signs of peripheral collapse.

A severe hypertensive crisis, sometimes fatal, may occur if a monoamine oxidase inhibitor is given simultaneously with some other drugs or cheese and certain other foods (see Precautions). These reactions are characterised by severe headache, a rapid and sometimes prolonged rise in blood pressure followed by intracranial haemorrhage or acute cardiac failure.

Seventy-four patients were treated with either phenelzine or imipramine in a double-blind study, at mean daily doses of 77 mg and 139 mg respectively, for 3 to 5 weeks. With the exception of significantly increased drowsiness in the phenelzine-treated group, the 2 groups did not differ in the frequency of autonomic, central nervous system, cardiovascular, or psychological side-effects. However, a significantly greater number of phenelzine-treated patients had to discontinue their treatment due to the severity of the side-effects.— D. L. Evans *et al.*, *J. clin. Psychopharmacol.*, 1982, *2*, 208.

EFFECTS ON THE BLOOD. Phenelzine has been reported to cause aplastic anaemia.— R. H. Girdwood, *Drugs*, 1976, *11*, 394.

EFFECTS ON THE CARDIOVASCULAR SYSTEM. Monoamine oxidase inhibitors are generally free of adverse cardiovascular effects, though orthostatic hypotension may be an occasional problem. However, the propensity of monoamine oxidase inhibitors to cause a hypertensive crisis in patients given direct-acting sympathomimetic amines or foods containing tyramine should not be forgotten.— M. L. Orme, *Br. med. J.*, 1984, *289*, 1.

In a study of 14 patients phenelzine produced both a significant decrease in lying systolic blood pressure and significant orthostatic hypotension. Two patients required modification of their treatment regimens due to orthostatic hypotension. Both the maximum orthostatic drop and the maximum decrease in lying systolic blood pressure occurred after 4 weeks on phenelzine, but it was suggested that the orthostatic effect may attenuate after 4 weeks.— M. H. Kronig *et al.*, *J. clin. Psychopharmacol.*, 1983, *3*, 307.

EFFECTS ON THE ENDOCRINE SYSTEM. Drug-induced hyperprolactinaemia may result from the administration of monoamine oxidase inhibitors (P.H. Baylis, *Adv. Drug React. Bull.*, 1986, *116*, 432) and this has led to galactorrhoea in women (M. Segal and R.F. Heys, *Br. med. J.*, 1969, *4*, 236). Occasionally, monoamine oxidase inhibitors may cause dilutional hyponatraemia due to a reduction in the renal excretion of free water mediated by both enhanced vasopressin release and increased antidiuretic action on the renal tubule (P.H. Baylis, 1986).

EFFECTS ON THE LIVER. Jaundice developed in 4 patients on 6 occasions following the administration of monoamine oxidase inhibitors. The drugs implicated were as follows: phenelzine 6.3 g over 5 months; pheniprazine, 2.5 g over 7 months, 560 mg over 60 days, 1.5 g—no time stated; nialamide 1.6 g over 3 weeks; iproniazid—no dose or time stated.— C. D. Holdsworth *et al.*, *Lancet*, 1961, *2*, 621.

A mention of 2 patients with hepatic failure, progressing to encephalopathy, attributed to a hypersensitivity reaction after administration of monoamine oxidase inhibitors.— S. P. Wilkinson *et al.*, *Br. med. J.*, 1974, *1*, 186.

Angiosarcoma of the liver in a 64-year-old woman who had taken phenelzine for 6 years was possibly drug-related; such a relationship had been reported in *mice*.— T. K. Daneshmend *et al.*, *Br. med. J.*, 1979, *1*, 1679.

EFFECTS ON THE NERVOUS SYSTEM. A myaesthenic syndrome of postoperative respiratory depression has been reported in patients taking phenelzine.— R. J. M. Lane and P. A. Routledge, *Drugs*, 1983, *26*, 124.

A report of sensorimotor peripheral neuropathy and pyridoxine deficiency in a 50-year-old woman treated with phenelzine 45 mg daily for 11 years.— C. A. Heller and P. A. Friedman, *Am. J. Med.*, 1983, *75*, 887.

Six patients developed symptoms of pyridoxine deficiency (numbness, paraesthesias, puffy hands) while taking phenelzine. All had low pyridoxine levels, 5 being abnormally low. In all patients, symptoms responded to the addition of pyridoxine while continuing phenelzine therapy. Electric shock-like sensations in 3 patients continued in 2 in spite of the addition of pyridoxine, but abated upon discontinuation of phenelzine.— J. W. Stewart *et al.*, *J. clin. Psychopharmacol.*, 1984, *4*, 225.

For further effects on the nervous system, see under Epileptogenic Effect and Extrapyramidal Effects, below.

EFFECTS ON SEXUAL FUNCTION. The monoamine oxidase inhibitors phenelzine, tranylcypromine, and isocarboxazid can produce both impotence and failure of ejaculation. Priapism has been reported with phenelzine (V.K. Yeragani and S. Gershon, *New Engl. J. Med.*, 1987, *317*, 117). There have also been several reports of anorgasmia in women attributed to monoamine oxidase inhibitors and, at least in the case of phenelzine, this effect seems to be dose-related (L. Beeley, *Adverse Drug React. Ac. Pois. Rev.*, 1984, *3*, 23). It should be remembered that loss of libido and impotence are common symptoms of depression, often making the role of drugs in producing sexual dysfunction difficult to assess. However, when due to depression, these symptoms usually improve with effective treatment (L. Beeley, 1984; *idem, Prescribers' J.*, 1982, *22*, 84).

Spermatogenesis. Monoamine oxidase inhibitors produce an initial transient increase in the sperm count, but this is followed by a profound drop almost to azoospermic levels, with a high percentage of abnormal cells.— B. H. Stewart, *Drug Ther.*, 1975, *156*, 42.

EPILEPTOGENIC EFFECT. A 46-year-old man with no history of epilepsy or predisposing factors experienced a grand mal seizure with tonic-clonic convulsions after 3 days of treatment with phenelzine 15 mg daily.— D. K. Bhugra and N. Kaye, *Br. J. clin. Pract.*, 1986, *40*, 173.

EXTRAPYRAMIDAL EFFECTS. A parkinsonian syndrome developed in a 42-year-old woman after the administration of phenelzine 15 mg twice daily for 2 weeks followed by 30 mg twice daily for 3 weeks. Symptoms resolved gradually over the 10 days following withdrawal of phenelzine.— M. A. Gillman and R. Sandyk, *Postgrad. med. J.*, 1986, *62*, 235.

LUPUS. A reversible lupus-like reaction developed in a 66-year-old woman who had been taking phenelzine sulphate for 8 months.— C. Swartz, *J. Am. med. Ass.*, 1978, *239*, 2693.

OVERDOSAGE. Monoamine oxidase inhibitors and tricyclic antidepressants can precipitate hyperthermia both singly, and more commonly in combination, especially when taken in overdose.— P. G. Blain and M. D. Rawlins, *Prescribers' J.*, 1981, *21*, 204.

Monoamine oxidase inhibitors in overdose rarely produce severe hypertension. More commonly the patient gradually develops widespread muscle spasms, trismus, and opisthotonus with widely dilated pupils and a hot and sweating skin. By approximately 16 to 24 hours after ingestion body temperature may increase to a point where hyperthermia can be fatal, unless neuromuscular blocking agents are given; temperatures of 42.1 to 43.8° have been recorded immediately before death. Disseminated intravascular coagulation, rhabdomyolysis, and acute tubular necrosis can also occur. It is recommended that the temperature of a patient who has taken an overdose of a monoamine oxidase inhibitor should be closely monitored, and if the rectal temperature increases to more than 39°, the trachea should be intubated and the patient's lungs ventilated using pancuronium bromide as a neuromuscular blocking agent; this produces a dramatic decrease in temperature.— J. A. Henry, *Br. J. Anaesth.*, 1986, *58*, 223.

A report of fatal disseminated intravascular coagulation following an overdose of phenelzine 450 mg.— T. E. McAlindon (letter), *Br. med. J.*, 1986, *293*, 1103.

Treatment of Adverse Effects

The stomach should be emptied by aspiration and lavage. Supportive therapy should be instituted, special care being taken with any drug therapy, in view of the many hazards of monoamine oxidase inhibitor interactions. In particular, sympathomimetic agents are not suitable for the treatment of hypotension, which should be managed with intravenous fluids and, in severe shock, intravenous hydrocortisone.

Chlorpromazine is indicated for restlessness and agitation, and also to combat hyperthermia unresponsive to mechanical cooling, but hypotension may occur. Severe hyperthermia may call for a muscle relaxant and intubation with assisted ventilation. Morphine, pethidine, and other opioid analgesics should be avoided.

Hypertensive crises associated with monoamine oxidase inhibitor overdosage or with a food or drug interaction, should be treated urgently with slow intravenous injection of phentolamine mesylate or phenoxybenzamine. Pentolinium has also been recommended, and chlorpromazine or tolazoline may be of value if more effective treatments are not available. It has been suggested that haemodialysis may be of value in very severely poisoned patients.

The acute effects of monoamine oxidase inhibitor overdosage may be followed by the delayed effects of monoamine oxidase inhibition which do not develop until several days later.

Reviews of monoamine oxidase inhibitor overdose and its treatment: C. H. Linden *et al.*, *Ann. emerg. Med.*, 1984, *13*, 1137; A. T. Proudfoot, *Prescribers' J.*, 1986, *26*, 97.

Labetalol hydrochloride 20 mg given intravenously over 5 minutes lowered blood pressure and reversed reflex bradycardia in a 33-year-old woman with severe, accelerated hypertension secondary to an interaction between a monoamine oxidase inhibitor and monoamine-containing food.— J. H. Abrams *et al.* (letter), *New Engl. J. Med.*, 1985, *313*, 52.

A 33-year-old man developed a fulminant hypermetabolic reaction with hyperpyrexia, diffuse muscle rigidity and diaphoresis following a drug overdose including up to 2.25 g of phenelzine. Haemodialysis decreased the patient's serum phenelzine concentration, but his clinical status did not improve, even after cooling blankets and paracetamol. Within 30 minutes of receiving an intravenous injection of dantrolene sodium 2.5 mg per kg body-weight however, muscle rigidity, trismus, tachycardia, hyperthermia, and metabolic acidosis dramatically resolved. The patient received the same dose of dantrolene sodium intravenously 6 hourly for 24 hours, then orally for another 18 hours, and subsequently recovered without evidence of any neurological deficit.— R. F. Kaplan *et al.*, *J. Am. med. Ass.*, 1986, *255*, 642.

It was suggested that patients who may have ingested a benzodiazepine concomitantly with a monoamine oxidase inhibitor in overdose should be observed for 36 hours, since the early signs of monoamine oxidase inhibitor toxicity (hyperreflexia, hypertension, tachycardia, hyperpyrexia) may be masked by the benzodiazepine.— S. Young and B. G. Walpole (letter), *Med. J. Aust.*, 1986, *144*, 166.

See also Overdosage under Adverse Effects.

Precautions

Phenelzine and other monoamine oxidase inhibitors should not be given to patients with liver disease or blood dyscrasias, or, because of their effects on blood pressure, to patients with cerebrovascular disease or phaeochromocytoma. They should be avoided or only used with great caution in patients with cardiovascular disease; masking of pain may occur in those with angina pectoris. Monoamine oxidase inhibitors should similarly be avoided or used with great caution in elderly or agitated patients or those with diminished renal function, who may be particularly susceptible to their adverse effects. They should be given with caution in epileptic patients since they may influence the incidence of seizures and affect anticonvulsant requirements; they may also affect insulin requirements in diabetic subjects.

Monoamine oxidase inhibitors may activate psychosis in susceptible patients and manic-depressive patients may switch to a manic phase; patients with suicidal tendencies should be carefully supervised during treatment.

Monoamine oxidase inhibitors have a prolonged action so patients should not take any of the foods or drugs known to cause reactions (see below) for at least 14 days after stopping treatment. A similar drug-free period should elapse before any patient undergoes surgery since it may involve the use of agents which can interact with monoamine oxidase inhibitors. Patients should carry cards giving details of their monoamine oxidase inhibitor therapy; they and their relatives should be fully conversant with the implications of food and drug interactions and the precautions to be taken.

Patients liable to take charge of vehicles or other machinery should be warned that monoamine oxidase inhibitors may modify behaviour and state of alertness. Patients affected by drowsiness should not drive or operate machinery. For further details of the effects of antidepressant therapy on driving see Amitriptyline Hydrochloride (p.353).

ECT. For a recommendation that treatment with monoamine oxidase inhibitors should be stopped 2 weeks prior to ECT, see Amitriptyline Hydrochloride, p.353.

GLAUCOMA. For a report suggesting that monoamine oxidase inhibitors are not contra-indicated in primary glaucomatous conditions, see Amitriptyline Hydrochloride, p.353.

INTERACTIONS. For interactions of monoamine oxidase inhibitors with foods and with other drugs, see below.

INTERFERENCE WITH DIAGNOSTIC TESTS. Abnormally low values of urinary 4-hydroxy-3-methoxymandelic acid and abnormally high values of urinary metadrenaline found in patients given monoamine oxidase inhibitors could affect adrenal medullary tests for phaeochromocytoma.— *Adverse Drug React. Bull.*, 1972, June, 104. See also *Drug & Ther. Bull.*, 1972, *10*, 69.

MANIA. Hypomania and mania can begin within a week of starting antidepressant therapy; the switch from depression into mania may be remarkably quick. It has been estimated that the risk of occurrence of hypomanic and manic reactions is 11% with monoamine oxidase inhibitors (tranylcypromine carries a greater risk that phenelzine), and about 8% with tricyclic antidepressants. It seems probable that serious manic reactions are mainly limited to those with bipolar predisposition.— H. A. McClelland, *Adverse Drug React. Bull.*, 1986, *119*, 444.

For a suggestion that the mania or hypomania caused by antidepressants may be refractory to lithium, see Lithium Carbonate p.367.

PORPHYRIA. Phenelzine was considered to be unsafe in patients with acute porphyrias because it has been shown to be porphyrinogenic in *animals* or *in vitro* systems.— M.R. Moore and K.E.L. McColl, *Porphyrias, Drug Lists*, Glasgow, Porphyria Research Unit, University of Glasgow, 1987.

PREGNANCY AND THE NEONATE. In a study in 836 infants with congenital malformations there was no significant difference in the maternal usage of monoamine oxidase inhibitors during the first trimester of pregnancy compared with the use in 836 controls.— G. Greenberg *et al.*, *Br. med. J.*, 1977, *2*, 853.

SURGERY. Monoamine oxidase inhibitors can predispose to hypertensive crisis if an opioid is given. Pethidine can also cause fatal hypotension and must not be given, but morphine may be used with great caution: a small intravenous test dose is given first (e.g. 10% of the required dose), and gradually increased until an effective dose is reached. Adrenaline, as a local vasoconstrictor, presents no extra risk in patients taking a monoamine oxidase inhibitor, but other sympathomimetic drugs are best avoided to prevent hypertensive crises. All these problems can be avoided by withdrawing the monoamine oxidase inhibitor for at least 2 weeks before surgery and substituting a different antidepressant. However, this may be considered undesirable for the chronically depressed patient who may respond only to a monoamine oxidase inhibitor and who has taken many months to stabilise. Changing to a tricyclic antidepressant may also be dangerous since the combination with a monoamine oxidase inhibitor can be hazardous.— *Drug & Ther. Bull.*, 1984, *22*, 73.

For a report of postoperative respiratory depression in patients taking phenelzine see Effects on the Nervous System under Adverse Effects, above.

TOLERANCE. Occasionally, patients will respond initially to a monoamine oxidase inhibitor, become refractory after several months, then derive further benefit from a dosage increase, often as high as 120 mg daily for phenelzine sulphate and 60 mg daily for tranylcypromine sulphate. Some may become completely refractory but will respond again if use of the monoamine oxidase inhibitor is discontinued for a month and then started again at a lower dosage.— D. S. Robinson, *J. Am. med. Ass.*, 1983, *250*, 2212.

For a further report of tolerance to antidepressants, including monoamine oxidase inhibitors, see Amitriptyline Hydrochloride, p.354.

WITHDRAWAL SYNDROMES. For a description of withdrawal syndromes seen after the discontinuation of monoamine oxidase inhibitors, and precautions to be taken to avoid such syndromes, see Amitriptyline Hydrochloride, p.354.

Interactions with Monoamine Oxidase Inhibitors and Foods

Reactions to foods rich in pressor amines can occur in patients being treated with monoamine oxidase inhibitors, producing hypertensive crises due to inhibition of the metabolism of the amines and enhancement of their pressor activity. Cheese, especially cheddar cheese, hydrolysed meat or yeast protein extracts such as Bovril, Marmite, or Oxo, which contain tyramine, and broad bean pods which contain levodopa have caused such reactions. Game contains tyramine and can also cause reactions, as can pickled herrings or liver that has been improperly stored. Patients should be warned not to eat any of these foods while being treated with a monoamine oxidase inhibitor and for at least 14 days after its discontinuation.

Any protein-containing food subject to hydrolysis, fermentation, pickling, smoking, or spoilage could contain tyramine derived from tyrosine as a result of these processes or of deterioration. Patients taking monoamine oxidase inhibitors should therefore be advised to eat protein-containing foods only if fresh.

Alcohol should be avoided, although some clinicians consider that small amounts of white wine or clear spirit are acceptable. Chianti has been implicated as a special risk because of its high tyramine content, but there are indications that this tyramine content has been reduced with modern production techniques.

It has been estimated that 6 to 25 mg of tyramine needs to be ingested to produce a reaction (D. Horwitz *et al.*, *J. Am. med. Ass.*, 1964, *188*, 1108; E. Marley and B. Blackwell, pp. 185-239 in *Advances in Pharmacology and Chemotherapy*, S. Garattini *et al.* (Eds), Vol. 8, London, Academic Press, 1970). Some foods will therefore only cause a reaction if large amounts are eaten, and foods may vary in tyramine content depending upon methods of manufacture and storage; isolated reports have implicated avocados, banana peel and rotten bananas, high protein foods such as Complan, nuts, soya sauce (M.M. Stewart, *Adv. Drug React. Bull.*, 1976, *Jun.*, 200), caviar (P. Isaac *et al.*, *Lancet*, 1977, *2*, 816), large quantities of New Zealand Prickly Spinach (A. Comfort, *Lancet*, 1981, *2*, 472), and nonalcoholic beer (R. Draper *et al.*, *Br. med. J.*, 1984, *289*, 308). Chocolate and some beverages now appear to be considered as risk factors because of their caffeine content.

Analyses of the amine content of foods: D. Horwitz *et al.*, *J. Am. med. Ass.*, 1964, *188*, 1108; N. P. Sen, *J. Fd Sci.*, 1969, *34*, 22; E. Marley and B. Blackwell, in *Advances in Pharmacology and Chemotherapy*, S. Garattini *et al.* (Eds), Vol. 8, London, Academic Press, 1970, pp. 185–239; D. G. Folks, *J. clin. Psychopharmacol.*, 1983, *3*, 249.

Interactions with Monoamine Oxidase Inhibitors and Other Drugs

Reactions to other drugs are very likely in patients treated with monoamine oxidase inhibitors.

Severe hypertensive reactions due to enhancement of pressor activity have followed the administration of sympathomimetic agents such as amphetamine, dopamine, ephedrine, levodopa, phenylephrine, and phenylpropanolamine. Reactions may also follow the use of anorectic agents and stimulants with sympathomimetic activity such as fenfluramine and methylphenidate. Adrenaline and noradrenaline in the usual doses of local anaesthetic solutions are no longer considered likely to cause hypertensive reactions in patients taking monoamine oxidase inhibitors unless they already have cardiovascular disease. Monoamine oxidase inhibitors also inhibit other drug-metabolising enzymes; they may enhance the effects of barbiturates and possibly other hypnotics, insulin and other hypoglycaemic agents, and possibly antimuscarinic agents. Alcohol metabolism may be altered and its effects enhanced. Antihypertensive agents including guanethidine, reserpine, and methyldopa should be given with caution; hypotensive and hypertensive reactions have been suggested with different agents; the hypotensive effects of thiazide diuretics may be enhanced.

Severe reactions have been reported in patients receiving tricyclic antidepressants such as amitriptyline while being treated with a monoamine oxidase inhibitor, though drugs from both groups have occasionally been used together; however, the concomitant administration of clomipramine with a monoamine oxidase inhibitor, particularly tranylcypromine, is especially hazardous. Fluvoxamine may potentiate the CNS effects of monoamine oxidase inhibitors. The administration of pethidine and other opioid analgesics to patients taking a monoamine oxidase inhibitor has also been associated with very severe and sometimes fatal reactions. Not every patient will react, so in cases where it is considered essential to use an opioid analgesic a test dose of morphine should be given. If this produces no untoward reaction, the dose of morphine can be gradually and carefully increased. Interactions can also occur between monoamine oxidase inhibitors themselves.

A review of the drug interactions with monoamine oxidase inhibitors.— S. Bazire, *Pharm. J.*, 1986, *1*, 418. Comment. Astemizole was not thought to interact with monoamine oxidase inhibitors.— E. W. Gascoigne and J. Griffiths (letter), *ibid.*, 545.

Alprazolam. For a possible hepatotoxic effect of alprazolam in association with phenelzine, see Alprazolam, p.712.

Antiparkinsonian therapy. For a report of hypertension following the administration of phenelzine to a patient receiving amantadine, see Amantadine, p.1008.

For the effect of monoamine oxidase inhibitors on levodopa therapy, see Levodopa, p.1017.

Dextromethorphan. The ingestion of a cough preparation containing dextromethorphan was probably the cause of death in a 26-year-old woman who had been treated with phenelzine 15 mg four times daily.— N. Rivers and B. Horner (letter), *Can. med. Ass. J.*, 1970, *103,* 85.

Doxapram. For the effect of a monoamine oxidase inhibitor on doxapram, see Doxapram, p.1442.

Hexamethylmelamine. For a report of severe orthostatic hypotension in patients receiving concurrent hexamethylmelamine and phenelzine, see Hexamethylmelamine, p.631.

Pyridoxine. For reports of peripheral neuropathy due to phenelzine-induced pyridoxine deficiency, see Effects on the Nervous System under Adverse Effects, above.

Tricyclic antidepressants. The combination of monoamine oxidase inhibitors with tricyclic antidepressants can result in agitation, delirium, hyperpyrexia, convulsions, and at times, hypertension.— B. H. Guzé and L. R. Baxter, *New Engl. J. Med.*, 1985, *313,* 163. See also E. Marley and K. M. Wozniak, *Psychol. Med.*, 1983, *13,* 735.

An 18-year-old girl being treated with trimipramine 150 mg at night and phenelzine 30 mg twice daily with no unwanted effects experienced nausea, disorientation, restlessness, shivering, hyperthermia, tachypnoea, tachycardia, mydriasis, and had extensor plantar reflexes when inadvertently given imipramine 150 mg instead of trimipramine.— P. M. Graham *et al.* (letter), *Lancet*, 1982, *2,* 440.

Pare *et al.* (*Lancet*, 1982, *2,* 183) found that the administration of amitriptyline greatly decreased the pressor response to intravenous tyramine in patients receiving monoamine oxidase inhibitors. Dothiepin and trimipramine, however, produced little change in sensitivity to tyramine. The safety of the concomitant administration was questioned by Spencer (*ibid.*, 385), who suggested that the combination could dramatically enhance the pressor and other cardiovascular effects of adrenaline and noradrenaline. Further work by Pare *et al.* (*J. Pharm. Pharmac.*, 1984, *36, Suppl.*, 65W) suggested that approximately half the patients receiving combined antidepressants would gain significant protection from oral tyramine, since the amount ingested orally was much greater than that given in the intravenous tyramine pressor test.

Tryptophan. When tryptophan was given by mouth in doses of 20 and 50 mg per kg body-weight concomitantly with a monoamine oxidase inhibitor, a reaction likened to inebriation persisted for several hours. Hyperreflexia and clonus had also occurred. The same dose of tryptophan given alone had produced no objective or subjective reaction.— A. Sjoerdsma *et al.*, *J. Pharmac. exp. Ther.*, 1959, *126,* 217. Further references: J. M. Thomas and E. H. Rubin, *Am. J. Psychiat.*, 1984, *141,* 281; H. G. Pope *et al.*, *ibid.*, 1985, *142,* 491; W. A. Price *et al.*, *J. clin. Pharmac.*, 1986, *26,* 77.

Absorption and Fate

Phenelzine is readily absorbed from the gastro-intestinal tract and is excreted in the urine almost entirely in the form of metabolites.

Although many of the actions of phenelzine are rapid in onset, several days elapse before maximum blockade of monoamine oxidase. Phenelzine itself blocks monoamine oxidase irreversibly but the blockade produced by some other monoamine oxidase inhibitors is reversible. The significance of monoamine oxidase inhibition in relation to the lifting of depression is not clear, but the adverse interactions liable to occur as a result of monoamine oxidase inhibition remain a hazard for about 14 days after discontinuation of the drug, i.e. until fresh supplies of the enzyme have been generated in the body.

There has been much controversy over the role of acetylator phenotype in the handling of phenelzine, but there is no convincing evidence that the drug is, in fact, significantly acetylated.— D. W. J. Clark, *Drugs*, 1985, *29,* 342.

Uses and Administration

Phenelzine is a hydrazine derivative and a non-selective monoamine oxidase inhibitor. Its mode of action in depression is not fully understood.

Phenelzine and other antidepressant monoamine oxidase inhibitors are used in the treatment of neurotic or atypical depression, particularly where phobic features are present, or in patients who have not responded to other antidepressants; they are probably less effective in endogenous depression. Associated anxiety may also respond, but concomitant administration of an anxiolytic, such as a benzodiazepine may also be necessary. Since up to a month may elapse before an antidepressant response is obtained, severely ill patients may require electroconvulsive therapy initially. After a response has been obtained maintenance therapy may need to be continued for several months to avoid relapse on withdrawal. Monoamine oxidase inhibitor therapy is not indicated for children and, where possible, should also be avoided in the elderly. Moreover, it is not suitable for patients considered unable to adhere to the strict dietary requirements necessary for its safe usage.

Phenelzine is given as the sulphate in doses equivalent to phenelzine 15 mg three times daily; if no response has been obtained after 2 weeks the dosage may be increased to 15 mg four times daily; severely depressed hospital patients may be given up to 30 mg thrice daily. Once a response has been obtained the dosage may be gradually reduced for maintenance therapy; some patients may continue to respond to 15 mg on alternate days.

Reviews of the actions and uses of monoamine oxidase inhibitors: *Drugs in Psychiatric Practice*, P.J. Tyrer (Ed.), London, Butterworths, 1982, p.249.; D.L. Murphy *et al.*, in *Pharmacotherapy of Affective Disorders: Theory and Practice*, W.G. Dewhurst and G.B. Baker (Eds), London, Croom Helm, 1985, p.238; B. Jarrott and F. J. E. Vajda, *Med. J. Aust.*, 1987, *146,* 634.

ADMINISTRATION. Monoamine oxidase inhibitors have been considered as ineffective or only weak antidepressants, but the doses previously used, for instance phenelzine 45 mg or isocarboxazid 30 mg daily are now considered too low. Studies of *post mortem* brains, suppression of REM sleep, and platelet monoamine oxidase all show that doses of approximately 75 mg daily for phenelzine and 50 mg daily for isocarboxazid are necessary to produce an adequate pharmacological response in man, and that these doses also result in good antidepressant effect.— C. M. B. Pare, *J. Pharm. Pharmac.*, 1984, *36, Suppl.*, 56W. See also F. M. Quitkin, *Br. J. Psychiat.*, 1985, *147,* 593.

ADMINISTRATION IN RENAL FAILURE. Phenelzine can be given in usual doses to patients with renal failure.— W. M. Bennett *et al.*, *Am. J. Kidney Dis.*, 1983, *3,* 155.

ANXIETY AND PHOBIAS. Monoamine oxidase inhibitors have been shown to provide effective treatment for panic attacks (L. Grunhaus *et al.*, *J. nerv. ment. Dis.*, 1981, *169,* 608; J.T. Brown *et al.*, *Ann. intern. Med.*, 1984, *100,* 558), and panic attacks associated with agoraphobia (J. Buigues and J. Vallejo, *J. clin. Psychiat.*, 1987, *48,* 55). In depressed patients with panic attacks, phenelzine has been shown to be as effective as amitriptyline (D.S. Robinson *et al.*, *Psychopharmac. Bull.*, 1985, *21,* 562) and imipramine (J. Davidson *et al.*, *J. clin. Psychiat.*, 1987, *48,* 143) in relieving depression, but more effective than either in reducing panic attacks. Monoamine oxidase inhibitors are also more effective than beta-blockers in treating recurrent panic attacks (*Med. Lett.*, 1984, *26,* 61).

Controlled studies of monoamine oxidase inhibitors in the treatment of agoraphobia have shown a small but definite benefit. However, patients often relapse on stopping treatment (*Drug & Ther. Bull.*, 1983, *21,* 61).

APHTHOUS STOMATITIS. A report of the successful treatment of aphthous stomatitis in 3 patients with phenelzine. Discontinuation of the drug resulted in recurrence of the lesions.— S. H. Rosenthal (letter), *New Engl. J. Med.*, 1984, *311,* 1442. Comment. The remission in aphthous stomatitis might have been due to the change in dietary habits required to avoid foodstuffs rich in monoamines in patients receiving monoamine oxidase inhibitors.— J. L. Lejonc and V. Fourestie (letter), *ibid.*, 1985, *312,* 859. Reply. Suppression of the ulceration appeared to be quite clearly related to the dose of phenelzine given, and similar preliminary dose-related effects were being seen in patients with herpes simplex. Further research into the potential antiviral properties of phenelzine should be encouraged.— S. H. Rosenthal (letter), *ibid.* Criticism. The lesions of aphthous stomatitis are not considered to be virally mediated. There have been scattered studies and anecdotal reports supporting psychological factors as being predisposing, and this may offer an explanation.— D. E. Becker (letter), *ibid.*, *313,* 330.

BEHAVIOUR DISORDERS. For a report suggesting that monoamine oxidase inhibitors may be useful alternatives to dexamphetamine in the treatment of attention deficit disorder in children, see Tranylcypromine Sulphate, p.381.

DEPRESSION. Reviews of the use of monoamine oxidase inhibitors in depression: G. D. Tollefson, *J. clin. Psychiat.*, 1983, *44,* 280; S. G. Bryant and C. S. Brown, *Clin. Pharm.*, 1986, *5,* 385.

Combination therapy with lithium. For a report of patients with depression refractory to phenelzine but responding with concomitant lithium therapy, see Lithium Carbonate, p.370.

Combination therapy with tricyclic antidepressants. For a report on the combined use of tricyclic antidepressants and monoamine oxidase inhibitors, see Amitriptyline Hydrochloride, p.355.

For comments on the hazards of giving tricyclic antidepressants with monoamine oxidase inhibitors, see under Interactions, above. See also under Amitriptyline Hydrochloride, Precautions, p.353.

Combination therapy with tricyclic antidepressants and central stimulants. For the successful use of combinations of monoamine oxidase inhibitors, tricyclic antidepressants, and central stimulants in treatment-resistant depression, see Amitriptyline Hydrochloride, p.355.

Depression in Alzheimer's disease. For a brief mention of the problem of orthostatic hypotension with the use of monoamine oxidase inhibitors in depressed patients with Alzheimer's disease, see Amitriptyline Hydrochloride, p.355.

Prophylaxis. Two placebo-controlled double-blind studies have found that continuing therapy with phenelzine after initial clinical improvement of depression was effective in preventing relapse or recurrence of depression within a few weeks (W. Harrison *et al.*, *J. clin. Psychiat.*, 1986, *47,* 346; D.S. Robinson *et al.*, *Psychopharmac. Bull.*, 1986, *22,* 553). The study of Robinson *et al.* is aimed at establishing the optimum length of continuation therapy.

EATING DISORDERS. For a review showing phenelzine to be superior to placebo in reducing bulimic symptoms, see Amitriptyline Hydrochloride, p.356.

HEADACHE. Twenty-five patients subject to frequent and severe attacks of migraine, who had not responded to conventional therapy, were treated with phenelzine sulphate 45 mg daily for up to 2 years. Reduction in headache frequency to less than one half of that of the preceding 12 months was noted by 20 patients.— M. Anthony and J. W. Lance, *Archs Neurol., Chicago*, 1969, *21,* 263.

HERPES INFECTION. In an open study, 29 patients with recurrent genital herpes experienced reduction in duration or termination of recurrences, reduced numbers of, and less painful blisters after taking phenelzine 30 to 60 mg daily.— S. H. Rosenthal and W. P. Fitch, *J. clin. Psychopharmacol.*, 1987, *7,* 119.

HYPOTENSION. For studies and comments on the merits and hazards of phenelzine and other monoamine oxidase inhibitors in the management of orthostatic hypotension, see Tyramine Hydrochloride, p.948.

OBSESSIVE COMPULSIVE DISORDERS. In a preliminary study of 7 patients with disabling obsessive thoughts but without major depression, 4 responded well to antidepressants (phenelzine, tranylcypromine, or imipramine).— M. A. Jenike *et al.*, *J. clin. Psychopharmacol.*, 1987, *7,* 33.

PAIN. For a brief mention of the usefulness of antidepressants, including monoamine oxidase inhibitors, in chronic pain, see Amitriptyline Hydrochloride, p.356.

See also under Headache, above.

PHOBIA. For comments on the role of monoamine oxidase inhibitors in the management of phobic states, see under Anxiety and Phobias, above.

PREMATURE EJACULATION. For a report of the successful use of a monoamine oxidase inhibitor in treating premature ejaculation, see Isocarboxazid, p.365.

Preparations

Phenelzine Sulfate Tablets *(U.S.P.).* Contain phenelzine sulphate. Potency is expressed in terms of the equivalent amount of phenelzine.

Phenelzine Tablets *(B.P.).* Tablets containing phenelzine sulphate. Potency is expressed in terms of the equivalent amount of phenelzine.

Proprietary Preparations

Nardil *(Parke, Davis, UK). Tablets,* phenelzine 15 mg (as sulphate).

Proprietary Names and Manufacturers

Nardelzine *(Belg.; Parke, Davis, Spain)*; Nardil *(Warner, Austral.; Parke, Davis, Canad.; Ital.; Warner, S.Afr.; Parke, Davis, UK; Parke, Davis, USA).*

13125-r

Pirandamine Hydrochloride *(USAN, rINNM).*

AY-23713. *NN*-Dimethyl-2-(1,3,4,9-tetrahydro-1-methylindeno[2,1-*c*]pyran-1-yl)ethylamine hydrochloride.

$C_{17}H_{23}NO,HCl=293.8$.

CAS — 42408-79-7 (pirandamine); 42408-78-6 (hydrochloride).

Pirandamine hydrochloride is a tricyclic antidepressant.

Proprietary Names and Manufacturers

Ayerst, USA.

13135-d

Pirlindole Hydrochloride *(rINNM).*

2,3,3a,4,5,6-Hexahydro-8-methyl-1*H*-pyrazino[3,2,1-*jk*]-carbazole hydrochloride.

$C_{15}H_{18}N_2,HCl=262.8$.

CAS — 60762-57-4 (pirlindole); 16154-78-2 (hydrochloride).

Pirlindole hydrochloride is reported to have antidepressant activity.

References: M. D. Mashkovsky and N. I. Andrejeva, *Arzneimittel-Forsch.*, 1981, *31*, 75.

Proprietary Names and Manufacturers

Lifril *(Casen Fisons, Spain)*; Pyrazidol *(USSR).*

13178-e

Propizepine Hydrochloride *(rINNM).*

UP-106 *(propizepine).* 6-(2-Dimethylaminopropyl)-6,11-dihydro-5*H*-pyrido[2,3-*b*][1,5]benzodiazepin-5-one hydrochloride.

$C_{17}H_{20}N_4O,HCl=332.8$.

CAS — 10321-12-7 (propizepine); 14559-79-6 (hydrochloride).

Propizepine hydrochloride is a tricyclic antidepressant with actions and uses similar to those of amitriptyline (p.354). It has been given by mouth in doses of 200 to 300 mg daily in the treatment of depression.

Proprietary Names and Manufacturers

Vagran 50 *(UPSA, Fr.).*

2534-j

Protriptyline Hydrochloride *(BANM, USAN, rINNM).*

MK-240. 3-(5*H*-Dibenzo[*a,d*]cyclohept-5-enyl)propyl(methyl)amine hydrochloride.

$C_{19}H_{21}N,HCl=299.8$.

CAS — 438-60-8 (protriptyline); 1225-55-4 (hydrochloride).

Pharmacopoeias. In *Br.* and *U.S.*

A white to yellowish odourless or almost odourless powder.

Soluble 1 in 2 of water, 1 in 3.5 to 4.5 of alcohol, and 1 in 3 of chloroform; practically insoluble in ether. A 1% solution in water has a pH of 5.0 to 6.5.

Store in well-closed containers.

Adverse Effects, Treatment, and Precautions

As for Amitriptyline Hydrochloride, p.351.

Anxiety, agitation, tachycardia, and hypotension may occur more frequently. Photosensitisation may be more of a problem with protriptyline and patients are recommended to avoid excessive exposure to sunlight or U.V. lamps.

Absorption and Fate

Protriptyline is well but slowly absorbed after oral administration, peak plasma concentrations being achieved after several hours. Since protriptyline slows gastro-intestinal transit-time, absorption can be further delayed in overdosage.

Paths of metabolism of protriptyline include *N*-oxidation and hydroxylation. Protriptyline is excreted in the urine, mainly in the form of its metabolites, either free or in conjugated form.

Protriptyline is widely distributed throughout the body and extensively bound to plasma and tissue protein. Protriptyline has been estimated to have a very prolonged half-life ranging from 55 to 198 hours, which may be further prolonged in overdosage.

Uses and Administration

Protriptyline is a tricyclic antidepressant with actions and uses similar to those of amitriptyline (p.354). It has considerably less marked sedative properties, and may have a stimulant effect; concomitant administration of a tranquilliser may be necessary, particularly in the early stages of therapy.

In the treatment of depression, protriptyline is given by mouth as the hydrochloride in doses of 5 to 10 mg three or four times daily; it has been suggested that dosage increases should be added to the morning dose first, and if insomnia occurs the last dose should be given no later than mid-afternoon; higher doses of up to 60 mg daily may be required in severely depressed hospital patients. A suggested initial dose for adolescents and the elderly is 5 mg three times daily; close monitoring of the cardiovascular system is required if the dose exceeds a total of 20 mg daily in elderly subjects. Since protriptyline has a prolonged half-life, once-daily dosage regimens are also suitable.

EATING DISORDERS. In a double-blind crossover study of 24 non-depressed obese females, protriptyline 5 mg daily by mouth was more effective than placebo in producing weight loss and controlling compulsive eating behaviour.— J. Box *et al.*, *J. psychiatr. Treat. Eval.*, 1983, *5*, 387.

SLEEP DISORDERS. *Narcolepsy.* Although it was found to have relatively poor REM sleep-suppressing properties, protriptyline 10 to 20 mg at bedtime had a beneficial effect in 5 patients with the narcolepsy-cataplexy syndrome and hypersomnia. Several patients noted a tendency for the drug to induce vivid dreaming, particularly in the first 2 weeks of therapy and in one patient the dreaming was sufficiently unpleasant for him to stop therapy.— H. S. Schmidt *et al.*, *Am. J. Psychiat.*, 1977, *134*, 183.

Sleep apnoea. In a double-blind crossover study of 5 men with obstructive sleep apnoea, protriptyline 20 to 30 mg daily markedly reduced daytime somnolence and improved nocturnal oxygenation with no change in body-weight, although the duration and frequency of sleep apnoea were not significantly decreased.— L. G. Brownell *et al.*, *New Engl. J. Med.*, 1982, *307*, 1037.

Protriptyline and other antidepressants reduce the amount of REM sleep, and thus the time during which obstructive apnoeic episodes can occur.— M. C. P. Apps, *Br. J. Hosp. Med.*, 1983, *30*, 339.

Protriptyline should be considered as an alternative to tracheostomy in patients with benign or moderately severe obstructive sleep apnoea, or when tracheostomy is refused. Tracheostomy remains the treatment of choice in patients not responding to protriptyline, despite optimal doses, and in cases of severe life-threatening sleep apnoea.— C. S. Conner, *Drug Intell. & clin. Pharm.*, 1983, *17*, 736.

Snoring. Protriptyline in an average dose of 10 mg taken at bedtime eliminated snoring in about 75% of patients.— J. A. Goldstein (letter), *New Engl. J. Med.*, 1983, *308*, 1602.

Preparations

Protriptyline Hydrochloride Tablets *(U.S.P.).* Store in airtight containers.

Protriptyline Tablets *(B.P.).* Tablets containing protriptyline hydrochloride.

Proprietary Preparations

Concordin *(Merck Sharp & Dohme, UK). Tablets* (Concordin-5), protriptyline hydrochloride 5 mg.

Tablets (Concordin-10), protriptyline hydrochloride 10 mg.

Proprietary Names and Manufacturers

Concordin *(Arg.; Merck Sharp & Dohme, Austral.; Belg.; Merck Sharp & Dohme, Denm.; Ital.; Neth.; MSD, Swed.; Merck Sharp & Dohme, UK)*; Concordine *(Fr.)*; Maximed *(Ger.)*; Triptil *(Austral.; Merck Sharp & Dohme, Canad.)*; Vivactil *(Merck Sharp & Dohme, USA).*

13204-x

Quinupramine *(rINN).*

LM-208. 10,11-Dihydro-5-(quinuclidin-3-yl)-5*H*-dibenz-[*b,f*]azepine.

$C_{21}H_{24}N_2=304.4$.

CAS — 31721-17-2.

Quinupramine is a tricyclic antidepressant with actions and uses similar to those of amitriptyline (p.354). It has been given by mouth in doses of 7.5 to 15 mg daily in the treatment of depression.

A brief mention of the actions and uses of quinupramine.— B. Blackwell and J. S. Simon, *Drugs Today*, 1986, *22*, 611.

Proprietary Names and Manufacturers

Kevopril *(Rhone-Poulenc, Belg.)*; Kinupril *(Fournier Frères, Fr.)*; Quinuprine *(Rhone, Spain).*

13218-m

Rolipram *(USAN, rINN).*

ZK-62711. 4-(3-Cyclopentyloxy-4-methoxyphenyl)pyrrolidin-2-one.

$C_{16}H_{21}NO_3=275.3$.

CAS — 61413-54-5.

Rolipram is reported to have antidepressant activity.

Proprietary Names and Manufacturers

Schering, Ger.

2535-z

Safrazine Hydrochloride

1-Methyl-3-(3,4-methylenedioxyphenyl)propylhydrazine hydrochloride.

$C_{11}H_{16}N_2O_2,HCl=244.7$.

CAS — 33419-68-0 (safrazine); 27849-94-1 (hydrochloride).

Safrazine is a monoamine oxidase inhibitor which has been used in the treatment of depression.

Proprietary Names and Manufacturers

Safra *(Ono, Jpn).*

18681-x

Sertraline Hydrochloride *(BANM, USAN, rINNM).*
CP-51974-01. (1*S*,4*S*)-4-(3,4-Dichlorophenyl)-1,2,3,4-tetrahydro-1-naphthyl(methyl)amine hydrochloride.
$C_{17}H_{17}Cl_2N,HCl=342.7$.

CAS — 79617-96-2 (sertraline); 79559-97-0.

Sertraline is an antidepressant which selectively inhibits the re-uptake of serotonin.

References: W. Guy *et al., Drug Dev. Res.,* 1986, *9,* 267.

Proprietary Names and Manufacturers
Pfizer, USA.

13295-c

Tametraline Hydrochloride *(USAN, rINNM).*
CP-24441-1. (1*R*,4*S*)-1,2,3,4-Tetrahydro-*N*-methyl-4-phenyl-1-naphthylamine hydrochloride.
$C_{17}H_{19}N,HCl=273.8$.

CAS — 52795-02-5 (tametraline); 52760-47-1 (hydrochloride).

Tametraline hydrochloride is reported to have antidepressant activity.

Proprietary Names and Manufacturers
Pfizer, USA.

13297-a

Tandamine Hydrochloride *(USAN, pINNM).*
AY-23946. 2-(9-Ethyl-1,3,4,9-tetrahydro-1-methylthiopyrano[3,4-*b*]indol-1-yl)-*NN*-dimethylethylamine hydrochloride.
$C_{18}H_{26}N_2S,HCl=338.9$.

CAS — 42408-80-0 (tandamine); 58167-78-5 (hydrochloride).

Tandamine hydrochloride is reported to have antidepressant properties.

References: R. S. B. Ehsanullah *et al., Psychopharmacology,* 1977, *52,* 73; I. Jirkovsky *et al., Arzneimittel-Forsch.,* 1977, *27,* 1642; B. Saletu *et al., Int. Pharmacopsychiat.,* 1977, *12,* 137.

Proprietary Names and Manufacturers
Ayerst, USA.

17007-n

Tianeptine *(rINN).*
7-[(3-Chloro-6,11-dihydro-6-methyldibenzo[*c,f*][1,2]thiazepin-11-yl)amino]heptanoic acid *S,S*-dioxide.
$C_{21}H_{25}ClN_2O_4S=437.0$.

CAS — 66981-73-5.

Tianeptine is reported to possess antidepressant activity.

2536-c

Tofenacin Hydrochloride *(BANM, USAN, rINNM).*
BS-7331 *(Tofenacin)*; Desmethylorphenadrine Hydrochloride. Methyl-2-(2-methylbenzhydryloxy)ethylamine hydrochloride.
$C_{17}H_{21}NO,HCl=291.8$.

CAS — 15301-93-6 (tofenacin); 10488-36-5 (hydrochloride).

Tofenacin is a derivative of orphenadrine (see p.539). It has been given as the hydrochloride in doses of 80 mg up to three times daily in the treatment of depression.

Proprietary Names and Manufacturers
Elamol *(Brocades, UK)*; Tofacine *(Belg.)*.

3229-y

Toloxatone *(rINN).*
5-(Hydroxymethyl)-3-*m*-tolyl-2-oxazolidinone.
$C_{11}H_{13}NO_3=207.2$.

CAS — 29218-27-7.

Toloxatone is an antidepressant which reversibly inhibits type A monoamine oxidase. It is given in doses of up to 600 mg daily.

The pharmacokinetics of toloxatone.— M. S. Benedetti *et al., Arzneimittel-Forsch.,* 1982, *32,* 276.

Toloxatone had been administered in doses of up to 1 g daily for 5 days to patients with Parkinson's disease receiving levodopa with a peripheral decarboxylase inhibitor with no significant variation in their blood pressure.— A. Cantagrel *et al., Thérapie,* 1986, *41,* 493.

Proprietary Names and Manufacturers
Humoryl *(Delalande, Fr.)*; Perenum *(Delalande, Ital.)*.

2537-k

Tranylcypromine Sulphate *(BANM, rINNM).*

SKF-385; Tranilcipromina *(base)*; Transamine Sulphate; Tranylcypromine Sulfate *(USAN)*.
(±)-*trans*-2-Phenylcyclopropylamine sulphate.
$(C_9H_{11}N)_2,H_2SO_4=364.5$.

CAS — 155-09-9 (tranylcypromine); 13492-01-8; 7081-36-9 (both sulphate).

Pharmacopoeias. In *Br.* and *U.S.*

A white or almost white crystalline powder; odourless or with a faint odour of cinnamaldehyde. Tranylcypromine sulphate 13.7 mg is approximately equivalent to 10 mg of tranylcypromine.

B.P. solubilities are: **soluble** 1 in 20 of water; very slightly soluble in alcohol and in ether; practically insoluble in chloroform. *U.S.P.* solubilities are: soluble 1 in 25 of water; very slightly soluble in alcohol and in ether; practically insoluble in chloroform. **Store** in well-closed containers.

Adverse Effects, Treatment, and Precautions

As for Phenelzine Sulphate, p.377.

Insomnia is a common side-effect if tranylcypromine is given in the evening.

Hypertensive reactions are more likely to occur with tranylcypromine than with phenelzine or other antidepressants derived from hydrazine, but severe liver damage occurs less frequently.

The concomitant administration of clomipramine with tranylcypromine is especially hazardous, see phenelzine sulphate (p.378).

PORPHYRIA. Tranylcypromine was considered to be unsafe in patients with acute porphyria because it has been shown to be porphyrinogenic in *animals* or *in vitro* systems.— M.R. Moore and K.E.L. McColl, *Porphyrias, Drug Lists,* Glasgow, Porphyria Research Unit, University of Glasgow, 1987.

PREGNANCY AND THE NEONATE. *Lactation.* Although tranylcypromine is transferred into breast milk, there were no reported effects on lactation or signs or symptoms in breast-fed infants.— *Pediatrics,* 1983, *72,* 375.

Absorption and Fate

Tranylcypromine is readily absorbed from the gastro-intestinal tract and excreted in the urine mainly in the form of metabolites.

In 9 depressed patients, tranylcypromine absorption was rapid after oral dosing. Absorption was biphasic in 7. Elimination was also rapid, with an elimination half-life of 1.54 to 3.15 hours. From 2 to 7 hours after dosing, standing systolic and diastolic blood pressures were lowered, and standing pulse was raised. The onset of the effect on standing systolic blood pressure correlated with the time of peak plasma tranylcypromine concentration. Maximum orthostatic drop of blood pressure and rise in pulse rate occurred 2 hours after dosing. Mean plasma tranylcypromine concentrations correlated with mean orthostatic drop of systolic blood pressure and rise of pulse rate. Patients experiencing clinically significant hypotensive reactions to tranylcypromine may benefit from changes in their dose regimen aimed at minimising peak concentrations.— A. G. Mallinger *et al., Clin. Pharmac. Ther.,* 1986, *40,* 444.

Uses and Administration

Tranylcypromine is a nonhydrazine monoamine oxidase inhibitor with actions and uses similar to those of phenelzine (p.379). Unlike phenelzine, it does not induce irreversible inhibition of monoamine oxidase, the activity of which is reported to recover within 3 to 5 days of withdrawing tranylcypromine.

Tranylcypromine is given as the sulphate in doses equivalent to tranylcypromine 10 mg in the morning and 10 mg at midday; if no response has been obtained after a week the midday dose may be increased to 20 mg; a dosage of 30 mg daily should only be exceeded with caution. Once a response has been obtained the dosage may be gradually reduced for maintenance; some patients may continue to respond to 10 mg daily.

BEHAVIOUR DISORDERS. In 14 boys aged 8 to 12 years with attention deficit disorder with hyperactivity, clorgyline, tranylcypromine sulphate, and dexamphetamine sulphate at mean daily doses of 12.13, 10.40, and 13.21 mg respectively were equally effective in improving restless, disruptive behaviour and attentional measures. Clinical effect was seen by the first week with all 3 drugs, and it was suggested that clorgyline and tranylcypromine may be useful alternative treatments in selected cases of attention deficit disorder.— A. Zametkin *et al., Archs gen. Psychiat.,* 1985, *42,* 962.

HYPOTENSION. For studies and comments on the merits and hazards of tranylcypromine and other monoamine oxidase inhibitors in the management of orthostatic hypotension, see Tyramine Hydrochloride, p.948.

Preparations

Tranylcypromine Sulfate Tablets *(U.S.P.).* Contain tranylcypromine sulphate. Potency is expressed in terms of the equivalent amount of tranylcypromine. Protect from light.

Tranylcypromine Tablets *(B.P.).* Contain tranylcypromine sulphate. Potency is expressed in terms of the equivalent amount of tranylcypromine.

Proprietary Preparations

Parnate *(Smith Kline & French, UK). Tablets,* tranylcypromine 10 mg (as sulphate).

Parstelin *(Smith Kline & French, UK). Tablets,* tranylcypromine 10 mg (as sulphate), trifluoperazine 1 mg (as hydrochloride).

Proprietary Names and Manufacturers

Parnate *(Smith Kline & French, Austral.; Canad.; Röhm, Ger.; Smith Kline & French, S.Afr.; Smith Kline & French, Spain; Smith Kline & French, UK; Smith Kline & French, USA)*; Tylciprine *(Théraplix, Fr.)*.

The following names have been used for multi-ingredient preparations containing tranylcypromine sulphate— Parstelin *(Smith Kline & French, Austral.; Smith Kline & French, UK)*.

2541-y

Trazodone Hydrochloride *(BANM, USAN, rINNM).*

AF-1161. 2-[3-(4-*m*-Chlorophenylpiperazin-1-yl)propyl]-1,2,4-triazolo[4,3-*a*]pyridin-3(2*H*)-one hydrochloride.
$C_{19}H_{22}ClN_5O,HCl=408.3$.

CAS — 19794-93-5 (trazodone); 25332-39-2 (hydrochloride).

Adverse Effects

Adverse effects associated with trazodone include drowsiness. Other side-effects occasionally reported include dizziness, headache, nausea and vomiting, weakness, weight loss, tremor, dry mouth, bradycardia or tachycardia, orthostatic hypotension, oedema, constipation, diarrhoea, blurred vision, restlessness, confusional states, insomnia, priapism, and skin rash.

Symptoms of overdosage include drowsiness, vomiting, priapism, respiratory arrest, seizures, and ECG changes.

Adverse reactions to trazodone.— P. E. Hayes and C. A. Kristoff, *Clin. Pharm.*, 1986, *5*, 471.

ANTIMUSCARINIC EFFECTS. For an estimate of the relative antimuscarinic potency of trazodone compared with the tricyclic antidepressants, see Amitriptyline Hydrochloride, p.351.

EFFECTS ON THE CARDIOVASCULAR SYSTEM. Trazodone in therapeutic doses has been associated with heart block in patients with ventricular conduction defects (J.L. Rausch *et al.*, *Am. J. Psychiat.*, 1984, *141*, 1472) or with no ECG abnormalities (S. Lippmann *et al.*, *ibid.*, 1983, *140*, 1383). Similarly, ventricular arrhythmias have been associated with therapeutic doses of trazodone both in patients with a history of cardiac problems (D. Janowsky *et al.*, *ibid.*, 796; S.C. Vlay and S. Friedling, *Am. Heart J.*, 1983, *106*, 604), and with no history of cardiac abnormalities (B.A. Johnson, *Br. J. Hosp. Med.*, 1985, *33*, 298). Atrial fibrillation has been reported following a daily dose of 300 mg of trazodone in an elderly woman with ischaemic heart disease (W.B. White and S.H.Y. Wong, *Archs gen. Psychiat.*, 1985, *42*, 424).

EFFECTS ON THE EYE. A 47-year-old man with resistant endogenous depression receiving clomipramine and trazodone by mouth noted excessive blinking whenever the dose of trazodone exceeded or equalled that of clomipramine. When trazodone, but not clomipramine, was withdrawn, blinking became normal within 3 weeks.— M. A. Cooper and T. R. Dening (letter), *Br. med. J.*, 1986, *293*, 1243.

EFFECTS ON THE LIVER. A mixed hepatocellular-cholestatic liver enzyme pattern with hyperbilirubinaemia has been seen following 2 to 3 weeks of trazodone treatment at doses of 50 to 500 mg daily, and resolving over 4 to 8 weeks following its discontinuation. Weekly liver enzyme monitoring for the first 4 weeks of trazodone treatment was advised (A.G. Chu *et al.*, *Ann. intern. Med.*, 1983, *99*, 128; K.H. Sheikh and A.S. Nies, *ibid.*, 572).

EFFECTS ON MENTAL FUNCTION. There have been reports of delirium in bulimics (M.F. Damlouji and J.M. Ferguson, *Am. J. Psychiat.*, 1984, *141*, 434), mania (M. Warren and P.A. Bick, *ibid.*, 1103; G.W. Arana and G.B. Kaplan, *ibid.*, 1985, *142*, 386) and paranoid psychosis with hallucinations (T.B. Kraft, *ibid.*, 1983, *140*, 1383) associated with the use of trazodone 50 to 400 mg daily.

EFFECTS ON SEXUAL FUNCTION. In the *USA* over 30 cases of priapism associated with the use of trazodone were known to the manufacturers. In most cases, priapism occurred during treatment with standard doses after 1 to 3 weeks of therapy. Several patients required surgery and recovery was not always complete.— Committee on Safety of Medicines, *Current Problems No. 13*, July, 1984.. See also *Med. Lett.*, 1984, *26*, 35.

A 51-year-old man experienced inhibition of ejaculation whilst taking trazodone 100 mg each night. Resolution of the problem occurred about 3 days after discontinuing trazodone.— S. D. Jones, *J. clin. Psychopharmacol.*, 1984, *4*, 279.

A report of 3 depressed women who experienced an increase in libido to above premorbid levels with therapeutic doses of trazodone.— N. Gartrell, *Am. J. Psychiat.*, 1986, *143*, 781.

EFFECTS ON THE SKIN. Leucocytoclastic vasculitis developed in a 62-year-old man within several days of starting trazodone 350 mg daily. His skin rash resolved within 10 days of stopping trazodone, and reappeared within 5 days of restarting the drug.— S. C. Mann *et al.* (letter), *J. Am. Acad. Derm.*, 1984, *10*, 669.

Erythema multiforme was associated with trazodone therapy in a 63-year-old woman.— H. E. Ford and M. A. Jenike, *J. clin. Psychiat.*, 1985, *46*, 294.

A 37-year-old man who had suffered from stable plaque psoriasis for 19 years was given trazodone hydrochloride 50 mg daily for depression accompanying the gradual worsening of his psoriasis. After 17 days, his psoriasis rapidly worsened, with skin tenderness and fever. Examination revealed generalised pustular psoriasis.— J. H. Barth and H. Baker, *Br. J. Derm.*, 1986, *115*, 629.

EPILEPTOGENIC EFFECT. A 50-year-old woman with no history of epilepsy experienced multiple tonic-clonic seizures after 18 days of treatment with trazodone 50 mg daily.— D. Lefkowitz *et al.* (letter), *Archs gen. Psychiat.*, 1985, *42*, 523. Another report. N. D. Bowdan (letter), *Am. J. Psychiat.*, 1983, *140*, 642.

OVERDOSAGE. A review of unpublished reports to the manufacturer indicated that the incidence of serious toxicity from trazodone overdose alone was low compared with tricyclic antidepressant overdose. Of 149 overdose cases, only 10 deaths had been reported. In only one case was trazodone the sole agent reported to be ingested; in this case autopsy revealed an acute myocardial infarction after the patient was stable. The remaining 9 patients also had histories of ingestion of unknown quantities of alcohol, benzodiazepines or other sedative-hypnotics that may have contributed to their demise. In the surviving 139 patients, 2 cases of respiratory arrest, one case of priapism, one occurrence of seizure, 2 cases of right bundle-branch block, one case of atrioventricular block, and one T-wave inversion were reported. The remaining patients had minor CNS-depressant effects.— E. Hassan and D. D. Miller, *Clin. Pharm.*, 1985, *4*, 97.

No fatalities occurred in 39 of 88 cases of trazodone overdosage where trazodone was ingested alone. However, a total of 9 deaths occurred in the remaining 49 cases where trazodone was co-ingested with other drugs or alcohol, suggesting trazodone overdosage may not be so benign when such co-ingestion is involved.— N. Babul and S. Rozek (letter), *J. Am. med. Ass.*, 1987, *257*, 2435. Further references: P. Crome and C. Ali, *Med. Toxicol.*, 1986, *1*, 411.

Precautions

Trazodone should be used with caution in patients with cardiovascular disorders, such as ischaemic heart disease and its use is not recommended in the immediate recovery phase after myocardial infarction. It should similarly be used with caution in patients with epilepsy and hepatic or renal insufficiency. Patients with suicidal tendencies should be carefully supervised during treatment. Patients developing inappropriate or prolonged penile erections should discontinue trazodone immediately.

Trazodone is considered unlikely to interact with monoamine oxidase inhibitors, although it is recommended that it should not be given to patients receiving monoamine oxidase inhibitors or for at least 14 days after their discontinuation. Similarly, trazodone is unlikely to diminish the effects of antihypertensive agents, such as guanethidine; some interaction may, however, occur with clonidine and, in general, blood pressure should be monitored when trazodone is prescribed with antihypertensive therapy. The sedative effects of trazodone may be enhanced by concurrent administration with alcohol or other central nervous system depressants.

Drowsiness is often experienced at the start of trazodone antidepressant therapy and patients if affected should not drive or operate machinery. For further details of the effects of antidepressant therapy on driving see amitriptyline hydrochloride (p.353).

INTERACTIONS. *Digoxin.* Trazodone therapy might have contributed to the increased serum digoxin concentrations seen in one case.— S. R. Kayser, *Drug Interact. News.*, 1985, *5*, 1.

Phenytoin. For the effect of trazodone on phenytoin, see Phenytoin Sodium, p.409.

Warfarin. For the effect of trazodone on warfarin therapy, see Warfarin Sodium, p.346.

PREGNANCY AND THE NEONATE. For a report showing no association between infant central nervous system defects and the administration of tetracyclic antidepressants during the trimester before the last menstrual period, and in the first trimester of pregnancy, see Amitriptyline Hydrochloride, p.354.

Lactation. In a study of 6 lactating women each given a single 50-mg dose of trazodone, it was concluded that exposure of babies to trazodone via breast milk is very small. However, trazodone has been reported to form an active metabolite and it was not known to what extent this metabolite distributed into breast milk.— R. K. Verbeeck *et al.*, *Br. J. clin. Pharmac.*, 1986, *22*, 367.

Absorption and Fate

Trazodone is rapidly absorbed from the gastro-intestinal tract and extensively metabolised. Paths of metabolism of trazodone include *N*-oxidation and hydroxylation. The metabolite *m*-chlorophenylpiperazine is active. Trazodone is excreted in the urine almost entirely in the form of its metabolites, either in free or in conjugated form. The elimination of trazodone is biphasic, with a terminal elimination half-life of 5 to 13 hours. Trazodone is excreted in breast milk.

There was an approximate two-fold increase in terminal phase half-life and significantly higher plasma concentrations of trazodone in 10 subjects aged 65 to 74 years compared with 12 subjects aged 23 to 30 years following a 100-mg dose of trazodone. It was suggested that there is an age-related reduction in the hepatic metabolism of trazodone.— A. J. Bayer *et al.*, *Br. J. clin. Pharmac.*, 1983, *16*, 371.

Uses and Administration

Trazodone is a triazolopyridine antidepressant. It does not appear to have very significant antimuscarinic properties, but has a marked sedative action. Unlike amitriptyline, it does not prevent the peripheral re-uptake of noradrenaline. It has been shown to be a selective inhibitor of central serotonin uptake and to decrease peripheral serotonin uptake. It also appears to increase the turnover of brain dopamine. The mode of action of trazodone in depression is not fully understood.

In the treatment of depression trazodone is given by mouth as the hydrochloride in doses of 150 mg daily initially, increased to 200 or 300 mg daily respectively after the first week. A suggested initial dose in elderly and other susceptible patients is 50 mg twice daily, and single doses above 100 mg should be avoided in these patients. The daily dosage may be divided throughout the day after food or given as a single dose at night. Divided daily dosages of up to 600 mg may be given in exceptionally severe depression.

Reviews of the actions and uses of trazodone: R. N. Brogden *et al.*, *Drugs*, 1981, *21*, 401; J. M. Davis and C. Vogel, *J. clin. Psychopharmacol.*, 1981, *1*, *Suppl.*, 27S.

ADMINISTRATION. Trazodone given as a single night time dose has been shown to be as effective in relieving depression as a divided daily dosage regimen (J.M. Mungavin and S.I. Ankier, *Clin. Trials J.*, 1983, *20*, 181); more side-effects were experienced with a divided daily dosage regimen (D. Brooks *et al.*, *Psychopharmacology*, 1984, *84*, 1) whereas the night time dose was better at improving sleep (D. Wheatley, *Pharmatherapeutica*, 1984, *3*, 607). However, although trazodone enhances the subjective quality of sleep, it does not prolong its duration (I. Montgomery *et al.*, *Br. J. clin. Pharmac.*, 1983, *16*, 139).

ADMINISTRATION IN THE ELDERLY. Although a low starting dose is recommended for elderly patients, a double-blind trial in 18 patients aged 60 to 78 years comparing a regimen of trazodone 25 mg three times daily with 50 mg three times daily found a faster antidepressant response with the higher dosage. Headache and nausea were more frequent in the high-dose group in the first 2 weeks, but at no time did adverse events outweigh therapeutic benefit.— P. K. Mukherjee and A. Davey, *J. int. med. Res.*, 1986, *14*, 279.

BEHAVIOUR DISORDERS. Combined treatment with trazodone 200 to 300 mg daily and tryptophan 2.5 to 3 g daily was successful in controlling aggressive behaviour and disrupted sleep in a 22-year-old retarded man with Cornelia de Lange syndrome (M. O'Neil *et al.*, *Lancet*, 1986, *2*, 859) and repetitive screaming and head and table banging in a 82-year-old woman with moderately advanced dementia (B.S. Greenwald *et al.*, *ibid.*, 1464). In 6 demented patients aged 70 to 90 years exhibiting very aggressive behaviour, combined treatment with trazodone and tryptophan resulted in improved behaviour in 3, reduction of symptoms in 1, and no improvement in 2 (G.K. Wilcock *et al.*, *ibid.*, 1987, *1*, 929). This treatment was considered to act by enhancing serotoninergic transmission.

DEPRESSION. In the treatment of depression trazodone has been shown to be as effective as amitriptyline (T.A. Kerr *et al.*, *Acta psychiat. scand.*, 1984, *70*, 573; S.A. Ather *et al.*, *Br. J. clin. Pract.*, 1985, *39*, 192), doxepin (J. Himmelhoch, *Curr. ther. Res.*, 1986, *39*, 1017), imipramine (S. Gershon *et al.*, *J. clin. Psychopharmacol.*, 1981, *1*, *Suppl.*, 39S), mianserin (E.H. Bennie *et al.*, *Curr. med. Res. Opinion*, 1984, *9*, 253), amoxapine, and maprotiline (D.S. Robinson *et al.*, *Curr. ther. Res.*, 1984, *35*, 549). See also under Administration, above.

Depression in medical patients. The use of tricyclic and tetracyclic antidepressants in depressed medical patients.— *Lancet*, 1986, *1*, 949.

TREMOR. Trazodone 100 to 150 mg daily produced significant improvement in 2 patients with marked essential tremor after 3 weeks of treatment.— N. A. McLeod and L. E. White (letter), *J. Am. med. Ass.*, 1986, *256*,

2675.

WITHDRAWAL SYNDROMES. Trazodone decreased cocaine craving and relieved withdrawal symptoms in a 32-year-old addict.— G. W. Small and J. J. Purcell, *Archs gen. Psychiat.*, 1985, *42*, 524. See also M. C. Rowbotham, *ibid.*, 1984, *41*, 895.

Proprietary Preparations

Molipaxin *(Roussel, UK). Capsules*, trazodone hydrochloride 50 and 100 mg.
Tablets, scored, trazodone hydrochloride 150 mg.
Liquid, trazodone hydrochloride 50 mg/5 mL.

Proprietary Names and Manufacturers

Deprax *(Farma-Lepori, Spain)*; Desyrel *(Bristol, Canad.; Bristol-Myers Products, USA)*; Manegan *(Arg.)*; Molipaxin *(Eire; Cassenne, S.Afr.; Roussel, UK)*; Pragmarel *(UPSA, Fr.)*; Thombran *(Thomae, Ger.)*; Tramensan *(Belg.; Medica, Fin.)*; Trittico *(Belg.; Angelini, Ital.; Angelini, Switz.)*.

2538-a

Trimipramine *(BAN, USAN, rINN).*

7162RP; IL-6001; Trimeprimine. Dimethyl-{3-(10,11-dihydro-5*H*-dibenz[*b,f*]azepin-5-yl-2-methyl)propyl}amine.

$C_{20}H_{26}N_2$=294.4.

CAS — 739-71-9.

2539-t

Trimipramine Maleate *(BANM, USAN, rINNM).*

Trimipramine Hydrogen Maleate; Trimipramini Maleas.

$C_{20}H_{26}N_2,C_4H_4O_4$=410.5.

CAS — 521-78-8.

Pharmacopoeias. In *Aust., Br., Eur., Fr., Ger., It., Neth.,* and *Swiss.*

A white or almost white crystalline powder. Trimipramine maleate 34.9 mg is approximately equivalent to 25 mg of trimipramine. Slightly **soluble** in water and alcohol; freely soluble in chloroform; practically insoluble in ether. **Store** in well-closed containers. Protect from light.

Adverse Effects, Treatment, and Precautions

As for Amitriptyline Hydrochloride, p.351.

INTERACTIONS. Interactions involving tricyclic antidepressants are discussed under amitriptyline (p.353). For a report of an adverse reaction to imipramine, but not trimipramine, in a patient receiving phenelzine, see phenelzine sulphate (p.379)

Absorption and Fate

Trimipramine is readily absorbed after oral administration. Since trimipramine slows gastro-intestinal transit-time, absorption can be delayed in overdosage.

Trimipramine is metabolised in the liver to its major metabolite desmethyltrimipramine. Trimipramine is excreted in the urine mainly in the form of its metabolites. It is extensively bound to plasma proteins.

In a study of 9 healthy subjects, the mean elimination half-life of trimipramine after a 50-mg oral dose was 24 hours. Trimipramine was more highly protein bound than other tricyclic antidepressants (average 94.9%), and it was suggested that it underwent high first-pass hepatic clearance, resulting in incomplete and variable systemic availability. On the basis of its elimination half-life, trimipramine could be administered on a twice-daily basis without marked interdose fluctuations in plasma concentrations.— D. R. Abernethy *et al.*, *Clin. Pharmac. Ther.*, 1984, *35*, 348.

Uses and Administration

Trimipramine is a tricyclic antidepressant with actions and uses similar to those of amitriptyline (p.354). Like amitriptyline, it has marked sedative properties. In the treatment of depression, trimipramine is given by mouth as the maleate in doses equivalent to 50 to 75 mg of trimipramine daily initially, gradually increased to 150 mg daily as necessary; higher doses of up to 300 mg daily may be required in severely depressed hospital patients. Maintenance doses are usually in the range of 75 to 150 mg daily. A suggested initial dose for adolescents and the elderly is 30 to 75 mg daily, gradually increased as necessary. Half the normal maintenance dose may be sufficient. Trimipramine may be given in divided doses during the day, but since it has a prolonged half-life, once-daily dosage regimens are also suitable, usually given at night, about 2 hours before bedtime.

Trimipramine has been given intramuscularly as the mesylate.

ANXIETY AND PHOBIAS. For a suggestion that antidepressants with secondary sedative properties, such as trimipramine, are the treatment of first choice in depressed patients with anxiety or agitation, see Amitriptyline Hydrochloride, p.355.

DEPRESSION. For a general review of the role of antidepressants in depression, see Amitriptyline Hydrochloride, p.355.

Combination therapy with monoamine oxidase inhibitors. For a report suggesting that trimipramine and amitriptyline are the tricyclic antidepressants least likely to produce side-effects in combination with monoamine oxidase inhibitors, see Amitriptyline Hydrochloride, p.355.

PAIN. *Musculoskeletal and joint pain.* In 36 patients with definite or classical rheumatoid arthritis, trimipramine 25 to 75 mg daily significantly reduced joint pain and tenderness, but depression scores remained unchanged.— J. G. Macfarlane *et al.*, *Curr. med. Res. Opinion*, 1986, *10*, 89.

For a report of the administration of amitriptyline resulting in no improvement in joint pain and tenderness in patients with rheumatoid arthritis, see Amitriptyline Hydrochloride, p.356.

PEPTIC ULCERATION. Trimipramine reduces gastric acid secretion (H.P. Mackay *et al.*, *J. int. med. Res.*, 1984, *12*, 303) and, at doses of 50 mg daily, has been shown to produce significantly faster healing of duodenal ulcers than placebo during the first 4 weeks of treatment (T.K. Daneshmend *et al.*, *Gut*, 1981, *22*, 1045; H.P. Mackay *et al.*, *Scand. J. Gastroenterol.*, 1984, *19*, 190), and to be as effective as cimetidine 1 g daily (K. Valnes *et al.*, *ibid.*, 1983, *18*, 33), although others have found it to be somewhat less effective than cimetidine (M. Miglioli *et al.*, *Curr. ther. Res.*, 1982, *31*, 7), with a slower healing rate (U. Becker *et al.*, *Scand. J. Gastroenterol.*, 1983, *18*, 137). At a dose of 25 mg each night, trimipramine was more effective than placebo in preventing recurrence of healed duodenal or prepyloric ulcers (K. Valnes *et al.*, *ibid.*, 1982, *17*, 1003), and as effective as cimetidine 400 mg daily (A. Berstad *et al.*, *ibid.*, 1981, *16*, 933), although a later study found trimipramine to be less effective than cimetidine and no better than placebo (U. Becker *et al.*, *ibid.*, 1984, *19*, 405).

Preparations

Trimipramine Tablets *(B.P.)*. Tablets containing trimipramine maleate. Potency is expressed in terms of the equivalent amount of trimipramine.

Surmontil *(May & Baker, UK). Capsules*, trimipramine 50 mg (as maleate).
Tablets, trimipramine 10 and 25 mg (as maleate).

Proprietary Names and Manufacturers of Trimipramine Salts

Stangyl *(Rhône-Poulenc, Ger.)*; Surmontil *(Arg.; May & Baker, Austral.; Belg.; Rhône-Poulenc, Canad.; Rhone-Poulenc, Denm.; Specia, Fr.; Carlo Erba, Ital.; Neth.; Rhône-Poulenc, Norw.; May & Baker, S.Afr.; Rhone, Spain; Leo Rhodia, Swed.; Rhone-Poulenc, Switz.; May & Baker, UK; Wyeth, USA)*; Tydamine *(Lennon, S.Afr.)*.

NOTE. The name Surmontil has also been used to denote trimipramine mesylate or trimipramine embonate in some countries.

664-p

Tryptophan *(USAN, pINN).*

L-Tryptophan. L-2-Amino-3-(indol-3-yl)propionic acid.

$C_{11}H_{12}N_2O_2$=204.2.

CAS — 73-22-3.

Pharmacopoeias. In *Cz., Jpn,* and *U.S. Fr.* includes DL-Tryptophan.

White to slightly yellowish-white crystals or crystalline powder. **Soluble** 1 in about 100 of water; slightly soluble in alcohol; practically insoluble in chloroform and ether; soluble in hot alcohol and solutions of dilute acids and alkali hydroxides. A 1% solution in water has a pH of 5.5 to 7.0. **Store** in well-closed containers. Protect from light.

Adverse Effects

Nausea, headache, light headedness, and drowsiness have been reported.

There have been occasional reports of sexual disinhibition, reversible dyskinesias, and reversible Parkinsonian-like rigidity in patients taking tryptophan with or after phenothiazines or benzodiazepines.

An increased incidence of bladder tumours has been reported in *mice* given L-tryptophan in association with cholesterol.

5-Hydroxytryptophan, an intermediate in the conversion of tryptophan to serotonin, has central stimulant activity as well as reported neurotoxic effects.

A loading dose of tryptophan caused striking increases in plasma-insulin concentrations in 13 patients when given 2 hours after a meal but in 6 fasting patients it had little or no effect.— B. Ajdukiewicz *et al.* (letter), *Lancet*, 1968, *1*, 92.

Reports concerning sexual disinhibition in patients taking tryptophan, sometimes in combination with phenothiazines: G. P. Egan and G. E. M. Hammad (letter), *Br. med. J.*, 1976, *2*, 701; R. P. Hullin and T. Jerram (letter), *ibid.*, 1010; A. D. Broadhurst and B. Rao (letter), *ibid.*, 1977, *1*, 51; I. Oswald (letter), *ibid.*, 1559; M. T. Hyyppä (letter), *ibid.*, 1073.

Precautions

Patients taking tryptophan may experience drowsiness and if affected they should not drive or operate machinery. For further details of the effects of antidepressant therapy on driving see amitriptyline hydrochloride (p.353). The concomitant administration of tryptophan and a monoamine oxidase inhibitor may enhance the effects of the monoamine oxidase inhibitor (see under Phenelzine Sulphate p.379).

INTERACTIONS. *Anticonvulsants.* Whole and free plasma-tryptophan concentrations were increased by carbamazepine and decreased by phenytoin.— J. A. Pratt *et al.*, *J. Neurol. Neurosurg. Psychiat.*, 1984, *47*, 1131.

Levodopa. For a report of tryptophan reducing blood concentrations of levodopa, see under Levodopa, p.1017.

Absorption and Fate

Tryptophan is readily absorbed from the gastro-intestinal tract. Tryptophan is extensively bound to serum albumin. It is metabolised by way of hydroxytryptophan to serotonin and other metabolites, including kynurenine derivatives, and excreted in the urine. Pyridoxine and ascorbic acid appear to be concerned in its metabolism.

The biological half-life of tryptophan was reported to be 15.8 hours.— W. A. Ritschel, *Drug Intell. & clin. Pharm.*, 1970, *4*, 332.

A comparison of the urinary metabolites of tryptophan in depressed and non-depressed patients did not indicate any increased excretion by the kynurenine route rather than the serotonin route in depressed patients.— A. Frazer *et al.*, *Archs gen. Psychiat.*, 1973, *29*, 528.

Pharmacokinetic factors in the clinical use of tryptophan.— R. J. Hedaya, *J. clin. Psychopharmacol.*, 1984, *4*, 347.

The pharmacokinetics of tryptophan in healthy subjects following its intravenous and oral administration.— A. R. Green *et al.*, *Br. J. clin. Pharmac.*, 1985, *20*, 317.

Uses and Administration

Tryptophan is an amino acid which is an essential constituent of the diet.

Tryptophan is a precursor of serotonin. Because CNS depletion of serotonin is considered to be involved in depression, tryptophan has been used in its treatment. Pyridoxine and ascorbic acid are considered to be involved in the metabolism of tryptophan to serotonin and are sometimes given concomitantly. A dose of 1 g of tryptophan three times daily by mouth, with food may be adequate in mild or moderate depression, increasing to 2 g three times daily if necessary. In severe depression tryptophan may be given with other antidepressants; tryptophan should not replace standard therapy in such cases. In patients receiving monoamine oxidase inhibitors the initial dose of tryptophan should be 500 mg daily for 1 week, followed by 1 g daily for 1 week, before normal doses are given. In patients receiving phenothiazines or benzodiazepines, or shortly after discontinuing treatment with phenothiazines, the initial dose of tryptophan should not exceed 1.5 g daily. It is recommended that treatment with tryptophan should be reviewed at 3-monthly intervals.

Tryptophan and DL-tryptophan are used as dietary supplements.

BEHAVIOUR DISORDERS. For the successful use of tryptophan in combination with trazodone for controlling aggressive behaviour, see under Trazodone Hydrochloride, p.382.

DEPRESSION. Studies have suggested that tryptophan in doses of 3 to 8 g daily by mouth may be as effective as, or more effective than ECT during the first 2 weeks of treatment. However, this advantage was lost by 4 weeks and tryptophan was not considered a suitable alternative to ECT (R.N. Herrington *et al.*, *Lancet*, 1974, *2*, 731; D.A. MacSweeney, *ibid.*, 1975, *2*, 510). Pretreatment with tryptophan shortened the duration of ECT seizures but did not affect the threshold to induce seizures (H. Raotma, *Acta psychiat. Scand.*, 1978, *57*, 253).

Reports have suggested that tryptophan in doses of 3 to 9 g daily by mouth might be as effective as therapeutic doses of tricyclic antidepressants in the treatment of depression (A. Coppen *et al.*, *Archs gen. Psychiat.*, 1972, *26*, 234; N.S. Kline and B.K. Shah, *Curr. ther. Res.*, 1973, *15*, 484; K. Jensen *et al.*, *Lancet*, 1975, *2*, 920; G. Chouinard *et al.*, *Br. med. J.*, 1978, *1*, 1422). This has been confirmed by some placebo-controlled studies (B. Rao and A.D. Broadhurst, *ibid.*, 1976, *1*, 460; J. Thomson *et al.*, *Psychol. Med.*, 1982, *12*, 741), although others have found tryptophan in doses of up to 16 g daily to be no more effective than placebo (J. Mendels *et al.*, *Archs gen. Psychiat.*, 1975, *32*, 22).

Combination therapy. In an attempt to enhance its antidepressant effect, tryptophan has been given with allopurinol to reduce its metabolism by the liver (B. Shopsin, *Lancet*, 1976, *1*, 1189) and also with pyridoxine hydrochloride and ascorbic acid, although these vitamins had no significant effect (A. Coppen, *ibid.*, 90). The concomitant administration of nicotinamide with tryptophan seemed to reduce the dose of tryptophan needed for an antidepressant effect (G. Chouinard *et al.*, *Br. med. J.*, 1978, *1*, 1422).

Combination therapy with antidepressants. The administration of tryptophan alone to patients with depression has been found to be less effective in relieving symptoms than combination therapy with amitriptyline (J. Thomson *et al.*, *Psychol. Med.*, 1982, *12*, 741), clomipramine (J. Wålinder *et al.*, *Archs gen. Psychiat.*, 1976, *33*, 1384), or tranylcypromine (A. Coppen *et al.*, *Lancet*, 1967, *2*, 1178). However, a review of the combined use of tryptophan with tricyclic antidepressants concluded that tryptophan did not enhance the antidepressant efficacy of tricyclics (S.L. Stern and J. Mendels, *J. clin. Psychiat.*, 1981, *42*, 368). In refractory depression, the use of tryptophan, clomipramine, and lithium in combination has been advocated, with substitution of phenelzine for clomipramine if the first combination is ineffective (D. Eccelston, *Br. J. Psychiat.*, 1981, *138*, 257; W.A. Barker and D. Eccleston, *ibid.*, 1984, *144*, 317).

Depression in parkinsonism. Tryptophan has been tried with variable success in the treatment of levodopa-induced depression in patients with parkinsonism. Improvement might be associated with a shorter duration of the disease (D.L. Murphy, *Am. J. Psychiat.*, 1972, *129*, 141; B.L. Beasley *et al.*, *Archs Neurol.*, *Chicago*, 1980, *37*, 155; R.C. Bryant *ibid.*, 677).

EATING DISORDERS. A preliminary study of tryptophan in bulimic patients concluded that tryptophan at a dose of 3 g daily by mouth was not significantly better than placebo at improving mood or decreasing binge eating.— D. Krahn and J. Mitchell (letter), *Am. J. Psychiat.*, 1985, *142*, 1130.

EXTRAPYRAMIDAL DISORDERS. *Myoclonus.* Post-anoxic action myoclonus responds, often dramatically, to tryptophan in combination with a monoamine oxidase inhibitor (D. Chadwick *et al.*, *Brain*, 1977, *100*, 455). However, this combination of drugs may also result in myoclonus, see Interactions with Monoamine Oxidase Inhibitors and Other Drugs under Phenelzine Sulphate (p.379).

Tardive dyskinesia. Drug-induced tardive dyskinesia, akathisia, and insomnia in a 66-year-old woman responded to treatment with tryptophan 2 to 8 g daily by mouth.— R. Sandyk *et al.* (letter), *New Engl. J. Med.*, 1986, *314*, 1257.

HEADACHE. Tryptophan 500 mg every 6 hours gave useful reduction in migraine symptoms in 4 of 8 patients.— P. Kangasniemi *et al.*, *Headache*, 1978, *18*, 161.

HEPATIC ENCEPHALOPATHY. For reference to the role of aromatic and branched-chain amino acids in the treatment of hepatic encephalopathy, see under Enteral and Parenteral Nutrition, p.1252.

MANIA AND MANIC DEPRESSION. A double-blind study in 5 patients with mania found tryptophan to be slightly superior to chlorpromazine (A.J. Prange *et al.*, *Archs gen. Psychiat.*, 1974, *30*, 56) and although a small placebo-controlled study found no benefit with tryptophan (C.A. Chambers and G.J. Naylor, *Br. J. Psychiat.*, 1978, *132*, 555), a larger double-blind placebo-controlled study demonstrated some therapeutic effect at doses of 12 g daily by mouth (G. Chouinard *et al.*, *Biol. Psychiat.*, 1985, *20*, 546). In patients with bipolar illness unresponsive to lithium therapy alone, the addition of tryptophan has controlled manic symptoms (G. Chouinard *et al.*, *Am. J. Psychiat.*, 1979, *136*, 719; B.D. Beitman and D.L. Dunner, *ibid.*, 1982, *139*, 1498; T.D. Brewerton and V.I. Reus, *ibid.*, 1983, *140*, 757).

PAIN. In a double-blind crossover study involving 5 patients with intractable pain, tolerance to the pain relief obtained by central grey stimulation (electrical stimulation of grey matter) was reversed in 4 by concurrent administration of tryptophan 750 mg four times daily. The fifth patient experienced acute gastric pain on ingestion of tryptophan and did not continue the study.— Y. Hosobuchi (letter), *Lancet*, 1978, *2*, 47.

Further references to the use of tryptophan for pain: R. B. King, *J. Neurosurg.*, 1980, *53*, 44.

Musculoskeletal and joint pain. Some patients with rheumatoid arthritis given tryptophan as an antidepressant had reduced rheumatic symptoms, with recurrence when tryptophan was withdrawn.— A. D. Broadhurst (letter), *Br. med. J.*, 1977, *2*, 456.

PHENYLKETONURIA. Treatment with tryptophan and tyrosine as a supplement to normal diet may be a therapeutic alternative in patients with phenylketonuria who cannot tolerate abandonment of dietary phenylalanine and where such dietary restriction is impracticable.— H. Lou (letter), *Lancet*, 1985, *2*, 150.

SLEEP DISORDERS. In 5 of 16 healthy young men, the delay in the onset of rapid-eye-movement sleep was reduced to less than 45 minutes when 5 to 10 g of tryptophan was given on retiring.— I. Oswald *et al.*, *Br. J. Psychiat.*, 1966, *112*, 391.

Rapid-eye-movement (REM) sleep decreased while delta-wave sleep and non-REM sleep increased in 5 healthy persons given tryptophan 7.5 g for 10 consecutive nights. Total sleep increased in all but 1 of 7 patients with insomnia given tryptophan. Tryptophan produced significant increases in non-REM sleep and decreases in REM sleep when given with fenclonine to block the metabolism of tryptophan to serotonin in 4 patients. It seemed that tryptophan produced its sleep effects through a non-serotonin mechanism.— R. J. Wyatt *et al.*, *Lancet*, 1970, *2*, 842.

Studies in 6 patients failed to show that tryptophan 7.5 g had any effect on the disturbed sleep pattern which had been induced by substituting a placebo for normal hypnotics.— V. Březinová *et al.* (letter), *Lancet*, 1972, *2*, 1086. See also M. H. Greenwood *et al.*, *Clin. Pharmac. Ther.*, 1974, *16*, 455.

Reviews of the use of tryptophan as a hypnotic: *Med. Lett.*, 1977, *19*, 108; E. L. Hartmann, *Archs intern. Med.*, 1977, *137*, 272; D. Schneider-Helmert and C. L. Spinweber, *Psychopharmacology*, 1986, *89*, 1.

Further references to the hypnotic effect of tryptophan: A. N. Nicholson and B. M. Stone, *Br. J. clin. Pharmac.*, 1979, *7*, 418P; J. G. Lindsley *et al.*, *Sleep*, 1983, *6*, 247; E. Hartmann, *J. Psychiat. Res.*, 1983, *17*, 107.

Proprietary Preparations

Optimax *(E. Merck, UK). Powder*, tryptophan 1 g, pyridoxine hydrochloride 10 mg, ascorbic acid 20 mg in sachets of 6 g.

Tablets, scored, tryptophan 500 mg, pyridoxine hydrochloride 5 mg, ascorbic acid 10 mg.

Tablets (Optimax WV), scored, tryptophan 500 mg.

Pacitron *(Rorer, UK). Tablets*, tryptophan 500 mg.

For proprietary preparations for enteral and parenteral nutrition containing tryptophan, see p.1289.

Proprietary Names and Manufacturers

Ardeytropin *(Ardeypharm, Ger.)*; Atrimon *(Asta Pharma, Ger.)*; Bikalm *(Promonta, Ger.)*; Biotonin *(UCB, Ger.)*; Dorphan *(Genera, Switz.)*; Kalma *(Fresenius, Ger.)*; Neurocalm *(Efeka, Ger.)*; Neuroremed *(Drug Houses Austral., Austral.)*; Optimax WV *(E. Merck, UK)*; Pacitron *(Rorer, UK)*; Sedanoct *(Woelm, Ger.)*; Trofan *(Upsher-Smith, USA)*; Tryptacin *(Arther, USA)*; Tryptan *(ICN, Canad.)*; Tryptocompren *(Cascan, Ger.)*.

The following names have been used for multi-ingredient preparations containing tryptophan— Optimax *(E. Merck, UK)*; Tryptoplex *(Tyson, USA)*.

2540-l

Viloxazine Hydrochloride *(BANM, USAN, rINNM)*.

ICI-58834. 2-(2-Ethoxyphenoxymethyl)morpholine hydrochloride.

$C_{13}H_{19}NO_3,HCl = 273.8$.

CAS — 46817-91-8 (viloxazine); 35604-67-2 (hydrochloride).

Adverse Effects

Nausea is commonly associated with viloxazine therapy, and vomiting and headache may also occur. Viloxazine has been associated with fewer antimuscarinic side-effects such as dry mouth, disturbance of accommodation, tachycardia, constipation, and difficulty with micturition than the tricyclic antidepressants. Exacerbation of anxiety, agitation, drowsiness, confusion, ataxia, dizziness, insomnia, tremor, paraesthesia, sweating, musculo-skeletal pain, mild hypertension, skin rashes, convulsions, and jaundice with elevated transaminases have also been reported.

Symptoms of overdosage have included drowsiness or coma, decreased reflexes, miosis, and hypotension. Tachycardia has occurred but, unlike amitriptyline, life-threatening cardiac arrhythmias do not appear to have been a problem.

In a study of 96 depressed patients taking viloxazine 200 to 400 mg daily, algorithms were used to differentiate between illness-related symptoms and side-effects. It was found that only a few instances of gastric disturbance and exacerbation of anxiety were probably viloxazine-related.— I. Maistrello *et al.*, *Eur. J. clin. Pharmac.*, 1983, *24*, 277.

EPILEPTOGENIC EFFECT. In a review of 6 cases of convulsive seizures during treatment with viloxazine notified to the *UK* Committee on Safety of Medicines, and 2 other cases from Japan, critical study of the patients' histories suggested a possible causal connection in only 2. It was concluded that even if viloxazine did possess convulsive properties like other antidepressants, it was probably less epileptogenic than conventional tricyclics and was not contra-indicated in epileptics.— J. G. Edwards and M. Glenn-Bott, *J. Neurol. Neurosurg. Psychiat.*, 1984, *47*, 960.

WEIGHT CHANGES. Mention of a tendency to weight loss associated with viloxazine therapy.— D. Nugent, *Clin. Trials J.*, 1979, *16*, 13.

Precautions

Although viloxazine appears to be less cardiotoxic than the tricyclic antidepressants, it should be used with caution in patients with cardiovascular disease and should be avoided in the immediate recovery phase after myocardial infarction. Viloxazine should also be avoided in patients with mania, impaired liver function, or a history of peptic ulcer. Caution is necessary in patients with epilepsy. Manic depressive patients may switch to a manic phase during viloxazine therapy, and patients with suicidal tendencies should be carefully supervised during treatment.

It is not recommended in patients who are breast-feeding.

Viloxazine should not be given to patients receiv-

ing monoamine oxidase inhibitors or for at least 14 days after their discontinuation. Viloxazine may diminish the effects of antihypertensive agents, such as guanethidine, debrisoquine, and bethanidine; some interaction may also occur with clonidine and, in general, blood pressure should be monitored when viloxazine is prescribed with antihypertensive therapy. Blood concentrations of phenytoin may be increased in patients concurrently given viloxazine and phenytoin dosage reduction may be necessary. Since viloxazine appears to have some influence on brain dopamine metabolism viloxazine should be given with caution to patients receiving levodopa. The central nervous system depressant action of alcohol may be enhanced by concurrent administration of viloxazine.
Withdrawal of viloxazine may occasionally be associated with malaise, headache, and vomiting.
Impaired alertness may be experienced at the start of viloxazine antidepressant therapy and patients, if affected, should not drive or operate machinery. For further details of the effects of antidepressant therapy on driving see amitriptyline hydrochloride (p.353).

INTERACTIONS. *Carbamazepine*. For a report of viloxazine resulting in increased serum concentrations of carbamazepine, see Carbamazepine, p.401.

MIGRAINE. Viloxazine may occasionally precipitate attacks in migrainous patients and in these circumstances should be discontinued.— S. Nightingale, *Prescribers' J.*, 1985, *25*, 129.

PORPHYRIA. Viloxazine hydrochloride was considered to be unsafe in patients with acute porphyrias because it has been shown to be porphyrinogenic in *animals* or *in vitro* systems.— M.R. Moore and K.E.L. McColl, *Porphyrias, Drug Lists*, Glasgow, Porphyria Research Unit, University of Glasgow, 1987.

Absorption and Fate

Viloxazine is readily absorbed from the gastrointestinal tract and extensively metabolised. The principal paths of metabolism of viloxazine include hydroxylation and conjugation. Viloxazine is excreted in the urine, mainly in the form of its metabolites, either free or in conjugated form.
Unlike the tricyclic antidepressants, viloxazine has a short plasma half-life of about 2 to 5 hours.
Viloxazine crosses the blood-brain barrier and is excreted in breast milk.

Uses and Administration

Viloxazine is an oxazine antidepressant and chemically distinct from the tricyclic and tetracyclic antidepressants. It does not have marked antimuscarinic or sedative properties and may have some stimulant action. Its properties include inhibitory effects on the re-uptake (and hence the inactivation) of biogenic amines in the central nervous system. Its mode of action in depression is not fully understood.
In the treatment of depression viloxazine is given by mouth as the hydrochloride in doses equivalent to viloxazine 300 mg daily, preferably taken as 200 mg in the morning and 100 mg at lunchtime. The last dose of the day should not be given later than 6 p.m. A maximum total daily dose of 400 mg should not be exceeded. A suggested initial dose for the elderly is 100 mg daily cautiously increased if necessary. Half the normal maintenance dose may be adequate.

DEPRESSION. In the treatment of depression viloxazine has been shown to be as effective as amitriptyline (G. Sedman, *Curr. med. Res. Opinion*, 1977, *5*, 217; W.M. Petrie *et al.*, *Int. Pharmacopsychiat.*, 1982, *17*, 280) and imipramine (B. Davies *et al.*, *Med. J. Aust.*, 1977, *1*, 521; O. Elwan, *J. Int. med. Res.*, 1980, *8*, 7).

For a general comment on the role of antidepressants in depression, see Amitriptyline Hydrochloride, p.355.

NOCTURNAL ENURESIS. Viloxazine was reported to be as effective as imipramine in children with nocturnal enuresis.— A. A. Attenburrow *et al.*, *Practitioner*, 1984, *228*, 99 and 545.

Proprietary Preparations

Vivalan *(ICI Pharmaceuticals, UK)*. *Tablets*, viloxazine 50 mg (as hydrochloride).

Proprietary Names and Manufacturers

Vicilan *(Arg.; ICI-Pharma, Ital.)*; Vivalan *(Belg.; I.C.I.-Pharma, Fr.; ICI, Ger.; ICI Pharmaceuticals, UK)*; Vivarint *(Aust.; ICI, Spain)*.

14028-v

Zimeldine Hydrochloride *(BAN, USAN, rINNM)*.

H-102/09; Zimelidine Hydrochloride. (*Z*)-4-Bromo-γ-(3-pyridyl)cinnamyldimethylamine dihydrochloride monohydrate.

$C_{16}H_{17}BrN_2,2HCl,H_2O=408.2$.

CAS — 56775-88-3 (zimeldine); 60525-15-7 (hydrochloride, anhydrous); 61129-30-4 (hydrochloride, monohydrate).

Zimeldine hydrochloride is an inhibitor of serotonin uptake and was formerly used in the treatment of depression in doses of 200 to 300 mg daily. It was withdrawn worldwide in September 1983 due to the risk of Guillain-Barré syndrome associated with its use.

Ten cases of Guillain-Barré syndrome in patients taking zimeldine had been reported worldwide (1 case in the *UK*) out of 200 000 prescriptions. The patients all recovered or were recovering. Patients who developed the Guillain-Barré syndrome had all previously had a hypersensitivity-like reaction to zimeldine, with influenza-like symptoms; many other patients had the hypersensitivity reaction without serious sequelae, but there was no way of predicting which patients were at risk.— *Pharm. J.*, 1983, *2*, 360.

The *UK* CSM received over 300 reports of adverse reactions associated with zimeldine although there had been fewer than 100 000 prescriptions. More than 60 of the reports were serious and included convulsions and liver damage, as well as neuropathies and the Guillain-Barré syndrome.— Committee on Safety of Medicines, *Current Problems No. 11*, August, 1983..

Proprietary Names and Manufacturers

Zelmid *(Astra, UK)*.

Antidiabetic Agents

7200-s

Diabetes mellitus is a state of chronic hyperglycaemia. Many factors may be involved, including those that are environmental, immunological, and genetic, and they may cause hyperglycaemia by reducing endogenous insulin or by opposing its action. The lack of insulin leads to abnormalties of carbohydrate, protein, and lipid metabolism.

The **classification of diabetes mellitus** and allied categories of glucose intolerance prepared by the World Health Organization (Report of a WHO Study Group, *Tech. Rep. Ser. Wld Hlth Org. No. 727*, 1985) has three clinical classes: diabetes mellitus, impaired glucose tolerance (IGT), and gestational diabetes mellitus. Diabetes mellitus is divided into insulin-dependent diabetes mellitus (IDDM), non-insulin-dependent diabetes mellitus (NIDDM), malnutrition-related diabetes mellitus (MRDM), and a fourth category, formerly termed secondary diabetes, which includes types associated with pancreatic disease and certain genetic syndromes, and with drug- or chemically-induced diabetes. Impaired glucose tolerance, formerly called asymptomatic diabetes, chemical diabetes, subclinical diabetes, borderline diabetes, or latent diabetes, is defined as a glycaemic response to a standard glucose challenge intermediate between normal and diabetic. Gestational diabetes is a form in which the onset or recognition is during pregnancy and which requires reclassification post partum. Comments are also made regarding the lack of agreement, and danger of confusion, over the use of the terms insulin-dependent, non-insulin-dependent, type 1, and type 2 diabetes mellitus. Insulin-dependent and non-insulin-dependent are clinical descriptions whereas types 1 and 2 represent different pathogenic mechanisms. The current use of the term type 1 implies the demonstration of certain immunological phenomena and genetic markers using methods that are rarely available and which lack standardisation. These phenomena and markers may also be found in some patients with non-insulin-dependent diabetes mellitus, impaired glucose tolerance, or normal glucose tolerance. There is, also, no definition of the term type 2, other than the absence of type 1 or other known causes of diabetes. Therefore the designations of type 1 and type 2 diabetes mellitus are not included in this classification but the report does recommend that, since the terms are at present widely used and in order to avoid confusion, they should be regarded as completely synonymous with insulin-dependent diabetes mellitus and non-insulin-dependent diabetes mellitus respectively.

Insulin-dependent diabetes has an onset typically in youth, although it may occur at any age, and was formerly termed juvenile-onset diabetes. Patients have little or no endogenous insulin, are prone to develop ketosis, and are dependent upon therapy with insulin (see p.391) for long-term survival. Brittle diabetes is usually used to describe diabetes where control is difficult and where problems of clinical management occur.

In **non-insulin-dependent diabetes** the onset is typically in later life, but again may occur at any age, and it was formerly called adult-onset or maturity-onset diabetes. In these patients endogenous insulin may be either depressed, normal, or elevated and many are obese. Treatment for non-insulin-dependent diabetes may be dietary modification, oral hypoglycaemic agents, or in certain circumstances, insulin. The two principal categories of oral hypoglycaemic agents are the sulphonylureas (see chlorpropamide, p.387) and the biguanides (now mainly metformin hydrochloride, p.397).

Also included in this section are agents such as acarbose (below) and guar gum (p.391) which have a hypoglycaemic effect only by interfering with the absorption of dietary monosaccharides. Other compounds which may have a similar action and which are under investigation include emiglitate and miglitol.

In many patients the progressive development of diabetes leads to several complications, such as diabetic neuropathy, diabetic nephropathy, diabetic retinopathy and cataracts, cardiovascular disease, and an increased risk of infection. Aldose-reductase inhibitors such as sorbinil (p.398) are being investigated for the management of some of these complications.

The immunological involvement in diabetes mellitus has led to the investigation of immunosuppression as a method of controlling the disease.

The **diagnosis of diabetes mellitus** and impaired glucose tolerance is based upon blood-glucose concentrations exceeding set values under specified conditions. It should be noted that glucose concentrations in venous plasma, venous whole blood, and capillary whole blood may be slightly different. In the presence of the classic symptoms of diabetes, a gross and unequivocal elevation of glucose concentration is usually considered sufficient for diagnosis. In other circumstances either repeated sampling for glucose concentration or the performance of the oral glucose tolerance test is necessary. The oral glucose tolerance test consists essentially of an overnight fast followed by measurement of the fasting blood-glucose concentration, the administration of glucose 75 g by mouth, and a further measurement of blood-glucose 2 hours after the glucose load. Further details concerning the diagnosis of diabetes, including values for glucose concentrations and the performance of the glucose tolerance test are given by the World Health Organization (*Tech. Rep. Ser. Wld Hlth Org. No. 727*, 1985).

A detailed report on diabetes mellitus including details on classification.— *Tech. Rep. Ser. Wld Hlth Org. No. 727* 1985.

DIETARY MODIFICATION. References to dietary modification in the management of diabetes mellitus, especially a reduction in fat intake with a compensating increase in high-fibre carbohydrate: *Pharm. J.*, 1982, *2*, 567; *Lancet*, 1983, *1*, 741; J. I. Mann, *Br. med. J.*, 1984, *288*, 1025.

MONITORING OF THERAPY. References to the self-monitoring of blood-glucose concentrations: P. F. W. Miller *et al.*, *Archs Dis. Childh.*, 1983, *58*, 294; P. M. Bell and K. Walshe, *Br. med. J.*, 1983, *286*, 1230; R. L. Gibbins *et al.*, *ibid.*, *287*, 801; *Med. Lett.*, 1983, *25*, 42 and 64; G. Petranyi *et al.*, *Br. med. J.*, 1984, *288*, 757; J. -L. Chiasson *et al.*, *Can. med. Ass. J.*, 1984, *130*, 38; M. A. V. Bosch and M. L. Hyneck, *Clin. Pharm.*, 1984, *3*, 291; G. Rayman *et al.*, *Practitioner*, 1984, *228*, 191; P. M. Bell and K. Walshe, *ibid.*, 197; S. Germer and I. W. Campbell, *Br. J. clin. Pract.*, 1985, *39*, 225; B. Rasaiah, *Can. med. Ass. J.*, 1985, *132*, 1357.

References to the measurement of glycosylated haemoglobin for the monitoring of therapy: I. Peacock, *J. clin. Path.*, 1984, *37*, 841; *Lancet*, 1984, *2*, 19; D. M. Nathan *et al.*, *New Engl. J. Med.*, 1984, *310*, 341; D. E. Goldstein, *ibid.*, 384; A. Marglin (letter), *ibid.*, 1746; J. M. May (letter), *ibid;* D. M. Nathan *et al.* (letter), *ibid;* M. A. Varnam and J. L. Skinner, *Practitioner*, 1984, *228*, 680.

References to the measurement of serum-fructosamine concentrations for the monitoring of therapy: J. R. Baker *et al.*, *Br. med. J.*, 1984, *288*, 1484; J. R. Baker *et al.*, *ibid.*, 1985, *290*, 352; E. J. Hindle *et al.*, *Archs Dis. Childh.*, 1986, *61*, 113.

References to the screening for microalbuminuria for the prediction of diabetic complications: A. H. Barnett *et al.* (letter), *Lancet*, 1985, *1*, 53; A. G. Davies *et al.* (letter), *ibid.*, 466; M. Marre *et al.* (letter), *ibid.*, 516; W. Gatling *et al.* (letter), *ibid.*, 875; G. Slama *et al.* (letter), *ibid.*, 1338; C. E. Mogensen *et al.* (letter), *ibid.*, 1512; R. E. J. Ryder *et al.* (letter), *ibid.*, 1513; A. S. Hutchison and D. St J. O'Reilly (letter), *ibid.*, *2*, 44; T. L. Dornan and S. R. Heller (letter), *ibid.*, 212.

12304-c

Acarbose *(BAN, USAN, rINN).*

Bay-g-5421. *O*-{4-Amino-4,6-dideoxy-*N*-[(1*S*,4*R*,5*S*,6*S*)-4,5,6-trihydroxy-3-hydroxymethylcyclohex-2-enyl]-α-D-glucopyranosyl}-(1→4)-*O*-α-D-glucopyranosyl-(1→4)-D-glucopyranose.

$C_{25}H_{43}NO_{18}$=645.6.

CAS — 56180-94-0.

Acarbose is an inhibitor of alpha glucosidase and through this action it reduces the increase in blood-sugar concentrations after a carbohydrate load. Its use in diabetes mellitus is under study.

Gastro-intestinal disturbances, particularly flatulence or meteorism, may occur and are reported to be due to gases from non-absorbed carbohydrate in the colon. A finding of renal adenomas in *rats* given acarbose led to the manufacturer extending toxicological studies.

Acarbose might help control insulin-dependent and non-insulin-dependent diabetes mellitus. It might control the symptoms of dumping syndrome. It has not yet demonstrated a therapeutic effect in hyperlipoproteinaemia or in obesity.— U. R. Fölsch, *Hepatogastroenterology*, 1982, *29*, 47.

Some references to acarbose given to diabetics: H. Vierhapper *et al.* (letter), *Lancet*, 1978, *2*, 1386; R. J. Walton *et al.*, *Br. med. J.*, 1979, *1*, 220; D. Sailer and G. Röder, *Arzneimittel-Forsch.*, 1980, *30*, 2182; H. Vierhapper *et al.* (letter), *Diabetologia*, 1981, *20*, 586; C. K. Lardinois *et al.*, *Archs intern. Med.*, 1984, *144*, 345; R. S. Scott *et al.*, *Aust. N.Z. J. Med.*, 1984, *14*, 649.

References to acarbose given in the dumping syndrome or for postprandial reactive hypoglycaemia after gastric surgery: J. C. McLoughlin *et al.*, *Lancet*, 1979, *2*, 603 and 808 (dumping syndrome); D. J. A. Jenkins *et al.* (letter), *ibid.*, 1982, *1*, 109 (dumping syndrome); P. A. J. Speth *et al.*, *Gut*, 1983, *24*, 798 (postprandial hypoglycaemia; with pectin).

Proprietary Names and Manufacturers

Bayer, UK.

7213-j

Acetohexamide *(BAN, USAN, rINN).*

1-(4-Acetylbenzenesulphonyl)-3-cyclohexylurea.

$C_{15}H_{20}N_2O_4S$=324.4.

CAS — 968-81-0.

Pharmacopoeias. In *Br.*, *Jpn* and *U.S.*

A white, odourless or almost odourless, crystalline powder. Practically **insoluble** in water and ether; soluble 1 in 230 of alcohol and 1 in 210 of chloroform; soluble in pyridine and dilute solutions of alkali hydroxides.

Adverse Effects, Treatment, and Precautions

As for chlorpropamide (p.387).

ADMINISTRATION IN RENAL FAILURE. Acetohexamide should be avoided in patients with renal failure whose glomerular filtration-rates are 50 mL per minute or less.— W. M. Bennett *et al.*, *Am. J. Kidney Dis.*, 1983, *3*, 155.

Absorption and Fate

Acetohexamide is readily absorbed from the gastro-intestinal tract and is extensively bound to plasma proteins. It is metabolised in the liver to hydroxyhexamide which also has hypoglycaemic activity. The plasma half-life of acetohexamide is about 1.3 hours and the half-life of its metabolite is about 5 hours. Both unchanged drug and metabolite are excreted in the urine.

Uses and Administration

Acetohexamide is a sulphonylurea hypoglycaemic agent with actions and uses similar to those of chlorpropamide (p.388). Its duration of action is 12 hours or more but is less prolonged than that of chlorpropamide. The usual initial dose by mouth in non-insulin-dependent diabetes mellitus is 250 mg daily before breakfast. This may then be increased by amounts of 250 to 500 mg daily at intervals of 5 to 7 days to a maintenance dose of up to 1.5 g daily; increasing the dose above 1.5 g does not usually lead to further benefit. Doses in excess of 1 g daily may be taken in 2 divided doses, before the morning and evening meals.

Acetohexamide had no antidiuretic effect but enhanced diuresis after water load in 7 subjects.— A. M. Moses *et al., Ann. intern. Med.*, 1973, *78*, 541.

For a recommendation to avoid acetohexamide in renal impairment, see above under Adverse Effects, Treatment, and Precautions.

Preparations

Acetohexamide Tablets *(B.P.)*

Acetohexamide Tablets *(U.S.P.)*

Proprietary Preparations

Dimelor *(Lilly, UK). Tablets,* scored, acetohexamide 500 mg.

Proprietary Names and Manufacturers

Dimelor *(Arg.; Austral.; Belg.; Lilly, Canad.; Lilly, Ital.; Lilly, S.Afr.; Lilly, UK)*; Dymelor *(Lilly, USA)*; Gamadiabet *(Salvat, Spain)*; Metaglucina *(Spain)*; Ordimel *(Neth.; Swed.)*.

16022-z

Alrestatin Sodium *(USAN, rINNM).*

AY-22284A. Sodium 1,3-dioxo-1*H*-benz[*de*]isoquinoline-2(3*H*)-acetate.

$C_{14}H_8NNaO_4$=277.2.

CAS — 51411-04-2 (alrestatin); 51876-97-2 (sodium salt).

Alrestatin sodium is an aldose-reductase inhibitor similar in action to sorbinil (p.398). It has been investigated for the treatment of diabetic neuropathy.

A double-blind study of alrestatin in 30 diabetic patients, 27 of whom had clinical signs of polyneuropathy. Alrestatin was given by mouth in a dose of 2 g daily for the first week, 4 g daily for the next 5 weeks, and 8 g daily for a further 6 weeks. Results indicated a beneficial effect on polyneuropathy; no improvement was found in retinopathy or cataracts. Side-effects noted were liver disturbance in 3 patients, mild constipation in 1, and nausea, reduced appetite, and weight loss in a further patient.— J. Fagius and S. Jameson, *J. Neurol. Neurosurg. Psychiat.*, 1981, *44*, 991. Other studies showing no significant benefit in diabetic neuropathy following oral or intravenous administration of alrestatin: K. H. Gabbay *et al., Metabolism*, 1979, *28, Suppl. 1*, 471; A. Culebras *et al., Archs Neurol., Chicago*, 1981, *38*, 133.

Proprietary Names and Manufacturers

Ayerst, USA.

7214-z

Buformin Hydrochloride *(pINNM).*

DBV *(buformin)*; W-37 *(buformin)*. 1-Butylbiguanide hydrochloride.

$C_6H_{15}N_5$,HCl=193.7.

CAS — 692-13-7 (buformin); 1190-53-0 (hydrochloride).

NOTE. Buformin is *USAN*.

Pharmacopoeias. In *Cz.* and *Jug.*

Buformin hydrochloride is a biguanide hypoglycaemic agent with actions and uses similar to those of metformin hydrochloride (p.397). It is given by mouth in non-insulin-dependent diabetes mellitus in doses of up to 300 mg daily.

Proprietary Names and Manufacturers

Diabrin *(Arg.)*; Silubin Retard *(Belg.; Grünenthal, S.Afr.; Andromaco, Spain; Grünenthal, Switz.)*; Sindiatil *(Bayer, Ital.)*.

7215-c

Carbutamide *(BAN, rINN).*

U-6987. 1-Butyl-3-sulphanilylurea.

$C_{11}H_{17}N_3O_3S$=271.3.

CAS — 339-43-5.

Pharmacopoeias. In *Fr., It.,* and *Nord.*

Carbutamide is a sulphonylurea hypoglycaemic agent with similar actions and uses to chlorpropamide (see below) but which is more toxic. It has been given by mouth in non-insulin-dependent diabetes mellitus in single daily doses of 0.5 to 1 g.

Proprietary Names and Manufacturers

Biouren *(Nessa, Spain)*; Carbutil *(Wasserman, Spain)*; Diabetin *(Diasan, Switz.)*; Diabetoplex *(Vaillant, Ital.)*; Diabutan *(Streuli, Switz.)*; Dia-Tablinen *(Beiersdorf, Ger.)*; Dibefanil *(Mepha, Switz.)*; Dicarbul *(Grossmann, Switz.)*; Glucidoral *(Servier, Fr.)*; Glucofren *(Cophar, Switz.)*; Insoral *(Valeas, Ital.)*; Invenol *(Hoechst, Ger.)*; Nadisan *(Boehringer, Arg.; Boehringer Mannheim, Belg.; Boehringer Mannheim, Ger.; Boehringer Mannheim, Spain; Boehringer Mannheim, Swed.; Boehringer Mannheim, Switz.)*.

7216-k

Chlorpropamide *(BAN, USAN, rINN).*

1-(4-Chlorobenzenesulphonyl)-3-propylurea.

$C_{10}H_{13}ClN_2O_3S$=276.7.

CAS — 94-20-2.

Pharmacopoeias. In *Br., Braz., Chin., Cz., Egypt., Fr., Ind., It., Jpn, Jug., Nord., Rus.,* and *U.S.*

A white, odourless or almost odourless, crystalline powder. *B.P.* **solubilities** are: insoluble in water; soluble 1 in 12 of alcohol, 1 in 5 of acetone, 1 in 9 of chloroform, and 1 in 200 of ether; soluble in solutions of alkali hydroxides. *U.S.P.* solubilities are: practically insoluble in water; soluble in alcohol; sparingly soluble in chloroform.

Adverse Effects

Among the mild adverse effects observed with sulphonylureas are gastro-intestinal disturbances such as nausea, vomiting, heartburn, anorexia, constipation, diarrhoea, and a metallic taste, and there may be headache, dizziness, weakness, paraesthesia, and tinnitus. These effects are usually dose-dependent. Skin rashes and pruritus may occur and photosensitivity has been reported. Rashes are usually allergic and may progress to more serious disorders.

Hypoglycaemia occurs with all hypoglycaemic agents and chlorpropamide has been associated with severe, prolonged, and sometimes fatal hypoglycaemia.

Other severe effects may be allergic in nature. They include cholestatic jaundice, leucopenia, thrombocytopenia, aplastic anaemia, agranulocytosis, haemolytic anaemia, erythema multiforme or the Stevens-Johnson syndrome, exfoliative dermatitis, and erythema nodosum.

Acute porphyrias may be exacerbated.

The sulphonylureas and particularly chlorpropamide may infrequently induce a syndrome of inappropriate secretion of antidiuretic hormone (SIADH)characterised by water retention, hyponatraemia, and central nervous system signs.

Work on tolbutamide has suggested that the sulphonylureas might be associated with an increase in cardiovascular mortality; this has been the subject of considerable debate (see p.399).

A review of the adverse effects of sulphonylurea drugs.— B. J. Paice *et al., Adverse Drug React. Ac. Pois. Rev.*, 1985, *4*, 23.

Sixty-one reports of reactions to chlorpropamide had been received by the Committee on Safety of Drugs; 25 related to skin reactions including the Stevens-Johnson syndrome, exfoliative dermatitis, eczema, photodermatitis, erythema nodosum, and purpuric and papular rashes. Blood disorders included aplastic anaemia (3), agranulocytosis (2), pancytopenia (3), leucopenia (4), thrombocytopenia (5), and haemolytic anaemia (2). Liver damage occurred in 8 patients and was mainly of the cholestatic type accompanied by jaundice.— E. L. Harris, *Br. med. J.*, 1971, *3*, 29.

EFFECTS ON THE EYES. When a diabetic patient who had experienced bilateral visual loss for several months and who had been taking chlorpropamide for one year stopped treatment, visual acuity improved and colour vision rapidly returned. A 5-day challenge with chlorpropamide resulted in a mild decrease in acuity followed by return to baseline values when treatment was again stopped. Drug-induced optic neuropathy was considered to have occurred.— J. Wymore and J. E. Carter, *Archs intern. Med.*, 1982, *142*, 381.

EFFECTS ON THE KIDNEY. A report in one patient of the nephrotic syndrome in association with chlorpropamide therapy. Serological testing and renal biopsy demonstrated that the glomerular lesions were of an immune-complex nature. Both the nephrotic syndrome and the glomerulonephritis resolved after treatment was stopped. The patient also developed a skin eruption, hepatitis, and eosinophilia.— G. B. Appel *et al., Am. J. Med.*, 1983, *74*, 337.

EFFECTS ON THE SKIN. A report of Stevens-Johnson syndrome in a woman given chlorpropamide. After one month's treatment she suddenly developed widespread skin and mouth lesions and chlorpropamide was at once stopped. The condition spread further despite prednisone treatment and there were typical target lesions of erythema multiforme. Progressive neutropenia also developed and she died on the fourth hospital day.— T. M. Kanefsky and S. J. Medoff, *Archs intern. Med.*, 1980, *140*, 1543.

HYPOGLYCAEMIA. A review of severe drug-induced hypoglycaemia or frank hypoglycaemic coma in 778 patients [excluding cases involving insulin alone], reported up to mid-1976. Sulphonylureas accounted for 465 of the cases; there were 46 deaths and 13 patients suffered serious sequelae. Phenformin or buformin were implicated in 8 episodes with 2 deaths. Restricted carbohydrate intake was by far the most frequent predisposing factor, followed by age: patients over 60 years were particularly at risk. Abnormal liver or kidney function were important contributing factors, depending on the drug administered. When treating the patient it was mandatory that intravenous glucose should not be stopped too soon if recurrent hypoglycaemia was to be guarded against.— H. S. Seltzer, *Compr. Ther.*, 1979, *5*, 21.

Of 204 episodes of severe hypoglycaemia in adults, recorded during a 1-year prospective survey of admissions to a hospital accident and emergency department, 200 occurred in insulin-treated diabetics, 3 in elderly patients receiving sulphonylureas, and 1 in a patient with insulinoma.— J. Potter *et al., Br. med. J.*, 1982, *285*, 1180. In a similar study, 2 of 77 episodes of hypoglycaemia occurred in patients taking oral hypoglycaemic drugs and the remainder in patients receiving insulin therapy.— R. G. Moses *et al., Med. J. Aust.*, 1985, *142*, 294.

A report of severe hypoglycaemia, at first thought to be due to insulinoma but later found to be due to adult nesidioblastosis [proliferation of the islet cells], in a woman covertly taking chlorpropamide.— G. Rayman *et al., J. clin. Path.*, 1984, *37*, 651.

Treatment of Adverse Effects

In acute poisoning the stomach should be emptied by aspiration and lavage. Hypoglycaemia should be treated; the general management of hypoglycaemia is described under insulin (p.393). The patient should be observed over several days in case hypoglycaemia recurs.

Evidence that activated charcoal adsorbs sulphonylureas and so may be of benefit in acute poisoning.— P. J. Neuvonen and S. Kärkkäinen, *Clin. Pharmac. Ther.*, 1983, *33*, 386 (healthy subjects). See also: P. J. Neuvonen *et al., Eur. J. clin. Pharmac.*, 1983, *24*, 243 (healthy subjects); H. Kannisto and P. J. Neuvonen, *J. pharm. Sci.*, 1984, *73*, 253 (study *in vitro*).

For reports of diazoxide being used in the treatment of chlorpropamide-induced hypoglycaemia, see p.478.

Precautions

Chlorpropamide and the other sulphonylureas should not be used in insulin-dependent diabetes mellitus. Use in non-insulin-dependent diabetes mellitus is contra-indicated in patients with ketoacidosis and in those with severe infection, stress, trauma, or other severe conditions where the sulphonylurea is unlikely to control the hyperglycaemia. Control may also be difficult in elderly subjects. Chlorpropamide should not be given in severe impairment of renal, hepatic, or thyroid function. Insulin is preferred for the treatment of pregnant patients. Care is necessary during excessive exercise as hypoglycaemia may be provoked. Chlorpropamide's antidiuretic effect may cause problems in patients with conditions associated with fluid retention.

INTERACTIONS. Many compounds have been reported to interact with chlorpropamide and the other sulphonylureas.

One interaction that does not fit into the usual pattern involves alcohol intolerance, mainly with chlorpropamide; this is similar to the disulfiram-alcohol interaction, although it is not clear whether the mechanism is the same. The main symptom is facial flushing and it has been proposed that this symptom could be used as a diagnostic test for non-insulin-dependent diabetes mellitus (R.D.G. Leslie and D.A. Pyke, *Br. med. J.*, 1978, *2*, 1519; D.A. Pyke and R.D.G. Leslie, *ibid.*, 1521; P.G. Wiles *et al.*, *ibid.*, 1984, *288*, 328). However, there have been reports of the test not being specific (N.E. de Silva *et al.*, *Lancet*, 1981, *1*, 128; S.N.T. Fui *et al.*, *Br. med. J.*, 1983, *287*, 1509) and despite a great deal having been published on the chloropropamide-alcohol flushing test (CPAF), its value is not clearly defined. Alcohol, as well as provoking a flushing reaction with chlorpropamide, has been reported both to increase and decrease the half-life of tolbutamide depending on whether the alcohol administration was acute or chronic (E.M. Sellers and M.R. Holloway, *Clin. Pharmacokinet.*, 1978, *3*, 440).

Most of the other interactions are due to the displacement of the sulphonylurea from plasma proteins, to alterations in the metabolism of the sulphonylurea, or to the interacting drug possessing its own activity on blood sugar. The overall effect of these interactions is to decrease or, more usually, increase the hypoglycaemic effect of the sulphonylurea.

Compounds that may *diminish the hypoglycaemic effect* and thus cause an increase in the dosage requirement of the sulphonylurea include:
rifampicin (E.K.G. Syvälahti *et al.*, *Lancet*, 1974, *2*, 232);
thiazide diuretics (P.C. Kansal *et al.*, *Sth. med. J.*, 1969, *62*, 1374).

There is a theoretical risk of a diminished hypoglycaemic effect with corticosteroids and with oral contraceptives.

Compounds that may *increase the hypoglycaemic effect* of sulphonylureas and cause a reduction in their dosage requirement include:
antibiotics or anti-infectives such as chloramphenicol (L.K. Christensen and L. Skovsted, *Lancet*, 1969, *2*, 1397) and sulphonamides including co-trimoxazole (W. Berger, *Schweiz. med. Wschr.*, 1971, *101*, 1013; L.M.H. Wing and J.O. Miners, *Br. J. clin. Pharmac.*, 1985, *20*, 482);
coumarin anticoagulants (W. Berger, *Schweiz. med. Wschr.*, 1971, *101*, 1013; J. Judis, *J. pharm. Sci.*, 1973, *62*, 232);
anti-inflammatory agents and analgesics including azapropazone, phenylbutazone, and salicylates (P.B. Andreasen, *et al.*, *Br. J. clin. Pharmac.*, 1981, *12*, 581; E.L. Harris, *Br. med. J.*, 1971, *3*, 29; E. Schulz, *Arch. klin. Med.*, 1968, *214*, 135);
lipid regulating agents such as clofibrate and halofenate (C. Ferrari *et al.*, *New Engl. J. Med.*, 1976, *294*, 1184; A.K. Jain *et al.*, *ibid.*, 1975, *293*, 1283).

Some of the other compounds implicated in increasing the hypoglycaemic effect of the sulphonylureas are:
cimetidine and ranitidine (J. Feely and N. Peden, *Br. J. clin. Pharmac.*, 1983, *15*, 607P; N.G. Dey *et al.*, *ibid.*, *16*, 438); R.S. MacWalter *et al.*, *ibid.*, 1985, *19*, 121P);
fenfluramine (M. Verdy *et al.*, *Int. J. Obes.*, 1983, *7*, 289);
indobufen (E. Elvander-Ståhl *et al.*, *Br. J. clin. Pharmac.*, 1984, *18*, 773);
methyldopa (B. Gachályi *et al.*, *Int. J. clin. Pharmac.*, 1980, *18*, 133);
miconazole (J.C. Meurice *et al.*, *Presse Méd.*, 1983, *12*, 1670);
sulphinpyrazone (D.J. Birkett *et al.*, *Br. J. clin. Pharmac.*, 1982, *14*, 574P).

Beta-blockers may mask some of the symptoms of hypoglycaemia. While there has been a report of beta-blockers reducing the hypoglycaemic action of glibenclamide (R. Zaman *et al.*, *Br. J. clin. Pharmac.*, 1982, *13*, 507) other studies have failed to observe an interaction with beta-blockers and glibenclamide or tolbutamide (I.B. Davies *et al.*, *ibid.*, 1984, *17*, 622P; J.O. Miners *et al.*, *ibid.*, *18*, 853).

It is considered that any interaction between sulphonylureas and calcium channel blockers such as nifedipine and verapamil is not significant (*Drug Interact. News.*, 1985, *5*, 27). Further details are provided under nifedipine (p.1510).

DRIVING. Hypoglycaemic events are the commonest cause of drug-induced acute illness while driving. Drivers needing insulin should not drive vocationally. Vocational drivers needing oral hypoglycaemic drugs have a difficult problem especially if they are on rotating shifts, if the amount of physical exercise varies greatly, or if they change jobs frequently. If they are to be allowed to drive they should be taking a biguanide or a short-acting sulphonylurea.— P. A. B. Raffle, *Prescribers' J.*, 1981, *21*, 197.

PORPHYRIA. Chlorpropamide was considered to be unsafe in patients with acute porphyria as it has been associated with acute attacks.— M.R. Moore and K.E.L. McColl, *Porphyrias, Drug Lists*, Glasgow, Porphyria Research Unit, University of Glasgow, 1987.

Absorption and Fate

Chlorpropamide is readily absorbed from the gastro-intestinal tract and is extensively bound to plasma proteins. The half-life in plasma is about 35 hours. It is partly metabolised in the liver to metabolites with some hypoglycaemic activity and metabolites and unchanged drug are excreted in the urine.

Although absorption is delayed by the presence of food, available evidence indicates that sulphonylureas are virtually completely absorbed after oral administration. They are avidly bound to plasma albumin. All sulphonylureas undergo varying degrees of hepatic metabolism; metabolites of some possess significant hypoglycaemic activity. Between 20 and 80% of an oral dose is eliminated by the kidneys within 24 hours in subjects with normal renal function.— A. C. Asmal and A. Marble, *Drugs*, 1984, *28*, 62. Another review of the clinical pharmacokinetics of sulphonylurea hypoglycaemic agents.— L. Balant, *Clin. Pharmacokinet.*, 1981, *6*, 215.

In a study of variations in serum-chlorpropamide concentrations in diabetic outpatients there was no correlation between dose or serum concentration and clinical state as assessed by blood or urine glucose concentrations. Furthermore, marked interindividual differences in serum-chlorpropamide concentrations were found between patients prescribed the same dose.— U. Bergman *et al.*, *Eur. J. clin. Pharmac.*, 1980, *18*, 165. A similar lack of correlation with tolbutamide.— A. Melander *et al.*, *Br. med. J.*, 1978, *1*, 142.

Uses and Administration

Chlorpropamide is a sulphonylurea hypoglycaemic agent which is given by mouth in the treatment of non-insulin-dependent diabetes mellitus. It is used to supplement treatment by diet modification when such modification has not proved effective on its own.

Chlorpropamide appears to have several modes of action. Initially, secretion of insulin by functioning islet beta cells is increased. However, when the insulin secretion falls again the hypoglycaemic effect persists and may be due to inhibition of hepatic glucose production and increased sensitivity to any available insulin; this may explain the observed clinical improvement in glycaemic control. The action of chlorpropamide is prolonged, allowing a once-daily dosage schedule. There are some reports of a duration of action of up to 72 hours.

Chlorpropamide is given in an initial daily dose of 250 mg as a single dose with breakfast. It is usual to adjust this dose after 5 to 7 days to achieve an optimum maintenance dose which is usually in the range 100 to 500 mg daily; increasing the dose above 500 mg is unlikely to produce further benefit.

Patients who do not respond to a sulphonylurea will need to be treated with insulin although sometimes treatment has been tried with a combination of a sulphonylurea and metformin. In such cases the dose of metformin hydrochloride is 500 mg twice daily, increased if necessary over several weeks to a maximum of 3 g daily in divided doses.

Chlorpropamide, though not the other sulphonylureas, is also sometimes used in mild diabetes insipidus. It has been reported to act by sensitising the renal tubules to antidiuretic hormone. The dose has to be carefully adjusted to minimise the risk of hypoglycaemia. A maximum of 350 mg daily has been recommended although doses of up to 500 mg daily have been used.

An extensive review of the actions and uses of sulphonylurea hypoglycaemic agents.— J. E. Jackson and R. Bressler, *Drugs*, 1981, *22*, 211 and 295. See also A. C. Asmal and A. Marble, *ibid.*, 1984, *28*, 62.

DIABETES MELLITUS. The mechanism of action of the sulphonylureas in diabetes mellitus is still unclear. There is an initial increase in the concentration of insulin in the blood, but this does not last, yet, despite the insulin concentration returning to pretreatment values, the blood glucose concentration is still reduced. There appears to be an extrapancreatic action with increases in the number of insulin receptors and an effect on insulin binding as well as on insulin resistance.

There is no 'best buy' in the sulphonylureas although the division into short-acting and long-acting drugs is useful. For convenience of dosage a long-acting sulphonylurea should be used in patients under the age of 65 with normal renal function. A shorter-acting drug is safer in those with declining renal function or with any difficulties in following dietary instructions. As patients grow older they may need to be switched to a short-acting sulphonylurea. Treatment should be started with the minimum dose. When control deteriorates there are doubts about the value of increasing the dose. Any benefits may be short-lived and the observation that the technique of insulin treatment is best learnt when the patient retains some manual dexterity has tended to lead towards earlier treatment with insulin.— M. Nattrass, *Br. med. J.*, 1986, *292*, 1033.

Further reviews of the sulphonylureas in diabetes mellitus: *Drug & Ther. Bull.*, 1981, *19*, 49; J. E. Gerich, *Mayo Clin. Proc.*, 1985, *60*, 439.

References to the actions of sulphonylureas: R. G. Judzewitsch *et al.*, *J. clin. Endocr. Metab.*, 1982, *55*, 321; R. A. DeFronzo and E. Ferrannimi, *Medicine, Baltimore*, 1982, *61*, 125; O. G. Kolterman *et al.*, *Diabetes*, 1984, *33*, 346.

Choice of therapy. The first report from the UK Prospective Study of Therapies of Maturity-Onset-Diabetes, a multicentre study planned to include up to 4000 patients and to continue until 1992, comparing the efficacy of diet, oral hypoglycaemics, or insulin. Patients were treated at first by diet. If, after 3 to 4 months their fasting plasma-glucose concentration remained above 6 mmol per litre, they were allocated to continuing diet alone, or additional oral therapy, or insulin. Results from a group of 286 patients who had been followed up for one year demonstrated that insulin and sulphonylurea therapy were equally effective in reducing glycaemia. End-points for the full study had been chosen with the aim of determining whether improved blood-glucose control would reduce disease complications and whether either drug therapy has deleterious side-effects.— *Diabetologia*, 1983, *24*, 404. See also R. C. Turner *et al.* (letter), *ibid.*, 1984, *27*, 419.

A study in 8 patients with non-insulin-dependent diabetes mellitus concluding that such patients have both increased rates of postabsorptive glucose production and decreased insulin-induced stimulation of glucose utilisation, and that therapy with either tolazamide or exogenous insulin resulted in similar improvements in both these abnormalities.— R. G. Firth *et al.*, *New Engl. J. Med.*, 1986, *314*, 1280.

A discussion on when to use insulin in patients with onset of diabetes in middle life: R. B. Tattersall and A. R. Scott, *Postgrad. med. J.*, 1987, *63*, 859.

Combination with insulin. For reviews and reports on

the use of sulphonylureas together with insulin, see Glibenclamide, below.

Diagnosis and testing. For a discussion of the chlorpropamide-alcohol flushing test, see above under Precautions.

Preparations

Chlorpropamide Tablets *(B.P.)*

Chlorpropamide Tablets *(U.S.P.)*

Proprietary Preparations

Diabinese *(Pfizer, UK). Tablets,* scored, chlorpropamide 100 and 250 mg.

Glymese *(DDSA Pharmaceuticals, UK). Tablets,* scored, chlorpropamide 250 mg.

Proprietary Names and Manufacturers

Bioglumin *(Spain)*; Catanil *(Ital.)*; Chloromide *(Canad.)*; Chloronase *(Canad.; Ger.; Neth.; Norw.)*; Clordiabet *(Carulla Vekar, Spain)*; Clordiasan *(Spain)*; Cloro-Hipoglucina *(Spain)*; Diabemide *(Guidotti, Ital.)*; Diabenal *(Norw.)*; Diabet *(Robert, Spain)*; Diabetal *(Swed.)*; Diabetasi *(Ital.)*; Diabetoral *(Ger.)*; Diabexan *(Crosara, Ital.)*; Diabines *(Pfizer, Swed.)*; Diabinese *(Arg.; Pfizer, Austral.; Belg.; Pfizer, Canad.; Pfizer, Fr.; Pfizer, Ital.; Neth.; Pfizer, Norw.; Pfizer, S.Afr.; Pfizer, Spain; Pfizer, Switz.; Pfizer, UK; Pfizer, USA)*; Diatron *(Ital.)*; Gliconorm *(Gentili, Ital.)*; Glucamide *(Lemmon, USA)*; Glucosulfina *(Spain)*; Glymese *(DDSA Pharmaceuticals, UK)*; Hypomide *(Lennon, S.Afr.)*; Insulase *(USA)*; Melisar *(Ital.)*; Melitase *(Berk Pharmaceuticals, UK)*; Mellinese *(Pfizer, Denm.; Ital.)*; Nogluc *(Arg.)*; Normoglic *(Salfa, Ital.)*; Normoglig *(Ital.)*; Novopropamide *(Novopharm, Canad.)*; Promide *(Protea, Austral.)*; Stabinol *(Canad.)*.

7217-a

Glibenclamide *(BAN, rINN).*

Glybenclamide; Glyburide *(USAN)*; Glycbenzcyclamide; HB-419; U-26452. 1-{4-[2-(5-Chloro-2-methoxybenzamido)ethyl]benzenesulphonyl}-3-cyclohexylurea.

$C_{23}H_{28}ClN_3O_5S=494.0$.

CAS — 10238-21-8.

NOTE. The name glibornuride has frequently but erroneously been applied to glibenclamide.

Pharmacopoeias. In *Br., Braz., Cz., Ind.,* and *Nord.*

A white or almost white, odourless or almost odourless, crystalline powder. Practically **insoluble** in water and ether; soluble 1 in 330 of alcohol, 1 in 36 of chloroform, and 1 in 250 of methyl alcohol.

Adverse Effects, Treatment, and Precautions

As for chlorpropamide (p.387). Unlike chlorpropamide, glibenclamide is reported to exert a mild diuretic action.

It has been suggested that interactions due to displacement from binding sites may be less likely with glibenclamide than with other sulphonylureas. However, it has also been stated that the absorption of glibenclamide from the gastro-intestinal tract may be reduced if it is taken together with guar gum.

There was a significant increase in nocturia in diabetic patients given glibenclamide compared with those given chlorpropamide, insulin, or dietary control.— K. M. Shaw *et al.* (letter), *Br. med. J.,* 1977, *1,* 1415.

A diabetic patient who was stabilised on glibenclamide 10 mg daily became comatose and also experienced intrahepatic cholestasis and a few cutaneous bullae; all these effects were reversible when treatment was withdrawn.— V. Wongpaitoon *et al., Postgrad. med. J.,* 1981, *57,* 244.

HYPOGLYCAEMIA. A review of 57 instances of hypoglycaemia associated with glibenclamide. The median age of patients affected was 70 years; only one was less than 60 years old. Median daily dosage was 10 mg. Coma or disturbed consciousness was observed in 46 patients and in 10 there was a fatal outcome. Those who died remained comatose despite alleviation of their hypoglycaemia; death occurred up to 20 days after presentation. In discussing their review, the authors reported that, including the present series of 57 cases, there have been published reports on 101 severe hypoglycaemias, 14 with a fatal outcome.— K. Asplund *et al., Diabetologia,* 1983, *24,* 412.

OVERDOSAGE. In a 16-year-old girl in coma after taking 50 glibenclamide tablets with suicidal intent, consciousness was rapidly restored after the infusion of glucose, but the blood-glucose concentration 64 hours after ingestion did not exceed 600 µg per mL despite almost continuous infusion of glucose.— S. Marigo *et al., Acta diabetol. latin.,* 1972, *9,* 688.

Absorption and Fate

Glibenclamide is readily absorbed from the gastro-intestinal tract and is extensively bound to plasma proteins. The half-life is about 10 hours. It is metabolised, almost completely, in the liver, the principal metabolite being only very weakly active. Approximately 50% of a dose is excreted in the urine and 50% via the bile into the faeces.

Uses and Administration

Glibenclamide is a sulphonylurea hypoglycaemic agent with similar actions and uses to chlorpropamide (p.388). It has a duration of action of up to 24 hours. The usual initial dose in non-insulin-dependent diabetes mellitus is 2.5 to 5 mg daily by mouth, with breakfast, adjusted every 7 days by increments of 2.5 mg daily up to 15 mg daily. Doses greater than 10 mg daily may be given in 2 divided doses.

Reviews of glibenclamide: B. D. Prendergast, *Clin. Pharm.,* 1984, *3,* 473; J. M. Feldman, *Am. J. Med.,* 1985, *79, Suppl.* 3B, 102.

ADMINISTRATION IN RENAL FAILURE. Although it has been reported that glibenclamide could be given in usual doses to patients with renal failure (W.M. Bennett *et al., Am. J. Kidney Dis.,* 1983, *3,* 155), it is generally recommended that like chlorpropamide it should not be used in patients with severe impairment of renal function.

DIABETES MELLITUS. *Combination with insulin.* Several studies have suggested that, in patients who have secondary failure of sulphonylurea treatment, combination therapy with insulin may provide better control of blood-glucose concentration. The rationale for such an approach is that secondary failure may have resulted from deterioration in islet beta cell function but that the sulphonylurea effect of improving insulin sensitivity may have persisted. Although appealing from a theoretical standpoint, such a combination should be viewed as experimental until definite benefits have been demonstrated. Certainly, for the patient with insulin-dependent disease, such a combination has not been shown to offer any advantage over insulin alone.— J. E. Gerich, *Mayo Clin. Proc.,* 1985, *60,* 439. See also M. Kyllästinen, *Ann. clin. Res.,* 1983, *15, Suppl.* 37, 29.

For some studies of glibenclamide or glipizide given together with insulin in non-insulin-dependent diabetes mellitus, see: H. Hamelbeck *et al., Dt. med. Wschr.,* 1982, *107,* 1581 (glibenclamide); L. Groop *et al., Acta endocr., Copenh.,* 1984, *106,* 97 (glibenclamide); K. Osei *et al., Am. J. Med.,* 1984, *77,* 1002 (glibenclamide); M. Kyllästinen and L. Groop, *Ann. clin. Res.,* 1985, *17,* 100 (glibenclamide); B. T. Allen *et al., Archs intern. Med.,* 1985, *145,* 1900 (glipizide).

Diabetic complications. For references to the effect of glibenclamide on platelet function in diabetes, see Gliclazide, p.390.

Preparations

Glibenclamide Tablets *(B.P.)*

Proprietary Preparations

Calabren *(Berk Generics, UK). Tablets,* glibenclamide 5 mg.

Daonil *(Hoechst, UK). Tablets* (Semi-Daonil), scored, glibenclamide 2.5 mg.
Tablets, scored, glibenclamide 5 mg.

Euglucon *(Roussel, UK). Tablets,* glibenclamide 2.5 mg.
Tablets, scored, glibenclamide 5 mg.

Malix *(Lagap, UK). Tablets,* glibenclamide 2.5 and 5 mg.

Proprietary Names and Manufacturers

Adiab *(Ital.)*; Azuglucon *(Azuchemie, Ger.)*; Bastiverit *(Bastian, Ger.)*; Betanase *(Cadila, Ind.)*; Calabren *(Berk Generics, UK)*; Daonil *(Alg.; Arg.; Hoechst, Austral.; Belg.; Hoechst, Denm.; Hoechst, Fr.; Hoechst, Ital.; Morocco; Neth.; Hoechst, Norw.; Hoechst, S.Afr.; Hoechst, Spain; Hoechst, Swed.; Hoechst, Switz.; Tun.; Hoechst, UK)*; Dia-Basan *(Sagitta, Ger.)*; Diaβeta *(Hoechst, Canad.; Hoechst, USA)*; Duraglucon *(Durachemie, Ger.)*; Euglucan *(Pierre Fabre, Fr.)*; Euglucon *(Reckitt & Colman, Austral.; Boehringer Mannheim, Canad.; Boehringer Mannheim, Norw.; Boehringer Mannheim, S.Afr.; Boehringer Mannheim, Spain; Roussel, UK)*; Euglucon or Semi-Euglucon *(Arg.; Belg.; Erco, Denm.; Boehringer Biochemia, Ital.; Boehringer Mannheim, Swed.)*; Gilemal *(Hung.)*; Gliben *(Klinge-Nattermann, Ger.; Gentili, Ital.)*; Gliboral *(Guidotti, Ital.)*; Glidiabet *(Spain)*; Glimidstada *(Stadapharm, Ger.)*; Glucolon *(Sabater, Spain)*; Gluconorm *(Wolff, Ger.)*; Gluco-Tablinen *(Beiersdorf, Ger.)*; Glukoreduct *(Midy, Ger.)*; Glukovital *(Wolff, Ger.)*; Glycolande *(Delalande, Ger.)*; Hemi-Daonil *(Alg.; Arg.; Belg.; Morocco; Neth.; Spain; Tun.)*; Hexaglucon *(Durascan, Denm.)*; Libanil *(Approved Prescription Services, UK)*; Malix *(Lagap, UK)*; Micronase *(Upjohn, USA)*; Miglucan *(Pierre Fabre, Fr.)*; Norglicem *(Gamir, Spain)*; Orabetic *(Dorsch, Ger.)*; Pira *(Arg.)*; Praeciglucon *(Pfleger, Ger.)*; Semi-Daonil *(Alg.; Arg.; Belg.; Denm.; Fr.; Ital.; Morocco; Neth.; Spain; Hoechst, Switz.; Tun.; Hoechst, UK)*.

7218-t

Glibornuride *(BAN, USAN, rINN).*

Ro-6-4563. 1-[(2*S*,3*R*)-2-Hydroxyborn-3-yl]-3-tosylurea; 1-[(2*S*,3*R*)-2-Hydroxyborn-3-yl]-3-*p*-tolylsulphonylurea.

$C_{18}H_{26}N_2O_4S=366.5$.

CAS — 26944-48-9.

NOTE. The name glibornuride has frequently but erroneously been applied to glibenclamide.

Adverse Effects, Treatment, and Precautions

As for chlorpropamide (p.387).

Absorption and Fate

Glibornuride is rapidly and almost completely absorbed from the gastro-intestinal tract. It is extensively bound to plasma proteins. The half-life is about 8 hours. It is extensively metabolised in the liver; the metabolites have little or no hypoglycaemic activity. It is excreted in the urine and bile.

Uses and Administration

Glibornuride is a sulphonylurea hypoglycaemic agent with actions and uses similar to those of chlorpropamide (p.388). Its duration of action is 8 hours or more. The usual initial dose by mouth in non-insulin-dependent diabetes mellitus is 12.5 mg taken with breakfast; this may be gradually increased, if necessary, up to a maximum of 75 mg daily. If a higher dose is required, it is recommended that 50 mg be taken in the morning and the remainder in the evening.

ADMINISTRATION IN RENAL FAILURE. Although it has been reported that glibornuride could be given in usual doses to patients with renal failure (W.M. Bennett *et al., Am. J. Kidney Dis.,* 1983, *3,* 155), it is generally recommended that like chlorpropamide it should not be used in patients with severe impairment of renal function.

Proprietary Names and Manufacturers

Glitrim *(Roche, Spain)*; Gluborid *(Grünenthal, Ger.; Neth.; Grünenthal, Switz.)*; Glutrid *(Arg.)*; Glutril *(Roche, Denm.; Roche, Fr.; Roche, Ger.; S.Afr.; Swed.; Roche, Switz.; Roche, UK)*.

7220-y

Gliclazide *(BAN, rINN).*

Glyclazide. 1-(3-Azabicyclo[3.3.0]oct-3-yl)-3-tosylurea; 1-(3-Azabicyclo[3.3.0]oct-3-yl)-3-*p*-tolylsulphonylurea.

$C_{15}H_{21}N_3O_3S=323.4$.

CAS — 21187-98-4.

Adverse Effects, Treatment, and Precautions

As for chlorpropamide (p.387).

Absorption and Fate

Gliclazide is readily absorbed from the gastro-intestinal tract; varying rates of absorption have been reported. It is extensively bound to plasma proteins. The half-life is about 10 to 12 hours. Gliclazide is extensively metabolised in the liver to metabolites without significant hypoglycaemic activity. Both unchanged drug and metabolites are excreted in the urine.

The pharmacokinetics of gliclazide in healthy subjects and diabetics.— K. Kobayashi *et al.*, *J. pharm. Sci.*, 1984, *73*, 1684.

Uses and Administration

Gliclazide is a sulphonylurea hypoglycaemic agent with actions and uses similar to those of chlorpropamide (p.388). Its duration of action is 12 hours or more. The usual initial dose by mouth in non-insulin-dependent diabetes mellitus is 40 to 80 mg daily, gradually increased, if necessary, up to 320 mg daily. It is suggested that doses of more than 160 mg daily should be given in 2 divided doses according to the main meals of the day.

A review of gliclazide including its effects on plasma lipids, platelet function, and fibrinolysis, and its possible effects on diabetic retinopathy.— B. Holmes *et al.*, *Drugs*, 1984, *27*, 301.

Results, based on the first 90 days' treatment, suggesting that the long-term effect of gliclazide may be due to persistent stimulation of insulin secretion rather than a predominantly extrapancreatic action.— B. L. Wajchenberg *et al.*, *Clin. Pharmac. Ther.*, 1980, *27*, 375.

Proceedings of a symposium, including reports of the effect of gliclazide on platelet aggregation, coagulation factors, and fibrinolysis.— *Gliclazide and the Treatment of Diabetes*, H. Keen *et al.*(Ed.), London, Royal Society of Medicine, 1980.

For a discussion of platelet function and diabetic vascular disease, the effects of gliclazide on these, and the view that, while there was strong *animal* data to suggest that gliclazide reduced platelet aggregability, human studies were less conclusive, see J. E. Jackson and R. Bressler, *Drugs*, 1981, *22*, 211.

Further references to possible beneficial effects of gliclazide on the vascular complications of diabetes.— Z. Rubinjoni *et al.*, *Curr. med. Res. Opinion*, 1978, *5*, 625 (platelet adhesiveness); L. J. Klaff *et al.*, *S. Afr. med. J.*, 1979, *56*, 247 (platelet aggregation; gliclazide and glibenclamide); R. C. Paton *et al.*, *Br. med. J.*, 1981, *283*, 1018 (no support for beneficial effect of gliclazide additional to glycaemic control); L. J. Klaff *et al.*, *Am. J. Med.*, 1981, *70*, 627 (platelet aggregation; gliclazide and glibenclamide); F. Violi *et al.*, *Curr. med. Res. Opinion*, 1982, *8*, 200 (platelet aggregation).

Proprietary Preparations

Diamicron *(Servier, UK)*. *Tablets*, scored, gliclazide 80 mg.

Proprietary Names and Manufacturers

Diabrezide *(Brocchieri, Ital.)*; Diamicron *(Servier, Austral.; Servier, Denm.; Servier, Fr.; Itherapia, Ger.; Servier, Ital.; Neth.; Servier, S.Afr.; Servier, Spain; Servier, Switz.; Servier, UK)*; Dramion *(Ital.)*.

7221-j

Gliflumide *(USAN, rINN).*

SH-3-1168. (−)-(*S*)-*N*-(5-Fluoro-2-methoxy-α-methylbenzyl)-2-[4-(5-isobutylpyrimidin-2-ylsulphamoyl)phenyl]acetamide.
$C_{25}H_{29}FN_4O_4S$=500.6.

CAS — 35273-88-2.

Gliflumide is a sulphonamidopyrimidine compound which has been used as a hypoglycaemic agent.

Proprietary Names and Manufacturers

Schering, Ger.

7222-z

Glipizide *(BAN, USAN, pINN).*

CP-28720; Glydiazinamide; K-4024. 1-Cyclohexyl-3-{4-[2-(5-methylpyrazine-2-carboxamido)ethyl]benzenesulphonyl}urea.
$C_{21}H_{27}N_5O_4S$=445.5.

CAS — 29094-61-9.

Pharmacopoeias. In *Br.*

A white or almost white, odourless or almost odourless crystalline powder. Practically **insoluble** in water and alcohol; sparingly soluble in acetone; soluble in chloroform. It dissolves in dilute solutions of alkali hydroxides.

Adverse Effects, Treatment, and Precautions

As for chlorpropamide (p.387).

Absorption and Fate

Glipizide is rapidly and completely absorbed from the gastro-intestinal tract. It is extensively bound to plasma proteins and has a half-life of approximately 3 to 4 hours. It is metabolised in the liver and excreted chiefly in the urine, largely as inactive metabolites.

Uses and Administration

Glipizide is a sulphonylurea hypoglycaemic agent with actions and uses similar to those of chlorpropamide (p.388).

Its hypoglycaemic effects may persist for up to 24 hours. The usual initial dose by mouth in the treatment of non-insulin-dependent diabetes mellitus is 2.5 to 5 mg daily given as a single dose before breakfast. Dosage may be adjusted at intervals of several days by amounts of 2.5 to 5 mg daily, to a maximum of 40 mg daily. Doses larger than 15 mg daily should be given in two divided doses before meals.

If glipizide alone does not produce control then it may be given concomitantly with a biguanide.

Reviews of glipizide.— R. N. Brogden *et al.*, *Drugs*, 1979, *18*, 329; B. D. Prendergast, *Clin. Pharm.*, 1984, *3*, 473.

Proceedings of a symposium on non-insulin-dependent diabetes and the role of glipizide in its treatment.— *Am. J. Med.*, 1983, *75*, *Suppl.* 5B, 1-99.

ADMINISTRATION IN RENAL FAILURE. Although it has been reported that glipizide could be given in usual doses to patients with renal failure (W.M. Bennett *et al.*, *Am. J. Kidney Dis.*, 1983, *3*, 155), it is generally recommended that like chlorpropamide it should not be used in patients with severe impairment of renal function.

DIABETES MELLITUS. *Combination with insulin.* For mention of glipizide used together with insulin in non-insulin-dependent diabetes mellitus, see Glibenclamide, p.389.

Diabetic complications. Results of a 3-year study indicated that glipizide could reverse one of the signs of early diabetic microangiopathy.— R. A. Camerini-Davalos *et al.*, *New Engl. J. Med.*, 1983, *309*, 1551.

Preparations

Glipizide Tablets *(B.P.)*

Proprietary Preparations

Glibenese *(Pfizer, UK)*. *Tablets*, scored, glipizide 5 mg.
Minodiab *(Farmitalia Carlo Erba, UK)*. *Tablets*, glipizide 2.5 mg.
Tablets, scored, glipizide 5 mg.

Proprietary Names and Manufacturers

Glibenese *(Belg.; Pfizer, Denm.; Pfizer, Fr.; Pfizer, Ger.; Neth.; Pfizer, Spain; Pfizer, Swed.; Mack, Switz.; Pfizer, UK)*; Glucotrol *(Roerig, USA)*; Mindiab *(Farmitalia, Denm.; Farmitalia, Norw.; Farmitalia Carlo Erba, Swed.)*; Minidiab *(Belg.; Farmitalia Carlo Erba, Fr.; Carlo Erba, Ital.; Farmitalia, NZ; Farmitalia Carlo Erba, S.Afr.)*; Minodiab *(Arg.; Farmitalia, Spain; Farmitalia Carlo Erba, UK)*.

7223-c

Gliquidone *(BAN, rINN).*

ARDF-26. 1-Cyclohexyl-3-{4-[2-(3,4-dihydro-7-methoxy-4,4-dimethyl-1,3-dioxo-2(1*H*)-isoquinolyl)ethyl]benzenesulphonyl}urea.
$C_{27}H_{33}N_3O_6S$=527.6.

CAS — 33342-05-1.

Adverse Effects, Treatment, and Precautions

As for chlorpropamide (p.387). Since renal excretion plays little part in gliquidone's elimination, it has been reported that it might be suitable in patients with reduced renal function.

Absorption and Fate

Gliquidone is readily absorbed from the gastro-intestinal tract and is extensively bound to plasma proteins. It is extensively metabolised in the liver, the metabolites having no significant hypoglycaemic effect, and is eliminated chiefly in the faeces via the bile; less than 5% of a dose is excreted via the kidneys.

Uses and Administration

Gliquidone is a sulphonylurea hypoglycaemic agent with actions and uses similar to those of chlorpropamide (p.388). It is given by mouth in the treatment of non-insulin-dependent diabetes mellitus in a usual initial dosage of 15 mg daily increased to 45 to 60 mg daily, given before meals in 2 or 3 divided doses. Single doses above 60 mg and daily doses above 180 mg are not recommended.

Proprietary Preparations

Glurenorm *(Winthrop, UK)*. *Tablets*, scored, gliquidone 30 mg.

Proprietary Names and Manufacturers

Glurenor *(Arg.; Guidotti, Ital.; Castejon, Spain)*; Glurenorm *(Thomae, Ger.; Neth.; Winthrop, UK)*.

12786-b

Glisentide *(pINN).*

Glipentide; Glypentide. 1-Cyclopentyl-3-[*p*-(2-*o*-anisamidoethyl)benzenesulphonyl]urea.
$C_{22}H_{27}N_3O_5S$=445.5.

CAS — 32797-92-5.

Glisentide is a sulphonylurea hypoglycaemic agent with actions and uses similar to chlorpropamide (p.387).

Proprietary Names and Manufacturers

Staticum *(Uriach, Spain)*.

12787-v

Glisolamide *(rINN).*

1-Cyclohexyl-3-{[*p*-[2-(5-methylisoxazole-3-carboxamido)ethyl]benzene]sulphonyl}urea.
$C_{20}H_{26}N_4O_5S$=434.5.

CAS — 24477-37-0.

Glisolamide is a sulphonylurea hypoglycaemic agent with actions and uses similar to chlorpropamide (p.387). It has been given by mouth in non-insulin-dependent diabetes mellitus in doses of 5 to 20 mg daily.

Proprietary Names and Manufacturers

Diabenor *(IFI, Ital.)*.

7224-k

Glisoxepide *(BAN, rINN).*

Glisoxepid. 1-(Perhydroazepin-1-yl)-3-{4-[2-(5-methylisoxazole-3-carboxamido)ethyl]benzenesulphonyl}urea.
$C_{20}H_{27}N_5O_5S$=449.5.

CAS — 25046-79-1.

Glisoxepide is a sulphonylurea hypoglycaemic agent with actions and uses similar to those of chlorpropamide (p.387). The usual dose by mouth in non-insulin-dependent diabetes mellitus is up to 16 mg daily in divided doses.

Proprietary Names and Manufacturers

Glisepin *(Bayer, Ital.)*; Glucoben *(Farmades, Ital.)*; Pro-Diaban *(Bayer, Ger.)*.

7225-a

Glybuzole *(rINN).*
Désaglybuzole. *N*-(5-*tert*-Butyl-1,3,4-thiadiazol-2-yl)benzenesulphonamide.
$C_{12}H_{15}N_3O_2S_2$=297.4.

CAS — 1492-02-0.

Glybuzole is an oral hypoglycaemic agent with a structure distinct from that of the sulphonylureas, biguanides, or sulphonamidopyrimidines.

Proprietary Names and Manufacturers
Gludiase *(Kyowa, Jpn).*

7226-t

Glyclopyramide *(rINN).*
1-(4-Chlorobenzenesulphonyl)-3-(pyrrolidin-1-yl)urea.
$C_{11}H_{14}ClN_3O_3S$=303.8.

CAS — 631-27-6.

Glyclopyramide is a sulphonylurea hypoglycaemic agent with actions and uses similar to those of chlorpropamide (p.387).

Proprietary Names and Manufacturers
Deamelin-S *(Jpn).*

7227-x

Glycyclamide *(rINN).*
Tolcyclamide. 1-Cyclohexyl-3-tosylurea; 1-Cyclohexyl-3-*p*-tolylsulphonylurea.
$C_{14}H_{20}N_2O_3S$=296.4.

CAS — 664-95-9.

Pharmacopoeias. In *Roum.*

Glycyclamide is a sulphonylurea hypoglycaemic agent with actions and uses similar to those of chlorpropamide (p.387). It is given by mouth in non-insulin-dependent diabetes mellitus in doses of 0.5 to 1.5 g daily.

Proprietary Names and Manufacturers
Diaborale *(Carlo Erba, Ital.).*

7228-r

Glymidine *(BAN).*

Glycodiazine; Glymidine Sodium *(USAN, rINN)*; SH-717. The sodium salt of *N*-[5-(2-methoxyethoxy)pyrimidin-2-yl]benzenesulphonamide.
$C_{13}H_{14}N_3NaO_4S$=331.3.

CAS — 3459-20-9; 339-44-6 (base).

Adverse Effects

Gastro-intestinal disturbances, skin eruptions and urticaria, leucopenia, and thrombocytopenic purpura have been reported. Hypoglycaemia may occur and require treatment as described under insulin (p.393).

Patients allergic to the sulphonylureas may not be sensitive to glymidine.

Precautions

As for chlorpropamide (p.387).

PORPHYRIA. Glymidine was considered to be unsafe in patients with acute porphyria because it has been shown to be porphyrinogenic in *animals* or *in vitro* systems.— M.R. Moore and K.E.L. McColl, *Porphyrias, Drug Lists*, Glasgow, Porphyria Research Unit, University of Glasgow, 1987.

Absorption and Fate

Glymidine is readily absorbed from the gastro-intestinal tract. It is extensively bound to plasma proteins; the half-life is about 4 hours. It is extensively metabolised in the liver and excreted in the urine chiefly as metabolites with a small proportion excreted in the faeces.

The demethylated metabolite of glymidine had hypoglycaemic activity comparable with that of glymidine.— M. Kramer *et al., Arzneimittel-Forsch.*, 1964, *14*, 377.

Uses and Administration

Glymidine is a sulphonamidopyrimidine hypoglycaemic agent with a short duration of action. It is given by mouth in non-insulin-dependent diabetes mellitus. Initial doses are 1.0 to 1.5 g daily, usually as a single daily dose. Maintenance doses are generally 0.5 to 1 g but may range to a maximum of 2 g, when it is recommended that 1.5 g be given with breakfast and 0.5 g be given in the late afternoon.

Proprietary Names and Manufacturers
Gondafon *(Schering, Austral.; Belg.; Ital.; Neth.; S.Afr.; Swed.; Switz.; Schering, UK)*; Lycanol *(Austral.; Swed.)*; Redul *(Schering, Ger.).*

5427-l

Guar Gum *(USAN).*

E412; Guar Flour; Jaguar Gum.

CAS — 9000-30-0.

Pharmacopoeias. In *Fr.* and *Ind.* Also in *U.S.N.F.*

A gum obtained from the ground endosperms of the seeds of *Cyamopsis psoraloides* (=*C. tetragonolobus*) (Leguminosae). It contains not less than 66% of a high molecular weight hydrocolloidal polysaccharide, a galactomannan, composed of galactan and mannan units combined through glycosidic linkages.

A white to yellowish-white almost odourless powder. **Dispersible** in hot or cold water to form a colloidal solution.

Adverse Effects and Precautions

Guar gum can cause gastro-intestinal disturbance with flatulence, diarrhoea, or nausea, particularly at the start of treatment.

It should not be used in patients with oesophageal or intestinal obstruction. There is a risk of guar gum affecting the absorption of other drugs.

For background toxicological information on guar gum in food, see *Fd Add. Ser. Wld Hlth Org. No. 5*, 1974.

Uses and Administration

Guar gum is used in diabetes mellitus as an adjunct to treatment with diet, insulin, or oral hypoglycaemics since it is considered to reduce the peak blood-glucose concentrations that occur following meals. It is given with or immediately before meals in doses of 5 g usually three times daily; each dose should be taken with about 200 mL of water. Guar gum is available in various formulations that attempt to overcome its unpalatability.

Guar gum is also used to slow gastric emptying in patients with the dumping syndrome.

Guar gum is also used as a thickening agent, emulsion stabiliser, and suspending agent.

DIABETES MELLITUS. A brief review of guar gum concluding that its contribution to the management of diabetic patients remains unproven.— *Drug & Ther. Bull.*, 1987, *25*, 65.

The postprandial increases in blood-glucose and -insulin concentrations in response to carbohydrate-containing meals were reduced in healthy subjects when they ate test meals containing guar gum, pectin, or both.— D. J. A. Jenkins *et al., Ann. intern. Med.*, 1977, *86*, 20. Mean urinary-glucose excretion fell markedly in diabetics when guar gum was added to their diet.— D. J. A. Jenkins *et al., Lancet*, 1977, *2*, 779. A conclusion that optimistic reports about fibre supplementation in the management of diabetes needed to be confirmed by careful long-term studies, following the authors' own negative findings in obese, poorly-controlled diabetics given guar gum or bran.— M. Cohen and F. I. R. Martin (letter), *Br. med. J.*, 1979, *1*, 616.

EFFECT ON SERUM LIPIDS. Guar gum given in a daily dose of 15 g for 2 weeks reduced the mean serum-cholesterol concentration in 10 patients with type II hyperlipidaemia.— D. J. A. Jenkins *et al., Am. J. clin. Nutr.*, 1979, *32*, 16.

Proprietary Preparations

Glucotard *(MCP Pharmaceuticals, UK). Mini-tablets,* guar gum 5 g per sachet.

Guarem *(Rybar, UK). Granules,* guar gum 5 g per sachet.

Guarina *(Norgine, UK). Granules,* guar gum 5 g per sachet.

Proprietary Names and Manufacturers
Decorpa *(Norgine, UK)*; Fibraguar *(Jorba, Spain)*; Glucotard *(Boehringer Mannheim, Ger.; Boehringer Mannheim, Switz.; MCP Pharmaceuticals, UK)*; Guarem *(Stroschein, Ger.; Rybar, UK)*; Guarina *(Norgine, Austral.; Norgine, UK)*; Lejguar *(Britannia Pharmaceuticals, UK)*; Lubo *(Kramer-Synthelabo, Switz.)*; Metabolite 2050 *(Robertson/Taylor, USA).*

The following names have been used for multi-ingredient preparations containing guar gum— Anorex-CCK *(Robertson/Taylor, USA).*

7202-e

Insulin

CAS — 9004-10-8 (insulin; neutral insulin); 11070-73-8 (bovine insulin); 12584-58-6 (porcine insulin); 11061-68-0 (human insulin); 8063-29-4 (biphasic insulin); 9004-21-1 (globin zinc insulin); 8049-62-5 (insulin zinc suspensions); 53027-39-7 (isophane insulin); 9004-17-5 (protamine zinc insulin); 9004-12-0 (dalanated insulin); 51798-72-2 (bovine insulin defalan); 11091-62-6 (porcine insulin defalan).

Insulin is a hormone produced by the beta cells of the islets of Langerhans of the pancreas and consists of 2 chains of amino acids, the A and B chains, connected by 2 disulphide bridges. Insulin produced by different species conforms to the same basic structure but has different sequences of amino acids in the chains. **Porcine insulin** ($C_{256}H_{381}N_{65}O_{76}S_6$ = 5777.6) differs from **human insulin** ($C_{257}H_{383}N_{65}O_{77}S_6$ = 5807.7) in only one amino acid in the B chain whereas **bovine insulin** ($C_{254}H_{377}N_{65}O_{75}S_6$ = 5733.6) differs from human insulin not only in this same amino acid in the B chain but also in 2 acids in the A chain.

The precursor of insulin in the pancreas is proinsulin which is a single polypeptide chain incorporating both the A and B chains of insulin connected by a peptide termed the C-peptide (or connecting-peptide). Although the insulins of various species may be similar in composition the proinsulins are not, in that the sequence and number of amino acids in the C-peptide may vary considerably.

Early commercial insulins were obtained by extraction from bovine or porcine or mixed bovine and porcine pancreases and were purified by recrystallisation only. Insulins obtained by such methods were often termed **'conventional insulins'** to distinguish them from insulins which have undergone further purification processes. An extract which has been recrystallised only once can be separated into 3 components or fractions termed the 'a', 'b', and 'c' components. The 'a' component consists of high molecular weight substances and is only usually found in very impure preparations since repeated recrystallisation will remove most of it. The 'b' component consists largely of proinsulin and insulin dimers, and the 'c' component consists of insulin, insulin esters, arginine insulin, and desamidoinsulin. Other pancreatic peptides such as glucagon, pancreatic polypeptide, somatostatin, and vasoactive intestinal peptide are also usually found in products which have not undergone further purification. Gel filtration will substantially reduce the content of proinsulin but will not significantly reduce the content of insulin derivatives or pancreatic peptides; products purified by gel filtration are often termed **'single-peak insulins'**. Addition of ion-exchange chromatography to the purification methods will further reduce the proinsulin content and also reduce the contamination by insulin derivatives and pancreatic peptides. In the *UK* **'highly purified insulins'** and **'monocomponent insulins'** are terms sometimes applied to insulins which have undergone both gel filtration and ion-exchange chromatography. In the *USA* the Food and Drugs Administration (FDA) has designated the term **'purified insulins'** for preparations containing less than 10 ppm of proinsulin.

Modification of the insulin molecule has resulted in such insulins as **dalanated insulin** (prepared by the removal of the C-terminal alanine from the B chain of insulin), **insulin defalan** (prepared by the removal of the terminal phenylalanine), and **sulphated insulin**.

A recent development in the evolution of insulin preparations is the production of insulin having an amino-acid sequence identical to that of human insulin. **Human insulin (emp)** is produced by the enzymatic modification of insulin obtained from the porcine pancreas; it is also sometimes called **semisynthetic human insulin**. **Human insulin (crb)** is produced by the chemical combination of A and B chains which have been obtained from bacteria genetically modified by recombinant DNA technology. **Human insulin (prb)** is produced from proinsulin obtained from bacteria genetically modified by recombinant DNA technology. **Human insulin (pyr)** is insulin produced from a precursor obtained from a yeast genetically modified by recombinant DNA technology. Human insulin obtained by recombinant DNA technology is sometimes termed **biosynthetic human insulin**.

Insulin *(B.P., Eur.P.)* is of either bovine or porcine origin, and contains not less than 26 units of insulin per mg (calculated on the dried basis). The *B.P.* recommends storage at a temperature not exceeding −20° in airtight containers and that it be protected from light. The *Eur. P.* recommends storage at 2° to 8° in airtight containers and that it be protected from light.

Human Insulin (*B.P.*) is produced either by the enzymatic modification of porcine insulin or by recombinant DNA technology in micro-organisms and contains not less than 26 units of human insulin per mg (calculated on the dried basis). The *B.P.* recommends storage at a temperature not exceeding −20° in an airtight container and that it be protected from light.

Insulin *(U.S.P.)* is of either bovine or porcine origin, or of mixed bovine and porcine origin, and contains not less than 26 units of insulin per mg. The *U.S.P.* recommends storage at no more than 8° in airtight containers and that it be protected from light.

Insulin Human*(U.S.P.)* is produced either by enzymatic modification of porcine insulin or by microbial synthesis and contains not less than 27.5 units of human insulin per mg. The *U.S.P.* recommends storage below 8° in airtight containers.

Crystalline insulin may be prepared for therapeutic use merely by making a solution, either of acidic or neutral pH, and such preparations are often referred to as **'regular insulin'** or **'unmodified insulin'**; these names reflect only the fact that the preparation has not been formulated in order to prolong the duration of action of the insulin and do not in any way reflect the degree of purity or the origin of the insulin. Insulin Injection (*B.P.*), Acid Insulin Injection (*B.P.*), and Insulin Injection (*U.S.P.*) are examples of formulations that are often referred to in this manner. Such formulations are described by the term **soluble insulins** in this chapter of *Martindale*.

In order to prolong the duration of action of insulin, preparations may be formulated as suspensions in 2 general ways. The first involves complexing insulin with a protein from which it is slowly released; examples are **protamine zinc insulin**, which contains an excess of protamine, and **isophane insulin**, which contains equimolecular amounts of insulin and protamine. The second method is by modifying the particle size of the insulin itself and the various **insulin zinc suspensions** are in this category. Again these names, in themselves, do not reflect degrees of purity nor origin of the insulin.

The *B.P.* and *U.S.P.* both recommend that official preparations of insulin be stored at 2° to 8° and that they should not be allowed to freeze. It is also stated that suspensions should be gently shaken before a dose is withdrawn.

ADSORPTION. Several studies have demonstrated that insulin is adsorbed onto glass and various plastics used in administration sets and that this adsorption may be reduced by the addition of albumin or polygeline to the solution.

References: C. Petty and N. L. Cunningham, *Anesthesiology*, 1974, *40*, 400; E. W. Kraegen *et al.*, *Br. med. J.*, 1975, *3*, 464; S. S. Weber *et al.*, *Am. J. Hosp. Pharm.*, 1977, *34*, 353; N. J. Goldberg and S. R. Levin (letter), *New Engl. J. Med.*, 1978, *298*, 1480; Z. J. Twardowski *et al.*, *Am. J. Hosp. Pharm.*, 1983, *40*, 583; M. Kanke *et al.*, *ibid.*, 1323; P. W. Niemiec and T. W. Vanderveen, *ibid.*, 1984, *41*, 893.

Insulin Syringes

A British Standard specifies requirements for re-usable hypodermic syringes for insulin injection. BS 1619: Part 1: 1962 covers specifications for syringes for use with insulin of strengths 20, 40, and 80 units per mL. BS 1619: Part 2: 1982 covers specifications for syringes for use with insulin of strength 100 units per mL only. Disposable syringes are readily available and are safer and more convenient for the patient.

A pre-set insulin syringe, for use by blind patients, is available.

Bilateral abscesses of the thigh in a diabetic patient associated with the use of surgical spirit instead of industrial methylated spirit for the storage of insulin syringes.— D. A. Leigh and G. W. Hough, *Br. med. J.*, 1980, *281*, 541.

References to the potential hazard of the dead space of syringes: J. A. H. Puxty *et al.*, *Br. med. J.*, 1983, *287*, 1762; G. H. Hall *et al.*, *ibid.*, 1984, *288*, 284; W. D. Alexander (letter), *ibid.*, 643; J. Sheldon (letter), *ibid.*, 720; G. H. Hall (letter), *ibid;* H. Keen and J. Jarrett (letter), *ibid.*

Units

The international unit of insulin is the activity contained in 0.04167 mg of the fourth International Standard Preparation for Bioassay (1958). The standard preparation is a mixture of 52% bovine and 48% porcine insulin, containing 24 units per mg.

Three international units of human insulin are contained in approximately 130 μg (with sucrose 5 mg) in one ampoule of the first International Reference Preparation for Immunoassay (1974).

Adverse Effects

The most frequent complication of insulin therapy is hypoglycaemia, the speed of onset and duration of which may vary according to the type of preparation used and the route of administration. It is usually associated with an excessive dosage of insulin, the omission of a meal by the patient, or increased physical activity, and has sometimes been reported in patients changing from bovine to other insulins. Symptoms of hypoglycaemia resulting from increased sympathetic activity include hunger, pallor, sweating, palpitations, anxiety, and tremulousness. Other symptoms include headache, visual disturbances such as blurred or double vision, slurred speech, paraesthesia of the mouth, alterations in behaviour, and impaired mental or intellectual ability. If untreated, hypoglycaemia may lead to convulsions and coma which should not be confused with hyperglycaemic coma. Some patients, especially the elderly or those with diabetes of long standing, may not experience the typical early warning symptoms of a hypoglycaemic attack.

Insulin, administered subcutaneously, may cause either lipoatrophy or lipohypertrophy. Lipoatrophy appears to occur less frequently with purified insulins than with conventional insulins; if it has occurred, it may be reversed by the injection of a purer animal insulin or human insulin into and around the atrophied site. Lipohypertrophy is usually associated with repeated injections at the same site and may usually be overcome by varying the site of injection, although it should be remembered that absorption of insulin may vary from different anatomical areas.

Insulin may occasionally cause local or systemic allergic reactions. Local reactions, characterised by erythema and pruritus at the injection site, usually disappear with continued treatment. Generalised allergy may produce urticaria, angioedema, and very rarely anaphylactoid reactions; if continued therapy with insulin is essential desensitisation procedures may need to be performed. Again, allergic reactions are observed less frequently with purified than with conventional insulins and porcine insulin is less immunogenic than bovine insulin. Although allergic reactions have been reported in patients receiving human insulin who were previously treated with animal insulins, there do not appear to be any reports of such reactions in patients treated exclusively with human insulin.

Many patients treated with insulin, either of animal origin or human insulin, develop antibodies but the significance of such antibody formation with regard to the clinical management of the patient is not entirely clear.

ALLERGY. Two diabetic patients were allergic to the zinc in their insulin preparations.— M. N. Feinglos and B. V. Jegasothy, *Lancet*, 1979, *1*, 122.

Allergy in one patient attributed to the protamine component of insulin injections.— M. B. Sánchez *et al.* (letter), *Lancet*, 1982, *1*, 1243.

Reports and comments on allergic reactions to human insulin in patients previously treated with or displaying allergy to animal insulins.— A. O. Carveth-Johnson *et al.* (letter), *Lancet*, 1982, *2*, 1287; A. W. Frankland (letter), *ibid.*, 1468; R. L. Blandford *et al.* (letter), *ibid;* J. J. Altman *et al.* (letter), *ibid.*, 1983, *2*, 524; P. G. Wiles *et al.*, *Br. med. J.*, 1983, *287*, 531; P. García-Ortega *et al.*, *ibid.*, 1984, *288*, 1271; J. S. Kristensen *et al.* (letter), *ibid.*, *289*, 1382; L. C. Grammer *et al.*, *J. Am. med. Ass.*, 1984, *251*, 1459; P. Silverstone, *Br. med. J.*, 1986, *292*, 933.

Following failure of standard desensitisation measures in a patient with cutaneous allergy to insulin, desensitisation was attempted by giving insulin by mouth with aspirin 1.3 g three times daily. After one week subsequent desensitisation using insulin by injection was successful. When the patient stopped taking aspirin after 6 months the original allergic reactions recurred; aspirin was then given permanently in a dose of 1.3 g twice daily.— I. M. Holdaway and J. D. Wilson, *Br. med. J.*, 1984, *289*, 1565. Comment on the mode of action of aspirin in such circumstances.— S. I. Asad *et al.*, *ibid.*, 1985, *290*, 473.

ANTIBODY FORMATION. A review of human insulin including a discussion on the clinical importance of insulin antibodies. Both pork and human insulin are definitely less immunogenic than beef insulin producing fewer circulating insulin antibodies, but several studies have indicated no detectable change in antibody concentrations on switching from pork to human insulin or *vice versa*. Antibodies cause lipoatrophy and are responsible for the substantial insulin resistance seen in some patients, but both events are rare now that purified pork insulin is in common use. Interest has recently been revived in the possible contribution of antibodies in modifying metabolic control. In the short term and under hospital conditions, they are known to prolong the intravenous half-life of injected insulin and to delay the appearance in the circulation of a subcutaneously administered bolus dose. Patients with moderate concentrations of antibodies are also reported to show delay in recovery from induced hypoglycaemia, but on the other hand to lose control less quickly after insulin withdrawal and thus may be relatively protected from ketoacidosis. Yet despite these findings, neither the amounts nor the binding characteristics of insulin antibodies can usually be linked with the degree of diabetic control in individual patients in ordinary conditions of life. The several other postulated adverse effects of insulin antibodies, such as causing or contributing to neonatal hypoglycaemia, have not been conclusively proved. However, recent studies do provide further evidence that the development of insulin antibodies in diabetic children is associated with a shortened 'honeymoon remission period', higher dosage of insulin, and impaired endogenous secretion of insulin.— J. Pickup, *Br. med. J.*, 1986, *292*, 155.

A study on the influence of insulin antibodies on the pharmacokinetics and bioavailability of beef and human insulin.— R. S. Gray *et al.*, *Br. med. J.*, 1985, *290*, 1687.

EFFECTS ON THE LIVER. Transient recurrent hepatomegaly associated with hypoglycaemia in a 12-year-old diabetic girl was associated with the surreptitious administration of additional insulin injections. It was considered that the excess of insulin had led to increased storage of glycogen in the liver which was reponsible for the hepatomegaly.— J. Asherov *et al.*, *Archs Dis. Childh.*, 1979, *54*, 148.

HYPOGLYCAEMIA. A discussion of the effects of hypoglycaemia on the nervous system.— *Lancet*, 1985, *2*, 759.

Results of a 1-year study of adult patients with severe hypoglycaemia presenting to an accident and emergency department. Of 204 episodes, one occurred in a patient with insulinoma, 3 in elderly diabetic patients receiving sulphonylureas, and 200 in 130 insulin-treated patients. A survey of diabetic clinics in the area, identifying all insulin-treated adults revealed that 9% had thus had episodes of hypoglycaemia severe enough to warrant admission to casualty. Precipitating causes were often difficult to assess and no definite cause could be found in over a third of patients. Comparison of patients with only one attack with those who suffered multiple attacks showed that missed or delayed meals accounted for 30% and 19% respectively, a recent increase in insulin dose for 14% and 13%, loss of warning symptoms for 4% and 11%, and exercise for 6% and 7%; other causes included carelessness, pregnancy, and intake of alcohol. Patients with single and multiple admissions differed in terms of the insulin dosage. Of those admitted more than once, 62% were receiving more than 1 unit per kg body-weight daily compared to 39% with only one attack; in those patients with multiple admissions the mean daily dose after 1 year had fallen to 0.8 units per kg compared to 1.1 units per kg at presentation. Only one of the 130 patients suffered any lasting ill-effect and this followed a suicide attempt.— J. Potter *et al.*, *Br. med. J.*, 1982, *285*, 1180. A similar study.— R. G. Moses *et al.*, *Med. J. Aust.*, 1985, *142*, 294.

See also Morning Hyperglycaemia, under Precautions.

OEDEMA. A report of generalised oedema in one patient about 7 days after being started on insulin; the condition was considered a rare example of insulin oedema.— N. R. Bleach *et al.*, *Br. med. J.*, 1979, *2*, 177. Reference to further cases of fluid retention.— J. R. Lawrence and M. G. Dunnigan (letter), *ibid.*, 445.

Treatment of Insulin-induced Hypoglycaemia

In the conscious and cooperative patient hypoglycaemia should be treated by the oral administration of a readily-absorbable form of carbohydrate, such as sugar lumps or a glucose-based drink.

If hypoglycaemic coma occurs, up to 50 mL of a 50% solution of glucose should be given intravenously and occasionally may need to be repeated. If after about one hour, blood-glucose concentrations are normal and the patient has failed to regain consciousness, the possibility of cerebral oedema should be considered. In situations where the intravenous administration of glucose is impractical or not feasible, glucagon 0.5 to 1 mg by subcutaneous or intramuscular injection may be given; intravenous injection may also be employed. If the patient fails to respond to glucagon, then glucose has to be given intravenously despite any impracticalities.

Following a return to consciousness, carbohydrates by mouth may need to be given until the action of insulin has ceased which, for preparations with a relatively long duration of action such as globin zinc insulin, isophane insulin, some insulin zinc suspensions, and protamine zinc insulin, may be several hours.

Reports of the treatment of insulin overdosage by excision of tissue at the site of injection.— I. W. Campbell and J. G. Ratcliffe, *Br. med. J.*, 1982, *285*, 408; D. F. Levine and C. Bulstrode (letter), *ibid.*, 974.

Precautions

Dosage requirements of insulin may be altered by many factors. Increased doses are usually necessary during infection, emotional stress, accidental or surgical trauma, puberty, and the latter two trimesters of pregnancy, and decreased doses are usually necessary in patients with impaired renal function or during the first trimester of pregnancy. Following initiation and stabilisation of therapy in newly-diagnosed diabetic patients, a temporary decrease in requirements may also occur (the so-called honeymoon period).

Concomitant drug therapy may also alter insulin requirements. Drugs which may decrease insulin requirements include alcohol, anabolic steroids, aspirin, beta blockers, fenfluramine, and monoamine oxidase inhibitors; there have been isolated reports of decreased insulin requirements with captopril, clofibrate, cyclophosphamide, guanethidine, mebendazole, methandienone, and oxytetracycline. Increased dosage requirements of insulin may occur with adrenaline, chlorpromazine, corticosteroids, oral contraceptives, thiazide diuretics, and thyroid hormones; there have also been isolated reports of increased insulin requirements or aggravation of hyperglycaemia with chlordiazepoxide, cyclophosphamide, dobutamine, and isoniazid. Beta blockers may also mask some of the symptoms due to hypoglycaemia caused by excessive doses of insulin.

Because of the possibility of differing responses to insulins of different species, care is recommended to avoid the inadvertent change from insulin of one species to another. Care is also necessary during excessive exercise as hypoglycaemia may be provoked.

The use of insulin necessitates monitoring of therapy, such as the testing of blood or urine for glucose concentrations and the urine for ketones, by the patient.

CAUTION. *Biphasic insulin, globin zinc insulin, insulin zinc suspensions, isophane insulin, and protamine zinc insulin should never be given intravenously and they are not suitable for the emergency treatment of diabetic ketoacidosis.*

In a study involving 11 insulin-dependent diabetic subjects, leg exercise accelerated insulin absorption from a subcutaneous injection site in the leg, whereas it had no effect on insulin absorption from the arm and reduced it from the abdomen.— V. A. Koivisto and P. Felig, *New Engl. J. Med.*, 1978, *298*, 79. Most exercise involved many muscle groups and increased absorption was still likely. Patients who developed hypoglycaemia were advised to take extra carbohydrate before exercise rather than decrease the insulin dose.— B. Zinman *et al.* (letter), *ibid.*, 1202. Studies in 5 subjects suggested that absorption was increased by exercise.— P. Dandona *et al.*, *Br. med. J.*, 1978, *1*, 479.

Studies in 8 insulin-dependent diabetic men indicated that a sauna accelerated insulin absorption from the subcutaneous injection site and that 2 hours after the sauna mean blood-glucose concentration was significantly lower than on the control day.— V. A. Koivisto, *Br. med. J.*, 1980, *280*, 1411. Comment.— H. J. Cüppers *et al.* (letter), *ibid.*, *281*, 307; V. A. Koivisto (letter), *ibid.*, 621. Hypoglycaemia and seizures in one patient following the use of a sunbed.— D. J. Husband and G. V. Gill (letter), *Lancet*, 1984, *2*, 1477.

DRIVING. Hypoglycaemic events are the commonest cause of drug-induced acute illness while driving, and the law treats these events as being under the influence of a drug in those on hypoglycaemic agents. Diabetics needing insulin should notify their disability to the licensing centre and should not drive vocationally.— P. A. B. Raffle, *Prescribers' J.*, 1981, *21*, 197.

INFECTIONS. Decreased requirements of insulin, added to the dialysate, occurred in 6 diabetic patients undergoing continuous ambulatory peritoneal dialysis for chronic renal failure during episodes of severe bacterial peritonitis. This was contrary to the increased insulin requirements exhibited by most diabetic patients during severe infections and probably resulted from increased absorption of insulin due to mesothelial damage.— I. S. Henderson *et al.*, *Br. med. J.*, 1985, *290*, 1474.

INTERACTIONS. Results of a retrospective survey indicating that patients receiving isophane insulin, which contains protamine, were subject to an increased risk of severe reactions simulating anaphylaxis when protamine was used to reverse systemic heparinisation after cardiac catheterisation.— W. J. Stewart *et al.*, *Circulation*, 1984, *70*, 788.

A range of compounds that have been reported to interact with insulin by increasing or decreasing insulin dosage requirements is listed above.

MENSTRUATION. Discussion on the control of diabetes during the menstrual cycle and the possible need to adjust insulin dosage regularly around the time of menstruation.— A. Magos and J. Studd, *Br. J. Hosp. Med.*, 1985, *33*, 68.

Of 200 women with diabetes 76 considered that the control of their diabetes changed with menstruation; effects ranged from hypoglycaemia to hyperglycaemia with ketoacidosis.— C. H. Walsh and J. M. Malins, *Br. med. J.*, 1977, *2*, 177.

MORNING HYPERGLYCAEMIA. Morning hyperglycaemia may be the result of mere waning of subcutaneously injected insulin. It may also be rebound hyperglycaemia (posthypoglycaemic hyperglycaemia or the Somogyi phenomenon) occurring after an episode of nocturnal hypoglycaemia. Morning hyperglycaemia has also been observed without antecedent hypoglycaemia even during constant intravenous infusion of insulin, when the waning of previously injected insulin would not be a factor and this is commonly referred to as the dawn phenomenon. Clinically, it is important to distinguish between the dawn phenomenon, simple waning of previously injected insulin, and rebound hyperglycaemia as a cause of early-morning hyperglycaemia because their treatment differs. Management of the dawn phenomenon and insulin waning generally consists of adjusting the evening dose of insulin to provide additional coverage between 4 a.m. and 7 a.m. Management of rebound hyperglycaemia consists of reducing insulin doses or providing additional late-evening carbohydrate, or both, to avoid nocturnal hypoglycaemia. Mistaking rebound hyperglycaemia for the dawn phenomenon or mere waning of injected insulin could result in more serious nocturnal hypoglycaemia, if evening doses of insulin were increased.— P. E. Cryer and J. E. Gerich, *New Engl. J. Med.*, 1985, *313*, 232.

Reviews, studies, and comments on nocturnal hypoglycaemia, the dawn phenomenon, and rebound hyperglycaemia.— D. E. Wilson, *Ann. intern. Med.*, 1983, *98*, 219; *Lancet*, 1984, *1*, 1333; J. G. Devlin (letter), *ibid.*, *2*, 237; G. B. Bolli and J. E. Gerich, *New Engl. J. Med.*, 1984, *310*, 746; G. B. Bolli *et al.*, *ibid.*, *311*, 1214; P. Orlander (letter), *ibid.*, 1985, *312*, 444; J. E. Gerich *et al.* (letter), *ibid*; P. J. Campbell *et al.*, *ibid.*, 1473; E. A. Chantelau *et al.* (letter), *ibid.*, *313*, 957; P. J. Campbell *et al.* (letter), *ibid.*, 958; S. Pramming *et al.*, *Br. med. J.*, 1985, *291*, 376; P. C. W. Lyn (letter), *ibid.*, 1047.

Studies of the effect of adjusting the timing of the evening dose of insulin on morning hyperglycaemia.— A. J. Francis *et al.*, *Br. med. J.*, 1983, *286*, 1173; F. R. J. Hinde and D. I. Johnston, *Archs Dis. Childh.*, 1985, *60*, 311; *idem*, 1986, *61*, 118.

PREGNANCY AND THE NEONATE. See Diabetes Mellitus under Uses.

RENAL FAILURE. References to the use of insulin, added to the dialysis fluid, in diabetic patients with end-stage renal disease undergoing continuous ambulatory peritoneal dialysis.— P. Amair *et al.*, *New Engl. J. Med.*, 1982, *306*, 625; L. Strom and R. R. Hallac (letter), *ibid.*, *307*, 1082; M. S. Neff *et al.* (letter), *ibid*; J. S. Najarian and D. E. R. Sutherland (letter), *ibid.*, 1083; B. Leibel *et al.* (letter), *ibid.*

A report of reduced insulin requirements in a diabetic who developed acute renal failure; requirements returned to previous levels after the patient recovered.— J. E. Naschitz *et al.*, *Postgrad. med. J.*, 1983, *59*, 269.

See also under Infections (above) and Surgery (below).

SURGERY. References to the management of diabetes during surgery.— P. J. Watkins, *Br. med. J.*, 1982, *285*, 361; P. J. Smail, *Archs Dis. Childh.*, 1986, *61*, 413.

Management of patients with diabetic nephropathy during renal transplantation and dialysis.— P. J. Watkins, *Br. med. J.*, 1982, *285*, 627.

TRAVELLING. Advice for the diabetic patient when travelling.— E. Walker and G. Williams, *Br. med. J.*, 1983, *286*, 1337.

Absorption and Fate

Insulin has no hypoglycaemic effect when administered by mouth since it is inactivated in the gastro-intestinal tract.

It is fairly rapidly absorbed from subcutaneous tissue following injection and although the half-life in blood is very short (being only a matter of minutes), the duration of action of most preparations is considerably longer due to their formulation (for further details see Uses and Administration, below). The rate of absorption from different anatomical sites may be different and may also be increased by exercise. The absorption of insulin after intramuscular administration is more rapid than that following subcutaneous administration.

Resistance to Insulin

The term insulin resistance has traditionally been used to describe a state in which diabetic patients exhibit considerably increased insulin requirements. It is now, however, used in a much wider sense, and is for instance also applied to patients in whom a subnormal biological response to insulin can be demonstrated, although many of these patients do not apparently present difficulties in their clinical management.

Insulin resistance of the type manifested by greatly increased insulin requirements may be due to a variety of factors, including antibody formation and inadequate absorption of insulin from subcutaneous sites.

Proposed definitions for the terms insulin resistance, insulin insensitivity, and insulin unreponsiveness. In the most general sense, insulin resistance may be said to exist whenever normal concentrations produce a less than normal biological response; insulin resistance should be regarded as a 'generic' term and may be applied to the entire organism, a single tissue, a single cell, or even a single metabolic pathway. In a hormone-resistant state both the maximal response and the dose-response may be changed; thus insulin-resistant states include decreased sensitivity, in which the maximal response is unchanged but greater than normal concentrations of insulin are required to elicit a quantitatively normal reponse; decreased responsiveness in which the maximal response to insulin is decreased but the dose-response relationship that exists between no effect and maximal effect is normal; and combinations of both decreased sensitivity and responsiveness. Causes of insulin resistance at the pre-receptor level would include factors that reduce free insulin concentration such as increased insulin degradation or binding of insulin to antibodies. At the receptor, alterations in receptor affinity or concentration would also result in a decrease in biological response.— C. R. Kahn, *Metabolism*, 1978, *27, Suppl.* 2, 1893.

In 6 patients with insulin requirements of 120 to 3000 units daily, diabetic control was improved by the use of intravenous infusions of insulin in doses of 50 to 63 units daily. It was considered that there was a defect in absorption from subcutaneous tissue.— P. Dandona *et al., Lancet*, 1978, *2*, 283. A reminder that the proper length of needle is necessary to ensure the subcutaneous deposition of insulin; if the injection is given into the fat pad, insulin will be absorbed neither rapidly nor completely. Three patients receiving insulin 80 to 100 units daily could be maintained on much smaller doses of 20 to 30 units daily following the use of needles of the right length.— R. Khardori (letter), *ibid.*, 742.

A report of massive insulin resistance treated by plasma exchange in a patient with autoantibodies to the insulin receptor.— M. Muggeo, *New Engl. J. Med.*, 1979, *300*, 477. Successful use of plasmaphaeresis in a patient with intractable insulin-resistant diabetes; administration of insulin by subcutaneous injection, continuous subcutaneous infusion, and intravenous and intramuscular infusions had all failed. The reason for the patient's resistance or how plasmaphaeresis worked was not known.— G. Antony *et al.* (letter), *Lancet*, 1983, *2*, 1148.

Control of severe brittle diabetes in 5 of 6 patients by continuous intramuscular infusion of insulin; they appeared to have impaired absorption of insulin given subcutaneously.— J. C. Pickup *et al., Br. med. J.*, 1981, *282*, 347.

A report of 5 patients resistant to high doses of insulin administered subcutaneously but who responded to small amounts given intravenously. In all patients subcutaneous insulin in conventional doses was immediately effective when mixed with aprotinin. The observations support the existence of excessive degradation or sequestration of insulin at the subcutaneous injection site and the efficacy of aprotinin suggests that the pathogenesis of this disorder is related to proteases. The use of aprotinin may thus be a reasonable temporary alternative to constant prolonged intravenous infusion of insulin but its use in the treatment of such patients remains experimental.— G. R. Friedenberg *et al., New Engl. J. Med.*, 1981, *305*, 363. Discussion, including emphasis on the hazards of anaphylaxis due to aprotinin: J. C. Pickup *et al.* (letter), *ibid.*, 1413; S. Colagiuri and H. Grunstein (letter), *ibid;* M. Berger *et al.* (letter), *ibid.*, 1414. Reply agreeing that caution is necessary. Since submission of the original report several patients with variants of the syndrome who have not responded to aprotinin have been identified. These patients pose a difficult problem in management as constant intravenous infusion of insulin with its associated complications is not a satisfactory solution.— G. R. Freidenberg *et al.* (letter), *ibid.*

The use of a computerised glucose-controlled system for the administration of intravenous insulin infusion in the control of insulin resistance in one patient.— H. Connor *et al., Br. med. J.*, 1982, *285*, 1316.

Continuous administration of insulin via an intraperitoneal catheter and open-loop peristaltic pump was used in a 28-year-old diabetic when intramuscular, continuous subcutaneous, and continuous intravenous administration had all failed to give adequate control. The technique achieved a metabolic improvement and a reduction in the daily insulin requirement although blood-glucose concentrations were still somewhat raised. The catheter was well tolerated for more than 120 days.— G. Pozza *et al., Br. med. J.*, 1983, *286*, 255.

Uses and Administration

Insulin is a hormone produced in the beta-cells of the islets of Langerhans in the pancreas. The main stimulus for its secretion is glucose, although many other factors including amino acids, catecholamines, cortisol, glucagon, growth hormone, and somatostatin, are involved in its regulation. The secretion of insulin is not therefore constant as peaks occur in response to the intake of food.

The major effects of insulin on carbohydrate homoeostasis follow its binding to specific cell-surface receptors on insulin-sensitive tissues, notably the liver, muscles, and adipose tissue. It inhibits hepatic glucose production and enhances peripheral glucose disposal thereby reducing blood-glucose concentration. It also inhibits lipolysis thereby preventing the formation of ketone bodies.

Therapy with insulin is essential for the long-term survival of all patients with insulin-dependent diabetes mellitus. It may also be necessary in some patients with non-insulin-dependent disease, especially during periods of severe infection, stress, or trauma, and during major surgery. Insulin is also usually the treatment chosen for all types of diabetes mellitus during pregnancy.

The different insulins described above are available in a variety of formulations; in the *UK* and also in many other countries the commercially available preparations have been standardised to a single strength containing 100 units per mL. They may all be given by subcutaneous injection, most by intramuscular injection, but only soluble insulins can be given by the intravenous route. The long-term management of diabetic patients usually involves the subcutaneous route.

The various formulations of insulin are often classified, according to their duration of action after subcutaneous injection, as short-, intermediate-, or long-acting. The exact duration of action for any particular preparation, however, is variable and may depend upon factors such as interindividual variation, the patient's antibody status, whether the insulin is of human or animal origin, the dose, and the site of injection. Short-acting insulins are the soluble insulins, which have an onset after about 30 minutes to 1 hour, a peak activity at about 2 to 5 hours, and a duration of about 6 to 8 hours. Intermediate-acting insulins include biphasic insulins, isophane insulins, and amorphous insulin zinc suspensions. In general these have an onset within about 2 hours, peak activity after about 4 to 12 hours, and a duration of up to 24 hours. Commercially available mixtures of soluble insulins and isophane insulins have activities which would normally place them within the intermediate-acting category. Mixed insulin zinc suspensions are sometimes classified as either intermediate- or long-acting as the duration of action may be up to 30 hours. Long-acting insulins include crystalline insulin zinc suspensions and protamine zinc insulins. These generally have an onset after about 4 hours and a duration of up to 36 hours. Following intramuscular injection, the onset of action of all insulins is generally more rapid and the duration of action shorter.

The particular insulin employed, such as human or animal, the type of formulation, the route of administration, and the frequency of administration must be chosen to suit the needs of the individual patient. The dosage of insulin must also be determined for each patient and although a precise dose range cannot be given a total dose in excess of about 80 units daily would be unusual and may indicate the presence of a form of insulin resistance. The dose should be adjusted as necessary according to the results of regular monitoring of blood or urine concentrations of glucose by the patient. The WHO has recommended that the glucose concentration of venous whole blood under fasting conditions should be kept within the range of 3.3 to 5.6 mmol per litre (60 to 100 mg per 100 mL) and after meals should not be allowed to exceed 10 mmol per litre (180 mg per 100 mL); blood-glucose concentrations should not be allowed to fall below 3 mmol per litre (55 mg per 100 mL). It should be remembered that the glucose concentrations in venous plasma, venous whole blood, and capillary whole blood may be slightly different. Insulin requirements may be altered by various factors (see Precautions, above). The aim of any regimen should be to achieve the best possible control of blood-glucose by attempting to mimic as closely as possible the pattern of optimum endogenous insulin secretion. Many regimens involve the use of a short-acting soluble insulin together with an intermediate-acting insulin, such as isophane insulin or mixed insulin zinc suspension. Such a combination is often given by subcutaneous injection twice daily with about two-thirds of the total daily requirement given before breakfast and the remaining third before the evening meal. It may sometimes be necessary, though, to give 3 or 4 injections daily to achieve good control and this typically involves the administration of a soluble insulin before meals together with an intermediate-acting insulin before breakfast or at bedtime. A once-daily injection of an intermediate- or long-acting insulin is now generally considered to be acceptable only for those patients with non-insulin-dependent diabetes mellitus who still retain some endogenous insulin secretion but nevertheless require insulin therapy or for those patients with insulin-dependent disease unable to cope satisfactorily with more intensive regimens. If a more intensive regimen than subcutaneous injections is desired, continuous subcutaneous insulin infusion may be employed. This technique involves the use of a small pump which delivers a constant basal infusion of insulin, providing about half of the total daily requirements, the remainder being provided by patient-activated bolus doses before each meal. Formulations in which the insulin is in suspension are not suitable for administration by continuous subcutaneous infusion.

Insulin is also an essential part of the emergency management of diabetic ketoacidosis. Only short-acting soluble insulins should be used. Treatment includes adequate fluid replacement, usually by infusing sodium chloride 0.9% initially, and the administration of potassium salts to prevent or correct hypokalaemia. If possible, insulin should be given by intravenous infusion and typical initial infusion rates range between 5 and 10 units per hour; alternatively intramuscular injection may be employed. Since insulin normally corrects hyperglycaemia before ketosis it is usually necessary to continue administration of insulin once normoglycaemia has been achieved but to change the rehydration fluid to glucose-saline so that the additional glucose prevents the development of hypoglycaemia.

ADMINISTRATION. *Continuous administration.* Continuous infusion of insulin is normally by either the subcutaneous or intravenous route. Open-loop delivery systems are simply an infusion pump with programmed or manual control of the infusion rate and blood-glucose monitoring must be performed manually. Such systems are now being used widely for continuous subcutaneous insulin infusion in the long-term management of some diabetic patients but their application for long-term intravenous use appears to be restricted by the problems of vascular complications such as infection and thrombosis. Closed-loop systems (the 'artificial pancreas') for intravenous administration also exist, and generally consist of a system for the infusion of insulin, a small computer, and an inbuilt glucose sensor, but their use is generally confined to research and experimental work. Administration of insulin by continuous intramuscular and intraperitoneal infusion has also been described but such techniques are not in general use.

A review and discussion of continuous subcutaneous insulin infusion. Continuous subcutaneous insulin infusion now has an established place in the treatment of diabetes. By providing continuous basal insulin infusion with preprandial boosts it aims at mimicking the physiological patterns of plasma-insulin concentrations more closely than those obtained with intermittent insulin injections. The chief benefit is the considerable improvement in lifestyle enjoyed by some patients and blood-glucose control is generally improved at the same time. Considerable flexibility for the patient, especially with regard to the timing of meals, is allowed and sometimes the dawn phenomenon is diminished with an improved sense of wellbeing. Disadvantages include the relative bulkiness of the apparatus, the risk of mechanical failures, obvious difficulties with vigorous physical activities, rapid development of ketoacidosis, some tendency to gain weight, and in some people, problems from skin infection. Problems from severe hypoglycaemia may decrease, but the overall incidence of such episodes is similar to that with conventional treatment; even exercise-induced hypoglycaemia may cause fewer problems, though reduction of the infusion rate may still be needed. Continuous subcutaneous insulin infusion is not suitable for all patients, and indeed many prefer to remain having conventional treatment. It does not provide a general solution for brittle diabetes, and is not suitable for emotionally or psychiatrically disturbed patients. It has obvious limitations, too, in very young diabetics. Patients receiving continuous subcutaneous insulin infusion must be well motivated, reliable, be able to monitor their own blood-glucose concentrations regularly, and have access to expert advice day and night.— P. J. Watkins, *Br. med. J.*, 1985, *290*, 655. See also.— F. K. Thorp, *J. Am. med. Ass.*, 1986, *255*, 645.

A discussion on the problems of infection, ketoacidosis, and hypoglycaemia that may arise acutely during continuous subcutaneous insulin infusion by portable pump.— *Lancet*, 1985, *1*, 911.

A review of insulin pharmacokinetics, with emphasis on those aspects relevant to subcutaneous insulin infusion devices.— E. W. Kraegen and D. J. Chisholm, *Clin. Pharmacokinet.*, 1985, *10*, 303.

Reports and comments on the use of continuous subcutaneous insulin infusion and its complications: R. S. Mecklenburg *et al.*, *New Engl. J. Med.*, 1982, *307*, 513; D. M. Nathan *et al.*, *Ann. intern. Med.*, 1982, *97*, 31; A. J. M. Boulton *et al.*, *Postgrad. med. J.*, 1983, *59*, 438; S. A. Greene *et al.*, *Archs Dis. Childh.*, 1983, *58*, 578; I. Lager *et al.*, *Br. med. J.*, 1983, *287*, 1661; J. C. Pickup *et al.*, *ibid.*, 1984, *288*, 796; A. G. Davies *et al.*, *Archs Dis. Childh.*, 1984, *59*, 1027; R. S. Mecklenburg *et al.*, *J. Am. med. Ass.*, 1984, *252*, 3265; S. M. Teutsch *et al.*, *New Engl. J. Med.*, 1984, *310*, 361; J. D. A. Clark *et al.* (letter), *ibid.*, *311*, 1052; S. M. Teutsch *et al.* (letter), *ibid.*, 1053; G. Knight *et al.*, *Br. med. J.*, 1985, *291*, 371; R. S. Mecklenburg *et al.*, *New Engl. J. Med.*, 1985, *313*, 465; S. J. Brink and C. Stewart, *J. Am. med. Ass.*, 1986, *255*, 617.

For references to the intraperitoneal administration of insulin, added to dialysis fluid, in patients undergoing peritoneal dialysis, see under Precautions.

For reports of the use of continuous administration of insulin by various routes in the management of brittle diabetes and insulin resistance, see under Resistance to Insulin.

For the role of continuous subcutaneous insulin infusion in the prevention or amelioration of diabetic complications, and in the management of diabetes during pregnancy, see under Diabetes Mellitus (below).

Intranasal administration. A report on the safety and efficacy of intranasal insulin in healthy subjects and insulin-dependent diabetics.— A. E. Pontiroli *et al.*, *Br. med. J.*, 1982, *284*, 303.

Results of studies involving 45 patients with type 1 diabetes and 9 healthy controls, demonstrated that intranasal insulin, given in a solution containing the surfactant laureth 9, rapidly crossed the nasal mucosa, reduced postprandial hyperglycaemia when given before a meal, and was a feasible long-term adjunct to subcutaneous insulin in type 1 diabetics. Intranasal insulin merits careful examination as an adjunct to subcutaneous insulin in the treatment of diabetes, but the extent of its usefulness will depend upon progress in the development of new surfactants.— R. Salzman *et al.*, *New Engl. J. Med.*, 1985, *312*, 1078. Comment.— D. S. Schade and R. P. Eaton, *ibid.*, 1120.

Jet injection. A review and discussion on the jet injection of insulin. Jet injection devices have been available for many years but have not been widely used.— *Lancet*, 1985, *1*, 1140. Comment that there is good experimental evidence to justify the reservations about the jet injection of insulin.— P. M. Gaylarde and I. Sarkany (letter), *ibid.*, 1513.

References to the administration of insulin by jet injection.— R. Worth *et al.*, *Br. med. J.*, 1980, *281*, 713; G. B. Pehling and J. E. Gerich, *Mayo Clin. Proc.*, 1984, *59*, 751.

Mixing of insulins. Evidence to suggest that mixing human neutral insulin injection with human crystalline insulin zinc suspension in the syringe results in the loss of the rapid hypoglycaemic effect of the soluble insulin component even when injected immediately after mixing.— I. Mühlhauser *et al.*, *Br. med. J.*, 1984, *289*, 1656. Similar results with a mixture of human neutral insulin injection and human insulin zinc suspension.— R. J. Heine *et al.*, *ibid.*, 1985, *290*, 204. The manufacturers report that their analysis of a study using mixtures (P.D. Home *et al.*, *Diabetic Med.*, 1984, *1*, 93) did not indicate a reduced effect.— M. Edwards *et al.* (letter), *ibid.*, 791. Since the study did not investigate the insulin pharmacokinetics, it could not be used to argue that there was no reduced effect from the mixture.— R. Heine (letter), *ibid.*, 1515.

Oral administration. Results in healthy subjects indicating that insulin by mouth can be absorbed from the intestine when taken in association with the α-chymotrypsin inhibitor FK-448.— M. Shinomiya *et al.* (letter), *Lancet*, 1985, *1*, 1092.

Timing of injections. Results of a study in adult diabetics suggested that an increase in the time between injection of insulin and eating to 45 minutes would be a simple and safe way of improving blood-glucose control, at least in those who currently allow less than 15 minutes.— M. E. J. Lean *et al.*, *Br. med. J.*, 1985, *290*, 105. Comment that from the evidence presented it would certainly appear undesirable to eat immediately after taking insulin, but that it is not justified to advocate a general extension of the delay to as much as 45 minutes. The currently recommended 30-minute delay seems quite sufficient.— S. D. Slater (letter), *ibid.*, 560.

Further references: A. L. Kinmonth and J. D. Baum, *Br. med. J.*, 1980, *280*, 604.

See also Morning Hyperglycaemia, under Precautions.

DIABETES MELLITUS. *Choice of insulin.* Mention that short-acting soluble insulins and medium-acting isophane insulin and insulin zinc suspensions are the main types of insulin in use. The long-acting crystalline insulin zinc suspension is sometimes of additional value, but the use of protamine zinc insulin is declining rapidly with the development of better formulations.— P. J. Watkins, *Br. med. J.*, 1983, *287*, 1571.

A review and discussion of human insulin. Both the *in vitro* and *in vivo* properties of intravenously administered human insulin have been reported to be virtually identical to those of purified pork insulin. Subcutaneously injected human insulin is, however, absorbed slightly more quickly than porcine insulin and this has been shown for both short-acting and intermediate-acting preparations; in some studies beef and human crystalline insulin zinc suspensions had a similar duration of action. Possibly the reason for the accelerated absorption of human insulin is that it is more soluble. In several clinical trials comparing the control of blood-glucose in diabetic patients treated with short- or intermediate-acting insulin of animal or human origin, differences have been shown but adjustments in the ratio and amounts of insulins given throughout the day usually allow comparable control to be achieved after a short while. Clinical trials of human insulin have also provided evidence that it can be less immunogenic. Human insulin seems a justifiable first choice in newly diagnosed diabetics and those needing short-term or intermittent treatment, such as gestational diabetics and type 2 diabetic patients during surgery. There is currently no good reason for transferring established diabetics, except perhaps those who have developed insulin allergy or those at risk or with a history of allergy, from pork to human insulin.— J. Pickup, *Br. med. J.*, 1986, *292*, 155. Comment.— P. Home (letter), *ibid.*, 625. Reply.— J. Pickup (letter), *ibid.*, 626.

A further review of human insulin: R. N. Brogden and R. C. Heel, *Drugs*, 1987, *34*, 350.

Comparisons of human and animal insulins in diabetic patients.— K. Egstrup and J. Olsen (letter), *Lancet*, 1982, *2*, 222 (human and porcine); A. J. L. Clark *et al.*, *ibid.*, 354 (human, bovine, and porcine); I. Peacock *et al.*, *ibid.*, 1983, *1*, 149 (human, bovine, and porcine); M. Castillo *et al.*, *Eur. J. clin. Pharmac.*, 1983, *25*, 767 (human and porcine); S. A. Greene *et al.*, *Br. med. J.*, 1983, *287*, 1578 (human and porcine); N. P. Mann *et al.*, *ibid.*, 1580 (human and porcine); R. R. Holman *et al.*, *ibid.*, 1984, *288*, 665 (human and bovine); P. S. Moffitt *et al.*, *Med. J. Aust.*, 1984, *140*, 200 (human and porcine); M. D. Hocking *et al.*, *Archs Dis. Childh.*, 1986, *61*, 341 (human and porcine).

Diabetic complications. Following the introduction of intensified insulin regimens to improve glycaemic control, much attention has been focussed on whether the use of continuous subcutaneous insulin infusion can modify the development or progression of diabetic complications. Several reports have been published including those of The Steno Study Groups on diabetic retinopathy and nephropathy (*Lancet*, 1982, *1*, 121; T. Lauritzen *et al.*, *ibid.*, 1983, *1*, 200; T. Lauritzen *et al.*, *ibid.*, 1445; *ibid.*, *2*, 178; B. Feldt-Rasmussen *et al.*, *New Engl. J. Med.*, 1986, *314*, 665; B. Feldt-Rasmussen *et al.*, *Lancet*, 1986, *2*, 1300), The Kroc Collaborative Study Group on diabetic retinopathy (*New Engl. J. Med.*, 1984, *311*, 365), and the Oslo Study Groups on diabetic retinopathy, nephropathy, and neuropathy (The Aker Diabetes Group, K. Dahl-Jørgensen *et al.*, *Br. med. J.*, 1985, *290*, 811; O. Brinchmann-Hansen *et al.*, *Am. J. Ophthal.*, 1985, *100*, 644; K. Dahl-Jørgensen *et al.*, *Br. med. J.*, 1986, *293*, 1195). Other workers have also published results concerning diabetic nephropathy (G.C. Viberti *et al.*, *Br. med. J.*, 1983, *286*, 598; M.J. Wiseman *et al.*, *New Engl. J. Med.*, 1985, *312*, 617; J.J. Bending *et al.*, *Br. med. J.*, 1986, *292*, 83) and diabetic neuropathy (A.J.M. Boulton *et al.*, *Diabetes Care*, 1982, *5*, 386; A. Samanta and A.C. Burden, *Lancet*, 1985, *1*, 348). All of these studies were of relatively short duration, being 2 years or less. In general terms they did not find initially that the improved metabolic control obtained with continuous subcutaneous insulin infusion had a beneficial effect although in studies in which 2 years of therapy was completed the results did appear to suggest that infusion may provide some protection. In a review Watkins (*Br. med. J.*, 1985, *290*, 655) has commented that since the usual evolution of diabetic complications is over 10 to 30 years no one should be surprised that studies using continuous subcutaneous insulin infusion and ranging from a few months to two years should not show an effect and that the answer can clearly come only from careful long-term observations.

A study in diabetic patients indicating that careful control of blood-glucose concentrations by using intravenous insulin infusions failed to improve the outcome after myocardial infarction.— D. J. Gwilt *et al.*, *Br. Heart J.*, 1984, *51*, 626. Conflicting results suggesting that the higher mortality in diabetic subjects compared to non-diabetic subjects following an acute myocardial infarction may be reduced by improved diabetic control.— R. S. Clark *et al.*, *Br. med. J.*, 1985, *291*, 303. Comments.— R. J. Jarrett (letter), *ibid.*, 677; G. A. Oswald and J. S. Yudkin (letter), *ibid;* R. S. Clark (letter), *ibid;* B. L. Pentecost *et al.* (letter), *ibid.*

Diabetic ketoacidosis. Guidelines for the management of diabetic ketoacidosis. Intravenous fluids should be given, the regimen being modified according to individual needs. A suitable regimen for most adult patients using sodium chloride intravenous infusion 0.9%, is, 1 litre in the first half-hour, 1 litre per hour over the next 2 hours, and 1 litre over each of the next successive 2-, 3-, and 4-hour periods (a total of 6 litres over 11.5 hours). Soluble insulin, diluted to a concentration of 1 unit per mL, should be started immediately and given intravenously by infusion pump set at a rate of 6 units per hour; children may be given 0.1 unit per kg body-weight per hour via a paediatric drip set. Higher infusion rates are rarely needed, but if necessary the rate may be doubled or quadrupled. When the blood-glucose concentration has fallen to less than 10 mmol per litre the insulin rate may be reduced to 3 units per hour (in adults) and the fluid should be changed from saline to glucose-saline. The insulin infusion should be continued until the patient is well enough to take food by mouth when subcutaneous insulin is given before and intravenous insulin discontinued after the meal. Alternatively, in adults, insulin may be given intramuscularly, with 20 units as a loading dose, then 6 units hourly until the blood-glucose concentration is less than 10 mmol per litre, and then every 2 hours. Potassium chloride administration should usually start at about the second hour and the exact amounts determined to maintain serum-potassium concentrations between 4 and 5 mmol per litre. Sodium bicarbonate is not given unless the blood pH is less than 7.1 or if the patient is shocked. Management of aketotic hyperosmolar states is the same as that for ketoacidosis except that sodium chloride intravenous infusion 0.45% is used if the serum-sodium concentration is greater than 150 mmol per litre and a lower rate of insulin infusion, such as 3 units per hour in adults, is often sufficient.— P. J. Watkins, *Br. med. J.*, 1982, *285*, 360.

A review and discussion on the metabolic derangements and treatment of diabetic ketoacidosis. Insulin is required for the treatment of diabetic ketoacidosis and in recent years investigators have been concerned primarily about the amount that should be given. Numerous studies indicate that doses considerably lower than those used before the early 1970's (usually 50 to 100 units given intravenously every hour to two hours) effectively reverse ketoacidosis. Initially, the use of low-dose regimens was promoted because the treatment was simple and hypoglycaemia and hypokalaemia were said to occur less frequently. Although there are now fewer claims for the superiority of low-dose schedules, their efficacy is still defended. If a low-dose schedule is to be followed at least 10 units per hour should be given. Regardless of the initial schedule chosen, large doses of insulin should be given without delay if there has been no fall in ketones or increase in pH within 3 to 4 hours after the start of therapy. It should be remembered that a major goal in the treatment of diabetic ketoacidosis is the complete clearance of ketone bodies from urine and plasma and since plasma-glucose almost invariably falls before reversal of ketogenesis, glucose should be infused as necessary during continued insulin treatment to avoid hypoglycaemia. It is a common error to slow or stop insulin infusion when acidosis or ketosis are still present simply because the glucose concentration is falling. Despite efforts to document the efficacy of intramuscular injections, it is clear that volume depletion and vascular collapse may impair absorption and thereby delay the response in some patients. Therefore it is recommended that intravenous therapy be used except in the absence of suitable veins. Although there has been extensive discussion about the relative merits of using 0.9% or 0.45% sodium chloride as the initial fluid, most investigators favour the former. About 1 litre per hour should be given for the first 2 to 3 hours, although slower rates may be appropriate depending on urine output and clinical response. Total body stores of potassium are depleted in patients with diabetic ketoacidosis but ordinarily potassium salts are not required until 2 to 4 hours after the start of therapy; however if the initial potassium concentration is low or normal, replacement must be started immediately. The administration of bicarbonate is a controversial practice. It seems wise to reserve bicarbonate for very severe acidosis (pH less than 7.0) and to stop administration when the pH reaches 7.2. Phosphate depletion in diabetic ketoacidosis is severe, but is usually clinically silent and shows up only in chemical measurements. Nevertheless, if the phosphate value before treatment is low, it seems reasonable to administer potassium phosphate when potassium is also needed.— D. W. Foster and J. D. McGarry, *New Engl. J. Med.*, 1983, *309*, 159. Comments.— H. R. de Vries (letter), *ibid.*, 1984, *310*, 199; T. Ring (letter), *ibid.*, 200.

Pregnancy and the neonate. A review of congenital malformations and blood-glucose control in diabetic pregnancy. Maternal hyperglycaemia causes measurable effects on the foetus, whose blood-glucose concentration closely reflects that of the mother. Poor diabetic control is associated with a raised foetal mortality, and ketoacidosis is often lethal. Maternal hyperglycaemia causes foetal hyperinsulinaemia which is responsible, at least in part, for increased deposition of fat in the infant. It also causes neonatal hypoglycaemia, a well-recognised condition in the newborn of diabetic mothers which is easily treated. Sporadic accounts have described an association between hyperglycaemia and the development of foetal congenital malformations and recently a large study came to the same conclusions. Unfortunately this study was retrospective and the finding cannot be regarded as conclusive. Nevertheless, additional evidence shows that foetal malformations occur less frequently in well-treated diabetics and first-trimester hyperglycaemia does seem to be associated with congenital malformations.— P. J. Watkins, *Br. med. J.*, 1982, *284*, 1357.

A review of diabetes and malformation. Congenital malformations are unhappily common and any possible relations between such a common event and a widely prevalent disease such as diabetes mellitus is therefore difficult to evaluate. In the investigations reported so far, a major problem is that few workers have studied the relevant phase of human gestation; the period before 7 to 8 weeks is clearly critical. If better control of diabetes offers a reduction of hazard to the embryo and foetus, it must clearly be started before conception.— *Lancet*, 1982, *2*, 587.

A short discussion on the management of diabetes during pregnancy. Women should be advised that if they plan a pregnancy diabetic control should be optimal at the time of conception and during the early weeks of pregnancy. Insulin injections are needed two or three times daily and the dose often increases substantially during pregnancy, sometimes to twice or three times that normally required. During labour, insulin and glucose should be given by intravenous infusion for all vaginal deliveries. During breast-feeding the mothers' diet should be increased by about 50 g of carbohydrate daily and ample fluids taken; if these measures are followed the dose of insulin is not usually affected. Women discovered to have diabetes during pregnancy should be given the same careful treatment as pregnant patients with established diabetes.— P. J. Watkins, *Br. med. J.*, 1982, *285*, 717.

A review and discussion on the care of the pregnant woman with insulin-dependent diabetes mellitus. Optimal therapy needs individualisation and combinations of intermediate (or long-acting) and regular insulin are usually employed. Early in gestation, injections twice daily may be adequate but after 24 to 28 weeks the authors use soluble insulin before each meal and additional longer-acting insulin at breakfast and supper or bedtime. The desirability of attempting to keep metabolism as close to normal as possible can no longer be disputed. Consensus also dictates that such efforts should be attempted before conception although there is still some controversy regarding the desired limits.— N. Freinkel *et al.*, *New Engl. J. Med.*, 1985, *313*, 96.

Further reviews on the management of diabetes in pregnancy: N. J. A. Vaughan, *Br. med. J.*, 1987, *294*, 558.

A comment that continuous subcutaneous insulin infusion has a limited place in planned pregnancies, when even the most conscientious patient may have difficulty with diabetic control, but in general it offers no advantage over conventional treatment and babies may still be very large.— P. J. Watkins, *Br. med. J.*, 1985, *290*, 655. A report of intra-uterine death during continuous subcutaneous insulin infusion. The mother had forgotten to prime the pump presumably causing ketoacidosis, which although not severe was sufficient to kill the baby.— J. M. Steel and C. P. West, *ibid.*, 1787.

Results of a study in 22 insulin-dependent diabetic pregnancies treated with either continuous subcutaneous insulin infusion or intensive conventional therapy consisting of multiple (two to four) subcutaneous injections of insulin daily suggested that there is no inherent advantage of one method over the other, provided that frequent monitoring and close medical supervision are practised. Both modes of therapy were associated with excellent metabolic control and a favourable outcome.— D. R. Coustan *et al.*, *J. Am. med. Ass.*, 1986, *255*, 631.

Reports and comments on foetal macrosomy and morphological abnormalities in placenta and foetus despite strict control of maternal blood-glucose.— G. Knight *et al.* (letter), *Lancet*, 1983, *2*, 1431; G. Russell *et al.* (letter), *ibid.*, 1984, *1*, 283 and 468; G. H. A. Visser *et al.* (letter), *ibid.*, 284; H. A. Verhaaren *et al.* (letter), *ibid.*, 285; P. Dandona *et al.* (letter), *ibid.*, 737; R. N. Laurini *et al.* (letter), *ibid.*, 800.

DIAGNOSIS AND TESTING. *Insulinoma.* References to the use of fish insulin for the diagnosis of insulinomas.— R. C. Turner and P. C. Johnson, *Lancet*, 1973, *1*, 1483; R. C. Turner and E. Harris, *ibid.*, 1974, *2*, 188.

Pituitary function. Insulin-induced hypoglycaemia has been used to provide a stressful stimulus in order to assess pituitary function. Administration of insulin alone has been used to stimulate release of growth hormone in tests of growth hormone deficiency (R.D.G. Milner and E.C. Burns, *Archs Dis. Childh.*, 1982, *57*, 944) although alternative tests have been proposed (J.M. King and D.A. Price, *Archs Dis. Childh.*, 1983, *58*, 220; N.C. Fraser *et al.*, *ibid.*, 355; P.C. Hindmarsh *et al.*, *Lancet*, 1985, *2*, 1033). A combined insulin test, using insulin, gonadorelin, and protirelin, has also been used to assess anterior pituitary function (P. Harsoulis *et al.*, *Br. med. J.*, 1973, *4*, 326) but again an alternative test has been suggested (L.M. Sandler *et al.*, *Br. med. J.*, 1986, *292*, 511).

GLYCOGEN STORAGE DISEASES. Injection of insulin was associated with improved growth, increased activity, and subjective improvement in 2 children with type I glycogen-storage disease.— O. Dulac *et al.* (letter), *Lancet*, 1978, *1*, 107.

LIVER DISORDERS. Initial results suggesting that intravenous infusions of insulin and glucagon may be a promising treatment for alcoholic hepatitis but that further investigations are needed.— A. L. Baker *et al.*, *Gastroenterology*, 1981, *80*, 1410.

A beneficial response, as assessed by a broad spectrum of hepatocellular function tests, in an obese woman with severe liver failure due to mild alcoholic cirrhosis and the superimposed hepatotoxic effect of a jejuno-ileal bypass following the introduction of intravenous infusions of insulin and glucagon.— J. B. Jaspan *et al.*, *Archs intern. Med.*, 1984, *144*, 2075.

TRAUMA. A review of the effects of therapeutic intervention on the metabolic responses to injury including the use of insulin with particular reference to its use in burns and after certain cardiac disorders.— I. W. Fellows and A. M. J. Woolfson, *Br. med. Bull.*, 1985, *41*, 287.

Preparations

Acid Insulin Injection *(B.P.)*. Acid Insulin. A sterile solution of bovine or porcine insulin. It is prepared from Insulin (*B.P.*). pH 3.0 to 3.5.

Biphasic Insulin Injection *(B.P.)*. Biphasic Insulin. A sterile suspension of crystals containing bovine insulin in a solution of porcine insulin. It is prepared from Insulin (*B.P.*) and may contain a suitable buffering agent. pH 6.6 to 7.2.

Biphasic Isophane Insulin Injection *(B.P.)*. Biphasic Isophane Insulin. A sterile buffered suspension of porcine or human insulin complexed with protamine sulphate or another suitable protamine, in a solution of porcine or human insulin respectively. It is prepared from Insulin (*B.P.*) or Human Insulin (*B.P.*). pH 6.9 to 7.5. It contains 300 to 600 µg of protamine sulphate per 100 units of insulin.

Extended Insulin Zinc Suspension *(U.S.P.)*. A sterile buffered aqueous suspension of Insulin (*U.S.P.*), modified by the addition of zinc chloride in a manner such that the solid phase of the suspension is predominantly crystalline. pH 7.0 to 7.8.

Insulin Human Injection *(U.S.P.)*. A sterile aqueous solution of Insulin Human (*U.S.P.*). pH 7.0 to 7.8.

Insulin Injection *(B.P.)*. Neutral Insulin; Neutral Insulin Injection; Soluble Insulin. A sterile solution of bovine, porcine, or human insulin. It is prepared from Insulin (*B.P.*) or Human Insulin (*B.P.*). pH 6.6 to 8.0.

Insulin Injection *(U.S.P.)*. A sterile acidified or neutral solution of Insulin (*U.S.P.*). pH of the acidified injection 2.5 to 3.5; pH of the neutral injection 7.0 to 7.8.

Insulin Zinc Suspension *(B.P.)*. IZS; Insulin Zinc Suspension (Mixed); Insulin Lente. A sterile neutral suspension of either bovine, porcine, or human insulin or a mixture of bovine and porcine insulin in the form of a complex obtained by the addition of a suitable zinc salt; the insulin is in a form insoluble in water. It is prepared from Insulin (*B.P.*) or Human Insulin (*B.P.*). pH 6.9 to 7.5.

Insulin Zinc Suspension *(U.S.P.)*. A sterile buffered aqueous suspension of Insulin (*U.S.P.*), modified by the addition of zinc chloride in a manner such that the solid phase of the suspension consists of a mixture of approximately 3 parts of amorphous insulin to 7 parts of crystalline insulin. pH 7.0 to 7.8.

Insulin Zinc Suspension (Amorphous) *(B.P.)*. Amorph. IZS; Insulin Semilente. A sterile neutral suspension of bovine or porcine insulin in the form of a complex obtained by the addition of a suitable zinc salt; the insulin is in a form insoluble in water. It is prepared from Insulin (*B.P.*). pH 6.9 to 7.5.

Insulin Zinc Suspension (Crystalline) *(B.P.)*. Cryst. IZS; Insulin Ultralente. A sterile neutral suspension of bovine or human insulin in the form of a complex obtained by the addition of a suitable zinc salt; the insulin is in the form of crystals insoluble in water. It is prepared from Insulin (*B.P.*) or Human Insulin (*B.P.*). pH 6.9 to 7.5.

Isophane Insulin Injection *(B.P.)*. Isophane Protamine Insulin Injection; Isophane Insulin; Isophane Insulin (NPH). A sterile suspension of bovine, porcine, or human insulin in the form of a complex obtained by the addition of protamine sulphate or another suitable protamine. It is prepared from Insulin (*B.P.*) or Human Insulin (*B.P.*). pH 6.9 to 7.5. It contains 300 to 600 µg of protamine sulphate per 100 units of insulin.

Isophane Insulin Suspension *(U.S.P.)*. A sterile buffered aqueous suspension of zinc-insulin crystals and protamine sulphate, combined in a manner such that the solid phase of the suspension consists of crystals composed of insulin, protamine, and zinc. The protamine sulphate is prepared from the sperm or from the mature testes of fish of *Oncorhynchus* spp. or *Salmo* spp. pH 7.0 to 7.8.

Prompt Insulin Zinc Suspension *(U.S.P.)*. A sterile buffered aqueous suspension of Insulin (*U.S.P.*), modified by the addition of zinc chloride in a manner such that the solid phase of the suspension is amorphous. pH 7.0 to 7.8.

Protamine Zinc Insulin Suspension *(U.S.P.)*. A sterile buffered aqueous suspension of Insulin (*U.S.P.*), modified by the addition of zinc chloride and protamine sulphate. The protamine sulphate is prepared from the sperm or from the mature testes of fish of *Oncorhynchus* spp. or *Salmo* spp. pH 7.1 to 7.4. It contains 1.0 to 1.5 mg of protamine per 100 units of insulin.

Proprietary Preparations

Human Actraphane *(Novo, UK)*. *Injection*, mixture of Insulin Injection (*B.P.*) (human, emp, monocomponent) 30% and Isophane Insulin Injection (*B.P.*) (human, emp, monocomponent) 70% 100 units/mL, in vials of 10 mL.

Human Actrapid *(Novo, UK)*. *Injection*, Insulin Injection (*B.P.*) (human, emp, monocomponent) 100 units/mL, in vials of 10 mL and also in Penfill cartridges of 1.5 mL for use in a specially designed injection device (Novopen).

Human Initard 50/50 *(Nordisk-UK, UK; Wellcome, UK)*. *Injection*, mixture of Insulin Injection (*B.P.*) (human, emp, highly purified) 50% and Isophane Insulin Injection (*B.P.*) (human, emp, highly purified) 50% 100 units/mL, in vials of 10 mL.

Human Insulatard *(Nordisk-UK, UK; Wellcome, UK)*. *Injection*, Isophane Insulin Injection (*B.P.*) (human, emp, highly purified) 100 units/mL, in vials of 10 mL.

Human Mixtard 30/70 *(Nordisk-UK, UK; Wellcome, UK)*. *Injection*, mixture of Insulin Injection (*B.P.*) (human, emp, highly purified) 30% and Isophane Insulin Injection (*B.P.*) (human, emp, highly purified) 70% 100 units/mL, in vials of 10 mL.

Human Monotard *(Novo, UK)*. *Injection*, Insulin Zinc Suspension (*B.P.*) (human, emp, monocomponent) 100 units/mL, in vials of 10 mL.

Human Protaphane *(Novo, UK)*. *Injection*, Isophane Insulin Injection (*B.P.*) (human, emp, monocomponent) 100 units/mL, in vials of 10 mL.

Human Ultratard *(Novo, UK)*. *Injection*, Insulin Zinc Suspension (Crystalline) (*B.P.*) (human, emp, monocomponent) 100 units/mL, in vials of 10 mL.

Human Velosulin *(Nordisk-UK, UK; Wellcome, UK)*. *Injection*, Insulin Injection (*B.P.*) (human, emp, highly purified) 100 units/mL, in vials of 10 mL.

Humulin I *(Lilly, UK)*. *Injection*, Isophane Insulin Injection (*B.P.*) (human, prb) 100 units/mL, in vials of 10 mL.

Humulin Lente *(Lilly, UK)*. *Injection*, Insulin Zinc Suspension (Crystalline) (*B.P.*) (human, prb) 100 units/mL, in vials of 10 mL.

Humulin M1 *(Lilly, UK)*. *Injection*, mixture of Insulin Injection (*B.P.*) (human, prb) 10% and Isophane Insulin Injection (*B.P.*) (human, prb) 90% 100 units/mL, in vials of 10 mL.

Humulin M2 *(Lilly, UK)*. *Injection*, mixture of Insulin Injection (*B.P.*) (human, prb) 20% and Isophane Insulin Injection (*B.P.*) (human, prb) 80% 100 units/mL, in vials of 10 mL.

Humulin M3 *(Lilly, UK)*. *Injection*, mixture of Insulin Injection (*B.P.*) (human, prb) 30% and Isophane Insulin Injection (*B.P.*) (human, prb) 70% 100 units/mL, in vials of 10 mL.

Humulin M4 *(Lilly, UK)*. *Injection*, mixture of Insulin Injection (*B.P.*) (human, prb) 40% and Isophane Insulin Injection (*B.P.*) (human, prb) 60% 100 units/mL, in vials of 10 mL.

Humulin S *(Lilly, UK)*. *Injection*, Insulin Injection (*B.P.*) (human, prb) 100 units/mL, in vials of 10 mL.

Humulin Zn *(Lilly, UK)*. *Injection*, Insulin Zinc Suspension (Crystalline) (*B.P.*) (human, prb) 100 units/mL, in vials of 10 mL.

Hypurin Insulin Injection (Soluble) *(CP Pharmaceuticals, UK)*. *Injection*, Acid Insulin Injection (*B.P.*) (bovine, highly purified) 100 units/mL, in vials of 10 mL.

Hypurin Isophane *(CP Pharmaceuticals, UK)*. *Injection*, Isophane Insulin Injection (*B.P.*) (bovine, highly purified) 100 units/mL, in vials of 10 mL.

Hypurin Lente *(CP Pharmaceuticals, UK)*. *Injection*, Insulin Zinc Suspension (*B.P.*) (bovine, highly purified) 100 units/mL, in vials of 10 mL.

Hypurin Neutral *(CP Pharmaceuticals, UK)*. *Injection*, Insulin Injection (*B.P.*) (bovine, highly purified) 100 units/mL, in vials of 10 mL.

Hypurin Protamine Zinc *(CP Pharmaceuticals, UK)*. *Injection*, protamine zinc insulin injection (bovine, highly purified) 100 units/mL, in vials of 10 mL.

Initard 50/50 *(Nordisk-UK, UK; Wellcome, UK)*. *Injection*, mixture of Insulin Injection (*B.P.*) (porcine, highly purified) 50% and Isophane Insulin Injection (*B.P.*) (porcine, highly purified) 50% 100 units/mL, in vials of 10 mL.

Insulatard *(Nordisk-UK, UK; Wellcome, UK)*. *Injection*, Isophane Insulin Injection (*B.P.*) (porcine, highly purified) 100 units/mL, in vials of 10 mL.

Lentard MC *(Novo, UK)*. *Injection*, Insulin Zinc Suspension (*B.P.*) (bovine with porcine, monocomponent) 100 units/mL, in vials of 10 mL.

Mixtard 30/70 *(Nordisk-UK, UK; Wellcome, UK)*. *Injection*, mixture of Insulin Injection (*B.P.*) (porcine, highly purified) 30% and Isophane Insulin Injection (*B.P.*) (porcine, highly purified) 70% 100 units/mL, in vials of 10 mL.

Rapitard MC *(Novo, UK)*. *Injection*, Biphasic Insulin Injection (*B.P.*) (bovine with porcine, monocomponent) 100 units/mL, in vials of 10 mL.

Semitard MC *(Novo, UK)*. *Injection*, Insulin Zinc Suspension (Amorphous) (*B.P.*) (porcine, monocomponent) 100 units/mL, in vials of 10 mL.

Velosulin *(Nordisk-UK, UK; Wellcome, UK)*. *Injection*, Insulin Injection (*B.P.*) (porcine, highly purified) 100 units/mL, in vials of 10 mL and also in cartridges of 5.7 mL for use in a specially designed subcutaneous infusion system (Nordisk Infuser).

Isophane Insulin Injection (*B.P.*) (bovine, purified), Insulin Injection (*B.P.*) (bovine, purified), and Insulin Zinc Suspension (*B.P.*) (bovine, purified) are also marketed in Great Britain by *Evans Medical, UK*.

Proprietary Names and Manufacturers

Actraphan *(Novo, Norw.; Novo, Swed.)*; Actraphane *(Novo, Ger.; Novo, S.Afr.; Novo, UK)*; Actrapid *(Commonwealth Serum Laboratories, Austral.; Novo, Denm.; Novo, Fr.; Novo, Ger.; Novo, Ital.; Novo, Norw.; Novo, S.Afr.; Novo, Spain; Novo, Swed.; Novo, UK; Squibb-Novo, USA)*; Bio-Insulin *(Guidotti, Ital.)*; Bitard *(Commonwealth Serum Laboratories, Austral.)*; H-Tronin *(Hoechst, Ger.)*; Huminsulin *(Lilly, Ger.; Lilly, Switz.)*; Humulin *(Lilly, Canad.; Lilly, Ital.; Lilly, Norw.; Lilly, S.Afr.; Lilly, Swed.; Lilly, UK; Lilly, USA)*; Humulina *(Lilly, Spain)*; Hypurin *(Weddel, Austral.; CP Pharmaceuticals, UK)*; Iletin *(Lilly, Canad.; Lilly, USA)*; Initard *(Nordisk Insulin, Canad.; Hormonchemie, Ger.; Nordisk, Swed.; Nordisk-UK, UK; Wellcome, UK)*; Insulatard *(Wellcome, Austral.; Nordisk Insulin, Canad.; Nordisk Gentofte, Denm.; Leo, Fr.; Hormonchemie, Ger.; Nordisk, Norw.; Nordisk, S.Afr.; Abello, Spain; Nordisk, Swed.; Nordisk-UK, UK; Wellcome, UK; Nordisk-USA, USA)*; Isotard *(Commonwealth Serum Laboratories, Austral.)*; Komb-Insulin *(Hoechst, Ger.)*; Lenta *(Novo, Ital.)*; Lentard *(Novo, S.Afr.; Novo, UK)*; Lente *(Commonwealth Serum Laboratories, Austral.; Novo, Fr.; Novo, Ger.; Novo, Norw.; Novo, Spain; Novo, Swed.)*; Mixtard *(Wellcome, Austral.; Nordisk Insulin, Canad.; Leo, Fr.; Hormonchemie, Ger.; Nordisk, Norw.; Nordisk, S.Afr.; Nordisk, Swed.; Nordisk-UK, UK; Wellcome, UK; Nordisk-USA, USA)*; Monophane *(Boots, UK)*; Monotard *(Commonwealth Serum Laboratories, Austral.; Novo, Denm.; Novo, Fr.; Novo, Ger.; Novo, Ital.; Novo, Norw.; Novo, S.Afr.; Novo, Spain; Novo, Swed.; Novo, UK; Squibb-Novo, USA)*; Neulente *(Wellcome, UK)*; Neuphane *(Wellcome, UK)*; Neusulin *(Wellcome, UK)*; Novolin *(Connaught Novo, Canad.; Squibb-Novo, USA)*; Nuralin *(Commonwealth Serum Laboratories, Austral.)*; Proptaphan *(Novo, Denm.)*; Protafan *(Novo, Spain)*; Protaphan *(Novo, Norw.; Novo, Swed.)*; Protaphane *(Commonwealth Serum Laboratories, Austral.; Novo, Fr.; Novo, S.Afr.; Novo, UK; Squibb-Novo, USA)*; Protophan *(Novo, Ger.)*; Quicksol *(Boots, UK)*; Rapitard *(Commonwealth Serum Laboratories, Austral.; Novo, Fr.; Novo, Ger.; Novo, Ital.; Novo, Norw.; Novo, S.Afr.; Novo, Spain; Novo, UK)*; Semilenta *(Novo, Ital.)*; Semilente *(Commonwealth Serum Laboratories, Austral.; Connaught Novo, Canad.; Novo, Fr.; Novo, Ger.; Novo, Norw.; Novo, Spain)*; Semitard *(Novo, S.Afr.; Novo, UK; Squibb-Novo, USA)*; Tempulin *(Boots, UK)*; Ultralent *(Novo, Spain)*; Ultralenta *(Novo, Ital.)*; Ultralente *(Commonwealth Serum Laboratories, Austral.; Connaught Novo, Canad.; Novo, Fr.; Novo, Ger.; Novo, Norw.)*; Ultratard *(Novo, Denm.; Novo, Fr.; Novo, Ger.; Novo, Norw.; Novo, S.Afr.; Novo, Swed.; Novo, UK; Squibb-Novo, USA)*; Velasulin *(Hormonchemie, Ger.)*; Velosulin *(Wellcome, Austral.; Nordisk Insulin, Canad.; Nordisk Gentofte, Denm.; Nordisk, Norw.; Nordisk, S.Afr.; Abello, Spain; Nordisk, Swed.; Nordisk-UK, UK; Wellcome, UK; Nordisk-USA, USA)*; Velosuline *(Leo, Fr.)*.

The proprietary names of commercially available insulins listed above are often qualified by various prefixes or suffixes which have not been given here. Also no attempt has been made to categorise them as human, bovine, or porcine, or into the type of formulation.

7229-f

Metahexamide *(BAN, rINN)*.
Glyhexylamide. 1-(3-Amino-*p*-tolylsulphonyl)-3-cyclohexylurea.
$C_{14}H_{21}N_3O_3S = 311.4$.
CAS — 565-33-3.

Metahexamide is a sulphonylurea hypoglycaemic agent with actions and uses similar to those of chlorpropamide (p.387). The usual dose by mouth in non-insulin-dependent diabetes mellitus is 100 to 200 mg daily.

Proprietary Names and Manufacturers
Isodiane *(Servier, Fr.)*.

7231-c

Metformin Hydrochloride *(BANM, pINNM)*.

LA-6023. 1,1-Dimethylbiguanide hydrochloride.
$C_4H_{11}N_5,HCl = 165.6$.
CAS — 657-24-9 (metformin); 1115-70-4 (hydrochloride).

NOTE. Metformin is *USAN*.

Pharmacopoeias. In *Br.*, *Nord.*, and *Roum.*

A white, odourless or almost odourless, hygroscopic, crystalline powder. **Soluble** 1 in 2 of water; slightly soluble in alcohol; practically insoluble in chloroform and ether. **Store** in well-closed containers.

Adverse Effects

Metformin causes gastro-intestinal adverse effects with anorexia, nausea, and vomiting; absorption of various substances including vitamin B_{12} may be impaired. Patients may experience a metallic taste and there may be weight loss, which in some diabetics could be an advantage.

Hypoglycaemia is less of a problem with metformin than with the sulphonylureas.

Lactic acidosis, sometimes fatal, has occurred but to a lesser extent than with phenformin and it is generally accepted that the lactic acidosis usually occurred in patients whose condition contra-indicated the use of metformin.

The biguanides, represented by phenformin, were implicated in the controversial reports of excessive cardiovascular mortality associated with oral hypoglycaemic therapy (see p.399).

A review of the adverse effects of biguanide therapy.— K. R. Paterson *et al.*, *Adverse Drug React. Ac. Pois. Rev.*, 1984, *3*, 173.

Megaloblastic anaemia due to vitamin B_{12} malabsorption in a 58-year-old woman was associated with long-term treatment with metformin.— T. S. Callaghan *et al.*, *Br. med. J.*, 1980, *280*, 1214.

Malabsorption of vitamin B_{12} was observed in 14 of 46 diabetics taking metformin or phenformin; metformin was more commonly to blame. Withdrawal of the drug resulted in normal absorption in only 7 of the 14.— J. F. Adams *et al.*, *Diabetologia*, 1983, *24*, 16.

A retrospective survey of diarrhoea in treated diabetic patients. In all, 30 treated patients among the 265 involved reported diarrhoea or alternating diarrhoea and constipation, comprising: 11 of 54 taking metformin; 9 of 45 taking metformin with a sulphonylurea; 3 of 53 taking a sulphonylurea only; 5 of 78 on insulin therapy; 2 of 35 on diet alone. Among 150 nondiabetic controls 12 reported diarrhoea.— P. Dandona *et al.*, *Diabetes Care*, 1983, *6*, 472.

LACTIC ACIDOSIS. It was estimated that there had only been 28 cases of lactic acidosis with metformin; at the time of this estimate the worldwide population receiving metformin was considered to be 650 000.— O. J. Lucis,

Can. med. Ass. J., 1983, *128*, 24.

A report of severe lactic acidotic coma, despite normal renal function, in a 35-year-old diabetic man taking metformin. He was taking various other drugs and on the previous day had drunk a considerable amount of alcohol.— R. E. J. Ryder, *Br. J. clin. Pract.*, 1984, *38*, 229.

Treatment of Adverse Effects

Acute poisoning with metformin calls for intensive supportive therapy. Lactic acidosis may require treatment with sodium bicarbonate as well as other measures.

Glucose or glucagon may be required for hypoglycaemia. For an outline of the general management of hypoglycaemia, see insulin (p.393).

Precautions

As for chlorpropamide (p.387).

In addition to the contra-indications described under chlorpropamide, metformin should not be used in patients with heart failure, dehydration, acute or chronic alcoholism, or any other condition likely to predispose to lactic acidosis.

Drug interactions are not a problem with metformin.

Absorption and Fate

Metformin hydrochloride is absorbed from the gastro-intestinal tract and is excreted, unchanged, in the urine.

References to some studies on the pharmacokinetics of metformin: C. R. Sirtori *et al.*, *Clin. Pharmac. Ther.*, 1978, *24*, 683; P. J. Pentikäinen *et al.*, *Eur. J. clin. Pharmac.*, 1979, *16*, 195; G. T. Tucker *et al.*, *Br. J. clin. Pharmac.*, 1981, *12*, 235.

Uses and Administration

Metformin hydrochloride is a biguanide hypoglycaemic agent used in non-insulin-dependent diabetes mellitus when diet control fails. It is sometimes given to patients no longer responding to the sulphonylureas. Overweight patients may experience a beneficial weight loss and this has sometimes been the rationale behind combining insulin and metformin in insulin-dependent diabetes.

Metformin's mode of action is not clear. It does not stimulate insulin release but does require that some insulin be present for it to exert a hypoglycaemic effect. It has been reported to increase blood-lipid concentrations.

Metformin hydrochloride is given by mouth in an initial dosage of 500 mg three times daily or 850 mg twice daily with meals, gradually increased if necessary to a maximum of 3 g daily.

Metformin has also been given as the chlorophenoxy acetate and as the embonate.

A review of biguanide hypoglycaemic agents, particularly metformin.— G. Schäfer, *Diabète Métab.*, 1983, *9*, 148. See also O. J. Lucis, *Can. med. Ass. J.*, 1983, *128*, 24.

DIABETES MELLITUS. Results indicating that metformin increases the number of low affinity insulin receptor binding sites on the erythrocytes of obese patients with type 2 diabetes.— J. M. Lord *et al.*, *Br. med. J.*, 1983, *286*, 830. Similar results using monocytes.— V. Trischitta *et al.*, *J. clin. Endocr. Metab.*, 1983, *57*, 713.

References to metformin in the treatment of non-insulin-dependent diabetes mellitus: B. F. Clarke and I. W. Campbell, *Br. med. J.*, 1977, *2*, 1576; O. Siitonen *et al.*, *Lancet*, 1980, *1*, 217.

Combination with insulin. Some references to the use of metformin together with insulin in insulin-dependent-diabetes: H. Gin *et al.*, *Diabetologia*, 1982, *23*, 34; G. Pagano *et al.*, *ibid.*, 1983, *24*, 351; C. Coscelli *et al.*, *Curr. ther. Res.*, 1984, *35*, 1058.

Preparations

Metformin Tablets *(B.P.)*. Tablets containing metformin hydrochloride.

Proprietary Preparations

Glucophage *(Lipha, UK)*. *Tablets*, metformin hydrochloride 500 and 850 mg.

Orabet *(Lagap, UK)*. *Tablets*, metformin hydrochloride 500 and 850 mg.

Proprietary Names and Manufacturers of Metformin Salts

Devian *(Farmacologico Milanese, Ital.)*; Dextin *(Rolab, S.Afr.)*; Diaberit *(IFI, Ital.)*; Diabetosan *(Brocchieri, Ital.)*; Diabex *(Difrex, Austral.)*; Diaformin *(Alphapharm, Austral.)*; Glucadal *(Ital.)*; Glucinan *(Anphar-Rolland, Fr.)*; Glucophage *(Riker, Austral.; Belg.; Canad.; Lipha, Denm.; Aron, Fr.; Lipha, Ger.; Ital.; Neth.; Lipha, Norw.; Script Intal, S.Afr.; CEPA, Spain; Lipha, Swed.; Lipha, Switz.; Lipha, UK)*; Glufagos *(Spain)*; Islotin *(Arg.)*; Mellitin *(Biosint, Ital.)*; Metforal *(Guidotti, Ital.)*; Metiguanide *(Carlo Erba, Ital.; Farmitalia Carlo Erba, UK)*; Orabet *(GEA, Denm.; Lagap, UK)*; Stagid *(Merck-Clévenot, Fr.)*.

7232-k

Phenformin Hydrochloride *(BANM, pINNM)*.

Fenformina Cloridrato. 1-Phenethylbiguanide hydrochloride.

$C_{10}H_{15}N_5,HCl=241.7$.

CAS — 114-86-3 (phenformin); 834-28-6 (hydrochloride).

Pharmacopoeias. In *Braz.*, *Egypt.*, *Ind.*, and *Nord.*

Phenformin hydrochloride is a biguanide hypoglycaemic agent that was formerly used in the treatment of non-insulin-dependent diabetes mellitus. It is associated with an unacceptably high incidence of lactic acidosis that has often proved fatal.

References to acute pancreatitis in patients taking phenformin: H. Wilde (letter), *Ann. intern. Med.*, 1972, *77*, 324; H. S. Chase and G. R. Mogan, *ibid.*, 1977, *87*, 314.

LACTIC ACIDOSIS. Reviews and discussions of lactic acidosis associated with phenformin: R. I. Misbin, *Ann. intern. Med.*, 1977, *87*, 591; *Br. med. J.*, 1977, *2*, 1436.

Further references to lactic acidosis: U. Bergman *et al.*, *Br. med. J.*, 1978, *2*, 464; T. Korhonen *et al.*, *Eur. J. clin. Pharmac.*, 1979, *15*, 407.

Proprietary Names and Manufacturers

Cronoformin *(Ital.)*; DBI *(Arg.; Belg.)*; Dibotin *(Winthrop, UK)*; Dipar *(S.Afr.; Spain; Hoechst, UK)*; Glucifrene *(Prats, Spain)*; Glucopostin *(Arg.; S.Afr.)*; Insoral *(Austral.; Continental Ethicals, S.Afr.)*; Meltrol *(Berk Pharmaceuticals, UK)*; Normoglucina *(Arg.)*.

19329-l

Ponalrestat *(BAN, pINN)*.

ICI-128436. 3-(4-Bromo-2-fluorobenzyl)-4-oxo-3*H*-phthalazin-1-ylacetic acid.

$C_{17}H_{12}N_2O_3BrF=391.2$.

CAS — 72702-95-5.

Ponalrestat is an aldose reductase inhibitor similar in action to sorbinil (below). It is under investigation for the treatment of diabetic complications including neuropathy.

Proprietary Names and Manufacturers

Statil;

Manufacturers include—*ICI Pharmaceuticals, UK.*

16992-t

Sorbinil *(BAN, USAN, rINN)*.

CP-45634. (*S*)-6-Fluorospiro(chroman-4,4′-imidazolidine)-2′,5′-dione.

$C_{11}H_9FN_2O_3=236.2$.

CAS — 68367-52-2.

Sorbinil inhibits the enzyme aldose reductase which catalyses the conversion of glucose to sorbitol. It has been suggested that accumulation of sorbitol in certain cells, occurring only in conditions of hyperglycaemia and resulting in a hyperosmotic effect, may be involved in the pathogenesis of some diabetic complications. Aldose reductase inhibitors have no influence on blood-glucose concentrations.

Sorbinil has been tried mainly in the treatment of diabetic neuropathy, with conflicting results.

Skin reactions have been reported.

The sorbitol pathway and the complications of diabetes.— K. H. Gabbay, *New Engl. J. Med.*, 1973, *288*, 831.

Aldose reductase and the complications of diabetes.— *Ann. intern. Med.*, 1984, *101*, 82.

Reviews of aldose reductase inhibitors.— P. F. Kador *et al.*, *J. med. Chem.*, 1985, *28*, 841; J. D. Ward, *Drugs*, 1986, *32*, 279; P. Benfield, *ibid.*, *Suppl.* 2, 43.

A double-blind crossover study of sorbinil 250 mg daily by mouth in diabetic patients with abnormal nerve conduction velocities but without symptomatic neuropathy. Small but significant increases in nerve conduction velocity were found during sorbinil treatment; the clinical applicability of this remained to be determined.— R. G. Judzewitsch *et al.*, *New Engl. J. Med.*, 1983, *308*, 119.

A study of sorbinil 250 mg daily by mouth in 11 patients with severely painful diabetic neuropathy. There was substantial pain relief in 8 patients and overall there was improvement in nerve conduction velocities; beneficial effects usually declined again after withdrawal of the drug.— J. Jaspan *et al.*, *Lancet*, 1983, *2*, 758. Criticisms.— R. J. Young *et al.* (letter), *ibid.*, 969; R. R. Abraham *et al.* (letter), *ibid.*

In a 16-week double-blind crossover study of sorbinil 200 mg daily in 15 patients with chronic painful diabetic neuropathy, pain was somewhat improved by treatment but of many nerve functions tested only 2 showed objective improvement. Erythematous, itchy, macular rashes occurred in 4 patients taking sorbinil; 3 of these also had oropharyngeal involvement including mucosal swelling and tenderness and 2 also had transient leucopenia or thrombocytopenia.— R. J. Young *et al.*, *Diabetes*, 1983, *32*, 938. No improvement in nerve function or pain could be demonstrated in a similar 8-week study of sorbinil in 12 patients. A febrile illness with rash and oral ulceration developed in one patient taking sorbinil.— I. G. Lewin *et al.*, *Diabetologia*, 1984, *26*, 445.

A report of improvement in joint mobility in 3 diabetic patients with an incapacitating hand syndrome given sorbinil 250 mg daily.— R. P. Eaton *et al.*, *J. Am. med. Ass.*, 1985, *253*, 1437.

ABSORPTION AND FATE. A study of the pharmacokinetics of sorbinil in healthy subjects demonstrating that it is rapidly absorbed after administration by mouth but slowly eliminated. Its kinetics make it suitable for once-a-day dosage.— G. Foulds *et al.*, *Clin. Pharmac. Ther.*, 1981, *30*, 693.

Proprietary Names and Manufacturers

Pfizer, USA.

7233-a

Tolazamide *(BAN, USAN, rINN)*.

U-17835. 1-(Perhydroazepin-1-yl)-3-tosylurea; 1-(Perhydroazepin-1-yl)-3-*p*-tolylsulphonylurea.

$C_{14}H_{21}N_3O_3S=311.4$.

CAS — 1156-19-0.

Pharmacopoeias. In *Br.* and *U.S.*

A white or almost white crystalline powder, odourless or with a slight odour. Very slightly **soluble** in water; slightly soluble in alcohol; soluble in acetone; freely soluble in chloroform. **Store** in airtight containers.

Adverse Effects, Treatment, and Precautions

As for chlorpropamide (p.387). Unlike chlorpropamide, tolazamide is reported to exert a mild diuretic action.

PORPHYRIA. Tolazamide was considered to be unsafe in patients with acute porphyria because it has been shown to be porphyrinogenic in *animals* or *in vitro* systems.— M.R. Moore and K.E.L. McColl, *Porphyrias, Drug Lists*, Glasgow, Porphyria Research Unit, University of Glasgow, 1987.

Absorption and Fate

Tolazamide is absorbed from the gastro-intestinal tract and is extensively bound to plasma proteins; it has a half-life of about 7 hours. It is metabolised in the liver to metabolites with some biological activity. It is excreted in the urine, chiefly as metabolites.

Uses and Administration

Tolazamide is a sulphonylurea hypoglycaemic

agent with actions and uses similar to those of chlorpropamide (p.388). Its duration of action is at least 10 hours and may be as much as 18 hours.

The usual initial dose in non-insulin-dependent diabetes mellitus is 100 to 250 mg daily by mouth given as a single dose with breakfast and increased if necessary at weekly intervals by 100 to 250 mg usually to a maximum of 1 g daily; no further benefit is likely to be gained with higher doses. Doses of 500 mg or more daily may be given in divided doses.

ADMINISTRATION IN RENAL FAILURE. Although it has been reported that tolazamide could be given in usual doses to patients with renal failure (W.M. Bennett *et al., Am. J. Kidney Dis.*, 1983, *3*, 155), it is generally recommended that like chlorpropamide it should not be used in patients with severe impairment of renal function.

Preparations

Tolazamide Tablets *(B.P.)*

Tolazamide Tablets *(U.S.P.)*

Proprietary Preparations

Tolanase *(Upjohn, UK). Tablets*, scored, tolazamide 100 and 250 mg.

Proprietary Names and Manufacturers

Diabewas *(IFI, Ital.; Spain; Switz.)*; Norglycin *(Upjohn, Ger.)*; Tolanase *(Upjohn, UK)*; Tolinase *(Upjohn, Austral.; Belg.; Neth.; Spain; Upjohn, Swed.; Switz.; Upjohn, USA)*; Tolisan *(Denm.)*.

7234-t

Tolbutamide *(BAN, USAN, rINN).*

Butamidum; Tolbutamidum; Tolglybutamide.

1-Butyl-3-tosylurea; 1-Butyl-3-*p*-tolylsulphonylurea.

$C_{12}H_{18}N_2O_3S$=270.4.

CAS — 64-77-7.

Pharmacopoeias. In *Arg., Aust., Belg., Br., Braz., Chin., Cz., Egypt., Eur., Fr., Ger., Ind., Int., It., Jpn, Jug., Neth., Nord., Pol., Roum., Rus., Swiss, Turk.*, and *U.S.* which also includes Sterile Tolbutamide Sodium.

A white or almost white, almost odourless, crystalline powder. Practically **insoluble** in water; soluble 1 in 10 of alcohol; soluble in acetone, chloroform, and dilute solutions of alkali hydroxides; slightly soluble in ether. **Store** in airtight containers.

Adverse Effects and Treatment

As for chlorpropamide (p.387).

Mortality from cardiovascular causes has been reported by the University Group Diabetes Program (UGDP) to be higher in patients receiving tolbutamide than in patients receiving insulin. While this has been accepted by the FDA, the association has been the subject of intense and continued debate.

Thrombophlebitis has occurred following the intravenous injection of tolbutamide sodium; too rapid injection may cause a transient sensation of heat in the vein.

Reactions to tolbutamide reported to the Committee on Safety of Drugs included 7 cases of rash including eczema and macular erythema, aplastic anaemia (2), jaundice with hepatocellular damage (1), and a syndrome resembling acute systemic lupus erythematosus.— E. L. Harris, *Br. med. J.*, 1971, *3*, 29.

EFFECTS ON THE CARDIOVASCULAR SYSTEM. A multicentre study carried out under the University Group Diabetes Program (UGDP) reported an increased incidence in mortality from cardiovascular complications in diabetics given tolbutamide; a similar increase was also noted in patients given phenformin (*J. Am. med. Ass.*, 1971, *218*, 1400; *ibid.*, *217*, 777). The reports from the UGDP have aroused prolonged controversy not entirely settled by detailed reassessment of relevant studies (*ibid.*, 1975, *231*, 583). Eventually in 1984 the FDA made it a requirement that sulphonylurea oral hypoglycaemics be labelled with a specific warning about the possibility of increased cardiovascular mortality associated with the use of these drugs (*FDA Drug Bull.*, 1984, *14*, 16).

A review of the clinical significance of the adverse effects of sulphonylureas.— R. Huupponen, *Med. Toxicol.*, 1987, *2*, 190.

OVERDOSAGE. Tolbutamide 25 to 30 g was taken by a non-diabetic woman with suicidal intent. Hypoglycaemic coma occurred with permanent brain damage and death from pneumonia some 5 months later without consciousness being regained.— J. Lazner, *Med. J. Aust.*, 1970, *1*, 327.

Precautions

As for chlorpropamide (p.387).

ADMINISTRATION IN RENAL FAILURE. See below under Uses.

INTERACTIONS. Tolbutamide may enhance the therapeutic or toxic effects of digoxin and phenytoin; information is contained within their respective monographs.

Details of sulphonylurea interactions are given under chlorpropamide (p.388).

PORPHYRIA. Tolbutamide was considered to be unsafe in patients with acute porphyria because it has been shown to be porphyrinogenic in *animals* or *in vitro* systems.— M.R. Moore and K.E.L. McColl, *Porphyrias, Drug Lists*, Glasgow, Porphyria Research Unit, University of Glasgow, 1987.

Absorption and Fate

Tolbutamide is readily absorbed from the gastro-intestinal tract and is extensively bound to plasma proteins; the half-life is generally within the range of 4 to 8 hours but may be considerably longer. Tolbutamide is metabolised in the liver and is excreted in the urine chiefly as metabolites.

For a lack of correlation between tolbutamide dose, serum concentrations, and effect, see Chlorpropamide (p.388).

Uses and Administration

Tolbutamide is a sulphonylurea hypoglycaemic agent with actions and uses similar to those of chlorpropamide (p.388). The duration of action is about 10 hours.

The usual initial dose by mouth in non-insulin-dependent diabetes mellitus may range from 1 to 2 g daily, given either as a single dose with breakfast or in divided doses. Maintenance doses may range from 0.25 to 2 g daily. Although it is unlikely that further response will be gained by increasing the dose further, daily doses of 3 g have been given.

Tolbutamide sodium has sometimes been used in the diagnosis of insulinoma as well as other pancreatic disorders including diabetes mellitus. The equivalent of 1 g of tolbutamide was given by intravenous injection as a 5% solution usually over 2 to 3 minutes.

ADMINISTRATION IN RENAL FAILURE. Although it has been reported that tolbutamide could be given in usual doses to patients with renal failure (W.M. Bennett *et al., Am. J. Kidney Dis.*, 1983, *3*, 155), it is generally recommended that like chlorpropamide it should not be used in patients with severe impairment of renal function.

Preparations

Tolbutamide Tablets *(B.P.)*

Tolbutamide Tablets *(U.S.P.)*

Proprietary Preparations

Glyconon *(DDSA Pharmaceuticals, UK). Tablets*, scored, tolbutamide 500 mg.

Rastinon *(Hoechst, UK). Tablets*, scored, tolbutamide 500 mg.

Proprietary Names and Manufacturers of Tolbutamide or Tolbutamide Sodium

Aglicem *(Spain)*; Aglycid *(IFI, Ital.)*; Arcosal *(Lundbeck, Denm.)*; Artosin *(Arg.; Reckitt & Colman, Austral.; Belg.; Boehringer Mannheim, Ger.; Neth.; Boehringer Mannheim, S.Afr.; Spain; Swed.)*; Butamel *(Adcock Ingram, S.Afr.)*; Chembutamide *(Canad.)*; Diaben *(Arg.)*; Diabeton Metilato *(Teknofarma, Ital.)*; Diasulfon *(Switz.)*; Diatol *(Protea, Austral.)*; Dolipol *(Alg.; Hoechst, Fr.; Morocco; Tun.)*; Fordex *(Spain)*; Glyconon *(DDSA Pharmaceuticals, UK)*; Guabeta *(OTW, Ger.)*; Insilange-D *(Jpn)*; Mellitol *(Canad.)*; Mobenol *(Horner, Canad.)*; Neo-Dibetic *(Canad.)*; Neo-Insoral *(Valeas, Ital.)*; Nigloid *(Jpn)*; Novobutamide *(Novopharm, Canad.)*; Oramide *(Canad.)*; Oribetic *(USA)*; Orinase *(Hoechst, Canad.; Upjohn, USA)*; Pramidex *(Berk Pharmaceuticals, UK)*; Proinsul *(Ital.)*; Rastinon *(Hoechst, Austral.; Belg.; Hoechst, Denm.; Hoechst, Ger.; Hoechst, Ital.; Neth.; Norw.; Hoechst, S.Afr.; Hoechst, Spain; Hoechst, Swed.; Hoechst, Switz.; Hoechst, UK)*; SK-Tolbutamide *(Smith Kline & French, USA)*; Tolbet *(Neth.)*; Tolbutone *(Canad.)*; Tydadex *(Lennon, S.Afr.)*.

17014-d

Tolrestat *(BAN, USAN, rINN).*

AY-27773. *N*-[6-Methoxy-5-trifluoromethyl-1-naphthyl(thiocarbonyl)]-*N*-methylglycine.

$C_{16}H_{14}F_3NO_3S$=357.4.

CAS — 82964-04-3.

Tolrestat is an aldose reductase inhibitor similar in action to sorbinil (see p.398). It is under investigation for the treatment of diabetic neuropathy.

The pharmacokinetics of tolrestat.— D. R. Hicks *et al., Clin. Pharmac. Ther.*, 1984, *36*, 493.

The effect of tolrestat on red blood cell concentrations of sorbitol in diabetic patients.— P. Raskin *et al., Clin. Pharmac. Ther.*, 1985, *38*, 625.

Proprietary Names and Manufacturers

Ayerst, USA.

Antiepileptics

6600-k

An epileptic seizure has been defined as a paroxysmal discharge of cerebral neurones accompanied by a clinical phenomenon apparent to the patient or to an observer and epilepsy as a condition characterised by a recurrence of such seizures.

There have been numerous attempts at classification; a proposed classification of epileptic seizures divides them into generalised and partial (focal). Generalised seizures include 'absences' (petit mal), tonic-clonic seizures (grand mal), and myoclonic seizures. Partial seizures may spread giving rise to secondarily generalised seizures.

The choice of antiepileptic agent for the treatment of epilepsy is determined by the type of seizure. For tonic-clonic seizures and partial seizures, phenytoin, carbamazepine, or valproic acid are generally the preferred agents with phenobarbitone or primidone as alternatives; for absence seizures usually ethosuximide or valproic acid are employed; for myoclonic seizures clonazepam, ethosuximide, or valproic acid are usually used. In general, therapy with a single antiepileptic agent is preferred unless seizures of a mixed type are present. Infantile spasms, not to be confused with childhood febrile convulsions, are generally unresponsive to the antiepileptic agents described in this section and management may involve the use of corticosteroids or corticotrophin. For further comments on the actions and relative merits of some of the antiepileptic drugs in the different forms of epilepsy see under phenytoin (p.410) as well as the individual drug monographs.

Publications relating to epilepsy and its treatment: *Antiepileptic Drugs*, 2nd Edn, D.M. Woodbury *et al.* (Ed.), New York, Raven Press, 1982; *Epilepsy Diagnosis and Management*, T.R. Browne and R.G. Feldman (Ed.), Boston, MA, Little, Brown & Co., 1983.

A discussion on the risk-benefit ratio of anticonvulsant drugs.— M. J. Eadie, *Med. Toxicol.*, 1987, *2*, 324.

Reviews and discussions of investigational antiepileptic agents including denzimol, felbamate, gabapentin, milacemide, nafimidone, stiripentol, and zonisamide.— *New Anticonvulsant Drugs*, B.S. Meldrum and R.J. Porter (Ed.), London, John Libbey & Co. Ltd, 1986.

6604-r

Beclamide *(BAN, pINN).*

Benzchlorpropamide. *N*-Benzyl-3-chloropropionamide.

$C_{10}H_{12}ClNO$=197.7.

CAS — 501-68-8.

Pharmacopoeias. In *Br.*

A white crystalline powder. Sparingly **soluble** in water; soluble in alcohol; freely soluble in chloroform. **Store** in well-closed containers.

Adverse Effects

Side-effects include dizziness, gastro-intestinal distress, loss of weight, skin rashes, transitory leucopenia, and renal disturbances.

Uses and Administration

Beclamide is reported to be an antiepileptic agent used for the control of tonic-clonic (grand mal) seizures and psychomotor epilepsy and for the management of behaviour disorders.

Beclamide is given in a dosage of 1.5 to 4 g daily in divided doses. Suggested doses for children are: less than 5 years of age, 0.75 to 1 g daily; 5 to 10 years of age, 1.5 g daily.

Preparations

Beclamide Tablets *(B.P.)*

Proprietary Preparations

Nydrane *(Lipha, UK). Tablets,* scored, beclamide 500 mg.

Proprietary Names and Manufacturers

Neuracen *(Promonta, Ger.)*; Nidrane *(Arg.)*; Nydrane *(Riker, Austral.; Lipha, UK)*; Posedrine *(Belg.; Aron, Fr.; Ital.; Lasa, Spain; Switz.)*; Seclar *(Arg.)*.

6605-f

Carbamazepine *(BAN, USAN, rINN).*

Carbamazepinum; G-32883. 5*H*-Dibenz[*b,f*]azepine-5-carboxamide.

$C_{15}H_{12}N_2O$=236.3.

CAS — 298-46-4.

Pharmacopoeias. In *Br., Braz., Cz., Eur., Ind., Jpn,* and *U.S.*

A white or almost white crystalline powder. Practically **insoluble** in water and ether; sparingly soluble in alcohol; soluble 1 in 10 of chloroform; soluble in acetone. **Store** in airtight containers.

Adverse Effects

Fairly common side-effects of carbamazepine, particularly in the initial stages of therapy, include dizziness, drowsiness, and ataxia. These effects may be minimised by starting therapy with a low dose. Drowsiness and disturbances of cerebellar and oculo-motor function (with ataxia, nystagmus, and diplopia) are also symptoms of excessive plasma concentrations of carbamazepine, and may disappear with continued treatment at reduced dosage.

Gastro-intestinal symptoms are reported to be less common, and include dry mouth, gastric distress and abdominal pain, nausea and vomiting, anorexia, and diarrhoea or constipation.

Generalised erythematous rashes, which may be severe, occur in about 3% of patients given carbamazepine, and may necessitate withdrawal of treatment. Photosensitivity reactions, urticaria, exfoliative dermatitis, erythema multiforme and the Stevens-Johnson syndrome, and lupus erythematosus have also been reported.

Occasional reports of blood disorders include agranulocytosis, aplastic anaemia, eosinophilia, leucopenia, leucocytosis, thrombocytopenia, and purpura. Abnormalities of liver and kidney function, and jaundice have occurred.

Other adverse effects reported include paraesthesia, headache, heart block, congestive heart failure, water intoxication, and dystonias and dyskinesias with asterixis.

Overdosage may be manifested by many of the adverse effects listed above, especially those on the nervous system, and may result in stupor, coma, and death.

Although congenital malformations have been reported in infants born to women who had received antiepileptic agents during pregnancy the direct causal role for some of these drugs has been debated due to the fact that combined therapy was often employed. For comments regarding the management of the pregnant epileptic patient see the section on epilepsy under the uses and administration of phenytoin.

ALLERGY. Reports of various allergic and hypersensitivity reactions to carbamazepine: S. A. Cullinan and G. C. Bower, *Chest,* 1975, *68,* 580 (eosinophilia, skin rash, and pulmonary infiltrates); W. C. Stephan *et al., ibid.,* 1978, *74,* 463 (acute hypersensitivity pneumonitis); C. R. Stewart *et al.* (letter), *New Engl. J. Med.,* 1980, *302,* 1262 (twice-daily fevers); T. Lee *et al., Br. med. J.,* 1981, *282,* 440 (eosinophilia and asthma); D. I. Bernstein *et al., Clin. Pediat.,* 1983, *22,* 524 (pseudo toxic shock syndrome); J. Tolmie *et al., Archs Dis. Childh.,* 1983, *58,* 833 (pulmonary eosinophilia); L. F. de Swert *et al., Acta paediat. scand.,* 1984, *73,* 285 (acute interstitial pneumonitis).

Suppression in 3 patients of a carbamazepine-induced skin rash with courses of prednisone.— N. A. Vick (letter), *New Engl. J. Med.,* 1983, *309,* 1193. Experience in one patient suggesting that corticosteroids may suppress a carbamazepine-associated drug rash but not necessarily other manifestations of hypersensitivity.— K. K. Hampton *et al.* (letter), *ibid.,* 1985, *313,* 959.

A report of successful desensitisation to carbamazepine in a 12-year-old boy who was sensitive to carbamazepine, sodium valproate, and phenytoin. Starting with a low dose of carbamazepine 0.1 mg daily the dose was doubled, generally every 2 days, up to a maintenance dose of 200 mg twice daily.— H. Smith and R. Newton (letter), *Lancet,* 1985, *1,* 753.

EFFECTS ON THE BLOOD. The annual review of suspected adverse drug reactions reported to the CSM during 1985 indicated that carbamazepine was one of the drugs most commonly reported to cause depressed peripheral white cell counts, there having been 10 reports in the year.— *Br. med. J.,* 1986, *293,* 688.

Agranulocytosis. A report of agranulocytosis associated with carbamazepine in a 61-year-old man. He had a positive reaction with anti-lymphoid leukaemia antiserum during recovery.— C. W. I. Owens *et al., Postgrad. med. J.,* 1980, *56,* 665. Fatal agranulocytosis in 1 patient attributed to the use of carbamazepine introduced about one month earlier.— D. J. Luchins, *Am. J. Psychiat.,* 1984, *141,* 687.

Aplastic anaemia. Details of aplastic anaemia in 2 patients given carbamazepine for trigeminal neuralgia.— G. W. K. Donaldson *et al., Br. J. clin. Pract.,* 1965, *19,* 699. See also J. D. Spillane, *Practitioner,* 1964, *192,* 71. Further references: W. R. Fellows, *Headache,* 1969, *9,* 92. Criticism of reports of carbamazepine-associated aplastic anaemia, and the view that a causative role of carbamazepine in the development of aplastic anaemia is not conclusively proved.— S. Livingston *et al., Neurology,* 1978, *28,* 101.

Leucopenia. Leucopenia in an immunosuppressed renal transplant patient appeared to be associated with carbamazepine therapy.— J. G. Gerber *et al., Sth. med. J.,* 1979, *72,* 81. A report of the development of leucopenia (neutropenia) in 2 patients after prolonged therapy with carbamazepine.— J. A. Rush and R. G. Beran, *Med. J. Aust.,* 1984, *140,* 426.

Thrombocytopenia. A 79-year-old woman who had taken carbamazepine 200 mg six-hourly for the pain of trigeminal neuralgia developed thrombocytopenia. When treatment was stopped the patient's platelet count returned to normal.— J. Pearce and M. A. Ron (letter), *Lancet,* 1968, *2,* 223. Profound isolated carbamazepine-induced thrombocytopenia in a young child.— J. M. Bradley *et al., Clin. Pharm.,* 1985, *4,* 221.

EFFECTS ON THE ENDOCRINE SYSTEM. Reports of and references to the adverse effects of hyponatraemia and water intoxication associated with the antidiuretic effect of carbamazepine: D. A. Henry *et al., Br. med. J.,* 1977, *1,* 83; W. P. Stephens *et al., ibid.,* 754; M. G. Ashton *et al., ibid.,* 1977, *1,* 1134; N. J. Smith *et al., ibid.,* 804; W. P. Stephens *et al., ibid.,* 1978, *1,* 1445; F. W. Ballardie and J. C. Mucklow, *Br. J. clin. Pharmac.,* 1984, *17,* 763; P. S. Sørensen and M. Hammer, *Eur. J. clin. Pharmac.,* 1984, *26,* 719.

EFFECTS ON THE EYES. On rare occasions lenticular opacities have been associated with carbamazepine.— *Med. Lett.,* 1976, *18,* 63.

EFFECTS ON THE HEART. Aggravation of a mild sick sinus syndrome in a 70-year-old woman after antiepileptic treatment was changed from pheneturide to carbamazepine. She experienced an increased frequency of cardiac syncope; failure to distinguish this from epileptic attacks might lead to increased carbamazepine dosage and further aggravation of symptoms.— K. A. Hewetson *et al., Postgrad. med. J.,* 1986, *62,* 497.

EFFECTS ON THE KIDNEYS. Renal failure in a patient taking 400 mg of carbamazepine four times daily. The renal failure was considered due to acute tubular necrosis. Three other cases of oliguria, dysuria, or haematuria had been reported.— D. P. Nicholls and M. Yasin (letter), *Br. med. J.,* 1972, *4,* 490.

The nephrotic syndrome with membranous glomerulopathy developed in a 25-year-old man who had been taking carbamazepine and phenobarbitone for 3 years. Improvement was seen as the carbamazepine was gradually withdrawn and replaced by sodium valproate. Acute tubulointerstitial nephritis had also previously been reported (R.J. Hogg *et al., J. Pediat.,* 1981, *98,* 830) in association with carbamazepine.— L. D. Hordon and J. H. Turney (letter), *Br. med. J.,* 1987, *294,* 375.

EFFECTS ON THE LIVER. Individual case-reports of adverse effects: I. D. Ramsay, *Br. med. J.,* 1967, *4,* 155 (jaundice); P. Zucker *et al., J. Pediat.,* 1977, *91,* 667 (hepatic encephalopathy, coma, and death); M. Levy *et al., Ann. intern. Med.*, 1981, *95*, 64 (granulomatous hepatitis).

EFFECTS ON THE NERVOUS SYSTEM. Carbamazepine was associated with decreased taste sensitivity in 1 patient.— H. Rollin, *Ann. Otol. Rhinol. Lar.*, 1978, *87*, 37.

Dyskinesias. Dystonia in brain-damaged children, associated with carbamazepine.— C. J. Crosley and P. T. Swander, *Pediatrics*, 1979, *63*, 612. A report of transient dystonia associated with treatment with carbamazepine in 4 patients.— D. Jacome (letter), *J. Am. med. Ass.*, 1979, *241*, 2263.

Continuous orofacial dyskinesia in a patient following the ingestion of an overdose of carbamazepine; symptoms had resolved a week later.— R. P. Joyce and C. H. Gunderson, *Neurology*, 1980, *30*, 1333.

A report of 3 patients who, following initiation of carbamazepine therapy, experienced either the onset of Tourette's syndrome or a worsening of tics and vocalisations; symptoms did not resolve following withdrawal of carbamazepine.— J. P. Neglia *et al., Pediatrics*, 1984, *73*, 841.

EFFECTS ON THE SKIN. Reports of adverse skin reactions associated with carbamazepine: S. M. Breathnach *et al., Clin. exp. Derm.*, 1982, *7*, 585 (toxic epidermal necrolysis); D. J. Godden and J. L. McPhie, *Postgrad. med. J.*, 1983, *59*, 336 (bullous eruption); S. Meisel and C. Q. North (letter), *Clin. Pharm.*, 1984, *3*, 15 (erythema multiforme); J. C. Delafuente, *Drug Intell. & clin. Pharm.*, 1985, *19*, 114 (erythema multiforme).

See also under Allergy, above.

LUPUS ERYTHEMATOSUS. Lupus erythematosus or dermatomyositis in one patient associated with carbamazepine.— J. R. Simpson, *Br. med. J.*, 1966, *2*, 1434. Further reports of systemic lupus erythematosus possibly associated with carbamazepine: D. E. Bateman, *Br. med. J.*, 1985, *291*, 632; B. McNicholl (letter), *ibid.*, 1126.

Treatment of Adverse Effects

The stomach should be emptied by lavage. The use of activated charcoal as an adjunct to gastric lavage has been suggested. Supportive therapy alone may then suffice for patients who are not severely poisoned; haemoperfusion has been suggested for the management of the more severely poisoned patient.

A report of a fatality due to self-poisoning with carbamazepine and a review of the treatment of overdosage. The following guidelines for the management of carbamazepine overdose were recommended. Patients who are suspected of taking a minor overdose or who are asymptomatic should undergo gastric lavage followed by the administration of activated charcoal into the stomach at the conclusion of the lavage; the patient should be admitted to hospital and monitoring of plasma concentrations and supportive medical and nursing care undertaken. In patients who have ingested large quantities of carbamazepine, who present with clinical features of poisoning, or who have high or rising plasma concentrations, gastric lavage with protection of the airway should be performed and activated charcoal should be administered through a nasogastric tube at 2-hourly intervals until the plasma concentration is within the therapeutic range with no evidence of accumulation; supportive medical and nursing care should be undertaken with cardiac monitoring and maintenance of fluid and electrolyte balance; an x-ray contrast medium should be instilled through the nasogastric tube to detect coagulated tablets and, if found to be present, gastrotomy should be considered; although the role of haemoperfusion is not fully established it should be used in patients with high and rising plasma concentrations or in patients with cardiovascular complications.— D. W. Denning *et al., Hum. Toxicol.*, 1985, *4*, 255.

A report of the use of charcoal haemoperfusion in a patient with carbamazepine poisoning.— P. J. Leslie *et al., Br. med. J.*, 1983, *286*, 1018.

Precautions

It has been recommended that carbamazepine should be avoided in patients with atrioventricular conduction abnormalities unless paced. Carbamazepine should be given with caution to patients with a history of blood disorders or of cardiac, hepatic, or renal disease.

Since carbamazepine has mild anticholinergic properties it has been suggested that caution should be observed in patients with raised intra-ocular pressure, and, owing to the similarity of its structure to that of phenothiazines, that patients should be examined periodically for eye changes.

Carbamazepine is extensively bound to plasma proteins and is therefore susceptible to interactions with drugs liable to compete for similar binding sites; for a comment on the relevance of this type of interaction, see the precautions section for phenytoin (p.408).

The metabolism of carbamazepine is reported to be less susceptible to inhibition by other drugs than that of phenytoin, nevertheless, dextropropoxyphene, erythromycin, isoniazid, and triacetyloleandomycin have been found to inhibit its metabolism, resulting in raised plasma concentrations and associated toxicity. Cimetidine, but not apparently ranitidine, has also been reported to inhibit the metabolism of carbamazepine but not all studies have shown that this results in increased concentrations of carbamazepine.

Carbamazepine is a hepatic enzyme inducer and induces its own metabolism as well as that of a number of other drugs, including some antibiotics (notably, doxycycline), anticoagulants, and sex hormones (notably, oral contraceptives). Carbamazepine and phenytoin may also mutually enhance one another's metabolism. The metabolism of carbamazepine is similarly enhanced by enzyme inducers such as phenobarbitone.

Because of the structural similarity to tricyclic antidepressants, it has been suggested that carbamazepine should not be given to patients taking a monoamine oxidase inhibitor or within 14 days of stopping such treatment.

For further reports of interactions in individual patients, see under Interactions (below).

Results of a study in 15 children suggesting that carbamazepine should be used with caution to treat a complex partial component of mixed seizure disorders since there is a risk of precipitating or exacerbating the generalised absence or atypical absence component.— O. C. Snead and L. C. Hosey, *New Engl. J. Med.*, 1985, *313*, 916.

DRIVING. For a comment on carbamazepine and driving, see Phenytoin, p.408.

INTERACTIONS. Reports of and references to the effects of carbamazepine on the following drugs may be found in their respective monographs: Doxycycline Hydrochloride and Warfarin Sodium.

Below are some reports of and references to interactions in which carbamazepine is affected by other agents.

Antidepressants. A patient receiving carbamazepine 200 mg three times daily became increasingly drowsy and lethargic over the 10 days following initiation of *viloxazine* therapy; serum-carbamazepine concentration rose to 44 µmol per litre. Treatment with viloxazine was stopped and she became alert, with restoration of normal concentration and mood.— J. H. B. Scarpello and N. Cottrell (letter), *Br. med. J.*, 1987, *294*, 1355.

Antiemetics. Neurotoxicity in 1 patient receiving carbamazepine and *metoclopramide* concurrently.— R. Sandyk (letter), *Br. med. J.*, 1984, *288*, 830.

Antiepileptics. In 7 patients receiving carbamazepine and *sodium valproate*, substitution of *valpromide* for valproate resulted in a marked increase in serum concentrations of carbamazepine-10,11-epoxide; 5 patients exhibited symptoms typical of carbamazepine intoxication during the period of increased epoxide concentrations, although carbamazepine concentrations did not increase.— J. W. A. Meijer *et al.* (letter), *Lancet*, 1984, *1*, 802. Results *in vitro* indicating that *valpromide* inhibits epoxide hydrolase and thereby the hydration of carbamazepine-10,11-epoxide whereas valproic acid does not.— G. M. Pacifici *et al.* (letter), *ibid.*, 1985, *1*, 397.

Antifungals. Malaise, myoclonus, and trembling, in 1 patient receiving carbamazepine developed following the addition of *miconazole* to therapy.— E. Loupi *et al., Thérapie*, 1982, *37*, 437.

Benzodiazepines. Reduction in dose of carbamazepine, due to increased blood concentrations, was needed for 7 of 8 patients when *clobazam* was added to existing anticonvulsant treatment which included carbamazepine.— M. Franceschi *et al., Clin. Trials J.*, 1983, *20*, 119.

Calcium antagonists. All of 6 patients with steady-state carbamazepine concentrations reported symptoms consistent with carbamazepine intoxication within 36 to 96 hours of the administration of the first dose of *verapamil*. In 5 patients, in whom plasma concentrations were measured, there was a mean increase of 46% in total carbamazepine and 33% in free carbamazepine; no effect on the plasma protein binding of carbamazepine was observed. The results suggested that verapamil inhibits the metabolism of carbamazepine to an extent likely to have important clinical repercussions.— G. J. A. MacPhee *et al., Lancet*, 1986, *1*, 700.

A report of 1 patient in whom *diltiazem*, but not *nifedipine*, precipitated carbamazepine neurotoxicity.— M. J. Brodie and G. J. A. MacPhee, *Br. med. J.*, 1986, *292*, 1170.

Lithium. In an investigation of an interaction suffered by a 22-year-old woman with bipolar affective disorder it was found that although the patient could tolerate either carbamazepine or lithium alone, the 2 drugs given together, in the doses previously used, resulted in symptoms of severe neurotoxicity. The 2 compounds might have acted synergistically; measured plasma concentrations did not indicate overdosage of either.— R. P. Chaudhry and B. G. H. Waters, *J. clin. Psychiat.*, 1983, *44*, 30. A report of severe neurotoxicity in a patient receiving lithium, carbamazepine, and haloperidol; previously the patient had received haloperidol with either lithium or with carbamazepine without toxic effects.— P. F. Andrus (letter), *ibid.*, 1984, *45*, 525.

PORPHYRIAS. For comments on the use of carbamazepine in porphyrias, see Phenytoin Sodium, p.409.

PREGNANCY AND THE NEONATE. For comments on the management of epilepsy in pregnancy, see Epilepsy under Uses and Administration of phenytoin (p.411).

Absorption and Fate

Carbamazepine is slowly but fairly completely absorbed from the gastro-intestinal tract.

Carbamazepine is extensively metabolised in the liver and one of its primary metabolites, carbamazepine-10,11-epoxide has been reported to have about one-third of the antiepileptic activity of carbamazepine. Carbamazepine is excreted in the urine almost entirely in the form of its metabolites.

Carbamazepine is widely distributed throughout the body and is extensively bound (about 75%) to plasma proteins. It has the property of inducing its own metabolism so that the plasma half-life after administration of single doses to previously untreated subjects may be considerably reduced on repeated administration. Estimation of the mean plasma half-life of carbamazepine on repeated administration is about 20 hours; it appears to be considerably shorter in children than in adults. Moreover, the metabolism of carbamazepine is readily induced by drugs which induce hepatic microsomal enzymes. For further comments on the relevance of the metabolism and protein binding, see Precautions.

Monitoring of plasma concentrations may be performed as an aid in assessing control and the therapeutic range of total plasma-carbamazepine is usually quoted as being 4 to 12.5 µg per mL (16 to 50 µmol per litre). It has been suggested by some but not all investigators that measurement of free carbamazepine concentrations in plasma may prove more reliable, and measurement of concentrations in saliva, which contains only free carbamazepine, has also been performed. It has been proposed that measurement of the metabolite, carbamazepine-10,11-epoxide, may in some circumstances, also be necessary.

Carbamazepine crosses the placental barrier and is excreted in breast milk.

An extensive review of the clinical pharmacokinetics of carbamazepine and its epoxide metabolite.— L. Bertilsson and T. Tomson, *Clin. Pharmacokinet.*, 1986, *11*, 177.

Uses and Administration

Carbamazepine is an antiepileptic agent used to control tonic-clonic (grand mal) and partial (focal) seizures. Its mode of action in epilepsy is not fully understood but some of its actions resemble those of phenytoin (p.409).

The dose of carbamazepine should be adjusted to the needs of the individual patient to achieve adequate control of seizures; this usually requires total plasma-carbamazepine concentrations of 4 to 12.5 μg per mL (16 to 50 μmol per litre). The suggested initial oral dose is 100 to 200 mg once or twice daily gradually increased to a usual maintenance dose of 0.8 to 1.2 g daily in 2 to 4 divided doses; up to 1.6 g daily may occasionally be necessary. Dosage increments of 200 mg daily are recommended. Suggested daily doses for children are: up to 1 year of age, 100 to 200 mg; 1 to 5 years, 200 to 400 mg; 5 to 10 years, 400 to 600 mg; 10 to 15 years, 600 mg to 1 g.

Since carbamazepine has a long plasma half-life, a twice-daily dosage regimen is usually adequate to maintain an effective plasma concentration and is preferred because improved compliance has been associated with twice-daily dosage regimens. A low initial dose of carbamazepine is recommended to minimise side-effects.

Withdrawal of carbamazepine or transition to or from another type of antiepileptic should be made gradually to avoid precipitating an increase in the frequency of seizures.

Carbamazepine is also used in the treatment of trigeminal neuralgia. The suggested initial dose is 100 mg twice daily increased by 200 mg daily (100 mg every 12 hours) to a maximum of 1.6 g daily. The usual maintenance dose is 400 to 800 mg daily in 2 to 4 divided doses; when pain relief has been obtained attempts should be made to reduce and ultimately discontinue the therapy, until another attack occurs.

Patients with manic depressive psychoses not responsive to lithium may respond to carbamazepine usually given in daily divided doses of 400 to 600 mg.

The time and manner of taking carbamazepine should be standardised for the patient since variations might affect absorption with consequent fluctuations in the plasma concentrations.

ADMINISTRATION IN RENAL FAILURE. Carbamazepine could be given in normal doses to patients with a glomerular filtration-rate of more than 10 mL per minute but doses should be reduced by 25% in those with a rate of less than 10 mL per minute.— W. M. Bennett *et al.*, *Am. J. Kidney Dis.*, 1983, *3*, 155.

DIABETES INSIPIDUS. Oral therapy with carbamazepine, which sensitises the kidney to the effects of vasopressin, has been used in diabetes insipidus but it is much less active than desmopressin and is not effective in severe forms.— J. S. Jenkins, *Practitioner*, 1979, *222*, 312.

See also under Adverse Effects, Effects on the Endocrine System, above.

EPILEPSY. For general comments concerning the use of carbamazepine in epilepsy, see under Phenytoin Sodium, p.410.

MULTIPLE SCLEROSIS. Favourable reports of the use of carbamazepine for various conditions in patients with multiple sclerosis: Y. Kuroiwa and H. Shibasaki (letter), *Lancet*, 1967, *1*, 116 (tonic spasms); M. L. E. Espir and M. E. Walker (letter), *ibid.*, 280 (dysarthria); M. L. Albert, *New Engl. J. Med.*, 1969, *280*, 1395 (pain); D. A. McFarling and J. O. Susac (letter), *J. Am. med. Ass.*, 1974, *230*, 962 (hiccup); P. O. Osterman, *Br. J. Derm.*, 1976, *95*, 555 (pruritus); D. E. Jacome, *Postgrad. med. J.*, 1985, *61*, 515 (coughing).

NEURALGIAS AND NEUROPATHIES. Reports, mostly favourable, of the use of carbamazepine in various neuralgias and neuropathies: F. G. Campbell *et al.*, *J. Neurol. Neurosurg. Psychiat.*, 1966, *29*, 265 (trigeminal neuralgia); K. A. Ekbom and C. E. Westerberg, *Archs Neurol., Chicago*, 1966, *14*, 595 (glossopharyngeal neuralgia); D. Alarcón-Segovia and M. A. Lazcano (letter), *J. Am. med. Ass.*, 1968, *203*, 57 (lightning pain in tabes dorsalis); J. M. Killian and G. H. Fromm, *Archs Neurol., Chicago*, 1968, *19*, 129 (trigeminal neuralgia and tabetic neuralgia; poor response or no benefit in postherpetic neuralgia and atypical facial pain); P. Rasmussen and J. Riishede, *Acta neurol. scand.*, 1970, *46*, 385 (trigeminal neuralgia and facial pain); K. Ekbom, *Archs Neurol., Chicago*, 1972, *26*, 374 (lightning pain in tabes dorsalis); M. L. Albert (letter), *New Engl. J. Med.*, 1974, *290*, 693 (painful paraesthesia); F. Elliott *et al.*, *New Engl. J. Med.*, 1976, *295*, 678 (phantom limb pain); Z. Zarday and R. J. Soberman (letter), *Ann. intern. Med.*, 1976, *84*, 296 (uraemic neuropathy); J. L. Bada *et al.* (letter), *New Engl. J. Med.*, 1977, *296*, 396 (painful paraesthesia in amyloidosis); J. R. Rees and P. G. Bicknell (letter), *Br. med. J.*, 1979, *1*, 754 (glossopharyngeal neuralgia); R. J. Guiloff, *ibid.*, *2*, 904 (metatarsophalangeal pain); J. C. Taylor *et al.*, *Postgrad. med. J.*, 1981, *57*, 16 (trigeminal neuralgia; long-term study); O. Lundvall *et al.*, *Eur. J. clin. Pharmac.*, 1983, *25*, 323 (restless leg syndrome); W. Telstad *et al.*, *Br. med. J.*, 1984, *288*, 444 (restless leg syndrome); K. A. Baker *et al.*, *Clin. Pharm.*, 1985, *4*, 93 (with baclofen in trigeminal neuralgia); E. J. Howard (letter), *J. Am. med. Ass.*, 1985, *253*, 2196 (postherpetic pudendal neuralgia).

PSYCHIATRIC DISORDERS. Carbamazepine's use in the management of a variety of psychiatric disorders has been the subject of several reviews: L.J. Birkhimer *et al.*, *Clin. Pharm.*, 1985, *4*, 425; R.W. Evans and C.T. Gualtieri, *Clin. Neuropharmacol.*, 1985, *8*, 221; *Drug & Ther. Bull.*, 1986, *24*, 59.

Some references to its antimanic and/or antidepressant activity in affective disorders: J.C. Ballenger and R.M. Post, *Am. J. Psychiat.*, 1980, *137*, 782; A. Kishimoto *et al.*, *Br. J. Psychiat.*, 1983, *143*, 327; M. Elphick, *ibid.*, 1985, *147*, 198; J. Fawcett and H.M. Kravitz, *J. clin. Psychiat.*, 1985, *46*, 58; R.M. Post *et al.*, *Am. J. Psychiat.*, 1986, *143*, 29.

Reports of carbamazepine being useful in the management of aggressive or violent psychotics: H.P.A. Hakola and V.A. Laulumaa, *Lancet*, 1982, *1*, 1358; V.M. Neppe, *ibid.*, *2*, 334; D.J. Luchins, *ibid.*, 1983, *1*, 766; J.A. Mattes, *ibid.*, 1984, *2*, 1164.

For reports of an interaction between carbamazepine and lithium, leading to neurotoxicity, see under Precautions, above.

TINNITUS. A short comment that several antiepileptic agents, including carbamazepine, have been tried in tinnitus and that although certain individuals may receive benefit, the response rate overall has been disappointing.— S. D. G. Stephens, *Br. med. J.*, 1986, *293*, 1162.

Some references to carbamazepine in tinnitus which when studied together support this opinion: P. S. Melding and R. J. Goodey, *J. Lar. Otol.*, 1979, *93*, 111; N. J. Marks *et al.*, *ibid.*, 1981, *95*, 941; I. Donaldson, *ibid.*, 947; R. Lechtenberg and A. Shulman, *ibid.*, 1984, *Suppl.* 9, 271.

Preparations

Carbamazepine Tablets *(B.P.)*

Carbamazepine Tablets *(U.S.P.)*

Proprietary Preparations

Tegretol *(Geigy, UK). Tablets*, scored, carbamazepine 100, 200, and 400 mg.
Oral liquid, carbamazepine 100 mg/5 mL.

Proprietary Names and Manufacturers

Biston *(Cz.)*; Carpaz *(Rolab, S.Afr.)*; Convuline *(Protea, Austral.)*; Degranol *(Lennon, S.Afr.)*; Hermolepsin *(Laakefarmos, Swed.)*; Karbamazepin *(DAK, Denm.)*; Mazepine *(ICN, Canad.)*; Nordotol *(Farmos, Denm.)*; Sirtal *(Labaz, Ger.)*; Tegretal *(Geigy, Ger.)*; Tegretol *(Arg.; Geigy, Austral.; Belg.; Geigy, Canad.; Geigy, Denm.; Geigy, Fr.; Geigy, Ital.; Neth.; Geigy, Norw.; Geigy, S.Afr.; Ciba, Spain; Geigy, Swed.; Geigy, Switz.; Geigy, UK; Geigy, USA)*; Temporol *(Orion, Denm.)*; Teril *(Alphapharm, Austral.)*; Timonil *(Desitin, Ger.; Desitin, Switz.)*; Trimonil Retard *(Rhone-Poulenc, Denm.)*.

6606-d

Clonazepam *(BAN, USAN, rINN).*

Ro-5-4023. 5-(2-Chlorophenyl)-1,3-dihydro-7-nitro-2*H*-1,4-benzodiazepin-2-one.
$C_{15}H_{10}ClN_3O_3$=315.7.

CAS — 1622-61-3.

Pharmacopoeias. In *It.* and *U.S.*

A light yellow powder with a faint odour. Practically **insoluble** in water; slightly soluble in alcohol and ether; sparingly soluble in acetone and chloroform. **Store** at room temperature in airtight containers. Protect from light.

Dependence

Prolonged use of clonazepam may lead to the development of dependence (see p.706).

It has a low liability for abuse.

Adverse Effects, Treatment, and Precautions

As for the benzodiazepines, p.706. Salivary or bronchial hypersecretion may cause respiratory problems in children.

Concomitant administration of hepatic enzyme inducers, such as phenobarbitone or phenytoin, may enhance the metabolism of clonazepam. Concomitant intake of alcohol may affect the patient's response to clonazepam. Clonazepam may enhance the effects of central nervous system depressants, and may reduce the patient's ability to drive vehicles or operate machinery.

EFFECTS ON THE ENDOCRINE SYSTEM. A report of precocious development of secondary sexual characteristics in a 15-month-old girl 2 months after starting treatment with clonazepam 500 μg twice daily for convulsions. Symptoms regressed upon withdrawal of clonazepam.— I. A. Choonara *et al.* (letter), *New Engl. J. Med.*, 1985, *312*, 185.

PORPHYRIAS. For comments on the use of benzodiazepines in porphyrias, see Phenytoin Sodium, p.409.

Absorption and Fate

For an account of the absorption and fate of a benzodiazepine, see Diazepam, p.730.

Clonazepam is extensively metabolised, its principal metabolite being 7-aminoclonazepam, which probably has little antiepileptic activity; minor metabolites are acetamide and hydroxylated derivatives. It is excreted in the urine almost entirely as its metabolites in free or conjugated form. It is about 50% bound to plasma protein and estimations of its plasma half-life range from about 20 to 40 hours, and occasionally up to 60 hours.

Unlike many of the other antiepileptic agents a therapeutic range of plasma concentrations has not been established.

Clonazepam crosses the placental barrier.

Uses and Administration

Clonazepam is a benzodiazepine compound similar to diazepam (p.731), with marked antiepileptic properties.

It may be used in the treatment of all types of epilepsy and seizures but its usefulness is sometimes limited by the development of tolerance and by sedation. Treatment is initiated with small doses which are progressively increased to an optimum dose according to the response of the patient. The usual daily doses, given in 3 or 4 divided doses, are: infants, 0.5 to 1 mg; children 1 to 5 years, 1 to 3 mg; children 5 to 12 years, 3 to 6 mg; adults, 4 to 8 mg.

Clonazepam may also be used as part of the emergency management of status epilepticus; it is given by slow intravenous injection over about 30 seconds. The usual dose is 500 μg for infants and children and 1 mg for adults, repeated if required. It may also be given by slow intravenous infusion, in sodium chloride 0.9% infusion, glucose 5 or 10% infusion, or sodium chloride 0.45% and glucose 2.5% infusion.

Withdrawal of clonazepam or transition to or from another type of antiepileptic therapy should be made gradually to avoid precipitating an increase in the frequency of seizures.

NEURALGIAS AND NEUROPATHIES. Favourable reports of the use of clonazepam in various neuralgias and neuropathies: S. Smirne and G. Scarlato, *Med. J. Aust.*, 1977, *1*, 93 (Sluder's syndrome and trigeminal neuralgia); W. B. Matthews (letter), *Br. med. J.*, 1979, *1*, 751 (restless leg syndrome); D. Boghen, *Ann. Neurol.*, 1980, *8*, 341 (restless leg syndrome); D. J. Read *et al.*, *Br. med. J.*, 1981, *283*, 885 (uraemic restless leg syndrome); P. Montagna *et al.*, *Acta neurol. scand.*, 1984, *69*, 428 (restless leg syndrome).

PSYCHIATRIC DISORDERS. Details of 50 patients with either panic disorder or agoraphobia with panic attacks who were treated with clonazepam; 41 had responded poorly to previous therapy. Response was seen in 39 patients and 34 continued to take the drug. It was suggested that further controlled investigation was desirable.— S. A. Spier *et al.*, *J. clin. Psychiat.*, 1986, *47*, 238.

TINNITUS. A study concluding that both clonazepam and oxazepam were more effective than other benzodiazepines, antihistamines, or carbamazepine for treating unremitting tinnitus.— R. Lechtenberg and A. Shulman, *J. Lar. Otol.*, 1984, *Suppl.* 9, 271.

Preparations

Clonazepam Tablets *(U.S.P.)*

Proprietary Preparations

Rivotril *(Roche, UK). Tablets*, scored, clonazepam 0.5 and 2 mg.
Injection, clonazepam 1 mg/mL, in ampoules of 1 mL, supplied with diluent.

Proprietary Names and Manufacturers

Clonopin *(Roche, USA)*; Iktorivil *(Roche, Swed.)*; Klonopin *(Roche, USA)*; Rivotril *(Arg.; Roche, Austral.; Belg.; Roche, Canad.; Roche, Denm.; Roche, Fr.; Roche, Ger.; Roche, Ital.; Neth.; Roche, Norw.; Roche, S.Afr.; Spain; Roche, Switz.; Roche, UK)*.

6610-t

Eterobarb *(BAN, USAN, rINN).*

Dimethoxymethylphenobarbital; DMMP; Eterobarbital; EX-12-095. 5-Ethyl-1,3-bis(methoxymethyl)-5-phenylbarbituric acid; 5-Ethyl-1,3-bis(methoxymethyl)-5-phenylperhydropyrimidine-2,4,6-trione.
$C_{16}H_{20}N_2O_5$=320.3.

CAS — 27511-99-5.

Eterobarb is a barbituric acid derivative which has been studied as an antiepileptic agent over a number of years.

References: B.B. Gallagher, Eterobarb, in *New Anticonvulsant Drugs*, B.S. Meldrum and R.J. Porter (Ed.), London, John Libbey & Co. Ltd, 1986, p.103.

Proprietary Names and Manufacturers

MacroChem, USA.

6611-x

Ethosuximide *(BAN, USAN, rINN).*

H-940; PM-671. 2-Ethyl-2-methylsuccinimide.
$C_7H_{11}NO_2$=141.2.

CAS — 77-67-8.

Pharmacopoeias. In *Br., Chin., Ind., Int., Jpn, Nord.*, and *U.S.*

A white or off-white, odourless or almost odourless, powder or waxy solid. **Soluble** 1 in 4.5 of water and 1 in less than 1 of alcohol, chloroform, and ether. **Store** in airtight containers.

Adverse Effects

Gastro-intestinal side-effects including nausea, vomiting, anorexia, gastric upset, and abdominal pain occur fairly frequently with ethosuximide. Other side-effects which may occur include headache, fatigue, lethargy, drowsiness, dizziness, ataxia, hiccup, and euphoria. Abnormal renal and liver function values, dyskinesias, personality changes, depression, psychosis, and skin rashes, and lupus erythematosus have also been reported. Blood disorders including eosinophilia, leucopenia, agranulocytosis, thrombocytopenia, pancytopenia, and aplastic anaemia have occasionally been reported. Erythema multiforme has also been reported.

Precautions

Ethosuximide should be used with extreme caution in patients with impaired hepatic or renal function; for suggested doses in patients with renal failure see Administration in Renal Failure under Uses (below).
Regular blood counts, tests of liver function, and examinations of the urine should be made during treatment with ethosuximide.

DRIVING. For a comment on anticonvulsant therapy and driving, see Phenytoin Sodium, p.408.

INTERACTIONS. *Antituberculous agents.* A report of psychotic behaviour in a patient stabilised on ethosuximide and sodium valproate, following the introduction of *isoniazid*. Serum-ethosuximide concentrations rose substantially until both ethosuximide and isoniazid were discontinued.— A. van Wieringen and C. M. Vrijlandt, *Neurology*, 1983, *33*, 1227.

PORPHYRIAS. For comments on the use of succinimides in porphyrias, see Phenytoin Sodium, p.409.

PREGNANCY AND THE NEONATE. Ethosuximide is recommended for the treatment of petit mal epilepsy in women of childbearing age because of its proven efficacy and relatively low teratogenic potential.— S. Fabro and N. A. Brown (letter), *New Engl. J. Med.*, 1979, *300*, 1280.

Absorption and Fate

Ethosuximide is readily absorbed from the gastro-intestinal tract and extensively hydroxylated in the liver to its principal metabolite which is reported to be inactive. It is excreted in the urine mainly in the form of its metabolites either free or in conjugated form but about 20% is also excreted as unchanged ethosuximide.
Ethosuximide is widely distributed throughout the body, but is not significantly bound to plasma proteins. A half-life of about 60 hours has been reported for adults with a shorter half-life of about 30 hours in children.
Monitoring of plasma concentrations has been suggested as an aid in assessing control and the therapeutic range of ethosuximide is usually quoted as being 40 to 100 µg per mL (about 300 to 700 µmol per litre); measurement of concentrations in saliva has also been performed.
Ethosuximide crosses the placental barrier, and is excreted in milk.

Uses and Administration

Ethosuximide is a succinimide antiepileptic agent used in the treatment of absence (petit mal) seizures; its mode of action is not fully understood. It may be used in conjunction with other antiepileptics when absences co-exist with other forms of epilepsy but occasionally this combined treatment may increase the incidence of tonic-clonic (grand mal) attacks, necessitating a readjustment of the medication used for controlling the major seizures. Change-over from existing medication should be made gradually.
A concentration of 40 to 100 µg per mL (about 300 to 700 µmol per litre) of plasma appears to be generally necessary. The initial dose for patients under 6 years of age is 250 mg daily and for patients of 6 years and over 500 mg daily . The dosage is then adjusted by increments, usually of 250 mg every 4 to 7 days, according to the response of the patient. Strict supervision is necessary if the dose exceeds 1 g daily for a child of up to 6 years or 1.5 g daily for an adult, although it has been stated that sometimes doses of up to 2 g may be necessary in an adult.

ADMINISTRATION IN RENAL FAILURE. Ethosuximide could be administered in normal doses to patients with a glomerular filtration-rate of 10 mL per minute or more but doses should be reduced by 25% in those with a rate of less than 10 mL per minute. A dose supplement should be given to patients undergoing haemodialysis.— W. M. Bennett *et al.*, *Am. J. Kidney Dis.*, 1983, *3*, 155.

Preparations

Ethosuximide Capsules *(B.P.)*

Ethosuximide Capsules *(U.S.P.)*

Ethosuximide Oral Solution *(B.P.)*. Ethosuximide Elixir. Store at a temperature not exceeding 25°.

Proprietary Preparations

Emeside *(Laboratories for Applied Biology, UK). Capsules*, ethosuximide 250 mg.
Syrup, ethosuximide 250 mg/5 mL.

Zarontin *(Parke, Davis, UK). Capsules*, ethosuximide 250 mg.
Syrup, ethosuximide 250 mg/5 mL.

Proprietary Names and Manufacturers

Emeside *(Laboratories for Applied Biology, UK)*; Ethymal *(Belg.; Neth.)*; Pétinimide *(Gerot, Switz.)*; Petinimid *(Switz.)*; Petnidan *(Desitin, Ger.)*; Pyknolepsinum *(ICI, Ger.)*; Simatin *(Inibsa, Spain; Switz.)*; Suxinutin *(Parke, Davis, Ger.; Parke, Davis, Swed.; Parke, Davis, Switz.)*; Thetamid *(Ital.)*; Zarondan *(Parke, Davis, Denm.; Parke, Davis, Norw.)*; Zarontin *(Arg.; Parke, Davis, Austral.; Belg.; Parke, Davis, Canad.; Substantia, Fr.; Parke, Davis, Ital.; Neth.; Parke, Davis, S.Afr.; Parke, Davis, Spain; Parke, Davis, UK; Parke, Davis, USA)*.

6612-r

Ethotoin *(BAN, rINN).*

3-Ethyl-5-phenylhydantoin.
$C_{11}H_{12}N_2O_2$=204.2.

CAS — 86-35-1.

Pharmacopoeias. In *Roum.*

Ethotoin is a hydantoin antiepileptic agent with general properties similar to those of phenytoin (p.406), but it is reported to be both less toxic and less effective.
Ethotoin is given in an initial dosage of 1 g daily, increased gradually at intervals of several days to 2 to 3 g daily, given in 4 to 6 divided doses after meals. A suggested maintenance dose for children is 0.5 to 1 g daily.

Proprietary Names and Manufacturers

Peganone *(Austral.; Abbott, Denm.; Abbott, Norw.; Swed.; Switz.; Abbott, UK; Abbott, USA)*.

18658-r

Lamotrigine *(BAN, rINN).*

430-C; BW-430C. 6-(2,3-Dichlorophenyl)-1,2,4-triazine-3,5-diyldiamine.
$C_9H_7Cl_2N_5$=256.1.

CAS — 84057-84-1.

Lamotrigine is a phenyltriazine compound chemically unrelated to other agents currently used in epilepsy. It is under study as an antiepileptic agent and has been tried in patients unresponsive to other therapy.

References: A.A. Miller *et al.*, Lamotrigine, in *New Anticonvulsant Drugs*, B.S. Meldrum and R.J. Porter (Ed.), London, John Libbey & Co. Ltd, 1986, p. 165.

Proprietary Names and Manufacturers

Wellcome, UK.

4047-z

Metharbitone *(BAN).*

Metharbital *(USAN)*. 5,5-Diethyl-1-methylbarbituric acid.
$C_9H_{14}N_2O_3$=198.2.

CAS — 50-11-3.

Pharmacopoeias. In *U.S.*

A white or almost white crystalline powder with a faint aromatic odour. **Soluble** 1 in 830 of water, 1 in 23 of alcohol, and 1 in 40 of ether. A saturated solution in water has a pH of about 6. **Store** in airtight containers.

Metharbitone is an antiepileptic agent with general properties similar to those of phenobarbitone (p.404); it is demethylated in the liver to barbitone. The usual initial dose is 100 mg one to three times daily.

Preparations

Metharbital Tablets *(U.S.P.)*. Tablets containing metharbitone.

Proprietary Names and Manufacturers

Gemonil *(Abbott, NZ; Abbott, USA)*.

6613-f

Methoin *(BAN).*

Mephenetoin; Mephenytoin *(USAN, rINN)*; Methantoin; Phenantoin. 5-Ethyl-3-methyl-5-phenylhydantoin.
$C_{12}H_{14}N_2O_2$=218.3.

CAS — 50-12-4.

Pharmacopoeias. In *Aust., Cz., Nord., Pol.*, and *U.S.*

A white crystalline powder. **Soluble** 1 in 1400 of water, 1 in 15 of alcohol, 1 in 3 of chloroform, and 1 in 90 of ether; soluble in aqueous solutions of alkali hydroxides.

Methoin is a hydantoin antiepileptic agent with general properties similar to those of phenytoin (p.406), but it is more toxic. Because of its potential toxicity it is given only to patients unresponsive to other treatment. Some of the side-effects of methoin may be due to the metabolite, 5-ethyl-5-phenylhydantoin (also termed nirvanol). Like phenytoin the rate of metabolism of methoin is subject to genetic polymorphism.
Methoin is given in a daily divided dosage beginning with 50 to 100 mg and increasing by about 50 mg

weekly until the optimum dose is reached, which is usually between 200 and 600 mg daily for an adult and 100 and 400 mg daily for a child.

Combined serum concentrations of methoin and its active metabolite, nirvanol, in the 25 to 40 μg per mL range are associated with good seizure control without clinical intoxication.— A. S. Troupin *et al.*, *Epilepsia*, 1976, *17*, 403.

Preparations

Mephenytoin Tablets *(U.S.P.)*. Tablets containing methoin.

Proprietary Names and Manufacturers

Mesantoin *(Sandoz, Austral.*; *Sandoz, Canad.*; *Sandoz, Swed.*; *Sandoz, Switz.*; *Sandoz, USA)*; Mesontoin *(Sandoz, UK)*; Sedantoinal *(Sandoz, Spain)*.

6614-d

Methsuximide *(BAN, USAN)*.

Mesuximide *(rINN)*; PM-396. *N*,2-Dimethyl-2-phenylsuccinimide.

$C_{12}H_{13}NO_2$=203.2.

CAS — 77-41-8.

Pharmacopoeias. In *U.S.*

A white to greyish-white crystalline powder; odourless or with a slight odour. M.p. 50° to 56°. **Soluble** 1 in 350 of water, 1 in 3 of alcohol, 1 in less than 1 of chloroform, and 1 in 2 of ether. **Store** in airtight containers.

Methsuximide is a succinimide antiepileptic agent with general properties similar to those of ethosuximide (p.403). It is usually only given to patients unresponsive to other treatment.

The usual initial dosage is a single dose of 300 mg daily by mouth, and this is increased by 300 mg at weekly intervals to an optimum dosage, according to the patient's response. The suggested maximum daily dose is 1.2 g.

Preparations

Methsuximide Capsules *(U.S.P.)*

Proprietary Names and Manufacturers

Celontin *(Parke, Davis, Austral.*; *Belg.*; *Parke, Davis, Canad.*; *Parke, Davis, Ital.*; *Parke, Davis, S.Afr.*; *Parke, Davis, UK*; *Parke, Davis, USA)*; Petinutin *(Parke, Davis, Ger.*; *Parke, Davis, Switz.)*.

4050-w

Methylphenobarbitone *(BAN)*.

Enphenemalum; Mephobarbital *(USAN)*; Methylphenobarbital *(rINN)*; Methylphenobarbitalum; Phemitone. 5-Ethyl-1-methyl-5-phenylbarbituric acid.

$C_{13}H_{14}N_2O_3$=246.3.

CAS — 115-38-8.

Pharmacopoeias. In *Aust.*, *Belg.*, *Br.*, *Eur.*, *Fr.*, *Ger.*, *It.*, *Jug.*, *Neth.*, *Nord.*, *Pol.*, *Port.*, *Swiss*, and *U.S.*

Odourless colourless crystals or a white crystalline powder. *B.P.* **solubilities** are: practically insoluble in water; very slightly soluble in dehydrated alcohol; slightly soluble in chloroform and ether. *U.S.P.* solubilities are: soluble 1 in more than 1000 of water, alcohol, and ether; soluble 1 in 50 of chloroform; soluble in solutions of ammonia and alkali hydroxides and carbonates. A saturated solution in water is acid to litmus.

Dependence

Prolonged use of methylphenobarbitone may lead to dependence (see p.706).

Adverse Effects, Treatment, and Precautions

As for Phenobarbitone, p.405.

Absorption and Fate

Methylphenobarbitone is incompletely absorbed from the gastro-intestinal tract. It is demethylated to phenobarbitone in the liver.

Uses and Administration

Methylphenobarbitone, like phenobarbitone, is used as an antiepileptic agent. It is given in usual doses of 200 to 400 mg daily; up to 600 mg daily may be given if required.

Preparations

Mephobarbital Tablets *(U.S.P.)*. Tablets containing methylphenobarbitone.

Proprietary Preparations

Prominal *(Winthrop, UK)*. *Tablets*, methylphenobarbitone 30, 60, and 200 mg.

Proprietary Names and Manufacturers

Mebaral *(Winthrop, Canad.*; *Winthrop-Breon, USA)*; Prominal *(Winthrop, Austral.*; *Belg.*; *Ital.*; *Igoda, Spain*; *Winthrop, UK)*; Prominalette *(Ital.)*.

The following names have been used for multi-ingredient preparations containing methylphenobarbitone— Ancatropine Gel *(Anca, Canad.)*; Mebroin *(Winthrop, Canad.)*.

19623-a

Oxcarbazepine *(pINN)*.

GP-47680. 10,11-Dihydro-10-oxo-5*H*-dibenz[*b,f*]azepine-5-carboxamide.

$C_{15}H_{12}N_2O_2$=252.3.

CAS — 28721-07-5.

Oxcarbazepine, which is closely chemically related to carbamazepine, is being studied as an antiepileptic agent. It has been tried in patients unresponsive to other therapy.

References: L. Gram and A. Philbert, Oxcarbazepine, in *New Anticonvulsant Drugs*, B.S. Meldrum and R.J. Porter (Ed.), London, John Libbey & Co. Ltd, 1986, p. 229.

6615-n

Paramethadione *(BAN, USAN, rINN)*.

5-Ethyl-3,5-dimethyloxazolidine-2,4-dione.

$C_7H_{11}NO_3$=157.2.

CAS — 115-67-3.

Pharmacopoeias. In *Ind.* and *U.S.*

A clear colourless liquid which may have an aromatic odour. Sparingly **soluble** in water; freely soluble in alcohol, chloroform, and ether. A 2.5% solution in water has a pH of about 6.0. **Store** in airtight containers.

Paramethadione is an oxazolidinedione antiepileptic agent with general properties similar to those of troxidone (p.412). Because of its potential toxicity it is given only to patients unresponsive to other treatment.

The initial dose of paramethadione is 900 mg daily in divided doses, increased by steps of 300 mg at intervals of one week, according to the patient's response, to a recommended maximum dose of 2.4 g daily. Suggested doses of paramethadione for children are 300 to 900 mg daily.

Preparations

Paramethadione Capsules *(U.S.P.)*

Paramethadione Oral Solution *(U.S.P.)*. A solution in dilute alcohol (63 to 67%) containing 282 to 318 mg of paramethadione in each mL. Protect from light.

Proprietary Names and Manufacturers

Paradione *(Austral.*; *Belg.*; *Canad.*; *Fr.*; *Abbott, UK*; *Abbott, USA)*.

6616-h

Phenacemide *(BAN, USAN, rINN)*.

Carbamidum Phenylaceticum. (Phenylacetyl)urea.

$C_9H_{10}N_2O_2$=178.2.

CAS — 63-98-9.

Pharmacopoeias. In *Pol.* and *U.S.*

An odourless or practically odourless, white or practically white, fine crystalline powder. Very slightly **soluble** in water, alcohol, chloroform, and ether; slightly soluble in acetone and methyl alcohol. **Store** in airtight containers.

Phenacemide is an acetylurea antiepileptic agent used in the treatment of epilepsy, especially in the psychomotor type of seizure. Because of its potential toxicity it should be employed only in patients whose seizures are impossible to control with other recognised antiepileptics.

The dosage of phenacemide is usually 500 mg three times daily, this dose being gradually increased until the symptoms are adequately controlled. The average dose for adults seldom exceeds 2 to 3 g daily. For children 5 to 10 years old, half the adult dose is suggested.

Severe adverse effects reported with phenacemide include personality changes, blood disorders including aplastic anaemia, and liver and kidney damage and extreme caution is advised in giving phenacemide to patients with a history of such disorders.

Withdrawal of phenacemide or transition to or from another type of therapy should be made gradually to avoid precipitating an increase in the frequency of seizures.

Preparations

Phenacemide Tablets *(U.S.P.)*

Proprietary Names and Manufacturers

Epiclase *(Bellon, Fr.)*; Phenurone *(Abbott, USA)*; Phetylureum *(Katwijk, Neth.)*.

6617-m

Pheneturide *(BAN, rINN)*.

Ethylphenacemide; S-46. (2-Phenylbutyryl)urea.

$C_{11}H_{14}N_2O_2$=206.2.

CAS — 90-49-3.

Pheneturide is an acetylurea antiepileptic agent which was formerly used in the treatment of tonic-clonic (grand mal) seizures and psychomotor epilepsy.

The suggested adult dose was 0.6 to 1 g daily. Suggested doses for children were: 6 months to 2 years, 50 mg daily; 2 to 5 years, 100 to 200 mg daily; 6 to 10 years, 200 to 600 mg daily.

Proprietary Names and Manufacturers

Benuride *(Vinas, Spain*; *Sapos, Switz.*; *Bengué, UK)*.

The following names have been used for multi-ingredient preparations containing pheneturide— Trinuride *(Bengué, UK)*.

4060-l

Phenobarbitone *(BAN)*.

Phenemalum; Phenobarbital *(USAN, rINN)*; Phenobarbitalum; Phenylethylbarbituric Acid; Phenylethylmalonylurea. 5-Ethyl-5-phenylbarbituric acid.

$C_{12}H_{12}N_2O_3$=232.2.

CAS — 50-06-6.

Pharmacopoeias. In *Arg.*, *Aust.*, *Belg.*, *Br.*, *Braz.*, *Chin.*, *Cz.*, *Egypt.*, *Eur.*, *Fr.*, *Ger.*, *Hung.*, *Ind.*, *Int.*, *It.*, *Jpn*, *Jug.*, *Mex.*, *Neth.*, *Nord.*, *Pol.*, *Port.*, *Roum.*, *Rus.*, *Span.*, *Swiss*, *Turk.*, and *U.S.* Also in *B.P. Vet.*

Colourless crystals or a white odourless crystalline powder. It may exhibit polymorphism.

Soluble 1 in 1000 of water and 1 in 10 of alcohol; sparingly soluble in chloroform; soluble in ether; soluble in aqueous solutions of alkali carbonates and hydroxides and ammonia. A saturated solution in water has a pH of about 5.

4061-y

Phenobarbitone Sodium *(BAN)*.

Phenemalnatrium; Phenobarbital Sodium *(USAN, rINN)*; Phenobarbitalum Natricum; Sodium Phenylethylbarbiturate; Soluble Phenobarbitone. Sodium 5-ethyl-5-phenylbarbiturate.

$C_{12}H_{11}N_2NaO_3$=254.2.

CAS — 57-30-7.

Pharmacopoeias. In *Arg.*, *Aust.*, *Belg.*, *Br.*, *Braz.*, *Chin.*, *Cz.*, *Egypt.*, *Ger.*, *Hung.*, *Ind.*, *Int.*, *It.*, *Jug.*, *Mex.*, *Nord.*, *Pol.*, *Roum.*, *Span.*, *Swiss*, *Turk.*, and *U.S.* Also in *B.P. Vet.*

A white odourless or almost odourless hygroscopic powder, granules, or flakes. It loses not more than 7% of its weight when dried.

Soluble 1 in 3 of water and 1 in 25 of alcohol; practically insoluble in chloroform and ether. A 10% solution in water has a pH of 9.2 to 10.2.

Phenobarbitone sodium is **incompatible** with many other drugs and phenobarbitone may be precipitated from mixtures containing phenobarbitone sodium. This precipitation is dependent upon the concentration and the pH, and also on the presence of other solvents. **Store** in airtight containers.

Dependence

Prolonged use of phenobarbitone may lead to dependence (see p.706).

Adverse Effects

Adverse effects of barbiturates include respiratory depression, sedation, and occasional allergic reactions, particularly affecting the skin (where an incidence of 1 to 3% has been reported for phenobarbitone). The skin rashes are most commonly of the maculopapular type, sometimes scarlatiniform; fixed-drug eruptions are commonly associated with barbiturates, and photosensitivity may occur. Purpura, exfoliative dermatitis, erythema multiforme (the Stevens-Johnson syndrome), and toxic epidermal necrolysis have occasionally been reported.

Nystagmus and ataxia may occur with excessive doses, and irritability and hyperexcitability may occur particularly in children or the elderly. Folate deficiency has developed during chronic administration of phenobarbitone and hypoprothrombinaemia has occurred in infants of mothers who have received phenobarbitone during pregnancy. Hepatitis and cholestasis have been associated with barbiturate administration.

The toxic effects of overdosage include prolonged coma, respiratory depression, and cardiovascular depression, with hypotension and shock leading to renal failure. Hypothermia is common, with associated pyrexia during recovery. Characteristic erythematous or haemorrhagic blisters (bullae) occur in about 6% of patients.

Owing to their extreme alkalinity necrosis has followed subcutaneous injection of sodium salts of barbiturates. Intravenous injections can be hazardous and cause hypotension, shock, laryngospasm, and apnoea.

Although congenital malformations have been reported in infants born to women who had received antiepileptic agents including phenobarbitone or primidone during pregnancy the direct causal role for some of these drugs has been debated due to the fact that combined therapy was often employed. For comments regarding the management of the pregnant epileptic patient see the section on epilepsy under the uses and administration of phenytoin.

ALLERGY. A report of hypersensitivity reactions in 7 children, occurring usually 1 to 2 weeks after initiation of phenobarbitone therapy. The condition began with fever, sometimes extreme, and was followed by an intensely pruritic rash; adenopathy or conjunctivitis was also seen in 5 patients. Lymphocyte studies *in vitro* suggested a cell-mediated reaction to phenobarbitone. It was considered that cross-reactivity among the major antiepileptic agents presented a real risk and that if a patient demonstrated a hypersensitivity reaction a chemically dissimilar drug should be substituted.— A. P. Knutsen *et al., J. Pediat.*, 1984, *105*, 558.

Treatment of Adverse Effects

Following the recent ingestion of an overdose of a barbiturate the stomach may be emptied by gastric lavage and aspiration. The prime objectives of management are then intensive symptomatic and supportive therapy with particular attention being paid to the maintenance of cardiovascular, respiratory, and renal functions and to the maintenance of the electrolyte balance.

Several methods aimed at the active removal of a barbiturate with a long elimination half-life such as phenobarbitone have been employed and include forced diuresis, haemodialysis, peritoneal dialysis, and charcoal haemoperfusion, but with the possible exception of charcoal haemoperfusion the hazards of such procedures are generally considered to outweigh any purported benefits.

Precautions

Phenobarbitone and other barbiturates should be used with care in children and elderly patients and in patients with impaired hepatic, renal, or respiratory function and are contra-indicated when the impairment is severe; for suggested doses for patients with renal failure, see Administration in Renal Failure under Uses (below). They are also contra-indicated in patients with acute intermittent porphyria.

Phenobarbitone and other barbiturates cause drowsiness and patients receiving them, if affected, should not take charge of vehicles or machinery where loss of attention could cause accidents. The effects of phenobarbitone and other barbiturates are enhanced by concurrent administration of other CNS depressants including alcohol. Valproic acid has been reported to cause rises in phenobarbitone (and primidone) concentrations in plasma.

Phenobarbitone and other barbiturates may reduce the activity of many drugs by increasing the rate of metabolism through induction of drug-metabolising enzymes in liver microsomes. Drugs which may be affected include carbamazepine, coumarin anticoagulants, cyclosporin, doxycycline, phenylbutazone, metronidazole, phenytoin, quinidine, theophylline, tricyclic antidepressants, and corticosteroids and other steroid hormones including oral contraceptives. Phenobarbitone may also reduce the activity of griseofulvin although the mechanism is not entirely clear.

INTERACTIONS. *Antibiotics.* Serum concentrations of phenytoin and phenobarbitone in a previously stabilised patient were increased when he took chloramphenicol concomitantly. Subsequent monitoring revealed a similar effect when chloramphenicol was taken with phenobarbitone alone.— J. R. Koup *et al., Clin. Pharmac. Ther.*, 1978, *24*, 571.

For the effect of phenobarbitone on serum-concentrations of chloramphenicol, see under Chloramphenicol, p.187.

Diuretics. Serum-phenobarbitone concentrations were raised in 8 of 10 epileptic patients taking phenobarbitone and additional antiepileptics when given frusemide 40 mg thrice daily for 4 weeks. This might have been the cause of drowsiness in 5 of 14 patients, 3 of whom had to discontinue frusemide.— S. Ahmad *et al., Br. J. clin. Pharmac.*, 1976, *3*, 621.

Vitamins. Pyridoxine reduced serum-phenobarbitone concentrations in 5 patients.— O. Hansson and M. Sillanpaa (letter), *Lancet*, 1976, *1*, 256.

PORPHYRIAS. For comments on the use of barbiturates in porphyrias, see Phenytoin Sodium, p.409.

PREGNANCY AND THE NEONATE. For comments on the management of epilepsy in pregnancy, see Epilepsy under Uses and Administration of phenytoin (p.411).

Absorption and Fate

Barbiturates are readily absorbed from the gastro-intestinal tract and most act within 30 minutes of ingestion, although the relatively lipid-insoluble barbitone and phenobarbitone may require an hour or longer. The sodium salts are a little more rapid in action.

The duration of action of barbiturates depends on their rate of inactivation in the liver and rate of excretion unchanged in the urine.

Phenobarbitone is only about 40% bound to plasma proteins and is only partly metabolised in the liver. About 25% of a dose is excreted in the urine unchanged. It has a plasma half-life of up to about 75 hours in children and 100 hours in adults; this is increased in the elderly, in overdosage, and in renal or hepatic disease.

Monitoring of plasma concentrations has been performed as an aid in assessing control and the therapeutic range of plasma-phenobarbitone is usually quoted as being 10 to 40 μg per mL (40 to 160 μmol per litre).

Phenobarbitone crosses the placental barrier and small amounts are excreted in breast milk.

Uses and Administration

Phenobarbitone is a barbiturate which may be used as an antiepileptic agent to control tonic-clonic (grand mal) and partial (focal) seizures.

The dose should be adjusted to the needs of the individual patient to achieve adequate control of seizures; this usually requires plasma concentrations of 10 to 40 μg per mL (40 to 160 μmol per litre). The usual dose by mouth is 60 to 180 mg daily, taken at night, and a suggested dose for children is up to 8 mg per kg body-weight daily.

Phenobarbitone sodium may be given parenterally as part of the emergency management of acute seizures or status epilepticus but doubts have been expressed as to the efficacy of the intramuscular route owing to the delay in achieving adequate blood concentrations, the subcutaneous route may cause tissue necrosis, and the intravenous route, even though the injection is given slowly and well diluted, is not without hazard; suggested parenteral doses have been around 200 mg for adults.

Barbexaclone ($C_{12}H_{12}N_2O_3$, $C_{10}H_{21}N$ = 387.5) which is a compound of phenobarbitone with (-)-propylhexedrine has also been used as an antiepileptic agent.

Withdrawal of phenobarbitone or transition to or from another type of antiepileptic therapy should be made gradually to avoid precipitating an increase in the frequency of seizures.

Phenobarbitone has also been used as a hypnotic and sedative but in general, more recently developed and safer drugs, such as the benzodiazepines, are usually preferred for such purposes.

Phenobarbitone stimulates the enzymes in hepatic microsomes responsible for the metabolism of some drugs and normal body constituents including bilirubin and for this reason has been used to reduce hyperbilirubinaemia in neonatal jaundice.

ADMINISTRATION IN RENAL FAILURE. Phenobarbitone could be administered to patients with renal failure by adjusting the dosage interval. A dosage interval of 12 to 16 hours was suggested for patients whose glomerular filtration-rate was less than 10 mL per minute. A dose supplement should be given to patients undergoing haemodialysis or peritoneal dialysis.— W. M. Bennett *et al., Am. J. Kidney Dis.*, 1983, *3*, 155.

CONVULSIONS. *Febrile convulsions.* Some brief comments on the management of the child with febrile convulsions. In general, children should be kept cool while the source of fever is sought and appropriate treatment given. At the onset of a febrile illness diazepam may be given rectally by the parent as soon as a fit is recognised, or intravenously by a doctor. It may be appropriate to try medium-term anticonvulsant prophylaxis in a child who already has neurodevelopmental delay, who has had several febrile convulsions, or who has suffered prolonged fits. Evidence that phenobarbitone daily is successful is not strong but this does not mean that alternative drugs are any better. An appropriate dose of phenobarbitone is 3 to 4 mg per kg body-weight daily or alternatively 5 mg per kg at night to minimise side-effects. Sodium valproate 15 to 30 mg per kg daily may also be used although there is the minimal risk of hepatotoxicity. Carbamazepine is not thought to be effective.— C. B. S. Wood, *Br. med. J.*, 1985, *291*, 1403. Similar guidelines for the management of febrile convulsions.— *Drug & Ther. Bull.*, 1987, *25*, 9.

Some studies and comments on the role of antiepileptic agents in febrile convulsions: J. Z. Heckmatt *et al., Br. med. J.*, 1976, *1*, 559 (phenobarbitone); S. M. Wolf and A. B. Forsythe (letter), *ibid.*, 1277 (phenobarbitone); J. Z. Heckmatt *et al., ibid* (phenobarbitone); S. M. Wolf *et al., Pediatrics*, 1977, *59*, 378 (phenobarbitone); S. J. Wallace and J. A. Smith, *Br. med. J.*, 1980, *280*, 353 and 612 (phenobarbitone or sodium valproate); A. Herxheimer (letter), *ibid.*, 642 (phenobarbitone or sodium valproate); J. B. P. Stephenson (letter), *ibid* (phenobarbitone or sodium valproate); P. M. Jeavons (letter), *ibid.*, 863 (phenobarbitone or sodium valproate); C. J. Bacon *et al., Lancet*, 1981, *2*, 600 and 704 (phenobarbitone); J. B. P. Stephenson (letter), *ibid.*, 1051 (phenobarbitone); J. A. Smith and S. J. Wallace, *Archs Dis. Childh.*, 1982, *57*, 104 (phenobarbitone or sodium valproate); J. H. Antony and S. H. B. Hawke, *Am. J. Dis. Child.*, 1983, *137*, 892 (phenobarbitone or carbamazepine); F. U. Knudsen, *Archs Dis. Childh.*, 1985, *60*, 1045 (diazepam).

EPILEPSY. For general comments concerning the use of phenobarbitone in epilepsy, see under Phenytoin Sodium, p.410.

INTRAVENTRICULAR HAEMORRHAGE. Two early reports by Donn *et al.* (*Lancet*, 1981, *2*, 215 and *ibid.*, 1982, *1*, 1240) showed promising results with phenobarbitone for the prevention of intraventricular haemorrhage in preterm infants and prompted several other sets of workers to perform further investigations. Most investigators (P.L. Hope *et al.*, *Lancet*, 1982, *1*, 444; M.E.I. Morgan and R.W.I. Cooke, *Lancet*, 1982, *1*, 558; A. Whitelaw *et al.*, *Lancet*, 1983, *2*, 1168; M. Anwar *et al.*, *Archs Dis. Childh.*, 1986, *61*, 196; K.C.K. Kuban *et al.*, *Pediatrics*, 1986, *77*, 443) consistently failed to find any beneficial effect. However Bedard *et al.* (*Pediatriacs*, 1984, *73*, 435) found that phenobarbitone reduced the severity but not the incidence of bleeding. Also Shankaran and colleagues (*Am. J. Obstet. Gynec.*, 1986, *154*, 53), who gave a single dose of phenobarbitone shortly before delivery to women less than 35 weeks gestation at imminent risk of delivery, reported apparent reduction in the severity of intraventricular haemorrhage. Another similar study by Morales and Koerten (*Obstet. Gynec.*, 1986, *68*, 295), in which successive doses were given first to the mother then to the neonate, also yielded encouraging results.

Preparations of Phenobarbitone and its Salts

Phenobarbital Elixir *(U.S.P.)*. Store in airtight containers. Protect from light.

Phenobarbitone Elixir *(B.P.)*. Phenobarbitone Oral Solution. A solution containing phenobarbitone 0.3% and alcohol 38%. Protect from light.

Phenobarbitone Sodium Mixture CF *(A.P.F.)*. Phenobarbitone sodium 15 mg, glycerol 1 mL, sorbitol 1.5 mL, concentrated chloroform water 0.1 mL or compound hydroxybenzoate solution 0.05 mL, water to 5 mL.

Phenobarbital Sodium Injection *(U.S.P.)*

Phenobarbitone Injection *(B.P.)*. Phenobarbitone Sodium Injection. A sterile solution of phenobarbitone sodium 20% in a mixture of propylene glycol 90% v/v and Water for Injections 10%. Sterilised by heating in an autoclave. pH 10 to 11.

Sterile Phenobarbital Sodium *(U.S.P.)*. Sterile phenobarbitone sodium suitable for parenteral use.

Phenobarbital Tablets *(U.S.P.)*. Tablets containing phenobarbitone.

Phenobarbital Sodium Tablets *(U.S.P.)*. Tablets containing phenobarbitone sodium.

Phenobarbitone Tablets *(B.P.)*

Phenobarbitone Sodium Tablets *(B.P.)*

Proprietary Preparations of Phenobarbitone and its Salts

Gardenal Sodium *(May & Baker, UK)*. *Injection*, phenobarbitone sodium 200 mg/mL, in ampoules of 1 mL.

Luminal *(Winthrop, UK)*. *Tablets*, phenobarbitone 15, 30, and 60 mg.

Proprietary Names and Manufacturers of Phenobarbitone and its Salts

Aphenylbarbit *(Switz.)*; Aphenyletten *(Switz.)*; Comizial *(Ogna, Ital.)*; Fenemal *(DAK, Denm.*; *NAF, Norw.*; *ACO, Swed.)*; Fenilcal *(Turon, Spain)*; Gardenal *(Belg.*; *Rhône-Poulenc, Canad.*; *Specia, Fr.*; *May & Baker, S.Afr.*; *Rhone, Spain*; *May & Baker, UK)*; Gardenale *(Farmitalia, Ital.)*; Gratusminal *(Farmasimes, Spain)*; Lethyl *(Lennon, S.Afr.)*; Lumcalcio *(Spain)*; Lumen *(Switz.)*; Luminal *(Arg.*; *Belg.*; *Winthrop, Canad.*; *Bayer, Ger.*; *Bayer, Spain*; *E. Merck, Switz.*; *Winthrop, UK*; *Winthrop-Breon, USA)*; Luminale *(Bracco, Ital.)*; Luminaletas *(Arg.*; *Spain)*; Luminalette *(Bracco, Ital.)*; Luminaletten *(Bayer, Ger.*; *Switz.)*; Luminalettes *(Belg.)*; Maliasin *(Knoll, Arg.*; *Knoll, Austral.*; *Knoll, Ger.*; *Knoll, Ital.*; *Knoll, Switz.)*; Mephabarbital *(Switz.)*; Nova-Pheno *(Canad.)*; Parabal *(Sinclair, UK)*; Phenaemal *(Woelm, Ger.)*; Phenaemaletten *(Woelm, Ger.)*; Phenobarbitone Spansule *(Smith Kline & French, UK)*; Sedadrops *(USA)*; Seda-Tablinen *(Ger.)*; Sedofèn *(Ital.)*; SK-Phenobarbital *(Smith Kline & French, USA)*; Solfoton *(Poythress, USA)*; Tequil *(Ital.)*.

The following names have been used for multi-ingredient preparations containing phenobarbitone and its salts—Alka-Donna P *(Carlton Laboratories, UK)*; Anaspaz PB *(Ascher, USA)*; Antrocol *(Poythress, USA)*; Arco-Lase Plus *(Arco, USA)*; Becosed *(Norton, UK)*; Belladenal *(Sandoz, Canad.*; *Wander, UK*; *Sandoz, USA)*; Belladenal-S *(Sandoz, USA)*; Bellergal *(Sandoz, Austral.*; *Sandoz, Canad.*; *Sandoz, UK*; *Sandoz, USA)*; Beplete *(Wyeth, UK)*; Bronkolixir *(Winthrop-Breon, USA)*; Bronkotabs *(Winthrop-Breon, USA)*; Cantil with Phenobarbitone *(MCP Pharmaceuticals, UK)*; Chardonna *(Rorer, USA)*; Climacteric Dellipsoids D19 *(Pilsworth, UK)*; Daricon PB *(Beecham Laboratories, USA)*; Diclophen *(Pro Doc, Canad.)*; Dilantin with Phenobarbitone *(Parke, Davis, USA)*; Donnatal *(Robins, Austral.*; *Robins, Canad.*; *Robins, UK*; *Robins, USA)*; Donnazyme *(Robins, Canad.*; *Robins, USA)*; Epanutin with Phenobarbitone *(Parke, Davis, UK)*; Franol Expect *(Winthrop, UK)*; Franyl; Garoin *(May & Baker, UK)*; Gustase Plus *(Geriatric Pharm. Corp., USA)*; Hybephen *(Beecham Laboratories, USA)*; Isuprel Compound Elixir *(Winthrop, Canad.*; *Breon, USA* : *Winthrop-Breon, USA)*; Kinesed *(Stuart Pharmaceuticals, USA)*; Levsin with phenobarbitone *(Kremers-Urban, USA* : *Rorer, USA)*; Levsinex with phenobarbitone *(Kremers-Urban, USA* : *Rorer, USA)*; Levsin-PB *(Kremers-Urban, USA* : *Rorer, USA)*; Maliasin *(Knoll, Switz.)*; Mudrane *(Poythress, USA)*; Mudrane GG *(Poythress, USA)*; Mudrane GG Elixir *(Poythress, USA)*; Neo-Tropine Alkaline *(Neolab, Canad.)*; Neuro-Spasex *(Beecham, Canad.)*; Neuro-Trasentin *(Ciba, Canad.*; *Ciba, UK)*; Pamol Supps for Babies *(Marshall's Pharmaceuticals, UK)*; Phazyme-PB *(Reed & Carnrick, USA)*; Phelantin *(Parke, Davis, Canad.)*; Phenaphen *(Robins, Canad.)*; Phenomet *(Woodward, UK)*; Phyldrox *(Carlton Laboratories, UK)*; Plexonal *(Sandoz, Canad.)*; Primatene P *(Whitehall, USA)*; Pro-Banthine with Phenobarbital *(Searle, USA)*; Quadrinal *(Knoll, USA)*; Sedative Tonic Dellipsoids D14 *(Pilsworth, UK)*; Seominal *(Winthrop, UK)*; Serpentinum and Theominal RS; Tedral *(Parke, Davis, Canad.*; *Parke, Davis, USA)*; T.E.P. *(Geneva, USA)*; T-E-P *(Schein, USA)*; Theogardenal *(May & Baker, UK)*; Theominal *(Winthrop, UK)*; Trinuride *(Bengué, UK)*; Tropinal *(Hamilton, Austral.)*; Valpin-PB *(Du Pont, USA)*; Veribid-VP *(Riker, UK)*; Viraxatone *(Faulding, Austral.)*.

NOTE. The names Franol and Franol Plus were formerly used to denote preparations containing phenobarbitone.

6618-b

Phensuximide *(BAN, USAN, rINN)*.

N-Methyl-2-phenylsuccinimide.

$C_{11}H_{11}NO_2$=189.2.

CAS — 86-34-0.

Pharmacopoeias. In *Cz.*, *Nord.*, and *U.S.* Also in *B.P.C. 1973.*

A white to off-white, odourless or almost odourless, crystalline powder. **Soluble** 1 in 210 of water, 1 in 11 of alcohol, 1 in less than 1 of chloroform, and 1 in 19 of ether. **Store** in airtight containers.

Phensuximide is a succinimide antiepileptic agent with general properties similar to those of ethosuximide (p.403), but it is reported to be less effective.

Phensuximide is given in usual doses of 0.5 to 1 g two or three times daily by mouth.

Preparations

Phensuximide Capsules *(U.S.P.)*

Proprietary Names and Manufacturers

Milontin *(Parke, Davis, Austral.*; *Parke, Davis, Canad.*; *Parke, Davis, UK*; *Parke, Davis, USA)*; Succitimal *(Katwijk, Neth.)*.

6601-a

Phenytoin *(BAN, USAN, rINN)*.

Fenitoína; Phenantoinum. 5,5-Diphenylhydantoin; 5,5-Diphenylimidazolidine-2,4-dione.

$C_{15}H_{12}N_2O_2$=252.3.

CAS — 57-41-0.

Pharmacopoeias. In *Aust.*, *Br.*, *Braz.*, *Cz.*, *Fr.*, *Ger.*, *Hung.*, *Int.*, *Jpn*, *Nord.*, *Roum.*, *Swiss*, *Turk.*, and *U.S.*

A white, or almost white, odourless or almost odourless, crystalline powder. Phenytoin 0.92 g is approximately equivalent to 1 g of phenytoin sodium. *B.P.* **solubilities** are: very slightly soluble in water; slightly soluble in chloroform and ether; soluble 1 in 70 of alcohol. *U.S.P.* solubilities are: practically insoluble in water; soluble in hot alcohol; slightly soluble in cold alcohol, chloroform, and ether. **Store** in airtight containers.

6602-t

Phenytoin Sodium *(BAN, USAN, rINNM)*.

Diphenin; Phenytoinum Natricum; Soluble Phenytoin.

$C_{15}H_{11}N_2NaO_2$=274.3.

CAS — 630-93-3.

Pharmacopoeias. In *Arg.*, *Aust.*, *Br.*, *Braz.*, *Chin.*, *Egypt.*, *Eur.*, *Fr.*, *Ger.*, *Ind.*, *Int.*, *It.*, *Jpn*, *Jug.*, *Mex.*, *Neth.*, *Pol.*, *Span.*, *Swiss*, and *U.S.* Also in *B.P. Vet.*

A white, odourless, slightly hygroscopic crystalline powder which on exposure to air absorbs carbon dioxide with the liberation of phenytoin. **Soluble** in water, the solution showing some turbidity due to partial hydrolysis and absorption of carbon dioxide; also soluble in alcohol; practically insoluble in chloroform and ether.

Solutions for injection have a pH of 10.0 to 12.3 and may be **sterilised** by filtration. **Store** in airtight containers.

INCOMPATIBILITY. Phenytoin sodium only remains in solution when the pH is considerably alkaline (about 10 to 12). The mixing of phenytoin sodium injection with other drugs or its addition to infusion solutions is not recommended.

Adverse Effects

Side-effects of phenytoin sodium are of fairly frequent occurrence, and include nausea, vomiting, constipation, ataxia, slurred speech, diplopia, nystagmus, and mental confusion, together with headache, dizziness, transient nervousness, and insomnia. Some of these effects may disappear with continued treatment at reduced dosage.

Tenderness and hyperplasia of the gums is a frequent occurrence particularly in younger patients; hirsutism is a less frequent effect, but is most noticeable in young females.

There have been a number of reports of rickets or osteomalacia in patients taking phenytoin, but the causative factors are complex and have been disputed. Polyarthropathy, fever, hepatitis, and lymphadenopathy have occasionally occurred. Hyperglycaemia may occur.

Leucopenia, thrombocytopenia, pancytopenia, granulocytopenia, and agranulocytosis have been reported. Megaloblastic anaemia following prolonged use usually responds to treatment with folic acid.

Skin rashes, sometimes accompanied by fever, are common, particularly in children; these may resemble measles. More serious skin reactions include lupus erythematosus and erythema multiforme, and the occurrence of bullous, exfoliative, or purpuric rash is an indication for withdrawing phenytoin.

Overdosage may lead to hypotension, coma, and respiratory depression.

Intravenous injections of phenytoin sodium are irritant and may cause phlebitis. Depression of cardiac conduction, and the occurrence of ventricular fibrillation and heart block have been reported. Rapid injection may also cause hypotension and central nervous system depression.

Although congenital malformations have been reported in infants born to women who had received antiepileptic agents including phenytoin or other hydantoins during pregnancy the direct causal role for some of these drugs has been debated due to the fact that combined therapy was often employed. For some references to individual case reports see below, and for comments regarding the management of the pregnant epileptic patient see epilepsy under the uses and administration section below.

ALLERGY. A review of 38 patients with phenytoin hypersensitivity. Thirty-five of the reactions occurred within the first 2 months of therapy, and were usually preceded by fever and dermatitis. In 25 patients, there was a licheniform or morbilliform eruption, which progressed to erythema multiforme or Stevens-Johnson syndrome in 7; in a further 3 erythema multiforme or Stevens-Johnson syndrome occurred without dermatitis preceding. Fever was the second most common manifestation (14 patients), followed by lymphadenopathy (9 patients), which was associated with a rash in all and with fever in all but one. Eosinophilia occurred in 8 patients and was associated with lymphadenopathy in all, with fever in 6, and with abnormal liver function tests in 6. Liver function tests were abnormal in 13 patients and blood counts were abnormal in 12 patients (leucopenia in 6, thrombocytopenia in 2, anaemia in 6, and increased atypical lymphocytes in 1). Two patients had serum sickness, 2 had albuminuria, and 1 had renal failure. It was concluded that prompt recognition of possible hypersensitivity reactions with early drug withdrawal and appropriate therapy, including corticosteroids when indicated, may reduce morbidity.— F. Haruda, *Neurology*, 1979, *29*, 1480.

A report of fatal systemic granulomatous vasculitis associated with phenytoin therapy in a 75-year-old black man. In a brief review of 7 additional cases of phenytoin-associated vasculitis, it was noted that 6 of the 7 had been black and 5 male.— C. M. Gaffey *et al.*, *Archs Path. lab. Med.*, 1986, *110*, 131.

Individual reports of allergic reactions possibly associated with phenytoin: S. R. Targan *et al.*, *Ann. intern. Med.*, 1975, *83*, 227 (disseminated intravascular coagulation with purpura fulminans, exfoliative dermatitis, hepatitis, cutaneous vasculitis, and microangiopathic haemolytic anaemia); A. S. Bayer *et al.* (letter), *Ann. intern. Med.*, 1976, *85*, 475 (miliary chest infiltrates and severe hypoxaemia, extensive dermatitis, hepatitis); J. R. Michael and W. E. Mitch, *J. Am. med. Ass.*, 1976, *236*, 2773; A. J. Wilensky (letter), *ibid.*, 1977, *237*, 2600 (both: reversible renal failure, myositis, fever, lymphadenopathy, exfoliative dermatitis, and hepatitis); B. N. Agarwal *et al.*, *Nephron*, 1977, *18*, 249 (acute renal failure with rash and fever); L. J. McCarthy and J. C. Aguilar (letter), *Lancet*, 1977, *2*, 932 (fatal hypersensitivity); K. J. Sheth *et al.*, *Pediatrics*, 1977, *91*, 438 (nephritis); L. R. Hyman *et al.*, *J. Pediat.*, 1978, *92*, 915 (nephritis); L. Fruchter and A. Laptook, *Ann. Allergy*, 1981, *47*, 453 (interstitial pulmonary infiltrates); R. Stalnikowicz *et al.*, *Neurology*, 1982, *32*, 1317 (fever, eosinophilia, and arthritis); S. Ting and E. H. Dunsky, *Ann. Allergy*, 1982, *48*, 331 (hepatitis); J. Harney and M. R. Glasberg, *Neurology*, 1983, *33*, 790 (hepatitis and myopathy); N. L. Harris and D. J. Widder (letter), *Archs Path. lab. Med.*, 1983, *107*, 663 (generalised lymphadenopathy); M. A. Lillie *et al.*, *Archs Derm.*, 1983, *119*, 415 (erythroderma and exfoliative dermatitis); C. P. Taliercio *et al.*, *Mayo Clin. Proc.*, 1985, *60*, 463 (myocarditis).

EFFECTS ON THE BLOOD. Subnormal serum-folate concentrations were found in one-half of 52 patients with chronic epilepsy who had been treated for 5 to 25 years with phenytoin 200 to 700 mg daily; most of the patients had also been given phenobarbitone and primidone. Twenty patients had neurological involvement. There was no significant difference in serum-folate concentrations between patients with or without neuropathy. Administration of folic acid 5 mg daily or a placebo for 3 months to 12 patients with nerve involvement produced no measurable improvement in their neuropathy.— S. J. Horwitz *et al.*, *Lancet*, 1968, *1*, 563.

In 75 children with epilepsy, most of whom were taking anticonvulsants, serum-folate concentrations and red-cell-folate concentrations were subnormal in 59% and 58% respectively. These low values correlated with hepatic microsomal enzyme activity (assessed by excretion of D-glucaric acid in urine) and with the daily dose of anticonvulsants. It was suggested that folate deficiency resulted from accelerated metabolism of folate consequent upon induction of liver enzymes by anticonvulsants. It might also explain the reduction in phenytoin concentrations (with consequent increase in the incidence of fits) in patients when given folic acid: prolonged administration of inducers (e.g. phenytoin) of liver enzymes would lead to increased demand for folate which might be a necessary cofactor for the metabolism of phenytoin. Folic acid supplements could then lead to increased metabolism of phenytoin.— J. D. Maxwell *et al.*, *Br. med. J.*, 1972, *1*, 297.

Although reduced folate values were detected in a study of 44 patients given phenytoin the effect was not found to be dose-dependent.— A. D. Korezyn *et al.*, *J. Neurol.*, 1974, *207*, 151.

Of 14 patients taking anticonvulsants (phenytoin in 13, usually with other anticonvulsants) 11 had evidence of megaloblastic erythropoiesis. Only 2 had evidence of vitamin B_{12} or folate deficiency, as assessed by abnormal suppression in the deoxyuridine test. Megaloblastic changes or macrocytosis were mediated by biochemical pathways other than the conversion of deoxyuridylate to thymidylate.— S. N. Wickramasinghe *et al.*, *Br. med. J.*, 1975, *4*, 136.

Inspection of the blood picture of 96 mentally handicapped patients receiving anticonvulsant drug therapy revealed that although a considerable proportion had low serum and red cell folate values, only 1 patient had macrocytic anaemia; folate depletion was not incriminated in 5 patients with hypochromic anaemia. The macrocytic anaemia sometimes noted in epileptic patients undergoing anticonvulsant therapy might represent inadequate nutrition rather than an effect of the anticonvulsants.— M. Rose and I. Johnson, *Lancet*, 1978, *1*, 1349. It has long been recognised that additional nutritional deficiency may sometimes precipitate megaloblastic anaemia, as may pregnancy. However, nutritional deficiency is not present in many patients and in view of the high incidence of macrocytosis, megaloblastic haemopoiesis, and low serum and red cell folate in non-anaemic treated epileptics, there can be little doubt that the drugs also play a role in the occasional anaemia.— E. H. Reynolds and M. Laundy (letter), *ibid.*, 1978, *2*, 682. Reply; the findings do not support the belief that long-term anticonvulsant therapy leads through a progression of abnormalities to megaloblastic anaemia due to folate depletion. The vast majority of such patients have low folates but neither anaemia nor macrocytosis, suggesting that we are dealing with something different.— M. Rose and I. Johnson (letter), *ibid.*, 994. Further comments and criticisms.— J. A. Child (letter), *ibid.*, 160; C. Hawkins (letter), *ibid.*, 317.

Further studies into folate deficiency and its relevance in patients receiving anticonvulsants: D. Labadarios *et al.*, *Br. J. clin. Pharmac.*, 1978, *5*, 167.

Agranulocytosis. A report of agranulocytosis with marked phagocytosis of myeloid precursors by marrow histiocytes associated with phenytoin 300 mg daily in one patient.— M. -F. Tan (letter), *Ann. intern. Med.*, 1976, *84*, 710. See also W. A. Parker and R. J. Gumnit, *Neurology*, 1974, *24*, 1178; R. D. Strickland *et al.*, *Oral Surg.*, 1983, *56*, 500.

Aplastic anaemia. A report of reversible pure red cell aplasia in a 19-year-old woman, probably associated with phenytoin therapy.— K. I. Pritchard *et al.*, *Can. med. Ass. J.*, 1979, *121*, 1491. See also Y. -G. Jeong *et al.*, *J. Am. med. Ass.*, 1974, *229*, 314; S. Livingston and L. L. Pauli (letter), *ibid.*, *230*, 211; P. C. Huijgens *et al.*, *Acta haemat.*, 1978, *59*, 31.

Leucopenia. A retrospective survey of the incidence and causes of neutropenia in hospitalised patients during 1973-78 in the Stockholm County region; patients with neutropenia induced by antineoplastic agents were excluded. Phenytoin was implicated in 2 of 84 episodes of drug-induced neutropenia.— P. Arneborn and J. Palmblad, *Acta med. scand.*, 1982, *212*, 289.

Thrombocytopenia. An analysis of blood dyscrasias reported to the Swedish Adverse Drug Reaction Committee for the 5-year period 1966-70 showed that thrombocytopenia attributable to phenytoin had been reported on 3 occasions. It was estimated that reported figures represented one-third of the true frequency.— L. E. Böttiger and B. Westerholm, *Br. med. J.*, 1973, *3*, 339.

After receiving phenytoin as single drug therapy for 8 years a patient developed thrombocytopenia. The phenytoin was stopped and the platelet count rose rapidly. Primidone was successfully substituted.— R. W. Fincham *et al.*, *Ann. Neurol.*, 1979, *6*, 370.

EFFECTS ON THE BONES. A review of the adverse effects of antiepileptic agents including comments regarding the effects on the skeletal system. Although there are numerous reports of antiepileptic drugs affecting the metabolism of vitamin D, the role of the antiepileptic is not clear and there have been only relatively rare reports of true clinical osteomalacia.— E. Beghi *et al.*, *Adverse Drug React. Ac. Pois. Rev.*, 1986, *5*, 63.

Further references: I. Fogelman *et al.*, *Scott. med. J.*, 1982, *27*, 136.

EFFECTS ON THE ENDOCRINE SYSTEM. Anticonvulsants diminish sexual potency and fertility in young male epileptics. Phenytoin is excreted in human semen in small quantities and this may possibly affect sperm morphology and motility.— *Br. med. J.*, 1979, *2*, 1118.

Plasma concentrations of free testosterone were reduced in male epileptics receiving anticonvulsants.— J. Dana-Haeri *et al.*, *Br. med. J.*, 1982, *284*, 85.

A report of gynaecomastia in 5 men receiving long-term antiepileptic treatment; one also complained of impotence but libido was stated to be normal in all 5. Phenytoin was a component of treatment in all patients and was the sole drug used in one.— J. P. Monson and D. F. Scott, *Br. med. J.*, 1987, *294*, 612.

EFFECTS ON THE KIDNEYS. For reference to nephritis and renal failure in patients given phenytoin, see Allergy, above.

EFFECTS ON THE LIVER. A cohort study of patients with very severe epilepsy and an increased mortality rate, provided no evidence of an increase in liver tumours.— S. J. White *et al.*, *Lancet*, 1979, *2*, 458. Updating of a previous 40-year review of the patients who died in 4 mental hospitals did not reveal an association between prolonged usage of various anticonvulsant and tranquillising drugs and liver cancer.— J. Jancar (letter), *ibid.*, 1980, *1*, 484.

Results of a study in 63 epileptic children indicated that phenobarbitone and phenytoin therapy may be continued despite transient elevations in transaminase values, and that liver biopsies are not warranted in such children.— H. W. Aiges *et al.*, *J. Pediat.*, 1980, *97*, 22.

Individual reports of adverse effects on the liver associated with phenytoin: U. Harinasuta and H. J. Zimmerman, *J. Am. med. Ass.*, 1968, *203*, 1015 (acute parenchymal hepatic disease); C. B. Campbell *et al.*, *Dig. Dis. Scis*, 1977, *22*, 255 (cholestatic liver disease); J. W. Taylor *et al.*, *Archs Neurol., Chicago*, 1984, *41*, 500 (cholestatic liver dysfunction).

See also under Allergy, above.

EFFECTS ON LYMPHOID TISSUE. Immunologic studies in a 28-year-old woman with phenytoin-induced pseudolymphoma syndrome did not support the suggestion that the syndrome resulted from a delayed hypersensitivity reaction.— E. N. Charlesworth, *Archs Derm.*, 1977, *113*, 477.

EFFECTS ON THE NERVOUS SYSTEM. Progressive neurological deterioration, thought at first to be a degenerative central nervous system disease, was observed in 9 patients receiving long-term hydantoin therapy. Symptoms included cerebellar signs of nystagmus and ataxia, and signs of more diffuse encephalopathy, including impaired intellectual performance, bizarre behaviour, increased seizure frequency, impaired speech, and EEG changes. On stopping the hydantoins, 6 patients improved neurologically and 3 did not deteriorate further.— J. M. Vallarta *et al.*, *Am. J. Dis. Child.*, 1974, *128*, 27.

A report of word reversal associated with phenytoin.— B. H. Fookes (letter), *Lancet*, 1975, *2*, 134.

A report of transient hemiparesis in a patient which appeared to have been precipitated by phenytoin intoxication.— R. Sandyk, *Postgrad. med. J.*, 1983, *59*, 601.

Marked cerebellar atrophy in a patient following an episode of acute severe phenytoin intoxication.— O. Lindvall and B. Nilsson, *Ann. Neurol.*, 1984, *16*, 258.

Dyskinesias. An account of a variety of dyskinesias in 6 epileptic patients with toxic plasma concentrations of phenytoin and other anticonvulsants, and a review of previously reported patients with anticonvulsant-induced dyskinesias. Phenytoin, carbamazepine, primidone, and phenobarbitone may cause asterixis. Phenytoin, but not other anticonvulsants, may cause orofacial dyskinesias, limb chorea, and dystonia in patients given excessive doses. These dyskinesias are similar to those induced by neuroleptics and may be related to the dopamine antagonist properties of phenytoin.— D. Chadwick *et al.*, *J. Neurol. Neurosurg. Psychiat.*, 1976, *39*, 1210.

Individual reports of dyskinesias (mainly choreoathetosis) in patients receiving phenytoin alone or with other anticonvulsants: E. Shuttleworth *et al.*, *J. Am. med. Ass.*, 1974, *230*, 1170; D. L. McLellan and M. Swash, *Br. med. J.*, 1974, *2*, 204; K. W. G. Heathfield (letter), *ibid.*, 507; M. H. Bellman and L. Haas (letter), *ibid.*, *3*, 256; E. G. Chalhub *et al.*, *Neurology*, 1976, *26*, 494; S. Zinsmeister and R. E. Marks, *Am. J. Dis. Child.*, 1976, *130*, 75; K. Luhdorf and M. Lund, *Epilepsia*, 1977, *18*, 409; S. Rasmussen and M. Kristensen, *Acta med. scand.*, 1977, *201*, 239; C. L. Opida *et al.*, *Ann. Neurol.*, 1978, *3*, 186; F. Mauguiere *et al.*, *Eur. Neurol.*, 1979, *18*, 116; R. J. Stark, *Med. J. Aust.*, 1979, *1*, 156; K. S. Krishnamoorthy *et al.*, *Pediatrics*, 1983, *72*, 831.

Ophthalmoplegia. Partial or total external ophthalmoplegia was reported in 3 patients after excessive doses of phenytoin and primidone. In a further patient, phenytoin only had been taken.— D. N. Orth *et al.*, *J. Am. med. Ass.*, 1967, *201*, 485. See also R. H. Spector *et al.*, *Neurology*, 1976, *26*, 1031; R. Sandyk, *S. Afr. med. J.*, 1984, *65*, 141.

Peripheral neuropathy. Patients receiving long-term phenytoin treatment may develop a predominantly sensory polyneuropathy that is usually mild and rarely causes symptoms. The incidence is uncertain, but signs of peripheral nerve disorders, such as depression of tendon reflexes, are found increasingly often in those receiving prolonged treatment.— Z. Argov and F. L. Mastaglia, *Br. med. J.*, 1979, *1*, 663. See also R. E. Lovelace and S. J. Horwitz, *Archs Neurol., Chicago*, 1968, *18*, 69; B. H. Dobkin, *Archs Neurol., Chicago*,

1977, *34*, 189 (reversible subacute peripheral neuropathy).

EFFECTS ON NEUROMUSCULAR TRANSMISSION. Myasthenia gravis associated with phenytoin.— J. Brumlik and R. S. Jacobs, *Can. J. neurol. Sci.*, 1974, *1*, 127.

EFFECTS ON THE SKIN. Individual reports of adverse skin reactions associated with phenytoin therapy: N. Hurwitz, *Br. med. J.*, 1969, *1*, 539 (erythema multiforme); R. B. Jenkins and A. C. Ratner (letter), *New Engl. J. Med.*, 1972, *287*, 148 (acne); J. A. Bosso and G. M. Chudzik, *Drug Intell. & clin. Pharm.*, 1973, *7*, 336 (Stevens-Johnson syndrome); K. P. Dawson, *Archs Dis. Childh.*, 1973, *48*, 239 (fatal morbilliform rash; macular rash); L. E. Gately and M. A. Lam, *Ann. intern. Med.*, 1979, *91*, 59 (fatal toxic epidermal necrolysis); S. J. Spechler *et al.*, *Ann. intern. Med.*, 1981, *95*, 455 (cholestasis and toxic epidermal necrolysis); D. Schmidt and W. Kluge, *Epilepsia*, 1983, *24*, 440 (fatal toxic epidermal necrolysis); H. L. Chan, *J. Am. Acad. Derm.*, 1984, *10*, 973 (toxic epidermal necrolysis); A. Maiche and L. Teerenhovi (letter), *Lancet*, 1985, *2*, 45 (Stevens-Johnson syndrome in 4 patients also receiving cerebral radiotherapy); M. S. Lewis-Jones *et al.*, *Br. med. J.*, 1985, *290*, 603 (zinc deficiency and acrodermatitis enteropathica).

LUPUS ERYTHEMATOSUS. Four children who had been taking anticonvulsants had lupus-like disease; 11 of 48 other asymptomatic children had significant antinuclear antibodies.— D. H. Beernink and J. J. Miller, *J. Pediat.*, 1973, *82*, 113.

PREGNANCY AND THE NEONATE. Some references to congenital abnormalities associated with phenytoin: J. W. Hanson and D. W. Smith, *J. Pediat.*, 1975, *87*, 285; J. W. Hanson *et al.*, *ibid.*, 1976, *89*, 662; R. W. Allen *et al.*, *J. Am. med. Ass.*, 1980, *244*, 1464; A. N. W. Evans *et al.*, *Practitioner*, 1980, *224*, 315; W. F. Taylor *et al.* (letter), *Lancet*, 1980, *2*, 481; W. E. Truog *et al.*, *J. Pediat.*, 1980, *96*, 112; L. T. Ehrenbard and R. S. K. Chaganti (letter), *Lancet*, 1981, *2*, 97; M. C. Phelan *et al.*, *New Engl. J. Med.*, 1982, *307*, 99.

Treatment of Adverse Effects

Treatment of poisoning with phenytoin tends to be supportive. Aspiration and lavage may be tried in severe cases.

The efficiency of haemodialysis in the treatment of a patient reported to have taken an overdose of 10 g of phenytoin was calculated to be 10%. Plasma concentrations reached a maximum of 34 µg per mL 6 hours after ingestion and did not change significantly for 24 hours, despite haemodialysis. About 350 mg of phenytoin was removed by haemodialysis and 1.05 g by gastric lavage.— D. Rubinger *et al.* (letter), *Br. J. clin. Pharmac.*, 1979, *7*, 405.

A review of data from 2 patients with phenytoin overdosage treated with charcoal haemoperfusion. Phenytoin has a relatively small volume of distribution, and haemoperfusion, particularly at high drug concentrations, should contribute significantly to total drug removal.— S. Pond *et al.*, *Clin. Pharmacokinet.*, 1979, *4*, 329. Lack of benefit.— R. W. Baehler *et al.*, *Archs intern. Med.*, 1980, *140*, 1466.

Peritoneal dialysis did not appreciably enhance the elimination of phenytoin in a 3-year-old boy with phenytoin intoxication. The effectiveness of peritoneal dialysis for phenytoin poisoning should be seriously questioned. The child died of septicaemia, which emphasises the potential hazards of peritoneal dialysis.— P. A. Czajka *et al.*, *J. clin. Pharmac.*, 1980, *20*, 565.

Precautions

Since phenytoin is extensively bound to plasma proteins it can be displaced by drugs competing for protein-binding sites, thus liberating more free (pharmacologically active) phenytoin into the plasma. Protein binding may also be reduced in certain disease states such as uraemia, and in certain patient populations such as the elderly. This elevation of free phenytoin is reported to be of little clinical significance, provided hepatic function is not impaired, because the free phenytoin is extensively distributed, metabolised, and excreted so that the actual concentration of free drug in the plasma remains more or less unchanged. Thus an alteration in protein binding would not necessarily require a change in dosage of phenytoin to be made but when plasma concentrations are being monitored, relatively lower total plasma-phenytoin concentrations will be found to be effective since there is less bound (pharmacologically inactive) phenytoin available for measurement. Drugs widely reported to displace phenytoin from plasma protein-binding sites include aspirin and some other salicylates, diazoxide, phenylbutazone, sulphinpyrazone, sulphonamides, tolbutamide, and valproic acid; drugs which affect lipid concentrations, such as clofibrate and heparin, may also influence binding by changing lipid availability.

A much more serious type of precaution and interaction stems from phenytoin's metabolism being saturable and thus susceptible to a relatively minor degree of inhibition. Toxic concentrations of phenytoin may readily develop in patients given drugs which inhibit phenytoin metabolism or in patients with impaired hepatic function. Drugs that have been widely reported to inhibit the metabolism of phenytoin include some antibiotics, some other anticonvulsants, cimetidine (but not apparently ranitidine), coumarin anticoagulants, disulfiram, isoniazid, some phenothiazines, phenylbutazone, and sulphinpyrazone. Particularly marked inhibition by chloramphenicol, dicoumarol, isoniazid, sulphaphenazole, and sulthiame has been reported. Phenylbutazone, sulphinpyrazone, and valproic acid appear both to inhibit phenytoin metabolism and to displace it from plasma proteins.

The metabolism of phenytoin may be induced or enhanced by other drugs and notably phenytoin and carbamazepine may mutually enhance one another's metabolism. Phenytoin is a potent enzyme inducer, and induces the metabolism of a number of drugs, including some antibiotics (notably, doxycycline), anticoagulants, corticosteroids, quinidine, and sex hormones (notably, oral contraceptives).

Benzodiazepines and phenobarbitone have been reported to alter phenytoin concentrations but the effect does not appear to be consistent.

Drugs with an epileptogenic potential, such as tricyclic antidepressants or phenothiazines may diminish the pharmacological action of phenytoin. The hypotensive properties of dopamine and the cardiac depressant properties of drugs such as lignocaine or propranolol may be dangerously enhanced by intravenous administration of phenytoin.

For further reports of interactions in individual patients, see under Interactions (below).

Intravenous phenytoin must be given slowly (for further details, see Uses) and extravasation must be avoided. Phenytoin should not be given intravenously to patients with bradycardia, heart block, or Stokes-Adams syndrome, and should be used with caution in patients with hypotension and severe myocardial insufficiency; monitoring of blood pressure and the ECG is recommended during intravenous therapy.

Phenytoin may cause decreased protein-bound iodine concentrations and thus interfere with some tests of thyroid function and it may also produce lower than normal values for dexamethasone and metyrapone tests.

DRIVING. Phenytoin, carbamazepine, and sodium valproate in appropriate doses may not as such impair driving skills, but epilepsy itself dictates the practice of driving.— T. Seppala *et al.*, *Drugs*, 1979, *17*, 389.

INFECTIONS. A 52-year-old woman previously well-controlled on phenytoin 400 mg daily suffered phenytoin toxicity after a viral infection; her plasma-phenytoin concentration was found to have increased from 16 µg per mL to 51 µg per mL. Six weeks later she had recovered and was re-stabilised on phenytoin 400 mg daily.— M. Levine and M. W. Jones (letter), *Can. med. Ass. J.*, 1983, *128*, 1270.

INTERACTIONS. A detailed review of drug interactions with phenytoin.— E. Perucca and A. Richens, *Drugs*, 1981, *21*, 120.

Phenytoin affects a number of other drugs including: carbamazepine, chlorpromazine hydrochloride, conjugated oestrogens, corticosteroids, dicoumarol, digoxin, disopyramide, doxycycline hydrochloride, frusemide, haloperidol, levodopa, lithium carbonate, methadone hydrochloride, methoxsalen, mexiletine hydrochloride, misonidazole, oral contraceptives, quinidine, streptozocin, thioridazine, and thyroxine sodium. Information about these interactions may be found under their respective monographs.

Below are some reports of and references to interactions in which phenytoin is affected by other agents.

Anaesthetic agents. A 10-year-old girl with epilepsy who had been treated with phenytoin 100 mg thrice daily for 5 years and who had lateral nystagmus developed symptoms of phenytoin intoxication following anaesthesia with *halothane*. The plasma concentration of phenytoin 72 hours after anaesthesia was 41 µg per mL. It was suggested that temporary liver dysfunction was responsible for impaired metabolism of phenytoin.— J. M. Karlin and H. Kutt, *J. Pediat.*, 1970, *76*, 941.

Analgesics. When *phenyramidol*, 400 mg thrice daily, was given to 5 healthy volunteers who were receiving phenytoin, 100 mg thrice daily, the mean biological half-life of phenytoin was increased from 26 to 55 hours; serum concentrations were correspondingly elevated from an average of 6.6 to 12 µg of phenytoin per mL 12 hours after administration.— H. M. Solomon and J. J. Schrogie, *Clin. Pharmac. Ther.*, 1967, *8*, 554.

Blood-phenytoin concentrations were elevated into the toxic range in a patient taking *dextropropoxyphene* concomitantly.— H. Kutt, *Ann. N.Y. Acad. Sci.*, 1971, *179*, 704. See also B. S. Hansen *et al.*, *Acta neurol. scand.*, 1980, *61*, 357.

Vertigo, anorexia, vomiting, and irreversible cerebellar damage in 2 patients receiving phenytoin, following concurrent administration of *phenylbutazone*.— M. B. Kristensen, *Clin. Pharmacokinet.*, 1976, *1*, 351. Treatment for 3 days with *aspirin, tolfenamic acid*, and *paracetamol* had no significant effect on serum concentrations of phenytoin or carbamazepine in 13 epileptic patients receiving continuous antiepileptic therapy. *Phenylbutazone* significantly lowered serum concentrations of phenytoin but not carbamazepine. When *phenylbutazone* was given for 2 weeks to 6 patients serum concentrations of phenytoin decreased in the first 2 days then increased and after 2 weeks were significantly higher than initial concentrations. It was concluded that aspirin, paracetamol, and tolfenamic acid could be used in moderate doses by epileptics taking phenytoin and carbamazepine. The use of phenylbutazone was not recommended although some patients did tolerate it well.— P. J. Neuvonen *et al.*, *Eur. J. clin. Pharmac.*, 1979, *15*, 263.

An epileptic woman stabilised on phenytoin and primidone developed phenytoin intoxication on receiving *azapropazone*. Azapropazone was considered to have competed for the hepatic metabolism of phenytoin.— C. J. C. Roberts *et al.*, *Postgrad. med. J.*, 1981, *57*, 191. A similar report of phenytoin toxicity in 1 patient following introduction of *azapropazone* and a study in 5 healthy subjects demonstrating raised plasma-phenytoin concentrations. Advice was given that the use of azapropazone should be avoided in patients treated with phenytoin.— D. P. Geaney *et al.*, *Br. med. J.*, 1982, *284*, 1373.

Increased phenytoin concentrations and toxicity in 1 patient previously stabilised on phenytoin after receiving *ibuprofen*. It was suggested that ibuprofen had an inhibitory effect on the hepatic degradation of phenytoin.— R. Sandyk (letter), *S. Afr. med. J.*, 1982, *62*, 592.

Anti-arrhythmics. Phenytoin toxicity with associated increase in serum concentrations occurred in 1 patient 4 weeks after the introduction of *amiodarone* therapy. A displacement of phenytoin from proteins and also a decrease in metabolism or clearance of phenytoin may have accounted for the interaction.— J. M. Gore *et al.*, *Am. J. Cardiol.*, 1984, *54*, 1145. A similar report of increases in phenytoin concentration in 3 patients, with toxicity in only 1, following addition of *amiodarone* to phenytoin therapy.— B. McGovern *et al.*, *Ann. intern. Med.*, 1984, *101*, 650.

Antibiotics. Following addition of *oxacillin* by mouth to the therapeutic regimen of a burnt epileptic woman who was taking phenytoin by mouth, her plasma-phenytoin concentrations showed a very marked drop and she developed status epilepticus. It was considered that the oxacillin might have interfered with the absorption of phenytoin.— R. W. Fincham *et al.*, *Neurology*, 1976, *26*, 879.

A report of decreased serum-phenytoin concentrations with recurrence of seizures in a patient controlled by phenytoin following the addition of *nitrofurantoin* to therapy; the changes were reversed after discontinuation of nitrofurantoin. It was suggested that both increased metabolism and decreased absorption of phenytoin might have taken place.— R. Heipertz and H. Pilz, *J. Neurol.*, 1978, *218*, 297.

Antidepressants. Plasma-phenytoin concentrations rose in 2 epileptic patients also receiving *imipramine* 75 mg daily for about 3 months for endogenous depression. In one patient the concentration gradually increased over several weeks to more than twice the pretreatment figure and he showed mild signs of phenytoin intoxication which remitted after imipramine was stopped.— E. Perucca and A. Richens (letter), *Br. J. clin. Pharmac.*, 1977, *4*, 485.

Increased serum-phenytoin concentration and phenytoin toxicity in one patient possibly precipitated by addition of *trazodone*.— J. M. Dorn, *J. clin. Psychiat.*, 1986, *47*, 89.

Antifungals. Reports of individual patients suffering phenytoin toxicity following the addition of *miconazole* to their therapies.— B. Bourgoin *et al.*, *Thérapie*, 1981, *36*, 347; E. Loupi *et al.*, *ibid.*, 1982, *37*, 437; P. E. Rolan *et al.*, *Br. med. J.*, 1983, *287*, 1760.

Antihistamines. A young woman developed drowsiness, ataxia, diplopia, tinnitus, and episodes of occipital headaches associated with vomiting after concomitant administration of phenytoin sodium and *chlorpheniramine*. Chlorpheniramine might have delayed the hepatic metabolism of phenytoin thereby increasing the plasma concentrations.— R. N. H. Pugh *et al.* (letter), *Br. J. clin. Pharmac.*, 1975, *2*, 173.

Antihypertensives and diuretics. In 2 patients plasma-phenytoin concentrations were raised by *frusemide* given concomitantly and in 1 patient by *propranolol*.— M. J. Eadie and J. H. Tyrer, *Anticonvulsant Therapy*, London, Churchill Livingstone, 1974, p. 64.

A report of severe osteomalacia in 2 active young women taking *acetazolamide* in association with phenytoin or primidone and phenobarbitone.— L. E. Mallette (letter), *New Engl. J. Med.*, 1975, *293*, 668. See also I. Matsuda *et al.*, *J. Pediat.*, 1975, *87*, 202; L. E. Mallette, *Archs intern. Med.*, 1977, *137*, 1013.

In 2 patients with hypoglycaemia associated with hyperinsulinism, therapeutic serum-phenytoin concentrations could not be achieved while they were also receiving *diazoxide*. It was suggested that an increased rate of metabolism, and possibly a decreased binding, of phenytoin induced by diazoxide might have been responsible.— T. F. Roe *et al.*, *J. Pediat.*, 1975, *87*, 480.

Antineoplastics. Plasma concentrations of phenytoin fell during antineoplastic therapy with *cisplatin* and *bleomycin*. Primidone and phenobarbitone concentrations were unaffected. Mucosal damage may have reduced the absorption of phenytoin.— R. W. Fincham and D. D. Schottelius, *Ther. Drug Monit.*, 1979, *1*, 277.

Decreased plasma-phenytoin concentrations with recurrence of seizures in 1 patient after treatment with chemotherapy consisting of *carmustine*, *methotrexate*, and *vinblastine*; concentrations of phenobarbitone were unchanged. It was suggested that impaired absorption of phenytoin, caused by methotrexate or vinblastine or both, was responsible.— P. Bollini *et al.*, *Epilepsia*, 1983, *24*, 75.

Antiprotozoals. Mention that in the author's experience several patients have had toxic phenytoin concentrations after *metronidazole* was added to the regimen.— E. H. Picard (letter), *Mayo Clin. Proc.*, 1983, *58*, 401.

Antituberculous agents. A report from the Boston Collaborative Drug Surveillance Program that about 25% of the recipients of phenytoin who also receive *isoniazid*, experience toxic effects on the CNS, whereas the frequency in patients receiving phenytoin without isoniazid is only about 3%. When isoniazid is added to the therapeutic regimen of a patient receiving phenytoin, a reduction in the dose of phenytoin should be anticipated.— R. R. Russell *et al.*, *Chest*, 1979, *75*, 356.

A patient stabilised on phenytoin experienced a generalised seizure 3 days after starting to take *rifampicin* in addition to vancomycin given intravenously; the blood-phenytoin concentration had fallen markedly.— J. C. Wagner, *Drug Intell. & clin. Pharm.*, 1984, *18*, 497. See also.— L. Kay *et al.*, *Br. J. clin. Pharmac.*, 1985, *20*, 323.

Calcium antagonists. Raised serum-phenytoin concentration with phenytoin toxicity in a patient who had been taking *nifedipine* in addition to phenytoin for 3 weeks; symptoms resolved completely after nifedipine withdrawal. The mechanism of interaction appeared to be complex.— S. Ahmad (letter), *J. Am. Coll. Cardiol.*, 1984, *3*, 1582.

Corticosteroids. Retrospective analysis showing that in a group of 23 patients receiving phenytoin and *dexamethasone* the mean serum-phenytoin concentration was higher (17.28 µg per mL) than that in a group of 15 receiving only phenytoin (12.48 µg per mL).— L. A. Lawson *et al.*, *Surg. Neurol.*, 1981, *16*, 23. Conflicting data from another retrospective study indicating that phenytoin concentrations were routinely lowered when dexamethasone was administered concurrently; in the patients studied the dosage of phenytoin had to be increased.— D. D. Wong *et al.* (letter), *J. Am. med. Ass.*, 1985, *254*, 2062.

Neuroleptics. Increased serum concentration of phenytoin in one patient given concomitant *chlorpromazine*, but no change in another 4.— G. W. Houghton and A. Richens, *Int. J. clin. Pharmac. Biopharm.*, 1975, *12*, 210.

A reduction of serum-phenytoin concentration was reported in 1 patient when he was given *loxapine succinate* 20 mg daily in addition to phenytoin 400 mg daily.— G. M. Ryan and P. A. Matthews (letter), *Drug Intell. & clin. Pharm.*, 1977, *11*, 428.

Toxic concentrations of phenytoin in 2 patients were associated with concomitant administration of *thioridazine*.— F. M. Vincent (letter), *Ann. intern. Med.*, 1980, *93*, 56.

Sulphonamides. In 6 patients the mean half-life of phenytoin was increased from 12.8 to 19.2 hours when *co-trimoxazole* was given concomitantly. Therapeutic doses of *sulphaphenazole, sulphadiazine*, and *sulphamethizole* inhibited the metabolism of phenytoin, but sulphadimethoxine, sulphamethoxypyridazine, and sulphamethoxydiazine did not.— J. M. Hansen *et al.* (letter), *Br. med. J.*, 1975, *2*, 684.

Sympathomimetics. The serum concentrations of phenytoin sodium and primidone were more than doubled in a 5-year-old boy when *methylphenidate* was added to his treatment. The serum concentration of phenobarbitone was also increased but to a lesser degree. No similar effect was seen in 2 other children who were receiving smaller doses of phenobarbitone and phenytoin.— L. K. Garrettson *et al.*, *J. Am. med. Ass.*, 1969, *207*, 2053. Methylphenidate 10 mg thrice daily given in a controlled study over 6-week periods to 11 epileptic patients aged 15 to 53 years was considered to have no significant effect on their plasma-anticonvulsant concentrations.— H. J. Kupferberg *et al.*, *Clin. Pharmac. Ther.*, 1972, *13*, 201.

Vaccines. A study in 16 patients receiving long-term phenytoin therapy showed no significant increases in mean serum-phenytoin concentrations after administration of an inactivated whole-virion trivalent *influenza vaccine* although temporary increases were seen in 4 patients.— M. Levine *et al.*, *Clin. Pharm.*, 1984, *3*, 505.

PORPHYRIAS. A comment that the porphyric patient with either acute or chronic convulsions presents a major therapeutic problem. Convincing clinical experience militates against the use of hydantoins (phenytoin, ethotoin, methoin), carbamazepine, and barbiturates for grand mal seizures, and against oxazolidinediones and succinimides for petit mal attacks. Although there is considerable evidence against the use of sodium valproate, it has sometimes been used without ill-effects. For the control of acute seizures, benzodiazepines, with the possible exception of chlordiazepoxide, could probably be used cautiously if necessary.— M. R. Moore and P. B. Disler, *Adverse Drug React. Ac. Pois. Rev.*, 1983, *2*, 149.

The severity and frequency of convulsive crises and symptoms of acute intermittent porphyria in a 14-year-old epileptic boy were both reduced when treatment with phenobarbitone and phenytoin was replaced by sodium valproate.— R. Biagini *et al.*, *Archs Dis. Childh.*, 1979, *54*, 644. A report of a young woman in whom an acute episode of acute intermittent porphyria was induced by sodium valproate.— J. A. Garcia-Merino and J. J. Lopez-Lozano (letter), *Lancet*, 1980, *2*, 856. Exacerbation in 1 patient of acute intermittent porphyria by valproate.— M. Doss *et al.* (letter), *ibid.*, 1981, *2*, 91.

A report of, and correspondence concerning, the induction of acute porphyria by carbamazepine.— A. A. C. Yeung Laiwah *et al.*, *Lancet*, 1983, *1*, 790; B. C. Shanley (letter), *ibid.*, 1229; A. C. Yeung Laiwah *et al.* (letter), *ibid.*, 1442; J. M. Rideout *et al.* (letter), *ibid.*, *2*, 464; M. R. Moore *et al.* (letter), *ibid.*, 846; M. Doss and H. -J. Schäfer (letter), *ibid.*, 1984, *1*, 1026.

PREGNANCY AND THE NEONATE. For comments on the management of epilepsy in pregnancy, see Epilepsy under Uses and Administration (below).

Absorption and Fate

Phenytoin is slowly but almost completely absorbed from the gastro-intestinal tract with most being absorbed from the upper intestine; the rate of absorption is variable and is reported to be increased by the presence of food. The bioavailability can differ markedly with different pharmaceutical formulations. Absorption from the intramuscular site is even slower than that from the gastro-intestinal tract.

Phenytoin is extensively metabolised in the liver to its primary metabolite, 5-(4-hydroxyphenyl)-5-phenylhydantoin, which is inactive. The rate of metabolism appears to be subject to genetic polymorphism and may also be influenced by racial characteristics. Phenytoin hydroxylation is also capacity-limited, and is therefore readily inhibited by agents which compete for its metabolic pathways. Phenytoin undergoes enterohepatic recycling and is excreted in the urine, mainly as its hydroxylated metabolite, in either free or conjugated form.

Phenytoin is widely distributed throughout the body and is extensively bound (about 90%) to plasma protein. It has a very variable, dose-dependent half-life, but the mean appears to be about 22 hours at steady-state; because phenytoin inhibits its own metabolism it may be several weeks before a steady-state plasma-phenytoin concentration is attained.

Monitoring of plasma concentrations may be performed as an aid in assessing control and the therapeutic range of total plasma-phenytoin is usually quoted as being 10 to 20 µg per mL (40 to 80 µmol per litre); some patients, however, are controlled at concentrations outside this range. It has been suggested that, because of differences in protein binding, measurement of free phenytoin concentrations in plasma may prove more reliable; measurement of concentrations in saliva, which contains only free phenytoin, has also been performed.

Phenytoin crosses the placental barrier and small amounts are excreted in breast milk.

Reviews of the pharmacokinetics of phenytoin: A. Richens, *Clin. Pharmacokinet.*, 1979, *4*, 153; *idem*, 1980, *5*, 402 (correction).

A discussion on the measurement of concentrations of antiepileptic agents.— A. S. Troupin, *Ann. intern. Med.*, 1984, *100*, 854. See also.— D. W. Chadwick, *Br. med. J.*, 1987, *294*, 723. For a study investigating the individual variation of the therapeutic concentrations of some antiepileptic agents, see Epilepsy under Uses (below).

Uses and Administration

Phenytoin is an antiepileptic agent used to control tonic-clonic (grand mal) and partial (focal) seizures; it has also been used for the prophylactic control of seizures developing during or after neurosurgery or following severe traumatic injury to the head. It is believed to stabilise rather than elevate the seizure threshold and to limit the spread of seizure activity.

The dose of phenytoin should be adjusted to the needs of the individual patient to achieve adequate control of seizures and calls for the monitoring of plasma concentrations; in many patients this usually requires total plasma-phenytoin concentrations of 10 to 20 µg per mL (40 to 80 µmol per litre), but some are satisfactorily controlled at concentrations outside this range. The suggested initial dose by mouth of phenytoin or phenytoin sodium is 100 mg three times daily progressively increased to 600 mg daily if necessary; the suggested interval between increments has ranged from about one week to about one month. The usual maintenance dose is 300 to 400 mg daily. A suggested initial dose for children is 5 mg per kg body-weight daily in 2 or 3 divided doses; a suggested maintenance dose is 4 to 8 mg per kg body-weight daily. Young children may require a higher dose per kg body-weight than adults due to more rapid metabolism.

Since phenytoin has a long plasma half-life, a twice-daily dosage regimen is adequate to maintain an effective plasma concentration and is preferred because of improved compliance. Once-daily regimens, usually given at night, are also suitable in some patients receiving formulations of phenytoin known to have a slow rate of dissolution. Different brands of phenytoin, as well as different formulations from the same manufacturer, can vary in their bioavailability and in their rates of dissolution; therefore patients should be maintained on the initial form used for stabilisation, and the need for restabilisation must be understood if a change is envisaged.

The practice of starting phenytoin therapy with initial small doses means that more than a week may be required before therapeutic plasma concentrations are attained; it has been reported that it may even be several weeks before a steady-state concentration is established. Some authorities therefore prefer to give an initial loading dose in order to reach the recommended plasma concentrations sooner. A suggested oral loading dose is 12 to 15 mg per kg body-weight divided into 2 or 3 doses given over about 6 hours, followed by 100 mg three times daily on the following days.

In order to lessen gastric irritation, phenytoin should be taken with at least half a tumblerful of water and may be taken with or after food. The time and manner of taking phenytoin should be standardised for the patient since variations might affect absorption with consequent fluctuations in the plasma concentrations.

If the patient is already taking other antiepileptic drugs, the transition to phenytoin should be made gradually, with some overlapping in dosage, since too rapid withdrawal of these drugs may lead to an increase in frequency of seizures; similarly if patients are transferred from phenytoin to another antiepileptic agent the transition should be gradual. Phenytoin may be given in association with other antiepileptic agents but single-drug therapy is generally preferred unless the patient is suffering from 2 different forms of epilepsy which require control by different drugs.

In the treatment of tonic-clonic status epilepticus a benzodiazepine such as diazepam is usually given initially intravenously followed by the administration of phenytoin sodium intravenously. A suggested dose of phenytoin sodium is 10 to 15 mg per kg body-weight which should be given by slow intravenous injection at a uniform rate of not more than 50 mg per minute; thereafter maintenance doses of 100 mg by mouth or intravenously should be given every 6 to 8 hours. The suggested intravenous dose for children and neonates has ranged from 10 to 20 mg per kg body-weight at a rate not exceeding 1 to 3 mg per kg per minute. Deaths have been caused by the over-rapid intravenous injection of phenytoin sodium and continuous monitoring of the electrocardiogram and blood pressure is recommended whenever phenytoin sodium is given intravenously.

Phenytoin sodium is only very slowly absorbed from the intramuscular site and therefore intramuscular injections are not appropriate for the emergency arrest of status epilepticus. They may, however, in certain situations, be used to maintain or establish therapeutic plasma concentrations of phenytoin in patients who are unconscious or otherwise unable to take phenytoin by mouth. Owing to the slower absorption of phenytoin from intramuscular sites, patients stabilised on the oral route require an increase in the intramuscular dose of about 50%; it is recommended that, if possible, intramuscular injections of phenytoin sodium should not be continued for longer than one week. On transfer back to the oral route the patient should receive 50% of the original oral dose for the same period of time as intramuscular injections were given to allow for continued absorption of the residual phenytoin in the intramuscular sites. In a patient who has not previously received phenytoin sodium a suggested intramuscular dose is 100 to 200 mg.

Phenytoin is also an anti-arrhythmic agent; it is used in the treatment of cardiac arrhythmias, particularly those associated with digitalis intoxication; it is of little or no value in cardiac arrhythmias caused by acute or chronic heart disease. The usual dose is 3.5 to 5 mg per kg body-weight administered by slow intravenous injection at a uniform rate of not more than 50 mg per minute; this dose may be repeated once if necessary.

ADMINISTRATION. *In children and neonates*. The pharmacokinetics of phenytoin given intravenously as the sodium salt to 30 newborn and young infants. The plasma half-life of phenytoin was prolonged and variable in premature infants. At term the half-life was less prolonged and less variable and this pattern of reduction continued in the children aged 2 to 96 weeks. Protein binding appeared to be diminished in infants under 12 weeks of age but thereafter binding was similar to that in the adult. Maintenance treatment with 4 mg per kg body-weight every 12 hours in the first week of life in full-term and premature infants produced some toxic plasma concentrations. No fixed dose could be recommended from these results for infants aged up to 2 weeks although some full-term infants could achieve therapeutic though variable plasma concentrations with 5.9 mg per kg every 24 hours. Most children aged 2 weeks or more would require doses of at least 8 mg per kg every 24 hours with the interval between doses being decreased from 12 to 6 or 8 hours.— P. M. Loughnan *et al.*, *Archs Dis. Childh.*, 1977, *52*, 302.

In the elderly. Pharmacokinetic studies in elderly patients have shown reduced binding to plasma protein which was not itself an indication for dosage change (M. Patterson *et al.*, *Br. J. clin. Pharmac.*, 1982, *13*, 423), but a study showing a decreased metabolism (L.A. Bauer and R.A. Blouin, *Clin. Pharmac. Ther.*, 1982, *31*, 301) did indicate that elderly patients may need lower doses of phenytoin than younger adults to maintain similar serum concentrations.

In hepatic and renal failure. For comments regarding the administration and dosage of phenytoin in hepatic and renal impairment, see Precautions.

Intravenous administration. The manufacturers of commercial preparations of phenytoin sodium do not recommend dilution of intravenous solutions of phenytoin sodium owing to the risk of precipitation of the crystals. Nevertheless, some sources report that they have diluted the intravenous preparation.

For a review of published studies relating to the dilution and administration of solutions of phenytoin sodium for intravenous infusion, see C. B. Tuttle, *Can. J. Hosp. Pharm.*, 1984, *37*, 137.

CONVULSIONS. *Alcohol withdrawal*. Results of a study involving 20 patients with a reliable history of previous alcohol-withdrawal seizures suggested that prophylaxis with phenytoin during alcohol withdrawal was not necessary provided a loading dose of diazepam by mouth was given. It was considered, however, that if a patient was already receiving phenytoin it should not be discontinued abruptly in favour of diazepam and that phenytoin may be indicated in patients with a history of seizures unrelated to alcohol withdrawal.— P. Devenyi and M. L. Harrison, *Can. med. Ass. J.*, 1985, *132*, 798.

EPILEPSY. General reviews on epilepsy and its treatment: D. L. W. Davidson, *Br. med. J.*, 1983, *286*, 2043; A. V. Delgado-Escueta *et al.*, *New Engl. J. Med.*, 1983, *308*, 1508 and 1576; D. Rosenbloom and A. R. M. Upton, *Can. med. Ass. J.*, 1983, *128*, 261; D. L. Schomer, *New Engl. J. Med.*, 1983, *309*, 536; M. J. Eadie, *Drugs*, 1984, *27*, 328; *idem*, *Med. J. Aust.*, 1984, *140*, 591; A. K. Scott, *Br. med. J.*, 1984, *288*, 986; G. Rylance, *Prescribers' J.*, 1986, *26*, 9; *Med. Lett.*, 1986, *28*, 91.

A review and discussion on decisions about when to start and stop treatment in patients with epilepsy. Antiepileptic treatment has sometimes been advocated as prophylaxis in patients with a high prospective risk of epilepsy after injury to the head and after craniotomy for various neurosurgical conditions but no evidence exists that such treatment is effective in either case. After a single seizure most neurologists in the *UK* appear not to treat patients and prefer to wait for evidence of recurrent seizures, whereas in the *USA* there is a greater tendency to treat patients after a single seizure although this appears to be based on defensive medicolegal considerations rather than on evidence of the value of such a policy. If 2 or more seizures occur within a short interval antiepileptic treatment is generally thought to be necessary, but problems arise in defining a short interval. The fact that antiepileptic drugs have been associated with various adverse effects is a potent argument for exploring the possibility of withdrawing drugs in patients who achieve remissions. Comparison of the few available studies that have been undertaken to determine the success of withdrawing treatment is difficult, but overall it seems that about 30% of patients achieving a remission of 2 or 3 years duration will have a recurrence of seizures on withdrawal; most seizures will occur either during the period of reduction in dosage or within 6 months to 1 year after drugs are stopped completely. Until the results of long-term, large, well-organised studies that shed light on the clinical course of epilepsy are known, it will remain uncertain as to what extent the prognosis of epilepsy is determined by its clinical course or by the effects of intervention with antiepileptic drugs.— D. Chadwick and E. H. Reynolds, *Br. med. J.*, 1985, *290*, 1885.

Studies in children with epilepsy to investigate the risk of relapse following withdrawal of therapy and concluding that withdrawal is usually successful except in reasonably well-defined sub-groups: J. H. Thurston *et al.*, *New Engl. J. Med.*, 1982, *306*, 831; S. Shinnar *et al.*, *ibid.*, 1985, *313*, 976.

Choice of antiepileptic agent. A study involving 181 previously untreated recently diagnosed patients with generalised or partial seizures randomised to receive either phenytoin, carbamazepine, or sodium valproate as monotherapy. High optimal serum concentrations were taken to be those in excess of 70 µmol per litre [17.5 µg per mL] for phenytoin, in excess of 30 µmol per litre [7.5 µg per mL] for carbamazepine, and in excess of 500 µmol per litre [71 µg per mL] for sodium valproate. In those patients with generalised tonic-clonic seizures without focal features, control was assessed as excellent (complete freedom from seizures) in 73%, 39%, and 59% receiving phenytoin, carbamazepine, or sodium valproate respectively; as good (greater than 50% reduction in seizure frequency) in 8%, 36%, and 19% respectively; and as poor (no response or less than 50% reduction in seizure frequency) in 19%, 25%, and 22% respectively. The corresponding figures for control in patients with partial seizures (with or without secondary generalised attacks) were: excellent in 57%, 35%, and 44% respectively; good in 19%, 39%, and 33% respectively; and poor in 24%, 26%, and 22% respectively. In 21 patients with a poor response to initial therapy re-randomisation to the second or even third drug was performed and in only 6 was it necessary to resort to combination therapy. It was concluded that all 3 drugs could be prescribed as an anticonvulsant of first choice but that, irrespective of the drug used, partial seizures are less responsive to treatment.— N. Callaghan *et al.*, *J. Neurol. Neurosurg. Psychiat.*, 1985, *48*, 639. Comments, particularly with regard to carbamazepine, stating that the measurement of peak rather than trough concentrations may have been of consequence and that failure to increase the dose of carbamazepine until a trough concentration of 50 µmol per litre [12.5 µg per mL] was attained, or until side-effects occurred, may explain the surprisingly poor performance of carbamazepine in patients with generalised seizures.— J. Duncan (letter), *ibid.*, 1986, *49*, 334. Reply that it was considered unlikely that a further increase in carbamazepine concentrations would have resulted in a significant further improvement but agreement, however, that some patients might have improved further if the dose had been increased to the limits of the patient's tolerance.— N. Callaghan (letter), *ibid.*, 335.

Results of a double-blind multicentre study to compare the efficacy and toxicity of phenytoin, carbamazepine, phenobarbitone, and primidone in patients with previously untreated or undertreated partial and secondarily generalised tonic-clonic seizures. Dosage of the drugs was increased gradually until control of seizures or toxicity occurred. Of 421 patients, 223 were considered to be drug failures due to continuing seizures alone in 11, toxicity alone in 85, or toxicity plus seizures in 127. Failure due to continuing seizures with or without side-effects was similar with all 4 drugs whereas failure due to toxicity alone was greatest with primidone. Acute primidone-induced toxicity was especially common and was associated with nausea, vomiting, dizziness, ataxia, and somnolence. Reports of decreased libido or impotence were also more frequent from patients receiving primidone and many patients refused to allow primidone to be re-instated or continued after their initial adverse experience. Phenobarbitone was associated with the lowest incidence of motor disturbance (ataxia, incoordination, nystagmus, and tremor) early in treatment and the strikingly different rates between the acute side-effects of primidone and phenobarbitone indicated that the two drugs have different actions despite the considerable conversion of primidone to phenobarbitone. Phenytoin caused more dysmorphic and idiosyncratic side-effects (including gum hypertrophy, hirsutism, acne, and rash) than the other drugs; carbamazepine caused no side-effects that were significantly worse than those associated with the other drugs. Comparing efficacy of seizure control, carbamazepine or phenytoin provided better control of partial seizures whereas control of tonic-clonic seizures was similar with all 4 drugs. In conclusion it was recommended that either carbamazepine or phenytoin should be chosen for the initial treatment of partial or secondarily generalised tonic-clonic seizures, but that in children, adolescents, or women, carbamazepine might be preferable because of the dysmorphic potential of phenytoin. If either of these 2 drugs failed then the other should be tried, or, alternatively, a barbiturate; primidone could be considered an alternative in patients who could tolerate the side-effects. It was stressed that overall the adequacy of seizure control in the patients studied was suboptimal even with expert neurological care and the outcome of the project underscored the unsatisfactory status of antiepileptic therapy with the medications currently available.— R. H. Mattson *et al.*, *New Engl. J. Med.*, 1985, *313*, 145.

A study involving 140 patients with previously untreated partial or tonic-clonic seizures showing no major difference in efficacy or in symptoms of toxicity between phenytoin and sodium valproate. Both drugs were relatively ineffective against partial seizures but appeared to suppress primary and secondary generalised seizures with equal efficacy.— D. M. Turnbull *et al.*, *Br. med. J.*, 1985, *290*, 815.

Pregnancy and the neonate. A review and discussion concerning the management of epilepsy in pregnancy. Facial clefts and cleft palate are among the most common foetal abnormalities associated with epilepsy and its treatment and, overall, studies have shown that the children of epileptic mothers taking drugs have approximately twice as many malformations as children of mothers in the population as a whole. Since it is unusual for seizures to recur during pregnancy after a prolonged seizure-free period, an epileptic woman who has had no seizures for two or three years should have antiepileptic therapy gradually withdrawn before any planned pregnancy. If drugs are necessary, the smallest dose compatible with control of seizures should be used but because of considerable changes in the pharmacokinetics during pregnancy this dose may be larger than that required in the non-pregnant state; serum or saliva concentrations should also be monitored regularly. With regard to individual antiepileptic agents, troxidone (now seldom used) has been reported to be strongly teratogenic with affected children having low-set, backwards-sloping ears, V-shaped eyebrows, anomalies of the palate, irregular teeth, and developmental delay. A foetal hydantoin (phenytoin) syndrome has also been reported with children suffering from craniofacial abnormalties, mental retardation, and limb defects such as digital hypoplasia. Similar dysmorphic features, however, have been observed in children of epileptic mothers treated with other drugs or not treated at all and the specificity of these 'syndromes' is in doubt; there is, however, good evidence of a genetic predisposition to congenital abnormalities induced by phenytoin. There is little doubt, though, that sodium valproate is particularly likely to result in neural tube defects. Although there have been few reports of foetal abnormality associated with carbamazepine, this may merely reflect the fact that the drug has been extensively used only in the past 12 years or so. Neonates born to mothers who have received antiepileptic therapy are at an increased risk of haemorrhage due to a deficiency of vitamin K but neonatal haemorrhage can be prevented by giving the mother vitamin K during pregnancy. Significant amounts of antiepileptic drugs do pass into breast milk, the ratio between the concentration in milk and serum being 0.19 for phenytoin, 0.41 for carbamazepine, 0.36 for phenobarbitone, and 0.70 for primidone. In practice, however, phenytoin and carbamazepine have little clinical effect on the neonate and most mothers taking antiepileptics may safely breast feed.— A. Hopkins, *Br. med. J.*, 1987, *294*, 497. For another review and discussion giving a similar overall view, see D. J. Dalessio, *New Engl. J. Med.*, 1985, *312*, 559.

Status epilepticus. A discussion on the management of status epilepticus and suggesting the following protocol for tonic-clonic and complex partial status epilepticus. To control seizures as quickly as possible, diazepam should be administered intravenously at a rate not exceeding 2 mg per minute until seizures stop or to a total of 20 mg. To prevent recurrence of seizures, phenytoin should be given simultaneously via another intravenous line at a rate not exceeding 50 mg per minute to a total of 18 mg per kg body-weight. If seizures persist either phenobarbitone or diazepam may then be employed, but *both* must *not* be used; phenobarbitone may be given intravenously at a rate not exceeding 100 mg per minute until seizures cease or to a loading dose of 20 mg per kg; diazepam may be diluted in a 5% glucose intravenous infusion to give a concentration of 200 µg per mL and administered at a rate of 40 mL per hour. If seizures are still continuing after 1 hour general anaesthesia, with halothane, and neuromuscular blockade are indicated. Alternatively, third-line drugs such as paraldehyde or lignocaine may be used whilst waiting for an anaesthetist. This protocol may be modified by the patient's history and phenytoin is indicated as the initial and sole drug in the management of patients where an alteration in the state of consciousness is contra-indicated. More clinical evaluation is needed to determine whether lorazepam can replace diazepam or phenytoin.— A. V. Delgado-Escueta *et al.*, *New Engl. J. Med.*, 1982, *306*, 1337. Correction.— *ibid.*, *307*, 68. Comments.— M. Blackstone *et al.* (letter), *ibid.*, 1145 (dosage and dilution of diazepam); H. -J. Priebe and C. Simon (letter), *ibid.*, 1146 (caution against the use of halothane and a suggestion for the use of thiopentone); T. J. Poulton (letter), *ibid* (caution against the use of neuromuscular blockade and comments on lorazepam); J. E. Walker and R. W. Homan (letter), *ibid* (lorazepam); S. J. Wilson and B. A. Krumholz (letter), *ibid.*, 1147 (special problems in pregnancy). Reply.— A. V. Delgado-Escueta (letter), *ibid.*

A report of the successful use of phenobarbitone and diazepam to control tonic-clonic status epilepticus in a previously healthy 5-year-old boy which developed after he had placed a Colorado River toad (*Bufo alvarius*) in his mouth. It was suggested that maybe some other cases of idiopathic childhood seizures may also be due to toad-kissing and that if you must kiss toads (to find your prince), then make sure that they are not bufos.— M. Hitt and D. D. Ettinger (letter), *New Engl. J. Med.*, 1986, *314*, 1517.

Therapeutic concentrations. Results of a study on the individual variation of the therapeutic plasma concentrations of phenytoin, carbamazepine, and phenobarbitone in relation to the seizure frequency and type; 84 patients whose epilepsy was completely controlled for at least one year with single-drug therapy were investigated. The plasma concentrations at which complete cessation of all seizures occurred were: phenytoin, a mean of 17.9 µg per mL (range, 3 to 50 µg per mL) in 53 patients; carbamazepine, a mean of 6.5 µg per mL (range, 4.8 to 9.7 µg per mL) in 11 patients; phenobarbitone, a mean of 24.5 µg per mL (range, 3 to 43 µg per mL) in 17 and 3 patients receiving primidone and phenobarbitone respectively. The clinical features in the group of 50 patients whose plasma concentrations were defined as being in the upper range (above 15 µg per mL, 6 µg per mL, and 25 µg per mL for phenytoin, carbamazepine, and phenobarbitone respectively) showed a relative excess of partial epilepsies and complex partial seizures whereas those patients defined as being in the lower range had a relative excess of generalised epilepsies and of generalised tonic-clonic seizures as the only type of seizure. The range of concentrations of carbamazepine and phenobarbitone were similar to those in earlier published reports but for phenytoin, 51% of the patients were controlled with plasma concentrations outside the usually accepted therapeutic range of 10 to 20 µg per mL; 21% needed concentrations below 10 µg per mL and 30% required concentrations above 20 µg per mL for seizure control, thus indicating that strict adherence to an arbitrary upper limit would have denied complete seizure control to these patients.— D. Schmidt and F. Haenel, *Neurology*, 1984, *34*, 1252.

HICCUP. Phenytoin 200 mg given intravenously over 5 minutes abolished persistent refractory hiccup within 1 hour. Treatment was continued with 100 mg four times daily intramuscularly then by mouth for 10 days without recurrence.— D. Petroski and A. N. Patel (letter), *Lancet*, 1974, *1*, 739.

PSYCHIATRIC DISORDERS. Of 10 patients with *compulsive eating* 9 showed improvement after treatment with phenytoin 100 mg two to four times daily. Nine of the 10 had EEG abnormalities.— R. S. Green and J. H. Rau, *Am. J. Psychiat.*, 1974, *131*, 428.

SKIN DISORDERS. *Epidermolysis bullosa.* A favourable but variable clinical response to phenytoin was achieved in patients with recessive dystrophic epidermolysis bullosa. Treatment with phenytoin was begun with a dose of about 3 mg per kg body-weight daily, taken by mouth in 2 divided doses, and the dose adjusted every 10 to 14 days until a blood concentration of at least 8 µg per mL was attained. A reduction in blisters and erosions of more than 45% was achieved in 12 of 17 patients. Studies *in vitro* suggested that the favourable response to phenytoin might result from an inhibition of collagenase expression.— E. A. Bauer *et al.*, *New Engl. J. Med.*, 1980, *303*, 776. Similar favourable reports of phenytoin in recessive dystrophic epidermolysis: T. W. Cooper and E. A. Bauer, *Archs Derm.*, 1984, *120*, 490 (a follow-up of the 17 patients and study of 5 more); M. Kero *et al.*, *Br. J. Derm.*, 1984, *110*, 177 (1 patient).

Preparations of Phenytoin and Phenytoin Sodium

Phenytoin Capsules *(B.P.).* Phenytoin Sodium Capsules

Extended Phenytoin Sodium Capsules *(U.S.P.)*

Prompt Phenytoin Sodium Capsules *(U.S.P.).* Not for once-daily dosing.

Phenytoin Injection *(B.P.).* Phenytoin Sodium Injection. A sterile solution of phenytoin sodium 4.75 to 5.25% containing propylene glycol 40% v/v and alcohol 10% v/v in water for injections. Store at a temperature not exceeding 25°. Protect from light. Solutions which have developed a haze or precipitate should not be used.

Phenytoin Sodium Injection *(U.S.P.).* A sterile solution of phenytoin sodium in propylene glycol, alcohol, and water for injections.

Sterile Phenytoin Sodium *(U.S.P.).* Sterile phenytoin sodium suitable for parenteral use.

Phenytoin Oral Suspension *(B.P.).* Phenytoin Mixture. pH 4.5 to 5.5.

Phenytoin Oral Suspension *(U.S.P.)*

Phenytoin Tablets *(B.P.).* Phenytoin Sodium Tablets. Tablets containing phenytoin sodium. They are either sugar-coated or film-coated.

Phenytoin Tablets *(U.S.P.).* They are to be chewed.

Proprietary Preparations of Phenytoin and Phenytoin Sodium

Epanutin *(Parke, Davis, UK). Capsules,* phenytoin sodium 25, 50, and 100 mg.
Infatabs, chewable tablets, scored, phenytoin 50 mg.
Suspension, phenytoin 30 mg/5 mL.

Epanutin Ready Mixed Parenteral *(Parke, Davis, UK). Injection,* phenytoin sodium 50 mg/mL, in ampoules of 5 mL. Do not add to intravenous infusion solutions.

Proprietary Names and Manufacturers of Phenytoin or Phenytoin Sodium

Antisacer *(Wander, Switz.)*; Citrullamon *(Südmedica, Ger.)*; Dantoin *(Canad.)*; Difhydan *(Leo, Denm.; Swed.)*; Di-Hydan *(Carrion, Fr.)*; Dilantin *(Parke, Davis, Austral.; Parke, Davis, Canad.; Parke, Davis, USA)*; Dintoina *(Recordati, Ital.)*; Diphantoine *(Belg.; Neth.)*; Diphenylan *(Lannett, USA)*; Ditan *(Mallard, USA)*; Epamin *(Parke, Davis, Arg.)*; Epanutin *(Belg.; Parke, Davis, Ger.; Neth.; Norw.; Parke, Davis, S.Afr.; Parke, Davis, Spain; Parke, Davis, Swed.; Parke, Davis, Switz.; Parke, Davis, UK)*; Epilantin *(Switz.)*; Epinat *(Nyco, Norw.)*; Fenantoin *(ACO, Swed.)*; Fenytoin *(Denm.; NAF, Norw.)*; Hydantol *(Jpn)*; Labopal *(Spain)*; Lehydan *(Ferrosan, Swed.)*; Lotoquis Simple *(Paylos, Arg.)*; Neosidantoina *(Squibb, Spain)*; Phénytoïne-Gerot *(Gerot, Switz.)*; Phenhydan *(Desitin, Ger.; Desitin, Switz.)*; Phenhytoin *(Austral.)*; Pyoredol *(Arg.; Roussel, Fr.)*; Solantyl *(Fr.)*; Tacosal *(Switz.)*; Toin Unicelles *(S.Afr.)*; Zentropil *(Nordmark, Ger.)*.

The following names have been used for multi-ingredient preparations containing phenytoin or phenytoin sodium— Dilantin with Phenobarbitone *(Parke, Davis, USA)*; Epanutin with Phenobarbitone *(Parke, Davis, UK)*; Garoin *(May & Baker, UK)*; Mebroin *(Winthrop, Canad.)*; Mysoline with Phenytoin *(ICI Pharmaceuticals, UK)*; Phelantin *(Parke, Davis, Canad.)*; Trinuride *(Bengué, UK)*.

6619-v

Primidone *(BAN, USAN, rINN).*

Hexamidinum; Primaclone. 5-Ethylperhydro-5-phenylpyrimidine-4,6-dione.
$C_{12}H_{14}N_2O_2$=218.3.

CAS — 125-33-7.

Pharmacopoeias. In *Arg., Br., Braz., Chin., Cz., Ind., Int., Jpn, Jug., Nord., Pol., Rus., Turk.,* and *U.S.* Also in *B.P. Vet.*

A white odourless or almost odourless crystalline powder. **Soluble** 1 in 2000 of water and 1 in 200 of alcohol; very slightly soluble or practically insoluble in most organic solvents.

Adverse Effects and Treatment

Side-effects caused by primidone include drowsiness, ataxia, nausea, vomiting, vertigo, irritability, headache, visual disturbances, and weakness or fatigue, and occasionally skin eruptions.

Adverse effects which occur only rarely include personality changes, oedema, thirst, polyuria, a lupus-like disorder, leucopenia, thrombocytopenia, megaloblastic anaemia, and impaired sexual function.

See also under phenobarbitone's adverse effects and their treatment (p.405) since phenobarbitone is one of the main metabolites of primidone.

It was noted that patients receiving primidone for essential tremor have a high incidence of acute adverse reactions following small initial doses. This could be due to the absence of induced hepatic enzymes in these patients previously not exposed to antiepileptics.— L. J. Findley *et al.*, *J. Neurol. Neurosurg. Psychiat.*, 1985, *48*, 911.

CRYSTALLURIA. There have been a few reports of crystalluria associated with acute primidone intoxication. Brillman *et al.* (*Archs Neurol., Chicago*, 1974, *30*, 255) observed masses of shimmering white crystals in the urine of 1 of 2 patients and van Heijst *et al.* (*J. Toxicol. clin. Toxicol.*, 1983, *20*, 307) saw glistening needle-like crystals in the urine of another.

EFFECTS ON THE NERVOUS SYSTEM. Severe flapping tremor, resembling uraemic encephalopathy, with drowsiness and cerebellar signs, was associated with high serum-primidone concentrations in an epileptic woman with poor renal function.— M. B. Forman *et al.* (letter), *Lancet*, 1979, *2*, 1250.

Precautions

As for Phenobarbitone, p.405.

There have been isolated case-reports indicating that metabolism of primidone may be inhibited by concomitant administration of isoniazid, and that acetazolamide may reduce the absorption of primidone.

PREGNANCY AND THE NEONATE. For comments on the management of epilepsy in pregnancy, see Epilepsy under Uses and Administration of phenytoin (p.411).

Absorption and Fate

Primidone is readily absorbed from the gastro-intestinal tract and is reported to have a relatively short plasma half-life compared with those of its principal metabolites phenylethylmalonamide and phenobarbitone.

Primidone is only partially bound to plasma protein; it has been suggested that it exhibits variable binding of about 20 to 25%. It crosses the placenta and is excreted in breast milk.

Uses and Administration

Primidone is an antiepileptic agent which is partially metabolised to phenobarbitone. It may be given by mouth to control tonic-clonic (grand mal) and partial (focal) seizures, and may also be given for some other forms of epilepsy.

Suggested initial doses are up to 125 mg daily increased, if necessary, by up to 125 mg every 3 days to a total of 500 mg daily; further increments, if necessary, every 3 days, of up to 250 mg or of up to 125 mg in children under 9 years of age, may then be given, up to a total dose of 1.5 to 2 g daily in adults or 1 g daily in children. Usual maintenance doses in adults and children over 9 years of age are 0.75 to 1.5 g daily. Suggested maintenance doses for children up to 2 years are 250 to 500 mg daily, for children aged 2 to 5 years 500 to 750 mg daily, and for children aged 6 to 9 years 0.75 to 1 g daily. Initial treatment is usually given as a single dose in the late evening; divided doses are used for maintenance treatment with primidone.

Withdrawal of primidone or transition to or from another type of antiepileptic therapy should be made gradually to avoid precipitating an increase in the frequency of seizures.

Primidone has been tried in the management of essential tremor.

ADMINISTRATION IN RENAL FAILURE. Primidone could be administered to patients with renal failure by adjusting the dosage interval. A dosage interval of 8 hours is suitable for patients whose glomerular filtration-rate exceeds 50 mL per minute; an interval of 8 to 12 hours between doses is advisable for rates of between 10 and 50 mL per minute; where the rate is less than 10 mL per minute, the dosage interval should be 12 to 24 hours. A dose supplement should be given to patients undergoing haemodialysis.— W. M. Bennett *et al.*, *Am. J. Kidney Dis.*, 1983, *3*, 155.

EPILEPSY. For general comments concerning the use of primidone in epilepsy, see under Phenytoin Sodium, p.410.

TREMOR. A review of essential tremor and its treatment. There is no completely satisfactory treatment; many mildly affected patients do not require regular medication and are content with reassurance. Traditionally drug treatment has relied on the use of sedatives and minor tranquillisers but their effect is nonspecific and proportional to the degree of sedation achieved. Phenobarbitone was one of the earliest treatments but there have been very few clinical studies to assess its efficacy. Several clinical studies, however, have established the usefulness of primidone in essential tremor (M.D. O'Brien *et al.*, *Br. med. J.*, 1981, *282*, 178; A. Chakrabarti and J.M.S. Pearce, *J. Neurol. Neurosurg. Psychiat.*, 1981, *44*, 650). Primidone though is poorly tolerated by a high proportion of patients; Findley *et al.* (*J. Neurol. Neurosurg. Psychiat.*, 1985, *48*, 911) while reporting a beneficial response with primidone in a placebo-controlled study also reported that 5 of 22 patients exhibited an acute toxic reaction after the first 62.5-mg dose.— L. J. Findley, *Br. J. Hosp. Med.*, 1986, *35*, 388.

In a dose-response study primidone reduced tremor amplitude, though not frequency, to a greater extent than did propranolol and patients reported subjective improvement; phenobarbitone was ineffective. It was recommended that treatment of essential tremor should start with primidone 50 mg at bedtime, increased gradually to 250 mg. Propranolol 40 mg three times daily should then be added and the dose increased to 320 mg daily if the response remained inadequate. This regimen frequently resulted in tremor reduction and increased functional abilities.— W. C. Koller and V. L. Royse, *Neurology*, 1986, *36*, 121.

Preparations

Primidone Oral Suspension *(B.P.)*. Primidone Mixture. A suspension of primidone in a suitable flavoured vehicle.

Primidone Oral Suspension *(U.S.P.)*. Contains 4.5 to 5.5% of primidone in a suitable aqueous vehicle; pH 5.5 to 7.0. Store in airtight containers. Protect from light.

Primidone Tablets *(B.P.)*

Primidone Tablets *(U.S.P.)*

Proprietary Preparations

Mysoline *(ICI Pharmaceuticals, UK)*. *Tablets*, scored, primidone 250 mg.
Suspension, primidone 250 mg/5 mL.

Proprietary Names and Manufacturers

Dilon *(Arg.)*; Liskantin *(Desitin, Ger.)*; Majsolin *(Jug.)*; Midone *(Protea, Austral.)*; Mylepsin *(ICI, Swed.)*; Mylepsinum *(ICI, Ger.)*; Mysoline *(ICI, Austral.; Belg.; Ayerst, Canad.; ICI, Denm.; I.C.I.-Pharma, Fr.; ICI-Pharma, Ital.; Neth.; ICI, Norw.; ICI, S.Afr.; ICI, Spain; ICI, Switz.; ICI Pharmaceuticals, UK; Ayerst, USA)*; Prosoline *(Israel)*; Resimatil *(Labaz, Ger.)*; Sertan *(Pharmascience, Canad.)*.

The following names have been used for multi-ingredient preparations containing primidone— Mysoline with Phenytoin *(ICI Pharmaceuticals, UK)*.

16968-t

Progabide *(BAN, USAN, rINN)*.

Halogabide; SL-76002. 4-(4'-Chloro-5-fluoro-2-hydroxybenzhydrylideneamino)butyramide.
$C_{17}H_{16}ClFN_2O_2$=334.8.

CAS — 62666-20-0.

Progabide is a GABA agonist and is used as an antiepileptic agent to control tonic-clonic (grand mal) and partial (focal) seizures. The usual dose by mouth for adults is 25 to 35 mg per kg body-weight daily in divided doses.

A review of progabide including studies in epilepsy, spasticity, and movement disorders.— K. J. Bergmann, *Clin. Neuropharmacol.*, 1985, *8*, 13.

Further references: P.L. Morselli *et al.*, Progabide, in *New Anticonvulsant Drugs*, B.S. Meldrum and R.J. Porter (Ed.), London, John Libbey & Co. Ltd, 1986, p.237.

Proprietary Names and Manufacturers

Gabrene *(Synthelabo, Fr.)*.

6621-f

Sulthiame *(BAN, USAN)*.

Sultiame *(rINN)*. 4-(Tetrahydro-2*H*-1,2-thiazin-2-yl)benzenesulphonamide *SS*-dioxide.
$C_{10}H_{14}N_2O_4S_2$=290.4.

CAS — 61-56-3.

Pharmacopoeias. In *Br.*

A white odourless or almost odourless crystalline powder. Very slightly **soluble** in water; slightly soluble in alcohol, chloroform, and ether.

Sulthiame is a carbonic anhydrase inhibitor that was formerly used as an antiepileptic agent in most forms of epilepsy except absence (petit mal) seizures. It was usually given in conjunction with other antiepileptic agents and it is believed that much of its activity was due to the inhibition of metabolism of the other agents. Sulthiame was given in initial doses of 100 mg twice daily gradually increased to 200 mg three times daily. A suggested dose for children was 3 to 5 mg per kg body-weight daily in equal divided doses, gradually increased to 10 to 15 mg per kg daily in equal divided doses. Adverse effects that were reported with sulthiame included paraesthesia, hyperpnoea, gastric disturbances, headache, and vertigo, and following overdosage, crystalluria and renal impairment. Caution was advised in giving sulthiame to patients with renal impairment.

Preparations

Sulthiame Tablets *(B.P.)*

Proprietary Names and Manufacturers

Ospolot *(Bayer, Austral.; Bayer, Denm.; Bayer, Ger.; Bayropharm, Ital.; Neth.; S.Afr.; Bayer, Spain; Bayer, UK)*.

6622-d

Troxidone *(BAN)*.

Trimethadione *(USAN, rINN)*; Trimethadionum; Trimethinum; Troxid. 3,5,5-Trimethyloxazolidine-2,4-dione.
$C_6H_9NO_3$=143.1.

CAS — 127-48-0.

Pharmacopoeias. In *Braz., Br., Cz., Egypt., Eur., Fr., Ind., Int., It., Jpn, Jug., Mex., Neth., Nord., Rus., Swiss, Turk.*, and *U.S.*

Colourless or white granular crystals with a slightly camphoraceous odour. M.p. 45° to 47°. **Soluble** 1 in 13 of water; freely soluble in alcohol, chloroform, and ether. **Store** in airtight containers. Protect from light.

Adverse Effects

Many adverse effects of troxidone are serious and call for prompt discontinuation of therapy. Common side-effects include drowsiness, which may subside on continuation of therapy, and photophobia and hemeralopia (blurring of vision in bright light), which is more frequent in adults and may respond to reduced dosage.

Other side-effects include nausea and vomiting, gastric distress, abdominal pain, anorexia, weight loss, hiccups, malaise, insomnia, vertigo, headache, alopecia, paraesthesias, changes in blood pressure, and personality changes. Blood disorders include neutropenia (which does not call for withdrawal of therapy providing it remains moderate), thrombocytopenia, pancytopenia, agranulocytosis, and aplastic anaemia. Lymphadenopathy, a lupus erythematosus syndrome, the nephrotic syndrome, and hepatitis may also occur. Skin rashes may lead to exfoliative dermatitis and erythema multiforme. A syndrome resembling myasthenia gravis has also been reported.

Symptoms of acute overdosage include drowsiness, nausea, dizziness, ataxia, visual disturbances, and coma.

Characteristic congenital malformations, termed the foetal troxidone syndrome, have been associated with the use of troxidone in pregnancy. For some references to individual case reports see below, and for comments regarding the management of the pregnant epileptic patient see the section on epilepsy under the uses and administration of phenytoin.

PREGNANCY AND THE NEONATE. An account of the offspring of 3 mothers who took troxidone during pregnancy. The children were considered to have a specific phenotype associated with intra-uterine exposure to troxidone which was termed 'the foetal troxidone syndrome'. Common features of the foetal troxidone syndrome included mild mental retardation, speech difficulty, V-shaped eyebrows, epicanthus, low-set backward sloped ears with anteriorly folded helix, palatal anomaly, and teeth irregularities. Less common features included intra-uterine growth retardation, short stature, microcephaly, cardiac anomaly, ocular anomaly, hypospadias, inguinal hernia, and simian crease.— E. H. Zackai *et al.*, *J. Pediat.*, 1975, *87*, 280.

Comment on the high incidence of congenital malformations associated with the use of troxidone in pregnancy. It is stressed that troxidone and paramethadione should be abandoned for petit mal epilepsy in the fecund woman.— S. Fabro and N. A. Brown (letter), *New Engl. J. Med.*, 1979, *300*, 1280.

Precautions

Troxidone is contra-indicated in patients with severe hepatic or renal disease or with severe blood disorders. It should be used with caution in patients with disease of the retina or optic nerve and should be withdrawn if scotomata occur.

Frequent examinations of blood, urine, and hepatic function should be carried out in patients receiving troxidone, and therapy should be withdrawn promptly at signs of renal or hepatic dysfunction, severe neutropenia or other blood disorders, or drug hypersensitivity. Patients receiving troxidone should be instructed to report immediately symptoms of infection or bleeding tendency, such as sore throat or easy bruising.

Troxidone should also be discontinued, at least temporarily, on the appearance of any skin disorder, however mild.

Administration of troxidone in pregnancy has been associated with a high incidence of congenital malformations.

PORPHYRIAS. For comments on the use of oxazolidinediones in porphyrias, see Phenytoin Sodium, p.409.

PREGNANCY AND THE NEONATE. For comments on the management of epilepsy in pregnancy, see Epilepsy under Uses and Administration of phenytoin (p.411).

Absorption and Fate

Troxidone is readily absorbed from the gastro-intestinal tract and extensively metabolised in the liver to its active metabolite, dimethadione, which is primarily responsible for the activity of troxidone on chronic administration.

Troxidone is very slowly excreted in the urine, over a period of several days, almost entirely in the form of dimethadione.

Troxidone is reported not to be significantly bound to plasma proteins.

Some correlation has been found between plasma concentrations of dimethadione exceeding 700 µg per mL and therapeutic response.

Uses and Administration

Troxidone is an oxazolidinedione antiepileptic agent used in the treatment of absence (petit mal) seizures. Because of its potential toxicity it is given only to patients unresponsive to other treatment.

The initial dose of troxidone is 900 mg daily in divided doses, increased by steps of 300 mg at intervals of one week, according to the patient's response, to a recommended maximum dose of 2.4 g daily. Suggested doses of troxidone for children are 300 to 900 mg daily.

Withdrawal of troxidone or transition to or from another type of antiepileptic therapy should be made gradually to avoid precipitating an increase in the frequency of seizures.

Suggested use of troxidone to dissolve pancreatic stones.— A. Noda *et al.* (letter), *Lancet*, 1984, *2*, 351.

Preparations

Trimethadione Capsules *(U.S.P.)*. Capsules containing troxidone.

Trimethadione Oral Solution *(U.S.P.)*. An aqueous solution of troxidone.

Trimethadione Tablets *(U.S.P.)*. Tablets containing troxidone.

Proprietary Names and Manufacturers

Tridione *(Austral.; Belg.; Denm.; Abbott, Ger.; S.Afr.; Spain; Switz.; Abbott, UK; Abbott, USA)*; Trimedone *(Canad.)*; Trioxanona *(Spain)*.

6623-n

Valproic Acid *(BAN, USAN, rINN)*.

Abbott-44089. 2-Propylvaleric acid; 2-Propylpentanoic acid.

$C_8H_{16}O_2$=144.2.

CAS — 99-66-1.

Pharmacopoeias. In *It.* and *U.S.*

A colourless to pale yellow, slightly viscous, clear liquid with a characteristic odour. Slightly **soluble** in water; freely soluble in acetone, alcohol, chloroform, ether, and methyl alcohol. **Store** in airtight glass containers.

16983-a

Semisodium Valproate *(BAN)*.

Abbott-50711; Divalproex Sodium *(USAN)*; Valproate Semisodium *(rINN)*. 2-Propylvaleric acid sodium 2-propylvalerate; Sodium hydrogen bis(2-propylvalerate).

$C_{16}H_{31}NaO_4$=310.4.

CAS — 76584-70-8.

6608-h

Sodium Valproate *(BANM, rINNM)*.

Abbott-44090; Valproate Sodium *(USAN)*. Sodium 2-propylvalerate; Sodium 2-propylpentanoate.

$C_8H_{15}NaO_2$=166.2.

CAS — 1069-66-5.

Pharmacopoeias. In *Br.*

A white or almost white, odourless or almost odourless, crystalline, deliquescent, powder. **Soluble** 1 in 5 of water and of alcohol. **Store** in well-closed containers.

2480-c

Valproate Pivoxil *(rINN)*.

Hydroxymethyl 2-propylvalerate pivalate.

$C_{14}H_{26}O_4$=258.4.

CAS — 77372-61-3.

6624-h

Valpromide *(rINN)*.

Dipropylacetamide. 2-Propylvaleramide.

$C_8H_{17}NO$=143.2.

CAS — 2430-27-5.

Adverse Effects

Nausea, vomiting, gastro-intestinal irritation, increased appetite and excessive weight gain, drowsiness, ataxia, oedema, and transient alopecia with regrowth of curly hair, have been reported with valproic acid or its sodium salt. Tremor, reversible prolongation of bleeding time, and thrombocytopenia may occur, particularly with high doses.

Liver dysfunction including hepatic failure has occasionally been reported, usually in the first few months of treatment, and necessitates withdrawal of valproic acid; there have been fatalities. Pancreatitis has also been reported.

Although congenital malformations have been reported in infants born to women who had received antiepileptic agents including valproic acid during pregnancy the direct causal role for some of these drugs has been debated due to the fact that combined therapy was often employed. For some references to individual case reports see below, and for comments regarding the management of the pregnant epileptic patient see the section on epilepsy under the uses and administration of phenytoin.

A review of the adverse effects of valproate.— D. M. Turnbull, *Adverse Drug React. Ac. Pois. Rev.*, 1983, *2*, 191.

A study of side-effects in 88 paediatric patients receiving sodium valproate monotherapy. Side-effects were present in 71 children and, although average doses in these patients were significantly higher than in the 17 with no side-effects, no difference in the plasma concentrations was observed between the 2 groups. Behavioural alterations were seen in 56 and included irritability, longer and deeper sleep, superficial sleep, hyperactivity, being more alert, lassitude, drowsiness, being more sociable, calmness, being happier, absent mindedness, being sadder, aggressiveness, being more skilful, and docility; it was emphasised that stimulatory reactions were as frequent as depressant effects. Digestive disorders occurred in 43 children with anorexia, abdominal pain, and nausea and vomiting being the most frequent; diarrhoea, constipation, an increase in appetite, and a gain in weight also occurred. Neurological changes in the form of tremor, paraesthesia, or ataxia, occurring in only 4 patients, were less frequent than either behavioural or digestive reactions. Miscellaneous reactions including polydipsia, polyuria, diaphoresis, enuresis, hair loss, change in hair colour or texture, and rash were seen in 23 children. Of the 71 children experiencing reactions therapy continued unchanged in 56, was changed either by altering the pharmaceutical formulation, by changing the frequency of dosing, or by reducing the dose in 6, and in the remaining 9 children valproate therapy was discontinued. None of the patients, with the exception of a temporary increase in plasma transaminase concentrations in 2, showed hepatic or pancreatic dysfunction.— J. L. Herranz *et al.*, *Epilepsia*, 1982, *23*, 203.

EFFECTS ON THE BLOOD. Pure red cell aplasia in 1 child on 2 occasions appeared to be associated with the administration of sodium valproate; in both instances the aplasia resolved promptly after drug withdrawal.— L. G. MacDougall, *J. Am. med. Ass.*, 1982, *247*, 53.

In a 1-year prospective study involving 45 patients receiving valproic acid absolute neutropenia developed in 12 and thrombocytopenia in 15 but in all cases the disorders were transient and self-limiting despite continued drug administration.— R. D. Barr *et al.*, *Archs Dis. Childh.*, 1982, *57*, 681. A report of severe neutropenia in a child which necessitated withdrawal of sodium valproate.— D. N. K. Symon and G. Russell (letter), *ibid.*, 1983, *58*, 235.

EFFECTS ON THE LIVER. A review of the hepatotoxicity of sodium valproate including analysis of the known 42 cases with fatal hepatitis, the 3 reported cases with a Reye's-like syndrome, and 22 instances of hyperammonaemia. In 19 clinical trials the incidence of abnormal serum aminotransferase activity has ranged from 0 to 44% with an overall incidence of 11% in the 1197 patients monitored; in the non-fatal cases activity was usually between one and three times the upper limit of normal and was not usually, except in the most severe cases, accompanied by rises in serum bilirubin or alkaline phosphatase. In the 42 cases of hepatitis with a fatal outcome the age at presentation ranged from 2.5 months to 34 years with 69% aged 10 years or less. Below the age of 15 years the proportion of males was 62.5% but above this age it was 30%; the disproportionate vulnerability of young individuals, particularly boys, does not appear to be a reflection of prescribing habits in that age group. In more than two-thirds of these patients with a fatal outcome, prodromal symptoms comprised anorexia and vomiting, loss of epilepsy control, impaired consciousness, and ataxia; in about one-third there were signs of liver damage with fever, jaundice, ascites, peripheral oedema, and easy bruising. In all of the patients hepatic coma developed. In 36 patients on whom data was available the onset of hepatic illness in one-third occurred between 1 and 2 months and in only 2 patients did the onset occur after more than 5 months. Of these 42 patients with fatal hepatotoxicity 36 had received other drugs, mostly anticonvulsants, concurrently. The 3 children with the Reye's-like syndrome all died within 3 weeks of the first occurrence of symptoms as a result of cerebral oedema (2) or aspiration pneumonia (1). In the 22 patients with symptomatic hyperammonaemia, characterised usually by impaired consciousness and ataxia, but without overt liver disease, withdrawal of valproate resulted in all becoming asymptomatic and biochemical abnormalties returned to normal. Hyperammonaemia has also been reported in asymptomatic patients. It was considered by the authors that measurement of serum aminotransferase would be of most value during the first three months of therapy and should be mandatory in the apparently predisposed patient with mental retardation, structural brain damage, or metabolic disorders and particular care should be given to those patients on multiple drug therapy. Testing at monthly intervals would then be reasonable and in those patients in whom an abnormality of aminotransferase developed the dose of valproate should be reduced and if values failed to normalise or continued to rise drug therapy should be withdrawn. It was felt likely though, that despite these precautions, a small number of severe reactions related to individual idiosyncrasy would not be prevented.— P. R. Powell-Jackson *et al.*, *Gut*, 1984, *25*, 673. A comment that, although the frequency of fatal liver failure has been previously estimated to be 1 in 20 000 patients, an analysis of cases in the southern part of West Germany revealed that the rate may be around 1 in 5 000. Until this recent estimate is shown to be wrong it is considered that it will be hard to justify the continued use of valproic acid as a drug of first choice in children with generalised epilepsies.— D. Scheffner (letter), *Lan-*

cet, 1986, *2*, 511. Analysis of cases in the *USA* over a 6-year period gave a total fatality-rate of 1 in 10 700, or 1 in 37 500 when valproate was the only drug used. The warning by Scheffner is inappropriate if the following precautions are taken: avoid polytherapy in children under 3 years if possible; avoid where there is a family history of childhood hepatic disease; use as low a dose as possible; avoid salicylates; do not give valproate to fasting children with intercurrent illness; maintain careful surveillance for untoward symptoms especially after febrile illness.— F. E. Dreifuss (letter), *ibid.*, 1987, *1*, 47.

EFFECTS ON THE NERVOUS SYSTEM. Tremor occurred in 4 patients taking sodium valproate and other anticonvulsants.— N. M. Hyman *et al.*, *Neurology*, 1979, *29*, 1177.

An extrapyramidal syndrome, unresponsive to benztropine or benzhexol, developed in a 52-year-old man with schizophrenia given a therapeutic trial of sodium valproate 1 to 2 g daily.— A. Lautin *et al.*, *Br. med. J.*, 1979, *2*, 1035. Administration of sodium valproate to a man with dystonic movements of the neck and spine produced a severe subjective and objective deterioration in his symptoms which returned to their previous severity on withdrawal of the drug.— D. J. Dick and M. Saunders (letter), *ibid.*, 1980, *280*, 189.

Description of a stuporous state associated with EEG abnormalities in 7 patients during valproic acid therapy for complex partial seizures. It was suggested that in certain forms of epilepsy valproic acid may exhibit a paradoxical epileptogenic effect.— C. Marescaux *et al.*, *Epilepsia*, 1982, *23*, 297.

EFFECTS ON THE PANCREAS. A report of pancreatitis associated with valproic acid therapy in 4 patients and a review of 10 previously published cases; none of the 14 patients suffered other symptoms of a toxic reaction to valproic acid. Pancreatitis was not a dose-related complication and had developed as early as one week and as late as 4.5 years following the introduction of therapy. Of the 14 patients 2 died; seven have been rechallenged with valproic acid and of these, 6 have had recurrence of pancreatitis. It would seem, therefore, that the development of valproic acid-induced pancreatitis is a relative contra-indication to further therapy but routine monitoring of serum-amylase concentrations in asymptomatic patients is not necessary.— E. Wyllie *et al.*, *Am. J. Dis. Child.*, 1984, *138*, 912.

Further reports of pancreatitis associated with valproic acid: L. H. P. Williams *et al.*, *Archs Dis. Childh.*, 1983, *58*, 543 (death of 1 child); A. M. Baskies, *J. med. Soc. New Jers.*, 1984, *81*, 399 (pancreatic pseudocyst secondary to pancreatitis in 1 adult).

EFFECTS ON THE SKIN. Five out of 250 patients developed curly hair during treatment with sodium valproate 1 g daily; in 3 patients this effect followed temporary alopecia.— P. M. Jeavons *et al.* (letter), *Lancet*, 1977, *1*, 359.

A report of valproate-induced nicotinic-acid deficiency with an associated pellagra-like syndrome in a young boy; the condition responded dramatically to the administration of nicotinamide.— M. A. Gillman and R. Sandyk (letter), *S. Afr. med. J.*, 1984, *65*, 986.

Reduced serum-zinc concentrations and cutaneous manifestations of zinc deficiency were found in 2 patients receiving antiepileptic drugs. It was postulated that deficiency occurred as a result of chelation by sodium valproate, and possibly phenytoin, in association with malabsorption and that, in one case, malabsorption was initiated by valproate.— M. S. Lewis-Jones *et al.*, *Br. med. J.*, 1985, *290*, 603.

ENURESIS. A report of nocturnal enuresis associated with sodium valproate therapy in 2 children. Remission of the enuresis was achieved either by reducing or redistributing the doses.— C. P. Panayiotopoulos (letter), *Lancet*, 1985, *1*, 980. Comment that several studies have recorded enuresis as a side-effect of valproate in children, the frequency being between 1 and 7%. The 2 most likely explanations are that it is secondary to a central effect on the thirst centre resulting in polydipsia or is a consequence of the increased depth of sleep associated with valproate.— I. A. Choonara (letter), *ibid.*, 1276.

HYPERGLYCINAEMIA. Hyperglycinaemia associated with sodium valproate.— J. Jaeken *et al.* (letter), *Lancet*, 1977, *2*, 617. See also K. Bartlett (letter), *ibid.*, 716; B. Wolf (letter), *Lancet*, 1978, *2*, 369. Nonketotic hyperglycinaemia should not be considered to be a contra-indication to the use of sodium valproate. Two patients with this condition received sodium valproate without any increase in the concentrations of glycine in the CSF (considered to be the cause of encephalopathy in nonketotic hyperglycinaemia).— K. MacDermot *et al.*, *Pediatrics*, 1980, *65*, 624.

PREGNANCY AND THE NEONATE. Pooled data from 13 study groups showed that neural tube defects occurred in 6 of 393 infants exposed to valproic acid compared to 6 of 1718 infants exposed to other antiepileptic agents. It was concluded that this collaborative study confirmed that exposure to valproic acid in the first trimester of pregnancy is causally associated with a considerably increased risk of neural tube defects and that the use of valproic acid during pregnancy should be avoided.— D. Lindhout and D. Schmidt (letter), *Lancet*, 1986, *1*, 1393.

Some further references to congenital abnormalities associated with valproic acid: E. Robert and P. Guibaud (letter), *Lancet*, 1982, *2*, 937; T. Bjerkedal *et al.* (letter), *ibid.*, 1096 and 1172; O. H. Stanley and T. L. Chambers (letter), *ibid.*, 1282; P. M. Jeavons (letter), *ibid;* E. Castilla (letter), *ibid.*, 1983, *2*, 683; E. Robert and F. Rosa (letter), *ibid.*, 1142; P. Mastroiacovo *et al.* (letter), *ibid.*, 1499; D. Lindhout and H. Meinardi (letter), *ibid.*, 1984, *2*, 396; E. Robert *et al.* (letter), *ibid.*, 1392; J. H. DiLiberti *et al.*, *Am. J. med. Genet.*, 1984, *19*, 473; A. S. Garden *et al.*, *Can. med. Ass. J.*, 1985, *132*, 933.

Treatment of Adverse Effects

The stomach should be emptied by aspiration and lavage, although it has been suggested that gastric lavage may be of limited value in view of the rapid absorption of valproic acid. Supportive therapy alone may then suffice for patients who are not severely poisoned.

A report of survival following supportive measures only for the treatment of severe self-poisoning with sodium valproate. Although a variety of active treatments including forced diuresis, naloxone, and haemodialysis or haemoperfusion have been advocated this case lends support to the view that questions the need for, and the efficacy of, such active measures.— M. Lakhani and M. E. T. McMurdo, *Postgrad. med. J.*, 1986, *62*, 409.

Precautions

Patients should be monitored for platelet function before and during valproic acid therapy and before elective surgery; valproic acid should be withdrawn if patients develop bruising or bleeding. Liver function tests should also be carried out before starting therapy, during the first 6 months of therapy, and when dosage is being increased. Valproic acid should be discontinued if signs of liver dysfunction occur, and should not be given to patients with pre-existing liver disease. It has also been recommended that pancreatic function be monitored.

Valproic acid is extensively bound to plasma proteins and is therefore susceptible to interactions with drugs liable to compete for similar binding sites; for a comment on the relevance of this type of interaction, see Phenytoin, Precautions, p.408. It should be noted, however, that the protein binding of valproic acid is saturable and thus shows concentration dependency with significant increases in free drug occurring at high total plasma concentrations.

Concomitant administration of hepatic enzyme inducers, such as phenytoin, carbamazepine, or phenobarbitone, may enhance the metabolism of valproic acid whereas, in turn, valproic acid has been reported to cause rises in phenobarbitone (and primidone) concentrations in plasma. The interaction between valproic acid and phenytoin is complex and involves inhibition of phenytoin metabolism as well as competition for protein binding sites. Unlike phenytoin and carbamazepine, valproic acid does not induce hepatic enzymes and is therefore unlikely to cause interactions which are dependent upon this mechanism of action. Caution is recommended when administering valproic acid with other drugs liable to interfere with blood coagulation, such as aspirin or warfarin.

Sodium valproate, because it is partly excreted in the form of ketone bodies, may cause false positives in urine tests for diabetes mellitus.

An opinion that valproic acid should not be given to patients with inherited disorders of straight-chain fatty acid metabolism as it is likely to be unusually toxic.— R. J. Pollitt, *Archs Dis. Childh.*, 1987, *62*, 6.

DRIVING. For a comment on valproate and driving, see Phenytoin, p.408.

INTERACTIONS. A review of drug interactions with valproic acid.— R. H. Levy and K. M. Koch, *Drugs*, 1982, *24*, 543.

PORPHYRIAS. For comments on the use of sodium valproate in porphyrias, see Phenytoin Sodium, p.409.

PREGNANCY AND THE NEONATE. For comments on the management of epilepsy in pregnancy, see Epilepsy under Uses and Administration of phenytoin (p.411).

Absorption and Fate

Valproic acid and its salts are rapidly and completely absorbed from the gastro-intestinal tract; the rate, but not the extent, of absorption is delayed by administration with or after food.

Valproic acid is extensively metabolised in the liver. It does not appear to have the property of enhancing its own metabolism, but metabolism may be enhanced by other drugs which induce hepatic microsomal enzymes. It is excreted in the urine almost entirely in the form of its metabolites.

Valproic acid is extensively bound (about 90%) to plasma protein. Reported half-lives for valproic acid have ranged from about 5 to 20 hours; the shorter half-lives have generally been recorded in epileptic patients receiving multiple drug therapy and the longer half-lives in healthy subjects or patients receiving valproate alone.

The therapeutic range of total plasma-valproic acid is usually quoted as being 40 to 100 μg per mL (280 to 700 μmol per litre) but routine monitoring of plasma concentrations is not generally considered to be of use as an aid to assessing control.

Valproic acid crosses the placental barrier and small amounts are excreted in breast milk.

Uses and Administration

Valproic acid is an antiepileptic agent used in the treatment of various forms of epilepsy, including absence (petit mal) seizures. Its mode of action in epilepsy is not fully understood but may involve a modification of the behaviour of gamma-aminobutyric acid in the brain.

Valproic acid can be given in a variety of forms including the sodium salts (semisodium valproate and sodium valproate), the amide derivative (valpromide), or as valproic acid itself. The dose should be adjusted to the needs of the individual patient to achieve adequate control of seizures; a limited correlation with plasma concentrations has indicated that total plasma concentrations of valproic acid of 40 to 100 μg per mL (approximately 280 to 700 μmol per litre) are usually necessary. A suggested initial oral dose of sodium valproate in the *UK* is 600 mg daily in divided doses, increased every 3 days by 200 mg daily to a usual range of 1 to 2 g daily (20 to 30 mg per kg body-weight daily); further increases to a maximum of 2.5 g daily may be necessary if adequate control has not been achieved. A suggested initial dose for children weighing more than 20 kg is 400 mg daily (irrespective of weight) in divided doses, gradually increased until control is achieved, with a usual range of 20 to 30 mg per kg daily; children weighing less than 20 kg may be given 20 mg per kg daily, which may be increased to 40 mg per kg in severe cases; it has been recommended that the dose of 40 mg per kg should only be exceeded in patients whose plasma concentrations, clinical chemistry, and haematological parameters are being monitored. In the *USA* doses are expressed in terms of valproic acid and in general appear to be higher than those recommended in the *UK*. A suggested initial dose in the *USA* is 15 mg per kg daily increased at one-week intervals by 5 to 10 mg per kg daily to a maximum of 60 mg per kg daily.

Sodium valproate may also be given by slow intravenous injection or infusion. The suggested initial dose for adults is up to 10 mg per kg body-weight followed by further doses, as necessary, up to a total of 2.5 g daily. The usual dose for children is in the range of 20 to 30 mg per kg daily.

Withdrawal of sodium valproate or valproic acid or transition to or from another type of anti-epileptic therapy should be made gradually to avoid precipitating an increase in the frequency of seizures.

Sodium valproate and valproic acid should be taken with or after food. A low initial dose is recommended to minimise gastric intolerance. The time of taking valproic acid and its salts should be standardised for the patient since variations might lead to inappropriate fluctuations in the plasma concentrations.

CONVULSIONS. *Febrile convulsions.* For the use of sodium valproate in the prophylaxis of febrile convulsions in children, see Phenobarbitone Sodium, p.405.

EPILEPSY. For general comments concerning the use of valproate in epilepsy, see under Phenytoin Sodium, p.410.

HICCUP. After courses of valproic acid, 4 of 5 patients with intractable hiccups were symptom-free for periods ranging from 3 to 12 months; the fifth patient was also markedly improved. Dosage began at 15 mg per kg body-weight daily and was increased by 250 mg daily at 2-weekly intervals until hiccups ceased or side-effects appeared.— P. L. Jacobson *et al.*, *Neurology*, 1981, *31*, 1458.

MULTIPLE SCLEROSIS. Sodium valproate suppressed nocturnal paroxysmal coughing attacks and greatly reduced diurnal attacks in a woman with multiple sclerosis.— D. E. Jacome, *Postgrad. med. J.*, 1985, *61*, 515.

PSYCHIATRIC DISORDERS. A review of alternative drug therapies, including valproate, for mania concluding that additional studies are needed before valproate can be considered an effective treatment.— M. W. Jann *et al.*, *Drug Intell. & clin. Pharm.*, 1984, *18*, 577.

Preparations of Valproic Acid and Valproates

Sodium Valproate Oral Solution *(B.P.)*. Sodium Valproate Elixir

Sodium Valproate Tablets *(B.P.)*

Valproic Acid Capsules *(U.S.P.)*

Valproic Acid Syrup *(U.S.P.)*

Proprietary Preparations of Valproic Acid and Valproates

Epilim *(Labaz Sanofi, UK)*. *Tablets*, scored, sodium valproate 100 mg.

Tablets, enteric-coated, sodium valproate 200 and 500 mg.

Oral liquid, sodium valproate 200 mg/5 mL.

Syrup, sodium valproate 200 mg/5 mL.

Injection (Epilim Intravenous), powder for reconstitution, sodium valproate 400 mg, supplied with solvent.

Epilim syrup changed colour going from red to yellow when diluted with syrup preserved with sulphur dioxide or sodium metabisulphite.— *Chemist Drugg.*, 1978, *210*, 444.

Proprietary Names and Manufacturers of Valproic Acid and Valproates

Convulex *(Belg.; Promonta, Ger.; Byk, Neth.; Gerot, Switz.)*; Convulexette *(Belg.)*; Depakene *(Abbott, Canad.; Jpn; Abbott, USA)*; Depakin *(Sigmatau, Ital.)*; Depakine *(Belg.; Labaz, Fr.; Neth.; Labaz, Spain; Labaz, Switz.)*; Depakote *(Abbott, USA)*; Depamide *(Labaz, Fr.; Sigmatau, Ital.; Sanofi Labaz, Neth.; Labaz, Spain)*; Deprakine *(Denm.; Orion, Norw.)*; Epilim *(Reckitt & Colman, Austral.; Labaz, S.Afr.; Labaz Sanofi, UK)*; Epival *(Abbott, Canad.)*; Ergenyl *(Labaz, Ger.; Orion, Swed.)*; Leptilan *(Geigy, Denm.; Geigy, Ger.)*; Leptilen *(Geigy, Swed.)*; Logical *(Arg.)*; Mylproin *(ICI, Ger.)*; Orfilept *(Leo Rhodia, Swed.)*; Orfiril *(Rhone-Poulenc, Denm.; Desitin, Ger.; Rhône-Poulenc, Norw.; Desitin, Switz.)*; Propymal *(Neth.)*; Valcote *(Abbott, Ger.)*; Vistora *(Vita, Spain)*.

17030-d

Vigabatrin *(BAN, USAN, rINN)*.

γ-Vinyl Aminobutyric Acid; γ-Vinyl-GABA; GVG; MDL-71754; RMI-71754. 4-Aminohex-5-enoic acid.

$C_6H_{11}NO_2$=129.2.

CAS — 60643-86-9.

Vigabatrin is an irreversible inhibitor of GABA-transaminase, the enzyme responsible for the catabolism of the neurotransmitter, GABA. It is being studied as an antiepileptic agent and has been tried in patients unresponsive to other therapy.

For a review and discussion concerning vigabatrin, see P.J. Schechter, Vigabatrin, in *New Anticonvulsant Drugs*, B.S. Meldrum and R.J. Porter (Ed.), London, John Libbey & Co. Ltd, 1986, p.265.

Studies on vigabatrin as an antiepileptic agent with encouraging results: E. M. Rimmer and A. Richens, *Lancet*, 1984, *1*, 189; L. Gram *et al.*, *Ann. Neurol.*, 1985, *17*, 262; P. Loiseau *et al.*, *Epilepsia*, 1986, *27*, 115; T. R. Browne *et al.*, *Neurology*, 1987, *37*, 184.

Beneficial results with vigabatrin in tardive dyskinesia.— C. A. Tamminga *et al.* (letter), *Lancet*, 1983, *2*, 97.

Proprietary Names and Manufacturers

Merrell Dow, USA.

Antifungal Agents

2560-c

Antifungal agents in common use include several macrolide antibiotics, other antifungal antibiotics (griseofulvin, pecilocin, and pyrrolnitrin), flucytosine, azole derivatives, and fatty acids.

The polyene macrolide class of antifungal agents comprises the *tetraenes* (amphotericin A, natamycin, and nystatin), the *heptaenes* (amphotericin B, candicidin, hachimycin, and hamycin), and the *pentaenes* (pentamycin).

Azole derivatives can be divided into the *imidazoles* (bifonazole, butoconazole, chlormidazole, clotrimazole, econazole, enilconazole, fenticonazole, isoconazole, ketoconazole, miconazole, oxiconazole, sulconazole, tioconazole), and the *triazoles* (fluconazole, itraconazole, and terconazole). There are many new azole derivatives under investigation, including the imidazoles Bay-L-9139 and zinoconazole, and the triazoles ICI-153066, and vibunazole.

Terbinafine is an antifungal agent under investigation which is related to naftifine.

The fatty acid antifungal agents include caprylic and propionic acids and their salts.

Most of the antifungal agents in this section are applied topically in the treatment of infections of the hair, mucous membranes, nails, or skin by *Candida* (candidiasis), dermatophyte fungi including *Epidermophyton, Microsporum,* and *Trichophyton* (tinea; ringworm), or *Malassezia furfur* (pityriasis versicolor).

Superficial candidal infection may be treated with local applications of azole or polyene antifungal agents, caprylic acid, sodium caprylate, ciclopirox olamine, or nifuroxime.

In tinea, the principal superficial infections are tinea capitis (head or scalp ringworm), tinea corporis (tinea circinata; body ringworm), tinea cruris (ringworm of the groin; jock itch), tinea pedis (athlete's foot; ringworm of the feet), and tinea unguium (ringworm of the nails).

Mild tinea infections may be treated with topical antifungal agents such as the azoles, fatty acids and their salts, buclosamide, chlorphenesin, ciclopirox olamine, loflucarban, fenticlor, fezatione, haloprogin, pecilocin, sulbentine, tolciclate, tolnaftate, or triacetin. The polyene antifungal agents are not effective in tinea. Infections not responding to topical therapy, extensive lesions, and lesions of the scalp or nails should be treated with a course of griseofulvin by mouth, the duration of treatment depending on the site of the infection.

Pityriasis versicolor may be treated by topical application of azole antifungal agents, ciclopirox olamine, haloprogin, tolciclate, or tolnaftate.

Systemic fungal infections are less common but may occur in the immunocompromised host and include infections due to *Aspergillus, Blastomyces, Candida, Coccidioides, Cryptococcus, Histoplasma,* and *Paracoccidioides.*

The principal drugs described in this section which are used in such infections are:

aspergillosis—amphotericin, flucytosine, natamycin

blastomycosis (North American)—amphotericin, hydroxystilbamidine, ketoconazole

candidiasis—amphotericin, flucytosine, ketoconazole, miconazole

coccidioidomycosis—amphotericin, ketoconazole, miconazole

chromomycosis—flucytosine

cryptococcosis—amphotericin, flucytosine, miconazole

histoplasmosis—amphotericin, ketoconazole

paracoccidioidomycosis—amphotericin, ketoconazole, miconazole

phycomycosis—amphotericin

sporotrichosis—amphotericin

Antifungal agents used in prophylactic regimens for the prevention of fungal infections include amphotericin, ketoconazole, and nystatin.

Other drugs used in the treatment of fungal infections which are not included in this section include benzoic acid (p.1355), crystal violet (p.959), potassium iodide (p.1186), selenium sulphide (p.932), sodium thiosulphate (p.855), and various disinfectants.

Reviews of various fungal infections: *Lancet,* 1982, *1,* 944 (cryptococcosis); *ibid.,* 1983, *2,* 323 (fungaemia); *ibid.,* 1066 (aspergilloma); *ibid.,* 1986, *1,* 1362 (phycomycosis).

General reviews of the uses of antifungal agents: J. Cohen, *Lancet,* 1982, *2,* 532; D. W. Warnock and D. C. E. Speller, *J. antimicrob. Chemother.,* 1982, *10,* 164; J. C. M. Stewart *et al., Br. med. J.,* 1983, *286,* 1802; R. J. Hay, *Med. J. Aust.,* 1985, *143,* 287.

Reviews of the treatment of systemic fungal infections: P. E. Hermans and T. F. Keys, *Mayo Clin. Proc.,* 1983, *58,* 223; J. R. Graybill and P. C. Craven, *Drugs,* 1983, *25,* 41; *Med. Lett.,* 1986, *28,* 41.

A review of the clinical pharmacokinetics of antifungal agents used in systemic infections.— T. K. Daneshmend and D. W. Warnock, *Clin. Pharmacokinet.,* 1983, *8,* 17.

For a report of a WHO meeting discussing mycotic diseases, their ecology, diagnosis, and treatment, see *EURO Reports and Studies No. 105, Mycotic diseases in Europe,* 1983.

ANTIFUNGAL ACTION. A review of the mechanisms of antifungal action of polyene and imidazole antifungal agents. The polyene macrolide antibiotics can be classified into small ring molecules, such as natamycin, whose fungistatic and fungicidal concentrations are indistinguishable, and large ring molecules, such as amphotericin, candicidin, and nystatin whose fungistatic and fungicidal concentrations differ. The imidazole antifungal agents show a dose-related inhibition of fungal growth, being fungicidal at high concentrations due to disruption of the fungal membrane. Members of this group differ in their ability to cause membrane damage, ketoconazole causing less membrane disruption than miconazole and tioconazole, and this has led to suggestions that they differ in their mode of action. Fungistatic concentrations of imidazoles inhibit biosynthesis of ergosterol but this is thought not to be the only mechanism of action.— A. H. Thomas, *J. antimicrob. Chemother.,* 1986, *17,* 269.

ANTIFUNGAL SENSITIVITY TESTING. Measurements of minimum inhibitory concentrations (MICs) for imidazole antifungal agents are dependent on the conditions of the test. Also, these drugs demonstrate partial inhibition of fungal growth over a wide concentration range. MICs may be obtained for responsive fungi which are above the attainable serum concentration, and standardised MIC tests have been unreliable in predicting the *in vivo* activity of imidazoles. To overcome these problems, ways of standardising MIC tests have been investigated, such as turbidimetric methods that avoid problems of inoculum variation and end-point determination (J.N. Galgiani and D.A. Stevens, *Antimicrob. Ag. Chemother.,* 1976, *10,* 721). Also, alternative methods for the assessment *in vitro* of antifungal activity have been developed, such as the measurement of relative inhibition factors (RIFs), or methods which measure the inhibition of processes considered to be important in the pathogenesis of fungal infections, such as germ-tube formation and elongation in *Candida albicans* (E.M. Johnson *et al., J. antimicrob. Chemother.,* 1983, *12,* 303). These new methods appear to have a clearer relationship to clinical efficacy, but have not yet been compared with activity in *animal* models.— D. C. E. Speller and D. W. Warnock, *J. antimicrob. Chemother.,* 1985, *15,* 514. The RIF of an antifungal agent was defined as the area under a fixed portion of dose-response curve, expressed as a percentage of the area under the dose-response curve for a theoretical non-inhibitory substance. Unlike MICs, areas under such curves take account of partial inhibitory effects. An RIF close to 0% would indicate considerable susceptibility of fungus to the drug; RIFs close to 100% would indicate resistance to the drug. When tested against yeast isolates, *Aspergillus* spp., and dermatophyte fungi, RIF data correlated well with MICs for nystatin, amphotericin, flucytosine, and griseofulvin and poorly with MICs for imidazole antifungals, indicating that RIF tests were expressing inhibitory effects in a manner different from MICs. The test for RIF appeared to offer the potential for more rapid and reliable prediction of antifungal activity *in vivo* than that provided by measurement of MICs.— F. C. Odds and A. B. Abbott, *J. antimicrob. Chemother.,* 1984, *13,* 31. RIF values were measured for 19 antifungal compounds against various yeast isolates, *Aspergillus* spp., and dermatophyte fungi. The RIFs of amphotericin, flucytosine, and ketoconazole against 8 yeasts were determined at a range of pH values; for amphotericin and ketoconazole the RIF fell as the pH rose, and for flucytosine the opposite trend was observed. The RIF values for the 14 azole antifungal agents tested appeared to reflect their activity *in vivo* more reliably than the MIC, which almost always predicted a lower antifungal activity, particularly for the so-called 'third generation' azoles (generally based on a triazole rather than imidazole structure). The RIF values measured for several of the new azole compounds tested agreed with published data of their relative activities against different fungi.— F. C. Odds *et al., J. antimicrob. Chemother.,* 1984, *14,* 105.

SUPERFICIAL FUNGAL INFECTIONS. A review of the treatment of superficial fungal infections including tinea, candidiasis, and pityriasis versicolor.— D. T. Roberts, *Prescribers' J.,* 1985, *25,* 40. A review of the use of topical imidazole antifungal agents in the treatment of superficial fungal infections.— S. E. Tett, *Aust. J. Pharm.,* 1986, *67,* 567.

A review of the use of topical combination preparations of antifungal agents and hydrocortisone. These may be considered in the treatment of tinea infections accompanied by severe inflammation, intertrigo, nappy rash, infected atopic eczema, and flexural seborrhoeic dermatitis although there is little published evidence to justify their use. They should not be used when diagnosis of the condition is uncertain.— *Drug & Ther. Bull.,* 1985, *23,* 83.

Candidiasis, oral. A review of the causes, diagnosis, and management of chronic atrophic candidiasis and denture stomatitis.— *Lancet,* 1986, *2,* 437.

Candidiasis, urinary. A review of urinary tract infections due to *Candida albicans.*— J. F. Fisher *et al., Rev. infect. Dis.,* 1982, *4,* 1107.

Candidiasis, vaginal. In a review of the management of recurrent vaginal candidiasis, oral treatment with polyene antifungal agents such as nystatin or amphotericin to prevent re-infection from the gastro-intestinal tract was considered to be disappointing; intestinal recolonisation often occurs after discontinuation of treatment. Prophylactic application of an antifungal cream to the perianal region and perineum may be more successful. Concomitant treatment of the male partner to reduce the risk of sexual re-infection has also been recommended but studies have not shown this to improve the results of treatment. Prolonged treatment periods have been advocated in patients with recurrent infection, and intermittent prophylactic treatment during each menstrual cycle has been shown to prevent symptomatic recurrence but not to prevent vaginal recolonisation. Studies using clotrimazole pessaries have shown single-dose treatment to be as effective as courses of 3 to 6 days in the treatment of acute episodes in such patients; this also appears to be effective for intermittent prophylactic treatment.— L. Forssman and I. Milsom, *Am. J. Obstet. Gynec.,* 1985, *152,* 959.

A summary of 5 studies of the treatment of acute vaginal candidiasis and one of the prophylaxis of chronic relapsing candidiasis carried out over 16 years. Similar failure and relapse rates were observed in all studies of treatment of acute infections, involving courses of nystatin or amphotericin pessaries for 15 days with or without concomitant oral nystatin therapy, nystatin pessaries for 6 days, tioconazole cream for 3 days, or single-dose therapy with econazole, clotrimazole, or isoconazole pessaries; there were few mycological relapses 7 days after completion of treatment, but there was a mycological relapse rate of 20% to 30% after 35 days.— L. Cohen, *Am. J. Obstet. Gynec.,* 1985, *152,* 961.

Further references to vaginal candidiasis and its treatment: M. W. Adler, *Br. med. J.,* 1983, *287,* 1611; J. D. Sobel, *Ann. intern. Med.,* 1984, *101,* 390; A. McMillan, *Br. med. J.,* 1986, *293,* 1357.

Dandruff. A review of the aetiology of dandruff including the possible role of the *Malassezia (Pityrosporum)* yeast. Nystatin and the imidazole antifungal agents were mentioned among the many agents useful in controlling dandruff.— *Lancet,* 1985, *2,* 703. See also S. Shuster, *Br. J. Derm.,* 1984, *111,* 235.

Tinea. A review of the aetiology of tinea pedis.— *Lancet,* 1985, *2,* 81.

2202-k

Acrisorcin *(USAN, rINN).*
Aminacrine 4-Hexylresorcinate; Sch-7056. 9-Aminoacridine compound with 4-hexylresorcinol.
$C_{13}H_{10}N_2,C_{12}H_{18}O_2$=388.5.

CAS — 7527-91-5.

Pharmacopoeias. In *U.S.*

A yellow odourless powder. **Soluble** 1 in 1000 of water, 1 in 18 of alcohol, 1 in 55 of acetone, 1 in 320 of chloroform, and 1 in 3 of dimethylformamide; very slightly soluble in ether. **Store** in well-closed containers.

Acrisorcin is an acridine derivative that has been used by topical application of a 0.2% cream in the treatment of tinea versicolor.
Skin irritation and photosensitivity may occasionally occur.

Preparations

Acrisorcin Cream *(U.S.P.).* Store in airtight containers.

Proprietary Names and Manufacturers

Akrinol *(Schering, USA).*

2562-a

Amphotericin *(BAN).*

Amphotericin B *(USAN, rINN)*; Anfotericina B.
A mixture of antifungal polyenes produced by the growth of certain strains of *Streptomyces nodosus* or by any other means. It consists largely of amphotericin B.
$C_{47}H_{73}NO_{17}$=924.1.

CAS — 1397-89-3.

Pharmacopoeias. In *Br., Braz., Chin., Cz., Egypt., Ind., It., Jpn,* and *U.S.*

It occurs as a yellow to orange, odourless or almost odourless powder. The *B.P.* material contains not less than 750 units per mg with reference to the dried substance and not more than 10% of tetraenes. The *U.S.P.* specifies not less than 750 μg of $C_{47}H_{73}NO_{17}$ per mg, and, for material intended for oral or topical use, not more than 15% of amphotericin A, both calculated on the dried substance.

B.P. **solubilities** are: practically insoluble in water, alcohol, and in ether; slightly soluble in dimethylformamide and methyl alcohol; soluble in dimethyl sulphoxide and propylene glycol. *U.S.P.* solubilities are: insoluble in water, dehydrated alcohol, benzene, ether, and toluene; slightly soluble in methyl alcohol; soluble in dimethylformamide, dimethyl sulphoxide, and propylene glycol. A 3% suspension in water has a pH of 6 to 8. In dilute solution it is sensitive to light, and inactivated at low pH.

Store at 2° to 8° in airtight containers. Protect from light. Under these conditions, it does not significantly deteriorate or lose potency for at least 1 year. Amphotericin is precipitated from solution by sodium chloride. Solutions for injection may be diluted with glucose injection adjusted, if necessary, to a pH above 4.2; they should be used immediately after preparation and protected from light during administration. If administered through an in-line filter, the pore diameter of the filter should not be less than 1 μm.

Due to the wide range of **incompatibilities** reported with amphotericin it is generally advisable not to mix it with any other drug. Most incompatibilities are caused by precipitation of amphotericin due to a change in pH or by the disruption of the colloidal suspension. Compounds reported to be incompatible with amphotericin include: amikacin sulphate, ampicillin, antihistamines, benzylpenicillin, calcium chloride, calcium gluconate, carbenicillin sodium, chlorpromazine hydrochloride, chlortetracycline hydrochloride, cimetidine, diphenhydramine hydrochloride, dopamine hydrochloride, gentamicin sulphate, kanamycin sulphate, lignocaine hydrochloride, metaraminol tartrate, methyldopate hydrochloride, nitrofurantoin sodium, oxytetracycline hydrochloride, polymyxin B sulphate, potassium chloride, preservatives, procaine hydrochloride, prochlorperazine mesylate, sodium calciumedetate, sodium chloride, streptomycin sulphate, tetracycline hydrochloride, verapamil hydrochloride, viomycin sulphate, and vitamins; and also with solutions for total parenteral nutrition. Solutions of amphotericin in glucose injection tend to be unstable (see above).

Units

One unit of amphotericin is contained in 0.001064 mg of the first International Standard Preparation (1963) which contains 940 units per mg.

Adverse Effects

Solutions of amphotericin irritate the venous endothelium and may cause pain and thrombophlebitis at the site of injection. Common adverse effects after intravenous infusion of amphotericin are headache, nausea, vomiting, chills, fever, malaise, muscle and joint pains, anorexia, diarrhoea, and gastro-intestinal cramp. Hypertension, hypotension, cardiac arrhythmias, ventricular fibrillation, cardiac arrest, skin rashes, blurred vision, tinnitus, vertigo, peripheral neuropathy, and convulsions have been occasionally reported. Amphotericin is nephrotoxic often resulting in a rise in blood urea, renal tubular acidosis, and hypokalaemia. This is usually reversible but degeneration of the renal tubules has been reported and is common with high doses in excess of 5 g. Hypomagnesaemia has also been observed, and anaemia is common. Thrombocytopenia, leucopenia, agranulocytosis, and anaphylactic reactions may occur.

After intrathecal injection amphotericin may also cause irritation of the meninges, neuropathy with pain, impaired vision, and retention of urine.

Topical application may produce local irritation, pruritus, and skin rash.

EFFECTS ON THE BLOOD. *Anaemia.* Amphotericin appeared to produce anaemia by inhibition of erythropoietin production rather than by suppressing bone-marrow activity directly.— R. R. MacGregor *et al., Antimicrob. Ag. Chemother.,* 1978, *14,* 270.

Thrombocytopenia. A patient with leukaemia developed thrombocytopenia after 4 weeks' therapy with intravenous amphotericin (2 weeks as single therapy, and 2 weeks in association with flucytosine) for the treatment of hepatic candidiasis. The platelet count rose 10 days after discontinuation of the antifungal agents, but declined again 2 weeks after amphotericin alone was restarted. However, therapy was continued without further depression of the platelet count, at a dosage of 55 mg on alternate days and with close monitoring, for a further 3 months. Within 2 weeks of cessation of therapy the platelet count rose to normal values. It was considered that amphotericin produced thrombocytopenia by suppressing platelet production.— C. S. P. Chan *et al., Ann. intern. Med.,* 1982, *96,* 332.

EFFECTS ON ELECTROLYTES. *Hypomagnesaemia.* Hypomagnesaemia due to renal magnesium wasting developed in 10 patients during the first 2 weeks of treatment with amphotericin for disseminated fungal infections; the effect was generally mild, requiring magnesium supplementation in only one patient, and appeared to plateau after 6 weeks' treatment. In 3 patients, assessed 1 year after discontinuation of amphotericin, serum-magnesium concentrations and magnesium excretion had returned close to pretreatment values.— C. H. Barton *et al., Am. J. Med.,* 1984, *77,* 471.

A woman with leukaemia developed tetany, hypocalcaemia, and hypokalaemia 8 days after starting therapy with the intravenous infusion of amphotericin for a *Candida albicans* infection. Daily intravenous infusions of potassium and intravenous injections of calcium gluconate did not produce symptomatic or biochemical improvement. Three days later severe hypomagnesaemia was detected; intravenous infusion of magnesium was begun and resulted in immediate resolution of tetany, and increase in serum concentrations of calcium and of potassium. Tests indicated an excessive urinary loss of magnesium, which was still evident 4 months later despite the administration of magnesium glycerophosphate daily by mouth; however tetany did not recur and serum concentrations of calcium and potassium remained within reference ranges. It was considered that amphotericin was a causative factor in the magnesium loss, although its effect might have been potentiated by prior administration of gentamicin or of antineoplastic agents.— S. V. Davies and J. A. Murray (letter), *Br. med. J.,* 1986, *292,* 1395.

EFFECTS ON THE LIVER. Amphotericin has only rarely been associated with adverse effects on the liver. Carnecchia and Kurtzke (*Ann. intern. Med.,* 1960, *53,* 1027) reported fatal liver failure in one patient after administration of a total dose of 4.82 g given intermittently over one year. Miller (*Can. med. Ass. J.,* 1984, *131,* 1245) reported abnormal liver function tests in a leukaemic patient after a total dose of 571 mg over 18 days; these values returned towards normal after withdrawal of amphotericin 3 days later. Treatment with amphotericin was begun again at a lower dose but liver function tests deteriorated yet again, necessitating amphotericin withdrawal. It was not known whether the toxicity, which appeared to involve the entire hepatobiliary system, was related to amphotericin or to sodium deoxycholate present to disperse the amphotericin. Abajo *et al.* (*Br. med. J.,* 1986, *293,* 1243) also reported a rise in liver enzyme values and hepatomegaly in one patient associated with the administration of amphotericin 1 mg per kg body-weight daily; as the dose was reduced to 0.5 mg per kg daily the raised values fell steadily.

EFFECTS ON THE NERVOUS SYSTEM. A report of delirium and depression associated with the intravenous administration of amphotericin.— W. W. Weddington, *Psychosomatics,* 1982, *23,* 1076.

Ellis *et al.* (*J. infect. Dis.,* 1982, *146,* 125) reported a high incidence of neurological dysfunction in a retrospective study of 14 patients who had received amphotericin methyl ester. Autopsies were performed, and the toxicity was attributed to a diffuse leucoencephalopathy. Hoeprich (*ibid.,* 173), however, considered that the adverse effects may be due to the drug itself, impurities present in the preparation, the mycosis being treated, or a combination of all three.

Parkinsonism. A clinical picture resembling advanced parkinsonism developed in a patient who received intraventricular amphotericin for 8 days for treatment of cryptococcal meningitis. Direct toxicity of amphotericin was considered to be responsible, but the possibility that it occurred as a result of cryptococcal involvement of the basal ganglia could not be discounted.— J. F. Fisher and J. Dewald, *J. antimicrob. Chemother.,* 1983, *12,* 97.

NEPHROTOXICITY. See under Treatment of Adverse Effects, (below).

Treatment of Adverse Effects

To reduce febrile reactions small doses of hydrocortisone may be given intravenously just before or during an infusion of amphotericin. Heparin has been given to reduce the incidence of thrombophlebitis. Both hydrocortisone sodium succinate and heparin have been added to the amphotericin infusion fluid itself (but see incompatibilities, above).

Amphotericin is not removed by haemodialysis.

For the possible reduction of the toxicity of amphotericin by encapsulation in liposomes see under Uses, (below).

NEPHROTOXICITY. A review of the postulated mechanisms of amphotericin nephrotoxicity and the possible measures for its prevention that have been investigated in *animals* and man. It was concluded that sodium loading may be effective in sodium-depleted patients, and that aminophylline, although not yet studied in humans, may have a role in patients where sodium loading is inappropriate. Treatment with mannitol or sodium bicarbonate is controversial and probably ineffective. Administration of amphotericin on alternate days is widely practised although it has never been proven to reduce nephrotoxicity.— J. Warda and S. L. Barriere, *Drug Intell. & clin. Pharm.,* 1985, *19,* 25. See also D. J. Yang and G. O. Rankin, *Adverse Drug React. Ac. Pois. Rev.,* 1985, *1,* 37.

Although there have been reports of a beneficial effect of intravenous infusions of mannitol in preventing the nephrotoxicity of amphotericin (J.J. Olivero *et al., Br. med. J.,* 1975, *1,* 550; J.M. Rosch *et al., J. Am. med. Ass.,* 1976, *235,* 1995 and *idem,* 1977, *237,* 27), a double-blind study in 11 patients (W.E. Bullock *et al., Antimicrob. Ag. Chemother.,* 1976, *10,* 555) failed to confirm this effect.

A report of 5 patients who developed impaired renal function early during the course of amphotericin for the treatment of systemic fungal infections, resulting in interruption of therapy in 4 patients. Correction of sodium depletion, present before or during therapy possibly as a result of a low-sodium diet, treatment with diuretics, or amphotericin-induced vomiting, allowed completion of amphotericin treatment without further loss of renal function.— H. T. Heidemann *et al.*, *Am. J. Med.*, 1983, *75*, 476.

THROMBOPHLEBITIS. Thrombophlebitis was decreased in one patient by the administration of amphotericin in glucose injection sterilised by filtration (final pH of 6.3) rather than by autoclaving (final pH of 5.0).— A. R. Tanser (letter), *Lancet*, 1966, *1*, 1102.

In a double-blind study of 15 patients receiving amphotericin in glucose injection with hydrocortisone sodium phosphate 25 mg added, the incidence and severity of phlebitis was not altered by filtration through a 1 µm membrane filter.— V. P. Gotz *et al.*, *Drug Intell. & clin. Pharm.*, 1985, *19*, 436.

Precautions

To reduce the risk of vein irritation, the rate of intravenous infusion of amphotericin should be slow, and the concentration of solutions should not exceed 100 µg per mL; the injection site should be changed frequently.

Tests of renal function should be performed regularly during treatment and treatment stopped if progressive impairment occurs. Concomitant administration of other nephrotoxic drugs and of antineoplastic agents should be avoided.

Blood counts, and serum-potassium concentrations should be monitored regularly.

The potassium-depleting effect of amphotericin may enhance the effects of neuromuscular blocking agents and may increase the toxicity of digitalis glycosides; corticosteroids may enhance the depletion of potassium.

A report of adrenal insufficiency considered to be precipitated by the administration of amphotericin in a patient being treated for blastomycosis.— P. T. Chandler, *Sth. med. J.*, 1977, *70*, 863.

Hyperkalaemia and ventricular fibrillation occurred on 2 occasions towards the end of a rapid infusion of amphotericin 1.4 mg per kg body-weight over 45 minutes in an anuric patient. Hyperkalaemia was probably due to release of intracellular potassium caused by high serum concentrations of amphotericin. It was recommended that anuric patients receive amphotericin during haemodialysis, and that azotaemic patients not being dialysed receive slow infusions with monitoring of serum-potassium concentrations.— P. C. Craven and D. H. Gremillion, *Antimicrob. Ag. Chemother.*, 1985, *27*, 868.

For reference to the possible effects of amphotericin on the immune system, see under Antimicrobial Action.

INTERACTIONS. The association of amphotericin and miconazole appeared to be less effective than either drug used alone.— L. P. Schacter *et al.* (letter), *Lancet*, 1976, *2*, 318.

On reviewing the records of 57 patients who had received leucocyte transfusions for 4 days or more, Wright *et al.* (*New Engl. J. Med.*, 1981, *304*, 1185) reported acute respiratory deterioration in 14 of 22 patients who also received amphotericin infusions, but only in 2 of 35 patients who received leucocytes alone. They therefore advised that the amphotericin infusion should be temporally separated from the leucocyte infusion as far as possible, that the amphotericin should be infused more slowly than usual, and the patient watched carefully. Bow *et al.* (*Can. med. Ass. J.*, 1984, *130*, 593) however, did not confirm these results in 32 granulocytopenic patients during 35 episodes of fever; pulmonary complications occurring in 12 of 21 patients who received both amphotericin and leucocytes, and in 6 of 14 who received leucocytes only. They considered the development of pulmonary complications to be related more to underlying fungal infections than to the combined use of amphotericin and leucocytes.

See also under Antimicrobial Action.

PREGNANCY AND THE NEONATE. A pregnant woman with blastomycosis was successfully treated with intravenous amphotericin and gave birth to a normal child. From a review of the literature of another 20 pregnant women treated with amphotericin there appears to be no incidence of teratogenesis or other persistent adverse effects in the infants, although amphotericin does diffuse into the foetal circulation.— M. A. Ismail and S. A. Lerner, *Am. Rev. resp. Dis.*, 1982, *126*, 350.

Antimicrobial Action

Amphotericin is a polyene antifungal antibiotic which interferes with the permeability of the cell membrane of sensitive fungi by binding to sterols, chiefly ergosterol. It is reported to be fungistatic at concentrations achieved clinically. It is active against *Absidia* spp., *Aspergillus* spp., *Basidiobolus* spp., *Blastomyces dermatitidis*, *Candida* spp., *Coccidioides immitis*, *Conidiobolus* spp., *Cryptococcus neoformans*, *Histoplasma capsulatum*, *Mucor* spp., *Paracoccidioides brasiliensis*, *Rhizopus* spp., *Rhodotorula* spp., and *Sporothrix schenckii*. Minimum inhibitory concentrations range from 0.03 to 1 µg per mL for many of these organisms. It is inactive against bacteria, rickettsias, and viruses but is reported to be effective against *Leishmania* protozoa.

Amphotericin was active *in vitro* against *Prototheca* spp. with MICs ranging from 0.09 to 3.12 µg per mL.— E. Segal *et al.*, *Antimicrob. Ag. Chemother.*, 1976, *10*, 75.

Sensitivity studies confirmed amphotericin as the most effective agent against *Naegleria fowleri*. Clotrimazole and miconazole were less active.— R. J. Duma and R. Finley, *Antimicrob. Ag. Chemother.*, 1976, *10*, 370.

Most fungi encountered in human mycoses, including *Candida* and *Cryptococcus* spp., can be expected to be sensitive to amphotericin, and laboratory sensitivity tests are generally only required with unusual fungi or recurrent isolations during treatment.— D. C. E. Speller and D. W. Warnock, *J. antimicrob. Chemother.*, 1985, *15*, 514.

In vitro and *animal* studies have shown amphotericin to have both immunostimulant and immunosuppressive properties. Roselle and Kauffman (*Antimicrob. Ag. Chemother.*, 1978, *14*, 398) suggested an immunosuppressive effect from studies using human lymphocytes, Thong and Ness (*Lancet*, 1977, *2*, 568) demonstrated an inhibition of chemotaxis by amphotericin using human neutrophils, and Abruzzo *et al.* (*Antimicrob. Ag. Chemother.*, 1986, *29*, 602) suggested a reduction in immune cell activity as measured by the chemiluminescence response of mouse spleen cells. Lin *et al.* (*ibid.*, 1977, *11*, 154) however, showed an increase in production and activity of macrophages in *mice* given amphotericin, and in a study by Bistoni *et al.* (*ibid.*, 1985, *27*, 625) *mice* given a single injection of amphotericin showed increased resistance to subsequent challenge with *Candida albicans*. The authors suggested that this immunostimulant effect may contribute to the therapeutic action of amphotericin. In a discussion on the effects of antimicrobial agents on host defence mechanisms, Oleske (*J. antimicrob. Chemother.*, 1984, *13*, 413) highlights some of the difficulties of investigating these effects.

For reports of the potentiation *in vitro* of the antiviral activity of acyclovir, see Acyclovir Sodium (p.690).

DIMINISHED ACTIVITY. *Ketoconazole. Candida albicans* became resistant to amphotericin *in vitro* in the presence of ketoconazole.— I. J. Sud and D. S. Feingold, *Antimicrob. Ag. Chemother.*, 1983, *23*, 185. Initial resistance in *Cryptococcus neoformans*, but then a synergistic effect. Amphotericin may enhance the penetration of ketoconazole into the fungal cells.— D. Smith *et al.*, *ibid.*, *24*, 851.

ENHANCED ACTIVITY. *Flucytosine.* See p.423.

Ketoconazole. See under Diminished activity, above.

Minocycline. In vitro studies have shown minocycline to increase the antifungal activity of amphotericin against various species of *Aspergillus* (C.E. Hughes *et al.*, *Antimicrob. Ag. Chemother.*, 1984, *26*, 837), various species of *Candida*, and *Cryptococcus neoformans* (M.A. Lew *et al.*, *ibid.*, 1978, *14*, 465). See also under Tetracycline (below).

Norfloxacin. For a report of norfloxacin enhancing the antifungal action of amphotericin against *Candida albicans in vitro*, see Norfloxacin (p.274).

Rifampicin. In vitro studies have shown rifampicin to increase the antifungal activity of amphotericin against various species of *Aspergillus* (M. Kitahara *et al.*, *Antimicrob. Ag. Chemother.*, 1976, *9*, 915; C.E. Hughes *et al.*, *ibid.*, 1984, *25*, 560), various species of *Candida* (R.M. Bannatyne and R. Cheung, *Curr. ther. Res.*, 1979, *25*, 71; J.E. Edwards *et al.*, *Antimicrob. Ag. Chemother.*, 1980, *17*, 484), *Coccidioides immitis* (D. Rifkind *et al.*, *ibid.*, 1974, *6*, 783), *Cryptococcus neoformans* (N.K. Fujita and J.E. Edwards, *ibid.*, 1981, *19*, 196) and *Leishmania tropica* (J. El-On *et al.*, *Ann. trop. Med. Parasit.*, 1984, *78*, 93).

Tetracycline. Lee *et al.* (*Antimicrob. Ag. Chemother.*, 1979, *16*, 217) demonstrated a synergistic action between both amphotericin and minocycline, and amphotericin and tetracycline *in vitro* against *Naegleria fowleri*, and this was confirmed for amphotericin and tetracycline by Thong *et al.* (*Med. J. Aust.*, 1978, *1*, 663) in experimental amoebic meningoencephalitis in *mice*.

RESISTANCE. The development of fungal resistance during therapy with amphotericin has been reported only rarely. Pappagianis *et al.* (*Antimicrob. Ag. Chemother.*, 1979, *16*, 123), reported the development of resistance by *Candida lusitaniae* in a leukaemic patient during treatment with systemic amphotericin; there was a 100-fold increase in the MIC of amphotericin to the organism over 20 days of therapy. Dick *et al.* (*Ann. intern. Med.*, 1985, *102*, 67) reported a similar increase in MIC of amphotericin to *C. guilliermondii* over 26 days of treatment in a patient with aplastic anaemia. In a study of yeast isolates from 308 patients, Dick *et al.* (*Antimicrob. Ag. Chemother.*, 1980, *18*, 158), had earlier recovered strains of *C. albicans*, *C. tropicalis*, and *C. glabrata* resistant to amphotericin in 6 patients all of whom had received extensive chemotherapy. All 3 reports considered the development of resistance to be due to a progressive depletion of ergosterol in the fungal membrane.

Absorption and Fate

There is little or no absorption of amphotericin from the gastro-intestinal tract. When administered intravenously in the colloidal form in the usual increasing dosage regimens (see Uses below), peak plasma concentrations of 0.5 to 3.5 µg per mL have been produced. Amphotericin is reported to be highly bound to plasma proteins, and to pass into the CSF only in small quantities. The plasma half-life has been reported to be about 24 hours.

Unchanged amphotericin is excreted in small amounts slowly in the urine. Traces have been reported to be present in the serum and urine several weeks after completion of treatment.

A review of the pharmacokinetics of amphotericin.— T. K. Daneshmend and D. W. Warnock, *Clin. Pharmacokinet.*, 1983, *8*, 17.

Values for the concentration of amphotericin in serum samples were generally lower when the assay had been carried out on a frozen sample than when an assay had been carried out immediately.— R. M. Bannatyne and R. Cheung, *Antimicrob. Ag. Chemother.*, 1977, *12*, 550.

The elimination half-lives of amphotericin were 14 and 16.5 days in 2 patients who had received long-term therapy with amphotericin.— A. J. Atkinson and J. E. Bennett, *Antimicrob. Ag. Chemother.*, 1978, *13*, 271.

Report of a study of 13 patients with haematological malignancies who received one amphotericin 10 mg lozenge, retained in the mouth until it dissolved (about 15 minutes), 3 or 4 times daily as prophylaxis against candidiasis. The approximate bioavailability (calculated on the assumption of a creatinine clearance rate of 30 mL per minute) was 8.3 and 9.9% respectively.— M. S. Ching *et al.*, *Br. J. clin. Pharmac.*, 1983, *16*, 106.

PREGNANCY AND THE NEONATE. For mention of the diffusion of amphotericin into the foetal circulation see under Precautions (above).

Uses and Administration

Amphotericin is administered by intravenous infusion in the treatment of severe systemic mycotic infections including aspergillosis, blastomycosis, candidiasis, coccidioidomycosis, cryptococcosis, histoplasmosis, paracoccidioidomycosis, phycomycosis, and sporotrichosis. It has also been given for the treatment of American mucocutaneous and cutaneous leishmaniasis, and for primary amoebic meningoencephalitis caused by *Naegleria* spp. Amphotericin may be used with flucytosine particularly in the treatment of cryptococcal meningitis.

It is applied topically in concentrations of 3% to treat cutaneous and mucocutaneous infections caused mainly by *Candida* spp. Amphotericin is also given by mouth in doses of up to 2 g daily for the suppression of oral or intestinal candidiasis, or for its prophylaxis in immunocompromised patients.

A colloidal form of amphotericin with sodium deoxycholate is used for injection and a crystalline form for topical or oral administration. A test dose of 1 mg intravenously is often given before embarking on intravenous therapy. For slow intravenous infusion a solution containing 100 µg of amphotericin per mL in glucose injection (with a pH greater than 4.2) should be given in an initial daily dose of up to 250 μg per kg body-weight. The dose may be increased gradually to a usual dose of 0.5 to 0.7 mg per kg daily or up to 1.5 mg per kg on alternate days. Children have been given similar doses. Severely ill patients may be given 1.5 mg per kg daily; this dose should not be exceeded. If for any reason treatment is interrupted for longer than 7 days, it should be resumed with the lowest initial dose. Therapy may need to be continued for several months depending on the infection.

Intrathecal injection is used for patients with severe meningitis especially when intravenous therapy has been ineffective. Commencing with 25 to 50 μg, the dose is gradually increased to the maximum that can be tolerated without excessive discomfort. The usual dosage is 0.25 to 1 mg every 2 or 3 days. It is administered as a solution containing 250 μg of amphotericin per mL, and the dose volume is diluted with cerebrospinal fluid. Doses should be reduced for children.

Amphotericin has also been administered into the bladder by irrigation, into the eye by subconjunctival or intravitreal injection, or into joint spaces by intra-articular injection.

The water-soluble methyl ester of amphotericin and some of its derivatives have been investigated.

Reviews of the actions and uses of amphotericin: J. Cohen, *Lancet*, 1982, *2*, 532; P. E. Hermans and T. F. Keys, *Mayo Clin. Proc.*, 1983, *58*, 223; J. R. Graybill and P. C. Craven, *Drugs*, 1983, *25*, 41; *Med. Lett.*, 1986, *28*, 41.

Fungal infection is an important cause of death among immunocompromised patients with cancer, however few studies have considered the place of antifungal therapy in empirical antimicrobial regimens for the treatment of febrile neutropenic patients. Pizzo *et al.* (*Am. J. Med.*, 1982, *72*, 101) studied 271 such patients in a paediatric oncology unit. In 652 episodes of fever and granulocytopenia all patients were given an empirical antibiotic regimen of cephalothin 170 mg per kg body-weight daily, gentamicin 6 mg per kg daily, and carbenicillin 500 mg per kg daily, all administered intravenously. In 323 episodes which appeared to have no infectious cause, fever and granulocytopenia remained in 50 patients after 7 days treatment. In 16 of these, antibiotic therapy was discontinued and the patient re-evaluated (Group 1), in 16 antibiotic therapy was continued (Group 2), and in 18 empirical intravenous amphotericin 500 μg per kg daily was added to antibiotic therapy (Group 3). Antimicrobial treatment was continued until fever and granulocytopenia had resolved. Infectious complications occurred in 6 patients in Group 1, (one fungal), 6 in Group 2, (5 fungal), and 2 in Group 3, (one fungal), and defervescence occurred in a median of 11, 8, and 6 days in the 3 groups respectively. Out of 329 episodes of fever which had a documented infectious cause, 22 patients still had fever and granulocytopenia after 7 days and had microbiological evidence of fungal colonisation of the gastro-intestinal tract. Empirical amphotericin was added to appropriate antibiotic therapy; 11 patients defervesced in a median of 3 days, and none of the 20 who received amphotericin within 2 weeks of the start of antibiotic therapy had evidence of subsequent fungal infection. The authors concluded that the addition of amphotericin to antibiotic therapy after 7 days of fever and granulocytopenia, with or without a proven focus of infection, appeared to be beneficial either by preventing fungal infections or by controlling clinically undetected fungal invasion. In a review of empirical treatment of infections in neutropenic patients with cancer, Klastersky (*Rev. infect. Dis.*, 1983, *5*, *Suppl.*, S21) considered that early antifungal therapy with amphotericin was appropriate in such patients who have no documented infection. He reported on preliminary results from a European Organisation for Research on Treatment of Cancer (EORTC) International Antimicrobial Therapy Project Group study in which treatment with amphotericin was begun after 4 days of antibiotic therapy if fever did not subside. There was some indication that early therapy with amphotericin prevented fatal fungal infection, although it seemed to have no effect on the overall mortality. In a discussion of these issues, Cohen (*J. antimicrob. Chemother.*, 1984, *13*, 409), considered that amphotericin was probably the antifungal agent of choice for such regimens, and should be continued for a full course of treatment in the case of a definite diagnosis of fungal infection, or until the neutrophil count is greater than 0.5×10^3 per mm^3 if no source of infection is found. The management of patients who remained febrile despite an adequate course of antifungal therapy (EORTC protocols require at least 500 mg amphotericin) was unclear. Cohen concluded that although present studies did not provide clear evidence of the efficacy of empirical antifungal therapy, such studies were difficult to assess because of the heterogeneity of the population investigated, and that the experience of many units showing the benefit of such therapy should be taken into consideration.

A review of 16 leukaemic patients with splenic abscesses due to *Aspergillus* or *Candida* spp. Ten received treatment with amphotericin alone, and 2 combined treatment with amphotericin and flucytosine usually in conjunction with surgery. Most patients recovered, but the importance of splenectomy was emphasised.— J. D. Johnson and M. J. Raff, *Archs intern. Med.*, 1984, *144*, 1987.

Endocarditis due to *Phialophora dermatitidis* (*Wangiella dermatitidis*) in an intravenous drug abuser was treated with intravenous amphotericin in association with ketoconazole and rifampicin both by mouth. Although blood cultures were negative after 8 weeks treatment, relapses occurred.— C. V. Vartian *et al.*, *Am. J. Med.*, 1985, *78*, 703.

In an outbreak of *Hansenula anomala* infection in a neonatal unit, 7 babies were successfully treated with amphotericin 100 μg per kg body-weight per day by infusion increasing to a maximum of 500 μg per kg per day over 5 days, in association with flucytosine 100 mg per kg per day intravenously at first, changing to enteral treatment when the baby was on feeds. Treatment was continued for 3 weeks.— N. Murphy *et al.*, *Lancet*, 1986, *1*, 291.

For a reference to the use of amphotericin methyl ester, see Effects on the Nervous System under Adverse Effects.

ADMINISTRATION. Amphotericin has been administered by rapid intravenous infusion; however, there are few studies on this form of administration which may be accompanied by complications such as hyperkalaemia.— D. J. Drutz, *Drugs*, 1983, *26*, 337. See also under Precautions, above.

Liposomal amphotericin has been shown to be effective in the prophylaxis and treatment of experimental fungal infections in *animals*, and is considered both to decrease the toxicity and enhance the activity of amphotericin. Liposomal amphotericin has been used in a preliminary study (G. Lopez-Berestein *et al. J. infect. Dis.*, 1985, *151*, 704) to treat systemic fungal infections in patients with cancer who had not responded to conventional treatment. The preparation was administered as an intravenous infusion over 15 to 45 minutes every 24 hours; 5 patients were cured, 7 responded partially, and in 5 there was no effect. The incidence of chills and fever was lower than is commmonly seen with amphotericin, and there was no further deterioration of renal function in patients who had received amphotericin or other nephrotoxic drugs.— G. Lopez-Berestein, *Ann. intern. Med.*, 1986, *105*, 130.

Intrathecal administration. Administration of amphotericin for fungal meningitis may be by the lumbar, cisternal, or intraventricular route. The most common route is into a lateral ventricle, most frequently via a subcutaneous reservoir (Ommaya reservoir). However, use of a reservoir may be complicated by misplacement of the ventricular catheter, obstruction of the system, or secondary bacterial infection; few patients complete therapy without at least one replacement of the reservoir, and the need for intervening intralumbar therapy.— D. J. Drutz, *Drugs*, 1983, *26*, 337.

Urinary-tract administration. A review of published reports of the use of amphotericin by direct administration into the bladder in the treatment of fungal urinary-tract infections. Most commonly it is given by continuous irrigation as a 0.005% solution of amphotericin in sterile water for at least 5 to 7 days, or by intermittent instillation for 8 to 14 days. The amphotericin may also be dispersed in glucose injection, but this may predispose patients to bacterial urinary-tract infections.— D. E. Nix *et al.*, *Drug Intell. & clin. Pharm.*, 1985, *19*, 299.

ADMINISTRATION IN RENAL FAILURE. Amphotericin can be administered in a usual dosage regimen to patients whose glomerular filtration-rate (GFR) is 10 mL per minute or more. In patients with GFR less than 10 mL per minute the dosage interval should be increased from 24 to 36 hours. Concentrations are not affected by haemodialysis or peritoneal dialysis.— W. M. Bennett *et al.*, *Am. J. Kidney Dis.*, 1983, *3*, 155. See also D. J. Morgan *et al.*, *Clin. Pharmac. Ther.*, 1983, *34*, 248.

Fungal infections are responsible for about 1 to 2% of cases of peritonitis associated with continuous ambulatory peritoneal dialysis, but the morbidity and mortality are high. Although infections have been successfully treated with the catheter *in situ*, catheter removal is generally advised. The treatment of choice is intravenous amphotericin. Amphotericin has been administered intraperitoneally by adding 5 mg to each litre of dialysis fluid but this route is painful. Intraperitoneal miconazole 20 mg per litre or flucytosine 50 mg per litre have also been used. Ketoconazole by mouth has been used but does not produce therapeutic levels in the dialysate.— British Society for Antimicrobial Chemotherapy, *Lancet*, 1987, *1*, 845.

See also under Precautions (above).

AMOEBIASIS. Although amphotericin is active *in vitro* against *Naegleria fowleri* and has been recommended for the treatment of primary amoebic meningoencephalitis caused by this amoeba, there have been few reports of survival after its use (J. Apley *et al.*, *Br. med. J.*, 1970, *1*, 596; K. Anderson and A. Jamieson, *Lancet*, 1972, *1*, 902). Seidel *et al.* (*New Engl. J. Med.*, 1982, *1*, 346) reported survival in one patient after treatment with amphotericin and miconazole both given intravenously and intrathecally, and rifampicin given by mouth. Ferrante (*Lancet*, 1986, *2*, 35) suggested that amphotericin disrupts the amoeba causing it to release substances toxic to mammalian cells, and therefore considered that it may be more successful if used in doses which only inhibit the mortality and phagocytic activity.

ASPERGILLOSIS. Aspergillosis is usually treated with amphotericin. It has been used with complete or partial success in patients with malignancies in total doses of up to 2.3 g, particularly when diagnosis is made early (J. Aisner, *Ann. intern. Med.*, 1977, *86*, 539). Ho *et al.* (*Br. J. Ophthal.*, 1984, *68*, 412) successfully treated a patient with endophthalmitis due to *Aspergillus fumigatus* with slow intravitreous injections of amphotericin 7.5 and 5 μg in association with vitreous surgery, followed by a total of 1.56 g amphotericin given intravenously over 34 days. The direct injection of an amphotericin paste has been reported to be successful in the treatment of aspergilloma (P. Krakówka *et al. Tubercle*, 1970, *51*, 184).

A decreased incidence of invasive aspergillosis was reported in an oncology unit after the use of prophylactic intranasal amphotericin in 34 patients. Amphotericin 10 mg three times daily was given for between 5 and 65 days as a 0.5% solution in sterile water by means of an atomiser.— F. Meunier-Carpentier *et al.* (letter), *New Engl. J. Med.*, 1984, *311*, 1056.

For reports of the use of amphotericin with flucytosine in the treatment of aspergillosis, see Flucytosine, p.424.

BLASTOMYCOSIS. Intravenous amphotericin has been considered the drug of choice for blastomycosis. Recent studies have, however, shown ketoconazole by mouth to be an effective alternative in immunocompetent patients with mild to moderately severe non-meningeal forms of the disease.— W. E. Dismukes, *New Engl. J. Med.*, 1986, *314*, 575.

Reports of the use of amphotericin in the treatment of blastomycosis: D. M. Skillrud, *Mayo Clin. Proc.*, 1985, *60*, 266.

CANDIDIASIS. A review of the use of oral amphotericin in the prophylaxis of invasive candidiasis in cancer patients.— F. Meunier-Carpentier, *Am. J. Med.*, 1984, *76*, 652.

For reports of the use of amphotericin with flucytosine in the treatment of systemic, including meningeal, candidiasis, see Flucytosine, p.424.

A review of 64 cases of endocarditis probably due to *Candida* spp. treated with antifungal agents, principally amphotericin, administered as a cardiac irrigation with a 0.1% solution before and after surgery, followed by long-term intravenous treatment.— M. S. Seelig *et al.*, *Postgrad. med. J.*, 1979, *55*, 632.

Ocular candidiasis. Reports of the treatment of candidal endophthalmitis with amphotericin: B. R. Meyers *et al.*, *Ann. intern. Med.*, 1973, *79*, 647 (intravenous); G. A. Stern *et al.*, *Archs Ophthal.*, *N.Y.*, 1977, *95*, 89 (intravitreal); H. L. Cantrill *et al.*, *J. Am. med. Ass.*, 1980, *243*, 1163 (intravenous and intravitreal, with flucytosine).

Oral candidiasis. In a retrospective study of 77 granulocytopenic patients who were receiving a regimen of selective decontamination of the gastro-intestinal tract which included amphotericin by mouth, addition of amphotericin 10 mg lozenges four times daily as prophylaxis or treatment of oropharyngeal candidiasis caused a further decrease in the mean growth density of *Candida* in throat swab cultures.— H. G. de Vries-Hospers *et al.*, *Infection*, 1982, *10*, 71.

For reference to the ability of amphotericin to inhibit the adherence of *Candida* spp. to denture acrylic, see

Nystatin p.432.

Urinary candidiasis. A report of the successful eradication of noninvasive candiduria in 37 of 40 patients treated by continuous bladder irrigation with a 0.005% aqueous suspension of amphotericin. Treatment was continued for 4 to 14 days, and there was no significant absorption of the drug through the bladder mucosa.— G. J. Wise *et al., J. Urol., Baltimore*, 1982, *128*, 82.

CHROMOMYCOSIS. Treatment of chromomycosis by intralesional administration of amphotericin with a pressure-gun.— D. A. Whiting, *Br. J. Derm.*, 1967, *79*, 345.

COCCIDIOIDOMYCOSIS. Amphotericin has been the treatment of choice in coccidioidomycosis for 25 years; only recently have alternative agents become available. Therefore there are few studies evaluating its efficacy or determining the optimum dosage regimen. The clinical impression is that it is effective in curing localised skin and soft-tissue infections, and that it prolongs survival and often cures coccidioidal meningitis. Coccidioidomycosis is more difficult to treat with amphotericin than comparable infections caused by other fungi, although its *in vitro* susceptibility is similar. In severe disseminated disease total doses of more than 12 to 15 g of amphotericin over several years have been required just to suppress the infection. Therefore, to reduce the renal damage that these doses will cause, courses of 1 to 3 g have been given to control the disease, with intervening out-patient maintenance infusions. In localised infection, intradermal, intra-articular, and inhalational administration have been used, although the value of this treatment has not been established; however, clinical experience has shown that in coccidioidal meningitis intrathecal in addition to intravenous treatment is essential. In patients with extensive lesions surgical excision is important to augment the efficacy of amphotericin. Dosage regimens of amphotericin for coccidioidomycosis vary according to the site and extent of infection, and on the immune status of the patient.— D. J. Drutz, *Drugs*, 1983, *26*, 337.

From experience of 7 patients with the acquired immune deficiency syndrome who developed coccidioidomycosis, initial treatment with intravenous amphotericin administered 3 or more times weekly up to a total dose of 1 to 2.5 g, followed by long-term therapy with ketoconazole at least 400 mg daily by mouth was suggested. It was considered, however, that the chronic administration of amphotericin at more prolonged intervals might prove to be as or more effective than treatment with ketoconazole in preventing recurrent symptoms.— D. A. Bronnimann *et al., Ann. intern. Med.*, 1987, *106*, 372.

For a report on the use of amphotericin with ketoconazole in the treatment of coccidioidal meningitis, see Ketoconazole p.429.

CRYPTOCOCCOSIS. Amphotericin is used in cryptococcal infections often in conjunction with flucytosine. For reports of this use see Flucytosine (p.424).

HISTOPLASMOSIS. For reference to the use of amphotericin for the treatment of histoplasmosis in patients with the acquired immune deficiency syndrome, see Ketoconazole p.429.

LEISHMANIASIS. In a comparison of 5 treatment regimens for mucosal leishmaniasis, amphotericin was used in 8 patients with good results. In patients who do not respond to antimony compounds amphotericin should be used.— R. N. R. Sampaio *et al.* (letter), *Lancet*, 1985, *1*, 1097.

PHYCOMYCOSIS. For reports of the treatment of phycomycosis with amphotericin see: R. K. Marwaha *et al., Postgrad. med. J.*, 1985, *61*, 733; M. O'Keefe *et al., Br. J. Ophthal.*, 1986, *70*, 634; G. Koren *et al., J. Infect.*, 1986, *12*, 165.

PREGNANCY AND THE NEONATE. For reference to the use of amphotericin during pregnancy, see under Precautions, above.

PROTOTHECOSIS. Amphotericin and transfer factor appeared to be successful in treating a patient with a systemic algal infection caused by *Prototheca*.— G. E. Cox *et al., Lancet*, 1974, *2*, 379.

Resolution of cutaneous protothecosis due to *Prototheca wickerhamii* in one patient after treatment with a combination of amphotericin and tetracycline.— F. R. Venezio *et al., Am. J. clin. Path.*, 1982, *77*, 485.

SPOROTRICHOSIS. A report of sporotrichosis arthritis in one patient which did not respond to maximum doses of intravenous amphotericin; the concentration of amphotericin in the joints was well below the established MIC. Marked clinical improvement was observed, however, after weekly intra-articular injection of amphotericin 10 mg for 4 weeks.— M. I. Khan *et al., S. Afr. med. J.*, 1983, *64*, 1099.

Preparations

Amphotericin B Cream *(U.S.P.)*

Amphotericin B for Injection *(U.S.P.)*. A sterile complex of amphotericin and sodium deoxycholate and one or more suitable buffers. pH of a 1% solution 7.2 to 8.0.

Amphotericin B Lotion *(U.S.P.)*. pH 5 to 7.

Amphotericin Lozenges *(B.P.)*. The content of tetraenes should not be more than 13.3% w/w of the stated amount of amphotericin.

Amphotericin B Ointment *(U.S.P.)*

Proprietary Preparations

Fungilin *(Squibb, UK)*. *Lozenges*, amphotericin 10 mg. *Tablets*, scored, amphotericin 100 mg. *Suspension*, amphotericin 100 mg/mL. *Cream*, amphotericin 3%. *Ointment*, amphotericin 3%.

Fungizone *(Squibb, UK)*. *Intravenous infusion*, powder for reconstitution, amphotericin 50 mg (as sodium deoxycholate complex).

Proprietary Names and Manufacturers

Amfostat Intravenoso *(Arg.)*; Ampho-Moronal *(Heyden, Ger.; Squibb, Switz.)*; Funganiline *(Med. y Prod. Quím., Spain)*; Fungilin *(Squibb, Austral.; Squibb, Denm.; Squibb, Ital.; Squibb, UK)*; Fungizona *(Squibb, Spain)*; Fungizone *(Squibb, Austral.; Belg.; Squibb, Canad.; Squibb, Fr.; Squibb, Ital.; Neth.; Novo, Norw.; Squibb, S.Afr.; Squibb, Swed.; Switz.; Squibb, UK; Squibb, USA)*.

The following names have been used for multi-ingredient preparations containing amphotericin— Mysteclin Syrup *(Squibb, UK)*; Mysteclin-F *(Squibb, USA)*; Resteclin *(Squibb, Canad.)*.

12428-v

Bensuldazic Acid *(BAN, rINN)*.

(5-Benzyl-6-thioxo-1,3,5-thiadiazin-3-yl)acetic acid.

$C_{12}H_{14}N_2O_2S_2$=282.4.

CAS — 1219-77-8; 1950-15-8 (sodium salt).

The sodium salt of bensuldazic acid is an antifungal agent used in veterinary medicine for the external treatment of ringworm.

Proprietary Veterinary Names and Manufacturers of Sodium Bensuldazate

Defungit *(Hoechst, UK)*.

2563-t

Benzoyl Disulphide

Bensulfene. Dibenzoyl disulphide.

$C_{14}H_{10}O_2S_2$=274.4.

CAS — 644-32-6.

Benzoyl disulphide is an antifungal agent which has been applied as a 10% cream.

Proprietary Names and Manufacturers

Thiocutol *(Rosa-Phytopharma, Fr.)*.

12444-v

Bifonazole *(BAN, USAN, rINN)*.

Bay-h-4502. 1-(α-Biphenyl-4-ylbenzyl)imidazole.

$C_{22}H_{18}N_2$=310.4.

CAS — 60628-96-8.

Bifonazole is an imidazole antifungal agent with a broad spectrum of antimicrobial activity. It is applied topically as a 1% cream, solution, gel, or powder in the treatment of tinea infections, pityriasis versicolor, candidiasis, and erythrasma.

Local reactions including burning and itching have been reported.

For a series of studies demonstrating the efficacy of bifonazole 1% solution or cream in the treatment of tinea infections or pityriasis versicolor, see Bifonazole Symposium Proceedings, *Adv. Therapy*, 1986, *3*, 250 to 317.

Further references: F. Soyinka, *Curr. med. Res. Opinion*, 1987, *10*, 390.

Proprietary Names and Manufacturers

Amycor *(Médicia, Fr.)*; Azolmen *(Menarini, Ital.)*; Bifazol *(Bayer, Ital.)*; Mycospor *(Bayer, Denm.; Bayer, Ger.; Bayer, S.Afr.; Bayer, Spain)*; Mycosporan *(Bayer, Swed.)*.

2212-t

Bromochlorosalicylanilide

5-Bromo-4′-chlorosalicylanilide; 5-Bromo-*N*-(4-chlorophenyl)-2-hydroxybenzamide.

$C_{13}H_9BrClNO_2$=326.6.

Bromochlorosalicylanilide is an antifungal agent applied topically in the prophylaxis and treatment of fungous infections. Photosensitivity has been reported. See also Bromsalans, (p.953).

Proprietary Names and Manufacturers

Multifungin *(Knoll, Arg.; Nordmark, Ger.; Knoll, Neth.; Knoll, Norw.; Knoll-Made, Spain)*.

2564-x

Buclosamide *(BAN, rINN)*.

N-Butyl-4-chlorosalicylamide; *N*-Butyl-4-chloro-2-hydroxybenzamide.

$C_{11}H_{14}ClNO_2$=227.7.

CAS — 575-74-6.

Adverse Effects

Allergic skin reactions and photosensitivity have occurred.

Uses and Administration

Buclosamide is an antifungal agent which has been applied topically in concentrations of 10% in association with salicylic acid in the treatment of dermatophytoses.

Proprietary Names and Manufacturers

The following names have been used for multi-ingredient preparations containing buclosamide— Jadit *(Hoechst, UK)*.

16554-x

Butoconazole Nitrate *(BANM, USAN, rINNM)*.

RS-35887; RS-35887-00-10-3. 1-[4-(4-Chlorophenyl)-2-(2,6-dichlorophenylthio)butyl]imidazole mononitrate.

$C_{19}H_{17}Cl_3N_2S,HNO_3$=474.8.

CAS — 64872-77-1; 64872-76-0 (butoconazole).

Butoconazole nitrate is an imidazole antifungal agent which is used as a 2% vaginal cream in the treatment of vaginal candidiasis.

Local reactions including burning and itching have been reported.

A brief review of the use of butoconazole nitrate in the treatment of vulvovaginal candidiasis. Studies have shown treatment with the 2% vaginal cream for 3 days to be as effective as treatment for 7 days with miconazole nitrate 2% vaginal cream or for 3 days with clotrimazole 200 mg pessaries.— *Med. Lett.*, 1986, *28*, 68.

Proprietary Names and Manufacturers

Femstat *(Syntex, Switz.; Syntex, USA)*.

2566-f

Candicidin *(BAN, USAN, rINN)*.

NSC-94219.

CAS — 1403-17-4.

Pharmacopoeias. In *U.S.*

A mixture of antifungal heptaenes produced by *Streptomyces griseus*. It occurs as a yellow to brown powder. It contains not less than 1000 µg per mg, calculated on the dried substance. **Soluble** 1 in 75 of water, 1 in 260 of alcohol, 1 in 10 000 of chloroform, 1 in 33 000 of ether, and 1 in 50 of dimethyl sulphoxide; very slightly soluble in acetone and butyl alcohol. A 1% aqueous suspension has a pH of 8 to 10. **Store** at 2° to 8° in airtight containers and protect from light.

Units

One unit of candicidin is contained in 0.0004766 mg of the first International Reference Preparation (1978) which contains 2098 units per mg.

Candicidin is a polyene antibiotic with antifungal actions similar to nystatin (p.432). It has been used in the treatment of vaginal candidiasis in a dosage of 3 mg twice daily for 2 weeks as pessaries or vaginal ointment. Slight irritation has occurred following vaginal application of candicidin.

Report of a double-blind study involving 41 patients with benign prostatic hyperplasia. Patients received candicidin 90 mg three times daily by mouth or placebo. There was no difference in the improvement of symptoms between the two groups after 4 or 6 months of treatment. However, there was an increase in the maximum flow rate, after correction for bladder volume, in the candicidin group only, after 6 months, although not after 4 months.— K. M. -E. Jensen and P. O. Madsen, *Urol. Res.*, 1983, *11*, 7.

Proprietary Names and Manufacturers
Candeptin *(Canad.; S.Afr.; Swed.; Pharmax, UK)*; Vanobid *(Merrell Dow, USA)*.

2597-g

Caprylic Acid

Octanoic Acid *(USAN, rINN)*; Octoic Acid.
$CH_3.(CH_2)_6.CO_2H$=144.2.

CAS — 124-07-2.

3004-t

Sodium Caprylate

Sodium Octoate. Sodium octanoate.
$C_8H_{15}NaO_2$=166.2.

CAS — 1984-06-1.

Caprylic acid and sodium caprylate have antifungal activity against dermatophytes and *Candida* spp. Caprylic acid has been given by mouth, and both caprylic acid and sodium caprylate are used topically often in combination with propionates or other antifungal agents.
Sodium caprylate is used to stabilise albumin against the effects of heat.

Proprietary Names and Manufacturers of Caprylic Acid and Sodium Caprylate
Candistat *(Advanced Medical Nutrition, USA)*; Caprystatin *(Ecological Formulas, USA)*.

The following names have been used for multi-ingredient preparations containing caprylic acid and sodium caprylate— Egomycol *(Ego, Austral)*.

2569-h

Chlormidazole Hydrochloride *(BANM, rINNM)*.

Clomidazole Hydrochloride. 1-(4-Chlorobenzyl)-2-methylbenzimidazole hydrochloride.
$C_{15}H_{13}ClN_2$,HCl=293.2.

CAS — 3689-76-7 (chlormidazole); 54118-67-1 (hydrochloride).

Chlormidazole is an imidazole antifungal agent which has been used in the treatment of fungal infections of the skin.

Proprietary Names and Manufacturers
Fungo-Polycid *(Medinsa, Spain)*.

2570-a

Chlorphenesin *(BAN, pINN)*.

3-(4-Chlorophenoxy)propane-1,2-diol.
$C_9H_{11}ClO_3$=202.6.

CAS — 104-29-0.

Pharmacopoeias. In *Ind.*

Chlorphenesin has antifungal properties, particularly against dermatophytes, and also has antibacterial properties. It is used mainly in the prophylaxis and treatment of tinea infections of the feet and other sites. It is applied topically as an ointment containing 0.5% and as a dusting-powder containing 1%. There have been reports of skin sensitisation to chlorphenesin.
Chlorphenesin carbamate is used as a muscle relaxant.

Proprietary Names and Manufacturers
Aero-Mycil *(Duncan, Flockhart, UK)*; Kolpicortin-sine *(Kade, Switz.)*; Mycil *(Glaxo, Austral.; Allen & Hanburys, Canad.; Glaxo, S.Afr.; Evans Medical, UK)*; Soorphenesin *(Kade, Ger.)*.

2572-x

Ciclopirox Olamine *(USAN)*.

HOE-296. The 2-aminoethanol salt of 6-Cyclohexyl-1-hydroxy-4-methyl-2-pyridone.
$C_{12}H_{17}NO_2,C_2H_7NO$=268.4.

CAS — 29342-05-0 (ciclopirox); 41621-49-2 (ciclopirox olamine).

Pharmacopoeias. In *U.S.*

A 1% aqueous solution has a pH of 8.0 to 9.0.

Adverse Effects
Irritation and pruritus have been reported rarely after topical application of ciclopirox olamine.

Antimicrobial Action
Ciclopirox olamine has a wide spectrum of antifungal activity and some antibacterial activity. It inhibits most *Candida*, *Epidermophyton*, *Microsporum*, and *Trichophyton* spp. at a concentration of 0.5 to 4.0 μg per mL. It is also active against *Malassezia furfur*.

Uses and Administration
Ciclopirox olamine is applied topically as a 1% cream or solution in the treatment of candidiasis, tinea, and pityriasis versicolor. It is also used as a 1% vaginal cream or pessaries of 50 or 100 mg in the treatment of vaginal candidiasis.

A review of the actions and uses of ciclopirox olamine. Limited studies have shown ciclopirox olamine 1% cream to be as effective as clotrimazole 1% cream in the treatment of superficial dermatophyte and candida infections. The use of the cream in association with a 1% solution in the treatment of onychomycosis, and the use of a 1% vaginal cream in the treatment of vaginal candidiasis has been encouraging.— S. G. Jue *et al.*, *Drugs*, 1985, *29*, 330.

Results of 2 multicentre double-blind studies involving 139 and 90 patients, demonstrating ciclopirox olamine 1% cream to be more effective than the vehicle alone, and as effective as clotrimazole 1% cream in the treatment of tinea corporis and tinea cruris.— H. Bogaert *et al.*, *J. int. med. Res.*, 1986, *14*, 210.

Preparations
Ciclopirox Olamine Cream *(U.S.P.)*. Store at 15° to 30°.

Proprietary Names and Manufacturers
Batrafen *(Hoechst, Braz.; Cassella-Riedel, Ger.; Albert-Farma, Ital.; Hoechst, Jpn; Hoechst, Switz.)*; Brumixol *(Bruschettini, Ital.)*; Ciclochem *(Novag, Spain)*; Fungowas *(Wasserman, Spain)*; Loprox *(Hoechst, Canad.; Hoechst, USA)*; Miclast *(Logifarm, Ital.)*; Micomicen *(ABC, Ital.)*; Micoxolamina *(Dompè, Ital.)*; Mycoster *(Pierre Fabre, Fr.)*.

2573-r

Clotrimazole *(BAN, USAN, rINN)*.

Bay-5097; FB-5097. 1-(α-2-Chlorotrityl)imidazole.
$C_{22}H_{17}ClN_2$=344.8.

CAS — 23593-75-1.

Pharmacopoeias. In *Br., Chin., Cz., Jpn,* and *U.S.*

A white to pale yellow crystalline powder. Practically **insoluble** in water; soluble 1 in 10 of alcohol and chloroform, and 1 in 100 of ether; freely soluble in acetone and methyl alcohol. **Store** in airtight containers. Protect from light.

Adverse Effects
Gastro-intestinal disturbance, urinary symptoms, elevation of liver enzymes, neutropenia, and mental depression have been reported after administration of clotrimazole by mouth. Local reactions including irritation and burning may occur in patients treated topically; contact allergic dermatitis has been reported.

Antimicrobial Action
Clotrimazole is an imidazole antifungal agent with similar antimicrobial action and activity to ketoconazole (p.427). It also has *in vitro* activity against *Cladosporium*, *Phialophora*, and *Mucor* spp. and against *Pseudallescheria boydii*. A high proportion of fungi sensitive to clotrimazole are inhibited by concentrations of 2 μg per mL although MICs of up to 10 μg per mL have been reported. *Trichomonas vaginalis* requires up to 100 μg per mL for inhibition. Clotrimazole is usually fungistatic in concentrations achieved clinically, however *Candida* spp. have been killed at concentrations of 2 μg per mL.

Review of the antimicrobial action and activity of clotrimazole.— R. J. Holt, in *Antifungal Chemotherapy*, D.C.E. Speller (Ed.), Chichester, John Wiley, 1980, p.114.

Absorption and Fate
Clotrimazole is absorbed from the gastro-intestinal tract. It is metabolised in the liver to inactive compounds and excreted in the faeces and urine. When applied topically clotrimazole penetrates the epidermis but there is little if any systemic absorption. Slight absorption has been reported following the administration of vaginal tablets.

Uses and Administration
Clotrimazole is applied topically as a 1% cream or solution in the treatment of candidiasis, tinea, and pityriasis versicolor; a 1% powder may be used in conjunction with the cream or solution and has been applied to prevent re-infection. It is given as a vaginal cream or pessaries in dosage regimens of 100 mg for 6 days, 200 mg for 3 days, or in a single dose of 500 mg in the treatment of candidal and trichomonal vaginitis.
Lozenges of clotrimazole 10 mg are used in the treatment or prophylaxis of oral candidiasis. Clotrimazole has also been administered by mouth or as eye-drops.

CANDIDIASIS. For a report of a comparative study of clotrimazole and econazole nitrate creams in the treatment of candidiasis, see Econazole Nitrate p.422.

Oral candidiasis. Clotrimazole 10 mg troches, dissolved in the mouth 5 times daily for 2 weeks had a beneficial effect on chronic oral candidiasis when compared with placebo in a double-blind study involving 20 patients.— C. H. Kirkpatrick and D. W. Alling, *New Engl. J. Med.*, 1978, *299*, 1201.

In a study involving 296 patients with cancer, clotrimazole 10 mg troches dissolved in the mouth 3 times daily were found to be effective prophylaxis against oropharyngeal candidiasis.— E. Yeo *et al.*, *J. clin. Oncol.*, 1985, *3*, 1668.

Vaginal candidiasis. In a double-blind study involving 72 women with vaginal candidiasis, treatment with a single clotrimazole 500 mg pessary was as effective as 200 mg for 3 nights as assessed clinically and mycologically 1 and 4 weeks after finishing the course.— I. Milsom and L. Forssman, *Br. J. vener. Dis.*, 1982, *58*, 124. In a study involving 110 women, treatment with a single dose of clotrimazole 10% vaginal cream was as effective as 2% vaginal cream used twice daily for 3 days, as assessed mycologically 1 and 5 weeks after treatment.— L. Cohen, *Curr. med. Res. Opinion*, 1985, *9*, 520.

A relapse of vaginal candidiasis occurring shortly after initial treatment requires a long course of treatment such as clotrimazole 100 mg pessaries inserted vaginally daily for 12 days increased if necessary to 200 mg daily for 12 days. Controversy exists as to whether this should be combined with nystatin by mouth to treat possible re-infection from the bowel.— M. W. Adler, *Br. med. J.*, 1983, *287*, 1611. In a study of 132 patients with vulvovaginal candidiasis there was no difference in clinical or mycological cure rate 4 weeks after treatment with clotrimazole pessaries given in dosage regimens of 100 mg for 4 or 6 days, 200 mg for 3 days, or 500 mg as a single dose. There was also no difference between cure rates in patients with primary infections and patients who had recurrent infections. It was considered that in the management of patients with recurrent vaginal candidiasis single-dose therapy with a clotrimazole 500 mg pessary was an alternative to traditional regimens in the treatment of acute infections, and would also ensure maximum compliance as prophylactic intermittent therapy. Oral treatment with antifungal agents may be of limited value, but an effective alternative to prevent recolonisation from the rectum was the perianal application of a topical antifungal. Topical treatment of the partner was considered to be of doubtful value.— L. Forssman and I. Milsom, *Am. J. Obstet. Gynec.*, 1985, *152*, 959.

For a comparative report of single-dose therapy with clotrimazole or isoconazole nitrate pessaries in the treatment of vaginal candidiasis, see Isoconazole Nitrate, p.426.

Preparations

Clotrimazole Cream *(B.P.)*

Clotrimazole Cream *(U.S.P.)*. Store at 2° to 30°.

Clotrimazole Lotion *(U.S.P.)*. Store at 2° to 30°. pH 5 to 7.

Clotrimazole Pessaries *(B.P.)*

Clotrimazole Topical Solution *(U.S.P.)*. Store at 2° to 30°.

Clotrimazole Vaginal Tablets *(U.S.P.)*

Clotrimazole and Betamethasone Dipropionate Cream *(U.S.P.)*

Proprietary Preparations

Canesten *(Baypharm, UK)*. *Cream*, clotrimazole 1%.
Pessaries, clotrimazole 100 and 200 mg.
Pessaries (Canesten 1), clotrimazole 500 mg.
Vaginal cream, clotrimazole 2%.
Duopak, combination pack, 6 clotrimazole 100 mg pessaries and clotrimazole 1% cream.
Topical powder, clotrimazole 1%.
Topical solution, clotrimazole 1%, in macrogol 400.
Topical spray, clotrimazole 1%, in isopropyl alcohol 30%.

Canesten 10% VC *(Baypharm, UK)*. *Vaginal cream*, clotrimazole 10%, in a pre-filled disposable applicator.

Canesten-HC *(Baypharm, UK)*. *Cream*, clotrimazole 1%, hydrocortisone 1%.

Proprietary Names and Manufacturers

Acnecolor *(Spirig, Switz.)*; Canastene *(Belg.)*; Candid *(Ind.)*; Canesten *(Bayer, Austral.; Miles, Canad.; Bayer, Denm.; Bayer, Ger.; Sigurtà, Ital.; Neth.; Bayer, Norw.; Bayer, S.Afr.; Bayer, Spain; Bayer, Swed.; Switz.; Baypharm, UK)*; Canestene *(Bayer, Switz.)*; Canifug *(Wolff, Ger.)*; Cutistad *(Stada, Ger.)*; Desamix Antimicotico *(Savoma, Ital.)*; Durafungol *(Durachemie, Ger.)*; Empecid *(Arg.; Jpn)*; Eparol *(Ger.)*; Fungiframan *(Oftalmiso, Spain)*; Fungizid *(Ratiopharm, Ger.)*; Gyne-Lotremin *(Essex, Austral.)*; Gyne-Lotrimin *(Schering, USA)*; Gyno-Canesten *(Sigurtà, Ital.)*; Lotremin *(Essex, Austral.)*; Lotrimin *(Schering, USA)*; Micomisan *(Hosbon, Spain)*; Micoter *(Cusi, Spain)*; Mono Baycuten *(Bayropharm, Ger.)*; Mycelex *(Miles Pharmaceuticals, USA)*; Mycelex-G *(Miles Pharmaceuticals, USA)*; Myclo *(Boehringer Ingelheim, Canad.)*; Mycofug *(Hermal, Ger.)*; Myko Cordes *(Ichthyol, Ger.)*; Panmicol *(Arg.)*; Pedisafe *(Sagitta, Ger.)*; Stiemazol *(Stiefel, Ger.)*; Tibatin *(DAK, Denm.)*; Trimysten *(Bellon, Fr.)*.

The following names have been used for multi-ingredient preparations containing clotrimazole— Canesten-HC *(Baypharm, UK)*; Lotriderm *(Kirby-Warrick, UK)*; Lotrisone *(Schering, USA)*.

2575-d

Diamthazole Hydrochloride *(BANM)*.

Amycazol Hydrochloride; Amycazolum; Diamthazole Dihydrochloride; Dimazole Hydrochloride *(pINNM)*; Ro-2-2453. 6-(2-Diethylaminoethoxy)-2-dimethylaminobenzothiazole dihydrochloride.
$C_{15}H_{23}N_3OS,2HCl=366.4$.

CAS — 95-27-2 (diamthazole); 136-96-9 (hydrochloride).

Pharmacopoeias. In *Rus.*

Adverse Effects

Diamthazole may produce local irritation. Ataxia, tremors, convulsions, and hallucinations have been reported in infants but this may possibly have been due to sucking the fingers or contaminated clothing rather than to percutaneous absorption.

Precautions

The use of diamthazole is contra-indicated in children under 6 years. Its use is not recommended during the acute or pyodermic phase of any fungal infection and it should not be applied to large areas of skin or mucous membranes.

Uses and Administration

Diamthazole has antifungal properties and is used as a tincture, powder, or ointment in a concentration of 5% in the treatment of tinea infections.

Proprietary Names and Manufacturers

Asterol *(Roche, Austral.; Roche, Ital.; Roche, Switz.; Roche, UK)*; Atelor *(Roche, Arg.)*.

2579-b

Econazole Nitrate *(BANM, USAN, rINNM)*.

C-C2470; R-14827; SQ-13050. 1-[2,4-Dichloro-β-(4-chlorobenzyloxy)phenethyl]imidazole nitrate.
$C_{18}H_{15}Cl_3N_2O,HNO_3=444.7$.

CAS — 27220-47-9 (econazole); 24169-02-6; 68797-31-9 (both nitrate).

Pharmacopoeias. In *Br.*

A white or almost white, odourless or almost odourless, crystalline powder. Very slightly **soluble** in water and in ether; slightly soluble in alcohol; soluble 1 in 60 of chloroform and 1 in 25 of methyl alcohol. **Store** in well-closed containers. Protect from light.

Adverse Effects

Local reactions including burning and irritation may occur when econazole nitrate is applied topically.

Contact dermatitis occurring in one patient after use of a cream containing econazole nitrate for 15 to 20 days.— R. Valsecchi *et al.*, *Contact Dermatitis*, 1982, *8*, 422.

Antimicrobial Action

Econazole is an imidazole antifungal agent with similar antimicrobial action and activity to ketoconazole (p.427).

A comparison *in vitro* of the antimicrobial activity of econazole and miconazole.— G. Schär *et al.*, *Chemotherapy, Basle*, 1976, *22*, 211.

Absorption and Fate

Absorption is not significant when econazole nitrate is applied to the skin or vagina.

Uses and Administration

Econazole nitrate is applied topically up to 3 times daily as a 1% cream, lotion, powder, or solution in the treatment of fungal infections such as candidiasis, tinea, and pityriasis versicolor. It is also used in the treatment of vaginal candidiasis as pessaries of 150 mg three times daily; a single dose of 150 mg daily has also been used.

Econazole nitrate has also been administered as eye-drops. Econazole, as the base, has been given by mouth and by intravenous infusion.

A detailed review of the actions and uses of econazole nitrate.— R. C. Heel *et al.*, *Drugs*, 1978, *16*, 177.

The treatment of trichonocardiosis palmellina with econazole nitrate spray.— H. Krause, *Arzneimittel-Forsch.*, 1978, *28*, 1804.

ADMINISTRATION. References to the use of econazole administered intravenously in doses of 200 to 300 mg up to three times daily.— D. Hantschke *et al.*, *Mykosen*, 1978, *Suppl.* 1, 230 (aspergillosis); D. T. McLeod *et al.*, *Br. med. J.*, 1982, *285*, 1166 (aspergillosis); H. N. Oguachuba and H. C. Gugnani, *J. trop. Med. Hyg.*, 1982, *85*, 259 (african histoplasmosis).

CANDIDIASIS. A study of 40 infertile patients showed the presence of vaginal and cervical candidiasis in 35, of whom 30 responded to treatment with econazole nitrate 150 mg given by pessary once daily for 3 days. Postcoital tests on cervical mucus showed some improvement in spermatozoal compatibility in 24 treated patients, and was followed by pregnancy in 9 of them.— P. A. Georgakopoulos, *Clin. Trials J.*, 1982, *19*, 191.

A double-blind study in 38 patients with intertriginous candidiasis demonstrating econazole nitrate 1% cream and clotrimazole 1% cream to be equally effective.— S. I. Cullen *et al.*, *Curr. ther. Res.*, 1984, *35*, 606.

A report of an open multicentre study of the use of econazole nitrate 150 mg pessaries for 3 days in 117 pregnant women with vaginal candidiasis. Further antifungal treatment before delivery was required in 20 women because of failure (13) or relapse (7) after the single course of treatment. One infant, born to a mother who was positive for *Candida* at the time of delivery developed oral candidiasis.— E. Goormans *et al.*, *Curr. med. Res. Opinion*, 1985, *9*, 371.

Preparations

Econazole Cream *(B.P.)*. Econazole Nitrate Cream

Econazole Pessaries *(B.P.)*. Econazole Nitrate Pessaries

Proprietary Preparations

Econacort *(Squibb, UK)*. *Cream*, econazole nitrate 1%, hydrocortisone 1%.

Ecostatin *(Squibb, UK)*. *Cream*, econazole nitrate 1%.
Pessaries, econazole nitrate 150 mg.
Twin pack, combination pack, 3 econazole nitrate 150 mg pessaries and econazole nitrate 1% cream.
Lotion, econazole nitrate 1%.
Topical powder, econazole nitrate 1%.
Topical powder spray, econazole nitrate 1%.
Topical spray, econazole nitrate 1%, in an alcoholic solution.

Ecostatin-1 *(Squibb, UK)*. *Pessaries*, econazole nitrate 150 mg, in a long-acting basis. For single-dose use.

Gyno-Pevaryl *(Ortho-Cilag, UK)*. *Cream*, econazole nitrate 1%.
Pessaries, econazole nitrate 150 mg.
Combipack, combination pack, 3 econazole nitrate 150 mg pessaries and econazole nitrate 1% cream.

Gyno-Pevaryl 1 *(Ortho-Cilag, UK)*. *Pessaries*, econazole nitrate 150 mg, in a polysaccharide basis. For single-dose use.
Combipack, combination pack, one Gyno-Pevaryl 1 pessary and econazole nitrate 1% cream.

Pevaryl *(Ortho-Cilag, UK)*. *Cream*, econazole nitrate 1%.
Lotion, econazole nitrate 1%.
Topical powder spray, aerosol, econazole nitrate 1%.

Proprietary Names and Manufacturers

Amicel *(Salus, Ital.)*; Chemionazolo *(Brocchieri, Ital.)*; Dermazol *(CT, Ital.)*; Eco Mi *(Geymonat, Ital.)*; Ecodergin *(Von Boch, Ital.)*; Ecorex *(Tosi-Novara, Ital.)*; Ecostatin *(Squibb, Austral.; Squibb, Canad.; NZ; S.Afr.; Squibb, UK)*; Ecotam *(Alacan, Spain)*; Epi-Pevaryl *(Cilag, Ger.)*; Etramon *(Johnson & Johnson, Spain)*; Gyno-Pevaryl *(Belg.; Cilag, Fr.; Cilag, Ger.; Neth.; Norw.; NZ; Fisons, S.Afr.; Pensa, Spain; Cilag, Switz.; Ortho-Cilag, UK)*; Gyno-Pevaryl 1 *(Ortho-Cilag, UK)*; Ifenec *(Italfarmaco, Ital.)*; Micofugal *(Biopharma, Ital.)*; Micogin *(Crosara, Ital.)*; Micos *(AGIPS, Ital.)*; Micosten *(Bergamon, Ital.)*; Microespec *(Centrum, Spain)*; Mycopevaryl *(Swed.)*; Pargin *(Gibipharma, Ital.)*; Pevaryl *(Smith Kline & French, Austral.; Belg.; Cilag-Chemie, Denm.; Cilag, Fr.; Cilag, Ital.; Neth.; Cilag-Chemie, Norw.; NZ; Fisons, S.Afr.; Pensa, Spain; Cilag, Swed.; Cilag, Switz.; Ortho-Cilag, UK)*; Pevaryl P.v. *(Cilag, Switz.)*; Skilar *(Bonomelli, Ital.)*; Spectazole *(Ortho Dermatological, USA)*.

12690-t

Enilconazole *(BAN, USAN, rINN)*.

R-23979. (±)-1-(β-Allyloxy-2,4-dichlorophenethyl)imidazole.
$C_{14}H_{14}Cl_2N_2O=297.2$.

CAS — 35554-44-0.

Enilconazole is an imidazole antifungal agent used in veterinary medicine as a 0.2% solution for the treatment of ringworm in cattle, horses, and dogs.

Proprietary Veterinary Names and Manufacturers

Imaverol *(Janssen, UK)*.

16641-t

Exalamide *(rINN)*.

o-(Hexyloxy)benzamide.
$C_{13}H_{19}NO_2=221.3$.

CAS — 53370-90-4.

Exalamide is an antifungal agent which is applied topically as a 5% ointment or solution in the treatment of superficial fungal infections.

Proprietary Names and Manufacturers

Hyperan *(S.S. Pharmaceuticals, Jpn)*.

2580-x

Fenticlor *(BAN, USAN, rINN).*
D-25; HL-1050; NSC-4112; Ph-549; S-7. 2,2′-Thiobis(4-chlorophenol).
$C_{12}H_8Cl_2O_2S$=287.2.

CAS — 97-24-5.

Fenticlor is an antifungal agent, reported to have some antibacterial activity, which is applied topically in concentrations of up to 5% in the treatment of dermatophyte infections. Sensitivity and photosensitivity reactions have been reported.

Proprietary Names and Manufacturers
ADT Spray *(Armour, UK)*; Antimyk *(Pfleger, Ger.)*.

16806-n

Fenticonazole Nitrate *(BANM, USAN, rINNM).*
Rec-15-1476. (±)-1-[2,4-Dichloro-β-{[*p*-(phenylthio)benzyl]oxy}phenethyl]imidazole mononitrate.
$C_{24}H_{20}Cl_2N_2OS,HNO_3$=518.4.

CAS — 73151-29-8; 72479-26-6 (fenticonazole).

Fenticonazole nitrate is an imidazole antifungal agent which is applied topically as a 2% cream, powder, or solution.

A brief review of the antimicrobial action of fenticonazole *in vitro* and in *animals*.— H. Koch, *Pharm. Int.*, 1982, *3,* 279.

Comparative studies of fenticonazole and miconazole in the treatment of fungal infections: H. Stetter, *Acta ther.*, 1984, *10,* 241 (dermatomycoses); A. Gastaldi, *Curr. ther. Res.*, 1985, *38,* 489 (vaginal candidiasis); T. A. M. Athow-Frost *et al.*, *Curr. med. Res. Opinion*, 1986, *10,* 107 (dermatomycoses and pityriasis versicolor).

Comparative studies of fenticonazole and clotrimazole: E. Brewster *et al.*, *J. int. med. Res.*, 1986, *14,* 306.

Proprietary Names and Manufacturers
Lomexin *(Recordati, Ital.)*.

2581-r

Fezatione *(rINN).*
Fezathione. 3-(4-Methylbenzylideneamino)-4-phenyl-4-thiazoline-2-thione.
$C_{17}H_{14}N_2S_2$=310.4.

CAS — 15387-18-5.

Fezatione is an antifungal agent which has been applied topically as an ointment containing 2% in the treatment of dermatophyte infections.

Proprietary Names and Manufacturers
Polyodin *(Takeda, Jpn)*.

18642-y

Fluconazole *(BAN, rINN).*
UK-49858. 2-(2,4-Difluorophenyl)-1,3-bis(1*H*-1,2,4-triazol-1-yl)propan-2-ol.
$C_{13}H_{12}F_2N_6O$=306.3.

CAS — 86386-73-4.

Fluconazole is a triazole antifungal agent used systemically in the treatment of candidiasis in doses of 50 mg daily by mouth for 7 to 14 days. A single oral dose of 150 mg is used in adult vaginal candidiasis.

References to fluconazole: M. J. Humphrey *et al.*, *Antimicrob. Ag. Chemother.*, 1985, *28,* 648 (pharmacokinetic studies); F. C. Odds *et al.*, *J. antimicrob. Chemother.*, 1986, *18,* 473 (antifungal activity); C. E. Hughes and W. H. Beggs, *ibid.*, 1987, *19,* 171 (antifungal activity).

Proprietary Names and Manufacturers
Diflucan *(Pfizer, UK)*.

2582-f

Flucytosine *(BAN, USAN, rINN).*

5-FC; Ro-2-9915. 5-Fluorocytosine; 4-Amino-5-fluoropyrimidin-2(1*H*)-one.
$C_4H_4FN_3O$=129.1.

CAS — 2022-85-7.

Pharmacopoeias. In *Br.*, *Jpn*, and *U.S.*

A white to off-white crystalline powder, odourless or with a slight odour. Sparingly **soluble** in water; slightly soluble in alcohol; practically insoluble in chloroform and ether. **Store** in airtight containers. Protect from light.

A solution of flucytosine for intravenous infusion should be stored between 15° and 20°. Precipitation may occur at lower temperatures and decomposition, with the formation of fluorouracil, at higher temperatures.

Studies of the hydrolysis of flucytosine in aqueous solution. Deamination occurs to fluorouracil; in acid solutions this is the final product, but in neutral and basic solutions this is converted to further products. Flucytosine is most stable at a pH of 6.4.— L. Biondi and J. G. Nairn, *J. parent. Sci. Technol.*, 1985, *39,* 200.

Report of stability studies of flucytosine as a 1% solution in glucose injection or sodium chloride injection, and as a 0.1% solution in an irrigating solution of sodium chloride 0.855% and sodium bicarbonate 0.375%. All preparations were stored for 8 weeks in plastic bags and glass bottles in conditions of light and dark. The concentration of flucytosine did not fall below 90% of the original for any of the solutions although it was considered to be less stable in the glucose injection. The pH of the solution in glucose injection decreased, possibly due to some decomposition of glucose.— *idem.*, *Can. J. Hosp. Pharm.*, 1986, *39,* 60.

Adverse Effects

Side-effects of flucytosine include nausea, vomiting, diarrhoea, and skin rashes. Less frequently observed side-effects include confusion, hallucinations, headache, sedation, vertigo, and eosinophilia. Alterations in liver function occur in about 5 to 10% of patients and appear to be dose-related and reversible; hepatomegaly may also occur. There have been a few reports of peripheral neuropathy, and of ulcerating enterocolitis.

Bone-marrow depression, especially leucopenia and thrombocytopenia, is associated with blood concentrations of flucytosine greater than 100 μg per mL. Fatal agranulocytosis and aplastic anaemia have been reported.

Leucopenia occurred in 4 of 15 patients receiving flucytosine. All 4 had peak serum-flucytosine concentrations of 125 μg or more per mL and 3 had renal impairment, of whom 1 (with a peak concentration of 500 μg per mL) developed marrow aplasia and died of pseudomonal sepsis. The bone-marrow depression was considered to be dose-related.— C. A. Kauffman and P. T. Frame, *Antimicrob. Ag. Chemother.*, 1977, *11,* 244.

A 60-year-old man developed crystalluria while receiving flucytosine 20 g per day (200 mg per kg body-weight). Reduction of the dosage to 10 g per day resulted in a marked decrease in the excretion of urinary gravel which was shown to be a co-precipitate of flucytosine and uric acid.— K. M. Williams *et al.*, *Med. J. Aust.*, 1979, *2,* 617.

Ulcerating enteritis in one patient associated with the administration of flucytosine by mouth.— C. A. White and J. Traube, *Gastroenterology*, 1982, *83,* 1127.

A report of photosensitivity associated with the administration of flucytosine for the treatment of sporotrichosis. Photosensitivity persisted throughout the 12-month course of flucytosine, and did not subside until 12 months after the drug was discontinued.— W. B. Shelley and P. A. Sica, *J. Am. Acad. Derm.*, 1983, *8,* 229.

For suggestions that some of the toxicity of flucytosine may be due to conversion to fluorouracil, see under Absorption and Fate (below).

Treatment of Adverse Effects

Flucytosine may be removed from the body by haemodialysis or peritoneal dialysis.

Precautions

Flucytosine should be administered with care to patients with renal or hepatic impairment, or with blood disorders or bone marrow depression. Blood concentrations should be checked regularly especially in patients with renal dysfunction and those also receiving amphotericin or other nephrotoxic drugs; concentrations should generally not exceed 100 μg per mL. Care should be taken in patients receiving other drugs which depress bone marrow. Tests for liver function and blood counts should be carried out routinely in all patients. It should be administered with great care to pregnant patients, especially since flucytosine may be metabolised partly to fluorouracil.

The topical use of flucytosine should be discouraged because of the risk of the development of resistant strains of fungi.

Flucytosine interfered with the measurement on one type of analyzer (the Ektachem) of serum creatinine concentrations in one patient.— E. K. Mitchell (letter), *Ann. intern. Med.*, 1984, *101,* 278. See also P. F. Souney and G. Mariani, *Am. J. Hosp. Pharm.*, 1985, *42,* 621.

ADMINISTRATION IN RENAL FAILURE. For dosage recommendations, see under Uses, below.

INTERACTIONS. Flucytosine has been reported to be inhibited competitively by cytarabine.— R. Y. Cartwright, *Br. med. J.*, 1978, *2,* 108.

See also under Antimicrobial Action, below.

Antimicrobial Action

Flucytosine is an antifungal agent which inhibits *Cryptococcus neoformans* and *Candida* spp. at concentrations of 0.5 to 8 μg per mL. Other sensitive fungi include *Phialophora* spp. and *Cladosporium carrionii*, but its spectrum of activity is less than that of amphotericin. Some *Aspergillus* spp. have also been reported to be sensitive.

Flucytosine is believed to act by interference with nucleic acid synthesis in fungal cells. Cytosine deaminase converts flucytosine to fluorouracil which may then be incorporated into fungal RNA. Further enzymatic conversions yield fluorodeoxyuridylic acid monophosphate which may inhibit synthesis of DNA.— J. Cohen, *Lancet*, 1982, *2,* 532.

Report of a Working Group of the British Society for Mycopathology on laboratory methods for flucytosine assays and sensitivity tests.— *J. antimicrob. Chemother.*, 1984, *14,* 1.

ENHANCED ACTIVITY. *Amphotericin.* Both *in vitro* and *in vivo* studies have demonstrated synergism between flucytosine and amphotericin against *Cryptococcus neoformans* and *Candida* spp. Initially it was suggested that amphotericin facilitated the penetration of flucytosine into the cell by a disruptive action on the cell membrane; this hypothesis would explain synergistic action against fungi resistant to flucytosine due to a deficiency of cytosine permease, the enzyme which allows entry of flucytosine into the cells. However, synergism has also been shown in yeast strains where transport via cytosine permease is not the rate-limiting step but where resistance is due to defects in intracellular enzymes, and in strains which are highly susceptible to flucytosine. It has been suggested that amphotericin may inhibit flucytosine transport, and hence its actions, and act alone until depleted. This is followed by suppression or killing by flucytosine of surviving organisms. Therefore, present evidence suggests the existence of at least two mechanisms of amphotericin-flucytosine synergism.— W. H. Beggs, *J. antimicrob. Chemother.*, 1986, *17,* 402.

Although Arroyo *et al.* (*Antimicrob. Ag. Chemother.*, 1977, *11,* 21) demonstrated a synergistic action of flucytosine and amphotericin against *Aspergillus fumigatus* infection in *mice*, Lauer *et al.* (*J. antimicrob. Chemother.*, 1978, *4,* 375) did not confirm these results against *Aspergillus* spp. *in vitro*. Lauer also found flucytosine to be active only against some strains of aspergillus.

Ketoconazole. In vitro studies generally demonstrated an additive or synergistic interaction between flucytosine and ketoconazole against *Candida* spp. including some strains showing flucytosine resistance.— W. H. Beggs and G. A. Sarosi, *Antimicrob. Ag. Chemother.*, 1982, *21,* 355.

Resistance

There is a high incidence of resistance to flucytosine among isolates of *Candida* spp. before treatment and resistance has developed during treatment. *Cryptococcus neoformans* may also develop resistance and cryptococci are considered to be resistant if the MIC exceeds 12.5 μg per mL. *Candida* spp. are considered to be resistant if the MIC exceeds 100 μg per mL. Sensitivity tests should be carried out before and during treatment.

Reviews of the incidence and possible mechanisms of primary and secondary resistance to flucytosine: H. J. Scholer, in *Antifungal Chemotherapy*, D.C.E. Speller(Ed.), Chichester, John Wiley, 1980, p.47; D.

Kerridge and R. O. Nicholas, *J. antimicrob. Chemother.*, 1986, *18, Suppl. B.*, 39.

Absorption and Fate

Flucytosine is absorbed rapidly and almost completely from the gastro-intestinal tract. After doses of 2 g, peak plasma concentrations of 30 to 40 µg per mL have been achieved within 2 to 4 hours; similar concentrations have been achieved but more rapidly, after an intravenous dose. About 90% of a dose is excreted by glomerular filtration and has been recovered unchanged from the urine. It is distributed widely through the body tissues and fluids and diffuses into the CSF; concentrations in the CSF have been reported to be 65 to 90% of those in serum. Flucytosine is reported to undergo negligible binding to plasma proteins, and to have a half-life of 3 to 6 hours. In some species flucytosine is metabolised to fluorouracil; this may also occur in man. Flucytosine may be removed by haemodialysis or peritoneal dialysis.

A review of the pharmacokinetics of flucytosine.— T. K. Daneshmend and D. W. Warnock, *Clin. Pharmacokinet.*, 1983, *8*, 17.

Diasio *et al.* (*Antimicrob. Ag. Chemother.*, 1978, *14*, 903) demonstrated the presence of fluorouracil in the serum of patients and healthy subjects given flucytosine. From *in vitro* studies Harris *et al.* (*ibid.*, 1986, *29*, 44) suggested that intestinal microflora can be induced by chronic exposure to flucytosine to convert flucytosine to fluorouracil. Both authors concluded that fluorouracil may account for some of the toxicity associated with flucytosine.

For references to the penetration of flucytosine into peritoneal fluid see under Uses, Administration in Renal Failure, below.

Uses and Administration

Flucytosine is used in the treatment of severe systemic and urinary-tract infections due to susceptible fungi including *Candida* and *Cryptococcus* spp. It has also been used in the treatment of aspergillosis and chromomycosis. To reduce the emergence of resistant strains flucytosine is most often used with amphotericin. Good excretion of flucytosine in the urine and penetration into body tissues and fluids makes it useful for localised infections. Flucytosine is given by mouth, by the intravenous infusion of a 1% solution over about 20 to 40 minutes, or by intraperitoneal infusion of a 1% solution. An ointment has been used, but see Precautions.

The usual dose by mouth for adults and children is 150 mg per kg body-weight daily in four divided doses. This dose is also used for intravenous or intraperitoneal administration. In some instances daily doses as high as 200 mg per kg or as low as 50 mg per kg have been used. To reduce toxic effects the plasma concentration of flucytosine should be maintained in the range of 25 to 100 µg per mL.

The dosage interval should be increased to 12 hours in patients with a creatinine clearance of 20 to 40 mL per minute, and to 24 hours in those with a clearance of 10 to 20 mL per minute. Where the creatinine clearance is less than 10 mL per minute the dosage interval should be adjusted to maintain plasma concentrations in the therapeutic range.

Reviews of the actions and uses of flucytosine.— H. J. Scholer, in *Antifungal Chemotherapy*, D.C.E. Speller (Ed.), Chichester, John Wiley, 1980, p.35; P. E. Hermans and T. F. Keys, *Mayo Clin. Proc.*, 1983, *58*, 223; J. R. Graybill and P. C. Craven, *Drugs*, 1983, *25*, 41.

For a report of the use of flucytosine and amphotericin in the treatment of fungal splenic abscesses, see Amphotericin, p.419.

For a report on the use of flucytosine with amphotericin in the treatment of infection due to *Hansenula anomala*, see Amphotericin, p.419.

ADMINISTRATION IN RENAL FAILURE. The normal half-life for flucytosine of 3 to 6 hours was increased to 75 to 200 hours in end-stage renal failure, thus the dosage interval should be increased in patients with renal impairment. Supplemental doses are required for patients on haemodialysis or peritoneal dialysis.— W. M. Bennett *et al.*, *Am. J. Kidney Dis.*, 1983, *3*, 155. See also T. K. Daneshmend and D. W. Warnock, *Clin. Pharmacokinet.*, 1983, *8*, 17.

Potentially toxic serum concentrations of flucytosine were achieved in one patient after the administration of 15 mg per kg body-weight every 6 hours by mouth for the treatment of fungal peritonitis associated with continuous ambulatory peritoneal dialysis. It was suggested that a more suitable dosage regimen for patients on peritoneal dialysis would be a loading dose of 15 mg per kg followed by a daily dose of 15 mg per kg.— C. M. Kerr *et al.*, *Ann. intern. Med.*, 1983, *99*, 334. Three patients with peritonitis due to *Candida albicans* or *Candida glabrata* associated with continuous ambulatory peritoneal dialysis were successfully treated with flucytosine by mouth in a dosage regimen of 40 mg per kg daily for 2 days, 30 mg per kg daily for the next 2 days, followed by a maintenance dose of 15 mg per kg daily. Peak serum concentrations were between 64 and 90 µg per mL, and concentrations in the peritoneal fluid were between 58 and 79 µg per mL. Resistance to flucytosine did not develop.— E. Cecchin *et al.* (letter), *ibid.*, 1984, *100*, 321.

For further reference to the use of flucytosine in the treatment of peritonitis associated with continuous ambulatory peritoneal dialysis, see Amphotericin p.419.

ASPERGILLOSIS. Treatment of invasive aspergillosis with a combination of amphotericin and flucytosine has been advocated and there have been reports of its successful use (S.D. Codish *et al.*, *J. Am. med. Ass.*, 1979, *241*, 2418). However, there is conflicting evidence of synergistic action between these agents *in vitro* and in *animal* studies, (see above under Antimicrobial Action).

CANDIDIASIS. A report of the treatment of urinary candidiasis in 225 patients with flucytosine 100 mg per kg body-weight daily by mouth, increased gradually to 200 mg per kg daily or until the serum concentration of flucytosine was 4 times the MIC of the *Candida* spp. The mean sensitivity level for *Candida* in these patients was 3.9 µg per mL; organisms with MICs greater than 12.5 µg per mL were considered to be resistant. Treatment for 21 to 28 days resulted in reduction of the mean colony count from 82 000 to 9 000 colonies per mL in the 124 patients with indwelling urethral catheters, and eradication of infection in all but 13 of the remainder. After 7 to 10 days of treatment, the MIC in 14 patients was greater than 12.5 µg per mL, considered by these authors to demonstrate secondary resistance to flucytosine. The infection in 4 of these improved with flucytosine alone; 4 required treatment with intravenous amphotericin and 6 with amphotericin by bladder irrigation.— G. J. Wise *et al.*, *J. Urol., Baltimore*, 1980, *124*, 70.

A report of the treatment of systemic candidiasis in 10 neonates. All babies were initially treated with flucytosine 100 to 215 mg per kg body-weight daily intravenously and/or by mouth. Intravenous amphotericin, 0.25 mg per kg daily increased gradually, if tolerated, to a maximum of 1 mg per kg daily, was added to the treatment of 2 patients within 48 hours when widespread dissemination of infection was apparent. Treatment was successful in 9 neonates who were treated for a duration of 5 to 18 days. In the tenth neonate treatment was delayed, and the infection did not respond to 3 separate courses of flucytosine and one of amphotericin. The authors concluded that flucytosine alone is appropriate treatment for candidiasis in babies who do not have a fulminating illness and in whom the diagnosis is made before multi-organ involvement occurs.— H. Smith and P. Congdon, *Archs Dis. Childh.*, 1985, *60*, 365. See also P. Duffty and D. J. Lloyd (letter), *ibid.*, 1983, *58*, 318.

A retrospective analysis of 17 patients with meningitis due to *Candida* spp. who were treated with a combination of amphotericin and flucytosine, 14 of whom had clinical and mycological cure. The authors concluded that combination therapy provided effective treatment, and that in the absence of a prospective controlled trial comparing it with amphotericin treatment alone, offered theoretical and practical advantages. These include synergistic activity against *Candida* spp. demonstrated *in vitro* and in *animals*, and the use of lower doses of amphotericin thereby reducing its toxicity.— R. A. Smego *et al.*, *Rev. infect. Dis.*, 1984, *6*, 791. See also S. Buchs and P. Pfister, *Mykosen*, 1983, *26*, 73.

CHROMOMYCOSIS. Treatment for 2 to 67 months with flucytosine by mouth cured 16 of 23 patients with chromomycosis. Resistance to flucytosine developed during treatment in 7 patients; it was suggested that resistance is less likely to develop when a dose of 200 mg per kg body-weight daily is given or when lesions are early and well localised.— C. F. Lopes *et al.*, *Int. J. Derm.*, 1978, *17*, 414.

CRYPTOCOCCOSIS. In a collaborative study of patients with cryptococcal meningitis, treatment with a 6-week course of amphotericin 300 µg per kg body-weight daily and flucytosine 150 mg per kg daily in divided doses every 6 hours was compared with a 10-week regimen of amphotericin alone, 400 µg per kg daily being given for 6 weeks then 800 µg per kg every other day for 4 weeks. Up to 3 intrathecal doses of amphotericin were allowed in either regimen. After 51 courses of treatment 16 of 24 patients were cured or improved by the combination treatment and 11 of 27 by amphotericin alone. Cerebrospinal fluid became sterile more rapidly in patients given the combination. Five patients on each regimen died during treatment. Side-effects attributed to flucytosine occurred in 11 of 34 patients originally randomised to receive the combination therapy and in 6 patients the side-effects were a major factor in the decision to discontinue flucytosine. Nine patients given the combination had leucopenia or thrombocytopenia or both, 3 had diarrhoea, and 3 an erythematous diffuse maculopapular rash. Most of the reactions began 10 to 26 days after starting flucytosine. Nevertheless the combination regimen was considered the treatment of choice in cryptococcal meningitis because of its equivalent or superior efficacy to amphotericin alone, more rapid sterilisation of the CSF, and shorter length of treatment.— J. E. Bennett *et al.*, *New Engl. J. Med.*, 1979, *301*, 126. A multicentre prospective study involving 91 patients with cryptococcal meningitis given either a 4-week or a 6-week regimen of flucytosine with amphotericin indicated that for selected patients a 4-week regimen was effective.— W. E. Dismukes *et al.*, *New Engl. J. Med.*, 1987, *317*, 334.

Successful treatment of cerebral cryptococcoma associated with cryptococcal meningitis with a combination of intravenous amphotericin and flucytosine by mouth.— P. Bayardelle *et al.*, *Can. med. Ass. J.*, 1982, *127*, 732.

A report of the successful treatment of systemic cryptococcosis in a patient on haemodialysis. Amphotericin 600 µg per kg body-weight was administered intravenously on alternate days during haemodialysis, and flucytosine 50 mg per kg was given by mouth after each haemodialysis. Treatment was necessary for a total of 10 weeks.— R. Banks *et al.*, *Postgrad. med. J.*, 1985, *61*, 745.

A report of the treatment of cryptococcal infection in 26 patients with the acquired immune deficiency syndrome (AIDS), most of whom had meningeal involvement. Ten patients received amphotericin 400 to 600 µg per kg body-weight daily by intravenous infusion; 14 received amphotericin 300 to 600 µg per kg daily in association with flucytosine 150 mg per kg daily by mouth. Only 2 from each group had sustained clinical improvement after the first course of treatment, and one receiving amphotericin alone after a relapse. Three patients also received intrathecal amphotericin in a total dose of 1.6 to 4.6 g, but treatment failed in all 3. Amphotericin was frequently associated with renal dysfunction, fevers and chills, but permanent discontinuation was not required in any patient. Flucytosine was discontinued during 7 courses of treatment in 6 patients due to leucopenia (6 episodes) and exacerbation of ulcerative colitis (1 episode).— J. A. Kovacs *et al.*, *Ann. intern. Med.*, 1985, *103*, 533. In a similar analysis of a further 26 AIDS patients with cryptococcosis, 14 received amphotericin 400 to 600 µg per kg daily by intravenous infusion, and 11 received amphotericin in association with flucytosine. Three patients also received intrathecal amphotericin. Flucytosine was given if renal function and peripheral leucocyte count were satisfactory. The addition of flucytosine to the treatment regimen was not considered to reduce the duration of therapy, reduce the total dose of amphotericin required, or have a significant effect on the relapse rate. Of 15 patients who were followed up after successful completion of the initial treatment course, 8 received no further treatment, 4 of whom relapsed within 6 months and died. The other 7 patients received maintenance treatment with intravenous amphotericin in a dose of either 100 mg weekly, or 40 mg twice weekly. None of these patients had a relapse.— A. Zuger *et al.*, *ibid.*, 1986, *104*, 234.

Most cases of cryptococcal meningitis in patients with AIDS have responded to treatment with systemic amphotericin and flucytosine without the need for intraventricular amphotericin via a subcutaneous reservoir; after a response to combined therapy is achieved the patient is treated with amphotericin once or twice a week indefinitely. Intraventricular administration of amphotericin is recommended by the author for severe cryptococcal meningitis in patients with neoplastic disease.— D. Armstrong *et al.*, *Ann. intern. Med.*, 1985, *103*, 738.

A retrospective study of 13 patients treated with a combination of amphotericin and flucytosine for first episodes of cryptococcal meningitis suggested that early intervention with intraventricular amphotericin in association with systemic therapy may be of benefit in patients known to have a poor prognosis from the outset of their disease. Complications of intraventricular therapy included those due to the subcutaneous reservoir, such as infection or clogging with proteinaceous material, or toxicity associated with the intraventricular administration of amphotericin, such as ventriculitis and tinnitus.— B. Polsky, *Am. J. Med.*, 1986, *81*, 24.

Preparations

Flucytosine Capsules *(U.S.P.)*

Flucytosine Tablets *(B.P.)*

Proprietary Preparations

Alcobon *(Roche, UK). Tablets*, scored, flucytosine 500 mg.

Infusion, flucytosine 10 mg/mL, in bottles of 250 mL. For intravenous or intraperitoneal administration.

Proprietary Names and Manufacturers

Alcobon *(NZ; Roche, S.Afr.; Roche, UK)*; Ancobon *(Roche, USA)*; Ancotil *(Arg.; Roche, Austral.; Roche, Canad.; Roche, Denm.; Roche, Fr.; Roche, Ger.; Roche, Ital.; Jpn; Roche, Norw.; Roche, Swed.; Switz.)*.

2561-k

Griseofulvin *(BAN, USAN, rINN)*.

Curling Factor; Griseofulvinum. (2*S*,4′*R*)-7-Chloro-2′,4,6-trimethoxy-4′-methylspiro[benzofuran-2(3*H*),3′-cyclohexene]-3,6′-dione.

$C_{17}H_{17}ClO_6$=352.8.

CAS — 126-07-8.

Pharmacopoeias. In *Aust., Br., Braz., Chin., Cz., Egypt., Eur., Fr., Ger., Ind., Int., It., Jpn, Jug., Neth., Nord., Roum., Rus., Swiss, Turk.,* and *U.S.* Also in *B.P. Vet.*

An antifungal substance produced by the growth of certain strains of *Penicillium griseofulvum*, or by any other means. It is a white to creamy- or yellowish-white, odourless or almost odourless powder. The *B.P.* specifies that the particles of the powder are generally up to 5 μm in maximum dimension, though larger particles, which may occasionally exceed 30 μm, may be present; *U.S.P.* describes material with a predominance of particles of the order of 4 μm in diameter.

The *B.P.* specifies 97 to 102% of $C_{17}H_{17}ClO_6$, calculated on the dried substance; the *U.S.P.* specifies not less than 900 μg of $C_{17}H_{17}ClO_6$ per mg.

B.P. **solubilities** are: practically insoluble in water; slightly soluble in alcohol and in methyl alcohol; soluble in chloroform; freely soluble in dimethylformamide and in tetrachloroethane. *U.S.P.* solubilities are: very slightly soluble in water; sparingly soluble in alcohol; soluble in acetone, chloroform, and dimethylformamide. **Store** in airtight containers.

Adverse Effects

Side-effects are usually mild and transient and consist of headache, skin rashes, dryness of the mouth, an altered sensation of taste, and gastro-intestinal disturbances. Angioedema, erythema multiforme, exfoliative dermatitis, proteinuria, leucopenia and other blood dyscrasias, candidiasis, paraesthesia, photosensitisation, and severe headache have been reported occasionally. Depression, confusion, dizziness, insomnia, and fatigue have also been reported.

Abnormalities of the sexual organs and breasts have occurred, especially in children. There have been a few reports of hepatotoxicity attributed to griseofulvin.

Report of a Type 1 (Lepra) 'downgrading' reaction, from borderline tuberculous leprosy to sub-polar lepromatous leprosy, associated with the administration of griseofulvin in one patient.— D. G. Shulman *et al.*, *Archs Derm.*, 1982, *118*, 909.

PREGNANCY AND THE NEONATE. Griseofulvin was embryotoxic and teratogenic in *rats*, and had caused primary hepatic carcinomas in *mice*. There was no present evidence of carcinogenicity in man where the latent periods might lie between 10 and 30 years.— *Med. Lett.*, 1976, *18*, 17.

For the only 2 sets of conjoined twins in the FDA teratogen information system, an association between maternal griseofulvin exposure in early pregnancy and this defect was postulated. Limited data indicated that most pregnancy outcomes after griseofulvin exposure early in pregnancy were normal, but there may be a moderate association with other defects, such as spontaneous abortion.— F. W. Rosa *et al.* (letter), *Lancet*, 1987, *1*, 171. The Hungarian register revealed no maternal use of griseofulvin in any of the 39 cases of conjoined twins.— J. Métneki and A. Czeizel (letter), *ibid.*, 1042.

Precautions

Griseofulvin is contra-indicated in patients with porphyria and liver failure, and should be used with extreme caution in patients with systemic lupus erythematosus.

Griseofulvin may diminish the effects of coumarin anticoagulants and oral contraceptives possibly by increasing their rate of metabolism. Phenobarbitone has been reported to decrease the gastro-intestinal absorption of griseofulvin, and therefore the effects of griseofulvin may be diminished by concurrent therapy with barbiturates. The use of griseofulvin in pregnancy is not recommended.

In a 22-year-old woman with a 6-year history of systemic lupus erythematosus, a fatal episode of the disease was associated with the administration of a total of not more than 1 g of griseofulvin over the 7 days preceding admission.— R. Madhok *et al.*, *Br. med. J.*, 1985, *291*, 249.

INTERACTIONS. The response to bromocriptine was blocked in a patient who was also receiving griseofulvin.— G. Schwinn *et al.*, *Eur. J. clin. Invest.*, 1977, *7*, 101.

For details of the inhibition of the anticoagulant activity of warfarin by griseofulvin, see Warfarin Sodium, p.346.

PORPHYRIA. Griseofulvin was considered to be unsafe in patients with acute porphyria as it has been associated with acute attacks.— M.R. Moore and K.E.L. McColl, *Porphyrias, Drug Lists*, Glasgow, Porphyria Research Unit, University of Glasgow, 1987.

Antimicrobial Action

Griseofulvin is an antifungal antibiotic which is reported to be deposited in keratin in fungistatic concentrations. It exerts an inhibitory action *in vitro* against the common dermatophytes, including *Epidermophyton floccosum, Microsporum* spp., and *Trichophyton* spp. The inhibitory action has been reported in concentrations of 0.14 to 5 μg per mL though 15 μg or more per mL has on occasion been necessary.

It is inactive against yeasts, such as *Cryptococcus neoformans*, yeast-like fungi such as *Candida albicans*, and against *Aspergillus* spp., *Blastomyces dermatitidis, Cladosporium carrionii, Coccidioides immitis, Geotrichum* spp., *Histoplasma capsulatum, Malassezia furfur* (*Pityrosporum orbiculare*), *Phialophora* spp., and *Sporotrichum schenckii*. It is also inactive against bacteria.

Absorption and Fate

Griseofulvin is irregularly absorbed from the gastro-intestinal tract. It is deposited in keratin precursor cells and is concentrated in the stratum corneum of the skin and in the nails and hair, thus preventing fungous invasion of newly formed cells. Griseofulvin is metabolised by the liver mainly to 6-demethylgriseofulvin which is excreted in the urine. A large amount of a dose of griseofulvin is excreted unchanged in the faeces and a small amount in the urine; some is excreted in the sweat.

The absorption of griseofulvin can be increased by administration with a fatty meal or a glass of milk, or by reducing its particle size.

Uses and Administration

Griseofulvin is administered by mouth in the treatment of tinea (ringworm) infections caused by various species of *Epidermophyton, Microsporum*, and *Trichophyton*. It is generally given for infections of the scalp, hair, and nails, and for infections of the skin which do not respond to topical treatment; however it is considered to be least effective against infections of the soles of the feet, the palms of the hands, and the toe-nails.

It is ineffective in the treatment of actinomycosis, aspergillosis, blastomycosis, coccidioidomycosis, cryptococcosis, histoplasmosis, chromomycosis, sporotrichosis, nocardiosis, candidiasis, and pityriasis versicolor.

The usual dose of griseofulvin is 0.5 to 1 g daily in single or divided doses; children may be given 10 mg per kg body-weight daily. These recommended doses have been reduced by one third when preparations, available in some countries, containing ultramicrocrystalline griseofulvin are used. Griseofulvin is probably best given with or after meals.

The duration of treatment depends on the thickness of the keratin layer: 2 to 6 weeks for infections of the hair and skin, 6 to 9 months for infections of the finger-nails, and 12 to 18 months for infections of the toe-nails.

ADMINISTRATION. *Topical use.* Reference to the topical use of griseofulvin in the treatment of superficial tinea infections.— H. Abdel-Aal, *J. int. med. Res.*, 1977, *5*, 382.

RAYNAUD'S SYNDROME. In a review of the management of Raynaud's syndrome, mention was made of several reports of successful treatment of the syndrome with griseofulvin administered by mouth. Improvement was more marked in patients with Raynaud's disease than in those with Raynaud's syndrome associated with systemic sclerosis. It was concluded, however, that long-term studies were required to establish whether griseofulvin offers a lasting clinical benefit in Raynaud's syndrome.— P. M. Dowd, *Br. J. Derm.*, 1986, *114*, 527.

TINEA. A 16-year-old girl whose tinea capitis had not responded to griseofulvin 1 g daily for 18 months was cured after receiving cimetidine 300 mg four times daily in association with griseofulvin 1.5 g daily for 2 months. The addition of cimetidine to griseofulvin allowed the patient's cell-mediated immunity to effect a cure.— S. E. Presser and H. Blank (letter), *Lancet*, 1981, *1*, 108.

Preparations

Griseofulvin Capsules *(U.S.P.)*. Capsules containing griseofulvin (microsize).

Griseofulvin Oral Suspension *(U.S.P.)*. A suspension containing griseofulvin (microsize); it contains one or more suitable diluents, preservatives, colouring, flavouring, and wetting agents. pH 6.5 to 7.5.

Griseofulvin Tablets *(B.P.)*

Griseofulvin Tablets *(U.S.P.)*. Tablets containing griseofulvin (microsize).

Ultramicrosize Griseofulvin Tablets *(U.S.P.)*. Tablets containing griseofulvin (ultramicrosize) dispersed in macrogol 6000 or by other suitable means.

Proprietary Preparations

Fulcin *(ICI Pharmaceuticals, UK). Tablets*, scored, griseofulvin 125 mg.

Tablets, griseofulvin 500 mg.

Suspension, griseofulvin 125 mg/5 mL.

Grisovin *(Glaxo, UK). Tablets*, griseofulvin 125 and 500 mg.

Proprietary Names and Manufacturers

Delmofulvina *(Coli, Ital.)*; Fulcin *(ICI, Austral.; Belg.; ICI, Denm.; ICI, Ger.; ICI-Pharma, Ital.; ICI, Norw.; S.Afr.; ICI, Spain; ICI, Swed.; ICI, Switz.; ICI Pharmaceuticals, UK)*; Fulcine *(I.C.I.-Pharma, Fr.)*; Fulvicin *(Schering, Canad.;Schering, USA)*; Fulvicina *(Interpharma, Spain)*; Fungivin *(Nyco, Norw.)*; Greosin *(Glaxo, Spain)*; Grifulvin *(Israel; Ortho Dermatological, USA)*; Grisactin *(Ayerst, USA)*; Grisaltin *(Canad.)*; Griséfuline *(Midy, Fr.)*; Griseostatin *(Essex, Austral.)*; Grisovin *(Glaxo, Austral.; Glaxo, S.Afr.; Glaxo, Swed.; Glaxo, Switz.; Glaxo, UK)*; Grisovina FP *(Glaxo, Ital.)*; Grisovine *(Greece)*; Grisovin-FP *(Glaxo, Canad.; Jpn)*; Gris-PEG *(Wander, Switz.; Herbert, USA)*; Lamoryl *(Leo, Denm.; Leo, Norw.; Lövens, Swed.)*; Likuden *(Cassella-Riedel, Ger.)*; Microcidal *(Lennon, S.Afr.)*; Neo-Fulcin; Polygris *(Essex, Ger.)*; Sulvina *(Dibios, Spain)*.

2583-d

Hachimycin *(BAN, pINN).*
Trichomycin; Trichomycinum. A mixture of heptaenes produced by the growth of *Streptomyces hachijoensis.* Approximate molecular formula: $C_{61}H_{84}N_2O_{20}$=1165.3.

CAS — 1394-02-1.

Pharmacopoeias. In *Jpn.*

Antimicrobial Action
Hachimycin is a polyene antibiotic with activity against some pathogenic fungi and yeasts including *Aspergillus* spp., *Candida* spp., *Trichophyton* spp., and against *Trichomonas vaginalis.*

Uses and Administration
Hachimycin is used in the treatment of vaginal candidiasis and trichomoniasis. It is used by topical application, as pessaries, and has also been given by mouth.

Proprietary Names and Manufacturers
Nipotracin *(Ralay, Spain)*; Trichimycin *(Fujisawa, Jpn)*; Trichomycine *(Syntex, Switz.)*; Tricomicin *(Inibsa, Spain).*

2585-h

Haloprogin *(USAN, rINN).*
M-1028; NSC-100071. 3-Iodoprop-2-ynyl 2,4,5-trichlorophenyl ether.
$C_9H_4Cl_3IO$=361.4.

CAS — 777-11-7.

Pharmacopoeias. In *U.S.*

Store in airtight containers and protect from light.

Adverse Effects
Local reactions may occur and include irritation, pruritus, and vesiculation. There may be increased maceration and exacerbation of existing lesions.

Reports of contact dermatitis with preparations of haloprogin being attributed to ethyl sebacate incorporated as a solubiliser: H. V. Moss, *Archs Derm.*, 1974, *109*, 572; A. R. Berlin and F. Miller, *ibid.*, 1976, *112*, 1563.

Antimicrobial Action
Haloprogin is reported to inhibit *Epidermophyton, Microsporum, Trichophyton,* and *Candida* spp. and *Malassezia furfur.*

Uses and Administration
Haloprogin is used in the treatment of tinea infections and pityriasis versicolor. It is applied topically as a 1% cream or solution.

Preparations

Haloprogin Cream *(U.S.P.).* Store at 15° to 30°.

Haloprogin Topical Solution *(U.S.P.).* Store at 15° to 30°.

Proprietary Names and Manufacturers
Halotex *(Westwood, Canad.; Westwood, USA)*; Mycanden *(Schering, Arg.; Schering, Denm.; Asche, Ger.; Schering, S. Afr.)*; Mycilan *(Belg.; Théraplix, Fr.)*; Polik *(Jpn).*

2586-m

Hamycin *(USAN, pINN).*
A polyene antimicrobial substance produced by the growth of *Streptomyces pimprina.*

CAS — 1403-71-0.

Hamycin has been reported to have antifungal and antitrichomonal properties. It has been administered topically and by mouth in a variety of fungal infections.

Separation by high-speed liquid chromatography indicated that hachimycin and hamycin were different antibiotics although minor components could be similar or even identical.— W. Mechlinski and C. P. Schaffner, *J. Chromat.*, 1974, *99*, 619.

Proprietary Names and Manufacturers
Imprina *(Lyka, Ind.)*;

2588-v

Hydroxystilbamidine Isethionate *(BANM, USAN).*
Hydroxystilbamidine Isetionate *(rINNM)*; Oxistilbamidine Isethionate. 2-Hydroxystilbene-4,4′-dicarboxamidine bis(2-hydroxyethanesulphonate).
$C_{16}H_{16}N_4O,2C_2H_6O_4S$=532.6.

CAS — 495-99-8 (hydroxystilbamidine); 533-22-2 (isethionate).

Pharmacopoeias. In *U.S.*

A fine, yellow, odourless, crystalline powder which decomposes on exposure to light. **Soluble** in water; slightly soluble in alcohol; practically insoluble in ether. A 1% solution in water has a pH of 4.0 to 5.5. **Store** in airtight containers. Protect from light.

INCOMPATIBILITY. A haze or precipitate was observed within an hour when an average dose of hydroxystilbamidine was mixed in glucose injection with heparin.— J. M. Meisler and M. W. Skolaut, *Am. J. Hosp. Pharm.*, 1966, *23*, 557.

Adverse Effects
The intravenous administration of hydroxystilbamidine isethionate may produce sudden hypotension if administered too rapidly. Dizziness, headache, nausea, vomiting, anorexia, diarrhoea, malaise, fever, breathlessness, tachycardia, pruritus, skin rash, and oedema can occur. Concentrated solutions may cause thrombophlebitis, particularly in small veins. Paraesthesia and hepatic dysfunction have also been reported. It is reported to be irritant when applied topically.
Side-effects may be diminished by administering the drug in dilute solution by slow infusion.

Precautions
Treatment with hydroxystilbamidine is probably best avoided in patients with impaired hepatic or renal function.

Antimicrobial Action
Hydroxystilbamidine isethionate has antifungal and antiprotozoal properties. It is effective against *Blastomyces dermatitidis* and *Leishmania.*

Uses and Administration
Hydroxystilbamidine isethionate has been used in the treatment of blastomycosis but the incidence of relapse can be high and it is considered less effective than amphotericin It also has been used in visceral leishmaniasis (kala-azar) and in the American mucocutaneous form.
Hydroxystilbamidine isethionate is usually administered in a dose of 225 or 250 mg daily by intravenous infusion over a period of 2 to 3 hours, the dose being dissolved, immediately before use, in 200 mL of sodium chloride 0.9% or glucose 5% injection. Children may be given 3 to 4.5 mg per kg body-weight daily. To avoid dangerous deterioration of the solution it must be protected from light during its administration. It has sometimes been given intramuscularly in similar doses but these injections are usually painful.

Preparations

Sterile Hydroxystilbamidine Isethionate *(U.S.P.).* Hydroxystilbamidine isethionate suitable for parenteral use.

Proprietary Names and Manufacturers
Merrell Dow, USA.

12868-g

Isoconazole Nitrate *(BANM, rINNM).*
R-15454. 1-[2,4-Dichloro-β-(2,6-dichlorobenzyloxy)phenethyl]imidazole nitrate.
$C_{18}H_{14}Cl_4N_2O,HNO_3$=479.1.

CAS — 27523-40-6 (isoconazole); 24168-96-5 (mononitrate); 40036-10-0 (xHNO₃).

NOTE. Isoconazole is *USAN.*

Isoconazole nitrate is an imidazole antifungal agent with a broad spectrum of antimicrobial activity including action against *Candida* spp., dermatophytes, and some bacteria. It is used in the treatment of vaginal mycoses, particularly due to *Candida* spp., in a single dose of 600 mg in the form of pessaries. It is often used in conjunction with the topical application of a 1% cream.

Local reactions including burning and itching have been reported.

A review of isoconazole nitrate used as a single dose of two 300 mg pessaries in the treatment of vaginal candidiasis. In a study in healthy subjects, little was absorbed systemically, and any drug that was absorbed appeared to be rapidly inactivated and excreted. In 7 open studies reported to date, a total of 17 700 women had been treated with this regimen; some also used isoconazole nitrate cream on the vulvo-perineal skin, and in some cases the partners also received topical treatment. When assessed 2 to 4 weeks after therapy, 80% to 90% of patients were clinically and mycologically cured.— *Drug & Ther. Bull.*, 1983, *21*, 3.

A summary of a double-blind study comparing single-dose therapy of acute vaginal candidiasis with two isoconazole [nitrate] 300 mg pessaries or one clotrimazole 500 mg pessary. The overall mycological cure rate was 78% and 74% respectively.— L. Cohen, *Am. J. Obstet. Gynec.*, 1985, *152*, 961.

Proprietary Preparations
Travogyn *(Schering, UK). Cream,* isoconazole nitrate 1%.
Pessaries, isoconazole nitrate 300 mg.

Proprietary Names and Manufacturers
Fazol *(Pharmuka, Fr.)*; Gyno-Travogène *(Schering, Switz.)*; Gyno-Travogen *(Schering, Austral.; Schering, Ger.; Schering, S.Afr.)*; Isogyn *(Crosara, Ital.)*; Travogen *(Schering, Austral.; Scherax, Ger.; Schering, Ital.; Schering, S.Afr.; Schering, Switz.)*; Travogyn *(Schering, UK).*

18657-x

Itraconazole *(BAN, USAN, rINN).*
Oriconazole; R-51211. (±)-2-*sec*-Butyl-4-[4-(4-{4-[(2R*,4S*)-2-(2,4-dichlorophenyl)-2-(1*H*-1,2,4-triazol-1-ylmethyl)-1,3-dioxolan-4-ylmethoxy]phenyl}-piperazin-1-yl)phenyl]-2,4-dihydro-1,2,4-triazol-3-one.
$C_{35}H_{38}Cl_2N_8O_4$=705.6.

CAS — 84625-61-6.

Itraconazole is a triazole antifungal agent under investigation. It may be administered by mouth or by topical application.

A review of the use of itraconazole administered by mouth for the treatment of various superficial and systemic fungal infections. Promising results have been obtained particularly in aspergillosis, chromomycosis, and sporotrichosis. Adverse effects reported have included nausea, headache, skin eruptions, and an asymptomatic rise in liver enzyme values.— G. Cauwenbergh and P. De Doncker, *Drug Dev. Res.*, 1986, *8*, 317.

Reports of the use of itraconazole by mouth: T. Heyl (letter), *Br. J. Derm.*, 1985, *112*, 728 (chromomycosis); J. Delescluse *et al., ibid.*, 1986, *114*, 701 (pityriasis versicolor); A. Del Palacio Hernanz *et al., ibid.*, *115*, 217 (pityriasis versicolor); M. A. Viviani *et al.* (letter), *Ann. intern. Med.*, 1987, *106*, 166 (cryptococcosis); G. Cauwenbergh, *Curr. ther. Res.*, 1987, *41*, 210 (vaginal candidiasis).

ADVERSE EFFECTS. Hair loss occurred in a 51-year-old woman 8 days after commencing treatment of madurомycosis with itraconazole 200 mg daily for 4 weeks. The dose was reduced to 100 mg daily for a further 6 weeks then stopped. Hair regrowth was observed, but due to progession of the infection itraconazole was reintroduced 5 weeks later at a dosage of 100 mg daily and hair loss recurred.— A. M. Heilesen (letter), *Br. med. J.*, 1986, *293*, 823.

Proprietary Names and Manufacturers
Janssen, Belg.

2589-g

Ketoconazole *(BAN, USAN, rINN).*
R-41400. (±)-*cis*-1-Acetyl-4-{4-[2-(2,4-dichlorophenyl)-2-imidazol-1-ylmethyl-1,3-dioxolan-4-ylmethoxy]phenyl}piperazine.
$C_{26}H_{28}Cl_2N_4O_4$=531.4.

CAS — 65277-42-1.

Pharmacopoeias. In *U.S.*

Adverse Effects
Gastro-intestinal disturbances including nausea

and vomiting, rash, pruritus, headache, dizziness, somnolence, and thrombocytopenia have been reported after the administration of ketoconazole by mouth. Gynaecomastia has occurred particularly after administration of high doses. Asymptomatic, transient elevations in serum concentrations of liver enzymes may occur. Hepatitis has also been reported; it is usually reversible on discontinuation of ketoconazole but fatalities have occurred.

After topical administration of ketoconazole, irritation, dermatitis, or a burning sensation has occurred.

A review of ketoconazole including adverse effects reported during treatment in 1361 patients with fungal infections.— R. C. Heel *et al.*, *Drugs*, 1982, *23*, 1.

ALLERGY. Severe angioedema occurred in 2 patients after a single dose of ketoconazole by mouth; one developed anaphylactic shock and the other dyspnoea and vomiting. One of the patients had previously shown an allergic reaction to miconazole administered topically.— C. P. H. van Dijke *et al.*, *Br. med. J.*, 1983, *287*, 1673.

EFFECTS ON ENDOCRINE FUNCTION. Pont *et al.* (*Ann. intern. Med.*, 1982, *97*, 370) demonstrated a decreased cortisol response to corticotrophin after administration of ketoconazole 400 or 600 mg by mouth to healthy male subjects. Bradbrook *et al.* (*Br. J. clin. Pharmac.*, 1985, *20*, 163) confirmed these results using tetracosactrin in 9 healthy female subjects given ketoconazole 200 mg twice daily for 5 days. In a study of 6 male patients taking ketoconazole 1.2 g daily for treatment of advanced prostatic carcinoma (M.C. White and P. Kendall-Taylor, *Lancet*, 1985, *1*, 44), all patients showed a decreased cortisol response to tetracosactrin 48 hours after commencing therapy, which was observed on occasions in 3 patients for up to 6 months. In 2 patients 24-hour urinary free cortisol concentrations also fell below normal. The authors concluded that relative corticosteroid deficiency may ensue in any subject treated with high-dose ketoconazole, and that replacement therapy should be considered, especially in the event of stress. Dandona *et al.* (*ibid.*, 227 and *J. clin. Path.*, 1985, *38*, 677), however, did not report suppression of adrenocortical secretion in 6 patients with haematological malignancies given ketoconazole 400 mg daily as long-term prophylaxis against fungal infection, and concluded that the dose-response relationship between ketoconazole and cortisol production needs confirmation. Symptomatic adrenal insufficiency, shown as hyponatraemia and confusion, was reported by Pillans *et al.* (*Lancet*, 1985, *1*, 821) in a man given ketoconazole 600 mg daily for 2½ months for the treatment of prostatic carcinoma. McCance *et al.* (*Lancet*, 1987, *1*, 573) also reported acute hypoadrenalism in a woman given ketoconazole 400 mg twice daily for 5 days.

Schürmeyer and Nieschlag (*Lancet*, 1982, *2*, 1098) demonstrated a reduction in serum and saliva concentrations of testosterone after administration of ketoconazole 400 mg by mouth to 5 healthy male subjects; the lowest values occurred 4 to 6 hours after ingestion and rose slowly reaching baseline values by the following morning. Pont *et al.* (*Archs intern. Med.*, 1984, *144*, 2150) observed a more prolonged decrease in serum-testosterone concentrations in male patients receiving ketoconazole 800 to 1200 mg daily. In 6 of 9 of these patients, who received ketoconazole for more than 4 months, sperm counts were below normal, and 2 of these were azoospermic. Out of 24 patients, 5 developed gynaecomastia, 5 impotence, and 3 decreased libido. DeFelice *et al.* (*Antimicrob. Ag. Chemother.*, 1981, *19*, 1073) reported the development of gynaecomastia in 3 out of 40 men treated with ketoconazole by mouth in doses of 200 to 1200 mg daily. Breast pain resolved after several weeks despite continued treatment although gynaecomastia persisted.

Hypothyroidism. Hypothyroidism developed in one patient during treatment of chronic mucocutaneous candidiasis with ketoconazole 200 mg twice daily by mouth decreased to 200 mg daily after 4 weeks. Hypothyroidism also developed in his 6-year-old son who received ketoconazole 100 mg daily for the treatment of oral candidiasis.— N. H. Kitching, *Br. med. J.*, 1986, *293*, 993. Comment that the hypothyroidism shown by this family may not be associated with administration of ketoconazole, but may be attributed to the 'candida endocrinopathy syndrome'. This is a syndrome of endocrine abnormalities commonly associated with chronic mucocutaneous candidiasis which may be inherited.— A. R. Tanner (letter), *ibid.*, 1987, *294*, 125.

EFFECTS ON THE LIVER. A review of all the cases of silent and symptomatic hepatic reactions occurring world wide during treatment with ketoconazole that had been reported to the manufacturer up to March 1982. Silent reactions (transient elevations of serum transaminases or alkaline phosphatase without symptoms of hepatic disease) had been observed during routine laboratory examination of patients on ketoconazole. These reactions occurred at any time during treatment and usually returned to normal despite continuation of therapy. In 1074 patients receiving ketoconazole in daily doses of 50 mg to 1 g for periods of up to 15 months, 8% had elevated serum liver enzymes before treatment, increasing to 11% during treatment, and decreasing to 6% towards the end of treatment. There were 31 reports of symptomatic hepatic reactions, 25 involving jaundice, in patients being treated with ketoconazole; viral aetiology could not be excluded in all of these. The majority of the patients were being treated for onychomycosis and symptoms occurred after a range of 1 to 24 weeks of treatment. Patients were aged between 5 and 90 years, 18 were women and 13 men. At least 9 had a history of idiosyncrasy to other drugs; 8 had a previous history of hepatitis; at least 14 had been treated with griseofulvin, and at least 19 were receiving concomitant drug therapy. Treatment was discontinued in 30 patients, all of whom recovered except one who died from hepatic necrosis. Two were retreated and both relapsed, one after approximately 2 weeks but the reaction was less severe than initially. The one patient in whom ketoconazole was not discontinued recovered uneventfully within one month while still taking the drug. By September 1982 a further 46 cases of symptomatic hepatic reactions, one fatal, had been reported, and the incidence of these reactions was estimated to be 1 in 12 000.— P. A. Janssen and J. E. Symoens, *Am. J. Med.*, 1983, *74*, 80.

Of 54 reports of alleged ketoconazole-induced hepatic injury received in the *USA* by the FDA and the manufacturer, 33 were considered likely to be caused by the administration of ketoconazole. These 33 reports occurred in 11 men and 22 women aged between 5 and 95 years, and receiving ketoconazole 100 to 400 mg daily. Jaundice occurred in 27 after treatment with ketoconazole for between 11 and 168 days. Thirty-two patients survived; in the 13 who were followed-up, it took between 1 and 16 weeks for jaundice to resolve and biochemical abnormalities to return to normal after discontinuation of ketoconazole. In the one patient who died of hepatic necrosis, therapy with ketoconazole had been continued. The hepatic damage was described as primarily hepatocellular in 18, primarily cholestatic in 5, a mixture of the two in 9, and unclear in one. It was considered that these hepatic reactions were idiosyncratic and were more likely to be due to a metabolite than to a hypersensitivity reaction. They did not appear to be dose-related.— J. H. Lewis *et al.*, *Gastroenterology*, 1984, *86*, 503.

Ketoconazole was introduced in the *UK* in 1981. By November 1984, 82 reports of possible hepatotoxicity associated with the drug, including 5 deaths, had been reported to the Committee on Safety of Medicines. In an analysis of 75 of these cases which had been adequately followed up, the reactions were classified as being probably (16 patients), possibly (48), or unlikely (5) to be related to treatment, or unclassifiable (6). The 16 patients in whom the relationship to ketoconazole treatment was probable were aged between 36 and 79 years, 11 were women, and the onset of jaundice occurred after 5 to 195 days of treatment with ketoconazole by mouth. The results of liver function tests suggested hepatocellular injury in 10 patients, and a mixed hepatocellular and cholestatic picture in the remainder. Death occurred in 3 patients; 2 had continued to receive ketoconazole after the development of symptoms, and one developed hepatic decompensation after having been asymptomatic for 2 months after treatment had been stopped. The characteristics of the 48 patients whose liver damage was possibly associated with use of ketoconazole were similar, although there was a higher incidence of mixed hepatocellular injury. Most patients in the analysis who had hepatic injury recovered when they stopped taking the drug, the results of liver function tests returning to normal after a range of 7 days to 6 months. It was concluded that the risk of hepatitis caused by ketoconazole is minimal with treatment of short duration (less than 10 days), but was greater with prolonged treatment. The reaction appears to be idiosyncratic, but is uncharacteristic of an immune-mediated reaction.— G. Lake-Bakaar *et al.*, *Br. med. J.*, 1987, *294*, 419.

Reports of fatal and non-fatal hepatitis associated with administration of ketoconazole by mouth: J. K. Heiberg and E. Svejgaard, *Br. med. J.*, 1981, *283*, 825; E. Svejgaard and L. Ranek (letter), *Ann. intern. Med.*, 1982, *96*, 788; C. P. H. van Dijke, *Pharm. Weekbl. Ned.*, 1983, *118*, 147; O. Rollman and L. Lööf (letter), *Br. J. Derm.*, 1983, *108*, 376; P. A. Duarte *et al.*, *Archs intern. Med.*, 1984, *144*, 1069; A. Svedhem, *Scand. J. infect. Dis.*, 1984, *16*, 123; E. Bercoff *et al.*, *Gut*, 1985, *26*, 636.

EFFECT ON LIPID METABOLISM. Results from a study in one patient receiving ketoconazole 400 mg daily by mouth demonstrating that ketoconazole may cause a decrease in serum-cholesterol concentrations by interfering with cholesterol synthesis. It was considered that this was a dose-dependent effect.— T. A. Miettinen and V. V. Valtonen (letter), *Lancet*, 1984, *2*, 1271.

Precautions

Since ketoconazole has been reported to cause hepatotoxicity it should not be administered to patients with pre-existing liver disease. Liver function tests should be performed before commencement of long-term treatment with ketoconazole and then at least monthly throughout treatment.

Ketoconazole has been shown to be teratogenic in *animal* studies and its use is generally not recommended during pregnancy.

Concomitant administration of drugs that reduce stomach acidity, such as anticholinergic agents, antacids, and H_2-receptor antagonists, may reduce the absorption of ketoconazole. If indicated, these drugs should be taken not less than 2 hours after ketoconazole. Ketoconazole has been shown to increase plasma concentrations of cyclosporin in patients receiving both drugs.

Reports of the effect of ketoconazole on phenazone kinetics in healthy subjects giving conflicting evidence for the inhibition of microsomal liver enzymes by ketoconazole: T. K. Daneshmend *et al.*, *Br. J. clin. Pharmac.*, 1983, *16*, 225P; G. T. Blyden *et al.*, *Clin. Pharmac. Ther.*, 1984, *35*, 229; A. P. D'Mello *et al.* (letter), *Lancet*, 1985, *2*, 209.

INTERACTIONS. *Alcohol.* Report of a reaction to alcohol, characterised by a rash on the face, upper chest, and back, occurring on 3 occasions while a patient was taking ketoconazole. The reaction had not recurred after ketoconazole therapy was discontinued.— A. J. Magnasco and L. D. Magnasco, *Clin. Pharm.*, 1986, *5*, 522.

Antituberculous agents. A report of failure of antifungal and antituberculous therapy in a child receiving ketoconazole, rifampicin, and isoniazid. Pharmacokinetic studies showed that serum concentrations of ketoconazole and rifampicin were both decreased when they were given concurrently and were undetectable when isoniazid, rifampicin, and ketoconazole were all given together. Concentrations of ketoconazole were also reduced when it was given concurrently with isoniazid alone. Although concentrations of ketoconazole were reduced when it was administered 12 hours apart from either antituberculous agent those of rifampicin were unaffected. This suggests these effects may have been due to alterations in the metabolism of ketoconazole and that ketoconazole interferes with the absorption of rifampicin.— D. Engelhard *et al.*, *New Engl. J. Med.*, 1984, *311*, 1681. See also N. Doble *et al.*, *Br. med. J.*, 1985, *291*, 849.

Antimicrobial Action

Ketoconazole is an imidazole antifungal agent which interferes with ergosterol synthesis and therefore alters the permeability of the cell membrane of sensitive fungi. It is reported to be fungistatic at concentrations achieved clinically. Ketoconazole has a wide spectrum of antimicrobial activity *in vitro* including activity against *Candida* spp., *Blastomyces dermatitidis*, *Coccidioides immitis*, *Cryptococcus neoformans*, *Histoplasma capsulatum*, *Paracoccidioides brasiliensis*, *Malassezia furfur*, *Aspergillus* spp., *Sporothrix schenckii*, most dermatophytes including *Epidermophyton floccosum*, *Microsporum canis*, *Trichophyton mentagrophytes*, and *T. rubrum*, and some bacteria. The MIC for many of these organisms ranges from 0.1 to 2 µg per mL, but values of up to 100 µg per mL have been reported for *Aspergillus* spp., *Sporothrix schenckii*, and some *Candida* spp. However, MIC values for ketoconazole are very dependent on the method used for their determination, and are not always predictive of *in vivo* activity.

A review of the antimicrobial activity and mechanism of action of ketoconazole.— R. C. Heel *et al.*, *Drugs*,

1982, *23*, 1.

The effects of ketoconazole on lymphocyte transformation responses may depend on the cell culture conditions employed and it remains to be determined whether ketoconazole would clinically act as an immunosuppressant.— J. P. Manzella and J. K. Clark (letter), *J. antimicrob. Chemother.*, 1984, *14*, 669.

For reports of the effect of ketoconazole and amphotericin on the antimicrobial activity of each other, see Amphotericin, p.418.

For a report of an additive or synergistic interaction between ketoconazole and flucytosine, see Flucytosine, p.423.

RESISTANCE. Horsburgh *et al.* (*Lancet*, 1982, *1*, 860) reported relapses during chronic therapy with ketoconazole for mucocutaneous candidiasis in 2 patients. They stated that *Candida albicans* isolates from the patients showed a high degree of *in vitro* resistance to ketoconazole, however Levine, (*ibid.*, *2*, 211) questioned this on the grounds that different methods were used to assess the MICs at the beginning and end of treatment. The isolates from these patients have been tested by a variety of methods (E.M. Johnson *et al.*, *J. antimicrob. Chemother.*, 1984, *13*, 547), and Speller and Warnock (*ibid.*, 1985, *15*, 514), have concluded that they were resistant to ketoconazole compared with the majority of isolates and have attributed this to a failure of uptake of ketoconazole by the cell. However they considered that it had not yet been shown conclusively that resistance emerged during treatment.

Absorption and Fate

The absorption of ketoconazole from the gastro-intestinal tract is variable and increases with decreasing stomach pH. Peak plasma concentrations of up to 7 µg per mL have been obtained 2 hours after administration of 200 mg by mouth. It is extensively bound to plasma proteins. Penetration into the cerebrospinal fluid is poor following oral administration. The elimination of ketoconazole is reported to be biphasic, with a terminal half-life of about 8 hours.

Ketoconazole is extensively metabolised in the liver to inactive metabolites. It is excreted as metabolites and unchanged drug chiefly in the faeces; some is excreted in the urine.

Reviews and studies of the pharmacokinetics of ketoconazole: C. Brass *et al.*, *Antimicrob. Ag. Chemother.*, 1982, *21*, 151; T. K. Daneshmend and D. W. Warnock, *Clin. Pharmacokinet.*, 1983, *8*, 17.

The pharmacokinetics of ketoconazole in severely immunocompromised patients receiving ketoconazole by mouth for the prophylaxis of fungal infection. Adults received 400 mg daily, and children 200 mg daily. Mean serum concentrations reached a peak of 5.14 µg per mL after 3 hours declining to 0.07 µg per mL after 12 hours. The mean ketoconazole concentration 2 hours after a dose remained at 3 to 5 µg per mL after prolonged therapy, except in those patients who were receiving an allogeneic bone marrow transplant in whom a marked drop in ketoconazole concentration was observed. This was considered to be related to impaired gastro-intestinal function seen in such patients.— I. M. Hann *et al.*, *J. antimicrob. Chemother.*, 1982, *10*, 489. A similar study assessing the pharmacokinetics of ketoconazole after dosage regimens of 200 mg every 6 or 12 hours.— A. W. Maksymiuk *et al.*, *Antimicrob. Ag. Chemother.*, 1982, *22*, 43.

ABSORPTION. In a study in 10 healthy subjects, Männistö *et al.* (*Antimicrob. Ag. Chemother.*, 1982, *21*, 730) reported a reduction in the absorption of ketoconazole when ingested immediately after a light breakfast. Although these results conflict with manufacturers' recommendations to take the drug with meals, the authors considered that this may be due to the low fat content of the meal used. Daneshmend *et al.* (*ibid.*, 1984, *25*, 1), however, reported that food did not reduce the absorption of ketoconazole using a meal of similar fat-content. There was a tendency for food to improve absorption at the 400- and 600-mg doses but this was not significant. There was also a delay in the time to reach peak serum concentrations at these doses but it was not considered of clinical importance.

DISTRIBUTION. Ketoconazole 200 mg by mouth with meals every 12 hours for 3 doses was given to 6 patients with infective peritonitis associated with continuous ambulatory peritoneal dialysis (CAPD). Absorption from the gastro-intestinal tract was poor and penetration into the CAPD fluid was negligible.— J. R. Chapman and D. W. Warnock (letter), *Lancet*, 1983, *2*, 510. See also C. M. Kerr *et al.*, *Ann. intern. Med.*, 1983, *99*, 334.

For a report of the penetration of ketoconazole into the CSF, see under Uses, Coccidioidomycosis.

Uses and Administration

Ketoconazole is an imidazole antifungal agent which is administered topically or by mouth. It is reported to be effective by mouth for the treatment of systemic blastomycosis, candidiasis, coccidioidomycosis, histoplasmosis, and paracoccidioidomycosis. It has also been reported to be effective by mouth in chronic mucocutaneous candidiasis, fungal infections of the gastro-intestinal tract, vaginal candidiasis, and tinea infections of the skin and nails. It has also been given for the prophylaxis of fungal infections in immunocompromised patients. However, it has been recommended that because of its erratic absorption, ketoconazole should not be used for the treatment of life-threatening fungal infections including fungal meningitis. In addition, use of ketoconazole in nonsystemic fungal infections tends to be restricted to serious infections resistant to other treatment because of the risk of hepatotoxicity.

The usual dose for treatment and prophylaxis of fungal infections is 200 mg once daily taken with food. This may be increased to 400 mg daily if an adequate response is not obtained. A dose of 400 mg once daily for 5 days is used for the treatment of chronic vaginal candidiasis. Children may be given approximately 3 mg per kg body-weight daily, or 50 mg for those aged 1 to 4 years and 100 mg for children aged 5 to 12 years.

The duration of treatment has not been established for most fungal infections, although it is considered that ketoconazole should be given for at least 6 months for systemic infections. Treatment should usually be continued for at least one week after symptoms have cleared and cultures have become negative, however, maintenance treatment may be required for some infections to prevent relapse.

Since high doses of ketoconazole have been reported to inhibit the synthesis of adrenal and testicular steroids, it has been investigated in the treament of various endocrine disorders and malignant neoplasms.

Ketoconazole is applied topically as a 2% cream in the treatment of candidial or tinea infections of the skin, or the treatment of pityriasis versicolor. It is applied once or twice daily and continued for at least a few days after the disappearance of symptoms.

Reviews and discussions of the actions and uses of ketoconazole: R. C. Heel *et al.*, *Drugs*, 1982, *23*, 1; J. R. Graybill and P. C. Craven, *Drugs*, 1983, *25*, 41; A. L. Hume and T. M. Kerkering, *Drug Intell. & clin. Pharm.*, 1983, *17*, 169; *Can. med. Ass. J.*, 1985, *133*, 1117; R. J. Hay, *Br. med. J.*, 1985, *290*, 260.

In a study of 72 neutropenic patients with malignancies or aplastic anaemia, 37 received ketoconazole 400 mg daily by mouth (200 mg daily for children) and 35 received amphotericin lozenges 10 mg four times daily in association with nystatin tablets 500 000 units and nystatin suspension 100 000 units both twice daily as prophylaxis against fungal infection. All patients received gut decontamination with neomycin sulphate and colistin, skin antiseptics, and co-trimoxazole by mouth. Prophylaxis with ketoconazole was considered to be more effective than amphotericin and nystatin. In the ketoconazole group, 11 had evidence of fungal infection, 5 had fungus, most frequently *Candida albicans*, persisting in the stools, and 3 had antibiotic-resistant fever which responded to antifungal therapy. Of the 4 patients in this group who died, none had evidence of fungal infection. In the amphotericin and nystatin group, 27 had evidence of fungal infection, 16 had fungus persisting in the stools, and 2 had antibiotic-resistant fever responding to antifungal therapy. Of the 9 patients who died in this group, 6 had concurrent fungal infection which was considered to be the primary cause of death in 2. Fungal infection was most often in oral, gastro-intestinal, or vaginal sites, but was systemic in 2 and 16 patients in the 2 groups respectively. Absorption of ketoconazole was impaired in patients receiving allogeneic bone marrow transplants, and may have contributed to a higher incidence of fungal infection in these patients receiving ketoconazole (see under Absorption and Fate, above).— I. M. Hann *et al.*, *Lancet*, 1982, *1*, 826. Of 43 patients with leukaemia or lymphoma who were treated with aggressive chemotherapy resulting in severe neutropenia, 20 received prophylaxis against fungal infection with ketoconazole 200 mg daily by mouth, and 23 received nystatin 500 000 units four times daily by mouth as a suspension. Of the 18 patients in each group who could be evaluated, fungal infections occurred in 3 and 9 patients given ketoconazole and nystatin respectively. In most cases these were localised infections, but one patient receiving ketoconazole developed disseminated aspergillosis.— P. G. Jones *et al.*, *Archs intern. Med.*, 1984, *144*, 549.

Reports of ketoconazole in the treatment of miscellaneous fungal infections: E. S. Mahgoub and S. A. Gumaa, *Trans. R. Soc. trop. Med. Hyg.*, 1984, *78*, 376 (eumycetoma due to *Madurella mycetomatis*); A. N. Cohen, *Ann. intern. Med.*, 1985, *103*, 480 (diarrhoea due to *Blastocystis hominis*).

For a report on the use of ketoconazole with amphotericin and rifampicin in the treatment of endocarditis due to *Phialophora dermatitidis* (*Wangiella dermatitidis*), see Amphotericin, p.419.

For a report of the use of ketoconazole with miconazole in the treatment of fungal keratitis, see Miconazole, p.430.

ADMINISTRATION IN RENAL FAILURE. Ketoconazole could be given in a usual dosage in renal failure. Concentrations were not affected by haemodialysis.— W. M. Bennett *et al.*, *Am. J. Kidney Dis.*, 1983, *3*, 155.

For reference to the use of ketoconazole in the treatment of peritonitis associated with continuous ambulatory peritoneal dialysis, see Amphotericin, p.419.

ASPERGILLOSIS. Results of a double-blind pilot study in 10 patients, of the use of ketoconazole in non-invasive pulmonary aspergillosis. Seven patients had allergic bronchopulmonary aspergillosis, and 3 had mycetoma. In the 6 patients who received ketoconazole 400 mg daily by mouth for one year a reduction in specific IgG antibody to *Aspergillus fumigatus* was evident after 3 months; the concentrations of total IgE and IgE specific for *A. fumigatus* in patients with allergic bronchopulmonary aspergillosis also decreased after one year. Patients with asthma reported an improvement in their symptoms although this was not supported by spirometry measurements or by decreased use of regular medication. It was concluded that long-term treatment of mycetoma, usually a benign condition, with ketoconazole may be inappropriate, but that further study of its use in allergic bronchopulmonary aspergillosis was warranted.— D. J. Shale *et al.*, *Thorax*, 1987, *42*, 26.

BLASTOMYCOSIS. Report of a multicentre study of the treatment of localised or disseminated blastomycosis or histoplasmosis in 134 patients. Patients with acute life-threatening or CNS disease were not included. Of 80 patients with blastomycosis 65 were treated for at least 6 months and followed up for a median of 17 months; 26 of 33 receiving 400 mg daily by mouth and all 32 receiving 800 mg daily were considered to be successfully treated. Of 54 patients with histoplasmosis, 39 were treated for at least 6 months and followed up for a median of 21 months; 23 of 25 receiving 400 mg daily and 10 of 14 receiving 800 mg daily were successfully treated. A total of 81 patients reported adverse effects necessitating withdrawal of therapy in 13. Adverse effects included gastro-intestinal disturbances, skin rash and pruritus, dryness of the skin and mucous membranes, raised liver enzymes, and endocrine effects including menstrual irregularities, impotence, and gynaecomastia. It was concluded that ketoconazole is effective treatment for immunocompetent patients with non-life-threatening non-meningeal forms of blastomycosis and histoplasmosis. Because of the higher frequency of adverse effects associated with the higher dose, ketoconazole therapy should be initiated at 400 mg daily.— *Ann. intern. Med.*, 1985, *103*, 861. Out of 44 patients with blastomycosis treated with ketoconazole 400 mg daily by mouth for at least 2 weeks, 35 were cured without relapse over a mean follow-up of 17 months. Ketoconazole was considered to be suitable initial treatment in compliant patients without life-threatening infections.— R. W. Bradsher *et al.*, *Ann. intern. Med.*, 1985, *103*, 872. The criteria for "cure" in systemic mycoses should include a minimum duration of good effect after stopping treatment of about 2 years for histoplasmosis and 4 years for blastomycosis (P.D. Hoeprich, *Ann. intern. Med.*, 1983, *98*, 105). He considered that the criteria used by Dismukes *et al.* (*ibid.*, 13), [and later by the National Institute of Allergy and Infectious Diseases Mycoses Study Group (*ibid.*, 1985, *103*, 861) and Bradsher *et al.* (*ibid.*, 872)] were not acceptable in systemic mycoses where the natural course of the disease is quite variable.

CANDIDIASIS. An outbreak of systemic candidiasis in an intensive care unit caused by a single strain of *Candida albicans* was controlled after all patients admitted to the unit were given prophylactic ketoconazole 400 mg daily by mouth until their discharge.— J. P. Burnie *et al.*, *Br. med. J.*, 1985, *291*, 1092.

Due to the slow improvement typically seen with ketoconazole, it is not considered effective for treatment of life-threatening systemic candidiasis.— *Med. Lett.*, 1986, *28*, 41.

In a study of 63 women with recurrent vulvovaginal candidiasis, all patients received ketoconazole 400 mg daily by mouth for 14 days, followed for 6 months by either placebo (21 patients), cyclical prophylaxis with ketoconazole 400 mg daily for 5 days at the beginning of the next 6 menstrual cycles (21), or continuous prophylaxis with ketoconazole 100 mg daily. All patients improved and had negative fungal cultures after the initial 14 days' treatment. During the next 6 months symptomatic and mycologically-proven recurrences of vaginal candidiasis occurred in 15, 6, and one patient of the 3 groups respectively. The mean time to clinical recurrence was 1.8 months in the patients receiving placebo and 3.6 months in those receiving cyclical prophylaxis. Six months after cessation of treatment however, a total of 16, 12, and 10 patients had suffered recurrences. It was concluded that long-term maintenance therapy with ketoconazole by mouth is more effective than cyclical prophylaxis in reducing the attack rate of vaginal candidiasis, but that relapse is common after withdrawal of the drug. However, because of the risk of hepatotoxicity caution is essential in selecting patients for long-term ketoconazole therapy and in following patients undergoing such treatment.— J. D. Sobel, *New Engl. J. Med.*, 1986, *315*, 1455.

COCCIDIOIDOMYCOSIS. A review of open studies carried out by 4 groups of investigators in a total of 214 patients on the use of ketoconazole by mouth in the treatment of coccidioidomycosis. Symptoms of pulmonary infections commonly improved but often only after several months of treatment with 400 mg or more daily. Skin and subcutaneous lesions were the most responsive soft-tissue infections observed. Lesions became quiescent in over 75% of patients frequently with a dosage of 200 mg daily, some response often occurring in the first month of treatment; however, lesions often harboured viable *Coccidioides immitis* organisms. Skeletal infections were slower to respond than pulmonary or soft-tissue infections. Improvement was observed in about two-thirds of patients and was more likely after 400 mg than 200 mg daily. Synovial disease appeared more likely to improve than osteomyelitis. It was concluded that ketoconazole may be a useful alternative antifungal agent for the treatment of serious coccidioidal infections although the optimum dosage and duration of therapy have yet to be established. Due to its variable absorption it may be most appropriate for the treatment of subacute or chronic infections.— J. N. Galgiani, *Drugs*, 1983, *26*, 355.

Beneficial effect of ketoconazole 800 mg daily by mouth in association with intrathecal amphotericin, or ketoconazole 1200 mg daily in the treatment of 5 patients with coccidioidal meningitis. At these doses ketoconazole could be detected in the CSF up to 24 hours after the dose; penetration was greater into the lumbar than ventricular fluid. However, it was considered that administration of ketoconazole may be required indefinitely to prevent relapse.— P. C. Craven *et al.*, *Ann. intern. Med.*, 1983, *98*, 160.

For further reference to the use of ketoconazole in the treatment of coccidioidomycosis, see Amphotericin, p.420.

ENDOCRINE DISORDERS AND MALIGNANT NEOPLASMS. Reports of the use of ketoconazole to decrease the production of steroid hormones in certain tumours and other endocrine disorders: A. Angeli and R. Frairia (letter), *Lancet*, 1985, *1*, 821 (cushing's disease); D. Carvalho *et al.* (letter), *ibid.*, *2*, 560 (hirsutism); P. Contreras *et al.* (letter), *ibid.*, 151 (malignant neoplasm of the adrenal cortex); L. D. Feldman (letter), *Ann. intern. Med.*, 1986, *104*, 123 (malignant neoplasm of the male breast); F. A. Shepherd *et al.*, *Archs intern. Med.*, 1985, *145*, 863 (small cell carcinoma of the lung with ectopic ACTH production).

Malignant neoplasm of the prostate. Two patients with advanced adenocarcinoma of the prostate relapsed after treatment with a luteinising-hormone-releasing hormone analogue (goserelin) despite maintenance of serum-testosterone concentrations below those observed after castration. There was improvement, however, after the addition of ketoconazole 200 to 400 mg four times daily by mouth. It was considered that the combination produced a total inhibition of androgen production.— J. M. Allen *et al.*, *Br. med. J.*, 1983, *287*, 1766.

Ketoconazole 400 mg by mouth was given every 8 hours to 15 patients with previously untreated advanced prostatic cancer. After 2 weeks' treatment pain had diminished in all 15 patients, and the need for analgesics was greatly reduced. Prostatic acid phosphatase concentrations fell rapidly in all 13 patients who had raised concentrations initially, and became normal in 9 after 6 weeks. Mean testosterone concentrations declined from 15 to 3.2 pmol per mL after 3 days and continued to decrease to 2.3 pmol per mL after 14 days; concentrations then however steadily increased, possibly due to a concurrent increase in concentrations of luteinising hormone. Adrenal androgens were suppressed or undetectable in 13 patients. In 13 patients who completed treatment for at least 6 months, bone scans at 6 months showed that no patient had any new lesions, and 9 had regression of some lesions. Adverse effects to treatment included transient rises in aspartate aminotransferase concentrations in 6 patients, mild transient nausea in 2, diminished libido or impotence in all, gynaecomastia in 3, and symptoms suggesting mild Addison's disease which responded to prednisone 5 mg daily in 2. A significant fall in serum-cholesterol concentrations was also observed with all patients. It was concluded that ketoconazole may be useful as sole therapy for prostate cancer in many patients.— J. Trachtenberg and A. Pont, *Lancet*, 1984, *2*, 433.

A study involving 20 patients with prostatic carcinoma that had relapsed following endocrine treatment and were subsequently given ketoconazole 200 mg or 400 mg by mouth every 8 hours. One patient withdrew due to persistent nausea while on ketoconazole treatment, and 8 died of progressive metastatic disease within 14 weeks of commencing treatment. Of the 11 alive at 6 months, one had a complete and 5 a partial response. Subjective improvement was observed in 10 patients within the first 3 months. At both doses, androstenedione concentrations decreased and there was a fall in concentrations of testosterone that were already at castrate concentrations before treatment. Ketoconazole may have a role in combination therapy to achieve total androgen ablation.— G. Williams *et al.*, *Br. J. Urol.*, 1986, *58*, 45.

Precocious puberty. A report of beneficial results with ketoconazole in 3 boys aged 3.3 to 3.9 years with precocious puberty unresponsive to buserelin. None of the patients responded to buserelin treatment given daily for 2 to 3 months, but within 24 hours of commencing therapy with ketoconazole 200 mg every 12 hours by mouth the serum-testosterone concentrations fell significantly in all patients; the mean serum-testosterone concentration after 5 days of therapy was 0.216 ng per mL, compared with 2.56 ng per mL before treatment. This was associated with striking behavioural improvements in 2; the third had only minor psychosocial problems which changed little with treatment.— F. J. Holland *et al.*, *New Engl. J. Med.*, 1985, *312*, 1023. Comment.— R. P. Kelch, *ibid.*, 1057.

HISTOPLASMOSIS. Beneficial response to ketoconazole by mouth in a 6-year-old girl with localised African histoplasmosis who did not respond to treatment with amphotericin.— D. C. W. Mabey *et al.*, *Trans. R. Soc. trop. Med. Hyg.*, 1983, *77*, 219.

A report of histoplasmosis occurring in patients with the acquired immune deficiency syndrome. It was concluded that in such patients amphotericin did not appear to be curative. Ketoconazole may be required to prevent recurrent dissemination following amphotericin treatment, but should not be used as primary therapy.— L. J. Wheat *et al.*, *Am. J. Med.*, 1985, *78*, 203.

For a report of the use of ketoconazole in the treatment of histoplasmosis, see under Blastomycosis, above.

LEISHMANIASIS. A report of 8 patients with cutaneous leishmaniasis due to *Leishmania major* treated with ketoconazole 400 mg daily by mouth for 28 days. Clinical and protozoological cure occurred in 5 patients 2 weeks after the end of treatment.— L. Weinrauch *et al.*, *Arch. dermatol. Res.*, 1983, *275*, 353. A similar dosage regimen given to 11 patients with cutaneous leishmaniasis due to *L. braziliensis guyanensis* resulted in clinical cure in 2 patients one and two months after the end of treatment.— J. -P. Dedet *et al.* (letter), *Trans. R. Soc. trop. Med. Hyg.*, 1986, *80*, 176.

PARACOCCIDIOIDOMYCOSIS. Forty-six patients with paracoccidioidomycosis were given ketoconazole 200 mg daily by mouth, increased to 400 mg daily in severe disseminated disease or in the event of an inadequate response, for 6 to 12 months. Five had failed to respond to prior treatment with sulphonamides and/or amphotericin. Four patients dropped out of the study and 4 died. Of the remaining 38, it was concluded from a scoring system that took into account clinical, radiological, and mycological indices, that none of the patients had deteriorated during therapy, the condition of one was unchanged, 2 had minor improvement, 30 had major improvement, and 5 had complete resolution of their condition. Of 10 patients who were followed up for 24 months and 28 who were followed up for less than or equal to 12 months, 2 relapsed 12 and 18 months after ceasing therapy.— A. Restrepo *et al.*, *Am. J. Med.*, 1983, *74*, 48.

PHYCOMYCOSIS. Beneficial effect on orbital mucormycosis in one patient treated with intravenous amphotericin followed by ketoconazole by mouth.— M. O'Keefe *et al.*, *Br. J. Ophthal.*, 1986, *70*, 634.

SEBORRHOEIC DERMATITIS AND PSORIASIS. Investigational studies demonstrating ketoconazole by mouth to be effective in seborrhoeic dermatitis (G.P. Ford *et al.*, *Br. J. Derm.*, 1984, *111*, 603) and scalp psoriasis (P.M. Farr *et al.*, *Lancet*, 1985, *2*, 921) have suggested an association between these conditions and colonisation with *Malassezia* (*Pityrosporum*) yeasts. Although ketoconazole by mouth is not recommended because of rapid relapse on cessation of treatment and the risk of hepatotoxicity, studies have shown a beneficial effect in seborrhoeic dermatitis after topical application of a 2% cream or shampoo (M.M. Carr *et al.*, *Br. J. Derm.*, 1987, *116*, 213; C.A. Green *et al.*, *ibid.*, 217).

Preparations

Ketoconazole Tablets *(U.S.P.)*

Proprietary Preparations

Nizoral *(Janssen, UK). Tablets*, scored, ketoconazole 200 mg.

Suspension, ketoconazole 100 mg/5 mL.

Cream, ketoconazole 2%. *Shampoo*, ketoconazole 2%.

Proprietary Names and Manufacturers

Fungarest *(Janssen, Spain)*; Fungo-Hubber *(Hubber, Spain)*; Fungoral *(Janssen Pharmaceutica, Swed.)*; Ketoderm *(Janssen, Fr.)*; Ketoisdin *(Isdin, Spain)*; Micoticum *(Vita, Spain)*; Nizoral *(Janssen, Austral.; Janssen, Canad.; Janssen, Denm.; Janssen, Fr.; Janssen, Ger.; Janssen, Ital.; Janssen, S.Afr.; Janssen, Switz.; Janssen, UK; Janssen, USA)*; Nizovules *(Janssen, S.Afr.)*; Panfungol *(Esteve, Spain)*.

2576-n

Loflucarban *(rINN)*.

Clofluonide; Dichlorofluorothiocarbanilide. 3,5-Dichloro-4′-fluorothiocarbanilide.

$C_{13}H_9Cl_2FN_2S=315.2$.

CAS — 790-69-2.

Loflucarban is an antibacterial and antifungal agent which is used as a 1% powder, or solution in the treatment of various forms of tinea and pyoderma.

Proprietary Names and Manufacturers

Fluonilid *(Searle, Arg.; Ascot, Austral.; Continental Pharma, Belg.)*.

2590-f

Mepartricin *(BAN, USAN, rINN)*.

Methylpartricin; SN-654; SPA-S-160. A mixture of the methyl esters of 2 related polyene antibiotics obtained from a strain of *Streptomyces aureofaciens* or by any other means.

CAS — 11121-32-7.

Mepartricin has antifungal and antiprotozoal activity and is used in candidal and trichomonal infections of the vagina as pessaries containing 25 000 units and as a vaginal cream. A cream and oral suspension are also available for the treatment of superficial and oral candidiasis.

A study *in vitro* comparing the antifungal activity of mepartricin and amphotericin.— M. A. Petrou and T. R. Rogers, *J. antimicrob. Chemother.*, 1985, *16*, 169.

Proprietary Names and Manufacturers

Ipertrofan *(SPA, Ital.)*; Montricin *(SPA, Ital.)*; Tricandil *(Prospa, Belg.; SPA, Ital.; Prospa, Switz.)*.

2591-d

Miconazole *(BAN, USAN, rINN).*

R-18134. 1-[2,4-Dichloro-β-(2,4-dichlorobenzyloxy)phenethyl]imidazole.
$C_{18}H_{14}Cl_4N_2O$=416.1.

CAS — 22916-47-8.

Pharmacopoeias. In *U.S.*

Protect from light.

2592-n

Miconazole Nitrate *(BANM, USAN, rINNM).*

Miconazoli Nitras; R-14889.
$C_{18}H_{14}Cl_4N_2O,HNO_3$=479.1.

CAS — 22832-87-7.

Pharmacopoeias. In *Br., Cz., Eur., Swiss,* and *U.S.*

A white or almost white, odourless or almost odourless, crystalline or microcrystalline powder. Very slightly **soluble** in water and ether; slightly soluble in alcohol and chloroform. **Store** in well-closed containers. Protect from light.

The concentration of miconazole in both castor and arachis oils had not decreased 3 months after dry heat sterilisation at 160° for 90 minutes. Castor oil was considered to be a suitable solvent for miconazole eye-drops which could be prepared by mixing the required amounts of miconazole and castor oil in the container followed by sterilisation by the above method.— R. L. H. Lee, *Aust. J. Hosp. Pharm.*, 1985, *15*, 233.

Adverse Effects

After the intravenous infusion of miconazole, phlebitis, nausea, vomiting, diarrhoea, anorexia, pruritus, rash, febrile reactions, flushes, drowsiness, and hyponatraemia have been reported. Effects on the blood include hyperlipidaemia, aggregation of erythrocytes, anaemia, and thrombocytosis. Transient tachycardia and cardiac arrhythmias have followed the rapid intravenous injection of miconazole. Rare adverse effects include acute psychosis, arthralgia, and anaphylaxis. Many of these adverse effects have been associated with the injection vehicle which contains Cremophor EL (see p.1246).

After intrathecal injection miconazole may cause irritation of the meninges.

Mild gastro-intestinal disturbances may occur when miconazole is taken by mouth.

Local irritation and sensitivity reactions may occur when miconazole nitrate is used topically; contact dermatitis has been reported.

Mention of haematuria after 22 infusions of miconazole in a 6-year-old boy.— J. Haapasaari *et al.*, *Br. med. J.*, 1982, *285*, 923.

A report of a generalised tonic-clonic convulsion in an infant occurring 10 to 15 minutes after infusion of miconazole. A dose of 500 mg rather than the prescribed dose of 50 mg had inadvertently been administered.— K. Coulthard *et al.* (letter), *Med. J. Aust.*, 1987, *146*, 57.

For a report of renal failure associated with the administration of miconazole, see under Uses, Administration in Renal Failure.

Treatment of Adverse Effects

The incidence and severity of phlebitis may be reduced by changing the site of infusion of miconazole every 2 to 3 days. Nausea and vomiting may be relieved by giving an antihistamine or anti-emetic drug before infusion, by slowing the rate of infusion, and by avoiding administration at mealtimes.

Precautions

When administered intravenously miconazole should be infused slowly over at least 30 minutes, especially in patients with cardiovascular disorders; blood values should be monitored regularly.

Miconazole given systemically may enhance the activity of anticoagulant or sulphonylurea hypoglycaemic drugs.

For reference to the immunosuppressant effects of miconazole, see under Antimicrobial Action.

ADMINISTRATION IN RENAL FAILURE. For dosage recommendations, see under Uses, below.

INTERACTIONS. The association of amphotericin and miconazole appeared to be less effective than either drug used alone.— L. P. Schacter *et al.* (letter), *Lancet*, 1976, *2*, 318.

A report of drug interactions with miconazole in 10 patients. These occurred with nicoumalone (2), phenindione (1), tioclomarol (1), ethyl biscoumacetate (1), gliclazide (2), glibenclamide (1), clomipramine (1), carbamazepine (1), phenytoin (1). In each case there was an enhanced effect of the interacting drug, which may be due to inhibition of its metabolism by miconazole.— E. Loupi *et al.*, *Thérapie*, 1982, *37*, 437.

See also under: phenytoin (p.409), warfarin sodium (p.346).

Antimicrobial Action

Miconazole is an imidazole antifungal agent with similar antimicrobial activity to ketoconazole. It also has *in vitro* activity against *Cladosporium*, *Madurella* and *Phialophora* spp. and against *Pseudallescheria boydii*, and Gram-positive bacteria including staphylococci and streptococci. A high proportion of fungi sensitive to miconazole are inhibited by concentrations of 2 μg per mL and killed by concentrations of 10 μg per mL.

Studies on the antimicrobial action of miconazole.— J. M. Van Cutsem and D. Thienpont, *Chemotherapy, Basle*, 1972, *17*, 392; M. Refai, *Mykosen*, 1973, *16*, 39; S. Shadomy *et al.*, *J. antimicrob. Chemother.*, 1977, *3*, 147; A. L. Costa *et al.*, *Mykosen*, 1977, *20*, 431.

Miconazole was effective *in vitro* against the amoeba *Naegleria fowleri*.— Y. H. Thong *et al.* (letter), *Lancet*, 1977, *2*, 876.

Miconazole inhibited *in vitro* the ability of neutrophils to reach the site of infection promptly (chemotaxis).— Y. H. Thong and D. Ness (letter), *Lancet*, 1977, *2*, 568.

Miconazole had marked immunosuppressive properties *in vitro*.— Y. H. Thong and B. Rowan-Kelly, *Br. med. J.*, 1978, *1*, 149.

The vehicle for miconazole (polyethoxylated castor oil, methyl-and propylhydroxybenzoates, and water) inhibited granulocyte adherence and leukotaxis *in vitro* at concentrations of 0.33% and above.— C. Lee and E. G. Maderazo, *Antimicrob. Ag. Chemother.*, 1978, *13*, 548.

ENHANCED ACTIVITY. A study *in vitro* indicating antimicrobial synergism of miconazole and benzoyl peroxide against *Staphylococcus* spp. and *Propionibacterium acnes*.— H. Vanden Bossche *et al.*, *Br. J. Derm.*, 1982, *107*, 343.

RESISTANCE. The development of miconazole resistance in *Candida albicans* causing a urinary-tract infection in a baby.— R. J. Holt and A. Azmi (letter), *Lancet*, 1978, *1*, 50.

Absorption and Fate

Miconazole is incompletely absorbed from the gastro-intestinal tract; peak plasma concentrations of about 1 μg per mL have been achieved 4 hours after a dose of 1 g. By intravenous infusion, doses above 9 mg per kg body-weight usually produce plasma concentrations above 1 μg per mL. Miconazole has a terminal half-life of about 24 hours. Over 90% is reported to be bound to plasma proteins. Penetration into the cerebrospinal fluid and sputum is poor but miconazole diffuses well into infected joints.

Miconazole is metabolised in the liver to inactive metabolites. From 10 to 20% of an oral or intravenous dose is excreted in the urine, mainly as metabolites, within 6 days; about 50% of an oral dose may be excreted mainly unchanged in the faeces.

Very little miconazole is removed by haemodialysis.

There is little absorption through skin or mucous membranes when miconazole nitrate is applied topically.

A review of the pharmacokinetics of miconazole.— T. K. Daneshmend and D. W. Warnock, *Clin. Pharmacokinet.*, 1983, *8*, 17.

Uses and Administration

Miconazole is administered by intravenous infusion in the treatment of severe systemic fungal infections including candidiasis, coccidioidomycosis, cryptococcosis, paracoccidioidomycosis, and infections due to *Pseudallescheria boydii*. Intravenous doses of miconazole range from 0.2 to 1.2 g three times daily. Each dose must be diluted in at least 200 mL of sodium chloride 0.9% or glucose 5% and infused slowly over 30 to 60 minutes. Children may be given 20 to 40 mg per kg body-weight daily but no more than 15 mg per kg of miconazole should be given at each infusion.

In fungal meningitis, intravenous treatment may be supplemented with intrathecal injections of miconazole; an adult dose of 15 to 20 mg has been recommended. An intravenous solution of miconazole has also been used for instillation into the bladder, trachea, and wounds. Solutions of miconazole have also been used for topical application into the eye.

Miconazole may be given by mouth in a dose of 125 to 250 mg as tablets or gel four times daily for the treatment of oral and intestinal candidiasis. It has also been given prophylactically to patients at high risk of opportunistic fungal infections. Children aged over 6 years may be given 125 mg four times daily; aged 2 to 6 years, 125 mg twice daily; under 2 years, 62.5 mg twice daily. For the treatment of oral lesions the tablets are dissolved in the mouth; a 2% w/w oral gel may also be used.

Miconazole nitrate is applied twice daily as a 2% cream, lotion, or powder in the treatment of fungal infections of the skin and nails including candidiasis, tinea, and pityriasis versicolor. In the treatment of vaginal candidiasis, 5 to 10 g of a 2% cream is inserted into the vagina once daily for 7 to 14 days, or tampons coated with miconazole nitrate 100 mg are inserted twice daily for 5 days. Miconazole nitrate pessaries may be inserted in dosage regimens of 100 mg daily for 7 to 14 days, 200 mg daily for 3 to 7 days, or in a single dose of 1200 mg.

A cream containing miconazole nitrate 2% and benzoyl peroxide 5% is used topically in the treatment of acne vulgaris.

Review of the actions and uses of miconazole.— J. R. Graybill and P. C. Craven, *Drugs*, 1983, *25*, 41.

In a study of 45 patients, miconazole 2% oral gel applied to the fitting surface of dentures after meals for 2 weeks was more effective than placebo in the treatment of denture stomatitis with or without associated angular cheilitis. Miconazole produced a greater decrease in *Candida albicans* isolated from imprint cultures and smears from dentures, and in inflammation of the palatal mucosa than placebo; there was also a greater decrease in the incidence of *Staphylococcus aureus* although this was not significant. The importance of effective brushing of dentures to prevent relapse of infection was emphasised. Two patients failed to complete treatment as they found the preparation to have a nauseating sweet taste.— C. J. Watson, *Br. dent. J.*, 1982, *152*, 403.

The use of intravenous miconazole in association with flucytosine by mouth in the treatment of fungal endophthalmitis in abusers of intravenous narcotic analgesics.— J. Gallo *et al.*, *Med. J. Aust.*, 1985, *142*, 386.

Fungal keratitis in 20 patients was treated initially with miconazole 5 mg by subconjunctival injection daily for 5 days, and also given topically every hour, in association with ketoconazole 200 mg daily by mouth in most cases. This was considered to be successful in 13 patients. In 3 patients organisms resistant to this regimen were isolated and treatment was successful after the use of alternative agents.— R. Fitzsimons and A. L. Peters, *Am. J. Ophthal.*, 1986, *101*, 605.

For reference to the use of miconazole in the treatment of primary amoebic meningoencephalitis, see Amphotericin, p.419.

ACNE. In a double-blind study involving 105 patients with moderate to severe acne, 53 received benzoyl peroxide 5% cream and 52 a cream containing benzoyl peroxide 5% in association with miconazole nitrate 2%. Both preparations were applied twice daily. After 12 weeks treatment, 3 and 15 patients were considered to be completely cured in the 2 groups respectively. Three patients did not complete the study, one due to an allergic reaction to benzoyl peroxide. Ten patients receiving benzoyl peroxide, and one receiving the combination preparation complained of irritation and drying of the skin.— H. Degreef and G. Vanden Bossche, *Dermatol-*

ogica, 1982, *164*, 201. See also under Antimicrobial Action (above).

ADMINISTRATION IN RENAL FAILURE. Miconazole could be given in a usual dosage in renal failure. Concentrations were not affected by haemodialysis or peritoneal dialysis.— W. M. Bennett *et al.*, *Am. J. Kidney Dis.*, 1983, *3*, 155. Renal failure was associated with miconazole 2.4 g daily given intravenously to a renal transplant patient. Renal function improved on reducing the dose. It would therefore seem wise to modify the dosage of miconazole when it is used in patients with chronic renal insufficiency.— K. N. Lai *et al.* (letter), *Lancet*, 1981, *2*, 48.

For reference to the use of miconazole in the treatment of peritonitis associated with continuous ambulatory peritoneal dialysis, see Amphotericin, p.419.

ASPERGILLOSIS. A patient with pulmonary aspergilloma received miconazole 5 to 10 mg in 20 mL sodium chloride 0.9% administered via a catheter into the cavity on 8 occasions in a period of 7 weeks. Sputum cultures became negative after the fourth instillation and small fragments of the fungus ball began to be expectorated after the seventh.— T. Hamamoto *et al.*, *Ann. intern. Med.*, 1983, *98*, 1030.

COCCIDIOIDOMYCOSIS. A review of the use of intravenous miconazole in the treatment of chronic pulmonary or meningeal coccidioidomycosis, or coccidioidal infections of the skin, soft tissues, or skeletal system. Coccidioidal meningitis was the least responsive and had the highest relapse rate in patients who did respond to the drug. Treatment with intrathecal and intravenous miconazole did not appear to have any advantage over treatment with intravenous miconazole alone. Coccidioidal arthritis responded more frequently than osteomyelitis, and in patients with chronic pulmonary disease the involvement of extrapulmonary sites was associated with a poor outcome. The authors concluded that with the intensive, relatively brief courses of miconazole that had been used, responses could be produced even in those who had failed to respond to amphotericin.— D. A. Stevens, *Drugs*, 1983, *26*, 347.

CRYPTOCOCCOSIS. Despite reported successes with miconazole in the treatment of cryptococcal meningitis, there was inadequate information to consider miconazole as appropriate treatment for this condition.— J. E. Bennett and J. S. Remington, *Ann. intern. Med.*, 1981, *94*, 708.

ECZEMA. The treatment of secondary bacterial infections, in atopic eczema, with miconazole plus hydrocortisone.— I. White and N. Blatchford, *Br. J. clin. Pract.*, 1983, *37*, 215.

SEBORRHOEIC DERMATITIS. In a double-blind study involving 70 patients with seborrhoeic dermatitis of the scalp, solutions of miconazole 2%, hydrocortisone 1%, or a combination of the two (Daktacort) applied each evening for 3 weeks were all effective, producing cure rates of 68%, 71%, and 90% respectively. Effective treatment was paralleled by a significant fall in the numbers of *Malassezia (Pityosporum) furfur* although this was less with hydrocortisone than with the other treatments. After cure, patients received the same treatment twice a month for 3 months as prophylaxis. Daktacort and miconazole were more effective prophylactic agents than hydrocortisone, 84%, 67%, and 18% of patients remaining clear of seborrhoeic dermatitis respectively. Recurrence was paralleled by a rise in numbers of *M. furfur*.— J. Faergemann, *Br. J. Derm.*, 1986, *114*, 695.

TINEA. In a double-blind study of 24 patients with tinea cruris or pedis, 12 responded better to treatment with a cream containing a combination of miconazole 2% and hydrocortisone 1%, than to miconazole 2% alone. Twelve patients showed no difference in response to the 2 medications.— A. Björnberg and E. Tegner, *Curr. ther. Res.*, 1986, *40*, 471.

Preparations

Miconazole Injection *(U.S.P.)*. Store at 15° to 30°.

Miconazole Cream *(B.P.)*. Miconazole Nitrate Cream

Miconazole Nitrate Cream *(U.S.P.)*. Store in airtight containers.

Miconazole Nitrate Vaginal Suppositories *(U.S.P.)*. Store at 15° to 30°.

Proprietary Preparations

Daktacort *(Janssen, UK)*. *Cream*, miconazole nitrate 2%, hydrocortisone 1%.
Ointment, miconazole 2%, hydrocortisone 1%.

Daktarin *(Janssen, UK)*. *Tablets*, scored, miconazole 250 mg.
Oral gel, miconazole 125 mg/5 mL.
Concentrate for intravenous infusion, miconazole 10 mg/mL, in a vehicle containing Cremophor EL 10%, in ampoules of 20 mL.
Cream, miconazole nitrate 2%.
Dusting-powder, miconazole nitrate 2%.
Twin pack, combination pack, miconazole nitrate 2% cream and miconazole nitrate 2% topical powder.
Topical powder spray, aerosol, miconazole nitrate 2%.

Dermonistat *(Ortho-Cilag, UK)*. *Cream*, miconazole nitrate 2%.

Gyno-Daktarin *(Janssen, UK)*. *Ovules* (Gyno-Daktarin 1), vaginal capsules, miconazole nitrate 1.2 g.
Pessaries, miconazole nitrate 100 mg.
Vaginal cream, miconazole nitrate 2%.
Combipack, combination pack, 14 miconazole nitrate 100 mg pessaries and miconazole nitrate 2% cream.
Tampons, coated with miconazole nitrate 100 mg.

Monistat *(Ortho-Cilag, UK)*. *Pessaries*, miconazole nitrate 100 mg.
Vaginal cream, miconazole nitrate 2%.

Proprietary Names and Manufacturers of Miconazole and Miconazole Nitrate

Albistat *(Belg.; Neth.)*; Andergin *(ISOM, Ital.)*; Brentan *(Janssen, Denm.)*; Daktar *(Janssen, Ger.; Janssen, Norw.; Janssen Pharmaceutica, Swed.)*; Daktarin *(Arg.; Janssen, Austral.; Belg.; Janssen, Fr.; Janssen, Ital.; Neth.; Janssen, S.Afr.; Esteve, Spain; Janssen, Switz.; Janssen, UK)*; Deralbine *(Arg.)*; Dermonistat *(Ortho-Cilag, UK)*; Epi-Monistat *(Cilag, Ger.)*; Funginazol *(Alcon, Spain)*; Fungisdin *(Isdin, Spain)*; Fungisidin *(Spain)*; Gyno-Daktar *(Janssen, Ger.)*; Gyno-Daktarin *(Arg.; Janssen, Austral.; Belg.; Janssen, Fr.; Neth.; Johnson & Johnson, S.Afr.; Janssen, UK)*; Gyno-Monistat *(Cilag, Ger.)*; Micatin *(McNeil, Canad.; Ortho Pharmaceutical, USA)*; Micoderm *(Logifarm, Ital.)*; Miconal *(Ecobi, Ital.)*; Micotef *(LPB, Ital.)*; Monistat *(Cilag, Austral.; Ortho, Canad.; Janssen, Switz.; Ortho-Cilag, UK; Janssen, USA; Ortho Pharmaceutical, USA)*; Monistat-Derm *(Cilag, Austral.; Ortho Dermatological, USA)*.

The following names have been used for multi-ingredient preparations containing miconazole and miconazole nitrate— Acnidazil *(Janssen, UK)*; Daktacort *(Janssen, UK)*.

12995-y

Naftifine Hydrochloride *(BANM, USAN, rINNM)*.

AW-105-843; Naftifungine Hydrochloride; SN-105-843 *(naftifine)*. *(E)*-*N*-Cinnamyl-*N*-methyl(1-naphthylmethyl)amine hydrochloride.
$C_{21}H_{21}N,HCl=323.9$.

CAS — 65473-14-5; 65472-88-0 (naftifine).

Naftifine hydrochloride is an antifungal agent which is applied topically as a 1% cream, gel, or solution in the treatment of fungal infections of the skin.

Studies of the antifungal activity of naftifine: A. Georgopoulos *et al.*, *Antimicrob. Ag. Chemother.*, 1981, *19*, 386 (*in vitro*); G. Petranyl *et al.*, *ibid.*, 390 (*in vivo*). A study *in vitro* indicating that the fungistatic action of naftifine against *Candida albicans* is due to inhibition of fungal ergosterol biosynthesis.— N. S. Ryder *et al.*, *ibid.*, 1984, *25*, 483.

Naftifine hydrochloride in the treatment of superficial dermatophyte infections.— U. Ganzinger *et al.*, *Clin. Trials J.*, 1982, *19*, 342.

Proprietary Names and Manufacturers
Exoderil *(Sandoz, Ger.)*.

2593-h

Natamycin *(BAN, USAN, pINN)*.

Antibiotic A-5283; CL-12625; Pimaricin. A polyene antibiotic produced by the growth of *Streptomyces natalensis*.
$C_{33}H_{47}NO_{13}=665.7$.

CAS — 7681-93-8.

Pharmacopoeias. In *U.S.*

An off-white to cream-coloured powder. It may contain up to 3 moles of water and has a potency of not less than 900 μg per mg calculated on the anhydrous basis.

Practically **insoluble** in water; slightly soluble in methyl alcohol; soluble in glacial acetic acid and dimethylformamide. A 1% aqueous suspension has a pH of 5.0 to 7.5. **Store** in airtight containers. Protect from light.

Preliminary studies indicated that natamycin eye-drops 5% underwent slight oxidative degradation during sterilisation at 116° for 30 minutes but were still satisfactory for use.— C. Alsop *et al.*, *Aust. J. Hosp. Pharm.*, 1984, *14*, 159.

Adverse Effects

Gastro-intestinal disturbances have occurred after the administration of large doses of natamycin by mouth. Topical application of natamycin has sometimes produced irritation.

Antimicrobial Action

Natamycin is a polyene antifungal agent with antimicrobial activity similar to that of nystatin. In addition it is active against *Trichomonas vaginalis*. The minimum inhibitory concentration of natamycin has been reported to range from 1 to 20 μg per mL.

Absorption and Fate

Natamycin is poorly absorbed from the gastro-intestinal tract. It is not absorbed through the skin or mucous membranes when applied topically.

Uses and Administration

Natamycin is used for the local treatment of candidiasis, trichomoniasis, and fungal keratitis. It has also been used in aspergillosis.

Natamycin has been given by mouth for the treatment of intestinal candidiasis in a dose of up to 400 mg daily in divided doses, often as enteric-coated tablets. For the treatment of oral candidiasis in infants, 4 drops of a 1% suspension of natamycin may be placed under the tongue after every feed; for older children and adults, 10 drops may be applied to the lesion after each meal. Pastilles have also been used.

For inhalation therapy in the treatment of infections of the lungs and respiratory tract caused by susceptible fungi and yeasts, a sterile suspension is administered by nebulisation in a dose equivalent to 2.5 mg of natamycin three times daily for 4 weeks and then twice daily until sputum cultures are consistently negative for the infecting organism.

For topical application to the skin and nail matrix a 2% cream is used. Pessaries containing natamycin 25 mg are used in the treatment of trichomonal and candidal infections of the vagina. One pessary is inserted nightly for 20 days, or twice daily for 10 days.

A 5% ophthalmic suspension of natamycin is used in the treatment of fungal infections of the eye, including those due to *Fusarium solani*.

When used in the treatment of allergy to house-dust mite, natamycin is sprayed onto the patient's mattress and pillow every 2 weeks for a period of 3 months and then again after a further 3 months to control the mould and hence the mite with which it is associated.

Natamycin has been used as a food additive in some countries.

A review of the properties and uses of natamycin.— W. P. Raab, *Natamycin (Pimaricin)*, Stuttgart, Georg Thieme, 1972.

Estimated acceptable daily intake of natamycin: up to 300 μg per kg body-weight.— Twentieth Report of the Joint FAO/WHO Expert Committee on Food Additives, *Tech. Rep. Ser. Wld Hlth Org. No. 599*, 1976.

It has been shown that the house-dust mite (*Dermatophagoides pteronyssinus*) depends on moulds, especially *Aspergillus penicilloides* for its growth and survival. This has prompted the investigation of natamycin in the control of the mite via its action on the mould. De Saint-Georges-Gridelet (*Acta Oecologica/Oecol. Applic.*, 1981, *2*, 117) demonstrated a decrease in the number of house-dust mites in samples of mattress dust inoculated with *A. penicilloides* when treated with natamycin 10% powder. As the frequency of treatment increased from 1 to 3 times in 4 weeks so the effect increased. In an open study (B. Van de Maele, *Pharmatherapeutica*, 1983, *3*,

441), 40 patients with allergy to house-dust mite whose condition was stable and unlikely to improve with current medication and standard measures of house-dust mite control, sprayed their mattress and pillow with at least 500 mg natamycin every 2 weeks for 3 months. Of 28 assessed by the physician, 15 were considered to be improved, 9 unchanged, and 4 deteriorated. Symptoms as recorded daily by 22 patients showed an overall improvement which was slightly more pronounced at night than during the daytime.

Preparations

Natamycin Ophthalmic Suspension *(U.S.P.)*. A sterile suspension of natamycin in a suitable aqueous vehicle; it contains one or more suitable preservatives. pH 5.0 to 7.5.

Proprietary Preparations

Pimafucin *(Brocades, UK)*. *Suspension*, natamycin 10 mg/mL.
Nebuliser suspension, natamycin 25 mg/mL.
Cream, natamycin 2%.
Pessaries, natamycin 25 mg.

Tymasil *(Brocades, UK)*. *Spray application*, aerosol, natamycin 625 mg/can. For use on the mattresses and pillows of patients with house-dust mite allergy.

Proprietary Names and Manufacturers

Natacyn *(Alcon, S.Afr.; Alcon Laboratories, USA)*; Natafucin *(Brocades, Ital.)*; Pimafucin *(Astra, Austral.; Belg.; Denm.; Basotherm, Ger.; Ital.; Neth.; Gist-Brocades, Norw.; S.Afr.; Gist-Brocades, Swed.; Switz.; Brocades, UK)*; Pimafucine *(Beytout, Fr.; Gist-Brocades, Switz.)*; Synogil *(Basotherm, Ger.)*; Tymasil *(Brocades, UK)*.

The following names have been used for multi-ingredient preparations containing natamycin— Pimafucort *(Astra, Austral.)*.

2594-m

Nifuroxime *(rINN)*.

5-Nitro-2-furaldehyde oxime.

$C_5H_4N_2O_4$=156.1.

CAS — 6236-05-1.

Nifuroxime is an antifungal agent which has been used with furazolidone to treat vaginitis due to *Candida albicans* or *Trichomonas vaginalis*.

Proprietary Names and Manufacturers

The following names have been used for multi-ingredient preparations containing nifuroxime— Tricofuron *(Norwich Eaton, USA)*.

13026-a

p-Nitrophenol

$C_6H_5NO_3$=139.1.

CAS — 100-02-7.

p-Nitrophenol is reported to have antifungal activity.

Proprietary Preparations

Phortinea *(Philip Harris, UK)*. *Liquid*, *p*-nitrophenol 2%.

2596-v

Nystatin *(BAN, USAN, rINN)*.

Fungicidin; Nistatina; Nystatinum.

Approximate molecular formula:
$C_{47}H_{75}NO_{17}$=926.1.

CAS — 1400-61-9.

Pharmacopoeias. In *Br., Braz., Eur., Ind., It., Swiss,* and *U.S.* which specify not less than 4400 units per mg, *Cz., Egypt., Hung., Int.,* and *Jug.* which specify not less than 3000 units per mg and *Turk.* which specifies not less than 2000 units per mg. *Roum.* specifies not less than 3500 units per mg. *Jpn* does not specify potency. Also in *B.P. Vet.*

An antifungal substance produced by the growth of certain strains of *Streptomyces noursei*. It contains mainly tetraenes, the principle component being nystatin A_1. It is a yellow to light brown hygroscopic powder with a characteristic odour suggestive of cereals, containing not less than 4400 units per mg of the dried substance. The *U.S.P.* states that nystatin intended for use in extemporaneous preparation of oral suspensions should contain not less than 5 000 units per mg.

B.P. **solubilities** are: very slightly soluble in water; practically insoluble in alcohol, chloroform, and ether; slightly soluble in methyl alcohol; freely soluble in dimethylformamide. *U.S.P.* solubilities are: very slightly soluble in water; slightly to sparingly soluble in alcohol, methyl alcohol, *n*-propyl alcohol, and *n*-butyl alcohol; insoluble in chloroform and ether. A 3% suspension in water has a pH of 6.5 to 8.0. **Store** at a temperature between 2 and 8° in airtight containers and protect from light.

Units

One unit of nystatin is contained in 0.0002059 mg of the second International Standard Preparation (1982) which contains 4855 units per mg.

Adverse Effects

Nausea, vomiting, and diarrhoea have occasionally been reported after the oral administration of nystatin. Irritation may occur rarely after the topical use of nystatin, and allergic contact dermatitis has been reported.

Although nystatin pastilles (Nystan Pastilles) contain sugar, a study in 100 dentate patients receiving the pastilles, usually for a period of 14 days and followed up for 10 to 12 months, did not find an increase in dental caries. This was attributed to the following factors: that the sugar is rapidly removed from the oral cavity after the 30 to 40-minute sucking period, that patients had received instructions on good dental hygiene, and that they were mostly in the 23- to 61-year age range which is less susceptible to dental caries.— P. Woods (letter), *Br. dent. J.*, 1985, *159*, 390.

Antimicrobial Action

Nystatin is a fungistatic and fungicidal polyene antibiotic which interferes with the permeability of the cell membrane of sensitive fungi by binding to sterols, chiefly ergosterol. Its main action is against *Candida* spp. It is also effective against *Aspergillus* spp., *Coccidioides immitis, Cryptococcus neoformans, Histoplasma capsulatum, Blastomyces dermatidis,* and other yeasts and fungi. The minimum inhibitory concentration of nystatin for most sensitive fungi has been reported to range from 1.56 to 6.25 µg per mL.

RESISTANCE. A report of a strain of *Candida albicans* causing oral candidiasis in a baby, resistant to nystatin but sensitive to amphotericin.— R. S. Illingworth (letter), *Archs Dis. Childh.*, 1978, *53*, 183.

Further references: J. D. Dick *et al.*, *Antimicrob. Ag. Chemother.*, 1980, *18*, 158.

Absorption and Fate

Nystatin is poorly absorbed from the gastro-intestinal tract. It is not absorbed through the skin or mucous membranes when applied topically.

Uses and Administration

Nystatin is used for the prophylaxis and treatment of candidiasis of the skin and mucous membranes, especially that caused by *Candida albicans*.

For the treatment of intestinal or oesophageal candidiasis, nystatin is given in doses of 500 000 or 1 000 000 units by mouth 3 or 4 times a day. In infants and children a dosage of 100 000 units or more may be given 4 times daily. For the prophylaxis of intestinal candidiasis in adults nystatin may be given in a dosage of 1 000 000 units daily. Nystatin is administered with non-absorbable antibiotics in various regimens to suppress the overgrowth of gastro-intestinal flora especially in immunocompromised patients.

For treatment of lesions of the mouth, pastilles or a suspension may be given in a dosage of 100 000 units four times daily. In the *US* doses of 400 000 to 600 000 units four times daily are used. Nystatin 100 000 units daily may be given to neonates for the prophylaxis of oral candidiasis.

For vaginal infections nystatin is administered in a dosage of 100 000 to 200 000 units daily as pessaries or vaginal cream. For cutaneous lesions, ointment, gel, cream, or dusting powder containing 100 000 units per g may be applied 2 to 4 times daily.

Nystatin has also been administered as eye-drops or as a bladder wash.

A discussion of the limitations of topically or orally administered nystatin in the prophylaxis of fungal infection in the immunocompromised host, including lack of evidence for its efficacy, and its poor activity against *Aspergillus* spp., *Mucor* spp., and *Pseudallescheria boydii*.— L. S. Young, *J. antimicrob. Chemother.*, 1982, *9*, 338. In a review of studies of oral nystatin in the prophylaxis of fungal infection in neutropenic patients, its efficacy in reducing oral and gastro-intestinal yeast colonisation and in preventing infection appeared to be unsubstantiated even when administered in doses of up to 30 million units daily.— F. Meunier-Carpentier, *Am. J. Med.*, 1984, *76*, 652.

For comparative reports of the use of nystatin as prophylaxis against fungal infections in the immunocompromised host, see Ketoconazole p.428.

For references to the use of nystatin as part of oral non-absorbable antibiotic regimens used to prevent colonisation and infection by the selective decontamination of the gastro-intestinal tract, and in the treatment of Crohn's disease, see Colistin Sulphomethate Sodium, p.205.

CANDIDIASIS. *Cutaneous.* Results of a study in 37 infants with candidial diaper dermatitis indicating that treatment with topical nystatin alone is as effective as combined oral and topical therapy. Initial treatment was given for 10 days, but about half the patients required topical treatment for 3 weeks.— D. Munz *et al.*, *J. Pediat.*, 1982, *101*, 1022.

Oral candidiasis. Mention of the use of nystatin ointment, 100 000 units per g applied thinly to the surfaces of dentures following their cleaning after meals, in the treatment of oral candidiasis.— K. D. Hay and P. C. Reade, *Drugs*, 1983, *26*, 268.

An *in vitro* study indicating that solutions of nystatin 25 000 to 200 000 units per mL or amphotericin 25 to 200 mg per mL inhibit the adherence of *Candida* spp. to denture acrylic. The results suggested, however, that soaking dentures in chlorhexidine gluconate 2% solution would be a more effective method of preventing colonisation of denture surfaces since it inhibited adherence for a significantly longer period.— J. McCourtie *et al.*, *J. antimicrob. Chemother.*, 1986, *17*, 575.

Mouth problems and drug treatment were investigated and mouth swabs taken weekly for up to 4 months in 140 hospice patients. Oral *Candida* and mouth symptoms were unaffected by nystatin given by mouth to 43 patients on clinical grounds. It was considered that candidal infection may be the result rather than the cause of mouth problems, indicating that general oral hygiene is more important than antifungal treatment.— I. G. Finlay, *Br. med. J.*, 1986, *292*, 592.

A study involving 50 patients with respiratory diseases who developed oropharyngeal candidiasis. In 45 of the patients this was confirmed microbiologically and was frequently associated with predisposing factors such as the wearing of dentures; administration of oral or inhaled corticosteroids, antibiotics, or sedatives; conditions or drugs such as atropine which decrease salivary flow; radiotherapy; diabetes; or cancer chemotherapy. Patients were given nystatin 100 000 units four times daily for 7 days as pastilles or suspension; no food or drink was taken for one hour after each dose. Dentures were soaked in 0.5% chlorhexidine and alcohol each night. Results showed the 2 formulations of nystatin to be equally efficacious both clinically and microbiologically. Significant improvement was observed in all 8 patients with chronic infections, 5 of whom had failed to respond to all other treatments. The concomitant chlorhexidine treatment of dentures, and the measures taken to enhance the retention of drug in the oropharynx were considered to be important factors contributing to the success of nystatin treatment.— P. J. Thompson *et al.*, *Br. med. J.*, 1986, *292*, 1699. Comments, and criticisms of the methodology of the study.— G. K. Crompton (letter), *ibid.*, *293*, 270; P. -J. Lamey and L. P. Samaranayake (letter), *ibid;* A. B. Mason and J. M. T. Willoughby (letter), *ibid.*, 564 and 699.

Vaginal candidiasis. Controversy exists as to whether relapsing vaginal candidiasis should be treated with nystatin 500 000 units every 8 hours by mouth for 1 to 2 weeks to treat possible re-infection from the bowel, in addition to a long course of topical antifungal therapy.— M. W. Adler, *Br. med. J.*, 1983, *287*, 1611.

Effective treatment of vulvovaginal candidiasis with the administration of a high-potency vaginal cream containing nystatin 1 million units per 2.5 g for 7 days.— N. L. Cassar, *Curr. ther. Res.*, 1983, *34*, 305.

PSORIASIS. Preliminary results in 4 patients suggesting that nystatin by mouth may be beneficial in the treatment of psoriasis.— N. Crutcher *et al.* (letter), *Archs Derm.*, 1984, *120*, 435.

Preparations

Nystatin Tablets *(B.P.).* Coated tablets. Store at a temperature not exceeding 25°.

Nystatin Tablets *(U.S.P.)*

Nystatin Oral Suspension *(B.P.).* Nystatin Mixture; Nystatin Oral Drops; Nystatin Suspension. A suspension of nystatin in a suitable flavoured vehicle. Store at a temperature not exceeding 15°.

Nystatin Oral Suspension *(U.S.P.).* A suspension of nystatin containing suitable preservatives, dispersing, flavouring, and suspending agents. pH 4.5 to 6.0 or, if it contains glycerol, 6.0 to 7.5.

Nystatin for Oral Suspension *(U.S.P.).* A dry mixture of nystatin with one or more suitable preservatives, diluents, colouring, flavouring, and suspending agents. pH of reconstituted suspension 4.9 to 5.5.

Nystatin Cream *(U.S.P.).* Store at a temperature not greater than 40°.

Nystatin Eye Drops *(A.P.F.).* Nystatin 1 g, sodium chloride 900 mg, chlorhexidine acetate 10 mg, Water for Injections to 100 mL. Prepared aseptically. The eye-drops must be freshly prepared. Store at 2° to 8°, and use within 7 days.

Nystatin Lotion *(U.S.P.).* pH 5.5 to 7.5. Store at 15° to 30°.

Nystatin Ointment *(B.P.)*

Nystatin Ointment *(U.S.P.).* Store at 15° to 30°.

Nystatin Pessaries *(B.P.)*

Nystatin Vaginal Tablets *(U.S.P.)*

Nystatin Vaginal Suppositories *(U.S.P.).* Store at 15° to 30°.

Nystatin Topical Powder *(U.S.P.)*

Nystatin and Clioquinol Ointment *(U.S.P.).* Store at 15° to 30°.

Nystatin, Neomycin Sulfate, Gramicidin, and Triamcinolone Acetonide Ointment *(U.S.P.)*

Nystatin, Neomycin Sulfate, Gramicidin, and Triamcinolone Acetonide Cream *(U.S.P.)*

Nystatin and Triamcinolone Acetonide Cream *(U.S.P.)*

Nystatin and Triamcinolone Acetonide Ointment *(U.S.P.)*

Proprietary Preparations

Multilind *(Squibb, UK). Ointment,* nystatin 100 000 units/g, zinc oxide 20%.

Nyspes *(DDSA Pharmaceuticals, UK). Pessaries,* nystatin 100 000 units.

Nystadermal *(Squibb, UK). Cream,* nystatin 100 000 units/g, triamcinolone acetonide 0.1%.

Nystaform *(Bayer, UK). Cream,* nystatin 100 000 units/g, chlorhexidine hydrochloride 1%.
Ointment, nystatin 100 000 units/g, chlorhexidine acetate 1%.

Nystaform-HC *(Bayer, UK). Cream,* nystatin 100 000 units/g, chlorhexidine hydrochloride 1%, hydrocortisone 0.5%.
Ointment, nystatin 100 000 units/g, chlorhexidine acetate 1%, hydrocortisone 1%.

Nystan *(Squibb, UK). Pastilles,* nystatin 100 000 units.
Tablets, nystatin 500 000 units.
Suspension, nystatin 100 000 units/mL.
Suspension, granules for reconstitution, nystatin 100 000 units/mL when reconstituted with water.
Cream, nystatin 100 000 units/g.
Gel, nystatin 100 000 units/g.
Ointment, nystatin 100 000 units/g.
Pessaries, nystatin 100 000 units.
Vaginal cream, nystatin 100 000 units/4-g application.
Triple pack, combination pack, 28 Nystavescent pessaries, 42 Nystan tablets, and Nystan gel.
Topical powder, nystatin 100 000 units/g.
Non-sterile powder, nystatin 3 000 000 units.
Sterile powder, nystatin 500 000 units.

Nystatin-Dome *(Lagap, UK). Suspension,* nystatin 100 000 units/mL.

Nystavescent *(Squibb, UK). Pessaries,* effervescent, nystatin 100 000 units.

Timodine *(Lloyd-Hamol, Reckitt & Colman Pharm., UK). Cream,* nystatin 100 000 units/g, hydrocortisone 0.5%, benzalkonium chloride solution 0.2%, dimethicone '350' 10%.

Tri-Adcortyl *(Squibb, UK). Cream, Ointment, Otic ointment,* nystatin 100 000 units, triamcinolone acetonide 1 mg, neomycin 2.5 mg (as sulphate), gramicidin 250 µg/g.

Proprietary Names and Manufacturers

Biofanal *(Pfleger, Ger.)*; Candex *(Miles Pharmaceuticals, USA)*; Candio-Hermal *(Hermal, Ger.; Neth.; Hermal, Switz.)*; Canstat *(S.Afr.)*; Diastatin *(G.P. Laboratories, Austral.)*; Fungistatin *(S.Afr.)*; Gyno-Nilstat *(Belg.)*; Korostatin *(Youngs, USA)*; Micostatin *(Arg.)*; Multilind *(Squibb, UK)*; Mycostatin *(Squibb, Austral.; Squibb, Canad.; Squibb, Denm.; Squibb, Ital.; Novo, Norw.; Squibb, S.Afr.; Squibb, Spain; Squibb, Swed.; Switz.; Squibb, USA)*; Mycostatine *(Squibb, Fr.; Labaz, Switz.)*; Nadostine *(Nadeau, Canad.)*; Nilstat *(Arg.; Lederle, Austral.; Belg.; Lederle, Canad.; Lederle, USA)*; Nyaderm *(Taro, Canad.)*; Nyspes *(DDSA Pharmaceuticals, UK)*; Nystan *(Squibb, UK)*; Nystatin-Dome *(Lagap, UK)*; Nystavescent *(Squibb, UK)*; Nystex *(Savage, USA)*; O-V Statin *(Squibb, USA)*.

The following names have been used for multi-ingredient preparations containing nystatin—Achrostatin *(Lederle, Austral.)*; Cobadex-Nystatin *(Cox, UK)*; Comycin *(Upjohn, Austral.)*; Dermovate-NN *(Glaxo, UK)*; Flagyl Compak *(May & Baker, UK)*; Flagystatin *(Rhône-Poulenc, Canad.)*; Gregoderm *(Unigreg, UK)*; Halcicomb *(Squibb, Canad.; Squibb, UK)*; Hiconcil-NS *(Bristol, S.Afr.)*; Kenacomb *(Squibb, Austral.; Squibb, Canad.)*; Lidecomb *(Syncare, Canad.)*; Mycolog *(Squibb, USA)*; Mycolog-II *(Squibb, USA)*; Myco-Triacet *(Lemmon, USA)*; Myco-Triacet-II *(Lemmon, USA)*; Mysteclin Tablets *(Squibb, UK)*; Mysteclin-V *(Squibb, Austral.)*; Mytrex *(Savage, USA)*; Mytrex-F *(Savage, USA)*; Nybadex *(Cox, UK)*; Nystadermal *(Squibb, UK)*; Nystaform *(Bayer, UK; Miles Pharmaceuticals, USA)*; Nystaform-HC *(Bayer, UK)*; Nyst-olone *(Schein, USA)*; Pentrex-F *(Bristol, S.Afr.)*; Terra-Cortril Nystatin *(Pfizer, UK)*; Tetrex-F *(Astra, Austral.)*; Timodine *(Lloyd-Hamol, Reckitt & Colman Pharm., UK)*; Tinaderm-M *(Kirby-Warrick, UK)*; Tri-Adcortyl *(Squibb, UK)*; Trimovate *(Glaxo, UK)*; Viaderm-KC *(Taro, Canad.)*.

16940-q

Oxiconazole Nitrate *(BANM, rINNM).*

Ro-13-8996/000 (oxiconazole); Ro-13-8996/001. 2′,4′-Dichloro-2-imidazol-1-ylacetophenone (*Z*)-*O*-(2,4-dichlorobenzyl)oxime mononitrate.
$C_{18}H_{13}Cl_4N_3O,HNO_3$=492.1.

CAS — 64211-46-7; 64211-45-6 (oxiconazole).

Oxiconazole nitrate is an imidazole antifungal agent which is applied topically as a cream, solution, or powder equivalent to oxiconazole 1% in the treatment of fungal infections of the skin.
Local reactions including burning and itching have been reported.

Proprietary Names and Manufacturers

Gyno-Myfungar *(Siegfried, Switz.)*; Myfungar *(Siegfried, Ger.; Siegfried, Switz.)*; Oceral *(Roche, Ger.; Sauter, Switz.)*;

2598-q

Pecilocin *(BAN, rINN).*

An antifungal substance produced by the growth of *Paecilomyces varioti* Bainier var. *antibioticus.* 1-[(2*E*,4*E*,6*Z*,8*R*)-8-Hydroxy-6-methyldodeca-2,4,6-trienoyl]pyrrolidin-2-one.
$C_{17}H_{25}NO_3$=291.4.

CAS — 19504-77-9.

Adverse Effects

Irritation may occur after the topical application of pecilocin. Contact dermatitis has been reported.

Antimicrobial Action

Pecilocin exerts an inhibitory effect on the growth of *Blastomyces, Cryptococcus, Epidermophyton, Microsporum,* and *Trichophyton* spp. It has no effect on *Candida albicans* or pathogenic bacteria.

Uses and Administration

Pecilocin is used in the treatment of various tinea infections, in the form of an ointment containing 3000 units per g or a solution containing 1500 units per mL.

Proprietary Names and Manufacturers

Leofungine *(Fr.)*; Supral *(Ger.)*; Variotin *(Denm.; Neth.; Leo, UK)*.

3000-z

Pentamycin

A polyene antibiotic obtained from *Streptomyces pentaticus.*
$C_{35}H_{58}O_{12}$=670.8.

CAS — 6834-98-6.

Pentamycin is an antifungal agent with reported activity *in vitro* against *Candida, Trichophyton* spp., and *Trichomonas vaginalis.* It is used as pessaries in the treatment of vaginitis.

Proprietary Names and Manufacturers

Cantricin *(Corvi, Ital.)*; Pentacin *(Farmaka, Ital.)*;

3001-c

Propionic Acid *(USAN).*

E280; E282 (calcium propionate); E283 (potassium propionate). Propanoic acid.
$C_2H_5.CO_2H$=74.08.

CAS — 79-09-4.

Pharmacopoeias. In *U.S.N.F.*

An oily liquid having a slight pungent, rancid odour. **Miscible** with water, alcohol, and various other organic solvents. **Store** in airtight containers.

3005-x

Sodium Propionate *(USAN).*

E281. Sodium propanoate.
$C_3H_5NaO_2$=96.06.

CAS — 137-40-6 (anhydrous); 6700-17-0 (hydrate).

Pharmacopoeias. In *Fr.* and *Nord.* Also in *B.P. Vet.* and *U.S.N.F.*

Colourless transparent crystals or white granular crystalline powder; odourless or with a slight characteristic odour. Deliquescent in moist air.
Soluble 1 in 1 of water, 1 in 0.65 of boiling water, and 1 in 24 to 25 of alcohol; practically insoluble in chloroform and ether. **Store** in airtight containers.

Propionic acid and its salts are antifungal agents effective against *Epidermophyton, Microsporum,* and *Trichophyton* spp.
Sodium propionate is used topically in concentrations of up to 10% alone, or often in combination with other propionates, caprylates, or other antifungal agents, in the form of ointments or solutions for the treatment of dermatophyte infections. Eye-drops containing sodium propionate 5% are also used. Sodium propionate is used in veterinary medicine.
The calcium and zinc salts have also been used as topical antifungal agents.
Propionic acid and its calcium, sodium, and potassium salts are used in the baking industry as inhibitors of moulds, and in the *UK* there are controls on the amounts that can be used as preservatives in foods.
In Great Britain the recommended exposure limits of propionic acid are 10ppm (long-term); 15ppm (short-term).

The use of propionic acid and its calcium, potassium, and sodium salts in food was limited only by good manufacturing practice.— Seventeenth Report of the Joint FAO/WHO Expert Committee on Food Additives, *Tech. Rep. Ser. Wld Hlth Org. No. 539*, 1974.

For background toxicological information of propionic acid and its calcium, potassium, and sodium salts, see *Fd Add. Ser. Wld Hlth Org. No. 5*, 1974.

Proprietary Names and Manufacturers of Propionic Acid and its Salts
C_3 *(Thilo, Ger.)*; Propionat *(Farmigea, Ital.)*.

The following names have been used for multi-ingredient preparations containing propionic acid and its salts— Amino-Cerv *(Milex, USA)*; Dermacide *(Sabex, Canad.)*; Egomycol *(Ego, Austral.)*; Mycoderm Cream and Powder *(Ego, Austral.)*; Oticane *(Rosken, Austral.)*; Prophyllin *(Rystan, USA)*.

3002-k

Pyrrolnitrin *(USAN, rINN)*.

52230; NSC-107654. An antifungal antibiotic isolated from *Pseudomonas pyrrocinia*. 3-Chloro-4-(3-chloro-2-nitrophenyl)pyrrole.
$C_{10}H_6Cl_2N_2O_2$=257.1.

CAS — 1018-71-9.

Pyrrolnitrin is an antifungal agent which is applied topically as a 1% cream, lotion, or powder in the treatment of superficial fungal infections. Erythema and skin eruptions may occur.

Proprietary Names and Manufacturers
Micutrin *(Belg.; Searle, Ital.; Sigma Tau, Spain)*; Pyroace *(Jpn)*.

3006-r

Sulbentine *(rINN)*.

Dibenzthion; Sulbentinum. 3,5-Dibenzyltetrahydro-2*H*-1,3,5-thiadiazine-2-thione.
$C_{17}H_{18}N_2S_2$=314.5.

CAS — 350-12-9.

Sulbentine is an antifungal agent applied topically in the form of a 3% ointment, gel, solution, or nail varnish or a 1% powder for treating dermatophyte infections of the skin and nails. Sensitivity reactions have been reported.

Proprietary Names and Manufacturers
Fungiplex *(Hermal, Ger.; Bruschettini, Ital.; Hermal, Swed.; Hermal, Switz.)*; Mycoplex *(Alcon-Couvreur, Belg.)*; Refungine *(Hermal, Neth.)*.

16999-m

Sulconazole Nitrate *(BANM, USAN, rINNM)*.

RS-44872; RS-44872-00-10-3. 1-[2,4-Dichloro-*β*-(4-chlorobenzyl)thiophenethyl]imidazole nitrate.
$C_{18}H_{15}Cl_3N_2S,HNO_3$=460.8.

CAS — 61318-90-9 (sulconazole); 61318-91-0 (nitrate).

Sulconazole nitrate is an imidazole antifungal agent with a broad spectrum of antimicrobial activity including action against dermatophytes, *Malassezia furfur*, *Candida albicans*, and some bacteria. It is applied topically as a 1% cream in the treatment of tinea infections, pityriasis versicolor, and candidiasis.
Local reactions including burning, itching, and erythema have been reported.

In a comparative study of sulconazole nitrate 1% cream and clotrimazole 1% cream, one patient developed an allergic reaction to sulconazole which was confirmed by patch testing.— A. Lassus *et al., Br. J. Derm.*, 1983, *108*, 195.

In a brief review of clinical studies of sulconazole nitrate 1% cream it was considered that although it was effective against dermatophyte infections, pityriasis versicolor, and cutaneous candidiasis, there was no evidence that it had any therapeutic advantage over other imidazole preparations such as clotrimazole 1% cream or miconazole nitrate 2% cream, and that further studies were required to establish long-term relapse rates.— *Drug & Ther. Bull.*, 1986, *24*, 67. See also S. A. Qadripur, *Curr. ther. Res.*, 1984, *35*, 753; P. Benfield and S. P. Clissold, *Drugs*, 1988, *35*, 143.

Proprietary Preparations
Exelderm *(ICI Pharmaceuticals, UK). Cream*, sulconazole nitrate 1%.

Proprietary Names and Manufacturers
Exelderm *(Degussa, Switz.; ICI Pharmaceuticals, UK)*.

13307-b

Terconazole *(BAN, USAN, rINN)*.

R-42470; Triaconazole. 1-{4-[[2-(2,4-Dichlorophenyl)-*r*-2-(1*H*-1,2,4-triazol-1-ylmethyl)-1,3-dioxolan-*c*-4-yl]methoxy]phenyl}-4-isopropylpiperazine.
$C_{26}H_{31}Cl_2N_5O_3$=532.5.

CAS — 67915-31-5.

Terconazole is a triazole antifungal agent reported to have a broad spectrum of antimicrobial activity. It is used in the treatment of vaginal candidiasis in a dosage of 40 mg for 5 days or 80 mg for 3 days in the form of a vaginal cream or pessaries.
Local reactions including burning and itching have been reported.

The anticandidal activity of terconazole.— E. L. Tolman *et al., Antimicrob. Ag. Chemother.*, 1986, *29*, 986.

Proprietary Names and Manufacturers
Gyno-Terazol *(Cilag, Switz.)*; Terazol *(Johnson & Johnson, S.Afr.)*; Tercospor *(Cilag, Ger.)*.

13348-y

Tioconazole *(BAN, USAN, rINN)*.

UK-20349. 1-[2,4-Dichloro-*β*-(2-chloro-3-thenyloxy)phenethyl]imidazole.
$C_{16}H_{13}Cl_3N_2OS$=387.7.

CAS — 65899-73-2.

Pharmacopoeias. In *U.S.*

Store in airtight containers.

Tioconazole is an imidazole antifungal agent with a broad spectrum of antimicrobial activity including action against dermatophytes, *Malassezia furfur*, *Candida albicans*, and some bacteria. It is applied topically as a 1% cream, lotion, or powder in the treatment of tinea infections, pityriasis versicolor, candidiasis, and erythrasma. When used for nail infections topical applications may have to continue for up to 6 or even 12 months. It is used in the treatment of vaginal candidiasis as pessaries or vaginal cream in a dosage regimen of 100 mg daily for 3 to 6 days or a single dose of 300 mg.
Local reactions including burning, itching, and erythema have been reported.

A detailed review of the actions and uses of tioconazole. Studies have indicated that tioconazole is absorbed only to a small extent after dermal or vaginal application. Topical formulations containing tioconazole 1% or 2% have been studied in various fungal infections of the skin, and superficial bacterial infections such as erythrasma and impetigo, and a formulation containing tioconazole 28% and undecenoic acid has been developed for the treatment of fungal infections of the nails. Vaginal formulations that have been investigated in vaginal candidiasis or trichomoniasis include a 2% cream, 6% ointment, and pessaries containing 100 or 300 mg; durations of treatment have ranged from 1 to 14 days. These studies have shown tioconazole to be at least as effective, and in some studies more effective, than other imidazole antifungal agents, however its place in therapy has not yet been established.— S. P. Clissold and R. C. Heel, *Drugs*, 1986, *31*, 29.

Further references: Gibbs. D.L. *et al., J. int. med. Res.*, 1987, *15*, 23 (use in infants and neonates).

Proprietary Preparations
Trosyl *(Pfizer, UK). Solution*, tioconazole 280 mg/mL, in a vehicle which penetrates the nail.

Proprietary Names and Manufacturers
Fungibacid *(Asche, Ger.)*; Gyno-Trosyd *(Pfizer, Fr.; Pfizer, S.Afr.; Pfizer, Switz.)*; Trosyd *(Pfizer, Canad.; Pfizer, S.Afr.; Pfizer, Switz.)*; Trosyl *(Pfizer, UK)*.

3008-d

Tolciclate *(USAN, rINN)*.

K-9147; KC-9147. *O*-(1,2,3,4-Tetrahydro-1,4-methano-6-naphthyl) *m,N*-dimethylthiocarbanilate.
$C_{20}H_{21}NOS$=323.5.

CAS — 50838-36-3.

Tolciclate is an antifungal agent with activity against *Epidermophyton*, *Microsporum*, and *Trichophyton* spp. It has been used as a 1% cream, lotion, or ointment, or as a 0.5% powder in the treatment of various tinea infections and in pityriasis versicolor.

Studies *in vitro* of the antifungal activity of tolciclate.— I. de Carneri *et al., Arzneimittel-Forsch.*, 1976, *26*, 769; A. Bianchi *et al., Antimicrob. Ag. Chemother.*, 1977, *12*, 429.

Studies suggesting the primary mechanism of action of tolnaftate and tolciclate to be inhibition of ergosterol biosynthesis.— N. S. Ryder *et al., Antimicrob. Ag. Chemother.*, 1986, *29*, 858.

Reports of the clinical use of tolciclate: L. C. Cucè *et al., J. int. med. Res.*, 1980, *8*, 144 (tinea and pityriasis versicolor); C. Intini *et al., Pharmatherapeutica*, 1980, *2*, 439 (tinea and pityriasis versicolor); A. Battaglia *et al., J. int. med. Res.*, 1982, *10*, 367 (candidiasis).

Proprietary Names and Manufacturers
Fungifos *(Basotherm, Ger.)*; Kilmicène *(Farmitalia Carlo Erba, Switz.)*; Tolmicen *(Carlo Erba, Ital.)*.

3009-n

Tolnaftate *(BAN, USAN, rINN)*.

Sch-10144. *O*-2-Naphthyl *m,N*-dimethylthiocarbanilate.
$C_{19}H_{17}NOS$=307.4.

CAS — 2398-96-1.

Pharmacopoeias. In *Br.*, *Egypt.*, and *U.S.*

A white to creamy-white fine powder, odourless or with a slight odour. Practically **insoluble** in water; very slightly soluble in alcohol; soluble 1 in 9 of acetone, 1 in 3 of chloroform, and 1 in 55 of ether. **Store** in airtight containers.

Adverse Effects

Skin reactions including irritation and pruritus may occur; contact dermatitis has been reported.

Antimicrobial Action

Tolnaftate inhibits the growth of *Epidermophyton*, *Microsporum*, *Trichophyton* spp., and *Malassezia furfur*, but is not active against *Candida* spp. or bacteria.

Studies *in vitro* of the comparative activity of undecenoic acid and tolnaftate against fungi usually present in tinea pedis infections.— L. P. Amsel *et al., J. pharm. Sci.*, 1979, *68*, 384.

Studies suggesting the primary mechanism of action of tolnaftate and tolciclate to be inhibition of ergosterol biosynthesis.— N. S. Ryder *et al., Antimicrob. Ag. Chemother.*, 1986, *29*, 858.

Uses and Administration

Tolnaftate is an antifungal agent used topically as a 1% solution, powder, or cream in the treatment or prophylaxis of various forms of tinea and of pityriasis versicolor. Infections due to *Trichophyton rubrum* may relapse and a second course of treatment may be required. It has been used with nystatin when candidal infections are present.
Tolnaftate is not considered suitable for deep infections in nail beds or hair follicles but it may be applied concomitantly with a systemic agent.

A brief discussion of the use of tolnaftate in the prevention and treatment of tinea pedis.— *Aust. J. Pharm.*, 1984, *65*, 99.

Preparations

Tolnaftate Cream *(U.S.P.)*
Tolnaftate Gel *(U.S.P.)*
Tolnaftate Powder *(U.S.P.)*
Tolnaftate Topical Aerosol Powder *(U.S.P.)*. A suspension of tolnaftate in suitable propellents in a pressurised container. Store at a temperature not exceeding 40°.
Tolnaftate Topical Solution *(U.S.P.)*

Proprietary Preparations

Mycil *(Evans Medical, UK). Ointment*, tolnaftate 1% with benzalkonium chloride.
Topical powder, tolnaftate 1% with chlorhexidine.
Timoped *(Reckitt & Colman Pharmaceuticals, UK). Cream*, tolnaftate 1%, triclosan 0.25%.
Tinaderm *(Kirby-Warrick, UK). Cream*, tolnaftate 1%.
Topical powder, tolnaftate 1%.
Topical powder spray, aerosol, tolnaftate 1%.
Topical solution, tolnaftate 1%, in a vehicle of macrogol 400.

Tinaderm-M *(Kirby-Warrick, UK). Cream,* tolnaftate 10 mg, nystatin 100 000 units/g.

Proprietary Names and Manufacturers
Aftate *(Plough, USA)*; Focusan *(Lundbeck, Norw.; Lundbeck, Swed.)*; Footwork *(Lederle, USA)*; Mycil *(Evans Medical, UK)*; Pediderm *(Nelson, Austral.)*; Pitrex *(Taro, Canad.)*; Sorgoa *(Scheurich, Ger.)*; Sporiderm *(Fr.)*; Sporiline *(Unicet, Fr.)*; Tinacidin *(Essex, Austral.)*; Tinactin *(Schering, Canad.; Switz.; Schering, USA)*; Tinaderm *(Arg.; Plough, Austral.; Essex, Ital.; Scherag, S.Afr.; Essex, Spain; Kirby-Warrick, UK)*; Tinatox *(Brenner, Ger.)*; Tonoftal *(Essex, Ger.)*; Zeasorb-AF *(Stiefel, USA)*.

3010-k

Triacetin *(USAN, rINN).*

Glyceryl Triacetate. 1,2,3-Propanetriol triacetate.
$C_9H_{14}O_6$=218.2.

CAS — 102-76-1.

Pharmacopoeias. In *U.S.*

A colourless somewhat oily liquid with a slight fatty odour. **Soluble** in water; slightly soluble in carbon disulphide; miscible with alcohol, chloroform, and ether. **Store** in airtight containers.

Triacetin is reported to possess fungistatic properties based on the liberation of acetic acid. It is applied topically as a 25% cream or ointment in the treatment of superficial fungal infections, particularly tinea.

Proprietary Names and Manufacturers
Enzactin *(Ayerst, Austral.; Ayerst, Ital.; Inibsa, Spain; Ayerst, USA)*; Fungacetin *(Harvey, Switz.; Blair, USA)*.

The following names have been used for multi-ingredient preparations containing triacetin— Fungoid *(Pedinol, USA)*.

2284-l

Tribromometacresol

2,4,6-Tribromo-*m*-cresol; 2,4,6-Tribromo-3-methylphenol.
$C_7H_5Br_3O$=344.8.

CAS — 4619-74-3.

Tribromometacresol is an antifungal agent used in the treatment of dermatomycoses. It has been applied topically as an aerosol spray containing 2%.

Proprietary Names and Manufacturers
Triphysan *(Dumex, Denm.)*; Tri-Physol *(Sigma, Austral.)*.

3012-t

Undecenoic Acid *(BAN).*

10-Hendecenoic Acid; Acidum Undecylenicum; Undecylenic Acid *(USAN)*. It consists mainly of undec-10-enoic acid.
$C_{11}H_{20}O_2$=184.3.

CAS — 112-38-9.

Pharmacopoeias. In *Arg., Aust., Belg., Br., Braz., Chin., Cz., Eur., Fr., Ger., Ind., Int., It., Neth., Nord., Swiss,* and *U.S.*

A colourless or pale yellow clear liquid or a white to very pale yellow crystalline mass with a characteristic odour.
B.P. **solubilities** are: practically insoluble in water; freely soluble in alcohol, chloroform, ether, and fixed and volatile oils. *U.S.P.* **solubilities** are: practically insoluble in water; miscible with alcohol, chloroform, ether, and fixed and volatile oils. **Store** in airtight containers at a temperature of 8 to 15°. Protect from light.

3014-r

Zinc Undecenoate *(BAN).*

Undecilinato de Zinco; Zinc Undecylenate *(USAN)*; Zinci Undecylenas. Zinc di(undec-10-enoate).
$(C_{11}H_{19}O_2)_2Zn$=431.9.

CAS — 557-08-4.

Pharmacopoeias. In *Arg., Aust., Br., Braz., Chin., Cz., Egypt., Eur., Fr., Ger., Ind., It., Neth., Nord., Swiss,* and *U.S.*

A fine white or almost white powder. Practically **insoluble** in water, alcohol, and ether. **Store** in well-closed containers. Protect from light.

Adverse Effects

Irritation may rarely occur after the topical application of undecenoic acid or its salts.

Antimicrobial Action

Undecenoic acid and zinc undecenoate are active against some pathogenic fungi, including *Epidermophyton, Trichophyton,* and *Microsporum* spp.

Uses and Administration

Undecenoic acid and its zinc salt are applied topically in the prophylaxis and treatment of dermatophytic infections of superficial areas. The calcium salt is used similarly.
Undecenoic acid is applied to the skin in concentrations of 2% to 10%, and zinc undecenoate in concentrations of up to 20%. They are used in creams, ointments, or powders, often in conjunction with each other.Calcium undecenoate is used as a 10% powder.
Compounds related to undecenoic acid, stated to have antifungal and antibacterial properties, are used in the form of shampoos for treatment of seborrhoeic dermatitis of the scalp.
Copper undecenoate has been used in veterinary practice.

Preparations of Undecenoic Acid and Zinc Undecenoate

Compound Undecylenic Acid Ointment *(U.S.P.).* Zinc undecenoate 18 to 22% and undecenoic acid 4.5 to 5.5% in a suitable ointment basis. Store at a temperature not exceeding 30° in airtight containers.

Zinc Undecenoate Dusting-powder *(B.P.C. 1973).* Zinc undecenoate 10 g, undecenoic acid 2 g, pumilio pine oil 0.5 mL, starch 50 g, sterilised light kaolin to 100 g.

Proprietary Preparations of Undecenoic Acid and Zinc Undecenoate

Mycota *(Crookes Healthcare, UK). Cream,* undecenoic acid 5%, zinc undecenoate 20%.
Topical powder, undecenoic acid 2%, zinc undecenoate 20%.
Spray application, aerosol, undecenoic acid 2.5%, dichlorophen 0.25%.

Tineafax *(Wellcome, UK). Ointment,* zinc undecenoate 8%, zinc naphthenate solution 8%.
Topical powder, zinc undecenoate 10%.

Proprietary Preparations of Related Compounds

Synogist *(Townendale, UK). Shampoo,* sodium sulphosuccinated undecenoic monoalkylolamide 2% ($C_{17}H_{27}NaNO_8$ = 396.4).

Proprietary Names and Manufacturers of Undecenoic Acid, its Salts, and Related Compounds

Arrow Fusscrème *(Switz.)*; Benzoderm *(Arzneimittel Huls, Ger.)*; Caldesene Powder *(Pharmacraft, USA)*; Cruex *(Pharmacraft, USA)*; Decylon *(Neth.)*; Desenex *(Pennwalt, Canad.)*; Mycodecyl *(Théraplix, Fr.)*; Mycota *(Crookes Healthcare, UK)*; Pedzyl *(Switz.)*; Pelsano *(Switz.)*; Rewocid DU 185 *(Rewo, UK)*; Rewocid SBU 185 *(Rewo, UK)*; Rewocid U 185 *(Rewo, UK)*; Synogist *(Townendale, UK)*; Tineafax Powder *(Wellcome, Austral.; Wellcome, UK)*; Undecilendermina *(Granata, Ital.)*; Vernpro *(Vernleigh, S.Afr.)*.

The following names have been used for multi-ingredient preparations containing undecenoic acid, its salts, and related compounds—Acnederm *(Ego, Austral.)*; Audicort *(Lederle, UK)*; Breezee *(Pedinol, USA)*; Ceanel Concentrate *(Quinoderm, UK)*; Egomycol *(Ego, Austral.)*; Genisol *(Key, Austral.; Fisons, UK)*; Monphytol *(Salmond & Spraggon, Austral.; Laboratories for Applied Biology, UK)*; Mycoderm Cream *(Ego, Austral.)*; Mycota Spray *(Crookes Healthcare, UK)*; Pedi-Dri *(Pedinol, USA)*; Pedi-Pro *(Pedinol, USA)*; Pedoz *(Hamilton, Austral.)*; Phytocil Powder *(Rorer, UK)*; Ringworm Ointment *(Wellcome, Austral.)*; Seborrol *(Ego, Austral.)*; Silderm *(Lederle, UK)*; Tineafax Ointment *(Wellcome, Austral.)*.

Antigout Agents

1000-f

Gout is the term used for a range of metabolic disorders associated with hyperuricaemia where the symptoms are caused by the deposition of monosodium urate in the joints and other tissues. In acute gout or acute gouty arthritis there is an intensely painful inflammation of a peripheral joint, often the great toe joint, caused by crystals of monosodium urate in the synovial fluid. Chronic gout is characterised by accumulations of urate (tophi) in soft tissue, particularly in the fingers and the ears, and deforming arthritis. Urate may also crystallise out in the kidneys causing either renal urate stones or chronic renal damage.

Plasma-urate concentrations are not normally distributed across the population and are generally higher in men. The upper limit of normal is generally taken as 420 µmol per litre (7 mg per 100 mL), but gout does not necessarily develop in individuals with plasma-uric-acid concentrations above this value.

Hyperuricaemia may be due to either overproduction of uric acid, which is the end product of purine metabolism in man, or to underexcretion by the kidneys. Overproduction or underexcretion can be either primary (genetic) or secondary (acquired). Causes of overproduction include enzyme disorders such as hypoxanthine-guanine phosphoribosyltransferase deficiency and increased purine intake or turnover due to myeloproliferative disorders, neoplastic diseases, cancer therapy, or psoriasis. Underexcretion is caused by renal disease, hypertension, lead nephropathy, lactic acidosis, ketosis, or drugs (especially diuretics and low doses of salicylates).

Asymptomatic hyperuricaemia is often treated conservatively or not treated at all unless there are special risk factors in the patients' environment or genetic background.

The treatment of gout is directed at ending acute attacks and preventing further attacks as well as joint and kidney damage from chronic gout. Colchicine is the classic treatment for acute gout, but has been largely superseded by indomethacin and other anti-inflammatory drugs because of its toxicity. The aim of treatment in chronic or recurrent acute gout is to reduce plasma-uric-acid concentrations. This can be achieved with drugs which inhibit the production of uric acid, such as allopurinol, or drugs which enhance renal excretion of uric acid, such as the uricosuric agents probenecid and sulphinpyrazone. Allopurinol is preferred in patients with impaired renal function, renal stones, and hyperuricaemia arising from diuretics, neoplastic disease, or antineoplastic treatment. Allopurinol and uricosuric agents may be given together in severe cases. Colchicine is also used prophylactically.

Acute gout attacks are precipitated by any sudden change in plasma concentrations of uric acid and prophylaxis with colchicine or an anti-inflammatory drug should be given during the initial stages of treatment with allopurinol or uricosurics. Treatment with allopurinol or uricosuric agents should not be started during an acute attack as they may prolong it indefinitely. If acute attacks do develop in patients receiving allopurinol or a uricosuric agent, treatment should continue at the same dosage while the acute attack is treated with other agents.

For reviews of the treatment of hyperuricaemia and gout, see P. A. Simkin, *Ann. intern. Med.*, 1979, *90*, 812; G. R. Boss and J. E. Seegmiller, *New Engl. J. Med.*, 1979, *300*, 1459; J. T. Scott, *Br. med. J.*, 1980, *281*, 1164; H. L. F. Currey, *Essentials of Rheumatology*, London, Pitman, 1983, 78; B. T. Emmerson, *Med. J. Aust.*, 1984, *141*, 31; J. T. Scott, *Prescribers' J.*, 1987, *27* (6), 7.

Evidence suggests that a conservative approach should be adopted to the treatment of asymptomatic hyperuricaemia. The risk of developing gout, azotaemia, or urolithiasis appears to be small and hyperuricaemia in itself does not appear to cause renal insufficiency. Studies have yielded conflicting results on the relationship of asymptomatic hyperuricaemia to cardiovascular disease but hyperuricaemia has not been shown to be an independent risk factor. Mild hyperuricaemia may safely be left untreated but opinion varies when urate concentrations are more than 540 µmol per litre. Some recommend that allopurinol should be used to treat this degree of hyperuricaemia but clinicians should remember that there is a risk from adverse effects and fatalities have occurred in patients treated for trivial or inadequate reasons.— J. T. Scott, *Br. med. J.*, 1987, *294*, 987.

Symptomless hyperuricaemia in a hypertensive patient who is receiving diuretic treatment should be ignored. There is no evidence that it will cause significant renal failure and the incidence of gout, whilst increased, is not enough to justify prophylaxis with uric-acid-lowering agents.— *Lancet*, 1987, *1*, 1124.

1004-m

Allopurinol *(BAN, USAN, rINN).*

Allopurinolum; BW-56-158; HPP; NSC-1390.
1*H*-Pyrazolo[3,4-*d*]pyrimidin-4-ol.
$C_5H_4N_4O$=136.1.

CAS — 315-30-0 (allopurinol); 17795-21-0 (sodium salt).

Pharmacopoeias. In *Br., Braz., Chin., Cz., Ind., Int., It., Jpn, Jug.,* and *U.S.*

A white or off-white, odourless or almost odourless, microcrystalline powder. Very slightly **soluble** in water and alcohol; practically insoluble in chloroform and ether; soluble in solutions of alkali hydroxides.

The stability of a suspension of allopurinol made by suspending two crushed 100-mg tablets in 10 mL of a flavoured methylcellulose gel was studied by the manufacturer of the tablets. Less than 3% of allopurinol in suspension decomposed during storage at ambient temperature or at 5° over 56 days.— J. B. Dressman and R. I. Poust, *Am. J. Hosp. Pharm.*, 1983, *40*, 616.

The development of prodrugs of allopurinol for parenteral and rectal administration.— H. Bundgaard and E. Falch, *Int. J. Pharmaceut.*, 1985, *23*, 223; *idem*, *24*, 307.

Adverse Effects

The most common side-effect of allopurinol is skin rash which may occur more frequently in patients with renal failure: the overall incidence has been put at about 10%. Rashes are generally maculopapular or pruritic, but more serious allergic reactions may occur and include exfoliative rashes, the Stevens-Johnson syndrome, and toxic epidermal necrolysis. It is therefore recommended that allopurinol be withdrawn immediately if a rash occurs. Further symptoms of allergy include fever, chills, leucopenia or leucocytosis, eosinophilia, arthralgia, and vasculitis leading to renal and hepatic damage. These reactions may be severe, even fatal, and patients with renal impairment or taking thiazide diuretics are at special risk. Renal damage may also result from deposition of xanthine or oxypurinol crystals, and hepatotoxicity and signs of altered liver function may be found in patients not exhibiting hypersensitivity. Other side-effects of a less serious nature include peripheral neuritis, alopecia, nausea, vomiting, abdominal pain, diarrhoea, headache, drowsiness, and vertigo. There have been reports of cataract formation.

In addition to these adverse effects patients may experience an increase in acute gouty attacks during the first few months of treatment.

A Boston Collaborative Drug Surveillance Program of 29 524 hospitalised patients revealed that, with the exception of skin reactions, of 1835 patients treated with allopurinol 33 (1.8%) experienced adverse effects. It appeared that although allopurinol is seldom associated with toxicity, when it does occur it can be of a serious nature. Adverse effects were dose-related and the most frequent were haematological (11 patients, 0.6%), diarrhoea (5 patients, 0.3%), and drug fever (5 patients, 0.3%). Hepatotoxicity was reported in 3 patients (0.2%). Two patients developed possible hypersensitivity reactions to allopurinol.— G. T. McInnes *et al.*, *Ann. rheum. Dis.*, 1981, *40*, 245. See also.— H. Jick and D. R. Perera (letter), *J. Am. med. Ass.*, 1984, *252*, 1411.

A review of 78 cases of severe toxicity to allopurinol; 16 of the patients died. Common symptoms included skin rash, fever, hepatitis, worsening renal function, and eosinophilia and were considered to be consistent with a diffuse vasculitis. A large proportion of patients had pre-existing renal insufficiency. Studies showed that renal clearance of oxypurinol was directly proportional to creatinine clearance and serum-oxypurinol half-life was inversely proportional to creatinine clearance. Steady-state serum-oxypurinol concentrations were also inversely proportional to creatinine clearance. Doses of allopurinol should be modified on the basis of the creatinine clearance.— K. R. Hande *et al.*, *Am. J. Med.*, 1984, *76*, 47.

Severe steatorrhoea induced by allopurinol in an 80-year-old man.— B. Chen *et al.* (letter), *Br. med. J.*, 1982, *284*, 1914.

A case of male subfertility associated with allopurinol.— E. J. Margalioth *et al.* (letter), *Lancet*, 1985, *2*, 275.

EFFECTS ON THE SKIN. It was reported that 87.4% of reports of adverse effects to allopurinol in Australia over a 16-year period related to the skin or mucous membranes.— C. Vinciullo (letter), *Med. J. Aust.*, 1984, *141*, 449.

Over a 5-year period toxic epidermal necrolysis was clearly associated with allopurinol in 5 patients and possibly associated with allopurinol in one. Despite appropriate treatment one patient died and 2 others suffered severe sequelae. There had been no therapeutic reason for prescribing allopurinol in any of the patients.— J. Auböck and P. Fritsch, *Br. med. J.*, 1985, *290*, 1969.

Fatal Stevens-Johnson syndrome associated with allopurinol in a 78-year-old man. The CSM had received 3 previous reports of deaths from this syndrome in patients taking allopurinol.— I. G. H. Renwick (letter), *Br. med. J.*, 1985, *291*, 485.

Analysis, by the Boston Collaborative Drug Surveillance Program, of data on 15 438 patients hospitalised between 1975 and 1982 detected 6 allergic skin reactions attributed to allopurinol among 784 recipients of the drug.— M. Bigby *et al.*, *J. Am. med. Ass.*, 1986, *256*, 3358.

Precautions

Allopurinol should not be used for the treatment of an acute attack of gout and administration of allopurinol should not be started during one. Treatment should be stopped if any skin reactions or other signs of allergy develop. A cautious re-introduction at a lower dose may be attempted when mild skin reactions have cleared. Allopurinol should be administered with care to patients with renal or hepatic impairment, and doses may need to be reduced. In all patients receiving allopurinol it is advisable to maintain a urinary output of not less than 2 litres a day and for the urine to be neutral or slightly alkaline.

It has been suggested that allopurinol should not be given to nursing mothers since it is excreted in the breast milk.

The metabolism of azathioprine and mercaptopurine is inhibited by allopurinol and their doses should be reduced to one-quarter to one-third of the usual dose when either of them is given with allopurinol. There may be an increase in the toxicity of cyclophosphamide and other antineoplastic drugs. Similarly, allopurinol can reduce the clearance of theophylline and other xanthines and their dosage might have to be reduced to avoid toxicity. An increase in allergic reactions, and possibly also other adverse effects, has been reported in patients receiving allopurinol with thiazide diuretics, particularly in patients with impaired renal function. Rare reports of an increased response to oral anticoagulants in patients taking allopurinol has led to the suggestion that patients receiving both treatments should be monitored for variations in anticoagulant response. A number of drugs increase uric acid concentrations and may require that the dose of allopurinol be adjusted.

INTERACTIONS. Although an increased incidence of skin rashes has been noted when allopurinol has been used with ampicillin or amoxycillin, data currently available is insufficient to confirm whether this is due to allopurinol or not. For further details see under Precautions in Ampicillin (p.117).

Captopril. Reports of apparent interactions with captopril resulting in allergic reactions in two patients with chronic renal failure: D. J. Pennell *et al.* (letter), *Lancet*, 1984, *1*, 463 (fatal Stevens-Johnson syndrome); A. Samanta and A. C. Burden (letter), *ibid.*, 679 (pyrexia, arthralgia, and myalgia).

Cyclophosphamide. For a report of an increased incidence of bone-marrow toxicity in patients given allopurinol and cyclophosphamide, see Cyclophosphamide, p.612.

Tamoxifen. A report of deterioration of hepatic function in a patient taking allopurinol after the addition of tamoxifen.— K. A. Shah *et al.*, *N.Y. St. J. Med.*, 1982, *82*, 1745.

Absorption and Fate

Allopurinol is absorbed from the gastro-intestinal tract after oral administration and is reported to have a plasma half-life of about 1 to 3 hours. It is converted primarily in the liver to oxypurinol (alloxanthine) which is also an inhibitor of xanthine oxidase with a reported half-life of 18 to 30 hours in patients with normal renal function, although this is prolonged by renal impairment. Allopurinol and oxypurinol are not bound to plasma proteins. Excretion is mainly through the kidney, but it is slow since oxypurinol undergoes glomerular filtration as well as tubular reabsorption. About 70% of a daily dose may be excreted as oxypurinol and 10% as allopurinol; prolonged administration may alter these proportions due to allopurinol inhibiting its own metabolism. The remainder of the dose is excreted in the faeces.

A review of the clinical pharmacokinetics of allopurinol.— G. A. C. Murrell and W. G. Rapeport, *Clin. Pharmacokinet.*, 1986, *11*, 343.

A study in 6 healthy subjects of the kinetics of allopurinol after intravenous, oral, and rectal administration. Bioavailability from the tablet was about 67% and no measurable plasma concentrations of allopurinol were obtained with the rectal suppository.— S. J. Appelbaum *et al.*, *Cancer Chemother. Pharmac.*, 1982, *8*, 93.

Restricting the protein intake in 6 healthy subjects given allopurinol reduced the clearance of its metabolite oxypurinol.— W. G. Berlinger *et al.*, *New Engl. J. Med.*, 1985, *313*, 771.

Uses and Administration

Allopurinol inhibits the action of xanthine oxidase, thus reducing the oxidation of hypoxanthine to xanthine and xanthine to uric acid. The urinary purine load, normally almost entirely uric acid, is thereby divided between hypoxanthine, xanthine, and uric acid, each with its independent solubility. This results in the reduction of uric acid concentrations in both plasma and urine, ideally to such an extent that deposits of uric acid are dissolved or prevented from forming. At low doses allopurinol which is an analogue of hypoxanthine acts as a competitive inhibitor of xanthine oxidase, but at higher doses both allopurinol and its active metabolite oxypurinol act as non-competitive inhibitors of the enzyme. Plasma concentrations of xanthine and hypoxanthine increase only slightly during treatment because renal clearance is rapid, but a high fluid intake and maintenance of neutral or alkaline urine is recommended to prevent the development of xanthine stones in the urinary tract, especially if initial uric acid concentrations are high.

Allopurinol is used to treat primary or secondary hyperuricaemia associated with chronic gout, uric acid nephropathy, recurrent uric acid stone formation, enzyme disorders, blood disorders, and cancer therapy. It may be used when uricosurics are ineffective or contra-indicated. Allopurinol is not used to treat acute gout although it may prevent attacks. However, in the first few months of treatment with allopurinol there may be an increase in acute attacks; it is therefore recommended that anti-inflammatory agents or colchicine should also be given during that period.

To reduce the possibility of precipitating acute gout a dose of 100 mg daily by mouth may be given initially, increased by 100 mg daily at weekly intervals until the concentration of uric acid in plasma is reduced to about 60 µg per mL. The average daily dose is 200 to 300 mg for those with mild gout and 400 to 600 mg for those with moderately severe gout. Up to 300 mg may be taken as a single daily dose; larger amounts should be taken in divided doses. Allopurinol is best taken after food.

When used for hyperuricaemia associated with cancer therapy 600 to 800 mg is given daily in divided doses generally for 2 or 3 days and starting 1 or 2 days before the cancer treatment. Maintenance doses of allopurinol are then given according to the response. When given concomitantly with azathioprine or mercaptopurine, the dose of the antineoplastic agent should be reduced to one-third to one-quarter of the usual dose. The suggested dose for children with malignant conditions and enzyme disorders varies; in the UK a dose of 10 to 20 mg per kg body-weight daily is recommended, while in the USA the dose is 150 mg daily for children under six and 300 mg daily for those aged 6 to 10 years, adjusted if necessary after 48 hours.

When changing treatment from a uricosuric agent reduce the dose of the uricosuric agent gradually and increase that of allopurinol gradually over several weeks.

Doses should be reduced in patients with impaired renal function; 100 to 200 mg daily should be used if the creatinine clearance is between 10 and 20 mL per minute and not more than 100 mg daily if the creatinine clearance is less. Allopurinol and its metabolite are removed by haemodialysis and doses should be adjusted accordingly or else a single dose of 300 to 400 mg should be given after each dialysis. Allopurinol is also used for the prophylaxis of calcium oxalate calculi, as well as those due to uric acid, and to prevent the hyperuricaemia that may develop during diuretic treatment (but see Adverse Effects). Allopurinol usually as the riboside has been shown to possess activity against leishmania and trypanosomes.

Allopurinol should only be used when there is clear evidence of therapeutic benefit such as in the treatment of gout. Because of occasional fatalities its use is not recommended for mild symptomless hyperuricaemia. Furthermore, in any patient presenting with gout or hyperuricaemia potential causes such as diet and drugs, particularly diuretics, should be sought and eliminated first. In men under 30 and women not taking diuretics specialist advice should be sought to exclude metabolic defects before beginning treatment with allopurinol. When allopurinol is used in conditions associated with gross purine overproduction including some malignant diseases and certain enzyme disorders there is a risk that xanthine may be precipitated in the kidney and urinary-tract; alkalinisation of the urine does not increase xanthine solubility.— J. S. Cameron and H. A. Simmonds, *Br. med. J.*, 1987, *294*, 1504.

For further reference to the management of asymptomatic hyperuricaemia, see p.436.

For a discussion on the use of allopurinol to reduce fluorouracil toxicity in patients receiving chemotherapy, see under Treatment of Adverse Effects in Fluorouracil, p.629.

ADMINISTRATION IN RENAL FAILURE. A suggested dose schedule for allopurinol in patients with renal impairment. A maintenance dose of 100 mg every 3 days was recommended for a patient with no creatinine clearance; 100 mg every 2 days for a clearance of 10 mL per minute; 100 mg daily for 20 mL per minute; 150 mg daily for 40 mL per minute; 200 mg daily for 60 mL per minute; 250 mg daily for 80 mL per minute; 300 mg daily for 100 mL per minute; 350 mg daily for 120 mL per minute; and 400 mg daily for 140 mL per minute.— K. R. Hande *et al.*, *Am. J. Med.*, 1984, *76*, 47.

CONTRACTURE. Preliminary clinical results have suggested that allopurinol may improve Dupuytren's contracture. Findings suggest that oxygen free radicals may be important in the pathogenesis of this condition and that any potential benefit of allopurinol may be due to it preventing their production from the action of xanthine oxidase on the abnormal concentrations of hypoxanthine found in the palmar fascia.— G. A. C. Murrell *et al.*, *Br. med. J.*, 1987, *295*, 1373.

EPILEPSY. The frequency of seizures was reduced in the majority of 41 patients receiving antiepileptic therapy when allopurinol was added to the treatment.— P. De Marco and P. Zagnoni, *Neurology*, 1986, *36*, 1538.

LEISHMANIASIS. A report of beneficial results in 5 patients with visceral leishmaniasis unresponsive to sodium stibogluconate following further treatment with allopurinol and sodium stibogluconate together.— C. N. Chunge *et al.*, *Trans. R. Soc. trop. Med. Hyg.*, 1985, *79*, 715.

For further information see under sodium stibogluconate (p.679).

MUSCULAR DYSTROPHY. Controversy has surrounded the use of allopurinol in Duchenne muscular dystrophy since the initial favourable report by Thomson and Smith (*Metabolism*, 1978, *27*, 151 and *New Engl. J. Med.*, 1978, *299*, 101) on 16 children. Allopurinol was used in an attempt to increase the ATP levels in muscle which are depleted in this muscular dystrophy. Castro-Gago *et al.* reported similar results, and suggested that treatment would be most effective if started early in the course of the disease (*Lancet*, 1980, *1*, 1358). Their findings were strongly criticised by Gardner-Medwin (*Lancet*, 1980, *2*, 92) on the grounds that the study was uncontrolled and that spurious spontaneous improvements were seen in children under 6 years of age. Among other studies, Bakouche *et al.* (*New Engl. J. Med.*, 1979, *301*, 785), Bretag *et al.* (*Lancet*, 1981, *1*, 276), and Bertorini *et al.* (*Neurology*, 1985, *35*, 61) have failed to show any benefit from treatment. In general patient numbers have been small.

RENAL CALCULI. Several studies have concluded that allopurinol is effective in preventing the recurrence of calcium oxalate calculi (F.L. Coe, *Ann. intern. Med.*, 1977, *87*, 404; M.J.V. Smith, *J. Urol., Baltimore*, 1977, *117*, 690). However, they have been criticised by Ettinger *et al.* (*New Engl. J. Med.*, 1986, *315*, 1386) for not being well-controlled or of sufficient duration and for treating patients without regard to the absence or presence of hyperuricosuria or hypercalciuria. Fellström *et al.* (*Br. J. Urol.*, 1985, *57*, 375) had found that the use of allopurinol with advice on diet and fluid intake was no more effective than the use of dietary advice alone in patients with hyercalciuria. Other workers (H.-G. Tiselius *et al.*, *J. Urol., Baltimore*, 1986, *136*, 50) considered that with the possible exception of hyperuricosuria or hyperuricaemia the indications for using allopurinol were weak. Ettinger (1986) therefore conducted a double-blind study designed to avoid the limitations of earlier studies. They concluded from their findings that even after allowing for the large reduction in stone formation found with placebo treatment, allopurinol 300 mg daily was effective in the prevention of calcium oxalate stones in patients with hyperuricosuria in the absence of hypercalciuria. However, there have also been some criticisms of this study (*Lancet*, 1987, *1*, 258; A. Ulmann, *New Engl. J. Med.*, 1987, *316*, 1415).

SARCOIDOSIS. Samuel *et al.* (*Br. J. Derm.*, 1984, *111*, *Suppl. 26*, 20) observed an improvement in 4 of 6 patients with sarcoidosis treated with allopurinol. There was no response in one patient reported by Jenkinson and Dawson (*ibid.*, 54).

Preparations

Allopurinol Tablets *(B.P.)*

Allopurinol Tablets *(U.S.P.)*

Proprietary Preparations

Aloral *(Lagap, UK)*. *Tablets*, scored, allopurinol 100 and 300 mg.

Aluline *(Steinhard, UK)*. *Tablets*, scored, allopurinol 100 and 300 mg.

Caplenal *(Berk Pharmaceuticals, UK)*. *Tablets*, scored, allopurinol 100 and 300 mg.

Cosuric *(DDSA Pharmaceuticals, UK)*. *Tablets*, allopurinol 100 and 300 mg.

Hamarin *(Nicholas, UK)*. *Tablets*, scored, allopurinol 100 and 300 mg.

Zyloric *(Calmic, UK)*. *Tablets*, allopurinol 100 mg. *Tablets* (Zyloric-300), allopurinol 300 mg.

Proprietary Names and Manufacturers
Abopur *(Benzon, Denm.)*; Adenock *(Jpn)*; Alinol *(USV, Austral.)*; Alloprin *(ICN, Canad.)*; Allopur *(Nyco, Norw.; GEA, Swed.; Max Ritter, Switz.)*; Allopurin *(Bicther, Spain)*; Alloremed *(Drug Houses Austral., Austral.)*; Allozym *(Jpn)*; Allural *(Ital.; Rovi, Spain)*; Allurit *(Rhone-Poulenc, Ital.)*; Aloral *(Lagap, UK)*; Alositol *(Jpn)*; Aluline *(Steinhard, UK)*; Anoprolin *(Jpn)*; Anzief *(Jpn)*; Aprinol *(Jpn)*; Apulonga *(Dorsch, Ger.)*; Apurin *(GEA, Denm.; Neth.)*; Apurol *(Sigamed, Switz.)*; Bleminol *(Desitin, Ger.)*; Caplenal *(Berk Pharmaceuticals, UK)*; Capurate *(Fawns & McAllan, Austral.)*; Cellidrin *(Hennig, Ger.)*; Cellidrine *(Sodip, Switz.)*; Cosuric *(DDSA Pharmaceuticals, UK)*; Dabroson *(Hoyer, Ger.)*; Embarin *(Diabetylin, Ger.)*; Epidropal *(Fresenius, Ger.)*; Foligan *(Henning Berlin, Ger.; Henning, Switz.)*; Hamarin *(Nicholas, UK)*; Ketanrift *(Jpn)*; Ketobun-A *(Jpn)*; Lopurin *(Boots, USA)*; Lo-uric *(Rolab, S.Afr.)*; Lysuron 300 *(Switz.)*; Masaton *(Jpn)*; Méphanol *(Mepha, Switz.)*; Milurit *(Hung.)*; Miniplanor *(Jpn)*; Monarch *(Jpn)*; Neufan *(Jpn)*; Novopurol *(Novopharm, Canad.)*; Progout *(Protea, Austral.)*; Puricos *(Lennon, S.Afr.)*; Purinol *(Horner, Canad.)*; Redurate *(Schwulst, S.Afr.)*; Remid *(TAD, Ger.)*; Riball *(Jpn)*; Sigapurol *(Siegfried, Ger.)*; Suspendol *(Merckle, Ger.)*; Takanarumin *(Jpn)*; Urbol-100 *(Ger.)*; Uribenz *(RAN, Ger.)*; Uric *(Jpn)*; Uricemil *(ICT-Lodi, Ital.)*; Uriconorme *(Streuli, Switz.)*; Urifugan *(IRBI, Ital.)*; Uripurinol *(Azupharma, Ger.)*; Uriscel *(Rorer, Ital.)*; Urobenyl *(Searle, Ger.)*; Urolit *(Ital.)*; Uroquad *(Arg.)*; Urosin *(Galenus Mannheim, Ger.)*; Urozyl-SR *(Restan, S.Afr.)*; Urtias *(Sagitta, Ger.)*; Vedatan *(Doppel, Ital.)*; Xanturat *(Ger.)*; Xanturic *(Roland-Marie, Fr.)*; Zyloprim *(Wellcome, Austral.; Wellcome, Canad.; Mex.; NZ; Wellcome, S.Afr.; Wellcome, USA)*; Zyloric *(Arg.; Belg.; Wellcome, Denm.; Wellcome, Fr.; Wellcome, Ger.; Wellcome, Ital.; Neth.; Wellcome, Norw.; Gayoso Wellcome, Spain; Wellcome, Swed.; Wellcome, Switz.; Calmic, UK)*.

1005-b

Benzbromarone *(BAN, USAN, rINN).*

Benzbromaronum; L-2214; MJ-10061. 3,5-Dibromo-4-hydroxyphenyl 2-ethylbenzofuran-3-yl ketone.

$C_{17}H_{12}Br_2O_3$=424.1.

CAS — 3562-84-3.

Pharmacopoeias. In *Swiss.*

Adverse Effects

Benzbromarone may cause gastro-intestinal side-effects, especially diarrhoea. Other side-effects occasionally reported include skin rash and allergic conjunctivitis. It may precipitate an acute attack of gout and renal symptoms of urate deposits.

Precautions

Benzbromarone should be used with caution in patients with impaired renal function. Like other uricosurics, treatment with benzbromarone should not be started during an acute attack of gout. Salicylates antagonise the effect of benzbromarone. Benzbromarone may increase the anticoagulant activity of oral anticoagulants.

Absorption and Fate

Benzbromarone is absorbed from the gastro-intestinal tract and absorption appears to be influenced by the particle size. It is metabolised in the liver to benzarone and bromobenzarone which are reported to have uricosuric activity. It is excreted mainly in the faeces; a small amount appears in the urine.

Uses and Administration

Benzbromarone is a uricosuric agent which reduces plasma concentrations of uric acid probably by blocking tubular reabsorption; it may also increase the intestinal elimination of uric acid. It is used in the treatment of hyperuricaemia in gout and thiazide-induced hyperuricaemia. The usual dose is 100 to 200 mg of non-micronised or 40 to 80 mg of micronised benzbromarone once daily. Colchicine may be given initially to reduce the risk of precipitating acute gout. An adequate fluid intake is recommended and the pH of the urine should be adjusted to reduce the risk of renal stones.

An extensive review of benzbromarone.— R. C. Heel *et al., Drugs,* 1977, *14,* 349.

Benzbromarone reduced serum concentrations of uric acid in 17 renal transplant patients with hyperuricaemia.— W. Flury *et al., Schweiz. med. Wschr.,* 1977, *107,* 1339.

Beneficial results of benzbromarone at doses ranging between 50 and 300 mg per day in 200 patients with gout or hyperuricaemia for up to 10 years.— A. Masbernard and C. P. Giudicelli, *S. Afr. med. J.,* 1981, *59,* 701.

Benzbromarone 100 mg daily compared favourably with allopurinol and probenecid in a short study of 6 hyperuricaemic patients.— G. W. Schepers, *J. int. med. Res.,* 1981, *9,* 511.

Proprietary Names and Manufacturers
Azubromaron *(Azupharma, Ger.)*; Désuric *(Labaz, Fr.; Labaz, Switz.)*; Desuric *(Labaz, Belg.; Sigmatau, Ital.; Labaz, Neth.)*; Harolan *(Merz, Ger.)*; Max-Uric *(Labinca, Arg.)*; Minuric *(Labaz, S.Afr.)*; Narcaricin *(Heumann, Ger.)*; Normurat *(Grünenthal, Ger.)*; Obaron *(Mepha, Switz.)*; Uricovac *(Labaz, Ger.)*; Urinome *(Jpn)*; Urinorm *(Labaz, Spain)*.

1001-d

Colchicine *(BAN, USAN).*

Colchicinum. (*S*)-*N*-(5,6,7,9-Tetrahydro-1,2,3,10-tetramethoxy-9-oxobenzo[*a*]heptalen-7-yl)acetamide.

$C_{22}H_{25}NO_6$=399.4.

CAS — 64-86-8.

Pharmacopoeias. In *Arg., Aust., Br., Braz., Chin., Cz., Egypt., Fr., Ind., Int., It., Jpn, Mex., Nord., Port., Span., Swiss, Turk.,* and *U.S.*
Chin. P. also has a monograph for colchicine amide.

An alkaloid obtained from the corm and seeds of the meadow saffron, *Colchicum autumnale* (Liliaceae) and other *Colchicum* spp. It occurs as pale yellow to greenish-yellow, odourless or almost odourless crystals or amorphous scales or powder. It may contain up to 10% of solvent and moisture and not more than 2 to 3% is lost on drying. It darkens on exposure to light.

B.P. **solubilities** are: freely soluble in water, alcohol, and chloroform; slightly soluble in ether; moderately concentrated aqueous solutions may deposit crystals of sesquihydrate, which is less soluble in cold water than the anhydrous alkaloid. *U.S.P.* solubilities are: soluble 1 in 25 of water, 1 in 220 of ether, freely soluble in alcohol and chloroform. Solutions are **sterilised** by autoclaving or by filtration. The *U.S.P.* injection may be prepared with the aid of sodium hydroxide and has a pH of 6.0 to 7.2. The injection should not be mixed with any fluid which would change the pH as precipitation may occur. **Store** in airtight containers. Protect from light.

Adverse Effects

The most frequent adverse effects of colchicine are those involving the gastro-intestinal tract and may be associated with its antimitotic action. Diarrhoea, nausea, vomiting, and abdominal pain are often the first signs of toxicity and are usually an indication that colchicine therapy should be stopped. Thrombophlebitis may occur rarely at the site of an intravenous injection and extravasation can cause local irritation.

Bone marrow depression with agranulocytosis, thrombocytopenia, and aplastic anaemia have occurred on prolonged treatment as have peripheral neuritis, myopathy, rashes, and alopecia.

Symptoms of overdosage do not appear for at least several hours. The first symptoms are nausea, vomiting, and diarrhoea. The diarrhoea may be severe and haemorrhagic, and can lead to metabolic acidosis, dehydration, hypotension, and shock. A burning sensation of the throat, stomach, and skin may also occur. Extensive vascular damage and acute renal toxicity with oliguria and haematuria have been reported. Bone marrow depression with leucopenia may be followed by rebound leucocytosis. The patient may develop convulsions, delirium, muscle weakness, neuropathy, and ascending paralysis of the CNS. Death may be due to respiratory depression, cardiovascular collapse, or bone-marrow depression. The lethal dose varies: 7 mg of colchicine has caused death, yet recovery has occurred after much larger doses.

There have been incidental reports of azoospermia (1 case; H.E. Merlin, *Fertil. Steril.,* 1972, *23,* 180) or oligospermia (11 cases; Y. Mizushima *et al., Lancet,* 1977, *2,* 1037) attributed to colchicine as well as a report that it had no effect on the sperm count or seminal hormone content of 7 men (W.J. Bremner and C.A. Paulsen, *New Engl. J. Med.,* 1976, *294,* 1384). However, Margalioth *et al.* (*Lancet,* 1985, *2,* 275) identified a patient who was taking colchicine who had a normal sperm count but an abnormal sperm penetration assay.

Analysis of the data on 12 patients who developed myopathy and neuropathy while receiving treatment with colchicine indicated that colchicine-induced myoneuropathy may be a common but unrecognised condition in patients with reduced renal function who receive usual doses of colchicine. Both skeletal muscles and peripheral nerves are affected but whereas the myopathy is most prominent the associated axonal neuropathy is mild. The condition usually presents with proximal muscle weakness and is always accompanied with elevations in serum creatine kinase concentrations. Withdrawal of colchicine leads to spontaneous remission of these symptoms within a few weeks but resolution of the polyneuropathy is slow. Examination of proximal muscles shows marked abnormal spontaneous activity and because of the features of the condition it is usually misdiagnosed as probable polymyositis or uraemic myopathy. Muscle biopsy has revealed distinctive vacuolation but no necrotic changes.— R. W. Kuncl *et al., New Engl. J. Med.,* 1987, *316,* 1562.

A report of a patient with normal renal function but chronic alcohol-induced liver disease who developed an unusual form of myoneuropathy after receiving colchicine. Unlike those patients in the report by Kuncl *et al.* this patient had only received a short course of colchicine. The microsomal enzyme-inhibiting activity of the tolbutamide she was also taking may have also contributed to her condition.— C. Besana *et al.* (letter), *Lancet,* 1987, *2,* 1271.

OVERDOSAGE. Some references to overdosage with colchicine.— R. N. Hill *et al.* (letter), *Ann. intern. Med.,* 1975, *83,* 523 (fatality following 150 mg of colchicine); D. Heaney *et al., Am. J. med. Sci.,* 1976, *271,* 233 (fatality with 35 mg); M. Besson-Leaud *et al., Annls Pédiat., Paris,* 1977, *24,* 363 (recovery in 3 infants and death in a fourth); A. J. Dodds *et al., Med. J. Aust.,* 1978, *2,* 91 (survival following 40 mg); S. S. Murray *et al., Mayo Clin. Proc.,* 1983, *58,* 528 (survival following 24 mg).

Treatment of Adverse Effects

Colchicine should be withdrawn or the dose reduced if adverse gastro-intestinal effects occur. In cases of overdosage or acute poisoning patients should be carefully monitored for some time to take account of the delayed onset of symptoms. In acute poisoning the stomach should be emptied by aspiration and lavage. Respiration may require assistance. The circulation should be maintained and fluid and electrolyte imbalance corrected. Morphine or atropine may be given to relieve severe abdominal cramps; symptomatic and supportive measures are used to treat other symptoms. Haemodialysis or peritoneal dialysis may be of value when kidney function is compromised.

An account of the symptoms and management of a 15-year-old girl who ultimately survived after ingesting an estimated 24 mg of colchicine. It was concluded that because of the transitory nature of the complications of acute colchicine toxicity, intensive medical support can lead to complete recovery despite failure of multiple organ systems. Advice on management included the recommendation to remove any remaining substance from the stomach because the recovery of even small amounts could greatly affect the prognosis, and the view that haemodialysis is not of substantial benefit.— S. S. Murray *et al., Mayo Clin. Proc.,* 1983, *58,* 528.

Precautions

Colchicine should be given with great care to old and debilitated patients and to those with cardiac, renal, or gastro-intestinal disease. Care should also be exercised if treating pregnant patients since there is a risk of foetal chromosome damage.

It should not be administered by subcutaneous or intramuscular injection.

Results of a study of 20 healthy subjects indicated that colchicine caused marked malabsorption of cyanocobalamin due to an effect primarily on the ileum.— D. I. Webb *et al.*, *New Engl. J. Med.*, 1968, *279*, 845.

Absorption and Fate

Colchicine is readily absorbed from the gastro-intestinal tract and reaches peak concentration in the plasma within 2 hours. It is partially deacetylated in the liver and the unchanged drug and its metabolites are excreted in the bile and undergo intestinal reabsorption. Colchicine is found in high concentrations in leucocytes, kidneys, the liver, and spleen. Most of the drug is excreted in the faeces but 10 to 20% is excreted in the urine and this proportion rises in patients with liver disorders.

A study of the kinetics of colchicine in patients with familial Mediterranean fever.— H. Halkin *et al.*, *Clin. Pharmac. Ther.*, 1980, *28*, 82.

Uses and Administration

Colchicine produces a dramatic response in acute gout probably by reducing the inflammatory reaction to urate crystals; this effect might be due to several actions including decreased leucocyte mobility. It is not an analgesic and has no effect on blood concentrations of uric acid, or on the excretion of uric acid. Colchicine also has an antimitotic action.

Colchicine is used for the relief of acute gout when the dramatic response can be diagnostic. Pain and swelling usually abate within 12 hours of starting colchicine therapy, and symptoms have usually disappeared after 48 to 72 hours. Colchicine is also used for the prophylaxis of recurrent gout and to prevent acute attacks during the first few months of treatment with allopurinol or uricosurics.

In acute gout the initial dose is 0.5 to 1.2 mg by mouth, followed by 0.5 to 0.65 mg every 1 to 2 hours or 1 to 1.3 mg every 2 hours to a maximum of 10 mg until relief is obtained or gastro-intestinal symptoms occur. The total amount required to relieve the attack is usually between 4 and 10 mg. A course should not be repeated within 3 days. Colchicine may be given by intravenous injection in a dose of 1 to 2 mg in sodium chloride injection injected over 2 to 5 minutes, with further doses of 0.5 to 1 mg at 6- to 12- hourly intervals to a total of 4 mg in 24 hours or in an attack. For prophylaxis of recurrent gout oral doses may range from 500 to 650 µg weekly to three times daily; 1 to 2 mg may be given by intravenous injection daily for several days.

Colchicine is also used for prophylaxis and treatment of familial Mediterranean fever (recurrent polyserositis), and has been used in some skin disorders.

Reference to evidence indicating that colchicine may produce beneficial results in patients with back pain associated with disk or spinal disorders.— M. R. Rask (letter), *J. Am. med. Ass.*, 1986, *255*, 2447.

ADMINISTRATION IN RENAL FAILURE. The dose of colchicine should be reduced by 50% in patients with a glomerular filtration-rate of less than 10 mL per minute. Prolonged use should be avoided if the glomerular filtration-rate is less than 50 mL per minute.— W. M. Bennett *et al.*, *Am. J. Kidney Dis.*, 1983, *3*, 155.

AMYLOIDOSIS. Although colchicine appears to ameliorate the effects of amyloidosis in familial Mediterranean fever it does not appear to improve survival of patients with primary systemic amyloidosis.— *Lancet*, 1986, *2*, 724.

See also below under Familial Mediterranean Fever.

BEHÇET'S DISEASE. An analysis on reports of 157 patients with Behçet's disease treated with colchicine showed that 46 patients were much improved, 58 showed some improvement, 42 showed no change, and 11 deteriorated.— Y. Mizushima *et al.* (letter), *Lancet*, 1977, *2*, 1037.

Cutaneous and ocular manifestations of Behçet's disease improved greatly in 5 patients within a month of starting colchicine 1 mg daily.— Y. Miyachi *et al.*, *Br. J. Derm.*, 1981, *104*, 67.

Signs of ocular inflammation were reduced in 8 of 18 patients with Behçet's disease treated with colchicine after 'resistance' to corticosteroid therapy had developed. The average duration of remission of symptoms was 3 months; the effect on prognosis was unclear.— D. Benezra and E. Cohen, *Br. J. Ophthal.*, 1986, *70*, 589.

CIRRHOSIS OF THE LIVER. In a review of the treatment of primary biliary cirrhosis Kaplan (*New Engl. J. Med.*, 1987, *316*, 521) concluded that there was still no satisfactory treatment for this condition and none of the agents currently used was totally effective. However, there is evidence to indicate that colchicine may slow the progression of the disease. Three prospective double-blind studies have found significant biochemical improvements (H. Bodenheimer *et al.*, *Hepatology*, 1986, *6*, 1172; M.M. Kaplan *et al.*, *New Engl. J. Med.*, 1986, *315*, 1448; T.W. Warnes *et al.*, *J. Hepatol.*, 1987, *5*, 1) in patients receiving colchicine. Kaplan *et al.* also found a higher rate of survival in those receiving colchicine 600 µg twice daily but there appears to have been no improvement in liver histology, symptoms, or physical findings.

ERYTHEMA NODOSUM LEPROSUM. Beneficial effects were seen in 10 patients with recurrent or chronic erythema nodosum leprosum during treatment with colchicine.— P. A. Sarojini and R. N. Mshana (letter), *Lepr. Rev.*, 1983, *54*, 151. Colchicine had little or no effect on corticosteroid requirements in patients with erythema nodosum leprosum.— J. N. A. Stanley *et al.* (letter), *Lepr. Rev.*, 1984, *55*, 317.

FAMILIAL MEDITERRANEAN FEVER. Complete remission of symptoms of familial Mediterranean fever was achieved in 46 of 47 patients treated with colchicine 500 µg per 25 kg body-weight daily.— M. Levy and M. Eliakim, *Br. med. J.*, 1977, *2*, 808.

A study involving 1070 patients with familial Mediterranean fever suggested that colchicine may prevent amyloidosis in this high risk population and that it could prevent further deterioration in patients with amyloidosis who have proteinuria but not in those who have nephrotic syndrome. Patients were given colchicine 1 to 2 mg daily and their progress followed for 4 to 11 years. Of the 960 patients who initially had no evidence of amyloidosis, proteinuria appeared in 4 patients who had adhered to the prophylactic schedule compared with proteinuria in 16 of 54 non-compliant patients. Life table analysis indicated the cumulative rate of proteinuria was 1.7% after 11 years in compliant patients and 48.9% after 9 years in noncompliant patients. Of 110 patients who already had proteinuria at the start of therapy, 5 patients had resolution of their proteinuria and 68 patients were stabilised for periods of up to 8 years or more. Renal function deteriorated in the remaining 13 patients and in all of the 24 patients with nephrotic syndrome or uraemia.— D. Zemer, *New Engl. J. Med.*, 1986, *314*, 1001.

Further references to the use of colchicine in familial Mediterranean fever: M. Eliakim and A. Licht (letter), *Lancet*, 1973, *2*, 1333; D. Zemer *et al.*, *New Engl. J. Med.*, 1974, *291*, 932; C. A. Dinarello *et al.*, *New Engl. J. Med.*, 1974, *291*, 934; D. G. Wright *et al.*, *Ann. intern. Med.*, 1977, *86*, 162; M. Ravid *et al.*, *Ann. intern. Med.*, 1977, *87*, 568.

IDIOPATHIC THROMBOCYTOPENIC PURPURA. Colchicine 600 µg two to four times a day caused partial or complete responses in 4 of 14 patients with idiopathic thrombocytopenic purpura refractory to splenectomy and corticosteroids.— S. V. Strother *et al.*, *Archs intern. Med.*, 1984, *144*, 2198.

PAGET'S DISEASE OF BONE. Pain was relieved in 5 patients with Paget's disease of bone treated with colchicine 600 µg three times a day. Improvement correlated with a reduction in values for serum alkaline phosphatase and urinary hydroxyproline.— A. Theodors *et al.*, *Clin. Ther.*, 1981, *3*, 365. See also A. J. Crisp and B. L. Hazleman (letter), *Clin. Rheumatol.*, 1985, *4*, 365.

PERICARDITIS. Administration of colchicine 1 mg daily produced an improvement in 3 patients who required corticosteroid therapy to control recurrent episodes of pericarditis. Corticosteroid therapy was withdrawn 2 months after starting treatment with colchicine and the patients had now been free of further attacks for up to 36 months. The maintenance dose had been reduced to 500 µg daily and no adverse effects had been reported.— A. Rodríguez De La Serna *et al.* (letter), *Lancet*, 1987, *2*, 1517.

SKIN DISORDERS. Reviews of the use of colchicine in dermatological disorders: F. D. Malkinson, *Archs Derm.*, 1982, *118*, 453; H. Aram, *Int. J. Derm.*, 1983, *22*, 566.

Rapid improvement was seen in 3 patients with acute febrile neutrophilic dermatosis (Sweet's syndrome) treated with colchicine.— S. Suehisa *et al.*, *Br. J. Derm.*, 1983, *108*, 99.

Colchicine 600 µg given twice daily produced beneficial results in 2 patients whose urticarial vasculitis had been unresponsive to other therapy.— J. C. Wiles *et al.*, *Archs Derm.*, 1985, *121*, 802.

Preparations

Colchicine Injection *(U.S.P.)*

Colchicine Tablets *(B.P.)*

Colchicine Tablets *(U.S.P.)*

Proprietary Names and Manufacturers

Colchicine Houdé *(Roussel, S.Afr.)*; Colchineos *(Houdé, Fr.)*; Colcin *(Knoll, Austral.)*; Colgout *(Protea, Austral.)*; Coluric *(Nelson, Austral.)*.

The following names have been used for multi-ingredient preparations containing colchicine— ColBenemid *(Merck Sharp & Dohme, UK; Merck Sharp & Dohme, USA)*; Verban *(Welcker-Lyster, Canad.)*.

1003-h

Colchicum

Colchique.

Pharmacopoeias. In *Arg.*, *Braz.*, *Egypt.*, *Fr.*, *Mex.*, *Port.*, *Span.*, and *Turk.* as the seed.

The dried ripe seeds or dried corm of the meadow saffron, *Colchicum autumnale*.

Colchicum which contains colchicine has been used similarly for the relief of pain in acute gout in various preparations such as colchicum and sodium salicylate mixture.

1006-v

Ethebenecid *(BAN)*.

Etebenecid *(rINN)*. 4-(Diethylsulphamoyl)benzoic acid.
$C_{11}H_{15}NO_4S$=257.3.

CAS — 1213-06-5.

Ethebenecid is a uricosuric agent that was formerly used similarly to probenecid in the treatment of gout and hyperuricaemia.

Proprietary Names and Manufacturers

Urelim *(WB Pharmaceuticals, UK)*.

12866-b

Isobromindione *(rINN)*.

5-Bromo-2-phenyl-indan-1,3-dione.
$C_{15}H_9BrO_2$=301.1.

CAS — 1470-35-5.

Isobromindione has been used in the treatment of hyperuricaemia. It appears to lack the anticoagulant activity of bromindione.

Proprietary Names and Manufacturers

Uridion *(Gentili, Ital.)*.

1008-q

Probenecid *(BAN, USAN, rINN)*.

Probenecidum. 4-(Dipropylsulphamoyl)benzoic acid.
$C_{13}H_{19}NO_4S$=285.4.

CAS — 57-66-9.

Pharmacopoeias. In *Br.*, *Braz.*, *Chin.*, *Cz.*, *Egypt.*, *Eur.*, *Fr.*, *Int.*, *It.*, *Jpn*, *Jug.*, *Neth.*, *Nord.*, *Swiss*, *Turk.*, and *U.S.*

A white or almost white, odourless or almost odourless, crystalline powder.

B.P. **solubilities** are: practically insoluble in water; sparingly soluble in alcohol and chloroform; soluble in acetone; slightly soluble in ether. *U.S.P.* solubilities are: practically insoluble in water and dilute acids; soluble in alcohol, acetone, chloroform, and in dilute alkali. **Store** in well-closed containers.

Adverse Effects

Probenecid is generally well tolerated, though nausea, vomiting, anorexia, headache, sore gums, flushing, dizziness, urinary frequency, and skin rashes may occasionally occur. Allergic reactions, with fever, dermatitis, pruritus and, rarely, anaphylaxis have occurred and there have been reports of hepatic necrosis, the nephrotic syndrome, and aplastic anaemia. Haemolytic anaemia has also occurred, and may be associated with glucose-6-phosphate dehydrogenase deficiency. When used in chronic gout, probenecid may precipitate an acute attack, and renal calculi or renal colic, with or without haematuria, may occur. In massive overdosage probenecid causes stimulation of the central nervous system, with convulsions and death from respiratory failure. Severe overdosage should be managed by emesis and lavage and symptomatic treatment.

ABUSE. It has been alleged that some athletes using banned anabolic steroids have also been taking probenecid in an attempt to inhibit the urinary excretion of steroid metabolites in order to avoid detection by urine screening tests.— *Pharm. J.*, 1987, *2*, 299.

Precautions

Probenecid therapy should not be started during an acute attack of gout and should not be given to patients with a history of renal uric acid calculi or blood dyscrasias. It is not recommended for children under 2 years of age or for the control of hyperuricaemia secondary to cancer therapy. It should be used with caution in patients with a history of peptic ulceration and also in patients with renal impairment when being used to block the tubular secretion of an antibiotic.

Interactions. Probenecid reduces the urinary excretion of a number of drugs by inhibiting tubular secretion. It is therefore given with some antimicrobial agents such as the penicillins and some cephalosporins to increase their effects. Increased concentrations resulting from altered excretion may be seen with other drugs including aminosalicylates, chlorpropamide, conjugated sulphonamides, dapsone, some non-steroidal anti-inflammatory agents such as indomethacin, and rifampicin. Although this may mean that the doses of some of these drugs could be reduced, as has been suggested for indomethacin, the effect is not generally considered to be clinically useful or significant. However, in some instances a reduction in dose is essential to counteract an increase in toxicity, as is the case with methotrexate. The dose of probenecid may need to be increased if patients are also given drugs such as diuretics which increase the blood concentration of uric acid. Reducing the urinary concentration of some drugs could diminish their activity in certain diseases as might happen with nitrofurantoin in urinary-tract infections and penicillamine in cystinuria. Salicylates and probenecid are mutually antagonistic and should not be given together.

A reducing substance has been found in the urine of some patients taking probenecid, and may give false positive results with some tests for glucose in the urine. Probenecid reduces the excretion of some iodinated contrast media and may interfere with laboratory tests by decreasing the excretion of aminohippuric acid, phenolsulphonphthalein, sulphobromophthalein, and 5-hydroxyindoleacetic acid.

INTERACTIONS. The half-life of probenecid was increased and its uricosuric effect reduced after prior treatment with pyrazinamide but protein binding was not affected. The excretion of probenecid was increased in alkaline urine.— T. F. Yü *et al.*, *Am. J. Med.*, 1977, *63*, 723.

PORPHYRIA. Probenecid was considered to be unsafe in patients with acute porphyria although there is conflicting experimental evidence on porphyrinogenicity.— M.R. Moore and K.E.L. McColl, *Porphyrias, Drug Lists*, Glasgow, Porphyria Research Unit, University of Glasgow, 1987.

Absorption and Fate

Probenecid is rapidly absorbed from the gastro-intestinal tract and is extensively bound to plasma proteins. It crosses the placenta. It is metabolised by the liver, and excreted in the urine mainly as metabolites. Excretion is increased in alkaline urine.

From 77 to 88% of a dose of probenecid was found in the urine of 2 healthy subjects after administration of 0.5 to 2 g in solution. The major metabolite was probenecid acyl glucuronide. The time required for elimination appeared to be dose dependent, and may have been due to delayed absorption of precipitated probenecid from the gastro-intestinal tract.— S. Melethil and W. D. Conway, *J. pharm. Sci.*, 1976, *65*, 861. Results achieved in 5 healthy subjects suggested that the dose-dependent elimination of probenecid was due to saturation of elimination mechanisms and was unlikely to be due to delayed absorption.— A. Selen *et al.*, *J. pharm. Sci.*, 1982, *71*, 1238. Re-evaluation of the data from the study by Melethil and Conway revealed that the elimination of probenecid followed 5 different parallel pathways. The elimination of its major metabolite the acyl glucuronide followed non-linear Michaelis-Menten kinetics and the elimination of its three oxidised metabolites followed dose-dependent pseudo first-order kinetics. Although progressive saturation of the glucuronidation pathway occurred with increasing doses a similar increase in product inhibition of the oxidative pathways counteracted this effect with the result that the relative amount of excreted metabolite is unchanged with changing dose.— J. C. Ho *et al.*, *ibid.*, 1986, *75*, 664. See also B.-M. Emanuelsson *et al.*, *Eur. J. clin. Pharmac.*, 1987, *32*, 395.

PROTEIN BINDING. The unbound fraction of probenecid in plasma, estimated using equilibrium dialysis, increased in a non-linear manner with increasing plasma concentrations reaching a maximum free fraction of 26%.— B.-M. Emanuelsson *et al.*, *Eur. J. clin. Pharmac.*, 1987, *32*, 395.

Uses and Administration

Probenecid is a uricosuric agent; in appropriate doses it promotes excretion of urates by inhibiting tubular reabsorption, which results in a lowering of the elevated concentrations of uric acid in the plasma with consequent dissolution of uric acid deposits in joints and tissues. Probenecid also inhibits the tubular secretion of a range of compounds that can be broadly classified as weak organic acids thus blocking their urinary excretion.

It is used in the treatment of chronic gout to reduce the incidence and severity of acute attacks; it may be some months before benefit is obtained. It is also used to prevent the effects of hyperuricaemia in patients taking diuretics or who are otherwise judged to be at risk; it is not used as an adjunct to cancer therapy. Probenecid has no analgesic or anti-inflammatory action and is of no value in acute gout, and treatment should not be initiated during, or for 2 to 3 weeks after, an acute attack. Acute attacks occurring during treatment with probenecid may be reduced by the concurrent administration of colchicine or a non-steroidal anti-inflammatory agent.

It is usual to start treatment with doses of 250 mg twice daily increased after a week to 500 mg twice daily and later, if the therapeutic effects are inadequate, by 500-mg increments every 4 weeks, up to 2 g daily. Probenecid may not be effective in chronic renal impairment particularly when the glomerular filtration rate is less than 30 mL per minute.

To reduce the risk of urolithiasis, an adequate fluid intake is required especially during the first few months of treatment, and, if necessary, sodium bicarbonate 3 to 7.5 g daily or potassium citrate 7.5 g daily may be given to render the urine alkaline.

When the patient has been free from acute attacks for at least 6 months, and providing the plasma concentration of uric acid is within acceptable limits, the daily dose may be gradually reduced, in stages of 500 mg every 6 months, to the lowest effective maintenance dose.

Probenecid is also used as an adjunct to antibiotic therapy to reduce the tubular excretion of penicillins and most cephalosporins when it may increase their plasma concentrations up to four-fold. It may also block the removal of penicillin from the CSF. Probenecid is used in conditions where very high or prolonged concentrations of penicillin or cephalosporin may be required, such as subacute bacterial endocarditis or the treatment of gonorrhoea. It is not used with cephaloridine. The usual dosage for reducing tubular excretion of penicillins and cephalosporins is 500 mg four times daily, or less in elderly patients with suspected renal impairment. The dosage for children over 2 years of age and weighing less than 50 kg is 25 mg per kg body-weight (700 mg per m² body-surface) initially, followed by 10 mg per kg (300 mg per m²) every 6 hours. When renal impairment is sufficient to retard the excretion of antibiotics, probenecid should not be given concurrently.

Single doses of probenecid 1 g are used in conjunction with antibiotics in the single-dose treatment of gonorrhoea. Probenecid is given at the same time as the antibiotic when the latter is given by mouth but is given 30 minutes before the antibiotic administered by injection.

CALCIFICATION DISORDERS. Reports of individual patients with calcification disorders benefitting from probenecid: C. E. Dent and T. C. B. Stamp, *Br. med. J.*, 1972, *1*, 216 (calcinosis circumscripta); R. MacKie (letter), *ibid.*, *2*, 768 (systemic sclerosis and calcification); D. Meyers, *Med. J. Aust.*, 1976, *2*, 457 (calcinosis circumscripta).

Probenecid 0.25 g increasing to 1 g twice daily was ineffective in 6 patients with chondrocalcinosis articularis.— E. E. Smith and A. St. J. Dixon (letter), *Lancet*, 1976, *2*, 376.

DIAGNOSTIC USE. The use of probenecid as a biochemical aid in the diagnosis of manic-depressive psychoses.— R. Sjöström, *Eur. J. clin. Pharmac.*, 1973, *6*, 75; B. -E. Roos *et al.*, *Eur. J. clin. Pharmac.*, 1980, *17*, 223.

Preparations

Probenecid and Colchicine Tablets *(U.S.P.)*

Probenecid Tablets *(B.P.)*

Probenecid Tablets *(U.S.P.)*

Proprietary Preparations

Benemid *(Merck Sharp & Dohme, UK). Tablets*, scored, probenecid 500 mg.

Proprietary Names and Manufacturers

Bénémide *(Théraplix, Fr.)*; Benemid *(Frosst, Austral.; Belg.; Merck Sharp & Dohme, Canad.; Ger.; Ital.; Neth.; Merck Sharp & Dohme, S.Afr.; Chibret, Switz.; Merck Sharp & Dohme, UK; Merck Sharp & Dohme, USA)*; Benuryl *(ICN, Canad.)*; Panuric *(Propan, S.Afr.)*; Probecid *(Astra, Norw.; Astra, Swed.)*; Probemid *(Spain)*; Proben *(SCS, S.Afr.)*; Probenid *(Belg.)*; Procid *(Protea, Austral.)*; SK-Probenecid *(Smith Kline & French, USA)*; Solpurin *(Salfa, Ital.)*; Uroben *(Ital.)*; Urocid *(Ist. Chim. Inter., Ital.)*.

The following names have been used for multi-ingredient preparations containing probenecid— Ampicin-PRB *(Bristol, Canad.)*; ColBenemid *(Merck Sharp & Dohme, UK; Merck Sharp & Dohme, USA)*; Polycillin-PRB *(Bristol, USA)*; Principen with Probenecid *(Squibb, USA)*; Pro-Biosan *(ICN, Canad.)*; Wycillin and Probenecid *(Wyeth, USA)*.

1009-p

Sulphinpyrazone *(BAN)*.

G-28315; Sulfinpyrazone *(USAN, rINN)*; Sulfinpyrazonum; Sulphoxyphenylpyrazolidine. 1,2-Diphenyl-4-(2-phenylsulphinylethyl)pyrazolidine-3,5-dione.

$C_{23}H_{20}N_2O_3S$=404.5.

CAS — 57-96-5.

Pharmacopoeias. In *Br.*, *Braz.*, *Egypt.*, and *U.S.*

A white, or off-white, odourless or almost odourless powder. *B.P.* **solubilities** are: practically insoluble in water and petroleum spirit, soluble 1 in 40 of alcohol, 1 in 2 of chloroform; slightly soluble in ether. *U.S.P.* solubilities are: practically insoluble in water and petroleum spirit, soluble in alcohol and acetone, and sparingly soluble in dilute solutions of alkalis. **Store** in well-closed containers.

Adverse Effects

The most frequent adverse effects of sulphinpyrazone involve the gastro-intestinal tract, and include nausea, vomiting, and abdominal pain. It may cause gastric bleeding and aggravate existing peptic ulcers. During the first few months of treatment acute attacks of gout may be more frequent and there is a risk of renal stones. Skin rashes have been reported, and may be associated with an allergic reaction. Anaemia, agranulocytosis, leucopenia, and thrombocytopenia have been reported rarely. Impaired renal function and occasionally renal failure may occur. Symptoms of overdosage include ataxia, laboured respiration, convulsions, and coma, as well as gastro-intestinal effects.

Oral challenge tests indicating that sulphinpyrazone can induce bronchospasm in patients with aspirin-induced asthma.— A. Szczeklik *et al.* (letter), *New Engl. J. Med.*, 1980, *303*, 702.

EFFECTS ON THE BLOOD. Three of 25 patients with gout who took sulphinpyrazone for 2.8 to 14 years and colchicine intermittently developed fatal acute myelomonocytic leukaemia (2) or multiple myeloma (1). Eight of 22 patients taking sulphinpyrazone for 5 months developed moderate granulocytopenia. Careful haematological control of sulphinpyrazone therapy was essential.— M. W. Witwer *et al.*, *Br. med. J.*, 1976, *2*, 89.

EFFECTS ON THE KIDNEY. Four cases of transient oliguric renal failure associated with the use of sulphinpyrazone in coronary disease.— J. Boelaert *et al.* (letter), *New Engl. J. Med.*, 1980, *303*, 49.

A report of sulphinpyrazone-induced acute renal failure with tubular necrosis in one patient being treated for gout.— D. S. Durham and L. S. Ibels, *Br. med. J.*, 1981, *282*, 609.

In a review of twenty-one patients with acute renal failure attributed to sulphinpyrazone, one had been treated for gout, one for thrombophlebitis, and in 18 it had been prescribed after a recent myocardial infarction. Most patients were taking 600 to 800 mg of sulphinpyrazone daily. Three possible mechanisms of renal damage were considered: acute uric acid nephropathy, acute interstitial nephritis, and inhibition of vasodilatory prostaglandins. There was evidence that interstitial nephritis had occurred in a minority of patients, but it was considered that inhibition of renal prostaglandin synthesis may at least partly mediate the changes in renal function, especially in infarction patients. It was suggested that sulphinpyrazone should be avoided during the first few weeks after a myocardial infarction.— J. Boelaert *et al.*, *Acta clin. belg.*, 1982, *37*, 368.

Acute renal failure developed within 7 days in 4 of 15 patients taking sulphinpyrazone 200 mg four times a day in a study in patients with recent myocardial infarction.— P. Lijnen *et al.*, *Clin. Nephrol.*, 1983, *19*, 143.

Precautions

Sulphinpyrazone should not be started during an acute attack of gout and should be given with care to patients with impaired renal function or a history of peptic ulcer or renal uric acid calculi. It should not be given to patients with active peptic ulcer or blood dyscrasias, nor to patients allergic to sulphinpyrazone or to other pyrazole derivatives such as phenylbutazone. Sulphinpyrazone should not be used to control hyperuricaemia secondary to the treatment of malignant diseases.

Interactions. Since sulphinpyrazone like probenecid inhibits the tubular secretion of weak organic acids interactions can be expected with drugs such as antibiotics and sulphonamides although the effect is not considered to be clinically useful. Sulphinpyrazone can also displace some drugs from binding sites; in some instances it can alter their metabolism. These effects can lead to an increase in activity. The most significant interaction of this type involves warfarin and possibly other coumarin anticoagulants; patients receiving sulphinpyrazone and such an anticoagulant should have their prothrombin times monitored. Phenytoin, tolbutamide, and possibly other sulphonylureas may be similarly affected. Sulphinpyrazone can also increase the metabolic clearance of some drugs and dosage increases may be required.

Sulphinpyrazone's tubular secretion is inhibited by probenecid and it has been reported that cholestyramine may bind sulphinpyrazone and delay its absorption. Doses of sulphinpyrazone may need to be adjusted if it is given with other drugs that increase uric acid concentrations. Sulphinpyrazone and salicylates are antagonistic and should not be used together.

Renal function tests may need to be carried out in some patients, but measurements involving aminohippuric acid or phenolsulphonphthalein may be invalidated.

INTERACTIONS. A review of the interactions of sulphinpyrazone with other drugs.— I. H. Stockley, *Pharm. J.*, 1983, *230*, 168.

Aspirin significantly increased plasma clearance of sulphinpyrazone following a single dose and at steady state in a study involving 6 subjects.— *Aust. J. Pharm.*, 1984, *65*, 794.

Conditions which alter the delivery of sulphinpyrazone to the lower gut or which alter gut flora might affect its antiplatelet activity by altering the formation of the active sulphide metabolite. While no significant changes were found in patients with quiescent Crohn's disease or a recent myocardial infarction only negligible amounts were formed in a patient who had undergone hemicolectomy and sulphide formation was almost completely suppressed in some, but not all, patients receiving antibiotics.— H. A. Strong *et al.*, *Clin. Pharmacokinet.*, 1986, *11*, 402.

For a study indicating that sulphinpyrazone can increase the plasma clearance of theophylline, see under Precautions in Theophylline, p.1529.

Absorption and Fate

Sulphinpyrazone is readily absorbed from the gastro-intestinal tract. About 98% of the sulphinpyrazone in the circulation is bound to plasma proteins. It has been reported to have a biological half-life of about 3 hours after intravenous injection. Two active metabolites have been identified; the *p*-hydroxide metabolite which is uricosuric and the sulphide which has been shown to have antiplatelet activity. Following oral administration about 50% of a dose has been reported to be excreted, largely unchanged, in the urine in 48 hours.

Sulphinpyrazone kinetics after intravenous and oral administration.— J. B. Lecaillon *et al.*, *Clin. Pharmac. Ther.*, 1979, *26*, 611; I. D. Bradbrook *et al.*, *Br. J. clin. Pharmac.*, 1982, *13*, 177.

Results suggesting that the gut microflora are the main site of reduction of sulphinpyrazone to its active sulphide metabolite.— P. J. Howarth *et al.*, *Br. J. clin. Pharmac.*, 1982, *14*, 599P.

Renal impairment had no appreciable effect in one patient on the pharmacokinetics of sulphinpyrazone after a single dose. Prolonged treatment resulted in evidence of self-induction of drug-metabolising enzymes, but there was no change in creatinine clearance and only slight changes in blood creatinine and blood urea nitrogen.— J. Godbillon *et al.* (letter), *Br. J. clin. Pharmac.*, 1984, *18*, 107.

Marked changes in the plasma concentration-time profile and pharmacokinetics of sulphinpyrazone occured in 9 healthy subjects after taking sulphinpyrazone for 23 days. The results suggested that sulphinpyrazone induces its own metabolism and that of its major metabolites. It was also suggested that induction of the gut bacteria responsible for the formation of the sulphide may have been responsible for some of the pharmacokinetic changes.— F. Schlicht *et al.*, *Eur. J. clin. Pharmac.*, 1985, *28*, 97.

Uses and Administration

Sulphinpyrazone, a derivative of phenylbutazone, is a uricosuric agent; it promotes excretion of urates by inhibiting tubular reabsorption. In appropriate doses it reduces elevated concentrations of uric acid in the blood and causes the slow depletion of urate deposits in the tissues. It is used in the treatment of recurrent and chronic gout; it has little analgesic or anti-inflammatory action and is of no value in acute gout nor is it used as an adjunct to cancer therapy. Treatment should not be initiated during or for 2 to 3 weeks following an acute attack.

The initial dose of sulphinpyrazone is 100 to 200 mg once or twice daily, taken with meals or milk. At the beginning of treatment acute episodes of gout may be precipitated. Colchicine or a non-steroidal anti-inflammatory drug may be given during the first few months of treatment to reduce the incidence of such attacks. The dosage of sulphinpyrazone may be gradually increased over 1 to 3 weeks until a daily dosage of 600 mg is reached; up to 800 mg daily may be given. After the plasma-urate concentration has been controlled, the daily maintenance dose may be reduced to as low as 200 mg.

To reduce the risk of urolithiasis, an adequate fluid intake is required and, if necessary, the urine should be rendered alkaline during the initial stages of therapy.

Sulphinpyrazone has been reported to lengthen platelet survival, to decrease platelet turnover, to inhibit platelet aggregation, and to inhibit prostaglandin synthesis by platelets. It has been investigated in myocardial infarction and other cardiovascular disorders, but the results of the studies are controversial.

CARDIOVASCULAR DISORDERS. Sulphinpyrazone has been shown to possess inhibitory platelet activity and affect thromboxane and prostacyclin biosynthesis (L. Viinikka *et al.*, *Br. J. clin. Pharmac.*, 1982, *14*, 456; A.K. Pedersen and G.A. FitzGerald, *Clin. Pharmac. Ther.*, 1985, *37*, 36). Early studies suggested that sulphinpyrazone could reduce the incidence of thrombotic episodes in arteriovenous shunts (A. Kaegi *et al.*, *New Engl. J. Med.*, 1974, *290*, 304; D.D. Michie and D.G. Wombolt, *Curr. ther. Res.*, 1977, *22*, 196) and there is some evidence of a protective effect against venous thrombosis (G. Evans and M. Gent in *Platelets, Drugs and Thrombosis*, J. Hirsh *et al.*, Basle, Karger, 1975, p.258). It has been tried in reducing the incidence of transient ischaemic attacks and stroke with conflicting results (P. Steel *et al.*, *Stroke*, 1977, *8*, 396; Canadian Cooperative Study Group, *New Engl. J. Med.*, 1978, *299*, 53).

The Anturane Reinfarction Trial (*New Engl. J. Med.*, 1978, *298*, 289; *ibid.*, 1980, *302*, 250) demonstrated a reduction in mortality in the 6 months following infarction in patients given sulphinpyrazone. Criticisms (R. Temple and G.W. Pledger, *ibid.*, 1488) stimulated further evaluation by the Pitt Committee (*ibid.*, 1982, *306*, 1005) that confirmed the earlier findings, although the trend to a reduction in mortality was less significant and it still left concern about the study (W.B. Hood, *ibid.*, 988). The Anturane Reinfarction Italian Study Group (*Lancet*, 1982, *1*, 237) demonstrated that sulphinpyrazone reduced the incidence of reinfarction but had no effect on mortality.

Sulphinpyrazone's platelet activity led Cairns *et al.* (*New Engl. J. Med.*, 1985, *313*, 1369) to study its activity in unstable angina. They found that it offered no benefit nor did it affect the activity of aspirin.

Preparations

Sulfinpyrazone Capsules *(U.S.P.)*
Sulfinpyrazone Tablets *(U.S.P.)*
Sulphinpyrazone Tablets *(B.P.)*

Proprietary Preparations

Anturan *(Geigy, UK)*. *Tablets*, sulphinpyrazone 100 and 200 mg.

Proprietary Names and Manufacturers

Antazone *(ICN, Canad.)*; Anturan *(Arg.; Geigy, Austral.; Belg.; Geigy, Canad.; Denm.; Ciba, Fr.; Geigy, S.Afr.; Spain; Geigy, Switz.; Geigy, UK)*; Anturane *(Ciba, USA)*; Anturano *(Ciba, Ger.)*; Enturen *(Ciba, Ital.; Neth.)*; Falizal *(Ciba, Spain)*; Novopyrazone *(Novopharm, Canad.)*; Sulfazone *(Lennon, S.Afr.)*; Zynol *(Horner, Canad.)*.

1010-n

Tisopurine *(rINN).*
MPP. 1*H*-Pyrazolo[3,4-*d*]pyrimidine-4-thiol.
$C_5H_4N_4S$=152.2.

CAS — 5334-23-6.

Tisopurine is used in the treatment of disorders associated with hyperuricaemia, including gout, in doses of 200 to 400 mg daily.

Proprietary Names and Manufacturers
Thiopurinol *(Bouchara, Fr.)*; Uricolyse *(Bago, Arg.)*.

14002-a

Urate Oxidase
CB-8129; Uricase.

CAS — 9002-12-4.

An enzyme obtained commercially from *Aspergillus flavus.*

Urate oxidase oxidises uric acid to allantoin and has been used in the treatment of hyperuricaemia.

The use of urate oxidase to treat hyperuricaemia.— P. Kissel *et al.* (letter), *Lancet*, 1975, *1*, 229.

The use of urate oxidase derived from *Candida utilis* and bound to polyethylene glycol to treat hyperuricaemia in 5 men with neoplastic disease, without producing antibodies.— S. Davis *et al.*, *Lancet*, 1981, *2*, 281.

Further references: A. Feuillu *et al.*, *Thérapie*, 1979, *34*, 743.

ADVERSE EFFECTS. Report of a patient who experienced an acute reaction with bronchospasm and hypertension soon after receiving the third injection of urate oxidase. Two other cases of severe anaphylactic reactions involving urate oxidase, one of which was fatal, had been reported to the French Service de Pharmacovigilance.— M. Leaustic *et al.* (letter), *Rev. Rhum.*, 1983, *50*, 553.

Proprietary Names and Manufacturers
Uricozyme *(Clin Midy, Fr.; Midy, Ital.)*.

Antihistamines

6100-x

Antihistamines are classified into two main groups according to the receptors that they affect: H_1 receptor antagonists or H_2 receptor antagonists. This section describes the H_1 antagonists; H_2 antagonists are described with the other gastro-intestinal agents (p.1073). The term 'antihistamine' is therefore used for the H_1 antagonists. Many of these antihistamines can be further classified into 5 groups based on their chemical structure:

Ethanolamines (e.g. diphenhydramine) which tend to have pronounced sedative and antimuscarinic effects.

Ethylenediamines (e.g. mepyramine) which have less central activity but may cause gastric disturbances and skin sensitisation.

Alkylamines (e.g. chlorpheniramine) which are potent H_1 antagonists but are prone to produce CNS stimulation.

Piperazines (e.g. meclozine) which also have anti-emetic properties.

Phenothiazines (e.g. promethazine) which have pronounced antimuscarinic and anti-emetic properties and also cause sedation and photosensitivity reactions.

Also included in this section is a description of treatment by specific desensitisation (p.463).

Adverse Effects of Antihistamines (H_1-Receptor Antagonists)

Side-effects with antihistamines vary in incidence and severity with each patient as much as with each drug, though some of the drugs give rise to more side-effects than others. The most common effect is sedation, varying from slight drowsiness to deep sleep, and including lassitude, dizziness, and inco-ordination. Sedative effects, when they occur, may diminish after a few days. Some antihistamines, for example astemizole and terfenadine, have predominantly peripheral activity and do not cause significant sedation.

Other side-effects include gastro-intestinal disturbances such as nausea, vomiting, diarrhoea or constipation, anorexia or increased appetite, and epigastric pain.

Antihistamines may also produce antimuscarinic effects including blurred vision, difficulty in micturition, dysuria, dryness of the mouth, and tightness of the chest. Other central effects include hypotension, muscular weakness, tinnitus, euphoria, and occasionally headache.

Paradoxical CNS stimulation may occur especially in children, with insomnia, nervousness, tachycardia, tremors, and convulsions. Antihistamines may precipitate epileptiform seizures in patients with focal lesions of the cerebral cortex. Extrapyramidal symptoms may develop with phenothiazine derivatives and have been reported with other antihistamines including oxatomide. For other adverse effects which may occur with the phenothiazine derivatives, see p.706.

Systemic or topical therapy may produce allergic reactions and cross-sensitivity to related drugs. Photosensitivity has also been reported, particularly with the phenothiazines. It is generally considered that local application of antihistamines carries an unacceptably high risk of skin sensitisation. Blood disorders, including agranulocytosis, leucopenia, and haemolytic anaemia, though rare, have been reported.

Systemic side-effects have been reported after topical application of antihistamines to large areas of the skin.

Various antihistamines have been associated with foetal abnormalities when taken during pregnancy, but a number of large studies have failed to demonstrate any strong associations.

Overdose may be fatal especially in infants and children in whom the main symptoms are CNS stimulation and antimuscarinic effects, including ataxia, excitement, hallucinations, muscle tremor, convulsions, dilated pupils, dry mouth, flushed face, and hyperpyrexia. Deepening coma, cardiorespiratory collapse, and death may occur within 18 hours. In adults, the usual symptoms are of CNS depression with drowsiness, coma, and convulsions. Hypotension may also occur. Elderly patients are more susceptible to the CNS depressant and hypotensive effects even at therapeutic doses.

Under laboratory conditions mean performance was impaired at 3 and 5 hours after ingestion of promethazine 10 mg or clemastine 1 mg and at 1.5 hours after chlorpheniramine 4 mg. There were no alterations in subjective assessments of performance. Improved alertness and wakefulness was reported after terfenadine 60 mg.— C. H. Clarke and A. N. Nicholson, *Br. J. clin. Pharmac.*, 1978, *6*, 31. In a multiple-dose study in 9 healthy subjects given carbinoxamine 12 mg, brompheniramine 12 mg or clemastine 1 mg at 12-hourly intervals, drowsiness occurred at 2 hours after carbinoxamine, 6 hours after brompheniramine and 12 hours after clemastine. There was less drowsiness on the second day despite increased plasma concentrations. Only brompheniramine and carbinoxamine tended to impair psychomotor skills, but results indicated that impairment may be more closely related to the subject's individual response than to pharmacokinetics. In general it was concluded that these antihistamines in the doses used were not detrimental to driving competence or operation of machinery.— T. Seppälä *et al.*, *ibid.*, 1981, *12*, 179. In a double-blind crossover study in 12 women triprolidine, taken for about 36 hours before a driving test, significantly reduced subjective and objective measures of mood and arousal, and impaired driving skills, while terfenadine had no such effect.— T. Betts *et al.*, *Br. med. J.*, 1984, *288*, 281 and 608.

ABUSE. For reports of abuse of antihistamines see under the individual antihistamine monographs.

EFFECTS ON THE SKIN. An opinion that the risk of sensitisation by topical antihistamines is small especially in patients with non-eczematous skin.— H. Baker (letter), *Lancet*, 1980, *2*, 863. An opinion that antihistamines should never be applied topically.— R. Lancaster, *Prescribers' J.*, 1983, *23*, 47.

EXTRAPYRAMIDAL SYMPTOMS. A review of the literature has indicated that oral dyskinesia after administration of antihistamines is rare but not unexpected.— R. P. Granacher (letter), *New Engl. J. Med.*, 1977, *296*, 516.

For possible exacerbation of dystonic glutethimide-withdrawal symptoms by antihistamines, see Glutethimide, p.742.

Tardive dyskinesia. Tardive dyskinesia developed in a 51-year-old man after 30 years' intermittent use of antihistamines.— C. Hale and T. Heins, *Med. J. Aust.*, 1978, *1*, 112.

For other reports of extrapyramidal symptoms following administration of antihistamines, see under the individual antihistamine monographs.

PREGNANCY AND THE NEONATE. Considerable controversy still surrounds the risk to the foetus of anti-emetic therapy during pregnancy. The most widely studied preparation is Debendox which contained doxylamine, dicyclomine, and pyridoxine, and was known as Bendectin in some countries. Dicyclomine was removed from the preparation in 1976 in the USA and subsequently in other countries, and the product was withdrawn from the market in 1983 because of threatened litigation. By that time Debendox had been used for over 27 years and in over 33 million pregnancies worldwide (*Lancet*, 1983, *1*, 1395).

Evidence against Debendox initially came from anecdotal reports of malformations in infants whose mothers had taken the preparation during pregnancy (D.C. Paterson, *Can. med. Ass. J.*, 1977, *116*, 1348; D. Donnai and R. Harris, *Br. med. J.*, 1978, *1*, 691; K. Frith, *ibid.*, 925; C.J.G. Menzies, *ibid.*), and later from animal studies (A.G. Hendrickx *et al.*, *Teratology*, 1985, *32*, 179 and *ibid.*, 191; W.G. McBride, *Med. J. Aust.*, 1984, *140*, 445). Eskenazi and Bracken (*Am. J. Obstet. Gynec.*, 1982, *144*, 919) found evidence of an association between prenatal exposure to the 3-component formulation of Bendectin and an increased risk of pyloric stenosis and defective heart valves in a study of 1369 malformed infants and 2968 healthy control cases. Other studies have shown increased incidence of amniotic band limb defects and oesophageal atresia (J.F. Cordero *et al.*, *J. Am. med. Ass.*, 1981, *245*, 2307), oral clefts (J. Golding *et al.*, *Hum. Toxicol.*, 1983, *2*, 63), gastro-intestinal atresia (H. Jick *et al.*, *J. Am. med. Ass.*, 1981, *246*, 343), and genital tract disorders (G.T. Gibson *et al.*, *Med. J. Aust.*, 1981, *1*, 410), but generally such increases have been small. No overall pattern of malformations appears to have emerged, and many other studies have failed to confirm such associations with specific malformations.

Large studies that have not demonstrated any increase in congenital malformations in infants exposed to doxylamine either alone or as either formulation of Debendox include those by Fleming *et al.* (*Br. med. J.*, 1981, *283*, 99), Harron *et al.* (*Br. med. J.*, 1980, *281*, 1379), Shapiro *et al.* (*Am. J. Obstet. Gynec.*, 1977, *128*, 480), Mitchell *et al.* (*J. Am. med. Ass.*, 1981, *245*, 2311 and *Am. J. Obstet. Gynec.*, 1983, *147*, 737) and Winship *et al.* (*Archs Dis. Childh.*, 1984, *59*, 1052). Milkovich and van den Berg (*Am. J. Obstet. Gynec.*, 1976, *125*, 244), in a prospective study of 11 481 pregnancies found no increased incidence of either severe congenital abnormalities or perinatal mortality rates in women who had been prescribed prochlorperazine, meclozine, cyclizine, or Bendectin during pregnancy, although there was some evidence of an excess number of congenital abnormalities in patients taking trimethobenzamide. The Collaborative Perinatal Project monitored the mothers of 50 282 children between 1958 and 1965 (O.P. Heinonen *et al.*, *Birth Defects and Drugs in Pregnancy*, 1977, Littleton MA, Publishing Sciences Group p.322). Of these, 5401 were exposed to antihistamines and 1309 to phenothiazines during the first 4 months of pregnancy. There was no evidence to suggest that exposure to these drugs was related to malformations, although there were slight suggestions of associations between respiratory malformations and pheniramine, inguinal hernia and meclozine, inguinal hernia or genito-urinary malformations and diphenhydramine, and cardiovascular deformities and phenothiazines. Slone *et al.* (*Am. J. Obstet. Gynec.*, 1977, *128*, 486), reporting on the same study, found no effects of phenothiazines on perinatal mortality, birth weight, or IQ scores at the age of 4 years.

Both the Committee on Safety of Medicines in the UK and the Food and Drugs Administration in the USA reviewed the available literature in 1981 and concluded that while the scientific evidence did not demonstrate an increase in birth defects with the Debendox combination, the risk of teratogenicity could not be completely excluded. More recently a study by M.A. Klebanoff and J. L. Mills did not indicate that vomiting itself was teratogenic (*Br. med. J.*, 1986, *292*, 724), but research in this field is continuing.

A number of other studies have been carried out on meclozine prompted by reports of foetal abnormalities in 10 patients associated with a preparation of meclozine and pyridoxine (G.I. Watson, *Br. med. J.*, 1962, *2*, 1446); these studies have not supported the 1962 reports (W. Lenz, *Sth. med. J.*, 1971, *64*, *Suppl.* 1, 41; G. Greenberg *et al.*, *Br. med. J.*, 1977, *2*, 853; S. Shapiro *et al.*, *ibid.*, 1978, *1*, 483).

Treatment of Adverse Effects

In severe overdosage with antihistamines the stomach should be emptied by aspiration and lavage. Emetics may be tried if the patient is alert and there are no symptoms of toxicity, but may be ineffective due to the anti-emetic activity of the antihistamine. Activated charcoal has been given, as have saline laxatives, especially if sustained-release preparations were involved. Convulsions may be controlled with diazepam given intravenously, although it has been suggested that sedatives should be avoided.

Other treatment is supportive and symptomatic and may include artificial respiration, external cooling for hyperpyrexia, and intravenous fluids. Vasopressors such as noradrenaline or phenylephrine may be used, but adrenaline must not be given as it can lower the blood pressure further. The use of physostigmine is considered to be controversial, although it may have some diagnostic value. Forced diuresis is of little value since antihistamines are rapidly metabolised and only traces are recovered in the urine.

Precautions for Antihistamines (H_1-Receptor Antagonists)

Antihistamines should not be given to premature infants or neonates, and are also contra-indicated during acute attacks of asthma. Topical preparations containing antihistamines should not be used for acute vesicular and exudative dermatoses due to an increased risk of allergic reactions. The topical use of antihistamines in general is widely considered to be inadvisable due to the risk of inducing sensitisation.

Because of their antimuscarinic properties antihistamines should be used with care in conditions such as narrow angle glaucoma, urinary retention, and prostatic hypertrophy. MAOIs may enhance the antimuscarinic effects of antihistamines, and antihistamines have an additive antimuscarinic action with other antimuscarinic drugs, such as atropine and tricyclic antidepressants.

Many antihistamines may cause drowsiness; patients so affected should not drive or operate machinery. Patients should abstain from alcohol.

Antihistamines may enhance the sedative effects of central nervous system depressants including alcohol, barbiturates, hypnotics, narcotic analgesics, sedatives, and tranquillisers.

It has been suggested that antihistamines could mask the warning signs of damage caused by ototoxic drugs such as aminoglycoside antibiotics.

Phenothiazine antihistamines should be used with caution in patients with hepatic or cardiovascular disorders. Some antihistamines have been associated with foetal abnormalities when taken during pregnancy, but a number of large studies have failed to demonstrate any strong associations, (see above).

Antihistamines may suppress positive skin test results and should be stopped several days before the test.

Antihistamines because of their antimuscarinic effects may aggravate nocturnal symptoms of gastro-oesophageal reflux if given in the late evening.— M. Atkinson, *Prescribers' J.*, 1982, *22*, 129.

Absorption and Fate

In general, antihistamines are readily absorbed from the gastro-intestinal tract, metabolised in the liver, and excreted usually mainly as metabolites in the urine.

An extensive review of the clinical pharmacokinetics of antihistamines including analytical methods, fundamental pharmacokinetic properties, the influence of various pathophysiological states, the relationship of serum or plasma concentration to therapeutic and adverse effects, and pharmacokinetic interactions. The antihistamines covered include astemizole, azatadine, brompheniramine, chlorpheniramine, cinnarizine, clemastine, cyclizine and chlorcyclizine, cyproheptadine, diphenhydramine, diphenylpyraline, doxylamine, flunarizine, hydroxyzine, oxatomide, pheniramine, promethazine, terfenadine, tripelennamine, and triprolidine.— D. M. Paton and D. R. Webster, *Clin. Pharmacokinet.*, 1985, *10*, 477.

Uses of Antihistamines (H_1-Receptor Antagonists)

Antihistamines diminish or abolish the main actions of histamine in the body by competitive, reversible blockade of histamine receptor sites on tissues; they do not inactivate histamine or prevent its synthesis or release. Histamine receptors are classified into two main groups. H_1 receptors are responsible for vasodilation, increased capillary permeability, flare and itch reactions in the skin, and to some extent for contraction of smooth muscle in the bronchi and gastro-intestinal tract. H_2 receptors are responsible for gastric secretions and contribute to vasodilation.

H_1 antagonists also possess antimuscarinic, adrenaline-enhancing and/or antagonising, serotonin-antagonising and local anaesthetic effects.

H_1 antagonists are used for the palliative treatment of allergic reactions. Allergic or hypersensitivity reactions may be immediate or delayed and are generally classified into 4 types (Types I to IV). The antihistamines in this section are mainly used in Type I and Type IV reactions.

Type I, anaphylactic or immediate reactions occur after exposure to an antigen in a sensitised subject. The subject has specific antibodies, mainly IgE, fixed to mast cells and basophils from the initial sensitisation. Subsequent exposure to the free allergen causes degranulation of the mast cells with release of histamine and other mediators. Local anaphylactic reactions include urticaria, angioedema, hay fever, and some gastro-intestinal allergies.

Type II, cytolytic reactions are caused by the interaction of circulating, not fixed, antibodies with antigens that are on the surfaces of cells such as erythrocytes. The reaction followed by complement fixation leads to cell lysis. Blood transfusion reactions and some drug reactions resulting in destruction of blood cells are caused by this type of hypersensitivity.

Type III, complex mediated or toxic precipitin reactions are caused by the interaction of antigen-stimulated antibodies, mostly IgG, with soluble free antigens such as serum proteins or with micro-organisms with complement activation of the resulting complex. Type III reactions are responsible for serum sickness, Type 2 Lepra reactions, and some local reactions to dust and micro-organisms particularly in the lungs.

Type IV, cell-mediated or delayed reactions are mediated by sensitised T-lymphocytes and macrophages in lymph nodes and at other sites and result in direct cytotoxicity or release of lymphokines. The reaction occurs 12 to 48 hours after contact with the allergen. This type of reaction is responsible for tuberculin reactions used for sensitivity testing and contact dermatitis to plants, industrial and domestic chemicals, and some drugs. Photosensitivity reactions and Type 1 Lepra reactions are also due to Type IV hypersensitivity.

The antihistamines are effective in relieving the symptoms of seasonal and perennial allergic rhinitis (Type I reactions). They relieve sneezing, rhinorrhoea, nasal itch, and conjunctivitis, but have little effect on nasal congestion. For optimum effectiveness in hay fever it is necessary to begin treatment before the start of the pollen season. Antihistamines are of little value in bronchial asthma since the bronchospasm is not solely mediated by histamine. The antimuscarinic action of many antihistamines may thicken the bronchial secretions and make expectoration more difficult.

Antihistamines may be used as an adjunct in the treatment of systemic anaphylactic reactions and angioedema, but adrenaline and corticosteroids form the main treatment as, again, histamine is not the only mediator involved. Mild allergic reactions to blood transfusions, but not ABO incompatibility, may be ameliorated with antihistamines.

Antihistamines are effective in allergic skin disorders including urticaria, pruritus, insect bites, dermographism, and some drug allergies and contact allergies to plants (Type I and Type IV reactions). Pruritus normally responds more rapidly than oedema. Topical application is not generally recommended due to the risk of inducing skin sensitisation. In serum sickness, antihistamines may be effective in reducing urticaria and oedema but fever and arthralgia respond less well.

There is little evidence that antihistamines are effective in reducing the symptoms of the common cold, although they are widely used in combination with decongestants, and in cough linctuses for their antitussive effects.

Although hyoscine is generally agreed to be the most effective treatment for motion sickness, some of the antihistamines, particularly the piperazine derivatives and dimenhydrinate are also effective although sedation can be a problem. These drugs also act as labyrinthine sedatives in Ménière's disease and related disorders. Some antihistamines, including promethazine may also be useful in nausea and vomiting due to other causes, possibly due to their central sedative activity.

Promethazine, diphenhydramine, mepyramine, and hydroxyzine are also used as hypnotics.

Antihistamines are normally given by mouth and should be taken with or after food to avoid gastric irritation. Some antihistamines are available in injectable formulations for use in severe allergic reactions, but are generally irritant and should only be given by deep intramuscular or slow intravenous injection.

A view that sustained-release formulations of antihistamines offer no therapeutic advantages over conventional formulations.— *Drug & Ther. Bull.*, 1984, *22*, 57.

An opinion that the sedative adverse effects of antihistamines can be substantially reduced by using controlled-release preparations.— A. H. Beckett (letter), *Pharm. J.*, 1984, *2*, 262.

A review of the clinical impact of the newer non-sedating antihistamines which do not cross the blood-brain barrier at usual therapeutic doses. Terfenadine and astemizole may be regarded as the most specific H_1-receptor antagonists currently available. Terfenadine has been found to be effective in allergic rhinitis, urticaria, and dermographism, and the new H_1 antagonists may relieve pruritus of peripheral origin but may not relieve itch of central origin. Mequitazine does not readily cross the blood-brain barrier, but does have some antimuscarinic activity and has been associated with some central effects at higher doses. The new non-sedating antihistamines are a valuable adjunct in the therapy of allergic patients and are replacing the older antihistamines initially for their non-sedative action.— M. L. Brandon, *Drugs*, 1985, *30*, 377.

ALLERGIC RHINITIS. Reviews and discussions of the treatment of allergic rhinitis.— *Br. med. J.*, 1981, *283*, 808; F. E. R. Simons and K. J. Simons, *Clin. Rev. Allergy*, 1984, *2*, 237.

SKIN DISORDERS. A combination of an H_1 antagonist with an H_2 antagonist was more effective than either treatment alone in the treatment of dermographism.— S. Kaur *et al.*, *Br. J. Derm.*, 1981, *104*, 185. Similar results in the management of chronic urticaria with dermographism.— J. Boyle and R. M. MacKie, *ibid.*, 1982, *107*, *Suppl.* 22, 18.

Some antihistamines, and particularly trimeprazine and hydroxyzine, have been found to relieve the itching associated with atopic eczema. Chlorpheniramine and brompheniramine are also useful but the non-sedating antihistamines terfenadine and astemizole have not been found to be helpful.— J. Verbov, *Practitioner*, 1984, *228*, 1013.

Antihistamines were considered to be the drugs of first choice in patients with mild or moderately severe recurrent or chronic urticaria.— K. P. Mathews, *Drugs*, 1985, *30*, 552.

16017-a

Acrivastine *(BAN, USAN, rINN).*

BW-825C. (*E*)-3-{6-[(*E*)-3-Pyrrolidin-1-yl-1-*p*-tolylprop-1-enyl]-2-pyridyl}acrylic acid.

$C_{22}H_{24}N_2O_2$=348.4.

CAS — 87848-99-5.

Acrivastine is an antihistamine. It has been reported to have few effects on the CNS. It is given by mouth in doses of 8 mg three times daily.

Acrivastine is a derivative of triprolidine. It was found to be a peripheral H_1-receptor antagonist with a potency and duration of action similar to triprolidine, but with minimal effects on the CNS.— A. F. Cohen *et al.*, *Br. J. clin. Pharmac.*, 1984, *17*, 647P.

In a study in 12 healthy subjects terfenadine 60 and 120 mg had a longer duration of action than acrivastine 2, 4, and 8 mg as measured by histamine-induced flare. Neither drug in the doses tested produced significant behavioural impairment or subjective drowsiness.— M. J. Hamilton *et al.*, *Br. J. clin. Pharmac.*, 1985, *20*, 283P.

Further references: J. R. Gibson *et al.*, *Dermatologica*, 1984, *169*, 179; A. F. Cohen *et al.*, *Clin. Pharmac. Ther.*, 1985, *38*, 381 (comparison with triprolidine); M. J. Hamilton *et al.*, *Br. J. clin. Pharmac.*, 1985, *19*, 585P (comparison with triprolidine).

Proprietary Names and Manufacturers
Semprex *(Wellcome, UK)*.

6104-n

Antazoline Hydrochloride *(BANM, rINNM)*.

Antazolini Hydrochloridum; Antazolinium Chloride; Imidamin Hydrochloride; Phenazolinum. *N*-Benzyl-*N*-(2-imidazolin-2-ylmethyl)aniline hydrochloride.
$C_{17}H_{19}N_3,HCl=301.8$.

CAS — 91-75-8 (antazoline); 2508-72-7 (hydrochloride).

Pharmacopoeias. In *Arg., Egypt., Fr., Int., Jug., Nord., Pol., Port., Swiss,* and *Turk.* Also in *B.P.C. 1973. It.* includes the sulphate.

A white or almost white, odourless or almost odourless, crystalline powder.
Soluble 1 in 50 of water and 1 in 16 of alcohol; slightly soluble in chloroform; practically insoluble in ether. A 1% solution in water has a pH of 5.0 to 6.5. **Store** in airtight containers. Protect from light.

6105-h

Antazoline Mesylate *(BANM)*.

Antazoline Mesilate *(rINNM)*; Antazoline Methanesulphonate.
$C_{17}H_{19}N_3,CH_3SO_3H=361.5$.

CAS — 3131-32-6.

Pharmacopoeias. In *Cz.* Also in *B.P.C. 1973.*

A white or almost white, odourless or almost odourless powder. It is slightly hygroscopic; significant amounts of moisture are absorbed at 20° at relative humidities above about 70%.
Soluble 1 in 6 of water, 1 in 7 of alcohol, and 1 in 12 of chloroform; practically insoluble in ether. A 1% solution in water has a pH of 4.0 to 6.5. **Store** in airtight containers. Protect from light.

6106-m

Antazoline Phosphate *(BANM, USAN, rINNM)*.

Antazolinium Biphosphate.
$C_{17}H_{19}N_3,H_3PO_4=363.4$.

CAS — 154-68-7.

Pharmacopoeias. In *U.S.*

A white to off-white crystalline powder. **Soluble** in water; sparingly soluble in methyl alcohol; practically insoluble in ether. A 2% solution in water has a pH of 4 to 5. **Store** in airtight containers.

Adverse Effects, Treatment, and Precautions
As for the antihistamines in general, p.443.
Allergic thrombocytopenic purpura has been reported.

Antazoline differs only slightly in chemical structure from xylometazoline, oxymetazoline, and naphazoline which are alpha-adrenoceptor agonists. Rebound congestion may follow withdrawal of nasal preparations containing these drugs. The over-enthusiastic use of nasal sprays or drops by adults has caused severe abnormalities of the cardiovascular and central nervous systems.— S. Chaplin, *Adverse Drug React. Bull.*, 1984, (Aug.), 396.

ALLERGY. A report of interstitial pneumonitis, with fever, rash, and dyspnoea, after antazoline; the condition recurred after challenge.— A. Pahissa *et al.*, *Br. med. J.*, 1979, *2*, 1328.

EFFECTS ON THE BLOOD. A report of immune haemolytic anaemia, thrombocytopenia, haemoglobinuria, and acute renal failure associated with antazoline administration.— U. Bengtsson *et al.*, *Acta med. scand.*, 1975, *198*, 223.

Uses and Administration
Antazoline is an ethylenediamine derivative with the properties and uses of the antihistamines (see p.444).
Antazoline sulphate and phosphate are used locally with a vasoconstrictor, such as naphazoline nitrate or xylometazoline hydrochloride, in nasal drops and eye-drops in a concentration of 0.5%, for nasal and ocular allergies.
The hydrochloride has been used systemically; it is also included in a cream.

Proprietary Preparations
Antistin-Privine *(Ciba Consumer, UK). Nasal drops,* antazoline sulphate 0.5%, naphazoline nitrate 0.025%. *Nasal spray,* antazoline sulphate 0.5%, naphazoline nitrate 0.025%.
RBC *(Rybar, UK). Cream,* antazoline hydrochloride 1.8%, calamine 8%, camphor 0.1%, cetrimide 0.5%.
Vasocon-A *(CooperVision, UK). Eye-drops,* antazoline phosphate 0.5%, naphazoline hydrochloride 0.05%.

Proprietary Names and Manufacturers of Antazoline Salts
Antasten *(Ciba, Swed.)*; Antistin *(Ger.; Switz.)*; Antistina *(Ciba, Denm.; Spain)*; Antistine *(Ciba, Canad.; Fr.; Ciba, Switz.)*.

The following names have been used for multi-ingredient preparations containing antazoline salts— Albalon A Liquifilm *(Allergan, Austral.; Allergan, Canad.)*; Antistine-Privine *(Zyma, Austral.)*; Antistin-Privine *(Ciba Consumer, UK)*; Otrivine Hay Fever Formula *(Ciba, UK)*; Otrivine Hay-Fever Formula *(Ciba-Geigy, Canad.)*; Otrivine-Antistin *(Ciba, UK; Zyma, UK)*; RBC *(Rybar, UK)*; Vasocon-A *(Coopervision, Canad.; CooperVision, UK)*; Zincfrin-A *(Alcon, Canad.)*.

12403-t

Astemizole *(BAN, USAN, rINN)*.

R-43512. 1-(4-Fluorobenzyl)-2-{[1-(4-methoxyphenethyl)-4-piperidyl]amino}benzimidazole.
$C_{28}H_{31}FN_4O=458.6$.

CAS — 68844-77-9.

Adverse Effects and Precautions
Astemizole may cause increased appetite and weight gain. Sedative effects are rare and antimuscarinic effects have not been reported.

Studies into the effects of astemizole on performance: A. N. Nicholson and B. M. Stone, *Br. J. clin. Pharmac.*, 1982, *13*, 199; A. N. Nicholson *et al.*, *ibid.*, *14*, 683; T. Seppälä and K. Savolainen, *Curr. ther. Res.*, 1982, *31*, 638.

INTERACTIONS. Astemizole 10 mg daily for 7 days had no significant effect on alcohol clearance or on the central effects of alcohol in 7 healthy subjects.— D. N. Bateman *et al.*, *Eur. J. clin. Pharmac.*, 1983, *25*, 567.

OVERDOSAGE. A 14-year-old girl who took astemizole 200 mg had no symptoms apart from slight drowsiness which lasted for 12 hours. Biochemical and haematological parameters remained normal. Peak plasma concentrations indicated that much of the stated dose had been absorbed despite prompt gastric lavage around 60 minutes after drug ingestion. The apparent plasma half-life was 31 hours.— J. C. Kingswood *et al.*, *Hum. Toxicol.*, 1986, *5*, 43.

Cardiac effects. Acute ventricular tachyarrhythmia with ECG recordings characteristic of torsade de pointes occurred in a patient after an overdose of 200 mg of astemizole. Seventeen episodes occurred despite treatment with lignocaine or amiodarone, 11 of which required DC cardioversion. Subsequent treatment with isoprenaline 1 µg per minute by intravenous infusion controlled the arrhythmias, and treatment was gradually reduced over 5 days.— T. M. Craft, *Br. med. J.*, 1986, *292*, 660. No ill-effects were observed in a child given 30 mg three times daily.— D. M. Salisbury (letter), *ibid.*, 961.

Absorption and Fate
Astemizole is readily absorbed from the gastro-intestinal tract and is extensively metabolised in the liver. It has a prolonged half-life and is highly protein bound. Excretion is mainly via the faeces. Astemizole does not appear to cross the blood-brain barrier to a significant extent.

Uses and Administration
Astemizole has the actions and uses of the antihistamines, p.444. It is reported to be a potent and long-acting histamine H_1 receptor antagonist with few central or antimuscarinic effects. It is used for allergic rhinitis, conjunctivitis, and skin disorders.
The dose for adults is 10 mg once daily, although up to 30 mg may be given once daily for the first 7 days if symptoms are particularly troublesome. Half the adult dose may be given to children aged 6 to 12 years.

A review of the pharmacodynamic properties and therapeutic efficacy of astemizole.— D. M. Richards *et al.*, *Drugs*, 1984, *28*, 38.

ALLERGY. Astemizole 40 mg produced greater inhibition of histamine-induced wheal and flare reactions than chlorpheniramine 16 mg, but had no effect on salivary flow or sedation. The antihistaminic effect of astemizole persisted for up to 32 days.— P. H. Chapman and M. D. Rawlins, *Br. J. clin. Pharmac.*, 1982, *13*, 593P. See also: D. N. Bateman *et al.*, *Eur. J. clin. Pharmac.*, 1983, *25*, 547.

Rhinitis. Beneficial responses of seasonal and perennial rhinitis to astemizole: J. D. Wilson and J. L. Hillas, *Clin. Allergy*, 1983, *13*, 131; P. H. Howarth *et al.*, *Br. J. clin. Pharmac.*, 1984, *18*, 1; J. P. Girard *et al.*, *J. int. med. Res.*, 1985, *13*, 102 (comparison with terfenadine).

Urticaria. Astemizole was slightly more effective than chlorpheniramine in the treatment of dermographic urticaria. The effects of astemizole lasted longer than those of chlorpheniramine, and were still apparent 4 weeks after treatment had been stopped, suggesting irreversible binding to the H_1 receptors.— L. B. Krause and S. Shuster, *Br. J. Derm.*, 1985, *112*, 447.

MASTOCYTOSIS. Astemizole was used successfully for skin symptoms of mastocytosis in a child. It was used alone or in combination with other drugs for more than 18 months and was well tolerated in doses of 30 mg three times daily (equivalent to 3 mg per kg body-weight daily). No alteration in liver function, sedation, or cardiac arrhythmias had been noted.— D. M. Salisbury (letter), *Br. med. J.*, 1986, *292*, 961.

Proprietary Preparations
Hismanal *(Janssen, UK). Tablets,* scored, astemizole 10 mg.
Suspension, astemizole 5 mg/5 mL.

Proprietary Names and Manufacturers
Hismanal *(Janssen, Canad.; Janssen, Denm.; Janssen, Fr.; Janssen, Ger.; Janssen, Spain; Janssen, Switz.; Janssen, UK)*; Histaminos *(Lesvi, Spain)*; Paralergin *(Vita, Spain)*; Retolen *(Elmu, Spain)*; Rimbol *(Esteve, Spain)*; Romadin *(Andromaco, Spain)*; Simprox *(Rocador, Spain)*.

6107-b

Azatadine Maleate *(BANM, USAN, rINNM)*.

Sch-10649. 6,11-Dihydro-11-(1-methyl-4-piperidylidene)-5*H*-benzo[5,6]cyclohepta[1,2-*b*]pyridine dimaleate.
$C_{20}H_{22}N_2,2C_4H_4O_4=522.6$.

CAS — 3964-81-6 (azatadine); 3978-86-7 (maleate).

Pharmacopoeias. In *U.S.*

Adverse Effects, Treatment, Precautions, and Absorption and Fate
As for the antihistamines in general, p.443.

In a study in 50 healthy subjects, azatadine maleate 1 mg twice daily and terfenadine 60 mg twice daily were not associated with decreased psychomotor performance. Azatadine appeared to increase the appetite after 26 hours from the start of treatment.— D. K. Luscombe *et al.*, *Pharmatherapeutica*, 1983, *3*, 370.

An acute dystonic reaction was reported in a patient who had taken azatadine maleate 20 to 30 mg over a 24-hour period. The condition was reversed by intravenous injection of benztropine 2 mg.— D. J. L. Joske (letter), *Med. J. Aust.*, 1984, *141*, 449.

Uses and Administration

Azatadine maleate has the actions and uses of the antihistamines (see p.444). It has a long duration of action. It also has antimuscarinic and antiserotonin properties.

Azatadine maleate is given for allergic disorders usually in doses of 1 mg twice daily; if necessary 2 mg twice daily may be given. In the *UK*, the recommended dose for children aged 6 to 12 years is 0.5 to 1 mg twice daily, and for children aged 1 to 6 years, 0.25 mg twice daily. However, in the *USA*, azatadine is not recommended for children under 12 years.

Azatadine inhibited the release of histamine and leukotriene C_4 from human lung mast cells *in vitro*. Azatadine applied as a nasal spray also suppressed the release of inflammatory mediators as well as the symptoms produced by nasal provocation with antigen in atopic volunteers.— A. G. Togias *et al.*, *J. Am. med. Ass.*, 1986, *255*, 225.

Preparations

Azatadine Maleate Tablets *(U.S.P.)*. Store in well-closed containers.

Proprietary Preparations

Congesteze *(Kirby-Warrick, UK)*. *Tablets*, azatadine maleate 1 mg, pseudoephedrine sulphate 60 mg in outer coating, pseudoephedrine sulphate 60 mg in sustained-release core.

Syrup, azatadine maleate 1 mg, pseudoephedrine sulphate 30 mg/5 mL.

Paediatric syrup, azatadine maleate 250 µg, pseudoephedrine sulphate 7.5 mg/5 mL.

Optimine *(Kirby-Warrick, UK)*. *Tablets*, scored, azatadine maleate 1 mg.

Syrup, azatadine maleate 500 µg/5 mL.

Proprietary Names and Manufacturers

Idulamine *(Arg.)*; Idulian *(Unicet, Fr.)*; Lergocil *(Juste, Spain)*; Optimine *(Schering, Canad.; Essex, Ger.; Neth.; Scherag, S.Afr.; Kirby-Warrick, UK; Schering, USA)*; Verbén *(Schering Corp., Denm.)*; Zadine *(Essex, Austral.)*.

The following names have been used for multi-ingredient preparations containing azatadine maleate— Congesteze *(Kirby-Warrick, UK)*; Trinalin *(Schering, Canad.; Schering, USA)*.

12413-r

Azelastine *(rINN)*.

A-5610; E-0659; W-2979M. 4-(4-Chlorobenzyl)-2-(perhydro-1-methylazepin-4-yl)phthalazin-1-one.

$C_{22}H_{24}ClN_3O$=381.9.

CAS — 58581-89-8; 79307-93-0 (hydrochloride).

NOTE. Azelastine Hydrochloride is *USAN*.

Azelastine is an antihistamine.

For a series of studies in *animals*, see *Arzneimittel-Forsch.*, 1981, *31*, 1184–1230.

6108-v

Bamipine *(BAN, rINN)*.

N-Benzyl-*N*-(1-methyl-4-piperidyl)aniline.

$C_{19}H_{24}N_2$=280.4.

CAS — 4945-47-5.

Bamipine has the general properties and uses of the antihistamines (see p.443). It has pronounced sedative effects.

It has been given as the hydrochloride in doses of 50 mg up to three times daily. Higher doses of up to 400 mg daily in divided doses have also been given. Bamipine has also been applied topically as the lactate.

Proprietary Names and Manufacturers

Soventol *(Knoll, Austral.; Knoll, Belg.; Knoll, Ger.; Knoll, Ital.; Knoll, Neth.; Knoll, S.Afr.; Knoll, Switz.)*; Taumidrine *(Biosédra, Fr.)*.

6109-g

Bromodiphenhydramine Hydrochloride *(BANM, USAN)*.

Bromazine Hydrochloride *(rINNM)*. 2-(4-Bromobenzhydryloxy)-*NN*-dimethylethylamine hydrochloride.

$C_{17}H_{20}BrNO,HCl$=370.7.

CAS — 118-23-0 (bromodiphenhydramine); 1808-12-4 (hydrochloride).

Pharmacopoeias. In *U.S.*

A white to pale buff-coloured, crystalline powder with a faint odour. **Soluble** 1 in less than 1 of water, 1 in 2 of alcohol and of chloroform, 1 in 31 of isopropyl alcohol, and 1 in 3500 of ether; practically insoluble in light petroleum. **Store** in airtight containers.

Bromodiphenhydramine hydrochloride is an ethanolamine derivative with the properties and uses of the antihistamines (see p.443). It is closely related to diphenhydramine p.452.

It is frequently used in combination preparations for the symptomatic relief of coughs and upper respiratory tract disorders in a dose of 12.5 to 25 mg every 4 to 6 hours. The recommended maximum dose in such preparations is 150 mg daily.

Preparations

Bromodiphenhydramine Hydrochloride Capsules *(U.S.P.)*

Bromodiphenhydramine Hydrochloride Elixir *(U.S.P.)*

Proprietary Names and Manufacturers

Ambodryl *(Belg.; Parke, Davis, UK; Parke, Davis, USA)*.

The following names have been used for multi-ingredient preparations containing bromodiphenhydramine hydrochloride— Ambenyl *(Parke, Davis, Canad.; Forest Pharmaceuticals, USA)*; Bromanyl *(Schein, USA)*.

6126-q

Dexbrompheniramine Maleate *(BANM, USAN, rINNM)*.

Dexbrompheniramine is the dextrorotatory isomer of brompheniramine which is racemic.

CAS — 132-21-8 (dexbrompheniramine); 2391-03-9 (maleate).

Pharmacopoeias. In *Braz.* and *U.S.*

A white odourless crystalline powder. **Soluble** 1 in 1.2 of water, 1 in 2.5 of alcohol, 1 in 2 of chloroform, and 1 in 3000 of ether. A 1% solution has a pH of about 5. **Store** in airtight containers. Protect from light.

6110-f

Brompheniramine Maleate *(BANM, USAN, rINNM)*.

Parabromdylamine Maleate. (±)-3-(4-Bromophenyl)-*NN*-dimethyl-3-(2-pyridyl)propylamine hydrogen maleate.

$C_{16}H_{19}BrN_2,C_4H_4O_4$=435.3.

CAS — 86-22-6 (brompheniramine); 980-71-2 (maleate); 32865-01-3 (maleate, ±).

Pharmacopoeias. In *U.S.*

A white odourless crystalline powder. **Soluble** 1 in 5 of water and 1 in 15 of alcohol and of chloroform; slightly soluble in ether. A 1% solution in water has a pH of 4.0 to 5.0. The *U.S.P.* injection has a pH of 6.8 to 7.0. **Store** in airtight containers. Protect from light.

Incompatibility has been reported with some diatrizoate, iodipamide, and iothalamate salts.

Adverse Effects, Treatment, Precautions, and Absorption and Fate

As for the antihistamines in general, p.443. Brompheniramine is contra-indicated in patients with known brain damage or epilepsy.

For a report of the effects of brompheniramine on performance see p.443.

Brompheniramine's effects on performance could be affected by variations in sustained-release formulations.— K. Millar and P. J. Standen, *Br. J. clin. Pharmac.*, 1982, *14*, 49.

EFFECTS ON THE BLOOD. Agranulocytosis in a 34-year-old alcoholic man was possibly associated with brompheniramine therapy.— A. S. Hardin and F. Padilla, *J. Ark. med. Soc.*, 1978, *75*, 206.

EFFECTS ON MENTAL STATE. For reports of psychotic episodes probably associated with the phenylpropanolamine content of preparations containing brompheniramine and phenylpropanolamine, see Phenylpropanolamine Hydrochloride, p.1476.

EXTRAPYRAMIDAL SYMPTOMS. Two patients developed oral and facial dyskinesias after long-term use of preparations for allergic rhinitis containing antihistamines (brompheniramine, chlorpheniramine, or phenindamine) and sympathomimetics. One patient improved when the preparations were discontinued. These cases best fit the category of late-onset, drug-induced (tardive) dyskinesia.— B. T. Thach *et al.*, *New Engl. J. Med.*, 1975, *293*, 486.

A report of an acute oral and facial dystonic reaction associated with the overdose of dexbrompheniramine maleate 24 mg and pseudoephedrine sulphate 480 mg in an 18-month-old girl.— D. A. Barone and J. Raniolo (letter), *New Engl. J. Med.*, 1980, *303*, 107.

OVERDOSAGE. A 2½-year-old boy who swallowed at least 25 tablets, each of 12 mg of brompheniramine maleate survived after gastric lavage and treatment with phenobarbitone.— E. Gilmore and B. H. Athreya, *New Engl. J. Med.*, 1960, *263*, 149 (see also the report under Extrapyramidal symptoms).

PREGNANCY AND THE NEONATE. Irritability, excessive crying, and disturbed sleep patterns occurred in a 3-month-old breast-fed infant whose mother was receiving a decongestant containing dexbrompheniramine and pseudoephedrine. Discontinuation of medication and substitution of an artificial feed were associated with resumption of normal behaviour in the infant within 12 hours.— E. A. Mortimer (letter), *Pediatrics*, 1977, *60*, 780.

Uses and Administration

Brompheniramine maleate is an alkylamine derivative with the actions and uses of antihistamines (see p.444).

Dexbrompheniramine is the dextrorotatory isomer of brompheniramine, which is racemic, and has approximately twice the activity of brompheniramine by weight.

Brompheniramine maleate is given by mouth usually in doses of 4 to 8 mg three or four times daily, or 12 mg every 12 hours as sustained-release preparations. It is also given as an ingredient of cough mixtures and decongestant preparations.

Children up to 3 years of age have been given 0.4 to 1 mg per kg body-weight over 24 hours in four divided doses. Children aged 3 to 6 years may be given 1 to 2 mg three or four times daily and those aged 6 to 12 years 2 to 4 mg three or four times daily. Children over 6 years may be given 8 to 12 mg as a sustained-release preparation every 12 hours.

Brompheniramine maleate has been given by subcutaneous, intramuscular, or slow intravenous injection in severe allergies; the dose is usually 5 to 20 mg every 6 to 12 hours as necessary and the total parenteral dose should not exceed 40 mg in 24 hours.

Dexbrompheniramine maleate is normally given as an ingredient of decongestant preparations containing pseudoephedrine. The dose of dexbrompheniramine maleate in these combinations is 2 mg four times a day or 4 mg three times a day, or as sustained-release formulations, 6 mg every 8 to 12 hours. The dose recommended for children over 6 years is 1 mg four times a day.

In the *UK*, the use of brompheniramine and its salts in cosmetics is prohibited by law.

MALE INFERTILITY. Brompheniramine by virtue of its antimuscarinic activity may be useful in the treatment of male infertility induced by diabetes mellitus.— W.-B. Schill and M. Michalopoulos, *Drugs*, 1984, *28*, 263.

URTICARIA. Brompheniramine maleate 12 mg twice a day in a sustained-release formulation was beneficial in the treatment of chronic urticaria with or without dermographism. The most troublesome adverse effect was drowsiness.— D. S. Jolliffe *et al.*, *Curr. med. Res. Opinion*, 1985, *9*, 394.

Preparations

Brompheniramine Maleate Elixir *(U.S.P.)*
Brompheniramine Maleate Injection *(U.S.P.)*
Brompheniramine Maleate Tablets *(U.S.P.)*

Proprietary Preparations

Dimotane *(Robins, UK)*. *Tablets*, scored, brompheniramine maleate 4 mg.
Elixir, brompheniramine maleate 2 mg/5 mL.

Dimotane Expectorant *(Robins, UK)*. *Oral liquid*, brompheniramine maleate 2 mg, guaiphenesin 100 mg, phenylephrine hydrochloride 5 mg, phenylpropanolamine hydrochloride 5 mg/5 mL.

Dimotane LA *(Robins, UK)*. *Tablets*, sustained-release, brompheniramine maleate 12 mg.

Dimotane Plus *(Robins, UK)*. *Oral liquid*, brompheniramine maleate 4 mg, pseudoephedrine hydrochloride 30 mg/5 mL.
Paediatric oral liquid, brompheniramine maleate 2 mg, pseudoephedrine hydrochloride 15 mg/5 mL.

Dimotane Plus LA *(Robins, UK)*. *Tablets*, sustained-release, brompheniramine maleate 12 mg, pseudoephedrine hydrochloride 120 mg.

Dimotane Co *(Robins, UK)*. *Oral liquid*, brompheniramine maleate 2 mg, pseudoephedrine hydrochloride 30 mg, codeine phosphate 10 mg/5 mL.
Paediatric oral liquid, brompheniramine maleate 2 mg, pseudoephedrine hydrochloride 15 mg, codeine phosphate 3 mg/5 mL.

Dimotapp *(Robins, UK)*. *Elixir*, brompheniramine maleate 4 mg, phenylephrine hydrochloride 5 mg, phenylpropanolamine hydrochloride 5 mg/5 mL.
Paediatric elixir, brompheniramine maleate 1 mg, phenylephrine hydrochloride 2.5 mg, phenylpropanolamine hydrochloride 2.5 mg/5 mL.

Dimotapp LA *(Robins, UK)*. *Tablets*, sustained-release, brompheniramine maleate 12 mg, phenylephrine hydrochloride 15 mg, phenylpropanolamine hydrochloride 15 mg.

Proprietary Names and Manufacturers of Brompheniramine or Dexbrompheniramine

Antial *(Ellem, Ital.)*; Bromolent *(Arg.)*; Dimegan *(Dexo, Fr.; Kreussler, Ger.; Dexo, Switz.)*; Dimetane *(Robins, Austral.; Robins, Canad.; S.Afr.; Spain; Robins, Swed.; Robins, USA)*; Dimotane *(Robins, UK)*; Drauxin *(Ital.)*; Ebalin *(Allergopharma, Ger.)*; Gammistin *(IBP, Ital.)*; Ilvin *(E. Merck, Ger.; Bracco, Ital.; E. Merck, Swed.)*; Probahist *(Legere, USA)*; Pyrimetane *(Arg.)*; Veltane *(Lannett, USA)*.

The following names have been used for multi-ingredient preparations containing brompheniramine or dexbrompheniramine— Atrohist *(Adams, USA)*; Biphetap *(USA)*; BPP *(Gen, Canad.)*; Brocon *(Forest Laboratories, USA)*; Bromfed *(Muro, USA)*; Bromfed-PD *(Muro, USA)*; Bromphen Compound *(Schein, USA)*; Bromphen DC *(Schein, USA)*; Bromphen Expectorant *(Schein, USA)*; Dallergy-JR *(Laser, USA)*; Dimedrine *(Robins, Canad.)*; Dimetane Expectorant *(Robins, Canad.)*; Dimetane Expectorant-C *(Robins, Canad.)*; Dimetane Expectorant-DC *(Robins, Canad.)*; Dimetane-DC *(Robins, USA)*; Dimetane-DX *(Robins, USA)*; Dimetapp *(Robins, Austral.; Robins, Canad.; Robins, USA)*; Dimetapp-A *(Robins, Canad.)*; Dimetapp-C *(Robins, Canad.)*; Dimetapp-DM *(Robins, Canad.)*; Dimotane Co *(Robins, UK)*; Dimotane Expectorant *(Robins, USA)*; Dimotane Expectorant DC *(Robins, UK)*; Dimotane Plus *(Robins, UK)*; Dimotane Plus LA *(Robins, UK)*; Dimotane with Codeine *(Robins, UK)*; Dimotapp *(Robins, UK)*; Dimotapp Elixir-Plus *(Robins, Austral.)*; Dimotapp P *(Robins, UK)*; Disobrom *(Geneva, USA)*; Disophrol *(Schering, USA)*; Drixoral *(Schering, Canad.; Schering, USA)*; Drixtab *(Schering, Canad.)*; Dura-Tap/PD *(Dura, USA)*; ENT Syrup *(Springbok, USA)*; E-Tapp *(Edwards, USA)*; Exyphen *(Norton, UK)*; Halin *(Nicholas, UK)*; Myphetapp *(Bay, USA)*; Poly-Histine CS *(Bock, USA)*; Poly-Histine DM *(Bock, USA)*; Poly-Histine Expectorant with Codeine *(Bock, USA)*; Poly-Histine-DX *(Bock, USA)*; Rynofen *(Charton, Canad.)*; Sequels *(Lederle, USA)*; S-T Decongest *(Scot-Tussin, USA)*; Tamine *(Geneva, USA)*.

6111-d

Buclizine Hydrochloride *(BANM, USAN, rINNM)*.

NSC-25141; UCB-4445. 1-(4-*tert*-Butylbenzyl)-4-(4-chlorobenzhydryl)piperazine dihydrochloride.
$C_{28}H_{33}ClN_2,2HCl=506.0$.

CAS — 82-95-1 (buclizine); 129-74-8 (hydrochloride).

Adverse Effects, Treatment, Precautions, and Absorption and Fate

As for the antihistamines in general, p.443.

Uses and Administration

Buclizine hydrochloride is a piperazine derivative with the actions of the antihistamines (see p.444). It is used mainly for its anti-emetic action and in vertigo due to labyrinthine disorders. It may also be used for the symptomatic treatment of allergic conditions. It is reported to have a prolonged antihistamine action.

The dose for nausea and vertigo is usually 25 to 50 mg up to three times a day. Buclizine is used in combination with analgesics for migraine, usually in doses of 12.5 mg of the hydrochloride.

Proprietary Preparations

Migraleve (also known as Migralift) *(International Laboratories, UK)*. *Tablets* (pink), buclizine hydrochloride 6.25 mg, paracetamol 500 mg, codeine phosphate 8 mg.
Tablets (yellow), paracetamol 500 mg, codeine phosphate 8 mg.
For migraine. *Dose*. 2 pink tablets at the start of an attack, then 2 yellow tablets every 4 hours if required; maximum daily dose, 2 pink tablets and 6 yellow tablets.

Proprietary Names and Manufacturers

Aphilan R *(UCB, Fr.)*; Bucladin-S *(Stuart Pharmaceuticals, USA)*; Longifene *(Belg.; Neth.; Vesta, S.Afr.; Switz.)*; Postafen *(Arg.)*.

The following names have been used for multi-ingredient preparations containing buclizine hydrochloride— Equivert *(Pfizer, UK)*; Migraleve Pink *(International Laboratories, UK)*; Migralift Pink *(International Laboratories, UK)*.

6113-h

Carbinoxamine Maleate *(BANM, USAN, rINNM)*.

2-[4-Chloro-α-(2-pyridyl)benzyloxy]-*NN*-dimethylethylamine hydrogen maleate.
$C_{16}H_{19}ClN_2O,C_4H_4O_4=406.9$.

CAS — 486-16-8 (carbinoxamine); 3505-38-2 (maleate).

Pharmacopoeias. In *U.S.*

A white odourless crystalline powder. **Soluble** 1 in less than 1 of water, and 1 in 1.5 of alcohol and of chloroform; very slightly soluble in ether. A 1% solution in water has a pH of 4.6 to 5.1. **Store** in airtight containers. Protect from light.

Adverse Effects, Treatment, and Precautions

As for the antihistamines in general, p.443.

For a report of comparative effects of carbinoxamine on performance see p.443.

Uses and Administration

Carbinoxamine maleate is an ethanolamine derivative with the actions and uses of the antihistamines (see p.444). The duration of action has been reported to be 3 to 6 hours.

Carbinoxamine maleate is usually given in doses of 4 to 8 mg three or four times daily. The dose for children, given 3 or 4 times daily, is: 1 to 3 years of age 2 mg, 3 to 6 years 2 to 4 mg, and children over 6 years 4 to 6 mg. It is also given in cough linctuses and decongestant preparations.

Preparations

Carbinoxamine Maleate Tablets *(U.S.P.)*

Proprietary Preparations

Davenol *(Wyeth, UK)*. *Linctus*, carbinoxamine maleate 2 mg, ephedrine hydrochloride 7 mg, pholcodine 4 mg/5 mL.

Proprietary Names and Manufacturers

Allergefon *(Lafon, Fr.)*; Clistin *(Arg.; Austral.; Ital.; McNeil Pharmaceutical, USA)*; Histex *(Austral.)*; Lergefin *(Spain)*; Polistin *(Trommsdorff, Ger.)*; Polistine *(Neth.)*; Ziriton *(Ital.)*.

The following names have been used for multi-ingredient preparations containing carbinoxamine maleate— Cardec DM *(Schein, USA)*; Davenol *(Wyeth, UK)*; Extil Compound *(Evans Medical, UK)*; Rondec *(Ross, USA)*; Rondec-DM *(Ross, USA)*; Tussafed *(Everett, USA)*.

6114-m

Chlorcyclizine Hydrochloride *(BANM, USAN, rINNM)*.

Chlorcyclizini Hydrochloridum; Chlorcyclizinium Chloride. (±)-1-(4-Chlorobenzhydryl)-4-methylpiperazine hydrochloride.
$C_{18}H_{21}ClN_2,HCl=337.3$.

CAS — 82-93-9 (chlorcyclizine); 1620-21-9; 14362-31-3 (both hydrochloride).

Pharmacopoeias. In *Arg., Br., Ind., Int., It., Turk.*, and *U.S.*

A white, odourless or almost odourless, crystalline powder.
Soluble 1 in 2 of water, 1 in 11 of alcohol, and 1 in 4 of chloroform; practically insoluble in ether. A 1% solution in water has a pH of 4.8 to 5.5. **Store** in airtight containers. Protect from light.

Chlorcyclizine hydrochloride is a piperazine derivative with the properties and uses of the antihistamines (see p.443).
Chlorcyclizine hydrochloride has been given by mouth in allergic conditions. A 2% cream or lotion has been used topically. The dibunate has also been used.

Proprietary Names and Manufacturers

Di-Paralene *(Abbott, Austral.; Abbott, Belg.; Abbott, Fr.; Abbott, Ital.; Abbott, Norw.; Abbott, Swed.)*; Tri-histan *(GEA, Denm.; Weiders, Norw.; Switz.)*.

The following names have been used for multi-ingredient preparations containing chlorcyclizine hydrochloride— Fedrazil *(Wellcome, USA)*; Histofax *(Wellcome, UK)*; Mantadil *(Wellcome, USA)*.

6115-b

Chloropyrilene Citrate *(BANM, rINNM)*.

Chloromethapyrilene Citrate; Chlorothen Citrate; Chlorpyrilen Citrate. *N*-(5-Chloro-2-thenyl)-*N'N'*-dimethyl-*N*-(2-pyridyl)ethylenediamine dihydrogen citrate.
$C_{14}H_{18}ClN_3S,C_6H_8O_7=488.0$.

CAS — 148-65-2 (chloropyrilene); 148-64-1 (citrate).

Pharmacopoeias. In *Arg.*

Chloropyrilene citrate is an ethylenediamine derivative with the properties and uses of the antihistamines (see p.443). It has been used for topical application as a 2.5% cream.

Proprietary Names and Manufacturers

Panta *(Valeas, Ital.)*.

The following names have been used for multi-ingredient preparations containing chloropyrilene citrate— Achrocidin *(Lederle, Canad.)*.

6127-p

Dexchlorpheniramine Maleate *(USAN, rINNM)*.

Dexchlorpheniramine is the dextrorotatory isomer of chlorpheniramine which is racemic.

CAS — 25523-97-1 (dexchlorpheniramine);

2438-32-6 (maleate).

Pharmacopoeias. In *Jpn, Nord.* and *U.S.*

A white odourless crystalline powder. **Soluble** 1 in 1.1 of water, 1 in 2 of alcohol, and 1 in 1.7 of chloroform; very slightly soluble in ether. A 1% solution in water has a pH of 4.0 to 5.0. **Store** in airtight containers. Protect from light.

6116-v

Chlorpheniramine Maleate *(BANM, USAN).*

Chlorphenamine Maleate *(rINNM)*; Chlorprophenpyridamine Maleate. (±)-3-(4-Chlorophenyl)-*NN*-dimethyl-3-(2-pyridyl)propylamine hydrogen maleate.

$C_{16}H_{19}ClN_2,C_4H_4O_4$=390.9.

CAS — 132-22-9 (chlorpheniramine); 42882-96-2 (chlorpheniramine, ±); 113-92-8 (maleate).

Pharmacopoeias. In *Arg., Br., Braz., Chin., Egypt., Eur., Ind., Int., Jpn, Neth., Swiss, Turk.,* and *U.S.*

A white odourless crystalline powder.

Soluble 1 in 4 of water and 1 in 10 of alcohol and of chloroform; slightly soluble in ether. A 1% solution in water has a pH of 4.0 to 5.0. Solutions are **sterilised** by autoclaving. **Store** in airtight containers. Protect from light.

Incompatibility has been reported with calcium chloride, kanamycin sulphate, noradrenaline acid tartrate, pentobarbitone sodium, and iodipamide meglumine.

Adverse Effects

As for the antihistamines in general, p.443.

Injections may be irritant and transient hypotension or stimulation of the CNS may occur during rapid intravenous injection.

Chlorpheniramine has been reported to affect the senses of smell and taste.— S. Schiffman, *New Engl. J. Med.*, 1983, *308*, 1275.

A 4-year-old child experienced visual hallucinations during treatment with high doses of a decongestant containing chlorpheniramine, phenylpropanolamine, and dextromethorphan.— H. Dungal and D. E. Griffiths (letter), *Can. med. Ass. J.*, 1984, *131*, 1186.

EFFECTS ON THE BLOOD. Chlorpheniramine given to an elderly woman to treat a wasp sting was probably responsible for agranulocytosis. She received a total of about 170 mg of chlorpheniramine.— G. Shenfield and C. J. F. Spry (letter), *Br. med. J.*, 1968, *2*, 52.

A report of chlorpheniramine-induced thrombocytopenic purpura in a 53-year-old man.— E. V. Eisner *et al.*, *J. Am. med. Ass.*, 1975, *231*, 735.

Pancytopenia in one patient was attributed to chlorpheniramine; thrombocytopenia developed rapidly after a challenge dose.— P. M. Deringer and A. Maniatis (letter), *Lancet*, 1976, *1*, 432. Doubts as to whether chlorpheniramine was responsible.— C. J. F. Spry (letter), *ibid.*, 545.

Aplastic anaemia was associated with prolonged chlorpheniramine use in 1 patient.— T. Kanoh *et al.* (letter), *Lancet*, 1977, *1*, 546.

EFFECTS ON THE EYES. A study indicating that usual therapeutic doses of dexchlorpheniramine interfere with colour vision.— J. Laroche and C. Laroche, *Annls pharm. fr.*, 1972, *30*, 433.

EXTRAPYRAMIDAL SYMPTOMS. Long-term use of chlorpheniramine caused progressive left-sided facial dyskinesia in a 57-year-old man. Dramatic improvement in the facial dyskinesia occurred within 6 weeks of discontinuing chlorpheniramine.— W. A. Davis (letter), *New Engl. J. Med.*, 1976, *294*, 113.

Treatment of Adverse Effects

As for the antihistamines in general, p.443.

Precautions

As for the antihistamines in general, p.444.

INTERACTIONS. For a report of the effect of chlorpheniramine on phenytoin, see Phenytoin Sodium, p.409.

Absorption and Fate

As for the antihistamines in general, p.444. Chlorpheniramine has been reported to undergo considerable first-pass metabolism. It is excreted partly unchanged in the urine.

A mean biological half-life for chlorpheniramine of 30.3 hours (range 20.6 to 42.5 hours), after the administration of chlorpheniramine maleate 8 mg by mouth to 5 fasting healthy subjects, was much longer than half-lives previously reported. Frequent dosing or the use of sustained-release preparations were considered unnecessary. A duration of effect of about 24 hours was predicted for most subjects.— W. L. Chiou *et al.* (letter), *New Engl. J. Med.*, 1979, *300*, 501.

In a review of the pharmacokinetics of chlorpheniramine, the bioavailability was reported to be incomplete, ranging from 25 to 50% of the oral dose in most studies. An extensive gut and hepatic first-pass effect had been observed. Considerable intersubject variation had been found in the metabolism and excretion of chlorpheniramine, and excretion was dependent on urinary pH and flow-rate. After single and multiple oral doses 21 and 34% of the doses were excreted unchanged, respectively. About 22% was excreted as the desmethyl metabolite, and 3% as the didesmethyl metabolite. In children there was evidence to suggest more rapid and complete oral absorption and faster clearance.— M. M. Rumore, *Drug Intell. & clin. Pharm.*, 1984, *18*, 701.

In a single-dose study, chlorpheniramine maleate 120 µg per kg body-weight was given to 11 children with allergic rhinitis. There was considerable variation in the elimination half-life, ranging from 6.3 hours to 23.1 hours. The rate of excretion of chlorpheniramine and two demethylated metabolites was dependent on urine flow-rate and pH.— K. J. Simons *et al.*, *J. pharm. Sci.*, 1984, *73*, 595.

Uses and Administration

Chlorpheniramine maleate is an alkylamine derivative with the actions and uses of the antihistamines (see p.444). It is one of the most potent of the antihistamines and causes a moderate degree of sedation.

Dexchlorpheniramine is the dextrorotatory isomer of chlorpheniramine, which is racemic, and has approximately twice the activity.

Chlorpheniramine maleate is given by mouth usually in doses of 4 mg three or four times daily. Higher doses of up to 36 mg daily have been given in sustained-release preparations. In the *UK*, the dose for children up to 1 year is 1 mg twice daily; for those aged 1 to 5 years, 1 to 2 mg three times daily; and for those aged 6 to 12 years, 2 to 4 mg three or four times daily. In the *USA*, the use of chlorpheniramine is not recommended in children under 2 years.

In severe allergies it may be given by intramuscular, subcutaneous, or, diluted with 5 to 10 mL of blood, by slow intravenous injection over a period of 1 minute. The usual dose is 10 to 20 mg and the total dose given by these routes in 24 hours should not normally exceed 40 mg. It has been administered prophylactically to persons with a history of transfusion reactions but should not be added to the blood being transfused. For children, doses of 87.5 µg per kg body-weight or 2.5 mg per m^2 body-surface subcutaneously have been suggested.

Dexchlorpheniramine maleate is given by mouth in doses of 2 mg up to 4- to 6-hourly as required. Children's doses are: 2 to 5 years, 0.5 mg every 4 to 6 hours up to a maximum of 3 mg in 24 hours; 6 to 11 years, 1 mg every 4 to 6 hours up to a maximum of 6 mg in 24 hours. Alternatively, adults may take up to 6 mg as a sustained-release formulation either at night or at 8- to 10-hourly intervals during the day.

Chlorpheniramine polistirex (a chlorpheniramine and sulphonated diethenylbenzene-ethenylbenzene copolymer complex) is also used.

ADMINISTRATION IN RENAL FAILURE. No dosage reduction of chlorpheniramine was considered necessary in patients with renal failure.— W. M. Bennett *et al.*, *Am. J. Kidney Dis.*, 1983, *3*, 155.

ASTHMA. Bronchodilatation was produced by nebulised chlorpheniramine in children with asthma.— R. C. Groggins *et al.*, *Archs Dis. Childh.*, 1979, *54*, 163.

IMMUNODEFICIENCY. A report, in a father and son, of a familial immunodeficiency disease, characterised by recurrent and persistent pyoderma, folliculitis, and atopic dermatitis; it was accompanied by abnormalities of lymphocyte and leucocyte function. The clinical manifestations and the disorders of lymphocyte and leucocyte function responded dramatically to administration of chlorpheniramine.— L. K. L. Jung *et al.*, *Lancet*, 1983, *2*, 185.

OTITIS MEDIA. Treatment with chlorpheniramine and pseudoephedrine given together had no beneficial effect in a double-blind controlled study in 553 children with otitis media with effusion.— E. I. Cantekin *et al.*, *New Engl. J. Med.*, 1983, *308*, 297 and 1599.

Preparations

Chlorpheniramine Oral Solution *(B.P.)*. Chlorpheniramine Elixir. A solution of chlorpheniramine maleate in a suitable flavoured vehicle.

Chlorpheniramine Maleate Syrup *(U.S.P.)*. A syrup containing 36 to 44 mg of chlorpheniramine maleate in each 100 mL.

Chlorpheniramine Injection *(B.P.)*. A sterile solution of chlorpheniramine maleate in Water for Injections free from dissolved air.

Chlorpheniramine Maleate Injection *(U.S.P.)*

Chlorpheniramine Maleate Tablets *(U.S.P.)*

Chlorpheniramine Tablets *(B.P.)*. Tablets containing chlorpheniramine maleate.

Dexchlorpheniramine Maleate Syrup *(U.S.P.)*

Dexchlorpheniramine Maleate Tablets *(U.S.P.)*

Proprietary Preparations

Alunex *(Steinhard, UK). Tablets*, scored, chlorpheniramine maleate 4 mg.

Haymine *(Pharmax, UK). Tablets*, sustained-release, chlorpheniramine maleate 10 mg, ephedrine hydrochloride 15 mg.

An evaluation of Haymine for the relief of hay fever symptoms.— *Drug & Ther. Bull.*, 1982, *20*, 40.

Piriton *(Allen & Hanburys, UK). Tablets*, chlorpheniramine maleate 4 mg.

Spandets, sustained-release tablets, chlorpheniramine maleate 12 mg.

Syrup, chlorpheniramine maleate 2 mg/5 mL.

Injection, chlorpheniramine maleate 10 mg/mL, in ampoules of 1 mL.

Proprietary Names and Manufacturers of Chlorpheniramine, Dexchlorpheniramine, and their Salts

Afeme *(Arg.)*; Alergitrat *(Fecofar, Arg.)*; Allergex *(Protea, Austral.; S.Afr.)*; Allergisan *(Swed.)*; Allerhist *(Vernleigh, S.Afr.)*; Allerton *(Ital.)*; AL-R *(Saron, USA)*; Alunex *(Steinhard, UK)*; Atalis-D *(Jpn)*; Bramahist *(Austral.)*; Chlor-100 *(Vortech, USA)*; Chloramin *(Eagle, Austral.)*; Chlor-Mal *(Rugby, USA)*; Chlormene *(USA)*; Chlorphen *(Pro Doc, Canad.)*; Chlorspan *(Vortech, USA)*; Chlortab *(Vortech, USA)*; Chlor-Trimeton *(Austral.; Schering, USA)*; Chlortrimeton *(Scherag, S.Afr.)*; Chlor-Tripolon *(Schering, Canad.)*; Cloro Trimeton *(Arg.)*; Clorten *(Panthox & Burck, Ital.)*; C-Meton-S *(Jpn)*; Colirio Llorens Antihistaminico *(Spain)*; Destral *(Tiber, Ital.)*; Dexchlor *(Schein, USA)*; Haynon *(R.P. Drugs, UK)*; Histaids *(Austral.)*; Histalon *(Canad.)*; Histamed *(Vernleigh, S.Afr.)*; Histaspan *(USA)*; Isomerine *(Essex, Arg.)*; Kelargine *(Belg.)*; Lentostamin *(SIT, Ital.)*; Lorphen *(USA)*; Methyrit *(Neth.)*; Niratron *(USA)*; Novopheniram *(Novopharm, Canad.)*; Phenamin *(Nyco, Norw.)*; Piriton *(Glaxo, Austral.; Allen & Hanburys, UK)*; Polaramin *(Schering, Denm.; Essex, Ital.; Schering, Norw.; Schering, Swed.)*; Polaramine *(Essex, Austral.; Schering, Belg.; Schering, Canad.; Unicet, Fr.; Essex, Neth.; Scherag, S.Afr.; Essex, Spain; Essex, Switz.; Schering, USA)*; Polaronil *(Essex, Ger.)*; Poracemin *(Jpn)*; Prof-N-4 *(Arg.)*; Teldrin *(Smith Kline & French, USA)*; Teledrin *(Austral.)*; Trimeton *(Essex, Ital.)*.

The following names have been used for multi-ingredient preparations containing chlorpheniramine, dexchlorpheniramine, and their salts—4-Way Tablets *(Bristol-Myers Products, USA)*; Alka-Seltzer Plus *(Miles Laboratories, USA)*; Allerest *(Pharmacraft, USA)*; Anafed *(Everett, USA)*; Anamine *(Mayrand, USA)*; Brexin LA *(Savage, USA)*; Cerose-DM *(Wyeth, USA)*; Chlorafed *(Hauck, USA)*; Chlor-Trimeton Decongestant *(Schering, USA)*; Chlor-Tripolon Decongestant *(Schering, Canad.)*; Citra Forte Capsules *(Boyle, USA)*; Codimal-L.A. *(Central Pharmaceuticals, USA)*; Cold Factor 12 *(Pharmacraft, USA)*;

Coldex *(Gen, Canad.)*; Comhist *(Norwich Eaton, USA)*; Comtrex *(Bristol-Myers Products, USA)*; Co-Pyronil *(Dista, USA)*; Coricidin *(Schering, Canad.)*; Coricidin D *(Schering, Canad.)*; Coricidin Pediatric Drops *(Schering, Canad.)*; Coricidin with Codeine *(Schering, Canad.)*; Corsym *(Pennwalt, Canad.; Pennwalt, USA)*; Coryban-D *(Pfipharmecs, USA)*; Cotaminol *(Gen, Canad.)*; Cotrol-D *(Beecham Laboratories, USA)*; CoTylenol *(McNeil Consumer, USA)*; CoTylenol, Children's *(McNeil Consumer, USA)*; Cremacoat 4 *(Richardson-Vicks, USA)*; Dallergy *(Laser, USA)*; Dallergy-D Capsules *(Laser, USA)*; Dallergy-D Syrup *(Laser, USA)*; Daribiol *(Cambridge Laboratories, Austral.)*; Dasikon *(Beecham Laboratories, USA)*; Deconamine *(Berlex, USA)*; Decotan *(Gen, Canad.)*; Dehist *(Forest Pharmaceuticals, USA)*; Demazin *(Schering, USA)*; Demazin Repetabs *(Schering, Austral.; Schering, USA)*; Demazin Syrup *(Schering, Austral.; Schering, USA)*; Demazin Tablets *(Schering, Austral.)*; Donatussin Drops *(Laser, USA)*; Dorcol Children's Cold Formula *(Dorsey Laboratories, USA)*; Dristan Advanced Formula *(Whitehall, Canad.; Whitehall, USA)*; Dristan Decongestant Tablets with Antihistamine*(Whitehall, UK)*; Drixine Cough Expectorant *(Essex, Austral.)*; Drixine Cough Suppressant *(Essex, Austral.)*; Drize *(Ascher, USA)*; Dura-Vent/A *(Dura, USA)*; Dura-Vent/DA *(Dura, USA)*; Eltor AF *(Dow, Canad.)*; ENT Tablets *(Springbok, USA)*; Expulin *(Galen, UK)*; Expurhin *(Galen, UK)*; Extendryl *(Fleming, USA)*; Fedahist *(Kremers-Urban, USA)*; Fedahist Expectorant *(Kremers-Urban, USA)*;
Haymine *(Pharmax, UK)*; Hista-Clopane *(Lilly, USA)*; Histadyl and A.S.A. *(Lilly, USA)*; Histalet *(Reid-Rowell, USA)*; Histalet DM *(Reid-Rowell, USA)*; Histalet Forte *(Reid-Rowell, USA)*; Histamic *(Metro Med, USA)*; Histaspan-D *(USV Pharmaceutical Corp., USA)*; Histaspan-P *(Rorer, Canad.)*; Histaspan-Plus *(USV Pharmaceutical Corp., USA)*; Histor-D *(Hauck, USA)*; Hycomine Compound *(Du Pont, USA)*; Iophen-C *(Schein, USA)*; Isoclor *(Fisons, USA)*; Juvatral *(Cambridge Laboratories, Austral.)*; Korigesic *(Trimen, USA)*; Kronofed-A *(Ferndale, USA)*; Kronohist *(Ferndale, USA)*; Metreton *(Schering, Canad.)*; Naldecon *(Bristol, USA)*; Neo-Nasol *(Neolab, Canad.)*; Neo-Tuss *(Neolab, Canad.)*; Nolamine *(Carnrick, USA)*; Novafed A *(Merrell Dow, USA)*; Novahistex Cold Capsules *(Dow, Canad.)*; Novahistine *(Lakeside, USA)*; Novahistine DH *(Lakeside, USA)*; Omni-Tuss *(Pennwalt, Canad.)*; Ornade *(Smith Kline & French, Canad.; Smith Kline & French, USA)*; Ornade Expectorant *(Smith Kline & French, Canad.)*; Ornade-DM *(Smith Kline & French, Canad.)*; Orthoxicol Expectorant *(Upjohn, Austral.)*; Papzans Modified *(Bowman, USA)*; Pediacare-2 *(McNeil Consumer, USA)*; Pediacare-3 *(McNeil Consumer, USA)*; Pediacof *(Winthrop-Breon, USA)*; Penntuss *(Pennwalt, Canad.; Pennwalt, USA)*; Phenate *(Mallard, USA)*; Polaramine Compound *(Essex, Austral.)*; Probahist Capsules *(Legere, USA)*; Promist HD *(Russ, USA)*; Protid *(Lasalle, USA)*; Pseudo-Hist *(Holloway, USA)*; Pseudo-Hist Expectorant *(Holloway, USA)*; P-V-Tussin Syrup *(Reid-Provident, USA)*; Quadrahist *(Schein, USA)*; Quelidrine *(Abbott, USA)*;
Resaid *(Geneva, USA)*; Rhinolar *(McGregor, USA)*; Rhinolar-EX *(McGregor, USA)*; Ru-Tuss 11 *(Boots, USA)*; Ru-Tuss Liquid *(Boots, USA)*; Ru-Tuss Plain *(Boots, USA)*; Ru-Tuss Tablets *(Boots, USA)*; Rynatan *(Wallace, USA)*; Rynatuss *(Wallace, USA)*; Sancos Co *(Sandoz, UK)*; Scot-Tussin Cough & Cold *(Scot-Tussin, USA)*; Sinarest *(Pharmacraft, USA)*; Singlet *(Lakeside, USA)*; Sinovan Timed *(Drug Industries, USA)*; Sinulin *(Carnrick, USA)*; Sinutab Antihistamine *(Warner, Austral.)*; Sinutab Extra Strength *(Parke, Davis, Canad.)*; Sinutab Tablets *(Parke, Davis, Canad.)*; Sinutab with Antihistamine and Pseudoephedrine *(Warner, Austral.)*; Sinutab with Codeine *(Parke, Davis, Canad.)*; Sudafed Plus *(Wellcome, USA)*; Symptrol *(Saron, USA)*; T-Dry *(T.E. Williams, USA)*; Teldrin *(Smith Kline & French, USA)*; Triaminic Cold *(Dorsey Laboratories, USA)*; Triaminic-12 *(Dorsey Laboratories, USA)*; Triaminicin *(Dorsey Laboratories, USA)*; Triaminicol *(Dorsey Laboratories, USA)*; Trind *(Mead Johnson Nutritional, USA)*; Trinex *(Mastar, USA)*; Triocos *(Sandoz, UK)*; Triolinctus *(Sandoz, UK)*; Triolix Night-Time *(Drug Houses Austral., Austral.)*; Tussar *(USV Pharmaceutical Corp., USA)*; Tussar DM *(USV Pharmaceutical Corp., USA)*; Tuss-Ornade *(Smith Kline & French, Canad.)*; Vasofrinic *(Trianon, Canad.)*; Vasofrinic DH *(Trianon, Canad.)*; Vasofrinic Plus *(Trianon, Canad.)*.

6118-q

Cinnarizine *(BAN, USAN, rINN).*

516-MD; R-1575; R-516. 1-Benzhydryl-4-cinnamylpiperazine.

$C_{26}H_{28}N_2$=368.5.

CAS — 298-57-7.

Adverse Effects, Treatment, Precautions, and Absorption and Fate

As for the antihistamines in general, p.443.

A report of immunologically-defined lichen planus pemphigoides in a 72-year-old woman taking cinnarizine. Lesions began to clear when treatment was stopped but challenge with cinnarizine provoked severe itching and reactivation of pigmented lesions.— S. Miyagawa *et al.*, *Br. J. Derm.*, 1985, *112*, 607.

Extrapyramidal symptoms have been associated with the administration of cinnarizine.— J. -R. Laporte and D. Capella, *Lancet*, 1986, *2*, 853; idem, 1987, *1*, 1324.

Cinnarizine was considered to be unsafe in patients with acute porphyria because it has been shown to be porphyrinogenic in *animals* or *in vitro* systems.— M.R. Moore and K.E.L. McColl, *Porphyrias, Drug Lists*, Glasgow, Porphyria Research Unit, University of Glasgow, 1987.

Uses and Administration

Cinnarizine is a piperazine derivative with the actions and uses of the antihistamines (see p.444); it also inhibits the transport of calcium ions across cell membranes. It is mainly used for the symptomatic treatment of nausea and vertigo due to Ménière's disease and other labyrinthine disturbances and for the prevention and treatment of motion sickness. Cinnarizine is reported to possess smooth muscle relaxant properties and to inhibit vasoconstriction, and is thus used in the management of various vascular disorders. Sedative effects are not marked.

The usual dose is 15 to 30 mg three times daily. Children aged 5 to 12 years may be given half the adult dose. For motion sickness a dose of 30 mg may be taken two hours before the start of the journey and 15 mg every 8 hours during the journey. For peripheral arterial disease doses of 75 mg may be given two or three times daily.

VASCULAR INSUFFICIENCY. A review of cinnarizine and of flunarizine in the treatment of peripheral vascular disease considered that they might be of help for some patients with intermittent claudication.— *Drug & Ther. Bull.*, 1981, *19*, 27.

A brief review of the clinical pharmacology and therapeutic efficacy of cinnarizine in cerebrovascular disorders. The results of four placebo-controlled trials had not confirmed beneficial effects claimed for a wide range of clinical symptoms.— A. Spagnoli and G. Tognoni, *Drugs*, 1983, *26*, 44.

VERTIGO AND LABYRINTHINE DISORDERS. Treatment of 63 patients suffering from vertigo with either cinnarizine 15 to 30 mg or prochlorperazine 5 to 10 mg, three times daily was compared in a double-blind, crossover, multicentre study. Both drugs gave good relief of symptoms. Side-effects were few with both drugs, but drowsiness or lassitude occurred in 8% on cinnarizine and in 3% on prochlorperazine.—Report No. 183 of the General Practitioner Research Group, *Practitioner*, 1973, *211*, 224.

Review of the use of cinnarizine in Ménière's disease and other labyrinthine disorders. Cinnarizine has been shown to be effective in the treatment of vertigo and Ménière's syndrome and in the prevention of motion sickness.— G. Towse, *J. Lar. Otol.*, 1980, *94*, 1009.

A brief evaluation of cinnarizine in the treatment of vestibular disorders including Ménière's disease concluded that cinnarizine was probably not superior to prochlorperazine, but could be worth trying in patients who had not responded to prochlorperazine.— *Drug & Ther. Bull.*, 1981, *19*, 17.

Proprietary Preparations

Marzine RF *(Wellcome, UK). Tablets*, cinnarizine 15 mg.

Stugeron *(Janssen, UK). Tablets*, scored, cinnarizine 15 mg.

Stugeron Forte *(Janssen, UK). Capsules*, cinnarizine 75 mg.

Proprietary Names and Manufacturers

Aplactan *(Jpn)*; Aplexal *(Jpn)*; Apomiterl *(Jpn)*; Apotomin *(Jpn)*; Apsatan *(Jpn)*; Artate *(Jpn)*; Carecin *(Jpn)*; Cerebolan *(Jpn)*; Cerepar *(Merckle, Ger.; Mepha, Switz.)*; Cero-Aterin *(Switz.)*; Cinaperazine *(Jpn)*; Cinazyn *(Italchimici, Ital.)*; Cinnacet *(Winthrop, Ger.)*; Cinnageron *(Streuli, Switz.)*; Cinnipirine *(Neth.)*; Corathiem *(Jpn)*; Cysten *(Jpn)*; Denapol *(Jpn)*; Dimitronal *(Belg.)*; Dismaren *(Arg.)*; Eglen *(Jpn)*; Folcodal *(Arg.)*; Giganten *(Tropon, Ger.)*; Glanil *(Janssen Pharmaceutica, Swed.)*; Hilactan *(Jpn)*; Hirdsyn *(Jpn)*; Ixertol *(Cimex, Switz.)*; Izaberizin *(Jpn)*; Katoseran *(Jpn)*; Marzine RF *(Wellcome, UK)*; Midronal *(Fr.)*; Natropas *(Arg.)*; Olamin *(Sigamed, Switz.)*; Pervasum *(Lesvi, Spain)*; Processine *(Jpn)*; Purazine *(Lennon, S.Afr.)*; Razlin *(Jpn)*; Roin *(Jpn)*; Sapratol *(Jpn)*; Sedatromin *(Jpn)*; Senoger *(Cilag, Ital.)*; Sepan *(Janssen, Denm.)*; Siptazin *(Jpn)*; Spaderizine *(Jpn)*; Stugeron *(Arg.; Belg.; Janssen, Ital.; Neth.; Janssen, S.Afr.; Esteve, Spain; Janssen, Switz.; Janssen, UK)*; Stutgeron *(Janssen, Ger.)*; Toliman *(Corvi, Ital.)*; Torizin *(Jpn)*.

6119-p

Clemastine Fumarate *(BANM, USAN, rINNM).*

Meclastine Fumarate; Mecloprodin Fumarate. (+)-(2*R*)-2-{2-[(*R*)-4-Chloro-α-methylbenzhydryloxy]ethyl}-1-methylpyrrolidine hydrogen fumarate.

$C_{21}H_{26}ClNO,C_4H_4O_4$=460.0.

CAS — 15686-51-8 (clemastine); 14976-57-9 (fumarate).

Pharmacopoeias. In *Jpn* and *U.S.*

Clemastine fumarate 1.34 mg is approximately equivalent to 1 mg of clemastine base.

Adverse Effects, Treatment and Precautions

As for the antihistamines in general, p.443. Drowsiness has been reported during clinical studies of clemastine although its sedative effect is claimed to be less pronounced than with some other antihistamines.

Report of an insulin-dependent diabetic who collapsed and remained unconscious for several days soon after starting a course of clemastine.— *Pharm. J.*, 1985, *2*, 109.

For a report on the comparative CNS sedative effects of clemastine with other antihistamines, see p.443.

EFFECTS ON THE EYES. A study indicating that usual therapeutic doses of clemastine interfere with colour vision.— J. Laroche and C. Laroche, *Annls pharm. fr.*, 1972, *30*, 433.

PORPHYRIA. Clemastine was considered to be unsafe in patients with acute porphyria because it has been shown to be porphyrinogenic in *animals* or *in vitro* systems.— M.R. Moore and K.E.L. McColl, *Porphyrias, Drug Lists*, Glasgow, Porphyria Research Unit, University of Glasgow, 1987.

PREGNANCY AND THE NEONATE. Drowsiness, irritability, and refusal to feed in a 10-week-old breast-fed baby occurred 12 hours after her mother started treatment with clemastine. Clemastine was detected in the mother's breast milk. The baby recovered and was feeding normally on the day after the drug was stopped.— T. H. H. G. Kok *et al.* (letter), *Lancet*, 1982, *1*, 914.

Absorption and Fate

As for the antihistamines in general, p.444.

In 12 healthy subjects given clemastine fumarate by mouth peak plasma concentrations occurred after 3 to 5 hours. After intravenous injection in 3 subjects a rapid decline in plasma concentration during the first 30 minutes occurred followed by a slow rise to peak concentration 2 to 3 hours after administration. In 5 subjects given clemastine fumarate the ability to inhibit histamine flares correlated well with plasma concentration.— R. Tham *et al.*, *Arzneimittel-Forsch.*, 1978, *28*, 1017.

Uses and Administration

Clemastine fumarate has the properties and uses of the antihistamines (see p.444). It is long acting and has been reported to have a duration of action of about 10 to 12 hours.

Clemastine fumarate is given by mouth for allergic conditions; the usual dose is the equivalent of 1 mg of clemastine base night and morning.

Higher doses may be required for dermatological symptoms. If necessary the equivalent of up to 6 mg daily may be given in divided doses. The dose for children up to 12 years is the equivalent of 0.5 mg night and morning increasing if necessary to 1 mg according to age.

It may be given by intramuscular or slow intravenous injection in a dose equivalent to 2 to 4 mg of clemastine daily in cases of acute allergy; for prophylaxis 2 mg is given by intravenous injection. The dose for children is 25 µg per kg body-weight by intramuscular injection.

Clemastine has also been used topically.

ASTHMA. In a study of 28 children with allergic bronchial asthma, clemastine syrup produced some initial prophylactic benefit. However, it did not offer substantial protection during prolonged treatment and was inferior to ketotifen.— Z. Hloušková *et al., J. int. med. Res.*, 1980, *8*, 408.

A study in 15 asthmatic children did not suggest that clemastine inhalation would be a useful addition to the management of their asthma although a bronchodilatory effect was seen.— R. L. Henry *et al., Archs Dis. Childh.*, 1983, *58*, 304.

URTICARIA. Clemastine 1 mg twice a day was beneficial in the treatment of chronic urticaria, with or without dermographism, in a crossover study involving 23 patients. Drowsiness occurred in 3 patients.— D. S. Jolliffe *et al., Curr. med. Res. Opinion*, 1985, *9*, 394.

Proprietary Preparations

Aller-eze *(Intercare, UK). Tablets*, scored, clemastine 1 mg (as fumarate).
Elixir, clemastine 500 µg (as fumarate)/5 mL.

Aller-eze Plus *(Intercare, UK). Tablets*, clemastine 500 µg (as fumarate), phenylpropanolamine hydrochloride 25 mg.

Tavegil *(Sandoz, UK). Tablets*, scored, clemastine 1 mg (as fumarate).
Elixir, clemastine 500 µg (as fumarate)/5 mL.

Proprietary Names and Manufacturers

Alagyl *(Jpn)*; Aller-eze *(Intercare, UK)*; Aloginan *(Jpn)*; Alphamin *(Jpn)*; Alusas *(Jpn)*; Anhistan *(Jpn)*; Benanzyl *(Jpn)*; Clemanil *(Jpn)*; Fuluminol *(Jpn)*; Fumaresutin *(Jpn)*; Histamedine *(Jpn)*; Inbestan *(Jpn)*; Kinotomin *(Jpn)*; Lacretin *(Jpn)*; Lecasol *(Jpn)*; Maikohis *(Jpn)*; Mallermin-F *(Jpn)*; Marsthine *(Jpn)*; Masletine *(Jpn)*; Natarilon *(Jpn)*; Piloral *(Jpn)*; Reconin *(Jpn)*; Tavegil *(Sandoz, Ger.; Sandoz, Ital.; Neth.; Sandoz, Spain; Sandoz, UK)*; Tavegyl *(Arg.; Sandoz, Austral.; Belg.; Sandoz, Denm.; Sandoz, Fr.; Hung.; Jpn; Sandoz, Norw.; Wander, S.Afr.; Sandoz, Swed.; Sandoz, Switz.)*; Tavist *(Ancalab, Canad.; Sandoz, USA)*; Telgin-G *(Jpn)*; Trabest *(Jpn)*; Xolamin *(Jpn)*.

The following names have been used for multi-ingredient preparations containing clemastine fumarate— Aller-eze Plus *(Intercare, UK)*; Tavist-D *(Sandoz, USA)*.

6120-n

Clemizole Hydrochloride *(BANM, rINNM).*
1-(4-Chlorobenzyl)-2-(pyrrolidin-1-ylmethyl)benzimidazole hydrochloride.
$C_{19}H_{20}ClN_3,HCl=362.3$.

CAS — 442-52-4 (clemizole); 1163-36-6 (hydrochloride).

Clemizole hydrochloride has the properties and uses of the antihistamines (see p.443). Clemizole hydrochloride has been given in doses of 20 to 40 mg two to four times daily. It has been applied topically as the hydrogen sulphate, and as the undecanoate in topical and rectal preparations combined with corticosteroids and local anaesthetics.

Proprietary Names and Manufacturers
Alercur *(Schering, Spain)*; Allercur *(Schering, Austral.; Schering, Switz.)*; Allerpant *(Lagap, Ital.)*; Pan-Allerg *(Borromeo, Ital.)*.

NOTE. The *UK* preparations Scheriproct and Ultraproct have been reformulated to exclude clemizole.

12583-c

Clocinizine Hydrochloride *(rINNM).*
Chlorcinnazine Dihydrochloride. 1-(4-Chlorobenzhydryl)-4-cinnamylpiperazine dihydrochloride.
$C_{26}H_{27}ClN_2,2HCl=475.9$.

CAS — 298-55-5 (clocinizine).

Clocinizine hydrochloride has the properties of the antihistamines (see p.443) and has been given in the treatment of rhinitis and in decongestant mixtures.

6121-h

Cyclizine *(BAN, USAN, rINN).*

1-Benzhydryl-4-methylpiperazine.
$C_{18}H_{22}N_2=266.4$.

CAS — 82-92-8.

Pharmacopoeias. In *Br.* and *U.S.*

A white or creamy-white almost odourless crystalline powder. M.p. 106° to 109°.

Practically **insoluble** in water; soluble 1 in 6 of alcohol and of ether, and 1 in 0.9 of chloroform. A saturated solution in water has a pH of 7.6 to 8.6. **Store** in airtight containers. Protect from light.

6122-m

Cyclizine Hydrochloride *(BANM, USAN, rINNM).*

Cyclizini Hydrochloridum; Cyclizinium Chloride.
$C_{18}H_{22}N_2,HCl=302.8$.

CAS — 303-25-3.

Pharmacopoeias. In *Br., Egypt., Ind., Int.*, and *U.S.*

A white, odourless or almost odourless, crystalline powder, or small colourless crystals. M.p. about 285° with decomposition.

B.P. **solubilities** are: slightly soluble in water and in alcohol; practically insoluble in ether. *U.S.P.* **solubilities** are: soluble 1 in 115 of water and alcohol, soluble 1 in 75 of chloroform; practically insoluble in ether. A 2% solution in alcohol 2 vol. and water 3 vol. has a pH of 4.5 to 5.5. **Store** in airtight containers. Protect from light.

6123-b

Cyclizine Lactate *(BANM, USAN, rINNM).*

$C_{18}H_{22}N_2,C_3H_6O_3=356.5$.

CAS — 5897-19-8.

The injection is prepared from cyclizine with the aid of lactic acid. The injection has a pH of 3.2 to 4.7. Solutions are **sterilised** by autoclaving. Cyclizine lactate injection is reported to be **incompatible** with oxytetracycline hydrochloride, chlortetracycline hydrochloride, penicillin injections, and solutions with a pH greater than 6.8.

Adverse Effects, Treatment, Precautions, and Absorption and Fate

As for the antihistamines in general, p.443. Cholestatic jaundice has been reported. Care should be taken when cyclizine is used postoperatively because of its hypotensive action.

Cyclizine given intravenously may increase the incidence of tremor and muscle movements if given before methohexitone anaesthesia.

ABUSE. Euphoria and hallucinations occurred in 3 youths who each took 750 mg of cyclizine. Physical symptoms included tachycardia, hypertension and dilated pupils, and convulsions in 1. The symptoms subsided within about 12 hours.— P. H. Gott, *New Engl. J. Med.*, 1968, *279*, 596.

A report of large quantities of cyclizine being taken, often by injection, by addicts in addition to prescribed methadone to enhance the effects of the opiate.— P. C. McLean; P. Casey, *Drugs in Psychiatric Practice*, P. J. Tyrer (Ed.), London, Butterworths, 1982, p.329. Evidence that dependency to cyclizine may occur when used with opiates in the treatment of chronic pain and complicate its management.— A. M. Hughes and J. Coote (letter), *Pharm. J.*, 1986, *1*, 130.

Further references to the abuse of cyclizine: T. H. Curry (letter), *Pharm. J.*, 1984, *1*, 310; A. Kahn and G. J. Harvey (letter), *ibid.*, 1985, *2*, 706; M. K. Atkinson (letter), *ibid.*, 773; *idem* (letter), 797.

ALLERGY. A fixed drug eruption occurred in a patient on 3 occasions within 12 hours after taking cyclizine 50 mg for motion sickness, and again after a challenge dose.— W. A. D. Griffiths and R. D. G. Peachey, *Br. J. Derm.*, 1970, *82*, 616.

EFFECTS ON THE BLOOD. Agranulocytosis occurred in 1 patient after six weeks of treatment with cyclizine 50 mg three times daily. The blood count returned to normal once cyclizine was withdrawn.— P. M. Collier, *Br. med. J.*, 1986, *292*, 174.

EFFECTS ON THE HEART. In a study of 11 patients with severe heart failure, cyclizine produced detrimental haemodynamic effects including increased systemic and pulmonary artery pressures and ventricular filling pressures, and negated the vasodilatory effects of diamorphine. It was suggested that the use of cyclizine should be avoided in patients with acute myocardial infarction or severe heart failure.— L. B. Tan *et al., Lancet*, 1988, *1*, 560.

EFFECTS ON THE LIVER. An 8-year-old girl developed jaundice on 2 occasions after taking cyclizine 25 mg daily. 'Hypersensitivity hepatitis' was considered responsible.— M. C. Kew *et al.* (letter), *Br. med. J.*, 1973, *2*, 307.

PREGNANCY AND THE NEONATE. For studies involving the use of cyclizine during pregnancy, see p.443.

Uses and Administration

Cyclizine is a piperazine derivative with the properties of the antihistamines (see p.444) but it is used mainly for its potent anti-emetic action. It has antimuscarinic activity. Sedative effects are not marked.

It is used for the prevention and treatment of motion sickness. It has also been used in irradiation sickness, postoperative vomiting, and drug-induced nausea and vomiting, and for the symptomatic treatment of vertigo due to Ménière's disease and other labyrinthine disturbances.

For the prevention of motion sickness cyclizine hydrochloride 50 mg is taken 20 to 30 minutes before departure; this dose may be repeated every 4 to 6 hours if necessary. Not more than 200 mg should be taken in a day. The dosage for children is 1 mg per kg body-weight or 33 mg per m^2 body-surface three times a day if necessary. Children aged 6 years and over may be given 25 mg three times a day if necessary.

Cyclizine is given by injection as the lactate in doses of 50 mg every 4 to 6 hours; for the prevention of postoperative vomiting it may be injected intramuscularly about 20 minutes before the anticipated end of surgery. A dose of 1 mg per kg or 33 mg per m^2 up to three times a day has been recommended for children under 12 years. Cyclizine tartrate is also used for injections.

In the *UK*, the use of cyclizine and its salts in cosmetics is prohibited by law.

ANAESTHESIA. Cyclizine 50 mg reduced pre- and postoperative nausea and vomiting caused by pethidine.— J. W. Dundee *et al., Br. J. Anaesth.*, 1966, *38*, 50.

Preparations

Cyclizine Hydrochloride Tablets *(U.S.P.)*

Cyclizine Tablets *(B.P.).* Tablets containing cyclizine hydrochloride.

Cyclizine Injection *(B.P.).* Cyclizine Lactate Injection

Cyclizine Lactate Injection *(U.S.P.)*

Proprietary Preparations

Valoid *(Calmic, UK). Tablets*, scored, cyclizine hydrochloride 50 mg.
Injection, cyclizine lactate 50 mg/mL, in ampoules of 1 mL.

Proprietary Names and Manufacturers of Cyclizine and its Salts

Echnatol *(Switz.)*; Maremal *(Spain)*; Marezine *(Wellcome, USA)*; Marzine *(Wellcome, Austral.; Wellcome, Canad.; Wellcome, Denm.; Wellcome, Fr.; Wellcome, Ital.; Neth.; Wellcome, Norw.; Wellcome, Swed.; Wellcome, Switz.*; Motozina *(Biomedica Foscama, Ital.)*;

Triazine *(Lennon, S. Afr.)*; Valoid *(Wellcome, S. Afr.; Calmic, UK)*.

The following names have been used for multi-ingredient preparations containing cyclizine and its salts.— Cyclimorph *(Calmic, UK)*; Diconal *(Calmic, UK)*; Migral *(Wellcome, Austral.)*; Migril *(Wellcome, UK)*; Wellconal.

NOTE. The *UK* preparation Marzine now contains cinnarizine instead of cyclizine.

6124-v

Cyproheptadine Hydrochloride *(BANM, USAN, rINNM)*.

Cyproheptadini Chloridum. 4-(5*H*-Dibenzo[*a,d*]-cyclohepten-5-ylidene)-1-methylpiperidine hydrochloride sesquihydrate.

$C_{21}H_{21}N,HCl,1\frac{1}{2}H_2O=350.9$.

CAS — 129-03-3 (cyproheptadine); 969-33-5 (hydrochloride, anhydrous); 41354-29-4 (hydrochloride, sesquihydrate).

Pharmacopoeias. In *Br., Ind., Jpn, Nord.,* and *U.S.*

A white to slightly yellow, odourless or almost odourless, crystalline powder. Anhydrous cyproheptadine hydrochloride 10 mg is approximately equivalent to 11 mg of cyproheptadine hydrochloride. The *U.S.P.* syrup has a pH of 3.5 to 4.5. **Soluble** 1 in 275 of water, 1 in 35 of alcohol, and 1 in 1.5 of methyl alcohol; soluble in chloroform; practically insoluble in ether.

Adverse Effects, Treatment, and Precautions

As for the antihistamines in general, p.443.

Increased appetite and weight gain may occur with cyproheptadine; this effect has been used clinically.

INTERFERENCE WITH DIAGNOSTIC TESTS. Cyproheptadine reduced hypoglycaemia-induced growth hormone secretion between 5 and 97% in 8 volunteers. It was suggested that if patients receiving cyproheptadine were given a pituitary function test which used growth hormone response to insulin-induced hypoglycaemia, then cyproheptadine therapy should be stopped before the test.— C. H. Bivens *et al., New Engl. J. Med.,* 1973, *289,* 236.

Absorption and Fate

As for the antihistamines in general, see p.444. Between 2 and 20% of the dose has been reported to be excreted in the faeces.

Uses and Administration

Cyproheptadine has the properties and uses of antihistamines (see p.443). It has potent antihistamine and serotonin-antagonist properties. It also has antimuscarinic activity and is reported to have calcium-channel blocking activity. It is used to suppress the symptoms of allergic reactions and is effective in cold urticaria. It has been used as an appetite stimulant particularly in anorexia nervosa. Other uses are the prophylaxis and treatment of vascular and migraine headaches and the treatment of Cushing's disease secondary to pituitary disorders. The mode of action of cyproheptadine is complex and not fully understood but part of its activity has been attributed to its anti-serotonin property.

The dose in adults, expressed as anhydrous cyproheptadine hydrochloride, is initially 4 mg three times a day increasing as necessary. The average dose requirement is 12 to 16 mg per day in three or four divided doses, but doses of up to 32 mg may occasionally be necessary. The dose for children aged 2 to 6 years is 2 mg two to three times a day increasing to a maximum of 12 mg per day and for children aged 7 to 14 years, 4 mg two or three times a day up to a maximum of 16 mg per day. Cyproheptadine is not recommended in children under 2 years of age, or in debilitated elderly patients. Doses from the lower end of each dose range have been used to stimulate the appetite. The pyridoxal phosphate salt of cyproheptadine dihexazine, has also been used as an appetite stimulant.

A review of the actions of serotonin on the vascular system and reference to the effects of cyproheptadine on migraine, arterial hypertension, and the carcinoid syndrome.— D. S. Houston and P. M. Vanhoutte, *Drugs,* 1986, *31,* 149.

ACANTHOSIS NIGRICANS. A favourable response to cyproheptadine 4 mg three times a day and topical corticosteroids in one patient with acanthosis nigricans associated with adenocarcinomas of the stomach and prostate and despite progression of metastatic disease.— R. Greenwood and F. C. Tring, *Br. J. Derm.,* 1982, *106,* 697.

ACROMEGALY. Cyproheptadine 4 mg every 6 hours for 2 days decreased plasma concentrations of growth hormone during oral glucose tolerance tests in 4 of 6 patients with acromegaly.— J. M. Feldman *et al., Clin. Endocr.,* 1976, *5,* 71.

ALDOSTERONISM. Suppression of aldosterone by cyproheptadine in idiopathic aldosteronism.— M. D. Gross *et al., New Engl. J. Med.,* 1981, *305,* 181.

ANOREXIA NERVOSA. There is conflicting evidence of the effectiveness of cyproheptadine in the management of anorexia nervosa. Vigersky and Loriaux (in *Anorexia Nervosa,* R.A. Vigersky (Ed.), New York, Raven, 1977, p.349) found no effect whereas Goldberg *et al.* (Br. J. Psychiat., 1979, *134,* 67) and Halmi *et al.* (Lancet, 1982, *1,* 1357) did. Despite these different findings, Herzog and Copeland (New Engl. J. Med., 1985, *313,* 295) considered cyproheptadine to be an attractive treatment of anorexia nervosa because of its relatively benign adverse effects.

CARCINOID SYNDROME. Cyproheptadine 4 mg three times a day and fenclonine 500 mg four times daily were given for 48 hours before hepatic arterial embolisation to 13 patients with severe symptoms of carcinoid syndrome to prevent complications arising from release of tumour metabolites. Treatment was discontinued four or five days after embolisation, and was successful in all but one patient.— P. N. Maton *et al., Br. med. J.,* 1983, *287,* 932 and 1664.

Two of 7 patients with carcinoid tumour or apudoma achieved objective remissions with regression of tumours when treated with cyproheptadine.— A. L. Harris and I. E. Smith, *Br. med. J.,* 1982, *285,* 475.

CUSHING'S DISEASE. Cushing's disease improved with cyproheptadine in incremental doses rising to 8 mg three times a day in 3 patients who had previously been treated surgically. Two patients who had had no previous treatment showed no improvement with cyproheptadine.— J. Marek *et al.* (letter), *Lancet,* 1977, *2,* 653.

Excellent clinical and biochemical response was obtained in a patient with Cushing's syndrome treated with cyproheptadine administered incrementally up to a dose of 24 mg daily. Treatment was continued for 22 months and the patient was still in continuing remission 40 months after stopping treatment. Although spontaneous remission could not be ruled out, there was reasonable circumstantial evidence that cyproheptadine had produced the remission in this patient.— D. N. Griffith and E. J. Ross (letter), *New Engl. J. Med.,* 1981, *305,* 893.

Nelson's syndrome. Reports of favourable responses to cyproheptadine in Nelson's syndrome.— W. Hartwig *et al.* (letter), *New Engl. J. Med.,* 1976, *295,* 394; D. T. Krieger (letter), *ibid;* N. Aronin and D. T. Krieger, *ibid.,* 1980, *302,* 453. No response.— J. Cassar *et al.* (letter), *Lancet,* 1976, *2,* 426.

DEPRESSION. Evidence that cyproheptadine may be effective for a subgroup of depressed patients with pituitary-adrenal disinhibition as demonstrated by dexamethasone suppression.— S. Bansal and W. A. Brown (letter), *Lancet,* 1983, *2,* 803.

GALACTORRHOEA-AMENORRHOEA SYNDROME. Beneficial results in 12 of 15 women with galactorrhoea-amenorrhoea syndrome treated with cyproheptadine 16 to 24 mg daily.— J. Wortsman *et al., Ann. intern. Med.,* 1979, *90,* 923. Cyproheptadine 16 to 24 mg per day did not cause significant decreases in serum prolactin concentrations in 5 patients with pituitary adenomas. Cyproheptadine was not considered to be the treatment of choice for galactorrhoea-amenorrhoea syndrome.— L. I. Dolman (letter), *Ann. intern. Med.,* 1979, *91,* 927.

MIGRAINE. Cyproheptadine has been used for prophylaxis of migraine in children, but is too sedating for most adults.— *Med. Lett.,* 1984, *26,* 95.

VIRILISING CONGENITAL ADRENAL HYPERPLASIA. In two adult patients with virilising congenital adrenal hyperplasia serum concentrations of androgens returned to normal and there was significant clinical improvement when cyproheptadine 16 mg daily in divided doses was added to the regular corticosteroid regimen.— T. -H. Hsu, *Ann. intern. Med.,* 1980, *92,* 628.

Preparations

Cyproheptadine Hydrochloride Syrup *(U.S.P.)*

Cyproheptadine Hydrochloride Tablets *(U.S.P.)*

Cyproheptadine Tablets *(B.P.).* Tablets containing cyproheptadine hydrochloride.

Proprietary Preparations

Periactin *(Merck Sharp & Dohme, UK). Tablets,* scored, cyproheptadine hydrochloride equivalent to anhydrous cyproheptadine hydrochloride 4 mg. *Syrup,* cyproheptadine hydrochloride equivalent to anhydrous cyproheptadine hydrochloride 2 mg/5 mL.

Proprietary Names and Manufacturers

Antegan *(Austral.)*; Cipractin *(Andromaco, Spain)*; Histatets *(Pharmadrug, Ger.)*; Ifrasarl *(Jpn)*; Nuran *(Frosst, Ger.)*; Périactine *(Merck Sharp & Dohme-Chibret, Fr.)*; Periactin *(Arg.; Frosst, Austral.; Belg.; Merck Sharp & Dohme, Canad.; Merck Sharp & Dohme, Denm.; Merck Sharp & Dohme, Ital.; Neth.; Merck Sharp & Dohme, Norw.; Merck Sharp & Dohme, S.Afr.; Sigma Tau, Spain; MSD, Swed.; Merck Sharp & Dohme, Switz.; Merck Sharp & Dohme, UK; Merck Sharp & Dohme, USA)*; Periactinol *(Frosst, Ger.)*; Peritol *(Hung.)*; Sigloton *(Spain)*; Vimicon *(Canad.)*.

The following names have been used for multi-ingredient preparations containing cyproheptadine hydrochloride— Perideca *(Merck Sharp & Dohme, UK)*.

12623-p

Danitracen *(rINN)*.

WA-335. 9,10-Dihydro-10-(1-methyl-4-piperidylidene)-9-anthrol.

$C_{20}H_{21}NO=291.4$.

CAS — 31232-26-5.

Danitracen, which is structurally related to cyproheptadine, has antihistamine and antiserotonin properties.

6125-g

Deptropine Citrate *(BANM, rINNM)*.

BS-6987; Dibenzheptropine Citrate. (1*R*,3*r*,5*S*)-3-(10,11-Dihydro-5*H*-dibenzo[*a,d*]cyclohepten-5-yloxy)tropane dihydrogen citrate.

$C_{23}H_{27}NO,C_6H_8O_7=525.6$.

CAS — 604-51-3 (deptropine); 2169-75-7 (citrate).

Deptropine citrate is an antihistamine with marked antimuscarinic action; it is mainly used in the treatment of asthma and bronchitis.

Deptropine citrate has been given by mouth in doses of 0.5 to 1 mg twice daily. It has also been given by aerosol inhalation.

Proprietary Names and Manufacturers

Brontin *(Formenti, Ital.)*; Brontina *(Brocades, UK)*; Brontine *(Belg.; Neth.)*.

The following names have been used for multi-ingredient preparations containing deptropine citrate— Brontisol *(Brocades, UK)*.

6128-s

Dimenhydrinate *(BAN, USAN, rINN)*.

Chloranautine; Diphenhydramine Theoclate; Diphenhydramini Teoclas. The diphenhydramine salt of 8-chlorotheophylline.

$C_{17}H_{21}NO,C_7H_7ClN_4O_2=470.0$.

CAS — 523-87-5.

Pharmacopoeias. In *Arg., Br., Braz., Chin., Egypt., Ind., Int., Jpn,* and *U.S.*

A white odourless crystalline powder. M.p. 102° to 107°.

Soluble 1 in 95 of water, 1 in 2 of alcohol, and 1

in 2 of chloroform; sparingly soluble in ether. The injection is a solution in a mixture of propylene glycol and water and is **sterilised** by maintaining at 98° to 100° for 30 minutes. The *B.P.* injection contains 5% benzyl alcohol and has a pH of 6.8 to 7.2. The *U.S.P.* injection has a pH of 6.4 to 7.2. **Store** in airtight containers.

Dimenhydrinate is reported in early studies to be **incompatible** in solution with a wide range of compounds; those most likely to be encountered with dimenhydrinate include: iodipamide, aminophylline, prednisolone sodium phosphate, hydroxyzine, hydrocortisone sodium succinate, phenothiazines, and soluble barbiturates.

Adverse Effects, Treatment, Precautions, and Absorption and Fate

As for the antihistamines in general, p.443.

Dimenhydrinate was considered to be unsafe for use in acute porphyrias and has been associated with clinical exacerbations of porphyria.— M. R. Moore and P. B. Disler, *Adverse Drug React. Ac. Pois. Rev.*, 1983, *2*, 149. See also M.R. Moore and K.E.L. McColl, *Porphyrias, Drug Lists*, Glasgow, Porphyria Research Unit, University of Glasgow, 1987.

EFFECTS ON THE EYES. Dimenhydrinate 100 mg 4 hourly was found to affect colour discrimination, night vision, reaction time, and stereopsis.— S. M. Luria *et al.*, *Br. J. clin. Pharmac.*, 1979, *7*, 585.

PREGNANCY AND THE NEONATE. Of 50 282 children born to mothers monitored by the Collaborative Perinatal Project, 5773 were found to have been exposed to xanthines at some time during the first 4 months of the pregnancy. Although no association was seen between malformations and exposures to xanthines in general a relationship between cardiovascular defects and inguinal hernia and dimenhydrinate exposure (319 children) was noted.— O. P. Heinonen *et al.*, *Birth Defects and Drugs in Pregnancy*, Littleton MA, Publishing Sciences Group, 1977, p. 366.

Uses and Administration

Dimenhydrinate is diphenhydramine theoclate and has the general properties of the antihistamines (p.444). It is used mainly as an anti-emetic in the prevention and treatment of motion sickness. It is also used for the symptomatic treatment of nausea and vertigo due to Ménière's disease and other labyrinthine disturbances.

For motion sickness, dimenhydrinate 50 to 100 mg is given by mouth at least 30 minutes before the journey. This dose may be repeated every 4 hours if required, but a total daily dose of 300 mg should not usually be exceeded. For the treatment of Ménière's disease, 50 mg has been given three times a day. Similar doses may be given rectally or by intramuscular injection. The doses for children are: 1 to 6 years, 12.5 to 25 mg two or three times daily; 7 to 12 years, 25 to 50 mg two or three times daily. In extreme emergency the injection may be diluted to 0.5% with sodium chloride injection and given by slow intravenous injection over 2 minutes. This dose may be repeated 4-hourly if necessary.

Preparations

Dimenhydrinate Injection *(B.P.)*
Dimenhydrinate Injection *(U.S.P.)*
Dimenhydrinate Syrup *(U.S.P.)*
Dimenhydrinate Tablets *(B.P., U.S.P.)*

Proprietary Preparations

Dramamine *(Searle, UK). Tablets*, scored, dimenhydrinate 50 mg.

Proprietary Names and Manufacturers

Amalmare *(Ital.)*; Amosyt *(Neth.; Leo, Swed.)*; Anautin *(DAK, Denm.)*; Andrumin *(Cilag, Austral.)*; Antemin *(Switz.)*; Aviomarine *(Pol.)*; Azules *(Spain)*; Biodramina *(Uriach, Spain)*; Contramareo *(Orravan, Spain)*; Dimate *(Reid-Provident, USA)*; Dramamine *(Searle, Austral.; Belg.; Canad.; Searle, Fr.; Searle, Ger.; Neth.; Searle, S.Afr.; Searle, Spain; Searle, Switz.; Searle, UK; Richardson-Vicks, USA)*; Dramarr *(Spain)*; Dramavir *(Spain)*; Dramocen *(Central Pharmaceuticals, USA)*; Dromyl *(Norw.)*; Epha-Retard *(Woelm, Ger.)*; Gravol *(Horner, Canad.; Pharmax, UK)*; Lomarin *(Geymonat, Ital.)*; Mareosan *(Cinfa, Spain)*; Mareozina Retard *(Spain)*; Marolin *(Spain)*; Nauseatol *(Sabex, Canad.)*; Nausicalm *(Brothier, Fr.)*; Neptusan *(Denm.)*; Nico-Vert *(Edwards, USA)*; Novodimenate *(Novopharm, Canad.)*; Novodramin *(Nessa, Spain)*; Novomina *(Ger.)*; Pastillas Azules *(Llano, Spain)*; Travamine *(ICN, Canad.)*; Travelgum *(Farmades, Ital.)*; Trawell *(Chemofux, Switz.)*; Valontan *(Recordati, Ital.)*; Vomex *(Searle, Ger.)*; Xamamina *(Zambeletti, Ital.)*.

The following names have been used for multi-ingredient preparations containing dimenhydrinate— Decadol *(Cambridge Laboratories, Austral.)*; Travacalm *(Hamilton, Austral.)*.

6129-w

Dimethindene Maleate *(BANM, USAN)*.

Dimethpyrindene Maleate; Dimethylpyrindene Maleate; Dimetindene Maleate *(rINNM)*; NSC-107677; Su-6518. *NN*-Dimethyl-2-{3-[1-(2-pyridyl)ethyl]-1*H*-inden-2-yl}ethylamine hydrogen maleate.
$C_{20}H_{24}N_2,C_4H_4O_4$=408.5.

CAS — 5636-83-9 (dimethindene); 3614-69-5 (maleate).

Dimethindene maleate is an alkylamine derivative with the properties and uses of the antihistamines (see p.443). It is given by mouth for the symptomatic treatment of allergic conditions in usual doses of 2.5 mg twice daily as a sustained-release preparation. It is also applied in nasal preparations.

Proprietary Preparations

Fenostil-Retard *(Zyma, UK). Tablets*, sustained-release, dimethindene maleate 2.5 mg.

Proprietary Names and Manufacturers

Fengel *(Zyma, Ital.)*; Fenistil *(Belg.; Zyma, Denm.; Zyma, Ger.; Zyma, Ital.; Neth.; Zyma, Norw.; Frumtost, Spain; Zyma, Swed.; Zyma, Switz.)*; Fenostil *(Zyma, Austral.; S.Afr.)*; Fenostil-Retard *(Zyma, UK)*; Forhistal *(Canad.; USA)*; Triten *(USA)*.

The following names have been used for multi-ingredient preparations containing dimethindene maleate— Vibrocil *(Zyma, UK)*.

6130-m

Dimethothiazine Mesylate *(BANM)*.

8599-R.P. *(dimethothiazine)*; Dimetotiazine Mesilate *(rINNM)*; Fonazine Mesylate *(USAN)*; IL-6302 *(dimethothiazine)*. 10-(2-Dimethylaminopropyl)-*NN*-dimethylphenothiazine-2-sulphonamide methanesulphonate.
$C_{19}H_{25}N_3O_2S_2,CH_3SO_3H$=487.6.

CAS — 7456-24-8 (dimethothiazine); 7455-39-2; 13115-40-7 (both mesylate).

Dimethothiazine mesylate is a phenothiazine derivative with the properties and uses of the antihistamines (see p.443). It has been used for allergies in doses equivalent to 20 mg of dimethothiazine three times daily, increasing if necessary. Total daily doses of up to 120 mg have been given. Dimethothiazine has also been used in the prophylaxis and treatment of migraine.

Proprietary Names and Manufacturers

Alius *(Scharper, Ital.)*; Banistyl *(Austral.; May & Baker, S.Afr.; May & Baker, UK)*; Bisbermin *(Jpn)*; Bonpac *(Jpn)*; Calsekin *(Jpn)*; Migrethiazin *(Jpn)*; Migristene *(Arg.; Belg.; Specia, Fr.; Ger.; Jpn; Rhone, Spain; Rhône-Poulenc, Switz.)*; Neomestin *(Jpn)*; Normelin *(Jpn)*; Promaquid *(Rhône-Poulenc, Canad.)*; Yoristen *(Jpn)*.

6131-b

Diphenhydramine Hydrochloride *(BANM, USAN, rINNM)*.

Benzhydramine Hydrochloride; Dimedrolum; Diphenhydramini Hydrochloridum; Diphenhydraminium Chloride. 2-Benzhydryloxy-*NN*-dimethylethylamine hydrochloride.
$C_{17}H_{21}NO,HCl$=291.8.

CAS — 58-73-1 (diphenhydramine); 147-24-0 (hydrochloride).

Pharmacopoeias. In *Aust., Belg., Br., Braz., Chin., Egypt., Eur., Fr., Ind., Int., It., Jpn, Jug., Mex., Neth., Nord., Pol., Port., Rus., Swiss, Turk.*, and *U.S. Jpn* also includes Diphenhydramine and Diphenhydramine Tannate. *U.S.* also includes Diphenhydramine Citrate.

A white or almost white, odourless or almost odourless, crystalline powder. It slowly darkens on exposure to light.

Soluble 1 in 1 of water, 1 in 2 of alcohol, 1 in 50 of acetone, and 1 in 2 of chloroform; very slightly soluble or practically insoluble in ether. A 5% solution in water has a pH of 4.0 to 6.0. **Store** in airtight containers. Protect from light.

Incompatibility has been reported with amphotericin, cephalothin sodium, hydrocortisone sodium succinate, some soluble barbiturates, some contrast media, and solutions of acids and alkalis.

Adverse Effects

As for the antihistamines in general, p.443. Diphenydramine has been reported to cause thrombocytopenia.

ABUSE. Abuse of diphenhydramine preparations has been reported in Scandinavia.— *Br. med. J.*, 1979, *1*, 459.

Report of abuse of diphenhydramine combined with butorphanol by injection.— S. G. Smith and W. M. Davis (letter), *J. Am. med. Ass.*, 1984, *252*, 1010.

A 34-year-old man took increasing doses of diphenhydramine over a six-month period up to 800 mg twice daily. Results of medical examinations were unremarkable except for a heart-rate of 114 beats per minute. A rapid tapering of the dose resulted in return of insomnia and increased daytime restlessness. Increased defaecation was the only muscarinic rebound effect noted.— M. D. Feldman and M. Behar (letter), *J. Am. med. Ass.*, 1986, *255*, 3119.

ALLERGY. An anaphylactoid reaction characterised by dizziness, weakness, tightness in the chest, severe shortness of breath, and a cough producing frothy red sputum occurred in a patient who received diphenhydramine hydrochloride 25 mg by intravenous injection over a period of about 10 seconds.— W. H. Lauderdale *et al.*, *Archs intern. Med.*, 1964, *114*, 693.

EFFECTS ON THE BLOOD. Diphenhydramine was reported to be a haemolytic agent in subjects deficient in glucose-6-phosphate dehydrogenase but only in conjunction with other factors such as infection.— M. E. Pembrey, *Practitioner*, 1974, *213*, 647. Diphenhydramine was considered to be probably safe when given in normal therapeutic doses to patients with glucose-6-phosphate dehydrogenase deficiency.— *Ann. intern. Med.*, 1985, *103*, 245.

EXTRAPYRAMIDAL SYMPTOMS. An acute dystonic reaction occurred in a 4-year-old boy 2 hours after being given a second dose of diphenhydramine hydrochloride 25 mg. Recovery occurred after discontinuation of the drug.— B. L. Lavenstein and F. K. Cantor, *J. Am. med. Ass.*, 1976, *236*, 291.

A report of trismus and subsequent laryngospasm following intramuscular injection of diphenhydramine.— K. A. Brait and A. J. Zagerman (letter), *New Engl. J. Med.*, 1977, *296*, 111. Comment.— R. Sovner (letter), *ibid.*, 633.

OVERDOSAGE. A 16-year-old girl developed a toxic psychosis resembling acute schizophrenia after she had ingested 500 mg of diphenhydramine hydrochloride. Throughout the reaction atropine-like autonomic symptoms were evident. She recovered her normal mental state within about 29 hours.— S. A. Nigro, *J. Am. med. Ass.*, 1968, *203*, 301.

Rhabdomyolysis developed in a patient following an overdose of diphenhydramine. There was no hypotension, shock, or physical damage to the muscle.— G. Hampel *et al.*, *Hum. Toxicol.*, 1983, *2*, 197.

Reports and comments on diphenhydramine overdosage and its treatment.— H. E. Hestand and D. W. Teske, *J. Pediat.*, 1977, *90*, 1017; M. Borkenstein and M. Haidvogl (letter), *ibid.*, 1978, *92*, 167; H. E. Hestand and D. W. Teske (letter), *ibid*; E. P. Krenzelok *et al.*, *Ann. emerg. Med.*, 1982, *11*, 212 (fatal massive overdose).

PREGNANCY AND THE NEONATE. Treatment with diphenhydramine during the first trimester of pregnancy was more frequent among mothers of children with cleft palate or clefts with other defects than among control mothers, although the incidence of nausea and the overall intake of anti-emetics did not differ.— I. Saxén (letter), *Lancet*, 1974, *1*, 407.

A report of perinatal death attributed to an interaction between diphenhydramine and temazepam.— G. A. Kargas *et al.* (letter), *New Engl. J. Med.*, 1985, *313*, 1417.

For further studies on the effects of diphenhydramine and other antihistamines during pregnancy, see p.443.

Neonatal dependence. A pregnant woman who was receiving diphenhydramine hydrochloride 150 mg daily for a pruritic rash gave birth to an infant who developed diarrhoea and generalised tremulousness 5 days later. The infant had a serum-diphenhydramine concentration of 7 µg per mL and the delay in appearance of withdrawal symptoms was considered to be due to absence of full activity of glucuronyl conjugating enzymes in the first few days of life. A response was obtained to phenobarbitone and the tremulousness did not recur on withdrawal of the phenobarbitone.— D. E. Parkin (letter), *J. Pediat.*, 1974, *85*, 580.

Treatment of Adverse Effects

As for the antihistamines in general, p.443.

The adsorption of diphenhydramine by activated charcoal, 50 g led to mean reductions in peak serum concentrations of 94.8% when administered 5 minutes after diphenhydramine and 12.3% when administered 60 minutes after diphenhydramine, in 6 healthy subjects. It was considered that activated charcoal had a potential value in the treatment of diphenhydramine overdose.— D. R. P. Guay *et al.*, *Int. J. clin. Pharmac. Ther. Toxic.*, 1984, *22*, 395.

Precautions

As for the antihistamines in general, p.444.

The effect of diphenhydramine on performance.— M. Burns and H. Moskowitz, *Eur. J. clin. Pharmac.*, 1980, *17*, 259.

LACTATION. Several reviews state that although small amounts of diphenhydramine are secreted into breast milk they do not have any clinical effects on breast-fed infants; reports of clinical studies are difficult to trace.

MYASTHENIA. Diphenhydramine interfered with neuromuscular transmission under experimental conditions and although it had not been implicated clinically it should be used with caution in patients with myasthenia.— Z. Argov and F. L. Mastaglia, *New Engl. J. Med.*, 1979, *301*, 409.

Absorption and Fate

As for the antihistamines in general, p.444.

Maximum plasma-diphenhydramine concentrations ranging from 81 to 159 ng per mL were obtained 2 to 4 hours after administration of diphenhydramine hydrochloride 100 mg by mouth to 4 healthy subjects. The plasma half-life calculated over the period 4 to 24 hours after administration ranged from about 5 to 8 hours. The plasma half-life calculated for total amines gave values of about 8 to 10 hours in 3 subjects indicating that the metabolites were eliminated less rapidly than unchanged diphenhydramine. Urinary excretion of diphenhydramine metabolites was about 64% of the dose after 96 hours. Following administration of diphenhydramine hydrochloride 50 mg four times daily for 13 doses to 4 subjects plasma-diphenhydramine concentrations reached a plateau after 2 or 3 days, total amines being about twice the concentration of unchanged diphenhydramine. After the last dose the plasma half-life was about 6 hours for diphenhydramine and about 8 for total amines; the mean recovery of urinary metabolites was about 50% of the total dose, with traces detected 2 to 3 days after the last dose.— A. J. Glazko *et al.*, *Clin. Pharmac. Ther.*, 1974, *16*, 1066.

Studies in 2 healthy subjects indicated that diphenhydramine exhibits a large first-pass effect, with about 50% metabolism occurring before the drug reaches the general circulation following oral administration.— K. S. Albert *et al.*, *J. Pharmacokinet. Biopharm.*, 1975, *3*, 159.

Diphenhydramine was reported to be 98% bound to plasma proteins.— W. M. Bennett *et al.*, *Am. J. Kidney Dis.*, 1983, *3*, 155.

The bioavailability of diphenhydramine after oral administration has been found to be 42 to 62%.— D. M. Paton and D. R. Webster, *Clin. Pharmacokinet.*, 1985, *10*, 477.

Uses and Administration

Diphenhydramine hydrochloride is an ethanolamine derivative with the actions and uses of the antihistamines (see p.444). It has pronounced sedative properties. It also has anti-emetic, antimuscarinic, and local anaesthetic properties.

Diphenhydramine hydrochloride is given in usual doses of 25 to 50 mg three or four times daily. A dose of 50 mg may be used as a hypnotic. The dose for children weighing more than 9.1 kg or 20 lb is 12.5 to 25 mg three or four times a day, or a total daily dose of 5 mg per kg body-weight or 150 mg per m^2 body-surface may be given in divided doses, up to a maximum of 300 mg daily. It has also been given in severe allergies by deep intramuscular or slow intravenous injection in usual doses of 10 to 50 mg.

Diphenhydramine hydrochloride has been used for the control of parkinsonian symptoms and drug-induced extrapyramidal reactions, and for the prevention and treatment of nausea and vomiting. It is also included in preparations for symptomatic relief of coughs and the common cold, and in some topical preparations. In the UK the use of diphenhydramine and its salts in cosmetics is prohibited by law.

The theoclate, dimenhydrinate, is also used, see p.452.

ADMINISTRATION. There was a direct relationship between the mean plasma concentration of diphenhydramine and its mean sedative and antihistaminic properties in 6 healthy subjects.— S. G. Carruthers *et al.*, *Clin. Pharmac. Ther.*, 1978, *23*, 375.

ADMINISTRATION IN RENAL FAILURE. The interval between doses of diphenhydramine should be extended from 6 hours in patients with a glomerular filtration-rate (GFR) greater than 50 mL per min to 6 to 9 hours in those with a GFR of 10 to 50 mL per min and to 9 to 12 hours in those with a GFR of less than 10 mL per min.— W. M. Bennett *et al.*, *Am. J. Kidney Dis.*, 1983, *3*, 155.

CARCINOID SYNDROME. For reports of the use of diphenhydramine in carcinoid syndrome, see Cimetidine, p.1085.

EXTRAPYRAMIDAL SYMPTOMS. For reference to the beneficial role of diphenhydramine in controlling dystonic reactions to metoclopramide, see Metoclopramide Hydrochloride, p.1098.

GALL STONES. Diphenhydramine enhanced dissolution of compressed cholesterol in sodium cholate solution and ox bile *in vitro*; this might indicate an application in gallstone dissolution.— R. O. King *et al.*, *Gut*, 1984, *25*, A575.

NAUSEA AND VOMITING. For mention of the use of diphenhydramine in combination with metoclopramide as an anti-emetic during cancer chemotherapy, see Metoclopramide Hydrochloride, p.1100.

PAIN. Diphenhydramine has been used in combination with paracetamol in a "Pain Cocktail".— G. M. Wyant, *Drugs*, 1983, *26*, 262.

Preparations

Diphenhydramine Capsules *(B.P.)*. Capsules containing diphenhydramine hydrochloride.

Diphenhydramine Hydrochloride Capsules *(U.S.P.)*

Diphenhydramine Oral Solution *(B.P.)*. Diphenhydramine Elixir. A solution of diphenhydramine hydrochloride in a suitable flavoured vehicle.

Diphenhydramine Elixir *(A.P.F.)*. Contains diphenhydramine hydrochloride 10 mg in 5 mL.

Diphenhydramine and Pseudoephedrine Elixir *(A.P.F.)*. Contains diphenhydramine hydrochloride 10 mg and pseudoephedrine hydrochloride 30 mg in 5 mL.

Diphenhydramine Hydrochloride Elixir *(U.S.P.)*

Diphenhydramine Hydrochloride Injection *(U.S.P.)*

Proprietary Preparations

Benadryl *(Parke, Davis, UK)*. *Capsules*, diphenhydramine hydrochloride 25 mg.

Benylin Day and Night Cold Treatment *(Warner-Lambert, UK)*. *Tablets* (yellow, day-time), paracetamol 500 mg, phenylpropanolamine hydrochloride 25 mg. *Tablets* (blue, night-time), diphenhydramine hydrochloride 25 mg, paracetamol 500 mg.

Benylin Decongestant *(Warner-Lambert, UK)*. *Syrup*, diphenhydramine hydrochloride 14 mg, pseudoephedrine hydrochloride 10 mg, sodium citrate 57 mg, menthol 1.1 mg/5 mL.

Benylin Expectorant *(Warner-Lambert, UK)*. *Syrup*, diphenhydramine hydrochloride 14 mg, ammonium chloride 135 mg, sodium citrate 57 mg, menthol 1.1 mg/5 mL.

Benylin Fortified *(Warner-Lambert, UK)*. *Linctus*, diphenhydramine hydrochloride 14 mg, dextromethorphan hydrobromide 6.5 mg, sodium citrate 57 mg, menthol 1.1 mg/5 mL.

Benylin Mentholated *(Warner-Lambert, UK)*. *Linctus*, diphenhydramine hydrochloride 14 mg, dextromethorphan hydrobromide 6.5 mg, pseudoephedrine hydrochloride 22.5 mg, menthol 1.75 mg/5 mL.

Benylin Paediatric *(Warner-Lambert, UK)*. *Syrup*, diphenhydramine hydrochloride 7 mg, sodium citrate 28.5 mg, menthol 550 µg/5 mL.

Benylin with Codeine *(Warner-Lambert, UK)*. *Syrup*, diphenhydramine hydrochloride 14 mg, codeine phosphate 5.7 mg, sodium citrate 57 mg, menthol 1.1 mg/5 mL.

Caladryl *(Warner-Lambert, UK)*. *Cream*, diphenhydramine hydrochloride 1%, calamine 8%, camphor 0.1%. *Lotion*, diphenhydramine hydrochloride 1%, calamine 8%, camphor 0.1%.

Guanor *(R.P. Drugs, UK)*. *Syrup*, diphenhydramine hydrochloride 14 mg, ammonium chloride 135 mg, sodium citrate 57 mg, menthol 1.1 mg/5 mL.

Guanor Paediatric *(R.P. Drugs, UK)*. *Syrup*, diphenhydramine hydrochloride 7 mg, sodium citrate 28.5 mg, menthol 550 µg/5 mL.

Histalix Expectorant *(Wallace Mfg Chem., UK)*. *Syrup*, diphenhydramine hydrochloride 14 mg, ammonium chloride 135 mg, sodium citrate 57 mg, menthol 1.1 mg/5 mL.
Paediatric syrup, diphenhydramine hydrochloride 7 mg, ammonium chloride 67.5 mg, sodium citrate 28.5 mg, menthol 550 µg/5 mL.

Histergan *(Norma, UK)*. *Tablets*, diphenhydramine hydrochloride 25 mg.
Syrup, diphenhydramine hydrochloride 10, 12.5, and 14 mg/5 mL.
Cream, diphenhydramine hydrochloride 2%.

Lotussin *(Searle, UK)*. *Linctus*, diphenhydramine hydrochloride 5 mg, dextromethorphan hydrobromide 6.25 mg, ephedrine hydrochloride 7.5 mg, guaiphenesin 50 mg/5 mL.

Proprietary Names and Manufacturers of Diphenhydramine Salts

Alergicap *(Austral.)*; Allerdryl *(ICN, Canad.; Legere, USA)*; Allergan *(Bouty, Ital.)*; Allergina *(De Angeli, Ital.)*; Amidryl *(Denm.)*; BayDryl *(Bay, USA)*; Benadryl *(Arg.; Parke, Davis, Austral.; Belg.; Parke, Davis, Canad.; Denm.; Ital.; Neth.; Parke, Davis, S.Afr.; Parke, Davis, Spain; Swed.; Parke, Davis, Switz.; Parke, Davis, UK; Parke, Davis, USA)*; Benocten *(Medinova, Switz.)*; Benylin *(Parke, Davis, Canad.; Substantia, Fr.; Parke, Davis, USA)*; Betasleep *(Restan, S.Afr.)*; Cathejell *(Switz.)*; Dermistina *(Ital.)*; Desentol *(Leo, Swed.)*; Dibadorm *(Kettelhack Riker, Ger.)*; Dihydral *(SCS, S.Afr.)*; Dobacen *(Switz.)*; Dolestan *(Ger.)*; Felben *(Switz.)*; Halbmond *(Ger.)*; Histergan *(Norma, UK)*; Insomnal *(Welcker-Lyster, Canad.)*; Lensen *(USA)*; Lipworth Sleepcaps *(Bovit, S.Afr.)*; Miles Nervine *(Miles Laboratories, USA)*; Neo-Synodorm *(Switz.)*; Pellisal *(Engelhard, Ger.)*; Pheramin *(Kanoldt, Ger.)*; S.8 *(Chefaro, Ger.)*; Sediat *(Pfleger, Ger.)*; Sekundal *(Rorer, Ger.)*; Selodorm *(Kanoldt, Ger.)*; Somenox *(Switz.)*; Somnium *(Canad.)*; Teldrin *(Ralay, Spain)*; Valdrene *(Vale, USA)*; Wehydryl *(Hauck, USA)*.

The following names have been used for multi-ingredient preparations containing diphenhydramine salts— Ambenyl *(Parke, Davis, Canad.)*; Benacine *(Parke, Davis, Austral.)*; Benadryl Decongestant *(Parke, Davis, USA)*; Benadryl Expectorant *(Parke, Davis, Austral.)*; Benafed *(Parke, Davis, UK)*; Benatuss *(Parke, Davis, Austral.)*; Benylets *(Parke, Davis, UK)*; Benylin Day and Night Cold Treatment *(Warner-Lambert, UK)*; Benylin Decongestant *(Parke, Davis, Canad.; Warner-Lambert, UK)*; Benylin Expectorant *(Parke, Davis, Canad.; Warner-Lambert, UK)*; Benylin Fortified *(Warner-Lambert, UK)*; Benylin Mentholated *(Warner-Lambert, UK)*; Benylin Paediatric *(Warner-Lambert, UK)*; Benylin with Codeine *(Warner-Lambert, UK)*; Benylin-DM *(Parke, Davis, Canad.)*; Benyphed *(Parke, Davis, Austral.)*; Bidramine *(Nelson, Austral.)*; Caladryl *(Parke, Davis, Canad.; Warner-Lambert, UK; Parke, Davis, USA)*; Calmasol *(Ethipharm, Canad.)*; Calmylin with codeine *(Technilab, Canad.)*; Delixir *(Hamilton, Austral.)*; Dolvan *(Norma, UK)*; Dytuss *(Lasalle, USA)*; Ephedramine *(Drug Houses Austral., Austral.)*; Ergodryl *(Parke, Davis, Austral.; Parke, Davis, Canad.; Parke, Davis, UK)*; Exedrin P.M. *(Bristol-Myers Products, USA)*; Globolotion *(R.P. Drugs, UK)*; Guanor *(R.P. Drugs, UK)*; Guanor Paediatric *(R.P. Drugs, UK)*;
Histalix Expectorant *(Wallace Mfg Chem., UK)*; Lotussin *(Searle, UK)*; Mandrax *(Roussel, Canad.; Roussel, UK)*; Noradran *(Norma, UK)*; Pharmidone *(Farmitalia Carlo Erba, UK)*; Propain *(Panpharma, UK)*; Sedu-Caps-D *(Lederle, Austral.)*; Ticipect *(Ticen, Eire)*; Tinol *(Ticen, Eire)*; Uniflu *(Unigreg, UK)*; Ziradryl *(Parke, Davis, Canad.; Parke, Davis, USA)*.

12669-f

Diphenhydramine Di(acefyllinate)
Bietanautine. Diphenhydramine bis(theophyllin-7-ylacetate).
$C_{17}H_{21}NO,2C_9H_{10}N_4O_4$=731.8.

CAS — 6888-11-5.

NOTE. The name Etanautine was formerly applied to diphenhydramine monoacefyllinate; it is now applied to ethylbenzhydramine, see p.532.

Diphenhydramine di(acefyllinate) is a derivative of diphenhydramine (p.452) which has been used as an anti-emetic.

Proprietary Names and Manufacturers
Nautamine *(Delagrange, Fr.).*

6132-v

Diphenylpyraline Hydrochloride *(BANM, USAN, rINNM).*

4-Benzhydryloxy-1-methylpiperidine hydrochloride.
$C_{19}H_{23}NO,HCl$=317.9.

CAS — 147-20-6 (diphenylpyraline); 132-18-3 (hydrochloride).

Pharmacopoeias. In *Br., Ind.,* and *U.S.*

A white or almost white, odourless or almost odourless, crystalline powder. **Soluble** 1 in 1 of water, 1 in 3 of alcohol, and 1 in 2 of chloroform; practically insoluble in ether. **Store** in airtight containers. Protect from light.

Adverse Effects, Treatment, Precautions, and Absorption and Fate
As for the antihistamines in general, p.443.

Uses and Administration
Diphenylpyraline hydrochloride is a piperidine derivative with the actions and uses of the antihistamines (see p.444). It is given in sustained-release preparations in doses of 5 to 10 mg twice daily. Children over 6 years of age have been given 5 mg daily in single or divided doses. The theoclate, known as piprinhydrinate, is also used (see p.458).
In the *UK* the use of diphenylpyraline and its salts in cosmetics is prohibited by law.

Preparations
Diphenylpyraline Hydrochloride Tablets *(U.S.P.)*

Proprietary Preparations
Histryl *(Smith Kline & French, UK). Spansules,* sustained-release capsules, diphenylpyraline hydrochloride 5 mg.
Paediatric spansules, sustained-release capsules, diphenylpyraline hydrochloride 2.5 mg.
Lergoban *(Riker, UK). Tablets,* sustained-release, diphenylpyraline hydrochloride 5 mg.

Proprietary Names and Manufacturers
Allerzine *(Faulding, Austral.)*; Anti-H *(Belg.)*; Anti-Hist *(Austral.)*; Dayfen *(Arg.)*; Diafen *(Riker, USA)*; Hispril *(Smith Kline & French, USA)*; Histalert *(Riker, Austral.; Riker, S.Afr.)*; Histryl *(Austral.; Belg.; S.Afr.; Smith Kline & French, UK)*; Kolton *(Ger.)*; Lergoban *(Belg.; Neth.; Riker, UK)*; Lyssipoll *(Ger.; Lyssia, Switz.).*

The following names have been used for multi-ingredient preparations containing diphenylpyraline hydrochloride—Biohisdex DHC *(Everest, Canad.)*; Biohisdex DM *(Everest, Canad.)*; Biohisdine *(Everest, Canad.)*; Biohisdine DHC *(Everest, Canad.)*; Biohisdine DM *(Everest, Canad.)*; Chemhisdex C *(Clark, Canad.)*; Chemhisdex-DHC *(Clark, Canad.)*; Chemhisdex-DHC-Expectorant *(Clark, Canad.)*; Chemhisdex-DM *(Clark, Canad.)*; Chemhisdine-DHC-Child *(Clark, Canad.)*; Chemhisdine-DHC-Expectorant *(Clark, Canad.)*; Chemhisdine-DM *(Clark, Canad.)*; Codalin *(Clark, Canad.)*; Coristine-DH *(Technilab, Canad.)*; Creo-Rectal *(Nadeau, Canad.)*; Eskornade *(Smith Kline & French, Austral.; Smith Kline & French, UK)*; Expansyl *(Smith Kline & French, UK)*; Novahistex DH *(Dow, Canad.)*; Novahistine DH *(Dow, Canad.)*; Sinuzets with Antihistamine *(Boots, Austral.).*

6133-g

Doxylamine Succinate *(BANM, USAN, rINNM).*

Doxylaminium Succinate; Histadoxylamine Succinate. *NN*-Dimethyl-2-[α-methyl-α-(2-pyridyl)benzyloxy] ethylamine hydrogen succinate.
$C_{17}H_{22}N_2O,C_4H_6O_4$=388.5.

CAS — 469-21-6 (doxylamine); 562-10-7 (succinate).

Pharmacopoeias. In *Arg.* and *U.S.*

A white or creamy-white powder with a characteristic odour. **Soluble** 1 in 1 of water, 1 in 2 of alcohol and of chloroform, and 1 in 370 of ether. **Protect** from light.

Adverse Effects, Treatment, Precautions, and Absorption and Fate
As for the antihistamines in general, p.443. The controversy surrounding the use in pregnancy of combination products of doxylamine is discussed on p.443.

Uses and Administration
Doxylamine succinate is an ethanolamine derivative with the properties and uses of the antihistamines (see p.444). It has pronounced sedative effects.
Doxylamine succinate has been given in doses of 25 mg every 4 to 6 hours. Children over 6 years of age have been given half this dose. It has also been used as a hypnotic in a night-time dose of 25 mg.
It is no longer used in the management of nausea and vomiting of early pregnancy.
In the *UK* the use of doxylamine and its salts in cosmetics is prohibited by law.

Preparations
Doxylamine Succinate Syrup *(U.S.P.)*
Doxylamine Succinate Tablets *(U.S.P.)*

Proprietary Names and Manufacturers
Alsadorm *(Woelm, Ger.)*; Decapryn *(Merrell, UK; Merrell Dow, USA)*; Doxised *(Corvi, Ital.)*; Gittalun *(Thomae, Ger.)*; Hoggar *(Stada, Ger.)*; Mereprime *(Inibsa, Spain)*; Mereprine *(Merrell Dow, Belg.; Merrell, Fr.; Merrell, Ger.; Merrell Dow, Switz.)*; Sanalepsi-N *(Sapos, Switz.)*; Sedaplus *(Chephasaar, Ger.)*; Somnil *(Lennon, S. Afr.)*; Unisom *(Leeming, USA).*

The following names have been used for multi-ingredient preparations containing doxylamine succinate—Bendectin *(Merrell Dow, USA)*; Calmydone *(Technilab, Canad.)*; Debendox *(Merrell, UK)*; Diclectin *(Duchesnay, Canad.)*; Fiorinal *(Sandoz, Austral.)*; Mersyndol *(Merrell Dow, Austral.; Merrell Dow, Canad.)*; Nethaprin Dospan *(Merrell, UK)*; Nethaprin Expectorant *(Merrell, UK)*; Nyquil *(Richardson-Vicks, Canad.)*; Quiactin *(Merrell Dow, Austral.)*; Syndol *(Merrell, UK)*; Vicks Formula 44 *(Richardson-Vicks, Canad.).*

6134-q

Embramine Hydrochloride *(BANM, rINNM).*
Mebrophenhydramine. 2-(4-Bromo-α-methylbenzhydryloxy)-*NN*-dimethylethylamine hydrochloride.
$C_{18}H_{22}BrNO,HCl$=384.7.

CAS — 3565-72-8 (embramine); 13977-28-1 (hydrochloride).

Pharmacopoeias. In Cz. which also has the theoclate.

Embramine hydrochloride is an ethanolamine derivative with the properties and uses of the antihistamines (see p.443). It was formerly given in doses of up to 120 mg daily.

Proprietary Names and Manufacturers
Bromadryl *(Cz.)*; Mebryl *(Smith Kline & French, UK)*; Medrin *(Cz.).*

12759-n

Flunarizine Hydrochloride *(BANM, USAN, rINNM).*

R-14950. *trans*-1-Cinnamyl-4-(4,4′-difluorobenzhydryl)piperazine dihydrochloride.
$C_{26}H_{26}F_2N_2,2HCl$=477.4.

CAS — 52468-60-7 (flunarizine); 30484-77-6 (hydrochloride).

Flunarizine is the difluorinated derivative of cinnarizine. It has antihistaminic and CNS depressant effects, but it is mainly used as an inhibitor of central and peripheral vasoconstriction. This effect appears to be due to calcium blockade.

An extensive review of flunarizine. Flunarizine prevents cell damage due to calcium overload by selectively blocking the entry of calcium into the cells of various tissues. It has been found to inhibit the contractions of vascular smooth muscle, and protect endothelial cells against damage by calcium overload, protect red blood cells from membrane rigidity, and protect brain cells from the effects of hypoxia. It is this latter action which is believed to be responsible for flunarizine's activity in migraine. It has also demonstrated vestibular depressive effects and antihistaminic, anticonvulsant, and anti-arrhythmic properties. Pharmacokinetic studies have demonstrated considerable interindividual variation in steady-state plasma concentrations which could indicate extensive first-pass hepatic metabolism. Beneficial results have been obtained in the prophylaxis of migraine, peripheral venous insufficiency, occlusive arterial disease and intermittent claudication. Flunarizine has also helped patients with vertigo of central or peripheral origin. Preliminary studies suggest that flunarizine may improve cognitive function in patients with cerebrovascular disorders, but these findings need confirmation. Further comparative studies are needed to clarify the relative efficacy of flunarizine. Drowsiness was the most frequently reported adverse effect. Asthenia has been reported to occur in 1.8% of patients; other adverse effects include weight gain, depression, and gastro-intestinal disturbances.— B. Holmes *et al., Drugs,* 1984, *27,* 6.

Extrapyramidal motor signs and psychic depression were reported in 12 patients who had received flunarizine 10 to 40 mg per day for between 3 weeks and 15 months. Symptoms included parkinsonism, orofacial tardive dyskinesia, and akathisia. Partial or complete improvement of symptoms occurred after withdrawal of flunarizine.— C. Chouza *et al., Lancet,* 1986, *1,* 1303. See also J. -R. Laporte and D. Capella, *ibid., 2,* 853; idem (letter), 1987, *1,* 1324.

CEREBROVASCULAR DISORDERS. A brief review of the pharmacology and clinical effectiveness of flunarizine in cerebrovascular disorders suggesting that there is no evidence that flunarizine has a beneficial effect on the mental symptoms of dementia.— A. Spagnoli and G. Tognoni, *Drugs,* 1983, *26,* 44.

MIGRAINE. Beneficial results with flunarizine 5 mg per day when given in the treatment of a 6-year-old child with alternating hemiplegia.— P. Casaer and M. Azou (letter), *Lancet,* 1984, *2,* 579. A similar report.— P. Curatolo and R. Cusmai (letter), *ibid.,* 980.

Further references to the effect of flunarizine on migraine: P. Louis and E. L. Spierings, *Cephalalgia,* 1982, *2,* 197 (comparison with pizotifen); S. Diamond and H. Schenbaum, *Headache,* 1983, *23,* 39.

URINARY INCONTINENCE. Flunarizine 20 mg at night reduced urgency and incontinence of urine in a study involving 14 patients with idiopathic detrusor instability.— J. H. Palmer *et al., Lancet,* 1981, *2,* 279.

Proprietary Names and Manufacturers
Flerudin *(Janssen, Spain)*; Flugeral *(Italfarmaco, Ital.)*; Flunagen *(Gentili, Ital.)*; Flurpax *(Hosbon, Spain)*; Fluxarten *(Zambeletti, Ital.)*; Gradient *(Polifarma, Ital.)*; Issium *(Lifepharma, Ital.)*; Sibelium *(Janssen, Fr.; Janssen, Ger.; Janssen, Ital.; Janssen, S.Afr.; Esteve, Spain; Janssen, Switz.)*; Vasculene *(Von Boch, Ital.).*

6135-p

Halopyramine Hydrochloride *(BANM).*
Chloropyramine Hydrochloride *(rINNM). N*-(4-Chlorobenzyl)-*N'N'*-dimethyl-*N*-(2-pyridyl)ethylenediamine hydrochloride.
$C_{16}H_{20}ClN_3,HCl=326.3$.

CAS — 59-32-5 (halopyramine); 6170-42-9 (hydrochloride).

Pharmacopoeias. In *Hung., Jug.,* and *Roum.*

Halopyramine hydrochloride is an ethylenediamine derivative with the properties and uses of the antihistamines (see p.443). It has been given in divided doses of up to 150 mg daily. It has also been given by injection.

Proprietary Names and Manufacturers
Synopen *(Padro, Spain)*; Synopène *(Geigy, Switz.)*; Synpen *(Geigy, Ger.).*

6136-s

Histapyrrodine Hydrochloride *(rINNM).*
N-Benzyl-*N*-phenyl-2-(pyrrolidin-1-yl)ethylamine hydrochloride.
$C_{19}H_{24}N_2,HCl=316.9$.

CAS — 493-80-1 (histapyrrodine); 6113-17-3 (hydrochloride).

Histapyrrodine hydrochloride is an ethylenediamine derivative with the properties and uses of the antihistamines (see p.443). It has been given in a dosage of 50 to 150 mg daily in divided doses.

Proprietary Names and Manufacturers
Domistan *(Servier, Fr.).*

6137-w

Homochlorcyclizine *(BAN, rINN).*
1-(4-Chlorobenzhydryl)perhydro-4-methyl-1,4-diazepine.
$C_{19}H_{23}ClN_2=314.9$.

CAS — 848-53-3.

Pharmacopoeias. Jpn includes the hydrochloride.

Homochlorcyclizine has the properties and uses of the antihistamines (see p.443). It has been given in doses of 10 to 20 mg three times daily. The hydrochloride has also been used in similar doses.

Proprietary Names and Manufacturers
Attackmin *(Jpn)*; Clomon-S *(Jpn)*; Curosajin *(Jpn)*; Homadamon *(Jpn)*; Homochlo *(Jpn)*; Homoclicin *(Jpn)*; Homoclizine *(Jpn)*; Homoclomin *(Jpn)*; Homocolzine *(Jpn)*; Homoradin *(Jpn)*; Homorestar *(Jpn)*; Noikohis *(Jpn)*; Puradenin *(Jpn)*; Rimskin *(Jpn)*; Sacronal *(Jpn)*; Sankumin *(Jpn)*; Wicron *(Jpn).*

12834-t

Hydroxyethylpromethazine Chloride
(2-Hydroxyethyl)dimethyl[1-methyl-2-(phenothiazin-10-yl)ethyl]ammonium chloride.
$C_{19}H_{25}ClN_2OS=364.9$.

CAS — 7647-63-4 (hydroxyethylpromethazine); 2090-54-2 (chloride).

Hydroxyethylpromethazine chloride is an antihistamine.

Proprietary Names and Manufacturers
Aprobit *(Kabi, Swed.)*; Histason *(Kabi, Swed.).*

6138-e

Hydroxyzine Embonate *(BANM, rINNM).*

Hydroxyzine Pamoate *(USAN).* 2-{2-[4-(4-Chlorobenzhydryl)piperazin-1-yl]ethoxy}ethanol 4,4'-methylenebis(3-hydroxy-2-naphthoate).
$C_{21}H_{27}ClN_2O_2,C_{23}H_{16}O_6=763.3$.

CAS — 68-88-2 (hydroxyzine); 10246-75-0 (embonate).

Pharmacopoeias. In *Jpn* and *U.S.*

A light yellow almost odourless powder. Hydroxyzine embonate 170 mg is approximately equivalent to 100 mg of hydroxyzine hydrochloride. Practically **insoluble** in water, chloroform, ether, and methyl alcohol; soluble 1 in 700 of alcohol and 1 in 10 of dimethylformamide; soluble 1 in 3.5 of 10M sodium hydroxide solution. **Store** in airtight containers.

6139-l

Hydroxyzine Hydrochloride *(BANM, USAN, rINNM).*

$C_{21}H_{27}ClN_2O_2,2HCl=447.8$.

CAS — 2192-20-3.

Pharmacopoeias. In *Belg., Jug.,* and *U.S.*

A white odourless powder.

Soluble 1 in 1 of water, 1 in 4.5 of alcohol, and 1 in 13 of chloroform; slightly soluble in acetone; practically insoluble in ether. The *U.S.P.* injection has a pH of 3.5 to 6.0. **Store** in airtight containers.

Incompatibility has been reported with aminophylline, benzylpenicillin salts, chloramphenicol sodium succinate, dimenhydrinate, thioridazine, and some soluble barbiturates.

A mixture of hydroxyzine hydrochloride, chlorpromazine hydrochloride, and pethidine hydrochloride stored in glass or plastic syringes was found to be stable for 366 days at 4° and 25°.— C. A. Conklin *et al., Am. J. Hosp. Pharm.,* 1985, *42,* 339.

Adverse Effects and Treatment

As for the antihistamines in general, p.443. Drowsiness, when it occurs, is usually mild and transitory.

Intramuscular injection of hydroxyzine has been reported to cause marked local discomfort. Intravenous administration has been associated with haemolysis.

For a discussion on early suggestions that foetal abnormalities might result from the use of hydroxyzine and similar compounds, see p.443.

Accidental intra-arterial injection of hydroxyzine led to necrosis of the extremity necessitating amputation of the digits of the affected limb.— W. H. Hardesty (letter), *J. Am. med. Ass.,* 1970, *213,* 872.

EFFECTS ON THE HEART. ECG abnormalities, particularly alterations in T-waves, were associated with anxiolytic doses of hydroxyzine hydrochloride, and, were similar to those produced by thioridazine and tricyclic antidepressants.— L. E. Hollister, *Psychopharmac. Comm.,* 1975, *1,* 61.

OVERDOSAGE. A 13-month-old child who took approximately 500 to 625 mg of hydroxyzine experienced generalised seizures, sinus tachycardia, mydriasis, intermittent apnoea, and mild pyrexia. She was semi-comatose on admission to hospital. The mean plasma-hydroxyzine concentration was reported as 102.7 µg per mL 8½ hours after ingestion. General supportive care and seizure control, initially with a combination of physostigmine, 0.5 mg and diazepam 1 mg, and later by physostigmine alone, resulted in complete recovery within 72 hours.— B. E. Magera *et al., Pediatrics,* 1981, *67,* 280.

Precautions

As for the antihistamines in general, p.444. Estimations of urinary 17-hydroxycorticosteroids may be falsely elevated in patients taking hydroxyzine.

Hydroxyzine was considered to be unsafe in patients with acute porphyria because it has been shown to be porphyrinogenic in *animals* or *in vitro* systems.— M.R. Moore and K.E.L. McColl, *Porphyrias, Drug Lists,* Glasgow, Porphyria Research Unit, University of Glasgow, 1987.

Absorption and Fate

As for the antihistamines in general, p.444. It has been reported that hydroxyzine and its metabolites are excreted in the bile in *animals.*

In 4 healthy subjects given a single dose of hydroxyzine hydrochloride 100 mg the mean peak plasma-hydroxyzine concentration was 82 ng per mL at a mean of 3 hours after administration. The mean half-lives of absorption and elimination were 1.02 and 2.97 hours respectively.— H. G. Fouda *et al., J. pharm. Sci.,* 1979, *68,* 1456.

Uses and Administration

Hydroxyzine is a piperazine derivative with the actions and uses of the antihistamines (see p.444). Its main use however is as an anxiolytic. It is also used as an anti-emetic, as an adjunct to pre- and post-operative medication, and in allergic conditions, particularly pruritus. Its actions develop within 15 to 30 minutes of oral administration and last for 4 to 6 hours.

The usual doses by mouth are the equivalent of 50 to 100 mg of the hydrochloride four times a day for anxiety, 25 mg three or four times a day as required for pruritus, and 50 to 100 mg for pre- or post-operative sedation. For children over 6 years the dose is 50 to 100 mg daily in divided doses, and 50 mg daily in divided doses for those under 6 years. The pre- or post-operative sedative dose in children is 600 µg per kg body-weight. Hydroxyzine hydrochloride may also be given by deep intramuscular injection. For prompt control of anxious or hysterical adults 50 to 100 mg is injected intramuscularly initially, and the dose may be repeated every four to six hours as required. For other indications when oral administration is not practical, the intramuscular dose is 25 to 100 mg for adults and 1.1 mg per kg for children. Hydroxyzine should not be given by intravenous injection since haemolysis may result. In the *UK* the use of hydroxyzine in cosmetics is prohibited by law.

ALCOHOL AND DRUG WITHDRAWAL. A study of hydroxyzine in alcohol withdrawal.— S. L. Dilts *et al., Am. J. Psychiat.,* 1977, *134,* 92.

ALLERGY. Results suggesting a favourable response to hydroxyzine in patients with allergic rhinitis compared to placebo.— L. Schaaf *et al., J. Allergy & clin. Immunol.,* 1979, *63,* 129.

ANAESTHESIA. The incidence of postoperative nausea in 60 outpatients undergoing general anaesthesia for therapeutic abortion was 20% in a control group, 15% in a diazepam group, and 5% in a hydroxyzine group; treatment being given pre-operatively. The incidence of pre-operative nausea was 45 to 50% in all groups.— R. K. Wadhwa and B. Tantisira (letter), *J. Am. med. Ass.,* 1974, *227,* 557.

Hydroxyzine 50 mg was found to be inferior to droperidol 2.5 or 5 mg as pre-operative medication when given with either morphine or pethidine.— P. Mehta *et al., Curr. ther. Res.,* 1984, *35,* 715.

Preparations of Hydroxyzine Salts

Hydroxyzine Hydrochloride Injection *(U.S.P.)*

Hydroxyzine Hydrochloride Syrup *(U.S.P.)*

Hydroxyzine Hydrochloride Tablets *(U.S.P.)*

Hydroxyzine Pamoate Capsules *(U.S.P.).* Capsules containing hydroxyzine embonate. Potency is expressed in terms of the equivalent amount of hydroxyzine hydrochloride.

Hydroxyzine Pamoate Oral Suspension *(U.S.P.).* A suspension of hydroxyzine embonate. Potency is expressed in terms of the equivalent amount of hydroxyzine hydrochloride. Protect from light.

Proprietary Preparations

Atarax *(Pfizer, UK). Tablets,* hydroxyzine hydrochloride 10 and 25 mg.
Syrup, hydroxyzine hydrochloride 10 mg/5 mL.

Proprietary Names and Manufacturers of Hydroxyzine Hydrochloride and Hydroxyzine Embonate

Atarax *(Arg.; Pfizer, Austral.; Belg.; Pfizer, Canad.; Denm.; UCB, Fr.; UCB, Ger.; UCB, Ital.; Neth.; UCB, Norw.; UCB, Spain; UCB, Swed.; UCB, Switz.; Pfizer, UK; Roerig, USA)*; Atazina *(Panthox & Burck, Ital.)*; Aterax *(UCB, S.Afr.)*; BayRox *(Bay, USA)*; Durrax *(Dermik, USA)*; Equipose *(Pfizer, UK)*; Masmoran *(Pfizer, Ger.)*; Multipax *(Rorer, Canad.)*; Neocalma *(Ital.)*; Neucalm *(Legere, USA)*; Neurozina *(Ital.)*; Orgatrax *(Organon, USA)*; Paxistil *(Belg.)*; Sedaril *(USA)*; Vistaril *(Roerig, Swed.; Pfizer, USA; Roerig, USA).*

The following names have been used for multi-ingredient preparations containing hydroxyzine hydrochloride and hydroxyzine embonate— Enarax *(Beecham Laboratories,*

USA); Marax *(Roerig, USA)*; T.E.H. *(Geneva, USA)*; Theozine *(Schein, USA)*; Vistrax *(Pfizer, USA)*.

6140-v

Isothipendyl Hydrochloride *(BANM, rINNM)*.
NN-Dimethyl-1-(pyrido[3,2-*b*][1,4]benzothiazin-10-ylmethyl)ethylamine hydrochloride.
$C_{16}H_{19}N_3S,HCl=321.9$.

CAS — 482-15-5 (isothipendyl); 1225-60-1 (hydrochloride).

Pharmacopoeias. In *B.P.C. 1973*

A fine white odourless or almost odourless crystalline powder. **Soluble** 1 in 5 of water, 1 in 60 of alcohol, and 1 in 10 of chloroform; practically insoluble in ether. Aqueous solutions are sensitive to heat and light but are most stable at pH 4.5 to 5.0. **Protect** from light.

Isothipendyl hydrochloride is an azaphenothiazine derivative with the properties and uses of the antihistamines (see p.443). It has been given by mouth in doses of 4 to 8 mg three times daily or 12 mg in controlled-release products two or three times daily. It has also been applied topically.

Preparations

Isothipendyl Tablets *(B.P.C. 1973)*. Isothipendyl Hydrochloride Tablets

Proprietary Names and Manufacturers

Andantol *(Homburg, Belg.; Gerda, Fr.; Degussa, Ger.; Rorer, Ital.; Remedia, S.Afr.; Degussa, Switz.)*; Andanton *(Lacer, Spain)*; Nilergex *(ICI, Austral.; ICI Pharmaceuticals, UK)*.

6141-g

Mebhydrolin Napadisylate *(BANM)*.

Diazolinum; Mebhydrolin Napadisilate *(rINNM)*; Mebhydrolin Naphthalenedisulphonate. 5-Benzyl-1,2,3,4-tetrahydro-2-methyl-γ-carboline naphthalene-1,5-disulphonate.
$(C_{19}H_{20}N_2)_2,C_{10}H_8O_6S_2=841.1$.

CAS — 524-81-2 (mebhydrolin); 6153-33-9 (napadisylate).

Pharmacopoeias. In *Rus.*

Mebhydrolin napadisylate 152 mg is approximately equivalent to 100 mg of mebhydrolin.

Adverse Effects, Treatment, Precautions, and Absorption and Fate

As for the antihistamines in general, p.443.
Granulocytopenia or agranulocytosis has been reported.

Uses and Administration

Mebhydrolin napadisylate has the actions and uses of the antihistamines (see p.444). It is given in doses equivalent to 50 to 100 mg of mebhydrolin base thrice daily. Children up to 10 years old may be given 50 to 200 mg of the base daily in divided doses.

Proprietary Preparations

Fabahistin *(Bayer, UK)*. *Tablets*, mebhydrolin 50 mg.
Suspension, mebhydrolin 50 mg (as napadisylate)/5 mL.

Proprietary Names and Manufacturers

Fabahistin *(Bayer, Austral.; Bayer, S.Afr.; Bayer, UK)*; Fabahistin TRT *(Bayer, S.Afr.)*; Incidal *(Bayropharm, Ital.; Neth.)*; Incidaletten *(Neth.)*; Omeril *(Tropon, Ger.)*.

The following names have been used for multi-ingredient preparations containing mebhydrolin napadisylate—Fabahistin Plus *(Bayer, Austral.)*.

6142-q

Meclozine Hydrochloride *(BANM, pINNM)*.

Meclizine Hydrochloride *(USAN)*; Meclizinium Chloride; Meclozini Hydrochloridum; Parachloramine Hydrochloride. 1-(4-Chlorobenzhydryl)-4-(3-methylbenzyl)piperazine dihydrochloride.
$C_{25}H_{27}ClN_2,2HCl=463.9$.

CAS — 569-65-3 (meclozine); 1104-22-9 (hydrochloride, anhydrous); 31884-77-2 (hydrochloride, monohydrate).

Pharmacopoeias. In *Br.* and *Int. Braz., Ind., Jug., Nord.,* and *U.S.* specify the monohydrate. *Nord.* also includes meclozine base.

A white or slightly yellowish, almost odourless, crystalline powder. *B.P.* **solubilities** are: slightly soluble in water, 1 in 25 of alcohol, and 1 in 5 of chloroform. *U.S.P.* solubilities are: practically insoluble in water and ether; freely soluble in chloroform, acid-alcohol-water mixtures, and pyridine; slightly soluble in dilute acids and alcohol. **Store** in airtight containers.

Adverse Effects, Treatment, Precautions, and Absorption and Fate

As for the antihistamines in general, p.443. For reports of the use of antihistamines, including meclozine, in pregnancy, see p.443.

Uses and Administration

Meclozine hydrochloride is a piperazine derivative with the properties of the antihistamines (see p.444). It is used for its anti-emetic action which may last for up to 24 hours. Sedative effects are not marked.

Meclozine hydrochloride is used for the prevention and treatment of motion sickness and for the symptomatic treatment of nausea and vertigo due to Ménière's disease and other labyrinthine disturbances. It has also been used in irradiation sickness, postoperative vomiting, drug-induced nausea and vomiting, and in severe vomiting of pregnancy.

The usual dosage for motion sickness is 25 to 50 mg by mouth taken 1 hour before commencing travel.

For severe nausea and vomiting a dose of 25 to 50 mg may be required 2 or 3 times daily. A dose of 25 to 100 mg per day in divided doses is given for vertigo and labyrinthine disturbances. Meclozine was also available in a preparation containing pyridoxine.

Preparations

Meclizine Hydrochloride Tablets *(U.S.P.)*. Tablets containing meclozine hydrochloride.

Meclozine Tablets *(B.P.)*. Tablets containing meclozine hydrochloride.

Proprietary Names and Manufacturers

Ancolan *(Glaxo, Austral.)*; Antivert *(Roerig, USA)*; Bonamina *(Arg.)*; Bonamine *(Pfizer, Canad.; Pfizer, Ger.)*; Bonine *(Leeming, USA)*; Calmonal *(Heyden, Ger.)*; Chiclida *(Torrens, Spain)*; Duremesan *(Switz.)*; Navicalm *(Vesta, S.Afr.; Spain)*; Neo-Istafene *(UCB, Ital.)*; Peremesin *(Heyden, Ger.; Switz.)*; Postafen *(UCB, Denm.; UCB, Ger.; UCB, Norw.; UCB, Swed.)*; Postafene *(Belg.; Neth.)*; Ru-Vert-M *(Reid-Provident, USA)*; Supermesin *(Med. y Prod. Quím., Spain)*; Suprimal *(Neth.)*.

The following names have been used for multi-ingredient preparations containing meclozine hydrochloride—Ancoloxin *(Duncan, Flockhart, UK)*; Antivert *(Pfizer, Canad.)*.

6143-p

Medrylamine *(rINN)*.
2-(4-Methoxybenzhydryloxy)-*NN*-dimethylethylamine.
$C_{18}H_{23}NO_2=285.4$.

CAS — 524-99-2.

Medrylamine is an ethanolamine derivative with the properties of the antihistamines (see p.443). It has been given by mouth in doses of 25 to 50 mg. It has also been given rectally and applied to the skin as a 2% ointment.

Proprietary Names and Manufacturers

Postafen *(UCB, Ger.)*.

6144-s

Mepyramine Maleate *(BANM, rINNM)*.

Mepyramini Maleas; Pyranisamine Maleate; Pyrilamine Maleate *(USAN)*. *N-p*-Anisyl-*N'N'*-dimethyl-*N*-(2-pyridyl)ethylenediamine hydrogen maleate.
$C_{17}H_{23}N_3O,C_4H_4O_4=401.5$.

CAS — 91-84-9 (mepyramine); 59-33-6 (maleate).

Pharmacopoeias. In *Arg., Br., Braz., Egypt., Eur., Fr., Ind., Int., It., Neth., Nord., Swiss, Turk.,* and *U.S.* Also in *B.P. Vet.*

A white or creamy-white, crystalline powder, odourless or with a slight odour. M.p. 99° to 103°. **Soluble** 1 in 0.5 of water, 1 in 2.5 to 3.0 of alcohol, 1 in 15 of dehydrated alcohol, and 1 in 1.5 to 2.0 of chloroform; slightly or very slightly soluble in ether. A 2% solution in water has a pH of 4.9 to 5.2. Solutions are **sterilised** by autoclaving. **Incompatible** with alkalis and oxidising agents. **Store** in airtight containers. Protect from light.

Adverse Effects, Treatment, Precautions, and Absorption and Fate

As for the antihistamines in general, p.443.

Uses and Administration

Mepyramine maleate is an ethylenediamine derivative with the actions and uses of the antihistamines (see p.444).

In the treatment of allergic conditions, mepyramine maleate is usually given in doses of 100 mg three times daily; the maximum daily dose should not exceed 1 g. Lower doses are used in the USA where the daily limit is 200 mg. A dose of 25 to 50 mg has been used as a hypnotic. The dose for children, given 3 or 4 times daily, is: under 3 years of age 12.5 to 25 mg, 3 to 7 years 25 to 50 mg, and older children 25 to 75 mg. Lower doses are also recommended for children in the USA where children 6 years of age or more may be given 12.5 to 25 mg every 6 to 8 hours.

A 2% cream has been employed locally for insect bites or stings, and for allergic and pruritic skin conditions, but may cause sensitisation. If large areas are treated, absorption through the skin may be sufficient to cause side-effects. The tannate has also been used.

In a double-blind study mepyramine maleate cream 2% was no more effective than placebo in reducing pruritus, erythema, and wheal size after skin testing with allergens.— C. J. Gibbs *et al.*, *Br. med. J.*, 1983, *287*, 1427.

Preparations

Mepyramine Tablets *(B.P.)*. Tablets containing mepyramine maleate.

Pyrilamine Maleate Tablets *(U.S.P.)*. Tablets containing mepyramine maleate.

Proprietary Preparations

Anthical *(May & Baker, UK)*. *Cream*, mepyramine maleate 1.5%, zinc oxide 15%.

Anthisan *(May & Baker, UK)*. *Tablets*, mepyramine maleate 50 mg.
Cream, mepyramine maleate 2%.

Proprietary Names and Manufacturers of Mepyramine and its Salts

Allergan *(Wiedenmann, Switz.)*; Allergon *(Pharmador, S.Afr.)*; Anthisan *(May & Baker, Austral.; Denm.; Norw.; May & Baker, S.Afr.; May & Baker, UK)*; Fluidasa *(Knoll-Made, Spain)*; Histamed *(Vernleigh, S.Afr.)*; Pymal *(S. Afr.)*.

The following names have been used for multi-ingredient preparations containing mepyramine and its salts— 4-Way Nasal Spray *(Bristol-Myers Products, USA)*; Albatussin *(Bart, USA)*; Anthical *(May & Baker, UK)*; Caldomine-DH *(Technilab, Canad.)*; Citra Forte Capsules *(Boyle, USA)*; Citra Forte Syrup *(Boyle, USA)*; Codimal DH *(Central Pharmaceuticals, USA)*; Codimal DM *(Central Pharmaceuticals, USA)*; Codimal PH *(Central Pharmaceuticals, USA)*; Fiogesic *(Sandoz, USA)*; Flavelix *(Pharmax, UK)*; Histalet Forte *(Reid-Rowell, USA)*; Hycomine *(Du Pont, Austral.; Du Pont, Canad.)*; IDM *(Rougier, Canad.)*; Kronohist *(Ferndale, USA)*; Larylgan *(Ayerst, USA)*; Midol PMS *(Sterling, Canad.; Glenbrook, USA)*; Neo-Diophen *(Hamilton, Austral.)*; Poly-Histine-D *(Bock, USA)*; Prefrin-A *(Allergan, Canad.; Allergan, USA)*; Primatene M *(Whitehall, USA)*; P-V-Tussin Syrup *(Reid-Provident, USA)*; Ru-Tuss with Hydrocodone *(Boots, USA)*; Rynatan *(Wallace, USA)*; Triaminic *(Ancalab, Canad.; Dorsey Laboratories, USA)*; Triaminic Expectorant *(Ancalab, Canad.)*; Triaminic Expectorant DH *(Ancalab, Canad.; Dorsey Laboratories, USA)*; Triaminic Infant Drops *(Dorsey Laboratories, USA)*; Triaminic TR *(Dorsey Laboratories, USA)*; Triaminic-DM Expectorant *(Ancalab, Canad.)*; Triaminicin *(Ancalab, Canad.)*; Triaminicol DM *(Ancalab, Canad.)*; Trisulfaminic *(Ancalab, Canad.)*; Tussaminic C *(Ancalab, Canad.)*; Tussaminic DH *(Ancalab, Canad.)*; Wans *(Webcon, USA)*.

NOTE. The *UK* preparation Triominic has been reformulated to exclude mepyramine maleate. The *UK* preparation Triotussic had been reformulated to exclude mepyramine maleate prior to its withdrawal from the market.

6145-w

Mequitazine *(BAN, rINN)*.

LM-209. 10-(Quinuclidin-3-ylmethyl)phenothiazine.
$C_{20}H_{22}N_2S$=322.5.

CAS — 29216-28-2.

Adverse Effects, Treatment, Precautions, and Absorption and Fate

As for the antihistamines in general, p.443.

As for all phenothiazine derivatives mequitazine should be used cautiously in patients with hepatic diseases.

Uses and Administration

Mequitazine is a phenothiazine derivative with the actions and uses of the antihistamines (see p.444). It is reported to cause less sedation than promethazine.

Mequitazine is given in usual doses of 5 mg twice daily.

Proprietary Preparations

Primalan *(May & Baker, UK)*. *Tablets*, mequitazine 5 mg.

Proprietary Names and Manufacturers

Instotal *(Arg.)*; Metaplexan *(Rhône-Poulenc, Ger.)*; Mircol *(Belg.; Neth.; Rhone, Spain)*; Primalan *(Spret-Mauchant, Fr.; Rorer, Ital.; May & Baker, UK)*; Vigigan *(Rhone-Poulenc, Switz.)*.

6146-e

Methapyrilene Fumarate *(BANM, rINNM)*.

NN-Dimethyl-*N'*-(2-pyridyl)-*N'*-(2-thenyl)ethylenediamine fumarate.
$(C_{14}H_{19}N_3S)_2,3C_4H_4O_4$=871.0.

CAS — 91-80-5 (methapyrilene); 33032-12-1 (fumarate).

A white or almost white crystalline powder with a faint odour. **Soluble** 1 in 20 of water and 1 in 30 of alcohol. A 5% solution in water has a pH of 3.0 to 4.0. **Store** at a temperature not exceeding 30° in airtight containers. Protect from light.

6147-l

Methapyrilene Hydrochloride *(BANM, rINNM)*.

Methapyrilenium Chloride; Thenylpyramine Hydrochloride.
$C_{14}H_{19}N_3S,HCl$=297.8.

CAS — 135-23-9.

Pharmacopoeias. In *Arg.*

A white or almost white crystalline powder with a faint odour. **Soluble** 1 in 0.5 of water, 1 in 5 of alcohol, and 1 in 3 of chloroform; practically insoluble in ether. A solution in water has a pH of about 5.5. **Store** in airtight containers. Protect from light.

Methapyrilene is an ethylenediamine derivative with the properties and uses of the antihistamines (see p.443). It has been given as the fumarate and as the hydrochloride but following reports of carcinogenicity in *rats* it is now little used.

Proprietary Names and Manufacturers

The following names have been used for multi-ingredient preparations containing methapyrilene hydrochloride or methapyrilene fumarate— Histadyl EC *(Lilly, UK)*.

6148-y

Methdilazine *(BAN, USAN, rINN)*.

10-(1-Methylpyrrolidin-3-ylmethyl)phenothiazine.
$C_{18}H_{20}N_2S$=296.4.

CAS — 1982-37-2.

Pharmacopoeias. In *U.S.*

A light tan crystalline powder with a characteristic odour. Methdilazine 7.2 mg is the equivalent of approximately 8 mg of methdilazine hydrochloride. Practically **insoluble** in water; soluble 1 in 2 of alcohol, 1 in 1 of chloroform, and 1 in 8 of ether; freely soluble in 3M hydrochloric acid; practically insoluble in 0.1M sodium hydroxide. **Store** in airtight containers. Protect from light.

6149-j

Methdilazine Hydrochloride *(BANM, USAN, rINNM)*.

$C_{18}H_{20}N_2S,HCl$=332.9.

CAS — 1229-35-2.

Pharmacopoeias. In *Ind.* and *U.S.*

A light tan crystalline powder with a slight characteristic odour. It darkens on exposure to light. **Soluble** 1 in 2 of water and of alcohol, and 1 in 6 of chloroform; practically insoluble in ether; soluble 1 in 1 of 0.1M hydrochloric acid and 0.1M sodium hydroxide solution. A 1% solution in water has a pH of 4.8 to 6. **Store** in airtight containers. Protect from light.

Methdilazine is a phenothiazine derivative with the properties and uses of the antihistamines (see p.443). Methdilazine and its hydrochloride are given for the symptomatic treatment of allergic conditions, particularly to control pruritus, in doses of 7.2 mg (base) or 8 mg (hydrochloride) 2 to 4 times daily. Children over 3 years of age have been given half the adult dose.

Preparations

Methdilazine Hydrochloride Syrup *(U.S.P.)*

Methdilazine Hydrochloride Tablets *(U.S.P.)*

Methdilazine Tablets *(U.S.P.)*

Proprietary Names and Manufacturers

Dilosyn *(Glaxo, Austral.; Allen & Hanburys, Canad.; Duncan, Flockhart, UK)*; Tacaryl *(Mead Johnson, Austral.; Pharmacia, Swed.; Westwood, USA)*; Tacryl *(Pharmacia, Denm.)*.

13006-j

Niaprazine *(rINN)*.

1709-CERM. *N*-[3-(4-*p*-Fluorophenylpiperazin-1-yl)-1-methylpropyl]nicotinamide.
$C_{20}H_{25}FN_4O$=356.4.

CAS — 27367-90-4.

Niaprazine is an antihistamine which has been used for its sedative and hypnotic properties.

Niaprazine 2 mg per kg body-weight was effective in the treatment of anxiety and sleep disorders in 20 children aged 2 to 14 years. The drug was generally well tolerated.— R. Besana *et al.*, *Curr. ther. Res.*, 1984, *36*, 58.

Proprietary Names and Manufacturers

Nopron *(Carrion, Fr.; Maggioni-Winthrop, Ital.)*.

13056-n

Oxatomide *(BAN, USAN, rINN)*.

R-35443. 1-[3-(4-Benzhydrylpiperazin-1-yl)propyl]benzimidazolin-2-one.
$C_{27}H_{30}N_4O$=426.6.

CAS — 60607-34-3.

Adverse Effects, Treatment, Precautions, and Absorption and Fate

As for antihistamines in general, p.443. Increased appetite and weight gain have been reported, particularly at higher doses.

Acute dystonic reactions and long-lasting impaired consciousness was associated with oxatomide therapy in 6 children. Impaired consciousness persisted for more than 2 days in three patients. Oxatomide plasma concentrations were found to be high in three patients, although two of these had been given the recommended dose.— M. Casteels-Van Daele *et al.* (letter), *Lancet*, 1986, *1*, 1204.

Uses and Administration

Oxatomide has the actions and uses of antihistamines in general, p.444. It has also been reported to have mast-cell stabilising properties.

Oxatomide is usually given by mouth in doses of 30 to 60 mg twice a day. Children aged 5 to 14 years may be given 15 to 30 mg twice a day.

A discussion of the use of oxatomide in the treatment of allergies. Oxatomide was reported to cause dose-dependent drowsiness.— *Drug & Ther. Bull.*, 1983, *21*, 35.

A review of the pharmacodynamic properties and therapeutic efficacy of oxatomide. In addition to its antihistamine activity, it displays some antiserotonin and antimuscarinic properties, and possibly antagonises slow-reacting substance of anaphylaxis. In common with some other antihistamines, oxatomide has also shown some mast-cell stabilising activity, although the contribution this action makes to the clinical activity of the drug is unknown. After oral administration peak-plasma concentrations are seen within 4 hours. It is excreted in the urine and the faeces, mainly as metabolites. Oxatomide has been found to be effective in the treatment of chronic urticaria and allergic rhinitis, but trials in adult asthma have shown the activity of oxatomide to be little different from that of placebo. Studies in children with asthma using high doses have been more encouraging, as have preliminary results in follicular conjunctivitis, atopic dermatitis, and food allergy. The most frequently reported adverse effect has been drowsiness.— D. M. Richards *et al.*, *Drugs*, 1984, *27*, 210.

Proprietary Preparations

Tinset *(Janssen, UK)*. *Tablets*, scored, oxatomide 30 mg.

Proprietary Names and Manufacturers

Cobiona *(Esteve, Spain)*; Tinset *(Janssen, Denm.; Janssen, Ger.; Formenti, Ital.; Janssen, S.Afr.; Janssen, Spain; Janssen, Switz.; Janssen, UK)*.

6151-p

Oxomemazine *(rINN)*.

RP-6847; Trimeprazine *SS*-Dioxide. 10-(3-Dimethylamino-2-methylpropyl)phenothiazine 5,5-dioxide.
$C_{18}H_{22}N_2O_2S$=330.4.

CAS — 3689-50-7.

6152-s

Oxomemazine Hydrochloride *(rINNM)*.

$C_{18}H_{22}N_2O_2S,HCl$=366.9.

CAS — 4784-40-1.

Pharmacopoeias. In *Fr.*

Oxomemazine hydrochloride 11.1 mg is approximately equivalent to 10 mg of oxomemazine.

Oxomemazine is a phenothiazine derivative with the properties and uses of the antihistamines (see p.443). It has been given both as the base and as the hydrochloride in doses equivalent to 10 to 40 mg of oxomemazine daily.

Proprietary Names and Manufacturers

Doxergan *(Rhone-Poulenc, Belg.; Specia, Fr.; Specia, Neth.; Rhone-Poulenc, Switz.)*; Imakol *(Rhône-Poulenc, Ger.)*.

6160-s

Parathiazine Theoclate
Parathiazine Teoclate *(pINNM)*; Parathiazone Theoclate; Pyrathiazine Theoclate. 10-(2-Pyrrolidin-1-ylethyl)phenothiazine 8-chlorotheophyllinate.
$C_{18}H_{20}N_2S,C_7H_7ClN_4O_2$=511.0.

CAS — 84-08-2 (parathiazine); 14006-99-6 (theoclate); 522-25-8 (hydrochloride).

Parathiazine theoclate is a phenothiazine derivative with the properties of the antihistamines (see p.443) but has been used mainly as an anti-emetic in the treatment of motion sickness and postoperative vomiting. It has been given in doses of up to 100 mg daily.

Proprietary Names and Manufacturers
Mediamer *(Spain).*

6153-w

Phenindamine Tartrate *(BANM, rINNM).*
Phenindamine Acid Tartrate; Phenindamini Tartras; Phenindaminium Tartrate. 1,2,3,4-Tetrahydro-2-methyl-9-phenyl-2-azafluorene hydrogen tartrate; 2,3,4,9-Tetrahydro-2-methyl-9-phenyl-1*H*-indeno[2,1-*c*]pyridine hydrogen tartrate.
$C_{19}H_{19}N,C_4H_6O_6$=411.5.

CAS — 82-88-2 (phenindamine); 569-59-5 (tartrate).

Pharmacopoeias. In *Arg., Br., Ind., Int.,* and *Turk.*

A white or almost white, almost odourless, voluminous powder. **Soluble** 1 in 70 of water; slightly soluble in alcohol; practically insoluble in chloroform and ether. A 1% solution in water has a pH of 3.4 to 3.9. **Store** in well-closed containers. Protect from light.

Adverse Effects, Treatment, Precautions, and Absorption and Fate
As for the antihistamines in general, p.443.
Unlike most other antihistamines phenindamine tartrate may have a stimulant effect; to avoid the possibility of insomnia patients may be advised to take the last dose of the day before 4 p.m.

Uses and Administration
Phenindamine tartrate has the actions and uses of the antihistamines (see p.444), however it may be mildly stimulating. It is given in doses of 25 to 50 mg up to three times daily. Children over 6 years of age have been given up to 75 mg daily in divided doses.

Preparations
Phenindamine Tablets *(B.P.).* Tablets containing phenindamine tartrate.

Proprietary Preparations
Thephorin *(Sinclair, UK). Tablets,* phenindamine tartrate 25 mg.

Proprietary Names and Manufacturers
Nolahist *(Carnrick, USA)*; Thephorin *(Austral.; Roche, S.Afr.; Sinclair, UK).*

The following names have been used for multi-ingredient preparations containing phenindamine tartrate— Nolamine *(Carnrick, USA)*; P-V-Tussin *(Reid-Provident, USA).*

6154-e

Pheniramine Maleate *(BANM, rINNM).*
Pheniraminium Maleate; Prophenpyridamine Maleate. *NN*-Dimethyl-3-phenyl-3-(2-pyridyl)propylamine hydrogen maleate.
$C_{16}H_{20}N_2,C_4H_4O_4$=356.4.

CAS — 86-21-5 (pheniramine); 132-20-7 (maleate).

Pharmacopoeias. In *Br.* and *Ind.*

A white or almost white crystalline powder odourless or with a slight odour. **Soluble** 1 in 0.3 of water, 1 in 2.5 of alcohol, and 1 in 1.5 of chloroform; very slightly soluble in ether. A 1% solution in water has a pH of 4.5 to 5.5. **Protect** from light.

Adverse Effects, Treatment, and Precautions
As for the antihistamines in general, p.443.

ABUSE. References to adverse effects following the abuse of pheniramine aminosalicylate: I. H. Jones *et al., Med. J. Aust.,* 1973, *1,* 382; E. R. Csillag and A. A. Landauer, *ibid.,* 653.

Absorption and Fate
As for the antihistamines in general, p.444.

The kinetics of pheniramine and its metabolites, *N*-desmethylpheniramine and *N*-didesmethylpheniramine, were investigated in 6 healthy subjects. After oral administration, peak-plasma concentrations were reached in 1 to 2.5 hours. The terminal half-life ranged between 8 and 17 hours after intravenous administration and 16 and 19 hours after oral administration. The total recovery of pheniramine as unchanged drug and metabolites from the urine was 68 to 94% of the intravenous dose and 70 to 83% of the oral dose.— P. U. Witte *et al., Int. J. clin. Pharmac. Ther. Toxic.,* 1985, *23,* 59.

Uses and Administration
Pheniramine is an alkylamine derivative with the actions and uses of the antihistamines (see p.444).
Pheniramine maleate, when used alone, is generally given in sustained-release preparations in doses of 75 mg once or twice daily or 150 mg at night if required.
Pheniramine is also administered as the aminosalicylate ($C_{16}H_{20}N_2,C_7H_7NO_3$ = 393.5) in usual doses of 25 to 50 mg three times daily. It has also been given as the tannate.

Proprietary Preparations
Daneral SA *(Hoechst, UK). Tablets,* sustained-release, pheniramine maleate 75 mg.

Owing to the risk of intestinal obstruction, sustained-release preparations such as Daneral SA, where the drug is released in transit, but the matrix ghost is often eliminated intact, should not be prescribed in patients with Crohn's disease or other intestinal disease in which strictures may form.— J. L. Shaffer *et al.* (letter), *Lancet,* 1980, *2,* 487.

Proprietary Names and Manufacturers of Pheniramine Maleate or other Salts of Pheniramine
Acovil *(Spain)*; Acoviletas *(Spain)*; Avil *(Hoechst, Austral.; Belg.; Albert-Roussel, Ger.; Neth.; Albert, S. Afr.)*; Aviletten *(Albert-Roussel, Ger.)*; Avilettes *(Hoechst, Austral.)*; Daneral SA *(Hoechst, UK)*; Fenamine *(Fawns & McAllan, Austral.)*; Inhiston *(Biomedica Foscama, Ital.).*

The following names have been used for multi-ingredient preparations containing pheniramine maleate or other salts of pheniramine— Ak-Vernacon *(Akorn, Canad.)*; Avil Decongestant *(Hoechst, Austral.)*; Caldomine-DH *(Technilab, Canad.)*; Citra Forte Capsules *(Boyle, USA)*; Citra Forte Syrup *(Boyle, USA)*; Coldex *(Gen, Canad.)*; Dristan Nasal Spray *(Whitehall, USA)*; Fiogesic *(Sandoz, USA)*; Muflin *(Concept Pharmaceuticals, UK)*; Naphcon-A *(Alcon, Canad.; Alcon Laboratories, USA)*; Opcon-A *(Charton, Canad.)*; Poly-Histine-D *(Bock, USA)*; Pulmorphan *(Riva, Canad.)*; Robitussin A-C *(Robins, Canad.)*; Robitussin AC *(Robins, UK)*; Ru-Tuss with Hydrocodone *(Boots, USA)*; Rynabond *(Fisons, UK)*; S-T Forte *(Scot-Tussin, USA)*; Syrtussar *(Armour, UK)*; Triaminic *(Ancalab, Canad.; Dorsey Laboratories, USA)*; Triaminic Expectorant *(Ancalab, Canad.)*; Triaminic Expectorant DH *(Ancalab, Canad.; Dorsey Laboratories, USA)*; Triaminic Infant Drops *(Dorsey Laboratories, USA)*; Triaminic TR *(Dorsey Laboratories, USA)*; Triminic-DM Expectorant *(Ancalab, Canad.)*; Triaminicin *(Ancalab, Canad.)*; Triaminicol DM *(Ancalab, Canad.)*; Triominic *(Sandoz, Austral.; Intercare, UK)*; Triotussic *(Beecham Research, UK)*; Trisulfaminic *(Ancalab, Canad.)*; Tussaminic C *(Ancalab, Canad.)*; Tussaminic DH *(Ancalab, Canad.)*; Tussirex *(Scot-Tussin, USA)*; Verstat *(Saron, USA).*

6155-l

Phenyltoloxamine Citrate *(BANM, rINNM).*
C 5581; Phenyltolyloxamine Citrate; PRN. 2-(2-Benzylphenoxy)-*NN*-dimethylethylamine dihydrogen citrate.
$C_{17}H_{21}NO,C_6H_8O_7$=447.5.

CAS — 92-12-6 (phenyltoloxamine); 1176-08-5 (citrate).

Phenyltoloxamine citrate is an ethanolamine derivative with the properties and uses of the antihistamines (see p.443). It is a structural isomer of diphenhydramine (see p.452). It has been given in doses of up to 50 mg three or four times daily.

Proprietary Names and Manufacturers of Phenyltoloxamine, its Salts and Complexes
The following names have been used for multi-ingredient preparations containing phenyltoloxamine, its salts and complexes— Atrohist *(Adams, USA)*; Comhist *(Norwich Eaton, USA)*; Histamic *(Metro Med, USA)*; Kutrase *(Kremers-Urban, USA)*; Magsal *(US Pharmaceutical, USA)*; Menoplex *(Fiske, USA)*; Mobigesic *(Ascher, USA)*; Naldecon *(Bristol, USA)*; Omni-Tuss *(Pennwalt, Canad.)*; Percogesic *(Richardson-Vicks, USA)*; Pholtex *(Riker, UK)*; Poly-Histine-D *(Bock, USA)*; Quadrahist *(Schein, USA)*; Rinurel Linctus *(Warner, UK)*; Rinurel Tablets *(Warner, UK)*; Sinubid *(Parke, Davis, USA)*; Sinutab SA *(Parke, Davis, Canad.)*; Sinutab with Codeine *(Warner, Austral.)*; Tussionex *(Pennwalt, Canad.; Pennwalt, USA).*

13118-f

Pimethixene *(rINN).*
BP-400. 9-(1-Methyl-4-piperidylidene)thioxanthene.
$C_{19}H_{19}NS$=293.4.

CAS — 314-03-4.

Pimethixene is reported to have antihistaminic properties and to be an inhibitor of serotonin. It has been used in the treatment of respiratory disorders in children.

Proprietary Names and Manufacturers
Calmixène *(Sandoz, Fr.)*; Muricalm *(Wander, Belg.)*; Sedosil *(Cooper, Switz.).*

6156-y

Piprinhydrinate *(BAN, rINN).*
Diphenylpyraline Theoclate. The diphenylpyraline salt of 8-chlorotheophylline; 4-Benzhydryloxy-1-methylpiperidine salt of 8-chlorotheophylline.
$C_{19}H_{23}NO,C_7H_7ClN_4O_2$=496.0.

CAS — 606-90-6.

Piprinhydrinate has the general properties and uses of the antihistamines (see p.443). It has been given in doses of 3 to 9 mg up to three times daily.

Proprietary Names and Manufacturers
Colton *(Byk Liprandi, Arg.)*; Kolton *(Promonta, Belg.; Promonta, Ger.).*

6157-j

Pizotifen Malate *(BANM, rINNM).*
BC-105 (base); Pizotyline Malate. 9,10-Dihydro-4-(1-methyl-4-piperidylidene)-4*H*-benzo-[4,5]cyclohepta[1,2-*b*]thiophene hydrogen malate.
$C_{19}H_{21}NS,C_4H_6O_5$=429.5.

CAS — 15574-96-6 (pizotifen); 5189-11-7 (malate).

NOTE. Pizotyline is *USAN.*

Pizotifen malate 145 mg is approximately equivalent to 100 mg of pizotifen.

Adverse Effects, Treatment, Precautions, and Absorption and Fate
As for the antihistamines in general, p.443.
Increased appetite and weight gain may occur. Drowsiness may be troublesome.

Of 47 patients with severe migraine given pizotifen 1 to 2 mg daily adverse effects were recorded in 22 patients.

These reactions included weight increase (15), muscle pain or cramps (3), heavy legs or restless legs (3), fluid retention (3), drowsiness (2), more frequent milder headaches (2), facial flushing (1), reduced libido (1), exacerbation of epilepsy (1), and dreaming (2). Adverse effects necessitating withdrawal from the study occurred in 11 patients. Advantageous effects were mood elevation in 3 and increased alertness in 6.— K. M. S. Peet, *Curr. med. Res. Opinion*, 1977, *5*, 192.

The ingestion of pizotifen during the first four to six weeks of pregnancy was not considered to be an indication for termination of the pregnancy.— J. O. Drife, *Br. med. J.*, 1984, *288*, 375.

Uses and Administration

Pizotifen malate has the actions of the antihistamines (see p.444). It is a strong serotonin antagonist, it antagonises the action of tryptamine, and it has weak antimuscarinic properties.

Pizotifen malate is used for the prophylaxis of recurrent vascular headaches including migraine. It is not effective in treating an acute attack.

The usual adult dose is 1.5 mg of pizotifen daily either in three divided doses or as a single dose at night. Doses should be adjusted according to the requirements of individual patients and may vary from 0.5 mg to 6 mg daily. Not more than 3 mg should be given as a single dose. In children aged over 5 years, doses of 1.5 mg daily in divided doses or up to 1 mg at night have been recommended.

Reviews and comments on the action and uses of pizotifen.— T. M. Speight and G. S. Avery, *Drugs*, 1972, *3*, 159; W. H. Aellig, *Eur. J. clin. Pharmac.*, 1983, *25*, 759; J. L. Elghozi *et al.*, *ibid.*, 1984, *27*, 191.

MIGRAINE. Pizotifen was considered to be the second most useful drug for the prophylaxis of migraine, after propranolol, although it is only effective in about two-thirds of patients. Side-effects include drowsiness and weight gain and may affect 60% of patients. In a small proportion of patients the effect of the drug diminishes after some months of treatment.— R. Peatfield, *Br. J. Hosp. Med.*, 1984, *31*, 142.

Pizotifen 1.5 to 3.0 mg daily was more effective than clonidine 100 to 150 µg daily in the prophylaxis of migraine in a study involving 44 patients. Pizotifen reduced the frequency, severity, duration, and the number of associated symptoms in most patients.— P. O. Behan, *Cephalalgia*, 1985, *5*, *Suppl.* 3, 524.

In a double-blind crossover study, pizotifen 0.5 mg three times a day and metoprolol 50 mg twice a day were both equally effective for the prophylaxis of migraine in 35 patients. Pizotifen had a greater effect on nausea than metoprolol, but adverse effects, particularly weight gain and drowsiness, were more troublesome.— S. Vilming *et al.*, *Cephalalgia*, 1985, *5*, 17.

Further references.— P. O. Behan, *Br. J. clin. Pract.*, 1982, *36*, 13 (single nocturnal dose therapy).

NAUSEA AND VOMITING. Pizotifen 500 µg three times a day prevented nausea and vomiting caused by calcitonin therapy in 3 patients.— A. J. Crisp (letter), *Lancet*, 1981, *1*, 775.

Cyclical vomiting. Pizotifen 1.5 mg at night was given prophylactically for 6 months to 7 children, aged 5 to 12 years, suffering from cyclical vomiting, with 4 to 7 attacks in the previous 12 months. While on pizotifen 6 children had no attacks and the seventh experienced a single mild attack. Apart from one child who had a minor attack 2 months after treatment ceased there have been no relapses. Two children have been attack-free and off all medication for 11 months and a further two for 9 months. A controlled study of pizotifen is considered warranted.— M. A. Salmon and D. D. Walters (letter), *Lancet*, 1985, *1*, 1036.

PRURITUS. Beneficial results with pizotifen in 6 of 9 patients with pruritus associated with polycythaemia vera.— E. J. Fitzsimons *et al.*, *Br. med. J.*, 1981, *283*, 277.

Proprietary Preparations

Sanomigran *(Sandoz, UK)*. *Tablets*, pizotifen 0.5 and 1.5 mg (as malate).
Elixir, pizotifen 250 µg (as malate)/5 mL.

Proprietary Names and Manufacturers

Mosegor *(Arg.; Belg.; Wander, Ger.; Sandoz, Spain; Wander, Switz.)*; Sandomigran *(Sandoz, Arg.; Sandoz, Austral.; Belg., Sandoz, Canad.; Sandoz, Ger.; Sandoz, Ital.; Neth.; Wander, S. Afr.; Sandoz, Spain; Sandoz, Switz.)*; Sandomigrin *(Sandoz, Denm.; Sandoz, Norw.; Sandoz, Swed.)*; Sanmigran *(Sandoz, Fr.)*; Sanomigran *(Sandoz, UK)*.

6101-r

Promethazine *(BAN, rINN)*.

1,*N*,*N*-Trimethyl-2-(phenothiazin-10-yl)ethylamine.

$C_{17}H_{20}N_2S = 284.4$.

CAS — 60-87-7.

6103-d

Promethazine Theoclate *(BAN)*.

Promethazine Teoclate *(rINN)*. The promethazine salt of 8-chlorotheophylline.

$C_{17}H_{20}N_2S,C_7H_7ClN_4O_2 = 499.0$.

CAS — 17693-51-5.

Pharmacopoeias. In *Br.* and *Ind.*

A white or almost white odourless or almost odourless powder. Promethazine theoclate 1.5 mg is approximately equivalent to 1 mg of promethazine hydrochloride.

Very slightly **soluble** in water; soluble 1 in 70 of alcohol and 1 in 2.5 of chloroform; practically insoluble in ether. **Store** in well-closed containers. Protect from light.

6102-f

Promethazine Hydrochloride *(BANM; USAN, rINNM)*.

Diprazinum; Proazamine Chloride; Promethazini Hydrochloridum; Promethazinium Chloride.

$C_{17}H_{20}N_2S,HCl = 320.9$.

CAS — 58-33-3.

Pharmacopoeias. In *Arg., Aust., Belg., Br., Braz., Chin., Cz., Egypt., Eur., Fr., Ger., Hung., Ind., Int., It., Jpn, Jug., Neth., Nord., Pol., Rus., Swiss, Turk.*, and *U.S.* Also in *B.P. Vet.*

A white or faintly yellow, odourless or almost odourless, crystalline powder. On prolonged exposure to air it is slowly oxidised, becoming blue in colour.

Soluble 1 in 0.6 of water, 1 in 9 of alcohol, and 1 in 2 of chloroform; very soluble in hot dehydrated alcohol; practically insoluble in acetone, ether, and ethyl acetate. A 10% solution in water has a pH of 4.0 to 5.0. The *B.P.* injection has a pH of 5.0 to 6.0. Solutions are **sterilised** by autoclaving. Promethazine has been reported to be **incompatible** with solutions of a number of compounds including aminophylline, barbiturates, benzylpenicillin salts, carbenicillin, heparin, hydrocortisone sodium succinate, morphine sulphate, alkalis, and some contrast media. **Store** in airtight containers. Protect from light.

ADSORPTION. The adsorption of promethazine hydrochloride onto PVC infusion bags in one week increased from 5% to 59% when the solution was buffered to pH 7.4.— E. A. Kowaluk *et al.*, *Am. J. Hosp. Pharm.*, 1981, *38*, 1308.

There was a 22% loss of promethazine by adsorption onto a plastic infusion set during a simulated infusion over 7 hours. Using a glass syringe and pump there was a loss of 5% with polyethylene tubing and 50% with silastic tubing in 1 hour.— E. A. Kowaluk *et al.*, *Am. J. Hosp. Pharm.*, 1982, *39*, 460.

A mixture of promethazine hydrochloride 25 mg, pethidine hydrochloride 50 mg, and atropine sulphate 0.4 mg was stable for 24 hours in plastic syringes.— R. S. Rhodes *et al.*, *Am. J. Hosp. Pharm.*, 1985, *42*, 112.

Adverse Effects

As for the antihistamines in general, p.443.

Cardiovascular side-effects are more commonly seen after injection, and bradycardia, tachycardia, transient minor increases in blood pressure, and occasional hypotension have been reported with promethazine. Jaundice and thrombocytopenic purpura have also been reported, and extrapyramidal effects may occur at high doses. Angioedema has been reported. Leucopenia and agranulocytosis occur rarely, and usually when promethazine is used in combination with other drugs. Photosensitivity reactions have followed its use by mouth or topical application.

Venous thrombosis has been reported at the site of intravenous injections, and arteriospasm and gangrene may follow inadvertent intra-arterial injection.

Following an initial report that 4 of 7 infants with sudden infant death syndrome (SIDS) had been given therapeutic doses of phenothiazines (trimeprazine or promethazine) before death (A. Kahn and D. Blum, *Lancet*, 1979, *2*, 364) and that a series of severe apnoeic crises had been observed in the twin of a SIDS victim also given promethazine, the same workers studied 52 SIDS victims, 36 near-miss infants and 175 control subjects to investigate the role of nasopharyngitis and phenothiazines (*Pediatrics*, 1982, *70*, 75). It was found that there was no difference in the incidence of nasopharyngitis between the 3 groups, but that the proportion of infants given phenothiazines was higher in both the SIDS group (23%) and the near-miss group (22%) than in the control group (2%). It was suggested that the SIDS victims may represent infants with excessive sensitivity to this group of drugs. In a subsequent study, Kahn *et al.* (*Pediatrics*, 1985, *75*, 844) found that the incidence of central and obstructive sleep apnoeas was increased in 4 healthy infants given promethazine for 3 days, although the duration of the attacks was unaltered and generally short, with a range of 3 to 10 seconds. Cockfield, reporting on behalf of the Commission of the European Communities, stated that no link between sudden deaths in infants and drug administration had been confirmed by national drug monitoring centres. It was likely that the risk of apnoea was associated with all sedative drugs, especially in overdose (*Off. J. E.E.C.*, 1986, *29*, C130/26). Previously Stanton (*Pediatrics*, 1983, *71*, 986) had proposed phenothiazine-induced hyperthermia as a contributory factor in SIDS.

For reports of the effects of promethazine on performance, see p.443.

EFFECTS ON THE EYES. A study indicating that usual doses of promethazine interfere with colour vision.— J. Laroche and C. Laroche, *Annls pharm. fr.*, 1972, *30*, 433.

EXTRAPYRAMIDAL SYMPTOMS. The Boston Collaborative Drug Surveillance Program monitored consecutively 32 812 medical inpatients. Drug-induced extrapyramidal symptoms occurred in 1 of 1194 patients given promethazine.— J. Porter and H. Jick, *Lancet*, 1977, *1*, 587.

Further references to extrapyramidal symptoms with promethazine.— M. E. Dodson and R. J. Eastley, *Br. J. Anaesth.*, 1978, *50*, 1059; T. L. Schwinghammer *et al.*, *Clin. Pharm.*, 1984, *3*, 83.

OVERDOSAGE. A toxic neurological syndrome which included CNS depression, acute excitomotor manifestations, ataxia and visual hallucinations, plus peripheral antimuscarinic effects developed in 2 children aged 44 months and 16 months after topical application of a 2% promethazine cream in doses between 12.9 and 26 mg per kg body-weight. The older child had also received hydroxyzine 10 mg 1 hour earlier.— D. H. Shawn and M. A. McGuigan, *Can. med. Ass. J.*, 1984, *130*, 1460.

A 27-year-old man died after taking a massive overdose of promethazine tablets. The drug concentrations in the body were 1000 times the therapeutic concentrations.— *Pharm. J.*, 1985, *1*, 529.

PREGNANCY AND THE NEONATE. In a study of 836 infants with congenital malformations there was no significant difference in the maternal usage of promethazine during the first trimester of pregnancy compared with the use in 836 controls.— G. Greenberg *et al.*, *Br. med. J.*, 1977, *2*, 853.

For further studies on the effects of antihistamines during pregnancy, see p.443.

Treatment of Adverse Effects

As for the antihistamines in general, p.443.

Precautions

As for the antihistamines in general, p.444.

As for all phenothiazine derivatives promethazine should be used cautiously in patients with cardiovascular or hepatic diseases.

Intravenous injections of promethazine hydrochloride must be given slowly and extreme care must be taken to avoid extravasation or inadvertent intra-arterial injection, due to the risk of severe irritation. Promethazine should not be

given by subcutaneous injection.
Promethazine is contra-indicated in comatose patients, and should be used with care in children, especially those who are acutely ill or dehydrated as these patients have an increased incidence of dystonias.
Like other phenothiazines, promethazine may potentiate the hypotensive effect of some antihypertensive agents. Some combinations of phenothiazines and tricyclic antidepressants have resulted in increased plasma concentrations of both drugs.
False negative and positive results have been reported with some pregnancy tests.

ADMINISTRATION IN RENAL FAILURE. A report of promethazine-induced toxic psychosis in a patient with chronic renal failure.— C. J. McAllister *et al.*, *Clin. Nephrol.*, 1978, *10*, 191.

ANAESTHESIA. In 8 healthy subjects promethazine 25 mg intravenously appeared to increase the incidence of gastro-oesophageal reflux and might therefore increase the risk of regurgitation and aspiration of gastric contents during induction of and recovery from anaesthesia.— J. G. Brock-Utne *et al.*, *Br. J. Anaesth.*, 1978, *50*, 295. See also B. R. Cotton and G. Smith, *ibid.*, 1984, *56*, 37.

PORPHYRIA. Promethazine was considered to be unsafe in patients with acute porphyria although there is conflicting experimental evidence on porphyrinogenicity.— M.R. Moore and K.E.L. McColl, *Porphyrias, Drug Lists*, Glasgow, Porphyria Research Unit, University of Glasgow, 1987.

Absorption and Fate

As for the antihistamines in general, p.444.

Promethazine had a mean oral bioavailability of 25% in 7 healthy subjects. The results strongly suggested extensive first-pass metabolism in the liver.— G. Taylor *et al.*, *Br. J. clin. Pharmac.*, 1983, *15*, 287.

PREGNANCY AND THE NEONATE. Promethazine rapidly diffused across the placenta and when 50 mg was given intravenously to 39 women before delivery, promethazine was found in umbilical vein blood in all cases. About 15 minutes after administration the maternal and foetal blood concentrations were the same. Some clinical depression of infants had been observed. Promethazine had been detected in foetal blood up to 4 hours after administration to the mother.— F. Moya and V. Thorndike, *Am. J. Obstet. Gynec.*, 1962, *84*, 1778.

Uses and Administration

Promethazine hydrochloride is a phenothiazine derivative with the actions and uses of the antihistamines (see p.444). The antihistamine action has been reported to last for between 6 and 12 hours. It also has some antimuscarinic, antiserotoninergic, and marked local anaesthetic properties.
Promethazine hydrochloride is usually given at night in a dose of 25 mg for allergic conditions because of its pronounced sedative effect. The UK manufacturers recommend that this dose may be increased to 50 or 75 mg if required. Alternatively, up to 60 mg a day may be given in divided doses. Doses for children are: 1 to 5 years 5 to 15 mg; 5 to 10 years 10 to 25 mg; if 2 doses are given in 24 hours the lower dose should be used.
Promethazine hydrochloride may also be given in severe allergies by deep intramuscular injection in doses of 25 to 50 mg; a dose of 100 mg should not be exceeded. In an emergency the injection may be diluted to 2.5 mg per mL with Water for Injections and given by slow intravenous injection or injected into the tubing of a freely running infusion at a rate not exceeding 25 mg per minute.
Doses of up to 50 mg have been given for sedation and hypnosis. The dose in children of 1 to 5 years of age is 15 to 20 mg and 6 to 10 years 20 to 25 mg. If administration by mouth is not possible half the oral dose may be given by deep intramuscular injection to children of 5 to 10 years.
Promethazine hydrochloride is also used for anaesthetic premedication and may be given by intramuscular injection with pethidine and atropine in a dose of 25 to 50 mg in adults.
As an antiemetic, either the hydrochloride or the theoclate may be used. For motion sickness a dose of 25 mg of either is usually sufficient, taken about an hour before travelling. This dose may be repeated once or twice daily as necessary. Children over 5 years may be given half the adult dose. Vomiting from other causes may require higher or more frequent doses, but it is usually unnecessary to exceed 100 mg in 24 hours. If vomiting is severe, the dose may be given by intramuscular injection.
Promethazine hydrochloride is used in compound cough linctuses.
Promethazine has been used locally for treatment of allergic skin conditions but systemic treatment is to be preferred. A 2% cream has been used for treatment of burns but it may delay healing and produce skin sensitisation.
In the *UK* the use of phenothiazine derivatives including promethazine in cosmetics is prohibited by law.

EXTRAPYRAMIDAL DISORDERS. Promethazine 10 to 15 mg by intravenous injection rapidly controls oculogyric crisis caused by metoclopramide treatment in children. It is recommended that a similar dose is given by intramuscular injection since a crisis may last longer than the effect of a single intravenous dose of promethazine.— J. Stonham and S. Ross, *Br. J. Hosp. Med.*, 1984, *31*, 354.

NAUSEA AND VOMITING. In a comparison with metoclopramide, promethazine was effective in preventing the increase in nausea and vomiting associated with pethidine administration during labour. However, the sedative effect of promethazine was considered to be a disadvantage and promethazine was also found to have an antianalgesic effect. Metoclopramide was preferred.— L. Vella *et al.*, *Br. med. J.*, 1985, *290*, 1173.

PREGNANCY AND THE NEONATE. Following initial studies which indicated that promethazine could modify the haemolytic process of antibody-coated foetal red blood cells, promethazine hydrochloride 150 mg daily was given to 21 mothers with severe rhesus isoimmunisation for 3 to 24 weeks of the pregnancy. Seven of 22 babies required intrauterine transfusions, a slightly lower figure than expected without promethazine pretreatment, but its value was not confirmed.— M. A. Stenchever, *Am. J. Obstet. Gynec.*, 1978, *130*, 665.

See also under Nausea and vomiting and under Adverse Effects.

RESPIRATORY DISORDERS. A study indicating that promethazine is of some benefit for breathlessness and exercise tolerance in pink and puffing patients with fixed airways obstruction.— A. A. Woodcock *et al.*, *Br. med. J.*, 1981, *283*, 343. A later comment by one of the authors that improvement was only slight and that the effects of promethazine were difficult to interpret.— D. M. Geddes, *Postgrad. med. J.*, 1984, *60*, 194.

Preparations

Promethazine Oral Solution *(B.P.)*. Promethazine Elixir; Promethazine Hydrochloride Elixir. A solution of promethazine hydrochloride in a suitable flavoured vehicle.

Promethazine Hydrochloride Syrup *(U.S.P.)*

Promethazine Injection *(B.P.)*. Promethazine Hydrochloride Injection

Promethazine Hydrochloride Injection *(U.S.P.)*

Promethazine Hydrochloride Tablets *(B.P.)*

Promethazine Hydrochloride Tablets *(U.S.P.)*

Promethazine Theoclate Tablets *(B.P.)*

Proprietary Preparations

Avomine *(May & Baker, UK). Tablets*, scored, promethazine theoclate 25 mg.

Phenergan *(May & Baker, UK). Tablets*, promethazine hydrochloride 10 and 25 mg.
Elixir, promethazine hydrochloride 5 mg/5 mL.
Injection, promethazine hydrochloride 25 mg/mL, in ampoules of 1 and 2 mL.

Phenergan Compound Expectorant *(May & Baker, UK). Linctus*, promethazine hydrochloride 5 mg, ipecacuanha liquid extract 0.01 mL, potassium guaiacolsulfonate 45 mg, citric acid 65 mg/5 mL.

Phensedyl *(May & Baker, UK). Linctus*, promethazine hydrochloride 3.6 mg, codeine phosphate 9 mg, ephedrine hydrochloride 7.2 mg/5 mL.

Sominex *(Beecham Proprietaries, UK). Tablets*, scored, promethazine hydrochloride 20 mg.

Tixylix *(May & Baker, UK). Linctus*, promethazine hydrochloride 1.5 mg, pholcodine 1.5 mg (as citrate)/5 mL.

Proprietary Names and Manufacturers of Promethazine and its Salts

Atosil *(Tropon, Ger.)*; Avomine *(May & Baker, Austral.; S.Afr.; May & Baker, UK)*; BayMeth *(Bay, USA)*; Daralix *(SCS, S.Afr.)*; Fargan *(Farmitalia, Ital.)*; Fellozine *(USA)*; Fenazil *(Sella, Ital.)*; Fenergan *(Arg.; Rhone, Spain)*; Ganphen *(Reid-Provident, USA)*; Histantil *(Pharmascience, Canad.)*; Lenazine *(S.Afr.)*; Lergigan *(Kabi, Swed.)*; Meth-zine *(Protea, Austral.)*; Pelpica *(Belg.)*; Phencen *(Central Pharmaceuticals, USA)*; Phenergan *(May & Baker, Austral.; Belg.; Rhône-Poulenc, Canad.; Rhone-Poulenc, Denm.; Specia, Fr.; Neth.; Rhône-Poulenc, Norw.; May & Baker, S.Afr.; Rhone-Poulenc, Switz.; May & Baker, UK; Wyeth, USA)*; Progan *(Nelson, Austral.)*; Prohist *(S.Afr.)*; Promet *(Legere, USA)*; Promine *(USA)*; Prothazine *(USV, Austral.)*; Quadnite *(Reid-Provident, USA)*; Remsed *(Du Pont, USA)*; Sayomol *(Cinfa, Spain)*; Sominex *(Beecham Proprietaries, UK)*; V-Gan *(Hauck, USA)*; ZiPan *(Savage, USA)*.

The following names have been used for multi-ingredient preparations containing promethazine or its salts—Maxigesic *(Mastar, USA)*; Medised *(Martindale Pharmaceuticals, UK : Panpharma, UK)*; Mepergan *(Wyeth, USA)*; Pamergan *(Rhône-Poulenc, Canad.)*; Pamergan AP100/25 *(Martindale Pharmaceuticals, UK)*; Pamergan P100 *(Martindale Pharmaceuticals, UK)*; Panadol Elixir with Promethazine *(Winthrop, Austral.)*; Panquil *(Rosken, Austral.)*; Phenergan Compound Expectorant Linctus *(May & Baker, UK)*; Phenergan Cream *(May & Baker, Austral.; May & Baker, UK)*; Phenergan Expectorant *(May & Baker, Austral.; Rhône-Poulenc, Canad.)*; Phenergan Expectorant with Codeine *(Rhône-Poulenc, Canad.)*; Phenergan VC *(Wyeth, USA)*; Phenergan VC Expectorant *(Rhône-Poulenc, Canad.)*; Phenergan VC Expectorant with Codeine *(Rhône-Poulenc, Canad.)*; Phenergan VC with Codeine *(Wyeth, USA)*; Phenergan with Codeine *(Wyeth, USA)*; Phenergan with Dextromethorphan *(Wyeth, USA)*; Phenergan-D *(Wyeth, USA)*; Phensedyl *(May & Baker, Austral.; May & Baker, UK)*; Promatussin *(Wyeth, Canad.)*; Prometh VC *(National Pharm., USA)*; Seda-Gel Suspension *(Nelson, Austral.)*; Sonergan *(May & Baker, UK)*; Tixylix *(May & Baker, Austral.; May & Baker, UK)*.

6158-z

Propiomazine Hydrochloride *(BANM, USAN, rINNM)*.

Wy-1359. 1-[10-(2-Dimethylaminopropyl)phenothiazin-2-yl]propan-1-one hydrochloride.
$C_{20}H_{24}N_2OS,HCl=376.9$.

CAS — 362-29-8 (propiomazine); 1240-15-9 (hydrochloride).

Pharmacopoeias. In *U.S.*

A yellow almost odourless powder. **Soluble** 1 in less than 1 of water, 1 in 6 of alcohol, and 1 in 2 of chloroform; practically insoluble in ether. A 2% solution has a pH of 4.6 to 5.6. **Store** in airtight containers. The *U.S.P.* injection should be stored at 15 to 30°.

6159-c

Propiomazine Maleate *(BANM, rINNM)*.

CB-1678; Propiomazine Hydrogen Maleate.
$C_{20}H_{24}N_2OS,C_4H_4O_4=456.6$.

CAS — 3568-23-8.

NOTE. Propiomazine is *USAN*.

Propiomazine maleate 1.3 mg is approximately equivalent to 1 mg of propiomazine and 1.1 mg of propiomazine hydrochloride.

Adverse Effects, Treatment, Precautions, and Absorption and Fate

As for the antihistamines in general, p.443. Local irritation may occur at the site of intravenous injection of propiomazine hydrochloride and there may be thrombophlebitis. As with all phenothiazine derivatives propiomazine should be used cautiously in patients with hepatic disease.

Uses and Administration
Propiomazine is a phenothiazine derivative with the properties of the antihistamines (see p.444).
It has been given by mouth as the maleate for sedation in doses equivalent to 25 mg of the base 2 to 4 times daily or 25 to 50 mg at night. It has also been given by intramuscular or intravenous injection in doses of 20 mg of the hydrochloride for anaesthetic premedication and during surgical and obstetric procedures; doses of up to 40 mg have been employed. Children weighing up to 27 kg have been given 0.55 to 1.1 mg per kg body-weight intramuscularly or intravenously. Those aged 2 to 4 years have been given 10 mg; 4 to 6 years 15 mg; older children, 25 mg.

Preparations
Propiomazine Hydrochloride Injection *(U.S.P.)*

Proprietary Names and Manufacturers
Largon *(Wyeth, USA)*; Propavan *(Pharmacia, Swed.)*; Serentin *(Midy, Ital.)*.

6161-w

Pyrrobutamine Phosphate *(BANM, USAN).*

1-[4-(4-Chlorophenyl)-3-phenylbut-2-enyl]pyrrolidine diphosphate.
$C_{20}H_{22}ClN,2H_3PO_4$=507.8.

CAS — 91-82-7 (pyrrobutamine); 135-31-9 (phosphate).

Pharmacopoeias. In *U.S.*

A white or almost white crystalline powder, usually with a faint odour. **Soluble** 1 in 10 of warm water; soluble 1 in 20 of alcohol; practically insoluble in chloroform and ether. **Store** in airtight containers. Protect from light.

Pyrrobutamine phosphate has the properties and uses of the antihistamines (see p.443). It has been given in usual doses of 15 mg two or three times daily.

Proprietary Names and Manufacturers
The following names have been used for multi-ingredient preparations containing pyrrobutamine phosphate—Co-Pyronil *(Lilly, UK)*.

13308-v

Terfenadine *(BAN, USAN, rINN).*

MDL-9918; RMI-9918. 1-(4-*tert*-Butylphenyl)-4-[4-(α-hydroxybenzhydryl)piperidino]butan-1-ol.
$C_{32}H_{41}NO_2$=471.7.

CAS — 50679-08-8.

Adverse Effects and Precautions

Terfenadine causes less drowsiness than the older antihistamines; in clinical studies the incidence of drowsiness has been similar to that seen with placebo. Other adverse effects that have been reported include headache, mild gastro-intestinal disturbances, increased appetite, sweating, and some skin rashes. The incidence of antimuscarinic effects is low.

Terfenadine 60 mg, 120 mg and 240 mg had no effect on psychomotor skills or subjective feelings, and 120 mg, did not influence the adverse effects of diazepam or alcohol in a study involving 20 healthy subjects.— L. Moser *et al., Eur. J. clin. Pharmac.,* 1978, *14,* 417.

In a study in 50 healthy subjects, azatadine maleate 1 mg twice daily and terfenadine 60 mg twice daily were not associated with decreased psychomotor performance. Azatadine appeared to increase the appetite after 26 hours from the start of treatment.— D. K. Luscombe *et al., Pharmatherapeutica,* 1983, *3,* 370.

Further reports of terfenadine not affecting performance: A. N. Nicholson and B. M. Stone, *Br. J. clin. Pharmac.,* 1982, *13,* 199; A. N. Nicholson *et al., ibid., 14,* 683.

See also p.443.

ALOPECIA. Hair loss was associated with terfenadine treatment in a 24-year-old patient. Regrowth occurred when treatment was stopped.— S. K. Jones and W. N. Morley (letter), *Br. med. J.,* 1985, *291,* 940.

EFFECTS ON THE LIVER. Three episodes of acute hepatitis with jaundice occurred in a patient taking terfenadine intermittently over a period of 17 months. Liver function tests returned to normal after interruption of the drug.— D. Larrey *et al.* (letter), *Ann. intern. Med.,* 1985, *103,* 634.

EFFECTS ON THE SKIN. Terfenadine administration was associated with 108 reports of skin reactions, including rashes, urticaria, angioedema, photosensitivity reactions and peeling of the skin of the hands or feet.— B. H. C. Stricker *et al., Br. med. J.,* 1986, *293,* 536.

PORPHYRIA. Terfenadine was considered to be unsafe in patients with acute porphyria because it has been shown to be porphyrinogenic in *animals* or *in vitro* systems.— M.R. Moore and K.E.L. McColl, *Porphyrias, Drug Lists,* Glasgow, Porphyria Research Unit, University of Glasgow, 1987.

Absorption and Fate

Terfenadine is well absorbed from the gastro-intestinal tract. It is extensively bound to plasma proteins. It is excreted in the urine and the faeces, mainly as metabolites.

Uses and Administration

Terfenadine has the actions and uses of the antihistamines p.444. However, it has little central sedative activity. It is used to relieve the symptoms of allergic rhinitis, conjunctivitis, and allergic dermatological disorders.
The usual dose in adults and children over 12 years is 60 mg twice a day. Alternatively for hay-fever, 120 mg may be taken in the morning. A dose of 30 mg twice a day has been recommended in children aged 6 to 12 years.

A single-dose study demonstrated circadian variation in the onset, duration, and degree of antihistamine action of terfenadine.— A. Reinberg *et al., Eur. J. clin. Pharmac.,* 1978, *14,* 245.

A review of the pharmacodynamic properties and therapeutic efficacy of terfenadine. Studies have shown that terfenadine binds preferentially to peripheral rather than central H_1-histamine receptors. This property may be responsible for terfenadine's apparent lack of CNS effects. Suppression of histamine-induced skin wheal lasts for at least 12 hours after administration. Terfenadine has been found to be as effective as other antihistamines in the treatment of allergic rhinitis and allergic dermatological disorders. The most frequently reported adverse effect has been drowsiness, but its incidence is comparable with that produced in patients taking placebo. Dry mouth has occurred in 2 to 5% of patients taking terfenadine compared with 4% in those taking placebo, and 3 to 8% in patients taking other antihistamines.— E. M. Sorkin and R. C. Heel, *Drugs,* 1985, *29,* 34.

Further short reviews of the uses and adverse effects of terfenadine: *Drug & Ther. Bull.,* 1984, *22,* 21; M. L. Brandon, *Drugs,* 1985, *30,* 377; *Med. Lett.,* 1985, *27,* 65.

For a comparison of terfenadine with acrivastine, see Acrivastine p.444.

Terfenadine was considered to be a particularly valuable antihistamine for use by divers because of its lack of sedation, especially when a nitrogen-oxygen breathing mixture is in use.— J. C. Betts, *Br. med. J.,* 1985, *291,* 592.

ALLERGY. *Dermographism.* In a 6-day double-blind placebo-controlled study terfenadine 60 mg twice daily reduced dermographic whealing and itch without subjective somnolence. These results were maintained in a subsequent long-term open study lasting 47 to 84 days.— L. B. Krause and S. Shuster, *Br. J. Derm.,* 1984, *110,* 73.

Rhinitis and hay fever. Terfenadine 60 mg twice daily was effective in controlling the symptoms of hay fever, particularly sneezing, running nose, and itching eyes. Increasing the dose to 120 mg twice daily did not improve the response. The mean onset of action was 72 minutes for the 60-mg dose and 59 minutes for the 120-mg dose.— J. C. Murphy-O'Connor *et al., J. int. med. Res.,* 1984, *12,* 333.

Terfenadine 60 mg twice a day was effective in relieving the symptoms of hay fever in a study involving 47 patients. The median onset of action was 3 hours for terfenadine compared with 2 days for astemizole 10 mg once daily. On the eighth day of treatment there were no differences in the effectiveness of the two treatments.— J. P. Girard *et al., J. int. med. Res.,* 1985, *13,* 102.

Terfenadine 60 mg by mouth twice daily and beclomethasone dipropionate aqueous nasal spray, 200 µg twice a day were both effective in relieving the symptoms of hay fever in a double-blind study in 40 patients, although there was greater relief of nasal symptoms with beclomethasone and of eye symptoms with terfenadine. Beclomethasone was considered to be superior in inhibiting the breakthrough of nasal symptoms when the pollen count was high.— K. B. J. Beswick *et al., Curr. med. Res. Opinion,* 1985, *9,* 560.

Further references to the use of terfenadine in allergic rhinitis: M. L. Brandon and M. Weiner, *Ann. Allergy,* 1980, *44,* 71; C. I. Backhouse *et al., Practitioner,* 1982, *226,* 347; J. P. Kemp *et al., Ann. Allergy,* 1985, *54,* 502.

Urticaria. A report of 24 patients with urticaria, some with associated angioedema, whose response to terfenadine 120 mg daily was insufficient. In most of them increasing the daily dose to 240 mg slightly increased the antihistamine effects but beyond this dose there was little or no improvement. None of the patients developed drowsiness but of 2 who took 960 mg daily one complained of slight dizziness.— R. P. Warin (letter), *Br. J. Derm.,* 1984, *111,* 121.

Beneficial responses were seen in 10 out of 14 patients with chronic idiopathic urticaria when treated with terfenadine 60 mg twice a day.— J. Ferguson *et al., Br. J. clin. Pharmac.,* 1985, *20,* 639.

ASTHMA. In 10 patients with exercise-induced asthma, terfenadine 120 or 180 mg by mouth offered protection against exercise-induced asthma in an exercise test 4 hours later; 3 patients showed good protection, 4 partial protection, and 3 no protection.— K. R. Patel, *Br. med. J.,* 1984, *288,* 1496.

PRURITUS. In 8 patients with pruritus due to liver disease cholestyramine (up to 8 g daily) and terfenadine (up to 180 mg daily) were each significantly more effective in relieving pruritus than chlorpheniramine (up to 12 mg daily) or placebo.— J. S. Duncan *et al., Br. med. J.,* 1984, *289,* 22.

Proprietary Preparations

Triludan *(Merrell, UK). Tablets,* scored, terfenadine 60 mg.
Suspension, terfenadine 30 mg/5 mL.

Proprietary Names and Manufacturers

Nebralin *(Gayoso Wellcome, Spain)*; Seldane *(Merrell Dow, Canad.; Merrell Dow, USA)*; Teldane *(Merrell, Fr.; Merrell, Ger.; Lepetit, Ital.; Merrell Dow, Switz.)*; Triludan *(Merrell Dow, Spain; Merrell, UK)*.

6164-y

Thenalidine Tartrate *(BANM, rINNM).*

Thenophenopiperidine Tartrate; Thenopiperidine Tartrate. *N*-(1-Methyl-4-piperidyl)-*N*-(2-thenyl)aniline hydrogen tartrate.
$C_{17}H_{22}N_2S,C_4H_6O_6$=436.5.

CAS — 86-12-4 (thenalidine); 16509-35-6 (tartrate).

Thenalidine tartrate has the properties and uses of the antihistamines (see p.443). There have been reports of agranulocytosis associated with its use.

Proprietary Names and Manufacturers
Sandosten *(Sandoz, S.Afr.)*.

6165-j

Thenyldiamine Hydrochloride *(BANM, rINNM).*

Thenyldiaminium Chloride. *NN*-Dimethyl-*N'*-(2-pyridyl)-*N'*-(3-thenyl)ethylenediamine hydrochloride.
$C_{14}H_{19}N_3S,HCl$=297.9.

CAS — 91-79-2 (thenyldiamine); 958-93-0 (hydrochloride).

Pharmacopoeias. In *Arg.*

Thenyldiamine hydrochloride is an ethylenediamine derivative with the properties and uses of the antihistamines (see p.443). Doses of 10 mg have been given by mouth three times daily. It has also been administered nasally. Thenyldiamine is an isomer of methapyrilene.

Proprietary Names and Manufacturers
The following names have been used for multi-ingredient preparations containing thenyldiamine hydrochloride—Hayphryn *(Winthrop, UK)*;
Neo-Synephrine Antihistamine Cold Tablets *(Winthrop, Austral.)*; NTZ *(Winthrop, Austral.)*; NTZ Superinone *(Winthrop, Austral.)*; Thenfacol *(Winthrop, Austral.)*.

NOTE. The *UK* preparations Bronchilator and Franol Plus have been reformulated to exclude thenyldiamine hydrochloride.

6166-z

Thiazinamium Methylsulphate
Methylpromethazinium Methylsulfuricum; Thiazinamium Metilsulfate *(rINN)*. Trimethyl[1-methyl-2-(phenothiazin-10-yl)ethyl]ammonium methyl sulphate.
$C_{19}H_{26}N_2O_4S_2$=410.5.

CAS — 2338-21-8 (thiazinamium); 58-34-4 (methylsulphate).

NOTE. Thiazinamium Chloride is *USAN*.

Pharmacopoeias. In *Fr.*

Thiazinamium methylsulphate is a phenothiazine derivative with the properties and uses of the antihistamines (see p.443). It has been given in doses of 0.6 to 1.2 g daily by mouth.

References to the absorption and fate of thiazinamium methylsulphate.— J. H. G. Jonkman *et al.*, *J. Pharm. Pharmac.*, 1974, *26, Suppl.*, 63P (oral and intramuscular administration); J. H. G. Jonkman *et al.* (letter), *Lancet*, 1976, *1*, 693 (intramuscular and intravenous administration); J. H. G. Jonkman *et al.*, *Clin. Pharmac. Ther.*, 1977, *21*, 457 (oral and intramuscular administration); J. H. G. Jonkman *et al.*, *Int. J. Pharmaceut.*, 1979, *3*, 55 (rectal administration); J. H. G. Jonkman *et al.*, *J. pharm. Sci.*, 1979, *68*, 69 (rectal administration).

Proprietary Names and Manufacturers
Multergan *(Belg.; Specia, Fr.; Specia, Neth.)*.

6167-c

Thonzylamine Hydrochloride *(BANM, rINNM)*.
N-p-Anisyl-*N'N'*-dimethyl-*N*-(pyrimidin-2-yl)ethylenediamine hydrochloride.
$C_{16}H_{22}N_4O,HCl$=322.8.

CAS — 91-85-0 (thonzylamine); 63-56-9 (hydrochloride).

Pharmacopoeias. In *Arg.*

Thonzylamine hydrochloride is an ethylenediamine derivative with the properties and uses of the antihistamines (see p.443). It has been used for nasal administration and has also been given by mouth in doses of 50 mg to 75 mg daily.

Proprietary Names and Manufacturers
Tonamil *(Ecobi, Ital.)*.

The following names have been used for multi-ingredient preparations containing thonzylamine hydrochloride— Biomydrin *(Warner, UK)*.

6168-k

Tolpropamine Hydrochloride *(BANM, rINNM)*.
NN-Dimethyl-3-phenyl-3-*p*-tolylpropylamine hydrochloride.
$C_{18}H_{23}N,HCl$=289.8.

CAS — 5632-44-0 (tolpropamine); 3339-11-5 (hydrochloride).

Tolpropamine hydrochloride is an alkylamine derivative with the properties of the antihistamines (see p.443). It has been used by topical application (1%) for the symptomatic relief of allergic and pruritic skin disorders.

Proprietary Names and Manufacturers
Pragman *(Hoechst, Austral.; Albert-Roussel, Ger.; Albert-Farma, Ital.)*; Pratalgin *(Spain)*.

6169-a

Trimeprazine Tartrate *(BANM, USAN)*.
Alimemazine Tartrate *(rINNM)*. *NN*-Dimethyl-2-methyl-3-(phenothiazin-10-yl)propylamine tartrate.
$(C_{18}H_{22}N_2S)_2,C_4H_6O_6$=747.0.

CAS — 84-96-8 (trimeprazine); 4330-99-8 (tartrate).

Pharmacopoeias. In *Br., Braz., Jpn*, and *U.S.* Also in *B.P. Vet.*

A white or slightly cream-coloured odourless or almost odourless crystalline powder. It darkens in colour on exposure to light. Trimeprazine tartrate 25 mg is approximately equivalent to 20 mg of trimeprazine. **Soluble** 1 in 2 to 4 of water, 1 in 20 to 30 of alcohol, 1 in 4 to 5 of chloroform, and 1 in 1800 of ether. A 2% solution has a pH of 5.0 to 6.5. **Store** in airtight containers. Protect from light.

Adverse Effects
As for the antihistamines in general, p.443. Depression of the CNS may be marked, especially at higher doses. Other effects include extrapyramidal symptoms, and, very rarely, agranulocytosis. Increases in appetite have been reported, and, as with other phenothiazines, photosensitivity reactions may occur. Malignant hyperpyrexia and convulsions have been reported in overdose.

Fatal malignant hyperpyrexia occurred in a 3-year-old child given 72 mg of trimeprazine tartrate.— D. G. Moyes, *Br. J. Anaesth.*, 1973, *45*, 1163.

Severe respiratory and CNS depression in 2 siblings given trimeprazine tartrate in doses of 2.4 and 2.9 mg per kg body-weight respectively.— N. P. Mann, *Archs Dis. Childh.*, 1981, *56*, 481.

Report of 4 children given trimeprazine 2.7 to 4.2 mg per kg body-weight by mouth as pre-operative medication who suffered severe hypotension with bradycardia within 90 minutes of administration.— W. B. Loan and D. Cuthbert, *Br. med. J.*, 1985, *290*, 1548.

For a report on the possible association between phenothiazine sedatives and sudden infant death, see promethazine p.459.

Treatment of Adverse Effects and Precautions
As for the antihistamines in general, p.443. Vomiting should not be induced. Particular attention should be paid to maintaining the blood pressure.

Absorption and Fate
As for the antihistamines in general, p.444.

Uses and Administration
Trimeprazine is a phenothiazine derivative related to chlorpromazine and with the properties of antihistamines (p.444). It has pronounced sedative and antihistaminic effects. It also has some antimuscarinic actions. It is used mainly for its marked effect in the relief of pruritus.

Trimeprazine tartrate is given by mouth for the relief of pruritis in doses of 10 mg two or three times daily for adults and doses of 2.5 to 5 mg at night or up to 4 times a day for children over 2 years. In severe cases adults have been given up to 100 mg daily. It may also be used for pre-operative medication of children. The usual recommended dose for children over 2 years, administered about 90 minutes before operation, is 2 to 4 mg per kg body-weight by mouth. When given with barbiturates or narcotics the dose of these should be reduced since their effect is enhanced.

Trimeprazine may also be used in cough linctuses.

ANAESTHESIA. When given with hyoscine as premedication in children, the effects of trimeprazine were most marked when the dose was given 2 hours before induction of anaesthesia. A dose of 4.4 mg per kg body-weight was more effective than 2.2 mg per kg in producing amnesia and in reducing salivation; its use was associated with a greater tendency to noisy delirium and with a high frequency of postoperative pallor. Sedation was unreliable but anti-emetic effects with doses of 2.2 or 4.4 mg of trimeprazine per kg were comparable.— D. R. Davies and A. Doughty, *Br. J. Anaesth.*, 1966, *38*, 878.

In a detailed study of a variety of drugs used pre- and postoperatively for vomiting after adenotonsillectomy, trimeprazine 4 mg per kg body-weight by mouth to a maximum of 100 mg with atropine 30 µg per kg given pre-operatively together with dihydrocodeine phosphate 1.0 to 1.5 mg per kg intramuscularly postoperatively was the most effective.— B. L. Smith and M. L. M. Manford, *Br. J. Anaesth.*, 1974, *46*, 373.

HYPNOTIC EFFECT. A regimen involving a short course of trimeprazine tartrate in high dosage in order to alter the sleep pattern of children with sleeping difficulties.— H. B. Valman, *Br. med. J.*, 1981, *283*, 422. For mention of excessive respiratory and CNS depression in children given trimeprazine, see above. A discussion of the treatment of night waking in children concluded that trimeprazine tartrate did not provide an answer to the problem of severe night waking.— *Lancet*, 1987, *2*, 948.

Preparations

Paediatric Trimeprazine Oral Solution *(B.P.)*. Paediatric Trimeprazine Tartrate Elixir; Paediatric Trimeprazine Elixir

Strong Paediatric Trimeprazine Oral Solution *(B.P.)*. Strong Paediatric Trimeprazine Elixir; Strong Paediatric Trimeprazine Tartrate Elixir

Trimeprazine Tartrate Syrup *(U.S.P.)*. Potency is expressed in terms of the equivalent amount of trimeprazine.

Trimeprazine Tablets *(B.P.)*. Tablets containing trimeprazine tartrate.

Trimeprazine Tartrate Tablets *(U.S.P.)*. Potency is expressed in terms of the equivalent amount of trimeprazine.

Proprietary Preparations

Vallergan *(May & Baker, UK)*. *Tablets*, trimeprazine tartrate 10 mg.
Syrup, trimeprazine tartrate 7.5 mg/5 mL.

Vallergan Forte *(May & Baker, UK)*. *Syrup*, trimeprazine tartrate 30 mg/5 mL.

Proprietary Names and Manufacturers
Nedeltran *(Neth.)*; Panectyl *(Rhône-Poulenc, Canad.)*; Repeltin *(Heilit, Ger.)*; Temaril *(Herbert, USA)*; Theralen *(Leo Rhodia, Swed.)*; Theralene *(Belg.; Théraplix, Fr.; Rhône-Poulenc, Ger.; Rhone-Poulenc, Switz.)*; Vallergan *(May & Baker, Austral.; Rhone-Poulenc, Denm.; Rhône-Poulenc, Norw.; May & Baker, S.Afr.; May & Baker, UK)*; Variargil *(Rhone, Spain)*.

The following names have been used for multi-ingredient preparations containing trimeprazine tartrate— Valledrine *(May & Baker, Austral.; May & Baker, UK)*; Vallex *(May & Baker, UK)*.

6170-e

Trimethobenzamide Hydrochloride
(USAN, rINNM).
N-[4-(2-Dimethylaminoethoxy)benzyl]-3,4,5-trimethoxybenzamide hydrochloride.
$C_{21}H_{28}N_2O_5,HCl$=424.9.

CAS — 138-56-7 (trimethobenzamide); 554-92-7 (hydrochloride).

Pharmacopoeias. In *U.S.*

A white crystalline powder with a slight phenolic odour. **Soluble** 1 in 2 of water, 1 in about 59 of alcohol, 1 in 67 of chloroform, and 1 in 720 of ether. The *U.S.P.* injection has a pH of 4.8 to 5.2.

Adverse Effects, Treatment, and Precautions
As for the antihistamines in general, p.443.
Pain at the site of injection and local irritation after rectal administration have been noted.

For a review of the effects of antihistamines, including trimethobenzamide, during pregnancy, see p.443.

Uses and Administration
Trimethobenzamide hydrochloride is an ethanolamine derivative with the properties of the antihistamines (see p.444) but it appears to have only weak antihistamine activity. It is used in the control of nausea and vomiting. It is of little or no value in the prevention and treatment of motion sickness or vertigo.
The usual dose is 250 mg by mouth or 200 mg by deep intramuscular injection 3 or 4 times daily. It has also been given rectally, as a suppository. Children have been given 15 mg per kg body-weight daily or, if over 15 kg in weight, 100 to 200 mg 3 or 4 times daily.

Preparations

Trimethobenzamide Hydrochloride Capsules *(U.S.P.)*

Trimethobenzamide Hydrochloride Injection *(U.S.P.)*

Proprietary Names and Manufacturers
Anaus *(Molteni, Ital.)*; Ibikin *(IBP, Ital.)*; Stemetic

(Legere, USA); Tigan *(Roche, Canad.; Beecham Laboratories, USA)*.

The following names have been used for multi-ingredient preparations containing trimethobenzamide hydrochloride— Tigan Suppositories *(Beecham Laboratories, USA)*.

6171-l

Tripelennamine Citrate *(BANM, USAN, rINNM)*.

Tripelennaminium Citrate. *N*-Benzyl-*N'N'*-dimethyl-*N*-(2-pyridyl)ethylenediamine dihydrogen citrate.

$C_{16}H_{21}N_3,C_6H_8O_7$=447.5.

CAS — 91-81-6 (tripelennamine); 6138-56-3 (citrate).

Pharmacopoeias. In *U.S.*

A white crystalline powder. Tripelennamine citrate 150 mg is approximately equivalent to 100 mg of tripelennamine hydrochloride. **Soluble** 1 in 1 of water; freely soluble in alcohol; very slightly soluble in ether; practically insoluble in chloroform. **Protect** from light.

6172-y

Tripelennamine Hydrochloride *(BANM, USAN, rINNM)*.

Tripelen. Hydrochlor.; Tripelennamini Hydrochloridum; Tripelennaminium Chloride.

$C_{16}H_{21}N_3$,HCl=291.8.

CAS — 154-69-8.

Pharmacopoeias. In *Braz., Fr., Ind., Int., Pol., Turk.,* and *U.S.*

A white odourless crystalline powder. It slowly darkens on exposure to light. **Soluble** 1 in 1 of water, 1 in 6 of alcohol and of chloroform, and 1 in 350 of acetone; practically insoluble in ether and ethyl acetate. **Protect** from light.

Adverse Effects, Treatment, Precautions, and Absorption and Fate

As for the antihistamines in general, p.443.

Blood dyscrasias have been reported with tripelennamine.

ABUSE. Some reports of the intravenous abuse of tripelennamine with pentazocine in the combination known as T's and blues.— C. V. Showalter, *J. Am. med. Ass.*, 1980, *244*, 1224; L. R. Caplan *et al.*, *Neurology*, 1982, *32*, 623.

OVERDOSAGE. A severe toxic reaction, including agitation and hallucinations, occurred in an 8-year-old child who was sprayed over the trunk and extremities with tripelennamine 2.1375 g in the treatment of severe poison ivy poisoning. It was likely that inhalation of the fine mist of the aerosol spray contributed to the reaction but in this patient the initial reaction began 3 hours after exposure suggesting that percutaneous absorption through the multiple skin lesions probably contributed significantly. The original reaction was prolonged by treatment with diphenhydramine and promethazine.— P. G. Schipior, *J. Pediat.*, 1967, *71*, 589.

Uses and Administration

Tripelennamine is an ethylenediamine derivative with the actions and uses of the antihistamines (see p.444). Antihistaminic activity lasts for 3 to 6 hours. It has antimuscarinic and marked local anaesthetic properties.

Tripelennamine hydrochloride is given in usual doses of 25 to 50 mg every 4 to 6 hours. Higher doses of up to 600 mg daily have been given. Alternatively a sustained release preparation containing 100 mg may be given every 8 to 12 hours. A recommended dose of the hydrochloride for children is 5 mg per kg body-weight daily in 4 to 6 divided doses; the citrate is used in equivalent doses in an elixir.

Tripelennamine hydrochloride has also been applied to the skin as a 2% cream.

In the *UK* the use of tripelennamine in cosmetics is prohibited by law.

Preparations

Tripelennamine Citrate Elixir *(U.S.P.)*

Tripelennamine Hydrochloride Tablets *(U.S.P.)*

Proprietary Names and Manufacturers of Tripelennamine and its Salts

Azaron *(Chefaro, Ger.; Chefaro, Neth.)*; PBZ *(Geigy, USA)*; Pyribenzamine *(Ciba-Geigy, Canad.)*; Sedilene *(Montefarmaco, Ital.)*.

6173-j

Triprolidine Hydrochloride *(BANM, USAN, rINNM)*.

(*E*)-2-[3-(Pyrrolidin-1-yl)-1-*p*-tolylprop-1-enyl]pyridine hydrochloride monohydrate.

$C_{19}H_{22}N_2$,HCl,H_2O=332.9.

CAS — 486-12-4 (triprolidine); 550-70-9 (hydrochloride, anhydrous); 6138-79-0 (hydrochloride, monohydrate).

Pharmacopoeias. In *Br.* and *U.S.*

A white crystalline powder, odourless or with a slight unpleasant odour. **Soluble** 1 in about 2 of water, 1 in 1.5 to 1.8 of alcohol, 1 in less than 1 of chloroform, and 1 in 2000 of ether. **Store** in airtight containers. Protect from light.

Adverse Effects, Treatment, and Precautions

As for the antihistamines in general, p.443.

For a comparison of the effects of triprolidine and terfenadine on driving skills, see p.443.

Absorption and Fate

As for the antihistamines in general, p.444.

In a study in 3 women of the excretion of triprolidine and pseudoephedrine, taken by mouth in a combined preparation, triprolidine was found to reach concentrations in breast milk similar to those found in plasma in one subject, and slightly lower than in plasma in the others. It was calculated that 0.06 to 0.2% of the ingested dose was excreted in breast milk over 24 hours. Concentrations of pseudoephedrine in breast milk exceeded those in plasma in all 3 women.— J. W. A. Findlay *et al.*, *Br. J. clin. Pharmac.*, 1984, *18*, 901.

Uses and Administration

Triprolidine hydrochloride has the actions and uses of the antihistamines (see p.444). It is given by mouth, the usual dose for adults being 2.5 to 5 mg three times daily. However, in the USA the recommended adult daily limit is 10 mg. The dose for children, which may be given three times daily, is up to 1 year of age 1 mg, 1 to 6 years 2 mg, and 6 to 12 years 3 mg. Once again lower doses are recommended in the USA.

A multicentre study in general practice in 189 children with otitis media showed that neither pseudoephedrine 30 mg twice daily nor triprolidine 2.5 mg twice daily given for 8 weeks were more effective than placebo in terms of relief of symptoms, time taken for symptoms to resolve, or recurrence-rate.— D. J. G. Bain, *Br. med. J.*, 1983, *287*, 654.

Triprolidine and pseudoephedrine were as effective when given alone as when given together in preventing nasal congestion produced by histamine challenge in 18 subjects with allergic rhinitis.— D. W. Empey *et al.*, *Br. J. clin. Pharmac.*, 1984, *18*, 86.

Preparations

Triprolidine Hydrochloride Syrup *(U.S.P.)*

Triprolidine and Pseudoephedrine Hydrochlorides Syrup *(U.S.P.)*

Triprolidine Hydrochloride Tablets *(U.S.P.)*

Triprolidine and Pseudoephedrine Hydrochlorides Tablets *(U.S.P.)*

Triprolidine Tablets *(B.P.)*. Triprolidine Hydrochloride Tablets.

Proprietary Preparations

Actidil *(Wellcome, UK)*. *Tablets*, scored, triprolidine hydrochloride 2.5 mg.
Elixir, triprolidine hydrochloride 2 mg/5 mL.

Pro-Actidil *(Wellcome, UK)*. *Tablets*, sustained-release, triprolidine hydrochloride 10 mg.

Proprietary Names and Manufacturers of Triprolidine Hydrochloride or another form of Triprolidine

Actidil *(Wellcome, Austral.; Canad.; Denm.; Wellcome, Ital.; S.Afr.; Wellcome, Swed.; Wellcome, UK; Wellcome, USA)*; Actidilon *(Arg.; Wellcome, Fr.)*; Actiphyll *(Gayoso Wellcome, Spain)*; Pro-Actidil *(Austral.; Wellcopharm, Ger.; Neth.; Wellcome, S.Afr.; Gayoso Wellcome, Spain; Switz.; Wellcome, UK)*; Pro-Actidilon *(Wellcome, Fr.)*; Venen *(Jpn)*.

The following names have been used for multi-ingredient preparations containing triprolidine hydrochloride or another form of triprolidine— Actifed *(Wellcome, Austral.; Wellcome, UK; Wellcome, USA)*; Actifed Compound Linctus *(Wellcome, UK)*; Actifed DM *(Wellcome, Canad.)*; Actifed Expectorant *(Wellcome, UK)*; Actifed with Codeine *(Wellcome, USA)*; Actifed-A *(Wellcome, Canad.)*; Actifed-C *(Wellcome, USA)*; Actifed-CC *(Wellcome, Austral.)*; CoActifed *(Wellcome, Canad.)*; CoActifed Expectorant *(Wellcome, Canad.)*; Linctifed *(Wellcome, UK)*; Sudafed Plus *(Calmic, UK)*; Triafed *(Schein, USA)*; Triafed-C *(Schein, USA)*; Trifed *(Geneva, USA)*; Vasylox Plus *(Wellcome, Austral.)*.

13384-k

Tritoqualine *(rINN)*.

L-554. 7-Amino-4,5,6-triethoxy-3-(5,6,7,8-tetrahydro-4-methoxy-6-methyl-1,3-dioxolo[4,5-*g*]isoquinolin-5-yl)phthalide.

$C_{26}H_{32}N_2O_8$=500.5.

CAS — 14504-73-5.

Tritoqualine is stated to inhibit histidine decarboxylase which catalyses the conversion of histidine to histamine. It has the uses of the antihistamines (see p.444) but is claimed to have no effects on the CNS.

Proprietary Names and Manufacturers

Hypohistamine *(Promesa, Spain)*; Hypostamine *(Promedica, Fr.; Zyma, Ital.)*; Inhibostamin *(Zyma, Ger.; Zyma, Switz.)*.

6175-c

Allergens and Specific Desensitisation

Units

100 000 units of house-dust mite extract (*Dermatophagoides pteronyssinus*) are contained in one ampoule of the First International Standard Preparation (1984).

100 000 units of short ragweed pollen extract are contained in the freeze-dried residue of 0.3 mL of an aqueous extract of the defatted pollen in one ampoule of the First International Standard Preparation (1983).

100 000 units of Timothy grass pollen extract are contained in the freeze-dried residue of 1 mL of an aqueous extract of the pollen in one ampoule of the First International Standard Preparation (1983).

Adverse Effects and Treatment

Adverse effects to prepared allergens can range from mild local reactions to severe generalised reactions which may be fatal. Severe reactions may be seen after skin tests in sensitive individuals as well as at any time during desensitisation, especially with insect venom. Aqueous solutions are more likely to provoke systemic reactions than preparations designed to give slower release rates. Severe reactions have also been attributed to tyrosine adsorbed vaccines which have a relatively short half-life.

Local reactions are normally limited to swelling and irritation. Systemic reactions, which may be immediate or delayed, include coughing, sneezing, rhinitis, urticaria, bronchospasm, laryngeal oedema, generalised anaphylaxis, and shock. Severe reactions normally occur within 30 minutes and should be treated promptly with adrenaline injection 1 in 1000, which should be immediately available when desensitising injections are being administered. Full supportive measures should be implemented and treatment with antihistamines and corticosteroids may be required for either immediate or delayed reactions. Further desensitisation should be stopped or continued at reduced dosage depending on the severity of the reaction and in accordance with the manufacturers recommendations.

Hypersensitivity has been reported to be induced in patients undergoing long-term therapy, particularly with aluminium-containing extracts.

A 19-year-old girl with allergic asthma and rhinitis who had received 14 desensitisation injections without reaction suffered an anaphylactic reaction and died following the fifteenth injection.— D. A. Rands, *Br. med. J.*, 1980, *281*, 854. A similar report.— R. C. H. Pollard (letter), *ibid.*, 1429.

The Committee on Safety of Medicines reported that desensitising vaccines have the potential to induce severe bronchospasm and anaphylaxis, and that these reactions had caused 26 deaths in the UK since 1957. In view of the risks, any desensitising agents should be used only where facilities for full cardiorespiratory resuscitation are immediately available and patients should be kept under medical observation for at least 2 hours after treatment.— *Br. med. J.*, 1986, *293*, 948.

Of twelve samples of *Aspergillus* extract used for desensitisation, 4 were found to contain aflatoxin, one being highly mutagenic as determined by the Ames' test. The results suggested that careful screening of commercially available mould extracts was warranted.— M. S. Legator *et al.*, (letter), *Lancet*, 1983, *2*, 915.

Precautions

Desensitising injections should not be given to patients with febrile conditions, serious immunological illness, or acute asthma. Allergen preparations should be avoided during pregnancy because of the risk to the foetus of any systemic reactions. Desensitising injections should only be administered where facilities for full cardiorespiratory resuscitation are immediately available. It has been recommended that patients should be observed for at least 2 hours after each injection. Strenuous exercise should be avoided for several hours following the injection. Whenever possible, the same batch of allergen should be used throughout the treatment course. Injections should be given subcutaneously and not by intravenous or intramuscular injection.

Antihistamines should be avoided for at least 24 hours before sensitivity testing is carried out; they have been given, during desensitisation, to very sensitive patients.

Diagnostic Use

Sensitivity testing can be used to confirm that suspected allergens are predominantly responsible for the symptoms of a suspected allergy. However, sensitivity testing should not form the sole basis of the treatment of allergic conditions.

Delayed hypersensitivity reactions such as contact dermatitis are normally tested using patch tests. A number of standard techniques are available, but in general they all involve maintaining a standard amount of the test substance in contact with the skin for 24 to 48 hours. A positive response is shown by erythema, swelling, or vesiculation. The sensitivity of different parts of the body varies, and this should be accounted for in applying test substances and controls. The test results are normally read half to one hour after removal of the patches to allow any pressure effects of the patches to subside.

Immediate hypersensitivity reactions such as allergic rhinitis, allergic asthma, and insect-sting allergy are tested using prick, scratch, or intradermal tests. Since the allergen is introduced through the skin in these tests the risk of systemic reactions is greater, and adrenaline injection should be kept available. This is particularly important for insect venoms. The test involves pricking or scratching the skin through a drop of allergen in solution, and comparing the result after 15 minutes with a control. The intradermal test is used if the prick test result does not agree with a strong clinical suspicion. The radioallergosorbent test (RAST) measures antigen-specific IgE, and can be used where skin tests are impractical, as in severe skin disorders or in apprehensive patients.

Recommendations of the subcommittee of the allergy section of the Canadian Paediatric Society on the use of diagnostic skin testing for allergy in children.— *Can. med. Ass. J.*, 1983, *129*, 828.

Desensitisation

The use of desensitising injections has become less popular following reports of severe and fatal anaphylactic reactions during therapy. Desensitisation with a specific allergen has been found to be useful in allergies to pollens, house-dust mite (*Dermatophagoides pteronyssinus*) and insect venom, particularly that of Hymenoptera. It is also used in allergies to a wide range of other substances including animal hair and dander, dusts and fungi. The mechanism of desensitisation is not fully understood; it may act partly by stimulating the production of IgG antibodies; these block the access of allergens to IgE attached to mast cells and thus reduce the degranulation of the mast cells with the resultant release of histamine and other mediators. Desensitisation is only a satisfactory treatment when a single allergen is predominantly responsible for the disorder. Desensitisation is not without danger, and it is often necessary to continue treatment for several years. Many patients may be adequately controlled on antihistamines or sodium cromoglycate and avoidance of the responsible allergens is also effective in some patients, although it is often difficult to achieve. Desensitisation has been found to be useful in hay fever and insect-venom allergy, but may be less effective in asthma. Desensitisation to pollens should be completed before the start of the pollen season.

The older units of measurement used for standardising allergen preparations such as percentage weight in volume and protein-nitrogen units (PNU) do not provide a reliable guide to the allergen content and for this reason great care must be taken if it is necessary to change to a different batch of allergen during a course of treatment. This problem is claimed to be overcome by the use of biological or activity units which are standardised on allergenic activity using RAST. Great care must be taken when desensitising to Hymenoptera sting not to confuse the older whole-body extracts which are practically inert with the highly allergenic purified venom extracts.

Desensitisation is normally carried out by subcutaneous injection of gradually increasing concentrations of allergen extract until a maintenance dose is achieved. The allergen must not be injected intramuscularly or intravenously. Stringent precautions must be taken whenever prepared allergens are being used. Dosage schedules vary, but the conventional method involves giving each injection at an interval of 7 to 14 days. Rush schedules are also used in which several injections are given daily on consecutive days, usually as a hospital inpatient.

The use of hyposensitisation therapy should be carefully controlled. Only insect venoms, grass pollens, and perhaps house dust mite extracts should be used. The modern extracts are potent, containing highly purified antigens, and therefore great care is required in using this treatment, particularly for patients with asthma. Full facilities for cardiopulmonary resuscitation must be immediately available, and patients must be carefully monitored before, during, and for two hours after injections.— J. O. Warner and J. W. Kerr, *Br. med. J.*, 1987, *294*, 1179. Further comments on the use of allergen extracts for desensitisation: H. Morrow Brown and A. W. Frankland (letter), *ibid.*, 1613; J. O. Warner and J. W. Kerr (letter), *ibid.*, 1614; S. M. Wood and R. D. Mann (letter), *ibid.*, *295*, 445.

Hyposensitisation to poison ivy had not been shown to be effective and could cause adverse effects that were often unpleasant and sometimes dangerous.— *Med. Lett.*, 1981, *23*, 40.

Rush hyposensitisation was successful in a woman with allergy to seminal plasma.— C. Frisch *et al.* (letter), *Lancet*, 1984, *1*, 1073.

ASTHMA. Desensitisation has proved disappointing in the treatment of asthma on the whole. However, there is a small group of patients in whom desensitisation, particularly to pollens, has produced a great improvement in their asthma.— S. G. F. Matts, *Br. J. clin. Pract.*, 1984, *38*, 205.

HOUSE-DUST ALLERGY. A review and discussion of the limited value of hyposensitisation to house-dust mites in adults.— *Br. med. J.*, 1980, *280*, 589.

A multicentre study of house-dust mite extract in bronchial asthma. Of 70 patients recruited at the start of the study, 56 were observed for at least 6 months; 24 of these were also taking corticosteroids. Of 43 patients who started injections of active material 7 had side-effects severe enough to necessitate withdrawal. In patients not receiving corticosteroids the treated group did a little better than the controls but no benefit was apparent by extending treatment beyond 18 weeks. In contrast patients receiving corticosteroids given placebo injections did a little better than the treated group. In view of the marginal benefit which was found only in the patients not receiving corticosteroids it seems doubtful whether treatment in this form is suitable for general use.—Mite Allergy Subcommittee of the Research Committee of the British Thoracic Association, *Br. J. Dis. Chest*, 1979, *73*, 260.

INSECT STINGS. A review of allergy to bee and wasp stings. There is no consistent pattern of reaction in patients who experience an allergic reaction to stings, and spontaneous cure rates of 40% have been reported. Cutaneous and respiratory reactions are among the most common reactions, and gastro-intestinal and visual symptoms, which are peculiar to insect-sting allergy. Diagnosis should be based largely on clinical history. Skin-prick and RAST tests can be used to confirm the clinical impression and to identify the insect. The choice of management is between treating allergic reactions symptomatically when they occur or hyposensitising the patient to prevent future reactions, and is highly controversial. Desensitisation is expensive and not without risk, although the use of pure venom extract is highly effective, and at present it is difficult to define criteria for its use.— P. W. Ewan, *J. R. Soc. Med.*, 1985, *78*, 234.

Further brief reviews of the use of bee and wasp venoms.— *Drug & Ther. Bull.*, 1981, *19*, 47; *Med. Lett.*, 1983, *25*, 53.

Proprietary Preparations of Allergens

Alavac-P *(Bencard, UK). Allergen extracts*, mixture, alum-precipitated, 12 grass pollens. For desensitisation.

Albay Pure Venom *(Dome/Hollister-Stier, UK). Allergen extract*, single, powder for reconstitution, lyophilised bee venom (*Apis mellifera*), supplied with diluent.
Allergen extract, single, powder for reconstitution, lyophilised wasp venom (*Vespula* spp.), supplied with diluent. For desensitisation.

Allpyral-G *(Dome/Hollister-Stier, UK). Allergen extracts*, mixture, alum-precipitated, 5 grass pollens. For desensitisation.

Allpyral-Specific *(Dome/Hollister-Stier, UK). Allergen extracts*, single or mixtures, alum-precipitated, individually formulated, specific allergens. For desensitisation.

Allpyral Stinging Insects *(Dome/Hollister-Stier, UK). Allergen extract*, single, alum-precipitated, whole body bee extract.
Allergen extract, single, alum-precipitated, whole body wasp extract. For desensitisation.

Alpha-Test (formerly known as Dialysed Allergen Extracts) *(Dome/Hollister-Stier, UK). Allergen extracts*, mixture, 2 grass pollens.
Allergen extract, single, house-dust mite (*Dermatophagoides pteronyssinus*.
For prick tests.

Bencard Skin Testing Solutions *(Bencard, UK). Allergen extracts*, single and mixtures, range of allergens. Glycerinated solutions for prick tests and buffered solutions for intradermal tests.

Conjuvac *(Dome/Hollister-Stier, UK). Allergen extracts*, mixture, sodium alginate-conjugated, powder for reconstitution, 2 grass pollens, supplied with diluent.
Allergen extract, single, sodium alginate-conjugated, powder for reconstitution, house-dust mite (*D. pteronyssinus*), supplied with diluent. For desensitisation.

DHS Skin Testing Solutions (formerly known as Glycerinated Skin Testing Solutions) *(Dome/Hollister-Stier, UK). Allergen extracts*, single and mixtures, range of allergens. For prick tests or nasal provocation.

Merck Skin Testing Solutions *(E. Merck, UK). Allergen extracts*, single and mixtures, range of allergens. For prick tests or nasal provocation.

Norisen *(E. Merck, UK). Allergen extracts*, single or mixtures, aluminium-adsorbed, individually formulated, specific allergens. For desensitisation.

Norisen Grass *(E. Merck, UK). Allergen extracts*, mixture, aluminium-adsorbed, 6 grass pollens. For desensitisation.

Pharmalgen *(Pharmacia, UK). Allergen extract*, single, powder for reconstitution, bee venom (*Apis mellifera*), supplied with diluent.
Allergen extract, single, powder for reconstitution, wasp venom (*Vespula* spp.), supplied with diluent. For desensitisation.

Pollinex *(Bencard, UK). Allergen extracts*, mixture, tyrosine-adsorbed, 12 grass pollens, in unit-dose prefilled syringes. For desensitisation.

Spectralgen *(Pharmacia, UK). Allergen extracts*, single, powder for reconstitution, 4 grass pollens and 3 tree pollens, supplied with diluent or depot diluent.
Allergen extracts, mixture, powder for reconstitution, 4 grass pollens, supplied with diluent or depot diluent.
Allergen extracts, mixture, powder for reconstitution, 3 tree pollens, supplied with diluent or depot diluent. For desensitisation.

Proprietary Names and Manufacturers of Allergens

A.D.L.; Alavac-P *(Bencard, UK)*; Alavac-S *(Bencard, Switz.; Bencard, UK)*; Albay Pure Venom *(Dome/Hollister-Stier, UK)*; Allogen-Ragweed *(Key, USA)*; Allpyral *(Miles, Austral.; Dome, Denm., Dome, Switz.)*; Allpyral Stinging Insects *(Dome/Hollister-Stier, UK)*; Allpyral-D *(Dome/Hollister-Stier, UK)*; Allpyral-G *(Dome/Hollister-Stier, UK)*; Allpyral-Mite Fortified House Dust *(Dome/Hollister-Stier, UK)*; Allpyral-Specific *(Dome/Hollister-Stier, UK)*; Alpha-Test *(Dome/Hollister-Stier, UK)*; Anjuvac *(Dome, Denm.)*; Aquagen *(ALK, Denm.)*; Bacterial Allergy Vaccine *(Commonwealth Serum Laboratories, Austral.)*; Bencard A; Bencard HDM; Bencard Skin Testing Solutions *(Bencard, S.Afr.; Bencard, UK)*; Conjuvac *(Dome/Hollister-Stier, UK)*; Coryza Vaccine Mixed *(Commonwealth Serum Laboratories, Austral.)*; DHS Skin Testing Solutions *(Dome/Hollister-Stier, UK)*; DHS-Alphatest *(Dome, Denm.)*; DHS-Betatest *(Dome, Denm.)*; Glycerinated Skin Testing Solutions *(Dome/Hollister-Stier, UK)*; Insect Allergen Extracts *(Commonwealth Serum Laboratories, Austral.)*; Merck Skin Testing Solutions *(E. Merck, UK)*; Migen *(Bencard, Switz.; Bencard, UK)*; Mite Allergen Extract *(Commonwealth Serum Laboratories, Austral.)*; Norisen *(E. Merck, UK)*; Norisen Grass *(E. Merck, UK)*; Paspat *(Luitpold, Austral.)*; Pharmalgen *(Pharmacia, Canad.; ALK, Denm.; Pharmacia, Switz.; Pharmacia, UK)*; Phazet *(Pharmacia, Denm.)*; Pollinex *(Beecham, Canad.; Bencard, UK)*; Polvac + *(Bencard, Switz.)*; Rhus All *(Barry, USA)*; Rhus Tox Antigen *(Lemmon, USA)*; S.D.L.; SDV *(Bencard, UK)*; S.D.V-R.; Soluprick *(ALK, Denm.)*; Spectralgen *(Pharmacia, UK)*; Tyrivac.

Antihypertensive Agents

850-w

Blood pressure is expressed in terms of the arterial systolic and diastolic pressures. Since many factors influence blood pressure it is not possible to define normality or abnormality precisely using only the figures for systolic and diastolic pressures. An arbitrary definition of normal adult blood pressure provided by the World Health Organization (WHO) is a systolic pressure equal to or below 140 mmHg (18.7 kPa) together with a diastolic (fifth Korotkoff phase) pressure equal to or below 90 mmHg (12.0 kPa). Hypertension in adults is also arbitrarily defined by WHO as a systolic pressure equal to or greater than 160 mmHg (21.3 kPa) and a diastolic pressure (fifth phase) equal to or greater than 95 mmHg (12.7 kPa). Blood pressure is still expressed in mmHg and this is the unit used throughout *Martindale.* The SI unit, the kilopascal (kPa), has not been generally accepted for expressing blood pressure.

The risks of elevated blood pressure are now well recognised as a result of studies such as those carried out at Framingham, and evidence has accumulated to show that reduction of elevated blood pressure reduces the risks of morbidity and mortality.

The drugs used in the treatment of hypertension belong to groups with distinct pharmacological actions, though the precise mode of action of some of them is not as yet fully understood. Major drugs used in the treatment of hypertension and described in other sections are diuretics (see p.973), beta-adrenoceptor blocking agents (see p.781), and calcium-channel blocking agents (see Nifedipine, p.1509). The antihypertensive drugs described in this section may be broadly classified as:

1. direct-acting vasodilators, which include: diazoxide (p.476), hydralazine (p.483), minoxidil (p.491), sodium nitroprusside (p.500);
2. centrally acting agents, which include: clonidine (p.472), guanabenz (p.480), methyldopa (p.487);
3. alpha-adrenoceptor blocking agents, which include: indoramin (p.485), phenoxybenzamine (p.493), phentolamine (p.494), prazosin (p.495);
4. adrenergic neurone blocking agents, which include: bethanidine (p.468), debrisoquine (p.476), guanethidine (p.481);
5. angiotensin-converting enzyme (ACE) inhibitors, which include: captopril (p.468), enalapril (p.478);
6. ganglion-blocking agents, which include: pentolinium (p.493), trimetaphan (p.503).

Other drugs used in the treatment of hypertension and described in this section include the rauwolfia alkaloids such as reserpine (p.498), the monoamine oxidase inhibitor pargyline (p.493), and the serotonin blocking agent ketanserin (p.486).

Arterial Hypertension, Report of a WHO Expert Committee, *Tech. Rep. Ser. Wld Hlth Org. No. 628,* 1978.

The question of whether diastolic or systolic blood pressure is the more important in predicting hypertensive complications is still the subject of debate. Fisher (*Lancet,* 1985, *2,* 1349) argued that while there was no evidence that diastolic pressure was of greater value than systolic, systolic pressure had been shown to have prognostic value in cardiovascular complications of hypertension. In addition, systolic pressure was easier to measure than diastolic, and measurement of systolic pressure by indirect methods was more accurate than diastolic. This view was supported by Gilston (*ibid.,* 1986, *1,* 209) although Ramsay and Waller (*ibid., 2,* 854) argued that diastolic pressure was much the better predictor of the risk of stroke and of the likely benefit from antihypertensive treatment. They based this assertion on a re-analysis of evidence presented in the MRC trial of treatment of mild hypertension (*Br. med. J.,* 1985, *291,* 97); their conclusions were criticised both by the original authors (S. Peart and G. Greenberg, *Lancet,* 1986, *2,* 1042) and by Wright (*ibid.,* 1041). In addition Wright considered systolic pressure to be a better predictor than diastolic of cardiovascular episodes in patients where systolic and diastolic pressures were not well correlated and pointed out that the measurement of diastolic pressure was subjective and that there was still no agreement as to whether the fourth or fifth Korotkoff sound should be used. However, Ramsay and Waller were supported by Venning (*ibid.,* 1338) who felt it would be premature to abandon diastolic pressure measurement until further information was available.

EFFECTS ON MORBIDITY AND MORTALITY. In the Multiple Risk Factor Intervention Trial on the mortality from coronary heart disease in 12 866 high-risk men, only a small and insignificant reduction in mortality was seen in patients who were treated for hypertension and given advice on smoking and reduction of blood lipid concentrations compared with controls.— *J. Am. med. Ass.,* 1982, *248,* 1465. Discussions: G. D. Lundberg, *ibid.,* 1501; P. M. Rautaharju, *Can. med. Ass. J.,* 1983, *128,* 113.

Results of the Medical Research Council study of treatment of mild hypertension indicated that active drug treatment was associated with a reduction in the rate of strokes. Treatment did not appear substantially to alter the overall risk of coronary heart disease. Treatment was with propranolol or bendrofluazide: neither treatment had a clear advantage over the other, although the diuretic appeared somewhat better at preventing stroke, while the beta-blocker may have prevented coronary events in non-smokers. For stroke and also for all cardiovascular events the difference between rates in smokers and non-smokers was greater than the effect of drug treatment.— Medical Research Council Working Party, *Br. med. J.,* 1985, *291,* 97. Discussion.— A. Breckenridge, *ibid.,* 89.

Results of the Hypertension Detection and Follow-up Program in 10 940 hypertensive patients indicated that antihypertensive treatment reduced the incidence of left ventricular hypertrophy and cardiomegaly and reversed pre-existing abnormalities of this type.— *Hypertension,* 1985, *7,* 105.

It was proposed that severe, possibly irreversible, restriction of coronary vascular reserve could explain the failure of antihypertensive therapy to reduce the incidence of coronary heart disease in patients with hypertension. Compensatory mechanisms in the brain could account for the observed reduction in the incidence of stroke in these patients.— S. Strandgaard and S. Haunsø, *Lancet,* 1987, *2,* 658.

See also under Hypertension in the Elderly, below.

Further references on the effects of the treatment of hypertension: Hypertension Detection and Follow-up Program Cooperative Group, *J. Am. med. Ass.,* 1979, *242,* 2562; *Lancet,* 1980, *1,* 1261; *New Engl. J. Med.,* 1982, *307,* 976; M. F. Oliver, *Br. med. J.,* 1982, *285,* 1065; D. C. Connolly *et al., Mayo Clin. Proc.,* 1983, *58,* 249; R. Callcott *et al., Med. J. Aust.,* 1984, *141,* 419; *J. Hypertens.,* 1985, *3,* 379.

RISKS AND BENEFITS OF TREATMENT. A discussion of the quality of life of treated hypertensives. The benefits of treating mild hypertensives at relatively low risk must be balanced against the adverse effects of detection and treatment on their wellbeing.— J. S. Gill and D. G. Beevers, *Br. med. J.,* 1983, *287,* 1490.

Review and discussion of studies of the treatment of mild hypertension. Although some benefits have been observed, the cost of treatment and the incidence of adverse effects probably do not justify the treatment of all patients with mild hypertension. In the absence of identifiable high-risk subgroups of patients the most reasonable course of action would seem to be a period of observation with treatment if the diastolic pressure is consistently 100 mmHg or more.— *Lancet,* 1985, *2,* 645. Comment on the cost of treating patients with mild hypertension.— P. C. Milner and I. S. Johnson (letter), *ibid.,* 1364.

A discussion of the risks of antihypertensive therapy concluded that non-drug treatment could be effective in mild hypertension and that with care the risks of antihypertensive therapy were considerably less than the benefits.— *Lancet,* 1986, *2,* 1075.

A discussion of how far blood pressure should be lowered. In most studies there has been no difficulty in demonstrating the beneficial effects of treatment of hypertension on the incidence of stroke, and there is now sufficient evidence to be fairly certain that drug treatment has a differential effect on stroke and heart attack. There is also evidence to suggest that excessive lowering of blood pressure may be harmful, perhaps as a result of decreased coronary perfusion, or possibly due to adverse effects of the drugs used unrelated to their hypotensive activity. However, these conclusions have generally been based on relatively small numbers of observations and it is also possible that a similar excess in mortality may be observed in untreated patients with low blood pressure.— *Lancet,* 1987, *2,* 251. Comment: J. M. Cruickshank *et al.* (letter), *ibid.,* 695 and 870; P. C. Waller *et al.* (letter), *ibid.,* 969. See also J. M. Cruickshank *et al., ibid., 1,* 581.

Adverse effects and precautions. Comment on the suggestion that antihypertensive therapy might impair physical and mental performance, and possible implications on driving skills.— *Lancet,* 1984, *1,* 87. Results of a study indicating that there was no evidence that the commonly-used antihypertensive drugs contribute to road traffic accidents, but suggesting an association with adrenergic blockers, particularly debrisoquine.— J. P. Deasy and L. E. Ramsay, *Br. J. clin. Pharmac.,* 1984, *18,* 269P.

A review of psychiatric reactions to antihypertensive agents.— H. A. McClelland, *Adverse Drug React. Bull.,* 1983, (Apr.), 364.

Report of 8 cases of focal cerebral ischaemia attributed to antihypertensive therapy.— G. J. Hankey and S. S. Gubbay, *Med. J. Aust.,* 1987, *146,* 412.

A review of sexual dysfunction caused by drugs including antihypertensive agents.— *Med. Lett.,* 1987, *29,* 65.

Further references to adverse effects to antihypertensive therapy: J. Poloniecki and M. Hamilton, *Hum. Toxicol.,* 1985, *4,* 287; J. D. Curb *et al., J. Am. med. Ass.,* 1985, *253,* 3263; S. Laganière *et al., Curr. ther. Res.,* 1986, *39,* 970.

Interactions. Non-steroidal anti-inflammatory drugs cause salt and water retention and could be expected to impair the action of antihypertensive agents. The mechanism is believed to involve a modification of renal prostaglandins.— M. J. Kendall, *Prescribers' J.,* 1986, *26,* 135.

Choice of Antihypertensive Treatment

In recent years a systematic approach to the treatment of hypertension has developed. During the initial assessment period and before any drug treatment patients are given advice on weight reduction and salt restriction, on reduction in cigarette smoking and alcohol intake, and on increased exercise. Such measures may be adequate in some patients with mild hypertension to control the blood pressure without the use of drugs. The decision to use drug treatment is based on the degree of hypertension, the adverse effects and potential benefits of treatment, and known risk factors. Factors which may indicate a higher risk of complications include male sex, black race, increasing age, abnormal blood lipids, cigarette smoking, obesity, diabetes mellitus, and existing cardiovascular disease, or a family history of cardiovascular complications. Patients with a diastolic pressure of about 105 mmHg or more generally require drug treatment, but in patients with mild hypertension, drug treatment is generally reserved for those in high-risk groups and those not responding to non-drug treatment.

Drug treatment is initiated by a stepped care approach. Although the final choice of drug will depend on the preferences of the physician and the characteristics of the patient there is broad agreement on the basic treatment. The standard approach is usually to give a thiazide diuretic or a beta blocker as the first step, but the calcium-channel blockers and ACE inhibitors are gaining in popularity as step 1 agents. If an adequate response is not achieved an alternative agent can be substituted or a second drug of a different type added. Traditionally, second-step therapy consists of a beta blocker and a thiazide diuretic given together but a number of combinations have been tried, the aim being to achieve an additive hypotensive effect while minimising side-effects. The third phase of treatment generally consists of a diuretic, a beta blocker, and either a vasodilator or a calcium-channel blocker or an ACE inhibitor. Patients resistant to triple therapy have been given a centrally acting agent or guanethidine in addition. The regimen should be kept as simple as possible and the majority of patients can be managed with once or twice daily dosing schedules. Fixed combination products may be useful once a patient has been stabilised on a regimen, but should not be used to initiate treatment.

Revised recommendations for classification and treatment of hypertension by the *US* Joint National Committee on Detection, Evaluation, and Treatment of High Blood Pressure.— *Archs intern. Med.*, 1984, *144*, 1045.

Report of the Canadian Hypertension Society's consensus conference on the management of mild hypertension.— A. G. Logan, *Can. med. Ass. J.*, 1984, *131*, 1053.

The 1986 Guidelines for the treatment of mild hypertension issued jointly by WHO and the International Society of Hypertension (WHO/ISH) recommended that effective antihypertensive measures should be started before symptoms appear. Mild hypertension in adults was defined as a diastolic pressure (fifth Korotkoff phase) persistently between 90 and 104 mm Hg (12 to 14 kPa) without obvious signs of left ventricular hypertrophy or damage to the heart or other organs. If the diastolic pressure remains on average below 100 mm Hg advice against smoking and appropriate non-drug treatment was recommended. Drug therapy should be started in patients with a diastolic pressure on average 100 mm Hg or above, and considered in patients with a diastolic pressure of 95 mm Hg or above despite non-drug treatment, and in high-risk patients. Factors which could influence the decision to begin drug treatment include the systolic pressure, age of the patient, cardiac signs, renal disease, unassociated potentially fatal disease, or a family history of stroke or heart disease.— *Bull. Wld Hlth Org.*, 1986, *64*, 31.

Further discussions of the treatment of mild hypertension: E. D. Freis, *New Engl. J. Med.*, 1982, *307*, 306; R. G. Wilcox *et al.*, *Br. med. J.*, 1986, *293*, 433; M. Moser *et al.*, *Drugs*, 1986, *31*, 279.

References on the choice of antihypertensive agent: G. Andrews *et al.*, *Br. med. J.*, 1982, *284*, 1523; *Lancet*, 1982, *2*, 1316; B. R. Walker, *Curr. ther. Res.*, 1984, *35*, 1; L. H. Opie, *Lancet*, 1984, *1*, 496; S. A. Smith and W. A. Littler, *J. clin. Hosp. Pharm.*, 1985, *10*, 113; *Med. Lett.*, 1987, *29*, 1.

ANTIHYPERTENSIVE THERAPY DURING ANAESTHESIA. Despite earlier concern on the risks of administering antihypertensive agents to patients about to undergo surgery, substantial subsequent data have confirmed that it is not only safe but probably preferable to continue such medication up to and including the morning of surgery.— L. Goldman, *Ann. intern. Med.*, 1983, *98*, 504. See also P. Ballard, *Br. J. Hosp. Med.*, 1987, *38*, 398.

A review of the use of induced hypotension during surgery.— W. R. MacRae, *Br. J. Hosp. Med.*, 1985, *33*, 341.

HYPERTENSION IN DIABETIC PATIENTS. A discussion of the choice of antihypertensive therapy in the diabetic patient. The information available about antihypertensive drugs in diabetes is limited and in some cases conflicting. Cardioselective beta blockers are acceptable first-line drugs in most hypertensive diabetics. A potassium-sparing diuretic would be a reasonable second-line choice in insulin-dependent patients without nephropathy, or prazosin or other vasodilators in non-insulin dependent patients. The main recommendation is that, once antihypertensive therapy is instituted, each patient should be reassessed for side-effects and for biochemical indices of blood glucose, potassium, and lipids.— A. D. Struthers, *Postgrad. med. J.*, 1985, *61*, 563.

HYPERTENSION IN THE ELDERLY. A study by the European Working Party on High Blood Pressure in the Elderly (EWPHE) involving 840 hypertensives over the age of 60 years. Treatment with diuretics with the addition of methyldopa if necessary was not associated with a reduction in overall mortality but was associated with a reduction in cardiovascular mortality-rate mainly due to a reduction in cardiac deaths with a smaller, statistically non-significant reduction in cerebrovascular mortality. Deaths from myocardial infarction were reduced.— A. Amery *et al.*, *Lancet*, 1985, *1*, 1349. Comment on the implications of the study. Reservations concerning the clinical applicability of the results included the lack of information on patient selection, the age and clinical characteristics of patients, and the rather unusual choice of treatment.— *ibid.*, 1369. A more detailed analysis of the data from the EWPHE study showed that cardiovascular mortality and morbidity were related to treatment, age, cardiovascular complications at randomisation, and systolic but not diastolic blood pressure. There was some evidence that treatment effects decreased with advancing age. Little or no benefit could be demonstrated in patients over the age of 80 years.— A. Amery *et al.*, *ibid.*, 1986, *2*, 589.

In a study involving 884 elderly hypertensive patients in general practice, stepwise antihypertensive treatment had no overall effect on mortality or on the incidence of fatal or non-fatal heart attacks, but there was a 42% reduction in the incidence of stroke and a 22% reduction in cardiovascular deaths, although this latter reduction was not statistically significant.— J. Coope and T. S. Warrender, *Br. med. J.*, 1986, *293*, 1145.

A statement on hypertension in the elderly by the Working Group on Hypertension in the Elderly including a brief review of clinical studies and recommendations for management. Dietary measures should be tried first as an alternative to drug therapy but care should be taken to ensure that the restricted diet is nutritionally adequate. If drug treatment is needed, a stepped-care approach should be used but initial doses of drugs should be lower, possibly no more than half the usual recommended dose, and the increments more gradual than for younger patients. Except when the blood pressure is alarmingly high or when it is causing dangerous symptoms, simultaneous introduction of two or more drugs is contra-indicated because of the increased sensitivity of some elderly patients to all antihypertensive agents.— *J. Am. med. Ass.*, 1986, *256*, 70.

Reviews and discussions of the treatment of hypertension in the elderly.— M. Chellingsworth and D. G. Beevers, *Postgrad. med. J.*, 1986, *62*, 1; *Drug & Ther. Bull.*, 1988, *26*, 9.

Recommendations from the Consensus Conference on Hypertension in the Elderly including comments on the need for more research.— P. Larochelle *et al.*, *Can. med. Ass. J.*, 1986, *135*, 741.

HYPERTENSION IN PREGNANCY. A discussion of the treatment of cardiovascular diseases including hypertension in pregnancy. Although the risks of maternal hypertension during pregnancy are clearly recognised, the benefits to the foetus of pharmacological intervention remain controversial. Results of controlled studies suggest that treatment of both chronic hypertension and pregnancy-induced hypertension is beneficial to the foetus, but the size of these studies limits the ability to draw definite conclusions. Recommendations about the level of blood pressure which warrants treatment during pregnancy is controversial, particularly since blood pressure is normally expected to fall to a nadir in the mid-trimester.— K. R. Lees and P. C. Rubin, *Br. med. J.*, 1987, *294*, 358.

References on the management of hypertension in pregnancy: W. F. Lubbe, *Drugs*, 1984, *28*, 170; A. Svensson, *Acta med. scand.*, 1985, *Suppl.* 695, 5-50; M. de Swiet, *Br. med. J.*, 1985, *291*, 365; P. C. Rubin, *Prescribers' J.*, 1985, *25*, 19; M. D. Lindheimer and A. I. Katz, *New Engl. J. Med.*, 1985, *313*, 675; M. Zinaman *et al.*, *Lancet*, 1985, *1*, 1245; J. N. Oats, *Med. J. Aust.*, 1985, *143*, 4; J. S. Horvath *et al.*, *ibid.*, 19; E. D. M. Gallery, *ibid.*, 23; P. Armstrong, *Br. J. Hosp. Med.*, 1986, *36*, 347.

NON-DRUG TREATMENT OF HYPERTENSION. A review of the non-drug treatment of hypertension, including weight reduction, sodium restriction, potassium, magnesium and calcium supplementation, dietary changes, exercise, relaxation, and the influence of alcohol, caffeine, and nicotine intake.— N. M. Kaplan, *Ann. intern. Med.*, 1985, *102*, 359. See also *Ann. intern. Med.*, 1983, *98*, 697-884.

Dietary fats and blood lipids. Results of a randomised study indicating that restriction of dietary fat was associated with a reduction in blood pressure. The fall in blood pressure was greater in hypertensive than in normotensive subjects.— P. Puska *et al.*, *Lancet*, 1983, *1*, 1.

Review of the effects of antihypertensive agents on serum lipids and lipoproteins.— R. P. Ames, *Drugs*, 1986, *32*, 335.

Mineral supplementation. Comment on dietary potassium and hypertension.— *Lancet*, 1985, *1*, 1308.

Comment on the influence of calcium on hypertension.— *Lancet*, 1986, *1*, 359.

Sodium restriction. Discussion of the effect of salt restriction in hypertension. Advising patients with hypertension to avoid salt was considered to do no harm, and a few studies had suggested that it may help some hypertensive patients. Whether it prevents the development of essential hypertension, or reduces its complications, remained unproven.— *Drug & Ther. Bull.*, 1986, *24*, 25.

Review of studies of the effects of salt restriction in hypertension suggesting that the effect is small and restricted largely to systolic blood pressure, and that salt restriction would only be of limited use in young patients with mild hypertension.— D. E. Grobbee and A. Hofman, *Br. med. J.*, 1986, *293*, 27. Comment that salt restriction is more effective in black than in white hypertensive patients.— M. R. Lee *et al.* (letter), *ibid.*, 266.

Further references on dietary sodium and hypertension: G. A. MacGregor, *Lancet*, 1983, *1*, 750; B. H. Scribner, *J. Am. med. Ass.*, 1983, *250*, 388; *Lancet*, 1984, *2*, 671; N. A. Boon and J. K. Aronson, *Br. med. J.*, 1985, *290*, 949.

For further references and discussions on salt intake and hypertension, see p.1023.

Urgent Treatment of Severe Hypertension

In patients with severe hypertension, sudden reduction of blood pressure may lead to cerebral or myocardial ischaemia or blindness. Oral therapy with a beta blocker, a calcium-channel blocker, a vasodilator, or an ACE inhibitor is normally adequate with the aim of lowering diastolic pressure to 100 to 110 mmHg over the first 24 to 48 hours. Parenteral therapy is only indicated when severe hypertension is associated with encephalopathy, gross ventricular failure as in dissecting aortic aneurysm, or eclampsia. Antihypertensive agents which may be given parenterally include sodium nitroprusside, diazoxide, labetalol, and hydralazine (which is widely used in eclampsia).

There is now increasing awareness of the hazards of over-rapid blood pressure reduction. Renal, cerebral, or myocardial infarction or blindness may be caused by precipitous drops in pressure. The malignant phase of hypertension is not itself an indication for parenteral therapy. Antihypertensive drugs should only be given by the parenteral route if there is severe left ventricular failure or hypertensive encephalopathy. In most malignant hypertensives blood pressure should be reduced over a period of days rather than hours or minutes.— D. G. Beevers, *Prescribers' J.*, 1984, *24*, 91.

A review of the management of hypertensive emergencies. Hypertensive emergencies are defined as life-threatening conditions which require prompt reduction of blood pressure within minutes to 1 hour. Hypertensive emergencies should be distinguished from hypertensive urgencies in which there is no immediate risk to vascular integrity and a slower reduction over a period of hours to several days is appropriate. In general, hypertensive emergencies are treated with parenteral hypotensive drugs with the aim of reducing arterial pressure to a safer level, generally to a range of 100 to 110 mmHg diastolic, and not to achieve normotension.— J. Y. Garcia and D. G. Vidt, *Drugs*, 1987, *34*, 263.

Further references to the urgent management of severe hypertension: B. N. J. Walters, *Br. J. Hosp. Med.*, 1984, *31*, 49; R. H. Ferguson and P. H. Vlasses, *J. Am. med. Ass.*, 1986, *255*, 1607; *Med. Lett.*, 1987, *29*, 18.

851-e

Alkavervir

A mixture of alkaloids obtained from green veratrum and standardised for total antihypertensive effect.

CAS — 8002-39-9 (see also under Veratrum, Green).

Alkavervir is a mixture of alkaloids derived from green veratrum and has the properties and uses described under White Veratrum (p.504).

Proprietary Names and Manufacturers

Veriloid *(Riker, UK)*.

The following names have been used for multi-ingredient preparations containing alkavervir—Rauwiloid + Veriloid *(Riker, UK)*; Thiaver *(Riker, UK)*; Veriloid-VP *(Riker, UK)*.

852-l

Alseroxylon
Selected alkaloid hydrochlorides of *Rauwolfia serpentina.*

CAS — 8001-95-4.

Alseroxylon has properties and uses similar to those described under reserpine (see p.498). For the treatment of hypertension the usual recommended dose is 4 mg daily initially, and maintenance doses of 2 mg daily, but some sources recommend an initial dose of 1 mg daily. Intervals of at least 10 days are recommended between dosage adjustments.

Proprietary Names and Manufacturers
Angioserpina *(Ital.)*; Iposalfa *(Ital.)*; Rauwan *(Lisapharma, Ital.)*; Rauwiloid *(Austral.; Norw.*; *Riker, UK*; *Riker, USA)*; Ra-Valeas *(Ital.)*.

The following names have been used for multi-ingredient preparations containing alseroxylon— Pentoxylon *(Riker, UK)*; Rauwiloid + Veriloid *(Riker, UK)*.

853-y

Azamethonium Bromide *(BAN, rINN).*
Pentamethazene Bromide; Pentaminum. 2,2′-Methyliminobis(diethyldimethylammonium) dibromide.
$C_{13}H_{33}Br_2N_3$=391.2.

CAS — 60-30-0 (azamethonium); 306-53-6 (bromide).

Pharmacopoeias. In *Rus.*

Azamethonium bromide is a ganglion-blocking agent that has been used in the treatment of hypertension.

Proprietary Names and Manufacturers
Pendiomid *(Ciba-Geigy, Switz.)*.

18951-m

Benazepril Hydrochloride *(pINNM).*
CGS-14824A. (3*S*)-3-{[(1*S*)-1-Carboxy-3-phenylpropyl]amino}-2,3,4,5-tetrahydro-2-oxo-1*H*-1-benzazepine-1-acetic acid hydrochloride, 3-ethyl ester; 1-Carboxymethyl-3-[1-ethoxycarbonyl-3-phenyl-(1*S*)-propylamino]-2,3,4,5-tetrahydro-1*H*-1(3*S*)-benzazepin-2-one hydrochloride.
$C_{24}H_{28}N_2O_5$,HCl.

CAS — 86541-75-5 (benazepril).

Benazepril is reported to be an angiotensin-converting-enzyme inhibitor.

References: M. D. Schaller *et al., Eur. J. clin. Pharmac.*, 1985, *28*, 267; G. Waeber *et al., ibid.*, 1987, *31*, 643.

Proprietary Names and Manufacturers
Ciba-Geigy, UK.

854-j

Bethanidine Sulphate *(BANM).*
Betanidine Sulphate *(pINNM)*; Betanidini Sulfas; Bethanidine Sulfate *(USAN)*. 1-Benzyl-2,3-dimethylguanidine sulphate.
$(C_{10}H_{15}N_3)_2,H_2SO_4$=452.6.

CAS — 55-73-2 (bethanidine); 114-85-2 (sulphate).

Pharmacopoeias. In *Br., Eur., Ind., It., Neth., Nord.,* and *Swiss.*

A white odourless powder. Freely **soluble** in water; sparingly soluble in alcohol; practically insoluble in ether.

Adverse Effects, Treatment, and Precautions
As for Guanethidine Monosulphate, p.481.
With bethanidine sulphate diarrhoea is rare. Postural hypotension with transient sweating and headache may occur.

Absorption and Fate
Bethanidine is rapidly but incompletely absorbed from the gastro-intestinal tract. It is excreted unchanged in the urine.

A study of the pharmacokinetics of bethanidine in 3 hypertensive subjects following intravenous and oral administration. Bethanidine was incompletely absorbed from the gastro-intestinal tract. It was excreted unchanged in the urine by active transport, and despite high renal clearance had an apparent half-life for the terminal urinary excretion phase of about 7 to 11 hours; this may be explained by a large apparent volume of distribution, suggesting that it is extensively bound to tissues, though not to plasma albumin.— D. Shen *et al., Clin. Pharmac. Ther.*, 1975, *17*, 363.

Uses and Administration
Bethanidine is an antihypertensive agent with actions and uses similar to those of guanethidine monosulphate (see p.482), but it causes less depletion of noradrenaline stores. It also has a more rapid onset, together with a shorter duration of action, than guanethidine.
The usual initial dose of bethanidine sulphate is 10 mg three times daily. The dosage is then increased by 5 mg three times daily at brief intervals according to the response of the patient. The maximum recommended dose is 200 mg daily. To reduce side-effects smaller doses of bethanidine may be given in conjunction with a thiazide diuretic and other antihypertensive agents.
In hypertensive heart disease, hypertensive crises, or malignant hypertension, an initial dose of 20 mg of bethanidine sulphate may be given and increased by 10 to 20 mg every 4 to 6 hours.

For a report of comparative antihypertensive effects and toxicity of guanethidine, bethanidine, and debrisoquine, see Guanethidine, Uses, p.482.

Preparations

Bethanidine Tablets *(B.P.)*. Tablets containing bethanidine sulphate.

Proprietary Preparations

Bendogen *(Lagap, UK). Tablets*, bethanidine sulphate 10 and 50 mg.

Esbatal *(Calmic, UK). Tablets*, scored, bethanidine sulphate 10 and 50 mg.

Proprietary Names and Manufacturers
Batel *(Gayoso Wellcome, Spain)*; Bendogen *(Lagap, UK)*; Benzoxine *(Jpn)*; Betaling *(Jpn)*; Esbaloid *(Canad.)*; Esbatal *(Arg.; Austral.; Belg.*; *Wellcome, Ital.*; *Neth.; Norw.*; *Wellcome, S.Afr.*; *Wellcome, Swed.*; *Calmic, UK)*; Eusmanid *(Aust.)*; Hypersin *(Jpn)*; Regulin *(Denm.; Norw.)*.

12443-b

Bietaserpine *(pINN).*
1-(2-Diethylaminoethyl)reserpine; DL-152; S-1210. Methyl 1-(2-diethylaminoethyl)-18-*O*-(3,4,5-trimethoxybenzoyl)reserpate.
$C_{39}H_{53}N_3O_9$=707.9.

CAS — 53-18-9.

Bietaserpine is an antihypertensive agent with properties and uses similar to reserpine (p.498). It is given as the tartrate in an initial dose of 10 mg twice daily for 2 to 4 weeks and a maintenance dose of 10 mg daily depending on the patients response.

Proprietary Names and Manufacturers
Pleiatensin Simplex *(Guidotti, Ital.)*; Tensibar *(Lefrancq, Fr.)*.

12464-s

Bufeniode *(rINN).*
Di-iodobuphenine; HF-241. 4-Hydroxy-3,5-di-iodo-α-{1-[(1-methyl-3-phenylpropyl)amino]ethyl}benzyl alcohol.
$C_{19}H_{23}I_2NO_2$=551.2.

CAS — 22103-14-6.

Bufeniode is used as an antihypertensive agent.

Proprietary Names and Manufacturers
Proclival *(Roussel, Arg.*; *Houdé, Fr.)*.

16559-h

Cadralazine *(rINN).*
ISF-2469. Ethyl 6-[ethyl(2-hydroxypropyl)amino]-3-pyridazinecarbazate.
$C_{12}H_{21}N_5O_3$=283.3.

CAS — 64241-34-5.

Cadralazine is a vasodilator with actions and uses in hypertension similar to those of hydralazine (p.484).

Studies of the haemodynamic effects of cadralazine: A. Semplicini *et al., Curr. ther. Res.*, 1983, *34*, 1038; J. A. Bouthier *et al., Clin. Pharmac. Ther.*, 1986, *39*, 82.

ABSORPTION AND FATE. Studies of the pharmacokinetics of cadralazine in healthy subjects.— S. A. Hauffe *et al., Eur. J. Drug Metab. Pharmacokinet.*, 1985, *10*, 217; H. Schütz *et al., ibid.*, 147.

USES. Studies of cadralazine in the treatment of hypertension: F. V. Costa *et al., Curr. ther. Res.*, 1983, *34*, 653; M. Catalano *et al., Eur. J. clin. Pharmac.*, 1983, *24*, 157; A. Pirrelli *et al., Curr. ther. Res.*, 1984, *36*, 712; M. Catalano *et al., Eur. J. clin. Pharmac.*, 1985, *28*, 135; A. Salvadeo *et al., Arzneimittel-Forsch.*, 1985, *35*, 623; M. Stornello *et al., Curr. ther. Res.*, 1986, *40*, 448; B. Persson *et al., Eur. J. clin. Pharmac.*, 1987, *31*, 513.

Proprietary Names and Manufacturers
ISF, Ital.; Ciba-Geigy, UK.

856-c

Captopril *(BAN, USAN, rINN).*
SQ-14225. 1-[(2*S*)-3-Mercapto-2-methylpropionyl]-L-proline.
$C_9H_{15}NO_3S$=217.3.

CAS — 62571-86-2.

Pharmacopoeias. In *U.S.*

A white or off-white crystalline powder which may have a characteristic sulphide-like odour. M.p. 104° to 110°. Freely **soluble** in water, in alcohol, in chloroform, and in methyl alcohol. **Store** in airtight containers.

Brief review of the stability of captopril.— W. Lund and H. J. Cowe (letter), *Pharm. J.*, 1986, *2*, 179.

Report of preformulation studies carried out by the manufacturers into the stability of captopril in aqueous solution. Degradation was pH-independent below pH4, but above pH4 the rate of degradation of captopril increased with increasing pH. Degradation was increased in the presence of metal ions.— P. Timmins *et al., Int. J. Pharmaceut.*, 1982, *11*, 329.

The manufacturer reported that an aqueous solution of captopril prepared from pulverised tablets with an initial concentration of 1 mg per mL contained 96.6% of its initial concentration when stored for 5 days at room temperature in a tightly closed glass container. The concentration of captopril disulphide was an average of 0.55% on formulation and rose to 5.3% by 5 days. The solution should be used within 2 days of preparation since it contains no preservative.— C. D. Andrews and A. Essex (letter), *Pharm. J.*, 1986, *2*, 734.

Adverse Effects
Captopril is generally well tolerated at doses below 150 mg daily. The commonest adverse effects are skin rashes which may be accompanied by pruritus, fever, and eosinophilia. A persistent dry cough has been reported. Taste disturbances may sometimes be associated with weight loss. Adverse effects tend to be dose-related and more frequent in patients with impaired renal function. Proteinuria has occurred mainly in patients with existing renal disease and some of these patients develop nephrotic syndrome. Evidence of deterioration in renal function, including increasing blood concentrations of urea and creatinine, and reversible acute renal failure have been reported in patients with existing renal dysfunction and may be aggravated by hypovolaemia. Captopril administration has also been associated with increases in blood potassium concentrations.
Neutropenia and agranulocytosis occur rarely in patients with normal renal function but have been reported in patients with renal failure and

collagen vascular disorders such as systemic lupus erythematosus and scleroderma. Thrombocytopenia and anaemia have also been reported.

Transient hypotension may occur at the start of therapy particularly in patients with congestive heart failure and in sodium- or volume-depleted patients. This can be minimised by starting with a low dose and giving the initial dose at night.

Other adverse effects reported with captopril include angioedema, tachycardia, lymphadenopathy, stomatitis, gastro-intestinal irritation, abdominal pain, and rare cases of hepatocellular injury and jaundice.

A review of the adverse reactions with angiotensin-converting-enzyme inhibitors. The high incidence of toxicity observed during early studies resulted from the high doses thought necessary at the time and the use of a patient population now recognised to be at increased risk of adverse effects including patients with renal disease, collagen vascular disease, and those on immunosuppressive therapy. As dosages have been reduced, there has been a reduction in the incidence of many side-effects previously described without loss of drug activity, and treatment with ACE-inhibitors has been shown to lack the metabolic and autonomic side-effects associated with conventional antihypertensive therapies.— R. Di Bianco, *Med. Toxicol.*, 1986, *1*, 122. See also C. R. W. Edwards and P. L. Padfield, *Lancet*, 1985, *1*, 30.

Results of a postmarketing surveillance study of 6737 hypertensive patients treated with captopril either alone or in combination with other antihypertensive drugs. In patients with normal renal function, dysgeusia occurred in 2.2% and rash in 4.3% of patients taking doses of 150 mg or less daily. The frequency was increased in patients with impaired renal function and in those taking higher doses. Symptoms of hypotension were reported in 5% of patients and were generally mild and transient. The frequency of discontinuation of therapy due to adverse effects was 5.8% at 12 months. Neutropenia occurred in 6 patients with severe renal impairment but was not reported in patients with normal renal function. Renal failure occurred in 33 patients; 20 with pre-existing progressive renal failure, 6 with renovascular hypertension or renal transplants, 1 with severe atherosclerosis and diabetes, and 3 with pre-existing renal failure. Proteinuria developed in 35 patients, 26 of whom had a history of renal disease.— A. C. Jenkins *et al.*, *J. cardiovasc. Pharmac.*, 1985, *7, Suppl.* 1, S96. Another postmarketing surveillance study.— I. R. Edwards *et al.*, *Br. J. clin. Pharmac.*, 1987, *23*, 529.

Report of lymphadenopathy in 2 patients treated with captopril.— H. Åberg *et al.*, *Br. med. J.*, 1981, *283*, 1297.

Cerebral symptoms occurred in 2 patients with arterial hypertension and carotid artery stenosis following administration of captopril 6.25 mg.— H. Jensen *et al.*, *Br. med. J.*, 1986, *293*, 1073.

ALLERGY. A report of an allergic reaction, resembling serum sickness in a patient taking captopril.— S. J. Hoorntje *et al.* (letter), *Lancet*, 1979, *2*, 1297.

Eosinophilia in 7 of 20 patients treated with captopril up to 350 mg daily for one year.— J. G. Kayanakis *et al.* (letter), *Lancet*, 1980, *2*, 923.

Fever, rash, and pericarditis were associated with captopril treatment in a 72-year-old man with ischaemic cardiomyopathy.— J. Zatuchni (letter), *J. Am. med. Ass.*, 1984, *251*, 343.

Angioedema and exacerbation of impaired renal function was associated with captopril therapy in a 57-year-old patient. The reaction recurred when the patient was subsequently treated with enalapril.— D. R. J. Singer and G. A. MacGregor (letter), *Br. med. J.*, 1986, *293*, 1243.

The Committee on Safety of Medicines had received reports of angioedema in 6 patients taking captopril between May 1981 and January 1986, and in 13 patients taking enalapril between January 1985 and January 1986.— S. M. Wood *et al.*, *Br. med. J.*, 1987, *294*, 91.

See also under Effects on the Skin.

APHTHOUS ULCERS. A report of severe aphthous ulcers in a woman taking captopril. The ulcers resolved when captopril was withdrawn and recurred when captopril was given again.— Y. K. Seedat (letter), *Lancet*, 1979, *2*, 1297.

Ulceration of the tongue was associated with captopril in doses up to 450 mg daily in a 72-year-old patient who also experienced loss of taste sensation.— M. G. Nicholls *et al.*, *Ann. intern. Med.*, 1981, *94*, 659.

Report of a scalded sensation of the oral mucosa in 3 patients during treatment with either captopril or enalapril.— P. H. Vlasses *et al.*, *Br. med. J.*, 1982, *284*, 1672.

COUGH. A brief discussion on cough and angiotensin-converting-enzyme inhibition. The Committee on Safety of Medicines in the *UK* has received 365 reports of cough related to ACE inhibitors. The cough is persistent and nonproductive, commoner in women and nonsmokers, has been reported as a side-effect of at least 4 ACE inhibitors, and is likely to be caused by all drugs of this class. The cause is not clear; accumulation of bradykinin, indirect effects on prostaglandin production, and stimulation of the cough reflex have been proposed. It is important to recognise that a patient's cough may be a side-effect of an ACE inhibitor and to attempt to confirm the relationship. It may be reasonable to continue treatment if the patient can tolerate the cough although in many the ACE inhibitor may have to be withdrawn; some patients may be helped by reducing the dose.— K. E. Berkin and S. G. Ball, *Br. med. J.*, 1988, *296*, 1279.

Analysis of 33 reports of cough associated with captopril and 26 associated with enalapril received by the New Zealand Medicines Adverse Reactions Centre as part of an intensive monitoring programme. Typical symptoms were a persistent, paroxysmal, dry cough that was sometimes severe enough to disturb sleep or cause vomiting. Symptoms were sufficiently severe to warrant withdrawal in 25 patients taking captopril and 23 taking enalapril. Seven of the patients who experienced cough with captopril also experienced it with enalapril. After treatment was stopped recovery seemed to be rapid and complete. The cough seemed to be sex-related, with a higher incidence in women. Analysis of prescriptions from one region indicated an incidence of spontaneous reporting of cough of 1.1% for captopril and 2.8% for enalapril. Results indicated that both the incidence and recovery time were appreciably greater with enalapril.— D. M. Coulter and I. R. Edwards, *Br. med. J.*, 1987, *294*, 1521.

Concurrent administration of sulindac reduced or abolished cough due to ACE-inhibitor therapy in 6 patients, supporting the theory that prostaglandins could be involved in the pathogenesis.— M. G. Nicholls and N. L. Gilchrist (letter), *Lancet*, 1987, *1*, 872.

Study indicating that cough during treatment with ACE inhibitors is caused by increased sensitivity of the cough reflex, although the cause of this remains obscure.— R. W. Fuller and N. B. Choudry, *Br. med. J.*, 1987, *295*, 1025. See also A. H. Morice *et al.*, *Lancet*, 1987, *2*, 1116.

EFFECTS ON THE KIDNEYS. Reversible renal failure has been associated with captopril treatment in renal transplant patients particularly when renal perfusion is reduced by renal artery stenosis (D. Hooke *et al.*, *Br. med. J.*, 1982, *285*, 1538; J.C. Mason and P.J. Hilton, *ibid.*, 1983, *286*, 145; J.F. De Plaen *et al.*, *ibid.*, 146; J.J. Curtis *et al.*, *New Engl. J. Med.*, 1983, *308*, 377) or by other causes (K.A. Nath *et al.*, *ibid.*, *309*, 666; J.C. Daving and P.M. Mahieu, *Lancet*, 1985, *1*, 820). Complete occlusion of stenotic renal arteries in the transplanted kidney has been reported by Turney (*Br. med. J.*, 1986, *292*, 1672) in a patient taking captopril and by Brown and Williams (*ibid.*, 732) in a patient taking enalapril and in non-transplanted patients taking captopril (W. H. L. Hoefnagels and T. Thien, *ibid.*, 24) or enalapril (G.G. Hartnell and D.J. Allison, *ibid.*, 410). Acute renal failure has also occurred in non-transplant patients with renal artery stenosis (D.E. Hricik *et al.*, *New Engl. J. Med.*, 1983, *308*, 373; M.J. Schreiber and L.S.T. Fang, *J. Am. med. Ass.*, 1983, *250*, 31). These individual reports were supported by studies by Silas *et al.*, (*Br. med. J.*, 1983, *286*, 1702) and Jackson *et al.* (*Hypertension*, 1986, *8*, 650).

Hooke *et al.* considered that the reduction in renal function was due to allergic interstitial nephritis, although the Captopril Collaborative Study Group (*Lancet*, 1982, *1*, 988) found ultrastructural and immunohistological abnormalities similar to those seen in patients on captopril in renal biopsy material from hypertensive patients not exposed to captopril. Changes in renal blood flow due to the action of captopril on the renin-angiotensin system were thought to be the most likely cause by De Plaen *et al.*, Mason and Hilton, Schreiber and Fang, and Hricik *et al.* Hricik (*Ann. intern. Med.*, 1985, *103*, 222) also suggested that the extracellular volume was an important factor in captopril-induced renal insufficiency and that sodium loading could attenuate the adverse effects of captopril on renal haemodynamics, although his interpretation of the results was challenged by Spital (*ibid.*, 1986, *104*, 126) and Andreucci *et al.* (*ibid.*, 283). In a study of 5 patients with severe bilateral renovascular disease, Watson *et al.* (*Lancet*, 1983, *2*, 404) found that renal function deteriorated during treatment with captopril and a diuretic but not with captopril alone. They suggested that mild sodium depletion by diuretics could adversely affect the haemodynamic response of the kidney to captopril. Packer *et al.* (*Ann. intern. Med.*, 1987, *106*, 346) found that functional renal insufficiency occurred during ACE inhibition in up to one third of 140 salt-restricted patients with severe chronic heart failure treated with diuretics. They found that drug-induced uraemia resolved after a reduction in diuretic dosage or liberalisation of salt intake without exacerbation of heart failure again suggesting that haemodynamic effects were responsible.

Jackson *et al.* (*Lancet*, 1984, *1*, 225) believed that a trial of an ACE inhibitor was still treatment of choice in renovascular hypertension where surgical correction or angioplasty was contra-indicated, provided that renal function was monitored closely. Burris *et al.* (*ibid.*, 1985, *1*, 1511) reported the successful long-term use of captopril without deterioration of renal function in a patient with renal artery stenosis in a solitary functioning kidney. However, Schalekamp and Wenting (*ibid.*, 1984, *1*, 464) considered that Jackson could have underestimated the incidence of renal failure in patients with a stenotic kidney since severe reductions in glomerular filtration-rate, as demonstrated by scintillation camera renography, were not accompanied by large increases in serum creatinine concentrations when only one kidney was affected.

EFFECTS ON THE LIVER. Reports of hepatic damage associated with captopril: M. Vandenburg *et al.* (letter), *Br. J. clin. Pharmac.*, 1981, *11*, 105 (hepatocellular jaundice with secondary cholestasis); A. Zimran *et al.* (letter), *Br. med. J.*, 1983, *287*, 1676 (cholestatic jaundice); W. A. Parker, *Drug Intell. & clin. Pharm.*, 1984, *18*, 234 (cholestatic jaundice); J. Rahmat *et al.*, *Ann. intern. Med.*, 1985, *102*, 56 (cholestatic jaundice in 1 patient and review of 13 additional cases of cholestatic and mixed cholestatic-hepatocellular jaundice).

EFFECTS ON THE NERVOUS SYSTEM. Report of encephalopathy and focal neurologic signs associated with captopril therapy in a 62-year-old patient with impaired renal function. Symptoms improved when captopril was stopped.— S. Rapoport and P. Zyman, *Ann. intern. Med.*, 1983, *98*, 1023.

Severe peripheral neuropathy developed in a 70-year-old diabetic patient after 6 months of treatment with captopril. Power and sensation returned when captopril was stopped.— A. Samanta and A. C. Burden, *Br. med. J.*, 1985, *291*, 1172.

Report of Guillain-Barré polyneuropathy associated with captopril treatment in a 57-year-old patient which resolved rapidly when captopril was discontinued.— T. K. Chakraborty and W. S. J. Ruddell, *Postgrad. med. J.*, 1987, *63*, 221.

EFFECTS ON THE SKIN. Profuse hyperhidrosis followed by stomatitis and neutropenia developed in a 49 year-old patient receiving captopril.— M. H. Morse, *Br. med. J.*, 1984, *289*, 1272.

A report of 4 patients who developed nail dystrophy (onycholysis) in association with captopril therapy.— C. D. Brueggemeyer and G. Ramirez (letter), *Lancet*, 1984, *1*, 1352. A further case.— J. V. Borders, *Ann. intern. Med.*, 1986, *105*, 305.

Report of a severe cutaneous reaction to captopril in 4 patients. The reaction was not dose-related and was considered to be allergic in origin.— M. J. Goodfield and L. G. Millard, *Br. med. J.*, 1985, *290*, 1111. Comment.— F. W. Fairhead, *ibid.*, 1592. A more extensive report.— P. N. Furness *et al.*, *J. clin. Path.*, 1986, *39*, 902. A similar rash occurring in a 74-year-old man taking captopril recurred when enalapril was substituted.— K. J. Misch, *Br. med. J.*, 1985, *290*, 1829.

Report of long-standing hyperpigmentation associated with captopril therapy in 2 children.— M. B. O'Neil *et al.*, *Br. med. J.*, 1987, *295*, 333.

PREGNANCY AND THE NEONATE. Administration of captopril to *sheep* and *rabbits* in doses analogous to those suitable for man, was associated with an increase in still-births.— F. B. Pipkin *et al.* (letter), *Lancet*, 1980, *1*, 1256.

Evidence of abnormalities in a foetus aborted following the administration of captopril during pregnancy.— P. C. Duminy and P. du T. Burger (letter), *S. Afr. med. J.*, 1981, *60*, 805.

A woman with nephrotic syndrome and arterial hypertension was treated throughout pregnancy with captopril and acebutolol. Intrauterine growth retardation was identified from the end of the third month and became progressively more severe. A male infant was delivered by caesarean section at 34 weeks. Respiratory arrest occurred 15 minutes after birth and mild to severe hypotension was present for the first 10 days. The infant also had a patent ductus arteriosus. The intrauterine growth retardation could have been due to the drugs or to the severe maternal nephropathy.— M. -J. Boutroy *et al.* (letter), *Lancet*, 1984, *2*, 935. A further report.— R. Fiocchi *et al.* (letter), *ibid.*, 1153.

A brief discussion of foetal anuria or oligoanuria reported in 2 premature infants whose mothers had taken captopril during pregnancy.— J. -P. Guignard and E. G. John, *Clin. Perinatol.*, 1986, *13*, 377.

Treatment of Adverse Effects

Volume expansion with an intravenous infusion of sodium chloride injection has been recommended for the treatment of hypotension. Captopril is removed by dialysis.

Precautions

Captopril should be used with great caution in patients with impaired renal function particularly if renovascular disease is present or suspected, and in patients with collagen vascular disorders such as systemic lupus erythematosus or scleroderma. Renal function should be assessed in all patients prior to administration of captopril. Patients with existing renal disease or taking high doses of captopril should be monitored regularly for proteinuria. Regular white blood cell counts should be made during the initial stages of therapy particularly in patients with collagen vascular disorders or impaired renal function and in patients receiving immunosuppressive therapy.

Patients with congestive heart failure and patients who are likely to be salt or water depleted due to concomitant treatment with diuretics or dialysis may experience symptomatic hypotension during the initial stages of captopril therapy: this may be minimised by starting with a low dose, preferably on retiring.

Since raised serum-potassium concentrations may develop potassium-sparing diuretics, potassium supplements, or potassium-containing salt substitutes should be used with caution. The hypotensive effect of captopril is enhanced by diuretics and other antihypertensive agents. Indomethacin has been shown to reduce or abolish the hypotensive action of captopril, and salicylates appear to produce a similar effect. Captopril may cause false positive results in tests for acetone in urine.

Captopril has been reported to produce harmful effects in *animal* foetuses following large maternal doses, and is secreted into breast milk in nursing mothers (see also under Pregnancy and the Neonate in Adverse Effects, above).

Life-threatening severe hypotension and pre-renal uraemia occurred in a patient taking captopril following a diarrhoeal illness. Captopril was considered to have blocked the normal homoeostatic responses to extracellular fluid volume loss.— J. McMurray and D. M. Matthews (letter), *Lancet*, 1985, *1*, 581. A similar report.— P. R. Benett and S. A. Cairns (letter), *ibid.*, 1105. See also J. McMurray and D. M. Matthews, *Postgrad. med. J.*, 1987, *63*, 385.

Administration of captopril 12.5 mg resulted in an increase in mean cerebral blood flow of 17% in 6 patients aged between 51 and 63, but in a decrease in mean cerebral blood flow of 13% in 3 patients aged 71 to 72 in a study of patients with severe congestive heart failure.— K. E. Britton *et al.*, *Lancet*, 1985, *2*, 1236.

A report of a woman with Huntington's disease whose condition deteriorated dramatically during treatment with captopril and improved on withdrawal of the drug.— J. Goldblatt and A. Bryer, *Br. med. J.*, 1987, *294*, 1659.

ADMINISTRATION IN RENAL FAILURE. Investigation of the adverse effects of captopril in patients with various grades of kidney dysfunction. In patients not undergoing haemodialysis the overall incidence of side-effects varied from 18% in patients with serum creatinine concentrations of less than 15 µg per mL to 75% in patients with serum creatinine concentrations of greater than 0.8 µg per mL.— K. Onoyama *et al.*, *Curr. ther. Res.*, 1986, *40*, 333.

DIABETES MELLITUS. Report of 3 cases of unexplained hypoglycaemia in insulin-dependent diabetic patients and 1 case in a non-insulin-dependent diabetic during captopril treatment. A subsequent study suggested that this effect may result from an enhancement of insulin sensitivity.— M. Ferriere *et al.*, *Ann. intern. Med.*, 1985, *102*, 134.

No evidence of hypoglycaemia had been seen in 38 diabetic patients receiving either captopril or enalapril for 6 to 24 months, or in a further 18 patients receiving enalapril.— P. Passa *et al.* (letter), *Lancet*, 1986, *1*, 1447.

Captopril had little effect on blood glucose control in 8 hypertensive insulin-dependent diabetics.— P. Winocour *et al.*, (letter), *Lancet*, 1986, *2*, 461.

FIRST DOSE EFFECT. Marked hypotension after a 25-mg dose of captopril in one patient with the hyponatraemic hypertensive syndrome. Captopril was subsequently reintroduced at a dose of 6.25 mg and a gradual reduction in blood pressure was achieved by gradually increasing the dose over 7 days.— A. B. Atkinson *et al.* (letter), *Lancet*, 1979, *1*, 557.

Precipitous falls in blood pressure occurred in 21 of 65 severely hypertensive patients after initial doses of captopril ranging from 6.25 to 25 mg. Predisposing factors appeared to be secondary hypertension and high pretreatment blood pressure: there was no evidence that the total body sodium value was involved. The extent of any first-dose effect cannot be easily predicted in patients with severe hypertension who have received other drugs; such patients should have close medical supervision for at least 3 hours.— G. P. Hodsman *et al.*, *Br. med. J.*, 1983, *286*, 832.

INTERACTIONS. A review of drug interactions with captopril.— *Drug Interact. News.*, 1985, *5*, 15.

Allopurinol. For reports of allergic reactions in patients taking captopril and allopurinol, see under Allopurinol, p.437.

Azathioprine. Leucopenia in a patient given captopril with azathioprine which resolved when either drug was given alone.— E. J. Kirchertz *et al.* (letter), *Lancet*, 1981, *1*, 1363. See also C. R. W. Edwards *et al.* (letter), *ibid.*, 723.

Cimetidine. Neuropathy in 2 patients receiving captopril in association with cimetidine.— A. B. Atkinson *et al.* (letter), *Lancet*, 1980, *2*, 36.

Digoxin. For reports of an increase in serum digoxin concentrations during captopril therapy, see under Digoxin p.828.

Diuretics. A discussion of the concomitant use of captopril and other ACE-inhibitors with diuretics.— *Drug Interact. News.*, 1987, *7*, 17.

Reports of impaired renal function in patients taking captopril and diuretics: B. F. Murphy *et al.*, *Br. med. J.*, 1984, *288*, 844; K. J. Hogg and W. S. Hillis (letter), *Lancet*, 1986, *1*, 501.

Heart block due to hyperkalaemia occurred in a patient taking captopril concomitantly with spironolactone and hydroflumethiazide.— T. C. N. Lo and R. J. Cryer (letter), *Br. med. J.*, 1986, *292*, 1672. A similar case in a patient taking enalapril.— M. Lakhani, *ibid.*, *293*, 271. A further report of hyperkalaemia in a patient taking captopril and a preparation containing frusemide with triamterene (Frusene).— B. Cook (letter), *Br. med. J.*, 1987, *295*, 1351.

Reports of pronounced hypotension in patients taking captopril and diuretics: J. S. Budd and M. A. R. Hoghton (letter), *Br. med. J.*, 1987, *295*, 612.

Naloxone. A study suggesting that the acute hypotensive effects of captopril in normotensive subjects could be attenuated by naloxone.— P. C. Rubin *et al.*, *Br. J. clin. Pharmac.*, 1984, *17*, 713. See also A. A. Ajayi *et al.*, *Clin. Pharmac. Ther.*, 1985, *38*, 560. A subsequent study in subjects with essential hypertension showing that naloxone did not modify the hypotensive effect of captopril during long-term therapy. The results suggest that different mechanisms may be involved in the hypotensive effect during acute and chronic administration.— A. A. Ajayi *et al.*, *Br. J. clin. Pharmac.*, 1986, *21*, 543.

PREGNANCY AND THE NEONATE. A study indicating that only very small amounts of captopril enter breast milk. Since the kidneys of neonates are immature, however, more accumulation may occur than in adults.— R. G. Devlin and P. M. Fleiss, *J. clin. Pharmac.*, 1981, *21*, 110.

See also under Adverse Effects, above.

WITHDRAWAL. Abrupt discontinuation of captopril therapy in patients with heart failure resulted in large increases in angiotensin II, but cardiac output was well maintained in the short term despite increases in arterial blood pressure, and myocardial reserve was not compromised.— A. H. Maslowski *et al.*, *Lancet*, 1981, *2*, 959.

Absorption and Fate

About 60 to 75% of a dose of captopril is absorbed from the gastro-intestinal tract. It is about 30% bound to plasma proteins. Transfer to breast milk is minimal but it crosses the placenta. It is largely excreted in the urine 40 to 50% as unchanged drug and as metabolites. The elimination half-life has been reported to be 2 to 3 hours but this is increased in renal failure. Captopril is removed by dialysis.

A review of the clinical pharmocokinetics of captopril and other ACE-inhibitors.— S. H. Kubo and R. J. Cody, *Clin. Pharmacokinet.*, 1985, *10*, 377.

The influence of chronic renal failure on the pharmacokinetics of captopril.— J. F. Giudicelli *et al.*, *Br. J. clin. Pharmac.*, 1984, *18*, 749. Comment: G. Deray (letter), *ibid.*, 1985, *20*, 90; J. F. Giudicelli and C. Richer (letter), *ibid.*, 91. The pharmacokinetics of captopril in uraemic patients on maintenance dialysis.— O. H. Drummer *et al.*, *Eur. J. clin. Pharmac.*, 1987, *32*, 267.

ABSORPTION. The bioavailability and peak plasma concentrations of captopril have been shown to be reduced by administration with food in single dose studies (G.M. Williams and A.A. Sugerman, *J. clin. Pharmac.*, 1982, *22*, 18A; S.M. Singhvi, *et al.*, *ibid.*, 135; H.-M. Müller *et al.*, *J. Hypertension*, 1985, *3*, *Suppl.* 2, S135) and with chronic dosing (K.P. Öhman *et al.*, *J. cardiovasc. Pharmac.*, 1985, *7*, *Suppl.* 1, S20). However, Izumi *et al.* (*Tohoku J. exp. Med.*, 1983, *139*, 279) found insignificant differences in these parameters between the fasting and nonfasting states, and their study as well as that by Müller *et al.*, indicated that food intake had no clinically significant effect on the antihypertensive effect of captopril.

Uses and Administration

Captopril inhibits angiotensin-converting enzyme (ACE; kininase II), the enzyme involved in the conversion of angiotensin I to angiotensin II and may also reduce the degradation of bradykinin. The pharmacological actions of captopril are thought to be primarily due to the inhibition of the renin-angiotensin-aldosterone system, but since it also effectively reduces blood pressure in patients with low renin concentrations other mechanisms are probably also involved. Captopril produces a reduction in total peripheral resistance and, in patients with congestive heart failure, a reduction in both preload and afterload. Following oral administration captopril produces a maximum effect within 1 to 2 hours, although the full effect may not develop for several weeks during chronic dosing. The duration of action is dose-dependent and may persist for 6 to 12 hours. Captopril is used as an adjunct to treatment with a thiazide diuretic in mild to moderate hypertension and in severe hypertension resistant to other treatment. It is also used as an adjunct to the treatment of severe congestive heart failure.

In the treatment of hypertension the initial dose is 12.5 mg twice daily by mouth, increased gradually according to the response. In mild to moderate hypertension the usual maintenance dose is 25 mg twice daily and should not exceed 50 mg twice daily; in severe hypertension a dose of 50 mg three times daily should not be exceeded. In the treatment of congestive heart failure an initial dose of 6.25 to 12.5 mg is given under close medical supervision; the usual maintenance dose is 25 mg three times daily and should not exceed 50 mg three times daily.

The first dose of captopril may cause a precipitous fall in blood pressure in patients with renal damage or receiving diuretics and it is recommended that all such patients should be given a test dose of 6.25 mg, preferably in hospital; when possible diuretics should be stopped for a few days before introducing captopril. The dose of captopril should be kept as low as possible in elderly patients and those with renal impairment.

For children an initial dose of 300 µg per kg body-weight increased gradually to a maximum of 6 mg per kg daily has been suggested.

A review of the actions and uses of angiotensin-converting enzyme (ACE) inhibitors including captopril. Although ACE inhibitors are specific for the enzyme which converts the inactive angiotensin I into the potent pressor agent angiotensin II, there has been considerable controversy over their mode of action, partly because ACE also degrades the potent vasodilator bradykinin. However, there is uncertainty about the effect of ACE inhibition on circulating bradykinin.

Early studies showed that the fall in blood pressure after ACE inhibition directly correlated with the pretreatment concentrations of circulating renin. However, captopril has been found to lower blood pressure in patients with normal or low renin concentrations especially when combined with a diuretic, suggesting that there are probably angiotensin II-independent mechanisms in the hypotensive effect. Reduction of angiotensin II concentrations may also affect neurogenic vasoconstriction although the clinical significance of this is uncertain. Captopril has also been shown to produce a reduction in plasma aldosterone although this is not maintained during prolonged captopril treatment and so is probably not critical to the antihypertensive effect. Thus the beneficial effects of ACE inhibitors are probably the result of several mechanisms, the relative importance of which varies depending on the condition being treated.

The efficacy of ACE inhibitors combined with their lack of central side-effects has revolutionised the treatment of many hypertensive patients. Captopril has been excellent treatment for most patients with renovascular hypertension, although reversible renal failure may occur in patients with renal artery stenosis. Treatment with captopril may also be of diagnostic value since it causes a greater rise in plasma renin activity in patients with renovascular hypertension than in patients with essential hypertension. In addition, the blood-pressure response to ACE inhibition may be a useful predictor of surgical curability in patients with renovascular hypertension. Numerous studies have shown the efficacy of captopril, usually in combination with a diuretic, in the treatment of severe hypertension, especially when this has been resistant to standard therapy. Care must be exercised in patients who are volume-depleted or taking adrenergic blocking drugs to avoid a precipitous drop in blood pressure. Captopril may also correct hypertension, hypokalaemia, and hyperaldosteronism in patients with primary aldosteronism not associated with a tumour.

Several studies have shown the efficacy of ACE inhibitors in lowering the blood pressure in essential hypertension. The pretreatment renin concentration does not appear to predict the hypotensive response, but there does seem to be a correlation with ACE inhibition. Most patients have required the addition of a thiazide diuretic to control blood pressure, and this combination considerably reduces the adverse effects of the diuretic although it is not known whether it can improve impotence.

Captopril has been shown to be effective in the treatment of congestive cardiac failure resistant to other drugs. The major advantage of ACE inhibitors over other vasodilators is that they do not induce sodium retention, and neither tachyphylaxis nor rebound effects occur when they are withdrawn. Acute haemodynamic studies have shown that captopril increases cardiac output and reduces mean arterial pressure, systemic vascular resistance, right arterial pressure, and pulmonary artery and capillary wedge pressures. The beneficial effects seem to relate to the pretreatment plasma renin activity. Long-term treatment with captopril has produced both subjective and objective improvement in patients with drug-resistant heart failure although it is unclear whether treatment with an ACE inhibitor changes the course of the disease. A wide variety of cardiac conditions have responded, including ischaemic and valvular heart disease and alcoholic and idiopathic cardiomyopathy, but captopril does not seem to be useful for primary pulmonary hypertension.

One major reason for the increasing popularity of ACE inhibitors, apart from their efficacy, is the feeling of well-being reported by many patients on these drugs. This was originally thought to relate to a central effect, but the euphoria now seems to result from stopping other drugs.— C. R. W. Edwards and P. L. Padfield, *Lancet*, 1985, *1*, 30. See also A. Breckenridge, *Br. med. J.*, 1988, *296*, 618.

Further reviews of captopril: S. G. Ball and J. I. S. Robertson, *Br. med. J.*, 1985, *290*, 180; *Aust. J. Pharm.*, 1987, *68*, 393.

A review of haemodynamic responses to specific renin-angiotensin inhibitors including ACE inhibitors in hypertension and congestive heart failure.— R. J. Cody, *Drugs*, 1984, *28*, 144.

A series of papers on the actions and uses of ACE inhibitors.— *Postgrad. med. J.*, 1986, *62*, *Suppl.* 1, 1-191.

Study of the haemodynamic effects of captopril during long-term therapy.— J. M. Sullivan *et al.*, *J. clin. Pharmac.*, 1982, *22*, 450.

A study in 10 hypertensive patients demonstrating a lack of correlation between plasma concentrations of captopril and the decrease in diastolic blood pressure. Captopril's biological and antihypertensive effects lasted at least 6 hours while captopril disappeared very rapidly from plasma.— C. Richer *et al.*, *Br. J. clin. Pharmac.*, 1984, *17*, 243.

In a study of 20 patients with mild to moderate hypertension, captopril with or without a thiazide diuretic reduced blood pressure without altering renal haemodynamics.— K. L. Duchin and D. A. Willard, *J. clin. Pharmac.*, 1984, *24*, 351.

A study in 18 hypertensive patients indicating that captopril caused no untoward effects on lipoprotein metabolism after 12 weeks of treatment.— J. Sasaki and K. Arakawa, *Curr. ther. Res.*, 1986, *40*, 898.

ADMINISTRATION IN RENAL FAILURE. In 15 patients with renal failure the concentration of unchanged captopril in blood was decreased and that of metabolites was increased. There was a linear relationship between individual overall elimination-rate constants and endogenous creatinine clearance.— A. J. Rommel *et al.*, *Clin. Pharmac. Ther.*, 1980, *27*, 282.

A study of 9 patients with chronic renal failure undergoing dialysis found that peak plasma concentrations of captopril were 2.5 times higher and peak concentrations of the disulphide metabolites were 4 times higher than in patients with normal renal function following a single dose of captopril. Peak concentrations occurred later in uraemic patients and the apparent half-life of total captopril was 46 hours in uraemic patients compared with 2.95 hours in patients with normal renal function. The results suggested that captopril disulphide conjugates contributed to the hypotensive effects of captopril, and that both dosage and frequency of administration of captopril should be reduced in renal failure.— O. H. Drummer *et al.*, *Eur. J. clin. Pharmac.*, 1987, *32*, 267.

ASCITES. Conflicting responses have been reported following the use of captopril in resistant ascites. Shepherd *et al.* (*Lancet*, 1983, *1*, 1391) reported a reduction in pulmonary oedema and ascites in a patient with liver disease with captopril 25 mg three times daily. However, Ring (*Lancet*, 1983, *2*, 165) suggested that in patients with cirrhosis captopril could cause a marked reduction in arterial pressure and severely compromise renal function since maintenance of glomerular filtration-rate might be mediated by angiotensin II in these patients. This theory was subsequently supported by Wood *et al.* (*Lancet*, 1985, *2*, 1008) who reported a reduction in glomerular filtration-rate in response to a fall in mean arterial pressure in 4 patients with resistant ascites secondary to hepatic cirrhosis. The fall in mean arterial pressure was associated with postural hypotension and increasing encephalopathy. Jørgensen *et al.* (*Lancet*, 1983, *2*, 405) reported severe confusion in 2 patients with cirrhosis during treatment with captopril 6.25 to 12.5 mg three times daily. More recently Noto *et al.* (*Curr. ther. Res.*, 1986, *40*, 733) reported that doses of captopril 300 mg daily reduced resistant ascites in a study of 10 patients; at these doses the effect appeared to be linked to reduced aldosterone secretion and not to the suppressed haemodynamic vascular effects induced by angiotensin II reported at lower doses.

BARTTER'S SYNDROME. Reports of beneficial responses to captopril in patients with Bartter's syndrome which is characterised by hypokalaemia, hyper-reninaemia, and, often, low blood pressure.— M. Aurell and A. Rudin (letter), *New Engl. J. Med.*, 1981, *304*, 1609; R. J. Hené *et al.*, *Br. med. J.*, 1982, *285*, 695; J. M. James and D. Davies, *ibid.*, 1984, *289*, 162; A. Savastano *et al.*, *Curr. ther. Res.*, 1986, *39*, 408.

CARDIAC DISORDERS. Dramatic resolution of heart failure and improvement in clinical condition of a neonate with hypertension secondary to renal artery thrombosis following treatment with captopril.— L. F. McGonigle *et al.*, *Archs Dis. Childh.*, 1987, *62*, 614.

Beneficial response to captopril in 3 patients with cardiogenic shock following myocardial infarction.— D. P. Lipkin *et al.* (letter), *Lancet*, 1987, *2*, 327.

Comment on the use of ACE inhibitors in the elderly. ACE inhibitors were considered to be an important form of treatment for heart failure and hypertension in the elderly. However elderly patients with cardiovascular disease could be at increased risk of adverse effects.— J. L. Reid, *Br. med. J.*, 1987, *295*, 943. Comment that the use of inappropriately high maintenance doses in elderly patients with heart failure may increase the potential for adverse reactions in this high-risk group.— J. P. Milnes and A. J. Shaw (letter), *ibid.*, 1209.

Heart failure. Review of pharmacological and clinical studies of captopril used for the treatment of congestive heart failure.— J. A. Romankiewicz *et al.*, *Drugs*, 1983, *25*, 6.

A discussion of the effects of vasodilator therapy including ACE inhibitors on mortality in congestive heart failure. Vasodilators improve left ventricular function by reducing afterload in patients with congestive heart failure and are widely used in patients who still have symptoms after treatment with diuretics. At present, ACE inhibitors are preferred to conventional vasodilators because they are usually better tolerated and are clinically more effective. Ideally, treatment should be started in hospital with a low dose because of the risk of profound hypotension and impaired renal function.— A. D. Timmis, *Br. med. J.*, 1987, *295*, 1225.

Further reviews and comments on the use of captopril in heart failure: L. H. Opie, *Lancet*, 1984, *1*, 496; *ibid.*, 1985, *2*, 811; G. H. Guyatt, *Drugs*, 1986, *32*, 538.

In a study comparing the effects of captopril and enalapril in 42 patients with severe chronic heart failure, captopril was preferred to enalapril since the prolonged duration of action of enalapril resulted in an increased risk of prolonged hypotension which could increase the risk of adverse cerebral and renovascular effects.— M. Packer *et al.*, *New Engl. J. Med.*, 1986, *315*, 847. Comment on the high fixed doses used in the study.— H. Feld and M. A. Greenberg (letter), *ibid.*, 1987, *316*, 879.

Reports of the beneficial response of patients with severe heart failure to intravenous captopril: M. Rademaker *et al.*, *Br. Heart J.*, 1986, *55*, 187; O. Boyd and J. E. F. Pohl (letter), *Lancet*, 1986, *1*, 1041.

A study indicating that captopril combined with frusemide corrects hyponatraemia in patients with severe congestive heart failure, but that this response may not occur with captopril used alone.— V. J. Dzau and N. K. Hollenberg, *Ann. intern. Med.*, 1984, *100*, 777. See also R. W. Hamilton and V. M. Buckalew, *ibid.*, 902.

Captopril improved symptomless ventricular dysfunction following myocardial infarction in a study of 60 patients compared with frusemide, which was no more effective than placebo.— N. Sharpe *et al.*, *Lancet*, 1988, *1*, 255.

The Captopril-Digoxin Multicenter Research Group found captopril to be a suitable alternative to digoxin in patients with mild to moderate heart failure on diuretic maintenance.— *J. Am. med. Ass.*, 1988, *259*, 539.

Further references on the use of captopril in heart failure: Captopril Multicenter Research Group, *J. Am. Coll. Cardiol.*, 1983, *2*, 755; J. Bayliss *et al.*, *Br. med. J.*, 1985, *290*, 1861; Captopril Multicenter Research Group, *Am. Heart J.*, 1985, *110*, 439; J. Bayliss *et al.*, *Br. Heart J.*, 1986, *55*, 265; M. Packer *et al.*, *Am. J. Cardiol.*, 1986, *57*, 1323; P. J. Murphy *et al.*, *Br. med. J.*, 1986, *293*, 239; A. J. Cowley *et al.*, *Lancet*, 1986, *2*, 770; A. Boccanelli *et al.* (letter), *ibid.*, 1331.

DIABETIC NEPHROPATHY. A prompt decrease in urinary protein occurred within 2 weeks of starting captopril treatment in 10 uraemic diabetic patients with heavy proteinuria. Serum creatinine increased in 2 patients and one of these was withdrawn from the study.— Y. Taguma *et al.*, *New Engl. J. Med.*, 1985, *313*, 1617. Comments and discussion: J. A. O'Hare (letter), *ibid.*, 1986, *315*, 515; E. A. Ross (letter), *ibid;* C. B. Sridhar and S. Lakshminarayan (letter), *ibid;* L. Elving *et al.* (letter), *ibid;* P. Sawicki *et al.* (letter), *ibid.*, 516; Y. Taguma *et al.* (letter), *ibid.* Correction J. A. O'Hare, *ibid.*, 1987, *316*, 52.

A study in 16 hypertensive diabetic patients showed that glomerular filtration rate was not dependent on angiotensin II concentrations in diabetic nephropathy, that albuminuria was pressure dependent to a large extent, and that captopril could be valuable in treating hypertensive type I diabetic patients with nephropathy.— E. Hommel *et al.*, *Br. med. J.*, 1986, *293*, 467.

A striking reduction in the rate of deterioration in the glomerular filtration rate was seen in 14 patients with type I diabetes with associated nephropathy treated with captopril for up to 3.5 years. Before treatment renal function showed a steady deterioration, whereas after 6 months of captopril treatment the glomerular filtration rate remained almost constant. No correlation was found between the effect on blood pressure and the reduction in the rate of deterioration of renal function.— S. Björck *et al.*, *Br. med. J.*, 1986, *293*, 471. Comment that control of hypertension was correlated with a reduction in proteinuria.— S. Ahmad (letter), *ibid.*, 1028.

No changes in renal haemodynamics or albumin excretion rate were found in a study of 8 hypertensive diabetic patients without nephropathy during 6 weeks of treatment with captopril.— P. H. Winocour *et al.* (letter), *Br. med. J.*, 1987, *295*, 391.

HYPERTENSION. Reviews of angiotensin converting enzyme inhibitors in the treatment of hypertension: C. I. Johnston *et al.*, *Drugs*, 1984, *27*, 271; E. D. Fröhlich *et al., Archs intern. Med.*, 1984, *144*, 1441; A. Nicholls, *Postgrad. med. J.*, 1984, *60*, 917; *Med. Lett.*, 1985, *27*, 103.

A series of papers on antihypertensive therapy with a combination of captopril and hydrochlorothiazide.— *Br. J. clin. Pharmac.*, 1987, *23*, *Suppl.* 1, 3S-103S.

In a study involving 495 hypertensive patients captopril, 37.5 mg daily was found to be as effective as 150 mg daily in reducing blood pressure. The addition of a thiazide diuretic enhanced the antihypertensive effect.— *Archs intern. Med.*, 1984, *144*, 1947.

Results of a post marketing surveillance study of 6737 hypertensive patients treated with captopril. Captopril was effective in the treatment of hypertension of various aetiology. The mean dose used was about 150 mg daily and there was no evidence of tolerance during long term treatment. At this dosage the frequency of adverse effects in patients with normal renal function was lower than that reported in earlier studies using doses of up to 450 mg daily.— A. C. Jenkins *et al., J. cardiovasc. Pharmac.*, 1985, *7*, *Suppl.* 1, S96.

A study indicating that adequate control of hypertension could be achieved with captopril administered as a single daily dose.— R. Fogari *et al., Curr. ther. Res.*, 1986, *40*, 500. Similar reports: J. A. Schoenberger and D. J. Wilson, *J. clin. Hypertens.*, 1986, *2*, 379; J. P. Deyoung *et al., Curr. ther. Res.*, 1987, *41*, 464.

In a study involving 620 men with essential hypertension, patients taking captopril with or without the addition of hydrochlorothiazide scored significantly higher on measures of general well-being, had fewer side-effects, and less sexual dysfunction than patients taking either methyldopa or propranolol. Scores for general well-being were substantially reduced by the addition of a diuretic. The rate of withdrawal because of adverse effects in the group treated with captopril was 40 to 60% lower than that in the other 2 groups and this may indicate that long-term noncompliance could be reduced in patients taking captopril.— S. H. Croog *et al., New Engl. J. Med.*, 1986, *314*, 1657. See also T. Rosenthal *et al., Curr. ther. Res.*, 1987, *41*, 614.

Further clinical studies of captopril in hypertension: Y. K. Seedat and R. Rawat, *Eur. J. clin. Pharmac.*, 1983, *25*, 9 (in combination with minoxidil, a beta-blocker and frusemide); A. C. Pessina *et al., Curr. ther. Res.*, 1984, *35*, 269 (in combination with minoxidil); L. Corea *et al., ibid.*, *36*, 347 (compared with diuretic therapy in the elderly); A. C. Jenkins *et al., Archs intern. Med.*, 1985, *145*, 2029 (in the elderly); B. L. Mirkin and T. J. Newman, *Pediatrics*, 1985, *75*, 1091 (in children); Y. M. Traub and J. B. Rosenfeld, *Israel J. med. Scis*, 1985, *21*, 737 (compared with propranolol); L. Andrén *et al., Acta med. scand.*, 1985, *217*, 155 (compared with atenolol in long-term treatment); J. F. Potter and D. G. Beevers, *J. clin. Pharmac.*, 1987, *27*, 410 (compared with nifedipine); O. M. Bhat *et al., Curr. ther. Res.*, 1986, *40*, 92 (compared with methyldopa); G. Garanin, *ibid.*, 567 (compared with enalapril); W. B. White *et al., Clin. Pharmac. Ther.*, 1986, *39*, 43 (in combination with nifedipine); A. M. Heagerty and J. D. Swales, *Pharmatherapeutica*, 1987, *5*, 21 (in combination with verapamil); G. A. MacGregor *et al., Br. med. J.*, 1987, *294*, 531 (in combination with moderate sodium restriction); P. C. Waller and G. T. McInnes (letter), *ibid.*, 769 (comment on MacGregor *et al.*'s study); A. Richardson *et al., Lancet*, 1987, *2*, 709 (compared with diuretic therapy); D. H. Roberts *et al., Lancet*, 1987, *2*, 650 (compared with atenolol, labetalol, and pindolol); R. Okun and J. Kraut, *Am. J. Med.*, 1987, *82*, *Suppl.* 1A, 58 (compared with prazosin).

Hypertensive emergencies. Captopril administered sublingually to 6 patients with symptoms of hypertensive crisis produced a fall in blood pressure of 62/23 mmHg after 10 minutes. This effect was maintained for at least 2 hours. No flushing or other side-effects were observed.— W. Tschollar and G. G. Belz (letter), *Lancet*, 1985, *2*, 34. A similar report.— J. H. Hauger-Klevene (letter), *ibid.*, 732. In a crossover study in 6 patients with severe hypertension, a hypotensive effect was seen 5 minutes after the administration of nifedipine 10 mg sublingually and 15 minutes after captopril 25 mg sublingually. The hypotensive effect persisted for 6 hours after captopril and for 4 hours after nifedipine. Captopril produced fewer side-effects and a smaller rise in heart-rate than nifedipine.— *idem* (letter), *ibid.*, 1986, *1*, 219.

Renovascular disease. Report of treatment of 45 hypertensive renal transplant patients with captopril. All patients also received frusemide, and two-thirds of them a beta-blocking agent. The mean dose of captopril was 102 mg daily. The blood pressure response was greater in patients given captopril within the first year after transplantation than in those given captopril later. Half the patients given captopril early also showed a decrease in serum creatinine during captopril treatment. Captopril was discontinued within 2 weeks in 2 patients who required surgery for renal artery stenosis and in 1 who developed hypotension.— H. Herlitz *et al.* (letter), *Lancet*, 1983, *2*, 1366.

Beneficial results with captopril in 7 of 8 patients with severe hypertension following renal transplantation. Hypertension had previously not been adequately controlled by standard therapy with a beta-blocker, a vasodilator, and a diuretic. All patients were maintained on diuretic therapy before and throughout treatment with captopril. Some continued to take beta-blockers but in reduced doses. The dose of captopril never exceeded 250 mg daily in 2 or 3 divided doses and the average daily dose was 89 mg. Apart from the initial dose effect of hypotension, which was severe enough to cause transient anuria in one patient, no adverse effects were reported with captopril.— M. K. Chan *et al., Postgrad. med. J.*, 1984, *60*, 132.

A retrospective study suggesting that captopril treatment may help to preserve renal function in patients with progressive renal failure compared with treatment with other antihypertensive agents.— J. Mann and E. Ritz (letter), *Lancet*, 1987, *2*, 622.

Diagnosis. A study suggesting that the response to long-term treatment with captopril in patients with renovascular hypertension could predict surgical outcome.— A. B. Atkinson *et al., Br. med. J.*, 1982, *284*, 689. Criticism and comment that age was a more accurate predictor of surgical outcome than response to captopril.— L. E. Ramsay (Letter), *ibid.*, 1120.

A study indicating that captopril improved the accuracy of renal vein catheterisation in the diagnosis of hypertension related to unilateral renal artery lesions.— M. Thibonnier *et al., J. Am. med. Ass.*, 1984, *251*, 56. Criticism.— C. E. Grim (letter), *ibid.*, 1985, *253*, 346. Reply.— M. Thibonnier (letter), *ibid.*

Scleroderma. A report of the dramatic reversal by captopril of vascular and renal crises in 2 patients with scleroderma.— J. A. Lopez-Ovejero *et al., New Engl. J. Med.*, 1979, *300*, 1417.

Captopril at a mean daily dose of 350 mg, controlled the blood pressure in 20 out of 23 patients with scleroderma renal crisis and reduced serum creatinine concentrations in 14. At follow-up after 21 to 36 months, 11 patients had continued good response, and 6 had died. Adverse effects were reported in 12 patients and captopril therapy was withdrawn in 2 of them.— R. H. Thurm and J. C. Alexander, *Archs intern. Med.*, 1984, *144*, 733.

In a study of 7 patients with scleroderma and combined hypertension and renal impairment treated with captopril, blood pressure was controlled in all 7 patients, and renal function stabilised or improved in 6. In these 6 patients, improvement was maintained for 1½ to nearly 3 years. However, no improvement was detected in other features of the disease.— V. L. Beckett *et al., Mayo Clin. Proc.*, 1985, *60*, 763.

Further reports of beneficial responses to captopril in scleroderma: L. B. Sorensen *et al., Arthritis Rheum.*, 1983, *26*, 797; C. D. Smith *et al., ibid.*, 1984, *27*, 826.

OEDEMA. In a 32-year-old woman with idiopathic oedema, all symptoms disappeared during treatment with captopril and resumed rapidly when placebo was given.— A. Mimran and R. Targhetta (letter), *New Engl. J. Med.*, 1979, *301*, 1289. A similar response in 4 patients. The patients were free of symptoms after 2 to 3 months of treatment.— D. Docci and F. Turci (letter), *ibid.*, 1983, *308*, 1102.

PERIPHERAL VASCULAR DISORDERS. A beneficial response to captopril in a patient with Raynaud's phenomenon.— S. Miyazaki *et al., Br. med. J.*, 1982, *284*, 310.

For a report of captopril in the treatment of peripheral ischaemia due to ergotamine, see p.1056.

PHAEOCHROMOCYTOMA. Report of successful treatment of hypertension due to phaeochromocytoma with captopril.— G. Loute *et al.* (letter), *Lancet*, 1984, *2*, 175. A similar report. After an initial response a gradual but moderate rise of blood pressure occurred despite continued treatment.— A. Israeli *et al.* (letter), *ibid.*, 1985, *2*, 278.

PULMONARY HYPERTENSION. Brief review of the use of captopril in primary pulmonary hypertension. Despite reports suggesting that inhibition of angiotensin-converting enzymes may attenuate experimentally induced pulmonary hypertension and isolated reports of the successful clinical use of captopril, investigations using large numbers of patients have failed to show a favourable effect in primary pulmonary hypertension.— M. Packer, *Ann. intern. Med.*, 1985, *103*, 258. See also A. A. McLeod and D. E. Jewitt, *Drugs*, 1986, *31*, 177.

RHEUMATOID ARTHRITIS. A preliminary open study of captopril in 15 patients with rheumatoid arthritis. A beneficial response was seen in 10 patients, poor responses in 3 patients, and 2 patients withdrew from the study because of adverse effects.— M. F. R. Martin *et al., Lancet*, 1984, *1*, 1325.

Proprietary Preparations

Acepril *(Duncan, Flockhart, UK). Tablets*, scored, captopril 12.5, 25, and 50 mg.

Acezide *(Duncan, Flockhart, UK). Tablets*, scored, captopril 50 mg, hydrochlorothiazide 25 mg.

Capoten *(Squibb, UK). Tablets*, captopril 25 mg. *Tablets*, scored, captopril 12.5 and 50 mg.

Capozide *(Squibb, UK). Tablets*, scored, captopril 50 mg, hydrochlorothiazide 25 mg.

Proprietary Names and Manufacturers

Acepril *(Duncan, Flockhart, UK)*; Alopresin *(Lafarquim, Spain)*; Capoten *(Squibb, Austral.; Squibb, Canad.; Squibb, Denm.; Squibb, Ital.; Novo, Norw.; Squibb, S.Afr.; Squibb, Spain; Squibb, Swed.; Squibb, UK; Squibb, USA)*; Captolane *(Théraplix, Fr.)*; Cesplon *(Esteve, Spain)*; Cor Tensobon *(Schwarz, Ger.)*; Dilabar *(Vita, Spain)*; Garranil *(Aristegui, Spain)*; Lopirin *(Heyden, Ger.; Squibb, Switz.)*; Lopril *(Squibb, Fr.)*; Tensobon *(Melusin, Ger.)*; Tensoprel *(Rubio, Spain)*.

The following names have been used for multi-ingredient preparations containing captopril— Acezide *(Duncan, Flockhart, UK)*; Capozide *(Squibb, UK; Squibb, USA)*.

12567-c

Ciclosidomine Hydrochloride *(BANM, rINNM)*.

PR-G-138-CL. *N*-(Cyclohexylcarbonyl)-3-morpholinosydnone imine hydrochloride.

$C_{13}H_{20}N_4O_3,HCl=316.8$.

CAS — 66564-16-7 (ciclosidomine).

Ciclosidomine hydrochloride is reported to be a peripheral vasodilator. It has been tried as an antihypertensive agent.

Ciclosidomine produced a reduction in systolic and diastolic blood pressure in 5 healthy subjects in the standing but not supine position. The accompanying increase in heart-rate could be prevented with propranolol.— R. G. Shanks *et al., Br. J. clin. Pharmac.*, 1984, *18*, 232.

Proprietary Names and Manufacturers
Boehringer Ingelheim, UK.

18620-q

Cilazapril *(BAN, USAN, rINN)*.

Ro-31-2848; Ro-31-2848/006. (1*S*,9*S*)-9-[(*S*)-1-Ethoxycarbonyl-3-phenylpropylamino]-10-oxoperhydropyridazino[1,2-*a*][1,2]diazepine-1-carboxylic acid.

$C_{22}H_{31}N_3O_5=417.5$.

CAS — 88768-40-5; 92077-78-6 (monohydrate).

Cilazapril is an angiotensin-converting enzyme inhibitor (see Captopril, p.470).

The pharmacodynamics and dose-response relationships of cilazapril in essential hypertension.— A. A. Ajayi *et al., Br. J. clin. Pharmac.*, 1986, *22*, 167.

Proprietary Names and Manufacturers
Inhibace *(Roche, USA)*.

857-k

Clonidine Hydrochloride *(BANM, USAN, rINNM)*.

2-(2,6-Dichloroanilino)-2-imidazoline Hydrochloride; 2-(2,6-Dichlorophenylimino)imidazolidine Hydrochloride; ST-155. 2,6-Dichloro-*N*-(imidazolidin-2-ylidene)aniline hydrochloride.

$C_9H_9Cl_2N_3,HCl=266.6$.

CAS — 4205-90-7 (clonidine); 4205-91-8 (hydrochloride).

Pharmacopoeias. In *Br., Chin., Eur., Ind., It., Swiss,* and *U.S.*

A white or almost white, crystalline powder. **Soluble** 1 in 13 of water; soluble in dehydrated alcohol; slightly soluble in chloroform. Solutions are **sterilised** by autoclaving. The *B.P.* states that a 5% solution in water has a pH of 4.0 to 5.0; the *U.S.P.* specifies 3.5 to 5.5; the *B.P.* Injection has a pH between 4.0 and 7.0. **Store** in airtight containers. Protect from light.

Adverse Effects

Drowsiness, dry mouth, dizziness, and headache commonly occur during the initial stages of therapy with clonidine. Fluid retention is often transient, but may be responsible for a reduction in the hypotensive effect during continued treatment. Constipation is also common, and other adverse effects which have been reported include depression, anxiety, fatigue, nausea, anorexia, parotid pain, sleep disturbances, vivid dreams, impotence, urinary retention or incontinence, slight orthostatic hypotension, and dry, itching, or burning sensations in the eye. Rashes and pruritus may occur, and are more common with the use of transdermal delivery systems. Less frequently, bradycardia, including sinus bradycardia with atrioventricular block, hallucinations, and transient abnormalities in liver function tests have been reported. Large doses have been associated with initial increases in blood pressure and transient hyperglycaemia, although these do not persist during continued therapy.

Symptoms of overdosage include transient hypertension or profound hypotension, bradycardia, sedation, miosis, respiratory depression, and coma. Treatment consists of general supportive measures. An alpha-adrenoceptor blocking agent may be given if necessary.

A transdermal clonidine "patch" dislodged during sleep was accidentally transferred to the skin of the patient's 9-month-old child who was sharing the bed. The child subsequently showed signs of somnolence, irritability, and increased fluid intake, presumably due to a dry mouth.— M. T. Reed and E. L. Hamburg (letter), *New Engl. J. Med.*, 1986, *314*, 1120.

Cerebral blood flow was reduced by up to 28% in 5 patients during treatment with intravenous clonidine for emergency reduction of severe high blood pressure.— O. Bertel *et al.*, *Br. med. J.*, 1983, *286*, 19.

For the effects of withdrawal of clonidine, see under Precautions, below.

EFFECTS ON BLOOD PRESSURE. Severe hypotension occurred in a patient 2 hours after a dose of clonidine 150 µg per m^2 body-surface area by mouth for a test for growth hormone deficiency. The patient recovered within half an hour following an intravenous infusion of plasma.— A. A. Massarano (letter), *Archs Dis. Childh.*, 1985, *60*, 399. See also B. D. Given *et al.*, *Archs intern. Med.*, 1983, *143*, 2195.

Postural hypotension occurred in a diabetic patient with symptoms of autonomic neuropathy during treatment with clonidine for diarrhoea and faecal incontinence.— B. Moffat, *Br. med. J.*, 1985, *290*, 822.

Report of paradoxical hypertension in 2 hypertensive diabetic patients. Autonomic neuropathy in these patients was considered to be a contributory factor.— E. Young *et al.*, *Ann. intern. Med.*, 1984, *101*, 282.

EFFECTS ON THE ENDOCRINE SYSTEM. Clonidine in low dosage impaired the response to glucose challenge in non-insulin-dependent diabetics but did not impair diabetic control over a 10-week period in a study of 10 patients.— G. P. Guthrie *et al.*, *Clin. Pharmac. Ther.*, 1983, *34*, 713.

Report of decreased insulin secretion and elevated blood glucose concentrations in a non-insulin-dependent diabetic during treatment with clonidine.— S. Okada *et al.*, *J. int. med. Res.*, 1986, *14*, 299.

EFFECTS ON THE GASTRO-INTESTINAL TRACT. A 26-year-old male renal transplant recipient suffered pseudo-obstruction of the bowel while receiving clonidine therapy. He recovered after withdrawal of clonidine despite continuing to take other antihypertensive agents.— R. Bear and K. Steer, *Br. med. J.*, 1976, *1*, 197. A further report.— G. E. Bauer and K. J. Hellestrand (letter), *ibid.*, 769.

Abdominal pain mimicking acute appendicitis occurred in a 48-year-old patient taking clonidine. The pain subsided 1 day after the drug was withdrawn and recurred when clonidine was restarted.— T. Mjörndal and G. Mellbring, *Br. med. J.*, 1986, *292*, 174.

EFFECTS ON THE HEART. A report on 2 patients with hypertension, that clonidine hydrochloride might have been associated with an atrioventricular conduction defect.— L. E. Kibler and P. C. Gazes, *J. Am. med. Ass.*, 1977, *238*, 1930. A further report of the development of atrioventricular dissociation in 1 patient who had received clonidine hydrochloride up to 200 µg every 8 hours for 10 days.— P. Abiuso and G. Abelow (letter), *ibid.*, 1978, *240*, 108.

EFFECTS ON MENTAL STATE. A 74-year-old man taking debrisoquine, bendrofluazide, and clonidine developed dementia, characterised by amnesia, unsteadiness of gait, drowsiness, aggressiveness, and urinary incontinence, 5 months after starting to take clonidine. He improved markedly a week after clonidine was withdrawn.— P. Lavin and C. P. Alexander (letter), *Br. med. J.*, 1975, *1*, 628.

Acute paranoid reactions associated with treatment for hypertension with clonidine were reported on 2 occasions with an interval of 18 months in a 54-year-old man. The reactions included delusions and auditory hallucinations and cleared on withdrawal of clonidine.— M. D. Enoch and G. E. M. Hammad, *Curr. med. Res. Opinion*, 1977, *4*, 670.

Visual hallucinations occurred in 2 patients and transient auditory hallucinations in a third during clonidine therapy. The visual hallucinations disappeared when the drug was withdrawn.— M. J. Brown *et al.*, *Ann. intern. Med.*, 1980, *93*, 456.

EFFECTS ON SEXUAL FUNCTION. The incidence of impotence in 59 hypertensive patients given clonidine was 24%; the incidence during a control period was 8%.— G. Onesti *et al.*, *Am. J. Cardiol.*, 1971, *28*, 74.

EFFECTS ON THE SKIN. Skin reactions have been reported in up to 38% of patients receiving clonidine by a transdermal delivery system. The highest occurrence was reported by Groth *et al.* (*Lancet* 1983, *2*, 850) in a study of 29 patients and was characterised by Type IV delayed local allergic reactions. McMahon and Weber (*ibid.*, 851) reported a 6% incidence of contact sensitisation in 85 patients, and Boekhorst (*ibid.*, 1031) reported local skin reactions including itching in 3 patients and erythema in 5 patients within 10 weeks of starting treatment in a study of 21 patients: allergic reactions were identified in 3 patients during continued therapy. In a brief review, Dick *et al.* (*ibid.*, 1987, *1*, 516) suggested that skin reactions became commoner when treatment was continued for several months, and reported that although only mild skin reactions had been observed in their trial of transdermal clonidine during 8 to 14 weeks of treatment in 15 patients, severe skin reactions occurred after an average of 20 weeks in 4 of 5 patients who continued treatment. Despite a claim that skin reactions were due to a component in the delivery system and not to clonidine itself (*Pharm. J.*, 1984, *2*, 16), Boekhorst and Groth obtained positive patch tests to clonidine in several of their patients.

Report of anogenital cicatricial pemphigoid associated with long-term therapy with clonidine.— Th. van Joost *et al.*, *Br. J. Derm.*, 1980, *102*, 715.

OVERDOSAGE. Analysis by the National Poisons Information Service of poisoning by clonidine in 133 children and 37 adults revealed the following percentage incidence of signs and symptoms: impaired consciousness 85 and 78% respectively, pallor 27 and 16%, bradycardia 24 and 49%, cardiac arrhythmias 5 and 0%, cardiac arrest 0 and 3%, hypotension 21 and 32%, depressed respiration 15 and 5%, apnoea 2 and 0%, miosis 14 and 8%, unreactive pupils 5 and 0%, hypotonia 11 and 5%, irritability 11 and 3%, hyporeflexia 4 and 3%, extensor plantar reflex 3 and 0%, hypertension 2 and 11%, dry mouth 2 and 11%. There were no deaths but clinical features were often severe. Supportive measures were usually adequate but atropine was often needed for severe and persistent bradycardia. Forced diuresis was not advised because hypotension could be enhanced and there was no evidence that excretion of clonidine was increased. The role of alpha-blockers was limited and unproven.— B. Stein and G. N. Volans, *Br. med. J.*, 1978, *2*, 667.

Two children, a boy aged 3.6 years and a girl aged 2.5 years, took between them 20 to 25 tablets of clonidine 25 µg three hours before arriving at hospital. The girl was unsteady, pale with peripheral vasoconstriction, and her conscious level fluctuated. There were episodes of bradycardia. Treatment consisted of gastric lavage and atropine 200 µg given intravenously on 5 occasions whenever the pulse-rate persisted at a low value. Four seizures occurred in the first 8 hours. The boy had less severe effects and no seizures. Neither child became hypotensive or hypothermic.— R. MacFaul and G. Miller (letter), *Lancet*, 1977, *1*, 1266.

Hypotension associated with clonidine poisoning in a 2½-year-old child responded temporarily to the second of 2 intravenous doses of tolazoline 5 mg administered at 15-minute intervals: a third 5 mg dose reversed all the symptoms of clonidine overdosage in this child, with the exception of bradycardia, which persisted for 16 hours.— J. E. Mendoza and M. Medalie, *Clin. Pediat.*, 1979, *18*, 123.

Recovery of 2 patients from overdoses of clonidine 25 mg.— J. A. O. Rotellar *et al.* (letter), *Lancet*, 1981, *1*, 1312.

Following ingestion of clonidine 100 mg by a previously healthy 28-year-old man, a hypertensive phase lasting 24 hours was followed by a hypotensive phase as plasma-clonidine concentrations fell. Associated with the hypertension were respiratory depression, bradycardia, ileus, mydriasis, and a mental status which ranged from coma to delirium characterised by agitation, disorientation to time and place, visual hallucinations, and paranoid ideas. During the fourth day when symptoms had appeared to clear, the patient suddenly exhibited tachycardia, hyperventilation, diaphoresis, anxiety, abdominal cramps, and a fine bilateral hand tremor. These symptoms lasted approximately 12 hours and were similar to those occurring during clonidine withdrawal.— L. E. Domino *et al.*, *Br. J. clin. Pharmac.*, 1986, *21*, 71.

Further reports of clonidine overdosage: M. A. Moore and P. Phillipi (letter), *Lancet*, 1976, *2*, 694; R. J. Anderson *et al.*, *Ann. emerg. Med.*, 1981, *10*, 107; J. M. Olsson and A. W. Pruitt, *J. Pediat.*, 1983, *103*, 646; M. Artman and R. C. Boerth, *Am. J. Dis. Child.*, 1983, *137*, 171.

TREATMENT OF ADVERSE EFFECTS. Naloxone did not reverse the hypotensive or bradycardiac effects of clonidine in a study of 6 patients.— J. F. Rodgers and L. X. Cubeddu, *Clin. Pharmac. Ther.*, 1983, *34*, 68.

Precautions

Clonidine should be used with caution in patients with cerebral, or coronary insufficiency, Raynaud's disease or thromboangiitis obliterans, or with a history of depression. The hypotensive effect may be antagonised by tricyclic antidepressants, and enhanced by thiazide diuretics. Clonidine causes drowsiness and patients should not drive or operate machinery where loss of attention could be dangerous. The effects of other central nervous system depressants may be enhanced.

Withdrawal of clonidine therapy should be gradual as sudden discontinuation may cause rebound hypertension which may be severe. Agitation, sweating, tachycardia, headache, and nausea may also occur. Beta-blockers can exacerbate the rebound hypertension and if clonidine is being given concurrently with a beta-blocking agent, clonidine should not be discontinued until several days after the withdrawal of the beta-blocker. It has been suggested that patients should be warned of the risk of missing a dose or stopping the drug without consulting their doctor and should carry a reserve supply of tablets.

Although hypotension may occur during anaesthesia in clonidine-treated patients clonidine should not be withdrawn, indeed if necessary it should be given intravenously during the operation to avoid the risk of rebound hypertension. Intravenous injections of clonidine should be given slowly to avoid a possible transient pressor effect especially in patients already receiving other antihypertensive agents such as guanethidine or reserpine.

INTERACTIONS. A review of the adverse interaction between clonidine and *tricyclic antidepressants* in 6 patients. Tricyclic antidepressants may antagonise the hypotensive effect of clonidine. The effect has usually occurred slowly over a week or more, but in 2 patients the blood pressure increased more rapidly. The mechanism of the interaction is unknown.— *Drug Interact. News.*, 1984, *4*, 13.

Results of a study in 8 healthy subjects suggesting that *maprotiline* did not alter the hypotensive effect of clonidine.— U. Gundert-Remy *et al.*, *Eur. J. clin. Pharmac.*, 1983, *25*, 595.

Administration of *mianserin* to patients taking clonidine did not affect the hypotensive action of clonidine following both acute and chronic dosing.— H. L. Elliott *et al.*, *Eur. J. clin. Pharmac.*, 1983, *24*, 15.

Acute, severe hypotension occurred in 2 agitated hypertensive patients following administration of clonidine and either *chlorpromazine* or *haloperidol*. Both patients had mitral insufficiency.— R. J. Fruncillo *et al.* (letter), *Am. J. Psychiat.*, 1985, *142*, 274.

For the effect of clonidine on *fluphenazine*, see Fluphenazine, p.740.

For a report of the inhibition of the therapeutic effect of *levodopa* by clonidine, see under Levodopa, Precautions p.1017.

The action of clonidine may be reduced by concurrent administration of non-steroidal anti-inflammatory drugs, see p.466.

ECT. Maximal ECT stimuli were unsuccessful in producing seizures in 4 of 7 treatment attempts in a 66-year-old patient receiving concomitant clonidine therapy. It was suggested that clonidine may elevate the seizure threshold.— R. L. Elliott, *Am. J. Psychiat.*, 1983, *140*, 1237.

PORPHYRIA. Clonidine was considered to be unsafe in patients with acute porphyria because it has been shown to be porphyrinogenic in *animals* or *in-vitro* systems.— M.R. Moore and K.E.L. McColl, *Porphyrias, Drug Lists*, Glasgow, Porphyria Research Unit, University of Glasgow, 1987.

WITHDRAWAL. A review of the clinical aspects of hypertensive crisis due to withdrawal of centrally acting antihypertensive agents including clonidine. The results of several prospective studies of the effects of sudden withdrawal of clonidine from hypertensive patients suggested that the severity of the underlying hypertension, the dose of clonidine, and possibly duration of treatment may influence the development of withdrawal symptoms and their severity. It was not possible to estimate the incidence of the withdrawal syndrome. The symptoms appear to be associated with a sudden increase in circulating catecholamine concentrations. Reintroduction of clonidine has been shown to reverse the withdrawal symptoms, but where this is clinically undesirable the simultaneous administration of an alpha-adrenoceptor antagonist and a beta-blocking agent may be useful.— L. Hansson, *Br. J. clin. Pharmac.*, 1983, *15, Suppl.* 4, 485S.

Further reviews of clonidine withdrawal and hypertension: *Drug & Ther. Bull.*, 1977, *15*, 99; E. B. Raftery, *Drugs*, 1984, *28*, 371; C. F. George, *Prescribers' J.*, 1985, *25*, 31.

Fatal rebound hypertension occurred after the abrupt withdrawal of clonidine and propranolol.— C. Vernon and A. Sakula, *Br. J. clin. Pract.*, 1979, *33*, 112.

Serious ventricular arrhythmias, including brief ventricular tachycardia, developed in 2 of 7 patients following abrupt withdrawal of clonidine. The development of arrhythmias seemed unrelated to age, dose, presence of withdrawal symptoms, initial heart rate, initial blood pressure, ECG abnormalities, or changes in urinary noradrenaline concentrations, although the episodes of tachycardia coincided with the highest urinary catecholamine concentrations. Both patients also had greater increases in systolic blood pressure and double product than the other patients.— R. W. Peters *et al.*, *Clin. Pharmac. Ther.*, 1983, *34*, 435.

Report of combined therapy with prazosin, atenolol, and chlordiazepoxide to reduce the withdrawal symptoms following clonidine therapy in 6 patients.— J. L. Reid *et al.*, *Hypertension*, 1984, *6*, *Suppl.* II, 71.

Absorption and Fate

Clonidine is well absorbed from the gastro-intestinal tract. Peak plasma concentrations are observed 3 to 5 hours after administration, declining with a half-life up to about 23 hours. Clonidine is metabolised in the liver. About 65% is excreted in the urine, partly as unchanged clonidine, and about 20% is excreted in the faeces.

A study of the pharmacokinetics and pharmacodynamics of clonidine in 7 healthy subjects. There was evidence to suggest that clonidine undergoes enterohepatic circulation.— D. Arndts *et al.*, *Eur. J. clin. Pharmac.*, 1983, *24*, 21.

Further studies of the pharmacokinetics of clonidine: D. S. Davies *et al.*, *Clin. Pharmac. Ther.*, 1977, *21*, 593; M. Frisk-Holmberg *et al.*, *Br. J. clin. Pharmac.*, 1981, *12*, 653; M. J. Hogan *et al.*, *Clin. Pharmac. Ther.*, 1981, *30*, 729; M. T. Velasquez *et al.*, *ibid.*, 1983, *34*, 341.

Study of the pharmacokinetics of clonidine administered by a transdermal delivery system. The plasma-clonidine concentrations correlated with the surface area of the system within individuals although there was some interindividual variation in the concentrations achieved. Steady-state plasma concentrations were maintained for at least 7 days: plasma concentrations remained constant for up to 11 days in 7 of 8 subjects with application to the arm and in 6 of 8 subjects with application to the chest. No substantial changes in plasma concentrations were seen during the 24-hour period following application of a replacement system during repeated administration.— T. R. MacGregor *et al.*, *Clin. Pharmac. Ther.*, 1985, *38*, 278.

Studies of the pharmacokinetics of clonidine following administration of sustained-release preparations: J. L. Shaffer *et al.* (letter), *Br. J. clin. Pharmac.*, 1985, *19*, 524; T. R. MacGregor *et al.*, *Arzneimittel-Forsch.*, 1985, *35*, 440.

Uses and Administration

Clonidine is an antihypertensive agent which appears to act centrally by stimulating alpha$_2$-adrenergic receptors and producing a reduction in sympathetic tone, resulting in a fall in diastolic and systolic blood pressure and a reduction in heart-rate. It also acts peripherally, and this peripheral activity may be responsible for the transient increase in blood pressure seen during rapid intravenous administration as well as contributing to the hypotensive effect during chronic administration. Peripheral resistance is reduced during continuous treatment. Cardiovascular reflexes remain intact so postural hypotension occurs infrequently. When given by mouth, its effects appear in about 30 to 60 minutes, reaching a maximum after 2 to 4 hours and lasting up to 8 hours.

Clonidine hydrochloride is used in the treatment of all grades of hypertension, although less toxic agents are now generally preferred. Tolerance to clonidine has been reported.

The usual initial dose of clonidine hydrochloride is 50 to 100 µg orally thrice daily increased every second or third day according to the response of the patient; the usual maintenance dose is 0.3 to 1.2 mg daily but doses of up to 1.8 mg or more daily may be required. To reduce side-effects, a smaller dose of clonidine may be given in conjunction with a thiazide diuretic but combination with a beta-blocking agent should be avoided where possible. Clonidine may also be given in a sustained-release formulation which enables twice-daily dosage, or by a transdermal delivery system which is applied once a week and delivers 100 to 300 µg daily at a constant rate.

Clonidine hydrochloride may be given by slow intravenous injection in hypertensive crises, usually in doses of 150 to 300 µg. The effect usually appears within 10 minutes, but transient hypertension may precede hypotension if the injection is made too rapidly. The hypotensive effect reaches a maximum about 30 to 60 minutes after administration and the duration is about 3 to 7 hours; up to 750 µg may be given intravenously over 24 hours. Although oral administration does not produce a sufficiently rapid hypotensive effect for use in an emergency situation, a dose of 100 to 200 µg initially followed by 50 to 100 µg every hour until control of blood pressure is achieved or a maximum of 500 to 800 µg is reached, has been recommended for the control of severe hypertension.

Clonidine hydrochloride is also used in lower doses for the prophylaxis of migraine or recurrent vascular headaches and in the treatment of menopausal flushing. The dose is 50 µg twice daily increased, if there is no remission after 2 weeks, to 75 µg twice daily. Clonidine has also been used in the symptomatic treatment of opiate withdrawal.

The pharmacology of centrally acting antihypertensive agents including clonidine.— P. A. van Zwieten *et al.*, *Br. J. clin. Pharmac.*, 1983, *15*, *Suppl.* 4, 455S.

A review and discussion of some non-cardiovascular actions of clonidine.— S. K. Kulkarni *et al.*, *Drugs Today*, 1984, *20*, 497.

A review of the therapeutic uses of clonidine.— D. B. Frewin, *Med. J. Aust.*, 1985, *142*, 254.

A depressor response to carotid sinus nerve stimulation in a patient during high-dose clonidine therapy suggested that the hypotensive effect of clonidine was mediated in part by its facilitation of the baroreceptor reflex.— M. G. Myers, *Br. med. J.*, 1977, *2*, 802.

Further references to the mechanism of the hypotensive activity of clonidine: G. P. Guthrie and T. A. Kotchen, *J. clin. Pharmac.*, 1983, *23*, 348; M. B. Murphy *et al.*, *Eur. J. clin. Pharmac.*, 1984, *27*, 23; P. R. Martin *et al.*, *Clin. Pharmac. Ther.*, 1984, *35*, 322.

Studies of the effect of clonidine on growth hormone: C. Ferrari *et al.* (letter), *Br. med. J.*, 1977, *2*, 123; B. Falkner *et al.*, *J. clin. Pharmac.*, 1981, *21*, 31; A. D. Struthers *et al.*, *Br. J. clin. Pharmac.*, 1985, *19*, 311.

Results of a study of 34 children suggested that clonidine could be useful in the treatment of short stature due to constitutional growth delay.— C. Pintor *et al.*, *Lancet*, 1987, *1*, 1226. See also C. Pintor *et al.*, *Lancet*, 1985, *1*, 1482.

Clonidine significantly stimulated linear growth velocity in a prepubertal child of normal stature during the first 6 months of treatment for hypertension.— O. Arisaka *et al.* (letter), *Lancet*, 1987, *2*, 344.

See under Diagnosis and Testing, below, for use as a growth hormone stimulation test.

Measurement of the clonidine-induced reduction in nocturnal secretion of melatonin could be used as a clinical test for inhibitory alpha-adrenoceptor function.— A. J. Lewy *et al.*, *J. Pharm. Pharmac.*, 1986, *38*, 555.

ADMINISTRATION IN RENAL FAILURE. The normal half-life of clonidine of 6 to 23 hours was increased to 39 to 42 hours in end-stage renal failure. The dose should be reduced to 50 to 75% in patients with a glomerular filtration-rate of less than 10 mL per minute. No dosage supplement was required for patients undergoing haemodialysis.— W. M. Bennett *et al.*, *Am. J. Kidney Dis.*, 1983, *3*, 155.

ASTHMA. Clonidine inhibited the antigen-induced histamine release from human basophils and mast cell preparations *in vitro*. The effect was possibly mediated through histamine H_2 receptors.— B. R. Lindgren *et al.*, *Arzneimittel-Forsch.*, 1987, *37*, 551.

Inhalation of clonidine 75 µg prior to a bronchoprovocation test markedly reduced the bronchoconstriction caused by an inhaled allergen in a study of 10 asthmatic patients.— B. R. Lindgren *et al.*, *Am. Rev. resp. Dis.*, 1986, *134*, 266.

CONTROLLED HYPOTENSION. Results of a study in 20 patients undergoing surgery suggesting that clonidine premedication potentiates isoflurane-induced hypotension.— T. E. Woodcock *et al.*, *Br. J. Anaesth.*, 1987, *59*, 1319P.

DIAGNOSIS AND TESTING. *Growth hormone stimulation test.* The oral clonidine test was one of 3 growth hormone stimulation tests for children recommended by the Health Services Human Growth Hormone Committee. The recommended dose of clonidine was 150 µg per m^2 body-surface area. It was recognised that this test as well as the other 2 (the intravenous arginine and intramuscular glucagon tests) has a false-positive and a false-negative response rate similar to that with the insulin tolerance test. [The clonidine test is based on stimulation of growth hormone release by clonidine, presumably due to a central adrenergic effect].— R. D. G. Milner and E. C. Burns, *Archs Dis. Childh.*, 1982, *57*, 944 (references to the action of clonidine on growth hormone are given above).

Report of studies of the reliability and safety of clonidine for growth hormone stimulation tests in children: I. Gil-Ad *et al.*, *Lancet*, 1979, *2*, 278; *Archs Dis. Childh.*, 1981, *56*, 852; N. C. Fraser *et al.*, *ibid.*, 1983, *58*, 355; R. Lanes *et al.*, *Am. J. Dis. Child.*, 1985, *139*, 87.

Results suggesting that the clonidine secretion test may not be suitable for adults.— C. Ferrari *et al.* (letter), *Lancet*, 1979, *2*, 796.

Phaeochromocytoma suppression test. The use of clonidine in a suppression test for phaeochromocytoma has been described by Bravo *et al.* (*New Engl. J. Med.*, 1981, *305*, 623). The test is based on the ability of clonidine to block the centrally-mediated secretion of catecholamines but not release of catecholamines from the tumour. Its main use is for excluding the diagnosis of phaeochromocytoma in patients with borderline symptoms (E.L. Bravo and R.W. Gifford, *ibid.*, 1985 *312*, 724). The utility of the test for patients with phaeochromocytoma and "near normal" plasma catecholamine concentrations has not been fully evaluated (E.L. Bravo, *ibid.*, 1982, *306*, 50; P.D. Levinson *et al.*, *Lancet*, 1983, *1*, 1216; P.-F. Plouin *et al.*, *New Engl. J. Med.*, 1985, *312*, 721). Difficulties in evaluating the results of the test have been encountered in patients with fluctuating catecholamine concentrations (J.B. Halter *et al.*, *ibid.*, 1982, *306*, 49; A.G. Dupont *et al.*, *ibid.*, 1984, *310*, 266), and the method used for estimating catecholamines can influence the results (D.C. Aron *et al.*, *Ann. intern. Med.*, 1983, *98*, 1023; W.J. Raum, *New Engl. J. Med.*, 1985, *312*, 723). Burris and D'Angelo (*ibid.*,

1982, *307*, 756) reported severe hypotension following the clonidine-suppression test in 2 patients who were concurrently taking other antihypertensive agents.

EPIDURAL ANALGESIA. Reports of the analgesic effect of epidural clonidine.— A. Tamsen and T. Gordh (letter), *Lancet*, 1984, *2*, 231; C. J. Glynn *et al.*, *ibid.*, 1986, *2*, 1249; J. C. D. Wells and P. A. J. Hardy (letter), *ibid.*, 1987, *1*, 108; A. J. Petros and R. M. B. Wright (letter), *ibid.*, 1034.

GASTRO-INTESTINAL DISORDERS. Preliminary report of response of ulcerative colitis to clonidine.— F. Lechin *et al.*, *J. clin. Pharmac.*, 1985, *25*, 219.

Clonidine reduced watery diarrhoea in a 74-year-old man with lung cancer.— K. E. McArthur *et al.*, *Ann. intern. Med.*, 1982, *96*, 323.

Clonidine therapy controlled diabetic diarrhoea for 6 to 24 months in 3 patients who had not responded to standard antidiarrhoeal agents.— R. N. Fedorak *et al.*, *Ann. intern. Med.*, 1985, *102*, 197. A report of topical (transdermal) clonidine used successfully to treat diabetic diarrhoea in 1 patient.— A. Sacerdote (letter), *ibid.*, 1986, *105*, 139.

HYPERHIDROSIS. Relief of diabetic gustatory sweating by clonidine.— H. U. Janka *et al.*, *Ann. intern. Med.*, 1979, *91*, 130.

Paroxysmal idiopathic localised hyperhidrosis was controlled in 2 patients with clonidine 250 µg three and five times daily.— A. Kuritzky *et al.*, *Archs Neurol., Chicago*, 1984, *41*, 1210.

HYPERTENSION. Treatment of hypertension with clonidine is best avoided because of the risk of rebound hypertension if doses are missed for any reason. It should never be prescribed with a beta-blocking agent. Parenteral preparations of clonidine are unsatisfactory for emergency blood pressure reduction because clonidine may cause an initial increase in blood pressure.— *Drug & Ther. Bull.*, 1984, *22*, 42.

Results of a study suggesting that clonidine given as a single dose at night in combination with a diuretic was as effective as half the dose given twice a day. Once-daily dosage produced fewer and less frequent adverse effects.— F. G. McMahon *et al.*, *Curr. ther. Res.*, 1983, *33*, 1041. See also M. Lilja *et al.*, *Acta med. scand.*, 1983, *214*, 111.

In a study of 98 patients with severe renal hypertension, combination therapy with clonidine and either propranolol or atenolol effectively reduced the blood pressure and was not associated with a greater risk of serious cardiovascular complications than other antihypertensive regimens.— R. Vanholder *et al.*, *Eur. J. clin. Pharmac.*, 1985, *28*, 125.

Comparisons of clonidine with other antihypertensive agents: W. M. Kirkendall *et al.*, *J. Am. med. Ass.*, 1978, *240*, 2553 (prazosin); E. Rodrigues and A. A. H. Lawson, *Curr. med. Res. Opinion*, 1982, *8*, 274 (propranolol); E. Kanniainen *et al.*, *Eur. J. clin. Pharmac.*, 1985, *28*, 35 (urapidil).

Hypertensive emergencies. Clonidine administered orally acts too slowly for most emergencies but can control blood pressure within 6 hours in patients who are less seriously ill. Sedation may be prominent and rebound hypertension can occur.— *Med. Lett.*, 1987, *29*, 18.

A review of the use of oral clonidine in the urgent or emergency treatment of hypertension. Rapid oral clonidine loading and titration was considered to be an easy, effective, and safe method of treatment to control severe hypertension in appropriately selected patients and in some patients with hypertensive emergencies. The average time to maximum reduction in blood pressure was 2.75 hours and the average response rate was 92.6%. A rapid, graded reduction in blood pressure started at 30 to 60 minutes after an oral dose, producing a maximum clinical effect at 2 to 4 hours and a duration of action of 8 to 12 hours. This gradual reduction in blood pressure allowed for careful titration to a blood pressure that does not fall below the critical perfusion pressure for vital organs. In hypertensive emergencies in which delay in treatment may result in progressive end-organ damage or death immediate blood pressure reduction with intravenous sodium nitroprusside is usually the preferred treatment.— M. C. Houston, *Archs intern. Med.*, 1986, *146*, 586. See also R. J. Anderson *et al.*, *J. Am. med. Ass.*, 1981, *246*, 848; G. N. Karachalios, *Eur. J. clin. Pharmac.*, 1986, *31*, 227; A. D. Marks *et al.*, *J. clin. Pharmac.*, 1987, *27*, 193.

Transdermal administration. A review of transdermal clonidine for hypertension. Once weekly transdermal clonidine may prove to be convenient and effective for treatment of mild to moderate hypertension, but it can be expensive. In addition, although adverse effects appear to be less severe and less frequent than with oral clonidine, skin reactions occur frequently.— *Med. Lett.*, 1985, *27*, 95.

A review and discussion of transdermal administration of clonidine. Transdermal clonidine had been found to be effective in all grades of hypertension. Control of blood pressure had been achieved in patients with a lower mean plasma concentration of clonidine compared with that achieved with oral therapy in the same patients. In addition the frequency and severity of adverse effects had generally been less with transdermal than with oral clonidine, but skin reactions had been reported with the transdermal system commonly within 3 to 9 months after the start of therapy.— M. A. Weber, *Am. Heart J.*, 1986, *112*, 906. See also *Lancet*, 1987, *1*, 79; M. S. Langley and R. C. Heel, *Drugs*, 1988, *35*, 123.

Transdermal clonidine successfully controlled the blood pressure of a 51-year-old patient with a history of chronic pancreatitis, malabsorption, and a subtotal gastrectomy not controlled by oral therapy with captopril and other antihypertensive agents.— W. B. White and J. C. Gilbert (letter), *New Engl. J. Med.*, 1985, *313*, 1418.

A study of 2769 patients with mild hypertension treated for at least 3 months with transdermal clonidine. Treatment with transdermal clonidine either alone or with a diuretic effectively controlled blood pressure in 75% of patients and was acceptable to physicians and patients. There was evidence to suggest that the use of the transdermal delivery system improved compliance. Treatment was discontinued in 7.6% of patients due to systemic adverse effects. Localised allergic dermatitis led to discontinuation of treatment by 12.9%; all but one patient were later treated with oral clonidine without a recurrence of the allergy.— J. Hollifield, *Am. Heart J.*, 1986, *112*, 900.

Further studies of transdermal clonidine in hypertension: M. A. Weber *et al.*, *Archs intern. Med.*, 1984, *144*, 1211; M. A. Weber *et al.*, *Lancet*, 1984, *1*, 9; J. F. Burris and W. J. Mroczek, *Pharmacotherapy*, 1986, *6*, 30; G. S. Kellaway and W. F. Lubbe, *N.Z. med. J.*, 1986, *99*, 711; S. Popli *et al.*, *Archs intern. Med.*, 1986, *146*, 2140; J. C. Boekhorst *et al.*, *Curr. ther. Res.*, 1987, *41*, 215.

MENOPAUSAL SYMPTOMS. In a double-blind crossover study in general practice, clonidine 25 to 75 µg twice daily was significantly more effective than a placebo in reducing the number of menopausal hot flushes in 86 patients. In general, side-effects occurred as often with the placebo as with clonidine but leg pain and ankle oedema were noted in 3 patients taking clonidine.— J. R. Clayden *et al.*, *Br. med. J.*, 1974, *1*, 409. See also L. R. Laufer *et al.*, *Obstet. Gynec.*, 1982, *60*, 583.

The decrease in subjective flushing induced by clonidine was mediated by a mechanism independent of factors affecting peripheral vascular reactivity or factors governing luteinising hormorne secretion.— T. Tulandi *et al.*, *Br. J. Obstet. Gynaec.*, 1983, *90*, 854.

See also under premenstrual syndrome, below.

MENTAL DISORDERS. *Mania*. Rapid and complete remission of symptoms occured 48 to 72 hours after the initiation of clonidine therapy in 1 bipolar and 2 manic patients. The 2 manic patients relapsed within 24 to 48 hours of discontinuation of clonidine and response returned when treatment was restarted.— G. S. Zubenko *et al.*, *Am. J. Psychiat.*, 1984, *141*, 1617.

Further references to the use of clonidine in mania: R. Jouvent *et al.*, *Am. J. Psychiat.*, 1980, *137*, 1275.

Schizophrenia. Clonidine in doses of up to 900 µg daily was as effective as standard antipsychotic treatment in reducing psychosis in 8 schizophrenic patients with co-existing drug-induced tardive dyskinesia.— R. Freedman *et al.*, *Acta psychiat. scand.*, 1982, *65*, 35.

MIGRAINE. Reviews and discussions on clonidine in migraine: *Med. Lett.*, 1976, *18*, 55; E. S. Johnson, *Postgrad. med. J.*, 1978, *54*, 231.

NERVOUS SYSTEM DISORDERS. *Gilles de la Tourette's syndrome*. Eight children with Tourette's syndrome, either uncontrolled by haloperidol or in whom it produced unacceptable side-effects, obtained control of their symptoms following administration of small doses of clonidine. In 7 of the children control of motor and phonic tics, compulsive actions, and other behavioural symptoms was obtained with doses of 50 to 150 µg daily; in a 14-year-old girl weighing 90 kg dramatic improvement followed doses of up to 600 µg daily. Some of the children have now taken clonidine for up to one year with continued relief of symptoms.— D. J. Cohen *et al.*, *Lancet*, 1979, *2*, 551.

In an open study of 68 patients with Gilles de la Tourette's syndrome, clonidine was generally less effective than neuroleptics, but clonidine may be beneficial in a small subgroup of patients.— A. K. Shapiro *et al.*, *Archs gen. Psychiat.*, 1983, *40*, 1235.

Beneficial responses to clonidine were seen in 6 of 13 children with Gilles de la Tourette's syndrome, and a further 6 children had an equivocal response during treatment for 8 weeks in a single-blind study. During long-term treatment 11 children showed a greater than 25% overall improvement after 12 months.— J. F. Leckman *et al.*, *Neurology*, 1985, *35*, 343.

Narcolepsy. Report of a beneficial response to clonidine in 2 patients with refractory narcolepsy.— R. Salin-Pascual *et al.*, *J. clin. Psychiat.*, 1985, *46*, 528.

Peripheral neuropathies. Symptomatic relief from disabling leg pain after treatment with clonidine in 3 diabetic patients.— Y. -M. Tan and J. Croese (letter), *Ann. intern. Med.*, 1986, *105*, 633.

Restless leg syndrome. Report of alleviation of restless leg syndrome by clonidine in 3 patients.— J. V. Handwerker and R. F. Palmer (letter), *New Engl. J. Med.*, 1985, *313*, 1228.

Spasticity. Clonidine reduced spasticity in 4 patients with both recent and long-term spinal cord injury.— P. W. Nance *et al.*, *Can. med. Ass. J.*, 1985, *133*, 41.

PREMENSTRUAL SYNDROME. Beneficial response to clonidine in 2 women with premenstrual tension.— W. A. Price and A. J. Giannini, *J. clin. Pharmac.*, 1984, *24*, 463.

Improvement of symptoms of premenstrual tension in 1 patient for 15 cycles during treatment with clonidine 25 µg three times a day for 17 days in each cycle.— L. C. Nilsson *et al.* (letter), *Lancet*, 1985, *2*, 549.

See also under menopausal symptoms, above.

WITHDRAWAL SYNDROMES. *Alcohol*. Discussion of the use of clonidine in alcohol withdrawal. Clonidine can relieve tremor, sweating, and tachycardia due to alcohol withdrawal, but there is no evidence that it can prevent delirium tremens.— *Med. Lett.*, 1986, *28*, 75. See also J. A. Steiner *et al.*, *Br. J. clin. Pharmac.*, 1983, *15*, 583P.

Opioids. Clonidine has been reported to be useful in controlling withdrawal symptoms following abrupt discontinuation of opioids. Treatment is required for about 10 days following methadone withdrawal and less for withdrawal from heroin (C. Cook *et al.*, *Br. med. J.*, 1986, *293*, 506). Most studies have reported favourable results (see also below), although studies by Preston *et al.* (*Clin. Pharmac. Ther.*, 1985, *38*, 219) and Jasinski *et al.* (*Archs gen. Psychiat.*, 1985, *42*, 1063) suggest that subjective response may be less favourable. However, the maximum dose of clonidine used by Preston *et al.* was 300 µg twice daily: Camí *et al.* (*Clin. Pharmac. Ther.*, 1985, *38*, 336) used initial doses of up to 1.35 mg daily and Washton *et al.* (*Lancet*, 1980, *1*, 1078) found that a dose of 100 to 200 µg every 4 to 6 hours was necessary: doses of up to 17 µg per kg body-weight have been used (M.S. Gold *et al.*, *ibid.*, *2*, 1078). The major drawback of clonidine therapy is the tendency to cause hypotension, and this may limit its usefulness in some patients.

Charney *et al.* (*Archs gen. Psychiat.*, 1982, *39*, 1327) reported the use of clonidine in combination with naltrexone to shorten the withdrawal syndrome and achieved withdrawal within 6 days. Subsequent modification to the regimen (D.S. Charney *et al.*, *Am. J. Psychiat.*, 1986, *143*, 831) allowed 38 of 40 patients addicted to methadone to withdraw completely in 4 to 5 days. Patients required a mean of 2.3 mg of clonidine on the first day which reduced but did not abolish symptoms. Further reports of the successful use of clonidine in managing opioid withdrawal syndromes: T. D. Scannell and M. Lipsedge (letter), *Br. med. J.*, 1984, *289*, 1538; C. Brewer (letter), *ibid.*, 1986, *293*, 391.

Neonatal opioid dependence. Clonidine 3 to 4 µg per kg body-weight daily in divided doses at 6-hourly intervals rapidly ameliorated symptoms of neonatal opioid-abstinence syndrome in 2 infants. Treatment was continued for 10 and 16 days.— E. L. Hoder *et al.* (letter), *New Engl. J. Med.*, 1981, *305*, 1284. See also E. L. Hoder *et al.*, *Psychiatry Res.*, 1984, *13*, 243.

Other psychotropic agents. A report of the successful use of clonidine in the management of lorazepam withdrawal in a 37-year-old man.— M. S. Keshavan and J. L. Crammer (letter), *Lancet*, 1985, *1*, 1325.

Smoking. Report of beneficial effects of clonidine on withdrawal effects from smoking.— K. I. Pearce (letter), *Lancet*, 1986, *2*, 810.

Preparations

Clonidine Injection *(B.P.)*. Clonidine Hydrochloride Injection

Clonidine Tablets *(B.P.)*. Clonidine Hydrochloride Tablets

Clonidine Hydrochloride Tablets *(U.S.P.)*
Clonidine Hydrochloride and Chlorthalidone Tablets *(U.S.P.)*

Proprietary Preparations

Catapres *(Boehringer Ingelheim, UK). Tablets*, scored, clonidine hydrochloride 100 and 300 µg.
Perlongets (Catapres PL), sustained release capsules, clonidine hydrochloride 250 µg.
Injection, clonidine hydrochloride 150 µg/mL, in ampoules of 1 mL.

Dixarit *(Boehringer Ingelheim, UK). Tablets*, clonidine hydrochloride 25 µg.

Proprietary Names and Manufacturers

Catapres *(Boehringer Ingelheim, Austral.; Boehringer Ingelheim, Canad.; Jpn; Boehringer Ingelheim, S.Afr.; Boehringer Ingelheim, UK; Boehringer Ingelheim, USA)*; Catapresan *(Arg.; Boehringer Ingelheim, Denm.; Boehringer Ingelheim, Ger.; Boehringer Ingelheim, Ital.; Neth.; Boehringer Ingelheim, Norw.; Boehringer Ingelheim, Spain; Boehringer Ingelheim, Swed.; Boehringer Ingelheim, Switz.)*; Catapressan *(Belg.; Boehringer Ingelheim, Fr.)*; Catapres-TTS *(Boehringer Ingelheim, USA)*; Clonilou *(Spain)*; Clonistada *(Stadapharm, Ger.)*; Dixarit *(Boehringer Ingelheim, Austral.; Belg.; Boehringer Ingelheim, Canad.; Neth.; Boehringer Ingelheim, S.Afr.; Boehringer Ingelheim, UK)*; Drylon *(Norw.)*; Hyposyn *(Denm.)*; Ipotensium *(Pierrel, Ital.)*; Isoglaucon *(Basotherm, Ger.; Boehringer Ingelheim, Ital.; Switz.)*; Tensinova *(Spain)*; Tenso-Timelets *(Temmler, Ger.)*.

The following names have been used for multi-ingredient preparations containing clonidine hydrochloride— Combipres *(Boehringer Ingelheim, Canad.; Boehringer Ingelheim, USA)*.

858-a

Cryptenamine Acetates

The acetate salts of alkaloids derived from an extract of green veratrum.

859-t

Cryptenamine Tannates

The tannate salts of alkaloids derived from an extract of green veratrum.

CAS — 1405-40-9.

Cryptenamine has the properties and uses described under White Veratrum, p.504. Cryptenamine tannates have been used for oral administration and cryptenamine acetates have been given by intravenous and intramuscular injection.

Proprietary Names and Manufacturers of Cryptenamine and its Salts

Unitensin *(Wallace, USA)*.

The following names have been used for multi-ingredient preparations containing cryptenamine and its salts— Diutensen *(Wallace, USA)*.

860-l

Debrisoquine Sulphate *(BANM, rINNM).*

Debrisoquin Sulfate *(USAN)*; Isocaramidine Sulphate; Ro-5-3307/1. 1,2,3,4-Tetrahydroisoquinoline-2-carboxamidine sulphate.
$(C_{10}H_{13}N_3)_2,H_2SO_4$=448.5.

CAS — 1131-64-2 (debrisoquine); 581-88-4 (sulphate).

Pharmacopoeias. In *Br.*

A white odourless or almost odourless crystalline powder. Debrisoquine sulphate 12.8 mg is approximately equivalent to 10 mg of debrisoquine. **Soluble** 1 in 40 of water; very slightly soluble in alcohol; almost insoluble in chloroform and ether. A 3% solution in water has a pH of 5.3 to 6.8. **Store** in well-closed containers. Protect from light.

Adverse Effects, Treatment, and Precautions

As for Guanethidine Monosulphate, p.481.
With debrisoquine sulphate diarrhoea is rare. Sweating and headache may occur. Abrupt cessation of treatment should be avoided as this may lead to rebound hypertension.
The metabolism of debrisoquine is subject to genetic polymorphism and non-metabolisers may show a marked response to doses that have little or no effect in metabolisers.

Absorption and Fate

Debrisoquine is rapidly absorbed from the gastro-intestinal tract. The major metabolite is 4-hydroxydebrisoquine; metabolism is subject to genetic polymorphism.

Pre-systemic metabolism of debrisoquine to its metabolite 4-hydroxydebrisoquine occurred in 15 patients with hypertension and 4 healthy subjects. Results indicated that debrisoquine or its metabolite could inhibit this metabolism and therefore increases in the dose of debrisoquine could produce disproportionate decreases in blood pressure. The estimated half-life of elimination for debrisoquine and 4-hydroxydebrisoquine ranged from 11.5 to 26 hours and from 5.8 to 14.5 hours respectively. A further study of one healthy subject indicated that debrisoquine was actively taken up by platelets and that this was responsible for its long half-life.— J. H. Silas *et al.*, *Br. J. clin. Pharmac.*, 1978, *5*, 27. See also J. H. Silas *et al.*, *ibid.*, 1980, *9*, 419 and 427.

A poor response to debrisoquine therapy was associated with extensive metabolism of the drug in a study of 12 patients.— J. H. Silas *et al.*, *Br. med. J.*, 1977, *1*, 422.

GENETIC POLYMORPHISM. A review of the therapeutic implications of genetically determined variations in oxidation. Polymorphic oxidation involving cytochrome P-450 enzymes was first clearly demonstrated with debrisoquine. Two distinct phenotypes were identified and characterised as "extensive" and "poor" metabolisers of debrisoquine. Subsequent work has shown that the major cause of variation in oxidation is under the control of a single gene. Poor metabolisers were subsequently shown to have an increased hypotensive response. Between 5 and 10% of Caucasian populations exhibit poor metabolism of debrisoquine and sparteine. Most studies indicate that the metabolism of both drugs appears to be controlled by identical or closely related genetic factors. Either debrisoquine or sparteine can be used to phenotype subjects for oxidation status. Poor metabolisers of debrisoquine or sparteine have been shown to exhibit altered pharmacokinetics of a number of other drugs, but the polymorphism does not affect the oxidation of all drugs oxidised by cytochrome P-450 isoenzymes.— D. W. J. Clark, *Drugs*, 1985, *29*, 342.

The determination of debrisoquine 'oxidiser status' was considered to be useful for detecting individuals potentially at increased risk of toxicity with some other drugs including metoprolol, phenacetin, and perhexiline, and in the evaluation of the relationship between metabolism and toxicity of new drugs.— *Adverse Drug React. Bull.*, 1987, Feb 456. Report of the use of dextromethorphan to determine debrisoquine-type hydroxylation phenotype: A. Küpfer *et al.* (letter), *Lancet*, 1984, *2*, 517. The use of methoxyphenamine and dextromethorphan in determining debrisoquine-type drug hydroxylation polymorphism.— S. D. Roy *et al.* (letter), *ibid.*, 1393. Result of a study suggesting that there would be little practical advantage in carrying out oxidation phenotyping for patients undergoing general medical admission for the purpose of identifying patients at increased risk of adverse drug reactions.— H. Wynne *et al.*, *Br. J. clin. Pharmac.*, 1985, *20*, 254P.

Studies of genetic and environmental factors determining debrisoquine hydroxylation polymorphism: T. P. Sloan *et al.*, *Br. J. clin. Pharmac.*, 1983, *15*, 443; E. Steiner *et al.*, *Clin. Pharmac. Ther.*, 1985, *38*, 394.

Studies of genetic polymorphism of debrisoquine in ethnic groups: K. Nakamura *et al.*, *Clin. Pharmac. Ther.*, 1985, *38*, 402; A. O. Iyun *et al.*, *ibid.*, 1986, *40*, 387; G. F. Peart *et al.*, *Br. J. clin. Pharmac.*, 1986, *21*, 465.

Further references to genetic polymorphism of debrisoquine: A. Mahgoub *et al.*, *Lancet*, 1977, *2*, 584; G. T. Tucker *et al.* (letter), *ibid.*, 718; D. S. Davies *et al.* (letter), *Br. J. clin. Pharmac.*, 1981, *11*, 89; G. C. Kahn *et al.*, *ibid.*, 1982, *13*, 594P; A. R. Boobis *et al.*, *ibid.*, *14*, 602P.

Uses and Administration

Debrisoquine sulphate is an antihypertensive agent with actions and uses similar to those of guanethidine monosulphate (see p.482), but it causes less depletion of noradrenaline stores. When administered by mouth, debrisoquine is reported to act within about 4 to 10 hours and to have effects lasting for 9 to 24 hours.
The usual initial dose is the equivalent of 10 to 20 mg of debrisoquine once or twice daily. The daily dose is then increased by 10 to 20 mg, according to the severity of the condition, every 3 or 4 days. The usual maintenance dose is 20 to 120 mg daily, but up to 300 mg or more daily may be given. To reduce side-effects smaller doses of debrisoquine may be given in conjunction with a thiazide diuretic and/or other antihypertensive agents.
For reference to the use of debrisoquine in identifying metabolic phenotypes, see under Genetic Polymorphism in Absorption and Fate, above.

For a report of comparative antihypertensive effects and toxicity of guanethidine, debrisoquine, and bethandine, see Guanethidine, Uses, p.482.

Preparations

Debrisoquine Tablets *(B.P.)*. Tablets containing debrisoquine sulphate. Potency is expressed in terms of the equivalent amount of debrisoquine.

Proprietary Preparations

Declinax *(Roche, UK). Tablets*, scored, debrisoquine 10 and 20 mg (as sulphate).

Proprietary Names and Manufacturers

Declinax *(Arg.; Roche, Austral.; Belg.; Roche, Canad.; S.Afr.; Switz.; Roche, UK)*; Equitonil *(Arg.)*; Redu-Pres *(Protea, Austral.)*.

2850-m

Delapril Hydrochloride *(USAN, rINNM).*

CV-3317; REV-6000A. Ethyl (*S*)-2-{[(*S*)-1-(carboxymethyl-2-indanylcarbamoyl)ethyl]amino}-4-phenylbutyrate hydrochloride.
$C_{26}H_{32}N_2O_5$,HCl=489.0.

CAS — 83435-67-0 (hydrochloride); 83435-66-9 (delapril).

Delapril is an antihypertensive agent which acts, similarly to captopril, as an angiotensin-converting enzyme inhibitor.

References to the actions and use of delapril: H. Shionoiri *et al.*, *Clin. Pharmac. Ther.*, 1987, *41*, 74.

Proprietary Names and Manufacturers

Takeda, Jpn; USV Pharmaceutical Corp., USA.

861-y

Deserpidine *(BAN, rINN).*

11-Demethoxyreserpine. Methyl 11-demethoxy-18-*O*-(3,4,5-trimethoxybenzoyl)reserpate.
$C_{32}H_{38}N_2O_8$=578.7.

CAS — 131-01-1.

An ester alkaloid isolated from the root of *Rauwolfia canescens*.

Deserpidine has properties and uses similar to those described under reserpine (see p.498). In the treatment of hypertension some sources have recommended an initial dose of 0.75 to 1 mg daily subsequently reduced to a maintenance dose of about 250 µg daily, while others have recommended an initial dose of 250 µg daily; intervals of 10 to 14 days are recommended between dosage adjustments.
In psychiatric conditions the average initial dose is 500 µg daily with a range of 0.1 to 1 mg.

Proprietary Names and Manufacturers

Harmonyl *(Belg.; Abbott, UK; Abbott, USA)*.

The following names have been used for multi-ingredient preparations containing deserpidine— Dureticyl *(Abbott, Canad.)*; Enduronyl *(Abbott, UK; Abbott, USA)*; Methyclodine *(Rugby, USA)*; Oreticyl *(Abbott, USA)*.

862-j

Diazoxide *(BAN, USAN, rINN).*

Diazoxidum; SRG-95213. 7-Chloro-3-methyl-2*H*-1,2,4-benzothiadiazine 1,1-dioxide.
$C_8H_7ClN_2O_2S$=230.7.

CAS — 364-98-7.

Pharmacopoeias. In *Br., Eur., Int.*, and *U.S.*

A white or creamy-white odourless or almost odourless crystalline powder. Practically **insoluble** to sparingly soluble in water, chloroform, and ether; slightly soluble in alcohol; very soluble in solutions of alkali hydroxides; freely soluble in dimethylformamide. Solutions of the sodium salt are **sterilised** by autoclaving. The injection is prepared with the aid of sodium hydroxide and has a pH of 11.2 to 11.9. Liquid preparations should be **stored** protected from light.

Adverse Effects

In addition to inappropriate hypotension and hyperglycaemia, side-effects during prolonged therapy frequently include oedema which may result in precipitation of congestive heart failure and hypertrichosis; nausea is also common in the initial stages of oral therapy. Other adverse effects which occur during prolonged therapy include anorexia, mild hyperuricaemia, extrapyramidal symptoms, allergic skin rashes, and leucopenia and thrombocytopenia.

During intravenous therapy, adverse effects may be associated with an inappropriately rapid reduction in the blood pressure: coronary ischaemia leading to cardiac arrhythmias, marked ECG changes, palpitations and bradycardia; cerebral ischaemia leading to neurological deficit; tachycardia, and symptoms of vasodilatation. Nausea and vomiting are also common. Symptoms of hyperglycaemia may range from very mild to ketoacidotic coma.

Alopecia has been reported in infants born to mothers taking diazoxide. Diazoxide may cause a burning sensation in the vein used for injection; extravasation of the alkaline solution is painful.

Side-effects of diazoxide in childhood hypoglycaemia included advancement of bone-age and depression of immunoglobulin.— L. Kollée and L. Monnens (letter), *Lancet*, 1978, *1*, 668.

Transplacental transfer of diazoxide was considered to be responsible for an inappropriately low plasma-insulin concentration in an infant whose mother had received diazoxide 150 mg daily for 47 days prior to delivery.— M. J. Smith *et al.*, *Br. med. J.*, 1982, *284*, 1234.

Evidence of raised serum androgen concentrations during oral diazoxide treatment in a 38-year-old woman. It was suggested that this could be at least partially responsible for the diazoxide-induced hirsutism seen in this patient.— B. Hallengren and B. Hökfelt (letter), *Lancet*, 1984, *2*, 1044.

EFFECTS ON THE BLOOD. A 26-year-old man with hypertension developed reversible haemolytic anaemia when treated with diazoxide by mouth on 3 separate occasions.— R. A. Best and H. M. Clink, *Postgrad. med. J.*, 1975, *51*, 402.

EFFECTS ON THE HEART. A 9-year-old girl given diazoxide 20 mg per kg body-weight per day for 6 months developed cardiomegaly possibly attributable to diazoxide.— W. J. Appleyard, *Proc. R. Soc. Med.*, 1968, *61*, 1257.

Cardiac failure in one infant and ataxia in another were attributed to the use of diazoxide for nesidioblastosis.— M. E. McGraw and D. A. Price, *Archs Dis. Childh.*, 1985, *60*, 62. Contributory factors in the development of cardiac failure during the treatment of nesidioblastosis include treatment with intravenous fluids and corticosteroids in addition to diazoxide.— D. R. N. Gillies (letter), *ibid.*, 500.

EXTRAPYRAMIDAL EFFECTS. In a study of 100 hypertensive patients receiving diazoxide, the incidence of extrapyramidal symptoms was 15%.— J. E. F. Pohl, *Am. Heart J.*, 1975, *89*, 401.

PANCREATITIS. Ten patients with severe hypertension and renal failure were treated with diazoxide in a last attempt to avert nephrectomy; 1 patient developed acute pancreatitis and another diabetic ketoacidosis. Both patients recovered from these effects when diazoxide was withdrawn.— M. De Broe *et al.* (letter), *Lancet*, 1972, *1*, 1397.

VOICE CHANGES. In addition to marked hypertrichosis, 2 children who had received diazoxide for several years were noted to have unusually deep (low-pitched) voices.— R. J. West (letter), *Br. med. J.*, 1978, *2*, 506.

Treatment of Adverse Effects

Hypotension may be treated by placing the patient in a supine position with the feet raised: severe hypotension can be controlled with infusions of electrolytes or sympathomimetics such as noradrenaline or dopamine. Severe hyperglycaemia may be corrected by giving intravenous fluids and insulin: less severe hyperglycaemia is reported to respond to tolbutamide. Antiparkinsonian agents, such as procyclidine, have been given to control extrapyramidal effects. Diazoxide can be removed from the body by dialysis but recovery is relatively low owing to extensive protein binding.

Precautions

Diazoxide should be used with care in patients with impaired cardiac or cerebral circulation and in patients with aortic coarctation, arteriovenous shunt, or other cardiac disorders in which an increase in cardiac output could be detrimental. During prolonged therapy blood-glucose concentrations should be monitored and the blood should be examined regularly for signs of leucopenia and thrombocytopenia, and, in children, bone and psychological maturation and growth should be regularly assessed.

If given during parturition, diazoxide may delay delivery unless oxytocin is given concomitantly. The hyperglycaemic, hyperuricaemic, and hypotensive actions of diazoxide may be enhanced by diuretics.

INTERACTIONS. A report of chlorpromazine enhancing the hyperglycaemic effect of diazoxide in a 2-year-old child.— A. Aynsley-Green and R. Illig (letter), *Lancet*, 1975, *2*, 658.

For the effect of diazoxide in displacing phenytoin from plasma protein binding sites, see Phenytoin, p.409.

For the effect of diazoxide, *in vitro*, in displacing warfarin from albumin binding sites, see Warfarin Sodium, p.346.

The action of diazoxide may be reduced by concurrent administration of non-steroidal anti-inflammatory drugs, see p.466.

PREGNANCY AND THE NEONATE. For a report of severe depression among infants born to mothers given both diazoxide and chlormethiazole edisylate for the treatment of toxaemia of pregnancy, see Chlormethiazole Edisylate, p.720.

See also under Uses (below).

Absorption and Fate

Diazoxide is readily absorbed from the gastro-intestinal tract and extensively bound to plasma proteins. Its plasma half-life has been estimated to range from about 20 to 45 hours but values of up to 60 hours have been reported. The half-life is reported to be prolonged in renal failure and shorter for children. The plasma half-life greatly exceeds the duration of vascular activity. Diazoxide is partly metabolised in the liver and is excreted in the urine both unchanged and in the form of metabolites; only small amounts are recovered from the faeces. It crosses the placenta and the blood-brain barrier.

A review of the metabolism and disposition of diazoxide.— P. G. Dayton *et al.*, *Drug Metab. & Disposit.*, 1975, *3*, 226.

A finding in severely hypertensive patients that metabolism may become the main route of elimination of diazoxide.— W. Sadee *et al.*, *J. Pharmacokinet. Biopharm.*, 1973, *1*, 295.

A pharmacokinetic study of diazoxide in 4 children with hypoglycaemia revealed a plasma half-life of 9.5 to 24 hours which is considerably shorter than that in adults.— A. W. Pruitt *et al.*, *Clin. Pharmac. Ther.*, 1973, *14*, 73.

PROTEIN BINDING. About 90% of a usual therapeutic dose of diazoxide was bound to plasma proteins. Repeated administration for a sustained hypotensive effect caused the accumulation of bound inactive diazoxide so that plasma concentration did not correlate well with intensity of hypotension. The hypotensive effect of diazoxide was dependent on the rate of injection.— E. M. Sellers and J. Koch-Weser, *New Engl. J. Med.*, 1969, *281*, 1141. Evidence of decreased protein binding in uraemia.— K. O'Malley *et al.*, *Clin. Pharmac. Ther.*, 1975, *18*, 53.

Uses and Administration

Diazoxide increases the concentration of glucose in the plasma; it inhibits the secretion of insulin by the beta cells of the pancreas, increases the release of catecholamines, and may increase the hepatic output of glucose. When administered intravenously, it produces a fall in blood pressure by a vasodilator effect on the arterioles and a reduction in peripheral resistance. Diazoxide is closely related structurally to the thiazide diuretics, but has an antidiuretic action and thus produces fluid and electrolyte retention.

Diazoxide is used in the treatment of intractable hypoglycaemia such as idiopathic hypoglycaemia of infancy or the hypoglycaemia resulting from functional islet cell tumours. Initially, 3 to 5 mg per kg body-weight daily is administered in 2 or 3 divided doses by mouth, then the dosage is adjusted according to the needs of the patient. Doses of up to 1 g daily have been used in adults with islet cell tumours. In children with leucine-sensitive hypoglycaemia a suggested maintenance dose is 15 to 20 mg per kg daily. The hyperglycaemic effect normally lasts for about 8 hours. Frusemide or ethacrynic acid may be required to reduce fluid retention.

Diazoxide is used intravenously for the treatment of severe hypertensive crises. Rapid bolus injection of 300 mg within 30 seconds produces a fall in blood pressure within 5 minutes and the effect usually lasts 4 to 6 hours, but may vary considerably. However, the rapid reduction in blood pressure produced may be deleterious and a rapid bolus injection of 1 to 3 mg per kg body-weight (maximum single dose of 150 mg) repeated after 5 to 15 minutes, if required, is now recommended. Diazoxide 0.4 to 1 g daily in 2 or 3 divided doses has also been given by mouth although it is rarely used for chronic treatment of hypertension because of the severity of the adverse effects produced during prolonged therapy.

A review of diazoxide including its mechanism of action, clinical use and indications, metabolism, and side-effects.— J. Koch-Weser, *New Engl. J. Med.*, 1976, *294*, 1271.

ADMINISTRATION IN RENAL FAILURE. Diazoxide was effective in the treatment of acute hypertension during haemodialysis in 13 patients.— G. Keusch *et al.*, *Eur. J. clin. Pharmac.*, 1983, *25*, 523.

For a report of reduced protein binding in uraemic patients, see under Absorption and Fate, above.

HYPERTENSION. It has been considered that rapid injection of diazoxide is necessary in the treatment of hypertensive crisis in order to produce adequate blood concentrations of unbound diazoxide. However, several studies have shown that acute severe hypertension could be controlled by repeated bolus injections of 25 mg (M. Velasco *et al.*, *Curr. ther. Res.*, 1976, *19*, 185) or 1 mg per kg body-weight (A. McNair *et al.*, *Eur. J. clin. Pharmac.*, 1983, *24*, 151) every 10 minutes or by slow intravenous infusion of 15 to 30 mg per minute (T.A. Thien *et al.*, *Clin. Pharmac. Ther.*, 1979, *25*, 795; B.N. Garrett and N.M. Kaplan, *Am. Heart J.*, 1982, *103*, 390; T.M. Huysmans *et al.*, *Archs intern. Med.*, 1983, *143*, 882). These regimens have been found to produce a gradual reduction in blood pressure without the risk of ischaemic damage to the heart and brain associated with the precipitous fall in blood pressure produced by rapid injection of large doses. Adequate control of blood pressure was shown by McNair *et al.* to be associated with plasma-diazoxide concentrations of 20 to 85 μg per mL.

In patients with severe hypertension and symptoms of hypertensive encephalopathy, resistant to treatment with frusemide 40 mg intravenously, a gradual reduction in blood pressure was produced by diazoxide 75 or 150 mg intravenously every 15 or 30 minutes or dihydralazine 6.25 mg initially then 12.5 mg every 30 minutes by intramuscular injection. No cerebral catastrophies occurred during treatment but 2 patients developed subendocardial infarctions secondary to abrupt blood pressure reduction. A dose of diazoxide 75 mg every 30 minutes was considered to produce an adequate response.— A. McNair *et al.*, *Acta med. scand.*, 1986, *220*, 15.

HYPOGLYCAEMIA. A review of the use of diazoxide in the treatment of hypoglycaemia. It would be useful in the treatment of hypoglycaemia due to hyperinsulinism, especially in infants and children, but should not be used for functional hypoglycaemia.— *Med. Lett.*, 1978, *20*, 110.

Drug-induced hypoglycaemia. Diazoxide was effective in controlling hypoglycaemia in a 9-year-old boy who had ingested about 5 g of chlorpropamide, about 5 g of methyldopa, and about 3 g of chlorothiazide. Infusions of glucose failed to control hypoglycaemia.— R. F. Jacobs *et al.*, *J. Pediat.*, 1978, *93*, 801.

Further references to the use of diazoxide in chlorpropamide-induced hypoglycaemia: S. F. Johnson *et al.*, *Am. J. Med.*, 1977, *63*, 799.

Diazoxide 100 mg by mouth every 6 hours was successful in controlling pentamidine-induced hypoglycaemia in a patient with *Pneumocystis carinii* pneumonia.— D. B. Fitzgerald and I. S. Young, *J. trop. Med. Hyg.*, 1984, *87*, 15.

PREGNANCY AND THE NEONATE. *Hypertension in pregnancy.* Blood pressure was successfully controlled in 34 patients with severe pre-eclampsia with diazoxide 30 mg intravenously every 1 to 2 minutes. The total dose required ranged from 90 to 150 mg and control was achieved in all patients within 5 to 10 minutes. No excessive hypotension occurred and the mean duration of effect was 4.8 hours. Eight infants had hypoglycaemia which was attributed to extreme prematurity.— D. K. L. Dudley, *Am. J. Obstet. Gynec.*, 1985, *151*, 196.

Further references to the use of diazoxide in pre-eclampsic hypertension: M. C. Macnaughton, *Prescribers' J.*, 1979, *19*, 52.

PULMONARY HYPERTENSION. A review of the use of diazoxide in primary pulmonary hypertension. Diazoxide has been shown to produce acute and long-term haemodynamic and clinical benefits in some studies, although the possibility of spontaneous remissions of the disorder could not be discounted. However, there have been reports of occasional catastrophic cardiovascular effects including severe hypotension, asystole, atrioventricular block, and death during acute administration of diazoxide, and exacerbation of pulmonary hypertension due to reflex sympathetic activity during short-term treatment. In addition, long-term therapy has been frequently associated with adverse effects.— M. Packer, *Ann. intern. Med.*, 1985, *103*, 258.

Preparations

Diazoxide Capsules *(U.S.P.)*

Diazoxide Injection *(B.P.)*

Diazoxide Injection *(U.S.P.)*

Diazoxide Oral Suspension *(U.S.P.)*

Diazoxide Tablets *(B.P.)*

Proprietary Preparations

Eudemine *(Allen & Hanburys, UK). Tablets*, diazoxide 50 mg.

Injection, diazoxide 15 mg/mL, in ampoules of 20 mL.

Proprietary Names and Manufacturers

Eudemine *(Allen & Hanburys, UK)*; Hyperstat *(Arg.; Essex, Austral.; Belg.; Schering, Canad.; Schering Corp., Denm.; Unicet, Fr.; Essex, Ital.; Neth.; Norw.; Scherag, S.Afr.; Essex, Spain; Schering, Swed.; Essex, Switz.; Medical Market, USA)*; Hypertonalum *(Essex, Ger.)*; Proglicem *(Unicet, Fr.; Essex, Ger.; Essex, Ital.; Neth.; Scherag, S.Afr.)*; Proglycem *(Schering, Canad.; Medical Market, USA)*.

863-z

Dicolinium Iodide *(rINN)*.

Dicolinum Iodide. 2-[2-(Diethylmethylammonio)ethoxycarbonyl]-1,1,6-trimethylpiperidinium di-iodide.
$C_{16}H_{34}I_2N_2O_2$=540.3.

CAS — 382-82-1.

Pharmacopoeias. In *Rus.*

Dicolinium iodide is a ganglion-blocking agent that has been used in the treatment of hypertension.

864-c

Dihydralazine Sulphate *(BANM, rINNM)*.

Dihydralazinum Sulfuricum; Dihydrallazine Sulphate. 1,4-Dihydrazinophthalazine sulphate.
$C_8H_{10}N_6,H_2SO_4$=288.3.

CAS — 484-23-1 (dihydralazine); 7327-87-9 (sulphate).

Pharmacopoeias. In *Cz. Jug. P.* and *Roum. P.* specify the dihydrate.

Dihydralazine sulphate is an antihypertensive agent with action and uses similar to those of hydralazine (see p.483). It has been given in doses of up to 150 mg daily in divided doses. The mesylate is given by injection.

References to the use of dihydralazine in hypertension: L. Pedrini *et al.*, *Curr. ther. Res.*, 1983, *33*, 1055; A. McNair *et al.*, *Acta med. scand.*, 1986, *220*, 15.

For a reference to the use of dihydralazine in hypertensive crises, see under Diazoxide, Uses p.477.

References to the use of dihydralazine in severe congestive heart failure: N. Reifart *et al.*, *Eur. Heart J.*, 1984, *5*, 568.

Proprietary Names and Manufacturers

Dihyzin *(Henning Berlin, Ger.)*; Dopatets *(Pharmadrug, Ger.)*; Nepresol *(Ciba, Belg.; Ciba, Denm.; Ciba, Fr.; Bristol, Ger.; Ciba, Ital.; Neth.; Ciba, Norw.; Ciba, S.Afr.; Ciba, Swed.; Ciba, Switz.)*.

The following names have been used for multi-ingredient preparations containing dihydralazine sulphate— Adelphane *(Ciba, Austral.)*.

16611-y

Doxazosin Mesylate *(BANM, USAN)*.

Doxazosin Mesilate *(rINNM)*; Doxazosin Methanesulphonate; UK-33274-27. 2-[4-(2,3-Dihydro-1,4-benzodioxin-2-ylcarbonyl)piperazin-1-yl]-6,7-dimethoxyquinazolin-4-ylamine methanesulphonate; 1-(4-amino-6,7-dimethoxyquinazolin-2-yl)-4-(1,4-benzodioxan-2-ylcarbonyl)piperazine methanesulphonate.
$C_{23}H_{25}N_5O_5,CH_3SO_3H$=547.6.

CAS — 77883-43-3 (mesylate); 74191-85-8 (doxazosin).

Doxazosin is an antihypertensive agent which blocks alpha$_1$-adrenergic receptors and has actions similar to prazosin (p.496). It has a longer half-life than prazosin .

A detailed review of doxazosin.— R. A. Young and R. N. Brogden, *Drugs*, 1988, *35*, 525.

References on the pharmacokinetics of doxazosin: P. A. Meredith *et al.*, *Br. J. clin. Pharmac.*, 1985, *19*, 541P; J. Vincent *et al.*, *ibid.*, *20*, 251P; J. Vincent *et al.*, *ibid.*, 1986, *21*, 521; R. V. Carlson *et al.*, *Clin. Pharmac. Ther.*, 1986, *40*, 561; J. K. Faulkner *et al.*, *Eur. J. clin. Pharmac.*, 1987, *31*, 685.

Studies and reviews of the pharmacological and clinical profile of doxazosin.— J. L. Reid and H. C. Davies, *Br. J. clin. Pharmac.*, 1986, *21*, *Suppl.* 1.

Further references to the actions and uses of doxazosin: L. X. Cubeddu *et al.*, *Clin. Pharmac. Ther.*, 1987, *41*, 439; J. Rosenthal, *Am. J. Cardiol.*, 1987, *59*, 40G; M. H. Frick *et al.*, *ibid.*, 61G; D. Torvik and H. P. Madsbu, *ibid.*, 68G.

Proprietary Names and Manufacturers

Pfizer, USA.

12969-e

Enalapril Maleate *(BANM, USAN, rINNM)*.

MK-421. *N*-{*N*-[(*S*)-1-Ethoxycarbonyl-3-phenylpropyl]-L-alanyl}-L-proline hydrogen maleate.
$C_{20}H_{28}N_2O_5,C_4H_4O_4$=492.5.

CAS — 75847-73-3 (enalapril); 76095-16-4 (maleate).

Adverse Effects

Enalapril has adverse effects similar to those of captopril (p.468); initial hypotension may be severe and prolonged, and renal failure has also been reported. However, enalapril does not contain the sulphydryl group thought to be responsible for some of the adverse effects of captopril and the incidence of skin rashes and taste disturbance may be lower with enalapril. Dizziness and headache are among the more frequently reported adverse effects; fatigue or lassitude has also been reported. Angioedema may occur and may be associated with laryngeal oedema and obstruction of the airway.

A review of enalapril. Enalapril has been generally well tolerated and serious adverse reactions have been rare but there has been considerable debate concerning the relative safety profiles of enalapril and captopril. Comparisons involving different studies are complicated by differences in patient populations. Captopril was initially used at high dosages in more severe, resistant forms of hypertension whereas enalapril has been used more often at relatively lower dosages in mild to moderate hypertension. In addition, patients treated with captopril more frequently had existing renal insufficiency or other diseases now known to predispose to adverse effects. However the evidence available tends to suggest that enalapril is better tolerated than captopril. Adverse effects which are associated with ACE inhibition such as acute hypotension and renal failure in patients with renal artery stenosis occur with a similar frequency with either drug. Proteinuria appears to occur more frequently with captopril even after excluding those patients who might be predisposed to renal complications. More experience is required in similar patient populations to determine whether the risk of renal toxicity and leucopenia is lower with enalapril.— P. A. Todd and R. C. Heel, *Drugs*, 1986, *31*, 198. See also *Drug & Ther. Bull.*, 1985, *23*, 89. and P. H. Vlasses *et al.*, *Clin. Pharm.*, 1985, *4*, 27.

Severe hypotension occurred after the first dose of enalapril in 3 patients during a study of 26 patients with heart failure. Short-term withdrawal of diuretic therapy prior to the introduction of enalapril did not prevent hypotension in 2 of these patients. Hypotension did not occur until at least 150 minutes after dosing.— J. G. F. Cleland *et al.*, *Br. med. J.*, 1985, *291*, 1309.

Report of hypotension in 4 of 14 patients taking diuretics following a single dose of enalapril.— J. Webster *et al.*, *Br. med. J.*, 1985, *290*, 1623.

Severe nasal obstruction was associated with enalapril treatment in a 45-year-old woman with a history of mild rhinorrhoea and sneezing. Symptoms cleared within 2 days of stopping enalapril and recurred on rechallenge.— A. Fennerty *et al.* (letter), *Lancet*, 1986, *2*, 1395.

Deafness was reported in 19 out of 12 543 patients taking enalapril, in a study of data derived from prescription event monitoring. Deafness had been reported only while patients were taking enalapril, there being no record of deafness after treatment.— W. H. W. Inman and N. S. B. Rawson (letter), *Lancet*, 1987, *1*, 872.

A post-marketing surveillance study of 11 710 hypertensive patients receiving enalapril for 6 weeks in general practice. An improvement in well-being was reported in 19.8% of patients. Serious adverse events occurred in 1.7% of patients. The authors considered that in subjects receiving enalapril the incidence rates of death (0.09%), stroke (0.11%), and myocardial infarction (0.15%) were compatible with rates which could be expected in hypertensive patients in this age range. Other events reported were hypotension (0.3%), angioneurotic oedema (0.03%), rash (0.5%), taste disturbance (0.2%), and cough (1.0%); 4.2% of patients withdrew from the study because of adverse effects.— W. D. Cooper *et al.*, *J. R. Coll. gen. Pract.*, 1987, *37*, 346.

ANGIOEDEMA. A study of enalapril by prescription event monitoring involving 10 500 patients indicated that the incidence of angioedema in patients taking enalapril was about 1 per 1000 patients per year overall, with an incidence of about half this for cases attributable to enalapril.— W. H. W. Inman and N. S. B. Rawson (letter), *Br. med. J.*, 1987, *294*, 578.

For reports of angioedema in patients taking enalapril, see under captopril, p.469.

COUGH. Cough, normally described as dry or unproductive, had been reported in 196 (2.4%) patients taking enalapril during a prescription event monitoring survey of 8299 patients. There was no underlying cause in 139 (1.7%) patients, 62% of whom continued with enalapril for the year of study despite the cough.— W. H. W. Inman (letter), *Lancet*, 1986, *2*, 1218.

Reports of coughing associated with enalapril therapy: D. Israel-Biet *et al.* (letter), *Lancet*, 1986, *2*, 918; D. Webb *et al.* (letter), *ibid.*, 1094.

For further reference to cough associated with enalapril and captopril see under captopril (p.469).

EFFECTS ON THE KIDNEYS. Uraemia and renal glycosuria were associated with enalapril treatment in a 42-year-old man.— M. D. Cressman *et al.* (letter), *Lancet*,

1982, *2*, 440.

Reversible renal failure in patients with renal artery stenosis during enalapril treatment.— L. N. Forbat and D. J. S. Carmichael, *Br. med. J.*, 1985, *291*, 450.

Reversible renal failure during enalapril treatment in a patient with chronic glomerulonephritis. Serum creatinine should be monitored in any patient with chronic renal disease with possible arterial involvement.— F. Brivet *et al.* (letter), *Lancet*, 1985, *1*, 1512.

Irreversible renal transplant failure after enalapril therapy.— A. R. Brown and P. F. Williams, *Br. med. J.*, 1986, *292*, 732.

EFFECTS ON THE SKIN. A patient who developed a mucocutaneous reaction to enalapril subsequently tolerated captopril without any adverse reaction.— S. H. Kubo and R. J. Cody (letter), *Ann. intern. Med.*, 1984, *100*, 616.

Report of nail changes in a 68-year-old patient taking enalapril.— S. Gupta *et al.* (letter), *Br. med. J.*, 1986, *293*, 140.

OVERDOSAGE. A 46-year-old woman who took enalapril 300 mg and oxazepam 225 mg with suicidal intent experienced hypotension and sustained total suppression of ACE activity, but suffered no serious complications.— B. Waeber *et al.*, *Br. med. J.*, 1984, *288*, 287.

Profound hypotension in a 56-year-old woman who had taken enalapril 440 mg and warfarin 42 mg was controlled by the rapid intravenous infusion of plasma and sodium chloride 0.9%. At 15 hours after ingestion the serum-enalapril concentration was 2.85 μg per mL and the angiotensin-converting-enzyme activity was completely suppressed. No effect on liver function was observed but renal function was impaired. The patient recovered from the acute episode of enalapril intoxication, but died 40 days later of intractable heart failure.— C. P. Lau (letter), *New Engl. J. Med.*, 1986, *315*, 197.

Precautions

As for Captopril (p.470).

Hypoglycaemia in 2 diabetic patients during enalapril treatment enabled withdrawal of sulphonylurea therapy in 1 patient and a reduction in insulin dosage in the other.— J. McMurray and D. M. Fraser (letter), *Lancet*, 1986, *1*, 1035. No changes in diabetic control or evidence of hypoglycaemia had been noticed in 18 insulin-dependent diabetic patients receiving enalapril or in a further 38 diabetic patients receiving either enalapril or captopril.— P. Passa *et al.* (letter), *ibid.*, 1447.

For a report of increased serum concentrations of enalapril in patients with impaired renal function see under Uses, below.

For a report of heart block due to hyperkalaemia in a patient taking enalapril concomitantly with spironolactone and frusemide, see under captopril (p.470).

For a report of toxic plasma concentrations of lithium during enalapril therapy, see under lithium carbonate (p.368).

Absorption and Fate

Approximately 55 to 75% of enalapril is rapidly absorbed from the gastro-intestinal tract following oral administration. Enalapril is extensively hydrolysed to its active form, enalaprilat. Enalapril and enalaprilat are excreted mainly in the urine and also in the faeces. Enalaprilat is removed by haemodialysis.

A review of the pharmacokinetics of the ACE inhibitors including enalapril. Following oral administration of enalapril, about 60 to 70% of the dose is absorbed. Enalapril is rapidly metabolised to enalaprilat, probably in the liver. Enalapril is almost undetectable in the plasma 4 hours after oral administration. The maximum concentration of enalaprilat occurs at about 4 hours, and enalaprilat is still detectable 96 hours after dosing. Excretion is primarily renal: 61% of the dose has been recovered from the urine, 18% as enalapril and 43% as enalaprilat; and 33% from the faeces.
The pharmacokinetics appear to be similar in hypertensive patients to those in healthy subjects. In patients with congestive heart failure, the half-life of enalaprilat was longer and clearance of enalapril slower than in healthy subjects.— S. H. Kubo and R. J. Cody, *Clin. Pharmacokinet.*, 1985, *10*, 377.

Uses and Administration

Enalapril is an angiotensin-converting enzyme inhibitor with properties and uses similar to captopril (see p.470). It owes its activity to enalaprilat to which it is converted after oral administration. The haemodynamic effects are seen within 1 hour of a single oral dose and the maximum effect occurs after about 4 to 6 hours, although the full effect may not develop for several weeks during chronic dosing. The haemodynamic action lasts for about 24 hours, allowing once-daily dosing. It is given by mouth as the maleate.
In the treatment of hypertension, an initial dose of 5 mg of enalapril maleate daily may be given to patients with normal renal function who are not receiving a diuretic. An initial dose of 2.5 mg daily should be given to patients with renal failure or who are receiving a diuretic; if possible, the diuretic should be withdrawn 2 or 3 days before enalapril is started. The dose should be titrated according to the response of the patient. The usual maintenance dose is 10 to 20 mg given once daily, although doses of up to 40 mg daily may be required in severe hypertension. It may be given in 2 divided doses if control is inadequate with a single dose.
As an adjunct to the treatment of congestive heart failure, an initial dose of 2.5 mg daily has been recommended; patients with congestive heart failure should be closely supervised during the initial stages of treatment and blood pressure and renal function should be monitored, both before and during treatment.
Enalaprilat (see below) has been given intravenously.

A review of the properties and uses of enalapril. Enalapril lowers blood pressure in patients with all grades of either essential or renovascular hypertension and appears as effective as usual doses of hydrochlorothiazide, propranolol, metoprolol, atenolol, or captopril. For a comparable reduction in diastolic pressure, enalapril produces a greater reduction in systolic pressure than beta blockers. In more severe forms of hypertension, many patients will respond to enalapril alone or in combination with hydrochlorothiazide, although a few patients may need the addition of a third agent such as a beta blocker. The use of enalapril can simplify complex drug regimens, and this is further aided by the once-daily administration of enalapril. This simplification of regimens and the avoidance of the use of potassium-sparing diuretics can reduce the incidence of adverse effects in hypertensive patients. Studies also indicate that enalapril is an effective alternative in patients with congestive heart failure.— P. A. Todd and R. C. Heel, *Drugs*, 1986, *31*, 198.

Further reviews of enalapril: R. O. Davies *et al.*, *Am. J. Med.*, 1984, *77*, 23; P. H. Vlasses *et al.*, *Clin. Pharm.*, 1985, *4*, 27; *Med. Lett.*, 1986, *28*, 53.

For reviews of the properties and actions of ACE inhibitors see Captopril, p.470.

Comparisons of enalapril and captopril.— *Drug & Ther. Bull.*, 1985, *23*, 89; A. Breckenridge, *Br. med. J.*, 1988, *296*, 618.

ADMINISTRATION IN RENAL FAILURE. Decreased renal function was associated with increased serum concentrations of enalaprilat. Reduced doses of enalapril would be required in patients with severely impaired renal function.— J. G. Kelly *et al.*, *Br. J. clin. Pharmac.*, 1986, *21*, 63. See also D. T. Lowenthal *et al.*, *Clin. Pharmac. Ther.*, 1985, *38*, 661.

DIABETIC NEPHROPATHY. Enalapril produced a reduction in albumin excretion rate associated with a reduction in blood pressure in a study of normotensive diabetic patients with persistent microalbuminuria. Further long-term studies are needed to confirm the beneficial effect of enalapril.— M. Marre *et al.*, *Br. med. J.*, 1987, *294*, 1448.

For reports of changes of diabetic control and hypoglycaemia in diabetic patients taking enalapril, see under Precautions, above.

HEART FAILURE. Enalapril produced beneficial haemodynamic and symptomatic responses over a 3-month period in a double-blind study of 36 patients with chronic heart failure who were already taking diuretics and digitalis.— D. N. Sharpe *et al.*, *Circulation*, 1984, *70*, 271.

The addition of enalapril to conventional therapy in patients with severe congestive heart failure was found to reduce mortality and improve symptoms. The Cooperative North Scandinavian Enalapril Survival Study known as the CONSENSUS study involved 127 patients taking enalapril up to 40 mg daily and 126 taking placebo in addition to conventional therapy with digitalis, diuretics, and vasodilators. The follow-up ranged from 1 day to 20 months with an average of 188 days. At 1 year mortality was 52% in the placebo group and 36% in the enalapril group. The study was terminated prematurely because of the consistent reduction in mortality in the enalapril group. At the end of the study 68 patients had died in the placebo group and 50 patients in the enalapril group, a reduction of 27%. The effect on survival was due to a reduction in mortality from the progression of heart failure. The treatment was well tolerated but it was considered important to initiate therapy with low doses of enalapril, particularly in high-risk patients.— *New Engl. J. Med.*, 1987, *316*, 1429.

In a study of enalapril in very elderly patients (mean age 82 years) with heart failure, 3 of the first 4 patients to enter the study had adverse reactions between 8 and 24 hours after the introduction of enalapril. In the remaining 11 patients the starting dose was reduced from 2.5 mg to approximately 1.25 mg. On this dose, 1 patient had hypotension and another developed reversible acute renal failure. In 10 patients maintained on enalapril, useful clinical improvements were seen.— M. A. Smith *et al.*, *Br. J. clin. Pharmac.*, 1987, *23*, 114P.

For a comparison of enalapril and captopril in severe chronic heart failure which suggested that the prolonged duration of action of enalapril could be disadvantageous, see under Captopril (p.471).

HYPERTENSION. A multicentre study involving 436 patients with essential hypertension showed that enalapril in doses of 20 or 40 mg was at least as effective as atenolol 50 or 100 mg or hydrochlorothiazide 25 or 50 mg. All three drugs were associated with an acceptable frequency of side-effects, but there were fewer reports of adverse reactions with enalapril than with atenolol or hydrochlorothiazide.— A. Helgeland *et al.*, *Lancet*, 1986, *1*, 872. Comments on the analysis and conclusions: P. C. Gøtzsche (letter), *ibid.*, *2*, 38; M. Safar (letter), *ibid.*, 39. Reply.— A. Helgeland *et al.* (letter), *ibid.*

In a pilot study, 20 elderly hypertensive patients aged 70 years or over received enalapril 10 or 20 mg daily for 9 weeks with the addition of hydrochlorothiazide 50 mg once daily if necessary. Enalapril alone was effective in 60% of patients and with the addition of hydrochlorothiazide was effective in a further 20%. Enalapril was well tolerated and no haematological or biochemical changes were observed.— J. Woo *et al.*, *Br. J. clin. Pract.*, 1987, *41*, 845.

Evidence that enalapril alone or in combination with hydrochlorothiazide maintained or improved renal function during the long-term treatment of hypertension in 23 patients.— J. H. Bauer *et al.*, *Archs intern. Med.*, 1987, *147*, 1397.

Further references to the use of enalapril in hypertension: *Br. J. clin. Pharmac.*, 1984, *18*, 51; A. Anderson *et al.*, *Med. J. Aust.*, 1987, *146*, 149; *Can. med. Ass. J.*, 1987, *137*, 803.

PHAEOCHROMOCYTOMA. Report of control of hypertension with enalapril in a patient with phaeochromocytoma.— R. Blum (letter), *Ann. intern. Med.*, 1987, *106*, 326.

SCLERODERMA. Enalapril controlled blood pressure, corrected biochemical anomalies, and improved the clinical status and renal function in a patient with scleroderma renal crisis.— S. R. Milsom and M. G. Nicholls, *Postgrad. med. J.*, 1986, *62*, 1059.

Proprietary Preparations

Innovace *(Merck Sharp & Dohme, UK)*. *Tablets*, scored, enalapril maleate 5 mg.
Tablets, enalapril maleate 2.5, 10, and 20 mg.

Proprietary Names and Manufacturers

Converten *(Neopharmed, Ital.)*; Enapren *(Merck Sharp & Dohme, Ital.)*; Innovace *(Merck Sharp & Dohme, UK)*; Naprilene *(Sigmatau, Ital.)*; Pres *(Dieckmann, Ger.)*; Renitec *(Merck Sharp & Dohme, Austral.; Merck Sharp & Dohme, Denm.; Merck Sharp & Dohme-Chibret, Fr.; Merck Sharp & Dohme, Norw.; Merck Sharp & Dohme, S.Afr.; MSD, Swed.)*; Reniten *(Merck Sharp & Dohme, Switz.)*; Vasotec *(Merck Sharp & Dohme, USA)*; Xanef *(Merck Sharp & Dohme, Ger.)*.

The following names have been used for multi-ingredient preparations containing enalapril maleate— Vaseretic *(Merck Sharp & Dohme, USA)*.

16618-x

Enalaprilat *(BAN, USAN, rINN).*
Enalaprilic acid; MK-422. *N*-{*N*-[(*S*)-carboxy-3-phenylpropyl]-L-alanyl}-L-proline.
$C_{18}H_{24}N_2O_5$=348.4.

CAS — 76420-72-9; 84680-54-6 (dihydrate).

Enalaprilat is the active form of the angiotensin-converting enzyme inhibitor enalapril (see above) and has similar actions and uses. It is not active by mouth, but is administered intravenously.

HYPERTENSION. Enalaprilat reduced blood pressure in 5 of 7 patients with severe hypertension one of whom was treated on 2 separate occasions. Enalaprilat was administered intravenously in doses of 1 mg followed after 30 minutes by 10 mg. An additional dose of 40 mg was administered after a further 40 minutes to 4 patients. Blood pressure decreased within 5 minutes of administration with a maximum reduction 30 minutes after the 10 mg dose. No further reduction of blood pressure occurred following the 40 mg dose. The hypotensive effect persisted for 12 hours in the responding patients. Marked reductions in blood pressure occurred in 3 patients, and 1 patient became normotensive 1 minute after receiving the 1 mg test dose.— D. J. DiPette *et al., Clin. Pharmac. Ther.*, 1985, *38*, 199.

A study in 11 patients with asymptomatic severe or accelerated hypertension. One patient responded fully to a test dose of enalaprilat 1 mg and required intravenous saline to prevent her blood pressure from falling to an undesirable level. One patient responded to enalaprilat 10 mg, but the remainder required frusemide 40 mg in addition. A subsequent injection of enalaprilat 40 mg in these patients did not decrease the blood pressure further, but prolonged the duration of the response to 6 hours or more. Overall, enalaprilat with or without a diuretic controlled the blood pressure in 6 of the 11 patients and partially decreased blood pressure in 4.— R. Strauss *et al., J. clin. Pharmac.*, 1986, *26*, 39.

Further references to the use of enalaprilat in hypertension: R. R. Evans *et al., J. clin. Pharmac.*, 1987, *27*, 415.

HEART FAILURE. An open pilot study of enalaprilat in 11 patients with left ventricular dysfunction. Enalaprilat 2.5 mg intravenously produced haemodynamic changes consistent with combined arterial and venodilatation. A small increase in cardiac output was seen. A rapid onset of action was observed with changes being evident during the first 5 minutes and maximum effects occurring 10 to 15 minutes after administration. The haemodynamic effects were sustained during the 1 hour of observation. Hypotension occurred in 3 patients but no other adverse effects were reported.— R. S. Hornung and W. S. Hillis, *Br. J. clin. Pharmac.*, 1987, *23*, 29.

Further references to the effect of enalaprilat in heart failure: P. Walinsky *et al., J. clin. Pharmac.*, 1985, *25*, 455; T. De Marco *et al., J. Am. Coll. Cardiol.*, 1987, *9*, 1131.

Proprietary Names and Manufacturers
Merck Sharp & Dohme, USA.

12688-h

Endralazine *(BAN, rINN).*
BQ-22-708. 6-Benzoyl-5,6,7,8-tetrahydropyrido[4,3-*c*]-pyridazin-3-ylhydrazine.
$C_{14}H_{15}N_5O$=269.3.

CAS — 39715-02-1 (endralazine); 65322-72-7 (mesylate).

NOTE. Endralazine Mesylate is *USAN.*

Endralazine is a vasodilator with properties similar to hydralazine (p.484) and has been used in the treatment of hypertension. It has been given by mouth, usually as the mesylate, in a dose of 5 to 20 mg daily.

Studies of the acute haemodynamic effects of endralazine: J. J. M. L. Hoffmann *et al., Br. J. clin. Pharmac.*, 1983, *16*, 39; E. E. van der Wall *et al., Postgrad. med. J.*, 1983, *59, Suppl.* 3, 42.

ABSORPTION AND FATE. A study of the pharmacokinetics of endralazine in healthy subjects and in hypertensive patients. The terminal elimination half-life of endralazine following a single dose was 2 to 3 hours in both groups. The bioavailability in normotensive subjects was about 75% suggesting that the drug was not subject to extensive first-pass metabolism. Following prolonged administration to hypertensive patients, the terminal half-life was prolonged to a mean of 448 minutes and there was also an increase in the absorption rate half-life. Despite these changes in kinetics, there was no evidence of endralazine accumulation during treatment for up to 3 months. There was no evidence of differences in the pharmacokinetics of endralazine in fast and slow acetylators in contrast to hydralazine.— P. A. Meredith *et al., Br. J. clin. Pharmac.*, 1983, *16*, 27. See also P. A. Reece *et al., Eur. J. clin. Pharmac.*, 1983, *25*, 553.

ADMINISTRATION IN RENAL FAILURE. The pharmacokinetics of endralazine were apparently altered in severe renal failure with a prolonged terminal elimination half-life. The haemodynamic effects were comparable to those reported in hypertensive patients and there was no evidence of increased cardiovascular responses in patients with renal impairment. It was considered unlikely that in practice renal impairment in itself would warrant a dosage reduction in the individual patient.— H. L. Elliott *et al., Eur. J. clin. Pharmac.*, 1984, *27*, 159.

USES. Studies of the use of endralazine in the treatment of hypertension. In general, endralazine, often in combination with antihypertensive agents, has been found to be well tolerated and effective in the treatment of hypertension. There have been no reports of lupus erythematosus developing in patients during endralazine therapy: J. C. Kingswood *et al., Postgrad. med. J.*, 1983, *59, Suppl.* 3, 173 (in patients with chronic renal failure); D. G. Holmes *et al., Lancet*, 1983, *1*, 670 (in combination with pindolol); W. A. J. L. Bogers and L. Meems, *Eur. J. clin. Pharmac.*, 1983, *24*, 301 (in combination with pindolol); M. D. C. Donaldson and T. L. Chambers (letter), *Lancet*, 1983, *2*, 635 (in children with renal disease); B. I. Chazan *et al., Curr. med. Res. Opinion*, 1986, *10*, 150 (compared with hydralazine).

Proprietary Names and Manufacturers of Endralazine and its Salts
Miretilan *(Sandoz, Neth.; Sandoz, Switz.).*

18878-w

Flosequinan *(BAN, rINN).*
BTS-49465. 7-Fluoro-1-methyl-3-methylsulphinyl-4-quinolone.
$C_{11}H_{10}FNO_2S$=239.3.

CAS — 76568-02-0.

Flosequinan is reported to be a vasodilator and has been tried in congestive heart failure and hypertension.

References on the actions and uses of flosequinan: A. J. Cowley *et al., J. Hypertens.*, 1984, *2, Suppl.* 3, 547; R. D. Wynne *et al., Eur. J. clin. Pharmac.*, 1985, *28*, 659; P. D. Kessler and M. Parker, *Am. Heart J.*, 1987, *113*, 137; A. J. Cowley *et al., Br. med. J.*, 1988, *297*, 169.

Proprietary Names and Manufacturers
Boots, UK.

12800-s

Guabenxan *(rINN).*
1-(1,4-Benzodioxan-6-ylmethyl)guanidine.
$C_{10}H_{13}N_3O_3$=207.2.

CAS — 19889-45-3.

Guabenxan is an antihypertensive agent with properties similar to guanethidine (see p.482). It is given as the sulphate normally in conjunction with a diuretic.

Proprietary Names and Manufacturers
The following names have been used for multi-ingredient preparations containing guabenxan— Tensigradyl *(Oberval, Fr.).*

865-k

Guanabenz Acetate *(USAN, rINNM).*
Wy-8678 (guanabenz). 1-(2,6-Dichlorobenzylideneamino)guanidine acetate.
$C_8H_8Cl_2N_4,C_2H_4O_2$=291.1.

CAS — 5051-62-7 (guanabenz); 23256-50-0 (acetate).

Pharmacopoeias. In *U.S.*

A white or almost white powder with not more than a slight odour. Sparingly **soluble** in water and in dilute hydrochloric acid; soluble in alcohol and in propylene glycol. A 0.7% solution in water has a pH of 5.5 to 7.0. **Store** in airtight containers. Protect from light.

Adverse Effects and Precautions
Guanabenz has adverse effects and precautions similar to those of Clonidine Hydrochloride, p.473.

WITHDRAWAL. Three of 4 hypertensive patients receiving guanabenz 48 mg daily developed a withdrawal syndrome of sympathetic overactivity within 16 to 48 hours of its abrupt discontinuation. None of 19 other patients, who had been receiving doses of 32 mg daily or less, developed the withdrawal syndrome. Guanabenz therapy should not be discontinued abruptly and, where possible, the dosage should be limited to less than 48 mg daily.— C. V. S. Ram *et al., J. clin. Pharmac.*, 1979, *19*, 148.

OVERDOSAGE. Report of 2 cases of overdosage with guanabenz. The main symptoms were lethargy, drowsiness, bradycardia, and hypotension. A 45-year-old woman who had taken 200 to 240 mg of guanabenz with alcohol recovered following gastric lavage and intravenous fluids: a 3-year-old child who had taken 12 mg of guanabenz responded to atropine and dopamine. Naloxone had little effect in either patient.— A. H. Hall *et al., Ann. intern. Med.*, 1985, *102*, 787. Further reports of overdosage with guanabenz: S. J. Rogers (letter) *ibid.*, 1986, *104*, 445.

Uses and Administration
Guanabenz is an antihypertensive agent with actions and uses similar to those of Clonidine Hydrochloride p.474. It is given in a usual dose of 4 mg twice a day initially increasing by increments of 4 to 8 mg per day every 1 to 2 weeks according to the patient's response. Doses of up to 32 mg twice daily have been used. Guanabenz may also be administered in conjunction with a thiazide diuretic.

A review of the pharmacodynamic properties and therapeutic efficacy of guanabenz. Guanabenz is an orally active central alpha$_2$-adrenoreceptor agonist with some structural similarities to clonidine. In clinical studies guanabenz 16 to 64 mg daily has been found to have similar antihypertensive efficacy to methyldopa 500 to 2000 mg and clonidine 450 to 900 µg. Guanabenz has been found to cause a higher incidence of drowsiness, dry mouth, and dizziness or weakness than methyldopa, although fluid retention, decreases in glomerular filtration, mental dysfunction, sexual dysfunction or positive coombs test have not been seen, and postural hypotension is rare. The antihypertensive effect of guanabenz is enhanced by concomitant administration of a diuretic.— B. Holmes *et al., Drugs*, 1983, *26*, 212.

Further reviews of guanabenz: *Med. Lett.*, 1983, *25*, 11.

Study of the pharmacokinetics of guanabenz.— R. H. Meacham *et al., Clin. Pharmac. Ther.*, 1980, *27*, 44.

HYPERTENSION. Studies of the hypotensive effect of guanabenz: F. G. McMahon *et al., Clin. Pharmac. Ther.*, 1977, *21*, 272; O. B. Holland *et al., J. clin. Pharmac.*, 1981, *21*, 133; B. R. Walker *et al., Clin. Ther.*, 1981, *4*, 217; J. H. Bauer, *Archs intern. Med.*, 1983, *143*, 1163; D. A. McCarron, *J. cardiovasc. Pharmac.*, 1985, *6, Suppl.* 5, S853; M. A. Weber and J. I. M. Drayer, *Sth. med. J.*, 1986, *79*, 323.

Comparisons of guanabenz with other antihypertensive agents: B. R. Walker *et al., Clin. Pharmac. Ther.*, 1977, *22*, 868 (methyldopa); P. Hirvonen *et al., Curr. ther. Res.*, 1980, *27*, 197 (methyldopa); Y. Kluyskens and J. Snoeck, *Curr. med. Res. Opinion*, 1980, *6*, 638 (clonidine); B. R. Walker *et al., J. int. med. Res.*, 1982, *10*, 6 (clonidine); C. Rosendorff, *S. Afr. med. J.*, 1982, *62*, 435 (methyldopa).

Study indicating a favourable effect of guanabenz on blood lipids.— N. M. Kaplan, *J. cardiovasc. Pharmac.*, 1984, *6, Suppl.* 5, S841.

OPIOID WITHDRAWAL. Symptoms of opioid withdrawal were controlled by guanabenz in a patient who had refused to complete detoxification with clonidine because of intolerable side-effects.— J. T. Mulry, *Drug Intell. & clin. Pharm.*, 1985, *19*, 32.

Preparations

Guanabenz Acetate Tablets *(U.S.P.)*

Proprietary Names and Manufacturers
Rexitene *(LPB, Ital.)*; Wytensin *(Wyeth, Ger.; Wyeth, USA).*

866-a

Guanacline Sulphate *(rINNM).*
B-1464; Cyclazenin Sulphate; FBA-1464; Guanacline Sulfate *(USAN).* 1-[2-(1,2,3,6-Tetrahydro-4-methylpyrid-1-yl)ethyl]guanidine sulphate dihydrate.
$C_9H_{18}N_4,H_2SO_4,2H_2O=316.4$.

CAS — 1463-28-1 (guanacline); 1562-71-6 (sulphate, anhydrous); 23389-32-4 (sulphate, dihydrate).

Guanacline sulphate is an antihypertensive agent with actions similar to those of guanethidine.

Proprietary Names and Manufacturers
Bayer, Ger.; Miles Pharmaceuticals, USA.

867-t

Guanadrel Sulphate *(rINNM).*

CL-1388R; Guanadrel Sulfate *(USAN)*; U-28288D. 1-(Cyclohexanespiro-2′-[1′,3′]dioxolan-4′-ylmethyl)guanidine sulphate; 1-(1,4-Dioxaspiro[4.5]dec-2-ylmethyl)guanidine sulphate.
$(C_{10}H_{19}N_3O_2)_2,H_2SO_4=524.6$.

CAS — 40580-59-4 (guanadrel); 22195-34-2 (sulphate).

Pharmacopoeias. In *U.S.*

A white to off-white crystalline powder. **Soluble** in water; sparingly soluble in methyl alcohol; slightly soluble in alcohol and in acetone.

Adverse Effects, Treatment, and Precautions
As for Guanethidine Monosulphate, below. Guanadrel may cause less diarrhoea and orthostatic hypotension on rising in the morning than guanethidine, although orthostatic symptoms seem to occur with a similar frequency during the day. Guanadrel has been reported to cause fewer CNS effects than methyldopa, but diarrhoea and orthostatic hypotension are more frequent.

Absorption and Fate
Guanadrel is rapidly absorbed from the gastro-intestinal tract. It is widely distributed throughout the body and about 20% is bound to plasma proteins. It is reported not to cross the blood-brain barrier. Plasma concentrations decline in a biphasic manner: the half-life in the initial phase is 1 to 4 hours, and in the terminal phase 5 to 45 hours. Guanadrel is metabolised in the liver and approximately 85% is excreted in the urine over 24 hours as the unchanged drug and its metabolites. About 40 to 50% of the drug is excreted unchanged.

Uses and Administration
Guanadrel sulphate is an antihypertensive agent with actions and uses similar to those of guanethidine monosulphate (see p.482). Following oral administration, guanadrel acts within 2 hours with the maximum effect after 4 to 6 hours. The hypotensive effect is reported to last for 4 to 14 hours following a single dose.

Guanadrel sulphate is used in the treatment of hypertension in patients who have not responded adequately to treatment with a diuretic or a beta blocker. The usual initial dose is 5 mg twice daily adjusted at weekly or monthly intervals according to the patient's response. The maintenance dose is normally in the range of 20 to 75 mg daily in two or more divided doses.

A review of the pharmacodynamic and pharmacokinetic properties and therapeutic use of guanadrel. Guanadrel had an antihypertensive effect similar to guanethidine and to methyldopa in studies in patients with hypertension not controlled by diuretics alone. Its use in patients not adequately controlled by other antihypertensive drugs has not been fully evaluated. As guanadrel has a rapid onset of action and is rapidly eliminated compared to guanethidine, titration of dosage can be achieved more readily than with guanethidine. Guanadrel appeared to be a useful alternative to other antihypertensive therapy for patients suffering unacceptable CNS side-effects or for whom other antihypertensive agents were unsuitable. It was considered probable that guanadrel would be used most often as second- or third-line drug therapy to treat patients with moderate to severe hypertension, and would usually be given with a diuretic.— F. A. Finnerty and R. N. Brogden, *Drugs*, 1985, *30*, 22.

Further reviews of guanadrel: J. D. Palmer and C. A. Nugent, *Pharmacotherapy*, 1983, *3*, 220; *Med. Lett.*, 1983, *25*, 95.

Further references to the use of guanadrel: C. A. Nugent *et al.*, *Pharmacotherapy*, 1982, *2*, 378; S. H. Malinow, *Clin. Ther.*, 1983, *5*, 284; R. D. Gore, *Clin. Ther.*, 1983, *6*, 86; W. J. Mroczek *et al.*, *Curr. ther. Res.*, 1984, *36*, 1004; A. Oren *et al.*, *J. clin. Pharmac.*, 1985, *25*, 343.

Proprietary Names and Manufacturers
Hylorel *(Pennwalt, USA).*

The following names have been used for multi-ingredient preparations containing guanadrel sulphate— Hyloride *(Upjohn, USA).*

12805-j

Guanazodine Sulphate *(rINNM).*
Egyt-739. 1-(Octahydroazocin-2-ylmethyl)guanidine sulphate monohydrate.
$C_9H_{20}N_4,H_2SO_4,H_2O=300.4$.

CAS — 32059-15-7 (guanazodine); 59252-59-4 (guanazodine); 42839-36-1 (sulphate, anhydrous).

Guanazodine sulphate is an antihypertensive agent.

Proprietary Names and Manufacturers
Sanegyt *(EGIS, Hung.).*

869-r

Guanethidine Monosulphate *(BANM, rINNM).*

Guanethidine Monosulfate *(USAN)*; Guanethidini Monosulfas. 1-[2-(Perhydroazocin-1-yl)ethyl]-guanidine monosulphate.
$C_{10}H_{22}N_4,H_2SO_4=296.4$.

CAS — 55-65-2 (guanethidine); 645-43-2 (monosulphate).

NOTE. The *U.S.P.* title for the hemisulphate is Guanethidine Sulfate.

Pharmacopoeias. In *Belg., Br., Cz., Eur., Fr., Ind., It., Jpn., Jug., Neth., Nord., Swiss,* and *U.S.*, which also includes the hemisulphate. *Braz.* and *Turk.* include the hemisulphate, $(C_{10}H_{22}N_4)_2,H_2SO_4$.

A colourless, white, or off-white, odourless, crystalline powder. *B.P.* **solubilities** are: 1 in 1.5 of water; practically insoluble in alcohol, chloroform, and ether. *U.S.P.* solubilities are: very soluble in water; sparingly soluble in alcohol; practically insoluble in chloroform. A 2% solution in water has a pH of 4.7 to 5.7. Solutions for injection are **sterilised** by autoclaving or by filtration. **Store** in well-closed containers. Protect from light.

Adverse Effects
The commonest side-effects with guanethidine are severe postural and exertional hypotension and diarrhoea which may be particularly troublesome during the initial stages of therapy and during the dose adjustment. Dizziness, syncope, muscle weakness, and lassitude are liable to occur, especially on rising from sitting or lying. Other frequent side-effects are bradycardia, failure of ejaculation, fatigue, and oedema which may be accompanied by breathlessness.

Nausea, vomiting, dry mouth, nasal congestion, parotid tenderness, blurring of vision, myalgia, muscle tremor, hair loss, dermatitis, disturbed micturition, aggravation or precipitation of asthma, and exacerbation of peptic ulcer have also been reported. It has been reported that guanethidine may possibly cause anaemia, leucopenia, and thrombocytopenia.

When guanethidine is used as eye-drops, common side-effects are conjunctival hyperaemia and miosis. Burning sensations and ptosis have also occurred. Superficial punctate keratitis has been reported particularly following prolonged administration of concentrated solutions.

Apnoea and syncope occurred in a 28-year-old man following regional intravenous injection of guanethidine 10 mg with heparin for treatment of reflex sympathetic dystrophy of the left arm. He recovered following mechanical ventilation and 100% oxygen.— R. L. Martin and S. E. Abram, *Reg. Anaesth.*, 1986, *11*, 39.

Treatment of Adverse Effects
If overdosage occurs the stomach should be emptied by aspiration and lavage. Withdrawal of guanethidine or reduction in dosage reverses many side-effects. Diarrhoea may be controlled by reducing dosage or giving codeine phosphate, or antimuscarinic agents, such as propantheline bromide. Severe hypotension may respond to placing the patient in the supine position with the feet raised. If hypotension is severe it may be necessary to give intravenous fluid replacement and small doses of vasopressor agents may be given cautiously. The patient must be observed for several days.

Precautions
Guanethidine should not be given to patients with phaeochromocytoma as it may cause a rise in blood pressure or to patients with heart failure not caused by hypertension. It should be used with caution in patients with renal, cerebral, or coronary insufficiency, or with a history of peptic ulceration or asthma. Exercise and heat may increase the hypotensive effect of guanethidine. Hypotension may occur during anaesthesia in patients being treated with guanethidine. There is an increased risk of cardiovascular collapse or cardiac arrest in patients undergoing surgery while taking guanethidine. Guanethidine should be discontinued before elective surgery: some authorities recommend for up to 2 or 3 weeks beforehand. In patients undergoing emergency procedures or where treatment has not been interrupted large doses of atropine should be given before induction of anaesthesia.

Patients taking guanethidine are sensitive to adrenaline, amphetamine, and other sympathomimetic agents. The hypotensive effects may also be antagonised by tricyclic antidepressants, monoamine oxidase inhibitors, and phenothiazine derivatives and related antipsychotic agents. It has been reported that oral contraceptives may reduce the hypotensive action of guanethidine. Concurrent administration of digitalis with guanethidine may cause excessive bradycardia. The hypotensive effects of guanethidine may be enhanced by thiazide diuretics, other antihypertensive agents, and levodopa. Alcohol may cause orthostatic hypotension in patients taking guanethidine.

Patients undergoing treatment with eye-drops containing guanethidine should be examined regularly for signs of conjunctival damage.

The intra-arterial blood pressure, pulse, and ECG were monitored continuously in 11 hypertensive patients being treated only with adrenergic neurone blocking agents (guanethidine, bethanidine, or debrisoquine). All experienced large sudden variations in blood pressure and all had severe postural hypotension. Three had ECG evidence of myocardial dysfunction during hypotensive episodes and 1 experienced right-sided weakness during exertion. It was considered that adrenergic neurone blocking agents might predispose patients to cerebral or myocardial infarction by alternately raising and lowering perfusion pressure in vessels damaged by atheromatous disease.— A. D. Goldberg and E. B. Raftery, *Lancet*, 1976, *2*, 1052.

The action of guanethidine may be reduced by concurrent administration of non-steroidal anti-inflammatory drugs, see p.466.

Absorption and Fate
Guanethidine is variably and incompletely absorbed from the gastro-intestinal tract with less than 50% of the dose reaching the systemic circulation. It is partially metabolised in the liver,

and is excreted in the urine as metabolites and unchanged guanethidine. It has a terminal half-life of several days. Guanethidine is actively transported into adrenergic neurones; it probably does not penetrate the blood-brain barrier. It is not bound to plasma proteins.

References to the absorption and fate of guanethidine: C. McMartin *et al.*, *Clin. Pharmac. Ther.*, 1970, *11*, 423; C. McMartin and P. Simpson, *ibid.*, 1971, *12*, 73; J. H. Hengstmann and F. C. Falkner, *Eur. J. clin. Pharmac.*, 1979, *15*, 121.

Uses and Administration

Guanethidine is an antihypertensive agent which acts by selectively inhibiting transmission in post-ganglionic adrenergic nerves. It is believed to act mainly by preventing the release of noradrenaline at nerve endings; it causes the depletion of noradrenaline stores in peripheral sympathetic nerve terminals and, unlike other common adrenergic neurone blocking agents, also causes significant depletion of tissue noradrenaline. It does not prevent the secretion of catecholamines by the adrenal medulla.

When administered by mouth its maximal effects take 1 to 2 weeks to appear on continued dosing and persist for 7 to 10 days after treatment has been stopped. It causes an initial reduction in cardiac output (which may be subsequently compensated by increased stroke volume despite continued bradycardia) but its main hypotensive effect is to cause peripheral vasodilatation; it reduces the vasoconstriction which normally results from standing up and which is the result of reflex sympathetic nervous activity.

Guanethidine is used in the treatment of hypertension when other drugs have proved inadequate, although it has largely been superseded by other drugs less likely to cause orthostatic hypotension. It is generally given in conjunction with a diuretic or beta blocker. In the majority of patients it reduces the standing blood pressure but has a less marked effect on the supine blood pressure. Tolerance to guanethidine has occurred in some patients; this may be countered by intensive diuretic therapy.

The usual initial dose of guanethidine monosulphate is 10 to 20 mg daily. This is increased by increments of 10 mg every 7 days according to the response of the patient although some authorities recommend intervals of 2 to 3 weeks between increments to avoid accumulation. The usual maintenance dose varies from 20 to 50 mg daily as a single dose but up to 300 mg daily may be given.

Children have been given 200 µg per kg bodyweight daily with increments of 200 µg per kg every 1 to 3 weeks until a satisfactory response is achieved; a dose of about 1.5 mg per kg daily may be required.

Smaller doses of guanethidine are needed when it is given concomitantly with other antihypertensive agents or diuretics which also reduce the oedema that sometimes occurs with guanethidine therapy.

Guanethidine has been given intramuscularly in the treatment of hypertensive crises, including toxaemia of pregnancy, but more suitable agents are available. An intramuscular dose of 10 to 20 mg is reported to produce a fall in blood pressure within 30 minutes, reaching a maximum in 1 to 2 hours and lasting for 4 to 6 hours. Intravenously, guanethidine produces an initial hypertensive effect.

Eye-drops containing guanethidine 5% are used in the treatment of lid retraction which may accompany thyrotoxicosis and in the treatment of glaucoma. Guanethidine is also used in lower concentrations, in conjunction with adrenaline in the treatment of glaucoma.

A review and discussion of the pharmacology of guanethidine.— R. A. Maxwell, *Br. J. clin. Pharmac.*, 1982, *13*, 35.

ADMINISTRATION IN RENAL FAILURE. The interval between guanethidine doses should be extended from 24 to up to 36 hours in patients with a glomerular filtration-rate of less than 10 mL per minute.— W. M. Bennett *et al.*, *Am. J. Kidney Dis.*, 1983, *3*, 155.

GLAUCOMA. Solutions of 1, 2, 3, 4, and 5% guanethidine were found to produce a fall in intra-ocular pressure. Despite twice daily instillation, this was not maintained and within a month little hypotensive effect remained. Instillation of 5% guanethidine solutions concurrently with 1% adrenaline gave a more prolonged fall in intra-ocular pressure.— G. D. Paterson and G. Paterson, *Br. J. Ophthal.*, 1972, *56*, 288.

In a double-blind crossover study of 20 patients with ocular hypertension, eye-drops containing guanethidine 1% in conjunction with adrenaline 1% were more effective at reducing ocular hypertension than adrenaline 1% alone. The effect lasted the full 8 weeks of the study. Adverse effects, which included headache, browache, red eye, pain, and blurred vision caused 5 patients to withdraw from treatment with the combination of guanethidine and adrenaline and 3 patients from treatment with adrenaline alone. Two of these patients could not tolerate either treatment.— R. A. Hitchings and D. Glover, *Br. J. Ophthal.*, 1982, *66*, 247.

Further references to the use of topical guanethidine in combination with adrenaline to reduce intra-ocular pressure: J. A. Roth, *Br. J. Ophthal.*, 1973, *57*, 507; K. B. Mills and A. E. Ridgway, *ibid.*, 1978, *62*, 320; J. Romano and G. Patterson, *ibid.*, 1979, *63*, 52; P. F. J. Hoyng and C. L. Dake, *ibid.*, 56; D. E. P. Jones *et al.*, *ibid.*, 813.

HYPERTENSION. A review of guanethidine therapy.— R. L. Woosley and A. S. Nies, *New Engl. J. Med.*, 1976, *295*, 1053.

A report on 229 hypertensive patients taking bethanidine, debrisoquine, or guanethidine, sometimes in association with a diuretic. Blood pressure was more effectively controlled by debrisoquine or guanethidine than by bethanidine. Symptoms of orthostatic or exertional hypotension were significantly more frequent in those taking guanethidine. Diarrhoea occurred in 23% on guanethidine, 4% on bethanidine, and 1% on debrisoquine.— S. Talbot *et al.* (letter), *Br. med. J.*, 1975, *2*, 278.

In a crossover study involving 7 hypertensive patients guanethidine was shown to further reduce blood pressure in patients who were uncontrolled on combination therapy with cyclopenthiazide, propranolol, and hydralazine in those patients able to tolerate treatment. However, guanethidine was less well tolerated than either methyldopa or prazosin.— M. J. Vandenburg *et al.*, *Br. J. clin. Pract.*, 1985, *39*, 17.

REGIONAL SYMPATHETIC BLOCKADE. A technique for producing regional sympathetic blockade by injecting guanethidine 10 to 20 mg with 500 units of heparin for the upper extremities and 20 mg with 1000 units of heparin for the lower extremities after applying a tourniquet.— J. G. Hannington-Kiff, *Lancet*, 1974, *1*, 1019.

The use of guanethidine sympathetic block for replacing a severed thumb.— K. H. Davies, *Br. med. J.*, 1976, *1*, 876.

Comment on the mode of action of guanethidine in the relief of causalgia.— *Lancet*, 1978, *2*, 462.

Relief of causalgia in 10 patients by regional intravenous block using guanethidine.— J. G. Hannington-Kiff, *Br. med. J.*, 1979, *2*, 367.

The use of sympathetic block using guanethidine for the relief of pain due to lesions of the central nervous system.— L. Loh *et al.*, *Br. med. J.*, 1981, *282*, 1026.

Regional sympathetic blockade with guanethidine was successfully used to increase the temperature and reduce cyanosis of the hand of a patient with severe frostbite.— R. Kaplan *et al.* (letter), *Lancet*, 1981, *2*, 940.

Report of experience with sympathetic blockade for painful nerve conditions over 8 years. A minimum of 3 blocks was considered necessary, and serial blocks were worth continuing if there was a slight response to treatment since the effect was cumulative. Some patients had received 12 or 20 blocks, and 3 patients had received over 30 blocks with long-lasting success. Full rehabilitation and follow-up were included as part of the programme. Recurrence of pain could be controlled by repeated treatments.— C. B. W. Parry and R. H. Withrington, *Postgrad. med. J.*, 1984, *60*, 869.

Regional intravenous guanethidine infusion relieved pain and increased pinch strength over 14 days in a double-blind placebo-controlled study involving 24 patients with active rheumatoid arthritis in the elbow, wrist, and/or fingers.— J. D. Levine *et al.*, *J. Rheumatol.*, 1986, *13*, 1040.

Further references: J. G. Hannington-Kiff, *Lancet*, 1977, *1*, 1132; N. N. S. McKay *et al.*, *Br. med. J.*, 1977, *1*, 1575.

Preparations

Guanethidine Monosulfate Tablets *(U.S.P.)*

Guanethidine Sulfate Tablets *(U.S.P.)*. Tablets containing guanethidine hemisulphate.

Guanethidine Tablets *(B.P.)*. Tablets containing guanethidine monosulphate.

Proprietary Preparations

Ganda *(Smith & Nephew Pharmaceuticals, UK)*. *Eye-drops* (1+0.2), guanethidine monosulphate 1%, adrenaline 0.2%.

Eye-drops (3+0.5), guanethidine monosulphate 3%, adrenaline 0.5%.

Ismelin *(Ciba, UK)*. *Tablets*, guanethidine monosulphate 10 and 25 mg.

Injection, guanethidine monosulphate 10 mg/mL, in ampoules of 1 mL.

Ismelin *(Zyma, UK)*. *Eye-drops*, guanethidine monosulphate 5%.

Proprietary Names and Manufacturers

Antipres *(Protea, Austral.)*; Dopom *(Ital.)*; Ipotidina *(Ital.)*; Ismelin *(Ciba, Austral.; Ciba, Canad.; Ciba, Denm.; Ciba, Ger.; Ciba, Ital.; Neth.; Ciba, Norw.; Ciba, S.Afr.; Spain; Ciba, Swed.; Dispersa, Switz.; Ciba, UK; Zyma, UK; Ciba, USA)*; Ismeline *(Belg.; Ciba, Fr.; Ciba, Switz.)*; Normoten *(Adcock Ingram, S.Afr.)*; Solo-ethidine *(S.Afr.)*; Visutensil *(Merck Sharp & Dohme, Ital.)*.

The following names have been used for multi-ingredient preparations containing guanethidine monosulphate— Esimil *(Ciba, USA)*; Ganda *(Smith & Nephew Pharmaceuticals, UK)*.

12806-z

Guanfacine Hydrochloride *(BANM, USAN, rINNM)*.

BS-100-141; LON-798. *N*-Amidino-2-(2,6-dichlorophenyl)acetamide hydrochloride.

$C_9H_9Cl_2N_3O,HCl = 282.6$.

CAS — 29110-47-2 (guanfacine); 29110-48-3 (hydrochloride).

Guanfacine hydrochloride 1.15 mg is approximately equivalent to 1 mg of guanfacine.

Adverse Effects

Guanfacine has adverse effects similar to those of clonidine (p.473). Dryness of the mouth and sedation are the effects most frequently reported especially in the initial stages of treatment.

A report on side-effects and withdrawal symptoms encountered in 580 hypertensive patients treated with guanfacine for 1 year and 169 patients who continued treatment for a second year. The most frequent side-effect was dryness of the mouth but the overall incidence of 60% during the first year had fallen to 15% by the end of the year. Sedation occurred in 33% of patients and had fallen to 5.7% by the end of the first year. Other side-effects reported during the first and second years respectively included orthostatic disturbances (15 and 6.5%), constipation (14 and 4.1%), male sexual dysfunction (4.6 and 0.6%), insomnia (5.5 and 2.2%), gastro-intestinal discomfort (4.1 and 2.2%), and sweating (5.3 and 1.7%). Sinus bradycardia was seen in only 12 patients and was transient in 9. The frequency and severity of adverse effects was dose-related and doses of 2 mg or less caused virtually no dry mouth. A withdrawal syndrome occurred in 2 to 4% of patients 2 to 7 days after discontinuation of guanfacine. No signs of tachyphylaxis or tolerance were seen.— P. Jerie, *Br. J. clin. Pharmac.*, 1980, *10*, *Suppl.* 1, 157S.

Rapid reduction of the guanfacine dosage resulted in rebound hypertension leading to generalised seizures and coma in a 47-year-old patient with renal failure who was receiving haemodialysis. There was evidence to suggest that concomitant administration of phenobarbitone enhanced metabolism of guanfacine and was considered to have contributed to the development of the withdrawal effect.— J. R. Kiechel *et al.*, *Eur. J. clin. Pharmac.*, 1983, *25*, 463.

Absorption and Fate

Guanfacine is rapidly and almost completely absorbed from the gastro-intestinal tract. It has a half-life reported to be between 10 and 30 hours.

Guanfacine is metabolised in the liver and excreted, partly as unchanged drug, in the urine.

A review of the pharmacokinetics and metabolism of guanfacine.— J. R. Kiechel, *Br. J. clin. Pharmac.*, 1980, *10, Suppl.* 1, 25S.

In 5 healthy subjects given the equivalent of 3 mg of guanfacine by mouth, peak plasma concentrations occurred at 1.5 to 4 hours and ranged from 9.2 to 11.7 ng per mL in 4 subjects, while the fifth subject had a much lower peak concentration of 4.5 ng per mL.— C. T. Dollery and D. S. Davies, *Br. J. clin. Pharmac.*, 1980, *10, Suppl.* 1, 5S.

Results in patients with normal and impaired renal function suggested that non-renal elimination of guanfacine plays an important role in patients with renal failure.— W. Kirch *et al., Br. J. clin. Pharmac.*, 1980, *10, Suppl.* 1, 33S.

In a study involving 8 patients with terminal renal failure undergoing haemodialysis clearance of guanfacine by dialysis was 53 mL per minute, representing about 15% of the total clearance. This result suggested that no adjustment of dosage intervals or maintenance doses of guanfacine would be required in patients undergoing intermittent haemodialysis.— W. Kirch *et al., Eur. J. Drug Metab. Pharmacokinet.*, 1982, *7,* 277.

Uses and Administration

Guanfacine is a centrally acting antihypertensive agent with actions and uses similar to those of clonidine (p.474). Guanfacine hydrochloride has been given by mouth in the treatment of hypertension in usual doses equivalent to 1 mg of guanfacine daily initially, increasing by 1 mg daily at intervals of several weeks to 3 mg daily if neccessary.

A review of the pharmacodynamics, pharmacokinetics, and therapeutic efficacy of guanfacine. The hypotensive action of guanfacine is primarily due to central stimulation of alpha$_2$-adrenoceptors resulting in decreased sympathetic tone and a reduction in peripheral resistance. Guanfacine is well absorbed from the gastro-intestinal tract and has a relatively long half-life ranging from 12.1 to 22.8 hours. Clinical studies have shown that guanfacine produces an antihypertensive effect comparable with that of clonidine and methyldopa. Adverse effects are generally related to the alpha-stimulant properties and are dose-dependent. Adverse effects due to guanfacine have generally occurred less frequently than with clonidine. A mild withdrawal syndrome has been reported following abrupt discontinuation of guanfacine in some studies.— E. M. Sorkin and R. C. Heel, *Drugs*, 1986, *31,* 301.

Further reviews of the actions and uses of guanfacine: *Med. Lett.*, 1987, *29,* 49.

Guanfacine had no influence on the lung function of 10 hypertensive patients with chronic obstructive lung disease.— A. M. J. Wever and P. van Brummelen, *Br. J. clin. Pharmac.*, 1983, *15, Suppl.* 4, 521S.

Studies on the actions of guanfacine: M. E. Safar *et al., J. clin. Pharmac.*, 1982, *22,* 385 (antihypertensive effect and plasma concentrations); R. Fariello *et al., Curr. ther. Res.*, 1984, *35,* 885 (effects on blood pressure, heart rate, and systolic time intervals at rest and after exercise); G. Pagani *et al., ibid.*, *36,* 155 (effect on glucose metabolism, plasma renin activity, and some anterior pituitary hormones); J. H. Hauger-Klevene *et al., Am. J. Cardiol.*, 1986, *57,* 27E (effect on blood lipids); M. Frisk-Holmberg and L. Wibell, *Clin. Pharmac. Ther.*, 1986, *39,* 169 (plasma concentrations for optimal antihypertensive effect).

Clinical studies of guanfacine in hypertension: P. Jerie, *Br. J. clin. Pharmac.*, 1980, *10, Suppl.* 1, 37S; B. J. Materson *et al., Am. J. Cardiol.*, 1986, *57,* 32E; R. E. Keenan *et al., ibid.*, 38E; P. Jerie, *ibid.*, 55E; A. G. Dupont *et al., Br. J. clin. Pharmac.*, 1987, *23,* 397.

Comparisons of guanfacine with other antihypertensive agents: M. S. Farooki *et al., Clin. Ther.*, 1985, *7,* 199 (methyldopa); M. F. Wilson *et al., Am. J. Cardiol.*, 1986, *57,* 43E (clonidine); J. M. Fillingim *et al., ibid.*, 50E (guanabenz).

Proprietary Names and Manufacturers

Entulic *(Sandoz, Swed.)*; Estulic *(Wander, Belg.; Sandoz, Eire; Sandoz, Fr.; Wander, Ger.; Sandoz, Greece; Sandoz, Neth.; Sandoz, Spain; Sandoz, Switz.)*; Tenex *(Robins, USA)*.

870-j

Guanoclor Sulphate *(BANM, rINNM).*

3-01029; Guanoclor Sulfate *(USAN)*. 1-[2-(2,6-Dichlorophenoxy)ethylamino]guanidine sulphate.

$(C_9H_{12}Cl_2N_4O)_2,H_2SO_4$=624.3.

CAS — 5001-32-1 (guanoclor); 551-48-4 (sulphate).

Guanoclor sulphate is an antihypertensive agent with actions similar to those of guanethidine, but it has also been reported to cause depletion of catecholamines in the central nervous system and inhibition of the enzymic conversion of dopamine to noradrenaline.

Proprietary Names and Manufacturers

Vatensol *(Pfizer, UK; Pfizer, USA)*.

12808-k

Guanoxabenz Hydrochloride *(rINNM).*

43-663 *(guanoxabenz)*. 1-(2,6-Dichlorobenzylideneamino)-3-hydroxyguanidine hydrochloride.

$C_8H_8Cl_2N_4O,HCl$=283.5.

CAS — 24047-25-4 (guanoxabenz); 7473-70-3 (guanoxabenz).

NOTE. Guanoxabenz is *USAN*.

Guanoxabenz hydrochloride is a centrally acting antihypertensive agent. It has been given in doses of up to 75 mg or exceptionally 150 mg daily.

Proprietary Names and Manufacturers

Benzérial *(Houdé, Fr.)*.

871-z

Guanoxan Sulphate *(BANM, rINNM).*

3-01003; Guanoxan Sulfate *(USAN)*. 1-(1,4-Benzodioxan-2-ylmethyl)guanidine sulphate.

$(C_{10}H_{13}N_3O_2)_2,H_2SO_4$=512.5.

CAS — 2165-19-7 (guanoxan); 5714-04-5 (sulphate).

Guanoxan has properties and uses similar to those of guanethidine p.481. Liver damage has followed treatment with guanoxan and it is now rarely used.

Of 96 patients treated with guanoxan, 26 had some derangement of liver function tests, severe in 10; four of these developed jaundice and 1 of the 4 patients died with chronic hepatic necrosis.— S. G. Cotton and E. Montuschi (letter), *Br. med. J.*, 1967, *3,* 174.

Proprietary Names and Manufacturers

Envacar *(Pfizer, USA)*.

873-k

Hexamethonium Bromide *(BAN, rINN).*

Hexamethonii Bromidum; Hexonium Bromide. *NN*-Hexamethylenebis(trimethylammonium) dibromide.

$C_{12}H_{30}Br_2N_2$=362.2.

CAS — 60-26-4 (hexamethonium); 55-97-0 (bromide).

Pharmacopoeias. In *Fr.*

Hexamethonium bromide is a quaternary ammonium ganglion-blocking agent with properties similar to those of trimetaphan (see p.503). The benzenesulphonate, chloride, iodide, and tartrate have also been used.

Proprietary Names and Manufacturers of Hexamethonium Salts

Vegolysen *(May & Baker, UK)*.

878-f

Hydralazine Hydrochloride *(BANM, USAN, rINNM).*

Apressinum; Cloridrato de Hidralazina; Hydralazini Hydrochloridum; Hydrallazine Hydrochloride; Idralazina. 1-Hydrazinophthalazine hydrochloride.

$C_8H_8N_4,HCl$=196.6.

CAS — 86-54-4 (hydralazine); 304-20-1 (hydrochloride).

NOTE. Hydralazine Polistirex is *USAN*.

Pharmacopoeias. In *Br., Braz., Ind., Int., Jpn, Nord., Rus.*, and *U.S.*

A white to off-white odourless or almost odourless crystalline powder. *B.P.* **solubilities** are: soluble in water; slighty soluble in alcohol and in methyl alcohol; practically insoluble in chloroform and in ether. *U.S.P.* solubilities are: 1 in 25 of water and 1 in 500 of alcohol; very slightly soluble in ether. A 2% solution in water has a pH of 3.5 to 4.2. Administration in solutions of glucose is inadvisable. **Store** in airtight containers.

Discoloration of hydralazine injection was observed on several occasions after storage in a syringe for up to 12 hours. Hydralazine reacts with metals and therefore the injection should be prepared using a non-metal filter and should be used as quickly as possible after being drawn through a needle into a syringe.— G. Enderlin (letter), *Am. J. Hosp. Pharm.*, 1984, *41,* 634.

A study of the rate of degradation of hydralazine hydrochloride, 1 mg per mL in sweetened, aqueous oral liquids showed that glucose, fructose, lactose, and maltose reduced the stability of the drug. In solutions containing mannitol or sorbitol, there was less than 10% degradation of hydralazine after 3 weeks.— V. Das Gupta *et al., J. clin. Hosp. Pharm.*, 1986, *11,* 215.

For a report of an incompatibility with ethacrynic acid, see Ethacrynic Acid, p.986.

Adverse Effects

Toxic effects occur frequently with hydralazine, particularly tachycardia, palpitations, angina pectoris, severe headache, anorexia, nausea, vomiting, and diarrhoea.

Side-effects which occur less frequently are postural hypotension, dizziness, fluid retention with oedema and weight gain, conjunctivitis, lachrymation, chills, fever, nasal congestion, and peripheral neuritis with numbness and tingling of the extremities. Occasionally, hepatitis, pruritus, skin rashes, constipation, paralytic ileus, depression, and anxiety occur.

A more serious toxic reaction which may occur following the prolonged use of large doses is a condition resembling systemic lupus erythematosus. The incidence is greater in slow acetylators, patients with renal impairment, and patients taking more than 100 mg of hydralazine daily. The rheumatic symptoms usually disappear when the drug is withdrawn; the severe erythematous condition may be controlled with corticosteroids. Following acute overdosage, hypotension, tachycardia, myocardial ischaemia, dysrhythmias, shock, and coma may occur.

Paradoxical hypertension in an 18-year-old woman following administration of hydralazine on 3 occasions.— D. B. Webb and J. P. White, *Br. med. J.*, 1980, *280,* 1582.

EFFECTS ON THE BLOOD. A 63-year-old man developed Coombs' positive haemolysis while receiving hydralazine 25 mg daily for mild hypertension. The Coombs' test was negative 11 weeks after withdrawal of hydralazine therapy which had continued for about 3 years.— A. A. Orenstein *et al.* (letter), *Ann. intern. Med.*, 1977, *86,* 450.

Pregnancy and the neonate. Report of 3 cases of neonatal thrombocytopenia in infants whose mothers had been treated with hydralazine for some months before delivery. The thrombocytopenia and bleeding was transient with full recovery occurring within a few weeks. No adverse effects were noticed in the mothers.— E. Widerlöv *et al.* (letter), *New Engl. J. Med.*, 1980, *303,* 1235.

EFFECTS ON THE KIDNEY. Rapidly progressive glomerulonephritis associated with hydralazine treatment has been reported by Muehrke and Kark (*Lancet*, 1966, *1,* 1148) in 1 patient, by Björk *et al.* (*ibid.*, 1983, *2,* 42 and *ibid.*, 1985, *1,* 392) in 15 patients, and by Kincaid-Smith and Whitworth (*ibid.*, 1983, *2,* 348) in 4 patients. The patients were managed by withdrawal of hydralazine, and immunosuppressive therapy.

EFFECTS ON THE LIVER. Reports of liver dysfunction in patients taking hydralazine: E. Bartoli *et al., Archs intern. Med.*, 1979, *139,* 698 (acute hepatitis with bridging necrosis); H. S. Forster (letter), *New Engl. J. Med.*, 1980, *302,* 1362 (hepatitis as part of a hypersensitivity reaction); D. B. Barnett *et al.*, *Br. med. J.*, 1980, *280*, 1165 (asymptomatic elevation of liver enzymes); G. W. Stewart *et al.* (letter), *Lancet*, 1981, *1*, 1207 (obstructive jaundice and pancytopenia); G. M. McKelvie *et al.*, *Hosp. Pharm.*, 1982, *17*, 562 (abnormal liver function tests); D. Rice and C. O. Burdick, *Archs intern. Med.*, 1983, *143*, 1077 (granulomatous hepatitis); J. L. Myers and N. A. Augur, *Gastroenterology*, 1984, *87*, 1185 (cholangitis).

EFFECT ON SEXUAL FUNCTION. A brief review of the effects of hydralazine on sexual function. Although there have been reports implicating hydralazine as a cause of sexual dysfunction, patients were often taking other antihypertensive drugs concurrently including thiazide diuretics and beta blockers, and it was often not possible to determine the offending agent. The incidence of hydralazine-induced sexual dysfunction appears to be rare.— J. G. Stevenson and G. S. Umstead, *Drug Intell. & clin. Pharm.*, 1984, *18*, 113.

EFFECTS ON THE SKIN. Pruritic skin rashes were associated with hydralazine therapy in 4 patients.— G. J. Schapel (letter), *Med. J. Aust.*, 1984, *141*, 765.

See also under Lupus Erythematosus, below.

LUPUS ERYTHEMATOSUS. A discussion of recent developments in drug-associated systemic lupus erythematosus with especial reference to hydralazine. Typically drug-induced lupus erythematosus is characterised by a delayed onset of between 1 month and 5 years of treatment, a non-deforming polyarthritis in 80 to 90% of patients, fever and myalgia in up to 50%, and pleuropulmonary features (in up to 30% of patients receiving hydralazine). Skin rashes occur in less than 25% and are less prominent than in idiopathic disease. Renal involvement has been reported with hydralazine, but CNS involvement does not appear to occur. Antinuclear antibodies occur in up to 50% of patients exposed to hydralazine, but only 1 to 3% develop clinical symptoms of lupus erythematosus. Slow acetylators develop antibodies earlier than fast acetylators. Studies of immunological factors have increased the understanding of one possible mechanism of hydralazine-induced lupus.— *Adverse Drug React. Bull.*, 1987, Apr., 460.

A study of the incidence of the lupus syndrome in 281 patients taking hydralazine. Of those treated for 1, 2, and 3 years the percentage incidence was 0.9, 5.5, and 6.7 respectively. In men the incidence was zero, 1.8, and 2.8 respectively, with an incidence of 1.9, 9.9, and 11.6 for women. There was clear dose-dependence and the 3-year incidence was nearly 20% in women taking hydralazine 200 mg daily. It was recommended that the dose of hydralazine should be limited to 100 mg daily and patients followed up closely. Prazosin may be preferable in women.— H. A. Cameron and L. E. Ramsay, *Br. med. J.*, 1984, *289*, 410.

Further references to the incidence of hydralazine-induced lupus-like syndrome: R. F. Bing *et al.*, *Br. med. J.*, 1980, *281*, 353; S. Freestone *et al.*, *Br. J. clin. Pharmac.*, 1982, *13*, 291P; R. Mansilla-Tinoco *et al.*, *Br. med. J.*, 1982, *284*, 936.

A brief discussion of the immunological processes concerned with hydralazine-induced lupus.— J. R. Batchelor and A. J. McMichael, *Br. med. Bull.*, 1987, *43*, 156.

A number of complications and symptoms associated with lupus erythematosus have been reported in patients taking hydralazine. Bernstein *et al.* (*Br. med. J.*, 1980, *280*, 156), Peacock and Weatherall (*ibid.*, 1981, *282*, 1121), and Finlay *et al.* (*ibid.*, 1703) reported cases of *cutaneous vasculitis* in patients taking hydralazine, and Neville *et al.* (*Postgrad. med. J.*, 1981, *57*, 378) reported a patient with *orogenital and cutaneous ulceration.* Doherty *et al.* (*Br. med. J.*, 1985, *290*, 675) observed *bilateral retinal vasculitis* in 2 patients; the retinal changes were not explicable in terms of hypertensive retinopathy alone and did not resolve when hydralazine was discontinued. *Reactive hypoglycaemia*, apparently due to the auto-immune insulin syndrome, developed in an 82-year-old patient taking hydralazine (P.J. Blackshear, *et al.*, *Ann. intern. Med.*, 1983, *99*, 182). Life-threatening *cardiac tamponade* was associated with hydralazine-induced lupus erythematosus in cases reported by Aylward *et al.* (*Aust. N.Z. J. Med.*, 1982, *12*, 546) and Anandadas and Simpson (*Br. J. clin. Pract.*, 1986 *40*, 305).

See also under Absorption and Fate.

Treatment of Adverse Effects

Withdrawal of hydralazine or reduction of the dosage causes the reversal of many side-effects. If overdosage occurs the stomach should be emptied by aspiration and lavage. Activated charcoal may be administered. Severe hypotension may respond to placing the patient in the supine position with the feet raised. The effects of gross overdosage may be treated by the infusion of plasma expanders. If a pressor agent is necessary, one should be chosen which will not cause tachycardia; adrenaline should not be used. Peripheral neuritis has been reported to be alleviated by pyridoxine.

Precautions

Hydralazine is contra-indicated in patients with tachycardia, rheumatic heart disease, or mitral valve disease. It should be used with caution in patients with coronary artery disease, or cerebrovascular disorders since it can increase ischaemia. The dose of hydralazine should be reduced in patients with impaired renal or hepatic function. Complete blood counts and antinuclear antibody determinations should be carried out periodically during long-term therapy.

Hydralazine is teratogenic in some species of *animals* and should therefore be avoided during the first half of pregnancy.

Adrenaline should not be given to antagonise the hypotensive effects of hydralazine since it enhances the cardiac-accelerating effect. The hypotensive effect may be enhanced by other agents with a hypotensive action. Severe hypotension may occur if hydralazine and diazoxide are given concurrently. However, some interactions with antihypertensive agents may be beneficial: thiazide diuretics also conteract the fluid retention caused by hydralazine, and beta-adrenoceptor blocking agents diminish the cardiac-accelerating effects.

INTERACTIONS. Indomethacin 100 mg daily was not found to attenuate the hypotensive effect of hydralazine in 9 healthy subjects (S.H.D. Jackson and H. Pickles, *Eur. J. clin. Pharmac.*, 1983, *25*, 303), but Cinquegrani and Chang-seng (*Clin. Pharmac. Ther.*, 1986, *39*, 564) subsequently showed that indomethacin 200 mg daily attenuated the hypotensive effect of hydralazine but not the effects on heart rate, renal or limb blood flow or plasma catecholamine concentration.

PORPHYRIA. Hydralazine was considered to be unsafe in patients with acute porphyria because it has been shown to be porphyrinogenic in *animals* or *in-vitro* systems.— M.R. Moore and K.E.L. McColl, *Porphyrias, Drug Lists*, Glasgow, Porphyria Research Unit, University of Glasgow, 1987.

Absorption and Fate

Hydralazine is rapidly absorbed from the gastro-intestinal tract but undergoes considerable first-pass hepatic metabolism. Peak concentrations have been reported to occur in the plasma after about one hour. It is metabolised by hydroxylation of the ring system and conjugation with glucuronic acid, and by *N*-acetylation. The rate of metabolism is genetically determined and depends upon the acetylator status of the individual. The bioavailability of hydalazine has been reported to be about 30% in slow acetylators and 50 to 55% in fast acetylators. The plasma half-life is also influenced by the ability to metabolise the drug: the average half-life is 2 to 4 hours with a reported range of 45 minutes to 8 hours. The half-life is prolonged in renal failure and may be up to 16 hours in patients with a creatinine clearance of less than 20 mL per minute.

Hydralazine is about 90% bound to plasma proteins. It is excreted mainly in the urine as metabolites. Hydralazine crosses the placenta and is excreted in the breast milk.

In a detailed review of studies on the clinical pharmacokinetics of hydralazine, Ludden *et al.* (*Clin. Pharmacokinet.*, 1982, *7*, 185) have emphasised their limitations, which include problems with the analytical procedures and the instability of hydralazine, as well as the paucity of studies in patients as against healthy subjects.

Although some workers (A.J. Jounela *et al.*, *Acta med. scand.*, 1975, *197*, 303; R. Zacest and J. Koch-Weser, *Clin. Pharmac. Ther.*, 1972, *13*, 420) have correlated the hypotensive effect of hydralazine with the serum concentrations, others (T. Talseth *et al.*, *Curr. ther. Res.*, 1977, *21*, 157) have been unable to do so. Moreover, the duration of hypotensive effect has been shown to exceed considerably that predicted from the rate of elimination (K. O'Malley *et al.*, *Clin. Pharmac. Ther.*, 1975, *18*, 581; A.M.M. Shepherd *et al.*, *ibid.*, 1980, *28*, 804). Possible explanations are the accumulation of hydralazine at its sites of action in the arterial walls (D. Moore-Jones and H.M. Perry, *Proc. Soc. exp. Biol. Med.*, 1966, *122*, 576) or the existence of active metabolites (K. Barron *et al.*, *Br. J. Pharmac.*, 1977, *61*, 345; K.D. Haegele *et al.*, *Br. J. clin. Pharmac.*, 1978, *5*, 489; P.A. Reece *et al.*, *J. pharm. Sci.*, 1978, *67*, 1150).

Concurrent intake of food has been found by Melander *et al.* (*Clin. Pharmac. Ther.*, 1977, *22*, 104) to enhance considerably the bioavailability of hydralazine but Shepherd *et al.* (*ibid.*, 1984, *36*, 14) demonstrated food-related reductions in plasma-hydralazine concentrations with reduced vasodilator effect. The discrepancy was thought to be due to the greater specificity of the assay used in the latter study (A.M.M. Shepherd *et al.*, *ibid.*, 1985, *38*, 475) and to differences in the timing of food and hydralazine administration in the two studies (A. Melander *et al.*, *ibid.*).

A review and discussion of the therapeutic implications of genetically determined variability in acetylation. There have been several reports that acetylator phenotype has an effect on serum concentrations of hydralazine. However, acetylator phenotype appears to have little influence on therapeutic response when hydralazine is given in a low dose in combination with other antihypertensive drugs.

Studies suggest that acetylator phenotype is a factor in the early development of systemic lupus erythematosus, although other factors such as gender, duration of treatment and HLA-DR antigens also contribute to the development of this adverse effect. It was concluded that determination of acetylator phenotype before commencing long-term hydralazine therapy may be useful in helping to predict those at greatest risk of developing systemic lupus erythematosus.— D. W. J. Clark, *Drugs*, 1985, *29*, 342.

Blood pressure was easier to control in slow acetylators than in fast acetylators in a study using hydralazine in doses of up to 200 mg daily. It was suggested that the acetylator status of patients who do not respond adequately to hydralazine 200 mg should be determined, and that the dosage may be safely increased in fast acetylators.— L. E. Ramsay *et al.*, *Eur. J. clin. Pharmac.*, 1984, *26*, 39.

Further references: D. W. Schneck *et al.*, *Clin. Pharmac. Ther.*, 1978, *24*, 714 (acetylation; lack of influence of procainamide); D. D. Shen *et al.*, *J. Pharmacokinet. Biopharm.*, 1980, *8*, 53 (pharmacokinetics); J. A. Timbrell *et al.*, *Clin. Pharmac. Ther.*, 1980, *28*, 350 (polymorphic acetylation); T. M. Ludden *et al.*, *Clin. Pharmac. Ther.*, 1980, *28*, 736 (hypertensive patients); P. A. Reece *et al.*, *Clin. Pharmac. Ther.*, 1980, *28*, 769 (polymorphic acetylation); A. M. M. Shepherd *et al.*, *Clin. Pharmac. Ther.*, 1980, *28*, 804 (pharmacokinetics); V. Facchini and J. A. Timbrell, *Br. J. clin. Pharmac.*, 1981, *11*, 345 (polymorphic acetylation); F. C. Phillips *et al.*, *Br. J. clin. Pharmac.*, 1982, *14*, 150P (polymorphic acetylation); A. Hanson *et al.*, *Eur. J. clin. Pharmac.*, 1983, *25*, 467 (pharmacokinetics in chronic heart failure); M. H. Crawford *et al.*, *Clin. Pharmac. Ther.*, 1985, *38*, 538 (systemic availablity in heart failure).

PREGNANCY AND THE NEONATE. Hydralazine concentrations were found to be similar in maternal and umbilical-cord blood in a study of 6 women being treated with hydralazine for pronounced hypertension during pregnancy. Hydralazine was determined in the breast milk of 1 mother, but amounts detected were unlikely to produce clinically relevant concentrations in the infant.— H. Liedholm *et al.*, *Eur. J. clin. Pharmac.*, 1982, *21*, 417.

For a report of thrombocytopenia occurring in neonates following maternal treatment with hydralazine during pregnancy, see under Adverse Effects, above.

Uses and Administration

Hydralazine is a vasodilator which acts predominantly on the arterioles. It reduces blood pressure and peripheral resistance and produces fluid retention. Tachycardia and an increase in cardiac output occur mainly as a reflex response to the reduction in peripheral resistance. Hydralazine tends to improve renal and cerebral blood flow and its effect on diastolic pressure is more marked than on systolic pressure. It is used for the treatment of moderate to severe hypertension usually in conjunction with a beta-adrenoceptor blocking agent and a thiazide diuretic. In addition to an additive antihypertensive effect, this combination reduces the reflex tachycardia and fluid retention caused by hydralazine.

The usual initial dose of hydralazine hydrochloride by mouth is 25 mg twice daily increased according to the patient's response, to a maximum of 100 mg daily in divided doses; higher doses are associated with an increased incidence of lupus erythematosus.

Hydralazine hydrochloride is given by slow intravenous injection or by intravenous infusion in a dose of 5 to 20 mg for hypertensive emergencies, but an over-rapid reduction in blood pressure may occur; the dose may be repeated after 20 to 30 minutes. A maximum fall in blood pressure is usually obtained within 10 to 80 minutes and the effect lasts for 2 to 8 hours. It has also been given by intramuscular injection.

Hydralazine polistirex (hydralazine and sulphonated diethenylbenzene-ethenylbenzene copolymer complex) is also used.

The use of hydralazine has increased since it became apparent that beta-blocking agents reduce some of the adverse effects when used concurrently. However, the high incidence of hydralazine-induced lupus limits the usefulness of the drug. Proposed methods of avoiding the risk of hydralazine-induced lupus include limiting the dosage, probably to a level where the antihypertensive effect would be negligible; testing the acetylator status before prescribing hydralazine, or monitoring the antinuclear factor during treatment, both of which are expensive, and the latter inaccurate. It is likely that the most practical suggestion is to use an alternative drug.— P. Kincaid-Smith, *Med. J. Aust.*, 1985, *142*, 337.

For a review of the therapeutic implications of genetically determined variations in acetylation of hydralazine, see under Absorption and Fate, above.

ADMINISTRATION IN RENAL FAILURE. The half-life of hydralazine was prolonged from 2 to 4.5 hours to 7 to 16 hours in patients with end-stage renal disease. An interval of 8 hours between doses of hydralazine is suitable for patients with glomerular filtration-rates above 10 mL per minute. The dosage interval for patients with glomerular filtration-rates of less than 10 mL per minute should be between 8 and 16 hours in fast acetylators and between 12 and 24 hours in slow acetylators.— W. M. Bennett *et al.*, *Am. J. Kidney Dis.*, 1983, *3*, 155.

HEART FAILURE. A review of vasodilator therapy in the treatment of severe chronic heart failure. Although hydralazine produces marked increases in cardiac output and decreases in systemic vascular resistance in patients with heart failure, the doses required to produce these effects are unpredictable, ranging from 150 mg to nearly 3 g daily. Furthermore, the haemodynamic responses to hydralazine are quite variable; patients with markedly dilated left ventricles who have marked degrees of secondary mitral regurgitation appear to respond best, but in others the drug may compromise peripheral perfusion without an improvement in cardiac performance. Haemodynamic and clinical tolerance on long-term therapy and the development of serious adverse reactions and myocardial ischaemia further limit the usefulness of hydralazine in the treatment of heart failure.— M. Packer, *Drugs*, 1986, *32*, *Suppl.5*, 13.

Further reviews of the use of hydralazine and other vasodilators in heart failure: *Drug & Ther. Bull.*, 1983, *21*, 50; *Med. Lett.*, 1984, *26*, 115; G. H. Guyatt, *Drugs*, 1986, *32*, 538.

A study of 11 patients with severe chronic heart failure who developed tolerance to the effects of hydralazine during long-term treatment. All the patients showed an initial favourable haemodynamic response to hydralazine, and 9 patients also showed initial clinical improvement. Six of these 9 patients subsequently had a recurrence of symptoms similar to those of the pretreatment state within 4 months of the start of therapy, and the remaining 3 showed clinical deterioration after 18 to 24 months. The clinical tolerance was generally not responsive to an increase in the dose of hydralazine or to the use of diuretics.— M. Packer *et al.*, *New Engl. J. Med.*, 1982, *306*, 57. Comment that a possible increase in the renal clearance of digoxin due to vasodilator therapy may contribute to the recurrence of heart failure in patients treated with hydralazine.— H. I. Bussey (letter), *New Engl. J. Med.*, 1982, *307*, 443.

In a study by the Veterans Administration Cooperative Study Group involving 642 men with stable chronic congestive heart failure who were taking digoxin and a diuretic, the results suggested that the addition of hydralazine and isosorbide dinitrate to the treatment regimen could have a favourable effect on left ventricular function and mortality. However, adverse effects were common in patients taking hydralazine and isosorbide dinitrate: in 19% of patients one or both drugs were discontinued due to adverse effects and only 55% were taking full doses of both drugs 6 months after the start of treatment.— J. N. Cohn *et al.*, *New Engl. J. Med.*, 1986, *314*, 1547. Criticisms of the study and comments that differences in the baseline characteristics of the patients could have influenced the outcome: C. P. Taliercio (letter), *ibid.*, *315*, 1227; O. Bertel (letter), *ibid;* R. H. Falk (letter), *ibid;* J. N. Cohn and D. G. Archibald (letter), *ibid.*, 1228.

Further references to the use of hydralazine in heart failure: K. Chatterjee *et al.*, *Ann. intern. Med.*, 1980, *92*, 600 (sustained beneficial haemodynamic effects); T. L. Biddle and H. W. Moses, *J. clin. Pharmac.*, 1981, *21*, 343 (comparison with dopamine and isosorbide dinitrate); D. J. Fitzgerald *et al.*, *Br. J. clin. Pharmac.*, 1982, *14*, 133P (comparison with captopril); G. I. C. Nelson *et al.*, *Br. J. clin. Pharmac.*, 1984, *17*, 205P (beneficial effects in combination with isosorbide dinitrate).

In children. Single intravenous injections of hydralazine 500 µg per kg body-weight produced increases in stroke volume index and cardiac index in 13 infants aged between 2 and 13 months with congestive heart failure and dilated cardiomyopathy. Oral hydralazine therapy was given to 10 of these infants in addition to treatment with digitalis and a diuretic. At a follow-up of 3 to 38 months, 8 patients were asymptomatic. One child showed no apparent improvement after 3 months of therapy, and one child died. It was concluded that hydralazine may be a beneficial adjunct to the management of congestive heart failure in young infants with dilated cardiomyopathy.— M. Artman *et al.*, *Am. Heart J.*, 1987, *113*, 144. Similar beneficial response was seen in 10 infants and children aged between 3 and 36 months with primary myocardial disease treated with oral hydralazine up to 4 mg per kg body-weight daily for up to 42 months.— P. S. Rao and W. G. Andaya, *J. Pediat.*, 1986, *108*, 530.

HYPERTENSION. Findings that administration of the same daily dosage of hydralazine in 2 doses rather than 4 gives equally effective blood pressure control and may increase patient compliance.— K. O'Malley *et al.*, *Clin. Pharmac. Ther.*, 1975, *18*, 581.

Hydralazine 100 mg twice daily as conventional tablets and as a 200 mg sustained-release tablet once daily gave satisfactory control of blood pressure for 24 hours in both fast and slow acetylators.— J. H. Silas *et al.*, *Br. med. J.*, 1982, *284*, 1602.

Evidence that guanfacine used in combination with hydralazine could counteract the hydralazine-induced increase in sympathetic nervous tone. — M. Velasco *et al.*, *Eur. J. clin. Pharmac.*, 1984, *27*, 393.

Studies of the efficacy of hydralazine in hypertension: Veterans Administration Cooperative Study Group on Antihypertensive Agents, *J. Am. med. Ass.*, 1977, *237*, 2303 (comparison with reserpine in combination therapy); M. J. Vandenburg *et al.*, *Br. J. clin. Pharmac.*, 1983, *16*, 537 (comparison with prazosin in third line therapy); G. I. Russell *et al.*, *Eur. J. clin. Pharmac.*, 1985, *28*, 119 (comparison with atenolol or methyldopa); L. E. Ramsay and L. Latham, *Br. J. clin. Pharmac.*, 1985, *20*, 524P (comparison with nifedipine and prazosin in third line therapy); D. Maclean, *ibid.*, 1986, *21*, 621 (comparison with felodipine as third line therapy); M. G. Myers *et al.*, *Clin. Pharmac. Ther.*, 1986, *39*, 409 (comparison with nifedipine in third line therapy); L. E. Ramsay *et al.*, *Postgrad. med. J.*, 1987, *63*, 99 (comparison with prazosin and nifedipine in third line therapy).

OESOPHAGEAL DISORDERS. Hydralazine 75 to 200 mg by mouth daily improved the symptoms of primary oesophageal motility disorders including decrease in chest pain and dysphagia in 4 patients. The clinical improvement was accompanied by significant decreases in the amplitude and duration of distal oesophageal contractions.— M. H. Mellow, *Gastroenterology*, 1982, *83*, 364.

PREGNANCY AND THE NEONATE. *Hypertension in pregnancy.* A discussion of the management of hypertension in pregnancy. If a beta blocker or methyldopa fails to control the blood pressure a vasodilator such as hydralazine may be added. In hypertensive crisis or eclampsia hydralazine may be administered by slow intravenous injection.— P. C. Rubin, *Prescribers' J.*, 1985, *25*, 19. See also B. N. J. Walters, *Br. J. Hosp. Med.*, 1984, *31*, 49.

PSORIASIS. Improvement of psoriasis was seen in 5 out of 10 patients treated with hydralazine 75 mg daily.— P. Isaac (letter), *Br. med. J.*, 1982, *285*, 744.

PULMONARY HYPERTENSION. A discussion of the use of hydralazine in the treatment of primary pulmonary hypertension. Conflicting evidence has been produced on the haemodynamic and clinical effectiveness of hydralazine in primary pulmonary oedema. It was suggested that response to hydralazine depends upon the degree of reversible vasoconstrictor tone in the pulmonary vascular bed. It is also possible that the response is dependent upon an increase in cardiac output, and it has been shown that the initial haemodynamic response to intravenous hydralazine may serve as a good indication of the effectiveness of continued oral therapy: a marked increase in cardiac output accompanied by no change or a reduction in pulmonary arterial pressure may indicate a beneficial response.— P. J. Kadowitz and A. L. Hyman, *New Engl. J. Med.*, 1982, *306*, 1357.

Preparations

Hydralazine Injection *(B.P.)*. Hydralazine Hydrochloride Injection

Hydralazine Hydrochloride Injection *(U.S.P.)*

Hydralazine Tablets *(B.P.)*. Hydralazine Hydrochloride Tablets. Store at a temperature not exceeding 25°. Protect from light.

Hydralazine Hydrochloride Tablets *(U.S.P.)*. Protect from light.

Proprietary Preparations

Apresoline *(Ciba, UK)*. *Tablets*, hydralazine hydrochloride 25 and 50 mg.

Injection, powder for reconstitution, hydralazine hydrochloride 20 mg.

Proprietary Names and Manufacturers

Alphapress *(Alphapharm, Austral.)*; Aprelazine *(Jpn)*; Apresolin *(Ciba, Denm.*; *Ciba, Ital.*; *Ciba, Norw.*; *Ciba, Swed.)*; Apresolina *(Ciba, Spain)*; Apresoline *(Ciba, Austral.*; *Ciba, Canad.*; *Neth.*; *Ciba, S.Afr.*; *Ciba, UK*; *Ciba, USA)*; Dralzine *(Lemmon, USA)*; Hydrapres *(Rubio, Spain)*; Hyperazin *(Jpn)*; Hyperex *(Propan, S.Afr.)*; Hyperphen *(Lennon, S.Afr.)*; Ipolina *(Lafare, Ital.)*; Rolazine *(Rolab, S.Afr.)*; Slow-Aprésoline *(Ciba, Switz.)*; Supres *(Protea, Austral.)*; Vasodur *(Pennwalt, USA)*.

The following names have been used for multi-ingredient preparations containing hydralazine hydrochloride—Apresazide *(Ciba, USA)*; Apresoline-Esidrix *(Ciba, USA)*; H-H-R *(Schein, USA)*; Hydral *(Reid-Provident, USA)*; Hydra-Zide *(Par, USA)*; Hyserp *(Reid-Provident, USA)*; Rezide *(Edwards, USA)*; Seragen *(Reid-Provident, USA)*; Ser-Ap-Es *(Ciba, Canad.*; *Ciba, USA)*; Serpasil-Apresoline *(Ciba, USA)*; Unipres *(Reid-Rowell, USA)*.

879-d

Indoramin Hydrochloride *(BANM, USAN, rINNM)*.

Wy-21901 (indoramin). *N*-[1-(2-Indol-3-ylethyl)-4-piperidyl]benzamide hydrochloride.

$C_{22}H_{25}N_3O,HCl = 383.9$.

CAS — 26844-12-2 (indoramin); 33124-53-7 (hydrochloride); 38821-52-2 (hydrochloride).

Adverse Effects and Precautions

Adverse effects reported for indoramin include sedation, dry mouth, nasal congestion, dizziness, depression, weight gain (almost certainly due to fluid retention), and failure of ejaculation.

As an alpha-adrenoceptor blocking agent indoramin would be expected to have a cardiac-accelerating action, but this has not been reported with therapeutic doses.

Indoramin should be avoided in patients with heart failure; it has been recommended that incipient heart failure should be controlled with diuretics and digitalis before giving indoramin, and that caution should be observed in patients with hepatic or renal insufficiency, or Parkinson's disease. Elderly patients may respond to lower doses.

It has been reported that the concomitant ingestion of alcohol can increase the rate and extent of absorption of indoramin and that indoramin should not be given to patients already receiving monoamine oxidase inhibitors.

Tachycardia and anxiety in a 56-year-old patient during treatment with indoramin and a diuretic (K.M. Mishra *et al., Practitioner*, 1984, *228*, 362) was considered to be related more to the diuretic than to indoramin (M. Cohen, *ibid.*).

EFFECTS ON MENTAL FUNCTION. Sleep disturbances and vivid dreams were reported during a study of indoramin in hypertensive patients already taking a thiazide diuretic and a beta-blocking agent.— A. J. Marshall *et al., Br. J. clin. Pharmac.*, 1980, *10*, 217.

EFFECTS ON SEXUAL FUNCTION. Failure of ejaculation in 6 of 9 men taking indoramin for migraine.— B. Pentland *et al., Br. med. J.*, 1981, *282*, 1433. See also B. A. Gould *et al.* (letter), *ibid.*, 1796.

Indoramin was shown to inhibit sperm motility *in vitro*.— R. B. Verma *et al.* (letter), *Br. J. clin. Pharmac.*, 1983, *15*, 127.

INTERACTIONS. *Alcohol.* Ingestion of alcohol caused a significant increase in the peak indoramin plasma concentration and the area under the plasma-concentration/time curve when administered with indoramin 50 mg by mouth.— S. M. L. Abrams *et al., Br. J. clin. Pharmac.*, 1984, *18*, 294P.

OVERDOSAGE. A 43-year-old woman with a long history of heavy alcohol intake died after taking 100 tablets of indoramin 25 mg. The main clinical features were deep sedation, respiratory depression, hypotension and convulsions. Although the hypotension was satisfactorily controlled the effects on the central nervous system were resistant to treatment and proved fatal. Other clinical features included areflexia, metabolic acidosis, tachycardia, and later bradyarrhythmias.— R. Hunter, *Br. med. J.*, 1982, *285*, 1011.

Treatment of Adverse Effects

If overdosage occurs the stomach should be emptied by aspiration and lavage. Severe hypotension may respond to placing the patient in the supine position with the feet raised. Ventilation should be monitored and assisted if necessary.

It has been recommended that the patient should be monitored for hypothermia and convulsions, in addition to hypotension.

Absorption and Fate

Indoramin is readily absorbed from the gastro-intestinal tract and undergoes extensive first-pass metabolism. It is reported to be about 90% bound to plasma proteins. It has a half-life of about 5 hours which is reported to be prolonged in elderly patients. It is extensively metabolised in the liver and is excreted mainly as metabolites in the urine and faeces. There is evidence to suggest that some metabolites may retain some α-receptor blocking activity.

The half-life of indoramin in 5 healthy elderly subjects following a single oral dose ranged from 6.6 to 32.8 hours with a mean of 14.7 hours. The increased half-life may have been caused by reduced clearance in elderly patients.— H. M. Norbury *et al., Eur. J. clin. Pharmac.*, 1984, *27*, 247.

Studies of the pharmacokinetics of indoramin in healthy subjects: G. H. Draffan *et al., Br. J. clin. Pharmac.*, 1976, *3*, 489; R. A. Franklin *et al., Eur. J. clin. Pharmac.*, 1983, *24*, 629; H. M. Norbury *et al., ibid.*, *25*, 243.

Uses and Administration

Indoramin is an antihypertensive agent which acts by competitive alpha$_1$-adrenoceptor antagonism (see Prazosin, Uses p.496); it is also reported to have membrane-stabilising properties. It is used in the treatment of mild to moderate hypertension either alone or in combination with a diuretic and a beta-blocker.

In the treatment of hypertension indoramin is given as the hydrochloride in initial doses equivalent to 25 mg of the base twice daily, increased in steps of 25 or 50 mg at intervals of 2 weeks to a maximum of 200 mg daily in 2 or 3 divided doses. A lower dose may be required in the elderly.

A review of the pharmacodynamics, pharmacokinetics, and therapeutic efficacy of indoramin. Indoramin has been shown to have selective postsynaptic alpha$_1$-adrenoceptor blocking and membrane-stabilising properties. It has also been shown to have a centrally mediated cardioregulatory effect, some class III anti-arrhythmic activity, and some beneficial effects on both cardiac preload and afterload. There has also been some evidence of elevations of plasma renin activity and effects on blood lipids although results have varied.

Indoramin has been shown to be effective in the treatment of mild to moderate hypertension both alone, and more commonly in combination with a thiazide diuretic. Additionally, moderate to moderately severe cases have responded to indoramin therapy given as a third agent in patients uncontrolled by a beta-blocker and a diuretic. A few small comparative studies have shown indoramin to be comparable in efficacy to methyldopa, propranolol, and prazosin when dosage was adjusted to individual requirements. The tolerability of indoramin has been shown to be similar to that of methyldopa and propranolol when studied under the same controlled conditions, but not as good as that of prazosin. Unlike prazosin, however, indoramin therapy has not been associated with first-dose syncope or orthostatic hypotension, or with tachycardia. Furthermore it has not been found to produce bronchospasm in predisposed patients nor to have any negative inotropic activity in patients, although this has been seen in *animal* studies.

Other potential uses of indoramin include Raynaud's phenomenon, migraine, nocturnal enuresis in children, and angina. However, consistent success has occurred only in a few studies in patients with Raynaud's phenomenon.— B. Holmes and E. M. Sorkin, *Drugs*, 1986, *31*, 467.

The absence of reflex tachycardia during indoramin therapy may be due to selective alpha$_1$-adrenoceptor blockade (D.P. Nicholls *et al., Br. J. clin. Pharmac.*, 1984, *17*, 719), prolongation of the duration of the cardiac action potential (D.W.G. Harron *et al., ibid.*, 1985, *19*, 266), and/or depression of baroreceptor sensitivity (A.H. Deering *et al., ibid.*, 1986, *22*, 231P).

In a study of 11 hypertensive patients, short-term indoramin therapy was associated with increases in glomerular filtration rate, effective renal plasma and renal blood flow, and a decrease in renal vascular resistance. Long-term indoramin therapy was associated with qualitatively similar renal effects.— J. H. Bauer *et al., Archs intern. Med.*, 1984, *144*, 308.

HEART FAILURE. In a study of 12 patients with chronic congestive heart failure, indoramin produced predominantly venodilatation after the initial dose. However, continuous dosing for 1 week resulted in a reduction in cardiac output and a decrease in exercise capacity. It was suggested that fluid retention and anti-adrenergic activity produced by indoramin could have contributed to the unfavourable haemodynamic response to prolonged treatment.— L. Seth *et al., Clin. Pharmac. Ther.*, 1986, *40*, 567.

No long-term clinical improvements were seen in a study involving 21 patients with congestive heart failure following treatment with indoramin up to 75 mg twice daily for 2 months.— C. V. Leier *et al., J. Am. Coll. Cardiol.*, 1987, *9*, 426.

HYPERTENSION. A review of indoramin in hypertension. Indoramin was as effective as prazosin and methyldopa in the treatment of hypertension and did not appear to cause orthostatic hypotension. In addition, it did not exacerbate bronchospasm or peripheral ischaemia. It could be used as an alternative third-line antihypertensive in combination therapy.— *Drug & Ther. Bull.*, 1982, *20*, 33.

Proprietary Preparations

Baratol *(Wyeth, UK). Tablets*, indoramin 25 mg (as hydrochloride).

Tablets, scored, indoramin 50 mg (as hydrochloride).

Proprietary Names and Manufacturers

Baratol *(Wyeth, S.Afr.; Wyeth, UK)*; Indorene *(Lusofarmaco, Ital.)*; Vidora *(Wyeth, Ital.)*; Wydora *(Wyeth, Ger.; Wyeth, Switz.)*.

12881-m

Ketanserin *(BAN, USAN, rINN).*

R-41468; R-49945 *(tartrate)*. 3-{2-[4-(4-Fluorobenzoyl)piperidino]ethyl}quinazoline-2,4(1*H*,3*H*)-dione.

$C_{22}H_{22}FN_3O_3$=395.4.

CAS — 74050-98-9.

Adverse Effects and Precautions

Ketanserin has been reported to cause sedation, dizziness, headache, dry mouth, and nausea.

Profound hypotension occurred in 2 patients one hour after taking ketanserin 40 mg by mouth. Both patients were also taking a beta-blocking agent which may have exacerbated the reaction.— P. C. Waller *et al., Postgrad. med. J.*, 1987, *63*, 305.

INTERACTIONS. The pharmacokinetics of ketanserin were not affected by concomitant administration of propanolol, nor the pharmacokinetics of propranolol by ketanserin in a single-dose study in healthy subjects.— F. M. Williams *et al., Br. J. clin. Pharmac.*, 1986, *22*, 301.

Study in healthy volunteers suggesting that therapeutic doses of ketanserin could impair the clearance of propranolol leading to increased area under the serum concentration curve and elevated peak serum concentrations.— H. R. Ochs *et al., Clin. Pharmac. Ther.*, 1987, *41*, 55.

Absorption and Fate

Ketanserin is rapidly absorbed from the gastro-intestinal tract but has a bioavailability of about 50% due to first-pass hepatic metabolism. The mean terminal half-life reported following single oral doses has been between 10 and 18 hours; following multiple doses the half-life has been between 19 and 29 hours. The metabolite ketanserol has a terminal half-life of 31 to 35 hours following multiple doses, and it has been suggested that reconversion of ketanserol to ketanserin may be responsible for the prolonged half-life of the parent compound during chronic administration.

In a study using plasma from healthy subjects a mean of 92.7% of ketanserin was bound to plasma proteins.— A. Johnston *et al., Br. J. clin. Pharmac.*, 1984, *17*, 230P.

References to the pharmacokinetics of ketanserin: I. W. Reimann *et al., Eur. J. clin. Pharmac.*, 1983, *25*, 73; M. Kurowski, *ibid.*, 1985, *28*, 411; A. Van Peer *et al., ibid.*, 1986, *31*, 339; J. Heykants *et al., ibid.*, 343; B. Persson *et al., ibid.*, 1987, *32*, 259.

Uses and Administration

Ketanserin blocks serotonin receptors with a high affinity for peripheral serotonin-2 (5-HT$_2$) receptors and thus inhibits serotonin-induced vasoconstriction, bronchoconstriction, and platelet aggregation. It also binds to alpha receptors, histamine H$_1$ receptors, and dopamine receptors, but the clinical significance of this is controversial. Ketanserin produces a hypotensive effect and has been tried both alone and in combination with other antihypertensive agents in the treatment of hypertension in doses of 20 mg twice daily increasing to 40 mg twice daily by mouth. It has also been given by intravenous injection.

Ketanserin has also been tried in peripheral vascular disorders.

The mechanism of the hypotensive action of ketanserin has been the subject of considerable debate. It was suggested (Wenting *et al., Br. med. J.*, 1982, *284*, 537 and *Lancet*, 1982, *2*, 859) that the hypotensive effect was due to 5-HT$_2$ receptor blockade, but this was refuted by Millar *et al.* (*ibid.*, 1154) who proposed D-receptor antagonism and alpha blockade as possible alternatives. The D-receptor theory was not supported by Van Nueten *et al.* (*ibid.*, 1983, *1*, 297) or by Williams and Bradley (*ibid.*, 703). Reimann and Frölich (*ibid.* and *Br. med. J.*, 1983, *287*, 381) presented evidence to support alpha$_1$ blockade as the mechanism of action which was further supported by Vermylen *et al.* (*ibid.*, 1551) but stimulated contradictory arguments from Ball *et al.* (*ibid.*, 1065) and Schalekamp and Wenting (*ibid.*, 1300).

Further references to the mechanism of action of ketanserin: J. M. Van Nueten *et al., J. Pharmac. exp. Ther.*, 1981, *218*, 217; C. Zoccali *et al., Br. J. clin. Pharmac.*, 1983, *16*, 305; I. W. Reimann *et al., Eur. J. clin. Pharmac.*, 1985, *28*, 273; D. J. Stott *et al., Br. J. clin. Pharmac.*, 1986, *21*, 84P; A. Berdeaux *et al., Eur. J. clin. Pharmac.*, 1987, *32*, 27.

CARCINOID SYNDROME. Reduction in symptoms in 5 out of 7 patients with carcinoid syndrome following treatment with ketanserin 40 to 160 mg daily.— J. Gustafsen *et al., Gut*, 1985, *26*, A556. For a fuller report of this study, see *idem, Scand. J. Gastroenterol.*, 1986, *21*, 816.

Mention of the use of ketanserin to alleviate flushing and reduce diarrhoea in patients with carcinoid syndrome.— B. Clarke and H. J. F. Hodgson, *Br. J. Hosp. Med.*, 1986, *35*, 146.

CARDIAC DISORDERS. Results of a preliminary study in

patients with heart failure indicating beneficial haemodynamic changes.— J. -C. Demoulin *et al.*, *Lancet*, 1981, *1*, 1186.

Single doses of ketanserin 20 to 40 mg had no significant effect on the rate-pressure product or exercise time to angina in 10 patients with stable angina uncontrolled by a beta blocker.— H. A. Cameron *et al.*, *Br. J. clin. Pharmac.*, 1986, *22*, 114.

HYPERTENSION. A number of studies have shown ketanserin to be effective in the treatment of mild to moderate hypertension, both alone (T. Hedner *et al.*, *Br. J. clin. Pharmac.*, 1983, *16*, 121; B. Persson *et al.*, *Eur. J. clin. Pharmac.*, 1983, *25*, 307; H. A. Cameron and L. E. Ramsay, *Postgrad. med. J.*, 1985, *61*, 583; A. Pettersson *et al.*, *Clin. Pharmac. Ther.*, 1985, *38*, 188; J. Staesson *et al.*, *J. cardiovasc. Pharmac.*, 1985, *7*, *Suppl.* 7, S140), and in combination with other antihypertensive agents including diuretics (H.A. Cameron and L.E. Ramsay), and beta blockers (T. Hedner and B. Persson, *Br. J. clin. Pharmac.*, 1984, *18*, 765; L.A. Ferrara *et al.*, *J. clin. Pharmac.*, 1985, *25*, 187; A. Pettersson *et al.*; H.A. Cameron and L.E. Ramsay). The antihypertensive action appears to be primarily due to a reduction of peripheral resistance (G.J. Wenting, *Br. med. J.*, 1982, *284*, 537; L. A. Ferrara *et al.*) and to affect both standing and supine blood pressure (J.C. McGourty *et al.*, *Br. J. clin. Pharmac.*, 1985, *20*, 37).

Ketanserin produced similar responses in supine, erect, postexercise and ambulatory blood pressure to prazosin. Neither drug significantly altered supine or erect pulse rates, body-weight, serum triglyceride concentrations, plasma renin activity, or urinary aldosterone excretion, and their side-effect profiles were similar. The only feature which distinguished the clinical effects of the two drugs was a reduction in serum cholesterol produced by prazosin but not by ketanserin.— G. S. Stokes *et al.*, *Clin. Pharmac. Ther.*, 1986, *40*, 56.

Intravenous ketanserin was not considered to be an agent of choice in the treatment of uncontrolled severe hypertension because it lowered blood pressure only briefly, was not effective in all patients treated, and produced a high incidence of neurological side-effects.— A. A. Jennings and L. H. Opie, *J. cardiovasc. Pharmac.*, 1987, *9*, 120.

For references on the use of ketanserin in pre-eclampsia, see under Pregnancy and the Neonate.

PERIPHERAL VASCULAR DISORDERS. A report of beneficial effects of ketanserin in intermittent claudication by De Cree *et al.* (*Lancet*, 1984, *2*, 775) was not supported by a subsequent study by Bounameaux *et al.* (*ibid.*, 1985, *2*, 1268). Comments on both studies: V. Fonseca *et al.* (letter), *ibid.*, 1984, *2*, 1212; L. E. Ramsay (letter), *ibid.*, 1986, *1*, 619.

Results of an open study involving 18 patients and a double-blind study involving 47 patients suggesting that ketanserin 40 mg twice daily may be of benefit in the early symptomatic treatment of acute superficial thrombophlebitis.— J. Porters *et al.*, *Curr. ther. Res.*, 1981, *30*, 499. See also J. de Roose and J. Symoens (letter), *Lancet*, 1982, *2*, 440.

Little long-term benefit was obtained with ketanserin by intravenous injection in the treatment of leg ulceration in a patient with scleroderma despite initial increases in transcutaneous oxygen pressure.— N. H. Cox and P. A. Dufton (letter), *Br. med. J.*, 1984, *289*, 1078.

Report of rapid healing in a patient with severe bilateral frostbite following treatment with ketanserin.— M. Vayssairat *et al.*, *Practitioner*, 1986, *230*, 406.

Raynaud's Syndrome. Reports of beneficial responses to ketanserin in Raynaud's phenomenon: E. Stranden *et al.*, *Br. med. J.*, 1982, *285*, 1069; O. K. Roald and E. Seem, *ibid.*, 1984, *289*, 577; J. R. Seibold and A. H. M. Jageneau, *Arthritis Rheum.*, 1984, *27*, 139.

No beneficial effects were observed in a single-blind study of 10 patients with secondary Raynaud's phenomenon.— W. Kirch *et al.*, *J. vasc. Dis.*, 1987, *16*, 77.

PREGNANCY AND THE NEONATE. *Hypertension in pregnancy.* Reports of the use of ketanserin in pre-eclamptic hypertension: C. P. Weiner *et al.*, *Am. J. Obstet. Gynec.*, 1984, *149*, 496; R. Montenegro *et al.*, *ibid.*, 1985, *153*, 130; V. A. Hulme and H. J. Odendaal, *ibid.*, 1986, *155*, 260.

Proprietary Names and Manufacturers
Sufrexal *(Janssen, Arg.; Janssen, Belg.)*.

16878-k

Lisinopril *(BAN, USAN, rINN).*
L-154826; MK-521. *N*-{*N*-[(*S*)-1-Carboxy-3-phenylpropyl]-L-lysyl}-L-proline.
$C_{21}H_{31}N_3O_5$=405.5.

CAS — 76547-98-3; 83915-83-7 (dihydrate).

Lisinopril is an angiotensin-converting enzyme inhibitor with properties and uses similar to captopril (see p.468).

Lisinopril is given once daily by mouth in the treatment of hypertension. Suggested doses are 2.5 mg initially, increased gradually according to response to a usual maintenance dose of 10 to 20 mg once daily. A dose of 40 mg daily is not generally exceeded.
It is also used as an adjunct to the treatment of congestive heart failure. Suggested doses are 2.5 mg initially, and 5 to 20 mg daily for maintenance.

A brief review of lisinopril.— *Med. Lett.*, 1988, *30*, 41.

References to the actions and uses of lisinopril: G. P. Hodsmans *et al.*, *Br. J. clin. Pharmac.*, 1984, *17*, 630P; J. P. Bussien *et al.*, *Curr. ther. Res.*, 1985, *37*, 342; E. B. Nelson *et al.*, *J. clin. Pharmac.*, 1985, *25*, 455; K. Dickstein *et al.*, *Am. Heart J.*, 1986, *112*, 121; M. S. Kochar *et al.*, *J. clin. Pharmac.*, 1987, *27*, 373.

References to the pharmacokinetics of lisinopril: A. A. Ajayi *et al.*, *Br. J. clin. Pharmac.*, 1984, *18*, 273P and 974; B. Beermann *et al.*, *J. clin. Pharmac.*, 1985, *25*, 455; B. A. M. van Schaik *et al.*, *Eur. J. clin. Pharmac.*, 1987, *32*, 11; J. G. Kelly *et al.*, *Br. J. clin. Pharmac.*, 1987, *23*, 629P.

Proprietary Preparations
Carace *(Morson, UK). Tablets*, lisinopril (as dihydrate) 2.5, 5, 10, and 20 mg.
Zestril *(ICI Pharmaceuticals, UK). Tablets*, lisinopril (as dihydrate) 2.5, 5, 10, and 20 mg.

Proprietary Names and Manufacturers
Carace *(Morson, UK)*; Prinivil *(Merck Sharp & Dohme, USA)*; Zestril *(ICI Pharmaceuticals, UK; Stuart Pharmaceuticals, USA)*.

12901-j

Lofexidine *(BAN, rINN).*
Ba-168; MDL-14042A; RMI-14042A. 2-[1-(2,6-Dichlorophenoxy)ethyl]-2-imidazoline.
$C_{11}H_{12}Cl_2N_2O$=259.1.

CAS — 31036-80-3 (lofexidine); 21498-08-8 (hydrochloride).

NOTE. Lofexidine Hydrochloride is *USAN*.

Lofexidine is an antihypertensive agent with properties similar to clonidine (p.472). It has also been studied in the control of opioid withdrawal symptoms.

HYPERTENSION. In a double-blind study involving 39 patients with mild or moderate hypertension lofexidine produced decreases in heart rate and blood pressure similar to those produced by clonidine.— H. S. Schultz *et al.*, *J. clin. Pharmac.*, 1981, *21*, 65.

Further references to the hypotensive effect of lofexidine. In general lofexidine appeared to be less potent than clonidine: W. St. J. LaCorte *et al.*, *Clin. Pharmac. Ther.*, 1981, *29*, 259; L. H. Wilkins *et al.*, *Clin. Pharmac. Ther.*, 1981, *30*, 752; T. C. Fagan *et al.*, *Br. J. clin. Pharmac.*, 1982, *13*, 405.

Study of haemodynamic and humoral effects of lofexidine.— F. M. Fouad *et al.*, *Clin. Pharmac. Ther.*, 1981, *29*, 498. See also N. D. Vlachakis *et al.*, *ibid.*, 1983, *34*, 764.

OPIOID WITHDRAWAL. Lofexidine in opioid withdrawal.— A. M. Washton *et al.* (letter), *Lancet*, 1981, *1*, 991; M. S. Gold *et al.* (letter), *ibid.*, 992.

Further references to the use of lofexidine in opioid withdrawal: A. M. Washton *et al.*, *J. clin. Psychiat.*, 1983, *44*, 335; J. Brunning *et al.*, *Alcohol Alcohol.*, 1986, *21*, 167.

Proprietary Names and Manufacturers
Nattermann, Ger.; Merrell Dow, USA.

880-c

Mecamylamine Hydrochloride *(BANM, USAN, rINNM).*
Mecamylamini Chloridum; Mecamylamini Hydrochloridum. *N*-Methyl-2,3,3-trimethylbicyclo[2.2.1]hept-2-ylamine hydrochloride.
$C_{11}H_{21}N,HCl$=203.8.

CAS — 60-40-2 (mecamylamine); 826-39-1 (hydrochloride).

Pharmacopoeias. In *Egypt.*, *Ind.*, *Int.*, *Turk.*, and *U.S.*

A white odourless or almost odourless crystalline powder. M.p. about 245° with decomposition. Freely **soluble** in water and in chloroform; soluble in isopropyl alcohol; practically insoluble in ether. **Store** in airtight containers.

Adverse Effects, Treatment, and Precautions
As for Trimetaphan Camsylate, p.503. The administration of mecamylamine may cause tremor, convulsions, choreiform movements, insomnia, sedation, dysarthria, and mental aberrations.

Absorption and Fate
Mecamylamine hydrochloride is almost completely absorbed from the gastro-intestinal tract. It diffuses across the placenta. About 50% of the dose is excreted unchanged in the urine over 24 hours, but the rate is diminished in alkaline urine.

Uses and Administration
Mecamylamine hydrochloride is a ganglion-blocking agent with actions and uses similar to those of trimetaphan (see p.503). The usual initial dosage is 2.5 mg twice daily, gradually increased or decreased, usually by increments of 2.5 mg at intervals of not less than 2 days, until a satisfactory response is obtained. Tolerance may develop.

Preparations
Mecamylamine Hydrochloride Tablets *(U.S.P.)*

Proprietary Names and Manufacturers
Inversine *(Merck Sharp & Dohme, UK; Merck Sharp & Dohme, USA)*; Mevasine *(Austral.; Neth.)*.

881-k

Methoserpidine *(BAN, rINN).*
10-Methoxydeserpidine. Methyl 11-demethoxy-10-methoxy-18-*O*-(3,4,5-trimethoxybenzoyl)reserpate.
$C_{33}H_{40}N_2O_9$=608.7.

CAS — 865-04-3.

Pharmacopoeias. In *Br.*

A cream-coloured, odourless or almost odourless, hygroscopic, microcrystalline powder. It darkens on exposure to light. Practically **insoluble** in water; soluble 1 in 60 of alcohol, 1 in 5 of chloroform, and 1 in 8 of dioxan. **Store** in well-closed containers. Protect from light.

Methoserpidine has properties and uses similar to those described under reserpine (see p.498).
In the treatment of mild or moderate hypertension the initial dose is 10 mg three times daily for at least a week. The dose is then adjusted by increments or decrements of 5 to 10 mg weekly according to the response of the patient. The maintenance dose is normally not more than 50 mg. Methoserpidine may also be given concomitantly with a diuretic.

Preparations
Methoserpidine Tablets *(B.P.)*

Proprietary Preparations
Decaserpyl *(Roussel, UK). Tablets*, scored, methoserpidine 5 and 10 mg.
Decaserpyl Plus *(Roussel, UK). Tablets*, scored, methoserpidine 10 mg, benzthiazide 20 mg.

Proprietary Names and Manufacturers
Decaserpyl *(Belg.; Fr.; Roussel, UK)*.

882-a

Methyldopa *(BAN, USAN, rINN).*
Alpha-methyldopa; Methyldopum; Methyldopum Hydratum; Metildopa; MK-351. (−)-3-(3,4-Dihydroxyphenyl)-2-methyl-L-alanine sesquihydrate; (−)-2-Amino-2-(3,4-dihydroxybenzyl)propionic acid sesquihydrate.
$C_{10}H_{13}NO_4,1\frac{1}{2}H_2O$=238.2.

CAS — 555-30-6 (anhydrous); 41372-08-1 (sesquihydrate).

Pharmacopoeias. In *Belg.*, *Br.*, *Braz.*, *Cz.*, *Egypt.*, *Eur.*,

Fr., Ind., Int., It., Jpn, Jug., Neth., Nord., Swiss, and *U.S.*

Colourless or almost colourless crystals or a white to yellowish-white odourless fine powder which may contain friable lumps. Methyldopa 1.13 g is approximately equivalent to 1 g of anhydrous methyldopa.

Slightly **soluble** in water and alcohol; practically insoluble in chloroform and ether; dissolves in dilute mineral acids. **Store** in well-closed containers. Protect from light.

Adverse Effects

The most common side-effect of methyldopa is drowsiness.

Other common side-effects include depression, psychic effects, impaired mental acuity, nightmares, nausea, dryness of the mouth, nasal stuffiness, weakness, dizziness, light-headedness, headache, oedema, and disorders of sexual function. More rarely, black or sore tongue, breast enlargement, lactation, hyperprolactinaemia, pancreatitis, salivary gland inflammation, paraesthesia, Bell's palsy, parkinsonism, gastro-intestinal upsets, diarrhoea, constipation, fever, mild arthralgia, myalgia, uraemia, myocarditis, and aggravation of angina pectoris may occur. There may be bradycardia and postural hypotension. Involuntary choreoathetotic movements have occurred in patients with severe bilateral cerebrovascular disease. Eczematous rashes and lichenoid and granulomatous skin eruptions have occurred.

Thrombocytopenia, leucopenia, granulocytopenia, and haemolytic anaemia have also been reported. A positive response to the direct Coombs' test may occur in 10 to 20% of patients on prolonged therapy, usually without evidence of haemolysis. Fever may occur within the first few weeks of therapy and may be accompanied by eosinophilia and abnormal liver function tests. Jaundice with or without fever may occur. Liver damage may also develop after long-term administration and, rarely, fatal hepatic necrosis has been reported. A condition resembling systemic lupus erythematosus has been reported.

Methyldopa may occasionally cause urine to darken on exposure to the air because of the breakdown of the drug or its metabolites.

During 1966–75 the Swedish Adverse Drug Reaction Committee received 308 reports of reactions to methyldopa including fever in 166, haemolysis in 67, hepatic effects in 29, allergic reactions in 23, gastro-intestinal symptoms in 17, and effects on the nervous system in 13. It was suggested that methyldopa should not be used as the drug of first choice in the treatment of benign hypertension.— A. -K. Furhoff, *Acta med. scand.*, 1978, *203*, 425.

A Boston Collaborative Drug Surveillance Program survey revealed that adverse reactions to methyldopa were reported by 149 of 1067 patients receiving methyldopa for hypertension. Most frequent side-effects were hypotension in 110, drowsiness in 26, depression in 5, and extrapyramidal signs and gastro-intestinal upsets in 4 each. Headaches, skin reactions, haemolytic anaemia, drug fever, bradycardia, and increase in blood-urea nitrogen occurred in 2 each, and altered liver function and disturbance in libido in 1 each. The findings suggested that methyldopa therapy should be commenced cautiously especially in younger patients, in the non-obese, and in those with impaired renal function.— D. H. Lawson *et al.*, *Am. Heart J.*, 1978, *96*, 572.

A report of asthma developing in a 27-year-old woman working in a factory where methyldopa tablets were manufactured. In a provocation test her FEV_1 fell by 30% eleven hours after exposure for 30 minutes to methyldopa dust.— M. G. Harries *et al.*, *Br. med. J.*, 1979, *1*, 1461.

EFFECTS ON THE BLOOD. An analysis of drug-induced blood dyscrasias reported to the Swedish Adverse Drug Reaction Committee for the 10-year period 1966-75 showed that haemolytic anaemia attributable to methyldopa had been reported on 69 occasions and had caused 3 deaths. This represented the vast majority of all the reports of drug-induced haemolytic anaemia.— L. E. Bottiger *et al.*, *Acta med. scand.*, 1979, *205*, 457.

Inhibition of suppressor-lymphocyte function was proposed as a cause for methyldopa-induced auto-immune haemolytic anaemia.— H. H. Kirtland *et al.*, *New Engl. J. Med.*, 1980, *302*, 825.

A study suggesting that in patients with methyldopa-induced anti-red-cell autoantibodies the absence of haemolysis is caused by impaired reticulo-endothelial function. It was considered likely that methyldopa was itself responsible for the impaired reticulo-endothelial function.— J. G. Kelton, *New Engl. J. Med.*, 1985, *313*, 596. Comment: R. P. Kimberly *et al.* (letter), *ibid.*, 1986, *314*, 248.

Reversible agranulocytosis associated with methyldopa in a 70-year-old patient was shown to be caused by the presence of methyldopa-dependent granulocyte antibodies with specificity for the drug absorbed onto the granulocytes and not for antigens on the granulocyte membrane. This mechanism differs from that postulated for auto-immune haemolytic anaemia and could explain why rapid recovery occurs when methyldopa is withdrawn.— S. P. Closs *et al.* (letter), *Lancet*, 1984, *1*, 1479.

Reports of individual cases of blood dyscrasias associated with methyldopa therapy: A. ten Pas *et al.* (letter), *Can. med. Ass. J.*, 1966, *95*, 322 (thrombocytopenia); K. G. A. Clark, *Br. med. J.*, 1967, *4*, 94 (auto-immune haemolysis and agranulocytosis); R. Greene and A. W. Spence (letter), *Br. med. J.*, 1967, *4*, 618 (neutropenia); N. G. Durgé *et al.* (letter), *Lancet*, 1968, *1*, 695 (fatal aplastic anaemia); J. M. Murdoch *et al.* (letter), *Lancet*, 1968, *1*, 207 (fatal aplastic anaemia); S. M. Manohitharajah *et al.*, *Br. med. J.*, 1971, *1*, 494 (severe thrombocytopenia with evidence of leucocyte and platelet antibodies); O. D. Polk *et al.*, *Sth. med. J.*, 1982, *75*, 374 (thrombocytopenia).

Haemolytic anaemia and hepatitis. Hepatitis and haemolytic anaemia developed in a patient taking methyldopa less than 1 g daily for over 7 years. Signs and symptoms of disease resolved when methyldopa was discontinued.— B. D. Breland and G. S. Hicks, *Drug Intell. & clin. Pharm.*, 1982, *16*, 489.

Further reports of haemolytic anaemia and hepatitis in patients taking methyldopa: O. Shalev *et al.*, *Archs intern. Med.*, 1983, *143*, 592.

EFFECTS ON THE ENDOCRINE SYSTEM. Report of 2 patients with amenorrhoea and hyperprolactinaemia associated with methyldopa. One patient also had galactorrhoea.— R. S. Arze *et al.*, *Br. med. J.*, 1981, *283*, 194.

EFFECTS ON THE GASTRO-INTESTINAL TRACT. Methyldopa produced severe colitis and hepatitis in a man on 2 occasions. Fever, rash, and eosinophilia were also present. Symptoms disappeared after discontinuing methyldopa.— H. L. Bonkowksy and J. Brisbane, *J. Am. med. Ass.*, 1976, *236*, 1602.

Reversible malabsorption in a 58-year-old man, with partial villous atrophy, inflammatory infiltrate of the mucosa, and giant-cell granuloma, was related to treatment with methyldopa.— J. M. Shneerson and B. G. Gazzard, *Br. med. J.*, 1977, *2*, 1456.

Report of 6 cases of colitis associated with methyldopa. An auto-immune mechanism was proposed.— C. F. Graham *et al.* (letter), *New Engl. J. Med.*, 1981, *304*, 1044.

Severe chronic diarrhoea was associated with methyldopa therapy for 2 years in a 62-year-old woman. Diarrhoea stopped immediately after discontinuation of methyldopa.— B. D. Quart and B. J. Guglielmo, *Drug Intell. & clin. Pharm.*, 1983, *17*, 462.

Pancreatitis. Increases in serum and urinary amylase activity accompanied by fever and suggestive of pancreatitis were associated with methyldopa in 2 patients. One patient also had symptoms of severe pancreatitis. Symptoms reappeared on rechallenge in both patients.— H. Van der Heide *et al.*, *Br. med. J.*, 1981, *282*, 1930.

Florid chronic pancreatitis with exocrine and endocrine insufficiency and heavy calcification over 30 months was associated with 2 periods of treatment with methyldopa. Symptoms during methyldopa treatment included diarrhoea, abdominal pain, and diabetic ketoacidosis.— L. E. Ramsay *et al.*, *Practitioner*, 1982, *226*, 1166.

A further case of acute pancreatitis associated with methyldopa therapy.— J. R. Anderson *et al.*, *Dig. Surg.*, 1985, *2*, 24.

EFFECTS ON THE HEART. *Myocarditis.* Five hypertensive patients being treated with methyldopa died suddenly. Autopsy revealed myocarditis in all and hepatitis in 4. Inflammatory changes were consistent with hypersensitivity. All patients had received or were receiving diuretics. Methyldopa was suspected of causing the hypersensitivity reactions.— F. G. Mullick and H. A. McAllister, *J. Am. med. Ass.*, 1977, *237*, 1699. Correction.— *ibid.*, *238*, 399.

A report of interstitial myocarditis in 6 hypertensive patients who had been treated with methyldopa in combination with other drugs. All 6 patients had died suddenly. Granulomatous pneumonitis was also diagnosed in 4 patients, and granulomatous hepatitis in 4 patients. A hypersensitivity reaction to methyldopa was suspected.— H. Seeverens *et al.*, *Acta med. scand.*, 1982, *211*, 233.

A brief discussion of the clinical features and management of myocarditis due to hypersensitivity to drugs including methyldopa.— *Lancet*, 1985, *2*, 1165.

Carotid sinus hypersensitivity. Carotid sinus hypersensitivity in 2 patients associated with methyldopa.— P. A. Alfino *et al.* (letter), *New Engl. J. Med.*, 1981, *305*, 344.

For further reports of carotid sinus hypersensitivity in patients taking methyldopa and digoxin concomitantly, see under Precautions, below.

EFFECTS ON THE LIVER. A 49-year-old woman developed granulomatous hepatitis after taking methyldopa 250 mg twice daily for only 2 days; her condition quickly improved when methyldopa was stopped and recurred when methyldopa was resumed.— A. C. Miller and W. M. Reid, *J. Am. med. Ass.*, 1976, *235*, 2001.

A report of 6 cases of hepatitis in patients taking methyldopa and a review of 77 cases from the literature. Most patients presented with nonspecific symptoms of hepatic injury including malaise, fatigue, anorexia, weight loss, nausea, and vomiting. Fever occurred in 28 of the 83 patients; rashes and eosinophilia occurred rarely. Symptoms usually began 1 to 4 weeks after the first dose of methyldopa. Clinically apparent jaundice occurred as early as 1 week and as late as 3 years after the initiation of therapy, although only 6 or 7 patients presented with jaundice later than 3 months. Liver damage was not dose-related and had features suggestive of an immunologically-mediated hypersensitivity reaction. The histological changes included chronic active hepatitis, massive fatal necrosis, and cirrhosis. — J. S. Rodman *et al.*, *Am. J. Med.*, 1976, *60*, 941.

In an analysis of 36 patients with liver damage due to methyldopa, hepatic injury tended to occur in 2 phases—acute and chronic. Acute liver damage developed within a few months of starting treatment with methyldopa, and was considered to be an allergic reaction to methyldopa metabolites. The chronic form usually occurred at least a year after starting methyldopa, and was characterised by an accumulation of fat in the liver. Recovery after withdrawal of methyldopa was directly related to duration of exposure and degree of liver damage. There was also a suggestion of genetic predisposition, as acute methyldopa-induced liver damage occurred in 4 members of a family.— E. A. Sotaniemi *et al.*, *Eur. J. clin. Pharmac.*, 1977, *12*, 429.

Investigation of the mechanisms involved in methyldopa-induced hepatotoxicity suggested that it was related to metabolic activation of methyldopa and the production of drug-associated antigen.— J. Neuberger *et al.*, *Gut*, 1985, *26*, 1232.

For reports of hepatitis in association with haemolytic anaemia, see under Effects on the Blood, above.

EFFECTS ON MEMORY. A study suggesting that methyldopa therapy was associated with serious verbal memory impairment.— S. Solomon *et al.*, *Archs gen. Psychiat.*, 1983, *40*, 1109.

EFFECTS ON THE NERVOUS SYSTEM. Methyldopa, 1 g daily increased after 22 days to 1.5 g daily for hypertension, caused involuntary choreoathetotic movements resembling those of Huntington's chorea in a 59-year-old man with cerebrovascular disease. He recovered when methyldopa therapy was withdrawn.— A. Yamadori and M. L. Albert (letter), *New Engl. J. Med.*, 1972, *286*, 610.

Bilateral choreiform movements associated with methyldopa occurred in a patient with deteriorating renal function but no history of cerebrovascular disease.— E. M. Neil and A. K. Waters, *Postgrad. med. J.*, 1981, *57*, 732.

EFFECTS ON SEXUAL FUNCTION. Seven of 27 men, aged 43 to 64 years, had some disorder of sexual function a few days after starting to take methyldopa 0.5 to 2 g daily; there were no similar effects in 22 comparable patients treated with a thiazide.— R. J. Newman and H. R. Salerno (letter), *Br. med. J.*, 1974, *4*, 106.

In 30 men taking methyldopa the incidence of failure of erection was 7% (volunteered) or 53% after specific questioning.— W. D. Alexander and J. I. Evans (letter), *Br. med. J.*, 1975, *2*, 501.

A brief review of the effects of methyldopa on sexual function. Effects reported in males included failure to maintain erection, decreased libido, ejaculatory difficulties, and gynaecomastia. In females, decreased libido, painful breast enlargement, and delayed orgasm or failure to achieve orgasm had been reported.— J. G.

Stevenson and G. S. Umstead, *Drug Intell. & clin. Pharm.*, 1984, *18*, 113. See also L. Beeley, *Adverse Drug React. Ac. Pois. Rev.*, 1984, *3*, 23.

EFFECTS ON THE SKIN AND MUCOUS MEMBRANES. Tongue ulceration with features of lichen planus was associated with methyldopa in 3 patients, and a fixed drug reaction in 1 patient.— J. N. Burry and J. Kirk (letter), *Br. J. Derm.*, 1974, *91*, 475.

Lichenoid eruption due to methyldopa in 1 patient.— P. J. A. Holt and A. Navaratnam, *Br. med. J.*, 1974, *3*, 234.

A review of 17 patients who had persistent oral ulceration while taking methyldopa. Relief and healing occurred after methyldopa was withdrawn but took several months in some patients.— K. D. Hay and P. C. Reade, *Br. dent. J.*, 1978, *145*, 195.

FEVER. Report of 78 cases of methyldopa-induced fever. Fever occurred 5 to 35 days after the first exposure to methyldopa in 77 patients and one day after recommencing methyldopa in the remaining patient. Rigors, headache, and myalgia were common accompanying symptoms, but eosinophilia and skin rashes were not seen. The majority of patients did not appear seriously ill, but 4 patients presented the picture of septic shock. Biochemical evidence of liver damage was found in 61% of patients but jaundice was uncommon. In the majority of patients, symptoms were relieved within 48 hours of the withdrawal of the drug.— P. Stanley and A. Mijch, *Med. J. Aust.*, 1986, *144*, 603.

A survey and retrospective analysis of 148 episodes of drug fever showed that methyldopa was responsible for the fever in 16 cases and was one of the most frequently cited agents.— P. A. Mackowiak and C. F. LeMaistre, *Ann. intern. Med.*, 1987, *106*, 728.

LUPUS ERYTHEMATOSUS. The incidence of antinuclear antibodies was 13% in 269 hypertensive patients taking methyldopa (irrespective of other medication), compared with 3.8% in 448 hypertensive patients not taking methyldopa. Apart from the occasional case of methyldopa-induced lupus, however, patients did not appear to be at risk.— J. D. Wilson *et al.*, *Br. med. J.*, 1978, *1*, 14.

A report of a lupus-like syndrome induced by methyldopa.— A. Dupont and R. Six, *Br. med. J.*, 1982, *285*, 693. See also T. H. Harrington and D. E. Davis, *Chest*, 1981, *79*, 696.

OVERDOSAGE. Ingestion of methyldopa 2.5 g produced coma, hypothermia, hypotension, bradycardia, and dry mouth in a 19-year-old man. The serum-methyldopa concentration 10 hours after ingestion was 19.2 µg per mL compared with serum concentrations of approximately 2 µg per mL in patients receiving therapeutic doses of methyldopa. The patient recovered following treatment with intravenous fluids.— Y. Shnaps *et al.*, *J. Toxicol. clin. Toxicol.*, 1982, *19*, 501.

RETROPERITONEAL FIBROSIS. A 60-year-old patient developed retroperitoneal fibrosis and a positive direct Coombs' test associated with methyldopa given in a daily dose of 750 mg with bendrofluazide 2.5 mg for about 5 years.— B. M. Iversen *et al.*, *Lancet*, 1975, *2*, 302. Further references: S. Ahmad, *Am. Heart J.*, 1983, *105*, 1037.

Treatment of Adverse Effects

Withdrawal of methyldopa or reduction in dosage causes the reversal of many side-effects. If overdosage occurs the stomach should be emptied by aspiration and lavage. Treatment is largely symptomatic, but if necessary, intravenous infusions may be given to promote urinary excretion, and pressor agents given cautiously. Methyldopa is dialysable.

Precautions

Methyldopa should be used with caution in patients with impaired kidney or liver function or with a history of liver disease or mental depression. It should not be given to patients with active liver disease and it is not recommended for phaeochromocytoma.

It is advisable to make blood counts and to perform liver-function tests at intervals during the first 6 to 12 weeks of treatment or if the patient develops an unexplained fever. Patients taking methyldopa may produce a positive response to a direct Coombs' test; if blood transfusion is required, prior knowledge of a positive direct Coombs' test reaction will aid cross matching.

Lower doses of general anaesthetics may be required in patients taking methyldopa. Methyldopa has been reported to aggravate porphyria. The hypotensive effects of methyldopa are enhanced by thiazide diuretics and other antihypertensive agents. Methyldopa may interfere with the measurement of urinary uric acid by the phosphotungstate method, serum creatinine by the alkaline picrate method, and AST (SGOT) by the colorimetric method. Interference with spectrophotometric methods for AST analysis has not been reported. Methyldopa fluoresces at the same wavelengths as catecholamines and may cause spurious reports of elevated urinary catecholamine concentrations. Tests which measure vanillylmandelic acid (VMA) by the conversion of VMA to vanillin are not affected.

Mention of tablets containing racemic methyldopa, which would be only partially effective, available in Nigeria.— O. Ogunyemi, *Br. med. J.*, 1983, *286*, 1956.

Results of a double-blind crossover study in 14 hypertensive patients with intermittent claudication demonstrated that peak hyperaemic calf blood flow was reduced by either metoprolol or methyldopa compared with placebo. Antihypertensive treatment should be used with care in patients with intermittent claudication.— M. Lepäntalo, *Br. J. clin. Pharmac.*, 1984, *18*, 90.

INTERACTIONS. *Alpha-adrenoceptor antagonists.* Urinary incontinence on concomitant administration of methyldopa and phenoxybenzamine in a patient who had undergone bilateral lumbar sympathectomy.— P. G. Fernandez *et al.*, *Can. med. Ass. J.*, 1981, *124*, 174.

Antipsychotic agents. A woman with systemic lupus erythematosus taking trifluoperazine up to 15 mg daily and prednisone up to 120 mg daily was given methyldopa up to 2 g and triamterene for high blood pressure. Her blood pressure rose further to 200/140 mmHg. After discontinuation of trifluoperazine blood pressure returned to 160/100 mmHg.— F. B. Westervelt and N. O. Atuk (letter), *J. Am. med. Ass.*, 1974, *227*, 557.

Two patients with essential hypertension who had been receiving methyldopa for 3 years and 18 months respectively developed symptoms of dementia within days of concurrent administration of haloperidol for anxiety. In both patients the symptoms resolved rapidly on discontinuation of haloperidol.— W. E. Thornton, *New Engl. J. Med.*, 1976, *294*, 1222.

Digoxin. A report of syncope associated with carotid sinus hypersensitivity possibly enhanced by methyldopa in a patient taking digoxin and chlorthalidone.— R. Bauernfeind *et al.*, *Ann. intern. Med.*, 1978, *88*, 214.

Symptomatic sinus bradycardia developed in 2 patients taking methyldopa and digoxin concomitantly.— J. C. Davis *et al.*, *J. Am. med. Ass.*, 1981, *245*, 1241.

Levodopa. For reference to a mutual interaction between methyldopa and levodopa see Levodopa, p.1017.

Lithium carbonate. For reference to the development of lithium toxicity on concurrent administration of methyldopa, see Lithium Carbonate, p.368.

Non-steroidal anti-inflammatory drugs. The action of methyldopa may be reduced by concurrent administration of non-steroidal anti-inflammatory drugs, see p.466.

Sympathomimetics. A 31-year-old man whose hypertension was well controlled with methyldopa and oxprenolol suffered a severe hypertensive episode when he took a preparation for a cold containing phenylpropanolamine.— E. H. McLaren, *Br. med. J.*, 1976, *2*, 283.

PORPHYRIA. Methyldopa was considered to be unsafe in patients with acute porphyria as it has been associated with acute attacks.— M.R. Moore and K.E.L. McColl, *Porphyrias, Drug Lists*, Glasgow, Porphyria Research Unit, University of Glasgow, 1987.

PREGNANCY AND THE NEONATE. Reduced blood pressure in the infants of mothers given methyldopa.— A. Whitelaw, *Br. med. J.*, 1981, *283*, 471.

Tremor in 7 infants was associated with maternal methyldopa therapy during pregnancy. Depressed cerebrospinal fluid noradrenaline concentrations were noted in the 3 infants examined leading to successful treatment of the other 4 infants with atropine: tremor was abolished in 2 and substantially reduced in the other 2 infants.— J. Bodis *et al.* (letter), *Lancet*, 1982, *2*, 498.

No evidence of developmental retardation was found in children whose mothers had received methyldopa prior to 21-weeks' gestation, at 4 years of age (M. Ounsted, *Lancet*, 1980, *1*, 705) and 7½ years of age (J. Cockburn *et al.*, *ibid.*, 1982, *1*, 647). There was also no difference in the blood pressure of children aged 7½ years whose mothers had received methyldopa during pregnancy compared with those who had received no specific treatment (M.K. Ounsted *et al.*, *Archs Dis. Childh.*, 1985, *60*, 631).

Absorption and Fate

Methyldopa is incompletely and variably absorbed from the gastro-intestinal tract. It is partly conjugated, mainly to the O-sulphate, and is excreted by the kidneys. Elimination follows a biphasic pattern with a half-life of about 1.7 hours during the initial phase. Plasma protein binding is reported to be minimal. It crosses the placenta and small amounts appear in breast milk.

A study of the pharmacokinetics of methyldopa in 5 healthy subjects.— Ø. Stenbaek *et al.*, *Eur. J. clin. Pharmac.*, 1977, *12*, 117.

Metabolic disposition of methyldopa in hypertensive and renal-insufficient children.— R. F. O'Dea and B. L. Mirkin, *Clin. Pharmac. Ther.*, 1980, *27*, 37.

Absorption of methyldopa was decreased in 10 patients with Crohn's disease compared with 10 healthy subjects. In 5 patients with coeliac disease methyldopa appeared to be absorbed normally, but the plasma concentrations of free and conjugated methyldopa were higher than expected.— A. G. Renwick *et al.*, *Br. J. clin. Pharmac.*, 1983, *16*, 77.

PREGNANCY AND THE NEONATE. Results of a preliminary study conducted around the time of delivery in 12 women who had received methyldopa 0.75 to 2 g daily for at least 4 weeks up to the time of delivery. Concentrations of both free and conjugated methyldopa were similar in maternal and foetal plasma but in the amniotic fluid total concentrations and the proportion of conjugated drug were generally higher than in the plasma. Milk samples collected from 3 women between 30 and 60 hours after delivery contained very small amounts of methyldopa, most of which was conjugated.— H. M. R. Jones and A. J. Cummings (letter), *Br. J. clin. Pharmac.*, 1978, *6*, 432.

Uses and Administration

Methyldopa is an antihypertensive agent which is thought to have a predominantly central action. It is decarboxylated in the CNS to alpha-methylnoradrenaline which stimulates alpha$_2$-adrenoceptors resulting in a reduction in sympathetic tone and a fall in blood pressure. Methyldopa reduces the tissue concentrations of dopamine, noradrenaline, adrenaline, and serotonin.

When administered by mouth its effects reach a maximum in 4 to 6 hours following a single dose, although the maximum hypotensive effect may not occur until the second day of continuous treatment; some effect is still usually apparent until 48 hours after withdrawal of methyldopa.

Methyldopa is used in the treatment of moderate to severe hypertension usually in combination with a diuretic or a beta-blocking agent. It reduces the standing blood pressure and also reduces the supine blood pressure.

The usual initial dose by mouth is the equivalent of 250 mg of anhydrous methyldopa two or three times daily for 2 days; this is then adjusted by small increments or decrements not more frequently than every 2 days according to the response of the patient. Although higher doses have been given it is generally considered that no advantage can be gained by giving doses larger than 3 g daily. The usual maintenance dosage is the equivalent of 0.5 to 2 g of anhydrous methyldopa daily.

To reduce side-effects smaller doses of methyldopa may be given in conjunction with a thiazide diuretic, which would also reduce the oedema that sometimes occurs with methyldopa therapy. Tolerance may develop.

A suggested initial dose for children is 10 mg per kg body-weight daily in 2 to 4 divided doses, increased as necessary to a maximum of 65 mg per kg or 3 g daily whichever is less.

For hypertensive crises, methyldopa has been given intravenously as methyldopate hydrochloride (see below).

An account of the development of methyldopa.— A. Sjoerdsma, *Br. J. clin. Pharmac.*, 1982, *13*, 45.

The pharmacology of centrally acting antihypertensive agents including methyldopa.— P. A. van Zwieten *et al.*, *Br. J. clin. Pharmac.*, 1983, *15*, *Suppl.* 4, 455S. See also E. D. Frohlich, *Archs intern. Med.*, 1980, *140*, 954.

In a study of 10 hypertensive diabetic patients methyldopa treatment produced no changes in the concentrations of high-density lipoproteins or cholesterol, but produced a reduction in free fatty acids and an increase in triglyceride concentrations.— G. F. A. Benfield and K. R. Hunter, *Br. J. clin. Pharmac.*, 1982, *13*, 219. Methyldopa reduced the high-density lipoprotein cholesterol concentration by about 10%, and increased the total cholesterol to high-density lipoprotein ratio in a study of 14 patients.— A. S. Leon *et al.*, *J. clin. Pharmac.*, 1984, *24*, 209. Further reference to the effects of methyldopa on plasma lipids: M. Velasco *et al.*, *Eur. J. clin. Pharmac.*, 1985, *28*, 513.

ADMINISTRATION IN RENAL FAILURE. Methyldopa could be administered to patients with renal failure by adjusting the dosage interval. A dosage interval of 6 hours is suitable for patients whose glomerular filtration-rates exceed 50 mL per minute; an interval of 9 to 18 hours between doses is advisable for rates between 10 and 50 mL per minute. Where the rate is less than 10 mL per minute, the dosage interval should be 12 to 24 hours. A dose supplement should be given to patients undergoing haemodialysis or peritoneal dialysis.— W. M. Bennett *et al.*, *Am. J. Kidney Dis.*, 1983, *3*, 155.

DYSKINESIAS. Methyldopa 250 mg three times daily for 2 weeks or a placebo was added to the usual neuroleptic medication of 15 psychogeriatric patients with severe dyskinesias. Tremor, rigidity, and dystonic spasms were significantly relieved but oro-facial dyskinesias, akinesia, and akathisia were not.— M. Viukari and M. Linnoila, *Curr. ther. Res.*, 1975, *18*, 417.

A double-blind study in 30 patients indicating that methyldopa 750 to 1500 mg daily or reserpine 0.75 to 1.5 mg daily were both effective in reducing the symptoms of tardive dyskinesia.— C. C. Huang *et al.*, *Psychopharmacology*, 1981, *73*, 359.

HYPERTENSION. Methyldopa may be used to control hypertension in patients in whom a diuretic alone is inadequate and a beta-blocker is contra-indicated, though many authorities would now use a calcium antagonist. Methyldopa is still used for the treatment of hypertension in pregnancy. Parenteral methyldopa acts too slowly to produce satisfactory reduction of blood pressure in an emergency.— *Drug & Ther. Bull.*, 1984, *22*, 42.

In a double-blind study of 9 patients with essential hypertension methyldopa was shown to reduce the tachycardia produced by hydralazine when used with hydralazine and a diuretic as part of "triple therapy".— J. D. Skehan *et al.*, *Br. J. clin. Pharmac.*, 1985, *19*, 134P. See also P. Ward and C. V. S. Ram, *Clin. Pharmac. Ther.*, 1984, *35*, 280.

Methyldopa 125 or 250 mg twice daily was effective in controlling mild to moderate hypertension in the majority of 30 patients.— L. Corea *et al.*, *Curr. ther. Res.*, 1983, *34*, 217.

Results of a crossover study in 7 patients with hypertension not controlled by concomitant administration of cyclopenthiazide, propranolol, and hydralazine. Further reduction in blood pressure could be achieved by the addition of methyldopa, guanethidine, or prazosin to existing treatment. Methyldopa was tolerated slightly better than prazosin, and guanethidine was least well tolerated.— M. J. Vandenburg *et al.*, *Br. J. clin. Pract.*, 1985, *39*, 17.

For the use of methyldopa in hypertension in pregnancy, see under Pregnancy and the Neonate, below.

Effect on plasma renin. In a study of 40 hypertensive patients classified as having high, normal, or low plasma-renin activity, the fall in blood pressure following administration of methyldopa was similar in all groups. Although a reduction in plasma-renin activity was observed in the majority of patients, plasma-renin activity did not appear to be of great value in predicting the effectiveness of methyldopa.— H. Gavras *et al.*, *J. clin. Pharmac.*, 1977, *17*, 372.

Results of a study indicating that methyldopa has a favourable effect on renal haemodynamics which may be beneficial in some situations.— P. L. Malini *et al.*, *Curr. ther. Res.*, 1983, *33*, 279.

Single bedtime dosage. In a preliminary double-blind crossover study of 14 hypertensive patients adequately controlled by methyldopa, the daily amount required was found to be as efficacious when given as a single dose at bedtime as when given as a three times daily regimen. A further 3 patients were dropped from the study: 1 owing to non-compliance, 1 owing to altered liver-function values, and 1 owing to an intolerable swimming sensation in her head and insomnia on taking what proved to be methyldopa 750 mg at night.— J. M. Wright *et al.*, *Clin. Pharmac. Ther.*, 1976, *20*, 733. Results of a study in 12 patients suggesting that single daily dosing of methyldopa could not be recommended for most patients. The antihypertensive effect of methyldopa reached a maximum after 6 to 9 hours and declined thereafter with a half-life of approximately 10 hours. Little hypertensive effect remained 24 to 26 hours after the dose.— J. M. Wright *et al.*, *Br. J. clin. Pharmac.*, 1982, *13*, 847. See also B. A. Gould *et al.*, *Clin. Pharmac. Ther.*, 1983, *33*, 438.

MENOPAUSAL SYMPTOMS. Methyldopa reduced the incidence of hot flushes in 26 of 28 menopausal women compared with placebo in a double-blind crossover study in general practice, but the incidence of side-effects and the lack of effect on the vaginal mucosa was considered to limit the usefulness of methyldopa in this condition.— B. -I. Nesheim and T. Saetre, *Eur. J. clin. Pharmac.*, 1981, *20*, 413.

Further references to the effects of methyldopa on menopausal flushes: T. Tulandi *et al.*, *Am. J. Obstet. Gynec.*, 1984, *150*, 709.

PREGNANCY AND THE NEONATE. *Hypertension in pregnancy.* Methyldopa was still considered the drug of first choice for treatment of hypertension during pregnancy.— *Drug & Ther. Bull.*, 1982, *20*, 1. See also P. C. Rubin, *Prescribers' J.*, 1985, *25*, 19.

In a randomised study of 100 pregnant women with mild to moderate hypertension treated with either methyldopa or oxprenolol no significant differences in final foetal outcome were shown, although methyldopa may have been superior to oxprenolol in controlling the blood pressure in those presenting early in pregnancy.— J. Fidler *et al.*, *Br. med. J.*, 1983, *286*, 1927.

Control of hypertension was equivalent in 183 pregnant women randomly allocated to treatment with either methyldopa or oxprenolol. However there was evidence of greater foetal benefit in patients treated with oxprenolol although the difference decreased with continuing treatment and there was no difference between the two groups after 10 weeks of treatment.— E. D. M. Gallery *et al.*, *Br. med. J.*, 1985, *291*, 563.

Further references to the use of methyldopa in pregnancy: C. W. G. Redman *et al.*, *Lancet*, 1976, *2*, 753.

See also under Precautions, above.

Preparations

Methyldopa Tablets *(B.P.)*

Methyldopa Tablets *(U.S.P.)*

Methyldopa and Chlorothiazide Tablets *(U.S.P.)*

Methyldopa and Hydrochlorothiazide Tablets *(U.S.P.)*

Methyldopa Oral Suspension *(U.S.P.)*

Proprietary Preparations

Aldomet *(Merck Sharp & Dohme, UK). Tablets*, methyldopa equivalent to anhydrous methyldopa 125, 250, and 500 mg.

Suspension, methyldopa equivalent to anhydrous methyldopa 250 mg/5 mL.

Dopamet *(Berk Pharmaceuticals, UK). Tablets*, methyldopa equivalent to anhydrous methyldopa 125, 250, and 500 mg.

Hydromet *(Merck Sharp & Dohme, UK). Tablets*, methyldopa equivalent to anhydrous methyldopa 250 mg, hydrochlorothiazide 15 mg.

Proprietary Names and Manufacturers

Aldomet *(Arg.; Merck Sharp & Dohme, Austral.; Merck Sharp & Dohme, Canad.; Denm.; Merck Sharp & Dohme-Chibret, Fr.; Merck Sharp & Dohme, Ital.; Neth.; Merck Sharp & Dohme, Norw.; Merck Sharp & Dohme, S.Afr.; Merck Sharp & Dohme, Spain; MSD, Swed.; Merck Sharp & Dohme, Switz.; Merck Sharp & Dohme, UK; Merck Sharp & Dohme, USA)*; Aldometil *(Merck Sharp & Dohme, Ger.)*; Alphamex *(S.Afr.)*; Baypresol *(Spain)*; Co-Caps Methyldopa *(DDSA Pharmaceuticals, UK)*; Dimal *(Protea, Austral.)*; Dopamet *(ICN, Canad.; Dumex, Denm.; Dumex, Norw.; Dumex, Swed.; Dumex, Switz.; Berk Pharmaceuticals, UK)*; Dopegyt *(Hung.)*; Elanpress *(Recordati, Ital.)*; Equibar *(Biogalenique, Fr.)*; Grospisk *(Jpn)*; Hyperpax *(Erco, Denm.; Neth.; Norw.; Ercopharm, Switz.)*; Hyperpaxa *(Swed.)*; Hypodopa *(Wilson, Pakistan)*; Hypolar *(Lagap, UK)*; Hy-po-tone *(Lennon, S.Afr.)*; Medimet-250 *(Canad.)*; Medomet *(DDSA Pharmaceuticals, UK)*; Medopa *(Jpn)*; Medopal *(Apothekernes Laboratorium, Norw.)*; Medopren *(Malesci, Ital.)*; Methopa *(USV, Austral.)*; Methoplain *(Jpn)*; Mulfasin *(Neth.)*; Normopress *(Schwulst, S.Afr.)*; Novomedopa *(Novopharm, Canad.)*; Presinol *(Belg.; Bayer, Ger.; Bayropharm, Ital.)*; Sembrina *(Boehringer Mannheim, Ger.; Boehringer Ingelheim, Ital.; Neth.; Boehringer Mannheim, Switz.)*; Sinepress *(Rolab, S.Afr.)*.

The following names have been used for multi-ingredient preparations containing methyldopa— Aldoclor *(Merck Sharp & Dohme, USA)*; Aldoril *(Merck Sharp & Dohme, Canad.; Merck Sharp & Dohme, USA)*; Apo-Methazide *(Apotex, Canad.)*; Dopazide *(Pharmascience, Canad.)*; Hydromet *(Merck Sharp & Dohme, UK)*; Novodoparil *(Novopharm, Canad.)*; Supres *(Frosst, Canad.)*.

883-t

Methyldopate Hydrochloride *(BANM, USAN)*.

Cloridrato de Metildopato. The hydrochloride of the ethyl ester of anhydrous methyldopa; Ethyl (−)-2-amino-2-(3,4-dihydroxybenzyl)propionate hydrochloride.

$C_{12}H_{17}NO_4,HCl=275.7$.

CAS — 2544-09-4 (methyldopate); 2508-79-4 (hydrochloride).

Pharmacopoeias. In *Br., Braz.,* and *U.S.*

A white or almost white, odourless or almost odourless, crystalline powder. **Soluble** 1 in 1 of water, 1 in 3 of alcohol, and 1 in 2 of methyl alcohol; slightly soluble in chloroform; practically insoluble in ether. A 1% solution in water has a pH of 3.0 to 5.0; the *B.P.* injection has a pH of 3.5 to 4.2. Solutions for injection are **sterilised** by filtration. **Protect** from light.

INCOMPATIBILITY. A haze developed over 3 hours when methyldopate hydrochloride 1 g per litre was mixed with amphotericin 200 mg per litre in glucose injection; crystals were produced with methohexitone sodium 200 mg per litre in sodium chloride injection, but a haze developed when they were mixed in glucose injection. A crystalline precipitate occurred with tetracycline hydrochloride 1 g per litre in glucose injection, and with sulphadiazine sodium 4 g per litre in glucose injection or sodium chloride injection.— B. B. Riley, *J. Hosp. Pharm.*, 1970, *28*, 228.

Adverse Effects, Treatment, and Precautions

As for Methyldopa p.488.

HYPERTENSION. Paradoxical hypertension occurred in a patient following the intravenous infusion of methyldopate 125 mg.— C. G. Zehnle, *Am. J. Hosp. Pharm.*, 1981, *38*, 1774.

Uses and Administration

Methyldopate hydrochloride has the actions described under methyldopa (see above) and has been administered by intravenous infusion in the treatment of hypertensive crises. The hypotensive effect may be obtained within 4 to 6 hours and last for 10 to 16 hours. A paradoxical pressor response may occasionally occur.

The usual dose is 250 to 500 mg in 100 mL of glucose injection administered over 30 to 60 minutes every 6 hours. It is suggested that the dose should not exceed 1 g every 6 hours. A suggested dose for children is 5 to 10 mg per kg body-weight every 6 hours. The maximum recommended daily dose for children is 65 mg per kg or 3.0 g, whichever is less.

Preparations

Methyldopate Injection *(B.P.)*. Contains methyldopate hydrochloride; not more than 10% of the declared content is due to methyldopa.

Methyldopate Hydrochloride Injection *(U.S.P.)*

Proprietary Preparations

Aldomet *(Merck Sharp & Dohme, UK). Injection*, methyldopate hydrochloride 50 mg/mL, in ampoules of 5 mL.

Proprietary Names and Manufacturers

Aldomet Injection *(Merck Sharp & Dohme, UK; Merck Sharp & Dohme, USA)*.

15325-f

Metirosine *(BAN, rINN).*

L-588357-0; Metyrosine *(USAN)*. (−)-α-Methyl-L-tyrosine.

$C_{10}H_{13}NO_3$=195.2.

CAS — 672-87-7; 620-30-4 (racemetirosine).

NOTE. The term α-methyltyrosine (α-MPT; α-MT; α-methyl-*p*-tyrosine) is used below since although metirosine, the (−)-isomer, is the active form the manufacturers state that some racemate (racemetirosine; (±)-α-methyl-DL-tyrosine) is produced during synthesis but that the material supplied contains mainly (−)-isomer with a small amount of (+)-isomer.

The code name MK 781, applied to earlier investigational material, may have described a racemate or a preparation containing a smaller proportion of (−)-isomer than the product now available commercially.

Potency of the proprietary preparation (Demser) is expressed in terms of metirosine.

Pharmacopoeias. In *U.S.*

Adverse Effects

Sedation occurs in the majority of patients receiving α-methyltyrosine. Extrapyramidal symptoms, anxiety, depression, and psychic disturbances including hallucinations, disorientation, and confusion, and diarrhoea have also been reported. Crystalluria, transient dysuria, and haematuria have been seen in a few patients. Other adverse effects reported occasionally include slight swelling of the breast, galactorrhoea, nasal stuffiness, decreased salivation, gastro-intestinal disturbances, headache, impotence or failure of ejaculation, and allergic reactions. Eosinophilia, raised serum aspartate aminotransferase, and peripheral oedema have been reported rarely.

Hypotension and cardiac arrhythmias may occur during surgery for phaeochromocytoma, when α-methyltyrosine is used pre-operatively. Life-threatening arrhythmias may require treatment with a beta-blocking agent or lignocaine.

Neuroleptic malignant syndrome occurred after the use of the dopamine-depleting agents tetrabenazine and α-methyltyrosine in a patient with Huntington's chorea.— R. E. Burke *et al., Neurology*, 1981, *31*, 1022.

Precautions

To minimise the risk of crystalluria, patients receiving α-methyltyrosine should have a fluid intake sufficient to maintain a urine volume of at least 2 litres daily and their urine should be examined regularly for the presence of crystals.

α-Methyltyrosine has sedative effects and patients should be warned of the hazards of driving a motor vehicle or operating machinery while receiving the drug. It may have additive effects with alcohol and other CNS depressants. The extrapyramidal effects of phenothiazines or haloperidol may be exacerbated. Symptoms of psychic stimulation and insomnia may occur when α-methyltyrosine is withdrawn.

When α-methyltyrosine is used pre-operatively in patients with phaeochromocytoma, blood pressure and the ECG should be monitored continuously during surgery. Blood volume must be maintained during and after surgery, particularly if an alpha-adrenoceptor blocking agent is used concurrently.

α-Methyltyrosine may cause spurious increases in urinary catecholamines because of the presence of metabolites of the drug.

Absorption and Fate

α-Methyltyrosine is well absorbed from the gastro-intestinal tract and is excreted mainly unchanged by the kidneys. A plasma half-life of 3.4 to 7.2 hours has been reported. Less than 0.5% of a dose may be excreted as the metabolites α-methyldopa, α-methyldopamine, α-methylnoradrenaline, and α-methyltyramine.

Uses and Administration

α-Methyltyrosine is an inhibitor of the enzyme tyrosine hydroxylase, and consequently of the synthesis of catecholamines. It is used to control the symptoms of excessive sympathetic stimulation in patients with phaeochromocytoma and decreases the frequency and severity of hypertensive attacks and related symptoms in most patients. It may be given for pre-operative preparation, to those patients for whom surgery is contra-indicated, or for long-term management in those with malignant phaeochromocytoma.

α-Methyltyrosine is given by mouth in a dose of 250 mg four times daily, increased daily by 250 mg or 500 mg to a maximum of 4 g daily in divided doses. The optimum dose, achieved by monitoring clinical symptoms and catecholamine excretion, is usually in the range of 2 to 3 g daily and when used pre-operatively it should be given for at least 5 to 7 days before surgery.

The concomitant use of alpha-adrenoceptor blocking agents may be necessary.

α-Methyltyrosine is not effective in controlling essential hypertension.

A review of the pharmacology and clinical use of α-methyltyrosine.— R. N. Brogden *et al., Drugs*, 1981, *21*, 81.

PHAEOCHROMOCYTOMA. Reviews of the use of α-methyltyrosine in phaeochromocytoma: *Lancet*, 1968, *2*, 1130; *Med. Lett.*, 1980, *22*, 28.

Long-term α-methyltyrosine therapy was associated with a reduction in the size of a functional pulmonary metastasis in a patient with malignant phaeochromocytoma.— O. Serri *et al.* (letter), *New Engl. J. Med.*, 1984, *310*, 1264.

SCHIZOPHRENIA. In a study of 10 patients with psychotic diseases given α-methyltyrosine up to 4 g daily, 5 of 7 of the patients with mania improved significantly and in 3 this continued after treatment was stopped. The 3 patients with depression became worse and improved when treatment was discontinued. Hypotension, lethargy, and day-time sedation occurred in patients given doses of over 2 g daily.— H. K. H. Brodie *et al., Clin. Pharmac. Ther.*, 1971, *12*, 218.

Preparations

Metyrosine Capsules *(U.S.P.)*. Capsules containing metirosine.

Proprietary Preparations

Demser *(Merck Sharp & Dohme, UK). Capsules*, metirosine 250 mg.

Proprietary Names and Manufacturers

Demser *(Neth.; Merck Sharp & Dohme, UK; Merck Sharp & Dohme, USA).*

884-x

Minoxidil *(BAN, USAN, rINN).*

Minoxidilum; U-10858. 2,6-Diamino-4-piperidinopyrimidine 1-oxide.

$C_9H_{15}N_5O$=209.3.

CAS — 38304-91-5.

Pharmacopoeias. In *U.S.*

A white or off-white crystalline powder. **Soluble** in alcohol and in propylene glycol; sparingly soluble in methyl alcohol; slightly soluble in water; practically insoluble in chloroform, in acetone, in ethyl acetate, and in light petroleum.

Adverse Effects and Treatment

Adverse effects commonly caused by minoxidil include reflex tachycardia, fluid retention accompanied by weight gain, oedema, and sometimes congestive heart failure and changes in the ECG. Reversible hypertrichosis is also very common and normally occurs within 3 to 6 weeks of the start of minoxidil therapy. Pericardial effusion, sometimes with associated tamponade, has been reported in about 3% of patients. Administration of minoxidil may aggravate or uncover angina pectoris. Other less frequent adverse effects include nausea, gynaecomastia and breast tenderness, polymenorrhoea, allergic skin rashes, and thrombocytopenia.

Reflex tachycardia can be overcome by the concomitant administration of a beta-blocking agent or methyldopa, and frusemide or a similar diuretic is used to reduce fluid retention. If excessive hypotension occurs, an intravenous infusion of electrolytes can be given to maintain the blood pressure. If a pressor agent is necessary, drugs such as adrenaline which can aggravate tachycardia should be avoided, and phenylephrine, vasopressin, or dopamine should be given only if there is evidence of inadequate perfusion of a vital organ. Minoxidil is dialysable.

Thrombocytopenia associated with the use of minoxidil.— S. J. Peitzman and C. Martin (letter), *Ann. intern. Med.*, 1980, *92*, 874.

A 2-year-old boy estimated to have taken 20 tablets of minoxidil 5 mg suffered no symptoms other than reflex tachycardia.— C. Isles *et al.* (letter), *Lancet*, 1981, *1*, 97.

EFFECTS ON BLOOD PRESSURE. Significant decreases in blood pressure were noted in 7 of 30 normotensive patients during the topical administration of a 3% minoxidil solution twice daily for alopecia.— R. E. Ranchoff and W. F. Bergfeld (letter), *J. Am. Acad. Derm.*, 1985, *12*, 586.

EFFECTS ON THE EYES. Bilateral optic neuritis and retinitis occurred in a patient during treatment with minoxidil for hypertension following a renal transplant. The patient was also taking prednisolone and azathioprine.— G. M. Gombos, *Ann. Ophthal.*, 1983, *15*, 259.

EFFECTS ON THE HEART. Pericardial effusions occurred in 7 of 18 patients given minoxidil for refractory hypertension; 6 of the 7 were symptom-free. Of the 7, four were on dialysis for terminal renal failure and 1 had moderate renal insufficiency. A review of the manufacturer's records on 1760 patients showed that 53 patients developed pericardial effusions of whom 36 had renal impairment or some other cause for their pericarditis. Effusion disappeared spontaneously without treatment in 5 of the remaining 17 patients despite their continuing minoxidil. Of 18 affected patients on haemodialysis 7 developed fatal tamponade. It was considered that pericardial effusions in patients without renal impairment might be part of the general fluid retention associated with minoxidil; their incidence might be reduced by controlling fluid weight gain.— A. Marquez-Julio and P. R. Uldall (letter), *Lancet*, 1977, *2*, 816. Pericardial effusion occurred in 9 out of 37 patients treated with minoxidil. Transient pericarditis occurred in a tenth patient. A causal relationship was suggested in 5 cases.— M. J. Reichgott, *Clin. Pharmac. Ther.*, 1981, *30*, 64.

It was considered that minoxidil-induced pericardial effusion in 1 patient was not attributable to salt and water retention or reduced renal function.— D. B. Webb and R. J. Whale, *Postgrad. med. J.*, 1982, *58*, 319.

Pericardial effusion was reported in a patient taking minoxidil whose only symptom was dysphagia.— B. A. Baker *et al.* (letter), *Drug Intell. & clin. Pharm.*, 1987, *21*, 753.

EFFECTS ON THE SKIN AND HAIR. A report of hair colour changes in 3 patients taking minoxidil. The dark hair of 2 patients became 'pepper and salt' and the completely white hair of a third patient became yellowish.— Y. M. Traub *et al., Israel J. med. Scis*, 1975, *11*, 991.

Report of erythema multiforme, the Stevens-Johnson syndrome associated with minoxidil administration. The symptoms disappeared when minoxidil was withdrawn and recurred on re-exposure to the drug.— D. J. DiSantis and T. Flanagan, *Archs intern. Med.*, 1981, *141*, 1515.

A report of increased hair loss, particularly noticeable at the temples in a 28-year-old black patient with end-stage renal failure and taking minoxidil. Red hair regrew after several months of treatment with minoxidil. Following withdrawal of minoxidil and its reinstatement there was a recurrence of alopecia, but no subsequent regrowth.— R. M. Ingles and T. Kahn, *Int. J. Derm.*, 1983, *22*, 120.

Precautions

Minoxidil is contra-indicated in phaeochromocytoma. It should be used with caution after a recent myocardial infarction, and in patients with pulmonary hypertension, angina pectoris, chronic congestive heart failure, and significant renal failure.

The antihypertensive effect may be enhanced by concomitant use of other hypotensive agents.

Severe orthostatic hypotension may occur if minoxidil and sympathetic blocking agents such as guanethidine or bethanidine are given concurrently.

PORPHYRIA. Minoxidil was considered to be unsafe in patients with acute porphyria because it has been shown to be porphyrinogenic in *animals* or *in-vitro* systems.— M.R. Moore and K.E.L. McColl, *Porphyrias, Drug Lists*, Glasgow, Porphyria Research Unit, University of Glasgow, 1987.

PREGNANCY AND THE NEONATE. A patient who took minoxidil, propranolol, and frusemide throughout pregnancy delivered a normal infant at 37 weeks. Pregnancy was uneventful. Subsequent studies showed that minoxidil was rapidly excreted into breast milk achieving similar concentrations to those in the plasma. No adverse effects were seen in the infant after 2 months but it was considered that prolonged exposure during breast feeding could be deleterious to the infant.— A. Valdivieso *et al.*, *Ann. intern. Med.*, 1985, *102*, 135.

Absorption and Fate

About 90% of an oral dose of minoxidil has been reported to be absorbed from the gastro-intestinal tract. The plasma half-life is about 4.2 hours although the haemodynamic effect may persist for up to 75 hours, presumably due to accumulation at its site of action. Minoxidil is not bound to plasma proteins. Minoxidil is extensively metabolised by the liver primarily by conjugation with glucuronic acid and is excreted in the urine mainly in the form of metabolites.

Minoxidil was shown to be poorly absorbed through the skin following topical application of formulations in vehicles containing water, alcohol, and propylene glycol. Urinary excretion ranged from 1.6 to 3.9% of the applied dose.— T. J. Franz, *Archs Derm.*, 1985, *121*, 203.

For a report of the excretion of minoxidil in breast milk, see under Precautions, above.

Uses and Administration

Minoxidil is an antihypertensive agent which acts predominantly by causing direct peripheral vasodilatation of the arterioles. It produces effects on the cardiovascular system similar to those of hydralazine, p.484. It is usually administered concurrently with other antihypertensive agents for the treatment of severe hypertension unresponsive to standard therapy. Following oral administration, the maximum hypotensive effect usually occurs after 2 to 3 hours. The action may persist for up to 75 hours. An initial dose of 5 mg daily is gradually increased at intervals of not less than 3 days to 40 to 50 mg daily according to the patient's response; in exceptional circumstances up to 100 mg daily has been given. The daily dose may be given as a single dose or in 2 divided doses. Beta-adrenoceptor blocking agents or methyldopa are used to diminish the cardiac-accelerating effects, and diuretics to control oedema. For children 12 years of age or under, the recommended initial dose is 200 µg per kg body-weight daily, increased in steps of 100 to 200 µg per kg at intervals of not less than 3 days, until control of blood pressure has been achieved or a maximum of 1 mg per kg or 50 mg daily has been reached.

Minoxidil has also been applied topically as a 1 to 5% lotion in the treatment of alopecia.

A review of the properties and uses of minoxidil. Minoxidil has been reserved for the treatment of severe or moderately severe hypertension in patients who do not respond to, or who are intolerant of, conventional treatment with up to 3 other antihypertensive agents. A beta-blocking agent is routinely given with minoxidil to control tachycardia and to aid reduction in blood pressure. A diuretic must also be given to reduce fluid retention. A thiazide diuretic may be sufficient if renal function is normal, but a more powerful "loop" diuretic such as frusemide is required if renal function is impaired or if oedema or weight gain appear when taking a thiazide diuretic. Oedema should be controlled before starting minoxidil and weight should be measured at each visit. With careful monitoring adverse effects are usually acceptable and many patients comment favourably on the lack of adverse effects including drowsiness, impairment of sexual function, or postural or exercise-induced hypotensive dizziness which are troublesome side-effects of other potent hypotensive agents.— G. D. O. Lowe, *Br. med. J.*, 1983, *286*, 1262.

Further reviews of minoxidil: V. M. Campese, *Drugs*, 1981, *22*, 257.

ADMINISTRATION IN RENAL FAILURE. Minoxidil could be administered to patients with renal failure in normal doses. A dose supplement should be given to patients undergoing haemodialysis.— W. M. Bennett *et al.*, *Am. J. Kidney Dis.*, 1983, *3*, 155.

ALOPECIA. A review of the use of topically applied minoxidil in the treatment of alopecia androgenetica and alopecia areata. The mode of action by which hair growth is stimulated is not fully understood but it may act by direct stimulation of the hair follicle epithelium. Studies have suggested the plasma-minoxidil concentration rarely exceeds 5 µg per litre following topical application of the lotion, indicating a low level of percutaneous absorption. Therapeutic studies of the use of minoxidil in alopecia androgenetica, or male-pattern baldness, have shown promising results with, in one multicentre study, up to one third of patients obtaining cosmetically acceptable hair regrowth using a 2% lotion, and a higher proportion of patients showing some regrowth of non-vellus hair. Some beneficial results have also been obtained in the treatment of alopecia areata with cosmetically acceptable response reported in up to 50% of patients, although the response rate has been variable. There was some indication of a dose-related response. In general, better results have been obtained in patients with less severe symptoms and a shorter duration of alopecia. A 2% lotion has been considered to give the most favourable risk-benefit ratio. Twice-daily application for periods of up to 6 months may be necessary before a response is obtained, and preliminary data suggest that continued therapy may be necessary to maintain hair growth. Treatment has been generally well tolerated, but some dermatological reactions have been reported. Topical minoxidil should probably be avoided in patients with hypertension or cardiovascular disease, although few adverse cardiovascular effects have been seen in normotensive patients.— S. P. Clissold and R. C. Heel, *Drugs*, 1987, *33*, 107.

Studies indicate that probably less than 10% of men treated with topical minoxidil for male-pattern baldness obtain a result that a neutral observer would find cosmetically acceptable: studies in which hair density has been measured showed that the density of new hair growth was considerably less than normal, and in one study, "moderate" growth achieved in 31% of patients was described as "mostly fluff". The costs of treatment are considerable, especially since the treatment apparently cannot be stopped without the loss of hair gained.— A. C. de Groot *et al.*, *Lancet*, 1987, *1*, 1019. Further reviews: J. A. Rumsfield *et al.*, *Clin. Pharm.*, 1987, *6*, 386; *Med. Lett.*, 1987, *29*, 87.

Results of a survey of 900 members of the American Academy of Dermatology indicated that 72% of the 552 respondents had prescribed topical minoxidil for hair loss: 69% of these had prescribed topical minoxidil for 10 or fewer patients during the previous 6 months and 9% were responsible for over half the patients treated during this period. Adverse effects other than local irritation were infrequent and were reported by only 8 respondents although this was suspected of being an underestimate of the true incidence.— R. S. Stern, *Archs Derm.*, 1987, *123*, 62.

Proceedings of a symposium on minoxidil lotion in the management of male-pattern baldness and alopecia areata: *J. Am. Acad. Derm.*, 1987, *16*, 647-750.

Studies of topical minoxidil in alopecia areata: D. A. Fenton and J. D. Wilkinson, *Br. med. J.*, 1983, *287*, 1015; V. C. Weiss *et al.*, *Archs Derm.*, 1984, *120*, 457; E. E. Vanderveen *et al.*, *J. Am. Acad. Derm.*, 1984, *11*, 416; J. P. Vestey and J. A. Savin, *Br. J. Derm.*, 1985, *113, Suppl.* 29, 35; V. C. Fiedler-Weiss *et al.*, *Archs Derm.*, 1986, *122*, 180; J. P. Vestey and J. A. Savin, *Acta derm.-vener., Stockh.*, 1986, *66*, 179.

Studies of topical minoxidil in male-pattern baldness: E. A. Olsen *et al.*, *J. Am. Acad. Derm.*, 1985, *13*, 185; R. L. De Villez, *Archs Derm.*, 1985, *121*, 197; Y. P. Shi, *Archs Derm.*, 1986, *122*, 506; J. S. Storer *et al.*, *Am. J. med. Sci.*, 1986, *291*, 328; A. Tosti, *Dermatologica*, 1986, *173*, 136; E. A. Olsen *et al.*, *J. Am. Acad. Derm.*, 1986, *15*, 30.

CONGESTIVE HEART FAILURE. Beneficial haemodynamic effects of a single dose of minoxidil in 6 patients with congestive heart failure.— J. A. Franciosa *et al.*, *Clin. Pharmac. Ther.*, 1980, *27*, 254.

Minoxidil produced sustained improvement in haemodynamic and left ventricular performance in 9 patients with chronic congestive heart failure. Despite these improvements, minoxidil did not affect exercise performance, symptomatic status, or clinical complications, and patients taking minoxidil encountered more clinical events including increased diuretic requirements, angina pectoris, ventricular arrhythmias, worsening heart failure, and death than patients taking placebo.— J. A. Franciosa *et al.*, *Circulation*, 1984, *70*, 63.

Further references to minoxidil in heart failure: C. R. McKay *et al.*, *Am. Heart J.*, 1982, *104*, 575.

HYPERTENSION. Reports of the use of minoxidil in the treatment of severe and refractory hypertension: P. K. Mehta *et al.*, *J. Am. med. Ass.*, 1975, *233*, 249; H. J. Dargie *et al.*, *Lancet*, 1977, *2*, 515; B. L. Devine *et al.*, *Br. med. J.*, 1977, *2*, 667; H. R. Brunner *et al.*, *ibid.*, 1978, *2*, 385.

Concomitant administration of small doses of minoxidil and captopril with a diuretic and a beta blocker controlled the blood pressure in 12 patients with severe hypertension who did not respond adequately to maximum doses of either minoxidil or captopril added to other drug combinations.— A. C. Pessina *et al.*, *Curr. ther. Res.*, 1984, *35*, 269. See also: Y. K. Seedat and R. Rawat, *Eur. J. clin. Pharmac.*, 1983, *25*, 9; Y. M. Traub and B. A. Levey, *Archs intern. Med.*, 1983, *143*, 1142.

Minoxidil was considered to be unsuitable for the treatment of moderate hypertension since low doses were ineffective and higher doses were associated with unacceptable adverse effects.— B. E. Westwood *et al.*, *Med. J. Aust.*, 1986, *145*, 151.

In children. Report of the use of minoxidil for periods of up to 77 months in the treatment of severe hypertension in 16 children with renal disease. The maximum doses in the 13 children who responded to minoxidil therapy ranged from 50 µg per kg body-weight per day to 1.88 mg per kg per day. Patients were also taking propranolol and those not on dialysis were treated with frusemide. Two patients had progressive transplant rejection and failed to respond to minoxidil and one discontinued therapy after 2 months because of hypertrichosis.— H. C. Puri *et al.*, *Am. J. Kidney Dis.*, 1983, *3*, 71.

A study involving 13 chronically hypertensive children suggested that single doses of minoxidil 200 µg per kg body-weight could be used to control severe hypertension within 4 hours in children already receiving diuretic and beta-blocker therapy.— C. F. Strife *et al.*, *Pediatrics*, 1986, *78*, 861.

Further reports of the use of minoxidil in hypertensive children: A. J. Pennisi *et al.*, *J. Pediat.*, 1977, *90*, 813.

Renal scleroderma. Malignant hypertension associated with oliguric renal failure in a 37-year-old man with scleroderma was successfully controlled when minoxidil 5 mg twice daily was given, although hydralazine 400 mg and propranolol 480 mg daily had been ineffective. After management of renal failure with haemodialysis for 6 months, renal function spontaneously improved. Dialysis was discontinued and blood pressure controlled with minoxidil 40 mg, propranolol 320 mg, and frusemide 400 mg daily. Nephrectomy had previously been advocated in this situation since antihypertensive therapy had frequently been reported to be ineffective and the renal failure in scleroderma considered irreversible.— P. D. Mitnick and P. U. Feig, *New Engl. J. Med.*, 1978, *299*, 871.

Preparations

Minoxidil Tablets *(U.S.P.)*. Store in airtight containers.

Proprietary Preparations

Loniten *(Upjohn, UK)*. *Tablets*, scored, minoxidil 2.5, 5, and 10 mg.

Regaine *(Upjohn, UK)*. *Topical solution*, minoxidil 20 mg/mL in a solution of alcohol, propylene glycol, and water.

Proprietary Names and Manufacturers

Alopexil *(Pierre Fabre, Fr.)*; Alostil *(Clin Midy, Fr.)*; Loniten *(Upjohn, Austral.; Upjohn, Canad.; Upjohn, Ital.; Upjohn, S.Afr.; Upjohn, Spain; Upjohn, Switz.; Upjohn, UK; Upjohn, USA)*; Lonolox *(Upjohn, Ger.)*; Lonoten *(Upjohn, Fr.)*; Minodyl *(Quantum, USA)*; Prexidil *(Bioindustria, Ital.)*; Regaine *(Upjohn, Eire; Upjohn, UK)*; Rogaine *(Upjohn, Canad.; Upjohn, USA)*.

13057-h

Oxdralazine *(rINN).*
L-6150 (dihydrochloride). *N*-(6-Hydrazinopyridazin-3-yl)-2,2′-iminodiethanol.
$C_8H_{15}N_5O_2$=213.2.

CAS — 17259-75-5 (oxdralazine); 27464-23-9 (dihydrochloride).

Oxdralazine is reported to have vasodilator and antihypertensive properties similar to hydralazine, p.484.

Study of the haemodynamic effects of oxdralazine in comparison with hydralazine in 7 patients with hypertension.— R. M. Moskowitz and J. N. Cohn, *Clin. Pharmac. Ther.*, 1980, *27*, 773.

Studies of oxdralazine in the treatment of hypertension in combination with other antihypertensive agents: A. Salvadeo *et al.*, *Arzneimittel-Forsch.*, 1979, *29*, 1753; E. Bartoli *et al.*, *J. clin. Pharmac.*, 1979, *19*, 751; A. Salvadeo *et al.*, *J. clin. Pharmac.*, 1983, *23*, 155.

Proprietary Names and Manufacturers
Lepetit, Ital.

886-f

Pargyline Hydrochloride *(BANM, USAN, rINNM).*

A-19120; MO-911. *N*-Methyl-*N*-prop-2-ynylbenzylamine hydrochloride.
$C_{11}H_{13}N,HCl$=195.7.

CAS — 555-57-7 (pargyline); 306-07-0 (hydrochloride).

Pharmacopoeias. In *U.S.*

A white or almost white crystalline powder with a slight odour. Sublimation occurs when kept at raised temperatures.

Soluble 1 in 0.6 of water, 1 in 5 of alcohol, and 1 in 7.2 of chloroform; very slightly soluble in acetone. Aqueous solutions are unstable. **Store** in airtight containers.

Adverse Effects

The toxic effects of pargyline are similar to those described for monoamine oxidase inhibitors under phenelzine, p.377. The most frequently occurring adverse effects are those associated with orthostatic hypotension. Constipation, dry mouth, difficulty in micturition, and drowsiness may also occur. Muscle twitching and acute extrapyramidal disorders have been reported. There have been reports of congestive heart failure in patients with reduced cardiac reserve. Hypoglycaemia has occurred in some patients.

Severe toxic reactions may occur if pargyline is taken simultaneously with certain other drugs or with cheese, yeast extract, and certain other foods—see under Precautions for Phenelzine Sulphate, p.378.

Manic psychosis occured in a patient a few months after beginning treatment with pargyline for depression and concurrent hypertension.— D. Folks and E. S. Arnold, *J. clin. Psychiat.*, 1983, *44*, 25.

OVERDOSAGE. About 15 hours after ingesting 150 or 175 mg of pargyline hydrochloride, a 2½-year-old child was anorectic, sleepless, lethargic, and mentally confused. Her eyes rolled, her teeth chattered, her speech was slurred, and she staggered. She complained of abdominal pain. Both pupils were dilated and responded only sluggishly to light; the accommodation reflex was absent and the eye movements hyperactive. After a day in hospital the child went into a short coma with Babinski reflexes and opisthotonos. Her subsequent behaviour alternated between extreme agitation and lethargy. The patient recovered following 12 hours of intermittent repeated peritoneal dialysis.— D. Lipkin and T. Kushnick, *J. Am. med. Ass.*, 1967, *201*, 57.

Treatment of Adverse Effects

If overdosage occurs the stomach should be emptied by aspiration and lavage. Mania or hyperexcitement may be treated with chlorpromazine. Severe hypotension may respond to placing the patient in the supine position with the feet raised. If pressor agents are required, they should be administered with extreme caution since an exaggerated pressor response may occur. Hypertension may be treated with alpha-adrenoceptor blocking agents such as phentolamine mesylate. External cooling has been recommended if hyperpyrexia occurs.

Precautions

Pargyline has precautions similar to those of other monoamine oxidase inhibitors: see Precautions for Phenelzine Sulphate, p.378, particularly with reference to other drugs and items of diet contra-indicated during therapy with monoamine oxidase inhibitors. Pargyline should not be given concomitantly with methyldopa or dopamine. Guanethidine or reserpine or other antihypertensive agents which may cause hypertensive reactions due to sudden release of catecholamines should not be given parenterally to patients taking pargyline or for at least 14 days after cessation of treatment with pargyline. The hypotensive effects of pargyline may be enhanced by thiazide diuretics. Concomitant administration of pargyline with other monoamine oxidase inhibitors may produce augmented pharmacological effects.

INTERACTIONS. A woman receiving pargyline developed vivid hallucinations on concomitant administration of *methyldopa*.— E. S. Paykel (letter), *Br. med. J.*, 1966, *1*, 803.

PORPHYRIA. Pargyline was considered to be unsafe in patients with acute porphyria because it has been shown to be porphyrinogenic in *animals* or *in vitro* systems.— M.R. Moore and K.E.L. McColl, *Porphyrias, Drug Lists*, Glasgow, Porphyria Research Unit, University of Glasgow, 1987.

Uses and Administration

Pargyline hydrochloride is a monoamine oxidase inhibitor which is occasionally used in the treatment of moderate to severe hypertension although less toxic agents are generally preferred. It has a more marked effect on the standing than the supine blood pressure. The maximum effect may not be achieved for between a few days and several weeks, and may persist for up to 3 weeks after pargyline is withdrawn. Tolerance to the effects of pargyline can develop during treatment. The usual initial dose is 25 mg daily gradually increased as necessary by 10-mg increments at intervals of not less than 7 days. The usual maintenance dose may be 25 or 50 mg daily; doses of more than 200 mg daily should not generally be exceeded. Dosages should be reduced in elderly patients. Smaller doses of pargyline may be given in conjunction with a thiazide diuretic, which would also reduce the oedema that sometimes occurs with pargyline. Pargyline may also be given with other antihypertensive agents, but see under Precautions, above.

Preparations

Pargyline Hydrochloride Tablets *(U.S.P.)*

Proprietary Names and Manufacturers
Eudatine *(Belg.)*; Eutonyl *(Abbott, UK; Abbott, USA).*

887-d

Pempidine Tartrate *(BANM, rINNM).*
1,2,2,6,6-Pentamethylpiperidine hydrogen tartrate.
$C_{10}H_{21}N,C_4H_6O_6$=305.4.

CAS — 79-55-0 (pempidine); 546-48-5 (tartrate).

Pempidine is a tertiary amine ganglion-blocking agent with properties similar to those of trimetaphan (p.503). Pempidine has been used in the treatment of severe or malignant hypertension, but has largely been superseded by drugs that do not produce the effects of parasympathetic blockade. Pempidine tosylate has also been used.

Proprietary Names and Manufacturers
Perolysen *(May & Baker, UK).*

889-h

Pentamethonium Bromide *(BAN, rINN).*
Dibromure de Pentaméthonium. *NN′*-Pentamethylenebis(trimethylammonium) dibromide.
$C_{11}H_{28}Br_2N_2$=348.2.

CAS — 2365-25-5 (pentamethonium); 541-20-8 (dibromide).

A ganglion-blocking agent which has been used in the treatment of hypertension. Pentamethonium iodide has also been used.

Proprietary Names and Manufacturers
Penthonium *(Delagrange, Fr.).*

891-t

Pentolinium Tartrate *(BAN).*
Pentapyrrolidinium Bitartrate; Pentolinio Tartrato; Pentolonium Tartrate *(rINN)*; Tartrate de Pyrroplégium.
NN′-Pentamethylenebis(1-methylpyrrolidinium) bis(hydrogen tartrate).
$C_{23}H_{42}N_2O_{12}$=538.6.

CAS — 144-44-5 (pentolinium); 52-62-0 (tartrate).

Pentolinium tartrate is a quaternary ammonium ganglion-blocking agent with properties similar to those of trimetaphan (see p.503).

Pentolinium tartrate has been given by intravenous or subcutaneous injection to produce controlled hypotension in patients undergoing surgical procedures and in hypertensive emergencies.

The use of pentolinium 2.5 mg by intravenous injection as a suppression test for the diagnosis of phaeochromocytoma.— M. J. Brown *et al.*, *Lancet*, 1981, *1*, 174. See also M. B. Murphy and R. Causon (letter), *ibid.*, 1983, *1*, 1216.

Severe hypotension occurred in a patient following a pentolinium suppression test.— K. S. Channer *et al.* (letter), *Lancet*, 1983, *1*, 988.

Proprietary Names and Manufacturers
Ansolysen *(May & Baker, Austral.; May & Baker, S.Afr.; May & Baker, UK)*; Pentio *(Estedi, Spain).*

729-s

Perindopril *(rINN).*
S-9490-3. (2*S*,3a*S*,7a*S*)-1-{(*S*)-*N*-[(*S*)-1-Carboxybutyl]-alanyl}-hexahydro-2-indolinecarboxylic acid, 1-ethyl ester.
$C_{19}H_{32}N_2O_5$=368.5.

CAS — 82834-16-0.

Perindopril is an antihypertensive agent which acts, similarly to captopril, as an angiotensin-converting enzyme inhibitor.

References: K. R. Lees *et al.*, *Br. J. clin. Pharmac.*, 1986, *22*, 233P; K. R. Lees and J. L. Reid, *ibid.*, 1987, *23*, 159; K. R. Lees and J. L. Reid, *Eur. J. clin. Pharmac.*, 1987, *31*, 519.

892-x

Phenoxybenzamine Hydrochloride *(BANM, USAN, rINNM).*

SKF-688A. *N*-(2-Chloroethyl)-*N*-(1-methyl-2-phenoxyethyl)benzylamine hydrochloride.
$C_{18}H_{22}ClNO,HCl$=340.3.

CAS — 59-96-1 (phenoxybenzamine); 63-92-3 (hydrochloride).

Pharmacopoeias. In *Br.*, *Chin.*, and *U.S.*

A white or almost white, odourless or almost odourless, crystalline powder.

B.P. **solubilities** are: sparingly soluble in water; soluble 1 in 9 of alcohol, and 1 in 9 of chloroform. *U.S.P.* solubilities are: soluble 1 in 25 of water, 1 in 6 of alcohol, 1 in 3 of chloroform, and 1 in more than 1000 of ether.

Adverse Effects and Treatment

The adverse effects of phenoxybenzamine are primarily due to its alpha-adrenoceptor blocking activity. They include postural hypotension and dizziness, reflex tachycardia, nasal congestion, and miosis. These effects may be minimised by using a low initial dose of phenoxybenzamine, and may diminish with continued administration, but the hypotensive effect can be exaggerated by exercise, heat, a large meal, or alcohol ingestion. Severe hypotension may occur in overdose and treatment includes support of the circulation by postural measures and parenteral fluid volume replacement. Sympathomimetic agents are considered to be of little value, and adrenaline is contra-indicated since it also stimulates beta-receptors causing increased hypotension and tachycardia. The use of noradrenaline has been suggested to overcome alpha-receptor blockade. Other side-effects include dryness of the mouth, drowsiness, sedation, and inhibition of ejaculation. Gastro-intestinal effects are usually slight. Phenoxybenzamine has been shown to be mutagenic in *in vitro* tests and carcinogenic in rodents.

Precautions

Phenoxybenzamine should be given with care to patients with congestive heart failure, coronary or cerebrovascular insufficiency or renal impairment. It should not be given in any conditions in which a fall in blood pressure would be dangerous. Phenoxybenzamine may aggravate the symptoms of respiratory infections.

Since phenoxybenzamine only blocks alpha-receptors, leaving the beta-receptors unopposed, concomitant administration of drugs, such as adrenaline, which also stimulate beta-receptors, may enhance the cardiac-accelerating and hypotensive action of phenoxybenzamine.

When given intravenously, phenoxybenzamine hydrochloride should always be diluted and given by infusion. Intravenous fluids must always be given beforehand to ensure an adequate circulating blood volume and to prevent a precipitous fall in blood pressure.

PORPHYRIA. Phenoxybenzamine was considered to be unsafe in patients with acute porphyria because it has been shown to be porphyrinogenic in *animals* or *in-vitro* systems.— M.R. Moore and K.E.L. McColl, *Porphyrias, Drug Lists*, Glasgow, Porphyria Research Unit, University of Glasgow, 1987.

Absorption and Fate

Phenoxybenzamine is incompletely absorbed from the gastro-intestinal tract. The maximum effect is attained in about 1 hour after an intravenous dose. Following oral administration the onset of action is gradual over several hours and persists for 3 or 4 days following a single dose. The plasma half-life is about 24 hours. Phenoxybenzamine is metabolised in the liver and excreted in the urine and bile, but small amounts remain in the body for several days. It has a prolonged action probably owing to stable covalent bonding.

Uses and Administration

Phenoxybenzamine is a powerful alpha-adrenoceptor blocking agent with a prolonged duration of action; it binds covalently to alpha-receptors to produce an irreversible ('non-competitive') blockade. A single large dose of phenoxybenzamine can cause alpha-adrenoceptor blockade for 3 days or longer.

It is used to control the hypertension caused by phaeochromocytoma during the pre-operative period and in patients whose tumours are inoperable. A beta-blocking agent may be given concomitantly to control tachycardia, but not before alpha blockade has completely suppressed the pressor effects of the phaeochromocytoma. The usual initial dose of phenoxybenzamine hydrochloride is 10 mg daily by mouth, increased gradually, according to the patient's response, to a usual dose of 1 to 2 mg per kg body-weight daily in 2 divided doses. It may be given intravenously for operative cover.

Phenoxybenzamine has been occasionally used, as an adjunct to other antihypertensive agents, in the treatment of some other forms of hypertension. It has also been used as an adjunct in the management of urinary retention due to a neurogenic bladder or prostatic hypertrophy and in the treatment of peripheral vascular disorders due to vasospasm.

CARCINOID SYNDROME. Phenoxybenzamine 10 to 20 mg four times daily may reduce flushes provoked by catecholamines or alcohol in patients with carcinoid syndrome although tolerance can occur.— B. Clarke and H. J. F. Hodgson, *Br. J. Hosp. Med.*, 1986, *35*, 146.

LEIOMYOMA. A 41-year-old woman with multiple cutaneous leiomyomas was treated with phenoxybenzamine 20 mg daily. After 10 days all the painful attacks were suppressed and benefit had continued over 7 months' treatment without noticeable side-effects.— P. Y. Venencie *et al.*, *Br. J. Derm.*, 1982, *107*, 483. Similar beneficial results in a 67-year-old patient were not maintained during long-term therapy.— R. Corbett, *ibid.*, 1984, *111, Suppl.* 26, 70.

PERIPHERAL VASCULAR DISORDERS. Phenoxybenzamine was more effective than orciprenaline, terbutaline, or prenalterol in a double-blind study in 12 patients with Raynaud's syndrome. The addition of propranolol to treatment with phenoxybenzamine did not reduce the beneficial effects of phenoxybenzamine and administration of phenoxybenzamine with a beta blocker may prevent the alpha-blocker side-effects of postural hypotension, excercise-induced hypotension, and tachycardia.— T. J. M. Cleophas *et al.*, *Angiology*, 1985, *36*, 219.

PHAEOCHROMOCYTOMA. A review of the management of phaeochromocytoma. Phenoxybenzamine has been widely used in the initial suppression of the pressor effects produced by catecholamines secreted by the tumour and was considered the first-choice vasodilator for the majority of patients. The non-competitive adrenergic blockade produced means that surges of catecholamine release cannot override the inhibition as may occur with a competitive blocker. However, since phenoxybenzamine blocks alpha$_2$-receptors as well as alpha$_1$-receptors it should be used with great caution in patients with marginal coronary perfusion with or without angina. Phenoxybenzamine was preferred to prazosin for the initial control of hypertension when the patient is intensely vasoconstricted and the plasma volume reduced since prazosin can cause severe initial hypotension. The treatment should be started at a low dose and increased gradually until the response is achieved: some patients have required 300 mg daily. If additional beta blockade is required, it should never be given until alpha blockade has completely suppressed the pressor effects of the tumour. Phenoxybenzamine was also considered to be the vasodilator of choice for the pre-operative preparation of patients with phaeochromocytoma.— C. J. Hull, *Br. J. Anaesth.*, 1986, *58*, 1453. See also E. L. Bravo and R. W. Gifford, *New Engl. J. Med.*, 1984, *311*, 1298.

Intravenous phenoxybenzamine in the operative management of phaeochromocytoma.— E. J. Ross *et al.*, *Br. med. J.*, 1967, *1*, 191.

Pregnancy and the neonate. Phenoxybenzamine could be used in the management of phaeochromocytoma during pregnancy and labour.— Z. M. van der Spuy and H. S. Jacobs, *Postgrad. med. J.*, 1984, *60*, 312.

SEXUAL DISORDERS. Preliminary report of the use of intracavernosal phenoxybenzamine to induce penile erection in erectile impotence.— G. S. Brindley, *Br. J. Psychiat.*, 1983, *143*, 332.

Report suggesting that phenoxybenzamine may be useful as a male oral contraceptive due to its effect of blocking ejaculation.— Z. T. Homonnai *et al.*, *Contraception*, 1984, *29*, 479.

SHOCK. Beneficial results with phenoxybenzamine hydrochloride administered intravenously to patients with septic shock who were unresponsive to fluid therapy and showed signs of sympathetic overactivity.— R. W. Anderson *et al.*, *Ann. Surg.*, 1967, *165*, 341.

URINARY DISORDERS. Overflow incontinence in the elderly could often be overcome with phenoxybenzamine which decreased the tone in the internal urethral sphincter.— M. E. Williams and F. C. Pannill, *Ann. intern. Med.*, 1982, *97*, 895.

A review of the use of phenoxybenzamine to alleviate symptoms of bladder neck obstruction, particularly those due to prostatic hypertrophy. Limited evidence from clinical studies suggested that phenoxybenzamine may alleviate urinary symptoms in about three quarters of patients with benign prostatic hypertrophy, although at least one-third can expect unwanted effects, mainly dizziness and tiredness. The drug did not replace prostatectomy but may help patients who were awaiting operation and were at immediate risk of urinary retention.— *Drug & Ther. Bull.*, 1983, *21*, 15. Selective α-adrenergic receptor antagonists such as prazosin might be expected to produce similar clinical results without the disadvantage of orthostatic hypotension seen with phenoxybenzamine, a nonspecific α-blocker.— *Lancet*, 1988, *1*, 1083.

In 30 women given morphine 4 mg by epidural injection after caesarean section 26 experienced difficulty in micturition, 14 had urinary retention, and 16 needed catheterisation. The incidence was reduced to 2, 3, and 3 respectively in 30 further women who also received 10 mg of phenoxybenzamine by mouth 24 and 2 hours before and 8 and 16 hours after surgery.— S. Evron *et al.*, *Br. med. J.*, 1984, *288*, 190.

Further references to the use of phenoxybenzamine in urinary disorders: S. A. Awad *et al.*, *Br. J. Urol.*, 1978, *50*, 336 (neurogenic bladder dysfunction).

Preparations

Phenoxybenzamine Capsules *(B.P.)*. Capsules containing phenoxybenzamine hydrochloride.

Phenoxybenzamine Hydrochloride Capsules *(U.S.P.)*

Proprietary Preparations

Dibenyline *(Smith Kline & French, UK)*. *Capsules*, phenoxybenzamine hydrochloride 10 mg.
Injection, phenoxybenzamine hydrochloride 50 mg/mL, in ampoules of 2 mL. To be diluted before use.

Proprietary Names and Manufacturers

Dibenyline *(Smith Kline & French, Austral.*; *Neth.*; *Smith Kline & French, S.Afr.*; *Smith Kline & French, UK)*; Dibenzyline *(Smith Kline & French, Switz.*; *Smith Kline & French, USA)*; Dibenzyran *(Röhm, Ger.)*.

893-r

Phentolamine Hydrochloride *(BANM, rINNM)*.
Cloridrato de Fentolamina; Phentolam. Hydrochlor.; Phentolamini Hydrochloridum; Phentolaminium Chloride. 3-[*N*-(2-Imidazolin-2-ylmethyl)-*p*-toluidino]-phenol hydrochloride.
$C_{17}H_{19}N_3O,HCl=317.8$.

CAS — 50-60-2 (phentolamine); 73-05-2 (hydrochloride).

Pharmacopoeias. In *Arg.*, *Braz.*, *Egypt.*, *Ind.*, and *Int.*

894-f

Phentolamine Mesylate *(BANM, USAN)*.

Phentolamine Mesilate *(rINNM)*; Phentolamine Methanesulphonate; Phentolamini Mesylas. 3-[*N*-(2-Imidazolin-2-ylmethyl)-*p*-toluidino]phenol methanesulphonate.
$C_{17}H_{19}N_3O,CH_4SO_3=377.5$.

CAS — 65-28-1.

Pharmacopoeias. In *Arg.*, *Br.*, *Chin.*, *Ind.*, *Int.*, *Turk.*, and *U.S.*

A white or off-white slightly hygroscopic, odourless or almost odourless, crystalline powder. **Soluble** 1 in 1 of water, 1 in 4 or 5 of alcohol, and 1 in 700 of chloroform. A freshly prepared 1% solution in water has a pH of 4.5 to 6.5; the *B.P.* injection has a pH of 3.5 to 5.0. Solutions are **sterilised** by filtration. Solutions slowly deteriorate on storage. **Store** in airtight containers. Protect from light.

Adverse Effects

Phentolamine may cause severe hypotension and tachycardia; myocardial infarction and cerebrovascular spasm or occlusion have been reported occasionally, usually in association with marked hypotension. Nausea, vomiting, and diarrhoea may also occur. Other side-effects include weakness, dizziness, flushing, and nasal stuffiness.

Reports of the death of a 21-year-old pregnant woman following administration of phentolamine mesylate for the diagnosis of a phaeochromocytoma (the presence of which was confirmed at autopsy). The patient developed profound vasomotor shock immediately after administration of the drug.— C. B. Roland, *J. Am. med. Ass.*, 1959, *171*, 1806.

Treatment of Adverse Effects

Severe hypotension should be treated by discontinuing treatment with phenotalamine and maintaining the patient in the supine position with the feet raised. Plasma expanders and noradrenaline may be given if necessary, but, as with other alpha-adrenoceptor blocking agents, adrenaline should be avoided.

Precautions

Phentolamine should not generally be given to patients with angina pectoris or coronary artery disease.

Uses and Administration

Phentolamine is an alpha-adrenoceptor blocking agent which also has a direct action on vascular smooth muscle. It produces vasodilatation, an increase in cardiac output, and has a positive inotropic effect, but is reported to have little effect on the blood pressure of patients with essential hypertension. The alpha-receptor blocking action is reported to be transient and incomplete; it is reversible ('competitive').

Phentolamine is used to prevent paroxysmal hypertension in patients with phaeochromocytoma and as prophylaxis against catecholamine-induced hypertensive crisis during surgery in these patients. Once alpha-blockade is achieved a beta-blocking agent may be given to reduce tachycardia. Phentolamine mesylate is given by intravenous or intramuscular injection in a dose of 5 to 10 mg 1 to 2 hours pre-operatively repeated during the operation if necessary. In children a dose of 1 to 5 mg may be given intravenously according to age.

Phentolamine mesylate has been employed for the differential diagnosis of phaeochromocytoma but it has been superseded by estimations of catecholamines in blood and urine.

A dose of 5 to 60 mg given by intravenous infusion over a period of 10 to 30 minutes at an infusion-rate of 0.1 to 2 mg per minute has been recommended for acute left ventricular failure (cardiogenic shock), particularly following myocardial infarction. If necessary 5 mg may be given over the first minute. The infusion-rate should be reduced if the systolic pressure falls below 100 mmHg.

Phentolamine has also been used for the management of hypertensive crisis due to overdosage with sympathomimetic agents, in patients taking monoamine oxidase inhibitors, and in patients with rebound hypertension due to clonidine withdrawal. It has been used to prevent dermal sloughing during intravenous infusions of noradrenaline and in the treatment of recent extravasation of noradrenaline or dopamine.

For the uses of phentolamine in the treatment of injury due to extravasation of catecholamines, see under Adrenaline p.1454.

CARDIOGENIC SHOCK. The use of phentolamine in cardiogenic shock has been limited by the production of excessive tachycardia in some patients.— K. Balakumaran and P. G. Hugenholtz, *Drugs*, 1986, *32*, 372.

PHAEOCHROMOCYTOMA. A review of the management of phaeochromocytoma. Phentolamine has been widely used in the initial suppression of the pressor effects produced by catecholamines secreted by the tumour, although the non-competitive alpha-adrenoceptor blockade produced by phenoxybenzamine was considered to be advantageous. Since phentolamine blocks $alpha_2$-receptors as well as $alpha_1$-receptors it should be used with great caution in patients with marginal coronary perfusion with or without angina. Phentolamine was considered to be less satisfactory than other vasodilators for the control of hypertension during surgery because tachycardia was an invariable problem, and tachyphylaxis could occur.— C. J. Hull, *Br. J. Anaesth.*, 1986, *58*, 1453.

PULMONARY HYPERTENSION. A brief review of the use of phentolamine in pulmonary hypertension. Some studies had shown beneficial haemodynamic and clinical responses, but this had not been confirmed by others.— M. Packer, *Ann. intern. Med.*, 1985, *103*, 258.

Further reviews mentioning the use of phentolamine in pulmonary hypertension: M. D. McGood and R. E. Vlietstra, *Mayo Clin. Proc.*, 1984, *59*, 672; A. A. McLeod and D. E. Jewitt, *Drugs*, 1986, *31*, 177.

SEXUAL DISORDERS. *Impotence.* For studies of the use of phentolamine in combination with papaverine by intracavernous injection to produce penile erection in organic and psychogenic impotence, see Papaverine, p.1598.

Preparations of Phentolamine and its Salts

Phentolamine Injection *(B.P.)*. A sterile solution of phentolamine mesylate in water for injections containing anhydrous glucose.

Phentolamine Mesylate for Injection *(U.S.P.)*. Sterile phentolamine mesylate or a sterile mixture of phentolamine mesylate with a suitable buffer or diluents.

Proprietary Preparations

Rogitine *(Ciba, UK)*. *Injection*, phentolamine mesylate 10 mg/mL, in ampoules of 1 and 5 mL.

Proprietary Names and Manufacturers of Phentolamine and its Salts

Regitin *(Ciba, Denm.; Ciba, Ger.; Ciba, Ital.; Ciba, Norw.; Ciba, Swed.; Switz.)*; Regitina *(Arg.)*; Regitine *(Ciba, Austral.; Belg.; Neth.; Ciba, S.Afr.; Ciba, Switz.; Ciba, USA)*; Rogitine *(Ciba, Canad.; NZ; Ciba, UK)*.

16954-y

Pinacidil *(USAN, rINN)*.

P-1134. (±)-2-Cyano-1-(4-pyridyl)-3-(1,2,2-trimethylpropyl)guanidine; (±)-*N''*-Cyano-*N*-4-pyridinyl-*N'*-(1,2,2-trimethylpropyl)guanidine.

$C_{13}H_{19}N_5$=245.3.

CAS — 60560-33-0 (anhydrous); 85371-64-8 (monohydrate).

Pinacidil is a vasodilator used in the treatment of hypertension.

References on the pharmacokinetics of pinacidil: J. W. Ward *et al.*, *Eur. J. clin. Pharmac.*, 1984, *26*, 603; A. McBurney *et al.*, *Br. J. clin. Pharmac.*, 1985, *19*, 91; O. Shaheen *et al.*, *Clin. Pharmac. Ther.*, 1986, *40*, 650; M. S. Laher and M. P. Hickey, *J. int. med. Res.*, 1985, *13*, 159.

References on the action and use of pinacidil: J. W. Ward, *Br. J. clin. Pharmac.*, 1984, *18*, 223; K. Koliopoulos *et al.*, *Eur. J. clin. Pharmac.*, 1984, *27*, 287; V. D'Arcy *et al.*, *ibid.*, 1985, *28*, 347; E. G. Breen *et al.*, *ibid.*, 375; *idem*, 381; M. P. Caruana *et al.*, *Br. J. clin. Pharmac.*, 1985, *20*, 140; L. R. Krusell *et al.*, *Eur. J. clin. Pharmac.*, 1986, *30*, 641; P. K. Zachariah *et al.*, *ibid.*, *31*, 133; R. L. Byyny *et al.*, *Clin. Pharmac. Ther.*, 1987, *42*, 50.

Proprietary Names and Manufacturers

Pindac *(Leo, Denm.)*.

918-j

Piperoxan Hydrochloride *(BANM, rINNM)*.

Benzodioxane Hydrochloride; Compound 933F; Fourneau 933; Piperoxane Hydrochloride. 2-Piperidinomethyl-1,4-benzodioxane hydrochloride.

$C_{14}H_{19}NO_2,HCl$=269.8.

CAS — 59-39-2 (piperoxan); 135-87-5 (hydrochloride).

Piperoxan hydrochloride is an alpha-adrenoceptor blocking agent with properties similar to those of phentolamine mesylate (p.494). It was formerly used for the diagnosis of phaeochromocytoma and for the control of hypertension during the surgical removal of the tumour.

896-n

Prazosin Hydrochloride *(BANM, USAN, rINNM)*.

CP-12299-1; Furazosin Hydrochloride. 1-(4-Amino-6,7-dimethoxyquinazolin-2-yl)-4-(2-furoyl)piperazine hydrochloride.

$C_{19}H_{21}N_5O_4,HCl$=419.9.

CAS — 19216-56-9(prazosin); 19237-84-4 (hydrochloride).

Pharmacopoeias. In *Br.* and *U.S.*

A white to tan-coloured, odourless or almost odourless, powder. Very slightly to slightly **soluble** in water and in alcohol; slightly soluble in methyl alcohol and in dimethylformamide; practically insoluble in chloroform and in acetone.

Store in airtight containers. Protect from light.

Adverse Effects

Severe postural hypotension with syncope can occur following the initial dose of prazosin, and may be preceded by tachycardia. This reaction can be avoided by starting treatment with a low dose, preferably at night (see Uses).

The more common side-effects include dizziness, drowsiness, headache, lack of energy, nausea and palpitations, and may diminish with continued prazosin therapy or with a reduction in dosage. Other adverse effects include postural hypotension, oedema, chest pain, dyspnoea, constipation, diarrhoea, vomiting, depression, vertigo, hallucinations, paraesthesia, nasal congestion, dryness of mouth, urinary frequency, reddened sclera, blurred vision, tinnitus, skin rashes, pruritus, and diaphoresis. Impotence has also been reported.

One patient developed 'flu-like' symptoms and arthritis 10 weeks after starting treatment with prazosin; the symptoms recurred when prazosin was given again.— S. A. Cairns and S. C. Jordan, *Br. med. J.*, 1976, *2*, 1424.

Hypothermia, recurring on challenge, in a woman given prazosin.— P. W. de Leeuw and W. H. Birkenhäger, *Br. med. J.*, 1980, *281*, 1181.

Urticaria and angioneurotic oedema were attributed to prazosin in a 70-year-old woman.— T. Ruzicka and J. Ring, *Lancet*, 1983, *1*, 473.

ANTINUCLEAR FACTOR. Antinuclear factor, without systemic lupus erythematosus, was detected in 19 of 57 patients treated with prazosin.— A. J. Marshall *et al.*, *Br. med. J.*, 1979, *1*, 165. The incidence of antinuclear factor was 9.8% in 132 hypertensive patients taking prazosin compared with 11.6% in 1087 patients taking other antihypertensive agents.— J. D. Wilson *et al.* (letter), *ibid.*, 553. None of 42 patients converted from negative to positive in antinuclear factor tests while under long-term prazosin treatment.— A. Melkild and P. I. Gaarder (letter), *ibid.*, 620. The association between prazosin and antinuclear factor was not proved.— B. Ø. Kristensen (letter), *ibid.*, 621.

EFFECTS ON MENTAL FUNCTION. Report of 3 patients who developed psychiatric symptoms including confusion, paranoia, and hallucinations associated with prazosin treatment. Two of the patients had chronic renal failure and the renal function of the third was mildly impaired.— D. K. F. Chin *et al.*, *Br. med. J.*, 1986, *293*, 1347.

OVERDOSAGE. A 19-year-old man who had taken about 200 mg of prazosin had a pulse-rate of 110 per minute and blood pressure of 120/80 mmHg after 90 minutes. Emesis was induced. Over the next 2 hours his pulse-rate rose to 140 per minute. He recovered after bed-rest for 36 hours with no serious after-effects.— W. J. McClean (letter), *Med. J. Aust.*, 1976, *1*, 592.

A report of acute poisoning in a 72-year-old patient following overdosage with prazosin 120 mg by mouth. The patient was comatose on admission, with a heart-rate of 100 beats per minute, blood pressure of 40/20 mmHg, and Cheyne-Stokes respiration. Worsening respiration, and the failure of dopamine 7.5 µg per minute per kg body-weight and angiotensin amide 0.1 µg per minute per kg to elevate blood pressure necessitated mechanical ventilation and gastric and gut lavage was started. Administration of a blood volume expander and dopamine 4 µg per minute per kg increased systolic pressure to 80 mmHg but heart-rate remained unchanged. Plasma concentration of prazosin was 47.6 ng per mL at this time, 11 hours after first admission. Following intravenous injection of atropine sulphate 500 µg, blood pressure rose to 160/80 mmHg and heart-rate to 150 beats per minute. Mechanical ventilation was discontinued 18 hours after ingestion.— K. Lenz *et al.*, *Hum. Toxicol.*, 1985, *4*, 53.

PRIAPISM. Reports of priapism in patients taking prazosin: A. K. Bhalla *et al.*, *Br. med. J.*, 1979, *2*, 1039; J. R. Burke and G. Hirst (letter), *Med. J. Aust.*, 1980, *1*, 382; J. M. Russell *et al.* (letter), *ibid.*, 1985, *143*, 321.

URINARY INCONTINENCE. Urinary incontinence in a 58-year-old woman was probably due to prazosin which appeared to cause alpha-adrenoceptor blockade.— T.

Thien *et al.*, *Br. med. J.*, 1978, *1*, 622. A further report.— G. H. Kiruluta *et al.*, *Urology*, 1981, *18*, 618.

Treatment of Adverse Effects

If overdosage occurs the stomach should be emptied by aspiration and lavage. Severe hypotension may respond to placing the patient in the supine position with the feet raised. The effects of gross overdosage may be treated by infusions of electrolytes or cautious intravenous infusion of a pressor agent. Prazosin is not removed by dialysis.

For reports of acute poisoning with prazosin, including treatment, see under Overdosage in Adverse Effects, above.

Precautions

Treatment with prazosin should be introduced cautiously because of the risk of sudden collapse following the initial dose.

Prazosin in not recommended for the treatment of congestive heart failure caused by mechanical obstruction, for example aortic or mitral valve stenosis, pulmonary embolism, and restrictive pericardial disease. It should be used with caution in patients with angina pectoris, and dosage should be reduced in patients with renal failure and in the elderly. Prazosin may cause drowsiness or dizziness; patients so affected should not drive or operate machinery.

The hypotensive effects of prazosin may be enhanced by the concomitant administration of diuretics and other antihypertensive agents.

Hypotension with disturbance of consciousness occurred in 3 patients with recent cerebral haemorrhage following an initial dose of prazosin 0.5 mg.— M. -S. Lin and W. -J. Hsieh, *Drug Intell. & clin. Pharm.*, 1987, *21*, 723.

INTERACTIONS. A patient who was taking chlorpromazine and amitriptyline developed acute agitation on receiving prazosin. The symptoms settled rapidly when prazosin was discontinued.— P. Bolli and F. O. Simpson (letter), *Br. med. J.*, 1974, *1*, 637.

Reduction of prazosin-induced hypotension by indomethacin in 4 of 9 subjects.— P. Rubin *et al.*, *Br. J. clin. Pharmac.*, 1980, *10*, 33.

The action of prazosin may be reduced by concurrent administration of non-steroidal anti-inflammatory drugs, see p.466.

The hypotensive effect of prazosin and verapamil administered concurrently was greater than could be accounted for by the additive effect of each drug given alone. This can be explained in part by an increase in plasma-prazosin concentration.— F. Pasanisi *et al.*, *Clin. Pharmac. Ther.*, 1984, *36*, 716. See also P. A. Meredith *et al.*, *Br. J. clin. Pharmac.*, 1986, *21*, 85P.

TOLERANCE. In a study involving 16 patients with congestive heart failure, a single dose of prazosin produced beneficial haemodynamic effects, but during long-term therapy there was no clinical benefit, despite sustained vasodilatation. This lack of effect was attributed to secondary activation of both the sympathetic and renin-angiotensin-aldosterone systems which was associated with fluid retention, despite increasing doses of frusemide in 4 patients.— J. Bayliss *et al.*, *Br. med. J.*, 1985, *290*, 1861.

Despite initially favourable responses to prazosin in a study of 27 patients with severe chronic heart failure, the effects became rapidly attenuated after 48 hours despite continued treatment: complete loss of haemodynamic efficacy was noted in 58% of 24 patients who completed the study. Long-term tolerance was not accompanied by changes in plasma renin activity or in body-weight and could not be prevented by concomitant treatment with aldosterone antagonists. Only 30 to 40% of patients with heart failure treated with prazosin showed notable long-term haemodynamic benefits.— M. Packer *et al.*, *J. Am. Coll. Cardiol.*, 1986, *7*, 671.

Absorption and Fate

Prazosin is readily absorbed from the gastro-intestinal tract. The bioavailability is variable and a range of 43 to 85% has been reported. Prazosin is highly bound to plasma protein. It is extensively metabolised in the liver and some of the metabolites are reported to have hypotensive activity. It is excreted as the metabolites and 5 to 11% as unchanged prazosin mainly in the faeces. Less than 10% is excreted in the urine. Its duration of action is longer than would be predicted from its relatively short plasma half-life of about 2 to 4 hours.

An extensive review of the clinical pharmacokinetics of prazosin.— P. Jaillon, *Clin. Pharmacokinet.*, 1980, *5*, 365.

In a study of 10 healthy subjects who received prazosin 5 mg by mouth after fasting overnight, peak plasma concentrations of about 23 ng per mL were reached after 2 or 3 hours. There was some variation in absorption rate: 2 subjects achieved peak concentrations after 1 hour, 1 after 4 hours, and 1 after 5 hours. There was less variation in the elimination rate, the mean plasma half-life being 3.8 hours. Prazosin had a marked effect on standing blood pressure without affecting supine blood pressure—subjects felt faint during the first 3 or 4 hours and 2 subjects felt too faint for nearly 6 and 10 hours respectively to allow standing blood pressure to be recorded.— A. J. Wood *et al.* (letter), *Br. J. clin. Pharmac.*, 1976, *3*, 199.

The elimination of prazosin was not impaired in patients with impaired renal function.— D. T. Lowenthal *et al.*, *Clin. Pharmac. Ther.*, 1980, *27*, 779.

The bioavailability of prazosin was significantly reduced in the elderly, about 40% less unchanged drug reaching the systemic circulation compared with the young. This was attributed to a reduction in the absorption from the gastro-intestinal tract. The half-life was also prolonged in the elderly and this was associated with an increase in the volume of distribution at steady state. However, it was considered unlikely that these effects would have major clinical significance.— P. C. Rubin *et al.*, *Br. J. clin. Pharmac.*, 1981, *12*, 401.

Evidence of accumulation of a metabolite of prazosin with some hypotensive activity during administration of prazosin 1 to 5 mg three times daily.— V. K. Piotrovskii *et al.*, *Eur. J. clin. Pharmac.*, 1984, *27*, 275.

Further references to the pharmacokinetics of prazosin: M. K. Dynon *et al.*, *Clin. Pharmacokinet.*, 1980, *5*, 583; N. P. Chau *et al.*, *Clin. Pharmac. Ther.*, 1980, *28*, 6; A. Grahnén *et al.*, *ibid.*, 1981, *30*, 439.

PROTEIN BINDING. Prazosin was extensively bound to plasma proteins; in 14 healthy subjects the mean free fraction was 0.051; this was increased to 0.064, 0.077, and 0.064 respectively in patients with cirrhosis, chronic renal failure, and congestive heart failure. The free fraction was not affected by propranolol.— P. Rubin and T. Blaschke, *Br. J. clin. Pharmac.*, 1980, *9*, 177.

Prazosin was highly bound to human serum albumin but less so to human alpha$_1$-acid glycoprotein *in vitro*. Binding *in vivo* will therefore be largely mediated by serum albumin, and alpha$_1$-acid glycoprotein might be less important for clinically significant changes in binding.— F. Brunner and W. E. Müller, *J. Pharm. Pharmac.*, 1985, *37*, 305.

Uses and Administration

Prazosin is an antihypertensive agent the mode of action of which is not fully established. It is thought to act by selective blockade of alpha$_1$-adrenoceptors producing peripheral dilatation of both arterioles and veins and reduction of peripheral resistance, usually without reflex tachycardia. It reduces both standing and supine blood pressure with a greater effect on the diastolic pressure. It is reported to have no effect on renal blood flow or glomerular filtration-rate, and has little effect on cardiac output in hypertensive patients. In patients with congestive heart failure, prazosin reduces both preload and afterload and produces an improvement in cardiac output. Tolerance may develop during the treatment of congestive heart failure, but is rarely observed during the treatment of hypertension.

Prazosin is used in the treatment of all grades of hypertension, often in conjunction with a diuretic and other antihypertensive agents. Following oral administration the hypotensive effect is seen within 2 to 4 hours and persists for 10 or more hours.

To lessen the risk of collapse which may occur in some patients after the first dose (see Adverse Effects) the usual initial dose of prazosin hydrochloride is 500 µg two or three times daily for 3 to 7 days, the starting dose being given in the evening; if tolerated the dose may then be increased to 1 mg three times daily for a further 3 to 7 days, and thereafter gradually increased, according to the patient's response, to a usual maximum of 20 mg daily in divided doses. Although sources in Great Britain recommend 20 mg as a maximum daily dose, sources in the *USA* report that a few patients may obtain benefit from up to 40 mg daily in divided doses. The usual maintenance dose is between 6 and 15 mg daily. Smaller doses are required in patients concurrently taking other antihypertensive agents or diuretics, the elderly, and patients with renal impairment.

In the treatment of congestive heart failure, prazosin hydrochloride is normally given in conjunction with a diuretic and an inotropic agent. Treatment is started with a low dose of 500 µg two to four times daily and increased gradually according to response; the usual maintenance dose is 4 to 20 mg daily.

Prazosin hydrochloride has also been used in the treatment of Raynaud's syndrome and as an adjunct in the symptomatic treatment of urinary obstruction caused by benign prostatic hypertrophy in an initial dose of 500 µg twice a day increasing to a maintenance dose not exceeding 2 mg twice a day.

A review of the properties and therapeutic use of prazosin. In numerous therapeutic studies, prazosin has been demonstrated to be effective in mild to moderate hypertension when given as a sole agent, and in more severe hypertension when given in combination with a beta-blocking agent and/or a diuretic, and other antihypertensive agents. Comparative studies have shown prazosin to be as effective as methyldopa, clonidine, hydralazine, atenolol, indoramin, minoxidil, tolamolol, propranolol, and labetalol in reducing blood pressure, and to be effective when added to treatment regimens which had not provided adequate blood pressure control. Data from follow-up of long-term prazosin use for periods of 2 to 5 years in patients with moderate to severe hypertension have demonstrated continued efficacy of the drug and acceptable patient compliance. Tachycardia and a significant increase in cardiac output were not commonly encountered. Prazosin has been used in patients with renal impairment, in pregnant patients, and in patients with respiratory disorders, left ventricular failure, or diabetes without any untoward effects. Prazosin has been generally accepted as a safe and well tolerated drug in patients with congestive heart failure. Studies involving small numbers of patients over several months have demonstrated the effectiveness of prazosin in providing sustained improvements in cardiac haemodynamics and exercise tolerance in patients with congestive heart failure refractory to adequate digitalis, diuretics, bed rest, and sodium restriction. Although an attenuation of initial effects has been observed with longer term therapy this had generally proved to be a reversible, transient phenomenon without clinically significant impact on the value of sustained ambulatory therapy with prazosin. In some patients delayed tolerance has been managed by prior administration of spironolactone, addition or increase of diuretic dosage, and by temporary dosage increases or interruption of prazosin treatment. Long-term studies were still needed.

Beneficial results have also been demonstrated in patients with myocardial infarction, aortic regurgitation, aortic stenosis, and Raynaud's phenomenon.— W. F. Stanaszek *et al.*, *Drugs*, 1983, *25*, 339.

Further reviews of prazosin: R. M. Graham and W. A. Pettinger, *New Engl. J. Med.*, 1979, *300*, 232.

The relation between plasma-prazosin concentration and blood pressure-lowering effect both after single and steady-state doses was not considered to be sufficiently informative to warrant routine measurement of plasma-prazosin concentrations. The maximal decrease in systolic blood pressure correlated with that after the first steady-state dose of 0.5 mg three times daily, indicating a possibility for early prediction of prazosin responders.— P. Seideman *et al.*, *Clin. Pharmac. Ther.*, 1981, *30*, 447. In a study of 11 patients, variability in the blood pressure response to prazosin was not related to the pharmacokinetic behaviour of the drug. Results suggested that patients who had a marked hypotensive response following the first dose of prazosin required a smaller dose to maintain the blood pressure reduction, whereas patients who had a minimal reduction in blood pressure following the first dose required higher doses of prazosin and demonstrated a correlation between the plasma-prazosin concentration and blood pressure reduction.— P. Larochelle *et al.*, *Hypertension*, 1982, *4*, 93.

Prazosin therapy was accompanied by decreases in serum cholesterol, insulin, and non-esterified fatty acids and an increase in high density lipoprotein-cholesterol fraction in a study of 20 hypertensive patients also taking hydrochlorothiazide.— M. Valesco *et al., Eur. J. clin. Pharmac.*, 1985, *28*, 513.

References to the actions of prazosin: C. V. S. Ram *et al., Clin. Pharmac. Ther.*, 1981, *29*, 719; C. Barbieri *et al., J. clin. Pharmac.*, 1981, *21*, 418; J. H. Bauer *et al., Archs intern. Med.*, 1984, *144*, 1196.

ADMINISTRATION IN RENAL FAILURE. Prazosin 2 to 6 mg daily added to the existing antihypertensive regimen of 7 patients with chronic renal failure and 5 patients with renal transplants who were also suffering from renal failure was an effective antihypertensive agent.— J. R. Curtis and F. J. A. Bateman, *Br. med. J.*, 1975, *4*, 432.

Prazosin could be given in usual doses to patients with renal failure, although patients with end-stage renal disease may respond to a lower dose.— W. M. Bennett *et al., Am. J. Kidney Dis.*, 1983, *3*, 155.

ASTHMA. Bronchodilator effect of prazosin in 2 subjects with asthma.— G. E. Marlin *et al.* (letter), *Lancet*, 1981, *1*, 225. Comment that the bronchodilatory effect could be related to the hypotensive effect.— P. Barnes (letter), *ibid.*, 391.

Further reports of bronchodilator activity of prazosin: G. E. Marlin *et al.* (letter), *Br. J. clin. Pharmac.*, 1982, *13*, 445; J. L. Black *et al., ibid.*, 1984, *18*, 349.

BITES AND STINGS. Prazosin was considered to be beneficial in the treatment of the cardiovascular manifestations of scorpion sting.— H. S. Bawaskar and P. H. Bawaskar (letter), *Lancet*, 1986, *1*, 510.

CARDIAC DISORDERS. *Heart failure.* A review of vasodilator therapy in the treatment of severe chronic heart failure. Although prazosin produces dramatic haemodynamic benefits with the administration of the first doses and is generally well tolerated, it has failed to produce consistent haemodynamic and clinical benefits in randomised, placebo-controlled studies. The main reason for the failure of prazosin in congestive heart failure is tolerance to the effects of the drug which develops rapidly in most patients and is generally not reversible.— M. Packer, *Drugs*, 1986, *32, Suppl.* 5, 13.

Further reviews of the use of vasodilators including prazosin in congestive heart failure: *Drug & Ther. Bull.*, 1983, *21*, 50; *Med. Lett.*, 1984, *26*, 115; G. H. Guyatt, *Drugs*, 1986, *32*, 538.

In a study examining the effects of vasodilator therapy in 642 patients with congestive heart failure, the addition of prazosin to existing therapy with digoxin and a diuretic did not reduce mortality after an average of about 2 years compared with placebo. No improvement in left ventricular ejection fraction was seen at either 8 weeks or 1 year.— J. N. Cohn *et al., New Engl. J. Med.*, 1986, *314*, 1547. A suggestion that the group taking prazosin may have had more advanced heart disease.— O. Bertel (letter), *ibid.*, *315*, 1227.

For references to the development of tolerance to prazosin during the treatment of congestive heart failure, see under Precautions, above.

Further references to the use of prazosin in heart failure: J. Bayliss *et al., Eur. Heart J.*, 1986, *7*, 877; G. A. J. Riegger *et al., Am. J. Cardiol.*, 1987, *59*, 906.

HYPERTENSION. A review of the treatment of hypertension. The advantages of prazosin included the absence of adverse effects on blood lipids, the maintenance of high cardiac output, and the lack of serious side-effects such as provocation of asthma, heart failure, or conduction block. Disadvantages were first-dose syncope, the wide range of total doses required, the need for multiple daily dosing, the possibility of tachyphylaxis, and adverse effects such as sexual or bladder dysfunction and postural hypotension.— L. H. Opie, *Lancet*, 1984, *1*, 496.

In a study of 23 hypertensive patients participating in the Oslo study, prazosin treatment was associated with a reduction in total serum cholesterol, low-density-lipoprotein plus very-low-density-lipoprotein cholesterol, and total triglycerides.— P. Leren *et al., Lancet*, 1980, *2*, 4. Further evidence of favourable effects of prazosin given alone or in combination with a beta-blocking agent or a diuretic on blood lipids.— J. Lowenstein, *Am. J. Cardiol.*, 1984, *53*, 21A.

Prazosin 10 to 20 mg twice daily in conjunction with atenolol and chlordiazepoxide was used successfully to control rebound hypertension associated with withdrawal of clonidine in 6 patients.— B. C. Campbell and J. L. Reid, *Br. J. clin. Pharmac.*, 1982, *14*, 578P.

Prazosin once daily was as effective in controlling blood pressure as prazosin twice daily in a study of 20 hypertensive patients. Dizziness and faintness occurred in 8 patients following the once daily but not the twice daily dose. It was suggested that these adverse effects could be overcome by administering the single dose at night, or by the development of a sustained-release preparation.— R. F. Westerman *et al., Eur. J. clin. Pharmac.*, 1985, *28*, 11. See also I. Soltero *et al., Curr. ther. Res.*, 1986, *40*, 739.

Beneficial responses have been reported to prazosin as third-line therapy for hypertension (M.J. Vandenburg *et al, Br. J. clin. Pharmac*, 1983, *16*, 537; L.E. Ramsay and L. Latham, *ibid*, 1985, *20* 524P; E. van der Veur *et al., Eur. J. clin. Pharmac.*, 1985, *28*, 507; L.E. Ramsay *et al., Postgrad. med. J.*, 1987, *63*, 99) and as fourth-line therapy (A.M. Heagerty *et al., Br. J. clin. Pharmac.*, 1982, *13*, 539; M.J. Vandenburg *et al., Br. J. clin. Pract.*, 1985, *39*, 17) although Ramsay *et al.* (*Postgrad. med. J.*, 1987, *63*, 99) considered that nifedipine might have some advantages over prazosin as a third-line drug.

Further references to studies of prazosin in hypertension: L. E. Ramsay, *Practitioner*, 1979, *222*, 127 (as second-line therapy); A. S. Nanivadekar and S. S. Kulkarni, *ibid.*, 1981, *225*, 1327 (comparison with methyldopa); *Circulation*, 1981, *64*, 772 (comparison with hydralazine); D. K. Falch and S. Solheim, *Curr. ther. Res.*, 1984, *35*, 863 (in combination with atenolol); A. Melkild, *Curr. med. Res. Opinion*, 1984, *9*, 219 (long-term therapy); G. S. Stokes *et al., Clin. Pharmac. Ther.*, 1986, *40*, 56 (comparison with ketanserin); R. Okun and J. Kraut, *Am. J. Med.*, 1987, *82, Suppl.* 1A, 58 (comparison with captopril); M. Mattarei *et al., Curr. ther. Res.*, 1987, *41*, 356 (comparison with nifedipine).

PERIPHERAL VASCULAR DISORDERS. Prazosin 2 mg daily reduced the number and duration of attacks of Raynaud's phenomenon in 5 out of 7 patients, but only 1 patient had complete relief from attacks. The effect tended to diminish during prolonged treatment.— S. L. Nielsen *et al., Eur. J. clin. Pharmac.*, 1983, *24*, 421.

Prazosin produced improvements in objective and subjective clinical symptoms in 30 patients with Raynaud's phenomenon. Beneficial effects were greater in patients with Raynaud's disease which has an idiopathic aetiology than in patients with Raynaud's syndrome in which factors other than vasospasm are involved.— C. Allegra *et al., Curr. ther. Res.*, 1986, *40*, 303.

Prazosin 3 mg daily produced a good response in 60% of 24 patients with Raynaud's phenomenon, with complete relief in 2 patients. No difference in response was seen between patients with Raynaud's disease and those with secondary Raynaud's phenomenon.— H. Wollersheim *et al., Clin. Pharmac. Ther.*, 1986, *40*, 219.

PHAEOCHROMOCYTOMA. A review of the management of phaeochromocytoma. Prazosin has been used successfully to overcome the pressor effects of catecholamines released by the tumour. Since it selectively blocks alpha$_1$-adrenoceptors, tachycardia following prazosin treatment is much less marked than following phentolamine or phenoxybenzamine and it may be of particular value in managing phaeochromocytoma crisis. However, the marked hypotensive effect is more pronounced than with other vasodilators such as phenoxybenzamine. Prazosin has also been advocated for control of hypertension during surgery, but its use is limited to the pre-operative phase of management because no parenteral preparation is available.— C. J. Hull, *Br. J. Anaesth.*, 1986, *58*, 1453. See also E. L. Bravo and R. W. Gifford, *New Engl. J. Med.*, 1984, *311*, 1298.

Studies of the use of prazosin in phaeochromocytoma: L. X. Cubeddu *et al., Clin. Pharmac. Ther.*, 1982, *32*, 156; J. P. Nicholson *et al., Ann. intern. Med.*, 1983, *99*, 477.

PORTAL HYPERTENSION. Portohepatic venous pressure gradient, an indirect measure of portal venous pressure, was measured in 24 patients with cirrhosis, portal hypertension, and oesophageal varices given propranolol, prazosin, or atenolol for 8 weeks. A sustained reduction in the gradient of about 25 and 18% was achieved with propranolol and prazosin respectively; a significant reduction with atenolol at 2 weeks was not sustained by 8 weeks.— P. R. Mills *et al., Gut*, 1984, *25*, 73.

PREGNANCY AND THE NEONATE. *Hypertension in pregnancy.* Prazosin 2 to 15 mg daily proved to be an effective antihypertensive agent in 8 women whose blood pressure had not responded to a beta-blocking agent alone. The perinatal outcome was generally satisfactory given that all women had high-risk pregnancies. Prazosin appeared to have a greater bioavailability in pregnant women than in men of similar age and it was possibly also eliminated more slowly.— P. C. Rubin *et al., Br. J. clin. Pharmac.*, 1983, *16*, 543.

URINARY-TRACT DISORDERS. Prazosin may be beneficial in the treatment of overflow incontinence by reducing outlet resistance and in reflex incontinence if treatment of the underlying cause is not possible or unsuccessful.— N. M. Resnick and S. V. Yalla, *New Engl. J. Med.*, 1985, *313*, 800.

In a double-blind placebo-controlled study in 55 men with prostatic obstruction, prazosin improved maximum urine flow rate and reduced voiding frequency.— R. S. Kirby *et al., Br. J. Urol.*, 1987, *60*, 136.

Comment that selective α_1-adrenergic antagonists such as prazosin seem certain to fulfil a role in the short-term management of benign prostatic hypertrophy.— *Lancet*, 1988, *1*, 1083.

Preparations

Prazosin Hydrochloride Capsules *(U.S.P.)*

Prazosin Tablets *(B.P.)*. Contain prazosin hydrochloride.

Proprietary Preparations

Hypovase *(Pfizer, UK). Tablets*, prazosin hydrochloride 500 µg.

Tablets, scored, prazosin hydrochloride 1, 2, and 5 mg. *Starter pack* combination pack, 8 tablets prazosin hydrochloride 500 µg and 32 tablets prazosin hydrochloride 1 mg.

Proprietary Names and Manufacturers

Duramipress *(Durachemie, Ger.)*; Eurex *(Labaz, Ger.)*; Hexapress *(Durascan, Denm.)*; Hypovase *(Pfizer, UK)*; Minipres *(Arg.; Pfizer, Spain)*; Minipress *(Pfizer, Austral.; Belg.; Pfizer, Canad.; Pfizer, Fr.; Pfizer, Ger.; Pfizer, Ital.; Neth.; Pfizer, S.Afr.; Pfizer, Switz.; Pfizer, USA)*; Peripress *(Pfizer, Denm.; Pfizer, Norw.; Pfizer, Swed.)*; Pratsiol *(Orion, Swed.)*; Prazac *(Erco, Denm.; Orion, Switz.)*; Sinetens *(Farmitalia Carlo Erba, UK)*.

The following names have been used for multi-ingredient preparations containing prazosin hydrochloride— Minizide *(Pfizer, USA)*.

13168-s

Prizidilol Hydrochloride *(BANM, USAN, rINNM)*.

SKF-92657-A. 1-*tert*-Butylamino-3-[2-(6-hydrazinopyridazin-3-yl)phenoxy]propan-2-ol dihydrochloride monohydrate.

$C_{17}H_{25}N_5O_2,2HCl,H_2O$=422.4.

CAS — 59010-44-5 (prizidilol); 63642-19-3 (hydrochloride, anhydrous); 73398-12-6 (hydrochloride, monohydrate).

Prizidilol hydrochloride is an antihypertensive agent reported to have vasodilator and beta-adrenoceptor blocking properties.

References to the action and uses of prizidilol in hypertension: D. W. Pitcher *et al., Br. J. clin. Pharmac.*, 1982, *13*, 711 (assessment of beta-adrenoceptor blockade); B. E. Karlberg *et al., Eur. J. clin. Pharmac.*, 1983, *25*, 179 (long-term efficacy, tolerance, and pharmacokinetics); O. Andersson *et al., ibid.*, 577 (cardiovascular response to exercise and regional haemodynamics); K. Boehringer *et al., Br. J. clin. Pharmac.*, 1983, *15*, 181 (effects on renal function); R. Eggertsen *et al., Curr. ther. Res.*, 1983, *34*, 1023 (comparison with propranolol in combination with hydralazine); P. L. Malini *et al., Br. J. clin. Pharmac.*, 1984, *17*, 251 (comparison with propranolol).

Proprietary Names and Manufacturers

Smith Kline & French, UK.

916-l

Protoveratrine A

Protoverine 6,7-diacetate 3(*S*)-(2-hydroxy-2-methylbutyrate) 15(*R*)-(2-methylbutyrate).

$C_{41}H_{63}NO_{14}$=793.5.

CAS — 143-57-7.

An alkaloid from white veratrum, *Veratrum album* (Liliaceae).

917-y

Protoveratrine B

Protoverine 6,7-diacetate 3(*S*)-(2,3-dihydroxy-2-methylbutyrate) 15(*R*)-(2-methylbutyrate).

$C_{41}H_{63}NO_{15}$=809.9.

CAS — 124-97-0 (Protoveratrine B); 8053-18-7 (Protoveratrines A and B).

Protoveratrines A and B have the properties and uses described under White Veratrum, p.504.

Proprietary Names and Manufacturers

Pro-Amid *(Amid, USA)*; Protalba *(Merrell Dow, USA)*; Puroverine *(Sandoz, UK)*.

491-m

Quinapril Hydrochloride *(USAN, rINNM).*
CI-906. (*S*)-2-{(*S*)-*N*-[(*S*)-1-Ethoxycarbonyl-3-phenylpropyl]alanyl}-1,2,3,4-tetrahydro-3-isoquinolinecarboxylic acid hydrochloride.
$C_{25}H_{30}N_2O_5,HCl=475.0$.

CAS — 90243-99-5 (hydrochloride); 85441-61-8 (quinapril).

Quinapril is an antihypertensive agent which acts, similarly to captopril, as an angiotensin-converting enzyme inhibitor.

In 8 patients with essential hypertension, doses of 2.5 mg of quinapril by mouth produced a clinically significant, though partial and short-lived, effect on blood pressure; doses of 5 and 10 mg reduced blood pressure by a mean of 26 and 25 mmHg respectively. Neither orthostatic hypotension nor tachycardia occurred.— I. Gavras *et al., J. clin. Pharmac.*, 1984, *24*, 343.

Results of a study involving 15 patients with severe congestive heart failure given single doses of quinapril 5 mg by mouth suggested that significant improvement in haemodynamic function had occurred; these single doses also appeared to have a similar time-course of effects to captopril.— P. Holt *et al., Eur. J. clin. Pharmac.*, 1986, *31*, 9.

Proprietary Names and Manufacturers
Parke, Davis, USA.

16975-a

Ramipril *(USAN, rINN).*
HOE-498. (2*S*,3a*S*,6a*S*)-1-{(*S*)-*N*-[(*S*)-1-Ethoxycarbonyl-3-phenylpropyl]alanyl}octahydrocyclopenta[*b*]pyrrole-2-carboxylic acid.
$C_{23}H_{32}N_2O_5=416.5$.

CAS — 87333-19-5.

Ramipril is an antihypertensive agent which acts, similarly to captopril, as an angiotensin-converting enzyme inhibitor.

A series of reports on the synthesis, biochemistry, pharmacology, and pharmacokinetics of ramipril, with reviews of the chemistry and pharmacology of inhibitors of the renin-angiotensin system: *Arzneimittel-Forsch.*, 1984, *34*, 1385–1454.

References on the pharmacokinetics and pharmacodynamics of ramipril: P. U. Witte *et al., Eur. J. clin. Pharmac.*, 1984, *27*, 577; H. Shionoiri *et al., Curr. ther. Res.*, 1986, *40*, 74.

References on the actions and uses of ramipril: P. J. O. Manhem *et al., Br. J. clin. Pharmac.*, 1985, *20*, 27; T. Lenz *et al., Arzneimittel-Forsch.*, 1986, *36*, 1693; E. R. Debusmann *et al., Am. J. Cardiol.*, 1987, *59*, 70D; P. W. De Leeuw and W. H. Birkenhäger, *ibid.*, 79D; Y. Kaneko *et al., ibid.*, 86D; P. U. Witte and U. Walter, *ibid.*, 115D; K. Fukiyama *et al., ibid.*, 121D; H. G. Predel *et al., ibid.*, 143D; P. A. De Graeff *et al., ibid.*, 164D; C. M. S. Dixon *et al., Br. J. clin. Pharmac.*, 1987, *23*, 91.

Proprietary Names and Manufacturers
Hoechst, Ger.

898-m

Rauwolfia Serpentina *(USAN).*
Chotachand; Rauvolfia; Rauwolfia; Rauwolfiae Radix; Rauwolfiawurzel.

CAS — 8063-17-0 (rauwolfia).

Pharmacopoeias. In *Egypt., Fr.* and *Ger.* (not less than 1% of total alkaloids); and *U.S.*
Also in *B.P.C. 1973* which also includes Rauwolfia Vomitoria (African Rauwolfia).

The dried roots of *Rauwolfia serpentina* (Apocynaceae). It contains not less than 0.15% of reserpine-rescinnamine group alkaloids calculated as reserpine.
Rauwolfia serpentina contains numerous alkaloids, the most active as hypotensive agents being the ester alkaloids, reserpine and rescinnamine. Other alkaloids present have structures related to reserpic acid, but are not esterified, and include ajmaline (rauwolfine), ajmalinine, ajmalicine, isoajmaline (isorauwolfine), serpentine, rauwolfinine, and sarpagine. **Store** at 15° to 30° in a dry place. Tablets containing powdered *Rauwolfia serpentina* should be stored in airtight containers protected from light.

The actions of rauwolfia serpentina are those of its alkaloids and it is used for the same purposes as reserpine, below. It is administered by mouth as the powdered whole root, in initial doses of 200 to 400 mg daily in 2 divided doses for 1 to 3 weeks, and maintenance doses of 50 to 300 mg daily depending on the response of the patient. Some sources suggest an initial dose of 50 mg. Lower doses are required if diuretics or other antihypertensive agents are given concomitantly. Preparations are also available with doses expressed in terms of the alkaloids; these doses of 2 mg should not be confused with the much larger doses used for the powdered whole root.

The crude drug has been used in India for centuries in the treatment of insomnia and certain forms of mental illness, in doses up to 1 to 2 g.

Preparations

Powdered Rauwolfia Serpentina *(U.S.P.).* Rauwolfia serpentina reduced to a fine or very fine powder and adjusted to contain 0.15 to 0.2% of reserpine-rescinnamine group alkaloids, calculated as reserpine.

Rauwolfia Serpentina Tablets *(U.S.P.).* Tablets containing powdered rauwolfia serpentina.

Proprietary Preparations

Hypercal *(Carlton Laboratories, UK). Tablets*, rauwolfia alkaloids 2 mg.

Hypercal-B *(Carlton Laboratories, UK). Tablets*, rauwolfia alkaloids 2 mg, amylobarbitone 15 mg.

Proprietary Names and Manufacturers
Bagoserfia *(Arg.)*; Hypercal *(Carlton Laboratories, UK)*; Hypertane *(Medo, UK)*; Hypertensan *(Medo, UK)*; Lesten *(Vernleigh, S.Afr.)*; Raudixin *(Squibb, Austral.; Squibb, Canad.; Squibb, UK; Princeton, USA)*; Rauserfia *(USA)*; Rauval *(Vale, USA)*; Rauverid *(Forest Pharmaceuticals, USA)*; Rauwolfinetas *(Spain)*; Rawlina *(Eagle, Austral.)*; Rivadescin *(Schaper & Brümmer, Ger.; Switz.)*; Serenol *(Austral.)*; Serpetin *(Jpn)*; Tensowolfia *(Spain)*; Wolfina *(Forest Pharmaceuticals, USA)*.

The following names have been used for multi-ingredient preparations containing rauwolfia serpentina— Hypercal-B *(Carlton Laboratories, UK)*; Hypertane Compound *(Medo, UK)*; Hypertane Forte *(Medo, UK)*; Mio-Pressin *(Smith Kline & French, UK)*; Rautractyl *(Squibb, Canad.)*; Rautrax *(Squibb, UK; Squibb, USA)*; Rautrax sine K *(Squibb, UK)*; Rautrax-N *(Squibb, USA)*; Rauzide *(Princeton, USA)*.

900-b

Rescinnamine *(BAN, rINN).*
Methyl 18-*O*-(3,4,5-trimethoxycinnamoyl)reserpate.
$C_{35}H_{42}N_2O_9=634.7$.

CAS — 24815-24-5.

An ester alkaloid isolated from the root of *Rauwolfia serpentina* or *R.vomitoria*.

Rescinnamine has properties and uses similar to those described under reserpine (see below). For the treatment of hypertension it is given in initial doses of 0.25 to 1 mg daily and maintenance doses of 250 to 500 µg daily according to the response of the patient.

Proprietary Names and Manufacturers
Anaprel *(Eutherapie, Belg.; Servier, UK)*; Cartric *(Jpn)*; Cinnasil *(Amfre-Grant, USA)*; Moderil *(Pfizer, USA)*; Rescimin *(Torlan, Spain)*.

13209-h

Reserpiline Hydrochloride
Methyl 16,17-didehydro-10,11-dimethoxy-19α-methyl-3β,20α-oxayohimban-16-carboxylate hydrochloride.
$C_{23}H_{28}N_2O_5,HCl=448.9$.

CAS — 131-02-2 (reserpiline); 63647-55-2 (hydrochloride).

Reserpiline, a rauwolfia alkaloid, is an antihypertensive agent similar to reserpine below. Dimethylaminoethyl reserpilinate has also been used.

Proprietary Names and Manufacturers of Reserpiline and its Salts
Andanol *(Nippon Shinyaku, Jpn)*; Belnalin *(Jpn)*; Dimeserpin *(Jpn)*; Grona *(Llorens, Spain)*; Hypertenis *(Jpn)*; Hypotensiol *(Green Cross Corp., Jpn)*; Moderyl *(Jpn)*; Morandamin *(Jpn)*; Paratensiol *(Latéma, Fr.; Yoshitomi, Jpn)*; Parenin *(Jpn)*; Perserin *(Jpn)*; Pilinate *(Jpn)*; Pullsmalin R *(Jpn)*; Redouline *(Belg.)*; Resporisan *(Jpn)*; Shinnabrein *(Jpn)*.

901-v

Reserpine *(BAN, USAN, rINN).*

Reserpinum. Methyl 11,17α-dimethoxy-18β-(3,4,5-trimethoxybenzoyloxy)-3β,20α-yohimbane-16β-carboxylate; Methyl 18-*O*-(3,4,5-trimethoxybenzoyl)reserpate.
$C_{33}H_{40}N_2O_9=608.7$.

CAS — 50-55-5.

Pharmacopoeias. In *Arg., Aust., Belg., Br., Braz., Chin., Cz., Egypt., Eur., Fr., Ger., Hung., Ind., Int., It., Jpn, Jug., Neth., Nord., Pol., Roum., Rus., Swiss, Turk.*, and *U.S.* Also in *B.P. Vet.*

An alkaloid obtained from the roots of certain species of *Rauwolfia* (Apocynaceae), mainly *Rauwolfia serpentina* and *R. vomitoria*, or by synthesis. The material obtained from natural sources may contain closely related alkaloids.
It occurs as odourless, small white or pale buff to slightly yellow-coloured crystals or crystalline powder. It darkens slowly on exposure to light but more rapidly when in solution.
B.P. **solubilities** are: practically insoluble in water and ether; soluble 1 in 6 of chloroform; slightly soluble in alcohol. *U.S.P.* solubilities are: insoluble in water; very slightly soluble in ether; soluble 1 in 1800 of alcohol and 1 in 6 of chloroform; freely soluble in acetic acid. The *U.S.P.* injection is prepared with the aid of a suitable acid and has a pH of 3.0 to 4.0. Reserpine is **unstable** in the presence of alkalis, particularly when the drug is in solution. Solutions may be **sterilised** by filtration. **Store** in airtight containers. Protect from light.
For a report of an incompatibility with ethacrynic acid, see Ethacrynic Acid, p.986.

Adverse Effects
Side-effects commonly include nasal congestion, CNS symptoms including depression, drowsiness, lethargy, nightmares, and symptoms of increased gastro-intestinal tract motility including diarrhoea, abdominal cramps, and, at higher doses, increased gastric acid secretion. Respiratory distress, cyanosis, anorexia, hypothermia, and lethargy may occur in infants whose mothers have received reserpine prior to delivery.
Higher doses may cause flushing, bradycardia, severe depression which may lead to suicide, and extrapyramidal effects. Hypotension, coma, respiratory depression and hypothermia also occur in overdosage. Hypotension is also more common in patients following a cerebrovascular accident.
Breast engorgement and galactorrhoea, gynaecomastia, increased prolactin concentrations, decreased libido, impotence, sodium retention, oedema, increased appetite, weight gain, miosis, dry mouth, sialorrhoea, and thrombocytopenic purpura have also been reported.
Reserpine has been shown to be tumorogenic in *rodents* following administration of large doses. Several reports have suggested that there might

be an association between the ingestion of reserpine and the development of neoplasms of the breast (see below) but other surveys have failed to confirm the association.

A 79-year-old woman developed fatigue, anorexia, fever, night sweats, and weight loss while taking reserpine, potassium chloride, hydrochlorothiazide, and ibuprofen. She was found to have generalised lymphadenopathy, hepatomegaly, and thrombocytopenia. She was Coombs' test positive, had raised platelet-associated IgG, and diffuse hypergammaglobulinaemia. Lymph node biopsy was diagnostic of angioimmunoblastic lymphadenopathy, a condition characterised by B-lymphocyte proliferation with associated autoimmune phenomena. Reserpine was discontinued and the syndrome resolved completely following treatment with corticosteroids. Reserpine, or an interaction between reserpine and another mutagen, was thought to have been responsible.— J. H. Entrican *et al.* (letter), *Lancet*, 1984, *2*, 820.

A brief review of the effects of reserpine on sexual dysfunction. Sexual dysfunction in patients taking reserpine may be due to sympatholytic effects, mental depression, and increased prolactin secretion. However, estimation of the incidence of reserpine-induced sexual dysfunction is complicated by concomitant administration of diuretics which may also produce disorders of sexual function.— J. G. Stevenson and G. S. Umstead, *Drug Intell. & clin. Pharm.*, 1984, *18*, 113.

NEOPLASMS OF THE BREAST. Despite a number of investigations the possible link between reserpine and an increased incidence of breast cancer remains unresolved. Epidemiological studies by the Boston Collaborative Drug Surveillance Program (*Lancet*, 1974, *2*, 669), Armstrong *et al.* (*ibid.*, 672), and Heinonen *et al.* (*ibid.*, 675) found that the incidence of breast cancer was up to 3 to 4 times greater in hypertensive women treated with rauwolfia preparations than in control groups, and the findings were subsequently supported by a further study by Armstrong *et al.* (*ibid.*, 1976, *2*, 8). The studies were criticised especially for the selections of control series (H. Immich, *ibid.*, 1974, *2*, 774; R.D. Mann *et al.*, *ibid.*, 966; C. Siegel and E. Laska, *ibid.*) although the validity of the criticisms was questioned by both the original authors (Boston Collaborative Drug Surveillance Program Research Group, *ibid.*, 1315; O.P. Heinonen and S. Shapiro, *ibid.*, 1316) and by Jick in an editorial (*J. Am. med. Ass.*, 1975, *233*, 896). Subsequent studies, however, have failed to find an association between reserpine and breast cancer (T.M. Mack *et al.*, *New Engl. J. Med.*, 1975, *292*, 1366; W.M. O'Fallon *et al.*, *Lancet* 1975, *2*, 292; E.M. Laska *et al.*, *ibid.*, 296; L.J. Christopher *et al.*, *Eur. J. clin. Pharmac.*, 1977, *11*, 409; D. R. Labarthe and W. M. O'Fallon, *J. Am. med. Ass.*, 1980, *243*, 2304; J.D. Curb *et al.*, *Hypertension*, 1982, *4*, 307; G.D. Friedman, *J. Chronic Dis.*, 1983, *36*, 367) although the difficulties in proving a negative correlation were discussed by Jick (*J. Am. med. Ass.*, 1975, *233*, 896).

An elevation of prolactin concentrations of about 50% in 15 women who had taken reserpine for at least 5 years compared with control groups was considered unlikely to greatly increase the risk of breast cancer.— R. K. Ross *et al.*, *Cancer Res.*, 1984, *44*, 3106.

Treatment of Adverse Effects

Withdrawal of reserpine or reduction of the dosage causes the reversal of many side-effects although mental disorders may persist for months and hypotensive effects may persist for weeks after the cessation of treatment. If overdosage occurs the stomach should be emptied by aspiration and lavage even if several hours have elapsed after ingestion. Treatment is generally supportive. Severe hypotension may respond to placing the patient in the supine position with the feet raised. Antimuscarinic agents such as atropine may be used to reduce bradycardia and other parasympathomimetic effects. Direct acting sympathomimetic agents may be effective for treatment of severe hypotension, but should be given with caution. The patient must be observed for at least 72 hours.

Concomitant administration of alprazolam reversed reserpine-induced depression in 2 patients.— R. J. Holt, *Drug Intell. & clin. Pharm.*, 1984, *18*, 311.

Precautions

Reserpine should not be used in patients with a history of mental depression, with active peptic ulcer, or with ulcerative colitis.

It should be used with caution in debilitated or elderly patients, and in the presence of cardiac arrhythmias, myocardial infarction, severe cardiac damage, renal insufficiency, gall-stones, epilepsy, or allergic conditions such as bronchial asthma.

If used in patients requiring electroconvulsive therapy an interval of at least 7 to 14 days should be allowed to elapse between the last dose of reserpine and the commencement of the shock treatment.

Although is is probably not necessary to discontinue treatment with reserpine during anaesthesia, the anaesthetist should be aware of the treatment. The effects of thiopentone and other CNS depressants may be enhanced by reserpine.

Patients taking reserpine are hypersensitive to adrenaline and other direct-acting sympathomimetic agents which should not be given except to antagonise reserpine. The effects of indirect-acting sympathomimetic agents such as ephedrine may be decreased by reserpine. The hypotensive effects of reserpine are enhanced by thiazide diuretics and other antihypertensive agents. Reserpine may cause excitation and hypertension in patients receiving monoamine oxidase inhibitors. Concurrent administration of digitalis or quinidine may cause cardiac arrhythmias. Reserpine has been reported to produce falsely low results in colorimetric methods of determining 17-hydroxycorticosteroids and may cause increases in the urinary excretion of 5-hydroxyindoleacetic acid, catecholamines, and vanillylmandelic acid (VMA).

The action of reserpine may be reduced by concurrent administration of non-steroidal anti-inflammatory drugs. See p.466.

Absorption and Fate

Reserpine is absorbed from the gastro-intestinal tract. It is extensively metabolised and is excreted slowly in the urine and faeces. About 8% has been reported to be excreted in the urine in the first 4 days, mainly as metabolite; about 60% has been reported to be excreted in the faeces in the first 4 days, mainly unchanged. Reserpine crosses the placental barrier and also appears in breast milk.

Uses and Administration

Reserpine is an antihypertensive agent which causes depletion of noradrenaline stores in peripheral sympathetic nerve terminals and depletion of catecholamine and serotonin stores in the brain, heart, and many other organs resulting in a reduction in blood pressure, bradycardia, and central nervous system depression. The hypotensive effect is mainly due to a reduction in cardiac output and a reduction in peripheral resistance. Cardiovascular reflexes are partially inhibited, but postural hypotension is rarely a problem at the doses used in hypertension. When given by mouth the full effect is only reached after several weeks of continued treatment and persists for up to 6 weeks after treatment is discontinued. It has a cumulative effect.

In the treatment of hypertension, reserpine is used in mild to moderate hypertension in patients who have not responded to a diuretic or a beta-blocker alone. The usual dosage for adults is 250 to 500 µg daily for about 2 weeks, then reduced to the lowest dose necessary to maintain the response. Some clinicians have recommended an initial dose of 100 µg. A maintenance dose of about 250 µg daily is usually adequate and 500 µg should not normally be exceeded. To reduce side-effects and tolerance smaller doses of reserpine may be given in conjunction with a thiazide diuretic. Reserpine has also been administered by intravenous and intramuscular injection.

Reserpine has been used as a sedative in anxiety states and chronic psychoses in daily doses of up to 2 mg, but for these purposes it has largely been replaced by safer and more effective agents. Reserpine has also been used in the treatment of Raynaud's syndrome.

ADMINISTRATION IN RENAL FAILURE. Reserpine could be given in normal doses to patients with a glomerular filtration-rate greater than 10 mL per minute, but should be avoided altogether in patients with a glomerular filtration-rate of less than 10 mL per minute. No dosage supplement was necessary during peritoneal or haemodialysis.— W. M. Bennett *et al.*, *Am. J. Kidney Dis.*, 1983, *3*, 155.

FAMILIAL MEDITERRANEAN FEVER. Treatment of 22 patients with familial Mediterranean fever with reserpine 200 to 300 µg daily fully suppressed attacks in 8 patients and produced a 75% improvement in the frequency and severity of attacks in a further 5 patients.— M. H. Barakat *et al.*, *J. Kuwait med. Ass.*, 1981, *15*, 3.

HYPERTENSION. A review of the drugs used for the treatment of chronic hypertension, including reserpine. Reserpine is an effective antihypertensive agent, but at doses unlikely to cause adverse reactions, reserpine alone is usually less effective than a diuretic. It should generally be used at a maximum dose of 250 µg daily with a thiazide diuretic.— *Med. Lett.*, 1984, *26*, 107.

In a double-blind study in 450 patients with mild hypertension propranolol, alone or in combination with hydrochlorothiazide and hydralazine was compared with reserpine with hydrochlorothiazide. Reduction of diastolic blood pressures to below 90 mmHg and a reduction of at least 5 mmHg from the initial blood pressure after 6 months' treatment was achieved in 92% of patients taking propranolol with hydrochlorothiazide and hydralazine, 88% taking reserpine and hydrochlorothiazide, 81% taking propranolol and hydrochlorothiazide, 72% taking propranolol and hydralazine, and 52% taking propranolol alone. No regimen had any advantage over any other with relation to side-effects.— Veterans Administration Cooperative Study Group on Antihypertensive Agents, *J. Am. med. Ass.*, 1977, *237*, 2303.

A double-blind, multicentre study involving 329 patients indicating that the dose of reserpine could be reduced to 125 µg daily with essentially no loss of antihypertensive activity and to 50 µg daily with only slight loss of effectiveness compared with standard doses of 250 µg daily, when administered concomitantly with chlorthalidone.— *J. Am. med. Ass.*, 1982, *248*, 2471.

Further references to the use of reserpine in hypertension: B. J. Materson *et al.*, *J. clin. Pharmac.*, 1985, *25*, 633.

HYPERTHYROIDISM. Thyroid storm responded to intramuscular doses of reserpine 2.5 mg given 4 to 8 hours apart in a patient who had not responded to propylthiouracil and propranolol. Full recovery was achieved with maintenance reserpine therapy.— E. Anaissie and J. F. Tohmé, *Archs intern. Med.*, 1985, *145*, 2248.

MENTAL DISORDERS. Mention of the use of reserpine as an adjunct to the treatment of acute mania in patients not responding to conventional antipsychotic therapy.— J. C. Cookson, *Br. J. Hosp. Med.*, 1985, *34*, 172. See also M. W. Jann *et al.*, *Drug Intell. & clin. Pharm.*, 1984, *18*, 577.

Further references to the use of reserpine in psychiatric disorders: A. Forsmen *et al.*, *Curr. ther. Res.*, 1983, *34*, 991.

RAYNAUD'S SYNDROME. A review of the treatment of peripheral vascular disease including a brief account of reserpine therapy. Reserpine 0.25 to 1 mg daily produces remarkable amelioration of symptoms in about 50% of patients with Raynaud's phenomenon. The author had given reserpine by intra-arterial injection only in the most severe cases and had found no difference from oral therapy.— J. D. Coffman, *New Engl. J. Med.*, 1979, *300*, 713.

Intra-arterial injection of reserpine 1 mg in 2 mL of saline given slowly over 1 minute increased basal skin blood flow in 7 patients with systemic sclerosis and severe Raynaud's phenomenon accompanied by peripheral ischaemia and ulceration. The effect usually lasted 1 to 3 weeks. Repeat injections of reserpine in 5 of the patients with ulcers of the fingers resulted in healing in 4.— K. H. Nilsen and M. I. V. Jayson, *Br. med. J.*, 1980, *280*, 1408.

Intra-arterial injections of reserpine were considered to be ineffective in the treatment of Raynaud's disease in a study of 24 patients. Administration of the drug by this route was associated with adverse cardiovascular effects which lasted for up to 6 weeks.— R. S. Surwit *et al.*, *Archs Derm.*, 1983, *119*, 733.

TARDIVE DYSKINESIA. A brief review of the management of tardive dyskinesia. Reserpine can help in the management of tardive dyskinesia, but its usefulness is limited by drowsiness, depression, and hypotension.— *Drug & Ther. Bull.*, 1986, *24*, 27.

Preparations

Reserpine Elixir *(U.S.P.)*

Reserpine Injection *(U.S.P.)*. A sterile solution of reserpine in Water for Injections, prepared with the aid of a suitable acid. It contains suitable antoxidants. pH 3 to 4.

Reserpine Tablets *(U.S.P.)*

Reserpine and Chlorothiazide Tablets *(U.S.P.)*

Reserpine and Hydrochlorothiazide Tablets *(U.S.P.)*

Reserpine, Hydralazine Hydrochloride, and Hydrochlorothiazide Tablets *(U.S.P.)*. Tablets containing, unless otherwise specified, reserpine 100 µg, hydralazine hydrochloride 25 mg, and hydrochlorothiazide 15 mg.

Proprietary Preparations

Abicol *(Boots, UK)*. *Tablets*, scored, reserpine 150 µg, bendrofluazide 2.5 mg.

Seominal *(Winthrop, UK)*. *Tablets*, scored, reserpine 200 µg, phenobarbitone 10 mg, theobromine 325 mg.

Serpasil *(Ciba, UK)*. *Tablets*, reserpine 100 µg. *Tablets*, scored, reserpine 250 µg.

Serpasil-Esidrex *(Ciba, UK)*. *Tablets*, scored, reserpine 150 µg, hydrochlorothiazide 10 mg.

Proprietary Names and Manufacturers

Lemiserp *(USA)*; Mephaserpin *(Switz.)*; Neo-Serp *(Canad.)*; Rausan *(Spain)*; Rau-Sed *(USA)*; Rauwita *(Spain)*; Resedril *(Spain)*; Rese-Lar *(Spain)*; Resercen *(USA)*; Reserfia *(Medic, Canad.)*; Reserpanca *(Canad.)*; Reserpine Dellipsoids D29 *(Pilsworth, UK)*; Reserpoid *(USA)*; Sandril *(Lilly, USA)*; Sedaraupin *(Arg.; Ger.)*; Serpasil *(Ciba, Austral.; Belg.; Ciba, Canad.; Ciba, Fr.; Ciba, Ger.; Ciba, Ital.; S.Afr.; Ciba, Swed.; Ciba, Switz.; Ciba, UK; Ciba, USA)*; Serpasol *(Arg.; Ciba, Spain)*; Serpate *(Vale, USA)*; Serpresan *(Maipe, Spain)*; SK-Reserpine *(Smith Kline & French, USA)*; Vio-Serpine *(USA)*.

The following names have been used for multi-ingredient preparations containing reserpine—Abicol *(Boots, UK)*; Adelphane *(Ciba, Austral.)*; Aquamox with Reserpine *(Lederle, Canad.)*; Chloroserpine *(Schein, USA)*; Demi-Regroton *(Rorer, USA)*; Diupres *(Merck Sharp & Dohme, USA)*; Diutensen-R *(Wallace, USA)*; H-H-R *(Schein, USA)*; Hydro-Fluserpine *(Schein, USA)*; Hydromox R *(Lederle, USA)*; Hydropres *(Merck Sharp & Dohme, Canad.; Merck Sharp & Dohme, USA)*; Hydroserpine *(Schein, USA)*; Hydrosine *(Major, USA)*; Hyserp *(Reid-Provident, USA)*; Metatensin *(Merrell Dow, USA)*; Naquival *(Schering, USA)*; Regroton *(USV Pharmaceutical Corp., USA)*; Renese-R *(Pfizer, USA)*; Rezide *(Edwards, USA)*; Salazide *(Major, USA)*; Salupres *(Merck Sharp & Dohme, UK)*; Salutensin *(Bristol, Canad.; Bristol, USA)*; Seominal *(Winthrop, UK)*; Seragen *(Reid-Provident, USA)*; Ser-Ap-Es *(Ciba, Canad.; Ciba, USA)*; Serpasil-Apresoline *(Ciba, USA)*; Serpasil-Esidrex *(Ciba, UK)*; Serpasil-Esidrex K *(Ciba, UK)*; Serpasil-Esidrix *(Ciba, Canad.; Ciba, USA)*; Tensanyl *(Leo, UK)*; Unipres *(Reid-Rowell, USA)*.

3157-y

Rilmenidine *(rINN)*.

S-3341. 2-[(Dicyclopropylemthyl)amino]-2-oxazoline.

$C_{10}H_{16}N_2O$=180.2.

CAS—54187-04-1.

Rilmenidine is an antihypertensive agent.

References: K. Weerasuriya *et al.*, *Eur. J. clin. Pharmac.*, 1984, *27*, 281.

Proprietary Names and Manufacturers
Servier, Fr.

902-g

Saralasin Acetate *(BANM, USAN, rINNM)*.

The acetate of 1-Sar-8-Ala-angiotensin; P-113. The hydrated acetate of Sar-Arg-Val-Tyr-Val-His-Pro-Ala; [1-(*N*-Methylglycine)-5-L-valine-8-L-alanine]-angiotensin II acetate hydrate.

$C_{42}H_{65}N_{13}O_{10}$, $x$$CH_3COOH$, $x$$H_2O$.

CAS — 34273-10-4 (saralasin); 39698-78-7 (acetate, hydrate); 54194-01-3 (anhydrous).

Saralasin acetate is a competitive antagonist of angiotensin II and thus blocks its pressor action. It is also a partial agonist and causes a transient initial rise in blood pressure. Saralasin has a short half-life and has been used in the differential diagnosis of renovascular hypertension: following intravenous administration, saralasin commonly causes a fall in blood pressure in patients with renovascular hypertension, whereas patients with low-renin essential hypertension may have a sustained pressor response. The reaction is affected by sodium balance and patients are normally mildly depleted of sodium before the test. False positive and false negative results are numerous, and the use of saralasin has largely been superseded by the ACE inhibitors.

A review of the use of saralasin for diagnosing renovascular hypertension. The incidence of false-negative results has been reported to be 19% and the incidence of false-positive results to be 30%. Adequate sodium depletion decreases the number of false-negative results but increases the number of false-positives. Rebound hypertension may occur in patients with a marked fall in blood pressure or with a history of hypertensive encephalopathy. Testing for renovascular hypertension using saralasin was not recommended as a screening procedure.— *Med. Lett.*, 1982, *24*, 3.

Further reviews and reports on the use of saralasin: E. T. Zawada *et al.*, *Archs intern. Med.*, 1984, *144*, 65; R. J. Cody, *Drugs*, 1984, *28*, 144.

Proprietary Names and Manufacturers
Sarenin *(Röhm, Ger.; Norwich Eaton, USA)*.

903-q

Sodium Nitroprusside *(BAN, USAN)*.

Disodium (*OC*-6-22)-Pentakis(cyano-*C*)nitrosylferrate Dihydrate; Sodium Nitroferricyanide Dihydrate; Sodium Nitroprussiate. Sodium nitrosylpentacyanoferrate(III) dihydrate.

$Na_2Fe(CN)_5NO$, $2H_2O$=298.0.

CAS — 14402-89-2 (anhydrous); 13755-38-9 (dihydrate).

Pharmacopoeias. In *Br.*, *Chin.*, *Egypt.*, *Eur.*, *It.*, and *U.S.*; *U.S.* also includes Sterile Sodium Nitroprusside.

Reddish-brown odourless or almost odourless crystals or powder. Freely **soluble** in water; slightly soluble in alcohol; very slightly soluble in chloroform. Aqueous solutions decompose when exposed to light. Solutions for injection are prepared immediately before use, by the addition of the requisite amount of glucose injection to the sterile contents of a container and dilution in further glucose injection.

Store in airtight containers. Protect from light.

CAUTION. *Solutions of sodium nitroprusside must be protected from light during infusion by wrapping the container with aluminium foil or some other light-proof material. Nitroprusside will react with minute quantities of organic and inorganic substances forming highly coloured products. If this occurs the solution should be discarded. Solutions should not be used more than 24 hours after preparation.*

STABILITY IN SOLUTION. The pH of a solution of sodium nitroprusside in water was 4.5 to 5 and its colour darkened from light orange on standing. Sodium nitroprusside was more stable in acid solutions and less stable in alkaline solutions. A 2% aqueous control solution of sodium nitroprusside of pH 4.7 did not discolour or precipitate for 13 days. By comparison, the addition of sodium metabisulphite, pH 9 buffer, or hydroxybenzoates reduced stability; 20% alcohol or propylene glycol had no effect, while other hydroxy compounds increased stability, to up to 51 days in the case of 50% glycerol. Sodium citrate 5% increased stability to more than 800 days. Other salts with anionic chelating potential such as sodium acetate or phosphate were also effective. Solutions containing sodium nitroprusside 2% and sodium citrate 5% were unchanged in colour and clarity after autoclaving for 60 minutes at 121°, but loss of potency was not determined.— G. E. Schumacher, *Am. J. Hosp. Pharm.*, 1966, *23*, 532.

A study of the degradation of 1% aqueous solutions of sodium nitroprusside demonstrated that light was essential for the change in colour from straw to orange which was independent of pH, whereas further degradation leading to the appearance of a blue precipitate required an acid pH. The appearance of a blue coloration should be taken to indicate that injections were unfit for use.— R. E. Hargrave, *J. Hosp. Pharm.*, 1974, *32*, 188.

The addition of dimethyl sulphoxide to solutions of sodium nitroprusside had a photoprotective effect.— A. F. Asker and R. Gragg, *Drug Dev. ind. Pharm.*, 1983, *9*, 837.

Sodium nitroprusside was stable over 48 hours in solution in glucose 5%, sodium chloride 0.9%, or lactated Ringer's solution in glass or plastic containers wrapped in aluminium foil. In addition, there was no decrease in the delivered potency of sodium nitroprusside solutions during simulated infusions lasting up to 24 hours.— C. Mahony *et al.*, *J. pharm. Sci.*, 1984, *73*, 838.

Sodium nitroprusside 0.5 to 1.67 mg per mL in glucose 5% injection was considered to be sufficiently stable for administration by motorised syringe pump over periods of up to 12 hours provided both the syringe and the intravenous line were wrapped with aluminium foil, and the syringe pump situated out of direct sunlight. Colour change was not considered to be a sufficiently sensitive or reliable indicator of degradation at these concentrations.— G. J. Sewell *et al.*, *J. clin. Hosp. Pharm.*, 1985, *10*, 351.

A study indicating that a light-protective amber intravenous administration set was as effective as a foil wrapped set in protecting solutions of sodium nitroprusside from the harmful effects of fluorescent light.— S. W. Davidson and D. Lyall, *Pharm. J.*, 1987, *2*, 599.

Further references: O. R. Leeuwenkamp *et al.*, *Int. J. Pharmaceut.*, 1985, *24*, 27.

Adverse Effects

Intravenous infusion of sodium nitroprusside may produce nausea and vomiting, apprehension, headache, dizziness, restlessness, perspiration, palpitations, retrosternal discomfort, abdominal pain, and muscle twitching, but these effects may be reduced by slowing the rate of infusion.

Sodium nitroprusside is metabolised rapidly to cyanide and then thiocyanate. High plasma concentrations of thiocyanate may occur if treatment is continued for several days and may cause mental confusion, tinnitus, blurred vision, nausea, fatigue, and ataxia. Cyanide toxicity could occur in overdosage or if endogenous thiosulphate (which converts cyanide to thiocyanate *in vivo*) is depleted. Metabolic acidosis may be the first sign of cyanide toxicity. Methaemoglobinaemia may also occur.

ACIDOSIS. Death attributed to sodium nitroprusside occurred in a 20-year-old man following anaesthesia during which he had received 750 mg of sodium nitroprusside. There was severe acidosis and hyperkalaemia but no chemical evidence of cyanide toxicity.— A. J. Merrifield and M. D. Blundell (letter), *Br. J. Anaesth.*, 1974, *46*, 324. Severe metabolic acidosis occurred on 1 of more than 600 occasions when sodium nitroprusside was used to induce hypotension during anaesthesia.— W. R. MacRae and M. Owen, *ibid.*, 795.

CYANIDE POISONING. A patient died of cyanide poisoning during an operation for which he had received 400 mg (10 mg per kg body-weight) of sodium nitroprusside to induce hypotension.— D. W. Davies *et al.*, *Can. Anaesth. Soc. J.*, 1975, *22*, 547.

Sodium nitroprusside toxicity was noted in a patient following administration by intravenous infusion at a maximum rate of 4.9 µg per kg body-weight per minute for 14 hours. It was suggested that prolonged infusion could result in accumulation of cyanide due to exhaustion of thiosulphate in the body which is necessary for the detoxification of cyanide.— A. B. Cetnarowski and D. R. Conti (letter), *Ann. intern. Med.*, 1986, *104*, 895.

EFFECTS ON THE BLOOD. *Methaemoglobinaemia.* Methaemoglobinaemia developed in a man whilst he was receiving sodium nitroprusside in a total dose of 321 mg over 4 days after extensive cardiac infarction.— P. J. Bower and J. N. Peterson, *New Engl. J. Med.*, 1975, *293*, 865.

Thrombocytopenia. Platelet counts decreased in 7 of 8 patients with congestive heart failure 1 to 6 hours after intravenous infusion of nitroprusside was started. The counts began to return to normal 24 hours after the infusion was stopped.— P. Mehta *et al.* (letter), *New Engl. J. Med.*, 1978, *299*, 1134.

EFFECTS ON INTRACRANIAL PRESSURE. Intracranial pressure rose significantly while the mean blood pressure was 90 or 80% of initial values in 14 normocapnic patients given an infusion of sodium nitroprusside to produce controlled hypotension prior to neurosurgery; values reverted towards normal at mean blood pressures of 70% of controls. A similar but insignificant trend occurred in 5 hypocapnic patients. The effect was considered to be due to vasodilatation increasing cerebral blood flow. Surgery was rendered difficult in some patients.— J. M. Turner *et al.*, *Br. J. Anaesth.*, 1977,

49, 419.

An increase in intracranial pressure was associated with sodium nitroprusside administration in a patient with metabolic encephalopathy.— W. R. Griswold *et al.*, *J. Am. med. Ass.*, 1981, *246*, 2679.

HYPOTENSION. A 50-kg patient with renal insufficiency, who had received about 13 mg of nitroprusside over 90 minutes, developed irreversible hypotension and died 2 hours after nitroprusside infusion was stopped. It was suggested that hypotension and death was probably due to cyanide toxicity and that hydroxocobalamin should be administered prophylactically to all patients receiving nitroprusside even in small doses.— J. Montoliu *et al.* (letter), *Am. Heart J.*, 1979, *97*, 541.

ILEUS. Postoperative adynamic ileus was reported in 5 out of 26 patients following the induction of controlled hypotension with sodium nitroprusside during surgery. It was suggested that diminished mesenteric arterial blood flow was the cause.— J. W. Chen *et al.* (letter), *J. Am. med. Ass.*, 1985, *253*, 633. A similar report possibly related to the concurrent use of opioids.— J. Lemmo and J. Karnes (letter), *ibid.*, *254*, 1721. An increase in catecholamine release accompanying sodium nitroprusside-induced hypotension could also have contributed to postoperative adynamic ileus.— S. Gelman (letter), *ibid.* See also: B. A. Lampert (letter), *ibid.*

PHLEBITIS. Acute transient phlebitis following sodium nitroprusside administration.— R. Miller and D. C. C. Stark (letter), *Anesthesiology*, 1978, *49*, 372.

Treatment of Adverse Effects

Side-effects due to excessive hypotension may be treated by slowing or discontinuing the infusion. For details of the treatment of cyanide poisoning see Hydrocyanic Acid, p.1350. Thiocyanate can be removed by dialysis. Hydroxocobalamin can be given to reduce cyanide concentrations, but is of little value in acute poisoning.

In a study involving 14 patients requiring nitroprusside hypotensive anaesthesia, blood-cyanide concentrations of those who concomitantly received an intravenous infusion of hydroxocobalamin 100 mg in 100 mL of glucose injection at a rate of 12.5 mg per 30 minutes throughout the duration of nitroprusside administration, were significantly decreased compared with those who received nitroprusside alone. They received a total of 87.5 to 100 mg of hydroxocobalamin and no significant adverse effects were noted other than transient pink discoloration of mucous membranes and urine.— J. E. Cottrell *et al.*, *New Engl. J. Med.*, 1978, *298*, 809.

Report of successful treatment of sodium nitroprusside-induced cyanide toxicity in a 58-year-old woman who had received a total dose of approximately 1 g sodium nitroprusside over 6 days. The blood-cyanide concentration was 5 µg per mL, approximately twice the toxic range reported in acute cyanide poisoning. Treatment consisted of sodium nitrite 300 mg and sodium thiosulphate 12.5 g. Haemodialysis resulted in significant removal of thiocyanate but not of cyanide, although the resulting shift in the concentration equilibrium substantially contributed to the indirect removal of cyanide from the body.— T. C. Marbury *et al.*, *J. Toxicol. clin. Toxicol.*, 1982, *19*, 475.

Report of the reduction of blood cyanide concentrations by sodium thiosulphate in patients receiving sodium nitroprusside.— P. V. Cole and C. J. Vesey, *Br. J. Anaesth.*, 1987, *59*, 531.

Precautions

Sodium nitroprusside should not be used in the presence of compensatory hypertension as in arteriovenous shunt or aortic coarctation. It should be used with caution in patients with impaired renal or hepatic function or cerebrovascular insufficiency, or in patients with low plasma-cobalamin concentrations or Leber's optic atrophy. The use of hydroxocobalamin before and during administration of sodium nitroprusside, has been advocated. Thiocyanate, a metabolite of sodium nitroprusside, inhibits iodine binding and uptake and sodium nitroprusside should be used with caution in patients with hypothyroidism. The plasma-thiocyanate concentration should be monitored if treatment continues for several days and should not exceed 100 µg per mL although toxicity may be apparent at lower thiocyanate concentrations. Thiocyanate concentrations do not reflect cyanide toxicity. The acid-base balance should also be monitored. Care should be taken to ensure that extravasation does not occur.

In a study in 26 anaesthetised patients sodium nitroprusside, infused throughout surgery, produced a marked reversible reduction in oxygen tension whether ventilation was spontaneous or artificial.— J. A. W. Wildsmith *et al.*, *Br. J. Anaesth.*, 1975, *47*, 1205.

Detailed recommendations for the safe use of sodium nitroprusside.— P. Cole, *Anaesthesia*, 1978, *33*, 473.

EFFECT ON THE LOWER OESOPHAGEAL SPHINCTER. Sodium nitroprusside causes a dose-dependent decrease in barrier pressure, maximal at 3 minutes after commencing the infusion.— B. R. Cotton and G. Smith, *Br. J. Anaesth.*, 1984, *56*, 37.

TACHYPHYLAXIS. A report of tachyphylaxis to sodium nitroprusside, associated with high plasma concentrations of cyanide but in the absence of metabolic acidosis, in 3 patients undergoing hypotensive anaesthesia.— J. E. Cottrell *et al.*, *Anesthesiology*, 1978, *49*, 141.

WITHDRAWAL. Rebound haemodynamic changes produced a profound but transient deterioration in cardiac performance 10 to 30 minutes after the discontinuation of an infusion of sodium nitroprusside in 20 patients.— M. Packer *et al.*, *New Engl. J. Med.*, 1979, *301*, 1193. See also J. E. Cottrell *et al.*, *Clin. Pharmac. Ther.*, 1980, *27*, 32.

Absorption and Fate

Sodium nitroprusside is converted in the erythrocytes to cyanide which is metabolised in the liver to thiocyanate by the enzyme rhodanase in the presence of thiosulphate and slowly excreted in the urine. The plasma half-life of thiocyanate is reported to be about 3 to 7 days and thiocyanate can accumulate to toxic concentrations if high doses of sodium nitroprusside are given for more than 3 days.

A review of the clinical pharmacokinetics of sodium nitroprusside, cyanide, thiosulphate, and thiocyanate.— V. Schulz, *Clin. Pharmacokinet.*, 1984, *9*, 239.

Metabolic studies in children.— D. W. Davies *et al.*, *Can. Anaesth. Soc. J.*, 1975, *22*, 553.

Uses and Administration

Sodium nitroprusside is a short-acting hypotensive agent with a duration of action of 1 to 10 minutes. It produces peripheral vasodilatation and reduces peripheral resistance by a direct action on both veins and arterioles and may be used in the treatment of hypertensive crises. It may also be used to produce controlled hypotension during general anaesthesia. It has also been used to reduce preload and afterload in severe congestive heart failure. Its effects appear within a few seconds of intravenous infusion and the blood pressure should be monitored closely during administration.

It is given by continuous infusion of a solution containing 50 to 200 µg per mL. The solution should be prepared immediately before use by dissolving sodium nitroprusside in 5% glucose injection and then diluting with 5% glucose or other suitable intravenous infusion fluid; the solution must be protected from light during administration. The initial dose is 0.3 to 1.0 µg per kg body-weight per minute increasing gradually under close supervision until the desired reduction in blood pressure is achieved. The average dose required to maintain the blood pressure 30 to 40% below the pretreatment diastolic blood pressure is 3 µg per kg per minute and the usual dose range is 0.5 to 6 µg per kg per minute. The maximum recommended rate is about 8 µg per kg per minute, and infusions should be stopped after 10 minutes if there is no response. It is only suitable for administration in the form of an infusion and care should be taken to prevent extravasation. Tachyphylaxis is rare and infusions may be continued for several days provided that the blood-thiocyanate concentration does not exceed 100 µg per mL. Alternative oral therapy should be introduced as soon as possible.

For the induction of hypotension during anaesthesia a maximum dose of 1.5 µg per kg body-weight per minute is recommended.

For the treatment of cardiac failure an initial dose of 10 to 15 µg per minute has been recommended increasing by increments of 10 to 15 µg per minute every 5 to 10 minutes until the initial response is seen. The usual dosage range is 10 to 200 µg per minute and the dose should not exceed 400 µg per minute or 6 µg per kg body-weight per minute.

Sodium nitroprusside is also used as a reagent for detecting ketones in urine.

There was evidence of cyanide toxicity when sodium nitroprusside was infused at doses not exceeding a maximum total of 1.5 mg per kg body-weight. It was recommended that for short infusions the dose of sodium nitroprusside should not exceed 500 µg per kg.— D. Aitken *et al.*, *Can. Anaesth. Soc. J.*, 1977, *24*, 651.

A suggested safe dose rate for long-term sodium nitroprusside of about 4 µg per kg body-weight per minute was recommended, with a maximum dose rate of less than 8 µg per kg per minute. In addition a maximum total dose of sodium nitroprusside in the region of 70 mg per kg for periods of less than 14 days in patients with adequate renal function was suggested. The administration of hydroxocobalamin will aid in cyanide detoxification and counteract any effects of thiocyanate on haematopoiesis, but the continuous infusion of thiosulphate is not a suitable cyanide antagonist during long-term sodium nitroprusside infusions since it will increase the rate of sodium nitroprusside accumulation and produce hypovolaemia.— C. J. Vesey and P. V. Cole, *Br. J. Anaesth.*, 1985, *57*, 148.

ADMINISTRATION IN RENAL FAILURE. Sodium nitroprusside could be given in usual doses to patients in renal failure but it was necessary to monitor thiocyanate concentrations to ensure they did not rise above 100 µg per mL.— W. M. Bennett *et al.*, *Am. J. Kidney Dis.*, 1983, *3*, 155.

CARDIAC DISORDERS. *Acute dissecting aneurysms.* Following worsening of 2 patients' conditions, and *animal* studies, the use of propranolol and nitroprusside to treat dissecting aneurysms of the aorta had been temporarily abandoned. Trimetaphan remained the drug of choice.— R. F. Palmer and K. C. Lasseter (letter), *New Engl. J. Med.*, 1976, *294*, 1403. Sodium nitroprusside was still the agent of choice.— J. N. Cohn (letter), *ibid.*, *295*, 567.

The successful use of sodium nitroprusside over 22 days in a patient with dissecting aortic aneurysm.— K. Hillman and J. Krapez, *Br. med. J.*, 1978, *2*, 799.

Myocardial infarction. In a review of the management of congestive heart failure in patients with acute myocardial infarction, glyceryl trinitrate was considered to be a more appropriate choice of vasodilator than sodium nitroprusside. Sodium nitroprusside may exacerbate ischaemia unless severe heart failure and/or severe hypertension are present, in which case improvement in haemodynamics can lead to an improved balance between myocardial oxygen supply and demand that may compensate for otherwise adverse effects of nitroprusside.— R. Genton and A. S. Jaffe, *J. Am. med. Ass.*, 1986, *256*, 2556.

Intravenous infusion of sodium nitroprusside within 24 hours of acute myocardial infarction in 163 patients resulted in a significant decrease in mortality in the nitroprusside group compared with 165 controls. The incidence of cardiogenic shock, clinical signs of left ventricular failure, and mean peak concentrations of creatine kinase isoenzyme MB were all reduced. The results indicated that infusion of nitroprusside in the early phase of acute infarction limited complications, possibly by reducing infarct size. The drug was particularly effective in anterior-wall infarction.— J. D. Durrer *et al.*, *New Engl. J. Med.*, 1982, *306*, 1121. In a study involving 812 patients sodium nitroprusside infusion did not reduce the mortality rates following presumed acute myocardial infarction. A deleterious effect on mortality was seen in patients whose infusions were started within 9 hours of the onset of pain although a beneficial effect was seen in those whose infusion was begun later. The results suggested that although nitroprusside should probably not be used routinely in patients with high left ventricular filling pressures after myocardial infarction, patients with persistent pump failure might receive sustained benefit from short-term nitroprusside therapy.— J. N. Cohn *et al.*, *ibid.*, 1129. In a discussion of the apparently contradictory findings of these two studies Passamani (*ibid.*, 1168) demonstrated that the clinical condition of the patients entered into each study was quite different: those in the Durrer study were largely without left ventricular failure and were treated early, but the patients in the Cohn study were treated later and had elevated filling pressure. The findings by Cohn of differences in mortality depending on the time of entry into the study could have been an artefact in the sub-group analysis. Thus the results suggest that nitroprusside probably does not affect mortality when given late to patients with left ventricular failure, but may be effective when given early to patients without left ventricular failure, although independent confirmation was considered necessary. Kern (*ibid.*, 1982, *307*, 1342) remarked on the more vigorous use of diuretics by Cohn, particularly in the control group, which may have influenced the outcome, and Cohn and Archibald (*ibid.*, 1343) in reply suggested that striking differences in mortality in the control groups could indicate further differences in the baseline characteristics in patients in the two studies.

ERGOTAMINE POISONING. For the use of sodium nitroprusside in the treatment of cyanosis of the extremities due to ergotamine overdosage, see Ergotamine Tartrate, p.1055.

HYPERTENSION. Sodium nitroprusside was considered to be the drug of first choice in the management of hypertensive crisis accompanied by pulmonary oedema (B.N.J. Walters, *Br. J. Hosp. Med.*, 1984, *31*, 49), severe hypertension accompanied by life-threatening left ventricular failure, and hypertensive encephalopathy (D.G. Beevers, *Prescribers' J.*, 1984, *24*, 91).

HYPERTENSION IN CHILDREN. An 11-year-old girl with refractory malignant hypertension received a continuous infusion of sodium nitroprusside for 28 days without evidence of toxicity.— J. R. Luderer *et al.*, *J. Pediat.*, 1977, *91*, 490.

Beneficial response to sodium nitroprusside infusion was reported in a study of 58 infants with life-threatening circulatory and pulmonary disorders which were refractory to conventional therapy.— W. E. Benitz *et al.*, *J. Pediat.*, 1985, *106*, 102.

NEUROLEPTIC MALIGNANT SYNDROME. Report of successful treatment of hypertension and hyperpyrexia with sodium nitroprusside in a patient with neuroleptic malignant syndrome who had not responded to dantrolene sodium.— M. G. Blue *et al.*, *Ann. intern. Med.*, 1986, *104*, 56.

PERIPHERAL VASCULAR DISORDERS. Sodium nitroprusside infusion may be useful in the management of acute attacks of Raynaud's syndrome.— E. C. Burns *et al.*, *Archs Dis. Childh.*, 1985, *60*, 537.

PHAEOCHROMOCYTOMA. Sodium nitroprusside was successfully used by infusion to prevent and control hypertensive episodes during arteriography and surgery in patients with phaeochromocytoma; 2 case reports were presented.— P. Daggett *et al.*, *Br. med. J.*, 1978, *2*, 311. Comment on the dosage.— J. Krapez and P. Cole (letter), *ibid.*, 1088. Adrenoceptor blockade makes the use of large doses of sodium nitroprusside unnecessary.— P. Daggett and I. Verner (letter), *ibid.*

Sodium nitroprusside was the most widely used drug for the control of hypertension in patients with phaeochromocytoma undergoing surgery, although avoidance of hypotension during quiescence between catecholamine surges can present considerable difficulty.— C. Hull, *Br. J. Anaesth.*, 1986, *58*, 1453.

PREGNANCY AND THE NEONATE. Sodium nitroprusside was successfully used during surgery for a cerebral aneurysm in a 25-year-old woman who was 7 months pregnant. A healthy baby was delivered 2 months later and at 2 years the child's development was normal.— Y. Donchin *et al.*, *Br. J. Anaesth.*, 1978, *50*, 849.

It was suggested that sodium nitroprusside should probably not be used to control hypertension during pregnancy unless control could not be achieved with any other drug since it may cause a 25% to 35% reduction in uterine blood flow.— B. N. J. Walters, *Br. J. Hosp. Med.*, 1984, *31*, 49.

PYREXIA. The intravenous infusion of sodium nitroprusside to induce peripheral vasodilatation was successfully used to treat extreme pyrexia in a 55-year-old man in whom conventional treatment had failed.— M. R. Katlic *et al.* (letter), *New Engl. J. Med.*, 1978, *299*, 154.

See also under Neuroleptic Malignant Syndrome, above.

RESPIRATORY DISTRESS SYNDROME. Beneficial response to sodium nitroprusside 0.2 to 5.0 μg per kg body-weight per minute intravenously was reported in 11 neonates with severe respiratory distress syndrome refractory to conventional therapy.— W. E. Benitz *et al.*, *J. Pediat.*, 1985, *106*, 102. See also T. R. Abbott *et al.*, *Br. med. J.*, 1978, *1*, 1113; D. W. Beverley *et al.* (letter), *Archs Dis. Childh.*, 1979, *54*, 403.

Preparations

Sodium Nitroprusside Intravenous Infusion *(B.P.)*

Proprietary Preparations

Acetest *(Ames, UK). Reagent tablets*, buffered sodium nitroprusside. Test for ketones in urine, plasma, or serum. In the *UK* these are described in the Drug Tariff as Nitroprusside Reagent Tablets (Rothera's Tablets).

Nipride *(Roche, UK). Infusion*, powder for reconstitution, sodium nitroprusside 50 mg, supplied with solvent.

Proprietary Names and Manufacturers

Acetest *(Ames, Canad.; Ames, UK)*; Hypoten *(Covan, S.Afr.)*; Nipride *(Roche, Austral.; Roche, Canad.; Roche, Denm.; Roche, Fr.; Ger.; Neth.; Roche, Swed.; Roche, Switz.; Roche, UK; Roche, USA)*; Nipruss *(Schwarz, Ger.; Neth.; Switz.)*; Nitropress *(Abbott, USA)*.

2542-j

Spirapril Hydrochloride *(BANM, USAN, rINNM).*

Sch-33844. (8*S*)-7{(*S*)-*N*-[(*S*)-1-Ethoxycarbonyl-3-phenylpropyl]-L-alanyl}-1,4-dithia-7-azaspiro[4.4]-nonane-8-carboxylic acid hydrochloride.

$C_{22}H_{30}N_2O_5S_2,HCl=503.1.$

CAS — 94841-17-5 (hydrochloride); 83647-97-6 (spirapril).

Spirapril is an antihypertensive agent which acts, similarly to captopril, as an angiotensin-converting enzyme inhibitor.

References: M. A. Weber *et al.*, *J. Hypertens.*, 1986, *4*, *Suppl.* 6, S171.

Proprietary Names and Manufacturers

Schering, USA.

905-s

Syrosingopine *(BAN, rINN).*

Methyl Carbethoxysyringoyl Reserpate. Methyl 18-*O*-(4-ethoxycarbonyloxy-3,5-dimethoxybenzoyl)reserpate.

$C_{35}H_{42}N_2O_{11}=666.7.$

CAS — 84-36-6.

Syrosingopine has properties and uses similar to those described under reserpine (see p.498). For the treatment of hypertension it has been given in doses of up to 3 mg daily.

Proprietary Names and Manufacturers

Aurugopin *(Jpn)*; Hipotensor Zambe Alfa *(Zambeletti, Spain)*; Londomin *(Jpn)*; Neoreserpan *(Panthox & Burck, Ital.)*; Novoserpina *(Ghimas, Ital.)*; Raunova *(Zambeletti,. Ital.)*; Seniramin *(Jpn)*; Siringina *(Toyo Jozo, Jpn)*; Siroshuten *(Jpn)*; Syrogopin *(Jpn)*.

906-w

Teprotide *(BAN, USAN, rINN).*

2-L-Tryptophan-3-de-L-leucine-4-de-L-proline-8-L-glutaminebradykinin potentiator B; BPF_{9a}; L-Pyroglutamyl-L-tryptophyl-L-prolyl-L-arginyl-L-prolyl-L-glutaminyl-L-isoleucyl-L-prolyl-L-proline; SQ-20881. 5-oxo-Pro-Trp-Pro-Arg-Pro-Gln-Ile-Pro-Pro.

$C_{53}H_{76}N_{14}O_{12}=1101.3.$

CAS — 35115-60-7.

Teprotide is a synthetic nonapeptide initially found in the venom of the pit-viper, *Bothrops jararaca*.

Teprotide is an angiotensin-converting enzyme inhibitor which preceded the orally active inhibitors such as captopril. It has been used as an investigational tool in hypertension. It is given parenterally and has a short duration of action.

Proprietary Names and Manufacturers

Squibb, UK.

13306-m

Terazosin Hydrochloride *(BANM, USAN, rINNM).*

Abbott-45975. 1-(4-Amino-6,7-dimethoxyquinazolin-2-yl)-4-(tetrahydro-2-furoyl)piperazine hydrochloride dihydrate.

$C_{19}H_{25}N_5O_4,HCl,2H_2O=459.9.$

CAS — 63590-64-7 (terazosin); 63074-08-8 (hydrochloride, anhydrous); 70024-40-7 (hydrochloride, dihydrate).

Terazosin hydrochloride is an antihypertensive agent with properties similar to those of prazosin (p.495). It is used in the treatment of mild to moderate hypertension either alone or in combination with a diuretic and/or other antihypertensive agents. Terazosin hydrochloride is given once daily by mouth in an initial dose equivalent to 1 mg of terazosin at bedtime, increasing gradually according to the patient's response to a maximum of 20 mg of terazosin daily. The usual maintenance dose is 2 to 10 mg daily.

A review of terazosin. Terazosin is chemically related to prazosin and acts primarily by blocking alpha$_1$-adrenoceptors. It has similar pharmacodynamic effects to prazosin but a longer duration of action which enables once daily dosing. Terazosin has also been shown to have neutral or possibly slightly beneficial effects on plasma lipids.

Terazosin is well absorbed from the gastro-intestinal tract with a reported bioavailability of 90% and little interindividual variability. It is 90 to 94% bound to plasma proteins, metabolised extensively in the liver, and excreted mainly in the bile. The elimination half-life in healthy subjects has ranged from about 10 to over 18 hours.

Terazosin appears to be as effective as prazosin in short-term studies in the treatment of mild to moderate hypertension, and has been used both alone and in combination with diuretics and other antihypertensive agents; experience of terazosin in long-term therapy is limited. Studies in small numbers of patients with congestive heart failure have shown beneficial haemodynamic changes but the therapeutic efficacy of terazosin has not been assessed.

Most adverse effects encountered during clinical studies have been of mild to moderate severity. The most frequent effects are dizziness, headache, asthenia, nasal congestion, and cold symptoms. Other adverse effects include somnolence, nausea, blurred vision, tachycardia, palpitations, chest pain, dyspnoea, and syncope. First-dose hypotension was largely avoided by limiting the initial dose of terazosin to 1 mg and giving it at bedtime, but a syncopal episode was reported in about 1% of patients at some time during therapy. Terazosin has no effect on renal function in patients with normal, or moderately or severely impaired renal function.— S. Titmarsh and J. P. Monk, *Drugs*, 1987, *33*, 461.

Further reviews of terazosin: *Med. Lett.*, 1987, *29*, 112.

For a series of papers on the actions and uses of terazosin see *Am. J. Med.*, 1986, *80*, *Suppl.* 5B.

Proceedings of a symposium on terazosin.— *Br. J. clin. Pract.*, 1987, *41*, *Suppl.* 54, 1–69.

Proprietary Preparations

Hytrin *(Abbott, UK). Tablets*, terazosin 1, 2, 5, and 10 mg (as hydrochloride).

Proprietary Names and Manufacturers

Heitrin *(Abbott, Ger.)*; Hytrin *(Abbott, UK; Abbott, USA)*; Hytrinex *(Abbott, Denm.)*.

907-e

Tetraethylammonium Bromide

TEAB; Tetramone Bromide; Tetrylammonium Bromide *(rINN)*.

$C_8H_{20}BrN=210.2.$

CAS — 71-91-0.

Tetraethylammonium bromide is a ganglion-blocking agent. It has been used in the treatment of hypertension but is now seldom employed. Tetraethylammonium chloride has also been used.

13336-s

Tiamenidine Hydrochloride *(BANM, USAN, rINNM).*
HOE-42-440; HOE-440. *N*-(2-Chloro-4-methyl-3-thienyl)-2-imidazolin-2-ylamine hydrochloride.
$C_8H_{10}ClN_3S,HCl=252.2$.

CAS — 31428-61-2 (tiamenidine); 51274-83-0 (hydrochloride); 31428-62-3 (hydrochloride).

Tiamenidine hydrochloride is an antihypertensive agent with properties and uses similar to those of clonidine, p.472.

In a study involving 4 hypertensive patients tiamenidine produced similar effects on blood and urinary catecholamine concentrations and on plasma renin activity to those produced by clonidine, and withdrawal was associated with clinically and biochemically similar rebound effects.— B. G. Hansson and B. Hökfelt, *Br. J. clin. Pharmac.*, 1981, *11*, 73.

Evidence of rebound hypertension following withdrawal of tiamenidine in 5 of 10 patients who had received tiamenidine for 1 year.— B. C. Campbell *et al.*, *Eur. J. clin. Pharmac.*, 1980, *18*, 449. See also B. P. Hamilton *et al.*, *Clin. Pharmac. Ther.*, 1984, *36*, 628.

ABSORPTION AND FATE. Study of the pharmacokinetics of tiamenidine in healthy and hypertensive subjects.— S. K. Puri *et al.*, *Clin. Pharmac. Ther.*, 1984, *35*, 267.

Proprietary Names and Manufacturers
Symcorad *(Hoechst, USA).*

The following names have been used for multi-ingredient preparations containing tiamenidine hydrochloride— Symcor *(Hoechst, USA).*

13358-z

Todralazine Hydrochloride *(BANM, pINNM).*
BT-621; CEPH; Ecarazine Hydrochloride; Todrazoline Hydrochloride. Ethyl 3-(phthalazin-1-yl)carbazate hydrochloride monohydrate.
$C_{11}H_{12}N_4O_2,HCl,H_2O=286.7$.

CAS — 14679-73-3 (todralazine); 3778-76-5 (hydrochloride, anhydrous).

Todralazine hydrochloride is an antihypertensive agent structurally related to hydralazine with similar properties (see p.483).

References: W. Reiterer and H. Czitober, *Arzneimittel-Forsch.*, 1977, *27*, 2163.

Proprietary Names and Manufacturers
Aperdor *(Tanabe, Jpn)*; Apiracohl *(Kyowa, Jpn)*; Apride *(Jpn)*; Atapren *(Sumitomo, Jpn)*; Binazin *(Biosedra, Arg.)*; Binazine *(Polfa, Pol.)*; Deprezid *(Jpn)*; Dypirecohl *(Jpn)*; Ecahain *(Jpn)*; Ecara *(Jpn)*; Hydrapron *(Jpn)*; Illcut *(Jpn)*; Marukunan *(Jpn)*; Propat *(Jpn)*; Prorazin *(Jpn)*; Seirof *(Jpn).*

909-y

Tolonidine Nitrate *(rINNM).*
ST-375. 2-(2-Chloro-*p*-toluidino)-2-imidazoline nitrate.
$C_{10}H_{12}ClN_3,HNO_3=272.7$.

CAS — 4201-22-3 (tolonidine); 57524-15-9 (nitrate).

Tolonidine nitrate is an antihypertensive agent with the actions and uses of clonidine (see p.472). It is given as an initial dose of 500 µg at night, increasing by increments of 125 µg according to the patient's response. Maintenance doses are usually between 500 and 1000 µg daily.

Pharmacology in *animals*.— D. Cosnier *et al.*, *Arzneimittel-Forsch.*, 1975, *25*, 1557, 1802, and 1926.

Proprietary Names and Manufacturers
Euctan *(Delalande, Fr.).*

910-g

Trimazosin Hydrochloride *(BANM, USAN, rINNM).*
CP-19106-1. 2-Hydroxy-2-methylpropyl 4-(4-amino-6,7,8-trimethoxyquinazolin-2-yl)piperazine-1-carboxylate hydrochloride monohydrate.
$C_{20}H_{29}N_5O_6,HCl,H_2O=490.0$.

CAS — 35795-16-5 (trimazosin); 35795-17-6 (hydrochloride, anhydrous); 53746-46-6 (hydrochloride, monohydrate).

Trimazosin is an antihypertensive agent which is chemically related to prazosin and appears to have vasodilatory properties.

HEART FAILURE. A review of the treatment of congestive heart failure with vasodilators including trimazosin. Some beneficial haemodynamic effects had been seen but clinical experience was very limited.— A. B. Schwartz and K. Chatterjee, *Drugs*, 1983, *26*, 148.

In a study of patients with chronic cardiac failure of varying cause and severity, trimazosin produced symptomatic improvement and a sustained increase in exercise tolerance and aerobic capacity.— K. T. Weber *et al.*, *New Engl. J. Med.*, 1980, *303*, 242.

HYPERTENSION. Trimazosin in doses of up to 900 mg daily led to blood pressure control in 16 of 25 patients with mild to moderate hypertension after 6 to 9 months of treatment. Control of blood pressure was also achieved in 5 of 7 patients unresponsive to trimazosin alone when polythiazide was added to the treatment.— M. A. Weber *et al.*, *Clin. Pharmac. Ther.*, 1982, *31*, 572.

Further references to the use of trimazosin in hypertension: H. L. Elliott *et al.*, *Clin. Pharmac. Ther.*, 1984, *35*, 156; C. K. van Kalken *et al.*, *Eur. J. clin. Pharmac.*, 1986, *31*, 63; L. P. Svetkey *et al.*, *Curr. ther. Res.*, 1986, *39*, 866; R. L. Byyny *et al.*, *J. clin. Pharmac.*, 1987, *27*, 101.

Proprietary Names and Manufacturers
Pfizer, USA.

911-q

Trimetaphan Camsylate *(BAN).*

Méthioplégium; Trimetaphan Camphorsulphonate; Trimetaphan Camsilate *(rINN)*; Trimetaphani Camsylas; Trimethaphan Camsylate *(USAN)*. 1,3-Dibenzylperhydro-2-oxoimidazo-[4,5-*c*]thieno[1,2-*a*]thiolium (+)-camphor-10-sulphonate; 4,6-Dibenzyl-1-thionia-4,6-diazatricyclo[6,3,0,$0^{3,7}$]undecan-5-one (+)-camphor-10-sulphonate.
$C_{22}H_{25}N_2OS,C_{10}H_{15}O_4S=596.8$.

CAS — 7187-66-8 (trimetaphan); 68-91-7 (camsylate).

Pharmacopoeias. In *Int.*, *It.*, *Jpn*, and *U.S.*

White crystals or white crystalline powder, odourless or with a slight odour.

Freely **soluble** in water, in alcohol and in chloroform; insoluble in ether. The *U.S.P.* injection has a pH of 4.9 to 5.6. **Incompatible** with thiopentone sodium, gallamine triethiodide, iodides, bromides, and strongly alkaline solutions. **Store** below 8° in airtight containers.

STABILITY. The manufacturer (*Roche, USA*) has reported that the stability of trimetaphan camsylate injection is maintained for up to 2 weeks at room temperature.— F. R. Vogenberg and P. F. Souney, *Am. J. Hosp. Pharm.*, 1983, *40*, 101.

Arfonad injection has been reported to be stable for up to 1 year when stored at room temperature.— P. W. Longland and P. C. Rowbotham, *Pharm. J.*, 1987, *1*, 147.

Adverse Effects and Treatment

The adverse effects of trimetaphan are mainly due to ganglionic blockade. A reduction in gastro-intestinal motility may result in constipation or paralytic ileus on prolonged administration. Urinary retention, cycloplegia, mydriasis, tachycardia, and gastro-intestinal disturbances may occur. Orthostatic hypotension may be severe in ambulatory patients. Rapid intravenous infusion at rates greater than 5 mg per minute can result in apnoea and respiratory arrest. Trimetaphan crosses the placenta and can cause paralytic or meconium ileus in neonates. Other adverse effects include raised intra-ocular pressure, dry mouth, anhydrosis, hypoglycaemia, hypokalaemia, weakness, urticaria, and itching.

If severe hypotension occurs, administration of trimetaphan should be stopped and the patient positioned with the head lower than the feet. A pressor agent may be given cautiously if necessary.

A sudden and dramatic reduction of intra-ocular pressure to very low levels was noted in 5 patients undergoing surgery when the systolic blood pressure was reduced to 60 mmHg with trimetaphan infusion.— P. L. R. Dias *et al.*, *Br. J. Ophthal.*, 1982, *66*, 721.

Precautions

Trimetaphan should be avoided in patients with severe arteriosclerosis, severe ischaemic heart disease, or pyloric stenosis and should only be used with extreme caution in those with impaired hepatic or renal function, degenerative disease of the central nervous system, Addison's disease, prostatic hypertrophy, glaucoma, cerebral or coronary vascular insufficiency, and diabetes. Owing to a histamine-liberating effect it should be used with caution in allergic subjects. Trimetaphan should also be used with caution in patients being treated with other antihypertensive agents, drugs which depress cardiac function, muscle relaxants, and in those taking corticosteroids. The hypotensive effect is enhanced by general anaesthetics.

For a reference to possible potentiation of neuromuscular blockade by trimetaphan, see suxamethonium (p.1239).

Uses and Administration

Trimetaphan is a ganglion-blocking agent which inhibits the transmission of nerve impulses in both sympathetic and parasympathetic ganglia. The sympathetic blockade produces peripheral vasodilatation. The parasympathetic block diminishes movement of the gastro-intestinal tract and bladder, reduces gastric and salivary secretions, and produces disturbances in visual accommodation. Trimetaphan also has a direct vasodilatory effect on peripheral blood vessels. It is used for inducing controlled hypotension during surgical procedures although sodium nitroprusside is usually preferred. It acts rapidly to produce a hypotensive response which persists for 10 to 30 minutes according to the amount given.

Trimetaphan camsylate is administered by the slow intravenous infusion of a solution usually containing 1 mg per mL. The infusion is started at the rate of 3 to 4 mg per minute and then adjusted according to the response of the patient. Similar doses have been recommended for children. A frequent check on the blood pressure is essential and this should be allowed to rise before wound closure.

Adrenaline should not be infiltrated locally at the site of incision when trimetaphan is being given since this may antagonise the effect of trimetaphan.

Trimetaphan has also been used for the emergency treatment of hypertensive crises, especially in association with pulmonary oedema or acute dissecting aortic aneurysms.

Although sodium nitroprusside is considered by many to be the most effective parenteral antihypertensive drug and can be used for most types of hypertensive emergency, trimetaphan is preferred for the treatment of hypertensive emergencies due to aortic dissection.— *Med. Lett.*, 1987, *29*, 18.

Preparations

Trimethaphan Camsylate Injection *(U.S.P.)*

Proprietary Preparations

Arfonad *(Roche, UK). Injection*, trimetaphan camsylate 50 mg/mL, in ampoules of 5 mL.

Proprietary Names and Manufacturers

Arfonad *(Roche, Austral.; Belg.; Roche, Canad.; Fr.; Roche, Ital.; Jpn; Neth.; Roche, S.Afr.; Roche, Spain; Roche, Swed.; Roche, UK; Roche, USA).*

912-p

Trimethidinium Methosulphate (*BAN*).

Trimethidinium Methosulfate (*rINN*). 1,3,8,8-Tetramethyl-3-(3-trimethylammoniopropyl)-3-azoniabicyclo-[3.2.1]octane bis(methylsulphate).
$C_{17}H_{36}N_2,2CH_3SO_4$=490.7.

CAS — 2624-50-2 (trimethidinium); 14149-43-0; 7009-82-7 (both methosulphate).

Trimethidinium methosulphate is a ganglion-blocking agent with properties similar to those of trimetaphan (see p.503).

Proprietary Names and Manufacturers
Ostensin *(Wyeth, USA).*

14001-k

Urapidil Hydrochloride (*BANM, rINNM*).

B-66256 (urapidil). 6-[3-(4-*o*-Methoxyphenylpiperazin-1-yl)propylamino]-1,3-dimethylpyrimidine-2,4(1*H*,3*H*)-dione hydrochloride.
$C_{20}H_{29}N_5O_3$,HCl=423.9.

CAS — 34661-75-1 (urapidil); 64887-14-5 (hydrochloride).

Urapidil is an antihypertensive agent which is reported to stimulate alpha$_2$-adrenoceptors and block alpha$_1$-adrenoceptors. It has been given as the hydrochloride by slow intravenous injection in an initial dose equivalent to 25 mg of base in the management of hypertensive emergencies, and by mouth in doses of 30 to 180 mg daily for less urgent treatment of hypertension.

Proceedings of a symposium on urapidil.— *Drugs*, 1988, *35, Suppl.* 6, 1–192.

References to the effects of urapidil in hypertensive patients: R. Evans *et al., J. clin. Pharmac.*, 1985, *25*, 455; E. Kanniainen *et al., Eur. J. clin. Pharmac.*, 1985, *28*, 35; V. L. Culbertson *et al., Clin. Pharmac. Ther.*, 1986, *39*, 690; R. Kirsten *et al., Eur. J. clin. Pharmac.*, 1987, *32*, 61.

Proprietary Names and Manufacturers
Ebrantil *(Byk, Aust.; Byk Gulden, Ger.; Byk Gulden, Switz.).*

913-s

Green Veratrum

American Hellebore; American Veratrum; Green Hellebore; Green Hellebore Rhizome; Veratro Verde; Veratrum Viride. The dried rhizome and roots of *Veratrum viride* (Liliaceae).

CAS — 8002-39-9 (see also under Alkavervir).

914-w

White Veratrum

European Hellebore; Veratrum Album; White Hellebore; White Hellebore Rhizome.

Pharmacopoeias. In *Cz.* and *Hung*, with not less than 1% of total alkaloids.

The dried rhizome and roots of *Veratrum album* (Liliaceae).

Adverse Effects
Veratrum alkaloids may cause nausea and vomiting at conventional therapeutic doses. Other adverse effects include epigastric and substernal burning, sweating, mental confusion, cardiac arrhythmias, dizziness, and hiccup. Profound hypotension and respiratory depression can occur at high doses.

Report of various symptoms of intoxication in 7 patients due to the use of a sneezing powder containing white veratrum alkaloids.— A. Fogh *et al., J. Toxicol. clin. Toxicol.*, 1983, *20*, 175.

Treatment of Adverse Effects
Following oral ingestion of veratrum alkaloids the stomach should be emptied by aspiration and lavage. Excessive hypotension with bradycardia or cardiac arrhythmias can be treated with atropine by intramuscular injection. The patient should be placed in a supine position with the feet raised.

Uses and Administration
White and green veratrum contain a number of pharmacologically active alkaloids. Protoveratrines which are obtained from white veratrum, cryptenamine, derived from green veratrum, and alkavervir, a mixture of alkaloids obtained from green veratrum, all produce centrally mediated peripheral vasodilatation and bradycardia. They have been used in the treatment of hypertension but are generally considered to produce an unacceptably high incidence of adverse effects and have largely been replaced by less toxic antihypertensive agents.
Both green and white veratrum have also been used as insecticides.

Proprietary Names and Manufacturers
Vera-67 *(Mallard, USA).*

Antimalarials

1370-h

Malaria is one of the most serious protozoal infections in man and is caused by infection by any of four species of *Plasmodium*: *P. falciparum* causes falciparum (malignant tertian or subtertian) malaria which is the most serious form of malaria and can be rapidly fatal in non-immune individuals if not treated promptly; *P. vivax* causes vivax (benign tertian) malaria which is widespread but rarely fatal, although symptoms during the primary attack can be severe; *P. malariae* causes quartan malaria which is generally mild but can cause fatal nephrosis; and *P. ovale* causes ovale (ovale tertian) malaria which is the least common type of malaria, and produces clinical features similar to *P. vivax*.

The life-cycle of the malaria parasite is complex, comprising a sexual phase (sporogony) in the mosquito (vector) and an asexual phase (schizogony) in man. Infection in man is caused by injection of *sporozoites* by the bite of a female anopheline mosquito. Some of the sporozoites rapidly enter liver parenchymal cells where they undergo *exoerythrocytic* or *pre-erythrocytic schizogony*, forming *tissue schizonts* which mature and release thousands of *merozoites* into the blood on rupture of the cell. Some of these merozoites enter erythrocytes where they transform into *trophozoites*. These produce *blood schizonts* which, as they mature, rupture and release merozoites into the circulation which can infect other erythrocytes. This is termed the *erythrocytic cycle* and it is this periodic release of merozoites which is responsible for the characteristic periodicity of the fever in malaria. After several erythrocytic cycles, depending on the type of malaria, some erythrocytic forms develop into sexual *gametocytes* which eventually give rise to the sexual cycle in the mosquito. In *P. vivax* and *P. ovale* infections, a proportion of sporozoites entering the liver cells are thought to enter a latent tissue stage in the form of *hypnozoites* which are responsible for relapses of malaria caused by these organisms: true relapses do not occur with falciparum or quartan malarias but recrudescences of malaria may occur due to persistent residual erythrocytic forms. Patients may sometimes be classified as non-immune if they have not previously or recently been exposed to plasmodium infection and as semi-immune or immune if they have a history of prolonged exposure.

Antimalarial drugs can be classified by the stage of the parasitic life-cycle they affect.

Blood schizontocides act on the erythrocytic stages of the parasite which are directly responsible for the clinical symptoms of the disease. They can produce a clinical cure or suppression of infection by susceptible strains of all four species of malaria parasite, but, since they have no effect on exoerythrocytic forms, do not produce a radical cure of relapsing forms of ovale or vivax malarias.

Tissue schizontocides act on the exoerythrocytic stages of the parasite and are used for causal prophylaxis to prevent invasion of the blood cells, or as antirelapse drugs to produce radical cures of vivax and ovale malarias.

Gametocyticides destroy the sexual forms of the parasite to interrupt transmission of the infection to the mosquito vector.

Sporonticides have no direct effect on the gametocytes in the human host but prevent sporogony in the mosquito.

The principal antimalarial drugs are conveniently classified by the chemical structure.

1. The *quinine salts* which are rapidly acting blood schizontocides with some gametocyticidal activity.
2. The *8-aminoquinolines* such as primaquine and quinocide. They are tissue schizontocides mainly used to prevent relapse of ovale and vivax malarias, and have gametocyticidal activity. They also have some activity at other stages of the parasites', life cycle.
3. The *9-aminoacridines* such as mepacrine, which is a blood schizontocide with some gametocyticidal activity.
4. The *4-aminoquinolines*, such as chloroquine and amodiaquine, are rapidly acting blood schizontocides with some gametocyticidal activity.
5. The *biguanides*, such as proguanil, have dihydrofolate reductase inhibitory activity. They are tissue schizontocides used mainly for causal prophylaxis of falciparum malaria. They also have some activity against blood schizonts.
6. The *diaminopyrimidines* such as pyrimethamine have actions similar to those of the biguanides.
7. The *sesquiterpine lactones* such as artemisinin which acts mainly as a blood schizontocide.

Other drugs with antimalarial activity include the sulphonamides, mefloquine, dapsone, and some antibiotics such as tetracycline and erythromycin. Various vaccines are under development and insecticides play a part in mosquito control.

References on malaria and its control: H. M. Gilles, *Br. med. J.*, 1981, *283*, 1382; Malaria control and national health goals, *Tech. Rep. Ser. Wld Hlth Org. No. 680*, 1982; D. J. Wyler, *New Engl. J. Med.*, 1983, *308*, 875 and 934; *Bull. Wld Hlth Org.*, 1984, *62, Suppl.*, 1–128; L. J. Bruce-Chwatt, Essential Malariology, Second Edition, London, Heinemann, 1985; W. Peters, *Lancet*, 1985, *2*, 144; Eighteenth Report of the WHO Expert Committee on Malaria, *Tech. Rep. Ser. Wld Hlth Org. No. 735*, 1986.

References to the use of antimalarial drugs: Advances in Malaria Chemotherapy, *Tech. Rep. Ser. Wld Hlth Org. No. 711*, 1984; D. M. James and H. M. Gilles, Human Antiparasitic Drugs: Pharmacology and Usage, Chichester, Wiley, 1985; *Chronicle Wld Hlth Org.*, 1985, *39*, 176; D. C. Warhurst, *Drugs*, 1987, *33*, 50.

For references to the use of tetracyclines and erythromycin in malaria, see p.319 and p.225 respectively.

ADVERSE EFFECTS OF ANTIMALARIAL DRUGS. A discussion of the problems of serious toxic reactions with antimalarial drugs. Chloroquine has been widely used throughout the tropics and subtropics for long periods, but partly or wholly resistant strains of *P. falciparum* have emerged over wide areas. Unfortunately resistance to the two alternative prophylactics, proguanil and pyrimethamine, has rendered them ineffective in these areas. The use of combination regimens including pyrimethamine with sulfadoxine or dapsone initially proved highly effective in areas of chloroquine resistance, but increasing concern about serious and sometimes fatal adverse reactions has limited their usefulness.— G. C. Cook, *J. Infect.*, 1986, *13*, 1.

Further references to adverse effects of antimalarial drugs: P. Winstanley, *Adverse Drug React. Bull.*, 1986, (Apr.), 436; *Br. med. J.*, 1986, *293*, 1163; A. Jaeger *et al.*, *Med. Toxicol.*, 1987, *2*, 242.

AIRPORT MALARIA. An Englishwoman developed malaria 12 days after travelling from London to Rome on an Ethiopian Airways flight. She had never been to a malarial zone and might have been bitten by a commuter mosquito on the aeroplane.— M. J. Smeaton *et al.* (letter), *Lancet*, 1984, *1*, 845. Report of a further 3 cases of malaria contracted in or around an airport in the *UK*.— D. C. Warhurst *et al.* (letter), *ibid.*, 1303. See also D. Whitfield *et al.*, *Br. med. J.*, 1984, *289*, 1607.

PREGNANCY AND THE NEONATE. In endemic areas, clinical episodes of malaria are more frequent and of greater severity during pregnancy. Falciparum malaria in pregnancy frequently constitutes a grave risk to the mother and the foetus. Pregnant women with falciparum malaria are particularly likely to develop severe manifestations and complications. It is generally agreed that malaria prophylaxis should be given during pregnancy to women both visiting and resident in malarious areas. If possible, women should be discouraged from visiting malarious areas during pregnancy. Chloroquine and proguanil are generally considered to be relatively safe during pregnancy. Pyrimethamine with or without a sulphonamide has been widely used without apparent adverse effects on the foetus, but its use is controversial and it is generally not recommended during pregnancy for malaria prophylaxis. Folate supplements should be given if any antifolate drugs are used. Tetracycline and primaquine are not recommended for use in pregnancy. References: L. J. Bruce-Chwatt, *Br. med. J.*, 1983, *286*, 1457; *Lancet*, 1983, *2*, 84; Advances in malaria chemotherapy, *Tech. Rep. Ser. Wld Hlth Org. No. 711*, 1984; Eighteenth Report of the WHO Expert Committee on Malaria, *Tech. Rep. Ser. Wld Hlth Org. No. 735*, 1986.

Report of meetings convened by the Ross Institute on malaria prevention in travellers from the United Kingdom, including advice for pregnant women. Although some manufacturers and national authorities recommend that combined antimalarials should not be used by pregnant women and infants, this is not practicable except in the case of neonates. The child of a British parent will not have protective antibodies but, owing to the immaturity of enzyme systems and the practical problems of giving the correct dose, only the least toxic antimalarials should be given prophylactically. Proguanil or chloroquine may be given in areas without resistance; mosquito nets should be used everywhere. Neither of the 2 antimalarial preparations appropriate for chloroquine-resistant areas (Maloprim or Fansidar) is considered by the manufacturers suitable for the first 6 weeks of life; several members of the committee would rely on proguanil and mosquito nets, treating any fever with Fansidar. It was universally thought that no entirely satisfactory strategy was currently available.— *Br. med. J.*, 1980, *283*, 214.

See also under Chloroquine p.511.

TRANSFUSION MALARIA. References to the detection and control of malaria parasites in donor blood: L. Wells and F. A. Ala, *Lancet*, 1985, *1*, 1317; L. J. Bruce-Chwatt (letter), *ibid.*, *2*, 271.

Prophylaxis and suppression of malaria

The spread of malaria in recent decades and the increasing prevalence of drug resistant strains particularly of *Plasmodium falciparum* (see below) have made recommendations for malaria prophylaxis difficult. The WHO has recommended that the widespread use of chemoprophylaxis in immune or semi-immune populations is no longer desirable and that chemoprophylaxis as a malaria control strategy should aim at reducing morbidity in groups that are at high risk from severe and complicated malaria, notably pregnant women and non-immune visitors. Since the protection afforded by many chemoprophylactic regimens is not absolute, travellers should be advised on methods of avoiding bites from infected mosquitoes such as the use of protective clothing, bed netting, and insecticides. Travellers should also be advised to regard any fever as possibly malaria even if chemoprophylaxis has been taken regularly.

Chemoprophylaxis may refer to absolute prevention of infection (*causal prophylaxis*) or to suppression of parasitaemia and its symptoms (*clinical prophylaxis*). Causal prophylaxis is provided by tissue schizontocides which destroy the exoerythrocytic forms of the parasite. Blood schizontocides produce suppression or clinical prophylaxis which, if continued until all exoerythrocytic forms of the parasite are destroyed, will ultimately produce a suppressive cure. In *P. falciparum* infections this would be achieved by about a month after the last infected bite, but infections with *P. vivax* and *P. ovale* may still recur after standard clinical prophylactic regimens due to the presence of latent exoerythrocytic forms.

Advice on chemoprophylaxis must be based on a knowledge of the occurrence and susceptibility of malaria strains in specific geographical areas. Local variations due to altitude, seasonal variations in temperature and rainfall, and the degree of urbanisation further complicate the issue. The WHO collate information provided by national health administrations and regularly publish this information to assist in advising international travellers on the current situation (see below), and similar information is provided at national level by local institutes specialising in tropical diseases. However the situation is so complex that advice is often conflicting. The toxicity of some chemoprophylactic regimens has further complicated the situation since the incidence of toxic reactions can approach or exceed the dangers of contracting malaria, particularly in visitors from Western Europe and North America to regions of relatively low malaria transmission. It is generally agreed that amodiaquine should not be used for prophylaxis and most experts, including the WHO, also agree that a combination of pyrimethamine with sulfadoxine (Fansidar) should not be used for prophylaxis. In regions where no safe and effective drug regimen is available, travellers will have to rely on protection against mosquito bites, and prompt medical attention in the event of infection.

In *areas of little or no chloroquine resistance*, chloroquine may still be used. Some experts suggest proguanil as an alternative. In *areas of low-grade chloroquine resistance*, chloroquine prophylaxis may still alleviate the infection, and travellers may keep a therapeutic dose of Fansidar or mefloquine or quinine in readiness in case a malaria attack occurs, although medical advice should be sought as soon as possible in this event. It has also been suggested that the curative dose should be taken in any case on leaving the malarious area. Proguanil may be given with chloroquine for enhanced prophylaxis, but a curative treatment course should still be held in readiness. Additional prophylaxis with primaquine should be considered in areas where *P. ovale* and *P. vivax* are endemic. In areas of *high-grade chloroquine resistance* in the past chloroquine with Fansidar was recommended but is now generally considered too toxic and in any case multidrug-resistant strains of malaria are increasingly widespread. Chloroquine plus pyrimethamine-dapsone (Maloprim) is a possible alternative, but the potential toxicity is again a problem. Less toxic regimens should be considered even if they are less effective, with adequate prompt medical assistance in the event of infection. Mefloquine may be useful if it is available, but there is concern that indiscriminate prophylactic use could induce mefloquine-resistance.

Whichever form of chemoprophylaxis is chosen it is generally recommended that prophylaxis should start a week before exposure to malaria, partly to ensure that the patient is not hypersensitive to the drug, and should continue for at least 4 to 6 weeks after leaving the malarious area.

A booklet published annually by the WHO containing up-to-date advice on malaria prophylaxis for travellers.— Vaccination Certificate Requirements and Health Advice for International Travel, Geneva, WHO.

A foreign travel guide published monthly with immunisation recommendations for individual countries.— *Pulse*.

Recommendations for malaria prophylaxis from the Centers for Disease Control in the *USA*.— *Morb. Mortal.*, 1985, *34*, 185.

Further publications of advice on malaria prophylaxis to travellers: *Med. Lett.*, 1987, *29*, 53; *ibid.*, 1988, *30*, 15.

A review of the problems of chemoprophylaxis against *Plasmodium falciparum*. The other malaria parasites remain sensitive to chloroquine and proguanil, so that prophylaxis against them is not difficult. The number of cases of falciparum malaria in the *UK* has been rising since 1970. The reasons for this increase include the expansion of international travel, failure of control programs in endemic areas for economic or administrative reasons, and increasing insecticide resistance in the mosquito population. Furthermore, since 1980 there has been a progressive increase in the incidence and geographical spread of drug-resistant, particularly chloroquine-resistant, falciparum malaria. In response alternative prophylactic regimens have been used, but reports of serious toxicity following antimalarial chemoprophylaxis have made the choice of drug very difficult.

A number of authors have reinforced the need for critical evaluation of individual risk of contracting malaria against the risk of drug toxicity to the traveller: the risk of contracting malaria is surprisingly low for many travellers and it is generally agreed that potentially more toxic agents should be reserved for situations of higher malarial risk. Many travellers are not aware of the need for malaria chemoprophylaxis and those who do take prophylaxis are ignorant of other useful preventive measures including the use of insect repellents, bed nets, and protective clothing. Compliance with prophylactic regimens is hindered by conflicting advice obtained from various advisory services and by the complexity of some of the advice received.— P. L. Chiodini, *J. antimicrob. Chemother.*, 1987, *20*, 297.

A discussion of the problems of advising Africans and Asians normally resident in the *UK* on malaria prophylaxis when returning to areas where malaria is endemic. Student populations and their families are especially vulnerable since their protection due to inherent immunity will have substantially diminished while they are not exposed to repeated infections. In hyperimmune adults, malaria antibody can remain high for some years. In children born in the *UK*, passive immunity derived from partially immune mothers is thought to last for several months. In semi-immune adults who have not been away from malarious areas for too long it is probably safe to allow immunity to be slowly regained from repeated sub-clinical attacks with prompt treatment of acute attacks. Children are, however, at risk of acquiring malaria and should probably be given continuous prophylaxis initially. The best form of prophylaxis is controversial, but proguanil is reasonably safe and effective.— *Lancet*, 1985, *2*, 871. A survey of 323 passengers from the *UK* to malarious areas indicated that non-white *UK* residents were less well informed of the need for malaria prophylaxis than white *UK* residents. The main cause of the problem was thought to be the fairly low proportion of travellers consulting health services before travelling. Insufficient emphasis was placed on forms of protection other than the use of drugs.— H. Campbell, *Br. med. J.*, 1985, *291*, 1013.

Further reviews and discussions on the problems of malaria prophylaxis: L. J. Bruce-Chwatt, *Br. med. J.*, 1982, *285*, 674; W. H. Wernsdorfer, *Chronicle Wld Hlth Org.*, 1983, *37*, 11; *Lancet*, 1983, *1*, 963; *Br. med. J.*, 1983, *287*, 1454.

Comparison of drug regimens for the prevention of malaria in travellers by means of risk-benefit analysis. The study confirmed the importance of measures to reduce mosquito contact and, using crude estimates of the relevant risk factors, concluded that in most cases a combination of chloroquine and proguanil provided the best protection. More toxic drugs were only rarely indicated, and only for high-risk travellers.— T. E. A. Peto and C. F. Gilks, *Lancet*, 1986, *1*, 1256.

VACCINES. Review of the current research towards the development of a vaccine against malaria. Current work is directed towards the three main types of vaccine: a sporozoite vaccine should prevent the development of liver schizonts and subsequent blood invasion; a merozoite vaccine should stop or limit the multiplication of malaria parasites and thus prevent or reduce clinical symptoms and the consequent mortality; the third type aims at blocking transmission of malaria in the community. Phase I studies in animals are under way, but considerable research in humans would be necessary before any clinical use was possible.— L. J. Bruce-Chwatt, *Lancet*, 1987, *1*, 371.

Further references to malaria vaccines: L. J. Bruce-Chwatt, *Br. med. J.*, 1985, *291*, 1072; S. L. Hoffmann *et al.*, *New Engl. J. Med.*, 1986, *315*, 601; L. H. Miller, *ibid.*, 640; J. B. Wyngaarden, *J. Am. med. Ass.*, 1987, *258*, 1139; *WHO Drug Inf.*, 1987, *1*, 14.

Resistance

Resistance of *Plasmodium falciparum* to most of the current antimalarial drugs has emerged as the main technical problem in malaria control. Drug resistance has been defined as the ability of a parasite strain to multiply or to survive in the presence of concentrations of a drug that normally destroy parasites of the same species or prevent their multiplication. Although drug resistance has been reported in other plasmodia species, it is the resistance of *P. falciparum* particularly to chloroquine which has caused most concern. The WHO has developed an arbitrary grading system to describe the relative degrees of resistance of strains of *P. falciparum* to chloroquine.

Sensitivity is defined as clearance of asexual parasitaemia within 7 days of initiation of treatment, without subsequent recrudescence.

RI resistance is defined as clearance of asexual parasitaemia as in sensitivity, followed by recrudescence.

RII resistance is defined as marked reduction of asexual parasitaemia, but no clearance.

RIII resistance is defined as no marked reduction in parasitaemia.

Chloroquine resistance developed almost simultaneously in Southern Asia and in South America at the end of the 1950s. Chloroquine resistance now affects most of Asia and the Western Pacific islands with evidence of a westward spread. It is well established in South and Central America. Major and alarming changes in susceptibility have occurred in Africa, south of the Sahara and in islands off the eastern coast and there are now reports of chloroquine resistance in West Africa. Resistance to proguanil and pyrimethamine first occurred in the early 1950s and is now apparent in many endemic areas. Cross resistance between proguanil and pyrimethamine may also occur.

Resistance to the alternative first line combination, pyrimethamine-sulfadoxine was first noted in the late 1970s in Thailand and has spread rapidly to other parts of the world including parts of South America and East Africa. Resistance to other drugs including quinine, amodiaquine, and mefloquine have also been noted, and multidrug-resistant strains are causing concern.

A knowledge of the extent of resistance in terms of the geographical distribution and degree of resistance is important for the selection of appropriate control measures and for the development of policies for the rational use of drugs. The use of subcurative doses of drugs contributes to the selection of resistance and radical curative treatment is probably the most reliable way of avoiding selective parasite survival. Mass drug administration for suppression should therefore be avoided. The use of combinations of drugs with similar half-lives may also delay the emergence of resistant strains.

Discussions on the development of drug-resistant malaria: *Lancet*, 1985, *1*, 1487; H. C. Spencer, *Trans. R. Soc. trop. Med. Hyg.*, 1985, *79*, 748.

Treatment of acute malaria

Falciparum malaria is a serious and potentially lethal disease which requires prompt and effective treatment. Serious or complicated falciparum malaria may require parenteral therapy. The agents of choice for both mild and severe disease are the blood schizontocides, but widespread resistance to chloroquine, which was formerly the drug of choice, has necessitated the development of alternative treatment regimens. Vivax and ovale malarias may produce less severe symptoms than falciparum malaria, but recurrent disease may occur months or years after the primary infection due to the presence of hypnozoites despite adequate treatment of parasitaemia. For radical cure of vivax and ovale malarias it is necessary to use a tissue schizontocide after initial treatment of parasitaemia with a blood schizontocide. In regions where malaria is not endemic, for example in travellers returning from a malarious area to a less malarious area, a gametocyticide or sporonticide may be given to reduce malaria transmission.

The treatment of acute malaria has been influenced by the development of drug-resistant strains of the malaria parasite and the choice of treatment will depend on the degree of drug resistance in any given geographical area. In areas where there is no known resistance or low grade resistance, chloroquine remains the drug of choice for treatment (Advances in malaria chemotherapy, *Tech. Rep. Ser. Wld Hlth Org. No. 711*, 1984; Eighteenth Report of WHO Expert Committee on Malaria, *Tech. Rep. Ser. Wld Hlth Org. No. 735*, 1986; *Med. Lett.*, 1988, *30*, 15) although it should be given in full curative doses of 25 mg of chloroquine base per kg bodyweight over 3 days even to semi-immune individuals for whom single doses of 10 mg per kg were formerly considered adequate (*Tech. Rep. Ser. Wld Hlth Org. No. 711* and *735*). Amodiaquine has been suggested as an alternative to chloroquine, but increasing concern over its safety in prophylaxis makes it a less popular choice even for treatment. Cook (*Lancet*, 1988, *1*, 32) commented that, in view of the widespread resistance to chloroquine, quinine is now almost always used. In regions of chloroquine resistance the choice of therapy lies between quinine (*Tech. Rep. Ser. Wld Hlth Org. No. 711*) or pyrimethamine with sulfadoxine (*Tech. Rep. Ser. Wld Hlth Org. No. 735*) or both (*Tech. Rep. Ser. Wld Hlth Org. No. 711*; *Med. Lett.*, 1988; G.C. Cook, *Lancet*, 1988). In some areas, pyrimethamine-sulfadoxine resistance is becoming a problem, and mefloquine, if available, may be useful either alone or in combination with other antimalarials, or alternatively quinine with tetracycline (*Tech. Rep. Ser. Wld Hlth Org. No. 711* and *735*; *Med. Lett.*, 1988) although tetracycline should not be given to pregnant women or children (p.315). Artemisinin (qinghaosu) may also be a useful alternative (G.C. Cook, *Lancet*, 1988). In areas of low malaria transmission or areas free of malaria, primaquine may be given sequentially with a blood schizonticide to reduce transmission of *P. falciparum* and to prevent relapse of vivax and ovale malarias (*Tech. Rep. Ser. Wld Hlth Org. No. 711* and *735*; *Med. Lett.*, 1988; G.C. Cook, *Lancet*, 1988). In areas with chloroquine-resistant *P. falciparum* where *P. vivax* may be present, a single dose of chloroquine with pyrimethamine-sulfadoxine may be given (*Tech. Rep. Ser. Wld Hlth Org. No. 711*).

In patients with **severe or complicated malaria** it is important to produce adequate blood concentrations of the chosen blood schizontocide as rapidly as possible, and parenteral therapy may be necessary in patients unable to take oral medication. Quinine is generally regarded as the drug of choice for parenteral therapy (*Tech. Rep. Ser. Wld Hlth Org. No. 711*; *Trans. R. Soc. trop. Med. Hyg.*, 1986, *80*, *Suppl.*; *Chemotherapy of Malaria*, L.J. Bruce-Chwatt (Ed), revised 2nd edition, 1986, Geneva, WHO), but alternatives include quinidine or chloroquine. There is no general agreement over the best route of administration for quinine, but slow intravenous infusion over 4 hours seems to be the most widely recommended regimen. A loading dose may be given if it is certain that the patient has not previously received quinine, but see under Quinine p.520 for the controversy surrounding the use of loading doses. Care should be taken when administering intravenous fluids since overhydration can precipitate pulmonary oedema (*Tech. Rep. Ser. Wld Hlth Org. No. 711*). The treatment of children with severe malaria can be problematical due to their apparent susceptibility to the toxic effects of parenteral therapy. While the WHO (*Tech. Rep. Ser. Wld Hlth Org. No. 711*) recommends intravenous quinine in both adults and children, Bruce-Chwatt (*Chemotherapy of Malaria*, 1986) states that parenteral quinine is strictly contra-indicated in children. Patients of all ages should in any case be closely monitored while undergoing parenteral antimalarial therapy.

For details of recommended dose regimens, see under individual monographs.

Discussion and recommendations for the clinical management of acute malaria in South-East Asia.— The Clinical Management of Acute Malaria, New Delhi, WHO Regional Publications, *South-East Asia Series No. 9*, 1986.

Further references to the treatment of malaria: G. C. Cook, *Q. J. Med.*, 1986, *61*, 1091.

1374-g

Amodiaquine Hydrochloride *(BANM, USAN, rINNM)*.

Amodiachin Hydrochloride; Amodiaquini Hydrochloridum; SN-10,751. 4-(7-Chloro-4-quinolylamino)-2-(diethylaminomethyl)phenol dihydrochloride dihydrate.

$C_{20}H_{22}ClN_3O,2HCl,2H_2O=464.8$.

CAS — 86-42-0 (amodiaquine); 69-44-3 (hydrochloride, anhydrous); 6398-98-7 (hydrochloride, dihydrate).

Pharmacopoeias. In *Arg.*, *Br.*, *Braz.*, *Egypt.*, *Fr.*, *Ind.*, *Int.*, and *U.S. U.S.* also includes Amodiaquine.

A yellow, odourless or almost odourless, crystalline powder. Amodiaquine base 200 mg is approximately equivalent to 260 mg of amodiaquine hydrochloride. **Soluble** 1 in about 22 of water and 1 in about 70 of alcohol; practically insoluble in chloroform and ether. A 2% solution in water has a pH of 3.6 to 4.6. **Store** in airtight containers.

For a report of reduced *in-vitro* activity against *P. falciparum* of amodiaquine hydrochloride solutions following membrane filtration, see Chloroquine p.508.

Adverse Effects

In therapeutic doses amodiaquine hydrochloride can give rise to side-effects similar to those of chloroquine (p.508). There have been several reports of agranulocytosis and these have limited its use in prophylaxis. Hepatitis and peripheral neuropathy have also been reported.

Four patients experienced involuntary movements, usually with speech difficulty, after large but not excessive doses of amodiaquine.— M. O. Akindele and A. O. Odejide, *Br. med. J.*, 1976, *2*, 214.

EFFECTS ON THE BLOOD. Sporadic cases of severe neutropenia were reported as early as 1953, but occurred more commonly in patients receiving the drug in anti-inflammatory doses for rheumatoid arthritis. However, in 1986, 7 cases were described in travellers returning to the *UK* who were taking amodiaquine for malaria prophylaxis. Sales figures for the use of amodiaquine in the *UK* suggested that the frequency of neutropenia among people taking the drug was about 1 in 2000. Further confirmation of the magnitude of the apparent risk was produced almost simultaneously when 5 further cases were reported among patients referred to a single medical centre in Switzerland within a period of 5 months. Some of these latter patients also had evidence of liver damage. In all, 23 cases of agranulocytosis associated with the use of amodiaquine were reported in the 12-month period ending in March 1986, of which 7 were fatal. Nearly all of these patients had used the drug at a dosage of 400 mg weekly and the periods of exposure ranged from 3 to 24 weeks. There was some speculation as to whether amodiaquine was safer taken alone, but further cases have since been reported in which there was no history of exposure to other antimalarials.— *WHO Drug Inf.*, 1987, *1*, 5.

Reports of severe neutropenia and agranulocytosis associated with amodiaquine: C. S. R. Hatton *et al.*, *Lancet*, 1986, *1*, 411; R. Carr (letter), *ibid.*, 556; K. A. Neftel *et al.*, *Br. med. J.*, 1986, *292*, 721; E. G. H. Rhodes *et al.*, *ibid.*, 717; *Morb. Mortal.*, 1986, *35*, 165.

EFFECTS ON THE EYES. Retinopathy, sometimes reversible, had been reported following treatment with amodiaquine hydrochloride 200 mg daily.— *Med. Lett.*, 1976, *18*, 63.

EFFECTS ON THE LIVER. Hepatitis developed in 7 patients taking amodiaquine for malaria prophylaxis for 4 to 15 weeks. Liver dysfunction recurred in 2 patients when amodiaquine was administered subsequently.— D. Larrey *et al.*, *Ann. intern. Med.*, 1986, *104*, 801.

Precautions

As for Chloroquine, p.509.

Absorption and Fate

Amodiaquine hydrochloride is readily absorbed from the gastro-intestinal tract. Amodiaquine is rapidly converted in the liver to the active metabolite desethylamodiaquine. Amodiaquine and desethylamodiaquine have been detected in the urine several months after administration.

References to the pharmacokinetics of amodiaquine: P. Winstanley *et al.*, *Br. J. clin. Pharmac.*, 1987, *23*, 1; N. J. White *et al.*, *ibid.*, 127.

Uses and Administration

Amodiaquine hydrochloride is an antimalarial drug which has an action similar to that of chloroquine (see p.510). It is at least as effective as chloroquine, and is effective against some chloroquine-resistant strains, although resistance to amodiaquine has been reported.

For treatment of acute attacks in non-immune subjects a dose equivalent to 600 mg of the base is given followed by 200 mg after 6 hours, then 400 mg daily on each of the 2 subsequent days. A number of variations of this regimen have been used. For partially immune subjects a single dose of 600 mg of the base is often sufficient.

Amodiaquine is not recommended for the prophylaxis of malaria because of reports of agranulocytosis associated with its use (see above).

Amodiaquine hydrochloride has been tried in the treatment of giardiasis and hepatic amoebiasis. It has also been tried, with variable success, in the treatment of lepra reactions, lupus erythematosus, rheumatoid arthritis, and urticaria.

Amodiaquine has been found to be effective in the treatment of chloroquine-resistant falciparum malaria: S. Noeypatimanond *et al.*, *Trans. R. Soc. trop. Med. Hyg.*, 1983, *77*, 338 (in combination with tetracycline); W. M. Watkins *et al.*, *Lancet*, 1984, *1*, 357 (used alone); H. C. Spencer *et al.* (letter), *ibid.*, 956 (used alone); P. Deleron *et al.*, *ibid.*, 1303 (used alone).

Favourable response to amodiaquine 10 mg base per kg body-weight given intravenously over 4 hours, then 5 mg per kg daily for 3 doses in 14 patients with moderately severe falciparum malaria.

In a study of 33 patients with uncomplicated falciparum malaria, erythromycin was not considered satisfactory as an alternative to tetracycline when added to oral amodiaquine therapy.— S. Looareesuwan *et al.*, *Lancet*, 1985, *2*, 805.

Preparations

Amodiaquine Hydrochloride Tablets *(U.S.P.)*

Amodiaquine Tablets *(B.P.)*. Tablets containing amodiaquine hydrochloride. Potency is expressed in terms of the equivalent amount of amodiaquine base.

Proprietary Preparations

Camoquin *(Parke, Davis, UK)*. *Tablets*, scored, amodiaquine 200 mg (as hydrochloride).

Proprietary Names and Manufacturers

Basoquin *(Parke, Davis, UK)*; Camoquin *(Parke, Davis, Spain*; *Parke, Davis, Switz.*; *Parke, Davis, UK)*; Flavoquine *(Roussel, Fr.)*.

12023-q

Artemisinin *(pINN)*.

Arteannuin; Artemisinine; Qinghaosu.

(3*R*,5a*S*,6*R*,8a*S*,9*R*,12*S*,12a*R*)-Octahydro-3,6,9-trimethyl-3,12-epoxy-12*H*-pyrano[4,3-*j*]-1,2-benzodioxepin-10(3*H*)-one.

$C_{15}H_{22}O_5=282.3$.

CAS — 63968-64-9.

A sesquiterpene derived from *Artemisia annua* (Compositae).

Artemisinin is a potent and rapidly acting blood schizontocide which has been reported to be particularly useful in the treatment of cerebral malaria. It is active against chloroquine-resistant strains of *Plasmodium falciparum* as well as chloroquine-sensitive *P. falciparum* and *P. vivax*. Artemisinin is reported to have a shorter half-life than some other antimalarial drugs, and this may account for the high rate of recrudescence seen in some studies. A number of semi-synthetic derivatives are under investigation: artemether and sodium artesunate are among the most promising.

A review of artemisinin and its derivatives. The activity of artemisinin has been shown to be potent and rapid against chloroquine-sensitive and chloroquine-resistant strains of *Plasmodium falciparum in vitro*, although *animal* studies suggest that it has no activity against exoerythrocytic forms of the malaria parasite. Overall the acute toxicity of artemisinin was found to be considerably less than that of chloroquine. However, there was evidence of a teratogenic effect in *rats*. In clinical studies the poor solubility of artemisinin has caused problems in choosing a route of administration. The tablet form produces rapid clearance of parasitaemia of both *P. vivax* and *P. falciparum*, but also a higher rate of recrudescence than intramuscular formulations. A number of semisynthetic derivatives have been tested and artemether and sodium artesunate are among the most promising.

The most striking clinical results with artemisinin and its derivatives are seen in the treatment of cerebral malaria, although high recrudescence rates necessitated the use of additional drugs such as sulfadoxine. Activity has also been demonstrated in infections with *Schistosoma* and *Clonorchis*.— D. L. Klayman, *Science*, 1985, *228*, 1049.

Further brief reviews and discussions on artemisinin: L. J. Bruce-Chwatt, *Br. med. J.*, 1982, *284*, 767; D. C. Warhurst, *J. antimicrob. Chemother.*, 1986, *18*, *Suppl.* B, 51; D. C. Warhurst, *Drugs*, 1987, *33*, 50. Artemisinin cleared parasitaemia more rapidly than oral mefloquine or intramuscular quinine in a study involving 40 patients with falciparum malaria; oral artemisinin acted more quickly than intramuscular artemisinin in aqueous suspension.— J. -B. Jiang *et al.*, *Lancet*, 1982, *2*, 285.

In a region of chloroquine-resistant malaria, artemisinin alone produced rapid parasite clearance with no side-effects but a high recrudescence rate in 20 patients with falciparum malaria. The addition of artemisinin to treatment with mefloquine and pyrimethamine-sulfadoxine greatly enhanced the rate of parasite clearance produced by mefloquine plus pyrimethamine-sulfadoxine alone.— G. Li *et al.*, *Lancet*, 1984, *2*, 1360. Comment that recrudescence after artemisinin therapy may be due to its short half-life and that prolonging the dosage regimen could result in an improved cure rate. The short half-life also makes artemisinin less than ideal for combination with drugs with longer half-lives like mefloquine and pyrimethamine-sulfadoxine.— T. E. A. Peto *et al.* (letter), *ibid.*, 1985, *1*, 216. Reply.— K. Arnold, *ibid.*, 704.

The semi-synthetic derivative of artemisinin, artemether, was found to be more effective than quinine in the treatment of complicated falciparum malaria in a study involving 31 pairs of patients. However, recrudescence occurred in 39% of the patients treated with artemether compared with 9% of those treated with quinine.— P. T. Myint and T. Shwe, *Trans. R. Soc. trop. Med. Hyg.*, 1987, *81*, 559.

References to the actions and *in-vitro* activity of artemisinin and its derivatives: Z. L. Li *et al.*, *Trans. R. Soc. trop. Med. Hyg.*, 1983, *77*, 522; S. Thaithong and G. H. Beale, *Bull. Wld Hlth Org.*, 1985, *63*, 617; A. N. Chawira *et al.*, *Trans. R. Soc. trop. Med. Hyg.*, 1986, *80*, 335; B. C. Elford *et al.*, *ibid.*, 1987, *81*, 434; S. R. Krungkrai and Y. Yuthavong, *ibid.*, 710.

1371-m

Chloroquine *(BAN, USAN, rINN).*

Cloroquina. 7-Chloro-4-(4-diethylamino-1-methylbutylamino)quinoline.

$C_{18}H_{26}ClN_3$=319.9.

CAS — 54-05-7.

Pharmacopoeias. In *Braz.* and *U.S.*

A white or slightly yellow odourless crystalline powder. Very slightly **soluble** in water; soluble in chloroform, ether, and dilute acids.

1372-b

Chloroquine Phosphate *(BANM, USAN, rINNM).*

Chingaminum; Chlorochinum Diphosphoricum; Chloroquine Diphosphate; Chloroquine Phos.; Chloroquini Diphosphas; Chloroquini Phosphas; Quingamine; SN-7618.

$C_{18}H_{26}ClN_3$, $2H_3PO_4$=515.9.

CAS — 50-63-5.

Pharmacopoeias. In *Arg., Aust., Br., Braz., Chin., Cz., Egypt., Eur., Fr., Hung., Ind., Int., It., Jug., Mex., Nord., Pol., Roum., Rus., Turk.,* and *U.S.*

A white or almost white, odourless or almost odourless powder which slowly discolours on exposure to light. Chloroquine base 100 mg is approximately equivalent to 161 mg of chloroquine phosphate.

Soluble 1 in 4 of water; very slightly soluble or practically insoluble in alcohol; practically insoluble in chloroform and ether. A 10% solution in water has a pH of 3.5 to 4.5. Solutions are **sterilised** by autoclaving.

An investigation of polymorphic behaviour of chloroquine phosphate.— P. Van Aerde *et al.*, *J. Pharm. Pharmac.*, 1984, *36*, 190.

Studies *in vitro* showing diminished activity after sterilisation by membrane filtration of solutions of amodiaquine hydrochloride, chloroquine phosphate, mefloquine hydrochloride, and quinine sulphate against *Plasmodium falciparum*. The reduced antimalarial activity was partially attributed to the drug binding to the membrane filters and also possibly to antagonism of the *in-vitro* activity by detergents or other materials present in the membrane. Loss of activity was overcome by increasing the drug concentration prior to filtration. It was recommended that, to prevent erroneous reporting of drug susceptibility studies, the drug solutions be filtered at high concentration and then aseptically diluted; alternatively the drug could be dissolved in alcohol initially, with subsequent serial dilutions performed aseptically.— J. K. Baird and C. Lambros, *Bull. Wld Hlth Org.*, 1984, *62*, 439.

Chloroquine phosphate was bound to soda glass but not to borosilicate glass. Binding was greater at concentrations below 0.25 µg per mL and at physiological pH than at pH values above or below this. Borosilicate glass should be used for chloroquine assays and sensitivity testing.— A. M. Yahya *et al.*, *Int. J. Pharmaceut.*, 1985, *25*, 217. A study of the binding of chloroquine phosphate to various plastics found that chloroquine was bound to cellulose propionate, methacrylate butadiene styrene, polypropylene, polyvinyl chloride, ethylvinyl acetate, and polyethylene, but not to polystyrene. The extent of binding was dependent on the pH of the solution, being greatest at higher pHs. Passing a 16 ng per mL chloroquine phosphate solution through cellulose acetate filters resulted in losses of up to 85% of chloroquine at pH 9.5.— A. M. Yahya *et al.*, *ibid.*, 1986, *34*, 137.

1373-v

Chloroquine Sulphate *(BANM, rINNM).*

Chloroquine Sulph.; Chloroquini Sulfas; RP-3377.

$C_{18}H_{26}ClN_3,H_2SO_4,H_2O$=436.0.

CAS — 132-73-0 (anhydrous).

Pharmacopoeias. In *Br., Egypt., Eur., Fr., Ind.,* and *Int.*

A white or almost white odourless or almost odourless crystalline powder. Chloroquine base 100 mg is approximately equivalent to 136 mg of chloroquine sulphate.

Soluble 1 in 3 of water; practically insoluble in alcohol; sparingly soluble in chloroform and ether. A 10% solution in water has a pH of 4.0 to 5.0. Solutions are **sterilised** by autoclaving.

Adverse Effects

Chloroquine is generally well tolerated when given in antimalarial doses and adverse effects are rare. The higher doses that may be used over prolonged periods for rheumatoid arthritis are more likely to produce adverse effects.

Side-effects occurring with antimalarial doses are usually reversible on withdrawal of the drug and include headache, gastro-intestinal disturbances such as nausea and vomiting, and diarrhoea, pruritus, and various skin eruptions. More rarely, a range of mental changes has been reported with chloroquine including psychotic episodes, anxiety, and personality changes. Visual disturbances including blurred vision and difficulties in focusing have occurred but are more common at high doses during prolonged treatment, when they may be associated with keratopathy or retinopathy. Keratopathy usually occurs in the form of corneal opacities and is normally reversible when treatment is withdrawn. Retinopathy constitutes the most severe adverse effect at high doses and may result in severe visual impairment which may progress even after chloroquine is discontinued and is generally irreversible. It has been suggested that the risk of retinopathy occurs when the total cumulative dose ingested exceeds 100 g but more recent evidence suggests that high daily doses are a greater risk factor. Hypotension and ECG changes may also occur at high doses. Other uncommon adverse effects from prolonged use include loss of hair, bleaching of hair pigment, bluish-black pigmentation of the mucous membranes and skin, photosensitivity, tinnitus, reduced hearing, nerve deafness, neuromyopathy, and myopathy.

Blood disorders have been reported rarely. They include aplastic anaemia, reversible agranulocytosis, thrombocytopenia, and neutropenia.

Overdosage with chloroquine is dangerous and may lead to death within a few hours. Small children seem to be particularly sensitive to the adverse effects of chloroquine, especially following parenteral administration. Acute overdosage or rapid intravenous injection in adults or children can cause headache, gastro-intestinal disturbances, drowsiness, dizziness, and a fall in blood pressure. Visual disturbances may be dramatic with a sudden loss of vision. The chief symptom of chloroquine overdosage is cardiovascular collapse progressing to convulsions, cardiac and respiratory arrest, and death. Cardiac arrhythmias may also occur.

Chloroquine was identified in the urine of a diamorphine addict although he had not been prescribed chloroquine. It was thought the diamorphine he was using had been adulterated by dilution with chloroquine in amounts which could have resulted in his ingestion of chloroquine 800 to 1000 mg over 5 days.— P. O'Gorman *et al.*, (letter), *Lancet*, 1987, *1*, 746.

EFFECTS ON THE BLOOD. Aplastic anaemia was associated with the use of chloroquine in 3 patients. Two patients had received treatment over several months and one of these was later found to have acute myeloblastic leukaemia after receiving chloroquine treatment initially for discoid lupus erythematosus, and later for cerebral malaria. In the third patient aplastic anaemia developed 3 weeks after a short course of chloroquine for malaria.— N. Nagaratnam *et al.*, *Postgrad. med. J.*, 1978, *54*, 108.

EFFECTS ON THE EYES. A review of adverse ocular reactions to drugs including chloroquine. The incidence of chloroquine keratopathy is high, with corneal deposits appearing in about 30 to 70% of treated patients and may be present after one or two months of treatment at full therapeutic doses. Chloroquine keratopathy is not related to the toxic retinopathy produced by chloroquine. It is often asymptomatic, and visual changes occur in less than 50% of patients with corneal changes. Chloroquine need not be withdrawn unless symptoms are present, but keratopathy is usually completely reversible on stopping treatment. Symptoms include haloes around lights, photophobia, and blurred vision.

Chloroquine-induced retinopathy can lead to progressive visual loss. The incidence of chloroquine retinopathy in different series has varied from less than 1% to more than 15% depending on diagnostic criteria and detection method. Chloroquine should be discontinued if any changes are detected in the central field during therapy. The daily dose is reported to be of greater importance than the duration of treatment or cumulative dose and should not exceed 250 mg daily for chloroquine or 200 mg daily for hydroxychloroquine. Visual symptoms include presbyopia, difficulty in reading, scotoma, defective colour vision, photophobia, and flashes of light. Symptoms do not run parallel to retinal changes. Improvement may follow discontinuation of chloroquine therapy in the early stages, but in many cases deterioration continues progressively. Patients with systemic lupus erythematosus are reported to be more susceptible than patients with rheumatoid arthritis.— M. A. Spiteri and D. G. James, *Postgrad. med. J.*, 1983, *59*, 343.

A discussion of factors contributing to adverse ocular reactions in patients taking chloroquine and hydroxychloroquine for the long-term therapy of rheumatoid arthritis. Doses of chloroquine 4.0 mg per kg body-weight daily or hydroxychloroquine 6.5 mg per kg daily were considered to be safe while the toxic threshold for retinopathy appears to be 5.1 and 7.8 mg per kg daily respectively.— A. H. Mackenzie, *Am. J. Med.*, 1983, *75*, 40.

No retinopathy had been detected in thousands of patients taking 500 mg of chloroquine weekly for suppression of malaria, but patients treated with 100 mg daily for other conditions had shown a perceptible rise in the retinal threshold for vision. All the reported cases of retinopathy had concerned patients who had taken 250 mg or more daily for many months, which suggested that doses not exceeding 200 mg daily might be safe for at least 1 year. The disturbing feature of reported cases was the possibility of retinopathy developing several years after chloroquine therapy had been discontinued.— *New Engl. J. Med.*, 1966, *275*, 730.

Maculopathy with impaired vision was present in 2% of 95 patients with rheumatoid arthritis who had taken a total of less than 100 g of chloroquine; in about 7% of 93 who had taken 101 to 300 g; in about 10% of 59 who had taken 301 to 600 g; and in 17% of 23 who had taken more than 600 g. Chloroquine retinopathy was present in one woman who had taken about 1000 g. It was considered that in patients under 50 years old taking a dose not higher than 250 mg daily for 10 months annually corresponding to chloroquine 4 mg per kg body-weight daily, the risk of chloroquine-induced retinal damage is small and regular ophthalmological checks should not be necessary.— A. Elman *et al.*, *Scand. J. Rheumatol.*, 1976, *5*, 161.

Retinal changes developed in 22 of 222 patients receiving long-term chloroquine phosphate treatment in a dose of not more than 250 mg daily. On stopping therapy deterioration of visual acuity occurred in only one and regression of macular changes occurred in 4; there was no progression of retinal changes in the other 17 who showed mild pigmentary disturbance of the macula. The frequency of retinopathy increased with the patients' ages and also with the total dose given (developing in only 10% of those given less than 200 g as against 50% of those receiving more than 600 g). These results indicated that the ocular hazards of long-term chloroquine therapy are low.— J. S. Marks and B. J. Power, *Lancet*, 1979, *1*, 371. A contrary view.— S. Ogawa *et al.* (letter), *ibid.*, 1408.

Delayed-onset chloroquine retinopathy developed in a 50-year-old patient 7 years after cessation of treatment with chloroquine for rheumatoid arthritis. The patient had received a total of 730 g at a dose of chloroquine 250 mg daily for 8 years.— M. Ehrenfeld *et al.*, *Br. J. Ophthal.*, 1986, *70*, 281.

EFFECTS ON GLUCOSE METABOLISM. Hypoglycaemia may occur in patients with malaria treated with chloroquine. White *et al.* (*Lancet*, 1987, *1*, 708 and *ibid.*, *2*, 281) considered that the malaria, rather than the chloroquine treatment, was responsible for the hypoglycaemia. Studies in healthy subjects (R.E. Phillips *et al.*, *Br. med. J.*, 1986, *292*, 1319; J.E. Ogbuokiri, *Lancet*, 1987, *2*, 281) have shown that single doses of chloroquine did not produce changes in blood-glucose concentrations and Brueton and Greenwood (*Lancet*, 1987, *2*, 281) found that severe hypoglycaemia could occur in untreated children with severe malaria. However Bamber and Redpath (*ibid.*, *1*, 1211) reported severe hypoglycaemia associated with chloroquine poisoning in a patient with no evidence of malaria.

See under Quinine p.519 for a report indicating a correlation between plasma-insulin and quinine concentrations.

EFFECTS ON THE HEART. A study in healthy subjects suggesting that the cardiovascular toxicity of parenteral chloroquine is related to transiently high plasma concentrations occurring early in the distribution phase and that the rate of administration is an important factor.— S. Looareesuwan *et al.*, *Br. J. clin. Pharmac.*, 1986, *22*, 31.

In 2 patients with cardiomyopathy associated with chloroquine or hydroxychloroquine therapy, endomycardial biopsy showed histological changes virtually identical to those seen in chloroquine-induced myopathy in skeletal muscle which were considered to be diagnostic of chloroquine cardiomyopathy.— N. B. Ratliff *et al.*, *New Engl. J. Med.*, 1987, *316*, 191.

Cardiac conduction abnormalities were found in 18 of 112 patients with lupus, including 5 patients with complete heart block. Lupus myocarditis was ruled out in 4 of these 5 patients: these 4 patients had been taking chloroquine for several years and the myocarditis was attributed to long-term chloroquine therapy.— J. -C. Piette *et al.* (letter), *New Engl. J. Med.*, 1987, *317*, 710.

EFFECTS ON MUSCLES. A review of adverse effects of drugs on muscles. Chloroquine-induced myopathy has developed insidiously after periods of therapy ranging from a few weeks to 4 years. The condition leads to progressive weakness and atrophy of proximal muscle groups often associated with mild sensory changes, depression of tendon reflexes, and abnormal nerve conduction studies suggestive of an associated peripheral neuropathy. In some cases there has been associated cardiomyopathy. The myopathy is reversible after the drug is stopped, but recovery is usually protracted and may take many months.— F. L. Mastaglia, *Drugs*, 1982, *24*, 304.

EFFECTS ON THE NERVOUS SYSTEM. Involuntary movements, often with protrusion of the tongue, occurred in 5 patients after treatment with chloroquine.— E. M. Umez-Eronini and E. A. Eronini, *Br. med. J.*, 1977, *1*, 945. Typical extrapyramidal symptoms occurred in 4 children treated with chloroquine.— S. Singhi *et al.* (letter), *ibid.*, *2*, 520.

Peripheral neuropathy and nystagmus occurred in a 49-year-old woman who had been taking chloroquine 250 mg daily for about 5 months.— J. S. Marks, *Postgrad. med. J.*, 1979, *55*, 569.

EFFECTS ON THE SKIN. A report of toxic epidermal necrolysis after the ingestion of one tablet of chloroquine.— A. J. Kanwar and O. P. Singh, *Indian J. Derm.*, 1976, *21*, 73.

A questionnaire survey of 550 Nigerian patients receiving chloroquine for malaria. Pruritus was reported in 81 of 109 respondents. The typical pruritic reaction had a latent period of about 11 hours, increased in intensity to a peak within about 25 hours, remained maximal for about 12 hours before gradually subsiding to full remission 55 hours after onset. Antihistamines were largely ineffective at relieving pruritus. It was suggested that the apparent racial predisposition among black patients could be associated with chloroquine binding to melatonin.— N. G. Osifo, *Archs Derm.*, 1984, *120*, 80.

Fatal Stevens-Johnson syndrome associated with chloroquine and pyrimethamine-sulfadoxine therapy in a 5-year-old boy.— M. G. Bamber *et al.*, *J. Infect.*, 1986, *13*, 31. Comment that the child had been given pyrimethamine-sulfadoxine twice weekly and that this high dose could have contributed to the reaction.— I. Lenox-Smith (letter), *ibid.*, 1987, *14*, 90.

Mention of a severe cutaneous adverse reaction in a patient taking chloroquine alone, and a case of erythema multiforme in which the patient gave a positive patch test to chloroquine, but no reaction with a rechallenge with pyrimethamine-sulfadoxine.— R. Steffen and B. Somaini (letter), *Lancet*, 1986, *1*, 610.

For a discussion of the possible association of chloroquine with the incidence of erythema multiforme in patients taking pyrimethamine-sulfadoxine, see under Pyrimethamine p.516.

PREGNANCY AND THE NEONATE. There has been concern about the potential teratogenic effects of chloroquine because of a few case reports including defects in hearing and vision. Two of 169 infants born to women who had received chloroquine 300 mg weekly throughout pregnancy had birth defects compared to 4 of 454 control infants whose mothers had not been exposed to antimalarials; the difference was not significant. The data suggested that chloroquine in the recommended prophylactic doses is not a strong teratogen and that its proved antimalarial benefits outweigh any possible risk of low-grade teratogenicity.— M. S. Wolfe and J. F. Cordero, *Br. med. J.*, 1985, *290*, 1466.

For a discussion of the prophylaxis and treatment of malaria during pregnancy, see under Uses, below.

Treatment of Adverse Effects

Since acute overdosage with chloroquine can be rapidly fatal, treatment should be commenced promptly. The stomach should be emptied by gastric lavage or emesis if ingestion has occurred recently. The administration of activated charcoal has been suggested to limit any further absorption. Treatment of toxic effects is symptomatic: respiratory and circulatory support may be necessary and diazepam may be used to treat convulsions. There is also evidence to suggest that diazepam may decrease the cardiotoxicity of chloroquine. Treatment of cardiovascular effects is similar to that for quinidine toxicity (see p.86). Peritoneal dialysis and exchange transfusions have been suggested to increase the elimination of chloroquine but are unlikely to be effective unless performed very early. Acidification of the urine with ammonium chloride has also been suggested to promote excretion.

A review of the clinical features and management of poisoning due to antimalarial drugs including chloroquine. Chloroquine overdosage is the most severe and frequent cause of intoxications with antimalarial drugs. It is frequently used for suicide attempts, particularly in Africa. Severe toxic manifestations may occur within 1 to 3 hours and deaths usually occur within 2 to 3 hours of drug ingestion. The major clinical symptoms are neurological, respiratory, and cardiovascular disorders. Chloroquine has a low safety margin: doses of 20 mg per kg body-weight are considered toxic, and 30 mg per kg may be fatal. The mortality rate in published studies has ranged from 10 to 30% and is among the highest in clinical toxicology.

Specific treatment of cardiovascular disturbances and hypokalaemia are discussed. Diazepam has been shown to decrease the toxicity of chloroquine in *animal* studies and beneficial responses have been observed in several clinical reports. The mechanism of the antagonistic action of diazepam is unclear but it has been suggested that competition for cardiac binding sites may be involved.

Early gastric lavage is indicated, but should be preceded by symptomatic treatment and intubation with artificial respiration in order to avoid sudden cardiac arrest and lung aspiration. There is no evidence that attempts to increase chloroquine elimination are effective in overdose. The clearances achieved by haemoperfusion or haemodialysis are low in comparison with the spontaneous total body clearance of chloroquine.— A. Jaeger *et al.*, *Med. Toxicol.*, 1987, *2*, 242.

Precautions

Regular examination for ocular disturbances should be carried out every 3 to 6 months in patients receiving long courses of treatment. Care is necessary in administering chloroquine to patients with impaired liver or renal function or with porphyria or psoriasis. Patients with glucose-6-phosphate dehydrogenase deficiency should be observed for haemolytic anaemia during chloroquine treatment. Ocular toxicity may render the patient unfit to take charge of vehicles or machinery. Although some adverse foetal effects have been reported with chloroquine, the dangers from malaria, especially the falciparum form, are usually considered to be greater and antimalarial treatment should not be withheld during pregnancy.

Report of the use of chloroquine and other bitter drugs applied to the nipples as a lotion to stop infants breast feeding among Ethiopian refugees in Sudan.— G. Barnabas and H. J. Lovel (letter), *Lancet*, 1982, *1*, 113.

INTERACTIONS. *Antacids*. Studies *in vitro* and *in vivo* have shown that antacids and kaolin can alter the absorption of chloroquine. It was recommended that doses of chloroquine and antacids should be separated by at least 4 hours.— P. F. D'Arcy and J. C. McElnay, *Drug Intell. & clin. Pharm.*, 1987, *21*, 607.

Antibiotics. For a report that chloroquine could reduce the gastro-intestinal absorption of ampicillin, see p.117.

PORPHYRIA. An opinion that chloroquine or quinine should be used in patients with porphyria if no alternative treatment for malaria is available despite concern about its safety in these patients.— M. R. Moore and P. B. Disler, *Adverse Drug React. Ac. Pois. Rev.*, 1983, *2*, 149.

Absorption and Fate

Chloroquine is readily absorbed from the gastro-intestinal tract and about 55% in the circulation is bound to plasma proteins. It accumulates in high concentrations in some tissues, such as the kidneys, liver, lungs, and spleen, and is strongly bound in melanin-containing cells such as those in the eyes and the skin. Chloroquine is eliminated very slowly from the body and it may persist in tissues for a prolonged period. Chloroquine is excreted mainly in the urine, with 70% as unchanged drug and about 25% as the desethyl metabolite. The rate of urinary excretion of chloroquine is increased at low pH values.

Comments on the measurement of chloroquine concentrations. Chloroquine is bound to platelets and granulocytes so that the plasma concentration is only 10 to 15% of that in whole blood. If these cells are not removed erroneously high plasma concentrations will be reported. To determine the true plasma concentrations a centrifugal force of 2000 *g* for 10 to 15 minutes is required to ensure that plasma is free of cells before the assay. Furthermore, chloroquine concentrations determined in serum are higher than those in plasma, probably because of the release of chloroquine from platelets during coagulation. It is crucial to state whether analysis has been done on whole blood, serum, or properly separated plasma.— L. L. Gustafsson *et al.* (letter), *Lancet*, 1983, *1*, 126. Following administration of chloroquine 100 mg daily for 10 days to healthy subjects, chloroquine concentrations varied considerably and were a mean of 1245 (± 598) nmol per litre in whole blood, 242 (± 105) nmol per litre in plasma, and 2068 (± 1147) nmol per litre in erythrocytes.— F. Verdier *et al.* (letter), *ibid.*, 1227.

The Dill Glazko eosin test, which has been recommended by the WHO, was found to be unreliable for detecting chloroquine in the urine in a study of 97 subjects.— F. Verdier *et al.* (letter), *Lancet*, 1985, *1*, 1282. See also L. Rombo *et al.* (letter), *ibid.*, 1509.

Concentrations of chloroquine in nail clippings could be used to help assess chloroquine intake for up to a year after administration, and could be obtained more easily than blood samples in the field.— D. Ofori-Adjei and O- Ericsson (letter), *Lancet*, 1985, *2*, 331.

A study indicating that determination of salivary chloroquine concentrations could be useful in assessing patient compliance and in therapeutic drug monitoring and determination of some pharmacokinetic parameters of chloroquine.— F. A. Ogubona *et al.*, *J. Pharm. Pharmac.*, 1986, *38*, 535.

Early studies suggesting that the pharmacokinetics of chloroquine were dose-dependent were refuted by later

weekly could result in sub-optimal blood concentrations if a dose was missed, or if diarrhoea and vomiting occurred. Travellers should be advised to take a further dose of chloroquine if diarrhoea and vomiting should occur and to repeat the dose if necessary two days later.— H. H. Neumann, *Lancet*, 1981, *2*, 1231.

Chloroquine base 300 mg weekly as used for malaria prophylaxis could be taken continuously for six and a half years before the total dose of 100 g, which is considered to be the safe upper limit, is reached. Then the safest advice is to replace chloroquine with another antimalarial prophylactic for at least a year before resuming regular prophylaxis with chloroquine again.— D. R. Bell, *Br. med. J.*, 1987, *294*, 300.

Transfusion malaria. In malarial zones a single dose of chloroquine 600 mg (calculated as the base) administered to the recipient 24 hours before or on the day of transfusion seemed to protect from induced malaria but it might be prudent to give all non-immune recipients a standard 3-day course of curative antimalarial treatment rather than rely on a single dose of chloroquine.— *Br. med. J.*, 1976, *1*, 542.

To prevent tranfusion-induced malaria the standard 3-day treatment course of chloroquine was given routinely to all blood recipients in Nigeria (a region of endemic malaria but with little, if any, chloroquine resistance). Prophylaxis was also given to all postoperative patients since surgery often activates latent malaria.— B. Camazine (letter), *Lancet*, 1985, *2*, 37.

Suggestion that chloroquine could be added routinely to donated blood in endemic areas.— N. J. White (letter), *Lancet*, 1987, *1*, 100. Comment that the addition of chloroquine to stored blood could adversely affect platelet function.— J. R. O'Brien (letter), *ibid.*, 455.

Treatment of mild to moderate malaria. In 41 Ethiopian patients with falciparum malaria treated with chloroquine 10 mg per kg body-weight as a single dose, recrudescence of asexual parasitaemia occurred in 11. All recovered after further treatment with chloroquine 25 mg per kg.— D. T. Dennis *et al.*, *Trans. R. Soc. trop. Med. Hyg.*, 1974, *68*, 241. In 23 of 24 and 12 of 27 children with heavy but asymptomatic *Plasmodium falciparum* infection in a semi-immune population of the United Republic of Tanzania, given chloroquine 5 or 10 mg per kg body-weight respectively by mouth as a single dose, asexual parasites were still present in the blood after 7 days. All of a further 25 children given 25 mg per kg over 3 days became negative on the day following the end of treatment and remained so during the remaining 6 days of follow-up. These results contrasted strongly with those of an earlier study (J. Lelijveld and F. Mzoo, *Bull. Wld Hlth Org.*, 1970, *42*, 471) which showed that chloroquine 5 mg per kg consistently produced a complete clearance of trophozoites within 72 hours of administration; the earlier study concluded that chloroquine 10 mg per kg was adequate for routine treatment of *P. falciparum* infections occurring in the semi-immune population of that area. The earlier study had also shown that asymptomatic infections were fully susceptible to a single dose of chloroquine 2.5 mg per kg and concluded that the long exposure to small chloroquine doses had not apparently induced the appearance of less sensitive strains. The present results have shown that the situation has changed significantly and the emergence of *P. falciparum* resistant to chloroquine among semi-immune subjects has several practical implications: chloroquine or amodiaquine can still be used for radical treatment of falciparum malaria provided they are given at the dosage of 25 mg per kg over a 3-day period; patients not responding to this treatment should be radically treated with either quinine or with a combination of sulfadoxine 1.5 g with pyrimethamine 75 mg for adults; in addition all these patients should receive an effective gametocyticide such as primaquine 30 to 45 mg as a single dose for adults.— E. Onori *et al.*, *Bull. Wld Hlth Org.*, 1982, *60*, 77. Findings indicating an exceptionally low humoral immunological response in the population. This reduction might be explained by the use of chloroquinised salt and easy access to chloroquine tablets but was so marked that other factors might have contributed to its establishment. It was recommended that further studies be conducted to assess the effects of chemosuppression on the immune response.— E. Onori *et al.*, *ibid.*, 899.

Doses of chloroquine base of up to 37.5 mg per kg body-weight were necessary to clear parasitaemia in an area of Indonesia with RII level chloroquine resistance.— S. L. Hoffman *et al.*, *Trans. R. Soc. trop. Med. Hyg.*, 1984, *78*, 175.

Treatment of severe and complicated malaria. Chloroquine base 18 mg per kg body-weight by intramuscular injection was administered to 11 patients with cerebral malaria for 1 to 2 days until neurological disturbances disappeared. One patient died compared with 4 of 30 patients treated with chloroquine base 10 mg per kg. The high dose was generally well tolerated except in one patient who suffered a cardiac arrest. High doses of chloroquine could be useful in cerebral malaria where there was a risk of RI chloroquine resistance and no alternative antimalarial drugs were available, but the higher risk of toxicity may not always justify their use.— S. Nuti and L. Savioli, *Trans. R. Soc. trop. Med. Hyg.*, 1983, *77*, 872.

Chloroquine 2.5 mg per kg intramuscularly every 6 hours was at least as effective as quinine 10 mg per kg intravenously every 12 hours in a study of 52 children with cerebral malaria in Zambia.— M. J. Maguire, *E. Afr. med. J.*, 1983, *60*, 260.

In a study of the pathogenesis of tropical splenomegaly syndrome, treatment of 14 patients with chloroquine 300 mg weekly for 9 to 26 months led to a partial reversal of immunological aberrations as well as marked clinical improvement.— S. L. Hoffman *et al.*, *New Engl. J. Med.*, 1984, *310*, 337.

Of 9 children presenting with severe malaria, chloroquine was detected in the serum of 7 before intramuscular treatment with chloroquine was commenced, presumably due to previous self-treatment. Only 2 patients admitted to using chloroquine before admission to hospital. In areas where chloroquine is freely available, its indiscriminate use increases the risk of chloroquine toxicity and may enhance the selection of drug-resistant strains of the malaria parasite.— D. Ofori-Adjei *et al.* (letter), *Lancet*, 1984, *1*, 1246. Comment on the increase in the already high risk of using parenteral chloroquine in children when chloroquine has been used for self-medication before admission to hospital. Intravenous quinine is recommended in children who cannot take chloroquine orally.— P. I. Trigg *et al.* (letter), *ibid.*, *2*, 288.

For references to blood concentrations achieved after parenteral administration of chloroquine and comments on minimising toxicity, see under Absorption and Fate, above.

For discussions of drug resistance in malaria and the prophylaxis and treatment of chloroquine-resistant malaria, see p.505.

PORPHYRIAS. There have been several reports of the beneficial effect of chloroquine therapy in patients with porphyria cutanea tarda. The demonstrated efficacy must be carefully weighed against the known hepatotoxicity of the drug in these patients. The mechanism of action of chloroquine appears to relate to its ability to form a water-soluble complex with hepatic porphyrin. This drug-porphyrin complex is then rapidly excreted in the urine. Associated with this rapid flushing of porphyrin from the liver may be fever, malaise, and abdominal pain with associated changes in hepatocellular enzymes. It has been suggested that administration of lower doses of antimalarial drugs may be therapeutically effective and obviate the toxic response seen in porphyria cutanea tarda. In the experience of the authors, low-dose chloroquine administration may be a useful alternative in patients unsuitable for phlebotomy, but toxicity is not always avoided.— M. E. Grossman *et al.*, *Am. J. Med.*, 1979, *67*, 277.

A study of low-dose chloroquine therapy in porphyria cutanea tarda. Seven patients with porphyria cutanea tarda were treated with chloroquine [sic] 125 mg twice weekly, or in one case 125 mg on alternate days. All 7 patients went into clinical and biochemical remission on ten separate occasions after 10 to 23 months. Relapses occurred in 4 patients on a total of 6 occasions at 3 to 35 months after completion of treatment. Three of the patients who relapsed were successfully retreated. Four patients remained in remission after 20 to 59 months. Treatment was considered to be well tolerated and was recommended for patients with mild disease, few signs of liver damage, reliable personalities, and stable social backgrounds.— R. E. Ashton *et al.*, *Br. J. Derm.*, 1984, *111*, 609. Low-dose chloroquine was considered to be a hazardous choice of treatment for porphyria cutanea tarda in view of potential hepatotoxicity.— E. Rocchi *et al.*, *ibid.*, 1986, *114*, 621. Comments: L. Malina (letter), *ibid.*, 1987, *116*, 139; E. Rocchi, *ibid.*

Further references to the use of chloroquine in porphyria cutanea tarda: J. J. F. Taljaard *et al.*, *Br. J. Derm.*, 1972, *87*, 261; M. J. Kowertz (letter), *J. Am. med. Ass.*, 1975, *233*, 22; G. Swanbeck and G. Wennersten, *Br. J. Derm.*, 1977, *97*, 77; V. Kordac *et al.* (letter), *New Engl. J. Med.*, 1977, *296*, 949; A. M. D. C. Batlle *et al.*, *Br. J. Derm.*, 1987, *116*, 407.

PREGNANCY AND THE NEONATE. The dangers of malaria infection during pregnancy are considered to far outweigh any potential adverse effects of malaria prophylaxis and treatment with chloroquine. Chloroquine is generally considered to be safe during pregnancy in the doses used for malarial prophylaxis, although exposure during the first trimester to chloroquine doses required to treat rheumatic disease has resulted in foetal sensorineural hearing loss (L.J. Bruce-Chwatt, *Br. med. J.*, 1983, *286*, 1457; *Lancet*, 1983, *2*, 84; *Br. med. J.*, 1984, *289*, 1296; R. Wise, *ibid.*, 1987, *294*, 42; M.A. Byron, *ibid.*, 236). Where chloroquine-resistant *Plasmodium falciparum* is found prophylaxis presents a problem: pyrimethamine-sulfadoxine and pyrimethamine-dapsone preparations are probably best avoided (R. Wise, 1987), particularly during the first 3 months and the last 2 weeks of pregnancy (*Br. med. J.*, 1984, *289*, 1296). Proguanil is probably safe in areas where it is still effective. Probably the best advice is to avoid travel to chloroquine-resistant areas during pregnancy, but if this is unavoidable, to give chloroquine prophylaxis and stress advice on precautions to avoid insect bites (L.J. Bruce-Chwatt, 1983; R. Wise, 1987).

For treatment of malaria chloroquine should be used but radical cure of *P. vivax* and *P. ovale* infections with primaquine should not be undertaken until after pregnancy (R. Wise, 1987). For the treatment of chloroquine-resistant *P. falciparum* infections Wise suggested quinine for 3 days followed by a single dose of pyrimethamine-sulfadoxine and, if asexual parasites are still present in a blood smear, a 7-day course of erythromycin.

RHEUMATIC DISORDERS. A review of the use and adverse effects of disease-modifying drugs in rheumatoid arthritis. Chloroquine and hydroxychloroquine are claimed to be less toxic than other disease-modifying drugs in rheumatoid arthritis, but are probably less effective than gold, penicillamine, and sulphasalazine.— *Drug & Ther. Bull.*, 1985, *26*, 101.

For a general outline of the treatment of rheumatoid arthritis, including the use of chloroquine see under analgesics and anti-inflammatory agents, p.1.

Palindromic rheumatism. Symptoms of palindromic rheumatism were alleviated in most of 18 patients treated with chloroquine phosphate 250 mg daily for 6 to 8 weeks.— D. N. Golding (letter), *Br. med. J.*, 1976, *2*, 1382.

Dramatic response to chloroquine in 3 patients with palindromic rheumatism.— M. R. Richardson and A. M. Zalin, *Br. med. J.*, 1987, *294*, 741. Comment.— P. Hanonen *et al.* (letter), *ibid.*, 1289.

SARCOIDOSIS. In a double-blind study 52 patients with pulmonary sarcoidosis received chloroquine sulphate, 600 mg daily for 8 weeks and then 400 mg daily for 8 weeks, or a placebo throughout. After 6 months, the chloroquine-treated patients showed significant improvement over the control group, but after 12 months there was no significant difference between them.—A report from the Research Committee of the British Tuberculosis Association, 1967, *Tubercle*, 1967, *47*, 257.

Chloroquine was effective in reducing concentrations of urinary calcium and serum concentrations of 1,25-dihydroxyvitamin D in 2 patients with chronic sarcoidosis. Serum 1,25-hydroxyvitamin D concentrations were unchanged.— T. J. O'Leary *et al.*, *New Engl. J. Med.*, 1986, *315*, 727.

Comment on the use of chloroquine in lupus pernio.— M. A. Spiteri *et al.*, *Br. J. Derm.*, 1985, *112*, 315.

Preparations of Chloroquine Salts

Chloroquine Hydrochloride Injection *(U.S.P.).* A sterile solution of chloroquine in Water for Injections prepared with the aid of hydrochloric acid; it contains in each mL 47.5 to 52.5 mg of $C_{18}H_{26}ClN_3,2HCl$, equivalent to approximately 38.7 to 42.8 mg of chloroquine base. pH 5.5 to 6.5.

Chloroquine Phosphate Injection *(B.P.).* Potency is expressed in terms of the equivalent amount of chloroquine base.

Chloroquine Sulphate Injection *(B.P.).* Potency is expressed in terms of the equivalent amount of chloroquine base. pH 4.0 to 5.5.

Chloroquine Phosphate Tablets *(B.P.)*

Chloroquine Phosphate Tablets *(U.S.P.)*

Chloroquine Sulphate Tablets *(B.P.)*

Proprietary Preparations of Chloroquine Salts

Avloclor *(ICI Pharmaceuticals, UK). Tablets*, scored, chloroquine phosphate 250 mg, equivalent to chloroquine base 155 mg.

Nivaquine *(May & Baker, UK). Tablets*, chloroquine sulphate 200 mg, equivalent to chloroquine base 150 mg. *Syrup*, chloroquine sulphate 68 mg equivalent to chloroquine base 50 mg/5 mL.

Proprietary Names and Manufacturers of Chloroquine Salts

Aralen *(Austral.*; *Winthrop, Canad.*; *Winthrop-Breon,*

USA); Avloclor *(ICI, Austral.; ICI Pharmaceuticals, UK)*; Chlorquin *(Protea, Austral.)*; Cidanchin *(Cidan, Spain)*; Delagil *(Hung.)*; Dichinalex *(Recordati, Ital.)*; Klorokinfosfat *(DAK, Denm.; NAF, Norw.)*; Lagaquin *(Lagap, Switz.)*; Malarex *(Dumex, Denm.)*; Malarivon *(Wallace Mfg Chem., UK)*; Malatets *(Pharmadrug, Ger.)*; Nivaquine *(Arg.; May & Baker, Austral.; Belg.; Specia, Fr.; Neth.; Norw.; May & Baker, S.Afr.; Spain; Rhone-Poulenc, Switz.; May & Baker, UK)*; Résochine *(Bayer, Switz.)*; Resochin *(Austral.; Denm.; Bayer, Ger.; Bayer, Ital.; Neth.; Norw.; Bayer, Spain; Switz.; Bayer, UK)*; Resochine *(Belg.)*.

The following names have been used for multi-ingredient preparations containing chloroquine salts— Aralen with Primaquine *(Winthrop-Breon, USA)*; Aralis *(Winthrop, UK)*; Elestol *(Bayer, UK)*; Milibis with Aralen *(USA)*; Nivembin *(May & Baker, UK)*.

1376-p

Chlorproguanil Hydrochloride *(BANM, rINNM).*
M5943. 1-(3,4-Dichlorophenyl)-5-isopropylbiguanide hydrochloride.
$C_{11}H_{15}Cl_2N_5,HCl=324.6$.

CAS — 537-21-3 (chlorproguanil); 15537-76-5 (hydrochloride).

Chlorproguanil is an antimalarial drug with actions and uses similar to those of proguanil (see p.515) but it is more active than proguanil and has a longer duration of action. Resistance has been reported in some areas.
It is given in doses of 20 mg at intervals of 7 days; administration should be continued for 4 weeks after leaving a malarious area.

Prophylaxis with chlorproguanil either alone or in combination with chloroquine did not prevent malaria infection in a study of semi-immune children living in a hyperendemic area where *Plasmodium falciparum* resistance to chloroquine, pyrimethamine, and cycloguanil had been demonstrated. There was no significant increase in efficacy when chlorproguanil was given in association with chloroquine.— M. H. Coosemans *et al., Trans. R. Soc. trop. Med. Hyg.*, 1987, *81*, 151.

A study of the pharmacokinetics of chlorproguanil and proguanil.— W. M. Watkins *et al., J. Pharm. Pharmac.*, 1987, *39*, 261.

Proprietary Names and Manufacturers
Lapudrine *(ICI Pharmaceuticals, UK).*

1377-s

Cycloguanil Embonate *(BAN, rINN).*
CI-501; Cycloguanil Pamoate *(USAN)*. Bis[1-(4-chlorophenyl)-1,2-dihydro-2,2-dimethyl-1,3,5-triazine-4,6-diamine] 4,4′-methylenebis(3-hydroxy-2-naphthoate).
$C_{11}H_{14}ClN_5,\frac{1}{2}(C_{23}H_{16}O_6)=445.9$.

CAS — 516-21-2 (cycloguanil); 609-78-9 (embonate).

Cycloguanil is the active metabolite of proguanil (see Proguanil Hydrochloride, p.515) and has similar actions and uses. An intramuscular injection of a suspension of fine particles of cycloguanil embonate in an oily basis provides protection for several months against infection. It may be given with a sulphone to delay the development of drug resistance. Cycloguanil embonate has also been used in the treatment of cutaneous leishmaniasis.

Proprietary Names and Manufacturers
Camolar.

19137-b

Enpiroline Phosphate *(USAN, rINNM).*
WR-180409. (±)-(R^*,R^*)-α-[2-(Trifluoromethyl)-6-(α,α,α-trifluoro-*p*-tolyl)-4-pyridyl]-2-piperidinemethanol phosphate.
$C_{19}H_{18}F_6N_2O,H_3PO_4=738.5$.

CAS — 66364-74-7 (phosphate); 66364-73-6 (enpiroline).

Enpiroline phosphate is an antimalarial drug which has been tried in the treatment of falciparum malaria.

References to the use of enpiroline in malaria: T. M. Cosgriff *et al., Am. J. trop. Med. Hyg.*, 1984, *33*, 767.

16829-p

Halofantrine Hydrochloride *(USAN, rINNM).*
WR-171669. 1,3-Dichloro-α-[2-(dibutylamino)ethyl]-6-trifluoromethyl-9-phenanthrene-methanol hydrochloride.
$C_{26}H_{30}Cl_2F_3NO,HCl=536.9$.

CAS — 69756-53-2 (halofantrine); 36167-63-2 (hydrochloride); 66051-63-6 (±-halofantrine).

Halofantrine is an antimalarial drug which has been tried in the treatment of falciparum malaria in doses of 1.0 to 1.5 g in divided doses.

References to the use of halofantrine in malaria: T. M. Cosgriff *et al., Am. J. trop. Med. Hyg.*, 1982, *31*, 1075; B. L. Robinson *et al., Trans. R. Soc. trop. Med. Hyg.*, 1986, *80*, 342; J. P. Couland *et al., ibid.*, 615; T. G. Geary *et al., ibid.*, 1987, *81*, 499; W. M. Watkins *et al., Lancet*, 1988, *2*, 247; J. Wirima *et al., ibid.*, 250.

1380-b

Hydroxychloroquine Sulphate *(BAN, rINNM).*

Hydroxychloroquine Sulfate *(USAN)*; Oxichlorochin Sulphate; Win-1258-2. 2-{*N*-[4-(7-Chloro-4-quinolylamino)pentyl]-*N*-ethylamino}ethanol sulphate.
$C_{18}H_{26}ClN_3O, H_2SO_4=433.9$.

CAS — 118-42-3 (hydroxychloroquine); 747-36-4 (sulphate).

Pharmacopoeias. In *Br.* and *U.S.*

A white or almost white odourless or almost odourless crystalline powder. Hydroxychloroquine sulphate 100 mg is approximately equivalent to 77 mg of hydroxychloroquine base. **Soluble** 1 in 5 of water; practically insoluble in alcohol, chloroform, and ether. A 1% solution in water has a pH of 3.5 to 5.5. **Protect** from light.

Adverse Effects, Treatment, and Precautions
As for Chloroquine, p.508.

EFFECTS ON THE EYES. Hydroxychloroquine was given in an average dose of 800 mg daily for up to 4½ years to 94 patients with lupus erythematosus, rheumatoid arthritis, or scleroderma. The patients had not previously received chloroquine, amodiaquine, mepacrine, or quinine. Corneal deposition occurred in 26 patients; it was reversible in 20, persistent in 3, and 3 were lost to follow-up. There was a rapid rise in incidence after 150 g had been given. One patient who had received 770 g over 26½ months developed retinopathy. A second case of probable retinopathy was subsequently seen in a further patient.— R. V. Shearer and E. L. Dubois, *Am. J. Ophthal.*, 1967, *64*, 245.

Ocular toxicity in 3 of 99 patients after long-term treatment with hydroxychloroquine.— R. I. Rynes *et al., Arthritis Rheum.*, 1979, *22*, 832.

A study suggesting that hydroxychloroquine may produce less retinal toxicity than chloroquine.— D. S. Finbloom *et al., J. Rheumatol.*, 1985, *12*, 692.

For further discussions of ocular toxicity associated with hydroxychloroquine including dosage recommendations, see under Chloroquine p.508.

EFFECTS ON THE SKIN. A report of marked exacerbation of psoriatic skin involvement in a patient with psoriatic arthritis after treatment with hydroxychloroquine.— M. J. Luzar, *J. Rheumatol.*, 1982, *9*, 462.

Generalised erythroderma and exfoliative dermatitis developed in a 31-year-old patient with psoriatic arthritis following treatment with hydroxychloroquine.— G. A. Slagel and W. D. James, *J. Am. Acad. Derm.*, 1985, *12*, 857.

PREGNANCY AND THE NEONATE. Hydroxychloroquine was detected in the breast milk of a lactating patient taking hydroxychloroquine 200 mg twice daily at 15 to 24 hours after the first dose, at a time when the maternal plasma concentration was slightly less than 100 ng per mL. The highest milk concentration of hydroxychloroquine was 10.6 ng per mL which occurred after 39 to 48 hours. A total of 480 ng of hydroxychloroquine was secreted into the breast milk during the first 24 hours from the start of treatment, and 2402 ng during the second 24-hour period.— M. Østensen *et al., Eur. J. clin. Pharmac.*, 1985, *28*, 357.

Further references to the secretion of hydroxychloroquine in breast milk: R. L. Nation *et al.* (letter), *Br. J. clin. Pharmac.*, 1984, *17*, 368.

Uses and Administration
Hydroxychloroquine sulphate has an antimalarial action similar to that of chloroquine (see p.510) but it is mainly used in the treatment of systemic and discoid lupus erythematosus and rheumatoid arthritis. Treatment is usually started with about 400 to 600 mg daily in divided doses with meals and the dose is reduced to about 200 to 400 mg when a response occurs. The minimum effective dose should be given which in any case should not exceed 6.5 mg per kg body-weight daily.
In malaria, a prophylactic dose of 400 mg every 7 days is used, and in treating an acute attack a dose of 800 mg has been used, followed after 6 to 8 hours by 400 mg and a further 400 mg on each of the 2 following days. Children may be given a weekly prophylactic dose equivalent to 5 mg of base (6.5 mg of sulphate) per kg body-weight, while for treatment an initial dose of 10 mg of base per kg may be given, followed by 5 mg per kg 6 hours later and again on the second and third days.
Hydroxychloroquine sulphate has been used in the treatment of polymorphous light eruptions. The dose is as for rheumatoid arthritis.
Hydroxychloroquine sulphate has also been suggested for prophylaxis of postoperative deep vein thrombosis at a dose of 200 mg every 6 to 8 hours.

POLYMORPHOUS LIGHT ERUPTIONS. Beneficial responses were seen in 13 patients with polymorphous light eruption treated with hydroxychloroquine compared with 15 control patients.— G. M. Murphy *et al., Br. J. Derm.*, 1987, *116*, 379.

PORPHYRIA CUTANEA TARDA. Hydroxychloroquine, 400 mg weekly for several months, had been reported to be safe and effective in the treatment of porphyria cutanea tarda.— F. De Matteis, *Br. J. Derm.*, 1972, *87*, 174.

In a study of 61 patients with porphyria cutanea tarda, hydroxychloroquine was more effective than phlebotomy at removing porphyrins, but the liver disease associated with porphyria cutanea tarda improved less with hydroxychloroquine than with phlebotomy.— T. Cainelli *et al., Br. J. Derm.*, 1983, *108*, 593.

RHEUMATOID ARTHRITIS. A review of drugs for rheumatoid arthritis. Hydroxychloroquine had been found to be effective for rheumatoid arthritis that had not responded adequately to non-steroidal anti-inflammatory drugs. Adverse effects were rare at recommended doses, but visual acuity should be monitored regularly and treatment discontinued promptly at the first signs of retinal toxicity.— *Med. Lett.*, 1987, *29*, 21. See also *Drug & Ther. Bull.*, 1985, *26*, 101.

Combination therapy with hydroxychloroquine, cyclophosphamide, and azathioprine in 17 patients with intractable rheumatoid arthritis had produced complete remission in 5 patients, near remission in 2, and partial disease suppression in 7. Disease suppression began within 3 to 16 months of the start of treatment. Adverse effects were common but mostly tolerable and transient.— D. J. McCarty and G. F. Carrera, *J. Am. med. Ass.*, 1982, *248*, 1718.

Hydroxychloroquine 2.2 mg per kg body-weight daily was less effective than penicillamine 7 mg per kg daily after 6 months of treatment, but 25% of patients receiving hydroxychloroquine derived prolonged benefit while the effects of penicillamine reduced with time.— T. W. Bunch *et al., Arthritis Rheum.*, 1984, *27*, 267.

A double-blind placebo-controlled study in 162 children with severe active juvenile rheumatoid arthritis failed to demonstrate that, in the presence of a non-steroidal anti-inflammatory drug, either hydroxychloroquine or penicillamine had any greater therapeutic effect than placebo.— E. J. Brewer *et al., New Engl. J. Med.*, 1986, *314*, 1269.

For comments on the use of hydroxychloroquine in rheumatoid disorders see under Chloroquine, p.511 and analgesics and anti-inflammatory agents, p.1.

THROMBO-EMBOLIC DISORDERS. Of 565 patients who underwent surgery 284 received an injection of hydroxychloroquine sulphate 200 mg with their premedication and then 200 mg eight-hourly by mouth or by injection until discharge from hospital. From postoperative observations and by phlebography it appeared that hydroxychloroquine could be useful in reducing the incidence of deep-vein thrombosis and pulmonary embolism.— A. E. Carter *et al., Br. med. J.*, 1971, *1*, 312.

The incidence of deep-vein thrombosis after surgery was 5% in 107 patients given hydroxychloroquine sulphate compared with 16% in 97 controls. The dose was 1.2 g by mouth in 3 divided doses in the 24 hours before surgery followed by 400 mg every 12 hours after surgery until discharge.— A. E. Carter and R. Eban, *Br. med. J.*, 1974, *3*, 94.

For discussions, see A. S. Gallus and J. Hirsh, *Drugs*, 1976, *12*, 132; A. G. G. Turpie and J. Hirsh, *Br. med. Bull.*, 1978, *34*, 183.

Preparations

Hydroxychloroquine Sulfate Tablets *(U.S.P.)*. Tablets containing hydroxychloroquine sulphate.

Hydroxychloroquine Tablets *(B.P.)*. Tablets containing hydroxychloroquine sulphate.

Proprietary Preparations

Plaquenil *(Sterling Research, UK). Tablets*, hydroxychloroquine sulphate 200 mg.

Proprietary Names and Manufacturers

Ercoquin *(Erco, Denm.; Nyco, Norw.; Erco, Swed.)*; Plaquenil *(Aust.; Winthrop, Austral.; Belg.; Winthrop, Canad.; Winthrop, Denm.; Fin.; Winthrop, Fr.; Iceland; Maggioni-Winthrop, Ital.; Neth.; Winthrop, Norw.; Sterling-Winthrop, Swed.; Winthrop, Switz.; Sterling Research, UK; Winthrop-Breon, USA)*; Quensyl *(Winthrop, Ger.)*.

1381-v

Mefloquine Hydrochloride *(BANM, USAN, rINNM)*.

Ro-21-5998/001; WR-142490 (mefloquine*)*.
(±)-α-[2,8-Bis(trifluoromethyl)-4-quinolyl]-α-(2-piperidyl)methanol hydrochloride.
$C_{17}H_{16}F_6N_2O,HCl=414.8$.

CAS — 53230-10-7 (mefloquine); 51773-92-3 (hydrochloride).

NOTE. Mefloquine is also *USAN*.

Mefloquine base 250 mg is approximately equivalent to mefloquine hydrochloride 274 mg.

For a report of reduced *in-vitro* activity against *P. falciparum* of mefloquine hydrochloride solutions following membrane filtration, see Chloroquine p.508.

Adverse Effects

Mefloquine is generally well tolerated at doses used for the prophylaxis and treatment of malaria. The most frequent adverse effects are nausea, dizziness, diarrhoea, vomiting, headache, and abdominal pain. Occasional patients have developed neuropsychiatric disturbances. Skin rashes, pruritus, and symptomless bradycardia have been reported rarely.

Precautions

Mefloquine should be given cautiously to patients with severe renal or hepatic dysfunction. Mefloquine should not be given in conjunction with quinine.

Absorption and Fate

Mefloquine is well absorbed from the gastro-intestinal tract and peak plasma concentrations occur 2 to 12 hours after a single oral dose. Mefloquine is about 98% bound to plasma proteins and high concentrations have been reported in red blood cells. It is widely distributed throughout the body. The mean elimination half-life has been reported to be 15 to 33 days. Mefloquine is excreted slowly, mainly in the faeces.

A review of the clinical pharmacokinetics of antimalarial drugs including mefloquine.— N. J. White, *Clin. Pharmacokinet.*, 1985, *10*, 187.

Study of the pharmacokinetics of mefloquine given alone and in combination with pyrimethamine-sulfadoxine in Thai subjects.— J. Karbwang *et al., Eur. J. clin. Pharmac.*, 1987, *32*, 173.

Study of the concentrations of mefloquine in plasma and whole blood during treatment with a combination of mefloquine, sulfadoxine, and pyrimethamine.— J. Karbwang *et al., Br. J. clin. Pharmac.*, 1987, *23*, 477.

Uses and Administration

Mefloquine is a rapidly acting blood schizontocide which is effective against all forms of malaria. In practice its use is restricted to the prophylaxis and treatment of chloroquine-resistant and multidrug-resistant falciparum malaria. In mixed malaria infections, vivax malaria may recur once mefloquine treatment finishes since exoerythrocytic forms are not affected. The usual dose for prophylaxis and suppression of falciparum malaria is 250 mg mefloquine base once every 7 days. It has been suggested that, until more is known about the long-term effects, weekly administration of mefloquine should not continue for more than 6 weeks. Persons staying in malarious areas for longer than this are advised to leave a two-week gap after every fourth dose of mefloquine. Alternatively the prophylactic dose could be halved once steady-state plasma concentrations have been reached after about 2 months. A suggested dose for children is 4 to 6 mg per kg body-weight weekly.

Although single doses of mefloquine 1.0 to 1.5 g have been reported to be effective in the treatment of falciparum malaria the dose normally recommended is mefloquine base 750 mg initially, then a further 500 mg after 6 to 8 hours. A dose of 25 mg per kg has been recommended for children.

There is experimental evidence to show that the emergence of resistance can be delayed by administering mefloquine in combination with pyrimethamine-sulfadoxine. This combination is available commercially in tablets containing mefloquine 250 mg, sulfadoxine 500 mg, and pyrimethamine 25 mg. For the treatment of malaria the usual dose is 3 tablets taken as a single dose. In order to delay the development of mefloquine resistance, the WHO are recommending that mefloquine should not be freely available and should be used only for chloroquine- and multidrug-resistant strains of *Plasmodium falciparum*. It may also be desirable to reserve mefloquine for treatment only.

For further discussions on the development of drug resistance and the treatment and prophylaxis of malaria, see p.505.

An extensive review of the development and clinical studies of mefloquine with recommendations for use in malaria prophylaxis and treatment.— Advances in malaria chemotherapy, *Tech. Rep. Ser. Wld Hlth Org. No. 711*, 1984, p.101.

Further reviews of mefloquine: *Bull. Wld Hlth Org.*, 1983, *61*, 169.

Clinical studies of the use of mefloquine in the treatment of malaria: K. E. Dixon *et al., Trans. R. Soc. trop. Med. Hyg.*, 1982, *76*, 664; F. Tin *et al., Bull. Wld Hlth Org.*, 1982, *60*, 913; T. Harinasuta *et al., ibid.*, 1983, *61*, 299; J. M. K. Ekue *et al., ibid.*, 713; J. -M. de Souza, *ibid.*, 815; K. E. Dixon *et al., Am. J. trop. Med. Hyg.*, 1985, *34*, 435; A. K. Alcantara *et al., S. E. Asian J. trop. med. publ. Hlth*, 1985, *16*, 534; J. M. de Souza *et al., Bull. Wld Hlth Org.*, 1985, *63*, 603; T. Harinasuta *et al., Lancet*, 1985, *1*, 885; L. Suebsaeng *et al., Bull. Wld Hlth Org.*, 1986, *64*, 759.

Studies of the use of mefloquine in combination with pyrimethamine-sulfadoxine in the treatment of malaria: J. M. Kofi Ekue *et al., Bull. Wld Hlth Org.*, 1985, *63*, 339; D. Botero *et al., ibid.*, 731; F. Tin *et al., ibid.*, 727.

Studies of the use of mefloquine in combination with pyrimethamine-sulfadoxine for malaria prophylaxis: K. Win *et al., Lancet*, 1985, *2*, 694.

For discussions on the prophylaxis and treatment of malaria, see p.505.

Proprietary Names and Manufacturers of Mefloquine or Mefloquine Hydrochloride

Lariam *(Roche, Fr.; Roche, Switz.)*; Mephaquine *(Mepha, Switz.)*.

The following names have been used for multi-ingredient preparations containing mefloquine or mefloquine hydrochloride— Fansimef *(Roche, Switz.)*.

1382-g

Mepacrine Hydrochloride *(rINNM)*.

Acrichinum; Acrinamine; Antimalarinae Chlorhydras; Chinacrina; Mepacrini Hydrochloridum; Quinacrine Hydrochloride *(USAN)*; Quinacrinium Chloride. 6-Chloro-9-(4-diethylamino-1-methylbutylamino)-2-methoxyacridine dihydrochloride dihydrate.
$C_{23}H_{30}ClN_3O,2HCl,2H_2O=508.9$.

CAS — 83-89-6 (mepacrine); 69-05-6 (dihydrochloride, anhydrous); 6151-30-0 (dihydrochloride, dihydrate).

Pharmacopoeias. In *Arg., Aust., Belg., Braz., Egypt., Eur., Fr., Hung., Int., It., Mex., Neth., Nord., Pol., Rus., Span., Turk.*, and *U.S.*

A bright yellow odourless crystalline powder. **Soluble** 1 in 35 of water; soluble in alcohol. A 1% solution in water has a pH of about 4.5. **Incompatible** with alkalis, nitrates, and oxidising agents. **Store** in airtight containers. Protect from light.

INCOMPATIBILITY. Mepacrine hydrochloride was incompatible with amaranth, benzylpenicillin, sodium alginate, sodium aminosalicylate, sodium carboxymethylcellulose, sodium lauryl sulphate, and thiomersal.— *J. Am. pharm. Ass., pract. Pharm. Edn*, 1952, *13*, 658.

Adverse Effects

Adverse effects which may occur following antimalarial doses of mepacrine are dizziness, headache, and mild gastro-intestinal disturbances. Most patients develop a yellow discoloration of the skin and urine during long-term administration and blue/black discoloration of the palate and nails has been reported. Large doses may give rise to nausea and vomiting and occasionally to transient acute toxic psychosis and CNS stimulation. A few patients develop chronic dermatoses after prolonged administration of the drug; these may be either lichenoid, eczematoid, or exfoliative in type. Deaths from exfoliative dermatitis and from hepatitis have been reported. The use of mepacrine over prolonged periods may give rise to aplastic anaemia. Corneal deposits resulting in visual disturbances have been reported.

The toxicity arising from prolonged administration has contributed to the decline in the use of mepacrine in malaria.

Two patients had convulsions a few hours after the intrapleural administration of mepacrine hydrochloride 400 mg for malignant effusions. One developed status epilepticus and died; the other was successfully controlled with phenobarbitone intravenously and phenytoin by mouth.— I. Borda and M. Krant, *J. Am. med. Ass.*, 1967, *201*, 1049.

EFFECTS ON THE BLOOD. Aplastic anaemia was reported to occur with an incidence of 1 in 20 000 users.— O. B. Eden, *Br. med. Bull.*, 1986, *42*, 191.

EFFECTS ON THE LIVER. Hepatitis was associated with mepacrine administration in a 37-year-old woman taking mepacrine up to 300 mg daily for 6 weeks. Liver function tests returned to normal within 2 months of stopping mepacrine.— W. Gibb *et al., Ann. rheum. Dis.*, 1985, *44*, 861.

EFFECTS ON MENTAL FUNCTION. Psychiatric disturbances, including anxiety, confusion, disorientation, and hallucinations were reported in 3 patients during treatment with mepacrine.— S. J. Weisholtz *et al., Sth. med. J.*, 1982, *75*, 359.

Symptoms of toxic psychosis occurred in a 63-year-old woman after taking mepacrine 100 mg twice daily for 14 days. Symptoms disappeared when mepacrine was withdrawn.— R. L. Evans *et al., Archs Derm.*, 1984, *120*, 765.

EFFECTS ON THE SKIN. A patient with rheumatoid arthritis treated with mepacrine hydrochloride for about 20 years had developed a blue-black discoloration of the hard palate, the nail beds, and the skin over the shins. The colour disappeared when mepacrine was stopped and reappeared when it was restarted.— M. J. Egorin *et al., J. Am. med. Ass.*, 1976, *236*, 385.

Treatment of Adverse Effects

As for Chloroquine, p.509.

Precautions

Mepacrine should be given with caution to patients over the age of 60 years, to patients with a history of psychosis, and to patients with hepatic disease or dysfunction. Mepacrine can cause exacerbations of psoriasis; it should be avoided in psoriatic patients. Mepacrine should not be given in conjunction with primaquine or other 8-aminoquinolines since this can result in high plasma concentrations of primaquine and enhanced toxicity.

Mepacrine might interfere with fluorimetric estimations of plasma hydrocortisone.— J. Millhouse, *Adverse Drug React. Bull.*, 1974, Dec., 164.

Mepacrine has been reported to cause minor disulfiram-like symptoms when taken with alcohol.— *Med. Lett.*, 1981, *23*, 33.

Absorption and Fate

Mepacrine is readily absorbed from the gastro-intestinal tract. It is widely distributed throughout the body. It accumulates in body tissues particularly the liver and is liberated slowly. It is excreted slowly in the urine, and is still detectable in the urine after 2 months. Mepacrine crosses the placenta.

Mepacrine hydrochloride was bound to serum proteins *in vitro*.— G. A. Lutty, *Toxic. appl. Pharmac.*, 1978, *44*, 225.

Uses and Administration

Mepacrine was formerly used for the suppression and treatment of malaria but it has been superseded for these purposes by chloroquine and other more recently introduced antimalarials. Usual doses were 100 mg daily for suppression and 2.8 g given over 7 days for treatment.

Mepacrine hydrochloride is used in the treatment of giardiasis at a dose of 100 mg three times daily for 5 to 7 days. A suggested dose for children is 2 mg per kg body-weight three times daily.

It has been used for the expulsion of tapeworms but successful treatment is dependent upon careful patient preparation and purgation. Duodenal intubation may be required for best results.

Instillations of mepacrine hydrochloride or mesylate are used in the symptomatic treatment of neoplastic effusions in the pleura or peritoneum but the treatment is associated with a high frequency of toxic effects.

GIARDIASIS. Mepacrine 100 mg three times daily for 5 to 7 days was usually effective in the treatment of giardiasis, although a second course might be required. The dose for children under 4 years old was one-quarter of the adult dose.— *Br. med. J.*, 1974, *2*, 347.

A 95% cure-rate was obtained in giardiasis after treatment with mepacrine hydrochloride 100 mg three times daily for 7 days.— M. S. Wolfe, *J. Am. med. Ass.*, 1975, *233*, 1362.

Mepacrine hydrochloride was considered to be the drug of choice for the treatment of giardiasis in the *USA*.— *Med. Lett.*, 1988, *30*, 15.

For discussions of the treatment of giardiasis and leishmaniasis including mention of mepacrine, see p.659.

MALIGNANT EFFUSIONS. A discussion of the treatment of malignant pleural effusions. Talc should be considered as a first-line treatment in patients with symptomatic effusions. Instillation of agents such as mepacrine was considered to be less effective than talc but may be of value in those patients unsuitable for talc pleurodesis.— I. S. Fentiman, *Br. J. Hosp. Med.*, 1987, *38*, 423.

Further references to mepacrine in malignant effusions: M. R. Dollinger *et al.*, *Ann. intern. Med.*, 1967, *66*, 249; E. R. Borja and R. P. Pugh, *Cancer*, 1973, *31*, 899; J. Mejer *et al.*, *Scand. J. resp. Dis.*, 1977, *58*, 319; D. P. Dhillon and S. G. Spiro, *Br. J. Hosp. Med.*, 1983, *29*, 506.

PNEUMOTHORAX. A patient with cystic fibrosis was treated for pneumothorax on the left side by the instillation of mepacrine hydrochloride 100 mg in 15 mL saline into the intrapleural space on 4 consecutive days. This procedure was repeated 12 months later for pneumothorax on the right. There was no recurrence of pneumothorax on either side before the patient died 11 months after the second treatment after several relapses of chronic pulmonary disease.— J. Kattwinkel *et al.*, *J. Am. med. Ass.*, 1973, *226*, 557. See also R. E. Jones and S. T. Giammona, *Am. J. Dis. Child.*, 1976, *130*, 777.

TAPEWORM INFECTIONS. Mepacrine may produce severe nausea and was considered less satisfactory for treating tapeworm than niclosamide.— F. Richards and P. M. Schantz, *Lancet*, 1985, *1*, 1264. Mepacrine is preferred by some clinicians for the treatment of *Taenia solium* infection because, unlike niclosamide, it expels the worm intact thus reducing the theoretical risk of cysticercosis.— *Med. Lett.*, 1988, *30*, 15.

Preparations

Quinacrine Hydrochloride Tablets *(U.S.P.)*. Tablets containing mepacrine hydrochloride.

Proprietary Names and Manufacturers

Atabrine *(Winthrop, Canad.; Winthrop-Breon, USA)*.

1384-p

Pamaquine Embonate

Gametocidum; Pamachin; Pamaquin; Pamaquine *(rINN)*; Pamaquine Naphthoate; Plasmoquinum; SN-971. 8-(4-Diethylamino-1-methylbutylamino)-6-methoxyquinoline 4,4′-methylenebis(3-hydroxy-2-naphthoate).

$C_{19}H_{29}N_3O,C_{23}H_{16}O_6=703.8$.

CAS — 491-92-9 (pamaquine); 635-05-2 (embonate).

Pamaquine embonate was formerly used in the treatment of malaria but has been superseded by primaquine phosphate.

1385-s

Pentaquine Phosphate *(BANM, rINNM)*.

Pentachini Phosphas. 8-(5-Isopropylaminopentylamino)-6-methoxyquinoline phosphate.

$C_{18}H_{27}N_3O,H_3PO_4=399.4$.

CAS — 86-78-2 (pentaquine); 5428-64-8 (phosphate).

Pharmacopoeias. In *Arg.* and *Mex.*

Pentaquine phosphate is an antimalarial with actions and uses similar to those of primaquine phosphate below.

1386-w

Plasmocid

Fourneau-710; Rhodoquine; SN-3115. 8-(3-Diethylaminopropylamino)-6-methoxyquinoline.

$C_{17}H_{25}N_3O=287.4$.

CAS — 551-01-9.

Pharmacopoeias. In *Rus.*

Plasmocid is an antimalarial drug with actions and uses similar to those of primaquine, below. It has been reported to be very toxic to the central nervous system.

1387-e

Primaquine Phosphate *(BANM, USAN, rINNM)*.

Primachin Phosphate; Primaquini Diphosphas; Primaquinium Phosphate; SN-13,272. 8-(4-Amino-1-methylbutylamino)-6-methoxyquinoline diphosphate.

$C_{15}H_{21}N_3O,2H_3PO_4=455.3$.

CAS — 90-34-6 (primaquine); 63-45-6 (phosphate).

Pharmacopoeias. In *Arg.*, *Br.*, *Braz.*, *Chin.*, *Egypt.*, *Fr.*, *Ind.*, *Int.*, *It.*, *Jug.*, *Nord.*, *Turk.*, and *U.S.*

An orange-red, odourless or almost odourless, crystalline powder. Primaquine base 7.5 mg is approximately equivalent to 13.2 mg of primaquine phosphate. **Soluble** 1 in about 16 of water; practically insoluble in chloroform, and ether. A 1% solution in water has a pH of 2.5 to 3.5. **Protect** from light.

STABILITY. Primaquine was rapidly destroyed in the course of the ordinary preparation of cooked food.— Chemotherapy of Malaria, *Tech. Rep. Ser. Wld Hlth Org. No. 266*, 1961, p. 56.

Adverse Effects

Primaquine is generally well tolerated at normal therapeutic doses. Adverse effects include abdominal cramps, gastric distress, nausea and vomiting, headache, visual disturbances, and pruritus. Methaemoglobinaemia, mild anaemia, and leucocytosis may occasionally occur. Primaquine may rarely produce leucopenia or agranulocytosis, usually following overdosage. Hypertension and cardiac arrhythmias have been reported. Acute, dose-dependent haemolytic anaemia may occur in persons with a deficiency of glucose-6-phosphate dehydrogenase (G6PD), particularly those of Mediterranean origin.

A discussion of the clinical problems associated with the use of primaquine. A wide range of side-effects has been reported following the ingestion of primaquine. Some effects, including pruritus and disturbances of visual accomodation, are inadequately documented or are doubtfully attributed to the drug, since other drugs or precipitating factors, including malaria itself, may have contributed to the symptoms. Abdominal pain or cramps commonly occur when primaquine is given on an empty stomach, and it is preferably taken after meals. Higher doses may induce anorexia, nausea, and vomiting. Primaquine, like other oxidant drugs, is able to convert haemoglobin to methaemoglobin, producing cyanosis when the methaemoglobin concentration exceeds around 10% of the normal level of haemoglobin. In severe cases, cyanosis can be treated with methylene blue or withdrawal of primaquine.
Acute intravascular haemolysis is the most serious toxic hazard of primaquine, especially in people with G6PD deficiency, other defects of the erythrocytic pentose phosphate pathway of glucose metabolism, or some types of haemoglobinopathy. In individuals with G6PD deficiency the severity of haemolysis is directly related to the degree of deficiency and to the quantity of primaquine administered. In patients with the African variant the standard course of primaquine generally produces a moderate and self-limiting anaemia, while in those with the Mediterranean and related Asian variants, haemolysis can result in progressive haemoglobinaemia and haemoglobinuria which can be fatal.
If possible, primaquine should not be given during the acute stage of malaria since it may induce haemolysis, and additive gastro-intestinal intolerance may result in vomiting of both primaquine and the blood schizontocide. Also it may have an immunosuppressive effect. Whenever possible the acute manifestations of the disease should be brought under control with a blood schizontocide before primaquine treatment is initiated.— D. F. Clyde, *Bull. Wld Hlth Org.*, 1981, *59*, 391.

Depression and confusion in a patient taking primaquine.— D. Schlossberg (letter), *Ann. intern. Med.*, 1980, *92*, 435.

Precautions

Primaquine should be administered cautiously to acutely ill patients with any serious systemic disease characterised by a tendency to granulocytopenia. In addition to producing haemolytic anaemia in patients with glucose-6-phosphate dehydrogenase deficiency (see above), primaquine can produce blood dyscrasias in patients with other erythrocyte enzyme defects such as methaemoglobinaemia in NADH methaemoglobin reductase deficiency. Primaquine should be withdrawn if signs of haemolysis occur and the blood count should be monitored periodically. The administration of other bone-marrow depressants or haemolytic agents should be avoided.

The metabolism of primaquine is diminished by mepacrine and its toxicity enhanced.

Absorption and Fate

Primaquine is readily absorbed from the gastro-intestinal tract. Peak plasma concentrations occur about 1 to 3 hours after a dose is taken and then rapidly diminish with a reported elimination half-life of 3 to 6 hours. It is rapidly metabolised; little unchanged drug is excreted. The principal metabolite is carboxyprimaquine.

References to the pharmacokinetics of primaquine: J. Greaves *et al*., *Trans. R. Soc. trop. Med. Hyg.*, 1979, *73*, 328; K. A. Fletcher *et al., Bull. Wld Hlth Org.*, 1981, *59*, 407; G. W. Mihaly *et al., Br. J. clin. Pharmac.*, 1985, *19*, 745; S. A. Ward *et al., ibid.*, 751; S. C. Bhatia *et al., Eur. J. clin. Pharmac.*, 1986, *31*, 205.

Uses and Administration

Primaquine is a tissue schizontocide effective against exoerythrocytic forms of the plasmodia parasite, and is a gametocyticide. It also has some activity against pre-erythrocytic forms, oocysts, and blood schizonts, although this latter activity is too slow to be of clinical use. It is used to produce radical cure and to prevent relapse of vivax and ovale malarias, and will also destroy gametocytes in falciparum malaria. A course of treatment with a schizontocide such as chloroquine is usually given to kill any erythrocytic parasites and this is given with or followed by a course of 14 daily doses of primaquine phosphate, each equivalent to 15 mg of the base, to kill the tissue forms. A suggested dose for children is 250 to 300 µg per kg body-weight daily for 14 days. Some *P. vivax* infections acquired in the south-west Pacific (the Chesson strain) may have some resistance to primaquine, and courses of treatment for up to 21 days have been recommended. Alternative regimens of 45 mg once every 7 days for 8 weeks or 30 mg once every 7 days for 15 weeks have been suggested to minimise haemolysis in patients with glucose 6-phosphate dehydrogenase deficiency (but see under Adverse Effects and Precautions, above).

A course of primaquine has also been given after prolonged exposure to *P. vivax* or *P. ovale* infection to prevent a delayed primary attack in travellers returning from a highly endemic area.

Primaquine has also been used to control parasitaemia in South American trypanosomiasis (Chagas disease), but is ineffective against intracellular parasites.

Review of the pharmacology of 8-aminoquinolines.— R. S. Grewal, *Bull. Wld Hlth Org.*, 1981, *59*, 397.

Studies of the use of liposomes as drug carriers to reduce the adverse effects of primaquine: A. Trouet *et al., Bull. Wld Hlth Org.*, 1981, *59*, 449; G. Lopez-Berestein, *Antimicrob. Ag. Chemother.*, 1987, *31*, 675.

MALARIA. Some 25% of patients with uncomplicated falciparum malaria given an antimalarial regimen incorporating primaquine 15 mg daily for 5 days (a regimen widely used in South-east Asia) remained potential gametocyte carriers for up to 21 days.— D. Bunnag *et al., Lancet*, 1980, *2*, 91.

Primaquine 45 mg weekly with chloroquine was used to treat a relapse of vivax malaria in a patient who had initially been treated with primaquine 15 mg daily for 14 days.— L. Savioli *et al., Br. med. J.*, 1985, *291*, 23.

For comments on the use of primaquine during pregnancy, see Chloroquine, p.511.

For discussions of the prophylaxis and treatment of malaria, see p.505.

Preparations

Primaquine Phosphate Tablets *(U.S.P.)*

Primaquine Tablets *(B.P.).* Tablets containing primaquine phosphate. Potency is expressed in terms of the equivalent amount of primaquine.

Proprietary Preparations

Primaquine Phosphate *(ICI Pharmaceuticals, UK). Tablets*, primaquine 7.5 mg (as phosphate).

Proprietary Names and Manufacturers

ICI Pharmaceuticals, UK; Winthrop, Canad.

The following names have been used for multi-ingredient preparations containing primaquine phosphate— Aralen with Primaquine *(Winthrop-Breon, USA).*

1388-l

Proguanil Hydrochloride *(BANM, rINNM).*

Bigumalum; Chloriguane Hydrochloride; Chloroguanide Hydrochloride; Proguanide Hydrochloride; Proguanili Hydrochloridum; RP-3359; SN-12,837. 1-(4-Chlorophenyl)-5-isopropylbiguanide hydrochloride.

$C_{11}H_{16}ClN_5,HCl = 290.2$.

CAS — 500-92-5 (proguanil); 637-32-1 (hydrochloride).

Pharmacopoeias. In *Arg., Br., Ind., Int., It., Rus.*, and *Turk.*

A white odourless or almost odourless crystalline powder. Slightly **soluble** in water, more soluble in hot water; soluble 1 in 40 of alcohol; practically insoluble in chloroform and ether. **Protect** from light.

Adverse Effects

Proguanil hydrochloride is well tolerated after usual doses; after large doses vomiting, epigastric discomfort, haematuria, and renal irritation may occur. Blood dyscrasias have been reported in patients with renal failure given proguanil.

Severe oral ulceration occurred in 7 of 150 people which appeared to be related to proguanil. In 2 cases withdrawal and re-introduction of proguanil on several occasions resulted in recurrence of mouth ulceration within 2 weeks of re-introduction.— A. M. Daniels (letter), *Lancet*, 1986, *1*, 269.

Report of a further case of mouth ulceration associated with proguanil.— N. McD. Davidson (letter), *ibid.*, 384.

Precautions

Proguanil should be used with caution in patients with severe renal impairment.

Absorption and Fate

Proguanil is well absorbed from the gastro-intestinal tract and peak concentrations in the circulation are attained about 3 hours after the dose is taken; about 75% in the plasma is bound to proteins and high concentrations occur in erythrocytes. About 50% of the administered dose is excreted in the urine, 60% as unchanged drug and 30% as the active metabolite cycloguanil.

References to the pharmacokinetics of proguanil: J. A. Kelly *et al., Trans. R. Soc. trop. Med. Hyg.*, 1986, *80*, 338; W. M. Watkins *et al., J. Pharm. Pharmac.*, 1987, *39*, 261.

Uses and Administration

Proguanil is metabolised in the body to the antimalarial drug cycloguanil which inhibits plasmodial dihydrofolate reductase thus indirectly inhibiting synthesis of nucleic acids in the parasite. Proguanil, like pyrimethamine, is active against pre-erythrocytic forms and is a slow blood schizontocide. It also has some sporonticidal activity, rendering the gametocytes non-infective to the mosquito vector.

It is used for causal prophylaxis of falciparum malaria, to suppress other forms of malaria, and to reduce transmission of infection. The schizontocidal activity of proguanil on erythrocytic forms is too slow for the treatment of acute malaria, and rapid blood schizontocides like chloroquine should be used. Proguanil can produce a clinical cure of relapsing malarias, but exoerythrocytic forms are not affected and further relapses may occur.

The usefulness of proguanil is limited by the rapid development of drug resistance.

For the causal prophylaxis and suppression of symptoms of acute malaria, doses of 100 to 200 mg are usually given daily and continued for 4 weeks after leaving the area of infection. A suggested dose for children is: up to 1 year 25 to 50 mg daily, 1 to 5 years 50 to 100 mg daily, 6 to 12 years 100 to 150 mg daily.

MALARIA. Dapsone 25 mg daily with proguanil 200 mg was more effective in the prophylaxis of chloroquine-resistant falciparum malaria in soldiers in Vietnam than proguanil alone. No cases of agranulocytosis were reported when dapsone was taken only during the months when *P. falciparum* was epidemic, although several cases were reported when it was taken throughout the year.— R. H. Black, *Med. J. Aust.*, 1973, *1*, 1265.

Proguanil was proposed for malaria prophylaxis in regions of multidrug resistance as an alternative to chloroquine.— V. V. Olsen (letter), *Lancet*, 1983, *1*, 649; L. Rombo *et al.* (letter), *ibid.*, 997; M. J. Colbourne and C. C. Draper (letter), *ibid.*, 1228.

Proguanil 200 mg daily with strict personal antimosquito measures produced safe and effective prophylaxis in 408 non-immune soldiers in Malaysia. Only a single case of vivax malaria occurred.— A. Henderson and J. A. Rixom, *Trans. R. Soc. trop. Med. Hyg.*, 1986, *81*, 981.

For discussions of drug-resistant malaria and the prevention and treatment of malaria, see p.505.

For reference to the use of proguanil during pregnancy see Chloroquine p.511.

TROPICAL SPLENOMEGALY SYNDROME. Proguanil 100 mg daily for 14 months or more, led to a marked improvement in 25 patients with the idiopathic tropical splenomegaly syndrome. Improvement in splenomegaly, hepatomegaly, and a rise in haemoglobin concentrations were first apparent after 3 months, but maximum effect took up to 42 months. A gain in weight was recorded in 16 of 18 patients. Relapse usually followed discontinuance of proguanil, but responded to retreatment.— E. J. Watson-Williams and N. C. Allan, *Br. med. J.*, 1968, *4*, 793.

Proguanil, 100 mg daily for at least 6 months, was given to 43 patients with an initial diagnosis of tropical splenomegaly syndrome. After 6 months' therapy, 32 patients showed a reduction in spleen size while in 11 patients no reduction or an increase in spleen size was noted. In those responding to treatment, serum IgM values were always very high before treatment, falling with the decrease in spleen size due to therapy. Of the other patients, those adequately followed developed identifiable diseases, usually malignant lymphoma or chronic lymphatic leukaemia.— A. -S. Sagoe, *Br. med. J.*, 1970, *3*, 378.

Four patients in whom the symptoms of tropical splenomegaly syndrome were controlled by proguanil relapsed when they defaulted in treatment; symptoms were again controlled when treatment recommenced.— A. S. David-West, *Br. med. J.*, 1974, *3*, 499.

Preparations

Proguanil Tablets *(B.P.).* Tablets containing proguanil hydrochloride.

Proprietary Preparations

Paludrine *(ICI Pharmaceuticals, UK). Tablets*, scored, proguanil hydrochloride 100 mg.

Proprietary Names and Manufacturers

Paludrine *(ICI, Austral.; Ayerst, Canad.; Neth.; Switz.; ICI Pharmaceuticals, UK)*; Paludrinol.

1389-y

Pyrimethamine *(BAN, USAN, rINN).*

BW-50-63; Pirimetamina; Pyrimethaminum; RP-4753. 5-(4-Chlorophenyl)-6-ethylpyrimidine-2,4-diamine.

$C_{12}H_{13}ClN_4 = 248.7$.

CAS — 58-14-0.

Pharmacopoeias. In *Br., Braz., Chin., Egypt., Eur., Fr., Ind., Int., It., Jug., Neth., Nord., Swiss.*, and *U.S.* Also in *B.P. Vet.*

A white or almost white, odourless, crystalline powder or colourless crystals. Practically **insoluble** in water; soluble 1 in 200 of alcohol and 1 in 125 of chloroform; slightly soluble in acetone; very slightly soluble in ether. **Store** in airtight containers. Protect from light.

Adverse Effects

Within the usual dose range side-effects are unlikely, but pyrimethamine given daily over a prolonged period may cause depression of haemopoiesis due to the interference of the drug in the metabolism of folic acid. Skin rashes may also occur.

With larger doses, megaloblastic anaemia, leucopenia, thrombocytopenia, agranulocytosis, pancytopenia, gastritis, and atrophic glossitis are more likely. Very large doses cause vomiting, convulsions, ataxia, tremor, and respiratory failure.

In a study of 8 children with CNS disease in acute leukaemia given pyrimethamine 75 mg per m^2 body-surface daily (maximum 100 mg) for 14 days, 2 withdrew because of convulsions or nausea and vomiting. Two of the remaining patients responded but the incidence of side-effects, which included exfoliative dermatitis, dizziness, nausea and vomiting, diarrhoea, and leucopenia, was considered intolerable.— A. H. Ragab (letter), *Lancet*, 1973, *1*, 1061.

Photosensitivity in a 9-year-old boy was attributed to pyrimethamine.— S. A. Craven (letter), *Br. med. J.*, 1974, *2*, 556.

Pyrimethamine had been reported to cause aplastic anaemia.— R. H. Girdwood, *Drugs*, 1976, *11*, 394.

OVERDOSAGE. A 14-month-old child who had ingested 450 mg of pyrimethamine developed vomiting, cyanosis, respiratory distress, unconsciousness, convulsions, tachycardia, and hyperpyrexia, together with blindness, deafness, and ataxia. Treatment included diazepam, oxygen, forced diuresis, and folic acid, and the child recovered. The blindness and deafness slowly regressed but there was residual mental retardation 2 years later. A 4-year-old child who had been given 50 mg of pyrimethamine weekly for 6 months developed severe folic acid-deficient megaloblastic anaemia which responded to blood transfusions and treatment (in the absence of folinic acid) with folic acid.— O. Akinyanju *et al.*, *Br. med. J.*, 1973, *4*, 147.

PREGNANCY AND THE NEONATE. Severe congenital defects in a stillborn male infant were attributed to pyrimethamine taken during early pregnancy with chloroquine and dapsone.— J. -P. Harpey *et al.* (letter), *Lancet*, 1983, *2*, 399. Comment on the non-specific nature of the abnormalities.— R. W. Smithells and S. Sheppard (letter), *ibid.*, 623.

For discussions of the use of pyrimethamine in pregnancy see under Uses, below.

PSEUDOLYMPHOMA. A report of fever and cervical, axillary, and inguinal lymphadenopathy in a 9-year-old boy after taking pyrimethamine and sulphadimidine; pyrimethamine was considered responsible. Histologically the neoplasm simulated malignant lymphoma.— J. M. Costello and D. M. O. Becroft, *N.Z. med. J.*, 1977, *86*, 430.

Adverse Effects of Drug Combinations containing Pyrimethamine

Pyrimethamine with sulfadoxine is generally well tolerated, but severe and sometimes fatal reactions have been reported. Severe cutaneous reactions include erythema multiforme, Stevens-Johnson syndrome, and toxic epidermal necrolysis. Blood dyscrasias have been reported rarely, and there have been isolated reports of hepatic toxicity.

Pyrimethamine with dapsone is also generally well tolerated at doses used for malaria prophylaxis, but agranulocytosis has occurred, particularly in patients who have received two doses weekly. Agranulocytosis has occasionally been fatal.

Further information on adverse effects due to the individual components can be found under pyrimethamine (above), dapsone (p.558) and sulphamethoxazole (p.306).

PYRIMETHAMINE WITH DAPSONE. A study of the haematological effects of long-term malaria prophylaxis with pyrimethamine-dapsone (Maloprim). No haematological abnormalities were found in 373 Papua New Guinean soldiers who had been taken Maloprim regularly for 5 years. Haematological abnormalities were seen in 9 of 159 white persons who had taken prophylactic Maloprim for more than 1 year. In addition, the total leucocyte count was lower in children taking Maloprim compared with children taking chloroquine, although counts remained within the normal range. These haematological changes were attributed to the difficulty in administering an accurate dose to children using an unscored tablet and the use of dosage based on age rather than on body-weight.— I. F. Cook and M. Y. Kish, *Med. J. Aust.*, 1985, *143*, 139.

Malaria prophylaxis with pyrimethamine-dapsone (Maloprim) was discontinued in 2 of 45 patients after 12 months because of unpleasant adverse effects. No serious adverse effects were seen in any patient in up to 7 years of treatment. No adverse effects were reported in patients who had taken Maloprim for more than 3 years.— K. O. Donovan (letter), *Med. J. Aust.*, 1985, *143*, 319.

A review of 21 cases of agranulocytosis associated with pyrimethamine-dapsone (Maloprim). Of the 18 individuals for whom dosage was certain, 12 were taking one tablet of Maloprim twice a week. The time of onset was 7 to 9 weeks after starting therapy in 16 of 19 cases where the duration of dosage was known. There were 9 deaths: 6 in patients taking one tablet twice weekly, 1 patient taking one tablet once weekly and 2 patients in whom the doses taken were uncertain. Agranulocytosis also occurs very rarely in patients taking pyrimethamine or dapsone alone. It was considered likely that dapsone, when given with other drugs, causes agranulocytosis in a very few individuals who may have a biochemical idiosyncrasy which renders them more susceptible to drug-induced destruction of the granulocyte series. In the case of Maloprim, the concomitant administration of pyrimethamine may exacerbate the situation, by inhibition of folate metabolism, thereby reducing recovery of granulopoiesis, or by displacing dapsone and its metabolites from plasma proteins.— D. B. A. Hutchinson *et al.*, *Hum. Toxicol.*, 1986, *5*, 221.

The risk of non-specific upper respiratory-tract infections was 64% higher in 8337 military recruits given antimalarial prophylaxis with pyrimethamine-dapsone than in 11 220 controls who received no prophylaxis. This result was considered to be a consequence of immunosuppression produced by pyrimethamine-dapsone, and suggested that travellers taking pyrimethamine-dapsone prophylaxis may be rendered more susceptible to common infections.— P. S. Lee and E. Y. L. Lau, *Br. med. J.*, 1988, *296*, 893.

PYRIMETHAMINE WITH SULFADOXINE. Report of severe adverse reactions in 3 patients taking pyrimethamine-sulfadoxine once weekly for malaria prophylaxis for 3 to 9 weeks. Reactions included drug fever and photodermatitis (1 patient), jaundice and toxic epidermal necrolysis (1 patient), and agranulocytosis (1 patient).— V. Vestergaard Olsen *et al.* (letter), *Lancet*, 1982, *2*, 994.

Fatal multisystem toxicity (including toxic epidermal necrolysis and hepatic and renal failure) in a 60-year-old woman following 3 weekly doses of pyrimethamine-sulfadoxine for malaria prophylaxis.— C. D. Selby *et al.*, *Br. med. J.*, 1985, *290*, 113.

Interim recommendations for malaria prophylaxis from the Centers for Disease Control in the *USA* in the light of the potential toxicity of pyrimethamine-sulfadoxine.— *J. Am. med. Ass.*, 1985, *253*, 483.

Effects on the liver. Granulomatous hepatitis in 2 patients was associated with malaria prophylaxis using pyrimethamine-sulfadoxine. The reaction was considered to be due to sulfadoxine.— H. P. Lazar *et al.* (letter), *Ann. intern. Med.*, 1985, *102*, 722.

Hepatitis was reported in 7 patients who had been taking pyrimethamine-sulfadoxine prophylaxis against malaria. Unintentional re-exposure to pyrimethamine-sulfadoxine in 1 patient 3 years after initial exposure produced recurrence of acute hepatitis.— R. Wejstal *et al.* (letter), *Lancet*, 1986, *1*, 854.

Fatal hepatic necrosis in a 15-year-old girl was associated with 4 weekly prophylactic doses of pyrimethamine-sulfadoxine and chloroquine. She also had extensive exfoliative dermatitis, diffuse lymphadenopathy, and evidence of hepatic encephalopathy with kernicterus.— B. J. Zitelli *et al.*, *Ann. intern. Med.*, 1987, *106*, 393.

Effects on the lungs. A report of pulmonary reactions (extensive, subpleural, localised, confluent alveolar infiltrates in the periphery of the lungs) associated with the use for about 6 weeks of Fansidar for malaria prophylaxis; another similar case had been reported to the manufacturers.— M. Svanbom *et al.*, *Br. med. J.*, 1984, *288*, 1876.

Effects on the skin. A review of the use of long-acting sulphonamides in antimalarial preparations. Initially there had been no reason to believe that the incidence of severe cutaneous adverse reactions with pyrimethamine-sulfadoxine (Fansidar) exceeded that ascribed to co-trimoxazole which was estimated to be about 1:100 000, of which 16 to 20% were fatal. By 1982 the manufacturer of Fansidar had received a total of only 10 notifications of serious suspected reactions by which time an estimated 1.5 million people had used the product for malaria prophylaxis. However, in late 1984 the Centers for Disease Control in the *USA* conducted a survey which indicated that severe reactions occurred in 1:5000 to 1:8000 users and that the risk of death was 1:11 000 to 1:25 000. All but one of these cases had also received chloroquine and it was suggested that this could have contributed to the adverse effect, but worldwide only 28 of 81 cases of severe cutaneous reactions had also received chloroquine, suggesting that apparent association with chloroquine was due to prescribing practices in the *USA* at the time. Evidence from other parts of the world has not supported the high incidence of adverse effects found in the *USA*: a report from Sweden reported the incidence of severe adverse reactions at less than 1:60 000 and a retrospective survey in Switzerland provided an estimated incidence of severe reactions of only 1:150 000 between 1974 and 1985 with no fatalities. In the light of the available findings the WHO has recommended that travellers to areas where chloroquine-resistant *Plasmodium falciparum* is prevalent should use mefloquine or pyrimethamine-sulfadoxine only if they develop a febrile reaction and if prompt medical attention is not available.— *WHO Drug Inf.*, 1987, *1*, 2. See also R. D. Pearson and E. L. Hewlett, *Ann. intern. Med.*, 1987, *106*, 714.

Comments on the incidence of severe toxic cutaneous reactions to pyrimethamine-sulfadoxine: R. Steffen and B. Somaini (letter), *Lancet*, 1986, *1*, 610 (in Switzerland); P. C. W. Lyn and E. Fernandez (letter), *Med. J. Aust.*, 1987, *146*, 335 (in Malaysia); U. Hellgren *et al.*, *Br. med. J.*, 1987, *295*, 365 (in Sweden).

Reports of Stevens-Johnson syndrome associated with pyrimethamine-sulfadoxine administration: D. Whitfield (letter), *Lancet*, 1982, *2*, 1272; O. P. Hornstein and K. W. Ruprecht (letter), *New Engl. J. Med.*, 1982, *307*, 1529; T. R. Navin *et al.* (letter), *Lancet*, 1985, *1*, 1332; S. J. Adams *et al.*, *Postgrad. med. J.*, 1985, *61*, 263; R. F. Jeffrey, *Postgrad. med. J.*, 1986, *62*, 893; M. G. Bamber *et al.*, *J. Infect.*, 1986, *13*, 31.

Erythroderma resembling Sézary syndrome in a patient after treatment with pyrimethamine-sulfadoxine and chloroquine.— J. A. A. Langtry *et al.*, *Br. med. J.*, 1986, *292*, 1107.

Treatment of Adverse Effects

The stomach should be emptied by aspiration and lavage. Convulsions should be cautiously controlled by the injection of diazepam 5 to 10 mg, and injections of calcium folinate should be given to counter folate deficiency. Respiration may require assistance.

Precautions

When doses high enough to interfere with folic acid metabolism are given as in the treatment of toxoplasmosis, white-cell and platelet counts should be made twice weekly. Subclinical folic acid deficiency may be aggravated by pyrimethamine and it should not be given to patients with megaloblastic anaemia associated with folate deficiency. The administration of folinic acid or folic acid has been recommended in order to prevent haematological toxicity due to pyrimethamine.

Pyrimethamine has caused foetal abnormalities in *animals*, and the use of folinic acid supplements, at least during the first trimester of pregnancy, have been recommended. High doses should be avoided during pregnancy unless folinic acid supplements are given. These do not interfere with the antimalarial action.

Administration of pyrimethamine with sulphonamides should be discontinued immediately if a rash occurs.

Pyrimethamine should be given with caution to patients with seriously impaired renal or hepatic function. Bone marrow depression may be enhanced if pyrimethamine is given concurrently with other folate antagonists such as co-trimoxazole or methotrexate.

Bone-marrow aplasia in a heterozygous beta-thalassaemic youth was attributed to pyrimethamine.— P. Malacarne *et al.* (letter), *Lancet*, 1974, *2*, 904.

GLUCOSE-6-PHOSPHATE DEHYDROGENASE DEFICIENCY. Pyrimethamine was not considered to cause clinically significant haemolytic anaemia in individuals with glucose-6-phosphate dehydrogenase deficiency under normal circumstances (e.g. in the absence of infection).— E. Beutler, *Pharmac. Rev.*, 1969, *21*, 73. Pyrimethamine did not cause haemolysis in Chinese patients with glucose-6-phosphate dehydrogenase deficiency.— T. K. Chan *et al.*, *Br. med. J.*, 1976, *2*, 1227. See also *Ann. intern. Med.*, 1985, *103*, 245.

INTERACTIONS. Mild liver toxicity occurred in several patients taking pyrimethamine and lorazepam concomitantly and was confirmed in 2 of 5 women who tolerated each drug without adverse effect when given separately.— M. Briggs and M. Briggs (letter), *Br. med. J.*, 1974, *1*, 40.

PORPHYRIA. Clinical experience has suggested that pyrimethamine could be used for malaria prophylaxis in patients with porphyria, although there is a report suggesting that problems could arise.— M. R. Moore and P. B. Disler, *Adverse Drug React. Ac. Pois. Rev.*, 1983, *2*, 149.

Absorption and Fate

Pyrimethamine is well absorbed from the gastro-intestinal tract and peak concentrations in the circulation are stated to occur about 2 hours after a dose is taken. It is mainly concentrated in the kidneys, lungs, liver, and spleen and is about 80% bound to plasma proteins. It is only slowly excreted, the average half-life in plasma being about 4 days; several metabolites appear in the urine. Pyrimethamine is present in the milk of nursing mothers being treated with the drug.

A review of the clinical pharmacokinetics of antimalarial drugs including pyrimethamine.— N. J. White, *Clin. Pharmacokinet.*, 1985, *10*, 187.

The concentration of pyrimethamine in saliva appeared to reflect the concentration of the unbound fraction of the drug in plasma.— R. A. Ahmad and H. J. Rogers (letter), *Br. J. clin. Pharmac.*, 1981, *11*, 101.

Significantly lower serum concentrations of pyrimethamine were found in Papua New Guineans than in caucasians taking pyrimethamine with dapsone for malaria prophylaxis.— I. F. Cook *et al.*, *Trans. R. Soc. trop. Med. Hyg.*, 1986, *80*, 897.

Uses and Administration

Pyrimethamine is an antimalarial drug which inhibits plasmodial dihydrofolate reductase thus indirectly blocking the synthesis of nucleic acids in the parasite. Pyrimethamine is active against primary tissue forms and is also a slow blood schizontocide. It also has some sporonticidal activity: it does not prevent the formation of gametocytes but renders them non-infective to the mosquito vector. It is mainly effective against *Plasmodium falciparum* but also has some activity against *P. vivax*.

It has been used alone for the causal prophylaxis and suppression of falciparum and sometimes vivax malaria in doses of 25 mg every 7 days, treatment being continued for at least 4 weeks after exposure to risk. Resistance has developed in several parts of the world and pyrimethamine is now normally used only in combination with other antifolate drugs, particularly the long-acting sulphonamides such as sulfadoxine and the sulphone, dapsone. These combinations produce an enhanced antimalarial effect, but their usefulness is limited by the development of multidrug-resistant strains of *P. falciparum* and the serious adverse effects which occasionally occur.

Pyrimethamine in combination with sulfadoxine in a fixed dose ratio of 1 to 20 is used for the treatment of mild or uncomplicated falciparum malaria particularly that caused by chloroquine-resistant strains of the parasite. A single dose of pyrimethamine 50 to 75 mg with sulfadoxine 1.0 to 1.5 g is usually effective, and may be given with a rapidly acting blood schizontocide such as quinine in more serious infections. The dose should not be repeated for at least 7 days.

Pyrimethamine with sulfadoxine has also been used for causal prophylaxis and suppression of malaria, but most authorities now agree that its toxicity makes it unsuitable for this purpose (see p.505 for a discussion of malaria prophylaxis in chloroquine-resistant areas). The usual dose for causal prophylaxis or suppression is sulfadoxine 500 mg with pyrimethamine 25 mg given every 7 days. A suggested weekly dose for children is: up to 4 years, one-quarter; 5 to 8 years, one-half; and 9 to 12 years, three-quarters of the adult dose. A similar combined regimen of pyrimethamine and dapsone is used for causal prophylaxis or suppression of malaria, particularly where strains resistant to pyrimethamine or proguanil are present. The usual dose is pyrimethamine 12.5 mg and dapsone 100 mg as a single weekly dose, with half this dose for children aged 5 to 10 years.

Toxoplasmosis may be controlled by the concurrent administration of high doses of pyrimethamine and a sulphonamide such as sulphadiazine. For this purpose pyrimethamine is given in a dose of 25 mg daily together with sulphadiazine 2 to 4 g daily, reduced according to the patient's response, after 1 to 3 weeks to about half these doses and continued for a further 3 to 4 weeks. Treatment for 6 months or more may be required in immunocompromised patients.

Pyrimethamine with sulfadoxine has also been tried for prophylaxis of *Pneumocystis carinii* pneumonia in patients with acquired immune deficiency syndrome (AIDS).

ISOSPORIASIS. A brief discussion of the use of pyrimethamine and a sulphonamide in the treatment of isosporiasis.— R. Knight and S. G. Wright, *Gut*, 1978, *19*, 940. See also WHO Scientific Working Group, *Bull. Wld Hlth Org.*, 1980, *58*, 819.

LEUKAEMIA. Experience from treating 12 patients with CNS leukaemia with either pyrimethamine or methotrexate or both indicated that the duration of remission was longer after pyrimethamine and that its haematological side-effects were reversible.— A. C. Boadella and R. P. P. Illa (letter), *Lancet*, 1973, *2*, 1330.

In the treatment of meningeal leukaemia, pyrimethamine should not be used immediately after methotrexate and the dose should not exceed 2 to 3 mg per kg body-weight daily.— J. Armata (letter), *Br. med. J.*, 1973, *4*, 783.

Eight patients in remission from meningeal leukaemia were given pyrimethamine 150 mg daily for 4 days every 3 weeks for a year and 5 sustained a complete remission. Side-effects were common and apart from 1 patient who withdrew because of severe vomiting, usually transitory and tolerable.— J. Hamers *et al.* (letter), *Lancet*, 1974, *1*, 310.

Of 17 adults with previously untreated acute lymphocytic leukaemia 9 achieved complete remissions after induction courses of thioguanine, vincristine, dexamethasone, and pyrimethamine. Seven of the 9 received consolidation and maintenance treatment; 6 of the 17 developed meningeal leukaemia; pyrimethamine provided inadequate prophylaxis for meningeal leukaemia.— A. C. Smyth and P. H. Wiernik, *Clin. Pharmac. Ther.*, 1976, *19*, 240.

MALARIA. Pyrimethamine-sulfadoxine is a valuable alternative to chloroquine in uncomplicated malaria due to chloroquine-sensitive and chloroquine-resistant *Plasmodium falciparum*. In recent years its usefulness has been limited by the progressive development of resistance in parts of South America and Asia. Pyrimethamine-sulfadoxine has a relatively slow action in malaria, and appears to act later in the parasite's development cycle than the more rapidly acting drugs. Thus it is not the drug of choice for use alone in severe or complicated falciparum malaria. It can, however, be used with a short course of quinine.

Adverse effects, which are due largely to the sulphonamide component, are known to occur when pyrimethamine-sulfadoxine is used both for weekly chemoprophylaxis and for single-dose therapy. If pyrimethamine-sulfadoxine is given for any prolonged period to patients who might develop folate deficiency (for example in pregnancy) folic acid or preferably folinic acid supplements should be given. Although a parenteral preparation of pyrimethamine-sulfadoxine is commercially available there is no place for this in the emergency treatment of severe malaria.

Other combinations of long-acting sulphonamides and pyrimethamine are probably equivalent to the sulfadoxine combination but these have been investigated less.

Pyrimethamine-dapsone is used for malaria prophylaxis but not for treatment.— *Trans. R. Soc. trop. Med. Hyg.*, 1986, *80, Suppl.*

Prophylaxis. Pyrimethamine and dapsone administered weekly in the malaria transmission season had proved completely active under conditions in which there was partial resistance to pyrimethamine.— G. Charmot, Anglo-French Symposium on Control of Tropical Endemic Diseases, May 1969, London,, per *Br. med. J.*, 1969, *2*, 568.

It had been suggested that young children in areas where falciparum malaria was endemic should be given pyrimethamine 25 mg once a month so that morbidity and mortality might be reduced while not completely suppressing parasitaemia, thus allowing protective antibodies to develop. In 36 Ugandan children this regimen did not prevent all episodes of severe malaria and was associated with low titres of malaria antibodies. It was uncertain whether the predominant cause for these low titres was the pyrimethamine regimen or the frequent courses of chloroquine which were prescribed for all febrile illnesses.— P. S. E. G. Harland *et al.*, *Trans. R. Soc. trop. Med. Hyg.*, 1975, *69*, 261.

Of 12 patients presenting with malaria in Papua New Guinea despite regular prophylaxis with pyrimethamine and dapsone (as demonstrated by blood concentrations), 10 had infections with *P. vivax* and 2 with *P. falciparum*. The 2 patients with *P. falciparum* infection had evidence of reduced drug concentrations due to poor bioavailability and rapid clearance. The failure of pyrimethamine-dapsone to suppress parasitaemia due to *P. vivax* was considered to be due to resistance of *P. vivax* to pyrimethamine.— I. F. Cook, *Med. J. Aust.*, 1985, *142*, 340.

Treatment. Recrudescences occurred in 17 of 21 patients with falciparum malaria treated with pyrimethamine 25 mg and dapsone 200 mg compared with 1 of 17 patients treated with sulfadoxine 1 g and pyrimethamine 50 mg. Two other patients in the latter group remained parasitaemic after treatment.— H. E. Segal *et al.*, *Trans. R. Soc. trop. Med. Hyg.*, 1975, *69*, 139.

For references to the use of pyrimethamine and sulfadoxine in combination with mefloquine, see under Mefloquine p.513.

For discussions of the prophylaxis and treatment of malaria, see p.505.

MYCETOMA. Pyrimethamine with sulfadoxine and streptomycin could provide a useful second-line therapy for actinomycetoma.— E. S. Mahgoub, *Bull. Wld Hlth Org.*, 1976, *54*, 303.

PNEUMOCYSTIS PNEUMONIA. Pyrimethamine with sulfadoxine has been reported to have some efficacy for pneumocystis pneumonia unrelated to AIDS. Preliminary results of a study into the prophylactic use against *Pneumocystis carinii* in AIDS patients suggest that pyrimethamine-sulfadoxine in a weekly dose is well tolerated and effective.— V. T. DeVita *et al.*, *Ann. intern. Med.*, 1987, *106*, 568.

Further references mentioning the use of pyrimethamine-sulfadoxine for pneumocystis pneumonia prophylaxis: A. Millar, *Br. med. J.*, 1987, *294*, 1334; I. V. D. Weller, *ibid.*, *295*, 200.

Reports of the use of pyrimethamine with a sulphonamide in pneumocystis pneumonia: H. B. Kirby *et al.*, *Ann. intern. Med.*, 1971, *75*, 505 (treatment with pyrimethamine and sulphadiazine); M. S. Gottlieb *et al.*, *Lancet*, 1984, *2*, 398 (prophylaxis with pyrimethamine-sulfadoxine); M. A. Fischl and G. M. Dickinson, *Ann. intern. Med.*, 1986, *105*, 629 (prophylaxis with pyrimethamine-sulfadoxine).

PREGNANCY AND THE NEONATE. Despite fears concerning the safety of pyrimethamine combinations during pregnancy, they have generally been found to be relatively safe. The administration of a folinic acid supplement to women taking antifolate malarials, at least during the first trimester of pregnancy, would seem a sensible precaution. However, several authorities recommend that pyrimethamine-sulfadoxine should be avoided during pregnancy.— *Lancet*, 1983, *2*, 1005 and 1378.

For a discussion of the use of antimalarial drugs during pregnancy, see p.505.

TOXOPLASMOSIS. The treatment of choice for toxoplasmosis in infants was pyrimethamine, 2 mg per kg body-weight daily for 3 days and then 1 mg per kg daily, with sulphadiazine 100 mg per kg daily together with calcium folinate 1 mg daily and fresh yeast 100 mg daily to overcome folate antagonism. For adults and children, 50 or 25 mg respectively of pyrimethamine was given daily for 3 days together with conventional doses of sulphadiazine and followed by one-half the dose of pyrimethamine daily thereafter, together with calcium folinate 5 to 15 mg and yeast. Treatment should be maintained for 1 month, provided that improvement occurred within the first 2 weeks. Counts of blood platelets and leucocytes should be performed at least twice weekly to detect early signs of folate antagonism.— H. A. Feldman, *New Engl. J. Med.*, 1968, *279*, 1431.

Comparison of treatment with corticosteroids alone or in conjunction with pyrimethamine and spiramycin in 69 patients with active toxoplasmic retinochoroiditis showed that, while pyrimethamine was the most effective drug, severe side-effects indicated that it should only be used when the lesions might cause permanent damage to the sight. Less severe cases might be treated with spiramycin.— J. Nolan and E. S. Rosen, *Br. J. Ophthal.*, 1968, *52*, 396.

Pyrimethamine with sulphonamides were generally considered to be too dangerous for the treatment of toxoplasmosis in pregnant women.— H. Williams, *Postgrad. med. J.*, 1977, *53*, 614.

Treatment with pyrimethamine 1 mg per kg body-weight daily with sulphadiazine 100 mg per kg daily for 30 days, given with a folinic acid supplement may be tried in toxoplasmosis during the second and third trimesters of pregnancy, although congenital infection may not always be prevented.— D. G. Fleck, *Archs Dis. Childh.*, 1981, *56*, 494.

Cardiac or cardiopulmonary transplant patients who developed infections with *Toxoplasma gondii* during immunosuppressive therapy were treated with pyrimethamine, spiramycin, and sulphonamides. In patients identified as being at increased risk, *T. gondii* infection did not occur in any of 7 patients given pyrimethamine for prophylaxis, but did occur in 4 of 7 patients who did not receive pyrimethamine.— M. Hakim *et al.*, *Br. med. J.*, 1986, *292*, 1108.

Pyrimethamine 25 mg daily plus trisulphapyrimidines 2 to 6 g daily for 3 to 4 weeks was considered the treatment of choice for toxoplasmosis in the *USA*.— *Med. Lett.*, 1988, *30*, 15.

Pyrimethamine with sulphadiazine was considered to be the treatment of choice for cerebral toxoplasmosis in patients with AIDS. Side-effects may necessitate stopping the sulphadiazine, but clindamycin had been used successfully as a substitute in uncontrolled studies. Relapse is common after treatment is stopped, and treatment should continue indefinitely.— I. V. D. Weller, *Br. med. J.*, 1987, *295*, 200.

Although some authorities mention doses of pyrimethamine as high as 75 mg per day for toxoplasmosis in AIDS patients, a common starting dose is 25 to 50 mg, followed by maintenance treatment with pyrimethamine 25 mg daily plus sulphadiazine 4 to 6 g. Alternative regimens of considerable promise include the combination of pyrimethamine with high-dose clindamycin, 900 to 1200 mg intravenously every 6 hours.— L. S. Young, *Lancet*, 1987, *2*, 1503. See also V. T. DeVita *et al.*, *Ann. intern. Med.*, 1987, *106*, 568.

Preparations

Pyrimethamine Tablets *(B.P.)*

Pyrimethamine Tablets *(U.S.P.)*

Sulfadoxine and Pyrimethamine Tablets *(U.S.P.)*

Proprietary Preparations

Daraprim *(Wellcome, UK). Tablets*, scored, pyrimethamine 25 mg.

Fansidar *(Roche, UK). Tablets*, scored, pyrimethamine 25 mg and sulfadoxine 500 mg.

Maloprim *(Wellcome, UK). Tablets*, scored, pyrimethamine 12.5 mg and dapsone 100 mg.

Proprietary Names and Manufacturers

Daraprim *(Arg.; Wellcome, Austral.; Belg.; Wellcome, Canad.; Denm.; Wellcome, Ger.; Neth.; Wellcome, S.Afr.; Gayoso Wellcome, Spain; Wellcome, Swed.; Switz.; Wellcome, UK; Wellcome, USA)*; Erbaprelina *(Ital.)*; Pirimecidan *(Cidan, Spain)*; Tindurin *(Hung.)*.

The following names have been used for multi-ingredient preparations containing pyrimethamine— Fansidar *(Roche, Austral.; Roche, Fr.; Roche, UK; Roche, USA)*; Fansimef *(Roche, Switz.)*; Maloprim *(Wellcome, Austral.; Wellcome, UK)*.

1398-j

Quinine *(BAN)*.

Chininum; Quinina. (8*S*,9*R*)-6′-Methoxycinchonan-9-ol; (α*R*)-α-(6-Methoxy-4-quinolyl)-α-[(2*S*,4*S*,5*R*)-(5-vinylquinuclidin-2-yl)]methanol.

$C_{20}H_{24}N_2O_2$=324.4.

CAS — 130-95-0 (anhydrous).

Pharmacopoeias. In *Fr. It.* and *Span.* have the trihydrate.

The chief alkaloid of various species of *Cinchona* (Rubiaceae). It is an optical isomer of quinidine. **Store** in airtight containers. Protect from light.

1391-q

Quinine Bisulphate *(BANM)*.

Chininum Bisulfuricum; Neutral Quinine Sulphate; Quinine Acid Sulphate.

$C_{20}H_{24}N_2O_2,H_2SO_4,7H_2O$=548.6.

CAS — 549-56-4 (anhydrous).

Pharmacopoeias. In *Aust., Br., Ind., Port.,* and *Span.*

Colourless, odourless or almost odourless crystals or white crystalline powder. It effloresces in dry air. Quinine bisulphate 169 mg is approximately equivalent to 100 mg of anhydrous quinine.

Soluble 1 in 8 of water, and 1 in 50 of alcohol. A 1% solution has a pH of 2.8 to 3.4 and has a blue fluorescence. **Store** in well-closed containers. Protect from light.

1393-s

Quinine Dihydrochloride *(BANM)*.

Chinini Bihydrochloridum; Neutral Quinine Hydrochloride; Quinine Acid Hydrochloride.

$C_{20}H_{24}N_2O_2,2HCl$=397.3.

CAS — 60-93-5.

Pharmacopoeias. In *Arg., Aust., Belg., Br., Braz., Chin., Ind., Mex., Port., Rus.,* and *Span.*

A white or almost white odourless or almost odourless powder. Quinine dihydrochloride 122 mg is approximately equivalent to 100 mg of anhydrous quinine.

Soluble 1 in 0.5 of water and 1 in 14 of alcohol. A 3% solution in water has a pH of 2.0 to 3.0. Solutions are **sterilised** by autoclaving. **Store** in well-closed containers. Protect from light.

1394-w

Quinine Ethyl Carbonate

Euquinina.

$C_{23}H_{28}N_2O_4$=396.5.

CAS — 83-75-0.

Pharmacopoeias. In *Arg., Fr., Jpn, Mex., Port.,* and *Span.*

Quinine ethyl carbonate 122 mg is approximately equivalent to 100 mg of anhydrous quinine.

1395-e

Quinine Hydrobromide

Basic Quinine Hydrobromide; Bromhydrate de Quinine; Chininum Hydrobromicum.

$C_{20}H_{24}N_2O_2,HBr,2H_2O$=441.4.

CAS — 549-49-5 (anhydrous).

Pharmacopoeias. In *Arg.* and *Belg.*, which specify $1H_2O$.

Quinine hydrobromide 136 mg is approximately equivalent to 100 mg of anhydrous quinine.

1396-l

Quinine Hydrochloride *(BANM)*.

Basic Quinine Hydrochloride; Chinini Hydrochloridum; Chininii Chloridum; Chininum Hydrochloricum; Quinini Hydrochloridum; Quininium Chloride.

$C_{20}H_{24}N_2O_2,HCl,2H_2O$=396.9.

CAS — 130-89-2 (anhydrous); 6119-47-7 (dihydrate).

Pharmacopoeias. In *Arg., Aust., Belg., Br., Braz., Cz., Eur., Fr., Ger., Hung., Int., It., Jpn, Jug., Mex., Neth., Nord., Pol., Port., Roum., Rus., Span., Swiss,* and *Turk.*

Colourless, fine, silky, acicular crystals. Quinine hydrochloride 122 mg is approximately equivalent to 100 mg of anhydrous quinine.

Soluble 1 in 23 of water; freely soluble in alcohol and in chloroform; very slightly soluble in ether. Solutions in chloroform may not be clear due to the formation of droplets of water. A 1% solution in water has a pH of 6.0 to 6.8. **Store** in well-closed containers. Protect from light.

MASKING THE TASTE. Doubling the usual concentration of flavouring agents and increasing the sugar content, adding salt to some flavoured syrups and an excess of citric acid to fruit flavours helped to disguise the taste of quinine hydrochloride. Increasing the viscosity of the solutions and diluting with skimmed or preferably homogenised milk instead of water helped to cover the taste. Cocoa syrup was the best agent for masking the bitter taste.— D. N. Entrekin and C. H. Becker, *J. Am. pharm. Ass., scient. Edn*, 1954, *43*, 693.

1390-g

Quinine Sulphate *(BANM)*.

Basic Quinine Sulphate; Chinini Sulfas; Chininum Sulfuricum; Quinine Sulfate *(USAN)*; Quinini Sulfas; Quininium Sulphate.

$(C_{20}H_{24}N_2O_2)_2,H_2SO_4,2H_2O$=782.9.

CAS — 804-63-7 (anhydrous); 6119-70-6 (dihydrate).

Pharmacopoeias. In *Arg., Aust., Belg., Br., Braz., Egypt., Eur., Fr., Ger., Hung., Ind., Int., It., Jpn, Mex., Neth., Pol., Port., Roum., Rus., Span., Swiss, Turk.,* and *U.S.*

Colourless or white, odourless, fine acicular crystals or a white or almost white crystalline powder, darkening on exposure to light. Quinine sulphate 121 mg is approximately equivalent to 100 mg of anhydrous quinine.

B.P. **solubilities** are: slightly soluble in water; sparingly soluble in boiling water and in alcohol; very slightly soluble in chloroform; practically insoluble in ether. *U.S.P.* solubilities are: soluble 1 in 500 of water and 1 in 120 of alcohol; sparingly soluble in boiling water; slightly soluble in chloroform and ether; freely soluble in a mixture of chloroform 2 and dehydrated alcohol 1 and in alcohol at 80°. A 1% suspension in water has a pH of 5.7 to 6.6. **Store** in well-closed containers. Protect from light.

For a report of reduced *in-vitro* activity against *P. falciparum* of quinine sulphate solutions following membrane filtration, see Chloroquine p.508.

Adverse Effects

The long-term administration of quinine in normal therapeutic doses may give rise to a train of symptoms known as cinchonism, characterised by tinnitus, headache, nausea, and disturbed vision in its mild form, with, in addition, vomiting, abdominal pain, diarrhoea, vertigo, fever, pruritus, and rashes in its more severe manifestations.

Some patients are hypersensitive to quinine and even small doses may give rise to cinchonism together with other hypersensitivity reactions including angio-oedema and asthma. Thrombocytopenia, hypoprothrombinaemia, and haemolysis may occur and agranulocytosis has been reported. Renal impairment may be due to an immune mechanism or to circulatory failure.

The symptoms of overdosage include gastro-intestinal, central nervous system, and cardiovascular disturbances. Visual disturbances are normally reversible but may be permanent, and may rarely include sudden blindness. Quinine can cause disturbances in cardiac conduction similar to those produced by quinidine, and reduction of blood pressure with syncope and circulatory failure: severe hypotension can also follow rapid injection of quinine. Severe poisoning can produce convulsions, coma, respiratory depression and death. The average fatal dose in adults has been reported to be about 8 g. Death may result in a few hours or may be delayed for 1 or 2 days.

Large doses of quinine can induce abortion, and congenital malformations, particularly of the optic and auditory nerves, have been reported after failure to induce abortion with quinine.

However, quinine should not be withheld from pregnant women with life-threatening malaria if other less hazardous agents are unavailable or inappropriate.

EFFECTS ON THE BLOOD. An analysis of blood dyscrasias reported to the Swedish Adverse Drug Reaction Committee for the 10-year period 1966–75 showed that thrombocytopenia attributable to quinine or quinidine had been reported on 43 occasions.— L. E. Böttiger *et al.*, *Acta med. scand.*, 1979, *205*, 457.

Quinine-induced agranulocytosis in a 64-year-old man was confirmed by the inhibition, *in vitro*, of bone-marrow cell cultures by therapeutic concentrations of quinine.— R. Sutherland *et al.*, *Br. med. J.*, 1977, *1*, 605.

Thrombocytopenia in a diamorphine addict was attributed to quinine which had been used to dilute the diamorphine.— D. J. Christie *et al.*, *Archs intern. Med.*, 1983, *143*, 1174.

Extensive bruising and bleeding due to thrombocytopenia was reported in a 53-year-old patient who had regularly taken 500 mL tonic water (containing about 40 mg quinine) daily over the previous 20 years for night cramps. Spontaneous bruising recurred after drinking a gin and tonic despite continued corticosteroid therapy.— C. C. Harland and P. J. Toghill (letter), *Br. med. J.*, 1985, *291*, 281 and 415.

EFFECTS ON THE EYES. Sudden loss of vision was reported in a 63-year-old woman following ingestion of 3 g of quinine. Sight slowly improved over 2 months but the visual fields were restricted, and colour and night vision were defective.— L. P. Fong *et al.*, *Med. J. Aust.*, 1984, *141*, 528.

Transient total blindness was associated with parenteral administration of quinine for malaria. At peak plasma-quinine concentrations of 90 nmol per mL the patient was blind and deaf, but recovered over the subsequent 3 days.— S. Migasena, *Ann. trop. Med. Parasit.*, 1985, *79*, 109.

See also under Overdosage, below.

EFFECTS ON GLUCOSE METABOLISM. In a study in Thailand of 151 patients with falciparum malaria hypoglycaemia associated with marked hyperinsulinaemia was noted in 17. Patients with severe life-threatening disease and pregnant women were identified as being at particular risk of developing hypoglycaemia. There was a significant correlation between plasma-insulin and quinine concentrations at the time of hypoglycaemia, although the majority of patients receiving quinine remained normoglycaemic.— N. J. White *et al.*, *New Engl. J. Med.*, 1983, *309*, 61.

Hypoglycaemia was associated with quinine given for muscle cramps in a patient without malaria.— N. Harats *et al.* (letter), *New Engl. J. Med.*, 1984, *310*, 1331.

Hypoglycaemia, defined as a plasma-glucose concentration of less than 2.8 mmol per litre, developed in 9 of 28 African patients during treatment with intravenous quinine for severe malaria.— W. Okitolonda *et al.*, *Br. med. J.*, 1987, *295*, 716.

See under Chloroquine p.509 for comments on the aetiology of hypoglycaemia during the treatment of malaria.

EFFECTS ON THE LIVER. Granulomatous hepatitis occurred in a woman who took quinine sulphate for nocturnal leg cramps. Challenge with quinine sulphate caused a recurrence of symptoms and abnormal biochemical values.— B. Katz *et al.*, *Br. med. J.*, 1983, *286*, 264. The diagnosis of granulomatous hepatitis was questioned and it was suggested that non-specific reactive hepatitis was a more accurate description based on the histological findings.— N. S. Nirodi (letter), *ibid.*, 647.

EFFECTS ON THE SKIN. Purpura was induced, in a patient previously sensitised to quinine, by drinking bitter lemon.— J. A. Murray *et al.*, *Br. med. J.*, 1979, *2*, 1551.

OVERDOSAGE. Loss of vision and hearing in 2 patients following overdoses of quinine 2 g and 4 g respectively. Hearing returned within a few days, but improvement in visual acuity was slow and incomplete.— S. B. Murray and J. L. Jay, *Br. med. J.*, 1983, *287*, 1700.

Severe visual loss accompanied by fixed dilated pupils was noted in a 3-year-old child following ingestion of up to 5.4 g of quinine when full consciousness returned after 2 days. Recovery appeared to be complete: treatment had included prompt stellate ganglion blockade.— S. Parker (letter), *Br. med. J.*, 1984, *288*, 152.

A review of the outcome of 165 patients with acute quinine poisoning. Symptoms occurred in 79% of patients: nausea in 47%, visual disturbances in 42%, tinnitus in 38%, other auditory disturbances in 23%, mild impairment of consciousness in 14%, sinus tachycardia in 23% and other ECG abnormalities in 8%. Deeper grades of coma were seen in 7 patients. Of the 5 patients who died, 4 developed intractable ventricular arrythmias and the fifth had a Jacksonian fit followed by cardiac arrest. Of the 70 patients who had visual disturbances 39 subsequently complained of total blindness and 31 of blurred vision only. Permanent visual deficits remained in 19 of the 39 patients with total visual loss although no patient was left with permanent bilateral blindness.— M. E. Boland *et al.*, *Lancet*, 1985, *1*, 384.

A review of 48 patients with acute quinine poisoning. Maximum plasma-quinine concentrations ranged from 4.0 to 23.5 mg per litre, and visual loss occurred in every patient with concentrations above 10 mg per litre.— E. H. Dyson *et al.*, *Br. med. J.*, 1985, *291*, 31.

For reviews of the clinical features and management of poisoning by quinine, see under Treatment of Adverse Effects, below.

PREGNANCY AND THE NEONATE. Jaundice not due to blood group incompatibility developed in a full-term infant with a deficiency of glucose-6-phosphate dehydrogenase born to a woman dependent on multiple daily injections of diamorphine mixed with quinine 30 to 50 mg.— L. Glass *et al.* (letter), *J. Pediat.*, 1973, *82*, 734.

In 104 children born to mothers monitored by the Collaborative Perinatal Project and found to have been exposed to quinine, and possibly other drugs, at some time during the first 4 months of pregnancy no evidence of a teratogenic effect was found.— O. P. Heinonen *et al.*, ***Birth Defects and Drugs in Pregnancy***, Littleton MA, Publishing Sciences Group, 1977, p. 296.

A study of 12 women in the third trimester of pregnancy treated with intravenous quinine for severe falciparum malaria. Quinine did not increase uterine contractions in patients already in labour and patients not in labour generally showed a decrease in frequency and amplitude of uterine contractions as they were cooled. No patient experienced sustained tetanic uterine contractions and none went into labour during quinine infusion. Hypoglycaemia and hyperinsulinaemia developed in 7 patients; in 2 before quinine was started. The important potential toxicity of quinine in late pregnancy was considered to be not an oxytocic effect but rather its capacity to release insulin.— S. Looareesuwan *et al.*, *Lancet*, 1985, *2*, 4.

Treatment of Adverse Effects

If large doses of quinine or its salts have been recently ingested, the stomach should be emptied by aspiration and lavage. Measures aimed at enhancing the elimination of quinine such as forced acid diuresis, haemodialysis, and haemoperfusion are largely ineffective since quinine is extensively metabolised in the liver with only a small proportion excreted unchanged in the urine. Blood pressure should be supported. Signs of haemolytic anaemia may be indicative of a need to treat acute renal failure. Assisted respiration may be necessary to combat respiratory failure. Cardiac rhythm should be monitored.

Vasodilators such as amyl nitrite and nicotinic acid have been given in attempts to reverse visual impairment; beneficial effects have been reported with stellate ganglion block if given promptly but some studies have failed to show any significant response.

The stomach should be emptied after any overdose of quinine. Considerable amounts of quinine may be removed even beyond the usual 4 hours due to the anticholnergic effects of the drug. The mainstay of treatment is full supportive care. Stellate ganglion block has only rarely produced dramatic improvements in vision and is no longer routinely recommended. Methods of increasing quinine elimination are generally ineffective, though haemoperfusion may improve the clinical condition of the patient.— M. Boland and G. Volans, *Br. med. J.*, 1984, *289*, 1361.

A detailed review of the clinical features and management of poisoning due to antimalarial drugs including quinine. The occurrence of ocular and cardiac toxicity is closely related to plasma quinine concentrations. In patients on long-term therapy, toxic effects generally occur at concentrations of 10 mg per litre or above. The use of vasodilator therapy and stellate ganglion block is based on the hypothesis that retinal arteriolar constriction was responsible for quinine-induced blindness. However, there is evidence for a direct toxic effect of quinine on the retina, and several clinical studies have failed to show that stellate ganglion block is effective. The value of gastric lavage is doubtful since quinine is rapidly absorbed and vomiting has often occurred before admission. Forced acid diuresis had been generally accepted as the mainstay of treatment of quinine overdose, but it had been shown not to greatly enhance the removal of quinine in patients with overdose and there was a possibility that the administration of acids could worsen cardiotoxic symptoms. Beneficial responses had been reported following haemodialysis and activated resin haemoperfusion, but kinetic studies had demonstrated a lack of benefit from either haemoperfusion, haemodialysis, or plasma exchange.— A. Jaeger *et al.*, *Med. Toxicol.*, 1987, *2*, 242.

An 18-month-old child who had become unconscious and convulsed after taking an unknown number of quinine sulphate tablets recovered completely after being given an exchange blood transfusion.— A. W. Burrows *et al.*, *Archs Dis. Childh.*, 1972, *47*, 304.

DIURESIS. Forced diuresis has a limited application in the management of drug overdosage to those few drugs that are excreted to a significant extent unchanged in the urine. Forced acid diuresis has been used for poisoning by basic drugs such as quinine but symptomatic treatment is usually adequate and is probably much safer. Forced diuresis should never be undertaken lightly. It is potentially lethal in elderly patients and in those with cardiac and renal disease. Other complications include electrolyte and acid-base disturbances, water intoxication, and cerebral oedema.— L. F. Prescott, Limitations of haemodialysis and forced diuresis, in *The Poisoned Patient: the role of the laboratory*, Ciba Foundation Symposium 26, Oxford, Elsevier, 1974, p. 269.

STELLATE GANGLION BLOCK. A 16-year-old girl who had taken 4.5 g of quinine sulphate with suicidal intent became virtually blind but responded promptly to bilateral stellate ganglion block using bupivacaine. Inhalation of amyl nitrite had produced flushing of the conjunctivae but no subjective visual improvement or fundal changes.— J. L. K. Bankes *et al.*, *Br. med. J.*, 1972, *4*, 85.

A 3-year-old child was completely blind 15 hours after the ingestion of quinine; 28 hours after ingestion he was given bilateral stellate block using bupivacaine, repeated 4½ hours later. After 12 hours central vision was normal but peripheral vision was poor. A month later there were residual pale optic disks and gross attenuation of the retinal vessels.— H. B. Valman and D. C. White, *Br. med. J.*, 1977, *1*, 1065.

Precautions

Quinine is contra-indicated in patients with a history of hypersensitivity to quinine, in the presence of haemolysis, and in patients with tinnitus or optic neuritis. It should be used with caution in patients with atrial fibrillation or other serious heart disease. Quinine may cause hypoprothrombinaemia and enhance the effects of anticoagulants. Quinine may aggravate the symptoms of myasthenia gravis and should be used with care if at all in such patients.

Pregnancy in a patient with malaria is not generally regarded as a contra-indication to the use of quinine.

Antimalarial agents and especially quinine, when given for prolonged periods, have been implicated in precipitating blackwater fever. However, in some cases deficiency of glucose-6-phosphate dehydrogenase may have been involved. Glucose-6-phosphate dehydrogenase-deficient patients with malaria may be at increased risk of haemolysis during quinine therapy.

As quinine has many of the adverse effects and actions of quinidine, see also under Quinidine Sulphate, p.85.

Chloroquine and quinine appeared to be antagonistic when given together for falciparum malaria.— A. P. Hall (letter), *Trans. R. Soc. trop. Med. Hyg.*, 1973, *67*, 425.

Quinine 2 g daily was not considered to cause clinically significant haemolytic anaemia in individuals with a deficiency of glucose-6-phosphate dehydrogenase under normal circumstances (e.g. in the absence of infection).— E. Beutler, *Pharmac. Rev.*, 1969, *21*, 73. See also D. J. Weatherall, *Practitioner*, 1978, *221*, 194 and *Ann. intern. Med.*, 1985, *103*, 245.

Diagnosis of malaria was hampered in a 22-year-old

patient by the consumption of soft drinks containing quinine.— D. Overbosch *et al.* (letter), *Lancet*, 1983, *1*, 539.

INTERACTIONS. Clearance of quinine was reduced and elimination half-life increased following administration of quinine to 6 healthy subjects pretreated with *cimetidine*. Ranitidine had no apparent effect on the clearance or half-life of quinine.— S. Wanwimolruk *et al.*, *Br. J. clin. Pharmac.*, 1986, *22*, 346.

For reports of increases in plasma-digoxin concentrations during quinine therapy, see under *Digoxin*, p.828.

For a report of quinine enhancing the anticoagulant effect of warfarin, see under *Warfarin*, p.346.

PREGNANCY AND THE NEONATE. A report of jitteriness in an infant, due to quinine withdrawal. The mother had taken quinine (as tonic water) for the last 17 weeks of pregnancy.— A. N. W. Evans *et al.*, *Practitioner*, 1980, *224*, 315.

See under Adverse Effects (above) for comments on congenital abnormalities following failed abortion with quinine.

Absorption and Fate

Quinine is rapidly and almost completely absorbed from the gastro-intestinal tract. Peak concentrations in the circulation are attained about 1 to 3 hours after ingestion and about 70% is bound to proteins in the plasma in healthy subjects rising to about 90% in patients with malaria. Quinine is widely distributed throughout the body. Concentrations attained in the CSF are about 2 to 7% of those in the plasma. Quinine is extensively metabolised in the liver and excreted in the urine. Estimates of the proportion of unchanged quinine excreted in the urine vary from less than 5% to 20%. Excretion is increased in acid urine. The elimination half-life is about 11 hours in healthy subjects but may be prolonged in patients with malaria. The pharmacokinetics of quinine are altered significantly by malaria infection, with reductions in both the apparent volume of distribution and clearance.

Quinine crosses the placenta and is excreted in the breast milk.

Reviews of the clinical pharmacokinetics of antimalarial drugs including quinine: N. J. White, *Clin. Pharmacokinet.*, 1985, *10*, 187; *Trans. R. Soc. trop. Med. Hyg.*, 1986, *80*, *Suppl.*

PREGNANCY AND THE NEONATE. The amount of quinine sulphate excreted in the milk of lactating mothers was too small to affect the child.— T. E. O'Brien, *Am. J. Hosp. Pharm.*, 1974, *31*, 844.

Further references to the pharmacokinetics of quinine during pregnancy and breast feeding: R. E. Phillips *et al.*, *Br. J. clin. Pharmac.*, 1986, *21*, 677.

Uses and Administration

Quinine is a rapidly acting blood schizontocide with activity against *Plasmodium falciparum*, *P. vivax*, *P. ovale*, and *P. malariae*. It is active against the gametocytes of *P. malariae* and *P. vivax*, but not against *P. falciparum* gametocytes. Since it has no activity against exoerythrocytic forms, quinine does not produce a radical cure in vivax or ovale malarias.

Quinine is used orally for the treatment of uncomplicated attacks of falciparum malaria due to chloroquine- or multidrug-resistant strains, and parenterally for severe or complicated malaria. Quinine is usually given by mouth as the sulphate or bisulphate and by infusion as the dihydrochloride, although other salts are used.

In the treatment of uncomplicated malaria, quinine sulphate 1.8 to 2 g (or the equivalent of another salt) is given daily in three divided doses for at least 7 days, either alone or more usually with pyrimethamine and a sulphonamide or with tetracycline, as appropriate. Treatment with primaquine will be needed to produce a radical cure in vivax or ovale malarias. For children, a dose of quinine sulphate 25 to 30 mg per kg body-weight daily in three divided doses has been recommended.

In severe or complicated malaria when the patient is unable to take oral medication quinine may be given by slow intravenous infusion. The most appropriate method of attaining effective plasma concentrations is still controversial. Some clinicians recommend the use of a loading dose of 20 mg quinine dihydrochloride (16.7 mg anhydrous base) per kg given by intravenous infusion over 4 hours provided that the patient has not recently taken quinine and reliable hospital facilities are available. This regimen has particularly been recommended in Thailand where there is evidence that the minimum inhibitory concentrations of quinine for *P. falciparum* are higher than in other parts of the world. However the potential toxicity of this dose has caused concern. The maintenance dose is 10 mg of quinine dihydrochloride (8.3 mg anhydrous base) per kg in 250 to 500 mL of diluent by intravenous infusion over 4 hours, repeated at 8 to 12 hourly intervals. Oral therapy should be substituted as soon as possible and a total of at least 7 days' therapy should be completed. After 72 hours it has been suggested that, if the patient is still seriously ill, the intravenous maintenance dose should be reduced by about one third to avoid cumulative toxicity. If intravenous infusion is not possible, quinine dihydrochloride may be given by intramuscular injection of 10 mg per kg (8.3 mg base), although this may cause pain and local irritation at the site of injection. Intravenous injection of quinine is no longer recommended because of the severe adverse cardiovascular effects.

Quinine is not generally used for malaria prophylaxis, but may be useful for multidrug-resistant strains. A dose of 325 mg of sulphate twice daily has been suggested.

For further discussions of the prophylaxis and treatment of malaria, see p.505.

Quinine is used to relieve nocturnal leg cramps in doses of 200 to 300 mg quinine sulphate or bisulphate at night.

Quinine has also been used as a bitter and a flavouring agent. It has mild analgesic and antipyretic properties but is not used for this purpose.

For references to the use of quinine with clindamycin in the treatment of babesiosis and cryptosporidiosis infections, see under Clindamycin, p.200.

CRAMPS. The incidence of cramp among patients during haemodialysis was reported to be less among those given quinine.— *Drug & Ther. Bull.*, 1982, *20*, 97.

A review of the treatment of muscle cramps. Early studies have shown beneficial responses to quinine in patients with nocturnal cramps and in diabetic patients, but less favourable results in a study in soldiers (mean age 24 years). In practice if quinine alleviates cramp it usually does so rapidly and should be stopped occasionally to see if it is still needed. Patients on long-term therapy should be monitored for adverse effects.— *Drug & Ther. Bull.*, 1983, *21*, 83.

Quinine sulphate, 300 mg at night, did not significantly reduce the incidence or severity of night cramps compared with placebo in a double-blind study of 25 patients.— S. H. Lim, *Br. J. clin. Pract.*, 1986, *40*, 462. A similar result in a double-blind crossover study in 22 patients.— A. Warburton *et al.*, *Br. J. clin. Pharmac.*, 1987, *23*, 459.

MALARIA. There has been considerable vehement debate over the most appropriate dosage regimen for intravenous quinine. Drs White and Warrell and their team showed that an initial loading dose of quinine dihydrochloride 20 mg per kg body-weight (equivalent to 16.7 mg of base) given by intravenous infusion over 4 hours followed by 10 mg per kg (8.3 mg of base) every 8 hours rapidly produced effective plasma concentrations without causing serious adverse effects (N.J. White *et al.*, *Am. J. trop. Med. Hyg.*, 1983, *31*, 1) in patients with cerebral malaria. They further commented that, in Thailand where quinine-resistant malaria was becoming more common, the minimum inhibitory concentration (MIC) of quinine for *Plasmodium falciparum* was approaching 10 mg per litre, so that higher plasma-quinine concentrations were needed than those that may be effective in areas of low quinine resistance (N.J. White, *Clin. Pharmacokinet.*, 1985, *10*, 187). Dr Hall favours a dose of 10 mg quinine base per kg every 12 hours and has criticised the higher doses used by White and Warrell (*New Engl. J. Med.*, 1982, *307*, 317; *Trop. Dis. Bull.*, 1984, *81*, 550; *ibid.*, 1985, *82*, 42; *Lancet*, 1985, *1*, 1453; *Br. med. J.*, 1985, *291*, 1146; *ibid.*, 1573; *Trop. Dis. Bull.*, 1986, *83*, R2) on the grounds of increased toxicity and a lack of evidence of decreased mortality at the higher dose, and also that fluid overload could increase the incidence of pulmonary oedema. The discrepancy appears to arise at least in part (A. Bryceson, *Br. med. J.*, 1985, *291*, 1719) from differences in the patient populations and clinical circumstances encountered by the two groups: Dr Hall bases his argument on experience in Thailand in the 1970's and subsequently on treatment in London of patients with African-acquired malaria, whereas Dr White is studying malaria in rural populations in Thailand where there is evidence of some degree of resistance to quinine. It seems unlikely that a definitive regimen will be developed to fit all circumstances, and the choice of dose should be based on the severity of the disease and the sensitivity of the organism to quinine, while being aware of the potential toxic effects of quinine and the need for careful maintenance of the fluid and electrolyte balance.

Intramuscular administration of quinine dihydrochloride 20 mg per kg body-weight initially, then 10 mg per kg every 8 hours to 8 patients with falciparum malaria produced therapeutic plasma concentrations 4 to 5 hours after injection. No serious adverse effects were seen: plasma concentrations increased steadily without dangerously high peaks. It was considered that intramuscular injection of quinine could be useful in the absence of the equipment or skills necessary for intravenous infusion.— Y. Wattanagoon *et al.*, *Br. med. J.*, 1986, *293*, 11 and 362.

For an account of the place of quinine in the treatment of malaria and its use in multidrug regimens, see p.506.

MYOTONIA. Mention that quinine has been shown to be effective for myotonia.— *Lancet*, 1987, *1*, 1242.

Preparations of Quinine and its Salts

Quinine Bisulphate Tablets *(B.P.)*

Quinine Sulfate Capsules *(U.S.P.)*. Capsules containing quinine sulphate.

Quinine Sulfate Tablets *(U.S.P.)*. Tablets containing quinine sulphate.

Quinine Sulphate Tablets *(B.P.)*

Proprietary Names and Manufacturers of Quinine and its Salts

Adaquin *(Nelson, Austral.)*; Adquin *(Adam, Austral.)*; Bi-chinine *(Drug Houses Austral., Austral.)*; Biquin *(Nelson, Austral.)*; Biquinate *(USV, Austral.)*; Chinine *(Drug Houses Austral., Austral.)*; Coquelusédal Quinine *(Elerte, Fr.)*; Dentojel *(Ayerst, Canad.)*; Grisotets *(Pharmadrug, Ger.)*; Kinin *(DAK, Denm.; ACO, Swed.)*; Kinine *(ICN, Canad.)*; Myoquin *(Fawns & McAllan, Austral.)*; Quinamm *(Merrell Dow, USA)*; Quinate *(USV, Austral.)*; Quinbisan *(Protea, Austral.)*; Quinbisul *(Alphapharm, Austral.)*; Quindan *(Danbury, USA)*; Quine *(Rowell, USA)*; Quinoctal *(Fawns & McAllan, Austral.)*; Quinoforme *(Vaillant-Defresne, Fr.)*; Quinsan *(Prosana, Austral.)*; Quinsul *(Alphapharm, Austral.)*; Quiphile *(Geneva, USA)*.

The following names have been used for multi-ingredient preparations containing quinine and its salts— Analgesic Dellipsoids D6 *(Pilsworth, UK)*; Q-Vel *(Rugby, USA)*; Rhinitis *(Lilly, USA)*; Vibrona *(Vine Products, UK)*.

1399-z

Quinocide Hydrochloride *(rINNM)*.

Chinocidum; CN-1115; Win-10,448. 8-(4-Aminopentylamino)-6-methoxyquinoline dihydrochloride. $C_{15}H_{21}N_3O,2HCl = 332.3$.

CAS — 525-61-1 (quinocide).

Pharmacopoeias. In *Rus.*

Quinocide, a structural isomer of primaquine, has actions and uses similar to those of primaquine phosphate p.514.

Experimental evidence suggested that the administration of 30 mg of quinocide could produce significant haemolysis in Negroes with a deficiency of glucose-6-phosphate dehydrogenase.— Standardisation of Procedures for the Study of Glucose-6-Phosphate Dehydrogenase, *Tech. Rep. Ser. Wld Hlth Org. No. 366*, 1967.

Quinocide, in total doses of 234 mg of base, given in conjunction with other schizontocidal drugs during the primary manifestations of induced vivax malaria, greatly reduced the number of relapses, especially long-term relapses.— N. A. Tiburskaia *et al.*, *Bull. Wld Hlth Org.*, 1968, *38*, 447.

1400-z

Totaquine
Totaquina.
CAS — 8014-53-7.

Pharmacopoeias. In *Mex.*

A mixture of alkaloids obtained from suitable species of *Cinchona* containing not less than 70% of crystallisable cinchona alkaloids of which not less than one-fifth is quinine.

Totaquine has been used as a substitute for quinine for the treatment of malaria. It has been given in doses of 600 mg three times daily.

Antimuscarinic Agents

330-s

Antimuscarinic agents are competitive inhibitors of the actions of acetylcholine at the muscarinic receptors of autonomic effector sites innervated by parasympathetic (cholinergic postganglionic) nerves, as well as being inhibitors to some extent of the action of acetylcholine on smooth muscle lacking cholinergic innervation. They are also described as parasympatholytic agents, atropinic agents, and as anticholinergic agents, although the latter term should encompass compounds with antinicotinic actions. At therapeutic doses antimuscarinics with a tertiary ammonium structure have little effect on the actions of acetylcholine at nicotinic receptors; however, the quaternary ammonium antimuscarinics exhibit a greater degree of antinicotinic potency, and some of their side-effects at high doses are due to ganglionic blockade.

Most currently available antimuscarinics do not appear to differentiate much in their actions between the proposed subtypes of muscarinic receptor, M_1 and M_2; for an example of an agent reported to have a selective action at M_1 receptors in the gastro-intestinal tract see Pirenzepine Hydrochloride, p.1103.

The peripheral antimuscarinic effects include increase in heart-rate, decreased production of saliva, sweat, and bronchial, nasal, gastric, and intestinal secretions, decreased intestinal motility, and inhibition of micturition.

The ocular effects include dilatation of the pupil, paralysis of ocular accommodation, and photophobia. The central effects normally consist of stimulation of the medulla and higher cerebral centres, manifested by mild central vagal excitation and respiratory stimulation, and depression of certain motor mechanisms, particularly those associated with the extrapyramidal tract.

The antimuscarinic actions of compounds related to atropine are qualitatively similar but differ quantitatively. In particular, the quaternary ammonium compounds are fully ionised in the pH range of body fluids and possess reduced lipid solubility. They thus penetrate cellular barriers less effectively and only pass across the blood-brain barrier or into the eye with difficulty. Accordingly they may display very considerably reduced central and ocular effects when given by oral or parenteral routes while otherwise demonstrating marked peripheral effects. In compounds of this nature gastro-intestinal absorption is also poor so that the oral dose is usually higher than the parenteral dose required to achieve the same effect; oral doses should normally be taken before food to maximise absorption.

In addition to the alkaloids atropine, hyoscine, and hyoscyamine, and their salts and galenical preparations, a number of synthetic antimuscarinic compounds have been developed which may be classified broadly into 3 groups according to whether they are used principally for their effects on the gastro-intestinal or urinary tract, for their depressant effects on the tremors and excessive salivation associated with the parkinsonian syndrome, or for their mydriatic and cycloplegic effects on the eye.

Patients should be warned that antimuscarinic agents will temporarily impair vision.

ASTHMA. A review of the treatment of asthma including discussion of antimuscarinic agents.— J. W. Paterson and R. A. Tarala, *Med. J. Aust.*, 1985, *143*, 390.

A detailed review of antimuscarinic bronchodilators.— N. J. Gross and M. S. Skorodin, *Am. Rev. resp. Dis.*, 1984, *129*, 856.

The proceedings of a symposium on antimuscarinic agents in airways disease.— *Postgrad. med. J.*, 1987, *63, Suppl. 1.*

EXTRAPYRAMIDAL DISORDERS. The mainstay of treatment of neuroleptic-induced parkinsonism has been the use of antimuscarinic agents, which have been employed both to treat symptoms when they appear and prophylactically, to try to prevent the emergence of acute dystonic reactions and parkinsonism. However, the routine therapeutic use of antimuscarinic agents in combination with neuroleptics is to be deprecated: the evidence for their effectiveness is less convincing than might be supposed, they may impair the antischizophrenic activity of neuroleptics, and there is strong concern that concurrent administration of antimuscarinics with neuroleptic drugs may increase the risk of developing tardive dyskinesia. Where a reduction in dosage of the offending neuroleptic, or substitution of another neuroleptic with a lesser propensity to cause parkinsonism is not feasible, then an antimuscarinic should be administered only until symptoms have abated to an acceptable level, and in any case not for longer than 3 months; longer periods of administration are unnecessary and ineffective.

In the treatment of acute dystonic reactions intravenous or intramuscular administration of an antimuscarinic can give dramatic and rapid relief of the movement disorder.

Antimuscarinic agents have no place in the management of tardive dyskinesia, which is exacerbated by their actions.

GASTRO-INTESTINAL DISORDERS. *Irritable bowel syndrome.* In a review of the value of antimuscarinics in the irritable bowel syndrome, Ivey (*Gastroenterology*, 1975, *68*, 1300) pointed out that, of 400 papers on 18 of the most commonly prescribed antimuscarinic agents, there was not a single well-controlled study showing any physiological effect on the colon of oral dosage, and in a condition in which a placebo is effective in over 35% of patients only placebo-controlled double-blind studies are of value. The evidence for clinical value of antimuscarinics was dubious at best although on a pathophysiological basis there seemed justification for trial in patients presenting with spastic colon, rather than nervous diarrhoea.

Drugs with an antispasmodic action, such as dicyclomine, or clidinium in association with chlordiazepoxide (Libraxin) have been found valuable in the subgroup of patients with colon spasm and pain (S.G.F. Matts, *Br. J. clin. Pract.*, 1985, *39*, 127) and it has been suggested (W.G. Thompson, *Gut*, 1984, *25*, 305) that antimuscarinic agents may be more effective when combined with a bulking agent; however, the majority of patients will not benefit from these drugs. Reassurance of the patient is probably the most valuable treatment: it has been shown (J. Svedlund *et al.*, *Lancet*, 1983, *2*, 589) that patients given psychotherapy in addition to medical therapy did significantly better than those receiving medical treatment alone.

Peptic ulcer. A review of the medical management of peptic ulcer. The adverse effects of antimuscarinic compounds have precluded their widespread use in the management of peptic ulcer.— J. J. Misiewicz, *Postgrad. med. J.*, 1984, *60*, 751.

OCULAR DISORDERS. The use of mydriatics to view the fundus. Tropicamide 0.5% eye-drops are almost ideal, because they produce a useful effect in about 20 minutes which peaks at 40 to 60 minutes and has passed off in 6 to 8 hours. Cyclopentolate 1% and homatropine 1% are less useful because their action lasts about 24 hours; the effect of atropine lasts for a week or more so it is rarely used for viewing the fundus. The individual response to all these drugs varies — it is poorest in the dark-brown (highly pigmented) iris.— C. I. Phillips, *Br. med. J.*, 1984, *288*, 1779.

PARKINSONISM. A review of drug therapy in parkinsonism. Adjunct therapy with antimuscarinic agents provided additional benefit in more than half the patients obtaining a beneficial effect with levodopa; although there were essentially no pharmacological differences between antimuscarinic agents some patients had marked preferences.— J. R. Bianchine, *New Engl. J. Med.*, 1976, *295*, 814. See also: N. P. Quinn, *Drugs*, 1984, *28*, 236; J. M. S. Pearce, *Br. med. J.*, 1984, *288*, 1777.

For further discussion of the treatment of parkinsonism, including reference to the role of antimuscarinic agents, see under Levodopa, p.1019.

See also under Extrapyramidal disorders, above.

336-z

Adiphenine Hydrochloride *(USAN, rINNM).*
Adiphenini Hydrochloridum; Cloridrato de Adifenina; NSC-129224; Spasmolytine. 2-Diethylaminoethyl diphenylacetate hydrochloride.
$C_{20}H_{25}NO_2$, HCl=347.9.

CAS — 64-95-9 (adiphenine); 50-42-0 (hydrochloride).

Pharmacopoeias. In *Pol.* and *Port. Swiss* has a monograph for Hexahydroadiphenine Hydrochloride

Adiphenine hydrochloride has been claimed to have weak peripheral effects similar to those of atropine (see p.524) together with a direct antispasmodic action and a local anaesthetic action and is used for the symptomatic relief of visceral spasms.

Proprietary Names and Manufacturers
The following names have been used for multi-ingredient preparations containing adiphenine hydrochloride— Neuro-Trasentin *(Ciba, Canad.; Ciba, UK).*

337-c

Ambutonium Bromide *(BAN).*
BL-700B; R-100. (3-Carbamoyl-3,3-diphenylpropyl)ethyldimethylammonium bromide.
$C_{20}H_{27}BrN_2O$=391.4.

CAS — 14007-49-9 (ambutonium); 115-51-5 (bromide).

Ambutonium bromide is a quaternary ammonium antimuscarinic agent with peripheral effects similar to those of atropine (see p.524). It is used as an adjunct to antacids in the treatment of peptic ulcer and gastritis in usual doses of 2.5 to 5 mg three or four times daily.

Proprietary Names and Manufacturers
The following names have been used for multi-ingredient preparations containing ambutonium bromide— Aludrox SA *(Wyeth, UK).*

338-k

Aprofene Hydrochloride *(rINNM).*
Aprophenum Hydrochloride 2-Diethylaminoethyl 2,2-diphenylpropionate hydrochloride.
$C_{21}H_{27}NO_2$, HCl=361.9.

CAS — 3563-01-7 (aprofene); 2589-00-6 (hydrochloride).

Pharmacopoeias. In *Rus.*

Aprofene hydrochloride is an antimuscarinic agent with a structure similar to that of adiphenine hydrochloride. It has been used as an antispasmodic in the *USSR* in doses of 25 mg by mouth 2 to 4 times daily; it has also been given by subcutaneous or intramuscular injection.

12406-f

Atromepine *(rINN).*
Levomepate, Tropine (—)-α-methyltropate; (1*R*,3*r*,5*S*)-Tropan-3-yl (—)-α-methyltropate.
$C_{18}H_{25}NO_3$=303.4.

CAS — 428-07-9.

Atromepine is an antimuscarinic agent with actions similar to those of atropine (see p.523).

Proprietary Names and Manufacturers
Analgispan *(Lepetit, Spain).*

331-w

Atropine *(USAN).*
(±)-Hyoscyamine. (1*R*,3*r*,5*S*)-Tropan-3-yl (±)-tropate.
$C_{17}H_{23}NO_3$=289.4.

CAS — 51-55-8.

Pharmacopoeias. In *Mex., Span., Swiss., Turk.,* and *U.S.* Also in *B.P.C. 1973.*

An alkaloid which may be obtained from solanaceous plants, or prepared by synthesis.
Odourless or almost odourless white crystals or

white crystalline powder. M.p. 114° to 118°. *U.S.P.* **solubilities** are: 1 in 460 of water, 1 in 2 of alcohol, 1 in 1 of chloroform, and 1 in 25 of ether. A saturated solution in water is alkaline to phenolphthalein. **Incompatible** with alkalis, mercury salts, and tannic acid. **Store** in airtight containers. Protect from light.

332-e

Atropine Methobromide *(BAN).*

Atropine Methylbromide; Methylatropine Bromide; Methylatropini Bromidum; Methylatropinium Bromatum; Mydriasine. (1*R*,3*r*,5*S*)-8-Methyl-3-[(±)-tropoyloxy]tropanium bromide.

$C_{18}H_{26}BrNO_3$=384.3.

CAS — 2870-71-5.

Pharmacopoeias. In *Aust., Br., Eur., Fr., Ger., It., Neth., Nord.,* and *Swiss.*

Colourless crystals or a white crystalline powder. Freely **soluble** in water, sparingly soluble in alcohol; practically insoluble in ether. **Incompatible** with alkalis, silver salts, and tannic acid. **Store** in well-closed containers and protect from light.

333-l

Atropine Methonitrate *(BAN, rINN).*

Atrop. Methonit.; Atropini Methonitras; Methylatropine Nitrate *(USAN)*; Methylatropini Nitras. (1*R*, 3*r*, 5*S*)-8-Methyl-3-[(±)-tropoyloxy]tropanium nitrate.

$C_{18}H_{26}N_2O_6$=366.4.

CAS — 52-88-0.

Pharmacopoeias. In *Aust., Br., Eur., Fr., Ger., Ind., Int., It., Neth., Span., Swiss,* and *Turk.*

Colourless crystals or a white crystalline powder. Freely **soluble** in water; soluble 1 in 13 of alcohol; practically insoluble in chloroform and in ether.

Aqueous solutions are unstable and should be freshly prepared. Stability is enhanced in acid solutions of pH below 6; solutions should be protected from alkalis. **Store** in well-closed containers and protect from light.

335-j

Atropine Sulphate *(BAN).*

Atrop. Sulph.; Atropine Sulfate *(USAN)*; Atropini Sulfas.

$(C_{17}H_{23}NO_3)_2, H_2SO_4, H_2O$=694.8.

CAS — 55-48-1 (anhydrous); 5908-99-6 (monohydrate).

Pharmacopoeias. In *Arg., Aust., Belg., Br., Braz., Chin., Cz., Egypt., Eur., Fr., Ger., Hung., Ind., Int., It., Jpn, Jug., Mex., Neth., Nord., Pol., Port., Roum., Rus., Span., Swiss, Turk.,* and *U.S.* Also in *B.P.Vet.*

Odourless colourless crystals or white crystalline powder. It effloresces in dry air.

Soluble 1 in 0.5 of water, 1 in 2.5 of boiling water, 1 in 5 of alcohol, and 1 in 2.5 of glycerol; practically insoluble in chloroform and ether. The *B.P.* states that a 2% solution in water has a pH of 4.5 to 6.2. Solutions are **sterilised** by autoclaving. **Incompatible** with alkalis, tannic acid, and mercury salts. **Store** in airtight containers. Protect from light.

For a study of the effect of the addition of water, alcohol, or dimethyl sulphoxide on the diffusion of atropine from different ointment bases, see C. W. Whitworth and R. E. Stephenson, *J. pharm. Sci.*, 1971, *60*, 48.

INCOMPATIBILITIES. During development of an assay for the atropine sulphate content of an oral mixture, incompatibility between the alkaloid and hydroxybenzoate preservatives was observed, resulting in a total loss of the atropine within 2 to 3 weeks of preparation.— T. Deeks (letter), *Pharm. J.*, 1983, *1*, 481.

For a report of an interaction between atropine sulphate and pralidoxime chloride solutions, see under Precautions, below.

PRESERVATIVE FOR EYE-DROPS. Benzalkonium chloride 0.01%, phenylmercuric nitrate 0.002%, or chlorhexidine acetate 0.01% were suitable preservatives for atropine methonitrate eye-drops sterilised by filtration.— Pharm. Soc. Lab. Rep., P/65/5, 1965.

Phenylmercuric borate 0.005% or chlorhexidine gluconate 0.02% were suitable preservatives for atropine methonitrate eye-drops sterilised by filtration.— M. Van Ooteghem, *Pharm. Tijdschr. Belg.*, 1968, *45*, 69.

STABILITY IN SOLUTION. The half-life of atropine in an ophthalmic solution at 120° had been reported to be about 1 hour at pH 6.8 and 60 hours at pH 5.0 (P. Zvirblis *et al., J. Am. pharm. Ass., scient. Edn*, 1956, *45*, 450 and A.A. Kondritzer and P. Zvirblis, *ibid.*, 1957, *46*, 531). It was therefore very important that only neutral glass or surface-treated soda-glass eye-drop bottles were used.— W. Lund and E. G. John, *Pharm. J.*, 1969, *2*, 217.

Adverse Effects

Side-effects of atropine and other antimuscarinic agents include dryness of the mouth with difficulty in swallowing and talking, thirst, dilatation of the pupils (mydriasis) with loss of accommodation (cycloplegia) and photophobia, flushing and dryness of the skin, transient bradycardia followed by tachycardia, with palpitations and arrhythmias, and urinary urgency, difficulty and retention, as well as reduction in the tone and motility of the gastro-intestinal tract leading to constipation. Occasionally vomiting, giddiness, and staggering may occur. Retrosternal pain may occur due to increased gastric reflux.

Toxic doses cause tachycardia, rapid respiration, hyperpyrexia, and CNS stimulation marked by restlessness, confusion, excitement, paranoid and psychotic reactions, hallucinations and delirium, and occasionally seizures or convulsions. A rash may appear on the face or upper trunk. In severe intoxication, central stimulation may give way to CNS depression, coma, circulatory and respiratory failure, and death.

There is considerable variation in susceptibility to atropine; recovery has occurred even after 1 g, whereas deaths have been reported from doses of 100 mg or less for adults and 10 mg for children.

Quaternary ammonium antimuscarinic agents, such as atropine methobromide and propantheline bromide, usually have some ganglion-blocking activity so that high doses may cause postural hypotension and impotence; in toxic doses non-depolarising neuromuscular block may be produced.

Systemic toxicity may be produced by the instillation of antimuscarinic eye-drops, particularly in infants. Prolonged administration of atropine to the eye may lead to local irritation, hyperaemia, oedema, and conjunctivitis. An increase in intra-ocular pressure may occur, especially in patients with closed-angle glaucoma.

Hypersensitivity to atropine is not uncommon and may occur as conjunctivitis or a skin rash.

EFFECTS ON BODY TEMPERATURE. Atropine poisoning with high fever (rectal temperature 41.9°) developed in a 2-year-old boy with catarrhal illness who was given atropine methonitrate in a dose of 400 µg with each feed for a week. Atropine and its derivatives should be used with caution especially when there is a pre-existing cause of fever, as in respiratory infections.— M. J. Purcell (letter), *Br. med. J.*, 1966, *1*, 738.

A report of acute hypothermia in a 14-year-old feverish patient following intravenous administration of atropine for bradycardia. Following subsequent administration of atropine premedication hypothermia again developed. In both cases the condition responded to treatment with warming blankets for several hours.— P. G. Lacouture *et al., Am. J. Dis. Child.*, 1983, *137*, 291.

For a report of fatal heat stroke in a patient receiving an antimuscarinic and a neuroleptic agent concomitantly, see under Benztropine Mesylate, p.528.

EFFECTS ON THE EYES. A 60-year-old man suffered complete blindness following intravenous injection of atropine 800 µg. After instillation of pilocarpine eye-drops his vision was gradually restored to its original level. Glaucoma was excluded on follow-up and this action of atropine was not fully understood.— J. M. Gooding and M. C. Holcomb, *Anesth. Analg. curr. Res.*, 1977, *56*, 872.

EFFECTS ON THE GASTRO-INTESTINAL TRACT. A report of paralytic ileus in a 77-year-old man with Parkinson's disease who had been receiving atropine sulphate by mouth to control excess salivation. The patient recovered following withdrawal of all drugs and treatment with nasogastric aspiration and intravenous fluid replacement.— N. Beatson, *Postgrad. med. J.*, 1982, *58*, 451. See also.— L. C. Wade and G. L. Ellenor, *Drug Intell. & clin. Pharm.*, 1980, *14*, 17 (reports of ileus during concomitant antimuscarinic and neuroleptic therapy).

EFFECTS ON THE HEART. Atropine sulphate to a total of 1 mg per 70 kg body-weight was given in 4 doses at 5-minute intervals to 79 patients aged 6 weeks to 79 years who had no cardiovascular disease and were undergoing elective surgery. Arrhythmias, which were associated with small rather than large doses, occurred in over 20% of patients and more frequently in the young. The cardiac accelerating effect of atropine was decreased in children and in adults over 60 years of age.— P. Dauchot and J. S. Gravenstein, *Clin. Pharmac. Ther.*, 1971, *12*, 274.

Following premedication including atropine by intramuscular injection in 25 patients, or glycopyrronium intramuscularly in a further 25, both groups had significantly greater incidences of tachycardia during anaesthetic induction and intubation compared with 25 controls who received no antimuscarinic drug. Patients who received glycopyrronium also had a higher incidence of tachycardia during surgery than the controls. No significant difference in bradycardia or extrasystoles was found in the atropine- or the glycopyrronium-treated patients.— E. A. Shipton and J. A. Roelofse, *S. Afr. med. J.*, 1984, *66*, 287.

A report of atrial fibrillation in 2 elderly glaucoma patients following post-surgical application of atropine ointment or eye-drops to the eye. A third patient who received atropine intramuscularly and intravenously pre- and post-operatively, as well as eye-drops prior to surgery, subsequently developed rapid supraventricular tachycardia.— G. J. Merli, *Archs intern. Med.*, 1986, *146*, 45.

EFFECTS ON THE SKIN. Therapeutic use of atropine had occasionally resulted in a violent eczema involving the whole face. Its action as a hapten antigen made it virtually impossible to desensitise to atropine.— J. S. Cant, *Practitioner*, 1969, *202*, 787.

OVERDOSAGE. A report of atropine poisoning in 9 infants due to inappropriate use of atropine methonitrate drops.— P. W. D. Meerstadt, *Br. med. J.*, 1982, *285*, 196. A further report of overdosage with atropine methonitrate oral drops and a report of a fixed dilated pupil, lasting 2 weeks, after an inadvertent drop into the eye.— C. M. Illingworth *et al.* (letter), *ibid.*, 650.

A report of acute poisoning in two 5-month-old identical twins following administration of 1 drop of atropine sulphate 0.5% solution into each eye.— J. J. Sanitato and M. J. Burke, *Ann. Ophthal.*, 1983, *15*, 380.

A 65-year-old patient who received more than 32 mg of atropine methonitrate instead of 2.25 mg, by inhalation as a nebulised solution, suffered no adverse effects other than transient headache and dry mouth. Unlike atropine sulphate, atropine methonitrate would appear to have a wide therapeutic margin owing to its poor absorption from mucosal surfaces.— N. J. Gross and M. S. Skorodin (letter), *Lancet*, 1985, *2*, 386.

For a report of toxicity in children administered atropine or homatropine eye-drops, see under Homatropine Methobromide, p.533.

Treatment of Adverse Effects

If overdoses of atropine have been taken by mouth the stomach should be emptied by aspiration and lavage, or by induction of emesis. The giving of activated charcoal to reduce absorption prior to lavage, has been suggested. Supportive therapy should be given as required.

Physostigmine has been tried in the treatment of atropine's central and peripheral adverse effects, but there is no evidence that it is superior to supportive management and its use is not generally recommended. Neostigmine or carbachol antagonises only the peripheral adverse effects.

For comments on the use of physostigmine to reverse antimuscarinic poisoning, see Physostigmine Sulphate, p.1334.

Use of promethazine to control agitation following atropine poisoning, as advocated by A.L. MacKenzie and J.F.G. Pigott (*Br. J. Anaesth.*, 1971, *43*, 1088) was unwise since promethazine, having antimuscarinic properties, might potentiate atropine toxicity.— D. J. Greenblatt and R. I. Shader (letter), *Br. J. Anaesth.*,

1972, *44*, 750.

Haemodialysis was thought to have contributed little to the management of a patient who had taken about 300 mg of atropine and who was also given anticholinesterases and routine supportive treatment. It was concluded that haemodialysis has no place in the treatment of atropine poisoning.— D. P. Worth *et al.*, *Br. med. J.*, 1983, *286*, 2023.

Precautions

Atropine should be used with caution in children and in geriatric patients, who may be more susceptible to its adverse effects. It is contra-indicated in patients with prostatic enlargement, in whom it may lead to urinary retention, and in those with paralytic ileus or pyloric stenosis. In patients with ulcerative colitis its use may lead to ileus or megacolon, and its effects on the lower oesophageal sphincter may exacerbate reflux. It is generally advisable to be cautious in giving atropine to any patient with diarrhoea. It should be used with extreme caution in myasthenia gravis.

Atropine should not be given to patients with closed-angle glaucoma or to patients with a narrow angle between the iris and the cornea, since it may raise intra-ocular pressure and precipitate an acute attack. The risk is greater in patients over 40 years of age and when the parenteral route is used. Systemic reactions have followed the absorption of atropine from eye-drops; overdosage is less likely if the eye ointment is used.

Due to the risk of provoking hyperpyrexia atropine should not be given to patients, especially children, when the ambient temperature is high. It should also be used cautiously in patients with fever.

Atropine and other antimuscarinic agents should be used with caution in conditions characterised by tachycardia such as thyrotoxicosis, cardiac insufficiency or failure, and in cardiac surgery, where it may further accelerate the heart-rate. Care is required in patients with acute myocardial infarction as ischaemia and infarction may be made worse.

Atropine may cause mental confusion, especially in elderly or brain-damaged patients. Reduced bronchial secretion caused by atropine may be associated with the formation of mucous plugs.

In the treatment of parkinsonism, increases in dosage and transfer to other forms of treatment should be gradual and antimuscarinic agents should not be withdrawn abruptly. Minor reactions may be controlled by reducing the dose until tolerance has developed.

Persons with Down's syndrome appear to have an increased susceptibility to the actions of atropine, whereas those with albinism may be resistant.

The effects of atropine and other antimuscarinic agents may be enhanced by the concomitant administration of other drugs with antimuscarinic properties, such as amantadine, some antihistamines, butyrophenones and phenothiazines, and tricyclic antidepressants. The reduction in gastric motility caused by antimuscarinic agents may affect the absorption of other drugs.

The ability of antimuscarinics to cause retrosternal pain due to increased oesophageal reflux had to be remembered because it had been confused with ischaemic heart pain.— D. W. Piper and T. R. Heap, *Drugs*, 1972, *3*, 366.

Dissolution of sublingual glyceryl trinitrate tablets had been noted to take over 5 minutes due to dry mouth in patients in a cardiac care unit who had received atropine shortly before, for severe bradycardia.— A. Kimchi (letter), *New Engl. J. Med.*, 1984, *310*, 1122.

Hypertensive crisis developed in a patient with malignant hypertension following intravenous administration of atropine 1 mg.— S. Sesoko *et al.* (letter), *Ann. intern. Med.*, 1984, *101*, 720.

INTERACTIONS. *Pralidoxime.* The effects of atropine sulphate intramuscularly on heart-rate were significantly delayed when it was mixed with pralidoxime chloride solution 300 mg per mL, whereas there was no delay when atropine sulphate was mixed with pralidoxime chloride 180 mg per mL. Absorption of atropine sulphate appeared to be delayed by solutions of higher osmolarity.— F. R. Sidell, *Clin. Pharmac. Ther.*, 1974, *16*, 711. Results of a study of 44 healthy subjects indicated that when pralidoxime mesylate 500 mg per mL and atropine sulphate 2 mg per mL were given intramuscularly mixed in the same syringe neither drug had a detrimental effect on the absorption of the other. A single injection emergency treatment of organophosphorus poisoning was feasible and possibly desirable.— P. Holland *et al.*, *Br. J. clin. Pharmac.*, 1975, *2*, 333.

Suxamethonium. Of 79 patients undergoing caesarean section, 44 received atropine 0.6 to 1 mg and 35 received hyoscine 600 to 800 µg intravenously immediately before induction of anaesthesia, suxamethonium being administered for intubation. The incidence of a rise of 30 mmHg or more in systolic and diastolic blood pressure was 4 to 5 times higher following atropine premedication than with hyoscine.— J. Shah and J. S. Crawford, *Br. J. Anaesth.*, 1969, *41*, 557. Analysis of 197 records of malignant hyperthermia showed that of the 139 patients with rigidity 108 had received atropine or hyoscine with suxamethonium. None of these compounds alone was associated with such a high incidence of rigidity.— W. Kalow and B. A. Britt (letter), *Lancet*, 1973, *2*, 390.

MYOCARDIAL INFARCTION. Three patients, 2 with acute myocardial infarction, were given atropine sulphate 1 mg intravenously for bradycardia. Tachycardia and ventricular fibrillation occurred in 2 patients and though defibrillation was successful, the patients died from left ventricular failure. The blood pressure of the third patient fell and numerous ectopic beats were recorded. However these effects disappeared within 15 minutes. It was suggested that the initial dose of intravenous atropine sulphate should be 300 to 600 µg in patients with ischaemic heart disease.— R. A. Massumi *et al.*, *New Engl. J. Med.*, 1972, *287*, 336. In 2 patients with myocardial infarction prophylactic administration of atropine sulphate 1 mg and 0.3 mg respectively resulted in tachycardia and an increase in ischaemia.— S. Richman, *J. Am. med. Ass.*, 1974, *228*, 1414. In a study of 30 patients with acute myocardial infarction and sinus bradycardia, atropine 600 µg given as a bolus injection intravenously increased the heart-rate and arrhythmias. When 300 µg was given as a slow infusion the bradycardia worsened.— N. G. Kounis and R. K. Chopra (letter), *Ann. intern. Med.*, 1974, *81*, 117.

Absorption and Fate

Atropine is readily absorbed from the gastro-intestinal tract and mucous membranes; it is also absorbed from the eye and to some extent through intact skin.

It is rapidly cleared from the blood and is distributed throughout the body. It crosses the blood-brain barrier. It is incompletely metabolised in the liver and is excreted in the urine as unchanged drug and metabolites.

Atropine crosses the placenta and traces appear in milk.

Quaternary ammonium salts of atropine, such as the methonitrate, are less readily absorbed by mouth. They are highly ionised in body fluids and being poorly soluble in lipids they do not readily cross the blood-brain barrier.

Plasma concentrations of atropine sulphate were determined by radioimmunoassay in 10 patients who received an intravenous or intramuscular injection of atropine sulphate 1 mg. Following intravenous injection there was a rapid reduction of initial plasma concentrations and it was calculated that after 10 minutes less than 5% of the administered dose was present in the circulation. Peak plasma concentrations occurred 30 minutes after intramuscular injection and atropine sulphate was still detectable after 240 minutes. Plasma concentrations after intramuscular and intravenous injection were comparable after one hour.— L. Berghem *et al.*, *Br. J. Anaesth.*, 1980, *52*, 597.

Pharmacokinetics of atropine were assessed in 8 anaesthetised subjects undergoing major gynaecological surgery, using a radioimmunoassay and a radioreceptor assay that measures only the active *l*-isomer. Following intravenous administration of atropine 20 µg per kg body-weight the mean elimination half-life was 4.3 hours by radioimmunoassay and 3.7 hours by radioreceptor assay. There was a tendency to a longer elimination half-life and slower clearance in patients over 55 years of age. Comparison of the results from the two assays suggested that the distribution of the *d*- and *l*-isomers was different.— L. Aaltonen *et al.*, *Eur. J. clin. Pharmac.*, 1984, *26*, 613.

A study of the pharmacokinetics and pharmacodynamics of atropine following the intravenous infusion of 1.35 and 2.15 mg of atropine, as the sulphate, over 3 minutes in 3 healthy subjects. Atropine had first-order elimination kinetics, but there was some evidence that the distribution kinetics might be dose-dependent. The mean elimination half-life was 132 minutes, and an average of 56.8% of the dose was excreted unchanged in the urine with the remainder mainly as tropine. Episodes of atrioventricular dissociation with synchronisation occurred 1 to 2 minutes after the start of infusion; heart-rate began to accelerate on average 1.5 minutes after infusion began and reached a maximum 7.5 minutes after termination. Saliva flow decreased shortly after drug administration and reached a minimum a mean of 7 minutes after termination of infusion. Both effects subsequently wore off gradually, but saliva flow recovered more slowly than heart-rate.— P. H. Hinderling *et al.*, *J. pharm. Sci.*, 1985, *74*, 703 and 711.

A study involving 9 patients who inhaled atropine sulphate 0.5 to 1.5 mg every 4 to 6 hours showed that while none of the patients had a measurable serum concentration of atropine after the first dose, 6 had detectable concentrations after multiple doses indicating that drug accumulation had occurred; in some of the patients the serum concentrations were high enough that they might have been expected to cause systemic side-effects.— W. A. Kradjan *et al.*, *Clin. Pharmac. Ther.*, 1985, *38*, 12.

PREGNANCY AND THE NEONATE. A study of the pharmacokinetics of atropine in mother and child in late pregnancy. Maximum concentrations of atropine in foetal cord blood were achieved about 5 minutes after intravenous injection of atropine 12.5 µg per kg body-weight in 16 women; concentrations were not significantly different from those in maternal blood. However the mean time to maximum effect on foetal heart-rate was 25.7 minutes whereas in the mothers, maximum blood concentration occurred at the same time as maximum pharmacological effect.— G. Barrier *et al.*, *Anesth. Analg. Réanim.*, 1976, *33*, 795. See also: I. Kivalo and S. Saarikoski, *Br. J. Anaesth.*, 1977, *49*, 1017.

Uses and Administration

Atropine is an antimuscarinic alkaloid with both central and peripheral actions, see p.522. It first stimulates and then depresses the central nervous system and has antispasmodic actions on smooth muscle and reduces secretions, especially salivary and bronchial secretions; it also reduces perspiration, but has little effect on biliary or pancreatic secretion. When given as its quaternary ammonium derivatives, such as the methonitrate, it has less effect on the CNS. Atropine methonitrate also has strong ganglion-blocking activity.

When given by mouth as the sulphate or methonitrate it reduces smooth-muscle tone and diminishes gastric and intestinal motility but has little effect on gastric secretion in usual therapeutic doses. Both the sulphate and the methonitrate have been used in the treatment of pylorospasm in infants and other spastic conditions of the gastro-intestinal tract. In the treatment of congenital hypertrophic pyloric stenosis where surgery is not possible, atropine methonitrate has been given in doses of 200 to 400 µg, as 1 or 2 drops of a 0.6% alcoholic solution 20 minutes before feeds; side-effects such as dry mouth, flushing of the skin, dilated pupils, or fever, call for an immediate reduction of the dose. If the patient responds to treatment the dose may be increased up to 600 to 800 µg at each feed, and maintained for the minimum period necessary, after which it may be gradually reduced.

Atropine has also been prescribed to alleviate the griping caused by vegetable laxatives, and in the treatment of smooth muscle spasm in conditions such as renal and biliary colic. The sulphate has also been tried as an adjunct to the treatment of gastric and duodenal ulcers. The antispasmodic action of atropine has been used to facilitate radiological examination of the gut.

Atropine has been used in the symptomatic treatment of idiopathic and postencephalitic parkinsonism. It reduces tremor and muscular rigidity, improves the gait, posture, and speech, and may have a favourable effect on oculogyric crises; it also reduces sialorrhoea. Other antimuscarinics such as benzhexol or orphenadrine are now preferred.

Atropine depresses the vagus and thereby increases the heart-rate although in infancy and old age this effect may be less marked. Atropine sulphate may be used during cardiopulmonary resuscitation to treat sinus bradycardia accompanied by hypotension or frequent ectopic beats, and may also be of value in lessening the degree of atrioventricular heart block. It has also been used in vagal syncope with bradycardia due to hyperactive carotid sinus reflex. In the treatment of bradycardia or asystole due to overdosage with parasympathomimetic agents doses of 1 to 2 mg by subcutaneous, intramuscular, or intravenous injection are employed; considerably higher doses may be required in the treatment of poisoning due to irreversible anticholinesterases such as organophosphorus insecticides (see Pralidoxime Chloride, p.851).

Atropine sulphate has been recommended, usually in initial doses of 300 to 600 µg intravenously, subsequently increased according to response, in the management of bradycardia of acute myocardial infarction; however, caution is required, as atropine may exacerbate ischaemia or infarction in these patients.

Atropine is given before the induction of general anaesthesia to diminish the risk of vagal inhibition of the heart and to reduce salivary and bronchial secretions. For premedication prior to anaesthesia 300 to 600 µg of atropine sulphate may be given by subcutaneous or intramuscular injection, usually in conjunction with 10 to 15 mg of morphine sulphate, about an hour before anaesthesia. Alternatively 300 to 600 µg may be given intravenously immediately before induction of anaesthesia.

Suitable paediatric premedication doses of the sulphate are: up to 65 µg subcutaneously for premature infants, 100 µg for full-term infants, 200 µg at 6 months to 1 year, and 10 to 20 µg per kg body-weight for older children, with reduced doses on hot days or for a febrile child.

It may be given with thiopentone sodium before electroconvulsive therapy. Atropine sulphate 0.6 to 1.2 mg is given by slow intravenous injection in conjunction with neostigmine methylsulphate to reverse the effects of non-depolarising muscle relaxants (see Neostigmine Methylsulphate, p.1332).

Atropine is used as a cycloplegic and mydriatic. Dilatation of the pupil occurs in half an hour following one local application and lasts for a week or more; marked paralysis of accommodation is obtained in 1 to 3 hours with recovery in 3 to 7 days. It is used in the treatment of iritis and uveitis to immobilise the ciliary muscle and iris and to prevent or break down adhesions. Because of its powerful cycloplegic action atropine is also used in the determination of refraction in children below the age of 6 and in children with convergent strabismus. Atropine may be used as oily eye-drops, or the sulphate or methonitrate may be used in aqueous eye-drops or eye ointments. The methobromide has also been used, dilatation of the pupil being reported to be less persistent than after the sulphate.

Atropine has been used in the form of liniment or belladonna plaster to relieve the pain of muscular rheumatism, sciatica, and neuralgia although there is no rationale for such usage.

The use of atropine or its salts and derivatives in cosmetics is prohibited in the *UK*.

Reports of antiviral activity of atropine *in vitro*: B. Alarcón *et al.*, *Antimicrob. Ag. Chemother.*, 1984, *26*, 702 (against herpes simplex); A. Sola *et al.*, *ibid.*, 1986, *29*, 284 (against African swine fever virus).

ANAESTHESIA. A review of some aspects of atropine premedication. Although children may be very sensitive to the effects of atropine, perhaps partly because of increased volume of distribution and prolonged elimination compared with adults, there are good reasons for the routine use of atropine in premedication in children. However, the use of atropine in the premedication of the healthy adult patient is controversial, particularly in view of the non-irritant nature of modern anaesthetics and the increased use of premedicants such as oral benzodiazepines rather than parenteral opioid analgesics. Routine use of atropine premedication in adults is not rational and should be avoided particularly in the elderly and during caesarean section; however, it is indicated in patients undergoing ophthalmic and otorhinolaryngological surgery, as well as in patients receiving opiates.— J. Kanto, *Int. J. clin. Pharmac. Ther. Toxic.*, 1983, *21*, 92.

A review of methods of increasing intragastric pH and reducing intragastric volume in patients undergoing general anaesthesia. Antimuscarinic agents only inhibit vagally-mediated gastric acid production and they are largely ineffective in raising intragastric pH. These drugs are unsuitable for use alone in the prevention of acid aspiration.— M. Morgan, *Br. J. Anaesth.*, 1984, *56*, 47. Antimuscarinic agents are powerful depressants of lower oesophageal sphincter tone, causing a reduction in barrier pressure; however, it appears that fortuitously the combination of neostigmine 2.5 mg and atropine 1.2 mg has a net negative effect on the sphincter. Nonetheless, the risk of gastro-oesophageal reflux is increased compared with healthy non-medicated subjects.— B. R. Cotton and G. Smith, *ibid.*, 37.

In children. Children under 2 years were more sensitive to atropine than adults; the dose required to produce dry mouth had been shown to be proportional to weight. Doses based on surface area might be excessive in children under the age of 2 years.— G. S. Robinson and V. S. Williams, *Practitioner*, 1970, *204*, 5.

In ECT. Commonly used doses of atropine—650 µg—were only of placebo value in preventing vagal inhibition before ECT.— J. L. Barton (letter), *Br. med. J.*, 1974, *3*, 409. Successful use of 1.2 mg intramuscularly 1 hour before ECT.— P. H. Gosling (letter), *ibid.*

In eye surgery. Experience in 140 children undergoing squint operations confirmed that atropine 10 µg per kg body-weight given intravenously protected patients from the oculocardiac reflex. The incidence of the reflex was 25% with a mean reduction in heart-rate of 2 beats per minute in 20 patients thus treated, compared with 70% and 17 beats per minute in 20 patients given atropine intramuscularly, and 90% and 30 beats per minute in 100 given no atropine.— J. P. Alexander, *Br. J. Ophthal.*, 1975, *59*, 518.

ANOXIC SEIZURES. Severe or frequent attacks of reflex anoxic seizures in 7 children were reduced in frequency by 93 to 100% following treatment with atropine, usually as an oral solution of the methonitrate. Antimuscarinic side-effects were seen in 2 patients and responded to a reduced dose given at more frequent intervals. Although treatment is seldom required for this condition atropine therapy may be offered for a limited period to allay parental anxiety or to maintain seizure control in children of school age.— R. C. McWilliam and J. B. P. Stephenson, *Archs Dis. Childh.*, 1984, *59*, 473. Another case report.— J. B. P. Stephenson (letter), *Lancet*, 1979, *2*, 955.

ANTICHOLINESTERASE POISONING. Atropine 2 mg given intramuscularly as an immediate measure before the patient reaches hospital may help to reverse the signs of poisoning with organophosphate insecticides. Larger doses of over 10 mg in the first 2 hours may be required.— J. Henry and G. Volans, *Br. med. J.*, 1984, *289*, 39.

The use of 19.59 g of atropine sulphate intravenously over 24 days in a patient with unusually severe organophosphate poisoning.— H. Golsousidis and V. Kokkas (letter), *Hum. Toxicol.*, 1985, *4*, 339. A similar report of a large dose being required: 11.442 g over 29 days.— G. Hopmann and H. Wanke, *Dt. med. Wschr.*, 1974, *99*, 2106.

Results in *mice* suggested that hyoscine might be more effective than atropine in the treatment of poisoning due to high doses of some centrally-acting anticholinesterases.— D. Janowsky *et al.* (letter), *Lancet*, 1984, *2*, 747. Criticism. Atropine and hyoscine were equally ineffective in the treatment of acute organophosphate poisoning in a study in *rats*.— C. M. Stein and P. Neill (letter), *ibid.*, 1985, *1*, 823. Comment. Atropine is a standard therapeutic agent in organophosphate poisoning; the results in *rats* would appear to be due to the choice of too low a dose of atropine.— D. M. Sanderson (letter), *ibid.*, 1168.

CARDIAC DISORDERS. In the sick sinus syndrome atropine generally produces side-effects which preclude the continued use either of atropine itself or of similar drugs, and it rarely speeds the bradycardia.— *Br. med. J.*, 1973, *2*, 677. Many patients with sick sinus syndrome have been saved from cardiac arrest by the timely administration of atropine: it does work, albeit with unpleasant side-effects.— D. H. Dighton (letter), *Lancet*, 1985, *1*, 1157.

Standards and guidelines for cardiopulmonary resuscitation and emergency cardiac care, including recommendations on the use of atropine.— National Conference on Cardiopulmonary Resuscitation and Emergency Cardiac Care, *J. Am. med. Ass.*, 1980, *244*, 453. Updated standards and guidelines.— *idem*, 1986, *255*, 2905.

In paroxysmal ventricular tachycardia interspersed with an underlying bradycardia atropine is the drug of first choice. A dose of 300 µg may be given intravenously, followed at 5-minute intervals if necessary by a further 300 µg and then by a final 600 µg until an appropriate rate is restored if possible to the underlying rhythm.— D. A. Chamberlain, *Prescribers' J.*, 1981, *21*, 153.

A report of the use of atropine methonitrate oral drops to treat bradycardia. Unlike atropine sulphate it does not cross the blood-brain barrier and has been found to be well tolerated and effective; its use has considerably lessened the requirement for insertion of pacemakers.— D. Mendel (letter), *Br. med. J.*, 1982, *285*, 1429.

A review of the management of acute arrhythmias. Sinus bradycardia, which is normally benign, should be treated if there is hypotension or reduced cerebral or renal perfusion. Atropine, given intravenously, is the drug of choice: 500 µg to 2.0 mg may be given in increments of 500 µg every 3 minutes. A single dose is usually effective but repeated doses may be necessary.— W. T. Brownlee, *Br. J. Hosp. Med.*, 1985, *33*, 138.

Patients with impending cardiac arrest caused by bradycardia with hypotension should be treated with atropine. The intravenous route is currently preferred by most practitioners but there has been a recent resurgence of interest in the intratracheal route in cardiopulmonary resuscitation; doses are essentially the same as those given intravenously and uptake is extremely rapid if doses are diluted to a volume of 10 mL.— P. J. F. Baskett, *Br. J. Hosp. Med.*, 1985, *34*, 345.

Myocardial infarction. A detailed review of the role of atropine in patients with acute myocardial infarction and sinus bradycardia. Atropine should not be administered routinely to the bradycardic patient and the potential deleterious effects should be weighed against its benefits.— P. Dauchot and J. S. Gravenstein, *Anesthesiology*, 1976, *44*, 501.

See also under Precautions, above.

GASTRO-INTESTINAL DISORDERS. *Atropine suppression test.* Tumour-produced pancreatic polypeptide concentrations in plasma were not significantly affected by atropine 1 mg intramuscularly in 12 patients with pancreatic endocrine tumours whereas there was a large fall in nontumour-produced concentrations in all control subjects. Testing with atropine may greatly help to detect early tumours in those patients who have an intermediate rise of plasma pancreatic polypeptide.— T. E. Adrian *et al.*, *Gut*, 1982, *23*, A905. See also T. W. Schwartz (letter), *Lancet*, 1978, *2*, 326.

Irritable bowel syndrome. For a discussion of the value of antimuscarinics in the treatment of irritable bowel syndrome, see under Antimuscarinics, p.522.

Nausea and vomiting. Both atropine and hyoscine have a useful anti-emetic action in anaesthetic practice, and this should not be forgotten now that their use as antisialogogues is diminishing.— R. S. J. Clarke, *Br. J. Anaesth.*, 1984, *56*, 19.

Pancreatitis. No evidence of benefit from atropine in mild to moderately severe pancreatitis.— J. L. Cameron *et al.*, *Surgery Gynec. Obstet.*, 1979, 148, 206.

Pyloric stenosis. The use of atropine in pyloric stenosis should be abandoned since Ramstedt's operation was curative and safe.— G. C. Robinson and V. S. Williams, *Practitioner*, 1970, *204*, 5.

Ulcer, peptic. Control of acid secretion was improved by addition of atropine 1.2 mg four times daily with food to cimetidine therapy in a study in patients with duodenal ulcer poorly responsive to cimetidine alone, but all patients experienced side-effects of dry mouth and blurred vision with the dose of atropine used.— T. Gledhill *et al.*, *Gut*, 1984, *25*, 1211.

HYPERHIDROSIS. Atropine sulphate 500 µg had a beneficial effect in 2 sisters with a new genetic syndrome of cold-induced profuse sweating over the chest and back. Propranolol in doses of up to 160 mg daily, had been ineffective.— E. Sohar *et al.*, *Lancet*, 1978, *2*, 1073.

Lack of specificity and short duration of action make atropine an unsuitable drug for hyperhidrosis, although propantheline may be worth trying; however, effective control of sweating is rarely possible without unacceptable side-effects.— W. A. D. Griffiths, *Prescribers' J.*, 1984, *24*, 38.

OCULAR DISORDERS. Atropine eye-drops 1% often gave great relief from pain in eye injuries; painful iris spasm could be relieved, as could the pain of arc eye.— P. A. Gardiner, *Br. med. J.*, 1978, *2*, 1347.

An outline of the ocular complications of leprosy. Iridocyclitis is the principal single cause of blindness in leprosy and is managed by the addition of atropine twice daily, as eye-drops or ointment, and corticosteroid therapy to antileprotic treatment. If intra-ocular pressure is elevated acetazolamide may be given, but pilocarpine should not be used as it counteracts the effect of the atropine.— V. C. Joffrion and M. E. Brand, *Lepr. Rev.*, 1984, *55*, 105.

Myopia. The possible arrest of myopia by the use of atropine eye-drops.— T. S. -B. Kelly *et al.*, *Br. J. Ophthal.*, 1975, *59*, 529. Comment.— *ibid.*, 527.

See also: R. L. Brenner, *Ann. Ophthal.*, 1985, *17*, 137.

Most paediatric ophthalmologists remain unconvinced by evidence published to date that any advantages of atropine treatment outweigh the disadvantages. The treatment of myopia with atropine requires further study before being accepted as standard clinical practice.— E. A. Palmer, *J. Am. med. Ass.*, 1985, *254*, 1374.

RESPIRATORY SYSTEM DISORDERS. *Emphysema*. Maximum increase in FEV_1 was seen after the second of 4 doses of atropine methonitrate 750 µg, inhaled hourly as a nebulised solution in isotonic saline, in a crossover study in 10 emphysemic patients; subsequent inhalation of salbutamol 360 µg produced no further increase. However, the increase in FEV_1 following inhalation of salbutamol 180 µg hourly did further improve after inhalation of atropine methonitrate 1.5 mg to the same level as that achieved with atropine alone. Doses were larger than those that would normally be given clinically but were well tolerated. The results suggest that there is a common cholinergic pathway for antimuscarinic and adrenergic bronchodilators in patients with emphysema, in the latter case indirect. Antimuscarinic agents provide a logical therapeutic approach worth exploring in these patients.— N. J. Gross and M. S. Skorodin, *New Engl. J. Med.*, 1984, *311*, 421. Comment.— J. A. Nadel, *ibid.*, 463. Criticism.— M. Kneussl and F. Kummer (letter), *ibid.*, 1379. Reply.— N. J. Gross and M. S. Skorodin (letter), *ibid.*

Pertussis. A review of the treatment of whooping cough. Symptomatic relief of whooping cough is still listed as an indication for atropine methonitrate, but there is no published evidence of its value.— J. Broomhall and A. Herxheimer, *Archs Dis. Childh.*, 1984, *59*, 185.

SPIDER BITE. Patients bitten by the black widow spider, *Latrodectus mactans*, responded well to treatment with atropine.— A. Gotlieb (letter), *Lancet*, 1970, *1*, 246.

Preparations

Atropine Eye Drops *(A.P.F.)*. Gutt. Atrop. Sulph. Contain atropine sulphate 1%. Sterilised by autoclaving.

Atropine Eye Drops *(B.P.)*. ATR. Contain atropine sulphate.

Atropine Sulfate Ophthalmic Solution *(U.S.P.)*. A sterile aqueous solution of atropine sulphate. pH 3.5 to 6.0.

Atropine Eye Ointment *(A.P.F.)*. Contains atropine sulphate 1% in a sterilised basis. Prepared aseptically.

Atropine Eye Ointment *(B.P.)*. Contains atropine sulphate in a sterilised basis.

Atropine Sulfate Ophthalmic Ointment *(U.S.P.)*. A sterile eye ointment containing atropine sulphate in a suitable basis.

Atropine Sulfate Injection *(U.S.P.)*. Contains atropine sulphate. pH 3.0 to 6.5.

Atropine Injection *(B.P.)*. Atropine Sulphate Injection. pH 2.8 to 4.5.

Atropine Sulfate Tablets *(U.S.P.)*. Contain atropine sulphate.

Atropine Tablets *(B.P.)*. Atropine Sulphate Tablets

Proprietary Preparations

Alcon Opulets Atropine 1% *(Alcon, UK)*. *Eye-drops*, atropine sulphate 1%, in single-use disposable applicators.

Isopto Atropine *(Alcon, UK)*. *Eye-drops*, atropine sulphate 1%, hypromellose 0.5%.

Min-I-Jet Atropine Sulphate *(IMS, UK)*. *Injection*, atropine sulphate 100 µg/mL, in single-use prefilled syringes of 5 and 10 mL.

Minims Atropine Sulphate *(Smith & Nephew Pharmaceuticals, UK)*. *Eye-drops*, atropine sulphate 1%, in single-use disposable applicators.

Proprietary Names and Manufacturers of Atropine, its Salts and Derivatives

Alcon Opulets Atropine 1% *(Alcon, UK)*; Atropin Minims *(Smith & Nephew, Norw.)*; Atropina Miro *(Spain)*; Atropinol *(Winzer, Ger.)*; Atropt *(Sigma, Austral.)*; Borotropin *(Winzer, Ger.)*; Cicloplegyl *(Arg.)*; Dosatropine *(Fr.)*; Eumydrin *(Winthrop, Austral.; S.Afr.; Winthrop, UK)*; Isopto Atropin *(Alcon, Swed.)*; Isopto Atropine *(Alcon, Canad.; S.Afr.; Alcon, UK)*; Liotropina *(SIFI, Ital.)*; Metylatropin *(DAK, Denm.)*; Midrioftal *(Arg.)*; Min-I-Jet Atropine Sulphate *(IMS, UK)*; Minims Atropine Sulphate *(Smith & Nephew, Austral.; Smith & Nephew, S.Afr.; Smith & Nephew Pharmaceuticals, UK)*; Ocean-A/S *(Fleming, USA)*; Skiatropine *(Novopharma, Switz.)*; SMP Atropine *(Coopervision, Canad.)*; Steropine *(Remedia, S.Afr.)*; Sulfatropinol *(Vera, Spain)*.

The following names have been used for multi-ingredient preparations containing atropine, its salts and derivatives— Actonorm Powder *(Wallace Mfg Chem., UK)*; Actonorm Tablets *(Wallace Mfg Chem., UK)*; Antrocol *(Poythress, USA)*; Arco-Lase Plus *(Arco, USA)*; Asma-Vydrin *(Lipomed, UK)*; Brovon *(Napp, UK)*; Brovon Pressurised Inhalant *(Napp, UK)*; Butabell *(Saron, USA)*; Contac *(Allergan, Austral.)*; Cyclopane *(Alcon, Austral.)*; Dasikon *(Beecham Laboratories, USA)*; Dasin *(Beecham Laboratories, USA)*; Diarsed *(Fr.)*; Di-Atro *(Legere, USA)*; Diban *(Robins, Canad.)*; Donnagel *(Robins, Austral.; Robins, Canad.)*; Donnagel with Neomycin *(Robins, Canad.; Robins, UK)*; Donnagel-PG *(Robins, USA)*; Donnalix *(Robins, Austral.)*; Donnatab *(Robins, Austral.)*; Donnatal *(Robins, Austral.; Robins, Canad.; Robins, UK; Robins, USA)*; Donnazyme *(Robins, Canad.; Robins, USA)*; Espasmotex *(Arlo, USA)*; Festalan *(Hoechst, USA)*; Hybephen *(Beecham Laboratories, USA)*; Kinesed *(Stuart Pharmaceuticals, USA)*; Lomotil *(Searle, Austral.; S.Afr.; Gold Cross, UK; Searle, USA)*; Lomotil with Neomycin *(Searle, UK)*; Lonox *(Geneva, USA)*; Lyspafen *(Protea, Austral.; Fisons, S.Afr.)*; Migranol *(Alcon, Austral.)*; Motofen *(McNeil Pharmaceutical, USA)*; Mydrapred *(Alcon, Canad.)*; Neo-Diophen *(Hamilton, Austral.)*; Pamergan AP100/25 *(Martindale Pharmaceuticals, UK)*; PIB *(Napp, UK)*; Prenomiser Plus *(Fisons, UK)*; Reasec *(Janssen, Austral.; Ital.; Switz.; Janssen, UK)*; Retardin *(Denm.; Norw.; Swed.)*; Riddobron Inhalant *(Seaford, UK)*; Riddobron Tablets *(Seaford, UK)*; Riddofan *(Seaford, UK)*; Riddovydrin Inhalant *(Seaford, UK)*; Ru-Tuss Tablets *(Boots, USA)*; Rybarvin *(Rybar, UK)*; Silbe *(Berk Pharmaceuticals, UK)*; SK-Diphenoxylate *(Smith Kline & French, USA)*; Trac Tabs *(Hyrex, USA)*; Tropinal *(Hamilton, Austral.)*; Urised *(Webcon, USA)*; Uroblue *(Geneva, USA)*; Urogesic *(Edwards, USA)*.

12417-h

Barbetonium Iodide

Diethyl[2-(5-ethylperhydro-2,4,6-trioxo-5-phenylpyrimidin-1-yl)ethyl]methylammonium iodide.
$C_{19}H_{28}IN_3O_3$=473.4.

CAS — 6191-48-6.

Barbetonium iodide is a quaternary ammonium antimuscarinic agent with peripheral actions similar to atropine (see p.524). It has been used as an adjunct in the treatment of peptic ulcer and to relieve visceral spasm.

Proprietary Names and Manufacturers

Defenale *(IBIS, Ital.)*.

339-a

Belladonna Herb *(BAN)*.

Bellad. Leaf; Belladone; Belladonna Leaf *(USAN)*; Belladonnae Folium; Belladonnae Herba; Deadly Nightshade Leaf; Hoja de Belladona; Tollkirschenblätter.

CAS — 8027-38-1 (belladonna).

Pharmacopoeias. In *Arg., Aust., Belg., Br., Braz., Chin., Cz., Egypt., Eur., Fr., Ger., Hung., Ind., Int., It., Jug., Mex., Neth., Nord., Pol., Port., Roum., Rus., Span., Swiss, Turk.,* and *U.S.* The *B.P.* also describes Powdered Belladonna Herb.

The dried leaves, or leaves and flowering tops of *Atropa belladonna* (Solanaceae). The *B.P.* specifies not less than 0.3% of total alkaloids, calculated as hyoscyamine; the *U.S.P.* specifies not less than 0.35% of alkaloids. The alkaloids consist mainly of those of the hyoscyamine—atropine group together with small quantities of hyoscine. **Store** in airtight containers. Protect from light.

NOTE. The *B.P.* directs that when Belladonna Herb or Belladonna Leaf is prescribed, Prepared Belladonna Herb is dispensed.

426-k

Prepared Belladonna Herb *(BAN)*.

Belladonnae Herbae Pulvis Standardisatus; Belladonnae Pulvis Normatus; Poudre Titrée de Belladone; Powdered Belladonna; Powdered Belladonna Leaf; Prep. Bellad.; Prepared Belladonna.

Pharmacopoeias. In *Br., Eur., Fr., Ger., Int., Neth.*, and *Turk.*

Belladonna herb, reduced to a powder and adjusted to contain 0.28 to 0.32% of alkaloids, calculated as hyoscyamine.

A greyish-green powder with a slightly nauseous odour. **Store** in airtight containers. Protect from light.

340-e

Belladonna Root

Bellad. Root; Belladonnae Radix; Deadly Nightshade Root.

Pharmacopoeias. In *Arg., Aust., Cz., Hung., Jpn, Pol.*, and *Roum.* Also in *B.P.C. 1973*. *Arg., Pol.*, and *Roum.* specify not less than 0.45% of alkaloids.

The dried root or root and rootstock of *Atropa belladonna*, containing not less than 0.4% of alkaloids, calculated as hyoscyamine. **Store** in a cool dry place.

STABILITY IN MIXTURES. Atropine in belladonna preparations was unstable at alkaline pH and would quickly be degraded in mixtures with a pH above 7. Such mixtures in the *B.P.C. 1968* [and *1973*] included Aluminium Hydroxide and Belladonna Mixture, Paediatric Belladonna and Ipecacuanha Mixture, Cascara and Belladonna Mixture, and Magnesium Trisilicate and Belladonna Mixture.— Pharm. Soc. Lab. Rep., P/71/9, 1971.

Adverse Effects, Treatment, and Precautions

As for Atropine Sulphate, p.523.

Belladonna had been designated by the FDA as a herb unsafe for use in foods, beverages, or drugs.— *Am. Pharm.*, 1984, *NS24* (Mar.), 20.

ABUSE. For reports of the abuse of belladonna and stramonium mixtures, see Stramonium, p.543.

POISONING. Severe poisoning, with subsequent recovery, in a 67-year-old woman following continued self-application of belladonna plasters to her back over a period of a month.— S. R. Sims, *Br. med. J.*, 1954, *2*, 1531.

Uses and Administration

Belladonna has the actions of atropine (see p.524). Belladonna herb and its preparations have been used in the treatment of intestinal and biliary colic, and as an adjunct in the management of peptic ulcer; they used to be given with laxatives with the aim of preventing griping. They have also been employed in the symptomatic management of parkinsonism, in particular in the treatment of sialorrhoea. Belladonna tincture was formerly used for the treatment of nocturnal enuresis.

Belladonna root has the same properties as the herb but is used chiefly in preparations for external use. Liniments and plasters have been used as counter-irritants for the relief of pain but there is little evidence that they have a beneficial effect and side-effects have occurred. Suppositories of belladonna have been employed to relieve the discomfort of haemorrhoids and anal fistulae.

Belladonna is used in homoeopathic medicine.

The use of belladonna and its compounds in cosmetics is prohibited in the *UK*.

Preparations

Belladonna Dry Extract *(B.P.)*. A dried and powdered percolate of belladonna herb with alcohol (70%). It is adjusted to contain 1% of alkaloids, calculated as hyoscyamine.

Store in small, wide-mouthed, well-closed containers.

Most pharmacopoeias include a similar extract and/or a

firm (pilular) extract, the specified content of alkaloids varying between 0.5 and 1.5%.

Belladonna Extract *(U.S.P.)*. It is adjusted to contain 1.25% of alkaloids. It may be in the form of a firm extract (Pilular Belladonna Extract) or a dry extract (Powdered Belladonna Extract). Store at a temperature not exceeding 30° in airtight containers.

Belladonna Liquid Extract *(B.P.C. 1973)*. Contains 0.75% of total alkaloids, calculated as hyoscyamine, in alcohol (80%).

Belladonna and Phenobarbitone Tablets *(B.P.C. 1973)*. Each contains belladonna dry extract 12.5 mg and phenobarbitone 25 mg. *Dose.* 1 tablet.

Belladonna Extract Tablets *(U.S.P.)*

Belladonna Tincture *(B.P.)*. Prepared from belladonna herb by alcoholic (70%) percolation and standardised to contain 0.03% of alkaloids calculated as hyoscyamine.
The *U.S.P.* preparation is similar. Store at a temperature not exceeding 40° in airtight containers.
Similar preparations are included in several pharmacopoeias.

Proprietary Preparations

Bellocarb *(Sinclair, UK)*. *Tablets* belladonna dry extract 10 mg, magnesium carbonate 300 mg, magnesium trisilicate 300 mg.

Proprietary Names and Manufacturers of Belladonna

Atrobel *(Fawns & McAllan, Austral.)*; Bellafit *(Switz.)*; Bellafolin *(Sandoz, Ger.; Switz.)*; Bellafolina *(Sandoz, Ital.; Spain)*; Locus Purgat *(Orravan, Spain)*; Tremoforat *(Klein, Ger.)*.

The following names have been used for multi-ingredient preparations containing belladonna—Alka-Donna *(Carlton Laboratories, UK)*; Alka-Donna P *(Carlton Laboratories, UK)*; Alophen *(Warner-Lambert, UK)*; Aluhyde *(Sinclair, UK)*; Aperient Dellipsoids D9 *(Pilsworth, UK)*; B & O Supprettes *(Webcon, USA)*; Becolyte *(McGloin, Austral.)*; Belladenal *(Sandoz, Canad.; Wander, UK; Sandoz, USA)*; Belladenal-S *(Sandoz, USA)*; Belladonna-Neutralon *(Schering, Austral.)*; Bellergal *(Sandoz, Austral.; Sandoz, Canad.; Sandoz, UK; Sandoz, USA)*; Bellocarb *(Sinclair, UK)*; Boldolaxine *(Simes, Austral.)*; Cafergot P-B *(Sandoz, USA)*; Cafergot-PB *(Sandoz, Austral.; Sandoz, Canad.)*; Carbellon *(Torbet Laboratories, UK)*; Chardonna *(Rorer, USA)*; Climacteric Dellipsoids D19 *(Pilsworth, UK)*; Fenobelladine *(Medo, UK)*; Neutradonna *(Nicholas, UK)*; Neutradonna Sed *(Nicholas, UK)*; Orgraine *(Organon, UK)*; Purgoids *(Evans Medical, UK)*; Rhinitis *(Lilly, USA)*; Stomachic Dellipsoids D20 *(Pilsworth, UK)*; Tussifans *(Norton, UK)*; Wigraine *(Organon, Canad.)*; Wigraine-PB *(Organon, USA)*; Wyanoids *(Wyeth, USA)*.

341-l

Benapryzine Hydrochloride *(BANM, USAN)*.

AP-1288; Benaprizine Hydrochloride *(rINNM)*; BRL-1288. 2-(*N*-Ethyl-*N*-propylamino)ethyl benzilate hydrochloride.
$C_{21}H_{27}NO_3$, HCl=377.9.

CAS — 22487-42-9 (benapryzine); 3202-55-9 (hydrochloride).

Benapryzine hydrochloride is an antimuscarinic agent with actions and uses similar to those of benzhexol (see p.527). It has been used in the symptomatic treatment of parkinsonism. It has also been used to alleviate the extrapyramidal syndrome induced by drugs such as the phenothiazine derivatives but is of no value against tardive dyskinesias, which may be exacerbated. Usual doses of 50 mg three or four times daily have been given.
Transition to or from benapryzine therapy should be gradual otherwise symptoms may be aggravated.

EXTRAPYRAMIDAL DISORDERS. For a review of the role of antimuscarinic agents in the treatment of drug-induced extrapyramidal disorders, see p.522.

Parkinsonism. For discussion of the treatment of parkinsonism, including reference to the role of antimuscarinic agents, see under Levodopa, p.1019.

Proprietary Names and Manufacturers
Brizin *(Beecham Research, UK)*.

342-y

Benzhexol Hydrochloride *(BANM)*.

Cloridrato de Triexilfenidila; Cyclodolum; Trihexyphenidyl Hydrochloride *(USAN, rINNM)*; Trihexyphenidyli Hydrochloridum; Trihexyphenidylium Chloratum. 1-Cyclohexyl-1-phenyl-3-piperidinopropan-1-ol hydrochloride.
$C_{20}H_{31}NO$, HCl=337.9.

CAS — 144-11-6 (benzhexol); 52-49-3 (hydrochloride).

Pharmacopoeias. In *Br., Braz., Chin., Cz., Egypt., Fr., Int., Jpn, Jug., Nord., Roum., Rus., Turk.,* and *U.S.*

A white or creamy-white, odourless or almost odourless, crystalline powder.
Slightly **soluble** in water; soluble 1 in 22 of alcohol, 1 in 15 of chloroform, and 1 in 10 of methyl alcohol. A saturated solution in water has a pH of 5.2 to 6.2. **Store** in airtight containers.

INCOMPATIBILITY. Benzhexol hydrochloride and thioridazine hydrochloride oral mixtures were physically compatible for approximately 30 minutes at 4° and 25°.— W. A. Parker, *Can. J. Hosp. Pharm.*, 1984, *37*, 133.

Adverse Effects and Treatment

As for Atropine Sulphate, p.523. In some patients benzhexol may produce severe mental disturbances, excitement, nausea, and vomiting. For minor reactions the dose may be reduced until tolerance has developed, but with more severe reactions administration of the drug should be discontinued and treatment at a lower dosage, or with another drug, resumed after several days.

ABUSE. Benzhexol hydrochloride had been abused by young schizophrenic patients. Several patients had presented with an acute brain syndrome after taking excessive amounts.— P. Marriott (letter), *Br. med. J.*, 1976, *1*, 152.

A study of 21 cases of benzhexol abuse to induce euphoria. Six of the abusers reported memory impairment and learning difficulty, persisting for several weeks after acute intoxication had cleared.— J. A. Crawshaw and P. E. Mullen, *Br. J. Psychiat.*, 1984, *145*, 300.

A report of 28 cases of abuse of antimuscarinic drugs among psychiatric patients. Benzhexol appeared to be the most commonly abused antimuscarinic; orphenadrine and biperiden were also popular; procyclidine and benztropine were the least abused. These preferences might reflect differences in the mood-elevating properties of the drugs or simply their availability.— G. P. Pullen *et al.*, *Br. med. J.*, 1984, *289*, 612.

DYSKINESIA. A report of 3 patients who were being treated for depression or psychoses with phenothiazines in whom benzhexol provoked or exacerbated tardive dyskinesia.— L. G. Kiloh *et al.*, *Med. J. Aust.*, 1973, *2*, 591. Choreiform movements induced in a 73-year-old man following long-term benzhexol therapy for Parkinsonism.— R. W. Warne and S. S. Gubbay, *ibid.*, 1979, *1*, 465.

EFFECTS ON MEMORY. Benzhexol 2 mg by mouth significantly impaired memory function compared with placebo in a study in 13 elderly patients.— G. Potamianos and J. M. Kellett, *Br. J. Psychiat.*, 1982, *140*, 470. In a study in 19 parkinsonian patients examined before, whilst, and after receiving benzhexol hydrochloride 5 mg or orphenadrine citrate 50 mg, both twice daily, results supported the theory that standard antimuscarinic therapy may have a deleterious effect on memory.— M. Sadeh *et al.*, *Archs Neurol., Chicago*, 1982, *39*, 666. See also: C. D. Marsden *et al.*, *J. Neurol. Neurosurg. Psychiat.*, 1984, *47*, 1166 (in children).

OVERDOSAGE. A 34-year-old woman took 300 mg of benzhexol hydrochloride with suicidal intent; 24 hours later she developed a toxic reaction with widely dilated pupils, dry skin, and visual hallucinations. After 3 to 4 days the hallucinations were replaced by illusions; complete recovery occurred after a week, with no special treatment.— J. V. Ananth *et al.* (letter), *Can. med. Ass. J.*, 1970, *103*, 771. See also G. F. Morgenstern, *ibid.*, 1962, *87*, 79.

Precautions

As for Atropine Sulphate, p.524.
Patients with arteriosclerosis or a history of idiosyncrasy to other drugs may be more likely to develop severe mental reactions to benzhexol.

INTERACTIONS. States of excitement, confusion, and hallucinations were precipitated in 3 elderly patients who took benzhexol 2 mg thrice daily in addition to imipramine or desipramine.— S. C. Rogers (letter), *Br. med. J.*, 1967, *1*, 500.

A patient experienced almost total loss of teeth resulting from extreme dryness of the mouth induced by concomitant administration of benzhexol, imipramine, and diphenhydramine.— J. A. Winer and S. Bahn, *Archs gen. Psychiat.*, 1967, *16*, 239.

The side-effects of benzhexol hydrochloride were enhanced by concomitant administration of amantadine causing nocturnal confusion and hallucinations typical of antimuscarinic overdose; reduction of dosage of either amantadine or the antimuscarinic agent alleviated the side-effects.— R. S. Schwab *et al.*, *J. Am. med. Ass.*, 1969, *208*, 1168.

For studies of the effect of benzhexol on the plasma concentrations of chlorpromazine, see Chlorpromazine, p.723.

Absorption and Fate

Benzhexol hydrochloride is well absorbed from the gastro-intestinal tract and has been stated to exert an action within 1 hour of a dose by mouth.

Uses and Administration

Benzhexol hydrochloride is an antimuscarinic agent with actions similar to those of atropine (see p.524). It also has a direct antispasmodic action on smooth muscle.
Benzhexol is employed mainly in the symptomatic treatment of parkinsonism; it is also used to alleviate the extrapyramidal syndrome induced by drugs such as phenothiazines, but is of no value against tardive dyskinesias, which may be exacerbated. The frequency and duration of oculogyric crises are reduced and antimuscarinic therapy may be of particular benefit in reducing sialorrhoea. It has been used in the treatment of spasmodic torticollis and other dyskinesias.
Benzhexol hydrochloride is given in 3 or 4 divided doses daily before or with food. The initial dose of 1 or 2 mg daily is gradually increased by 2-mg increments to 6 to 10 mg daily according to the response of the patient; for advanced cases, 12 to 15 mg or even more may be needed daily. As a rule, postencephalitic patients tolerate and require the larger doses; elderly patients may require smaller doses. Once maintenance dosage has been established benzhexol hydrochloride may also be given as controlled-release capsules once or twice daily.
Antimuscarinic treatment of parkinsonism should never be terminated suddenly and it is usual when changing from one drug to another to withdraw the one in small amounts while gradually increasing the dose of the other.
Benzhexol hydrochloride may be given with other drugs used for the relief of parkinsonism, such as other antimuscarinic agents, levodopa, and amantadine; reduced dosage may be needed.

ADMINISTRATION IN RENAL FAILURE. The normal half-life for benzhexol of 13 hours was prolonged in end-stage renal failure. Benzhexol could be given in usual doses to patients with renal failure.— W. M. Bennett *et al.*, *Am. J. Kidney Dis.*, 1983, *3*, 155.

DYSTONIAS. A patient with severe hemidystonia that was temporarily relieved by nicotine chewing-gum subsequently achieved amelioration of his spasms, lasting for about 4 hours, with benzhexol 2 mg daily.— A. J. Lees (letter), *Lancet*, 1984, *2*, 871.

In a crossover study in 31 patients with torsion dystonia 22 were considered to have had a clinically significant response to benzhexol in doses up to 30 mg daily (7.5 mg four times daily), and despite the high dose benzhexol was generally well tolerated. On follow-up for a mean of 2.4 years, 21 continued to take benzhexol at a mean daily dose of 40 mg, and 13 were considered to have obtained considerable or dramatic benefit from the drug. Although benzhexol is effective, it only provides symptomatic therapy and there is no evidence that it affects the course of dystonia.— R. E. Burke *et al.*, *Neurology*, 1986, *36*, 160.

See also: *Lancet*, 1985, *1*, 321.

EXTRAPYRAMIDAL DISORDERS. For a review of the role of antimuscarinic agents in the treatment of drug-induced extrapyramidal disorders see p.522.

Parkinsonism. For discussion of the treatment of parkinsonism, including reference to the role of antimuscarinic agents, see under Levodopa, p.1019.

Preparations

Benzhexol Tablets *(B.P.)*. Contain benzhexol hydrochloride.

Trihexyphenidyl Hydrochloride Elixir *(U.S.P.)*. An elixir containing benzhexol hydrochloride 37.2 to 42.8 mg in each 100 mL with 4.5 to 5.5% of alcohol. pH 2 to 3.

Trihexyphenidyl Hydrochloride Extended-release Capsules *(U.S.P.)*. Contain benzhexol hydrochloride.

Trihexyphenidyl Hydrochloride Tablets *(U.S.P.)*. Contain benzhexol hydrochloride.

Proprietary Preparations

Artane *(Lederle, UK)*. *Tablets*, scored, benzhexol hydrochloride 2 and 5 mg.

Bentex (formerly known as Artilan) *(Steinhard, UK)*. *Tablets*, scored, benzhexol hydrochloride 2 and 5 mg.

Broflex *(Bio-Medical, UK)*. *Syrup*, benzhexol hydrochloride 5 mg/5 mL.

Proprietary Names and Manufacturers

Anti-Spas *(Protea, Austral.)*; Aparkane *(ICN, Canad.)*; Apo-Trihex *(Apotex, Canad.)*; Artane *(Lederle, Austral.; Belg.; Lederle, Canad.; Denm.; Théraplix, Fr.; Cyanamid-Novalis, Ger.; Cyanamid, Ital.; Neth.; Norw.; Lederle, S.Afr.; Cyanamid, Spain; Swed.; Lederle, Switz.; Lederle, UK; Lederle, USA)*; Artilan *(Steinhard, UK)*; Bentex *(Steinhard, UK)*; Broflex *(Bio-Medical, UK)*; Novohexidyl *(Novopharm, Canad.)*; Paralest *(Neth.)*; Pargitan *(Kabi, Swed.)*; Parkinane Retard *(Lederle, Fr.)*; Peragit *(GEA, Denm.; Nyco, Norw.)*; Peragit Gea *(Ital.)*; Pipanol *(Ital.)*; Tremin *(Schering, USA)*; Trixyl *(Canad.)*.

343-j

Benzilonium Bromide *(BAN, USAN, rINN)*.

CI-379; CN-20172-3; PU-239. 3-Benziloyloxy-1,1-diethylpyrrolidinium bromide.
$C_{22}H_{28}BrNO_3$=434.4.

CAS — 1050-48-2.

Benzilonium bromide is a quaternary ammonium antimuscarinic agent with peripheral effects similar to those of atropine (see p.524). It is used as an adjunct in the treatment of peptic ulcer and to relieve visceral spasms. The usual initial dose is 10 mg by mouth three times daily before food, increasing according to the patient's need. Doses of 35 mg twice daily as sustained-release tablets have also been given.

The use of benzilonium bromide in cosmetics is prohibited in the *UK*.

Proprietary Names and Manufacturers

Ortyn Retard *(Parke, Davis, Norw.)*; Portyn *(Belg.; Parke, Davis, UK)*; Ulcoban *(Parke, Davis, Denm.; Parke, Davis, Norw.; Parke, Davis, Swed.)*.

344-z

Benztropine Mesylate *(BANM, USAN)*.

Benzatropine Mesilate *(rINNM)*; Benzatropine Methanesulfonate. (1*R*,3*r*,5*S*)-3-Benzhydryloxytropane methanesulphonate.
$C_{21}H_{25}NO,CH_4O_3S$=403.5.

CAS — 86-13-5 (benztropine); 132-17-2 (mesylate).

Pharmacopoeias. In *Br.*, *Nord.*, and *U.S.*

A white, odourless or almost odourless, slightly hygroscopic, crystalline powder.

Soluble 1 in 0.7 of water and 1 in 1.5 of alcohol; practically insoluble in ether. Solutions for injection are **sterilised** by autoclaving. The *B.P.* and *U.S.P.* injections have a pH of 5.0 to 8.0. **Store** in airtight containers.

Adverse Effects and Treatment

As for Atropine Sulphate, p.523. Drowsiness may be severe in some patients (see also Precautions). In some patients benztropine may produce severe mental disturbances and excitement. For minor reactions the dose may be reduced until tolerance has developed, but with more severe reactions administration of the drug should be discontinued and treatment at a lower dosage, or with another drug, resumed later.

ABUSE. For a report of abuse of antimuscarinic agents, including benztropine, in psychiatric patients, see under Benzhexol Hydrochloride, p.527.

EFFECTS ON BODY TEMPERATURE. For reports of fatal heat stroke in patients receiving benztropine and antipsychotic drugs concomitantly, see Interactions, under Precautions, below.

EFFECTS ON THE GASTRO-INTESTINAL TRACT. For a report of ileus in 2 patients taking benztropine and mesoridazine concomitantly, see Interactions, under Precautions, below.

Precautions

As for Atropine Sulphate, p.524.

Benztropine causes drowsiness and patients so affected should not drive or operate machinery. Patients should abstain from alcohol.

INTERACTIONS. A report of paralytic ileus developing in 2 patients (fatal in one) taking benztropine mesylate and mesoridazine concomitantly.— L. C. Wade and G. L. Ellenor, *Drug Intell. & clin. Pharm.*, 1980, *14*, 17.

A report of fatal heat stroke in a patient receiving benztropine mesylate concomitantly with chlorpromazine, following exposure to an ambient temperature of 35° (95°F).— A. N. Stadnyk and J. D. Glezos, *Can. med. Ass. J.*, 1983, *128*, 957. A similar report in a patient receiving benztropine mesylate, methotrimeprazine, and fluphenazine decanoate concomitantly.— F. Tyndel and R. Labonté (letter), *ibid.*, *129*, 680.

Uses and Administration

Benztropine mesylate is an antimuscarinic agent with actions and uses similar to those of benzhexol (see p.527); it also has antihistaminic and local anaesthetic properties. Following an oral dose its action has been stated to occur in 1 to 2 hours and last for 24 hours. Its actions in parkinsonism are cumulative, and may not be manifest for several days after beginning therapy.

It is used for the symptomatic treatment of parkinsonism. It is also used to alleviate the extrapyramidal syndrome induced by drugs such as the phenothiazine derivatives but is of no value against tardive dyskinesias, which may be exacerbated.

Benztropine mesylate is given by mouth in a usual initial daily dose of 0.5 to 1 mg in idiopathic parkinsonism. Patients with post-encephalitic parkinsonism often tolerate an initial dose of 2 mg. The dose may be gradually increased by 500 µg every 5 to 6 days until the optimum dose for each individual patient is reached. This is usually 2 to 6 mg a day, and may be given as a single dose, usually at bedtime, or in divided doses according to the requirements and tolerance of the patient.

In the management of drug-induced extrapyramidal disorders doses of 1 to 4 mg once or twice daily have been given orally or parenterally.

In emergency, benztropine mesylate may be injected intramuscularly or intravenously in a dose of 1 to 2 mg; intramuscular administration is reported to produce an effect as quickly as intravenous administration, so the latter is rarely necessary. Transition to or from benztropine therapy should be gradual otherwise symptoms may be aggravated.

The use of benztropine mesylate in cosmetics is prohibited in the *UK*.

EXTRAPYRAMIDAL DISORDERS. For a review of the role of antimuscarinic agents in the treatment of drug-induced extrapyramidal disorders, see p.522.

Parkinsonism. Results in *mice* suggesting that benztropine might be able to prevent parkinsonism induced by 1-methyl-4-phenyl-1,2,3,6-tetrahydropyridine (MPTP)— A. J. Bradbury *et al.* (letter), *Lancet*, 1985, *1*, 1444.

For discussion of the treatment of parkinsonism, including reference to the role of antimuscarinic agents, see under Levodopa, p.1019.

Preparations

Benztropine Injection *(B.P.)*. Contains benztropine mesylate.

Benztropine Mesylate Injection *(U.S.P.)*

Benztropine Mesylate Tablets *(U.S.P.)*

Benztropine Tablets *(B.P.)*. Contain benztropine mesylate.

Proprietary Preparations

Cogentin *(Merck Sharp & Dohme, UK)*. *Tablets*, scored, benztropine mesylate 2 mg.
Injection, benztropine mesylate 1 mg/mL, in ampoules of 2 mL.

Proprietary Names and Manufacturers

Bensylate *(ICN, Canad.)*; Cogentin *(Merck Sharp & Dohme, Austral.; Belg.; Merck Sharp & Dohme, Canad.; Merck Sharp & Dohme, Denm.; Neth.; Merck Sharp & Dohme, Norw.; MSD, Swed.; Merck Sharp & Dohme, UK; Merck Sharp & Dohme, USA)*; Cogentine *(Fr.)*; Cogentinol *(Astra, Ger.)*.

345-c

Bevonium Methylsulphate *(BAN)*.

Bevonium Metilsulfate *(rINN)*; Bevonum Metylsulfat; CG-201; Piribenzil Methyl Sulphate. 2-Benziloyloxymethyl-1,1-dimethylpiperidinium methylsulphate.
$C_{22}H_{28}NO_3,CH_3O_4S$=465.6.

CAS — 33371-53-8 (bevonium); 5205-82-3 (methylsulphate).

Bevonium methylsulphate is a quaternary ammonium antimuscarinic agent with peripheral effects similar to those of atropine (see p.524). It has been given in the symptomatic treatment of visceral spasms.

Proprietary Names and Manufacturers

Acabel *(Grünenthal, Ger.; Sigmatau, Ital.; Grünenthal, S.Afr.)*; Dalys *(Arg.)*; Spalgo *(Scharper, Ital.)*.

346-k

Biperiden *(BAN, USAN, rINN)*.

1-(Bicyclo[2.2.1]hept-5-en-2-yl)-1-phenyl-3-piperidinopropan-1-ol.
$C_{21}H_{29}NO$=311.5.

CAS — 514-65-8.

Pharmacopoeias. In *U.S.*

A white or almost white, odourless or almost odourless, crystalline powder. Practically **insoluble** in water; sparingly soluble in alcohol; freely soluble in chloroform. **Store** in well-closed containers. Protect from light.

347-a

Biperiden Hydrochloride *(BANM, USAN, rINNM)*.

$C_{21}H_{29}NO,HCl$=347.9.

CAS — 1235-82-1.

Pharmacopoeias. In *U.S.*

A white, almost odourless, crystalline powder. Slightly **soluble** in water, alcohol, chloroform, and ether; sparingly soluble in methyl alcohol. **Store** in airtight containers. Protect from light.

348-t

Biperiden Lactate *(BANM, USAN, rINNM)*.

$C_{21}H_{29}NO,C_3H_6O_3$=401.5.

CAS — 7085-45-2.

Pharmacopoeias. The *U.S.P.* includes Biperiden Lactate Injection.

Solutions for injection have a pH of 4.8 to 5.8. They should be **protected** from light.

Adverse Effects, Treatment, and Precautions

As for Atropine Sulphate, p.523.

Parenteral administration may be followed by slight transient hypotension.

Biperiden may cause drowsiness and patients so affected should not drive or operate machinery. Patients should abstain from alcohol.

ABUSE. For a report of abuse of antimuscarinic agents, including biperiden, in psychiatric patients, see under Benzhexol Hydrochloride, p.527.

Uses and Administration

Biperiden is an antimuscarinic agent with actions and uses similar to those of benzhexol (see p.527) but with more potent antinicotinic properties.

It is used in the symptomatic treatment of parkinsonism. It may also be used to alleviate the extrapyramidal syndrome induced by drugs such as the phenothiazine derivatives but is of no value against tardive dyskinesias, which may be exacerbated.

Biperiden is administered by mouth as the hydrochloride and by injection as the lactate.

The initial dose by mouth is 1 mg of the hydrochloride twice daily, gradually increased over several days according to the needs of the patient. The usual optimum maintenance dosage varies from 1 to 4 mg three times daily.

For a rapid effect in acute drug-induced dystonic reactions biperiden lactate 2 mg may be given by intramuscular or slow intravenous injection and repeated every 30 minutes if needed up to a maximum of 4 doses; higher doses of up to 5 mg have been given.

Transition to or from biperiden therapy should be gradual, otherwise symptoms may be aggravated.

ABSORPTION AND FATE. In a study of the pharmacokinetics and pharmacodynamics of biperiden following doses of 4 mg by mouth in 6 healthy subjects, peak plasma concentrations of between 3.9 and 6.3 ng per mL occurred after 1.5 hours and subsequently declined with a mean elimination half-life of 18.4 hours. Bioavailability was estimated at 29%. Effects on the CNS, as assessed by a self-rating score were maximal 2.5 hours after taking the dose but effects on the eye did not reach a maximum until after 5 to 6 hours and lasted 6 to 8 hours.— M. Hollmann *et al., Eur. J. clin. Pharmac.*, 1984, *27*, 619.

EXTRAPYRAMIDAL DISORDERS. For a review of the role of antimuscarinic agents in the treatment of drug-induced extrapyramidal disorders, see p.522.

Parkinsonism. For discussion of the treatment of parkinsonism, including reference to the role of antimuscarinic agents, see under Levodopa, p.1019.

Preparations

Biperiden Hydrochloride Tablets *(U.S.P.)*

Biperiden Lactate Injection *(U.S.P.)*. Biperiden Injection. A sterile solution in Water for Injections prepared from biperiden and lactic acid.

Proprietary Preparations

Akineton *(Abbott, UK). Tablets*, scored, biperiden hydrochloride 2 mg.

Injection, biperiden lactate 5 mg/mL, in ampoules of 1 mL.

Proprietary Names and Manufacturers of Biperiden Salts

Akineton *(Arg.; Schering, Austral.; Belg.; Knoll, Canad.; Knoll, Denm.; Biosédra, Fr.; Nordmark, Ger.; Knoll, Ital.; Neth.; Knoll, Norw.; Knoll, S.Afr.; Knoll-Made, Spain; Knoll, Swed.; Knoll, Switz.; Knoll, USA)*; Akineton Ampoules *(Abbott, UK)*; Akineton Tablets *(Abbott, UK)*; Akinophyl *(Fr.)*; Tasmolin *(Jpn)*.

349-x

Bornaprine Hydrochloride *(BANM, rINNM)*.

3-Diethylaminopropyl 2-phenylbicyclo[2.2.1]heptane-2-carboxylate hydrochloride.

$C_{21}H_{31}NO_2,HCl=365.9$.

CAS — 20448-86-6 (bornaprine); 26908-91-8 (hydrochloride).

Bornaprine hydrochloride is an antimuscarinic agent with actions and uses similar to those of benzhexol (see p.527) but it is claimed to be mainly effective against tremor. It is used in initial doses of 2 mg daily gradually increased to 6 to 12 mg daily according to the response of the patient.

Proprietary Names and Manufacturers

Sormodren *(Nordmark, Ger.; Knoll, Ital.; Knoll-Made, Spain)*.

350-y

Butropium Bromide *(rINN)*.

(−)-(1*R*,3*r*,5*S*)-8-(4-Butoxybenzyl)-3-[(*S*)-tropoyloxy]-tropanium bromide.

$C_{28}H_{38}BrNO_4=532.5$.

CAS — 29025-14-7.

Butropium bromide is a quaternary ammonium antimuscarinic agent with peripheral effects similar to those of atropine (see p.524). It has been used in the symptomatic treatment of visceral spasms in a dose of 10 mg three times daily by mouth; it has also been given in a dose of 4 mg daily subcutaneously.

Proprietary Names and Manufacturers

Coliopan *(Eisai, Jpn)*.

351-j

Buzepide Metiodide *(rINN)*.

Diphexamide Iodomethylate; FI-6146; Metazepium Iodide; R-661. 1-(3-Carbamoyl-3,3-diphenylpropyl)-1-methylperhydroazepinium iodide.

$C_{23}H_{31}IN_2O=478.4$.

CAS — 15351-05-0.

Buzepide metiodide is a quaternary ammonium antimuscarinic agent with peripheral effects similar to those of atropine (see p.524). It has been given with other compounds for the relief of visceral spasms and of rhinitis.

352-z

Caramiphen Hydrochloride *(BANM, rINNM)*.

2-Diethylaminoethyl 1-phenylcyclopentane-1-carboxylate hydrochloride.

$C_{18}H_{27}NO_2,HCl=325.9$.

CAS — 77-22-5 (caramiphen); 125-85-9 (hydrochloride).

Uses and Administration

Caramiphen hydrochloride is a weak antimuscarinic agent with actions similar to those of benzhexol (see p.527). It has been used similarly in the treatment of parkinsonism.

The edisylate is claimed to be antitussive and is given with a sympathomimetic in preparations for the symptomatic relief of coughs and colds.

Proprietary Names and Manufacturers of Caramiphen Edisylate

The following names have been used for multi-ingredient preparations containing caramiphen edisylate— Rescaps-D *(Geneva, USA)*; Tuss-Ade *(Schein, USA)*; Tuss-Ornade *(Smith Kline & French, Canad.; Smith Kline & French, USA)*.

353-c

Chlorphenoxamine Hydrochloride *(BANM, USAN, rINNM)*.

2-(4-Chloro-α-methylbenzhydryloxy)-*NN*-dimethylethylamine hydrochloride.

$C_{18}H_{22}ClNO,HCl=340.3$.

CAS — 77-38-3 (chlorphenoxamine); 562-09-4 (hydrochloride).

Pharmacopoeias. In *U.S.*

A white crystalline powder. **Soluble** 1 in 2 of water, 1 in 1.8 of alcohol, and 1 in 1.5 of chloroform; very soluble in methyl alcohol; soluble in acetone; practically insoluble in ether. **Store** in airtight containers. Protect from light.

Adverse Effects, Treatment, and Precautions

As for Atropine Sulphate, p.523. See also Adverse Effects of Antihistamines, p.443.

Absorption and Fate

Chlorphenoxamine is absorbed from the gastro-intestinal tract and has an onset of action after about 30 minutes and a duration of action of about 4 hours.

Uses and Administration

Chlorphenoxamine, a congener of diphenhydramine, has weak antimuscarinic actions; it also has antihistaminic, local anaesthetic, and skeletal muscle-relaxant properties. It has been used similarly to benzhexol (see p.527) in the symptomatic treatment of parkinsonism.

Transition to or from chlorphenoxamine therapy should be gradual, otherwise symptoms may be aggravated.

Chlorphenoxamine is also used for its antihistaminic properties in the symptomatic treatment of allergic conditions.

PARKINSONISM. For discussion of the treatment of parkinsonism, including reference to the role of antimuscarinic agents, see under Levodopa, p.1019.

Preparations

Chlorphenoxamine Hydrochloride Tablets *(U.S.P.)*

Proprietary Names and Manufacturers

Clorevan *(Evans Medical, UK)*; Phenoxene *(Dow, Canad.; Dow, USA: Merrell Dow, USA)*; Systral *(Asta, Belg.; Asta, Denm.; Lucien, Fr.; Degussa, Ger.; Asta, Neth.; Degussa, Switz.)*; Systraletten *(Asta, Ger.)*.

354-k

Clidinium Bromide *(BAN, USAN, rINN)*.

Ro-2-3773. 3-Benziloyloxy-1-methylquinuclidinium bromide.

$C_{22}H_{26}BrNO_3=432.4$.

CAS — 7020-55-5 (clidinium); 3485-62-9 (bromide).

Pharmacopoeias. In *U.S.*

A white or nearly white almost odourless crystalline powder. **Soluble** in water and alcohol; slightly soluble in ether. **Store** in airtight containers. Protect from light.

Adverse Effects, Treatment, and Precautions

As for Atropine Sulphate, p.523.

Patients taking clidinium with chlordiazepoxide may experience sedation and should not take charge of vehicles or operate machinery where loss of attention may lead to accidents.

Uses and Administration

Clidinium bromide is a quaternary ammonium antimuscarinic agent with peripheral effects similar to those of atropine (see p.524). It is used alone or in conjunction with chlordiazepoxide in the symptomatic treatment of peptic ulcer and other gastro-intestinal disorders. The usual dose of clidinium bromide is 2.5 mg three or four times a day before meals and at bedtime; this may be increased to 5 mg four times a day if necessary.

Preparations

Clidinium Bromide Capsules *(U.S.P.)*

Proprietary Names and Manufacturers

Quarzan *(Roche, USA)*.

The following names have been used for multi-ingredient preparations containing clidinium bromide— Apo-Chlorax *(Apotex, Canad.)*; Clipoxide *(Schein, USA)*; Corium *(ICN, Canad.)*; Librax *(Roche, Austral.; Roche, Canad.; Roche, USA)*; Libraxin *(Roche, UK)*.

355-a

Cyclopentolate Hydrochloride *(BANM, USAN, rINNM).*

Cloridrato de Ciclopentolato. 2-Dimethylaminoethyl 2-(1-hydroxycyclopentyl)-2-phenylacetate hydrochloride.

$C_{17}H_{25}NO_3,HCl = 327.9$.

CAS — 512-15-2 (cyclopentolate); 5870-29-1 (hydrochloride).

Pharmacopoeias. In *Br., Braz.,* and *U.S.*

A white crystalline powder, odourless or with an odour of phenylacetic acid. **Soluble** 1 in less than 1 of water and 1 in 5 of alcohol; practically insoluble in ether. A 1% solution in water has a pH of 4.5 to 5.5. Solutions may be **sterilised** by filtration. **Store** at a temperature not exceeding 8° in airtight containers.

Adverse Effects, Treatment, and Precautions

As for Atropine Sulphate, p.523.

Eye-drops of cyclopentolate hydrochloride may cause temporary irritation.

Of 66 patients who received one drop of 2% cyclopentolate eye-drops in each eye, 10 developed systemic toxicity of mild to moderate severity. The manifestations were: physical weakness, nausea, light-headedness, changes in emotional attitude, unprovoked weeping, and loss of equilibrium; tachycardia was always present but changes in blood pressure were insignificant. Nine of the 10 were female and spontaneous recovery occurred within 1 hour to several days. It is recommended that concentrations of cyclopentolate eye-drops above 1% should only be used when absolutely necessary.— K. J. Awan, *Ann. Ophthal.*, 1976, *8*, 695. For a report of fatal gastro-intestinal toxicity in 1 of 2 premature infants following the ocular administration of cyclopentolate 3 mg, as 6 drops of a 1% eye-drop solution, see C. R. Bauer *et al.*, *J. Pediat.*, 1973, *92*, 501.

Uses and Administration

Cyclopentolate hydrochloride is an antimuscarinic agent with actions similar to those of atropine (see p.524). It is used as eye-drops to produce cycloplegia and mydriasis. It acts more quickly than atropine and has a shorter duration of action; the maximum effect is produced 30 to 60 minutes after instillation; accommodation recovers within 24 hours but may be hastened if 1 or 2 drops of a 2% solution of pilocarpine are instilled.

For refraction, 1 drop of a 0.5% solution repeated after about 5 to 15 minutes is usually sufficient, but more deeply pigmented eyes may require a 1% solution. In some countries, higher strengths have been used.

Studies *in vivo* and *in vitro* showed that the mydriatic activity of the racemate of cyclopentolate hydrochloride was almost entirely due to the laevo-isomer.— S. A. Smith, *Br. J. clin. Pharmac.*, 1976, *3*, 503.

Cyclopentolate often gave great relief from pain in eye injuries; painful iris spasm could be relieved.— P. A. Gardiner, *Br. med. J.*, 1978, *2*, 1347.

Cyclopentolate eye-drops could be used in association with corticosteroid eye-drops to treat the chronic uveitis that occurred in approximately 10% of children with juvenile chronic arthritis.— A. W. Craft, *Prescribers' J.*, 1985, *25*, 75.

Preparations

Cyclopentolate Eye Drops *(B.P.).* CYC. Contain cyclopentolate hydrochloride.

Cyclopentolate Hydrochloride Ophthalmic Solution *(U.S.P.).* pH 3.0 to 5.5. Store at 15° to 30° in airtight containers.

Proprietary Preparations

Alcon Opulets Cyclopentolate *(Alcon, UK). Eye-drops,* cyclopentolate hydrochloride 1%, in single-use disposable applicators.

Minims Cyclopentolate Hydrochloride *(Smith & Nephew Pharmaceuticals, UK). Eye-drops,* cyclopentolate hydrochloride 0.5 and 1%, in single-use disposable applicators.

Mydrilate *(Boehringer Ingelheim, UK). Eye-drops,* cyclopentolate hydrochloride 0.5 and 1%.

Proprietary Names and Manufacturers

Ak-Pentolate *(Akorn, Canad.)*; Alcon Opulets Cyclopentolate *(Alcon, UK)*; Ciclolux *(Allergan, Ital.)*; Ciclopegic *(Llorens, Spain)*; Colircusi Ciclopejico *(Spain)*; Colirio Oculos Cicloplegic *(Spain)*; Cyclogyl *(Alcon, Austral.; Alcon, Canad.; Alcon, Denm.; Neth.; Alcon, S.Afr.; Alcon, Swed.; Alcon, Switz.; USA)*; Cyclopen *(Austral.)*; Cyclopentol Colircusi *(Belg.)*; Cyclopentolat Minims *(Smith & Nephew, Norw.; Smith & Nephew, Swed.)*; Cyplegin *(Jpn)*; Minims Cyclopentolate Hydrochloride *(Smith & Nephew, Austral.; Smith & Nephew, S.Afr.; Smith & Nephew Pharmaceuticals, UK)*; Mydplegic *(Canad.)*; Mydrilate *(Austral.; Boehringer Ingelheim, UK)*; Skiacol *(POS, Fr.)*; Zyklolat *(Mann, Ger.)*.

356-t

Cycrimine Hydrochloride *(BANM, rINNM).*

Cycriminium Chloride. 1-Cyclopentyl-1-phenyl-3-piperidinopropan-1-ol hydrochloride.

$C_{19}H_{29}NO,HCl = 323.9$.

CAS — 77-39-4 (cycrimine); 126-02-3 (hydrochloride).

Cycrimine hydrochloride is an antimuscarinic agent which has been used similarly to benzhexol (see p.527) in the symptomatic treatment of parkinsonism.

Proprietary Names and Manufacturers

Pagitan *(Lilly, Arg.)*; Pagitane *(Lilly, Austral.; Lilly, Ital.; Lilly, USA)*.

358-r

Dexetimide Hydrochloride *(BANM, rINNM).*

Dexbenzetimide Hydrochloride; Dexetimide Monohydrochloride; R-16470. (+)-(*S*)-2-(1-Benzyl-4-piperidyl)-2-phenylglutarimide hydrochloride; (+)-(*S*)-3-(1-Benzyl-4-piperidyl)-3-phenylpiperidine-2,6-dione hydrochloride.

$C_{23}H_{26}N_2O_2,HCl = 398.9$.

CAS — 21888-98-2 (dexetimide); 21888-96-0 (hydrochloride).

NOTE. Dexetimide is *USAN.*

Dexetimide hydrochloride 1.1 mg is approximately equivalent to 1 mg of dexetimide.

Dexetimide is a long-acting antimuscarinic agent with actions similar to those of benzhexol (see p.527). It has been used as the hydrochloride to alleviate neuroleptic-induced parkinsonism.

Proprietary Names and Manufacturers

Tremblex *(Johnson, Arg.; Janssen, Aust.; Janssen, Belg.; Gedeon Richter, Hung.; Brocades, Ital.; Janssen, Neth.; Janssen, Switz.)*.

360-z

Dicyclomine Hydrochloride *(BANM, USAN).*

Cloridrato de Dicicloverina; Dicycloverine Hydrochloride *(rINNM)*. 2-Diethylaminoethyl bicyclohexyl-1-carboxylate hydrochloride.

$C_{19}H_{35}NO_2,HCl = 346.0$.

CAS — 77-19-0 (dicyclomine); 67-92-5 (hydrochloride).

Pharmacopoeias. In *Br., Braz.,* and *U.S.*

A white or almost white, odourless or almost odourless, crystalline powder.

B.P. **solubilities** are: 1 in 20 of water, 1 in 5 of alcohol, and 1 in 2 of chloroform; practically insoluble in ether. The *U.S.P.* has: soluble 1 in 13 of water and 1 in 50 of acetone.

Adverse Effects, Treatment, and Precautions

As for Atropine Sulphate, p.523.

A report of severe apnoea following single doses of dicyclomine 10 mg (Merbentyl syrup) by mouth in 2 infants aged 5 and 6 weeks. The indiscriminate use of this drug for all manner of feeding problems is to be condemned.— J. Williams and R. Watkin-Jones, *Br. med. J.*, 1984, *288*, 901. Further reports: P. D. L. Edwards (letter), *ibid.*, 1230; H. Spoudeas and S. Shribman (letter), *ibid* (dicyclomine with dimethicone (Ovol drops)). During 1984 fourteen cases of respiratory distress, including apnoea, were reported worldwide in infants 3 months of age or younger in association with the administration of dicyclomine liquid preparations; there were several deaths. Although cause and effect had not been established Merrell Dow had contra-indicated Merbentyl syrup in infants under 6 months of age and it was no longer indicated in the treatment of infant colic.— P. M. Altman (letter), *Med. J. Aust.*, 1985, *142*, 579. Comment. Dicyclomine has been widely used for infantile colic for the past 30 years: it could be assumed that it is a 'safe' drug, but some individuals may always be hypersensitive to a particular drug, resulting in adverse effects or even death.— W. McBride (letter), *ibid.*, 620.

PREGNANCY AND THE NEONATE. For a review of the risks to the foetus of anti-emetic therapy during pregnancy, with particular reference to Debendox (Bendectin: dicyclomine with doxylamine and pyridoxine) see under Adverse Effects of Antihistamines, p.443.

Uses and Administration

Dicyclomine hydrochloride is an antimuscarinic agent with effects similar to but much weaker than those of atropine (see p.524); it also has a direct antispasmodic action.

Dicyclomine is used in gastro-intestinal spasm, particularly that associated with the irritable bowel syndrome, and is also given in association with antacids as an adjunct in the treatment of peptic ulcer. For adults, 10 to 20 mg of dicyclomine hydrochloride may be given 3 or 4 times daily; in the *USA*, subsequent increase to a maximum of 40 mg four times daily has been recommended where adverse effects permit. Children aged 6 months to 2 years may be given 5 to 10 mg 3 or 4 times daily, to a total daily dose not exceeding 40 mg; doses are usually given 15 minutes before feeds. Children aged 2 to 12 years may be given 10 mg three times daily. Dicyclomine hydrochloride is contra-indicated in children below the age of 6 months (see also under Adverse Effects, above).

Dicyclomine hydrochloride has been given intramuscularly in doses of 20 mg given 4 times daily to patients in whom oral therapy was temporarily impractical.

Dicyclomine also used to be given with an antihistamine and pyridoxine for the nausea and vomiting of early pregnancy, but there was no evidence of its effectiveness in such a combination which is now no longer in use (see p.443).

COLIC. Colic was eliminated in 15 of 24 infants receiving dicyclomine but only in 6 given placebo in a double-blind study. However there was no evidence that the effectiveness of dicyclomine resulted in improved temperament or sleep patterns.— M. Weissbluth *et al.*, *J. Pediat.*, 1984, *104*, 951. In a crossover study in 30 colicky infants with an average age of 4.5 weeks, 25 were considered to have improved while receiving dicyclomine hydrochloride 5 mg four times daily, and 17 while receiving placebo. Dicyclomine reduced, but did not abolish, crying in some colicky babies but it was the impression of the experimenters that reduction of symptoms was often limited and that psychological support may in many instances offer similar relief: the decision to prescribe dicyclomine to these otherwise healthy babies should be carefully considered.— C. P. Hwang and B. Danielsson, *Br. med. J.*, 1985, *291*, 1014.

For reports of adverse effects in infants aged less than 6 months given dicyclomine, including the view that such treatment should not be used, see under Adverse Effects, above.

URINARY INCONTINENCE. Reports of the use of dicyclomine in the management of incontinence: S. A. Awad *et al.*, *J. Urol., Baltimore*, 1977, *117*, 161; C. P. Fischer *et al.*, *ibid.*, 1978, *120*, 328.

Preparations

Dicyclomine Hydrochloride Capsules *(U.S.P.)*

Dicyclomine Hydrochloride Syrup *(U.S.P.).* Store in airtight containers.

Dicyclomine Hydrochloride Injection *(U.S.P.)*

Dicyclomine Hydrochloride Tablets *(U.S.P.)*

Dicyclomine Oral Solution *(B.P.).* Dicyclomine Elixir. Contains dicyclomine hydrochloride.

Dicyclomine Tablets *(B.P.).* Contain dicyclomine hydrochloride.

Proprietary Preparations

Merbentyl *(Merrell, UK). Tablets,* dicyclomine hydro-

chloride 10 and 20 mg.
Syrup, dicyclomine hydrochloride 10 mg/5 mL.

Proprietary Names and Manufacturers
Ametil *(Corvi, Ital.)*; Atumin *(Ger.)*; Babypasmil *(Arg.)*; Benacol *(USA)*; Bentyl *(Lepetit, Ital.; Lakeside, USA)*; Bentylol *(Merrell Dow, Canad.; Merrell Dow, Spain)*; Clomin *(SCS, S.Afr.)*; Colix *(S.Afr.)*; Cyclobec *(Canad.)*; Formulex *(ICN, Canad.)*; Icramin *(Jpn)*; Incron *(Jpn)*; Lomine *(Riva, Canad.)*; Mamiesan *(Jpn)*; Menospasm *(Canad.)*; Merbentyl *(Merrell Dow, Austral.; Mer-National, S.Afr.; Merrell, UK)*; Nomocramp *(S.Afr.)*; Or-Tyl *(Ortega, USA)*; Panakiron *(Jpn)*; Pasmin *(USA)*; Procyclomin *(Austral.)*; Protylol *(Pro Doc, Canad.)*; Sawamin *(Jpn)*; Spasmoban *(Trianon, Canad.)*; Tarestin *(Dibios, Spain)*; Viscerol *(Medic, Canad.)*; Wyovin *(NZ)*.

The following names have been used for multi-ingredient preparations containing dicyclomine hydrochloride—Abacid Plus *(Ticen, Eire)*; Debendox *(Merrell, UK)*; Diarrest *(Galen, UK)*; Diclophen *(Pro Doc, Canad.)*; Infacol-C *(Rosken, Austral.)*; Kolanticon *(Merrell, UK)*; Kolantyl *(Merrell, UK)*; Ovol *(Pharmax, UK)*.

NOTE. The name Bendectin has been used to denote a preparation containing dicyclomine hydrochloride.

361-c

Diethazine Hydrochloride *(BANM, rINNM)*.

Diaethazinium Chloratum; Eazamine Hydrochloride; RP-2987. 10-(2-Diethylaminoethyl)phenothiazine hydrochloride.
$C_{18}H_{22}N_2S,HCl=334.9$.

CAS — 60-91-3 (diethazine); 341-70-8 (hydrochloride).

Pharmacopoeias. In *Cz.* and *Fr.*

Diethazine hydrochloride is an antimuscarinic agent with actions and uses similar to those of ethopropazine hydrochloride (see p.532) but it is more toxic and bone marrow depression may occur.
In the treatment of parkinsonism 150 mg to 1.5 g has been given daily in divided doses by mouth according to response.

362-k

Difemerine Hydrochloride *(rINNM)*.

UP-57. 2-Dimethylamino-1,1-dimethylethyl benzilate hydrochloride.
$C_{20}H_{25}NO_3,HCl=363.9$.

CAS — 80387-96-8 (difemerine); 70280-88-5 (hydrochloride).

Difemerine hydrochloride is an antimuscarinic agent with effects similar to those of atropine (see p.524); it has also been claimed to possess a local anaesthetic action. It is used as an adjunct in the treatment of peptic ulcer and in the symptomatic treatment of visceral spasms, in doses of 7.5 to 10 mg daily by mouth. It has been given intramuscularly in doses of 1 to 3 mg daily and rectally in doses of 15 to 30 mg daily; it has also been given by the intravenous route.

Proprietary Names and Manufacturers
Luostyl *(UPSA, Fr.)*.

363-a

Dihexyverine Hydrochloride *(USAN, rINNM)*.

Dihexiverine Hydrochloride; JL-1078. 2-Piperidinoethyl bicyclohexyl-1-carboxylate hydrochloride.
$C_{20}H_{35}NO_2,HCl=358.0$.

CAS — 561-77-3 (dihexyverine); 5588-25-0 (hydrochloride).

Dihexyverine hydrochloride is an antimuscarinic agent with effects similar to those of atropine (see p.524). It is given in the symptomatic treatment of visceral spasms in doses of 10 to 50 mg by mouth or 50 to 150 mg rectally daily. It has also been given in doses of 10 mg by intramuscular injection.

Proprietary Names and Manufacturers
Diverine *(Ital.)*; Metaspas *(ICN, Canad.)*; Seclin *(Panthox & Burck, Ital.)*; Spasmodex *(Crinex, Fr.)*; Spasmolevel *(Level, Spain)*.

12668-r

Dipenine Bromide *(BAN)*.

Diponium Bromide *(rINN)*; HL-267; SA-267. 2-(Dicyclopentylacetoxy)ethyltriethylammonium bromide.
$C_{20}H_{38}BrNO_2=404.4$.

CAS — 2001-81-2.

Dipenine bromide is a quaternary ammonium antimuscarinic agent with peripheral actions similar to those of atropine (see p.524). It has been used in the symptomatic treatment of visceral spasms.

References: G. Partsch *et al., Int. J. clin. Pharmacol. Res.*, 1983, *3*, 55.

Proprietary Names and Manufacturers
Unospaston *(Belg.)*.

364-t

Diphemanil Methylsulphate *(BAN)*.

Diphemanil Methylsulfate *(USAN)*; Diphemanil Metilsulfate *(rINN)*; Diphenmethanil Methylsulphate; Vagophemanil Methylsulphate. 4-Benzhydrylidene-1,1-dimethylpiperidinium methylsulphate.
$C_{20}H_{24}N,CH_3SO_4=389.5$.

CAS — 62-97-5.

Pharmacopoeias. In *U.S.*

A white or almost white, hygroscopic, crystalline powder with a faint characteristic odour.
Soluble 1 in 33 of water, of alcohol, and of chloroform. A 1% solution in water has a pH of 4 to 6. **Store** in airtight containers.

Adverse Effects, Treatment, and Precautions
As for Atropine Sulphate, p.523.

Absorption and Fate
Diphemanil methylsulphate is poorly absorbed from the gastro-intestinal tract. Its effects appear within 1 or 2 hours of a dose being taken, and last approximately 4 hours. It is excreted mainly in the urine; unabsorbed drug is excreted in the faeces.

Uses and Administration
Diphemanil methylsulphate is a quaternary ammonium antimuscarinic agent with peripheral effects similar to those of atropine (see p.524).
It is used as an adjunct in the treatment of peptic ulcer, and to relieve visceral spasms.
The usual dose is 100 mg given 3 or 4 times a day, adjusted according to the patient's needs. It has also been given in doses of 15 to 25 mg by subcutaneous or intramuscular injection.
Diphemanil methylsulphate is also used topically in the treatment of excessive sweating as a 2% cream or powder.

Preparations
Diphemanil Methylsulfate Tablets *(U.S.P.)*. Contain diphemanil methylsulphate.

Proprietary Names and Manufacturers
Prantal *(Essex, Austral.; Unicet, Fr.; Essex, Ital.; Schering, USA)*; Prentol *(Essex, Spain)*.

365-x

Emepronium Bromide *(BAN, rINN)*.

Ethyldimethyl(1-methyl-3,3-diphenylpropyl)ammonium bromide.
$C_{20}H_{28}BrN=362.4$.

CAS — 27892-33-7 (emepronium); 3614-30-0 (bromide).

18635-j

Emepronium Carrageenate *(BAN)*.

Adverse Effects, Treatment, and Precautions
As for Atropine Sulphate, p.523.
To avoid oesophageal ulceration, tablets of emepronium bromide should always be swallowed with an adequate volume of water, and patients should always be in the sitting or standing position while, and for 10 to 15 minutes after, taking the tablets. Emepronium is contra-indicated in patients with symptoms or signs of oesophageal obstruction or with pre-existing oesophagitis.
The carrageenate is claimed to have less of an irritant effect on the oesophagus than the bromide.

BUCCAL AND OESOPHAGEAL ULCERATION. Because of the hygroscopic nature of emepronium bromide tablets they should be swallowed with water to prevent any tablet sticking to the oesophageal mucosa with possible risk of ulceration. Patients with difficulties in swallowing tablets should take emepronium bromide tablets as a slurry in water.— Å. Pilbrant, *Kabi, Swed.* (letter), *Lancet*, 1977, *1*, 749.

When an irritant medication is held up in the oesophagus oesophagitis develops which may progress to oesophageal ulceration and even stricture, but oesophagitis caused by emepronium bromide usually heals without stricture formation and no deaths have been reported.— *Drug & Ther. Bull.*, 1981, *19*, 33. and *ibid.*, 1985, *23*, 73. Emepronium bromide is known to cause stricturing in addition to producing a self-perpetuating lesion. In 3 patients in the author's experience emepronium produced such a violent reaction of the germinal layer of the squamous epithelium that the cells were mistaken for those of squamous carcinoma.— D. A. W. Edwards, *Postgrad. med. J.*, 1984, *60*, 737.

A report of extensive oral ulceration in an elderly patient receiving emepronium bromide 100 mg three times daily. The lesions resolved on withdrawal of emepronium and treatment with chlorhexidine gluconate mouthwash to control secondary infection.— A. J. Duxbury and E. P. Turner, *Br. dent. J.*, 1982, *152*, 94.

Absorption and Fate
Emepronium is incompletely absorbed from the gastro-intestinal tract and is mainly excreted unchanged in the urine and faeces. It does not cross the blood-brain barrier in therapeutic doses.

In 4 healthy men given an intramuscular injection of emepronium bromide 25 mg, the maximum serum concentration (about 450 ng per mL) was reached after 15 minutes and the serum half-life was 1½ to 2¼ hours. Between 70 and 90% of the dose was excreted unchanged in faeces and urine. In 5 subjects given 0.15, 0.6, or 1.2 g of emepronium bromide by mouth, the peak serum concentrations were 8 to 100 ng per mL, 99 to 301 ng per mL, and 174 to 802 ng per mL respectively; only about 1 to 2% of the dose appeared in the urine suggesting that only 2.5 to 5% of the dose had been absorbed.— A. Sundwall *et al., Eur. J. clin. Pharmac.*, 1973, *6*, 191.

Uses and Administration
Emepronium is a quaternary ammonium antimuscarinic agent with peripheral effects similar to those of atropine (see p.524).
It is mainly used to reduce the muscular tone of the urinary bladder in postoperative vesical tenesmus and in urinary frequency. The usual dose is 200 to 250 mg of the bromide, or its equivalent as the carrageenate, 3 times daily; in nocturnal frequency 200 to 500 mg of the bromide or its equivalent is given in the evening before bed. The bromide has also been given by subcutaneous or intramuscular injection in a dose of 25 mg three times daily.

Emepronium bromide is the best known of the antimuscarinic drugs used in urinary incontinence. It is effective by injection but is poorly and irregularly absorbed by mouth and it has been questioned whether it does anything at all by the oral route.— B. Isaacs, *Prescribers' J.*, 1981, *21*, 285.

In a crossover study in 19 women with urge incontinence emepronium bromide 200 mg, flavoxate hydrochloride 200 mg or placebo were taken 4 times daily but only placebo treatment resulted in a significant reduction in episodes of incontinence and nocturia; comparisons between the three treatments failed to show significant differences. Nine of the patients preferred the placebo treatment, whereas 4 preferred emepronium, and 3, flavoxate. The results suggest that placebo rather than active drug may be the treatment of choice in these patients.— H. H. Meyhoff *et al., Br. J. Urol.*, 1983, *55*, 34.

A review of cancer pain, including the view that emepronium is of value in bladder or urethral spasm secondary to tumour, infection, or catheter.— M. J. Baines, *Postgrad. med. J.*, 1984, *60*, 852.

For a study comparing the effectiveness of emepronium in urinary frequency, urgency, and incontinence with that of terodiline, see under Terodiline p.543.

Proprietary Names and Manufacturers of Emepronium Salts

Cetiprin *(Denm.; Eire; Neth.; KabiVitrum, Norw.; Kabi, S.Afr.; Kabi, Swed.; KabiVitrum, Switz.; KabiVitrum, UK)*; Detrulisin *(Bonomelli, Ital.)*; Hexanium *(Fides, Spain)*; Uro-Ripirin *(Kabi, Ger.)*.

367-f

Ethopropazine Hydrochloride *(BANM, USAN)*.

Cloridrato de Profenamina; Isothazine Hydrochloride; Profenamine Hydrochloride *(rINNM)*; Profenamini Hydrochloridum; Prophenamini Chloridum. 10-(2-Diethylaminopropyl)phenothiazine hydrochloride.

$C_{19}H_{24}N_2S,HCl=348.9$.

CAS — 522-00-9 (ethopropazine); 1094-08-2 (hydrochloride).

Pharmacopoeias. In *Braz., Egypt., Ind., Int.,* and *U.S.*

A white or slightly off-white, odourless, crystalline powder; it darkens in colour on exposure to light. **Soluble** 1 in 225 of water, 1 in 35 of alcohol, and 1 in 7 of chloroform; sparingly soluble in acetone; practically insoluble in ether. **Store** in airtight containers. Protect from light.

Adverse Effects, Treatment, and Precautions

As for Atropine Sulphate, p.523.

Drowsiness and confusion are common in patients taking ethopropazine; patients should not take charge of vehicles or operate machinery where loss of attention may lead to accidents. Ethopropazine may also cause muscle cramps, paraesthesia, and a sense of heaviness in the limbs, epigastric discomfort, and nausea.

Ethopropazine is a phenothiazine derivative— for adverse effects associated with phenothiazines, see p.706.

PREGNANCY AND THE NEONATE. Ethopropazine was excreted in the milk of lactating mothers in amounts too small to affect the baby.— J. J. Rowan (letter), *Pharm. J.*, 1976, *2*, 184.

Uses and Administration

Ethopropazine hydrochloride is a phenothiazine derivative with antimuscarinic, adrenergic-blocking, slight antihistaminic, local anaesthetic and ganglion-blocking properties. It has been used in the symptomatic treatment of parkinsonism. It can also be used to alleviate the extrapyramidal syndrome induced by drugs such as other phenothiazine compounds but is of no value against tardive dyskinesias, which may be exacerbated.

It has been used in a usual dose of 50 mg once or twice daily initially gradually increased to 500 or 600 mg daily in divided doses, according to the response of the patient; higher doses have been given. Transition to or from ethopropazine therapy should be gradual, otherwise symptoms may be aggravated.

Ethopropazine has also been tried in the symptomatic treatment of hepatolenticular degeneration and congenital athetosis.

The hybenzate has been used similarly.

The use of ethopropazine and its salts in cosmetics is prohibited in the *UK*.

EXTRAPYRAMIDAL DISORDERS. For a review of the role of antimuscarinic agents in the treatment of drug-induced extrapyramidal disorders, see p.522.

Parkinsonism. For discussion of the treatment of parkinsonism, including reference to the role of antimuscarinic agents, see under Levodopa, p.1019.

Preparations

Ethopropazine Hydrochloride Tablets *(U.S.P.)*

Proprietary Names and Manufacturers

Lysivane *(May & Baker, Austral.; May & Baker, UK)*; Parkin *(Jpn)*; Parsidol *(Sévenet, Fr.; Parke, Davis, USA)*; Parsitan *(Rhône-Poulenc, Canad.)*; Parsotil *(Spain)*.

368-d

Ethybenztropine Hydrobromide *(BANM)*.

Etybenzatropine Hydrobromide *(rINNM)*; Tropethydryline Hydrobromide; UK-738. (1*R*,3*r*,5*S*)-3-Benzhydryloxy-8-ethylnortropane hydrobromide.

$C_{22}H_{27}NO,HBr=402.4$.

CAS — 524-83-4 (ethybenztropine); 24815-25-6 (hydrobromide).

NOTE. Ethybenztropine is *USAN*.

Ethybenztropine hydrobromide 6.25 mg is approximately equivalent to 5 mg of ethybenztropine.

Ethybenztropine hydrobromide is an antimuscarinic agent with actions and uses similar to those of benzhexol (see p.527). It also has antihistaminic properties and patients receiving it should not take charge of vehicles or operate machinery where loss of attention may lead to accidents as it may cause sedation.

It has been used for the symptomatic treatment of parkinsonism and of the drug-induced extrapyramidal syndrome in doses equivalent to 5 to 30 mg of ethybenztropine daily. The hydrochloride has also been given by injection.

Proprietary Names and Manufacturers

Ponalid *(Sandoz, Aust.; Sandoz, Spain)*; Ponalide *(Sandoz-Wander, Belg.; Sandoz, Fr.)*.

12709-j

Ethylbenzhydramine Hydrochloride

β-Diethylaminoethylbenzhydryl Ether Hydrochloride; Diethylaminoethoxydiphenylmethane Hydrochloride; Etanautine Hydrochloride. 2-(Benzhydryloxy)triethylamine hydrochloride.

$C_{19}H_{25}NO,HCl=319.9$.

CAS — 642-58-0 (ethylbenzhydramine); 86-24-8 (hydrochloride).

NOTE. The name Etanautine was formerly applied to diphenhydramine monoacefyllinate.

Ethylbenzhydramine hydrochloride is an antimuscarinic agent with actions and uses similar to those of benzhexol (see p.527). It has been given by mouth in the symptomatic treatment of parkinsonism.

Proprietary Names and Manufacturers

PKM *(Montavit, Switz.)*.

369-n

Eucatropine Hydrochloride *(BANM, USAN, rINNM)*.

Clorhidrato de Euftalmina; Eucatropinium Chloride. 1,2,2,6-Tetramethyl-4-piperidyl mandelate hydrochloride.

$C_{17}H_{25}NO_3,HCl=327.9$.

CAS — 100-91-4 (eucatropine); 536-93-6 (hydrochloride).

Pharmacopoeias. In *Arg., Egypt., Mex.,* and *U.S.*

A white odourless granular powder. Very **soluble** in water; freely soluble in alcohol and chloroform; practically insoluble in ether. Solutions in water are neutral to litmus; the *U.S.P.* Ophthalmic Solution has a pH of 4 to 5. **Store** in airtight containers. Protect from light.

Eucatropine hydrochloride is an antimuscarinic agent with mydriatic properties similar to those of atropine (see p.524). It has little or no effect on accommodation. It has been applied as a 10% solution.

Preparations

Eucatropine Hydrochloride Ophthalmic Solution *(U.S.P.)*

370-k

Fentonium Bromide *(rINN)*.

Fa-402; Fentonii Bromidum; *N*-(4-Phenylphenacyl)-1-hyoscyaminium Bromide; Ketoscilium; Z-326. (−)-(1*R*,3*r*,5*S*)-8-(4-Phenylphenacyl)-3-[(*S*)-tropoyloxy]tropanium bromide.

$C_{31}H_{34}BrNO_4=564.5$.

CAS — 5868-06-4.

Fentonium bromide is a quaternary ammonium antimuscarinic agent with peripheral effects similar to those of atropine (see p.523). It is used as an adjunct in the treatment of peptic ulcer, and to relieve visceral spasms. It has been given in a usual dose of 20 mg by mouth three or four times daily; it has also been given intramuscularly.

Proprietary Names and Manufacturers

Ulcesium *(Inpharzam, Ger.; Zambon, Ital.)*.

371-a

Glycopyrronium Bromide *(BAN, rINN)*.

AHR 504; Glycopyrrolate *(USAN)*. 3-(α-Cyclopentylmandeloyloxy)-1,1-dimethylpyrrolidinium bromide.

$C_{19}H_{28}BrNO_3=398.3$.

CAS — 596-51-0.

Pharmacopoeias. In *Nord.* and *U.S.*

A white odourless crystalline powder. **Soluble** 1 in 4.2 of water and 1 in 30 of alcohol; slightly soluble in chloroform; practically insoluble in ether. **Incompatible** with alkalis. The *U.S.P.* injection has a pH of 2 to 3. **Store** in airtight containers.

The compatibility of glycopyrronium bromide with infusion solutions and additives. The stability of glycopyrronium bromide is questionable above a pH of 6, due to ester hydrolysis: the pH of infusion fluids and additives should be determined before mixing with glycopyrronium.— T. S. Ingallinera *et al.*, *Am. J. Hosp. Pharm.*, 1979, *36*, 508.

Adverse Effects, Treatment, and Precautions

As for Atropine Sulphate, p.524.

Absorption and Fate

Glycopyrronium bromide is a quaternary ammonium compound and is poorly absorbed from the gastro-intestinal tract. About 10 to 25% has been stated to be absorbed following a dose by mouth, and is excreted in bile and urine as unchanged drug and metabolites. Like other quaternary ammonium compounds it penetrates the blood-brain barrier only poorly.

A study of 6 postoperative patients given glycopyrronium bromide 200 μg intravenously showed that 90% of the dose had disappeared from the circulation in 5 minutes and was rapidly excreted in bile and urine, mainly as the free drug.— E. Kaltiala *et al.*, *J. Pharm. Pharmac.*, 1974, *26*, 352.

Uses and Administration

Glycopyrronium bromide is a quaternary ammonium antimuscarinic agent with peripheral effects similar to those of atropine (see p.524). It is used as an adjunct in the treatment of peptic ulcer and to relieve visceral spasms.

The usual dose is 1 to 4 mg two or three times daily. Doses of 100 to 200 μg have been given by subcutaneous, intramuscular, or intravenous injection 3 or 4 times daily.

Glycopyrronium bromide is also used similarly to atropine in anaesthetic practice. For anaesthetic premedication it is given in doses of 200 to 400 μg intravenously or intramuscularly before the induction of anaesthesia; alternatively, it may be given in a dose of 4 to 5 μg per kg bodyweight to a maximum of 400 μg. If necessary, similar or lower doses may be given intravenously during the operation and repeated if required. A suggested dosage for premedication in children is 4 to 8 μg per kg intravenously or intramuscularly to a maximum of 200 μg.

Glycopyrronium bromide is given in conjunction with anticholinesterases to reverse the effects of non-depolarising muscle relaxants (see Neostigmine Methylsulphate, p.1332). The dose is glycopyrronium bromide 200 μg intravenously per 1 mg of neostigmine (or the equivalent dose of pyridostigmine); alternatively, it may be given in a dose of 10 to 15 μg per kg intravenously with neostigmine 50 μg per kg. A suggested dosage for children is 10 μg per kg intravenously with neostigmine 50 μg per kg. Glycopyrronium bromide can be administered mixed in the same syringe with the anticholinesterase, and it has been suggested that greater cardiovascular stability results from this method of administration.

Glycopyrronium bromide is also used as a 0.05% solution in the iontophoretic treatment of hyperhidrosis.

ANAESTHESIA. A double-blind comparison of glycopyrronium bromide 200 µg with atropine 600 µg given intramuscularly as the antimuscarinic component of premedication was made in 200 patients undergoing surgery. Although glycopyrronium bromide was associated with a smaller increase in heart-rate, there was no difference between the drugs in respect of cardiac arrhythmia, change in arterial pressure, control of secretions in the upper respiratory tract, frequency of nausea and vomiting after operation, or the subjective well-being of the patients.— T. D. McCubbin *et al.*, *Br. J. Anaesth.*, 1979, *51*, 885.

Glycopyrronium bromide 200 µg produced less tachycardia, pyrexia, nausea and vomiting, and blurred vision than atropine sulphate 600 µg when used for premedication in a double-blind study in 90 patients undergoing surgery. The sedative effect of glycopyrronium bromide was less than that of hyoscine hydrobromide 400 µg. The antisialogogue actions of the 3 drugs were similar.— A. Sengupta *et al.*, *Br. J. Anaesth.*, 1980, *52*, 513.

For a study indicating that glycopyrronium premedication is associated with increased incidences of tachycardia during surgery see under Adverse Effects of Atropine Sulphate, p.523.

Studies involving 84 patients about to undergo coronary artery surgery demonstrated that glycopyrronium bromide was as effective as atropine in correcting bradycardia and approximately twice as potent.— D. Preiss and P. Berguson, *Br. J. clin. Pharmac.*, 1983, *16*, 523.

Reversal of neuromuscular blockade. Neuromuscular blockade in 20 patients was reversed by atropine 1.2 mg with neostigmine 2.5 mg, and in 20 patients by glycopyrronium 500 µg and neostigmine 2.5 mg. The latter treatment avoided the tachycardia present initially in the atropine group, and the antisialogogue effect of glycopyrronium was considered superior to that of atropine. Transient arrhythmias in the 2 groups were comparable.— R. K. Mirakhur *et al.*, *Br. J. Anaesth.*, 1977, *49*, 825.

Glycopyrronium bromide 10 or 15 µg per kg bodyweight gave protection against the bradycardic and sialogogic effects of neostigmine administered to reverse pancuronium-induced neuromuscular blockade in surgical patients, but doses of 5 µg per kg failed to do so. When glycopyrronium was administered before the neostigmine it produced dose-related tachycardia, an increase in heart-rate of over 30% being observed at the highest dose, but the increase was minimal when administered concurrently. The results indicate that glycopyrronium should be administered simultaneously with neostigmine for the reversal of neuromuscular blockade.— J. W. Dundee *et al.*, *Br. J. clin. Pharmac.*, 1981, *11*, 417P.

On occasion the onset of action of glycopyrronium is too slow so that if it is given mixed with neostigmine a short but marked bradycardia may ensue. If the glycopyrronium is given first and the neostigmine given on the first sign of a rising heart-rate this problem does not occur.— C. J. Hull, *Br. J. Hosp. Med.*, 1983, *30*, 273.

BRAIN SCANNING. Glycopyrronium bromide was considered a useful adjunct in brain scanning using pertechnetate (^{99m}Tc).— R. A. Holmes and C. N. Luth, *J. nucl. Med.*, 1975, *16*, 819.

GOUT. Glycopyrronium bromide increased the excretion of uric acid in 8 of 19 patients with hyperuricaemia or gout.— A. E. Postlethwaite *et al.*, *Archs intern. Med.*, 1974, *134*, 270.

GUSTATORY SWEATING. In studies involving 22 patients with the Frey syndrome (localised flushing and sweating on eating) glycopyrronium bromide as 1, and 2% cream or roll-on solution gave good control of symptoms; patients tended to prefer the roll-on lotion as it was easier to apply. Topical hyoscine as 0.25, 1 or 3% solution or cream also gave control of sweating, but was associated with a much higher incidence of side-effects.— L. L. Hays *et al.*, *Otolaryngol. Head Neck Surg.*, 1982, *90*, 419.

HYPERHIDROSIS. Prolonged anhidrosis resulted from iontophoresis of glycopyrronium bromide into palmar and plantar skin but results with axillary treatment were disappointingly transient. Antimuscarinic symptoms were usually mild and transient.— E. Abell and K. Morgan, *Br. J. Derm.*, 1974, *91*, 87.

Glycopyrronium bromide iontophoresis has given excellent results in palmar and plantar hyperhidrosis. Treatment is required at approximately 4-week intervals. Careful calibration of the equipment should avoid serious antimuscarinic effects although some systemic effects, such as difficulty in swallowing and blurred vision are common in the first 24 to 48 hours after treatment.— W. A. D. Griffiths, *Prescribers' J.*, 1984, *24*, 38.

PREGNANCY AND THE NEONATE. Administration of glycopyrronium intravenously to 20 patients in labour had no significant effect on foetal heart-rate or foetal heart-rate variability. Glycopyrronium appeared to be more suitable than atropine during pregnancy since it did not cross the placental barrier.— T. Abboud *et al.*, *Anesthesiology*, 1980, *53*, S316.

Preparations

Glycopyrrolate Injection *(U.S.P.)*. A sterile solution of glycopyrronium bromide in Water for Injections.

Glycopyrrolate Tablets *(U.S.P.)*. Contain glycopyrronium bromide.

Proprietary Preparations

Robinul *(Robins, UK)*. *Tablets*, scored, glycopyrronium bromide 2 mg.
Injection, glycopyrronium bromide 200 µg/mL, in ampoules of 1 and 3 mL.
Topical solution, powder for reconstitution, glycopyrronium bromide.

Robinul-Neostigmine *(Robins, UK)*. *Injection*, glycopyrronium bromide 500 µg, neostigmine methylsulphate 2.5 mg/mL, in ampoules of 1 mL.

Proprietary Names and Manufacturers

Asécryl *(Fr.)*; Nodapton *(Switz.)*; Robanul *(Spain)*; Robinul *(Robins, Austral.; Robins, Canad.; Robins, Denm.; Brenner, Ger.; Neth.; Robins, Norw.; Continental Ethicals, S.Afr.; Robins, Swed.; Robins, Switz.; Robins, UK; Robins, USA)*; Tarodyl *(Lundbeck, Denm.)*; Tarodyn *(Lundbeck, Swed.)*.

372-t

Hexocyclium Methylsulphate *(BAN)*.

Hexocyclium Metilsulfate *(rINN)*. 4-(β-Cyclohexyl-β-hydroxyphenethyl)-1,1-dimethylpiperazinium methylsulphate.

$C_{20}H_{33}N_2O,CH_3O_4S=428.6$.

CAS — 6004-98-4 (hexocyclium); 115-63-9 (methylsulphate).

Hexocyclium methylsulphate is a quaternary ammonium antimuscarinic agent with peripheral effects similar to those of atropine (see p.523). It is used as an adjunct in the treatment of peptic ulcer, and to relieve visceral spasms. It has been given in an initial dose of 100 mg daily in divided doses by mouth, adjusted according to the response of the patient.

Proprietary Names and Manufacturers

Tral *(Abbott, Ital.; Abbott, Switz.; Abbott, USA)*; Traline *(Odopharm, Fr.; Abbott, Ger.)*.

373-x

Homatropine

(1*R*,3*r*,5*S*)-Tropan-3-yl (±)-mandelate.

$C_{16}H_{21}NO_3=275.3$.

CAS — 87-00-3.

374-r

Homatropine Hydrobromide *(BAN, USAN)*.

Bromidrato de Homatropina; Homatr. Hydrobrom.; Homatropini Hydrobromidum; Homatropinium Bromide; Homatropinum Bromatum; Omatropina Bromidrato; Oxtolyltropine Hydrobromide; Tropyl Mandelate Hydrobromide.

$C_{16}H_{21}NO_3,HBr=356.3$.

CAS — 51-56-9.

Pharmacopoeias. In *Arg., Aust., Belg., Br., Braz., Cz., Egypt., Eur., Fr., Ger., Hung., Ind., Int., It., Jpn, Jug., Mex., Neth., Nord., Pol., Rus., Span., Swiss, Turk.*, and *U.S.* Also in *B.P.Vet.*

Colourless odourless crystals or a white crystalline powder.

B.P. **solubilities** are: soluble 1 in 6 of water and 1 in 60 of alcohol; slightly soluble in chloroform; very slightly soluble in ether. *U.S.P.* solubilities are: soluble 1 in 6 of water, 1 in 40 of alcohol, and 1 in 420 of chloroform; practically insoluble in ether. The *B.P.* specifies that a 5% solution in water has a pH of 5.0 to 6.5. The *U.S.P.* specifies that a 2% solution in water has a pH between 5.7 and 7.0. The *U.S.P.* ophthalmic solution has a pH of 2.5 to 5.0. **Store** in airtight containers. Protect from light.

375-f

Homatropine Methobromide

Brometo de Metil-Homatropina; Homatropine Methylbromide *(USAN, rINN)*; Methylhomatropinium Bromatum; Methylhomatropinium Bromide. (1*R*,3*r*,5*S*)-3-[(±)-Mandeloyloxy]-8-methyltropanium bromide.

$C_{16}H_{21}NO_3,CH_3Br=370.3$.

CAS — 80-49-9.

Pharmacopoeias. In *Aust., Braz., Hung.*, and *U.S.*

A white odourless powder that slowly darkens on exposure to light. Very **soluble** in water; freely soluble in alcohol; practically insoluble in acetone and ether. A 1% solution in water has a pH of 4.5 to 6.5. **Store** in airtight containers. Protect from light.

Adverse Effects, Treatment, and Precautions

As for Atropine Sulphate, p.523.

A report of acute toxicity in 5 children, 4 of whom had received homatropine hydrobromide eye-drops and 1 atropine sulphate eye-drops. Symptoms included severe ataxia, restlessness, excitement, and hallucinations and suggested primarily CNS involvement. Four of the cases occurred in the summer, during periods of high heat and humidity.— D. Hoefnagel, *New Engl. J. Med.*, 1961, *264*, 168.

Uses and Administration

Homatropine is an antimuscarinic agent with effects similar to, but weaker than, those of atropine (see p.524); when applied to the eye its cycloplegic and mydriatic actions are more rapid and of shorter duration, and for this reason it may be preferred to atropine for these purposes. However, it is not a reliable cycloplegic in very young people because of their strong accommodative reserve; they may require a more powerful drug such as atropine to produce complete paralysis of accommodation. Homatropine is sometimes used with cocaine, which enhances its mydriatic effect.

It is generally used as a 2 or 5% solution of the hydrobromide; for the determination of refraction one or two drops of a 2% solution may be instilled, repeated if necessary 5 or 10 minutes later. In the treatment of uveitis, one or two drops of a 2 or 5% solution may be given, usually 2 or 3 times daily.

Homatropine has also been used as the quaternary ammonium methobromide derivative, as an adjunct in the treatment of peptic ulcer, and in the treatment of gastro-intestinal spasm. Usual oral doses of homatropine methobromide have been 5 or 10 mg 3 or 4 times daily.

MYDRIASIS. A study was made of the mydriatic effects of 4 drugs in the concentrations in which they were used in ophthalmology. Homatropine hydrobromide and phenylephrine hydrochloride produced comparable mydriasis but the effect of homatropine lasted longer. Tropicamide had the shortest latency period and produced the greatest dilatation in the shortest time. Hydroxyamphetamine hydrobromide was the least effective.— H. D. Gambill *et al.*, *Archs Ophthal., N.Y.*, 1967, *77*, 740.

TEST FOR GLAUCOMA. A description of a provocative outflow test for detecting open-angle glaucoma, which utilised 2% homatropine eye-drops and drinking water.— D. A. Leighton *et al.*, *Br. J. Ophthal.*, 1970, *54*, 19.

Preparations

Homatropine Eye Drops *(A.P.F.)*. Gutt. Homatrop. Contain homatropine hydrobromide 2%. Sterilised by autoclaving.

Homatropine Eye Drops *(B.P.)*. HOM. Contain homatropine hydrobromide.

Homatropine Hydrobromide Ophthalmic Solution *(U.S.P.)*. pH 2.5 to 5.0.

Homatropine Methylbromide Tablets *(U.S.P.)*. Contain homatropine methobromide.

For eye preparations of homatropine hydrobromide with cocaine, see under Cocaine Hydrochloride, p.1215.

Proprietary Preparations

Minims Homatropine Hydrobromide *(Smith & Nephew Pharmaceuticals, UK)*. *Eye-drops*, homatropine hydrobromide 2%, in single-use disposable applicators.

Proprietary Names and Manufacturers of Homatropine and its Salts

Allergan Homatropine (Homat) *(Allergan, Austral.)*; Dallapasmo *(Dallas, Arg.)*; Homapin *(Mission Pharmacal, USA)*; Isopto Homatropine *(Alcon, Austral.; Alcon, Canad.; Alcon, S.Afr.)*; Mesopin *(Fulton, Ital.)*; Minims Homatropine Hydrobromide *(Smith & Nephew, Austral.; Smith & Nephew, S.Afr.; Smith & Nephew Pharmaceuticals, UK)*; Novatrin *(Ayerst, USA)*; Novatropina *(Chinoin, Ital.; Promesa, Spain)*; Paratropina *(Lazar, Arg.)*; Pasmolona *(Paylos, Arg.)*; SMP Homatropine *(Armour, UK)*.

The following names have been used for multi-ingredient preparations containing homatropine and its salts—Acidobyl *(Desbergers, Canad.)*; Acidobyl with Cascara *(Desbergers, Canad.)*; Ancatropine Infant Drops *(Anca, Canad.)*; APP Stomach Preparations *(Consolidated Chemicals, UK)*; Bustase Plus *(Geriatric Pharm. Corp., USA)*; Hycodan *(Du Pont, USA)*; Hycomine *(Du Pont, Austral.)*; Neo-Tropine Alkaline *(Neolab, Canad.)*; Neuro-Spasex *(Beecham, Canad.)*.

376-d

Hyoscine Butylbromide *(BAN)*.

Butylscopolamine Bromide; Butylscopolamonii Bromidum; Hyoscine-*N*-Butyl Bromide; *N*-Butylscopolammonium Bromide; Scopolamine Butylbromide; Scopolamine *N*-Butyl Bromide. (−)-(1*S*,3*s*,5*R*,6*R*,7*S*)-8-Butyl-6,7-epoxy-3-[(*S*)-tropoyloxy]tropanium bromide.
$C_{21}H_{30}BrNO_4$=440.4.

CAS — 51-34-3 (hyoscine); 149-64-4 (butylbromide).

Pharmacopoeias. In *Br., Cz.*, and *Roum.*

A white or almost white, odourless or almost odourless, crystalline powder. **Soluble** 1 in 1 of water, 1 in 50 of alcohol, and 1 in 5 of chloroform. A 10% solution in water has a pH of 5.5 to 6.5. The *B.P.* injection has a pH of 3.7 to 5.5. **Store** in well-closed containers. Protect from light.

377-n

Hyoscine Hydrobromide *(BAN)*.

Bromhidrato de Escopolamina; Hyoscini Hydrobromidum; Ioscina Bromidrato; Scopolamine Bromhydrate; Scopolamine Hydrobromide *(USAN)*; Scopolamini Hydrobromidum. (−)-(1*S*,3*s*,5*R*,6*R*,7*S*)-6,7-Epoxytropan-3-yl (*S*)-tropate hydrobromide trihydrate.
$C_{17}H_{21}NO_4,HBr,3H_2O$=438.3.

CAS — 114-49-8 (anhydrous); 6533-68-2 (trihydrate).

Pharmacopoeias. In *Arg., Aust., Belg., Br., Chin., Cz., Egypt., Eur., Fr., Ger., Hung., Ind., Int., It., Jpn, Jug., Mex., Neth., Nord., Pol., Port., Roum., Rus., Span., Swiss, Turk.*, and *U.S.*

Efflorescent odourless, colourless, crystals or white crystalline powder.

B.P. **solubilities** are: 1 in 3.5 of water and 1 in 30 of alcohol; practically insoluble in chloroform and ether. The *U.S.P.* has soluble 1 in 1.5 of water and 1 in 20 of alcohol; slightly soluble in chloroform; practically insoluble in ether. A 5% solution in water has a pH of 4.0 to 5.5. The *U.S.P.* injection has a pH of 3.5 to 6.5 and the *U.S.P.* ophthalmic solution a pH of 4.0 to 6.0. **Incompatible** with alkalis, silver salts, and tannic acid. **Store** below 15° in well-filled airtight containers of small capacity. Protect from light.

NOTE. Hyoscine is the *l*-isomer; the racemic mixture (*dl*-hyoscine) is known as atroscine.

378-h

Hyoscine Methobromide *(BAN)*.

Epoxymethamine Bromide; Hyoscine Methylbromide; Methscopolamine Bromide *(USAN)*; Scopolamine Methobromide; Scopolamine Methylbromide. (−)-(1*S*,3*s*,5*R*,6*R*,7*S*)-6,7-Epoxy-8-methyl-3-[(*S*)-tropoyloxy]tropanium bromide.
$C_{18}H_{24}BrNO_4$=398.3.

CAS — 155-41-9.

Pharmacopoeias. In *U.S.*

White crystals or a white or almost white, odourless or almost odourless crystalline powder. Freely **soluble** in water; slightly soluble in alcohol; practically insoluble in acetone and chloroform. The *U.S.P.* injection has a pH of 4.5 to 6.0. **Store** in airtight containers. Protect from light.

379-m

Hyoscine Methonitrate *(BAN)*.

Hyoscine Methylnitrate; Methscopolamine Nitrate; Methylhyoscini Nitras; Methylscopolamini Nitras; Scopolamine Methonitrate; Scopolamine Methylnitrate. (−)-(1*S*,3*s*,5*R*,6*R*,7*S*)-6,7-Epoxy-8-methyl-3-[(*S*)-tropoyloxy]tropanium nitrate.
$C_{18}H_{24}N_2O_7$=380.4.

CAS — 6106-46-3.

Pharmacopoeias. In *Aust., Fr., It., Neth., Nord.*, and *Swiss.*

Adverse Effects, Treatment, and Precautions

As for Atropine Sulphate, p.523. Central stimulation sometimes precedes depression, especially after large doses of hyoscine or in severe pain, but the main central symptom is drowsiness leading to coma. Bradycardia is more likely than with atropine. Idiosyncratic reactions to hyoscine are more common than to atropine and alarming effects may occur at therapeutic doses.

Hyoscine should be used with care in patients receiving other central depressants concomitantly as CNS depression may be enhanced. Caution has also been advised in patients with impaired metabolic, liver, or kidney function, as adverse CNS effects have been stated to be more likely in these patients.

The quaternary derivatives, such as the butylbromide, methobromide, or methonitrate do not readily cross the blood-brain barrier, so central effects are rare.

CAUTION. *Hyoscine may cause drowsiness; patients so affected should not drive or operate machinery. Patients should abstain from alcohol.*

EFFECTS ON THE EYE. *Anisocoria.* A report of fixed dilated pupil, on the side of the head on which a hyoscine transdermal drug delivery system had been affixed to a patient for 6 hours to prevent motion sickness. The effect was noted 48 hours after removal of the system, and had worn off 24 hours later.— J. S. Chiaramonte (letter), *New Engl. J. Med.*, 1982, *306*, 174. Comment. Although bilateral mydriasis has been observed concomitant with the use of transdermal hyoscine a unilateral fixed dilated pupil might have been caused by contamination of a finger with hyoscine in applying the device, and then rubbing the eye.— F. E. Lepore (letter), *ibid.*, 824.

Further reports of and comments on anisocoria associated with finger-to-eye contamination with hyoscine from transdermal patches: J. A. McCrary and N. R. Webb, *J. Am. med. Ass.*, 1982, *248*, 353; R. A. Bienia *et al.* (letter), *Ann. intern. Med.*, 1983, *99*, 572; B. H. Price (letter), *J. Am. med. Ass.*, 1985, *253*, 1561; D. C. Love, *ibid.*, *254*, 1720; W. Davenport (letter), *ibid;* B. H. Price (letter), *ibid.*

Glaucoma. A report of 2 cases of closed-angle glaucoma precipitated by transdermal hyoscine.— F. T. Fraunfelder (letter), *New Engl. J. Med.*, 1982, *307*, 1079. See also.— M. B. Hamill *et al.*, *Ann. Ophthal.*, 1983, *15*, 1011.

EFFECTS ON MENTAL FUNCTION. Of the remedies for travel sickness hyoscine is said to impair driving skills less than antihistamines, but antimuscarinic drugs may also cause drowsiness and can lead to difficulties in visual accommodation which may reduce driving ability.— H. Ashton, *Adverse Drug React. Bull.*, 1983, (Feb.), 360.

Results of studies involving 58 healthy subjects suggested that hyoscine hydrobromide significantly impaired psychomotor performance, but in practice, with moderate oral doses, preferably less than 0.9 mg, the impairment is relatively mild in the majority of patients. Administration in association with ephedrine 25 mg allowed the use of a smaller dose of hyoscine and antagonised some of hyoscine's cardiovascular side-effects.— E. Nuotto, *Eur. J. clin. Pharmac.*, 1983, *24*, 603.

In a study in 10 healthy subjects hyoscine delivered from a transdermal system had no significant effect on psychomotor performance.— C. H. Gleiter *et al.*, *Psychopharmacology*, 1984, *83*, 397.

Psychosis. A report of ataxia and hallucinations in a child who had received cyclopentolate and hyoscine eye-drops.— M. K. Wang and J. R. Tatane, *Br. med. J.*, 1974, *1*, 453.

Reports of psychotic reactions associated with the transdermal administration of hyoscine: R. K. Osterholm and J. K. Camoriano (letter), *J. Am. med. Ass.*, 1982, *247*, 3081; K. J. Rodysill and J. B. Warren (letter), *Ann. intern. Med.*, 1983, *98*, 561; J. G. Cairncross, *Ann. Neurol.*, 1983, *13*, 582; P. Johnson *et al.* (letter), *New Engl. J. Med.*, 1984, *311*, 468; R. C. Steer (letter), *ibid;* G. W. MacEwan, *Can. med. Ass. J.*, 1985, *133*, 431; R. T. Paasuke (letter), *ibid.*, 956.

INTERACTIONS. Hyoscine butylbromide 20 mg by intravenous injection significantly delayed oesophageal transit of hard gelatin capsules in 48 healthy subjects compared with 48 controls.— K. S. Channer *et al.*, *Br. J. clin. Pharmac.*, 1983, *15*, 560.

OVERDOSAGE. Report of acute hyoscine poisoning in 3 subjects. All 3 responded to gastric lavage and supportive treatment.— M. M. Kaplan *et al.*, *Clin. Toxicol.*, 1974, *7*, 509.

PORPHYRIA. A detailed review of drug-induced porphyrias. Hyoscine butylbromide had been reported by at least 3 people to be associated with clinical exacerbations of porphyria.— M. R. Moore and P. B. Disler, *Adverse Drug React. Ac. Pois. Rev.*, 1983, *2*, 149.

PREGNANCY AND THE NEONATE. A report of hyoscine toxicity in a neonate born to a mother who had received a total of 1.8 mg of hyoscine in divided doses with pethidine and levorphanol prior to delivery. The neonate was lethargic, barrel chested, and had a heart-rate of 200. Symptoms subsided following physostigmine 100 µg given intramuscularly.— R. P. Evens and J. C. Leopold (letter), *Pediatrics*, 1980, *66*, 329.

WITHDRAWAL. Mention of dizziness and nausea three days after removal of a hyoscine transdermal delivery system. The patient had been using the transdermal patches during a 10-day cruise to prevent sea-sickness.— R. H. B. Meyboom (letter), *New Engl. J. Med.*, 1984, *311*, 1377. Comment. A warning of the possibility of withdrawal symptoms had been added to the data sheet.— R. C. Steer (letter), *ibid.*

X-RAY EXAMINATION. Administration of hyoscine butylbromide intramuscularly 10 to 15 minutes before radiological examination of the stomach to slow peristaltic movements was recommended only when detailed examination was to be carried out, otherwise deformity of the stomach due to linear and multiple ulcers might be obscured.— T. F. Solanke *et al.*, *Gut*, 1969, *10*, 436.

Absorption and Fate

Hyoscine is readily absorbed from the gastro-intestinal tract following oral doses of the hydrobromide. It is almost entirely metabolised, probably in the liver; only a small proportion of an oral dose has been reported to be excreted unchanged in the urine. It crosses the blood-brain barrier and has been stated to cross the placenta. Hyoscine is also well absorbed following application to the skin.

The quaternary derivatives, such as the butylbromide or methobromide, are poorly absorbed from the gastro-intestinal tract and do not readily pass the blood-brain barrier.

In a controlled double-blind study in groups of 8 subjects, measurements were made of saliva flow, heart-rate, pupil diameter, and mental alertness for up to 8 hours after intramuscular injection of 50, 100, 200, and 400 μg of hyoscine hydrobromide. Peak activity was achieved 1 to 2 hours after the dose, with a gradual decline over the 8-hour period.— J. J. Brand, *Br. J. Pharmac. Chemother.*, 1969, *35*, 202.

After 50 to 100 mg of hyoscine butylbromide was given to 6 male volunteers, by mouth or by intra-intestinal infusion, very little hyoscine butylbromide was absorbed from the upper small intestine and none appeared in the plasma. About 2% and 90% of the dose appeared in the urine and faeces respectively. After intravenous administration of 8 mg to 1 volunteer, 42% was eliminated in the urine and 37% in faeces.— K. Hellström *et al.*, *Scand. J. Gastroenterol.*, 1970, *5*, 585.

Studies in 2 patients showed that hyoscine butylbromide had an enterohepatic circulation.— H. Vapaatalo *et al.*, *J. Pharm. Pharmac.*, 1975, *27*, 542.

Urinary excretion of hyoscine was determined using a radioligand binding assay in 9 healthy subjects following administration of approximately 450 μg of the drug over 64 hours via a transdermal delivery system. During the time of medication and 48 hours thereafter, a mean total of 156 μg of hyoscine was excreted in urine, of which 21% was as unchanged drug and the remainder mainly as glucuronide or sulphate conjugates. Steady-state urinary concentrations were achieved about 12 hours after applying the medication. Concentrations in plasma were below the detectable level of 1.2 ng per mL.— M. Scheurlen *et al.*, *J. pharm. Sci.*, 1984, *73*, 561. See also.— C. Muir and R. Metcalfe, *J. pharm. biomed. Anal.*, 1983, *1*, 363 (comparison of plasma concentrations after oral and transdermal administration).

Uses and Administration

Hyoscine is an antimuscarinic agent with central and peripheral actions. It is a more powerful suppressant of salivation than atropine, and usually slows rather than increases heart-rate, especially in low doses. Its central action differs from that of atropine in that it depresses the cerebral cortex, especially the motor areas, and produces drowsiness and amnesia.

As a premedicant, hyoscine hydrobromide is injected subcutaneously in doses of 400 μg, usually in association with papaveretum 20 mg, or with morphine or pethidine, about half to one hour before induction of general anaesthesia; these doses may be halved or reduced in elderly patients and others who may be more sensitive to its actions.

Hyoscine is effective in the prevention and control of motion sickness and has also been given as an anti-emetic in the prophylactic treatment of other forms of nausea. Hyoscine hydrobromide 300 μg may be taken by mouth 30 minutes before a journey to prevent motion sickness; followed by 300 μg every 6 hours if required. Children aged 4 to 10 years may be given 75 to 150 μg and those over 10 years, 150 to 300 μg. Hyoscine has also been given to prevent motion sickness via a transdermal delivery system supplying 500 μg over 3 days.

Hyoscine hydrobromide may also be given by subcutaneous or intramuscular injection in a dose of 200 μg.

Hyoscine hydrobromide was formerly used in obstetrics, in conjunction with morphine or pethidine, to produce a condition of amnesia and partial analgesia known as 'twilight sleep'. It has also been employed alone or with morphine as a sedative in acute mania and delirium, particularly delirium tremens.

Hyoscine has been given as its quaternary ammonium derivatives in conditions associated with visceral spasm, in usual doses of 20 mg of the butylbromide intramuscularly or intravenously, repeated after 30 minutes if necessary, or 20 mg by mouth four times daily. The methobromide, methonitrate, and methylsulphate have also been used as adjuncts in the treatment of peptic ulcer.

Hyoscine hydrobromide has been used in the eye for its cycloplegic and mydriatic actions. It has a shorter duration of action than atropine.

Hyoscine has been employed in the treatment of parkinsonism, but has largely been supplanted by other drugs when antimuscarinic agents are required.

The use of hyoscine and its salts and derivatives in cosmetics is prohibited in the *UK*.

In normal subjects, a rapid intravenous injection of hyoscine hydrobromide, 25 to 200 μg per 70 kg body-weight, decreased the heart-rate by 12 to 15 beats per minute within 10 minutes. Doses of 300 to 600 μg first increased then decreased the heart-rate. Atropine, 200 μg per 70 kg intravenously, given 180 minutes after 300 to 600 μg of hyoscine increased the heart-rate but had no effect when given after lower doses of hyoscine hydrobromide.— J. S. Gravenstein and J. I. Thornby, *Clin. Pharmac. Ther.*, 1969, *10*, 395.

Hyoscine methobromide appeared to be more reliable than atropine in causing dose-related increments in heart-rate; it could be safely administered in doses of 150 μg or less, intravenously every 5 or 10 minutes until the desired heart-rate had been obtained.— J. B. Neeld *et al.*, *Clin. Pharmac. Ther.*, 1975, *17*, 290.

Hyoscine butylbromide had restored sinus rhythm for periods of up to one hour to hearts affected by arrhythmias associated with pancuronium and halothane. It had also restored normal cardiac rhythm in 2 cases of nodal bradycardia and hypotension, in 3 cases of multiple ventricular extrasystoles, and in one case of atrioventricular dissociation within one minute of intravenous injection.— E. N. S. Fry (letter), *Br. med. J.*, 1979, *2*, 1075.

In a study in 6 healthy subjects hyoscine butylbromide in doses of 1 to 16 mg by intravenous injection induced tachycardia at all doses whereas atropine sulphate induced bradycardia at lower doses and tachycardia at higher; however, the dose-response curve of hyoscine butylbromide was flatter, suggesting that it had ganglion-blocking action in addition to its antimuscarinic activity.— S. L. Grainger and S. E. Smith, *Br. J. clin. Pharmac.*, 1983, *16*, 623.

ANAESTHESIA. In a comparison of the efficacy of drugs commonly used in pre-anaesthetic medication, a double-blind study was made of (1) papaveretum 20 mg with hyoscine 400 μg, (2) pethidine 100 mg with atropine 600 μg, (3) promethazine 50 mg with atropine 600 μg, and (4) hyoscine alone, 400 μg, all given intramuscularly. The majority of patients were neither asleep nor sleepy before operation. Papaveretum with hyoscine produced most sedation and greatest relief of anxiety. Atropine produced greater tachycardia than hyoscine. There was a high incidence of hypotension with the papaveretum-hyoscine and the pethidine-atropine mixtures. Dry throat was commonest after premedication which included hyoscine.— S. A. Feldman, *Anaesthesia*, 1963, *18*, 169.

In 49 patients who had undergone general anaesthesia for an obstetric or gynaecological procedure and who had received hyoscine 800 μg pre-operatively, no incidence of awareness during operation was reported, but 18 of 229 patients who received atropine 0.6 to 1 mg reported awareness, while 2 of 12 patients who received neither reported awareness. When atropine was used, dreams recalled were nearly always described as horrifying and accompanied by a feeling of dizziness, while with the use of hyoscine dreaming was less pronounced and was always pleasant.— J. S. Crawford *et al.* (letter), *Br. med. J.*, 1969, *1*, 508.

Amnesia. Hyoscine, 600 μg by intravenous injection, produced amnesia in up to 50% of patients studied. The maximum incidence of amnesia occurred at 50 to 80 minutes but effects were still evident in some patients after 120 minutes.— J. W. Dundee and S. K. Pandit, *Br. J. Pharmac.*, 1972, *44*, 140.

ANOXIC SEIZURES. Report of the use of transdermal hyoscine, administered as half a standard skin patch applied every 3 days, to relieve frequent reflex anoxic seizures in 2 children.— L. Palm and G. Blennow, *Acta paediat. scand.*, 1985, *74*, 803.

ANTICHOLINESTERASE POISONING. For the suggestion that hyoscine might be more effective than atropine in the treatment of central anticholinesterase poisoning, see under Atropine, p.525.

GASTRO-INTESTINAL DISORDERS. A study of the effects of hyoscine butylbromide on gut motility. In 6 of 7 healthy subjects 8 mg intravenously reduced motility, as assessed by bowel sounds, for 15 to 30 minutes whereas 200 mg by mouth had no effect over a 3-hour period. Reduced motility was followed by increased sounds. The 7th subject had increased motility after both oral and intravenous doses.— J. -P. Guignard *et al.*, *Clin. Pharmac. Ther.*, 1968, *9*, 745. See also: E. N. S. Fry and S. Deshpande (letter), *Br. med. J.*, 1976, *1*, 646.

For a study demonstrating that hyoscine butylbromide by mouth delayed oesophageal transit of capsules, see Interactions, under Adverse Effects and Precautions, above.

Intestinal obstruction. In a study on the medical management of intestinal obstruction in 38 patients with advanced malignant disease, 29 patients reported colic that was severe or moderate in 17. Hyoscine 300 to 600 μg was given sublingually to relieve occasional spasms or before meals for the prophylaxis of attacks precipitated by food. Persistent severe colic was managed by hyoscine 800 μg to 2 mg by continuous subcutaneous infusion via a syringe driver. Loperamide was used for persistent colic in patients who were not vomiting.— M. Baines *et al.*, *Lancet*, 1985, *2*, 990.

Ulcer, duodenal. In a study in 5 patients with duodenal ulcer in remission hyoscine methobromide administered via a transdermal delivery system significantly reduced mean overnight acid output to 1.7 mmol per hour, compared with 6.8 mmol per hour with placebo. There was no significant change in hydrogen ion concentration. The results suggested that transdermal hyoscine methobromide had potential value as a maintenance treatment for healed duodenal ulcers.— R. P. Walt *et al.*, *Br. med. J.*, 1982, *284*, 1736. Similar results with transdermal hyoscine in patients scheduled for selective proximal vagotomy.— C. H. Gleiter *et al.* (letter), *New Engl. J. Med.*, 1984, *311*, 1378.

GUSTATORY SWEATING. Hyoscine hydrobromide applied as a 3% cream was successful in reducing gustatory sweating, consisting of flushing and sweating over the right mandible during eating, in a patient who had previously undergone surgical excision of the right submandibular salivary gland.— B. M. W. Bailey and D. E. Pearce, *Br. dent. J.*, 1985, *158*, 17.

NAUSEA AND VOMITING. For a detailed preliminary review of the properties and uses of transdermally delivered hyoscine, see S. P. Clissold and R. C. Heel, *Drugs*, 1985, *29*, 189.

For references to adverse effects associated with transdermal hyoscine see under Adverse Effects and Precautions, above.

In chemotherapy. A study in 45 cancer patients receiving cisplatin therapy found that transdermal hyoscine was no more effective than placebo in alleviating cisplatin-induced emesis.— D. L. Longo, *Cancer Treat. Rep.*, 1982, *66*, 1975.

In postoperative emesis. A review of nausea and vomiting. Both atropine and hyoscine have a useful anti-emetic action in anaesthetic practice which should not be forgotten when their role as antisialogogues is diminishing. Hyoscine is the more effective of the two, due to its greater central sedative action. Their main role is probably to reduce postoperative emesis due to opiates but their protective action is considerably shorter in duration than the emetic effect of morphine.— R. S. J. Clarke, *Br. J. Anaesth.*, 1984, *56*, 19.

In a study completed by 38 patients undergoing gynaecological surgery transdermal hyoscine was significantly more effective than placebo in reducing postoperative nausea and vomiting only during the first 24 hours; however, there was no such difference in the number of doses of additional anti-emetics given to each group, and 13 of 19 patients given active drug still experienced severe nausea and vomiting in this period. Transdermal hyoscine alone is unlikely to be the answer to postoperative nausea and vomiting.— J. Uppington *et al.*, *Anaesthesia*, 1986, *41*, 16. Comment. Further studies of the efficacy of transdermal hyoscine are required. Until more evidence becomes available the use of hyoscine either intramuscularly or by transdermal patch should not be regarded as a first-line approach in the prevention of postoperative nausea and vomiting.— J. K. Aronson and J. W. Sear, *ibid.*, 1.

Motion sickness. In a study by the Army, Navy, Air Force Motion Sickness Team (*J. Am. med. Ass.*, 1956, *160*, 755) single doses of hyoscine hydrobromide 1 mg, followed by 500 μg three times daily failed to give good protection against motion sickness of long duration and had distressing side-effects. However, later studies, using much lower doses of hyoscine, have shown benefit: Brand *et al.* (*Br. J. Pharmac. Chemother.*, 1967, *30*, 463) found that hyoscine hydrobromide in doses equivalent to 100 μg of base protected 75% of susceptible volunteers from motion sickness with minimal side-effects, while Wood and Greybiel (*Aerospace Med.*, 1972, *43*, 249) found hyoscine 600 μg by mouth the most effective of 14 anti-motion sickness drugs assessed in a placebo-controlled study. It has been concluded that hyoscine is probably the drug of choice in motion sickness, despite its side-effects (D.N. Bateman, *Prescribers' J.*, 1985, *25*, 81).

In an attempt to maintain therapeutic blood concentrations over prolonged periods, and reduce side-effects, interest has been focussed on the transdermal administration of hyoscine from controlled-release skin patches. In a series of studies, Price *et al.* (*Clin. Pharmac. Ther.*, 1981, *29*, 414) found transdermal hyoscine, from a patch designed to deliver 500 µg over 3 days, to be more effective than oral dimenhydrinate or placebo in protecting against motion sickness over a 7 to 8 hours journey; the effect was greater if the patch were applied 16 hours rather than 4 hours before motion. Similarly, Dahl *et al.* (*ibid.*, 1984, *36*, 116) found transdermal hyoscine superior to oral meclozine or placebo in the prevention of motion sickness induced in 36 subjects over a 90 minute period. In both studies the most significant adverse effect associated with transdermal hyoscine was dry mouth. In a study of the prevention of longer-term sea sickness (W.F. van Marion *et al.*, *ibid.*, 1985, *38*, 301), transdermal hyoscine 500 µg over the first 3 days of a 7-day period of exposure to heavy or moderate seas significantly reduced nausea compared to a placebo in the first 2 days. However, vomiting was significantly greater in the active drug group 3 days after removal of the delivery system, perhaps due to a delay in adaptation to motion because of the use of hyoscine.

SUPPRESSION OF SALIVATION. Mention of the use of transdermal hyoscine hydrobromide to inhibit salivation in players of recorders, reducing accumulation of moisture in the instrument and the concomitant loss of sound quality.— C. E. Dettman (letter), *New Engl. J. Med.*, 1984, *310*, 1396.

VERTIGO. A study of the effects of transdermal hyoscine involving 30 patients with vertigo. In general, results suggested that a single transdermal patch was a reasonable alternative to other forms of treatment for acute peripheral vertigo; further comparative investigations should be undertaken.— T. Rahko and P. Karma, *J. Lar. Otol.*, 1985, *99*, 653.

See also: T. J. Balkany, *Ann. Otol. Rhinol. Lar.*, 1984, *93*, 25 (comparison with meclozine).

Preparations

Scopolamine Hydrobromide Ophthalmic Ointment (*U.S.P.*). A sterile eye ointment containing hyoscine hydrobromide in a suitable basis.

Hyoscine Eye Drops (*B.P.*). HYO. Contain hyoscine hydrobromide.

Scopolamine Hydrobromide Ophthalmic Solution (*U.S.P.*). A sterile solution containing hyoscine hydrobromide. pH 4 to 6.

Hyoscine Butylbromide Injection (*B.P.*). Sterilised by autoclaving. pH 3.7 to 5.5.

Hyoscine Injection (*B.P.*). Hyoscine Hydrobromide Injection. Contains hyoscine hydrobromide. Sterilised by autoclaving.

Methscopolamine Bromide Injection (*U.S.P.*). A sterile solution of hyoscine methobromide. pH 4.5 to 6.0.

Scopolamine Hydrobromide Injection (*U.S.P.*). A sterile solution of hyoscine hydrobromide. pH 3.5 to 6.5.

Hyoscine Butylbromide Tablets (*B.P.*)

Hyoscine Tablets (*B.P.*). Contain hyoscine hydrobromide.

Methscopolamine Bromide Tablets (*U.S.P.*). Contain hyoscine methobromide.

Scopolamine Hydrobromide Tablets (*U.S.P.*). Contain hyoscine hydrobromide.

Proprietary Preparations

Buscopan (*Boehringer Ingelheim, UK*). *Tablets*, hyoscine butylbromide 10 mg.
Injection, hyoscine butylbromide 20 mg/mL, in ampoules of 1 mL.

Proprietary Names and Manufacturers of Hyoscine Derivatives

Blocan (*Estedi, Spain*); Boro-Scopol (*Winzer, Ger.*); Buscapina (*Arg.*; *Boehringer Ingelheim, Spain*); Buscopan (*Boehringer Ingelheim, Austral.*; *Belg.*; *Boehringer Ingelheim, Canad.*; *Boehringer Ingelheim, Denm.*; *Delagrange, Fr.*; *Boehringer Ingelheim, Ger.*; *Boehringer Ingelheim, Ital.*; *Neth.*; *Boehringer Ingelheim, Norw.*; *S.Afr.*; *Boehringer Ingelheim, Swed.*; *Boehringer Ingelheim, Switz.*; *Boehringer Ingelheim, UK*); Butibol (*Jpn*); Butylmido (*Jpn*); Diaste-M (*Jpn*); Holopon (*Byk, Belg.*; *Byk Gulden, Ger.*); Hyospan (*Jpn*); Hyospasmol (*Lennon, S.Afr.*); Isopto Hyoscine (*S.Afr.*); Minims Hyoscine Hydrobromide (*Smith & Nephew Pharmaceuticals, UK*); Pamine (*Upjohn, Austral.*; *Upjohn, Canad.*; *Upjohn, UK*; *Upjohn, USA*); Reladan (*Jpn*); Salfalgin (*Ital.*); Scop (*Ciba, Austral.*); Scopoderm (*Ciba, Denm.*; *Ciba, Fr.*; *Ciba, Norw.*; *Ciba, Swed.*); Scopoderm TTS (*Ciba, Ger.*; *Ciba, S.Afr.*; *Geigy, Switz.*; *Ciba, UK*); Scopos (*Spret-Mauchant, Fr.*); Scordin (*Jpn*); Scordin-B (*Jpn*); Skopyl (*Pharmacia, Denm.*; *Pharmacia, Ger.*; *Pharmacia, Swed.*; *Pharmacia, UK*); Spasmamina (*Ital.*); Transcop (*Recordati, Ital.*); Transderm Scop (*Ciba, USA*); Transderm-V (*Ciba-Geigy, Canad.*); Vorigeno (*Inibsa, Spain*).

The following names have been used for multi-ingredient preparations containing hyoscine derivatives—Benacine (*Parke, Davis, Austral.*); Butabell (*Saron, USA*); Contac (*Allergan, Austral.*); Dallergy (*Laser, USA*); Diban (*Robins, Canad.*); Donnagel (*Robins, Austral.*; *Robins, Canad.*); Donnagel with Neomycin (*Robins, Canad.*; *Robins, UK*); Donnagel-PG (*Robins, USA*); Donnalix (*Robins, Austral.*); Donnatab (*Robins, Austral.*); Donnatal (*Robins, Austral.*; *Robins, Canad.*; *Robins, UK*; *Robins, USA*); Donnazyme (*Robins, Canad.*; *Robins, USA*); Dura-Vent/DA (*Dura, USA*); Extendryl (*Fleming, USA*); Histaspan-D (*USV Pharmaceutical Corp., USA*); Histor-D (*Hauck, USA*); Hybephen (*Beecham Laboratories, USA*); Kinesed (*Stuart Pharmaceuticals, USA*); Omnopon-Scopolamine (*Roche, Austral.*; *Roche, UK*); Paminal (*Upjohn, UK*); Plexanal (*Sandoz, Canad.*); Rhinolar (*McGregor, USA*); Ru-Tuss Tablets (*Boots, USA*); Sedol (*Rhône-Poulenc, Canad.*); Sinovan Timed (*Drug Industries, USA*); Travacalm (*Hamilton, Austral.*); Urogesic (*Edwards, USA*).

381-x

Hyoscyamine (*USAN*).

l-Hyoscyamine; (−)-Hyoscyamine. (−)-1*R*,3*r*,5*S*)Tropan-3-yl (*S*)-tropate.
$C_{17}H_{23}NO_3$=289.4.

CAS — 101-31-5.

Pharmacopoeias. In *U.S.*

An alkaloid obtained from various solanaceous plants. It is the laevo-isomer of atropine into which it can be converted by heating or by the action of alkali. A white crystalline powder, m.p. 106° to 109°. Slightly **soluble** in water and in benzene; freely soluble in alcohol, chloroform, and dilute acids; sparingly soluble in ether. A solution in water is alkaline to litmus. **Store** in airtight containers. Protect from light.

382-r

Hyoscyamine Hydrobromide (*USAN*).

Bromidrato de Hiosciamina; Hyoscyamine Bromhydrate.
$C_{17}H_{23}NO_3,HBr$=370.3.

CAS — 306-03-6.

Pharmacopoeias. In *Braz.*, *Span.*, and *U.S.*

White, odourless crystals or crystalline powder. M.p. not less than 149°.
Freely **soluble** in water; soluble 1 in 2.5 of alcohol, 1 in 1.7 of chloroform, and 1 in 2300 of ether. A 5% solution in water has a pH of about 5.4. **Store** in airtight containers. Protect from light.

383-f

Hyoscyamine Sulphate (*BAN*).

Hyoscyamine Sulfate (*USAN*); Hyoscyamini Sulfas; Hyoscyaminum Sulfuricum; Iosciamina Solfato.
$(C_{17}H_{23}NO_3)_2,H_2SO_4,2H_2O$=712.9.

CAS — 620-61-1 (anhydrous); 6835-16-1 (dihydrate).

Pharmacopoeias. In *Aust.*, *Br.*, *Eur.*, *Fr.*, *Ger.*, *It.*, *Neth.*, *Swiss*, and *U.S.*

White, odourless crystals or a white deliquescent crystalline powder. *B.P.* **solubilities** are: very soluble in water; sparingly soluble to soluble in alcohol; practically insoluble in chloroform and ether. *U.S.P.* solubilities are: soluble 1 in 0.5 of water and 1 in 5 of alcohol; practically insoluble in ether. The *B.P.* specifies that a 2% solution in water has a pH of 4.5 to 6.2. The *U.S.P.* states that a 1% solution in water has a pH of about 5.3. The *U.S.P.* injection and other dosage forms have a pH of 3.0 to 6.5. **Incompatibilities** as for Atropine Sulphate, p.523. **Store** at 15° to 30° in airtight containers. Protect from light.

For a study on the stability of hyoscyamine in some *B.P.C.* mixtures, see S. A. H. Khalil and S. El-Masry, *J. Pharm. Pharmac.*, 1978, *30*, 664.

Adverse Effects, Treatment, and Precautions

As for Atropine Sulphate, p.523.

Uses and Administration

Hyoscyamine is an antimuscarinic agent with the actions of atropine (see p.524) which is ±-hyoscyamine, but has approximately twice the potency of atropine since the dextro-isomer has only very weak antimuscarinic action. It is used as an adjunct in the treatment of peptic ulcer and in the relief of conditions associated with visceral spasm. It has also been given to relieve the symptoms of parkinsonism.

Hyoscyamine is given in usual doses of 150 to 300 µg four times daily, but it is more usually employed as the sulphate or hydrobromide. In the *USA* suggested doses of hyoscyamine sulphate are 125 to 250 µg three or four times daily, or 375 µg twice daily as a sustained-release capsule; in the *UK* recommended doses are: 400 to 600 µg of the sulphate twice daily as a sustained-release tablet, up to a maximum of 1 mg three times daily if required. Hyoscyamine sulphate has also been given by injection, particularly as an alternative to atropine for premedication before general anaesthesia or in the treatment of the adverse effects of anticholinesterases.

Preparations

Hyoscyamine Sulfate Elixir (*U.S.P.*). Contains hyoscyamine sulphate.

Hyoscyamine Sulfate Injection (*U.S.P.*). Contains hyoscyamine sulphate.

Hyoscyamine Sulfate Oral Solution (*U.S.P.*). Contains hyoscyamine sulphate.

Hyoscyamine Sulfate Tablets (*U.S.P.*). Contain hyoscyamine sulphate.

Hyoscyamine Tablets (*U.S.P.*)

Proprietary Preparations

Peptard (*Riker, UK*). *Tablets*, sustained-release, hyoscyamine sulphate 200 µg.

Proprietary Names and Manufacturers of Hyoscyamine or its Salts

Anaspaz (*Ascher, USA*); Cystospaz (*Webcon, USA*); Cystospaz-M (*Webcon, USA*); Duboisine (*Martinet, Fr.*); Egacen (*S.Afr.*; *Switz.*); Egacene (*Neth.*); Egazil (*Hässle, Denm.*; *Hässle, Norw.*; *Hässle, Swed.*); Levsin (*Canad.*; *Kremers-Urban, USA*); Levsinex (*Kremers-Urban, USA*); Peptard (*Riker, UK*).

The following names have been used for multi-ingredient preparations containing hyoscyamine or its salts—Anaspaz PB (*Ascher, USA*); Arco-Lase Plus (*Arco, USA*); Butabell (*Saron, USA*); Contac (*Allergan, Austral.*); Diban (*Robins, Canad.*); Donnagel (*Robins, Austral.*; *Robins, Canad.*); Donnagel with Neomycin (*Robins, Canad.*; *Robins, UK*); Donnagel-PG (*Robins, USA*); Donnalix (*Robins, Austral.*); Donnatab (*Robins, Austral.*); Donnatal (*Robins, Austral.*; *Robins, Canad.*; *Robins, UK*; *Robins, USA*); Donnazyme (*Robins, Canad.*; *Robins, USA*); Hybephen (*Beecham Laboratories, USA*); Kinesed (*Stuart Pharmaceuticals, USA*); Kutrase (*Kremers-Urban, USA*); Levsin with Phenobarbital (*Kremers-Urban, USA*); Levsinex with Phenobarbital (*Kremers-Urban, USA*); Levsin-PB (*Kremers-Urban, USA*); Natirose (*Lipomed, UK*); Pyridium Plus (*Parke, Davis, USA*); Ru-Tuss Tablets (*Boots, USA*); Trac Tabs (*Hyrex, USA*); Urised (*Webcon, USA*); Uroblue (*Geneva, USA*); Urogesic (*Edwards, USA*).

384-d

Hyoscyamus Leaf (*BAN*).

Banotu; Bilsenkrautblätter; Feuilles de Jusquiame; Giusquiamo; Henbane Leaves; Hojas de Beleño; Hyoscy.; Hyoscyami Folium; Hyoscyami Herba; Hyoscyamus; Jusquiame Noire; Meimendro.

Pharmacopoeias. In *Arg.*, *Aust.*, *Belg.*, *Br.*, *Eur.*, *Fr.*, *Ger.*, *Hung.*, *Int.*, *Mex.*, *Neth.*, *Rus.*, *Span.*, and *Turk.* *Port.* specifies not less than 0.065% alkaloids, *Roum.* not less than 0.04%, *Swiss* not less than 0.05%. *Br.* also includes Powdered Hyoscyamus Leaf. *Chin.* specifies only the seeds.
Belg., *Egypt.*, and *Int.* include Hyoscyamus Muticus (Egyptian Henbane, Herbe de Jusquiame d'Egypte, Aegyptisches Bilsenkraut).

The dried leaves, or leaves, flowering tops, and occasionally fruits of *Hyoscyamus niger* (Solanaceae), containing not less than 0.05% of alkaloids calculated as hyoscyamine. The alkaloids consist of those of the hyoscyamine—atropine group together with hyoscine in varying proportions. The odour is nauseous and disagreeable. **Store** in airtight containers. Protect from light.

428-t

Prepared Hyoscyamus (*BAN*).

Hyoscyami Pulvis Normatus; Poudre Titrée de Jusquiame; Prep. Hyoscy.

Pharmacopoeias. In *Aust.*, *Br.*, *Eur.*, *Fr.*, *Ger.*, and *Neth.*

Hyoscyamus leaf reduced to a powder and adjusted to

contain 0.05 to 0.07% of alkaloids calculated as hyoscyamine. A grey to grey-green powder with a slightly nauseous odour. **Store** in airtight containers. Protect from light.

Adverse Effects, Treatment, and Precautions
As for Atropine Sulphate, p.523.

Hyoscyamus had been designated by the FDA as a herb unsafe for use in foods, beverages, or drugs.— *Am. Pharm.*, 1984, *NS24* (Mar.), 20.

Uses and Administration
Hyoscyamus leaf and preparations of hyoscyamus have peripheral and central effects similar to those of atropine sulphate (see p.524). Hyoscyamus leaf has been used to counteract griping due to strong purgatives and to relieve spasms of the urinary tract.

Preparations

Hyoscyamus Dry Extract *(B.P.)*. A dried and powdered percolate of hyoscyamus leaf with alcohol (70%), adjusted to contain 0.3% of alkaloids calculated as hyoscyamine. Store in small wide-mouthed well-closed containers.

Hyoscyamus Liquid Extract *(B.P.C. 1973)*. Contains 0.05% of alkaloids calculated as hyoscyamine in alcohol(70%). *Dose*. 0.2 to 0.5 mL.

386-h

Ipratropium Bromide *(BAN, USAN, rINN)*.

Sch-1000. (1*R*,3*r*,5*S*,8*r*)-8-Isopropyl-3-[(±)-tropoyloxy]tropanium bromide monohydrate.
$C_{20}H_{30}BrNO_3,H_2O$=430.4.

CAS — 22254-24-6 (anhydrous); 66985-17-9 (monohydrate).

Adverse Effects, Treatment, and Precautions
As for Atropine Sulphate, p.523.

In 3 atopic patients with reversible airway obstruction inhalation of ipratropium bromide as a nebulised solution or from an inhaler resulted in an apparent increase in obstruction and consequent deterioration in condition. The effect might be due to increased sputum viscosity.— C. K. Connolly (letter), *Br. med. J.*, 1982, *285*, 934. Comment. The paradoxical bronchoconstrictor response might alternatively be due to a change in the reactivity of bronchial smooth muscle to antimuscarinic agents in some atopic asthmatics, as even large doses of ipratropium bromide had been reported by Francis *et al.* (*Postgrad. med. J.*, 1975, *51*, Suppl. 7, 110) to have no adverse effect on bronchial mucus flow.— O. M. P. Jolobe (letter), *ibid.*, 1425. A report of pronounced bronchoconstriction following inhalation of ipratropium bromide as an isotonic nebuliser solution by an atopic asthmatic. A similar severe bronchoconstriction was produced by an isotonic solution of sodium bromide but atropine methonitrate solution produced bronchodilatation. The bronchoconstrictor response to ipratropium bromide was unlikely to be due to changes in sputum viscosity or altered response to antimuscarinic agents as there was no similar response to atropine. The results suggest that in this patient bronchoconstriction was related to an adverse reaction to bromide.— K. R. Patel and W. M. Tullett, *ibid.*, 1318. A further report of profound bronchoconstriction in an atopic asthmatic in response to nebulised ipratropium bromide; bronchoconstriction could be reversed by inhalation of salbutamol. Inhalation of nebulised sodium cromoglycate 30 minutes before challenge with ipratropium bromide converted the bronchoconstrictor response to a mild bronchodilator response.— P. H. Howarth (letter), *ibid.*, 1825. In 8 subjects showing paradoxical bronchoconstriction after inhaling ipratropium bromide, the reduction in FEV_1 was 55.5% after inhaling hypo-osmotic placebo, 48% after commercially available hypo-osmotic ipratropium, 12.5% after iso-osmotic ipratropium, and 8.4% after iso-osmotic placebo. The paradoxical response was considered due to hypo-osmolality.— J. S. Mann *et al.*, *ibid.*, 1984, *289*, 469. The manufacturers have now replaced the hypotonic formulation of the nebuliser solution (Atrovent) with an isotonic formulation; it is hoped that bronchoconstriction due to hypotonicity will no longer occur.— J. K. Dewhurst (letter), *ibid.*, 833. Although hypotonicity has been shown to be one factor in bronchoconstriction induced by ipratropium bromide, in the author's original report one case involved a rapid idiosyncratic response to a metered-dose inhaler, and subsequent studies have shown deterioration in peak expiratory flow rate with ipratropium where the effect could not have been due to hypotonicity. Ipratropium bromide is a good and effective drug in certain cases but its effect on airway conductance is unpredictable and it should always be used with caution.— C. K. Connolly (letter), *ibid.*

BUCCAL ULCERATION. A report of inflammation and ulceration of the buccal mucosa associated with the use of an ipratropium bromide inhaler.— P. A. Spencer, *Br. med. J.*, 1986, *292*, 380.

EFFECTS ON THE EYES. A report of closed-angle glaucoma in a patient receiving nebulised ipratropium bromide and salbutamol, via a face-mask. It is likely that acute glaucoma was caused by the topical effect of nebuliser solution escaping from the face-mask; salbutamol may have aggravated the effects of the ipratropium.— G. E. Packe *et al.* (letter), *Lancet*, 1984, *2*, 691. Studies in healthy subjects failed to demonstrate any ocular effects due to nebulised ipratropium bromide administered either via carefully applied or deliberately misplaced face-mask.— P. R. Farrow and G. J. Fancourt, *Hum. Toxicol.*, 1986, *5*, 53.

EFFECTS ON SPUTUM VISCOSITY. Long-term management of asthma with ipratropium bromide carries the danger of increasing sputum viscosity - a highly undesirable complication in a disease in which severe attacks are characterised by mucus plugging of the bronchi.— G. K. Crompton (letter), *Lancet*, 1982, *1*, 1243. Criticism. There is no evidence that the use of antimuscarinic drugs shown to be effective in asthma causes dry tenacious secretions or mucus plugging.— D. Pavia *et al.* (letter), *ibid.*, *2*, 332; J. A. Nadel (letter), *ibid.*, 823.

See also above.

Absorption and Fate
Ipratropium bromide is poorly absorbed from the gastro-intestinal tract. It has been reported to be partly metabolised following oral administration and to be excreted in the urine and faeces as unchanged drug and metabolites. Little or none is absorbed from the lungs following inhalation.

After administration of ipratropium bromide by mouth, intravenously, and by inhalation, cumulative renal excretion was 9.3, 72.1 and 3.2% respectively and faecal excretion was 88.5, 6.3 and 69.4% respectively. The half-life of elimination from plasma was 3.2 to 3.8 hours for all methods of administration. Comparison of results following oral administration and inhalation leads to the conclusion that the pharmacokinetics of inhaled ipratropium bromide is due to the swallowed portion of the dose.— J. Adlung *et al.*, *Arzneimittel-Forsch.*, 1976, *26*, 1005.

Uses and Administration
Ipratropium bromide is a quaternary ammonium antimuscarinic agent with peripheral effects similar to those of atropine (see p.524). It is used by inhalation as a bronchodilator in the treatment of chronic reversible airways obstruction, particularly in chronic bronchitis. The usual dose is 20 or 40 µg (1 or 2 puffs of a metered-dose inhaler) three or four times daily by inhalation; single doses of up to 80 µg have been required during the initial stages of treatment. In children aged 6 to 12 years the usual dose is 20 or 40 µg three times daily, and below 6 years the usual dose is 20 µg three times daily.

Ipratropium bromide has also been administered by inhalation as a nebulised solution.

A review of antimuscarinic bronchodilators, with particular reference to ipratropium.— N. J. Gross and M. S. Skorodin, *Am. Rev. resp. Dis.*, 1984, *129*, 856.

Studies with ipratropium bromide administered via inhalation show it to be at least as effective as, and possibly superior to, commonly used $beta_2$-adrenoceptor agonists in chronic bronchitis, but it appears to be less effective than these agents in asthma. Maximum bronchodilation occurs after 1.5 to 2 hours, suggesting it would be more appropriate for prophylaxis rather than treatment of attacks of acute dyspnoea.

Combination of ipratropium bromide with a $beta_2$-agonist or theophylline has resulted in an enhanced bronchodilator effect over the individual agents alone, although studies have not always shown the increase to be significant.

Ipratropium bromide appears to be indicated primarily in the management of chronic obstructive airways disease as an alternative in patients who fail to respond adequately to sympathomimetics; it may also be useful in patients unable to tolerate therapeutic doses of $beta_2$-agonists, or in combination regimens in patients who fail to respond to single-drug regimens.— K. L. Massey and V. P. Gotz, *Drug Intell. & clin. Pharm.*, 1985, *19*, 5.

Earlier reviews: G. E. Pakes *et al.*, *Drugs*, 1980, *20*, 237; *Drug & Ther. Bull.*, 1980, *18*, 59.

The proceedings of a symposium on antimuscarinic drugs, including ipratropium, in airways disease.— *Postgrad. med. J.*, 1987, *63 Suppl. 1*.

ASTHMA. A nebulised beta-stimulant remains first-line treatment in *acute asthma*, but nebulised ipratropium bromide should be added if appropriate, the two being given alternately at 60 to 120 minute intervals.— J. Rees, *Br. med. J.*, 1984, *288*, 1747. Administration of nebulised ipratropium bromide with or after a $beta_2$-adrenoceptor agonist should remove any risk of ipratropium-induced bronchoconstriction, and can give useful additional bronchodilatation in patients with *acute asthma*.— *Lancet*, 1986, *1*, 131.

In *chronic asthma*, ipratropium bromide is most effective in very young children and older patients, and least effective in those in their 'teens and twenties. The dose delivered by the standard inhaler is probably too low and ipratropium bromide has taken second place as a bronchodilator, except when tremor is troublesome with $beta_2$-adrenoceptor stimulants.— J. Rees, *Br. med. J.*, 1984, *288*, 1819.

A review of the use of ipratropium bromide in association with $beta_2$-adrenoceptor agonist bronchodilators. The information in the published literature has borne out the suggestion that such a combination might offer greater efficacy and longer duration of action in patients with chronic bronchitis and emphysema, who are generally older, but the case for giving such treatment to younger asthmatic patients perhaps needs more evaluation before any definite recommendation can be made.— M. Rudolf, *Postgrad. med. J.*, 1984, *60*, *Suppl.* 1, 9.

Reviews and comments on a fixed-dose combination inhaler containing ipratropium bromide with fenoterol hydrobromide (Duovent): V. J. Phillips, *Postgrad. med. J.*, 1984, *60*, *Suppl.* 1, 13; *Drug & Ther. Bull.*, 1985, *23*, 3. There is no justification whatsoever for using the combined preparation of fenoterol hydrobromide and ipratropium bromide unless the response to each component is assessed separately.— C. K. Connolly, *Br. med. J.*, 1984, *289*, 833. In a variable disease such as asthma where treatment should be regularly tailored to the state of the disease it seems particularly illogical to use fixed-dose combinations which restrict flexibility of treatment.— J. Rees, *ibid.*, *288*, 1819.

In a crossover study involving 14 patients with *chronic asthma*, high-dose ipratropium bromide 160 µg at night, inhaled alone or with salbutamol 200 µg, was significantly more effective than the same dose of salbutamol alone in reducing the morning 'dip' of peak expiratory flow rate and in improving nocturnal symptoms, although there was no significant difference with respect to morning wheezing. Ipratropium in association with salbutamol was no more effective than ipratropium alone. Dry mouth was reported in 3 patients and an unpleasant taste in 5 following ipratropium.— I. D. Cox *et al.*, *Postgrad. med. J.*, 1984, *60*, 526. In an earlier study in 12 asthmatic patients administered either nebulised salbutamol 5 mg, followed 1 hour later by ipratropium bromide 1 mg, or the other way around, both drugs produced a significant increase in peak expiratory flow rate when given first, but a further increase with the second drug occurred only with salbutamol following ipratropium. The results suggest that to obtain a synergistic action the sympathomimetic should be given after ipratropium.— B. C. Leahy *et al.*, *Br. J. Dis. Chest*, 1983, *77*, 159.

In a crossover study in 9 *chronic asthmatics* significant increases in FEV_1 occurred following high doses of ipratropium bromide 80, 200, or 400 µg by metered-dose inhaler, and the higher doses appeared to produce greater bronchodilation and a longer duration of action. Further studies with high doses of this drug are warranted to evaluate their clinical usefulness in the management of asthma.— B. Hockley and N. M. Johnson, *Br. J. Dis. Chest*, 1985, *79*, 379.

In children. If treatment for distress associated with wheezing in children under 18 months of age is required, inhaled nebulised ipratropium bromide sometimes temporarily relieves the bronchoconstriction; infants of this age are relatively unresponsive to beta agonists, which are more effective in children over 18 months old.— J. Reiser, *Br. J. Hosp. Med.*, 1985, *33*, 196. See also J. Reiser and J. O. Warner, *Archs Dis. Childh.*, 1986, *61*, 88.

In 138 children admitted to hospital because of asthma and given either salbutamol alone or salbutamol in association with ipratropium bromide, via a nebuliser, severe airways obstruction responded better to salbutamol alone than to combined treatment. There were no significant differences between the groups in length of hospital stay or number of doses received. In the light of these results, the addition of ipratropium to treatment regimens in acute severe childhood asthma cannot be recommended.— J. Storr and W. Lenney, *Archs Dis. Childh.*, 1986, *61*, 602.

BRONCHITIS AND BRONCHIOLITIS. A study involving 25 sleeping infants aged 5 to 48 weeks with acute severe bronchiolitis administered salbutamol 5 mg or ipratropium bromide 250 µg, via a nebuliser, showed that after salbutamol there was effectively no change in the work of breathing per litre of air, and a mean deterioration of 21.8% in work of breathing per minute; whereas following ipratropium bromide there was a mean fall of 16% in work of breathing per litre and of 18.2% in work of breathing per minute. The study indicates that ipratropium bromide can sometimes reduce airways obstruction in acute bronchiolitis.— G. M. Stokes *et al.*, *Archs Dis. Childh.*, 1983, *58*, 279. A subsequent double-blind study from the same unit involving 66 children with acute bronchiolitis failed to find any evidence that treatment with ipratropium bromide 250 µg as a nebulised solution had any significant benefit over placebo; in 2 cases ipratropium bromide might actually have prolonged the illness.— R. L. Henry *et al.*, *ibid.*, 925.

Results of a placebo-controlled study in 20 patients with chronic bronchitis demonstrated that nebulised ipratropium bromide 500 µg or nebulised salbutamol 5 mg both acted within 15 minutes and produced similar degrees of bronchodilatation; used together they produced bronchodilatation of greater magnitude than either agent alone and of greater duration than salbutamol. Individual responses varied, suggesting that some, but not all, patients would benefit from addition of ipratropium bromide to their therapy.— C. S. Chan *et al.*, *Br. J. clin. Pharmac.*, 1984, *17*, 103.

Ipratropium bromide and salbutamol were equipotent when inhaled in maximal doses in a crossover study in 11 patients with chronic obstructive lung disease and there was no further advantage when the other drug was added as a second agent.— P. A. Easton *et al.*, *New Engl. J. Med.*, 1986, *315*, 735.

Studies of ipratropium bromide in association with fenoterol in patients with obstructive airways disease including chronic bronchitis: G. E. Packe *et al.*, *Postgrad. med. J.*, 1984, *60*, *Suppl.* 1, 18; O. T. Tang and M. Flatley, *ibid.*, 24; O. Morton, *ibid.*, 32.

See also under Asthma, above.

CYSTIC FIBROSIS. A review of the management of cystic fibrosis. Improved expiratory flow has been shown in some patients after inhalation of ipratropium bromide, and this drug should be tried if there is no response to beta$_2$-adrenoceptor stimulants.— M. B. Mearns, *Archs Dis. Childh.*, 1985, *60*, 272.

RHINITIS. Intranasal ipratropium bromide 40 µg to each nostril 4 times daily significantly reduced chronic watery rhinorrhoea in a crossover study in 20 patients, but had no significant effect on nasal obstruction or sneezing.— N. P. von Haacke *et al.*, *Br. med. J.*, 1983, *287*, 1258.

In a study in 24 patients with allergic or non-allergic rhinitis, pretreatment with ipratropium bromide 40 µg to each nostril resulted in a lower volume of nasal secretion and fewer sneezes, following challenge with nasal methacholine, than did placebo treatment. Intranasal ipratropium may have a place in the treatment of nasal hypersecretion and sneezing in allergic as well as non-allergic patients suffering from rhinitis.— S. Sanwikarja *et al.*, *Ann. Allergy*, 1986, *56*, 162.

Proprietary Preparations

Atrovent *(Boehringer Ingelheim, UK). Inhaler*, aerosol, ipratropium bromide 18 µg/metered inhalation.
Nebuliser solution, ipratropium bromide 250 µg/mL.

Atrovent Forte *(Boehringer Ingelheim, UK). Inhaler*, aerosol, ipratropium bromide 36 µg/metered inhalation.

Proprietary Names and Manufacturers

Atem *(Chiesi, Ital.)*; Atrovent *(Boehringer Ingelheim, Austral.*; *Belg.*; *Boehringer Ingelheim, Canad.*; *Boehringer Ingelheim, Denm.*; *Boehringer Ingelheim, Fr.*; *Boehringer Ingelheim, Ger.*; *Neth.*; *Boehringer Ingelheim, Norw.*; *Boehringer Ingelheim, S.Afr.*; *Spain*; *Boehringer Ingelheim, Swed.*; *Boehringer Ingelheim, Switz.*; *Boehringer Ingelheim, UK*; *Boehringer Ingelheim, USA)*; Disne-Asmol *(Berenguer-Beneyto, Spain)*; Itrop *(Boehringer Ingelheim, Ger.)*.

387-m

Isopropamide Iodide *(BAN, USAN, rINN)*.

Iodeto de Isopropamida. (3-Carbamoyl-3,3-diphenylpropyl)di-isopropylmethylammonium iodide.
$C_{23}H_{33}IN_2O$=480.4.

CAS — 7492-32-2 (isopropamide); 71-81-8 (iodide).

Pharmacopoeias. In *Braz.* and *U.S.*

A white to pale yellow crystalline powder. Isopropamide iodide 1.36 mg is approximately equivalent to 1 mg of isopropamide. **Soluble** 1 in 50 of water, 1 in 10 of alcohol, and 1 in 5 of chloroform; very slightly soluble in ether. **Protect** from light.

Isopropamide is a quaternary ammonium antimuscarinic agent with peripheral effects similar to those of atropine (see p.524). It is used as an adjunct in the treatment of peptic ulcer in doses of isopropamide iodide equivalent to 5 to 10 mg of isopropamide every 12 hours. It has also been used in the relief of visceral spasms.

The use of isopropamide iodide in cosmetics is prohibited in the *UK*.

Preparations

Isopropamide Iodide Tablets *(U.S.P.)*

Proprietary Names and Manufacturers

Darbid *(Smith Kline & French, Canad.*; *Smith Kline & French, USA)*; Dipramid *(Ital.)*; Priamide *(Janssen, Belg.*; *Janssen, Denm.*; *Delalande, Fr.*; *Janssen, Ger.*; *Janssen, Neth.)*; Tyrimide *(Smith Kline & French, Austral.*; *Smith Kline & French, UK)*.

The following names have been used for multi-ingredient preparations containing isopropamide iodide—Combid *(Smith Kline & French, Canad.*; *Smith Kline & French, USA)*; Prochlor-Iso *(Schein, USA)*; Pro-Iso *(Geneva, USA)*; Stelabid *(Smith Kline & French, Austral.*; *Smith Kline & French, Canad.*; *Smith Kline & French, UK)*.

389-v

Lachesine Chloride

E-3; Laches. Chlor.; Lachesine. (2-Benziloyloxyethyl)ethyldimethylammonium chloride.
$C_{20}H_{26}ClNO_3$=363.9.

CAS — 1164-38-1.

Pharmacopoeias. In *B.P.C. 1973.*

Adverse Effects, Treatment, and Precautions

As for Atropine Sulphate, p.523.

Lachesine is not recommended in old people as the subsequent response to miotics is slower than after homatropine.

Uses and Administration

Lachesine chloride is a quaternary ammonium antimuscarinic agent with cycloplegic and mydriatic properties similar to, but less prolonged than, those of atropine (see p.524). It has been used as eye-drops containing 1% as a substitute for atropine or homatropine in patients with hypersensitivity to these drugs.

Preparations

Lachesine Eye-drops *(B.P.C. 1973)*. LAC. A sterile solution containing up to 1% of lachesine chloride in water. The solution is sterilised by autoclaving or by filtration or by maintaining at 98° to 100° for 30 minutes; it is adversely affected by alkalis.

12914-t

Mazaticol Hydrochloride *(rINNM)*.

KAO-264; PG-501. 6,6,9-Trimethyl-9-azabicyclo[3.3.1]-non-3β-yl di(2-thienyl)glycolate hydrochloride monohydrate.
$C_{21}H_{27}NO_3S_2,HCl,H_2O$=460.1.

CAS — 42024-98-6 (mazaticol).

Mazaticol hydrochloride is an antimuscarinic agent with actions and uses similar to those of benzhexol (see p.527). It has been used by mouth in the symptomatic treatment of parkinsonism and of the drug-induced extrapyramidal syndrome.

Proprietary Names and Manufacturers

Pentona *(Tanabe, Jpn)*.

390-r

Mepenzolate Bromide *(BAN, USAN, rINN)*.

Mepenzolate Methylbromide; Mepenzolone Bromide. 3-Benziloyloxy-1,1-dimethylpiperidinium bromide.
$C_{21}H_{26}BrNO_3$=420.3.

CAS — 25990-43-6 (mepenzolate); 76-90-4 (bromide).

Pharmacopoeias. In *Jpn* and *U.S.*

A white or light cream-coloured powder. **Soluble** 1 in 110 of water, 1 in 120 of dehydrated alcohol, 1 in 630 of chloroform, and 1 in about 8 of methyl alcohol; practically insoluble in ether. **Store** in airtight containers.

Adverse Effects, Treatment, and Precautions

As for Atropine Sulphate, p.523.

Mepenzolate may cause gastric pain, which should be distinguished from the pain of the visceral spasms that it is used to treat.

Uses and Administration

Mepenzolate bromide is a quaternary ammonium antimuscarinic agent with peripheral actions similar to those of atropine (see p.524). It is given in the symptomatic treatment of peptic ulcer, and in the relief of visceral spasms in doses of 25 to 50 mg three or four times daily.

ABSORPTION AND FATE. About 14% of a dose of 25 or 30 mg of mepenzolate bromide was absorbed from the gastro-intestinal tract and excreted in the urine over 4 to 5 days.— H. L. Friedman and R. I. H. Wang, *J. pharm. Sci.*, 1972, *61*, 1663.

Preparations

Mepenzolate Bromide Syrup *(U.S.P.)*. Mepenzolate Bromide Solution; Mepenzolate Bromide Oral Solution. Protect from light.

Mepenzolate Bromide Tablets *(U.S.P.)*

Proprietary Preparations

Cantil *(MCP Pharmaceuticals, UK). Tablets*, scored, mepenzolate bromide 25 mg.
Elixir, mepenzolate bromide 12.5 mg/5 mL.

Proprietary Names and Manufacturers

Cantil *(Sigma, Austral.*; *Bellon, Fr.*; *Draco, Swed.*; *MCP Pharmaceuticals, UK*; *Merrell Dow, USA)*; Cantril *(Ital.)*; Colibantil *(Ital.)*; Colum *(Ital.)*; Eftoron *(Jpn)*; Gastropidil *(Ital.)*; Tralanta *(Jpn)*.

The following names have been used for multi-ingredient preparations containing mepenzolate bromide— Cantil with Phenobarbitone *(MCP Pharmaceuticals, UK)*; Neo-cantil *(MCP Pharmaceuticals, UK)*.

391-f

Methanthelinium Bromide *(BAN, pINN)*.

Dixamonum Bromidum; Methantheline Bromide *(USAN)*; MTB-51; SC-2910. Diethylmethyl[2-(xanthen-9-ylcarbonyloxy)ethyl]ammonium bromide.
$C_{21}H_{26}BrNO_3$=420.3.

CAS — 5818-17-7 (methanthelinium); 53-46-3 (bromide).

Pharmacopoeias. In *Arg.*, *Port.*, and *U.S.*

A white, or almost white, almost odourless powder. **Soluble** 1 in less than 5 of water, alcohol, and chloroform, and 1 in 390 of acetone; practically insoluble in ether. A solution in water has a pH of about 5. Aqueous solutions hydrolyse slowly.

Adverse Effects, Treatment, and Precautions

As for Atropine Sulphate, p.523.

Skin rashes, including exfoliative dermatitis, have been reported in patients receiving methanthelinium.

Uses and Administration

Methanthelinium bromide is a quaternary ammonium antimuscarinic agent with peripheral effects similar to those of atropine (see p.524). It has been largely replaced in clinical practice by its more potent derivative, propantheline bromide (see p.542). Doses of 50 to 100 mg have been given four times daily as an adjunct in the treatment of peptic ulcer, and in the relief of visceral spasms. It has also been used in the management of neurogenic bladder.

Preparations

Methantheline Bromide Tablets *(U.S.P.)*. Contain methanthelinium bromide.

Sterile Methantheline Bromide *(U.S.P.)*. Methanthelinium bromide suitable for parenteral use.

Proprietary Names and Manufacturers
Banthine *(Searle, Arg.; Searle, Denm.; Searle, USA)*; Broneg *(Ital.)*; Evogal *(Zambeletti, Ital.)*; Frenogastrico *(Vera, Spain)*; Probantim *(Lusofarmaco, Ital.)*; Ulcuwas Antiespasmodico *(Spain)*; Vagantin *(Brunnengräber, Ger.)*; Vaxantene *(Boniscontro & Gazzone, Ital.)*; Xantenol *(Janus, Ital.)*.

392-d

Methixene Hydrochloride *(BAN, USAN)*.

Methixene Hydrochloride Monohydrate; Metixene Hydrochloride *(rINNM)*; NSC-78194; SJ-1977. 9-(1-Methyl-3-piperidylmethyl)thioxanthene hydrochloride monohydrate.
$C_{20}H_{23}NS,HCl,H_2O=364.0$.

CAS — 4969-02-2 (methixene); 1553-34-0 (hydrochloride, anhydrous); 7081-40-5 (hydrochloride, monohydrate).

Adverse Effects, Treatment, and Precautions
As for Atropine Sulphate, p.523.

Absorption and Fate
Methixene is absorbed from the gastro-intestinal tract and is excreted in the urine, partly unchanged and partly as its isomeric sulphoxides or their metabolites.

Uses and Administration
Methixene hydrochloride is an antimuscarinic agent with actions similar to those of atropine (see p.524); it also has antihistaminic and direct antispasmodic properties. It is used for the symptomatic treatment of parkinsonism. Unlike some other antimuscarinic antiparkinsonian drugs, it is claimed to be more effective in controlling the tremors than in reducing the rigidity of this syndrome.
The usual dose of methixene hydrochloride is 2.5 mg three times daily initially, gradually increased according to the response of the patient to a total of 15 to 60 mg daily in divided doses. Transition to or from methixene therapy should be gradual otherwise symptoms may be aggravated.
Methixene hydrochloride has been used as an adjunct in the treatment of peptic ulcer, and to relieve visceral spasms in usual doses of 1 or 2 mg three times daily.

PARKINSONISM. For discussion of the treatment of parkinsonism, including reference to the role of antimuscarinic agents, see under Levodopa, p.1019.

Proprietary Preparations
Tremonil *(Sandoz, UK)*. *Tablets*, scored, methixene hydrochloride 5 mg.

Proprietary Names and Manufacturers
Methyloxan *(Jpn)*; Tremaril *(Belg.; Sandoz, Denm.; Sandoz, Ital.; Neth.; S.Afr.; Sandoz, Spain; Wander, Switz.)*; Tremarit *(Wander, Ger.)*; Tremonil *(Austral.; Sandoz, UK)*; Tremoquil *(Astra, Swed.)*; Trest *(USA)*.

12945-m

Methscopolamine Methylsulphate

N-Methyl Hyoscine Methylsulphate. (−)-(1*S*,3*s*,5*R*,6*R*,7*S*)-6,7-Epoxy-8-methyl-3-[(*S*)-tropoyloxy]tropanium methyl sulphate.
$C_{18}H_{24}NO_4,CH_3O_4S=429.5$.

CAS — 13265-10-6 (methscopolamine); 18067-13-5 (methylsulphate).

Methscopolamine methylsulphate is a quaternary ammonium antimuscarinic agent with peripheral effects similar to those of atropine; it shares the general properties of salts of *N*-methyl hyoscine (see Hyoscine Methobromide, p.534). It is used as an adjunct in the treatment of peptic ulcer and to relieve visceral spasms, in doses of 1 or 2 mg by mouth 3 or 4 times daily; doses of 2 mg have also been given twice daily as sustained-release capsules.

Proprietary Names and Manufacturers
Daipin *(Jpn)*; Sandrix *(Sanders-Probel, Belg.)*; Ulix *(Substantia, Fr.)*.

393-n

Octatropine Methylbromide *(BAN, rINN)*.

Anisotropine Methobromide; Anisotropine Methylbromide *(USAN)*. (1*R*,3*r*,5*S*)-8-Methyl-3-(2-propylvaleryloxy)tropanium bromide.
$C_{17}H_{32}BrNO_2=362.4$.

CAS — 80-50-2.

Octatropine methylbromide is a quaternary ammonium antimuscarinic agent with peripheral actions similar to those of atropine (see p.524). It is used in doses of 10 mg three or four times daily by mouth to relieve visceral spasms; in the *USA* it is used in doses of 50 mg three times daily as an adjunct in the treatment of peptic ulcer.

Proprietary Names and Manufacturers
Valpin *(Du Pont, Austral.; Endo, Canad.; Crinos, Ital.; Endo, S.Afr.; Du Pont, USA)*; Vapin *(Lacer, Spain)*.

The following names have been used for multi-ingredient preparations containing octatropine methylbromide—Valpin-PB *(Du Pont, USA)*.

394-h

Orphenadrine Citrate *(BANM, USAN, rINNM)*.

Mephenamine Citrate; Orphenadin Citrate.
$C_{18}H_{23}NO,C_6H_8O_7=461.5$.

CAS — 83-98-7 (orphenadrine); 4682-36-4 (citrate).

Pharmacopoeias. In *Br.* and *U.S.*

A white or almost white, odourless or almost odourless, crystalline powder. Orphenadrine citrate 100 mg is approximately equivalent to 66 mg of orphenadrine hydrochloride.
Soluble 1 in 70 of water; slightly soluble in alcohol; practically insoluble in chloroform and ether. The *U.S.P.* injection has a pH between 5 and 6. **Store** in airtight containers. Protect from light.

395-m

Orphenadrine Hydrochloride *(BANM, rINNM)*.

BS-5930; Mephenamine Hydrochloride; Orphenadin Hydrochloride. *NN*-Dimethyl-2-(2-methylbenzhydryloxy)ethylamine hydrochloride.
$C_{18}H_{23}NO,HCl=305.8$.

CAS — 341-69-5.

Pharmacopoeias. In *Br.*

A white or almost white, odourless or almost odourless, crystalline powder.
Soluble 1 in 1 of water and of alcohol, and 1 in 2 of chloroform; practically insoluble in ether. **Store** in well-closed containers. Protect from light.

Adverse Effects and Treatment
As for Atropine Sulphate, p.523.

ABUSE. A 23-year-old schizophrenic man, whose treatment included orphenadrine 100 mg thrice daily, obtained illicit supplies and increased the dose for euphoric effect. On one occasion he had an epileptic convulsion after a 600-mg dose.— M. E. Shariatmadari (letter), *Br. med. J.*, 1975, *3*, 486.
See also under Benzhexol Hydrochloride, p.527.

OVERDOSAGE. A 25-year-old man who had ingested an estimated 1.2 to 1.5 g of orphenadrine citrate was successfully treated by intravenous injection of physostigmine 1 mg. The patient had been severely mentally agitated but within 5 minutes of injection was alert, orientated and cooperative, and his heart-rate had gone down from 150 beats per minute to 75. He required no further treatment with physostigmine.— B. D. Synder *et al.* (letter), *New Engl. J. Med.*, 1976, *295*, 1435. Criticism. Since cardiotoxic problems were the direct cause of death in orphenadrine intoxication, and the antimuscarinic side-effects of relatively minor importance, the administration of physostigmine was not indicated and could be dangerous. Only after at least 12 hours and when the extent of cardiac involvement had been assessed should administration of physostigmine be considered.— B. Sangster *et al.* (letter), *ibid.*, 1977, *296*, 1006.
Orphenadrine was considered to be a dangerous drug when given in large doses or when overdoses are taken and 3 deaths are reported. Toxic effects can occur rapidly within 2 hours with convulsions, cardiac dysrhythmias, and death; these effects are considered to be very similar to those of tricyclic antidepressants. Eleven patients suffering from the toxic effects of orphenadrine had been admitted to the Regional Poisoning Treatment Centre in Edinburgh in the first 6 months of 1977 and 1 of these patients had died.— W. M. Millar (letter), *Lancet*, 1977, *2*, 566.
A report of acute poisoning with orphenadrine following massive overdosage in a schizophrenic patient, who responded to intensive supportive treatment, including huge doses of adrenaline, dopamine, and dobutamine to restore blood pressure following asystole. Between 1977 and 1980 twelve deaths due to orphenadrine were recorded by the National Poisons Unit at Guy's Hospital: drugs such as orphendrine should be prescribed carefully and only in small amounts to patients in whom it is considered that there is a real risk of self-poisoning.— B. Clarke *et al.* (letter), *Lancet*, 1985, *1*, 1386. Agreement. Other antimuscarinic agents are to be preferred in such patients as they are usually less toxic when ingested in overdose.— B. Sangster (letter), *ibid.*, *2*, 280. Criticism. The antimuscarinics available for drug-induced parkinsonism have similar pharmacological effects; although there is a risk of self-poisoning, it is not restricted to orphenadrine.— C. J. Mugglestone (letter), *ibid.*, 617.

Precautions
As for Atropine Sulphate, p.524.

A suggested interaction between orphenadrine and dextropropoxyphene was open to question.— R. E. Pearson and F. J. Salter (letter), *New Engl. J. Med.*, 1970, *282*, 1215. See also W. H. Puckett and J. A. Visconti (letter), *ibid.*, *283*, 544. Criticism.— W. Renforth (letter), *ibid.*, 998.

PORPHYRIA. Orphenadrine was considered to be unsafe in patients with acute porphyria because it has been shown to be porphyrinogenic in *animals* or *in vitro* systems.— M.R. Moore and K.E.L. McColl, *Porphyrias, Drug Lists*, Glasgow, Porphyria Research Unit, University of Glasgow, 1987.

Absorption and Fate
Orphenadrine is readily absorbed from the gastro-intestinal tract. It is rapidly distributed in tissues and most of a dose is metabolised and excreted in the urine along with a small proportion of unchanged drug. A half-life of 14 hours has been reported.

Uses and Administration
Orphenadrine, which is a congener of diphenhydramine without sharing its soporific effect, is an antimuscarinic agent with actions and uses similar to those of benzhexol (see p.527). It also has weak antihistaminic and local anaesthetic properties.
Orphenadrine is used as the hydrochloride in the symptomatic treatment of parkinsonism. It is also used to alleviate the extrapyramidal syndrome induced by drugs such as the phenothiazine derivatives but is of no value against tardive dyskinesias, which may be exacerbated. The initial dose is 150 mg daily in divided doses gradually increased by 50 mg every 2 or 3 days according to the response of the patient; some patients may require a total of up to 400 mg daily. In emergency, orphenadrine hydrochloride may be given intramuscularly in a dose of 20 to 40 mg. Transition to or from orphenadrine therapy should be gradual otherwise symptoms may be aggravated.
Orphenadrine is also used as the citrate to relieve pain due to spasm of skeletal muscle. The usual dose of orphenadrine citrate is 100 mg twice or three times daily by mouth, adjusted according to the patient's response, or 60 mg every 12 hours by intramuscular or slow intravenous injection (over a period of about 5 minutes).

EXTRAPYRAMIDAL DISORDERS. For a review of the role of antimuscarinic agents in the treatment of drug-induced extrapyramidal disorders, see p.522.

MUSCULAR PAIN. Reports and studies on the use of orphenadrine alone or in association with analgesics to relieve pain associated with skeletal muscle spasm: T. Tervo *et al.*, *Br. J. clin. Pract.*, 1976, *30*, 62; E. N. S. Fry (letter), *Br. J. Anaesth.*, 1978, *50*, 205; R. H. Gold, *Curr. ther. Res.*, 1978, *23*, 271; L. Winter and A. Post, *J. int. med. Res.*, 1979, *7*, 240; B. W. McGuinness, *ibid.*, 1983, *11*, 42; H. O. Høivik and N. Moe, *Curr. med. Res. Opinion*, 1983, *8*, 531.

PARKINSONISM. For discussion of the treatment of parkinsonism, including reference to the role of antimuscarinic agents, see under Levodopa, p.1019.

RESTLESS LEG SYNDROME. Orphenadrine was effective in the treatment of restless legs in some patients who could not tolerate diazepam.— L. K. Morgan (letter), *Med. J. Aust.*, 1975, *2*, 753.

Preparations of some Orphenadrine Salts

Orphenadrine Citrate Injection *(U.S.P.)*
Orphenadrine Hydrochloride Tablets *(B.P.)*

Proprietary Preparations of some Orphenadrine Salts

Biorphen *(Bio-Medical, UK)*. *Oral liquid*, orphenadrine hydrochloride 25 mg/5 mL.

Disipal *(Brocades, UK)*. *Tablets*, orphenadrine hydrochloride 50 mg.
Injection, orphenadrine hydrochloride 20 mg/mL, in ampoules of 2 mL.

Norflex *(Riker, UK)*. *Injection*, orphenadrine citrate 30 mg/mL, in ampoules of 2 mL.

Proprietary Names and Manufacturers of Orphenadrine Salts

Biorphen *(Bio-Medical, UK)*; Brocadisipal *(Denm.)*; Disipal *(Riker, Austral.; Belg.; Riker, Canad.; Gist-Brocades, Denm.; Beytout, Fr.; Brocades, Ital.; Neth.; Gist-Brocades, Norw.; Brocades, S.Afr.; Gist-Brocades, Swed.; Gist-Brocades, Switz.; Brocades, UK; Riker, USA)*; Distalene *(Arg.)*; Euflex *(Ital.)*; Lysantin *(GEA, Denm.)*; Mefeamina *(Morrith, Spain)*; Myotrol *(Legere, USA)*; Norflex *(Riker, Austral.; Belg.; Riker, Canad.; Riker, Denm.; Kettelhack Riker, Ger.; Riker, S.Afr.; Riker, Swed.; Riker 3M, Switz.; Riker, UK; Riker, USA)*; Orpadrex *(Protea, Austral.; S.Afr.)*; Orphenate *(Hyrex, USA)*; Tega-Flex *(USA)*; X-Otag *(Reid-Provident, USA)*.

The following names have been used for multi-ingredient preparations containing orphenadrine salts— Norgesic *(Riker, Austral.; Riker, Canad.; Riker, UK; Riker, USA)*.

13048-n

Otilonium Bromide *(rINN)*.

Diethylmethyl{2-[4-(2-octyloxybenzamido)benzoyloxy]-ethyl}ammonium bromide.
$C_{29}H_{43}BrN_2O_4$=563.6.

CAS — 26095-59-0.

Otilonium bromide is a quaternary ammonium antimuscarinic agent with peripheral actions similar to those of atropine (see p.524). It is used in the symptomatic treatment of visceral spasms; doses of 20 to 40 mg by mouth 2 or 3 times daily, or 20 mg up to 3 times daily by the rectal route have been recommended.

Proprietary Names and Manufacturers
Spasmoctyl *(Menarini, Spain)*; Spasmomen *(Menarini, Ital.)*.

13053-r

Oxapium Iodide *(rINN)*.

Cyclonium Iodide; SH-100. 1-(2-Cyclohexyl-2-phenyl-1,3-dioxolan-4-ylmethyl)-1-methylpiperidinium iodide.
$C_{22}H_{34}INO_2$=471.4.

CAS — 6577-41-9.

Oxapium iodide is a quaternary ammonium antimuscarinic agent with peripheral actions similar to those of atropine (see p.524). It has been used for the symptomatic treatment of visceral spasm.
Oxapium has also been given as the bromide.

Proprietary Names and Manufacturers
Esperan *(Toyama, Jpn)*.

13065-h

Oxitropium Bromide *(BAN, rINN)*.

BA-253. 6,7-Epoxy-8-ethyl-3-[(*S*)-tropoyloxy]tropanium bromide.
$C_{19}H_{26}BrNO_4$=412.3.

CAS — 30286-75-0.

Oxitropium bromide is a quaternary ammonium antimuscarinic agent with peripheral actions similar to those of atropine (see p.524). It is used similarly to ipratropium bromide, to which it is structurally related, in the treatment of chronic reversible airways obstruction; doses of 200 µg (2 puffs) by inhalation from a metered-dose aerosol have been given 2 to 3 times daily.

Oxitropium bromide is a quaternary ammonium compound derived from hyoscine. In a study in 20 atopic asthmatics oxitropium bromide 200 µg by inhalation was as effective as ipratropium bromide 80 µg in increasing peak expiratory flow rate over placebo values.— G. Anderson, *Postgrad. med. J.*, 1983, *59*, *Suppl.* 3, 64. See also: A. Taytard *et al.*, *Eur. J. clin. Pharmac.*, 1984, *26*, 429 (use in asthmatic patients); E. T. Peel *et al.*, *Eur. J. resp. Dis.*, 1984, *65*, 106 (comparison with ipratropium bromide).

The proceedings of a symposium on antimuscarinic drugs, including oxitropium, in airways disease.— *Postgrad. med. J.*, 1987, *63*, *Suppl.1*.

Proprietary Names and Manufacturers
Oxivent *(Boehringer Ingelheim, Belg.)*; Tersigat *(Boehringer Ingelheim, Fr.)*; Ventilat *(Dieckmann, Ger.)*.

396-b

Oxybutynin Hydrochloride *(BANM, rINNM)*.

MJ-4309-1; Oxybutynin Chloride *(USAN)*. 4-Diethylaminobut-2-ynyl α-cyclohexylmandelate hydrochloride.
$C_{22}H_{31}NO_3$,HCl=394.0.

CAS — 5633-20-5 (oxybutynin); 1508-65-2 (hydrochloride).

Pharmacopoeias. In *U.S.*

Oxybutynin hydrochloride is an antimuscarinic agent with effects similar to those of atropine (see p.524); it has also been reported to possess direct effects on smooth muscle, antihistaminic, and local anaesthetic properties.
It is used in the management of urgency and incontinence associated with neurogenic bladder in usual doses of 5 mg two or three times daily by mouth.
Oxybutynin hydrochloride has also been tried in the symptomatic treatment of visceral spasms.

In a study involving 30 patients with detrusor instability, 23 completed a 28-day course of oxybutynin hydrochloride 5 mg three times daily, and 17 of these had symptomatic improvement, although improvement was demonstrated only in 9 on urodynamic assessment. These results were significantly better than those with placebo, particularly in view of the fact that the patients included some with established, advanced neurological disease unresponsive to other regimens. Five patients were unable to complete the course due to side-effects, chiefly dry mouth.— C. U. Moisey *et al.*, *Br. J. Urol.*, 1980, *52*, 472.

A review of the management of urinary incontinence in the elderly. Oxybutynin 5 to 20 mg daily in divided doses is frequently successful in patients with urge incontinence; combination in lower doses with an agent with complementary actions, such as imipramine, may be beneficial.— N. M. Resnick and S. V. Yalla, *New Engl. J. Med.*, 1985, *313*, 800.

Preparations
Oxybutynin Chloride Syrup *(U.S.P.)*
Oxybutynin Chloride Tablets *(U.S.P.)*

Proprietary Names and Manufacturers
Cystrin *(Tillotts, UK)*; Ditropan *(Norwich-Eaton, Canad.; Debat, Fr.; Scharper, Ital.; Marion Laboratories, S.Afr.; Inofarma, Spain; Marion Laboratories, USA)*; Dridase *(Pharmacia Arzneimittel, Ger.)*.

397-v

Oxyphencyclimine Hydrochloride *(BANM, USAN, rINNM)*.

1,4,5,6-Tetrahydro-1-methylpyrimidin-2-ylmethyl α-cyclohexylmandelate hydrochloride.
$C_{20}H_{28}N_2O_3$, HCl=380.9.

CAS — 125-53-1 (oxyphencyclimine); 125-52-0 (hydrochloride).

Pharmacopoeias. In *U.S.*

A white odourless crystalline powder. **Soluble** 1 in 100 of water, 1 in 75 of alcohol, 1 in 500 of chloroform; soluble in methyl alcohol; very slightly soluble in ether. **Store** in airtight containers.

Oxyphencyclimine hydrochloride is an antimuscarinic agent with effects similar to those of atropine (see p.524). It is used as an adjunct in the treatment of peptic ulcer in usual doses of 5 to 10 mg by mouth twice daily. It has also been given for the relief of visceral spasms.

Preparations
Oxyphencyclimine Hydrochloride Tablets *(U.S.P.)*

Proprietary Names and Manufacturers
Daricol *(Pfizer, Swed.)*; Daricon *(Pfizer, Austral.; Roerig, Belg.; Pfizer, Denm.; Roerig, Neth.; Pfizer, Norw.; Pfizer, Spain; Pfizer, UK; Beecham Laboratories, USA)*; Enteromex *(Pharmadrug, Ger.)*; Madil *(Ital.)*; Manir *(Valpan, Fr.)*; Oximin *(Norw.)*; Sedomucol *(Spain)*; Vagogastrin *(Benvegna, Ital.)*.

The following names have been used for multi-ingredient preparations containing oxyphencyclimine hydrochloride— Daricon-PB *(Beecham Laboratories, USA)*; Enarax *(Beecham Laboratories, USA)*; Vistrax *(Pfizer, USA)*.

398-g

Oxyphenonium Bromide *(BAN, rINN)*.

Oxphenonii Bromidum; Oxyphenonium Bromatum. 2-(α-Cyclohexylmandeloyloxy)ethyl-diethylmethylammonium bromide.
$C_{21}H_{34}BrNO_3$=428.4.

CAS — 14214-84-7 (oxyphenonium); 50-10-2 (bromide).

Pharmacopoeias. In *Cz., Ind., Jug.,* and *Pol.*

Oxyphenonium bromide is a quaternary ammonium antimuscarinic agent with peripheral effects similar to those of atropine (see p.524). It is used as an adjunct in the treatment of peptic ulcer, and to relieve visceral spasms, in usual doses of 5 to 10 mg by mouth 4 times daily; it has also been given in smaller doses by subcutaneous, intramuscular, or intravenous injection.
A 1% solution of oxyphenonium bromide has been used as eye-drops for the mydriatic effect.

Proprietary Names and Manufacturers
Antrenil *(Ciba, Ital.)*; Antrenyl *(Ciba, Austral.; Ciba, Belg.; Ciba, Ger.; Ciba, Neth.; Ciba, S.Afr.; Ciba, Spain; Ciba, Switz.; Ciba, UK; Ciba, USA)*; Spastrex *(Propan, S.Afr.)*.

400-q

Parapenzolate Bromide *(USAN, rINN)*.

Sch-3444. 4-Benziloyloxy-1,1-dimethylpiperidinium bromide.
$C_{21}H_{26}BrNO_3$=420.3.

CAS — 5634-41-3.

Parapenzolate bromide is a quaternary ammonium antimuscarinic agent and a structural isomer of mepenzolate bromide (see p.538). It has peripheral actions similar to those of atropine (p.524) and is used for the relief of visceral spasms in usual doses of 500 µg twice daily by mouth or 1 to 2 mg daily rectally; doses of 100 to 200 µg daily have been recommended by intramuscular or intravenous injection.
Parapenzolate bromide has also been used as an adjunct in the treatment of peptic ulcer.

Proprietary Names and Manufacturers
Neupran *(Essex, Arg.)*; Spacine *(Unicet, Fr.)*; Vagopax *(Essex, Ital.)*.

3910-q

Pargeverine Hydrochloride *(rINNM).*
2-(Dimethylamino)ethyldiphenyl(2-propynyloxy)acetate hydrochloride.
$C_{21}H_{23}NO_3,HCl=373.9$.

CAS — 13479-13-5 (pargeverine).

Pargeverine is reported to possess antimuscarinic and smooth-muscle relaxant properties and has been used in the treatment of gastro-intestinal and smooth muscle spasm in doses of 5 mg by mouth three times daily as the hydrochloride. Similar doses have been given by injection.

Proprietary Names and Manufacturers
Terisal *(IBYS, Spain).*

401-p

Pentapiperide Methylsulphate *(BANM).*
Pentapiperium Methylsulfate *(USAN)*; Pentapiperium Methylsulphate; Pentapiperium Metilsulfate *(rINN)*; Pentapiperium Metilsulphate; Valpipamate Methylsulphate. 1,1-Dimethyl-4-(3-methyl-2-phenylvaleryloxy)piperidinium methylsulphate.
$C_{19}H_{30}NO_2,CH_3O_4S=415.6$.

CAS — 7009-54-3 (pentapiperide); 26372-86-1 (pentapiperium); 7681-80-3 (pentapiperide methylsulphate or pentapiperium methylsulphate).

NOTE. Pentapiperide is rINN. NOTE. Pentapiperide methylsulphate and pentapiperium methylsulphate are identical but pentapiperide differs from pentapiperium in having one less methyl group.

Pentapiperide methylsulphate is a quaternary ammonium antimuscarinic agent with peripheral effects similar to those of atropine (see p.524). It is used as an adjunct in the treatment of peptic ulcer and to relieve visceral spasms. Doses of 20 to 30 mg are given daily by mouth. The hydrogen fumarate has also been used.

Proprietary Names and Manufacturers
Crilin *(Ayerst, Ital.)*; Crylène *(Auclair, Fr.).*

402-s

Penthienate Bromide *(BANM).*
Penthienate Methobromide. 2-[2-Cyclopentyl-2-(2-thienyl)glycoloyloxy]ethyldiethylmethylammonium bromide.
$C_{18}H_{30}BrNO_3S=420.4$.

CAS — 22064-27-3 (penthienate); 60-44-6 (bromide).

Penthienate bromide is a quaternary ammonium antimuscarinic agent with peripheral effects similar to those of atropine (see p.524). It is used as an adjunct in the treatment of peptic ulcer and to relieve visceral spasms in usual doses of 5 mg or less by mouth 3 or 4 times daily adjusted according to the needs of the patient to a maximum total dose of 40 mg daily.

Proprietary Names and Manufacturers
Monodral *(Winthrop, Austral.; Belg.; Norw.; Sterling Research, UK).*

403-w

Phenglutarimide Hydrochloride *(BANM, rINNM).*
2-(2-Diethylaminoethyl)-2-phenylglutarimide hydrochloride; 3-(2-Diethylaminoethyl)-3-phenylpiperidine-2,6-dione hydrochloride.
$C_{17}H_{24}N_2O_2,HCl=324.9$.

CAS — 1156-05-4 (phenglutarimide); 1674-96-0 (hydrochloride).

Phenglutarimide hydrochloride is an antimuscarinic agent with actions and uses similar to those of benzhexol (see p.527). It was formerly used in the treatment of parkinsonism.

Proprietary Names and Manufacturers
Aturban *(Ciba-Geigy, Switz.)*; Aturbane *(Ciba, UK).*

404-e

Pipenzolate Bromide *(BAN, rINN).*
Pipenzolate Methylbromide. 3-Benziloyloxy-1-ethyl-1-methylpiperidinium bromide.
$C_{22}H_{28}BrNO_3=434.4$.

CAS — 13473-38-6 (pipenzolate); 125-51-9 (bromide).

Pipenzolate bromide is a quaternary ammonium antimuscarinic agent with peripheral actions similar to those of atropine (see p.524). It is used as an adjunct in the treatment of peptic ulcer, and to relieve visceral spasms. The usual dose is 5 mg by mouth three times daily and 5 to 10 mg at bedtime.

Proprietary Preparations
Piptal *(MCP Pharmaceuticals, UK). Tablets,* pipenzolate bromide 5 mg.
Piptalin *(MCP Pharmaceuticals, UK). Elixir,* pipenzolate bromide 4 mg, activated dimethicone 40 mg/5 mL.

Proprietary Names and Manufacturers
Piper *(Panthox & Burck, Ital.)*; Piptal *(Sigma, Austral.; Bellon, Fr.; Rhone-Poulenc, Ital.; Switz.; MCP Pharmaceuticals, UK).*

405-l

Piperidolate Hydrochloride *(BANM, rINNM).*
1-Ethyl-3-piperidyl diphenylacetate hydrochloride.
$C_{21}H_{25}NO_2,HCl=359.9$.

CAS — 82-98-4 (piperidolate); 129-77-1 (hydrochloride).

Piperidolate hydrochloride is an antimuscarinic agent with effects similar to those of atropine (see p.524). It is given in the symptomatic treatment of visceral spasms in a dose of 50 mg four times daily by mouth.

Proprietary Preparations
Dactil *(MCP Pharmaceuticals, UK). Tablets,* piperidolate hydrochloride 50 mg.

Proprietary Names and Manufacturers
Dactil *(Bellon, Fr.; Ger.; Ital.; MCP Pharmaceuticals, UK).*

13123-t

Pipethanate Ethobromide *(rINNM).*
Ethylpipethanate Bromide; Piperilate Ethobromide. 1-(2-Benziloyloxyethyl)-1-ethylpiperidinium bromide.
$C_{23}H_{30}BrNO_3=448.4$.

CAS — 4546-39-8 (pipethanate); 23182-46-9 (ethobromide); 4544-15-4 (hydrochloride).

Pipethanate ethobromide is an antimuscarinic agent with properties similar to those of atropine (see p.524). It has been used in the symptomatic treatment of visceral spasm.
The hydrochloride has also been used; it has been reported to possess tranquillising properties.

Proprietary Names and Manufacturers
Panpurol *(Nippon Shinyaku, Jpn).*

13136-n

Piroheptine Hydrochloride *(rINNM).*
3-(10,11-Dihydro-5*H*-dibenzo[*a,d*]cyclohepten-5-ylidene)-1-ethyl-2-methylpyrrolidine hydrochloride.
$C_{22}H_{25}N,HCl=339.9$.

CAS — 16378-21-5 (piroheptine); 16378-22-6 (hydrochloride).

Piroheptine is structurally related to the tricyclic antidepressants (see p.350) and has been used in the treatment of parkinsonism and drug-induced extrapyramidal symptoms.

Proprietary Names and Manufacturers
Trimol *(Fujisawa, Jpn).*

406-y

Platyphylline Acid Tartrate
Platyphylline Bitartrate; Platyphyllini Hydrotartras. 1,2-Dihydro-12-hydroxysenecionan-11,16-dione hydrogen tartrate.
$C_{18}H_{27}NO_5,C_4H_6O_6=487.5$.

CAS — 480-78-4 (platyphylline); 1257-59-6 (acid tartrate).

Pharmacopoeias. In *Rus.*

The acid tartrate of platyphylline, a pyrrolizidine alkaloid occurring in *Senecio platyphyllus* and other *Senecio* spp.

Platyphylline acid tartrate has actions similar to those of atropine (see p.524) and it has been used in the *USSR* for similar purposes.

407-j

Poldine Methylsulphate *(BAN).*

IS-499; McN-R-72647; Poldine Methosulphate; Poldine Methylsulfate *(USAN)*; Poldine Metilsulfate *(pINN)*. 2-Benziloyloxymethyl-1,1-dimethylpyrrolidinium methylsulphate.
$C_{21}H_{26}NO_3,CH_3O_4S=451.5$.

CAS — 596-50-9 (poldine); 545-80-2 (methylsulphate).

Pharmacopoeias. In *Br.* and *Cz.*

A white odourless or almost odourless crystalline powder. **Soluble** 1 in 1 of water, 1 in 20 of alcohol; slightly soluble in chloroform. A 1% solution in water has a pH of 5.0 to 7.0.

Adverse Effects, Treatment, and Precautions
As for Atropine Sulphate, p.523.

Uses and Administration
Poldine methylsulphate is a quaternary ammonium antimuscarinic agent with peripheral actions similar to those of atropine (see p.524). It is used as an adjunct in the treatment of peptic ulcer, and dyspepsia associated with hyperacidity. The usual initial dose is 2 to 4 mg four times a day, subsequently adjusted according to the response of the patient. In the treatment of nocturnal enuresis in children 2 mg has been given at bedtime.

ABSORPTION AND FATE. Following repeated administration of poldine methylsulphate by mouth to *rats* nearly 70% of the administered dose was excreted in the faeces unchanged or as metabolites; a proportion of this might have been due to enterohepatic cycling.— P. F. Langley *et al., Biochem. Pharmac.,* 1966, *15,* 1821.

PEPTIC ULCER. A discussion of drug therapy for gastric and duodenal ulcers including the view that antimuscarinic agents such as poldine are limited in value by their side-effects and are no longer first-line treatments.— M. J. S. Langman and C. J. Hawkey, *Prescribers' J.,* 1984, *24,* 106.

Preparations

Poldine Tablets *(B.P.).* Contain poldine methylsulphate.

Proprietary Names and Manufacturers

Nactate *(Denm.; Neth.)*; Nacton *(Bencard, UK)*; Poldina *(Landerlan, Spain).*

The following names have been used for multi-ingredient preparations containing poldine methylsulphate— Nactisol *(Bencard, UK).*

409-c

Prifinium Bromide *(rINN).*
PDB; Pyrodifenium Bromide. 3-Diphenylmethylene-1,1-diethyl-2-methylpyrrolidinium bromide.
$C_{22}H_{28}BrN=386.4$.

CAS — 10236-81-4 (prifinium); 4630-95-9 (bromide).

Prifinium bromide is a quaternary ammonium antimuscarinic agent with the peripheral actions of atropine (see p.524). It is structurally related to diphemanil methylsulphate.
Prifinium bromide is used as an adjunct in the treatment of peptic ulcer and to relieve visceral spasms. By mouth, 45 to 120 mg has usually been given in divided doses daily; in some countries it has been given as sustained-release tablets. Prifinium bromide has also been administered rectally, or, in a dose of 7.5 mg, by subcutaneous, intramuscular, or intravenous injection.

References: H. Noguchi *et al.*, *Int. J. clin. Pharmac. Ther. Toxic.*, 1983, *21*, 213 (pharmacokinetics); T. Sasaki *et al.*, *Clin. Ther.*, 1985, *7*, 512 (use in irritable bowel syndrome); D. Sasaki *et al.*, *ibid.*, 190 (irritable bowel syndrome).

Proprietary Names and Manufacturers
Padrin *(Jpn)*; Riabal *(Gador, Arg.; Logeais, Fr.; Ibi, Ital.; Fujisawa, S.Afr.; Made, Spain).*

410-s

Procyclidine Hydrochloride *(BANM, USAN, rINNM).*

Procyclidini Hydrochloridum. 1-Cyclohexyl-1-phenyl-3-(pyrrolidin-1-yl)propan-1-ol hydrochloride.
$C_{19}H_{29}NO,HCl=323.9$.

CAS — 77-37-2 (procyclidine); 1508-76-5 (hydrochloride).

Pharmacopoeias. In *Br.*, *Egypt.*, *Int.*, and *U.S.*

A white crystalline powder odourless or with a slight characteristic odour.
B.P. **solubilities** are: 1 in 40 of water, and 1 in 15 of alcohol; practically insoluble in acetone or ether. The *U.S.P.* has: soluble 1 in 35 of water, 1 in 9 of alcohol, and 1 in 6 of chloroform. The *B.P.* states that a 1% solution in water has a pH of 4.5 to 6.5, the *U.S.P.* that it has a pH between 5.0 and 6.5. Solutions for injection may be **sterilised** by autoclaving or filtration. **Store** in a dry place in airtight containers. Protect from light.

INCOMPATIBILITY. Procyclidine hydrochloride and thioridazine hydrochloride oral mixtures were physically compatible for approximately 30 minutes at 4 and 25°, but not for 1 hour.— W. A. Parker, *Can. J. Hosp. Pharm.*, 1984, *37*, 133.

Adverse Effects, Treatment, and Precautions
As for Atropine Sulphate, p.523.

ABUSE. A report of 2 cases of abuse of procyclidine by adolescents.— R. B. McGucken *et al.* (letter), *Lancet*, 1985, *1*, 1514.

See also under Benzhexol Hydrochloride, p.527.

Absorption and Fate
Procyclidine hydrochloride is absorbed from the gastro-intestinal tract and disappears rapidly from the tissues. Procyclidine given intravenously acts within 5 to 20 minutes and has a duration of effect of up to 4 hours.

A study of the pharmacokinetics and pharmacodynamics of procyclidine. Mean terminal half-life in 5 of 6 healthy subjects given procyclidine hydrochloride 10 mg by slow intravenous injection was 11.5 hours; following oral administration of the same dose the mean elimination half-life for all 6 was 12.6 hours. Absorption was generally rapid following oral dosage and time to maximum plasma concentration was a mean of 1.1 hours in 5 subjects; the other subject gave a value of 8 hours. Oral procyclidine had a calculated bioavailability of 75.2%. The pharmacodynamics were sustained, consistent with the plasma half-life of the drug, and maximum effects correlated well with plasma concentration.— P. D. Whiteman *et al.*, *Eur. J. clin. Pharmac.*, 1985, *28*, 73.

Uses and Administration
Procyclidine hydrochloride is an antimuscarinic agent with actions and uses similar to those of benzhexol (see p.527). It is mainly used for the symptomatic treatment of parkinsonism. It controls rigidity more effectively than tremor. It may also be used to alleviate the extrapyramidal syndrome induced by drugs such as the phenothiazine derivatives but is of no value against tardive dyskinesias, which may be exacerbated.
The initial dose of 2.5 mg three times daily after meals may be increased gradually by 2.5 mg daily until the optimum maintenance dose, usually 20 to 30 mg daily in 3 or 4 divided doses, is reached; daily doses of up to 60 mg have occasionally been required. In emergency, 5 to 10 mg may be given by intravenous injection; the intramuscular route has also been used.
Transition to or from procyclidine therapy should be gradual otherwise symptoms may be aggravated.

EXTRAPYRAMIDAL DISORDERS. For a review of the role of antimuscarinic agents in the treatment of drug-induced extrapyramidal disorders, see p.522.

Parkinsonism. For discussion of the treatment of parkinsonism, including reference to the role of antimuscarinic agents, see under Levodopa, p.1019.

Preparations

Procyclidine Hydrochloride Tablets *(U.S.P.)*

Procyclidine Injection *(B.P.C. 1973).* Procyclidine Hydrochloride Injection. Contains procyclidine hydrochloride. pH 4.5 to 7.0. Store at a temperature not exceeding 25° and avoid freezing.

Procyclidine Tablets *(B.P.).* Contain procyclidine hydrochloride.

Proprietary Preparations

Arpicolin *(R.P. Drugs, UK). Syrup*, procyclidine hydrochloride 2.5 and 5 mg/5 mL.

Kemadrin *(Wellcome, UK). Tablets*, scored, procyclidine hydrochloride 5 mg.
Injection, procyclidine hydrochloride 5 mg/mL, in ampoules of 2 mL.

Proprietary Names and Manufacturers
Arpicolin Syrup *(R.P. Drugs, UK)*; Kémadrine *(Wellcome, Fr.)*; Kemadren *(Gayoso Wellcome, Spain)*; Kemadrin *(Wellcome, Austral.; Belg.; Wellcome, Canad.; Wellcome, Denm.; Wellcome, Ital.; Neth.; Wellcome, Norw.; S.Afr.; Wellcome, Swed.; Wellcome, Switz.; Wellcome, UK; Wellcome, USA)*; Osnervan *(Wellcopharm, Ger.)*; Procyclid *(ICN, Canad.).*

411-w

Propantheline Bromide *(BAN, USAN, rINN).*

Bromuro de Propantelina; Propanthelini Bromidum. Di-isopropylmethyl[2-(xanthen-9-ylcarbonyloxy)ethyl]ammonium bromide.
$C_{23}H_{30}BrNO_3=448.4$.

CAS — 298-50-0 (propantheline); 50-34-0 (bromide).

Pharmacopoeias. In *Arg.*, *Br.*, *Braz.*, *Chin.*, *Egypt.*, *Fr.*, *Ind.*, *Int.*, *Jpn*, *Jug.*, *Nord.*, *Turk.*, and *U.S.*

A white or yellowish-white odourless or almost odourless slightly hygroscopic powder.
Very **soluble** in water, alcohol, and in chloroform; practically insoluble in ether. **Store** in well-closed containers.

Propantheline bromide was shown to exist in 2 polymorphic forms.— L. Borka, *Acta pharm. suec.*, 1983, *20*, 155.

Adverse Effects, Treatment, and Precautions
As for Atropine Sulphate, p.523.
Toxic doses of propantheline bromide may produce non-depolarising neuromuscular blocking effects with paralysis of voluntary muscle. Contact dermatitis has been reported following topical application.
Like other antimuscarinic agents, propantheline may slow the transit of other drugs through the intestine, with variable effects on absorption: the absorption of nitrofurantoin and of digoxin has been reported to be enhanced and that of paracetamol reduced and retarded.
The absorption of propantheline from the gastro-intestinal tract is reportedly reduced by food: doses should be taken 30 minutes to 1 hour before meals.

BUCCAL AND OESOPHAGEAL ULCERATION. Severe buccal mucosal ulceration, which developed in a 95-year-old woman as a result of retaining emepronium bromide tablets in her mouth, recurred on administration of propantheline bromide tablets.— G. J. Huston *et al.*, *Postgrad. med. J.*, 1978, *54*, 331.

EFFECTS ON SEXUAL FUNCTION. Impotence followed treatment for about 1 year with propantheline bromide.— D. Manners (letter), *Med. J. Aust.*, 1966, *2*, 436.

Absorption and Fate
Propantheline bromide is a quaternary ammonium compound and is incompletely absorbed from the gastro-intestinal tract: it has been estimated that only about 10% of a dose by mouth is absorbed as active drug.
It is extensively metabolised, in part in the small intestine before absorption, and is eliminated mainly in the urine as metabolites and a small amount of unchanged drug. The duration of action is about 6 hours. There is some evidence of enterohepatic recycling.

Uses and Administration
Propantheline bromide is a quaternary ammonium antimuscarinic agent with peripheral effects similar to those of atropine (see p.524). It is used as an adjunct in the treatment of peptic ulcer. The usual initial dose is 15 mg three times daily before meals and 30 mg at bedtime, subsequently adjusted according to the response of the patient. A suggested dose for children is 375 µg per kg body-weight 4 times daily.
It has been used in the treatment of gastritis, acute pancreatitis, and spasm of the gastro-intestinal, biliary, and urinary tract. For rapid relief of pain, 30 mg dissolved in 10 mL of sodium chloride injection may be injected intravenously.
As an adjunct to X-ray examination of the gastro-intestinal tract or endoscopic examinations, 30 mg has been given by mouth or intramuscularly before the procedure. Because of the poor oral absorption of propantheline bromide, parenteral doses may result in considerably higher plasma concentrations than the equivalent doses given by mouth.
Propantheline is also used in the treatment of enuresis, 15 to 45 mg being given at bedtime.
Propantheline has also been used in the treatment of hyperhidrosis.

EFFECTS ON BLOOD GLUCOSE. Administration of propantheline 30 mg forty-five minutes before administration of glucose to stimulate insulin-release, prevented hypoglycaemic symptoms in 7 patients with reactive hypoglycaemia. It was considered that antimuscarinic agents might be useful adjuncts in the therapy of reactive hypoglycaemia, and that for ordinary meals doses of propantheline as low as 7.5 mg might control the symptoms of reactive hypoglycaemia.— M. A. Permutt *et al.*, *Diabetes*, 1977, *26*, 121.

Propantheline 45 mg by mouth at bedtime, in association with a reduced dose of long-acting insulin resulted in a fall in mean blood glucose levels in 4 insulin-dependent diabetics from 2.38 mg per mL at bedtime to 1.54 mg per mL in the morning, associated with a considerable reduction in sleep-related peaks of growth hormone secretion. When the same dose of insulin was given alone mean blood glucose concentrations were 1.88 and 2.00 mg per mL at night and in the morning respectively. Antimuscarinic agents without central effects may be of clinical value in diabetes since inhibition of growth hormone secretion may favourably influence the course of retinopathy and reduce the hyperglycaemic effects of growth hormone stimulated by sleep, stress, poor metabolic control, and exercise.— B. Davis and K. Davis (letter), *Lancet*, 1986, *1*, 1382.

HYPERHIDROSIS. A lotion containing propantheline bromide 5% in a mixture of alcohol and glycerol, pH about 5.5, applied to the skin of 16 men with hyperhidrosis inhibited sweating.— E. A. Knudsen and C. H. K. Meier, *Acta derm.-vener., Stockh.*, 1963, *43*, 154.

Propantheline bromide 15 mg by mouth 2 to 4 times daily is worth trying in patients with hyperhidrosis, but effective control of sweating is rarely possible without unacceptable side-effects.— W. A. D. Griffiths, *Prescribers' J.*, 1984, *24*, 38.

INFLAMMATORY BOWEL DISEASE. Antimuscarinics, such as propantheline bromide, 15 mg three or four times daily by mouth, might be valuable in reducing abdominal pain and lessening diarrhoea in ulcerative colitis. However large doses of antimuscarinics might predispose to acute dilatation of the colon, which was dangerous.— S. C. Truelove, *Br. med. J.*, 1968, *2*, 539.

PEPTIC ULCER. A study in 9 duodenal ulcer patients indicated that propantheline bromide 15 mg was as effective as near toxic doses (average 48 mg) in suppressing food-stimulated gastric acid secretion; additive inhibition of gastric acid secretion was noted on concurrent administration of propantheline bromide 15 mg and cimetidine 300 mg.— M. Feldman *et al.*, *New Engl. J. Med.*, 1977, *297*, 1427. Results of a placebo-controlled study involving 58 patients with symptomatic gastric, prepyloric or duodenal ulcers indicated that addition of propantheline bromide 15 mg three times daily to cimetidine therapy offered no significant advantage in terms of healing rates or relief from pain compared with cimetidine alone.— A. Paerregaard *et al.*, *Acta med. scand.*, 1983, *213*, 195.

A discussion of drug therapy for gastric and duodenal ulcers including the view that antimuscarinic agents such as propantheline are limited in value by their side-effects and are no longer first-line treatments.— M. J. S. Langman and C. J. Hawkey, *Prescribers' J.*, 1984, *24*, 106.

SYNCOPE. In 12 patients with a history of syncope or near-syncope associated with abnormalities of vagal tone, treatment with propantheline bromide 7.5 to 15 mg three or four times daily was associated with a decrease in frequency of attacks from a median of 7 per patient over 10.5 months to 1 per patient over 22.5 months.— C. J. McLaran *et al.*, *Br. Heart J.*, 1986, *55*, 53. See also *Lancet*, 1986, *1*, 594.

URINARY INCONTINENCE. A review of urinary incontinence in the elderly. Treatment of the uninhibited neurogenic bladder is by antimuscarinic or other drugs which may prevent uninhibited contractions or reduce bladder excitability: propantheline bromide 15 mg every 6 hours is in common use.— J. C. Brocklehurst, *Practitioner*, 1984, *228*, 275. An earlier review. Although no reports describing the use of propantheline in the incontinent elderly are available, 30% of younger patients treated with this agent or similar drugs developed side-effects.— M. E. Williams and F. C. Pannill, *Ann. intern. Med.*, 1982, *97*, 895.

Propantheline is probably the most widely used drug for urge incontinence, where the patient is unable to delay voiding long enough to reach a toilet or toilet substitute.— P. A. L. Haber, *Ann. intern. Med.*, 1986, *104*, 429.

Preparations

Propantheline Bromide Tablets *(U.S.P.)*

Propantheline Tablets *(B.P.)*. Contain propantheline bromide.

Sterile Propantheline Bromide *(U.S.P.)*. Propantheline bromide suitable for parenteral use.

Proprietary Preparations

Pro-Banthine *(Gold Cross, UK)*. *Tablets*, propantheline bromide 15 mg.

Proprietary Names and Manufacturers

Banlin *(Canad.)*; Corrigast *(Searle, Ger.)*; Enteromex-PB *(Pharmadrug, Ger.)*; Ercarol *(Ego, Austral.)*; Ercorax *(Ercopharm, Switz.)*; Ercoril *(Erco, Denm.)*; Ercotina *(Erco, Swed.)*; Mephathelin *(Switz.)*; Pantheline *(Protea, Austral.)*; Pervagal *(Ital.)*; Pro-Banthine *(Searle, Austral.; Belg.; Searle, Canad.; Searle, Denm.; Neth.; Norw.; Searle, S.Afr.; Searle, Spain; Searle, Swed.; Searle, Switz.; Gold Cross, UK; Searle, USA)*; Probanthine *(Searle, Fr.)*; Propanthel *(ICN, Canad.)*; SK-Propantheline Bromide *(Smith Kline & French, USA)*; Suprantil *(Ital.)*.

The following names have been used for multi-ingredient preparations containing propantheline bromide— Pro-Banthine with Dartalan *(Searle, UK)*; Pro-Banthine with Phenobarbital *(Searle, USA)*; Silocalm *(Concept Pharmaceuticals, UK)*.

412-e

Propyromazine Bromide *(rINN)*.

LD-335. 1-Methyl-1-[1-(phenothiazin-10-ylcarbonyl)ethyl]pyrrolidinium bromide.
$C_{20}H_{23}BrN_2OS=419.4$.

CAS — 145-54-0.

Propyromazine bromide is a quaternary ammonium antimuscarinic agent with peripheral effects similar to those of atropine (see p.524). It is given in the symptomatic treatment of visceral spasms in a dose of 50 mg one to three times daily by mouth; it is also given in a dose of 20 mg by subcutaneous, intramuscular, or slow intravenous injection.

Proprietary Names and Manufacturers
Diaspasmyl *(Diamant, Fr.; Farmabion, Spain)*.

413-l

Stramonium Leaf *(BAN)*.

Datura; Figueira do Inferno; Hoja de Estramonio; Jamestown Weed; Jimson Weed; Stechapfelblatt; Stramoine; Stramonii Folium; Stramonii Herba; Stramonium; Thornapple Leaf.

Pharmacopoeias. In *Arg., Aust., Belg., Br., Braz., Eur., Fr., Ger., Int., Mex., Neth., Pol., Port., Roum., Rus.,* and *Swiss. Egypt., Hung.,* and *Span.* specify not less than 0.2% of alkaloids. *Br.* also includes Powdered Stramonium Leaf.

The dried leaves and flowering tops and, occasionally, fruits of *Datura stramonium* and its varieties (Solanaceae), containing not less than 0.25% of alkaloids calculated as hyoscyamine. The alkaloids consist mainly of those of the hyoscyamine—atropine group together with hyoscine. It has an unpleasant odour. **Store** in airtight containers. Protect from light.

414-y

Prepared Stramonium *(BAN)*.

Poudre Titrée de Datura; Prep. Stramon.; Stramonii Pulvis Normatus.

CAS — 8063-18-1 (stramonium).

Pharmacopoeias. In *Aust., Br., Eur., Fr., Ger., Neth.,* and *Swiss.*

Stramonium leaf reduced to a powder and adjusted to contain 0.23 to 0.27% of alkaloids, calculated as hyoscyamine. A grey to greenish-grey powder. **Store** in airtight containers. Protect from light.

Adverse Effects, Treatment, and Precautions
As for Atropine Sulphate, p.523.

Stramonium had been designated by the FDA as a herb unsafe for use in foods, beverages, or drugs.— *Am. Pharm.*, 1984, *NS24* (Mar.), 20.

ABUSE. In an analysis of 212 cases of stramonium and belladonna abuse, identifiable hallucinatory episodes were obtained by 99 subjects, 5 of whom died as a result of actions provoked by their mental state. Patients showed a marked tendency to aggressive behaviour. Recovery from the acute phase usually occurred within 24 hours although the mydriasis might persist for 7 days. Treatment was best limited to supportive and protective measures.— J. M. Gowdy, *J. Am. med. Ass.*, 1972, *221*, 585.

Reports of poisoning following abuse of *Datura stramonium* or its preparations: D. A. Mahler (letter), *J. Am. med. Ass.*, 1975, *231*, 138 (acute poisoning following ingestion of the *seeds* by 5 adolescents); E. A. Harrison and D. H. Morgan (letter), *Br. med. J.*, 1976, *2*, 1195 (ingestion of a decoction prepared from asthma cigarettes); R. K. Siegel, *J. Am. med. Ass.*, 1976, *236*, 473 (2 cases due to smoking herbal cigarettes); R. G. H. Bethel (letter), *Br. med. J.*, 1978, *2*, 959 (ingestion of herbal cigarettes); R. E. Shervette *et al.*, *Pediatrics*, 1979, *63*, 520 (report of 29 cases due to ingestion by adolescents); W. Klein-Schwartz and G. M. Oderda, *Am. J. Dis. Child.*, 1984, *138*, 737 (report on 59 cases of stramonium intoxication in adolescents).

EFFECTS ON THE EYE. A report of anisocoria in a patient following accidental entry of a piece of jimson weed (*Datura stramonium*) into the eye while gardening.— D. L. Savitt *et al.* (letter), *J. Am. med. Ass.*, 1986, *255*, 1440.

Uses and Administration
Stramonium leaf and preparations of stramonium have the actions of atropine (see p.524). It is very similar to belladonna and has been given to relieve spasm of the bronchioles in asthma, for which purpose it has been given in tablets or in mixtures. It has also been smoked in cigarettes or burnt in powders and the fumes inhaled but the irritation produced by the fumes may aggravate the bronchitis.

Stramonium leaf has also been used to control the salivation and muscular spasm in idiopathic and postencephalitic parkinsonism.

The seed has also been used.

Preparations

Compound Lobelia and Stramonium Mixture *(B.P.C. 1973)*. Mist. Lobel. et Stramon. Co.; Mistura Lobeliae Composita. Contains stramonium tincture 10% and lobelia ethereal tincture 5%. It should be recently prepared. *Dose.* 10 mL. 5 mL contains 125 µg of stramonium alkaloids.

Stramonium and Potassium Iodide Mixture *(B.P.C. 1973)*. Contains stramonium tincture 12.5% and potassium iodide 2%. It should be recently prepared. *Dose.* 10 mL. 5 mL contains approximately 156 µg of stramonium alkaloids.

Proprietary Names and Manufacturers of Stramonium
The following names have been used for multi-ingredient preparations containing stramonium— Ephedramine *(Drug Houses Austral., Austral.)*.

416-z

Sultroponium *(rINN)*.

A-118. (1*R*,3*r*,5*S*)-8-(3-Sulphopropyl)-3-[(±)-tropoyloxy]tropanium inner salt.
$C_{20}H_{29}NO_6S=411.5$.

CAS — 15130-91-3.

Sultroponium is a quaternary ammonium antimuscarinic agent with peripheral effects similar to those of atropine (see p.524). It has been given as an adjunct in the treatment of peptic ulcer, and to relieve visceral spasms. It has also been given by injection.

Proprietary Names and Manufacturers
Sultroponium B *(Biothérax, Fr.)*.

13310-f

Terodiline Hydrochloride

N-tert-Butyl-1-methyl-3,3-diphenylpropylamine hydrochloride.
$C_{20}H_{27}N,HCl=317.9$.

CAS — 15793-40-5 (terodiline); 7082-21-5 (hydrochloride).

Adverse Effects, Treatment, and Precautions
As for Atropine Sulphate, p.523. Following overdosage, if calcium antagonist effects with associated bradycardia and hypotension, should be predominant, then intravenous infusion of calcium gluconate has been suggested.

Uses and Administration
Terodiline hydrochloride is an antimuscarinic agent with actions similar to those of atropine (see p.524); it is also reported to possess calcium-channel blocking activity.

It is used for the relief of urinary frequency, urgency, and incontinence in patients with motor urge incontinence and neurogenic bladder, in doses of 12.5 to 25 mg by mouth twice daily.

Terodiline hydrochloride has also been used for its calcium-channel blocking properties in the treatment of angina pectoris.

In a study involving 9 healthy subjects given terodiline 12.5 or 20 mg intravenously, or 12.5 or 25 mg by mouth, terodiline was found to be almost completely absorbed from the gastro-intestinal tract, with a mean bioavailability of 92%, but there were considerable variations in serum concentrations and clearance between subjects following both oral and intravenous administration. The elimination half-life was prolonged, with a mean value of 65 hours, suggesting that dosage once or twice daily would be adequate, but that steady-state serum concentrations would not be achieved at the standard maintenance dose until after 2 weeks of therapy.— B. Karlén *et al.*, *Eur. J. clin. Pharmac.*, 1982, *23*, 267.

In a crossover study involving 23 women suffering from urinary frequency, urgency, and incontinence, terodiline 25 mg twice daily and emepronium 200 mg three times daily both reduced micturition frequency compared to placebo, particularly in those patients initially most severely affected; this reduction was greater after terodiline than emepronium. Of 16 patients showing symptomatic improvement with terodiline, 12 also showed cystometric improvement, compared with 6 of 11 receiving emepronium. Further work comparing terodiline with emepronium at their maximal tolerated doses will help to clarify terodiline's place in the management of patients with detrusor instability.— G. M. Sole and D. G. Arkell, *Scand. J. Urol. & Nephrol.*, 1984, *Suppl.* 87, 55.

A further study: U. Ulmsten *et al.*, *Am. J. Obstet. Gynec.*, 1985, *153*, 619.

Proprietary Preparations

Terolin *(KabiVitrum, UK). Tablets*, terodiline hydrochloride 12.5 mg.

Proprietary Names and Manufacturers

Bicor *(Swed.)*; Mictrol *(KabiVitrum, Denm.*; *Kabi, Swed.)*; Terolin *(KabiVitrum, UK)*.

417-c

Thiphenamil Hydrochloride *(USAN)*.

Thiphenum; Tifenamil Hydrochloride *(rINNM)*; Tiphen Hydrochloride. *S*-(2-Diethylaminoethyl) diphenylthioacetate hydrochloride.

$C_{20}H_{25}NOS,HCl = 364.0$.

CAS — 82-99-5 (thiphenamil); 548-68-5 (hydrochloride).

Pharmacopoeias. In *Rus.*

Thiphenamil hydrochloride has been described as a weak antimuscarinic agent with actions similar to those of atropine (see p.524); it has also been claimed to exert a direct antispasmodic effect on smooth muscle and a local anaesthetic effect. It has been used for the relief of visceral spasms in a dose of 400 mg by mouth, repeated after 4 hours as necessary. Lower doses have been given in the *USSR*.

Proprietary Names and Manufacturers

Trocinate *(Poythress, USA)*.

418-k

Tiemonium Iodide *(BAN, rINN)*.

TE-114. 4-[3-Hydroxy-3-phenyl-3-(2-thienyl)propyl]-4-methylmorpholinium iodide.

$C_{18}H_{24}INO_2S = 445.4$.

CAS — 6252-92-2 (tiemonium); 144-12-7 (iodide).

Tiemonium iodide is a quaternary ammonium antimuscarinic agent with peripheral effects similar to those of atropine (see p.524). It is used as an adjunct in the treatment of peptic ulcer, and to relieve visceral spasms. Doses of 100 to 300 mg have been given daily, in divided doses by mouth, and 5 to 10 mg has been given by subcutaneous, intramuscular, or intravenous injection. Doses of 20 mg have also been administered rectally as suppositories. Tiemonium has also been used as the methylsulphate.

Proprietary Names and Manufacturers

Ottimal *(ICT-Lodi, Ital.)*; Visceralgin *(Fawns & McAllan, Austral.)*; Visceralgina *(SIT, Ital.)*; Visceralgina Jarabe *(Liade, Spain)*; Visceralgine *(Sanders-Probel, Belg.*; *Riom, Fr.*; *Provita, Switz.)*.

419-a

Tigloidine Hydrobromide *(BANM, rINNM)*.

Tiglylpseudotropine Hydrobromide. (1*R*,3*s*,5*S*)-3-(3-Methylmethacryloyloxy)tropane hydrobromide.

$C_{13}H_{21}NO_2,HBr = 304.2$.

CAS — 495-83-0 (tigloidine); 22846-83-9 (hydrobromide).

Tigloidine was first isolated from *Duboisia myoporoides* (Solanaceae) but is now synthesised.

Adverse Effects, Treatment, and Precautions

As for Atropine Sulphate, p.523. The antimuscarinic side-effects of tigloidine hydrobromide are claimed to be slight.

Uses and Administration

Tigloidine hydrobromide is chemically similar to atropine. It has been used in the relief of muscular spasm, rigidity, and spasticity, including that due to lesions of the upper motor neurones or spinal cord. It has also been used in patients with parkinsonism. The usual dose is 1 to 2 g daily in 3 divided doses with meals.

Proprietary Names and Manufacturers

Tiglyssin *(Duncan, Flockhart, UK)*.

13346-e

Timepidium Bromide *(rINN)*.

SA-504. 3-[Di-(2-thienyl)methylene]-5-methoxy-1,1-dimethylpiperidinium bromide

$C_{17}H_{22}BrNOS_2 = 400.4$.

CAS — 35035-05-3.

Timepidium bromide is a quaternary ammonium antimuscarinic agent with peripheral actions similar to those of atropine (see p.524). It has been used for the symptomatic treatment of visceral spasms.

Proprietary Names and Manufacturers

Mepidium *(Recordati, Ital.)*; Sesden *(Tanabe, Jpn)*.

421-l

Tridihexethyl Chloride *(BAN, USAN)*.

(3-Cyclohexyl-3-hydroxy-3-phenylpropyl)triethylammonium chloride.

$C_{21}H_{36}ClNO = 354.0$.

CAS — 60-49-1 (tridihexethyl); 4310-35-4 (chloride); 125-99-5 (iodide).

NOTE. Tridihexethyl Iodide is rINN.

Pharmacopoeias. In *U.S.*

A white odourless crystalline powder. **Soluble** 1 in 3 of water and of alcohol, 1 in 2 of chloroform; freely soluble in methyl alcohol; practically insoluble in acetone and ether. pH of an aqueous solution for injection is 5.0 to 7.5. **Store** in airtight containers.

Tridihexethyl chloride is a quaternary ammonium antimuscarinic agent with peripheral effects similar to those of atropine (see p.524). It is used as an adjunct in the treatment of peptic ulcer and to relieve visceral spasms. Doses of 25 to 75 mg are given three or four times daily by mouth; 10 to 20 mg has also been administered every 6 hours by subcutaneous, intramuscular, or intravenous injection.

Tridihexethyl has also been given as the iodide.

Preparations

Tridihexethyl Chloride Injection *(U.S.P.)*. A sterile solution in Water for Injections.

Tridihexethyl Chloride Tablets *(U.S.P.)*

Proprietary Names and Manufacturers

Duoesetil *(Dessy, Ital.)*; Pathilon *(Lederle, USA)*.

The following names have been used for multi-ingredient preparations containing tridihexethyl chloride— Pathibamate *(Lederle, USA)*.

422-y

Tropacine Hydrochloride

Tropacinum; Tropazine Hydrochloride; Tropine Diphenylacetate Hydrochloride. (1*R*,3*r*,5*S*)-Tropan-3-yl diphenylacetate hydrochloride.

$C_{22}H_{25}NO_2, HCl = 371.9$.

CAS — 6878-98-4 (tropacine); 548-64-1 (hydrochloride).

Pharmacopoeias. In *Rus.*

Tropacine is an antimuscarinic agent which has been employed in the *USSR* in the treatment of parkinsonism in a maximum daily dose of 100 mg.

13385-a

Tropatepine Hydrochloride *(rINNM)*.

SD-1248-17. 3-(Dibenzo[*b*,*e*]thiepin-11(6*H*)-ylidene)tropane hydrochloride.

$C_{22}H_{23}NS,HCl = 370.0$.

CAS — 27574-24-9 (tropatepine); 27574-25-0 (hydrochloride).

Tropatepine hydrochloride is an antimuscarinic agent with actions and uses similar to those of benzhexol (see p.527). It is used in the treatment of parkinsonism and of drug-induced extrapyramidal syndromes, in doses of 2.5 mg by mouth daily initially, gradually increased according to the response of the patient, to a usual total dose of 10 to 20 mg daily.

Proprietary Names and Manufacturers

Lepticur *(Diamant, Fr.)*.

423-j

Tropenziline Bromide *(rINN)*.

MTS-263. (1*R*,3*s*,5*R*)-3-Benziloyloxy-6-methoxy-8-methyltropanium bromide.

$C_{24}H_{30}BrNO_4 = 476.4$.

CAS — 6732-80-5 (tropenziline); 143-92-0 (bromide).

Tropenziline bromide is a quaternary ammonium antimuscarinic agent with peripheral effects similar to those of atropine (see p.524). It has been given in the symptomatic treatment of visceral spasms in doses of 20 to 40 mg three times daily by mouth; it has also been given rectally, and by intramuscular or intravenous injection.

424-z

Tropicamide *(BAN, USAN, rINN)*.

Bistropamide; Ro-1-7683. *N*-Ethyl-*N*-(4-pyridylmethyl)tropamide.

$C_{17}H_{20}N_2O_2 = 284.4$.

CAS — 1508-75-4.

Pharmacopoeias. In *Br.*, *Jpn*, and *U.S.*

A white or almost white, odourless or almost odourless, crystalline powder. Slightly **soluble** in water; soluble 1 in 3.5 of alcohol, and 1 in 2 of chloroform; freely soluble in solutions of strong acids. Solutions for ophthalmic use have a pH of 4.0 to 5.8. **Store** in airtight containers. Protect from light.

The effect of different ophthalmic vehicles on the activity of tropicamide. Bioavailability of tropicamide generally increased with increasing viscosity of the vehicle.— M. F. Saettone *et al.*, *J. Pharm. Pharmac.*, 1980, *32*, 519.

Adverse Effects, Treatment, and Precautions

As for Atropine Sulphate, p.523.

Uses and Administration

Tropicamide is an antimuscarinic agent with actions similar to those of atropine (see p.524), but its cycloplegic and mydriatic effects have a more rapid onset and a shorter duration of effect. Mydriasis is produced within 15 to 20 minutes of instillation and usually lasts for about 7 hours; cycloplegia is maximal after about 20 minutes and is short lasting, with complete recovery of accommodation normally within 2 to 6 hours.

To produce mydriasis, 1 or 2 drops of a 0.5% solution are instilled prior to examination of the eye. To produce cycloplegia 1 or 2 drops of a 1% solution are required, repeated after 5 minutes; a further drop may be necessary to prolong the effect after 20 to 30 minutes. Tropicamide has been reported to be inadequate for cycloplegia in children: more powerful cycloplegics may be required.

MYDRIASIS. Tropicamide 0.5% was the drug of choice for pupillary dilatation for ophthalmoscopy because of its rapid, short-lasting mydriatic effect with minimal effect on accommodation.— S. Davidson (letter), *Br. med. J.*, 1979, *1*, 821.

Tropicamide 0.5% failed to produce satisfactory mydriasis in diabetics in a study involving 41 diabetic patients and 20 healthy subjects; diabetics who had received laser photocoagulation treatment were particularly unresponsive. However, instillation of 2 drops of phenylephrine 10% eye-drops 30 minutes before tropicamide resulted in adequate pupil dilatation in all diabetics receiving it; the increment in pupil diameter associated with phenylephrine in healthy subjects was significantly less than in diabetics. The combination of tropicamide and phenylephrine provides effective and comfortable mydriasis in diabetic patients without the need for excessive dosage of more powerful mydriatic agents.— M. J. E. Huber, *Br. J. Ophthal.*, 1985, *69*, 425. See also S. E. Smith and S. A. Smith (letter), *Br. med. J.*, 1984, *289*, 111.

For a study comparing the mydriatic effects of tropicamide with other mydriatic agents see under Homatropine Methobromide, p.533.

TEST FOR GLAUCOMA. The use of tropicamide in provocative tests to determine patients likely to develop closed-angle glaucoma.— R. Mapstone, *Br. J. Ophthal.*, 1976, *60*, 115.

Preparations

Tropicamide Eye Drops *(B.P.)*. TRO. Store at a temperature of 8° to 15°.

Tropicamide Ophthalmic Solution *(U.S.P.)*. Avoid freezing.

Proprietary Preparations

Minims Tropicamide *(Smith & Nephew Pharmaceuticals, UK)*. *Eye-drops*, tropicamide 0.5 and 1%, in single-use disposable applicators.

Mydriacyl *(Alcon, UK)*. *Eye-drops*, tropicamide 0.5 and 1%.

Proprietary Names and Manufacturers

Alcon-Mydril *(Arg.)*; Minims Tropicamide *(Smith & Nephew, Austral.; Smith & Nephew, S.Afr.; Smith & Nephew Pharmaceuticals, UK)*; Mydriacyl *(Alcon, Austral.; Alcon, Canad.; Alcon, Denm.; Alcon, S.Afr.; Alcon, Swed.; Alcon, UK)*; Mydrian *(Dispersa, Norw.)*; Mydriaticum *(Belg.; Merck Sharp & Dohme-Chibret, Fr.; Roche, Ger.; Neth.; Dispersa, Switz.)*; Tropicacyl *(Akorn, Canad.)*; Tropikamid Minims *(Smith & Nephew, Norw.; Smith & Nephew, Swed.)*; Tropimil *(Farmigea, Ital.)*; Visumidriatic *(Merck Sharp & Dohme, Ital.)*.

The following names have been used for multi-ingredient preparations containing tropicamide— Phenyltrope *(Akorn, Canad.)*.

425-c

Valethamate Bromide

Diethylmethyl[2-(3-methyl-2-phenylvaleryloxy)ethyl]-ammonium bromide.

$C_{19}H_{32}BrNO_2$=386.4.

CAS — 16376-74-2 (valethamate); 90-22-2 (bromide).

Valethamate bromide is a quaternary ammonium antimuscarinic agent with peripheral effects similar to those of atropine (see p.524). It is used in the symptomatic treatment of visceral spasms. Doses of 10 to 20 mg have been given three or four times daily by mouth; it has also been given by intramuscular or intravenous injection.

Proprietary Names and Manufacturers

Epidosan *(Raffo, Arg.)*; Epidosin *(Kali-Chemie, Ger.; Farmades, Ital.; Kali-Farma, Spain)*; Frenant *(Jpn)*; Narest *(Jpn)*.

Antimycobacterial Agents

7550-p

The agents described in this section are those used in the treatment of infections due to mycobacteria including tuberculosis, leprosy, and opportunistic infections due to the atypical mycobacteria.

Tuberculosis and Antituberculous Agents

Tuberculosis is caused by *Mycobacterium tuberculosis, M. africanum,* or *M. bovis*, and the most usual site of primary infection is the lungs, although extrapulmonary sites may be involved. Tuberculous infection occurs as a result of the inhalation of infected droplets or, in the case of *M. bovis*, by drinking infected milk and may be diagnosed in asymptomatic patients by use of a tuberculin test (p.947). The term tuberculosis is used when the infected person has a disease process involving one or more parts of the body. In generalised miliary tuberculosis, bacilli are disseminated through the blood and give rise to discrete tubercles scattered throughout the lungs and other tissues.

Compounds used in the treatment or prophylaxis of tuberculosis and described in this section include aminosalicylic acid and its salts and derivatives, the antibiotics capreomycin, cycloserine, and rifampicin, hydrazides such as isoniazid, thioamides such as ethionamide and prothionamide, and ethambutol, pyrazinamide, and thiacetazone. Other antibiotics used include kanamycin (p.251) and streptomycin (p.298).

The addition of corticosteroids or corticotrophin to antituberculous therapy may lead to earlier improvement in the patient's condition and in the radiographic clearing of shadows, but generally the slight long-term benefit is not considered to justify their routine use. However, they may be of benefit to seriously ill patients or in the treatment of severe hypersensitivity reactions.

Adverse Effects of Antituberculous Agents

Side-effects may be a particular problem when antituberculous agents are given for prolonged periods; chronic toxicity may be reduced with intermittent and short-term treatment schedules. Although adverse effects associated with antituberculous agents are dealt with under the individual monographs it may be difficult to attribute toxicity to specific agents since the treatment of tuberculosis involves the use of 2 or more drugs.

Reviews of the adverse effects of antituberculous agents.— D. J. Girling, *Drugs*, 1982, *23*, 56.

ALLERGY. *Desensitisation.* Minor hypersensitivity reactions may only require treatment with antihistamines and treatment need not be interrupted. However, if more severe reactions occur all treatment should be withdrawn. Once the reaction has subsided daily challenge doses to the drugs of the regimen should be started. The aim is to resume adequate chemotherapy as soon as possible using not less than 2 drugs by challenging the patient first with those drugs which are least likely to have caused the reaction. If there is no reaction to the initial dose a larger dose is given on day two and if there is still no reaction the agent may be continued in full dosage. Agents should be tested using the following sequence and doses: isoniazid 50 mg initially then 300 mg; rifampicin 75 mg then 300 mg; pyrazinamide 250 mg then 1 g; ethionamide or prothionamide 125 mg then 375 mg; cycloserine 125 mg then 250 mg; ethambutol 100 mg then 500 mg; aminosalicylic acid 1 g then 5 g; thiacetazone 25 mg then 50 mg; streptomycin or other aminoglycosides 125 mg then 500 mg. If the initial hypersensitivity reaction was severe one-tenth of the first dose should be used. Desensitisation to a drug should only be attempted if it is necessary for resumption of adequate chemotherapy and should be carried out under the cover of at least 2 antituberculous agents. Corticosteroids should be given if the initial reaction was severe, or if the patient is hypersensitive to more than one drug, or if administration needs to be resumed rapidly. Desensitisation should not be attempted, even in conjunction with corticosteroids, in patients with severe exfoliative dermatitis. If a reaction occurred with the first challenge dose then desensitisation doses should start with one-tenth of the first challenge dose otherwise the first challenge dose is given. Doses should be given twice daily, each dose being double the previous one. If a reaction occurs the dose is again reduced and increased more gradually thereafter.— D. J. Girling, *Drugs*, 1982, *23*, 56.

EFFECTS ON THE LIVER. The hepatotoxic effects of antituberculous regimens.— D. J. Girling *et al.*, *Tubercle*, 1978, *59*, 13.

EFFECTS ON MENTAL STATE. A brief discussion of the role of tuberculostatics in causing depression.— F. A. Whitlock and L. E. J. Evans, *Drugs*, 1978, *15*, 53.

EFFECTS ON THE NERVOUS SYSTEM. The neurotoxicity of antituberculous agents.— M. R. Holdiness, *Med. Toxicol.*, 1987, *2*, 33. See also S. R. Snavely and G. R. Hodges, *Ann. intern. Med.*, 1984, *101*, 92.

PREGNANCY AND THE NEONATE. For reference to the adverse effects and safety of antituberculous agents during pregnancy and breast feeding, see under Treatment of Tuberculosis, p.548.

Antimicrobial Action and Resistance of Antituberculous Agents

The activity of antituberculous agents can be considered under 3 different topics according to Mitchison (*Tubercle*, 1985, *66*, 219): prevention of resistance, early bactericidal activity, and sterilising activity.

Prevention of Resistance

Antituberculous agents may be graded according to their ability to prevent the emergence of resistance to isoniazid or a second drug. Isoniazid and rifampicin are both highly active in this respect, ethambutol and streptomycin are the next most active, while pyrazinamide and thiacetazone appear to have low activity.

Early Bactericidal Activity

This is a measure of the rate of killing of actively dividing bacteria during the first few days of treatment. Isoniazid has the greatest early bactericidal activity and increases considerably the activity of other agents. Ethambutol and rifampicin are the next most active but add nothing to the activity of other drugs. Streptomycin, pyrazinamide, and thiacetazone are only just bactericidal. However, the early bactericidal activity of an agent has little bearing on its use in therapy except perhaps as an indication of the period during which a patient remains infectious.

Sterilising Activity.

The sterilising activity of an antituberculous agent is the ability to kill all or virtually all of the tuberculous bacilli in lesions as rapidly as possible. It measures the speed with which the last few viable bacilli are killed and indicates the effect an agent will have on the duration of treatment. It may be used to assess an agent's suitability for use in short-term therapy. Rifampicin and pyrazinamide have the greatest sterilising activity; isoniazid is less active and takes longer to sterilise lesions. Although less active than isoniazid, streptomycin or thiacetazone when added to an antituberculous regimen may increase its overall sterilising activity slightly. Ethambutol appears to have virtually no sterilising activity.

These characteristics can be used for the selection of appropriate therapy in patients with various bacterial populations. Proposed populations are:

Population A. This comprises the majority of tubercle bacilli that before treatment are growing actively. Agents with early bactericidal activity are active against these organisms and in therapy isoniazid kills the majority of them within the first few days.

Population B. This covers semi-dormant bacilli found mainly within cells and inhibited by an acid environment. These bacilli are readily killed by pyrazinamide which is only active at a pH of 5.5 or less.

Population C. This covers semi-dormant organisms that have occasional brief spurts of metabolism that may only last a few hours. These organisms are most effectively killed by rifampicin, not because it is highly bactericidal but because it rapidly kills during the short periods of metabolism before isoniazid has a chance to act. These organisms may be in a neutral or acid environment and therefore there may be some overlap between group B and C bacterial populations.

Population D. This covers organisms that are completely dormant and are unaffected by all agents.

It has also been proposed (Mitchison 1985) that pH and inflammation have a role in modifying the growth of tubercle bacilli during treatment. At the start of therapy most population A organisms are in a mildly acid extracellular environment in which isoniazid is active but streptomycin is only weakly bactericidal. However, the pH is not sufficiently low for pyrazinamide to be bactericidal. The inflammatory response produced by these organisms reduces the pH and inhibition produces population B and C organisms. Pyrazinamide and rifampicin are then more active than isoniazid; streptomycin is completely inactive. After a steady transfer of bacilli from population A to population B the inflammatory response dies down, the pH becomes less acidic, and pyrazinamide is again inactive. However, if inflammation recurs due to growth of isoniazid-resistant organisms, the pH rises producing population B organisms which are again killed by pyrazinamide. Population C bacilli remain as 'persistors' and are killed by rifampicin or more slowly by isoniazid or streptomycin if rifampicin is absent.

Reviews of the antimicrobial action of antituberculous agents in short-term chemotherapy of pulmonary tuberculosis.— J. Costello, *Postgrad. med. J.*, 1983, *59*, *Suppl.* 3, 181; D. A. Mitchison, *Tubercle*, 1985, *66*, 219.

RESISTANCE. For reviews and discussions of drug resistance and drug tolerance in mycobacteria, see B. G. Guernsey and M. R. Alexander, *Am. J. Hosp. Pharm.*, 1978, *35*, 690; R. Urbanczik, *Bull. int. Un. Tuberc.*, 1983, *58*, 245; D. A. Mitchison, *Br. med. Bull.*, 1984, *40*, 84; T. Shimao, *Tubercle*, 1987, *68*, *Suppl.*, 5; E. S. Hershfield, *ibid.*, 17.

Examination of the results of 12 clinical studies carried out in collaboration with the British Medical Research Council indicated that the failure-rate after 4 months' treatment in patients with tuberculosis initially resistant to isoniazid, streptomycin, or both was 32% in regimens using streptomycin, isoniazid, and pyrazinamide and 17% in regimens containing isoniazid and rifampicin. The failure-rate decreased as the number of drugs in the regimen was increased and the duration of rifampicin therapy was prolonged. Treatment failed in 2% of patients receiving isoniazid and rifampicin with 2 or 3 additional agents. Relapse-rates after treatment indicated that even in the presence of initial resistance to isoniazid or streptomycin, rifampicin or pyrazinamide is capable of producing the full or almost full sterilising activity of a regimen. However, isoniazid has some sterilising activity as continuation phases containing just isoniazid only need to be prolonged by 2 months to obtain results similar to those containing rifampicin. Ethambutol appears to be ineffective as a sterilising agent but useful in the initial phase to prevent failure due to initial resistance. Initial resistance to rifampicin often occurred with resistance to isoniazid, streptomycin, or both and had a more serious effect on outcome with 8 of 11 patients being treatment failures or relapsing after treatment.— D. A. Mitchison, *Bull. int. Un. Tuberc.*, 1985, *60*, 38. See also D. A. Mitchison and A. J. Nunn, *Am. Rev. resp. Dis.*, 1986, *133*, 423.

Incidence of resistance. Of 12 157 isolates of tubercle bacilli collected in the *USA* between 1975 and 1982 from previously untreated tuberculosis patients, 6.9% were resistant to one or more antituberculous agents. Resistance to individual agents was 4% for isoniazid,

3.8% for streptomycin, and 1.1% for ethionamide. Less than 1% of isolates were resistant to aminosalicylic acid, rifampicin, ethambutol, kanamycin, capreomycin, or cycloserine. Large differences were found for the incidence of resistance in different areas and different racial and ethnic groups, the highest percentage of resistant strains being isolated from Asian and Hispanic patients. There was also a significant inverse relationship between the age of the patient and the incidence of resistance; 14% of isolates from patients up to 10 years of age displayed resistance.— *Morb. Mortal.*, 1983, *32*, 521.

A survey of drug-resistant tuberculosis in children treated in one hospital in New York between 1961 and 1984 indicated an increasing incidence of primary drug resistance to rifampicin in recent years.— P. Steiner *et al.*, *Am. Rev. resp. Dis.*, 1986, *134*, 446.

Of 555 previously untreated patients with tuberculosis examined from 1978 to 1980 in Tanzania, 10.1% had a strain of *M. tuberculosis* resistant to one or more antituberculous agents, 7.6% being resistant to isoniazid, 0.7% to streptomycin, and 1.8% resistant to both agents. Overall resistance was similar to that found in a similar survey in 1969 but initial resistance to isoniazid had increased from 6.3% in 1969 to 9.4% in 1978–80. This may indicate a true increase in resistance due to a build up of excretors of resistant strains in the community or it may be due to previously treated patients presenting as new cases.— Tanzanian/British Medical Research Council Collaborative Study, *Tubercle*, 1985, *66*, 161.

The results of the national survey of tuberculosis notifications in England and Wales have been compared for the years 1978–9 and 1983. In sensitivity tests to isoniazid, streptomycin, ethambutol, and rifampicin, 3% of 1070 strains of tubercle bacilli isolated from patients in 1978–9 had resistance to one or more agents compared with 4.6% of 855 strains in 1983. Resistance to one agent only occurred in 2.2% and 3.4% of the strains respectively and 0.7% and 1.2% of the strains respectively were resistant to isoniazid and streptomycin. In 1978–9 one strain was resistant to rifampicin, streptomycin, and isoniazid but in 1983 no strains were resistant to rifampicin. While there was no resistance to ethambutol in 1978–9 one strain was resistant in 1983. There was no change in the incidence of resistant strains isolated from white patients (1.6%) between the 2 surveys but in patients from the Indian subcontinent the incidence increased from 7.5% to 12.8%.— MRC Tuberculosis and Chest Diseases Unit, *Tubercle*, 1987, *68*, 19. Further surveys of drug resistance in tuberculosis in England and Wales.— M. D. Yates *et al.*, *ibid.*, 1982, *62*, 55 (South-east England, 1977–80); H. E. Thomas and J. G. Ayres, *ibid.*, 1986, *67*, 179 (Birmingham, 1956–83); L. P. Ormerod *et al.*, *Thorax*, 1986, *41*, 946 (Blackburn).

Further references to resistance in different countries: Second East African/British MRC Kenya Tuberculosis Survey Follow-Up 1979, *Tubercle*, 1979, *60*, 125 (Kenya); M. Janowiec *et al.*, *ibid.*, 233 (Poland); N. J. Nielsen, *ibid.*, 239 (Eastern Botswana); E. S. Hershfield *et al.*, *Int. J. clin. Pharmac. Biopharm.*, 1979, *17*, 387 (Canada); F. D. Pien *et al.*, *Am. Rev. resp. Dis.*, 1982, *126*, 928 (Hawaii); A. E. Pitchenik *et al.*, *New Engl. J. Med.*, 1982, *307*, 162 (Haitians in the *USA*); M. L. Blancarte *et al.*, *Salud públ. Méx.*, 1982, *24*, 321 (Mexico); M. T. Valenzuela *et al.*, *Bull. int. Un. Tuberc.*, 1984, *59*, 191 (Chile); U. D. Hardas and V. S. Jayaraman, *Indian J. Tuberc.*, 1984, *31*, 168 (India); J. Gibson, *Tubercle*, 1986, *67*, 119 (Sierra Leone).

Prophylaxis of Tuberculosis

Prophylaxis is intended to prevent the occurrence of acute tuberculosis in patients with tuberculous infection and in susceptible contacts, and to curb its spread through the community. Chemoprophylaxis with isoniazid is more widely used in the *USA* than in the *UK* and other countries where vaccination with BCG vaccine is employed (see p.1157). Isoniazid is usually given for 12 months, but 6 months of therapy may be equally effective. Rifampicin with or without ethambutol has been suggested for contacts of isoniazid-resistant tuberculosis. A regimen of isoniazid with ethambutol given for 6 to 9 months has also been recommended, although some authorities do not consider ethambutol to be suitable for prophylaxis.

In the *USA* where isoniazid prophylaxis is widely used controversy still exists over the benefits and risks of its use in various patient groups. The American Thoracic Society and the Centers for Disease Control (*Am. Rev. resp. Dis.*, 1986, *134*, 355) have issued detailed recommendations for prophylactic treatment of tuberculosis: Prophylaxis with isoniazid for 6 to 12 months is generally recommended for the following categories of patients, in order of priority, who exhibit a positive tuberculin skin test; the potential toxicity of isoniazid should be borne in mind:

1) Household members and other close associates of potentially infectious tuberculosis patients. As children are considered to be especially at risk it may be prudent to treat those with non-significant skin tests for 3 months. The skin test should be repeated after 3 months and if positive, therapy should be continued or initiated in those not already being treated.

2) Newly infected patients whose skin tests have become positive within the past 2 years.

3) Persons with past tuberculosis who have not previously received adequate chemotherapy.

4) Persons with abnormal chest X-rays. These patients should be treated for 12 months.

5) Prophylaxis is also recommended for some patients in special clinical situations such as those with silicosis, diabetes mellitus, leukaemia, Hodgkin's disease, end-stage renal failure, or those receiving immunosuppressive therapy or patients with acquired immunodeficiency syndrome or a positive test for HIV virus. Prophylaxis may also be required for patients with conditions associated with rapid weight loss or chronic undernutrition including intestinal bypass surgery, postgastrectomy state, chronic peptic ulcer disease, chronic malabsorption syndromes, and those with carcinoma of the upper gastro-intestinal tract. Patients receiving prolonged therapy with corticosteroids should also be considered for prophylactic treatment and although there is insufficient data categorically to recommend isoniazid for persons treated with less than the equivalent of 15 mg of prednisone daily or alternate day therapy, it may be prudent to consider some of these patients.

6) Persons under 35 years of age.

To rule out the possibility of progressive disease all positive skin reactors should be given a chest X-ray. Patients who have already received an adequate course of isoniazid should also be excluded. Prophylactic therapy with isoniazid is contra-indicated in patients with a history of severe adverse reactions or hepatic injury associated with isoniazid or acute liver disease. Isoniazid therapy for pregnant women should be delayed until after delivery except in cases of recent infection when prophylaxis should start immediately but after the first trimester. The neonate of a mother with current tuberculosis should be treated with isoniazid for 2 to 3 months or at least until the mother is smear and culture negative. If after 3 months of treatment the mother is sputum negative and the infant is tuberculin-negative and has a normal chest X-ray, isoniazid may be discontinued. If the infant has a significant tuberculin reaction and an abnormal chest X-ray, a second drug such as rifampicin should be added to treatment. In high risk situations BCG vaccination should be considered for long-term protection after a course of isoniazid.

It is also considered reasonable to use rifampicin with or without ethambutol for 1 year in children or adults at high risk who are intolerant to isoniazid or in contact with isoniazid-resistant tuberculosis. BCG vaccine is recommended only for prophylaxis when isoniazid cannot be used; it may be considered for those who have no reaction to a tuberculin skin test and who are repeatedly exposed to infectious cases.

Some of these recommendations have been challenged. Taylor *et al.* (*Ann. intern. Med.*, 1981, *94*, 808) had already concluded, from a decision analysis study, that the benefits of prophylaxis with isoniazid did not clearly outweigh the risks for tuberculin-positive patients between 20 and 34 years of age. However, Rose *et al.* (*J. Am. med. Ass.*, 1986, *256*, 2709) considered that Taylor had underestimated the effectiveness of isoniazid and using similar methods found that isoniazid prophylaxis would be of benefit for all the ages analysed between 10 and 80 years old, though the margin would be small for those over 65. Although patients between 50 and 65 years of age risked a higher incidence of hepatitis there was still a lower likelihood of fatal illness. Furthermore Stead *et al.* (*New Engl. J. Med.*, 1985, *312*, 1483) in an epidemiological study of 223 nursing homes in Arkansas found that elderly patients in these institutions were at greater risk of developing tuberculosis and considered isoniazid prophylaxis might be indicated. However, many clinicians still recommend that isoniazid should not be given to tuberculin-positive patients 35 or more years old unless other factors, such as recent tuberculin conversion, indicate a high risk (*Med. Lett.*, 1986, *28*, 6). Rose *et al.* (*Mt Sinai J. Med.*, 1985, *52*, 253) had also applied decision analysis to evaluate the risk in diabetics and considered that the benefits were minimal for asymptomatic tuberculin-positive diabetics. Likewise, Thomas (*Archs Surg., Chicago*, 1979, *114*, 597) considered that routine prophylaxis was not justified in patients with kidney transplants.

The International Union against Tuberculosis (IUAT) and the World Health Organization (WHO) considered that chemoprophylaxis for tuberculosis has virtually no role in developing countries. Preventative treatment would not be an appropriate part of any tuberculosis control programme unless resources could be allocated without compromising the ability to provide curative treatment to all tuberculosis patients (*Tech. Rep. Ser. Wld Hlth Org. No. 671*, 1982).

Chemoprophylaxis is sometimes employed in the *UK*. Cole (*Prescribers' J.*, 1985, *25*, 110) reported that its main justification is among contacts in whom tuberculin conversion is likely to have occurred recently, particularly children up to 5 years of age with grade 2 to 4 reactions to the Heaf multiple puncture skin test and those between 5 and 15 years with grade 3 or 4 reactions. It is also recommended for contacts of an Asian index case with reaction of grades 2 to 4 up to the age of 15 years, and can also be justified up to the age of 35 years if compliance is assured.

There has also been some debate over the duration of therapy required. Results of a 5-year follow-up study, conducted under the auspices of the IUAT in 7 Eastern European countries (*Bull. Wld Hlth Org.*, 1982, *60*, 555), involving nearly 28 000 tuberculin-positive patients with fibrotic pulmonary lesions showed that the risk of developing tuberculosis was reduced by 21, 65, and 75% in those given isoniazid prophylaxis for 12, 24, or 52 weeks respectively when compared with placebo. Hepatitis developed in 0.5% of patients treated with isoniazid, nearly half of the cases occurring during the first 12 weeks, compared with 0.1% in those receiving placebo. Although the risk of dying from tuberculosis in this study was calculated to be greater than that of dying from isoniazid-induced hepatitis it was considered that the benefit to risk ratio could be improved as the 3 deaths due to isoniazid-induced hepatitis were in patients who continued therapy despite clinical signs of liver involvement (*Lancet*, 1983, *1*, 395). Preliminary reports of the 8 to 10 year follow-up results (A. Krebs, *Bull. int. Un. Tuberc.*, 1982, *57*, 81 and *idem*, 1983, *58*, 167) indicate that the 12-week regimen was only temporarily effective and that 24 weeks of treatment was as effective as 52 weeks. Using data from this study Snider *et al.* (*J. Am. med. Ass.*, 1986, *255*, 1579) calculated that 24 weeks of treatment was more cost-effective than 12 or 52 weeks. Comstock (*Ann. intern. Med.*, 1983, *98*, 663) recommended that patients with fibrotic lesions of the lungs consistent with pulmonary tuberculosis, and who have not completed a full course of antituberculous therapy should receive isoniazid prophylaxis; efforts to achieve compliance should be concentrated during the first 6 months. A suggestion has also been made (*Lancet*, 1983, *1*, 395) that these patients could be given 24 weeks of treatment increased to a year if the fibrotic lesions were more than 2 cm^2 in size. However, there have been criticisms of the true efficacy of isoniazid in the IUAT study and comments that the number of cases prevented was small (K.P. Goldman, *Lancet*, 1983, *1*, 592; H.T. Foley and R.F. Donohoe, *Ann. intern. Med.*, 1983, *99*, 409). Goldman considered that the efficacy of 24 weeks of treatment was too low and that apart from patients at increased risk of breakdown of lesions, such as Asian immigrants or patients taking immunosupressive drugs, isoniazid prophylaxis was undesirable and unnecessary.

When compliance is a problem Bailey *et al.* (*Chest*, 1985, *87*, *Suppl.*, 128S) suggested that when using isoniazid for prophylactic treatment, lapses in therapy for less than one month can probably be ignored. For longer periods of non-compliance, it was recommended that consideration should be given to terminating treatment if the patient has already received more than 6 months of treatment. If the patient had received less than 6 months of treatment, therapy should be re-started and continued for a further 6 months. When compliance with daily therapy cannot be assured twice-weekly supervised administration of isoniazid at a dosage of 15 mg per kg body-weight for one year may be considered.

For references on the management and prophylaxis of tuberculosis in patients undergoing dialysis, see Administration in Renal Failure, under Treatment of Tuberculosis, below.

Treatment of Tuberculosis

A rationale for the selection of appropriate schedules of treatment for tuberculosis is discussed above under the section on Antimicrobial Action.

Isoniazid is the mainstay of regimens used for the treatment of tuberculosis and in an attempt to reduce the risk of failure due to initial drug resistance or to emergence of resistance during therapy it is always administered with one or more other antituberculous agents. Treatment is usually divided into two phases. The initial phase consists of intensive treatment with the aim of controlling the disease by reducing the bacterial population as soon as possible and usually lasts for 2 or more months or until the results of drug sensitivity tests are known. Treatment in the continuation phase is less intensive and administration of some of the agents may be stopped, but it should consist of at least two agents, one of which should always be isoniazid. The aim of the continuation phase is to eradicate the remaining bacilli or to continue treatment until the disease dies out. The total duration of therapy varies according to the number and nature of the antituberculous agents used. Antituberculous agents of first choice, often referred to as primary or 'first-line' agents include isoniazid, rifampicin, ethambutol, pyrazinamide, and streptomycin. Thiacetazone is also used as a primary agent in some developing countries. Other drugs used in the treatment of tuberculosis, such as capreomycin, cycloserine, ethionamide, prothionamide, and kanamycin, are considered to be secondary agents and are generally only used if resistance or toxicity to primary drugs develops during therapy. Although the aminosalicylates were once widely used as primary agents they are now generally regarded as of secondary importance.

Prolonged and sometimes unpalatable therapy is associated with poor patient compliance and has led to the development of intermittent and of short-term regimens. With the first of these developments the aim has been to devise regimens in which treatment is still effective when given intermittently so that administration of doses may be supervised. Intermittent administration is usually employed during the continuation phase of treatment though some regimens are intermittent throughout. Doses are usually given twice or three times weekly though once weekly administration has been used. Individual doses used in intermittent therapy are generally higher than the usual daily doses. However, in rapid acetylators once weekly administration of isoniazid may not be effective and slow-release preparations have been tried to produce a sustained therapeutic effect. Although intermittent administration of rifampicin has been associated with serious adverse effects it has been used following careful adjustment of dosage. However, the use of rifampicin intermittently or only in the continuation phase may necessitate increasing the duration of therapy.

With the second of the developments the availability of the potent bactericidal agent rifampicin has allowed the length of treatment to be reduced, because in addition to producing a rapid reduction in the bacterial population when used with isoniazid it also produces a sterilising effect by eliminating those semi-dormant or 'persisting organisms' associated with late relapse. Addition of pyrazinamide to the initial phase of treatment has increased the 'sterilising activity' of regimens since it is particularly active against organisms inhibited by an acid environment and this has allowed the duration of therapy to be reduced even further.

There are now a number of highly effective short-term regimens of 6 to 9 months duration which are based on an initial phase of rifampicin, isoniazid, and pyrazinamide supplemented by ethambutol or streptomycin followed by a continuation phase of rifampicin and isoniazid. Regimens may consist of daily administration in both phases or may be intermittent in the continuation phase. A number of fully intermittent short-term regimens have also been tried. Shorter regimens are constantly being devised and studied and since many developing countries do not have the resources to administer rifampicin throughout therapy, the effectiveness of regimens which utilise less rifampicin are also being studied.

The various regimens are discussed in detail below.

Reviews of antituberculous agents.— R. E. Van Scoy and C. J. Wilkowske, *Mayo Clin. Proc.*, 1983, *58*, 233; *Med. Lett.*, 1988, *30*, 43.

A review of the clinical pharmacokinetics of antituberculous agents.— M. R. Holdiness, *Clin. Pharmacokinet.*, 1984, *9*, 511.

As there are few controlled studies on the treatment of extrapulmonary tuberculosis, therapy has largely been based on regimens of proven efficacy in pulmonary tuberculosis. Therefore following the successful application of short-term chemotherapy to the treatment of pulmonary tuberculosis short-term regimens are also being tried in the treatment of extrapulmonary tuberculosis. However, results of controlled studies are becoming available (see *Lancet*, 1986, *1*, 1423 and below) and there is already some evidence of effectiveness from retrospective surveys. Dutt *et al.* (*Ann. intern. Med.*, 1986, *104*, 7) have reviewed their experience treating 350 patients with extrapulmonary tuberculosis and found that rifampicin and isoniazid given daily for one month followed by rifampicin and isoniazid twice weekly for a further 8 months was successful in 95% of the patients. A survey by Monie *et al.* (*Br. med. J.*, 1982, *285*, 415), conducted in Wales in 1976–78, found that despite there being no recommendations for use in the *UK* many patients with extrapulmonary tuberculosis were already being treated with short-term regimens. Furthermore in the *US* some authorities have already endorsed the use of short-term chemotherapy (Committee on Chemotherapy of Tuberculosis, *Chest*, 1985, *87*, *Suppl.*, 117S; Joint Statement of the American Thoracic Society and the Centers for Disease Control, *Am. Rev. resp. Dis.*, 1986, *134*, 355). It has been suggested that patients who have received adequate chemotherapy for initially sensitive organisms should be followed-up for 2 years (*Lancet*, 1986, *1*, 1423).

See also below under individual sites of infection.

There is limited experience in the treatment of tuberculosis in patients with AIDS, but most patients appear to respond to standard antituberculous agents though therapy may have to be administered for longer periods than in hosts with normal immune function. The Centers for Disease Control (*Ann. intern. Med.*, 1987, *106*, 254) have recommended a regimen of isoniazid and rifampicin given with either ethambutol or pyrazinamide for the first 2 months. A fourth drug may be indicated in serious infections or if resistance to isoniazid is suspected. Treatment should continue for a minimum of 9 months and for at least 6 months after culture conversion. If regimens not including rifampicin or isoniazid are used it is recommended that treatment should continue for a minimum of 18 months and for at least 12 months after culture conversion. Consideration should also be given to the presence of other mycobacterial infections, especially those due to the *Mycobacterium avium* complex, which may influence the choice of therapy (see p.553). Maintenance therapy is often required and isoniazid and possibly rifampicin are given in conjunction with other antimicrobial agents as prophylaxis against opportunistic infections.

Some reviews on tuberculosis treatment in patients with AIDS.— I. H. Frazer and B. P. Mulhall, *Med. J. Aust.*, 1986, *145*, 524; A. J. Pinching, *Tubercle*, 1987, *68*, 65; C. U. Tuazon and A. M. Labriola, *Drugs*, 1987, *33*, 66.

ADMINISTRATION. Observed serum concentrations of rifampicin, streptomycin, ethambutol, and pyrazinamide in an obese patient were within the expected range for lean patients when dosage was based on ideal body-weight rather than total body-weight.— P. J. Geiseler *et al.*, *Am. Rev. resp. Dis.*, 1985, *131*, 944.

ADMINISTRATION IN THE ELDERLY. The rate of non-compliance was high among the elderly. Treatment should be fully supervised and intermittent chemotherapy, at least in the second phase of treatment, is preferable.— *Tubercle*, 1983, *64*, 69.

ADMINISTRATION IN RENAL FAILURE. References to the treatment of tuberculosis in renal transplant patients.— *Tubercle*, 1979, *60*, 193; H. Riska and B. Kuhlback, *Bull. int. Un. Tuberc.*, 1979, *54*, 165.

Provided that there is little likelihood of initial drug resistance to isoniazid, patients with tuberculosis and renal failure should receive standard doses of rifampicin and isoniazid with pyridoxine for a minimum of 9 months, although patients with a creatinine clearance of less than 10 mL per minute will require a reduction in the dosage of isoniazid to 200 mg daily. If substitution of any of these agents is indicated, streptomycin or ethambutol might be considered, but both require careful dosage regulation. Patients receiving ethambutol would also require regular ophthalmological evaluations.— R. B. Cole, *Prescribers' J.*, 1985, *25*, 110. See also *Lancet*, 1980, *1*, 909.

Discussions and studies on the prophylaxis and management of tuberculosis in patients undergoing dialysis: A. P. Lundin *et al.*, *Am. J. Med.*, 1979, *67*, 597; O. T. Andrew *et al.*, *ibid.*, 1980, *68*, 59; *Br. med. J.*, 1980, *280*, 349; D. A. Mitchison and G. A. Ellard (letter), *ibid.*, 1186 and 1533.

MILIARY TUBERCULOSIS. Cryptic miliary tuberculosis is a cause of pyrexia of unknown origin and can be diagnosed by a therapeutic response to narrow-spectrum antimicrobial agents such as ethambutol plus isoniazid.— *Lancet*, 1986, *1*, 1423.

PLEURAL EFFUSION. A favourable report on the use of a regimen consisting of aminosalicylic acid, isoniazid, and streptomycin with or without corticosteroid therapy in the treatment of 113 patients with tuberculous pleural effusion.— B. O. Onadeko, *Tubercle*, 1978, *59*, 269.

A discussion on experience with short-term chemotherapy for the treatment of pleural tuberculosis.— A. K. Dutt *et al.*, *Chest*, 1986, *90*, 112. See also *idem*, *Ann. intern. Med.*, 1986, *104*, 7.

PREGNANCY AND THE NEONATE. There have been 2 large surveys of mothers who received isoniazid, ethambutol, rifampicin, and streptomycin alone or in combination for all or part of their pregnancy (D.J. Scheinhorn and V.A. Angelillo, *West. J. Med.*, 1977, *127*, 195; D.E. Snider *et al.*, *Am. Rev. resp. Dis.*, 1980, *122*, 65). Routine therapeutic abortion for pregnant women receiving first-line antituberculous drugs is not medically indicated since apart from streptomycin, which produced an increase in auditory and vestibular disturbances, there was no significant increase in congenital abnormalities with these agents. Current opinion is that isoniazid is safe in pregnancy provided that pyridoxine is given simultaneously and a combination of isoniazid and ethambutol has been considered to be the most suitable combination for use during pregnancy. Ethionamide should not be used because of teratogenicity. Similar effects can be expected with prothionamide. Some consider that pyrazinamide should be avoided because of lack of teratogenicity data. The gastro-intestinal effects of aminosalicylic acid and the effects of cycloserine on the nervous system make their use during pregnancy undesirable (D. Snider, *Chest*, 1984, *86*, *Suppl.*, 10S). Opinions also differ on the use of rifampicin during pregnancy because of evidence of teratogenicity in *animals* given large doses (p.572). Regimens comprising isoniazid and rifampicin given for 9 months possibly supplemented with ethambutol for the initial phase have been recommended by some clinicians (American Thoracic Society and Centers for Disease Control, *Am. Rev. resp. Dis.*, 1986, *134*, 355; R. Wise, *Br. med. J.*, 1987, *294*, 42). While others consider that rifampicin should be withdrawn if pregnancy occurs during therapy unless there is isoniazid-resistance or very extensive disease. Treatment should then continue with at least 2 and preferably 3 agents, such as isoniazid, ethambutol, and pyrazinamide, during the initial 2-month phase and with isoniazid and ethambutol during the continuation phase. If rifampicin is re-introduced once the pregnancy is over the total duration of treatment and surveillance may need to be extended (R.B. Cole, *Prescribers' J.*, 1985, *25*, 110).

Breast-feeding. From a review of studies of the excretion of antituberculous drugs into breast milk, Snider and Powell (*Archs intern. Med.*, 1984, *144*, 589) estimated that the amount of the usual therapeutic dose for infants that would be ingested by a breast-fed infant would be: isoniazid 6.4% to 20%; rifampicin 0.57%; streptomycin sulphate 9.5%; kanamycin sulphate 0.95%; cycloserine 11.3%; ethambutol hydrochloride 3.4 to 5.7%. Holdiness (*Archs intern. Med.*, 1984, *144*, 1888) later estimated that the equivalent amounts of pyrazinamide and aminosalicylic acid that would be ingested were far below the therapeutic range. Snider and Powell concluded that the small number of subjects studied prevented definite conclusions being made about the risk of toxicity to breast-fed infants but considered that mothers taking antituberculous agents can safely nurse their infants if the following precautions are taken: the infants should be periodically examined for adverse effects but routine monitoring of drug concentrations in milk or in the infants' blood and urine is considered unnecessary; the mother should take her antituberculous treatment immediately after breast feeding and a bottle substituted for the next feed; mothers should not breast feed if the child also requires antituberculous therapy.

PULMONARY TUBERCULOSIS. The present state and development of short-course chemotherapy for pulmonary tuberculosis has been the subject of several reviews (Sister M. Aquinas, *Drugs*, 1982, *24*, 118; J.H. Angel,

Drugs, 1983, *26*, 1; D. Larbaoui, *Bull. int. Un. Tuberc.*, 1985, *60*, 17; W. Fox, *ibid.*, 40). Extensive clinical studies over the past few decades have enabled more effective and increasingly shorter treatment regimens to be introduced.

A study by the British Thoracic Association (*Lancet*, 1980, *1*, 1182 and *ibid.*, *2*, 272) conducted under routine clinic conditions found that a 9-month regimen of isoniazid and rifampicin supplemented by ethambutol or streptomycin for the first 2 months was almost 100% effective, the only 2 relapses to treatment occurring 4 to 5 years after the end of therapy. Similar results were also obtained in French studies. This regimen was recommended as the treatment of choice in Britain; it has also been widely used in many other countries. Similar regimens have been endorsed in the *USA* by the American Thoracic Society and the Centers for Disease Control (*Am. Rev. resp. Dis.*, 1986, *134*, 355) but it is considered that ethambutol may be omitted unless isoniazid resistance is suspected. Another 9-month regimen recommended by these *US* authorities, in which isoniazid and rifampicin are given daily for one month and then twice weekly for 8 months also appear to be effective (A.K. Dutt *et al.*, *Am. J. Med.*, 1984, *77*, 233).

Numerous studies have been conducted on regimens lasting 6 months. Most of these and shorter regimens have utilised a 4-drug initial intensive phase. The use of daily rifampicin with isoniazid alone for 6 months had been considered to be inadequate in an United States Public Health Service Co-operative study (D.E. Snider *et al.*, *Am. Rev. resp. Dis.*, 1984, *129*, 573) and although addition of streptomycin to this regimen had reduced the relapse-rates to 2 to 3% under study conditions (East African/British MRCs, *Lancet*, 1974, *2*, 237 and *Am. Rev. resp. Dis.*, 1976, *114*, 471) the use of this regimen under routine clinic conditions in Britain and France produced relapse rates regarded as unacceptably high in developed countries (British Thoracic Association, *Lancet*, 1980, *1*, 1182 and *ibid.*, *2*, 272). However, the British Thoracic Society [formerly Association] (*Br. J. Dis. Chest*, 1984, *78*, 330) found that 6-month regimens of daily isoniazid and rifampicin supplemented for the first 2 months with pyrazinamide and streptomycin or pyrazinamide and ethambutol were as effective as the 9-month regimen they had recommended previously. The relapse rate at the 36-month follow-up was 1.7% for the regimen containing streptomycin and 3.1% for the totally oral regimen containing ethambutol. Similar results have been obtained by other workers using the streptomycin regimen (East and Central African/British MRC Fifth Collaborative Study, *Tubercle*, 1986, *67*, 5) and the ethambutol regimen (M. Berkani *et al.*, Algerian Working Group/British MRC, *Revue fr. mal. Resp.*, 1986, *3*, 73). These two regimens together with the 9-month regimens were therefore recommended by the British Thoracic Society as the treatments of choice for pulmonary tuberculosis. Although the need for ethambutol or streptomycin in these 6- or 9-month regimens remains to be resolved (*Drug & Ther. Bull.*, 1988, *26*, 1), regimens recommended by the American Thoracic Society and the Centers for Disease Control in the *USA* (*Am. Rev. resp. Dis.*, 1986, *134*, 355) omit ethambutol when treatment is for patients with fully susceptible organisms. Preparations containing isoniazid, rifampicin, and pyrazinamide have been introduced to aid compliance and their use has been the subject of both pharmacokinetic and clinical studies (G. Acocella *et al.*, *Am. Rev. resp. Dis.*, 1985, *132*, 510; G.A. Ellard, *ibid*, 1986, *133*, 1076; L. J. Geiter, United States Public Health Service, *Tubercle*, 1987, *68*, *Suppl.*, 41). Relapse rates of 1 to 2% have been obtained at the 24-month follow-up for modified forms of these regimens in which 4 or 5 agents were administered three times weekly (Hong Kong Chest Service/British MRC, *Tubercle*, 1982, *63*, 89). Favourable results have also been obtained in some studies of 6-month regimens consisting of 2 months of daily isoniazid, rifampicin, pyrazinamide, and streptomycin followed by a 4-month continuation phase of two or three times weekly administration of isoniazid and rifampicin (Singapore Tuberculosis Service/British MRC, *Am. Rev. resp. Dis.*, 1985, *132*, 374; D.E. Snider *et al.*, *Eur. J. resp. Dis.*, 1986, *68*, 12). Treatment had been found to be inadequate when the continuation phase had consisted of twice weekly dosing of either isoniazid, pyrazinamide, and streptomycin or isoniazid, ethambutol, and streptomycin, given for four months; some workers have obtained acceptable results when this phase was given for 5 or 6 months (Hong Kong Chest Service/British MRC, *Tubercle*, 1979, *60*, 201; Tuberculosis Research Centre, Madras, India, *Tubercle*, 1983, *64*, 73). In a series of studies in East Africa relapse-rates have sometimes appeared to be unacceptably high when the same initial phase has been followed by a 4-month continuation phase of isoniazid and thiacetazone (East African/British MRCs, *Tubercle*, 1980, *61*, 59; Tanzania/British MRCs, *Am. Rev. resp. Dis.*, 1985, *131*, 727) though the relapse rate at the 24-month follow-up has been reduced to zero by prolongation of the continuation phase to 6 months. In the treatment of patients who are difficult to supervise, such as prisoners and drug addicts, a highly intensive 6-month regimen consisting of daily isoniazid, rifampicin, pyrazinamide, and ethambutol supplemented with streptomycin for the first 3 months has produced good results with a surprisingly low frequency of adverse reactions (Hong Kong Chest Service/British MRC, *Tubercle*, 1983, *64*, 265).

Relapse rates of about 4 to 5.5% have also been obtained at 24-month follow-up of partially intermittent 5-month regimens using isoniazid, rifampicin, pyrazinamide, and streptomycin for 2 or 3 months followed by isoniazid, pyrazinamide, and streptomycin given twice weekly for the duration of therapy (Tuberculosis Research Centre, Madras, India, *Tubercle*, 1983, *64*, 73; Tuberculosis Research Centre, Madras, India, and National Tuberculosis Institute, Bangalore, India, *Am. Rev. resp. Dis.*, 1986, *134*, 27).

A number of 4-month regimens employing the same 2-month initial phase followed by various agents in the continuation phase have also been evaluated but results have largely been disappointing (East African and British MRC, *Am. Rev. resp. Dis.*, 1981, *123*, 165; Singapore Tuberculosis Service and British MRC, *Tubercle*, 1981, *62*, 95 and *Am. Rev. resp. Dis.*, 1986, *133*, 779). Relapse-rates at the 24-month follow-up ranged from 8 to 11% for the regimen with a continuation phase of isoniazid and rifampicin to over 30% for regimens in which rifampicin was omitted from the continuation phase. Pyrazinamide added to the continuation phase appeared to add little or nothing to the effectiveness of these regimens. However, administration of the same 4 drugs throughout the course of treatment has produced more favourable results (S. Perdrizet *et al.*, *Bull. int. Un. Tuberc.* 1984, *59*, 11).

Relapse-rates have also been high in patients given isoniazid, rifampicin, pyrazinamide, and streptomycin daily for 3 months (Tuberculosis Research Centre, Madras, and National Tuberculosis Institute, Bangalore, India, *Am. Rev. resp. Dis.*, 1986, *134*, 27) although Mehrotra *et al.* (*Am. Rev. resp. Dis.*, 1984, *129*, 1016) considered that addition of an extra 1½ months of treatment with isoniazid and rifampicin may produce an effective regimen; they had obtained a relapse-rate of 2% at the 24-month follow-up.

Isoniazid, rifampicin, pyrazinamide, and streptomycin given daily for 2 to 3 months has been found to be inadequate in smear-negative patients with radiologically active pulmonary tuberculosis, who were culture-positive as well as in those who were culture-negative (Hong Kong Chest Service, Tuberculosis Research Centre, Madras, India, and British MRC, *Am. Rev. resp. Dis.*, 1984, *130*, 23). A considerable proportion of the relapses occurred more than 24 months after the end of therapy. At the 60-month follow-up, of those patients with initially drug-sensitive strains, relapse had occurred in 32% of those treated for 2 months and 13% treated for 3 months compared with 5% of patients treated with a 12-month 'standard' regimen. Results were similar for patients with resistant organisms. In culture-negative patients the relapse-rates were 11%, 7%, and 2% respectively. The need for treatment of smear-negative culture-negative tuberculosis was demonstrated by the fact that of those patients who were initially untreated 57% later required treatment after confirmation of active disease. However, results of another study in similar patients given the same regimen three times weekly for 3, 4, or 6 months have been promising at the 24-month follow-up but as already demonstrated longer assessment is required (S.L. Chan, Hong Kong Chest Service, Tuberculosis Research Centre, Madras, India, British MRC, *Bull. int. Un. Tuberc.*, 1985, *60*, 106). Furthermore, the relapse rate 4 years after the end of therapy was about 1% in smear- and culture-negative patients given 4 months of daily rifampicin and isoniazid supplemented with pyrazinamide for the first 2 months (T. Nurmela *et al.*, *Bull. int. Un. Tuberc.*, 1986, *61*, (Sept.), 47).

Longer or standard length regimens may sometimes be preferred. Good results have been achieved through improved compliance and supervision in Hong Kong by using a 12-month regimen comprising of an initial 2-month phase of daily rifampicin, isoniazid, pyrazinamide, ethambutol, and streptomycin with pyrazinamide being dropped from the continuation phase during which all agents are administered once weekly for 10 months (Hong Kong Chest Service/British MRC, *Tubercle*, 1984, *65*, 5).

Definitions of successful treatment and other terms of reference used in the investigation of short-course chemotherapy for pulmonary tuberculosis were inadequate or flawed. Stricter definitions would invalidate nearly all existing studies of short-course chemotherapy.— H. A. Buechner (letter), *Lancet*, 1982, *1*, 1462. See also.— *Lancet*, 1982, *1*, 1163.

Some regimens using rifampicin with a preparation containing dapsone, isoniazid, and prothionamide (Isoprodian) have been found to be effective in the treatment of pulmonary tuberculosis (H. Kittel, *Dt. med. Wschr.*, 1979, *104*, 477; H.H. Kleeberg, *Chemotherapy, Basle*, 1987, *33*, 219) but efficacy and acceptability were considered to be poor when the same preparation was administered with rifampicin and pyrazinamide (M.E. Langton and R.L. Cowie, *S. Afr. med. J.*, 1985, *68*, 881).

Treatment of pulmonary tuberculosis due to *Mycobacterium bovis* using short-term chemotherapy.— W. J. O'Donohue *et al.*, *Archs intern. Med.*, 1985, *145*, 703.

References to the treatment of pulmonary tuberculosis associated with pneumoconiosis or silicosis.— F. L. Jones, *Am. Rev. resp. Dis.*, 1982, *125*, 681; B. C. Escreet *et al.*, *S. Afr. med. J.*, 1984, *66*, 327.

For reports that levamisole enhances the recovery of patients receiving antituberculous chemotherapy for pulmonary tuberculosis, see p.57.

Administration in children. Reviews and discussions on the treatment of pulmonary tuberculosis in children.— M. I. Lorin *et al.*, *Pediat. Clins N. Am.*, 1983, *30*, 333; R. F. Jacobs and R. S. Abernathy, *Pediatr. infect. Dis.*, 1985, *4*, 513; E. L. Kendig, *Pediatrics*, 1985, *75*, 684.

Discussion on the treatment of congenital tuberculosis.— *Tubercle*, 1984, *65*, 81.

See also under Recommendations for Treatment of Pulmonary Tuberculosis, below.

Follow-up. Except for patients with high-risk factors, the routine follow-up of patients believed to have taken adequate 'standard' chemotherapy for pulmonary tuberculosis was originally abandoned in the *UK* following a recommendation from the British Thoracic and Tuberculosis Association Joint Tuberculosis Committee (*Br. med. J.*, 1975, *2*, 28). Follow-up is still considered to be unnecessary with the currently recommended 9- and 6-month regimens since relapse is very unlikely in fully-compliant patients. Nevertheless it has been stressed that the discharged patient must be encouraged to report any symptoms indicative of relapse. Where there has been initial drug resistance or any doubt about the patient's compliance with therapy, it is considered better to review the patient occasionally for 2 years following the end of therapy since relapse is most likely to occur within this time (R.B. Cole, *Prescribers' J.*, 1985, *25*, 110). Recommendations in the *US* are similar except for patients treated with a 6-month regimen for whom a 6- and possibly a 12-month follow-up has been recommended (Joint Statement of the American Thoracic Society and the Centers for Disease Control, *Am. Rev. resp. Dis.*, 1986, *134*, 355).

In the treatment of extrapulmonary tuberculosis it has been suggested that patients who have received adequate short-term chemotherapy for initially sensitive organisms should be followed-up for 2 years (*Lancet*, 1986, *1*, 1423).

Infectivity. Concern was expressed by some clinicians following recommendations that the routine isolation of patients with pulmonary tuberculosis who were being treated should be abandoned. Although active disease has been produced in *guinea-pigs* injected with sputum from patients who have received up to 8 weeks of antituberculous chemotherapy (S.G. Jenkinson *et al.*, *Am. Rev. resp. Dis.*, 1979, *119*, *Suppl.* 1, 403; L. Clancy *et al.*, *Bull. int. Un. Tuberc.*, 1986, *61*, (Sept.), 73), it is considered that the outcome from the usual route of transmission is likely to differ considerably (*Br. med. J.*, 1980, *280*, 962). The Joint Tuberculosis Committee of the British Thoracic Society in their Code of Practice for Control and Prevention of Tuberculosis (*Br. med. J.*, 1983, *287*, 1118) consider that for practical purposes the only source of tuberculous infection is a person whose sputum is positive on direct examination and recommend that such patients should be regarded as noninfectious after 2 weeks of therapy which includes rifampicin. They stress that patients will only remain noninfectious if regular and adequate chemotherapy is continued. Their recommendations do not apply to patients with acquired drug-resistance. Longer periods of avoidance may also be required when close contacts include infants or children; a period of a month had previously been suggested, assuming any cough had ceased (*Br. med. J.*, 1980, *281*, 434) but this has been criticised (R.G. Townshend, *Br. med. J.*, 1980, *281*, 942). The British Thoracic Society have also stated that patients with nonpulmonary tuberculosis should be regarded as noninfectious (*Br. med. J.*, 1983, *287*, 1118).

With the abandonment of routine isolation it is considered that a strict and effective organisation for examining contacts, as set out by the British Thoracic Association (*Tubercle*, 1978, *59*, 245), is all the more important. Snider *et al.* (*Am. Rev. resp. Dis.*, 1985, *132*, 125) have also recommended that investigation of contacts of patients excreting drug-resistant tubercle bacilli should be given high priority. Previous opinion had been that resistant bacilli were significantly less infectious. However, they had shown in a study involving nearly 800 patients with previously untreated tuberculosis that there was no difference in the risk of infection among contacts of patients infected with bacilli resistant to isoniazid and/or streptomycin or of those infected with drug-sensitive organisms.

Recommendations for treatment of pulmonary tuberculosis. In Great Britain the British Thoracic Society (*Br. J. Dis. Chest.*, 1984, *78*, 330) have recommended that in the treatment of pulmonary tuberculosis regimens of rifampicin, isoniazid, pyrazinamide, and ethambutol or streptomycin given daily for 2 months followed by rifampicin and isoniazid daily for 4 months are acceptable alternatives to the use of the previously recommended 9-month regimen which consisted of daily isoniazid and rifampicin supplemented with ethambutol or streptomycin for the first 2 months (*Lancet*, 1980, *1*, 1182 and *ibid.*, *2*, 272). Similar recommendations have also been issued in the *USA* by the American Thoracic Society and the Centers for Disease Control (*Am. Rev. resp. Dis.*, 1986, *134*, 355) except that it is considered that ethambutol may be omitted for patients with fully susceptible organisms. It is also considered that in the continuation phase administration may be continued twice weekly instead of daily. The Centers for Disease Control have also suggested that for the homeless, when supervision and compliance would be a problem, the use of a regimen of thrice weekly administration with larger doses should be considered (*Morb. Mortal.*, 1987, *36*, 257). The American authorities also considered that children should be treated in essentially the same way as adults using appropriately adjusted doses.

In developing countries the inexpensive regimens recommended by the WHO (*Tech. Rep. Ser.*, 1974, No.552) such as isoniazid, thiacetazone, and streptomycin given daily or intermittently for at least 12 months can produce excellent results if properly supervised. Although an IUAT/WHO Study Group (*Tech. Rep. Ser.*, 1982, No.671) affirmed that these still remained the basic regimens for use under programme conditions in many developing countries, the aim should be to make effective short-course regimens available in all countries. At the XIVth Conference of the Far East Region of the IUAT in Nepal, 1985 (*Bull. int. Un. Tuberc.*, 1986, *61*, (Mar.-Jun.), 72) it was pointed out that short-term chemotherapy with its higher compliance-rate and smaller danger of relapse in early defaulters might in fact be more economical in the long run. It was considered that only regimens of proven efficacy should be used and suggested that to avoid confusion no country should adopt more than 2 alternative regimens. The following regimens were considered to be suitable: an initial 2-month phase of daily rifampicin, isoniazid, and pyrazinamide followed by 4 to 6 months of rifampicin and isoniazid given daily or twice weekly; the same initial 2-month phase followed by 6 months of daily isoniazid and thiacetazone with or without a supplement of streptomycin in the initial phase; the same initial 2-month phase supplemented by streptomycin and followed by 6 months of isoniazid and streptomycin given twice weekly. In cases of intolerance streptomycin can be replaced by ethambutol. Rifampicin and pyrazinamide can also be replaced by ethambutol but the duration of therapy should be prolonged to 12 months. It was stressed that intermittent regimens could be dangerous unless fully supervised.

Treatment of relapse. It appears that modern short-course regimens are nearly as effective in patients whose strains are initially resistant to isoniazid or streptomycin, or both, as in patients with fully sensitive strains (*Bull. Wld Hlth Org.*, 1985, *63*, 653— see also under Antimicrobial Action, p.546). Furthermore, in patients who relapse after completing short-course regimens containing isoniazid and rifampicin, initially susceptible organisms usually remain susceptible and the American Thoracic Society and the Centers for Disease Control (*Am. Rev. resp. Dis.*, 1986, *134*, 355) consider that these patients can be managed by the re-institution of the regimen previously used. However, in the presence of resistance to isoniazid, they have recommended that a regimen of rifampicin and ethambutol, possibly supplemented by pyrazinamide in the initial phase, should be given for 12 months. From a review of the literature, Moulding (*Am. Rev. resp. Dis.*, 1981, *123*, 262) found that the data on the value of isoniazid in retreatment regimens for isoniazid-resistant tuberculosis was conflicting. A controlled study indicated that there was no benefit when isoniazid was added to treatment in a dosage of 300 mg daily, but in an uncontrolled study doses of 1 to 1.5 g daily significantly improved therapeutic outcome. Snider *et al.* (*Chest*, 1985, *87, Suppl.*, 117S) have also recommended a number of regimens for treating drug-resistant tuberculosis which vary in duration and content according to the pattern of resistance. They recommend that for retreatment of tuberculosis resistant to rifampicin and ethambutol, the patient should be treated for 24 months with a 3-drug regimen selected on the basis of susceptibility studies. If resistance to all first-line antituberculous agents has been acquired a regimen of ethionamide, cycloserine, and capreomycin or kanamycin can be used but is relatively toxic.

TUBERCULOSIS OF THE ABDOMEN. Regimens used in the treatment of abdominal tuberculosis usually include 3 drugs in the initial phase while sensitivity of the organisms is being tested. Isoniazid with rifampicin and pyrazinamide are the agents of choice but ethambutol or streptomycin may be substituted for one or other of these drugs. Once sensitivities are available the patient can be managed on 2 appropriate agents for the remainder of treatment. Courses lasting 9 to 12 months are considered to be adequate.— P. F. Schofield, *Gut*, 1985, *26*, 1275.

TUBERCULOSIS OF BONES AND JOINTS. BCG osteomyelitis in a child was successfully managed with sodium aminosalicylate, isoniazid, and streptomycin.— M. Pauker *et al.*, *Archs Dis. Childh.*, 1977, *52*, 330.

An 11-year-old child with proptosis due to tuberculosis of the orbit made a full recovery after receiving isoniazid with rifampicin for 18 months supplemented with streptomycin for the first 6 weeks.— A. Oakhill *et al.*, *Br. J. Ophthal.*, 1982, *66*, 396.

Reports of polyarthritis associated with tuberculosis (Poncet's disease) responding to antituberculous chemotherapy.— A. G. Wilkinson and S. Roy, *Tubercle*, 1984, *65*, 301; S. K. Malik and S. D. Deodhar (letter), *ibid.*, 1985, *66*, 152.

A study of three 6-month regimens for the treatment of tuberculosis of the bones and joints.— M. R. Martini *et al.*, *Bull. int. Un. Tuberc.*, 1986, *61*, (Sept.), 40.

Spinal tuberculosis. A series of controlled studies, organised by the British MRC Working Party on Tuberculosis of the Spine, of different methods of management of patients with spinal tuberculosis, has been carried out in Korea, Zimbabwe, Hong Kong, and South Africa (see Eighth Report— *J. Bone Jt Surg.*, 1982, *64-B*, 393 and the Ninth Report— ibid., 1985, *67-B*, 103 for 10-year follow-up assessments). Chemotherapy with isoniazid and aminosalicylic acid daily for 18 months, with or without streptomycin daily for the first 3 months has been highly effective in arresting spinal disease in patients fully ambulant from the start of treatment. No extra benefit has been derived from plaster jackets or bed-rest in hospital. Supplementation with streptomycin was considered necessary only in those patients who have previously received chemotherapy for a long period or who live in areas where there is a high initial level of drug resistance (Fifth Report— *J. Bone Jt Surg.*, 1976, *58-B*, 399). In countries lacking the resources to perform radical resection of the tuberculous focus, ambulant chemotherapy is the treatment of choice. There was also no significant difference between the response obtained when 2 different methods of surgical management (radical resection or debridement) were used in addition to standard chemotherapy (Seventh Report— *Tubercle*, 1978, *59*, 79). Studies are also being conducted to assess the effectiveness of short-term chemotherapy with isoniazid and rifampicin given for 6 or 9 months with or without streptomycin. Preliminary results (Tenth Report— *Tubercle*, 1986, *67*, 243) indicate that these regimens are as effective as the previous long-term therapy.

Further references: A. K. Dutt *et al.*, *Ann. intern. Med.*, 1986, *104*, 7.

TUBERCULOSIS OF THE CENTRAL NERVOUS SYSTEM. Surgical excision has been favoured in the past as the most desirable form of treatment for intracranial tuberculoma and there has been controversy over the relative efficacy of antituberculous chemotherapy used alone. However, Harder *et al.* (*Am. J. Med.*, 1983, *74*, 570) considered that chemotherapy was the treatment of choice after studying the outcome in 10 patients managed with isoniazid, rifampicin, and ethambutol for about 12 months and 10 similar patients treated by craniotomy and antituberculous chemotherapy. Tandon and Bhargava (*Tubercle*, 1985, *66*, 85) using computerised tomography to assess response in 50 patients considered that in the absence of raised intracranial pressure threatening life or vision, surgical treatment should be reserved for those failing to respond to chemotherapy. Corticosteroids have been used to reduce intracranial pressure (A.J. Lees *et al. Lancet*, 1980, *1*, 1208 and 1372; J. Lebas *et al.*, *ibid.*, *2*, 84) although it has been suggested that their use may aid the development of tuberculomas by depressing the immune mechanism (J.F. Warner, *Lancet*, 1980, *2*, 84). Paradoxical expansion of intracranial tuberculomas has been reported during antituberculous chemotherapy (S.T. Chambers *et al.*, *Lancet*, 1984, *2*, 181) but it is considered that if the patient's general condition is satisfactory, alteration of treatment is not indicated (*Lancet*, 1984, *2*, 204). It has been proposed that the effect might have an immunological basis (J. Colover, *Lancet*, 1984, *2*, 471) while Clezy (*Lancet*, 1984, *2*, 750) has suggested that it might be related to liquefaction of the lesion for which simple aspiration might be considered.

See also under Tuberculous Meningitis, below.

TUBERCULOSIS OF THE GENITO-URINARY TRACT. Isoniazid and aminosalicylic acid given for 18 months or 2 years, supplemented with streptomycin for the first 120 days has produced a cure in up to 89% of female patients with tuberculosis of the genito-urinary tract (A.M. Sutherland, *Tubercle*, 1985, *66*, 79). A regimen using ethambutol instead of aminosalicylic acid has proved to be less effective.

Short-term chemotherapy is still under evaluation. Preliminary results of a regimen using isoniazid and rifampicin daily for 1 year supplemented with ethambutol for the first 3 months indicate that after an average of 2.5 years 97% of patients are cured (A.M. Sutherland, *Tubercle*, 1985, *66*, 79). However, only one relapse had occurred in 106 patients followed-up for at least 45 months after a 6-month regimen consisting of isoniazid, rifampicin, and pyrazinamide daily for 2 months followed by isoniazid and rifampicin for a further 4 months (V. Skutil *et al.*, *Eur. Urol.*, 1985, *11*, 170). Good results have also been reported after reducing the length of treatment to 4 months using a regimen consisting of daily isoniazid, rifampicin, and pyrazinamide, with or without streptomycin, given for 2 months followed by intermittent isoniazid and rifampicin for a further 2 months (J.G. Gow and S. Barbosa, *Br. J. Urol.*, 1984, *56*, 449). Some clinicians, however, prefer a 9-month regimen especially if there is suspicion of active disease elsewhere (*Lancet*, 1986, *1*, 1423) and Wong *et al.* (*Br. J. Urol.*, 1984, *56*, 349) consider that the duration of treatment should be adjusted for individual patients according to the degree of infection and any surgical procedures used.

The treatment of male genital tuberculosis has been reviewed by Gorse and Belshe (*Rev. infect. Dis.*, 1985, *7*, 511). Recommended durations of therapy using 2 or 3 drug regimens have ranged from 12 to 24 months, but Gorse and Belshe considered that 18 months' therapy with isoniazid and rifampicin would be effective in the majority of patients.

TUBERCULOSIS OF THE LIVER. Reports of the use of antituberculous chemotherapy in conjunction with surgery in the management of tuberculosis of the liver.— R. D. Rosin, *Tubercle*, 1978, *59*, 47; C. T. Spiegel and C. U. Tuazon, *ibid.*, 1984, *65*, 127.

TUBERCULOSIS OF THE LYMPH NODES. A study conducted under the auspices of the British Thoracic Association (I.A. Campbell and A.J. Dyson, *Tubercle*, 1977, *58*, 171 and 1979, *60*, 95) has shown that 18 months of chemotherapy alone can achieve good results in the treatment of lymph-node tuberculosis and that therapeutic resection is not essential. Regimens consisting of isoniazid and rifampicin or isoniazid and ethambutol, both given with streptomycin for the first 2 months, were found to be equally effective after 18 months of follow-up of 90 patients. In a later study conducted by the British Thoracic Society (*Br. med. J.*, 1985, *290*, 1106) involving 113 patients, short-term chemotherapy with rifampicin and isoniazid given for 9 months, supplemented with ethambutol for the first 8 weeks, was compared with the same regimen, but with rifampicin and isoniazid continued for a further 9 months. At follow-up, 3 years after the start of the study, response to the 9-month regimen was considered to be adequate but these results needed confirmation after a longer period of follow-up. There was no evidence that surgical removal of nodes was advantageous. However, the experience of Malik and Behera (*Br. med. J.*, 1985, *291*, 139) in 35 patients indicated that treatment with isoniazid, rifampicin, and ethambutol given for 36 weeks does not satisfactorily resolve the underlying disease in tubercular lymphadenitis. Some patients only responded after a further 12 weeks of therapy while others required surgical treatment and a full 18 months of chemotherapy.

Lymph nodes may appear or enlarge during and after chemotherapy but this is not due to microbiological relapse; the effect may have an immunological basis (*Lancet*, 1986, *1*, 1423).

Further references: R. Amrane *et al.*, *Bull. int. Un. Tuberc.*, 1986, *61*, (Sept.), 40 (6- and 9-month regimens).

TUBERCULOUS MENINGITIS. The major factor influencing a poor outcome in tuberculous meningitis is not the failure of antituberculous therapy but the delay in the commencement of treatment, and the World Health Organization considers (*Bull. Wld Hlth Org.*, 1985, *63*, 653) that efforts should be focussed on early diagnosis and intensive treatment.

There appears to be no generally accepted regimen for the treatment of tuberculous meningitis but the choice of agents will be influenced by their ability to diffuse across the meninges. The pharmacokinetics of antituberculous agents in the CSF has been reviewed by Holdiness (*Clin. Pharmacokinet.*, 1985, *10*, 532). Isoniazid penetrates well into the CSF and is considered to be essential to all regimens. Ethionamide, pyrazinamide, and cycloserine also achieve therapeutic concentrations in the CSF but are considered to be relatively toxic (R.J. Fallon, *J. antimicrob. Chemother.*, 1978, *4*, 1). Rifampicin, ethambutol, streptomycin, and kanamycin may only penetrate well when the meninges are inflamed. The role of intrathecal administration of streptomycin in the treatment of tuberculous meningitis is still contentious.

Most clinicians use 3 drugs in the initial phase of treatment and regimens of isoniazid, aminosalicylic acid, and streptomycin given for 18 months have been successfully used in the past. Ethambutol has sometimes been used in place of aminosalicylic acid. Some workers (N.I. Girgis *et al.*, *J. trop. Med. Hyg.*, 1978, *81*, 246; E.J. Haas *et al.*, *Archs intern. Med.*, 1977, *137*, 1518) have found that replacing aminosalicylic acid or ethambutol with rifampicin did not appear to improve the prognosis. Other studies have shown that the response is better and the resulting sequelae fewer with regimens incorporating rifampicin (N.N. Rahajoe *et al.*, *Tubercle*, 1979, *60*, 245; P. Latorre *et al.*, *Eur. J. Clin. Pharmac.*, 1984, *26*, 583). Although some clinicians have suggested that suitable regimens should include isoniazid and rifampicin given for 12 months supplemented with ethionamide or pyrazinamide for the first 2 or 3 months, Molavi and LeFrock (*Med. Clins N. Am.*, 1985, *69*, 315) consider that a 9-month regimen of isoniazid and rifampicin would be adequate supplemented with ethambutol or streptomycin for the first 2 months in severe cases. It has also been suggested that 4 agents may be required if drug-resistance is suspected. The use of corticosteroids to prevent or treat raised intracranial pressure has been recommended by some clinicians (*Lancet*, 1986, *1*, 1423; American Thoracic Society and Centers for Disease Control, *Am. Rev. resp. Dis.*, 1986, *134*, 355).

Ramachandran *et al.* (*Tubercle*, 1986, *67*, 17) compared the efficacy of three regimens of antituberculous therapy in 180 children with tuberculous meningitis: (1) an initial phase of isoniazid, rifampicin, and streptomycin for the first 2 months followed by a continuation phase of 10 months of isoniazid and ethambutol supplemented with streptomycin for the first 4 months; (2) as in (1) but pyrazinamide was added to the initial phase and streptomycin dropped from the continuation phase; (3) as in (2) but rifampicin given twice weekly. Some patients in regimen (1) received isoniazid in a dosage of 20 mg per kg body-weight though this was later reduced to 12 mg per kg after 39% of the patients developed jaundice. Other agents were given in the following doses: rifampicin 12 mg per kg, ethambutol 17.5 mg per kg, pyrazinamide 30 mg per kg, and streptomycin 40 mg per kg. All patients also received corticosteroids. This study confirmed that early diagnosis and initiation of therapy is more important than the choice of drug regimen. At follow-up 12 months later the efficacy was considered to be similar for all regimens and despite the inclusion of rifampicin 44 patients died (27%) and 64 (39%) had neurological sequelae. However, regimen (3) was considered to be the most suitable since only 5% of patients developed jaundice during the first 2 months of treatment compared with 21% of patients receiving regimen (2) and 16% of patients receiving regimen (1).

TUBERCULOUS PERICARDITIS. A discussion on experience of short-term chemotherapy for the treatment of tuberculous pericarditis.— A. K. Dutt *et al.*, *Bull. int. Un. Tuberc.*, 1986, *61*, (Sept.), 42. See also *idem*, *Ann. intern. Med.*, 1986, *104*, 7.

TUBERCULOSIS OF THE SKIN. Seven patients with tuberculosis verrucosa cutis were cleared of lesions within 6 months by treatment, twice weekly, with streptomycin 1 g intramuscularly and isoniazid 14 mg per kg.— V. S. Rajan and Y. S. Goh, *Br. J. Derm.*, 1972, *87*, 270.

A favourable report of the use of streptomycin, isoniazid and rifampicin in the treatment of 4 patients with tuberculosis of the skin.— N. G. Kounis and K. Constantinidis, *Practitioner*, 1979, *222*, 390.

Although there have been no controlled studies isoniazid given by mouth appears to have been successfully used in the treatment of local reactions to BCG vaccination (G.R.M. de Souza *et al.*, *Tubercle*, 1983, *64*, 23). Hanley *et al.* (*Br. med. J.*, 1985, *290*, 970) also found that isoniazid and erythromycin produced similar results in the treatment of these reactions but expressed doubt as to whether either drug had any effect on the natural resolution of the lesions. However, Goldman (*Tubercle*, 1985, *66*, 158) considered that, although placebo-controlled studies are required, it would be reasonable to use a short course of either of these agents. Some clinicians have used local applications of isoniazid or aminosalicylic acid powder following incision for the treatment of abscesses while others prefer to use a 3% chlortetracycline cream or ointment for abscesses or ulceration (J. Verbov, *Practitioner*, 1984, *228*, 1069). Rifampicin is usually also active against BCG vaccine and there have been 2 reports of its use in the treatment of local reactions, resulting from accidental BCG inoculation, which have failed to respond to isoniazid. An abscess in one patient that had failed to respond to isoniazid alone healed when rifampicin was added to the treatment (J.P. Warren *et al.*, *Lancet*, 1984, *2*, 289). Lesions in another patient were cleared following the use of rifampicin with ethambutol (B. Lorber *et al.*, *J. Am. med. Ass.*, 1977, *238*, 55).

Leprosy and Antileprotic Agents

According to their immunological response persons suffering from leprosy (Hansen's disease) can be placed into 6 different categories ranging from those with no natural defence mechanisms who carry massive body-loads of *Mycobacterium leprae* (lepromatous leprosy) to those with high defence and a sparse body-load (tuberculoid leprosy). The categories are: polar lepromatous (LLp); sub-polar lepromatous (LLs); borderline lepromatous (BL); borderline (BB); borderline tuberculoid (BT); tuberculoid (TT). In patients with lepromatous leprosy the lepromin test (see under Lepromin, p.942) is negative whereas at the tuberculoid end of the spectrum it is strongly positive. An early transitory stage, called indeterminate leprosy is also described.

Shifts between these leprosy categories cause leprosy reactions, which are responsible for much of the disability suffered by leprosy patients. Patients with other than polar lepromatous (LLp) or tuberculoid (TT) forms of leprosy may develop a Type 1 reaction (or Type 1 Lepra reaction) which is equivalent to a Type IV hypersensitivity reaction; in untreated patients it involves a 'downgrading' towards the lepromatous end of the spectrum and in treated patients a 'reversal' or 'upgrading' towards the tuberculoid end. Patients with lepromatous forms of leprosy may develop a Type 2 reaction (sometimes termed erythema nodosum leprosum, ENL, or Type 2 Lepra reaction); this is equivalent to a Type III hypersensitivity reaction, it generally occurs as a result of drug therapy and is associated with the massive body-load of dead bacteria. The treatment of leprosy is thus directed not only at eradicating the *Mycobacterium leprae* but also at avoiding or alleviating the reactional states.

Antimicrobial Action and Resistance of Antileprotic Agents

All antileprotic agents currently recommended for use in combined regimens for the treatment of leprosy are considered to have some bactericidal activity against *Mycobacterium leprae*; rifampicin has the greatest bactericidal activity, ethionamide and prothionamide are considered to have intermediate bactericidal activity, and dapsone and clofazimine are considered to be weakly bactericidal. Other agents that have been used in the treatment of leprosy, including thiacetazone, thiambutosine, and some sulphonamides, are only bacteriostatic against *M. leprae* and are considered by some to be unsuitable for use in the relatively short-term multidrug regimens currently recommended. Secondary (acquired) dapsone resistance in *M. leprae* is widespread and its prevalence is increasing. Primary dapsone resistance has also been reported with increasing frequency in areas with secondary resistance. In addition, secondary resistance to other agents bactericidal to *M. leprae* such as rifampicin, clofazimine, and ethionamide has also been reported.

In lepromatous leprosy present chemotherapeutic agents appear to be incapable of eradicating all sensitive bacilli from some patients; these persisting organisms are sometimes called 'persisters'. Patients with lepromatous forms of leprosy may therefore relapse during treatment (due to the emergence of resistant bacilli) or on the termination of years of therapy (due to the multiplication of persisting viable bacilli).

Measures to arrest the emergence of resistance in *M. leprae* include improved means of identifying resistant strains, the use of combined drug regimens, and the avoidance of irregular medication.

RESISTANCE. A review of drug resistance in leprosy.— B. Ji, *Lepr. Rev.*, 1985, *56*, 265.

Studies in 67 patients with lepromatous leprosy (resistant in 65 to dapsone) showed that treatment with rifampicin, usually 600 mg daily, produced a rapid initial clinical improvement but viable bacteria persisted in 7 of 12 patients treated for at least 5 years. Persistence of viable bacteria seemed to be reduced in patients treated with rifampicin plus dapsone 100 mg daily.— M. F. R. Waters *et al.*, *Br. med. J.*, 1978, *1*, 133.

At the 12th International Leprosy Congress, Delhi, 1984, it was reported that organisms with a low degree of resistance to dapsone have been encountered in as many as 50% of patients with previously untreated lepromatous leprosy. Persistent *Mycobacterium leprae* have been detected in significant proportions of patients treated by a variety of multidrug regimens among them regimens consisting of rifampicin, dapsone, and clofazimine or prothionamide, each drug administered continuously in full dosage for 2 years. Although this suggests that no multidrug regimen is likely to eliminate persisting *M. leprae* it is not certain that cure of multibacillary leprosy requires that all persisting bacteria be killed. No relapses were noted amongst 100 multibacillary patients followed up for 8 to 9 years after receiving dapsone monotherapy of variable duration followed by 2 years of multidrug therapy compared with a relapse rate of 1% per year in 300 multibacillary patients released from control after 20 years of well-supervised dapsone monotherapy.— *Lepr. Rev.*, 1984, *55*, 191.

Treatment of Leprosy

By virtue of its cheapness, relative nontoxicity, and high activity against *Mycobacterium leprae* monotherapy with dapsone remained the mainstay of leprosy treatment for several decades. However, because of an increasing incidence of both primary and secondary resistance to dapsone it is now generally recommended that it should be administered in association with other antileprotic agents such as rifampicin (p.574), clofazimine (p.556), and ethionamide (p.563) or prothionamide (p.568).

Multidrug regimens based on the same principles as those determining the treatment of tuberculosis have been recommended for use in all forms of leprosy. The exact regimen used is primarily determined by the bacillary load of the patient and patients with a multibacillary form of leprosy (lepromatous, borderline lepromatous, or borderline leprosy) generally receive more intensive therapy and for longer periods than patients with a paucibacillary form (borderline tuberculoid, tuberculoid, or indeterminate leprosy). Long-term studies are in progress to determine the optimum multidrug regimens. As well as delaying or preventing the emergence of resistance, it is hoped that the more intensive treatment will allow a reduction in the duration of therapy required, thereby aiding patient compliance.

Other drugs used in the treatment of leprosy have included certain sulphonamides and thiacetazone (p.578). It is not yet certain how leprosy is transmitted but infectivity is mainly associated with untreated or lapsed multibacillary forms of leprosy. Treatment of leprosy damages or kills solid-staining viable bacilli, rendering them non-viable with a fragmented or granular appearance. The 'bacterial index' is a measure of the number of organisms per unit volume of tissue whereas the 'morphological index' is a measure of their viability. Leprosy patients with a morphological index of zero are accordingly noninfectious, regardless of their bacterial index. Usually a patient achieves a morphological index of zero within about 6 months of effective therapy with dapsone and this period can be reduced to a few weeks by supplementation with rifampicin.

In areas where leprosy is endemic, prophylactic treatment with dapsone or related drugs (described as sulphones) has reduced the incidence of new cases but such prophylaxis has not been considered practical for large-scale routine programmes. Bacillus Calmette-Guérin vaccine, p.1158, has also been given for leprosy prophylaxis. The development and use of vaccines with greater specificity against *Mycobacterium leprae* is being studied.

In the late 1970's it became apparent that chemotherapeutic methods being used for the treatment of lepromatous leprosy were failing both to prevent the emergence of resistant *Mycobacterium leprae* and to eradicate persisting viable bacilli. Consequently patients relapsed either during treatment or on termination of a prolonged course of treatment. In an attempt to develop more effective therapeutic measures the Programme of Research on Chemotherapy of Leprosy (THELEP) prepared a standard protocol (*Lepr. Rev.*, 1978, *49*, 69) for the study of multidrug regimens in the treatment of lepromatous leprosy. At about the same time a WHO Expert Committee on Leprosy (*Tech. Rep. Ser. Wld Hlth Org. No. 607*, 1977) recommended that patients with lepromatous, borderline lepromatous, or borderline leprosy should receive dapsone treatment combined with clofazimine or rifampicin. Dapsone given alone was still considered to be sufficient for patients with bacteriologically negative tuberculoid or borderline tuberculoid leprosy or indeterminate leprosy. However, in 1982 a WHO Study Group (*Tech. Rep. Ser. Wld Hlth Org. No. 675*, 1982) expressed concern over the failure of leprosy control programmes to implement the recommended regimens and by then the widespread prevalence of both primary and secondary resistance to dapsone precluded the recommendation of the use of dapsone plus one additional drug for patients with multibacillary leprosy (lepromatous, borderline lepromatous, or borderline leprosy) since this would be likely to give rise to multiple drug resistance.

The 1982 WHO Study Group reviewed the agents available for treatment of leprosy and concluded that, although those with bacteriostatic activity against *M. leprae* might be considered for life-long treatment of leprosy, only bactericidal drugs were suitable for multidrug regimens to be administered for limited periods. Only rifampicin, dapsone, clofazimine, and ethionamide or prothionamide could be recommended. It was also recommended that in the treatment of multibacillary leprosy at least two additional drugs should be combined with dapsone, one of which should always be rifampicin. Since there was no evidence to indicate that the efficacy of monthly treatment with rifampicin was inferior to that of daily treatment and because of the dangers of unsupervised use, it was recommended that rifampicin should be given monthly in a supervised dose.

The WHO Study Group expressed the opinion that since multidrug therapy can prevent or overcome resistance in all patients there was no justification for attempting to diagnose dapsone-resistant leprosy by means of a period of supervised dapsone monotherapy. Even if mouse-foot-pad testing could be accomplished, multidrug therapy should be started immediately. The WHO-recommended standard regimen in *multibacillary leprosy* is: rifampicin 600 mg once a month for patients of more than 35 kg body-weight and 450 mg for those weighing less; dapsone 100 mg (1 to 2 mg per kg) daily, self-administered; clofazimine 300 mg once a month and 50 mg daily, self-administered. All doses are to be given by mouth and each monthly dose should be supervised. This regimen may be supplemented by the addition of 500 mg (5 to 10 mg per kg) of ethionamide or prothionamide given monthly under supervision, but further study is required to assess the potential contribution of such an addition. Where clofazimine is unacceptable due to discoloration of the skin, consideration should be given to replacing it with self-administered daily doses of 250 to 375 mg of ethionamide or prothionamide. This combined therapy should be given for at least 2 years and be continued wherever possible up to smear negativity. However, a follow-up study of the Malta-Project (W.H. Jopling *et al.*, *Lepr. Rev.*, 1984, *55*, 247) raised doubts as to the practicality of this recommendation since some patients treated with dapsone, rifampicin, prothionamide, and isoniazid together were still smear-positive 10 or more years after the initiation of therapy and 4 or more years after stopping therapy. Jopling *et al.* considered that further follow-up might indicate that if 'persisters' were not killed after 2 to 3 years of treatment no useful purpose would be served by continuing to bacterial negativity. At the 12th International Leprosy Congress, Delhi, 1984 (*Lepr. Rev.*, 1984, *55*, 191) it was stated that patients should be considered to have completed treatment if they had taken 24 supervised monthly doses within a period of 36 months. It was also recommended that surveillance should be continued for at least 5 years after the course of treatment.

In order to avoid the risk of rifampicin resistance in patients wrongly diagnosed as paucibacillary, the WHO Study Group recommended that combined therapy with rifampicin and dapsone should be given to all patients diagnosed as having paucibacillary leprosy (tuberculoid, borderline tuberculoid, or indeterminate leprosy). The WHO-recommended standard regimen for *paucibacillary leprosy* is: rifampicin 600 mg for patients of more than 35 kg body-weight and 450 mg for those weighing less, given once a month under supervision for 6 months with dapsone 100 mg (1 to 2 mg per kg) self-administered daily for 6 months. If relapse occurs the regimen should be restarted. If treatment is interrupted the regimen should be recommenced at the point at which it was interrupted and the course finished. The regimen should not be interrupted if reversal reactions occur. At the 12th International Leprosy Congress it was considered that patients had completed treatment if they had taken 6 supervised monthly doses within a period of 9 months; it was recommended that surveillance should be continued for at least 2 years after the course of treatment.

Because of the risk of rifampicin-resistant *Mycobacterium tuberculosis* developing the WHO Study Group recommended that patients also having active tuberculosis should be given appropriate antituberculous chemotherapy in addition to these regimens.

Long-term studies of the regimens recommended by the WHO and some of those suggested by THELEP are in progress to determine the optimum multidrug regimens.

Current American recommendations for the treatment of leprosy in the USA (R.R. Jacobson, *Hosp. Formul.*, 1982, *17*, 1076) differ significantly from those of the WHO. The regimens of the WHO are considered by some (W.R. Levis, *Bull. N.Y. Acad. Med.*, 1984, *60*, 696) to be a compromise in that they do not take advantage of the highly bactericidal activity of rifampicin and consequently in the USA recommendations include the use of rifampicin 600 mg daily instead of monthly. However, Yawalkar *et al* (*Lancet*, 1982, *1*, 1199) have shown in a single-blind study that regimens consisting of dapsone 50 mg given daily with rifampicin 1200 mg once monthly or 450 mg daily are of similar efficacy.

In the USA regimens for the treatment of *lepromatous, borderline lepromatous* or *borderline leprosy* consist of dapsone 100 mg daily with rifampicin 600 mg daily with or without clofazimine 100 mg daily for at least 2 years followed by dapsone monotherapy for life after inactivity of the patient's disease has been obtained. However, since clofazimine is frequently unacceptable in the USA the resulting dual therapy is used in conjunction with mouse foot-pad tests for resistance. It is considered that ethionamide may be used as an alternative to clofazimine but because of an increased incidence of hepatotoxicity when used with rifampicin this combination is used only in patients with sulphone-resistant leprosy who refuse one of the regimens containing clofazimine. *Sulphone-resistant borderline lepromatous* or *lepromatous leprosy* is usually treated with clofazimine and rifampicin or clofazimine and ethionamide for at least 2 years followed by clofazimine monotherapy or rifampicin with ethionamide for life after an inactive disease status has been obtained. Patients with *indeterminate* or *tuberculoid leprosy* are treated with dapsone monotherapy, 50 or 100 mg daily for at least 2 years after inactive disease status has been obtained and patients with *borderline tuberculoid leprosy* are given dapsone monotherapy for at least 5 years after obtaining inactive status.

LEPRA has made the following recommendations for children's doses of antileprosy agents for use in multidrug regimens recommended by WHO. Children up to 5 years of age: dapsone 25 mg daily unsupervised; rifampicin 150 to 300 mg monthly supervised; clofazimine 100 mg once weekly unsupervised and 100 mg monthly supervised. Children 6 to 14 years: dapsone 50 to 100 mg daily unsupervised; rifampicin 300 to 450 mg monthly supervised; clofazimine 150 mg once weekly unsupervised and 150 to 200 mg monthly supervised. Children over 15 years: dapsone 100 mg daily unsupervised; rifampicin 600 mg monthly supervised; clofazimine 50 mg daily unsupervised and 300 mg monthly supervised. The dosages for dapsone and rifampicin are suitable for use in paucibacillary and multibacillary leprosy and those for clofazimine for use in multibacillary leprosy. It is assumed that clofazimine will be acceptable for all children and that no child will therefore require ethionamide or prothionamide.— *Lepr. Rev.*, 1984, *55*, 309.

A study of relapses in patients who had received dapsone monotherapy for paucibacillary leprosy indicated that 50% of relapses would occur during the first 3 years after stopping treatment. This figure was considered to be relevant also for multidrug regimens since this type of therapy would only influence the duration of treatment and not the incubation time of relapse.— S. R. Pattyn, *Lepr. Rev.*, 1984, *55*, 115.

Despite finding an unexpectedly low relapse-rate during follow-up of patients with lepromatous leprosy (LL and BL) who had received long-term therapy with sulphones it was recommended that these patients should receive a course of multidrug therapy before release from control.— M. F. R. Waters *et al.*, *Lepr. Rev.*, 1986, *57*, 101.

Preliminary reports on some multidrug-treatment programmes based on WHO recommendations for the treatment of leprosy.— P. Rose, *Lepr. Rev.*, 1984, *55*, 143 (paucibacillary leprosy); M. C. Birch, *ibid.*, 255 (multibacillary and paucibacillary leprosy); N. M. Samuel *et al.*, *ibid.*, 265 (multibacillary and paucibacillary leprosy); R. F. Keeler, *ibid.*, 391 (multibacillary and paucibacillary leprosy).

A report on the favourable results obtained using rifampicin with a preparation containing prothionamide, dapsone, and isoniazid (Isoprodian) in the treatment of leprosy.— G. Depasquale, *Lepr. Rev.*, 1986, *57, Suppl.* 3, 29.

A review of Diuciphon, an antileprotic drug synthesised and investigated in the USSR.— W. H. Jopling, *Lepr. Rev.*, 1981, *52*, 104. See also.— N. M. Goloshchapov *et al.*, *Vest. Derm. Vener.*, 1983, 4, 67.

Further references: M. F. R. Waters, *Tubercle*, 1983, *64*, 221.

INFECTIVITY AND PROPHYLAXIS. Guidelines for the prophylaxis of leprosy and the management of household contacts of leprosy patients.— *Memorandum on Leprosy*, London, HM Stationery Office, 1977; G. A. Filice and D. W. Fraser, *Ann. intern. Med.*, 1978, *88*, 538.

A discussion on when leprosy patients should be considered as 'cured'. A patient's morale can be improved if he is told when he is considered to be no longer infective to others; a zero morphological index might be a better indication than the WHO definition which includes negative bacteriological findings. Patients who are no longer infective should be regarded as in no way different from any other sick person, and should be subject to no hospital, employment, or social restrictions.— T. F. Davey, *Lepr. Rev.*, 1978, *49*, 1.

Reviews, discussions, and studies on the immunology of leprosy with implications for immunotherapy and immunoprophylaxis.— W. C. Van Voorhis *et al.*, *New Engl. J. Med.*, 1982, *307*, 1593; C. C. Shepard, *ibid.*, 1640; J. Convit *et al.*, *Lepr. Rev.*, 1983, 47S; G. A. W. Rook, *Tubercle*, 1983, *64*, 297; B. R. Bloom and T. Godal, *Rev. infect. Dis.*, 1983, *5*, 765; W. van Eden and R. R. P. de Vries, *Lepr. Rev.*, 1984, *55*, 89.

PREGNANCY AND THE NEONATE. Recurrent pregnancies provide periods of physiological suppression of cell-mediated immunity and this suppression could be a factor in contributing to dapsone resistance among women with leprosy. The suppression of cell-mediated immunity during pregnancy is also probably responsible for the extremely rapid deterioration observed during the third trimester of pregnancy. The possibility of giving supplementary chemotherapy in effective dosage during pregnancy and lactation might be considered. Clofazimine 100 mg given at least three times a week for one year starting at the beginning of the second trimester would probably be the most suitable drug and would have the additional advantage of possibly reducing the amount of Type 2 (ENL) reactions during pregnancy and lactation.— M. E. Duncan *et al.*, *Lepr. Rev.*, 1981, *52*, 263.

Leprosy Reactions

It is generally considered that antileprotic therapy should be continued in full dosage during leprosy reactions as long as the reactions can be effectively treated. The main drugs used to alleviate reactions in leprosy include clofazimine (p.556), corticosteroids (p.875), and thalidomide (p.1621).

Symptoms of mild reactions may usually be controlled with analgesics such as aspirin. Control of the acute phase of more severe leprosy reactions may be achieved with corticosteroids in both Type 1 (Lepra) and Type 2 (ENL) reactions and with thalidomide in Type 2 (ENL) reactions. Thalidomide is of no benefit in the Type 1 (Lepra) reaction but although it must be avoided in fertile women with a potential for pregnancy it is considered by some to be the treatment of choice in Type 2 (ENL) reactions in suitable patients. Prednisolone has been given in a dosage of 30 to 40 mg daily for the initial control of symptoms but some consider that 60 to 80 mg is an appropriate starting dose. The dosage should be tapered gradually thereafter to the minimum required to control symptoms or if possible until complete withdrawal can be achieved. Some patients may require long-term maintenance with relatively high doses. Thalidomide is usually given in an initial dose of up to 400 mg daily reduced over a period of about 2 weeks to a daily maintenance dose of 50 to 100 mg.

Clofazimine does not appear to be as effective as thalidomide or corticosteroids in the treatment of leprosy reactions and since it takes several weeks for its beneficial effects to appear it may be necessary to administer it with corticosteroids or thalidomide until the acute phase is controlled. However, the use of clofazimine may permit the gradual withdrawal of corticosteroids in steroid-dependent cases. It has been used for the treatment of leprosy reactions in an initial dosage of 300 mg daily gradually reduced to a minimum maintenance dose as soon as possible. There is evidence that clofazimine may be ineffective in Type 1 (Lepra) reactions.

If iridocyclitis develops local treatment with corticosteroids and mydriatic eye drops such as homatropine has been recommended.

A review of reactions in leprosy.— G. Bjune, *Lepr. Rev.*, 1983, 61S.

Discussions on the treatment of reactions in leprosy.— M. F. R. Waters, *Lepr. Rev.*, 1974, *45*, 337; D. S. Jolliffe, *Br. J. Derm.*, 1977, *97*, 345; W. R. Levis, *Bull. N.Y. Acad. Med.*, 1984, *60*, 696.

Clofazimine should not be recommended for the management of Type 1 (reversal) reactions until definite evidence of effectiveness is available.— W. F. Ross, *Lepr. Rev.*, 1980, *51*, 197. Evidence that clofazimine is not effective in Type 1 Lepra reactions.— F. M. J. H. Imkamp, *ibid.*, 1981, *52*, 135.

A Type 1 leprosy reversal reaction which occurred after treatment for 4 months with rifampicin 600 mg, dapsone 100 mg, and clofazimine 100 mg all daily in a 24-year-old man with borderline lepromatous leprosy was unresponsive to an increase in dose of clofazimine to 400 mg daily and introduction of prednisolone 1 mg per kg body-weight but did respond to plasma exchange on 5 successive days; his condition again improved after a second identical Type 1 leprosy reversal reaction following plasma exchange.— F. Lucht *et al.*, *Br. med. J.*, 1984, *289*, 1647.

For reference to the concurrent administration of rifampicin and corticosteroids exacerbating rather than alleviating neuritis in tuberculoid leprosy and a warning that rifampicin may reduce the efficacy of corticosteroids when used in the treatment of leprosy reactions, see p.874.

For a report suggesting that colchicine may have a beneficial effect in erythema nodosum leprosum, see Colchicine, p.439.

Atypical Mycobacterial Infections

Mycobacteria other than *M. tuberculosis, M. africanum, M. bovis,* and *M. leprae* have been referred to as atypical, nontuberculous, tuberculoid, opportunistic, or MOTT mycobacteria (mycobacteria other than tuberculous) and a common name remains to be agreed. Diseases due to these organisms differ from tuberculosis and leprosy in that they are rarely, if ever, transmitted from person to person but are acquired from the environment. The most common diseases produced include pulmonary infections, lymphadenitis, and skin and soft-tissue infections though disseminated infections may develop rapidly in immunocompromised patients such as those with AIDS.

The course of treatment depends on the site and nature of infection and in some cases surgery is the treatment of choice either alone or in conjunction with chemotherapy. Response to chemotherapy is often difficult to predict as *in vitro* sensitivity of the organisms may not reflect the response obtained *in vivo*. Clinical improvements may still be achieved despite resistance *in vitro* to the individual agents used in a regimen and selection of agents is often on the basis of the best activity *in vitro*. Most assessments of treatment have been based on retrospective surveys of empirical therapy and anecdotal reports.

As an aid to selecting appropriate treatment Bailey (*Chest*, 1983, *84*, 5) suggested that atypical mycobacteria could be divided into 3 groups. The first group contains organisms which may be considered to be non-pathogens as they rarely produce infection in humans. These include *Mycobacterium gordonae* (but see below), *M. gastri, M. terrae* complex, *M. flavescens, M. smegmatis, M. vaccae,* and *M. parafortuitum* complex.

The second group contains pathogenic organisms that Bailey considered were easy to treat with standard antimycobacterial therapy and includes *M. kansasii, M. xenopi, M. marinum,* and *M. szulgai.* Pulmonary infections due to *M. kansasii, M. xenopi, M. malmoense* have all responded to regimens including isoniazid, rifampicin, and ethambutol given for up to 24 months (J. Banks *et al.*, *Thorax*, 1983, *38*, 271; M.J. Smith and K.M. Citron, *ibid.*, 373; J. Banks *et al.*, *Tubercle*, 1985, *66*, 197). Some clinicians advocate the use of streptomycin if there is intolerance to one of the first choice agents or if there is a lack of response. Although some consider that short-term therapy may be unsuitable, Schraufnagel *et al.* (*Can. med. Ass. J.*, 1984, *130*, 34) obtained a good outcome using short-term chemotherapy in patients with pulmonary infections due to *M. kansasii.* Three out of the following agents: isoniazid, rifampicin, ethambutol, streptomycin, or pyrazinamide selected according to activity *in vitro*, were given until patients had been smear- and culture-negative for 9 to 12 months. Preliminary results of a study by the British Thoracic Society (I.A. Campbell, *Bull. int. Un. Tuberc.*, 1986, *61*, *Sept.*, 43) suggest that 9 months of treatment with rifampicin and ethambutol may be adequate for *M. kansasii* pulmonary infections. Rifampicin with ethambutol given for up to 12 months may be effective for skin lesions due to *M. marinum* (J.P. Bailey *et al.*, *J. Am. med. Ass.*, 1982, *247*, 1314; S.T. Donta *et al.*, *Archs intern. Med.*, 1986, *146*, 902) though some authorities (*Med. Lett.*, 1986, *28*, 33) consider minocycline to be the agent of choice; co-trimoxazole has also been used. A patient with cutaneous lesions and osteomyelitis due to *M. szulgai* was free of disease 17 months after therapy for 24 months with isoniazid, ethambutol, and rifampicin (G.M. Cross *et al.*, *Archs Derm.*, 1985, *121*, 247). Although Bailey included *M. ulcerans* in this group treatment is often difficult and controversial; clofazimine has been tried (p.557).

The last group contains pathogenic mycobacteria which Bailey considered were difficult to treat using standard antimycobacterial therapy. The group may be divided into two sub-groups. One sub-group contains mycobacteria that have a similar susceptibility pattern to *M. avium intracellulare* and also includes *M. scrofulaceum* and *M. simiae.* Although *M. avium intracellulare* is usually resistant *in vitro* to standard antituberculous agents, infections do sometimes respond to combination chemotherapy. *M. avium intracellulare* is of increasing importance as a cause of infection in patients with AIDS. Empirical regimens of 5 or 6 antituberculous agents given for up to 2 years have been used and good results have been obtained with isoniazid, rifampicin, and ethambutol (A.M. Hunter *et al.*, *Thorax*, 1981, *36*, 326; J.B. Bass, *Am. Rev. resp. Dis.*, 1986, *134*, 431) with or without streptomycin. Regimens including rifabutin and clofazimine have been suggested for use in disseminated infections (Centers for Disease Control, *Ann. intern. Med.*, 1987, *106*, 254), although some consider that these 2 agents have not lived up to early expectations based on *in vitro* activity (A.J. Pinching, *Tubercle*, 1987, *68*, 65). Chemotherapy appears to be of limited value in lymphadenitis due to *M. scrofulaceum* and *M. avium intracellulare* and surgical excision is the treatment of choice (M.P. White *et al.*, *Archs Dis. Childh.*, 1986, *61*, 368).

The other sub-group contains mycobacteria which are usually resistant to antituberculous agents but which may be susceptible to some standard antibiotics and includes *M. fortuitum* and *M. chelonei.* Combinations of the following drugs have been used or recommended: amikacin, doxycycline, erythromycin, cefoxitin, and co-trimoxazole (R.J. Wallace *et al.*, *J. infect. Dis.*, 1985, *152*, 500; *Med. Lett.*, 1986, *28*, 33).

Some further references to the treatment of atypical mycobacterial infections:

Mycobacterium avium complex: H.C. Engbaek *et al.*, *Eur. J. resp. Dis.*, 1984, *65*, 411; R.J. O'Brien *et al.*, *Bull. int. Un. Tuberc.*, 1986, *61*, (Sept.), 11; L.S. Farer, *ibid.*, (Mar.-Jun.), 63; C.C. Hawkins *et al.*, *Ann. intern. Med.*, 1986, *105*, 184; C.R. Horsburgh and D.L. Cohn, *ibid.*, 968; C. Pedersen and J.O. Nielsen, *ibid.*, 1987, *106*, 165.

M. chelonei: B.S. Azadian *et al.*, *Tubercle*, 1981, *62*, 281 (co-trimoxazole, erythromycin and doxcycline); P.G. Jackson *et al.*, *Tubercle*, 1981, *62*, 277 (co-trimoxazole and erythromycin).

M. fortuitum: M.J. Rivron *et al.*, *Archs Dis. Childh.*, 1979, *54*, 312 (cervical lymphadenitis; management with surgery and ethionamide with gentamicin); J. Santamaría-Jaúregui *et al.*, *Am. Rev. resp. Dis.*, 1984, *130*, 136 (meningitis responsive to isoniazid, co-trimoxazole, and surgery).

M. gordonae: Lorber and Suh, *Am. Rev. resp. Dis.*, 1983, *128*, 565 (isoniazid and rifampicin); P. Kurnik *et al.*, *Am. J. med. Sci.*, 1983, *285*, 45 (isoniazid, rifampicin, and ethambutol); P. McIntyre *et al.*, *J. Infect.*, 1987, *14*, 71 (suggested empirical regimen of amikacin, ethambutol, rifampicin, and co-trimoxazole).

Some reviews and discussions on the treatment of atypical mycobacterial infections: W.C. Bailey, *Chest*, 1983, *84*, 625; American Thoracic Society and Centers for Disease Control, *Am. Rev. resp. Dis.*, 1983, *127*, 790; R.A. Benn and A.J. Woolcock, *Med. J. Aust.*, 1985, *143*, 602; J.M. Grange and M.D. Yates, *J. R. Soc. Med.*, 1986, *79*, 226; Centers for Disease Control, *Ann. intern. Med.*, 1987, *106*, 254.

Shaffer *et al.* (*Gut*, 1984, *25*, 203) in a controlled study of 27 patients found that rifampicin with ethambutol was of no benefit in Crohn's disease and considered that it was unlikely that *Mycobacterium kansasii* was aetiologically significant in this disease. However, Warren *et al.* (*New Engl. J. Med.*, 1986, *314*, 182) still considered that atypical mycobacteria may be causally associated with Crohn's disease as they had reported remission of long-standing disease in a patient who had received rifampicin, ethambutol, isoniazid, and pyrazinamide in the initial phase of treatment for coincidental tuberculosis. Other case reports have also shown improvement (M.G. Schultz *et al.*, *Lancet*, 1987, *2*, 1391; A. Picciotto *et al.*, *ibid.*, 1988, *1*, 536) although the 2 patients treated by Picciotto *et al.* relapsed while still taking their antituberculous agents but then responded to conventional treatment for inflammatory bowel disease.

6551-n

Acedapsone *(BAN, USAN, rINN).*

CI-556; DADDS. Bis(4-acetamidophenyl) sulphone.

$C_{16}H_{16}N_2O_4S=332.4$.

CAS — 77-46-3.

Pharmacopoeias. In *Braz.*

Acedapsone is a sulphone and has the actions and uses of dapsone (see p.558) to which it is metabolised. It is given intramuscularly and in the treatment of leprosy it may be of use as part of a multidrug regimen to supplement dapsone when compliance to oral treatment is likely to be poor. It is also used in prophylaxis. If it is administered in a dose of 225 mg every 70 to 77 days (or 5 times yearly), plasma-dapsone concentrations can be maintained above a minimum of 10 ng per mL.

LEPROSY PROPHYLAXIS. During a 3½ year study of children who were household contacts of patients with active multibacillary leprosy 22 of 348 children who received acedapsone for prophylaxis developed leprosy compared with 42 of 351 untreated children. Protection appeared to be higher in the younger age groups. Acedapsone had been administered every 10 weeks with children 1 to 5 years of age receiving 150 mg and older children 225 mg.— P. N. Neelan *et al.*, *Indian J. med. Res.*, 1983, *78*, 307.

Proprietary Names and Manufacturers

Hansolar *(Parke, Davis, USA).*

6552-h

Achyranthes Aspera

Apamarga; Latjira. The whole plant of *Achyranthes aspera* (Amaranthaceae).

NOTE. Achyranthes *(Jpn. P.)* is the root of *Achyranthes fauriei* and *A. bidentata. Chin. P.* contains a monograph on the root of *A. bidentata*.

A decoction of *Achyranthes aspera* has been tried in the treatment of leprosy and of reactional states in leprosy.

References: D. Ojha *et al., Lepr. Rev.*, 1966, *37*, 115; D. Ojha and G. Singh, *ibid.*, 1968, *39*, 23.

7551-s

Aminosalicylic Acid *(USAN).*

4-Aminosalicylic Acid; Aminosalylum; Para-aminosalicylic Acid; PAS; Pasalicylum. 4-Amino-2-hydroxybenzoic acid.

$C_7H_7NO_3$=153.1.

CAS — 65-49-6.

NOTE. Distinguish from 5-aminosalicylic acid (Mesalazine, p.1097) which is used in the treatment of ulcerative colitis.

Pharmacopoeias. In *Arg., Aust., Braz., Hung., Pol., Span., Turk.*, and *U.S.*

A white or almost white, bulky powder which darkens on exposure to air and light; it is odourless or has a slight acetous odour.

Slightly **soluble** in water and ether; soluble in alcohol. A saturated solution in water has a pH of 3.0 to 3.7.

Aqueous solutions are unstable. The *U.S.P.* directs that a solution must not be used if it is darker in colour than a freshly prepared solution. **Store** at a temperature not exceeding 30° in airtight containers. Protect from light.

7552-w

Calcium Aminosalicylate

Aminosalicylate Calcium *(USAN)*; Calcii Para-aminosalicylas; Calcium PAS. Calcium 4-amino-2-hydroxybenzoate trihydrate.

$(C_7H_6NO_3)_2Ca,3H_2O$=398.4.

CAS — 133-15-3 (anhydrous).

Pharmacopoeias. In *Arg.* (anhydrous); in *Aust., Braz., Egypt., Fr., Ind., Neth.*, and *U.S.*; in *Nord.* (½H_2O); in *Port.* (½ or $3H_2O$); and in *Jpn* ($7H_2O$).

A white or cream-coloured, odourless, hygroscopic, crystalline powder. Calcium aminosalicylate trihydrate 1.3 g is approximately equivalent to 1 g of aminosalicylic acid. **Soluble** 1 in 7 of water and slightly soluble in alcohol. A 2% solution in water has a pH of 6 to 8. Aqueous solutions are unstable and darken in colour. The *U.S.P.* directs that solutions should be prepared within 24 hours of administration and that a solution must not be used if it is darker in colour than a freshly prepared solution. **Store** in airtight containers. Protect from light.

7553-e

Calcium Benzamidosalicylate *(BAN, rINN).*

Benzoylpas Calcium *(USAN)*; Bepascum; Calcii Benzamidosalicylas. Calcium 4-benzamido-2-hydroxybenzoate pentahydrate.

$(C_{14}H_{10}NO_4)_2Ca,5H_2O$=642.6.

CAS — 13898-58-3 (4-benzamidosalicylic acid); 528-96-1 (calcium salt, anhydrous); 5631-00-5 (calcium salt, pentahydrate).

Pharmacopoeias. In *Rus.*

Calcium benzamidosalicylate 2.1 g is approximately equivalent to 1 g of aminosalicylic acid.

7564-j

Phenyl Aminosalicylate *(BAN, USAN).*

Fenamisal *(rINN)*; FR-7; Phenyl PAS. Phenyl 4-amino-2-hydroxybenzoate.

$C_{13}H_{11}NO_3$=229.2.

CAS — 133-11-9.

Phenyl aminosalicylate 1.5 g is approximately equivalent to 1 g of aminosalicylic acid.

7566-c

Potassium Aminosalicylate

Aminosalicylate Potassium. Potassium 4-amino-2-hydroxybenzoate.

$C_7H_6KNO_3$=191.2.

CAS — 133-09-5.

Each g of potassium aminosalicylate represents approximately 5.23 mmol of potassium. Potassium aminosalicylate 1.25 g is approximately equivalent to 1 g of aminosalicylic acid.

7571-y

Sodium Aminosalicylate *(BAN).*

Aminosalicylate Sodium *(USAN)*; Aminosalylnatrium; Natrii Aminosalicylas; Natrii Para-aminosalicylas; Pasalicylum Solubile; Sodium Para-aminosalicylate; Sodium PAS. Sodium 4-amino-2-hydroxybenzoate dihydrate.

$C_7H_6NNaO_3,2H_2O$=211.1.

CAS — 133-10-8 (anhydrous); 6018-19-5 (dihydrate).

Pharmacopoeias. In *Arg., Aust., Braz., Chin., Cz., Egypt., Fr., Hung., Ind., It., Jug., Neth., Pol., Port., Roum., Rus., Span., Swiss, Turk.*, and *U.S.*

White to cream-coloured practically odourless crystalline powder. Each g of sodium aminosalicylate represents approximately 4.74 mmol of sodium. Sodium aminosalicylate 1.38 g is approximately equivalent to 1 g of aminosalicylic acid.

Soluble 1 in 2 of water; sparingly soluble in alcohol; very slightly soluble in chloroform and in ether. A 2% solution in water has a pH of 6.5 to 8.5.

Aqueous solutions are unstable and should be freshly prepared. The addition of sodium metabisulphite 0.1% retards oxidation and darkening of the solution. The *U.S.P.* directs that solutions should be prepared within 24 hours of administration and that a solution must not be used if it is darker in colour than a freshly prepared solution. Tablets that have turned brown should not be used. **Store** at a temperature not exceeding 40° in airtight containers. Protect from light.

Solutions of sodium aminosalicylate 5% and 20% containing 25% glycerol were less quickly degraded to *m*-aminophenol than those with syrup or sorbitol but were more quickly discoloured. Solutions with 25% propylene glycol, whilst slightly less stable than those with glycerol, discoloured at a slower rate than any of the solutions.— M. I. Blake *et al., Am. J. Hosp. Pharm.*, 1973, *30*, 441.

A paediatric mixture containing isoniazid 10 g, sodium aminosalicylate 27.5 g, pyridoxine 25 mg, and vehicle for Isoniazid Elixir *B.P.C. 1973* to 100 mL was examined for stability. The pH of the freshly-prepared mixture was 6.2. Overnight storage in a refrigerator resulted in formation of a copious deposit. After storage for 1 week at room temperature the *B.P.C.* limit for 3-aminophenol in isoniazid dry granules (0.3%) was exceeded.— Pharm. Soc. Lab. Rep. P/75/17, 1975.

Adverse Effects

Aminosalicylic acid and its salts may cause the side-effects of salicylates (see p.3) and of the *p*-aminophenyl group which is also formed during the metabolism of such compounds as the sulphonamides and sulphones. Cross-sensitivity may occur between the aminosalicylates and related compounds.

Gastro-intestinal side-effects are common and include nausea, vomiting, and diarrhoea; they may be reduced by giving doses with food or in association with an antacid but occasionally may be severe enough that therapy has to be withdrawn. Alteration of gastro-intestinal function may lead to malabsorption of vitamin B_{12}, folate, and protein, associated with steatorrhoea; hypokalaemia may also develop. Salts of aminosalicylic acid may be better tolerated than the acid. Tolerance in children is better than in adults.

Allergic reactions have been reported in 5 to 10% of adults, usually during the first few weeks of treatment, and include fever, skin rashes, arthralgia, lymphadenopathy, hepatosplenomegaly, and, more rarely, a syndrome resembling infectious mononucleosis. Other adverse effects which have been attributed to an allergic reaction to aminosalicylate include jaundice, necrosis of the liver, encephalitis, and renal failure. Blood disorders reported include haemolytic anaemia, agranulocytosis, eosinophilia, leucopenia, and thrombocytopenia and these may also have an immunological basis. Psychosis may occasionally occur. Prolonged treatment may induce goitre and hypothyroidism.

ALLERGY. Hypersensitivity reactions to sodium aminosalicylate are often associated with fever and gastro-intestinal symptoms. The rash takes the form of macular or morbilliform exanthema. Findings such as lachrymation, lymphadenopathy, splenomegaly, and leucocytosis might closely simulate infective mononucleosis. Exfoliative dermatitis is a possible complication more common with sodium aminosalicylate than the other tuberculostatics.— N. Thorne, *Practitioner*, 1973, *211*, 606.

A lymphoma-like syndrome, suggestive of Hodgkin's lymphoma, developed in a 40-year-old man receiving aminosalicylic acid as part of antituberculous therapy. Complete regression occurred on withdrawal of therapy. It was suggested that drug hypersensitivity might have triggered an underlying abnormal immune state into an exaggerated response.— N. Nagaratnam *et al., Postgrad. med. J.*, 1982, *58*, 729.

See also under Effects on the Heart, below.

EFFECTS ON THE EYE. Sodium aminosalicylate could cause optic neuritis.— P. A. MacFaul, *Prescribers' J.*, 1973, *13*, 68.

EFFECTS ON THE GASTRO-INTESTINAL TRACT. For a brief review of aminosalicylic acid-induced malabsorption, see G. F. Longstreth and A. D. Newcomer, *Mayo Clin. Proc.*, 1975, *50*, 284.

EFFECTS ON THE HEART. Pericarditis which developed in a patient who took aminosalicylic acid and isoniazid for 9 months may have been due to hypersensitivity to aminosalicylic acid. Therapy with isoniazid and pyrazinamide was continued without ill effect after aminosalicylic acid was withdrawn.— M. D. R. Morris, *Tubercle*, 1970, *51*, 192.

For a report of pericarditis considered to be a complication of the lupoid syndrome in a patient treated with isoniazid and aminosalicylic acid see under Lupus in Isoniazid, p.564.

EFFECTS ON THE LIVER. Drug-induced hepatitis occurred in 0.32% of 7492 patients receiving antituberculous drugs; aminosalicylic acid was the most common cause among the 38 patients analysed. Patients with aminosalicylate induced hepatitis had lower serum aspartate aminotransferase (SGOT) values than those in whom it was uncertain whether aminosalicylate or isoniazid was responsible.— J. E. Rossouw and S. J. Saunders, *Q. J. Med.*, 1975, *44*, 1. See also *Br. med. J.*, 1975, *2*, 522.

EFFECTS ON THE METABOLISM. Two episodes of hypoglycaemic coma occurred in a diabetic patient taking aminosalicylic acid 12 to 18 g daily.— P. Dandona *et al., Postgrad. med. J.*, 1980, *56*, 135.

LUPUS. See under Isoniazid, p.564.

PREGNANCY AND THE NEONATE. See under Adverse Effects in Isoniazid, p.564.

Treatment of Adverse Effects

Although it may be safer to substitute other anti-tuberculous agents such as ethambutol for aminosalicylic acid when hypersensitivity occurs desensitisation may be attempted if the use of aminosalicylic acid is considered essential for the provision of adequate chemotherapy (see p.546).

Concentrations of aminosalicylate in the blood are affected by haemodialysis.

The percentage of a dose of aminosalicylic acid adsorbed by activated charcoal varied according to the ratio of the amounts of the two drugs involved. To avoid saturation of the adsorptive capacity of activated charcoal in acute poisoning with aminosalicylic acid, large doses of 50 to 100 g of charcoal should be used.— K. T. Olkkola, *Br. J. clin. Pharmac.*, 1985, *19*, 767.

Precautions

Aminosalicylic acid and its salts should be administered with great care to patients with impaired renal function. They should also be used with caution in diabetics and patients with gastric ulcer. Use of the sodium salt should be avoided in conditions where sodium restriction is desirable and likewise the calcium salt should be avoided in conditions associated with hypercalcaemia.

The adverse effects of aminosalicylates and salicylates

may be additive. Probenecid may also increase toxicity by delaying renal excretion and enhancing plasma concentrations of aminosalicylate.
Aminosalicylates interfere with tests for glycosuria using copper reagents.

EFFECT OF DISEASE STATES. There was an approximate 20% increase in the free fraction of aminosalicylic acid in the serum of patients with kwashiorkor. About 15% was bound to plasma proteins in healthy subjects.— N. Buchanan and L. A. Van der Walt, *S. Afr. med. J.*, 1977, *52*, 522.

EFFECTS ON LABORATORY ESTIMATIONS. Aminosalicylic acid has been reported to interfere with Coombs' test (P.D. Hansten, *Am. J. Hosp. Pharm.*, 1971, *28*, 629), urine estimations for bilirubin, ketones, urobilinogen, and porphobilinogen, and serum estimations of serum aspartate aminotransferase (SGOT) (*Drug & Ther. Bull.*, 1972, *10*, 69).

INTERACTIONS. For references to granules of aminosalicylic acid reducing the absorption of rifampicin, see Rifampicin, p.572.

PREGNANCY AND THE NEONATE. For a discussion on the use of antituberculous agents during pregnancy and for recommendations on precautions to be taken by nursing mothers receiving antituberculous therapy, see under Treatment of Tuberculosis, p.548.

For reference to the clastogenic activity of aminosalicylic acid used with isoniazid and advice to avoid conception during use of this drug combination, see under Precautions in Isoniazid, p.566.

Antimicrobial Action and Resistance

Aminosalicylic acid is bacteriostatic and is active only against mycobacteria. It has a relatively weak action compared with other antituberculous drugs but most strains of *Mycobacterium tuberculosis* have been reported to be inhibited by 1 µg per mL. Resistance emerges slowly.

Absorption and Fate

When given by mouth, aminosalicylic acid and its salts are readily absorbed, and peak plasma concentrations occur after about 1 to 2 hours. Half-lives of about 0.75 to 1.0 hours have been reported. The benzoyl derivative, calcium benzamidosalicylate is absorbed more slowly from the gastro-intestinal tract and is slowly hydrolysed to produce lower though more prolonged plasma concentrations of aminosalicylate. Aminosalicylate diffuses widely through body tissues and fluids, producing high concentrations in the kidneys, lungs, and liver. Diffusion into the cerebrospinal fluid occurs only if the meninges are inflamed.
Urinary excretion of aminosalicylate is rapid, and 80% or more of a dose is excreted within 24 hours; 50% or more of the dose is excreted in the acetylated form. Though aminosalicylate is acetylated in the body, the rate of the process is not genetically determined as is the case for isoniazid. Aminosalicylate is excreted into breast milk.

Comparative studies of the pharmacokinetics of aminosalicylic acid and its salts: S. H. Wan *et al.*, *J. pharm. Sci.*, 1974, *63*, 708; *idem*, *J. Pharmacokinet. Biopharm.*, 1974, *2*, 1.
Some 58 to 73% of aminosalicylic acid was bound in the body to serum proteins.— C. M. Kunin, *Ann. intern. Med.*, 1967, *67*, 151. About 15% of aminosalicylic acid was bound to plasma proteins in healthy subjects.— N. Buchanan and L. A. Van der Walt, *S. Afr. med. J.*, 1977, *52*, 522.

PREGNANCY AND THE NEONATE. The peak concentration of aminosalicylic acid in breast milk of a 27-year-old woman was 1.1 µg per mL 3 hours after administration of a 4-g dose of aminosalicylic acid. The peak plasma concentration was 70.1 µg per mL after 2 hours.— M. R. Holdiness (letter), *Archs intern. Med.*, 1984, *144*, 1888.

Uses and Administration

Aminosalicylic acid and its salts were widely used with isoniazid and streptomycin in the primary treatment of pulmonary tuberculosis but have been largely replaced by more effective agents which allow the implementation of shorter courses of treatment. However, aminosalicylates are still used in some developing countries and may be valuable when bacterial resistance is a problem—see Treatment of Tuberculosis, p.547. They may also be of use in young children in whom ethambutol should be avoided.
The usual daily dosage for adults is 12 g by mouth in divided doses given with or after food. Doses of up to 20 g daily have been used but may be badly tolerated. Children may be given 200 to 300 mg per kg bodyweight daily in divided doses. Aminosalicylates have also been used in intermittent treatment regimens.
Aminosalicylic acid has been used as the sodium, calcium, and potassium salts which have been administered in a wide range of dosage forms in an attempt to overcome their bulk and exceedingly unpleasant taste. The salts appear to be better tolerated than the free acid and solutions in iced water prepared immediately before use may be less unpleasant to take. Several derivatives of aminosalicylic acid have also been used in the treatment of tuberculosis including the phenyl ester, the calcium salt of the benzoyl derivative, and a hydrazide derivative (pashydrazide, $C_7H_9N_3O_2$ = 167.2). An equimolecular salt of isoniazid and aminosalicylate (see Isoniazid Aminosalicylate, (p.568) has also been used.

ADMINISTRATION IN RENAL FAILURE. Many clinicians recommend that aminosalicylic acid should be avoided in patients with renal failure because it can exacerbate symptoms of uraemia and acidosis (J.S. Cheigh, *Am. J. med.*, 1977, *62*, 555; G.B. Appel and H.C. Neu, *New Engl. J. Med.*, 1977, *296*, 663). If it cannot be avoided, Bennett *et al.* (*Ann. intern. Med.*, 1977, *86*, 754) have suggested a schedule of dosage reductions although Held and Fried (*Chemotherapy, Basle*, 1977, *23*, 405) considered that the dosage should not be reduced if therapeutic concentrations are to be maintained. Blood concentrations of aminosalicylic acid are affected by haemodialysis (P. Sharpstone, *Br. med. J.*, 1977, *2*, 36).

DIAGNOSIS AND TESTING. Use of aminosalicylic acid in the bentiromide test for pancreatic function replaces the need for administration of radio-labelled aminobenzoic acid and makes the test more widely applicable.— I. M. Chesner *et al.*, *Gut*, 1986, *27*, A1260. See also F. J. Hoek *et al.*, *ibid.*, 1987, *28*, 468.

HYPOLIPIDAEMIC ACTION. Studies and discussions on the hypolipidaemic action of a highly purified form of aminosalicylic acid, obtained by recrystallisation with ascorbic acid (PAS-C): P. J. Barter *et al.*, *Ann. intern. Med.*, 1974, *81*, 619; *J. Am. med. Ass.*, 1974, *228*, 961; P. T. Kuo *et al.*, *Circulation*, 1976, *53*, 338; B. Vessby *et al.*, *Clin. Pharmac. Ther.*, 1978, *23*, 651.

TUBERCULOSIS. For the use of aminosalicylic acid and other antituberculosis agents in the treatment of tuberculosis, see under Treatment of Tuberculosis, p.547.

Tuberculosis of the skin. For reference to the use of local applications of aminosalicylic acid powder for the treatment of local reactions to BCG vaccination, see under Tuberculosis of the Skin in Treatment of Tuberculosis, p.551.

ULCERATIVE COLITIS. Rectally administered aminosalicylic acid and mesalazine were found to be equally effective in the treatment or maintenance of ulcerative colitis in a double-blind randomised study involving 63 patients. Aminosalicylic acid may be a useful alternative to mesalazine because of its superior stability.— M. Campieri *et al.*, *Gastroenterology*, 1984, *86*, 1039.

Preparations

Aminosalicylic Acid Tablets *(U.S.P.)*

Aminosalicylate Sodium Tablets *(U.S.P.)*

Proprietary Names and Manufacturers of Aminosalicylic Acid, its salts and derivatives

Aluminonippas Calcium *(Tanabe, Jpn)*; Apir Pas *(IBYS, Spain)*; B-Pas *(Wander, Spain)*; Eupasal Sodico *(Stholl, Ital.)*; Gamirpas *(Gamir, Spain)*; Italpas Sodico *(Isola-Ibi, Ital.)*; Na-PAS *(Ferrosan, Swed.)*; Nemasol *(ICN, Canad.)*; Nippas Calcium *(Tanabe, Jpn)*; Paramisan Sodium *(Smith & Nephew Pharmaceuticals, UK)*; Parasal Sodium *(Panray, USA)*; Parispas *(Parisis, Spain)*; Pasalba *(Fawns & McAllan, Austral.)*; Pasdrazide *(Bruco, Ital.)*; Paskalium *(Glenwood, UK)*; Salf-Pas *(Salf, Ital.)*; Teebacin *(Consolidated Midland, USA)*; Therapas *(Smith & Nephew Pharmaceuticals, UK)*; Vadrine *(Inibsa, Spain)*.

The following names have been used for multi-ingredient preparations containing aminosalicylic acid, its salts and derivatives— Dantyl *(Leo, UK)*; Inapasade *(Smith & Nephew Pharmaceuticals, UK)*; Pasinah-D *(Wander, UK)*.

7554-l

Capreomycin Sulphate *(BANM, rINNM)*.

Capreomycin Sulfate *(USAN)*; Capromycin Sulphate.

CAS — 11003-38-6 (capreomycin); 1405-37-4 (sulphate).

Pharmacopoeias. In *Br.* *U.S.* includes Sterile Capreomycin Sulfate.

A mixture of the sulphates of the polypeptide antimicrobial substances produced by certain strains of *Streptomyces capreolus* and containing not less than 90% of capreomycin I. The *B.P.* specifies that it contains not less than 700 units per mg.
Capreomycin I consists of capreomycin IA ($C_{25}H_{44}N_{14}O_8$=668.7) and capreomycin IB ($C_{25}H_{44}N_{14}O_7$=652.7) which predominates. Capreomycin II which makes up about 10% of the mixture consists of capreomycin IIA and capreomycin IIB.
A white or almost white solid or amorphous powder. One million units of capreomycin is approximately equivalent to 1 g of capreomycin. **Soluble** 1 in 1 of water; practically insoluble in alcohol, chloroform, ether, and most other organic solvents. A 3% solution in water has a pH of 4.5 to 7.5. **Store** at a temperature not exceeding 15° in airtight containers. Solutions for injection may be stored for 48 hours at 20° and for up to 14 days at 2 to 8°.

The structure of capreomycin IB. The capreomycins were closely related in structure to viomycin.— B. W. Bycroft *et al.*, *Nature*, 1971, *231*, 301.

Units

One unit of capreomycin is contained in 0.001087 mg of the first International Reference Preparation (1967) of capreomycin sulphate which contains 920 units per mg.

Adverse Effects

The effects of capreomycin on the kidney and eighth cranial nerve are like those of the aminoglycosides (p.236). Nitrogen retention and progressive renal damage may occur. Severe tubular dysfunction may lead to alkalosis and disturbances of calcium, magnesium, and potassium excretion. Vertigo, tinnitus, and occasionally hearing loss may also occur and are sometimes irreversible. Abnormalities in liver function have been reported when capreomycin has been adminstered with other antituberculous agents. Hypersensitivity reactions including urticaria, maculopapular rashes, and sometimes fever have been reported. Leucocytosis and leucopenia have also been observed. Eosinophilia commonly occurs with capreomycin. Loss of visual acuity has been reported rarely. Capreomycin also has a neuromuscular blocking action. There may be pain, induration, and excessive bleeding at the site of intramuscular injection; sterile abscesses may also form.

Precautions

Capreomycin should be given with care and in reduced dosage to patients with impaired renal function. Care is also essential in patients with signs of cranial nerve damage or a history of allergy, especially to drugs. It is advisable to carry out checks on renal and auditory function and on blood-potassium concentrations in all patients before and during therapy with capreomycin. It has also been suggested that liver function should be monitored.
Care should be taken when capreomycin is used with other drugs that have neuromuscular blocking activity. It should not be administered with other drugs which are ototoxic or nephrotoxic.

Antimicrobial Action and Resistance

Capreomycin is bacteriostatic against various mycobacteria. An MIC of 10 µg per mL has been reported for *Mycobacterium tuberculosis*, though this varies greatly with the media used. Resistance develops readily if capreomycin is used alone. It shows cross-resistance with kanamycin, neomycin, and viomycin, but cross-resistance has not been reported between capreomycin and other antituberculous agents.

Absorption and Fate

Capreomycin is poorly absorbed from the gastro-intestinal tract. A dose of 1 million units of capreomycin (approximately equivalent to 1 g) administered intramuscularly has been reported to give a peak serum concentration of about 30 μg per mL after 1 or 2 hours. About 50% of a dose is excreted by glomerular filtration unchanged in the urine within 12 hours.

Capreomycin is considered to be unable to penetrate to the cavities in fibro-sclerotic lesions in patients with pulmonary tuberculosis.— M. Tsukamura, *Tubercle*, 1972, *53*, 47.

Uses and Administration

Capreomycin sulphate is a secondary antituberculous agent and is used in treatment regimens as described under Treatment of Tuberculosis, p.547, when primary agents have been ineffective or when their use is precluded due to intolerance or the presence of resistant organisms. It is preferred to kanamycin or viomycin because the incidence of severe side-effects is less.

Capreomycin sulphate is administered by deep intramuscular injection. The usual dose is 1 million units, equivalent to about 1 g of capreomycin, with a maximum of 20 000 units (20 mg) per kg body-weight given daily for 2 to 3 months, then two or three times a week for the remainder of therapy.

Preparations

Capreomycin Injection *(B.P.)*. Contains capreomycin sulphate.

Sterile Capreomycin Sulfate *(U.S.P.)*. The disulphate of capreomycin.

Proprietary Preparations

Capastat *(Dista, UK)*. *Injection*, powder for reconstitution, capreomycin sulphate 1 million units.

Proprietary Names and Manufacturers

Capastat *(Lilly, Arg.*; *Lilly, Canad.*; *Lilly, S.Afr.*; *Dista, Spain*; *Lilly, Swed.*; *Lilly, Switz.*; *Dista, UK*; *Lilly, USA)*; Caprocin *(Lilly, Austral.)*; Ogostal *(Lilly, Ger.)*.

6553-m

Clofazimine *(BAN, USAN, rINN)*.

B-663; G-30320. 3-(4-Chloroanilino)-10-(4-chlorophenyl)-2,10-dihydro-2-phenazin-2-ylideneisopropylamine.

$C_{27}H_{22}Cl_2N_4$=473.4.

CAS — 2030-63-9.

Pharmacopoeias. In *Br.* and *Ind.*

A fine reddish-brown, odourless or almost odourless powder. Practically **insoluble** in water; soluble 1 in 15 of chloroform; slightly soluble in alcohol; very slightly soluble in ether.

Adverse Effects

Adverse effects to clofazimine are dose-related, the most common being red to brown discoloration of the skin especially on areas exposed to sunlight. Discoloration tends to be more pronounced at leprotic lesions which may become mauve to black. These changes are more noticeable in light-skinned people and may limit its acceptance. The conjunctiva may also show some signs of red to brown pigmentation. The generalised discoloration may disappear within a year of stopping therapy with clofazimine although it may take 5 years before the patient is free of the discoloration at the lesions. Discoloration of hair, tears, sweat, sputum, breast milk, urine, and faeces may occur and production of tears and sweat may be reduced.

Gastro-intestinal effects are uncommon for doses of clofazimine less than 100 mg daily and usually they are not severe. Symptoms of nausea, vomiting, and abdominal pain experienced shortly after the start of treatment may be due to direct irritation of the gastro-intestinal tract and such symptoms usually disappear on dose reduction or withdrawal of treatment. Administration of large doses for several months sometimes produces abdominal pain, diarrhoea, weight loss, and in severe cases the small bowel may become oedematous and symptoms of bowel obstruction may develop. This may be due to deposition of crystals of clofazimine in the wall of the small bowel and in the mesenteric lymph nodes. Symptoms may slowly regress on withdrawal of treatment.

Clofazimine may produce a dryness of the skin and ichthyosis. Pruritus, acneform eruptions, skin rashes, and photosensitivity reactions have also been reported.

The incidence of side-effects experienced with clofazimine was reviewed in 34 patients receiving up to 700 mg per week (group A), in 23 patients receiving more than 700 mg per week (group B), and in 8 patients who had discontinued treatment with clofazimine (group C). Length of treatment ranged from 1 to 83 months. Side-effects on the skin included discoloration in 20% of patients (13 patients), pigmentation in 64.6% (42), dry skin in 35.4% (23), and pruritus in 4.6% (3). Ocular side-effects experienced were conjunctival pigmentation in 49.2% of patients (32), dimness of vision in 12.3% (8), and dry eyes, burning and other ocular irritation in 24.6% (16). Gastro-intestinal side-effects included abdominal pain in 33.8% of patients (22), nausea in 9.2% (6), diarrhoea in 9.2% (6), and weight loss, vomiting, or loss of appetite in 13.8% (9). Groups A and B generally had similar incidences of side-effects but no evaluation of significance was performed. However, dimness of vision was reported more frequently in group A. A few patients related subsidence or disappearance of some of the symptoms on decreasing the dose of clofazimine. Skin pigmentation in patients in group C disappeared on average 8.5 months after stopping therapy, the maximum time required being one year. Side-effects of clofazimine were generally well tolerated and no patient stopped treatment because of them.— V. J. Moore, *Lepr. Rev.*, 1983, *54*, 327.

EFFECTS ON THE EYES. Preliminary observations from 57 leprosy patients treated with clofazimine for periods of 3 to 26 months suggested that no significant untoward effect on the eyes was directly attributable to clofazimine, except corneal sub-epithelial brown-red pigmentation.— A. D. Nêgrel *et al.*, *Lepr. Rev.*, 1984, *55*, 349 (See also the report by V.J. Moore, above).

EFFECTS ON THE GASTRO-INTESTINAL TRACT. A report of a fatal syndrome of abdominal pain, malabsorption, and intra-abdominal deposition of clofazimine crystals in one patient.— R. F. Harvey *et al.*, *Br. J. Derm.*, 1977, *97*, *Suppl.* 15, 19. A 46-year-old woman experienced weight loss, diarrhoea, and abdominal pain 10 months after receiving a 6-month course of clofazimine 300 mg given daily for prurigo nodularis. Abdominal symptoms were initially relieved by a gluten-free diet but returned 22 months after withdrawal of clofazimine. Laparotomy showed crystal deposition in the chorion of intestinal villi and in the mesenteric lymph nodes.— P. Belaube *et al.*, *Int. J. Lepr.*, 1983, *51*, 328.

SPLENIC INFARCTION. Splenic infarction and tissue accumulation of clofazimine in a patient receiving clofazimine for the treatment of pyoderma gangrenosum.— A. C. McDougall *et al.*, *Br. J. Derm.*, 1980, *102*, 227.

Precautions

Because of dose-related adverse effects on the gastro-intestinal tract it has been recommended that daily doses of 300 mg or more of clofazimine should not be administered for more than 3 months.

As clofazimine crosses the placental barrier and is excreted in breast milk, neonates of women receiving clofazimine may have skin discoloration at birth or from breast-feeding.

PREGNANCY AND THE NEONATE. Although 2 pregnant patients received clofazimine without any adverse effects to the foetus, 3 neonatal deaths had been reported in 15 pregnancies in patients given clofazimine. Further evaluation of the perinatal consequences of clofazimine therapy in patients with leprosy is needed.— H. Farb *et al.*, *Obstet. Gynec.*, 1982, *59*, 122.

Urinary-oestrogen excretion, which can be used as an index of foeto-placental function, was reduced in women with lepromatous leprosy receiving clofazimine.— M. E. Duncan and R. E. Oakey (letter), *Int. J. Lepr.*, 1983, *51*, 112.

Antimicrobial Action and Resistance

Clofazimine is weakly bactericidal against *Mycobacterium leprae*. Using the mouse foot-pad technique the minimum inhibitory concentration for *Mycobacterium leprae* has been estimated to lie between 0.1 and 1 μg per gram; more accurate estimation is hindered by the marked accumulation of clofazimine in the tissues.

Clofazimine has been shown to be active *in vitro* against various species of *Mycobacterium*. Some references: P. Damle *et al.*, *Tubercle*, 1978, *59*, 135; J. B. Greene *et al.*, *Ann. intern. Med.*, 1982, *97*, 539; T. E. Kiehn *et al.*, *J. clin. Microbiol.*, 1985, *21*, 168.

RESISTANCE. A patient experienced a clinical and bacteriological relapse after 7½ years of monotherapy with clofazimine. Isolates of *Mycobacterium leprae* exhibited resistance to clofazimine in the mouse foot-pad sensitivity test.— T. Warndorff-van Diepen, *Int. J. Lepr.*, 1982, *50*, 139.

Absorption and Fate

Clofazimine is incompletely absorbed from the gastro-intestinal tract; absorption is influenced by particle size. It disappears rapidly from the blood stream to become deposited in most body tissues, from which it is then slowly released. Clofazimine has been estimated to have a half-life in the body of about 70 days. It is excreted in the bile; probably less than 1% of a dose is excreted in the urine daily. It is also excreted through sebaceous and sweat glands and in milk.

Distribution and tissue concentrations of clofazimine. Highest concentrations were observed in tissues with a high fat content and in the bile. This suggests that some proportion of drug recovered from the faeces may represent excretion in the bile rather than incomplete absorption from the gastro-intestinal tract. Concentrations were also high in tissues with a reticuloendothelial component and in the liver and gall bladder. Relatively high concentrations were also found in the kidney.— R. E. Mansfield, *Am. J. trop. Med. Hyg.*, 1974, *23*, 1116.

Quantitative assessment of clofazimine at autopsy demonstrated heavy accumulation of the drug particularly in the reticuloendothelial system and in the intestines. Very low concentrations in the kidneys indicated that accumulation was proportional to the number of macrophages in the organ or tissue. Clofazimine was found in all organs studied except the brain, indicating that it did not cross the blood-brain barrier.— K. V. Desikan and S. Balakrishnan, *Lepr. Rev.*, 1976, *47*, 107.

Identification of 2 metabolites of clofazimine in urine.— P. C. C. Feng *et al.*, *Drug Metab. & Disposit.*, 1981, *9*, 521.

Uses and Administration

Clofazimine, an iminophenazine dye, is an antileprotic agent. It is less liable than dapsone to provoke leprosy reactions and because of its anti-inflammatory properties it is used to alleviate them (see p.552).

When used in the treatment of leprosy, clofazimine should be used in association with other antileprotic agents to prevent the emergence of resistance. It is usually given with food in doses adjusted according to body-weight and the activity of the disease. A dose of 300 mg once-monthly plus 50 mg daily or 100 mg on alternate days has been recommended for the treatment of multibacillary forms of leprosy.

Clofazimine is used in the management of leprosy reactions, but since the beneficial effect takes several weeks to appear, initial control of symptoms is usually obtained with corticosteroids or, in Type 2 (ENL) reactions, with thalidomide. Administration of clofazimine may permit the withdrawal of corticosteroids in steroid-dependent cases as well as suppressing recurrent episodes and increasing tolerance to dapsone. Clofazimine may not be effective in Type 1 (Lepra) reactions. A dose of 300 mg daily has been suggested for the treatment of leprosy reactions, but this dosage should not be administered for more than 3 months. The dose should be gradually reduced, as soon as the reaction has been brought under control, to a minimum suppressant dose.

It has also been tried in the treatment of Buruli ulcer due to *Mycobacterium ulcerans* (but see below).

Studies suggest that the most probable mechanisms of clofazimine-mediated anti-inflammatory activity are inhibition of polymorphonuclear leucocyte migration and

T-lymphocyte responsiveness to antigens which may control Type 2 (ENL) and reversal immunity reactions respectively. Although clofazimine is therapeutically useful both as an anti-inflammatory and as an antimicrobial agent, it may still precipitate adverse immunological reactions in susceptible individuals by antigen release mechanisms.— R. Anderson, *Lepr. Rev.*, 1983, *54*, 139.

ADMINISTRATION IN CHILDREN. For recommendations for children's doses of clofazimine for use in multidrug regimens in the treatment of multibacillary leprosy, see p.552.

ATYPICAL MYCOBACTERIAL INFECTIONS. For the use of clofazimine and other antimycobacterial agents in the treatment of atypical mycobacterial infections, see p.553.

FUNGAL INFECTIONS. Clinical improvement in 3 patients with Lobo's disease (a chronic tropical mycosis) after treatment with clofazimine.— D. Silva, *Bull. Soc. Path. exot.*, 1978, *71*, 409.

GASTRO-INTESTINAL DISORDERS. Encouraging results from a preliminary study of clofazimine in the treatment of Crohn's disease. Clofazimine produced clinical and histological improvement and allowed proctocolectomy to be deferred in 4 patients who had severe acute ulcerative colitis refractory to corticosteroids and sulphasalazine.— D. Kelleher *et al.*, *Gut*, 1982, *23*, A449.

LEISHMANIASIS. A report of beneficial effects in 6 of 10 patients with American leishmaniasis, following clofazimine therapy.— O. Rotta *et al.*, *Anais bras. Derm. Sif.*, 1975, *50*, 197.

LEPROSY. For some recommended multidrug regimens including clofazimine in the treatment of leprosy, see p.552.

Reactions. For comments on the use of clofazimine in the control of leprosy reactions, see p.553.

LUPUS ERYTHEMATOSUS. Clofazimine in doses of up to 200 mg daily for 6 months produced improvement in 17 of 26 patients with discoid lupus erythematosus.— J. P. Mackey and J. Barnes, *Br. J. Derm.*, 1974, *91*, 93. No response in 6 patients with discoid lupus erythematosus and 2 patients with diffuse photosensitive systemic lupus erythematosus lesions after receiving up to 100 mg of clofazimine daily for 5 days a week for a mean of 25 weeks.— J. T. Jakes *et al.* (letter), *Ann. intern. Med.*, 1982, *97*, 788.

SKIN DISORDERS. Various skin disorders have improved with clofazimine and include: psoriasis (T. Chuaprapaisilp and T. Piamphongsant, *Br. J. Derm.*, 1978, *99*, 303); pyoderma gangrenosum (G. Michaëlsson *et al.*, *Archs Derm.*, 1976, *112*, 344); Sweet's syndrome (acute febrile neutrophilic dermatosis) (N. Saxe and W. Gordon, *S. Afr. med. J.*, 1978, *53*, 253); vitiligo (S. Bor, *S. Afr. med. J.*, 1973, *47*, 1451).

ULCERS. Although there have been some reports of benefit in Buruli ulcer, due to *Mycobacterium ulcerans*, following treatment with clofazimine (H.F. Lunn and R.J.W. Rees, *Lancet*, 1964, *1*, 247; J.H.S. Pettit *et al.*, *Br. J. Derm.*, 1966, *78*, 187), Revill *et al.* (*Lancet*, 1973, *2*, 873) concluded from a double-blind study that clofazimine was ineffective either alone or in conjunction with surgical treatment.

Preparations

Clofazimine Capsules *(B.P.)*

Proprietary Preparations

Lamprene *(Geigy, UK). Capsules*, clofazimine 100 mg.

Proprietary Names and Manufacturers

Lampren *(Neth.)*; Lamprene *(Geigy, Austral.; Geigy, S. Afr.; Ciba, Spain; Geigy, Switz.; Geigy, UK; Ciba-Geigy, USA).*

7555-y

Cyacetazide *(BAN).*

Cyacetacide *(rINN)*; Cyanoacetic Acid Hydrazide. Cyanoacetohydrazide.

$C_3H_5N_3O$=99.09.

CAS — 140-87-4.

Pharmacopoeias. In *Nord.*

Cyacetazide is a hydrazide derivative and has actions similar to those of isoniazid (p.563). It was formerly used in the treatment of tuberculosis in conjunction with other antituberculous agents. The aminosalicylate has also been used.

In veterinary medicine, it has been used as an anthelmintic in the treatment of lungworm infestations.

Proprietary Names and Manufacturers

Armazal *(Spain)*; Cianpas *(Infale, Spain).*

64-q

Cycloserine *(BAN, USAN, rINN).*

Cicloserina; Cycloserinum; D-Cycloserin. (+)-(*R*)-4-Aminoisoxazolidin-3-one.

$C_3H_6N_2O_2$=102.1.

CAS — 68-41-7.

Pharmacopoeias. In *Br., Cz., Egypt., Ind., It., Jpn, Jug.,* and *U.S. Hung.* has the hydrogen tartrate.

An antimicrobial substance produced by the growth of certain strains of *Streptomyces orchidaceus* or *S. garyphalus*, or obtained by synthesis.

A white or pale yellow, hygroscopic, crystalline powder, odourless or with a slight odour. Its activity diminishes on absorbing water.

Soluble 1 in 10 of water and 1 in 50 of alcohol; slightly soluble in chloroform and ether. The *B.P.* states that a 10% solution in water has a pH of 5.7 to 6.3; the *U.S.P.* specifies 5.5 to 6.5. **Store** at a temperature not exceeding 25° in airtight containers.

Adverse Effects

Adverse effects are common with cycloserine and mainly include dose-related neurological reactions. It has been reported that at therapeutic doses of 500 mg daily up to 30% of patients have experienced side-effects within 2 weeks of starting therapy; symptoms usually disappear on discontinuation. Adverse effects frequently encountered include anxiety, confusion, disorientation, depression, psychoses, possibly with suicidal tendencies, aggression, irritability, and paranoia. Vertigo, headache, drowsiness, speech difficulties, tremor, paresis, and hyperreflexia may also occur. Peripheral neuropathies, coma, and convulsions, occur more rarely. Toxic reactions may be reduced by keeping plasma concentrations below 30 μg per mL.

Allergic skin reactions and photosensitivity occur rarely. Serum aminotransferase values may be raised, especially in patients with a history of liver disease. Folate and pyridoxine deficiency, megaloblastic anaemia, and sideroblastic anaemia have been reported occasionally when cycloserine has been administered with other antituberculous agents. Cardiac arrhythmias have occurred in patients receiving doses of 1 g or more daily.

Treatment of Adverse Effects

Convulsions and other toxic effects on the central nervous system usually disappear when treatment is withdrawn, but specific treatment may be necessary. Although pyridoxine has been employed to diminish side-effects during treatment its value is unproven and severe toxic effects are most effectively prevented by adjusting the dose so as to avoid high blood concentrations of cycloserine.

Overdosage may require gastric lavage and symptomatic treatment. Peritoneal dialysis has been tried.

Desensitisation may be attempted following hypersensitivity reactions if the use of cycloserine is considered essential for the provision of adequate chemotherapy (see p.546).

Precautions

Cycloserine is contra-indicated in epileptics and mentally unstable patients. It has been reported that cycloserine may enhance the toxic effects of alcohol on the CNS and it should therefore be administered with great care to alcoholics.

As cycloserine has a low therapeutic index relatively small rises in serum concentrations may greatly increase the risk of developing adverse reactions. Dosage should therefore be reduced in patients with renal impairment and serum concentrations monitored at least weekly; it is recommended that its use be avoided if the patient has severe renal impairment. Monitoring is also advised for patients receiving doses of more than 500 mg daily and in patients exhibiting symptoms resembling those of CNS toxicity. Administration should be discontinued or the dosage reduced if adverse effects develop.

Cycloserine appeared to enhance the toxic effects of alcohol on the CNS in 2 patients.— F. Glass *et al.*, *Arzneimittel-Forsch.*, 1965, *15*, 684.

Dizziness and drowsiness experienced by 9 of 11 subjects receiving cycloserine with high-dosage isoniazid was thought to be due to the additive CNS toxicity of the two drugs. Isoniazid did not consistently modify serum concentrations of cycloserine.— M. J. Mattila *et al.*, *Scand. J. resp. Dis.*, 1969, *50*, 291.

PORPHYRIA. Cycloserine was considered to be unsafe in patients with acute porphyria because it has been shown to be porphyrinogenic in *animals* or *in vitro* systems.— M.R. Moore and K.E.L. McColl, *Porphyrias, Drug Lists*, Glasgow, Porphyria Research Unit, University of Glasgow, 1987.

PREGNANCY AND THE NEONATE. It was estimated that a breast-fed infant of a mother receiving cycloserine would ingest about 11.3% of the usual therapeutic dose for an infant.— D. E. Snider and K. E. Powell, *Archs intern. Med.*, 1984, *144*, 589.

For a recommendation that cycloserine is best avoided during pregnancy and for precautions to be taken by nursing mothers receiving antituberculous therapy, see under Treatment of Tuberculosis, p.548.

Antimicrobial Action and Resistance

Cycloserine is active against *Mycobacterium tuberculosis* and other mycobacteria including *M. kansasii*. Cross-resistance to other anti-tuberculous agents has not been demonstrated. Minimum inhibitory concentrations *in vitro* for *M. tuberculosis* range from 5 to 20 μg per mL.

Cycloserine has some activity against Gram-negative bacteria, including *Escherichia coli* and *Enterobacter*, and against Gram-positive bacteria including some strains of *Staphylococcus aureus*. Although minimum inhibitory concentrations for *E. coli* are usually greater than 50 μg per mL these concentrations are readily achieved in the urine with therapeutic doses.

Cycloserine interferes with bacterial cell wall synthesis by competing with D-alanine for incorporation into the cell wall. The antimicrobial action of cycloserine is therefore antagonised by D-alanine.

Fludalanine (3-fluoro-2-deutero-D-alanine) enhanced the activity of cycloserine *in vitro* against rapidly growing mycobacteria so that *Mycobacterium fortuitum* and *M. phlei* were inhibited at cycloserine concentrations attainable in serum. Fludalanine had little effect on the activity of cycloserine against slowly growing mycobacteria, including *M. tuberculosis*.— J. M. Dickinson and D. A. Mitchison, *Tubercle*, 1985, *66*, 109.

Isolates of *Mycobacterium avium-M. intracellulare* from patients with AIDS were significantly more susceptible to cycloserine at concentrations of 30 and 60 μg per mL than isolates from non-AIDS patients (C.R. Horsburgh *et al.*, *Antimicrob. Ag. Chemother.*, 1986, *30*, 955 and *ibid.*, 1987, *31*, 969).

Absorption and Fate

Cycloserine is readily and almost completely absorbed from the gastro-intestinal tract when administered by mouth. Peak plasma concentrations of 10 μg per mL have been obtained 3 to 4 hours after a dose of 250 mg. Cycloserine accumulates to some extent and repeated doses produce considerably higher concentrations. The plasma half-life is about 10 hours.

Cycloserine is widely distributed in body tissues and fluids and diffuses into cerebrospinal, pleural, and ascitic fluids in concentrations similar to those obtained in serum. It also diffuses across the placenta and is excreted in breast milk.

Cycloserine is excreted by glomerular filtration and high concentrations are obtained in the urine. About 50% of a dose is excreted unchanged in the urine within 12 hours and about 70% is excreted within 72 hours. As negligible amounts of cycloserine appear in the faeces it is assumed that the remainder of a dose is metabolised to unidentified metabolites.

Less than 20% of cycloserine was bound to serum proteins.— M. J. Mattila *et al.*, *Arzneimittel-Forsch.*, 1972, *22*, 1769.

Uses and Administration

Cycloserine is a secondary antituberculous agent and is used in treatment regimens, as described under Treatment of Tuberculosis (p.547), when primary agents have been ineffective or when their use is precluded due to intolerance or the presence of resistant organisms. It is also used in the treatment of urinary-tract infections unresponsive to other therapy.

Cycloserine is administered by mouth in doses of 250 mg once or twice daily. This can be increased to 250 mg three or four times daily if necessary. However, the total daily dose should not exceed 1 g and plasma concentrations should be kept below 30 µg per mL. Children have been given up to 10 mg per kg body-weight daily in divided doses, adjusted according to the blood concentration.

Preparations

Cycloserine Capsules *(B.P., U.S.P.)*

Cycloserine Tablets *(B.P.)*

Proprietary Preparations

Cycloserine, Lilly *(Lilly, UK)*. *Capsules*, cycloserine 125 and 250 mg.

Proprietary Names and Manufacturers

Ciclovalidin *(Bracco, Ital.)*; Closina *(Commonwealth Serum Laboratories, Austral.)*; Cycloserine, Lilly *(Lilly, UK)*; Farmiserina *(Farmitalia, Spain)*; Micoserina *(Ital.)*; Seromycin *(Lilly, USA)*; Setavax *(Mabo, Spain)*.

6554-b

Dapsone *(BAN, USAN, rINN)*.

DADPS; Dapsonum; DDS; Diaphenylsulfone; Disulone; Sulphonyldianiline. Bis(4-aminophenyl) sulphone.

$C_{12}H_{12}N_2O_2S$=248.3.

CAS — 80-08-0.

Pharmacopoeias. In *Belg., Br., Braz., Chin., Egypt., Eur., Fr., Ind., Int., It., Neth., Turk., Swiss,* and *U.S.* Also in *B.P. Vet.*

A white or slightly yellowish-white odourless crystalline powder. *B.P.* **solubilities** are: very slightly soluble in water; soluble 1 in 30 of alcohol; freely soluble in acetone. *U.S.P.* solubilities are: very slightly soluble in water, freely soluble in alcohol and soluble in acetone. Both pharmacopoeias state soluble in dilute mineral acids. **Protect** from light.

DAPSONE INJECTION. (*Univ. Coll. Hosp.*). Dapsone 5 g, dehydrated alcohol 40 mL, benzyl alcohol 5 mL, propylene glycol to 100 mL.

Sterilised by autoclaving; it should be tested for sterility before use. No significant loss of potency or therapeutic effect was found after storage in the dark for 9 months, though slight darkening occurred.— T. M. French, *Lepr. Rev.*, 1968, *39*, 171.

Adverse Effects

Most side-effects caused by dapsone are dose-related and uncommon at the low doses of up to 100 mg daily that have usually been given to treat leprosy. They include anorexia, nausea, vomiting, headache, dizziness, tachycardia, nervousness, and insomnia. Hypersensitivity reactions, often referred to as the dapsone syndrome, develop rarely and tend to occur during the first 6 weeks of therapy. Symptoms may include fever, eosinophilia, mononucleosis, lymphadenopathy, leucopenia, jaundice with hepatitis, and exanthematous skin eruptions which may progress to exfoliative dermatitis, toxic epidermal necrolysis, or Stevens-Johnson syndrome. Although patients usually improve if dapsone is withdrawn fatalities have occurred. Some patients may respond to desensitisation. Fixed drug eruptions occur in dark-skinned people. Although agranulocytosis has been reported rarely with dapsone when used alone reports have been more common when dapsone has been used with other agents in the prophylaxis of malaria.

Peripheral neuritis has been reported and there have been occasional reports of psychosis.

Varying degrees of dose-related haemolysis and methaemoglobinaemia are the most frequently reported adverse effects of dapsone and occur in most subjects given more than 200 mg daily; doses of up to 100 mg daily do not cause significant haemolysis but subjects deficient in glucose-6-phosphate dehydrogenase are affected by doses above about 50 mg daily. These adverse effects on the blood are probably caused by hydroxylamine derivatives produced during metabolism.

Reactions which occur during therapy of leprosy with dapsone may be difficult to distinguish from those of the disease but leprosy reactions, which may complicate therapy, are not toxic effects of dapsone but changes in the category of leprosy; for further details, see p.552.

ALLERGY. Findings of anti-dapsone antibodies in patients receiving dapsone.— P. K. Das *et al.* (letter), *Lancet*, 1980, *1*, 1309.

A report of a fatal hypersensitivity reaction in a 17-year-old boy, three weeks after the start of therapy with dapsone 100 mg daily for erythema nodosum leprosum. The clinical symptoms and progression of illness conformed well to the 'dapsone syndrome'. The soundness of beginning dapsone therapy in full dosage in patients with lepromatous leprosy is questioned.— H. M. Frey *et al.*, *Ann. intern. Med.*, 1981, *94*, 777.

Some reports of hypersensitivity reactions to dapsone.— K. J. Tomecki and C. J. Catalano, *Archs Derm.*, 1981, *117*, 38; N. P. Kromann *et al.*, *ibid.*, 1982, *118*, 531; T. E. Gan and M. B. Van Der Weyden, *Med. J. Aust.*, 1982, *1*, 350; K. N. Mohamed, *Lepr. Rev.*, 1984, *55*, 385; M. S. Joseph, *ibid.*, 1985, *56*, 315.

CARCINOGENICITY. A survey of 1678 patients admitted for treatment of histologically confirmed leprosy to the National Hansen's Disease Center in Carville between 1939 and 1977 indicated that, although dapsone has been implicated as a carcinogen *in animals*, the use of sulphones, including dapsone, did not appear to affect significantly the risk of any cancer in these patients.— L. A. Brinton *et al.*, *J. natn. Cancer Inst.*, 1984, *72*, 109.

EFFECTS ON THE BLOOD. Red-cell hypoplasia and agranulocytosis in a 23-year-old woman taking dapsone 100 mg with pyrimethamine 12.5 mg (Maloprim) weekly for antimalarial prophylaxis.— M. D. Nicholls and A. J. Concannon, *Med. J. Aust.*, 1982, *2*, 564. A further report of red-cell hypoplasia. The patient was taking pyrimethamine 25 mg with dapsone 100 mg (Deltaprim) for malaria prophylaxis.— M. Gelfand and E. H. Froese, *Cent. Afr. J. Med.*, 1983, *29*, 181.

Aplastic anaemia occurred in a patient receiving dapsone 50 mg daily for lepromatous leprosy.— J. Foucauld *et al.* (letter), *Ann. intern. Med.*, 1985, *102*, 139.

Agranulocytosis. Agranulocytosis has been reported in patients receiving dapsone alone: P. H. Levine and L. R. Weintraub, *Ann. intern. Med.*, 1968, *68*, 1060; F. C. Firkin and A. F. Mariani, *Med. J. Aust.*, 1977, *2*, 247; B. McConkey (letter), *Lancet*, 1981, *2*, 525; P. Barss, *Lepr. Rev.*, 1986, *57*, 63.

For a review of reported cases of agranulocytosis associated with the use of Maloprim (dapsone plus pyrimethamine) in the prophylaxis of malaria, see under Pyrimethamine, p.516.

Reports of agranulocytosis in patients receiving dapsone with other antimalarial agents.— A. J. Ognibene, *Ann. intern. Med.*, 1970, *72*, 521; *idem* (letter), 1972, *77*, 153 (with chloroquine and primaquine); B. A. Smithhurst *et al.*, *Med. J. Aust.*, 1971, *1*, 537 (with proguanil).

EFFECTS ON THE EYES. See Overdosage, below.

EFFECTS ON FERTILITY. The fertility of 2 male patients was abolished during dapsone therapy and restored some time after the drug was stopped.— J. Grieve (letter), *Lancet*, 1979, *2*, 464.

HYPOALBUMINAEMIA. Severe hypoalbuminaemia developed in 2 men with dermatitis herpetiformis after treatment for 3 and 11 years with dapsone in doses of 100 mg daily and 150 mg daily respectively. Both patients deteriorated to a point when they seemed unlikely to survive, with symptoms including massive ascites, oedema, and circulatory failure. On withdrawal of dapsone they made a rapid and complete recovery.— J. G. C. Kingham *et al.*, *Lancet*, 1979, *2*, 662 and 1018. A similar fatal case possibly due to dapsone.— S. Young and J. M. Marks (letter), *ibid.*, 908.

Significant hypoalbuminaemia developed in a woman with dermatitis herpetiformis after 32 months of therapy with dapsone 100 mg daily. She died 10 days after dapsone was withdrawn.— P. N. Foster and C. H. J. Swan (letter), *Lancet*, 1981, *2*, 806.

EFFECTS ON MENTAL STATE. In the early 1970s there was some discussion about dapsone inducing psychoses. Jopling (*Br. med. J.*, 1971, *4*, 366) considered that dapsone given in low doses to leprosy patients did not cause psychoses while Browne (*Br. med. J.*, 1971, *4*, 558) argued that psychoses could occur in a small proportion of patients given 100 mg or less daily. In 1983 Fine *et al.* (*J. Am. Acad. Derm.*, 1983, *9*, 274) reported a psychiatric reaction in one patient given 25 to 150 mg daily for dermatitis herpetiformis and suggested that the adverse effect was not dose-dependent.

See also under Overdosage, below.

EFFECTS ON THE NERVOUS SYSTEM. Motor neuropathy is the most common neurological effect of dapsone in patients with diseases other than leprosy. Symptoms usually include weakness of hands and limbs. Sensory impairment is less common but paraesthesia of digits, hands, and limbs has occurred. Although recovery is usually complete upon discontinuation some patients may never regain full function. The onset of recovery may range from a few weeks to a few months or longer. The mechanism of dapsone-induced neuropathy is unknown and opinion varies as to whether the effect is dose-related or an idiosyncratic reaction. It also appears that dapsone can produce neuropathy in patients with leprosy and that the incidence may be greater than that previously recognised. Movement disorders have been reported in children, though not in adults, following acute poisoning. Cerebral anoxia has been suggested as a likely mechanism. Symptoms do not persist or recur after recovery from poisoning. There have been only 2 reports of visual impairment in patients receiving dapsone and both may have been secondary to vascular damage.— T. K. Daneshmend, *Adverse Drug React. Ac. Pois. Rev.*, 1984, *3*, 43.

OVERDOSAGE. Three boys took large single doses of dapsone in an attempt to simplify their treatment regimens. One aged about 10 years took 500 mg without ill effect, a second aged about 16 years took 1.45 g and died about 4 days later after suffering vomiting, severe abdominal pains, haematuria, jaundice, and coma. The third, who was also about 16 years old, took 1.2 g and suffered similar symptoms but recovered within a week.— J. Sturt, *Papua New Guin. med. J.*, 1967, *10*, 97.

Permanent retinal damage occurred in a man who took 7.5 g of dapsone in a suicide attempt.— D. J. Kenner *et al.*, *Br. J. Ophthal.*, 1980, *64*, 741. Blindness (optic atrophy) and motor neuropathy after overdosage with dapsone; the conditions were not resolved 6 months later.— M. Homeida *et al.*, *Br. med. J.*, 1980, *281*, 1180. The motor neuropathy had resolved completely over the last 14 months but optic atrophy and visual impairment persisted.— T. K. Daneshmend and M. Homeida (letter), *ibid.*, 1981, *283*, 311. No evidence of impaired retinal blood flow in 7 patients taking therapeutic doses of dapsone for dermatitis herpetiformis. One patient was taking 600 mg daily.— J. N. Leonard *et al.* (letter), *Lancet*, 1982, *1*, 453.

A report of toxic delirious psychosis in a 5-year-old child who ingested 400 mg of dapsone.— K. Krishna Murthy and K. K. Raja Babu, *Lepr. India*, 1980, *52*, 443.

A report of delayed sulphaemoglobinaemia in a 22-year-old patient following acute intoxication with 3 g of dapsone.— M. Lambert *et al.*, *J. Toxicol. clin. Toxicol.*, 1982, *19*, 45.

See also under Treatment of Adverse Effects (below).

Treatment of Adverse Effects

In severe overdosage the stomach should be emptied by aspiration and lavage. Administration of activated charcoal by mouth has been shown to enhance the elimination of dapsone and its monoacetyl metabolite. Methaemoglobinaemia has been treated with slow intravenous injections of methylene blue 1 to 2 mg per kg body-weight repeated after one hour if necessary. Ascorbic acid 0.5 to 2 g may be given in addition by intravenous injection or by mouth; it should not normally be used alone because of its slow speed of action, but may be of use in patients deficient in glucose-6-phosphate dehydrogenase in whom methylene blue will be ineffective. Haemolysis has been treated by infusion of concentrated human red blood cells to replace the damaged cells. Supportive therapy includes administration of oxygen to alleviate hypoxia, and administration of fluids to maintain renal flow and promote the elimination of dapsone.

Decreases in serum methaemoglobinaemia and resolution of cyanosis were obtained within 64 hours in an 18-month-old child, who had ingested 100 mg of dapsone, by administering activated charcoal 10 g every 6 hours. Cyanosis had reappeared after an initial response to methylene blue 1 mg per kg body-weight given intravenously.— J. R. Reigart *et al.*, *J. Toxicol. clin. Toxicol.*, 1982-83, *19*, 1061.

Charcoal haemoperfusion was successfully used to treat acute dapsone intoxication in a 22-year-old female who was admitted to hospital 2 hours after taking 4 g of dapsone. Initial treatment included gastric lavage and activated charcoal, mannitol, and intravenous fluids. However, 15½ hours after ingestion serum concentrations of dapsone were still rising and despite treatment with 2 infusions of methylene blue there was haemolysis and progressive methaemoglobinaemia and clinical deterioration. Charcoal haemoperfusion and sequential haemodialysis successfully accelerated dapsone removal resulting in clinical improvement. The use of dialysis was later considered to have been unnecessary.— Z. H. Endre *et al.*, *Aust. N.Z. J. Med.*, 1983, *13*, 509.

DESENSITISATION. Dapsone desensitisation was successfully carried out in 48 of 52 patients. Gradually increasing doses of solapsone and then dapsone were used.— S. G. Browne, *Br. med. J.*, 1963, *2*, 664.

Precautions

In order to avoid permanent disability, rapid and adequate treatment is essential for leprosy patients who develop leprosy reactions during treatment with dapsone (for further details, see p.552).

Dapsone should not be used in patients with severe anaemia. It is recommended that regular blood counts be performed during treatment. Patients deficient in glucose-6-phosphate dehydrogenase are more susceptible to the haemolytic effects of dapsone. Patients with cardiac or pulmonary disease do not easily tolerate the effects of haemolysis and methaemoglobinaemia. It is now generally considered that the benefits of dapsone in the treatment of leprosy outweigh any potential risk to the pregnant patient.

Excretion of dapsone is reduced and plasma concentrations increased by concurrent administration of probenecid. Rifampicin has been reported to increase the plasma clearance of dapsone.

INTERACTIONS. The efficacy of dapsone in preventing patency of mosquito-induced infection was reduced when potassium aminobenzoate was given concurrently in a dose of 4 g daily.— R. L. DeGowin *et al.*, *Bull. Wld Hlth Org.*, 1966, *34*, 671.

Reports that concurrent administration of rifampicin shortens the plasma half-life of dapsone.— R. H. Gelber and R. J. W. Rees, *Am. J. trop. Med. Hyg.*, 1975, *24*, 963; S. Balakrishnan and P. S. Sheshadri, *Lepr. India*, 1979, *51*, 54. Doubt as to the clinical significance of the interaction between dapsone and rifampicin.— G. Acocella and R. Conti, *Tubercle*, 1980, *61*, 171.

There had been 2 reports to the Committee on Safety of Medicines of oral contraceptive failure in women also receiving dapsone.— D. J. Back *et al.*, *Drugs*, 1981, *21*, 46.

PORPHYRIA. Dapsone was considered to be unsafe in patients with acute porphyria because it has been shown to be porphyrinogenic in *animals* or *in vitro* systems.— M.R. Moore and K.E.L. McColl, *Porphyrias, Drug Lists*, Glasgow, Porphyria Research Unit, University of Glasgow, 1987.

PREGNANCY AND THE NEONATE. From a review of 62 pregnancies in patients being treated for leprosy it appeared that sulphones may be safely used during pregnancy. There was a low incidence of congenital malformations but an unusually high incidence of twins. The cause was unknown. It was considered that patients with inactive disease who continue to be treated with sulphone therapy have a low incidence of disease and pregnancy complications. Patients with tuberculoid disease who are successfully being treated also appear to have a low incidence of problems. An increased incidence of complications and reactions in patients with active borderline or lepromatous leprosy appears to be more of a problem in untreated patients. Patients with active disease should be on a well-established treatment programme before pregnancy is considered. The newborn need not be removed from the mother who has active disease as long as she is being treated with chemotherapy.— J. N. Maurus, *Obstet. Gynec.*, 1978, *52*, 22.

Mild haemolytic anaemia occurred in the breast-fed neonate of a mother who was receiving dapsone 50 mg daily for dermatitis herpetiformis. Concentrations of dapsone and monacetyldapsone detected in the infant's serum indicated that dapsone is absorbed from breast milk.— S. W. Sanders *et al.*, *Ann. intern. Med.*, 1982, *96*, 465.

Antimicrobial Action

Dapsone is active against a wide range of bacteria but it is mainly employed for its action against *Mycobacterium leprae*. It is usually considered to be bacteriostatic against *M. leprae* although it may also possess weak bactericidal activity. It is also active against *Plasmodium*. Its mechanism of action is probably similar to that of the sulphonamides since they both have a similar range of antimicrobial activity and both are antagonised by *p*-aminobenzoic acid. Using the mouse foot-pad technique the minimum inhibitory concentration for *M. leprae* has been reported to be less than 10 ng per mL; the minimum inhibitory concentration in man has been estimated to be up to 30 ng per mL.

References to the activity of dapsone against *Mycobacterium leprae*: J. H. Peters *et al.*, *Antimicrob. Ag. Chemother.*, 1975, *8*, 551; L. Levy and J. H. Peters, *ibid.*, 1976, *9*, 102.

Resistance

Secondary (acquired) dapsone resistance of *Mycobacterium leprae* is wide-spread and is steadily increasing. Primary dapsone resistance has also been reported with increasing frequency in areas with secondary resistance. Resistance of *M. leprae* to dapsone should be suspected whenever a patient relapses clinically and bacteriologically or fails to improve during supervised treatment with dapsone.

Reviews of sulphone resistance in leprosy.— J. M. H. Pearson, *Lepr. Rev.*, 1983, 85S. Comment.— J. G. Almeida and C. J. G. Chacko (letter), *ibid.*, 1984, *55*, 183; B. Ji, *ibid.*, 1985, *56*, 265.

Some reports of secondary resistance to dapsone.— G. Baquillon *et al.*, *Lepr. Rev.*, 1983, *54*, 19; B. Ji *et al.*, *Lepr. Rev.*, 1983, *54*, 197; J. Bourland *et al.*, *Lepr. Rev.*, 1983, *54*, 239; J. G. Almeida *et al.*, *Int. J. Lepr.*, 1983, *51*, 366; T. W. van Diepen *et al.*, *Lepr. Rev.*, 1984, *55*, 149; S. R. Pattyn *et al.*, *Lepr. Rev.*, 1984, *55*, 361.

Reports of primary resistance to dapsone: L. Janssens (letter), *Lepr. Rev.*, 1983, *54*, 77; R. Utji *et al.*, *ibid.*, 193; R. H. Gelber, *Int. J. Lepr.*, 1984, *52*, 471; N. M. Samuel *et al.*, *Indian J. Lepr.*, 1984, *56*, 819; *Lepr. Rev.*, 1987, *58*, 209.

Absorption and Fate

Dapsone is almost completely absorbed from the gastro-intestinal tract with peak plasma concentrations occurring from 1 to 8 hours after a dose. Plasma concentrations in the region of 2 μg per mL have been reported after administration of 100 mg daily but these are subject to wide variations. Steady-state concentrations are not obtained until after at least 8 days of daily administration. The plasma half-life is also subject to variation with reports ranging from 10 to 50 hours with an average of 28 hours. About 50 to 80% of dapsone in the circulation is bound to plasma proteins and nearly 100% of its monoacetylated metabolite is bound.

Dapsone is metabolised by acetylation and *N*-oxidation, together with glucuronic acid and sulphate conjugation; acetylation exhibits genetic polymorphism and slow, intermediate, and rapid acetylators have been identified. It is widely distributed throughout the body and is subject to enterohepatic recycling.

About 70 to 85% of a dose is excreted in the urine of which about 20% is unchanged drug. Small amounts are found in the faeces. It is excreted in breast-milk in clinically significant amounts and it may be found in the serum of breast-fed infants.

A review of the clinical pharmacokinetics of dapsone.— J. Zuidema *et al.*, *Clin. Pharmacokinet.*, 1986, *11*, 299.

INTRAMUSCULAR ADMINISTRATION. A study of the pharmacokinetics of a long-acting intramuscular injection of dapsone, consisting of an aqueous suspension of dapsone crystals, given in doses of 900 and 1200 mg. Following administration of the 900-mg dose, the mean peak serum concentration of 2.28 μg per mL obtained in the first week in men had fallen to 0.11 μg per mL after 4 weeks while in women the mean peak concentration of 1.04 μg per mL only fell to 0.42 μg per mL after 4 weeks. The large discrepancies between the serum concentration curves in men and women were probably due to differences in thickness of gluteal fat.— E. S. M. Modderman *et al.*, *Int. J. Lepr.*, 1983, *51*, 359. See also.— E. S. M. Modderman *et al.*, *Int. J. clin. Pharmac. Ther. Toxic.*, 1982, *20*, 51.

Uses and Administration

By virtue of its cheapness, relative nontoxicity and high activity against *Mycobacterium leprae*, dapsone remains the principal drug used in the treatment of all forms of leprosy; it is now generally used with other drugs. The recommended dosage is 1 to 2 mg per kg body-weight daily by mouth (about 50 to 100 mg daily, with children receiving correspondingly less). Treatment may last for several years in multibacillary leprosy. Regimens involving initial low doses have been considered to reduce the incidence of leprosy reactions but doubts have been cast on the need for this, providing prompt measures are available to control the reactions; also any merits of low-dose administration must be balanced against the increased risk of encouraging dapsone resistance, especially in the multibacillary (lepromatous) forms.

Dapsone may also be given by intramuscular injection in a dosage of 300 to 400 mg twice weekly or 600 mg weekly; such injections are painful and can cause abscess formation.

Dapsone has also been used in the prophylaxis of leprosy and in the management of household contacts of leprosy patients.

In addition to its use in leprosy, dapsone has been found of value in dermatitis herpetiformis and other dermatoses. The dose required for the treatment of dermatitis herpetiformis has to be titrated for individual patients but it is usual to start with 50 mg daily by mouth gradually increased to 300 mg daily or more if required. This dose should be reduced to a minimum as soon as possible. Maintenance doses of as little as 50 mg weekly may be adequate but sometimes as much as 400 mg daily has been required. Maintenance dosage can often be reduced or even eventually omitted in patients receiving a gluten-free diet. The prompt response to treatment with dapsone has been used as a definitive test in the diagnosis of dermatitis herpetiformis.

Dapsone is also used in combination regimens in the treatment and prophylaxis of malaria (see under Antimalarials, p.505).

It is suggested that dapsone is pro-inflammatory and may contribute to Type 2 (ENL) reactions and reversal immunity reactions by stimulating polymorphonuclear leucocyte motility and lymphocyte responsiveness to antigens respectively. Its well-documented anti-inflammatory activity in a variety of dermatological conditions may seem difficult to reconcile with this, but it is possible that in patients with lepromatous leprosy and a high antigen load the immunostimulatory and pro-inflammatory activities of dapsone are dominant.— R. Anderson, *Lepr. Rev.*, 1983, *54*, 139.

ADMINISTRATION IN CHILDREN. For recommendations on children's doses of dapsone for use in multidrug regimens in the treatment of leprosy, see p.552.

AIDS. There are conflicting reports of the value of dapsone in Kaposi's sarcoma in AIDS patients. Poulsen *et al.* (*Lancet*, 1984, *1*, 560) reported improvement in 1 patient whereas Hruza *et al.* (*Lancet*, 1985, *1*, 642 and 998) obtained no response in 9 patients. However, Poulsen *et al.* (*Acta derm.-vener., Stockh.*, 1984, *64*, 561) have achieved a response in 4 of 6 non-AIDS patients.

Pneumocystis carinii has been shown to be susceptible to dapsone in a *mouse* model (W.T. Hughes and B.L. Smith, *Antimicrob. Ag. Chemother.*, 1984, *26*, 436). Although dapsone alone may not be as effective as conventional therapy in treating *Pneumocystis carinii* pneumonia (J. Mills *et al.*, *Clin. Res.*, 1986, *34*, 101A) dapsone 100 mg daily with trimethoprim 20 mg per kg body-weight daily has produced encouraging results (G.S. Leoung *et al.*, *Ann. intern. Med.*, 1986, *105*, 45) and appears to be as effective as co-trimoxazole (I. Medina *et al.*, *Program and Abstracts of the Interscience Conference on Antimicrobial Agents and Chemotherapy*, Oct. 1987, *27*, 261). Edelson *et al.* (*Ann. intern. Med.*, 1985, *103*, 963) assessed dapsone's safety in 14 AIDS patients and considered that it could be used safely even in those who had reacted adversely to co-trimoxazole.

BEHÇET'S SYNDROME. See Rheumatic and Connective Tissue Disorders, below.

CHONDRITIS. See Rheumatic and Connective Tissue Disorders, below.

DETERMINATION OF ACETYLATOR PHENOTYPE. Dapsone could be used as a determinant of the acetylator phenotype. The assessment could be carried out using plasma (K. Carr *et al.*, *Br. J. clin. Pharmac.*, 1978, *6*, 421; P.A. Philip *et al.*, *ibid.*, 1984, *17*, 465) or saliva (K. Lammintausta *et al.*, *Int. J. clin. Pharmac. Biopharm.*, 1979, *17*, 159). Assessment using saliva was considered however to be unreliable by Peters *et al.* (*Pharmacology*, 1981, *22*, 162) because concentrations of the monoacetyl metabolite were so low. Also Weber and Hein (*Pharmac. Rev.*, 1985, *37*, 25) considered dapsone to be a poorer discriminant than sulphadimidine.

FUNGAL INFECTIONS. Dapsone has been used successfully in the treatment of a few cases of mycetoma (H.F. Vismer and J.G.L. Morrison, *S. Afr. med. J.*, 1974, *48*, 433; R.S. Rogers and S.A. Muller, *Archs Derm.*, 1974, *109*, 529; E. S. Mahgoub, *Bull. Wld Hlth Org.*, 1976, *54*, 303. Nair (*Laryngoscope*, 1979, *89*, 291) used dapsone successfully in the prophylaxis of rhinosporidiosis to prevent recurrence of the infection following surgical treatment.

GASTRO-INTESTINAL DISORDERS. Dapsone in doses of 50 mg daily or 50 and 100 mg on alternate days produced remissions in 4 of 6 patients with Crohn's disease with a fistula or rectal involvement and which had not responded to conventional treatment.— M. Ward and J. P. A. McManus (letter), *Lancet*, 1975, *1*, 1236. A similiar report.— C. Prantera *et al.* (letter), *ibid.*, 1988, *1*, 536.

KAPOSI'S SARCOMA. See under AIDS, above,

LEPROSY. For background information on the changing role of dapsone in the treatment of leprosy and details of its use in multidrug treatment regimens, see p.551.

Monitoring of therapy. Various methods of checking dapsone compliance are used or have been suggested. Estimation of the dapsone-creatinine ratio in urine was one way (S.J.M. Low and J.M.H. Pearson, *Lepr. Rev.*, 1974, *45*, 218). Enzyme-linked immunosorbent assay (ELISA) was another (H. Huikeshoven, *Lepr. Rev.*, 1979, *50*, 275). Huikeshoven has also described a simple urine spot test (*Bull. Wld Hlth Org.*, 1986, *64*, 279). Isoniazid has been suggested as a marker for compliance testing (J.N.A. Stanley *et al.*, *Lepr. Rev.*, 1983, *54*, 317).

Prophylaxis. Guidelines for the use of dapsone in the prophylaxis of leprosy and the management of household contacts of leprosy patients.— *Memorandum on Leprosy*, London, HM Stationery Office, 1977; G. A. Filice and D. W. Fraser, *Ann. intern. Med.*, 1978, *88*, 538.

Reactions. For reference to the management of patients suffering leprosy reactions while undergoing sulphone therapy, see p.552.

LUPUS ERYTHEMATOSUS. See Rheumatic and Connective Tissue Disorders, below.

PNEUMOCYSTIS CARINII PNEUMONIA. See AIDS, above.

PULMONARY TUBERCULOSIS. For reference to the use of rifampicin with a preparation containing dapsone, isoniazid, and prothionamide in the treatment of pulmonary tuberculosis, see under Treatment of Tuberculosis p.549.

RHEUMATIC AND CONNECTIVE TISSUE DISORDERS. Dapsone has been used in a number of inflammatory disorders. Various reports demonstrate that dapsone can produce improvement in rheumatoid arthritis (D.R. Swinson *et al.*, *Ann. rheum. Dis.*, 1981, *40*, 235; P.D. Fowler *et al.*, *ibid.*, 1984, *43*, 200) although Fowler *et al.* considered that it should be reserved for those who could not tolerate or did not respond to chloroquine. Some clinicians consider that the principal limitation of dapsone is its weak action and not its toxicity and that it is therefore worth considering for use before more potent and potentially more toxic agents such as gold, penicillamine, or sulphasalazine (B. McConkey and R.D. Situnayake, *Prescribers' J.*, 1987, *27* (1), 27). Relapsing polychondritis has responded to dapsone (V.P. Barranco *et al.*, *Archs Derm.*, 1976, *112*, 1286; L.R. Espinoza *et al.*, *Am. J. Med.*, 1981, *71*, 181) as has Behçet's syndrome (K.E. Sharquie, *Br. J. Derm.*, 1984, *110*, 493; S. Handfield-Jones *et al.*, *ibid.*, 1985, *113*, 501) and lupus erythematosus (T. Ruzicka and G. Goerz, *Br. J. Derm.*, 1981, *104*, 53; R.P. Hall *et al.*, *Ann. intern. Med.*, 1982, *97*, 165). Vasculitic syndromes have also responded to dapsone (D.M. Thompson, *Br. J. Derm.*, 1973, *88*, 117; J.A. Ledermann and B.I. Hoffbrand, *J. R. Soc. Med.*, 1983, *76*, 613); its use in other skin disorders is discussed below.

SKIN DISORDERS. Dapsone produces a rapid response in dermatitis herpetiformis although why it does so is not clear (J. Marks, *Br. med. J.*, 1983, *286*, 1331). Linear IgA disease, which could be considered as a dermatosis distinct from dermatitis herpetiformis, has also responded (J.N. Leonard *et al.*, *Br. J. Derm.*, 1982 *107*, 301).

Various other skin disorders have improved with dapsone and include:

erythema elevetum dilutinum (S.I. Katz *et al.*, *Medicine, Baltimore*, 1977, *56*, 443);

miliary lupus (K. Kumano *et al.*, *Br. J. Derm.*, 1983, *109*, 57);

pemphigoid and pemphigus (C.I. Harrington and I.B. Sneddon, *Br. J. Derm.*, 1979, *100*, 441; R.S. Rogers *et al.*, *J. Am. Acad. Derm.*, 1982, *6*, 215);

psoriasis (R.D.G. Peachey, *Br. J. Derm.*, 1977, *97*, *Suppl.* 15, 64; A. Saunders and G. Johnson, *Aust. J. Hosp. Pharm.*, 1985, *15*, 192);

pyoderma gangrenosum (L.D. Soto, *Int. J. Derm.*, 1979, *9*, 293);

Sweet's syndrome (acute febrile neutrophilic dermatosis) (H. Aram, *Archs Derm.*, 1984, *120*, 245).

SPIDER BITES. A prospective clinical study of 31 patients with brown recluse spider bites indicated that treatment with dapsone followed by delayed surgical intervention if necessary reduced the incidence of wound complications and residual scarring compared with treatment by immediate surgical excision. [The dose of dapsone in a preliminary report (L.E. King and R.S. Rees, *J. Am. med. Ass.*, 1983, *250*, 648) was 100 mg twice daily for 14 days].— R. S. Rees *et al.*, *Ann. Surg.*, 1985, *202*, 659.

Preparations

Dapsone Tablets *(B.P.)*

Dapsone Tablets *(U.S.P.)*

Proprietary Names and Manufacturers

Avlosulfon *(ICI, Austral.; Ayerst, Canad.; ICI, Denm.; ICI, Swed.)*; D.A.P.S. *(Sintyal, Arg.)*; Dermosone *(Wilson, Pakistan)*; Dubronax *(Belg.)*; Servidapson *(Servipharm, Switz.)*; Sulfona Oral *(Esteve, Spain)*;

The following names have been used for multi-ingredient preparations containing dapsone— Isoprodian *(Kolassa, Aust.; Saarstickstoff-Fatol, Ger.; Saarstickstoff-Fatol, S. Afr.)*; Maloprim *(Wellcome, Austral.; Wellcome, UK)*.

12691-x

Enviomycin *(rINN)*.

Tuberactinomycin N. Stereoisomer of 9,12-bis(hydroxymethyl)-15-(3,6-diamino-4-hydroxyhexanamido)-3-(hexahydro-2-iminopyrimidin-4-yl)-2,5,8,11,14-pentaoxo-1,4,7,10,13-pentaazacyclohexadec-6-ylidenemethylurea.

$C_{25}H_{43}N_{13}O_{10}$=685.7.

CAS — 33103-22-9.

An antibiotic produced by *Streptomyces griseoverticillatus* var. *tuberacticus*.

Enviomycin is an antibiotic which has been used, as the sulphate, in the treatment of pulmonary tuberculosis.

Proprietary Names and Manufacturers

Tuberactin *(Toyo Jozo, Jpn)*.

7556-j

Ethambutol Hydrochloride *(BANM, USAN, rINNM)*.

(+)-(*R,R*)-*NN'*-Ethylenebis(2-aminobutan-1-ol) dihydrochloride.

$C_{10}H_{24}N_2O_2$,2HCl=277.2.

CAS — 74-55-5 (ethambutol); 1070-11-7 (hydrochloride).

Pharmacopoeias. In *Br., Braz., Chin., Eur., Egypt., Ind., Int., It., Jpn, Jug., Nord.*, and *U.S.*

A white, odourless or almost odourless crystalline powder. *B.P.* **solubilities** are: soluble 1 in 1 of water, 1 in 4 of alcohol; slightly soluble in chloroform; practically insoluble in ether. *U.S.P.* solubilities are: freely soluble in water; soluble in alcohol and in methyl alcohol; slightly soluble in chloroform and in ether. **Store** in well-closed containers.

Adverse Effects

Adverse effects to ethambutol appear to be uncommon with doses of 15 mg per kg body-weight. The most important adverse effect of ethambutol is retrobulbar neuritis with a reduction in visual acuity, constriction of visual field, central or peripheral scotoma, and green-red colour blindness. One or both eyes may be affected. The degree of visual impairment appears to depend on the dose and duration of therapy and may be associated with progressive depletion of zinc in the eye. Ocular complications can occur many months after the start of therapy. Recovery of vision usually takes place over a period of a few weeks or months but in rare cases it may take up to one year or more or the effect may be permanent. Retinal haemorrhage has occurred rarely.

Renal clearance of urate may be reduced in about 50% of patients receiving ethambutol and acute gout has been precipitated in patients with gout or impaired renal function.

Other adverse effects occur infrequently or rarely but since ethambutol is never given alone, other antituberculous agents may be responsible. Allergic reactions including skin rashes, pruritus, leucopenia, fever, and joint pains appear to be rare with ethambutol. Other adverse effects which have been reported include confusion, disorientation, hallucinations, headache, dizziness, malaise, jaundice or transient liver dysfunction, peripheral neuritis, and gastro-intestinal disturbances such as metallic taste, nausea, vomiting, anorexia, and abdominal pain.

Teratogenicity has been observed in *animals*.

EFFECTS ON THE BLOOD. Neutropenia in a 75-year-old man treated with isoniazid, ethambutol, and rifampicin. Neutropenia was induced, on challenge, by each of the 3 agents.— P. F. Jenkins *et al.*, *Br. med. J.*, 1980, *280*, 1069.

Substitution of ethambutol for isoniazid was considered to be responsible for thrombocytopenia in a 71-year-old woman who had been receiving isoniazid and rifampicin for tuberculosis.— M. Rabinovitz *et al.*, *Chest*, 1982, *81*, 765.

EFFECTS ON THE EYE. A report of open-angle glaucoma of the hypersecretion type occurring in a study of 17 patients given ethambutol 25 mg per kg body-weight daily for 4 months.— S. S. Bhola and S. D. Purohit, *Indian J. Chest Dis. Allied Sci.*, 1976, *18*, 189.

Although ethambutol given in high doses can induce optic neuropathy recent large clinical studies indicate that optic neuropathy is virtually unknown when ethambutol is given in doses of up to 15 mg per kg body-weight and is rare at doses of up to 25 mg per kg. Oculotoxicity appears to be more common in patients suffering from alcoholism or diabetes mellitus in association with pulmonary tuberculosis or in patients with renal tuberculosis.— A. L. Crombie, *Prescribers' J.*, 1981, *21*, 222.

A patient developed rapid progressive deterioration of vision only 3 days after beginning therapy with ethambutol 800 mg daily by mouth (about 15 mg per kg body-weight) as part of combination chemotherapy for pulmonary tuberculosis. The patient remained blind over one year after the initial reaction.— A. M. Karnik *et al.*, *Postgrad. med. J.*, 1985, *61*, 811.

Subclinical impairment of colour discrimination was found to be relatively common in 54 patients receiving about 14.7 mg per kg body-weight of ethambutol daily as part of antituberculous chemotherapy when compared with 50 patients receiving other antituberculous agents. Differences in the areas of colour vision affected were indicative of early and late manifestations of ethambutol oculotoxicity.— P. H. Joubert *et al.*, *Br. J. clin. Pharmac.*, 1986, *21*, 213.

See also under Effects on the Nervous System, below.

EFFECTS ON THE KIDNEYS. Ethambutol might have caused renal failure in 2 patients.— J. Collier *et al.*, *Br. med. J.*, 1976, *2*, 1105.

A report of acute diffuse interstitial nephritis in 3 patients attributed to antituberculous therapy and especially isoniazid and/or ethambutol.— W. J. Stone *et al.*, *Antimicrob. Ag. Chemother.*, 1976, *10*, 164.

EFFECTS ON THE LIVER. A review indicating that retreatment regimens for tuberculosis based on rifampicin with ethambutol carry a very low risk of hepatitis.— D. J. Girling, *Tubercle*, 1978, *59*, 13.

Ethambutol was considered to be the cause of jaundice which developed in a patient also receiving isoniazid and streptomycin. Liver-enzyme values which had failed to improve on withdrawal of isoniazid returned to normal when all treatment was stopped and further deteriorated when ethambutol or ethambutol and streptomycin were re-administered. Subsequent treatment with isoniazid and streptomycin was uneventful.— M. Gulliford *et al.*, *Br. med. J.*, 1986, *292*, 866.

EFFECTS ON THE NERVOUS SYSTEM. Peripheral neuropathy considered to be due to ethambutol was found in 3 tubercular patients who had received ethambutol 13 to 50 mg per kg body-weight, among other drugs. In each case there was improvement and some reversal of damage when ethambutol was discontinued.— P. Tugwell and S. L. James, *Postgrad. med. J.*, 1972, *48*, 667.

A report of a 57-year-old woman who developed peripheral neuropathy several months before optic neuritis suggests that peripheral neuropathies may serve as an early warning for more serious visual toxicity.— V. S. Nair *et al.*, *Chest*, 1980, *77*, 98.

EFFECTS ON THE SKIN. A generalised erythematous macular and papular eruption developed in a 23-year-old woman about 8 days after starting to take ethambutol; challenge confirmed that ethambutol was responsible.— J. S. Pasricha and A. J. Kanwar, *Archs Derm.*, 1977, *113*, 1122.

A report of toxic epidermal necrolysis associated with the use of ethambutol in one patient.— P. S. Pegram *et al.*, *Archs intern. Med.*, 1981, *141*, 1677.

For a report of the Stevens-Johnson syndrome, associated with rifampicin therapy, possibly being triggered by ethambutol, see Rifampicin, p.571.

HYPERURICAEMIA. Hyperuricaemia has been found in up to 66% of patients receiving ethambutol (A.E. Postlethwaite *et al.*, *New Engl. J. Med.*, 1972, *286*, 761; B.K. Khanna *et al.*, *Tubercle*, 1984, *65*, 195) and there have been reports of acute gouty arthritis precipitated by ethambutol in some patients (T.H. Self *et al.*, *Chest*, 1977, *71*, 561). Khanna *et al.* found that significant increases of serum-uric-acid concentrations occurred within 2 weeks in the majority of patients.

OVERDOSAGE. Post-mortem findings following a fatal overdose of rifampicin and ethambutol.— D. B. Jack *et al.* (letter), *Lancet*, 1978, *2*, 1107.

A patient who took ethambutol 20 g, rifampicin 9 g, and isoniazid 6 g made an uneventful recovery after haemodialysis and treatment with pyridoxine.— J. Ducobu *et al.* (letter), *Lancet*, 1982, *1*, 632.

PREGNANCY AND THE NEONATE. Two pregnant patients were treated with ethambutol; 1 delivered a normal infant and in the other, pregnancy was terminated and the foetus was found to be normal. Published reports listed 18 pregnant women who were given ethambutol and no adverse effect was seen on the foetus.— S. Keidan (letter), *Tubercle*, 1973, *54*, 84. See also J. M. Shneerson and R. S. Francis, *Tubercle*, 1979, *60*, 167.

Treatment of Adverse Effects

Overdosage with ethambutol should be treated with gastric lavage. Concentrations in the blood are reduced by haemodialysis or peritoneal dialysis.

Desensitisation may be attempted following hypersensitivity reactions if the use of ethambutol is considered essential for provision of adequate chemotherapy (see p.546).

Reference to the use of hydroxycobalamin for ethambutol-induced optic neuropathy. *Animal* studies are required to confirm efficacy.— R. Guerra and L. Casu (letter), *Lancet*, 1981, *2*, 1176.

Precautions

Ethambutol is generally contra-indicated in patients with optic neuritis. It should be given in reduced dosage to patients with impaired kidney function. It should be used with great care in patients with visual defects, the elderly, and in children in whom evaluation of changes in visual acuity may be difficult; it should not be used in children under at least 6 years and some consider it should not be used in patients with visual defects. Ocular examination is recommended before treatment with ethambutol and some consider that regular examinations are necessary during treatment especially in children. Patients should be advised to report visual disturbances immediately and ethambutol should be withdrawn if vision deteriorates. Ethambutol may precipitate attacks of gout.

INTERACTIONS. Results of a crossover study involving 13 tuberculous patients suggest that concomitant administration of aluminium hydroxide may delay and reduce absorption of ethambutol in some patients. No effect was seen in 6 healthy subjects.— M. J. Mattila *et al.*, *Br. J. clin. Pharmac.*, 1978, *5*, 161.

PREGNANCY AND THE NEONATE. For reference to the opinion that ethambutol is considered suitable for use during pregnancy and for a discussion on the use of other antituberculous agents during pregnancy, see under Treatment of Tuberculosis, p.548.

Snider and Powell (*Archs intern. Med.*, 1984, *144*, 589) had received 2 communications about concentrations of ethambutol in breast milk of women receiving ethambutol. The concentration of ethambutol in one sample of breast milk collected during a 2-hour period after a dose of 15 mg per kg body-weight was 1.4 µg per mL. Another woman had had simultaneous concentrations of 4.62 and 4.60 µg per mL in plasma and milk respectively, but no dose had been specified. From this limited data Snider and Powell estimated that a breast-fed infant would receive about 3.4 to 5.7% of the usual therapeutic dose for an infant.

For recommendations on precautions to be taken by nursing mothers receiving antituberculous therapy, see under Treatment of Tuberculosis, p.548.

See also under Adverse Effects above.

Antimicrobial Action and Resistance

Ethambutol is bacteriostatic. It is effective against *Mycobacterium tuberculosis* and *M. bovis* with an MIC of 0.5 to 8 µg per mL but possesses little sterilising activity (see p.546). It is also active against some atypical mycobacteria including *M. kansasii* (see p.553). Activity against other micro-organisms has not been reported. It is effective against tubercle bacilli resistant to other antituberculous agents. Cross-resistance has not been reported.

Primary resistance to ethambutol is uncommon in developed countries but resistant strains of *M. tuberculosis* are readily produced if ethambutol is used alone.

The precise mode of action of ethambutol against mycobacteria is unknown. Takayama *et al.* (*Antimicrob. Ag. Chemother.*, 1979, *16*, 240) proposed that ethambutol inhibits cell wall synthesis by preventing the incorporation of mycolic acids. However, Pöso *et al.* (*Lancet*, 1983, *2*, 1418 and *ibid.*, 1984, *1*, 178) suggested that its activity against *Mycobacterium* spp. but not other bacteria may be due to inhibiton of spermidine synthesis specifically in mycobacteria. The same workers (L.G. Paulin *et al.*, *Antimicrob. Ag. Chemother.*, 1985, *28*, 157) also demonstrated that inhibition of spermidine synthesis only occurred with the active antimycobacterial dextro isomer.

See also under Antimicrobial Action of Antituberculous Agents, p.546.

Absorption and Fate

About 80% of an oral dose of ethambutol is absorbed from the gastro-intestinal tract, and the remainder appears in the faeces unchanged. Absorption is not significantly impaired by food. After a single dose of 25 mg per kg body-weight, peak plasma concentrations of up to 5 µg per mL appear within 4 hours, and are less than 1 µg per mL by 24 hours. Ethambutol is partially metabolised in the liver to the aldehyde and dicarboxylic acid derivatives and then excreted in the urine. Most of a dose appears in the urine within 24 hours as unchanged drug and 8 to 15% as the inactive metabolites.

Ethambutol diffuses readily into red blood cells and into the cerebrospinal fluid when the meninges are inflamed. It has been reported to cross the placenta and is excreted in breast milk.

In 6 healthy subjects given a single dose of ethambutol 15 mg per kg body-weight as an aqueous solution and as a commercial tablet preparation mean peak plasma concentrations of 4.45 and 4.01 µg per mL occurred in a mean of 1.91 and 2.83 hours respectively after administration. For plasma concentration measured up to 12 hours after administration the apparent mean elimination half-life was 4.78 and 4.06 hours respectively which increased to about 10 hours for 24 to 72-hour samplings. About 54 to 67% of the dose was excreted unchanged in the urine within 72 hours. The results of studies with pooled human plasma and in 3 subjects indicated that approximately 20 to 30% of ethambutol was bound to plasma proteins.— C. S. Lee *et al.*, *Clin. Pharmac. Ther.*, 1977, *22*, 615. When ethambutol 15 mg per kg was given intravenously or by mouth as tablets or solution a mean of 79.2%, 63.4%, and 61.1% respectively of the administered dose was excreted in the urine unchanged within 72 hours.— C. S. Lee and L. Z. Benet, *J. pharm. Sci.*, 1978, *67*, 470.

Pharmacokinetic studies of ethambutol in elderly patients with tuberculosis.— L. M. O. Omer, *Prax. Klin. Pneumol.*, 1978, *32*, 252.

Pharmacokinetics of ethambutol in renal failure.— A. Varughese *et al.*, *J. clin. Pharmac.*, 1984, *24*, 410.

DIFFUSION. *Into cerebrospinal fluid.* In a study of the absorption of ethambutol given in a dose of 25 mg per kg body-weight to 13 healthy subjects and to 21 patients with tuberculous meningitis, mean serum concentrations measured at 3 hours were 4.1 µg per mL (range 2.6 to 6.6) and 4.9 µg per mL (range 3.4 to 8) respectively. A CSF concentration of 0.07 µg per mL was measured at 3 hours in 2 of 5 healthy subjects, no ethambutol being detected in the other 3. The mean CSF concentration at 3 hours was 0.48 µg per mL (0.05 to 1.6) in 4 of 5 patients, no ethambutol being detected in the fifth.— J. A. Pilheu *et al.*, *Tubercle*, 1971, *52*, 117. See also U. Gundert-Remy *et al.*, *Eur. J. clin. Pharmac.*, 1973, *6*, 133.

Into joints. Synovial fluid concentrations of ethambutol in 2 patients were 2.1 and 3.3 µg per mL respectively 3 hours after administration of a 1-g dose. Simultaneous plasma concentrations were 2.6 µg per mL.— D. Mouries *et al.*, *Nouv. Presse méd.*, 1975, *4*, 2734.

PREGNANCY AND THE NEONATE. For reference to concentrations of ethambutol in breast milk of nursing mothers, see under Precautions.

Uses and Administration

Ethambutol hydrochloride is used with other antituberculous agents in the primary treatment of pulmonary and extrapulmonary tuberculosis as described under Treatment of Tuberculosis, p.547. As ethambutol is only bacteriostatic and has little or no sterilising activity its main role in current antituberculous therapy is to suppress emergence of resistance to the other agents used in the regimens. It is also used with rifampicin in re-treatment regimens, following failure of primary therapy, when resistance to isoniazid is present (see p.550).

For initial treatment it is given by mouth in a single daily dose of 15 mg per kg body-weight. In re-treatment it is given in a single daily dose of 25 mg per kg for 60 days then 15 mg per kg daily. A dose of 50 mg per kg has been given twice weekly in intermittent treatment regimens. Children over the age of 6 years have been given doses similar to those used for adults.

Ethambutol has also been administered by injection.

ADMINISTRATION. *Intravenous use.* Reference to the slow intravenous injection of ethambutol.— F. Mandler *et al.*, *Farmaco, Edn prat.*, 1972, *27*, 369.

ADMINISTRATION IN GASTRO-INTESTINAL DISORDERS. Results suggesting that adequate serum concentrations can be obtained in patients with jejunoileal bypass after a dose of ethambutol of 15 to 25 mg per kg body-weight.— R. E. Polk *et al.* (letter), *Ann. intern. Med.*, 1978, *89*, 430. See also T. M. Griffiths *et al.*, *Br. J. Dis. Chest*, 1982, *76*, 286.

ADMINISTRATION IN RENAL FAILURE. The dose of ethambutol should be reduced in patients with impaired renal function. Doses of 15 to 25 mg per kg body-weight daily could be given to those with a glomerular filtration-rate (GFR) of 25 to 50 mL per minute; 7.5 to 15 mg per kg to those with a GFR of 10 to 25 mL per minute, and 5 mg per kg for those with a GFR of less than 10 mL per minute or on haemodialysis or peritoneal dialysis.— J. S. Cheigh, *Am. J. Med.*, 1977, *62*, 555.

Data for predicting removal of ethambutol by conventional haemodialysis.— T. P. Gibson and H. A. Nelson, *Clin. Pharmacokinet.*, 1977, *2*, 403. See also C. S. Lee *et al.*, *J. Pharmacokinet. Biopharm.*, 1980, *8*, 69.

Ethambutol could be administered to patients with renal failure by adjusting the dosage interval. A dosage interval of 24 hours is suitable for patients whose glomerular filtration-rates exceed 50 mL per minute, an interval of 24 to 36 hours between doses is advisable for rates between 10 and 50 mL per minute. Where the rate is less than 10 mL per minute, the dosage interval should be 48 hours. A dose supplement should be given to patients undergoing haemodialysis or peritoneal dialysis.— W. M. Bennett *et al.*, *Am. J. Kidney Dis.*, 1983, *3*, 155.

See also under Treatment of Tuberculosis, p.548.

TUBERCULOSIS. For the use of ethambutol and other antituberculous agents in the treatment of tuberculosis, see p.547.

Preparations

Ethambutol Hydrochloride Tablets *(U.S.P.)*

Ethambutol Syrup. The following formula has been recommended by the manufacturers of ethambutol. Ethambutol powder 500 mg, citric acid 100 mg, orange tincture 0.3 mL, syrup 2.5 mL, and double-strength chloroform water to 5 mL. Stable for 1 month. Isoniazid should not be added to this syrup.—Personal Communication, *Lederle*, 1987.

Ethambutol Tablets *(B.P.)*. Tablets containing ethambutol hydrochloride.

Proprietary Preparations

Myambutol *(Lederle, UK)*. *Tablets*, ethambutol hydrochloride 100 and 400 mg.
Oral powder, ethambutol hydrochloride.

Mynah *(Lederle, UK)*. *Tablets* (Mynah 200), ethambutol hydrochloride 200 mg, isoniazid 100 mg.
Tablets (Mynah 250), ethambutol hydrochloride 250 mg, isoniazid 100 mg.
Tablets (Mynah 300), ethambutol hydrochloride 300 mg, isoniazid 100 mg.
Tablets (Mynah 365), ethambutol hydrochloride 365 mg, isoniazid 100 mg.

Proprietary Names and Manufacturers

Afimocil *(Prodes, Spain)*; Anvital *(Cheminova, Spain)*; Cidanbutol *(Cidan, Spain)*; Dexambutol *(Sobio, Fr.)*; Ebutol *(Kaken, Jpn; Infar, Port.)*; EMB-Fatol *(Saarstickstoff-Fatol, Ger.)*; Esanbutol *(Lederle, Jpn)*; Etambin *(Wasserman, Spain)*; Etambutyl *(Stholl, Ital.)*; Etapiam *(Piam, Ital.)*; Etibi *(ICN, Canad.; Saarstickstoff-Fatol, Ger.; Zoja, Ital.)*; Farmabutol *(Llorente, Spain)*; Fimbutol *(Spain)*; Inagen *(Morgens, Spain)*; Miambutol *(Cyanamid, Ital.)*; Myambutol *(Lederle, Arg.; Lederle, Austral.; Cyanamid, Belg.; Lederle, Canad.; Lederle, Denm.; Lederle, Fr.; Cyanamid-Lederle, Ger.; Lederle, Neth.; Lederle, S.Afr.; Cyanamid, Spain; Lederle, Swed.; Lederle, Switz.; Lederle, UK; Lederle, USA)*; Mycobutol *(Cadila, Ind.; ICI-Pharma, Ital.)*; Servambutol *(Servipharm, Switz.)*; Sural *(Chinoin, Hung.)*; Tibutolo *(Bracco, Ital.)*; Tisiobutol *(Capitol, Spain)*.

The following names have been used for multi-ingredient preparations containing ethambutol hydrochloride—Mynah *(Lederle, S.Afr.; Lederle, UK)*.

7557-z

Ethionamide *(BAN, USAN, rINN)*.

Ethionamidum; Etionamide; TH-1314. 2-Ethylpyridine-4-carbothioamide.

$C_8H_{10}N_2S$=166.2.

CAS — 536-33-4.

Pharmacopoeias. In *Br., Braz., Cz., Egypt., Eur., Fr., Hung., Ind., It., Jpn, Jug., Neth., Roum., Swiss,* and *U.S.*

Yellow crystals or a yellow crystalline powder, darkening on exposure to light, with a slight sulphide-like odour. The *B.P.* specifies practically **insoluble** in water while the *U.S.P.* states slightly soluble. Soluble 1 in 30 of alcohol; slightly soluble in chloroform, and in ether; soluble in methyl alcohol; sparingly soluble in propylene glycol. A 1% suspension in water has a pH of 6 to 7. **Store** in airtight containers.

Adverse Effects

Many patients cannot tolerate therapeutic doses of ethionamide and have to discontinue treatment. The most common adverse effects are dose-related: gastro-intestinal disturbances, including anorexia, excessive salivation, a metallic taste, nausea, vomiting, stomatitis, and diarrhoea. Dizziness, drowsiness, headache, postural hypotension, and asthenia may also occur occasionally. Although jaundice is rare hepatitis may occur in about 5% of patients receiving ethionamide.

Other side-effects reported include acne, allergic reactions, alopecia, convulsions, deafness, dermatitis (including photodermatitis), visual disturbances, tremor, gynaecomastia, impotence, menstrual disturbances, olfactory disorders, peripheral and optic neuropathy, thrombocytopenia, and rheumatic pains. Mental disturbances, including depression, anxiety, and psychosis have been provoked. A pellagra-like syndrome with encephalopathy has been reported rarely. A tendency towards hypoglycaemia may occur and could be of significance in patients with diabetes mellitus. Hypothyroidism has also occurred. Racial differences in tolerance may occur; Chinese and Africans are often more tolerant of ethionamide than are Europeans.

Teratogenic effects have been reported in *animals*.

EFFECTS ON THE EYE. Ethionamide had been reported to cause optic neuritis and optic atrophy but these rarely occurred when recommended doses were used.— *Med. Lett.*, 1976, *18*, 63.

EFFECTS ON THE LIVER. Abnormalities of liver function, but no jaundice, occurred in 12 of 80 patients treated with ethionamide as part of antituberculous chemotherapy. However 10 of these patients were also taking pyrazinamide. The use of these 2 agents together may increase the risk of hepatotoxicity and should be avoided.— J. M. Schless *et al.*, *Am. Rev. resp. Dis.*, 1965, *91*, 728.

A girl developed acute hepatic necrosis and died after treatment with ethionamide, isoniazid, and aminosalicylic acid. It was considered that ethionamide was the most likely cause.— K. Hollinrake, *Br. J. Dis. Chest*, 1968, *62*, 151.

The use of rifampicin with the thioamides ethionamide or prothionamide as part of the regimens recommended by WHO (see p.552) for the treatment of multibacillary leprosy has been associated with an unexpectedly high incidence of hepatotoxicity. Pattyn *et al.* (*Int. J. Lepr.*, 1984, *52*, 1) have reported an incidence of 4.5% in 596 patients treated with these regimens. Hepatotoxicity appeared to be associated with the daily administration of rifampicin during initial treatment as hepatotoxicity did not occur when rifampicin was given twice weekly throughout therapy. Other workers have reported even higher rates of hepatotoxicity. Cartel *et al.* (*Int. J. Lepr.*, 1983, *51*, 461) found an incidence of 13% in 54 patients while Ji *et al.* (*Lepr. Rev.*, 1984, *55*, 283) reported hepatotoxicity in 22% of 50 patients treated with rifampicin and an incidence of 56% in 39 patients given another rifamycin antibiotic.

EFFECTS ON MENTAL STATE. For reports of psychological changes associated with ethionamide, see F. S. Lansdown *et al.*, *Am. Rev. resp. Dis.*, 1967, *95*, 1053; R. K. Narang, *Tubercle*, 1972, *53*, 137; G. S. Sharma *et al.*, *Tubercle*, 1979, *60*, 171.

EFFECTS ON THE NERVOUS SYSTEM. A report of encephalopathy with pellagra-like symptoms occurring in association with ethionamide in 2 patients and with ethionamide and cycloserine in 1. Treatment was with nicotinamide and compound vitamin preparations.— M. Swash *et al.*, *Tubercle*, 1972, *53*, 132.

EFFECTS ON THE THYROID. It was suggested that ethionamide had caused a disturbance in the synthesis of thyroid hormone in 2 patients, resulting in hypothyroidism.— T. Moulding and R. Fraser, *Am. Rev. resp. Dis.*, 1970, *101*, 90. See also D. Drucker, *Ann. intern. Med.*, 1984, *100*, 837.

Treatment of Adverse Effects

It is suggested that pyridoxine should be given to patients taking ethionamide or prothionamide for prophylaxis of peripheral neuropathies. Anti-emetics may be of value in the treatment of severe nausea and vomiting.

Desensitisation may be attempted following hypersensitivity reactions if the use of ethionamide or prothionamide is considered essential for the provision of adequate chemotherapy (see p.546).

Precautions

Ethionamide should not be given to patients with severe liver disease. Liver function tests should be carried out before and during treatment with ethionamide.

Caution is necessary in administering ethionamide to patients with depression or other psychiatric illness, chronic alcoholism, or epilepsy. As there have been reports of goitre and hypothyroidism associated with the use of ethionamide it should also be administered with care to patients requiring treatment for hypothyroidism. Difficulty may be experienced in controlling diabetes when ethionamide is given to diabetics. The side-effects of other tuberculostatic agents may be increased when ethionamide is administered concomitantly. Ethionamide is best avoided during pregnancy.

Until there has been further evaluation of cross-resistance it would be preferable not to give multidrug regimens containing prothionamide or ethionamide to patients previously treated with thiacetazone or thiambutosine for more than 2 years.— B. Ji, *Lepr. Rev.*, 1985, *56*, 265.

PORPHYRIA. Ethionamide was considered to be unsafe in patients with acute porphyria because it has been shown to be porphyrinogenic in *animals* or *in vitro* systems.— M.R. Moore and K.E.L. McColl, *Porphyrias, Drug Lists*, Glasgow, Porphyria Research Unit, University of Glasgow, 1987.

Antimicrobial Action and Resistance

Ethiomanide is only active against mycobacteria including *Mycobacterium tuberculosis*, *M. bovis*, *M. kansasii*, and *M. leprae*. It is bacteriostatic against *M. tuberculosis* at therapeutic concentrations, but may be bactericidal at higher concentrations. Most susceptible organisms are inhibited by 10 µg or less per mL. It is considered to be bactericidal against *M. leprae* and an MIC of 0.05 µg per mL has been reported in *mice*.

Resistance develops rapidly if used alone and there is complete cross-resistance between ethionamide and prothionamide. Despite the structural similarity cross-resistance does not occur with isoniazid but may occur with thiacetazone and thiambutosine.

Clinical isolates of *Mycobacterium avium-M. intracellulare* from patients with AIDS were found to be significantly more susceptible to ethionamide at concentrations of 10 and 15 µg per mL than were isolates from non-AIDS patients.— C. R. Horsburgh *et al.*, *Antimicrob. Ag. Chemother.*, 1986, *30*, 955. See also *idem* (letter), 1987, *31*, 969.

Absorption and Fate

Ethionamide is readily absorbed from the gastro-intestinal tract, and peak plasma concentrations occur 2 to 3 hours after a dose. Half-lives of 2 to 3 hours have been reported. It is widely distributed throughout body tissues and fluids. It crosses the placenta and penetrates the uninflamed meninges, appearing in the CSF in concentrations equivalent to those in serum. Ethionamide is extensively metabolised, probably in the liver, to the active sulphoxide and other inactive metabolites and less than 1% of a dose appears in the urine as unchanged drug.

Peak plasma concentrations of about 3 µg per mL could be expected 2 hours after a 500-mg dose of ethionamide by mouth.— P. J. Jenner and G. A. Ellard, *J. Chromat-*

ogr. biomed. Appl., 1981, *225*, 245.

Jenner *et al.* (*J. antimicrob. Chemother.*, 1984, *13*, 267) had found plasma concentrations of ethionamide and its sulphoxide metabolite to be higher than those of prothionamide and its corresponding metabolite after administration of similar oral doses. However, from the results of a later study of oral and intravenous administration Jenner and Smith (*Lepr. Rev.*, 1987, *58*, 31) concluded that the differences between the pharmacokinetics of ethionamide and prothionamide are slight and not of clinical significance; other factors would be more important in selecting which thioamide should be used in the treatment of leprosy.

Uses and Administration

Ethionamide is a thioamide derivative which has been used with other antituberculous agents for the treatment of tuberculosis, generally when resistance to primary agents has developed (see Treatment of Tuberculosis, p.547). Ethionamide is also used in multidrug regimens for the treatment of leprosy (see p.552).

The usual adult dose in tuberculosis is 0.5 to 1 g daily in divided doses with meals. Treatment has been given as a single dose at night. The usual dose for children is 12 to 15 mg per kg body-weight daily to a maximum of 750 mg daily in divided doses. Some children have received 20 mg per kg daily.

Doses of 250 to 375 mg (5 to 10 mg per kg) daily have been recommended for use in the treatment of leprosy.

Ethionamide has also been administered as rectal suppositories; the hydrochloride has been given intravenously.

ATYPICAL MYCOBACTERIAL INFECTIONS. For the use of antimycobacterial agents in the treatment of atypical mycobacterial infections, see p.553.

LEPROSY. For reference to the use of ethionamide in multidrug treatment regimens in leprosy, see p.552.

TUBERCULOSIS. Use of ethionamide in the treatment of resistant pulmonary tuberculosis.— P. A. L. Horsfall, *Tubercle*, 1972, *53*, 166.

See also under Treatment of Tuberculosis, p.547.

Preparations

Ethionamide Tablets *(U.S.P.)*

Proprietary Names and Manufacturers

Ethatyl *(SCS, S.Afr.)*; Etiocidan *(Cidan, Spain)*; Panathide *(Propan, S.Afr.)*; Regenicide *(Gedeon Richter, Hung.)*; Thioniden *(Kaken, Jpn)*; Trecator *(Belg.; Théraplix, Fr.)*; Trecator-SC *(Wyeth, USA)*; Trescatyl *(May & Baker, S.Afr.; May & Baker, UK)*; Tubenamide *(Meiji, Jpn)*.

12776-h

Furonazide

2′-(α-Methylfurfurylidene)isonicotinohydrazide.

$C_{12}H_{11}N_3O_2$=229.2.

CAS — 3460-67-1.

Furonazide is a derivative of isoniazid that has been used in the treatment of tuberculosis.

Proprietary Names and Manufacturers

Clitizina *(Menarini, Belg.)*; Menazone *(Menarini, Ital.)*.

12789-q

Gluconiazide

D-Glucuronic acid γ-lactone 1-(isonicotinoylhydrazone).

$C_{12}H_{13}N_3O_6$=295.3.

CAS — 3691-74-5.

Gluconiazide is a derivative of isoniazid that has been used in the treatment of tuberculosis.

Proprietary Names and Manufacturers

Glucazide *(Stholl, Ital.)*; Gluronazid *(Hormonchemie, Ger.; Switz.)*; Guidazide *(Guidotti, Ital.)*.

6556-g

Hydnocarpus Oil

Chaulmoogra Oil; Oleum Hydnocarpi.

CAS — 8001-74-9.

Pharmacopoeias. In *Int.* Similar oils are included in *Port., Span.,* and *Turk.*

The fixed oil expressed from the fresh ripe seeds of *Hydnocarpus wightiana, H. anthelmintica, H. heterophylla,* and other species of *Hydnocarpus* and also *Taraktogenos kurzii* (Flacourtiaceae).

Hydnocarpus oil, its ethylesters, and sodium hydnocarpate were formerly employed in the treatment of leprosy.

7559-k

Isoniazid *(BAN, USAN, pINN).*

INAH; INH; Isoniazidum; Isonicotinic Acid Hydrazide; Isonicotinylhydrazide; Isonicotinylhydrazine; Tubazid. Isonicotinohydrazide.

$C_6H_7N_3O$=137.1.

CAS — 54-85-3.

NOTE. The name Isopyrin, which has been applied to isoniazid, has also been applied to isopropylaminophenazone.

Pharmacopoeias. In *Arg., Aust., Br., Braz., Chin., Cz., Egypt., Eur., Fr., Ger., Hung., Ind., Int., It., Jpn, Jug., Neth., Nord., Pol., Port., Roum., Rus., Span., Swiss, Turk.,* and *U.S.*

Colourless, odourless crystals, or white crystalline powder.

Soluble 1 in 8 of water, 1 in 50 of alcohol; slightly soluble in chloroform; very slightly soluble in ether. The *B.P.* specifies that a 5% solution in water has a pH of 6.0 to 8.0; the *U.S.P.* specifies that a 10% solution has a pH of 6.0 to 7.5. The *B.P.* injection has a pH of 5.6 to 6.0; the *U.S.P.* injection has a pH between 6.0 and 7.0. Solutions are **sterilised** by autoclaving.

Incompatible with sugars. **Store** in airtight containers. Protect from light.

It was recommended that sugars such as glucose, fructose, and sucrose should not be used in isoniazid preparations because the absorption of the drug was impaired by the formation of a condensation product. Sorbitol might be a suitable substitute.— K. V. N. Rao *et al., Bull. Wld Hlth Org.*, 1971, *45*, 625.

STABILITY. Isoniazid and its metabolite *N*-acetylisoniazid were stable for at least 5 weeks in human plasma when stored at −70°. Clinical samples should be maintained at this temperature during transport and storage.— A. Hutchings *et al., Br. J. clin. Pharmac.*, 1983, *15*, 263.

For a report of instability in a mixture containing isoniazid and sodium aminosalicylate, see p.554.

Adverse Effects

It has been reported that isoniazid has relatively low toxicity and only about 5% of patients may experience some form of adverse effect during treatment if pyridoxine is administered concurrently. Many of the adverse effects of isoniazid are related to hypersensitivity or to the use of large doses. Hypersensitivity reactions may include various skin eruptions, fever, lymphadenopathy, and vasculitis. Patients who are slow inactivators may experience a greater incidence of toxicity.

Peripheral neuropathy may be common if pyridoxine is not administered concurrently. Pellagra, which is also probably related to isoniazid-induced pyridoxine deficiency, occurs rarely. Optic neuritis and atrophy have also been reported rarely. Transient elevations of liver enzymes commonly occur during the first few months of therapy and usually return to normal despite continued treatment. However, severe progressive liver damage sometimes occurs especially in patients over the age of 35 and in those consuming alcohol regularly. Fatalities have occurred following liver necrosis.

Other adverse effects may include nausea, vomiting, and other gastro-intestinal effects. Hyperglycaemia and metabolic acidosis have also occurred. Blood disorders reported following the use of isoniazid have included haemolytic, aplastic, and sideroblastic anaemias, agranulocytosis, thrombocytopenia, and eosinophilia. There have been occasional reports of lupus-like reactions, a rheumatic syndrome, and gynaecomastia. Urinary retention may occur in the elderly and there have been reports of convulsions and psychotic reactions, especially in patients with a history of these conditions. Some patients may experience slight euphoria when taking isoniazid.

Symptoms of overdosage include slurred speech, metabolic acidosis, hyperglycaemia, hallucinations, respiratory and CNS depression, convulsions, and coma.

Reviews of the clinical consequences of acetylator status in relation to the therapeutic and adverse effects of isoniazid: W. W. Weber *et al., Fedn Proc.*, 1983, *42*, 3086; G. A. Ellard, *Tubercle*, 1984, *65*, 211; D. W. J. Clark, *Drugs*, 1985, *29*, 342; W. W. Weber and D. W. Hein, *Pharmac. Rev.*, 1985, *37*, 25.

Giddiness characterised by onset at about 12 hours after dosage, and persisting for about 24 hours was reported among 16% of 75 slow inactivators given a slow-release preparation of isoniazid (matrix isoniazid) 45 mg per kg body-weight. Among rapid inactivators giddiness was reported by 6% of 72 patients given 37.5 to 45 mg per kg and by 25% of 65 patients given 52.5 mg of matrix isoniazid per kg. The incidence was 2% among a total of 101 control patients given isoniazid 15 mg per kg plus matrix base.— R. Parthasarathy *et al., Tubercle*, 1976, *57*, 115. See also T. Santha *et al., ibid.*, 123 (matrix isoniazid with streptomycin).

ABUSE. Isoniazid in doses of 3 to 5 g has been abused for its hallucinogenic properties.— C. V. Brown (letter), *Lancet*, 1972, *1*, 743.

ALLERGY. See Effects on the Liver, Effects on the Skin, and Lupus, below.

CARCINOGENICITY. Concern about the carcinogenicity of isoniazid arose in 1974 when Miller (*J. Am. med. Ass.*, 1974, *230*, 1254) reported an increased risk of bladder cancer in patients treated with isoniazid. A later study by Kerr and Chipman (*Am. J. Epidem.*, 1976, *104*, 335) also found an increased risk of bladder cancer and Miller *et al.* (*J. chron. Dis.*, 1978, *31*, 51) confirmed their earlier findings but found that the risk only applied to female patients. Cancer of the bile duct was also reported in two patients treated with isoniazid (A.B. Lowenfels and J. Norman, *J. Am. med. Ass.*, 1978, *240*, 434). However, no evidence to support a carcinogenic effect of isoniazid was found in more than 25 000 patients followed up for 9 to 14 years in studies organised by the *US* Public Health Service (J.L. Glassroth *et al., Am. Rev. resp. Dis.*, 1977, *116*, 1065) and in 3842 patients followed up for 16 to 24 years in the *UK* (H. Stott *et al., Tubercle*, 1976, *57*, 1). Several other studies, including one by Boice and Fraumeni in female patients (*Am. J. publ. Hlth*, 1980, *70*, 987), also failed to show an increased risk in patients treated with isoniazid. Furthermore 2 studies in children (E.C. Hammond *et al., Br. med. J.*, 1967, *2*, 792; B.M. Sanders and G.J. Draper, *Br. med. J.*, 1979, *1*, 717) have failed to support any association between the administration of isoniazid during pregnancy and the subsequent development of cancer in childhood. However, Tuman *et al.* (*Lancet*, 1980, *2*, 362), who reported a mesothelioma in a 9-year-old boy whose mother had received isoniazid during pregnancy, considered that the length of follow-up in these 2 studies was too short to allow one to conclude that isoniazid was not a carcinogen.

EFFECTS ON THE BLOOD. Bleeding occurred in a patient receiving isoniazid, owing to an acquired inhibitor of fibrin stabilisation associated with isoniazid therapy.— P. T. Otis *et al., Blood*, 1974, *44*, 771.

A report of disseminated intravascular coagulation associated with isoniazid-induced hepatitis in one patient.— J. J. Stuart and H. R. Roberts (letter), *Ann. intern. Med.*, 1976, *84*, 490.

Further reports on the effects of isoniazid on the blood.— G. H. Tomkin, *Practitioner*, 1973, *211*, 773 (sideroblastic anaemia); P. F. Jenkins *et al., Br. med. J.*, 1980, *280*, 1069 (neutropenia); R. A. Claiborne and A. K. Dutt, *Am. Rev. resp. Dis.*, 1985, *131*, 947 (red cell aplasia); C. R. Lewis and A. Manoharan, *Postgrad. med. J.*, 1987, *63*, 309 (red cell aplasia).

EFFECTS ON BONES AND JOINTS. For evidence that isoniazid may have an adverse effect on vitamin D metabolism and could induce metabolic bone diseases, see under Precautions, below.

EFFECTS ON THE KIDNEY. A report of acute diffuse interstitial nephritis in 3 patients attributed to antituberculous therapy and especially isoniazid and/or ethambutol.— W. J. Stone, *Antimicrob. Ag. Chemother.*, 1976, *10*, 164.

EFFECTS ON THE LIVER. In an extensive review of the hepatotoxicity of antituberculosis regimens including isoniazid, especially those used in the controlled studies of the British MRC, Girling (*Tubercle*, 1978, *59*, 13) stressed that hepatitis occurring during antituberculosis chemotherapy may be attributed to other causes such as the disease itself, alcoholism, cirrhosis, or infectious hepatitis. When treatment is definitely implicated it may not be clear which drug or combination of drugs is responsible. Isoniazid alone is widely used prophylactically in the *US* and a survey by the *US* Public Health Service (M. Black *et al., Gastroenterology*, 1975, *69*, 289; D.E. Kopanoff *et al., Am. Rev. resp. Dis.*, 1978, *117*, 991) indicates that there is a definite risk of hepatitis during isoniazid prophylaxis, especially in patients over 35 years of age and in those who consume alcohol daily.

Studies of standard first-line treatment regimens based on isoniazid in Great Britain, Africa, and Asia show that the incidence of hepatitis is about 2% or less and this risk is considered acceptable. In Africans many episodes could be attributed to underlying chronic liver disease. Drug-induced hepatitis often appeared to be caused by aminosalicylic acid or thiacetazone rather than by isoniazid. Early reports of a higher incidence of hepatitis with regimens based on isoniazid and rifampicin have not been confirmed in later studies; Baron and Bell (*Tubercle*, 1974, *55*, 115) found that transient increases in serum concentrations of liver enzymes were common in the early weeks of antituberculosis therapy but that they rarely implied serious toxicity. However, there has been some concern over reports of severe hepatotoxic reactions in children receiving isoniazid with rifampicin (see below). Grönhagen-Riska *et al.* (*Am. Rev. resp. Dis.*, 1978, *118*, 461) have identified elderly women, alcoholics, slow acetylators, and patients with previous liver or biliary disease as being at particular risk from hepatotoxicity induced by combined treatment with isoniazid and rifampicin. However, Cross *et al.* (*Am. Rev. resp. Dis.*, 1980, *122*, 349) considered that treatment with isoniazid and rifampicin was not contra-indicated in alcoholics unless there were clinically significant and persistent pretreatment abnormalities in hepatic function.

The addition of pyrazinamide to regimens of isoniazid with rifampicin does not appear to be associated with an increased incidence of hepatotoxicity (D.J. Girling, *Tubercle*, 1978, *59*, 13– See also under pyrazinamide, p.569). The mechanism of isoniazid-induced hepatotoxicity remains to be determined. Black *et al.* (*Gastroenterology*, 1975, *69*, 289) attributed the liver damage to a direct toxic effect of isoniazid metabolites but the expected association between isoniazid dosage and hepatitis has not been demonstrated. Israel (*Gastroenterology*, 1975, *69*, 539) considered it to be a hypersensitivity reaction but few studies have found any evidence of a possible immunological basis (R.J. Warrington *et al. Clin. Allergy*, 1982, *12*, 217). Furthermore, many patients have resumed an isoniazid regimen uneventfully after only a short interruption.

Mitchell *et al.* (*Clin. Pharmac. Ther.*, 1975, *18*, 70) suggested that isoniazid might be more hepatotoxic for rapid rather than slow acetylators; in healthy subjects amounts of acetylisoniazid and isonicotinic acid in the urine were higher in the rapid acetylators. *Animal* work reported by Nelson *et al.* (*Science*, 1976, *193*, 901) provided evidence that acetylisoniazid can be converted to acetylhydrazine which is further metabolised to a highly reactive compound capable of causing liver necrosis. However, Timbrell *et al.* (*Clin. Pharmac. Ther.*, 1977, *22*, 602) found that although rapid acetylators produced more acetylhydrazine than slow acetylators they also acetylated comparatively more of this metabolite to diacetylhydrazine before toxic metabolites could be produced. Lauterberg *et al.* (*Clin. Pharmac. Ther.*, 1985, *38*, 566) also demonstrated that slow acetylators metabolise more isoniazid via a pathway associated with the production of toxic metabolites and others (I.W. Beever *et al., Br. J. clin. Pharmac.*, 1982, *13*, 599P; I.A. Blair *et al., Hum. Toxicol.*, 1985, *4*, 195) have shown that concentrations of free and total hydrazine were significantly higher in slow rather than rapid acetylators. There was also accumulation of free hydrazine in slow acetylators after 2 weeks of administration of isoniazid. While some clinical studies have failed to find any significant effect for acetylator status on isoniazid-induced hepatitis (P. Gurumurthy *et al., Am. Rev. resp. Dis.*, 1984, *129*, 581) others indicate a greater incidence of hepatitis in slow acetylators (D.S. Dickinson *et al., J. clin. Gastroenterol.*, 1981, *3*, 271).

There have been suggestions that the enzyme-inducing ability of rifampicin might affect the rate of formation of hepatotoxic metabolites of isoniazid. Despite evidence of microsomal enzyme induction Timbrell *et al.* (*Hum. Toxicol.*, 1985, *4*, 279) failed to find any significant effect for rifampicin on the metabolism of isoniazid. However, Sarma *et al.* (*Am. Rev. resp. Dis.*, 1986, *133*, 1072) later showed that rifampicin increased the metabolism of isoniazid to isonicotinic acid and hydrazine, the effect being greater in slow rather than rapid acetylators. They considered that the increased formation of hydrazine might explain the higher frequency of hepatitis reported in slow acetylators treated with rifampicin and isoniazid (C. Grönhagen-Riska *et al., Am. Rev. resp. Dis.*, 1978, *118*, 461).

Further references to liver toxicity and isoniazid: J. D. Boice and J. F. Fraumeni, *Am. J. publ. Hlth*, 1980, *70*, 987; R. Parthasarathy *et al., Tubercle*, 1986, *67*, 99.

Hepatotoxicity in children. Although liver enzyme values may be raised in children receiving isoniazid (P. Spyridis *et al., Archs Dis. Childh.*, 1979, *54*, 65) reports of overt hepatotoxicity have been rare (S.H. Walker and J.O. Park-Hah, *J. Pediat.*, 1977, *91*, 344; M.T. Stein, *Pediatrics*, 1979, *64*, 499). Therefore, following anecdotal reports of severe hepatic reactions in infants and children receiving treatment with rifampicin and isoniazid (M. Casteels-Van Daele *et al., J. Pediat.*, 1975, *86*, 739; L. Gutman, *J. antimicrob. Chemother.*, 1978, *4*, 283) the Centers for Disease Control conducted a retrospective study to determine the risk of combined therapy with isoniazid and rifampicin in children (R.J. O'Brien *et al., Pediatrics*, 1983, *72*, 491). A total of 16 hepatotoxic reactions was noted in 874 children treated for tuberculosis between 1977 and 1979. Hepatotoxic reactions occurred in 14 of 430 (3.3%) children treated concurrently with isoniazid and rifampicin. This rate was considered to be comparable to that in adults. As half of the reactions occurred during the first month of therapy and 75% within 10 weeks it was suggested that the frequency of biochemical monitoring could be reduced after the first 2 months. Furthermore, since the risk of hepatotoxicity appeared to be related to the severity of the disease it was considered that if the dose of isoniazid was limited to 10 mg per kg body-weight and that of rifampicin to 15 mg per kg routine monitoring may not be necessary in children with mild disease or normal pre-treatment liver function. Martinez-Roíg *et al.*. (*Pediatrics*, 1986, *77*, 912) have also found that acetylator phenotype appears to have no significant effect on the incidence of hepatotoxicity in children receiving isoniazid with rifampicin.

EFFECTS ON THE NERVOUS SYSTEM. *Convulsions.* Pyridoxine-responsive convulsions occurred in a 17-day-old infant receiving isoniazid 20 mg twice a day (13 mg per kg body-weight daily) from birth. Doses in excess of 10 mg per kg daily are considered to be dangerous.— S. A. McKenzie *et al., Archs Dis. Childh.*, 1976, *51*, 567.

The Boston Collaborative Drug Surveillance Program monitored consecutively 32 812 medical inpatients. Drug-induced convulsions occurred in 1 of 906 patients given isoniazid.— J. Porter and H. Jick, *Lancet*, 1977, *1*, 587. The small number of patients with seizures made it difficult to draw conclusions. Of 3155 patients evaluated in a San Francisco Hospital between 1973 and 1982 for seizures, isoniazid was the causative agent in 10 of the 51 patients with drug-induced seizures.— R. O. Messing *et al., Neurology*, 1984, *34*, 1582.

Epileptiform seizures occurred in 2 patients after a single 300-mg dose of isoniazid and recurred on rechallenge. Desensitisation was tried in one patient but was unsuccessful and administration of pyridoxine 100 mg daily failed to prevent the seizures.— S. K. Gupta *et al., Indian J. Tuberc.*, 1984, *31*, 19.

Encephalopathy. Severe aseptic purulent meningoencephalitis in a 27-year-old man resulted from the prophylactic administration of isoniazid for 3 days, and repeated a few months later for 3 days. He rapidly improved after treatment with methylprednisolone sodium succinate 10 mg every 4 hours intramuscularly and ampicillin sodium 1 g intravenously every 2 hours.— V. F. Garagusi *et al., J. Am. med. Ass.*, 1976, *235*, 1141.

A 38-year-old man in chronic renal failure developed encephalopathy when he was mistakenly given isoniazid 300 mg three times daily. An altered mental status became apparent on the fourth day of treatment. Isoniazid was discontinued and the patient recovered after treatment with pyridoxine and dialysis.— R. L. Gibson and W. J. Stone, *Dialysis Transplant.*, 1979, *8*, 276.

A report of pellagra encephalopathy, undiagnosed clinically and found at necropsy, in patients treated with isoniazid. Pellagra should be suspected whenever patients receiving isoniazid develop mental or neurological symptoms. As isoniazid-induced pellagra responds well to nicotinamide, pyridoxine and nicotinamide should be administered to patients with mental symptoms and the response observed.— N. Ishii and Y. Nishihara, *J. Neurol. Neurosurg. Psychiat.*, 1985, *48*, 628.

EFFECTS ON THE SKIN. Young adults taking isoniazid might develop an acneform syndrome, and pruritus without skin eruption was not unusual. Occasionally urticaria, purpura, and a lupus erythematosus-like syndrome have been reported.— N. Thorne, *Practitioner*, 1973, *211*, 606.

Toxic epidermal necrolysis (Lyell's syndrome) occurred in a pregnant patient given isoniazid and streptomycin for the prophylaxis of pulmonary tuberculosis.— J. Kvasnička *et al., Br. J. Derm.*, 1979, *100*, 551.

Analysis, by the Boston Collaborative Drug Surveillance Program, of data on 15 438 patients hospitalised between 1975 and 1982 detected 1 allergic skin reaction attributed to isoniazid among 180 recipients of the drug.— M. Bigby *et al., J. Am. med. Ass.*, 1986, *256*, 3358.

Further reports of skin and related reactions to isoniazid.— B. S. Bomb *et al., Tubercle*, 1976, *57*, 229 (Stevens-Johnson syndrome); M. A. Rosin and L. E. King, *Sth. med. J.*, 1982, *75*, 81 (exfoliative dermatitis); R. Yamasaki *et al.* (letter), *Br. J. Derm.*, 1985, *112*, 504 (pustular dermatosis).

LUPUS. Antinuclear antibodies have been reported to occur in up to 22% of patients receiving isoniazid for prolonged periods either alone or in combination with other antituberculous agents (A. Cannat and M. Seligmann, *Lancet*, 1966, *1*, 185; N.F. Rothfield *et al., Ann. intern. Med.*, 1978, *88*, 650; 0. Hüscher *et al., ibid.*, *89*, 1011). Although patients are usually asymptomatic there have been rare reports of an overt lupoid syndrome (N. Debeyere *et al., Sem. Hôp. Paris*, 1967, *43*, 3063; M.A. Masel, *Med. J. Aust.*, 1967, *2*, 738; J.H. Greenberg and C.L. Lutcher, *J. Am. med. Ass.*, 1972, *222*, 191). The incidence of antibody induction has been reported to be higher in slow acetylators than in fast acetylators (D. Alarcón-Segovia *et al., Arthritis Rheum.*, 1971, *14*, 748) and Sim *et al.*, (*Lancet*, 1984, *2*, 422) have demonstrated that the syndrome appeared to be due to isoniazid itself rather than its metabolite acetylisoniazid. However, while Weber *et al.* (*Fedn proc.*, 1983, *42*, 3086) concluded, from a review of the literature, that slow acetylators appeared to be more susceptible to drug-induced lupus erythematosus in general others consider that the risk from isoniazid therapy is only slight (D.W.J. Clark, *Drugs*, 1985, *29*, 342).

A 39-year-old man developed a lupoid syndrome after the treatment of tuberculosis with isoniazid and aminosalicylic acid. Pericarditis which progressed to cardiac tamponade was considered to be a complication of the lupoid syndrome. The data was insufficient to determine if one or both agents were responsible for the reaction. However, drug-induced cell positivity has not been encountered in patients taking aminosalicylic acid alone or aminosalicylic acid with other drug combinations, other than isoniazid.— J. H. Greenberg and C. L. Lutcher, *J. Am. med. Ass.*, 1972, *222*, 191.

For a report of pericarditis considered to be due to hypersensitivity to aminosalicylic acid in a patient treated with isoniazid and aminosalicylic acid, see under Effects on the Heart in Sodium Aminosalicylate, p.554.

PELLAGRA. Pellagra, unresponsive to pyridoxine supplementation or therapy, has been reported in individuals with low dietary intakes of tryptophan and nicotinic acid receiving isoniazid (C.I. Harrington, *Practitioner*, 1977, *218*, 716; D.A. Bender and R. Russell-Jones, *Lancet*, 1979, *2*, 1125; R.H.M. Thomas *et al., Br. med. J.*, 1981, *283*, 287). Isoniazid appears to interfere with the conversion of tryptophan to nicotinic acid by inhibiting the action of pyridoxal phosphate. Thomas *et al.* considered that populations with a high prevalence of vegetarian diet and slow acetylator phenotypes, such as Indians, were at particular risk and should be considered for nicotinic acid supplementation.

See also under Effects on the Nervous System, above.

PREGNANCY AND THE NEONATE. There was no difference between isoniazid and placebo in the frequency of conception, birth-rates, sex ratios, or birthweights in a 5-year controlled study of prophylaxis with isoniazid in 2435 male and female patients.— J. Ludford *et al., Am. Rev. resp. Dis.*, 1973, *108*, 1170.

Results from the Collaborative Perinatal Project suggesting an almost twofold increase in the malformation-rate in children exposed to isoniazid (85) or aminosalicylic acid (43) at some time during the first 4 months of the mothers' pregnancy need independent confirmation before conclusions can be made regarding the possible teratogenicity of these drugs.— O. P. Heinonen *et al.*, *Birth Defects and Drugs in Pregnancy*, Littleton MA, Publishing Sciences Group, 1977, p. 296.

See also under Carcinogenicity, p.563, and under Treatment of Tuberculosis, p.548.

Treatment of Adverse Effects

Peripheral neuritis has been treated with pyridoxine hydrochloride; 10 mg daily is the dose recommended in the *UK* for prophylaxis though some authorities have suggested using up to 50 mg daily; a dose of 100 to 200 mg daily has been suggested for treatment if peripheral neuritis develops.

Desensitisation may be attempted following hypersensitivity reactions if the use of isoniazid is considered essential for the provision of adequate chemotherapy (see p.546).

Treatment of overdosage consists of gastric lavage following intubation and the control of convulsions by anticonvulsants given intravenously as well as the intravenous injection of large doses of pyridoxine. Metabolic acidosis is corrected with sodium bicarbonate. Haemodialysis or peritoneal dialysis has been used.

Standal *et al.* (*Am. J. clin. Nutr.*, 1974, *27*, 479) found that pyridoxine 50 mg given daily was adequate to maintain a satisfactory pyridoxine status in patients receiving high dosage therapy with isoniazid; Atkins (*Am. Rev. resp. Dis.*, 1982, *126*, 714) obtained similar results in pregnant patients given 52 to 60 mg. However, neither of these studies tried to determine the minimum dose required and pyridoxine in a dose of 6 mg daily has been shown to prevent peripheral neuropathy in patients receiving isoniazid (Tuberculosis Chemotherapy Centre, Madras, *Bull. Wld Hlth Org.*, 1963, *29*, 457; D.V. Krishnamurthy *et al.*, *ibid.*, 1967, *36*, 853). Some consider that the dosage of pyridoxine should not exceed 10 mg daily as McCune *et al.* (*Am. Rev. Tuberc. pulm. dis.*, 1957, *76*, 1100) have demonstrated that large doses may interfere with the antibacterial activity of isoniazid. However, Riemensnider and Mitchell (*Am. rev. resp. Dis.*, 1960, *82*, 412) found that pyridoxine has no effect on the antibacterial action or serum concentrations of isoniazid. In a review of the use of pyridoxine supplementation in isoniazid therapy Snider (*Tubercle*, 1980, *61*, 191) considered that pyridoxine was not given routinely to all patients probably because peripheral neuropathy occurs infrequently with standard doses of isoniazid and when it does occur it is usually reversible following withdrawal of isoniazid and treatment with pyridoxine 100 to 200 mg daily. However Cawano and Davis (*Drug Intell. & clin. Pharm.*, 1978, *12*, 112 and 297) have warned that pyridoxine is not always effective when peripheral neuropathy has become established. Cost and compliance were considered to be other factors influencing the use of supplementation. Most programmes usually reserved pyridoxine prophylaxis for the following high risk patients: those with nutritional deficiency, especially alcoholics and aged patients, pregnant women, and uraemic and diabetic patients. Snider also considered that pyridoxine should be routinely administered to all patients with a history of seizure disorder who are prescribed isoniazid.

OVERDOSAGE. From a review of the treatment of acute isoniazid toxicity Sievers and Herrier (*Am. J. Hosp. Pharm.*, 1975, *32*, 202) recommended a regimen for the management of isoniazid overdosage based partly on work by Brown (*Am. Rev. resp. Dis.*, 1972, *105*, 206) using pyridoxine given intravenously in a dose of 1 g for each gram of isoniazid estimated to have been ingested. An adequate airway should first be established and gastric lavage performed. Sodium bicarbonate is given as needed to correct metabolic acidosis. Studies in *animals* (L. Chin *et al.*, *Toxic. appl. Pharmac.*, 1978, *45*, 713 and L. Chin *et al.*, *ibid.*, 1981, *58*, 504) suggest that anticonvulsants act synergistically with pyridoxine in antagonising isoniazid-induced convulsions and preventing death from isoniazid overdosage and it has been reported that when required diazepam appears to be the most effective anticonvulsant available. Miller *et al.* (*Am. J. Dis. Child.*, 1980, *134*, 290) considered that the use of phenytoin should be avoided in isoniazid poisoning because of the potential for interaction. Patients asymptomatic after isoniazid overdosage should be observed for at least 4 hours and pyridoxine should be administered intravenously as early as possible even if seizures have not occurred. All patients should initially receive 5 g of pyridoxine administered over a period of 3 to 5 minutes and repeated at 5 to 20 minute intervals until the dose greatly exceeds that of isoniazid, the seizures cease, or consciousness is regained. If the estimated amount of isoniazid ingested exceeds 200 mg per kg body-weight it may be desirable to administer 5 g of pyridoxine as an infusion over 2 hours repeated as necessary. Wason *et al.* (*J. Am. med. Ass.*, 1981, *246*, 1102) reported that seizures were controlled and the depth of coma was reduced within 2 hours if the total dose of pyridoxine was administered in a single dose given over 30 to 60 minutes by intravenous infusion. Pyridoxine also appears to control acidosis unresponsive to sodium bicarbonate. However, Schaumburg (*New Engl. J. med.*, 1984, *310*, 198) considers that such high-dose treatment should be undertaken with caution as studies in *animals* have shown that large doses of pyridoxine can have adverse effects on dorsal root ganglion cells.

Some workers have found forced diuresis to be of use (Brown 1972). Haemodialysis and peritoneal dialysis have also been tried in the treatment of isoniazid overdosage but it is considered by some (W.M. Cameron, *Can. med. Ass. J.*, 1978, *118*, 1413) that if adequate treatment with pyridoxine is given there is little indication for their use. Glogner *et al.* (*Dt. med. Wschr.*, 1971, *96*, 1307) found that more isoniazid was excreted via the kidneys than was removed by dialysis and recommended that dialysis should only be used in patients who have ingested more than 5 g or in those with impaired renal function. Königshausen *et al.* (*Vet. hum. Toxicol.*, 1979, *21*, *Suppl.*, 12) have reported on the use of haemoperfusion in one patient. A study by Scolding *et al.* (*Hum. Toxicol.*, 1986, *5*, 285) indicated that activated charcoal was unlikely to be of value if given more than one hour after overdosage and its use should not replace the need for specific treatment with pyridoxine.

A patient who took rifampicin 9 g, ethambutol 20 g, and isoniazid 6 g made an uneventful recovery after haemodialysis and treatment with pyridoxine.— J. Ducobu *et al.* (letter), *Lancet*, 1982, *1*, 632.

Precautions

Isoniazid should not be given to patients who have experienced severe adverse reactions to it including drug-induced liver disease. Care should be taken in giving isoniazid to patients suffering from convulsive disorders, diabetes mellitus, chronic alcoholism, or impaired liver or kidney function or to patients taking other potentially hepatotoxic agents. If symptoms of hepatitis such as malaise, fatigue, anorexia, and nausea develop isoniazid should be discontinued immediately.

There may be an increased risk of liver damage in patients receiving rifampicin and isoniazid but liver enzymes are generally raised only transiently.

Some patients, particularly those at risk from peripheral neuropathies, may require additional treatment with pyridoxine (see under Treatment of Adverse Effects). It has also been suggested that supplements of vitamin D may be indicated for patients at risk of developing metabolic bone disease (see below).

Isoniazid is an inhibitor of hepatic drug-metabolism and may therefore enhance the effects of some drugs taken concomitantly. Inhibition of metabolism may be sufficient with some drugs to produce toxic concentrations and adverse reactions have occurred when isoniazid has been given with antiepileptics such as phenytoin, primidone, carbamazepine, and ethosuximide. However, there have been reports that isoniazid increases the metabolism of some drugs, see below.

Death due to fulminant hepatitis occurred in an epileptic patient receiving phenobarbitone and other anticonvulsant agents, 9 days after starting antituberculous therapy with isoniazid and rifampicin and 7 days after receiving halothane anaesthesia during thoracotomy. The risk of hepatotoxicity from isoniazid is increased when given with drugs that induce microsomal enzymes.— A. K. M. Bartelink *et al.*, *Tubercle*, 1983, *64*, 125.

If antituberculous therapy is to be given on a daily, thrice-or twice-weekly basis, there is no need to determine the patients' acetylator phenotypes prior to treatment, even in patients with renal failure. Phenotype assessment is unlikely to be of value in establishing whether side-effects during treatment are due to isoniazid or not. Furthermore, simple tests for compliance (see below) can be of value in the management of patients who fail to respond to potentially effective regimens despite indications that the tubercle bacilli are still sensitive to isoniazid.— G. A. Ellard, *Tubercle*, 1984, *65*, 211.

Studies have shown that 10 to 20% of persons receiving isoniazid will develop some mild abnormalities of liver function values usually within the first 6 months of treatment. In most patients these abnormalities tend to resolve even if isoniazid is continued and only occasionally do progressive liver damage and clinical hepatitis occur. It is not recommended that liver function tests be performed routinely to monitor preventive therapy for individuals younger than 35 years of age but because of the higher frequency of isoniazid-associated hepatitis in persons older than this, serum transaminase values should be obtained before and periodically during the course of therapy in persons older than 35 years of age. If any of these tests exceed 3 to 5 times the normal upper limit, discontinuation of isoniazid should be strongly considered. Liver function tests are not a substitute for monthly clinical evaluations.—Joint statement: American Thoracic Society and Centers for Disease Control, *Am. Rev. resp. Dis.*, 1986, *134*, 355.

Concern was expressed about the effects of antituberculous therapy on calcium and vitamin D metabolism when in a series of studies Brodie *et al.* found that rifampicin (*Clin. Pharmac. Ther.*, 1980, *27*, 810; *Br. J. clin. Pharmac.*, 1980, *9*, 286P) and isoniazid (*Clin. Pharmac. Ther.*, 1981, *30*, 363; *Br. J. clin. Pharmac.*, 1981, *11*, 422P) reduced serum concentrations of 25-hydroxycholecalciferol. Isoniazid appeared to have a different mechanism of action to rifampicin as it also reduced serum concentrations of calcium and 1,25-dihydroxycholecalciferol and increased concentrations of parathyroid hormone. In a later study (*Clin. Pharmac. Ther.*, 1982, *32*, 525; *Br. J. clin. Pharmac.*, 1982, *14*, 144P) Brodie *et al.* found that the effect of combination therapy with rifampicin and isoniazid appeared to be less than either drug used alone. Osteomalacia had already been reported in an Indian patient receiving therapy with rifampicin and ethambutol (S.C. Shah *et al.*, *Tubercle*, 1981, *62*, 207) and a hypocalcaemic effect had been noted in a study of a 6-month antituberculous regimen containing isoniazid and rifampicin (British Thoracic Association, *Br. J. Dis. Chest.*, 1981, *75*, 141). Patients most often affected appeared to be mainly Asian or to be already suffering from osteomalacia. Perry *et al.* (*J. R. Soc. Med.*, 1982, *75*, 533) considered that 18 months of antituberculous therapy with isoniazid and rifampicin had no significant effect on calcium metabolism and Williams *et al.* (*Tubercle*, 1985, *66*, 49) came to a similar conclusion after a study of a 9-month regimen. Perry *et al.* concluded that if there was a clinical effect it was a small one and in relation to osteomalacia in patients at risk, such as Asians, it could be adequately overcome by daily administration of 900 units of ergocalciferol. However, Brodie and Hillyard (*J. R. Soc. med.*, 1982, *75*, 919) stated that the data did not support Perry *et al.*'s conclusion that the effect was insignificant. Davis *et al.* (*Tubercle*, 1985, *66*, 151) also criticised the lack of matched control subjects and any reference to seasonal variations during treatment in the study by Williams *et al.* (1985). On the other hand Davis *et al.* considered that the effect was important as they had found in a controlled study of the effects of a 9-month antituberculous regimen containing isoniazid and rifampicin (*Thorax*, 1985, *40*, 197) that concentrations of 25-hydroxycholecalciferol were maintained at a low level in patients who had low pre-treatment concentrations and that seasonal rises were suppressed. They considered that patients with very low serum concentrations of 25-hydroxycholecalciferol, such as those of Asian descent, who had received prolonged antituberculous therapy may be at risk of developing metabolic bone diseases.

EFFECT ON DRIVING. Administration of 750 mg of isoniazid (about 10 mg per kg body-weight) affected skills connected with driving.— M. Linnoila and M. J. Mattila, *J. clin. Pharmac.*, 1973, *13*, 343.

INTERACTIONS. Although isoniazid appears to have some monoamine oxidase inhibiting activity, reports of interactions of the type associated with the 'classical' monoamine oxidase inhibitors (see Phenelzine, p.378) have been rare.

Alcohol. The metabolism of isoniazid may be increased and its clinical effect reduced in some patients with chronic alcohol abuse.— *Med. Lett.*, 1981, *23*, 33.

Antacids. Aluminium hydroxide mixture delayed and depressed the absorption of isoniazid. It is recommended that isoniazid be given at least 1 hour before the antacid.— A. Hurwitz and D. L. Schlozman, *Am. Rev. resp. Dis.*, 1974, *109*, 41.

Anticoagulants. For a reference to isoniazid enhancing the effect of warfarin, see Warfarin Sodium, p.345.

Antimycobacterial agents. Plasma concentrations of isoniazid were increased and its half-life extended when it was given concomitantly by mouth with aminosalicylic acid. The effect was more pronounced among rapid inactivators.— G. Boman *et al.*, *Acta pharmac. tox.*, 1970, *28, Suppl.* 1, 15.

For a report of the additive CNS toxicity of isoniazid and cycloserine used together, see under Precautions in Cycloserine, p.557.

Benzodiazepines. Studies by Ochs *et al.* (*Clin. Pharmac. Ther.*, 1981, *29*, 671 and *Br. J. clin. Pharmac.*, 1983, *16*, 743) have shown that isoniazid prolongs the half-life of diazepam and triazolam but appears to have no effect on the pharmacokinetics of oxazepam.

Corticosteroids. Administration of prednisolone 20 mg to 13 slow acetylators and 13 fast acetylators receiving isoniazid 10 mg per kg body-weight reduced plasma concentrations of isoniazid by 25 and 40% respectively. The renal clearance of isoniazid was also enhanced in both acetylator phenotypes and the rate of acetylation increased in slow acetylators only. Although rifampicin 12 mg per kg body-weight had no effect on the biodisposition of isoniazid, when prednisolone was given with rifampicin to the same patients receiving isoniazid, plasma concentrations of isoniazid were only reduced by 15% in slow acetylators while there was no significant effect in rapid acetylators. However, since response to antituberculous regimens containing corticosteroids had been excellent, it was considered that these decreases in isoniazid plasma concentrations may not be of therapeutic significance unless smaller doses of isoniazid are being used.— G. R. Sarma *et al.*, *Antimicrob. Ag. Chemother.*, 1980, *18*, 661.

Disulfiram. In 1969 Whittington and Grey (*Am. J. Psychiat.*, 1969, *125*, 1725) reported that 7 alcoholic patients with tuberculosis who were receiving isoniazid showed changes in behaviour and coordination when treatment with disulfiram was started. The numbers affected constituted less than a third of the total number of patients given both drugs. Interference with dopamine metabolism in the CNS by both isoniazid and disulfiram was proposed as a possible cause of the effects. Although Whittington and Grey discounted the possible role of chlordiazepoxide being taken by some of the patients (they reproduced the effects in a further 4 patients receiving only isoniazid), it has been shown that disulfiram can inhibit the metabolism of chlordiazepoxide (E.M. Sellers *et al.*, *Clin. Pharmac. Ther.*, 1977, *21*, 117; S.M. MacLeod, *ibid.*, 1978, *24*, 583). Rothstein (*J. Am. med. Ass.*, 1972, *219*, 1216) has reported a patient with chronic alcoholism who received rifampicin, isoniazid, disulfiram and later chlordiazepoxide without signs of an interaction.

Enflurane. For a report suggesting that isoniazid might enhance the toxicity of enflurane by increasing metabolism to inorganic fluoride, see p.1115.

Food. Adverse reactions have been reported during therapy with isoniazid after ingestion of certain types of food rich in tyramine including: cheese (C.K. Smith and D.T. Durack, *Ann. intern. Med.*, 1978, *88*, 520; J.L. Lejonc *et al.*, *ibid.*, 1979, *91*, 793; C.G. Uragoda and S.C. Lodha, *Tubercle*, 1979, *60*, 59), red wine (M.J. Hauser and H. Baier, *Drug. Intell. & clin. Pharm.*, 1982, *16*, 617; M. Toutoungi *et al.*, *Lancet*, 1985, *2*, 671) and certain types of fish with a high histamine content including skipjack fish (N. Senanayake *et al.*, *Br. med. J.*, 1978, *2*, 1127; C.G. Uragoda and S.R. Kottegoda, *Tubercle*, 1977, *58*, 83), tuna fish (C.G. Uragoda, *Am. Rev. resp. Dis.*, 1980, *121*, 157), other scombroid fish and certain other tropical species. It has become standard practice in some countries to instruct patients receiving isoniazid to exclude these from their diets. Symptoms have been somewhat similar after each type of food and commonly include palpitations, skin flushing, headache, conjunctival irritation, and itching. The patient reported by Senanayake *et al.* also experienced a cerebrovascular accident. Although isoniazid inhibits monoamine and diamine oxidases, Hauser and Baier considered that since some cheeses contain both tyramine and histamine it remained to be determined whether these adverse effects were due to the potentiation of the effects of tyramine or histamine.

All types of food, especially those containing carbohydrates, significantly impaired the absorption of isoniazid in both slow and rapid acetylators. Isoniazid should be taken on an empty stomach.— P. Männisto *et al.*, *J. antimicrob. Chemother.*, 1982, *10*, 427. See also A. Melander *et al.*, *Acta med. scand.*, 1976, *200*, 93.

Ketoconazole. For a report of failure of antifungal and antituberculous therapy resulting from reduced concentrations of rifampicin and ketoconazole in a patient receiving ketoconazole, rifampicin, and isoniazid, see under Precautions in Ketoconazole, p.427.

Levodopa. A hypertensive reaction and severe tremor occurred when isoniazid was given to a patient receiving levodopa; it was not known whether isoniazid was acting as a monoamine oxidase inhibitor.— J. P. Morgan (letter), *Ann. intern. Med.*, 1980, *92*, 434.

Oral contraceptives. There is little clinical evidence to support the view that isoniazid may impair the efficacy of oral contraceptives.— *Drug Interact. News.*, 1983, *3*, 7.

Pethidine. A patient receiving antituberculous therapy which included isoniazid became hypotensive and lethargic 20 minutes after an intramuscular injection of pethidine. The reaction may have been due to isoniazid acting experimental evidence of porphyrinogenicity.— M. R. *al.* (letter), *Ann. intern. Med.*, 1983, *99*, 415.

Propranolol. The clearance of isoniazid was significantly reduced in 6 healthy subjects by pretreatment with propranolol 40 mg given three times daily for 3 days. The mechanism of the interaction was unknown but was unlikely to be an effect on liver-blood flow.— B. Santoso, *Int. J. clin. Pharmac. Ther. Toxic.*, 1985, *23*, 134.

Sodium salicylate. The half-life of isoniazid was shortened by sodium salicylate, and its antimicrobial action *in vitro* was antagonised when concentrations of isoniazid were low.— M. J. Mattila *et al.*, *Arzneimittel-Forsch.*, 1972, *22*, 1769.

PORPHYRIA. Isoniazid was considered to be unsafe in patients with acute porphyria although there is conflicting experimental evidence of porphyrinogenicity.— M.R. Moore and K.E.L. McColl, *Porphyrias, Drug Lists*, Glasgow, Porphyria Research Unit, University of Glasgow, 1987.

PREGNANCY AND THE NEONATE. The use of isoniazid is considered to be safe during pregnancy provided that pyridoxine is given simultaneously (R.B. Cole, *Prescribers' J.*, 1985, *25*, 110). See also under Treatment of Tuberculosis, p.548.

Isoniazid is excreted into breast milk in significant amounts. Snider and Powell (*Archs intern. Med.*, 1984, *144*, 589) have estimated that a breast-fed infant of a mother receiving isoniazid would ingest about 6 to 20% of the usual therapeutic dose for an infant. Because of the risk of neurotoxicity it has been recommended that nursing mothers and breast-fed infants should receive prophylactic treatment with pyridoxine (*Drug & Ther. Bull.*, 1983, *21*, 5). For further precautions to be taken by nursing mothers receiving antituberculous therapy, see under Treatment of Tuberculosis, p.548.

Although isoniazid has been shown to be non-clastogenic, combinations of isoniazid with thiacetazone or aminosalicylic acid, with or without streptomycin have been found to increase lymphocyte chromosome damage in patients with tuberculosis when compared with untreated healthy subjects (M. Jaju *et al.*, *Hum. Genet.*, 1983, *64*, 42). However, Goulding (*Hum. Toxicol.*, 1985, *4*, 221) considered that the significance to humans of these chromosome changes had not been proven and that the advice to avoid these combinations was unreasonable and needed qualifying. Jaju (*Hum. Toxicol.*, 1985, *4*, 222) pointed out that several other equally effective combinations of antituberculous agents had been shown to be non-clastogenic in humans and since the chromosomal damage appeared to be transient, conception need only be avoided during therapy.

See also under Adverse Effects, above and Absorption and Fate, below.

Antimicrobial Action and Resistance

Isoniazid is highly active against *Mycobacterium tuberculosis* which it inhibits *in vitro* at concentrations of 0.02 to 0.2 µg per mL. In tuberculous patients it has some activity against both intracellular and extracellular bacilli. Although it is rapidly bactericidal against actively dividing organisms it is considered to be only bacteriostatic against semi-dormant organisms and has less sterilising activity than rifampicin or pyrazinamide. Isoniazid appears to be highly effective in preventing emergence of resistance to other antituberculous agents (see also p.546). Isoniazid may have activity against some strains of other mycobacteria including *M. kansasii*.

Although the incidence of primary drug resistance is generally low in developed countries mycobacteria rapidly become resistant to isoniazid used alone. For this reason it is usually given in conjunction with other antituberculous drugs, except in prophylaxis.

For further information see p.546.

Absorption and Fate

Isoniazid is readily absorbed from the gastro-intestinal tract. Peak concentrations appear in blood 1 to 2 hours after a dose by mouth. Isoniazid is not considered to be bound appreciably to plasma proteins and diffuses into all body tissues and fluids, including the cerebrospinal fluid; it appears in foetal blood if given during pregnancy and in the milk of nursing mothers.

Elimination of isoniazid from the body is dependent on the rate of acetylation. In patients with normal renal function 70% or more of a dose appears in the urine in 24 hours, partly unchanged but mainly as metabolites. The primary metabolic route is the acetylation of isoniazid to acetylisoniazid by *N*-acetyltransferase found in the liver and small intestine. Acetylisoniazid is then hydrolysed to isonicotinic acid and monoacetylhydrazine; isonicotinic acid is conjugated with glycine to isonicotinyl glycine (isonicotinuric acid) and monoacetylhydrazine further acetylated to diacetylhydrazine. Some unacetylated isoniazid is also conjugated to hydrazones. The metabolites of isoniazid have no tuberculostatic activity and apart possibly from monoacetylhydrazine they are also less toxic. The rate of acetylation of isoniazid and monoacetylhydrazine is genetically determined and there is a bimodal distribution of persons who acetylate them either slowly or rapidly. Various ethnic groups, especially Eskimos, Japanese, and Chinese, are predominantly rapid acetylators whereas in populations of Caucasians, Negroes, and Indians (Madras), proportions of slow and rapid acetylators are similar. Rapid acetylators have been reported to acetylate isoniazid about 5 times more rapidly than slow acetylators. The half-life of isoniazid has been reportd to be 0.5 to 1.5 hours in rapid acetylators and 2 or more hours in slow acetylators.

Although rapid acetylators of isoniazid have relatively low serum concentrations of free drug and excrete a smaller proportion of free isoniazid in the urine than do slow acetylators, therapeutic efficacy appears only to be affected in patients on intermittent treatment regimens given once weekly.

A review of the clinical pharmacokinetics of isoniazid.— W. W. Weber and D. W. Hein, *Clin. Pharmacokinet.*, 1979, *4*, 401.

Pharmacokinetic studies of isoniazid in neonates and children.— W. A. Olson *et al.*, *Pharmacologist*, 1976, *18*, 153; *idem*, *Pediatrics*, 1981, *67*, 876; J. N. Miceli *et al.*, *Develop. Pharmac. Ther.*, 1981, *2*, 235; *idem*, *Fedn Proc.*, 1983, *42*, 1140.

A study in 20 healthy subjects indicated that the elimination pharmacokinetics of isoniazid are dose-dependent within the therapeutic dose range.— B. Santoso and M. D. Rawlins, *Br. J. clin. Pharmac.*, 1983, *15*, 137P.

Pharmacokinetic studies of slow-release preparations of isoniazid which have been developed in an attempt to maintain therapeutic blood concentrations in rapid acetylators after once-weekly intermittent therapy for tuberculosis.— G. A. Ellard *et al.*, *Lancet*, 1972, *1*, 340; G. A. Ellard *et al.*, *Tubercle*, 1973, *54*, 57; L. Eidus *et al.*, *Am. Rev. resp. Dis.*, 1974, *110*, 34; L. Eidus and M. M. Hodgkin, *Arzneimittel-Forsch.*, 1975, *25*, 1077; G. R. Sarma *et al.*, *Tubercle*, 1975, *56*, 314; G. A. Ellard, *Bull. int. Un. Tuberc.*, 1976, *51*, 144; M. M. Hodgkin and B. Eidus, *ibid.*, 1979, *54*, 55; M. M. Hodgkin *et al.*, *Res. Commun. chem. Path. Pharmac.*, 1979, *24*, 349.

ABSORPTION. For the effect of food and of aluminium hydroxide mixture on the absorption of isoniazid, see Precautions above.

DIFFUSION. *Into cerebrospinal fluid.* Mean cerebrospinal fluid concentrations of isoniazid in a patient with tuberculous meningitis were 2 µg per mL 3 to 6 hours after doses of 600 mg by mouth and were about 90% of concentrations found in the serum.— R. Forgan-Smith *et al.* (letter), *Lancet*, 1973, *2*, 374. Concentrations of isoniazid in the serum and CSF of a child were 4.0 and 4.4 µg per mL respectively, 9 hours after administration of isoniazid 5.9 mg per kg body-weight.— J. N. Miceli *et al.*, *Fedn Proc.*, 1983, *42*, 1140.

Into joints. Therapeutic concentrations of isoniazid have been obtained in synovial fluid.— D. Mouries *et al.*, *Nouv. Presse méd.*, 1975, *4*, 2734.

Into saliva. Therapeutic drug monitoring in saliva including details of studies on saliva-isoniazid concentrations.— M. Danhof and D. D. Breimer, *Clin. Pharmacokinet.*, 1978, *3*, 39.

EFFECTS OF DISEASE STATES. Children with Down's syndrome had higher serum concentrations of isoniazid than control children given the same dose. The difference was probably due to a defect in acetylation in children with Down's syndrome.— R. Turpin *et al.* (letter), *Lancet*, 1967, *2*, 1369.

METABOLISM. Evidence for a trimodal pattern of acetylation of isoniazid in uraemic patients who were classified as slow, intermediate, or rapid acetylators.— D. J. Chapron *et al.*, *J. pharm. Sci.*, 1978, *67*, 1018.

For the effect that acetylator phenotype has on the incidence of hepatotoxicity in patients taking isoniazid, see p.564.

Determination of acetylator phenotype. Isoniazid has been the drug traditionally used to determine acetylator phenotype and although Ellard and Gammon (*Br. J. clin. Pharmac.*, 1977, *4*, 5) found isoniazid and sulphadimidine to be equally accurate some (G.A. Ellard, *Tubercle*, 1984, *65*, 211; W.W. Weber and D.W. Hein, *Pharmac. Rev.*, 1985, *37*, 25) now consider that when available sulphadimidine is more convenient to use. Procedures have been based on determination of isoniazid and/or acetylisoniazid in plasma or urine or on the rate of elimination of isoniazid from plasma. Determinations were originally performed from plasma samples after intravenous or oral administration but various methods have been developed since to determine the phenotype from urine samples after administration intravenously (G.A. Ellard *et al.*, *Tubercle*, 1973, *54*, 201), intramuscularly (P. Venkataraman *et al.*, *Tubercle*, 1972, *53*, 84), or by mouth (L. Eidus *et al.*, *Bull. Wld Hlth Org.*, 1973, *49*, 507). Ellard *et al.* (*Tubercle*, 1973, *54*, 57) have also described a method suitable for use with slow-release matrix isoniazid. A sensitive fluorometric assay has been developed by Scott *et al.*, (*J. clin. Invest.*, 1969, *48*, 1173) and further modified by Miceli *et al.*, (*Biochem. Med.*, 1975, *12*, 348) to improve its sensitivity for use in determining the acetylator status of neonates.

Distribution of acetylator phenotypes. The incidence of rapid acetylators of isoniazid varies according to the racial and geographic origins of populations and is particularly high in some Far Eastern populations. Reports range from an incidence of about 95% in Canadian Eskimos to 20% or less in Egyptians and certain Jewish groups.— W. W. Weber and D. W. Hein, *Clin. Pharmacokinet.*, 1979, *4*, 401.

PREGNANCY AND THE NEONATE. Isoniazid has been shown to reach the foetus within 15 minutes of administration by mouth. Foetal blood concentrations might exceed maternal blood concentrations of isoniazid. The possibility of adverse effects on the central nervous system from prolonged exposure of the foetus to isoniazid should be considered.— F. Moya and V. Thorndike, *Am. J. Obstet. Gynec.*, 1962, *84*, 1778.

Excretion in breast milk. In a study of 3 lactating mothers Ricci and Copaitich (*Rass. Clin. Ter.*, 1954, *53*, 209) reported that peak concentrations of isoniazid in breast milk were about 5.5 and 10.6 µg per mL 3 hours after administration of 300- and 600-mg doses respectively. However, in a later study of one mother conducted by Berlin and Lee (*Fedn Proc.*, 1979, *38*, 426) a peak concentration of 16.6 µg per mL was obtained in breast milk 3 hours after a 300-mg dose of isoniazid. Berlin and Lee also reported that peak concentrations of the acetyl metabolite of 3.76 µg per mL were obtained in breast milk after 5 hours. Concentrations of isoniazid were twice those in plasma at 5 and 12 hours and were still detectable after 24 hours. From these 2 studies Snider and Powell (*Archs intern. Med.*, 1984, *144*, 589) estimated that a breast-fed infant of a mother receiving isoniazid would ingest about 6 to 20% of the usual therapeutic dose for an infant.

Uses and Administration

Isoniazid is a hydrazide derivative which is still the mainstay of primary treatment of pulmonary and extrapulmonary tuberculosis. It is administered in a variety of regimens with other antituberculous agents as described under Treatment of Tuberculosis, p.547. Isoniazid is also used in high risk subjects for the prophylaxis of tuberculosis. Pyridoxine is often given in conjunction with isoniazid to avert its neurotoxicity (see under Treatment of Adverse Effects).

The usual dose of isoniazid in tuberculosis is 5 mg per kg body-weight daily given by mouth in single or divided doses to a maximum of 300 mg daily; up to 10 mg per kg daily may be given particularly during the first few weeks of treatment of tuberculous meningitis. A dose of 15 mg per kg has been given twice weekly in intermittent treatment regimens. Once-weekly administration has also been tried but may be less effective in patients who are rapid acetylators of isoniazid. Slow-release preparations of isoniazid have also been used in such regimens in an attempt to achieve sustained therapeutic concentrations, especially in patients who are rapid acetylators of isoniazid. Recommendations on the dosage of isoniazid for children vary. In the *UK* a dose of 6 mg per kg daily has been recommended whereas in the *US* doses of 10 to 20 mg per kg, up to a maximum of 500 mg have been used.

Similar doses to those used orally may be given by intramuscular injection when isoniazid cannot be taken by mouth; it may also be given intravenously. Although it is distributed into the CSF on oral administration, isoniazid has sometimes been given intrathecally in doses of 25 to 50mg daily for adults and 10 to 20 mg daily for children to supplement treatment by mouth. Doses of 50 to 250 mg have been instilled intrapleurally after the removal of pus.

In tuberculosis prophylaxis, daily doses of 300 mg have usually been given for up to 1 year, although shorter courses of isoniazid, given either alone or in combination with ethambutol, have also been recommended (see under Prophylaxis of Tuberculosis, p.547). The prophylactic dose for children is 5 to 10 mg per kg daily to a maximum of 300 mg daily in single or divided doses.

Tuberculin testing after treatment with isoniazid has produced variable results. While some workers have reported that positive reactions have reverted to negative, Hsu (*Am. J. Dis. Child.*, 1983, *137*, 1090) found in 221 children followed-up for 3 to 10 years that, although there may be some fluctuation in intensity, reversion to negative was rare. Tager *et al.*, (*Am. Rev. resp. Dis.*, 1985, *131*, 214) have also reported that some reactions that have reverted to negative may later become positive. Hsu considered the persistence of a positive tuberculin reaction to be an asset since with the risk of endogenous disease removed by treatment, the patient gains cell-mediated immunity to protect against future exogenous re-infections.

ADMINISTRATION. After a review of several controlled clinical studies of intermittent antituberculous chemotherapy using isoniazid Ellard (*Tubercle*, 1984, *65*, 211) concluded that the effect of isoniazid acetylator phenotype on therapeutic outcome was only of importance if isoniazid was administered once-weekly as rapid acetylators then responded less satisfactorily. Such regimens were considered to be unsuitable for general use, especially in populations with predominantly rapid acetylators. However, a study in Czechoslovakia (WHO Collaborating Centre for Tuberculosis Chemotherapy, Prague *Tubercle*, 1977, *58*, 129) indicated that slow acetylators could be given isoniazid once-weekly in the continuation phase while rapid acetylators could receive isoniazid twice weekly.

For pharmacokinetic studies of slow-release isoniazid preparations developed in an attempt to overcome low concentrations in rapid acetylators and further references to acetylator status, see Absorption and Fate.

ADMINISTRATION IN THE ELDERLY. While some studies have found no significant differences between the pharmacokinetic parameters for isoniazid in young and elderly patients (F. Farah *et al.*, *Br. med. J.*, 1977, *2*, 155; C. Advenier *et al.*, *Br. J. clin. Pharmac.*, 1980, *10*, 167) results of a study by Pilheu (*Bull. int. Un. Tuberc.*, 1986, *61*, 109) suggest that isoniazid and rifampicin may be given to elderly patients with tuberculosis in reduced dosage without loss of efficacy. However, confirmation with clinical evidence is needed. This effect may only be significant for isoniazid in slow acetylators (M.F. Kergueris *et al.*, *Thérapie*, 1986, *41*, 19).

ADMINISTRATION IN GASTRO-INTESTINAL DISORDERS. Results suggesting that adequate serum concentrations can be reliably obtained in patients with jejuno-ileal bypass after a dose of isoniazid of 300 mg.— R. E. Polk *et al.* (letter), *Ann. intern. Med.*, 1978, *89*, 430. See also T. M. Griffiths *et al.*, *Br. J. Dis. Chest*, 1982, *76*, 286.

ADMINISTRATION IN INFANTS AND CHILDREN. Some authorities recommend higher doses of isoniazid for children than for adults. However, serum concentrations achieved in some preliminary studies on the pharmacokinetics of isoniazid in children suggest that the use of different dosages is not justified (I. Miceli *et al.*, *Bull. int. Un. Tuberc.*, 1986, *61*, 109; J.T. Steensma *et al.*, *ibid.*, 110). Steensma also considered that because isoniazid had excellent penetration through the uninflamed or inflamed meninges doses should not exceed 10 mg per kg body-weight even in the treatment of meningitis. Miceli *et al.* (*Fedn Proc.*, 1983, *42*, 1140) found wide inter-individual variations in absorption, serum concentrations, and elimination half-life in children and recommended that serum concentrations should be monitored in children to avoid potential toxicity and to maintain concentrations in the therapeutic range. Paire *et al.* (*Thérapie*, 1984, *39*, 625) have devised a method for calculating isoniazid dosage in children, that is based on the inactivation index, and consider it to be easier to use and more suitable than using the acetylator phenotype.

For neonates McKenzie *et al.* (*Archs Dis. Childh.*, 1976, *51*, 567) also consider that doses greater than 10 mg per kg body-weight are dangerous. Peonides (*Archs Dis. Childh.*, 1977, *52*, 165) has suggested that a daily dose of 3 to 5 mg per kg might be suitable for the first two months of life.

O'Brien *et al.* (*Pediatrics*, 1983, *72*, 491) from the Centers for Disease Control recommend that to minimise the risk of hepatotoxic reactions when isoniazid and rifampicin are used together in children the dose of isoniazid should be limited to 10 mg per kg and that of rifampicin to 15 mg per kg.

See also under Tuberculosis Prophylaxis, below.

ADMINISTRATION IN LIVER DISEASE. In patients with chronic active liver disease requiring absolutely necessary prophylaxis with isoniazid, serum aspartate aminotransferase concentrations should be monitored weekly and treatment stopped if any rise in concentration persists for longer than 4 weeks or if other signs of toxicity develop.— R. K. Roberts *et al.*, *Drugs*, 1979, *17*, 198.

Isoniazid dosage may require adjustment in patients with acute or chronic liver disease.— M. R. Holdiness, *Clin. Pharmacokinet.*, 1984, *9*, 511.

See also under Precautions, above.

ADMINISTRATION IN MALNUTRITION. Buchanan *et al.* (*S. Afr. med. J.*, 1979, *56*, 299) found that the half-life of isoniazid in children with kwashiorkor was significantly reduced as nutritional status improved. They considered that the effect was probably not significant in children receiving divided daily doses but a dosage adjustment may be required in malnourished adults receiving a once daily dosage. Thom *et al.* (*Br. J. clin. Pharmac.*, 1981, *11*, 423P) demonstrated a similar effect in healthy adults after administration of glucose.

ADMINISTRATION IN RENAL FAILURE. From the results of a controlled study of 10 patients with chronic renal failure, the recommended daily dosage of isoniazid for patients with a serum-creatinine concentration less than 120 µg per mL was 300 mg. Patients with more severe renal failure who were rapid acetylators would need no reduction but in slow acetylators the dose should be reduced so that serum-isoniazid concentrations were less than 1 µg per mL 24 hours after the preceding dose. Doses would seldom need to be reduced to less than 200 mg daily.— D. W. Bowersox *et al.*, *New Engl. J. Med.*, 1973, *289*, 84.

The normal half-life for isoniazid of 2 to 4 hours in slow acetylators and of 0.5 and 1.5 in rapid acetylators was increased to 10 and 2 hours respectively in end-stage renal failure. Patients with a glomerular filtration-rate of less than 10 mL per minute might require a reduction in the dose to between 66 and 75% of the normal dose. A dose supplement should be given to patients undergoing haemodialysis or peritoneal dialysis.— W. M. Bennett *et al.*, *Am. J. Kidney Dis.*, 1983, *3*, 155.

Studies have shown that the half-life of isoniazid is only increased by about 30% (in slow acetylators) in the event of almost complete renal failure reflecting the small amount of unmetabolised isoniazid normally excreted in the urine. Such an increase is unlikely to result in significantly elevated toxicity, and dosage reduction is unnecessary and could lead to ineffective treatment. There is also no reason to determine the patients' acetylator phenotype.— G. A. Ellard, *Tubercle*, 1984, *65*, 211.

Further references: M. M. Reidenberg *et al.*, *Am. Rev. resp. Dis.*, 1973, *108*, 1426; C. H. Gold *et al.*, *Clin. Nephrol.*, 1976, *6*, 365.

See also under Treatment of Tuberculosis, p.548.

ATYPICAL MYCOBACTERIAL INFECTIONS. For the use of isoniazid and other antimycobacterial agents in the treatment of atypical mycobacterial infections, see p.553.

COMPLIANCE MARKER. Isoniazid has been suggested as a

marker for compliance testing in patients receiving antileprotic chemotherapy (J.N.A. Stanley *et al.*, *Lepr. Rev.*, 1983, *54*, 317; *idem.*, 1986, *57*, 9) and psychiatic patients receiving psychotropic drugs (S.R. Bazire, *Pharm. J.*, 1985, *1*, 95; *ibid.*, *2*, 473).

LEISHMANIASIS. For reports of beneficial effects with rifampicin and isoniazid in some patients with leishmaniasis, see Rifampicin, p.576.

LEPROSY. For references to a favourable report on the use of a preparation containing dapsone, isoniazid, and prothionamide (Isoprodian) concurrently with rifampicin, see under Treatment of Leprosy, p.552.

NERVOUS SYSTEM DISORDERS. Isoniazid given in large doses has been shown to increase brain concentrations of gamma-aminobutyric acid (GABA) and it has therefore been tried in the treatment of various neurological disorders which may be due to deficiency of this neurotransmitter.

Chorea. In 1979 Perry *et al.* (*Neurology*, 1979, *29*, 370) reported that a slight to marked improvement had been obtained in 5 of 6 patients with Huntington's chorea. But when Perry *et al.* (*Neurology*, 1982, *32*, 354) conducted a double-blind placebo controlled crossover study they found that despite increased GABA concentrations in CSF only 1 of 9 patients improved after 4 months of isoniazid treatment. However, because of the good clinical condition of one of the patients from the original open study after 7 years of therapy with isoniazid, they considered that isoniazid might still be worth trying on selected patients with Huntington's chorea. Doses of isoniazid had ranged from 10 to 21 mg per kg body-weight supplemented with pyridoxine 100 mg daily. Other double-blind studies have found no improvement in adventitous movement and that any beneficial effects of isoniazid are offset by its adverse effects (B.V. Manyam *et al.*, *Ann. Neurol.*, 1981, *10*, 35; D.R. McLean, *Neurology*, 1982, *32*, 1189).

Multiple sclerosis. Following a report from Sabra *et al.* (*Neurology*, 1982, *32*, 912) of significant improvement of postural tremor in 4 patients with multiple sclerosis given isoniazid, some double-blind crossover studies have been conducted to assess its role in the management of multiple sclerosis. Isoniazid was generally given in daily divided doses of up to 1.2 g usually with pyridoxine 100 mg. In one study (M. Hallett *et al.*, *Neurology*, 1985, *35*, 1374), some clinical improvement was obtained in postural tremor in 6 patients with multiple sclerosis and in another (C.B. Bozek *et al.*, *Neurology*, 1984, *34*, *Suppl.* 1, 128) 6 of 8 patients had limited improvement in intention tremor. However, Duquette *et al.* (*Neurology*, 1985, *35*, 1772) considered that the improvement obtained in 10 of 12 patients with postural or intention tremor did not result in significant functional improvement and that side-effects were common with the dosage used. Furthermore, although Francis *et al.* (*J. Neurol. Neurosurg. Psychiat.*, 1986, *49*, 87) detected a reduction in action tremor using polarised light goniometry when standard methods of assessment showed only marginal improvement, they still considered that the results did not justify recommending isoniazid in the management of multiple sclerosis.

Spasmodic torticollis. Combination therapy with diazepam, isoniazid, pyridoxine and levoglutamide improved involuntary spasmodic torticollis to varying degrees in 7 of 14 patients whose condition was refractory to previous forms of therapy; dyskinesias became worse in 2 patients. However, treatment was later discontinued in 5 of the patients with improvement either due to adverse effects or because the degree of improvement was not sufficient to warrant the complex regimen.— J. Korein *et al.*, *Ann. Neurol.*, 1981, *10*, 247.

TUBERCULOSIS. For the use of isoniazid and other antituberculous agents in the treatment of tuberculosis, see p.547.

TUBERCULOUS MENINGITIS. Retrospective analysis of the treatment of 143 adults and children with tuberculous meningitis indicated that isoniazid should be given in a daily dose no lower than 8 mg per kg body-weight.— P. Latorre *et al.*, *Eur. J. clin. Pharmac.*, 1984, *26*, 583.

For the use of antituberculous agents in the treatment of tuberculous meningitis, see Treatment of Tuberculosis, p.551.

TUBERCULOSIS PROPHYLAXIS. Following diagnosis of sputum-positive tuberculosis in a member of the medical staff of a paediatric department 82 infants who had been in the baby care unit during the 8 weeks before diagnosis received prophylactic isoniazid therapy in a dosage of 8 mg per kg body-weight daily for 8 weeks. None developed tuberculosis.— C. J. Stewart, *Br. med. J.*, 1976, *1*, 30.

For recommendations on the prophylactic use of isoniazid see Prophylaxis of Tuberculosis, p.547.

Preparations

Isoniazid Elixir *(B.P.C. 1973).* Isoniazid Syrup. Isoniazid 50 mg, citric acid monohydrate 12.5 mg, sodium citrate 60 mg, concentrated anise water 0.05 mL, compound tartrazine solution 0.05 mL, glycerol 1 mL, double-strength chloroform water 2 mL, water to 5 mL. Store at a temperature not exceeding 25° in well-filled airtight containers. Protect from light. Under these conditions it may be expected to retain its potency for 1 year. Not more than a month's supply should be dispensed at a time. When a dose less than 5 mL is prescribed the elixir should be diluted to 5 mL with chloroform water. Such dilutions must be freshly prepared and not used more than 2 weeks after issue. Syrup must not be used as the diluent.

Isoniazid Elixir (*B.P.C. 1973*) is not adequately preserved against microbial spoilage as assessed by the *B.P.* challenge test.— T. R. R. Kurup and L. S. C. Wan, *Pharm. J.*, 1986, *2*, 761.

Isoniazid Syrup *(U.S.P.)*

Isoniazid Injection *(B.P.)*

Isoniazid Injection *(U.S.P.).* If crystals have formed they should be redissolved by warming before use.

Isoniazid Tablets *(B.P., U.S.P.)*

Proprietary Preparations

Rimifon *(Roche, UK). Injection*, isoniazid 25 mg/mL, in ampoules of 2 mL.

Proprietary Names and Manufacturers

Anidrasona *(Hortel, Spain)*; Bacikoch *(IBYS, Spain)*; Cemidon *(Gayoso Wellcome, Spain)*; Cin Vis *(Vis, Ital.)*; Dardex *(Llorente, Spain)*; Diazid *(Nippon Shinyaku, Jpn)*; Fimazid *(Wasserman, Spain)*; Hidrafasa *(Sabater, Spain)*; Hidranic *(Spain)*; Hidranison *(Cheminova, Spain)*; Hidrasolco *(Inibsa, Spain)*; Hidrastol *(Sur De Espana, Spain)*; Hidrazida *(Cronofar, Spain; Rovi, Spain)*; Hidrulta *(Euroulta, Spain)*; Hiperazida *(Spain)*; Hydra; Hydronsan *(Chugai, Jpn)*; Idrazil *(Bracco, Ital.)*; Iscontin *(Daiichi, Jpn)*; Iso-Dexter *(Spain)*; Isotamine *(ICN, Canad.)*; Isotinyl *(USV, Austral.)*; Isozid *(Saarstickstoff-Fatol, Ger.)*; Kridan Simple *(Cidan, Spain)*; Laniazid *(Lannett, USA)*; Lefos *(Spain)*; Lubacida *(Spain)*; Midral *(Orravan, Spain)*; Neoteben *(Bayer, Ger.)*; Nicazide *(IFI, Ital.)*; Nicizina *(Farmitalia, Ital.)*; Nicotibina *(Lepetit, Arg.)*; Nicotibine *(Belg.)*; Nicozid *(Piam, Ital.)*; Nydrazid *(Squibb, USA)*; Panazid *(US Products, USA)*; Pyreazid *(Salvat, Spain)*; Rimifon *(Roche, Belg.; Roche, Canad.; Roche, Fr.; Roche, Ger.; Roche, Port.; Roche, Spain; Roche, Switz.; Roche, UK)*; Sumifon *(Sumitomo, Jpn)*; Tb-Phlogin *(Heyl, Ger.)*; Tebesium-s *(Hefa-Frenon, Ger.)*; Tibinide *(Ferrosan, Swed.)*; Tibizina *(Ital.)*; Tuberon *(Shionogi, Jpn)*; Vivo Niplen *(Tanabe, Jpn)*; Zidafimia *(Santos, Spain)*; Zideluy *(Spain)*.

The following names have been used for multi-ingredient preparations containing isoniazid— Inapasade *(Smith & Nephew Pharmaceuticals, UK)*; Isoprodian *(Kolassa, Aust.; Saarstickstoff-Fatol, Ger.; Saarstickstoff-Fatol, S.Afr.)*; Mynah *(Lederle, UK)*; Pasinah-D *(Wander, UK)*; Rifamate *(Merrell Dow, USA)*; Rifater *(Merrell, UK)*; Rifinah *(Merrell, UK)*; Rimactazid *(Ciba, UK)*.

7560-w

Isoniazid Aminosalicylate

GEWO-339; Pasiniazid *(pINN)*. Isonicotinohydrazide 4-amino-2-hydroxybenzoate.
$C_6H_7N_3O,C_7H_7NO_3=290.3$.

CAS — 2066-89-9.

Isoniazid aminosalicylate has the actions and uses of isoniazid (p.563) and sodium aminosalicylate (p.554) and has been given in a dose of 10 to 20 mg per kg body-weight daily in divided doses in the treatment of tuberculosis.

Proprietary Names and Manufacturers

Dipasic *(Gamaprod, Austral.; Belg.; Gewo, Ger.; Ital.; Geistlich, Neth.; Inibsa, Spain)*; Paraniazide *(Anphar-Rolland, Fr.)*; PAS Hidral-Grey *(Orravan, Spain)*; Pasison *(Jean-Marie, Hong Kong)*; Propasal *(Llorente, Spain)*; Vitasic-S *(Inibsa, Spain)*.

7562-l

Methaniazide *(rINN).*

Isoniazid Mesylate; Isoniazid Methanesulfonate. 2-isonicotinoylhydrazinomethanesulphonic acid.
$C_7H_9N_3O_4S=231.2$.

CAS — 13447-95-5 (methaniazide); 6059-26-3 (calcium salt); 3804-89-5 (sodium salt).

Methaniazide is a derivative of isoniazid (p.563) with similar actions and uses. It has been administered as the sodium or calcium salt.

Proprietary Names and Manufacturers

Neo-Iscontin *(Daiichi, Hong Kong)*; Neolscotin *(Daiichi, Jpn)*; Neo-Tizide *(Carlo Erba, Ital.)*.

7563-y

Morinamide *(pINN).*

Morphazinamide. *N*-Morpholinomethylpyrazine-2-carboxamide.
$C_{10}H_{14}N_4O_2=222.2$.

CAS — 952-54-5.

Morinamide is an antituberculous agent which is chemically related to pyrazinamide (see p.569); cross-resistance between the 2 drugs has been reported. Morinamide has been given by mouth and by intravenous injection. Morinamide hydrochloride has also been used.

In 4 subjects given morinamide 3 g by mouth, peak plasma concentrations of about 60 µg per mL were attained after 1 hour. The half-life was about 3.5 hours. The activity of morinamide *in vitro* was not due to the formation of pyrazinamide.— T. C. Bravo *et al.*, *Tubercle*, 1975, *56*, 211.

A study of the use of morinamide in short-term chemotherapy of pulmonary tuberculosis.— A. Bouslama *et al.*, *Bull. int. Un. Tuberc.*, 1985, *60*, *March-June*, 27.

Proprietary Names and Manufacturers

Morfomide *(Infar, Port.)*; Piazofolina *(Bracco, Ital.)*; Piazolina *(Bracco, S.Afr.; Vinas, Spain)*; Piazoline *(Beytout, Fr.)*.

7567-k

Prothionamide *(BAN).*

Protionamide *(rINN)*; RP-9778; Th-1321. 2-Propylpyridine-4-carbothioamide.
$C_9H_{12}N_2S=180.3$.

CAS — 14222-60-7.

Pharmacopoeias. In *Br.* and *Jpn.*

Odourless or almost odourless, yellow crystals or crystalline powder. Practically **insoluble** in water; soluble 1 in 30 of alcohol; slightly soluble in chloroform and in ether; soluble 1 in 16 of methyl alcohol. **Protect** from light.

Absorption and Fate

Prothionamide is readily absorbed from the gastro-intestinal tract and produces peak plasma concentrations about 2 hours after a dose by mouth. It is widely distributed throughout body tissues and fluids, including the CSF. Prothionamidc is metabolised to the active sulphoxide and other inactive metabolites and less than 1% of a dose appears in the urine as unchanged drug.

For a comparison of the pharmacokinetics of prothionamide and ethionamide, see under Absorption and Fate in ethionamide, p.563.

Uses and Administration

Prothionamide is a thioamide derivative considered to be virtually interchangeable with ethionamide (p.563) although it appears to be better tolerated. Complete cross-resistance occurs between the two agents. Prothionamide is administered by mouth in doses similar to those used for ethionamide. It has also been administered as rectal suppositories; prothionamide hydrochloride has been given intravenously.

LEPROSY. For reference to the use of prothionamide in multidrug treatment regimens in leprosy, see p.552.

Preparations

Prothionamide Tablets *(B.P.)*

Proprietary Names and Manufacturers

Ektebin *(Hefa-Frenon, Ger.)*; Peteha *(Saarstickstoff-Fatol, Ger.)*; Tebeform *(Gedeon Richter, Hung.)*; Trevintix *(Commonwealth Serum Laboratories, Austral.*; *May & Baker, Austral.*; *Belg.*; *Théraplix, Fr.*; *May & Baker, S.Afr.*; *Spain*; *May & Baker, UK)*; Tuberamin *(Meiji, Jpn)*; Tuberex *(Shionogi, Jpn)*.

The following names have been used for multi-ingredient preparations containing prothionamide— Isoprodian *(Kolassa, Aust.*; *Saarstickstoff-Fatol, Ger.*; *Saarstickstoff-Fatol, S.Afr.)*.

7568-a

Pyrazinamide *(BAN, USAN, rINN).*

Pyrazinamidum; Pyrazinoic Acid Amide. Pyrazine-2-carboxamide.

$C_5H_5N_3O$=123.1.

CAS — 98-96-4.

Pharmacopoeias. In *Br.*, *Cz.*, *Egypt.*, *Ind.*, *Jpn*, *Jug.*, *Nord.*, and *U.S.*

A white or almost white, odourless or almost odourless, crystalline powder.

B.P. **solubilities** are: soluble 1 in 70 of water; slightly soluble in alcohol; soluble 1 in 70 of chloroform; very slightly soluble in ether. *U.S.P.* solubilities are: soluble 1 in 67 of water, 1 in 175 of dehydrated alcohol, 1 in 135 of chloroform, 1 in 1000 of ether, and 1 in 72 of methyl alcohol. **Store** in well-closed containers.

Adverse Effects

Hepatotoxicity is the most serious side-effect of pyrazinamide therapy and its frequency appears to be related to dose and duration of treatment. With doses of 3 g daily up to 15% of patients may show signs of liver damage, though the incidence is reported to be lower with currently recommended daily doses. Hepatomegaly, splenomegaly, and jaundice may develop and in rare cases fulminating acute yellow atrophy and death have occurred.

Other side-effects are anorexia, nausea, vomiting, arthralgia, malaise, fever, sideroblastic anaemia, and dysuria. Photosensitivity and skin rashes have been reported on rare occasions.

Hyperuricaemia commonly occurs and may lead to attacks of gout.

EFFECTS ON THE LIVER. The risk of hepatitis with antituberculous regimens containing pyrazinamide is now considered to be lower than suggested by early studies, in which large doses were used, often for long periods. There have been no reports of unacceptable rates of hepatotoxicity with currently recommended doses (D.J. Girling, *Tubercle*, 1978, *59*, 13 and 1984, *65*, 1). In 3 studies of short-course regimens conducted under the auspices of the British Medical Research Council Tuberculosis and Chest Diseases Unit the rate of hepatitis in regimens employing pyrazinamide ranged from 0.2% to 2.8%. These and later studies (M. Zierski and E. Bek, *Tubercle*, 1980, *61*, 41; British Thoracic Society, *Br. J. Dis. Chest.*, 1984, *78*, 330; R. Parthasarathy *et al.*, *Tubercle*, 1986, *67*, 99) have shown that hepatoxicity is not increased when pyrazinamide is added to the initial phase of short-term chemotherapy containing rifampicin and isoniazid. Findings by Pilheu *et al.* (*Bull. int. Un. Tuberc.*, 1984, *59*, 144) suggest that regimens containing 2 months of treatment with pyrazinamide in the initial phase may be suitable for use in alcoholic patients. However, despite the low incidence of hepatitis Cohen *et al.* (*S. Afr. med. J.*, 1983, *63*, 960) still considered that pyrazinamide was the major cause of hepatitis in patients they had treated with antituberculous therapy.

EFFECTS ON THE NERVOUS SYSTEM. Convulsions which developed in a 2-year-old child receiving antituberculous therapy appeared to be due to pyrazinamide. Pyrazinamide had been administered in a dose of 250 mg daily.— P. Herlevsen *et al.*, *Tubercle*, 1987, *68*, 145.

HYPERURICAEMIA. Arthralgia during therapy with pyrazinamide may be due to inhibition of uric acid excretion by pyrazinoic acid the main metabolite of pyrazinamide (G.A. Ellard and R.M. Haslam, *Tubercle*, 1976, *57*, 97). Zierski and Bek (*Tubercle*, 1980, *61*, 41) found that serum-urate concentrations were increased in 56% of patients receiving antituberculous regimens containing pyrazinamide. However, Jenner *et al.* (*Tubercle*, 1981, *62*, 175) have also shown that serum concentrations of uric acid in patients who developed arthralgia while taking pyrazinamide were similar to those in matched controls without arthralgia. The incidence of arthralgia appears to be lower with regimens employing intermittent rather than daily administration of pyrazinamide (Hong Kong Tuberculosis Treatment Services/British MRC, *Tubercle*, 1976, *57*, 81). While Jenner *et al.* (1981) considered that the incidence of arthralgia during daily treatment with regimens containing pyrazinmide was uninfluenced by rifampicin other workers (S.P. Tripathy, *Bull. int. Un. Tuberc.*, 1979, *54*, 28; Tuberculosis Research Centre, Madras, *Tubercle*, 1983, *64*, 73) found it to be considerably less in patients receiving rifampicin concomitantly. Sarma *et al.* (*Tubercle*, 1983, *64*, 93) subsequently found that while rifampicin had no effect on either the metabolism or excretion of pyrazinamide it did enhance the renal excretion of uric acid.

PELLAGRA. Pellagra, probably due to pyrazinamide developed in a 26-year-old woman receiving antituberculous therapy. Symptoms regressed, without stopping therapy, on administration of nicotinamide.— J. Jørgensen, *Int. J. Derm.*, 1983, *22*, 44.

Treatment of Adverse Effects

Treatment of overdosage with pyrazinamide consists of gastric lavage and supportive therapy.

If hyperuricaemia with acute gouty arthritis occurs pyrazinamide should generally be withdrawn although a uricosuric agent such as probenecid has been given—but see under Precautions below.

Precautions

Pyrazinamide is contra-indicated in patients with liver damage. Liver function should be assessed before and regularly during treatment. Caution should be observed in patients with impaired renal function or a history of gout. Increased difficulty has been reported in controlling diabetes mellitus when diabetics are given pyrazinamide.

EFFECT ON DIAGNOSTIC TESTS. Pyrazinamide could interfere with the Acetest and Ketostix qualitative urine tests for ketones to produce a pink-brown colour.— *Drug & Ther. Bull.*, 1972, *10*, 69.

INTERACTIONS. A study of the complex interactions occurring when pyrazinamide and probenecid are given to patients with gout. Urinary excretion of urate depends on the relative size and timing of doses of the two drugs. Probenecid is known to block the excretion of pyrazinamide.— T. F. Yü *et al.*, *Am. J. Med.*, 1977, *63*, 723.

PORPHYRIA. Pyrazinamide was considered to be unsafe in patients with acute porphyria as it has been associated with acute attacks.— M.R. Moore and K.E.L. McColl, *Porphyrias, Drug Lists*, Glasgow, Porphyria Research Unit, University of Glasgow, 1987.

PREGNANCY AND THE NEONATE. For a discussion on the use of antituberculous agents during pregnancy and for recommendations on precautions to be taken by nursing mothers receiving antituberculous therapy, see under Treatment of Tuberculosis, p.548.

Antimicrobial Action and Resistance

Pyrazinamide has a bactericidal effect on *M. tuberculosis* but is only effective in an acid environment when an MIC of 20 µg per mL has been reported *in vitro*. It appears to have no activity against other mycobacteria or microorganisms including *M. bovis*. Pyrazinamide possesses high sterilising activity in that it is active against persisting tubercle bacilli inhibited in an acid environment, but is relatively ineffective in preventing the emergence of resistance to other antituberculous agents (see p.546). Resistance rapidly develops when used alone.

A simple method for detecting pyrazinamide resistance.— E. Brander, *Tubercle*, 1972, *53*, 128.

Mycobacterium bovis lacks the amidase enzyme necessary for converting pyrazinamide into active pyrazinoic acid.— E. G. L. Wilkins and C. Roberts (letter), *Lancet*, 1986, *2*, 458.

Kantor *et al.* (*Bull. int. Un. Tuberc.*, 1986, *61*, 60) confirmed the findings of other workers that the determination of pyrazinamidase activity was a fairly reliable substitute for the qualitative determination of pyrazinamide susceptibility in strains of *Mycobacterium tuberculosis*. Butler and Kilburn (*Antimicrob. Ag. Chemother.*, 1983, *24*, 600) had found the test to be of limited value.

Absorption and Fate

Pyrazinamide is readily absorbed from the gastro-intestinal tract. Peak serum concentrations occur about 2 hours after a dose by mouth and have been reported to be about 35 µg per mL after 1.5 g, and 66 µg per mL after 3 g. The half-life has been reported to be about 9 to 10 hours. Pyrazinamide is widely distributed in body fluids and tissues and diffuses into the CSF. It is metabolised primarily in the liver by hydrolysis to the major active metabolite pyrazinoic acid which is subsequently hydroxylated to the major excretory product 5-hydroxypyrazinoic acid. It is excreted through the kidney mainly by glomerular filtration. About 70% of a dose appears in the urine within 24 hours mainly as metabolites and 4 to 14% as unchanged drug.

Pyrazinamide is excreted in breast milk.

The pharmacokinetics of pyrazinamide administered alone or in combination with isoniazid and rifampicin.— F. Boulahbal *et al.*, *Archs Inst. Pasteur Algér.*, 1978, *53*, 165.

Further references: K. D. Stottmeier *et al.*, *Am. Rev. resp. Dis.*, 1968, *98*, 70; G. A. Ellard, *Tubercle*, 1969, *50*, 144; I. M. Weiner and J. P. Tinker, *J. Pharmac. exp. Ther.*, 1972, *180*, 411; G. A. Ellard and R. M. Haslam, *Tubercle*, 1976, *57*, 97.

DIFFUSION. Pyrazinamide was given to 28 patients with suspected tuberculous meningitis in doses of 34 to 41 mg per kg body-weight. The mean concentration of pyrazinamide in the CSF 2 hours after administration was 38.6 µg per mL and represented about 75% of that in serum; concentrations at 5 and 8 hours were 44.5 and 31.0 µg per mL respectively and were about 10% higher than those in serum.— G. A. Ellard *et al.*, *Br. med. J.*, 1987, *294*, 284.

The use of corticosteroids did not appear to influence the penetration of pyrazinamide into the cerebrospinal fluid of patients with tuberculous meningitis.— J. Woo *et al.*, *Curr. ther. Res.*, 1987, *42*, 235.

Further references: R. Forgan-Smith *et al.* (letter), *Lancet*, 1973, *2*, 374.

PREGNANCY AND THE NEONATE. The peak concentration of pyrazinamide in breast milk of a 29-year-old woman was 1.5 µg per mL 3 hours after administration of a 1-g dose of pyrazinamide. The peak plasma concentration was 42 µg per mL after 2 hours.— M. R. Holdiness (letter), *Archs intern. Med.*, 1984, *144*, 1888.

Uses and Administration

The high incidence of hepatotoxicity associated with early regimens employing large doses of pyrazinamide given for prolonged periods led to pyrazinamide being considered to be unsuitable for the primary treatment of tuberculosis. Its use was largely reserved for re-treatment regimens for drug-resistant tuberculosis and for initial therapy in developing countries where the incidence of primary resistance is high. However, recent studies have shown that currently recommended doses are considerably safer and because of its unique activity against tubercle bacilli in an acid environment, pyrazinamide is now considered to be an important first-line agent in the intensive phase of short-term antituberculous regimens (see under Treatment of Tuberculosis p.547).

Recommended doses by mouth for adults range from 15 to 35 mg per kg body-weight to a maximum of 3 g daily given in 3 or 4 equally spaced doses. Doses of 20 mg per kg have been used for children when there is no satisfactory alternative.

A review and criticism of the value of pyrazinamide for assessing urate secretion.— T. H. Steele, *Ann. intern. Med.*, 1973, *79*, 734.

ADMINISTRATION. The currently recommended dosages of pyrazinamide are 35 mg per kg body-weight daily, 45 mg per kg three times a week, or 70 mg per kg twice a week. In routine pratice, adults weighing less than 50 kg are given 1.5 g daily, 2.0 g three times a week, or 3.0 g twice a week and heavier patients are given 2.0 g daily, 2.5 g three times a week or 3.5 g twice a week. In short-course regimens, pyrazinamide in these dosages has not been reported to cause unacceptable rates of hepatotoxicity.— D. J. Girling, *Tubercle*, 1984, *65*, 1. The daily dose of pyrazinamide for patients weighing 75 kg or more is 2.5 g.— R. B. Cole, *Prescribers' J.*, 1985, *25*, 110.

TUBERCULOSIS. Pyrazinamide is uniquely active against persisting tubercle bacilli inhibited by an acid environment but lacks the ability to suppress all bacilli continuously. It is therefore an important sterilising drug but relatively ineffective in preventing the emergence of resistance. The important sterilising role of pyrazinamide has been demonstrated in controlled studies by its ability to increase the culture-negativity rate at 2 months and to reduce the relapse rate after chemotherapy. Inclusion of pyrazinamide for 2 months in regimens containing isoniazid and rifampicin throughout with ethambutol or streptomycin in the initial phase has produced highly effective short-term regimens which prevent failure associated with the emergence of resistance during chemotherapy and which are followed by negligible relapse rates. These regimens are highly effective in the presence of initial resistance to isoniazid, streptomycin or both, and are likely to cure a high proportion of even early defaulters. Addition of pyrazinamide has also permitted the duration of therapy to be reduced from 9 to 6 months. Pyrazinamide should be included in primary chemotherapy for pulmonary tuberculosis unless there are specific contra-indications such as gout.— D. J. Girling, *Tubercle*, 1984, *65*, 1.

See also under Treatment of Tuberculosis, p.547.

TUBERCULOSIS PROPHYLAXIS. Pyrazinamide was substituted for rifampicin, in a renal transplant patient also receiving isoniazid as prophylactic antituberculous therapy, after rifampicin reduced the efficacy of cyclosporin immunosuppresive therapy.— R. A. Coward *et al.* (letter), *Lancet*, 1985, *1*, 1342. Comment that prophylaxis with isoniazid alone is satisfactory.— W. A. Jurewicz *et al.* (letter), *ibid.*, 1343.

Preparations

Pyrazinamide Tablets *(B.P., U.S.P.)*

Proprietary Preparations

Zinamide *(Merck Sharp & Dohme, UK). Tablets*, scored, pyrazinamide 500 mg.

Proprietary Names and Manufacturers

Isopas *(Lennon, S.Afr.)*; Pezetamid *(Hefa-Frenon, Ger.)*; Piraldina *(Bracco, Ital.)*; Pirilene *(Lepetit, Fr.)*; Pyrafat *(Saarstickstoff-Fatol, Ger.)*; Pyrazide *(SCS, S.Afr.)*; Rozide *(Rolab, S.Afr.)*; Tebrazid *(Continental Pharma, Belg.; ICN, Canad.)*; Zinamide *(Commonwealth Serum Laboratories, Austral.; Merck Sharp & Dohme, UK)*.

The following names have been used for multi-ingredient preparations containing pyrazinamide— Rifater *(Merrell, UK)*.

16512-w

Rifabutin *(rINN)*.

Ansamicin; Ansamycin; LM-427; Rifabutine.
(9*S*,12*E*,14*S*,15*R*,16*S*,17*R*,18*R*,19*R*,20*S*,21*S*,22*E*,24*Z*)-6,16,18,20-Tetrahydroxy-1′-isobutyl-14-methoxy-7,9,15,17,19,21,25-heptamethylspiro[9,4-(epoxypentadeca[1,11,13]trienimino)-2*H*-furo-[2′,3′:7,8]-naphth[1,2-*d*]imidazole-2,4′-piperidine]-5,10,26-(3*H*,9*H*)-trione 16-acetate.
$C_{46}H_{62}N_4O_{11}$=847.0.

CAS — 72559-06-9.

Rifabutin is a rifamycin antibiotic. It is being studied particularly for the treatment of infections caused by *Mycobacterium* spp.

ANTIMICROBIAL ACTIVITY. Rifabutin was one of the most active of a range of antibiotics tested *in vitro* against *Campylobacter jejuni*. The MIC ranged from 0.31 to 0.62 μg per mL.— P. Van der Auwera and B. Scorneaux, *Antimicrob. Ag. Chemother.*, 1985, *28*, 37.

Activity of rifabutin in combination with other antimicrobial agents against *Staphylococcus aureus*.— P. Van der Auwera and P. Joly, *J. antimicrob. Chemother.*, 1987, *19*, 313.

Activity against Mycobacteria. Evidence that rifabutin shows activity against *Mycobacterium leprae* in mouse foot-pad infections.— R. C. Hastings and R. R. Jacobson (letter), *Lancet*, 1983, *2*, 1079. Correction.— *ibid.*, 1210. Rifabutin was active against rifampicin-resistant *M. leprae*.— R. C. Hastings *et al.* (letter), *ibid.*, 1984, *1*, 1130.

Although rifabutin had good *in-vitro* activity against *Mycobacterium intracellulare*, it had only very poor activity in *mice* infected with this organism. Serum and tissue extracts failed to show any *in-vitro* activity.— V. K. Perumal *et al.*, *Bull. int. Un. Tuberc.*, 1986, *61*, *Sept.*, 11.

A comparative study of the activity *in vitro* of rifampicin and the rifamycin derivatives rifabutin, rifapentine, CGP-29861, CGP-7040, CGP-27557, and FCE-22250. Twenty-three strains of *Mycobacterium tuberculosis* tested were sensitive to rifampicin (MIC of less than 1.25 μg per mL). All the rifamycin derivatives had lower MICs than rifampicin for these strains; about four times lower for rifapentine and CGP-27557, and about eight times lower for rifabutin, CGP-29861, and CGP-7040. FCE-22250 was less stable during incubation than rifampicin and the results were not reported. Of 35 strains of *M. tuberculosis* resistant to rifampicin 11 were sensitive to rifabutin, but only between 1 and 4 strains were sensitive to the other rifamycins. A strain was considered sensitive if it had an MIC of less than 1.25 μg per mL.

The rifamycins were also tested against 26 strains of *Mycobacterium avium/intracellulare/scrofulaceum* complex. A strain was considered sensitive if the MIC was less than 0.6 μg per mL. The number of strains sensitive were as follows: rifampicin (9 strains), rifabutin and rifapentine (18), CGP-29861 (22), CGP-7040 (24), and CGP-27557 (13).— J. M. Dickinson and D. A. Mitchison, *Tubercle*, 1987, *68*, 177. Studies *in vitro* of the bactericidal activity of these rifamycin derivatives against *M. tuberculosis*.— *idem*, 183.

Further references: M. H. Cynamon, *Antimicrob. Ag. Chemother.*, 1985, *28*, 440 (activity against *Mycobacterium intracellulare*); L. B. Heifets *et al.*, *ibid.*, 570 (activity against *M. avium* complex).

For a discussion on the treatment of atypical mycobacterial infections including the use of regimens containing rifabutin for infections due to *M. avium intracellulare* see under Atypical Mycobacterial Infections, p.553.

Activity against viruses. Rifabutin blocks the *in-vitro* infectivity and replication of HIV.— R. Anand *et al.* (letter), *Lancet*, 1986, *1*, 97.

USES. During the period October 1983 to July 1985, 821 patients with life-threatening mycobacterial disease were treated with rifabutin. These included patients with AIDS and disseminated *Mycobacterium avium* complex (MAC) disease (604 patients), other immunosuppressed patients with disseminated MAC disease (36), patients with disabling, progressive MAC pulmonary disease (138), and those with rifampicin-resistant tuberculosis (43). Patients received rifabutin in a dose of either 300 or 150 mg, and other antimicrobial agents could be given. Death occurred in 347 patients and suspected adverse reactions to rifabutin leading to cessation of treatment in 51. Although one-third of patients with disseminated disease showed clinical improvement during therapy, documented eradication of MAC in these patients was uncommon. Sputum culture conversion occurred in 15% of patients with pulmonary MAC disease and 29% of patients with rifampicin-resistant tuberculosis.— R. J. O'Brien *et al.*, *Bull. int. Un. Tuberc.*, 1986, *61*, *Sept.*, 11.

Beneficial response to therapy with isoniazid, ethambutol, rifabutin, and clofazimine in a man with AIDS and associated *Mycobacterium avium* complex infection.— C. R. Horsburgh and D. L. Cohn (letter), *Ann. intern. Med.*, 1986, *105*, 968.

In a preliminary study, 13 AIDS patients with *Mycobacterium avium-Mycobacterium intracellulare* bacteraemia were treated with rifabutin and clofazimine by mouth. Both the bacteriological and clinical response were poor, and in some cases isolates became resistant to rifabutin.— H. Masur *et al.*, *J. infect. Dis.*, 1987, *155*, 127.

Proprietary Names and Manufacturers

Farmitalia Carlo Erba, UK.

7569-t

Rifampicin *(BAN, rINN)*.

Ba-41166/E; L-5103; NSC-113926; Rifaldazine; Rifampicinum; Rifampin *(USAN)*; Rifamycin AMP. 3-(4-Methylpiperazin-1-yliminomethyl)rifamycin SV; (12*Z*,14*E*,24*E*)-(2*S*,16*S*,17*S*,18*R*,19*R*,20*R*,21*S*,22*R*,23*S*)-1,2-Dihydro-5,6,9,17,19-pentahydroxy-23-methoxy-2,4,12,16,18,20,22-heptamethyl-8-(4-methylpiperazin-1-yliminomethyl)-1,11-dioxo-2,7-(epoxypentadeca[1,11,13]trienimino)naphtho-[2,1-*b*]furan-21-yl acetate.
$C_{43}H_{58}N_4O_{12}$=823.0.

CAS — 13292-46-1.

Pharmacopoeias. In *Belg., Br., Braz., Chin., Cz., Egypt., Eur., Fr., Ind., It., Jpn, Neth., Roum., Swiss,* and *U.S.*

A practically odourless brick red to reddish brown crystalline powder. *B.P.* **solubilities** are: slightly soluble in water, acetone, alcohol, and ether; freely soluble in chloroform; soluble in methyl alcohol. *U.S.P.* solubilities very slightly soluble in water; freely soluble in chloroform; soluble in ethyl acetate and methyl alcohol. A 1% suspension in water has a pH of 4.5 to 6.5. **Store** at a temperature not exceeding 15° in airtight containers in an atmosphere of nitrogen. Protect from light.

The solubility of rifampicin in aqueous solutions is increased at low pH values, but aqueous solutions are relatively unstable. At an acid pH part of the rifampicin in solution is decomposed by hydrolysis, whereas in alkaline solutions in the presence of atmospheric oxygen rifampicin is oxidised. Oxidation may be inhibited by the addition of sodium ascorbate. Lyophilised preparations for intravenous administration are stable for at least 2 years before reconstitution.— M. T. Kenny and B. Strates, *Merrell Dow, Drug Metab. Rev.*, 1981, *12*, 159.

Adverse Effects

Rifampicin is usually well tolerated. Adverse effects are more common during intermittent therapy or after restarting interrupted treatment. Gastro-intestinal side-effects have sometimes been severe enough to necessitate withdrawal. There have been rare reports of pseudomembranous colitis associated with the use of rifampicin.

Rifampicin produces abnormalities in liver function. Jaundice may be associated with the concomitant use of other agents, including isoniazid, and fatalities have been reported in patients with pre-existing liver disorders or who had also taken other potentially hepatotoxic agents; alcoholic patients may also be at risk. Some patients experience a febrile reaction with influenza-like symptoms which may have an immunological basis. Alterations in kidney function and renal failure have also occurred. Skin reactions, eosinophilia, transient leucopenia, thrombocytopenia, purpura, haemolysis and shock have also occurred.

Other side-effects reported include confusion, drowsiness, headache, muscular weakness, ataxia, dizziness, generalised numbness, visual disturbances, and menstrual irregularities. Post-natal haemorrhage has been reported in mothers and neonates following therapy with rifampicin during the last trimester of pregnancy. Thrombophlebitis has occurred when rifampicin has been given intravenously for long periods.

Adverse reactions to daily or intermittent treatment with rifampicin include cutaneous and gastro-intestinal reactions, liver dysfunction, and thrombocytopenic purpura. *Cutaneous reactions* are usually mild and transient and start early in treatment. Typically they consist of flushing of the face and neck sometimes with itching or a rash which may be generalised; up to 5% of patients may be affected. There may be redness and watering of the eyes. Occasionally patients with severe cutaneous reactions may require desensitisation before treatment with rifampicin can be resumed (see p.546). *Gastro-intestinal reactions* are rarely serious and usually consist of anorexia, nausea, and mild abdominal pain; vomiting may occur and, less frequently, diarrhoea. They can often be prevented by giving rifampicin during or immediately after a meal but a few patients seem unable to tolerate rifampicin, in which case it should be withdrawn. There may be transient disturbances of *liver function* during the early weeks of treatment with rifampicin. Hepatitis is uncommon, occurring in up to 1% of patients, and is more likely in alcoholics and patients with pre-existing liver disease. If hepatitis occurs treatment should be stopped, liver-function tests carried out, and supportive treatment given if necessary. Rifampicin may usually be resumed once liver function is normal but should be stopped and alternative chemotherapy used if it becomes abnormal again. *Thrombocytopenic purpura* is very uncommon but if it occurs rifampicin should be withdrawn immediately and never given again.

Some reactions to rifampicin have usually only been reported with intermittent treatment, particularly once-weekly or twice-weekly regimens, and include the 'flu' syndrome, shock, shortness of breath, haemolytic anaemia, and renal failure. They are unlikely to occur when rifampicin is given thrice-weekly or only once a month as in leprosy. The *'flu' syndrome* consists of episodes of fever, chills, and malaise, sometimes with headache, dizziness, and bone pain, starting one to two hours after each dose of rifampicin and lasting for up to 8 hours. The syndrome usually appears after at least 3 months of treatment and may occur in up to 20% of patients receiving once-weekly regimens including rifampicin in a dose of 20 mg or more per kg body-weight. It is more common in women than in men and may be stopped by reducing the dose or changing to daily administration. Circulating rifampicin-dependent antibodies are associated with the occurrence of the 'flu' syndrome which suggests that the symptoms described have an immunological basis. *Shock, shortness of breath, acute haemolytic anaemia,* and *renal failure* have been reported rarely during intermittent therapy but if any of these reactions occur rifampicin should be withdrawn and never given again. When rifampicin is resumed after an interval of several weeks severe reactions have occasionally been experienced by patients who have previously had no reaction or only minor reactions. Treatment should therefore be re-introduced gradually beginning with a daily dose of 75 mg and increasing by 75 mg daily until the required dosage is reached. Despite the potentially dangerous reactions with rifampicin, especially with intermittent regimens, it has been possible to minimise the risks by adjustment of treatment regimens in the light of results from controlled studies.— D. J. Girling, *J. antimicrob. Chemother.*, 1977, *3*, 115; D. J. Girling and K. L. Hitze, *Bull. Wld Hlth Org.*, 1979, *57*, 45. See also J. Grosset and S. Leventis, *Rev. infect. Dis.*, 1983, *5*, *Suppl.* 3, S440.

There is no need to assess the titre of rifampicin-dependent antibodies since no matter how high the titre in patients with reactions, rifampicin can usually be continued without risk by changing to a daily dose. A higher serum-rifampicin concentration was detected in patients experiencing adverse reactions than in patients who did not. Although intermittent treatment can give a higher incidence of side-effects, there is a lower incidence with a twice-weekly than a once-weekly schedule and the incidence with once-weekly rifampicin can be reduced if the schedule is preceded by 2 months of daily treatment.— D. J. Girling *et al.* (letter), *Br. med. J.*, 1974, *3*, 114.

A suggestion that some of the adverse reactions associated with rifampicin may be attributed to its metabolite desacetylrifampicin.— H. Nakagawa *et al.*, *Bull. int. Un. Tuberc.*, 1979, *54*, 171.

The 'flu' syndrome or other adverse effects are unlikely to be a problem in patients receiving short courses of rifampicin 900 mg daily for 7 to 10 days. Rifampicin-specific antibodies were not formed in 8 healthy subjects who had received rifampicin 900 mg daily in combination with trimethoprim 240 mg for one week and a challenge dose of 900 mg of rifampicin given 3 months later failed to induce antibody formation. No untoward effect had been experienced by 8 patients who had been treated with a second course of rifampicin with trimethoprim.— W. Brumfitt *et al.* (letter), *Lancet*, 1981, *2*, 865.

Administration of rifampicin three times weekly, in association with other antituberculous agents, did not appear to be associated with an increased incidence of adverse effects when compared with daily therapy in 86 adults and children.— C. M. Mukerjee and D. K. McKenzie, *Aust. N.Z. J. Med.*, 1985, *15*, 226.

A report of 'flu' syndrome in 1 patient receiving rifampicin once monthly as part of antileprotic chemotherapy. This regimen had been recommended by WHO on the basis that 'flu' syndrome would be unlikely to occur with once-monthly administration.— B. Naafs and B. O. Matemera (letter), *Lepr. Rev.*, 1986, *57*, 271.

CARCINOGENICITY. A report of nasopharyngeal lymphoma developing in a 41-year-old man following treatment with isoniazid, ethambutol, and rifampicin for 2 years. It was thought this might be due to the immunosuppressive effects of rifampicin following long-term treatment.— R. Rate *et al.* (letter), *Ann. intern. Med.*, 1979, *90*, 276.

Reports suggesting that rifampicin may facilitate tumour growth in the lung: D. Rodescu *et al.* (letter), *Lancet*, 1981, *2*, 983; L. Sebba *et al.* (letter), *ibid.*, 1982, *2*, 105.

EFFECTS ON THE BLOOD. *Agranulocytosis.* Mention of a case of fatal aplastic anaemia or agranulocytosis probably due to rifampicin.— W. H. W. Inman, *Br. med. J.*, 1977, *1*, 1500.

Haemorrhage. A patient who experienced a major episode of bleeding when treated with rifampicin and teicoplanin was found to have a circulating inhibitor of factor VIII. Although the inhibitor may have been produced by sensitisation to teicoplanin or rifampicin other causes could not be excluded.— J. C. Legrand *et al.* (letter), *J. antimicrob. Chemother.*, 1987, *19*, 850.

For reports of haemorrhage in mothers and their neonates after administration of rifampicin, see under Pregnancy and the Neonate in Precautions (p.572).

Leucopenia. A 75-year-old man treated with isoniazid, ethambutol, and rifampicin developed neutropenia which was re-induced, on challenge, by each of the 3 agents.— P. F. Jenkins *et al.*, *Br. med. J.*, 1980, *280*, 1069.

Van Assendelft (*Eur. J. resp. Dis.*, 1984, *65*, 251) originally reported differences between the frequency of leucopenia occurring with 2 different preparations of rifampicin. Of 140 patients treated with Rimapen (*Orion, Fin.*) 11 (7.9%) developed leucopenia compared with 1 of 132 (0.8%) patients who received Rimactan (*Ciba-Geigy, Switz.*). However, in a later randomised study (*J. antimicrob. Chemother.*, 1985, *16*, 407) involving 150 patients Van Assendelft found no difference in the incidence. Although the total frequency of leucopenia in the second study (2.4%) was lower than that in the earlier study (4.4%) it was higher than that previously reported (0.08%) in the literature.

EFFECTS ON BONE. For the effect of rifampicin and isoniazid on vitamin D metabolism and a report of osteomalacia in a patient treated with rifampicin, see under Precautions of Isoniazid, p.565.

EFFECTS ON THE EYE. A 34-year-old man suffering from pulmonary tuberculosis developed reversible exudative conjunctivitis as a result of rifampicin therapy.— F. E. Cayley and S. K. Majumdar, *Br. med. J.*, 1976, *1*, 199. Conjunctival reactions to rifampicin such as redness and watering of the eyes are not uncommon.— D. J. Girling (letter), *ibid.*, 585.

EFFECTS ON THE GASTRO-INTESTINAL TRACT. There have been rare reports of pseudomembranous colitis associated with the use of rifampicin. The condition was usually mild and responsive to withdrawal of rifampicin or to treatment with vancomycin. Although isolates of *Clostridium difficile*, a common cause of antibiotic-associated pseudomembranous colitis, are usually highly susceptible to rifampicin, resistant strains have been isolated in studies in *hamsters* and in humans.— R. Fekety *et al.*, *Rev. infect. Dis.*, 1983, *5*, *Suppl.* 3, S524.

EFFECTS ON THE KIDNEY. After experience of rifampicin-induced renal failure in 2 patients and a review of 83 other reported cases Cohn *et al.* (*Tubercle*, 1985, *66*, 289) concluded that intermittent or interrupted therapy appeared to be a risk factor for this complication. Many cases were mild and severe oliguric renal failure appeared to be uncommon. Most patients recover with appropriate supportive care. However, it has been recommended (D.J. Girling, *J. antimicrob. Chemother.*, 1977, *3*, 115; H. Riska and T. Tornroth, *Bull. int. Un. Tuberc.*, 1984, *59*, 147) that rifampicin should be discontinued and never be re-administered to patients with rifampicin-induced renal failure. Other clinicians (M.D. Katz and E. Lor, *Drug Intell. & clin. Pharm.*, 1986, *20*, 789) consider that patients who are noncompliant with rifampicin should be changed to less toxic antituberculous agents. The mechanism of renal failure is as yet unknown but it is sometimes associated with shock and acute haemolysis and may have an immunological basis in some patients. Renal biopsies in some patients have found evidence of tubular necrosis, tubulo-interstitial lesions, cortical necrosis, mild tubular damage or glomerulonephritis.

EFFECTS ON THE LIVER. The hepatotoxicity of antituberculous regimens containing rifampicin has been reviewed by Girling (*Tubercle*, 1978, *59*, 13). For a discussion on the hepatoxicity of regimens containing isoniazid with rifampicin, see under Isoniazid, p.564. Also for evidence suggesting that rifampicin may potentiate the hepatotoxicity of the thioamides, see under Ethionamide, p.562.

Hepatotoxicity in children. Hepatitis occurred in a child treated with rifampicin and ethambutol. Additional symptoms included polyarthritis and the presence of anti-native DNA antibodies.— D. M. Grennan and R. D. Sturrock, *Tubercle*, 1976, *57*, 259.

For a discussion on hepatotoxicity in children receiving rifampicin and isoniazid, see under Isoniazid, p.564.

EFFECTS ON MENTAL STATE. Rifampicin administered daily to a 60-year-old man was associated with the development of an acute organic brain syndrome in which he became confused, disorientated, agitated, and incoherent and suffered hallucinations and delusions.— T. H. Pratt, *J. Am. med. Ass.*, 1979, *241*, 2421.

Further references.— C. W. L. Jeanes *et al.*, *Can. med. Ass. J.*, 1972, *106*, 884.

EFFECTS ON METABOLISM. Early phase hyperglycaemia following oral administration of glucose was observed in patients with pulmonary tuberculosis receiving rifampicin and might be due to increased intestinal absorption of glucose. However, overt diabetes mellitus or diabetic ketoacidosis has not been seen in patients treated with rifampicin for periods longer than one year.— N. Takasu *et al.*, *Am. Rev. resp. Dis.*, 1982, *125*, 23.

EFFECTS ON MUSCLES. Myopathy in one patient induced by rifampicin.— P. Jenkins and P. A. Emerson, *Br. med. J.*, 1981, *283*, 105.

EFFECTS ON THE PANCREAS. Pancreatitis associated with rifampicin therapy might be connected with raised concentrations of the lysosomal enzymes β-glucuronidase and β-*N*-acetyl-glucosaminidase.— W. Perry *et al.* (letter), *Lancet*, 1979, *1*, 492.

EFFECTS ON THE SKIN. Chronic papular acneform lesions developed on the face, neck, and shoulders of 8 patients after taking rifampicin, isoniazid, and thiacetazone for about 5 weeks; the lesions disappeared when rifampicin was gradually withdrawn after 12 to 18 weeks of treatment.— U. Nwokolo (letter), *Br. med. J.*, 1974, *3*, 473.

A 40-year-old African man with tuberculosis given rifampicin, streptomycin, and isoniazid developed the Stevens-Johnson syndrome when ethambutol was added 4 weeks later. All drugs were withdrawn and he responded to treatment with corticosteroids. The condition recurred when rifampicin was again added. Ethambutol had possibly triggered the reaction.— R. Nyirenda and G. V. Gill, *Br. med. J.*, 1977, *2*, 1189.

A report of erythema multiforme bullosum due to rifampicin.— P. Nigam *et al.*, *Lepr. India*, 1979, *51*, 249.

Itching of the face and hands and contact dermatitis occurred in staff preparing and administering an intravenous formulation of rifampicin. As with other antibiotics parenteral formulations of rifampicin should be prepared in an aspirator that removes airborne particles. Gloves should be worn to avoid contact with the skin.— N. Anker and F. Da Cunha Bang, *Eur. J. resp. Dis.*, 1981, *62*, 84.

Pemphigus. Pemphigus occurring in a 65-year-old woman after about 9 months of treatment with rifampicin, isoniazid, and ethambutol was attributed to rifampicin.— R. W. Gange *et al.*, *Br. J. Derm.*, 1976, *95*, 445.

Pemphigus foliaceus which developed in a patient receiving isoniazid and rifampicin cleared completely within 5 weeks on withdrawal of rifampicin without need for systemic therapy.— C. W. Lee *et al.*, *Br. J. Derm.*, 1984, *111*, 619.

An acute exacerbation of pemphigus was precipitated by rifampicin in a patient whose condition was usually controlled by betamethasone. Rifampicin-induced metabolism of betamethasone was considered to be responsible. Patients with active tuberculosis and pemphigus should be treated with isoniazid and ethambutol.— S. Miyagawa *et al.*, *Br. J. Derm.*, 1986, *114*, 729.

OVERDOSAGE. Acute overdosage with rifampicin has produced a characteristic bright-red discoloration of the skin and mucous membranes sometimes referred to as "the red-man syndrome". This pigmentation is susceptible to removal by washing or scrubbing. The sclera may also sometimes be affected. Other adverse effects have included facial oedema, generalised pruritus, vomiting, and transient liver-enzyme abnormalities. Although recovery has generally been uneventful in adults and adolescents ingesting up to 12 g of rifampicin (R.W. Newton and A.R.W. Forrest, *Scott. med. J.*, 1975, *20*, 55; P. Wong *et al.*, *J. Pediat.*, 1984, *104*, 781) and in children given 100 mg per kg body-weight (G. Bolan *et al.*, *Pediatrics*, 1986, *77*, 633) a fatal outcome has been reported after ingestion of 14 g (T.A. Plomp *et al.*, *Arch. Tox.*, 1981, *48*, 245), and 60 g (R.O. Broadwell *et al.*, *J. Am. med. Ass.*, 1978, *240*, 2283). Although a fatality has also been reported after ingestion of unspecified amounts of rifampicin and ethambutol (D.B. Jack *et al.*, *Lancet*, 1978, *2*, 1107) a patient who took rifampicin 9 g, ethambutol 20 g, and isoniazid 6 g made an uneventful recovery after haemodialysis and treatment with pyridoxine (J. Ducobu *et al.*, *Lancet*, 1982, *1*, 632).

Treatment of Adverse Effects

Overdosage with rifampicin should be treated with gastric lavage and intensive supportive measures. Activated charcoal following gastric lavage may be of some help.

Desensitisation may be attempted following hypersensitivity reactions if the use of rifampcin is considered essential for the provision of adequate chemotherapy (see p.546).

Precautions
Rifampicin is generally contra-indicated in patients who are hypersensitive to rifamycins; desensitisation has been employed where there is no alternative to its use. It should not be given to patients with jaundice and should be used with caution in alcoholics and other patients with impaired liver function, especially when given with isoniazid (p.565) or other hepatotoxic drugs. Hypersensitivity reactions including nephrotoxicity appear to be associated with the intermittent use of rifampicin; if treatment with rifampicin is interrupted it should be re-introduced cautiously. Some authorities consider that it can be used with caution during pregnancy. Faeces, saliva, sputum, sweat, tears, urine, and other body-fluids may be coloured orange-red. Soft contact lenses worn by patients receiving rifampicin may become permanently stained.

It has been suggested that supplements of vitamin D may be indicated for certain patients at risk of developing metabolic bone disease when receiving rifampicin (see under Isoniazid, p.565).

Interactions. Rifampicin accelerates the metabolism of some drugs by inducing microsomal liver enzymes and possibly by interfering with hepatic uptake. A number of drugs have been reported to be affected but the clinical significance of some of these interactions remains to be determined. Although most drugs involved may require an increase in dosage to maintain effectiveness patients taking oral contraceptives should be advised to use other forms of contraception. Other drugs reported to be affected include chloramphenicol, clofibrate, corticosteroids, coumarin anticoagulants, cyclosporin, dapsone, diazepam, hexobarbitone, ketoconazole, methadone, oral hypoglycaemic agents, phenytoin, sulphasalazine, theophylline, and several cardiovascular drugs including beta-adrenoceptor blocking agents, digitoxin, digoxin, and antiarrhythmic agents such as disopyramide, lorcainide, mexiletine, quinidine, and verapamil. For further details see under the individual drugs mentioned and below.

Rifampicin may also interfere with a number of diagnostic tests and may reduce biliary excretion of contrast media used for visualisation of the gall bladder.

Rises in the serum concentration of testosterone in 8 healthy male subjects given rifampicin for 2 weeks may have been due to an increase in the binding capacity of sex hormone binding globulin. However, rifampicin may induce the synthesis of oestradiol.— M. J. Brodie *et al.* (letter), *Br. J. clin. Pharmac.*, 1981, *12*, 431.

The bile of 4 patients became supersaturated with cholesterol during treatment with rifampicin. Administration of rifampicin may predispose patients to formation of cholesterol gallstones.— K. von Bergmann *et al.*, *Antimicrob. Ag. Chemother.*, 1981, *19*, 342.

Rifampicin should be given with caution to patients receiving thyroid-hormone replacement therapy or to those with decreased thyroid reserve. A patient with primary hypothyroidism receiving thyroxine replacement therapy developed biochemical hypothroidism during treatment with rifampicin. There was a decrease in serum-thyroxine concentrations and the free thyroxine index and a rise in serum-thyrotrophin concentrations. Although other workers (E.E. Onhaus and H. Studer, *Br. J. clin. Pharmac.*, 1980, *9*, 285P) have demonstrated similar reductions in healthy subjects given rifampicin, the reason why healthy subjects do not develop hypothyroidism may be because with intact thyroid function serum concentrations of thyrotrophin remain unchanged.— W. L. Isley, *Ann. intern. Med.*, 1987, *107*, 517.

For precautions to be observed by persons preparing or administering intravenous formulations of rifampicin, see under Effects on the Skin in Adverse Effects (p.571).

EFFECTS ON LABORATORY ESTIMATIONS. Sulphobromophthalein sodium tests for liver function cannot be interpreted until at least 24 hours after rifampicin has been discontinued.— P. Capelle *et al.*, *Gut*, 1972, *13*, 366.

Toxic serum concentrations of rifampicin, but not therapeutic concentrations, interfered with the total serum bilirubin assay.— S. Meisel *et al.*, *Antimicrob. Ag. Chemother.*, 1980, *18*, 206.

Samples for estimates of vitamin B_{12} or folate should be taken 24 to 48 hours after the last dose of rifampicin to avoid erroneously low results.— C. F. Stanford and A. Bittles (letter), *Tubercle*, 1982, *62*, 236.

IMMUNOSUPPRESSION. Although intracellular concentration of rifampicin may facilitate elimination of intracellular organisms concern has been expressed that any effects on granulocyte function could be detrimental to patients suffering from immunodeficiencies. Some studies have shown that rifampicin may depress immune specific response by reducing polymorphonuclear leucocyte function (J.M. Oleske, *J. antimicrob. Chemother.*, 1984, *13*, 413). However, Humber *et al.* (*Am. Rev. resp. Dis.*, 1980, *122*, 425) were unable to demonstrate in a double-blind study that usual dosages of rifampicin had any detrimental immunosuppressive effect in otherwise healthy patients with pulmonary tuberculosis or in tuberculosis contacts.

A decline in reactivity to skin tests with tuberculin PPD in 8 of 11 patients was associated with rifampicin.— P. Mukerjee *et al.*, *Antimicrob. Ag. Chemother.*, 1973, *4*, 607.

INTERACTIONS. Studies have shown that rifampicin is a potent inducer of drug metabolism and causes a proliferation of the smooth endoplasmic reticulum and an increase in the cytochrome P-450 content of the liver. It also appears that rifampicin is a selective inducer of oxidative drug metabolism (D.D. Breimer *et al.*, *Clin. Pharmac. Ther.*, 1977, *21*, 470; M.W.E. Teunissen *et al.*, *Br. J. clin. Pharmac.*, 1984, *18*, 701) and therefore not all drugs metabolised by oxidation will be affected. There is also evidence that enzyme induction may be impaired in the elderly (Y. Twum-Barima *et al.*, *Br. J. clin. Pharmac.*, 1984, *17*, 595). For some reviews and discussions of pharmacokinetic interactions with rifampicin, see Zilly *et al.*, *Clin. Pharmacokinet.*, 1977, *2*, 61; Acocella, *ibid.*, 1978, *3*, 108; Acocella and Conti, *Tubercle*, 1980, *61*, 171; Baciewicz and Self, *Archs intern. Med.*, 1984, *144*, 1667.

For the effect of rifampicin and isoniazid on vitamin D metabolism, see under Precautions in Isoniazid, p.565.

See also under Antimicrobial Action.

Antacids. The bioavailability of rifampicin was significantly reduced when administered simultaneously with magnesium trisilicate, aluminium hydroxide, or sodium bicarbonate; change in gastric pH, chelation with aluminium ions, and binding by magnesium trisilicate may be implicated. Although the clinical significance was not assessed it might be prudent to avoid concurrent administration of rifampicin and antacids.— S. A. H. Khalil *et al.*, *Int. J. Pharmaceut.*, 1984, *20*, 99.

Antimycobacterial agents. Clofazimine reduced the rate of absorption of rifampicin and increased the time required to reach peak serum-rifampicin concentrations in a study involving 18 patients with leprosy. Dapsone had no significant effect on pharmacokinetic parameters for rifampicin, but when clofazimine and dapsone were administered together serum-rifampicin concentrations at one hour and the area under the serum concentration-time curve were reduced.— J. Mehta *et al.*, *Lepr. Rev.*, 1986, *57*, *Suppl.* 3, 67.

The reduction in rifampicin absorption reported after administration with aminosalicylic acid (G. Boman *et al.*, *Lancet*, 1971, *1*, 800; *idem*, *Eur. J. clin. Pharmac.*, 1974, *7*, 217) was shown to be due to the absorption of rifampicin by the bentonite used in the aminosalicylic acid granules (G. Boman *et al.*, *Eur. J. clin. Pharmac.*, 1975, *8*, 293). This could be overcome by administering the drugs separately at an interval of 8 to 12 hours.

It has been shown that there is little significant pharmacokinetic interaction between rifampicin and isoniazid (G. Acocella *et al.*, *Gut*, 1972, *13*, 47). Although Mouton *et al.* (*J. antimicrob. Chemother.*, 1979, *5*, 447) found that isoniazid had an unfavourable effect on rifampicin blood concentrations it was considered to be of doubtful clinical significance. Despite evidence of microsomal enzyme induction Timbrell *et al.* (*Hum. Toxicol.*, 1985, *4*, 279) also failed to find any significant effect on the metabolism of isoniazid. However, Sama *et al.* (*Am. Rev. resp. Dis.*, 1986, *133*, 1072) later showed that rifampicin increased the metabolism of isoniazid to isonicotinic acid and hydrazine, the effect being greater in slow rather than rapid acetylators. They considered that the increased formation of hydrazine might explain the higher frequency of hepatitis in slow acetylators treated with rifampicin and isoniazid.

For references to the effect of rifampicin on the pharmacokinetics of dapsone, see Dapsone Precautions, p.559.

Corticosteroids. There have been several reports of rifampicin reducing the effectiveness of corticosteroid therapy (see p.874). Acute adrenal crisis has also been precipitated by rifampicin in patients with adrenal insufficiency (E.H. Elansary and J.E. Earis, *Br. med. J.*, 1983, *286*, 1861) and induction of microsomal enzymes may be enough to compromise even patients with mildly impaired cortisol production. Critical hypotension has also developed in non-Addisonian patients within a week to 10 days of starting rifampicin therapy (G. Boss *et al.*, *Br. med. J.*, 1983, *287*, 62). However, it has not been necessary to suspend the use of rifampicin during subsequent treatment with corticosteroids.

For reference to the concurrent administration of rifampicin and corticosteroids exacerbating rather than alleviating neuritis in tuberculoid leprosy, see under Precautions for Corticosteroids, p.874.

Ketoconazole. For a report of failure of antifungal and antituberculous therapy resulting from reduced concentrations of rifampicin and ketoconazole in a patient receiving ketoconazole, rifampicin, and isoniazid, see under Precautions in Ketoconazole, p.427.

Probenecid. Although a study by Kenwright and Levi (*Lancet*, 1973, *2*, 1401) showed that concomitant administration of probenecid could increase serum-rifampicin concentrations, Fallon *et al.* (*Lancet*, 1975, *2*, 792) subsequently found that the effect was uncommon and inconsistent and concluded that probenecid had no place as an adjunct to routine rifampicin therapy.

PORPHYRIA. Porphyria cutanea tarda (J.W. Millar, *Br. J. Dis. Chest.*, 1980, *74*, 405) and porphyria variegata (J.-P. Igual *et al.*, *Nouv. Presse méd.*, 1982, *11*, 2846) have been precipitated by rifampicin. Moore and McColl (*Porphyrias, Drug Lists*, Glasgow, Porphyria Research Unit, University of Glasgow, 1987) consider rifampicin to be unsafe for use in patients with acute porphyria.

PREGNANCY AND THE NEONATE. The manufacturers had contra-indicated the use of rifampicin in pregnancy based on dose-dependent teratogenicity in *rats* and *mice* (J.S.M. Steen and D.M. Stainton-Ellis, *Lancet*, 1977, *2*, 604). In an unpublished report, referred to by Steen and Stainton-Ellis, Pagani provided data on 226 women (229 conceptions) who had taken rifampicin during pregnancy. There were 179 babies considered morphologically normal, 9 with malformations, 10 with haemorrhagic tendencies, 4 died in infancy but had no altered morphology, 5 infants died *in utero* (the foetuses showed no abnormalities), and there were 22 abortions, 17 of them induced. The incidence of malformations at birth was 4.3% compared with 1.8% for infants exposed to tuberculosis and 6.5% for infants exposed to other antituberculous regimens. As no follow-up was done on the 179 apparently healthy babies and as not all abnormalities could be detected at birth the incidence of 4.3% of malformations was expected to rise.

There have been further reports of haemorrhage associated with vitamin K deficiency in mothers and their neonates after administration of rifampicin during pregnancy (J.P. Chouraqui *et al.*, *Thérapie*, 1982, *37*, 447; J. Lissens *et al.*, *Tijdschr. Geneeskd.*, 1983, *39*, 277). Prophylactic treatment with vitamin K and blood coagulation tests have been proposed for both mothers and their offspring if rifampicin is used especially during the last few weeks of pregnancy.

Summers (*Lepr. Rev.*, 1986, *57*, 274) on reviewing the implications for the use of rifampicin in leprosy in developing countries considered that the use of rifampicin during pregnancy might be justified for the treatment of lepromatous leprosy but not in non-lepromatous leprosy. Futhermore the risk of haemorrhage was considered to be less acceptable in developing countries where appropriate treatment could not be assured. As Snider and Powell (*Archs intern. Med.*, 1984, *144*, 589) had estimated that a breast-fed infant of a nursing mother receiving rifampicin would ingest only about 0.57% of the usual therapeutic dose for an infant Summers considered that their recommendations for minimising ingestion of rifampicin in breast milk (see p.548) may be inappropriate. In most leprosy endemic areas the risks of artificial feeds far outweigh any small theoretical risks from rifampicin.

Although the possibility of rifampicin and isoniazid causing genetic damage seems unlikely it is considered wise for a potential father to refrain from parenthood while receiving these drugs.— D. M. Stainton-Ellis, *Practitioner*, 1977, *219*, 432.

See also under Treatment of Tuberculosis, p.548.

Antimicrobial Action and Resistance
Rifampicin is bactericidal against a wide range of micro-organisms and interferes with their synthesis of nucleic acids by inhibiting DNA-dependent RNA polymerase. It has the ability to kill

intracellular organisms. It is active against mycobacteria, including *Mycobacterium tuberculosis* and *M. leprae* and, having high sterilising activity against these organisms, it possesses the ability to eliminate semi-dormant or persisting organisms (see p.546 and p.551). Several of the atypical mycobacteria are also sensitive to rifampicin (see p.553). Rifampicin is active against Gram-positive bacteria, especially staphylococci, but less active against Gram-negative organisms. The most sensitive Gram-negative bacteria include *Neisseria meningitidis, N. gonorrhoeae, Haemophilus influenzae*, and *Legionella* spp. Rifampicin also has activity against *Chlamydia trachomatis* and some anaerobic bacteria. At high concentrations it is active against some viruses. Rifampicin has no effect on fungi but has been reported to enhance the antifungal activity of amphotericin.

Minimum inhibitory concentrations tend to vary with the medium used but Gram-positive organisms are usually inhibited by 0.5 µg or less per mL, mycobacteria by 0.005 to 2 µg per mL, and susceptible Gram-negative micro-organisms by up to 4 µg per mL. The concomitant use of other antimicrobial agents may enhance the bactericidal activity of rifampicin.

As with other antituberculous compounds resistant mycobacteria rapidly emerge if rifampicin is used alone. Resistance has also been reported in other organisms. There does not appear to be cross-resistance apart from that between rifampicin and other rifamycins.

A discussion on the mechanisms of action of rifampicin.— W. Wehrli, *Rev. infect. Dis.*, 1983, *5, Suppl.* 3, S407.

A review of the antibacterial spectrum of rifampicin.— C. Thornsberry *et al., Rev. infect. Dis.*, 1983, *5, Suppl.* 3, S412.

Studies demonstrating the intracellular activity of rifampicin.— G. L. Mandell, *Rev. infect. Dis.*, 1983, *5, Suppl.* 3, S463.

Isolates of *Mycobacterium avium-M. intracellulare* from patients with AIDS were significantly less susceptible to rifampicin at concentrations of 5 and 10 µg per mL (C.R. Horsburgh *et al., Antimicrob. Ag. Chemother.*, 1986, *30*, 955 and *ibid.*, 1987, *31*, 969) than isolates from non-AIDS patients.

Some other reports of the activity of rifampicin *in vitro*: H. Werner, *Arzneimittel-Forsch.*, 1972, *22*, 1043 (Gram-negative anaerobic bacteria); R. M. Bannatyne and R. Cheung, *Antimicrob. Ag. Chemother.*, 1982, *21*, 666 (*Bordetella pertussis*); Y. R. Bilgeri *et al., ibid.*, *22*, 686 (*Haemophilus ducreyi*).

Rifampicin had significant activity *in vitro* against *Giardia lamblia* and may deserve consideration for clinical evaluation of efficacy.— A. A. Crouch *et al., Trans. R. Soc. trop. Med. Hyg.*, 1986, *80*, 893.

ACTIVITY AGAINST BRUCELLA. All of 95 clinical isolates of *Brucella melitensis* were inhibited by rifampicin 4 µg per mL, doxycycline 0.25 µg per mL, tetracycline 0.5 µg per mL, ciprofloxacin 0.5 µg per mL, streptomycin 1 µg per mL, ceftriaxone 1 µg per mL, and co-trimoxazole 10 µg per mL.— J. Bosch *et al., J. antimicrob. Chemother.*, 1986, *17*, 459.

ACTIVITY AGAINST CHLAMYDIA. Rifampicin is generally more active than erythromycin, tetracyclines, and chloramphenicol *in vitro* against *Chlamydia trachomatis* (H.J. Blackman *et al., Antimicrob. Ag. Chemother.*, 1977, *12*, 673; A. Mourad *et al., ibid.*, 1980, *18*, 696; S.J. How *et al., J. antimicrob. Chemother.*, 1985, *15*, 399) but resistance may develop rapidly (A.J. Davies and D.A. Lewis, *Br. med. J.*, 1984, *289*, 3).

ACTIVITY AGAINST HAEMOPHILUS. Of 98 strains of *H. influenzae* type b, all were inhibited by rifampicin 0.5 µg per mL.— R. M. Bannatyne and R. Cheung, *Antimicrob. Ag. Chemother.*, 1978, *13*, 969.

Rifampicin 1 µg per mL inhibited 90% of 83 clinical isolates of *H. influenzae* of various types that were resistant to both ampicillin and chloramphenicol.— J. Campos and S. Garcia-Tornel, *J. antimicrob. Chemother.*, 1987, *19*, 297.

ACTIVITY AGAINST LEGIONELLA. Rifampicin appears to be one of the most active antimicrobial agents *in vitro* against *Legionella* spp. including *L. pneumophila* and *L. micdadei*. Minimum inhibitory concentrations have been reported to be 0.01 µg or less per mL against *L. pneumophila* (C. Thornsberry *et al., Antimicrob. Ag. Chemother.*, 1978, *13*, 78) and less than 0.0625 µg per mL against *L. micdadei* (A.W. Pasculle *et al., Antimicrob. Ag. Chemother.*, 1981, *20*, 793). Although many other antimicrobial agents are active *in vitro* against *Legionella* spp. at concentrations achievable in serum, efficacy in experimental infections in *animals* has been poor compared with rifampicin and erythromycin (A.W. Pasculle *et al., Antimicrob. Ag. Chemother.*, 1985, *28*, 730; R.B. Fitzgeorge, *J. Infect.*, 1985, *10*, 189). This may be due partly to the superior intracellular penetration of rifampicin and erythromycin.

ACTIVITY AGAINST MENINGOCOCCI. All of 60 strains of meningococci resistant to sulphadiazine sodium 10 µg per mL were sensitive to rifampicin 0.125 µg per mL.— M. Hassan-King *et al., Trans. R. Soc. trop. Med. Hyg.*, 1979, *73*, 567.

Further references.— A. O'Beirne and J. A. Robinson, *Am. J. med. Sci.*, 1971, *262*, 33; W. Brown and R. J. Fallon, *J. antimicrob. Chemother.*, 1980, *6*, 91.

ACTIVITY AGAINST STAPHYLOCOCCI. Rifampicin is extremely active against staphylococci *in vitro*. Sabath *et al.* (*Antimicrob. Ag. Chemother.*, 1976, *9*, 962) found that it was more active than 64 other antimicrobial agents with antistaphylococcal activity when tested *in vitro* against *Staph. aureus* and *Staph. epidermidis*. All strains were inhibited by concentrations of 0.005 µg or less per mL. High activity has also been demonstrated against methicillin-resistant strains (K.E. Aldridge *et al., Antimicrob. Ag. Chemother.*, 1985, *28*, 634).

Further references S. Dixson *et al., J. antimicrob. Chemother.*, 1984, *13, Suppl.* C, 7.

ACTIVITY WITH OTHER ANTIMICROBIAL AGENTS. The activity of rifampicin has been tested *in vitro* with many other antimicrobial agents against a range of organisms. Findings have not always been consistent and results often depend on the method and concentrations used. Combinations exhibiting enhanced activity in one study may show no effect or antagonism in another and results are sometimes a poor indication of activity in vivo and clinical efficacy. Furthermore, because of the risk of selection of resistant organisms some clinicians consider that the use of rifampicin should be limited to the treatment of tuberculosis and leprosy.

There has been some controversy about the activity of rifampicin used with trimethoprim. Enhanced activity was initially reported by Kerry *et al.* (*J. antimicrob. Chemother.*, 1975, *1*, 417) against a wide range of organisms, but findings, including antagonism against *Klebsiella aerogenes* and *Enterococcus faecalis*, led Harvey (*J. antimicrob. Chemother.*, 1978, *4*, 315) to suggest that this combination was unsuitable for use. However, these findings have been criticised and disputed (V. Arioli and M. Berti, *J. antimicrob. Chemother.*, 1979, *5*, 113; D.L. Steward and J.N. Eble, *ibid.*, 114; W. Brumfitt and J.M.T. Hamilton-Miller, *ibid.*, 311). Other workers have also demonstrated enhanced activity for rifampicin with trimethoprim against urinary pathogens (R.N. Grüneberg and A.M. Emmerson, *J. antimicrob. Chemother.*, 1977, *3*, 453; W. Farrell *et al., ibid.*, 459; B.P. Goldstein *et al., Antimicrob. Ag. Chemother*, 1979, *16*, 736) and this combination has been tried in the treatment of urinary-tract infections (see p.577). Despite encouraging activity *in vitro* (L.K. McDougal and C. Thornsberry, *J. antimicrob. Chemother.*, 1982, *9*, 369) clinical results do not appear to justify the addition of trimethoprim to treatment with rifampicin for nasal carriers of *Haemophilis influenzae* (see p.576).

Although rifampicin has no activity on its own against fungi, it has been reported to enhance the antifungal activity of amphotericin.

Some references to studies of the activity of rifampicin with other antimicrobial agents:

Staphylococcus aureus, including methicillin resistant strains—C.U. Tuazon *et al., Antimicrob. Ag. Chemother.*, 1978, *13*, 759 (enhanced activity with nafcillin, vancomycin); C. Watanakunakorn and J.C. Guerriero, *Antimicrob. Ag. Chemother.*, 1981, *19*, 1089 (antagonism with vancomycin); C. Watanakunakorn and J.C. Tisone, *Antimicrob. Ag. Chemother.*, 1982, *22*, 920 (antagonism with nafcillin, oxacillin); A.S. Bayer and J.O. Morrison, *Antimicrob. Ag. Chemother.*, 1984, *26*, 220 (variable effect with vancomycin); T.J. Walsh *et al., J. antimicrob. Chemother.*, 1986, *17*, 75 (enhanced activity with novobiocin); C. Watanakunakorn, *J. antimicrob. Chemother.*, 1985, *16*, 335 (indifferent effect with clindamycin); C.J. Hackbarth *et al., Antimicrob. Ag. Chemother.*, 1986, *29*, 611 (enhanced activity with clindamycin, erythromycin).

Staph. epidermidis, inclucing methicillin resistant strains—M.E. Ein *et al., Antimicrob. Ag. Chemother.*, 1979, *16*, 655 (enhanced activity with vancomycin, cephalothin, cephamandole); F.D. Lowy *et al., Antimicrob. Ag. Chemother.*, 1983, *23*, 932 (enhanced activity with gentamicin, vancomycin); V.L. Yu *et al., J. antimicrob. Chemother.*, 1984, *14*, 359 (enhanced activity with vancomycin with gentamicin or dicloxacillin with fusidic acid).

Enterococcus faecalis—C. Watanakunakorn and J.C. Tisone, *Antimicrob. Ag. Chemother.*, 1982, *22*, 915 (some antagonism with vancomycin, mainly indifference).

Group B streptococci—S.M. Smith *et al., Antimicrob. Ag. Chemother.*, 1982, *22*, 522 (antagonism with ampicillin).

Listeria monocytogenes—C.U. Tuazon *et al., Antimicrob. Ag. Chemother.*, 1982, *21*, 525 (enhanced activity with ampicillin and other penicillins); D.L. Winslow *et al., Antimicrob. Ag. Chemother.*, 1983, *23*, 555 (antagonism with penicillins).

Pseudomonas aeruginosa—J.J. Zuravleff *et al., J. Lab. clin. Med.*, 1984, *103*, 878 (enhanced activity with ticarcillin with tobramycin); K.P. Fu *et al., J. antimicrob. Chemother.*, 1985, *15*, 579 (enhanced activity with cefsulodin); J. Korvick *et al., J. antimicrob. Chemother.*, 1987, *19*, 847 (enhanced activity with imipenem but indifference with several antipseudomonal agents including tobramycin).

Serratia marcescens—R.C. Ostenson *et al., Antimicrob. Ag. Chemother.*, 1977, *12*, 655 (enhanced activity with polymyxin B).

Bacteroides fragilis—E.D. Ralph and Y.E. Amatnieks, *Antimicrob. Ag. Chemother.*, 1980, *17*, 379 (enhanced activity with metronidazole); K.P. Fu *et al., J. antimicrob. Chemother.*, 1985, *15*, 579 (enhanced activity with cefsulodin).

Some reports of enhanced activity for amphotericin with rifampicin against fungi:

Aspergillus spp.—M. Kitahara *et al., Antimicrob. Ag. Chemother.*, 1976, *9*, 915; C.E. Hughes *et al., ibid.*, 1984, *25*, 560.

Blastomyces and *Histoplasma*—M. Kitahara *et al., J. infect. Dis.*, 1976, *133*, 663.

Candida spp.—W.H. Beggs *et al., J. infect. Dis.*, 1976, *133*, 206; R.M. Bannatyne and R. Cheung, *Curr. ther. Res.*, 1979, *25*, 71; J.E. Edwards *et al., Antimicrob. Ag. Chemother.*, 1980, *17*, 484.

Rhizopus spp.—J.C. Christenson *et al., Antimicrob. Ag. Chemother.*, 1987, *31*, 1775.

RESISTANCE. A short discussion on the mechanism of resistance to rifampicin.— W. Wehrli, *Rev. infect. Dis.*, 1983, *5, Suppl.* 3, S407.

Resistance of Haemophilus. All strains of *Haemophilus influenzae* isolated from nasopharyngeal swabs were susceptible to rifampicin before wide-spread chemoprophylaxis using rifampicin for children or minocycline followed by rifampicin for adults. Of strains isolated 1 and 9 weeks after prophylaxis 10.3% and 7.5% respectively were resistant to rifampicin.— L. E. Nicolle *et al., Antimicrob. Ag. Chemother.*, 1982, *21*, 498.

Resistance of Mycobacteria. Primary resistance to rifampicin in *Mycobacterium tuberculosis* is still uncommon in developed countries but appears to occur more frequently in developing countries. In a 6-year survey conducted in the *UK* by Collins and Yates (*Thorax*, 1982, *37*, 526) rifampicin-resistant tubercle bacilli were isolated from 0.15% of patients with European names compared with 1.0% of patients with non-European names. They considered that the very low incidence amongst Europeans may have been due to the implementation of stricter antituberculous regimens. They also found that the majority of rifampicin-resistant strains were also resistant to other antituberculous agents. Other workers have also reported multiple-resistance involving rifampicin. Siddiqi *et al.* (*J. clin. Path.*, 1981, *34*, 927) found that all of 55 strains of rifampicin-resistant tubercle bacilli they had examined were resistant to isoniazid as well. Racial and ethnic differences for resistance similar to those in the *UK* have also been reported by the Centers for Disease Control in the *USA* for antituberculous agents in general (*Morb. Mortal.*, 1983, *32*, 521). An increasing incidence of primary resistance to rifampicin in children has also been observed in the *USA* (P. Steiner *et al., Am. Rev. resp. Dis.*, 1986, *134*, 446).

Because of the fear of emergence of primary resistance to rifampicin in *M. tuberculosis* there have been calls for the use of rifampicin to be restricted to the treatment of mycobacterial infections. Although some studies have indicated an increasing incidence of resistance in Gram-negative organisms (E.P. Trallero *et al., Lancet*, 1977, *1*, 956) a review of resistance patterns of *M. tuberculosis* in countries where the use of rifampicin was restricted to tuberculosis and in countries where it had wider use did not reveal any difference in the incidence of resistance (G. Acocella *et al., Thorax*, 1980, *35*, 788).

Since the first report of rifampicin-resistant leprosy made by Jacobson and Hastings (*Lancet*, 1976, *2*, 1304) there have been several reports of resistance of *Mycobacterium leprae* in patients receiving rifampicin. It appears that when used as monotherapy, secondary resistance to rifampicin occurs earlier than with dapsone. Resistance had developed within 3 to 5 years in 4 of 16 patients receiving monotherapy with rifampicin 300 or 600 mg daily (B. Ji, *Lepr. Rev.*, 1985, *56*, 265). Resistance has also been reported in a further 9 patients (C.-C. Guelpa-Lauras *et al.*, *Int. J. Lepr.*, 1984, *52*, 101) and Sreevatsa *et al.* (*Jpn. J. Lepr.*, 1984, *53*, 28) claim to have demonstrated primary resistance to rifampicin in 3 patients with secondary resistance to dapsone.

Strains of *Mycobacterium kansasii* resistant to rifampicin were isolated from 2 patients after rifampicin had been added to treatment regimens that had been ineffective for their *M. kansasii* infections.— P. T. Davidson and R. Waggoner, *Tubercle*, 1976, *57*, 271.

See also p.546 and p.551.

Resistance of Neisseria. A report of resistance *in vitro* of gonococci and meningococci to rifampicin.— H. Schneider *et al.*, *Br. J. vener. Dis.*, 1972, *48*, 500.

Resistance of staphylococci. Resistance to rifampicin appears to develop readily in methicillin-susceptible and methicillin-resistant strains of *Staphylococcus aureus in vitro* when rifampicin is tested alone. There have been reports of resistance to rifampicin developing in patients receiving rifampicin and vancomycin for infections due to *Staph. aureus* (J.F. Acar *et al.*, *Rev. infect. Dis.*, 1983, *5*, *Suppl.* 3, S502; G.L. Simon *et al.*, *ibid.*, S507) and *Staph. epidermidis* (B. Chamovitz *et al.*, *J. Am. med. Ass.*, 1985, *253*, 2867). Eng *et al.* (*J. antimicrob. Chemother.*, 1985, *15*, 201) also found that vancomycin was less effective than nafcillin *in vitro* in preventing the emergence of resistance to rifampicin and recommended that patients receiving rifampicin with vancomycin should be monitored for rifampicin resistance during therapy.

Absorption and Fate

Rifampicin is readily absorbed from the gastro-intestinal tract and peak plasma concentrations of about 7 to 9 µg per mL have been reported 2 to 4 hours after a dose of 600 mg but there may be considerable interindividual variation. Food may reduce and delay absorption. Half-lives for rifampicin have been reported to range initially from 2 to 5 hours, the longest elimination times occurring after the largest doses. However, as rifampicin induces its own metabolism, elimination time may decrease by up to 40% during the first 2 weeks resulting in half-lives of about 2 to 3 hours. The half-life is prolonged in patients with liver disease. Rifampicin may be highly bound to plasma proteins.

Rifampicin, but not its main metabolite, undergoes enterohepatic circulation. It is widely distributed in body tissues and fluids and diffuses into the cerebrospinal fluid when the meninges are inflamed.

Rifampicin is rapidly metabolised in the liver mainly to active desacetylrifampicin and is excreted in the bile and about 60% of a dose eventually appears in the faeces. The amount excreted in the urine increases with increasing doses and up to 30% of a dose of 900 mg may be excreted in the urine, about half of it within 24 hours. The metabolite formylrifampicin is also excreted in the urine.

Rifampicin crosses the placenta and is excreted in breast milk.

Detailed reviews of the clinical pharmacokinetics of rifampicin.— G. Acocella, *Clin. Pharmacokinet.*, 1978, *3*, 108; M. T. Kenny and B. Strates, *Drug Metab. Rev.*, 1981, *12*, 158; G. Acocella, *Rev. infect. Dis.*, 1983, *5*, *Suppl.* 3, S428.

Pharmacokinetic studies on rifampicin with trimethoprim.— J. M. T. Hamilton-Miller and W. Brumfitt, *J. antimicrob. Chemother.*, 1976, *2*, 181; G. Acocella and R. Scotti, *ibid.*, 271; A. M. Emmerson *et al.*, *ibid.*, 1978, *4*, 523.

A single dose of rifampicin 600 mg intravenously given to 2 patients produced peak serum-rifampicin concentrations of 6.82 and 12.85 µg per mL respectively after 2 hours and in a third patient the peak concentration was 7.72 µg per mL after 4 hours. In 5 patients rifampicin 600 mg daily intravenously for 1 week gave similar concentrations in serum to those reported after oral administration but concentrations in urine were lower.— G. Acocella *et al.*, *Arzneimittel-Forsch.*, 1977, *27*, 1221. See also V. Nitti *et al.*, *Chemotherapy, Basle*, 1977, *23*, 1.

The pharmacokinetics of rifampicin in infants and children.— G. H. McCracken *et al.*, *Pediatrics*, 1980, *66*, 17.

Peak serum concentrations of rifampicin have been estimated to be 8.52, 14.91, and 21.45 µg per mL after doses of 5 to 10, 11 to 15, and 16 to 20 mg per kg body-weight given by mouth (M.T. Kenny and B. Strates, *Drug Metab. Rev.*, 1981, *12*, 159). However, Ganiswarna *et al.* (*Int. J. clin. Pharmac. Ther. Toxic.*, 1986, *24*, 60) in a study of the bioavailability of rifampicin 'caplets' obtained much higher peak plasma concentrations in healthy Indonesian male subjects. In subjects weighing more than 50 kg body-weight, who were given 600 mg (mean 11 mg per kg body-weight), the mean peak plasma concentration was 20.0 µg per mL while a peak of 17.6 µg per mL was obtained after a 450-mg dose in subjects weighing less than 50 kg. The reason for the difference was unclear although a racial effect cannot be excluded.

DIFFUSION. Rifampicin is widely distributed in body tissues and fluids following oral or intravenous administration. Therapeutic concentrations have been demonstrated in bile (I.J. Kiss *et al.*, *Int. J. clin. Pharmac. Biopharm.*, 1978, *16*, 105), bone (B. Roth, *Chemotherapy, Basle*, 1984, *30*, 358), cardiac valves (G.L. Archer *et al.*, *Antimicrob. Ag. Chemother.*, 1982, *21*, 800), pancreatic juices (P. Pederzoli *et al.*, *J. antimicrob. Chemother.*, 1985, *16*, 129), pleural fluid (G. Boman and A.-S. Malmborg, *Eur. J. clin. Pharmac.*, 1974, *7*, 51) and saliva and gingival fluid (K.W. Stephen *et al.*, *Br. J. clin. Pharmac.*, 1980, *9*, 51). Rifampicin is also able to penetrate into polymorphonuclear leucocytes to kill intracellular pathogens (R.C. Prokesch and W.L. Hand, *Antimicrob. Ag. Chemother.*, 1982, *21*, 373). Rifampicin does not appear to diffuse well through the uninflamed meninges (J.E. Sippel *et al.*, *Am. Rev. resp. Dis.*, 1974, *109*, 579) but therapeutic concentrations have been attained in the CSF following daily doses of 600 and 900 mg when the meninges are inflamed (J.J.G. D'Oliveira, *Am. rev. Resp. Dis.*, 1972, *106*, 432; R. Forgan-Smith *et al.*, *Lancet*, 1973, *2*, 374); concentrations in the CSF are about 10 to 20% of simultaneous serum concentrations, and approximately represent the fraction unbound to plasma proteins. Administration of corticosteroids does not appear to influence the penetration of rifampicin into the CSF of patients with tuberculous meningitis (J. Woo *et al.*, *Curr. ther. Res.*, 1987, *42*, 235).

EXCRETION. For doses of rifampicin greater than 300 mg the excretory capacity of the liver is saturated, rifampicin concentrations rise in the serum and the drug appears in the urine (D.J. Girling, *J. antimicrob. Chemother.*, 1977, *3*, 115). Brechbühler *et al.* (*Arzneimittel-Forsch.*, 1978, *28*, 480) found that the percentage of rifampicin plus desacetylrifampicin excreted in the urine within 24 hours increased from 4% after a 150-mg dose to 18% after a 900-mg dose.

PREGNANCY AND THE NEONATE. Rifampicin concentrations in maternal blood, placenta, foetus, and liquor after oral administration.— I. Rocker (letter), *Lancet*, 1977, *2*, 48.

PROTEIN BINDING. Published values for the binding of rifampicin by serum proteins have ranged from 4 to 92% depending on the procedure used. The ultracentrifugation technique which has been found to be more reliable for other antimicrobial agents has yielded values in the range of 57 to 80% protein binding.— M. T. Kenny and B. Strates, *Drug Metab. Rev.*, 1981, *12*, 159.

Uses and Administration

Rifampicin belongs to the rifamycin group of antibiotics (p.109) and is used primarily in the treatment of infections due to mycobacteria. It is usually the most effective drug for administration in association with isoniazid in the primary treatment of pulmonary tuberculosis and has also been used successfully with ethambutol for the re-treatment of pulmonary tuberculosis resistant to other antituberculous agents. The use of rifampicin with other antituberculous agents is described under Treatment of Tuberculosis, p.547. Rifampicin is also used in association with other antileprotics such as dapsone and clofazimine, in the treatment of leprosy (see p.551).

Rifampicin is used to eradicate nasal carriage of *Neisseria meningitidis* as prophylaxis against meningococcal meningitis; in the *US* it is used similarly to eliminate nasal carriage of *Haemophilus influenzae* in patients at risk. It has also been increasingly used in a variety of non-tuberculous conditions caused by susceptible organisms despite fears that this may compromise its effectiveness in the treatment of tuberculosis and leprosy.

The usual dose of rifampicin in tuberculosis is 8 to 12 mg per kg body-weight given daily before food; patients weighing less than 50 kg body-weight are often given 450 mg daily while patients more than 50 kg in weight receive 600 mg. Children may be given 10 to 20 mg per kg to a maximum daily dose of 600 mg. In patients with impaired liver function the dose should generally not exceed 8 mg per kg daily. Intermittent schedules are often employed although this may increase the incidence of side-effects, depending on the schedule adopted; doses of up to 900 mg have been given twice weekly.

Doses similar to those used in tuberculosis are also used in the treatment of leprosy (see p.552).

In the treatment of meningococcal carriers, rifampicin is usually given in a dose of 600 mg two times daily for two days; in the *UK* recommended doses to be given to children twice daily are 10 mg per kg for children between 1 and 12 years of age and 5 mg per kg for children between 3 and 12 months; in the *US* suggested doses for children are 10 mg per kg for children between 1 month and 12 years of age and 5 mg per kg for neonates less than 1 month old. For prophylaxis against meningitis due to *Haemophilus influenzae* authorities in the *US* have recommended a dose of 20 mg per kg for adults and children older than one month to be given once daily for 4 days with a maximum daily dose of 600 mg.

Rifampicin has also been given intravenously in doses of up to 20 mg per kg or a maximum total daily dose of 600 mg.

Although studies by Acocella *et al.* (*Thorax*, 1980, *35*, 788) suggest that the risk of increasing the incidence of rifampicin-resistant strains of *Mycobacterium tuberculosis* is probably small when short courses of the antibiotic are used for non-tuberculous diseases, many clinicians consider that there is no sound clinical reason to take this risk when alternative antibiotics are available. Nevertheless rifampicin has been used in combination with other antibacterial agents in an attempt to achieve enhanced activity and reduce the risk of resistance. Although the potential problems of toxicity and development of resistance are sufficient to preclude its routine use Davis and Lewis (*Br. med. J.*, 1984, *289*, 3) consider that rifampicin could be useful as a prophylactic and therapeutic agent in non-mycobacterial infections. They stressed that when it is employed care should be taken to use it with another antimicrobial agent with similar pharmacological and antibacterial properties. Experience of the use of rifampicin in combination therapy of non-mycobacterial infections has been reviewed by Kissling and Bergamini (*Chemotherapy, Basle*, 1981, *27*, 368); similar experience in paediatric patients has been reviewed by Naveh (*Curr. ther. Res.*, 1980, *27*, 272). The use of rifampicin in non-tuberculous infections has also been the subject of a symposium (*Rev. infect. Dis.*, 1983, *5*, *Suppl.* 3, S399-S632) and its use as an anti-staphylococcal agent was discussed as part of the 13th International Congress of Chemotherapy (*J. antimicrob. Chemother.*, 1984, *13*, *Suppl.* C).

Since rifampicin is extremely active against *Staphylococcus aureus* and appears in high concentrations in nasal secretions (M.W. Casewell and R.L.R. Hill, *J. antimicrob. Chemother.*, 1986, *18*, *Suppl.* A, 1) it has been used for the treatment of nasal carriers of staphylococci especially in the control of nosocomial infections due to methicillin-resistant strains. It has been reported to be effective when used alone or with other antimicrobial agents such as co-trimoxazole (T.T. Ward *et al.*, *Infect. Control.*, 1981, *2*, 453) or cloxacillin (L.J. Wheat *et al.*, *Rev. infect. Dis.*, 1983, *5*, *Suppl.* 3, S459). Results of a 5-year controlled study by Yu *et al.* (*New Engl. J. Med.*, 1986, *315*, 91) indicated that whereas neither vancomycin nor bacitracin were efficacious in eradicating nasal carriage, rifampicin with bacitracin was effective for up to about 3 months after treatment. However, McAnally *et al.* (*Antimicrob. Ag. Chemother.*, 1984, *25*, 422) had already shown that treatment with rifampicin alone was more effective than rifampicin with bacitracin.

A double-blind placebo-controlled study in 101 patients with infection due to *Staph. aureus* indicated that addition of rifampicin to therapy with oxacillin or vancomycin might only be beneficial for severely ill patients.— P. Van der Auwera *et al.*, *Antimicrob. Ag. Chemother.*, 1985, *28*, 467.

The use of rifampicin with erythromycin or flucloxacillin for the treatment of catheter-associated exit-site and tunnel infections due to *Staphylococcus aureus* had reduced the need for catheter removal during continuous ambulatory peritoneal dialysis.— A. R. Morton *et al.* (letter), *Lancet*, 1987, *1*, 1258.

Reference to the use of rifampicin as part of therapy for recurrent peritonitis due to coagulase-negative staphylococci in patients undergoing continuous ambulatory peritoneal dialysis.— S. J. Pickering *et al.* (letter), *Lancet*, 1987, *1*, 1258.

For further references to the use of rifampicin as an antistaphylococcal agent, especially against methicillin-resistant strains, see below under individual diseases. See also Resistance in Methicillin, p.259.

Despite being used with erythromycin or fusidic acid, resistance to rifampicin developed when it was used to eradicate nasal carriage of penicillin-resistant *Streptococcus pneumoniae*. This may have been due to the poor penetration of fusidic acid into respiratory secretions.— M. R. Jacobs *et al.*, *New Engl. J. Med.*, 1978, *299*, 735.

Addition of rifampicin to treatment produced a favourable response in 4 patients with infections due to *Pseudomonas aeruginosa* who were deteriorating despite receiving therapy with a carboxypenicillin and an aminoglycoside antibiotic.— V. L. Yu *et al.*, *Antimicrob. Ag. Chemother.*, 1984, *26*, 575.

ADMINISTRATION. Sex-linked differences in rifampicin kinetics would enable a 10% reduction to be made in the dosage for female patients without loss of efficacy even with intermittent administration.— H. Iwainsky *et al.*, *Scand. J. resp. Dis.*, 1976, *57*, 5. See also R. Scotti, *Chemotherapy, Basle*, 1973, *18*, 205.

Red coloration of the urine cannot be relied upon as evidence of dosage compliance with rifampicin as it does not indicate that therapeutic concentrations have been achieved (R. Gabriel, *Br. med. J.*, 1983, *286*, 1749). A sensitive microbiological test for detection of rifampicin in urine has been described by Mitchison *et al.* (*Tubercle*, 1974, *55*, 245).

Dosage alterations may not be necessary for rifampicin in undernourished patients. Increased free-drug concentrations in serum, due to reduced plasma protein-binding, may compensate for reduced absorption and lower peak serum concentrations.— K. Polasa *et al.*, *Br. J. clin. Pharmac.*, 1984, *17*, 481.

Parenteral use. Report on the experience of parenteral administration of rifampicin in 237 patients with tuberculous or severe non-mycobacterial infections. Although long-term intravenous administration appeared to be safe, thrombophlebitis might develop if treatment is continued for more than 30 days.— M. Kissling *et al.*, *Chemotherapy, Basle*, 1982, *28*, 229.

ADMINISTRATION IN THE ELDERLY. Results suggesting that elderly patients with tuberculosis can take isoniazid and rifampicin in reduced dosage without loss of efficacy. Confirmation with clinical evidence is needed.— J. A. Pilheu, *Bull. int. Un. Tuberc.*, 1986, *61*, 109.

ADMINISTRATION IN GASTRO-INTESTINAL DISORDERS. Although absorption may be delayed, blood concentrations of rifampicin following oral administration appear to be adequate in patients with coeliac or Crohn's disease (R.L. Parsons, *J. antimicrob. Chemother.*, 1975, *1*, 39; P.G. Welling and F.L.S. Tse, *J. clin. Hosp. Pharm.*, 1984, *9*, 163), gastrectomized patients (C.-H.H. Hagelund, *Scand. J. resp. Dis.*, 1977, *58*, 241), and patients who have undergone massive small bowel resection (P.N. Wake *et al.*, *Tubercle*, 1980, *61*, 109). However, Griffiths *et al.* (*Br. J. Dis. Chest*, 1982, *76*, 286) found it necessary to double the dose of rifampicin from 600 to 1200 mg to obtain therapeutic serum concentrations in a patient with jejunoileal bypass.

ADMINISTRATION IN INFANTS AND CHILDREN. Pharmacokinetic data indicated that doses of rifampicin higher than 10 mg per kg body-weight need to be given in infants and should possibly be based on body-surface. In newborn infants, a dose of 10 mg per kg should definitely not be exceeded and should probably be reduced.— G. Acocella, *Clin. Pharmacokinet.*, 1978, *3*, 108.

To minimise the risk of hepatotoxic reactions when isoniazid and rifampicin are used together in children the dose of rifampicin should be limited to 15 mg per kg body-weight and that of isoniazid to 10 mg per kg.— R. J. O'Brien *et al.*, *Pediatrics*, 1983, *72*, 491.

For recommendations on children's doses of rifampicin for use in multidrug regimens in the treatment of leprosy, see p.552.

ADMINISTRATION IN LIVER DISEASE. Serum concentrations of rifampicin are higher and the biological half-life increased in patients with impaired liver function (G. Acocella, *Clin. Pharmacokinet.*, 1978, *3*, 108). Knop *et al.* (*Dt. med. Wschr.*, 1977, *102*, 1913) have recommended that in chronic liver disease the dose of rifampicin should be less than 10 mg per kg body-weight. McConnell *et al.* (*Q. J. Med.*, 1981, *50*, 77) have suggested that for patients with cirrhosis, bilirubin concentrations exceeding 0.05 µmol per mL should be an indication for reduction in rifampicin dosage.

See also below under Liver Disease.

ADMINISTRATION IN RENAL FAILURE. Reduced renal clearance of rifampicin in patients with renal impairment is compensated to some extent by increased biliary elimination. From a review of data from pharmacokinetic studies Kenny and Strates (*Drug Metab. Rev.*, 1981, *12*, 159) consider that a dose of 600 mg daily does not need to be reduced in patients with renal insufficiency whose liver function is normal. However, Appel and Neu (*New Engl. J. Med.*, 1977, *296*, 663) have recommended that the dose of rifampicin should be reduced to 300 mg daily in patients with a creatinine clearance of 10 mL or less per minute. Although rifampicin is dialysable, Bennett *et al.* (*Am. J. Kidney Dis.*, 1983, *3*, 155) consider that dosage supplements are unnecessary for patients undergoing haemodialysis. Data for predicting the removal of rifampicin by conventional haemodialysis has been presented by Gibson and Nelson (*Clin. Pharmacokinet.*, 1977, *2*, 403).

See also p.548.

AMOEBIASIS. Rifampicin has been shown to have some activity *in vitro* against *Naegleria fowleri*, the causative agent of primary amoebic meningoencephalitis, and to enhance the activity of amphotericin in infected *animals* (Y.H. Thong, *New Engl. J. Med.*, 1982, *306*, 1295). For reference to the successful treatment of primary amoebic meningoencephalitis in a patient treated with amphotericin, rifampicin, and miconazole, see under Uses in Amphotericin, p.419.

ATYPICAL MYCOBACTERIAL INFECTIONS. For the use of rifampicin and other antimycobacterial agents in the treatment of atypical mycobacterial infections, see p.553.

BONE AND JOINT INFECTIONS. Studies of experimental osteomyelitis in *animals* suggest that addition of rifampicin to vancomycin enhances the efficacy of treatment (C.W. Norden and M. Shaffer, *J. infect. Dis.*, 1983, *147*, 352) even in the presence of antagonism *in vitro*. Beam (*Lancet*, 1979, *2*, 227) attributed the response to addition of rifampicin to treatment, in a patient with osteomyelitis refractory to nafcillin alone, to the ability of rifampicin to kill intracellular organisms. Some clinicians consider that rifampicin with another antibiotic such as a penicillin may be of use in the treatment of osteomyelitis and bacterial arthritis due to staphylococci and streptococci that is unresponsive to conventional antimicrobial therapy (A.S. Dickie, *Drugs*, 1986, *32*, 458).

Further reports on the use of rifampicin in combination therapy of bone and joint disorders.— R. A. Cluzel *et al.*, *J. antimicrob. Chemother.*, 1984, *13*, *Suppl.* C, 23.

BRUCELLOSIS. Although rifampicin has produced favourable results when used alone in the treatment of brucellosis it has been recommended that it should be used with another antimicrobial agent. The regimen of choice currently recommended by WHO for the treatment of brucellosis is rifampicin 600 to 900 mg with doxycycline 200 mg both given daily in the morning as a single dose for at least 6 weeks (Sixth Report of the Joint FAO/WHO Expert Committee on Brucellosis, *Tech. Rep. Ser. Wld Hlth Org. No. 740*, 1986). Administration of doxycycline and rifampicin for 30 days has been found by some workers (J. Ariza *et al.*, *Antimicrob. Ag. Chemother.*, 1985, *28*, 548) to result in higher relapse-rates than those for the regimen of tetracycline and streptomycin previously recommended by WHO. Resistance to rifampicin has emerged following therapy despite administration with doxycycline (Y.M. De Rautlin De La Roy *et al.*, *J. antimicrob. Chemother.*, 1986, *18*, 648). Rifampicin has also been administered with co-trimoxazole and this regimen has been reported to be effective in the treatment of children (J. Llorens-Terol and R.M. Busquets, *Archs Dis. Childh.*, 1980, *55*, 486).

For the treatment of brucellosis during pregnancy WHO recommends rifampicin as the drug of choice and that co-trimoxazole or tetracycline should only be given if rifampicin is unavailable; streptomycin is contra-indicated. In the treatment of neurobrucellosis the length of therapy also appears to be of critical importance; relapses may occur after treatment lasting only 2 to 3 weeks and a regimen of tetracycline 2 g daily and rifampicin 600 to 900 mg daily given for 8 to 12 weeks supplemented with streptomycin 1 g daily for 6 weeks has consequently been recommended by some (R.A. Shakir, *Postgrad. med. J.*, 1986, *62*, 1077). There have also been reports of the successful use of similar triple therapy in the treatment of endocarditis due to *Brucella melitensis* (D.S. Pratt *et al.*, *Am. J. Med.*, 1978, *64*, 897; Z. Farid and B. Trabolsi, *Br. med. J.*, 1985, *291*, 110).

CHANCROID. *Haemophilus ducreyi* was rapidly eliminated from genital ulcers with subsequent healing of ulcers and buboes in most of the 54 patients evaluated in a controlled randomised study after receiving rifampicin 600 mg daily for 3 days either alone or with trimethoprim 160 mg. Therapy failed in 1 and ulcers recurred in 2 of the 32 patients treated with combination therapy, whereas there were no relapses or failure following rifampicin alone. Genital ulcers culture negative for *H. ducreyi* in 16 further patients responded favourably to either treatment. Also, in an uncontrolled open study, ulcers and buboes had resolved in 17 of 18 with genital ulcers positive for *H. ducreyi* within 14 days of receiving a single dose of rifampicin 600 mg with trimethoprim 160 mg.— F. A. Plummer *et al.*, *Rev. infect. Dis.*, 1983, *5*, *Suppl.* 3, S565.

ENDOCARDITIS. Rifampicin is extremely active *in vitro* against staphylococci including methicillin-resistant strains of *Staphylococcus aureus* and *Staph. epidermidis* and although the effect of rifampicin and vancomycin on each other's activity *in vitro* is variable (see under Activity with other Antimicrobial Agents in Antimicrobial Action), this combination has been recommended by some as an initial choice for the treatment of methicillin-resistant staphylococcal endocarditis; others however, consider that they should not be used together (see p.96). While some clinicians (J.G. Morris and J.H. Tenney, *Ann. intern. Med.*, 1983, *99*, 283) have successfully used this regimen, despite the presence of antagonism *in vitro*, Chamovitz *et al.* (*J. Am. med. Ass.*, 1985, *253*, 2867) have reported its failure in 3 patients with prosthetic valve endocarditis due to *Staph. epidermidis* which developed resistance to rifampicin during therapy. Although Auger *et al.* (*Can. med. Ass. J.*, 1982, *127*, 609) have described a patient with staphylococcal endocarditis who only responded when rifampicin was added to cephalosporin therapy, Karchmer *et al.* (*Ann. intern. Med.*, 1983, *98*, 447) found that generally the cure-rate was little improved when rifampicin was added to therapy with beta-lactam antibiotics.

There have been isolated reports of rifampicin being used with erythromycin in staphylococcal endocarditis (M.C. Peard *et al.*, *Br. med. J.*, 1970, *4*, 410; N.D. Burman *et al.*, *Postgrad. med. J.*, 1973, *49*, 920) and Suter *et al.* (*J. antimicrob. Chemother.*, 1984, *13*, *Suppl.* C, 57) have obtained favourable results with rifampicin and aminoglycoside antibiotics in 2 patients.

Since rifampicin is more active *in vitro* against *Coxiella burnetti* than the tetracyclines, a regimen of rifampicin and co-trimoxazole has been suggested for use in Q fever endocarditis unresponsive to standard treatment (A.M. Geddes, *Br. med. J.*, 1983, *287*, 927). However, Subramanya *et al.* (*Br. med. J.*, 1982, *285*, 343) had reported that this regimen failed to control Q fever endocarditis in a patient who was unable to tolerate tetracycline.

Further reports on the use of rifampicin in the treatment of endocarditis: A. G. Jariwalla *et al.*, *Br. med. J.*, 1980, *280*, 155 (*Chlamydia psittaci*); A. J. Davies *et al.*, *J. Infect.*, 1986, *12*, 169 (amoxycillin and rifampicin; *Lactobacillus* endocarditis).

For a report on the use of rifampicin with amphotericin and ketoconazole in the treatment of endocarditis due to *Phialophora dermatidis* (*Wangiella dermatitidis*), see Amphotericin, p.419.

See also under Brucellosis, above.

ENTERIC INFECTIONS. Treatment of 11 infants with rifampicin 10 to 12 mg per kg body-weight daily in 2 divided doses for 7 days eradicated dysentery due to *Shigella flexneri* which had failed to respond to previous antimicrobial therapy; stool cultures remained negative at follow-up 1 month later.— Y. Naveh *et al.*, *Archs Dis. Childh.*, 1977, *52*, 960.

Further references.— Y. Naveh and A. Friedman, *Postgrad. med. J.*, 1974, *50*, 707 (gastro-enteritis in infants due to *Escherichia coli*).

GONORRHOEA. Although gonorrhoea has been treated successfully with rifampicin WHO (*Tech. Rep. Ser. Wld Hlth Org. No. 736*, 1986) consider that the use of rifampicin for sexually transmitted infections could threaten its usefulness for treating tuberculosis or leprosy. In order to avoid the emergence of resistance some clinicians have used rifampicin with other antimicrobial agents and a single dose of erythromycin 1 g with rifampicin 900 mg has produced favourable results in the treatment of gonorrhoea including infections due to penicillinase-producing strains of *Neisseria gonorrhoeae* in both men and women (A.J. Boakes *et al.*, *Br. J. vener. Dis.*, 1984, *60*, 309; K. Panikabutra *et al.*, *J. med. Ass. Thailand*, 1985, *68*, 579). Belli *et al.* (*J. int. med. Res.*, 1983, *11*, 32) also considered that rifampicin alone in a single dose of 1.2 g was effective and did not produce resistance in mycobacterial species.

GRANULOMATOUS DISEASE. Rifampicin has the ability to penetrate leucocytes and kill organisms therein (G. Ezer and J.F. Soothill, *Archs Dis. Childh.*, 1974, *49*, 463). It has been used successfully for infections due to staphylococci (B. Lorber, *New Engl. J. Med.*, 1980, *303*, 111) and *Legionella pneumophila* (A.G. Peerless *et al.*, *J. Pediat.*, 1985, *106*, 783) in patients with chronic granulomatous disease.

LEGIONNAIRES' DISEASE. Therapy with erythromycin is usually considered to be the treatment of choice for legionella infections but rifampicin should be added when there is no response to erythromycin alone (*Med. Lett.*, 1986, *28*, 33). As the role of therapy appears to be the suppression of bacterial growth while an effective immune defence develops, treatment should be continued for 3 weeks to prevent relapse. Failure of therapy with erythromycin and rifampicin has been reported in immunocompromised patients (A. Mercatello *et al.*, *J. Infect.*, 1985, *10*, 282). There have also been isolated reports of the successful use of rifampicin with oxytetracycline or co-trimoxazole in patients who have not responded to erythromycin with rifampicin (L. Dodds, *Pharm. J.*, 1986, *1*, 728).

For reference to the use of rifampicin in a patient with legionella pneumonia and chronic granulomatous disease, see under Granulomatous Disease, above.

LEISHMANIASIS. There have been reports that rifampicin alone or with isoniazid may be effective in treating cutaneous leishmaniasis due to *Leishmania mexicana amazonensis* (W. Peters *et al.*, *Lancet*, 1981, *1*, 1122) and *L. tropica* (J.L. Pace, *Archs Derm.*, 1982, *118*, 880; R. Livshin *et al.*, *Int. J. Derm.*, 1983, *22*, 61) and has limited therapeutic action against *L. aethiopica* (J. van der Meulen *et al.*, *Lancet*, 1981, *2*, 197). However, antituberculous agents do not appear to be effective *in vivo* against *L. donovani* the causative agent of visceral leishmaniasis (J.-K.M.E. Schattenkerk *et al.*, *Lancet*, 1981, *2*, 304).

LEPROSY. A review of the use of rifampicin in leprosy.— W. E. Bullock, *Rev. infect. Dis.*, 1983, *5*, *Suppl.* 3, S606.

For the use of rifampicin in multidrug regimens in the treatment of leprosy, see under Treatment of Leprosy, p.551.

LIVER DISEASE. Although hepatic drug metabolism is stimulated by rifampicin in patients with liver disease there is, unlike phenobarbitone, no improvement in liver function (W. Zilly *et al.*, *Eur. J. clin. Pharmac.*, 1977, *11*, 287). However, Hoensch *et al.* (*Eur. J. clin. Pharmac.*, 1985, *28*, 475) have found that enzyme induction reduces serum concentrations of bile acids and ameliorates pruritus in patients with primary biliary cirrhosis.

MENINGITIS AND VENTRICULITIS. There have been occasional reports of patients with non-tuberculous meningitis refractory to conventional antimicrobial chemotherapy responding when rifampicin is added to treatment. Ryan *et al.* (*Am. J. Med.*, 1980, *68*, 449) have successfully used rifampicin with vancomycin in such a patient with enterococcal meningitis. Lewis and Priestley (*Br. med. J.*, 1986, *292*, 448) and Haines and Patfield (*Br. med. J.*, 1986, *292*, 900) reported that addition of rifampicin 20 mg per kg body-weight to treatment produced a prompt response in 2 infants with meningitis and ventriculitis due to *Haemophilus influenzae* type B. Salour (*Advances in Antimicrobial and Antineoplastic Chemotherapy*, Vol. 1/2, M. Hejzlar *et al.* (Ed.), London, University Park Press, 1972, p.1203) has obtained favourable results with the use of rifampicin as part of antimicrobial therapy for meningococcal meningitis. There have also been some reports of ventriculitis due to infection of CSF shunts with staphylococci responding to antimicrobial therapy only after oral therapy with rifampicin has been added to the treatment (J.C. Ring *et al.*, *J. Pediat.*, 1979, *95*, 317; G.L. Archer *et al.*, *J. Am. med. Ass.*, 1978, *240*, 751; T.V. Stanley and V. Balakrishnan, *Aust. paediat. J.*, 1982, *18*, 200). However, Kelsey *et al.* (*Eur. J. clin. Microbiol.*, 1982, *1*, 138) attributed failure of therapy with a combination of rifampicin and erythromycin in a patient with ventriculitis due to *Flavobacterium meningosepticum* to inadequate antimicrobial concentrations in the CSF.

For the suggestion that the use of ampicillin with rifampicin should be avoided in listeria infections, see under Meningitis, in Uses of Ampicillin (p.120).

Tuberculous meningitis. Intraventricular administration of rifampicin was effective in the treatment of a patient with tuberculous meningitis which had been unresponsive to oral therapy with rifampicin, isoniazid, ethambutol, ethionamide, pyrazinamide, and corticosteroids. Rifampicin 5 mg in 5 mL of sodium chloride injection (0.9%) was injected daily during the first week followed by 3 mg every other day in order to obtain a minimum concentration in the CSF that exceeded 15 µg per mL.— P. Dajez *et al.*, *J. Neurol.*, 1981, *225*, 153.

For the use of antituberculous agents in the treatment of tuberculous meningitis, see Treatment of Tuberculosis, p.551.

MENINGITIS PROPHYLAXIS. *Haemophilus influenzae meningitis prophylaxis. Haemophilus influenzae* type b is the commonest cause of meningitis in the *USA* and although detailed recommendations on rifampicin prophylaxis for contacts of infected patients have been issued by the American Academy of Pediatrics [AAP] (*Pediatrics*, 1984, *74*, 301) and the Immunization Practices Advisory Committee [ACIP] of the Centers for Disease Control (*Morb. Mortal.*, 1986, *35*, 170), such prophylaxis is still controversial and has not been widely accepted. Several workers have shown that rifampicin 20 mg per kg body-weight given for 4 days will eradicate nasopharyngeal carriage in 90 to 95% of contacts of patients with *H. influenzae* type b (U.B. Schaad, *J. antimicrob. Chemother.*, 1985, *15*, 131; D.T. Casto and D.L. Edwards, *Clin. Pharm.*, 1985, *4*, 637). Rifampicin 10 mg per kg given for 2 to 4 days appears to be less effective and the addition of trimethoprim to rifampicin has not produced the increase in efficacy required to warrant their routine use together (R.S. Daum *et al.*, *Antimicrob. Ag. Chemother.*, 1983, *24*, 658; T. Jadavji *et al.*, *Can. med. ass. J.*, 1986, *135*, 328; M.P. Glode *et al.*, *Rev. infect. Dis.*, 1983, *5*, *Suppl.* 3, S549). From the results of a randomised placebo-controlled study Band *et al.* (*J. Am. med. Ass.*, 1984, *251*, 2381) considered that rifampicin 20 mg per kg body-weight given for 4 days was effective in reducing not only carriage but also the risk of developing disease in both household and day-care contacts but Osterholm and Murphy (*J. Am. med. Ass.*, 1984, *251*, 2408) stated that the study was biased towards demonstrating rifampicin efficacy and suggested that it was premature to accept the use of rifampicin prophylaxis as standard practice for either group of patients. Concern has also been expressed that eradication appears to be less effective in children under 5 years of age (M.P. Glode *et al.*, *Rev. infect. Dis.*, 1983, *5*, *Suppl.* 3, S549; T.V. Murphy *et al.*, *Am. J. Dis. Child.*, 1983, *137*, 627) and that there are reports of resistance to rifampicin (T.V. Murphy *et al.*, *J. Pediat.*, 1981, *99*, 406) and of meningitis developing in patients who have received appropriate prophylaxis (E.G. Boies *et al.*, *Pediatrics*, 1982, *70*, 141). However, the AAP and the ACIP have recommended that all household contacts should receive rifampicin prophylaxis if one of the contacts is under 4 years of age. Treatment should be for 4 days with adults receiving 20 mg per kg body-weight (maximum 600 mg) once daily; neonates under 1 month of age may be given 10 mg per kg.

Since the antimicrobial agents used to treat meningitis often do not eliminate nasopharyngeal carriage it is recommended that prophylaxis is also given to patients treated for active meningitis. Although some workers (K.I. Li and E.R. Wald, *Am. J. Dis. Child.*, 1986, *140*, 381) consider that rifampicin prophylaxis is effective if given with or after active treatment it is recommended that prophylaxis should be withheld until therapy has been completed since rifampicin has been reported to reduce serum concentrations of chloramphenicol.

The status of prophylaxis for contacts in day-care classrooms is less well established and the benefits have been questioned by some clinicians. When updating their recommendations the AAP excluded any definite guidelines for prophylaxis in day-care contacts but the ACIP have suggested that its use should be considered for all children and staff if one of the contacts is under 2 years of age. Some studies have indicated that rifampicin prophylaxis may not be appropriate in this setting since the risk of contacts of these patients developing *Haemophilus* disease was found to be lower than that previously reported (M.T. Osterholm *et al.*, *New. Engl. J. Med.*, 1987, *316*, 1; T.V. Murphy *et al.*, *ibid.*, 5). However, despite this relatively low incidence the Centers for Disease Control still considered that the reduction in the risk of acquiring a potentially fatal disease was worthwhile (C.V. Broome *et al.*, *New Engl. J. Med.*, 1987, *316*, 1226).

Some clinicians consider that the American experience with rifampicin prophylaxis may have limited application in the *UK* (H.P. Lambert, *Br. med. J.*, 1984, *288*, 739; H. Smith, *Archs Dis. Childh.*, 1986, *61*, 4). Although the incidence is increasing, meningitis due to *H. influenzae* is less common in the *UK* and the overall mortality rate appears to be lower than in the *US*. Prophylaxis might be indicated for contacts under 4 years of age but must not be regarded as a substitute for careful surveillance.

Meningococcal meningitis prophylaxis. Rifampicin can eradicate pharyngeal colonisation with meningococci in more than 80% of those receiving therapy (U.B. Schaad, *J. antimicrob. Chemother.*, 1985, *15*, 131; M. Whitby and R. Finch, *Drugs*, 1986, *31*, 266). Because of the incidence of sulphonamide-resistance and the vestibular side-effects of minocycline, rifampicin is considered to be the agent of choice for prophylaxis in contacts of patients with meningococcal disease unless the isolates from the infected patient are sensitive to sulphonamides (H. Smith, *Archs Dis. Childh.*, 1986, *61*, 4; Immunization Practices Advisory Committee, Centers for Disease Control, *Drug Intell. & clin. Pharm.*, 1985, *19*, 615). Immediate prophylactic treatment is recommended for all those who were in household or intimate contact with the index patient in the week prior to the development of the infection, but is not generally required following normal social or medical contact except when there has been mouth-to-mouth contact. Adults should be given rifampicin 600 mg every 12 hours for 48 hours; in the *US* it has been suggested that children older than 1 month may be given 10 mg per kg body-weight every 12 hours while those less than 1 month old may be given 5 mg per kg. In the *UK* recommended doses to be given to children twice daily are 10 mg per kg for children between 1 and 12 years of age and 5 mg per kg for children between 3 and 12 months. However, there have been instances of rifampicin failing to prevent meningococcal disease in contacts (E.R. Cooper, *J. Pediat.*, 1986, *108*, 93). Although resistance to rifampicin has occurred following prophylaxis Broome (*J. antimicrob. Chemother.*, 1986, *18*, *Suppl.* A, 25) considered that it had not been a problem. However, some consider that it may be prudent to use rifampicin with another agent (A.J. Davies and D.A. Lewis, *Br. med. J.*, 1984, *289*, 3). Studies on the efficacy of rifampicin, used alone or with other agents such as minocycline, in eradicating carriage and preventing meningococcal disease have been reviewed by Broome (1986). As antimicrobial agents used to treat meningococcal meningitis often do not eliminate nasopharyngeal carriage (*Lancet*, 1986, *2*, 551) it is recommended that patients treated for active meningitis should also receive prophylactic therapy prior to discharge.

MYCETOMA. For reference to rifampicin being used with streptomycin in the treatment of mycetoma, see E. S. Mahgoub, *Bull. Wld Hlth Org.*, 1976, *54*, 303.

PHARYNGITIS. Failure of penicillins to eradicate group A streptococci during outbreaks of pharyngitis may be due to treatment failures being streptococcal carriers and not acutely infected individuals (A.S. Gastanduy *et al.*, *Lancet*, 1980, *2*, 498). Addition of rifampicin during the final 4 days of therapy with phenoxymethylpenicillin improved the cure rate in children with streptococcal pharyngitis (S. Chaudhary *et al.*, *J. Pediat.*, 1985, *106*, 481) when compared with the use of the penicillin alone and use of this combination cured some patients retreated after failure of the penicillin therapy. Although routine use of this combination is not recommended it might be justified in certain groups of patients. Tanz *et al.* (*J. Pediat.*, 1985, *106*, 876) also found in a controlled study that addition of rifampicin to benzathine penicillin improved the eradication of chronic pharyngeal carriage of group A streptococci in children. However, Tanz *et al.* stressed that this combination was not indicated for routine use in all carriers.

PNEUMONIA. Rifampicin has good activity against *Staphylococcus aureus* in sputum and is a suitable adjunct to antibiotics such as flucloxacillin or vancomycin in staphylococcal pneumonia.— J. Symonds, *Br. med. J.*, 1987, *294*, 1181.

See also under Legionnaires' disease, above.

Pneumocystis carinii pneumonia. Szychowska *et al.* (*Lancet*, 1983, *1*, 935) have suggested that rifampicin may be effective in the treatment of *Pneumocystis carinii* pneumonia after reporting the successful use of rifampicin in 4 children with pneumonia apparently due to *Pneumocystis carinii*. However, Hughes (*Lancet*, 1983, *2*, 162) called for caution as the pneumonitis in these children might have been due to *Chlamydia trachomatis* and he had already found rifampicin to be ineffective in *Pneumocystis carinii* pneumonia in *animal* studies.

PROSTATITIS. While lipid-soluble antibiotics such as rifampicin and trimethoprim are able to diffuse across prostatic epithelium into prostatic fluid in therapeutic concentrations, antimicrobial agents such as sulphonamides achieve low concentrations. Some clinicians therefore consider the use of rifampicin with trimethoprim to be more suitable in the treatment of prostatitis than therapy with co-trimoxazole (*Lancet*, 1983, *1*, 393; A.J. Davies and D.A. Lewis, *Br. med. J.*, 1984, *289*, 3). Although bacterial prostatitis is usually due to Gram-negative organisms Giamarellou *et al.* (*J. Urology*, 1982, *128*, 321) have reported the successful use of rifampicin with trimethoprim in chronic prostatitis due mainly to *Staphylococcus aureus*.

PSORIASIS. Psoriasis in 9 patients, associated with chronic carriage of streptococci and previously unresponsive to treatment with phenoxymethylpenicillin or erythromycin responded favourably when rifampicin was added for the final 5 days of a 10- to 14-day course of treatment.— E. W. Rosenburg *et al.*, *J. Am. Acad. Derm.*, 1986, *14*, 761.

TUBERCULOSIS. For the use of rifampicin and other antituberculous agents in the treatment of tuberculosis, see p.547.

TRACHOMA. Although rifampicin and tetracyclines, applied as 1% ophthalmic ointments three times daily for 6 weeks have produced similar beneficial results in double-blind studies of the treatment of paratrachoma (sexually-transmitted trachoma-inclusion conjunctivitis) and hyperendemic trachoma (trachoma transmitted from eye to eye) (S. Darougar *et al.*, *Br. J. Ophthal.*, 1980, *64*, 37 and 1981, *65*, 549) tetracyclines are usually the agents of choice. The use of rifampicin in chlamydial infections has been reviewed by Schachter (*Rev. infect. Dis.*, 1983, *5*, *Suppl.* 3, S562).

For reference to rifampicin being effective in chlamydial infections unresponsive to treatment with tetracyclines, see under Urinary-tract Infections, below.

URINARY-TRACT INFECTIONS. Although rifampicin is effective in chlamydial urethritis tetracyclines or erythromycin are usually the agents of choice. WHO also consider that it cannot be recommended for use in non-gonococcal urethritis since it is inactive against *Ureaplasma urealyticum* and because of its potential for producing resistant strains of *Chlamydia trachomatis* (*Bull. Wld Hlth Org.*, 1986, *64*, 481). Furthermore, the use of rifampicin in sexually transmitted infections could threaten its usefulness for treating tuberculosis or leprosy (*Tech. Rep. Ser. Wld Hlth Org. No. 736*, 1986). However, Midulla *et al.* (*Br. med. J.*, 1987, *294*, 742) have reported the successful use of rifampicin in 3 patients with chlamydial infections of the pharynx, conjunctiva, and urogenital tract who failed to respond to treatment with tetracycline and then doxycycline. The use of rifampicin in chlamydial infections has been reviewed by Schachter (*Rev. infect. Dis.*, 1983, *5*, *Suppl.* 3, S562).

With trimethoprim. Rifampicin administered with trimethoprim appears to be more effective than co-trimoxazole in the treatment of urinary-tract infections (T. Adachi and T.R. de Almeida, *J. int. med. Res.*, 1979, *7*, 132; J. Kosmidis *et al.*, *J. antimicrob. Chemother.*, 1983, *11*, 239) but some clinicians (A.J. Davies and D.A. Lewis, *Br. med. J.*, 1984, *289*, 3) consider that the availability of other effective antimicrobial agents and the risk of adverse effects with rifampicin make the use of this combination unnecessary for uncomplicated infections. However, although they do not advocate the widespread use of rifampicin outside tuberculosis, Brumfitt *et al.* (*Rev. infect. Dis.*, 1983, *5*, *Suppl.* 3, S573) concluded from their own studies and evaluation of the clinical experience of other workers, that rifampicin with trimethoprim would be a valuable alternative for the treatment of recurrent urinary-tract infection, especially in patients with renal involvement.

Preparations

Rifampicin Capsules (*B.P.*)

Rifampin Capsules (*U.S.P.*). Capsules containing rifampicin.

Rifampin and Isoniazid Capsules (*U.S.P.*). Capsules containing rifampicin and isoniazid.

Rifampicin Oral Suspension (*B.P.*). pH 4.2 to 4.8.

Proprietary Preparations

Rifadin (*Merrell, UK*). *Capsules*, rifampicin 150 and 300 mg.
Syrup, rifampicin 100 mg/5 mL.
Intravenous infusion, powder for reconstitution, rifampicin 600 mg, supplied with solvent.

Rimactane (*Ciba, UK*). *Capsules*, rifampicin 150 and 300 mg.
Syrup, rifampicin 100 mg/5 mL.
Intravenous infusion, powder for reconstitution, rifampicin 300 mg, supplied with solvent.

Rifater (*Merrell, UK*). *Tablets*, rifampicin 120 mg, isoniazid 50 mg, pyrazinamide 300 mg. *Dose.* for patients less than 40 kg body-weight, 3 tablets daily as a single dose; for patients weighing 40 to 49 kg, 4 tablets daily; for patients weighing 50 to 64 kg, 5 tablets daily; for patients weighing 65 kg or more, 6 tablets daily.

Rifinah (*Merrell, UK*). *Tablets* (Rifinah 150), rifampicin 150 mg, isoniazid 100 mg.
Tablets (Rifinah 300), rifampicin 300 mg, isoniazid 150 mg. *Dose.* Rifinah 150: for patients less than 50 kg body-weight, 3 tablets daily as a single dose; Rifinah 300: for patients over 50 kg body-weight, 2 tablets daily.

Rimactazid (*Ciba, UK*). *Tablets* (Rimactazid 150), rifampicin 150 mg, isoniazid 100 mg.
Tablets (Rimactazid 300), rifampicin 300 mg, isoniazid 150 mg. *Dose.* Rimactazid 150: for patients less than 50 kg body-weight, 3 tablets daily as a single dose; Rimactazid 300: for patients over 50 kg body-weight, 2 tablets daily.

Proprietary Names and Manufacturers

Aptecin (*Jpn*); Archidyn (*Ital.*); Chibro-Rifamycine (*Chibret, Switz.*); Diabacil (*Hosbon, Spain*); Eremfat (*Saarstickstoff-Fatol, Ger.*); Fenampicin (*Antibioticos, Spain*); Feronia (*Spain*); Fimizina (*IBYS, Spain*); Rifa (*Grünenthal, Ger.*); Rifadin (*Lepetit, Arg.; Merrell Dow, Austral.; Merrell Dow, Canad.; Lepetit, Ital.; Neth.; Ferrosan, Norw.; Mer-National, S.Afr.; Ferrosan, Swed.; Merrell, UK; Merrell Dow, USA*); Rifadine (*Merrell Dow, Belg.; Lepetit, Fr.*); Rifagen (*Morgens, Spain*); Rifaldin (*Merrell Dow, Spain*); Rifampicin-hefa (*Hefa-Frenon, Ger.*); Rifapiam (*Piam, Ital.*); Rifaprodin (*High Noon, Pakistan; Prodes, Spain*); Rifex (*Infar, Port.*); Rifocina (*Lepetit, Arg.*); Rifoldin (*Merrell, Ger.*); Rifoldine (*Merrell Dow, Switz.*); Rifonilo (*Spain*); Riforal (*Spain*); Rimactan (*Ciba, Arg.; Ciba, Belg.; Ciba, Denm.; Ciba, Fr.; Ciba, Ger.; Ciba, Ital.; Neth.; Ciba, Norw.; Ciba, Spain; Ciba, Swed.; Ciba, Switz.*); Rimactane (*Ciba, Austral.; Ciba, Canad.; Ciba, S.Afr.; Ciba, UK; Ciba, USA*); Rimapen (*Orion, Fin.*); Rimpacin (*Cadila, Ind.*); Rimycin (*Alphapharm, Austral.*); Rofact (*ICN, Canad.*); Seamicin (*Galepharma, Spain*); Tibirim (*Ranbaxy, Ind.*); Tugaldin (*Bicther, Spain*).

The following names have been used for multi-ingredient preparations containing rifampicin— Rifamate (*Merrell Dow, USA*); Rifaprim (*Lepetit, Arg.; Lepetit, Ital.*); Rifater (*Merrell, UK*); Rifinah (*Merrell, UK*); Rimactazid (*Ciba, UK*).

16978-r

Rifapentine (*BAN, USAN, rINN*).

DL-473; DL-473-IT; L-11473; MDL-473. 3-[*N*-(4-Cyclopentyl-1-piperazinyl)formimidoyl]rifamycin.
$C_{47}H_{64}N_4O_{12}$=877.0.

CAS — 61379-65-5.

Rifapentine is a rifamycin antibiotic.

A study in 6 healthy subjects concluding that, like rifampicin, rifapentine is a potent inducer of mixed function oxidase activity in man.— D. Vital Durand *et al.*, *Br. J. clin. Pharmac.*, 1986, *21*, 1.

ANTIMICROBIAL ACTIVITY. A study comparing the *in-vitro* antibacterial activity of rifapentine with that of rifampicin, ampicillin, and vancomycin. Rifapentine had poor activity against Enterobacteriaceae, and against *Pseudomonas* and *Acinetobacter* spp. It had good activity, though less than rifampicin, against staphylococci, streptococci, *Listeria* and *Bacteroides* spp.— H. C. Neu, *Antimicrob. Ag. Chemother.*, 1983, *24*, 457.

Further references to the antibacterial activity of rifapentine: G. L. Ridgway and J. D. Oriel (letter), *J. antimicrob. Chemother.*, 1979, *5*, 483 (activity against *Chlamydia trachomatis*); J. Korvick *et al.* (letter), *ibid.*, 1987, *19*, 847 (interaction of rifapentine with other antimicrobial agents against *Pseudomonas aeruginosa*).

Activity against Mycobacteria. Rifapentine had very similar *in-vitro* activity to rifampicin against a range of *Mycobacteria* spp.— M. D. Yates and C. H. Collins, *J. antimicrob. Chemother.*, 1982, *10*, 147.

Results in experimental tuberculosis in *mice* have shown rifapentine given once a week to be as effective as rifampicin given 6 days a week.— J. Grosset *et al.*, *Bull. int. Un. Tuberc.*, 1983, *58*, 90.

Rifapentine was usually more active than rifampicin, but less active than rifabutin *in vitro* against *Mycobacterium intracellulare*.— M. H. Cynamon, *Antimicrob. Ag. Chemother.*, 1985, *28*, 440.

The MICs of rifapentine against *Mycobacterium tuberculosis* were 2 to 4 times lower than those of rifampicin. The bactericidal activity, however, was equal to or slightly lower than that of rifampicin.— J. M. Dickinson and D. A. Mitchison, *Tubercle*, 1987, *68*, 113.

For reference to comparative studies of 6 rifamycin derivatives, including rifapentine, against *Mycobacterium tuberculosis* and *M. avium/intracellulare/scrofulaceum* complex, see Rifabutin, p.570.

Activity against staphylococci. Rifapentine generally had similar inhibitory activity to rifampicin against methicillin-susceptible and -resistant staphylococci, and there appeared to be cross-resistance between the 2 antibiotics. In combination with a range of other antimicrobial agents active against staphylococci, both drugs demonstrated mainly indifference but also some degree of synergy depending on the test method used.— P. E. Varaldo *et al.*, *Antimicrob. Ag. Chemother.*, 1985, *27*, 615. See also C. S. F. Easmon and J. P. Crane, *J. antimicrob. Chemother.*, 1984, *13*, 585.

Proprietary Names and Manufacturers

Lepetit, Ital.; Merrell Dow, USA.

6558-p

Sodium Acetosulphone

Acetosulfone Sodium (*USAN*); Sulfadiasulfone Sodium (*rINN*). Sodium 2-*N*-acetylsulphamoyl-4,4′-diaminodiphenyl sulphone.
$C_{14}H_{14}N_3NaO_5S_2$=391.4.

CAS — 80-80-8 (acetosulphone); 128-12-1 (sodium salt).

Sodium acetosulphone is a sulphone and has actions and uses similar to those of dapsone (see p.558), but only about 25% of a dose is absorbed from the gastro-intestinal tract. It was formerly used in the treatment of leprosy and also in the treatment of dermatitis herpetiformis.

Proprietary Names and Manufacturers

Promacetin (*Parke, Davis, USA*).

6559-s

Sodium Glucosulphone

Glucosulfone Sodium (*rINNM*). Disodium bis[4-(*N*-1-sulphoglucosylamino)phenyl] sulphone.
$C_{24}H_{34}N_2Na_2O_{18}S_3$=780.7.

CAS — 551-89-3 (glucosulphone); 554-18-7 (disodium salt).

Sodium glucosulphone is a sulphone and has the actions and uses of dapsone (see p.558) to which it is converted in the body. It is not well tolerated by mouth and was usually given by intravenous injection in the treatment of leprosy.

Proprietary Names and Manufacturers

Promin (*Parke, Davis, USA*).

6561-m

Solapsone (*BAN*).

Solasulfone (*pINN*); Solasulfonum; Solusulfone. Tetrasodium 3,3′-diphenyl-4,4′-sulphonylbis(1-anilinopropane-1,3-disulphonate).
$C_{30}H_{28}N_2Na_4O_{14}S_5(+xH_2O)$=892.8.

CAS — 133-65-3 (anhydrous).

Pharmacopoeias. In *It.*

Solapsone is a sulphone and has the actions and uses of dapsone (see p.558) to which it is partially metabolised. It has been given by mouth in the treatment of leprosy but was more commonly given by subcutaneous or intramuscular injection.

Pharmacokinetic studies of solapsone.— R. H. Gelber *et al.*, *Lepr. Rev.*, 1974, *45*, 308; *idem*, 1975, *46*, 124; J. H. Peters *et al.*, *ibid.*, 171.

Proprietary Names and Manufacturers

Sulphetrone.

6562-b

Sulfoxone Sodium *(USAN).*
Aldesulfone Sodium *(rINN)*; Sodium Sulfoxone; Sulfoxydiasulfone Sodium. Disodium [sulfonylbis(*p*-phenyleneimino)]dimethanesulfinate.
$C_{14}H_{14}N_2Na_2O_6S_3$=448.4.

CAS — 144-76-3 (sulfoxone); 144-75-2 (disodium salt).

Pharmacopoeias. In *Arg.* and *U.S.*

A white to pale yellow powder with a characteristic odour, containing 73 to 81% of $C_{14}H_{14}N_2Na_2O_6S_3$ with suitable buffers and inert ingredients.
Soluble 1 in about 14 of water yielding a clear to hazy pale yellow solution; very slightly soluble in alcohol, chloroform, and ether. A 10% solution in water has a pH of 10.5 to 11.5. **Store** at −10° to −20° in an atmosphere of nitrogen in airtight containers. Protect from light.

Sulfoxone sodium is a sulphone and has the actions and uses of dapsone (see p.558) to which it is hydrolysed in the gastro-intestinal tract. It has been given to patients who experience severe gastro-intestinal side-effects with dapsone but absorption is erratic. For the treatment of leprosy it has been given by mouth as enteric-coated tablets, 330 mg daily being roughly equivalent to dapsone 50 mg daily. Higher doses have been given for dermatitis herpetiformis.

Pharmacokinetics of sulfoxone sodium.— J. H. Peters *et al., Lepr. Rev.*, 1975, *46*, 171.

A report of peripheral neuropathy in a patient receiving sulfoxone sodium for dermatitis herpetiformis.— G. Volden, *Br. med. J.*, 1977, *1*, 1193.

Preparations

Sulfoxone Sodium Tablets *(U.S.P.).* Enteric-coated tablets of sulfoxone sodium.

Proprietary Names and Manufacturers

Diasone *(Abbott, Norw.; Abbott, Swed.)*; Diasone Sodium *(Abbott, USA).*

7572-j

Thiacetazone *(BAN).*

Amithiozone; TBI/698; Tebezonum; Thioacetazone *(rINN)*. 4-Acetamidobenzaldehyde thiosemicarbazone.
$C_{10}H_{12}N_4OS$=236.3.

CAS — 104-06-3.

Pharmacopoeias. In *Ind.* and *Span.*

Adverse Effects

Gastro-intestinal disorders, hypersensitivity reactions including skin rashes, and vertigo are the side-effects most frequently reported with thiacetazone although the incidence appears to vary from country to country. Toxic epidermal necrolysis, exfoliative dermatitis, which has sometimes been fatal, and the Stevens-Johnson syndrome have been reported. Thiacetazone may cause bone-marrow depression with leucopenia, agranulocytosis, and thrombocytopenia. Acute haemolytic anaemia may occur and a large percentage of patients will have some minor degree of anaemia. Hepatotoxicity with jaundice may also develop especially when thiacetazone is given with isoniazid. Cerebral oedema has been reported.

Thiacetazone was administered in a double-blind study in doses of 150 mg increasing by increments of 75 mg to 600 mg for 2589 doses. The incidence of side-effects was 2.3% for thiacetazone and 1.6% for placebo given for 568 doses. All doses of thiacetazone were well tolerated.— W. Fox *et al., Tubercle*, 1974, *55*, 29.

In a 10-year series of 1212 Nigerian patients with tuberculosis who were treated with a regimen of streptomycin, isoniazid, and thiacetazone, 171 (14%) had adverse reactions associated with thiacetazone and in 134 of these aminosalicylic acid had to be substituted for thiacetazone. The most common side-effects were giddiness (10%), occurring mainly in association with streptomycin, and skin rashes (3%) including exfoliation and the Stevens-Johnson syndrome. Despite these adverse effects the advantages of this regimen, in Nigeria, are considered to outweigh the disadvantages providing adequate precautions are taken.— C. A. Pearson, *J. trop. Med. Hyg.*, 1978, *81*, 238.

Further references: A. B. Miller *et al., Bull. Wld Hlth Org.*, 1970, *43*, 107; *idem*, 1972, *47*, 211.

EFFECTS ON BONES AND JOINTS. A report of osteomalacia and/or osteoporosis in Asian patients who had been taking an antituberculous regimen of thiacetazone, isoniazid, and streptomycin for 12 to 24 months.— B. M. Kallan, *Bull. int. Un. Tuberc.*, 1986, *61*, *Sept.*, 77.

EFFECTS ON THE NERVOUS SYSTEM. Acute peripheral neuropathy which occurred in a 50-year-old man on 2 separate occasions within 15 minutes of administration of thiacetazone may have been due to an allergic reaction.— P. K. Gupta *et al., Indian J. Tuberc.*, 1984, *31*, 126.

EFFECTS ON THE SKIN. Hypertrichosis in 2 children associated with the use of thiacetazone.— L. V. Nair and P. Sugathan, *Indian J. Derm. Vener.*, 1982, *48*, 161.

GYNAECOMASTIA. Gynaecomastia in 7 patients associated with the use of thiacetazone.— B. Chunhaswasdikul, *J. med. Ass. Thailand*, 1974, *57*, 323.

Precautions

The efficacy and toxicity of a regimen of treatment which includes thiacetazone should be determined in a community before it is used widely since there appears to be a geographical difference in response.

Thiacetazone should not be given to patients with liver impairment. It has also been suggested that because thiacetazone has a low therapeutic index and is excreted mainly in the urine, it should not be given to patients with renal failure. Thiacetazone should generally be discontinued if the patient develops hypersensitivity reactions but desensitisation may be attempted if the use of thiacetazone is considered essential for the provision of adequate chemotherapy (see p.546).

Thiacetazone may enhance the ototoxicity of streptomycin.

PREGNANCY AND THE NEONATE. For advice that patients receiving isoniazid with thiacetazone should avoid conception, see under Isoniazid, p.566.

Antimicrobial Action and Resistance

Thiacetazone is bacteriostatic. It is effective against *Mycobacterium tuberculosis, M. bovis*, and *M. leprae* although the sensitivity of strains may vary in different parts of the world.

Its ability to prevent resistance developing to other antituberculous agents appears to be poor but its use may help to increase the overall sterilising activity of a regimen (see p.546). Cross-resistance can develop between thiacetazone and thiambutosine, thiocarlide, ethionamide, or prothionamide. Resistance to thiacetazone develops when used alone.

Whereas 0.5 µg per mL of thiacetazone inhibited all isolates of *Mycobacterium tuberculosis* from Kenyan patients this concentration produced only partial inhibition in 77% of isolates from patients in Hong Kong.— G. A. Ellard *et al., Tubercle*, 1974, *55*, 41.

The minimum inhibitory concentration of thiacetazone against *M. leprae* had been estimated from *mouse* foot-pad studies to be 0.2 µg per mL.— M. J. Colston *et al., Lepr. Rev.*, 1978, *49*, 101.

Absorption and Fate

Thiacetazone is absorbed from the gastro-intestinal tract and peak plasma concentrations of 1 to 2 µg per mL have been obtained about 4 to 5 hours after a 150-mg dose. About 20% of a dose is excreted unchanged in the urine. A half-life of about 12 hours has been reported.

References: G. A. Ellard *et al., Tubercle*, 1974, *55*, 41; P. J. Jenner *et al., Lepr. Rev.*, 1984, *55*, 121.

Uses and Administration

Thiacetazone is used, in tolerant populations in developing countries, in the primary treatment of pulmonary tuberculosis with isoniazid supplemented in the initial phase of treatment, with streptomycin.

The usual adult dose is 150 mg daily. It may be preferable to start treatment with lower doses, gradually increasing over 1 to 2 weeks to the maximum tolerated dose. Thiacetazone has also been administered in intermittent regimens.

Thiacetazone has been used in the treatment of leprosy in daily doses similar to those used in tuberculosis.

A review of the actions and uses of thiacetazone.— J. Leowski, *Indian J. Chest Dis. Allied Sci.*, 1982, *24*, 184.

LEPROSY. Thiacetazone is only bacteriostatic against *Mycobacterium leprae* and is therefore considered to be unsuitable for inclusion in short-term multi-drug regimens used in the treatment of leprosy.— Report of a WHO Study Group on Chemotherapy of Leprosy for Control Programmes, *Tech. Rep. Ser. Wld Hlth Org. No. 675*, 1982.

Thiacetazone cannot be recommended for general use in the multidrug treatment of lepromatous leprosy as poor compliance would seriously impair therapeutic efficacy. Pharmacokinetic studies had indicated that concentrations of thiacetazone inhibitory against *Mycobacterium leprae* would only be maintained for 3 days following cessation of regular daily treatment with 150-mg doses.— P. J. Jenner *et al., Lepr. Rev.*, 1984, *55*, 121.

TUBERCULOSIS. *Pulmonary tuberculosis.* In a pilot study carried out in East Africa with the collaboration of the East African and British MRCs, a regimen consisting of streptomycin sulphate 1 g with thiacetazone 150 mg and isoniazid 300 mg daily for 4 weeks followed by thiacetazone 450 mg with isoniazid 15 mg per kg bodyweight twice weekly for 48 weeks was compared with a second regimen in which the initial intensive phase was continued for 8 weeks and the twice-weekly phase for 44 weeks. After 1 year 20 of 25 (80%) in the first group compared with 22 of 24 (92%) in the second group had responded favourably.— *Tubercle*, 1974, *55*, 211.

Further reports.— *Tubercle*, 1973, *54*, 169 (East African/British MRC Fifth Thiacetazone Investigation, 1970); *Tubercle*, 1974, *55*, 251 (Singapore Tuberculosis Services/Brompton Hospital/British MRC).

See also under Treatment of Tuberculosis, p.547.

Proprietary Names and Manufacturers

Tebewas *(Spain)*; Thetazone *(Propan, S.Afr.)*; Thioparamizone *(Smith & Nephew Pharmaceuticals, UK).*

6563-v

Thiambutosine *(BAN, rINN).*
DPT; Su-1906. 1-(4-Butoxyphenyl)-3-(4-dimethylaminophenyl)thiourea.
$C_{19}H_{25}N_3OS$=343.5.

CAS — 500-89-0.

Thiambutosine was formerly used in the treatment of leprosy but its value was limited by the development of resistance within 1 or 2 years. Thiambutosine was usually given in initial doses of 500 mg daily by mouth gradually increased to 1.5 to 2 g daily but doses of 3 g daily have been given. Thiambutosine has also been given by deep intramuscular injection as a 20% suspension in oil in an initial dose of 200 mg weekly gradually increased to 1 g weekly.

In contrast to dapsone, thiambutosine has a very short half-life and its peak serum concentration does not exceed its MIC. Since thiambutosine is bacteriostatic, its serum concentrations need to be maintained in excess of its MIC in order continuously to inhibit multiplication of *Mycobacterium leprae*. Thiambutosine is therefore unsuitable for multidrug therapy of leprosy.— Report of a WHO Study Group on Chemotherapy of Leprosy for Control Programmes, *Tech. Rep. Ser. Wld Hlth Org.* No. 675, 1982.

Proprietary Names and Manufacturers

Ciba-1906 *(Ciba, Austral.; Ciba, UK).*

6564-g

Thiazosulphone
Thiazolsulfone; Thiazosulfone *(rINN)*. 4-Aminophenyl 2-aminothiazol-5-yl sulphone.
$C_9H_9N_3O_2S_2$=255.3.

CAS — 473-30-3.

Thiazosulphone is a sulphone with the actions of dapsone (p.558). It was formerly used in the treatment of leprosy, but was found to be less effective than other sulphones. Prolonged treatment with thiazosulphone has caused thyroid enlargement and, in young persons, the development of secondary sexual characteristics before puberty.

7573-z

Thiocarlide *(BAN)*.
Tiocarlide *(rINN)*. 4,4'-Bis(isopentyloxy)thiocarbanilide; 1,3-Bis(4-isopentyloxyphenyl)thiourea.
$C_{23}H_{32}N_2O_2S$=400.6.

CAS — 910-86-1.

Thiocarlide is an antituberculous agent that has been used for the treatment of pulmonary tuberculosis in conjunction with other antituberculous agents, generally in patients who could not tolerate or who had not responded to other treatments.

Proprietary Names and Manufacturers
Datanil *(Spain)*; Isoxyl *(Fawns & McAllan, Austral.; Continental Pharma, Belg.; Lusofarmaco, Ital.; Continental Pharma, Neth.; Inibsa, Spain; Continental Pharma, Switz.; Lipha, UK)*.

7574-c

Viomycin Sulphate *(BANM, pINNM)*.
Tuberactinomycin B.
$C_{25}H_{43}N_{13}O_{10}(+xH_2SO_4)$=685.7.

CAS — 32988-50-4 (viomycin); 37883-00-4 (sulphate).

The sulphate of an antimicrobial polypeptide base produced by certain strains of *Streptomyces griseus* var. *purpureus* or by any other means.

Units
One unit of viomycin is contained in 0.0012285 mg of the second International Reference Preparation (1969) of viomycin sulphate which contains 814 units per mg.

Adverse Effects and Precautions
As for Capreomycin Sulphate, p.555 but its adverse effects are considered to be more severe.

Viomycin should not be given to patients with impaired renal function.

Uses and Administration
Viomycin sulphate has similar actions and uses to capreomycin (p.556) and has generally been replaced by it.

It is given only by deep intramuscular injection. Doses of 1 to 2 g of viomycin given in 2 equal portions 12 hours apart have been administered two or three times weekly.

Proprietary Names and Manufacturers
Viocina *(Pfizer, Spain)*; Viocine *(Pfizer, Belg.)*.

Antineoplastic Agents and Immunosuppressants

1800-p

Antineoplastic agents (also known as cytotoxic agents) are used in the treatment of malignant disease when surgery or radiotherapy is not possible or has proved ineffective, as an adjunct to surgery or radiotherapy, or, as in leukaemia, as the initial treatment. Therapy with antineoplastic agents is notably successful in a few malignant conditions and may be used to palliate symptoms and prolong life in others.

The two main groups of drugs used in the treatment of malignant disease are the alkylating agents and the antimetabolites. Nitrogen mustards, ethyleneimine compounds, and alkyl sulphonates are the main *alkylating agents*. Other compounds with an alkylating action are the various nitrosoureas. Cisplatin and dacarbazine appear to act similarly.

All the effective alkylating agents appear to act by alkylating and cross-linking guanine and possibly other bases in deoxyribonucleic acid thus arresting cell division; they are described as cell-cycle nonspecific agents. Not only malignant cells are affected but also other actively dividing cells such as those of bone marrow, skin, gastro-intestinal mucosa, and foetal tissues.

The *antimetabolites* combine with the same enzymes as physiologically occurring cellular metabolites but prevent the metabolic process. Usually, the synthesis of nucleic acid is affected by folic acid, purine, or pyrimidine antagonists. They are described as cell-cycle specific agents.

Several *antibiotics* interfere with nucleic acids and are effective as antineoplastic agents.

Although streptozocin is an antibiotic it is usually classed as a nitrosourea (above).

Some plant *alkaloids* are used as antineoplastics, such as the vinca alkaloids, while the antineoplastic agents etoposide and teniposide are derivatives of podophyllotoxin.

Also described in this section are other agents which act by various routes to affect the growth and proliferation of malignant cells. They include: aminoglutethimide, colaspase, hydroxyurea, mitotane, procarbazine, razoxane, and tamoxifen.

Glucocorticoids (see Corticosteroids, p.875) are used in association with antineoplastic agents in the treatment of malignant disease, especially in acute leukaemias and lymphomas. Other agents used in antineoplastic therapy include sex hormones (p.1383) and radiopharmaceuticals (p.1377). Treatment may also be immunological and newer approaches involve the use of antibodies.

Adverse Effects with Antineoplastic Agents and Immunosuppressants

The toxicity of the compounds described in this chapter is generally a function of their therapeutic activity. Although they may have differing modes of action, their antineoplastic effect is dependent on a cytotoxic action which is not selective for malignant cells but may affect all rapidly dividing cells. The spectrum of adverse effects occurring with antineoplastic agents is therefore similar, but there may be marked quantitative differences and the speed of onset of adverse effects is variable. However, some adverse effects appear to be specific for individual agents, such as the cardiotoxicity of the anthracyclines, doxorubicin and daunorubicin, and may not be related to their principal effect on dividing cells. Also it may be difficult to attribute many of the adverse effects seen in patients with cancer to a specific agent because of the nature of the disease and the complexity of treatment.

Despite its toxicity, cancer chemotherapy is valuable in some instances where malignant cells are slightly more sensitive than normal cells, and in general malignant cells surviving treatment recover less readily than do normal cells surviving treatment. In addition, toxicity may be minimised by careful control of the size and timing of doses of individual antineoplastic agents and by using drugs with different dose-limiting adverse effects in combination chemotherapy regimens.

Adverse effects common to all antineoplastic agents to a varying extent may be divided into acute effects occurring shortly after administration, delayed effects occurring days or weeks after administration, and long-term effects which may not become evident for years. Acute effects include anorexia, nausea and vomiting, allergic reactions, and local irritant effects. Nausea and vomiting are common to most antineoplastic agents, are often central in origin, and may occur, with varying severity, minutes or hours after an injection. Allergic reactions include skin rashes, pruritus, and erythema, often of areas previously irradiated, as well as symptoms such as fever, headache, hypotension, malaise, and weakness; anaphylaxis has been reported, particularly with colaspase. Many antineoplastic agents have vesicant or irritant effects on the skin and mucous membranes and may cause thrombophlebitis when injected intravenously.

Delayed or long-term adverse effects may result from the action of antineoplastic agents on rapidly dividing normal cells in the bone marrow, lymphoreticular tissue, gastro-intestinal mucosa, skin, gonads, and foetus. The most common serious effect is probably bone-marrow depression with leucopenia, anaemia, and thrombocytopenia and bleeding, as well as an immunosuppressant effect involving both antibody and cell-mediated immunity. The attendant increased risks of infection and haemorrhage can be life-threatening although the severity of myelosuppression varies for individual agents and may occur days or weeks after administration. Some agents, including the nitrosoureas carmustine, lomustine, and semustine, may cause cumulative delayed bone-marrow depression leading to prolonged severe pancytopenia.

Adverse effects on the gastro-intestinal tract have included stomatitis, mouth ulcers, oesophagitis, abdominal pain, haemorrhage, diarrhoea, and intestinal ulceration and perforation.

The active cells of the hair follicles are susceptible to most antineoplastic agents, but especially cyclophosphamide and doxorubicin, and reversible alopecia may occur. Wound healing may be delayed.

Antineoplastic chemotherapy may lead to suppression of ovarian and testicular function resulting in amenorrhoea and the inhibition of spermatogenesis. Gynaecomastia has been reported. The majority of antineoplastic agents are potentially mutagenic and teratogenic. Administration in the first trimester of pregnancy in particular may result in foetal abortion, stunting, or malformation. Second malignancies may develop in patients who have previously undergone successful cancer chemotherapy, particularly where the alkylating agents were used. This carcinogenic effect has been linked with the ability of antineoplastic agents to induce mutations and with the effects of prolonged immunosuppression but it is not possible entirely to separate the effects of chemotherapy from those of radiation, and the underlying defects associated with the disease state.

Other adverse effects occurring with antineoplastic agents include hyperuricaemia and acute renal failure due to uric acid nephropathy which may result from the lysis of large numbers of cells and the breakdown of nucleoproteins; nephrotoxicity may also occur, notably with cisplatin and cyclosporin. Hyperphosphataemia and other disturbances of electrolyte balance have also been reported. Pigmentation of the skin and nails occurs with several antineoplastic agents and may occasionally be part of an Addisonian syndrome. Jaundice and abnormal liver-function tests may sometimes be a manifestation of the disease rather than its treatment. Effects on the lung, culminating in pulmonary fibrosis, and neurotoxicity, both central and peripheral, occur variably.

Reviews of the adverse effects of antineoplastic agents.— M. H. Cullen, *Prescribers' J.*, 1979, *19*, 42; *Drug & Ther. Bull.*, 1983, *21*, 45.

A review of the long-term effects of treatment for malignant disease.— L. A. Price, *Br. J. Hosp. Med.*, 1983, *30*, 8. See also: *Lancet*, 1982, *1*, 1108.

CARCINOGENICITY. Broadly speaking, the risk of induced neoplasia appears relatively low with antimetabolites such as methotrexate. On the other hand alkylating agents such as chlorambucil, cyclophosphamide, and carmustine, antibiotic antineoplastics such as doxorubicin, bleomycin, and mitomycin, and certain other agents including cisplatin and procarbazine are either proven or strongly suspected to be carcinogens (*Lancet*, 1984, *1*, 261). In a survey of the literature, Lien and Ou (*J. clin. Hosp. Pharm.*, 1985, *10*, 223) found reports of carcinogenicity (mostly in *animals*) for 16 alkylating agents, 8 antimetabolites, and 4 antibiotic antineoplastics.

Varying reports have been made of the risk associated with chemotherapy, not all of which are strictly comparable. Althouse *et al.* (*Br. med. J.*, 1979, *1*, 1630) have suggested that over a period of 10 years from 5 to 15% of patients given alkylating agents will develop cancer while Boice *et al.* (*New Engl. J. Med.*, 1983, *309*, 1079) in a study in 3633 patients with gastro-intestinal cancer found a cumulative risk of developing leukaemia of 4% in patients surviving 6 years after treatment with semustine; a relative risk, compared to other forms of treatment, of 12.4.

In an evaluation involving over 440 000 patients, 34 cases of acute non-lymphoblastic leukaemia occurred in 70 764 patients known to have received chemotherapy for previous malignancies; this compared with an expected value of 7.6 and gave an overall relative risk of 4.5. Excesses of acute non-lymphoblastic leukaemia were seen in patients who had received chemotherapy for breast cancer, ovarian cancer, and multiple myeloma, with relative risk factors of 8.1, 22.2, and 9.5 respectively. There was also an increased risk of acute leukaemia associated with radiotherapy alone (relative risk 2.5), and in patients with renal cancer (relative risk 2.2) regardless of treatment (R.E. Curtis *et al.*, *J. natn. Cancer Inst.*, 1984, *72*, 531).

The likelihood of developing secondary malignancy appears to be linked to the cumulative dose. Boice *et al.* (*New Engl. J. Med.*, 1986, *314*, 119) have shown evidence of a dose-response relationship between alkylating agent therapy with semustine in patients with gastro-intestinal cancer, and subsequent development of leukaemia. Patients in whom a leukaemic disorder developed received an average cumulative dose of 809 mg of semustine per m^2 body-surface area, compared with an average of 647 mg per m^2 in the group as a whole.

Risk appears to be increased in patients who receive both radiotherapy and chemotherapy. A study in 579 patients with Hodgkin's disease who received radiotherapy, chemotherapy, or both, indicated that the actuarial risk of developing a secondary non-Hodgkin's lymphoma, or acute myelocytic leukaemia was 15.2% and 3.9% respectively at 10 years in patients given both MOPP and radiotherapy, compared with 4.4% and 2.0% risks in the group as a whole (J.G. Krikorian *et al.*, *New Engl. J. Med.*, 1979, *300*, 452). However, there is some evidence that the period of increased risk is not indefinite; analysis of secondary neoplasms developing among 192 patients given combined chemotherapy and radiotherapy for Hodgkin's disease (D.W. Blayney *et al.*, *ibid.*, 1987, *316*, 710) demonstrated that there appeared to be a 'critical window' for development of secondary leukaemia of from about 2 to 12 years after first treatment. The peak incidence of leukaemia-related complications occurred 6 years after first treatment. Similar results have been reported by Pedersen-Bjergaard *et al.*, (*Lancet*, 1987, *2*, 83). However, such a 'window' does not appear to apply to solid tumours, for the risk of such tumours after therapy for Hodgkin's disease has been observed to continue to increase with time by Tucker *et al.* whose study on second cancers covered a period of 15 years (*New Engl. J. Med.*, 1988,

318, 76).

There is also evidence that age may be a risk factor. Pedersen-Bjergaard and Larsen (*New Engl. J. Med.*, 1982, *307*, 965) found a highly increased risk of leukaemic complications in patients aged over 40 years in a study in patients given chemotherapy, with or without radiotherapy, for Hodgkin's disease.

A discussion on the role of immunosuppression in the development of malignant neoplasms. Skin cancers and lymphomas have been reported to account for about two thirds of all malignancies in transplant patients reported to the Denver Transplant Tumour Registry (I. Penn, *Transplant Proc.*, 1975, *7*, 323). Skin cancers in renal transplant patients occur primarily on areas exposed to the sun and the risk of developing them increases with the length of immunosuppression. The majority of these skin cancers are squamous cell carcinomas and in immunosuppressed patients the progression of solar keratoses to squamous cell carcinomas appears to be accelerated. Immunosuppressants may also act as co-carcinogens with u.v. light in the induction of skin cancers but the potentiation of viral oncogenesis by immunosuppression seems an unlikely explanation for these cancers. Undue exposure to the sun should be avoided in patients receiving long-term immunosuppressant therapy and the skin should be examined regularly.— J. C. Maize, *J. Am. med. Ass.*, 1977, *237*, 1857.

In 3823 patients who had undergone renal transplantation and were taking azathioprine, cyclophosphamide, or chlorambucil the incidence of deaths from non-Hodgkin's lymphoma was 26 times that expected, with a 10-fold increase in squamous-cell skin cancer. The incidence of non-Hodgkin's lymphoma and squamous-cell skin cancer was increased about 60-fold and 23-fold respectively. In 1349 patients without transplants who had taken the immunosuppressants for at least 12 weeks for non-malignant conditions the incidence of the 2 neoplasms was significantly increased but to a lesser degree. Other rare neoplasms, including mesenchymal tumours, were increased in transplant and non-transplant patients. There was no evidence that common [other] neoplasms were increased.— L. J. Kinlen *et al.*, *Br. med. J.*, 1979, *2*, 1461. The mechanism of induction of malignant change is almost certainly unrelated to immunosuppression even though the incidence of some types of malignant tumours does increase in patients who are immunosuppressed.— J. M. A. Whitehouse, *ibid.*, 1985, *290*, 261.

Effects on chromosomes. Visible chromosome gaps, breaks, and structural rearrangements are found in blood lymphocytes from patients who have received substantial doses of combination chemotherapy, and the changes persist for years after the end of treatment. A more sensitive, if transient, measure of genetic damage is the increased rate of sister chromatid exchange (SCE) that occurs with even quite small doses of cytotoxic drugs. Evidence from a study by Palmer *et al.* in patients given chlorambucil (*Lancet*, 1984, *1*, 246) suggests that as the dose increases so the capacity of the cells to cope with induced genetic damage is progressively exceeded, and thus SCE frequency reflects cumulative toxicity throughout the course of treatment.

See also under Effects on Reproductive Potential (below).

EFFECTS ON THE BLADDER. Cyclophosphamide (see p.611) is the antineoplastic agent most frequently associated with adverse effects on the bladder, but see also Busulphan, p.604, and Chlorambucil, p.606.

EFFECTS ON THE BLOOD. *Bone-marrow depression.* The formation and development of blood cells takes place in the bone-marrow. A common progenitor, the pluripotent stem cell, gives rise to 3 major cell lines, from which red cells, white cells, and platelets are derived. The development of each of these cell-types takes about a week but their half-lives in the circulation are very different. Red cells circulate for about 120 days and platelets for 8 to 10 days; the half-life of granulocytes is about 7 hours.

Bone-marrow depression or myelosuppression, is common to the majority of antineoplastic agents and is the single most important dose-limiting adverse effect. Involvement of all cellular elements may result in pancytopenia. However, depression is often selective and in any event white cells and platelets tend to be affected before red cells since they have a more rapid turnover in the circulation. The most usual manifestation of bone-marrow depression is leucopenia, followed by thrombocytopenia and anaemia; anaemia may be characterised by falling haemoglobin concentrations and megaloblastic changes in the bone marrow. The degree and duration of myelosuppression varies greatly with different antineoplastic agents and they may be graded according to the severity of their effect on leucocyte and platelet counts and according to the time of onset, nadir, and recovery time of their depressive effect. The cytotoxic effect on haematopoietic cells, relative to that on other normal or malignant cells, varies for different agents. Marrow aplasia is generally transient and may last from 5 to 10 days but with agents such as busulphan it may be prolonged or even permanent; nitrosoureas such as carmustine are known to have a cumulative delayed myelosuppressive effect. A few agents such as bleomycin, mitotane, and tamoxifen do not appear to be myelosuppressive in therapeutic doses and suppression may be relatively mild with colaspase and vincristine. Specific differences in their effects on bone marrow are discussed under the individual antineoplastic agents.

See also under Effects on Immune Response (below).

For reports of lithium reducing the incidence and degree of neutropenia in patients receiving cancer chemotherapy, see Lithium Carbonate, p.370.

EFFECTS ON BODY TEMPERATURE. Hypothermia occurred in 3 patients with Hodgkin's disease and fever when given multiple chemotherapy.— M. J. Jackson *et al.*, *Br. med. J.*, 1983, *286*, 1183. A similar report. The hypothermia of Hodgkins's disease does not appear to be a direct effect of specific drugs associated with treatment but rather to a disease-associated disorder of thermoregulation wherein pharmacological or endogenous influences can lead to thermal lability.— R. V. Buccini (letter), *New Engl. J. Med.*, 1985, *312*, 244.

EFFECTS ON BONES AND JOINTS. Several reports have indicated that avascular necrosis of bone may be a complication of combination chemotherapy for cancer. In cases reported so far there has been a preponderance of Hodgkin's disease and of men aged 30 to 50 years, the former possibly related to the length of the chemotherapy cycle, which extends over 2 weeks. Avascular necrosis is a well-recognised complication of long-term corticosteroid treatment; it is possible that administration with cytotoxic agents increases the chance of the condition developing.— *Lancet*, 1982, *1*, 433. See also: R. Obrist *et al.* (letter), *ibid.*, 1978, *1*, 1316 (aseptic bone necrosis in a woman given cyclophosphamide, methotrexate, and fluorouracil); P. G. Harper *et al.*, *Br. med. J.*, 1984, *288*, 267 (avascular necrosis probably related to treatment with bleomycin and vinblastine).

See also under Hyperuricaemia, below.

EFFECTS ON ELECTROLYTES. Hyperphosphataemia (due to drug-induced release of phosphorus from destroyed malignant lymphoblasts) and acute renal failure in a patient given antineoplastic agents for lymphoma.— A. Kanfer *et al.*, *Br. med. J.*, 1979, *1*, 1320.

A report of hypocalcaemia and hypomagnesaemia in 9 patients undergoing chemotherapy and radiotherapy for acute leukaemias. All 9 were found to be in a state of absolute or relative hypoparathyroidism.— D. B. Freedman, *Br. med. J.*, 1982, *284*, 700.

Aggressive cancer chemotherapy and its complicating opportunistic infection is exposing some patients to a combination of treatments likely to produce hypomagnesaemia, including: drug-induced loss of appetite and increased gastro-intestinal magnesium loss due to vomiting and diarrhoea; impaired intestinal absorption due to drug-induced mucosal damage; and a direct magnesium-losing effect on the kidney of certain drugs such as cisplatin and some antibiotics.— D. P. Brenton and T. E. Gordon, *Br. J. Hosp. Med.*, 1984, *32*, 60.

For a report of cardiac arrest due to hyperkalaemia and hyperuricaemia following chemotherapy for leukaemia, see Effects on the Heart (below).

EFFECTS ON THE GASTRO-INTESTINAL TRACT. Reports of effects on the gastro-intestinal mucosa: J. M. Merrill *et al.*, *Lancet*, 1976, *1*, 1105 (inflammatory anorectal lesions associated with radiotherapy and combined chemotherapy for lung cancer); L. Lubitz and H. Ekert (letter), *ibid.*, 1979, *2*, 532 (severe, but reversible, changes in the duodenal mucosa and profuse diarrhoea associated with high-dose cytotoxic chemotherapy); D. Cunningham *et al.*, *J. clin. Path.*, 1985, *38*, 265 (functional and structural changes in the jejunum after cytotoxic therapy).

Effects on the mouth. Cytotoxic drugs are capable of causing many clinical oral disorders including generalised inflammatory changes of the gingival and oral mucosa, ulceration, erythema multiforme, lichenoid reactions, vesiculobullous lesions, and xerostomia with its associated problems including increased dental caries.— K. D. Hay and P. C. Reade, *Drugs*, 1983, *26*, 268.

EFFECTS ON THE HEART. Cardiac arrest due to hyperkalaemia in association with hyperuricaemia following successful chemotherapy for acute lymphoblastic leukaemia with a large tumour burden and despite allopurinol cover. Haemodialysis was required to clear the uric acid and the patient survived.— D. Wilson *et al.*, *Cancer*, 1977, *39*, 2290.

EFFECTS ON IMMUNE RESPONSE. Lymphocytes are produced by stem cells in the bone marrow and at other sites, including the thymus, and are involved in humoral and cell-mediated immunity. The majority of agents described in this chapter have a depressant effect on bone marrow (see Effects on the Blood, above) and many have immunosuppressant properties although the degree of suppression varies considerably and may depend on the dose and schedule of administration used. Immunosuppression decreases the patient's resistance to infection and has also been implicated in the development of malignancies (see Carcinogenicity, above).

Immunisation of 53 patients with Hodgkin's disease and 10 controls, using dodecavalent pneumococcal vaccine, indicated that antibody response was profoundly impaired in patients who had received intensive radiotherapy and/or chemotherapy. Impairment persisted for at least 4 years after the completion of intensive therapy.— G. R. Siber *et al.*, *New Engl. J. Med.*, 1978, *299*, 442.

For a discussion on the effects of immunosuppressant therapy on the immune response and the infections associated with it, see Corticosteroids, p.873.

See also under Activation of Infection in Precautions (below).

EFFECTS ON THE KIDNEYS. Nephropathies associated with antineoplastic agents and immunosuppressants include: inappropriate secretion of antidiuretic hormone with the vinca alkaloids and cyclophosphamide; acute interstitial nephritis with azathioprine and mercaptopurine; and acute tubular necrosis with cisplatin, doxorubicin, and methotrexate.— J. R. Curtis, *Br. J. Hosp. Med.*, 1980, *24*, 29.

For a report of acute renal failure associated with hyperphosphataemia, see Effects on Electrolytes (above).

EFFECTS ON THE LIVER. A detailed review of antineoplastic and immunosuppressant agents and the liver. Although it is difficult to incriminate the drugs as causes of liver dysfunction, assessment of the available reports suggested that methotrexate, mercaptopurine, azathioprine, cytarabine, carmustine, streptozocin, colaspase, and plicamycin could probably be classified as hepatotoxic. There was considered to be insufficient evidence to classify fluorouracil, cyclophosphamide, busulphan, dacarbazine, the anthracyclines, the vinca alkaloids, and the podophyllum derivatives as hepatotoxic, but more comprehensive experience might well demonstrate that some of the drugs assessed were either more or less hepatotoxic than suggested by this classification.— D. B. Ménard *et al.*, *Gastroenterology*, 1980, *78*, 142.

Data from the Boston Collaborative Drug Surveillance Program revealed 11 cases of liver disease considered to be due to drugs received for the first time by hospitalised patients, of which 1 was associated with cyclophosphamide, 1 with chlorambucil, and 2 with mercaptopurine; one of the latter pair also received oxymetholone. The total number of patients receiving each antineoplastic was 559, 144, and 52, respectively.— H. Jick *et al.*, *J. clin. Pharmac.*, 1981, *21*, 359.

A report of liver damage in 3 nurses following exposure to antineoplastics for several years on an oncology ward.— E. A. Sotaniemi *et al.*, *Acta med. scand.*, 1983, *214*, 181.

Liver disorders due to venous occlusive disease have been reported in patients receiving cytotoxic therapy.— S. Sherlock, *Lancet*, 1986, *2*, 440.

EFFECTS ON MENTAL STATE. Increased psychiatric morbidity in women given cyclophosphamide, methotrexate, and fluorouracil after mastectomy compared with those given melphalan or receiving no chemotherapy after surgery.— C. P. Maguire *et al.*, *Br. med. J.*, 1980, *281*, 1179. Patients receiving cancer chemotherapy inevitably suffer emotional distress, associated in part with coming to terms with a severe and possibly fatal disease, but in part by the adverse effects of treatment. Patients should be fully informed of aims and likely outcomes of treatment, and adverse effects minimised, in order to keep emotional distress to a minimum.— D. Brinkley, *Br. med. J.*, 1983, *286*, 663.

A report of acute psychosis in 2 adolescents with acute lymphoblastic leukaemia following induction therapy with vincristine and prednisone. Both patients returned to normal when the corticosteroid was discontinued.— J. M. Ducore *et al.*, *J. Pediat.*, 1983, *103*, 477.

EFFECTS ON THE NERVOUS SYSTEM. Antineoplastics commonly affect the nervous system owing to interference with neural metabolism. The alkylating agents, as well as antimetabolites, antimitotics, and antibiotics, are known to produce peripheral neuropathies that regress after drug discontinuation. Treatment with vincristine may cause peripheral neuropathy which may be associated with a painful proximal myopathy.— Report of a WHO Study Group on Peripheral Neuropathies, *Tech. Rep. Ser. Wld Hlth Org. No. 654*, 1980, p.79. See also: H. D. Weiss *et al.*, *New Engl. J. Med.*, 1974, *291*, 75 and 127; Z. Argov and F. L. Mastaglia, *Br. med. J.*, 1979, *1*, 663; I. D. Goldberg *et al.*, *J. Am. med. Ass.*, 1982, *247*, 1437.

Doxorubicin, methotrexate, azathioprine, carmustine, and vincristine had all been reported to cause alterations in the senses of taste or smell.— S. S. Schiffman, *New Engl. J. Med.*, 1983, *308*, 1275.

Peripheral neuropathy with vincristine is dose-limiting and is discussed on p.655. The intrathecal administration of methotrexate (p.637), and occasionally cytarabine, may be associated with damage to the central nervous system.

EFFECTS ON REPRODUCTIVE POTENTIAL. *Chromosomes.* If patients are fertile after treatment with antineoplastics, no significant increase has been seen in foetal chromosome damage, foetal abnormality, or the abortion rate. In a study in 217 women who had received chemotherapy for gestational trophoblastic tumours Rustin *et al.* (*Br. med. J.*, 1984, *288*, 103) found no significant increase in miscarriage rate and incidence of congenital abnormality in a total of 368 pregnancies. Similarly there were no abnormal findings in 286 pregnancies in 146 patients, 77 of whom received cytotoxic chemotherapy, treated for a variety of cancers in childhood (F.P. Li *et al.*, *J. natn. Cancer Inst.*, 1979, *62*, 1193) nor in 93 conceptions in 29 women and the spouses of 19 men who had been treated for Hodgkin's disease (G.E. and F.F. Holmes, *Cancer*, 1978, *41*, 1317), although women who had received both chemotherapy and irradiation did have an apparently increased risk of producing abnormal offspring. However, there have been individual reports of congenital malformations in the offspring of men previously given antineoplastics (e.g. J.A. Russell *et al.*, *Br. med. J.*, 1976, *1*, 1508) and Schilsky *et al.* (*Ann. intern. Med.*, 1980, *93*, 109) suggest that the available evidence does not allow an adequate assessment of the risk at present.

Advice that women should delay conception for a year from the cessation of chemotherapy, which may permit mature ova, damaged by exposure to cytotoxic agents, to be eliminated.— P. A. M. Walden and K. D. Bagshawe (letter), *Lancet*, 1979, *2*, 1241.

For references to chromosomal aberrations with antineoplastic agents, see Carcinogenicity (above).

See also under Pregnancy and the Neonate.

Gonads. In **men**, cytotoxic drugs predominantly affect the germinal epithelium of the testis, producing aplasia with oligospermia or azoospermia and elevated concentrations of follicle-stimulating hormone. Leydig cell function is relatively less affected, and testosterone concentrations are usually normal, but luteinising hormone values are sometimes elevated indicating compensated Leydig cell damage.

Alkylating agents are believed to be the most toxic to the testis. The extent of gonadal damage depends on the dose and duration of treatment. Irreversible azoospermia has been reported in patients treated with cyclophosphamide or chlorambucil, but recovery from complete azoospermia can occur even more than a year after treatment has stopped, and severe damage can be avoided altogether by using small doses. Methotrexate appears less toxic than the alkylating agents. Doxorubicin, even in high doses, appears not to have a permanent effect on human germ cells.

Combination chemotherapy regimens as used to treat Hodgkin's disease produce complete azoospermia in all patients during treatment, usually after only 1 or 2 cycles. Azoospermia persists in over 80% of patients; recovery of spermatogenesis is more likely to occur in patients who are under 30 years of age when treated. The most intensively studied regimens are mustine, vincristine, procarbazine, and prednisone (MOPP) and mustine, vinblastine, procarbazine, and prednisone (MVPP). Mustine and procarbazine are thought to be mainly responsible for the infertility produced, but vincristine and vinblastine may have a potentiating effect. Regimens that do not contain an alkylating agent are less toxic, and return of fertility has been described after the use of vinblastine, bleomycin, and cisplatin for disseminated testicular teratoma.

In **women**, cytotoxic drugs act on the ovary to produce loss of primordial follicles with failure of ovulation, oligomenorrhoea or amenorrhoea, and failure of endocrine function resulting in loss of libido and menopausal symptoms. The degree of damage and its reversibility depend partly on the drug and its dose but more on the age of the woman at the time of treatment, probably a reflection of the decrease in oocyte numbers with age. Ovarian failure appears to be progressive, but pregnancy can occur despite ovarian damage that subsequently progresses to ovarian failure.

As with men, alkylating agents appear to be the most toxic and ovarian failure has been described after single-agent therapy with busulphan, chlorambucil, or cyclophosphamide. However, methotrexate chemotherapy for choriocarcinoma appears to carry a good prognosis for ovarian function, despite the use of cyclophosphamide as well in some of these patients.

In **children**, results have been conflicting. Early studies suggested that the prepubertal testis was relatively resistant to damage by cytotoxic drugs but this is probably not true. Cyclophosphamide and cytarabine appear to produce the most severe damage. During puberty the testis may become more susceptible and combination chemotherapy with MOPP has been reported to produce both germinal aplasia and Leydig cell failure; regimens that do not contain an alkylating agent are less toxic.

The ovaries of prepubertal girls are relatively resistant to cytotoxic drugs, probably because follicular activity is low before puberty. There is good evidence however that cytotoxic drugs can produce gonadal damage if enough is given. The long-term effects of ovarian damage in childhood are unknown. The impaired follicular development may be reversible but premature menopause is a possible sequel.— L. Beeley, *Adverse Drug React. Ac. Pois. Rev.*, 1984, *3*, 23. See also under Sexual Function, below. Further reference: R. L. Schilsky *et al.*, *Ann. intern. Med.*, 1980, *93*, 109.

Gynaecomastia occurred in 9 of 13 pubertal boys (11 to 16 years) an average of 28 months after the onset of combination chemotherapy for Hodgkin's disease with mustine, vincristine, procarbazine, and prednisone. Increased plasma concentrations of FSH and LH, low plasma-testosterone concentrations, and the results of testicular biopsies in 6 boys confirmed that germ-cell depletion had occurred.— R. J. Sherins *et al.*, *New Engl. J. Med.*, 1978, *299*, 12.

Reduced function, not severe enough to suggest infertility, in men treated during childhood with a single course of cyclophosphamide for nephrotic syndrome.— R. S. Trompeter *et al.*, *Lancet*, 1981, *1*, 1177.

See also Pregnancy and the Neonate.

Sexual function. A retrospective study on fertility and gonadal function was carried out on 74 men aged 17 to 72 years who had received cyclical combination chemotherapy consisting of mustine, vinblastine, procarbazine, and prednisolone, to treat Hodgkin's disease; 8 of the men had also received doxorubicin, bleomycin, and dacarbazine. Results of a questionnaire indicated that 40 of 54 men noted a decrease in libido and sexual performance during therapy which persisted in 25 on completion of therapy. Semen analysis of 64 of the men revealed that all were azoospermic 1 to 14 months after stopping therapy; of those investigated later only 5 produced samples containing viable motile sperm, but 1 had become azoospermic in subsequent investigation. The wives of 2 of the other 4 patients became pregnant and one had given birth to a normal infant. Hormone estimations indicated that median follicle-stimulating hormone concentrations were consistently raised, median luteinising-hormone concentrations were around the upper limit of normal, and median testosterone concentrations were consistently normal; the range of prolactin concentrations was wide but median values were mainly within normal limits. The data obtained did not support the suggestion by H.P. Roeser *et al.* (*Aust. N.Z. J. Med.*, 1978, *8*, 250) that declining follicle-stimulating hormone concentrations may indicate return of spermatogenesis. No relationship was noted between depressed libido and testosterone concentrations. It was concluded that patients receiving such therapy should be warned about possible changes in sexual activity and its possible effect on personal relationships, and since infertility is certain with recovery unlikely, such patients should be offered sperm-storage facilities and advice on contraceptive practice.— R. M. Chapman *et al.*, *Lancet*, 1979, *1*, 285.

EFFECTS ON RESPIRATORY FUNCTION. Interstitial pneumonitis and pulmonary fibrosis have been reported with the alkylating agents, busulphan, chlorambucil, cyclophosphamide, melphalan, and uramustine; the nitrosoureas, carmustine and semustine; the antineoplastic antibiotics, bleomycin, mitomycin, and zinostatin; the antimetabolites, mercaptopurine and methotrexate; and with procarbazine. Pulmonary toxicity occurs frequently with bleomycin and, with more awareness of the problem, is being diagnosed and reported more often with other agents. Symptoms include tachypnoea, dyspnoea, and nonproductive cough. Chest X-rays show interstitial infiltrates which are usually bilateral, and pulmonary-function tests show hypoxaemia and ventilation-perfusion dysfunction. Other causes of pneumonitis such as infection should be ruled out; the surest method of diagnosis is lung biopsy. However, the only effective control is to stop the offending treatment at the first hint of pulmonary toxicity. Once pneumonitis becomes apparent clinically it is often fatal and treatment with corticosteroids is generally ineffective. There may be enhanced toxicity when more than one drug is used concomitantly and when a drug is used in association with thoracic irradiation or with high oxygen concentrations in inspired air. Further studies are needed to define risk factors, dose relationships, and methods of control or prevention of pulmonary toxicity.— R. B. Weiss and F. M. Muggia, *Am. J. Med.*, 1980, *68*, 259. See also: W. M. Castle, *Adverse Drug React. Bull.*, 1985, (Oct.), 424.

A review of drug-induced pulmonary disease. The cytotoxic reaction associated with bleomycin, which is marked histologically by enlargement and bizarre nucleation of type II alveolar lining cells, has also been reported with azathioprine, busulphan, chlorambucil, cyclophosphamide, hydroxyurea, melphalan, mitomycin, the nitrosoureas, and procarbazine. The lung injury develops in approximately 10% of patients receiving bleomycin, and death occurs in 1 to 2%. Non-cytotoxic reactions occur with some antineoplastic drugs, notably methotrexate. Such reactions produce no bizarre appearance in type II cells, are often self-limiting and rarely fatal. They have been reported with bleomycin and procarbazine although both are primarily associated with cytotoxic reactions. Noncardiac pulmonary oedema, often fatal, has also been reported in patients given cytarabine, or intrathecal methotrexate.— E. C. Rosenow *et al.*, *Mayo Clin. Proc.*, 1985, *60*, 473.

Diffuse alveolar damage, fibrosis, and fatal respiratory failure following chemotherapy with etoposide, cisplatin, and bleomycin, in a patient with extensive pulmonary metastases, might have been due to lysis of the tumour, and consequent release of enzymes, vasoactive peptides, and oxygen radicals, rather than being a direct toxic effect of the chemotherapy.— J. H. Phipps *et al.* (letter), *Lancet*, 1985, *1*, 1505.

The pulmonary toxicity of antineoplastic agents is also discussed under the individual monographs.

EFFECTS ON THE SKIN. A review of the cutaneous side-effects of antineoplastic agents. The mouth is sensitive to antimitotic agents as the turnover rate of mucosal epithelium approaches that of many tumours. Stomatitis or mucositis is seen with many chemotherapeutic agents but occurs most frequently with methotrexate, fluorouracil, doxorubicin and daunorubicin, actinomycin D, and amsacrine. Alopecia also occurs, and may be severe with doxorubicin, the nitrosoureas, and cyclophosphamide. The alkylating agents and some antibiotic antineoplastics are often associated with hyperpigmentation, most commonly of skin, although pigmentation of nails, hair, and teeth has occurred. Certain drugs may interact with ultraviolet light or x-ray radiation to enhance its effects on the skin and may cause radiation recall, photosensitivity, or, in the case of methotrexate, reactivation of ultraviolet burns. Hypersensitivity to antineoplastics may produce cutaneous reactions including allergic rashes, angioedema, and pruritus. In addition to the above there may be local reactions to irritant and vesicant drugs following extravasation. Finally, certain drugs are associated with specific dermatological reactions: bleomycin may produce hyperkeratotic and sclerotic lesions, actinomycin D is associated with an erythematous papular or pustular rash mimicking septic emboli, fluorouracil may produce inflammation of solar keratoses, and plicamycin is associated with a distinctive flushing phenomenon.— A. K. Bronner and A. F. Hood, *J. Am. Acad. Derm.*, 1983, *9*, 645.

GYNAECOMASTIA. Gynaecomastia may occur when the testis is damaged by infections, physical agents, or chemical agents such as antineoplastic drugs.— A. P. Forbes, *New Engl. J. Med.*, 1978, *299*, 42.

A report of 6 cases of gynaecomastia in men receiving combination chemotherapy.— D. L. Trump *et al.*, *Archs intern. Med.*, 1982, *142*, 511.

See also Effects on Reproductive Potential, Gonads.

HYPERURICAEMIA. Gout is now well recognised as a complication of treatment with cytotoxic drugs.— D. M. Davies, *Adverse Drug React. Bull.*, 1985, (Jun.), 416.

For a report of cardiac arrest due to hyperkalaemia in association with hyperuricaemia see under Effects on the Heart, above.

LOCAL TOXICITY. Local toxicity due to intravenous cancer chemotherapy may include local irritation, extravasation necrosis, and hypersensitivity. Venous irritation, presenting as vasospasm and pain or endothelial chemical burn of the vessel, resulting in a painful, streaky, long-lasting sterile phlebitis, may be due to the drug, or, as with carmustine, due to the diluent (alcohol). Irritation and phlebitis have been reported particularly with fluorouracil, carmustine, bisantrene, and

mustine.
Up to 6% of patients treated with peripheral intravenous chemotherapy may experience extravasation, usually with pain, erythema, and swelling at the site of injection. Severe necrosis requiring surgical intervention may develop, particularly with antibiotic antineoplastics such as doxorubicin. Alkylating agents, vinca alkaloids, and etoposide have also been associated with ulceration and necrosis following extravasation.
Local hypersensitivity reactions, usually self-limiting, may occur: it is important to distinguish such reactions from extravasation. In contrast to the latter, there is no swelling at the injection site, and pain is felt as a dull ache along the course of the vein, as opposed to the stinging commonly noted following extravasation.— M. L. Brigden and J. B. Barnett, *Can. J. Hosp. Pharm.*, 1986, *39*, 96.

NAUSEA AND VOMITING. For a series of papers on chemotherapy-induced nausea and vomiting, see *Drugs*, 1983, *25*, *Suppl.* 1.

The nausea associated with cancer chemotherapy may provoke the development of conditioned responses in which any mention, sound, sight, or smell which reminds the patient of treatment can cause reflex panic, nausea, and vomiting.— R. Maguire, *Br. J. Hosp. Med.*, 1985, *34*, 100.

Most antineoplastic agents are capable of inducing nausea and vomiting which may be severe with agents such as cisplatin, and for some drugs, such as dacarbazine, streptozocin, actinomycin D, mitotane, fluorouracil, and hexamethylmelamine, it may be dose-limiting. For further details, see under individual monographs, and in Treatment of Adverse Effects, below.

PREGNANCY AND THE NEONATE. A large number of cytotoxic drugs have been associated in one or more cases with the birth of malformed children. Such drugs include aminopterin, busulphan, chlorambucil, cyclophosphamide, fluorouracil, mercaptopurine, methotrexate, mustine, procarbazine, vinblastine, and vincristine. Such compounds can be potent teratogens and must be considered capable, when given in the first trimester of pregnancy, of causing serious malformations.— H. Kalter and J. Warkany, *New Engl. J. Med.*, 1983, *308*, 491. Many alkylating agents and antimetabolites are teratogenic. The highest risk is associated with folic acid antagonists, reaching over 40% with aminopterin. Various malformations may be produced, including defects of the central nervous system, limbs, and kidneys. The incidence of spontaneous abortion is also increased and is estimated at 70% in patients treated with aminopterin.— H. Ashton, *Adverse Drug React. Bull.*, 1983, (Aug.), 372.

The risks of maternal administration of antineoplastic drugs to the growth and development of the offspring do not appear to be as great as sometimes anticipated.— P. Gal and M. K. Sharpless, *Drug Intell. & clin. Pharm.*, 1984, *18*, 186.

Occupational exposure. A retrospective study of 545 pregnancies in 139 nurses and 429 controls indicated that there was a significant association between occupational exposure in the first trimester to antineoplastics and foetal loss. Women who experienced foetal loss were 2.3 times more likely to have had first-trimester exposure to antineoplastic drugs than were women who gave birth. However, no association between foetal loss and cumulative exposure was found.— S. G. Selevan *et al.*, *New Engl. J. Med.*, 1985, *313*, 1173. Comments and criticisms of the study's conclusions: E. Bingham, *ibid.*, 1220; H. Kalter (letter), *ibid.*, 1986, *314*, 1048; J. J. Mulvihill and K. R. Stewart (letter), *ibid.*, 1049; B. A. Chabner (letter), *ibid.*

See also under Precautions, below.

Treatment of the Adverse Effects of Antineoplastic Agents

Anti-emetic therapy should be given in an attempt to prevent or control nausea and vomiting.

In bone-marrow depression, transfusions of blood products may be required and active measures may be necessary to combat infection. Hyperuricaemia is avoided by the addition of allopurinol to treatment schedules and measures such as alkalinisation of the urine and hydration may also be adopted.

Techniques attempting to prevent the occurrence of alopecia have met with varying success. Scalp tourniquets and ice-packs (see Doxorubicin, p.624) have been used to minimise concentrations of antineoplastic agents in the scalp after intravenous injection. However, such methods may allow the development of a cancer-cell sanctuary and should not be used in patients with leukaemia or other conditions with circulating malignant cells.

The treatment of extravasation is controversial. Warm moist soaks or ice-packs have been applied and a corticosteroid may sometimes be instilled into the affected area.

A scalp tourniquet placed immediately below the hairline 5 minutes before the intravenous injection of doxorubicin, cyclophosphamide, vincristine, or teniposide and maintained in position for a further 20 minutes reduced the frequency and extent of alopecia in 37 patients when compared with 31 controls. Five patients could not tolerate the tourniquet.— A. Pesce *et al.* (letter), *New Engl. J. Med.*, 1978, *298*, 1204.

An improved method of scalp cooling, using a thermocirculator to pump coolant through a plastic cap, for prevention or reduction of chemotherapy-induced hair loss.— R. Guy *et al.*, *Lancet*, 1982, *1*, 937.

EXTRAVASATION. If, despite precautionary measures, extravasation occurs, as much as possible of the infiltrating drug should be aspirated. In the authors' opinion, cold in the form of ice packs should be applied to the area for at least 1 hour, longer if pain persists, to improve cellular survival by lowering metabolic rate. However, extravasation of the vinca alkaloids should be treated with hot compresses to promote systemic drug uptake.
Local infiltration of dexamethasone 4 mg or hydrocortisone 100 mg may be of benefit although efficacy has not been proven. If the overlying skin is red and inflamed 1% hydrocortisone cream may be applied locally.
The use of specific antidotes is controversial. Infiltration of 5 mL of an 8.4% (1 mmol per mL) solution of sodium bicarbonate has been advocated for the anthracyclines and for carmustine and bisantrene. Dimethyl sulphoxide applications have been tried for doxorubicin extravasation, and sodium thiosulphate injections for drugs such as mustine, mitomycin, and cisplatin; injection of hyaluronidase is recommended for the vinca alkaloids to enhance uptake from the skin.
Once an evolving ulcer is apparent, early surgical consultation is imperative. A widespread excision followed by skin grafting is usually required to minimise further spread to the surrounding healthy tissues.— M. L. Brigden and J. B. Barnett, *Can. J. Hosp. Pharm.*, 1986, *39*, 96. See also: R. Smith, *Br. J. parent. Ther.*, 1985, *6*, 114; R. Bacovsky, *Can. J. Hosp. Pharm.*, 1986, *39*, 27.

NAUSEA AND VOMITING. The mechanisms whereby cytotoxic drugs induce vomiting are unknown and the variable interval between dosing and symptoms suggests it may vary for different agents. The principal group of anti-emetic drugs used are dopamine antagonists (including phenothiazines, such as prochlorperazine, as well as haloperidol, domperidone, and metoclopramide) but optimum regimens have yet to be established. High doses of intravenous metoclopramide are effective in severe nausea, although sedation and extrapyramidal effects may occur, and metoclopramide infusions may be of value. Cannabinoids are also of use, although their spectrum of adverse effects makes them more appropriate for younger patients than the elderly. However the current optimum regimen consists of a dopamine receptor antagonist such as metoclopramide in high dose, a benzodiazepine such as lorazepam, and high-dose corticosteroids.— D. N. Bateman, *Prescribers' J.*, 1985, *25*, 81. Further reviews: J. H. Kearsley and M. H. N. Tattersall, *Med. J. Aust.*, 1985, *143*, 341; C. L. Fortner *et al.*, *Drug Intell. & clin. Pharm.*, 1985, *19*, 21.

Precautions for Antineoplastic Agents

These agents should only be used as immunosuppressants in life-threatening situations. Immunosuppression and bone-marrow depression are features of the majority of the agents described in this chapter and their use is associated with an increased risk of infections caused by pathogenic bacteria or opportunistic micro-organisms including fungi, viruses, and protozoa, and a reduced capacity to cope with them. Those agents which are immunosuppressant should not be given, where possible, to patients with acute infections and dosage reduction or withdrawal should be considered if infection develops, until the infection has been controlled. Special care is necessary in debilitated patients. There may also be a risk that prolonged immunosuppression may stimulate the development of neoplasms (see Carcinogenicity, under Adverse Effects, p.580).

Blood counts and measurement of haemoglobin concentrations should be carried out routinely to help predict the onset of bone-marrow depression and antineoplastic agents should be given with extreme caution when the marrow is already depressed following radiotherapy or therapy with other antineoplastic agents.

Although positive evidence of teratogenicity in humans is not available for all antineoplastic agents, it is considered that they are best avoided during pregnancy, especially during the first trimester, and should not be used in mothers who are breast-feeding.

Many antineoplastic drugs, particularly the alkylating agents, are vesicant or irritant. They must be handled with great care and contact with skin and eyes avoided; they should not be inhaled. Care must be taken to avoid extravasation since severe pain and tissue damage may ensue. In the *UK*, official guidelines on precautions for the safe handling of cytotoxic drugs have been issued.

See under Treatment of Adverse Effects for the caution required when attempting to prevent alopecia.

Of 94 renal transplant patients receiving long-term immunosuppressant therapy, cases of actinic keratoses (7 patients) and squamous cell carcinoma (2) were confined to the 17 who had a history of high sun exposure. Viral warts were also significantly more common in this group than in patients with normal sun exposure or controls. Patients receiving long-term immunosuppressive therapy should be advised on the use of sunscreens and be carefully monitored to detect cutaneous malignancies at an early stage.— J. Boyle *et al.*, *Lancet*, 1984, *1*, 702. Correction.— *ibid.*, 864.

AIDS. Use of conventional cytotoxic therapy to treat Kaposi's sarcoma in patients with the acquired immune deficiency syndrome (AIDS) has resulted in unexpectedly severe myelosuppression, and there is some evidence that chemotherapy further damages the immune system, increasing the risk of opportunistic infections.— P. A. Volberding, *Ann. intern. Med.*, 1985, *103*, 729.

CONTRACEPTION. Immunosuppressive treatment contra-indicates the use of an intra-uterine device for contraception.— *Drug & Ther. Bull.*, 1986, *24*, 73.

DOWN'S SYNDROME. Results suggesting that children with Down's syndrome may tolerate myelosuppressive chemotherapy less well than other children, possibly due to abnormalities of drug metabolism, particularly of methotrexate.— J. Blatt *et al.* (letter), *Lancet*, 1986, *2*, 914.

HANDLING AND DISPOSAL. Most antineoplastic agents can cause local toxic or allergic reactions if handled without due care. The potential risks of carcinogenicity and mutagenicity should also be borne in mind. The manufacturers generally advise that contact with injection solutions should be avoided by wearing gloves and eye protection and, where appropriate, a mask to prevent inhalation of powder. However, K. Thomson and H.I. Mikkelsen (*Contact Dermatitis*, 1975, *1*, 268) reported that rubber or polyethylene gloves allowed penetration of mustine and that only polyvinyl chloride gloves provided any protection. R. S. Knowles and J. E. Virden, *Br. med. J.*, 1980, *281*, 589. See also: P. F. D'Arcy, *Drug Intell. & clin. Pharm.*, 1983, *17*, 532. Concern about the potential hazards of handling cytotoxic drugs is increasing, and although few dispute the need for care with these agents controversy surrounds the mutagenic risks to hospital staff. Although the evidence suggests that hospital staff who prepare and administer cytotoxic drugs are at risk from mutagenicity, it is not conclusive. Ideally the preparation of intravenous cytotoxic drugs should be carried out only in hospital pharmacies where staff are experienced and safety equipment is available.— C. J. Williams, *Br. med. J.*, 1985, *291*, 1299. The Committee on the Review of Medicines had drawn up guidelines which it would like to see included in both data sheets and package inserts for cytotoxic drugs:
a) trained personnel should reconstitute the drugs
b) reconstitution should be carried out in designated areas
c) protective clothing, including gloves, should be worn
d) the eyes should be protected and means of first aid specified
e) pregnant staff should not handle cytotoxic drugs
f) adequate care should be taken in the disposal of waste material, including syringes, containers, and absorbent material.— W. Asscher (letter), *ibid.*, 1986, *292*, 59.

Guidelines for the handling of cytotoxic drugs: *Pharm. J.*, 1983, *1*, 230 (Report of a Working Party to the Pharmaceutical Society of Great Britain); *Procedures for Handling Cytotoxic Drugs*, Bethesda, American Society of Hospital Pharmacists, 1983; *Am. J. Hosp. Pharm.*, 1985, *42*, 131 (Technical Assistance Bulletin of the American Society of Hospital Pharmacists); *J. Am. med. Ass.*, 1985, *253*, 1590 (A Report from the Council on Scientific Affairs of the AMA); *Am. J. Hosp. Pharm.*, 1986, *43*, 1193 (OSHA work-practice guidelines for personnel dealing with antineoplastic drugs).

Recommendations for the disposal of antineoplastics: P. L. Vaccari *et al.*, *Am. J. Hosp. Pharm.*, 1984, *41*, 87. Correction.— *ibid.*, 450.

Recommendations on handling body wastes from patients receiving cytotoxic drugs: J. Harris and L. J. Dodds, *Pharm. J.*, 1985, *2*, 289.

INTERACTIONS. *With drugs.* Absorption of other drugs given in association with antineoplastic agents may be impaired as a result of damage to the gastro-intestinal mucosa.

Hepatic dysfunction was reported in 13 patients who had received daunorubicin 180 to 450 mg per m^2 body-surface. Eleven of the patients had also received thioguanine, cytarabine, or vincristine or combinations of these antineoplastic agents. A study in *rabbits* suggested that doxorubicin might modify the metabolism of mercaptopurine and thereby increase blood-mercaptopurine concentrations (F. Pannuti *et al.*, *Riv. Patol. Clin.*, 1974, *29*, 169). A previous study by R.A. Minow *et al.* (*Cancer*, 1976, *38*, 1524) indicated that the hepatotoxicity of mercaptopurine might be enhanced by doxorubicin in leukaemic patients. It is therefore suggested that a similar interaction could be involved in the possible hepatotoxicity of daunorubicin, thioguanine, cytarabine and other antineoplastic agents.— J. S. Penta *et al.* (letter), *Ann. intern. Med.*, 1977, *87*, 247.

Results in *rats* suggested that dronabinol and cyclophosphamide enhanced one anothers immunosuppressive effects. Clinical studies of the effects of cannabinoids on immune function, when superimposed on immunomodulating chemotherapy, are required.— R. Ader and L. J. Grota, *New Engl. J. Med.*, 1981, *305*, 463.

With radiation. Interactions with radiotherapy include enhanced pulmonary toxicity of antineoplastic agents (see Effects on Respiratory Function, p.582), and enhanced toxicity or susceptibility to radiation in patients receiving actinomycin D or the anthracyclines. See also under the individual monographs.

LOCAL TOXICITY. Chemotherapeutic agents are thrombogenic and irritant to vessels. They are best administered through a wide-bore centrally-sited catheter such as a Hickman. Such cannulae are suitable for repeated courses of chemotherapeutic agents even for over a year.— J. S. P. Lumley, *Br. J. Hosp. Med.*, 1984, *32*, 244. For reports of extravasation associated with administration of antineoplastics via venous access ports, see W. P. Reed *et al.*, *Ann. intern. Med.*, 1985, *102*, 788; J. J. Lokich and C. Moore (letter), *ibid.*, 1986, *104*, 124.

For discussions of the prevention and management of extravasation see under Treatment of Adverse Effects, above.

PREGNANCY AND THE NEONATE. See under Adverse Effects, above.

RESISTANCE. A discussion of acquired resistance to cancer chemotherapy. Commonly acquired resistance seems to be due to biochemical changes within the tumour cells, and the cellular basis for experimentally-induced drug resistance is known at least in part for many anticancer drugs. Mechanisms include failure of drug uptake or activation, increased drug efflux or catabolism, mutant target enzymes, or increased repair of DNA. Much interest has also been focused on alterations in the cell membrane which appear to induce pleomorphic resistance to several drugs of different groups. However the relevance of these mechanisms to clinical practice is as yet uncertain.

Methods for overcoming or avoiding the acquisition of drug resistance have met limited success. The use of drug combinations and intermittent dose schedules may be beneficial. Progressive rises in dosage are usually limited by normal tissue tolerance but high doses of alkylating agents appear to be effective against some apparently resistant tumours. Understanding of biochemical resistance mechanisms should provide more useful therapeutic ideas—for example, resistance due to increased quantities of target enzyme, as with methotrexate, might be countered with new agents activated by that enzyme. However early clinical experience seems to support the view that resistance may be best avoided by the early use of alternating drug combinations which may not induce cross-resistance.— P. Selby, *Br. med. J.*, 1984, *288*, 1252. See also G. Kolata, *Science*, 1986, *231*, 220 (genetic basis of multiple drug resistance).

Choice of Antineoplastic Agent

Antineoplastic agents are used for the primary treatment of choriocarcinoma, leukaemia, myeloma, and other conditions responsive to chemotherapy where surgery or radiotherapy is impracticable. Permanent remissions are possible in choriocarcinoma and in acute lymphoblastic leukaemia. Chemotherapy alone or with surgery and/or radiotherapy may also be effective in Burkitt's lymphoma, Hodgkin's disease, retinoblastoma, some tumours of the testis, and Wilms' tumour; survival may be prolonged in other conditions including histiocytic lymphoma, acute myeloid leukaemia, sarcomas, and carcinomas of the breast and lung. In advanced malignant disease chemotherapy is widely used and produces varying degrees of remission or palliation.

Adjuvant chemotherapy is given following surgery and/or radiotherapy in diseases such as breast cancer in an attempt to eradicate micrometastases. Surgery and radiotherapy only remove localised and regional malignancy and a tumour may often be microscopically disseminated at diagnosis.

Immunotherapy with non-specific immunostimulants such as BCG vaccine (p.1157), *Corynebacterium parvum* (p.610), and levamisole (p.56) has been tried as a adjunct to the treatment of cancer in an attempt to stimulate the patient's own defences against his disease.

Most of the antineoplastic agents are very toxic and should only be used where there is a reasonable chance of success. Treatment is generally best carried out in hospitals with staff experienced in the treatment of malignant disease.

Antineoplastic agents do not all act at the same sites and at the same stages in the mitotic cycle. Treatment with several agents together or in sequence, with breaks in the treatment to allow for recovery of normal cell function, is usually more effective than treatment with a single agent; the likelihood of resistance to a particular agent may also be reduced. Also, since not all agents have the same toxicity, combination therapy can give a lower spread of side-effects rather than the crippling toxicity that can occur with high doses of some single agents.

Although some measures of efforts to control cancer appear to show substantial progress, some show substantial losses, and others, little change. If age-adjusted mortality-rate for all forms of cancer combined is used (considered to be probably the single best measure of progress) then the war against cancer is being lost. Age-adjusted mortality-rates for cancer in the *USA* have shown a steady increase over several decades, with no evidence of a recent downward trend. Substantial increases in understanding of the nature and properties of cancer have not led to a corresponding fall in mortality-rate because of the lack of any substantial recent improvement in treating the most common forms of the disease. On the basis of past experience with other diseases it is suggested that the most promising areas may be in cancer prevention rather than treatment (J.C. Bailar and E.M. Smith, *New Engl. J. Med.*, 1986, *314*, 1226). Similar views have been expressed elsewhere, although not without controversy (P.M. Boffey, *Med. J. Aust.*, 1984, *2*, 743). Milsted *et al.* (*Lancet*, 1980, *1*, 1343) concluded in summary that the widespread use of cancer chemotherapy was not justified outside well-conducted clinical trials or specialist cancer centres. In a critical review Kearsley (*Br. med. J.*, 1986, *293*, 871) suggested that treatment of the most common adult tumours by cytotoxic chemotherapy is still disappointing; that reliable criteria for assessing both tumour response and palliation, or quality of life, are required; that there is a need for better designed clinical trials and a less pragmatic approach to the use of cytotoxic drugs; that there is a need for identification of those subgroups of patients likely to benefit from a cytotoxic regimen, and for newer agents with a more favourable therapeutic ratio.

A critical review of adjuvant chemotherapy. Adjuvant drug treatment after surgery or radiotherapy has not led to the dramatic breakthroughs expected.— S. K. Carter, *Drugs*, 1986, *31*, 337.

Reviews of antineoplastic agents: P. Davey and G. R. Tudhope, *Br. med. J.*, 1983, *287*, 110; *Med. Lett.*, 1985, *27*, 13.

Reviews of the treatment of childhood malignancies: C. C. Bailey, *Br. J. Hosp. Med.*, 1984, *31*, 36; A. Goldman and J. Pritchard, *Prescribers' J.*, 1985, *25*, 2; B. H. Kaufman, *Mayo Clin. Proc.*, 1986, *61*, 269.

ACTION. A discussion of the concepts for systemic treatment of micrometastases to achieve a total tumour cell kill, a probable requirement for the cure of at least some tumours. Micrometastases containing up to 10^6 viable tumour cells are generally undetectable and therefore unsuitable for surgery or radiotherapy. The fraction of viable cells undergoing active cell replication is inversely related to population size and micrometastases should be more sensitive to cell cycle specific agents than the primary tumour. First-order cell kill kinetics characterise effective drug kill of tumour cells and when micrometastases are likely, drug treatment should be started as soon after the end of radiotherapy or surgery as possible, using cell cycle specific agents (antimetabolites) or cell cycle stage-specific agents (cytarabine, hydroxyurea, vinblastine, and vincristine). Cell cycle nonspecific agents (alkylating agents and antibiotics) have steep dose-response curves and the relatively high doses required prolong normal cell recovery times. Combination chemotherapy aimed at avoiding or controlling the selection of drug-resistant tumour cells is important.— F. M. Schabel, *Cancer*, 1975, *35*, 15.

A review of tumour cell kinetics and response to treatment. Growth rates of solid tumours affect response to therapy and tumours may be classified into 3 groups according to cell-population doubling time. The minimum detectable body burden of tumour in man is of the order of 1×10^9 cells, equivalent to about 1 g of tissue, and represents about 30 doublings. The lethal body tumour burden is reached when the tumour cell mass approaches or exceeds 1×10^{12} cells, equivalent to about 1 kg and representing 40 doublings. Ewing's sarcoma, testicular carcinoma, and non-Hodgkin's lymphomas (primarily histiocytic lymphoma) have mean doubling times that are shorter than 30 days; Hodgkin's disease, osteogenic sarcoma, and fibrosarcoma have intermediate growth rates with mean doubling times ranging from 30 to 70 days. Adenocarcinoma, squamous cell and small cell carcinomas of the lung, adenocarcinoma of the colon, and advanced breast cancer have mean doubling times which exceed 70 days. Doubling time distributions for individual tumour types are quite wide, adenocarcinoma of the lung has a reported doubling time of 15 to 960 days. Correlations between tumour doubling time and patient survival patterns suggest that the rate of tumour cell proliferation is a major determinant of therapeutic response; median survival is not considered the best measure of therapeutic effectiveness. The relationship between a cytotoxic drug and a tumour cell population can be described as a first-order kinetic process; a given dose or course of therapy kills a given fraction of the cell population rather than a number of cells. Thus, treatment of rapidly growing tumours produces a high initial fractional cell kill with frequent clinical complete responses and perhaps eradication of the last tumour cell in many patients. Rapidly growing tumours in advanced stages will undergo growth retardation on treatment but with a critical reduction in fractional cell kill. Fractional cell kills are also small in slowly growing tumours explaining the partial responses and shallow complete responses to treatment. In the treatment of slowly growing tumours the fractional tumour cell kills achieved at maximum tolerated therapeutic intensity were not sufficient to produce high complete response rates or durable responses without associated toxicity from long-term therapy. Clinical studies based on cell kinetic principles would improve therapeutic results in patients with responsive tumours but protocols for the treatment of patients with slowly growing tumours require reappraisal.— S. E. Shackney *et al.*, *Ann. intern. Med.*, 1978, *89*, 107.

ADMINISTRATION. Apart from the routine methods of administration special techniques have been designed to improve effectiveness. Antineoplastic agents may be injected directly into the tumour or body cavity or they may be administered by isolated regional perfusion or intra-arterial infusion. Isolated regional perfusion entails isolation of a tumour and its blood supply in an extracorporeal circulation so that the antineoplastic agent can be given in sufficiently high dosage to destroy the tumour. This is more easily carried out in the limbs, but in tumours of the abdomen or pelvis there is a risk of leakage and an alternative is to employ continuous intra-arterial infusion into an artery as close as possible to the tumour. When giving intravenous therapy the problems of long-term venous access, particularly in children, may be overcome through the use of central venous catheters. Implanted subcutaneous administration systems have also been employed for continuous or bolus administration of antineoplastic agents.

Reviews of some methods of administering antineoplastic agents: R. W. Carlson and B. I. Sikic, *Ann. intern. Med.*, 1983, *99*, 823 (continuous intravenous infusion); R. F. Ozols *et al.*, *ibid.*, 1984, *101*, 118 (intraperitoneal administration); K. C. Okafor and S. C. Adams, *Infusion*, 1985, *9*, 51 (intrathecal administration).

A study on the circadian timing of cancer chemotherapy involving 31 women with advanced ovarian cancer; administration of doxorubicin in the morning followed by cisplatin, 12 hours later, in the evening produced fewer complications, dose reductions, and treatment delays than administration of doxorubicin in the evening and cisplatin in the morning.— W. J. M. Hrushesky, *Science*, 1985, *228*, 73. See also under Cisplatin, p.609.

A discussion of cancer in the elderly including reference to factors affecting administration of antineoplastics.— *Ann. intern. Med.*, 1985, *102*, 218.

For a discussion of intravesicular chemotherapy in bladder cancer see under Malignant Neoplasms of the Bladder, below.

BLOOD DISORDERS, NON-MALIGNANT. *Polycythaemia vera.* Polycythaemia vera is a chronic myeloproliferative disorder in which red cell count, packed cell volume, and haemoglobin are increased. It may be treated by venesection, chemotherapy, or radiotherapy. Busulphan or chlorambucil are the drugs most commonly used but neither appears to be very satisfactory. Treatment with phosphorus-32 remains the method of choice, especially in older patients and those with severe disease.— S. M. Lewis, *Br. J. Hosp. Med.*, 1976, *16*, 125. In a prospective randomised study of 431 patients with polycythaemia vera, chlorambucil offered no advantage over phosphorus-32 and was associated with a significant increase in the incidence of acute leukaemia when compared with phlebotomy or phosphorus-32. The use of chlorambucil for the long-term management of polycythaemia vera has been discontinued.— P. D. Berk *et al.*, *New Engl. J. Med.*, 1981, *304*, 441 (Polycythaemia Vera Study Group). In a study involving 118 patients half of whom had received no previous myelosuppressive therapy, treatment with hydroxyurea produced good control of polycythaemia in 37 of the previously untreated and 30 of the previously treated patients. Cumulative 1-year failure-free survival was 73% and 59% respectively. Doses of hydroxyurea were 30 mg per kg body-weight daily by mouth for 1 week, subsequently halved to 15 mg per kg but the high loading dose was associated with a higher incidence of toxicity, and it was now recommended that therapy be initiated at a dose of 15 to 20 mg per kg daily. Two patients developed acute leukaemia during the study and a third subsequently did so; long-term assessment of hydroxyurea's mutagenic potential is required, particularly since treatment must be continued indefinitely to maintain remission.— P. B. Donovan *et al.*, *Am. J. Hematol.*, 1984, *17*, 329.

BURKITT'S LYMPHOMA. Although surgery, and possibly, with newer techniques and dose schedules, radiotherapy, may have a role to play, systemic chemotherapy is the treatment of choice in Burkitt's lymphoma. Initial chemotherapy must contain high doses of cyclophosphamide given intermittently for 3 to 6 courses. A number of drug combinations employing vincristine, methotrexate, or cytarabine, appear to lower the relapse rate and prevent systemic tumour recurrence, while a more aggressive regimen employs cyclophosphamide, vincristine, doxorubicin, and prednisone, with intermittent courses of high-dose methotrexate, augmented by intrathecal methotrexate and cytarabine (CHOMP). The weight of available data suggests that maintenance therapy is of little value and that the patient should receive only 1 or 2 courses beyond complete remission and then stop. The treatment of patients who have a relapse soon after induction of remission ('early relapse') is frustrating as such patients have only transient responses to the agents used initially; there is a high incidence of CNS involvement and prognosis is poor. However, some patients with relapse have responded to very high doses of alkylating agents along with bone marrow transplants and intensive supportive care. Late relapse occurring more than 3 months after remission, responds readily to reinduction chemotherapy with no evidence of resistance, and often a prolonged second remission.— J. L. Ziegler, *New Engl. J. Med.*, 1981, *305*, 735.

Cyclophosphamide alone, or with vincristine and methotrexate are currently the preferred drugs in Burkitt's lymphoma but carmustine and ifosfamide have also been investigated.— *Med. Lett.*, 1983, *25*, 1.

CARCINOID SYNDROME. Uncontrolled studies have shown a reduction in tumour size using a variety of regimens. However, in general, chemotherapy is not effective in either producing symptomatic relief or prolonging life. Cytotoxic therapy may produce crises due to release of tumour products from necrotic cells. There is no evidence that intra-arterial chemotherapy is more effective than intravenous. Patients with mild symptoms require no treatment, while when symptoms become more troublesome codeine phosphate, cyproheptadine, or in severe cases fenclonine or methysergide, are used to control diarrhoea. Ketanserin may be of value in alleviating flushing. When patients become resistant to pharmacological therapy tumour embolisation should be considered.— B. Clarke and H. J. F. Hodgson, *Br. J. Hosp. Med.*, 1986, *35*, 146. See also: *Br. med. J.*, 1978, *1*, 1572; G. P. Stathopoulos *et al.* (letter), *New Engl. J. Med.*, 1981, *305*, 52 (tamoxifen); M. D. King *et al.*, *Archs Dis. Childh.*, 1985, *60*, 269 (prednisolone, streptozocin, and fluorouracil in a 9-year-old).

In a comparison involving 210 evaluable patients with carcinoid tumours, treatment with doxorubicin or with fluorouracil in association with streptozocin produced overall response rates of 20 and 23% respectively. Of 33 patients who failed the combination regimen and crossed over to doxorubicin therapy the response rate was 18% and of 35 patients failing doxorubicin the response rate on crossing to combination therapy was 29%, thus demonstrating that both regimens had activity. However, since median durations of response were short at 31 weeks for combined therapy and 26 weeks for doxorubicin, and since there were only 3 complete responses (2 to combined and one to single-agent therapy), it is unlikely that either regimen contributed significantly to survival in these patients, and neither should be considered standard in patients with carcinoid tumour.— P. F. Engstrom *et al.*, *J. clin. Oncol.*, 1984, *2*, 1255.

GESTATIONAL TROPHOBLASTIC TUMOURS. The most effective single agents in the treatment of gestational trophoblastic tumours are methotrexate, actinomycin D, and etoposide. Other useful agents include cisplatin, alkylating agents (cyclophosphamide appears to have fewest disadvantages), vincristine, mercaptopurine, hydroxyurea, doxorubicin, bleomycin, and fluorouracil. In low-risk patients, intramuscular methotrexate (with folinic acid), or intravenous actinomycin D is recommended. Medium-risk patients may be given a combination of these agents with cyclophosphamide (MAC III) or etoposide followed by hydroxyurea, methotrexate, and mercaptopurine, then actinomycin D, then vincristine with cyclophosphamide, with the sequence then being repeated (EHMMAC). High-risk patients may be given a more toxic regimen such as hydroxyurea, vincristine, methotrexate, cyclophosphamide, actinomycin D and doxorubicin (CHAMOCA) or preferably etoposide, actinomycin D, methotrexate, vincristine and cyclophosphamide in the EMA-Co regimen. Methotrexate in adequate doses is also of prime importance in the prophylaxis and treatment of brain metastases.— Report of a WHO Scientific Group on Gestational Trophoblastic Diseases, *Tech Rep. Ser. Wld Hlth Org. No. 692*, 1983, p.53. See also: Report of a WHO Expert Committee on Chemotherapy of Solid Tumours, *Tech. Rep. Ser. Wld Hlth Org. No. 605*, 1977, p. 47 (choriocarcinoma); *Med. Lett.*, 1983, *25*, 1 (choriocarcinoma); L. A. Hansen and B. D. Clayton, *Drug Intell. & clin. Pharm.*, 1984, *18*, 569 (trophoblastic tumours).

HISTIOCYTIC SYNDROMES, NON-MALIGNANT. The term histiocytosis X [Langerhans-cell histiocytosis] refers to a group of rare syndromes, Letterer-Siwe disease, Hand-Schüller-Christian disease, and eosinophilic granuloma, that share certain histopathological features, namely granulomatous formation with infiltration and proliferation of histiocytes. The clinical manifestations can range from a solitary eosinophilic granuloma in the medullary cavity of bone to acute disseminated fulminant disease. The standard treatment of chemotherapy or radiotherapy or both is similar to that used in the treatment of cancer.— M. E. Osband *et al.*, *New Engl. J. Med.*, 1981, *304*, 146.

Vinblastine alone is claimed to be successful in the treatment of systemic Langerhans-cell histiocytosis, and has been claimed to be the treatment of choice, but one child, with skin involvement only at diagnosis, developed pulmonary infiltration despite vinblastine therapy, and only responded when given prednisone, vinblastine, cyclophosphamide, and doxorubicin. A further case, with multiple organ involvement including the lungs, has shown good response to this quadruple chemotherapy.— E. A. Bingham *et al.*, *Br. J. Derm.*, 1982, *106*, 205.

In patients with single system disease, who have a good prognosis with a high rate of spontaneous remission, local injection of methylprednisolone is used for lesions in weight-bearing bones with a risk of spontaneous fracture, or those causing pain or disfigurement. Radiotherapy, with its risk of secondary malignancies, is reserved for lesions inaccessible to local injection which threaten vital structures such as spinal cord or optic nerve. Management of children with multisystem disease is much more controversial, and as with single system disease spontaneous remission can occur. During the period when Langerhans-cell histiocytosis was believed to be a malignancy, treatment was with a variety of cytotoxic drugs, alone or in combination, but whatever regimen is used the total response-rate is 50 to 70% with only marginal effects on mortality, and side-effects may outweigh benefits. High-dose prednisolone is as effective as combinations of cytotoxic drugs and has less severe side-effects, especially in relatively short courses of 2 to 3 months: maintenance treatment probably has little advantage and leads to extra morbidity.— V. Broadbent and J. Pritchard, *Archs Dis. Childh.*, 1985, *60*, 605.

Recommendations for a new classification of histiocytic syndromes. Langerhans-cell histiocytosis, previously known as histiocytosis X, remains unclear in its aetiology and pathogenesis. Only a few patients have progressive disease that responds poorly to current therapy, while the remainder require only minimum treatment.— The Writing Group of the Histiocyte Society, *Lancet*, 1987, *1*, 208.

HODGKIN'S DISEASE AND OTHER LYMPHOMAS. Reviews of the classification and management of the lymphomas: T. A. Lister; J. S. Malpas *Postgrad. med. J.*, 1983, *59*, 219 (lymphomas); T. J. McElwain, *Br. J. Hosp. Med.*, 1984, *31*, 10 (lymphomas); B. C. Behrens *et al.*, *Drugs*, 1985, *30*, 355 (Hodgkin's disease); T. A. Lister, *Postgrad. med. J.*, 1985, *61*, 103 (Hodgkin's disease in adults); J. G. McVie and R. Somers, *Br. med. J.*, 1985, *290*, 950 (chemotherapy in Hodgkin's disease); W. N. Hait *et al.*, *J. Am. med. Ass.*, 1985, *253*, 1431 (non-Hodgkin's lymphomas); G. M. Mead and J. M. A. Whitehouse, *Br. med. J.*, 1986, *293*, 577 (non-Hodgkin's lymphomas).

Hodgkin's disease. Hodgkin's disease can be treated by radiotherapy or chemotherapy or both, and the choice of treatment depends on the volume and histological subtype of the tumour, the age of the patient, but particularly the stage of the disease. The Ann Arbor classification recognises 4 stages:

Stage I, with involvement of a single lymph node region or extralymphatic site;

Stage II, in which spread is restricted to lymph nodes and sites on one side of the diaphragm only;

Stage III, involving spread on both sides of the diaphragm with possible splenic and extralymphatic involvement;

Stage IV, where the patient has diffuse or disseminated disease in one or more extralymphatic organs or tissues.

Stages are subclassified A or B according to the absence or presence of symptoms of fever, night sweats, or weight loss, which carry a poorer prognosis.

Radiotherapy is usually the treatment of choice in stage I or II disease, and total nodal irradiation may be used to treat small volume stage IIIA disease; however, a review of studies carried out by the British National Lymphoma Investigation (J.L. Haybittle *et al.*, *Lancet*, 1985, *1*, 967) has concluded that radiotherapy should be reserved for IA and IIA disease and that chemotherapy should be used from the start in all other patients, including those with stage IB or IIB disease. The 5-year disease-free survival rate is about 80 to 90% in patients with stage I or IIA disease treated with radiotherapy alone.

Chemotherapy is generally considered to be the treatment of choice in advanced disease. Many agents have been tried both singly and in combination regimens, but the commonest treatment remains combination chemo therapy with mustine, vincristine, procarbazine, and prednisone (MOPP) introduced by DeVita *et al.* (*Ann. intern. Med.*, 1970, *73*, 881). Mustine 6 mg per m^2 body-surface and vincristine 1.4 mg per m^2 are given intravenously on days 1 and 8 and procarbazine 100 mg per m^2 and prednisone 40 mg per m^2 are taken by mouth on days 1 to 14, courses being repeated every 4 weeks, usually for at least 6 courses; prednisolone is often used instead of prednisone. No combination regimen has been conclusively shown to be more effective than MOPP, but a number of MOPP-variant regimens exist which may be as effective and less toxic; these include substitution of chlorambucil for mustine (LOPP), vinblastine for vincristine (MVPP), and both of these changes in one regimen (ChlVPP).

Chemotherapy with MOPP has been reported to produce complete remission in 80% of patients, with an overall 10-year disease-free survival rate of 63% (V.T. DeVita *et al.*, *ibid.*, 1980, *92*, 587) but prognosis is poorer in patients with more advanced stages of disease and may be closer to 50% disease-free at 5 years in patients with stage IIIB or IV disease. Although it has been emphasised that the effectiveness of MOPP therapy depends upon optimum dose scheduling and administration of a minimum of 6 cycles of chemotherapy, Fermé *et al.* (*Nouv. Presse méd.*, 1983, *12*, 2031) reported that 3 cycles were as effective as 6 in a group of patients given MOPP and radiotherapy with disease stages IB to III.

A number of regimens have been tried in patients with disease resistant to MOPP. A combination of doxorubicin, bleomycin, vinblastine, and dacarbazine (ABVD), introduced by Bonadonna *et al.* (*Cancer*, 1975, *36*, 252) was claimed to exhibit no cross-resistance with MOPP. Good results have also been reported with a regimen containing streptozocin, lomustine, doxorubicin, and bleomycin, (SCAB); this gave results comparable with those achieved with MOPP when used for initial therapy of Hodgkin's disease in a group of patients with advanced disease, although at the cost of substantial toxicity (C.H. Diggs *et al.*, *Cancer*, 1981, *47*, 224).

In an effort to improve remission rates in patients with stage IV disease, alternation of non-cross-resistant regimens is being tried. Santoro *et al.* (*New Engl. J. Med.*, 1982, *306*, 770) reported that a regimen alternating MOPP and ABVD produced remission in 34 (92%) of 37 patients with stage IV disease, compared with 27 (71%) of 38 similar patients given MOPP alone; subsequent results after 8 years (G. Bonadonna *et al.*, *Ann. intern. Med.*, 1986, *104*, 739) have been claimed to bear out the superiority of the alternating combination regimen. However, the very small sample size, and the fact that patients receiving only MOPP did not all receive the suggested 6 cycles, mean that statistically valid conclusions cannot be drawn from this study. Large-scale studies of alternating MOPP and ABVD and MOPP and SCAB are being undertaken, but no definitive results have yet emerged (R.J. Mayer, *New Engl. J. Med.*, 1982, *306*, 800; J.H. Glick and A. Tsiatis, *Ann. intern. Med.*, 1986, *104*, 876).

Administration of a polyvalent pneumococcal vaccine is recommended for all patients with Hodgkin's disease, to be given before or after splenectomy, but before specific immunosuppressive therapy is started.— J. E. Addiego *et al.*, *Lancet*, 1980, *2*, 450. See also: M. L. Brigden (letter), *Can. med. Ass. J.*, 1985, *133*, 1108.

Non-Hodgkin's lymphomas. A working formulation devised by the *US* National Cancer Institute for classification of non-Hodgkin's lymphomas.— A. H. T. Robb-Smith, *Lancet*, 1982, *2*, 432.

Non-Hodgkin's-lymphomas can be divided into groups, based on the prognosis. Patients with lymphomas that have a good prognosis, such as poorly differentiated lymphocytic nodular lymphoma, may remain well despite extensive disease for years and require no treatment while asymptomatic.

Patients with stage I and II nodal disease may be cured by radiotherapy, or at least survive a long time before relapse, but most patients require chemotherapy which may range from very gentle to intensive depending on the histological subtype and clinical circumstances. The most effective single drugs are alkylating agents such as cyclophosphamide, chlorambucil, mustine, carmustine, and lomustine. Corticosteroids may be used alone for lymphomas with good prognosis and are included in most combinations for the bad prognostic group.

Patients with disseminated good-prognostic lymphomas should be treated with low-dose alkylating agents, with or without corticosteroids. There is no evidence that combination therapy prolongs survival beyond that achieved with single agents in the good prognostic group, although response to a combination may be more rapid. The median survival is about 5 years and some patients live 20 years or more.

Patients with disseminated bad-prognosis lymphomas benefit from treatment with combination chemotherapy, the aim being to induce complete remission, which is associated with prolonged survival. The combinations are similar to those employed in Hodgkin's disease. There is good evidence that combinations containing doxorubicin give higher remission rates than those without; the commonest such regimen is cyclophosphamide, doxorubicin, vincristine, and prednisone (CHOP) which gives complete remission in about 65% of patients with diffuse histiocytic lymphoma.

Non-Hodgkin's lymphomas in children have a bad prognosis if untreated. Treatment is often the same as for patients with poor-prognosis acute lymphoblastic leukaemia, including intrathecal chemotherapy and cranial irradiation.— T. J. McElwain, *Br. J. Hosp. Med.*, 1984, *31*, 10. An earlier review. Until the present, only a minority of patients with unfavourable-prognosis lymphomas have shown obvious benefit from intensive combination chemotherapy but for them the benefit has been massive. Although this minority represents only about 30% of the total in adults and 50 to 70% in children presenting with advanced disease, it is encouraging since the natural history of the disease is of an inexorable progression towards death in months. In addition, as with the low-grade lymphomas, experimental approaches involving the use of intensive chemotherapy, with bone-marrow transplantation after 'clean-up' with specific antisera, may alter the prognosis markedly.— T. A. Lister and J. S. Malpas, *Postgrad. med. J.*, 1983, *59*, 219. See also R. G. MacKenzie and J. J. Rusthoven, *Can. med. Ass. J.*, 1985, *133*, 559.

Early reports of first generation chemotherapy regimens in the treatment of large-cell non-Hodgkin's lymphomas: V. T. DeVita *et al.*, *Lancet*, 1975, *1*, 248 (C-MOPP (mustine or cyclophosphamide, vincristine, procarbazine and prednisone)); R. I. Fisher *et al.*, *Am. J. Med.*, 1977, *63*, 177 (similar results with MOPP, C-MOPP, and BACOP (bleomycin, doxorubicin, cyclophosphamide, vincristine, and prednisone)); T. A. Lister *et al.*, *Br. med. J.*, 1978, *1*, 533 (unsatisfactory results with chlorambucil or CVP (cyclophosphamide, vincristine, prednisolone)); D. L. Sweet *et al.*, *Ann. intern. Med.*, 1980, *92*, 785 (COMLA (cyclophosphamide, vincristine, methotrexate with folinic acid rescue, and cytarabine)).

In a multicentre study involving 234 children with non-Hodgkin's lymphomas patients received either a 4-drug regimen of cyclophosphamide, vincristine, methotrexate, and prednisone (COMP) or a modified LSA_2-L_2 regimen employing cyclophosphamide, vincristine, prednisone, daunorubicin, methotrexate, cytarabine, thioguanine, colaspase, hydroxyurea, and carmustine. Treatment results did not differ according to regimen in patients with localised disease but among children with non-localised disease 76% of those with lymphoblastic lymphoma were disease-free at 24 months after LSA_2-L_2 compared to 26% of those given COMP: conversely, in the group with nonlymphoblastic lymphoma those treated with COMP had a significantly higher disease-free survival rate of 57% compared to 28% at 24 months in those who had been given the other regimen.— J. R. Anderson *et al.*, *New Engl. J. Med.*, 1983, *308*, 559. Comment.— H. J. Weinstein (letter), *ibid.*, *309*, 310. Reply.— J. R. Anderson and R. D. T. Jenkin (letter), *ibid.*, 311.

Alternating therapy with MOPP and ProMACE (prednisone, methotrexate, doxorubicin, cyclophosphamide, and etoposide) achieved complete remission in 55 (74%) of 74 patients with various diffuse aggressive non-Hodgkin's lymphomas, with only 10 of the complete responders relapsing in 2½ years of follow-up. ProMACE-MOPP chemotherapy appears to have significantly improved the previous remission rate of 46% in patients with advanced stages of diffuse aggressive lymphomas.— R. I. Fisher *et al.*, *Ann. intern. Med.*, 1983, *98*, 304.

Complete response occurred in 51 (84%) of 61 patients with diffuse large-cell lymphomas, and partial response in 10 (16%), following 12 weeks of therapy with MACOP-B, a novel regimen employing methotrexate with folinic acid rescue, doxorubicin, cyclophosphamide, vincristine, prednisone, and bleomycin, with antibiotic prophylaxis. On follow-up, 5 of the complete responders relapsed, 4 within the first 6 months. Results suggest that MACOP-B therapy can achieve results in these patients similar or superior to other regimens of longer duration.— P. Klimo and J. M. Connors, *Ann. intern. Med.*, 1985, *102*, 596. Comment. The first generation chemotherapy combinations introduced in the 1970's, including CHOP, HOP, and COMLA all produced survival plateaux or prolonged disease-free survival rate of 35 to 45%. In the late 1970's, with the advent of the notion that intensity, timing, and placement of drugs might be critical to the success of therapy, a second generation of studies was initiated with regimens such as ProMACE-MOPP, COP-BLAM (cyclophosphamide, vincristine, prednisone, bleomycin, doxorubicin, procarbazine), and M-BACOD (methotrexate with folinic acid rescue, bleomycin, doxorubicin, cyclophosphamide, vincristine, and dexamethasone). Most of these regimens are characterised by increasing numbers of drugs, with cycles of myelosuppressive drugs as frequently as every 3 weeks, due to the realisation that bone-marrow toxicity was ameliorated by that time, and non-marrow-toxic drugs in the cytopenic phases. With these regimens survival plateaux of 55 to 60% were achieved, and complete remissions proved durable and long-lasting. Further application of the principles behind these regimens has produced third generation regimens such as COPBLAM III, in which the vincristine and bleomycin are given by infusion, ProMACE-CytaBOM, in which the ProMACE regimen is alternated with cytarabine, bleomycin, vincristine, and methotrexate with folinic acid rescue, and the MACOP-B regimen. These regimens are producing survival plateaux of approximately 70%, and in contrast to some of the second generation regimens have mostly fared well in the presence of poor prognostic characteristics such as bulky or advanced (stage IV) disease, B symptoms, and immunoblastic histological subtype. However, few of the third (or even the second) generation regimens have been studied in prospective controlled randomised trials, and many of the concepts advanced for the newer regimens have never been established beyond any doubt. It is still too early, and the numbers are too small to conclude that the third generation regimens are better.— M. Coleman, *ibid.*, *103*, 140.

Although patients with large-cell lymphomas and risk factors such as bulky disease and B symptoms would probably benefit from new therapeutic approaches, patients without these factors respond well to CHOP therapy and need not be treated with more intensive regimens until an advantage is proved.— A. Pereira *et al.* (letter), *Ann. intern. Med.*, 1986, *105*, 631.

See also under Burkitt's Lymphoma (above) and Mycosis Fungoides (below).

Bone-marrow transplantation.
Mentions of the use of high-dose chemotherapy and bone-marrow transplantation in the management of non-Hodgkin's lymphomas: T. Philip *et al.* (letter), *Lancet*, 1984, *1*, 391; P. Ricci *et al.* (letter), *ibid.*, 686; G. L. Phillips *et al.*, *New Engl. J. Med.*, 1984, *310*, 1557.

Prophylaxis of CNS-relapse.
Studies suggesting that CNS prophylactic therapy may be warranted in patients with lymphoblastic and diffuse undifferentiated lymphomas: C. J. Hawkey and P. J. Toghill, *Postgrad. med. J.*, 1983, *59*, 283; G. J. Johnson *et al.*, *Lancet*, 1984, *2*, 685. Correction.— *ibid.*, 996.

LEUKAEMIA, ACUTE. *Acute lymphoblastic leukaemia.* Treatment of acute lymphoblastic leukaemias may be divided into several phases: induction of remission, prevention of CNS disease, and maintenance, or consolidation, or intensification therapy.

Induction of remission.
In patients classified as having standard risk, vincristine and corticosteroids form the basis of induction of remission. Vincristine 1 to 1.5 mg per m² body-surface area by intravenous injection weekly, plus prednisone 40 mg per m² daily by mouth can induce haematological remission in over 90% of children, and in about 50% of adults. In an attempt to improve the remission rates in adults more intensive induction regimens are employed, with addition of a third agent, usually colaspase or an anthracycline, and sometimes both or further agents as well. In a randomised study Gottlieb *et al.* (*Blood*, 1984, *64*, 267) found that addition of daunorubicin to induction therapy with vincristine, prednisone, and colaspase improved remission rates from 47% to 83% in similar groups of adult patients.

Studies in a number of centres have provided circumstantial evidence that, despite the greater toxicity involved, more intensive induction therapy is also of benefit in children, as it prolongs the duration of remission, particularly in those with high-risk disease, by reducing the risk of bone-marrow relapse. Results from West Germany (H. Riehm *et al.*, *Am. J. pediatr. Hematol. Oncol.*, 1980, *2*, 299) indicate that by use of an intensive induction regimen, with additional treatment for children deemed at high risk of relapse, patients with unfavourable prognostic indicators such as male sex and high white cell count can achieve the same 70% chance of disease-free survival at 5 years as children in the best prognostic group. An analysis of results from a series of studies carried out in the *UK* for the Medical Research Council (UKALL Trials II to VIII) appears to confirm the value of an intensive sustained regimen (*Lancet*, 1986, *1*, 408).

CNS therapy.
The majority of children who achieve an initial remission will subsequently relapse with meningeal involvement unless CNS therapy directed at the sanctuary sites in the meninges is undertaken. Standard therapy consists of a combination of cranial irradiation (2400 rad) with intrathecal methotrexate; however, such a combination does carry some risk of serious sequelae, including leucoencephalopathy, and particularly when high doses of methotrexate are given. Effective prophylaxis can reduce the incidence of CNS relapse to well below 10% (*Lancet*, 1985, *1*, 1196). Some studies (D.M. Komp *et al.*, *Cancer*, 1982, *50*, 1031; M.P. Sullivan *et al.*, *Blood*, 1982, *60*, 948) have indicated that intrathecal therapy with methotrexate, hydrocortisone, and cytarabine may be as effective as combined radio- and chemotherapy. The role of CNS prophylaxis in adult acute lymphoblastic leukaemia has not been precisely determined.

Consolidation.
Once remission has been achieved, further chemotherapy is indicated to prevent relapse. Two strategies have been used: consolidation or intensification, and maintenance. Consolidation or intensification therapy involves continuation of intensive chemotherapy regimens after the achievement of complete remission. Randomised studies have not demonstrated any benefit for such an approach in children with standard risk factors but there is some evidence for an advantage in children with high-risk disease. Results in adults have been contradictory but appear to suggest a longer duration of remission with intensive consolidation therapy (A.D. Jacobs and R.P. Gale, *New Engl. J. Med.*, 1984, *311*, 1219).

Maintenance.
Maintenance therapy is generally given for some 2½ to 3 years after remission; mercaptopurine, usually in doses of 50 to 75 mg per m^2 daily, and methotrexate 15 to 20 mg per m^2 weekly are commonly used. Many protocols also employ periodic administration of vincristine and a corticosteroid; some have provided periods of intensive consolidation therapy alternating with periods of mercaptopurine and methotrexate maintenance.
It is generally agreed that patients who maintain remission for 4 years after the end of maintenance therapy are at little risk of relapse and may be regarded as effectively cured. Between 50% and 70% of children entering remission may now expect to be cured. Age of less than 2 or greater than 10 at presentation, male sex (in part because of the risk of testicular relapse), high white cell count, presence of a mediastinal mass, and CNS disease at presentation are all high-risk factors, possibly reflecting the presence of different biological species of acute lymphoblastic leukaemia with different treatment requirements (D. Pinkel, *Postgrad. med. J.*, 1985, *61*, 93). Cure rates in adults have been relatively poor until recently, but with intensive chemotherapy are starting to approach those in children; the data suggest that 20 to 50% may now be cured (Jacobs and Gale, 1984).
Second remission.
Patients who relapse after stopping treatment can usually be brought to second remission, often by a repeat of their original induction therapy. However, relapse during treatment carries a poor prognosis, and if second remission is achieved it is likely to be short lived. Some extension of second remission may be obtained through therapy with teniposide and cytarabine; G.K. Rivera *et al.*, in a Paediatric Oncology Group Study (*New Engl. J. Med.*, 1986, *315*, 273) concluded that intensive chemotherapy including consolidation with intravenous teniposide and cytarabine in early remission could produce durable second remissions in about half the patients whose initial remissions had lasted 18 months or more. Although bone marrow transplantation has been advocated in patients in second remission with a suitable donor, and some studies have indicated better results than with chemotherapy (F.L. Johnson and E.D. Thomas, *New Engl. J. Med.*, 1984, *310*, 263), a study by Chessells *et al.* has suggested that the role of bone marrow transplantation is limited (*Lancet*, 1986, *1*, 1239) and it has been pointed out by J.R. Hobbs (*ibid.*, *2*, 862) that salvage, already difficult, is likely to become more so in the future for the smaller numbers of children who relapse from new chemotherapy protocols.

Differences in prognosis for boys and girls with acute lymphoblastic leukaemia.— H. Sather *et al.*, *Lancet*, 1981, *1*, 739.

Differences in response to treatment in children and adults appear to be related to the differing proportions of leukaemia subgroups. The incidence of common acute lymphoblastic leukaemia (ALL) is higher in children. Adults with common ALL have a prognosis superior to that of adults with null-cell ALL, T-cell ALL, or B-cell ALL and results with chemotherapy can approach those in children with common ALL.— M. F. Greaves and T. A. Lister (letter), *New Engl. J. Med.*, 1981, *304*, 119.

A study in 118 children receiving maintenance chemotherapy for acute lymphoblastic leukaemia suggested that disease-free survival was significantly better in those given methotrexate and mercaptopurine in the evening rather than the morning.— G. E. Rivard *et al.*, *Lancet*, 1985, *2*, 1264. Correction.— *idem*, 1986, *1*, 1161. See also under Administration, above.

Acute non-lymphoblastic leukaemia. The acute non-lymphoblastic leukaemias (ANLL's), also known as acute myeloid, or acute myelogenous leukaemias include, under the French-American-British (FAB) classification myeloblastic and monocytic leukaemias, as well as erythroleukaemia. In contrast to the progress in childhood acute lymphoblastic leukaemia, long-term survival in patients with this group of diseases is still poor.
Induction of remission.
Induction of remission is usually possible with intensive chemotherapy. A combination of daunorubicin, cytarabine, and thioguanine (TAD or DAT: R.P. Gale and M.J. Cline, *Lancet*, 1977 *1*, 497 ; J.K.H. Rees and F.G.J. Hayhoe, *ibid.*, 1978, *1*, 1360) is commonly used, but amsacrine and high-dose cytarabine may also be useful. Remission has been stated to be achievable in some 60 to 80% of patients, but patients suffer severe neutropenia during induction and remission rate is to some extent dependent upon the standard of supportive care.
It has been suggested that reported improvements in chemotherapy for acute non-lymphoblastic leukaemias may reflect inadvertent exclusions and refinements in leukaemia classification rather than true improvement in treatment results: in a study involving 272 patients the Toronto Leukemia Study Group (*Lancet*, 1986, *1*, 786) demonstrated that remission rate varied between 43.8 and 85.3% depending on the exclusion criteria used.
Maintenance.
Maintaining remission once achieved has proved difficult. CNS treatment does not prolong bone marrow remissions in these patients and its use is reserved for young patients with acute monoblastic leukaemia. Results of maintenance chemotherapy and immunotherapy have been disappointing, and the role of consolidation chemotherapy is likewise controversial (R.P. Gale, *Ann. intern. Med.*, 1984, *101*, 702).
A number of studies have failed to show an advantage for routine use of maintenance therapy. Bell *et al.* (*Br. med. J.*, 1982, *284*, 1221) and Champlin *et al.* (*Lancet*, 1984, *1*, 894) found that patients given early intensive treatment could achieve prolonged duration of remission without further maintenance. A study from the Swiss Group for Clinical Cancer Research (C. Sauter *et al.*, *Lancet*, 1984, *1*, 379) compared patients given maintenance therapy after remission induction and consolidation with those given no maintenance and found no significant differences in either duration of remission or survival between the groups. Although the conclusions of this study have been questioned, and contrary results cited from other studies (T. Büchner *et al. ibid.*, 571 ; *idem*, 1985, *1*, 1224), the consensus appears to be that maintenance chemotherapy is of little if any value in the treatment of acute non-lymphoblastic leukaemias. Powles (*ibid.*, 800) has postulated that this may be because the leukaemic cells are capable of a limited degree of maturation during remission and may then be insensitive to the agents normally used in treatment.
Consolidation.
The relative value of consolidation or intensification therapy in these patients is also uncertain. In the UK Medical Research Council's 8th Acute Myeloid Leukaemia Trial (J. K. H. Rees *et al.*, *Lancet*, 1986, *2*, 1236) consolidation with 6 courses of DAT had a small but non-significant advantage in terms of survival and freedom from relapse over consolidation with 2 courses. In the same study, late intensification therapy with cyclophosphamide, vincristine, cytarabine, and prednisolone (COAP) was calculated to produce a non-significant improvement in 5-year survival from 31 to 47% and in 5-year relapse-free survival from 24 to 37%. The studies by Bell *et al.*, Champlin *et al.*, and Sauter *et al.* cited above reported moderately encouraging results with brief, high-dose consolidation therapy; however, a subsequent study by Champlin *et al.* (*Ann. intern. Med.*, 1985, *102*, 285) suggested that allogeneic bone-marrow transplantation from an HLA-identical sibling was superior in terms of actuarial 4-year relapse rate (40% versus 71%) to consolidation chemotherapy with azacitidine and doxorubicin, and a repeat of the TAD induction regimen. The MRC trial found the results of allogeneic bone-marrow transplantation to be disappointing due to a high incidence of treatment-related complications.
Although median duration of remission remains less than 2 years, results of recent studies have been taken by Gale (*ibid.*, 1984, *101* , 702) to indicate that some 10 to 40% of those achieving remission will have extended disease-free survival, and some may be cured. The outlook is better in younger patients.
Second remission.
In patients who relapse prognosis is extremely poor. Few patients achieve second remission with standard chemotherapy, but some benefit may be obtained from newer regimens such as MAZE (amsacrine, azacitidine, and etoposide: A.M. Worsley *et al. Lancet*, 1984, *1*, 1232) or high-dose cytarabine with mitozantrone (W. Hiddemann *et al. ibid.*, 1985, *2*, 508).
Allogeneic bone-marrow transplantation has been advocated in relapse: Santos *et al.* (*New Engl. J. Med.*, 1983 *309*, 1347) reported a 2-year survival rate of 29% in 17 patients in second or third remission, or early relapse, given infusions of HLA-identical sibling marrow after treatment with high doses of busulphan and cyclophosphamide. Unfortunately, the majority of patients lack related HLA-matched donors but a subsequent study (A.M. Yeager *et al.*, *ibid.*, 1986, *315*, 141) indicated that infusion of the patient's own marrow, collected in remission and treated with 4-hydroperoxycyclophosphamide to purge leukaemic cells, compared favourably with the results of allogeneic or syngeneic transplantation, with an actuarial survival calculated at 43%.

Reviews of the treatment of acute non-lymphoblastic leukaemias: R. P. Gale, *New Engl. J. Med.*, 1979, *300*, 1189; C. D. Bloomfield, *Ann. intern. Med.*, 1980, *93*, 133; J. A. Whittaker, *Br. med. J.*, 1980, *281*, 960; K. A. Foon and R. P. Gale, *Am. J. Med.*, 1982, *72*, 963.

LEUKAEMIA, CHRONIC. *Chronic granulocytic leukaemia.* Chronic granulocytic or chronic myeloid leukaemia is a rare disease, occurring usually in older patients, and representing less than a quarter of all adult leukaemias (G.P. Canellos, *New Engl. J. Med.*, 1979, *300*, 360). It is associated in over 95% of cases with the presence in blood cells of an abnormal chromosome, the Philadelphia chromosome (Ph^1).
During the chronic phase, which may last for several years, the patient may be asymptomatic and require no treatment. Where symptoms arise a course of palliative therapy with busulphan, usually in doses of 4 mg daily by mouth, normally suffices to bring elevated white cell counts, splenomegaly, and hepatomegaly under control. Patients poorly controlled by busulphan may be given hydroxyurea 500 mg to 2 g daily.
The onset of the subsequent transformed phase is unpredictable and may present as rapid onset of a blast cell crisis with the behaviour of an acute leukaemia, or a more gradual appearance of blast cells accompanied by gradual resistance to previous treatment. Transformation may produce lymphoblastic or myeloblastic cells. Lymphoblastic patients may respond well for a time to vincristine and prednisone in similar doses to those used in acute lymphoblastic leukaemia. In myeloblastic transformation limited success has been achieved with a regimen of thioguanine, daunorubicin, cytarabine, methotrexate, prednisolone, cyclophosphamide, vincristine, and colaspase (TRAMPCOL), as advocated by Spiers *et al.* (*Br. med. J.*, 1974, *3*, 77) but it has been suggested that so toxic a regimen is unjustified in patients whose outlook is so poor and some sources have advocated treatment with hydroxyurea, which may also be of benefit in more chronic transformed disease.
The median survival for patients with Ph^1-positive disease is about 3 years, while in Ph^1-negative disease, which carries a worse prognosis, median survival is about 1 year. Chemotherapy has not substantially improved survival. There is, however, some evidence (A. Fefer *et al.*, *New Engl. J. Med.*, 1982, *306*, 63; B. Speck *et al.*, *Lancet*. 1984, *1*, 665; A. Gratwohl *et al.*, *ibid.*, 1985, *2*, 1290; J.M. Goldman *et al.*, *New Engl. J. Med.*, 1986, *314*, 202) that chemoradiotherapy followed by allogeneic bone-marrow transplantation may be curative, particularly when performed in the chronic phase. New therapies may also improve the prognosis of the myeloid blast phase. Koller and Miller (*ibid.*, 1433) have reported a return to the chronic phase in 6 such patients treated with combined plicamycin and hydroxyurea.

The drug currently preferred for the stable phase of chronic myelocytic leukaemia was busulphan; in the acute phase a regimen of daunorubicin, cytarabine, vincristine, and prednisone, sometimes with thioguanine, was preferred. Other drugs with activity reported in stable disease were mitobronitol, hydroxyurea, mercaptopurine, thioguanine, and melphalan; amsacrine, azacitidine, and vindesine had been reported as having some value in the acute phase.— *Med. Lett.*, 1983, *25*, 1.

Chronic lymphatic leukaemia. Chronic lymphatic leukaemia accounts for approximately 30% of all cases of leukaemia in the *US* and Europe, although it is rare in the Far East. The clinical course is variable and many patients may require no treatment, at least for several years. Most physicians initiate systemic therapy with radiation, alkylating agents, corticosteroids, or a combination of the three, for patients with organomegaly or cytopenias.
Initial therapy is usually chlorambucil, in standard doses of 100 to 200 µg per kg body-weight daily by mouth, reduced once the disease is under control, or, better, 400 to 600 µg per kg every 2 to 4 weeks. A response rate of 60% is common, with 10% to 20% complete remissions. Some studies indicate a potential slight advantage to the combination of prednisone and chlorambucil over chlorambucil alone. Patients unresponsive to chlorambucil may reasonably be given a combination of cyclophosphamide, vincristine, and prednisone. Combination therapy with other chemotherapeutic agents should be reserved for refractory patients. It is uncertain whether combination of chemotherapy with total body irradiation improves responses. Interferons have proved of little value to date but it is hoped that newer biological therapies such as gamma-interferon and monoclonal antibodies will prove useful.— R. P. Gale and K. A. Foon, *Ann. intern. Med.*, 1985, *103*, 101.

The 2-year survival rates were better in 30 poor prognosis patients (Binet Stage C) with chronic lymphatic leukaemia who were given cyclophosphamide, doxorubicin, vincristine, and prednisone (CHOP) than in 29 similar patients given the same regimen without doxorubicin (COP): rates were 77 and 44% respectively. There were no significant differences in survival among good prognosis patients (Stage A) randomised to receive chlorambucil or no treatment or among intermediate-prognosis patients (Stage B) given either chlorambucil or COP therapy.— French Co-operative Group on Chronic Lymphocytic Leukaemia, *Lancet*, 1986, *1*, 1346.

Hairy-cell leukaemia. Hairy-cell leukaemia is a chronic lymphoproliferative disorder marked by the presence of white blood cells with prominent cytoplasmic villi, pancytopenia, and splenomegaly. Splenectomy corrects pancytopenia in most patients and improves survival in some but about 80% of patients require other forms of treatment at some stage. Chlorambucil was formerly popular but has now been superseded by interferon. Interferon given daily or 3 times a week by the intramuscular or subcutaneous route produces normal blood counts in most patients after 3 to 6 months; complete elimination of hairy cells from the bone marrow and correction of fibrosis require treatment for a year or more. Treatment with interferon confers benefit in close to 100% of cases. Good results have also been reported with pentostatin. At low dosage it induces complete remissions in hairy-cell leukaemia without the toxicity caused at the higher dosage used in lymphoblastic leukaemia. In contrast to interferon the duration of treatment required to obtain complete bone marrow remission is relatively short and prolonged remissions without maintenance have been recorded in some patients.— D. Catovsky, *Br. med. J.*, 1986, *292*, 786.

For a review of the use of interferons in malignant neoplasms, including hairy-cell leukaemia, see under Interferons, p.699.

Myelodysplasia. A review of the management of myelodysplastic syndromes. These disorders are characterised by anaemia, neutropenia, or thrombocytopenia in various combinations and have been described as smouldering leukaemia; progression to acute non-lymphoblastic leukaemia occurs in some patients. Patients are often elderly, and management is generally conservative. Many patients survive for a period with transfusions and antibiotic therapy alone, and there is often reluctance to introduce cytotoxic therapy. Paradoxically a less toxic regimen may be selected to avoid morbidity when more intensive treatment would offer greater likelihood of remission and extended survival. Encouraging results have been reported in recent years with the use of isotretinoin or low-dose cytarabine (20 mg per m^2 body-surface area daily) to induce cellular differentiation but clinical studies are needed to provide better guidelines for the management of these patients.— R. A. Larson, *Ann. intern. Med.*, 1985, *103*, 136. See also: *Lancet*, 1984, *1*, 943; G. T. Mufti *et al.* (letter), *ibid.*, 1187; A. Jacobs, *J. clin. Path.*, 1985, *38*, 1201; *Lancet*, 1986, *2*, 436; E. J. Watts (letter), *ibid.*, 754.

MALIGNANT EFFUSIONS. Malignant effusions often complicate the course of cancer. Tumours can cause effusions by increasing the permeability of pleural or pericardial surfaces, obstructing lymphatics, or blocking veins. Systemic chemotherapy for the tumour is the treatment of choice for asymptomatic malignant effusions but when systemic therapy fails to give control, local treatment can be useful. Temporary relief of dyspnoea due to pleural effusions may often be obtained by thoracentesis; patients who benefit are likely to respond to subsequent intracavitary therapy with a sclerosing agent—usually a nonspecific irritant; a cytotoxic agent such as mustine, thiotepa, fluorouracil, or bleomycin; or a radionuclide. The preferred intracavitary agent is tetracycline. Pericardial effusions may require emergency drainage, a pericardial window, or pericardiectomy; if the effusion recurs, tetracycline can be used.— *Med. Lett.*, 1981, *23*, 59. See also: *Lancet*, 1981, *1*, 198.

The success or failure of intracavitary sclerosing agents for malignant pleural effusions depends to a considerable extent on the method of instillation of the agent. Ideally the 2 pleural surfaces should be held in apposition following the instillation. The largest possible thoracotomy tube is inserted, the effusion evacuated to dryness, and the sclerosing agent in 50 mL of solvent flushed through the tube with another 50 mL of saline. Adequate analgesia must be given before and after administration as the intended pleurisy is painful. Following administration the tube is clamped and the patient rotates 90° every 10 minutes for 40 minutes. The tube is subsequently unclamped and suction applied for 48 hours to ensure pleural apposition.— D. P. Dhillon and S. G. Spiro, *Br. J. Hosp. Med.*, 1983, *29*, 506.

The management of malignant pericardial effusion and tamponade. Mustine, fluorouracil, thiotepa, and bleomycin are among the compounds that have been instilled for the long-term management of pericardial effusion, although tetracycline is probably the drug of choice for sclerotherapy. However, surgical treatment is probably preferable.— O. W. Press and R. Livingston, *J. Am. med. Ass.*, 1987, *257*, 1088.

MALIGNANT NEOPLASMS OF THE BLADDER. The chemotherapy of bladder carcinoma has not been intensively studied. Overall response-rates of 35% and 27% have been reported for fluorouracil and doxorubicin respectively but, because of discouraging results in a placebo-controlled study, fluorouracil cannot be recommended for primary treatment. The intracavitary instillation of thiotepa appears to be beneficial in the treatment of small multiple superficial papillary tumours and has been used prophylactically in patients with multiple tumour recurrences. Other drugs with some activity in bladder cancer include mitomycin, teniposide, and cisplatin.— Report of a WHO Expert Committee on Chemotherapy of Solid Tumours, *Tech. Rep. Ser. Wld Hlth Org. No. 605*, 1977, p. 49.

A brief review of intravesical instillation of antineoplastics for superficial bladder cancer. Most experience is available with thiotepa. Following weekly instillation, usually as 30 to 60 mL of a 1 mg per mL solution for 6 to 8 weeks, approximately one third of patients experience complete clearance of tumour and another third partial clearance; large and multiple tumours respond to a lesser degree. Thiotepa may also have some prophylactic value against recurrence, as may mitomycin and doxorubicin, which have also been given by intravesical instillation. Other agents which have been tried by this route are bleomycin and cisplatin and promising results have been obtained with BCG.— J. T. Spaulding, *Cancer Chemother. Pharmac.*, 1983, *11*, *Suppl* S5.

Local laser treatment will be a great improvement in the treatment of papillomata, but in the treatment of more advanced disease there has been no significant improvement in outlook. Following surgery and radiotherapy the 5-year survival rate is 65% in those with superficial and 20% in those with deeply infiltrating tumours: half the patients with deeply invasive tumours will be dead in 18 months despite treatment. Cytotoxic agents have been tried both locally, by instillation of drugs such as thiotepa, doxorubicin, and ethoglucid, and more recently by systemic administration of cisplatin or methotrexate, but despite some encouraging results in palliation, no significant advances in the cure of bladder carcinoma have been made in the last 20 years.— J. B. Garland, *Practitioner*, 1984, *228*, 725.

Intravesical chemotherapy is likely to be most effective when fluid intake is restricted for 12 hours before treatment, the drug is instilled at the highest concentration that does not produce unacceptable local or systemic toxicity, and the patient retains the instillate as long as possible. Response rates are likely to improve further when additional factors such as pH and osmolality are regulated.— J. R. W. Masters (letter), *Lancet*, 1986, *1*, 740.

Cisplatin has achieved an overall response rate of 30% and seems to be slightly more active than other single agents in the management of metastatic transitional cell bladder cancer. Rates of response to combination regimens are generally slightly higher than to single agents but few studies have been randomised and it is questionable whether combination regimens offer any benefit over cisplatin alone, especially in view of the morbidity involved; indeed it remains unproved whether chemotherapy can reliably offer clinically useful palliation or extension of survival in the majority of patients with metastatic bladder cancer. However, recent results (D. Raghavan *et al.*, *J. Urol.*, 1985, *133*, 399) suggest considerable benefits from the use of cisplatin induction chemotherapy prior to surgery or radiotherapy for locally advanced disease.— J. H. Kearsley, *Br. med. J.*, 1986, *293*, 871.

Further discussions of chemotherapy in bladder cancer: T. F. Sandeman, *Med. J. Aust.*, 1984, *140*, 253; T. B. Hargreave, *Br. med. J.*, 1985, *290*, 338; *Lancet*, 1986, *1*, 479.

MALIGNANT NEOPLASMS OF THE BONE. Osteosarcoma, chondrosarcoma, and fibrosarcoma are the 3 basic types of primary malignant tumour of bone. Others such as Ewing's tumour and malignant myeloma arise in the marrow rather than the bone itself.— R. Sweetnam, *Br. J. Hosp. Med.*, 1980, *24*, 452.

See also under Sarcoma (below).

MALIGNANT NEOPLASMS OF THE BRAIN. Glioblastoma multiforme constitutes 31 to 64% of all the gliomas. Cerebral oedema surrounding the tumour can have the same effect as the expanding tumour mass and survival may be prolonged if increased intracranial pressure is alleviated by surgical decompression or the use of corticosteroids (see under Dexamethasone, p.887). Regional chemotherapy with methotrexate has been attempted in order to overcome the blood-brain barrier and lipid-soluble antineoplastic agents are sought. The nitrosoureas are highly lipid-soluble and are probably the only drugs that are genuinely active; a response-rate of 46% with definite prolongation of survival has been reported with carmustine and similar results have been seen with lomustine and semustine. Preliminary results suggest that procarbazine and teniposide may also be active against glioblastoma. There have been few attempts at combination chemotherapy because of the limited number of active agents available.— Report of a WHO Expert Committee on Chemotherapy of Solid Tumours, *Tech. Rep. Ser. Wld Hlth Org. No. 605*, 1977, p. 66.

Tests *in vitro* on cells from patients with malignant glioma showed that while cells from 7 of 8 patients aged 50 or under were sensitive to carmustine, in only 1 of 8 aged over 50 years were cells similarly sensitive. This was reflected in median survival after initial surgery followed by radiotherapy and chemotherapy; which was more than 54 weeks in the younger patients, whereas all those over 50 had died within 37 weeks. Modifications in treatment based on the different responsiveness of cells from young and old patients could lead to improved treatment of patients with malignant gliomas.— M. L. Rosenblum *et al.*, *Lancet*, 1982, *1*, 885.

Carmustine or lomustine were currently preferred for the drug treatment of malignant neoplasms of the brain, although semustine, procarbazine, doxorubicin, and vincristine may also be tried. In the treatment of medulloblastoma, combination therapy with vincristine, carmustine, and sometimes mustine and methotrexate is preferred; alternatively MOPP (mustine, vincristine, procarbazine, and prednisone) may be used.— *Med. Lett.*, 1983, *25*, 1.

For a study of the relative benefits of radiotherapy and nitrosoureas in the postsurgical treatment of malignant glioma, see Carmustine, p.606. For a report of complete remission of brain metastases following chemotherapy in a patient with small-cell lung cancer, see under Malignant Neoplasms of the Bronchus and Lung, below.

MALIGNANT NEOPLASMS OF THE BREAST. Cancer of the breast is the most common malignant tumour of women. The clinical course is extremely variable: certain types of breast cancer such as lobular carcinoma and intraduct carcinoma carry a better prognosis, as do small tumour size, absence of axillary lymph node and skin involvement, postmenopausal status, and presence of sex hormone receptors in the tumour. The appropriate treatment varies with disease stage and prognosis.

A statement issued by a UK Consensus Development Conference on the Treatment of Primary Breast Cancer (*Br. med.J.*, 1986, *293*, 946) states that in the past the main treatment for breast cancer was radical mastectomy but that in recent years there has been a trend towards less radical surgery, often in combination with radiotherapy or systemic drug therapy.

Chemotherapy has 3 distinct potential roles in the treatment of breast cancer. In early disease it may be given as adjuvant treatment in addition to surgery or radiotherapy. It may also be given first for locally advanced disease to reduce disease bulk, thus simplifying subsequent surgery or radiotherapy. Finally it may be given palliatively in metastatic (stage IV) disease. It is important to remember the appropriate aims when selecting therapy (A. Coates, *Drugs*, 1984, *28*, 93). However, in this as in other aspects of the treatment of breast cancer there is controversy: it has been suggested (see R. Ghys, *Can. med. Ass. J.*, 1986, *135*, 17) that there is little real evidence of the curative value of cytotoxic chemotherapy and that it should be restricted to clinical research, and then used solely in premenopausal women with cancerous lymph nodes.

Reviews and discussions on the treatment of breast cancer: I. C. Henderson and G. P. Canellos, *New Engl. J. Med.*, 1980, *302*, 17; *idem*, 78; I. E. Smith, *Postgrad. med. J.*, 1985, *61*, 117; N. O'Higgins, *Br. J. Hosp. Med.*, 1986, *35*, 404; G. N. Brodie and A. Elefanty, *Drugs*, 1988, *35*, 584.

A report of the management of breast cancer by initial chemotherapy, followed by surgery, in patients with large, poor-prognosis operable tumours (T_2 and T_{3A}). Patients received endocrine therapy with aminoglutethimide plus hydrocortisone, tamoxifen, a gonadorelin analogue, or oophorectomy; or else chemotherapy with cyclophosphamide, doxorubicin, vincristine, and prednisolone (CHOP). Patients in whom endocrine therapy failed to prevent disease progression had their treatment changed to chemotherapy. Response to endocrine therapy occurred in 11 of 23 patients but was not striking and was slower than the response seen in metastatic disease or than that in 12 of 13 given chemotherapy. By contrast response to chemotherapy was substantial and in 5 patients the subsequent surgery, after 3 months chemotherapy, revealed no histological evidence of any remaining tumour. The regimen may prove valuable, but the results may not apply to all invasive breast cancers.— A. P. M. Forrest *et al.*, *Lancet*, 1986, *2*, 840.

Early breast cancer. There is no single right therapy for

patients with early breast cancer. In the author's own practice radical surgery alone, limited surgery combined with radiotherapy, limited surgery or radiotherapy alone, and, in certain elderly patients, endocrine therapy alone may be used, according to the circumstances of the individual patient. Adjuvant endocrine or cytotoxic therapy may be given after primary treatment, usually when histological examinations after mastectomy reveal more extensive disease than had been anticipated. In the future there is every reason to expect that sympathetic endocrine therapy will figure increasingly in the treatment of breast cancer, and it may ultimately supplant surgery, radiotherapy, and cytotoxic chemotherapy in the majority of patients, even those with early disease.— I. Burn, *Practitioner,* 1984, *228,* 563.

See also under Adjuvant Therapy, below.

Advanced breast cancer. Advanced breast cancer refers to stages of the disease not curable by conventional surgical methods, and may be described by the Manchester clinical classification of stage III, locally advanced disease, and stage IV, metastatic disease (M. Baum, *Br. J. Hosp. Med.*, 1980, *23,* 32). Stage III disease is conventionally treated by radiotherapy, either preceded or followed by adjuvant systemic therapy, but there is some divergence of opinion as to the correct management of patients with stage IV disease.

Advanced disease cannot be cured, but the accurate selection of the best treatment remains a worthwhile goal, the aim being maximal tumour response, for as long as possible, with minimal side-effects. Many patients will respond to one or all of the treatments available and it is necessary to select an appropriate sequence of treatments (C. Williams and R. Buchanan, *Br. med. J.*, 1982, *285,* 1444).

In the *UK* many authorities have adopted a cautious approach to the use of aggressive cytotoxic regimens. In a review of controversies in the medical management of breast cancer, Smith (*Postgrad. med. J.*, 1985, *61,* 117) has advocated use of chemotherapy as a first-line treatment only in patients with rapidly progressive metastatic disease occurring after a short disease-free interval, and particularly in patients with visceral (e.g. liver) metastases. For most patients an initial trial of endocrine therapy is indicated and tamoxifen is now probably the treatment of choice in both pre- and post-menopausal patients. It is not necessary to know the hormone-receptor status of the tumour, as a therapeutic trial is simpler, cheaper, and more accurate. In patients responding to tamoxifen, second-line endocrine therapy should be considered at relapse. About 30% of patients respond to endocrine therapy and a further 15 to 20% achieve disease stabilisation. Remission may last several years. Bone metastases may respond better to aminoglutethimide than to tamoxifen, but the former drug is ineffective in premenopausal patients (R. Stuart-Harris, *Prescribers' J.*, 1984, *24,* 133).

In patients in whom metastases progress despite endocrine therapy, a trial of chemotherapy should be undertaken, and stopped after 2 courses if there is no evidence of therapeutic benefit. Combinations achieve higher response rates than single agents. Responses are seen in around 60% of patients given combination chemotherapy but few patients sustain response for more than a year.

Although first-line chemotherapy continues to have its proponents (L.A. Price, *Br. med. J.*, 1982, *285,* 1741; *idem,* 1983, *286,* 643), approaches recognisably similar to that generally advocated in the *UK* have been proposed in a number of countries including, in the light of recent results, the *US* (J.N. Ingle, *Mayo Clin. Proc.*, 1984, *59,* 232). Initial use of endocrine therapy is particularly useful in elderly patients (S.G. Taylor, *et al.*, *Ann. intern. Med.*, 1986, *104,* 455).

A number of studies have addressed the potential value of combined endocrine and chemotherapeutic treatment, generally with negative results. In a study by the Swiss Group for Clinical Cancer Research (F. Cavalli *et al.*, *Br. med. J.*, 1983, *286,* 5) concomitant chemotherapy and endocrine therapy (oophorectomy in premenopausal patients; tamoxifen in postmenopausal patients) was evaluated in 207 patients, and compared with endocrine therapy alone, followed by chemotherapy only if necessary, in 199. No overall statistical advantage of concomitant therapy emerged, and in postmenopausal patients with less aggressive tumour, survival was significantly reduced by administration of cytotoxic drugs with the tamoxifen. It has been suggested that the overall lack of benefit shown in many studies derives from failure to identify a sub-group who benefit from such concomitant therapy: Kiang *et al.* (*New Engl. J. Med.*, 1985, *313,* 1241) reported improved response rates and survival times in patients with tumours rich in oestrogen receptors when given combined cytotoxic and stilboestrol therapy, as compared with stilboestrol alone. However, combined therapy offered no apparent benefit over cytotoxic therapy alone in receptor-poor patients.

Adjuvant cytotoxic therapy. Many patients given local treatment for apparently localised breast cancer subsequently develop metastases from which they will die. The aim of adjuvant therapy is to eradicate occult systemic disease (micrometastases).

Considerable controversy attaches to the value or otherwise of adjuvant antineoplastic therapy, and the form that it should take. Although the results of initial chemotherapeutic studies had a short follow-up time, and no survival data were given, great enthusiasm was generated, which has not generally been justified by subsequent results (I.E. Smith, *Postgrad. med. J.*, 1985, *61,* 117). In a substantial review of the subject, Carter (*Drugs,* 1986, *31,* 337) has advocated that adjuvant chemotherapy in breast cancer should still be viewed as an experimental approach which has not yet reached its full potential and in which interpretation of the available data should be viewed as changeable in the light of new data.

Among the earliest studies of cytotoxic adjuvant chemotherapy was that carried out by the National Cancer Institute in Milan, in women given cyclophosphamide, methotrexate, and fluorouracil (CMF). Long-term analysis (G. Bonadonna *et al.*, *Lancet,* 1985, *1,* 976) indicated that overall survival at 10 years, as well as relapse-free survival, was better in premenopausal women given CMF (59 and 48.3% respectively) than in those given surgery alone (45 and 31%); no significant differences in relapse-free or overall survival were detected between CMF and control groups in postmenopausal women. In general the few adequately designed studies have shown a benefit of cytotoxic adjuvant therapy only in premenopausal women with 3 or fewer involved axillary nodes (S.K. Carter, 1986).

The efficacy of adjuvant cytotoxic therapy appears to depend in part upon dosage: Bonadonna has suggested (*Br. J. Hosp. Med.*, 1980, *23,* 40; G. Bonadonna and P. Valagussa, *New Engl. J. Med.*, 1981, *304,* 10) that failure of cytotoxic chemotherapy to achieve benefit in older women may be because fewer have received full therapeutic doses compared with younger patients. However, 12 cycles of chemotherapy, as originally given in the Milan study, may not be necessary: Bonadonna *et al.* could demonstrate no significant difference at 6 years in relapse-free and total survival between women given 6 and 12 cycles of CMF (*Lancet,* 1983, *1,* 1157).

Adjuvant cytotoxic therapy has been widely accepted in some countries. In the *USA*, the guidelines issued by the NIH Consensus Conference on Adjuvant Chemotherapy for Breast Cancer (*J. Am. med. Ass.*, 1985, *254,* 3461) state that combination chemotherapy should become standard care for premenopausal women with axillary lymph node involvement, and should be considered in high-risk premenopausal women with negative nodes, in postmenopausal women with positive nodes but low or absent endocrine receptor levels in the tumour, and in a few high-risk postmenopausal women with negative nodes.

In other countries, notably the *UK* and Australia, acceptance has been tempered by concern for the serious morbidity sometimes associated with complex chemotherapy regimens, and genuine doubt as to the value, in terms of patient survival, of adjuvant therapy. No study has yet addressed the important question of whether adjuvant treatment offers any survival benefit over reserving the same adjuvant cytotoxics for the treatment of symptomatic secondary deposits, and it has been suggested that patients who 'fail' adjuvant chemotherapy may have a significantly shorter median survival than previously untreated women. Given the morbidity and mortality associated with treatment a realistic argument can be made for not routinely administering adjuvant cytotoxic chemotherapy outside studies conducted for clinical research; even in such research there is no longer any justification for the absence of a control (surgery-only) arm (J.H. Kearsley, *Br. med. J.*, 1986, *293,* 871).

Adjuvant endocrine therapy. The role of adjuvant endocrine chemotherapy cannot be fully evaluated as yet, either alone or combined with cytotoxic chemotherapy, but follow-up for up to 6 years in a large multicentre randomised study, carried out by the Nolvadex Adjuvant Trial Organisation (*Lancet,* 1985, *1,* 836), has yielded some encouraging results. Treatment with tamoxifen 10 mg twice daily as sole adjuvant, for 2 years after total mastectomy with axillary node clearance or sampling, was associated with a 34% reduction in number of deaths among 562 evaluable patients, compared with 567 controls. In this trial significant increase in the disease-free interval, and in survival, was shown regardless of menopausal, nodal, or oestrogen receptor status.

Other studies, however, have suggested that adjuvant tamoxifen therapy is most likely to benefit patients with tumours rich in oestrogen receptors (C. Rose *et al.*, *Lancet,* 1985, *1,* 16; H.J. Stewart and R. Prescott, *ibid.*, 573). Nonetheless the case remains unproven: there is some doubt as to the clinical usefulness of oestrogen receptor measurement as a practical means of selecting patients for adjuvant tamoxifen therapy (R.P. A'Hern *et al.*, *ibid.*, 976), and at least one study (G.M. Clark *et al.*, *New Engl. J. Med.*, 1983, *309,* 1343) has suggested that the presence of progesterone receptors is a better prognostic indicator of response to endocrine therapy than that of oestrogen receptors.

Overall analysis of some 43 studies of adjuvant therapy, involving 16 000 women, suggests that a year or two of tamoxifen treatment reduced the number of early deaths in postmenopausal women by about one-sixth (*Lancet,* 1984, *2,* 1193); if the mechanism of action is essentially cytostatic, prolonged treatment for 5 years, or until disease recurrence, might be expected to produce an even greater benefit and should be free of serious side-effects (C. Furnival, *Med. J. Aust.*, 1985, *142,* 496). A randomised multicentre study addressing this question, and involving 1312 evaluable patients, has reported preliminary results (*Lancet,* 1987, *2,* 171). The study, administered by the Scottish Cancer Trials Office of the MRC, compared the value of adjuvant tamoxifen 20 mg daily for 5 years (or until relapse), with a policy of observation only and tamoxifen as the preferred treatment on relapse. The initial results, after administration of tamoxifen for a median duration of 47 months in the adjuvant therapy group, indicate a pronounced benefit from prolonged adjuvant therapy over the use of tamoxifen for first recurrence. The benefit was maintained regardless of menopausal, nodal, or oestrogen receptor status, although benefit was greatest in patients with the highest tumour concentrations of oestrogen receptors.

In the *USA* in particular, a number of studies have investigated combined cytotoxic and endocrine chemotherapy. A study in 1891 patients carried out by the National Surgical Adjuvant Breast and Bowel Project (NSABP) compared treatment with melphalan plus fluorouracil (PF), with the same regimen plus tamoxifen (PFT). Fisher *et al.* (*J. Clin. Oncol.*, 1983, *1,* 227) found that in women under 50, overall survival results favoured those who had not received tamoxifen, although there was no difference in relapse-free survival; and those with low progesterone receptor content in their tumours actually had inferior survival when given the PFT regimen. Similar results were seen in women aged 50 to 59; however, in those aged 60 to 70, PFT was superior to PF regardless of hormone receptor status. Although it is difficult to draw conclusions from these results, they do suggest that tamoxifen is not necessarily safe to give empirically as adjuvant therapy, particularly in younger women (S.K. Carter, *Drugs,* 1986, *31,* 337). Multicentre studies carried out by the Ludwig Breast Cancer Study Group (*Lancet,* 1984, *1,* 1256) found that although both combined cytotoxic and endocrine therapy (cyclophosphamide, methotrexate, and fluorouracil (CMF) plus prednisone and tamoxifen), and endocrine therapy alone, improved 3-year relapse-free survival probability (72% and 59% respectively, against 40% for control) only the combined cytotoxic and endocrine therapy reduced the incidence of distant as against local and regional recurrences. Nonetheless, neither treatment showed an overall survival advantage against control, and any advantage of the combined regimen must therefore be weighed against the higher frequency of toxic effects.

Interestingly, Padmanabhan *et al.* (*Lancet,* 1986, *2,* 411) in a controlled study of CMF adjuvant therapy produced results suggesting that adjuvant cytotoxic chemotherapy may well act primarily by indirect endocrine effects. In this study relapse-free and overall survival were significantly better in the 61% of treated premenopausal women who became amenorrhoeic, and in those whose tumours were positive for progesterone receptors. The effects of CMF appeared to be secondary to ovarian ablation, although a smaller direct cytotoxic effect could not be excluded. However, these results have been disputed (P. Valagussa and G. Bonadonna, *ibid.*, 1035), and remain to be reproduced.

A controlled study of oestrogen use in postmenopausal patients with breast cancer.— R. K. Ross *et al.*, *J. Am. med. Ass.*, 1980, *243,* 1635. See also P. Meier and R. L. Landau, *ibid.*, 1658.

MALIGNANT NEOPLASMS OF THE MALE BREAST. A report of the treatment of 18 male patients with advanced breast cancer, using single- or multiple-drug regimens.— H. -Y. Yap *et al.*, *J. Am. med. Ass.*, 1980, *243,* 1739.

Favourable responses to tamoxifen therapy without prior orchiectomy in 2 men. Since the disease is too rare to allow controlled studies, further case reports are needed to confirm the efficacy of primary tamoxifen treatment and delayed orchiectomy in men with advanced breast cancer.— R. Becher *et al.* (letter), *New Engl. J. Med.*,

1981, *305*, 169.

MALIGNANT NEOPLASMS OF THE BRONCHUS AND LUNG. A re-appraisal of the prevention and control of lung cancer. A classification that discriminates between small-cell and non-small-cell (squamous cell, large-cell, or adenocarcinoma) types is essential. Small-cell lung cancer has usually become a systemic disease at the time of diagnosis, and accordingly systemic combination chemotherapy is the main mode of treatment. The most active agents include cyclophosphamide, etoposide, doxorubicin, vincristine, lomustine, and methotrexate: most treatment schedules include 3 or 4 of these drugs. If disease progression is noted within 2 months of treatment it should be discontinued, but should be maintained in responders for at least 6 months. Current data suggest no advantage in short-term survival from concomitant radiotherapy, even prophylactic cranial irradiation to prevent cranial metastases. In patients with non-small-cell carcinoma surgical treatment is the preferred form of therapy where the tumour is resectable. In patients who cannot tolerate surgery, radiotherapy may be considered, but it remains to be proved that chemotherapy is superior to supportive care. There is no scientific evidence at present that immunotherapy is of any benefit and it is not recommended.— Bull. Wld Hlth Org., 1982, *60*, 809. See also: Report of a WHO Expert Committee on Chemotherapy of Solid Tumours, *Tech. Rep. Ser. Wld Hlth Org. No 605*, 1977, p. 30; D. C. Flenley, *Postgrad. med. J.*, 1983, *59*, 1; S. G. Spiro, *ibid.*, 1984, *60*, 218.

The 15-year findings of a study involving 726 patients given daily busulphan, cyclophosphamide, or placebo following surgical resection for carcinoma of the bronchus indicated no significant differences between survival curves for the 3 treatments or different histological types. Single-drug postoperative treatment does not appear to influence survival in these patients, or offer any benefit over early surgical resection with adequate staging procedures.— D. J. Girling *et al.*, *Br. J. Cancer*, 1985, *52*, 867.

Non-small-cell lung cancer. The relative success of chemotherapy in small-cell lung cancer has tended to overshadow the more common yet intractable problem of non-small-cell lung cancer. Data on the efficacy of the many combination chemotherapy regimens studied have been difficult to interpret because of the heterogeneity of patients and treatment. Adenocarcinoma and squamous cell carcinoma appear to be more chemosensitive than the large-cell type. Highest response rates in adenocarcinoma have been reported with vindesine alone, while for squamous cell carcinoma the most active regimen seems to be a combination of vindesine and cisplatin. However, there is still a lack of evidence that the use of cytotoxic drugs either alone, or in combination improves median survival or quality of life in large, unselected series of patients with non-small-cell lung cancer. Until new agents can be identified, chemotherapy for non-small-cell lung cancer should be largely considered to be experimental.— J. H. Kearsley, *Br. med. J.*, 1986, *293*, 871.

Small-cell lung cancer. Untreated small-cell lung cancer is rapidly fatal, median survial being only 3 months in patients with limited disease and 1.5 months in patients with extensive disease. Although single agent chemotherapy confers a modest survival advantage in both categories of patients, appreciable long-term survival, i.e. greater than 18 months, is generally achieved only with moderately intensive combinations of cytotoxic agents such as doxorubicin, cisplatin, etoposide, vincristine, and methotrexate. Such combinations have led to a four- or five-fold improvement in median survival compared with untreated patients: complete response occurs in 20 to 25% of patients with extensive disease and up to 60% of those with limited disease. However of the 5 to 10% of patients who achieve long-term survival more than one-third will die of recurrent disease. Intensive induction regimens have generally failed to improve median or overall survival.— J. H. Kearsley, *Br. med. J.*, 1986, *293*, 871. See also: S. G. Spiro, *Br. med. J.*, 1985, *290*, 413.

A study indicating that sequential chemotherapy may be as effective as combination regimens in patients with limited small-cell carcinoma. Complete tumour response occurred in 29 of 55 patients who received methotrexate 100 mg per m^2 body-surface area by intravenous injection on days 0 and 14, followed by radiotherapy over 10 days, and then, after a 10-day interval intravenous cyclophosphamide in doses of 1.5 g per m^2, 2.5 g per m^2, and 3.5 g per m^2 at 21-day intervals. Most complete responses occurred within 2 months of the last cyclophosphamide dose, and median duration of complete response was 4 months, with 1 and 2 year survivals of 74 and 37% respectively, compared with 24 and 0% among patients not responding completely. The results show that a relatively short regimen with a low incidence of side-effects can produce prolonged survival in some patients with small-cell bronchogenic carcinoma, with results apparently similar to prolonged combination chemotherapy.— N. Thatcher *et al.*, *Lancet*, 1982, *1*, 1040.

The results of the MRC's Third Small-Cell Study in 186 patients with limited small-cell carcinoma of the bronchus failed to find any survival or tolerance advantages for either of 2 regimens: RC, in which radiotherapy was followed by 10 pulses of chemotherapy with cyclophosphamide and methotrexate, lomustine being added on alternate pulses; and CRC, in which 2 pulses of chemotherapy preceded radiotherapy, which was then followed by the remaining 8 pulses. At 3 years, only 7 of 91 given RC, and 1 of 95 randomised to CRC were still alive. Age was of no prognostic significance but 6 of 38 patients initially classified as in excellent condition were still alive at 3 years. The results suggest that better chemotherapy is needed for this condition.— Report to the MRC by its Lung Cancer Working Party, *Br. J. Cancer*, 1983, *48*, 755.

A report of remission of brain metastases in a patient with small-cell lung cancer following treatment with cyclophosphamide 7 g per m^2 body-surface area and etoposide 900 mg per m^2, followed by etoposide 1.5 g per m^2 for 4 monthly courses. Until now no effective antitumour therapy was available for patients with brain metastases recurring after previous radiotherapy. High-dose etoposide might potentially be incorporated into standard treatment as prophylaxis for central nervous system metastases, for example as part of a late intensification regimen.— P. E. Postmus *et al.* (letter), *Ann. intern. Med.*, 1984, *101*, 717.

Twenty-eight of 252 patients with small-cell lung cancer were alive and cancer-free 30 months after initiation of therapy with combination chemotherapy, combined in some cases with chest radiotherapy. Of the 28, 14 were alive and without cancer at 6 or more years from the start of treatment, representing 12 of 103 with limited stage and 2 of 149 with extensive disease. However, neuropsychiatric testing revealed abnormalities of mental function, gait, or coordination in 10 of 13 survivors; there was some evidence suggesting that abnormal mental status was more likely in patients given cranial irradiation. Results suggest that up to 12% of patients with limited small-cell lung cancer and occasional patients with extensive stage disease may be cured by currently available therapy. Although the long-term impairments seen in these patients are of concern the authors consider that the marked survival benefits and modest curative potential of such therapy outweigh the disadvantages.— B. E. Johnson *et al.*, *Ann. intern. Med.*, 1985, *103*, 430.

A review of survival among 101 patients with limited stage small-cell lung cancer. Patients received surgical therapy, or chemotherapy and/or radiotherapy initially; those who relapsed were subsequently given chemotherapy or radiotherapy. In patients treated with chemotherapy initially the complete remission rate was 12% and the rate of partial remission 26%, but response to chemotherapy in patients who progressed after initial therapy was poor, with no complete remissions. Only 18 of the original 101 patients were still alive at 2.5 years, and when the group who had received initial surgical treatment were excluded, long-term survival fell to 12%. With only modest remission rates, ineffective long-term palliation, and few disease-free survivors beyond 2 to 3 years, no treatment can be considered standard in limited-stage small-cell lung cancer.— T. K. George *et al.*, *Cancer*, 1986, *58*, 1193.

MALIGNANT NEOPLASMS OF THE CERVIX. Chemotherapy has moderate activity in the treatment of cervical cancer, currently preferred drugs being cisplatin, sometimes in combination with methotrexate and/or bleomycin. Other drugs with reported activity are cyclophosphamide, vincristine, and mitomycin.— *Med. Lett.*, 1983, *25*, 1.

A review of the treatment of cervical cancer. Stage I lesions are usually treated by surgery and stage II by radiotherapy. Stage III are also treated by radiotherapy but chemotherapy, usually with cisplatin, may be given before and after for poorly differentiated or aggressive lesions. Stage IV disease is treated with radiotherapy and chemotherapy. Chemotherapy for cervical cancer has been slow to evolve because this tumour was thought resistant to cytotoxic drugs but it has now been shown that response rates of 10 to 40% can be obtained with several drugs and that cisplatin can produce regression in previously irradiated disease where other agents have little effect. Other agents such as cyclical high-dose methotrexate are also being studied and the combination of chemotherapy with radical radiotherapy may ultimately offer the best prospect for patients with poor-risk cervical carcinoma.— L. M. A. Shaw *et al.*, *Practitioner*, 1984, *228*, 555.

The giving of chemotherapy is logical as many women have micrometastasis outside the pelvic treatment area at initial therapy. Single agent treatment with cisplatin, doxorubicin, or bleomycin has been employed, or combinations such as doxorubicin with semustine, methotrexate, or cyclophosphamide; mitomycin with bleomycin or vincristine; or cisplatin with doxorubicin or mitomycin. There is an urgent need for controlled studies of chemotherapy in these patients.— A. Singer, *Br. J. Hosp. Med.*, 1986, *35*, 178. See also B. G. Ward *et al.*, *Br. med. J.*, 1985, *290*, 1301.

MALIGNANT NEOPLASMS OF THE ENDOMETRIUM. A review of carcinoma of the endometrium. Surgical removal by total hysterectomy and bilateral salpingo-oophorectomy remains standard therapy in early (stage I and II) disease: experience to date suggests that the combination of adequate surgery, selective adjuvant radiotherapy and unselective oral progesterone therapy will produce close to 100% cure rates in early disease. However, such treatment has provided small success in controlling advanced disease. Response of stage III or IV lesions is around 15% to progesterone alone, but this may be increased to an apparent 30% by addition of tamoxifen. Most of the known antineoplastic agents have been tried in advanced disease. A full clinical response is rare, although it has been claimed for doxorubicin therapy, but there has been a disappointing lack of success with cisplatin. Combination chemotherapy offers no apparent advantages.— A. P. Bond, *Br. J. clin. Pract.*, 1986, *40*, 157. Although experience with cytotoxic chemotherapy in endometrial cancer is limited, because of the efficacy of surgery and the sensitivity of the disease to progesterone, cytotoxic drugs appear only modestly effective in the palliation of advanced disease. Doxorubicin or cisplatin appear to achieve the highest response rates as single agents; results of combination therapy with these agents have been conflicting.— J. H. Kearsley, *Br. med. J.*, 1986, *293*, 871.

Earlier reports. Chemotherapy has mainly been used in the management of invasive adenocarcinoma of the endometrium. Progestational agents are generally given and achieve a regression-rate of about 30% in advanced disease. Experience with antineoplastic agents is meagre but a response-rate of 23% has been reported with fluorouracil. Responses have also been achieved with cyclophosphamide or doxorubicin but not with chlorambucil.— Report of a WHO Expert Committee on Chemotherapy of Solid Tumours, *Tech. Rep. Ser. Wld Hlth Org. No. 605*, 1977, p. 45. In patients with endometrial cancer whose aortic lymph nodes are involved a treatment regimen including cyclophosphamide, doxorubicin, fluorouracil, and megestrol acetate has been found useful.— S. B. Gusberg, *New Engl. J. Med.*, 1980, *302*, 729.

MALIGNANT NEOPLASMS OF THE EYE. See Retinoblastoma (below).

MALIGNANT NEOPLASMS OF THE GASTRO-INTESTINAL TRACT. A review of 20 studies of the treatment of gastro-intestinal cancer carried out by the Southeastern Cancer Study Group between 1979 and 1983, involving a total of 1087 patients. The percentage of responses to various agents has been variable but it is apparent that none of the new agents tested nor any of the combinations studied has produced any significant benefit, while toxicity has been substantial in many studies. No useful result was obtained in studies with doxorubicin, anguidine, BCG vaccine, bleomycin, cisplatin, cytarabine, colaspase, maytansine, methotrexate, mitoguazone, mitomycin, amsacrine, mitozantrone, razoxane, semustine, thioguanine, vincristine, or fluorouracil. More promising results from other groups using fluorouracil, doxorubicin, and mitomycin have yet to be accepted. It is clear that much work remains to be done before the common gastro-intestinal cancers can be approached with any optimism.— G. J. Hill *et al.*, *Sth. med. J.*, 1986, *79*, 1197.

Malignant neoplasms of the oesophagus. Bleomycin is the only agent with any marked activity in cancer of the oesophagus; response-rates of about 30% have been reported but the duration of response is extremely short.— Report of a WHO Expert Committee on Chemotherapy of Solid Tumours, *Tech. Rep. Ser. Wld Hlth Org. No. 605*, 1977, p. 32.

Further references to the chemotherapy of oesophageal cancer: A. Y. Rostom *et al.* (letter), *Lancet*, 1980, *2*, 912 (methotrexate, bleomycin, fluorouracil, and vincristine); R. B. Buchanan and R. E. Lea (letter), *ibid.*, 1134 (vincristine, bleomycin, and methotrexate).

Malignant neoplasms of the stomach. The prospects for cure in patients with cancer of the stomach are still poor. Surgical resection produces high 5-year survival rates in patients with early disease, but in those with more advanced disease 5-year survival is only 10%, and the majority (65%) of tumours are found to be inoperable at the time of surgery.

Chemotherapy has been attempted in patients with unresectable gastric cancers but its value is disputable. Fluorouracil has been most widely used, but mitomycin, doxorubicin, and the nitrosoureas have also been employed. In the *US*, combination chemotherapy with fluorouracil, doxorubicin, and either mitomycin (comprising the FAM regimen), or semustine, has been preferred (*Med. Lett.*, 1983, *25*, 1). However, Cullinan *et al.* (*J. Am. med. Ass.*, 1985, *253*, 2061) studied 151 patients with gastric and 144 with pancreatic cancer and found no significant advantages for treatment with FAM or FA (fluorouracil with doxorubicin) over fluorouracil alone.

The value of adjuvant chemotherapy after resection also remains unproven. Results of studies of single-agent therapy with thiotepa or floxuridine have been disappointing, and the few studies of combination adjuvant chemotherapy have produced equivocal results to date (S.K. Carter, *Drugs*, 1986, *31*, 337).

Malignant neoplasms of the colon and rectum. The treatment of colorectal cancer is largely surgical: its effectiveness depends upon the extent of disease at the time of resection. Chemotherapy has been tried in patients with inoperable advanced or metastatic disease, and as adjuvant therapy after surgery, but no uniformly effective regimen has been found. Fluorouracil has been the most frequently used agent, either alone or in combination with other agents such as the nitrosoureas. Some evidence suggests that adjuvant chemotherapy may be of benefit in certain patients with rectal, but not colonic cancer (see below).

A randomised study involving 572 evaluable patients who had undergone surgical resection of carcinoma of the colon (Dukes stage B_2 or C) failed to demonstrate any significant difference in disease-free survival time or overall survival between those given adjuvant chemotherapy or immunotherapy or both, compared with untreated controls. The chemotherapy regimen comprised fluorouracil 325 mg per m^2 body-surface area intravenously for 5 days every 5 weeks, with semustine 130 mg per m^2 by mouth on the first day of alternate courses; immunotherapy was performed with a methanol extraction residue of bacillus Calmette-Guérin. Seven of the patients assigned to one of the chemotherapy arms subsequently developed leukaemia. At present there are no data that support the indiscriminate use of fluorouracil alone or in conjunction with semustine as a routine treatment for patients who have undergone resection for colonic carcinoma.—Gastrointestinal Tumor Study Group, *New Engl. J. Med.*, 1984, *310*, 737. The possibility remains that adjuvant therapy may be of benefit to some subsets of patients with regional lymph node involvement; further trials, and improved staging to identify subsets of patients who may benefit, are needed.— J. J. DeCosse, *ibid.*, 782.

In a study involving 202 evaluable patients who underwent resection for adenocarcinoma of the rectum, patients were assigned to receive chemotherapy with fluorouracil and semustine; radiotherapy; or both combined, or else no further treatment. Combined chemoradiotherapy produced a significant prolongation of disease-free interval compared with untreated controls or patients given radiotherapy alone; no other significant differences were demonstrated between treatments. However the benefit of combined therapy was not demonstrated in terms of survival and it was associated with significantly greater toxicity than either form of therapy alone. Unlike the companion trial in colon carcinoma this study has shown some benefit for chemotherapy, particularly in patients given combined therapy: radiotherapy and chemotherapy appear to reduce the rates of local and distant recurrence respectively. Although the price paid by the patient is high in terms of toxicity, it was considered acceptable.— Gastrointestinal Tumor Study Group, *New Engl. J. Med.*, 1985, *312*, 1465. Comment. It is difficult to recommend widespread application of a combination treatment that is associated with serious toxicity and does not improve overall patient survival; however, it is possible that such an improvement occurred but that the statistical power of the study was insufficient to show it.— S. A. Rosenberg, *ibid.*, 1512.

A review of adjuvant chemotherapy, including the adjuvant treatment of colorectal cancer. In total there have been 6 randomised studies of fluorinated pyrimidines (floxuridine or fluorouracil) as adjuvant chemotherapy in colorectal cancer, and none has been positive. More recent studies have involved the combination of semustine with fluorouracil but with hind sight it is now clear that this combination has no superiority to fluorouracil alone, and is more toxic.— S. K. Carter, *Drugs*, 1986, *31*, 337.

Most studies of single-agent palliative, as opposed to adjuvant, therapy continue to confirm the relative chemoresistance of advanced colorectal cancer. Of the agents that have been tried, fluorouracil is probably the most acceptable, with an overall response-rate of 15% and only moderate toxicity. Combination chemotherapy with regimens such as semustine, vincristine, fluorouracil, and streptozocin (MOF-Strep) has yet to be proved superior to fluorouracil alone.— J. H. Kearsley, *Br. med. J.*, 1986, *293*, 871.

For the treatment of hepatic metastases see under Malignant Neoplasms of the Liver, below.

See also Malignant Neoplasms of the Pancreas, below.

MALIGNANT NEOPLASMS OF THE HEAD AND NECK. In recent years many studies of induction chemotherapy before surgery and/or radiotherapy have been carried out in patients with advanced squamous-cell carcinoma of the head and neck. Uncontrolled studies have shown complete response in 20 to 60% of patients, the most promising results being with a combination of cisplatin and fluorouracil, but randomised studies have generally failed to confirm the apparent superiority of induction regimens. Some results have indicated that the high initial response rates of primary and nodal disease were partially negated by the early development of metastases; whether induction chemotherapy will be of long-term benefit in terms of survival remains uncertain. Results of treatment of advanced or recurrent disease are discouraging. The standard regimen is methotrexate in intravenous doses of 25 to 50 mg per m^2 body-surface area weekly, which yields a response rate of 25 to 35% for a median of 3 months. Similar response rates are obtained with cisplatin, but methotrexate is better tolerated. Increasing the dosage of methotrexate does not appear to improve response. Combination chemotherapy tends to result in higher response rates, especially when it includes cisplatin, but improvements are short-lived, toxicity is substantial, and overall survival is not extended. J. H. Kearsley, *Br, med. J.*, 1986, *293*, 871.

Reviews and studies of chemotherapy in the treatment of head and neck cancer: P. Clifford *et al.* (letter), *Lancet*, 1982, *2*, 708 (SECOG Head and Neck Trial: vincristine, bleomycin, methotrexate, with or without fluorouracil, and radiotherapy); W. K. Hong and R. Bromer, *New Engl. J. Med.*, 1983, *308*, 75 (review); P. M. Stell *et al.* (letter), *Lancet*, 1983, *1*, 1205 (lack of value of bleomycin, alone or combined with cisplatin); G. M. Mead and J. M. A. Whitehouse, *Br. med. J.*, 1984, *288*, 585 (limitations of chemotherapy of solid tumours); L. A. Price and B. T. Hill (letter), *ibid.*, 1089 (a contrary view).

MALIGNANT NEOPLASMS OF THE KIDNEY. See Wilm's Tumour, p.594.

MALIGNANT NEOPLASMS OF THE LIVER. At present, surgical resection offers the only chance of cure for hepatocellular carcinoma, but only a minority of patients are operable. The disease is resistant to radiotherapy, and cytotoxic therapy has usually produced disappointing results.— M. C. Kew, *Postgrad. med. J.*, 1983, *59*, *Suppl.* 4, 78. Chemotherapy with drugs such as fluorouracil and mitomycin, particularly intra-arterially, can be shown to alter the progression of hepatocellular carcinoma but prolongation of survival is minimal, at most a month or two. Some form of tumour regression can be induced in about one quarter of patients given doxorubicin; less than 10% obtain complete symptomatic remission but median survival of those who do is nearly 2 years. Likelihood of remission can be foretold by a fall in alpha-fetoprotein concentrations: if these continue to rise after 2 cycles of therapy, doxorubicin is unlikely to be effective.— H. J. F. Hodgson, *Br. J. Hosp. Med.*, 1983, *29*, 240.

A review of hepatic arterial chemotherapy for colorectal cancer metastatic to the liver. Current data suggest that continuous hepatic arterial infusion of floxuridine is the most effective current treatment.— R. J. Stagg *et al.*, *Ann. intern. Med.*, 1984, *100*, 736. There is no convincing evidence from many reports on the subject that worthwhile clinical benefit can be obtained from either single agent or combination chemotherapy in most patients with colorectal liver metastases. Reported results of response rate to infusion of fluorouracil into the hepatic artery vary between 12 and 90%, and lack of standardisation of the site of catheter placement, drug and dose delivered, duration of infusion, response criteria, and survival analysis preclude adequate comparison of reported results between studies.— J. H. Kearsley, *Br. med. J.*, 1986, *293*, 871.

MALIGNANT NEOPLASMS OF THE NERVES. Combined therapy with cyclophosphamide, vincristine, doxorubicin, and dacarbazine (cyVADIC) produced complete remissions in 2 patients with metastic malignant schwannoma.— R. L. Goldman *et al.*, *Cancer*, 1977, *39*, 1955.

See also under Neuroblastoma (below).

MALIGNANT NEOPLASMS OF THE OVARY. The treatment of advanced ovarian cancer. Most patients present with tumours extending beyond the pelvis, and although it has been suggested that radiotherapy may be beneficial in up to stage III disease, patients with more extensive disease have usually been given chemotherapy. Response rates to single-agent alkylating therapy range from 36 to 65% but duration of response is only 10 to 14 months and 5-year survival is only 0.9%. Combination regimens that include cisplatin have proved highly effective, if toxic, even in advanced disease, but long-term survival benefit remains uncertain. Initial surgical management may be crucial in removing as much of the tumour as possible: patients with minimal residual disease after surgery may justifiably be given intensive chemotherapy with cisplatin-containing regimens, provided there are no complications. About half these patients achieve complete remission but relapse is common on stopping treatment. Intraperitoneal administration of platinum compounds may be an advance in patients with minimal residual disease but the role of carboplatin is debatable. Managing advanced ovarian cancer remains difficult and a simple solution is unlikely to emerge in the foreseeable future.— R. W. Burslem and P. M. Wilkinson, *Br. med. J.*, 1986, *293*, 972. Disagreement.— J. W. Sweetenham *et al.* (letter), *ibid.*, 1435.

Earlier reviews of the treatment of ovarian cancer: *Lancet*, 1980, *2*, 1010; J. S. Scott, *Br. med. J.*, 1983, *286*, 824; F. M. Muggia *et al.*, *Ann. intern. Med.*, 1985, *103*, 79; G. S. Richardson *et al.*, *New Engl. J. Med.*, 1985, *312*, 474.

In a prospective randomised study of patients with advanced ovarian adenocarcinoma, combination chemotherapy with hexamethylmelamine, cyclophosphamide, methotrexate, and fluorouracil produced complete remission in 13 of 40 patients, compared with 6 of 37 given melphalan alone. Median survival was 29 months in the group given combination chemotherapy compared with 17 months in those receiving melphalan; however, side-effects were more frequent in the combination chemotherapy group.— R. C. Young *et al.*, *New Engl. J. Med.*, 1978, *299*, 1261.

A randomised study in patients with stage III or IV epithelial ovarian cancer found that therapy with a cisplatin-containing regimen (CHAP-5) was significantly better than a standard combination regimen (Hexa-CAF) in terms of remission rate and duration of survival. Patients assigned to CHAP-5 received in each 35-day cycle: cisplatin 20 mg per m^2 body-surface area, by intravenous infusion on days 1 to 5; doxorubicin 35 mg per m^2 by intravenous injection on day 1; and oral hexamethylmelamine 150 mg per m^2 with cyclophosphamide 100 mg per m^2 on days 15 to 28. The Hexa-CAF regimen consisted of: methotrexate 40 mg per m^2 and fluorouracil 600 mg per m^2, both given intravenously on days 1 and 8; and hexamethylmelamine with cyclophosphamide in the same doses as above on days 1 to 14 of a 28-day cycle. Doses were modified when myelosuppression occurred. Of the patients evaluable for response, 25 of 84 given CHAP-5 had complete remission compared with 15 of 88 given Hexa-CAF. Overall survival for the 2 groups was 30.7 and 19.6 months respectively. Although it is rather toxic, CHAP-5 appears to be one of the most effective regimens currently available for the treatment of ovarian cancer.— J. P. Neijt *et al.*, *Lancet*, 1984, *2*, 594. Further data. Some 60% of all patients who achieved complete remission were still alive at 5-year follow-up, and there was no difference between those who had received Hexa-CAF and those given CHAP-5. Patients who had shown microscopic disease at second examination, who had received at least 2 further cycles of chemotherapy, had a similar survival rate, suggesting that patients with 'complete remission' also had some microscopic disease which was not seen at biopsy.— J. P. Neijt *et al.* (letter), *ibid.*, 1986, *1*, 1028.

A study by the North Thames Cooperative Group comparing single-agent alkylating therapy, using cyclophosphamide, with cisplatin therapy, in patients with advanced epithelial ovarian cancer, found that 31 of 49 patients given cisplatin treatment achieved complete clinical response, compared with only 14 of 37 given cyclophosphamide. Patients treated with cisplatin survived significantly longer than those given cyclophosphamide, median survival being 19 and 12 months respectively. The quality of life of patients achieving complete response was good. The results suggest that cisplatin rather than an alkylating agent may be the drug of choice when single-agent therapy is given for the treatment of advanced ovarian cancer.— H. E. Lambert and R. J. Berry, *Br. med. J.*, 1985, *290*, 889. Comments. The conclusions of the study remain unconfirmed.— B. G. Ward and M. L. Slevin (letter), *ibid.*, 1351; C. J. Williams and J. M. Whitehouse (letter), *ibid.*

In a multicentre open study in 531 women with advanced ovarian epithelial cancer 174 patients received cisplatin 50 mg per m^2 body-surface per cycle; 182 also received cyclophosphamide 650 mg per m^2; and a further 175 were given doxorubicin 50 mg per m^2 in addition to the other 2 drugs (CAP regimen). Cycles were repeated every 28 days for 6 courses; doses were modified according to the degree of myelosuppression. The evaluable patients in each group numbered 173, 174, and 169 respectively, and of these 89, 107, and 120 had some response. Complete pathological response (no lesions apparent on laparotomy and random biopsy) occurred in 35 of those given cisplatin alone (20.2%) compared with 36 of those also given cyclophosphamide (20.7%) and 44 of those receiving CAP (26.0%). Survival curves over 4 years were not significantly different between treatment arms. These results cast doubt on the superiority of polychemotherapy with CAP over cisplatin alone in advanced ovarian cancer.— Gruppo Interegionale Cooperativo Oncologico Ginecologia, *Lancet*, 1987, *2*, 353. Comment. Higher doses of cyclophosphamide, as well as of cisplatin, could have been given, and it is possible that there is a threshold dose below which cyclophosphamide's contribution is not apparent. Mustards such as cyclophosphamide have a long track record in the treatment of ovarian carcinoma and should not be dispensed with before residual questions about optimum dose intensity and long survival are answered.— G. A. Omura (letter), *ibid.*, 689.

MALIGNANT NEOPLASMS OF THE PANCREAS. Surgery offers the only possibility of cure in adenocarcinoma of the pancreas and although chemotherapy has had a palliative effect in some patients in general it has not been successful. Fluorouracil has a reported overall response-rate of 38% which is probably an overestimate and similar results have been achieved with mitomycin. About half of patients with islet cell carcinoma of the pancreas have responded to streptozocin. Survival gains with fluorouracil in association with carmustine have not been significant but beneficial results have been achieved with fluorouracil in association with radiotherapy when compared with radiotherapy alone.— Report of a WHO Expert Committee on Chemotherapy of Solid Tumours, *Tech. Rep. Ser. Wld Hlth Org. No. 605*, 1977, p.36. See also G. R. Giles and J. de Mello, *Br. J. Hosp. Med.*, 1981, *25*, 15; M. J. O'Connell, *Mayo Clin. Proc.*, 1983, *58*, 47.

For a reference to the use of fluorouracil with doxorubicin and mitomycin in patients with pancreatic cancer, see under Malignant Neoplasms of the Stomach, above.

MALIGNANT NEOPLASMS OF THE PROSTATE. Although there is considerable debate concerning the best therapy for the different stages of prostatic cancer the role of cytotoxic chemotherapy is small. Localised disease may be treated with radiotherapy or surgery; patients with asymptomatic early disease may require no treatment. In patients with metastatic disease orchiectomy or some other form of hormonal therapy is given (oestrogens, anti-androgens such as cyproterone, gonadorelin analogues (buserelin and goserelin), or high-dose ketoconazole). Cytotoxic agents that have been tried include cyclophosphamide, doxorubicin, cisplatin, fluorouracil, and estramustine. Therapy with aminoglutethimide has ben reported to produce palliation in some patients with advanced disease.

Reviews and discussions of the treatment of prostatic cancer: F. M. Torti and S. K. Carter, *Ann. intern. Med.*, 1980, *92*, 681; G. D. Chisholm, *Prescribers' J.*, 1981, *21*, 278; D. Kirk, *Br. med. J.*, 1985, *290*, 875; *Drug & Ther. Bull.*, 1986, *24*, 85.

Results in 28 patients referred to a medical oncology unit with metastatic cancer of the prostate, in most cases refractory to hormone therapy, showed no survival benefit from a variety of intensive cytotoxic treatments and suggested that once resistance to hormonal manoeuvres develops, prostatic cancer takes a more adverse course.— L. B. Schneider and A. S. D. Spiers (letter), *Lancet*, 1984, *1*, 400. Cytotoxic drugs with some efficacy in metastatic prostatic cancer resistant to hormones include doxorubicin, fluorouracil, cyclophosphamide, and cisplatin, which individually have achieved overall response rates of up to 40%, but criteria defining response to treatment have been difficult to agree on. Response rates and duration of response with combination regimens have not been clearly superior to those achieved with single agents.— J. H. Kearsley, *Br. med. J.*, 1986, *293*, 871.

A review of cytotoxic treatment of metastatic prostatic cancer. Complete and partial responses occur rarely, and there is no convincing evidence that chemotherapy is of benefit to a meaningful proportion of patients with this disease. Furthermore the potential for toxicity in patients with extensive bony metastases is high. Chemotherapy should not be regarded as part of the standard management of prostatic cancer.— I. F. Tannock, *J. clin. Oncol.*, 1985, *3*, 1013.

MALIGNANT NEOPLASMS OF THE SKIN. The most common skin cancers are basal cell carcinomas and squamous cell carcinomas and topical treatment with fluorouracil has sometimes been used. Bleomycin has also been given systemically.— Report of a WHO Expert Committee on Chemotherapy of Solid Tumours, *Tech. Rep. Ser. Wld Hlth Org. No. 605*, 1977, p.57.

A report of the use of cisplatin, bleomycin, and methotrexate followed by calcium folinate rescue, to treat squamous cell carcinoma of the skin complicating hidradenitis suppurativa in a 35-year-old patient.— M. K. Sparks *et al.*, *Archs Derm.*, 1985, *121*, 243.

See also under Melanoma, Mycosis Fungoides, and Kaposi's Sarcoma (below).

MALIGNANT NEOPLASMS OF THE TESTIS. Testicular tumours vary in their response to treatment; seminomas are particularly responsive to radiotherapy, while embryonal carcinomas and teratomas are more responsive to chemotherapy with a variety of agents which can produce very high response rates and prolonged remissions (Report of a WHO Expert Committee on Chemotherapy of Solid Tumours, *Tech. Rep. Ser. Wld Hlth Org. No. 605*, 1977, p.51). Various agents have been given for metastatic disease, including actinomycin D, vinblastine, cisplatin, bleomycin, melphalan, chlorambucil, cyclophosphamide, doxorubicin, etoposide, methotrexate, and plicamycin (*Med. Lett.*, 1983, *25*, 1). Einhorn and Donohue (*Ann intern. Med.*, 1977, *87*, 293) demonstrated that addition of cisplatin to combination chemotherapy with vinblastine and bleomycin (PVB) produced complete remission in 35 of 47 evaluable patients with metastatic non-seminomatous germ-cell tumours; 27 of the 50 patients (54%) survived for 7 years (L.H. Einhorn and S.D. Williams, *Lancet*, 1983, *1*, 1335). Toxicity with this regimen was considerable and there were 2 treatment-related deaths in this series. This has led to a search for equally effective but less toxic regimens. A study carried out by M.J. Peckham *et al.* (*Br. J. Cancer*, 1983, *47*, 613) achieved complete remission of disease in 30 of 36 patients (83%) with metastatic germ-cell tumours given a regimen combining bleomycin, etoposide, and cisplatin (BEP). This diseease-free group included 15 of 19 men with large-volume disease which has been associated with a poor prognosis. In the *UK*, it has been recommended (M. Ellis and K. Sikora, *Br. med. J.*, 1986, *292*, 672) that the PVB regimen should be abandoned in favour of a regimen containing etoposide, of which BEP is the most widely used.

Some centres have advocated sequential combination chemotherapy: E.S. Newlands *et al.* (*Lancet*, 1983, *1*, 948) used a regimen of vincristine, methotrexate with folinic acid rescue, bleomycin, and cisplatin, alternating with actinomycin D, cyclophosphamide, and etoposide (POMB/ACE) to induce remission in 69 patients with metastatic malignant teratoma. Sixty of these patients were alive at follow-up for a mean of 16.5 months and projected survival was 83%, which was superior to results reported with PVB. However, this comparison may not be valid as more recent studies of PVB have reported survival rates 77% and haematological toxicity comparable to that reported for POMB/ACE therapy (L.H. Einhorn and S.D. Williams, *Lancet*, 1983, *1*, 1335).

In general, the results of treatment with combination regimens have improved with experience in their use, particularly with experience and judgement in timing and the necessary dosage adjustments to avoid deaths related to drug toxicity (R. T. D. Oliver, *Postgrad. med. J.*, 1985, *61*, 123).

A multicentre study of prognostic factors involving 458 patients treated with chemotherapy between 1976 and 1982 for non-seminomatous germ-cell testicular tumours showed that the 3-year survival rate was 75% overall. 180 patients in the low-risk category had a survival rate of 91%; 205 intermediate risk patients had a survival rate of 72%, and the 73 high-risk patients had a survival rate of 47%. However, when only those patients treated between 1980 and 1982 were considered, survival rates for the 3 groups were 95, 85, and 54% respectively. These results may be explained by more appropriate use of chemotherapy and post-chemotherapy surgery.— Report from the MRC Working Party on Testicular Tumours, *Lancet*, 1985, *1*, 8.

Reports of late relapse (up to 5 years) after chemotherapy for testicular cancer: L. J. Geier *et al.* (letter), *Lancet*, 1983, *1*, 1049; S. Y. T. Chan *et al.* (letter), *ibid.*, 1985, *2*, 773. Emphasis on the importance of surgery after chemotherapy to remove residual disease masses.— R. E. Taylor (letter), *ibid.*, 1125 (See also R.T.D. Oliver, *ibid.*).

The routine use of CNS prophylaxis with intrathecal methotrexate, as advocated by Newlands *et al.* (*Lancet*, 1983, *1*, 948) in POMB/ACE therapy of patients with metastatic malignant teratoma, must be questioned. Of 276 consecutive patients at Indiana University, only 13 have had brain metastases during or after therapy. Brain metastases as the sole cause of death occurred in only 2.— L. H. Einhorn and S. D. Williams (letter), *Lancet*, 1983, *1*, 1335. Reply. Most of the patients in the authors' series had pulmonary metastases and/or raised serum concentrations of human chorionic gonadotrophin, both of which are associated with CNS spread. For the chemotherapy defined, no patients have died of brain metastases as the sole cause of death. Although the advantage of CNS prophylaxis is small it is to be expected that only by attention to this type of detail will further improvements in survival be obtained.— E. S. Newlands *et al.* (letter), *ibid.*, *2*, 163.

Seminoma. It is now clear that the response of seminoma to cisplatin alone or in combination with bleomycin and etoposide (BEP) is excellent. Chemotherapy with a regimen containing cisplatin should be used as primary treatment for patients with bulky or extensive seminoma, instead of large-field irradiation. Radiotherapy should be confined to sites of bulky disease reduced in volume by chemotherapy.— M. Ellis and K. Sikora, *Br. med. J.*, 1986, *292*, 672. Disagreement. For patients in stage IIB disease (node mass 2 to 5 cm) retroperitoneal node irradiation would appear to be effective. Although metastatic seminoma is very sensitive to cisplatin-based chemotherapy, long-term follow-up is not available. Seminoma metastases are extremely sensitive to even modest doses of radiation, and retroperitoneal node irradiation would appear to be effective therapy for those with stage IIB disease, allowing chemotherapy to be reserved for those patients with bulky abdominal nodes at presentation and for the minority who relapse following radiotherapy.— R. E. Taylor (letter), *ibid.*, 901.

MALIGNANT NEOPLASMS OF THE THYMUS. Report of the use of combination chemotherapy comprising vincristine, cyclophosphamide, and lomustine in 9 patients with malignant thymoma. Six patients also received prednisone; some had undergone partial resection of the tumour, radiotherapy, or both. Complete response was seen in 4 patients, lasting a median of 37 months. The results are encouraging enough to continue with this regimen, possibly with the addition of cisplatin, which is effective as a single agent, but further studies are needed to show the role of combination chemotherapy when integrated with surgery and radiotherapy.— G. Daugaard *et al.*, *Ann. intern. Med.*, 1983, *99*, 189. Comment. The addition of cisplatin seems appropriate. Previous series have found objective responses primarily in non-irradiated patients which also applied to 3 of the 4 complete responders cited by Daugaard *et al.* Based on limited experience, the best approach in patients with large invasive thymomas would appear to be chemotherapy first, followed by consolidation radiotherapy and then consideration of surgical exploration and resection of residual tumours.— A. P. Chahinian *et al.* (letter), *ibid.*, 736.

MALIGNANT NEOPLASMS OF THE THYROID. Iodine-131 is the mainstay of treatment following thyroidectomy in thyroid cancer; doxorubicin and cyclophosphamide have been known to produce occasional regressions.— Report of a WHO Expert Committee on Chemotherapy of Solid Tumours, *Tech. Rep. Ser. Wld Hlth Org. No. 605*, 1977, p. 57.

Nine of 14 patients with advanced anaplastic thyroid carcinoma unresponsive to surgery, external radiotherapy, and radioactive iodine derived some benefit from chemotherapy with doxorubicin, vincristine, and bleomycin (ABC). After some modification the regimen given to 8 patients was: doxorubicin 60 mg per m^2 body-surface in association with vincristine 2 mg, both given intravenously, followed 4 to 6 hours later by 30 mg of bleomycin given intramuscularly, the cycle being repeated every 3 to 4 weeks.— M. Sokal and C. L. Harmer, *Clin. Oncol.*, 1978, *4*, 3.

MELANOMA. Surgery is usually curative in superficial melanoma but of all cancers originating in the skin, it has the greatest potential for dissemination with a propensity to metastasise to the brain. Chemotherapy is used in advanced disease. Dacarbazine is the agent most extensively studied in malignant melanoma but semustine appears to be as effective. A variety of combination regimens has been tested but none can definitely be recommended.— Report of a WHO Expert Committee on Chemotherapy of Solid Tumours, *Tech. Rep. Ser. Wld Hlth Org. No. 605*, 1977, p. 59.

Treatment with the antineoplastic agent vindesine has achieved objective response-rates in advanced malignant melanoma similar to those seen with dacarbazine and is far better tolerated. Beneficial results are possible with dexamethasone, cranial irradiation, and combination chemotherapy including lomustine in patients with cerebral metastases.— S. Retsas, *Practitioner*, 1980, *224*, 1019.

Review of the value of high-dose chemotherapy with autologous marrow transplantation in patients with melanoma. Of 103 cases reviewed, plus a further 2 reported here, responses were noted in 48, and in 17 cases the response was complete. In the majority of cases treatment was with a single drug, usually an alkylating agent: the role of high-dose combination chemotherapy remains to be demonstrated.— A. Kessinger, *J. Am. Acad. Derm.*, 1985, *12*, 337.

A prospective randomised study involving 761 evaluable patients with malignant melanoma was carried out by the WHO International Melanoma Group. Following radical surgery patients received either chemotherapy with dacarbazine, immunotherapy with BCG vaccine, or both; or else no adjuvant therapy. No significant difference could be demonstrated between groups in disease-free and overall survival: either such a difference did not exist or it was of limited clinical importance.— U. Veronesi *et al.*, *New Engl. J. Med.*, 1982, *307*, 913.

MESOTHELIOMA. Response rates in small numbers of patients suggest that doxorubicin and the alkylating agents, including cyclophosphamide, probably have activity as single agents against mesothelioma. Azacitidine and fluorouracil may also be effective. Response rates of up to 30 or 40% have been reported with doxorubicin-containing combination regimens, with palliation of symptoms and longer median survival times in responding patients.— K. H. Antman, *New Engl. J. Med.*, 1980, *303*, 200.

See also under Sarcoma (below).

MYCOSIS FUNGOIDES. A brief report on treatment protocols for mycosis fungoides from the Dutch Mycosis Fungoides Study Group. Topical application of mustine is one of the alternatives in early stages of the disease. In more advanced stages combination chemotherapy with cyclophosphamide, vincristine, and prednisone (COP) or with mustine, vincristine, procarbazine, and prednisone (MOPP) is used, often in association with topical treatment.— L. Hamminga and W. A. van Vloten, *Br. J. Derm.*, 1980, *102*, 477. Since 1974, 17 patients with mycosis fungoides and lymph node involvement have been treated with the COP regimen; 10 also received electron beam irradiation. Seven patients achieved complete remission, with a median disease-free interval of 5 months on follow-up.— H. J. Sentis *et al.*, *ibid.*, 1985, *112*, 232.

MYELOMA. Progress in the treatment of multiple myeloma has been disappointingly slow. Since multiple myeloma is not curable, treatment should be delayed until evidence of progression develops, the patient becomes symptomatic, or treatment is needed to prevent imminent complications.

Although radiation is appropriate for localised plasmacytoma, chemotherapy is the preferred initial treatment for overt multiple myeloma. The standard approach is the use of melphalan with prednisone, the author preferring melphalan 150 µg per kg body-weight by mouth daily and prednisone in a dose of 15 mg four times daily, for a 7-day period every 6 weeks. This therapy should be given for at least 3 courses unless the disease progresses rapidly; the daily dose of melphalan should be increased in patients who do not absorb melphalan adequately. Maximal improvement may not be forthcoming for many months.

Because of the shortcomings of melphalan and prednisone, various combination regimens have been tried. High response rates have been reported for the M-2 (VBMCP) protocol, which employs vincristine, carmustine, cyclophosphamide, melphalan, and prednisone, but in a randomised study comparing standard melphalan and prednisone therapy with M-2, Oken *et al.* (*Proc. Am. Soc. clin. Oncol.*, 1984, *3*, 270) found that although response rates were higher with the more intensive regimen (74% as against 53%) the median survival was not significantly different. Although other combinations of chemotherapeutic agents appear to produce results superior to those achieved with melphalan and prednisone this difference has not been proved conclusively. The duration of chemotherapy is controversial, but a reasonable approach is to continue chemotherapy for 2 years, then discontinue if the patient's response was satisfactory and tumour burden low.

Some patients do not respond initially to alkylating agents, and the remainder eventually become resistant. Combinations of carmustine, doxorubicin, vincristine, and prednisone are beneficial in about 40% of these patients. Vindesine, cisplatin, chlorozotocin, amsacrine, hexamethylmelamine, pentostatin, and interferons have also been tried, but with limited success. The biology of myeloma must be better understood before major progress can be made in the disease.— R. A. Kyle, *New Engl. J. Med.*, 1984, *310*, 1382.

Reviews and discussions of the treatment of multiple myeloma: J. E. Oakley and I. M. Franklin, *J. clin. Hosp. Pharm.*, 1984, *9*, 15; D. E. Bergsagel, *Postgrad. med. J.*, 1985, *61*, 109.

Treatment with a regimen combining intermittent high-dose dexamethasone with infusions of vincristine and doxorubicin (VAD) produced rapid reduction in tumour mass of greater than 75% in 17 of 29 patients with multiple myeloma refractory to alkylating agents, a result superior to that achieved with previous salvage regimens. The regimen consisted of vincristine 400 µg daily and doxorubicin 9 mg per m^2 body-surface area daily, given as 4-day continous infusions via an indwelling catheter, plus dexamethasone 40 mg daily by mouth for 4 days beginning on day 1, 9, and 17 of each cycle. VAD chemotherapy was repeated until a maximum reduction in myeloma protein occurred or for 4 cycles after its disappearance. Fourteen of 20 patients refractory to melphalan and prednisone and 3 of 9 also resistant to previous doxorubicin combinations responded; survival was significantly longer in responders than non-responders. The major side-effect was infection, partly associated with the steroid component: omission of the second and third dexamethasone pulse in every second course of VAD has resulted in less frequent infection.— B. Barlogie *et al.*, *New Engl. J. Med.*, 1984, *310*, 1353. Results in these and a further 10 patients treated with VAD were compared with 49 consecutive patients with resistant myeloma given only the intermittent high-dose dexamethasone. Of the 39 patients given VAD, 7 of 22 who had never responded to previous therapy but 11 of 17 who relapsed from prior remission were responsive to VAD. Comparable figures with dexamethasone were 8 of 30 and 4 of 19. The findings suggest that previously unresponsive patients responded as well to the glucocorticoid alone (27%) as to the full VAD regimen (32%). However, in patients who had acquired drug resistance addition of vincristine and doxorubicin more than doubled the response rate achieved with dexamethasone alone (65% versus 21%). There was no significant difference in survival between the regimens; median survival in responders was 22 months. Despite the small number of patients the results appear to justify the early use of dexamethasone in patients with unresponsive myeloma and prompt use of the VAD regimen in patients with relapsing disease.— R. Alexanian *et al.*, *Ann. intern. Med.*, 1986, *105*, 8.

It has become clear that prognosis in myeloma is related to the attainment of a kinetically characteristic plateau phase. Chemotherapy does not prolong this state, in which the myeloma cells are kinetically hypoactive. Potentially leukaemogenic cytotoxic therapy is not indicated in patients who are clearly in plateau phase at presentation nor in those who have established plateau phase after chemotherapy. These medications should be stopped as soon as plateau phase is reached since continuation may do more harm than good.— D. E. Joshua *et al.* (letter), *Lancet*, 1985, *2*, 210. See also: B. G. M. Durie *et al.*, *ibid.*, 1980, *2*, 65.

NEUROBLASTOMA. A review of neuroblastoma and its treatment. Although children with neuroblastoma represent only 7% of the total cases of childhood cancer diagnosed each year, 15% of cancer deaths in children are due to this tumour. The stage of disease at diagnosis affects the prognosis, patients with localised (Stage I or II) disease generally have good long-term survival but those with widespread metastatic disease (stage IV) are rarely alive and disease-free 2 years from diagnosis. In general, younger patients have a better prognosis than older ones. Stage I or II disease is treated by surgical excision with radiotherapy for any residual tumour: chemotherapy has not had any beneficial effect in these patients. For stages III or IV, multimodal therapy is used. Stage III patients undergo excision of the tumour and associated lymph nodes, followed by local irradiation and systemic chemotherapy. Agents active against advanced neuroblastoma include cyclophosphamide, melphalan, vincristine, doxorubicin, dacarbazine, teniposide, and cisplatin. Most patients have stage IV disease at diagnosis, and in these primary treatment is with combination chemotherapy, which yields a complete response in 30 to 40% and partial response in a further 30%. However, recurrence is frequent within a year, and the 2-year disease-free survival in these patients is less than 10%. New therapeutic directions are urgently needed for patients with stage III or IV disease, and approaches under investigation include high-dose melphalan, or chemotherapy and radiotherapy, followed by bone-marrow rescue. Preclinical studies with monoclonal antibodies, and with retinoic acid, may lead to the development of new therapies. The exception to the poor prognosis in stage IV are those patients, usually under 1 year of age, classified as IV-S, in whom little or no treatment is usually necessary, and in whom chemotherapy with low-dose cyclophosphamide, with or without vincristine, is usually reserved for those with progressive tumour growth.— R.C. Seeger (moderator), *Ann. intern. Med.*, 1982, *97*, 873. See also C. C. Bailey, *Br. J. Hosp. Med.*, 1984, *31*, 36.

Encouraging preliminary results with purged autologous bone-marrow transplantation and high-dose chemotherapy in 25 patients with very poor prognosis neuroblastoma. The high-dose regimen comprised vincristine 4 mg per m^2 body-surface area as a continuous infusion over 5 days with melphalan 180 mg per m^2 on day 6, together with total body irradiation. The bone marrow was purged by Asta Z (an active derivative of cyclophosphamide), or oxidopamine, or by immunomagnetic depletion. Of 13 patients with progressive disease or in partial remission, 8 achieved complete remission, of whom 2 remain in remission at 445 and 453 days after transplantation. Two of the remaining 12, who were in complete remission at the time of therapy, died of side-effects; 3 have relapsed and the remaining 7 were alive at a median of 158 days after transplantation.— T. Philip *et al.* (letter), *Lancet*, 1985, *1*, 576.

RETINOBLASTOMA. Chemotherapy had moderate activity in the treatment of retinoblastoma; the currently preferred drugs were doxorubicin in combination with cyclophosphamide.— *Med. Lett.*, 1983, *25*, 1.

Retinoblastoma is highly radiosensitive, and large tumours are effectively treated by radiotherapy and smaller tumours by photocoagulation or cryotherapy alone. It is an eminently curable cancer of childhood with an overall 5-year survival rate in excess of 85% in the *UK*. In most cases metastatic disease is initially responsive to vincristine and cyclophosphamide, but the relapse rate is high and there are no published reports of long-term survival. A combination of vincristine, cyclophosphamide, cisplatin, and etoposide, originally used in children with disseminated neuroblastoma has recently been used with some success in children with metastatic retinoblastoma. For ectopic intracranial retinoblastoma, intrathecal methotrexate should be considered, in combination with surgery and radiotherapy; a case could also be made for the administration of intensive systemic chemotherapy in addition.— J. E. Kingston *et al.*, *Br. J. Ophthal.*, 1985, *69*, 742.

SARCOMA. *Bone sarcoma.* Chemotherapy has major activity in the treatment of *Ewing's sarcoma*. Preferred drugs were cyclophosphamide with doxorubicin and vincristine. Actinomycin D has also been reported to possess activity in this condition.— *Med. Lett.*, 1983, *25*, 1.

Earlier references to the chemotherapy of Ewing's sarcoma: S. Seeber *et al.*, *Dt. med. Wschr.*, 1979, *104*, 804; R. A. Abrams *et al.*, *Lancet*, 1980, *2*, 385.

Despite the findings of Taylor *et al.* (*Mayo Clin. Proc.*, 1985, *60*, 91) that survival has improved significantly for patients with *osteosarcoma* treated with surgery alone, and that chemotherapy does not influence this outcome, the use of adjuvant chemotherapy in osteosarcoma continues to have powerful advocates. Spectacularly successful results have been reported with a combination regimen (T10) in which postoperative chemotherapy was individually tailored according to the response of resected tumour to a pre-operative course. It is hoped that further studies using cisplatin, doxorubicin, and high-dose methotrexate, which appear to be the most active agents in this condition, will confirm that appropriate drugs and doses administered at specialised centres improve the outlook for patients with this aggressive tumour.— *Lancet*, 1985, *2*, 131.

A review of progress in the treatment of osteosarcoma. Studies have demonstrated that intensive multi-drug adjuvant chemotherapy has increased the disease-free and overall survival rates of patients with non-metastatic osteosarcoma from 20% to 60 to 80% in 1985. Recent advances with intra-arterial cisplatin, intra-arterial doxorubicin combined with radiotherapy, and hyperthermia also offer hope that increased numbers of patients may become eligible for limb-sparing operations as their primary tumours become easier to resect after such therapy.— A. M. Goorin *et al.*, *New Engl. J. Med.*, 1985, *313*, 1637. A contrary review. The case for adjuvant chemotherapy of osteogenic sarcoma, an extremely heterogeneous disease, has not been made.— S. K. Carter, *Drugs*, 1986, *31*, 337. Preliminary results of the Multi-Institutional Osteosarcoma Study (MIOS), a partly-randomised multicentre study of the value of adjuvant chemotherapy in patients with osteosarcoma. Following surgery, 18 patients were assigned to chemotherapy with a regimen of bleomycin, cyclophosphamide, actinomycin D, high-dose methotrexate plus folinic acid rescue, doxorubicin, and cisplatin; the remaining 18 received no adjuvant therapy and acted as controls. A further 59 patients who declined randomisation received adjuvant therapy, and 18 similar patients were observed as controls. On follow-up, 12 of 18 and 43 of 59 patients who received chemotherapy remained relapse-free, compared with 3 of 18 controls in both cases. The 2-year actuarial relapse-free survivals were calculated to be, among randomised patients, 66% for those treated versus 17% for controls; among the unrandomised patients, the figures were 67% versus 9% respectively. Two patients died wholly or partly from treatment-related toxicity; the remaining toxic effects were moderate and readily managed. From these results the favourable effect of adjuvant chemotherapy in patients with osteosarcoma of the extremity appears incontrovertible; however, at a median follow-up of only 2 years, no significant difference in overall survival has yet been demonstrated.— M. P. Link *et al.*, *New Engl. J. Med.*, 1986, *314*, 1600. See also G. Rosen *et al.*, *J. Cancer Res. clin. Oncol.*, 1983, *106, Suppl.*, 55.

Kaposi's sarcoma. Preliminary observations in 12 patients with Kaposi's sarcoma associated with AIDS suggested that recombinant interferon alfa might be useful treatment.— S. E. Krown *et al.*, *New Engl. J. Med.*, 1983, *308*, 1071. The reported response rate of about 42%, including only 3 patients with complete response, is not reason for optimism. Reported response rates to vinblastine or actinomycin D or both in the management of generalised Kaposi's sarcoma in African patients range from 89 to 100%, and there is no reason to expect that the nature of the disease in homosexual men is different from the classic disease.— P. Kondlapoodi (letter), *ibid.*, *309*, 923. Reply. Results of recent chemotherapy trials suggest that the form of Kaposi's sarcoma in homosexual men does differ in its drug sensitivity from the classical form of the disease: although overall response rate of classic Kaposi's sarcoma to vinblastine has been estimated at 89%, only 1 complete and 6 partial responses were seen in a series of 19 evaluable patients with Kaposi's sarcoma and AIDS treated with this agent, a response rate of 37%. In 2 trials with a combination of doxorubicin, vinblastine, and bleomycin objective responses were seen in over 80% of the patients but treatment was associated with a high rate of opportunistic infection. Recombinant interferon alfa should be tried in combination with other cytoreductive or immunomodulatory agents in the treatment of this disease.— S. E. Krown *et al.* (letter), *ibid.*

About 34% of patients with AIDS have developed Kaposi's sarcoma, and nearly 28% of these patients have died. The treatment of the non-epidemic forms of Kaposi's sarcoma has generally been radiotherapy, since most patients have localised disease, and this achieves a complete response in 93 to 100% of patients. Those patients with more aggressive or advanced disease have shown high response rates to a variety of antineoplastic agents. However the treatment of the epidemic form associated with AIDS has not been so successful. Responses to single-agent or combination chemotherapy are common, but there have been no long-term disease-free survivors.— D. L. Longo, in A. S. Fauci (Moderator), *Acquired Immunodeficiency Syndrome, Ann. intern. Med.*, 1984, *100*, 92.

Soft-tissue sarcoma. Soft-tissue sarcomas are a group of tumours consisting of a variety of malignancies derived from mesenchymal tissue. Most types of soft-tissue sarcomas respond to a regimen of doxorubicin with dacarbazine, cyclophosphamide, and vincristine, but chondrosarcomas and mesotheliomas do poorly. Soft-tissue sarcomas are often very bulky and may be reduced pre-operatively by intensive chemotherapy, with or without radiotherapy.— Report of a WHO Expert Committee on Chemotherapy of Solid Tumours, *Tech. Rep. Ser. Wld Hlth Org. No. 605*, 1977, p. 63.

A report of complete response of congenital *fibrosarcoma* in a 5-month-old child to a regimen of ifosfamide, vincristine, and actinomycin D (IVA).— N. Delepine *et al.* (letter), *Lancet*, 1986, *2*, 1453.

Rhabdomyosarcoma accounts for approximately 8 to 10% of childhood malignancies. Two histological types exist in children, alveolar and embryonal. The former is most commonly seen in distal lesions of the limbs, and carries a relatively poor prognosis; treatment is by radiotherapy and adjuvant chemotherapy with vincristine, actinomycin D, doxorubicin, and cyclophosphamide. Therapy of embryonal rhabdomyosarcoma has to be tailored to the site of the tumour, and as with the alveolar type consists mainly of radiotherapy and chemotherapy. Embryonal rhabdomyosarcoma of the orbit carries an excellent prognosis, and genito-urinary tumours also do well, while tumours in the nasopharynx and trunk do less well.— C. C. Bailey, *Br. J. Hosp. Med.*, 1984, *31*, 36.

A report of remission of metastatic rhabdomyosarcoma in a 3-year-old patient given intensive chemotherapy with vincristine, bleomycin, methotrexate, doxorubicin, actinomycin D, and cyclophosphamide. Relapse-free survival is now more than 58 months suggesting that effective chemotherapy may produce long-term survival in rhabdomyosarcoma without the use of radiotherapy.— S. S. N. De Graaf *et al.*, *Archs Dis. Childh.*, 1985, *60*, 482.

WILMS' TUMOUR. Although chemotherapy is considered ineffective by some authorities in the treatment of renal cancer, it does have major activity in Wilms' tumour, actinomycin D plus vincristine being the drugs currently preferred; doxorubicin or cyclophosphamide also have reported activity.— *Med. Lett.*, 1983, *25*, 1.

Wilms' tumour accounts for approximately 8% of childhood malignancies. The treatment and prognosis is related to the histological appearance of the tumour and its stage at diagnosis. Children with stage I disease (limited to 1 kidney) have an excellent prognosis following excision of the tumour and postoperative treatment with vincristine alone or with actinomycin D. Stages II and III receive postoperative radiotherapy together with vincristine and actinomycin D; addition of doxorubicin to this regimen is being studied. The 2-year disease-free survival in these children is approximately 75%. In stage IV (haematogenous metastatic disease), and all stages with unfavourable histology, good responses are obtained with a regimen comprising vincristine, actinomycin D, doxorubicin, and cyclophosphamide; a probable 2-year disease-free survival of about 40% can be attained.— C. C. Bailey, *Br. J. Hosp. Med.*, 1984, *31*, 36.

Use of Immunosuppressants

Antilymphocyte and antithymocyte immunoglobulins, cyclosporin, and azathioprine are used as immunosuppressants mainly to prolong the survival of organ and tissue transplants. Azathioprine and some antineoplastic agents that possess immunosuppressant properties are also used in a variety of auto-immune disorders including those affecting the skin, kidneys, and joints.

These agents may be given in association with corticosteroids (p.873), the other main group of immunosuppressants, to permit a reduction in the dosage of corticosteroids. They are also used in conditions refractory to corticosteroids and other therapy.

AMYLOIDOSIS. Because of the grave prognosis in monoclonal protein amyloidosis, a trial of antineoplastic agents appears warranted especially when an associated immunocyte dyscrasia can be documented. Antineoplastic agents have also been used to treat reactive amyloidosis associated with collagen vascular diseases.— G. G. Glenner, *New Engl. J. Med.*, 1980, *302*, 1333.

A report of the resolution of amyloidosis and acquired factor X deficiency in a patient treated with melphalan in association with prednisone.— J. K. Camoriano *et al.*, *New Engl. J. Med.*, 1987, *316*, 1133.

DIABETES MELLITUS. Summary of a workshop on immunosuppression in the management of type I (insulin-dependent) diabetes mellitus. Recent evidence that type I diabetes may have an important auto-immune component in some cases has led to efforts to suppress, abort, or reverse this response, using agents such as antilymphocyte immunoglobulin, corticosteroids, and immunosuppressants such as azathioprine and cyclosporin. The outcomes in patients appear to be variable and still too preliminary to warrant anything other than further research. Some consider that immunotherapy is premature or even contra-indicated until the importance of the immune component and the question of heterogeneity in the origin of the disease is resolved. More specific guidelines must await the demonstration of a more definitive risk/benefit ratio than has so far been demonstrated.— Diabetes Research Program, National Institutes of Health, *New Engl. J. Med.*, 1983, *309*, 1199.

Further references to the immunotherapy of type I diabetes mellitus: H. Kolb *et al.* (letter), *Lancet*, 1982, *2*, 97; *ibid.*, 1983, *1*, 104; A. A. Rossini, *New Engl. J. Med.*, 1983, *308*, 333.

GASTRO-INTESTINAL DISORDERS. For the use of immunosuppressants in inflammatory diseases of the bowel, see Azathioprine, p.600.

HEPATIC DISORDERS. For reference to the use of immunosuppressants in chronic active hepatitis, see Azathioprine, p.601.

NEUROLOGICAL DISORDERS. *Multiple sclerosis.* A double-blind controlled study of combined immunosuppressive treatment with antilymphocyte immunoglobulin, prednisolone, and azathioprine in patients with multiple sclerosis. Significant changes indicating a beneficial effect of the treatment were seen in the *in-vitro* immune response of lymphocytes from treated patients, and in their visual evoked potentials. However, clinical improvement was marginal and the small differences between treated patients and controls in terms of relapse rates and deterioration were not significant. It is possible that improvements of the immunosuppression regimen may lead to improved clinical results.— J. Mertin *et al.*, *Lancet*, 1982, *2*, 351. There is no evidence of immunological abnormality in multiple sclerosis, and it has been emphasised that this preoccupation with immunosuppression has led to neglect of the vascular features of the disease. Furthermore, in a recent controlled trial, Lhermitte *et al.* (letter, *Lancet*, 1984, *1*, 276) have shown an increased risk of cancer in multiple sclerosis patients taking azathioprine.— P. James (letter), *Br. med. J.*, 1984, 288, 1831. Comment. The relative risk of developing malignancy appears small and must be balanced against the overall risk of developing severe disability in multiple sclerosis.— W. I. McDonald and J. Mertin (letter), *ibid.*, 1914.

The British and Dutch multiple sclerosis azathioprine trial group found no clear benefit with azathioprine over placebo.— *Lancet*, 1988, *2*, 179.

Myasthenia gravis. For a review of the treatment of myasthenia gravis, including the role of immunosuppressants, see Neostigmine Methylsulphate, p.1333.

ORGAN AND TISSUE TRANSPLANTATION. For the role of immunosuppressants in transplantation see under the individual monographs and under Corticosteroids, p.879.

RENAL DISORDERS. References to the use of immunosuppressants in the treatment of renal disorders: Arbeitsgemeinschaft für Pädiatrische Nephrologie, *New Engl. J. Med.*, 1982, *306*, 451 (cyclophosphamide or chlorambucil with tapered prednisone in frequently relapsing nephrotic syndrome); M. Levin *et al.*, *Archs Dis. Childh.*, 1983, *58*, 697 (prednisolone with cyclophosphamide and azathioprine in Goodpasture's syndrome); S. Carette *et al.*, *Ann. intern. Med.*, 1983, *99*, 1 (azathioprine or cyclophosphamide plus prednisone better than prednisone alone in moderate chronic lupus nephritis); C. R. K. Hind *et al.*, *Lancet*, 1983, *1*, 263 (plasma exchange, corticosteroids, and cytotoxic drugs in crescentic glomerulonephritis); N. W. Boyce, *Med. J. Aust.*, 1984, *140*, 775 (prednisolone alone as effective as prednisolone with azathioprine in lupus nephritis); C. O. S. Savage *et al.*, *Br. med. J.*, 1986, *292*, 301 (corticosteroids, cytotoxic drugs, and plasma exchange used in antiglomerular basement membrane nephritis).

See also under Corticosteroids, p.880.

RHEUMATIC DISORDERS. The chronicity of the condition coupled with its relentless progress may encourage the use of drastic measures in patients with severe rheumatoid arthritis who have failed to respond to second-line agents such as sulphasalazine, antimalarials, gold, or penicillamine. In patients with refractory disease an attempt at immunological modification may be attractive though the rationale is muddled: drugs used have included azathioprine, cyclophosphamide, methotrexate, chlorambucil, levamisole, cyclosporin, and thymopentin. Azathioprine is probably the immunosuppressant of choice since it appears to be less toxic and is easier to handle than methotrexate or cyclophosphamide. Cyclophosphamide may be the most effective of the immunosuppressant drugs but also has the most potent side-effects, while there is little evidence of the efficacy of methotrexate in controlled studies in rheumatoid disease. Chlorambucil is probably best reserved for late rheumatoid arthritis in the elderly. Bed rest and pulsed steroids should be tried before resorting to cytotoxic agents.— V. Wright, *Br. med. J.*, 1986, *292*, 431. See also *Lancet*, 1982, *2*, 748 (systemic vasculitis).

Children. A review of the managment of chronic arthritis in children. Cytotoxic and immunosuppressive drugs such as azathioprine and chlorambucil are only rarely indicated, e.g. for very severe progressive disease unresponsive to other measures. Their serious adverse effects such as secondary malignancy and infertility outweigh any advantage in most circumstances.— A. W. Craft, *Prescribers' J.*, 1985, *25*, 75. See also idem, *Br. J. Hosp. Med.*, 1985, *33*, 188.

See also under Methotrexate, p.640.

SKIN AND CONNECTIVE-TISSUE DISORDERS. The use of immunosuppressants in dermatology. Immunosuppressants are clearly of value in diseases such as pemphigus, severe psoriasis and Wegener's granulomatosis, but have also been tried in conditions such as granuloma annulare, pityriasis rubra, systemic lupus erythematosus, and lichen planus where the risk-to-benefit ratio is less clear. In view of the potential toxicity of present immunosuppressants, especially the potential for long term complications, including carcinogenesis, these agents should be limited to life-threatening or disabling conditions in which standard therapy has either failed or is likely to produce intolerable side-effects.— I. Bell and G. D. Weinstein, *Archs Derm.*, 1985, *121*, 195.

Behçet's syndrome. In a study in 49 patients with the ocular type of Behçet's syndrome, 16 of 20 responded to treatment with chlorambucil; average remission was approximately 6 months, but 2 of the responding patients had no relapses for 24 and 25 months respectively. In contrast only 8 of 18 responded to colchicine, for a relatively short period, and only 1 of 4 patients given azathioprine had a decrease in ocular inflammatory signs. All patients had initially responded to high doses of corticosteroids; the 7 patients maintained on this treatment responded with an average remission of 8 months. Despite the favourable responses to chlorambucil or corticosteroids the long-term prognosis for vision remains very poor.— D. BenEzra and E. Cohen, *Br. J. Ophthal.*, 1986, *70*, 589.

Dermatomyositis. Seven young patients with dermatomyositis who had failed to respond to treatment with corticosteroids showed clinical improvement following treatment with methotrexate or cyclophosphamide.— A. El-Ghobarey *et al.*, *Postgrad. med. J.*, 1978, *54*, 516.

A review of the treatment of 29 children with dermatomyositis. Primary treatment was with corticosteroids but some patients received treatment with azathioprine, alone or with chlorambucil, or else cyclophosphamide alone, in addition to prednisolone therapy. Although the efficacy and steroid-sparing effect of immunosuppressants has been previously documented, the authors have not been convinced that they make much difference in individual cases. The use of azathioprine has been favoured, as it seems to have the least toxicity, but only to achieve a reduction in corticosteroid dosage where there is dependency or unacceptable corticosteroid toxicity. The authors' experience with other immunosuppressants such as cyclophosphamide and methotrexate is limited.— G. Miller *et al.*, *Archs Dis. Childh.*, 1983, *58*, 445.

Pemphigus. Methotrexate or azathioprine act rather slowly and are not suitable for the initial control of pemphigus and pemphigoid. They remain a useful adjunct to maintenance therapy especially when the side-effects of corticosteroids become serious.— J. A. Savin, *Practitioner*, 1977, *219*, 847.

A retrospective review of patients seen between 1968 and 1975 showed that of 57 patients with active bullous pemphigoid and of 51 with active cicatricial pemphigoid a number had been maintained on treatment with antineoplastic agents including azathioprine and cyclophosphamide, usually in conjunction with corticosteroids.— J. R. Person and R. S. Rogers, *Mayo Clin. Proc.*, 1977, *52*, 54.

Psoriasis. A discussion of the treatment of psoriasis. Methotrexate deserves a prime place among systemic treatments for life-threatening or life-ruining psoriasis not responding to other remedies; however, evidence of liver damage must be sought by liver biopsies every year or 2. Hydroxyurea is less effective, more toxic to bone marrow, but virtually lacks the liver problems, and is a useful drug in patients with bad psoriasis who have alcohol problems. Other cytotoxic and immunosuppressant drugs have only occasional uses, although thioguanine shows some promise.— R. H. Champion, *Br. med. J.*, 1986, *292*, 1693.

Systemic lupus erythematosus. For reference to the use of immunosuppressant drugs in the treatment of the renal lesions of systemic lupus erythematosus (lupus nephritis) see under Renal Disorders, above.

Takayasu's arteritis. For the suggestion that cyclophosphamide may be of benefit in patients with Takayasu's arteritis unresponsive to corticosteroids, see under Cyclophosphamide, p.614.

WEGENER'S GRANULOMATOSIS. A study on the angiitides and granulomatous diseases of the lung in 35 patients. These disorders can be classified into Wegener's granulomatosis, lymphomatoid granulomatosis, and benign lymphocytic angiitis and granulomatosis of the lung. They appear to result from a hypersensitivity or immunologically mediated process but respond differently to various immunosuppressant chemotherapeutic regimens. Wegener's granulomatosis, a systemic disease characterised by necrotising granulomatous vasculitis of the upper and lower airways, glomerulonephritis, and disseminated small vessel vasculitis, is very sensitive to cyclophosphamide and in most cases long-term remissions and even cures can be achieved. Cyclophosphamide was effective in 7 of 8 patients with Wegener's granulomatosis but azathioprine was of no value in 4 similar patients and the disease progressed in one patient given prednisone. Lymphomatoid granulomatosis on the other hand, is refractory to cyclophosphamide in advanced disease and is usually fatal despite combination chemotherapy. Benign lymphocytic angiitis and granulomatosis were formerly included in the previous two categories but have been classified as a separate group because they are mainly limited to the lungs and are consistently responsive to chlorambucil. Azathioprine and cyclophosphamide are also effective.— H. L. Israel *et al.*, *Ann. intern. Med.*, 1977, *87*, 691.

During the past decade, treatment with cyclophosphamide, usually combined with steroids, has transformed the outlook in Wegener's granulomatosis: Fauci *et al.* (*Ann. intern. Med.*, 1983, *98*, 76) have claimed a remission induction-rate of 93%, and 75 of 85 patients were alive after an average follow-up of 4 years. However, despite an high initial response-rate the long-term outlook for patients with severe renal impairment remains grim; 7 of 18 patients reported by Pinching *et al.* (*Q. J. Med.*, 1983, *52*, 435) died during the early phase of intensive therapy and by 3 years only 8 of the original 18 were still alive. These results emphasise the importance of starting treatment before irrevocable damage has occurred.— *Lancet*, 1984, *1*, 260.

For a report of the induction of remission in patients with lymphomatoid granulomatosis given cyclophosphamide and prednisone, see under Cyclophosphamide, p.614.

12305-k

Aceglatone *(rINN).*
2,5-Di-*O*-acetyl-D-glucaro-1,4:6,3-dilactone.
$C_{10}H_{10}O_8$=258.2.

CAS — 642-83-1.

Aceglatone inhibits the activity of β-glucuronidase and has an anti-inflammatory action. It has been given by mouth to prevent relapse after surgery of carcinoma of the bladder. Adverse effects have included anorexia, gastric discomfort, dry skin, and pigmentation.

Proprietary Names and Manufacturers
Glucaron *(Chugai, Jpn).*

12317-r

Acivicin *(USAN, rINN).*
AT-125; NSC-163501; U-42126. (αS,5S)-α-Amino-3-chloro-2-isoxazolin-5-ylacetic acid.
$C_5H_7ClN_2O_3$=178.6.

CAS — 42228-92-2.

Acivicin is an antineoplastic antibiotic that is believed to act by interfering with glutamine metabolism. It has been tried by intravenous infusion or injection in a variety of solid tumours. Bone-marrow depression and central neurotoxicity may be dose-limiting.

Proprietary Names and Manufacturers
Upjohn, USA.

12318-f

Aclarubicin Hydrochloride *(rINNM).*
Aclacinomycin A Hydrochloride; NSC-208734. The hydrochloride of an anthracycline antineoplastic antibiotic isolated from *Streptomyces galilaeus.*
$C_{42}H_{53}NO_{15}$,HCl=848.3.

CAS — 57576-44-0 (aclarubicin).

NOTE. Aclarubicin is *USAN.*

Aclarubicin hydrochloride 1.04 mg is approximately equivalent to 1 mg of aclarubicin.

In a study of the stability of anthracycline antineoplastic agents in 4 infusion fluids— glucose injection (5%), sodium chloride injection (0.9%), lactated Ringer's injection, and a commercial infusion fluid— aclarubicin hydrochloride was stable in all 4, the percentage remaining after 24 hours being 96.7%, 98.1%, 95.8%, and 92.4% respectively. Stability appeared to be partly related to pH; aclarubicin was most stable in sodium chloride injection, with a pH of 6.2, and any increase or decrease in pH appeared to affect stability adversely.— G. K. Poochikian *et al.*, *Am. J. Hosp. Pharm.*, 1981, *38*, 483.

Adverse Effects, Treatment, and Precautions
As for Doxorubicin Hydrochloride, p.623. The cardiotoxic effects of aclarubicin may be less pronounced than those of other anthracyclines.

In a study involving 22 patients with advanced solid tumours, intravenous aclarubicin was given in doses up to 30 mg per m^2 body-surface area by infusion, daily for 5 days every 4 weeks. Bone-marrow suppression, and particularly thrombocytopenia, was the major dose-limiting toxicity; the other major adverse effect was nausea and vomiting at the higher doses. One patient developed atrial fibrillation, and one developed congestive heart failure. Cardiac toxicity was considered to be minimal, although most patients in the study had only received low cumulative doses. There was no evidence of hepatotoxicity in these patients.— P. V. Woolley *et al.*, *J. clin. Pharmac.*, 1982, *22*, 359.

See also under Uses, below.

Uses and Administration
Aclarubicin is an anthracycline antibiotic with antineoplastic actions similar to those of the other anthracyclines (see Doxorubicin Hydrochloride, p.624).

It may be given as the hydrochloride in the treatment of malignant blood disorders, such as acute myeloid leukaemia, in usual doses equivalent to 15 to 20 mg of the base per m^2 body-surface area daily by intravenous infusion, up to a total dose of 300 to 600 mg of base per m^2.

A review of the development and uses of aclarubicin. Studies in patients with relapsed acute non-lymphoblastic leukaemia have confirmed the activity of aclarubicin, with reported complete remission rates of the order of 12 to 24%. Doses have varied from 10 to 30 mg per m^2 body-surface daily to higher doses of 75 to 120 mg per m^2 for 2 to 4 days; in general a total dose of about 300 mg per m^2 appears to be necessary to induce remission. Less information is available concerning activity in acute lymphoblastic leukaemia, but response rates have been lower than those in acute non-lymphoblastic leukaemia. Results in the malignant lymphomas have been generally disappointing. It has become apparent in the course of clinical studies that aclarubicin is not devoid of cardiotoxicity. A strikingly high incidence of ECG changes has been observed but although acute cardiotoxicity occurs the chronic cardiomyopathy classically associated with the anthracyclines appears to be a rare event. Alopecia is also rare, although gastro-intestinal disturbances and mucositis are as common or more common than with doxorubicin. R. P. Warrell, *Drugs exp. & clin. Res.*, 1986, *12*, 275. Other reviews of aclarubicin: K. Ota, *ibid.*, 1985, *11*, 17; H. -J. Röthig *et al.*, *ibid.*, 123.

A study of the use of aclarubicin in patients with acute myeloid leukaemia. Aclarubicin hydrochloride was given in daily doses equivalent to 10 to 30 mg of base per m^2 body-surface area intravenously to 13 patients, up to a maximum of 300 mg per m^2 or until toxicity became unacceptable; a further 25 patients were assigned to a cyclic regimen of the equivalent of aclarubicin 15 mg per m^2 daily for 10 days followed by a 10-day interval and then repeated. Two of 13 patients on the first regimen and 11 of 25 receiving the second regimen achieved complete remission. Toxicity was more severe with the first regimen and 9 of the 13 patients had to have therapy discontinued. Further clinical studies are required to establish the most suitable dosage regimen and the value of aclarubicin in combination therapy.— D. Machover *et al.*, *Cancer Treat. Rep.*, 1984, *68*, 881.

Further references to the use of aclarubicin: A. Y. Bedikian *et al.*, *Am. J. clin. Oncol.*, 1983, *6*, 187; J. Pedersen-Bjergaard *et al.*, *Cancer Treat. Rep.*, 1984, *68*, 1233.

Proprietary Names and Manufacturers
Aclacinomycine *(Bellon, Fr.)*; Aclaplastin *(Behringwerke, Ger.)*; Jaclacin *(Lundbeck, Denm.)*;
Manufacturers also include—*Bristol, USA.*

1802-w

Actinomycin D *(BAN).*
Dactinomycin *(USAN, rINN)*; Meractinomycin; NSC-3053.
$C_{62}H_{86}N_{12}O_{16}$=1255.4.

CAS — 8052-16-2 (actinomycin C); 50-76-0 (actinomycin D).

Pharmacopoeias. In *Braz.*, *Chin.*, and *U.S.*

An antineoplastic antibiotic produced by the growth of *Streptomyces chrysomallus* and *S. antibioticus*. It is a bright red, somewhat hygroscopic, crystalline powder. It has a potency of not less than 900 μg per mg, calculated on the dried basis.

Soluble in water at 10°, slightly soluble in water at 37°, freely soluble in alcohol; very slightly soluble in ether. The *U.S.P.* directs that a solution of Dactinomycin for Injection has a pH between 5.5 and 7.5 on reconstitution. **Store** at a temperature not exceeding 40° in airtight containers. Protect from light.

Actinomycin C (cactinomycin; HBF-386; NSC-18268) is a mixture of actinomycin D (10%), actinomycin C_2 (45%), and actinomycin C_3 (45%).

CAUTION *Actinomycin D is irritant; avoid contact with skin and mucous membranes.*

Actinomycin D binds to cellulose filters; such filtration should be avoided.— P. F. D'Arcy, *Drug Intell. & clin. Pharm.*, 1983, *17*, 532. See also M. Kanke *et al.*, *Am. J. Hosp. Pharm.*, 1983, *40*, 1323.

Actinomycin D should not be given by continuous or intermittent infusion as adsorption to glass and plastic occurs with loss of significant amounts of drug. The diluent should be sterile water without preservatives.— R. P. Rapp *et al.*, *Drug Intell. & clin. Pharm.*, 1984, *18*, 218.

Adverse Effects, Treatment, and Precautions

For an outline of the adverse effects experienced with antineoplastic agents and immunosuppressants, general guidelines for their treatment, and precautions, see Antineoplastic Agents, p.580, p.583.

Actinomycin D is given in short, intermittent courses because of its potential for severe toxicity. Apart from nausea and vomiting adverse effects are often delayed, occurring days or weeks after the completion of a course of treatment. Bone-marrow depression is apparent 1 to 7 days after therapy and may be manifest first as thrombocytopenia; agranulocytosis and pancytopenia have been reported. There have been fatalities. Other adverse effects include oral and gastro-intestinal effects such as stomatitis, diarrhoea, and proctitis; fever, malaise, hypocalcaemia, erythema, myalgia, alopecia, and kidney and liver abnormalities. Actinomycin D is very irritant and extravasation results in severe tissue damage.

The effects of radiotherapy are enhanced by actinomycin D and severe reactions may follow the concomitant use of high doses. Erythema and pigmentation of the skin may occur in areas previously irradiated. Actinomycin D should not be given to patients with varicella as severe and even fatal systemic disease may occur. Its use is best avoided in infants under 1 year who are reported to be highly susceptible to the toxicity of actinomycin D.

Nausea and vomiting were the acute dose-limiting effects of actinomycin D; other acute effects included diarrhoea, local toxicity and phlebitis, and anaphylactoid reactions. Delayed dose-limiting effects were bone-marrow depression, stomatitis, and oral ulceration; alopecia, folliculitis, and dermatitis in previously irradiated areas were other delayed toxic effects.— *Med. Lett.*, 1985, *27*, 13.

EFFECTS ON THE LIVER. Abnormalities in liver function and an enlarged liver were associated with actinomycin D and radiotherapy in a 5-year-old child with Wilms' tumour.— S. Jayabose *et al.* (letter), *J. Pediat.*, 1976, *88*, 898. Five of 40 children with stage I or II Wilms' tumour developed profound hepatotoxicity following administration of actinomycin D 60 μg per kg body-weight as a single dose as part of a pulsed/intensive regimen. One child, who had complicating factors, succumbed. However, on examination of the records it seemed that in all 5 cases factors in the management or clinical course might have contributed to the toxicity, and the initial impression is that the liver will tolerate this dosage if no additional demands are made on it. The National Wilms' Tumor Study Committee has changed the single dose of actinomycin D in the intensive arm of the study from 60 to 45 μg per kg.— G. J. D'Angio (letter), *Lancet*, 1987, *2*, 104.

Absorption and Fate

Following intravenous administration actinomycin D is rapidly distributed and extensively bound to body tissues. It undergoes only minimal metabolism and is slowly excreted in urine and bile. It does not cross the blood-brain barrier but is thought to cross the placenta.

In a study of the distribution and excretion of actinomycin D in 3 adult patients with malignant melanoma actinomycin D was found to be slightly metabolised; it was concentrated in nucleated cells, and did not readily penetrate the blood-brain barrier. The slow phase of the plasma disappearance of actinomycin D had a half-life of about 36 hours although results in 1 patient who had received doses on each of the 4 previous days indicated that prior administration of actinomycin D altered drug clearance. Substantial amounts were found in the granulocytes and leucocytes of 1 patient 9 days after administration; this might impair their ability to repair irradiation damage which could explain why marked local reaction to irradiation had been noted in patients receiving radiotherapy several weeks after actinomycin D.— M. H. N. Tattersall *et al.*, *Clin. Pharmac. Ther.*, 1975, *17*, 701.

Uses and Administration

Actinomycin D is a highly toxic antibiotic with antineoplastic properties. It inhibits the proliferation of cells in a cell-cycle nonspecific way by forming a stable complex with DNA and interfering with DNA-dependent RNA synthesis. It may enhance the cytotoxic effects of radiotherapy (but see also Adverse Effects, above). Actinomycin D also has immunosuppressant properties.

It has been used in the treatment of Wilms' tumour, rhabdomyosarcoma, and tumours of the uterus and testis, and also in Ewing's sarcoma, osteogenic sarcoma, Kaposi's sarcoma, and other solid tumours. In Wilms' tumour actinomycin D is given in conjunction with radiotherapy and vincristine and, in more severe disease, with doxorubicin and cyclophosphamide. Agents such as cyclophosphamide, vincristine, and doxorubicin are also used with actinomycin D in the treatment of rhabdomyosarcoma. Combination chemotherapy including actinomycin D has been given to patients with neoplasms of the testis but is not the treatment of choice. Beneficial results have also been achieved in patients with choriocarcinoma. See also under Choice of Antineoplastic Agent, p.584.

The usual adult dose is 500 μg intravenously, daily, for a maximum of 5 days and this course may be repeated after 3 or more weeks if there are no signs of residual toxic effects.

The usual dose for children is 15 μg per kg body-weight daily for 5 days; alternatively, a total of 2.5 mg per m^2 of body-surface may be given over a period of 7 days.

Great care must be taken to avoid extravasation. An isolation-perfusion technique has also been used.

SARCOMA. For reference to the use of actinomycin D in various sarcomas see under Choice of Antineoplastic Agent, p.593.

Kaposi's sarcoma. A review of 23 Zambian patients presenting with Kaposi's sarcoma in 1983. Ten of the patients presented with classic disease, similar to that seen previously in East Africa, which responded to treatment with actinomycin D 1 to 1.5 mg per m^2 body-surface area as a bolus injection every 3 weeks, and vincristine 2 mg intravenously every week for 6 weeks, and thereafter with each dose of actinomycin D. Responses were maintained although only 1 patient was known to have achieved a complete response. Of the remaining 13, who presented with atypical aggressive disease similar to that described in immunosuppressed homosexuals, 12 had a satisfactory initial response to chemotherapy but this was maintained only in 3. The remaining 9 deteriorated rapidly and 8 had died by the end of 1983.— A. C. Bayley, *Lancet*, 1984, *1*, 1318.

WILMS' TUMOUR. For reference to the use of actinomycin D in the treatment of Wilms' tumour see under Choice of Antineoplastic Agent, p.594.

Preparations

Dactinomycin for Injection *(U.S.P.)*. A sterile mixture of actinomycin D 500 μg and mannitol in each container.

Proprietary Preparations

Cosmegen, Lyovac *(Merck Sharp & Dohme, UK)*. *Injection*, powder for reconstitution, actinomycin D 500 μg. Also available as Cosmegen in many other countries.

12335-d

Alanosine *(rINN)*.
NSC-153353; L-Alanosine. L-3-(Hydroxynitrosoamino)alanine; (-)-(*S*)-2-Amino-3-(hydroxynitrosoamino)propionic acid.
$C_3H_7N_3O_4$=149.1.

CAS — 5854-93-3.

It may be prepared from *Streptomyces alanosinicus*.

Alanosine is an antineoplastic antibiotic that inhibits purine synthesis. It has been tried in acute leukaemias as well as in malignant melanoma and other tumours. Doses of 250 mg per m^2 body-surface area daily have been given intravenously for 3 days every 3 weeks. Stomatitis may be severe and dose-limiting.

12352-n

Ametantrone Acetate *(USAN, rINNM)*.
CI-881; NSC-287513. 1,4-Bis[2-(2-hydroxyethylamino)ethylamino]anthraquinone diacetate.
$C_{22}H_{28}N_4O_4,2C_2H_4O_2$=532.6.

CAS — 64862-96-0 (ametantrone); 70711-40-9 (diacetate).

Ametantrone acetate is an antineoplastic agent structurally related to doxorubicin (p.623) and with reportedly similar actions. It has been tried in the treatment of a variety of malignant neoplasms in doses of 140 mg per m^2 body-surface area intravenously, as a single dose or divided over several days. The dose may be repeated every 3 weeks. Myelotoxicity may be dose-limiting; gastro-intestinal disturbances, alopecia, thrombophlebitis, and blue-grey skin discoloration have been reported.

Proprietary Names and Manufacturers
Parke, Davis, USA.

1803-e

Aminoglutethimide *(BAN, USAN, rINN)*.

Ba-16038. 2-(4-Aminophenyl)-2-ethylglutarimide; 3-(4-Aminophenyl)-3-ethylpiperidine-2,6-dione.
$C_{13}H_{16}N_2O_2$=232.3.

CAS — 125-84-8.

Pharmacopoeias. In *U.S.*

A white or creamy-white, fine, crystalline powder. Very slightly **soluble** in water; readily soluble in most organic solvents. It forms water-soluble salts with strong acids. The pH of a 0.1% solution in dilute methyl alcohol (1 in 20) is between 6.2 and 7.3.

Adverse Effects

Adverse effects reported with aminoglutethimide include drowsiness, lethargy, ataxia, fever, skin rashes, and gastro-intestinal disturbances; most side-effects diminish after the first 6 to 8 weeks of therapy due to enhanced metabolism of the drug. Bone-marrow depression, with leucopenia, agranulocytosis, or severe pancytopenia has occurred rarely. There have been reports of endocrine disturbances including hypothyroidism, and virilisation. Orthostatic hypotension may occur in some patients.

Overdosage may lead to CNS depression and impairment of consciousness, electrolyte disturbances, and respiratory depression.

EFFECTS ON THE BLOOD. A report of fatal irreversible thrombocytopenia in a patient receiving aminoglutethimide with corticosteroid supplementation.— M. W. Kissin and A. E. Kark, *Cancer Treat. Rep.*, 1983, *67*, 849. Severe thrombocytopenia developed in 2 patients 3 and 5 weeks respectively after the start of aminoglutethimide therapy, but there was a rapid recovery within 3 to 5 days of stopping treatment. In a third patient severe leucopenia occurred 7 weeks after the start of therapy but myelosuppression did not recur when aminoglutethimide was restarted 2 weeks later.— A. U. Buzdar *et al.* (letter), *Ann. intern. Med.*, 1984, *100*, 159.

Agranulocytosis developed in 3 of 161 patients receiving adjuvant aminoglutethimide with corticosteroid supplementation, 5 to 8 weeks after starting therapy. One patient died of septicaemia. By February 1985 the Committee on the Safety of Medicines had documented 4 cases of marrow depression and aplasia, 7 of agranulocytosis and granulocytopenia, and 1 of thrombocytopenia. The manufacturers have reported 36 similar cases of bone-marrow failure between 1962 and 1984.— M. D. Vincent *et al.*, *Br. med. J.*, 1985, *291*, 105. See also G. Caldwell *et al.* (letter), *ibid.*, 970 (pancytopenia).

EFFECTS ON THE LIVER. A report of cholestatic jaundice, with pruritus and a macular rash, in a patient who had been receiving aminoglutethimide for 2 months. The symptoms probably represented an idiosyncratic hypersensitivity reaction, possibly indicating a latent direct hepatotoxic potential of aminoglutethimide.— S. B. Gerber and K. B. Miller (letter), *Ann. intern. Med.*, 1982, *97*, 138. A similar report. Symptoms recurred on rechallenge with aminoglutethimide. The increasing use of aminoglutethimide warrants recognition of this potentially severe toxicity and indicates a need for monitoring liver function tests in all patients receiving aminoglutethimide who develop fever and eruptions.— D. J. Perrault and E. Domovitch (letter), *ibid.*, 1984, *100*, 160.

EFFECTS ON THE LUNG. Pulmonary infiltrates in a patient who developed progressive dyspnoea on commencing therapy with aminoglutethimide were found to be due to diffuse alveolar damage and haemorrhage; thrombocytopenia was present but prothrombin and bleeding times were normal. The patient's gas exchange and chest radiographs improved on discontinuation of aminoglutethimide and institution of corticosteroid therapy.— D. M. Rodman *et al.* (letter), *Ann. intern. Med.*, 1986, *105*, 633.

LUPUS. A report of systemic lupus erythematosus induced by aminoglutethimide in one patient.— M. McCraken *et al.*, *Br. med. J.*, 1980, *281*, 1254.

Precautions

Aminoglutethimide inhibits adrenal steroid production and the adrenal response to stress may be impaired; supplementary glucocorticoid therapy with hydrocortisone must normally be given although supplementation may not be necessary in patients with Cushing's syndrome. Some patients also require a mineralocorticoid. Blood counts and serum electrolytes should be regularly monitored during aminoglutethimide therapy.

Aminoglutethimide should not be given during pregnancy as pseudohermaphroditism may occur in the foetus.

The rate of metabolism of some drugs is increased by aminoglutethimide; patients receiving concomitant therapy with warfarin or other coumarin anticoagulants, or with oral hypoglycaemic agents, may require increased dosages of these drugs. The metabolism of dexamethasone is also accelerated, and it should not be used for corticosteroid supplementation in patients receiving aminoglutethimide.

Cholesterol concentrations were raised in all of 9 breast cancer patients receiving aminoglutethimide 1 g daily in divided doses, and in 68% of a further 42 patients who received 500 mg daily. In 7 patients whose post-treatment cholesterol was measured, serum-cholesterol values returned to normal a few weeks after aminoglutethimide therapy was stopped. In the setting of adjuvant therapy, such hypercholesterolaemia might predispose to atherosclerosis in patients whose life-expectancy is good.— J. Bonneterre *et al.* (letter), *Lancet*, 1984, *1*, 912. Comment. In 50 similar women, given aminoglutethimide 1 g daily for 2 months total cholesterol concentrations also rose significantly, as did γ-glutamyltransferase and alkaline phosphatase values, while uric acid and indirect bilirubin concentrations decreased. To suggest that attention be paid to serum cholesterol values seems overly simplistic.— G. Ceci *et al.* (letter), *ibid.*, *2*, 358. Aminoglutethimide did not appear to provoke hypercholesterolaemia in patients with Cushing's disease.— A. Kasperlik-Zaluska and B. Migdalska (letter), *ibid.*

PORPHYRIA. Aminoglutethimide was considered to be unsafe in patients with acute porphyria because it has been shown to be porphyrinogenic in *animals* or *in-vitro* systems.— M.R. Moore and K.E.L. McColl, *Porphyrias, Drug Lists*, Glasgow, Porphyria Research Unit, University of Glasgow, 1987.

Absorption and Fate

Aminoglutethimide is rapidly and completely absorbed following oral administration. It is metabolised in the liver and excreted in the urine as unchanged drug and metabolites.

Results of a pharmacokinetic study in 13 women with metastatic breast carcinoma, who were given aminoglutethimide 1 g and hydrocortisone 40 mg daily over one year, indicated that aminoglutethimide increases its own metabolism which may explain why adverse effects diminish during treatment. In 6 of the patients mean half-lives of aminoglutethimide fell from about 13.3 hours at the start of therapy to about 7.3 hours after 6 to 32 weeks; conversely, mean clearance-rates increased. Serum concentrations of aminoglutethimide in 7 patients were similar throughout treatment with a mean value of 11.5 µg per mL.— F. T. Murray *et al.*, *J. clin. Pharmac.*, 1979, *19*, 704.

A report of the characterisation of 4 new minor metabolites in the urine of patients undergoing therapy with aminoglutethimide. These are in addition to the two major metabolites, acetylaminoglutethimide and hydroxylaminoglutethimide, and 2 minor metabolites, *p*-nitroglutethimide and formylaminoglutethimide, which have been previously reported.— A. B. Foster *et al.*, *Drug Metab. & Disposit.*, 1984, *12*, 511. See also W. W. Weber and D. W. Hein, *Pharmac. Rev.*, 1985, *37*, 25 (role of acetylation).

A study of the single- and multiple-dose pharmacokinetics of aminoglutethimide in 17 patients. Following oral administration of radiolabelled drug to 4 patients, absorption was almost complete; a mean of 90.1% of the radioactivity was recovered in urine over 3 days. Peak plasma concentrations of aminoglutethimide were reached between 1 and 4 hours after administration. The plasma half-life had a mean value of 15.5 hours after single-dose administration but fell to 8.9 hours during multiple-dose therapy. This marked reduction in half-life could largely be attributed to a decrease in the volume of distribution; auto-induction of metabolism may be of less importance in decreasing half-life than has been previously suggested.— P. E. Lønning *et al.*, *Clin. Pharmacokinet.*, 1985, *10*, 353.

Characterisation of the plasma protein binding of aminoglutethimide. There was no significant difference between the protein binding in 10 healthy males and 10 healthy females given aminoglutethimide, the percentage bound being 25 and 22% respectively, nor between these and 5 breast cancer patients in whom aminoglutethimide was found to be 23% bound to plasma protein.— P. D. Dalrymple and P. J. Nicholls, *Br. J. clin. Pharmac.*, 1985, *20*, 295P.

Uses and Administration

Aminoglutethimide is an analogue of glutethimide (p.742) and was formerly used for its weak anticonvulsant properties. By its inhibitory action on the adrenal cortex and on peripheral aromatase, aminoglutethimide blocks the production of adrenal steroids and the conversion of androgens to oestrogens, and produces a state of 'medical' adrenalectomy. It is used in the treatment of metastatic breast cancer in post-menopausal or oophorectomised women, and as palliative treatment in patients with advanced prostatic cancer, in doses of 250 mg up to four times daily by mouth. Replacement therapy with a corticosteroid must also be given, usually hydrocortisone 40 mg daily in divided doses.

Aminoglutethimide is used in similar doses in the treatment of Cushing's syndrome.

Reviews of aminoglutethimide: *Med. Lett.*, 1981, *23*, 71.

CUSHING'S SYNDROME. Proper treatment of Cushing's syndrome depends on a correct definition of its cause. Adrenal adenomas and micronodular hyperplasia are always cured by surgery but surgical results in adrenal carcinoma are poor and malignant tumours in the ectopic ACTH syndrome are often unresectable: in these cases hypercortisolaemia can be controlled with aminoglutethimide or metyrapone. In patients with indolent tumours 'medical' adrenalectomy with mitotane should be considered. Aminoglutethimide and metyrapone may also be used as adjuvants to control hypercortisolism in patients with Cushing's disease awaiting the results of radiotherapy.— D. N. Orth, *New Engl. J. Med.*, 1984, *310*, 649.

MALIGNANT NEOPLASMS OF THE BREAST. Administration of aminoglutethimide 250 mg four times daily to 40 oophorectomised or postmenopausal women with metastatic breast carcinoma was at least as effective as surgical adrenalectomy in producing beneficial responses. Of 20 patients who responded, 2 relapsed after 6 months, 1 after 11, and the other 17 were still receiving treatment after 3 to 17 months. In particular, rapid and sometimes dramatic relief of bone pain was obtained in 19 of 36 patients with bony metastases, which confirmed previous experience with adrenalectomy. A response was most common in patients who had previously responded to other forms of endocrine therapy. Cortisone acetate 25 mg twice or three times daily was given concurrently to prevent symptoms of adrenal insufficiency.— I. E. Smith *et al.*, *Lancet*, 1978, *2*, 646. A review of clinical experience with aminoglutethimide in 129 postmenopausal patients with breast cancer. Overall, 37% of patients experienced tumour regression; among women whose tumours were oestrogen receptor-positive, 49% experienced regression. Skin and soft tissue lesions responded most frequently, followed by bone and lung. Regression lasted an average of 30 months in complete responders and 14.5 months in partial responders. Side-effects are considerable, but can be managed; the current regimen used by the authors initiates treatment with aminoglutethimide 250 mg twice daily and hydrocortisone 100 mg daily to reduce initial adverse effects. After 2 weeks, aminoglutethimide is increased to 250 mg four times a day and the dose of hydrocortisone reduced to 40 mg in divided doses daily.— R. J. Santen *et al.*, *Ann. intern. Med.*, 1982, *96*, 94.

Comparable effects with aminoglutethimide and tamoxifen.— I. E. Smith *et al.*, *Br. med. J.*, 1981, *283*, 1432. No additive effect.— I. E. Smith *et al.*, *ibid.*, 1983, *286*, 1615. Comment on the higher incidence of adverse effects with aminoglutethimide. However, the response rate of bone metastases to aminoglutethimide appears to be higher than for tamoxifen.— R. Stuart-Harris, *Prescribers' J.*, 1984, *24*, 133.

A study of low-dose aminoglutethimide in patients with advanced breast cancer showed that aminoglutethimide in doses of 62.5 to 125 mg by mouth twice daily, given without hydrocortisone, was as effective as conventional doses of aminoglutethimide with hydrocortisone in reducing serum-oestrogen concentrations in postmenopausal patients; this appeared to be due to peripheral aromatase inhibition, and adrenal suppression was slight. Eleven of 57 evaluable patients had an objective tumour response, although this was complete only in 1. Disappointingly, however, toxicity was still significant at the lower doses, possibly due to the absence of hydrocortisone. The combination of low-dose aminoglutethimide with hydrocortisone may prove a more acceptable alternative to conventional treatment than low-dose therapy alone.— R. Stuart-Harris *et al.*, *Lancet*, 1984, *2*, 604.

A further study of aminoglutethimide as second-line hormonal therapy in advanced breast cancer. There were 2 complete and 12 partial responses among 64 postmenopausal patients who were able to tolerate therapy with aminoglutethimide in doses of 250 mg two or three times daily, in association with hydrocortisone. Median duration of response was 10 months. An additional 10 patients were withdrawn from the study due to toxicity, and 1 further patient died of drug-induced agranulocytosis. Side-effects were greater in patients aged over 65, 1 in 3 of whom could not tolerate the drug.— N. P. Rowell *et al.*, *Hum. Toxicol.*, 1987, *6*, 227. Comment. Aminoglutethimide is not a panacea for prostate and breast cancer. In the former it has no therapeutic indications, and in the latter it has a limited role as second-line therapy which may soon be eclipsed by more specific aromatase inhibitors. In the elderly aminoglutethimide is probably no longer indicated.— P. N. Plowman, *ibid.*, 187.

See also under Choice of Antineoplastic Agent, p.589.

MALIGNANT NEOPLASMS OF THE PROSTATE. Based on previous evidence of objective response in 7 of 26 patients with advanced prostatic cancer who were treated with aminoglutethimide, stilboestrol, and corticosteroids it seems imperative that studies be done to reassess the value of aminoglutethimide in this condition.— M. R. G. Robinson, *Br. J. Urol.*, 1980, *52*, 328.

Aminoglutethimide 0.5 to 1 g daily together with glucocorticoid replacement produced an objective response in 11 of 23 evaluable patients with advanced prostatic cancer, 1 of whom had complete response and remains disease-free on therapy after 275 weeks. The remaining 12 patients suffered disease progression. Survival was significantly longer in patients who responded. The results were considered comparable to those with chemotherapy but present therapy of advanced prostatic carcinoma remains palliative at best with discouraging results.— T. J. Worgul *et al.*, *J. Urol., Baltimore*, 1983, *129*, 51.

But see also under Malignant Neoplasms of the Breast, above.

Preparations

Aminoglutethimide Tablets *(U.S.P.)*

Proprietary Preparations

Orimeten *(Ciba, UK). Tablets*, scored, aminoglutethimide 250 mg.

Proprietary Names and Manufacturers

Cytadren *(Ciba, Austral.; Ciba, Canad.; Ciba, USA)*; Oriméténe *(Ciba, Fr.; Ciba, Switz.)*; Orimeten *(Ciba, Ger.; Ciba, Ital.; Ciba, S.Afr.; Ciba, Spain; Ciba, Swed.; Ciba, UK)*.

12374-q

Amsacrine *(BAN, USAN, pINN).*

Acridinyl Anisidide; CI-880; *m*-AMSA; NSC-249992. 4′-(Acridin-9-ylamino)methanesulphon-*m*-anisidide.

$C_{21}H_{19}N_3O_3S$=393.5.

CAS — 51264-14-3.

Amsacrine is reported to be **incompatible** with sodium chloride and other chloride solutions.

Amsacrine reacted with plastics and should be given by glass syringes. It was unstable in chloride-containing solutions; precipitation might occur.— P. F. D'Arcy, *Drug Intell. & clin. Pharm.*, 1983, *17*, 532.

Adverse Effects, Treatment, and Precautions

For an outline of the adverse effects experienced with antineoplastic agents and immunosuppressants, general guidelines for their treatment, and precautions, see Antineoplastic Agents, p.580, p.583.

Bone-marrow depression is usually dose-limiting and may be severe. The nadir of the white cell count has been reported at about 12 days after treatment, with recovery usually by the 25th day. Pancytopenia may occur. Gastro-intestinal disturbances, including severe stomatitis, grand mal seizures, renal dysfunction, and hepatotoxicity, which may be fatal, have been reported. Cardiac arrhythmias may occur, especially in patients with pre-existing hypokalaemia. Amsacrine is irritant: there may be phlebitis and local tissue necrosis associated especially with administration of high intravenous doses.

It should be given with caution to patients with liver disease, who may require dosage adjustments.

Absorption and Fate

Amsacrine is poorly absorbed following oral administration. When given intravenously it is cleared from the blood in a biphasic manner with a reported terminal half-life of about 7 hours. It is metabolised in the liver and excreted primarily in the bile, mostly as metabolites.

Uses and Administration

Amsacrine is an antineoplastic agent that acts by intercalation with DNA and inhibition of nucleic acid synthesis. It may also exert an action on cell membranes.

It is used for the induction and maintenance of remission in adult acute leukaemias, particularly acute non-lymphoblastic leukaemia. See also under Choice of Antineoplastic Agent, p.587.

Amsacrine is prepared as a solution in lactic acid and dimethylacetamide, and is given, diluted in glucose injection (5%), by intravenous infusion over 1 to 2 hours.

For the induction of remission, amsacrine is given in doses of 90 to 120 mg per m^2 body-surface area daily for 5 to 8 days, depending on toxicity. Courses may be repeated at 2- to 4-week intervals. Maintenance doses of 150 mg per m^2 as a single dose or divided over 3 consecutive days have been given every 3 to 4 weeks, adjusted if necessary according to response. The granulocyte and platelet counts should be allowed to recover to more than 1500 per mm^3 and 100 000 per mm^3 respectively between courses. Complete blood counts should be performed regularly, and cardiac, liver, kidney, and CNS function should be monitored. Doses should be reduced by 20 to 30% in patients with impaired hepatic or renal function.

Reviews: J. Hornedo and D. A. Van Echo, *Pharmacotherapy*, 1985, *5*, 78.

LEUKAEMIAS, ACUTE. Amsacrine produces a remission rate of 17 to 28% in patients with acute non-lymphoblastic leukaemia when given as a single agent in doses of between 0.45 and 1 g per m^2 body-surface area per course; in acute lymphoblastic leukaemia where the dose per course has ranged from 0.225 to 1.2 g per m^2, rates of 9% to 42% have been reported. In general, however, remission duration is short, with a mean of about 4 months. Various combination regimens with drugs such as cytarabine, etoposide, and thioguanine have been investigated in acute non-lymphoblastic leukaemia, and have produced higher remission rates than with amsacrine alone. Further investigation is required of amsacrine with high-dose cytarabine and amsacrine with azacitidine in particular.— Z. A. Arlin, *Cancer Treat. Rep.*, 1983, *67*, 967.

See also under Choice of Antineoplastic Agent, p.587.

Proprietary Preparations

Amsidine *(Parke, Davis, UK). Concentrate for intravenous infusion*, amsacrine 50 mg/mL, in ampoules of 2 mL, supplied with diluent.

Proprietary Names and Manufacturers

Amekrin *(Parke, Davis, Denm.; Parke, Davis, Norw.; Parke, Davis, Swed.)*; Amsa *(Parke, Davis, Canad.)*; Amsidine *(Substantia, Fr.; Parke, Davis, UK)*; Amsidyl *(Parke, Davis, Austral.; Gödecke, Ger.)*;

1824-c

Ancitabine Hydrochloride *(rINNM).*

Ancytabine Hydrochloride; Cyclocytidine Hydrochloride; NSC-145668. 2,2′-Anhydro-1-β-D-arabinofuranosylcytosine hydrochloride.

$C_9H_{11}N_3O_4$,HCl=261.7.

CAS — 31698-14-3 (ancitabine); 10212-25-6 (hydrochloride).

Ancitabine hydrochloride is an antineoplastic agent which is hydrolysed slowly to cytarabine (p.619) *in vivo.* It has been used in acute non-lymphoblastic leukaemia and other malignant diseases and has been given intravenously in doses of 8 to 20 mg per kg body-weight daily.

References: N. Movassaghi *et al.*, *Med. pediat. Oncol.*, 1984, *12*, 352.

Proprietary Names and Manufacturers

Cyclo C *(Jpn).*

1805-y

Antilymphocyte Serum

ALS; Lymphocytic Antiserum. Native serum prepared by injecting viable lymphoid cells into suitable animals and collecting the sera.

1806-j

Antilymphocyte Immunoglobulin (Horse) *(BAN).*

AHLG; ALG; Anti-human Lymphocyte Immunoglobulin; Anti-lymphocytic Globulin; Lymphocytic Antiglobulin. A purified preparation of horse immunoglobulins containing antibodies to human lymphocytes and obtained from antilymphocyte serum.

Adverse Effects

Fever, shivering, nausea, tachycardia, and hypotension can occur shortly after administration. Allergic reactions are common; anaphylaxis may occur. There may be a decrease in the incidence of reactions with antilymphocyte immunoglobulin compared with the serum. As well as lymphocytopenia patients may experience leucopenia and thrombocytopenia. Nephrotoxicity has been reported. Thrombophlebitis is common following intravenous administration.

Precautions

Antilymphocyte immunoglobulin and serum are contraindicated in hypersensitive patients. Patients should always be tested for hypersensitivity.

Uses and Administration

Antilymphocyte immunoglobulin and serum act against lymphocytes to produce immunosuppression without greatly affecting the development of immunity to infection and are used mainly to prolong the survival of organ and tissue transplants. They have also been used similarly to azathioprine (see p.600) in the treatment of various auto-immune disorders. See also under Use of Immunosuppressants, p.594.

Following a test dose, antilymphocyte immunoglobulin is administered by intravenous infusion in usual doses of 10 to 30 mg of immunoglobulin per kg body-weight daily. The daily dose of antilymphocyte immunoglobulin is diluted in 250 to 500 mL of sodium chloride injection (0.9%) and infused slowly over 1 to 2 hours.

BLOOD DISORDERS, NON-MALIGNANT. *Aplastic anaemia.* Antilymphocyte immunoglobulin with or without allogeneic bone-marrow infusions produced a beneficial response in 17 of 29 patients with severe aplastic anaemia. Serum sickness developed in 20 patients 10 days after immunoglobulin treatment and resolved with prednisone. Doses ranged from 15 mg per kg body-weight daily for 4 or 5 days to 40 mg per kg daily for 4 days. Survival was similar to that achieved with bone-marrow transplantation with cyclophosphamide but bone-marrow recovery was considered to be less complete.— B. Speck *et al.*, *Lancet*, 1977, *2*, 1145. In a study in 50 patients treatment of severe aplastic anaemia with antilymphocyte globulin and norethandrolone, with or without bone-marrow infusion, was more effective than bone-marrow transplantation.— *idem*, *Br. med. J.*, 1981, *282*, 860.

DIABETES MELLITUS. For reference to the use of antilymphocyte immunoglobulin with azathioprine and prednisolone in diabetes mellitus, see under Azathioprine, p.600.

Proprietary Preparations

Pressimmune *(Hoechst, UK). Injection*, concentrate for intravenous infusion, antilymphocyte immunoglobulin 50 mg per mL, in ampoules of 10 mL.

Proprietary Names and Manufacturers

Immossar *(Fr.; Italfarmaco, Ital.)*; Lymphoglobuline *(Merieux, Ital.)*; Lymphoser *(Berna, Spain; Berna, Switz.)*; Pressimmun *(Behringwerke, Ger.; Istituto Behring, Ital.)*; Pressimmune *(Hoechst, UK)*; Uman-Gal E *(Biagini, Ital.)*.

1807-z

Antithymocyte Serum
Antithymitic Serum; Thymitic Antiserum. Native serum prepared by injecting thymus cells into suitable animals and collecting the sera.

1808-c

Antithymocyte Immunoglobulin (Equine)
Antithymocyte Gammaglobulin; Antithymocyte Globulin; ATG; ATGAM. A purified preparation of horse immunoglobulins from antithymocyte serum.

Adverse Effects and Precautions
As for Antilymphocyte Immunoglobulin, p.598.

A study in renal transplant patients given an immunosuppressive regimen comprising azathioprine and prednisone, with or without antithymocyte immunoglobulin, found that those who received antithymocyte immunoglobulin were more likely to have herpesvirus infections and inverted T-cell subset ratios.— R. T. Schooley *et al.*, *New Engl. J. Med.*, 1983, *308*, 307.

A report of the development of multiple myeloma in a patient given antithymocyte immunoglobulin for aplastic anaemia.— G. S. Beyer *et al.* (letter), *New Engl. J. Med.*, 1986, *314*, 247.

Uses and Administration
Antithymocyte immunoglobulin and serum have properties and uses similar to those of antilymphocyte immunoglobulin and serum (above).

Guidelines for the preparation and use of antithymocyte immunoglobulin. Immunoglobulin raised in *goats* is consistently more potent and less toxic than that from *horses* and the authors prefer to manufacture their own rather than use the commercial equine preparation.— D. C. Mears *et al.*, *Aust. J. Hosp. Pharm.*, 1985, *15*, 153.

BLOOD DISORDERS, NON-MALIGNANT. A report of beneficial results with antithymocyte immunoglobulin in patients with moderate or severe aplastic anaemia who were not considered candidates for bone-marrow transplantation. Equine antithymocyte immunoglobulin was given by intravenous infusion in a dose of 20 mg per kg body-weight daily for 8 days. Each dose was diluted in 250 to 500 mL of sodium chloride injection (0.9%) and infused over 4 to 6 hours. Eleven of 21 patients randomised to receive antithymocyte immunoglobulin had haematological improvement within 3 months and 2 improved 4.5 and 5 months, respectively, after treatment. None of 21 control patients who received only supportive care improved within 3 months; 12 of these controls were subsequently given antithymocyte immunoglobulin and 6 improved within 3 months. Patients responding to treatment generally had only a partial response with peripheral blood counts typically remaining unchanged for 1 to 3 months and then slowly increasing and stabilising in the lower normal or mildly pancytopenic range. Survival in patients who received immediate antithymocyte immunoglobulin tended to be superior to that of the control group although the difference was not statistically significant. Antithymocyte immunoglobulin treatment was associated with fever, chills, rash, thrombocytopenia, and serum sickness in all patients and 3 patients had transient hypotension during the infusion. Further studies are needed to determine the optimum dosage, schedule, and method of administration of antithymocyte immunoglobulin.— R. Champlin *et al.*, *New Engl. J. Med.*, 1983, *308*, 113. The view that good results are obtained in patients with aplastic anaemia by the use of thymostimulin, an immunomodulator that specifically increases the number of T-cells with the helper phenotype. Immunomodulating treatment is better tolerated than immunosuppression with antithymocyte immunoglobulin, and lacks the latter's severe side-effects.— P. Guglielmo *et al.* (letter), *ibid.*, 1362.

A retrospective study of 13 patients treated with antithymocyte immunoglobulin for aplastic anaemia suggested that the effects were related to dose. All of 5 patients given a total dose of more than 100 mg per kg improved or returned to normal, whereas only 1 of 5 given between 70 and 100 mg per kg and none of 5 given less than 60 mg per kg did so. Two of those who failed to respond to a lower dose subsequently improved when given a second course to a total dose greater than 100 mg per kg. This experience suggests that doses higher than 100 mg per kg divided over 6 to 8 days, are necessary to produce remission in aplastic anaemia.— B. Coiffier *et al.* (letter), *Lancet*, 1983, *2*, 100.

A report of a dramatic response to antithymocyte immunoglobulin in a patient with amegakaryocytic thrombocytopenic purpura given a total dose of 150 mg per kg body-weight over 7 days. Four days after the end of treatment, platelet counts rose dramatically and subsequently fell to normal levels; the patient was still in remission at 7 months.— A. Khelif *et al.* (letter), *Ann. intern. Med.*, 1985, *102*, 720.

See also under Skin and Connective-tissue Disorders, below.

LYMPHOMAS. The beneficial effect of antithymocyte immunoglobulin in a patient with mycosis fungoides classified as a T-cell lymphoma.— R. L. Edelson *et al.* (letter), *Lancet*, 1977, *2*, 249. Failure of this treatment in 1 patient.— D. J. Gould *et al.* (letter), *ibid.*, 1365.

A 63-year-old man with a T-cell lymphoma who had not responded to chemotherapy experienced a 75% reduction in adenopathy and complete resolution of skin erythema after 7 daily infusions of antithymocyte serum 825 mg. Despite continuing tumour regression the patient died of an intracerebral haemorrhage, secondary to thrombocytopenia.— R. I. Fisher *et al.*, *Ann. intern. Med.*, 1978, *88*, 799.

ORGAN AND TISSUE TRANSPLANTATION. *Kidney*. The use of antithymocyte immunoglobulin and corticosteroids for immunosuppression in patients given total lymphoid irradiation (TLI) prior to renal transplantation: B. Levin *et al.*, *Lancet*, 1985, *2*, 1321 (results comparable to those with cyclosporin). See also M. Waer *et al.* (letter), *ibid.*, 1354.

SKIN AND CONNECTIVE-TISSUE DISORDERS, NON-MALIGNANT. Administration of antithymocyte immunoglobulin 15 mg per kg body-weight daily for 10 days, together with oral prednisone, to a patient with aplastic anaemia, also resulted in resolution of his scleroderma. Both conditions had been unresponsive to corticosteroids alone.— E. P. Balaban *et al.*, *Ann. intern. Med.*, 1987, *106*, 56.

Proprietary Names and Manufacturers
Atgam *(Upjohn, Austral.; Upjohn, Canad.; Upjohn, Spain; Wyeth, USA)*.

1809-k

Azacitidine *(USAN, rINN)*.
5-Azacytidine; Ladakamycin; NSC-102816; U-18496; WR-183027. 4-Amino-1-β-D-ribofuranosyl-1,3,5-triazin-2(1*H*)-one.
$C_8H_{12}N_4O_5$=244.2.

CAS — 320-67-2.

STABILITY IN SOLUTION. Azacitidine is very unstable in aqueous solutions, with a 10% loss of drug in 2 to 3 hours at room temperature in lactated Ringer's injection. Degradation is complex, with an initial reversible formation of an intermediate formyl product which then undergoes slower irreversible change to produce further degradation products. Loss of azacitidine is rapid initially, but as the intermediate accumulates reversal of the first reaction slows down the apparent loss of azacitidine. Misunderstanding of the kinetics has led to erroneously long 90% stability times being quoted in the literature.— D. C. Chatterji (letter), *Am. J. Hosp. Pharm.*, 1982, *39*, 1638. See also D. C. Chatterji and J. F. Gallelli, *J. pharm. Sci.*, 1979, *68*, 822.

A study of the stability of azacitidine in infusion fluids at 25°. The mean time for a reduction to 90% of original concentration, for a 200 μg per mL solution in glass bottles, was 1.9 hours in sodium chloride injection (0.9%), 1.93 hours in lactated Ringer's injection, and 1.87 hours in a commercial fluid (Normosol-R). The drug appeared to be less stable in glucose injection (5%), with a 90% stability time of 0.8 hours. The drug was more stable as a 2 mg per mL solution, with 90% stability times of 2.4, 2.87, 3.03, and 3.0 hours respectively; this might be due to the pH of the solutions which ranged from 6.4 to 7.0, the range in which azacitidine is most stable. When polyvinyl chloride containers were used for the non-proprietary solutions there was no evidence of an effect on stability in sodium chloride or Ringer's injection but there was enhanced degradation of the solution in glucose injection. The results suggest that azacitidine should be administered immediately after preparation; dilution in glucose injection (5%) at lower drug concentrations is not recommended.— Y. -W. Cheung *et al.*, *Am. J. Hosp. Pharm.*, 1984, *41*, 1156.

Adverse Effects, Treatment, and Precautions
For an outline of the adverse effects experienced with antineoplastic agents and immunosuppressants, general guidelines for their treatment, and precautions, see Antineoplastic Agents, p.580, p.583. Nausea and vomiting with azacitidine may be severe, especially after rapid injection. Bone-marrow suppression is usually dose-limiting, and is manifested by leucopenia, thrombocytopenia, and anaemia. Gastro-intestinal disturbances, neuromuscular effects, fever, rashes, liver disorders, and hypotension have occurred.

Uses and Administration
Azacitidine is an antineoplastic agent which acts similarly to cytarabine (p.620). It also inhibits cellular pyrimidine synthesis. It has been used mainly in the treatment of acute non-lymphoblastic leukaemia and may be given by continuous intravenous infusion in a dose of 50 to 400 mg per m^2 body-surface daily for 5 days. Azacitidine is unstable in solution and it has been suggested that infusions should be freshly prepared every 3 to 4 hours. It has also been given subcutaneously.

BLOOD DISORDERS, NON-MALIGNANT. *Haemoglobinopathies*. Following results in *animals* suggesting that azacitidine could activate the genes responsible for production of haemoglobin F (foetal haemoglobin), it was given to a patient with beta-thalassaemia in an attempt to ameliorate the symptoms of the disease. The patient received azacitidine 2 mg per kg body-weight daily for 7 days as a continuous intravenous infusion. Treatment produced a temporary increase in haemoglobin concentration and absolute reticulocyte count, and an improvement in bone pain. Immediately before therapy 1.6% of the patient's haemoglobin was haemoglobin F; this figure rose to 20.8% after 40 days and then declined on reinstitution of transfusion therapy. This prolonged effect was presumably due to transient production of red cells with a more normal haemoglobin content and thus improved survival in the circulation. Further study of the drug will be required to determine a regimen of therapeutic benefit to patients, and in view of the potential risks such therapy should not be used until controlled studies of efficacy and safety have been carried out.— T. J. Ley *et al.*, *New Engl. J. Med.*, 1982, *307*, 1469. Comment. There could be no obvious lasting benefit to the patient from such therapy and the use of such a potent drug and potential carcinogen in patients with beta-thalassaemia, where more conventional supportive therapy has much to offer, seem premature.— *Lancet*, 1983, *1*, 36. Reply. Conventional supportive therapy for sickle-cell anaemia and beta-thalassaemia is neither ideal nor without severe adverse effects of its own. Furthermore a precedent exists for the use of cytotoxic agents in other severe non-malignant disorders such as psoriasis. Azacitidine therapy represents an attempt to find a new therapeutic approach in a group of patients with incapacitating or fatal diseases but it is still experimental and should not be routinely recommended.— T. J. Ley *et al.* (letter), *ibid.*, 467. Further criticism.— J. B. Clegg *et al.* (letter), *ibid.*, 536.

See also *Science*, 1984, *223*, 470 (discussion of the use of cytotoxic agents in haemoglobinopathies).

LEUKAEMIAS, ACUTE. For mention of the use of azacitidine with amsacrine and etoposide (MAZE) to treat acute non-lymphoblastic leukaemia in relapse, see under Choice of Antineoplastic Agent, p.587.

Proprietary Names and Manufacturers
Mylosar *(Upjohn, USA)*.

1810-w

Azaribine *(BAN, USAN, rINN)*.
CB-304; NSC-67239; Triacetyl Azauridine. 2-β-D-Ribofuranosyl-1,2,4-triazine-3,5(2*H*,4*H*)-dione 2′,3′,5′-triacetate; 6-Azauridine 2′,3′,5′-triacetate.
$C_{14}H_{17}N_3O_9$=371.3.

CAS — 2169-64-4.

Azaribine is a derivative of azauridine (p.601) and has the same general properties. It was formerly used in the treatment of mycosis fungoides and psoriasis but was withdrawn from the market in the *USA* after reports of serious thrombosis.

1812-l

Azathioprine *(BAN, USAN, rINN)*.
Azathioprinum; BW-57322; NSC-39084. 6-(1-Methyl-4-nitroimidazol-5-ylthio)purine.
$C_9H_7N_7O_2S$=277.3.

CAS — 446-86-6.

Pharmacopoeias. In *Br., Braz., Cz., Eur., It., Jpn, Jug., Neth., Swiss,* and *U.S. U.S.* also includes Azathioprine Sodium for Injection.

A pale yellow odourless powder. Practically **insoluble** in water, alcohol, and in chloroform; sparingly soluble in dilute mineral acids; dissolves in dilute solutions of alkali hydroxides. Solutions of azathioprine sodium for injection have a pH of 9.8 to 11.0; they are prepared by dissolving in Water for Injections, immediately before use. **Store** in airtight containers. Protect from light. The *U.S.P.* preparation for injection should be stored at 15° to 30°.

Adverse Effects and Treatment

For an outline of the adverse effects experienced with antineoplastic agents and immunosuppressants and general guidelines for their treatment, see Antineoplastic Agents, p.580 and p.583.

Depression of the bone marrow, commonly manifest as leucopenia and less often thrombocytopenia, is dose related and may be delayed. Other side-effects associated with azathioprine include gastro-intestinal disturbances, joint pains, rashes, drug fever, liver damage, and pancreatitis. Solutions for injection are irritant.

A review of the adverse effects of azathioprine.— D. H. Lawson *et al.*, *Adverse Drug React. Ac. Pois. Rev.*, 1984, *3*, 161.

ALLERGY AND ANAPHYLAXIS. Reports of allergic reactions associated with azathioprine.— M. D. Lockshin and L. J. Kagen (letter), *New Engl. J. Med.*, 1972, *286*, 1321 (meningitic reactions); N. B. Hershfield (letter), *Can. med. Ass. J.*, 1973, *109*, 1082 (polyarthritis and fever); L. J. Brandt, *Ann. intern. Med.*, 1977, *87*, 458 (formication); J. S. Sergent and M. Lockshin (letter), *J. Am. med. Ass.*, 1978, *240*, 529 (meningitic reaction); M. J. G. Farthing *et al.*, *Br. med. J.*, 1980, *280*, 367 (fever, arthralgia, polyneuritis); G. F. Watts, *Postgrad. med. J.*, 1984, *60*, 362 (fever, rigors, dysphagia, dysarthria, and increased weakness in a myasthenic patient also allergic to mercaptopurine).

See also under Effects on the Vascular System, below.

CARCINOGENICITY. For reference to the role of immunosuppression in the development of secondary malignancy see Adverse Effects of Antineoplastic Agents, p.581.

EFFECTS ON THE BLOOD. Severe megaloblastic anaemia in a patient taking azathioprine was associated with abnormal metabolism of the drug.— L. Lennard *et al.*, *Br. J. clin. Pharmac.*, 1984, *17*, 171. See also J. L. Maddocks *et al.* (letter), *Lancet*, 1986, *1*, 156.

EFFECTS ON THE LIVER. A review of drug-related hepatotoxicity. Azathioprine has been associated with hepatocanalicular cholestasis, in which the interference with bile flow is combined with hepatocyte damage, and with several hepatic vascular disorders, including focal sinusoidal dilatation, peliosis, and veno-occlusive disease.— S. Sherlock, *Lancet*, 1986, *2*, 440.

EFFECTS ON THE VASCULAR SYSTEM. Pronounced hypotension in 2 patients with rheumatoid arthritis given azathioprine.— T. Cunningham *et al.*, *Br. med. J.*, 1981, *283*, 823. Comment. Pancreatitis may be implicated in such reactions.— A. L. Pozniak *et al.* (letter), *ibid.*, 1548. Profound circulatory collapse requiring inotropic support occurred in a patient hypersensitive to azathioprine on re-exposure.— E. Rosenthal, *Postgrad. med. J.*, 1986, *62*, 677.

A report of fast atrial fibrillation and fever in a patient given azathioprine for psoriasis.— H. J. Dodd *et al.*, *Br. med. J.*, 1985, *291*, 706. Criticism. The atrial fibrillation may have been due to the fever rather than the drug.— P. C. Chijioke (letter), *ibid.*, 1049. Further criticism.— G. Nikolic (letter), *ibid.* A similar case in which atrial fibrillation has persisted.— G. Murphy *et al.* (letter), *ibid.*

For controversy concerning the relative incidence of thromboembolic disorders in patients given azathioprine and those given cyclosporin, see Cyclosporin, p.615.

Precautions

For reference to the precautions necessary with antineoplastic agents and immunosuppressants, see Antineoplastic Agents, p.583.

Azathioprine should be used with care in patients with liver damage or a history of liver disease.

The effects of azathioprine are enhanced by allopurinol and the dose of azathioprine should be reduced to about one-quarter when allopurinol is given concomitantly. Reduced doses may be required in patients with impaired renal function.

PREGNANCY AND THE NEONATE. From a detailed analysis of successful pregnancies notified to the European Dialysis and Transplant Association, only 7 of 110 babies born to 97 women with renal transplants had congenital abnormalities, one of them being a congenital cytomegalovirus infection. Abnormalities were trivial in 3 babies. Chromatid breaks were found in 2 of 16 babies who underwent chromosome analysis. Mothers of the 7 babies with abnormalities had taken significantly higher daily doses of azathioprine (a mean of 2.64 mg per kg body-weight) compared with those who had normal babies (a mean of 2.02 mg per kg). There was no significant difference in the daily dose of prednisone. This congenital abnormality-rate is probably not excessive when compared with a reported figure of 2% for all births.—The Registration Committee of the European Dialysis and Transplant Association, *Br. J. Obstet. Gynaec.*, 1980, *87*, 839. A view that foetal growth retardation was more common in women who had undergone kidney transplantation and who continued to receive azathioprine and prednisolone during pregnancy.— Y. Pirson *et al.* (letter), *New Engl. J. Med.*, 1985, *313*, 328. Factors other than immunosuppression may influence growth of the foetus in renal transplant recipients.— S. Hou (letter), *ibid.*

There is little evidence that azathioprine is teratogenic in humans.— M. J. Whittle and K. P. Hanretty, *Br. med. J.*, 1986, *293*, 1485. Despite the lack of evidence for foetal damage associated with azathioprine, it seems prudent to avoid its use in pregnancy if possible.— M. de Swiet, *Prescribers' J.*, 1979, *19*, 59.

Absorption and Fate

Azathioprine is well absorbed from the gastro-intestinal tract when given by mouth. After oral or intravenous administration it disappears rapidly from the circulation and is extensively metabolised to mercaptopurine (see p.635). Both azathioprine and mercaptopurine are about 30% bound to plasma proteins. About 10% of a dose is reported to be split between the sulphur and the purine ring to give 1-methyl-4-nitro-5-thioimidazole. Small amounts of unchanged azathioprine and mercaptopurine are eliminated in the urine.

Uses and Administration

Azathioprine is an immunosuppressant (see p.594) and antineoplastic agent with similar actions to those of mercaptopurine (p.635), to which it is slowly converted in the body. Its effects may not be seen for several weeks after administration. It is given by mouth; in patients in whom oral administration is not feasible it may be given intravenously as azathioprine sodium, by slow intravenous injection or by infusion, diluted in glucose or sodium chloride injections.

Azathioprine is mainly used as an immunosuppressant for facilitating the survival of organ and tissue transplants. The dose for this purpose varies from 1 to 5 mg per kg body-weight daily and depends partly on whether other drugs, such as a corticosteroid, or radiotherapy are employed at the same time. The dose may be increased if there is incipient rejection of the graft, but withdrawal of the drug, with concomitant likelihood of rejection, may be necessary if toxicity occurs.

It is also used in a wide variety of conditions such as lupus erythematosus, rheumatoid arthritis, renal disorders, chronic active hepatitis, and some severe skin disorders which are considered to be auto-immune in character and for which corticosteroid therapy is often tried. Its use in conjunction with a corticosteroid (see p.875) may allow a lower dose of both drugs to be used, thus reducing side-effects. The usual dose of azathioprine in these conditions is in the range of 1 to 2.5 mg per kg body-weight daily by mouth in adults and children.

Blood counts should be carried out regularly during treatment and azathioprine withdrawn or the dosage reduced at the first indication of bone-marrow depression.

A review of azathioprine.— A. R. Ahmed and R. Moy, *Int. J. Derm.*, 1981, *20*, 461.

ADMINISTRATION IN HEPATIC INSUFFICIENCY. For a recommendation on dosage restriction in patients with chronic active hepatitis, see under Hepatic Disorders, below.

ADMINISTRATION IN RENAL INSUFFICIENCY. The interval between doses of azathioprine should be extended from 24 hours to 36 hours, or the dose reduced to 75%, in patients with a glomerular filtration-rate of less than 10 mL per minute. Concentrations of azathioprine are affected by haemodialysis.— W. M. Bennett *et al.*, *Am. J. Kidney Dis.*, 1983, *3*, 155.

DIABETES MELLITUS. During a study in *rats* it was found that azathioprine may have an antidiabetogenic effect.— A. S. Serra *et al.* (letter), *Lancet*, 1979, *1*, 1292.

Results of a study in newly-diagnosed insulin-dependent (type I) diabetics suggested that immunosuppressant treatment with azathioprine increased the rate of remission. Seven of 13 patients who were assigned to treatment with azathioprine 2 mg per kg body-weight in addition to their insulin had a remission, compared to only 1 of 11 untreated patients. Treatment was continued for 6 months or a year in 11 patients but was stopped in 2 because of side-effects. Remissions were not sustained in the 1 to 2 years following treatment but patients who relapsed had lower insulin requirements.— L. C. Harrison *et al.*, *Diabetes*, 1985, *34*, 1306.

Intensive immunosuppression with azathioprine, prednisolone, and antilymphocyte immunoglobulin did not cure diabetes in 5 newly-diagnosed insulin-dependent diabetics. Although 3 patients temporarily came off insulin, one with normal glucose tolerance, this was considered indistinguishable from the common "honeymoon period".— R. D. G. Leslie *et al.* (letter), *Lancet*, 1985, *1*, 516.

For further controversy concerning the role of immunosuppressants in diabetes mellitus, see Cyclosporin, p.617.

GASTRO-INTESTINAL DISORDERS, NON-MALIGNANT. A patient with *coeliac disease* inadequately controlled by prednisone in doses as high as 20 mg daily was effectively treated with azathioprine 2 mg per kg body-weight daily. It was possible to reduce the dose of prednisone to 2.5 mg daily.— J. D. Hamilton *et al.*, *Lancet*, 1976, *1*, 1213.

Sensorineural hearing loss in a patient receiving sulphasalazine maintenance for *ulcerative colitis* in remission was considered to be an extra-intestinal manifestation of the disease. Hearing rapidly improved on addition of prednisolone 60 mg daily, but deteriorated whenever the dose was reduced below 40 mg daily. The addition of azathioprine 2 mg per kg body-weight daily allowed the steroid treatment to be slowly reduced and then stopped without appreciable deterioration in hearing. The hearing loss remained stable over nine months despite an exacerbation of ulcerative colitis. Such sensorineural deafness should be immediately treated with a combination of azathioprine and prednisolone.— A. Dowd and W. D. W. Rees, *Br. med. J.*, 1987, *295*, 26.

Villous atrophy unresponsive to gluten withdrawal in 3 patients was dramatically improved by replacement of prednisolone by azathioprine 2 mg per kg body-weight daily. Azathioprine is a useful alternative therapy in this potentially fatal disease when prednisolone has failed or where the dose of prednisolone required to maintain remission causes unacceptable side-effects.— T. S. Sinclair *et al.*, *Gut*, 1983, *24*, A494.

Reports of a favourable influence of azathioprine and mercaptopurine in *Crohn's disease* are unexplained and not universally accepted.— J. B. Kirsner and R. G. Shorter, *New Engl. J. Med.*, 1982, *306*, 775.

While resolution of symptoms of *Crohn's disease* may follow treatment with azathioprine, good evidence to support its widespread use is lacking. However, in children with symptomatic Crohn's disease the authors' current practice is to start azathioprine 1 to 2 mg per kg body-weight daily at the same time that corticosteroid treatment is begun and to continue after the reduction and probable cessation of steroids in the hope of exerting a steroid-sparing effect or prolonging remission in the absence of corticosteroids.— I. W. Booth and J. T. Harries, *Gut*, 1984, *25*, 188.

Results from a study involving 42 patients with *Crohn's disease* given long-term azathioprine treatment suggested that the drug had a favourable influence on the clinical course of the disease, with remission in 11, which has persisted in 10 for a mean of 40 months without therapy.— M. Nyman *et al.*, *Scand. J. Gastroenterol.*, 1985, *20*, 1197.

The indications for a trial of azathioprine in *ulcerative colitis* appear to be chronic, active, steroid-dependent disease for which surgical treatment is inappropriate. The dose used is 2 to 2.5 mg per kg body-weight. About 10% of patients are unable to take the drug because of side-effects, but marrow depression is rare at this dose. The drug exerts a steroid-sparing effect but it appears to act slowly over weeks or months and an effective corticosteroid dose should be maintained for at least a month before attempts are made at reduction. No data are available to suggest the optimal duration of such treatment.— J. E. Lennard-Jones, *Postgrad. med. J.*, 1984, *60*, 797. Azathioprine has only a modest therapeutic benefit which rarely justifies the risk of marrow suppression.— J. M. Rhodes, *Prescribers' J.*, 1986, *26*, 1.

HEPATIC DISORDERS, NON-MALIGNANT. *Chronic active hepatitis*. Chronic active hepatitis may be associated with hepatitis B infection or may present as an autoimmune condition; in the latter case, if disease is severe enough to warrant treatment, the use of corticosteroids, with or without azathioprine, has been recommended.

The precise role of azathioprine in chronic active hepatitis is contentious. Most authorities have regarded corticosteroids as the drugs of choice, with azathioprine being given to permit a reduction in steroid dosage. However, there is some evidence that azathioprine is effective in its own right. Giusti *et al.* retrospectively compared treatment regimens among 394 patients with chronic active hepatitis negative for hepatitis B surface antigen (HBsAg) (*Hepatogastroenterology*, 1984, *31*, 24). Relative improvement rates were: 32.1% among 28 treated with azathioprine 50 to 100 mg daily; 39.1% among 152 given prednisone or prednisolone 10 to 30 mg daily; and 53.7% among 95 given combined corticosteroid and azathioprine therapy. These were higher rates than the 18.5% of 119 untreated patients who improved, but the difference was significant only for the combination and corticosteroid regimens. In the same retrospective study 473 patients positive for HBsAg were also included. Azathioprine therapy (in 57) or corticosteroids (in 135) each produced significantly more frequent improvement than no treatment in 134 patients (40.3% and 41.5%, as against 21%) but did not arrest deterioration in others. Combined therapy with azathioprine and corticosteroids was the most effective in this group, with a 52.4% improvement rate among 147 patients, and a lower deterioration rate than the untreated patients.

Other studies have confirmed the value of azathioprine in combination therapy. Vegnente *et al.* (*Archs Dis. Childh.*, 1984, *59*, 330) found that 18 of 26 children with chronic active hepatitis had inadequate response to prednisolone alone but improved when azathioprine was added to the regimen. A study in 50 patients by Stellon *et al.* (*Lancet*, 1985, *1*, 668) also compared azathioprine and prednisolone with prednisolone alone for the maintenance of disease remission; 23 patients remained on the combined regimen while 27 had the azathioprine component withdrawn and were maintained with prednisolone only. Over a follow-up period of 3 years, relapse occurred in 8 of the patients who had had azathioprine withdrawn but in only 1 of those receiving combined therapy, a cumulative risk of relapse of 32% and 6% respectively. Increasing prednisolone dosage and re-introducing azathioprine were effective in re-inducing remission in patients who relapsed.

Although the above study showed a clear benefit for azathioprine given with a corticosteroid the authors concluded that it became effective in chronic active hepatitis only after corticosteroid treatment had improved liver function adequately enough to permit metabolic activation of the azathioprine. However, this view has been queried by Brunner and Hopf (*Lancet*, 1985, *1*, 1216) who suggest that the use of a higher dose of azathioprine (2 mg per kg body-weight daily) gives good results from azathioprine therapy alone. However, in view of the ability of azathioprine to cause liver damage it has been suggested in some quarters that the dose in patients with chronic active hepatitis should not exceed about 1.5 mg per kg daily.

It was recommended that the dose of azathioprine should be restricted to 75 to 100 mg daily when used with prednisolone in the treatment of active chronic hepatitis.— *Br. med. J.*, 1973, *2*, 193.

Results in 52 patients assigned to maintenance therapy of chronic active hepatitis with either azathioprine and prednisolone combined, or with azathioprine alone, suggested that prednisolone suppressed autoantibody formation against the liver-specific lipoprotein complex, whereas azathioprine might act directly on killer cells involved in the reactions that produce liver damage.— J. J. Keating *et al.*, *Gut*, 1986, *27*, A1239.

Primary biliary cirrhosis. A review of primary biliary cirrhosis. Although initial results of controlled studies indicated that azathioprine, in doses of 1 to 2 mg per kg body-weight daily, had no therapeutic value in primary biliary cirrhosis, the most recent results (E. Christensen *et al.*, *Gastroenterology*, 1985, *89*, 1084) suggest that it may prolong survival and retard the rate of clinical deterioration. Nonetheless, no satisfactory treatment for primary biliary cirrhosis yet exists.— M. M. Kaplan, *New Engl. J. Med.*, 1987, *316*, 521.

NEUROLOGICAL DISORDERS. *Multiple sclerosis*. For reference to the use of immunosuppressants, including azathioprine, in the management of multiple sclerosis, see under Use of Immunosuppressants, p.594.

Myasthenia gravis. For a detailed review of the treatment of myasthenia gravis, including the role of azathioprine, see under Neostigmine Methylsulphate, p.1333.

OCULAR DISORDERS, NON-MALIGNANT. When azathioprine 1.5 mg per kg body-weight daily was added to the normal treatment of thyrotoxicosis in 109 patients with Graves' disease who were expected to develop malignant exophthalmos because of a positive leucocyte migration test, no clinical signs of exophthalmos developed.— R. Winand and P. Mahieu (letter), *Lancet*, 1973, *1*, 1196. See also *ibid.*, 1982, *2*, 1378.

Some patients with Graves' disease do not develop eye changes and in most patients the eye signs are mild and do not require treatment. Where severe ophthalmopathy occurs, however, azathioprine has not been as successful as corticosteroids.— R. Wilkinson, *Prescribers' J.*, 1984, *24*, 97.

ORGAN AND TISSUE TRANSPLANTATION. For studies comparing the use of azathioprine with that of cyclosporin in transplant recipients see under Cyclosporin, p.617.

RHEUMATIC DISORDERS. In a multicentre study completed by 134 patients, patients with rheumatoid arthritis unresponsive to gold therapy were assigned to treatment with azathioprine 1.25 to 1.5 mg per kg body-weight daily, or with penicillamine 10 to 12 mg per kg daily, for 24 weeks. None of the 70 patients given azathioprine or the 64 given penicillamine experienced remission but both drugs improved joint pain and swelling in about 40% of patients. Although both agents were considered equally effective, azathioprine was better tolerated and might be preferred for this reason.— H. E. Paulus *et al.*, *Arthritis Rheum.*, 1984, *27*, 721. A critical evaluation of 17 published studies on long-acting agents in the treatment of rheumatoid arthritis. There was insufficient evidence for an effect of azathioprine or penicillamine in retarding the radiographic progression of joint damage.— L. Iannuzzi *et al.*, *New England J. Med.*, 1983, *309*, 1023.

The management of rheumatoid arthritis. Immunosuppressants, of which azathioprine is the most widely used in the *UK*, are reserved for older patients, or those who have failed to respond to other agents. Azathioprine in a dose of 1.5 mg per kg body-weight daily is reportedly about as effective as gold. Regular monitoring of blood counts and liver function is required during therapy.— H. A. Bird, *Br. J. Hosp. Med.*, 1986, *35*, 374.

For preliminary results suggesting that striking improvement can be attained in refractory rheumatoid arthritis with an experimental regimen combining hydroxychloroquine, cyclophosphamide, and azathioprine, see Cyclophosphamide, p.613.

SKIN AND CONNECTIVE-TISSUE DISORDERS, NON-MALIGNANT. *Dermatitis*. A report of the use of azathioprine 2.5 mg per kg body-weight daily in 25 patients with eczema. The best response was seen in patients with discoid eczema and actinic reticuloid; in each case 5 of 6 patients had clearance of lesions, although in the latter group the effect was slower and toxicity temporarily interrupted treatment in 2 patients and ended it in a third. Patients with atopic eczema responded less well and treatment in 4 patients with chronic erythrodermic eczema was rapidly ended by toxicity.— P. J. August, *Br. J. Derm.*, 1982, *107*, *Suppl.* 22, 23.

Nine of 14 patients with chronic actinic dermatitis were found to have benefited from treatment with azathioprine in a retrospective review. Patients received azathioprine 100 to 200 mg daily for up to 33 months; complete clearance was seen in 5 and improvement in 4. A further patient cleared initially and then relapsed and there was no benefit in 2. A further 2 discontinued treatment because of adverse effects. The results were considered encouraging enough to justify further study.— I. M. Leigh and J. L. M. Hawk, *Br. J. Derm.*, 1984, *110*, 691.

Systemic lupus erythematosus. For comparison of immunosuppressant therapy with azathioprine and with cyclophosphamide in the management of lupus nephritis, see under Cyclophosphamide, p.613.

Preparations

Azathioprine Sodium for Injection *(U.S.P.)*. A sterile solid prepared by freeze-drying an aqueous solution of azathioprine and sodium hydroxide. Potency is expressed in terms of the equivalent amount of azathioprine.

Azathioprine Tablets *(B.P., U.S.P.)*

Proprietary Preparations

Azamune *(Penn, UK)*. *Tablets*, scored, azathioprine 50 mg.

Imuran *(Calmic, UK)*. *Tablets*, azathioprine 50 mg. *Injection*, powder for reconstitution, azathioprine 50 mg (as sodium salt).

Proprietary Names and Manufacturers of Azathioprine and Azathioprine Sodium

Azamune *(Penn, UK)*; Azanin *(Jpn)*; Azapress *(Lennon, S.Afr.)*; Imuran *(Arg.*; *Wellcome, Austral.*; *Belg.*; *Wellcome, Canad.*; *Wellcome, Ital.*; *Neth.*; *S.Afr.*; *Calmic, UK*; *Wellcome, USA)*; Imurek *(Aust.*; *Wellcome, Ger.*; *Wellcome, Switz.)*; Imurel *(Wellcome, Denm.*; *Wellcome, Fr.*; *Wellcome, Norw.*; *Gayoso Wellcome, Spain*: *Well--come, Swed)*; Thioprine *(Alphapharm, Austral.)*.

1813-y

Azauridine

6-Azauracil Riboside; 6-Azauridine; AzUR; NSC-32074.
2-β-D-Ribofuranosyl-1,2,4-triazine-3,5(2*H*,4*H*)-dione.
$C_8H_{11}N_3O_6$=245.2.

CAS — 54-25-1.

Azauridine is an antineoplastic agent which acts as an antimetabolite (see p.580) and interferes with pyrimidine biosynthesis to retard the formation of cell nucleic acids. It was formerly tried in the treatment of acute leukaemia.

14036-v

Azelaic Acid *(rINN)*.

Anchoic acid; Lepargylic acid; ZK-62498. Nonanedioic acid; Heptane-1,7-dicarboxylic acid.
$C_9H_{16}O_4$=188.2.

CAS — 123-99-9.

Azelaic acid has been applied as a 15% or 20% cream to the lesions of malignant melanoma; it has also been given by mouth. A cytotoxic effect on the malignant melanocyte has been reported. Azelaic acid has also been tried in the treatment of acne.

A review of azelaic acid. The drug is relatively non-toxic, and non-teratogenic; up to 20 g daily can be tolerated as an oral dose. It has also been administered as the sodium salt intravenously, intra-arterially, and intralymphatically without apparent adverse effects. Following a dose by mouth about 60% is excreted unchanged in the urine; metabolism is partly by beta-oxidation. Azelaic acid appears to act primarily on malignant or hyperactive melanocytes, apparently by affecting the mitochondria of the cell; it has little or no effect on other skin cells or normal melanocytes. In the treatment of lentigo maligna it has been applied as a 15 to 20% cream. Despite the view that surgery is the only justifiable treatment in this condition, the authors have successfully treated 51 cases with topical azelaic acid, and are of the opinion that it provides a satisfactory form of therapy. A 20% cream, combined with oral azelaic acid therapy, has also been tried in primary cutaneous melanoma, with a lesser degree of benefit; later studies have suggested that the benefit of oral therapy is minimal. Further studies in this condition would appear justified; however, results of last resort intravenous infusion in patients with disseminated melanoma have been disappointing, probably because of the failure to achieve and maintain adequate drug concentrations at disease sites. Azelaic acid has also been tried in non-malignant dermatological conditions. Benefit has been demonstrated following topical application of a 15% cream in patients with acne vulgaris, including severe nodulo-cystic forms. There is some evidence both for an effect on sebum secretion (although this has been disputed) and for an antibacterial effect. It is clear that azelaic acid and other dicarboxylic acids have definite potential as therapeutic agents for a number of conditions.— A. S. Breathnach *et al.*, *Br. J. Derm.*, 1984, *111*, 115.

Both *Staphylococcus epidermidis* and *Propionibacterium acnes* were moderately sensitive to azelaic acid *in vitro*, but *Malassezia ovalis* (*Pityrosporum ovale*) exhibited slight sensitivity. The bactericidal effect was considerably reduced when azelaic acid was dissolved in nutrient broth rather than buffer.— J. P. Leeming *et al.*, *Br. J. Derm.*, 1986, *115*, 551.

SKIN AND CONNECTIVE-TISSUE DISORDERS, NON-MALIG-

NANT. *Acne vulgaris.* A report of significant improvement in acne vulgaris in 100 patients using azelaic acid 15% cream by topical application twice daily for 3 to 9 months.— M. Nazzaro-Porro *et al., Br. J. Derm.*, 1983, *109*, 45.

In a double-blind study in male acne patients, tetracycline 1 g daily by mouth in 22 and azelaic acid as a 20% cream in 17 were both effective in reducing the number of lesions. After 6 months the median facial acne grade was reduced by 66% in the azelaic acid-treated group and by 77% in the tetracycline-treated group. Azelaic acid, but not tetracycline, significantly reduced the density of the skin microflora. Six of the 23 patients originally assigned to receive azelaic acid did not complete the study, in 5 because of poor response or compliance; 4 of these subsequently responded well to tetracycline and benzoyl peroxide. Side-effects of both azelaic acid and tetracycline were mild and transient; minor erythema and scaling were observed in some patients receiving azelaic acid. In a further 11 patients also given topical azelaic acid 20% cream for physiological acne, treatment had no significant effect on sebum excretion rate. Azelaic acid was clearly beneficial in these patients, but appears to be marginally less effective clinically than tetracycline. Further work on delivery and mode of action may lead to the successful use of azelaic acid as a topical treatment for acne vulgaris.— P. T. Bladon *et al., Br. J. Derm.*, 1986, *114*, 493.

Proprietary Names and Manufacturers
Schering, Ger.

1815-z

Bleomycin Sulphate *(BANM, pINNM)*.

Bleomycin Sulfate *(USAN)*. The sulphates of a mixture of basic antineoplastic glycopeptide antibiotics, obtained by the growth of *Streptomyces verticillus* or by any other means. It has a mol. wt of about 1400.

CAS — 11056-06-7 (bleomycin); 9041-93-4 (sulphate).

Pharmacopoeias. U.S. includes Sterile Bleomycin Sulfate. *Jpn* includes Bleomycin Hydrochloride.

A cream-coloured amorphous powder. It loses not more than 6% of its weight when dried. Very **soluble** in water. The *U.S.P.* states that a solution in water containing 10 units per mL has a pH of 4.5 to 6.0.

Sterile Bleomycin Sulfate (*U.S.P.*) contains between 55% and 70% of bleomycin A_2; between 25% and 32% of bleomycin B_2; the content of bleomycin B_4 is not more than 1%. The combined percentage of bleomycin A_2 and B_2 is not less than 85%.

Bleomycin sulphate could be given by continuous intravenous infusion, as well as by intravenous injection or intermittent infusion, but should be infused from a glass bottle to avoid drug loss due to absorption by plastic.— R. P. Rapp *et al., Drug Intell. & clin. Pharm.*, 1984, *18*, 218. See also J. Adams *et al.* (letter), *Am. J. Hosp. Pharm.*, 1982, *39*, 1636.

INCOMPATIBILITY. There was a loss of bleomycin activity when bleomycin solutions were mixed with solutions of carbenicillin, cephazolin or cephalothin sodium, nafcillin sodium, benzylpenicillin sodium, methotrexate, mitomycin, hydrocortisone sodium succinate, aminophylline, ascorbic acid, or terbutaline.— R. T. Dorr *et al., J. Med.*, 1982, *13*, 121.

Bleomycin chelates divalent and trivalent cations, and should not be mixed with solutions containing these ions, especially copper. It may be precipitated by hydrophobic anions. Solutions of bleomycin should not be mixed with solutions of essential amino acids, riboflavine, ascorbic acid, dexamethasone, aminophylline, or frusemide. Bleomycin is inactivated by compounds containing sulphydryl groups such as glutathione.— P. F. D'Arcy, *Drug Intell. & clin. Pharm.*, 1983, *17*, 532.

Units

8910 units of bleomycin complex A_2/B_2 are contained in 5 mg of bleomycin complex in one ampoule of the first International Reference Preparation (1980).

These units differ from those of the *U.S.P.*: Sterile Bleomycin Sulfate (*U.S.P.*) contains 1.5 to 2.0 units of bleomycin in each mg. Doses in the *US* are now expressed in terms of these units and one such unit can be considered to be equivalent to 1 mg of active bleomycin.

Adverse Effects and Treatment

For an outline of the adverse effects experienced with antineoplastic agents and immunosuppressants and general guidelines for their treatment, see Antineoplastic Agents, p.580 and p.583.

The most frequent side-effects with bleomycin involve the skin and mucous membranes and include rash, erythema, pruritus, vesiculation, hyperkeratosis, nail changes, alopecia, hyperpigmentation, striae, and stomatitis. There is little depression of the bone marrow. Local reactions, thrombophlebitis, and fever may follow parenteral administration.

The most serious delayed effect is pulmonary toxicity; interstitial pneumonitis and fibrosis occurs in about 10% of patients and produces an overall mortality-rate of 1% of patients treated with bleomycin. Acute anaphylactoid reactions with hyperpyrexia and cardiorespiratory collapse have been reported in patients with lymphoma.

A report of hyperpyrexia and hypotension, culminating in respiratory arrest, coma, and death, in a patient with lymphoma given chemotherapy including bleomycin.— J. J. Carter *et al., Am. J. Med.*, 1983, *74*, 523.

EFFECTS ON THE EARS. Bleomycin may be ototoxic when it is given in high dosage.— J. Ballantyne, *Audiology*, 1973, *12*, 325. See also R. J. M. Lane and P. A. Routledge, *Drugs*, 1983, *26*, 124.

EFFECTS ON THE NAILS. A patient developed blistering and ulceration after injection of bleomycin into periungual warts, and many nails fell off. A previous set of injections, 1 month before, had caused only mild pain. Two years later the patient still had complete loss of the nail in one finger, which had also developed Raynaud's phenomenon, and partial loss of nails on 3 other digits.— D. Czarnecki (letter), *Med. J. Aust.*, 1984, *141*, 40.

EFFECTS ON RESPIRATORY FUNCTION. Lung injury develops in approximately 10% of all patients who receive bleomycin and death occurs in 1 to 2%. Changes in the lung are diffuse and include fibrosis of the alveolar septa, chronic pneumonitis with lymphocytes in the interstitium, and enlargement of the type II alveolar lining cells with bizarre alterations in the nucleus. Clinically, the reaction presents as insidious onset of nonproductive cough, dyspnoea, and fever over a period of days to weeks. Pulmonary reactions are dose-related, being more likely when more than 450 units have been given, although reactions have occurred with doses of less than 150 units; reactions are also more common in patients over 70 years of age. Radiotherapy or administration of oxygen exacerbates the reaction and it has been suggested that lung injury is mediated by drug-induced peroxide and superoxide oxygen radicals.— E. C. Rosenow *et al., Mayo Clin. Proc.*, 1985, *60*, 473. For results suggesting that combination with other antineoplastic agents may enhance the pulmonary toxicity of bleomycin, see K. A. Bauer *et al., Am. J. Med.*, 1983, *74*, 557.

Three patients developed hypersensitivity pneumonitis after treatment with bleomycin. Since all the patients responded to therapy with prednisone it was suggested that hypersensitivity pneumonitis induced by bleomycin should be regarded as a separate entity from interstitial pneumonitis which seldom responds to treatment with corticosteroids.— P. Y. Holoye *et al., Ann. intern. Med.*, 1978, *88*, 47.

EFFECTS ON THE VASCULAR SYSTEM. Raynaud's symptoms developed in a patient 3 and 7 months after treatment with bleomycin and radiotherapy.— B. Sundstrup (letter), *Med. J. Aust.*, 1978, *2*, 266. Raynaud's phenomenon developed in a 71-year-old patient given bleomycin alone for the treatment of Kaposi's sarcoma. The patient had received a total of 240 mg of bleomycin.— D. Adoue and P. Arlet (letter), *Ann. intern. Med.*, 1984, *100*, 770.

Raynaud's phenomenon in patients receiving vinblastine and bleomycin.— N. J. Vogelzang *et al., Ann. intern. Med.*, 1981, *95*, 288; J. J. Grau *et al.* (letter), *ibid.*, 1983, *98*, 258.

See also Effects on the Nails, above.

Precautions

For reference to the precautions necessary with antineoplastic agents and immunosuppressants, see Antineoplastic Agents, p.583.

Bleomycin should be given with extreme caution to patients with renal impairment or pulmonary incapacity, in whom the risk of pulmonary toxicity is increased. Respiratory function should be monitored in all patients. Because of the risk of anaphylaxis patients with lymphomas should receive low doses initially. Elderly patients should also receive low doses.

Toxicity may be enhanced when bleomycin is given in association with radiotherapy and doses may need to be reduced.

There may be an enhanced risk of pulmonary toxicity in patients given oxygen.

In *dogs* and *monkeys* bleomycin caused skin lesions at pressure sites. It is therefore desirable to watch pressure sites carefully in patients treated with bleomycin.— J. R. Baker *et al., Toxic. appl. Pharmac.*, 1973, *25*, 190.

Protective clothing should be worn when handling urine from patients who had received bleomycin for up to 72 hours previously.— J. Harris and L. J. Dodds, *Pharm. J.*, 1985, *2*, 289.

INTERACTIONS. A report of the development of fatal pulmonary toxicity in a patient with cisplatin-induced acute renal failure given bleomycin. Renal function should be carefully monitored when bleomycin and cisplatin are given together, and the dose of bleomycin reduced as dictated by the degree of renal impairment. Administration of bleomycin by constant infusion rather than intermittent bolus may increase the therapeutic window under such circumstances.— W. M. Bennett *et al., Cancer Treat. Rep.*, 1980, *64*, 921. A further report.— P. W. C. van Barneveld *et al., Oncology*, 1984, *41*, 4.

Absorption and Fate

Bleomycin is thought to be poorly absorbed from the gastro-intestinal tract. Following parenteral administration some 60 to 70% of a dose has been reported to be excreted in urine as active drug. Most tissues, but not lung or skin, are capable of enzymic degradation of bleomycin. Bleomycin does not cross the blood-brain barrier.

Continuous intravenous infusions of bleomycin 30 mg daily for 4 to 5 days resulted in an average steady state plasma concentration of 146 ng per mL, generally in 24 hours, in 6 cancer patients and initial and terminal half-lives of 1.3 and 8.9 hours respectively were found after the termination of infusions. A similar patient, but with impaired renal function, attained a steady state plasma concentration of about 1 μg per mL and half-lives of 2 and 33 hours respectively. In patients with normal renal function about 60% of the administered dose was eliminated in the urine, probably by glomerular filtration up to 48 hours after infusion. Low concentrations of bleomycin were found in the saliva of 2 patients. Since overall plasma clearance was generally greater than renal clearance a non-renal mechanism is also important in bleomycin elimination.— A. Broughton *et al., Cancer*, 1977, *40*, 2772.

A study of the pharmacokinetics of bleomycin given by intravenous bolus injection to 9 patients with advanced cancer in a mean dose of 15 mg per m^2 body-surface. Eight patients had normal renal function and mean initial and terminal plasma half-lives were 24 minutes and 4 hours respectively; 24-hour urinary excretion accounted for about 45% of the dose in 7 patients. In one patient with moderately severe renal failure (serum creatinine of 1.5 mg per 100 mL) plasma half-lives were 74 and 624 minutes and only 12% of the dose was excreted in the urine in 24 hours.— D. S. Alberts *et al., Cancer Chemother. Pharmac.*, 1978, *1*, 177.

A study of the disposition of bleomycin in 14 children. Concentrations of bleomycin in body fluids were measured using a radioimmunoassay. After intravenous bolus injections, the mean total plasma clearance in 8 older children was similar at 44.8 mL per minute per m^2 to the figures previously reported in adults. However, the mean total plasma clearance was significantly greater at 70.5 mL per minute per m^2 in 3 children less than 3 years old. Elimination half-lives for the 2 groups were 3.1 and 3.5 hours respectively. Elimination half-life following prolonged intravenous infusion in 6 older children was 2.1 hours, and 7.9 hours in 1 with impaired renal function; total plasma clearances were a mean of 57.1, and 4.8 mL per minute per m^2. The results suggest that although the pharmacokinetics of bleomycin are the same in older children as in adults, younger children eliminate the drug significantly more rapidly.— G. C. Yee *et al., Clin. Pharmac. Ther.*, 1983, *33*, 668.

The pharmacokinetics of a suspension of bleomycin in sesame oil were compared with those of bleomycin in saline following intramuscular administration in 6 patients. Both formulations were rapidly absorbed, with mean absorption half-lives of 22 and 7 minutes respectively, to produce mean peak levels that were not significantly different. However, the elimination half-life for the oily formulation was biphasic, with a prolonged terminal half-life of 10.8 hours, whereas the saline formulation had a single mean elimination half-life of 2.5 hours, which was similar to the first phase elimination half-life after the oily suspension (1.9 hours). The clinical significance of the difference is unknown.— M. L. Slevin *et al.*, *Br. J. clin. Pharmac.*, 1983, *16*, 215P.

Uses and Administration

Bleomycin is an antineoplastic antibiotic which binds to DNA and causes strand scissions. It is used in squamous cell carcinomas, including those of the cervix and external genitalia, oesophagus, skin, and head and neck, in Hodgkin's disease and other lymphomas, and in malignant neoplasms of the testis. It has also been tried in carcinoma of the bladder, lung, and thyroid, and in the treatment of malignant effusions. Bleomycin is often used in association with other antineoplastic agents. In Hodgkin's disease it has been given with doxorubicin, vinblastine, and dacarbazine. Treatment schedules of bleomycin, vinblastine, and cisplatin are used in testicular tumours. See also under Choice of Antineoplastic Agent, p.584.

Tumour localisation may be carried out with a complex of bleomycin and indium-111; a complex with cobalt-57 has also been used.

Bleomycin sulphate may be administered by subcutaneous, intramuscular, intravenous, or intra-arterial injection; it has also been instilled intrapleurally or intraperitoneally. In the treatment of squamous cell carcinoma and testicular tumours, the usual *UK* dose is 15 to 60 mg of bleomycin weekly in divided doses depending on age, elderly patients being given doses in the lower range. A continuous intravenous infusion of 15 mg per 24 hours for up to 10 days, or 30 mg per 24 hours for up to 5 days has also been used. Patients with lymphomas may be given 15 mg by intramuscular injection once or twice a week, up to a total dose of 225 mg; these doses should be reduced in the elderly. See also under Precautions, above.

In the *US*, doses are expressed in units that can be considered to be equivalent to milligrams of bleomycin; recommended doses are 0.25 to 0.5 units per kg body-weight, or 10 to 20 units per m^2 body-surface area, given once or twice weekly. In patients with Hodgkin's disease once a 50% response has been achieved it may be maintained with 1 unit of bleomycin daily, or 5 units weekly.

Doses may require adjustment when given in combination with other antineoplastic agents, or with radiotherapy.

If intramuscular injections are painful they may be given in a 1% solution of lignocaine.

Reviews of bleomycin: H. Umezawa, *Lloydia*, 1977, *40*, 67; J. M. Bennett and S. D. Reich, *Ann. intern. Med.*, 1979, *90*, 945.

ACTION. The influence of acronine, bleomycin, and cytarabine, alone and combined with radiation, on the cell cycle.— S. B. Reddy *et al.*, *Arzneimittel-Forsch.*, 1977, *27*, 1549.

Lowering of copper concentrations does not affect the toxicity of bleomycin towards whole cells, therefore an alternate explanation must be found for enhancement of the cytotoxic effect of bleomycin by prior administration of penicillamine.— J. Lunec and A. D. Nunn (letter), *Lancet*, 1979, *2*, 739. The effects of iron, copper, cobalt, and their chelators on bleomycin cytotoxicity.— P. -S. Lin *et al.*, *Cancer Res.*, 1983, *43*, 1049.

Heat enhances the effect of some cytotoxic drugs, such as bleomycin *in vivo* and *in vitro*. If heating can be confined to the tumour then theoretically this combination could provide selective toxicity. The results so far reported with radiofrequency hyperthermia are sufficiently promising to merit further investigation.— *Lancet*, 1984, *1*, 885.

An assay for the quantitative measurement of single- and double-strand breakage of DNA in *Escherichia coli* incubated with bleomycin or the structurally related compound talisomycin.— C. K. Mirabelli *et al.*, *Antimicrob. Ag. Chemother.*, 1985, *27*, 460.

ADMINISTRATION. *In renal failure.* The dose of bleomycin should be reduced to 50% when the glomerular filtration-rate is less than 10 mL per minute. Bleomycin is not removed by haemodialysis.— W. M. Bennett *et al.*, *Am. J. Kidney Dis.*, 1983, *3*, 155. Lung toxicity has occurred at low total doses of bleomycin in patients with transient minor episodes of renal dysfunction. Substitution of bleomycin for methotrexate in the treatment of large-cell lymphoma with the MACOP-B regimen (methotrexate, doxorubicin, cyclophosphamide, vincristine, prednisone, bleomycin) in patients with a creatinine clearance of less than 60 mL per minute was considered to be unwise.— V. J. Harvey and P. I. Thompson (letter), *Ann. intern. Med.*, 1986, *105*, 976.

BLOOD DISORDERS, NON-MALIGNANT. Autoimmune cytopenia in 2 patients with lymphomas in remission was successfully treated with bleomycin after conventional therapy had failed.— E. A. Phillips *et al.* (letter), *New Engl. J. Med.*, 1980, *302*, 1031.

HYPERCALCAEMIA. Bleomycin was associated with rapid normalisation of serum-calcium concentrations when administered either as a continuous intravenous infusion or an intravenous bolus injection to 3 patients with hypercalcaemia due to malignancies (metastatic squamous cell carcinoma or lymphoma). In one patient the resulting normalisation of serum calcium was maintained for about 5 months. The results suggest that bleomycin may be a potent anti-hypercalcaemic agent; this action was not linked to any effect on tumour progression.— T. Nijjar and L. J. Brandes (letter), *New Engl. J. Med.*, 1983, *308*, 655.

MALIGNANT EFFUSIONS. Preliminary results of a multicentre study involving 153 patients indicate that bleomycin is well tolerated and is effective as palliative treatment of malignant effusions. Aspiration of effusions was followed by an intracavitary injection of 30 to 150 mg of bleomycin in 100 mL of physiological saline; the most usual dose was 60 mg. An overall response-rate of 58% was attained in 117 evaluable patients; pleural effusions responding better (63%) than peritoneal effusions (49%). The two most common side-effects were fever (8%) and pain at the the site of injection (10%).— M. J. Ostrowski and G. M. Halsall (letter), *Br. med. J.*, 1980, *281*, 64. Intracavitary administration of bleomycin, in total doses of 15 to 240 mg, is painless, relatively nontoxic, but expensive; tetracycline is probably the agent of choice.— D. P. Dhillon and S. G. Spiro, *Br. J. Hosp. Med.*, 1983, *29*, 506.

See also under Choice of Antineoplastic Agent, p.588.

MALIGNANT NEOPLASMS. A report of the treatment of verrucous squamous-cell carcinoma of the oesophagus with intravenous bleomycin. Bleomycin produced prompt relief of symptoms and a reduction in tumour size; the total dose administered was 150 mg.— T. Sakurai *et al.*, *Postgrad. med. J.*, 1983, *59*, 578.

SKIN DISORDERS. References to the use of bleomycin in skin disorders: M. Hagedorn *et al.*, *Archs Derm.*, 1978, *114*, 1083 (florid oral papillomatosis); W. G. Watring *et al.*, *Cancer*, 1978, *41*, 10 (topical application for Paget's disease of the vulva); S. Sayama and H. Tagami, *Br. J. Derm.*, 1983, *109*, 449 (intralesional bleomycin to treat keratoacanthoma).

TRYPANOSOMIASIS. Bleomycin or eflornithine alone were ineffective in curing *mice* infected with *Trypanosoma brucei brucei* and with CNS involvement, but a combination of bleomycin with eflornithine 1% achieved 100% cure-rate.— A. B. Clarkson *et al.*, *Proc. natn. Acad. Sci. U.S.A.*, 1983, *80*, 5729.

WARTS. A report of the successful use of intralesional injections of bleomycin in the treatment of warts. An overall cure-rate of more than 99% was achieved when bleomycin was injected into the base of 1052 warts, including mosaic, plantar, common, plane, and eponychial warts. An injection of 0.1 mL of a solution of bleomycin 1 mg per mL in physiological saline was repeated every 4 weeks, if necessary, to a maximum total dose of 2 mg.— P. H. Shumack and M. J. Haddock, *Aust. J. Derm.*, 1979, *20*, 41. In a study involving 62 patients, 0.1 mL of a solution of bleomycin 0.1% in physiological saline, or in oil, injected into 22 and 36 warts respectively, and repeated 3 times at 2-weekly intervals achieved cure rates of only 18 and 23%, compared with 42% for saline alone and 43% for oil alone. Adverse effects, including dullness, pain, swelling, and bleeding were observed in 19 of 62 patients. The use of bleomycin in the treatment of warts could not be recommended.— M. Munkvad *et al.*, *Dermatologica*, 1983, *167*, 86.

Bleomycin sulphate solution injected in very small doses into resistant warts has proved highly successful. Systemic side-effects have not been experienced and would not be expected with the doses used. The pain associated with the haemorrhagic necrosis of the wart can be tolerated with the aid of an analgesic, and careful injections leave no scarring. Isolated cases of local complications have been reported but are not generally experienced.— M. H. Bunney, *Br. med. J.*, 1986, *293*, 1045.

Further references to the use of bleomycin in the treatment of warts: M. H. Bunney *et al.*, *Br. J. Derm.*, 1984, *111*, 197 (intralesional injection); M. Takigawa *et al.*, *Archs Derm.*, 1985, *121*, 1108 (use of pressure-sensitive adhesive tape containing bleomycin sulphate).

Preparations

Sterile Bleomycin Sulfate *(U.S.P.)*. Bleomycin sulphate suitable for parenteral use. It contains 1.5 to 2 units of bleomycin per mg.

Proprietary Names and Manufacturers

Blenoxane *(Bristol-Myers, Austral.; Bristol, Canad.; Bristol, S. Afr.; Bristol-Myers Oncology, USA)*; Bleo Oil *(Jpn)*; Bleo-S *(Jpn)*; Blocamicina *(Arg.)*; Verbublen *(Canad.)*. Manufacturers also include — *Lundbeck, UK.*

1816-c

Broxuridine *(rINN)*.

BUDR; NSC-38297. 5-Bromo-2′-deoxyuridine; 5-Bromo-1-(2-deoxy-β-D-ribofuranosyl)pyrimidine-2,4(1*H*,3*H*)-dione.

$C_9H_{11}BrN_2O_5$=307.1.

CAS — 59-14-3.

Broxuridine is a thymidine analogue which exerts its antineoplastic action by interfering with normal DNA synthesis. It is claimed to enhance the effects of radiotherapy. It is also reported to possess antiviral activity.

Broxuridine has been given by intra-arterial infusion, in association with radiotherapy and other antineoplastic agents, in the treatment of tumours of the brain, head, and neck. It has also been given by the intraventricular route.

Broxuridine was given as a radiosensitiser in doses of 350 to 700 mg per m^2 body-surface daily to 8 patients with malignant gliomas. Each dose was given by intravenous infusion over 12 hours and repeated daily for up to 14 days; the course was repeated after 2 weeks. The patients underwent concomitant radiotherapy over a 7-week period. Some antitumour response was noted but overall efficacy was low, and dose-limiting myelotoxicity occurred in almost all patients; however there was evidence from bone-marrow samples of radiation enhancement by up to a factor of 2.2 at high plasma concentrations. Results suggested that intra-carotid arterial infusion would be more effective than intravenous infusion providing that new technology could overcome the complications of prolonged intra-arterial administration.— A. Russo *et al.*, *Cancer Res.*, 1984, *44*, 1702.

Proprietary Names and Manufacturers

Radibud *(Takeda, Jpn)*.

1817-k

Busulphan *(BAN)*.

Busulfan *(USAN, rINN)*; Busulfanum; CB-2041; GT-41; Myelosan; NSC-750; WR-19508. Tetramethylene di(methanesulphonate); Butane-1,4-diol di(methanesulphonate).

$C_6H_{14}O_6S_2$=246.3.

CAS — 55-98-1.

Pharmacopoeias. In *Br., Chin., Cz., Egypt., Eur., Fr., Ind., Int., It., Jpn, Jug., Nord., Rus., Turk.*, and *U.S.*

A white crystalline powder. The *B.P.* states that it is **soluble** in water and in alcohol; soluble 1 in 25 of acetone. The *U.S.P.* gives a solubility of 1 in 45 of acetone.

Store in airtight containers. Protect from light.

CAUTION. *Busulphan is irritant; avoid contact with skin and mucous membranes.*

Adverse Effects and Treatment

For an outline of the adverse effects experienced with antineoplastic agents and immunosuppressants and general guidelines for their treatment, see Antineoplastic Agents, p.580 and p.583.

The most important side-effects of busulphan in high dosage are leukopenia, thrombocytopenia, and haemorrhage symptoms. Large doses may also cause irreversible or extremely prolonged bone-marrow depression which may not become apparent for several months after the initiation of therapy. The nadir of granulocytes has been reported at 11 to 30 days with recovery occurring over up to 5 months.

Interstitial pulmonary fibrosis, known as 'busulphan lung', and cataract formation can occur on prolonged treatment as can hyperpigmentation which may be part of a syndrome simulating Addison's disease.

Busulphan may result in impaired fertility and gonadal function. As with other alkylating agents, it is potentially carcinogenic and teratogenic.

EFFECTS ON THE BLADDER. Haemorrhagic cystitis occurred in a patient who had received prolonged therapy with busulphan.— D. Pode *et al., J. Urol., Baltimore,* 1983, *130,* 347.

EFFECTS ON THE EYES. Busulphan is known to cause cataracts in *animals;* posterior subcapsular lens opacities and early lens changes in patients with chronic granulocytic leukaemia have been associated with the duration of disease and treatment with busulphan.— S. M. Podos and G. P. Canellos, *Am. J. Ophthal.,* 1969, *68,* 500. See also M. P. Ravindranathan *et al., Br. med. J.,* 1972, *1,* 218 (bilateral cataracts in a patient given busulphan for about 4 years); Y. Sidi *et al., J. Am. med. Ass.,* 1977, *238,* 1951 (bilateral cataracts and severe sicca syndrome in a patient given busulphan for 9 years).

EFFECTS ON THE LIVER. Jaundice in the terminal phase of chronic granulocytic leukaemia in a 31-year-old man was attributed to busulphan which had been taken for 6 years.— J. C. E. Underwood *et al.* (letter), *Br. med. J.,* 1971, *1,* 556.

Busulphan toxicity involving the liver, with 'busulphan lung', in an elderly man who had taken busulphan for 54 months for myeloid leukaemia, might have been a contributory factor in the development of portal hypertension.— M. D. Foadi *et al., Postgrad. med. J.,* 1977, *53,* 267.

EFFECTS ON THE NERVOUS SYSTEM. Two of 5 patients given high-dose busulphan as part of a conditioning regimen before bone-marrow transplantation had central complications, with loss of consciousness in one and convulsions in the other. The use of anticonvulsants is recommended in regimens containing high-dose busulphan.— R. E. Marcus and J. M. Goldman (letter), *Lancet,* 1984, *2,* 1463. Experience with children given high doses of busulphan suggests that prophylactic anticonvulsants are not needed routinely.— K. Hugh-Jones and P. J. Shaw (letter), *ibid.,* 1985, *1,* 220. Control of convulsions with phenytoin.— B. Thalayasingam (letter), *ibid.,* 818. A report of the development of myoclonic epilepsy in a patient given high-dose busulphan.— R. W. Martell *et al.* (letter), *Ann. intern. Med.,* 1987, *106,* 173.

Precautions

For reference to the precautions necessary with antineoplastic agents and immunosuppressants, see Antineoplastic Agents, p.583.

Since secondary gout occurred in up to 10% of patients with polycythaemia vera given busulphan, allopurinol was recommended for routine prophylaxis.— *Drug & Ther. Bull.,* 1975, *13,* 73.

Severe cutaneous reactions occurred in patients given radiotherapy at least 30 days after combined chemotherapy with high-dose busulphan.— G. Vassal *et al.* (letter), *Lancet,* 1987, *1,* 571.

HANDLING AND DISPOSAL. Protective clothing was probably unnecessary when handling urine and faeces from patients who were receiving busulphan.— J. Harris and L. J. Dodds, *Pharm. J.,* 1985, *2,* 289.

PORPHYRIA. Busulphan was considered to be unsafe in patients with acute porphyria because it has been shown to be porphyrinogenic in *animals* or *in-vitro* systems.— M.R. Moore and K.E.L. McColl, *Porphyrias, Drug Lists,* Glasgow, Porphyria Research Unit, University of Glasgow, 1987.

Absorption and Fate

Busulphan is readily absorbed from the gastro-intestinal tract and rapidly disappears from the blood. It is largely excreted in the urine as sulphur-containing metabolites.

Studies of the pharmacokinetics of busulphan: P. W. Feit and N. Rastrup-Anderson, *J. pharm. Sci.,* 1973, *62,* 1007 (metabolism); H. Ehrsson *et al., Clin. Pharmac. Ther.,* 1983, *34,* 86 (study of the pharmacokinetics using gas chromatography); H. Ehrsson and M. Hassan, *J. Pharm. Pharmac.,* 1984, *36,* 694 (protein-binding).

Uses and Administration

Busulphan is an antineoplastic agent, with a cell-cycle nonspecific alkylating action unlike that of the nitrogen mustards, and having a selective depressant action on bone marrow. In small doses, it depresses granulocytopoiesis and to a lesser extent thrombocytopoiesis but has little effect on lymphocytes. With larger doses, severe bone-marrow depression eventually ensues.

Because of its selective action, busulphan is used in the palliative treatment of chronic granulocytic (myeloid) leukaemia. It provides symptomatic relief with a reduction in spleen size and a general feeling of well-being. The fall in leucocyte count is usually accompanied by a rise in the haemoglobin concentration. Permanent remission is not induced.

Busulphan has been used in patients with polycythaemia vera who are resistant to phosphorus-32, and in some patients with myelofibrosis and primary thrombocythaemia.

See also under Choice of Antineoplastic Agent, p.584.

The usual dosage of busulphan in chronic myeloid leukaemia is 60 µg per kg body-weight daily by mouth, up to a maximum single dose of 4 mg. This is continued until the white cell count has fallen to between 20 000 and 25 000 per mm^3. It should be discontinued earlier if the platelet count falls below 100 000 per mm^3. Higher doses may be given if the response after 3 weeks is inadequate; 6 to 8 mg or more daily has been given in refractory cases but this increases the risk of irreversible damage to the bone marrow and calls for special vigilance. Children may be given 60 µg per kg once daily.

Large doses cause a rapid fall in granulocytes but with small doses this may not occur for several weeks. Complete blood counts should be made every week and the trends followed closely; if haemorrhagic tendencies occur or there is a steep fall in the white cell count indicating severe bone-marrow depression, busulphan should be withdrawn until marrow function has returned.

Maintenance treatment with doses of 0.5 to 2 mg daily may be given, especially when remission is shorter than 3 months, the aim being to maintain a white cell count of 10 000 to 15 000 per mm^3. Alternatively treatment may be discontinued until the count reaches 50 000 per mm^3.

ADMINISTRATION IN RENAL INSUFFICIENCY. Busulphan could be given in usual doses to patients with renal insufficiency.— W. M. Bennett *et al., Am. J. Kidney Dis.,* 1983, *3,* 155.

LEUKAEMIAS, CHRONIC. For the use of busulphan in the treatment of chronic granulocytic leukaemia, see Choice of Antineoplastic Agent, p.587.

MYELOPROLIFERATIVE DISORDERS. For reference to the use of busulphan and thioguanine in patients with myelofibrosis, see thioguanine, p.652.

ORGAN AND TISSUE TRANSPLANTATION. For a report of the use of high-dose busulphan and cyclophosphamide for bone-marrow conditioning before bone-marrow transplantation for beta-thalassaemia, see under Cyclophosphamide, p.613.

Preparations

Busulfan Tablets *(U.S.P.).* Tablets containing busulphan.

Busulphan Tablets *(B.P.)*

Proprietary Preparations

Myleran *(Calmic, UK). Tablets,* busulphan 0.5 and 2 mg.

Proprietary Names and Manufacturers

Misulban *(Ital.; Techni-Pharma, Mon.);* Myleran *(Wellcome, Austral.; Belg.; Wellcome, Canad.; Wellcome, Denm.; Wellcome, Ger.; Wellcome, Ital.; Neth.; Wellcome, Norw.; Wellcome, S.Afr.; Wellcome, Swed.; Wellcome, Switz.; Calmic, UK; Wellcome, USA).*

16564-f

Carboplatin *(BAN, USAN, rINN).*

CBDCA; JM-8; NSC-241240. *cis*-Diammine(cyclobutane-1,1-dicarboxylato)platinum.

$C_6H_{12}N_2O_4Pt$=371.3.

CAS — 41575-94-4.

Adverse Effects and Precautions

As for cisplatin (p.607); nephrotoxicity and gastrointestinal toxicity are reported to be less severe than with cisplatin. A reversible myelosuppression is the dose-limiting toxicity; platelet counts reach a nadir between 14 and 21 days after a dose, with recovery within 35 days, but recovery from leucopenia may be slower.

Analysis by the manufacturers of the adverse effects of carboplatin, in studies involving 710 patients. Myelosuppression was the dose-limiting toxicity: leucopenia occurred in 55% of the evaluable patients. Leucopenia and thrombocytopenia result in symptomatic events such as infection or bleeding in a minority of patients. Anaemia was frequent (59%) and required transfusional support in about one-fifth of the patients. Nephrotoxicity and serum electrolyte loss were extremely reduced in intensity; no high-volume fluid hydration or electrolyte supplementation was given during treatment. Vomiting occurred in about half the patients, and a further 25% had nausea without vomiting. Peripheral neurotoxicity was reported in 6% of evaluable patients and clinical ototoxicity occurred in only 8 cases (about 1%). Increases in liver enzyme values have also been reported, as well as, more rarely, alopecia, skin rash, a flu-like syndrome, and local effects at the injection site.— R. Canetta *et al., Cancer Treat. Rev.,* 1985, *12, Suppl.* A, 125.

Uses and Administration

Carboplatin is an analogue of cisplatin with similar actions and uses (see p.608). It is used in the treatment of advanced ovarian cancers and of small-cell lung cancer, both alone and combined with other antineoplastic agents. It has also been tried in other solid tumours, including those of the bladder, cervix, and testes.

Carboplatin is given in usual doses of 400 mg per m^2 body-surface area by intravenous infusion over 15 minutes to 1 hour. Doses should not be given more frequently than every 4 weeks, and should be reduced in patients at risk of myelosuppression. Lower doses may also be given as part of combination regimens.

Reviews and studies of carboplatin: A. H. Calvert *et al., Cancer Chemother. Pharmac.,* 1982, *9,* 140; M. Rozencweig *et al., J. clin. Oncol.,* 1983, *1,* 621; A. H. Calvert *et al., Cancer Treat. Rev.,* 1985, *12, Suppl.* A, 51; R. Canetta *et al., ibid.,* 125; *Drug & Ther. Bull.,* 1987, *25,* 67.

ABSORPTION AND FATE. Following administration of radiolabelled carboplatin to 4 patients the majority of the dose was rapidly cleared from the blood, and largely excreted in urine within 6 hours. The remaining activity was eliminated in a biphasic manner, with mean half-lives of 2.5 hours and about 5 days. The rate of binding to plasma protein was significantly lower than that which occurs with cisplatin, perhaps accounting for the greater proportion of free material available for rapid excretion; the degree of urinary excretion indicates less organ retention than cisplatin.— H. Sharma *et al., Cancer Chemother. Pharmac.,* 1983, *11,* 5.

The pharmacokinetics of carboplatin in patients with normal and impaired renal function. Total and renal clearance of free platinum were strongly correlated with glomerular filtration-rate and patients with impaired renal function (glomerular filtration-rate less than 60 mL per minute) should have the dose of carboplatin reduced to avoid undue toxicity.— S. J. Harland *et al., Cancer Res.,* 1984, *44,* 1693.

ADMINISTRATION IN RENAL FAILURE. The manufacturers recommended that carboplatin should not be given to patients whose creatinine clearance rate is 20 mL per minute or below.

See also under Absorption and Fate, above.

MALIGNANT NEOPLASMS OF THE CERVIX. Preliminary results of an ongoing multicentre study comparing carboplatin 400 mg per m^2 with iproplatin 300 mg per m^2, both given as a 30-minute intravenous infusion every 4 weeks, indicated that both agents had activity against recurrent or metastatic cervical carcinoma.— F. M. Muggia *et al.*, *Cancer Treat. Rev.*, 1985, *12, Suppl.* A, 93.

MALIGNANT NEOPLASMS OF THE LUNG. Five of 56 patients achieved complete response and 18 a partial response following treatment with carboplatin in doses of 250 to 400 mg per m^2 every 4 weeks for small-cell lung cancer. Three of those achieving complete response and 15 of those achieving partial response were among the 30 who had not received previous chemotherapy. The median duration of response was 4.5 months for both previously treated and untreated patients and the longest response was for more than 20 months; median duration of survival was 5 months overall, but 8 months in previously untreated patients. The results suggest that carboplatin may be an important new drug in the treatment of small-cell lung cancer.— I. E. Smith *et al.*, *Cancer Treat. Rep.*, 1985, *69*, 43. In a subsequent study, 36 patients received intravenous combination chemotherapy with carboplatin 300 mg per m^2 on day 1, and etoposide 100 mg per m^2 on days 1 to 3, repeated monthly for 4 courses. Of the 23 patients with limited disease, who also received local radiotherapy or surgery, 7 achieved complete response and 13 a partial response. Of the remaining 13 patients, who had extensive disease, 12 achieved a response but there were no complete remissions; median duration of response was 6 months. The median duration of response in patients with limited disease has not yet been reached.— I. E. Smith and B. D. Evans, *Cancer Treat. Rev.*, 1985, *12, Suppl.* A, 73.

MALIGNANT NEOPLASMS OF THE NERVES. A report of a striking response to carboplatin treatment in a patient with metastatic paraganglioma, a rare tumour arising from the paraganglionic cells of the autonomic nervous system.— F. Cairnduff and I. E. Smith (letter), *Lancet*, 1986, *2*, 982.

See also under Neuroblastoma, below.

MALIGNANT NEOPLASMS OF THE OESOPHAGUS. Two of 30 patients with epidermoid carcinoma of the oesophagus achieved complete remission following treatment with carboplatin 400 mg per m^2 by intravenous infusion over 1 hour once a month. Infusion of 500 mL of 5% glucose in 0.45% sodium chloride solution was carried out before and after therapy, and the dose of carboplatin was reduced to 300 mg per m^2 in patients who had received previous therapy, due to thrombocytopenia. Although the response rate was low, achievement of 2 complete remissions, which are rare in these patients, and which lasted 7 and 16 months respectively, suggest that carboplatin warrants further study in combination with other agents.— C. Sternberg *et al.*, *Cancer Treat. Rep.*, 1985, *69*, 1305.

MALIGNANT NEOPLASMS OF THE OVARY. In a phase II study in patients with advanced ovarian carcinoma comprising 33 patients with recurrent disease who had received previous chemotherapy, including cisplatin, and a further 3 with no previous treatment, patients received carboplatin in doses of 200 to 300 mg per m^2 repeated at monthly intervals up to a maximum of 9 courses. Of the pretreated patients 28 were evaluable: 2 of these achieved complete response and 5 a partial response, while one of the previously untreated patients achieved a complete and one a partial response. Duration of responses was between 3 and 7 months. The response rate of 25% overall in heavily pretreated patients suggests that carboplatin is active in advanced ovarian cancer. The fact that 4 of the responders had not responded to previous cisplatin suggests that carboplatin may sometimes be effective against cisplatin-resistant tumours.— B. D. Evans *et al.*, *Cancer Treat. Rep.*, 1983, *67*, 997.

Early results of a prospective randomised study comparing cisplatin therapy with carboplatin 400 mg per m^2 monthly for 10 months in patients with advanced ovarian carcinoma. Three of 21 patients given cisplatin and 3 of 18 given carboplatin had achieved a complete response; figures for partial response were 8 and 6 respectively. Although the response rates were similar with both drugs carboplatin appeared to be much better tolerated.— E. Wiltshaw *et al.* (letter), *Lancet*, 1983, *1*, 587.

MALIGNANT NEOPLASMS OF THE TESTIS. Encouraging preliminary results with carboplatin alone or combined with bleomycin, and etoposide or vinblastine, in patients with a variety of advanced testicular germ-cell tumours.— M. J. Peckham *et al.*, *Cancer Treat. Rev.*, 1985, *12, Suppl.* A, 101.

NEUROBLASTOMA. A report of the use of carboplatin, in doses of 200 to 500 mg per m^2, in the treatment of 3 children with neuroblastoma. The drug was generally well tolerated, and no deterioration in renal or auditory function was noted, but treatment was stopped because of disease progression.— J. Pritchard *et al.* (letter), *Lancet*, 1987, *1*, 214.

Proprietary Preparations

Paraplatin *(Bristol-Myers, UK). Injection,* powder for reconstitution, carboplatin 150 mg.

Proprietary Names and Manufacturers

Paraplatin *(Bristol, Canad.; Bristol-Myers, UK)*; Paraplatine *(Bristol, Switz.)*.

1818-a

Carboquone *(rINN)*.

Carbazilquone. 2,5-Bis(aziridin-1-yl)-3-(2-hydroxy-1-methoxyethyl)-6-methyl-*p*-benzoquinone carbamate.

$C_{15}H_{19}N_3O_5$=321.3.

CAS — 24279-91-2.

Carboquone is an alkylating agent (see p.580) which has been used in the treatment of malignant diseases.

Proprietary Names and Manufacturers

Esquinon *(Sankyo, Jpn)*.

18912-t

Carmofur *(rINN)*.

HCFU. 5-Fluoro-*N*-hexyl-3,4-dihydro-2,4-dioxo-1-(2*H*)-pyrimidinecarboxamide.

$C_{11}H_{16}FN_3O_3$=257.3.

CAS — 61422-45-5.

Carmofur is a derivative of fluorouracil (see p.628) and has similar actions. It is given by mouth in the treatment of malignant neoplasms of the gastro-intestinal tract.

Reference: T. Taguchi, *Recent Results Cancer Res.*, 1980, *70*, 125.

Proprietary Names and Manufacturers

Mifurol *(Mitsui, Jpn)*; Yamaful *(Yamanouchi, Jpn)*.

1819-t

Carmustine *(BAN, USAN, rINN)*.

BCNU; NSC-409962; WR-139021. 1,3-Bis(2-chloroethyl)-1-nitrosourea.

$C_5H_9Cl_2N_3O_2$=214.1.

CAS — 154-93-8.

The manufacturers state that carmustine must be stored at 2° to 8°. It has a low melting-point (approximately 27°) and exposure to this or higher temperatures will cause the drug to liquefy and decompose.

Solutions for injection may be prepared by dissolving 100 mg of carmustine in 3 mL of absolute alcohol and adding 27 mL of Water for Injections to produce a clear colourless solution with a pH of 5.6 to 6.0. When reconstituted as directed and stored at room temperature approximately 6% of the drug solution decomposes in 3 hours; storage at 4° increases stability with about 4% decomposition in 24 hours. When further diluted with sodium chloride injection (0.9%) or glucose injection (5%) the resulting solution is stated to be stable for 48 hours if protected from light and stored at 4°.

There was no appreciable decomposition of carmustine 100 µg per mL in sodium chloride (0.9%) or glucose (5%) injections when stored for 90 minutes at room temperature; however, addition of 10 mmol of sodium bicarbonate increased the rate of degradation, so that only approximately 73% of the active drug remained after 90 minutes. The results indicate that carmustine should not be admixed with sodium bicarbonate infusions or given through a common line with such infusions.— M. Colvin *et al.*, *Am. J. Hosp. Pharm.*, 1980, *37*, 677.

Adverse Effects and Treatment

For an outline of the adverse effects experienced with antineoplastic agents and immunosuppressants and general guidelines for their treatment, see Antineoplastic Agents, p.580 and p.583.

Delayed and cumulative bone-marrow depression is the most frequent and serious side-effect of carmustine. Platelets and leucocytes are affected with platelet nadirs occurring at 4 to 5 weeks after administration and leucocyte nadirs at 5 to 6 weeks after administration; although thrombocytopenia is usually more severe, leucopenia may also be dose-limiting. Other side-effects reported include pulmonary fibrosis, renal and hepatic damage, and optic neuritis. Venous irritation may follow intravenous injection and transient hyperpigmentation has been noted after contact of a solution with the skin. Flushing of the skin and suffusion of the conjunctiva may occur following rapid intravenous infusion.

As with other alkylating agents, carmustine is potentially carcinogenic, mutagenic, and teratogenic.

CARCINOGENICITY. A report of 2 cases of acute nonlymphoblastic leukaemia among 1628 patients treated with carmustine for brain tumours, a more than 24-fold increase over the expected figure. No leukaemic disorders were observed in patients treated with surgery, with or without radiation, or with other chemotherapeutic agents. The results suggest that carmustine is a leukaemogen.— M. H. Greene *et al.* (letter), *New Engl. J. Med.*, 1985, *313*, 579. A report of a patient with carmustine-induced myelodysplasia. The nitrosoureas should be added to the list of drugs considered leukaemogenic in humans and should be used with caution.— S. M. Lichtman and P. Schulman (letter), *Ann. intern. Med.*, 1985, *103*, 964.

EFFECTS ON THE EYES. A report of ocular toxicity in 2 of 50 patients given high-dose intravenous carmustine, and in 7 of 10 given intra-arterial infusions via the carotid.— B. J. Shingleton *et al.*, *Archs Ophthal., N.Y.*, 1982, *100*, 1766. A further report of severe retinal toxicity and blindness in patients receiving intra-arterial carotid infusions of carmustine. The incidence of ocular toxicity was reduced from 38% to 7% when the alcohol concentration in the diluent was reduced.— H. S. Greenberg *et al.*, *J. Neurosurg.*, 1984, *61*, 423.

EFFECTS ON RESPIRATORY FUNCTION. A review of pulmonary fibrosis associated with the nitrosoureas. Carmustine is now well established as a potentially fatal pulmonary toxin and should be viewed with the same caution as bleomycin. The cumulative dose at which toxicity becomes a serious risk is 1.2 to 1.5 g per m^2 body-surface but patients on a high-dose regimen are at greater risk. Pre-existing lung disease, thoracic irradiation, oxygen therapy, and concomitant administration of other drugs with a toxic effect on the lung increase the risk, but age does not appear to be a risk factor. Few cases of toxicity with semustine have been reported, and none with lomustine, perhaps because patients have not received high-enough cumulative doses to cause it. Fibrosing alveolitis and interstitial pneumonitis have been reported for chlorozotocin but not with streptozocin. It is likely that some pulmonary toxicity will be seen with PCNU as more experience is gained.— R. B. Weiss *et al.*, *Cancer Treat. Rev.*, 1981, *8*, 111.

Precautions

For reference to the precautions necessary with antineoplastic agents and immunosuppressants, see Antineoplastic Agents, p.583.

A suggestion that, if the long-term use of nitrosoureas is being considered, creatinine clearance should be measured periodically and renal size monitored frequently.— W. E. Harmon *et al.* (letter), *New Engl. J. Med.*, 1979, *301*, 662.

HANDLING AND DISPOSAL. A study of the permeability of latex and polyvinyl chloride gloves to carmustine concluded that the materials tested offered only limited protection against contact exposure to carmustine. Permeation increased with time, and the mean amount of carmustine that passed through a single thickness of glove material by 90 minutes ranged from 53 to 86 µg. No one type of glove was clearly superior, but when two thicknesses of gloves were used the thicker polyvinyl chloride gloves were slightly better.— T. H. Connor *et al.*, *Am. J. Hosp. Pharm.*, 1984, *41*, 676. See also P. H. Thomas and V. Fenton-May, *Pharm. J.*, 1987, *1*, 775.

INTERACTIONS. Reductions in white cell counts and platelet counts well below those normally attributed to treatment with carmustine alone were seen in 6 of 8 patients receiving their first course of carmustine and steroids in association with cimetidine given prophylactically.— R. G. Selker *et al.* (letter), *New Engl. J. Med.*, 1978, *299*, 834.

Absorption and Fate

Carmustine is readily absorbed from the gastro-intestinal tract. It is rapidly metabolised, with an estimated half-life of less than 15 minutes; metabolites have a much longer half-life. It is excreted in the urine, mostly as metabolites; some is also excreted as carbon dioxide, via the lungs. Carmustine diffuses very readily into the cerebrospinal fluid, appearing almost immediately after intravenous injection. Very small amounts have been detected in the faeces.

A review of the pharmacokinetics of some antineoplastic agents, including the nitrosoureas carmustine, lomustine, and semustine.— F. M. Balis *et al.*, *Clin. Pharmacokinet.*, 1983, *8*, 202.

Uses and Administration

Carmustine is a cell-cycle phase nonspecific antineoplastic agent belonging to the nitrosourea group of compounds, which are considered to function as alkylating agents. It has been used in the treatment of brain tumours, and has also been tried as an adjunct in meningeal leukaemia, and in combination chemotherapy for multiple myeloma, Hodgkin's disease, and other lymphomas. See also under Choice of Antineoplastic Agent, p.584.

Carmustine is given intravenously as a single dose of 200 mg per m^2 body-surface or divided into doses of 100 mg per m^2 given on 2 successive days. Lower doses are given in combination therapy. Doses are repeated every 6 weeks provided that blood counts have returned to acceptable levels, that is, platelets above 100 000 per mm^3 and leucocytes above 4 000 per mm^3. Subsequent doses must be adjusted according to the haematological response. Reconstituted solutions are further diluted with sodium chloride (0.9%) or glucose (5%) injection and infused over 1 to 2 hours.

MALIGNANT NEOPLASMS OF THE BRAIN. A report by M.D. Walker *et al.* (*J. Neurosurg.*, 1978, *49*, 333) concluded that patients with malignant glioma who received radiotherapy, with or without carmustine, had a significantly improved survival over those receiving only carmustine or only supportive care. In the randomised study now reported the relative benefits of radiotherapy and nitrosoureas, after surgery, were investigated further and 4 treatment regimens, semustine alone, radiotherapy alone, carmustine and radiotherapy, and semustine and radiotherapy, were compared in 358 patients. The results confirmed the benefits of radiotherapy in the treatment of malignant glioma and suggested that carmustine remains the drug of choice for chemotherapy. Semustine alone was inferior to regimens that included radiotherapy, as was carmustine previously, and semustine in combination with radiotherapy provided no advantage over carmustine and radiotherapy. Whether nitrosourea combined with radiotherapy is better than radiotherapy alone is not certain. Corticosteroids are virtually mandatory for symptomatic control in patients with malignant brain tumours but an oncolytic effect has not yet been demonstrated; preliminary results of a study of intermittent high-dose methylprednisolone, with or without carmustine, have not shown any survival benefit. On the basis of the results so far it appears best to use radiotherapy in the treatment of malignant glioma and to continue the search for chemotherapy regimens to use in association with radiotherapy.— M. D. Walker *et al.*, *New Engl. J. Med.*, 1980, *303*, 1323.

MYCOSIS FUNGOIDES. The use of topical carmustine, usually as a 0.2% solution or 0.4% ointment, in mycosis fungoides. Over a 10-year period 86 patients had been treated in this way, and complete remission was achieved in 21 of 25 with less than 10% skin involvement (stage IA), and in 11 of 21 patients in whom there was greater than 10% involvement (stage IB). Among patients with more advanced disease the degree of involvement was also predictive of response, and those with predominantly superficial lesions responded better than those with infiltrating plaque lesions. Erythema and telangiectasia were troublesome side-effects but severe cutaneous reactions were generally rare with current dosage schedules. The results confirm that topical carmustine is an effective treatment for mycosis fungoides and related cutaneous T-cell lymphomas.— H. S. Zackheim *et al.*, *J. Am. Acad. Derm.*, 1983, *9*, 363.

Topical application of carmustine solution resulted in a reduction in the number and size of lesions in 7 patients with lymphomatoid papulosis. Erythematous reactions occurred in all patients but were generally limited in extent and duration and there was no histologic evidence of premalignant change.— H. S. Zackheim *et al.*, *Archs Derm.*, 1985, *121*, 1410.

WALDENSTRÖM'S MACROGLOBULINAEMIA. Meningeal involvement in a woman with Waldenström's macroglobulinaemia was successfully treated with combined intraventricular chemotherapy and intravenous carmustine with oral prednisone.— J. J. Torrey and S. B. Katakkar, *Ann. intern. Med.*, 1984, *101*, 345.

Proprietary Preparations

BiCNU *(Bristol-Myers Pharmaceuticals, UK). Injection,* powder for reconstitution, carmustine 100 mg, supplied with diluent.

Proprietary Names and Manufacturers

Becenun *(Bristol-Myers, Denm.; Bristol, Norw.; Bristol, Swed.)*; BiCNU *(Bristol, Canad.; Bristol, Fr.; Bristol-Myers Pharmaceuticals, UK; Bristol-Myers Oncology, USA)*; Carmubris *(Bristol, Ger.)*; Nitrumon *(Simes, Ital.)*.

12534-q

Carubicin Hydrochloride *(USAN, rINNM).*

Carminomycin Hydrochloride; NSC-180024. (1*S*,3*S*)-3-Acetyl-1,2,3,4,6,11-hexahydro-3,5,10,12-tetrahydroxy-6,11-dioxonaphthacen-1-yl 3-amino-2,3,6-trideoxy-α-L-lyxopyranoside hydrochloride.

$C_{26}H_{27}NO_{10},HCl=550.0$.

CAS — 39472-31-6; 50935-04-1 (both carubicin); 52794-97-5 (hydrochloride).

Carubicin hydrochloride is an anthracycline antibiotic with antineoplastic actions similar to those of doxorubicin (p.623). It has been tried in the treatment of patients with acute leukaemias and some solid tumours.

In a study involving 44 patients with various nonhaematological cancers, carubicin was given in doses of 15, 20, 22.5 or 25 mg per m^2 body-surface intravenously, at four-week intervals. Moderate to severe thrombophlebitis occurred in 50% of patients, but the major dose-limiting toxicity was granulocytopenia. Three of 9 patients given total doses of 100 mg per m^2 or more developed changes in cardiac function, and one, who had received a total dose of 160 mg per m^2, developed congestive heart failure. Nausea and vomiting were mild and alopecia was less pronounced than with doxorubicin. Carubicin was found to be rapidly metabolised to an active metabolite, carubicinol (carminomycinol), with mean elimination half-lives of about 6 to 10 hours and 50 hours respectively. Partial responses to chemotherapy were seen in 2 of 7 previously untreated patients with non-small cell lung cancer, and in 1 of 3 patients with squamous cell carcinoma of the head and neck.— R. L. Comis *et al.*, *Cancer Res.*, 1982, *42*, 2944.

Further references S. K. Carter, *Drugs*, 1980, *20*, 375; R. C. Young *et al.*, *New Engl. J. Med.*, 1981, *305*, 139; *Drugs of the Future*, 1985, *10*, 414.

Proprietary Names and Manufacturers

Bristol, USA.

1820-l

Chlorambucil *(BAN, USAN, rINN).*

CB-1348; Chlorambucilum; Chloraminophene; Chlorbutinum; NSC-3088; WR-139013. 4-[4-Bis(2-chloroethyl)aminophenyl]butyric acid.

$C_{14}H_{19}Cl_2NO_2=304.2$.

CAS — 305-03-3.

Pharmacopoeias. In *Br., Cz., Egypt., Eur., Fr., It., Jug., Neth., Rus., Swiss, Turk.,* and *U.S.*

A white or off-white crystalline or granular powder. Practically **insoluble** in water; soluble 1 in 1.5 of alcohol, 1 in 2 of acetone, and 1 in 2.5 of chloroform; soluble in dilute solutions of alkali hydroxides. **Store** in airtight containers. Protect from light.

CAUTION. *Chlorambucil is irritant; avoid contact with skin and mucous membranes.*

Adverse Effects and Treatment

For an outline of the adverse effects experienced with antineoplastic agents and immunosuppressants and general guidelines for their treatment, see Antineoplastic Agents, p.580 and p.583.

A reversible progressive lymphocytopenia tends to develop during treatment with chlorambucil. Neutropenia may continue to develop up to 10 days after the last dose. Irreversible bone-marrow depression can occur particularly when the total dosage for the course approaches 6.5 mg per kg body-weight.

Other reported adverse effects include gastro-intestinal disturbances, hepatotoxicity, skin rashes, and central neurotoxicity, including seizures. Interstitial pneumonia and pulmonary fibrosis have occurred; the latter is usually reversible but fatalities have been recorded.

Chlorambucil in high doses may produce azoospermia and amenorrhoea; sterility has developed particularly when chlorambucil has been given to boys at or before puberty.

Overdosage may result in pancytopenia and in neurotoxicity, including agitation, ataxia, and grand mal seizures.

Chlorambucil is mutagenic, teratogenic, and carcinogenic, and an increased incidence of acute leukaemias and other secondary malignancies has been reported in patients who have received the drug.

EFFECTS ON THE BLADDER. Chlorambucil-induced cystitis was reported in a 73-year-old woman given 2 mg daily for over 2 years for the treatment of lymphocytic lymphoma.— D. Daoud *et al.* (letter), *Drug Intell. & clin. Pharm.*, 1977, *11*, 491.

EFFECTS ON THE NERVOUS SYSTEM. Chlorambucil has been reported to cause a peripheral neuropathy of the sensorimotor type.— R. J. M. Lane and P. A. Routledge, *Drugs*, 1983, *26*, 124.

Precautions

For reference to the precautions necessary with antineoplastic agents and immunosuppressants, see Antineoplastic Agents, p.583. Chlorambucil should not be administered for at least 4 weeks after treatment with radiotherapy or other antineoplastic agents unless only low doses of radiation have been given to parts remote from the bone marrow and the neutrophil and platelet counts are not depressed. The dose should be reduced if there is lymphocytic involvement of the bone marrow or if it is hypoplastic. Chlorambucil should be given with care to patients with impaired renal function; the manufacturers state that consideration should also be given to dose reduction in patients with gross hepatic dysfunction.

HANDLING AND DISPOSAL. Protective clothing should be worn for up to 48 hours after therapy when handling urine from patients given chlorambucil.— J. Harris and L. J. Dodds, *Pharm. J.*, 1985, *2*, 289.

PORPHYRIA. Chlorambucil was considered to be unsafe in patients with acute porphyria because it has been shown to be porphyrinogenic in *animals* or *in vitro* systems.— M.R. Moore and K.E.L. McColl, *Porphyrias, Drug Lists*, Glasgow, Porphyria Research Unit, University of Glasgow, 1987.

Absorption and Fate

Chlorambucil is rapidly and almost completely absorbed from the gastro-intestinal tract following oral doses and is reported to have a terminal half-life in plasma of about 1.5 hours. It is extensively metabolised in the liver, primarily to active phenylacetic acid mustard, which like chlorambucil also undergoes some spontaneous degradation to further derivatives. Chlorambucil and its metabolites are extensively protein bound. It is excreted in the urine almost entirely as metabolites with less than 1% unchanged.

The rate of absorption of chlorambucil 40 mg by mouth was decreased in 5 patients when given following a standard breakfast compared with absorption in the fasting state. Mean peak plasma concentration of drug was reduced and the time to peak was increased but the bioavailability was not affected; peak plasma concentrations of the major metabolite, phenylacetic acid mustard were not affected by food, although the peak was delayed. The elimination half-life of the metabolite was

2.03 hours compared with 0.94 hours for chlorambucil and it was estimated that about 20% of the metabolite, compared with about 5% of chlorambucil, was involved in alkylation reactions. Further studies of the antineoplastic activity of phenylacetic acid mustard in man are needed.— H. Ehrsson *et al.*, *Eur. J. clin. Pharmac.*, 1984, *27*, 111.

Earlier references: D. S. Alberts *et al.*, *Cancer Treat. Rev.*, 1979, *6*, *Suppl.*, 9; A. McLean *et al.*, *ibid.*, 33.

Uses and Administration

Chlorambucil is an antineoplastic agent derived from mustine (p.645) and has a similar mode of action. It acts on lymphocytes and to a lesser extent on neutrophils and platelets. Chlorambucil is most valuable in those conditions associated with the proliferation of white blood cells, especially lymphocytes, and is used in the treatment of chronic lymphocytic leukaemia and lymphomas, including Hodgkin's disease. It is also used in Waldenström's macroglobulinaemia and in carcinoma of the breast, ovary, and testis. Chlorambucil has immunosuppressant properties and has been given in various auto-immune disorders. See also under Choice of Antineoplastic Agent, p.584.

Chlorambucil is better tolerated than mustine hydrochloride and serious bone-marrow toxicity is not usually a problem with normal doses. Chlorambucil is administered by mouth in usual doses of 100 to 200 µg per kg body-weight daily for 3 to 6 weeks, as a single dose before food. A dose of 100 µg per kg daily may be adequate for the treatment of lymphosarcoma or chronic lymphocytic leukaemia; in Hodgkin's disease, 200 µg per kg daily is usually required. If lymphocytic infiltration of the bone marrow is present or if the bone marrow is hypoplastic, the daily dose should not exceed 100 µg per kg. Alternatively, chlorambucil may be given intermittently, usually in an initial dose of 400 µg per kg increased by 100 µg per kg at each 2-week dose interval until control of lymphocytosis is achieved or toxicity occurs.

Once a remission has been established the patient may receive continuous maintenance with 30 to 100 µg per kg body-weight daily. However, short interrupted maintenance courses appear to be safer and are generally preferred for maintenance.

Total and differential white-cell counts and haemoglobin examinations should be made each week during treatment with chlorambucil.

LIVER DISORDERS, NON-MALIGNANT. A review of primary biliary cirrhosis. Chlorambucil has been evaluated prospectively in some patients with primary biliary cirrhosis, and produced improvement in some symptoms after 2 years but without any decrease in hepatic fibrosis or stage of disease. Concern about the long-term toxicity of chlorambucil has prevented the start of a prospective randomised trial.— M. M. Kaplan, *New Engl. J. Med.*, 1987, *316*, 521.

RENAL DISORDERS, NON-MALIGNANT. Chlorambucil has been successfully used in frequently-relapsing children with minimal-change nephrotic syndrome but does not seem to be superior to cyclophosphamide. Although short-term toxicity seems to be less with chlorambucil than with other alkylating agents, long-term effects may turn out to be disastrous. The occurrence of acute leukaemia, renal carcinoma, and fatal viral infections suggest that exposure to chlorambucil can only be justified in those with serious corticosteroid toxicity.— R. S. Trompeter, *Archs Dis. Childh.*, 1986, *61*, 727.

Preparations

Chlorambucil Tablets *(B.P.)*

Chlorambucil Tablets *(U.S.P.)*

Proprietary Preparations

Leukeran *(Calmic, UK)*. *Tablets*, chlorambucil 2 and 5 mg.

NOTE. The manufacturers recommend that the tablets be stored at 2° to 8°.

Proprietary Names and Manufacturers

Leukeran *(Wellcome, Austral.; Belg.; Wellcome, Canad.; Wellcome, Denm.; Wellcome, Ger.; Wellcome, Ital.; Neth.; Wellcome, Norw.; Wellcome, S. Afr.; Gayoso Wellcome, Spain; Wellcome, Swed.; Wellcome, Switz.; Calmic, UK; Wellcome, USA)*; Linfolysin *(ISM, Ital.)*.

1821-y

Chlorozotocin

DCNU; NSC-178248. 2-[3-(2-Chloroethyl)-3-nitrosoureido]-2-deoxy-D-glucopyranose.

$C_9H_{16}ClN_3O_7$=313.7.

CAS — 54749-90-5.

Chlorozotocin is an analogue of the antineoplastic agent streptozocin (p.649) and has been reported not to have a diabetogenic effect.

Progressive normochromic normocytic anaemia was noted in a 46-year-old woman who had been given chlorozotocin 120 mg per m² body-surface intravenously every 6 weeks during the previous 12 months, for the treatment of bronchoalveolar carcinoma. Therapy was continued for a further 6 months, when a total dose of 2.1 g had been given. Over the following 4 to 6 weeks progressive renal failure developed from which the patient died.— J. J. Baker *et al.* (letter), *New Engl. J. Med.*, 1979, *301*, 662.

Proprietary Names and Manufacturers

Dome, USA.

1822-j

Cisplatin *(BAN, USAN, rINN).*

CDDP; Cis-platinum; DDP; *cis*-DDP; NSC-119875; Peyrone's Salt; Platinum Diamminodichloride. *cis*-Diamminedichloroplatinum.

$(NH_3)_2.PtCl_2$=300.0.

CAS — 15663-27-1.

Pharmacopoeias. In *U.S.*

INCOMPATIBILITY. A report of a chemical reaction between cisplatin and sodium bisulfite. Such antoxidants might inactivate cisplatin before administration if they are present in intravenous fluids.— A. A. Hussain *et al.*, *J. pharm. Sci.*, 1980, *69*, 364. There was total loss of cisplatin in 30 minutes at room temperature when mixed with metoclopramide and sodium metabisulphite in concentrations equivalent to those that would be found on mixing with a commercial formulation (Reglan Injectable) of metoclopramide.— K. W. Garren and A. J. Repta, *Int. J. Pharmaceut.*, 1985, *24*, 91.

Cisplatin was incompatible with aluminium, which had been used in the design of a dispensing pin intended to aid antineoplastic drug preparation. On inspection, a solution of cisplatin in contact with a part-aluminium needle underwent immediate reaction resulting in the formation of gas and a black precipitate.— G. S. Ogawa *et al.* (letter), *Am. J. Hosp. Pharm.*, 1985, *42*, 1042.

STABILITY IN SOLUTION. Studies on the stability of cisplatin in aqueous solution indicated that when reconstituted with sodium chloride injection (0.9%) it was stable for 24 hours at room temperature. It was not necessary to prepare a solution immediately before use provided it was protected from light. If stored at refrigerator temperatures the concentration should be less than 600 µg per mL to prevent precipitation.— R. F. Greene *et al.*, *Am. J. Hosp. Pharm.*, 1979, *36*, 38.

The rate of loss of cisplatin in aqueous parenteral solutions was dependent on the concentration present and was not affected by glucose or mannitol; cisplatin stability was decreased in the presence of sodium bicarbonate, but enhanced by sodium chloride.— A. A. Hincal *et al.*, *J. parent. Drug Ass.*, 1979, *33*, 107.

Based on the results of stability tests by the manufacturer (*Bristol*, *USA*), it was recommended that admixtures of cisplatin with mannitol (to minimise nephrotoxicity) and magnesium sulphate (to prevent hypomagnesaemia) in either glucose (5%) or sodium chloride (0.9%) injection, and containing 50 or 200 µg cisplatin per mL, should be used within 48 hours if stored in polyvinyl chloride bags at 25°. The mixtures could be stored at 4° for 4 days or be frozen at −15° for up to 30 days, in which cases they would remain stable for a further 48 hours at 25°.— J. M. LaFollette *et al.* (letter), *Am. J. Hosp. Pharm.*, 1985, *42*, 2652.

Adverse Effects

For an outline of the adverse effects experienced with antineoplastic agents and immunosuppressants see Antineoplastic Agents, p.580.

Severe nausea and vomiting occur in most patients during treatment with cisplatin.

Serious toxic effects on the kidneys, bone marrow, and ears have been reported in about one third of patients given a single dose of cisplatin; the effects are generally dose-related and cumulative. Damage to the renal tubules may be evident during the second week after a dose of cisplatin and renal function must return to normal before further cisplatin is given. Electrolyte disturbances, particularly hypomagnesaemia and hypocalcaemia, may occur, possibly as a result of renal tubular damage. Hyperuricaemia is common.

Bone-marrow depression may be severe with higher doses of cisplatin. Nadirs in platelet and leucocyte counts occur between days 18 and 23 and most patients recover by day 39; anaemia is commonly seen.

Ototoxicity may be more severe in children. It can be manifest as tinnitus, loss of hearing in the high frequency range, and occasionally deafness. Other neurological effects reported include peripheral neuropathies including optic neuritis, papilloedema, cerebral blindness, and seizures.

Anaphylactoid reactions and cardiac abnormalities have occurred.

An anaphylactic reaction attributed to drug absorption was reported in 7 of 67 patients receiving cisplatin by intravesical instillation. All patients developing the reaction were among the 50 who had received at least 8 instillations, over a period of 4 months. Symptoms consisted of pruritus, rash, and hypotensive shock, and required treatment with corticosteroids and plasma expanders in 3 patients. The frequency and gravity of these systemic reactions to intravesical administration may be more serious than first thought.— L. Denis (letter), *Lancet*, 1983, *1*, 1378. In contrast, intraperitoneal or intrapleural administration of cisplatin was not associated with a risk of allergic reaction greater than that seen with systemic delivery.— M. Markman (letter), *ibid.*, 1984, *2*, 1164.

Further references to allergic reactions to cisplatin: D. D. Von Hoff *et al.* (letter), *Lancet*, 1976, *1*, 90; R. F. U. Ashford *et al.* (letter), *ibid.*, 1980, *2*, 691.

EFFECTS ON THE BLOOD. Findings which suggest that cisplatin-induced anaemia probably has 2 mechanisms, the more usual being destruction of the erythroid stem-cell pool and the less usual being haemolysis.— S. A. Rothmann and J. K. Weick (letter), *New Engl. J. Med.*, 1981, *304*, 360.

EFFECTS ON THE EARS. A report of positional vertigo developing in a patient given a single dose of cisplatin. Peripheral labyrinthine impairment was confirmed by vestibular function tests. In addition to the recognised side-effects of tinnitus and high-tone sensorineural deafness 3 cases of vestibular toxicity associated with cisplatin have been recorded by the manufacturers, 2 of which were in patients with pre-existing vestibular problems. Toxicity appears to be dose-related.— A. O. Keith and U. K. Mallick, *Br. med. J.*, 1985, *291*, 1542.

For the view that ototoxicity may be enhanced in children with brain tumours see under Precautions, below.

EFFECTS ON ELECTROLYTES. In a retrospective study of 37 patients who had received cisplatin 70 mg per m² body-surface by intravenous injection every 3 weeks, 21 patients developed hypomagnesaemia while receiving cisplatin, which eventually returned to normal in 10 patients, and a further 8 developed hypomagnesaemia after cisplatin was withdrawn. Symptomatic hypomagnesaemia requiring hospitalisation occurred in 2 patients, while inappropriate renal magnesium loss occurred in 4 patients. In a prospective study of a further 7 patients who received a standard liquid diet for 4 days before cisplatin administration, 2 developed hypomagnesaemia.— R. L. Schilsky and T. Anderson, *Ann. intern. Med.*, 1979, *90*, 929. A report of severe hypomagnesaemic-hypocalcaemic tetany with marked hypokalaemia in a woman undergoing cisplatin therapy. The electrolyte losses were replaced and chemotherapy continued satisfactorily.— C. F. Winkler *et al.* (letter), *ibid.*, *91*, 502. A report of tetany in a 23-year-old man receiving cisplatin without concurrent administration of a diuretic. Serum magnesium and calcium concentrations should be monitored in patients receiving cisplatin so that replacement therapy can be started promptly.— R. Stuart-Harris *et al.* (letter), *Lancet*, 1980, *2*, 1303. Further references: F. C. Clark, *Adverse Drug React. Bull.*, 1982, (Apr.), 340; D. P. Brenton and T. E. Gordon, *Br. J. Hosp. Med.*, 1984, *32*, 60; J. E. Scoble *et al.* (letter), *Lancet*, 1987, *1*, 276.

For effects associated with altered electrolyte homoeostasis, see under Effects on the Kidney and Effects on the Mental State, below.

EFFECTS ON THE EYES. Retinal toxicity, manifest mainly as blurred vision and altered colour perception, was associated with the administration of high-dose cisplatin.— G. Wilding *et al.*, *J. clin. Oncol.*, 1985, *3*, 1683.

EFFECTS ON THE HEART. Bradycardia, associated with vertigo and weakness, following repeated administration of cisplatin as part of a combination regimen, in a patient with mouth cancer.— F. Schlaeffer *et al.*, *Drug Intell. & clin. Pharm.*, 1983, *17*, 899.

See also under Effects on the Vascular System, below.

EFFECTS ON THE KIDNEY. A review of the nephrotoxic effects of cisplatin. Cisplatin may produce azotaemia and acute renal failure, with tubular necrosis primarily in the distal portions of the nephron. It has been shown that most patients whose renal function is impaired by cisplatin never regain their pretreatment level of function. Selective renal wasting of magnesium is not unusual and may be commoner than azotaemia as an expression of nephrotoxicity: hypocalcaemia and hypokalaemia may result. These findings probably result from a specific membrane or transport-system defect. The nephrotoxic effects of cisplatin are cumulative, and increase with total dose and duration of treatment: adequate hydration and urine volumes greater than 2 litres daily reduce the frequency of renal insufficiency as may simultaneous infusion of mannitol, and the use of chloride-containing vehicles such as sodium chloride injection rather than glucose.— J. D. Blachley and J. B. Hill, *Ann. intern. Med.*, 1981, *95*, 628.

Substantial concentrations of lead were found in the kidneys of 4 of 10 patients receiving cisplatin: tissue concentrations ranged between 222 and 813 μg per g, the latter representing a massive and quite unprecedented lead burden. Subsequent measurements in 3 of the patients 1 to 3 months later revealed much lower or undetectable lead concentrations. It appears that cisplatin may mobilise lead accumulated in bone and cause temporary accumulation in the kidney. Such mobilisation and release might be sufficient to induce toxic effects.— A. M. El-Sharkawi *et al.*, *Lancet*, 1986, *2*, 249. Comment. Cisplatin may be mobilising lead from adipose tissue rather than bone stores.— W. L. Marcus *et al.* (letter), *ibid.*, 1098.

See also Administration, below.

EFFECTS ON MENTAL STATE. Disorientation, paranoia, and agitation had been attributed to drug-induced magnesium deficiency in one patient receiving cisplatin.— *Med. Lett.*, 1986, *28*, 81.

EFFECTS ON THE NERVOUS SYSTEM. Repeated convulsions followed cisplatin 100 mg per m^2 body-surface in a patient with ovarian cancer, who had received 3 previous courses. Although the convulsions were eventually controlled the patient did not recover consciousness and died 10 hours later. The patient had also received a transfusion of concentrated red blood cells, which may have contributed to the convulsions.— A. M. Smith (letter), *Br. med. J.*, 1982, *285*, 733.

Administration of very high doses of cisplatin (200 mg per m^2 body-surface over 5 days) in hypertonic sodium chloride solution as suggested by Ozols *et al.* (*Ann. intern. Med.*, 1984, *100*, 19) resulted in severe and disabling neuropathy when given as part of a combination regimen to 4 patients with ovarian cancer. Symptoms became marked in 1 patient after 3, and in the remainder after 4 cycles of treatment, and were severe enough for the patients to require assistance to walk. On 4 to 6 months follow-up there was only minimal neurological improvement to date.— C. M. Bagley *et al.* (letter), *Ann. intern. Med.*, 1985, *102*, 719. Comment. Although the regimen used has a lower incidence of renal toxicity it does not prevent other toxic effects of cisplatin, including neurotoxicity, which was also seen in 4 of the 6 patients in the original study. Cisplatin-induced neurotoxicity is primarily sensory, with loss of proprioception and vibratory sense in a stocking-glove distribution; although motor function is not significantly affected the severe proprioceptive loss can lead to ataxia. Although patients given this high-dose regimen in hypertonic saline often have some mild neuropathy as early as the second cycle of therapy the severity increases with the fourth cycle and can progress after completion of therapy. The authors now administer a fourth cycle only if there is evidence of residual ovarian cancer after 3 cycles, and only if the patient has minimal neurotoxicity.— R. F. Ozols and R. C. Young (letter), *ibid.*

EFFECTS ON THE VASCULAR SYSTEM. Acute arterial occlusive events, comprising myocardial infarction in 2 patients and cerebrovascular accidents in a further 2, occurred following administration of cisplatin-based combination chemotherapy to 23 patients with testicular tumours. Hypoperfusion resulting from arterial vasospasm or thrombosis probably underlies the acute ischaemic complications.— D. C. Doll *et al.*, *Ann. intern. Med.*, 1986, *105*, 48.

LOCAL TOXICITY. For a report of local necrosis following cisplatin extravasation, see M. Leyden and J. Sullivan, *Cancer Treat. Rep.*, 1983, *67*, 199.

Treatment of Adverse Effects

For general guidelines, see Antineoplastic Agents, p.583.

Cisplatin nephrotoxicity may be reduced by adequate hydration and intravenous administration of mannitol, which increase the urinary volume and thus decrease the effective urinary concentration of platinum: for regimens designed to minimise nephrotoxicity, see under Administration, below. For a brief review of strategies for preventing cisplatin-induced nephrotoxicity, see R. S. Finley *et al.*, *Drug Intell. & clin. Pharm.*, 1985, *19*, 362.

Injection of sodium thiosulphate 7.5 g per m^2 body-surface as an intravenous loading dose, followed by 2.13 g per m^2 per hour by intravenous infusion over 12 hours, reduced the incidence of nephrotoxicity associated with intraperitoneal cisplatin in 17 patients. When cisplatin 90 mg per m^2 was given by instillation into the peritoneum, there was an average rise in serum creatinine of 55% above pretreatment values, whereas this rise averaged only 9% when the same dose was given with thiosulphate. As a result of the effectiveness of thiosulphate protection the dose of cisplatin could be increased to 270 mg per m^2 without evidence of nephrotoxicity. Nausea and vomiting occurred after all courses of cisplatin and was not affected by thiosulphate; myelosuppression was transient and tolerable and there was no evidence of peripheral neuropathy or hearing loss.— S. B. Howell *et al.*, *Ann. intern. Med.*, 1982, *97*, 845.

NAUSEA AND VOMITING. For reviews and discussions of the treatment of antineoplastic-induced nausea and vomiting, see under Antineoplastic Agents, p.583.

A report of reduced emetic side-effects in patients given electroacupuncture treatment either before or soon after the start of cisplatin infusion.— J. W. Dundee *et al.* (letter), *Lancet*, 1987, *1*, 1083.

Precautions

For reference to the precautions necessary with antineoplastic agents and immunosuppressants, see Antineoplastic Agents, p.583. Cisplatin should not be given to patients with a history of hypersensitivity to platinum-containing compounds. It is generally contra-indicated in patients with renal or hearing impairment. Renal function and hearing should be monitored during treatment and adequate hydration and urinary output maintained before, and for 24 hours after, administration. Neurotoxicity may be irreversible and cisplatin should be stopped in patients who develop signs of peripheral neuropathies. The concomitant use of other nephrotoxic or ototoxic drugs should be avoided.

Enhanced cisplatin neurotoxicity in paediatric patients with brain tumours. Severe and early hearing loss developed in 5 of 6 such patients, perhaps due to an interaction with the adverse effects of cranial irradiation.— L. Granowetter *et al.*, *J. Neurooncol.*, 1983, *1*, 293. See also D. H. Mahoney *et al.* (letter), *J. Pediat.*, 1983, *103*, 1006.

HANDLING AND DISPOSAL. Methods for the destruction of cisplatin wastes by reduction with zinc powder under acidic conditions or by reaction with sodium diethyldithiocarbamate. The former method is recommended for solutions in water-miscible organic solvents (but may also be used for solid wastes, which should be dissolved to produce a solution of the appropriate strength), for aqueous solutions, and for water used to clean contaminated glassware. Sulphuric acid should be added to produce the equivalent of cisplatin 0.06% in sulphuric acid 2 mol per litre, and the solution reacted with 3 g of zinc powder for every 100 mL: it may then be neutralised with sodium hydroxide, and discarded. The second method is recommended for solid waste, which should be dissolved in water, for aqueous solutions, glassware and spillages, and involves reaction with 3 mL of an approximately 1% sodium diethyldithiocarbamate solution per 100 mg of cisplatin, an equal volume of saturated sodium nitrate solution being added. Contaminated glassware may be immersed in a mixture of equal parts of sodium diethyldithiocarbamate solution and saturated sodium nitrate solution, and a similar mixture may be used to neutralise material used to absorb rinse water from spillages, prior to discarding it. Residue produced by the degradation of cisplatin by either method showed no mutagenicity *in vitro*.— IARC Scientific Publications No. 73, *Laboratory Decontamination and Destruction of Carcinogens in Laboratory Wastes: Some Antineoplastic Agents*, M. Castegnaro *et al.* (Eds), Lyon, International Agency for Research on Cancer, 1985, pp. 89 and 97.

Protective clothing should be worn for up to 7 days after therapy when handling urine from patients given cisplatin.— J. Harris and L. J. Dodds, *Pharm. J.*, 1985, *2*, 289.

INTERACTIONS. A report of nephrotoxicity in a patient given cisplatin and antihypertensive therapy with frusemide, hydralazine, diazoxide, and propranolol. On 2 subsequent occasions the same dose of cisplatin given alone had no effect on renal function.— M. Markman and D. L. Trump (letter), *Ann. intern. Med.*, 1982, *96*, 257.

Absorption and Fate

After intravenous administration cisplatin disappears from the plasma in a biphasic manner and half-lives of 25 to 49 minutes and 58 to 73 hours have been reported. The majority of a dose is rapidly bound to plasma protein. Cisplatin is concentrated in the liver, kidneys, and large and small intestines. Penetration into the central nervous system appears to be poor. Excretion is mainly in the urine but is incomplete and prolonged: up to 43% of a dose has been reported to be excreted in urine over 5 days. Cisplatin is well absorbed following intraperitoneal administration.

A review of the pharmacokinetics of some antineoplastic agents, including cisplatin. Most pharmcokinetic studies have measured total platinum but cisplatin is believed to be non-enzymatically transformed into 1 or more metabolites, which are protein bound; only the non-bound fraction has more than minimal cytotoxic activity. Protein-bound platinum species represent more than 90% of the dose by 2 to 4 hours after administration. Although total platinum has a bi-exponential decline with a prolonged terminal half-life of 58 to 96 hours the non-bound active form has a much more rapid decline with an initial phase half-life of 8 to 30 minutes and a terminal half-life of 40 to 48 minutes. By 4 to 5 hours, unbound cisplatin accounts for less than 2 to 3% of the total circulating platinum. Excretion is primarily renal, with an initial period of rapid output followed within 4 hours by a decline in renal clearance due to protein binding. There is evidence to suggest that the unbound drug may be actively secreted by the renal tubules. The fraction of a dose excreted in urine increases with increased length of infusion. Faecal excretion is probably insignificant, although the drug is found in bile.— F. M. Balis *et al.*, *Clin. Pharmacokinet.*, 1983, *8*, 202.

In a patient given an infusion of cisplatin, 0.21% of the total dose administered was recovered from the bile over 3 days via a cholecystostomy, compared with 47.0% from urine. There was no evidence of enterohepatic recycling in this patient.— M. D. Shelley *et al.*, *Antimicrob. Ag. Chemother.*, 1985, *27*, 275.

Uses and Administration

The antineoplastic agent cisplatin is a platinum-containing complex which may act similarly to the alkylating agents (p.580). Its antineoplastic actions are cell-cycle nonspecific and are dependent upon the *cis* configuration: the *trans* isomer is inactive. It also causes immunosuppression which is reported to be followed by an increase in the host immune response and may contribute to the effect of cisplatin against tumours.

Cisplatin is of value in the treatment of metastatic tumours of the testis, usually as a major component of combination chemotherapy regimens, and particularly in combination with bleomycin and vinblastine. It is also used in metastatic ovarian tumours and advanced bladder cancer, and has been reported to be active against other solid tumours including those of the cervix, lung, and head and neck.

See also under Choice of Antineoplastic Agent, p.584.

Cisplatin is administered intravenously, not more frequently than every 3 to 4 weeks. It is given as a single dose of 50 to 120 mg per m^2 body-surface, alternatively 15 to 20 mg per m^2 may be given daily for 5 days. In combination chemotherapy regimens, lower doses may be given, ranging from 20 mg per m^2 upwards every 3 to 4 weeks. A dose of 20 mg per m^2 daily for 5 days every 3 weeks is often employed in combination with bleomycin and vinblastine in the treatment of testicular tumours.

The reconstituted injection is administered in 2 litres of sodium chloride (0.9%) injection or glucose 4% and sodium chloride 0.18% injection and infused over 6 to 8 hours. To aid diuresis and protect the kidneys, 37.5 g of mannitol may be added to the infusion. In order to initiate diuresis the patient is usually hydrated by the infusion of 1 to 2 litres of a suitable fluid for 8 to 12 hours before the administration of cisplatin. Adequate hydration must also be maintained for 24 hours after a dose. Renal, auditory, and neurological function should be monitored during therapy, and administration adjusted accordingly.

Cisplatin has also been administered by the intra-arterial and intraperitoneal routes, and by instillation into the bladder.

Reviews of cisplatin: *Lancet*, 1982, *1*, 374; P. J. Loehrer and L. H. Einhorn, *Ann. intern. Med.*, 1984, *100*, 704.

ACTION. The cytotoxicity of cisplatin appears to be related to its hydrolysis in the body. The aquated form, *cis*-$Pt(NH_3)_2(H_20)(OH)^+$, is very reactive, and can also form hydroxyl-bridged dimers and trimers. Selective killing of tumour cells is probably due to attack on the guanine- and cytosine-rich regions of DNA, producing damage which is repairable by normal cells. Platinum crosslinks between DNA strands are not now thought to be important cytotoxic events. It has also been suggested that platinum binding to guanine activates the base so that it can form abnormal base pairs, resulting in unwinding of DNA.— P. J. Sadler, *Chem. in Br.*, 1982, *18*, 182.

ADMINISTRATION. Results of a study in 11 patients indicated that the circadian timing of administration had a pronounced effect on the kinetics and toxicity of cisplatin. When cisplatin was given at 6.00 a.m., with doxorubicin at 6.00 p.m., peak urine production was delayed and the amplitude of the rhythm of urine production markedly flattened, compared to those in the same patients given the opposite regimen (cisplatin in the evening, doxorubicin in the morning), or before treatment. These findings imply that renal function, as gauged by recovery of the normal circadian rhythm of urine production, recovers less completely when cisplatin is given in the morning rather than the evening. The benefit of tailoring administration to circadian rhythms requires further study.— W. J. M. Hrushesky *et al.*, *Clin. Pharmac. Ther.*, 1982, *32*, 330.

See also under Choice of Antineoplastic Agent, p.585.

Administration of cisplatin in hypertonic saline, accompanied by vigorous hydration, permitted the use of high doses of cisplatin without any increased nephrotoxicity in 17 patients with poor-prognosis nonseminomatous testicular cancer. Patients, who were all previously untreated, received cisplatin 40 mg per m^2 body-surface daily for 5 days, by intravenous infusion over 30 minutes in 250 mL of 3% saline as part of a combination regimen with vinblastine, etoposide, and bleomycin (PVeBV). Intensive hydration with 250 mL per hour of 0.9% saline, containing in addition potassium chloride 20 mmol per litre, was started 12 hours before the first dose of cisplatin and continued until 12 hours after the last dose. All patients were monitored for signs and symptoms of fluid overload. Of 15 patients completing either 3 or 4 cycles of this therapy, none had a significant decrease in creatinine clearance. A similar regimen of cisplatin, given to 6 patients with refractory ovarian cancer who had previously received standard doses, produced transient raised serum-creatinine concentrations in 2. Hypertonic saline did not protect against the nonrenal adverse effects of cisplatin.— R. F. Ozols *et al.*, *Ann. intern. Med.*, 1984, *100*, 19.

For a report of neurotoxicity associated with high-dose cisplatin, see Effects on the Nervous System, above.

For the use of sodium thiosulphate in the prevention of nephrotoxicity with high-dose intraperitoneal cisplatin, see under Treatment of Adverse Effects, above.

Administration of cisplatin as a 24-hour continuous intravenous infusion was well tolerated in a study involving 96 cancer patients. Patients received a continuous infusion of cisplatin 20 mg per m^2 body-surface daily for 5 days every 4 to 6 weeks, either alone or with other agents. Patients were adequately hydrated for 12 hours before, and during the course of, treatment, but no mannitol or other diuretics were given. Only 4 of 81 evaluable patients developed nephrotoxicity, and nausea and vomiting were markedly reduced or absent. In view of this minimal toxicity the therapeutic efficacy of this regimen should be assessed.— P. Salem *et al.*, *Cancer*, 1984, *53*, 837.

In renal failure. The dose of cisplatin should be reduced to 75% in patients with a glomerular filtration-rate of between 10 and 50 mL per minute, and to 50% in patients in whom the rate is less than 10 mL per minute. The terminal half-life of cisplatin is increased from between 2 and 72 hours up to 240 hours in patients with end-stage renal disease.— W. M. Bennett *et al.*, *Am. J. Kidney Dis.*, 1983, *3*, 155.

MALIGNANT NEOPLASMS. Cisplatin has a major role in the treatment of testicular and ovarian cancer, and also has moderate activity in other tumours of the genitourinary system. It is one of the most active drugs in metastatic bladder cancer, with response-rates ranging from 33 to 57% and a median duration of remission of 4 to 6 months. It is also reportedly effective in metastatic squamous cell carcinoma of the penis but appears to have no significant role in hormone-refractory prostate cancer. It has activity in cervical cancer, and responses have been seen in endometrial carcinoma but it is clearly inactive in previously treated patients with this condition. Despite a response-rate of only 10 to 15% in untreated patients, cisplatin is one of the most active agents available for the treatment of non-small-cell lung cancer, and may have a role with etoposide for late intensification in small-cell lung cancer. The role of cisplatin therapy in head and neck cancer remains to be proven but it has established itself as an effective treatment in osteosarcoma and has modest activity in oesophageal and gastric cancer.— P. J. Loehrer and L. H. Einhorn, *Ann. intern. Med.*, 1984, *100*, 704.

See also under Choice of Antineoplastic Agent, p.584.

TRYPANOSOMIASIS. Cisplatin had significant activity against *Trypanosoma rhodesiense* infections in *mice*.— K. E. Kinnamon *et al.*, *Antimicrob. Ag. Chemother.*, 1979, *15*, 157.

Treatment with cisplatin intraperitoneally for 7 days was effective in curing *T. rhodesiense* infection in *mice*, but highly toxic: hydration and oral disulfiram could minimise nephrotoxicity.— M. S. Wysor *et al.*, *Science*, 1982, *217*, 454.

Preparations

Cisplatin for Injection *(U.S.P.)*

Proprietary Preparations

Platosin *(Nordic, UK)*. *Injection*, powder for reconstitution, cisplatin 10, 25, or 50 mg.

Proprietary Names and Manufacturers

Cisplatyl *(Bellon, Fr.; Rhone-Poulenc, Swed.)*; Citoplatino *(Rhone-Poulenc, Ital.)*; Neoplatin *(Bristol-Myers, Spain; Bristol-Myers Pharmaceuticals, UK)*; Placis *(Wasserman, Spain)*; Platamine *(Farmitalia Carlo Erba, S.Afr.)*; Platiblastin *(Farmitalia, Ger.)*; Platinex *(Bristol, Ger.; Bristol Italiana Sud, Ital.; Bristol-Myers Pharmaceuticals, UK)*; Platinol *(Bristol-Myers, Austral.; Bristol, Belg.; Bristol, Canad.; Bristol-Myers, Denm.; Lux.; Bristol, Norw.; Bristol, S.Afr.; Bristol, Swed.; Bristol, Switz.; Bristol-Myers Oncology, USA)*; Platistil *(Farmitalia, Spain)*; Platistin *(Farmitalia, Denm.; Farmitalia, Norw.; Farmitalia Carlo Erba, Swed.)*; Platosin *(Nordic, UK)*.

Manufacturers also include—*Bull, UK; Farmitalia Carlo Erba, UK; Lederle, UK.*

1823-z

Colaspase *(BAN)*.

Asparaginase *(USAN)*; NSC-109229; L-Asparaginase; L-Asparagine Amidohydrolase.

CAS — 9015-68-3.

An enzyme obtained from cultures of *Escherichia coli* ATCC 9637. *E. coli* produces two colaspase iso-enzymes of which only one, EC-2, has antineoplastic activity.

Crisantaspase (*BAN*) is the name used for L-asparagine amidohydrolase obtained from *Erwinia chrysanthemi* (*E. carotovora*).

Although colaspase was routinely kept under refrigeration, information from the manufacturer (Merck Sharp & Dohme) indicated that it would remain stable for 48 hours at 15° to 30°.— F. R. Vogenberg and P. F. Souney, *Am. J. Hosp. Pharm.*, 1983, *40*, 101.

Units

One unit of colaspase splits 1 μmol of ammonia from L-asparagine in 1 minute under standard conditions.

Adverse Effects

Colaspase may produce anaphylaxis and other allergic reactions due to its protein nature; there does not appear to be cross-sensitivity between colaspase derived from *Escherichia coli* and that from *Erwinia chrysanthemi*. Chills and pyrexia have been attributed to the presence of bacterial endotoxins in the product. Liver disorders occur in many patients, and there may be hyperammonaemia, decreased blood concentrations of fibrinogen and clotting factors, alterations in blood lipids and cholesterol, hypoalbuminaemia, uraemia, and occasionally renal failure. Pancreatitis may occur and may be fatal: there may also be hyperglycaemia due to decreased insulin production, and death from diabetic ketoacidosis has occurred. Nausea and vomiting, anorexia, weight loss, and CNS disturbances, including depression, coma, hallucinations, and a Parkinson-like syndrome, have also been reported. Bone-marrow depression is rare, but acute leucopenia has occurred.

EFFECTS ON BODY TEMPERATURE. Extreme hyperpyrexia, with a temperature of 42.6°, developed in a boy following administration of colaspase as part of a combination regimen for relapsing acute lymphocytic leukaemia. The patient was successfully treated with ice packs and intravenous dantrolene.— W. A. Smithson *et al.*, *Cancer Treat. Rep.*, 1983, *67*, 318.

EFFECTS ON THE BLOOD. A 55-year-old man with acute lymphoblastic leukaemia developed iliofemoral vein thrombosis 3 days after completing a course of colaspase therapy. His plasma antithrombin III concentration was only 56% before heparin therapy began; a month later it was 81%. More detailed observations in a second patient revealed a rapid and dramatic fall in plasma antithrombin III concentration associated with colaspase therapy. Venous thrombosis may be associated with reduced antithrombin concentrations; the rarity of this complication during colaspase therapy may be explained by a concomitant decrease in coagulation factors.— W. R. Pitney *et al.* (letter), *Lancet*, 1980, *1*, 493. The fall in antithrombin III associated with colaspase therapy may be the explanation for reports of pulmonary embolism following colaspase therapy.— E. Vellenga *et al.* (letter), *ibid.*, 649. See also J. Conard *et al.* (letter), *ibid.*, 1091.

A report of a syndrome of thrombosis and haemorrhage in children receiving colaspase for leukaemia.— J. R. Priest *et al.*, *J. Pediat.*, 1982, *100*, 984. Stroke occurred in an adult when colaspase was added to combination chemotherapy for acute lymphocytic leukaemia. Fibrinogen and antithrombin III concentrations were depressed and the intracranial haemorrhage was believed to be secondary to an imbalance in the coagulation process.— G. S. Lederman (letter), *New Engl. J. Med.*, 1982, *307*, 1643.

Precautions

For reference to the precautions necessary with antineoplastic agents and immunosuppressants, see Antineoplastic Agents, p.583.

Colaspase is contra-indicated in patients with pancreatitis. It should be given cautiously to patients with impaired liver function. Test doses should always be administered at the start of treatment to check for hypersensitivity, as described below under Uses. Re-treatment with colaspase may be associated with an increased risk of allergic reactions.

Colaspase has been reported to interfere with tests of thyroid function by transient reduction of concentrations of thyroxine-binding globulin.

Absorption and Fate

Following intravenous injection the plasma half-life has varied from 8 to 48 hours. It is found in the lymph at about 20% of the concentration in plasma. There is virtually no diffusion into the CSF. Little is excreted in the urine.

Uses and Administration

Colaspase is an enzyme which acts as an antineoplastic agent by breaking down the amino acid L-asparagine to aspartic acid and ammonia. It interferes with the growth of those malignant cells which, unlike most healthy cells, are unable to synthesise L-asparagine for their metabolism. Its action is reportedly specific for the G_1 phase of the cell cycle.

Colaspase is used mainly for the induction of remissions in children with acute lymphoblastic leukaemia. See also under Choice of Antineoplastic Agent, p.586. It may be given intravenously in a dose of 1000 units per kg body-weight daily for 10 days following treatment with vincristine and prednisone or prednisolone, or intramuscularly in a dose of 6000 units per m^2 body-surface given every third day for 9 doses during treatment with vincristine and prednisone or prednisolone. Colaspase is not generally used alone as an induction agent but doses of 200 units per kg daily have been given intravenously for 28 days to adults and children. Children appear to tolerate colaspase better than adults. Although not entirely reliable, a test dose of about 2 units should be given intradermally before treatment with colaspase, or where more than a week has elapsed between doses, and the injection site observed for at least an hour for evidence of a positive reaction; desensitisation has been advocated if no alternative antineoplastic treatment is available.

When administered intravenously a solution of colaspase in Water for Injections or sodium chloride injection (0.9%) should be given over not less than 30 minutes through a running infusion of sodium chloride injection or glucose injection (5%). When given intramuscularly no more than 2 mL of a solution in sodium chloride injection should be injected at a single site.

ADMINISTRATION. Colaspase from *Erwinia chrysanthemi* conjugated with dextran had a half-life approximately 20-fold greater than unmodified enzyme when injected into 3 patients with acute lymphoblastic leukaemia. In one patient the conjugate was able to deplete plasma asparagine for 100 days, compared to 7 days with a comparable dose of unmodified enzyme, suggesting that a single dose could replace the multiple doses given at present and thus reduce the risk of a hypersensitivity reaction. The conjugate also had enhanced glutaminase activity; further evaluation of its metabolic activity was needed.— T. Wileman *et al.*, *J. Pharm. Pharmac.*, 1983, *35*, 762. Conjugates of colaspase with oxidised dextrans of molecular weights 10 000 to 250 000 had reduced antigenicity, as well as prolonged half-life, in *animals*. In general terms, antigen reactivity *in vivo* fell with an increase in the size of the dextran attached.— T. E. Wileman *et al.*, *ibid.*, 1986, *38*, 264.

Proprietary Preparations

Erwinase *(Porton, UK)*. *Injection*, Powder for reconstitution, 10 000 units colaspase (crisantaspase).

Proprietary Names and Manufacturers

Crasnitin *(Bayer, Denm.; Bayer, Ger.; Bayer, Ital.; Bayer, Norw.; Bayer, UK)*; Crasnitine *(Bayer, Belg.; Bayer, Switz.)*; Elspar *(Merck Sharp & Dohme, USA)*; Erwinase *(Porton, UK)*; Kidrolase *(Rhône-Poulenc, Canad.; Bellon, Fr.)*; Laspar *(MPS Lab., S.Afr.)*; Leucogen *(Bayer, Spain)*; Leunase *(May & Baker, Austral.)*.

12609-w

Corynebacterium parvum

C. parvum; *Propionibacterium acnes*; NSC-220537. A species of Gram-positive bacteria.

Corynebacterium parvum is available as a preparation containing inactivated freeze-dried organisms. Commercial preparations are **stored** at 2° to 8°. Protect from light.

Adverse Effects and Precautions

Fever has been reported in 10 to 60% of patients following intracavitary injection and abdominal pain or discomfort in 20% following intraperitoneal injection. Nausea and vomiting may occur and leakage into tissues may result in local discomfort.

The incidence and severity of side-effects may be enhanced if it is given intrapleurally within 10 days of thoracic surgery.

Side-effects arising from *Corynebacterium parvum* have included hypotension, fever, and malaise. Premedication with hydrocortisone, chlorpromazine and promethazine has reduced the hypotension and malaise. Dyspnoea, hyperaesthesia, and transient hemiparesis have occurred causing infusions of *C. parvum* to be stopped.— I. H. McIntosh *et al.* (letter), *Lancet*, 1976, *2*, 803.

Three of 87 patients receiving antineoplastic regimens involving intravenous administration of *Corynebacterium parvum* developed a syndrome of nephrotoxicity with renal failure which resolved on withdrawal of *Corynebacterium parvum*. A fourth patient with *Corynebacterium parvum*-induced renal failure was identified in another hospital.— G. M. Dosik *et al.*, *Ann. intern. Med.*, 1978, *89*, 41.

Uses and Administration

Inactivated *Corynebacterium parvum* has been used in the treatment of malignant effusions. Usual doses of 7 to 14 mg of inactivated freeze-dried *Corynebacterium parvum* in 10 to 20 mL of sodium chloride injection (0.9%) are injected into the pleural or peritoneal cavity immediately after the effusion has been aspirated. If necessary injections may be repeated every 1 to 4 weeks.

Corynebacterium parvum has immunostimulant activity and has been tried as an adjuvant to cancer chemotherapy. It has been injected subcutaneously, intramuscularly, intravenously, and into tumours.

MALIGNANT EFFUSIONS. A review of the use of *Corynebacterium parvum* in the treatment of malignant effusions.— *Drug & Ther. Bull.*, 1983, *21*, 79.

See also under Choice of Antineoplastic Agent, p.588.

Proprietary Preparations

Coparvax *(Calmic, UK)*. *Injection*, powder for reconstitution, *Corynebacterium parvum*, 7 mg.

1825-k

Cyclophosphamide *(BAN, USAN, rINN)*.

B-518; NSC-26271; WR-138719. 2-[Bis(2-chloroethyl)amino]perhydro-1,3,2-oxazaphosphorine 2-oxide monohydrate.

$C_7H_{15}Cl_2N_2O_2P,H_2O = 279.1$.

CAS — 6055-19-2; 50-18-0 (anhydrous).

Pharmacopoeias. In *Br., Braz., Chin., Egypt., Fr., Ind., It., Jpn, Jug., Rus., Turk.,* and *U.S.*

A fine, white crystalline powder. M.p. 49.5° to 53°. It liquefies upon loss of its water of crystallisation. **Soluble** 1 in 25 of water and 1 in 1 of alcohol; slightly soluble in ether. The *B.P.* states that a freshly prepared 2% solution in water has a pH of 4.0 to 6.0. The *U.S.P.* requires that a 1% solution should have a pH of 3.9 to 7.1 when determined 30 minutes after preparation. Solutions deteriorate on storage. Aqueous solutions may be kept for a few hours at temperatures up to 25°. At temperatures above 30° hydrolysis occurs with removal of chlorine.

Solutions for injection are prepared by dissolving, immediately before use, the sterile contents of a sealed container in Water for Injections. **Store** at 2° to 30° in airtight containers. The *U.S.P.* recommends that preparations should be stored at a temperature not exceeding 25°, although they will withstand brief exposure to temperatures up to 30°; it requires preparations to be protected from temperatures above 30°.

INCOMPATIBILITY. The calculated rate constant for decomposition of cyclophosphamide in water preserved with benzyl alcohol was significantly larger than the value for cyclophosphamide in sterile Water for Injection.— D. Brooke *et al.*, *Am. J. Hosp. Pharm.*, 1973, *30*, 134.

ISOMERISM. For the suggestion that the (−)-enantiomer of cyclophosphamide may be more active, see Action, under Uses and Administration, below.

STABILITY IN SOLUTION. Solutions of cyclophosphamide reconstituted with water and diluted to 4 mg per mL with sodium chloride injection (0.9%) lost about 3.5% potency in 24 hours and 11.9% in 1 week when stored at 25°. When protected from light and stored at 5° the loss was 0.55% after 1 week and 1% after 4 weeks.— J. F. Gallelli, *Am. J. Hosp. Pharm.*, 1967, *24*, 425.

Warming vials of cyclophosphamide to facilitate dissolution could result in decreased potency.— D. Brooke *et al.*, *Am. J. Hosp. Pharm.*, 1975, *32*, 44.

A study of the stability of cyclophosphamide injection in polypropylene syringes and polyvinyl chloride infusion bags when stored either refrigerated or frozen and subsequently thawed by microwaving. Only a small degree of degradation occurred when cyclophosphamide injection, reconstituted under strict aseptic conditions with Water for Injections was stored at 4° or −20° for 4 weeks. Storage in polypropylene syringes at −20° was not recommended however, since at the relatively high concentrations used (about 20 mg per mL) precipitation readily occurred during thawing and despite redissolving by vigorous shaking there was a risk that particulate cyclophosphamide might be given to the patient; there was also a marked reversible contraction of the syringe plungers during freezing, resulting in seepage of injection fluid. The results suggest that when cyclophosphamide injection is prepared as described and stored at 4° the expiry date may be extended to 4 weeks.— B. Kirk *et al.*, *Br. J. parent. Ther.*, 1984, *5*, 90.

Adverse Effects and Treatment

For an outline of the adverse effects experienced with antineoplastic agents and immunosuppressants and general guidelines for their treatment, see Antineoplastic Agents, p.580 and p.583. The major dose-limiting effect is myelosuppression which is chiefly manifest as leucopenia. Following single doses the maximum depression of the white cell count may occur in around 1 to 2 weeks with full recovery usually in 3 to 4 weeks. Thrombocytopenia and anaemia may occur but tend to be less common and less severe.

Urinary complications considered to be associated with the excretion of active metabolites in urine include cystitis, which is often severe and haemorrhagic, and may be life-threatening. Adequate hydration to maintain urine output or administration of mesna (see p.842) have been tried in an attempt to reduce urotoxicity.

Alopecia, usually reversible, occurs in about 20% of patients within 3 weeks of starting treatment at normal doses and in practically all patients given high doses. Hyperpigmentation of skin, especially that of the palms and soles, and of the nails, has been reported.

Other reported adverse effects include gastro-intestinal disturbances, hepatotoxicity, inappropriate secretion of antidiuretic hormone, disturbances of carbohydrate metabolism, gonadal suppression, occasionally resulting in sterility, interstitial pulmonary fibrosis, and, especially at high doses, cardiotoxicity.

Cyclophosphamide, in common with other alkylating agents, has carcinogenic, mutagenic, and teratogenic potential and secondary malignancies have occurred in patients given previous antineoplastic therapy including cyclophosphamide.

ALLERGY AND ANAPHYLAXIS. Analysis of data by the Boston Collaborative Drug Surveillance Program detected only one allergic skin reaction among 210 patients given cyclophosphamide, resulting in a calculated incidence of 4.8 reactions per 1000 recipients.— M. Bigby *et al.*, *J. Am. med. Ass.*, 1986, *256*, 3358.

CARCINOGENICITY. There is considerable evidence for an increased incidence of bladder and lymphoproliferative or myeloproliferative malignancies in patients who have received cyclophosphamide. A number of studies have attempted to quantify the risk: Baltus *et al.* (*Ann. rheum. Dis.*, 1983, *42*, 368) suggested that the risk of malignancy in 81 patients treated with cyclophosphamide for rheumatoid arthritis was 4.1 times greater than that in 81 controls. A follow-up study carried out by Pedersen-Bjergaard *et al.* (*Ann. intern. Med.*, 1985, *103*, 195) in 602 former lymphoma patients 7 years after beginning treatment, found that 9 had developed overt acute leukaemia or preleukaemia: the estimated cumulative risk was 6% and the relative risk was 76 times greater than a normal population, and was of similar magnitude to that with other alkylating agents. However, another study involving 333 women treated with cyclophosphamide for ovarian cancer (M.H. Greene *et al.*, *ibid.*, 1986, *105*, 360) estimated the cumulative 10-year risk of acquiring a leukaemic disorder at 5.4%, which was considerably less than 11.2% in 605 women who had received melphalan. This study suggested a correlation between the dose of cyclophosphamide received and the risk of secondary malignancy, which was highest 5 to 6 years after chemotherapy and subsequently declined. In view of the potential risk, Elliott *et al.* (*Br. med. J.*, 1982, *284*, 1160), reporting on 2 women who developed invasive bladder carcinoma following cyclophosphamide treatment of lupus nephritis concluded that its use in this condition was not justified by the results and that its use in other auto-immune conditions and also in malignant disease should be carefully evaluated to ensure that the benefits outweighed the long-term risk before being accepted as standard treatment.

EFFECTS ON THE BLADDER. Sterile haemorrhagic cystitis, believed to be secondary to renal excretion of alkylating metabolites, occurs following high-dose infusions of cyclophosphamide or, more commonly, with prolonged low-dose administration. The cystitis appears to result from chronic inflammation leading to fibrosis and telangiectasia of the bladder epithelium; haemorrhage may be life-threatening if drug administration is continued. Forced diuresis during high-dose infusions of cyclophosphamide has been attempted to minimise the risk of haemorrhagic cystitis but severe impairment of water excretion has been reported, leading to hyponatraemia, weight gain, and inappropriately concentrated urine.— R. A. Bender *et al.*, *Drugs*, 1978, *16*, 46.

In a study of 54 patients with systemic lupus erythematosus or rheumatoid arthritis treated with oral cyclophosphamide, 7 episodes of acute haemorrhagic cystitis were reported, and 2 patients developed carcinoma of the bladder. The use of cyclophosphamide in the treatment of nonmalignant inflammatory rheumatic conditions should be limited.— P. H. Plotz *et al.*, *Ann. intern. Med.*, 1979, *91*, 221.

Limited fluid intake following her daily dose of cyclophosphamide, which had been taken at the evening meal, may have contributed to the development of severe haemorrhagic cystitis in a 17-year-old girl who had taken cyclophosphamide 100 mg daily, gradually reduced to 25 mg daily over 4 years. The drug was withdrawn and haematuria and anaemia slowly resolved during the following 4 months.— M. D. Bischel (letter), *J. Am. med. Ass.*, 1979, *242*, 238.

Haemorrhagic cystitis in 3 men was attributed to treatment with cyclophosphamide which had been discontinued 3 to 6 months earlier.— B. Armstrong *et al.* (letter), *New Engl. J. Med.*, 1979, *300*, 45.

A report of haemorrhagic cystitis in 4 patients given cyclophosphamide in relatively low doses. No common risk factor could be detected in these patients. In one patient, who failed to respond to aminocaproic acid, or intravesical dimethyl sulphoxide, instillation of formalin 4% (1.6% formaldehyde) was effective in arresting bleeding: previous instillation of 1% formalin (0.4% formaldehyde) had produced only a transient reduction in haematuria.— A. S. D. Spiers *et al.* (letter), *Lancet*, 1983, *1*, 1213.

Haemorrhagic cystitis developed in 4 patients receiving very high dose cyclophosphamide, despite concurrent administration of mesna, when the brand of cyclophosphamide they had been receiving was substituted with another. The apparent difference in activity of the 2 brands might be due to a different ratio of the enantiomers in the 2 preparations. When prescribing high doses it is important to stick to one brand of cyclophosphamide or regulate the dosage of the drug and of mesna according to the preparation used.— I. C. Shaw *et al.* (letter), *Lancet*, 1983, *1*, 709. Comment. The manufacturers found no evidence that the 2 brands mentioned were other than identical racemic mixtures. However, the more active brand had its strength specified in terms of the anhydrous substance and the less active as the monohydrate, despite the fact that both were present as the monohydrate; thus, although a vial is specified as 1 g cyclophosphamide, one contains 6.4% more active substance than the other. The results mentioned by Shaw *et al.* appear to be solely explicable by the higher dose administered.— P. Hilgard *et al.* (letter), *ibid.*, 1436.

Massive recurrent bladder haemorrhage may occur in up to 40% of patients given cyclophosphamide, as well as in patients given other cancer treatments such as irradiation. Bleeding may be controlled with 5 to 10% formalin but this is systemically absorbed, leading to potential toxicity and may cause mucosal damage and ureteric fibrosis. Alum may be beneficial, given as a bladder irrigation, in some cases of bladder haemorrhage; steroids, aminocaproic acid, silver nitrate, phenol, and vasopressin have also been tried with little success or severe adverse effects. Diathermy may be of benefit.— N. Bullock and R. H. Whitaker, *Br. med. J.*, 1985, *291*, 1522. Comment. The incidence of bladder haemorrhage has decreased dramatically in patients given cyclophosphamide since the introduction of mesna, and is now exceptional rather than being 40% as stated.— J. de Kraker (letter), *ibid.*, 1986, *292*, 628.

See also, Mesna, p.842 and under Treatment of Adverse Effects, below.

EFFECTS ON ELECTROLYTES. A report of water intoxication in 6 patients following administration of intravenous cyclophosphamide in doses of 15 to 20 mg per kg.— R. B. Bressler and D. P. Huston, *Archs intern. Med.*, 1985, *145*, 548.

EFFECTS ON THE EYES. Blurred vision of varying onset and duration occurred in 5 of 29 children after the intravenous administration of cyclophosphamide.— G. Kende *et al.*, *Cancer*, 1979, *44*, 69.

EFFECTS ON THE LIVER. Hepatitis, marked by abnormal liver enzyme values and jaundice, occurred in a patient given cyclophosphamide 1.5 mg per kg body-weight daily for systemic lupus erythematosus. Symptoms resolved on stopping cyclophosphamide and recurred on restarting at a dose of 50 mg daily.— A. M. Bacon and S. A. Rosenberg, *Ann. intern. Med.*, 1982, *97*, 62.

EFFECTS ON REPRODUCTIVE POTENTIAL. *Gonads.* Azoospermia has been reported to occur after cumulative doses of cyclophosphamide 6 to 10 g, whereas lower doses may be associated with depressed spermatogenesis without complete azoospermia. However it is difficult to separate the effect of the total dose administered from the duration of exposure. Recovery from cyclophosphamide-induced infertility is variable; generally, the larger the dose, the less likely that fertility will return, but many studies claiming infertility to be permanent did not follow patients for long enough to substantiate the claim. Cyclophosphamide therapy in women has resulted in cases of disrupted menstrual cycles and amenorrhoea. Doses that have been associated with "irreversible" sterility in men frequently have a less profound effect on gonadal function in women, with a more rapid time to the return of fertility. Cyclophosphamide-induced infertility in young males appears to be dose-related and there is evidence suggesting that those entering puberty may be particularly sensitive; adolescent and pre-adolescent females are also susceptible but gonadal effects may not be manifested at the same doses that cause testicular damage in boys. It has been reported that exposure to doses up to 17 and 18 g in pubertal and prepubertal females respectively causes no ovarian damage while higher doses have adverse reproductive effects.— J. F. Buchanan and L. J. Davis, *Drug Intell. & clin. Pharm.*, 1984, *18*, 122.

A study of the long-term effects of cyclophosphamide on testicular function. Of 30 men studied a mean of 12.8 years after treatment with cyclophosphamide 2 to 3 mg per kg body-weight daily for a mean of 280 days, 17 had normal sperm counts, 9 were oligospermic, and 4 were azoospermic. There was a significant inverse correlation betweeen sperm density and the dose and duration of cyclophosphamide therapy. None of the patients who were treated for less than 112 days and received less than 10 g of the drug had an abnormal sperm count. Thirteen of the patients had undergone semen analysis over 5 years previously; 9 remained in the same categories (3 azoospermic, 2 oligospermic, 4 normospermic) but 3 previously oligospermic and 1 azoospermic patient had recovered normal sperm counts. However, all patients studied, including those with normal sperm counts, had hormonal evidence of testicular damage, and in particular of compensated Leydig cell failure.— A. R. Watson *et al.*, *Br. med. J.*, 1985, *291*, 1457.

See also under Adverse Effects of Antineoplastics, p.582.

EFFECTS ON RESPIRATORY FUNCTION. Insidiously progressive fibrosis may occur in patients on long-term therapy with cyclophosphamide or similar drugs that damage alveolar endothelial cells directly causing intra-alveolar exudation of fibrinous fluid.— S. J. Pearce, *Adverse Drug React. Bull.*, 1982, (Jun.), 344.

A report of progressive, and ultimately fatal, pulmonary fibrosis in 2 patients given cyclophosphamide. Progression to respiratory failure occurred despite withdrawal of the drug and conservative treatment.— D. A. Burke *et al.*, *Br. med. J.*, 1982, *285*, 696.

A report of early-onset pneumonitis in 4 lymphoma patients receiving cyclophosphamide. Lung biopsies revealed diffuse interstitial pneumonitis in 3 who had received total cyclophosphamide doses of 6.3, 4.9, and 3.6 g; the fourth, who had received 6 g, showed nonspecific alveolar changes. Resolution of symptoms and signs occurred within 1 to 3 weeks of discontinuing cyclophosphamide and treatment with prednisone in 3. These patients, and a further 3 previously reported (J.I. Spector and H. Zimbler, *J. Am. med. Ass.*, 1979, *242*, 2852) subsequently received further chemotherapy without cyclophosphamide and had no recurrence of pneumonitis. It is possible that cyclophosphamide may be interacting with a factor peculiar to lymphoma patients to produce pneumonitis.— J. I. Spector and H. Zimbler (letter), *New Engl. J. Med.*, 1982, *307*, 251.

Results in *rats* suggested that the reactive metabolite acrolein was at least partly responsible for cyclophosphamide-induced lung toxicity.— J. M. Patel *et al.*, *Toxic. appl. Pharmac.*, 1984, *76*, 128.

EFFECTS ON THE THYROID. Reversible hypothyroidism could be caused by treatment with cyclophosphamide.— P. H. Baylis, *Adverse Drug React. Bull.*, 1986, (Feb.), 432.

TREATMENT OF ADVERSE EFFECTS. Evidence that autologous bone-marrow rescue is unnecessary after cyclophosphamide even in very high doses of 7 g per m^2 body-surface over 12 hours.— I. E. Smith *et al.* (letter), *Lancet*, 1983, *1*, 76.

A study indicating that disulfiram could be used similarly to mesna to protect against cyclophosphamide-induced bladder toxicity.— W. B. Ershler *et al.* (letter), *Cancer Treat. Rep.*, 1983, *67*, 1145.

Instillation of dinoprostone 750 μg in 200 mL of sodium chloride injection (0.9%) daily for 5 days was effective in arresting haematuria in a patient with severe chronic haemorrhagic cystitis induced by cyclophosphamide.— J. Mohiuddin *et al.* (letter), *Ann. intern. Med.*, 1984, *101*, 142.

For the use of mesna in the prevention of cyclophosphamide-induced bladder toxicity, see Mesna, p.842. See also under Effects on the Bladder, above.

Precautions

For reference to the precautions necessary with antineoplastic agents and immunosuppressants, see Antineoplastic Agents, p.583.

Cyclophosphamide should not be given to patients with haemorrhagic cystitis, acute urinary infection, or drug- or radiation-induced urothelial toxicity. It should be given with care to those with diabetes mellitus. Reduced doses may need to be employed in elderly or debilitated patients, or those with renal or hepatic failure. Liberal fluid intake and frequent micturition are advised to reduce the risk of cystitis but care must be taken to avoid water retention and intoxication.

Since cyclophosphamide must undergo metabolism before it is active, interactions are possible with drugs which either inhibit or stimulate the enzymes responsible. There may be an increased risk of cardiotoxicity in patients who have also received doxorubicin or other cardiotoxic anthracyclines, or have had irradiation to the area of the heart.

Cyclophosphamide has teratogenic and mutagenic potential; its use in pregnancy should be avoided where possible. Mothers taking cyclophosphamide should avoid breast-feeding.

HANDLING AND DISPOSAL. A method for the destruction of cyclophosphamide or ifosfamide using alkaline hydrolysis in the presence of dimethylformamide. Refluxing 100 mg of either drug with 10 mL of a 12% sodium hydroxide solution (about 3 molar) and 20 mL of dimethylformamide, for 4 hours, results in complete degradation of the drug. Aqueous solutions should be diluted with 40% sodium hydroxide to achieve a maximum drug content of 1% and a minimum sodium hydroxide concentration of 12% and then added to twice their volume of dimethylformamide and refluxed. The method may also be used for solutions of up to 2% cyclophosphamide or ifosfamide in dimethyl sulphoxide, by addition of an equal volume of dimethylformamide and enough 12% sodium hydroxide to achieve a 4% concentration of alkali and not more than 0.5% of drug. Glassware should be rinsed with 12% sodium hydroxide and then with water and the combined rinsings may be treated as for aqueous solutions while the area of a spillage, once the bulk has been collected and dealt with, should be rinsed with excess 12% sodium hydroxide and the rinsings taken up on absorbent material, immersed in a 2:1 mixture of dimethylformamide and 12% sodium hydroxide, and refluxed. Residues by degradation of either drug by this method showed no mutagenicity *in vitro*. However, an alternative method exists, involving refluxing of cyclophosphamide with molar hydrochloric acid 40 mL per g of drug, neutralising to pH 6 and then reacting with 6 g of sodium thiosulphate per g in a strongly alkaline environment for 1 hour. This method is effective for the degradation of cyclophosphamide, but residues from ifosfamide were still highly mutagenic *in vitro* and this second method should therefore not be used to degrade ifosfamide.— IARC Scientific Publications No. 73, *Laboratory Decontamination and Destruction of Carcinogens in Laboratory Wastes: Some Antineoplastic Agents*, M. Castegnaro *et al.* (Eds), Lyon, International Agency for Research on Cancer, 1985, p. 57.

When handling urine and faeces from patients receiving cyclophosphamide protective clothing should be worn for up to 72 hours and 5 days (after an oral dose) respectively after therapy. As cyclophosphamide was present in sweat and saliva, protective clothing was advised for 72 hours after a dose when bathing the patient or carrying out oral procedures.— J. Harris and L. J. Dodds, *Pharm. J.*, 1985, *2*, 289.

See also under Absorption and Fate, below.

INTERACTIONS. *Allopurinol.* The incidence of bone-marrow depression in 95 patients with neoplastic diseases other than leukaemia who received cyclophosphamide or other cytotoxic drugs was 12.6%. There was a significantly higher incidence of bone-marrow depression (33.8%) in 65 patients who also received allopurinol.— Boston Collaborative Drug Surveillance Program, *J. Am. med. Ass.*, 1974, *227*, 1036.

Antibacterial agents. Administration of chloramphenicol prior to cyclophosphamide prolonged the mean cyclophosphamide serum half-life from 7.5 to 11.5 hours and reduced the peak activity in all of 5 subjects. Administration of sulphaphenazole prior to cyclophosphamide significantly inhibited the rate of biotransformation of cyclophosphamide in 2 of 7 subjects and enhanced it in 2; it remained unchanged in 3.— O. K. Faber *et al.*, *Br. J. clin. Pharmac.*, 1975, *2*, 281.

Barbiturates. Although patients receiving cyclophosphamide developed higher peak plasma concentrations of active cyclophosphamide metabolites when given enzyme-inducing agents such as barbiturates, the active metabolites also disappeared rapidly.— C. M. Bagley *et al.*, *Cancer Res.*, 1973, *33*, 226.

Corticosteroids. A suggestion that since corticosteroids appear to inhibit the enzyme systems which activate cyclophosphamide, doses should be reduced when concomitant treatment with corticosteroids is withdrawn.— S. R. Kaplan and P. Calabresi, *New Engl. J. Med.*, 1973, *289*, 952. Doubts about this conclusion. Single doses of prednisone have been found to inhibit the activation of cyclophosphamide but after longer-term treatment the rate of activation has increased.— O. K. Faber and H. T. Mouridsen (letter), *ibid.*, 1974, *291*, 211.

Digoxin. Cardiac arrhythmias during combination chemotherapy in a patient with atrial fibrillation previously well controlled with digoxin might have been due to an interaction between cyclophosphamide and digoxin.— H. Echizen and T. Ishizaki, *Br. med. J.*, 1985, *291*, 1172.

Suxamethonium. For reference to a possible interaction between cyclophosphamide and suxamethonium, see under Suxamethonium Chloride, p.1239.

PORPHYRIA. Cyclophosphamide was considered to be unsafe in patients with acute porphyria because it has been shown to be porphyrinogenic in *animals* or *in-vitro* systems.— M.R. Moore and K.E.L. McColl, *Porphyrias, Drug Lists*, Glasgow, Porphyria Research Unit, University of Glasgow, 1987.

PREGNANCY AND THE NEONATE. The American Academy of Pediatrics recommended that cyclophosphamide be contra-indicated during breast-feeding.— *Pediatrics*, 1983, *72*, 375.

Absorption and Fate

Following oral administration, cyclophosphamide is absorbed from the gastro-intestinal tract; absorption has been reported to be incomplete after high doses. Peak concentrations in plasma occur about 1 hour after an oral dose. Cyclophosphamide is widely distributed in the tissues. It undergoes activation by the mixed function oxidase systems in the liver. The initial metabolites are 4-hydroxycyclophosphamide and its acylic tautomer, aldophosphamide; both undergo further metabolism to active compounds including nor-nitrogen mustard and phosphoramide mustard. Acrolein is also produced. Cyclophosphamide is excreted principally in urine, as metabolites and some unchanged drug.

It crosses the placenta, and is found in breast milk.

A detailed review of the pharmacokinetics of some antineoplastic agents, including cyclophosphamide. Cyclophosphamide has been estimated to be 97% absorbed following an oral dose of 100 mg and 74% absorbed following 300 mg. It is metabolised in the liver to the 4-hydroxy derivative which is in spontaneous equilibrium with aldophosphamide. The latter can spontaneously eliminate acrolein to form phosphoramide mustard but both primary metabolites may also be further oxidised to 5-ketocyclophosphamide and carboxyphosphamide, the major urinary metabolites. Cyclophosphamide itself is reportedly 12 to 14% protein bound but its alkylating metabolites are more extensively bound. Its disposition is biexponential following intravenous doses, with a terminal half-life variously reported as from 1.8 to 12.4 hours, the mean value being 6.5 hours. The half-life in children appears to be shorter with a mean of 4.1 hours. Half-life decreases with daily exposure, suggesting that it induces its own metabolism. Cyclophosphamide is excreted in urine, about 6.5 to 20% of a dose reportedly unchanged, the rest as active and inactive metabolites.— F. M. Balis *et al.*, *Clin. Pharmacokinet.*, 1983, *8*, 202. See also: L. B. Grochow and M. Colvin, *ibid.*, 1979, *4*, 380.

Cyclophosphamide was detected in the urine of 5 patients following application to intact skin, demonstrating that cyclophosphamide can be absorbed via this route. Absorption continued after the site of application had been cleaned, suggesting that cyclophosphamide had penetrated subcutaneous lipid and was slowly released to the circulation from this depot. Cyclophosphamide was also identified in the urine of 2 oncology nurses but appeared more quickly than in patients, suggesting a faster route of absorption, perhaps by inhalation of aerosols generated during dissolution of the drug.— M. Hirst *et al.*, *Lancet*, 1984, *1*, 186.

DISTRIBUTION. Cyclophosphamide was identified in the blood, cerebrospinal fluid, milk, saliva, sweat, synovial fluid, and urine of patients receiving cyclophosphamide for malignant disease or for rheumatoid arthritis.— J. H. Duncan *et al.*, *Toxic. appl. Pharmac.*, 1973, *24*, 317.

Results in 3 patients following short intravenous infusions of cyclophosphamide indicated that although pharmacokinetics varied widely between patients the ratio of the unchanged drug concentration in saliva and plasma was consistent at 62%. Measurement of salivary concentrations may offer a simple non-invasive method to measure cyclophosphamide plasma concentrations.— W. A. Ritschel *et al.*, *J. clin. Pharmac.*, 1981, *21*, 461.

Uses and Administration

Cyclophosphamide is an antineoplastic agent which is converted in the body to an active alkylating metabolite with properties similar to those of mustine (p.645). It also possesses marked immunosuppressant properties.

Cyclophosphamide is widely used, often in combination with other agents, in the treatment of a variety of malignant diseases including Burkitt's lymphoma, Hodgkin's disease and other lymphomas, acute and chronic lymphoblastic leukaemia, acute non-lymphoblastic leukaemia, multiple myeloma, and mycosis fungoides. It is also used in the treatment of various solid tumours such as carcinoma of the breast, cervix, lung, and ovary; neuroblastoma; retinoblastoma; and sarcomas. The immunosuppressant properties of cyclophosphamide are used in Wegener's granulomatosis and in prolonging the survival of homografts, such as in kidney transplantation. It has also been used in the management of auto-immune disorders such as systemic lupus erythematosus, the nephrotic syndrome, and rheumatoid arthritis. See also under Choice of Antineoplastic Agent, p.584.

Cyclophosphamide is given by mouth or intravenous injection; it is not a tissue irritant or vesicant. The dosage given depends on the malignant disease being treated, the condition of the patient including the state of the bone marrow, and the concomitant use of radiotherapy or other chemotherapy. Regimens used include: cyclophosphamide 2 to 6 mg per kg body-weight daily as a single intravenous dose or in divided doses by mouth; 10 to 15 mg per kg weekly as a single intravenous dose; 20 to 40 mg per kg as a single intravenous dose every 10 to 20 days. Much higher doses have been used.

In the *USA*, an initial dose of 40 to 50 mg per kg has been advocated, given intravenously in divided doses over 2 to 5 days. Alternatively, 1 to 5 mg per kg daily has been given orally. Maintenance therapy may be carried out with doses of 1 to 5 mg per kg daily, orally or intravenously, or by intravenous doses of 3 to 5 mg per kg twice weekly or 10 to 15 mg per kg every seven to ten days.

Children have been given initial doses of 2 to 8 mg per kg daily by intravenous injection or by mouth and maintenance doses of 2 to 5 mg per kg twice weekly by mouth.

A daily dose of 2 to 3 mg per kg body-weight has been used in children with the nephrotic syndrome in whom corticosteroids have been unsuccessful.

In the *B.P.* the potency of Cyclophosphamide Injection is expressed in terms of the equivalent amount of anhydrous cyclophosphamide whereas the potency of Cyclophosphamide Tablets is given in terms of the monohydrate; the *U.S.P.* expresses potency in terms of anhydrous cyclophosphamide for both injection and tablets.

Cyclophosphamide has also been given intramuscularly, intraperitoneally, intrapleurally, and intra-arterially, and by local perfusion (but see Absorption and Fate). A liquid preparation of cyclophosphamide for oral use may be prepared using the powder for injection.

Regular blood counts are essential during therapy with cyclophosphamide and in general treatment should be withdrawn or delayed if leucopenia or thrombocytopenia becomes severe.

A review of the actions and uses of cyclophosphamide.— A. R. Ahmed and S. H. Hombal, *J. Am. Acad. Derm.*, 1984, *11*, 1115.

ACCELERATION OF BONE-MARROW RECOVERY. Bone-marrow recovery of 7 patients who received cyclophosphamide 500 mg intravenously one week before a high dose of melphalan (140 mg per m^2) was more rapid than that of 4 controls who received smaller doses of melphalan (60 to 125 mg per m^2) without previous cyclophosphamide therapy. The role of cyclophosphamide priming to accelerate bone-marrow recovery after high doses of alkylating agents appears to merit further study.— D. W. Hedley *et al.*, *Lancet*, 1978, *2*, 966.

ACTION. There is some evidence to suggest that cyclophosphamide could be better employed if the (−)-enantiomer was used. Although the toxicity of the two enantiomers is equivalent the cytotoxic activity of the (−)-enantiomer is twice as great as that of the (+)-enantiomer. The former thus has a therapeutic index approximately twice that of the latter and about 1.3 times greater than that of the racemate, implying that it would have less toxicity in clinical practice.— K. Williams and E. Lee, *Drugs*, 1985, *30*, 333.

ADMINISTRATION IN RENAL INSUFFICIENCY. Doses of cyclophosphamide should be halved and the interval between doses extended from 12 hours to 18 to 24 hours in patients with a glomerular filtration-rate of less than 10 mL per minute. Concentrations of cyclophosphamide are affected by haemodialysis.— W. M. Bennett *et al.*, *Am. J. Kidney Dis.*, 1983, *3*, 155.

A study indicating that significant amounts of cyclophosphamide are removed by dialysis.— L. H. Wang *et al.*, *Clin. Pharmac. Ther.*, 1981, *29*, 365.

ADMINISTRATION IN HEPATIC INSUFFICIENCY. The mean half-life of cyclophosphamide was 12.5 hours in 7 patients with severe liver failure compared to 7.6 hours in 10 patients with normal hepatic function, following administration to both groups of cyclophosphamide 15 mg per kg body-weight intravenously. The total body clearance was significantly reduced in patients with impaired hepatic function, suggesting that cyclophosphamide might accumulate in patients with liver disease.— F. D. Juma, *Eur. J. clin. Pharmac.*, 1984, *26*, 591.

BLOOD DISORDERS, NON-MALIGNANT. *Aplastic anaemia.* Two of 6 patients with aplastic anaemia resistant to anabolic steroids had obtained a beneficial response to cyclophosphamide therapy with almost complete remission after 5 months of therapy.— J. Pizzuto *et al.* (letter), *New Engl. J. Med.*, 1978, *298*, 164.

Aplastic anaemia in a patient with systemic lupus erythematosus responded to treatment with cyclophosphamide 1 g intravenously. The bone marrow aplasia had not responded to previous treatment with prednisolone and azathioprine. The patient subsequently remained well on prednisolone therapy.— M. J. Walport *et al., Br. med. J.*, 1982, *285*, 769. High-dose cyclophosphamide and methylprednisolone had no discernible effect in a similar case.— D. W. Milligan and I. W. Delamore (letter), *ibid.*, 1352. See also R. Storb *et al., New Engl. J. Med.*, 1983, *308*, 302.

LEUKAEMIA, ACUTE. The use of cyclophosphamide and total body irradiation followed by transplantation of unpurged autologous bone marrow in patients with acute myeloid leukaemia in first remission. Patients were brought to remisssion with standard induction and consolidation chemotherapy. Bone marrow was subsequently collected, and the patients given cyclophosphamide 60 mg per kg body-weight on 2 occasions, 2 and 22 hours after collection. Total body irradiation was then carried out and the unpurged bone marrow re-infused. Seven of 12 patients so treated remain in remission between 26 and 140 weeks after autograft, without maintenance therapy, and the 3-year estimated remission rate is 58%. One patient required cystectomy for haemorrhagic cystitis, and one developed fatal respiratory failure. The duration of remission and exemption from graft-versus-host disease are encouraging, and although the numbers are too small to draw a definite conclusion the study suggests that even with unpurged bone marrow the technique may offer prolonged remission to a significant proportion of patients.— A. K. Burnett *et al., Lancet*, 1984, *2*, 1068. Comment. Comparable results had also been obtained following high-dose melphalan and autologous marrow transplantation, a less aggressive and perhaps less toxic approach than cyclophosphamide and total body irradiation.— D. Maraninchi *et al.* (letter), *ibid.*, 1401.

Further references: R. Storb *et al., New Engl. J. Med.*, 1986, *314*, 729; J. Chang *et al., Lancet*, 1986, *1*, 294.

LUPUS ERYTHEMATOSUS. Since 1965, cyclophosphamide had been used in the treatment of 42 patients (37 female, 5 male) with systemic lupus erythematosus. Prednisolone, 15 to 60 mg daily, was given initially. Cyclophosphamide 400 mg was given intravenously once a week, then 100 mg by mouth 4 times a week; some patients continued to take small doses of prednisolone. Treatment had continued for 6 to 84 months and in some patients was no longer required; 16 patients had complete clinical and biochemical remissions and 12 had minimal residual clinical and biochemical involvement.— P. H. Feng *et al., Br. med. J.*, 1973, *2*, 450. See also W. J. McCune *et al., New Engl. J. Med.*, 1988, *318*, 1423.

Lupus nephritis. Immunosuppressant drugs have been used in the treatment of systemic lupus erythematosus, normally combined with prednisolone, the major indications being severe active lupus nephritis, and to permit reduction of corticosteroid dosage. Because of its toxicity, cyclophosphamide has normally been reserved for severely-ill patients unresponsive to other drugs.

There has been considerable debate as to the value of such immunosuppressant therapy in lupus nephritis, and a number of studies have failed to show a clinical benefit. However, a review of pooled data from published studies, carried out by Felson and Anderson (*New Engl. J. Med.*, 1984, *311*, 1528) concluded that immunosuppressive therapy with cyclophosphamide or azathioprine, combined with corticosteroids, was significantly superior to corticosteroids alone in preventing renal functional deterioration, end-stage renal failure, and nephritis-related death, and that previous clinical studies had been too small to demonstrate a statistically significant effect. Balow *et al.* in a study involving 62 patients (*ibid.*, 491) were able to demonstrate that conventional high-dose prednisone treatment did not prevent the progression of renal scarring, whereas no progression appeared in patients given cyclophosphamide (oral or intravenous), azathioprine, or both. The same group subsequently found (H.A. Austin *et al., ibid.*, 1986, *314*, 614) immunosuppressive treatment with intermittent high-dose cyclophosphamide, given by intravenous infusion in doses of 0.5 to 1 g per m^2 body-surface every 3 months, together with low-dose prednisone, to be significantly superior to high-dose prednisone alone in reducing the probability of progression to end-stage renal failure. Although this study suggested that the intravenous cyclophosphamide regimen was more effective than oral cyclophosphamide or azathioprine, or both, the statistical validity of the latter conclusion has been criticised: there is no real evidence that one immmunosuppressant regimen is better than another (D.T. Felson and J. Anderson., *ibid.*, *315*, 458). However, while this is true, the intravenous regimen has shown evidence of reduced toxicity in terms of malignancy, cystitis, and bone-marrow suppression (H.A. Austin *et al., ibid.*, 459). Toxicity, and in particular the risk of subsequent malignancies, remains a major consideration of such therapy (see also under Adverse Effects above) and the decision to employ it must be made with care in patients in whom the benefits are likely to outweigh the risks (J.F. Fries, *ibid.*, 1985, *312*, 921).

MALIGNANT NEOPLASMS OF THE BREAST. See under Choice of Antineoplastic Agent, p.588.

MALIGNANT NEOPLASMS OF THE BRONCHUS AND LUNG. Encouraging results from a pilot study of very high dose cyclophosphamide (150 to 200 mg per kg body-weight) and autologous bone-marrow transplantation in patients with small cell carcinoma of the bronchus. Of 25 patients given a single high-dose course, 16 achieved complete response; median survival was 66 weeks.— R. L. Souhami *et al., Cancer Chemother. Pharmac.*, 1982, *8*, 31.

See also under Choice of Antineoplastic Agent, p.590.

MALIGNANT NEOPLASMS OF THE OVARY. For a study indicating that cyclophosphamide is less effective than cisplatin in the single-agent therapy of advanced ovarian cancer, see Choice of Antineoplastic Agent, p.591.

MULTIPLE SCLEROSIS. References to the use of cyclophosphamide in multiple sclerosis: S. L. Hauser *et al., New Engl. J. Med.*, 1983, *308*, 173; K. H. Fischbeck (letter), *ibid.*, *309*, 239; D. P. Huston *et al.* (letter), *ibid.*, 240; S. L. Hauser *et al.* (letter), *ibid.*, 241; *Lancet*, 1983, *1*, 909; B. Giesser, *Drugs*, 1985, *29*, 88.

MYELOMA. Cyclophosphamide has been used in the treatment of multiple myeloma, in doses of 50 mg daily by mouth, increased according to bone-marrow toxicity. More recently it has been given intravenously as a single weekly dose of 300 mg per m^2 body-surface. Side-effects include nausea and thinning of hair, but these tend to improve with time. The median duration of survival is about 2 years from starting treatment, which is comparable to melphalan therapy.— J. E. Oakley and I. M. Franklin, *J. clin. Hosp. Pharm.*, 1984, *9*, 15.

OCULAR DISORDERS, NON-MALIGNANT. The symptoms of Graves' ophthalmopathy were improved in 2 patients by treatment with cyclophosphamide 150 mg daily for 15 months and 85 mg daily for 5 months by mouth. Similar symptoms improved in another patient receiving cyclophosphamide 700 mg intravenously each month for 12 months to treat ovarian carcinoma.— S. T. Bigos *et al., Ann. intern. Med.*, 1979, *90*, 921. See also R. Wilkinson, *Prescribers' J.*, 1984, *24*, 97.

ORGAN AND TISSUE TRANSPLANTATION. The use of cyclophosphamide and busulphan to prepare children with beta-thalassaemia for bone-marrow transplantation. Patients were given high-dose busulphan 3.5 or 4 mg per kg body-weight in divided doses by mouth for 4 days, followed by cyclophosphamide 50 mg per kg intravenously for a further 4 days. Allogeneic marrow was infused 36 hours after the last dose of cyclophosphamide. Post-transplant immunosuppression was with methotrexate alone or combined with cyclophosphamide. Of 30 patients engraftment was achieved in 27, of whom 22 were still alive and free of thalassaemia on evaluation 64 to 762 days after transplantation; a further 4 were living but developed a recurrence of disease, while one patient died of graft-versus-host disease. The overall incidence of acute graft-versus-host disease was 23%.— G. Lucarelli *et al., Lancet*, 1985, *1*, 1355.

For reference to the use of cyclophosphamide in bone-marrow transplantation to prolong remissions in leukaemia patients see Leukaemia, Acute, above.

PARAQUAT POISONING. Fifty-two of 72 patients severely poisoned with paraquat survived following treatment with cyclophosphamide and dexamethasone in addition to forced diuresis and inactivation of remaining paraquat in the gut.— E. Addo and T. Poon-king, *Lancet*, 1986, *1*, 1117. Comment. Although the results are encouraging only 25 patients had had the plasma concentration of paraquat assessed; in 6 it was indetectible, indicating that an insignificant amount had been ingested, while of the 19 remaining, 12 with very high plasma concentrations all died, and it is uncertain how many of the remaining 7 would have survived without the intensive regimen. For the moment, cyclophosphamide treatment cannot be recommended.— *ibid.*, *2*, 375.

RENAL DISORDERS, NON-MALIGNANT. Cyclophosphamide 3 mg per kg body-weight was compared with azathioprine 2.5 to 3 mg per kg in the treatment of 24 Nigerian children with the nephrotic syndrome mainly associated with quartan malaria and generally considered to be corticosteroid-resistant. Both drugs were given daily for 12 weeks and 12 additional patients acted as controls. Complete clinical remission occurred in 2 children treated with cyclophosphamide, and considerable improvement in 6, but there was a high incidence of adverse effects and the 5-year survival-rate was not improved. Complete clinical remission occurred in 2 children treated with azathioprine, but there was increased mortality due to renal failure. No remissions were noted in the control group. It was recommended that cyclophosphamide could be used to treat West African children with a short history of nephrotic syndrome and relatively mild histological lesions, and that azathioprine was contra-indicated.— A. Adeniyi *et al., Archs Dis. Childh.*, 1979, *54*, 204.

From the results of a study involving 55 children with minimal-change nephrotic syndrome, cyclophosphamide 2.5 mg per kg body-weight daily for 8 weeks appeared to be a safe, effective, and justifiable alternative in the few children with minimal-change disease who would otherwise need an unacceptably high cumulative corticosteroid dose.— J. Feehally *et al., New Engl. J. Med.*, 1984, *310*, 415. Comment. Daily administration of cyclophosphamide puts the patient at daily risk of bladder complications, infections, and chromosomal abnormalities. The more self-limited the disease, the fewer the risks that should be taken with the drug.— A. D. Steinberg, *ibid.*, 458. Further comment and criticism. In view of the potential for development of malignancy in patients given cyclophosphamide the use of this drug in children with minimal-change nephrotic syndrome is unjustifiable.— H. W. Grünwald and F. Rosner (letter), *ibid.*, *311*, 126. Reply. Minimal-change disease is not benign, and 35% of patients died before drug treatment was available. Furthermore, cyclophosphamide is not offered to patients who respond to corticosteroids and do not relapse. Its cautious use generally spares appropriate patients from the need to take steroids over a prolonged period, and has been an important clinical advance, and in view of the evidence that side-effects are related to dose this low-dose regimen should continue to be viewed as a justifiable alternative in such patients.— N. P. Mallick (letter), *ibid.*

Further references to the use of cyclophosphamide in minimal-change disease: R. S. Trompeter, *Archs Dis. Childh.*, 1986, *61*, 727; J. S. Lilleyman (letter), *ibid.*, 1987, *62*, 214.

See also under Wegener's Granulomatosis, below.

RESPIRATORY DISORDERS, NON-MALIGNANT. Cryptogenic fibrosing alveolitis may be treated with cyclophosphamide when corticosteroids fail, usually with a dose of 2 mg per kg body-weight daily. Improvement tends to occur slowly over 3 to 6 months and treatment is normally continued for this time before accepting failure. If haematuria occurs it is the author's current practice to change to azathioprine.— M. E. H. Turner-Warwick, *Postgrad. med. J.*, 1984, *60*, 183.

RHEUMATIC DISORDERS. In a study in 17 patients with severe rheumatoid arthritis unresponsive to gold treatment, treatment for an average of 27 months with an experimental regimen combining low-dose hydroxychloroquine, cyclophosphamide, and azathioprine produced striking improvement in 7, 5 of whom were considered to have achieved complete remission. A further 7 had some improvement, while 3 had little or no change in disease status. The mean daily doses of drugs taken were cyclophosphamide 550 µg per kg body-weight, azathioprine 780 µg per kg, and hydroxychloroquine 3.15 mg per kg. All patients continued to receive salicylates during treatment; 10 also received prednisone, 5 of whom were subsequently able to discontinue it due to improved disease status. Side-effects were relatively mild in these patients, but a further 4 were withdrawn from the study due to infections, haemorrhagic cystitis, or oral ulceration and leukopenia. Three of these patients had been receiving high doses of corticosteroids and had evidence of Cushing's syndrome. These promising results should be regarded as experimental until a controlled blinded study of this regimen has been carried out.— D. J. McCarty and G. F. Carrera, *J. Am. med. Ass.*, 1982, *248*, 1718.

Treatment with intermittent cyclophosphamide 100 mg by mouth every 2 to 4 days was effective in abolishing disease symptoms in 3 patients with rheumatoid arthritis.— K. Hørslev-Petersen *et al., Br. med. J.*, 1983, *287*, 711. See also *idem*, 1717.

A review of published studies, including 4 studies of the use of cyclophosphamide, suggested that it could retard radiographic deterioration in patients with rheumatoid arthritis.— L. Iannuzzi *et al., New Engl. J. Med.*, 1983, *309*, 1023.

SKIN AND CONNECTIVE-TISSUE DISORDERS, NON-MALIGNANT. Reports on the use of cyclophosphamide in the treatment of severe skin diseases: A. Medved and I. Maxwell, *Can. med. Ass. J.*, 1974, *111*, 245 (pemphigus vulgaris and bullous pemphigoid); J. S. Pasricha *et al., Br. J. Derm.*, 1975, *93*, 573 (pemphigus); J. G. L. Morrison and E. J. Schulz, *Br. J. Derm.*, 1978, *98*, 203 (eczema); *J. Am. med. Ass.*, 1979, *241*, 2475 (ichythyosis linearis circumflexa and poikiloderma congenitale); L. M. Newell and F. D. Malkinson, *Archs Derm.*, 1983, *119*, 495 (pyoderma gangrenosum); D. A. Paslin, *Archs Derm.*, 1985, *121*, 236 (lichen planus).

Takayasu's arteritis. In a study in 20 patients with Takayasu's arteritis (a large vessel arteritis) 16 were considered to have active disease and were treated initially with prednisone 1 mg per kg body-weight daily by mouth. Seven patients failed to respond to corticosteroids and had cyclophosphamide 2 mg per kg daily by mouth added to their regimen; the corticosteroid dose was reduced to an alternate day regimen, and discontinued altogether in 1 patient. All patients given the combined regimen had either symptomatic improvement (in 2) or arrest of disease progression, although progression subsequently occurred in 2 at 30 and 48 months after starting therapy. Although drug therapy appeared to have produced a more favourable outcome in these patients than has previously been reported, the uncertainty as to the natural history of the disease in these patients makes it difficult to know whether cortisteroids, cyclophosphamide, or both will be effective in the long-term preservation of organ function and prolongation of life.— J. H. Shelhamer *et al.*, *Ann. intern. Med.*, 1985, *103*, 121. Comparable results with prednisone alone.— S. Hall and G. G. Hunder (letter), *ibid.*, 1986, *104*, 288. Cyclophosphamide 1 mg per kg by mouth daily was ineffective in a patient with advanced Takayasu's arteritis.— J. Jiménez-Alonso *et al.* (letter), *Drug Intell. & clin. Pharm.*, 1985, *19*, 477.

Vasculitic syndromes. Complete, sometimes dramatic, remissions were achieved in 13 of 16 patients with severe systemic necrotising vasculitis when they took cyclophosphamide 2 mg per kg body-weight daily, and in one patient who took the same dose of azathioprine; 3 patients died although 2 were in remission. Within 2 weeks of starting treatment with cyclophosphamide, the corticosteroid regimens which 16 patients had been on previously were tapered; 6 remained on alternate-day therapy and corticosteroids were eventually stopped in 7. The cyclophosphamide dose was continually titrated and readjusted to maintain the total neutrophil count at not less than 1000 to 1500 per mm^3. There were no relapses during treatment with cyclophosphamide and remissions ranged from 2 to 61 months.— A. S. Fauci *et al.*, *New Engl. J. Med.*, 1979, *301*, 235.

A discussion of the treatment of systemic vasculitis, including the role of cyclophosphamide.— *Lancet*, 1985, *1*, 1252.

Comment on the treatment of vasculitis of the central nervous system. Two patients with primary angiitis of the CNS were treated with cyclophosphamide and high-dose prednisone. Cerebral angiography after 6 months demonstrated complete resolution; cyclophosphamide was discontinued and prednisone therapy slowly tapered off. The patients had remained disease-free for 6 months and 2 years respectively. The optimum length of this therapy for uncomplicated primary angiitis of the CNS should be about 6 months or less if signs and symptoms have resolved.— L. H. Calabrese and J. A. Mallek (letter), *J. Am. med. Ass.*, 1987, *258*, 778. Reply. Patients should certainly be restudied at about 6 months but the decision about duration of treatment should be based on the angiographic findings.— G. M. Kammer (letter), *ibid.*

See also under Wegener's Granulomatosis, below.

WEGENER'S GRANULOMATOSIS. Prospective experience of the use of low-dose cyclophosphamide and alternate-day corticosteroids in patients with Wegener's granulomatosis. A total of 85 patients have been treated over 21 years with a regimen comprising cyclophosphamide 2 mg per kg body-weight and prednisone 1 mg per kg, both given daily by mouth initially. The prednisone was gradually reduced to an alternate-day regimen, and after at least a year the cyclophosphamide dosage was lowered by 25-mg decrements every 2 to 3 months until it could be discontinued or a disease flare occurred. Dosage adjustments were made when necessary to avoid severe neutropenia. Complete remissions were obtained and maintained in 79 patients, with a mean duration of remission of 48 months; 23 patients were able to stop all therapy. Twenty-five patients who achieved remission underwent some degree of relapse; one died, but the remainder had remission successfully re-induced. Results in the 23 patients who also received azathioprine during the study suggested it was less effective than cyclophosphamide in inducing remission of disease. Side-effects included alopecia, gonadal dysfunction, and haemorrhagic cystitis, but only in 1 patient did a malignancy (lymphoma) develop. Cyclophosphamide was discontinued in 13 patients because of cystitis, and was substituted with azathioprine in 9 of these. The study has shown that a high rate of long-term remissions can be obtained without life-threatening complications, in what was once a fatal disease.— A. S. Fauci *et al.*, *Ann. intern. Med.*, 1983, *98*, 76. Comment. Improvements in diagnosis have meant that life expectancy has improved in untreated patients with Wegener's granulomatosis. A comparison with less toxic and potentially more effective therapies is mandatory.— A. D. Steinberg (letter), *ibid.*, 1026. Reply, and a reminder that Wegener's granulomatosis is still uniformly fatal within 5 months of the onset of clinically detectable renal disease if untreated, and within 12 months if treated with corticosteroids alone.— A. S. Fauci *et al.* (letter), *ibid.*, 1027.

See also under Renal Disorders, Non-malignant, above.

See also under Use of Immunosuppressants, p.594.

Lymphomatoid granulomatosis. Treatment in 13 patients with lymphomatoid granulomatosis using the same regimen of prednisone and cyclophosphamide employed in patients with Wegener's granulomatosis (see above) produced complete remission in 7, with a mean total duration of remission of 5.2 years. In the remaining 6, disease progressed to malignant lymphoma and all subsequently died despite combination chemotherapy.— A. S. Fauci *et al.*, *New Engl. J. Med.*, 1982, *306*, 68.

Preparations

Cyclophosphamide for Injection *(U.S.P.).* A sterile mixture of cyclophosphamide and sodium chloride for reconstitution.

Cyclophosphamide Injection *(B.P.).* To be prepared immediately before use.

Cyclophosphamide Tablets *(B.P.)*

Cyclophosphamide Tablets *(U.S.P.)*

Proprietary Preparations

Endoxana *(Boehringer Ingelheim, UK). Tablets*, cyclophosphamide 10 and 50 mg.
Injection, powder for reconstitution, cyclophosphamide 0.107, 0.214, 0.535, and 1.069 g (equivalent to anhydrous cyclophosphamide 0.1, 0.2, 0.5, and 1.0 g).

Proprietary Names and Manufacturers

Carloxan *(Farmitalia, Denm.)*; Cycloblastin *(Austral.)*; Cyclostin *(Farmitalia, Ger.)*; Cyclostine *(Farmitalia Carlo Erba, Switz.)*; Cytoxan *(Bristol, Canad.*; *Bristol-Myers Oncology, USA)*; Endoxan *(Arg.*; *Bristol-Myers, Austral.*; *Lucien, Fr.*; *Asta Pharma, Ger.*; *Schering, Ital.*; *Neth.*; *Noristan, S.Afr.*; *Degussa, Switz.)*; Endoxana *(Boehringer Ingelheim, UK)*; Enduxan *(Braz.)*; Genoxal *(Funk, Spain)*; Neosar *(Adria, USA)*; Procytox *(Horner, Canad.)*; Sendoxan *(Asta, Denm.*; *Asta, Norw.*; *Asta-Werke, Swed.)*.
Manufacturers also include—*Farmitalia Carlo Erba, UK.*

1882-m

Cyclosporin *(BAN).*

Ciclosporin *(rINN)*; Cyclosporin A; Cyclosporine *(USAN)*; OL-27-400. Cyclo{-[4-(*E*)-but-2-enyl-*N*,4-dimethyl-L-threonyl]-L-homoalanyl-(*N*-methylglycyl)-(*N*-methyl-L-leucyl)-L-valyl-(*N*-methyl-L-leucyl)-L-alanyl-D-alanyl-(*N*-methyl-L-leucyl)-(*N*-methyl-L-leucyl)-(*N*-methyl-L-valyl)-}.
$C_{62}H_{111}N_{11}O_{12}$=1202.6.

CAS — 59865-13-3.

Pharmacopoeias. In *U.S.*

Store in airtight containers. Protect from light.

Adverse Effects and Treatment

Nephrotoxicity is the major adverse effect of cyclosporin and occurs in approximately one-third of all patients. It is related to drug-plasma concentrations and is usually reversible on reduction of the dose. Hypertension and electrolyte disturbances, notably hyperkalaemia, have occurred.

Other adverse effects include gastro-intestinal disturbances, hepatotoxicity, hirsutism and acne, hypertrophy of the gums, and neurotoxicity. Tremor is common, and hallucinations and convulsions have been reported, the latter possibly related to hypomagnesaemia.

Anaphylactoid reactions have occurred following intravenous administration; it has been suggested that these represent a reaction to the polyethoxylated castor oil vehicle of the intravenous preparation.

There is an increased incidence of development of lymphomas in patients receiving cyclosporin therapy.

ALLERGY AND ANAPHYLAXIS. Reports of anaphylactic reactions in patients given the intravenous formulation of cyclosporin: B. D. Kahan *et al.* (letter), *Lancet*, 1984, *1*, 52; K. M. L. Leunissen *et al.* (letter), *ibid.*, 1985, *1*, 636; R. J. Ptachcinski *et al.* (letter), *ibid;* B. Chapuis *et al.* (letter), *New Engl. J. Med.*, 1985, *312*, 1259.

CARCINOGENICITY. A report by Calne *et al.* (*Lancet*, 1979, *2*, 1033 and 1202) of the disturbing occurrence of 3 lymphomas, one in a patient receiving only cyclosporin in a study of 34 transplant patients over only 15 months was followed by a similar report in *primate* allograft recipients whose postoperative treatment included cyclosporin (C.P. Bieber *et al.*, *ibid.*, 1980, *1*, 43). The association has been confirmed by subsequent reports. The manufacturers (*Sandoz*) have stated that of an estimated 5550 transplant patients who had been treated with cyclosporin by February 1984, lymphoproliferative disorders had been reported in 40, an overall incidence of 0.7%. The incidence was increased in patients who received cyclosporin combined with other immunosuppressants compared with those given cyclosporin alone or with low-dose corticosteroids. It was concluded that there was no clear evidence that the risk with cyclosporin was greater than for other immunosuppressants (T. Beveridge *et al.*, *Lancet*, 1984, *1*, 788).

It has been suggested that these lymphomas represent proliferation of B-cells under the influence of Epstein-Barr virus, a process normally prevented by the T-cells which are specifically inhibited by cyclosporin. However, considerable doubt has been raised as to whether the resultant, usually polyclonal, lymphoproliferative tumours are truly analogous to naturally-occurring lymphomas (*Lancet*, 1984, *1*, 601). This may have important implications for management. Starzl *et al.* (*ibid.*, 583), studying 17 transplant patients with lymphoproliferative disorders, demonstrated that reduction or discontinuation of their cyclosporin and corticosteroid regimen resulted in prompt regression of the lesions, in most cases without graft loss. Furthermore, use of lower dose cyclosporin regimens appears to maintain normal elimination of Epstein-Barr virus-infected B-cells by specific T-cells (D.H. Crawford and J.M.B. Edwards, *ibid.*, 1982, *1*, 1469) and may lead to a reduced incidence of lymphoma compared with earlier results.

The problem should be borne in perspective. Calne *et al.* (*Br. med. J.*, 1980, *280*, 43) have stressed that an increased incidence of lymphoma is reported with all immunosuppressants, that transplant patients are suffering from lethal diseases, and that cyclosporin has enabled previously hopeless patients to receive transplants.

Reports of *skin cancer* in patients receiving cyclosporin: P. S. Mortimer *et al.*, *J. R. Soc. Med.*, 1983, *76*, 786; J. F. Thompson *et al.* (letter), *Lancet*, 1985, *1*, 158; P. L. Bencini *et al.* (letter), *Br. J. Derm.*, 1985, *113*, 373; M. L. Price *et al.* (letter), *New Engl. J. Med.*, 1985, *313*, 1420.

DYSMORPHIC CHANGES. There was pronounced coarsening of facial features in 11 children who were treated with prednisone and cyclosporin for renal transplantation and followed up for more than 6 months. The changes resembled those seen with phenytoin therapy.— V. M. Reznik *et al.*, *Lancet*, 1987, *1*, 1405.

EFFECTS ON THE BLOOD. A report of haemolytic-uraemic syndrome developing in a patient given cyclosporin for a liver transplant. The patient recovered when cyclosporin was withdrawn and alternative immunosuppressants substituted.— R. S. Bonser *et al.* (letter), *Lancet*, 1984, *2*, 1337. Erythraemia associated with cyclosporin.— A. J. Tatman *et al.* (letter), *Lancet*, 1988, *1*, 1279.

For reports of thrombo-embolic disorders in patients given cyclosporin see under Effects on the Vascular System, below.

Effects on the bone marrow. A report of profound leucopenia in a patient given cyclosporin.— F. Michel *et al.* (letter), *Lancet*, 1986, *2*, 304.

EFFECTS ON ELECTROLYTES. Sustained hyperkalaemia developed in 7 of 43 cyclosporin-treated patients compared with only 1 of 28 given azathioprine with prednisolone. The raised serum-potassium concentrations did not appear to be a direct consequence of renal impairment but were apparently associated with hyperchloraemic acidosis and hypoaldosteronism.— D. Adu *et al.*, *Lancet*, 1983, *2*, 370. A report of persistent hyperkalaemia associated with cyclosporin therapy in a renal transplant patient which was successfully treated with fludrocortisone acetate 100 µg twice daily. This response is consistent with the suggestion that hypoaldosteronism plays a role in cyclosporin-induced hyperkalaemia.— K. C. Petersen *et al.* (letter), *ibid.*, 1984, *1*, 1470.

EFFECTS ON GLUCOSE TOLERANCE. Following a change from azathioprine to cyclosporin immunosuppression 4 patients who had received pancreas transplants developed impaired glucose tolerance. A rise in C peptide concentrations suggested that the effect might be due to induction of insulin resistance. The effect was reversible on discontinuing cyclosporin; in 2 patients who continued to receive the drug the effect did not worsen.— R. Gunnarsson *et al.* (letter), *Lancet,* 1983, *2,* 571.

A report of the development of insulin-dependent diabetes in a renal transplant patient given cyclosporin. The condition slowly resolved over several months following reduction of the cyclosporin dose.— J. J. Bending *et al., Br. med. J.,* 1987, *294,* 401.

EFFECTS ON THE KIDNEY. A review of cyclosporin nephrotoxicity. Clinical use of cyclosporin is associated with reversible, dose-related increases in blood-urea-nitrogen and serum-creatinine concentrations, and with decreased creatinine clearance. Some nephrotoxicity has been reported to occur in almost 80% of renal transplant patients in some studies. Elevated creatinine concentrations have been considered to imply no permanent kidney damage, with return to baseline on stopping cyclosporin even after 1 year of therapy, but such conclusions remain tentative. It is extremely difficult to distinguish renal transplant rejection from cyclosporin nephrotoxicity; the only definitive means of diagnosis in these patients is that in the latter case renal function improves on dose reduction. Monitoring cyclosporin concentrations is considered essential, but the relative merits of radioimmunoassay (less specific) and high-performance liquid chromatography remain controversial. Plasma trough levels have been suggested as a simple index of whole-blood concentrations. Although high steady-state trough values generally correlate with nephrotoxicity, which is more frequent at values above 400 ng per mL, no clear cause-and-effect relationship with renal dysfunction has been established. Furthermore, a concentration of only 200 ng per mL is probably not enough to avoid rejection, making for a narrow therapeutic window which is difficult to maintain in practice. Cyclosporin should be used with caution, particularly in renal transplantation.— W. M. Bennett and J. P. Pulliam, *Ann. intern. Med.,* 1983, *99,* 851.

A study comparing 17 heart-transplant patients who received cyclosporin for at least 1 year with 15 similar patients given azathioprine found that the former group had a significantly reduced glomerular filtration-rate of 51 mL per minute as against 93 mL per minute in the latter. There was evidence that patients receiving cyclosporin had undergone a progressive elevation in serum-creatinine concentrations despite maintenance of mean trough plasma-cyclosporin concentrations below 400 ng per mL. Two of the cyclosporin-treated patients subsequently developed end-stage renal failure. Although cyclosporin-induced nephrotoxicity is widely held to be fully reversible this may not be so when the drug is given for a long time. Cyclosporin should be used only when its potential benefits clearly outweigh the risk of irreversible renal failure.— B. D. Myers *et al., New Engl. J. Med.,* 1984, *311,* 699. Comment. Switching from initial cyclosporin to other immunosuppressants, or using much lower doses than those previously thought to be effective may offer strategies for the safer use of cyclosporin.— T. B. Strom and R. Loertscher, *ibid.,* 728.

Results in 34 patients given cyclosporin for 3 months and then switched to azathioprine and prednisolone indicated that the nephrotoxic effects of cyclosporin were largely reversible with this regimen. Mean serum-creatinine concentrations began to rise significantly from day 28 of cyclosporin therapy to between 200 and 228 nmol per mL compared with 144 to 156 nmol per mL in 28 similar patients treated with azathioprine and prednisolone alone; however, 14 days after conversion of cyclosporin to the second regimen the 2 groups had similar concentrations. Serum-uric acid concentrations were similarly affected.— J. R. Chapman *et al., Lancet,* 1985, *1,* 128.

A suggestion that some of the symptoms of cyclosporin-induced nephrotoxicity may be due to interference with prostacyclin synthesis.— R. Duarte (letter), *Ann. intern. Med.,* 1985, *102,* 420. Further evidence of possible effects on prostaglandin metabolism: D. Adu *et al.* (letter), *ibid., 103,* 303; R. A. K. Stahl *et al.* (letter), *ibid.,* 474. Results suggesting that nephrotoxicity is caused by metabolites of cyclosporin. Nephrotoxicity developed in a patient whose dosage had been adjusted to give trough plasma concentrations of 0.15 µg per mL measured by high-performance liquid chromatography. However, the trough concentration when measured by radioimmunoassay, which also measures metabolites, was 1.06 µg per mL, suggesting that it is trough concentrations of metabolites which correlate with kidney damage.— K. M. L. Leunissen *et al.* (letter), *Lancet,* 1986, *2,* 1398.

For results in *rats* indicating that nephrotoxicity may be reduced by administration at an optimal stage of the daily circadian cycle, see under Administration, below.

EFFECTS ON THE NERVOUS SYSTEM. Serious neurotoxicity was associated with the use of cyclosporin in 5 of 64 patients. Symptoms included ataxia, drowsiness, confusion, and paresis. All 5 had also received cyclophosphamide, intrathecal methotrexate, and radiotherapy as part of a marrow transplant regimen. Signs and symptoms were reversed when cyclosporin was stopped, or the dose reduced. It is possible that the neurotoxicity was cumulative, with intrathecal medication and irradiation contributing, but it is important to be aware that serious neurological complications may be associated with cyclosporin.— K. Atkinson *et al.* (letter), *New Engl. J. Med.,* 1984, *310,* 527. Coma lasting 44 days developed 20 days after renal transplantation in a patient receiving cyclosporin and prednisone. There was some evidence of leucoencephalopathy. Cyclosporin was replaced by azathioprine and the patient eventually recovered.— J. H. M. Berden *et al.* (letter), *Lancet,* 1985, *1,* 219. In 2 patients with cyclosporin toxicity following bone-marrow transplantation there was disturbance of the blood-brain barrier. This may be a mechanism for CNS damage by rendering the brain susceptible to injurious substances from which it is normally protected.— J. P. Sloane *et al.* (letter), *ibid.,* 2, 280.

Reports and discussions of convulsions in patients receiving cyclosporin: S. Durrant *et al.* (letter), *Lancet,* 1982, *2,* 829 (with high-dose methylprednisolone); M. A. Boogaerts *et al.* (letter), *ibid.,* 1216 (with high-dose methylprednisolone); D. Shah *et al., Br. med. J.,* 1984, *289,* 1347 (convulsions associated with high cyclosporin blood concentrations; treatment with phenytoin); P. H. Whiting *et al.* (letter), *ibid.,* 1985, *290,* 162 (phenytoin for convulsions may interact with cyclosporin); M. Beaman *et al., ibid.,* 139 (grand mal seizures associated with high blood concentrations; the need for regular monitoring); M. L. P. Gross *et al.* (letter), *ibid.,* 555 (convulsions may be associated with transplant rejection rather than cyclosporin); T. Velu *et al.* (letter), *Lancet,* 1985, *1,* 219 (fatal convulsions in a patient with a family history of epilepsy); D. H. Adams *et al., ibid.,* 1987, *1,* 949 (grand mal, myoclonic, and focal seizures in liver transplant patients).

Evidence that cyclosporin neurotoxicity is associated with hypomagnesaemia. Of 7 patients who had grand mal seizures all were significantly hypomagnesaemic, with a mean serum-magnesium concentration of 0.56 µmol per mL compared with 0.77 µmol per mL in controls and in the same patients before starting cyclosporin. All patients were given an anti-epileptic initially; when patients were given magnesium supplements there were no further seizures. A further 5 patients with other signs of neurotoxicity (ataxia, tremor, depression, and transient aphasia) were also markedly hypomagnesaemic and responded to magnesium replacement therapy. Neurotoxic effects are probably due to renal magnesium wasting which may account for their lower prevalence in renal transplant patients. Prevention of hypomagnesaemia seems likely to reduce the risk of associated neurotoxicity in patients receiving cyclosporin.— C. B. Thompson *et al., Lancet,* 1984, *2,* 1116. Comment. Hypomagnesaemia cannot necessarily be incriminated as the cause of neurological disorders in patients treated with cyclosporin and may simply reflect co-existing nephrotoxicity.— R. D. Allen *et al.* (letter), *ibid.,* 1985, *1,* 1283. See also I. A. Borland *et al.* (letter), *ibid.,* 103; N. Schmitz *et al.* (letter), *ibid.,* 104; J. P. O'Connor *et al.* (letter), *ibid.*

Results suggesting that subclinical aluminium overload may render patients prone to seizures when given cyclosporin.— K. P. Nordal *et al.* (letter), *Lancet,* 1985, *2,* 153.

EFFECTS ON THE VASCULAR SYSTEM. In a retrospective study, thrombo-embolic complications, comprising 10 pulmonary emboli, 1 renal-vein thrombosis, 3 deep-vein thromboses, and 3 haemorrhoidal thromboses, occurred in 13 of 90 renal transplant patients given cyclosporin and low-dose corticosteroids. In 90 similar patients given azathioprine, antilymphocyte immunoglobulin, and high-dose corticosteroids there was only a single thrombo-embolic event, a case of superficial thrombophlebitis at an injection site. Clotting factors and platelet aggregation were increased in blood samples from those receiving cyclosporin over both patients receiving azathioprine and untreated controls. Results indicate an increased incidence of thrombosis in patients receiving cyclosporin; consideration should be given to prophylactic anticoagulant therapy in these patients.— Y. Vanrenterghem *et al., Lancet,* 1985, *1,* 999. Comment. Thrombo-embolic complications are also common in patients treated with azathioprine and prednisolone.— J. Zazgornik *et al.* (letter), *ibid.,* 2, 102. Further comments and criticisms: A. W. Thomson *et al.* (letter), *ibid., 1,* 1396; S. -E. Bergentz *et al.* (letter), *ibid;* F. J. Echternacht (letter), *ibid.,* 1397; N. Choudhury *et al.* (letter), *ibid., 2,* 606; K. V. Rao (letter), *ibid.*

A report of a *lower* incidence of venous thrombosis in patients receiving cyclosporin compared with those given azathioprine.— R. D. Allen *et al.* (letter), *Lancet,* 1985, *2,* 1004.

Severe irreversible hypertension in a patient given cyclosporin for Graves' disease.— J. J. Sennesael *et al.* (letter), *Ann. intern. Med.,* 1986, *104,* 729.

A report of 2 cases of Raynaud's phenomenon in patients treated with cyclosporin for uveitis.— G. Deray *et al.* (letter), *Lancet,* 1986, *2,* 1092.

OVERDOSAGE. A report of accidental administration of cyclosporin 250 mg, equivalent to a dose of about 6.25 mg per kg body-weight, by rapid injection over less than 30 minutes. The patient rapidly developed anxiety, diarrhoea, vomiting, and perspiration, with weak and irregular pulse. The patient subsequently developed atrial fibrillation, which was treated with digoxin, and in the following 36 hours showed signs of slight renal insufficiency. Two days later no adverse effects were apparent.— P. E. Wallemacq and M. L. Lesne, *Drug Intell. & clin. Pharm.,* 1985, *19,* 29.

There were no adverse renal, hepatic, or neurological effects in a patient who took 25 g of cyclosporin over 8 days. There was a mild increase in blood pressure. Other symptoms included mouth upset, disturbances of the extremities, facial flushing, and gastro-intestinal disturbances. Symptoms resolved within 2 weeks of stopping cyclosporin.— R. W. Baumhefner *et al.* (letter), *Lancet,* 1987, *2,* 332.

See also under Treatment of Adverse Effects, below.

TREATMENT OF ADVERSE EFFECTS. Results in renal transplant patients suggesting that diltiazem may reduce cyclosporin's nephrotoxic effects.— K. Wagner and H. -H. Neumayer (letter), *Lancet,* 1985, *2,* 1355.

Despite the suggestion that administration of co-dergocrine mesylate counteracts the nephrotoxicity of cyclosporin, treatment with 1 mg three times daily was no more effective than placebo in a crossover study in 10 patients with cyclosporin-induced nephrotoxicity who had been receiving cyclosporin for an average of 35 months. The failure might be due to the dosage of co-dergocrine used, or to the irreversible kidney changes associated with prolonged cyclosporin therapy.— R. B. Nussenblatt *et al.* (letter), *Lancet,* 1986, *1,* 1220. Higher doses of co-dergocrine were also of no value in improving renal function. Glomerular filtration-rate and effective renal plasma flow did not improve in 3 cyclosporin-treated patients given 4 weeks treatment with co-dergocrine mesylate 6 mg and 12 mg daily.— T. L. Kho *et al.* (letter), *ibid.,* 2, 394.

A report of beneficial results with activated charcoal in the management of acute oral cyclosporin overdosage.— N. Honcharik and S. Anthone (letter), *Lancet,* 1985, *1,* 1051.

Precautions

For reference to the precautions necessary with immunosuppressants, see Antineoplastic Agents, p.583. Care is needed if cyclosporin is given with other potentially nephrotoxic drugs such as the aminoglycoside antibiotics.

Cyclosporin is metabolised in the liver: phenytoin, phenobarbitone, rifampicin, and other inducers of hepatic enzymes may cause lowered plasma concentrations of cyclosporin. Increased plasma concentrations have been reported following concurrent administration of ketoconazole, amphotericin, erythromycin, and corticosteroids.

A report of cyclosporin malabsorption in a patient with Crohn's disease.— J. D. Williams *et al.* (letter), *Lancet,* 1987, *1,* 914.

INFECTIONS. Comment on the development of *Pneumocystis carinii* pneumonia in patients receiving cyclosporin therapy. Whether patients given cyclosporin are more likely than other immunosuppressed persons to develop *Pneumocystis* pneumonia is still controversial.— M. B. Markus (letter), *Med. J. Aust.,* 1985, *143,* 91. Some studies have reported a disturbingly high incidence of *Pneumocystis carinii* pneumonia in patients given cyclosporin and corticosteroids.— F. W. Ballardie *et al.* (letter), *Lancet,* 1984, *2,* 638. Recipients of a regimen comprising cyclosporin in association with azathioprine and prednisolone were more prone to infections than those given cyclosporin alone, with prednisolone added for rejection episodes. Although triple therapy may be safe for uncomplicated cases, poor-risk patients or those who require further anaesthetics for surgical complications have a high risk of dying.— J. R. Salaman and P. J. A.

Griffin (letter), *ibid.*, 1985, *2*, 1066. A contrary view.— C. Hiesse *et al.* (letter), *ibid.*, 1355. Seventy-two heart-transplant patients who received cyclosporin and corticosteroids were retrospectively compared with 38 historical controls given the previous immunosuppressant regimen of azathioprine, antithymocyte immunoglobulin, and corticosteroids. There were 105 infections in 51 patients in the cyclosporin group (2.1 per patient) compared with 99 infections in 34 controls (2.9 per patient) and the rates of infection-related death were 11% and 39% respectively. There were fewer bacterial infections in the cyclosporin-treated group and fewer cases of *Pneumocystis carinii* pneumonia but visceral cytomegalovirus and herpes simplex infections, candidal infections, and toxoplasmosis were not significantly different in incidence between groups. It was concluded that there was a significant reduction in infection and associated mortality in patients given cyclosporin immunosuppression for heart transplants.— J. M. Hofflin *et al.*, *Ann. intern. Med.*, 1987, *106*, 209.

INTERACTIONS. *Calcium-channel blockers.* Administration of diltiazem to a patient receiving cyclosporin resulted on 2 separate occasions in an increase in serum-cyclosporin trough concentrations and a reversible deterioration in renal function.— J. M. Pochet and Y. Pirson (letter), *Lancet*, 1986, *1*, 979. A similar report.— J. M. Griño *et al.* (letter), *ibid.*, 1387. Criticism.— H. -H. Neumayer and K. Wagner (letter), *ibid.*, *2*, 523.

Further references to increased cyclosporin concentrations with concurrent administration of calcium-channel blockers: B. Bourbigot *et al.* (letter), *Lancet*, 1986, *1*, 1447 (with nicardipine but not nifedipine); A. Lindholm and S. Henricsson (letter), *ibid.*, 1987, *1*, 1262 (with verapamil).

Corticosteroids. Cyclosporin interfered with the metabolism of prednisolone, perhaps by competing for cytochrome P-450 in the liver.— L. Öst (letter), *Lancet*, 1984, *1*, 451. Cyclosporin plasma concentrations rose strikingly in 22 of 33 renal transplant patients given high-dose methylprednisolone for rejection episodes. The mean trough plasma concentration in these patients while receiving cyclosporin maintenance therapy, together with prednisolone, was 205 ng per mL by radioimmunoassay; this rose to peaks of 482 ng per mL during or immediately after intravenous methylprednisolone injections.— G. Klintmalm and J. Säwe (letter), *ibid.*, 731.

Diuretics. A report of deterioration in renal function, without elevation of cyclosporin blood concentrations, in a patient who had low-dose metolazone added to his regimen, for oedema following renal transplantation.— P. Christensen and M. Leski (letter), *Br. med. J.*, 1987, *294*, 578.

Melphalan. For a report of a potentially dangerous interaction between cyclosporin and melphalan, see under Melphalan, p.634.

Sex hormones. Inappropriately high whole-blood concentrations of cyclosporin in a patient converted from azathioprine to cyclosporin immunosuppression were thought to be due to concurrent administration of methyltestosterone for hypogonadism. The cyclosporin dosage was reduced from 15 to 9 mg per kg body-weight daily without any effect on blood concentrations, and signs of both nephrotoxicity and hepatotoxicity persisted until both drugs were withdrawn. Pharmacokinetic studies indicated the half-life of cyclosporin to be prolonged to about 4 days compared with a normal half-life of about 12 hours. These observations suggest that administration of androgens with cyclosporin is probably contra-indicated.— B. B. Møller and B. Ekelund (letter), *New Engl. J. Med.*, 1985, *313*, 1416.

Introduction of danazol to the therapeutic regimen in a 15-year-old patient resulted in increases in previously stable cyclosporin concentrations, with raised serum creatinine. Substitution of norethisterone for danazol resulted in a fall in serum creatinine but not in the cyclosporin concentration, which remained high until norethisterone was also withdrawn. Since some sex hormones are weak inhibitors of hepatic microsomal enzymes caution is required when they are introduced or withdrawn in patients taking cyclosporin.— W. B. Ross *et al.* (letter), *Lancet*, 1986, *1*, 330.

Severe hepatotoxicity was associated with re-introduction of an oral contraceptive containing levonorgestrel and ethinyloestradiol in a woman who had stopped taking it 2 months before beginning cyclosporin therapy. Concurrent administration also resulted in increased plasma-cyclosporin trough values. Liver function should be monitored when oral contraceptives are given to patients on cyclosporin.— G. Deray *et al.* (letter), *Lancet*, 1987, *1*, 158.

Sulphonamides. Cyclosporin serum trough concentrations fell dramatically to unmeasurable values in a patient given intravenous sulphadimidine and trimethoprim for *Pneumocystis* infection. The dose of cyclosporin was increased from 10 to 18 mg per kg body-weight daily but serum concentrations remained low at 80 to 140 ng per mL, compared with a previous range of 250 to 700 ng per mL. The patient subsequently developed a severe rejection episode; substitution of oral for intravenous sulphonamide therapy subsequently permitted maintenance of adequate cyclosporin concentrations for immunosuppression.— J. Wallwork *et al.* (letter), *Lancet*, 1983, *1*, 366. A report of 4 further cases in which an interaction between intravenous sulphadimidine and cyclosporin resulted in inadequate cyclosporin immunosuppression. Cyclosporin concentrations must be closely monitored when a patient receiving this immunosuppressant is given concomitant treatment with a sulphonamide.— D. K. Jones *et al.*, *Br. med. J.*, 1986, *292*, 728.

Vaccines. Discussion of the potential interactions of cyclosporin with vaccines and toxoids. Efficacy of immunoprophylaxis may be expected to be diminished during cyclosporin therapy, and administration of live virus vaccines, in particular, is contra-indicated in an immunocompromised host. Further, there is some evidence that antigens administered during cyclosporin therapy may induce tolerance, which might result in increased susceptibility to the diseases one wishes to protect against.— J. D. Grabenstein and J. R. Baker (letter), *Drug Intell. & clin. Pharm.*, 1985, *19*, 679.

PORPHYRIA. Cyclosporin was considered to be unsafe in patients with acute porphyria because it has been shown to be porphyrinogenic in *animals* or *in-vitro* systems.— M.R. Moore and K.E.L. McColl, *Porphyrias, Drug Lists*, Glasgow, Porphyria Research Unit, Univeristy of Glasgow, 1987.

PREGNANCY AND THE NEONATE. A report of successful pregnancy in a renal-transplant patient who conceived while taking cyclosporin and continued to receive it during pregnancy.— G. J. Lewis *et al.*, *Br. med. J.*, 1983, *286*, 603.

Absorption and Fate

Absorption of cyclosporin from the gastro-intestinal tract is variable and incomplete, with a reported absolute bioavailability of about 20 to 50%. Peak plasma concentrations are achieved about 3½ hours after an oral dose and are reported to be approximately 1 ng per mL for each mg given; whole-blood concentrations are roughly 1.4 to 2.7 ng per mL for each mg. It is widely distributed throughout the body. In the blood, approximately 50% is found in erythrocytes, 40% in plasma, and 10% in leucocytes; the proportion found in plasma is almost completely protein bound, mostly to lipoproteins. Clearance from the blood is biphasic with a reported terminal elimination half-life of 10 to 27 hours.

Cyclosporin is extensively metabolised in the liver and primarily excreted, as metabolites, in the bile. About 6% of a dose is reported to be excreted in urine, less than 0.1% of it is unchanged.

Cyclosporin is reported to cross the placenta and to be distributed into breast milk.

Reviews of the pharmacokinetics of cyclosporin, and the problems of monitoring therapeutic concentrations: S. M. Faynor *et al.*, *Mayo Clin. Proc.*, 1984, *59*, 571; W. S. Burkle, *Drug Intell. & clin. Pharm.*, 1985, *19*, 101; R. J. Ptachcinski *et al.*, *Clin. Pharmacokinet.*, 1986, *11*, 107; R. J. Ptachcinski *et al.*, *J. clin. Pharmac.*, 1986, *26*, 358.

Plasma concentrations of cyclosporin were higher, as measured by radioimmunoassay, when the same blood sample was stored at 37° than when it was stored at 21°, the ratio being 1 to 0.68: possibly leucocytes and red-blood cells absorb more of the drug at lower temperatures. Constant temperatures should be maintained for plasma or serum separation before assay.— H. Dieperink (letter), *Lancet*, 1983, *1*, 416. Comment. Correct maintenance of temperature is difficult and may produce variable results. It is more practical and perhaps more useful to measure concentrations in whole blood.— G. Bandini *et al.* (letter), *ibid.*, 762.

The lack of specificity of the current radioimmunoassay may well account for the apparent lack of correlation between drug concentrations and efficacy and toxicity. Clinicians using cyclosporin should have access to high pressure liquid chromatographic (HPLC) assays; in the absence of these, a method for extraction and purification of cyclosporin prior to performing radioimmunoassay is described.— Z. Varghese *et al.* (letter), *Lancet*, 1984, *1*, 1407. Recommending the use of HPLC or modified radioimmunoassay to titrate cyclosporin dosage presupposes that renal toxicity is related only to the concentration of the parent drug and not the metabolites, which may not be the case. Furthermore, there are practical advantages in terms of cost and efficiency to the use of the standard radioimmunoassay which make it premature to dismiss its use for cyclosporin measurement.— D. W. Holt and D. J. G. White (letter), *ibid.*, *2*, 228. Satisfactory results from the use of radioimmunoassay.— J. D. M. Albano *et al.* (letter), *ibid.*, 408. The view that HPLC data are essential for patients with liver transplants, in whom cyclosporin metabolism and excretion depends on graft function, but that either HPLC or radioimmunoassay may be used in kidney transplant patients if appropriate reference scales are used.— W. Woloszczuk *et al.* (letter), *ibid.*, 638.

For a report that nephrotoxicity is correlated with plasma concentrations of cyclosporin measured by radioimmunoassay but not by HPLC, and the suggestion that nephrotoxicity is caused by cyclosporin metabolites, see under Effects on the Kidney, above.

Cyclosporin pharmacokinetics are known to vary considerably between patients: a study in 69 patients aged 10 months to 56 years showed a significant inverse relationship between age and both volume of distribution and total systemic clearance. Patients received intravenous doses of 2.6 to 3.5 mg per kg body-weight of cyclosporin after allogeneic bone-marrow transplants, and plasma and whole blood concentrations were measured using high-performance liquid chromatography. The mean total systemic clearance was 82.2 mL per minute per kg in 12 patients aged up to 10 years, compared with 43.0 and 20.2 mL per minute per kg in those aged between 11 and 40 (48 patients) and over 40 (9 patients) respectively. The mean steady-state volume of distribution in the same groups was 34.4, 20.6, and 4.7 litres per kg. The results indicate that because infants and children have more rapid clearance and a larger volume of distribution than adults they require proportionately larger doses to achieve comparable serum concentrations; conversely, older patients may be at more risk of nephrotoxicity. However, as other factors affect pharmacokinetics, dosage modifications cannot be based on age alone.— G. C. Yee *et al.*, *Clin. Pharmac. Ther.*, 1986, *40*, 438.

Uses and Administration

Cyclosporin is a powerful immunosuppressant which appears to act specifically on lymphocytes, mainly helper T-cells, and inhibits the production of lymphokines including interleukin-2, resulting in a depression of cell-mediated immune response. Unlike most other immunosuppressants it has little effect on bone marrow.

It is used, usually combined with corticosteroids, in organ and tissue transplantation for the prophylaxis and treatment of graft rejection. It has also been tried in a number of auto-immune diseases.

Cyclosporin is given by mouth as an oily solution, which may be diluted with milk or orange juice immediately before administration to improve palatability. The usual initial dose is 14 to 18 mg per kg body-weight daily, beginning 4 to 12 hours before transplantation, and continued for 1 to 2 weeks. Dosage may subsequently be reduced gradually to a daily maintenance dose of 5 to 10 mg per kg or less.

Kidney and liver function should be determined regularly, as well as blood or plasma concentrations of cyclosporin (for discussion of the methods used to determine concentration see under Absorption and Fate, above). Dosage should be adjusted in patients who show signs of deterioration in renal or hepatic function. It has been suggested that maintenance of whole-blood trough concentrations of 250 ng to 1 μg per mL or plasma concentrations of 50 to 200 ng per mL, as measured by radioimmunoassay, produces satisfactory immunosuppression and minimises adverse effects.

Cyclosporin may also be given intravenously, at one-third of the oral dose, in patients in whom oral administration is not feasible. It is given by slow intravenous infusion over 2 to 6 hours, the 5% concentrate being diluted 1:20 to 1:100 in sodium chloride injection (0.9%) or glucose injection (5%), to give a 0.05% to 0.25% solution of cyclosporin. Because of the risk of anaphylaxis, patients should be transferred to oral therapy as soon as possible.

Reviews of cyclosporin: A. Laupacis *et al.*, *Can. med. Ass. J.*, 1982, *126*, 1041; M. Field, *J. R. Soc. Med.*, 1984, *77*, 701; D. J. Cohen *et al.*, *Ann. intern. Med.*, 1984, *101*, 667; R. J. Ptachcinski *et al.*, *Drug Intell. & clin. Pharm.*, 1985, *19*, 90; P. J. Miach, *Med. J. Aust.*, 1986, *145*, 146.

Comparisons of cyclosporin with its analogue, cyclosporin G (NVA²-cyclosporin): R. Y. Calne *et al.* (letter), *Lancet*, 1985, *1*, 1342 (in *dogs*); J. I. Duncan *et al.* (letter), *ibid.*, *2*, 1004 (in *rats*); St J. Collier *et al.* (letter), *ibid.*, 1986, *1*, 216 (in *rats*).

ACTION. The immunosuppressive effects of cyclosporin occur at an early stage of the immune response, but only after the recipient has been exposed to antigens: pretreatment with cyclosporin does not influence the development of response and it does not appear to be effective once an immune response has commenced. Although the drug may inhibit antibody formation in some situations its predominant effect appears to be on the helper subset of T lymphocytes. It interferes with T-helper-cell activation and results in the inhibition of the production and release of lymphokines, notably interleukin-2, which activate cytotoxic T-cells. The precise mechanism of its action is not yet known.— P. J. Miach, *Med. J. Aust.*, 1986, *145*, 146.

Results suggesting that cyclosporin inhibits prolactin stimulation of ornithine decarboxylase synthesis in lymphocytes, thus inhibiting mitosis.— D. H. Russell *et al.*, *Clin. Pharmac. Ther.*, 1984, *35*, 271.

Cyclosporin was shown to bind *in vitro* to calmodulin, a protein that binds calcium and is essential to normal cell function. Interruption of the T-lymphocyte activation pathway by cyclosporin may occur by inactivation of calmodulin thus preventing the activation of second messengers necessary for synthesis of proteins, nucleic acids, and prostaglandins.— P. M. Colombani *et al.*, *Science*, 1985, *228*, 337.

ADMINISTRATION. Comment on the importance of blood concentration monitoring, especially when changing the route of administration. A patient originally given intravenous cyclosporin had subtherapeutic trough blood concentrations when given oral doses of 12.5 to 14.1 mg per kg body-weight. A subsequent oral dose of 23.4 mg per kg produced therapeutic blood concentrations and was gradually reduced to 9.2 mg per kg without producing excessively low drug concentrations. This gradual improvement in bioavailability has been observed in other patients and could have led to excessive blood concentrations if the dosage had not been adjusted according to monitoring results.— J. H. Glerum *et al.* (letter), *Lancet*, 1985, *1*, 1447.

Results in *rats* demonstrated that intraperitoneal cyclosporin was twice as toxic when given during the waking, active phase of the circadian cycle as when it was given during the usual resting or sleeping phase.— W. J. M. Hrushesky (letter), *New Engl. J. Med.*, 1985, *313*, 184.

For discussion of the relative merits of prolonged cyclosporin administration and conversion to other immunosuppressant regimens see under Organ and Tissue Transplantation, below.

ADMINISTRATION IN HEPATIC INSUFFICIENCY. Cyclosporin is thought to be excreted in the bile and abnormalities of liver function probably interfere with absorption and excretion of the drug.— R. Y. Calne *et al.*, *Lancet*, 1979, *2*, 1033 and 1202.

ADMINISTRATION IN RENAL INSUFFICIENCY. A study of the pharmacokinetics of cyclosporin in 4 patients with advanced renal failure indicated that elimination of cyclosporin was apparently not markedly different from that reported in healthy subjects; no important modification of the initial dosage regimen appeared necessary in patients with impaired renal function, although toxicity should be suspected and the dosage reduced in any patient with rising serum creatinine.— F. Follath *et al.*, *Clin. Pharmac. Ther.*, 1983, *34*, 638.

AIDS. Reference to the use of cyclosporin in the treatment of AIDS. No significant alterations in immunological parameters were seen in 11 patients given the drug.— E. G. Sandström and J. C. Kaplan, *Drugs*, 1987, *34*, 372. See also R. B. Stricker (letter), *Lancet*, 1987, *2*, 796.

BLOOD DISORDERS, NON-MALIGNANT. Severe aplastic anaemia in a patient unresponsive to platelet transfusions, corticosteroids, and antithymocyte immunoglobulin responded to treatment with cyclosporin 6 mg per kg twice daily by mouth. The dose was subsequently reduced to a total of 7 mg per kg daily because of toxicity. No clear correlation between dosage and platelet counts could be seen.— P. A. Stryckmans *et al.* (letter), *New Engl. J. Med.*, 1984, *310*, 655. A similar report.— F. Wisløff and H. C. Godal (letter), *ibid.*, 1985, *312*, 1193.

A report of the use of cyclosporin, alone or in combination with low-dose prednisolone to induce and maintain remission in 4 patients with acquired or congenital (Blackfan-Diamond syndrome) pure red-cell aplasia.— T. H. Tötterman *et al.* (letter), *Lancet*, 1984, *2*, 693.

The successful treatment of refractory amegakaryocytic thrombocytopenic purpura in an 80-year-old patient with cyclosporin. Treatment with cyclosporin 15 mg per kg body-weight by mouth was given for 14 days. One week after cessation of cyclosporin therapy, the platelet counts began to rise and continued to approach normal values over several weeks; the patient has had complete remission for 21 months.— W. Hill and R. Landgraf (letter), *New Engl. J. Med.*, 1985, *312*, 1060.

For the use of cyclosporin to treat the neutropenia of Felty's syndrome, see under Rheumatic Disorders, below.

DIABETES MELLITUS. Considerable interest in immunosuppressant treatment for diabetes mellitus has followed the increasing evidence that type I diabetes is associated with an immunological mechanism. Uncontrolled studies by Stiller *et al.* (*Science*, 1984, *223*, 1362) and Assan *et al.* (*Lancet*, 1985, *1*, 67) suggested that when given to newly-diagnosed type I diabetics cyclosporin could restore insulin independence (frequently defined as "complete remission") or at least reduce insulin requirements ("partial remission"). However, in view of the 'honeymoon effect', the temporary improvement in insulin requirements often seen in the early months of diabetes, these results were inconclusive. A controlled double-blind study by Feutren *et al.* (*Lancet*, 1986, *2*, 119) found that at 6 months insulin treatment was not required in 16 of 63 newly-diagnosed type I diabetics given cyclosporin, compared with 11 of 59 given placebo; at 9 months, 13 of 54 in the cyclosporin group but only 3 of 52 given placebo were still insulin-independent. Although this is evidence of an effect it has been pointed out that cyclosporin has prolonged the honeymoon period in no more than a fifth of patients and that the patients remained hyperglycaemic whilst on a diet; it is uncertain if cyclosporin treatment would provide any benefit that outweighed the risks of such therapy (*Lancet*, 1986, *2*, 140). It has been suggested (A.H. Rubenstein and D. Pyke, *Lancet*, 1987, *1*, 436) that by the time type I diabetes is diagnosed it may be too late for immunosuppression to be effective. It is generally thought that about 90% of beta-cells are lost by the time of diagnosis; even if further loss were halted by immunosuppression, the remaining 10% might be too little to maintain normality of blood glucose. Although controlled studies of cyclosporin have shown an effect in preserving residual beta-cell function it is not great enough to justify clinical use, and there is little point in further studies unless new treatment regimens are employed.

EYE DISORDERS, NON-MALIGNANT. A report of rapid objective improvement in 2 patients with Graves' ophthalmopathy treated with cyclosporin 5 and 10 mg per kg body-weight daily, the higher dose being chosen because sight was threatened. Long-term follow-up and studies of more patients are required to consolidate these findings.— A. P. Weetman *et al.*, *Lancet*, 1983, *2*, 486. Cyclosporin therapy returned the disturbed immunological status almost to normal in 3 patients with long-standing Graves' ophthalmopathy but did not produce any clinical improvement.— G. Brabant *et al.* (letter), *ibid.*, 1984, *1*, 515. Cyclosporin therapy failed to produce an objective improvement in proptosis, eye movements or extra-ocular muscle size in a further 3 patients, and in 2 of these therapy had to be discontinued because of a further deterioration in visual acuity, which subsequently responded to more conventional treatments.— T. A. Howlett *et al.* (letter), *ibid.*, *2*, 1101. Four of 11 patients had an objective response when given cyclosporin for Graves' ophthalmopathy; more information is required in order to define more clearly those most likely to benefit.— A. M. McGregor *et al.* (letter), *J. R. Soc. Med.*, 1985, *78*, 511.

In a pilot study, cyclosporin had a rapidly beneficial effect in 7 of 8 patients with bilateral sight-threatening posterior uveitis, including 2 with Behçet's disease.— R. B. Nussenblatt *et al.*, *Lancet*, 1983, *2*, 235.

See also Behçet's syndrome, under Skin and Connective Tissue Disorders, Non-malignant, below.

A report of excellent responses to cyclosporin in 3 patients with Mooren's ulcer, a chronic progressive ulceration of the cornea. Cyclosporin was given initially in a dose of 8 mg per kg body-weight daily in 2 divided doses by mouth, for 2 days, and subsequently reduced to 3 to 4 mg per kg daily, the dose being adjusted to maintain trough serum concentrations of 200 to 400 ng per mL; treatment was tailed off and stopped after 6 weeks. All patients had rapid relief of the severe pain, and the ulcers ceased to progress and showed evidence of healing within a week of beginning therapy. At follow-up of 12 to 16 months there has been no recurrence of disease.— J. C. Hill and P. Potter, *Br. J. Ophthal.*, 1987, *71*, 11.

GASTRO-INTESTINAL DISORDERS. A patient with Crohn's disease unresponsive to sulphasalazine, and who developed an acute psychotic reaction while receiving prednisolone, had a prompt response to therapy with cyclosporin. The patient received cyclosporin 16 mg per kg body-weight daily by mouth for 1 month and 8 mg per kg daily for a further month, and received no other treatment during these 8 weeks; her general health gradually improved with a loss of abdominal pain and a return of normal bowel function.— M. C. Allison and R. E. Pounder (letter), *Lancet*, 1984, *1*, 902. Of 2 patients with Crohn's disease given cyclosporin 5 mg per kg twice daily by mouth, subsequently reduced to 3 mg per kg twice daily, one had a positive response but the other, with a severe lesion, did not.— P. A. Bianchi *et al.* (letter), *ibid.*, 1242.

Ulcerative colitis in an elderly patient was treated with cyclosporin 12 mg per kg body-weight daily. There was a gradual improvement over 6 weeks, with a return to normal of rectal histology. The patient was discharged on cyclosporin 8 mg per kg daily, but took this irregularly. Symptoms subsequently recurred, but again responded to treatment with the original dosage. Cyclosporin might be considered for the management of irritable bowel disease unresponsive to conventional therapy; further studies seem indicated.— S. Gupta *et al.* (letter), *Lancet*, 1984, *2*, 1277.

Results in 11 patients with active Crohn's disease treated with cyclosporin were disappointing; cyclosporin appeared to be of low efficacy and had only a limited place in the treatment of Crohn's disease.— H. R. Parrott *et al.*, *Gut*, 1986, *27*, A1277.

HEPATIC DISORDERS. A report of rapid improvement in a patient with autoimmune chronic active hepatitis treated with low-dose cyclosporin.— S. P. Mistilis *et al.*, *Med. J. Aust.*, 1985, *143*, 463.

Cyclosporin was being evaluated in the treatment of primary biliary cirrhosis, a chronic, progressive, and often fatal cholestatic liver disease.— M. M. Kaplan, *New Engl. J. Med.*, 1987, *316*, 521.

MYASTHENIA GRAVIS. Preliminary results suggesting that treatment with cyclosporin may be of benefit in patients with myasthenia gravis.— R. S. A. Tindall *et al.*, *New Engl. J. Med.*, 1987, *316*, 719. Comment. On balance, cyclosporin appears to have moderate potential for use in myasthenia gravis, but its ultimate value will depend upon comparison of its benefits and toxicity with those of currently used and effective drugs.— D. B. Drachman, *ibid.*, 743.

ORGAN AND TISSUE TRANSPLANTATION. *Bone marrow.* A discussion of graft-versus-host disease (GVHD) after bone-marrow transplantation. Early studies with cyclosporin suggested little value against established gut disease, and in the prevention of skin manifestations, but mortality was none-the-less impressively low. Uncontrolled evidence of prophylactic value was supported by the observation that when the drug was stopped after 6 months graft-versus-host disease developed in about half the patients and was controlled by reintroduction of cyclosporin. Other means of preventing graft-versus-host disease are under investigation but although graft-versus-host disease develops in up to 70% of cyclosporin-treated patients the morbidity is slight and all but 5% recover; other regimens will not easily improve on these results.— *Lancet*, 1984, *1*, 491.

A comparison of methotrexate and cyclosporin with cyclosporin alone for the prevention of graft-versus-host disease following bone-marrow transplantation. All of 93 leukaemic patients received cyclophosphamide, followed in 89 by total-body irradiation, prior to transplantation of HLA-identical marrow grafts from siblings. Following transplantation 43 patients were randomly assigned to treatment with methotrexate in a dose of 15 mg per m^2 intravenously on day 1, and 10 mg per m^2 on days 3, 6, and 11 after grafting, in addition to cyclosporin. Cyclosporin was begun the day before transplantation at a dose of 1.5 mg per kg body-weight every 12 hours until the patient recovered from initial chemotherapy; thereafter 6.25 mg per kg was given every 12 hours until the 50th day, unless toxicity forced a dose reduction. Fifty patients received the cyclosporin regimen alone. All patients with acute nonlymphoblastic leukaemia also received intrathecal methotrexate for CNS protection. The combination of methotrexate and cyclosporin was superior to cyclosporin alone in preventing acute graft-versus-host disease: grade II to IV disease occurred in 14 of 43 on the combined regimen and 27 of 50 receiving cyclosporin alone. However chronic graft-versus-host disease occurred equally in both groups. Projected survival at 1½ years was 80% among patients given the combined regimen and 55% among those given cyclosporin alone but the follow-up period was short and more time was required to assess the risk of leukaemic relapse associated with the lower incidence of graft-versus-host disease following combined therapy.— R. Storb *et al.*, *New Engl. J. Med.*, 1986, *314*, 729. Combined cyclosporin and methotrexate therapy was also more effective than methotrexate alone in preventing graft-versus-host disease.— R. Storb *et al.*, *Blood*, 1986, *68*, 119.

Heart. Improved results in cardiac allograft recipients treated with cyclosporin have been striking. In addition to a lower incidence of rejection, the process when it does occur appears to progress slowly and have fewer haemodynamic consequences. As a result episodes of rejection have been less dangerous and easier to treat and both survival and rehabilitation have improved markedly in cyclosporin-treated patients, with a projected 2-year survival of 75% compared with 58% after conventional immunosuppression, and a reduction in length of hospital stay. The major toxic effect is impaired renal function; it is to be hoped that the continuing development of cyclosporin analogues will eventually yield a compound of comparable immunosuppressive potency but less toxicity.— W. G. Austen and A. B. Cosimi, *New Engl. J. Med.*, 1984, *311*, 1436.

Results at the 2 *UK* cardiac transplant centres had been greatly improved by the introduction of cyclosporin, which had reduced the frequency and severity of both rejection and infective episodes; the 1-year actuarial survival of patients treated with cyclosporin was now about 75%.— A. Pomerance and P. G. I. Stovin, *J. clin. Path.*, 1985, *38*, 146.

Reports of the use of cyclosporin, in combination with other immunosuppressants, in heart-lung transplants: B. A. Reitz *et al.*, *New Engl. J. Med.*, 1982, *306*, 557; C. M. Burke *et al.*, *Lancet*, 1986, *1*, 517.

Kidney. Cyclosporin has been widely investigated for use in preventing and treating rejection following kidney transplantation. Various centres have compared its efficacy with that of azathioprine combined with corticosteroids. In a multicentre study, the European Multicentre Trial Group (*Lancet*, 1983, *2*, 986) reported a 1-year graft survival of 72% in 117 recipients of renal allografts given cyclosporin compared with 52% in 115 similar patients given the conventional regimen; on follow-up this benefit was maintained, with survival figures of 66% and 42% respectively for the 2 groups at 3 years (R.Y. Calne and A.J. Wood, *ibid.*, 1985, *2*, 549) and 55% and 40% at 5 years (R.Y. Calne, *ibid.*, 1987, *2*, 506). A similar study carried out by the Canadian Multicentre Transplant Study Group reported an actuarial graft survival of 77.5% among 142 patients receiving cyclosporin with prednisone, compared to 69.8% among 149 patients given azathioprine and prednisone, with or without antilymphocyte immunoglobulin (C.R. Stiller *New Engl. J. Med.*, 1984, *310*, 1464). The 3-year analysis of this study (*ibid.*, 1986, *314*, 1219 and 1652) reported graft survival rates of 69% and 58% respectively, with patient survival rates of 90% and 82% respectively; it was concluded that despite poorer renal function in cyclosporin-treated patients, such patients had benefited significantly from cyclosporin therapy.

However, other studies have failed to demonstrate superiority of cyclosporin therapy over conventional immunosuppressive regimens in terms of patient and graft survival (B.M. Hall *et al.*, *Med. J. Aust.*, 1985, *142*, 179; R.M. Merion *et al.*, *New Engl. J. Med.*, 1984, *310*, 148) and in view of the risks to renal function with long-term cyclosporin therapy, and its cost, it has been suggested (A.J.F. D'Apice, *Med. J. Aust.*, 1985, *142*, 172) that azathioprine and low-dose corticosteroids should remain the treatment of choice for most patients; however, those centres involved in the European multicentre study have adopted cyclosporin as first-choice immunosuppressive therapy for patients with functioning renal allografts.

It has been suggested that the effectiveness of cyclosporin immunosuppression may depend on the cause of the renal failure requiring transplantation. Cats *et al.* (*Lancet*, 1985, *1*, 490) analysed data from 133 centres and concluded that patients with underlying glomerulonephritis did better on cyclosporin than conventional therapy whereas no significant difference was seen in patients with renal failure due to other causes. However, the statistical analysis in this paper has been severely criticised (S.M. Gore, *ibid.*, 755) and Opelz has stated that data from 206 centres in the Collaborative Transplant Study do not confirm such an analysis (*ibid.*). Furthermore, Turney *et al.* (*Lancet*, 1986, *1*, 1104) have reported recurrence of glomerulonephritis in a renal transplant patient given cyclosporin and suggest that this may cast doubt on the potential value of cyclosporin in the treatment of glomerulonephritis.

Because of concern over potential nephrotoxicity associated with long-term cyclosporin therapy a number of centres have investigated initial immunosuppression with cyclosporin followed by subsequent *conversion* to a conventional regimen.

Hoitsma *et al.* (*Lancet*, 1987, *1*, 584) investigated therapy with cyclosporin for 3 months after cadaveric renal transplantation in 72 patients, followed by conversion to azathioprine and prednisone, compared with azathioprine and prednisone from the day of transplantation in a further 71. During the initial 3 months patients receiving cyclosporin had far fewer rejection episodes but had impaired renal function and a higher incidence of hypertension. After conversion, renal function improved immediately; there were only 5 acute rejection episodes, perhaps due to an increase in prednisone dosage on conversion, and all were easily reversible. Graft survival at 1 year was 10% higher in the cyclosporin group; it was concluded that cyclosporin use could be safely restricted to the early post-transplant period. However, a similar study by Morris *et al.* (*ibid.*, 586), although concurring that conversion at 90 days leads to better function of the transplanted kidney and reduces cost, reported 1 graft loss due to acute rejection following conversion, 1 because of acute-on-chronic rejection, and 2 due to chronic rejection, among 38 converted patients. The risk of losing the kidney has to be weighed against the advantages of conversion.

Paul *et al.* (*Lancet*, 1987, *1*, 917) compared conversion to azathioprine with continuation of cyclosporin; although there was no significant difference in the number of rejection episodes, graft function was superior at 12 months in converted patients than in those given continuous cyclosporin. In contrast, Adu *et al.* (*Lancet*, 1985, *1*, 392) reported stable renal function in 7 transplant patients who continued to receive cyclosporin; results in a further 5 who were converted at 11 weeks to azathioprine (with a 1-week overlap) were disastrous, with several cases of infection, one fatal, and acute rejection episodes in 3. The reasons for the differing outcomes in these studies are unknown.

A number of reports have suggested that since the introduction of cyclosporin, matching of HLA antigens is no longer necessary in renal transplantation. However there is evidence from other studies as well as data from the authors' own unit to support the view that HLA matching improves graft survival further in patients treated with cyclosporin.— P. J. Morris *et al.*, *Br. med. Bull.*, 1987, *43*, 184.

Support for the continued value of HLA-typing in cyclosporin-treated renal allograft recipients: S. Cats *et al.* (letter), *New Engl. J. Med.*, 1984, *311*, 675; P. A. Dyer *et al.* (letter), *Lancet*, 1985, *2*, 212; J. Cicciarelli *et al.* (letter), *ibid.*, 1986, *1*, 267; B. A. Bradley *et al.* (letter), *ibid.*, *2*, 568; G. G. Persijn *et al.* (letter), *ibid.*, 915.

Analyses suggesting that HLA matching is of no value in renal-transplant patients given cyclosporin: K. R. Harris *et al.*, *Lancet*, 1985, *2*, 802; G. Lundgren *et al.*, *ibid.*, 1986, *2*, 66.

Comment on the value of pre-graft blood transfusion in renal transplant recipients treated with cyclosporin. The findings of the European Multicentre Trial Group (*Lancet*, 1983, *2*, 986) produced no evidence of a beneficial effect of blood transfusion in cyclosporin-treated patients, in contrast to previous findings in patients on immunosuppression with azathioprine and prednisolone. However, in other studies the authors have noted significantly better graft survival at one year in transfused cyclosporin-treated patients than in non-transfused (87% versus 58%). It would seem prudent not to assume that the beneficial effects of pre-graft blood transfusion can be ignored if cyclosporin is to be used for immunosuppression.— P. J. Morris *et al.* (letter), *Lancet*, 1984, *1*, 98. Transfusions given at the time of transplantation improved the success of second, but not of first, kidney transplants, with or without the use of cyclosporin.— K. Tokunaga and P. I. Terasaki (letter), *ibid.*, 1986, *2*, 634.

Discussions of the difficulty in distinguishing kidney graft rejection from cyclosporin nephrotoxicity, and suggested methods for doing so: W. A. Jurewicz *et al.* (letter), *Lancet*, 1983, *1*, 998 (platelet uptake index); J. R. Salaman and P. J. A. Griffin, *ibid.*, *2*, 709 (fine-needle intrarenal manometry); P. A. Lear *et al.* (letter), *ibid.*, 1985, *1*, 922 (intrarenal manometry of value during the first 3 postoperative months); C. P. Gibbons *et al.* (letter), *ibid.*, 1269 (intrarenal manometry may be unreliable in the more difficult cases); G. H. Neild *et al.*, *J. clin. Path.*, 1986, *39*, 152 (morphological differences in biopsy specimens).

Liver. Twelve-month survival rates in both children and adults after liver transplantation exceed 50%, with 3-year survival rates in the region of 40%, and some of this improvement in survival is due to the introduction of cyclosporin; however, better surgical techniques and more careful patient selection have also contributed.— *Lancet*, 1985, *1*, 27.

Unlike kidney transplantation, where cyclosporin can be used as the sole immunosuppressant, use of either cyclosporin or corticosteroids alone in liver transplant recipients leads to rapid graft rejection; however, combined therapy has contributed to improved overall graft survival and a reduction in the frequency of acute rejection. Although there is much to learn about the optimal use of cyclosporin the route of administration appears to be important: a high frequency of rejection has been found in patients with liver transplants when the drug is administered intravenously.— G. M. Danovitch, in R.W. Busuttil (Moderator), *Liver Transplantation Today*, *Ann. intern. Med.*, 1986, *104*, 377.

Evidence from the clinical course of 29 liver transplant recipients that although cyclosporin was an effective immunosuppressant and allowed subsequent withdrawal of corticosteroid therapy in many patients, its severe side-effects could lead to withdrawal in up to a quarter of patients.— A. Blackburn *et al.*, *Gut*, 1985, *26*, A554.

Lung. A report of successful unilateral lung transplantation in 2 patients with pulmonary fibrosis. Patients received postoperative immunosuppression with cyclosporin by mouth and intravenous azathioprine; azathioprine was subsequently discontinued and oral prednisone therapy begun. Rejection episodes were treated with methyl prednisolone and antilymphocyte immunoglobulin. The patients remained able to lead normal lives 14 and 26 months respectively after transplantation.— Toronto Lung Transplant Group, *New Engl. J. Med.*, 1986, *314*, 1140.

See also under Heart, above.

Pancreas. A discussion of pancreatic transplantation. Cyclosporin is the lynchpin of every regimen but is now rarely used alone; most centres use additional azathioprine and prednisolone, often as an initial high-dose regimen, reducing to very-low-dose maintenance. Of 309 patients thus treated reported to the world registry, 85% survived more than 1 year. Rejection is mostly treated by antilymphocyte immunoglobulin or monoclonal T-cell antibodies; if a second episode of rejection occurs patient survival is improved by removal of the graft and re-institution of insulin therapy.— R. A. Sells and H. Brynger, *Lancet*, 1987, *1*, 1024.

Skin. References to the use of cyclosporin in extending the survival of skin allografts in burn patients: B. M. Achauer *et al.*, *Lancet*, 1986, *1*, 14; J. D. Frame (letter), *ibid.*, 1987, *1*, 154.

RENAL DISORDERS, NON-MALIGNANT. References to the use of cyclosporin with idiopathic nephrotic syndrome: A. Meyrier *et al.*, *Br. med. J.*, 1986, *292*, 789 (adults); P. F. Hoyer *et al.* (letter), *Lancet*, 1986, *2*, 335 (children); C. Lagrue *et al.* (letter), *ibid.*, 692 (adults).

The use of cyclosporin in IgA nephropathy.— K. N. Lai *et al.*, *Br. med, J.*, 1987, *295*, 1165.

RHEUMATIC DISORDERS. Cyclosporin 5 mg per kg body-weight daily by mouth produced improvement of profound neutropenia in a patient with Felty's syndrome; polymorphonuclear leucocyte counts began to rise 4 weeks after beginning therapy and approached normal after 2 months, subsequently permitting a reduction in the patient's corticosteroid dosage. The patient's polyarthralgia was also improved, with an increase in the ability to walk.— B. Coiffier (letter), *New Engl. J. Med.*, 1986, *314*, 184.

In a multicentre study, cyclosporin therapy had a significantly greater effect in 17 patients with refractory rheumatoid arthritis than placebo in 19 similar patients. Patients received cyclosporin 10 mg per kg body-weight daily by mouth for 2 months, reduced to 7.5 mg per kg and then 5 mg per kg, each for 2 months. Increased creatinine concentrations in 13 cyclosporin and 5 placebo recipients led to the withdrawal of 2 patients from the cyclosporin group.— A. W. A. M. Van Rijthoven *et al.*, *Ann. rheum. Dis.*, 1986, *45*, 726.

SARCOIDOSIS. Beneficial results with cyclosporin in 3 patients with pulmonary sarcoidosis (*Lancet*, 1984, *1*, 1174) had not been borne out by subsequent findings in a further 6 patients. Corticosteroids remain the mainstay of therapy for active sarcoidosis.— A. S. Rebuck *et al.* (letter), *Lancet*, 1987, *1*, 1486.

SKIN AND CONNECTIVE-TISSUE DISORDERS, NON-MALIGNANT. *Alopecia.* Application of 0.5 mL daily of an oily solution containing cyclosporin 100 mg per mL to half the scalp resulted in the growth of terminal hairs in 7 of 22 patients with severe alopecia areata after 2 to 6 months of treatment, but not in any of 21 controls treated with a placebo solution. Diffuse vellus hair, predominantly on the treated side, appeared in 5 patients receiving cyclosporin and 3 controls. Although regrowth was mild, delayed in onset, and incomplete the results should encourage further studies.— Y. de Prost *et al.* (letter), *Lancet*, 1986, *2*, 803. Similar results in 2 of 7 men with alopecia areata who applied cyclosporin 5% oily solution to a localised area of scalp. Folliculitis occurred in 3, requiring topical corticosteroid treatment in 1 case. These effects are consistent with the inhibitory action of cyclosporin on T-cells and the postulated role of T-cells in alopecia areata.— A. W. Thomson *et al.* (letter), *ibid.*, 971.

Behçet's syndrome. Complete clinical remission occurred within a week in a patient with Behçet's disease given cyclosporin 10 mg per kg daily by mouth. The drug was withdrawn after 10 days due to evidence of impaired kidney function, and symptoms returned; re-institution at a dose of 5 mg per kg again brought remission but skin pustules and arthralgia returned after 3 weeks.— C. Ffrench-Constant *et al.* (letter), *Lancet*, 1983, *2*, 454.

Cyclosporin in 3-month courses of 10 mg per kg daily by mouth, reduced to 6 to 8 mg per kg if necessary because of side-effects, was given to 8 patients with Behçet's disease. The drug was considered to have been effective in arresting inflammatory ocular activity, resulting in an improvement in visual acuity, and a reduction in inflammatory activity in mucocutaneous symptoms. All patients but one experienced acute exacerbations of disease on withdrawal of the drug; to gain any lasting benefit a long-term treatment regimen would have to be considered.— A. U- Müftüoglu, *Br. J. Ophthal.*, 1987, *71*, 387.

See also under Eye Disorders, Non-malignant, above.

Dermatomyositis. A report of a beneficial effect of cyclosporin in a 15-year-old girl with an unusually acute form of dermatomyositis. Although the patient subsequently died of aspiration pneumonia there was definite remission of the primary auto-immune disease.— P. Zabel *et al.* (letter), *Lancet*, 1984, *1*, 343.

Weakness and muscle pain in 2 patients with polymyositis responded to treatment with cyclosporin 7.5 to 10 mg per kg body-weight daily. Irreversible muscle damage may be preventable in patients with myositis unresponsive to conventional therapy by the prompt administration of cyclosporin.— K. Bendtzen *et al.* (letter), *Lancet*, 1984, *1*, 792.

Ichthyosis. Striking improvement in lifelong autosomal dominant ichthyosis vulgaris was attributed to cyclosporin therapy following transplantation in a kidney graft recipient.— P. J. Velthuis and R. F. M. Jesserun (letter), *Lancet*, 1985, *1*, 335. Ichthyosis in another patient resolved completely following kidney transplantation but the improvement was attributed to a return to normal renal function rather than to cyclosporin.— J. M. D. Nightingale and S. L. Atkin (letter), *ibid.*, 1987, *1*, 743.

Pemphigus. Two patients with bullous pemphigoid and 2 with pemphigus all responded to treatment with cyclosporin 6 mg per kg body-weight daily by mouth, adjusted to obtain a plasma concentration of 80 to 180 ng per mL. In 3 of the patients cyclosporin was added to treatment with prednisone, which had proved unsatisfactory; after 2 or 3 months on cyclosporin the prednisone was withdrawn without relapse. In the fourth patient, given cyclosporin alone, bullous pemphigoid lesions cleared within 4 weeks and the patient remained healed after 2 months without treatment.— J. Thivolet *et al.* (letter), *Lancet*, 1985, *1*, 334.

Psoriasis. Preliminary results suggesting that the skin lesions of psoriasis can be beneficially affected by cyclosporin. Psoriatic plaques almost disappeared 5 days after the start of treatment with cyclosporin 900 mg daily then 450 mg daily in a 64-year-old woman with widespread psoriasis and progressive psoriatic arthropathy. A beneficial effect was also seen in 3 similar patients, with less severe joint changes, given 300 to 450 mg daily for about a week. The lesions gradually returned in all patients about 2 weeks after stopping cyclosporin.— W. Mueller and B. Herrmann (letter), *New Engl. J. Med.*, 1979, *301*, 555.

Further reports of beneficial results in psoriatic patients given oral cyclosporin: J. I. Harper *et al.* (letter), *Lancet*, 1984, *2*, 981 (dramatic response in a patient with extensive plaque psoriasis and psoriatic arthropathy); J. P. van Hooff *et al.* (letter), *ibid.*, 1985, *1*, 335 (in 1 patient); C. N. Ellis *et al.*, *J. Am. med. Ass.*, 1986, *256*, 3110 (superior to placebo in a double-blind study); J. Marks (letter), *Br. med. J.*, 1986, *293*, 509 (response to low doses of 1 to 5 mg per kg daily by mouth); C. E. M. Griffiths *et al.*, *ibid.*, 731 (complete clearance of psoriasis in 5 of 10 given 3 mg per kg daily).

A report of a patient in whom cyclosporin appeared to induce psoriasis. The case should act as a warning to those considering employing cyclosporin as a therapeutic agent in psoriasis.— B. E. Monk (letter), *Br. J. Derm.*, 1986, *115*, 249.

In a double-blind study, cyclosporin was no more effective than placebo when applied topically to 6 patients with chronic plaque psoriasis.— C. E. M. Griffiths *et al.* (letter), *Lancet*, 1987, *1*, 806. Criticism.— A. W. Thomson *et al.* (letter), *ibid.*, 1212.

Treatment with cyclosporin 2 to 3 mg per kg body-weight daily for 12 weeks in 6 patients with severe psoriasis resulted in a substantial decrease in numbers of helper and suppressor T-cells in the skin and selectively depleted the DR+6- subset of dendritic cells found only in lesional epidermis; this depletion correlated closely with reduction in the area and severity of the lesions. At the end of 12 weeks treatment the skin of 4 patients was clear and there was 85% reduction in surface area involved in the other 2 patients. The results provide strong support for the concept that T-cells play a central role in the pathogenesis of psoriasis.— B. S. Baker *et al.*, *Br. J. Derm.*, 1987, *116*, 503.

Pyoderma gangrenosum. Healing of leg ulceration in a patient with pyoderma gangrenosum commenced within 3 weeks of starting treatment with cyclosporin 10 mg per kg body-weight daily by mouth. Dosage of cyclosporin was gradually reduced over 4 months; some ulceration recurred at 3 mg per kg but healed when the dose was temporarily increased to its original value. Both legs now remain healed on cyclosporin 4 mg per kg daily.— R. K. Curley *et al.*, *Br. J. Derm.*, 1985, *113*, 601.

Systemic lupus erythematosus. Of 5 patients with systemic lupus erythematosus, who were given a total of 6 courses of cyclosporin in liquid form at a dose of 10 mg per kg body-weight daily, only 2 patients, both with severe arthralgia, benefited and no patient could tolerate the drug for longer than 7 weeks. Side-effects included nausea, vomiting, a burning sensation in the skin, increasing alopecia, renal toxicity, and angio-oedema. The angio-oedema occurred in 3 patients, began about 2 weeks after the start of treatment, and persisted for up to 2 weeks after treatment was stopped.— D. A. Isenberg *et al.* (letter), *New Engl. J. Med.*, 1980, *303*, 754.

Preparations

Cyclosporine Concentrate for Injection *(U.S.P.)*. A sterile solution of cyclosporin in a mixture of alcohol and a suitable vegetable oil. To be diluted before use. For intravenous infusion.

Cyclosporine Oral Solution *(U.S.P.)*. A solution of cyclosporin in a mixture of alcohol and a suitable vegetable oil.

Proprietary Preparations

Sandimmun *(Sandoz, UK)*. *Capsules*, cyclosporin 25 and 100 mg.
Oral solution, cyclosporin 100 mg/mL, in bottles of 50 mL.
Concentrate for intravenous infusion, oily, cyclosporin 50 mg/mL (in a basis containing polyoxyethylated castor oil), in ampoules of 1 and 5 mL.

Proprietary Names and Manufacturers

Sandimmun *(Sandoz, Austral.; Sandoz, Denm.; Sandoz, Fr.; Sandoz, Ger.; Sandoz, Ital.; Sandoz, Norw.; Sandoz, S.Afr.; Sandoz, Spain; Sandoz, Swed.; Sandoz, Switz.; Sandoz, UK)*; Sandimmune *(Sandoz, Canad.; Sandoz, USA)*.

1826-a

Cytarabine *(BAN, USAN, rINN)*.

Arabinosylcytosine; Ara-C; Cytosine Arabinoside; NSC-63878 *(hydrochloride)*; U-19 920; WR-28453. 1-β-D-Arabinofuranosylcytosine; 4-Amino-1-β-D-arabinofuranosylpyrimidin-2(1*H*)-one.

$C_9H_{13}N_3O_5$=243.2.

CAS — 147-94-4.

Pharmacopoeias. In *Br.*, *Fr.*, *Swiss*, and *U.S. Chin.* includes the hydrochloride.

An odourless white to off-white crystalline powder. **Soluble** 1 in 10 of water; very slightly soluble in alcohol and chloroform. A 1% solution in water has a pH of 4 to 8. **Store** at a temperature not exceeding 15° in well-closed containers. Protect from light.

INCOMPATIBILITY. Cytarabine was incompatible with solutions of fluorouracil and methotrexate.— P. F. D'Arcy, *Drug Intell. & clin. Pharm.*, 1983, *17*, 532. (But see under Stability in Solution, below).

STABILITY IN SOLUTION. Cytarabine was stable for 24 hours at 25° in Elliott's B solution (artificial spinal fluid), sodium chloride injection (0.9%), glucose injection (5%), and Lactated Ringer's Injection (*U.S.P.*). When mixed with methotrexate sodium and hydrocortisone sodium succinate in each of the 4 fluids, mixtures could be stored for up to 24 hours at room temperature without substantial loss of potency or precipitation.— Y. -W. Cheung *et al.*, *Am. J. Hosp. Pharm.*, 1984, *41*, 1802.

Cytarabine was stable for at least 48 hours at 8 and 25° when added at a concentration of 50 µg per mL to a paediatric parenteral nutrient solution.— J. R. Quock and R. I. Sakai, *Am. J. Hosp. Pharm.*, 1985, *42*, 592.

Adverse Effects and Treatment

For an outline of the adverse effects experienced with antineoplastic agents and immunosuppressants and general guidelines for their treatment, see Antineoplastic Agents, p.580 and p.583.

The major adverse effect of cytarabine is bone-marrow depression, manifest as leucopenia, particularly granulocytopenia, thrombocytopenia, and anaemia, sometimes with striking megaloblastic changes. Granulocytopenia is biphasic, with a nadir at 7 to 9 days after a dose and another, more severe, at 15 to 24 days. The nadir of the platelet count occurs at about 12 to 15 days. Recovery generally occurs in a further ten days.

Gastro-intestinal disturbances may occur: nausea and vomiting may be more severe when doses are given rapidly. Other adverse effects reported include hepatic dysfunction, renal dysfunction, neurotoxicity (particularly via the intrathecal route), rashes, oral and anal ulceration, gastro-intestinal haemorrhage, oesophagitis, and conjunctivitis. A 'flu-like' syndrome has been reported, which may be treated with corticosteroid therapy if severe. Anaphylactoid reactions have occurred.

High-dose therapy has been associated with particularly severe gastro-intestinal and central nervous system effects, including severe ulceration of the gastro-intestinal tract, pneumatosis cystoides leading to peritonitis, necrotising colitis and bowel necrosis, personality changes, somnolence, and coma. There may also be corneal toxicity and haemorrhagic conjunctivitis, sepsis, liver abscess, severe skin rash leading to desquamation, alopecia, and cardiac disorders. Pulmonary oedema, sometimes fatal, has occurred.

There may be local pain, cellulitis, and thrombophlebitis at the site of injection.

Deoxycytidine was reported to antagonise the toxic as well as some antitumour effects of cytarabine.— V. M. Buchman *et al.* (letter), *Lancet*, 1977, *1*, 1061.

A report of transient myelosuppression with disproportionate erythroid aplasia in a patient receiving low-dose cytarabine. Such a response has not been previously described with a low-dose regimen.— M. -S. Lee *et al.* (letter), *New Engl. J. Med.*, 1984, *310*, 1328.

EFFECTS ON THE EYES. Four patients who had received high-dose cytarabine for 6 days, together with prophylactic dexamethasone eye-drops developed pain, photophobia, lachrymation, and visual loss 5 to 7 days after therapy. Examination revealed bilateral diffuse punctate keratitis. Discontinuation of the corticosteroid eye-drops and substitution of antibiotic ointment, with cold compresses and dim illumination, gave some symptomatic relief. The keratitis cleared in 1 to 2 weeks. Keratitis developed in these patients despite the use of corticosteroids, and may be the major abnormality accounting for eye-symptoms in patients on high-dose cytarabine; the prophylactic use of corticosteroids is inappropriate in this setting.— M. G. Gressel and R. L. Tomsak (letter), *Lancet*, 1982, *2*, 273. Contrary results. In 11 patients receiving high-dose cytarabine therapy for 6 days, one eye was treated with prednisolone eye-drops, beginning the day before chemotherapy and continuing for 10 days. Signs of decreased visual acuity, conjunctival hyperaemia, and superficial punctate keratitis were almost invariably observed in the untreated eyes, together with foreign-body sensation, intense photophobia, redness, lachrymation, and blurred vision. Treated eyes developed only mild irritation and redness. The treated eyes were asymptomatic within 1 week of finishing cytarabine whereas corneal changes persisted in some untreated eyes after a month. A topical corticosteroid was recommended for the prophylaxis of cytarabine-induced keratitis.— J. H. Lass *et al.*, *Am. J. Ophthal.*, 1982, *94*, 617.

EFFECTS ON THE HEART. Acute pericarditis with cardiac tamponade, presenting as acute chest pain and dyspnoea, were associated with administration of high-dose intermittent cytarabine therapy in a patient with acute lymphocytic leukaemia. There was no evidence of myocardial damage and the patient recovered following pericardiocentesis.— L. Vaickus and L. Letendre, *Archs intern. Med.*, 1984, *144*, 1868.

EFFECTS ON THE NERVOUS SYSTEM. A report of cytarabine-induced cerebellar syndrome.— R. K. Sylvester *et al.*, *Drug Intell. & clin. Pharm.*, 1987, *21*, 177.

EFFECTS ON THE SKIN. Palmar-plantar skin toxicity, identical to that reported by Lokich and Moore (*Ann. intern. Med.*, 1984, *101*, 798) in patients receiving combination chemotherapy, had been seen in patients given high-dose cytarabine. In 2 patients inadvertently given high-dose cytarabine doses as rapid intravenous boluses rather than infusions both developed unusually severe palmar and plantar skin toxicity, including large bullae involving both surfaces of one patient's palms. This palmar-plantar erythrodysesthesia syndrome may be associated with transient high peak drug concentrations. The syndrome may be treated with topical agents useful in burn therapy and with systemic corticosteroids if the process is less than 96 hours old. Cooling of the extremities might help to attenuate toxicity. M. R. Baer *et al.* (letter), *Ann. intern. Med.*, 1985, *102*, 556. Comment. The syndrome described by Lokich and Moore appears to be distinct from the skin toxicity of high-dose cytarabine.— N. J. Vogelzang and M. J. Ratain (letter), *ibid.*, *103*, 303. The palmar-plantar erythodysesthesia syndrome had occurred in 8 of 85 courses of intermediate- or high-dose cytarabine therapy. The syndrome developed in 6 patients during the last 2 days of the course and 4 and 5 days after the end of the course in 2 patients. Clinical signs consisted of dysesthesias in the palms and soles, pain, erythema, bulla formation, and desquamation. These skin changes disappeared as the peripheral granulocyte count recovered, and did not recur when therapy was re-instituted. Patients who also received corticosteroid treatment did not develop the syndrome.— W. G. Peters and R. Willemze (letter), *ibid.*, 805.

EFFECTS ON THE VASCULAR SYSTEM. A fatal Budd-Chiari-like illness or toxic veno-occlusive disease of the liver developed in 2 adult male patients during treatment with thioguanine. Both patients had also received cytarabine. There were 4 further reports of veno-occlusive disease of the liver in children with acute myelogenous leukaemia during maintenance therapy with thioguanine and daunorubicin; all had been previously treated with cytarabine.— P. F. Griner *et al.*, *Ann. intern. Med.*, 1976, *85*, 578.

Precautions

For reference to the precautions necessary with antineoplastic agents and immunosuppressants, see Antineoplastic Agents, p.583.

Cytarabine should be given with care to patients with impaired liver function. Blood-uric acid should be monitored and adequate fluid intake maintained because of the risk of hyperuricaemia.

Cytarabine is teratogenic in *animals*.

A report of acute pancreatitis in patients receiving cytarabine who had previously received colaspase therapy.— A. J. Altman *et al.*, *Cancer*, 1982, *49*, 1384.

PREGNANCY AND THE NEONATE. A report of limb and ear deformities in the infant of a woman given cytarabine at the estimated time of conception and at an estimated 4 to 8 weeks after conception.— V. M. Wagner *et al.* (letter), *Lancet*, 1980, *2*, 98. Of 20 cases reported, including 3 women who conceived while taking cytarabine and 2 who received it at 10 to 12 weeks after conception, no congenital abnormalities were noted in any of the 17 normal infants, 5 therapeutic abortions, and one stillbirth (following pre-eclamptic toxaemia).— G. Morgenstern (letter), *ibid.*, 259.

Absorption and Fate

Cytarabine is not effective by mouth, less than 20% of a dose is absorbed from the gastro-intestinal tract. After intravenous injection it disappears rapidly from the plasma. It is converted to an active form by phosphorylation which is rapidly deaminated, mainly in the liver and the kidneys, to inactive 1-β-D-arabinofuranosyluracil (uracil arabinoside). The majority of an intravenous dose is excreted in the urine as the inactive metabolite within 24 hours.

There is only moderate diffusion of cytarabine across the blood-brain barrier but, because of low deaminase activity in the cerebrospinal fluid, concentrations achieved after continuous intravenous infusion or intrathecal injection are maintained for longer in the CSF than are those in plasma.

Single doses of 47 mg to 3 g per m^2 body-surface of tritiated cytarabine given intravenously to 8 patients produced total plasma concentrations which decreased in a biphasic pattern with a mean half-life for the 1st phase of 12 minutes and for the 2nd of 111 minutes. Most of the activity was accounted for by cytarabine and uracil arabinoside; after the 1st phase over 80% of the radioactivity in the plasma and urine was due to uracil arabinoside. Red blood cell and liver concentrations were detected in patients and higher red blood cell concentrations occurred in patients with solid tumours. A dose of 112 mg per m^2 daily given by constant infusion produced a steady plasma concentration of 50 to 100 ng per mL. When 400 mg per m^2 was given, the plasma concentration increased to nearly 500 ng per mL and 1 patient maintained a steady CSF concentration of 200 ng per mL. The intrathecal administration of 50 mg per m^2 to 1 patient produced a CSF concentration which decreased exponentially with a half-life of 2 hours; after 7 hours only 10% was in the form of uracil arabinoside. Following parenteral administration between 70 and 84% of the dose was excreted in the urine within 24 hours, 7 to 8% as cytarabine, but in 3 patients given their dose by mouth only 14% was excreted in 24 hours and less than 3% was as cytarabine.— D. H. W. Ho and E. Frei, *Clin. Pharmac. Ther.*, 1971, *12*, 944. A study of the pharmacokinetics of cytarabine following bolus intravenous injections in 14 patients with acute myeloid leukaemia. Following the initial half-life phase of about 1 to 2 minutes, the plasma half-life of the second phase was 6.6 to 18.9 minutes which agreed with Momparler *et al.* (*Cancer Res.*, 1972, *32*, 408) and Baguley and Falkenhaug (*Eur. J. Cancer*, 1975, *11*, 43) and suggested that the mean initial phase of 12 minutes found by Ho and Frei (*Clin. Pharmac. Ther.*, 1971, *12*, 944) might correspond to the second phase with their second-phase finding of 111 minutes possibly indicating a third phase of about 2 hours. Variations in elimination or degradation might be important in predicting the results of chemotherapy since a complete remission was obtained in 9 of the patients with an average second-phase half-life of 15.1 minutes whereas therapy failed in the other 5 whose average was 9.6 minutes. Push injections with an increased dose or continuous infusions might improve the results in patients with a short half-life.— R. van Prooijen *et al.*, *Clin. Pharmac. Ther.*, 1977, *21*, 744. A further study in which most patients showed a biphasic or triphasic decline in plasma concentrations with terminal half-lives ranging from 7 to 107 minutes. The pharmacokinetics of cytarabine varied markedly from patient to patient and a wide range of plasma concentrations was associated with therapeutic response. Unless plasma concentrations can be related to tissue concentrations of active metabolites, individualisation of therapy will remain difficult.— A. L. Harris *et al.*, *Br. J. clin. Pharmac.*, 1979, *8*, 219. See also F. M. Balis *et al.*, *Clin. Pharmacokinet.*, 1983, *8*, 202.

Cytarabine was well absorbed following subcutaneous injection of 100 mg per m^2 body-surface in 5 patients with acute non-lymphoblastic leukaemia. The mean half-life of absorption was 3.4 minutes, and the subsequent decline in plasma concentrations was biphasic, with mean initial and terminal half-lives of 15.7 minutes and 1.4 hours. The pharmacokinetics of subcutaneous administration were considered to approximate those of an intravenous bolus.— M. L. Slevin *et al.*, *Br. J. clin. Pharmac.*, 1981, *12*, 507.

Uses and Administration

Cytarabine, a pyrimidine nucleoside analogue, is an antineoplastic agent which inhibits the synthesis of deoxyribonucleic acid. Its actions are specific for the S phase of the cell cycle. It also has antiviral and immunosuppressant properties.

Cytarabine is used mainly in the treatment of leukaemia, especially acute non-lymphoblastic leukaemia in adults when it is often given in association with thioguanine and doxorubicin or daunorubicin (see p.587).For the induction of remission in adults and children with acute non-lymphoblastic leukaemias doses of 100 to 200 mg per m^2 body-surface or 2 to 6 mg per kg body-weight may be given daily by intravenous infusion over 1 to 24 hours, or by intravenous injection, for 5 to 7 days or until bone-marrow hypoplasia occurs. Courses may be repeated after 7 to 14 days or once bone-marrow recovery has occurred.

In the treatment of refractory disease high-dose regimens have been employed, with cytarabine given in doses of up to 3 g per m^2 by continuous intravenous infusion every 12 hours for 6 days.

For maintenance 1 to 1.5 mg per kg may be given intravenously, intramuscularly, or subcutaneously once or twice weekly; other regimens have been used.

In leukaemic meningitis cytarabine has been given intrathecally, often in a dose of 30 mg per m^2 body-surface every 4 days; it has also been used prophylactically.

White cell and platelet counts should be determined regularly during treatment with cytarabine and therapy should be stopped immediately if the count falls rapidly or to low values.

A review of the actions of cytarabine.— M. G. Pallavicini, *Pharmac. Ther.*, 1984, *25*, 207.

Further references: *Lancet*, 1987, *2*, 717.

ADMINISTRATION. *Low-dose regimens.* Following evidence *in vitro* that low doses of cytarabine could induce differentiation and maturation of leukaemic cells, there have been a number of attempts to treat acute myeloid leukaemia, myelodysplasia, and other myeloproliferative disorders with low-dose cytarabine therapy. There has been particular enthusiasm for this method in frail or elderly patients who might not tolerate more intensive regimens, and in those with refractory disease or conditions such as myelodysplastic states that do not respond well to the usual therapy. Results have been variable, and at present it is not clear which kinds of myeloproliferative disease respond to low-dose cytarabine, nor which regimen is most effective (J.F. Desforges, *New Engl. J. Med.*, 1983, *309*, 1637).

In the majority of cases, doses of around 10 to 20 mg per m^2 body surface have been given twice daily by subcutaneous injection, or intravenously. Manoharan *et al.* (*Med. J. Aust.*, 1984, *141*, 643) reported complete remission in 6 of 20 patients with acute non-lymphoblastic leukaemia and partial remission in 9, following cytarabine 10 mg per m^2 every 12 hours for 14 to 21 days. The periods of survival of responding patients ranged from 2 to 15 months.

Harousseau *et al.* (*Lancet*, 1984, *2*, 288) have compared the effectiveness of low-dose cytarabine (10 mg/m^2 every 12 hours for 7 to 21 days) with a conventional combination regimen (standard dose cytarabine and zorubicin) in elderly patients with acute non-lymphoblastic leukaemia. Complete remission was achieved in 15 of 30 patients given the low dose and 18 of 32 given the conventional regimen: the latter figure included 2 of 3 patients who failed to respond to low-dose cytarabine. Seven and 9 of the complete responders respectively were still in complete remission a median of 10 and 16.5 months later -there were no significant differences between the regimens in remission rate and median survival. These figures were considered to confirm the role of low-dose cytarabine as initial treatment of acute non-lymphoblastic leukaemia in elderly patients.

Beneficial responses were also reported by Wisch *et al.* (*New. Engl. J. Med.*, 1983, *309*, 1599) in 6 of 8 patients with preleukaemia, or preleukaemia in evolution to acute leukaemia, who were given 20 mg per m^2 daily by continuous intravenous infusion for 7 to 21 days. Patients who responded had a marked decrease in bone-marrow and peripheral blood blasts and an increase in peripheral blood counts which markedly decreased transfusion requirements.

Beneficial effects of low-dose therapy have also been reported in patients with acute myelofibrosis (S. Whitehead and C.G. Geary, *Br. J. Haematol.*, 1984, *58*, 375) and in refractory anaemia secondary to myelodysplastic syndromes (J.H. Gallo and M.C. Rozenberg, *Aust. N.Z. J. Med.*, 1986, *16*, 231). Interesting preliminary results have also been seen in patients with sickle-cell anaemia—see under Hydroxyurea, p.631.

In general, low-dose cytarabine appears to be well tolerated, although most studies have reported a transient cytopenia in treated patients. Harousseau *et al.* (1984) reported cytopenia in 27 of 30 patients given a low-dose regimen, but none had the life-threatening side-effects responsible for 9 treatment-related deaths among patients receiving intensive conventional chemotherapy. However, Mufti *et al.* (*New Engl. J. Med.*, 1983, *309*, 1653) have reported a profound reduction in the blood-count of 6 patients with myelodysplastic syndrome who were given 10 to 20 mg [per m^2] twice daily subcutaneously for 12 to 21 days. This cytopenia was fatal in 3 despite intensive haematological support.

As a result of bone-marrow suppression even at low doses, some centres have treated patients with so-called **very-low-dose** regimens. Worsley *et al.* (*Lancet*, 1986, *1*, 966) have treated 8 patients with myelodysplastic syndromes or acute non-lymphoblastic leukaemia with cytarabine 3 mg per m^2 twice daily for 21 days. Complete remission occurred in 3 and improvement in a further 3 and clinical impressions were that this regimen was safer than, and at least as effective as, low-dose cytarabine. However, even at these doses haematological toxicity may occur: Pesce *et al.* (*ibid.*, 1436), while confirming the effectiveness of a similar very-low-dose regimen reported bone-marrow suppression in 5 of 16 patients with acute non-lymphoblastic leukaemia and in 4 of 11 with acute transformation of refractory anaemia with excess of blasts.

In addition to disagreement as to the appropriate dose there is also controversy as to the mode of action of low-dose cytarabine. Although much of the early work was stimulated by reports that low-dose cytarabine might induce differentiation of myeloid leukaemic cells, some subsequent investigators have suggested that the effects of the low-dose regimen imply a cytotoxic action (see Manoharan, 1984). However, Tilly and co-workers (*New Engl. J. Med.*, 1986, *314*, 246) have reported the persistence of a marker for a leukaemic clone in a patient in clinical remission after low-dose therapy, suggesting an action, at least in part, via differentiation, and the question remains to be resolved.

High-dose regimens. Cytarabine is the mainstay of current treatment for acute non-lymphoblastic leukaemia, and is associated with a remission rate of more than 50%. However, resistance to cytarabine may develop at any point during the course of the disease. In an effort to improve the remission rate in patients with resistant disease one effective manoeuvre has been to increase the dose of the drug approximately 15-fold— the so-called high-dose cytarabine regimen. This approach has been shown to improve the remission rate but it also increases toxicity and may lead to enhanced gastro-intestinal, hepatic, and CNS toxicity.— J. F. Desforges, *New Engl. J. Med.*, 1983, *309*, 1637.

References to the use of high-dose intravenous cytarabine regimens: R. H. Herzig *et al.*, *Blood*, 1983, *62*, 361 (refractory acute non-lymphoblastic leukaemia); H. D. Preisler *et al.*, *New Engl. J. Med.*, 1983, *308*, 21 (secondary acute nonlymphoblastic leukaemia following previous cancer therapy); M. A. Shipp *et al.*, *Am. J. Med.*, 1984, *77*, 845 (non-Hodgkin's lymphoma); M. Markham (letter), *Ann. intern. Med.*, 1984, *101*, 398 (acute myeloid leukaemia with extreme leucocytosis); R. E. Marcus *et al.* (letter), *Lancet*, 1985, *1*, 1384 (with mitozantrone in relapsed acute myeloid leukaemia); W. Hiddemann *et al.* (letter), *ibid.*, *2*, 508 (with mitozantrone in refractory acute myeloid leukaemia).

The administration of thymidine with cytarabine in an attempt to enhance the activity of the latter in patients with acute leukaemias.— R. Zittoun *et al.*, *Cancer Res.*, 1985, *45*, 5186.

ADMINISTRATION IN RENAL INSUFFICIENCY. Cytarabine could be given in usual doses to patients with renal failure.— W. M. Bennett *et al.*, *Am. J. Kidney Dis.*, 1983, *3*, 155.

ANTIVIRAL ACTION. References to the antiviral action of cytarabine: B. E. Juel-Jensen, *Prescribers' J.*, 1983, *23*, 126; D. L. Swallow and G. L. Kampfner, *Br. med. Bull.*, 1985, *41*, 322.

LEUKAEMIAS, ACUTE. For reference to the use of cytarabine in the treatment of acute leukaemia, see under Choice of Antineoplastic Agent, p.587. See also under Administration, above.

SKIN DISORDERS, NON-MALIGNANT. A report of the virtual resolution of extensive psoriasis refractory to conventional treatment in a patient given low-dose cytarabine for acute leukaemia.— A. S. Duncombe and T. C. Pearson, *Br. med. J.*, 1986, *292*, 450.

Preparations

Cytarabine Injection *(B.P.)*. To be prepared immediately before use.

Sterile Cytarabine *(U.S.P.)*. Cytarabine suitable for parenteral use.

Proprietary Preparations

Alexan *(Pfizer, UK)*. *Injection*, cytarabine 20 mg/mL in ampoules of 2 and 5 mL.
Injection, (Alexan 100) hypertonic solution, cytarabine 100 mg/mL, in ampoules of 1 and 10 mL.

Cytosar *(Upjohn, UK)*. *Injection*, powder for reconstitution, cytarabine 100 and 500 mg, supplied with solvent.

Proprietary Names and Manufacturers

Alexan *(Belg.; Mack, Illert., Ger.; Byk Gulden, Ital.; Neth.; Spain; Mack, Switz.; Pfizer, UK)*; Arabitin *(Jpn)*; Aracytin *(Arg.; Upjohn, Ital.)*; Aracytine *(Upjohn, Fr.)*; Cytosar *(Upjohn, Austral.; Belg.; Upjohn, Canad.; Upjohn, Denm.; Jpn; Neth.; Upjohn, Norw.; S.Afr.; Upjohn, Swed.; Upjohn, Switz.; Upjohn, UK; Upjohn, USA)*; Erpalfa *(INTES, Ital.)*; Iretin *(Jpn)*; Udicil *(Upjohn, Ger.)*.

1827-t

Dacarbazine *(BAN, USAN, rINN)*.

DIC; DTIC; Imidazole Carboxamide; NSC-45388; WR-139007. 5-(3,3-Dimethyl-1-triazeno)imidazole-4-carboxamide.

$C_6H_{10}N_6O = 182.2$.

CAS — 4342-03-4.

Pharmacopoeias. In *Br.* and *U.S.*

A colourless or pale-yellow crystalline powder. Slightly **soluble** in water and in alcohol. **Store** in airtight containers at 2° to 8°. Protect from light.

Solutions for injection are prepared by dissolving the sterile contents of a sealed container in Water for Injections. Such solutions, containing the equivalent of dacarbazine 10 mg per mL, have a pH of 3 to 4 and are stable for up to 8 hours at room temperature or for 72 hours at 4°.

CAUTION. *Dacarbazine is irritant; avoid contact with skin and mucous membranes.*

INCOMPATIBILITY. Dacarbazine is incompatible with hydrocortisone sodium succinate.— P. F. D'Arcy, *Drug Intell. & clin. Pharm.*, 1983, *17*, 532.

STABILITY IN SOLUTION. Solutions of pure dacarbazine are sensitive to light and rapidly photolyse to 5-diazoimidazole-4-carboxamide and then to 2-azahypoxanthine, both of which are biologically active. Photodegradation of the commercial product, which when reconstituted contains dacarbazine citrate and mannitol, differs significantly from that of pure dacarbazine. A dilute aqueous solution of DTIC-Dome 1 mg in 100 mL is completely transformed within one minute to 5-diazoimidazole-4-carboxamide in direct sunlight and after 30 minutes 5-hydroxyimidazole-4-carboxamide and not 2-azahypoxanthine has been identified. A concentrated aqueous solution of DTIC-Dome 100 mg in 50 mL evolves gas and turns red when exposed to sunlight. Dacarbazine should be protected from light at all times.— M. F. G. Stevens and L. Peatey, *J. Pharm. Pharmac.*, 1978, *30*, *Suppl.*, 47P.

The stability of dacarbazine solutions in the presence of a range of cytotoxic agents was monitored by ultra violet and visible spectrometry both in the dark and in ambient laboratory light. No detectable interaction occurred with actinomycin D, bleomycin, carmustine, cyclophosphamide, cytarabine, doxorubicin, fluorouracil, lomustine, methotrexate, or vinblastine. The only notable chemical change was the photo-decomposition of dacarbazine itself.— J. K. Horton and M. F. G. Stevens, *J. Pharm. Pharmac.*, 1979, *31*, *Suppl.*, 64P.

The manufacturers state that following reconstitution of dacarbazine as a solution for injection the solution may be further diluted with glucose (5%) or sodium chloride (0.9%) injections, and the resulting solution may be stored at 4° for up to 24 hours. The undiluted reconstituted solution may be stored at 4° for 72 hours or at normal room temperature for up to 8 hours.

Adverse Effects, Treatment, and Precautions

For an outline of the adverse effects experienced with antineoplastic agents and immunosuppressants, general guidelines for their treatment and precautions, see Antineoplastic Agents, p.580, p.583.

Leucopenia and thrombocytopenia with dacarbazine may be severe and the maximum effect may not be seen for 3 to 4 weeks. Anorexia, nausea, and vomiting are very common. Other side-effects include hepatotoxicity, skin reactions, alopecia, an influenza-like syndrome, and facial flushing and paraesthesia. Extravasation produces pain and tissue damage. Anaphylaxis has occurred occasionally.

Local venous pain and systemic side-effects such as nausea, vomiting, and hepatic toxicity after injection of dacarbazine might be due to photodegradation products. After reconstituting and rapidly injecting the drug at a concentration of 100 mg in 10 mL in a room lit only with a red photographic light, 3 patients received a total of 14 injections with no pain or only minor discomfort during the first few seconds. Nausea and vomiting also seemed to be reduced.— G. M. Baird and M. L. N. Willoughby (letter), *Lancet*, 1978, *2*, 681.

EFFECTS ON THE LIVER. Fatal hepatic vascular lesions associated with dacarbazine.— M. A. Greenstone *et al.*, *Br. med. J.*, 1981, *282*, 1744.

Based on experience in more than 100 patients it was reported that the spectrum of adverse hepatic effects with dacarbazine was broader than previously thought, and necrosis may be associated with venous thrombosis or occur without signs of inflammation; granulomatous hepatitis has occurred, as has a case of acute toxic hepatitis during the first course of dacarbazine. Morphological studies suggested that dacarbazine may exert a toxic effect on the microfilamentous cytoskeleton of the hepatocytes.— H. Dancygier *et al.*, *Gut*, 1982, *23*, A447.

EFFECTS ON THE SKIN. Dacarbazine had frequently been reported to cause photosensitivity reactions.— *Med. Lett.*, 1986, *28*, 51.

INTERACTIONS. A report that BCG injected into *rats* reduced the activity of liver enzymes which metabolise dacarbazine.— T. L. Loo *et al.*, *Cancer Treat. Rep.*, 1976, *60*, 149.

PREGNANCY AND THE NEONATE. Studies in *rats* and *rabbits* indicated that dacarbazine was toxic to mother and foetus; a marginal effect on spermatozoal integrity was also noted.— D. J. Thompson *et al.*, *Toxic. appl. Pharmac.*, 1975, *33*, 281.

Absorption and Fate

Dacarbazine is poorly absorbed from the gastro-intestinal tract. Following intravenous injection it is rapidly distributed with an initial plasma half-life of about 20 minutes; the terminal half-life is reported to be about 5 hours. Only about 5% is bound to protein. Penetration into the cerebrospinal fluid is poor. Dacarbazine is extensively metabolised in the liver; the major metabolite appears to be 5-aminoimidazole-4-carboxamide (AIC). About half of a dose is excreted unchanged in the urine by tubular secretion.

Uses and Administration

Dacarbazine is a cell-cycle nonspecific antineoplastic agent which may function as an alkylating agent (see p.580) after it has been activated in the liver. It has minimal immunosuppressant activity. Dacarbazine is used mainly in the treatment of metastatic malignant melanoma, with a response rate of about 20%. It is also given to patients with refractory Hodgkin's disease, notably in association with doxorubicin, bleomycin, and vinblastine (ABVD), and has been given in the treatment of soft-tissue sarcomas and other tumours. See also under Choice of Antineoplastic Agent, p.584.

It is given intravenously in doses of 2 to 4.5 mg per kg body-weight daily for 10 days and repeated after intervals of 4 weeks or 250 mg per m^2 body-surface daily for 5 days and repeated after intervals of 3 weeks. In the treatment of Hodgkin's disease doses of 150 mg per m^2 daily for 5 days, or 375 mg per m^2 every 15 days have been given in association with other agents. Injections may be given over one to two minutes. In an attempt to prevent pain along the injected vein the reconstituted solution has been further diluted with glucose injection (5%) or sodium chloride injection (0.9%) and given by infusion.

MALIGNANT NEOPLASMS OF THE PANCREAS. Reports of the successful use of dacarbazine in the treatment of malignant glucagonoma: G. M. Strauss *et al.*, *Ann. intern. Med.*, 1979, *90*, 57; S. P. Marynick *et al.*, *ibid.*, 1980, *93*, 453; L. A. Duncan and S. P. Marynick (letter), *ibid.*, 1982, *97*, 930; T. Kurose *et al.* (letter), *Lancet*, 1984, *1*, 621.

MELANOMA. For references to the use of dacarbazine in melanoma see Choice of Antineoplastic Agent, p.592.

Preparations

Dacarbazine for Injection *(U.S.P.)*

Dacarbazine Injection *(B.P.)*

Proprietary Preparations

DTIC-Dome *(Bayer, UK). Injection*, powder for reconstitution, dacarbazine 100 and 200 mg.

Proprietary Names and Manufacturers

Deticene *(Bellon, Fr.; Medac, Ger.; Rhone-Poulenc, Ital.; Neth.; Rhone-Poulenc, Switz.)*; DTIC-Dome *(Miles, Austral.; Miles, Canad.; Ital.; Neth.; NZ; Bayer, S.Afr.; Miles Martin, Spain; Dome, Swed.; Dome, Switz.; Bayer, UK; Miles Pharmaceuticals, USA)*.

1828-x

Daunorubicin Hydrochloride *(BANM, USAN, rINNM)*.

Daunomycin Hydrochloride; FI-6339 *(daunorubicin)*; NDC-0082-4155; NSC-82151; RP-13057 *(daunorubicin)*; Rubidomycin Hydrochloride.

(1*S*,3*S*)-3-Acetyl-1,2,3,4,6,11-hexahydro-3,5,12-trihydroxy-10-methoxy-6,11-dioxonaphthacen-1-yl 3-amino-2,3,6-trideoxy-α-L-lyxopyranoside hydrochloride.

$C_{27}H_{29}NO_{10},HCl=564.0$.

CAS — 20830-81-3 (daunorubicin); 23541-50-6 (hydrochloride).

Pharmacopoeias. In *Fr., It.,* and *U.S.*

The hydrochloride of an antineoplastic anthracycline antibiotic produced by *Streptomyces coeruleorubidus* or *S. peucetius.* It has a potency equivalent to 842 to 1030 µg of the base per mg. A 0.5% solution has a pH of 4.5 to 6.5. **Store** at a temperature not exceeding 40° in airtight containers. Protect from light.

CAUTION. *Daunorubicin hydrochloride is irritant; avoid contact with skin and mucous membranes.*

INCOMPATIBILITY. Daunorubicin is incompatible with heparin sodium.— P. F. D'Arcy, *Drug Intell. & clin. Pharm.*, 1983, *17*, 532.

Daunorubicin was incompatible with aluminium, which had been used in the design of a dispensing pin intended to aid antineoplastic drug preparation. On inspection, a solution of daunorubicin hydrochloride in contact with a part-aluminium needle darkened to ruby red, and black patches appeared on the aluminium surface after 12 to 24 hours. A similar reaction occurred with a solution of doxorubicin hydrochloride.— G. S. Ogawa *et al.* (letter), *Am. J. Hosp. Pharm.*, 1985, *42*, 1042.

Daunorubicin hydrochloride solution has also been reported to be incompatible with a solution of dexamethasone sodium phosphate. The manufacturer recommends that daunorubicin hydrochloride should not be administered mixed with other drugs.

STABILITY IN SOLUTION. In a study of the stability of anthracycline antineoplastic agents in 4 infusion fluids (glucose injection (5%), sodium chloride injection (0.9%), lactated Ringer's injection, and a commercial infusion fluid) daunorubicin hydrochloride was stable in all 4, the percentage remaining after 24 hours being 98.5%, 97.4%, 94.7%, and 95.4% respectively. Stability appeared to be partly related to pH; daunorubicin was more stable as the pH of the mixture became more acidic, with the best stability in glucose injection (5%) with a pH of 4.5.— G. K. Poochikian *et al.*, *Am. J. Hosp. Pharm.*, 1981, *38*, 483.

Adverse Effects, and Treatment

As for Doxorubicin, p.623.

Cardiotoxicity is more likely when the total dose of daunorubicin exceeds 550 mg per m^2 body-surface in adults, or 300 mg per m^2 in children.

Transient red discoloration of the urine may occur.

EFFECTS ON THE HEART. A retrospective analysis of risk factors for the development of daunorubicin cardiotoxicity. Of the 5613 patients studied, 65 developed congestive heart failure. The incidence of congestive heart failure was clearly dose-related, and was calculated at 4% in patients receiving cumulative doses up to and including 550 mg per m^2 but at 14% in patients receiving a total dose of 1050 mg per m^2. In addition, the risk appeared to be higher in children than in adults from 15 to 40 years of age (6% versus 1.3% at a total dose of 550 mg per m^2). As well as these patients, a further 45 patients had electrocardiographic changes without any of the signs or symptoms of heart failure. These changes were not dose-related and did not presage the development of drug-induced congestive heart failure.— D. D. Von Hoff and M. Layard, *Cancer Treat. Rep.*, 1981, *65, Suppl.* 4, 19. See also D. D. Von Hoff *et al.*, *Ann. intern. Med.*, 1979, *91*, 710; P. C. Adams, *Adverse Drug React. Bull.*, 1982, (Feb.), 336.

EFFECTS ON THE SKIN. A report of the development of red-brown erythematous hyperpigmentation in a patient given a 3-day course of daunorubicin; the pigmentation subsequently lightened and disappeared within 6 weeks, but recurred on subsequent re-administration of the drug.— T. M. Kelly *et al.*, *Archs Derm.*, 1984, *120*, 262.

For the management of skin damage induced by extravasation of daunorubicin hydrochloride, see R. F. Cox, *Am. J. Hosp. Pharm.*, 1984, *41*, 2410.

See also Local Toxicity, under Adverse Effects of Antineoplastic Agents, p.582 and Extravasation, under Treatment of Adverse Effects, p.583.

Precautions

As for Doxorubicin Hydrochloride, p.624.

HANDLING AND DISPOSAL. For a method for the destruction of daunorubicin in wastes see under Doxorubicin Hydrochloride, p.624.

Absorption and Fate

After intravenous injection, daunorubicin is rapidly distributed into body tissues, particularly the liver, lungs, kidneys, spleen, and heart. It is metabolised mainly in the liver and excreted in bile and urine. The major metabolite, daunorubicinol, has antineoplastic activity. Up to 25% of a dose is excreted in urine in an active form over several days; an estimated 40% is excreted in bile. Daunorubicin does not appear to cross the blood-brain barrier, but crosses the placenta.

A review of the pharmacokinetics of some antineoplastic agents, including daunorubicin. The terminal half-lives of daunorubicin and daunorubicinol were reported to be 18.5 and 26.7 hours respectively. Blood concentrations of the anthracyclines and their active metabolites may be very useful in selection of the individual's maximum tolerated dose.— F. M. Balis *et al.*, *Clin. Pharmacokinet.*, 1983, *8*, 202.

A study of the cellular pharmacokinetics of daunorubicin in 6 leukaemic subjects given intravenous doses of 40 to 70 mg per m^2 body-surface. Daunorubicin concentrations in leukaemic cells in plasma or bone marrow were considerably higher than those in plasma. Maximum concentrations were achieved soon after the end of the infusion, the values in plasma after a uniform dose of 45 mg per m^2 being calculated as 12.3 to 38.3 ng per mL after 2 hours; the intracellular concentrations in peripheral blood were calculated at 2.99 to 17.00 µg per g, an average of about 350 times higher. Plasma and intracellular concentrations subsequently declined, the former more rapidly than the latter: in consequence, the ratio between intracellular and plasma concentrations had increased to a mean of about 700 at 24 hours. Concentrations of daunorubicin in leukaemic cells in bone marrow, which could be determined in only 4 patients, were even higher than those in cells in peripheral blood. Determination of intracellular concentrations of daunorubicin should prove more useful than a simple assay in plasma as an index of the therapeutic action.— V. Trillet *et al.*, *Eur. J. clin. Pharmac.*, 1985, *29*, 127.

Uses and Administration

Daunorubicin is an antineoplastic antibiotic closely related to doxorubicin (p.623). It forms a stable complex with DNA and interferes with the synthesis of nucleic acids. Daunorubicin is a cell-cycle nonspecific agent, but its cytotoxic effects are most marked on cells in the S phase. Daunorubicin also has antibacterial and immunosuppressant properties. It is used with other antineoplastic agents to induce remissions in acute leukaemias. Daunorubicin hydrochloride is given in association with vincristine and prednisone or prednisolone in acute lymphoblastic leukaemia and with cytarabine and thioguanine in acute non-lymphoblastic leukaemias. See also under Choice of Antineoplastic Agent, p.586. It has also been tried in lymphomas, and in neuroblastoma.

In treatment regimens for acute non-lymphoblastic leukaemia, daunorubicin hydrochloride is given in doses equivalent to 30 to 60 mg of base per m^2 body-surface daily for 3 to 5 days, by injecting a solution in sodium chloride injection (0.9%) into a fast-running infusion of sodium chloride or glucose. Courses may be repeated after 3 to 6 weeks. A dose equivalent to 25 mg of base per m^2 has been given intravenously once a week, in combination with vincristine and prednisone or prednisolone, to children with acute lymphoblastic leukaemia. The maximum total dose in adults should not exceed 550 mg per m^2; in patients who have received radiotherapy to the chest it may be advisable to limit the total dose to about 450 mg per m^2.

Blood counts should be determined frequently during treatment as daunorubicin has a potent effect on bone-marrow function. Electrocardiogram examination should be made at regular intervals to detect signs of cardiotoxicity.

LEUKAEMIA, ACUTE. For reference to the use of daunorubicin with other agents in the treatment of acute lymphoblastic leukaemia and acute non-lymphoblastic leukaemia, see Choice of Antineoplastic Agent, p.586.

Di Guglielmo's disease. Nine patients with Di Guglielmo's syndrome, an erythroleukaemia considered resistant to chemotherapy, were treated with daunorubicin 1 mg per kg body-weight daily by rapid intravenous infusion for 5 days, and concomitant prednisone. Four patients obtained complete remission and 3 patients partial remission 3 to 8 weeks after the start of therapy; all patients with no prior treatment responded. The duration of remission was from 2 to 16 months with a median duration of survival of 12 months. Maintenance therapy was instituted with other cytotoxic agents; following relapse only 1 patient responded to daunorubicin and prednisone.— C. D. Bloomfield *et al.*, *Ann. intern. Med.*, 1974, *81*, 746.

TRYPANOSOMIASIS. Daunorubicin has an extremely potent trypanocidal action *in vitro* but was inactive *in vivo*, as was daunorubicin bound to ferritin or bovine serum albumin by a stable non-covalent linkage; however, conjugates of daunorubicin with bovine serum albumin or ferritin, in which the linkage was labile, were active in *mice* infected with *Trypanosoma rhodesiense*.— J. Williamson *et al.*, *Nature*, 1981, *292*, 466. Evidence that the labile daunorubicin-bovine serum albumin complex (D-BSAG) acts as a delivery system for slow intracellular release of the drug within the trypanosome, where it then acts on the nucleus.— L. Golightly *et al.*, *J. Pharm. Pharmac.*, 1985, *37*, *Suppl.*, 145P.

Preparations

Daunorubicin Hydrochloride for Injection *(U.S.P.)*. A sterile mixture of daunorubicin hydrochloride and mannitol. Potency is expressed in terms of the equivalent amount of daunorubicin.

Proprietary Names and Manufacturers

Cerubidin *(May & Baker, Austral.; Rhone-Poulenc, Denm.; Rhône-Poulenc, Norw.; May & Baker, S.Afr.; Leo Rhodia, Swed.; May & Baker, UK)*; Cerubidine *(Rhone-Poulenc, Belg.; Rhône-Poulenc, Canad.; Bellon, Fr.; Specia, Neth.; Rhone-Poulenc, Switz.; Wyeth, USA)*; Daunoblastin *(Farmitalia, Ger.)*; Daunoblastina *(Farmitalia, Ital.; Farmitalia, Spain)*.

12635-l

Detorubicin *(rINN)*.

A glyoxylic acid ester of doxorubicin.

$C_{33}H_{39}NO_{14}=673.7$.

CAS — 66211-92-5.

Detorubicin is an analogue of doxorubicin (p.623) under study as an antineoplastic agent.

References: S. K. Carter, *Drugs*, 1980, *20*, 375.

12640-s

Dianhydrogalactitol

DAG; Dianhydrodulcitol; NSC-132313. 1,2:5,6-Dianhydrogalactitol; 1,2:5,6-Diepoxyhexane-3,4-diol.
$C_6H_{10}O_4$=146.1.

CAS — 23261-20-3.

Dianhydrogalactitol is an antineoplastic agent which is reported to function by alkylation (see p.580) and has been tried in the management of various solid neoplasms. Bone-marrow suppression is reported to be dose-limiting.

References: B. Hoogstraten and C. Haas, *Clin. Pharmac. Ther.*, 1976, *19*, 108; R. T. Eagan *et al.*, *J. Am. med. Ass.*, 1979, *241*, 2046.

Proprietary Names and Manufacturers
Chinoin, Hung.

1830-j

Dichlorodiethylsulphide

Mustard Gas; Sulphur Mustard; Yellow Cross Liquid. Bis(2-chloroethyl)sulphide.
$C_4H_8Cl_2S$=159.1.

CAS — 505-60-2.

Dichlorodiethylsulphide has even more severe vesicant and irritant properties than its nitrogen analogue, mustine (p.645). It was formerly used topically in the treatment of psoriasis.

A report of 11 cases of exposure to dichlorodiethylsulphide in fishermen who accidentally retrieved corroded and leaking gas shells from underwater dumps. The patients presented with very inflamed skin, especially in the axillary and genitofemoral regions, yellow blisters on the hands and legs, painful irritation of the eyes, and transient blindness. Two developed pulmonary oedema. There was evidence of a mutagenic effect and in view of the increased risk of lung cancer in soldiers and workers exposed to the gas it is reasonable to assume that fishermen heavily exposed to dichlorodiethylsulphide also have an increased cancer risk.— H. C. Wulf *et al.* (letter), *Lancet*, 1985, *1*, 690.

19107-r

Doxifluridine *(rINN).*

5′-Deoxy-5-fluorouridine; 5-DFUR; FUDR; Ro-21-9738.
$C_9H_{11}FN_2O_5$=246.2.

CAS — 3094-09-5.

Adverse Effects, Treatment, and Precautions

As for fluorouracil, p.628. Side-effects are reported to be less severe than after the same dose of fluorouracil.

Uses and Administration

Doxifluridine is an antineoplastic agent which probably acts through its conversion in the body to fluorouracil (p.628). It has been tried in the management of malignant neoplasms of the breast and gastro-intestinal tract, and of other solid tumours, in doses of 1 to 4 g per m^2 body-surface daily for 5 days by intravenous injection. Single doses of up to 15 g have also reportedly been given weekly by slow intravenous infusion. Doxifluridine has also been given by mouth.

Activity in rectosigmoid adenocarcinoma.— R. Abele *et al.*, *J. clin. Oncol.*, 1983, *1*, 750.

ABSORPTION AND FATE. The pharmacokinetics and metabolism of doxifluridine in patients given up to 15 mg per m^2 weekly by intravenous infusion. Doxifluridine was metabolised to fluorouracil and 5,6-dihydrofluorouracil; plasma concentrations of fluorouracil were approximately 6% of those of doxifluridine.— J. -P. Sommadossi *et al.*, *Cancer Res.*, 1983, *43*, 930.

Proprietary Names and Manufacturers
Furtulon *(Roche, Jpn).*

1831-z

Doxorubicin Hydrochloride *(BANM, USAN, rINNM).*

14-Hydroxydaunorubicin Hydrochloride; 3-Hydroxyacetyldaunorubicin Hydrochloride; Adriamycin Hydrochloride; FI-106 *(doxorubicin)*; NSC-123127. (1*S*,3*S*)-3-Glycoloyl-1,2,3,4,6,11-hexahydro-3,5,12-trihydroxy-10-methoxy-6,11-dioxonaphthacen-1-yl 3-amino-2,3,6-trideoxy-α-L-lyxopyranoside hydrochloride.
$C_{27}H_{29}NO_{11}$, HCl=580.0.

CAS — 23214-92-8 (doxorubicin); 25316-40-9 (hydrochloride).

Pharmacopoeias. In *It.* and *U.S.*

The hydrochloride of an anthracycline antineoplastic antibiotic isolated from *Streptomyces peucetius* var. *coesius.* It has a potency of 900 to 1100 μg per mg, calculated on the dried basis. An orange-red hygroscopic crystalline powder. **Soluble** in water and methyl alcohol; practically insoluble in chloroform, ether, and other organic solvents. A 0.5% solution in water has a pH of 4.0 to 5.5. **Store** in airtight containers.

CAUTION. *Doxorubicin hydrochloride is irritant; avoid contact with skin and mucous membranes.*

INCOMPATIBILITY. Doxorubicin is incompatible with heparin sodium and may be incompatible with aluminium, aminophylline, cephalothin sodium, dexamethasone, fluorouracil, and hydrocortisone.— P. F. D'Arcy, *Drug Intell. & clin. Pharm.*, 1983, *17*, 532.

A solution of doxorubicin hydrochloride containing a piece of aluminium changed colour to a darker ruby red over 24 hours, and the pH altered from 4.8 to 5.2. A control solution, and solutions containing stainless steel needles with steel or plastic hubs, underwent no colour change during this period and pH altered from 4.8 to 4.9. However, assays of the potency of the aluminium-containing and control doxorubicin solutions showed no loss of potency at 6 hours; after 3 days, the 2 solutions contained 91.9 and 94.4% of their original doxorubicin concentrations respectively. Doxorubicin does react with aluminium but the reaction is slow and does not result in substantial loss of potency. Syringes containing doxorubicin solutions should not be capped with aluminium-hubbed needles for storage, but such needles may safely be used for injection of doxorubicin. — M. J. Williamson *et al.* (letter), *Am. J. Hosp. Pharm.*, 1983, *40*, 214.

For a report of incompatibility between a solution of doxorubicin hydrochloride and an aluminium segment from a dispensing pin see under Daunorubicin Hydrochloride, p.622.

STABILITY IN SOLUTION. The stability of refrigerated and frozen solutions of doxorubicin hydrochloride.— D. M. Hoffman *et al.*, *Am. J. Hosp. Pharm.*, 1979, *36*, 1536.

Studies indicating that doxorubicin in solution is photodegradable and that at concentrations lower than 500 μg per mL appreciable loss of biochemical activity occurs if exposure to light is not prevented. However as higher concentrations (2 mg per mL) are usually prepared for administration to patients with cancer special precautions do not appear to be necessary to protect freshly prepared solutions from light during intravenous administration.— N. Tavoloni *et al.*, *J. Pharm. Pharmac.*, 1980, *32*, 860. See also J. M. C. Gutteridge and S. Wilkins, *J. biol. Stand.*, 1983, *11*, 359.

In a study of the stability of anthracycline antineoplastic agents in 4 infusion fluids (glucose injection (5%), sodium chloride injection (0.9%), lactated Ringer's injection, and a commercial infusion fluid) doxorubicin hydrochloride was stable in all 4, the percentage remaining after 24 hours being 97.9%, 94.5%, 92.3%, and 90.1% respectively. Stability appeared to be partly related to pH; doxorubicin becomes more stable as the pH of the mixture becomes more acidic with optimum stability in glucose injection (5%) with a pH of 4.5.— G. K. Poochikian *et al.*, *Am. J. Hosp. Pharm.*, 1981, *38*, 483.

A further study. Doxorubicin and its 4′-congeners underwent considerable degradation when stored in the dark as solutions in lactated Ringer's solution (pH 6.8) or 0.9% sodium chloride solution (pH 7); the time taken for a 10% loss of doxorubicin to occur was 1.7 and 6 days respectively. However, solutions in 5% glucose (pH 4.7) or 3.3% glucose and 0.3% sodium chloride (pH 4.4) were stable for at least 4 weeks.— J. H. Beijnen *et al.*, *J. parent. Sci. Technol.*, 1985, *39*, 220.

Adverse Effects

For an outline of the adverse effects experienced with antineoplastic agents, see Antineoplastic Agents, p.580.

Doxorubicin causes pronounced bone-marrow depression with leucopenia at a maximum 10 to 15 days after administration; blood counts recover about 21 days after a dose.

The anthracyclines may produce cardiac toxicity, both as an acute, usually transient disturbance of cardiac function, and as a delayed, sometimes fatal, chronic congestive heart failure. Severe cardiotoxicity is more likely in adults receiving total cumulative doses greater than 550 mg per m^2 body-surface area of doxorubicin, and may occur up to 6 months after administration.

Gastro-intestinal disturbances, stomatitis, and, more rarely, facial flushing, conjunctivitis, and lachrymation may occur. Doxorubicin is very irritant and thrombophlebitis has been reported following injection. Alopecia occurs in the majority of patients. The urine may be coloured red.

Reduction of doxorubicin toxicity by liposomal entrapment.— R. A. Sells *et al.* (letter), *Lancet*, 1987, *2*, 624.

ALLERGY. A report of 3 patients who developed systemic hypersensitivity reactions following administration of doxorubicin. Reactions were limited to urticarial lesions and localised pruritus; changes in blood pressure were mild to moderate and did not require treatment. Such reactions should be distinguished from the erythematous flare which has been reported along the vein being infused and which may have been due in the past to the low tonicity of infusates reconstituted in water rather than saline.— D. A. Solimando and J. P. Wilson, *Drug Intell. & clin. Pharm.*, 1984, *18*, 808. See also: L. Souhami and R. Feld, *J. Am. med. Ass.*, 1978, *240*, 1624; J. E. Maldonado (letter), *New Engl. J. Med.*, 1979, *301*, 386; C. Cordonnier *et al.* (letter), *Ann. intern. Med.*, 1982, *97*, 783; J. A. Collins, *Drug Intell. & clin. Pharm.*, 1984, *18*, 402.

EFFECTS ON THE GASTRO-INTESTINAL TRACT. Oesophagitis, sometimes progressing to oesophageal strictures, has occurred in patients receiving radiotherapy and doxorubicin; doxorubicin may enhance the toxic effect of the radiotherapy.— A. Horwich *et al.* (letter), *Lancet*, 1975, *2*, 561; F. A. Greco *et al.*, *Ann. intern. Med.*, 1976, *85*, 294.

EFFECTS ON THE HEART. The therapeutic potential of doxorubicin and daunorubicin is limited by the development of cardiac failure in up to 5% of patients due to cardiomyopathy. Microscopic changes occur even in patients with no evidence of cardiac decompensation. Mild degrees of damage are reversible but this does not appear to be so in more severe cases, and the prognosis of established heart failure is poor with over 50% of patients dying. The cumulative likelihood of failure is related to total dose, rising from 3% at a total dose of 400 mg per m^2 body-surface area to 20% at 700 mg per m^2. Previous mediastinal irradiation increases the risk, as does age, the young and the old being more vulnerable, and possibly the concurrent use of other cytotoxic agents such as cyclophosphamide and the vinca alkaloids. Many workers discontinue treatment once a total dose of about 500 mg per m^2 is reached, although patients have tolerated higher doses; some doctors rely on appearance of a third heart sound and a change in heart size on chest radiographs before ceasing treatment.— P. C. Adams, *Adverse Drug React. Bull.*, 1982, (Feb.), 336. See also: I. C. Henderson and E. Frei, *New Engl. J. Med.*, 1979, *300*, 310; D. D. Von Hoff *et al.*, *Ann. intern. Med.*, 1979, *91*, 710.

Recommendations for the prevention of cardiotoxicity during treatment with doxorubicin: (1) if the absolute QRS voltage of the 6 limb leads of the ECG decreased by 30% or more during therapy, doxorubicin should be discontinued. (2) No matter what the ECG reading might be the cumulative dose should not exceed 550 mg per m^2 body-surface in most patients. (3) As cyclophosphamide and radiotherapy to the heart appeared to enhance the cardiotoxicity of doxorubicin, the cumulative dose in such cases should not exceed 450 mg per m^2. (4) The dose should also be limited to 450 mg per m^2 where it has to be used in patients with associated heart disease that might increase cardiac work-load. (5) There should be early diagnosis of cardiotoxicity with prompt withdrawal of doxorubicin.— R. A. Minow *et al.*, *Cancer*, 1977, *39*, 1397. In studies on 33 patients, doxorubicin produced dose-related myocardial degeneration which began before abnormalities in left ventricular function could be detected clinically. Heart failure occurred at cumulative doses ranging from 330 to 545 mg per m^2.— M. R. Bristow *et al.*, *Ann. intern. Med.*, 1978, *88*, 168. New clinical indices of left ventricular function offered an improved sensitivity to contractile anomalies in patients treated with doxorubicin, allowing early detection of left ventricular dysfunction, at a stage where it appears to be reversible. In addition, these end-systolic indices may be useful in evaluating approaches for reducing anthracycline cardiotoxicity such as low weekly or continuous infusion dosage schedules, use of new analogues, and addition of ameliorating agents such as vitamin E, ubidecarenone, or vasoactive antagonists.— K. M. Borow *et al.*, *ibid.*, 1983, *99*, 750.

For the use of a weekly dosage schedule to reduce cardiotoxicity associated with doxorubicin administration see Administration, under Uses, below.

Ventricular arrhythmia occurred during infusion of doxorubicin in a 21-year-old man.— T. M. Cosgriff (letter), *Ann. intern. Med.*, 1980, *92*, 434. Experimental data suggest that doxorubicin-associated dysrhythmias may be commoner than presently appreciated.— R. A. Levandowski (letter), *ibid.*, 866.

Myocardial infarction occurred twice in a patient given combination therapy for multiple myeloma; the infarctions were thought possibly to have been caused by the doxorubicin component, despite the fact that it was given by continuous infusion.— J. M. Carter and P. S. Bergin (letter), *New Engl. J. Med.*, 1986, *314*, 1118.

EFFECTS ON THE LIVER. A report of 6 cases of hepatitis and non-specific hepatocellular damage in patients receiving doxorubicin as part of combination therapy. Liver function tests returned to normal on withdrawal of therapy but abnormal liver function values recurred in 4 on rechallenge with doxorubicin.— A. Aviles *et al.*, *Archs Path. lab. Med.*, 1984, *108*, 912.

A characteristic hepatotoxicity can be produced by the combination of radiotherapy with doxorubicin. The liver enlarges in the irradiated site, and liver scans show a localised defect. The syndrome may progress to cirrhosis; there is also a danger that it can be misinterpreted as showing liver metastases.— L. A. Price, *Br. J. Hosp. Med.*, 1983, *30*, 8.

EFFECTS ON THE NERVOUS SYSTEM. Doxorubicin was neurotoxic when perfused through the cerebrospinal fluid spaces in *rhesus monkeys*. Its intrathecal use is not recommended.— P. C. Merker *et al.*, *Toxic. appl. Pharmac.*, 1978, *44*, 191.

LOCAL TOXICITY. For local toxicity following injection of doxorubicin, and the treatment of extravasation see under Adverse Effects of Antineoplastic Agents, p.582 and Treatment of Adverse Effects, p.583.

Treatment of Adverse Effects

For general guidelines, see Antineoplastic Agents, p.583.

Digoxin appeared to have a protective effect against doxorubicin cardiotoxicity. ECG abnormalities were present in 5 of 6 patients who had received doxorubicin in a dose of at least 400 mg per m^2 body-surface area but not (apart from abnormalities due to digoxin) in 16 given digoxin 250 µg daily starting 7 days before doxorubicin. The incidence of muscle weakness fell from 58 to 8%. Ouabain appeared to have some protective value but its short half-life made digoxin preferable. Oxytetracycline, with a structure similar to that of doxorubicin, had been used empirically in treatment in 2 patients.— D. Guthrie and A. L. Gibson, *Br. med. J.*, 1977, *2*, 1447. Ten patients who received prophylactic treatment with digoxin during treatment for acute myeloid leukaemia did not develop significant changes in the ratio of the pre-ejection period to left-ventricular-ejection time, in contrast to results in 8 controls, despite total dosages of doxorubicin greater than 400 mg per m^2 body-surface area. The results suggested that digoxin might protect the heart against damage induced by doxorubicin. Prophylactic vitamin E administration in a further 7 patients had no significant effect.— J. A. Whittaker and S. A. D. Al-Ismail, *Br. med. J.*, 1984, *288*, 283.

Further references to the treatment and prevention of doxorubicin cardiotoxicity: G. C. Carlon *et al.*, *Chest*, 1980, *77*, 570 (prazosin); V. De Leonardis *et al.*, *Int. J. clin. Pharmacol. Res.*, 1985, *5*, 137 (carnitine).

Results in *mice* supported the hypothesis that methylene blue might reduce the toxic effects of doxorubicin, by interfering with its *in vivo* reduction and blocking or slowing free radical production, without reducing antineoplastic activity.— W. J. M. Hrushesky *et al.*, *Lancet*, 1985, *1*, 565.

See also under Acetylcysteine, p.904.

ALOPECIA. Hypothermia of the scalp provided good protection against alopecia throughout all cycles of treatment in 20 of 33 cancer patients who were receiving chemotherapy with doxorubicin by intravenous injection. Ice-packs were applied to the scalp 5 minutes before each injection of doxorubicin and were left in place for 35 minutes. The protective effect of hypothermia was inversely related to the dose of doxorubicin. It was considered later that the ice should be applied for 10 minutes before injection; the technique should not be used in leukaemias or other neoplastic diseases in which numerous tumour stem cells may be present in the scalp.— J. C. Dean *et al.*, *New Engl. J. Med.*, 1979, *301*, 1427. Ice-packs held in place for 20 minutes before and after injection of doxorubicin prevented alopecia in 2 patients despite almost total loss of hair in the pubic and axillary regions.— A. R. Timothy *et al.* (letter), *Lancet*, 1980, *1*, 663.

Ten of 24 patients receiving high-dose doxorubicin showed satisfactory hair retention when scalp cooling was undertaken before injection of doxorubicin, and maintained for a further 30 to 40 minutes. These results compare favourably to those reported in other high-dose studies, probably because of the delay in administering doxorubicin until maximal scalp cooling had been reached. Scalp temperature varied between patients from 18.5 to 28.5°, but was consistent for any given patient. When frequent pulses of high-dose doxorubicin are used it appears that scalp temperature must be reduced below 22° before injection, and this temperature maintained for 20 minutes to prevent alopecia.— R. P. Gregory *et al.*, *Br. med. J.*, 1982, *284*, 1674.

A study involving 25 patients failed to confirm the report of Wood (*New Engl. J. Med.*, 1985, *312*, 1060) that *dl*-alpha tocopherol 1600 units daily, beginning 7 days before chemotherapy, was effective in preventing alopecia induced by doxorubicin.— M. Martin-Jimenez *et al.* (letter), *New Engl. J. Med.*, 1986, *315*, 894.

EXTRAVASATION. For the management of doxorubicin extravasation, see under Antineoplastic Agents, p.583.

Precautions

For reference to the precautions necessary with antineoplastic agents and immunosuppressants, see Antineoplastic Agents, p.583.

Doxorubicin is generally contra-indicated in patients with heart disease. Doses should not be repeated when there is bone-marrow depression or ulceration of the mouth. It should be given with great care in reduced doses to elderly patients and to those with hepatic impairment. Extravasation results in severe tissue damage and doxorubicin should not be given by intramuscular or subcutaneous injection. The adverse effects of irradiation may be enhanced by doxorubicin and skin reactions previously induced by radiotherapy may recur.

For precautions in the administration of doxorubicin to patients with impaired cardiac function, see under Administration, p.625.

Acute haemolytic anaemia developed in a patient with glucose-6-phosphate dehydrogenase deficiency after receiving doxorubicin.— D. C. Doll, *Br. med. J.*, 1983, *287*, 180.

HANDLING AND DISPOSAL. A method for the destruction of doxorubicin or daunorubicin wastes using sulphuric acid and potassium permanganate. A solution of doxorubicin or daunorubicin 0.3% in dilute sulphuric acid (3 mol per litre) can be destroyed in 2 hours by addition of potassium permanganate 100 mg per mL. Solid waste should be dissolved to produce a solution of the appropriate strength, and aqueous solutions diluted. Solutions of either drug in volatile organic solvents should have the solvent evaporated off and be redissolved in water before degradation. A solution of potassium permanganate in sulphuric acid may also be used to clean contaminated glassware, or decontaminate spillages. In the latter case excess solution should be used; the area may subsequently be decolourised with ascorbic acid or sodium bisulphite and neutralised with solid sodium carbonate. Residues produced by degradation of daunorubicin by this method showed no mutagenicity *in vitro*; some mutagenicity was seen with high concentrations of residues from doxorubicin.—IARC Scientific Publications No.73, *Laboratory Decontamination and Destruction of Carcinogens in Laboratory Wastes: Some Antineoplastic Agents*, M. Castegnaro *et al.* (Eds), Lyon, International Agency for Research on Cancer, 1985, p.25.

Protective clothing should be worn for up to 7 days after therapy when handling urine and faeces from patients receiving doxorubicin.— J. Harris and L. J. Dodds, *Pharm. J.*, 1985, *2*, 289.

INTERACTIONS. Side-effects due to doxorubicin were increased when doxorubicin and streptozocin were given together. Streptozocin apparently caused enough liver damage to slow down the metabolism of doxorubicin.— P. Chang *et al.*, *J. Am. med. Ass.*, 1976, *236*, 913.

The toxicity of doxorubicin was enhanced in a patient with osteogenic sarcoma when it was given after methotrexate rather than before.— J. H. Robertson *et al.*, *Br. med. J.*, 1976, *1*, 23.

Absorption and Fate

Following intravenous injection, doxorubicin is rapidly cleared from the blood, and distributed into tissues including lungs, liver, heart, spleen, and kidneys. It undergoes rapid metabolism in the liver to metabolites including the active metabolite doxorubicinol (adriamycinol). About 40 to 50% of a dose is stated to be excreted in bile within 7 days, of which about half is as unchanged drug. Only about 5% of a dose is excreted in urine within 5 days. It does not cross the blood-brain barrier but may cross the placenta.

A study in cancer patients with or without hepatomas, who were treated with doxorubicin, indicated that plasma profiles of doxorubicin were similar. Formation and elimination of the major active metabolite, adriamycinol, appeared to be impaired in hepatoma patients.— K. K. Chan *et al.*, *Cancer Res.*, 1980, *40*, 1263.

A review of the pharmacokinetics of some antineoplastic agents, including doxorubicin. Binding of the anthracyclines to tissue and plasma proteins is rapid and extensive, the highest concentration of doxorubicin after an intravenous bolus being located in the liver. The hepatobiliary system is also the primary route of excretion; in studies of hepatic artery infusion, 50% of a doxorubicin dose could be extracted in a single pass through the liver. Plasma elimination is triphasic, the terminal elimination half-life having been reported by Benjamin *et al.* (*Cancer Res.*, 1977, *37*, 1416) as 29.6 hours. Patients with hepatic dysfunction indicated by elevated serum bilirubin have uniformly elevated and prolonged concentrations of doxorubicin and its metabolites; other liver function abnormalities are reportedly not predictive.— F. M. Balis *et al.*, *Clin. Pharmacokinet.*, 1983, *8*, 202.

Doxorubicin was excreted in detectable amounts in saliva.— L. A. Celio *et al.*, *Eur. J. clin. Pharmac.*, 1983, *24*, 261.

A study of the pharmacokinetics of doxorubicin given by intravenous infusion to 21 patients. For a given dose, the peak plasma concentration was markedly reduced when the infusion time was prolonged: a 4-hour infusion was calculated to reduce peak plasma concentration 25-fold compared with the same dose by intravenous bolus. Since much of the toxicity, but not the efficacy, of doxorubicin, is believed to depend upon the concentration reached in plasma, prolonged infusion offers a way to increase its therapeutic index.— S. Eksborg *et al.*, *Eur. J. clin. Pharmac.*, 1985, *28*, 205.

PREGNANCY AND THE NEONATE. Neither doxorubicin nor its major metabolite, doxorubicinol, were found in the amniotic fluid of a pregnant woman who required treatment with doxorubicin at 20 weeks' gestation. This suggests that doxorubicin is not transferred transplacentally to the foetus at this age.— J. Roboz *et al.* (letter), *Lancet*, 1979, *2*, 1382. Doxorubicin was not detectable in amniotic fluid from a patient receiving ABVD therapy (doxorubicin, bleomycin, vinblastine, and dacarbazine) who had an abortion at 17 weeks' gestation. However, high concentrations of doxorubicin, up to 10 times those in maternal plasma, were found in foetal liver, kidney, and lung. The absence of a chemical agent in amniotic fluid should not be taken as proof of the absence of transplacental passage.— M. D'Incalci *et al.* (letter), *ibid.*, 1983, *1*, 75.

Uses and Administration

Doxorubicin is an antineoplastic antibiotic which may act by forming a stable complex with DNA and interfering with the synthesis of nucleic acids. It is a cell-cycle nonspecific agent but is most active against cells in S phase. It also has actions on cell membranes, and immunosuppressant properties. It is an effective antineoplastic against a wide range of tumours. Doxorubicin is used, often in association with other antineoplastic agents, in the treatment of acute leukaemias, lymphomas, sarcomas, neuroblastoma, Wilms' tumour, and malignant neoplasms of the bladder, breast, lung, ovary, and thyroid. It has also been used in other tumours including those of the cervix, endometrium, stomach, and testis. See also under Choice of Antineoplastic Agent, p.584.

Doxorubicin hydrochloride is administered intravenously by injecting a solution in Water for

Injections, or, preferably, sodium chloride injection (0.9%), into a fast-running infusion of sodium chloride or glucose injection (5%). It is given in doses of 60 to 75 mg per m^2 body-surface, or 1.2 to 2.4 mg per kg body-weight, as a single dose every 3 weeks; alternatively, doses of 20 to 30 mg per m^2 may be given daily for 3 days every 3 to 4 weeks. A regimen of 20 mg per m^2 as a single weekly dose has also been tried and is reported to be associated with a lower incidence of cardiotoxicity.

Doses may need to be reduced if doxorubicin is given with other antineoplastic agents: a dose of 30 to 40 mg per m^2 every 3 weeks has been suggested. Doses should also be halved in patients with moderate liver dysfunction (serum-bilirubin concentrations of 12 to 30 μg per mL) and those with severe impairment (serum bilirubin greater than 30 μg per mL) should be given a quarter of the usual dose.

The maximum total dose should not exceed 550 mg per m^2; in patients who have received radiotherapy to the chest, or other cardiotoxic drugs, it may be advisable to limit the total dose to about 450 mg per m^2.

Doxorubicin has also been given by intra-arterial injection. Great care must be taken to avoid extravasation. In the treatment of non-invasive tumours of the bladder, solutions of doxorubicin hydrochloride have been instilled into the bladder.

Blood counts should be made routinely during treatment with doxorubicin and electrocardiograms should be examined at regular intervals for early signs of cardiotoxicity.

ADMINISTRATION. Doxorubicin is reported to be neurotoxic in animals. It should not be given by intrathecal injection.— P. C. Merker *et al.*, *Toxic. appl. Pharmac.*, 1978, *44*, 191.

A review of alterations in dose scheduling to reduce cardiotoxicity in patients receiving doxorubicin. Recent studies have reported a very low incidence of heart failure when doxorubicin is administered on a weekly intravenous schedule, or by continuous intravenous infusion. Altered dose schedules have been combined with tests of cardiac function such as radionuclide ejection fractions and endomyocardial biopsies to reduce cardiotoxicity and exceed the empirical dose limit of 450 to 550 mg per m^2 body-surface. The evidence suggests that the therapeutic efficacy of weekly or continuous infusion doxorubicin is at least as great as when administered by the conventional three-weekly regimen. B. L. Lum *et al.*, *Drug Intell. & clin. Pharm.*, 1985, *19*, 259.

A comparative study of the cardiotoxicity and efficacy of doxorubicin given by prolonged continuous intravenous infusion and by standard intravenous regimens. Doxorubicin 60 mg per m^2 body-surface was given by prolonged infusion via a central venous catheter every 3 weeks to 11 patients with metastatic breast cancer, and as part of combination chemotherapy to 10 patients with metastatic sarcomas. The duration of infusion was increased from 24 hours initially to 48 or 96 hours. A further 30 patients, most of whom had metastatic lung cancer, received standard doses of doxorubicin by intravenous injection. Cardiac monitoring, including radionuclide ejection fractions and endomyocardial biopsy was carried out in all patients. Despite the fact that 13 of the patients receiving continuous infusion were given total doses greater than 550 mg per m^2 (mean cumulative dose 660 mg per m^2) compared with only 4 of those given conventional dosage (mean cumulative dose 470 mg per m^2) none of the former group developed congestive heart failure, whereas one of the latter did so. Furthermore, only 2 of the patients given continuous infusions had marked cardiac changes at biopsy, compared with 14 of the standard-dose group. Radionuclide ejection fractions proved to be a relatively insensitive predictor of the severity of cardiac changes. The therapeutic efficacy of doxorubicin did not appear to be compromised by continuous infusion, and in addition to reduced cardiotoxicity there was a significant reduction in nausea and vomiting with this regimen, which increased patient acceptance. Myelotoxicity and mucositis were not reduced. Although administration by continuous infusion may appear more difficult than conventional schedules, outpatient treatment is feasible, and the use of a central venous catheter eliminates the complications of extravasation.— S. S. Legha *et al.*, *Ann. intern. Med.*, 1982, *96*, 133.

A study in 27 patients assigned to receive doxorubicin 20 mg per m^2 body-surface weekly, combined with other antineoplastics in 5, found severe cardiac damage in only 3 out of 41 endomyocardial biopsies, and none of the patients developed congestive heart failure. In comparison, severe damage was seen in 38 of 119 biopsies carried out on 98 patients assigned to a conventional regimen of approximately 60 mg per m^2 every 3 weeks as part of combination chemotherapy and 13 patients developed congestive heart failure. It was calculated that approximately 168 mg per m^2 more doxorubicin could be given to reach the same biopsy score when delivered on the weekly rather than the 3-weekly schedule, a difference equivalent to about 2 additional months of treatment: this would probably extend the duration of safe treatment for most patients beyond the point where doxorubicin remains an effective drug.— F. M. Torti *et al.*, *Ann. intern. Med.*, 1983, *99*, 745.

A study in *mice* suggested that doxorubicin formulated in fibrinogen microspheres was more effective against Ehrlich ascites carcinoma than the free drug.— S. Miyazaki *et al.*, *J. Pharm. Pharmac.*, 1986, *38*, 618.

Studies in *mice* of the toxicity and efficacy of doxorubicin entrapped in cardiolipin liposomes: A. Rahman *et al.*, *Cancer Chemother. Pharmac.*, 1986, *16*, 22; A. Rahman *et al.*, *Br. J. Cancer*, 1986, *54*, 401.

In cardiovascular disorders. A retrospective study in 29 cancer patients with abnormal heart function (baseline left-ventricular-ejection fraction under 55%) given doxorubicin 30 to 50 mg per m^2 body-surface every 3 to 4 weeks. In the 17 patients who received a cumulative dose of less than 350 mg per m^2 there was no significant difference between the baseline and final left-ventricular-ejection fractions, as measured by sequential radionuclide angiocardiography, but in the 12 who received a cumulative dose of 350 mg per m^2 or more there was a significant reduction from a mean of 48% to 43%. Doxorubicin probably should not be used where baseline left-ventricular-ejection fraction is less than 30%; at 30 to 54%, sequential studies should be obtained before each dose or alternate doses, and before each dose when the cumulative dose reaches 350 mg per m^2.— B. W. Choi *et al.*, *Am. Heart J.*, 1983, *106*, 638.

In children. Doxorubicin was given in low doses of 10 or 20 mg per m^2 body-surface weekly or biweekly to a maximum of 500 mg per m^2 for remission maintenance in solid tumours in 6 children. Three children were disease-free over 1 year later. This schedule was considered to avoid the serious toxicity of doxorubicin.— E. V. Hvizdala *et al.*, *Cancer*, 1977, *39*, 2411.

In hepatic insufficiency. For references to the impaired metabolism of doxorubicin in patients with hepatoma, see Absorption and Fate (above).

In renal insufficiency. The dose of doxorubicin should be reduced to 75% in patients with a glomerular filtration-rate of less than 10 mL per minute. W. M. Bennett *et al.*, *Am. J. Kidney Dis.*, 1983, *3*, 155.

LEUKAEMIAS, ACUTE. For reference to the use of doxorubicin with other agents in the treatment of acute lymphoblastic leukaemia and in acute and chronic myeloid leukaemia, see Choice of Antineoplastic Agent, p.586.

MALIGNANT EFFUSIONS. Doxorubicin 30 mg in 30 to 100 mL of physiological saline had been injected intracavitarily, after diagnostic or therapeutic aspiration of the malignant effusion, in 12 patients; probably at least 500 mL of residual effusion remained at the time of drug administration in all cases. Doxorubicin appears to be a safe, and sometimes effective, local treatment for malignant disease.— M. H. N. Tattersall *et al.* (letter), *Lancet*, 1979, *1*, 390. Caution is needed in interpreting the absolute value of topical doxorubicin or other chemotherapeutic agents. Three untreated patients had been noted to have satisfactory results in terms of effusions which might have been ascribed to therapy had it been given. Results from an initial 14 patients in a controlled study had shown no systemic or topical toxicity probably because a dose of only 10 mg in 15 mL of saline is being used.— S. D. Desai and A. Figueredo (letter), *ibid.*, 872. See also R. F. Kefford *et al.*, *Med. J. Aust.*, 1980, *2*, 447.

See also Choice of Antineoplastic Agent, p.588.

MALIGNANT NEOPLASMS OF THE BLADDER. Intravesicular instillation of doxorubicin 50 mg, in 50 mL of 0.9% sodium chloride solution was performed twice in the first week, then weekly for 1 month, and monthly for 1 year thereafter, in 82 patients with superficial transitional cell carcinoma of the bladder. Tumours recurred in 32 patients, progressing to highly invasive lesions in 5, but treatment was considered effective in preventing recurrence in the remaining 50.— C. C. Schulman *et al.*, *Cancer Chemother. Pharmac.*, 1983, *11*, *Suppl.*, S32.

Prophylactic intravesicular doxorubicin therapy was given following resection to 27 patients with multiple recurrent superficial transitional cell carcinoma of the bladder, 12 of whom had disease unresponsive to intravesicular thiotepa. Doses of 60 mg were given, increased to a maximum of 90 mg, in 40 or 50 mL of 0.9% sodium chloride solution, administered every 3 weeks for 8 doses; thereafter 2 doses were given at 6-week and 2 at 12-week intervals. Complete remission was maintained in 15 of the patients; disease recurrence occurred in 9. The median duration of response was 12 months. Adverse effects including dysuria, haematuria, and bladder spasms were not sufficiently severe to require discontinuation of therapy.— M. B. Garnick *et al.*, *J. Urol., Baltimore*, 1984, *131*, 43.

See also under Choice of Antineoplastic Agent, p.588.

MALIGNANT NEOPLASMS OF THE LIVER. Chemotherapy can be shown to alter the progression of hepatocellular carcinoma, particularly when given parenterally and intra-arterially. The most encouraging results have been reported by Johnson *et al.* (*Lancet*, 1978, *1*, 1006) with doxorubicin 60 mg per m^2 intravenously every 3 weeks. This regimen induces some form of tumour regression in about one quarter of patients unsuitable for surgery; less than 10% of patients have a complete remission, but in this group median survival is nearly 2 years. It is possible to foretell by monitoring alpha-fetoprotein concentrations whether remission will recur, and if the alpha-fetoprotein concentration continues to rise after 2 cycles of treatment doxorubicin is unlikely to be effective.— H. J. F. Hodgson, *Br. J. Hosp. Med.*, 1983, *29*, 240. In a study involving 50 patients doxorubicin in doses up to 70 mg per m^2 body-surface intravenously, as a single dose at 4-week intervals, was not effective in the treatment of primary liver cell carcinoma, particularly for patients with stage III disease.— Y. M. Fakunle *et al.*, *Clin. Trials J.*, 1983, *20*, 347.

MALIGNANT NEOPLASMS OF THE OVARY. The development of doxorubicin resistance by tumour cells could be completely or partially reversed by verapamil, which prevented the enhanced efflux of the antineoplastic from the cell. These results have stimulated a study of the combination in patients with refractory ovarian cancer.— A. M. Rogan *et al.*, *Science*, 1984, *224*, 994.

For the use of combination chemotherapy including doxorubicin in the treatment of ovarian carcinoma, see under Choice of Antineoplastic Agent, p.591.

MALIGNANT NEOPLASMS OF THE THYROID. Eleven of 30 patients with malignant neoplasm of the thyroid refractory to surgery or radiotherapy achieved partial remission with doxorubicin after an average of 3 courses at a starting dose of 75 mg per m^2 of body-surface. Doxorubicin-induced cardiomyopathy, fatal in 1 case, developed in 3 patients who had received a total dose of doxorubicin in excess of 550 mg per m^2.— J. A. Gottlieb and C. S. Hill, *New Engl. J. Med.*, 1974, *290*, 193.

In 21 patients with metastasising thyroid carcinoma given chemotherapy, 2 achieved full remission and 5 partial remission. Treatment consisted of doxorubicin 75 mg per m^2 body-surface intravenously every 3 weeks (to a total dose of 550 mg per m^2) and bleomycin 30 mg intramuscularly every week (to a total dose of 360 mg).— G. Benker *et al.*, *Dt. med. Wschr.*, 1977, *102*, 1908.

Further references: A. G. Katsas (letter), *New Engl. J. Med.*, 1980, *302*, 467.

PREGNANCY AND THE NEONATE. Two women given doxorubicin from the 22nd and 24th weeks of pregnancy respectively were delivered of apparently healthy infants. Doxorubicin given in late pregnancy does not appear to be a serious hazard to the foetus.— J. S. Tobias *et al.* (letter), *Lancet*, 1980, *1*, 776 and 836. See also M. Khurshid and M. Saleem (letter), *Lancet*, 1978, *2*, 534.

SARCOMA. Twenty-four patients with osteogenic sarcoma were treated with doxorubicin to a maximum cumulative dose of 540 mg per m^2 body-surface, starting about 8 weeks after surgery. Of these, 13 remained free of pulmonary metastases or local recurrences for from 9 to more than 40 months.— E. P. Cortes *et al.*, *New Engl. J. Med.*, 1974, *291*, 998.

Doxorubicin seems to be one of the most active agents against osteosarcoma.— *Lancet*, 1985, *2*, 131.

In a study in patients with uterine sarcomas, doxorubicin 60 mg per m^2 body-surface intravenously, plus cyclophosphamide 500 mg per m^2, was given to 66 patients every 3 weeks; a further 66 received only the doxorubicin. Doses were modified according to toxicity, and therapy was stopped when the total dose of doxorubicin reached 480 mg per m^2. Of 54 evaluable patients given the combined regimen, 26 had measurable disease, and only 2 of these had a complete response, lasting 5.4 and 5.7 months respectively. Three of the 26 had a partial response. Of the 50 evaluable patients given doxorubicin alone, 26 had measurable disease which showed complete response, lasting more than 13 months in only 1; 4 patients had partial responses. Approximately 80% of the patients had died within 2 years, and in approximately 90% the disease had recurred or progressed. The study failed to show any benefit to combined therapy over doxorubicin alone; the overall prognosis for patients with uterine sarcoma remains poor.— H. B. Muss *et al.*, *Cancer*, 1985, *55*, 1648.

See also under Choice of Antineoplastic Agent, p.593.

Preparations

Doxorubicin Hydrochloride for Injection *(U.S.P.).* A sterile mixture of doxorubicin hydrochloride and lactose.

Proprietary Preparations

Adriamycin *(Farmitalia Carlo Erba, UK). Injection,* powder for reconstitution, doxorubicin hydrochloride 10 and 50 mg.

A preparation known as Doxorubicin Rapid Dissolution is also available.

Proprietary Names and Manufacturers

Adriamycin *(Austral.; Adria, Canad.; Farmitalia, Norw.; Farmitalia Carlo Erba, Swed.; Farmitalia Carlo Erba, UK; Adria, USA)*; Adriblastin *(Farmitalia, Ger.)*; Adriblastina *(Arg.; Belg.; Farmitalia, Ital.; Neth.; Farmitalia Carlo Erba, S.Afr.)*; Adriblastine *(Bellon, Fr.; Farmitalia Carlo Erba, Switz.)*; Farmiblastina *(Farmitalia, Spain)*.

19135-h

Enocitabine *(rINN).*

Behenoyl Cytarabine; Behenoylcytosine Arabinoside; BH-AC; NSC-239336. *N*-(1-β-D-Arabinofuranosyl-1,2-dihydro-2-oxo-4-pyrimidinyl)docosanamide.

$C_{31}H_{55}N_3O_6$=565.8.

CAS — 55726-47-1.

Enocitabine is an antineoplastic agent that acts as a pro-drug of cytarabine (p.619). It has been used similarly in the treatment of acute leukaemias.

A report of the use of enocitabine in the combination chemotherapy of acute non-lymphoblastic leukaemia. Twenty previously untreated patients received the BH-AC-DMP regimen, comprising enocitabine 170 mg per m² body-surface daily as a 3-hour intravenous infusion together with daunorubicin, mercaptopurine, and prednisolone, for 5 to 14 days. Doses were adjusted according to response. Patients who achieved complete remission were given a further 3 courses as consolidation therapy. Complete remission was achieved in 17 of 20 patients, 16 of whom were below 59 years of age. On follow up, 14 of the 17 patients were still in remission after a period of 8 months or more. The results were considered extremely encouraging. Myelotoxicity was the main adverse effect, but hepatotoxicity, fatal in one patient, also occurred.— K. Yamada *et al.*, *Acta Haemat. Jpn.*, 1980, *43*, 1080.

Proprietary Names and Manufacturers

Sunrabin *(Toyo Jozo, Jpn)*.

16631-k

Epirubicin Hydrochloride *(BANM, USAN, rINNM).*

4′-Epiadriamycin Hydrochloride; 4′-Epidoxorubicin Hydrochloride; IMI-28; Pidorubicin Hydrochloride. (8*S*,10*S*)-10-(3-Amino-2,3,6-trideoxy-α-L-*arabino*-hexopyranosyloxy)-8-glycolloyl-7,8,9,10-tetrahydro-6,8,11-trihydroxy-1-methoxynaphthacene-5,12-dione hydrochloride.

$C_{27}H_{29}NO_{11}$,HCl=580.0.

CAS — 56420-45-2 (epirubicin); 56390-09-1 (hydrochloride).

Adverse Effects, Treatment, and Precautions

As for Doxorubicin Hydrochloride, p.623.

Cardiotoxicity is more likely when the cumulative dose exceeds 700 mg per m² body-surface, and left-ventricular failure may occur particularly in patients who have received more than 1 g per m².

A report of primary Sjögren's syndrome following 3 cycles of administration of epirubicin to a patient with breast cancer. The repeated relation between administration of the drug and development of the symptoms suggested that epirubicin contributed to the syndrome.— A. Oxholm *et al.* (letter), *Lancet*, 1986, *2*, 629.

EFFECTS ON THE HEART. Results in 101 patients given epirubicin 50 to 90 mg per m² body-surface at intervals of 3 weeks or more to a total cumulative dose of up to 630 mg per m² indicated that compared with previous results in 78 patients given doxorubicin, the incidence of early cardiotoxic activity was lower. However, there was no significant difference between the groups in the incidence of delayed cardiotoxicity, although none of the patients receiving epirubicin developed signs of congestive heart failure.— F. Villani *et al.*, *Int. J. clin. Pharmac. Ther. Toxic.*, 1983, *21*, 203.

Absorption and Fate

Following intravenous administration epirubicin is rapidly and extensively distributed into body tissues, and undergoes metabolism in the liver. The major metabolite, epirubicinol (13-hydroxy-epirubicin) has antineoplastic activity. Epirubicin is eliminated mainly in bile, with a terminal plasma elimination half-life of about 40 hours.

The pharmacokinetics of epirubicin in patients with normal and impaired renal function and with hepatic metastases.— C. M. Camaggi *et al.*, *Cancer Treat. Rep.*, 1982, *66*, 1819. See also C. M. Camaggi *et al.*, *Br. J. clin. Pharmac.*, 1986, *21*, 95P.

Uses and Administration

Epirubicin is an anthracycline antibiotic with antineoplastic actions similar to those of doxorubicin (p.624). It has been tried, alone or in combination with other antineoplastic agents, in acute leukaemias, lymphomas, multiple myeloma, and in solid tumours, including cancer of the breast, ovary, and gastro-intestinal tract.

Epirubicin hydrochloride is administered intravenously by injecting a solution in Water for Injections into a fast-running infusion of sodium chloride (0.9%) over 3 to 5 minutes. It is given in usual doses of 75 to 90 mg per m² body-surface as a single dose every 3 weeks; this dose may be divided over 2 days if desired. Doses should be reduced if epirubicin is given with other antineoplastic agents, and should be halved in patients with moderate liver dysfunction (serum bilirubin concentrations of 12 to 30 μg per mL), while those with severe liver impairment (serum bilirubin greater than 30 μg per mL) should be given a quarter of the usual dose. Reduced doses are also recommended in the elderly, and in patients who have received previous chemotherapy or radiotherapy.

A total cumulative dose of 700 mg per m² should probably be exceeded only with caution, because of the risk of cardiotoxicity; in some countries the maximum total dose has been stated to be 900 mg per m².

A summary of 1 year's experience in the use of epirubicin for malignant disease. Of 9 patients with non-Hodgkin's lymphomas, malignant thymoma, or angiosarcoma of the liver there were 5 remissions and 2 objective responses (in the 2 patients with thymoma). Patients received a total dose of up to 300 mg per m² epirubicin, and cardiotoxicity appeared to be lower than with doxorubicin.— H. Lunt and P. J. Dady (letter), *N.Z. med. J.*, 1985, *98*, 1057.

References to the use of epirubicin in the treatment of malignant disease: E. Berman *et al.*, *Cancer Treat. Rep.*, 1984, *68*, 679 (malignant melanoma); J. A. Ajani *et al.*, *ibid.*, 1507 (metastatic colorectal cancer); E. Campora *et al.*, *ibid.*, 1285 (advanced breast cancer); W. G. Jones and W. Mattsson, *ibid.*, 675 (advanced breast cancer in postmenopausal women); R. A. Joss *et al.*, *Eur. J. Cancer clin. Oncol.*, 1984, *20*, 495 (advanced squamous adenocarcinoma and large cell carcinoma of the lung); S. Eridani *et al.*, *Oncology*, 1984, *41*, 383 (acute leukaemias and non-Hodgkin's lymphoma); A. Martoni *et al.*, *Cancer Treat. Rep.*, 1984, *68*, 1391 (with cisplatin in advanced ovarian cancer); M. J. Magee *et al.*, *ibid.*, 1985, *69*, 125 (head and neck cancer); F. J. Meyers *et al.*, *ibid.*, 143 (advanced colorectal cancer).

Proprietary Preparations

Pharmorubicin *(Farmitalia Carlo Erba, UK). Injection,* powder for reconstitution, epirubicin hydrochloride 10, 20, and 50 mg.

Proprietary Names and Manufacturers

Farmarubicine *(Farmitalia Carlo Erba, Fr.)*; Farmorubicin *(Farmitalia, Denm.; Farmitalia, Ger.; Farmitalia Carlo Erba, S.Afr.)*; Farmorubicina *(Farmitalia, Ital.; Farmitalia, Spain)*; Farmorubicine *(Farmitalia Carlo Erba, Fr.; Farmitalia Carlo Erba, Switz.)*; Pharmorubicin *(Austral.; Adria, Canad.; Farmitalia Carlo Erba, UK)*.

19147-g

Esorubicin *(rINN).*

4′-Deoxydoxorubicin; 4′-DXDX; IMI-58; NSC-267469. (8*S*,10*S*)-10-{[(2*S*,4*R*,6*S*)-4-Aminotetrahydro-6-methyl-2*H*-pyran-2-yl]oxy}-8-glycoloyl-7,8,9,10-tetrahydro-6,8,11-trihydroxy-1-methoxy-5,12-naphthacenedione.

$C_{27}H_{29}NO_{10}$=527.5.

CAS — 63521-85-7.

NOTE. Esorubicin hydrochloride is *USAN*.

Esorubicin is a derivative of doxorubicin (p.623) which has been tried in the management of various malignant neoplasms by intravenous injection. It is claimed to be less cardiotoxic than doxorubicin.

1832-c

Estramustine Sodium Phosphate *(BANM, rINNM).*

Estramustine Phosphate Sodium *(USAN)*; NSC-89199 *(estramustine phosphate)*; Ro-21-8837/001. Estra-1,3,5(10)-triene-3,17β-diol 3-[bis(2-chloroethyl)carbamate] 17-(disodium phosphate); Disodium 3-[bis(2-chloroethyl)-carbamoyloxy]estra-1,3,5(10)-trien-17β-yl orthophosphate.

$C_{23}H_{30}Cl_2NNa_2O_6P$=564.4.

CAS — 2998-57-4 (estramustine); 4891-15-0 (phosphate); 52205-73-9 (sodium phosphate).

Pharmacopoeias. In *Br.*

A white or almost white powder. Freely **soluble** in water and in methyl alcohol; very slightly soluble in dehydrated alcohol and in chloroform. A 0.5% solution in water has a pH of 8.5 to 10.0. **Store** in well-closed containers at 2° to 8°. Protect from light.

Adverse Effects, Treatment, and Precautions

As for Mustine Hydrochloride, p.645. Side-effects related to the oestrogenic activity of estramustine, such as gynaecomastia and cardiovascular effects, may also occur.

It is contra-indicated in patients with peptic ulceration and severe hepatic or cardiovascular disease.

The most frequent dose-limiting toxicities in patients receiving estramustine are nausea and vomiting, followed by anorexia, oedema, and cardiovascular complications. Other side-effects, similar to those of other oestrogenic substances are diarrhoea, impotence, gynaecomastia, skin rashes, and abnormal liver enzyme values; bone marrow depression may occur. It should be used with caution in men with a history of thrombo-embolic disorders, in whom there may be an increased risk of thrombosis. It should also be used with care in patients with cerebrovascular or coronary artery disease or conditions affected by fluid retention such as congestive heart failure, epilepsy, and kidney disorders. Hypertension and diabetes mellitus may be exacerbated, and since the drug may influence calcium and phosphate metabolism patients with hypercalcaemia should be carefully monitored.— A. R. Hauser and R. Merryman, *Drug Intell. & clin. Pharm.*, 1984, *18*, 368.

Absorption and Fate

About 75% of a dose of estramustine sodium phosphate is absorbed from the gastro-intestinal tract. It is concentrated in prostatic tissue. The phosphate moiety appears to be lost in the gastro-intestinal tract, liver, and phosphatase-rich tissue such as the prostate. Following breakage of the carbamate linkage the oestrogenic and alkylating moieties are excreted independently.

Uses and Administration

Estramustine is a combination of oestradiol and normustine and has weaker oestrogenic activity than oestradiol and weaker antineoplastic activity than mustine (p.645) and most other alkylating agents. Estramustine phosphate is given by mouth as the disodium salt in the treatment of advanced prostatic carcinoma; it has been used with meglumine by injection.

The usual initial dosage by mouth is the equivalent of 560 mg to 1.12 g of estramustine phosphate daily, with meals; the dose may later be adjusted to between 140 mg and 1.4 g daily according to the response and gastro-intestinal tolerance. In the *US* a dose of 14 mg per kg body-weight is employed.

The equivalent of 150 to 450 mg of estramustine phosphate has been given daily by slow intravenous injection for about 3 weeks, followed by maintenance doses of 150 to 300 mg twice weekly.

Reviews of the use of estramustine sodium phosphate in prostate cancer: *Med. Lett.*, 1982, *24*, 74; A. R. Hauser and R. Merryman, *Drug Intell. & clin. Pharm.*, 1984, *18*, 368.

Of those patients with prostatic carcinoma who respond to oestrogen therapy the majority subsequently relapse, and in these patients it may be worth changing to estramustine phosphate, if tolerable, and supplementing this with prednisolone 5 mg three times daily.— J. B. Garland, *Practitioner*, 1984, *228*, 725.

See also under Choice of Antineoplastic Agent, p.592.

Preparations

Estramustine Phosphate Capsules *(B.P.).* Estramustine Sodium Phosphate Capsules. Potency is expressed in terms of the equivalent amount of estramustine phosphate.

Proprietary Preparations

Estracyt *(Lundbeck, UK). Capsules*, estramustine phosphate 140 mg (as estramustine sodium phosphate).

Proprietary Names and Manufacturers

Emcyt *(Roche, Canad.; Roche, USA)*; Estracyt *(Lundbeck, Denm.; Roche, Fr.; Pharmacia Arzneimittel, Ger.; Roche, Ital.; Neth.; Mekos, Norw.; MPS Lab., S.Afr.; Abello, Spain; Leo, Swed.; Leo Suede, Switz.; Lundbeck, UK).*

1833-k

Ethoglucid *(BAN).*

Etoglucid *(rINN)*; ICI-32865; Triethyleneglycol Diglycidyl Ether. 1,2:15,16-Diepoxy-4,7,10,13-tetraoxahexadecane.

$C_{12}H_{22}O_6$=262.3.

CAS — 1954-28-5.

CAUTION. *Ethoglucid is irritant; avoid contact with skin and mucous membranes.*

The manufacturers state that some plastic materials interact with ethoglucid and that therefore glass irrigation syringes are recommended for the preparation and administration of ethoglucid solutions.

Stability of ethoglucid in plastic disposable syringes.— M. G. Lee (letter), *Pharm. J.*, 1981, *2*, 651.

Solutions of ethoglucid were stable for 16 hours, 2 days, and 14 days when stored at temperatures of 37°, 20°, and 4° respectively. Storage in glass bottles, polypropylene syringes or polyvinyl chloride bags had no effect on stability and it was concluded that ethoglucid was not absorbed from solution in polypropylene or polyvinyl chloride containers.— M. G. Lee, *Pharm. J.*, 1985, *2*, 563.

Adverse Effects and Treatment

For an outline of the adverse effects experienced with antineoplastic agents and immunosuppressants and general guidelines for their treatment, see Antineoplastic Agents, p.580 and p.583.

Following intracavitary instillation of ethoglucid urinary frequency or dysuria, cystitis, and mucosal changes have been reported. A fall in white cell counts has occurred in some patients.

Precautions

For reference to the precautions necessary with antineoplastic agents and immunosuppressants, see Antineoplastic Agents, p.583.

HANDLING AND DISPOSAL. Diluted solutions of ethoglucid could be inactivated by addition of 1 volume of concentrated hydrochloric acid to every 3 volumes of ethoglucid solution and allowing to react for 30 minutes while stirring. The resultant liquid could be neutralised with sodium hydroxide solution and washed away. Undiluted ethoglucid could be similarly reacted with an equal volume of 10% hydrochloric acid. Both these operations should be carried out in a fume cupboard. Containers should be washed out with 10% hydrochloric acid and then with water, the washings amalgamated, and allowed to stand for 30 minutes before neutralisation of pH and disposal.— S. J. Wilson, *J. clin. Hosp. Pharm.*, 1983, *8*, 295.

Uses and Administration

Ethoglucid is an antineoplastic agent which acts by alkylation (see p.580). It must be diluted before administration and is used mainly for the treatment of non-invasive tumours of the bladder by the instillation of a solution containing 1 or 2% v/v of ethoglucid in water or sodium chloride solution. The patient's fluid intake should be restricted beforehand. Treatment may be repeated daily for 2 weeks, and then at less frequent intervals.

Ethoglucid has also been given by intra-arterial and intravenous injection in the treatment of a variety of malignant disorders.

Proprietary Preparations

Epodyl *(ICI Pharmaceuticals, UK). Bladder instillation*, sterile, ethoglucid 1 mL (1.13 g).

Proprietary Names and Manufacturers

Epodyl *(ICI, Austral.; Neth.; ICI, S.Afr.; ICI Pharmaceuticals, UK).*

1834-a

Etoposide *(BAN, USAN, rINN).*

EPEG; NSC-141540; VP-16; VP-16-213. 4′-*O*-Demethyl-1-*O*-(4,6-*O*-ethylidene-β-D-glucopyranosyl)epipodophyllotoxin; (5*S*,5a*R*,8a*S*,9*R*)-9-(4,6-*O*-Ethylidene-β-D-glucopyranosyloxy)-5,8,8a,9-tetrahydro-5-(4-hydroxy-3,5-dimethoxyphenyl)-isobenzofuro[5,6-*f*][1,3]benzodioxol-6(5a*H*)-one.

$C_{29}H_{32}O_{13}$=588.6.

CAS — 33419-42-0.

NOTE. The trivial name epipodophyllotoxin has occasionally been used incorrectly for this derivative.

Etoposide injection dissolved single-use cellulose filters when being transferred into an infusion bag, apparently because of the macrogol used as a solubilising agent in the injection formulation.— S. C. Forrest (letter), *Pharm. J.*, 1984, *1*, 88.

Adverse Effects, Treatment, and Precautions

For an outline of the adverse effects experienced with antineoplastic agents and immunosuppressants, general guidelines for their treatment, and precautions, see Antineoplastic Agents, p.580, p.583.

The dose-limiting toxicity with etoposide is myelosuppression, predominantly manifesting as leucopenia, but also thrombocytopenia, and rarely anaemia. Nausea and vomiting are common; there may also be anorexia, diarrhoea, and stomatitis. Gastro-intestinal toxicity is more common after oral administration. Reversible alopecia may occur in up to half of all patients.

Disturbances of liver function, peripheral neuropathy, effects on the CNS, and anaphylactoid reactions have been reported rarely. Local irritation and thrombophlebitis may occur at the site of injection.

Following rapid intravenous administration hypotension may occur; etoposide should be given by infusion over at least 30 minutes. Care should be taken to avoid extravasation. Etoposide should not be given by intrapleural or intraperitoneal injection, and should not be given to patients with severe hepatic dysfunction.

Some of the adverse effects associated with intravenous administration of etoposide may be due to the formulation of the vehicle.

HANDLING AND DISPOSAL. When handling urine and faeces from patients receiving etoposide protective clothing should be worn for up to 4 and 7 days respectively after therapy.— J. Harris and L. J. Dodds, *Pharm. J.*, 1985, *2*, 289.

Absorption and Fate

Following administration by mouth about 50% of the dose of etoposide is absorbed. It is rapidly distributed, and concentrations in plasma fall in a biphasic manner, with a terminal half-life of 3 to 15 hours. It is extensively bound to plasma protein (about 94%). Etoposide is excreted in urine and faeces as unchanged drug and metabolites: about 45% of a dose is reported to be excreted in urine over 72 hours, two-thirds as unchanged drug. It penetrates the CNS poorly, with concentrations in CSF from 1 to 10% of those in plasma.

Following administration of etoposide 100 mg as oral solution or capsules to 6 patients, the mean bioavailability was 66.7% and 54.8% respectively but there was marked variation between patients in plasma concentrations achieved. Results in a further 6 patients suggested that bioavailability from capsules was not significantly different when a single dose was given than when the dose was divided and administered at hourly intervals for 4 hours.— V. J. Harvey *et al.*, *Br. J. clin. Pharmac.*, 1984, *17*, 204P.

Studies *in vitro* suggested that metabolic activation of etoposide by oxidation into the *O*-quinone derivative might play an essential role in its activity against DNA.— J. M. S. van Maanen *et al.*, *Hum. Toxicol.*, 1986, *5*, 136.

Uses and Administration

Etoposide is a semi-synthetic derivative of podophyllotoxin with antimitotic and antineoplastic properties; it inhibits DNA synthesis and is most active against cells in the late S and G_2 phases of the cell cycle.

It is used, usually in combination with other antineoplastic agents, in the treatment of refractory tumours of the testis, and cancers of the lung. It has been tried in other solid tumours, in lymphomas and acute non-lymphoblastic leukaemias, and in the treatment of Kaposi's sarcoma associated with the acquired immune deficiency syndrome (AIDS).

It is given by slow intravenous infusion, as a solution in sodium chloride (0.9%) or glucose (5%) injection, in usual doses of 50 to 120 mg per m^2 body-surface daily for 5 days. Alternatively, 100 mg per m^2 has been given on alternate days to a total of 300 mg per m^2. Double the dose given intravenously may be given when etoposide is taken by mouth. Courses may be repeated after 3 to 4 weeks.

In the treatment of Kaposi's sarcoma, intravenous doses of 150 mg per m^2 daily for 3 days have been employed.

When given intravenously, infusion should be over 30 to 60 minutes to avoid the risk of hypotension (see Adverse Effects, above); the concentration of the infusion should be below 400 μg per mL, and preferably below 250 μg per mL, to avoid the risk of the drug crystallising out of solution.

Reviews of etoposide: N. J. Vogelzang *et al.*, *Am. J. Med.*, 1982, *72*, 136; J. A. Sinkule, *Pharmacotherapy*, 1984, *4*, 61; *Med. Lett.*, 1984, *26*, 48; P. J. O'Dwyer *et al.*, *New Engl. J. Med.*, 1985, *312*, 692; P. I. Clark and M. L. Slevin, *Clin. Pharmacokinet.*, 1987, *12*, 223.

For the role of an etoposide-containing regimen in the treatment of non-Hodgkin's lymphomas, see p.586, and for the use of etoposide in acute non-lymphoblastic leukaemias, see p.587.

GESTATIONAL TROPHOBLASTIC TUMOURS. Etoposide has important clinical activity in metastatic gestational trophoblastic disease.— T. W. Montag (letter), *New Engl. J. Med.*, 1985, *313*, 518.

See also under Choice of Antineoplastic Agent, p.585.

MALIGNANT NEOPLASMS OF THE BRONCHUS AND LUNG. The full potential of etoposide has not yet been realised in small-cell lung cancer. Both the dose-response relationship and the use of high-dose etoposide with autologous bone-marrow transplantation are being explored, although preliminary data have not indicated a higher response rate when the dose has been double. Novel regimens incorporating etoposide, cisplatin, and radiotherapy, or including etoposide in non-cross-resistant schedules are being investigated in the hope of improving survival.— P. J. O'Dwyer *et al.*, *New Engl. J. Med.*, 1985, *312*, 692.

See also under Choice of Antineoplastic Agent, p.590.

MALIGNANT NEOPLASMS OF THE TESTIS. For the role of etoposide in the combination chemotherapy of testicular cancer, see Choice of Antineoplastic Agent, p.592.

Proprietary Preparations

Vepesid *(Bristol-Myers Pharmaceuticals, UK). Capsules*, etoposide 50 and 100 mg.
Injection, etoposide 20 mg/mL, in ampoules of 5 mL.

Proprietary Names and Manufacturers

Etopol *(Jug.)*; Vepesid *(Bristol-Myers, Austral.*; *Bristol, Canad.*; *Bristol-Myers, Denm.*; *Bristol, Ger.*; *Bristol Italiana Sud, Ital.*; *Bristol, Norw.*; *Bristol, S.Afr.*; *Bristol-Myers, Spain*; *Bristol, Swed.*; *Bristol, Switz.*; *Bristol-Myers Pharmaceuticals, UK*; *Bristol-Myers Oncology, USA)*.

1835-t

Floxuridine *(USAN, rINN)*.

5-Fluorouracil Deoxyriboside; 5-FUDR; NSC-27640; WR-138720. 2′-Deoxy-5-fluorouridine; 5-Fluoro-2′-deoxyuridine; 1-(2-Deoxy-β-D-ribofuranosyl)-5-fluoropyrimidine-2,4(1*H*,3*H*)-dione.

$C_9H_{11}FN_2O_5$=246.2.

CAS — 50-91-9.

Pharmacopoeias. In *U.S.*

A white to off-white odourless powder. **Soluble** 1 in 3 of water, 1 in 12 of alcohol, 1 in 43 of isopropyl alcohol, and 1 in 7 of methyl alcohol; practically insoluble in chloroform, ether, and petroleum spirit. A 2% solution in water has a pH of 4.0 to 5.5. **Store** in airtight containers. Protect from light. The *U.S.P.* states that reconstituted solutions of Sterile Floxuridine may be stored at 2° to 8° for not more than 2 weeks.

Adverse Effects, Treatment, and Precautions

As for Fluorouracil, below. Local reactions, including erythema and stomatitis, are more common than systemic effects following intra-arterial infusion. There have also been signs of liver dysfunction.

EFFECTS ON THE LIVER. A report of fatal, progressive cirrhosis of the liver, without previous overt cholestasis, in a patient receiving long-term hepatic artery infusion of floxuridine.— J. Pettavel *et al.* (letter), *Lancet*, 1986, *2*, 1162.

Sclerosing cholangitis has resulted from hepatic arterial infusion of floxuridine, and acalculous cholecystitis may also be associated with such therapy. Serious biliary toxicity has been noted in 56% of patients receiving this treatment.— S. Sherlock, *Lancet*, 1986, *2*, 440. Because of the incidence of biliary disorders associated with continuous hepatic arterial infusion of floxuridine some surgeons routinely remove the gallbladder at the time of infusion pump implantation.— *Med. Lett.*, 1984, *26*, 89.

Absorption and Fate

Floxuridine is poorly absorbed from the gastro-intestinal tract and it is usually given by injection. Floxuridine is metabolised mainly in the liver to fluorouracil following rapid injection. When given by slow intra-arterial infusion it is reported to be converted to active floxuridine monophosphate. It is excreted as carbon dioxide via the lungs; some is excreted, as unchanged drug and metabolites, in urine. Floxuridine crosses the blood-brain barrier to some extent and is found in CSF.

Uses and Administration

Floxuridine is an antineoplastic agent which acts as an antimetabolite similarly to fluorouracil. When it is administered by rapid injection it acts as fluorouracil, but when infused slowly, usually intra-arterially, it is converted to floxuridine monophosphate (F-dUMP) which leads to enhanced inhibition of DNA synthesis.

Floxuridine is used in the palliative treatment of malignant neoplasms of the liver and gastro-intestinal tract. It has also been tried in the management of tumours of the head and neck, and other solid neoplasms. Doses of 100 to 600 µg per kg body-weight daily are given by continuous arterial infusion, usually with the aid of an infusion pump, until toxicity occurs.

It used to be given by intravenous injection in doses of 30 mg per kg body-weight daily for up to 5 days, followed by a lower maintenance dose. White cell and platelet counts should be carried out regularly during therapy and treatment should be stopped if the white cell count falls rapidly or falls to below 3 500 per mm^3, if the platelet count falls below 100 000 per mm^3, or if adverse effects occur.

Preparations

Sterile Floxuridine *(U.S.P.)*

Proprietary Names and Manufacturers

Roche, USA.

1836-x

Fluorouracil *(BAN, USAN, rINN)*.

5-Fluorouracil; 5-FU; NSC-19893; Ro-2-9757; WR-69596. 5-Fluoropyrimidine-2,4(1*H*,3*H*)-dione.

$C_4H_3FN_2O_2$=130.1.

CAS — 51-21-8.

Pharmacopoeias. In *Br.*, *Braz.*, *Chin.*, *Egypt.*, *Ind.*, *It.*, *Jpn*, and *U.S.*

A white to almost white, odourless, crystalline powder. Sparingly **soluble** in water; slightly soluble in alcohol; practically insoluble in chloroform and ether. A 1% solution has a pH of 4.3 to 5.3; the *U.S.P.* injection has a pH of 8.6 to 9.0 and the *B.P.* injection has a pH of 8.5 to 9.1. **Store** in airtight containers. Protect from light. The *B.P.* injection should be stored at a temperature between 10° and 30°, and **sterilised** by filtration. The *U.S.P.* injection and topical solution should be stored similarly.

CAUTION. *Fluorouracil is irritant; avoid contact with skin and mucous membranes.*

INCOMPATIBILITY. Fluorouracil is reportedly incompatible with cytarabine, diazepam, doxorubicin and other anthracyclines, and probably with methotrexate. Formulated solutions are alkaline and it is recommended that admixture with acidic drugs or preparations should be avoided.

STABILITY IN SOLUTION. When fluorouracil dissolved in glucose injection (5%) was stored in polyvinyl chloride bags there was a 10% loss of drug from solution in 43 hours; the same amount was lost in 7 hours when the solution was stored in glass containers.— J. A. Benvenuto *et al.*, *Am. J. Hosp. Pharm.*, 1981, *38*, 1914. A contrary study. Fluorouracil was stable in glucose injection for at least 16 weeks when stored at 5° in polyvinyl chloride or elastomeric drug reservoirs from delivery systems. When stored at room temperature, however, there was a progressive increase in fluorouracil concentration during the 16-week observation period, presumably because of evaporation of water. There was no evidence of degradation of fluorouracil.— E. J. Quebbeman *et al.*, *ibid.*, 1984, *41*, 1153.

Adverse Effects and Treatment

For an outline of the adverse effects experienced with antineoplastic agents and immunosuppressants and general guidelines for their treatment, see Antineoplastic Agents, p.580 and p.583.

The toxic effects of fluorouracil may be severe and sometimes fatal. The main adverse effects are on the bone marrow and the gastro-intestinal tract. Leucopenia, stomatitis, gastro-intestinal ulceration and bleeding, or severe diarrhoea, are signs that treatment should be stopped. The nadir of the white-cell count may occur from 7 to 20 days after a dose, and counts usually return to normal after about 30 days. Thrombocytopenia is usually at a maximum 7 to 17 days after a dose. Anaemia may also occur. Nausea and vomiting, effects on the skin including rashes and hyperpigmentation, alopecia, central neurotoxicity (notably cerebellar ataxia), and myocardial ischaemia have occurred. Reducing the rate of injection to a slow infusion over several hours can decrease the toxicity but this may be less effective than administration by rapid injection.

Local inflammatory and photosensitivity reactions have occurred following topical use.

EFFECTS ON THE EYES. Excessive watering of the eyes was associated with fluorouracil in 6 patients, one of whom had symptoms consistent with fibrosis of the tear duct. Only one patient improved when fluorouracil was discontinued.— D. J. Haidak *et al.*, *Ann. intern. Med.*, 1978, *88*, 657. Fluorouracil can be detected in the tear fluid and may produce local irritation of the tear duct.— N. Christophidis *et al.* (letter), *ibid.*, *89*, 574.

A report of recurrent episodes of optic neuropathy, culminating in near blindness, following administration of fluorouracil as part of a combination regimen in a patient with breast cancer.— J. W. Adams *et al.* (letter), *Cancer Treat. Rep.*, 1984, *68*, 565.

EFFECTS ON THE HEART. Severe chest pain and electrocardiographic changes in a patient receiving fluorouracil by intravenous infusion were relieved following discontinuation of fluorouracil and administration of nitrate vasodilators. Cardiac catheterisation revealed normal coronary arteries and left-ventricular function. The results strongly support a diagnosis of coronary artery spasm induced by fluorouracil. As coronary artery spasm may initiate myocardial infarction patients who develop cardiotoxicity with fluorouracil should be given vasodilators if further therapy is necessary.— C. Sponzilli *et al.*, *Br. med. J.*, 1987, *294*, 125.

Earlier reports of cardiotoxicity associated with fluorouracil: M. E. Carpenter (letter), *Br. med. J.*, 1972, *2*, 595 (tachycardia, controlled by quinidine given immediately before fluorouracil); R. G. Dent and I. McColl (letter), *Lancet*, 1975, *1*, 347 (angina pectoris); D. L. Stevenson *et al.* (letter), *ibid.*, 1977, *2*, 406 (chest pain, tachycardia, breathlessness, and pulmonary oedema; protection with prednisolone and glyceryl trinitrate was generally effective); A. Pottage *et al.*, *Br. med. J.*, 1978, *1*, 547 (severe chest pain and ECG changes possibly related to previous radiotherapy); M. Soukop *et al.* (letter), *ibid.*, 1422 (severe chest pain and fatal myocardial infarction).

EFFECTS ON THE NERVOUS SYSTEM. A brief discussion on cerebral ataxia associated with fluorouracil. Although in general fewer than 1% of patients receiving fluorouracil will have manifestations of cerebellar dysfunction, the incidence increases when high doses or intensive daily treatment regimens are used. It is important to differentiate between this reversible and rarely serious neurotoxicity and metastatic involvement of the cerebellum.— H. D. Weiss *et al.*, *New Engl. J. Med.*, 1974, *291*, 75.

A report of an 'organic brain syndrome', with acute confusion, emotional lability, disorientation, and impaired memory and intellectual function which followed fluorouracil treatment in an elderly patient. Mental status slowly returned to normal after cessation of the therapy.— H. T. Lynch *et al.*, *Dis. Colon Rectum*, 1981, *24*, 130.

Severe neurotoxicity in a patient given fluorouracil, manifest as sluggish speech, cerebellar ataxia, and confusion progressing to semi-coma, was associated with a previously undetected familial disorder of pyrimidine metabolism.— M. Tuchman *et al.*, *New Engl. J. Med.*, 1985, *313*, 245.

EFFECTS ON THE SKIN. A report of dermatitis and erosions in 4 patients due to the inappropriate use of topical fluorouracil.— E. Epstein (letter), *J. Am. med. Ass.*, 1983, *249*, 1565.

A report of a syndrome of paraesthesia and pain, erythema, and swelling of the palms and soles in patients receiving continuous infusions of fluorouracil or doxorubicin. In all patients the syndrome was progressive if the infusion was continued and receded over a 7- to 10-day period on interruption of the infusion.— J. J. Lokich and C. Moore, *Ann. intern. Med.*, 1984, *101*, 798. A similar report in a patient given bolus injections of fluorouracil.— J. N. Atkins (letter), *ibid.*, 1985, *102*, 419. See also L. D. Feldman and J. A. Ajani, *J. Am. med. Ass.*, 1985, *254*, 3479; *idem.*, 1986, *255*, 3116.

A report of melanonychia associated with topical application of fluorouracil in a 69-year-old patient. Pigmentation occurred on all the finger nails although the drug was applied to the proximal nail folds of only 2 fingers.— R. Baran and P. Laugier, *Br. J. Derm.*, 1985, *112*, 621.

Fluorouracil could cause photosensitivity reactions.— *Med. Lett.*, 1986, *28*, 51.

TREATMENT OF ADVERSE AFFECTS. A number of studies have suggested that allopurinol might reduce the toxicity of fluorouracil. Fox *et al.* (*Lancet*, 1979, *1*, 677) reported that allopurinol 300 mg three times daily by mouth in 13 patients permitted an increase in the dose of fluorouracil given concurrently by continuous 24-hour infusion to up to 2.9 g per m^2 body-surface daily, an approximately 2-fold increase. No patients evinced tumour response at doses below 1.5 g per m^2, but there were 5 objective responses at doses above 2 g per m^2 daily. These results were questioned by Tisman and Wu (*ibid.*, 1353) who suggested that allopurinol might prefentially protect tumour cells rather than normal tissue at anything less than the very high doses used. However, a number of other studies of the protective value of allopurinol have been subsequently carried out. Howell *et al.* confirmed the results reported by Fox and colleagues in a study in 23 patients (*Cancer*, 1981, *48*, 1281) in whom allopurinol 300 mg by mouth was given every 8 hours commencing 2 hours before beginning continuous 5-day infusions of fluorouracil. These patients were also able to tolerate fluorouracil doses of 2 g per m^2 and the protective effects of allopurinol were noted to be exerted on oral and gastro-intestinal epithelia, and on bone marrow.

Earlier studies were concerned with the protective effect of allopurinol when fluorouracil was given by continuous infusion, and some doubt has been raised as to the value of allopurinol given with bolus doses of fluorouracil: the findings of Garewal and Ahmann (*New Engl. J. Med.*, 1985, *312*, 587) suggested that although allopurinol provided moderate protection against the myelotoxicity of bolus fluorouracil it was unlikely to be of clinical help, in contrast to the dose escalations that were possible with continuous infusion of fluorouracil when allopurinol was given. Similar findings were reported by Campbell *et al.* (*Cancer Treat. Rep.*, 1982, *66*, 1723) who found that neurotoxicity, against which allopurinol did not protect, limited the usefulness of a high-dose bolus fluorouracil and allopurinol regimen, and the tumour response rate was low.

Allopurinol has also been used locally in the management of fluorouracil toxicity. Clark and Slevin treated 6 patients who had developed mucositis during previous dosage cycles of fluorouracil with a mouthwash of allopurinol 0.1% in 3% methylcellulose. The mouthwash was given immediately after injection of fluorouracil and repeated three times at hourly intervals; the solution remained in the mouth for a few seconds on each occasion. All patients experienced a decrease in mucositis of 1 to 2 grades (WHO). Taste abnormalities in 2 patients were also improved. (*Eur. J. surg. Oncol.*, 1985, *11*, 267).

Reference to the use of high-dose uridine in the management of fluorouracil toxicity: A. Leyva *et al.*, *Cancer Res.*, 1984, *44*, 5928.

Precautions

For reference to the precautions necessary with antineoplastic agents and immunosuppressants, see Antineoplastic Agents, p.583. Fluorouracil should be given with care to weak or malnourished patients or to those with hepatic or renal insufficiency.

Painful burns around the parts of the face where spectacle frames rested in a patient treated with topical fluorouracil were probably due to occlusion of the drug by the frame, increasing the absorption and irritation of the treatment.— *J. Am. med. Ass.*, 1985, *253*, 3166.

HANDLING AND DISPOSAL. Protective clothing should be worn when handling urine and faeces from patients receiving fluorouracil and this precaution should continue for up to 48 hours and 5 days (after an oral dose) respectively after therapy.— J. Harris and L. J. Dodds, *Pharm. J.*, 1985, *2*, 289.

INTERACTIONS. Pretreatment with cimetidine for 4 weeks led to increased plasma concentrations of fluorouracil following intravenous and oral administration in 6 patients. The effect was probably due to a combination of hepatic enzyme inhibition and reduced hepatic blood flow. No such effect was seen following single doses of cimetidine in 5 or pretreatment for just 1 week in 6. Care is required in patients taking both drugs simultaneously.— V. J. Harvey *et al.*, *Br. J. clin. Pharmac.*, 1984, *18*, 421.

With diagnostic tests. Fluorouracil could interfere with diagnostic tests of thyroid function by causing rises in total thyroxine and liothyronine due to increased globulin binding.— I. Ramsay, *Postgrad. med. J.*, 1985, *61*, 375.

Absorption and Fate

Absorption of fluorouracil from the gastro-intestinal tract is unpredictable and fluorouracil is usually given intravenously. Little is absorbed when fluorouracil is applied to healthy skin.

After intravenous injection fluorouracil is cleared rapidly from plasma. It is distributed throughout body tissues and fluids including the cerebrospinal fluid and malignant effusions, and disappears from the plasma within about 3 hours. Fluorouracil is converted to active nucleotide metabolites within the target cell itself. About 15% of an intravenous dose is excreted unchanged in the urine within 6 hours. The remainder is inactivated primarily in the liver and is catabolised similarly to endogenous uracil. A large amount is excreted as respiratory carbon dioxide; urea is also produced.

A detailed review of the pharmacokinetics of some antineoplastic agents, including fluorouracil. Following oral administration there is marked inter- and intra-patient variation in bioavailability, apparently due more to first-pass hepatic metabolism than poor gastro-intestinal absorption. Once absorbed, fluorouracil distributes throughout the body, including the brain, entering cells by passive diffusion. With oral or bolus intravenous administration bone-marrow concentrations of drug are equivalent to those in plasma but after slow intravenous infusion bone-marrow concentrations are 50- to 1000-fold lower, correlating with the clinical impression that slow infusions are less myelosuppressive. Within the target cell fluorouracil is converted to 5-fluorouridine monophosphate and floxuridine monophosphate (5-FUMP and 5-FdUMP), the former being further phosphorylated to the triphosphate which can be incorporated into RNA, while the latter inhibits thymidylate synthetase. The drug is cleared primarily by hepatic metabolic degradation, with less than 15% of the drug excreted intact in the urine. Up to 95% of a slow hepatic artery infusion is extracted on first passage through the liver. High intravenous doses have been associated with lower clearance values suggesting saturation of the hepatic enzymes mediating detoxification. The plasma decline is generally agreed to be monoexponential, although biexponential curves have been reported in a few patients. A half-life for plasma clearance of 10 to 20 minutes has been reported and after 2 to 3 hours plasma concentrations are no longer detectable by conventional assay; more sensitive assays have purported to demonstrate a prolonged terminal elimination phase with a half-life of 20 hours.— F. M. Balis *et al.*, *Clin. Pharmacokinet.*, 1983, *8*, 202.

Fluorouracil was present in detectable quantities in parotid saliva following intravenous administration of doses ranging from 0.6 to 1 g to 11 patients.— L. A. Celio *et al.*, *Eur. J. clin. Pharmac.*, 1983, *24*, 261.

For a report that fluorouracil is present in tear fluid see under Effects on the Eyes, in Adverse Effects, above.

A study of fluorouracil metabolites in colorectal cancer tissue.— G. R. Giles *et al.*, *Gut*, 1986, *27*, 176.

Uses and Administration

Fluorouracil, a pyrimidine analogue, is an antineoplastic agent which acts as an antimetabolite to uracil. After intracellular conversion to the active deoxynucleotide it interferes with the synthesis of DNA by blocking the conversion of deoxyuridylic acid to thymidylic acid by the cellular enzyme thymidylate synthetase. It can also interfere with RNA synthesis. It also has immunosuppressant properties.

Fluorouracil is used alone or in combination in the palliation of inoperable malignant neoplasms, especially those of the gastro-intestinal tract, breast, liver, genito-urinary system, and pancreas. It is often used with cyclophosphamide and methotrexate in the combination chemotherapy of breast cancer. See also Choice of Antineoplastic Agent, p.588.

A usual dose by intravenous injection is 12 mg per kg body-weight daily to a maximum of 1 g daily for 3 or 4 days. If there is no evidence of toxicity, this is followed after 1 day by 6 mg per kg on alternate days for 3 or 4 further doses. Doses should be halved in patients with poor nutritional status, impaired bone-marrow, hepatic, or renal function, and after major surgery.

An alternative schedule is to give 15 mg per kg intravenously once a week throughout the course. The course may be repeated after 1 month or maintenance doses of 5 to 15 mg per kg may be given weekly. Fluorouracil may also be given by intravenous infusion, 15 mg per kg daily, to a maximum of 1 g daily, being infused in 500 mL of glucose injection (5%) over 4 hours and repeated on successive days until toxicity occurs or a total of 12 to 15 g has been given. The course may be repeated after 4 to 6 weeks. Fluorouracil has also been given by intra-arterial infusion in doses of 5 to 7.5 mg per kg daily, and by mouth.

The white cell count should be determined daily during treatment with fluorouracil and therapy stopped immediately if the count falls rapidly or falls to below 3500 per mm^3, if the platelet count falls below 100 000 per mm^3, or if adverse effects occur.

Fluorouracil is used topically in the treatment of solar or actinic keratoses and other tumours and premalignant conditions of the skin including Bowen's disease and superficial basal cell carcinomas. It is usually applied as a 5% cream or ointment or as a 1 to 5% solution in propylene glycol.

The use of fluorouracil in cosmetics is prohibited in the *UK*.

ADMINISTRATION. Co-administration of fluorouracil with various agents has been tried in an effort to enhance its effects. Au *et al.* (*Cancer Res.*, 1982, *42*, 2930) found no improvement in the response-rate of colorectal cancer treated with fluorouracil and *thymidine*. Pretreatment with *sparfosic acid* (E.S. Casper *et al.*, *ibid.*, 1983, *43*, 2324) also had little apparent value and when given in high doses of 1 to 2 g per m^2 body-surface prevented the use of fluorouracil in full doses. However, more promising results were reported by O'Connell *et al.* (*J. clin. Oncol.*, 1984, *2*, 1133) with sequential administration of sparfosate sodium, thymidine and fluorouracil and these results were particularly encouraging in patients with aggressive or highly anaplastic carcinomas. Another combination is that of high-dose *calcium folinate* with fluorouracil, which was reported by Madajewicz *et al.* (*Cancer Res.*, 1984, *44*, 4667) to be effective in patients with colorectal cancer resistant to fluorouracil alone.

For the administration of allopurinol with fluorouracil, see under Treatment of Adverse Effects, above.

The use of intraperitoneal infusions of fluorouracil in patients with colonic or gastric cancer.— J. W. Gyves *et al.*, *Clin. Pharmac. Ther.*, 1984, *35*, 83.

Synergistic activity has been reported when methotrexate is given before fluorouracil. In a phase I study involving 39 patients with a variety of metastatic neoplasms, patients were given an initial bolus of methotrexate 30 mg per m^2 body-surface followed by 15 mg per m^2 per hour by constant infusion for 36 hours. Fluorouracil 62.5 mg per m^2 per hour was given for 24 hours, beginning after 24 hours of the methotrexate infusion so that the two infusions overlapped for 12 hours. All patients also received folinic acid rescue. Cycles were administered every 2 weeks. Of 34 evaluable patients 11 had a response although there were no complete responses. Therapy was generally well tolerated, with mucositis and diarrhoea the most frequent toxicity. Results in 3 patients suggested that the dose of fluorouracil could be increased by doubling the infusion time to 48 hours, but beyond this dose mucositis occurred. The regimen was considered deserving of further evaluation, particularly in patients with adenocarcinoma.— C. Benz *et al.*, *Cancer Res.*, 1985, *45*, 3354.

In renal insufficiency. Fluorouracil could be given in usual doses to patients with renal failure. Concentrations of fluorouracil are affected by haemodialysis.— W. M. Bennett *et al.*, *Am. J. Kidney Dis.*, 1983, *3*, 155. The manufacturers recommend dosage reduction in patients with renal insufficiency. See also under Uses, above.

LARYNGEAL PAPILLOMAS. Comment on the role of fluorouracil in the adjuvant treatment of laryngeal papillomas.— *Lancet*, 1981, *1*, 367.

MALIGNANT NEOPLASMS OF THE BLADDER. See under Choice of Antineoplastic Agent, p.588.

MALIGNANT NEOPLASMS OF THE BREAST. See under Choice of Antineoplastic Agent, p.589.

MALIGNANT NEOPLASMS OF THE GASTRO-INTESTINAL TRACT. See under Choice of Antineoplastic Agent, p.590.

MALIGNANT NEOPLASMS OF THE HEAD AND NECK. See under Choice of Antineoplastic Agent, p.591.

MALIGNANT NEOPLASMS OF THE LIVER. Adjuvant therapy with fluorouracil and semustine failed to produce any evidence of improved survival among 26 patients who had undergone hepatic resection for colorectal carcinoma metastatic to the liver, when compared with 26 controls.— M. J. O'Connell *et al.*, *Mayo Clin. Proc.*, 1985, *60*, 517.

A beneficial response in a patient with multiple liver metastases treated with diathermy and liver perfusion with fluorouracil.— R. H. Grace and K. W. M. Scott, *Br. med. J.*, 1987, *295*, 637. See also R. M. Barone *et al.*, *Cancer*, 1982, *50*, 850.

See also under Choice of Antineoplastic Agent, p.591.

MALIGNANT NEOPLASMS OF THE OVARY. See under Choice of Antineoplastic Agent, p.591.

MALIGNANT NEOPLASMS OF THE PANCREAS. Islet-cell carcinoma, which is quite uncommon is usually responsive to chemotherapy with streptozocin and fluorouracil; however adenocarcinoma of the exocrine pancreas is much less responsive to chemotherapy. Single-agent therapy with fluorouracil has produced a 15% response rate in this latter disease among patients at the Mayo Clinic but responses to single-agent therapy are typically partial rather than complete. A median survival of 24 weeks has been reported in patients with fluorouracil alone; no greater survival advantage has yet been reported for combination chemotherapy, although reported objective response rates have been higher in general than with single-agent therapy. Radiotherapy combined with fluorouracil is more effective than radiotherapy alone in patients with locally unresectable disease and has been shown to improve longevity.— M. J. O'Connell, *Mayo Clin. Proc.*, 1983, *58*, 47.

See also under Choice of Antineoplastic Agent, p.592.

MALIGNANT NEOPLASMS OF THE PROSTATE. See under Choice of Antineoplastic Agent, p.592.

MALIGNANT NEOPLASMS OF THE SKIN. Topical fluorouracil is widely used in the treatment of actinic keratoses, with excellent results. Other conditions for which fluorouracil treatment has been employed include Bowen's disease, leucoplakia, and genital carcinoma *in situ* (erythroplasia of Queyrat). Isolated lesions may be better treated with curettage or cryotherapy, but fluorouracil is usually employed for multiple keratoses.

Local fluorouracil treatment has also been increasingly used in the treatment of superficial basal cell and squamous cell carcinomas of the skin, particularly for recurrent or multiple lesions; however, surgery and/or radiotherapy remain the primary treatment. The advantages of topical cytotoxic therapy include the possibility of repeated use where necessary and its value in the treatment of large areas of carcinoma *in situ* where other methods of treatment are unsuitable because of the extent. Fluorouracil is not usually recommended for thick or invasive lesions.

Actinic (solar) keratoses. A collodion-based varnish containing fluorouracil 5% and salicylic acid 5, 8, or 10% was used in the treatment of solar keratoses in 20 patients, 6 of whom had been previously treated with fluorouracil ointment 5%. The varnish adhered to the skin for 2 to 3 weeks and lesions were therefore treated only every 3 weeks. Those on the face required 1 to 5 applications and those of 2 patients on the hands 7 and 9. There was no dermatitis or photosensitisation. The varnish appeared to be superior to the ointment except where a rapid response was required or the lesions were very numerous.— J. C. A. Goncalves, *Br. J. Derm.*, 1975, *92*, 85. The morning application of tretinoin 0.1% and the evening application of fluorouracil cream 5% eradicated all keratoses on the forearms and hands of 20 patients. Tretinoin was discontinued after 8 to 14 days when inflammation developed. Fluorouracil cream alone was effective against keratoses of the face, some of the forearms, but ineffective against those on the hands.— T. A. Robinson and A. M. Kligman, *ibid.*, 703. A further study. Tretinoin 0.05% cream applied nightly was more effective than a placebo cream in enhancing the effect of twice daily applications of 5% fluorouracil cream for the treatment of solar keratoses in 19 patients.— L. Bercovitch, *ibid.*, 1987, *116*, 549.

Basal cell carcinoma. Following experience gained in treating 103 patients, the topical treatment of invasive basal cell carcinoma of the face with fluorouracil was not recommended since it often produced the appearance of control by superficial inhibition of the tumour while the deeper extensions continued to grow.— F. E. Mohs *et al.*, *Archs Derm.*, 1978, *114*, 1021.

The use of 25% fluorouracil paste in soft paraffin to treat thin basal cell carcinomas. The 5-year cumulative recurrence-rate in 44 carcinomas treated with the paste under an occlusive dressing for 3 weeks was 21%. In a second series of 244 lesions, light curettage followed by the fluorouracil paste produced a 5-year recurrence-rate of only 6%. Cosmetic results were considered good to excellent in 80% or more cases in both series. The results show that topical fluorouracil treatment combined with curettage can produce cure-rates as good as other more conventional means of treatment.— E. Epstein, *Archs Derm.*, 1985, *121*, 207.

RETINAL DETACHMENT. A report of the use of subconjunctival and intravitreal injection of fluorouracil to prevent further retinal detachment in patients with proliferative vitreoretinopathy who had undergone retinal re-attachment surgery. Patients received 10 mg subconjunctivally or 1 mg intravitreally or both, repeated up to 5 times if necessary. Treatment was successful in preventing detachment in 12 of 20 patients followed for 6 months.— M. Blumenkranz *et al.*, *Ophthalmology*, 1984, *91*, 122.

SKIN DISORDERS, NON-MALIGNANT. Fluorouracil has been tried in various skin disorders, including refractory psoriasis and keratoacanthoma.

See also under Malignant Neoplasms of the Skin, above.

The use of fluorouracil 5% cream daily for about 7 days under an occlusive dressing resulted in the successful repigmentation of previously-abraded lesions of vitiligo in 18 of 28 patients.— T. Tsuji and T. Hamada, *Archs Derm.*, 1983, *119*, 722.

WARTS. Fluorouracil has been used in wart treatment as a 5% cream, which should be applied accurately to the wart daily and covered with a waterproof dressing. It is not always successful and should be used, with care, only under exceptional circumstances. Some authorities have claimed success using fluorouracil without a covering in the treatment of plane warts.— F. E. Anderson, *Drugs*, 1985, *30*, 368.

Variable results have been reported for the use of fluorouracil as a 5% cream or a 1% alcoholic solution in the treatment of genital warts (condylomata acuminata) but controlled studies are lacking. Present studies suggest that fluorouracil has side-effects and is not superior to podophyllin.— M. W. Adler and A. Mindel, *Br. med. Bull.*, 1985, *41*, 361.

Fluorouracil cream is sometimes successful with widespread vaginal and cervical warts.— M. H. Bunney, *Br. med. J.*, 1986, *293*, 1045.

Preparations

Fluorouracil Cream *(B.P.)*

Fluorouracil Cream *(U.S.P.)*. It may also contain sodium hydroxide to adjust the pH.

Fluorouracil Injection *(B.P.)*. Prepared by the interaction of fluorouracil and sodium hydroxide.

Fluorouracil Injection *(U.S.P.)*. A sterile solution in Water for Injections, prepared with the aid of sodium hydroxide. It contains 45 to 55 mg of fluorouracil in each mL. If a precipitate forms, redissolve by warming to 60°, with shaking, and cool.

Fluorouracil Topical Solution *(U.S.P.)*

Proprietary Preparations

Efudix *(Roche, UK)*. *Cream*, fluorouracil 5%.

Roche, UK also supply ampoules and capsules as Fluorouracil.

Proprietary Names and Manufacturers

Adrucil *(Adria, Canad.; Adria, USA)*; Arumel *(Jpn)*; Carzonal *(Jpn)*; Effluderm *(Allergan, Ger.)*; Efudex *(Roche, Canad.; Roche, USA)*; Efudix *(Roche, Austral.; Belg.; Roche, Fr.; Roche, Ger.; Roche, Ital.; Jpn; Neth.; Roche, S.Afr.; Roche, Spain; Roche, Switz.; Roche, UK)*; Fluoroplex *(Allergan, Austral.; Canad.; Herbert, USA)*; Fluorouracil *(Austral.; Belg.; Roche, Denm.; Neth.; Roche, Norw.; Roche, S.Afr.; Roche, Swed.; Roche, Switz.; Roche, UK)*; Fluoro-Uracile *(Roche, Fr.)*; Fluroblastin *(Farmitalia, Ger.; Farmitalia Carlo Erba, S.Afr.)*; Fluroblastine *(Farmitalia Carlo Erba, Switz.)*; Timazin *(Jpn)*; ULUP *(Jpn)*.

Manufacturers also include—*Bull, UK*.

12780-r

Gallium Nitrate

NSC-15200; WR-135675.

$Ga(NO_3)_3,9H_2O=417.9$.

CAS — 13494-90-1 (anhydrous).

Adverse Effects, Treatment, and Precautions

For an outline of the adverse effects experienced with antineoplastic agents and immunosuppressants, general guidelines for their treatment, and precautions, see Antineoplastic Agents, p.580, p.583.

Gallium nitrate may produce serious nephrotoxicity, especially when given as a brief intravenous infusion; administration by continuous infusion, with adequate hydration, may reduce the incidence of renal damage. Concomitant administration of other nephrotoxic drugs, such as aminoglycosides, should be avoided, and it should be given with great care and in reduced doses, if at all, to patients with existing renal dysfunction.

Bone-marrow toxicity, optic neuritis, and hypocalcaemia have also been reported.

Uses and Administration

Gallium nitrate is an inorganic antineoplastic agent that has been tried in the management of Hodgkin's disease and other lymphomas refractory to standard therapy. It has also been tried in patients with advanced malignant melanoma and in malignant disease metastatic to bone. Doses of 100 to 300 mg per m^2 body-surface daily have been given by intravenous infusion for 7 days.

References: B. J. Foster *et al.*, *Cancer Treat. Rep.*, 1986, *70*, 1311.

12791-n

Glutaminase

AGA; Glutaminase-asparaginase.

CAS — 9001-47-2.

An enzyme obtained from *Acinetobacter* spp, which hydrolyses glutamine and asparagine; it has also reportedly been obtained from *Achromobacter* spp.

Glutaminase has been tried, similarly to colaspase (p.609), in the treatment of acute leukaemias.

References: R. P. Warrell *et al.*, *Cancer Treat. Rep.*, 1982, *66*, 1479 (in adult leukaemia); J. Holcenberg *et al.*, *Cancer Res.*, 1983, *43*, 1381 (intraperitoneally with melphalan in patients with abdominal metastatic disease).

19285-c

Harringtonine

The 2-(methoxycarbonylmethyl)-2,5-dihydroxy-5-methylhexanoate ester of cephalotaxine derived from *Cephalotaxus harringtonia* (Cephalotaxaceae) and related species.

$C_{28}H_{37}NO_9=531.6$.

19300-f

Homoharringtonine

NSC-141633. The 2-(methoxycarbonylmethyl)-2,6-dihydroxy-5-methylheptanoate ester of cephalotaxine derived from *Cephalotaxus harringtonia* (Cephalotaxaceae) and related species.

$C_{29}H_{39}NO_9=545.6$.

Adverse Effects

Severe hypotension may occur, particularly after injection of homoharringtonine, and may be dose limiting. Tachycardia and cardiac arrhythmias, bone-marrow toxicity, gastro-intestinal disturbances, neurotoxicity, alopecia, and hyperglycaemia have also been reported.

Uses and Administration

Homoharringtonine and its congener harringtonine and the related compounds isoharringtonine and deoxyharringtonine, have each been tried as antineoplastic agents in the treatment of acute leukaemias and other neoplastic disorders. Doses of 2 to 4 mg homoharringtonine per m^2 body-surface daily have been given for 5 days by intravenous infusion; similar doses of harringtonine have been tried.

Homoharringtonine was given to 49 patients with refractory acute lymphoblastic or non-lymphoblastic leukaemias, or chronic myelocytic leukaemia, in total cumulative doses of 35 to 49 mg per m^2 divided over 7 or 9 days. None of the the patients given the lowest dose achieved complete remission although 3 had absence of leukaemic blasts from the bone marrow. Of the 38 patients given cumulative doses of 45 to 49 mg per m^2, 7 of 28 with primary acute non-lymphoblastic disease achieved complete remission and 19 of 27 evaluated had clearance of leukaemic blasts from bone marrow. There were no complete remissions among the 10 with acute lymphoblastic or secondary disease although 3 had clearance of leukaemic blasts. Homoharringtonine appears to be an effective drug for the treatment of patients with acute non-lymphoblastic leukaemia and appears not to be cross-resistant with the agents usually used in this disorder.— R. P. Warrell *et al.*, *J. clin. Oncol.*, 1985, *3*, 617.

A report of the use of harringtonine to prolong survival in an elderly patient with acute myeloid leukaemia. Infusion of harringtonine 2 mg daily over 6 hours, subsequently increased to 4 mg daily, up to a cumulative dose of 24 mg, was well tolerated and was followed by complete remission.— J. Sullivan and M. Leyden, *Med. J. Aust.*, 1985, *142*, 693.

Further references to homoharringtonine: T. Ohnuma and J. F. Holland, *J. clin. Oncol.*, 1985, *3*, 604; P. J. O'Dwyer *et al.*, *ibid.*, 1986, *4*, 1563.

1838-f

Hexamethylmelamine

Altretamine *(rINN)*; HMM; NSC-13875; WR-95704. 2,4,6-Tris(dimethylamino)-1,3,5-triazine.
$C_9H_{18}N_6$=210.3.

CAS — 645-05-6.

CAUTION. *Hexamethylmelamine is irritant; avoid contact with skin and mucous membranes.*

Adverse Effects, Treatment, and Precautions

For an outline of the adverse effects experienced with antineoplastic agents and immunosuppressants, general guidelines for their treatment, and precautions, see Antineoplastic Agents, p.580, p.583.

The neurotoxicity of hexamethylmelamine may be manifest both centrally and as peripheral neuropathies. Nausea and vomiting may be dose-limiting.

INTERACTIONS. *Antidepressants.* Severe and potentially life-threatening orthostatic hypotension developed in 3 patients who received amitriptyline or imipramine concurrently with hexamethylmelamine, and in a fourth patient who took phenelzine and hexamethylmelamine concurrently. One patient was able to tolerate a combination of the antineoplastic with nortriptyline.— H. W. Bruckner and S. J. Schleifer, *Cancer Treat. Rep.*, 1983, *67*, 516.

Metoclopramide. For reference to an acute fatal dystonic reaction in a patient receiving hexamethylmelamine and metoclopramide, see Metoclopramide, p.1098.

Absorption and Fate

Variable absorption of hexamethylmelamine has been reported from the gastro-intestinal tract. It is demethylated in the body to pentamethylmelamine and other metabolites which are excreted in urine.

Uses and Administration

Hexamethylmelamine is an antineoplastic agent structurally similar to tretamine (p.653) although its mode of action may not be attributed to alkylation only. It has been given by mouth in the treatment of ovarian carcinoma and other solid tumours in doses ranging from 4 to 12 mg per kg body-weight, or 150 to 320 mg per m^2 body-surface daily.

A review of hexamethylmelamine. Although originally thought to be an alkylating agent this has been demonstrated not to be its mode of action, which has yet to be clearly defined. It is a valuable agent for combination therapy because myelotoxicity is relatively mild. The average tolerable dose is 8 mg per kg body-weight daily, given as a 21-day course. Many combination regimens give 100 to 200 mg per m^2 body-surface for 14 days each month, but dosage reduction is frequently necessary due to gastro-intestinal, neurological, or haematological toxicity. It is used particularly as a second-line treatment in ovarian cancer, as a component of regimens such as HexaCAF (with cyclophosphamide, methotrexate, and fluorouracil) and CHAP (with cyclophosphamide, doxorubicin, and cisplatin): combinations with cisplatin are particularly effective. It has also been used in small-cell lung cancer, with encouraging results, and has been tried in the treatment of endometrial and prostatic carcinomas and in some types of lymphoma.— D. A. Hahn, *Drug Intell. & clin. Pharm.*, 1983, *17*, 418.

Further references: R. B. Weiss, *Gynecol. Oncol.*, 1981, *12*, 141.

Proprietary Names and Manufacturers

Hexastat *(Rhône-Poulenc, Canad.; Rhone-Poulenc, Denm.; Bellon, Fr.; Rhone-Poulenc, Ital.; Rhone-Poulenc, Switz.)*; Hexinawas *(Wasserman, Spain)*.

1839-d

Hydroxyurea *(BAN, USAN)*.

Hydroxycarbamide *(rINN)*; NSC-32065; SQ-1089; WR-83799.
$HO.NH.CO.NH_2$=76.05.

CAS — 127-07-1.

Pharmacopoeias. In *Br.*, *Fr.*, and *U.S.*

A white to off-white, odourless or almost odourless, crystalline powder. It is hygroscopic and decomposes in the presence of moisture. Freely **soluble** in water and hot alcohol. **Store** in airtight containers in a dry atmosphere.

Adverse Effects and Treatment

For an outline of the adverse effects experienced with antineoplastic agents and immunosuppressants and general guidelines for their treatment, see Antineoplastic Agents, p.580 and p.583.

Bone-marrow suppression, including megaloblastic changes, is the main adverse effect of hydroxyurea. The erythema caused by irradiation may be exacerbated by hydroxyurea. Other side-effects reported have included gastro-intestinal disturbances, impairment of renal function, pulmonary oedema, mild dermatological reactions, and neurological reactions such as headache, dizziness, drowsiness, disorientation, hallucinations, and convulsions.

If anaemia occurs, it may be corrected by transfusions of whole blood without stopping therapy. Megaloblastic changes are usually self-limiting.

EFFECTS ON THE LIVER. A report of self-limited hepatitis and a flu-like syndrome in a patient receiving hydroxyurea. Symptoms recurred when the patient was rechallenged with the drug.— R. Heddle and A. F. Calvert, *Med. J. Aust.*, 1980, *1*, 121.

EFFECTS ON THE VASCULAR SYSTEM. Acral erythema occurred in a patient given hydroxyurea as part of the treatment of chronic myelogenous leukaemia. Symptoms resolved on discontinuation of hydroxyurea and treatment with indomethacin, but recurred with greater severity when hydroxyurea was restarted at a lower dose.— F. S. Silver *et al.* (letter), *Ann. intern. Med.*, 1983, *98*, 675.

Precautions

For reference to the precautions necessary with antineoplastic agents and immunosuppressants, see Antineoplastic Agents, p.583.

Hydroxyurea should be used with caution in patients with impaired renal function. The elderly may be more sensitive to the adverse effects of hydroxyurea. Pre-existing anaemia should be corrected before beginning therapy with hydroxyurea.

HANDLING AND DISPOSAL. Protective clothing should be worn for up to 48 hours after therapy when handling urine from patients receiving hydroxyurea.— J. Harris and L. J. Dodds, *Pharm. J.*, 1985, *2*, 289.

Absorption and Fate

Hydroxyurea is readily absorbed from the gastro-intestinal tract and distributed throughout the body. Peak plasma concentrations are reached within 2 hours. Hydroxyurea is metabolised by the liver, and excreted in urine as urea and unchanged drug. Some is excreted as carbon dioxide via the lungs. About 80% of a dose is reported to be excreted in the urine within 12 hours. It crosses the blood-brain barrier.

Uses and Administration

Hydroxyurea is an antineoplastic agent which may act by inhibition of DNA synthesis. It is S-phase specific. Hydroxyurea is used in the treatment of chronic myeloid leukaemia though busulphan is usually preferred. It has also been used in the treatment of malignant melanoma and inoperable tumours of the ovary. Beneficial results have been obtained with radiotherapy and hydroxyurea in squamous cell carcinomas of the head and neck and this combination has also been tried in cancer of the cervix and the lung.

It is given by mouth in a single dose of 20 to 30 mg per kg body-weight daily or in a single dose of 80 mg per kg every third day. If a beneficial effect is evident after 6 weeks, therapy may be continued indefinitely.

The haemoglobin concentration, white cell and platelet counts, and hepatic and renal function should be determined repeatedly during treatment. Treatment should be interrupted if the white cell count drops to 2500 per mm^3 or the platelet count to 100 000 per mm^3.

ADMINISTRATION IN RENAL FAILURE. The dose of hydroxyurea should be reduced to 50% in patients with a glomerular filtration-rate of less than 10 mL per minute.— W. M. Bennett *et al.*, *Am. J. Kidney Dis.*, 1983, *3*, 155.

BLOOD DISORDERS, NON-MALIGNANT. Hydroxyurea has been useful in patients with the hypereosinophilic syndrome. It is presumed that it reduced eosinophil production and thereby the degree of tissue injury.— *Lancet*, 1983, *1*, 1417.

For a report of beneficial results with hydroxyurea in patients with corticosteroid-resistant hypereosinophilia, see Corticosteroids, p.877. For the use of hydroxyurea to treat polycythaemia vera, see Choice of Antineoplastic Agent, p.585.

Haemoglobinopathies. Results in *animals* given high doses of hydroxyurea showed that it could enhance foetal haemoglobin production. Further research might lead to useful treatment of some patients with haemoglobinopathies.— N. L. Letvin *et al.*, *New Engl. J. Med.*, 1984, *310*, 869. Comment. Stimulation of the gamma-globin gene responsible for the production of foetal haemoglobin offers a hopeful approach in the treatment of haemoglobinopathies such as sickle cell anaemia and beta-thalassaemia. If agents such as hydroxyurea can be used to achieve sustained elevations in foetal haemoglobin (haemoglobin F) in such patients then a prospective study of their effects will possible.— J. W. Adamson, *ibid.*, 917.

Treatment with hydroxyurea 36 to 50 mg per kg body-weight daily for 3 days produced haematological changes reflecting cytoreduction and regeneration in 2 patients with sickle cell anaemia, but single weekly doses of 50 mg per kg in one had no such effect. Both patients also responded dramatically when given cytarabine in doses between 10 and 40 mg per m^2 body-surface daily by intravenous infusion for 3 days. Treatment produced marked increases in blood concentrations of foetal haemoglobin. Whether treatment with cytarabine or hydroxyurea can produce effects sufficient to ameliorate the clinical course of sickle cell anaemia remains to be determined.— R. Veithe *et al.*, *New Engl. J. Med.*, 1985, *313*, 1571.

SKIN DISORDERS, NON-MALIGNANT. Hydroxyurea has been used in doses of 1 to 2 g daily by mouth in the treatment of psoriasis but response is slower and less complete than with methotrexate, and resistance may develop more frequently. In a review of over 100 patients treated with hydroxyurea no serious toxicity was attributed to the drug but response was excellent in only 18% of patients and worthwhile in another 45%. The virtues of hydroxyurea are its gastro-intestinal tolerance and lack of hepatotoxicity, but careful monitoring of blood counts is necessary during therapy; rare side-effects include vasculitis, hypersensitivity rashes, cutaneous erosions, and loss of libido.— E. M. Farber and L. Nall, *Drugs*, 1984, *28*, 324.

See also under Use of Immunosuppressants, p.595.

Preparations

Hydroxyurea Capsules *(B.P.)*
Hydroxyurea Capsules *(U.S.P.)*

Proprietary Preparations
Hydrea *(Squibb, UK). Capsules,* hydroxyurea 500 mg.

Proprietary Names and Manufacturers
Hydrea *(Squibb, Austral.; Belg.; Squibb, Canad.; Squibb, Fr.; Ital.; Neth.; Squibb, S.Afr.; Squibb, UK; Squibb, USA)*; Litalir *(Rhône-Poulenc, Ger.)*; Onco-Carbide *(Simes, Ital.; Spain)*.

19335-w

Idarubicin *(rINN)*.

4-Demethoxydaunorubicin; IMI-30 (base or hydrochloride); NSC-256439; SC-33428. (1*S*,3*S*)-3-Acetyl-1,2,3,4,6,11-hexahydro-3,5,12-trihydroxy-6,11-dioxo-1-naphthacenyl 3-amino-2,3,6-trideoxy-α-L-*lyxo*-hexopyranoside.
$C_{26}H_{27}NO_9$=497.5.

CAS — 58957-92-9.

NOTE. Idarubicin Hydrochloride is *USAN.*

Idarubicin is an analogue of doxorubicin (p.623) which is active when given by mouth. It has been tried in the management of acute leukaemias and a variety of solid tumours. Bone-marrow toxicity is dose-limiting; the drug is claimed to be less cardiotoxic than doxorubicin.

A preliminary review of idarubicin. Unlike doxorubicin or daunorubicin it is active when given by mouth. Following intravenous or oral administration it is metabolised to an active metabolite, idarubicinol, which has a prolonged life in the body. Phase II clinical studies of idarubicin in patients with refractory or relapsed adult acute non-lymphoblastic leukaemias have shown clinical effect with doses of 8 to 12 mg per m^2 body-surface daily, intravenously for 3 days or 7 to 8 mg per m^2 daily for 5 days. There was also some evidence of activity when the drug was given by the oral route in doses of 20 to 30 mg per m^2 daily for 3 days. Idarubicin has also been investigated in combination with other agents, notably cytarabine and etoposide. Idarubicin has also been investigated in the management of solid tumours; some activity has been reported with oral doses of 35 to 45 mg per m^2 given every 3 to 4 weeks, or 15 mg per m^2 daily for 3 days every 3 to 4 weeks in patients with advanced breast cancer.— F. Ganzina *et al., Invest. New Drugs,* 1986, *4,* 85.
The pharmacokinetics of idarubicin.— H. C. Gillies *et al., Br. J. clin. Pharmac.,* 1987, *23,* 303.

1840-c

Ifosfamide *(BAN, USAN, rINN)*.

Iphosphamide; Isophosphamide; MJF-9325; NSC-109724; Z-4942. 3-(2-Chloroethyl)-2-(2-chloroethylamino)perhydro-1,3,2-oxazaphosphorinane 2-oxide.
$C_7H_{15}Cl_2N_2O_2P$=261.1.

CAS — 3778-73-2.

Store below 25°.

For the physical properties, including stability and storage, of ifosfamide, see L. A. Trissel *et al., Drug Intell. & clin. Pharm.,* 1979, *13,* 340.
Evidence that mesna and ifosfamide do not react when mixed in an infusion bag.— I. C. Shaw and J. W. P. Rose (letter), *Lancet,* 1984, *1,* 1353. Similar results with polypropylene syringes prefilled with a mixture of mesna and ifosfamide and stored for 4 weeks at room temperature and at 4°. No significant changes could be detected in the mesna concentration; the ifosfamide concentration fell by about 3% in 7 days and 12% in 4 weeks under both storage conditions. As a result of these findings patients are provided with 7 days' supply of the mixture, prefilled into syringes; there have been no incidents to date.— C. G. Rowland *et al.* (letter), *ibid.,* 2, 468.

Adverse Effects, Treatment, and Precautions

As for Cyclophosphamide, p.610. Toxic effects on the urinary tract may be more severe with ifosfamide. Central nervous system side-effects have been reported, especially confusion and lethargy.

For the use of mesna to reduce ifosfamide-induced bladder toxicity, see Mesna, p.842.
Severe hypokalaemia in 4 patients (fatal in 1) associated with treatment with ifosfamide and mesna.— D. J. Husband and S. W. Watkin (letter), *Lancet,* 1988, *1,* 1116.

EFFECTS ON THE KIDNEYS. Therapy with ifosfamide may be associated with life-threatening nephrotoxicity. Results in *rats* suggested that the mechanism might involve generation of toxic metabolites within the kidney.— M. I. Graham *et al., Hum. Toxicol.,* 1985, *4,* 545.

EFFECTS ON THE NERVOUS SYSTEM. For a discussion of severe encephalopathy associated with the administration of ifosfamide with mesna, see Mesna, p.842. The nomogram proposed by Meanwell *et al.* (*Lancet,* 1986, *2,* 406) for prediction of patients at risk from encephalopathy was derived from a 24-hour infusion schedule. Experience in patients given 6-hour infusions suggests that encephalopathy becomes apparent in these patients at lesser degrees of renal and hepatic impairment and modification of the recommendations for exclusion is required.— T. J. Perren *et al.* (letter), *Lancet,* 1987, *1,* 390. Serious central neurotoxicity occurred in 3 of 27 patients receiving mesna with ifosfamide as part of the combination chemotherapy of small-cell lung cancer. All patients had limited disease only and were predicted from the nomogram as having a 90% or better probability of remaining free from encephalopathy. This method of prediction, which has proved useful in other patients, may have little application in evaluating patients with lung cancer.— A. K. McCallum (letter), *ibid.,* 987.

Absorption and Fate

The pharmacokinetics of ifosfamide are similar to those of cyclophosphamide (p.612). Ifosfamide must be metabolised in the liver before it is active.

References to the absorption and fate of ifosfamide: P. J. Creaven *et al., Clin. Pharmac. Ther.,* 1974, *16,* 77; L. M. Allen and P. J. Creaven, *Clin. Pharmac. Ther.,* 1975, *17,* 492; L. M. Allen *et al., Cancer Treat. Rep.,* 1976, *60,* 451; R. L. Nelson *et al., Clin. Pharmac. Ther.,* 1976, *19,* 365.

Uses and Administration

Ifosfamide is used similarly to cyclophosphamide (p.612) in the treatment of a variety of solid tumours.
Ifosfamide is given intravenously, either by injection as a solution diluted to less than 4%, or by infusion. It is usually given in a total dose of 8 to 10 g per m^2 divided over 5 days; alternatively, courses comprising 5 to 6 g per m^2, to a maximum of 10 g, have been given as a single 24-hour infusion. Courses may be repeated at intervals of 2 to 4 weeks, depending on the blood count.
Ifosfamide should be administered in association with mesna (see p.842), and adequate hydration should be maintained, to avoid urological toxicity.

MALIGNANT NEOPLASMS OF THE BRONCHUS AND LUNG. Despite the suggestion that ifosfamide is active in the single agent therapy of non-small-cell lung cancer none of 17 patients obtained a complete response when treated with ifosfamide 5 g per m^2 body-surface as a 24-hour infusion. Ifosfamide was given concurrently with mesna 3 g per m^2; a further 3 g of mesna per m^2 was given over the ensuing 12 hours. There were 2 partial responses in patients with squamous-cell tumours but 6 patients had progressive disease. The median survival was only 5½ months which is very similar to that previously described for untreated patients. In view of these disappointing results ifosfamide cannot be recommended as a single agent in non-small-cell cancer.— M. D. Peake and D. Parker (letter), *Lancet,* 1985, *2,* 496.

Proprietary Preparations

Mitoxana *(Boehringer Ingelheim, UK). Injection,* powder for reconstitution, ifosfamide 0.5, 1, or 2 g.

Proprietary Names and Manufacturers

Holoxan *(Lucien, Fr.; Asta Pharma, Ger.; Schering, Ital.; Neth.; Degussa, Switz.)*; Mitoxana *(Boehringer Ingelheim, UK)*; Tronoxal *(Funk, Spain)*.

12846-d

Improsulfan Tosylate

864T; Improsulfan Tosilate *(rINNM)*; NSC-140117.
Iminodipropyl dimethanesulphonate 4-toluenesulphonate.
$C_8H_{19}NO_6S_2,C_7H_8O_3S$=461.6.

CAS — 13425-98-4 (improsulfan); 32784-82-0 (tosylate).

Improsulfan is an alkylating agent structurally related to busulphan (p.603). It has been used as the tosylate in the management of chronic granulocytic (myeloid) leukaemia. The usual initial dose is 30 to 90 mg of the tosylate by mouth daily in 3 divided doses, adjusted according to response and haematological toxicity. Doses of 20 to 60 mg daily have been given for maintenance therapy.

Proprietary Names and Manufacturers
Protecton *(Jpn)*.

16854-s

Interleukin-2

Epidermal Thymocyte Activating Factor; ETAF; IL-2; T-cell Growth Factor. A naturally-occurring 133-amino-acid glycoprotein with a molecular weight of about 15 000. It is available from natural sources or as a product of recombinant DNA technology (rIL-2).

Units
100 units of human interleukin-2 are contained in one ampoule of the first International Standard Preparation (1987).

Adverse Effects

Decreased vascular resistance and increased capillary permeability occur in patients given interleukin-2; fluid replacement may be necessary to treat the resultant hypovolaemia. Hypotension, fluid retention and weight gain, renal abnormalities including uraemia and oliguria, hyperbilirubinaemia, gastro-intestinal disturbances, fever, rashes, anaemia and thrombocytopenia, headache, confusion, disorientation, and drowsiness are relatively common, particularly at high doses. Cardiac disorders, including myocardial infarction, have occurred. Toxicity is dose-related and may be severe; fatalities have been recorded.

A study of the effects of interleukin-2 on renal function. Interleukin-2 therapy in 99 consecutive patients was associated with varying degrees of acute renal dysfunction in almost all patients. The clinical syndrome of hypotension, oliguria, fluid retention and associated azotaemia with intense tubular avidity for filtered sodium all support prerenal acute renal failure as the cause of renal dysfunction. However, renal function values returned to baseline levels within 7 days in 62% of patients and in 95% by 30 days. Patients with elevated pretreatment serum-creatinine values, particularly those aged over 60 years, and those who had previously undergone a nephrectomy, were at risk of more severe and prolonged changes in renal function, and might be particularly vulnerable to the use of indomethacin for associated fever and chills, which might potentiate renal impairment through its effects on intrarenal prostaglandin production.— A. Belldegrun *et al., Ann. intern. Med.,* 1987, *106,* 817.

Uses and Administration

Interleukin-2 is a lymphokine which stimulates the proliferation of T-lymphocytes and thus amplifies immune response to an antigen; it also has actions on B-lymphocytes, and induces the production of interferon-γ and the activation of natural killer cells.
Interleukin-2 has been investigated in the adoptive immunotherapy of various malignant neoplasms. It has been given together with lymphokine-activated killer cells (LAK) in usual doses of 100 000 units per kg body-weight intravenously every 8 hours.
Interleukin-2 has also been tried in patients with the acquired immune deficiency syndrome (AIDS) in an attempt to restore immune response.
Other lymphokines such as teceleukin (*N*-methionylinterleukin-2), interleukin-1, and interleukin-3 are under investigation (see also p.1580).

Reviews of the use of lymphokines and immunomodulators, including interleukin-2: D. W. Horohov and J. P. Siegel, *Drugs,* 1987, *33,* 289; *Ann. intern. Med.,* 1987, *106,* 257; *ibid.,* 421.

AIDS. Interleukin-2 partially restored proliferation response and natural killer cell activity of lymphocytes from AIDS patients *in vitro*. Clinical trials appear warranted.— J. D. Lifson *et al.*, *Lancet.*, 1984, *1*, 698.

Interleukin-2 might be used with suramin in patients with AIDS.— S. Broder *et al.*, *Lancet*, 1985, *2*, 627.

Studies in patients with AIDS given up to 2.5 million units of recombinant interleukin-2 daily by continuous 24-hour infusion, for 5 days per week over 4 to 8 weeks, found a temporary elevation in the numbers of T_4 lymphocytes, an increase in spontaneous lymphocyte proliferation, decreased isolation of the human immunodeficiency virus (HIV), and minor regressions of Kaposi's sarcoma. Although no patient has had a long-lasting reconstitution of the immune response it is thought that a combination of antiretroviral therapy with appropriate immunological enhancement, whether bone-marrow transplantation, lymphocyte transfusion, or treatment with biological response modifiers such as interleukin 2 holds the best hope of controlling the disease in patients with full-blown AIDS.— A. S. Fauci, in V.T. DeVita (Moderator), *Developmental Therapeutics and the Acquired Immunodeficiency Syndrome, Ann. intern. Med.*, 1987, *106*, 568.

MALIGNANT NEOPLASMS. A report of the use of interleukin-2 and lymphokine-activated killer cells in 25 patients with metastatic cancer resistant to conventional therapy. Patients underwent daily leucaphaeresis, usually for 5 days, and the cells were cultured with interleukin-2 to produce lymphokine-activated killer cells, which were subsequently infused intravenously over 3 days. Recombinant interleukin-2 diluted in 50 mL of sodium chloride injection (0.9%) containing 5% human serum albumin was given in doses of 10 000, 30 000, or 100 000 units per kg body-weight by intravenous infusion every 8 hours, beginning at the time of the first cell infusion, and continued for several days, depending on tolerance. The 2-week cycle of leucaphaeresis and reinfusion was repeated, beginning in the third week, in most patients. The cumulative doses received varied from 280 000 to 3 320 000 units of interleukin-2 per kg, and from 1.8 to 18.4×10^{10} killer cells. Measurable tumour regression occurred in 11 patients; complete response occurred in 1 patient with malignant melanoma, who has remained disease-free for 10 months. Although toxicity was severe, adverse effects disappeared promptly after interleukin-2 treatment ended. The results offer the hope of an effective new therapy against a wide variety of tumours.— S. A. Rosenberg *et al.*, *New Engl. J. Med.*, 1985, *313*, 1485. A further progress report in 108 consecutive patients, including the 25 reported on above, treated with interleukin-2 and killer cells and 49 treated with interleukin-2 alone. Of the 106 evaluable patients given the combined treatment, 8 had total regression of all cancer, 15 had a partial response of more than 50% tumour reduction, and 10 had a 25% to 50% tumour reduction. There was some evidence of a variation in response with type of cancer: responses were seen in 12 of 36 patients with renal-cell cancer, 6 of 26 with melanoma, 3 of 26 with colorectal cancer and both of 2 with non-Hodgkin's lymphoma. Of the 46 evaluable patients given interleukin-2 alone 1 had a complete response, 5 a partial response, and 1 a minor response. Toxic effects were severe but transient. Until the ultimate role of this therapy, if any, in the treatment of cancer is determined it should be regarded as an experimental approach in selected patients for whom no effective therapy is available.— S. A. Rosenberg *et al.*, *ibid.*, 1987, *316*, 889. Severe criticism. The demonstrated anticancer activity of this regimen is less than sensational, and the criteria used for regression were less stringent than they might have been. Furthermore, the toxicity is severe, and the cost prohibitive, and in view of the marginal therapeutic gain this specific adoptive immunotherapy would not seem to merit further clinical application.— C. G. Moertel (letter), *ibid.*, 274.

In a study in 40 patients with metastatic cancer refractory to standard therapy recombinant interleukin-2 was given by continuous intravenous infusion over 24 hours in 5-day cycles, accompanied, after the first priming cycle, by lymphokine-activated killer cells cultured after leucaphaeresis. Patients received doses of interleukin-2 of between 1000 000 and 7000 000 units per m^2 body-surface daily; an initial dose of 3000 000 units per m^2 appeared to produce optimal lymphocytosis for leucaphaeresis and the most beneficial regimen appeared to comprise 2 cycles of interleukin-2 beginning at this dose and increased to 5000 000 units per m^2, with 1 day of rest and 4 days of leucaphaeresis intervening. These cycles were repeated after 2 to 4 weeks rest. There were 13 partial and 2 minor responses among patients so treated. Administration of interleukin-2 by constant infusion rather than as a bolus appears to yield antineoplastic responses without such severe toxicity as seen with the latter method.— W. H. West *et al.*, *New Engl. J. Med.*, 1987, *316*, 898.

Enormous interest and controversy have surrounded the use of adoptive immunotherapy for cancer. The responses reported have been substantial, in cancers notorious for resistance to standard therapy, and although toxicity is also severe the experience with continuous infusion is encouraging. The reports so far do not describe practical approaches suitable for widespread application but if lymphokine-activated killer cells are truly contributing to the responses observed, as they appear to be, then this therapy represents a successful manipulation of the cellular immune system to treat malignant disease, and may open the way to effective immunotherapy of cancer.— J. R. Durant, *New Engl. J. Med.*, 1987, *316*, 939.

VIRAL INFECTIONS. A report of the response of chronic active Epstein-Barr virus infection to treatment with recombinant interleukin-2.— K. Kawa-Ha *et al.* (letter), *Lancet*, 1987, *1*, 154.

See also under AIDS, above.

18653-c

Iproplatin *(BAN, USAN, rINN).*

CHIP; JM-9; NSC-256927. *bc*-Dichloro-*af*-dihydroxy-*de*-bis(isopropylamino)platinum.
$C_6H_{20}Cl_2N_2O_2Pt = 418.2$.

CAS — 62928-11-4.

Adverse Effects and Precautions

As for Cisplatin, p.607. Nephrotoxicity is reportedly less severe than with cisplatin.

Uses and Administration

Iproplatin is an analogue of cisplatin (p.607) with antineoplastic properties, that has been investigated in the treatment of a variety of malignant neoplasms in doses of 180 to 350 mg per m^2 body-surface intravenously every 4 weeks.

References: W. S. F. Wong *et al.*, *J. R. Soc. Med.*, 1985, *78*, 203 (malignant neoplasms of the fallopian tube).

For mention of the use of iproplatin in cervical cancer, see under Carboplatin, p.605.

Proprietary Names and Manufacturers

Bristol-Myers, UK.

1841-k

Lomustine *(BAN, USAN, rINN).*

CCNU; NSC-79037; RB-1509; WR-139017. 1-(2-Chloroethyl)-3-cyclohexyl-1-nitrosourea.
$C_9H_{16}ClN_3O_2 = 233.7$.

CAS — 13010-47-4.

Pharmacopoeias. In *Br.*

A yellow crystalline powder. M.p. 88 to 90°. Practically **insoluble** in water; soluble in alcohol; freely soluble in acetone and in chloroform.

Adverse Effects, Treatment, and Precautions

As for Carmustine, p.605, although bone-marrow depression may be even more delayed with lomustine. Neurological reactions such as confusion and lethargy have been reported.

EFFECTS ON THE LUNGS. For a review of pulmonary fibrosis associated with the nitrosoureas, including lomustine, see under Carmustine, p.605.

INTERACTIONS. *Theophylline.* Leucopenia and thrombocytopenia in a 45-year-old woman are believed to have been secondary to an interaction between theophylline and lomustine.— P. M. Zeltzer and S. A. Feig (letter), *Lancet*, 1979, *2*, 960.

Absorption and Fate

Lomustine is absorbed from the gastro-intestinal tract and is rapidly metabolised; metabolites have a prolonged plasma half-life reported to range from 16 to 48 hours. Active metabolites readily cross the blood-brain barrier and appear in the cerebrospinal fluid. About half a dose is excreted as metabolites in the urine within 24 hours but less than 75% is excreted within 4 days.

For a review of the pharmacokinetics of the nitrosoureas, see under Carmustine, p.606.

Uses and Administration

Lomustine is a nitrosourea with actions and uses similar to those of carmustine (p.606). It has been used in the treatment of brain tumours and Hodgkin's disease, and also lung cancer, malignant melanoma, and various solid tumours.

Lomustine is given by mouth to adults and children as a single dose of 130 mg per m^2 body-surface. A dose of 100 mg per m^2 should be given to patients with compromised bone-marrow function. Doses are also generally reduced when lomustine is given as part of a combination regimen. Providing blood counts have returned to acceptable levels, that is, platelets above 100 000 per mm^3 and leucocytes above 4000 per mm^3, doses may be repeated every 6 weeks, and should be adjusted according to the haematological response.

MALIGNANT NEOPLASMS OF THE KIDNEY. Lomustine produced an objective remission lasting from 3 to 6 months in 4 of 20 patients with renal cell carcinoma.— A. Mittelman *et al.*, *J. Am. med. Ass.*, 1973, *225*, 32.

Preparations

Lomustine Capsules *(B.P.)*

Proprietary Preparations

CCNU Lundbeck *(Lundbeck, UK). Capsules*, lomustine 10 and 40 mg.

Proprietary Names and Manufacturers

Belustine *(Bellon, Fr.; Rhone-Poulenc, Ital.)*; CCNU *(Rhône-Poulenc, Ger.; Lundbeck, UK)*; Cecenu *(Belg.; Medac, Ger.; Neth.)*; CeeNU *(Bristol-Myers, Austral.; Bristol, Canad.; Bristol, S.Afr.; Bristol-Myers Pharmaceuticals, UK; Bristol-Myers Onocology, USA)*; CiNU *(Bristol, Switz.)*; Lucostine *(Lundbeck, Denm.; Lundbeck, Norw.; Lundbeck, Swed.)*.

1842-a

Mannomustine Hydrochloride *(BANM, rINNM).*

BCM; Mannitol Mustard; NSC-9698. 1,6-Bis(2-chloroethylamino)-1,6-dideoxy-D-mannitol dihydrochloride.
$C_{10}H_{22}Cl_2N_2O_4,2HCl = 378.1$.

CAS — 576-68-1 (mannomustine); 551-74-6 (hydrochloride).

Pharmacopoeias. In *B.P.C 1973.*

Mannomustine hydrochloride is an antineoplastic agent with the general properties of mustine, p.645. It has been given in the treatment of various malignant diseases by intravenous injection in doses of 50 to 100 mg daily or on alternate days. It has also been given as an intravenous infusion in doses of 100 to 200 mg on alternate days.

It has also been given by mouth in doses of 50 to 100 mg.

Preparations

Mannomustine Injection *(B.P.C. 1973).* Mannomustine Hydrochloride Injection. A sterile solution of mannomustine hydrochloride prepared by dissolving, shortly before use, the sterile contents of a sealed container in sodium chloride injection (0.9%). The injection deteriorates on storage and it must be used within 24 hours of preparation.

Proprietary Names and Manufacturers

Degranol *(Landerlan, Spain; Sinclair, UK).*

1843-t

Melphalan *(BAN, USAN, rINN).*

CB-3025; NSC-8806 *(hydrochloride)*; PAM; Phenylalanine Nitrogen Mustard; WR-19813. 4-Bis(2-chloroethyl)amino-L-phenylalanine.
$C_{13}H_{18}Cl_2N_2O_2 = 305.2$.

CAS — 148-82-3.

NOTE. Merphalan (CB-3007; NSC-14210; sarcolysine) is the racemic form of melphalan; Medphalan (CB-3026; NSC-35051) is the D-isomer of melphalan.

Pharmacopoeias. In *Br.* and *U.S.* Sarcolysini Hydrochloridum (*Int. P.*) and Sarcolysinum (*Rus. P.*) are the hydrochlorides of merphalan. *Chin. P.* includes Formylmerphalanum, and Methoxymerphalanum.

A white to buff-coloured powder, odourless or with a faint odour. It loses not more than 7% of its weight on drying.

Practically **insoluble** in water, chloroform, and ether; slightly soluble in alcohol and methyl alcohol; dissolves in dilute mineral acids. **Store** at a temperature not exceeding 25° in airtight containers. Protect from light.

STABILITY IN SOLUTION. A study of the stability of melphalan 40 and 400 μg per mL in infusion fluids. The time for a 10% loss of drug at 20° in sodium chloride injection (0.9%) was 4.5 hours, compared with 2.9 hours in lactated Ringer's injection, which has a considerably lower chloride ion content, and only 1.5 hours in glucose injection (5%). At 25° the corresponding figures were 2.4, 1.5, and 0.6 hours, and at 37° they were 0.6, 0.4, and 0.3 hours. It was concluded that melphalan is sufficiently stable at 20° in sodium chloride injection to permit infusion, but that increased temperature and decreased chloride ion concentration were associated with faster degradation rates: when heated perfusate is used the extent and time of pre-heating must be considered in dose determination.— S. E. Tabibi and J. C. Cradock, *Am. J. Hosp. Pharm.*, 1984, *41*, 1380.

A further study of stability of melphalan. There was a 5% loss of activity from a solution containing 20 μg per mL when it was stored for 1.5 hours at 21.5°; however when stored at -7° the time for a 5% loss was about 20 to 30 days and it was calculated that at -20° and -35° the time to 5% loss would be 14.3 and 10.9 months respectively. Freezing and thawing of the solution had minimal effect on melphalan concentration, as did filtration. It was suggested that melphalan be handled at temperatures greater than 5° for the minimum of time but that solutions can be stored for at least 6 or possibly up to 12 months at -20° without significant deterioration.— A. G. Bosanquet, *J. pharm. Sci.*, 1985, *74*, 348.

Adverse Effects and Treatment

For an outline of the adverse effects experienced with antineoplastic agents and immunosuppressants and general guidelines for their treatment, see Antineoplastic Agents, p.580 and p.583.

The onset of neutropenia and thrombocytopenia is variable; maximum bone-marrow depression has been reported 2 to 3 weeks after starting treatment with melphalan but has also occurred after only 5 days. Recovery may be prolonged.

Skin rashes and allergic reactions may occur. Haemolytic anaemia, vasculitis, and pulmonary fibrosis have been reported. As with other alkylating agents, melphalan also has carcinogenic, mutagenic, and teratogenic potential.

Adverse effects resulting from regional perfusion include oedema, neurotoxicity, and vesiculation of the skin.

CARCINOGENICITY. For reference to a study suggesting that melphalan may be more likely to induce secondary leukaemias than cyclophosphamide, see Cyclophosphamide, p.610.

EFFECTS ON THE REPRODUCTIVE SYSTEM. A report of primary ovarian failure in 3 adolescents given high-dose melphalan.— S. J. Kellie and J. E. Kingston (letter), *Lancet*, 1987, *1*, 1425.

OVERDOSAGE. A 12-month old child given melphalan 140 mg (a 10-fold overdose) intravenously developed pronounced lymphopenia within 24 hours but had no other significant adverse effects until the 7th day, when neutropenia, thrombocytopenia, oral ulceration, and diarrhoea developed. Bone marrow recovered within 40 days. Treatment was by vigorous hyperalimentation and close surveillance during the period of suppression and the patient has subsequently remained well 9 months afterwards, without complications.— T. D. Coates (letter), *Lancet*, 1984, *2*, 1048.

Precautions

For reference to the precautions necessary with antineoplastic agents and immunosuppressants, see Antineoplastic Agents, p.583.

When melphalan is given to patients with impaired renal function, urea concentrations should be monitored and dosage reduction considered.

HANDLING AND DISPOSAL. When handling urine and faeces from patients receiving melphalan protective clothing should be worn for up to 48 hours, and 7 days (after an oral dose), respectively, after therapy.— J. Harris and L. J. Dodds, *Pharm. J.*, 1985, *2*, 289.

INTERACTIONS. Severe renal failure developed in 13 of 17 patients given high-dose intravenous melphalan followed by standard oral doses of cyclosporin. There were no cases of renal failure in 7 similar patients given high-dose melphalan alone, and nephrotoxicity with cyclosporin alone is generally mild or moderate. The mechanism of the interaction was unknown but it was potentially dangerous.— G. R. Morgenstern (letter), *Lancet*, 1982, *2*, 1342.

With diagnostic tests. Melphalan could produce a false positive response to the Coombs' test.— P. D. Hansten, *Am. J. Hosp. Pharm.*, 1971, *28*, 629.

Absorption and Fate

Absorption of melphalan from the gastro-intestinal tract is reported to be variable. Following absorption it is rapidly distributed throughout body water and has been reported to be inactivated mainly by spontaneous hydrolysis. It is excreted in the urine, about 10% as unchanged drug. About 50 to 60% of an absorbed dose has been stated to be protein bound initially, increasing to 80 to 90% after 12 hours.

In a study involving 9 cancer patients, melphalan rapidly disappeared from the plasma after the intravenous injection of 600 μg per kg body-weight. Composite plasma α-half-life was 7.7 minutes and β-half-life was 107.6 minutes. The mean 24-hour urinary excretion of melphalan was 13% of the administered dose. The results differ from those reported by M.H.N. Tattersall *et al.* (*Eur. J. Cancer*, 1978, *14*, 507). In 2 patients given labelled melphalan, monohydroxy and dihydroxy melphalan products made up a large portion of the drug found in plasma and urine samples up to 24 hours after administration.— D. S. Alberts *et al.*, *Clin. Pharmac. Ther.*, 1979, *26*, 73. A further study in 14 cancer patients given single doses of 600 μg per kg by mouth or intravenously. The systemic availability of melphalan given as tablets or oral solution was extremely variable, the first appearance in plasma ranging from a few minutes to 6 hours after a dose. In one patient melphalan did not appear in the plasma or urine. Monohydroxy and dihydroxy derivatives were detected in the plasma within 30 minutes of an oral dose. Spontaneous degradation rather than enzymatic metabolism may be the major determinant of plasma half-life. The mean plasma terminal phase half-life for 12 patients given melphalan by mouth was 90 minutes and mean 24-hour urinary excretion was 10.9% of the total dose; the mean peak plasma concentration was 280 ng per mL (range 70 to 630 ng per mL). In 5 of the patients half-lives after administration of melphalan by mouth were similar to those achieved after intravenous injection but the mean area under the plasma concentration time curve was less than 60% of that after an intravenous dose; 24-hour urinary excretion was 28% of the oral dose and 56.4% of the intravenous dose. It is considered that variability in the bioavailability of oral melphalan might help to explain the variability in response to treatment and, if there is no evidence of myelosuppression or antitumour effect after increased dosage, melphalan should be given intravenously or replaced by another alkylating agent.— D. S. Alberts *et al.*, *Clin. Pharmac. Ther.*, 1979, *26*, 737.

Uses and Administration

Melphalan is an antineoplastic agent derived from mustine (p.645) and has a similar mode of action. It is used mainly in the treatment of multiple myeloma. Melphalan is also given to patients with carcinoma of the breast and ovary and has been administered by intra-arterial regional perfusion for malignant melanoma and soft-tissue sarcomas. It has immunosuppressant properties and has been used in the treatment of auto-immune disorders. Melphalan is usually given by mouth; it is also administered intravenously.

See also under Choice of Antineoplastic Agent, p.584.

Numerous regimens have been tried for the treatment of multiple myeloma and there is still controversy as to the best schedule. Oral dosage regimens include: 150 μg per kg body-weight daily for 4 to 7 days, combined with prednisone 40 to 60 mg daily; or melphalan 250 μg per kg for 4 to 5 days; or 6 mg daily for 2 to 3 weeks. Courses are followed by a rest period of up to 6 weeks to allow recovery of haematological function and are then either repeated, or maintenance therapy is instituted, usually with a daily dose of 2 to 4 mg, or 50 μg per kg. For optimum effect, therapy is usually adjusted to produce a moderate leucopenia, with white cell counts in the range 3000 to 3500 per mm^3.

In the treatment of breast cancer, suggested doses of melphalan are 200 to 300 μg per kg daily or 6 mg per m^2 body-surface daily for 4 to 6 days, repeated every 3 to 6 weeks. Doses of 200 μg per kg for 5 days every 4 to 6 weeks, have been given to patients with ovarian carcinoma.

Melphalan should not be given if the platelet count falls below 75 000 per mm^3 or the neutrophil count below 2000 per mm^3. During administration of melphalan, frequent blood counts are essential, especially during continuous administration. It should not be given with radiotherapy or if the neutrophil count has recently been depressed by chemotherapy or radiotherapy.

Melphalan is also given intravenously; a single dose of 1 mg per kg, repeated in 8 weeks if the platelet and neutrophil counts are normal has been given in ovarian adenocarcinoma. It may be infused in sodium chloride injection (0.9%) or injected into the tubing of a fast-running drip; when given by infusion the same solution should not be used for more than 2 hours and prolonged infusions should be carried out with several batches of solution, each freshly prepared.

ACCELERATION OF BONE-MARROW RECOVERY. For reference to the accelerating effect of cyclophosphamide priming on bone-marrow recovery following high doses of melphalan, see Cyclophosphamide, p.612.

ADMINISTRATION. A report of the intraperitoneal administration of melphalan to 19 patients with gastro-intestinal or ovarian tumours involving the peritoneal cavity. Doses of 30 mg per m^2 body-surface were given initially, in 2 litres of sodium chloride injection (0.9%) and allowed to dwell in the abdominal cavity for 4 hours before being drained. The dose was repeated every 4 weeks or when toxicity permitted and was increased in 10 mg per m^2 increments. Myelosuppression was the dose-limiting toxicity, and the maximum tolerable dose was found to be 70 mg per m^2. Total drug exposure was on average 65 times greater for the peritoneal cavity than for plasma. However, of 14 evaluable patients, all with ovarian carcinoma, only 1 had a response, and further studies are required to see whether the pharmacological advantage of the route will produce a clinical advantage.— S. B. Howell *et al.*, *Ann. intern. Med.*, 1984, *101*, 14.

In renal failure. Melphalan may be given in normal doses to patients with renal failure.— W. M. Bennett *et al.*, *Am. J. Kidney Dis.*, 1983, *3*, 155. But see Precautions (above).

AMYLOIDOSIS. Discussions of the treatment of amyloidosis with reference to the use of melphalan with prednisone: R. A. Kyle and P. R. Greipp, *Mayo Clin. Proc.*, 1983, *58*, 665; M. A. Gertz and R. A. Kyle, *ibid.*, 1986, *61*, 218. See also R. A. Sheehan-Dare and A. V. Simmons, *Postgrad. med. J.*, 1987, *63*, 141 (prednisolone and melphalan in combined amyloidosis and myeloma).

BONE DISORDERS, NON-MALIGNANT. A patient with fibrogenesis imperfecta ossium, a progressive abnormality of bone structure leading to bone pain and fractures, responded to treatment with melphalan 10 mg and prednisolone 20 mg daily, in 7-day courses.— T. C. B. Stamp *et al.* (letter), *Lancet*, 1985, *1*, 582.

MALIGNANT NEOPLASMS OF THE BREAST. In a study involving 370 patients who had undergone surgery for breast cancer, adjuvant therapy with melphalan in 187 had no significant effect on survival, regardless of menopausal status or axillary node involvement, when compared with no adjuvant treatment in the remainder. Patients receiving melphalan were given 6 mg per m^2, to a maximum of 10 mg, daily for 5 days, by mouth. This was repeated every 6 weeks for 16 cycles. The results indicate that melphalan has no place in the adjuvant therapy of early breast cancer.— R. D. Rubens *et al.*, *Lancet*, 1983, *1*, 839. Comment. Nearly 80% of the patients in the study did not experience myelosuppression, suggesting that absorption of the drug may have been incomplete and hence the dosage absorbed inadequate. At the authors' institution dosage of adjuvant melphalan is now routinely adjusted to produce myelosuppression. Without an analysis of patients who experienced myelosuppression compared with those who did not, conclusions about the efficacy of adjuvant melphalan may be premature.— J. T. Carpenter and W. A. Maddox (letter), *ibid.*, *2*, 450.

MYELOMA. A report of the use of high-dose intravenous melphalan in 8 patients with myeloma and 1 with plasma-cell leukaemia. Patients received melphalan 100 to 140 mg per m^2 body-surface intravenously. Five of the 9 patients had not received previous chemotherapy and 3 of these, including the patient with plasma-cell leukaemia, achieved complete remission. Results were less striking in patients who had had previous treatment but 2 had a distinct improvement in disease that had been resistant to conventional drugs. All patients with bone pain had rapid and lasting relief. A longer period will be required to assess the durability of remissions; however the patient with plasma-cell leukaemia has survived 30 months from initial treatment, despite relapse and re-induction of remission, which compares with a median survival of 2 months reported for conventional treatment.— T. J. McElwain and R. L. Powles, *Lancet*, 1983, *2*, 822. Comment, and mention of the use of high-dose oral melphalan for multiple myeloma.— M. Cavo *et al.* (letter), *ibid.*, 1194.

See also under Choice of Antineoplastic Agent, p.593.

Preparations

Melphalan Injection *(B.P.)*. A sterile solution of melphalan hydrochloride prepared immediately before use by completely dissolving the contents of a sealed container containing melphalan in the required amount of alcohol (96%) containing 2% of hydrogen chloride, and diluting the resulting solution with the requisite amount of a solution containing dibasic potassium phosphate 1.2% dissolved in a solution of propylene glycol 60% v/v in water for injections. A 1% injection has a pH of 6 to 7. It deteriorates on storage. Potency is expressed in terms of the equivalent amount of anhydrous melphalan.

Melphalan Tablets *(B.P., U.S.P.)*

Proprietary Preparations

Alkeran *(Calmic, UK)*. *Tablets*, melphalan 2 and 5 mg. *Injection*, powder for reconstitution, melphalan 100 mg, supplied with solvent and diluent.

Proprietary Names and Manufacturers

Alkeran *(Wellcome, Austral.; Belg.; Wellcome, Canad.; Wellcome, Denm.; Wellcome, Fr.; Wellcome, Ger.; Wellcome, Ital.; Neth.; Wellcome, Norw.; Wellcome, S.Afr.; Wellcome, Swed.; Wellcome, Switz.; Calmic, UK; Wellcome, USA)*; Alkerana *(Arg.)*.

1844-x

Mercaptopurine *(BAN, USAN, rINN)*.

6MP; Mercaptopurinum; NSC-755; Purinethiol; WR-2785. 6-Mercaptopurine monohydrate; Purine-6-thiol monohydrate; 1,7-Dihydro-6*H*-purine-6-thione monohydrate.

$C_5H_4N_4S,H_2O = 170.2$.

CAS — 6112-76-1; 50-44-2 (anhydrous).

Pharmacopoeias. In *Belg., Br., Chin., Cz., Egypt., Eur., Fr., Ind., Int., It., Jpn, Jug., Neth., Nord., Rus., Swiss, Turk.*, and *U.S.*

A yellow, odourless or almost odourless, crystalline powder.

Practically **insoluble** in water, acetone, and ether; slightly soluble in alcohol; soluble in hot alcohol and in solutions of alkali hydroxides; slightly soluble in M sulphuric acid. **Store** in well-closed containers. Protect from light.

Adverse Effects and Treatment

For an outline of the adverse effects experienced with antineoplastic agents and immunosuppressants and general guidelines for their treatment, see Antineoplastic Agents, p.580 and p.583.

Bone-marrow depression with mercaptopurine may be delayed; hypoplasia may occur. Mercaptopurine is less toxic to the gastro-intestinal tract than the folic acid antagonists or fluorouracil. Hepatotoxicity has been reported, with cholestatic jaundice and necrosis, sometimes fatal. Crystalluria with haematuria has been observed rarely as have skin disorders. Fever may occur.

Mercaptopurine is potentially carcinogenic and mutagenic; an increased incidence of abortion has occurred in women given mercaptopurine during the first trimester of pregnancy.

ALLERGY AND ANAPHYLAXIS. For a report of fever and rigors in a patient taking mercaptopurine, see Azathioprine, p.600.

EFFECTS ON THE BLOOD. The degree of neutropenia in 22 children receiving mercaptopurine correlated with the erythrocyte concentration of the metabolite thioguanine nucleotide.— L. Lennard *et al.*, *Br. J. clin. Pharmac.*, 1983, *16*, 359. Measurement of thioguanine nucleotide in erythrocytes from patients receiving azathioprine, mercaptopurine, and thioguanine now permits prediction of bone-marrow toxicity when using these drugs.— J. L. Maddocks *et al.* (letter), *Lancet*, 1986, *1*, 156.

EFFECTS ON THE SKIN. Multiple pigmented naevi occurred in 4 children given mercaptopurine as part of a combination regimen.— H. Ippen and G. Prindull (letter), *Br. med. J.*, 1984, *289*, 734.

OVERDOSAGE. A 15-year-old 75-kg girl who had been taking mercaptopurine and prednisone for 2½ years for chronic hepatitis took an alleged overdose of twenty tablets of mercaptopurine 75 mg (a total of 1.5 g). About 80 minutes later her only symptoms were dizziness, frontal headache, and right-upper-quadrant pain. They soon resolved and physical examination revealed nothing abnormal. She had a marginal increase in serum bilirubin but her white blood cell count remained normal. Ipecacuanha induced vomiting 90 minutes after the overdose but no tablet fragments were seen; 5½ hours after the overdose she was given sodium sulphate, charcoal, and oral fluids. Mercaptopurine was removed from her treatment regimen and 9 months after the incident she appeared to be in good health with no exacerbation of her hepatitis and no adverse reaction to the drug overdose. A similar lack of toxic manifestations was noted by Carney *et al.* (*Am. J. med.*, 1974, *56*, 133) in a patient who received 7.5 g of azathioprine. Aggressive measures do not seem to be warranted in mercaptopurine or azathioprine overdosage.— D. Hendrick and B. L. Mirkin (letter), *Lancet*, 1984, *1*, 277.

Precautions

For reference to the precautions necessary with antineoplastic agents and immunosuppressants, see Antineoplastic Agents, p.583.

Mercaptopurine should be used with care in patients with impaired hepatic or renal function. The effects of mercaptopurine are enhanced by allopurinol and the dose of mercaptopurine should be reduced to about one-quarter when allopurinol is given concomitantly.

Results in 12 boys and 10 girls receiving mercaptopurine as part of maintenance therapy for lymphoblastic leukaemia suggested that girls developed mercaptopurine-mediated cytotoxicity more readily and more predictably than boys.— J. S. Lilleyman *et al.*, *Br. J. Cancer*, 1984, *49*, 703.

HANDLING AND DISPOSAL. When handling urine and faeces from patients receiving mercaptopurine protective clothing should be worn for up to 48 hours and 5 days respectively after therapy.— J. Harris; L. J. Dodds, *Pharm. J.*, 1985, *2*, 289.

INTERACTIONS. *Allopurinol.* Mercaptopurine plasma concentrations were markedly increased by allopurinol when mercaptopurine was given by mouth but not when it was given intravenously. The results appear to indicate that allopurinol inhibits the first-pass metabolism of mercaptopurine.— S. Zimm *et al.*, *Clin. Pharmac. Ther.*, 1983, *34*, 810. See also: J. J. Coffey *et al.*, *Cancer Res.*, 1972, *32*, 1283.

Anticoagulants. For a report of mercaptopurine diminishing the activity of warfarin, see Warfarin Sodium, p.346.

Interactions with diagnostic tests. Mercaptopurine has been reported to produce elevated results for determinations of serum alanine aminotransferase and bilirubin, and falsely to decrease values for uric acid determinations.

PORPHYRIA. Mercaptopurine was considered to be unsafe in patients with acute porphyria because it has been shown to be porphyrinogenic in *animals* or *in vitro* systems.— M.R. Moore and K.E.L. McColl, *Porphyrias, Drug Lists*, Glasgow, Porphyria Research Unit, University of Glasgow, 1987.

PREGNANCY AND THE NEONATE. *First trimester.* When given mercaptopurine during pregnancy, 7 women produced normal infants and so did 3 women on busulphan, but 1 woman given both mercaptopurine and busulphan in the first trimester produced an infant with multiple deformities.— J. Sokal and E. Lessmann, *J. Am. med. Ass.*, 1960, *172*, 1765. A woman who was receiving treatment with mercaptopurine, 50 mg twice daily for acute myeloblastic leukaemia, became pregnant and while continuing treatment with mercaptopurine and prednisone gave birth at 32 weeks to an infant with no malformations but with an abnormal blood picture similar to micro-angiopathic haemolytic anaemia. This gradually improved and he made good progress.— J. B. McConnell and R. Bhoola, *Postgrad. med. J.*, 1973, *49*, 211.

See also Adverse Effects, above.

Absorption and Fate

Mercaptopurine is variably and incompletely absorbed from the gastro-intestinal tract; about 50% of an oral dose has been reported to be absorbed, but the absolute bioavailability is somewhat lower, probably due to gastro-intestinal or first-pass metabolism. Once absorbed it is widely distributed throughout body water and tissues. Plasma half-lives ranging from about 10 to 90 minutes have been reported after intravenous injection and the drug is not found in plasma after about 8 hours. Mercaptopurine is activated intracellularly by conversion to nucleotide derivatives. It is rapidly and extensively metabolised in the liver, by methylation and oxidation as well as by the formation of inorganic sulphates. Considerable amounts are oxidised to thiouric acid by the enzyme xanthine oxidase. It is excreted in urine as metabolites and some unchanged drug; about half an oral dose has been recovered in 24 hours. A small proportion is excreted over several weeks.

Mercaptopurine crosses the blood-brain barrier to some extent and is found in the cerebrospinal fluid, but only in subtherapeutic concentrations.

Mean bioavailability of oral mercaptopurine was only 16% in 7 patients given 75 mg per m^2 by mouth and intravenously. Bioavailability and peak plasma concentration were highly variable in these patients.— S. Zimm *et al.*, *New Engl. J. Med.*, 1983, *308*, 1005. Comment and the view that it is premature to recommend the administration of mercaptopurine intravenously in standard regimens. The biochemical pharmacology of mercaptopurine, which requires activation by conversion to thiopurine nucleotides (a process shown to vary widely between patients) may be more important than pharmacokinetic data for the parent drug.— R. W. Rundles and G. B. Elion (letter), *ibid.*, 1984, *310*, 929.

Plasma concentrations of mercaptopurine did not appear to be useful in monitoring the effectiveness of mercaptopurine therapy in a study in 19 children. However, measurement of thioguanine nucleotide concentrations in red blood cells may identify those patients who are likely to fail because of suboptimal therapy.— L. Lennard *et al.*, *Clin. Pharmac. Ther.*, 1986, *40*, 287.

See also under Effects on the Blood, above and Administration, below.

Uses and Administration

Mercaptopurine is an antineoplastic agent which acts as an antimetabolite (p.580). It is an analogue of the natural purines, hypoxanthine and adenine. After the intracellular conversion of mercaptopurine to active nucleotides, including thioinosinic acid, it interferes with nucleic acid synthesis. It also has immunosuppressant properties.

Mercaptopurine is used, usually with other agents, in the treatment of leukaemia. It induces remissions in acute lymphoblastic and non-lymphoblastic leukaemias but other agents are generally preferred and mercaptopurine is chiefly employed in maintenance programmes. It may also be effective in chronic myeloid leukaemia. See also Choice of Antineoplastic Agent, p.587.

There is cross-resistance between mercaptopurine and thioguanine (p.652). Mercaptopurine has been used for its immunosuppressant properties in the treatment of various auto-immune disorders but has been largely replaced by azathioprine.

Mercaptopurine is administered by mouth. The usual initial dose for children and adults is 2.5 mg per kg body-weight daily but the dosage varies according to individual response and tolerance. If there is no clinical improvement and no evidence of white cell depression after 4 weeks, the dose may be cautiously increased up to 5 mg per kg daily. In maintenance schedules the dose may vary from 1.5 to 2.5 mg per kg daily. Blood counts should be taken at least once a week and if there is a steep fall in the white cell count or severe bone-marrow depression the drug should be withdrawn immediately. Therapy may be resumed carefully if the white cell count remains constant for 2 or 3 days or rises.

It has been administered intravenously as mercaptopurine sodium.

ADMINISTRATION. For the low bioavailability associated with oral administration, and the warning that intravenous administration may not be warranted, see under Absorption and Fate, above.

Evidence that some children with acute lymphoblastic leukaemia are more resistant to the effects of mercaptopurine. Failure to induce mild toxicity could lead to inadvertent underdosage in some patients and enable residual leukaemic cells to survive and ultimately re-emerge. For future regimens simple titration in each patient until myelosuppression occurred, rather than administering a ceiling dose could perhaps avoid this.— L. Lennard and J. S. Lilleyman, *Lancet*, 1987, *2*, 785.

ADMINISTRATION IN HEPATIC INSUFFICIENCY. Side-effects which occurred in 8 patients with active chronic hepatitis who were treated with mercaptopurine in daily doses of from 50 to 125 mg included anaemia, hepatic coma, jaundice, leucopenia, and thrombocytopenia. Hepatic coma and jaundice occurred in 4 and 6 patients respectively after only 2 to 3 weeks' treatment. It was suggested that the initial dose in chronic hepatitis should be 25 mg daily increased by small increments if no toxic effects occurred.— W. P. Fung and S. P. Mistilis, *Gut*, 1967, *8*, 198.

GASTRO-INTESTINAL DISORDERS, NON-MALIGNANT. *Crohn's disease.* The results of a 2-year randomised double-blind crossover study indicated that mercaptopurine was more effective than placebo in the treatment of patients with chronic Crohn's disease in whom conventional treatment had failed. The mean initial dose of mercaptopurine was 1.5 mg per kg body-weight, subsequently adjusted according to blood counts. The crossover study was completed by 39 patients and of those who improved 26 (67%) had been taking mercaptopurine during their better year and 3 (8%) had been taking placebo. Mercaptopurine was also more effective than placebo in the 33 patients who completed 2 full years of the study without crossover and was more effective in closing fistulas. Treatment with corticosteroids could be discontinued or reduced and clinical improvement maintained in 28 of 44 patients (64%) during mercaptopurine therapy compared with only 6 of 39 patients (15%) during placebo therapy. The onset of improvement with mercaptopurine was often delayed; the mean time of response was 3.1 months with a range of 2 weeks to 9 months. Treatment with mercaptopurine was stopped in 7 of 68 patients because of reversible adverse effects; the majority of patients had mild leucopenia at some time but only 2 had substantial bone-marrow depression.— D. H. Present *et al.*, *New Engl. J. Med.*, 1980, *302*, 981. Correction.— *ibid.*, *303*, 537. Comment.— M. H. Sleisenger, *ibid.*, *302*, 1024.

Preparations

Mercaptopurine Tablets *(B.P., U.S.P.)*

Proprietary Preparations

Puri-Nethol *(Calmic, UK)*. *Tablets*, scored, mercaptopurine 50 mg.

Proprietary Names and Manufacturers

Ismipur *(ISM, Ital.)*; Puri-Nethol *(Belg.; Wellcome, Denm.; Wellcome, Ger.; Neth.; Wellcome, Norw.; Wellcome, S.Afr.; Wellcome, Swed.; Wellcome, Switz.; Calmic, UK)*; Purinethol *(Wellcome, Austral.; Wellcome, Canad.; Wellcome, Fr.; Wellcome, Ital.; Wellcome, USA)*.

1845-r

Methotrexate *(BAN, USAN, rINN)*.

4-Amino-10-methylfolic Acid; 4-Amino-10-methylpteroyl-L-glutamic Acid; 4-Amino-4-deoxy-10-methylpteroyl-L-glutamic Acid; α-Methopterin; Amethopterin; CL-14377; Methotrexatum; MTX; NSC-740; WR-19039. *N*-{4-[(2,4-Diaminopteridin-6-ylmethyl)methylamino]benzoyl}-L(+)-glutamic acid.

$C_{20}H_{22}N_8O_5$=454.4.

CAS — 59-05-2.

Pharmacopoeias. In *Aust., Br., Braz., Chin., Egypt., Eur., Fr., Ind., It., Jpn, Jug., Neth., Swiss,* and *U.S.*

The *U.S.P.* permits a mixture of 4-amino-10-methylfolic acid and related substances and specifies not less than 94% of $C_{20}H_{22}N_8O_5$, calculated on the anhydrous basis. It contains not more than 12% of water. A yellow to orange-brown crystalline powder.

Practically **insoluble** in water, alcohol, chloroform, and ether; dissolves in solutions of mineral acids and in dilute solutions of alkali hydroxides and carbonates. The *B.P.* injection is **sterilised** by filtration; the *B.P.* and *U.S.P.* injections have a pH of 8 to 9. **Store** in airtight containers. Protect from light.

CAUTION. *Methotrexate is irritant; avoid contact with skin and mucous membranes.*

STABILITY IN SOLUTION. Methotrexate 2.5 mg per mL was stable for 7 days at room temperature and at 30° in Elliott's B solution, sodium chloride injection, or lactated Ringer's injection.— J. C. Cradock *et al.*, *Am. J. Hosp. Pharm.*, 1978, *35*, 402.

The stability of methotrexate at a concentration of 750 μg per mL was determined in an intravenous preparation containing glucose 5% with sodium bicarbonate 0.05 mmol per mL. When stored at 4° to 5° and protected from light there was a mean decrease in the methotrexate concentration of 1.4% after 72 hours, and 6.1% after one week. The mean decrease in methotrexate concentrations in the preparations stored at room temperature and exposed to light were 6.2 and 14.9% respectively, while the mean decrease in 24 hours was 4.2%.— A. Humphreys *et al.*, *Aust. J. Hosp. Pharm.*, 1978, *8*, 66.

A study of the degradation kinetics of methotrexate in aqueous solution and in the absence of light. The pH-degradation rate profile from first-order kinetic plots suggested maximum stability at pH 6.6 to 8.2; the presence of acetate, phosphate, borate, or bicarbonate buffers appeared to catalyse degradation. At pH above 6.5 the only degradation product observed was N^{10}-methylfolic acid but at lower pH the route of degradation was more complex. The results suggested that an isotonic buffer-free solution at an initial pH of 8.5 would lose 10% of its potency in 4.5 years if stored at 25°; if stored at 4° the time to a 10% loss of potency was calculated to be over 80 years.— J. Hansen *et al.*, *Int. J. Pharmaceut.*, 1983, *16*, 141.

Methotrexate sodium was stable for 24 hours at 25° in Elliott's B solution (artificial spinal fluid), sodium chloride injection (0.9%), glucose injection (5%), or Lactated Ringer's Injection (*U.S.P.*). No precipitation was observed when methotrexate was mixed with cytarabine and hydrocortisone sodium succinate in any of the fluids and stored for 8 hours at 25°, but storage for several days resulted in precipitation. The stability of each of the drugs did not appear to be affected by the presence of the others and the admixtures could be stored for up to 24 hours at room temperature without precipitation or substantial loss of potency.— Y. -W. Cheung *et al.*, *Am. J. Hosp. Pharm.*, 1984, *41*, 1802.

Adverse Effects

For an outline of the adverse effects experienced with antineoplastic agents and immunosuppressants, see Antineoplastic Agents, p.580.

Early signs of toxicity with methotrexate include leucopenia, thrombocytopenia, anaemia, ulceration of the mouth, and gastro-intestinal effects; stomatitis or diarrhoea are signs that treatment should be interrupted, otherwise haemorrhagic enteritis and intestinal perforation may follow. Bone-marrow depression may occur abruptly; megaloblastic anaemia has been reported. Methotrexate is immunosuppressant and hypogammaglobulinaemia may occur. Liver damage has been reported, especially in patients given high-dose therapy or long-term treatment; it may occur in the absence of other signs of methotrexate toxicity. Kidney damage, osteoporosis, effects on skin and nails, and pulmonary reactions, including interstitial pneumonitis, have developed. Fatalities have occurred. Methotrexate may cause defective oogenesis and spermatogenesis, and fertility may be impaired. Metabolic alterations, including precipitation of diabetes, have been reported.

Neurotoxic reactions may occur, especially after the intrathecal use of methotrexate. Teratogenic effects and foetal deaths have been reported.

ALLERGY AND ANAPHYLAXIS. A report of anaphylactic reactions in 2 patients given high-dose methotrexate.— P. Klimo and E. Ibrahim, *Cancer Treat. Rep.*, 1981, *65*, 725.

CARCINOGENICITY. A view that there is no justification for describing methotrexate as carcinogenic.— C. Turnbull and M. Roach (letter), *Br. med. J.*, 1980, *281*, 808.

A follow-up study in women treated with methotrexate and other antineoplastic agents for gestational trophoblastic tumours suggested that methotrexate chemotherapy was not carcinogenic in the medium term. Of 457 long-term survivors, at a mean of 7.8 years after beginning treatment, only 2 had developed secondary malignancies, which is less than the statistical likelihood of 3.5 cases. All but 2 had received methotrexate and 261 had received other cytotoxic drugs.— G. J. S. Rustin *et al.*, *New Engl. J. Med.*, 1983, *308*, 473.

A study involving 11 patients receiving methotrexate for non-malignant skin disorders and a further 10 receiving hydroxyurea (4) or azathioprine (6) found morphological abnormalities in the bone marrow of 16 patients. One patient receiving methotrexate had some evidence of chromosome abnormalities. Despite the absence of malignancy in this group so far, patients receiving cytotoxic drugs for non-malignant disorders should be closely monitored.— P. V. Harrison *et al.* (letter), *Lancet*, 1984, *1*, 966.

See also under Antineoplastic Agents, p.580.

For a report of the synergistic carcinogenicity of methotrexate and PUVA therapy see under Precautions, below.

EFFECTS ON BODY TEMPERATURE. Fever developed in 3 patients with acute myeloid leukaemia given intrathecal methotrexate. None was neutropenic or received antibiotics and all subsequently received methotrexate without problems. Fever is a cause for concern in leukaemic patients and it should be recognised that intrathecal methotrexate may cause fever in the absence of infection.— S. O'Rahilly and R. E. Marcus, *Br. med. J.*, 1984, *289*, 84.

EFFECTS ON THE BLOOD. A report of 4 cases of megaloblastic anaemia in elderly patients receiving long-term weekly methotrexate therapy. The patients had been receiving methotrexate for between 16 months and 15 years. Anaemia was preceded by marked macrocytosis; mean corpuscular volumes were 108 to 115 fL compared with an average of 95 fL in 61 other psoriatic patients receiving methotrexate. Although macrocytosis *per se* is not an indication to stop methotrexate it is suggested that therapy should be withdrawn should the mean corpuscular volume exceed 106 fL.— H. J. Dodd *et al.* (letter), *Br. J. Derm.*, 1985, *112*, 630. Severe megaloblastic anaemia in a patient who had been taking methotrexate for 6 years without ill effects was precipitated by the patient embarking on a weight-reducing diet poor in folate. All patients, especially the elderly, who are receiving methotrexate, should be encouraged to maintain a proper diet during treatment.— R. A. Fulton (letter), *ibid.*, 1986, *114*, 267.

See also under Treatment of Adverse Effects, below.

EFFECTS ON BONES AND JOINTS. Osteoporosis, predominantly in knees, ankles, and feet but also affecting the pelvis, and radiological changes suggesting a combination of stress fractures and bone infarction, occurred in an elderly man who had been receiving long-term therapy with methotrexate for psoriasis.— G. Ansell *et al.* (letter), *Br. med. J.*, 1983, *287*, 762.

EFFECTS ON THE GASTRO-INTESTINAL TRACT. In a study in 18 children with acute lymphoblastic leukaemia, absorption of D-xylose was reduced in 14 who had been taking methotrexate, compared with 4 studied before methotrexate was given; in those who had taken methotrexate within the last 7 days the reduction in absorption was significant. Reduction in absorption was progressive and related to the total cumulative dose of methotrexate.— A. W. Craft *et al.*, *Br. med. J.*, 1977, *2*, 1511. A suggestion that once-weekly treatment might be too frequent.— A. W. Craft and W. Aherne, *Archs Dis. Childh.*, 1978, *53*, 262.

Severe methotrexate enteropathy (presenting as chronic diarrhoea and anorexia) in a 6-year-old leukaemic child was considered to be due to enterohepatic recycling. Abnormal gut toxicity may be related to abnormally efficient biliary excretion of methotrexate.— G. M.

Baird and J. F. B. Dossetor (letter), *Lancet*, 1981, *1*, 164. Comment. Such severe enteropathy is rare, and could conceivably be related to pre-existing folate deficiency or other contributary factors.— C. R. Pinkerton and J. F. T. Glasgow (letter), *ibid.*, 996.

A report of severe enteropathy in 7 children receiving weekly methotrexate as part of a maintenance regimen for acute leukaemia. All presented with weight loss, anorexia and vomiting, bowel disturbances including steatorrhoea, and abdominal distension. Five had definite folate deficiency and a sixth had megaloblastic marrow changes; dietary folate deficiency probably played a part in exacerbating the disorder, as did concurrent administration of co-trimoxazole.— I. J. Lewis *et al.*, *Archs Dis. Childh.*, 1982, *57*, 663.

A report of toxic megacolon in a patient receiving methotrexate for psoriasis.— L. D. Atherton *et al.*, *Gastroenterology*, 1984, *86*, 1583.

EFFECTS ON THE KIDNEYS. Methotrexate in high doses may rarely cause renal failure by intrarenal tubular obstruction due to precipitation of crystals of methotrexate.— D. Adu, *Prescribers' J.*, 1984, *24*, 46.

EFFECTS ON THE LIVER. Methotrexate produces a zone-I (periportal) fibrosis, resulting from a toxic metabolite of microsomal origin which induces fibrosis and ultimately cirrhosis. This can be reduced by giving the drug only at weekly intervals. Repeated tests of liver function with an occasional liver biopsy are needed to monitor treatment.— S. Sherlock, *Lancet*, 1986, *2*, 440. For an earlier review, see D. B. Ménard *et al.*, *Gastroenterology*, 1980, *78*, 143.

Twenty-two of 29 patients with rheumatoid arthritis, who were receiving low-dose pulsed methotrexate therapy, developed liver abnormalities but cirrhosis did not ensue in any patient. Isolated elevations of liver enzyme values did not predict liver disease, neither did the absence of elevation ensure the absence of disease; however, serial elevations of these values were diagnostic for the development of liver disorders. In these patients, severe liver disease was associated with more than 2 years of therapy, or with a cumulative dose of methotrexate in excess of 1.5 g.— K. G. Tolman *et al.*, *J. Rheumatol.*, 1985, *12*, *Suppl.* 12, 29.

EFFECTS ON MENTAL FUNCTION. Results in 23 children who had received intrathecal methotrexate to a maximum of 12 mg, together with cranial irradiation, for the prophylaxis of CNS leukaemia, indicated a significant intellectual deficit compared with their siblings. The mean intelligence quotient (IQ) in patients was 99.1, compared with 108.4 in the siblings. Since there is evidence that brothers and sisters have correlated IQ's it was estimated that the mean IQ of patients before treatment would have been 104.3. There was no corresponding significant reduction in IQ in a group of 19 children who had received systemic chemotherapy, and radiotherapy (in 17), when compared with their sibling controls. The results suggest that intrathecal methotrexate and cranial irradiation cause intellectual problems, particularly on the higher, more complex and integrated intellectual functions, and that the repercussions are greater in younger children. Although CNS prophylaxis cannot be omitted from the treatment of acute lymphoblastic leukaemia the current reduction of the radiation dose from 24 to 18 Gray may help. The extent of damage remains unclear; longer term observation of these children will be necessary.— V. Twaddle *et al.*, *Archs Dis. Childh.*, 1983, *58*, 949. Subsequent results indicated that the lowering of IQ in the leukaemia patients had persisted but had not progressed since the original study.— V. Twaddle *et al.*, *ibid.*, 1986, *61*, 700.

A study in 20 patients who had been receiving intermittent methotrexate therapy for psoriasis for between 6 months and 10 years found no evidence of psychological impairment in 19; 1 elderly patient had mild senile dementia which did not worsen over the following year despite continued administration of the drug. The blood-brain barrier appears to provide protection against methotrexate-induced brain damage.— P. Duller and P. C. M. van de Kerkhof (letter), *Br. J. Derm.*, 1985, *113*, 503.

EFFECTS ON THE NERVOUS SYSTEM. Intrathecal methotrexate is associated with a spectrum of neurotoxic reactions. Acute arachnoiditis and meningismus can develop within hours of administration. The incidence is dose-related and usually subsides within a few days. A subacute form of toxic reaction, characterised by varying degrees of paresis, is generally associated with multiple intrathecal injections and apparently results from prolonged elevation of methotrexate concentrations in the CSF. Paraplegia has been reported, but appears to be rare, and decreasing in incidence with improved drug preparation and monitoring of drug concentrations in CSF. There is also a more delayed syndrome, occurring months to years after treatment, and characterised by necrotising leucoencephalopathy. The syndrome may begin insidiously, and progress to dementia, confusion, ataxia, seizures, and eventual stupor. The effects are dose-related and occur particularly when intrathecal methotrexate in doses greater than 50 mg is combined with cranial irradiation and systemic methotrexate therapy. A late feature may be calcification of the necrotic brain tissue. Not all patients develop this severe encephalopathy but minor neurological injuries, presenting as mild ataxia, seizures, or perceptual disorders, have been reported in at least half the patients in some studies.— I. D. Goldberg *et al.*, *J. Am. med. Ass.*, 1982, *247*, 1437.

See also under Effects on Mental Function, above.

EFFECTS ON RESPIRATORY FUNCTION. A review of pneumonitis associated with methotrexate. Both allergic and cytotoxic effects have been implicated in methotrexate-induced pulmonary disease. Predominant symptoms are non-productive cough, dyspnoea, and fever. The chest radiograph usually demonstrates diffuse, extensive bilateral infiltrates. Pleural effusion may occur rarely. There are non-specific histological changes, including granulomatous pneumonitis which may evolve to diffuse pulmonary fibrosis. Four of 36 recorded cases died, in 1 case due to superimposed bacterial infection, and some patients develop persistent abnormalities of pulmonary function. Treatment with corticosteroids may hasten recovery.— H. D. Sostman *et al.*, *Medicine, Baltimore*, 1976, *55*, 371. See also S. J. Pearce, *Adverse Drug React. Bull.*, 1982, (Jun.), 344.

A study of pulmonary function in 10 psoriatic patients taking long-term low-dose methotrexate failed to show any changes indicative of early pulmonary damage on comparison with 10 similar patients not receiving methotrexate. The authors have recently seen 2 patients who developed pulmonary complications (pneumonitis, and irreversible progressive pulmonary fibrosis) after taking long-term low-dose methotrexate for psoriasis.— T. J. Phillips *et al.*, *Br. J. Derm.*, 1986, *115*, *Suppl.* 30, 13.

EFFECTS ON THE SKIN. A report of skin ulceration and necrosis in 6 patients receiving weekly methotrexate for psoriasis. One patient developed bullae. Three patients had other symptoms of methotrexate toxicity, fatal in one; of the 5 surviving patients withdrawal of methotrexate (permanently in one, temporarily in 3), or dose reduction, produced resolution of symptoms.— C. M. Lawrence and M. G. C. Dahl, *Br. J. Derm.*, 1982, *107*, *Suppl.* 22, 24. Intramuscular injection of methotrexate 15 mg in a psoriatic patient was followed by erythema, maceration, and skin breakdown. The patient recovered but was subsequently given oral methotrexate, and developed bullae and skin necrosis, ulceration, and skin changes consistent with toxic epidermal necrolysis.— K. M. Reed and A. J. Sober, *J. Am. Acad. Derm.*, 1983, *8*, 677.

An erythematous, desquamating rash of the hands developed in 3 cancer patients after treatment with high-dose methotrexate.— L. A. Doyle *et al.*, *Ann. intern. Med.*, 1983, *98*, 611.

Small vessel vasculitis, manifest as small, purpuric skin lesions, and in 1 patient, erythema, occurred in 8 patients being treated for arthritis with weekly methotrexate. Five patients had had cutaneous reactions to previous therapy.— C. R. Marks *et al.* (letter), *Ann. intern. Med.*, 1984, *100*, 916. Leucocytoclastic vasculitis in a patient with osteogenic sarcoma was ascribed to treatment with high-dose methotrexate.— M. Navarro *et al.* (letter), *ibid.*, 1986, *105*, 471.

Methotrexate could cause photosensitivity reactions.— *Med. Lett.*, 1986, *28*, 51.

Treatment of Adverse Effects

For general guidelines, see Antineoplastic Agents, p.583.

Folinic acid neutralises the immediate toxic effects of methotrexate on the bone marrow. It is given as calcium folinate by mouth, intramuscularly, by intravenous bolus injection, or by infusion. When overdosage is suspected the dose of calcium folinate should be at least as high as that of methotrexate and should be administered within the first hour; further doses are given as required. When average doses of methotrexate have an adverse effect, the equivalent of 6 to 12 mg of folinic acid may be given intramuscularly every 6 hours for 4 doses. See also under Calcium Folinate, p.1264.

Folinic acid may also be given in association with high-dose methotrexate regimens to prevent damage to normal tissue and this is discussed in the Uses section below.

Eighteen of 33 psoriatic patients receiving methotrexate had lowered red cell- and plasma-folate concentrations, and red cell macrocytosis (mean corpuscular volume greater than 95 fL) when compared with 33 psoriatic controls. Addition of folic acid 10 mg daily to the treatment regimen produced a prompt fall in mean corpuscular volume, leading to the conclusion that some patients on methotrexate require folate supplements to prevent bone-marrow depression.— M. G. C. Dahl, *Br. J. Derm.*, 1984, *111*, *Suppl.* 26, 18.

In a patient who received a massive intrathecal overdose of 625 mg of methotrexate immediate lumbar puncture and subsequent ventriculolumbar perfusion over 4 hours were effective in removing 606 mg, or 97% of the instilled dose. The perfusion was carried out with 550 mL of sodium chloride injection (0.9%), the final 100 mL containing in addition calcium folinate. The patient was also given high-dose systemic calcium folinate rescue, and subsequently continuous intravenous infusion of thymidine 8 g per m^2 body-surface daily. The patient remained comatose for 24 hours and required assisted ventilation but subsequently recovered without apparent neurological or mental deficit.— R. J. Spiegel *et al.*, *New Engl. J. Med.*, 1984, *311*, 386. Comment. Although folinic acid and thymidine are able to prevent systemic toxicity due to methotrexate their role in preventing neurotoxicity resulting from intrathecal overdose remains speculative.— D. G. Poplack, *ibid.*, 400.

Comments on the management of patients with very high plasma-methotrexate concentrations. Measuring plasma concentrations at 24 and 48 hours identifies patients with dangerously high methotrexate concentrations due to renal failure but it is essential to use these measured concentrations to determine the increased dosage of folinic acid rescue required. Toxicity is determined by both plasma-methotrexate concentration and duration of exposure so increased rescue must start immediately and continue until concentrations fall below 0.1 μmol per litre. Attempts to remove methotrexate from the circulation by peritoneal dialysis, haemodialysis, or charcoal haemoperfusion cause transient falls, but the drug is protein-bound and highly ionised and these efforts have been largely ineffective. Alternative rescue techniques, including plasmaphaeresis. thymidine, and carboxypeptidase, are no substitute for early folinic acid rescue at increased dosage.— C. J. Twelves (letter), *Lancet*, 1986, *1*, 737. Evidence that effective salvage may be achieved with charcoal haemoperfusion or exchange transfusion.— E. Bouffet *et al.* (letter), *ibid.*, 1497.

Precautions

For reference to the precautions necessary with antineoplastic agents and immunosuppressants, see Antineoplastic Agents, p.583.

Methotrexate should be used with great care in patients with hepatic or renal impairment. It should also be used cautiously in alcoholics or those with ulcerative disorders of the gastro-intestinal tract. With high-dose regimens, plasma concentrations of methotrexate and urinary excretion should be monitored. Regular monitoring of liver function is advisable. Precipitation of methotrexate or its metabolites in the renal tubules may be prevented by alkalinisation of the urine using sodium bicarbonate and maintaining an adequate urine flow. Pleural or ascitic effusions may act as a depot for methotrexate and produce enhanced toxicity.

The effects of methotrexate may be enhanced by concurrent administration of aminobenzoic acid, chloramphenicol, phenylbutazone, phenytoin, probenecid, salicylates, sulphonamides, and tetracyclines. Fatal toxicity has occurred in patients given nonsteroidal anti-inflammatory drugs concurrently with methotrexate.

Methotrexate is a potent teratogen and should be avoided in pregnancy.

Studies of alternatives to serial liver biopsies in detecting methotrexate-induced liver damage in psoriatic patients: J. A. Miller *et al.*, *Br. J. Derm.*, 1985, *113*, 699 (ultrasound scanning); E. A. Bingham *et al.*, *Gut*, 1985, *26*, A1101 (dynamic liver scanning with ^{99}Tc-colloid); D. M. Mitchell *et al.*, *ibid.*, 1986, *115*, *Suppl.* 30, 29 (sequential assay of the aminoterminal peptide of type III procollagen in serum).

DOWN'S SYNDROME. For the suggestion that children

with Down's syndrome are less able to tolerate methotrexate see Antineoplastic Agents, p.583.

HANDLING AND DISPOSAL. Methods for the destruction of methotrexate wastes by oxidation with potassium permanganate and sulphuric acid, by oxidation with aqueous alkaline potassium permanganate, or by oxidation with sodium hypochlorite. The first method may also be used for dichloromethotrexate. A solution of methotrexate 0.5%, or dichloromethotrexate 0.1%, in dilute sulphuric acid (3 mol per litre) can be destroyed in 1 hour by addition of potassium permanganate 50 mg per mL. This method is recommended for solutions in dimethyl sulphoxide or dimethylformamide which should be diluted with water to a solvent concentration of not more than 20% and not more than 2.5 mg per mL of drug. The second method is recommended for solid wastes and aqueous solutions, which should be dissolved or diluted as appropriate to produce a 0.1% solution of drug in 4% sodium hydroxide: 1% potassium permanganate solution is then added until the purple colour persists for 30 minutes and 1% sodium bisulphite solution then added to decolourise the resultant liquid. This method is also recommended for solutions in volatile organic solvents which should first have the solvent evaporated off before dissolving as above. Glassware may be decontaminated by immersing it in a 1% solution of potassium permanganate in 4% sodium hydroxide for 30 minutes and then cleaning by immersion in sodium bisulphite solution. The third method is recommended for solid spills which should be taken up and dissolved in 4% sodium hydroxide to give up to a 0.05% solution: about 10 mL of sodium hypochlorite solution (5%) should be added for each 50 mg of methotrexate and allowed to react for 30 minutes. The area of the spill should be rinsed with sodium hypochlorite solution and the rinse discarded. Aqueous spills may be taken up on absorbent material and reacted with sodium hypochlorite solution as above. Residues produced by the degradation of methotrexate by these methods showed no mutagenicity *in vitro*.—IARC Scientific Publications No. 73, *Laboratory Decontamination and Destruction of Carcinogens in Laboratory Wastes: Some Antineoplastic Agents*, M. Castegnaro *et al.* (Eds), Lyon, International Agency for Research on Cancer, 1985, p.33.

When handling urine and faeces from patients receiving methotrexate protective clothing should be worn for up to 72 hours and 7 days respectively after therapy.— J. Harris and L. J. Dodds, *Pharm. J.*, 1985, *2*, 289.

INTERACTIONS. *With drugs.* Reports of severe or fatal toxicity in patients given *nonsteroidal anti-inflammatory drugs* concurrently with methotrexate: A. Thyss *et al.*, *Lancet*, 1986, *1*, 256 (with ketoprofen; 3 fatalities); A. G. Maiche (letter), *ibid.*, 1390 (with indomethacin); R. R. Singh *et al.* (letter), *ibid* (with naproxen; death); H. M. Daly *et al.*, *Br. J. Derm.*, 1986, *114*, 733 (with azapropazone); A. Gabrielli *et al.* (letter), *Br. med. J.*, 1987, *294*, 776 (with indomethacin and diclofenac; death).

Cisplatin significantly decreased methotrexate elimination in 14 patients treated with a combination regimen for osteosarcoma, particularly following a high cumulative cisplatin dose. Appropriate monitoring and intervention with escalated folinic acid doses were essential to prevent serious toxicity.— W. R. Crom *et al.*, *Drug Intell. & clin. Pharm.*, 1985, *19*, 467.

When methotrexate was given 6 hours before *cytarabine* to *mice* inoculated with lymphoma cells, no antitumour effect was seen. Both compounds were shown to increase survival if given separately, together, or if cytarabine was given 6 hours before methotrexate.— M. H. N. Tattersall *et al.* (letter), *Lancet*, 1972, *2*, 1378.

A report of the development of acute megaloblastic anaemia following high-dose *co-trimoxazole* therapy in a patient who had been receiving methotrexate for graft-versus-host-disease.— N. L. Kobrinsky and N. K. C. Ramsay, *Ann. intern. Med.*, 1981, *94*, 780.

Evidence that *nitrous oxide* may increase the side-effects of methotrexate therapy and reduce the therapeutic benefit.— P. M. Ueland *et al.* (letter), *New Engl. J. Med.*, 1986, *314*, 1514. Comment. Results in *rats* suggest that nitrous oxide enhances the therapeutic effect of methotrexate, as well as its toxicity.— A. C. M. Kroes (letter), *ibid.*, *315*, 895. See also Ludwig Breast Cancer Study Group, *Lancet*, 1983, *2*, 542; A. Goldhirsch *et al.* (letter), *Lancet*, 1987, *2*, 151.

A report of toxicity in 2 patients given *packed red cells* immediately after 24-hour infusion of methotrexate. Neither patient exhibited signs of toxicity when methotrexate was given without red cell transfusions. Methotrexate accumulates in erythrocytes and tends to leave slowly so that erythrocytes may act as a reservoir for methotrexate. Great care should be exercised whenever packed red blood cells and methotrexate are administered concurrently.— A. K. L. Yap *et al.* (letter), *Lancet*, 1986, *2*, 641.

An increase in plasma-methotrexate concentrations in a patient given methotrexate and *etretinate* for psoriasis.— P. V. Harrison *et al.* (letter), *Lancet*, 1987, *2*, 512. Severe drug-induced hepatitis occurred in 2 of 10 patients treated with methotrexate and etretinate.— H. Zachariae, *ibid.*, 1988, *1*, 422.

For discussion of the effects of probenecid on methotrexate excretion see Precautions, under Probenecid, p.440. For the suggestion that vidarabine might enhance the risks of methotrexate therapy see Vidarabine Phosphate p.702.

With PUVA. Of a total of 94 patients with psoriasis and 38 with mycosis fungoides treated with PUVA therapy (methoxsalen and ultraviolet light) 2 psoriatics who received concomitant methotrexate and PUVA therapy have developed subsequent skin cancers. It was suggested that the combination of methotrexate and PUVA may be synergistic in inducing cutaneous malignancy.— C. P. Fitzsimons *et al.* (letter), *Lancet*, 1983, *1*, 235.

With radiation. Analysis of neutrophil counts for 18 months in children with acute lymphoblastic leukaemia, some of whom were given CNS irradiation, showed that methotrexate was the main agent associated with severe neutropenia. Methotrexate-induced neutropenia was significantly greater in patients given CNS irradiation and was considered to have contributed to 3 of 5 deaths during remission.—Report to the MRC of the Working Party on Leukaemia in Childhood, *Br. med. J.*, 1975, *3*, 563.

For the role of cranial irradiation and intrathecal methotrexate in producing neurotoxicity see Effects on the Nervous System, above.

PORPHYRIA. Methotrexate was considered to be unsafe in patients with acute porphyria because it has been shown to be porphyrinogenic in *animals* or *in-vitro* systems.— M.R. Moore and K.E.L. McColl, *Porphyrias, Drug Lists*, Glasgow, Porphyria Research Unit, University of Glasgow, 1987.

PREGNANCY AND THE NEONATE. An infant born to a woman who had conceived within 6 months of completing treatment with methotrexate, had desquamating fibrosing alveolitis. The rarity of this pulmonary disorder, particularly in childhood, and the fact that methotrexate can be retained in the tissues of both animals and man, suggest that it may have been a causative factor.— P. A. M. Walden and K. D. Bagshawe (letter), *Lancet*, 1979, *2*, 1241.

Methotrexate was contra-indicated during breast feeding.— *Pediatrics*, 1983, *72*, 375.

See also Adverse Effects, above, and Absorption and Fate and Uses and Administration, below.

Absorption and Fate

When given in low doses, methotrexate is rapidly absorbed from the gastro-intestinal tract, but higher doses are less well absorbed. It is also rapidly and completely absorbed following intramuscular administration. Methotrexate is distributed to tissues and extracellular fluid; it penetrates ascitic fluid and effusions which may act as a depot and thus enhance toxicity. It enters the cells in part by an active transport mechanism and is bound as polyglutamate conjugates: bound drug may remain in the body for several months, particularly in the liver. Only small or insignificant amounts cross the blood-brain barrier and enter CSF following oral or parenteral administration although this may be increased by giving higher doses; however, following intrathecal doses there is significant passage into the systemic circulation. It is about 50% bound to plasma protein.

Methotrexate does not appear to undergo significant metabolism at low doses; following high-dose therapy the 7-hydroxy metabolite has been detected. Methotrexate may be partly metabolised by the intestinal flora before absorption. It is excreted primarily in the urine, and some undergoes active tubular secretion by the kidney. Small amounts are excreted in bile and found in faeces; there is some evidence for enterohepatic recirculation.

Methotrexate has been detected in very small amounts in saliva and breast milk. It crosses the placenta.

Considerable interindividual variation exists in the pharmacokinetics of methotrexate: those patients in whom absorption or elimination are prolonged are at increased risk of toxicity.

A review of the clinical pharmacokinetics of methotrexate. Following intramuscular injection of methotrexate absorption is rapid and complete and more sustained serum concentrations are achieved than those following rapid intravenous administration. Gastro-intestinal absorption is dose-dependent, peak serum concentrations occurring 1 to 2 hours after doses below 30 mg per m^2 body-surface. A slowing in the rate of absorption has been noted during a 6-week course of therapy in some patients. Absorption has been reduced to 50 to 70% at doses above 80 mg per m^2. Plasma clearance of methotrexate is reported to be biphasic or triphasic. Although plasma concentrations are roughly proportional to dose, methotrexate elimination may be saturable at very high doses.

Methotrexate is transported across cellular membranes by a carrier-mediated active-type process. With high doses the carrier route becomes saturated and passive diffusion becomes more important. Being highly ionised at physiological pH little methotrexate penetrates the blood-brain barrier in general but persisting and high concentrations in the CSF can be achieved with high-dose intravenous infusions, at the cost of increased systemic toxicity. After the intrathecal injection of methotrexate, a half-life in CSF of 12 to 18 hours was reported by Bleyer *et al.* (*New Engl. J. Med.*, 1973, *289*, 770). Shapiro *et al.* (*New Engl. J. Med.*, 1975, *293*, 161) found considerable variation in peak intraventricular concentrations after the administration of methotrexate by lumbar puncture; more consistent concentrations were achieved with an indwelling intraventricular-subcutaneous reservoir.

About 80% of a dose is excreted in the urine by glomerular filtration and active renal tubular secretion. Intratubular precipitation of methotrexate is possible with high doses. A peak concentration in urine of 5 mg per mL has been reported in patients receiving high doses. This exceeds the saturation concentration of methotrexate at low urinary pHs and routine administration of fluid and/or bicarbonate is therefore recommended. Methotrexate may be contaminated with byproducts of its synthesis or with degradation products and these impurities may be confused with methotrexate metabolites.— D. D. Shen and D. L. Azarnoff, *Clin. Pharmacokinet.*, 1978, *3*, 1. See also F. M. Balis *et al.*, *ibid.*, 1983, *8*, 202.

The clinical pharmacokinetics of methotrexate in children. Age appears to exert a dominant effect on the pharmacokinetics of high-dose methotrexate therapy, with a greater distribution and elimination of methotrexate in younger patients. This increased distribution and elimination results in a lower plasma concentration of drug at the same dose. Younger patients appear to tolerate high-dose methotrexate regimens better than older patients.— Y. -M. Wang and T. Fujimoto, *Clin. Pharmacokinet.*, 1984, *9*, 335.

An assessment of changes in the transfer-rate of methotrexate from spinal fluid to plasma in adults and children receiving intrathecal injections. Two patterns were identified: the 'slow' type in which plasma concentrations reached a rather low maximum followed by a relatively slow decline and the 'fast' type in which plasma concentrations increased rapidly to a high value followed by a relatively rapid biphasic decline. The incidence of 'fast' type increased progressively with the number of intrathecal injections and might be attributed to facilitated leakage from the spinal fluid possibly resulting from damage caused by repeated injections, the effects of radiotherapy, or altered circulation of the spinal fluid. Therapeutic efficacy in the CNS is likely to be less for the 'fast' type whereas systemic toxicity is expected to be higher in the 'slow' type.— J. Lankelma *et al.*, *Clin. Pharmacokinet.*, 1980, *5*, 465.

Results of a pilot study in 9 children suggested that an estimate of methotrexate concentration in CSF after high intravenous doses could be made by measuring the concentration in saliva. Salivary concentration was closely correlated with concentration in CSF, but not with plasma-methotrexate concentration.— G. M. Baird *et al.*, *Br. J. clin. Pharmac.*, 1981, *11*, 112P.

The kinetics of high-dose methotrexate infusions: M. Luyckx *et al.*, *Eur. J. clin. Pharmac.*, 1985, *28*, 457; A. K. L. Yap *et al.*, *Br. J. clin. Pharmac.*, 1985, *20*, 297P. See also I. G. Kerr *et al.*, *Clin. Pharmac. Ther.*, 1983, *33*, 44 (test dose to predict the kinetics of high-dose infusion). A reminder that when measuring serum concentrations of methotrexate assays should be used that are capable of measuring concentrations approaching the minimal cytotoxic concentration of the drug. Failure to do so had resulted in unnecessary therapy and hospitalisation in 2 patients.— C. J. Allegra *et al.* (letter), *New Engl. J. Med.*, 1985, *313*, 184.

A study of methotrexate kinetics and folate storage in circulating erythrocytes during methotrexate therapy for psoriasis. In 5 patients receiving their first oral dose, there was an initial peak in the erythrocyte concentration of methotrexate which was related to the peak in plasma concentration and was probably due to diffusion; however, after 3 to 4 days methotrexate re-appeared in significant amounts in erythrocytes despite the fact that the plasma concentration remained below the level of detection, suggesting an energy dependent uptake process. Erythrocyte concentrations steadily increased until a steady-state concentration was achieved after the fourth to sixth weekly dose. The concentration was maintained during 6 months of observation and there was no change in erythrocyte-folate concentration during this period. In 25 further patients who had been receiving long-term methotrexate therapy there was no linear correlation between methotrexate accumulation in erythrocytes and folate concentration, although patients with high methotrexate accumulation tended to have lower erythrocyte-folate concentrations, probably reflecting overall folate depletion with long-term methotrexate therapy.— J. Hendel and A. Nyfors, *Eur. J. clin. Pharmac.*, 1984, *27*, 607.

In a study involving 108 children given high-dose methotrexate intravenously and intrathecally as part of the maintenance therapy of acute lymphoblastic leukaemia methotrexate clearance varied widely between individuals from 44.7 to 132.1 mL per minute per m^2. When the group was subdivided by creatinine clearance and liver function (as measured by abnormal liver-enzyme values) it became apparent that the observed interpatient variability in clearance was not totally random but was related in part to differences in renal and hepatic function. There was also some evidence that in patients with the slowest creatinine clearance and abnormal liver-enzyme values, boys may have faster methotrexate clearance than girls.— W. R. Crom *et al.*, *Clin. Pharmac. Ther.*, 1986, *39*, 592.

For studies suggesting that methotrexate clearance influences the probability of relapse in patients with acute lymphoblastic leukaemia see under Uses, below.

Uses and Administration

Methotrexate is an antineoplastic agent which acts as an antimetabolite (p.580) of folic acid. It also has immunosuppressant properties. Within the cell, folic acid is reduced to dihydrofolic and then tetrahydrofolic acid. Methotrexate competitively inhibits the enzyme dihydrofolate reductase and prevents the formation of tetrahydrofolate which is necessary for purine and pyrimidine synthesis and consequently the formation of DNA and RNA. It is most active against cells in the S phase of the cell cycle but its actions on protein and nucleic acid synthesis slow the entry of cells into S phase and so are to some extent self-limiting. Folinic acid, the 5-formyl derivative of tetrahydrofolic acid, or the nucleoside thymidine, have been given after high doses to bypass the block in tetrahydrofolate production in normal cells and prevent the adverse effects of methotrexate. A suggested schedule for *folinic acid rescue* is described under Calcium Folinate, p.1264. (See also under Treatment of Adverse Effects, above). Methotrexate, in very high doses, followed by folinic acid rescue, is being investigated in a number of malignant diseases. High doses may be used to try and overcome the development of resistance. Resistant cells may have greatly increased concentrations of dihydrofolate reductase, and the use of high drug doses may permit intracellular concentrations of methotrexate sufficient to inactivate even these elevated amounts of enzyme. Resistance may also occur due to impaired entry of methotrexate into the cell, or the production of resistant enzyme.

Methotrexate is used in the management of acute lymphoblastic leukaemia. It is seldom used for the induction of remission but is employed in maintenance programmes and in the prophylaxis and treatment of meningeal leukaemia. It is effective in the treatment of choriocarcinoma and other trophoblastic tumours and is used, often in association with other antineoplastic agents, in the treatment of a variety of malignant diseases including lymphosarcoma, Burkitt's lymphoma, mycosis fungoides, osteogenic sarcoma, and tumours of the bladder, brain, breast, cervix, head and neck, lung, ovary, and testis. See also under Choice of Antineoplastic Agent, p.584.

Methotrexate is of value in the treatment of psoriasis but because of the risks associated with this use, it should only be given when the disease is severe and has not responded to other forms of treatment. It has been used as an immunosuppressant (see p.594) in other non-malignant diseases.

Methotrexate may be given by mouth, or by injection as methotrexate sodium. The doses and regimens employed vary widely, and may need to be adjusted according to the bone-marrow or other toxicity. In general, courses of treatment are not given more frequently than every 1 to 2 weeks. Doses larger than 100 mg are usually given partly or wholly by intravenous infusion over not more than 24 hours and it has been recommended that when doses in excess of 70 mg per m^2 are given folinic acid rescue should be employed.

A common dose for maintenance therapy of acute lymphoblastic leukaemia is 15 to 30 mg per m^2 body-surface once or twice weekly, by mouth or intramuscularly, with other agents such as mercaptopurine. Alternatively, 2.5 mg per kg body-weight may be given intravenously every 14 days. Meningeal leukaemia may be treated by the intrathecal injection of 12 mg per m^2 body-surface, to a maximum of 15 mg, once or twice weekly. Similar doses have been given prophylactically to patients with lymphoblastic leukaemia, sometimes in association with intrathecal cytarabine and hydrocortisone. For reference to the use of intrathecal methotrexate and radiotherapy for CNS prophylaxis see p.586. Methotrexate in intravenous doses of about 500 mg per m^2, followed by folinic acid rescue, may also produce effective concentrations in the CSF.

In advanced lymphosarcoma 3 to 30 mg per kg, or about 90 to 900 mg per m^2, has been given intravenously, with folinic acid rescue when required. In the *USA*, doses of 0.625 to 2.5 mg per kg daily have been suggested in combination with other antineoplastic agents. For Burkitt's lymphoma, 10 to 25 mg of methotrexate may be given daily by mouth for 4 to 8 days, repeated after an interval of 7 to 10 days, while patients with mycosis fungoides may be given 2.5 to 10 mg daily by mouth to induce remission; alternatively 50 mg may be given weekly as a single dose or two divided doses, by intramuscular injection.

Choriocarcinoma has been treated with doses of 15 to 30 mg daily by mouth or intramuscularly for 5 days, at intervals of 1 to 2 weeks, for 3 to 5 courses. Alternatively 0.25 to 1 mg per kg body-weight up to a maximum of 60 mg has been given intramuscularly every 48 hours for 4 doses, followed by folinic acid rescue, and repeated at intervals of 7 days. Combination chemotherapy may be necessary in patients with metastases. A range of doses of methotrexate has been used in the management of solid tumours. Very high doses, in the range 1 to 9 g per m^2 or more, have been given by intravenous infusion, followed by folinic acid, in patients with osteogenic sarcoma and carcinoma of the lung and of the head and neck.

Single weekly doses of 10 to 25 mg may be given by mouth or by intramuscular or intravenous injection in the treatment of psoriasis. Alternatively 2.5 mg has been administered by mouth every 12 hours for 3 doses or every 8 hours for 4 doses each week or 2.5 mg may be given daily by mouth for 5 days out of 7. A weekly dosage regimen appears to be less hepatotoxic than a daily one.

It is essential that examinations of blood and tests of renal and liver function should be made before, during, and after each course of treatment with methotrexate. If there is a severe fall in the white cell or platelet counts, methotrexate should be withdrawn.

Reviews of the actions and uses of methotrexate: J. Jolivet *et al.*, *New Engl. J. Med.*, 1983, *309*, 1094.

ACTION. The critical result produced by methotrexate's inhibition of dihydrofolate reductase is depletion of intracellular pools of reduced folate. The reaction most sensitive to folate depletion is thymidylate synthesis, which is brought to a halt at concentrations of 1×10^{-8} M of methotrexate. Cessation of purine synthesis occurs at concentrations of methotrexate approximately 10-fold greater. The lack of thymidylate or purine blocks synthesis of DNA. The polyglutamate derivatives to which methotrexate is extensively converted within the cell have an affinity for dihydrofolate reductase at least as great as the parent drug, and their inhibition is less readily reversible; in addition they inhibit other enzymes, including thymidylate synthetase and enzymes involved in purine synthesis, which are not directly affected by methotrexate.— J. Jolivet *et al.*, *New Engl. J. Med.*, 1983, *309*, 1094.

A discussion of resistance to methotrexate and vincristine. Methotrexate resistance may occur by several mechanisms. Influx of drug to the cell may be impaired by alterations in the affinity of the carrier that actively transports the drug. Alternatively increased amounts of dihydrofolate reductase may be produced, in some cases by gene amplification (increased expression of the enzyme-producing gene). A third alternative is the production of variant forms of dihydrofolate reductase that are less sensitive to methotrexate. Results *in vitro* suggest that the first mechanism produces a relatively low order of resistance, while the second and third are associated with increasingly high orders of resistance.— B. T. Hill, *J. antimicrob. Chemother.*, 1986, *18*, *Suppl.* B, 61. See also G. A. Curt *et al.*, *New Engl. J. Med.*, 1983, *308*, 199.

ADMINISTRATION. Studies of methotrexate-induced malabsorption in children with acute lymphoblastic leukaemia indicated that prolonged administration may lead to slower absorption and lower peak blood concentrations and that once-weekly dosage may be too frequent.— A. W. Craft and W. Aherne, *Archs Dis. Childh.*, 1978, *53*, 262. A study in 10 similar children indicated that methotrexate absorption is delayed by food, particularly milk. Peak plasma-methotrexate concentrations were reduced. For maximum absorption it is therefore recommended that methotrexate should not be taken at meal times.— C. R. Pinkerton *et al.*, *Lancet*, 1980, *2*, 944. Xylose absorption studies should not be used to predict methotrexate absorption.— *idem*, 1981, *282*, 1276.

The rate of clearance of methotrexate had a significant effect on the probability of relapse in a study in 108 children with standard-risk acute lymphoblastic leukaemia receiving intermediate-dose methotrexate (1 g per m^2 for 15 doses) as part of their maintenance therapy. When patients were divided into 36 with slow clearance, 37 with medium clearance and 35 with fast clearance there were 3 haematological and 3 CNS relapses in the first group, 5 and 2 in the second, and 6 and 3 in the third. There was a significant difference between the fast and slow clearance groups in the probability of relapse, though not between slow and medium, or medium and fast clearance groups. Serum-methotrexate concentrations in the fast clearance group were consistently below 20 nmol per mL, the concentration which has been reported to be necessary for substantial passive uptake of methotrexate by human lymphoblastoid cells. The use of higher doses of methotrexate with folinic acid rescue might be necessary to ensure adequate exposure even in patients with fast clearance.— W. E. Evans *et al.*, *Lancet*, 1984, *1*, 359. See also W. E. Evans *et al.*, *New Engl. J. Med.*, 1986, *314*, 471. A study involving 144 children in remission from acute lymphoblastic leukaemia indicated that oral methotrexate was [illegible] effective as intramuscular dosage in maintaining [illegible] mission. Seventy-five patients were randomised [illegible] and 69 [illegible] hotrexate 20 mg per m^2 weekly by [illegible] injection; received the same dose by intra[illegible] ristine, and patients also received mercaptop[illegible] difference in prednisolone. There was no s[illegible] and 30 in the incidence of relapse, with 27 [illegible] se-free survival intramuscular group and a[illegible] up and 51.2% in at 6 years was 63.9% in th[illegible] patients receiving the latter. Convulsions w[illegible] d to intramuscular oral methotrexate and [illegible] leucoencephalopa- therapy; there was s[illegible] and 3 of the 5 on thy in one of the [illegible] y suggests that intra- intramuscular tre[illegible] er, and perhaps more muscular meth[illegible] le in the maintenance harmful, tha[illegible] lymphoblastic leukae- treatment [illegible] *Archs Dis. Childh.*, 1987, mias.— J[illegible]

62, 172.

In renal failure. Doses of methotrexate should be reduced to 50% of normal in patients with a glomerular filtration-rate (GFR) of 10 to 50 mL per minute, and should be avoided altogether in those with a GFR of less than 10 mL per minute.— W. M. Bennett *et al.*, *Am. J. Kidney Dis.*, 1983, *3*, 155.

BURKITT'S LYMPHOMA. For reference to methotrexate in the treatment of Burkitt's lymphoma, see Choice of Antineoplastic Agent, p.585.

CHOLANGITIS. A report of 2 patients with primary sclerosing cholangitis, a rare, inflammatory, progressive fibrosis of the bile ducts, who responded to low-dose oral therapy with methotrexate. One patient received 2.5 mg, the other 5 mg, both given 3 times weekly at 12-hour intervals. Both patients have remained in remission while on methotrexate and liver histology has returned to normal. Further studies of this phenomenon are required.— M. M. Kaplan *et al.*, *Ann. intern. Med.*, 1987, *106*, 231.

ECTOPIC PREGNANCY. A report of the use of a local injection of methotrexate, together with transvaginal aspiration, to treat ectopic pregnancy.— W. Feichtinger and P. Kemeter (letter), *Lancet*, 1987, *1*, 381. See also D. E. Robertson *et al.*, *ibid.*, 975.

GESTATIONAL TROPHOBLASTIC TUMOURS. For reference to methotrexate in the treatment of choriocarcinoma, see Choice of Antineoplastic Agent, p.585.

IMMUNOSUPPRESSION. For the use of methotrexate as an immunosuppressant see under the headings for non-malignant disorders in this section and under Use of Immunosuppressants, p.594.

LEUKAEMIA, ACUTE. For the role of methotrexate in the treatment of acute leukaemias see under Choice of Antineoplastic Agent, p.586. For the effect of drug clearance on intermediate-dose methotrexate therapy for acute lymphoblastic leukaemia, see under Administration, above.

High-dose methotrexate therapy with folinic acid rescue has been reported to have limited effectiveness in patients with acute myelogenous leukaemia.— R. P. Gale, *New Engl. J. Med.*, 1979, *300*, 1189.

Meningeal leukaemia. A comparison of "prophylactic" post-induction therapy for acute lymphoblastic leukaemia using combined intermediate-dose intravenous methotrexate and intrathecal methotrexate with a conventional regimen of intrathecal methotrexate plus cranial irradiation. On completion of induction therapy, 506 children and adolescents were randomised to receive one of the 2 regimens. Intermediate-dose methotrexate was administered at a dose of 500 mg per m^2 body-surface once every 3 weeks for 3 doses, and followed by folinic acid rescue; administration of one-third of the dose was by intravenous bolus and the remainder was infused over 24 hours. Intrathecal methotrexate 12 mg per m^2 to a maximum of 15 mg was given concurrently. The alternative regimen comprised a total of 24 Gy of cranial irradiation and the same dose of intrathecal methotrexate. On completion of prophylaxis all patients received the same maintenance therapy and were re-evaluated after 3 years. Overall continuous complete remission was similar in both groups but intermediate-dose methotrexate gave better protection to the bone marrow and to the testes in male patients, while cranial irradiation gave better protection against CNS relapse. More intensive intermediate-dose and intrathecal methotrexate therapy, although not without its own risks, might give adequate protection to the CNS and avoid the long-term toxicity inherent in cranial irradiation.— A. I. Freeman *et al.*, *New Engl. J. Med.*, 1983, *308*, 477.

See also under Effects on the Nervous System in Adverse Effects (above).

MALIGNANT NEOPLASMS OF THE BREAST. For the use of methotrexate with cyclophosphamide and fluorouracil in the ad[illegible] therapy of breast cancer, see under Choice of Anti[illegible]tic Agent, p.589.

MALIGNANT NEOPLASMS OF THE BRONCHUS AND LUNG. For refe[illegible]he use of methotrexate in lung cancer, see under [illegible] Antineoplastic Agent, p.590.

MALIGNANT NEOPLASMS OF THE GASTRO-INTESTINAL TRACT. In [illegible] with metastatic colorectal cancer treatment [illegible]th methotrexate 40 mg per m^2 body-surface [illegible]us injection, followed by fluorouracil 700 [illegible] and allopurinol. Cycles were repeated every [illegible] a 200 mg escalation in fluorouracil dose [illegible] far as toxicity allowed. Results in 26 p[illegible] for at least 8 weeks were 7 partial remiss[illegible]re than 65 weeks duration. In 8 patien[illegible]ed stable and in 11 it progressed. The [illegible]te was 27% but in those who had received no previous treatment it was 39%. Results suggest that this sequential regime with allopurinol "rescue" is well tolerated and might achieve results better than those with fluorouracil alone.— P. C. Raich *et al.*, *Clin. Pharmac. Ther.*, 1984, *35*, 268.

MALIGNANT NEOPLASMS OF THE HEAD AND NECK. An 89-year-old patient with a fungating squamous cell carcinoma at the base of the neck was successfully treated by local infiltration of methotrexate 5 mg in 10 mL sodium chloride injection (0.9%), weekly for 6 weeks to reduce tumour bulk; the remaining fungating tissue was treated with daily applications of fluorouracil ointment and the resultant scar excised to avoid recurrence. Local treatment offers a safe and simple alternative for treating squamous cell carcinoma in the elderly.— I. Walker (letter), *Med. J. Aust.*, 1984, *140*, 183.

ORGAN AND TISSUE TRANSPLANTATION. For comparison of methotrexate with cyclosporin in bone-marrow transplantation, see under Cyclosporin, p.617.

PREGNANCY AND THE NEONATE. *First trimester*. See Adverse Effects, above.

Second trimester. An apparently normal infant girl was born to a woman in whom acute leukaemia was diagnosed when she was 16 weeks pregnant, and who was treated with a regimen including methotrexate.— M. Khurshid and M. Saleem (letter), *Lancet*, 1978, *2*, 534.

RHEUMATIC DISORDERS. Because efficacy has also been claimed for methotrexate in conditions such as Reiter's syndrome and polymyositis it has been tried in rheumatoid arthritis. Methotrexate therapy has been evaluated by the oral, intramuscular, and intravenous routes, generally in the lowest feasible therapeutic concentrations, for refractory disease. Improvement has been reported for all 3 routes and there is some evidence that patients with the HLA-Dr2 haplotype do particularly well. However, despite the trend to lower doses it is not yet possible to judge whether the risk/benefit ratio is acceptable, whether the drug is as effective as gold therapy and penicillamine, whether the interaction with aspirin will prove a handicap in practice, and whether erosive radiological progression can be arrested.— *Lancet*, 1986, *1*, 74.

Further reviews of the use of methotrexate in rheumatoid arthritis: R. F. Willkens, *Ann. intern. Med.*, 1985, *103*, 612; W. S. Wilke and A. H. Mackenzie, *Drugs*, 1986, *32*, 103; P. Tugwell *et al.*, *Ann. intern. Med.*, 1987, *107*, 358; Health and Public Policy Committee, *ibid.*, 418.

A study of the value of intravenous methotrexate in rheumatoid arthritis. Of 14 patients with persistent arthritis unresponsive to other therapy 11 showed objective evidence of improvement within 2 months of starting therapy with methotrexate in doses between 10 and 50 mg weekly by intravenous injection. Four patients required modification of the maximum dose of 50 mg because of toxicity and 3 of these were subsequently withdrawn from therapy.— R. M. Michaels *et al.*, *Arthritis Rheum.*, 1982, *25*, 339.

A double-blind crossover study of the efficacy of intramuscular pulsed weekly doses of methotrexate in 12 patients with active refractory rheumatoid arthritis. Patients were randomly assigned to methotrexate or placebo. In the former group, following a test dose of 5 mg, therapy was begun with 10 mg of methotrexate weekly, increased if necessary by 5 mg every 3 weeks up to 25 mg weekly. After 14 weeks patients crossed over to the alternative therapy. Marked clinical improvement in joint swelling and tenderness, as well as in subjective scores, was seen following methotrexate. In 11 patients the maximum dose was required; the other was maintained on 20 mg weekly. There was no consistent improvement after placebo and patients crossing from methotrexate to placebo experienced rapid flaring of disease. Two patients developed mild signs of toxicity (rash and stomatitis) during methotrexate, but were able to continue therapy. A thirteenth patient, with renal insufficiency, developed pancytopenia and was excluded from the study. Tests of immune function suggested that methotrexate was not acting via immunosuppression in these patients. The results indicate that weekly intramuscular methotrexate is effective in patients with refractory rheumatoid arthritis but that exclusion of high-risk patients (e.g. with impaired renal function), and careful monitoring of therapy, is essential.— P. A. Andersen *et al.*, *Ann. intern. Med.*, 1985, *103*, 489.

A double-blind crossover study of the efficacy of low-dose oral methotrexate therapy in refractory rheumatoid arthritis. Patients were assigned to receive either placebo or methotrexate 2.5 mg three times weekly, increased to 5 mg three times weekly if necessary, and crossed over after 12 weeks. The study involved 33 patients of whom 28 completed both arms. Methotrexate therapy was associated with a significant improvement in disease activity; of the 8 patients who were considered to show the most substantial response to methotrexate, 4 were of the HLA-Dr2 haplotype, compared with only 3 of the remaining 25 evaluated. Adverse reactions, including elevated serum concentrations of aminotransferases, occurred in 17 patients while receiving methotrexate whereas only 5 patients reported adverse effects during the placebo period. There was a significant disease flare in patients who switched from methotrexate to placebo.— M. E. Weinblatt *et al.*, *New Engl. J. Med.*, 1985, *312*, 818. Comment. There is now considerable evidence that methotrexate is superior to placebo in the management of rheumatoid arthritis but in view of the risk of hepatic fibrosis it might be prudent to undertake liver biopsies when the cumulative dose of methotrexate reached 1.5 g.— J. H. Klippel and J. L. Decker, *ibid.*, 853. See also H. J. Williams *et al.*, *Arthritis Rheum.*, 1985, *28*, 721; L. E. Boh *et al.*, *Clin. Pharm.*, 1986, *5*, 503.

For the use of methotrexate in vasculitis secondary to rheumatoid arthritis, see under Skin and Connective-tissue Disorders, Non-malignant, below.

SARCOIDOSIS. In the treatment of sarcoidosis methotrexate 25 mg once weekly initially, reduced gradually if improvement occurred, cleared cutaneous lesions in 12 of 16 patients and uveal lesions in 3 of the 4 patients in whom the eyes were also involved. The effect on hilar node, lung, and other sarcoidosis lesions was less certain.— N. K. Veien and H. Brodthagen, *Br. J. Derm.*, 1977, *97*, 213. Methotrexate should only be used if corticosteroids are contra-indicated.— B. L. Fanburg, *Am. J. Hosp. Pharm.*, 1979, *36*, 351. Methotrexate was an alternative in the treatment of chronic fibrotic persistent disease.— D. G. James, *Postgrad. med. J.*, 1984, *60*, 234.

See also Lupus Pernio, under Skin and Connective-tissue Disorders, Non-malignant, below.

SKIN AND CONNECTIVE-TISSUE DISORDERS, NON-MALIGNANT. *Lupus pernio*. Methotrexate is a valuable adjunct in the treatment of lupus pernio (cutaneous sarcoidosis) in doses of 25 mg weekly by mouth, for courses of 3 months. The drug may be given in combination with corticosteroids and antimalarials.— M. A. Spiteri *et al.*, *Br. J. Derm.*, 1985, *112*, 315.

Lymphomatoid papulosis. Control of lymphomatoid papulosis was achieved in 3 patients given methotrexate 5 to 25 mg weekly by mouth. Results in the 2 who had obtained partial remission following PUVA therapy indicated that methotrexate might be more effective.— G. L. Wantzin and K. Thomsen, *Br. J. Derm.*, 1984, *111*, 93.

Psoriasis. A review of the treatment of psoriasis. Methotrexate has been used in refractory or disabling disease. The clinician must constantly supervise patients, and therapy must be discontinued if toxicity develops. Methotrexate is best given either as a single weekly dose of 10 to 20 mg by mouth or in 3 doses of 2.5 to 7.5 mg at 12-hour intervals once a week. Experience has shown that the drug gives significant symptomatic relief; however, a few weeks after withdrawal psoriasis recurs and may be more severe than before.— E. M. Farber and L. Nall, *Drugs*, 1984, *28*, 324.

A retrospective study involving 98 patients indicated that methotrexate therapy was effective in maintaining remission from psoriasis when used after Ingram therapy (tar baths, ultraviolet radiation, and dithranol). Patients were chosen for maintenance therapy because of a history of relapse or a slow response to Ingram therapy. Methotrexate was given initially in doses of 5 mg at three 12-hourly intervals weekly, and was subsequently reduced where possible or when side-effects occurred. The average duration of methotrexate treatment was 29 months and methotrexate considerably lengthened the remission period when compared with previous courses of treatment in some of the same group of patients.— P. C. M. van de Kerkhof and J. W. H. Mali, *Br. J. Derm.*, 1982, *106*, 623. The remission rate in 61 patients with severe psoriasis given Ingram therapy, but no maintenance treatment, was only 24% after 1 year. In 37 who were given subsequent PUVA maintenance therapy, and 108 given methotrexate, the 1-year remission rates were 82% and 96% respectively, and 83% of the methotrexate-treated group were still in remission 3 years later. However, on stopping methotrexate therapy a rapid relapse followed whereas after stopping PUVA many patients remained in remission for months.— P. C. M. van de Kerkhof *et al.*, *ibid.*, 605.

See also under Use of Immunosuppressants, p.595.

For reference to the use of methotrexate with etretinate in severe erythrodermic psoriasis see Etretinate, p.922.

Vasculitis. Methotrexate 10 mg weekly as a single dose by mouth in 8 patients produced complete resolution of skin ulcers resulting from vasculitis secondary to rheumatoid arthritis, after an average of 12 weeks' treatment. The dose was subsequently reduced and remission was maintained for between 6 and 48 months.— L. R. Espinoza *et al.*, *J. Am. Acad. Derm.*, 1986, *15*, 508.

Preparations

Methotrexate Injection *(B.P.)*. Contains methotrexate and sodium hydroxide. When intended for intrathecal use it contains no preservative.

Methotrexate Sodium Injection *(U.S.P.)*. A sterile solution of methotrexate in Water for Injections prepared with the aid of sodium hydroxide.

Methotrexate Tablets *(B.P.)*

Methotrexate Tablets *(U.S.P.)*

Proprietary Preparations

Emtexate *(Ferring, UK)*. *Tablets*, methotrexate 10 mg. *Injection*, methotrexate 2.5 mg (as methotrexate sodium)/mL, in ampoules of 2 mL, 25 mg (as methotrexate sodium)/mL, in vials of 2, 10, 20, 40, and 200 mL, and 100 mg (as methotrexate sodium)/mL, in vials of 10 and 50 mL.

Injection, powder for reconstitution, methotrexate 0.5, 1, and 5 g (as methotrexate sodium).

Maxtrex *(Farmitalia Carlo Erba, UK)*. *Tablets*, scored, methotrexate 2.5 and 10 mg.

Injection, methotrexate 2.5 mg (as methotrexate sodium)/mL, in vials of 2mL, and methotrexate 25 mg (as methotrexate sodium)/mL, in vials of 2, 20, 40, and 200 mL.

Proprietary Names and Manufacturers of Methotrexate and Methotrexate Sodium

Emtexate *(Ger.; Switz.; Nordic, UK)*; Emthexat *(Nyco, Norw.; Nycomed, Swed.)*; Emthexate *(Neth.)*; Farmitrexat *(Farmitalia, Ger.)*; Farmotrex *(Farmos, Denm.)*; Folex *(Adria, USA)*; Ledertrexate *(Belg.; Lederle, Fr.; Neth.)*; Maxtrex *(Farmitalia Carlo Erba, UK)*; Methotrexat *(Ger.)*; Metotrexato *(Arg.)*; Metrexan *(Pharmacia, Denm.)*; Mexate *(Bristol-Myers Oncology, USA)*; Tremetex *(Laakefarmos, Swed.)*.

Manufacturers also include—*Bull, UK; Lederle, UK; Lederle, USA.*

12966-p

Misonidazole *(BAN, USAN, rINN)*.

NSC-261037; Ro-7-0582. 3-Methoxy-1-(2-nitroimidazol-1-yl)propan-2-ol.

$C_7H_{11}N_3O_4$=201.2.

CAS — 13551-87-6.

Adverse Effects, Treatment, and Precautions

Peripheral neuropathy occurs frequently in patients given misonidazole, and is dose-related; concurrent administration of dexamethasone may reduce the incidence. High total doses of misonidazole have been associated with severe and sometimes fatal encephalopathy.

INTERACTIONS. Phenytoin and phenobarbitone induced the metabolism of misonidazole in a study in 12 healthy subjects. Pretreatment with phenytoin 300 mg daily or phenobarbitone 200 mg daily, by mouth, for 7 days, significantly reduced the mean elimination half-life of misonidazole from 10.8 to 7.9 and from 11.5 to 8.9 hours respectively; this was associated with an increase in misonidazole clearance, and increased presence of the major metabolite desmethylmisonidazole. Pretreatment with ascorbic acid in a further 6 patients had little effect on misonidazole kinetics. The results show that total tissue exposure to misonidazole is reduced in patients pretreated with phenytoin or phenobarbitone.— K. Williams *et al.*, *Clin. Pharmac. Ther.*, 1983, *33*, 314. Evidence from a study of the kinetics of misonidazole enantiomers that phenytoin and phenobarbitone preferentially increase the clearance of the (+)-enantiomer of misonidazole.— K. M. Williams, *ibid.*, 1984, *36*, 817.

TREATMENT OF ADVERSE EFFECTS. The use of dexamethasone to reduce the incidence of misonidazole-induced neuropathy: R. C. Urtasun *et al.*, *Int. J. Radiat. Oncol. Biol. Phys.*, 1982, *8*, 365; H. Tanasichuk *et al.*, *ibid.*, 1984, *10*, 1735.

Absorption and Fate

Pharmacokinetic studies in 6 patients indicated that the time to peak plasma concentration varies greatly in patients receiving misonidazole. The absorption half-life ranged from 4 to 125 minutes and the time to peak plasma concentration from 0.5 to 6.5 hours; the longest time was in a patient with liver cancer, who also had the longest elimination half-life of 11.4 hours, reflecting the major role of hepatic metabolism in the elimination of this drug. The usual clinical practice of irradiating the tumour 4 hours after misonidazole administration is probably not valid for all patients. The time to achieve peak concentration in saliva was similar to that in plasma, although the correlation between concentrations was not high; salivary peak time could probably be used to predict the individual peak time and consequently the optimal time for irradiation.— I. Matheson *et al.*, *Hum. Toxicol.*, 1984, *3*, 29.

The pharmacokinetics of misonidazole and its major metabolite, desmethylmisonidazole in patients receiving radiotherapy.— P. G. Meering *et al.*, *Hum. Toxicol.*, 1985, *4*, 425.

See also under Interactions, above.

Uses and Administration

Misonidazole is structurally related to metronidazole (p.667) and shares some of the same properties. It has been given to sensitise resistant, hypoxic tumour cells to the effects of irradiation. Doses of 1 to 5 g per m^2 body-surface have been given by mouth, 4 to 6 hours before radiotherapy. Desmethylmisonidazole has also been investigated as a radiosensitiser.

Hypoxic cells in tumours are up to 3 times more resistant to radiation than aerobic cells, and compounds such as misonidazole can mimic oxygen and thus sensitise these cells. The phase I studies of this compound, together with more recent experience have led to a dose recommendation of 6 g per m^2 over 1 week, 10.5 g per m^2 over 2 to 3 weeks or 12 g per m^2 over 6 weeks. Neurotoxicity is dose-limiting, and other related compounds which enter the CNS less readily, are under examination.— T. L. Phillips *et al.*, *Cancer*, 1981, *48*, 1697. A trial of misonidazole in radiotherapy for cervical carcinoma.— Report from the MRC Working Party on Misonidazole for Cancer of the Cervix, *Br. J. Radiol.*, 1984, *57*, 491.

Proprietary Names and Manufacturers

Roche, UK.

1847-d

Mitobronitol *(BAN, rINN)*.

DBM; Dibromomannitol; NSC-94100; R-54; WR-220057. 1,6-Dibromo-1,6-dideoxy-D-mannitol.

$C_6H_{12}Br_2O_4$=308.0.

CAS — 488-41-5.

Pharmacopoeias. In *Br.*

A white or almost white crystalline solid. Slightly **soluble** in water, alcohol, and acetone; practically insoluble in chloroform. **Store** in well-closed containers. Protect from light.

Adverse Effects, Treatment, and Precautions

For an outline of the adverse effects experienced with antineoplastic agents and immunosuppressants, general guidelines for their treatment, and precautions, see Antineoplastic Agents, p.580, p.583.

Bone-marrow depression during treatment with mitobronitol may be severe.

Absorption and Fate

Mitobronitol is readily absorbed from the gastro-intestinal tract and is excreted through the liver into the bile with reabsorption in the small intestine. It is eliminated in the urine, partly as bromine-containing metabolites.

Uses and Administration

Mitobronitol is an antineoplastic agent which appears to act as an alkylating agent (p.580), perhaps by epoxide formation. It has been used in the management of thrombocythaemia, both primary, and secondary to chronic myeloid leukaemia or polycythaemia vera.

The usual dose is 250 mg daily by mouth until the platelet count falls to acceptable levels. Intermittent dosage has been given for maintenance therapy, adjusted according to the blood count. Frequent examination of the blood should be performed during treatment.

Long-term follow-up of a co-operative study involving 350 patients with polycythaemia vera and treated with mitobronitol. In general one course of mitobronitol consisted of a total of 1.5 to 3.5 g by mouth given over 3 to 6 days, with 2 to 3 courses being given per year; patients over 70 years of age received smaller doses at least on the first occasion. Of 113 patients followed for over 10 years 68 have survived, and there were no deaths due to acute non-lymphoblastic leukaemia; among the 168 living and 69 dead patients who had been followed for between 2 and 10 years there were 7 cases of acute non-lymphoblastic leukaemia. The frequency of this leukaemia was less than that observed with other chemotherapy regimens and it is possible that mitobronitol has an advantage not only over the already discarded chlorambucil but also over phosphorus-32 or busulphan in rarely inducing acute non-lymphoblastic leukaemia.— E. Kelemen *et al.* (letter), *Lancet*, 1987, *2*, 625.

Preparations

Mitobronitol Tablets *(B.P.)*

Proprietary Preparations

Myelobromol *(Sinclair, UK)*. *Tablets*, mitobronitol 125 mg.

Proprietary Names and Manufacturers

Myebrol *(Jpn)*; Myelobromol *(Ger.; Switz.; Sinclair, UK)*.

1848-n

Mitoguazone *(rINN)*.

Methyl-GAG; Methylglyoxal Bisguanylhydrazone; NSC-32946 *(dihydrochloride)*. 1,1′-[(Methylethanediylidene)dinitrilo]diguanidine.

$C_5H_{12}N_8$=184.2.

CAS — 459-86-9 (mitoguazone); 7059-23-6 (dihydrochloride).

Adverse Effects, Treatment, and Precautions

For an outline of the adverse effects experienced with antineoplastic agents and immunosuppressants, general guidelines for their treatment, and precautions, see Antineoplastic Agents, p.580, p.583.

Adverse effects reported with mitoguazone include hypoglycaemia, fatigue, weakness, peripheral neuropathies, and myopathy, which may be dose-limiting. Granulocytopenia and thrombocytopenia are generally reversible on stopping treatment. Gastro-intestinal effects frequently occur. Ventricular arrhythmias have been reported in some patients.

Uses and Administration

Mitoguazone is an antineoplastic agent which may exert its cytotoxic effects by its ability to inhibit polyamine biosynthesis. It has been given as the dihydrochloride, by intravenous infusion in doses of 80 to 300 mg daily, for 3 to 5 days, in the treatment of acute myeloid leukaemias. It may also be given by intramuscular injection. Mitoguazone has also been tried, as the dihydrochloride or the acetate, in the treatment of solid tumours.

Proprietary Names and Manufacturers

Riom, Fr.

1849-h

Mitolactol *(rINN)*.

DBD; Dibromodulcitol; NSC-104800; WR-138743. 1,6-Dibromo-1,6-dideoxy-D-galactitol.

$C_6H_{12}Br_2O_4$=308.0.

CAS — 10318-26-0.

Adverse Effects, Treatment, and Precautions

For an outline of the adverse effects experienced with antineoplastic agents and immunosuppressants, general guidelines for their treatment, and precautions, see Antineoplastic Agents, p.580, p.583.

Myelosuppression is the most significant adverse effect of mitolactol. Pulmonary and hepatic complications have also sometimes occurred.

Uses and Administration

Mitolactol is an antineoplastic agent which may act by alkylation (p.580). It has been given by mouth in the treatment of metastatic breast carcinoma, malignant melanoma, and other solid tumours, and has also been tried in leukaemia and lymphomas. Doses of about 3 mg per kg body-weight, or of 130 mg per m^2 body-surface have been given daily. Blood counts should be taken regularly during treatment and mitolactol withdrawn if bone-marrow depression occurs.

Proprietary Names and Manufacturers

Elobromol *(Chinoin, Hung.)*.

1850-a

Mitomycin *(BAN, USAN, rINN).*

Mitomycin C; Mitomycine C; NSC-26980. 6-Amino-1,1a,2,8,8a,8b-hexahydro-8-hydroxymethyl-8a-methoxy-5-methylazirino[2′,3′:3,4]-pyrrolo[1,2-*a*]indole-4,7-dione carbamate; (1*R*,2*R*,9*R*,9a*S*)-7-Amino-2,3,5,8,9,9a-hexahydro-9a-methoxy-6-methyl-5,8-dioxo-1,2-epimino-1-*H*-pyrrolo[1,2-*a*]indol-9-ylmethyl carbamate.

$C_{15}H_{18}N_4O_5$=334.3.

CAS — 50-07-7.

Pharmacopoeias. In *Fr., Jpn,* and *U.S.*

An antineoplastic antibiotic produced by the growth of *Streptomyces caespitosus.* It has a potency of not less than 900 μg per mg.

It occurs as a blue-violet crystalline powder. **Soluble** in water, acetone, methyl alcohol, butyl acetate, and cyclohexanone. A 0.5% solution in water has a pH of 6 to 8. **Store** in airtight containers. Protect from light.

STABILITY IN SOLUTION. A study of the degradation of mitomycin in acidic solutions.— J. H. Beijnen and W. J. M. Underberg, *Int. J. Pharmaceut.*, 1985, *24,* 219.

Mitomycin was less stable as a solution in glucose injection (5%) than in sodium chloride injection (0.9%); following storage for 12 hours at 5°C in a refrigerator 33% of the initial concentration of mitomycin was lost in the former mixture, compared with 10% loss in the latter. When stored at room temperature, less than 26% of the initial mitomycin concentration remained in the glucose admixture after 12 hours. In contrast when mitomycin solutions were mixed with glucose or sodium chloride injections buffered to pH 7.7 to 7.8 they remained stable for 15 days at room temperature and for at least 120 days when refrigerated. The results suggest that unbuffered solutions of mitomycin should not be administered by prolonged intravenous infusion because of the rapid degradation of mitomycin.— E. J. Quebbeman *et al., Am. J. Hosp. Pharm.*, 1985, *42,* 1750. Comment by a manufacturer (*Bristol, USA*). These results are substantially different from those generated by the manufacturers which suggest that mitomycin is stable for 48 hours at 25° as an unbuffered solution in glucose injection (5%) and for 6 days at this temperature as a solution in sodium chloride injection (0.9%). The difference may be because the authors used a different product.— J. H. Keller (letter), *ibid.*, 1986, *43,* 59. Reply, and the suggestion that the assay used by the manufacturer may not be specific for the undegraded drug.— E. J. Quebbeman and N. E. Hoffman (letter), *ibid.*, 64. A further reference to poor stability in glucose injection (5%).— J. A. Benvenuto *et al., ibid.*, 1981, *38,* 1914.

Adverse Effects, Treatment, and Precautions

For an outline of the adverse effects experienced with antineoplastic agents and immunosuppressants, general guidelines for their treatment, and precautions, see Antineoplastic Agents, p.580.

The main adverse effect of mitomycin is delayed cumulative bone-marrow suppression. Profound leucopenia and thrombocytopenia occurs after about 4 weeks with recovery in about 8 weeks after a dose. Blood counts may not recover in about one-quarter of patients. Other serious adverse-effects include renal damage and pulmonary reactions; a potentially fatal haemolytic-uraemic syndrome has been reported in some patients. Gastro-intestinal toxicity, dermatitis, alopecia, fever, and malaise may also occur. Local tissue necrosis, ulceration, and cellulitis may occur following extravasation.

Mitomycin is contra-indicated in patients with impaired renal function or coagulation disorders.

EFFECTS ON THE BLADDER. A report of severe bladder contracture following intravesical administration of mitomycin.— Z. Wajsman *et al., J. Urol., Baltimore,* 1983, *130,* 340.

Eight of 160 patients given mitomycin by intravesical instillation following resection of superficial bladder cancers developed indolent, symptomless ulcers at the site of resection. No treatment was required, and the lesion eventually appears to heal but biopsy was man[illegible]ry to distinguish such lesions from infiltrating blad[illegible]cer.— B. Richards and D. Tolley (letter), *Lan*[illegible] 45. A similar report. Ulcers were seen in 13 of 43 patients given intravesical mitomycin. In 5, the ulcer disappeared within 3 months of the start of treatment and in a further 3 after 8 to 10 months; in the remaining 5 invasive tumour was found at 3 to 8 months.— J. W. Hetherington and P. Whelan (letter), *ibid.*, 324.

EFFECTS ON THE KIDNEYS. Evidence that long-term therapy with mitomycin and fluorouracil is hazardous, in that it appears to produce a low-grade haemolytic-uraemic state. Attempts to correct this by compatible blood transfusions in 2 patients led to exacerbation of the haemolytic process, with schistocytes in the peripheral blood, rapidly progressive renal failure, and death. Treatment with corticosteroids, antiplatelet drugs, and fresh frozen plasma had no significant effect in the patient in whom these were tried. The therapeutic regimen of mitomycin with fluorouracil should be terminated at the first sign of intravascular haemolysis, persistent proteinuria, and rising serum-urea concentrations.— B. G. Jones *et al., Lancet,* 1980, *1,* 1275. Dose correction, and report of a patient who had a rash while on chemotherapy, followed, 2 months after his last dose of mitomycin, by nephritis, renal insufficiency, haemolysis, and severe hypertension.— D. A. Karlin and J. R. Stroehlein (letter), *ibid., 2,* 534.

Chronic haemolysis and progressive renal impairment following a prolonged course of fluorouracil, doxorubicin, and mitomycin. This patient also deteriorated clinically following red cell transfusion. Limited success was obtained after one plasmaphaeresis (the platelet count increased, but the azotaemia and anaemia got worse) but the patient died before the efficacy could be adequately assessed.— K. D. Lempert (letter), *Lancet,* 1980, *2,* 369.

Haemolysis and renal failure in a woman treated with mitomycin without fluorouracil. Once again, the symptoms got worse with blood transfusion, and there was a latency period of about 4 months after the last mitomycin treatment.— K. W. Rumpf *et al.* (letter), *Lancet,* 1980, *2,* 1037.

A report of 25 cases of mitomycin-induced nephrotoxicity. All patients had received mitomycin in total doses of 70 mg or more and developed a haemolytic-uraemic syndrome, of which 6 patients died. Treatment consisted of cessation of chemotherapy and symptomatic management. The value of plasma exchange was uncertain but might have some benefit in the long-term.— D. Cordonnier *et al., Néphrologie,* 1985, *6,* 19.

EFFECTS ON THE LIVER. Hepatic veno-occlusive disease developed in 6 of 29 patients given intensive mitomycin therapy and autologous bone-marrow transplantation. The effect was manifest as abdominal pain, hepatomegaly, and ascites, and liver failure was progressive and fatal in 3. A further patient, who had no symptoms, was found to have veno-occlusive disease at post mortem.— H. M. Lazarus *et al., Cancer,* 1982, *49,* 1789.

EFFECTS ON RESPIRATORY FUNCTION. A retrospective study found evidence of mitomycin-related lung disease in 6 of approximately 200 patients.— S. R. Gunstream *et al., Cancer Treat. Rep.*, 1983, *67,* 301.

EFFECTS ON THE SKIN. A report of irritation and acute vesicular eczema on the palms and soles in a patient receiving intravesicular mitomycin; symptoms resolved on stopping mitomycin.— V. S. Neild *et al., J. R. Soc. Med.*, 1984, *77,* 610.

EXTRAVASATION. Injection of 4 mL of a 10% solution of sodium thiosulphate with 6 mL of water had been suggested as an antidote to the adverse effects of extravasation of mitomycin. The mechanism of the antidote would be direct inactivation of mitomycin.— M. E. MacCara, *Drug Intell. & clin. Pharm.*, 1983, *17,* 713.

The manufacturers recommend treatment of mitomycin extravasation by infiltration of the area with sodium bicarbonate, local dexamethasone injection, and systemic injection of pyridoxine.

INTERACTIONS. For a report of mitomycin possibly enhancing the cardiotoxicity of doxorubicin, see A. U. Buzdar *et al., Cancer Treat. Rep.*, 1978, *62,* 1005.

For reports of acute bronchospasm following injection of a vinca alkaloid in patients pretreated with mitomycin, see Vinblastine Sulphate, p.654.

Absorption and Fate

Mitomycin disappears rapidly from the blood after intravenous injection. It is widely distributed but does not appear to cross the blood-brain barrier. Mitomycin is metabolised mainly but not exclusively in the liver. Following normal doses about 10% of a dose is excreted unchanged in the urine; small amounts are also present in bile and faeces.

Uses and Administration

Mitomycin is a highly toxic antibiotic with antineoplastic properties. It acts as an alkylating agent (p.580) after activation *in vivo* and also suppresses the synthesis of nucleic acids.It is a cell-cycle nonspecific agent, but is most active in the late G_1 and early S phases.

Mitomycin is used, with other antineoplastic agents, in the palliative treatment of gastric and pancreatic adenocarcinomas. It has also been given to patients with other solid tumours including those of the bladder, colon and rectum, lung, cervix, and breast and has been tried in patients with leukaemias. The usual initial dose is 10 to 20 mg per m^2 body-surface given as a single dose through a running intravenous infusion and repeated every 6 to 8 weeks. Alternatively it may be given intravenously in divided doses of 2 mg per m^2 daily for 5 days, repeated after 2 days. Subsequent doses are adjusted according to the effect on bone marrow and treatment should not be repeated until the leucocyte count is above 3000 per mm^3 and the platelet count above 75 000 per mm^3.

Mitomycin is also used as a bladder instillation: 4 to 10 mg is instilled one to three times a week in the prevention of recurrent bladder tumours and 10 to 40 mg is instilled in the treatment of bladder tumours.

ADMINISTRATION. Intra-arterial infusion of ethylcellulose microcapsules of mitomycin in total doses of 10 to 90 mg, alone, or with gelatine sponge to induce complete vascular occlusion, produced objective tumour reduction in 20 of 33 and 13 of 18 tumours respectively in a study involving 56 patients with a variety of malignant neoplasms. Of the remaining 18 tumours 13 showed some degree of response. Most patients had symptomatic improvement. Tumour reduction facilitated surgical procedures in 18 of 22 patients. These preliminary, uncontrolled results suggest that the use of mitomycin microcapsules in this way to combine chemotherapeutic and embolic effects (chemoembolisation) is effective as a pre-operative and palliative measure in the treatment of locally-advanced carcinoma and helpful in the control of intractable symptoms such as haemorrhage or pain.— T. Kato *et al., J. Am. med. Ass.*, 1981, *245,* 1123. Comment. The lower doses of mitomycin may have been insufficient to exert a cytotoxic effect, although there might have been a synergistic effect with the embolisation.— V. P. Chuang and S. Wallace, *ibid.*, 1151. See also T. Kato *et al.* (letter), *Lancet,* 1979, *2,* 479; J. W. Gyves *et al., Clin. Pharmac. Ther.*, 1983, *34,* 259.

MALIGNANT NEOPLASMS. A review of mitomycin. The contribution of mitomycin to combination regimens for gastric, pancreatic, and lung cancer has not been determined but it does appear to have demonstrable activity in the treatment of superficial bladder cancer and may be of some benefit in patients with refractory carcinoma of the breast.— D. C. Doll *et al., J. clin. Oncol.*, 1985, *3,* 276.

For a report of the use of mitomycin with vindesine in patients with lung cancer, see under Vindesine Sulphate, p.656.

MALIGNANT NEOPLASMS OF THE BLADDER. Follow-up in 48 patients given instillations of mitomycin following resection of superficial bladder cancer appeared to confirm that mitomycin treatment reduced the recurrence rate to approximately 10%, compared with about 50% in 31 controls. Survival-rate in treated patients was 100% over 2.5 years, but was only 84% in the controls. Mitomycin treatment, consisting of instilllation of 20 mg of mitomycin in 20 mL of water, fortnightly for 1 year and then monthly for 2 years, was well tolerated, with only minimal side-effects.— H. Hulland *et al., J. Urol., Baltimore,* 1984, *132,* 27.

In 23 patients with superficial bladder cancer, instillation of mitomycin 20 mg in 20 mL of water, for a total of 21 instillations over 7 weeks produced complete disappearance of the tumour in 17, and partial response in 4. On follow-up for 2 years in 22 of the patients, 18 were still alive, of whom 7 were free of recurrence, 9 had endoscopically controlled disease and 6 had progressed to invasive cancer. Four patients had died, 3 of invasive bladder cancer. Despite the excellent short-term results, the subsequent results in this group were disappointing, and care is needed in patients with carcinoma *in situ*, in whom initial symptomatic relief was maintained even in those who subsequently developed invasive disease.— J. J. F. Somerville *et al., Br. J. Urol.*, 1985, *57*, 686.

MALIGNANT NEOPLASMS OF THE BREAST. A detailed review of mitomycin in the treatment of advanced breast cancer. Response rates of 23% to 38% have been reported when mitomycin is given as initial single-agent therapy, and of 18% when mitomycin was used in patients who had previously received treatment with cyclophosphamide, methotrexate, and fluorouracil. Mitomycin has also been used in various combination regimens, notably with doxorubicin, and response rates of 42 to 66% have been reported, with median durations of response of 5 to 15 months. Mitomycin-containing regimens may also have a role in salvage therapy.— S. S. Legha, *Clin. Ther.*, 1985, *7*, 286.

Preparations

Mitomycin for Injection *(U.S.P.)*. A dry mixture of mitomycin and mannitol.

Proprietary Preparations

Mitomycin-C Kyowa *(Martindale Pharmaceuticals, UK)*. *Injection*, powder for reconstitution, mitomycin 2, 10, and 20 mg.

Proprietary Names and Manufacturers

Amétycine *(Choay, Fr.)*; Mitomycin-C *(Sigma, Austral.; MPS Lab., S.Afr.; Martindale Pharmaceuticals, UK)*; Mitomycine *(Belg.)*; Mutamycin *(Bristol, Canad.; Bristol, Norw.; Bristol, Swed.; Bristol, Switz.; Bristol-Myers Oncology, USA)*.

1852-x

Mitotane *(USAN, rINN)*.

CB-313; *o,p'*DDD; NSC-38721; WR-13045. 1,1-Dichloro-2-(2-chlorophenyl)-2-(4-chlorophenyl)ethane.
$C_{14}H_{10}Cl_4$=320.0.

CAS — 53-19-0.

Pharmacopoeias. In *U.S.*

A white crystalline powder with a slight aromatic odour. Practically **insoluble** in water; soluble in alcohol, ether, petroleum spirit, and in fixed oils. **Store** in airtight containers. Protect from light.

Adverse Effects

Almost all patients given mitotane experience anorexia, nausea and vomiting, and sometimes diarrhoea, and about 40% suffer some central toxicity with dizziness, vertigo, sedation, lethargy, and mental depression. Permanent brain damage may develop with prolonged dosage. Ocular side-effects may occur with blurred vision, diplopia, lenticular opacities, and retinopathy. Other side-effects include allergic reactions, albuminuria, skin rashes, fever, myalgia, haemorrhagic cystitis, flushing, hypertension, and orthostatic hypotension.

Precautions

Mitotane inhibits the adrenal cortex and adrenal insufficiency may develop during treatment. In trauma or shock the drug should be temporarily withdrawn and corticosteroids should be given systemically. Mitotane should be given with care to patients with liver disease. Patients should not take charge of vehicles or machinery where loss of attention may lead to accidents. Behavioural and neurological assessments should be carried out regularly in patients who have been receiving treatment for 2 years or more.

INTERACTIONS. Administration of mitotane up to 3 g daily to a 65-year-old patient with Cushing's syndrome appeared to be ineffective and did not produce the side-effects usually associated with mitotane whilst the patient was also receiving treatment with spironolactone.— J. Wortsman and N. G. Soler, *J. Am. med. Ass.*, 1977, *238*, 2527.

With diagnostic tests. Mitotane inhibited the binding of thyroid hormones to binding globulins and could interfere with tests of thyroid function.— I. Ramsay, *Postgrad. med. J.*, 1985, *61*, 375. See also *Med. Lett.*, 1981, *23*, 30.

Absorption and Fate

Up to 40% of a dose of mitotane is absorbed from the gastro-intestinal tract. After daily doses of 5 to 15 g, concentrations in the blood of 7 to 90 µg per mL of unchanged drug and 29 to 54 µg per mL of metabolite have been reported. Mitotane has been detected in the blood 10 weeks after stopping treatment. It is widely distributed and appears to be stored mainly in fatty tissues. It is metabolised in the liver and other tissues and excreted as metabolites in urine and bile. From 10 to 25% of a dose has been recovered in the urine as a water-soluble metabolite.

Uses and Administration

Mitotane is an antineoplastic agent with a selective inhibitory action on adrenal cortex activity. It is given in the treatment of inoperable adrenocortical tumours and has also been used in patients with Cushing's syndrome. The usual initial dosage is 8 to 10 g, or 6 to 15 mg per kg body-weight, daily by mouth in 3 or 4 divided doses, adjusted to the maximum tolerated dose which may range from 2 to 16 g daily. Slightly lower doses have usually been given to patients with Cushing's syndrome. Patients may require replacement therapy with corticosteroids during mitotane treatment.

CUSHING'S SYNDROME. Mitotane 4 to 12 g daily was given for an average of 8 months (range 3 to 34 months) to 62 patients with Cushing's syndrome. Cobalt irradiation of the pituitary was also carried out in 16 of the patients before or during treatment with mitotane. Remissions were achieved in 38 of the 46 patients who received only mitotane and in all of the 16 who also received irradiation. Relapses occurred in 20 of the 38 an average of 17 months later and further treatment was required; in 14 patients Cushing's syndrome was still controlled 6 to 80 months later. Overall, the syndrome had been controlled in 63% of the patients and surgery avoided so far.— J. P. Luton *et al., New Engl. J. Med.*, 1979, *300*, 459. Criticism of the use of mitotane and the view that trans-sphenoidal resection of pituitary adenomas is the treatment of choice for Cushing's disease.— P. R. Cooper and W. A. Shucart (letter), *ibid.*, *301*, 48. In some cases the alternative of adrenalectomy or mitotane may still be the therapeutic choice.— H. Bricaire *et al.* (letter), *ibid.*, 49.

Remission was achieved in 29 of 36 patients with Cushing's disease who were given low doses of mitotane in association with irradiation of the pituitary. Remission was maintained after treatment was discontinued in 17 patients. Initial doses of 4 g daily in divided doses were gradually reduced during the first 3 to 4 months to 1.5 to 2 g daily. After sustained suppression of cortisol concentrations for many months and with remission of the disease, the dose was decreased to as low as 500 mg twice weekly in some patients. The longest duration of treatment at these low doses was 7 years.— D. E. Schteingart *et al., Ann. intern. Med.*, 1980, *92*, 613.

Proper treatment of Cushing's syndrome depends on a correct definition of its cause. Surgical results with adrenal carcinomas are poor, and although they occasionally respond to mitotane there is no effective chemotherapy, the tumours are radioresistant, and survival is usually brief. Most patients with the ectopic ACTH syndrome have nonresectable malignant tumours but in those with indolent tumours 'medical adrenalectomy' with mitotane, or surgical adrenalectomy should be considered. Cushing's disease itself is always curable, although initial treatment may fail. Irradiation combined with a 6-month course of mitotane cures about 80% of adults, but the preferred treatment is surgery.— D. N. Orth, *New Engl. J. Med.*, 1984, *310*, 649.

Preparations

Mitotane Tablets *(U.S.P.)*

Proprietary Names and Manufacturers

Lysodren *(Bristol, Canad.; Bristol-Myers Oncology, USA)*.

12967-s

Mitozantrone Hydrochloride *(BANM)*.

CL-232315; DHAD; Dihydroxyanthracenedione Dihydrochloride; Mitoxantrone Hydrochloride *(USAN, rINNM)*; NSC-301739. 1,4-Dihydroxy-5,8-bis[2-(2-hydroxyethylamino)ethylamino]-anthraquinone dihydrochloride.
$C_{22}H_{28}N_4O_6$,2HCl=517.4.

CAS — 65271-80-9 (mitozantrone); 70476-82-3 (hydrochloride).

Mitozantrone solutions should be stored at room temperature, as refrigeration may cause a precipitate to form. The manufacturer states that solutions of mitozantrone hydrochloride are incompatible with heparin, and should not be given in the same infusion with other drugs.

Adverse Effects and Treatment

As for Doxorubicin Hydrochloride, p.623. Mitozantrone is reported to be better tolerated than doxorubicin.

Transient blue-green coloration of the urine, and occasionally the sclerae, may occur.

ALLERGY AND ANAPHYLAXIS. A report of 3 patients with allergic reactions to mitozantrone, including vasculitis, facial oedema and skin rashes, and in one, breathlessness, tachypnoea, cyanosis, and unrecordable pulse and blood pressure. However, allergic reactions to the drug appear to be rare.— W. B. Taylor *et al.* (letter), *Lancet*, 1986, *1*, 1439.

ALOPECIA. Two patients receiving therapy with mitozantrone developed selective alopecia of white but not of dark hair.— Z. A. Arlin *et al.* (letter), *New Engl. J. Med.*, 1984, *310*, 1464.

EFFECTS ON THE HEART. Two of 78 patients receiving mitozantrone developed congestive heart failure, after cumulative doses of 174 and 243 mg per m^2. In both, heart failure responded to diuretic therapy. Of the 9 other patients receiving more than 100 mg per m^2 1 had an increase in cardiac diameter, necessitating withdrawal, and 3 had significant falls in ejection fractions on serial radionuclide scanning after doses of 144 mg per m^2 or more. One further patient, who had previously received 313 mg per m^2 of doxorubicin had a significant fall in stress ejection fraction after only 47 mg per m^2 of mitozantrone. Caution is urged with mitozantrone in cumulative doses of more than 140 mg per m^2, and possibly at even lower doses in patients heavily pretreated with doxorubicin.— R. Stuart-Harris *et al.* (letter), *Lancet*, 1984, *2*, 219.

Pooled data from 3360 patients treated with mitozantrone include 88 reports with details of cardiac events, including 29 cases of congestive heart failure and 25 of decreased left ventricular ejection fraction. The major predisposing factor appeared to be prior treatment with an anthracycline, and congestive heart failure seemed to be more likely in patients exposed to a cumulative mitozantrone dose of 160 mg per m^2 body-surface or 120 mg per m^2 in those who had already received anthracyclines.— R. J. Crossley, *Cancer Treat. Rev.*, 1983, *10*, *Suppl.* B, 29. See also R. J. Crossley, *Semin. Oncol.*, 1984, *11*, *Suppl.* 1, 54.

EFFECTS ON THE LIVER. Transient abnormalities in liver function were seen in 11 of 26 patients given mitozantrone, including elevated serum bilirubin in one. In 7 patients enzyme concentrations returned to normal a median of 8 days later but in 3 the abnormalities persisted. In a further 19 patients receiving combination chemotherapy including mitozantrone, elevations of hepatic enzyme values and bilirubin concentrations occurred after treatment in 20 of 25 courses.— P. S. Paciucci and N. T. Sklarin (letter), *Ann. intern. Med.*, 1986, *105*, 805.

EFFECTS ON THE NERVOUS SYSTEM. Following intrathecal administration of mitozantrone to a patient with CNS leukaemia, severe leg pain followed by paraplegia subsequently developed. The patient remains paraplegic 4 months later. Although intrathecal mitozantrone is effective in treating resistant CNS disease in leukaemia, it should be used with caution.— A. K. Lakhani *et al.* (letter), *Lancet*, 1986, *2*, 1393. The manufacturers discourage administration by this route. At this early stage, in view of the reports of CNS problems that have been received, mitozantrone should not be administered intrathecally or intracranially.— P. G. Brock, *Pharm. J.*, 1987, *1*, 86.

EFFECTS ON SKIN. Four of 18 patients developed pruritus and skin desquamation associated with excessive skin dryness (asteatosis) while receiving chemotherapy with mitozantrone plus cytarabine. Treatment with emollients, moisturisers, and antihistamines resulted in only moderate improvement. Clinicians should be aware of this distressing potential side-effect, particularly in patients aged over 40.— F. Dharmasena *et al.* (letter), *Lancet*, 1985, *2*, 101.

LOCAL TOXICITY. A report of complications following 2 of 6 cases of extravasation of mitozantrone infusions. One patient developed an ulcer, which healed with conservative treatment, but the other developed severe induration and flexion deformity of the elbow, requiring surgery. Extravasation of mitozantrone has been reported to cause a transient blue discoloration of tissue but cellulitis or necrosis have not been previously reported: patients should be supervised to minimise the risk of extravasation.— G. G. Khoury, *Br. med. J.*, 1986, *292*, 802. Comment. The manufacturers accept that extravasation of mitozantrone may lead to tissue necrosis, but this is extremely rare.— A. Man, *ibid.*, *293*, 140.

Precautions

As for Doxorubicin Hydrochloride, p.624.

For the dangers associated with intrathecal administration of mitozantrone, and a warning that this route should not be used, see under Effects on the Nervous System, above.

For precautions in extravasation, see under Local Toxicity, above.

HANDLING AND DISPOSAL. Protective clothing should be worn for up to 7 days after therapy when handling urine and faeces from patients receiving mitozantrone.— J. Harris and L. J. Dodds, *Pharm. J.*, 1985, *2*, 289.

KAPOSI'S SARCOMA. Six patients with AIDS-related Kaposi's sarcoma, 5 of whom had advanced disease, experienced severe myelosuppression following treatment with mitozantrone, with neutropenia but no thrombocytopenia. All patients experienced disease progression during therapy. AIDS patients appear to have poor bone-marrow reserve, and the myelosuppression seen in these patients was greater than that in non-AIDS patients given mitozantrone. Treatment of AIDS-related Kaposi's sarcoma with mitozantrone should be discouraged.— L. Kaplan and P. A. Volberding (letter), *Lancet*, 1985, *2*, 396.

Absorption and Fate

Following intravenous administration mitozantrone is rapidly and extensively distributed to body tissues, and slowly excreted in urine and bile as unchanged drug and metabolites. Between 6 and 11% of a dose has been recovered from urine, and 13 to 25% in faeces, within 5 days of administration. It does not appear to cross the blood-brain barrier.

A study, involving 8 patients, of the disposition of radio-labelled mitozantrone following a single intravenous dose of 12 mg per m^2 body-surface. Pharmacokinetics in the majority of patients were best described by a 3-compartment model, with a mean terminal plasma half-life of 42.6 hours. The total drug related material recovered after excretion averaged 28% of the dose in 5 days, 10.1% in urine and 18% in faeces. Chromatography of urine revealed up to 3 polar metabolites. Postmortem analysis of organ samples from one patient revealed relatively high mitozantrone concentrations in tissues 35 days after administration, the highest concentration being in the liver, followed by bone marrow, heart, lungs, spleen, kidney, and thyroid: the total amount remaining in tissue was estimated at up to 15% of the dose.— D. S. Alberts *et al.*, *Cancer Treat. Rev.*, 1983, *10*, *Suppl.* B, 23.

Uses and Administration

Mitozantrone is an antineoplastic agent structurally related to doxorubicin (p.623). Its mode of action has not been fully established.

It is used in the treatment of advanced breast cancer, and of non-Hodgkin's lymphomas, alone or in combination with other agents. It may also be given to treat relapses of adult acute non-lymphoblastic leukaemias, and has been used in patients with hepatocellular carcinoma.

In the treatment of breast cancer and lymphomas, mitozantrone is given as the hydrochloride in an initial dose equivalent to 14 mg of base per m^2 body-surface, repeated every 3 weeks, by injecting a solution diluted in sodium chloride (0.9%) or glucose (5%) injection into a freely-running intravenous infusion of either, over at least 3 minutes. Subsequent doses may be adjusted according to the degree of myelosuppression produced and dosage may need to be reduced to 12 mg per m^2 initially in debilitated patients or those who have had previous chemotherapy. Doses should also probably be reduced when mitozantrone is given as part of a combination regimen: an initial dose of 10 to 12 mg per m^2 has been suggested.

In the treatment of patients with relapses of acute non-lymphoblastic leukaemia a dose of 12 mg per m^2 daily for 5 days may be given to induce remission.

Cardiac examinations are recommended in all patients who receive a cumulative dose of mitozantrone greater than 160 mg per m^2.

Reviews of mitozantrone: I. E. Smith, *Cancer Treat. Rev.*, 1983, *10*, 103; *Lancet*, 1984, *2*, 265; T. D. Shenkenberg and D. D. Von Hoff, *Ann. intern. Med.*, 1986, [illegible]05, 67.

[illegible]ntrone has produced responses both alone and [illegible] agents as initial chemotherapy in patients with breast cancer, and has also produced responses in acute myeloblastic and acute lymphoblastic leukaemia, including relapsed or refractory disease. Prelimary data suggest that mitozantrone with cytarabine may be effective in relapsed refractory myeloblastic leukaemia. Mitozantrone has also proved effective in previously treated patients with malignant lymphomas and has shown activity in primary hepatocellular cancer, but not in other tumours. Its place in treatment has not yet been defined: its spectrum of activity is narrower than that of doxorubicin, and it appears slightly less effective in breast cancer. However, its lesser toxicity makes it suitable in patients, such as the elderly, who tolerate chemotherapy poorly.— *Drug & Ther. Bull.*, 1986, *24*, 71.

ACTION. The mode of action of mitozantrone is not completely defined. Preliminary evidence *in vitro* suggests that mitozantrone binds to nucleic acids by intercalation, and it is a potent inhibitor of DNA and RNA synthesis. Unlike classical intercalators mitozantrone also induces non-protein-associated breaks in single-stranded DNA and it has been suggested that it may bind to DNA by non-intercalative electrostatic interactions. Cells in S phase are most sensitive but cell killing induced by mitozantrone is not cell-cycle specific.— T. D. Shenkenberg and D. D. Von Hoff, *Ann. intern. Med.*, 1986, *105*, 67.

ADMINISTRATION. A report of the intrathecal use of mitozantrone to treat refractory CNS involvement in a patient with lymphoblastic lymphoma. The patient received mitozantrone 0.8 or 1 mg twice weekly initially; subsequently 2 mg twice weekly was given by Ommaya reservoir for 4 weeks. The patient subsequently died of systemic disease refractory to chemotherapy but without recurrence of neurological symptoms; 1 month before death he developed paraplegia but the relationship to intrathecal mitozantrone therapy was unknown.— J. P. Laporte *et al.* (letter), *Lancet*, 1985, *2*, 160. Mitozantrone 2 mg twice weekly via an Ommaya reservoir resulted in a remarkable reduction in the number of blasts in CSF in a patient with CNS leukaemia resistant to intrathecal methotrexate and cytarabine.— A. Zuiable *et al.* (letter), *ibid.*, 1060.

For a further report of paraplegia following intrathecal mitozantrone, and a warning that this route should not be used, see under Effects on the Nervous System, above.

HODGKIN'S DISEASE AND OTHER LYMPHOMAS. In a Southwest Oncology Group study, 1 of 13 evaluable patients with Hodgkin's disease and 2 of 37 evaluable patients with non-Hodgkin's lymphomas had a complete response to therapy with mitozantrone in initial doses of 12 mg per m^2 body-surface, repeated every 3 weeks. There were also 2 partial responses among the patients with Hodgkin's disease and 7 partial responses among the group with non-Hodgkin's lymphomas. All patients had received previous combination chemotherapy. The median duration of response was 169 days in Hodgkin's and 232 days in non-Hodgkin's patients. The results were not remarkable but in view of the fact that the patients were heavily pretreated, and that severe toxicity was minimal, further studies with mitozantrone in combination in non-Hodgkin's lymphomas were planned.— C. A. Coltman *et al.*, *Cancer Treat. Rev.*, 1983, *10*, *Suppl.* B, 73.

Preliminary results of multicentre studies suggested that response rate to mitozantrone in patients with non-Hodgkin's lymphomas was higher when given in doses of 14 mg per m^2 by intravenous infusion every 3 weeks than as a weekly infusion of 5 mg per m^2. Toxicity also appeared less with the former regimen.— R. A. Gams *et al.*, *Cancer Treat. Rev.*, 1983, *10*, *Suppl.* B, 69.

LEUKAEMIA, ACUTE. Of 21 leukaemic patients treated with mitozantrone 10 mg per m^2 body-surface by intravenous infusion daily for 5 days, repeated if necessary, 5 had complete and 5 had partial responses: this included 1 complete and 2 partial responses among 7 patients with acute lymphoblastic leukaemia and 4 complete and 2 partial responses among 11 with acute myeloblastic leukaemia. Only 1 of 3 patients with chronic myeloid leukaemia in myeloid transformation achieved a partial response. Short-term toxicity was relatively mild.— H. G. Prentice *et al.*, *Cancer Treat. Rev.*, 1983, *10*, *Suppl.* B, 57. Five of 12 patients with acute lymphoblastic leukaemia achieved complete remission following treatment with mitozantrone in intravenous doses between 8 and 16 mg per m^2 daily for 5 days: 4 of these had previously failed to respond to re-induction, and 1 to initial induction chemotherapy. Two of the responding patients relapsed and subsequently achieved further complete remissions on treatment with mitozantrone. The duration of response varied between 3 and 30 weeks. Of the 7 patients remaining, 4 failed to respond and 3 died of sepsis before bone-marrow recovery. The drug appeared to be well-tolerated.— P. A. Paciucci *et al.*, *ibid.*, 65.

Sixteen patients with relapsed acute myeloid leukaemia (13 in first relapse and 3 in second), and 2 with primary disease refractory to treatment, were given mitozantrone 12 mg per m^2 body-surface by intravenous infusion daily for 5 days, together with cytarabine 1 g per m^2 by infusion twice daily for 3 days. Complete remission was achieved in 1 of the 2 patients with refractory acute myeloid leukaemia, in 6 of those in first relapse and in all 3 in second relapse; partial response occurred in 1 patient with refractory disease and 2 in first relapse. Six patients achieved complete remission after 1 course of chemotherapy only. Chemotherapy was generally well-tolerated, nausea being the most serious adverse effect. All patients had previously received anthracyclines and cardiac toxicity was seen in 2 who had received high doses. In a further 4 patients with previously untreated acute myeloid leukaemia treatment with mitozantrone and cytarabine produced complete remission in all after a single course. This combination is both effective and well-tolerated and deserves a wider trial both in relapsed patients and as part of the intensive consolidation therapy of acute myeloid leukaemia.— R. E. Marcus *et al.* (letter), *Lancet*, 1985, *1*, 1384. Similar results from a multicentre study in patients with refractory acute myeloid leukaemia. Complete remission was achieved in 8 of 20 patients given cytarabine 3 g per m^2 by infusion twice daily for 4 days, plus mitozantrone, initially in doses of 12 mg per m^2 by intravenous infusion on days 3, 4, and 5 of a cycle, but in later patients in a dose of 10 mg per m^2 on days 2 to 5. Partial remission was achieved in 4 patients. One patient died suddenly 12 hours after the first dose of mitozantrone, possibly due to cardiac toxicity, but toxicity was otherwise mild to moderate.— W. Hiddemann *et al.* (letter), *ibid.*, *2*, 508.

MALIGNANT NEOPLASMS OF THE BREAST. In patients with breast cancer mitozantrone produces responses in about 33% of patients when it is used as a first-line single agent. This rate is similar to that with doxorubicin currently considered the most active single agent in the treatment of advanced breast cancer. Comparative trials have thus far shown no significant difference in efficacy of the 2 agents. Combination regimens have apparently improved response rates over mitozantrone alone, and have lower toxicity than regimens containing doxorubicin.— T. D. Shenkenberg and D. D. Von Hoff, *Ann. intern. Med.*, 1986, *105*, 67.

An objective response was seen in 19 of 62 evaluable patients with advanced breast cancer given mitozantrone 12 or 14 mg per m^2 body-surface by intravenous infusion, repeated at 3-week intervals; a response rate of 31%. One patient achieved complete remission. The response rate in patients who had received no previous chemotherapy was 35% compared with 22% in those who had had previous treatment. Two patients developed reversible cardiac failure after prolonged treatment, at cumulative doses of 240 and 175 mg per m^2, and 2 more had falls in ventricular ejection fraction, but other toxicities were mild. In a further 9 patients given combination chemotherapy with mitozantrone 12 mg per m^2, methotrexate 30 mg per m^2, and vincristine 1.4 mg per m^2, repeated every 3 weeks, objective tumour responses were seen in 2.— I. E. Smith *et al.*, *Cancer Treat. Rev.*, 1983, *10*, *Suppl.* B, 37.

In an ongoing comparative study involving 51 evaluable patients with advanced breast cancer, patients were randomised to receive either doxorubicin 60 mg per m^2 or mitozantrone 12 mg per m^2 initially, repeated every 3 weeks, and adjusted to minimise leucopenia. Patients with progression after 2 courses or progression after initial response, and patients failing to achieve partial response after 4 courses were crossed over to receive the other agent. Ten of 25 given initial doxorubicin and 7 of 26 given mitozantrone achieved a partial response; a further 2 of 12 crossed to doxorubicin and 2 of 15 crossed to mitozantrone as secondary therapy achieved partial response. Results to date indicated no significant difference between the treatments in response rate and response duration (median of 84 days with doxorubicin and of 96 days with mitozantrone) but final conclusions could not yet be drawn.— J. A. Neidhart *et al.*, *Cancer Treat. Rev.*, 1983, *10*, *Suppl.* B, 41.

Further studies of mitozantrone in breast cancer: H. T. Mouridsen *et al.*, *Cancer Treat. Rev.*, 1983, *10*, *Suppl.* B, 47 (as first-line cytotoxic therapy in advanced disease); H. Y. Yap *et al.*, *ibid.*, 53 (with cyclophosphamide and fluorouracil).

MALIGNANT NEOPLASMS OF THE LIVER. Mitozantrone was given in initial doses of 12 mg per m^2 body-surface intravenously every 3 weeks to 40 patients with primary hepatocellular carcinoma; doses were subsequently modified according to toxicity and tolerance. Five patients to date had achieved partial remissions, the longest being of 21 weeks duration, and a further 4 had stable disease.— A. A. Dunk *et al.*, *Gut*, 1984, *25*, A1131.

Proprietary Preparations

Novantrone *(Lederle, UK)*. *Injection*, mitozantrone 2 mg (as hydrochloride)/mL, in vials of 10, 12.5, and 15 mL.

Proprietary Names and Manufacturers

Novantron *(Cyanamid-Lederle, Ger.; Lederle, Switz)*; Novantrone *(Lederle, Austral.; Lederle, Canad.; Lederle, Fr.; Lederle, S. Afr.; Lederle, UK)*.

12975-s

Mopidamol *(BAN, rINN)*.

Ra-233. 2,2′,2″,2‴-(4-Piperidinopyrimido[5,4-*d*]pyrimidine-2,6-diyldinitrilo)tetraethanol.
$C_{19}H_{31}N_7O_4$=421.5.

CAS — 13665-88-8.

Mopidamol is an antineoplastic agent used for the postoperative prophylaxis of metastases in patients undergoing surgery for primary sarcoma or malignant lymphomas of the head and neck. It has been given by slow intravenous injection on the day of operation, and for up to 10 days following, in doses of 150 mg two to three times daily. It has also been given by mouth in recommended doses of 500 mg three times daily.

Proprietary Names and Manufacturers

Rapenton *(Thomae, Ger.)*.

3278-f

Muromonab-CD3

OKT3. A murine monoclonal antibody comprising a purified IgG_{2a} immunoglobulin with a heavy chain having a molecular weight of about 50 000 and a light chain with a molecular weight of approximately 25 000.

Adverse Effects, Treatment, and Precautions

Potentially fatal pulmonary oedema has been reported following the first dose of muromonab-CD3 in patients with fluid overload; it is contra-indicated in patients who have undergone a greater than 3% weight gain in the week preceding therapy, or who have radiographic evidence of fluid overloading.

Allergic reactions, fever and chills, dyspnoea and wheezing, chest pain, diarrhoea, nausea and vomiting, and tremor have also frequently occurred. Concomitant administration of corticosteroids may reduce adverse reactions to the first dose (see under Uses and Administration, below).

Muromonab-CD3 should not be given to patients with pre-existing fever, or in patients hypersensitive to products of murine origin.

Concurrent administration with cyclosporin is not recommended.

A report of fever, cephalgia (in 3), and photophobia (in 2) associated with pleocytosis of the cerebrospinal fluid in 4 patients receiving muromonab-CD3. Meningismus occurred in 1 of the 4. There was no evidence of CNS infection in any of the patients. Symptoms resolved on withdrawal of muromonab-CD3.— C. Emmons *et al.* (letter), *Lancet*, 1986, *2*, 510.

Uses and Administration

Muromonab-CD3 is a murine monoclonal antibody to the T3 (CD3) antigen of human T-lymphocytes, which is essential to antigen recognition and response; the antibody thus specifically blocks T-cell generation and function without affecting the bone marrow.

It is used in the treatment of acute allograft rejection in renal transplant recipients, in doses of 5 mg daily by intravenous injection for 10 to 14 days, usually in association with azathioprine and corticosteroids. The first dose may be preceded by intravenous administration of methylprednisolone sodium succinate 1 mg per kg body-weight and followed, after 30 minutes, by intravenous hydrocortisone sodium succinate 100 mg, in order to decrease the incidence of reactions. Patients should be monitored closely for 48 hours after the first dose.

Reviews: G. Goldstein, *Transplantn Proc.*, 1986, *18*, 927; *Med. Lett.*, 1986, *28*, 97.

Muromonab-CD3 was significantly more effective than conventional high-dose corticosteroid treatment in reversing episodes of acute graft rejection in a prospective multicentre study involving 123 renal transplant recipients. Acute rejection was reversed in 58 of 62 patients given muromonab-CD3 5 mg daily for a mean of 14 days; continued immunosuppression with prednisone and azathioprine was given at reduced dosage during muromonab-CD3 treatment. This reversal rate was significantly higher than the 45 of 60 patients who were given methylprednisolone 500 mg daily for up to 3 days, followed by prednisone, in addition to continuation of their previous immunosuppressive therapy. Among patients in whom rejection was reversed the mean time to reversal was shorter in the antibody treated group, at 3.3 days, than in those given corticosteroids (4.9 days). The incidence of further rejection was similar in both groups. On 1-year follow-up, kidney survival rates were calculated at 62% in those treated with muromonab-CD3 and 45% in those given conventional antirejection therapy. Antibodies to muromonab-CD3 frequently developed shortly after therapy: if it is to be used for the treatment of subsequent episodes of rejection it will be necessary to develop protocols for preventing antibody formation or give sufficiently high doses to overcome host antibody concentrations.— Ortho Multicenter Transplant Study Group, *New Engl. J. Med.*, 1985, *313*, 337.

Proprietary Names and Manufacturers

Orthoclone OKT3 *(Ortho Pharmaceutical, USA)*.

1853-r

Mustine Hydrochloride *(BANM)*.

Chlorethazine Hydrochloride; Chlormethine Hydrochloride *(rINNM)*; HN2 *(mustine)*; Mechlorethamine Hydrochloride *(USAN)*; Nitrogen Mustard; NSC-762; WR-147650. *NN*-Bis(2-chloroethyl)methylamine hydrochloride; 2,2′-Dichloro-*N*-methyldiethylamine hydrochloride.
$C_5H_{11}Cl_2N,HCl$=192.5.

CAS — 51-75-2 (mustine); 55-86-7 (hydrochloride).

Pharmacopoeias. In *Br., Chin., Egypt., Fr., Int., Jug.,* and *U.S.*

A white or almost white, hygroscopic, vesicant, crystalline powder or mass. Very **soluble** in water. A 0.2% solution in water has a pH of 3 to 5. The U.S.P. injection which is a 2% solution also has a pH of 3 to 5. Solutions lose their activity very rapidly. Solutions for injections are prepared by dissolving, immediately before use, the sterile contents of a sealed container in Water for Injections.

Store at a temperature of 8° to 15° in airtight containers. Protect from light.

CAUTION. *Mustine hydrochloride is a strong vesicant; avoid contact with skin and mucous membranes.*

STABILITY IN SOLUTION. Conflicting reports of the stability of mustine hydrochloride solution have been largely derived from studies using non-specific assays. A study using an assay specific for mustine found that a 0.1% solution in Water for Injections or sodium chloride injection (0.9%) underwent a loss of approximately 10% when stored for 6 hours at room temperature, and of approximately 4 to 6% when stored for the same period at 4°; similar results were obtained whether the solution was stored in glass vials or plastic syringes. Solutions in 500 mL of sodium chloride or glucose (5%) injection and stored in PVC infusion bags were still less stable, with 15% and 10% degradation respectively after 6 hours at room temperature.— B. Kirk, *Br. J. parent. Ther.*, 1986, *7*, 86.

Adverse Effects

For an outline of the adverse effects experienced with antineoplastic agents and immunosuppressants, see Antineoplastic Agents, p.580.

Mustine hydrochloride is extremely toxic and its use is invariably accompanied by side-effects. Severe nausea and vomiting may commence within an hour of injection of the drug and last for some hours. It causes varying degrees of bone-marrow depression depending on the dose. When the total dose for a single course exceeds 400 µg per kg body-weight there is a risk of severe and possibly fatal depression with anaemia, lymphocytopenia, granulocytopenia, and thrombocytopenia with consequent haemorrhage. Depression of lymphocytes may be apparent within 24 hours of the administration of mustine hydrochloride and maximum suppression of granulocytes and platelets occurs within 7 to 21 days; haematological recovery may be adequate after 4 weeks.

Tinnitus, vertigo, and deafness have been reported. Skin reactions to mustine hydrochloride include maculopapular rashes. There is a high incidence of hypersensitivity when topical preparations are used in conditions such as psoriasis. Mustine hydrochloride has a powerful vesicant action on the skin and mucous membranes and great care must be taken to avoid contact with the eyes. Extravasation of the injection causes severe irritation and even sloughing. Thrombophlebitis is a potential hazard of mustine if it is not sufficiently diluted.

Mustine hydrochloride may produce temporary or permanent inhibition of fertility. There is some evidence of teratogenicity.

ALLERGY AND ANAPHYLAXIS. A preliminary study of the use of prior ultraviolet light or PUVA therapy to delay contact sensitivity to mustine hydrochloride. Only 1 of 15 patients so treated became sensitive within the first 30 days, compared with 12 of 28 controls.— K. M. Halprin *et al.*, *Br. J. Derm.*, 1981, *105*, 71. A subsequent report. The method failed to prevent sensitisation in a patient being treated for mycosis fungoides.— F. A. Vega *et al.*, *ibid.*, 1982, *106*, 361.

EFFECTS ON THE NERVOUS SYSTEM. Neuropathy has been reported following intra-arterial infusion of cytotoxic agents such as mustine hydrochloride.— R. J. M. Lane and P. A. Routledge, *Drugs*, 1983, *26*, 124.

Treatment of Adverse Effects

For general guidelines, see Antineoplastic Agents, p.583.

The administration of anti-emetics and sedation before injection of mustine hydrochloride may help to control severe nausea and vomiting.

If extravasation occurs during injection, the involved area should be infiltrated with an isotonic 4% solution of sodium thiosulphate, followed by the application of an ice compress intermittently for 6 to 12 hours. A 1% lignocaine solution may also be infiltrated.

For reference to the use of ultraviolet light in delaying contact sensitivity to mustine, see under Allergy and Anaphylaxis, above.

Precautions

For reference to the precautions necessary with antineoplastic agents and immunosuppressants, see Antineoplastic Agents, p.583.

HANDLING AND DISPOSAL. Protective clothing should be worn for up to 48 hours after therapy when handling urine from patients receiving mustine.— J. Harris and L. J. Dodds, *Pharm. J.*, 1985, *2*, 289.

The manufacturers state that unused injection solutions may be neutralised by mixing with an equal volume of a solution containing sodium thiosulphate 2.5% and sodium bicarbonate 2.5% and allowing to stand for 45 minutes. Equipment used in the preparation and administration of mustine hydrochloride solutions may be treated similarly.

Absorption and Fate

Mustine is only partially absorbed from serous surfaces. Following intravenous injection, it is rapidly converted to a reactive ethyleneimmonium ion. It usually disappears from the blood in a few minutes. A very small proportion is excreted unchanged in the urine.

Uses and Administration

Mustine belongs to the group of antineoplastic drugs described as alkylating agents (see p.580). It also possesses weak immunosuppressant properties.

Mustine hydrochloride is used in the treatment of advanced Hodgkin's disease, usually in conjunction with a vinca alkaloid, procarbazine, and prednisone or prednisolone. It may also be used in other lymphomas and has been tried in chronic leukaemias and polycythaemia vera, as well as in carcinoma of the lung and other solid tumours. In mycosis fungoides with extensive skin involvement, very dilute solutions of mustine have been applied topically.

See also under Choice of Antineoplastic Agent, p.584.

The usual dose of mustine hydrochloride is 400 μg per kg body-weight, preferably as a single dose, although it may be divided into 2 or 4 equal doses on successive days. It is given by intravenous injection in a strength of 1 mg per mL in Water for Injections or sodium chloride injection (0.9%). Rapid injection into the tubing of a fast running intravenous infusion of sodium chloride injection or glucose injection may reduce the incidence of thrombophlebitis. Doses of 6 mg per m^2 body-surface are used in the combination schedules for Hodgkin's disease.

The response should be assessed by the trend of the blood counts. Treatment with mustine may be repeated when the bone-marrow function has recovered.

Intracavitary injections of 200 to 400 μg per kg have been given in the treatment of malignant, especially pleural, effusions.

MYCOSIS FUNGOIDES. Epithelial neoplasms other than actinic keratoses were found in 14 of 202 patients with mycosis fungoides who had received topical treatment with mustine hydrochloride and had been followed for up to 9 years. From preliminary observations these neoplasms were considered to be easily treated and application of mustine was still recommended as a not inappropriate treatment for a condition requiring early treatment, while still limited to the skin.— A. du Vivier *et al.*, *Br. J. Derm.*, 1978, *99*, 61.

Treatment with topical mustine, as a 20% aqueous solution, alone or in combination with PUVA therapy produced clearance of visible disease in 20 patients with early and 5 with advanced mycosis fungoides; however, whereas maintenance therapy with mustine appeared to prolong remission in patients with early disease, all 5 with late disease relapsed while receiving maintenance therapy. Similar treatment was also of benefit in 3 patients with chronic superficial scaly dermatitis. Thirteen patients developed contact sensitivity, but topical desensitisation permitted resumption of treatment in 10.— B. E. Monk *et al.*, *Br. J. Derm.*, 1982, *107*, *Suppl.* 22, 25.

RENAL DISORDERS. Prolonged remission has been reported in children with minimal change nephrotic syndrome treated with mustine. A report by M.J. Schoeneman *et al.* (*Am. J. Kidney Dis.*, 1983, *2*, 526) indicated a sustained remission of 46% 27 months after treatment in 12 children with steroid-responsive disease given mustine 100 μg per kg body-weight daily for 4 days. However the role of mustine, as of other alkylating agents, is not established and in view of the excellent long-term prognosis of this non-malignant condition the use of cytotoxic drugs must remain controversial.— R. S. Trompeter, *Archs Dis. Childh.*, 1986, *61*, 727.

Preparations

Mechlorethamine Hydrochloride for Injection *(U.S.P.)*. A sterile mixture of mustine hydrochloride with sodium chloride or other suitable diluent. A 2% solution has a pH of 3 to 5.

Mustine Injection *(B.P.)*. Contains mustine hydrochloride. To be prepared immediately before use.

Proprietary Names and Manufacturers

Caryolysine *(Delagrange, Fr.)*; Cloramin *(Ital.)*; Erasol *(Denm.)*; Mustargen *(Merck Sharp & Dohme, Canad.; Merck Sharp & Dohme, Switz.; Merck Sharp & Dohme, USA)*.

Manufacturers also include—*Boots, UK*.

13019-t

Nimustine *(rINN)*.

ACNU; NSC-245382; Pimustine. 1-(4-Amino-2-methylpyrimidin-5-ylmethyl)-3-(2-chloroethyl)-3-nitrosourea.
$C_9H_{13}ClN_6O_2$=272.7.

CAS — 42471-28-3.

Nimustine is a nitrosourea antineoplastic agent with actions and uses similar to of those of carmustine (see p.605). It has been given as the hydrochloride, in doses of 2 to 3 mg per kg body-weight intravenously.

Proprietary Names and Manufacturers
ACNU *(Asta Pharma, Ger.)*; Nidran *(Sankyo, Jpn)*.

1856-n

Novembichine

Novoembichin. *NN*-Bis(2-chloroethyl)-2-chloropropylamine hydrochloride.
$C_7H_{14}Cl_3N,HCl$=255.0.

CAS — 1936-40-9.

Pharmacopoeias. In *Rus.*

Novembichine is an antineoplastic agent with properties similar to those of mustine (p.645). It has been used in a maximum dose of 10 mg intravenously, not more frequently than once every 2 days.

2297-k

Pentamethylmelamine Hydrochloride

NSC-118742.
$C_8H_{16}N_6,HCl$=232.7.

CAS — 16268-62-5 (pentamethylmelamine); 16268-63-6 (hydrochloride).

Pentamethylmelamine is a water-soluble metabolite of hexamethylmelamine (p.631), that has been investigated for its antineoplastic properties. It has been given by intravenous infusion as the hydrochloride.

A review of pentamethylmelamine. Dose-limiting toxicities include gastro-intestinal and central nervous system disturbances, which are severe enough when given by 2- or 24-hour or 10-day infusion to infer that the drug offers little advantage over hexamethylmelamine. In patients with liver dysfunction the plasma clearance of pentamethylmelamine and its metabolites decreases, with a consequent increase in central neurotoxicity. In general, the maximum tolerated dose from Phase I trials appears to be in the range of 1.5 g per m^2 when given as a 24-hour infusion.— D. A. Hahn, *Drug Intell. & clin. Pharm.*, 1983, *17*, 418. See also J. R. F. Muindi *et al.*, *Br. J. Cancer*, 1983, *47*, 27.

16946-y

Pentostatin *(USAN, rINN)*.

2′-Deoxycoformycin; CI-825; Co-vidarabine; NSC-218321. (*R*)-3-(2-Deoxy-β-D-*erythro*-pentofuranosyl)-3,6,7,8-tetrahydroimidazo[4,5-*d*][1,3]diazepin-8-ol.
$C_{11}H_{16}N_4O_4$=268.3.

CAS — 63677-95-2.

Adverse Effects

Central neurotoxicity and nephrotoxicity have been reported in patients treated with pentostatin, and may be dose-limiting. Respiratory failure, arthralgia, myalgia, photophobia, conjunctivitis, and peripheral lymphopenia have also occurred.

Pentostatin was considered an agent that should be administered with extreme caution. Severe toxic effects had been observed in patients with leukaemia (although not to the same extent in patients with hairy-cell leukaemia). Severe and unusual infections may occur even in the absence of neutropenia, and the drug may be fatal in the presence of established infection or poor performance status. The incidence of haematological side-effects is also high.— A. S. D. Spiers *et al.*, *New Engl. J. Med.*, 1987, *316*, 825.

Uses and Administration

Pentostatin is a potent inhibitor of the enzyme adenosine deaminase that probably exerts its cytotoxic actions through the interruption of normal purine metabolism and DNA synthesis. It enhances the antiviral and antineoplastic actions of vidarabine, which is normally rapidly metabolised by adenosine deaminase.

Pentostatin has been given in the treatment of refractory acute leukaemias, and particularly hairy-cell leukaemia, in usual doses of 100 to 500 μg per kg body-weight intravenously daily for 5 days. It has been given in association with vidarabine.

A review of pentostatin.— P. J. O'Dwyer *et al.*, *Ann. intern. Med.*, 1988, *108*, 733.

In a study involving 27 patients with hairy-cell leukaemia carried out by the Eastern Co-operative Oncology Group, pentostatin was given initially in doses of 5 mg per m^2 body-surface by intravenous injection on 3 consecutive days every 4 weeks; this schedule was later modified to 5 mg per m^2 on 2 consecutive days every 2 weeks— i.e. 2 days of treatment followed by a 12-day interval. Complete remission was achieved in 16 patients and partial remission in 10, with a median time of 99.5 days to achieve remission after beginning therapy. At the time of writing all patients who had achieved complete remission were still alive; 10 had been in complete remission for more than 6 months. Side-effects included one death from multiple infections and 1 patient stopped treatment because of severe myalgias. The relative roles of splenectomy, interferon, and pentostatin in hairy-cell leukaemia remain to be determined but pentostatin is clearly effective in patients with good performance status.— A. S. D. Spiers *et al.*, *New Engl. J. Med.*, 1987, *316*, 825.

Further references to the use of pentostatin: H. G. Prentice *et al.*, *Lancet*, 1980, *2*, 170 (acute lymphoblastic leukaemia); A. S. D. Spiers and S. J. Parekh (letter), *ibid.*, 1984, *1*, 1080 (hairy-cell leukaemia); C. E. Dearden *et al.*, *Br. med. J.*, 1987, *295*, 873 (T-cell malignancies).

Proprietary Names and Manufacturers
Parke, Davis, USA.

13092-v

Peplomycin Sulphate *(rINNM)*.

NK-631; Pepleomycin Sulphate; Peplomycin Sulfate *(USAN)*. N^1-{3-[(*S*)-(α-Methylbenzyl)amino]propyl-}bleomycinamide sulphate.
$C_{61}H_{88}N_{18}O_{21}S_2,H_2SO_4$=1571.7.

CAS — 68247-85-8 (peplomycin); 70384-29-1 (sulphate).

Peplomycin is an antineoplastic agent derived from bleomycin (p.602) and claimed to produce a lower incidence of pulmonary toxicity. It has been tried as the sulphate in the treatment of malignant neoplasms of the prostate and lung.

Proprietary Names and Manufacturers
Pepleo *(Nippon Kayaku, Jpn)*.

1857-h

Pipobroman *(USAN, pINN)*.

A-8103; NSC-25154. 1,4-Bis(3-bromopropionyl)piperazine.
$C_{10}H_{16}Br_2N_2O_2$=356.1.

CAS — 54-91-1.

Pharmacopoeias. In *U.S.*

A white or almost white, crystalline powder with a slightly sharp fruity odour. M.p. 101° to 105°.

Soluble 1 in 230 of water, 1 in 35 of alcohol, 1 in 4.8 of chloroform, and 1 in 530 of ether; soluble in acetone.

Adverse Effects, Treatment, and Precautions

For an outline of the adverse effects experienced with antineoplastic agents and immunosuppressants, general guidelines for their treatment, and precautions, see Antineoplastic Agents, p.580, p.583.

The principal adverse effect is moderate bone-marrow depression, which may be delayed. Anaemia may be marked at higher doses and is usually accompanied by leucopenia. Thrombocytopenia and haemolysis have occurred.

Uses and Administration

Pipobroman is an antineoplastic agent which appears to act by alkylation (see p.580). It has been used in the treatment of polycythaemia vera, particularly in patients resistant to conventional therapy, and in chronic myeloid leukaemia resistant to busulphan and radiotherapy.

The usual dose initially is 1 to 1.5 mg per kg body-weight by mouth daily, according to the patient's response, increased to 3 mg per kg, if necessary. Maintenance dosage is 100 to 200 μg per kg daily for polycythaemia vera and from 7 to 175 mg daily in chronic myeloid leukaemia.

In the initial stages of treatment, white cell counts should be determined on alternate days and complete blood counts once or twice weekly. Doses should be discontinued if the white cell count is below 3,000 per mm^3 or the platelet count below 150,000 per mm^3.

The use of pipobroman in polycythaemia vera.— A. Najman *et al.*, *Blood*, 1982, *59*, 890.

Preparations

Pipobroman Tablets *(U.S.P.)*

Proprietary Names and Manufacturers
Amedel *(Jpn)*; Vercite 25 *(Abbott, Ital.)*; Vercyte *(Abbott, Belg.; Abbott, Canad.; Abbott, Fr.; Abbott, USA)*.

1846-f

Plicamycin *(BAN, USAN, rINN).*

A-2371; Aureolic Acid; Mithramycin; NSC-24559; PA-144.

$C_{52}H_{76}O_{24}$=1085.2.

CAS — 18378-89-7.

Pharmacopoeias. In *U.S.*

An antineoplastic antibiotic produced by the growth of *Streptomyces argillaceus*, *S. plicatus* and *S. tanashiensis*. It is a yellow, odourless, hygroscopic, crystalline powder, with a potency of not less than 900 µg per mg, calculated on the dry basis. It loses not more than 8% of its weight when dried. Slightly **soluble** in water and methyl alcohol; very slightly soluble in alcohol; freely soluble in ethyl acetate. A 0.05% solution in water has a pH of 4.5 to 5.5. The *U.S.P.* states that Plicamycin for Injection has a pH of 5.0 to 7.5 when reconstituted. **Store** at 2° to 8° in airtight containers. Protect from light.

Plicamycin was bound to cellulose filters used for inline filtration of intravenous infusions. Following passage of 1 litre infusions containing plicamycin 2.5 µg per mL in glucose injection (5%), or in sodium chloride injection (0.9%), at a rate of 120 mL per hour, there was a loss of 14.3% and 9.9% of the dose respectively. Equilibrium binding studies confirmed that more drug was likely to be lost from glucose than from sodium chloride injection at the low concentrations of drug used in therapy. Given slow flow-rates, short-term administration, or both, a substantial percentage of the intended dose of drugs such as plicamycin may be retained by the cellulose ester filter, possibly altering the patient's therapeutic response.— L. D. Butler *et al.*, *Am. J. Hosp. Pharm.*, 1980, *37*, 935. See also M. Kanke *et al.*, *ibid.*, 1983, *40*, 1323.

INCOMPATIBILITY. Plicamycin readily chelates divalent cations, especially iron. Admixture with trace element solutions should be avoided.— P. F. D'Arcy, *Drug Intell. & clin. Pharm.*, 1983, *17*, 532.

Adverse Effects and Treatment

For an outline of the adverse effects experienced with antineoplastic agents and immunosuppressants and general guidelines for their treatment, see Antineoplastic Agents, p.580.

The major adverse effect of plicamycin is a bleeding syndrome, manifest initially as epistaxis, which may progress to haematemesis and potentially fatal haemorrhage. Effects on clotting factors in the blood are thought to contribute to this syndrome. Severe thrombocytopenia may also occur due to bone-marrow depression.

Gastro-intestinal effects are common during treatment with plicamycin. Other side-effects include fever, malaise, drowsiness, lethargy and weakness, headache, depression, skin rashes, facial flushing, and reduced serum concentrations of calcium, phosphorus, and potassium. There may also be reversible impairment of renal and hepatic function.

Extravasation of plicamycin solutions may cause local irritation, cellulitis, and phlebitis. Application of moderate heat to the site of extravasation may aid dispersal of plicamycin and minimise discomfort and local irritation.

EFFECTS ON THE KIDNEY. A report of reversible oliguria and deterioration of renal function occurring on 2 occasions in a patient given single doses of plicamycin.— R. G. Benedetti *et al.*, *Am. J. Nephrol.*, 1983, *3*, 277.

EFFECTS ON THE SKIN. Toxic epidermal necrolysis occurring in a 22-year-old man was attributed to treatment with plicamycin.— D. Purpora *et al.* (letter), *New Engl. J. Med.*, 1978, *299*, 1412.

EXTRAVASATION. Disodium edetate had been suggested as an antidote to local toxicity following extravasation of plicamycin.— M. E. MacCara, *Drug Intell. & clin. Pharm.*, 1983, *17*, 713.

Precautions

For reference to the precautions necessary with antineoplastic agents and immunosuppressants, see Antineoplastic Agents, p.583.

Plicamycin should only be given with great care to patients with impaired hepatic or renal function. It should not be administered to patients with depressed bone-marrow function or coagulation disorders.

Uses and Administration

Plicamycin is a highly toxic antibiotic with antineoplastic and hypocalcaemic properties. It may act by inhibiting synthesis of ribonucleic acid.

It has been used in the treatment of inoperable metastatic neoplasms of the testis which cannot be treated by radiotherapy. The usual dose is 25 to 30 µg per kg body-weight daily by slow intravenous infusion over 4 to 6 hours in a litre of glucose injection (5%) or sodium chloride injection (0.9%) for not more than 10 doses. Individual daily doses should not exceed 30 µg per kg. Doses have also been given on alternate days. Courses may be repeated at monthly intervals.

It is also used for the symptomatic treatment of hypercalcaemia and hypercalciuria. The usual dose is 25 µg per kg daily by slow intravenous infusion for 3 or 4 days. To achieve calcium balance further doses may be given at intervals of a week or more.

Blood cell counts, bleeding time, prothrombin time, and hepatic and renal function should be determined frequently during treatment and for several days after, and treatment stopped if there is any sudden change.

Plicamycin was successfully used to reverse the hypoglycaemia which occurred in a 59-year-old woman with metastatic islet-cell carcinoma. After the first dose of 1 mg, given intravenously, serum-insulin concentration was rapidly reduced. A further 4 doses for mild episodes of hypoglycaemia were well tolerated.— D. T. Kiang *et al.*, *New Engl. J. Med.*, 1978, *299*, 134.

ADMINISTRATION IN RENAL INSUFFICIENCY. Doses of plicamycin should be reduced to 75% in patients with a glomerular filtration-rate of 10 to 50 mL per minute and to 50% when the rate is less than 10 mL per minute.— W. M. Bennett *et al.*, *Am. J. Kidney Dis.*, 1983, *3*, 155.

HYPERCALCAEMIA. Plicamycin 20 µg per kg given intravenously over 6 hours usually produces a substantial fall in plasma calcium commencing in 12 to 36 hours and lasting 1 to 2 weeks. The effect is probably a direct toxic one on osteoclasts. Plicamycin is a useful drug in the treatment of hypercalcaemia, but very toxic: there is usually evidence of mild liver damage at the doses used.— R. A. Evans, *Drugs*, 1986, *31*, 64.

Plicamycin, which inhibits osteoclastic bone resorption, is the only available uniformly effective drug for treating hypercalcaemia but it has to be given intravenously and is usually used only in severe hypercalcaemia. The duration of effect is unpredictable; in some patients the response lasts several days and in others several weeks. Repeated doses carry a risk of marrow suppression or of damage to the kidneys or liver.— R. Wilkinson, *Br. med. J.*, 1984, *288*, 812. Plicamycin has a calcium-lowering effect in malignant hypercalcaemia, but this is not immediate, which limits usefulness in acute states, and its hepatic, renal, and platelet toxicity largely precludes its use, particularly when the patient may later need other cytotoxic regimens.— J. C. Stevenson, *ibid.*, 1985, *291*, 421.

For reports of the use of plicamycin in the treatment of hypercalcaemia of malignancy, see Disodium Aminohydroxypropylidenediphosphonate, p.1340, and Disodium Etidronate, p.1342.

For a report of the effect of plicamycin in association with disodium clodronate on the paraparesis caused by carcinoma of the prostate, see Disodium Clodronate, p.1341.

MYELOMA. Plicamycin may be given to maintain calcium homoeostasis in patients with hypercalcaemia secondary to uncontrolled myeloma. It may also be of value in controlling bone pain in occasional patients with end stage myeloma.— J. E. Oakley and I. M. Franklin, *J. clin. Hosp. Pharm.*, 1984, *9*, 15.

PAGET'S DISEASE OF BONE. A review of the treatment of Paget's disease of bone. Plicamycin has been shown to be an effective agent in the treatment of Paget's disease but because of its cytotoxicity is not usually used as a first-line treatment. It should be considered in cases refractory to treatment with other agents such as calcitonin and the biphosphonates, or when a rapid response is desired. Doses used have ranged from 10 to 25 µg per kg body-weight by intravenous infusion over 8 to 24 hours. The author has usually used 15 µg per kg but 10 µg per kg has been reported to be fully effective. The dose is repeated daily for 5 to 10 days. Plicamycin produces a rapid fall in plasma alkaline phosphatase and urinary hydroxyproline concentrations within a few days of the start of treatment, ultimately to about 25% of their initial values. There is a great decrease in osteoclast numbers. The improvement produced may last several months to several years. The use of plicamycin with disodium etidronate is under evaluation for a cure in Paget's disease with encouraging preliminary results.— R. A. Melick, *Med. J. Aust.*, 1985, *143*, 394.

Conflicting views on the use of plicamycin for Paget's disease of bone. Russell (*Lancet*, 1980, *1*, 884) has reported the successful use of low doses of plicamycin for the pain of Paget's disease. Doses of about 10 µg per kg body-weight were given daily by intravenous injection for 10 days and complete relief of pain was achieved by 4 or 5 days. Although this regimen was reported to be safe, Evans and Stevenson (*ibid.*, 1093) have criticised the use of such a potentially toxic drug when there is a safe alternative in calcitonin. Nagant de Deuxchaisnes *et al.* (*ibid.*, 1193) consider that, unlike calcitonin, it has not been proved that plicamycin can strengthen bone and control the disease process while relieving pain. The toxicity of plicamycin necessitates extensive monitoring of the patient during treatment and calcitonin is considered preferable.

A patient who had received plicamycin treatment for Paget's disease of bone was still in remission in 1984 having received no further treatment since 1972 and it was considered reasonable to suppose that she had been cured of her disease.— W. G. Ryan and E. W. Fordham (letter), *Ann. intern. Med.*, 1984, *100*, 771.

Preparations

Plicamycin for Injection *(U.S.P.)*. A sterile dry mixture of plicamycin and mannitol. It may contain a suitable buffer.

Proprietary Preparations

Mithracin *(Pfizer, UK)*. *Injection*, powder for reconstitution, plicamycin 2.5 mg.

Proprietary Names and Manufacturers

Mithracin *(Pfizer, Austral.; Pfizer, Norw.; Pfizer, UK; Miles Pharmaceuticals, USA)*; Mithracine *(Pfizer, Fr.; Pfizer, Switz.)*.

1859-b

Prednimustine *(USAN, rINN).*

Leo-1031; NSC-134087. 11β,17,21-Trihydroxypregna-1,4-diene-3,20-dione 21-(4-{4-[bis(2-chloroethyl)amino]-phenyl}butyrate).

$C_{35}H_{45}Cl_2NO_6$=646.6.

CAS — 29069-24-7.

Adverse Effects, Treatment, and Precautions

As for Chlorambucil, p.606. The myelosuppressive effects of prednimustine are stated to be relatively weak.

Uses and Administration

Prednimustine is the prednisolone ester of chlorambucil, (p.606) and is used in the treatment of various malignant diseases including chronic lymphocytic leukaemia and non-Hodgkin's lymphomas.

It has been given by mouth in doses of 200 mg daily for 5 consecutive days, repeated after an interval of at least 9 days. Prednimustine has also been given continuously in a dose of 20 to 30 mg daily.

In a study of the pharmacokinetics of predn[illegible] and chlorambucil Newell *et al.* (*Br. J. clin. Pharmac.*, 1983, *15*, 253) found that the former appeared to [illegible]e poorly absorbed, with indetectable concentrations [illegible] drug or metabolites in the plasma of 6 patients [illegible]n an oral dose of 20 mg, compared with clearly [illegible]ble concentrations of chlorambucil and its m[illegible]te following 10 mg of chlorambucil. They sugg[illegible]at chlorambucil, with or without prednisolone, [illegible]erable to prednimustine. The manufacturers, [illegible]bsequent letter, (G.P. Forshell *et al.*, *ibid.*, [illegible]pointed out that evidence of alkylating activi[illegible]a exists for prednimustine, and that highe[illegible] 40 to 60 mg daily continuously or 100 mg [illegible]as part of an intermittent dose schedul[illegible]mmended. However, Newell *et al.* point o[illegible]*id.*, 762) that there is still no evidence th[illegible]tine is acting as anything other than a [illegible] prodrug of chlorambucil, and therefor[illegible]mbucil and prednisolone therapy is indic[illegible]ugs should continue to be given separat[illegible]

Proprietary Names and Manufacturers
Mostarina *(Abello, Spain)*; Stéréocyt *(Bellon, Fr.)*; Sterecyt *(Pharmacia Arzneimittel, Ger.; Leo Suede, Switz.)*.

1860-x

Procarbazine Hydrochloride *(BANM, USAN, rINNM)*.

Ibenzmethyzin; NSC-77213; Ro-4-6467. *N*-Isopropyl-*α*-(2-methylhydrazino)-*p*-toluamide hydrochloride.
$C_{12}H_{19}N_3O,HCl=257.8$.

CAS — 671-16-9 (procarbazine); 366-70-1 (hydrochloride).

Pharmacopoeias. In *Braz., Chin.,* and *U.S.*

A white to pale yellow crystalline powder with a slight odour. Procarbazine hydrochloride 116 mg is approximately equivalent to 100 mg of procarbazine. Freely **soluble** in water; soluble in methyl alcohol; sparingly soluble in alcohol; slightly soluble in chloroform; practically insoluble in ether. Solutions in water are unstable and acid to litmus. **Store** in airtight containers. Protect from light.

Adverse Effects and Treatment

For an outline of the adverse effects experienced with antineoplastic agents and immunosuppressants and general guidelines for their treatment, see Antineoplastic Agents, p.580 and p.583.

The most common adverse effects associated with procarbazine are gastro-intestinal disturbances such as nausea and vomiting (although patients may soon become tolerant), and bone-marrow depression. Leucopenia and thrombocytopenia may be delayed and recovery protracted. Anaemia, haemolysis, and bleeding tendencies have been reported. Neurotoxicity is also common, with central effects such as somnolence, depression, agitation, psychoses, and dizziness, and peripheral neuropathies including paraesthesias and decreased reflexes. Tremors, convulsions, and coma have occasionally occurred.

Other side-effects reported with procarbazine include a 'flu-like' syndrome, pulmonary, genito-urinary, and skin reactions, tachycardia, orthostatic hypotension, ocular defects, and impaired liver function.

CARCINOGENICITY. For a discussion of the carcinogenic effects of antineoplastic agents, including mention of procarbazine, see Adverse Effects of Antineoplastic Agents, p.580. See also under Effects on the Liver, below.

EFFECTS ON THE LIVER. A suggestion that ingestion of substituted hydrazines, such as procarbazine, may have a role in the development of hepatic angiosarcoma.— T. K. Daneshmend and J. W. B. Bradfield (letter), *Lancet*, 1979, *2*, 1249.

EFFECTS ON THE SKIN. Procarbazine could cause photosensitivity reactions.— *Med. Lett.*, 1986, *28*, 51.

Precautions

For reference to the precautions necessary with antineoplastic agents and immunosuppressants, see Antineoplastic Agents, p.583.
Procarb[azine] should be used with caution in patients [wi]th impaired liver or kidney function, phaeochr[omo]cytoma, epilepsy, or cardiovascular or cerebr[ovasc]ular disease.
Procarbaz[ine is] a weak monoamine oxidase inhibitor [and inter]actions with other drugs and food, altho[ugh ve]ry rare, must be borne in mind—for [details o]f such reactions see under Phenelzine, p.378. Procarbazine may enhance the effects of other CNS depressants. A [hyper]tensive agonist-like reaction has been reported with [...] and the effects of anti-hypertensive ag[ents ...] enhanced.

HANDLING AND DIS[POSAL] ... [protec]tive clothing should be worn for up to 48 [hours after th]erapy when handling urine from patients [receiving proca]rbazine.— J. Harris and L. J. Dodds, *Pharm. J.*, 1985, *2*, 289.

PREGNANCY AND THE NEONATE. Reference to a theoretical risk of induction of the foetal-alcohol syndrome following concurrent ingestion of procarbazine and alcohol during pregnancy.— P. M. Dunn *et al.* (letter), *Lancet*, 1979, *2*, 144.

Absorption and Fate

Procarbazine is readily absorbed from the gastro-intestinal tract. It crosses the blood-brain barrier and diffuses into the cerebrospinal fluid. A plasma half-life of about 10 minutes has been reported. Procarbazine is rapidly metabolised and only about 5% is excreted unchanged in the urine. The remainder is oxidised to *N*-isopropylterephthalamic acid and excreted in the urine, about 25 to 42% of a dose being excreted in 24 hours. Some of the drug is excreted as carbon dioxide and methane via the lungs. During oxidative breakdown in the body hydrogen peroxide and hydroxyl radicals are formed which may account for some of the drug's actions.

Uses and Administration

Procarbazine hydrochloride is an antineoplastic agent which appears to inhibit protein and nucleic acid synthesis and suppress mitosis. It is unrelated to the other antineoplastic agents and it may be effective when other agents have become ineffective. Procarbazine also has some immunosuppressant activity.

Its main use is the treatment of Hodgkin's disease when it is usually given in association with other drugs such as mustine, vincristine, and prednisone (the MOPP regimen). Procarbazine has also been used in the treatment of other lymphomas and in malignant neoplasms of the brain and lung. See also under Choice of Antineoplastic Agent, p.585. To reduce nausea and vomiting, the usual initial dose in the *UK* is the equivalent of 50 mg of procarbazine daily, increased daily by 50 mg to 250 or 300 mg daily in divided doses. Alternatively, in the *USA*, initial doses equivalent to about 2 to 4 mg of procarbazine per kg body-weight have been given, subsequently increased to the equivalent of about 4 to 6 mg per kg, with maintenance doses of the equivalent of 1 to 2 mg per kg; doses are given to the nearest 50 mg. This dose is continued until the maximum response is obtained or until the white cell or platelet counts fall below 4000 or 100 000 per mm^3 respectively, or there are other signs of toxicity. A maintenance dose of 50 to 150 mg daily may be given. In children, initial daily doses of the equivalent of 50 mg have been suggested, increased to 100 mg per m^2 body-surface, then adjusted according to the white cell and platelet response.

In the combination regimens procarbazine has been given to adults and children in doses of 100 mg per m^2 body-surface on days 1 to 14 of each 4- or 6-week cycle.

The haematological status of the patient should be determined every 3 or 4 days and hepatic and renal function determined weekly.

Preparations

Procarbazine Hydrochloride Capsules *(U.S.P.)*

Proprietary Preparations

Natulan *(Roche, UK)*. *Capsules*, procarbazine 50 mg (as hydrochloride).

Proprietary Names and Manufacturers

Matulane *(Roche, USA)*; Natulan *(Arg.; Roche, Austral.; Belg.; Roche, Canad.; Roche, Fr.; Roche, Ger.; Roche, Ital.; Neth.; Roche, Norw.; Roche, S.Afr.; Roche, Spain; Roche, Switz.; Roche, UK)*; Natulanar *(Roche, Denm.; Roche, Swed.)*.

13181-g

Prospidium Chloride *(rINN)*.

3,12-Bis(3-chloro-2-hydroxypropyl)-3,12-diaza-6,9-diazoniadispiro[5.2.5.2]hexadecane dichloride.
$C_{18}H_{36}Cl_4N_4O_2=482.3$.

CAS — 23476-83-7.

Prospidium chloride is reported to have antineoplastic activity and has been given by injection in doses of up to 600 mg daily.

References: P. Grohn *et al.*, *Cancer Treat. Rep.*, 1984, *68*, 915.

Proprietary Names and Manufacturers
Prospidin *(Casen Fisons, Spain)*.

1861-r

Razoxane *(BAN, rINN)*.

ICI-59118; ICRF-159; NSC-129943. (±)-4,4′-Propylenebis(piperazine-2,6-dione).
$C_{11}H_{16}N_4O_4=268.3$.

CAS — 21416-87-5.

Adverse Effects, Treatment, and Precautions

For an outline of the adverse effects experienced with antineoplastic agents and immunosuppressants, general guidelines for their treatment, and precautions, see Antineoplastic Agents, p.580, p.583.

The principal adverse effects of razoxane include bone-marrow depression, gastro-intestinal disturbances, skin reactions, and alopecia. It may enhance the adverse effects of radiotherapy.

Razoxane therapy has been associated with the development of secondary malignancies: it is contra-indicated in the treatment of non-malignant conditions.

CARCINOGENICITY. References to the development of malignant neoplasms in patients treated with razoxane: R. Joshi *et al.* (letter), *Lancet*, 1981, *2*, 1343 (acute myelomonocytic leukaemia); J. J. Horton *et al.*, *Br. J. Derm.*, 1983, *109*, 675 (epithelioma in psoriatic patients); S. Lakhani *et al.* (letter), *Lancet*, 1984, *2*, 288 (acute myeloid leukaemia after treatment of psoriasis); J. J. Horton *et al.* (letter), *Br. J. Derm.*, 1984, *110*, 633 (acute myeloid leukaemia); E. A. Caffrey *et al.*, *ibid.*, 1985, *113*, 131 (acute myeloid leukaemia).

Absorption and Fate

Absorption of razoxane from the gastro-intestinal tract is reported to be variable.

Uses and Administration

Razoxane is an antineoplastic agent with inhibitory activity during the pre-mitotic and early mitotic phases of cell growth (G_2-M). It also has some immunosuppressant activity. It is used in association with radiotherapy in the treatment of sarcomas. Razoxane has also been tried in other malignant diseases including acute leukaemias, non-Hodgkin's lymphomas, and some solid tumours including colorectal carcinoma.

In the treatment of sarcomas it has generally been given by mouth in doses of 125 mg twice daily; higher doses have been given in the management of acute leukaemias and Kaposi's sarcoma, up to a maximum of 1 g per m^2 body-surface daily in divided doses for 3 days every 3 weeks in the latter condition. The white cell count should be monitored during treatment.

Mention of razoxane and its D-isomer (ICRF-187) preventing metastasis and discussion of their value in the prophylaxis of doxorubicin-induced cardiotoxicity.— *Lancet*, 1987, *2*, 721.

ACTION. Razoxane had mutagenic acitivity in animal cell assays *in vitro* but this was not shown in bacterial assays.— R. Albanese *et al.*, *Hum. Toxicol.*, 1985, *4*, 106. A further study. Razoxane and its analogues ICRF-202, ICRF-187, and ICRF-154 produced dose-dependent increases in chromosome damage and polyploid cells in human lymphocyte cultures.— R. Albanese, *ibid.*, 542.

SKIN DISORDERS, NON-MALIGNANT. Razoxane has been used in the systemic treatment of psoriasis, and has been found to be extremely effective, with an initial response rate of 97% overall. It has been found to be of use in all forms of cutaneous psoriasis and psoriatic arthropathy and has been advocated as the drug of first choice in the systemic treatment of psoriasis (J.J. Horton and R.S. Wells, *Br. J. Derm.*, 1983, *109*, 669). However, the development of acute myeloid leukaemias and other malignancies in patients given razoxane (see under Adverse Effects, above) has led to its being contra-indicated in non-malignant conditions. A survey by Cerio *et al.* (*ibid.*, 1985, *113*, *Suppl.* 29, 27) in 30 patients withdrawn from razoxane therapy found severe psychological problems, including refusal to stop therapy and 7 patients subsequently indicated a desire to resume razoxane therapy despite knowledge of the potential consequences. Griffiths (*Br. med. J.*, 1985, *290*, 555) has pointed out that such therapy can transform the life of patients with crippling psoriasis and suggested that the relative risks and benefits should be carefully weighed even in non-malignant conditions.

Proprietary Preparations

Razoxin *(ICI Pharmaceuticals, UK)*. *Tablets*, scored, razoxane 125 mg.

1863-d

Semustine *(USAN, rINN)*.

Methyl Lomustine; Methyl-CCNU; NSC-95441; WR-220076. 1-(2-Chloroethyl)-3-(4-methylcyclohexyl)-1-nitrosourea.

$C_{10}H_{18}ClN_3O_2$=247.7.

CAS — 13909-09-6.

Adverse Effects, Treatment, and Precautions

As for Carmustine, p.605.

CARCINOGENICITY. For a review of the carcinogenicity of antineoplastics, including references to semustine, see Adverse Effects of Antineoplastics, p.580.

EFFECTS ON THE KIDNEYS. In a retrospective study, from two centres, of 17 children with brain tumours given semustine after radiotherapy, all 6 who had received a total dose of 1500 mg per m^2 body-surface over at least 17 months had severe renal damage. During treatment there was no evidence by blood urea nitrogen or creatinine determinations that the patients were losing renal function. A decrease in kidney size occurred in 2 patients who received lower total doses. The use of semustine should be limited to lower doses given for short periods until its toxicity is clarified.— W. E. Harmon *et al.*, *New Engl. J. Med.*, 1979, *300*, 1200. In a retrospective review of 857 patients treated with semustine over the past 6 years, there were only 4 patients with delayed renal insufficiency that was considered to have been related possibly to semustine.— W. C. Nichols and C. G. Moertel (letter), *ibid.*, *301*, 1181.

Absorption and Fate

Semustine is well absorbed from the gastro-intestinal tract following oral doses, and is rapidly metabolised. The metabolites are reported to possess prolonged plasma half-lives, and cross the blood-brain barrier into the cerebrospinal fluid. It is excreted in urine as metabolites.

For a review of the pharmacokinetics of the nitrosoureas, see Carmustine, p.606.

Uses and Administration

Semustine is a nitrosourea with actions and uses similar to those of carmustine (p.606) and lomustine (p.633). It has been given by mouth in single doses of 200 mg per m^2 body-surface, repeated every 6 weeks if blood counts recover adequately.

ADMINISTRATION IN RENAL INSUFFICIENCY. Nephrotoxicity has been associated with total doses of semustine above 1200 mg per m^2 body-surface. Its use should be avoided in patients with a glomerular filtration-rate below 10 mL per minute.— W. M. Bennett *et al.*, *Ann. intern. Med.*, 1980, *93*, 286.

MALIGNANT NEOPLASMS OF THE LIVER. For mention of the use of fluorouracil and semustine after surgical resection of liver metastases from colorectal carcinoma, see Fluorouracil, p.630.

Proprietary Names and Manufacturers

National Institutes of Health, USA.

13243-b

Sodium Bromebrate *(BANM, rINNM)*.

MBBA; NSC-104801; WR-149912. The sodium salt of (*E*)-3-*p*-anisoyl-3-bromoacrylate.

$C_{11}H_8BrNaO_4$=307.1.

CAS — 5711-40-0 (bromebric acid); 21739-91-3 (sodium salt).

Pharmacopoeias. In *Cz.*

Sodium bromebrate is an antineoplastic agent which has been administered intravenously. It has immunosuppressant activity.

Proprietary Names and Manufacturers

Cytembena *(Cz.)*.

16995-f

Sparfosic Acid *(rINN)*.

PALA. *N*-Phosphonoacetyl-L-aspartic acid.

$C_6H_{10}NO_8P$=255.1.

CAS — 51321-79-0.

12022-g

Sparfosate Sodium *(USAN, rINNM)*.

CI-882; NSC-224131; PALA Disodium. The disodium salt of sparfosic acid.

$C_6H_8NNa_2O_8P$=299.1.

CAS — 66569-27-5.

Adverse Effects and Precautions

Stomatitis, gastro-intestinal disturbances, and effects on the skin have been found to be dose-limiting in patients receiving sparfosic acid. Central neurotoxicity has been reported, with seizures and encephalopathy.

Care should be taken to avoid extravasation.

Uses and Administration

Sparfosic acid is an antineoplastic agent that prevents the first step of pyrimidine biosynthesis by inhibition of the enzyme aspartate transcarbamylase.

It has been tried with limited success in the management of various solid tumours, alone or in combination with other agents such as fluorouracil.

For reference to the use of sparfosic acid to enhance the antineoplastic activity of fluorouracil see p.629.

SKIN DISORDERS, NON-MALIGNANT. A report of the response of skin lesions in patients with psoriasis who were receiving sparfosic acid for various malignant neoplasms.— R. H. Earhart *et al.* (letter), *Lancet*, 1981, *1*, 1257. Sparfosic acid 625 mg per m^2 body-surface daily intravenously was given for 5 consecutive days every 4 weeks to 7 patients with refractory psoriasis. This dose was doubled if there was no improvement after a month. Three patients showed definite improvement at the higher dose but the response was ultimately judged unsatisfactory or of short duration in all patients, and treatment was stopped. One patient developed progressive erythroderma requiring hospitalisation. It seems unlikely that sparfosic acid will have a major role in the treatment of psoriasis.— J. A. Doyle *et al.*, *J. Am. Acad. Derm.*, 1984, *10*, 21.

Proprietary Names and Manufacturers

Parke, Davis, USA.

13265-w

Spirogermanium Hydrochloride *(BANM, USAN, rINNM)*.

NSC-192965. 3-(8,8-Diethyl-2-aza-8-germaspiro[4.5]-dec-2-yl)-*NN*-dimethylpropylamine dihydrochloride.

$C_{17}H_{36}GeN_2$,2HCl=414.0.

CAS — 41992-23-8 (spirogermanium); 41992-22-7 (hydrochloride).

Adverse Effects, Treatment, and Precautions

For an outline of the adverse effects experienced with antineoplastic agents and immunosuppressants, general guidelines for their treatment, and precautions, see Antineoplastic Agents, p.580, p.583.

Neurotoxicity, both central and peripheral, is usually dose-limiting. Grand mal seizures have been reported following overdosage. Gastro-intestinal disturbances, elevation of liver enzyme values and renal toxicity have occurred; myelotoxicity is claimed to be slight.

Uses and Administration

Spirogermanium hydrochloride is an antineoplastic agent that inhibits protein and nucleic acid synthesis, and which has been tried in the management of a variety of malignant neoplasms. Doses of 80 to 200 mg per m^2 body-surface daily have been given by intravenous infusion over at least 1 hour.

Spirogermanium also possesses immunosuppressant and antiprotozoal actions and has been investigated in the management of conditions such as multiple sclerosis and rheumatoid arthritis, and in the treatment of malaria.

Proprietary Names and Manufacturers

Boehringer Ingelheim, UK; Unimed, USA.

18684-d

Spiroplatin *(BAN, USAN, rINN)*.

NSC-311056; TNO-6. *cis*-(Cyclohexylidenedimethylenediamine-*N,N'*)(sulphato)platinum.

$C_8H_{18}N_2O_4PtS$=433.4.

CAS — 74790-08-2.

Spiroplatin is an analogue of cisplatin (p.607) that has been investigated for its antineoplastic properties in the treatment of malignant neoplasms.

Proprietary Names and Manufacturers

Bristol-Myers, UK.

1864-n

Streptozocin *(USAN, rINN)*.

NSC-85998; Streptozotocin; U-9889. 2-Deoxy-2-(3-methyl-3-nitrosoureido)-D-glucopyranose.

$C_8H_{15}N_3O_7$=265.2.

CAS — 18883-66-4.

An antineoplastic antibiotic produced by the growth of a *Streptomyces achromogenes* variant or by synthesis. Very **soluble** in water; soluble in alcohol. **Store** at 2° to 8°. Protect from light.

Adverse Effects and Treatment

For an outline of the adverse effects experienced with antineoplastic agents and immunosuppressants and general guidelines for their treatment, see Antineoplastic Agents, p.580 and p.583.

Cumulative nephrotoxicity is common with streptozocin and may be severe. Fatal irreversible renal failure has been reported. Other side-effects include severe nausea and vomiting and alterations in liver function. Myelosuppression may occur but is rarely severe.

Streptozocin may affect glucose metabolism. A diabetogenic effect has been reported; hypoglycaemia attributed to the release of insulin from damaged cells has also occurred.

Streptozocin is irritant to tissues and extravasation may lead to local ulceration and necrosis.

A report of an acute febrile reaction in a patient given streptozocin. Eight hours after an infusion of streptozocin 500 mg per m^2 body-surface the patient developed rigors, confusion, hypotension, somnolence, and a rise in rectal temperature to 41.4°. Symptoms recurred following rechallenge 6 days later.— M. B. Garnick *et al.* (letter), *New Engl. J. Med.*, 1984, *311*, 798.

Precautions

For reference to the precautions necessary with antineoplastic agents and immunosuppressants, see Antineoplastic Agents, p.583.

Streptozocin should be used with extreme care in patients with renal or hepatic impairment. Care should be taken to avoid extravasation, which may lead to local tissue necrosis.

INTERACTIONS. A suggestion that, since phenytoin appeared to protect the beta cells of the pancreas from the cytotoxic effects of streptozocin, its concomitant use with streptozocin should be avoided in patients being treated for pancreatic tumours.— L. Koranyi and L. Gero (letter), *Br. med. J.*, 1979, *1*, 127.

Absorption and Fate

Following intravenous administration streptozocin is rapidly cleared from the blood and distribute to body tissues, particularly the liver, kidneys, intestines, and pancreas. It is extensively metabolised, mainly in the liver, and excreted principally in the urine as metabolites and a small amount of unchanged drug. Approximately 60 to 70% of an intravenous dose is excreted in urine within 24 hours. Some is also excreted via the lungs. Streptozocin itself does not cross the blood-brain barrier but its metabolites are found in the CSF.

Studies in cancer patients given a single intravenous dose of streptozocin 1.5 g per m^2 body-surface suggested that the plasma half-life was about 40 minutes, and the elimination half-life about 13 minutes.— A. B. Adolphe *et al.*, *J. clin. Pharmac.*, 1977, *17*, 379.

Uses and Administration

Streptozocin is an antibiotic antineoplastic agent belonging to the nitrosoureas (see Carmustine, p.606) and is used, alone or in combination with other antineoplastic agents, mainly in the treatment of islet-cell tumours of the pancreas. It has been tried in the carcinoid syndrome and other tumours and in combination regimens for Hodgkin's disease (see p.585). It has been given by intravenous injection or infusion in doses of 1 g per m^2 body-surface weekly, increased if necessary after 2 weeks to up to 1.5 g per m^2. Alternatively doses of 500 mg per m^2 may be given daily for 5 days and repeated every 6 weeks.

Streptozocin has also been given by intra-arterial infusion.

Renal and hepatic function tests should be performed routinely during treatment.

ADMINISTRATION IN RENAL FAILURE. Doses of streptozocin should be reduced to 75% in patients with a glomerular filtration-rate of 10 to 50 mL per minute and to 50% in those in whom the rate was less than 10 mL per minute.— W. M. Bennett *et al.*, *Am. J. Kidney Dis.*, 1983, *3*, 155.

CARCINOID SYNDROME. For a study comparing the effects of fluorouracil plus streptozocin against doxorubicin in patients with carcinoid tumours see Choice of Antineoplastic Agent, p.585.

MALIGNANT NEOPLASMS OF THE PANCREAS. Streptozocin is active against both functioning and nonfunctioning islet-cell tumours; endocrine-secreting tumours may respond both biochemically and with measurable tumour regression, and patients with hypoglycaemia due to insulin-secreting tumours often improve dramatically.— *Med. Lett.*, 1982, *24*, 100.

Results in 15 patients with metastatic islet-cell carcinoma not amenable to surgery treated with streptozocin 500 mg per m^2 body-surface intravenously on alternate days for 5 days. Of 7 patients with vasoactive intestinal-polypeptide-secreting tumours, 4 responded with long-term disappearance of symptoms, 2 had partial symptomatic and biochemical responses, and 1 failed to respond; reduction in tumour size occurred in only 2 of the 7. One of 4 patients with glucagonoma remained in total remission 6 years after treatment, and 1 had a partial response with a 50% fall in plasma glucagon, the remaining 2 failing to respond. There was also no response in 2 patients with pancreatic-polypeptide-secreting tumours. Of 2 patients with non-functioning tumours one had dramatic tumour regression, the other did not respond. Mild proteinuria occured in 50% of patients but none had significant impairment in renal function; other side-effects included nausea and vomiting in all patients.— S. M. Woods *et al.*, *Gut*, 1983, *24*, A596.

Further references: C. R. Kahn *et al.*, *New Engl. J. Med.*, 1975, *292*, 941 (intra-arterial streptozocin in pancreatic-cholera syndrome and non-beta islet-cell carcinoma); L. Sadoff and D. Franklin (letter), *Lancet*, 1975, *2*, 504 (Zollinger-Ellison syndrome); C. B. H. Lamers and J. H. M. van Tongeren (letter), *ibid.*, 1150 (lack of response in gastrinoma with hepatic metastases); J. R. Hayes *et al.*, *Gut*, 1976, *17*, 285 (response to intra-arterial but not intravenous streptozocin in gastrinoma); D. N. Danforth *et al.*, *New Engl. J. Med.*, 1976, *295*, 242 (glucagonoma); R. G. Wiggans *et al.*, *Cancer*, 1978, *41*, 387 (with fluorouracil and mitomycin (SMF) in pancreatic adenocarcinoma); C. G. Moertel *et al.*, *New Engl. J. Med.*, 1980, *303*, 1189 (alone or with fluorouracil in islet-cell tumours).

[illegible]HAEOCHROMOCYTOMA. References to the use of strepto[illegible] in patients with malignant phaeochromocytoma: J. [illegible]an, *Archs intern. Med.*, 1983, *143*, 1799; D. J. [illegible](letter), *ibid.*, 1985, *145*, 367.

Proprietary Names and Manufacturers

Zanosar *(Upjohn, Canad.; Upjohn, Fr.; Upjohn, USA)*.

1865-h

Tamoxifen Citrate *(BANM, USAN, rINNM)*.

ICI-46474. (*Z*)-2-[4-(1,2-Diphenylbut-1-enyl)phenoxy]-*NN*-dimethylethylamine citrate.

$C_{26}H_{29}NO,C_6H_8O_7 = 563.6$.

CAS — 10540-29-1 (tamoxifen); 54965-24-1 (citrate).

Pharmacopoeias. In *Br.* and *U.S.*

A white or almost white crystalline powder. Slightly **soluble** in water and acetone; soluble in methyl alcohol; very slightly soluble in chloroform. It contains not more than 1% of the *E*-isomer. **Store** in well-closed containers. Protect from light.

Tamoxifen citrate 15.2 mg is approximately equivalent to 10 mg of tamoxifen.

Adverse Effects and Precautions

Adverse effects with tamoxifen include hot flushes, oedema, vaginal bleeding, pruritus vulvae, gastro-intestinal upsets, dizziness, rashes, and tumour pain and flare. Transient thrombocytopenia and leucopenia have been reported. There have also been reports of headache, depression, fatigue, confusion, leg cramps, and dry skin. There may be an increased tendency to develop deep vein thromboses; pulmonary embolism has occurred. Hypercalcaemia may develop in patients with bony metastases.

Blurred vision and loss of visual acuity, corneal opacities, and retinopathies have occurred, mostly following administration of very high doses.

Tamoxifen should not be given during pregnancy and should be used with caution in women with functioning ovaries; the latter may also develop menstrual irregularities and cystic ovarian swelling.

EFFECTS ON THE LIVER. A report of peliosis hepatis and massive and fatal liver haemorrhage in a patient who had received tamoxifen for 2 years. The patient was also receiving warfarin, and thyroxine with liothyronine (Liotrix).— G. N. Loomus *et al.*, *Am. J. clin. Path.*, 1983, *80*, 881.

A report of cholestasis and increased liver enzyme values following administration of tamoxifen to a 75-year-old-patient. Enzyme activity rose again on rechallenge with tamoxifen.— A. M. Blackburn *et al.*, *Br. med. J.*, 1984, *289*, 288.

EFFECTS ON THE NERVOUS SYSTEM. Depression, dizziness, syncope, and left-sided cerebellar dysfunction developed in a patient receiving tamoxifen as part of an adjuvant regimen. Cerebellar symptoms resolved within 48 hours of discontinuing tamoxifen, and depression in 7 to 10 days; when tamoxifen therapy was re-instituted, symptoms recurred.— J. L. Pluss and N. J. DiBella, *Ann. intern. Med.*, 1984, *101*, 652.

INTERACTIONS. For a report of deterioration of hepatic function in a patient given tamoxifen concurrently with allopurinol see Allopurinol, p.437.

PORPHYRIA. Tamoxifen was considered to be unsafe in patients with acute porphyria because it has been shown to be porphyrinogenic in *animals* or *in-vitro* systems.— M.R. Moore and K.E.L. McColl, *Porphyrias, Drug Lists*, Glasgow, Porphyria Research Unit, University of Glasgow, 1987.

Absorption and Fate

Peak plasma concentrations of tamoxifen occur 4 to 7 hours after an oral dose. Plasma clearance is reported to be biphasic and the terminal half-life may be longer than 7 days. It is extensively metabolised, the major serum metabolite being N-desmethyltamoxifen, and is excreted slowly in the faeces, mainly as conjugates. Small amounts are excreted in urine. Tamoxifen appears to undergo enterohepatic circulation.

A study of the steady-state pharmacokinetics of tamoxifen and its metabolites in breast cancer patients. Patients received 20 mg of one of two brands of tamoxifen twice daily for 8 weeks and were then crossed over to the other brand for a further 8 weeks. The major metabolite was *N*-desmethyltamoxifen, which was present in plasma at concentrations on average 77% higher than those of tamoxifen, whereas those of *N,N*-desdimethyltamoxifen, and metabolite Y (a side-chain primary alcohol metabolite) were on average 21% and 16% of the concentration of the parent drug. The hydroxylated metabolite 4-hydroxytamoxifen was generally present at concentrations below the level of detection of 2.5 ng per mL. There were no significant differences between the preparations. Tamoxifen and N-desmethyltamoxifen were present in urine, the latter at a concentration 2.5 times higher than that of the former. The total amount excreted in urine was below 1% of the dose. The study confirms that demethylation is the major route of metabolism.— K. Soininen *et al.*, *J. int. med. Res.*, 1986, *14*, 162.

When tamoxifen was given rectally to 6 healthy subjects as a 40 mg suppository the mean relative bioavailability was only 28% compared with the same dose given by mouth. When the suppositories were formulated in a base containing lecithin relative bioavailability was even lower with a mean value of 13% of that by mouth. The low rectal bioavailability might be partly due to low solubility of tamoxifen in rectal mucus. Rectal administration of tamoxifen cannot be recommended at present.— J. J. Tukker *et al.*, *J. Pharm. Pharmac.*, 1986, *38*, 888.

Uses and Administration

Tamoxifen citrate is an oestrogen antagonist with actions similar to those of clomiphene citrate (p.1394). It is used as an alternative to androgens and oestrogens in the management of breast cancer in doses equivalent to 10 to 20 mg of tamoxifen twice daily by mouth. See also under Choice of Antineoplastic Agent, p.589.

Tamoxifen citrate is also used to stimulate ovulation in anovulatory infertility. The usual dose is the equivalent of tamoxifen 10 mg twice daily on days 2, 3, 4, and 5 of the menstrual cycle, increased if necessary in subsequent cycles up to 40 mg twice daily. In women with irregular menstruation the initial course may be begun on any day, and a second course begun at a higher dose after 45 days if there has been no response. If the patient responds by menstruation, subsequent courses may begin on day 2 of the cycle.

Reviews of tamoxifen: *Lancet*, 1983, *1*, 1199; B. J. A. Furr and V. C. Jordan, *Pharmac. Ther.*, 1984, *25*, 127.

CARCINOID SYNDROME. In contrast to the marked response to tamoxifen reported by Myers *et al.* (*Ann. intern. Med.*, 1982, *96*, 383) in a patient with the carcinoid syndrome, results in 16 patients with metastatic carcinoid tumours and the carcinoid syndrome were negative. Patients received tamoxifen 20 to 40 mg daily in 2 divided doses: none had any objective improvement in malignant disease, and only 3 claimed any degree of symptomatic improvement. No patient had complete improvement of symptoms.— C. G. Moertel *et al.*, *Ann. intern. Med.*, 1984, *100*, 531.

GYNAECOMASTIA. Relief of gynaecomastia in 3 men (2 with lung cancer) after treatment with tamoxifen.— D. B. Jefferys, *Br. med. J.*, 1979, *1*, 1119. Gynaecomastia associated with puberty in 2 boys responded to treatment with tamoxifen 10 mg two or three times daily.— P. D. Hooper, *J. R. Coll. gen. Pract.*, 1985, *35*, 142.

INFERTILITY. Tamoxifen was as effective as clomiphene in treating anovulatory infertility in a crossover study in 46 women. Patients received tamoxifen 20 mg daily or clomiphene 50 mg daily on day 5 of uterine bleeding, continued for 5 days; if no ovulation occurred, dosage was increased in each cycle to a maximum of 80 mg daily of tamoxifen or 200 mg daily of clomiphene. Overall, 32 women ovulated both after tamoxifen and after clomiphene, 3 after tamoxifen alone, 6 after clomiphene alone; 5 patients did not ovulate after either drug. It was noted that the ovulation rate was higher in the 16 women who had received clomiphene prior to the study (77.8% after both drugs) than in those who had not (46.7% after tamoxifen, 56.4% after clomiphene). Lengths of ovulatory cycles and luteal phases were similar after both drugs.— I. E. Messinis and S. J. Nillius, *Acta obstet. gynec. scand.*, 1982, *61*, 377.

Results in infertile women with deficient postcoital tests (indicating that the cervical mucus was acting as a barrier to spermatozoa) suggested that tamoxifen might be preferable to clomiphene in treating this type of infertility. Following clomiphene there was an overproduction of 17-β-oestradiol which did not result in an improvement of cervical mucus characteristics; the pH of endocervical mucus was lowered. In contrast, after tamoxifen, serum concentrations of 17-β-oestradiol were approximately normal, and spermatozoal penetration of the cervical mucus was improved; there was no corresponding fall in the pH of endocervical mucus.— F. J. M. E. Roumen *et al.*, *Fert. Steril.*, 1984, *41*, 237.

Male infertility. Doses of 10 to 20 mg daily of tamoxifen have been given to infertile men, with oligospermia. Treatment schedules vary from 2 to 24 months. Plasma-testosterone concentrations rise in most patients shortly after treatment, and 55 to 80% of patients are reported to show a significant increase in sperm output, generally after 3 or more months.— A. A. Templeton, *Prescribers' J.*, 1985, *25*, 91. See also W-B. Schill and M. Michalopoulos, *Drugs*, 1984, *28*, 263; *Ann. intern. Med.*, 1985, *103*, 906.

MASTALGIA. In a double-blind study involving 60 patients with severe breast pain, tamoxifen 20 mg daily for 3 months relieved pain in 22 of 31 patients, compared with 11 of 29 taking placebo (71% and 38% respectively). Only 3 of the tamoxifen group had non-cyclical pain, and pain was relieved in 2 of these. Side-effects were severe enough to interrupt treatment in 6 patients from each group. Of the 9 patients not responding to tamoxifen, 6 were subsequently given a 3-month course of placebo, and 2 responded; 12 patients not responding to placebo were given tamoxifen, and relief of symptoms was obtained in 8. The study confirms that in women with severe mastalgia tamoxifen is an effective treatment.— I. S. Fentiman *et al.*, *Lancet*, 1986, *1*, 287. Comment. There is very limited knowledge of the effects of tamoxifen in premenopausal women, who form the largest sub-group of mastalgia patients, those with cyclical pronounced mastalgia. In addition, prescription of tamoxifen for benign breast disease may diminish its usefulness in those patients who subsequently get breast cancer.— *ibid.*, 305. Further comment. There are theoretical objections to the use of tamoxifen in benign disease in premenopausal women, and any study of tamoxifen should be restricted to severe cases that have failed first-line treatment.— J. A. Smallwood and I. Taylor (letter), *ibid.*, 680. Reply, and agreement. Tamoxifen is not a first-line treatment in mastalgia and until the results of further work become available it should be used only in cases of severe prolonged pain.— I. S. Fentiman *et al.* (letter), *ibid.*, 681.

Further references: I. S. Fentiman, *Drugs*, 1986, *32*, 477.

MALIGNANT NEOPLASMS. Tamoxifen was ineffective in arresting progressive pulmonary insufficiency in a patient with lymphangioleiomyomatosis, a rare disease found in women of child-bearing age, but this might be because it was used at a very late stage: further studies alone or with oophorectomy, were recommended.— A. Tomasian *et al.* (letter), *New Engl. J. Med.*, 1982, *306*, 745.

Reports of excellent response in 2 patients with non-Hodgkin's lymphoma who were given tamoxifen 10 mg twice daily; one, who also received combination chemotherapy, had maintained partial remission from her refractory disease for 15 months. A third patient with chronic lymphocytic leukaemia refractory to combination therapy had responded to treatment with the same dose of tamoxifen in association with prednisone 10 mg on alternate days.— P. Narasimhan (letter), *New Engl. J. Med.*, 1984, *311*, 1258.

MALIGNANT NEOPLASMS OF THE BREAST. For a discussion of the treatment of breast cancer, including the role of tamoxifen, see p.588. For the role of adjuvant endocrine therapy see p.589.

In 61 patients in whom breast cancer progressed despite tamoxifen, withdrawal of the drug produced complete remission in 1 and partial remission in 4; 1 patient had stabilisation of previously progressive disease. These withdrawal responses occurred only among the 28 patients who had initially responded to tamoxifen therapy, and only in soft-tissue disease. It is possible that the weak oestrogenic properties of tamoxifen may produce tumour stimulation in patients who have relapsed. Patients who have shown some response to tamoxifen should be observed for a withdrawal response, where clinical condition permits, before further active hormonal manipulation is initiated.— P. A. Canney *et al* (letter), *Lancet*, 1987, *1*, 36.

Prophylaxis. Discussion of the potential role of tamoxifen in the prophylaxis of breast cancer in women at high risk. Available evidence suggests that the amount of free oestrogen is a key factor in the development of breast cancer, and in view of the effectiveness of tamoxifen in established disease its use in a preventive study in very high-risk groups would be logical.— J. Cuzick *et al.*, *Lancet*, 1986, *1*, 83. See also J. Cuzick and M. Baum (letter), *ibid.*, 1985, *2*, 282. Further mention of tamoxifen in the prophylaxis of breast cancer. J. C. Gazet (letter), *ibid.*, 1119. Comment. The goal is laudable but great caution is required, particularly in premenopausal women: pilot toxicity studies should be considered first. Long-term studies in postmenopausal patients, who are in any case at increased risk, might be better.— V. C. Jordan (letter), *ibid.*, 1986, *1*, 105. Further discussion, and criticisms of the proposed studies of prophylactic therapy: J. - C. Gazet (letter), *ibid.*, 263 (recruitment for a randomised study); V. E. Basco *et al.* (letter), *ibid* (need for contraception in premenopausal women); M. J. Daly (letter), *ibid* (risk of tamoxifen resistance if patients develop breast cancer); W. Wong (letter), *ibid.*, 264 (possible development of resistance); M. C. Pike and M. P. Coleman (letter), *ibid* (doubt as to the prophylactic value of tamoxifen); P. Milner *et al.* (letter), *ibid* (cost of prophylactic therapy); H. W. Simpson and W. Candlish (letter), *ibid.*, 265 (prophylaxis should be carried out in younger women).

MALIGNANT NEOPLASMS OF THE MALE BREAST. Tamoxifen 20 mg daily in 24 patients with breast cancer, 4 of whom were given a loading dose of 160 mg, produced complete response in 5 and partial responses in a further 4. The duration of response ranged from 8 months to 60 months with a mean of 21 months. A further 2 patients had stabilisation of disease for a 24 months, but disease progressed in the remaining 13. There was an apparent correlation between good clinical response of the tumour and a positive assay for oestrogen and progesterone receptors. There were no side-effects of therapy, and in view of the response rate of 37.5%, which is comparable to that achieved with stilboestrol, it would seem that tamoxifen is a reasonable drug to try in this condition before attempting orchidectomy or adrenalectomy.— G. G. Ribeiro, *Clin. Radiol.*, 1983, *34*, 625.

See also under Choice of Antineoplastic Agent, p.589.

MALIGNANT NEOPLASMS OF THE ENDOMETRIUM. In a pilot study of tamoxifen 10 mg twice daily for the treatment of advanced endometrial carcinoma, 4 of 7 patients responded.— K. D. Swenerton *et al.* (letter), *New Engl. J. Med.*, 1979, *301*, 105. See also M. Slavik *et al.*, *Cancer Treat. Rep.*, 1984, *68*, 809.

MALIGNANT NEOPLASMS OF THE PROSTATE. A report of encouraging results with tamoxifen in drug-resistant advanced prostatic carcinoma.— M. O. El-Arini (letter), *Lancet*, 1979, *2*, 588. Tamoxifen had no activity against advanced prostatic cancer in a study in 17 patients given doses of 10 to 50 mg by mouth twice daily.— F. M. Torti *et al.*, *Cancer*, 1984, *54*, 739.

MELANOMA. Four of 26 patients with advanced malignant melanoma had an objective response to treatment with tamoxifen 20 to 40 mg daily. The 4 who responded all had soft-tissue disease. Adverse effects were generally mild although some men reported decreased sexual performance and one woman had moderate alopecia.— R. A. Nesbit *et al.* (letter), *New Engl. J. Med.*, 1979, *301*, 1241. See also R. O. Mirimanoff *et al.* (letter), *Lancet*, 1981, *1*, 1368. Comment. It was doubtful if tamoxifen had a significant place in the therapy of melanoma.— C. M. Furnival *et al.* (letter), *ibid.*, *2*, 374.

Preparations

Tamoxifen Citrate Tablets *(U.S.P.)*

Tamoxifen Tablets *(B.P.)*. Tamoxifen Citrate Tablets. Potency is expressed in terms of the equivalent amount of tamoxifen.

Proprietary Preparations

Noltam *(Lederle, UK)*. *Tablets*, tamoxifen 10 mg (as citrate).
Tablets, scored, tamoxifen 20 mg (as citrate).

Nolvadex *(ICI Pharmaceuticals, UK)*. *Tablets*, tamoxifen 10 mg (as citrate).
Tablets, (Nolvadex-D), tamoxifen 20 mg (as citrate).
Tablets, (Nolvadex-Forte), tamoxifen 40 mg (as citrate).

Tamofen *(Tillotts, UK)*. *Tablets*, scored, tamoxifen 10 mg (as citrate).
Tablets, tamoxifen 20 and 40 mg (as citrate).

Proprietary Names and Manufacturers

Istubol *(Chile)*; Kessar *(Farmitalia Carlo Erba, Fr.; Farmitalia, Ger.; Farmitalia Carlo Erba, S.Afr.; Farmitalia Carlo Erba, Switz.; Farmitalia Carlo Erba, UK)*; Noltam *(Lederle, UK)*; Nolvadex *(Arg.; ICI, Austral.; Belg.; ICI, Canad.; ICI, Denm.; I.C.I.-Pharma, Fr.; ICI, Ger.; ICI-Pharma, Ital.; Neth.; ICI, Norw.; ICI, S.Afr.; ICI, Spain; ICI, Swed.; ICI, Switz.; ICI Pharmaceuticals, UK; Stuart Pharmaceuticals, USA)*; Tamaxin *(Farmos, Denm.; Laakefarmos, Swed.)*; Tamofen *(Rhône-Poulenc, Canad.; Rhone-Poulenc, Denm.; Rhône-Poulenc, Ger.; Rhône-Poulenc, Norw.; Rhone-Poulenc, Swed.; Tillotts, UK)*; Tamoxasta *(Asta Pharma, Ger.)*; Zitazonium *(Hung.)*.

1866-m

Tegafur *(BAN, USAN, rINN)*.

FT-207; Ftorafur; MJF-12264; NSC-148958; WR-220066. 5-Fluoro-1-(tetrahydro-2-furyl)uracil; 5-Fluoro-1-(tetrahydro-2-furyl)pyrimidine-2,4(1*H*,3*H*)-dione. $C_8H_9FN_2O_3$=200.2.

CAS — 17902-23-7.

Adverse Effects, Treatment, and Precautions

As for fluorouracil (p.628). Bone-marrow depression may be less severe with tegafur but central neurotoxicity is more common.

Results in *animals* suggested that co-administration of uracil with tegafur reduced the latter's cardiotoxic and neurotoxic effects.— J. Yamamoto *et al.*, *J. pharm. Sci.*, 1984, *73*, 212.

Absorption and Fate

Tegafur is well absorbed from the gastro-intestinal tract after oral administration. Following an intravenous dose it is reported to have a prolonged plasma half-life of 6 to 16 hours, and to be slowly metabolised to fluorouracil. It crosses the blood-brain barrier and is found in the CSF.

References: J. L. Au *et al.*, *Cancer Treat. Rep.*, 1979, *63*, 343.

Uses and Administration

Tegafur is an antineoplastic agent which appears to act by the release of fluorouracil (p.628) in the body. It has been used in the management of malignant neoplasms of the breast and gastro-intestinal tract. Doses of 1 to 3 g per m^2 body-surface daily for 5 or more days have been administered intravenously every 4 weeks. Tegafur has also been given by mouth.

Proprietary Names and Manufacturers

Citofur *(Lusofarmaco, Ital.)*; Coparogin *(Jpn)*; Exonal *(Jpn)*; Fental *(Jpn)*; FH *(Jpn)*; Franroze *(Jpn)*; Fulaid *(Jpn)*; Fulfeel *(Jpn)*; Fultol-P *(Jpn)*; Furafuluor *(Jpn)*; Furofutran *(Jpn)*; Futraful *(Jpn)*; Helpa *(Jpn)*; Icalus *(Jpn)*; Lamar *(Jpn)*; Lifril *(Jpn)*; Lunacin *(Jpn)*; Neberk *(Jpn)*; Nitobanil *(Jpn)*; Pharmic *(Jpn)*; Richina *(Jpn)*; Riol *(Jpn)*; Sinoflurol *(Jpn)*; Tefsiel-C *(Jpn)*; Torafurine *(Morrith, Spain)*; Utefos *(Almirall, Spain)*.

1867-b

Teniposide *(BAN, USAN, rINN)*.

ETP; NSC-122819; PTG; VM-26. (5*S*,5a*R*,8a*S*,9*R*)-5,8,8a,9-Tetrahydro-5-(4-hydroxy-3,5-dimethoxyphenyl)-9-(4,6-*O*-thenylidene-β-D-glucopyranosyloxy)isobenzofuro[5,6-*f*][1,3]benzodioxol-6(5a*H*)-one. $C_{32}H_{32}O_{13}S$=656.7.

CAS — 29767-20-2.

Adverse Effects, Treatment, and Precautions

As for Etoposide, p.627.

A report of renal failure with acute tubular necrosis, and haemolytic anaemia, due to an antibody to teniposide.— B. Habibi *et al.*, *New Engl. J. Med.*, 1982, *306*, 1091.

Uses and Administration

Teniposide is an antineoplastic agent with the general properties of etoposide (p.627). It has been given alone or with other antineoplastic agents in the treatment of lymphomas and solid tumours of the bladder and brain. Doses of 30 mg per m^2 body-surface have been administered daily for 5 days by intravenous infusion as a single agent. In combination chemotherapy, teniposide has been given in doses of 50 to 100 mg daily by slow intravenous infusion, dissolved in sodium chloride injection (0.9%) or glucose injection (5%). Infusion should be carried out over 45 to 60 minutes.

A review of teniposide.— P. J. O'Dwyer *et al.*, *Cancer Treat. Rep.*, 1984, *68*, 1455.

The successful use of teniposide in induction therapy of familial erythrophagocytic lymphohistiocytosis (FEL), a rare, usually fatal disease of childhood characterised by fever, hepatosplenomegaly, and pancytopenia, with non-malignant lymphohistiocytic infiltration and erythrophagocytosis in reticuloendothelial organs. Three of 4 children were given intravenous teniposide 30 mg per m² body-surface daily for 5 days, with oral prednisolone, the course being repeated every other week for 8 weeks. Intrathecal methotrexate was also given. The other child received teniposide 100 mg per m^2 twice weekly for 4 weeks, because of a less rapid response. All 4 patients responded during the first week of therapy, with return to normal body temperature and a reduction in spleen size. The effects of teniposide therapy were very promising, and a suitable maintenance therapy was being sought.— J. - I. Henter *et al.* (letter), *Lancet*, 1986, *2*, 1402.

Proprietary Names and Manufacturers

Véhem *(Sandoz, Fr.)*; Vumon *(Bristol-Myers, Austral.*; *Bristol, Canad.*; *Bristol Italiana Sud, Ital.*; *Bristol, S.Afr.*; *Bristol-Myers, Spain*; *Bristol, Swed.*; *Bristol, Switz.)*.

1868-v

Thioguanine *(BAN, USAN)*.

6-TG; 6-Thioguanine; NSC-752; Tioguanine *(rINN)*; WR-1141. 2-Aminopurine-6(1*H*)-thione; 2-Amino-6-mercaptopurine; 2-Aminopurine-6-thiol.

$C_5H_5N_5S=167.2$.

CAS — 154-42-7 (anhydrous); 5580-03-0 (hemihydrate).

Pharmacopoeias. In *Br. Braz.* and *U.S.* permit anhydrous or hemihydrate.

A pale yellow, odourless or almost odourless, crystalline powder. Practically **insoluble** in water, alcohol, and chloroform; dissolves in dilute solutions of alkali hydroxides. **Store** in airtight containers.

Adverse Effects, Treatment, and Precautions

As for Mercaptopurine, p.635.

In some patients, gastro-intestinal reactions are reported to be less frequent than with mercaptopurine. Normal doses of thioguanine may be employed when it is used with allopurinol.

EFFECTS ON THE BLOOD. For the view that bone-marrow depression by thioguanine may now be predictable, see under Mercaptopurine, p.635.

EFFECTS ON THE LIVER. Reports of hepatic veno-occlusive disease attributed to thioguanine.— R. A. Gill *et al.*, *Ann. intern. Med.*, 1982, *96*, 58; N. Krivoy *et al.* (letter), *ibid.*, 788.

Absorption and Fate

Thioguanine is incompletely and variably absorbed from the gastro-intestinal tract. It is rapidly activated in the body by intracellular conversion to its nucleotide, thioguanosine 5′-phosphate (thioguanine ribose phosphate). Very little unchanged thioguanine has been detected circulating in the blood but the half-life of the nucleotide in the tissues is prolonged. Thioguanine is inactivated primarily by methylation to aminomethylthiopurine; small amounts are deaminated to thioxanthine, and may go on to be oxidised by xanthine oxidase to thiouric acid, but inactivation is essentially independent of xanthine oxidase and is not affected by inhibition of the enzyme. About 40% of a dose has been reported to be excreted in the urine within 24 hours as metabolites; only negligible amounts of thioguanine have been detected. Thioguanine does not appear to cross the blood-brain barrier to a significant extent; very little is found in cerebrospinal fluid after normal clinical doses. It crosses the placenta.

A study of the absorption and fate of thioguanine in 24 cancer patients given thioguanine by mouth and intravenously as the sodium salt. After an intravenous dose plasma half-lives of 25 to 240 minutes (a median of 80 minutes) were achieved and about 77% of the dose (range 41 to 81%) was excreted in the urine in 24 hours, entirely as metabolites after 2 hours. After oral doses only metabolites were detected in the urine; 24 to 46% of a dose was excreted in 24 hours. Blood concen[illegible]ions and incorporation into bone-marrow DNA were [illegible]t on the dose and primarily on the state of the [illegible]v. Incorporation into DNA of the bone marrow was slight after one dose but after 5 daily doses thioguanine had almost replaced guanine in the DNA indicating that most cells were stimulated to enter DNA synthesis during that time.— G. A. LePage and J. P. Whitecar, *Cancer Res.*, 1971, *31*, 1627.

Uses and Administration

Thioguanine is an analogue of the naturally occurring purine, guanine, and is an antineoplastic agent with actions and uses similar to those of mercaptopurine (see p.635). It appears to cause fewer gastro-intestinal reactions but cross-resistance exists between it and mercaptopurine so that patients who do not respond to one are unlikely to respond to the other.

Thioguanine is given by mouth with other agents, usually cytarabine and an anthracycline, in the induction and maintenance of remissions in acute non-lymphoblastic leukaemia. It has also been used in acute lymphoblastic leukaemia and chronic myeloid leukemia.

A dose of 2 to 2.5 mg per kg body-weight daily increased after 4 weeks, if there is no response or toxicity allows, to 3 mg per kg daily may be given to adults and children. Alternatively, doses up to 100 mg per m^2 body-surface every 12 hours have been given for 5 to 7 days as part of a combined induction regimen. See also under Choice of Antineoplastic Agent, p.587.

Blood counts should be made daily during induction and when thioguanine is given with other antineoplastic agents, or weekly when given on its own for maintenance. Therapy should be withdrawn at the first sign of severe bone-marrow depression.

It has been administered intravenously as thioguanine sodium.

MYELOPROLIFERATIVE DISORDERS. Twelve patients with myelofibrosis characterised by anaemia, splenomegaly, or constitutional symptoms such as fever, weight-loss, and night sweats were treated with busulphan 2 to 4 mg daily (in 9) or thioguanine 20 to 40 mg daily (in 3). Both therapies achieved a significant reduction in the size of spleen and liver, and were effective in resolving constitutional symptoms. In 5 patients in whom marrow examinations were carried out chemotherapy also had achieved reduction of bone-marrow fibrosis. Therapy was well tolerated by all patients, none of whom developed any major or troublesome adverse effects. The question as to whether single agent chemotherapy would alter prognosis in patients with myelofibrosis can only be answered by a much larger and longer term study, but present results suggest that in patients with symptomatic disease thioguanine or busulphan are effective and safe alternatives to splenectomy, which carries a high postoperative mortality-rate without necessarily prolonging survival.— A. Manoharan and W. R. Pitney, *Scand. J. Haemat.*, 1984, *33*, 453.

Preparations

Thioguanine Tablets *(B.P.)*

Thioguanine Tablets *(U.S.P.)*

Proprietary Preparations

Lanvis *(Calmic, UK). Tablets*, scored, thioguanine 40 mg.

Proprietary Names and Manufacturers

Lanvis *(Wellcome, Austral.*; *Belg.*; *Wellcome, Canad.*; *Neth.*; *Wellcome, S.Afr.*; *Wellcome, Swed.*; *Wellcome, Switz.*; *Calmic, UK)*.

1870-f

Thioinosine

Mercaptopurine Riboside; Tioinosine. 9-*β*-D-Ribofuranosyl-9*H*-purine-6-thiol.

$C_{10}H_{12}N_4O_4S=284.3$.

CAS — 574-25-4.

Thioinosine is the riboside of mercaptopurine (see p.635) and has been used similarly in the treatment of leukaemia.

Proprietary Names and Manufacturers

Thioinosie *(Morishita, Jpn)*.

1869-g

Thiotepa *(BAN, USAN, rINN)*.

NSC-6396; TESPA; Thiophosphamide; Triethylene Thiophosphoramide; TSPA; WR-45312. Phosphorothioic tri(ethyleneamide); Tris(aziridin-1-yl)phosphine sulphide.

$C_6H_{12}N_3PS=189.2$.

CAS — 52-24-4.

Pharmacopoeias. In *Br.*, *Chin.*, *Egypt.*, *Fr.*, *Jpn*, *Rus.*, and *U.S.*

Fine white, odourless or almost odourless, crystalline flakes. M.p. 52° to 57°. The *B.P.* states that it is **soluble** 1 in 8 of water, 1 in 2 of alcohol, and 1 in 2 of chloroform; *U.S.P.* solubilities are 1 in 13 of water, 1 in about 8 of alcohol, 1 in about 2 of chloroform, and 1 in about 4 of ether. A 0.75% solution for injection has a pH of 7.0 to 8.2. **Store** at 2° to 8° in airtight containers. At higher temperatures it polymerises and becomes inactive. Protect from light.

CAUTION. *Thiotepa is irritant; avoid contact with skin and mucous membranes.*

Adverse Effects, Treatment, and Precautions

For an outline of the adverse effects experienced with antineoplastic agents and immunosuppressants, general guidelines for their treatment, and precautions, see Antineoplastic Agents, p.580, p.583.

Thiotepa is very toxic to the haemopoietic system; maximum depression of the bone marrow may occur up to 30 days after therapy has been discontinued and irreversible hypoplastic anaemia may occur. The relation between dosage and toxicity is highly variable and extreme caution is always required. Headache and dizziness, allergy, and impaired fertility have also been reported. As with other alkylating agents, thiotepa is potentially mutagenic, teratogenic, and carcinogenic.

Thiotepa should be given with extreme care, if at all, to patients with pre-existing impairment of hepatic, renal, or bone-marrow function.

CARCINOGENICITY. A report of acute nonlymphoblastic leukaemia in an 83-year-old patient who had completed 39 months of treatment wth thiotepa bladder instillations. Although intramuscular administration of thiotepa has been associated with development of leukaemia this is believed to be the first such report following intravesical administration.— M. A. Poon; D. J. Easton, *Can. med. Ass. J.*, 1983, *129*, 578.

EFFECTS ON THE BLOOD. Ten of 25 consecutive patients given instillations of thiotepa into the bladder had at least one episode of acute dose-related myelosuppression, occurring most often within the first 3 months of treatment. One of the 25, and 4 further patients developed chronic myelosuppression. Thrombocytopenia was the most common abnormality. The 2 forms of myelosuppression were not related and there was no way of predicting which patients will develop chronic myelosuppression. A treatment schedule averaging 90 mg of thiotepa monthly during the first 3 months, reduced to 45 mg monthly over longer periods, is recommended.— D. Hollister and M. Coleman, *J. Am. med. Ass.*, 1980, *244*, 2065.

EFFECTS ON THE KIDNEYS. A 76-year-old man developed ureteral obstruction and renal failure after topical treatment with thiotepa following bladder resection.— P. F. Schellhammer, *J. Urol., Baltimore*, 1973, *110*, 498.

Absorption and Fate

The absorption of thiotepa from the gastro-intestinal tract is incomplete and unreliable; variable absorption also occurs from intramuscular injection sites. Absorption through serous membranes such as the bladder and pleura occurs to some extent. Only traces of unchanged thiotepa and triethylene phosphoramide are excreted in the urine, together with a large proportion of metabolites.

Uses and Administration

Thiotepa is an ethyleneimine compound whose antineoplastic effect is related to its alkylating action (see p.580). It has a spectrum of activity similar to that of mustine (p.645) but has gene-

rally been replaced by cyclophosphamide (p.612) or other agents. It is not a vesicant and may be given by all parenteral routes, as well as directly into tumour masses. Thiotepa may be used in the palliation of carcinoma of the breast and ovary and has been given in the treatment of various lymphomas. Instillations of thiotepa are used in the treatment of superficial tumours of the bladder and in the control of malignant effusions. It has been given intrathecally to patients with malignant meningeal disease. It has also been used as an adjunct to the surgical removal of pterygium, to prevent recurrence. Thiotepa has some immunosuppressant activity.
See also under Choice of Antineoplastic Agent, p.584.
Thiotepa is given in a variety of dosage schedules. In general, initial doses to suit the individual patient are followed by maintenance doses given at intervals of one to 4 weeks. Blood counts are recommended before administration and if there is leucopenia the dose should be reduced. Thiotepa should not be given if the white cell count falls below 3000 per mm^3 or the platelet count below 150 000 per mm^3.
Up to 60 mg in single or divided doses may be given by intramuscular injection or by instillation in adults and children over 12 years. Intravenous doses of up to 30 mg may be given every one to 4 weeks. Alternatively, 300 to 400 µg per kg body-weight every 1 to 4 weeks, or 200 µg per kg for 4 to 5 days every 2 to 4 weeks have been suggested.
A solution containing 1 mg of thiotepa per mL has been injected intrathecally in doses of up to 10 mg; in the *USA*, doses of 1 to 10 mg per m^2 have been suggested.
Following dehydration for 8 to 12 hours, up to 60 mg of thiotepa in 30 to 60 mL of sterile water may be instilled into the bladder, where it is retained for 2 hours if possible, and the instillation repeated weekly for 4 weeks; single-dose instillations of 90 mg in 100 mL of sterile water have been used prophylactically as an adjunct to surgery.
Malignant effusions may be treated by the instillation of 10 to 30 mg or more of thiotepa in 20 to 60 mL of sterile water, following aspiration; a dose of 600 to 800 µg per kg has been suggested in the *USA*. Similar doses have also been injected directly into tumours.
Thiotepa for local use has been mixed with solutions of procaine and adrenaline.
A 0.05% solution has been instilled as eye-drops every 3 hours for up to 8 weeks following surgical removal of pterygium in order to reduce the likelihood of recurrence.

Preparations

Thiotepa for Injection *(U.S.P.)*

Thiotepa Injection *(B.P.)*. Prepared immediately before use. If solid particles separate, the solution should not be used.

Proprietary Names and Manufacturers

Ledertepa *(Belg.; Neth.)*; Onco Tiotepa *(Spain)*; Tifosyl *(Norw.; Swed.)*.
Manufacturers also include—*Lederle, UK; Lederle, USA.*

1871-d

Treosulfan *(BAN, rINN).*

Dihydroxybusulphan; NSC-39069. L-Threitol 1,4-dimethanesulphonate.
$C_6H_{14}O_8S_2$=278.3.

CAS — 299-75-2.

Adverse Effects, Treatment, and Precautions

As for Busulphan, p.603.

Uses and Administration

Treosulfan is an antineoplastic agent which is reported to act by alkylation (see p.580) after conversion *in vivo* to epoxide compounds. It is used palliatively or as an adjunct to surgery mainly in the treatment of ovarian cancer.
Treosulfan 1 g daily is given by mouth in 4 divided doses for 2 or 4 weeks followed by the same period without treatment. Alternatively 1.5 g daily in 3 divided doses may be given for 1 week, followed by 3 weeks without therapy. The cycle is then repeated, the dose being adjusted if necessary according to the effect on bone marrow. Lower doses should be used if treatment with other antineoplastic drugs or radiotherapy is being given concomitantly. Treosulfan may also be given intravenously in doses of 5 to 15 g every one to three weeks.

Proprietary Names and Manufacturers

Leo, UK.

1872-n

Tretamine *(BAN, rINN).*

NSC-9706; TEM; Tretaminum; Triethanomelamine; Triethylenemelamine. 2,4,6-Tris(aziridin-1-yl)-1,3,5-triazine.
$C_9H_{12}N_6$=204.2.

CAS — 51-18-3.

Pharmacopoeias. In *Jug.*

CAUTION. *Tretamine is irritant; avoid contact with skin and mucous membranes.*

Tretamine is an ethyleneimine compound with properties similar to those of thiotepa (p.652). It was formerly given by mouth in the palliative treatment of malignant neoplasms.

13373-j

Triazinate

BAF; Baker's Antifol; NSC-139105; WR-219427. 3-[2-Chloro-4-(4,6-diamino-2,2-dimethyl-1,3,5-triazin-1(2*H*)-yl)phenoxymethyl]-*NN*-dimethylbenzamide.
$C_{21}H_{25}ClN_6O_2$=428.9.

CAS — 48223-06-9 (triazinate); 41191-04-2 (esylate).

Triazinate is a folate antagonist which has been tried as the esylate in neoplastic disease.

13382-z

Trimetrexate *(BAN, USAN, rINN).*

CI-898. 5-Methyl-6-(3,4,5-trimethoxyanilinomethyl)quinazoline-2,4-diyldiamine.
$C_{19}H_{23}N_5O_3$=369.4.

CAS — 52128-35-5.

Trimetrexate is a folate-inhibitor (see Methotrexate, p.639) and is reported to have antineoplastic activity. It has been tried in the management of malignant neoplasms of the lung and other solid tumours. It has also been reported to possess activity against *Pneumocystis carinii* pneumonia.

References: P. J. O'Dwyer *et al., Invest. New Drugs*, 1985, *3*, 71; D. H. W. Ho *et al., Clin. Pharmac. Ther.*, 1987, *42*, 351.

A study of the use of trimetrexate to treat *Pneumocystis carinii* pneumonia in patients with AIDS. Trimetrexate 30 mg per m^2 body-surface was given as an intravenous bolus daily for 21 days together with folinic acid rescue (20 mg per m^2 every 6 hours for 23 days). Treatment resulted in survival in 11 of 16 patients resistant or intolerant to other treatment as well as in 14 of 16 given trimetrexate as initial therapy. A further 17 patients also received sulphadiazine by mouth and 12 of these responded to the combined therapy. Toxicity of trimetrexate was minimal and easily managed; in patients in whom cytopenia developed the trimetrexate dose was halved for an average of four days. Trimetrexate appears to be a safe and effective treatment when given in this way to patients with pneumocystis pneumonia; comparison with standard therapy appears warranted.— C. J. Allegra *et al., New Engl. J. Med.*, 1987, *317*, 978.

Proprietary Names and Manufacturers

Parke, Davis, USA.

1875-b

Trofosfamide *(rINN).*

NSC-109723; Trilophosphamide; Trophosphamide; Z-4828. 3-(2-Chloroethyl)-2-[bis(2-chloroethyl)amino]-perhydro-1,3,2-oxazaphosphorine-2-oxide.
$C_9H_{18}Cl_3N_2O_2P$=323.6.

CAS — 22089-22-1.

Trofosfamide is a derivative of cyclophosphamide (see p.610) and has the same general properties. It is used in the treatment of a variety of malignant disorders in usual initial doses of 300 to 400 mg daily by mouth. Doses of 50 to 150 mg daily have been given for maintenance therapy.

Proprietary Names and Manufacturers

Ixoten *(Asta Pharma, Ger.; Schering, Ital.; Asta, Neth.; Noristan, S.Afr.).*

1876-v

Uramustine *(BAN, rINN).*

NSC-34462; U-8344; Uracil Mustard *(USAN).*
5-Bis(2-chloroethyl)aminouracil; 5-[Bis(2-chloroethyl)amino]pyrimidine-2,4(1*H*,3*H*)-dione.
$C_8H_{11}Cl_2N_3O_2$=252.1.

CAS — 66-75-1.

Pharmacopoeias. In *U.S.*

An off-white odourless crystalline powder. Very slightly **soluble** in water; soluble 1 in 150 of alcohol; slightly soluble in acetone; practically insoluble in chloroform. Unstable in the presence of water. **Store** in airtight containers.

CAUTION. *Uramustine is irritant; avoid contact with skin and mucous membranes.*

Adverse Effects, Treatment, and Precautions

For an outline of the adverse effects experienced with antineoplastic agents and immunosuppressants, general guidelines for their treatment, and precautions, see Antineoplastic Agents, p.580, p.583.
Maximum depression of the bone marrow may not occur until 2 to 4 weeks after uramustine has been discontinued and if the total dosage approaches 1 mg per kg body-weight, the cumulative damage to the bone marrow may be irreversible.

Uses and Administration

Uramustine is an antineoplastic agent derived from mustine (p.645) and has a similar mode of action but it has largely been replaced by more effective agents. It has been given by mouth in the treatment of chronic lymphocytic leukaemia and malignant lymphomas and has occasionally been used in mycosis fungoides, polycythaemia vera, thrombocytosis, and as an adjunct in carcinoma of the ovary and lung.
A suggested initial dosage is 150 µg per kg body-weight weekly, as a single dose, for 4 weeks. Alternatively, patients have been given 1 to 2 mg daily until a clinical response or bone-marrow depression occurs. When the bone marrow recovers or the patient deteriorates treatment is reinstituted with 1 mg daily for 3 weeks, followed by 1 week's rest, and then repeated courses for several months. Another scheme of administration is to give 3 to 5 mg daily for 7 days, followed by 1 mg daily for 3 weeks out of 4. The total dose in the first week should not be more than 500 µg per kg body-weight. Total and differential white-cell counts, platelet counts, and haemoglobin examinations should be made once or twice weekly and the dosage adjusted according to the patient's response.

Preparations

Uracil Mustard Capsules *(U.S.P.)*. Capsules containing uramustine.

Proprietary Names and Manufacturers

Upjohn, UK; Upjohn, USA.

1877-g

Urethane *(rINN)*.
Ethylurethane; NSC-746; Urethanum. Ethyl carbamate.
$NH_2.CO.O.C_2H_5$=89.09.

CAS — 51-79-6.

Pharmacopoeias. In *Arg., Belg., Hung., Int., Mex., Nord., Pol., Port., Roum., Span.,* and *Turk.*

Urethane is an antineoplastic agent formerly used in the treatment of chronic myeloid leukaemia. It is also a mild hypnotic and has been employed as an anaesthetic for small animals.

1878-q

Vinblastine Sulphate *(BANM, rINNM)*.

LE-29060; NSC-49842; Vinblastine Sulfate *(USAN)*; Vincaleucoblastine Sulphate; Vincaleukoblastine Sulphate; VLB *(vinblastine)*. The sulphate of an alkaloid, vincaleukoblastine, extracted from *Vinca rosea* (*Catharanthus roseus*) (Apocynaceae).
$C_{46}H_{58}N_4O_9,H_2SO_4$=909.1.

CAS — 865-21-4 (vinblastine); 143-67-9 (sulphate).

Pharmacopoeias. In *Br., Chin., Cz., Egypt., Jug.,* and *U.S.*

A white to slightly yellow, odourless, very hygroscopic, amorphous or crystalline powder. It loses not more than 17% of its weight on drying. **Soluble** 1 in 10 of water and 1 in 50 of chloroform; very slightly soluble in alcohol; practically insoluble in ether. A 0.15% solution in water has a pH of 3.5 to 5.0 and a 0.3% solution is clear. **Store** at 2° to 8° in airtight containers. Protect from light.

Adverse Effects and Treatment

For an outline of the adverse effects experienced with antineoplastic agents and immunosuppressants and general guidelines for their treatment, see Antineoplastic Agents, p.580 and p.583.

Bone-marrow depression, especially leucopenia, is the most common adverse effect with vinblastine and tends to be dose-limiting. Maximum depression occurs 4 to 10 days after administration with recovery in a further 1 to 3 weeks. Gastro-intestinal effects may occur; nausea and vomiting respond to treatment with anti-emetics.

Neurological effects that can also involve the autonomic nervous system include malaise, dizziness, weakness, headache, depression, psychoses, paraesthesia and numbness, neuromyopathy, loss of deep tendon reflexes, ataxia, peripheral neuritis, constipation and adynamic ileus, parotid gland pain, and convulsions. Overdosage has caused permanent damage to the central nervous system.

Other reported effects include skin reactions, alopecia, ischaemic cardiac toxicity. A syndrome of inappropriate secretion of antidiuretic hormone has occurred, and may be relieved by fluid restriction.

Vinblastine is irritant to the skin and mucous membranes and extravasation may cause necrosis, cellulitis, and sloughing. The application of warmth and local injection of hyaluronidase may be of benefit in relieving the effects of extravasation.

EFFECTS ON RESPIRATORY FUNCTION. Pulmonary oedema occurred in a 64-year-old woman 2 hours after the intravenous administration of vinblastine.— R. H. Israel and J. P. Olson (letter), *J. Am. med. Ass.*, 1978, *240*, 1585.

See also under Interactions, below.

EFFECTS ON THE SKIN. Vinblastine could cause photosensitivity reactions.— *Med. Lett.*, 1986, *28*, 51.

LOCAL TOXICITY. Corneal changes were apparent in a doctor 24 hours after he had accidentally sprayed his face with a solution of vinblastine sulphate. Over the next 8 days he experienced increasing blepharospasm, photophobia, epiphora, swelling of the eyelids, and a fall in visual acuity. Topical treatment with corticosteroids was required and subepithelial corneal changes persisted.— B. F. McLendon and A. J. Bron, *Br. J. Ophthal.*, 1978, *62*, 97.

Precautions

For reference to the precautions necessary with antineoplastic agents and immunosuppressants, see Antineoplastic Agents, p.583.

Vinblastine should not be injected into an extremity with impaired circulation because of an increased risk of thrombosis.

HANDLING AND DISPOSAL. A method for the destruction of vincristine or vinblastine wastes using sulphuric acid and potassium permanganate. A solution of vincristine or vinblastine sulphate 0.1% in dilute sulphuric acid (3 mol per litre) can be destroyed in 2 hours by addition of 50 mg of potassium permanganate per mL. Solid waste should be dissolved to produce a solution of the appropriate strength and aqueous solutions diluted if necessary. Solutions of either drug in volatile organic solvents should have the solvent evaporated off and be redissolved in water before degradation. A solution of potassium permanganate in sulphuric acid may also be used to clean contaminated glassware and to inactivate rinsings taken up on absorbent material after spillages. Residues produced by degradation of either drug by this method showed no mutagenicity *in vitro*.—IARC Scientific Publications No. 73, Laboratory Decontamination and Destruction of Carcinogens in Laboratory Wastes: Some Antineoplastic Agents, M. Castegnaro *et al.* (Eds), Lyon, International Agency for Research on Cancer, 1985, p.73.

When handling urine and faeces from patients receiving vinblastine protective clothing should be worn for up to 4 and 7 days respectively after therapy.— J. Harris and L. J. Dodds, *Pharm. J.*, 1985, *2*, 289.

INTERACTIONS. A warning from the manufacturer (*Lilly, USA*) that acute bronchospasm may occur following injection of a vinca alkaloid, particularly in patients who have been treated with mitomycin.— R. W. Dyke (letter), *New Engl. J. Med.*, 1984, *310*, 389. A report of acute respiratory distress and pulmonary infiltration associated with vinblastine as part of a combination regimen with mitomycin. A second patient had an episode of acute bronchitis, with the development of acute pulmonary insufficiency, cyanosis, and dyspnoea. P. H. Konits *et al.*, *Cancer*, 1982, *50*, 2771. Five of 13 patients given a regimen comprising vinblastine, mitomycin, and progesterone (MVP) developed respiratory distress with interstitial pulmonary infiltrates, and 2 subsequently died of respiratory complications.— R. F. Ozols *et al.*, *Cancer Treat. Rep.*, 1983, *67*, 721.

Absorption and Fate

Vinblastine is not reliably absorbed from the gastro-intestinal tract. Following intravenous administration it is rapidly cleared from the blood and distributed to tissues; it is reported to be concentrated in blood platelets. It is extensively protein bound. Vinblastine is metabolised in the liver to an active metabolite, desacetylvinblastine, and is excreted in bile and urine as unchanged drug and metabolites. It does not cross the blood-brain barrier in significant amounts.

For a review of the clinical pharmacokinetics of commonly used antineoplastic agents, including vinblastine, see F. M. Balis *et al.*, *Clin. Pharmacokinet.*, 1983, *8*, 202.

PROTEIN BINDING. A study in 6 healthy subjects indicated that although vinblastine and prednisolone were both highly protein bound (99.7% and 95% respectively) there was no apparent competition for binding sites and the percentage protein bound for each was the same when the two drugs were given in combination.— W. H. Steele *et al.*, *Br. J. clin. Pharmac.*, 1982, *13*, 595P. See also W. H. Steele *et al.*, *Eur. J. clin. Pharmac.*, 1983, *24*, 683 (protein binding of vinblastine in Hodgkin's disease).

Uses and Administration

Vinblastine sulphate is an antineoplastic agent which apparently acts by binding to the microtubular proteins of the spindle and arresting mitosis at the metaphase; it also interferes with amino acid metabolism and nucleic acid synthesis. It also has some immunosuppressant activity. Cross-resistance with vincristine has not been reported although pleiotropic resistance may occur.

Vinblastine sulphate is mainly used, in association with other antineoplastic agents, in the treatment of Hodgkin's disease and other lymphomas, including mycosis fungoides. It is also of use in the treatment of some inoperable malignant neoplasms including those of the breast and testis and in neuroblastoma, choriocarcinoma, Kaposi's sarcoma, and histiocytosis X. In the treatment of Hodgkin's disease it is often given with cyclophosphamide or mustine, procarbazine, and prednisone (CVPP or MVPP), or with doxorubicin, bleomycin, and dacarbazine (ABVD). In carcinoma of the testis vinblastine is given with bleomycin and cisplatin. See also under Choice of Antineoplastic Agent, p.592.

Vinblastine sulphate is given by intravenous injection as a solution containing 1 mg per mL in sodium chloride injection (0.9%). Care should be taken to avoid extravasation and the injection may be given into a freely running infusion of sodium chloride injection if preferred. The suggested dosage scheme is as follows: weekly injections starting with 100 µg per kg body-weight or 3.7 mg per m^2 body-surface, raised by increments of 50 µg per kg or 1.8 mg per m^2 to a maximum weekly dose of 500 µg per kg or 18.5 mg per m^2; or until the white cell count has fallen to 3000 per mm^3. Most patients respond to 150 to 200 µg per kg or 5.5 to 7.4 mg per m^2 weekly. A maintenance dose is then given every 7 to 14 days and should be one increment smaller than the maximum dose that the patient is able to tolerate without serious leucopenia occurring. An alternative maintenance regimen has consisted of 10 mg given once or twice a month.

Children may be given vinblastine sulphate in an initial dose of 2.5 mg per m^2 body-surface intravenously, increased by 1.25 mg per m^2 weekly to a usual maximum weekly dose of 7.5 mg per m^2. Doses of up to 12.5 mg per m^2 per week have been given.

White cell counts should be made before each injection and a repeat dose should never be given unless the count has risen to 4000 per mm^3.

ADMINISTRATION IN RENAL INSUFFICIENCY. Vinblastine can be given in usual doses to patients with impaired renal function.— W. M. Bennett *et al.*, *Am. J. Kidney Dis.*, 1983, *3*, 155.

BLOOD DISORDERS, NON-MALIGNANT. Infusions of vinblastine, bound to platelets by incubation, were given to 11 patients with refractory idiopathic thrombocytopenic purpura in an attempt to achieve selective delivery of large amounts of the drug to the macrophages. All patients had been treated previously with vinca alkaloids by conventional injection but responses had been short-lived. Six patients achieved complete remission, which was maintained for at least 5 months in 3 of them, and 3 achieved partial remission. Side-effects were reversible and included neutropenia, mild confusion, alopecia, jaw pain, and burning tongue.— Y. S. Ahn *et al.*, *New Engl. J. Med.*, 1978, *298*, 1101. Subsequent reports have suggested that the technique may be less effective than had been thought, partly because the binding of vinblastine to platelets is easily reversible and thus for therapy to be selectively delivered to macrophages platelets must be cleared very rapidly from the circulation. Although the technique has also been used successfully in 3 of 4 patients with refractory auto-immune haemolytic anaemia (Y.S. Ahn *et al.*, *J. Am. med. Ass.*, 1983, *249*, 2189), and other disorders, it has not become a popular method of treating auto-immune disease: in the first place the technique is cumbersome, and furthermore it has never been clearly shown to be superior to simple infusion of the vinca alkaloids.— W. F. Rosse, *ibid.*, 1984, *310*, 1051. Vincristine is more stably bound to platelets and clinical and *in vitro* results suggest that the use of vincristine rather than vinblastine might renew earlier enthusiasm for this approach.— G. Agnelli *et al.* (letter), *ibid.*, *311*, 599. Reply. Since loading of platelets with vinblastine or vincristine is cumbersome, expensive, and not generally available it will never be popular, but a place remains for its use. Overall, 68% of patients with chronic refractory idiopathic thrombocytopenc purpura were helped, 38% had lasting remissions and some have been cured. The technique has been extended to haemolytic anaemias, drug-induced thrombocytopenia, leukaemias, and other malignancies. When needed, vinca-alkaloid-loaded platelets seem to have more than fulfilled their early promise.— Y. S. Ahn *et al.* (letter), *ibid.*, 600.

The use of slow infusions of vinca alkaloids to treat idiopathic thrombocytopenic purpura. Intravenous infusion of vinblastine 100 µg per kg body-weight, or vincristine 20 µg per kg was carried out over 6 to 8 hours in 24 patients with refractory idiopathic thrombocytopenic purpura. Initially, vincristine and vinblastine were given alternately if prolonged treatment was anticipated, but latterly vinblastine was used exclusively. Treatment was repeated every 5 to 10 days at first; when the platelet count became normal the interval was increased. Thirteen of the patients had excellent responses, and 4 had a good response; therapy was well tolerated. When results were compared with previous responses to bolus injections and infusion of vinca-loaded-platelets, slow infusion appeared more effective than the former, but less effective as a single treatment than the latter, more treatments being needed with slow infusion than with platelets. However, slow infusion of the alkaloid was better tolerated than the platelet infusion, and is best suited to long-term management of patients with refractory disease in whom glucocorticoids, danazol, and splenectomy have failed.— Y. S. Ahn *et al.*, *Ann. intern. Med.*, 1984, *100*, 192. Further comments and references: A. Manoharan (letter), *ibid.*, 921; M. V. Pillai *et al.* (letter), *ibid.*, *101*, 149; Y. S. Ahn *et al.* (letter), *ibid.*

See also under Vincristine Sulphate (below).

HODGKIN'S DISEASE AND OTHER LYMPHOMAS. For mention of the use of vinblastine with other agents in the treatment of lymphomas, see Choice of Antineoplastic Agent, p.585.

KAPOSI'S SARCOMA. Vinblastine in initial doses of 4 mg weekly by slow intravenous injection, and adjusted so that the leucocyte count remained above about 2500 per mm^3, was given to 38 patients with Kaposi's sarcoma associated with AIDS. The median weekly dosage was 6 mg with a range of 3 to 8 mg. One patient had a complete and 9 a partial response; disease was stable in 19 and progressed in only 9. Median duration of response was 13 weeks; patients often relapsed after initially responding to therapy. Toxicity was minimal and no patient required discontinuation of therapy. Vinblastine is an effective but weak agent in the treatment of syndrome-related Kaposi's sarcoma.— P. A. Volberding *et al.*, *Ann. intern. Med.*, 1985, *103*, 335.

MALIGNANT NEOPLASMS OF THE TESTIS. For reports on the use of vinblastine with bleomycin and cisplatin in malignant neoplasms of the testis, see Choice of Antineoplastic Agent, p.592.

Preparations

Sterile Vinblastine Sulfate *(U.S.P.)*. Vinblastine sulphate suitable for parenteral use.

Vinblastine Injection *(B.P.)*. Contains vinblastine sulphate in sodium chloride intravenous infusion (0.9%).

Proprietary Preparations

Velbe *(Lilly, UK)*. *Injection*, powder for reconstitution, vinblastine sulphate 10 mg, supplied with solvent.

Proprietary Names and Manufacturers

Velban *(Lilly, USA)*; Velbe *(Arg.; Lilly, Austral.; Belg.; Lilly, Canad.; Lilly, Denm.; Lilly, Fr.; Lilly, Ger.; Lilly, Ital.; Neth.; Lilly, Norw.; S.Afr.; Lilly, Swed.; Switz.; Lilly, UK)*.

Manufacturers also include—*Bull, UK; Lederle, UK.*

1879-p

Vincristine Sulphate *(BANM, rINNM)*.

22-Oxovincaleukoblastine Sulphate; Leurocristine Sulphate; NSC-67574; Vincristine Sulfate *(USAN)*. The sulphate of an alkaloid, 22-oxovincaleukoblastine, obtained from *Vinca rosea* (*Catharanthus roseus*) (Apocynaceae).

$C_{46}H_{56}N_4O_{10},H_2SO_4$=923.0.

CAS — 57-22-7 (vincristine); 2068-78-2 (sulphate).

Pharmacopoeias. In *Br., Braz., Chin., Cz., Egypt., Jug.,* and *U.S.*

A white to slightly yellow, odourless, very hygroscopic, amorphous or crystalline powder. It loses not more than 12% of its weight on drying. **Soluble** 1 in 2 of water and 1 in 30 of chloroform; slightly soluble in alcohol; soluble in methyl alcohol; practically insoluble in ether. A 0.1% solution in water has a pH of 3.5 to 4.5. **Store** at 2° to 8° in airtight containers. Protect from light.

Adverse Effects and Treatment

As for Vinblastine Sulphate, p.654.

Bone-marrow depression occurs less commonly than with vinblastine but neurological and neuromuscular effects are more severe with vincristine and are dose limiting. Walking may be impaired and the neurological effects may not be reversed for several months after the drug is discontinued. Convulsions, often with hypertension, have occurred. There may be constipation and abdominal pain. Acute uric acid nephropathy has occurred and alopecia is common.

Adverse effects occur less frequently when the weekly dosage is kept below 100 µg per kg body-weight.

Folinic acid has been given for the treatment of overdosage: suggested doses are 15 mg of folinic acid every 3 hours for 24 hours, then every 6 hours for at least 48 hours.

Severe headache, followed by bladder paresis, neurological disorders, respiratory paralysis, and death in a 5-year-old child accidentally given an intrathecal dose of vincristine.— J. Manelis *et al.*, *J. Neurol.*, 1982, *228*, 209. Further reports of fatalities from intrathecal administration of vincristine: M. E. Williams *et al.*, *Cancer*, 1983, *51*, 2041; W. G. Gaidys *et al.*, *ibid.*, *52*, 799.

EFFECTS ON THE EYES. A report of bilateral optic atrophy and blindness in a patient given vincristine.— A. S. Awidi (letter), *Ann. intern. Med.*, 1980, *93*, 781.

See also under Effects on the Nervous System, below.

EFFECTS ON THE MUSCLES. Vincristine could produce a necrotising myopathy.— P. G. Blain, *Adverse Drug React. Bull.*, 1984, (Feb.), 384.

EFFECTS ON THE NERVOUS SYSTEM. A review of vincristine neurotoxicity. In its most typical form, neurotoxicity manifests as a mixed sensorimotor neuropathy of the distal type. The earliest symptoms are sensory changes in the form of paraesthesias, accompanied by impairment and ultimately loss of deep tendon reflexes. In more severe forms, impairment of motor function occurs with wrist drop and foot drop, ataxia and gait abnormalities, and occasionally progressive quadriparesis. In contrast to these peripheral neuropathies which are usually associated with long-term usage there may be short-term autonomic neuropathy resulting in constipation and occasionally ileus, abdominal pain, atony of the urinary bladder (which may lead to urinary retention), postural hypotension, and rarely, impotence. There may be effects on the cranial nerves, resulting in ptosis, hoarseness (due to laryngeal nerve paralysis), or optic neuropathies. Effects on the CNS are rare, probably in part because of poor penetration into CSF, but include excessive release of antidiuretic hormone and consequent hyponatraemia. Toxicity is related to both the cumulative and the individual dose. It usually begins in adults after receiving a total of 5 to 6 mg, and is significant by the time a cumulative dose of 15 to 20 mg is reached. If individual doses are low (less than 2 mg) or intervals between doses are longer than the usual week, patients can tolerate higher cumulative doses. Children tolerate vincristine better than adults, but the elderly are particularly prone to neurotoxicity. There is no good treatment for the effects of vincristine on the nervous system: symptoms are largely reversible once administration is interrupted, and should be managed with appropriate symptomatic care.— S. S. Legha, *Med. Toxicol.*, 1986, *1*, 421.

Reports suggesting an increased incidence of neurotoxicity with ready-to-use solutions of vincristine compared with the reconstituted lyophilised preparation: A. M. Arnold *et al.* (letter), *Lancet*, 1985, *1*, 346; S. Jalihal and N. Roebuck (letter), *ibid.*, 637; C. E. Davies *et al.* (letter), *ibid;* R. P. Warrier and R. Ducos (letter), *ibid.*, 980. Comment by the manufacturer (*Lilly*). The association with the ready-to-use solution is not yet established.— B. A. Gennery (letter), *ibid.*, *2*, 385.

Reports of severe neurotoxicity following vincristine therapy in patients with neurological disorders: C. M. Hogan-Dann *et al.*, *J. Am. med. Ass.*, 1984, *252*, 2862 (in Charcot-Marie-Tooth syndrome); B. R. Miller (letter), *ibid.*, 1985, *253*, 2045 (in a former poliomyelitis victim); T. R. Chauncy (letter), *ibid.*, *254*, 507 (Charcot-Marie-Tooth syndrome); J. D. Griffiths *et al.*, *Med. J. Aust.*, 1985, *143*, 305 (Charcot-Marie-Tooth syndrome).

Precautions

For reference to the precautions necessary with antineoplastic agents and immunosuppressants, see Antineoplastic Agents, p.583.

Because severe constipation and impaction of faeces often occur with vincristine, enemas or purgatives may be necessary. Vincristine should be given with caution to patients with pre-existing neuromuscular disease and is contra-indicated in patients with the demyelinating form of Charcot-Marie-Tooth syndrome (see under Effects on the Nervous System, above). Doses may need to be adjusted in patients with impaired liver function. Care should also be taken in elderly patients, who may be more susceptible to neurotoxicity.

The warning has been given that intrathecal administration of vincristine is invariably fatal (see also under Adverse Effects, above).

Patients with lymphoma appear more likely than patients with other cancers to develop neuropathy when treated with vincristine.— R. J. M. Lane and P. A. Routledge, *Drugs*, 1983, *26*, 124.

HANDLING AND DISPOSAL. When handling urine and faeces from patients receiving vincristine protective clothing should be worn for up to 4 and 7 days respectively after therapy.— J. Harris and L. J. Dodds, *Pharm. J.*, 1985, *2*, 289.

For a method for the destruction of vincristine wastes, see under Vinblastine Sulphate, p.654.

Absorption and Fate

Vincristine is not reliably absorbed from the gastro-intestinal tract. After intravenous injection it disappears rapidly from the blood. It is extensively protein bound and is reported to be concentrated in blood platelets. It is metabolised in the liver and excreted primarily in the bile—about 70% of a dose is found in faeces, as unchanged drug and metabolites, over 72 hours. Some also appears in the urine. Vincristine does not appear to cross the blood-brain barrier in significant amounts.

A review of the clinical pharmacokinetics of some commonly used antineoplastic agents, including vincristine.— F. M. Balis *et al.*, *Clin. Pharmacokinet.*, 1983, *8*, 202.

Uses and Administration

Vincristine sulphate is an antineoplastic agent which may act similarly to vinblastine (above) by arresting mitosis at the metaphase. It also has some immunosuppressant activity. Cross-resistance with vinblastine has not been reported although pleiotropic resistance may occur.

It is used principally in combination chemotherapy regimens for acute leukaemia and Hodgkin's disease and other lymphomas, including Burkitt's lymphoma. It is also used in the treatment of Wilm's tumour, neuroblastoma, and sarcomas, and in tumours of the breast, brain, and lung. Remissions are induced in acute lymphoblastic leukaemia with vincristine in association with prednisone alone or with daunorubicin (or doxorubicin) or colaspase. In Hodgkin's disease, vincristine is given with mustine, procarbazine, and prednisone (MOPP) and similar regimens have been used in other lymphomas. See also under Choice of Antineoplastic Agent, p.585.

Vincristine sulphate is administered by intravenous injection and solutions containing 0.01 to 1 mg per mL in sodium chloride injection (0.9%) have been used. Care should be taken to avoid extravasation and the injection may be given into a freely-running intravenous infusion of sodium chloride injection if preferred.

In acute leukaemia the weekly dose of vincristine sulphate for children is 1.5 to 2 mg per m^2 body-surface or 50 µg per kg body-weight increasing by weekly increments of 25 µg per kg to a maximum of 150 µg per kg. Adults may be

given about 1.4 mg per m^2 or 25 to 75 μg per kg weekly. For other malignancies 25 μg per kg may be given weekly and reduced to 5 to 10 μg per kg for maintenance.
Blood counts should be carried out before giving each dose.

ADMINISTRATION IN RENAL FAILURE. Vincristine can be given in usual doses to patients with renal failure.— W. M. Bennett *et al.*, *Am. J. Kidney Dis.*, 1983, *3*, 155.

BLOOD DISORDERS, NON-MALIGNANT. A follow-up study of 8 of 10 patients with refractory auto-immune thrombocytopenia who were treated with a series of 1 to 6 intravenous injections of vincristine. Of the 4 patients with idiopathic thrombocytopenia, followed up for an average of 3.5 years, 2 responded completely to treatment, 1 responded partially, and 1 did not respond. All 3 patients with collagen vascular disorders, followed up for about 3 years, were complete responders. One patient with drug-induced thrombocytopenia, followed up for 2.5 years, also responded completely. The continued use of vincristine in refractory immune thrombocytopenia appears to be justified.— G. M. Rogers and C. A. Ries (letter), *New Engl. J. Med.*, 1980, *303*, 585.

A report of 5 patients with thrombotic thrombocytopenic purpura who responded to intravenous injection of vincristine sulphate. No progression of symptoms occurred in these patients following vincristine administration and complete remission occurred 2 to 4 weeks after therapy was initiated. Based on this experience, doses of 2 mg of vincristine initially, followed by 1 mg every 4 days were recommended, continued for at least 2 weeks after evidence of haematological remission. Relapses subsequently occurred in 2 patients but responded to further vincristine therapy. In view of the seriousness of the condition, vincristine would seem worthy of further evaluation in its management.— L. A. Gutterman and T. D. Stevenson, *J. Am. med. Ass.*, 1982, *247*, 1433.

A patient with haemolytic-uraemic syndrome, including evidence of early hepatocellular abnormalities, had completely recovered within 1 month of beginning intravenous vincristine therapy. The results suggest that vincristine may have activity in this syndrome and further evaluation seems warranted.— L. A. Gutterman *et al.*, *Ann. intern. Med.*, 1983, *98*, 612.

A report of the use of slow infusions of vincristine to treat childhood immune thrombocytopenic purpura.— A. Manoharan (letter), *Lancet*, 1986, *1*, 317. Criticism. The vast majority of children with this condition remit spontaneously or maintain an adequate circulating platelet mass without treatment. They should not be unnecessarily exposed to risks, and any treatment must be shown to be effective.— J. S. Lilleyman (letter), *ibid.*, 499.

For references to the use of vincristine by slow infusion or by platelet loading in the management of idiopathic thrombocytopenic purpura, see Vinblastine Sulphate, p.654.

KAPOSI'S SARCOMA. The treatment of Kaposi's sarcoma with vincristine in patients with AIDS. Of 18 evaluable patients given vincristine 2 mg weekly by rapid intravenous infusion for 2 to 5 weeks, then every 2 weeks as tolerated, 11 had a partial response and 7 only a minor response; none had a complete response. The median duration of partial responses was more than 4 months at the time of writing. In 3 patients with co-existing thrombocytopenia there was an increase in platelet count, sustained for several months in 2. The main toxicity seen was peripheral neuropathy, requiring dose reduction in 6 patients and discontinuation in 2. Myelotoxicity was minimal. In the light of its marrow-sparing effects and antitumour efficacy, vincristine may be a reasonable drug to include in the combination therapy of the epidemic form of Kaposi's sarcoma, in patients with AIDS.— D. M. Mintzer *et al.*, *Ann. intern. Med.*, 1985, *102*, 200.

LEUKAEMIA. For reference to the use of vincristine with other agents in acute lymphoblastic leukaemia, acute myeloid leukaemia, and chronic myeloid leukaemia, see Choice of Antineoplastic Agent, p.586.

NEUROBLASTOMA. For references to the use of vincristine in the treatment of neuroblastoma see Choice of Antineoplastic Agent, p.593.

PAIN. Mention of the administration of vincristine by iontophoresis to relieve postherpetic neuralgia. Vincristine is thought to block axon transmission and thereby relieve pain. Rashes have occurred following treatment, which may need to be carried out daily for 4 weeks [illegible]re beneficial results are seen.— P. N. Robinson and [illegible]her, *J. R. Coll. gen. Pract.*, 1986, *36*, 24.

Preparations

Vincristine Injection *(B.P.)*

Vincristine Sulfate Injection *(U.S.P.)*.

Vincristine Sulfate for Injection *(U.S.P.)*

Proprietary Preparations

Oncovin *(Lilly, UK)*. *Injection*, vincristine sulphate 1 mg/mL, in vials of 1 and 2 mL.
Injection, powder for reconstitution, vincristine sulphate 1, 2, and 5 mg, supplied with solvent.

Proprietary Names and Manufacturers

Kyocristine *(Jpn)*; Oncovin *(Arg.; Lilly, Austral.; Belg.; Lilly, Canad.; Lilly, Denm.; Lilly, Fr.; Neth.; Lilly, Norw.; S.Afr.; Lilly, Swed.; Lilly, Switz.; Lilly, UK; Lilly, USA)*; Pericristine *(S. Afr.)*; Vincasar *(Adria, USA)*; Vincrisul *(Lilly, Spain)*.
Manufacturers also include—*Bull, UK; Lederle, UK.*

1880-n

Vindesine Sulphate *(BANM, rINNM)*.

Compound 112531 *(vindesine)*; Desacetyl Vinblastine Amide Sulfate; LY-099094; NSC-245467; Vindesine Sulfate *(USAN)*. 3-Carbamoyl-4-*O*-deacetyl-3-de(methoxycarbonyl)vincaleukoblastine.
$C_{43}H_{55}N_5O_7,H_2SO_4=852.0$.

CAS — 53643-48-4 (vindesine); 59917-39-4 (sulphate).

A synthetic vinca alkaloid derived from vinblastine sulphate.

The manufacturer states that vindesine sulphate should be stored between 0° and 6°. Reconstituted solutions are stated to retain their potency for 30 days when stored in this fashion.

Adverse Effects, Treatment, and Precautions

As for Vinblastine Sulphate, p.654.
The main dose-limiting effect of vindesine is granulocytopenia. Although neurotoxicity occurs it may be less severe than that seen with vincristine (p.655). Alopecia is the most common side-effect.
Folinic acid has been suggested for the treatment of overdosage.
Vindesine should not be given by the intrathecal route, as this may produce fatal toxicity. Care should be taken if acute abdominal pain occurs: further administration may result in paralytic ileus.

A report of drowsiness, weakness, diplopia, and neurological symptoms in a 10-year-old child who was accidentally given an intrathecal injection of vindesine. Treatment with folinic acid and dexamethasone produced transient recovery but symptoms subsequently recurred and the patient died of progressive ascending paralysis. The CNS showed changes at necropsy similar to those seen following intrathecal administration of vincristine.— G. Robbins (letter), *Br. med. J.*, 1985, *291*, 1094.

Absorption and Fate

The pharmacokinetics of vindesine are similar to those of the other vinca alkaloids. After intravenous administration elimination from the blood is triphasic; the drug is rapidly distributed to body tissues. It is metabolised primarily in the liver and excreted in bile and urine.

A review of the clinical pharmacokinetics of the vinca alkaloids, including vindesine, and some other antineoplastic agents.— F. M. Balis, *Clin. Pharmacokinet.*, 1983, *8*, 202.

Uses and Administration

Vindesine sulphate is an antineoplastic agent derived from vinblastine (p.654); like the other vinca alkaloids it causes mitotic arrest in metaphase by binding to microtubular protein. It has been used in the treatment of acute lymphoblastic leukaemia resistant to other drugs, in lymphomas, in blastic crises of chronic myeloid leukaemia, and in refractory malignant melanoma. It has also been tried in malignant neoplasms of the breast and lung. See also under Choice of Antineoplastic Agent, p.584.
Vindesine sulphate is given weekly by intravenous injection as a solution containing 1 mg per mL in sodium chloride injection (0.9%). Care should be taken to avoid extravasation and it may be given into a fast-running infusion of sodium chloride, glucose (5%), or glucose-saline injection. The usual starting dose for adults is 3 mg per m^2 body-surface which may be raised by increments of 500 μg per m^2 weekly providing that the neutrophil count does not fall below 1500 per mm^3, the platelet count does not fall below 100 000 per mm^3, and acute abdominal pain is not experienced; weekly doses are usually between 3 and 4 mg per m^2. Children may be given 4 mg per m^2 initially, with weekly doses usually ranging between 4 and 5 mg per m^2. Blood counts should be made before each injection.

A review of vindesine sulphate.— W. J. Dana, *Drug Intell. & clin. Pharm.*, 1980, *14*, 28.

Vindesine was used, with prednisone and sometimes other agents, in the treatment of 26 patients with a variety of refractory malignant blood disorders (1 with Hodgkin's disease; 6 with non-Hodgkin's lymphomas; 2 with acute myeloblastic and 4 with acute lymphoblastic leukaemia; a further 2 with acute undifferentiated leukaemia; 3 with chronic granulocytic leukaemia in blast transformation; 3 with multiple myeloma; 2 with chronic lymphatic leukaemia; and 1 each with myeloid dysplasia, systemic mastocytosis, and Waldenström's macroglobulinaemia). None of the patients with acute leukaemic conditions achieved true remission although there was a significant fall in blast-cell count in all cases; 2 patients in the acute phase of chronic granulocytic leukaemia had a dramatic resolution of bone pain but the disease subsequently became refractory to vindesine therapy. One patient with a non-Hodgkin's lymphoma in relapse had a complete remission after therapy with vindesine, cyclophosphamide, and prednisone, and stable disease was documented in the patient with Waldenström's macroglobulinaemia given the same 3 compounds, but the remaining patients had no lasting response to therapy.— G. A. R. Young *et al.*, *Med. J. Aust.*, 1985, *142*, 189.

MALIGNANT NEOPLASMS OF THE BRONCHUS AND LUNG. In a study in 81 patients with advanced squamous cell or adenocarcinoma of the lung, patients received vindesine 3 mg per m^2 weekly with cisplatin either in a dose of 60 or 120 mg per m^2 at intervals of 4 to 6 weeks. Three of 41 patients receiving the lower-dose regimen obtained complete remission, and 16 had partial remission; of the 40 on the higher-dose regimen, 5 had complete and 11 had partial responses. There were no significant differences in response rate between the regimens, but the median duration of response was 12 months for patients treated with high-dose cisplatin, compared with 5.5 months for the other patients. The major side-effect was peripheral neuropathy which was related to the total dose of vindesine given. The results demonstrate that chemotherapy with vindesine and cisplatin can produce results in non-small-cell lung cancer superior to those achieved with standard combinations or with either agent used alone.— R. J. Gralla *et al.*, *Ann. intern. Med.*, 1981, *95*, 414.

Of 84 patients with non-small-cell lung cancer treated with vindesine and mitomycin, 2 had a complete and 9 a partial response; a further 14 were considered to have improved. Of these 25 responders, 20 were among the 55 patients who received no previous chemotherapy including both complete responders. The regimen used comprised vindesine 3 mg per m^2 intravenously every week for 5 weeks and then every 2 weeks, with mitomycin 10 mg per m^2 intravenously on days 1, 21, and 57, then every 6 weeks for 2 further doses, then every 8 weeks. The median duration of response to this regimen was 5.8 months in patients with no previous chemotherapy and 6.5 months among those who had received previous chemotherapy. These results compared with those previously reported for either agent alone suggest that the combination is superior to single-agent therapy. Further randomised studies of the combination seem warranted.— M. G. Kris *et al.*, *Chest*, 1985, *87*, 368.

See also under Choice of Antineoplastic Agent, p.590.

Proprietary Preparations

Eldisine *(Lilly, UK)*. *Injection*, powder for reconstitution, vindesine sulphate 5 mg, supplied with solvent.

Proprietary Names and Manufacturers
Eldisine *(Lilly, Austral.; Lilly, Canad.; Lilly, Fr.; Lilly, Ger.; Lilly, Ital.; Lilly, S.Afr.; Lilly, Swed.; Lilly, Switz.; Lilly, UK)*; Enison *(Lilly, Spain)*.

14018-m

Vinzolidine Sulphate *(rINNM)*.

LY-104208; Vinzolidine Sulfate *(USAN)*.
$C_{48}H_{58}ClN_5O_9,H_2SO_4$=982.5.

CAS — 67699-40-5 (vinzolidine); 67699-41-6 (sulphate).

Vinzolidine sulphate is structurally related to vinblastine sulphate and is reported to have antineoplastic activity when given by mouth.

References: G. Sarna *et al.*, *Cancer Chemother. Pharmac.*, 1985, *14*, 12.

Proprietary Names and Manufacturers
Lilly, USA.

1881-h

Zinostatin *(USAN, rINN)*.

Neocarzinostatin; NSC-157365 (formerly NSC-69856).
An antineoplastic antibiotic obtained from *Streptomyces carzinostaticus*.

CAS — 9014-02-2.

Aqueous solutions should be **stored** at 2° to 8°. Protect from light.

Zinostatin is an antibiotic with antineoplastic activity and has been used in the treatment of acute leukaemia and malignant neoplasms including those of the stomach and pancreas.

Proprietary Names and Manufacturers
Neocarzinostatin *(Jpn)*.
Manufacturers also include—*Bristol, USA*.

14032-n

Zorubicin Hydrochloride *(USAN, rINNM)*.

NSC-164011; RP-22050 (zorubicin). Benzoic acid (2*S*,4*S*)-{1-[4-(3-amino-2,3,6-trideoxy-α-L-lyxopyranosyloxy)-1,2,3,4,6,11-hexahydro-2,5,12-trihydroxy-7-methoxy-6,11-dioxonaphthacen-2-yl]ethylidene}hydrazide hydrochloride.
$C_{34}H_{35}N_3O_{10}$,HCl=682.1.

CAS — 54083-22-6 (zorubicin); 36508-71-1 (hydrochloride).

In a study of the stability of anthracycline antineoplastic agents in 4 infusion fluids, zorubicin base was stable in a commercial fluid (Normosol-R), with a pH of 7.4, but not in glucose injection (5%), sodium chloride injection (0.9%), or lactated Ringer's injection which had pH's of 4.5, 6.2, and 6.3 respectively. The percentage of zorubicin remaining in the mixture after 24 hours was 89.1% in Normosol-R, 0% in glucose injection, 34.3% in sodium chloride injection, and 50.9% in lactated Ringer's injection. In contrast to doxorubicin and daunorubicin, zorubicin, which contains an acid-sensitive hydrazone linkage, becomes more stable as the pH of the mixture rises.— G. K. Poochikian *et al.*, *Am. J. Hosp. Pharm.*, 1981, *38*, 483.

Adverse Effects, Treatment, and Precautions
As for Doxorubicin Hydrochloride, p.623. Cardiotoxicity is reported to be more likely when the cumulative dose exceeds 1.8 g per m^2 body-surface.

Uses and Administration
Zorubicin is an anthracycline antibiotic derived from daunorubicin (p.622) and with antineoplastic actions similar to those of doxorubicin (p.624). It is used as the hydrochloride in the treatment of acute lymphoblastic and non-lymphoblastic leukaemias. Zorubicin hydrochloride is administered intravenously by injection into a fast-running infusion in doses of 3 to 5 mg per kg daily for 4 to 8 days, up to a total dose of 20 to 25 mg per kg.

Proprietary Names and Manufacturers
Rubidazone *(Bellon, Fr.)*.

Antiprotozoal Agents

4750-z

The drugs described in this section are those used primarily in the treatment of parasitic protozoal infections including amoebiasis, giardiasis, leishmaniasis, trichomoniasis, and trypanosomiasis. Metronidazole and related nitroimidazole derivatives are also important in the treatment of anaerobic bacterial infections. Some veterinary antiprotozoal drugs are included. Drugs used in the treatment of malaria are described in the Antimalarials section.

Protozoal infections such as trichomoniasis occur worldwide whereas many others have generally been limited to tropical areas. However, protozoal infections are being seen increasingly in immunocompromised individuals living in temperate climates.

Brief reviews of parasitic protozoal infections and their management.— H. Most, *New Engl. J. Med.*, 1984, *310*, 298; A. P. Hall, *Br. J. Hosp. Med.*, 1986, *35*, 420.

A review of the choice and dosage of drugs in parasitic protozoal infections.— *Med. Lett.*, 1986, *28*, 9.

African Trypanosomiasis

African trypanosomiasis (sleeping sickness) is caused by subspecies of the protozoan *Trypanosoma brucei*, transmitted by the bite of infected tsetse flies (*Glossina* spp.). Gambian or West African sleeping sickness is caused by *T. brucei gambiense*, carried by riverine tsetse flies, and Rhodesian or East African sleeping sickness is caused by *T. brucei rhodesiense*, carried by savannah tsetse flies. *T. brucei brucei* does not infect man. Infection can follow blood transfusion and congenital trypanosomiasis has also occurred. Trypanosomiasis due to *T. brucei gambiense* develops slowly over several years and is characterised by infection of the blood stream and lymph nodes followed by infection of the central nervous system. In *T. brucei rhodesiense* infections involvement of the central nervous system rapidly follows infection of the blood stream and death frequently occurs within a year if the disease is untreated.

The principal drugs used in the treatment of the haemolymphatic phase are pentamidine and suramin; for CNS involvement melarsoprol is generally used.

African trypanosomiasis, or sleeping sickness, is endemic in 36 countries of sub-Saharan Africa within the areas where the vector, the tsetse fly, occurs. It is almost always fatal if left untreated and remains a threat to many rural communities in Africa. The frequency of signs and symptoms may vary according to whether the parasite is *Trypanosoma brucei gambiense* or *T.b. rhodesiense* and may also vary from region to region. Early symptoms of *T.b. rhodesiense* infection are more severe and acute; a chancre is frequently seen within a few days of the bite of an infected *Glossina* (tsetse fly), but seldom in *T.b. gambiense* disease. The haematolymphatic stage includes intermittent fever which is characteristic of the early stage of the disease, enlarged lymph nodes, pruritus, skin rash, oedema, anaemia, cardiovascular disorders, endocrinological disorders, albuminuria, and intercurrent infections. In the meningoencephalitic stage neurological symptoms include disorders of consciousness and sleep patterns which can lead to permanent hypersomnia and may end in coma.

Standard guidelines for treatment are not yet possible, but the following broad recommendations are made.

In *early-stage disease*, where there is no detectable involvement of the CNS, treatment with pentamidine or suramin is given. Pentamidine is used for the early stages of *T. b. gambiense* infection except in areas where it has been widely employed for chemoprophylaxis; suramin may be used as an alternative in areas where pentamidine resistance exists. Suramin is used for the early stages of *T.b rhodesiense* infection; pentamidine should not be used since primary resistance to it has been found in some areas. Pentamidine is given intramuscularly as the isethionate or mesylate in a dose of 4 mg of pentamidine base per kg body-weight daily or on alternate days to a total of 7 to 10 injections [but see Uses of pentamidine, p.676, for comment on expression of the dose]. Suramin is given intravenously, commonly in a dose of 20 mg per kg every 5 to 7 days; courses usually comprise 5 injections and should not exceed 7. Because of the risk of hypersensitivity reactions it is advisable to give a test dose of 4 mg per kg before embarking on full treatment with suramin.

In *late-stage disease* with CNS involvement, melarsoprol is the drug of choice; it should not be used in the early stage because of the risk of serious side-effects. The usual course of treatment comprises 3 or 4 series of intravenous injections of melarsoprol given daily for 3 or 4 days, each series being separated by an interval of at least a week; doses are increased gradually to a maximum of 3.6 mg per kg daily. The number of courses and total dose may be standard or may be based on the leucocyte count and protein levels in the cerebrospinal fluid. In late-stage *T.b. rhodesiense* infection parasitaemias are usually much higher than in *T.b. gambiense* infection and the course of melarsoprol is often preceded by 2 or 3 injections of suramin (5, 10, and 20 mg per kg, respectively) in order to reduce the risk of Herxheimer-type reactions. In late-stage *T.b. gambiense* infection pretreatment with 1 or 2 injections of pentamidine 4 mg per kg can be given to sterilise the blood. Corticosteroids have been given for prevention of fatal complications during treatment with melarsoprol, but there is no conclusive evidence of their value and routine use is not recommended. In certain areas relapses can occur after melarsoprol treatment and nitrofurazone, which is highly toxic, has been the only compound available with proven activity against infections refractory to melarsoprol. More recently nifurtimox and eflornithine, both of which are given by mouth, have shown promise although further studies are needed.

After treatment for African trypanosomiasis patients should be followed up for at least 2 years to ascertain that they are cured.

Prophylaxis with pentamidine was introduced in the 1950's and an intramuscular dose of 4 mg per kg was assumed to protect against trypanosome infections for several months. However, it can no longer be recommended since the prophylactic dose is subcurative and there is a risk of masking undetected infections; the prophylactic use of pentamidine has also provoked resistance in several areas.—Report of a WHO Expert Committee on Epidemiology and Control of African Trypanosomiasis. *Tech. Rep. Ser. Wld Hlth Org. No. 739*, 1986.

Further reviews: W. E. Gutteridge, *Br. med. Bull.*, 1985, *41*, 162.

American Trypanosomiasis

South American trypanosomiasis (Chagas' disease) is caused by *Trypanosoma cruzi*, carried by reduviid or triatomine bugs which feed on human blood. Infected bugs defaecate on the human host while feeding and metacyclic trypanosomes are shed and enter the host via skin abrasions or by direct penetration of mucous membranes such as the conjunctiva. Trypomastigotes circulate in the blood, eventually penetrate tissue cells, and transform into amastigotes. Those multiply to produce further trypomastigotes which are liberated into the blood and re-invade the tissues; those in the blood may infect further blood-sucking bugs. Transmission by blood transfusion and congenital infections also occurs.

Infection with *T. cruzi* is found throughout South and Central America and has been recorded in Mexico and Texas. Three phases of the disease are recognised. In the early acute phase of infection parasites are present in the blood; this phase may be asymptomatic or there may be a swelling or chagoma at the site of infection, allergic reactions, and more rarely acute heart failure or meningo-encephalitis. In the intermediate phase, infection may be present in tissue for years without clinical manifestations. Classical features of the chronic phase are cardiomyopathy, megacolon, and mega-oesophagus. Parasites are rarely found in the blood after the acute phase.

Available treatment is generally unsatisfactory, but, despite their toxicity, nifurtimox or benznidazole are of value especially in the acute phase; benefit in the chronic phase is less certain. The efficacy of treatment varies from country to country and may be linked to variations in the sensitivity of different strains of *T. cruzi*.

Amoebiasis

Amoebiasis is defined as an infection with the protozoan parasite *Entamoeba histolytica*, with or without clinical manifestations. The reservoir of infection is man. Transmission is by the faeco-oral route and infection results from the ingestion of cysts, usually in contaminated food and drink. The cysts transform to trophozoites in the intestines and reproduction occurs by fission of the trophozoites. Further cysts develop and are excreted in the faeces. Amoebiasis occurs throughout the world. It is more prevalent and severe in the tropics and subtropics, but is more closely related to sanitation and socio-economic status than to climate. The majority of people infected with *E. histolytica* are asymptomatic cyst passers and nonpathogenic trophozoites live as commensals in the large intestine. In others, the trophozoites invade the wall of the large intestine causing ulceration and may migrate to other tissues, especially the liver, where they continue to divide and destroy tissue. Factors increasing susceptibility to tissue invasion include malnutrition, immunosuppression, and pregnancy.

In 1969, the WHO classified amoebiasis as asymptomatic or symptomatic, with symptomatic amoebiasis further divided into intestinal or extra-intestinal amoebiasis. Intestinal amoebiasis comprises two main states, amoebic dysentery and non-dysenteric amoebic colitis; amoeboma, a localised form of intestinal amoebiasis, and amoebic appendicitis may also occur. Hepatic amoebiasis, the most common form of extra-intestinal amoebic disease, may present as acute non-suppurative disease or as amoebic liver abscess. Amoebiasis may also involve the skin or organs such as the lungs, brain, and spleen.

Drugs used in the treatment of amoebiasis may be classified according to their site of action.

Luminal amoebicides acting principally in the bowel lumen have included:

diloxanide furoate and other dichloroacetamide derivatives such as clefamide, etofamide, and teclozan;

di-iodohydroxyquinoline and other halogenated hydroxyquinoline derivatives such as broxyquinoline and halquinol;

acetarsol and other arsenical derivatives such as bismuth glycollylarsanilate, carbarsone, and difetarsone.

Diloxanide furoate is generally the luminal amoebicide of choice. The arsenicals are toxic and no longer used and, although some authorities still recommend di-iodohydroxyquinoline, most oral preparations of halogenated hydroxyquinolines have been withdrawn since the association between clioquinol and subacute myelo-opticoneuropathy (SMON) was established. The antibiotics paromomycin (see p.280) and tetracycline (see p.313) have also been used.

Tissue or *systemic amoebicides* acting principally in the intestinal wall and liver include the alkaloid emetine, and its synthetic derivative dehydroemetine, and the antimalarial chloroquine (see p.508) which acts principally in the liver.

Mixed amoebicides act at all sites of infection, that is within the intestinal lumen and in the intestinal wall and other tissues, and include metronidazole and other 5-nitroimidazole derivatives such as nimorazole, ornidazole, secnidazole, and tinidazole. However, because of their rapid absorption from the gastro-intestinal tract, the nitroimidazoles are less effective against parasites in the lumen.

In non-endemic areas, patients with asymptomatic intestinal amoebiasis (cyst passers) are generally treated with a luminal amoebicide such as diloxanide furoate or alternatively, di-iodohydroxyquinoline or paromomycin. Invasive amoebiasis (amoebic dysentery; hepatic amoebiasis) requires treatment with a systemically absorbed amoebicide followed by a luminal amoebicide to eradicate any surviving organisms from the lumen of the large intestine and prevent relapse. The treatment of choice is generally metronidazole followed by diloxanide furoate. Alternatively emetine or dehydroemetine, together with chloroquine in hepatic amoebiasis, followed by a luminal amoebicide may be used. Tetracycline has been added to treatment regimens in severe amoebic dysentery.

Mass treatment with metronidazole or diloxanide has been tried in population groups where invasive disease is common, although a 1985 report of a WHO meeting on strategies for control of amoebiasis concluded that there was no acceptable chemoprophylaxis for amoebiasis at that time. Visitors to the tropics should not attempt chemoprophylaxis.

References: Report of a WHO Expert Committee on Amoebiasis, *Tech. Rep. Ser. Wld Hlth Org. No. 421*, 1969; Report of a WHO Scientific Group on Intestinal Protozoan and Helminthic Infections, *Tech. Rep. Ser. Wld Hlth Org. No. 666*, 1981; *Bull. Wld Hlth Org.*, 1985, *63*, 417. Findings from a study in India on *Entamoeba histolytica* cyst passers suggesting that the organism is not responsible for many of the gastro-intestinal symptoms comprising non-dysenteric amoebic colitis and that the classification of intestinal amoebiasis should be revised. Invasive amoebiasis did not develop in any of the cyst passers and their routine treatment was not considered justifiable in countries where amoebiasis is endemic.— R. Nanda *et al.*, *Lancet*, 1984, *2*, 301.

Comments on the varying pathogenicity of different strains of *Entamoeba histolytica* and discussion as to whether asymptomatic carriers including homosexuals, who frequently harbour the parasite, should be treated.— *Lancet*, 1985, *1*, 732; D. J. Krogstad, *New Engl. J. Med.*, 1986, *315*, 390; *Lancet*, 1986, *2*, 1133.

Balantidiasis

Infection with the ciliate protozoan *Balantidium coli* results from the ingestion of cysts, the commonest source of which is *pigs*. Water-borne epidemics of balantidiasis have been reported. Most infections are asymptomatic and the organism lives in the large intestine as a luminal commensal. Those with symptoms have diarrhoea. Colonic ulceration resulting in a severe dysenteric syndrome resembling amoebic dysentery may occur in some individuals, especially those who are malnourished. Treatment is with metronidazole or tetracycline; di-iodohydroxyquinoline and paromomycin have also been used.

Giardiasis

Infection with *Giardia intestinalis* (*G. lamblia*; *Lamblia intestinalis*) occurs throughout the world and is one of the commonest intestinal protozoal infections. Transmission is generally by the faeco-oral route with infection resulting from the ingestion of cysts in contaminated food and water. Cysts are transformed in the small intestine to trophozoites which become attached to the intestinal mucosa. The trophozoites divide by binary fission, undergo encystment in the gut lumen, and are excreted in the faeces. Person-to-person transmission can occur in crowded living conditions such as institutions. Giardiasis is a frequent cause of traveller's diarrhoea and is also recognised as a cause of diarrhoea in male homosexuals. Infected patients may have acute or chronic diarrhoea or they may be asymptomatic. Treatment is with metronidazole or other nitroimidazole derivatives such as tinidazole. Mepacrine and furazolidone have also been given but may be more toxic. Cure-rates of over 80% have been reported, although treatment may sometimes need to be repeated.

References: Report of a WHO Scientific Group on Intestinal Protozoan and Helminthic Infections, *Tech. Rep. Ser. Wld Hlth Org. No. 666*, 1981.

Leishmaniasis

Leishmaniasis is a collection of diseases caused by various species and subspecies of the protozoan parasite *Leishmania*. Treatment varies according to the clinical form of the disease. The drugs used include the pentavalent antimonials meglumine antimonate and sodium stibogluconate, pentamidine, and amphotericin (see the section on Antifungal Agents).

The spread and occurrence of leishmaniases in the world is increasing and current efforts to control these diseases are insufficent. All forms of leishmaniasis are transmitted by the bite of female phlebotomine sandflies infected with *Leishmania*. In man, *Leishmania* occur as intracellular parasites known as amastigotes that multiply in macrophages and other phagocytic cells of the reticuloendothelial system. Leishmanial infection induces both humoral and cellular immune responses, but the balance of their expression varies with the type of disease. The clinical forms of leishmaniasis are widely diverse.

Visceral leishmaniasis is caused by *L. donovani* and its subspecies. The reticuloendothelial hyperplasia that follows infection affects the spleen, liver, mucosa of the small intestine, bone marrow, lymph nodes, and other lymphoid tissues. Darkening of the skin of the face, hands, feet, and abdomen is common in endemic visceral leishmaniasis in India (kala-azar = black sickness). The pentavalent antimonials meglumine antimonate and sodium stibogluconate are the standard first-line drugs for the treatment of visceral leishmaniasis. Most patients seem to respond rapidly to treatment, but relapse-rates differ in various parts of the world. Second-line drugs currently available for relapsed and unresponsive patients are pentamidine, amphotericin, and allopurinol.

Cutaneous leishmaniasis is caused by various species of *Leishmania* and a wide variety of clinical presentations is possible. A 'classical' lesion starts as a nodule at the site of inoculation. A crust develops centrally which may fall away exposing an ulcer which heals gradually. Satellite nodules at the edge of the lesion are charcteristic. Cutaneous leishmaniasis of the Old World is normally caused by *L. tropica*, *L. major*, or *L. aethiopica*, although cutaneous lesions due to *L. donovani* are reported from Africa and the Mediterranean basin. Cutaneous leishmaniasis of the New World is caused by numerous species and subspecies of *Leishmania* including *L. braziliensis*, *L. mexicana*, and *L. peruviana*. Early noninflamed nodular lesions due to *L. tropica*, *L. major*, *L. mexicana*, or *L. peruviana* may be treated with intralesional injections of mepacrine, sodium stibogluconate, or meglumine antimonate; a systemic pentavalent antimonial drug should be given in more severe disease. Cutaneous leishmaniasis due to *L. aethiopica* is unresponsive to antimonials at conventional doses and until better drugs are available most sores should be left to heal spontaneously; mucocutaneous lesions justify the use of pentamidine. In cutaneous leishmaniasis due to *L. braziliensis* lymphatic involvement is common early in the disease and prolonged systemic treatment with a pentavalent antimonial is indicated in order to prevent the later development of mucocutaneous leishmaniasis; lesions due to *L. braziliensis guyanensis* are particularly slow to respond and liable to relapse, but these lesions respond well to pentamidine.

Diffuse cutaneous leishmaniasis is also caused by various species and subspecies of *Leishmania* and is characterised by widely disseminated thickening of the skin in plaques, papules, or multiple nodules, especially on the face and exterior surfaces of the limbs. There is no ulceration or mucosal involvement. The disease does not heal spontaneously and there tends to be relapse after treatment since patients lack specific cellular immunity to *Leishmania* and seldom acquire it. That due to *L. aethiopica* is treated with pentamidine. In the New World, diffuse cutaneous leishmaniasis is usually due to *L. mexicana amazonensis* and responds initially to pentavalent antimony. The apparent failure of pentamidine makes amphotericin the second choice. Recently one patient responded to a combination of rifampicin and isoniazid.

Mucocutaneous leishmaniasis of the New World or *espundia* is caused by *L. braziliensis braziliensis* and possibly by *L. b. panamensis* and *L. b. guyanensis*. A few cases of mucocutaneous leishmaniasis have been reported from the Old World, caused by *L. aethiopica* in Ethiopia and probably *L. donovani* in the Sudan. In mucocutaneous leishmaniasis the primary lesions are similar to other types of cutaneous leishmaniasis but do not heal spontaneously. Metastatic spread to the oronasal/pharyngeal mucosa may occur during the presence of the primary lesions or up to 30 years later. Ulceration and erosion progressively destroy the soft tissue and cartilage of the oronasal/pharyngeal cavity. Suffering and mutilation are severe and death occurs as a result of bronchopneumonia or malnutrition. The treatment of choice is pentavalent antimony, usually meglumine antimonate; failure to respond is an indication for the use of amphotericin or pentamidine. Nifurtimox has been shown to be effective in some cases of mucocutaneous leishmaniasis, although its role as a second-line drug or in combination with pentavalent antimony has not yet been established.— Report of a WHO Expert Committee on the Leishmaniases, *Tech. Rep. Ser. Wld Hlth Org. No. 701*, 1984.

Further reviews of leishmaniasis: P. D. Marsden, *Trans. R. Soc. trop. Med. Hyg.*, 1986, *80*, 859 (mucocutaneous leishmaniasis).

Pneumocystis Carinii Pneumonia

The protozoan *Pneumocystis carinii* is generally only pathogenic in immunocompromised individuals in whom it causes pneumonia. Standard treatment is with co-trimoxazole (see p. 210) or with pentamidine.

For a review of pentamidine in the treatment of *Pneumocystis carinii* pneumonia, see pentamidine, p.676.

Trichomoniasis

Infection by the protozoan *Trichomonas vaginalis* is treated principally with metronidazole or other nitroimidazole derivatives. For further details, see under metronidazole, p.672.

4752-k

Acetarsol *(BAN, rINN).*

Acetaminohydroxyphenylarsonsäure; Acetarsone; Acetphenarsinum; Osarsolum. 3-Acetamido-4-hydroxyphenylarsonic acid.

$C_8H_{10}AsNO_5$=275.1.

CAS — 97-44-9.

Pharmacopoeias. In *Fr.*, *Int.*, *Nord.*, *Pol.*, *Port.*, *Rus.*, *Span.*, and *Turk. Fr.* and *Span.* also include Acetarsol Sodium.

Acetarsol, a pentavalent organic arsenical derivative, is a luminal amoebicide and also has antitrichomonal activity. It was formerly administered orally in the treatment of intestinal amoebiasis (see Amoebiasis, p.658) and vaginally in the treatment of trichomoniasis, but has been superseded by less toxic drugs.

INFLAMMATORY BOWEL DISEASES. Suppositories each containing acetarsol 250 mg are a traditional remedy for proctitis and in a controlled study (A.M. Connell *et al.*, *Lancet*, 1965, *1*, 238) were found to be as effective as a steroid suppository. They are, however, no longer available commercially.— J. E. Lennard-Jones, *Postgrad. med. J.*, 1984, *60*, 797.

Proprietary Names and Manufacturers

Acetylarsan *(May & Baker, UK)*; Gynoplix *(Théraplix, Fr.; Vaillant, Ital.)*; Neo-Vagex *(Neolab, Canad.)*; RVC *(Lennon, S.Afr.)*; Stovarsol *(Fr.)*; SVC *(May & Baker, S.Afr.; May & Baker, UK)*; Vagoflor *(Switz.)*.

4754-t

Acinitrazole *(BAN).*

Aminitrozole *(rINN)*; CL-5279; Nithiamide *(USAN)*. *N*-(5-Nitrothiazol-2-yl)acetamide.

$C_5H_5N_3O_3S$=187.2.

CAS — 140-40-9.

Pharmacopoeias. In *Cz.*

Acinitrazole has been given by mouth in the treatment of trichomoniasis.

Proprietary Names and Manufacturers

Tricomon *(Wasserman, Spain)*; Tricosil *(Panthox & Burck, Ital.)*; Trigamma *(IBP, Ital.)*.

12332-x

Aklomide *(BAN, USAN, rINN).*
2-Chloro-4-nitrobenzamide.
$C_7H_5ClN_2O_3$=200.6.

CAS — 3011-89-0.

Aklomide is an antiprotozoal agent which has been used in veterinary practice for the control of coccidiosis in poultry.

Proprietary Veterinary Names and Manufacturers
Salsbury, UK.

12355-b

Amicarbalide Isethionate *(BANM).*
Amicarbalide Isetionate *(rINNM)*; M & B-5062A.
3,3′-Diamidinocarbanilide isethionate; 1,3-Bis(3-amidinophenyl)urea bis(2-hydroxyethanesulphonate).
$C_{15}H_{16}N_6O, 2C_2H_6O_4S$=548.6.

CAS — 3459-96-9 (amicarbalide); 3671-72-5 (isethionate).

Amicarbalide isethionate is an antiprotozoal agent used in veterinary practice in the treatment of bovine babesiosis.

Proprietary Veterinary Names and Manufacturers
Diampron *(May & Baker, UK).*

12372-v

Amprolium Hydrochloride *(BANM, rINNM).*
1-(4-Amino-2-propylpyrimidin-5-ylmethyl)-2-methylpyridinium chloride hydrochloride.
$C_{14}H_{19}ClN_4$,HCl=315.2.

CAS — 121-25-5 (amprolium); 137-88-2 (hydrochloride).

NOTE. Amprolium is *USAN.*

Pharmacopoeias. In *B.P. Vet.* Also in *Fr.* and *U.S.*, for veterinary use only.

A white or almost white, odourless or almost odourless powder. **Soluble** 1 in 2 of water; slightly soluble in alcohol; very slightly soluble in ether; practically insoluble in chloroform.

Amprolium hydrochloride is an antiprotozoal agent used in veterinary practice, usually in conjunction with other agents such as ethopabate, pyrimethamine, or sulfaquinoxaline, for the control of coccidiosis in poultry.

Beneficial results with amprolium in 2 AIDS patients with severe diarrhoea, one with *Isospora belli* infection and the other with cryptosporidiosis. However, one patient developed polyneuropathy while receiving amprolium 90 mg per kg body-weight daily and the other had a rapidly reversible cardiomyopathy and reversible neurological symptoms while receiving 200 mg per kg daily. It is suggested that the daily dose should be below 50 mg per kg to avoid severe side-effects.— S. J. O. Veldhuyzen van Zanten *et al.* (letter), *Lancet*, 1984, *2*, 345.

Proprietary Veterinary Names and Manufacturers
Merck Sharp & Dohme, UK.

12015-q

Arprinocid *(BAN, USAN, rINN).*
9-(2-Chloro-6-fluorobenzyl)adenine.
$C_{12}H_9ClFN_5$=277.7.

CAS — 55779-18-5.

Arprinocid is an antiprotozoal agent used in veterinary practice for the prevention of coccidiosis in poultry.

Proprietary Veterinary Names and Manufacturers
Arpocox *(Merck Sharp & Dohme, UK).*

12411-t

Azanidazole *(BAN, USAN, rINN).*
F-4. 4-[(*E*)-2-(1-Methyl-5-nitroimidazol-2-yl)vinyl]-pyrimidin-2-ylamine.
$C_{10}H_{10}N_6O_2$=246.2.

CAS — 62973-76-6.

Azanidazole is a 5-nitroimidazole derivative similar to metronidazole and is used in the treatment of trichomoniasis.

Proprietary Names and Manufacturers
Triclose *(Schwarz, Ital.).*

4756-r

Benznidazole *(rINN).*

Ro-7-1051. *N*-Benzyl-2-(2-nitroimidazol-1-yl)acetamide.
$C_{12}H_{12}N_4O_3$=260.3.

CAS — 22994-85-0.

Adverse Effects

Nausea, vomiting, abdominal pain, peripheral neuropathy, and severe skin reactions have been reported following the administration of benznidazole.

A study involving 20 patients with chronic American trypanosomiasis given benznidazole 5 mg per kg body-weight daily had to be stopped because of the high incidence of skin rashes and neurological symptoms.— W. Apt *et al.* (letter), *Trans. R. Soc. trop. Med. Hyg.*, 1986, *80*, 1010.

Absorption and Fate

Benznidazole is absorbed from the gastro-intestinal tract following administration by mouth.

Peak plasma concentrations of 2.22 to 2.81 (average 2.54) µg per mL of benznidazole were obtained in 6 healthy subjects 3 to 4 hours after administration of a single 100-mg dose of benznidazole. The half-life of elimination ranged from 10.5 to 13.6 (average 12) hours. Benznidazole was about 44% bound to plasma proteins.— J. Raaflaub and W. H. Ziegler, *Arzneimittel-Forsch.*, 1979, *29*, 1611.

Uses and Administration

Benznidazole is a 2-nitroimidazole derivative with antiprotozoal activity. It is of value in the treatment of South American trypanosomiasis (Chagas' disease) due to infection with *Trypanosoma cruzi* , especially the early acute stage of the disease. Benznidazole has been given by mouth in a dose of 5 mg per kg body-weight daily for 30 to 60 days.

TRYPANOSOMIASIS. Benznidazole has been claimed to be effective in curing more than 80% of both acute and chronic cases of South American trypanosomiasis at doses of 5 mg per kg body-weight daily for 60 days in adults or 10 mg per kg daily for children. Initial clinical studies with benznidazole used higher doses and serious side-effects such as polyneuropathy and progressive purpuric dermatitis were seen. It is still not clear whether benznidazole has any advantage over nifurtimox in terms of efficacy or toxicity.— W. E. Gutteridge, *Br. med. Bull.*, 1985, *41*, 162.

Reports of beneficial results with benznidazole in the treatment of acute or chronic American trypanosomiasis: C. A. Barclay *et al.*, *Current Chemotherapy, Vol. 1*, W. Siegenthaler and R. Luthy (Ed.), Washington, American Society for Microbiology, 1978, 158; J. A. Cerisola *et al.*, *ibid.*, 159; J. R. Coura *et al.*, *ibid.*, 161.

For a brief description of South American trypanosomiasis, see p.658.

Proprietary Names and Manufacturers

Radanil *(Roche, Arg.*; *Roche, Switz.)*; Rochagan *(Roche, Braz.).*

4759-n

Bismuth Glycollylarsanilate *(BAN).*
Glycobiarsol *(USAN, rINN).* (Hydrogen *N*-glycoloylarsanilato)oxobismuth; Bismuthyl 4-glycolamidophenylarsonic acid.
$C_8H_9AsBiNO_6$=499.1.

CAS — 116-49-4.

Pharmacopoeias. In *U.S.*

An odourless, yellowish-white to beige-pink-coloured, amorphous powder. It decomposes on heating.
Very slightly **soluble** in water and alcohol; practically insoluble in chloroform and ether. **Protect** from light.

Bismuth glycollylarsanilate, a pentavalent organic arsenical derivative, is a luminal amoebicide formerly given by mouth in the treatment of intestinal amoebiasis. It has been superseded by less toxic drugs (see Amoebiasis, p.658).

Preparations

Glycobiarsol Tablets *(U.S.P.).* Tablets containing bismuth glycollylarsanilate.

Proprietary Names and Manufacturers
Milibis *(Winthrop-Breon, USA)*; Wintodon *(Winthrop, Arg.).*

The following names have been used for multi-ingredient preparations containing bismuth glycollylarsanilate— Aralis *(Winthrop, UK.*

4760-k

Broxaldine *(pINN).*
Brobenzoxaldine. 5,7-Dibromo-2-methyl-8-quinolyl benzoate.
$C_{17}H_{11}Br_2NO_2$=421.1.

CAS — 3684-46-6.

Broxaldine was formerly used in conjunction with broxyquinoline in the treatment of intestinal infections (see below).

Proprietary Names and Manufacturers
The following names have been used for multi-ingredient preparations containing broxaldine— Intestopan *(Sandoz, Switz.).*

4761-a

Broxyquinoline *(rINN).*
Broxichinolinum. 5,7-Dibromoquinolin-8-ol.
$C_9H_5Br_2NO$=303.0.

CAS — 521-74-4.

Broxyquinoline and broxaldine are halogenated hydroxyquinolines with properties similar to those of clioquinol (p.661). They were formerly used together in the treatment of intestinal infections including amoebiasis.

Proprietary Names and Manufacturers
Colipar *(Fr.)*; Diromo *(Spain).*

The following names have been used for multi-ingredient preparations containing broxyquinoline— Intestopan *(Sandoz, Switz.).*

4762-t

Carbarsone *(USAN, pINN).*
Aminarsonum. *N*-Carbamoylarsanilic acid; 4-Ureidophenylarsonic acid.
$C_7H_9AsN_2O_4$=260.1.

CAS — 121-59-5.

Pharmacopoeias. In *Int.*, *It.*, *Jug.*, *Mex.*, *Rus.*, *Turk.*, and *U.S.*

A white almost odourless powder.
Slightly soluble in water and alcohol; very slightly soluble in chloroform and ether; soluble in solutions of alkali hydroxides and carbonates. A saturated solution in water is acid to litmus.

Carbarsone, a pentavalent organic arsenical derivative, is a luminal amoebicide which has been given by mouth in the treatment of intestinal amoebiasis in a dose of 250 mg two or three times daily for 10 days. It has been superseded by less toxic drugs (see Amoebiasis, p.658).

Preparations

Carbarsone Capsules *(U.S.P.)*

Proprietary Names and Manufacturers

Leucarsone *(May & Baker, UK; Lilly, USA).*

4763-x

Carnidazole *(BAN, USAN, pINN).*

R-25831; R-28096 (hydrochloride). *O*-Methyl [2-(2-methyl-5-nitroimidazol-1-yl)ethyl]thiocarbamate.
$C_8H_{12}N_4O_3S$=244.3.

CAS — 42116-76-7.

Carnidazole is a 5-nitroimidazole derivative similar to metronidazole. It is employed in veterinary practice in the treatment and control of trichomoniasis in pigeons.

Proprietary Veterinary Names and Manufacturers

Spartrix *(Harkers, UK).*

1601-n

Chlorquinaldol *(BAN, rINN).*

5,7-Dichloro-2-methylquinolin-8-ol.
$C_{10}H_7Cl_2NO$=228.1.

CAS — 72-80-0.

Pharmacopoeias. In *Roum.*

Chlorquinaldol is a halogenated hydroxyquinoline with properties similar to those of clioquinol (below). It has been applied topically in infected skin conditions and in vaginal infections.

Proprietary Names and Manufacturers

Gyno-Stérosan *(Geigy, Switz.)*; Gyno-Sterosan *(Ger.; Neth.; Norw.)*; Gynothérax *(Bouchard, Fr.; Switz.)*; Siogen *(Neth.; Switz.)*; Siogeno *(Ger.)*; Siosteran *(Neth.; Switz.)*; Stérosan *(Geigy, Switz.)*; Sterosan *(Geigy, Denm.; Ger.; Neth.; Swed.)*; Steroxin *(Geigy, Austral.; Geigy, UK; Geigy, USA).*

The following names have been used for multi-ingredient preparations containing chlorquinaldol—Locoid C *(Brocades, UK)*; Steroxin-Hydrocortisone *(Geigy, UK).*

4769-m

Clefamide *(BAN, rINN).*

Chlorphenoxamide. 2,2-Dichloro-*N*-(2-hydroxyethyl)-*N*-[4-(4-nitrophenoxy)benzyl]acetamide.
$C_{17}H_{16}Cl_2N_2O_5$=399.2.

CAS — 3576-64-5.

Pharmacopoeias. In *B.P.C. 1973.*

A lemon-yellow, odourless or almost odourless, crystalline powder. Practically **insoluble** in water; soluble 1 in 100 of alcohol, 1 in 80 of chloroform, and 1 in 40 of ethyl acetate.

Clefamide, a dichloroacetamide derivative, is a luminal amoebicide with actions and uses similar to those of diloxanide furoate (see p.663). It is available in some countries as tablets of 250 mg for use in the treatment of intestinal amoebiasis, and has been given in a dosage of 1.5 g daily in divided doses, for 10 days.

Proprietary Names and Manufacturers

Mebinol *(Carlo Erba, Ital.).*

4770-t

Clioquinol *(BAN, USAN, rINN).*

Chinoform; Chloroiodoquine; Cliochinolum; Iodochlorhydroxyquin; Iodochlorhydroxyquinoline; Quiniodochlor. 5-Chloro-7-iodoquinolin-8-ol.
C_9H_5ClINO=305.5.

CAS — 130-26-7.

Pharmacopoeias. In *Aust., Br., Egypt, Hung., Ind., It., Jug., Mex., Port., Swiss,* and *U.S.*

A yellowish-white to brownish-yellow, voluminous powder with a slight characteristic odour. M.p. about 180° with decomposition. It darkens on exposure to light.

Practically **insoluble** in water and alcohol; soluble 1 in 120 of chloroform; very slightly soluble in ether; soluble in dimethylformamide, hot ethyl acetate, and hot glacial acetic acid. **Store** in airtight containers. Protect from light.

Aqueous creams containing clioquinol are **incompatible** with aluminium.

Adverse Effects

Clioquinol may rarely cause iodism in sensitive patients. Local application of clioquinol in ointments or creams may occasionally cause severe irritation and there may be cross-sensitivity with other halogenated hydroxyquinolines. Clioquinol stains clothing and linen yellow on contact and may stain the skin and discolour fair hair.

Clioquinol given by mouth has been associated with severe neurotoxicity. In Japan, the epidemic development of subacute myelo-opticoneuropathy (SMON) in the 1960's was associated with the ingestion of normal or high doses of clioquinol for prolonged periods and the sale of clioquinol and related hydroxyquinolines was subsequently banned in Japan. Symptoms of subacute myelo-opticoneuropathy are principally those of peripheral neuropathy, including optic atrophy, and myelopathy. Abdominal pain and diarrhoea often precede neurological symptoms such as paraesthesias in the legs progressing to paraplegia in some patients and loss of visual acuity sometimes leading to blindness. A characteristic green pigment, a chelate of clioquinol with iron, is often seen on the tongue and in the urine and faeces. Cerebral disturbances, including confusion and retrograde amnesia, have also been reported. Although many patients improved when clioquinol was withdrawn, others had residual disablement.

It was suggested that the Japanese epidemic might be due to genetic susceptibility, but a few similar cases of subacute myelo-opticoneuropathy have been reported from several other countries in association with clioquinol or related hydroxyquinoline derivatives, such as broxyquinoline or di-iodohydroxyquinoline. Oral preparations of clioquinol have now been banned worldwide.

In view of their neurotoxicity the worldwide withdrawal of all oral products containing halogenated hydroxyquinolines is advocated.— O. Hansson and A. Herxheimer (letter), *Lancet*, 1984, *2*, 864.

Absorption of clioquinol through the skin has been noted following topical application (T. Fischer and P. Hartvig, *Lancet*, 1977, *1*, 603; S.J. Stohs *et al.*, *J. invest. Derm.*, 1984, *82*, 195). Significant toxicity was found in *dogs* treated with 5 g of a 3% clioquinol topical preparation for 28 days (F. W. Ezzedeen *et al.*, J. pharm. Sci., 1984, *73*, 1369) and representations have been made requesting that all products containing clioquinol be removed from the market because of their potential danger.

ABNORMAL COLORATION. Topical application of a clioquinol-containing corticosteroid preparation was associated with intense red discoloration of white hair in 2 patients with generalised dermatitis.— H. -J. Bandmann and U. Speer, *Contact Dermatitis*, 1984, *10*, 113.

ALLERGY. Over the 2-year period 1976-1977, primary irritant dermatitis was noted in 7 patients compared with contact allergy in 35, following the topical application of clioquinol. Irritant dermatitis was associated with clioquinol concentration rather than crystal size.— M. Kero *et al.*, *Contact Dermatitis*, 1979, *5*, 115.

Classification of clioquinol as a contact allergen which can commonly cause sensitisation, especially when applied to eczematous skin; chlorquinaldol can also cause sensitisation, but less frequently. It is important to include clioquinol and chlorquinaldol in routine patch testing since the clinical reaction may be relatively mild and sensitivity easily missed, particularly in the presence of a corticosteroid which suppresses or attenuates the reaction.— *Drug & Ther. Bull.*, 1986, *24*, 57.

Absorption and Fate

Much of a dose of clioquinol passes through the gastro-intestinal tract without being absorbed, but a variable degree of absorption does occur. Some absorption occurs through the skin when clioquinol is applied topically (see Adverse Effects).

The absorption of halogenated hydroxyquinolines was assessed in 6 healthy subjects. Mean excretion in the urine, as glucuronide, during the 10 hours following a single oral dose was: clioquinol 250 mg, 12.6% of the dose; di-iodohydroxyquinoline 300 mg, 4.6%; broxyquinoline 250 mg, 10.2%; and chlorquinaldol 200 mg, 34.9%.— L. Berggren and O. Hansson, *Clin. Pharmac. Ther.*, 1968, *9*, 67.

Uses and Administration

Clioquinol, a halogenated hydroxyquinoline, is a luminal amoebicide formerly given by mouth in the treatment of intestinal amoebiasis. It was also formerly used for the prophylaxis and treatment of traveller's diarrhoea and similar infections but was of doubtful value. Oral preparations have now been withdrawn worldwide because of neurotoxicity (see Adverse Effects).

Clioquinol has antibacterial and antifungal activity and is used in creams and ointments, usually containing 3%, in the treatment of skin infections. It is also applied together with a corticosteroid in inflammatory skin conditions complicated by bacterial or fungal infections.

Vaginal insufflations usually containing 25% of clioquinol were formerly used in the treatment of trichomonal vaginitis.

Preparations

Clioquinol Cream *(B.P.)*

Clioquinol Cream *(U.S.P.)*

Clioquinol Cream Aqueous *(A.P.F.).* Iodochlorhydroxyquin Cream Aqueous

Clioquinol Ointment *(U.S.P.)*

Compound Clioquinol Powder *(U.S.P.).* Clioquinol 25 g, lactic acid 2.5 g, zinc stearate 20 g, and lactose 52.5 g.

Hydrocortisone Acetate and Clioquinol Cream *(B.P.)*

Hydrocortisone and Clioquinol Ointment *(B.P.)*

Zinc Paste, Calamine, and Clioquinol Bandage *(B.P.).* See under Zinc Oxide, p.936.

Proprietary Preparations

Barquinol HC *(Fisons, UK). Cream*, clioquinol 3%, hydrocortisone acetate 0.5%.

Oralcer *(Vitabiotics, UK). Lozenges*, clioquinol 35 mg, ascorbic acid 6 mg.

Vioform-Hydrocortisone *(Zyma, UK). Cream* and *Ointment*, clioquinol 3%, hydrocortisone 1%.

Proprietary Names and Manufacturers

Budoform *(Austral.)*; Cremo-Quin *(Austral.)*; Enteritan *(Switz.)*; Entero-Valodon *(Wallace Mfg Chem., UK)* Entero-Vioform *(Austral.; Canad.; Ger.; Neth.; S.Afr.; Ciba, UK)*; Entero-Vioformio *(Ital.)*; Entero-Vioformo *(Arg.; Spain)*; Linola *(Wolff, Ger.)*; Oralcer *(Vitabiotics, UK)*; Silic C *(Ego, Austral.)*; Vioform *(Ciba, Austral.; Ciba, Canad.; Zyma, Ger.; S.Afr.; Ciba, UK; Ciba, USA)*; Vioforme *(Ciba, Switz.).*

The following names have been used for multi-ingredient preparations containing clioquinol—Aristoform *(Lederle, Canad.)*; Barquinol HC *(Fisons, UK)*; Betnovate-C *(Glaxo, Austral.; Glaxo, UK)*; Dioderm C *(Dermal Laboratories, UK)*; Haelan-C *(Dista, UK)*; HCV Creme *(Saron, USA)*; Hydroform *(Dermacare, Austral.)*; Hysone *(Mallard, USA)*; Iodo-Cortifair *(Pharmafair, USA)*; Locacorten-Vioform *(Ciba, Austral.; Ciba, Canad.)*; Locorten-Vioform *(Ciba, UK)*; Pedi-Cort V *(Pedinol, USA)*; Phen-Oris *(Stickley, Canad.)*; Pricort Cream and Lotion *(Arlo, USA)*; Propaderm-C *(Allen & Hanburys, UK)*; Quinaband *(Seton, UK: Bateman-Jackson, UK)*; Synalar-C *(ICI Pharmaceuticals, UK)*; Vioform-Hydrocortisone *(Ciba, Austral.; Ciba, Canad.; Ciba, UK; Ciba, USA).*

NOTE. The *UK* preparations Nystaform and Nystaform-HC have been reformulated to exclude clioquinol.

12589-f

Clopidol *(BAN, USAN, rINN).*
Clopindol; Meticlorpindol. 3,5-Dichloro-2,6-dimethylpyridin-4-ol.
$C_7H_7Cl_2NO$=192.0.

CAS — 2971-90-6.

Clopidol is an antiprotozoal agent used in veterinary practice for the prevention of coccidiosis in poultry and rabbits.

Proprietary Veterinary Names and Manufacturers
Coyden *(Dow Agriculture, UK).*

12626-e

Decoquinate *(BAN, USAN, rINN).*
HC-1528; M & B-15497. Ethyl 6-decyloxy-7-ethoxy-4-hydroxyquinoline-3-carboxylate.
$C_{24}H_{35}NO_5$=417.5.

CAS — 18507-89-6.

Pharmacopoeias. In *B.P. Vet.*

A cream to buff-coloured, odourless or almost odourless, microcrystalline powder. **Insoluble** in water; practically insoluble in alcohol; very slightly soluble in chloroform and ether.

Decoquinate is an antiprotozoal agent used in veterinary practice for the control of coccidiosis in poultry and sheep.

Proprietary Veterinary Names and Manufacturers
Deccox *(RMB Animal Health, UK).*

4773-f

Dehydroemetine Hydrochloride *(BANM, rINNM).*

2,3-Dehydroemetine Hydrochloride; BT-436; DHE; Ro-1-9334. 2,3-Didehydro-6′,7′,10,11-tetramethoxyemetan dihydrochloride; 3-Ethyl-1,6,7,11b-tetrahydro-9,10-dimethoxy-2-(1,2,3,4-tetrahydro-6,7-dimethoxy-1-isoquinolylmethyl)-4*H*-benzo[*a*]quinolizine dihydrochloride.
$C_{29}H_{38}N_2O_4$,2HCl=551.6.

CAS — 4914-30-1 (dehydroemetine); 2228-39-9 (hydrochloride).

Pharmacopoeias. In *Ind.*

Dehydroemetine, a synthetic derivative of emetine (p.664), is a tissue amoebicide with similar actions and uses. It has also been used as an anthelmintic in the treatment of schistosomiasis and fascioliasis.

Dehydroemetine is reported to be more rapidly eliminated from the body than emetine; the risk of accumulation is thus reduced and it is probably less toxic than emetine. For this reason dehydroemetine may be preferred to emetine in the treatment of severe intestinal amoebiasis and hepatic amoebiasis, although both drugs are being replaced by metronidazole which is less toxic.

In the treatment of amoebiasis, dehydroemetine hydrochloride is given by deep subcutaneous or intramuscular injection in a dose of 1 to 1.5 mg per kg body-weight daily, but no more than 90 mg daily, generally for up to 5 days; in children it should be given in 2 divided doses daily.

Dehydroemetine hydrochloride has also been given by mouth as enteric-coated tablets.

FASCIOLIASIS. Dehydroemetine hydrochloride is an alternative to bithionol in the treatment of fascioliasis (infection with the liver fluke *Fasciola hepatica*). It is given intramuscularly in a dosage of 1 mg per kg body-weight daily for 10 days together with chloroquine base 150 mg three times daily by mouth for 21 days.— S. C. Glover, *Br. J. Hosp. Med.*, 1983, *30*, 169.

Proprietary Names and Manufacturers
Dametine *(E. Merck, Ger.)*; Dehydroemetine *(Roche, Switz.).*

NOTE. The name D.H.E. 45 has been used to denote a preparation of dihydroergotamine mesylate.

12641-w

Diaveridine *(BAN, USAN, rINN).*
BW-49-210; NSC-408735. 5-Veratrylpyrimidine-2,4-diyldiamine.
$C_{13}H_{16}N_4O_2$=260.3.

CAS — 5355-16-8.

Pharmacopoeias. In *B.P. Vet. Cz.* includes Diaveridine for veterinary use.

A white or creamy-white, odourless powder. Very slightly **soluble** in water and alcohol; slightly soluble in chloroform.

Diaveridine is an antiprotozoal agent and has been used in veterinary practice for the control of coccidiosis in poultry.

Proprietary Veterinary Names and Manufacturers
May & Baker, UK.

4775-n

Difetarsone Sodium *(BANM, rINNM).*
Diphetarsone; RP-4763. Disodium *NN*′-ethylenebis(4-aminophenylarsonate) decahydrate.
$C_{14}H_{16}As_2N_2Na_2O_6,10H_2O$=684.3.

CAS — 3639-19-8 (difetarsone); 515-76-4 (sodium salt, anhydrous).

Difetarsone sodium, a pentavalent organic arsenical derivative, is a luminal amoebicide. It has been used in some countries in the treatment of intestinal amoebiasis, but in general the arsenical amoebicides have been superseded by less toxic drugs (see Amoebiasis, p.658). Difetarsone has also been used in the treatment of whipworm and threadworm infection.

Cure-rates of 97 to 100% were achieved with difetarsone 500 mg three times daily for 10 days in 89 patients who were either asymptomatic *Entamoeba histolytica* cyst passers or were infected with non-pathogenic amoebae including *Dientamoeba fragilis* and *Endolimax nana*, or with *Trichuris trichiura* [whipworm]. Side-effects noted were: swelling of mouth (1 patient), lightheadedness (2), nausea and flatulence (3), diarrhoea (2), and headache (1). Five patients had transient elevation of liver enzymes which suggested that difetarsone should be contra-indicated in patients with severe liver disease. Commenting on these results and experience gained in over 10 000 patients treated with difetarsone since 1971 it was noted that, although most North American physicians have shied away from using arsenicals to treat amoebiasis because they have been associated with encephalopathy, polyneuritis, visual disturbances, and severe dermatitis, none of these problems has been reported specifically with difetarsone.— J. S. Keystone *et al., Trans. R. Soc. trop. Med. Hyg.*, 1983, *77*, 84.

A report of generalised angioedema which developed during treatment with difetarsone.— L. McIntyre *et al., Trop. geogr. Med.*, 1983, *35*, 49.

Proprietary Names and Manufacturers
Bémarsal *(Specia, Fr.).*

4777-m

Di-iodohydroxyquinoline *(BAN).*

Diiodohydroxyquin; Diiodohydroxyquinoline *(rINN)*; Di-iodoxychinolinum; Diiodoxyquinoléine; Iodoquinol *(USAN)*. 5,7-Di-iodoquinolin-8-ol.
$C_9H_5I_2NO$=397.0.

CAS — 83-73-8.

Pharmacopoeias. In *Egypt., Fr., Ind., Int.*, and *U.S.*

A light yellowish to tan-coloured, microcrystalline powder, not readily wetted in water, odourless or with a slight odour.

Practically **insoluble** in water; sparingly soluble in alcohol and ether.

Adverse Effects

As for Clioquinol, p.661.

In addition to occasional reports of optic neuritis, optic atrophy, and peripheral neuropathy, especially in children given high doses long term, the oral administration of di-iodohydroxyquinoline has been associated with gastro-intestinal effects such as abdominal cramps, nausea, and diarrhoea. Adverse effects which may be attributable to the iodine content of di-iodohydroxyquinoline include pruritus ani, skin eruptions, and enlargement of the thyroid gland. Fever, chills, headache, and vertigo have also occurred.

Precautions

Di-iodohydroxyquinoline is contra-indicated in patients known to be hypersensitive to iodine or halogenated hydroxyquinolines and in those with impaired kidney or liver function. It should be used with caution in thyroid disease and may interfere with determinations of protein-bound iodine for up to 6 months in tests for thyroid function. Its use is best avoided in patients with neurological disorders.

Absorption and Fate

Di-iodohydroxyquinoline is partly and irregularly absorbed from the gastro-intestinal tract.

For a comparison of the absorption of halogenated hydroxyquinolines, including di-iodohydroxyquinoline, see Clioquinol, p.661.

Uses and Administration

Di-iodohydroxyquinoline, a halogenated hydroxyquinoline, is a luminal amoebicide acting principally in the bowel lumen and is used in the treatment of intestinal amoebiasis, although a dichloroacetamide derivative such as diloxanide furoate is usually preferred. It is given alone in the treatment of asymptomatic cyst-passers and in conjunction with an amoebicide that acts in the tissues, such as metronidazole or dehydroemetine, in patients with symptomatic intestinal amoebiasis or with hepatic amoebiasis.

For a description of amoebiasis and its treatment, see p.658.

Di-iodohydroxyquinoline has also been given in the treatment of balantidiasis and infections with *Dientamoeba fragilis* or *Blastocystis hominis*.

Di-iodohydroxyquinoline was formerly used in the treatment of acrodermatitis enteropathica; it is reported to act by enhancing zinc absorption and has now been superseded by oral zinc therapy.

The usual dosage in the treatment of amoebiasis is 630 or 650 mg three times daily by mouth for 20 days; children may be given 30 to 40 mg per kg body-weight daily in divided doses.

Di-iodohydroxyquinoline has antibacterial and antifungal activity and has been used topically in various skin conditions, usually together with a corticosteroid. It also has some antitrichomonal activity.

Preparations

Iodoquinol Tablets *(U.S.P.).* Tablets containing di-iodohydroxyquinoline.

Proprietary Names and Manufacturers
Diodoquin *(Searle, Canad.; Searle, UK)*; Dioxiquin *(Spain)*; Direxiode *(Austral.; Belg.; Delalande, Fr.; Switz.)*; Drioquilen *(Arg.)*; Embequin *(May & Baker, UK)*; Floraquin *(Arg.; Searle, Austral.; Belg.; Searle, S.Afr.; Searle, Spain; Searle, UK)*; Moebiquin *(USA)*; Ovoquinol *(Nadeau, Canad.)*; Searlequin *(Arg.)*; Yodoxin *(Glenwood, USA).*

The following names have been used for multi-ingredient preparations containing di-iodohydroxyquinoline—Cor-Tar-Quin *(Lagap, UK)*; Vytone *(Dermik, USA).*

4779-v

Diloxanide Furoate *(BANM, rINNM).*

4-(*N*-Methyl-2,2-dichloroacetamido)phenyl 2-furoate.
$C_{14}H_{11}Cl_2NO_4$=328.2.

CAS — 579-38-4 (diloxanide); 3736-81-0 (diloxanide furoate).

Pharmacopoeias. In *Br.* and *Ind.*

A white or almost white, odourless, crystalline powder. Very slightly **soluble** in water; slightly soluble in alcohol and in ether; soluble 1 in 2.5 of chloroform. **Protect** from light.

Adverse Effects

Flatulence is the most common adverse effect during treatment with diloxanide furoate. Vomiting, pruritus, and urticaria may occasionally occur.

Absorption and Fate

Diloxanide furoate is hydrolysed before absorption from the gastro-intestinal tract. The resulting diloxanide is readily absorbed and excreted mainly in the urine; less than 10% of a dose appears in the faeces.

Uses and Administration

Diloxanide furoate, a dichloroacetamide derivative, is a luminal amoebicide acting principally in the bowel lumen and is used in the treatment of intestinal amoebiasis. It is given alone in the treatment of asymptomatic cyst-passers and in conjunction with an amoebicide that acts in the tissues, such as metronidazole or dehydroemetine, in patients with symptomatic intestinal amoebiasis or with hepatic amoebiasis. Diloxanide furoate has also been used with metronidazole in the treatment of *Entamoeba polecki* infection.

For a description of amoebiasis and its treatment, see p.658.

Diloxanide furoate is administered by mouth in a dosage of 500 mg three times daily for 10 days; children may be given 20 mg per kg body-weight daily, in divided doses, for 10 days. The course of treatment may be repeated if necessary.

Preparations

Diloxanide Tablets *(B.P.).* Diloxanide Furoate Tablets

Proprietary Preparations

Entamizole *(Boots, UK). Tablets,* scored, diloxanide furoate 250 mg, metronidazole 200 mg.

Furamide *(Boots, UK). Tablets,* scored, diloxanide furoate 500 mg.

Proprietary Names and Manufacturers

Entamide *(Boots, UK)*; Furamide *(Boots, Austral.; Boots, UK)*.

12662-z

Dimetridazole *(BAN, pINN).*

1,2-Dimethyl-5-nitroimidazole.
$C_5H_7N_3O_2$=141.1.

CAS — 551-92-8.

Pharmacopoeias. In *B.P. Vet. Cz.* includes Dimetridazole for veterinary use only. *Fr.* includes Dimetridazole and Dimetridazole Mesylate for veterinary use only.

An almost white to brownish-yellow, odourless or almost odourless powder which darkens on exposure to light. Slightly **soluble** in water; soluble 1 in 30 of alcohol and 1 in 5 of chloroform; slightly soluble in ether. **Protect** from light.

Dimetridazole is a 5-nitroimidazole derivative similar to metronidazole. It is used in veterinary practice for the prevention and treatment of blackhead (histomoniasis) in turkeys and other poultry and for the control of swine dysentery in pigs and trichomoniasis in pigeons.

Proprietary Veterinary Names and Manufacturers
Dazole *(Peter Hand, UK)*; Emtryl *(RMB Animal Health, UK)*; Unizole *(Cheminex, UK)*.

4780-r

Diminazene Aceturate *(BANM, rINNM).*

1,3-Bis(4-amidinophenyl)triazene bis(*N*-acetylglycinate).
$C_{22}H_{29}N_9O_6$=515.5.

CAS — 536-71-0 (diminazene); 908-54-3 (aceturate, anhydrous).

Diminazene aceturate, an aromatic diamidine derivative related to pentamidine, is an antiprotozoal agent which has been used in veterinary medicine in the treatment of trypanosomiasis and babesiosis. It has also been tried in human infections.

BABESIOSIS. A patient infected with *Babesia microti* who had failed to respond to chloroquine had a rapid clinical and parasitologic response after administration of diminazene. However the patient developed Guillain-Barré syndrome after treatment and it was suggested that pentamidine might be preferable to diminazene in severe cases of human babesiosis.—T. K. Ruebush and A. Spielman, *Ann. intern. Med.*, 1978, *88*, 263.

TRYPANOSOMIASIS. In a retrospective study of 99 patients successfully treated for early-stage African trypanosomiasis with 3 doses of diminazene aceturate 5 mg per kg body-weight, given intramuscularly at intervals of 1 or more days, all patients were in good physical health 12 to over 109 months after receiving treatment. Five patients who had complained of numbness of the legs immediately after treatment were found to be well. It is suggested that diminazene should be considered as an alternative to suramin in the treatment of early-stage African trypanosomiasis.— D. E. Abaru *et al.*, *Tropenmed. Parasit.*, 1984, *35*, 148.

Proprietary Names and Manufacturers
Ganaseg.

Proprietary Veterinary Names and Manufacturers
Berenil *(Hoechst, UK)*.

12665-a

Dinitolmide *(BAN, rINN).*

Dinitrotoluamide; Methyldinitrobenzamide. 3,5-Dinitro-*o*-toluamide.
$C_8H_7N_3O_5$=225.2.

CAS — 148-01-6.

Pharmacopoeias. In *Fr.* Also in *B.P. Vet.*

A cream-coloured to light tan-coloured odourless powder. Practically **insoluble** in water; soluble 1 in 100 of alcohol and 1 in 15 of acetone; slightly soluble in chloroform and ether.

Dinitolmide is an antiprotozoal agent used in veterinary practice for the prevention of coccidiosis in poultry.

Proprietary Veterinary Names and Manufacturers
Salcostat *(Salsbury, UK)*; Unicox *(Cheminex, UK)*.

16604-j

Eflornithine Hydrochloride *(BANM, USAN, rINNM).*

α-Difluoromethylornithine Hydrochloride; DFMO; MDL-71782; MDL-71782A; RMI-71782 (hydrochloride). 2-(Difluoromethyl)-DL-ornithine monohydrochloride monohydrate.
$C_6H_{12}F_2N_2O_2,HCl,H_2O$=236.6.

CAS — 96020-91-6; 67037-37-0 (eflornithine).

Eflornithine hydrochloride is an irreversible inhibitor of ornithine decarboxylase, the rate-limiting enzyme in polyamine biosynthesis, and has antiprotozoal and antineoplastic activity. It may be administered by mouth or intravenously and has been given in the treatment of African trypanosomiasis and *Pneumocystis carinii* pneumonia. Eflornithine is also under study for use in cancer chemotherapy.

A review of eflornithine and the chemotherapeutic implications of polyamine biosynthesis inhibition. Polyamines have important roles in cellular phenomena such as replication and differentiation and eflornithine is an irreversible inhibitor of ornithine decarboxylase, the key enzyme in polyamine biosynthesis; the enzyme decarboxylates ornithine to produce putrescine which is then converted to the higher polyamines spermidine and spermine. Eflornithine has been found to have antineoplastic and antiprotozoal activity. The dramatic antitumour effects noted in *rodents* have not yet been demonstrated unequivocally in clinical studies in cancer patients. In these patients tolerance of eflornithine has been excellent and serious toxicity uncommon. Thrombocytopenia, leucopenia, and hearing loss, all reversed on discontinuing therapy, have been reported. Tolerance is better when eflornithine is administered intravenously; diarrhoea tends to limit dosage by the oral route. Antiprotozoal activity has been demonstrated, in experimental infections or *in vitro*, against parasitic protozoa including some *Trypansoma* and *Plasmodium* spp. and *Eimeria tenella* (coccidiosis) and there have been dramatic responses to eflornithine in clinical cases of African trypanosomiasis. Other analogues of ornithine, including α-monofluoromethylornithine (MFMO), and putrescine analogues are also under study.— A. Sjoerdsma and P. J. Schechter, *Clin. Pharmac. Ther.*, 1984, *35*, 287.

ABSORPTION AND FATE. The kinetics of eflornithine, administered as the hydrochloride, were studied in 6 healthy subjects following single doses of 5 and 10 mg per kg body-weight intravenously and 10 and 20 mg per kg by mouth and were found to follow a dose-linear model. Eflornithine was well absorbed and mean peak plasma concentrations of 39.1 and 76.8 nmol per mL were achieved 4 hours after oral doses of 10 and 20 mg per kg, respectively. The plasma-concentration decay phase had an average half-life of 199 minutes. Eflornithine was eliminated mainly by the kidneys. The amount of unchanged drug excreted in the urine in 24 hours was 46.9% and 40.3% of the 10 mg per kg and 20 mg per kg oral doses, respectively, and 78% and 81% of the 5 mg per kg and 10 mg per kg intravenous doses. Depending on the method used, bioavailability of the 10 mg per kg oral dose was estimated as 58% or 54%.— K. D. Haegele *et al.*, *Clin. Pharmac. Ther.*, 1981, *30*, 210.

For reference to the penetration of eflornithine into the CSF, see under Trypanosomiasis (below).

ADVERSE EFFECTS. Fatal cardiac arrest occurred in an AIDS patient with *Pneumocystis carinii* pneumonia during the intravenous infusion of eflornithine 100 mg per kg body-weight over 1 hour. Although a causal relationship cannot yet be established, sudden death after infusion of eflornithine has occurred recently in several other critically ill patients with AIDS.— R. A. Barbarash *et al.* (letter), *Ann. intern. Med.*, 1986, *105*, 141.

CRYPTOSPORIDIOSIS. Brief mention that eflornithine has been tried in the treatment of cryptosporidiosis in AIDS patients with inconclusive results.— D. Armstrong *et al.*, *Ann. intern. Med.*, 1985, *103*, 738.

PNEUMOCYSTIS CARINII PNEUMONIA. Eflornithine was effective in 4 of 10 AIDS patients with *Pneumocystis carinii* pneumonia who were refractory or intolerant to conventional therapy with co-trimoxazole or pentamidine. Treatment was with eflornithine 400 mg per kg body-weight daily in 4 divided doses given intravenously for 10 days, then reduced to 300 mg per kg daily, given intravenously for 4 days and by mouth thereafter. The duration of oral therapy ranged from 8 to 39 days. One patient received a reduced dose of 200 mg per kg daily throughout treatment because of renal impairment. The commonest side-effects were gastro-intestinal disturbances and, although anorexia, diarrhoea, and nausea are common in patients with *Pn. carinii* pneumonia and AIDS, eflornithine did appear to cause or exacerbate gastro-intestinal symptoms in some patients. The most serious adverse effect was bone marrow suppression and anaemia, leucopenia, and thrombocytopenia were noted; frequent monitoring of erythrocyte, leucocyte, and platelet counts is indicated. Other adverse effects noted were elevated serum transaminase, creatine kinase, and lactic dehydrogenase levels, alopecia, and dysgeusia.— T. M. Gilman *et al.* (letter), *J. Am. med. Ass.*, 1986, *256*, 2197.

Comment on drugs, including eflornithine, being evaluated on an experimental basis for the treatment of *Pneumocystis carinii* pneumonia in AIDS patients. Eflornithine has been released on a compassionate-use basis by the manufacturer to more than 100 patients, 33% of whom responded, but a randomised clinical trial is needed to evaluate its efficacy and toxicity.— V. T. DeVita *et al.*, *Ann. intern. Med.*, 1987, *106*, 568.

Further references: J. A. Golden *et al.*, *West. J. Med.*, 1984, *141*, 613.

TRYPANOSOMIASIS. In a preliminary study in the Sudan in 20 patients with African trypanosomiasis due to *Trypanosoma brucei gambiense*, eflornithine appeared to be remarkably effective in treating early- and late-stage infection, including late-stage infection refractory to arsenical treatment. Eflornithine hydrochloride was administered orally approximately every 6 hours and doses were chosen empirically. In 13 patients with late-stage refractory disease, treatment with 400 mg per kg body-weight daily for at least a month (32 to 44 days) resulted in a consistent decrease in CSF white blood cell count and protein concentration and the disappearance of parasites. Side-effects were frequent and included diarrhoea (13 patients), abdominal discomfort (10), vomiting (3), dizziness (2), arthralgia (2), and numbness of the limbs (1); convulsions in 2 patients were probably related to the disease. Erythrocyte counts decreased more than 30% in 3 of the 10 patients in which they were measured. Relapses were seen at 3, 7, and 10.5 months in 3 of the 11 patients followed for up to 23 months. Of 2 patients with late-stage infection without previous treatment, one relapsed 10 weeks after receiving eflornithine hydrochloride 258 mg per kg daily for 44 days and the other was still free of parasites 23 months after the end of treatment with 266 mg per kg daily for 37 days. In 2 patients with early-stage infection without previous treatment eflornithine hydrochloride 218 mg per kg daily for 42 days or 203 mg per kg daily for 45 days, respectively, eliminated parasites and reversed clinical symptoms; no side-effects were noted. Additional clinical studies are necessary to establish optimal dosage for each stage of the disease.— S. Van Nieuwenhove *et al.*, *Trans. R. Soc. trop. Med. Hyg.*, 1985, *79*, 692.

A report of the successful use of eflornithine hydrochloride 400 mg per kg body-weight daily by continuous intravenous infusion for 14 days followed by 75 mg per kg every 6 hours by mouth for 30 days in a patient with late-stage African trypanosomiasis due to *Trypanosoma brucei gambiense*.— C. di Bari *et al.* (letter), *Ann. intern. Med.*, 1986, *105*, 803.

Eflornithine proved effective in 2 patients with early-stage and 3 patients with late-stage African trypanosomiasis due to *Trypanosoma brucei gambiense*. It was administered either by continuous intravenous infusion at a dosage not exceeding 30 g daily (range, 350 to 600 mg per kg body-weight) or by mouth as a powder dissolved in water or fruit juice at an initial dosage of 15 to 20 g daily (range, 175 to 300 mg per kg) in divided doses; the dose was reduced if necessary according to digestive tolerance. Four patients received eflornithine intravenously initially, followed by oral therapy; the fifth received oral therapy only. Improvement was particularly impressive in one patient with terminal-stage disease who made an almost complete recovery. Side-effects were negligible and spontaneously reversible, and included loose stools in 3 patients and anaemia and hearing loss in 1. Pharmacokinetic studies in 3 patients demonstrated good absorption of eflornithine from the gastro-intestinal tract and diffusion into the CSF. Penetration of eflornithine into the CSF appeared to be more or less proportional to the degree of CNS involvement since the highest concentration was obtained in the most severe form of the disease. It was concluded that large clinical trials of eflornithine are warranted to establish optimal treatment regimens in early- and late-stage disease.— H. Taelman *et al.*, *Am. J. Med.*, 1987, *82*, 607.

Further references: J. Pepin *et al.*, *Lancet*, 1987, *2*, 1431.

For a brief description of African trypanosomiasis and WHO guidelines for its treatment, see p.658.

Proprietary Names and Manufacturers
Merrell Dow, USA.

4782-d

Emetine Hydrochloride *(BANM, USAN).*

Cloridrato de Emetina; Emet. Hydrochlor.; Emetine Dihydrochloride; Emetine Hydrochloride Heptahydrate; Emetini Chloridum; Emetini Hydrochloridum; Emetini Hydrochloridum Heptahydricum; Ipecine Hydrochloride; Methylcephaëline Hydrochloride. 6′,7′,10,11-Tetramethoxyemetan dihydrochloride heptahydrate; (2*S*,3*R*,11b*S*-)-3-Ethyl-1,3,4,6,7,11b-hexahydro-9,10-dimethoxy-2-[(1*R*)-1,2,3,4-tetrahydro-6,7-dimethoxy-1-isoquinolylmethyl]-2*H*-benzo[*a*]quinolizine dihydrochloride heptahydrate.
$C_{29}H_{40}N_2O_4,2HCl,7H_2O=679.7$.

CAS — 483-18-1 (emetine); 316-42-7 (hydrochloride, anhydrous); 7083-71-8 (hydrochloride, hydrate); 79300-08-6 (hydrochloride, heptahydrate).

Pharmacopoeias. In *Arg., Aust., Belg., Br., Braz., Cz., Eur., Egypt., Fr., Ger., Ind., Int., It., Jug., Mex., Neth., Nord., Port., Roum., Rus., Span., Swiss,* and *Turk. Belg., Eur., Fr., Neth.,* and *Swiss* also have a monograph for Emetine Hydrochloride Pentahydrate. *It.* permits the heptahydrate or pentahydrate. *U.S.* has a monograph for the anhydrous salt. Many others specify a variable proportion of water of crystallisation.

The dihydrochloride of an alkaloid obtained from ipecacuanha, or prepared by methylation of cephaëline (another alkaloid present in ipecacuanha), or prepared synthetically.

A white or slightly yellow odourless crystalline powder.

Freely **soluble** in water, alcohol, and chloroform. A 2% solution in water has a pH of 4.0 to 6.0. The *B.P.* injection has a pH of 2.7 to 4.0; the *U.S.P.* injection has a pH of 3.0 to 5.0. Solutions are **sterilised** by heating in an autoclave. **Store** in a well-closed container. Protect from light.

The stability of emetine hydrochloride in solution: C. Schuyt *et al.*, *Pharm. Weekbl. Ned.*, 1977, *112*, 1125; *idem*, 1979, *114*, 186.

Adverse Effects

Administration of emetine hydrochloride is commonly associated with aching, tenderness, stiffness, and weakness of the muscles in the area of the injection site; there may be necrosis and abscess formation. After injection diarrhoea and nausea and vomiting, sometimes accompanied by dizziness and headache, are common. There may be generalised muscle weakness and muscular pain, especially in the neck and limbs, and, more rarely, mild sensory disturbances. Eczematous, urticarial, and purpuric skin lesions have been reported.

Cardiovascular effects are considered the most serious and include precordial pain, dyspnoea, tachycardia, and hypotension. Changes in the ECG, particularly flattening or inversion of the T-wave and prolongation of the Q-T interval, occur in many patients. Emetine accumulates in the body and large doses or prolonged administration may cause lesions of the heart, gastro-intestinal tract, kidneys, liver, and skeletal muscle. Severe acute degenerative myocarditis may occur and may give rise to sudden cardiac failure and death. In some patients cardiotoxic effects have appeared after the completion of treatment with therapeutic doses.

Emetine hydrochloride is very irritant and contact with mucous membranes should be avoided.

Precautions

Emetine is contra-indicated in cardiac, renal, or neuromuscular disease. Its use should be avoided during pregnancy and it should not be given to children, except in severe amoebic dysentery unresponsive to other drugs. It should be used with great caution in old or debilitated patients. Patients receiving emetine should be closely supervised; ECG monitoring is advisable during treatment.

Absorption and Fate

After injection emetine hydrochloride is concentrated in the liver. Appreciable concentration occurs also in kidney, lung, and spleen. Excretion is slow and detectable concentrations may persist in urine 40 to 60 days after treatment has been discontinued. Cumulation may occur.

Uses and Administration

Emetine, an alkaloid of ipecacuanha, is a tissue amoebicide acting principally in the bowel wall and in the liver. It is used in the treatment of severe intestinal amoebiasis and hepatic amoebiasis although metronidazole, which is less toxic, is generally preferred. In patients with symptomatic intestinal amoebiasis emetine is administered in conjunction with an amoebicide that acts in the bowel lumen (a luminal amoebicide), such as diloxanide furoate, and in those with hepatic amoebiasis it is given in conjunction with a luminal amoebicide and chloroquine. For a description of amoebiasis and its treatment, see p.658.

Emetine hydrochloride is administered by deep subcutaneous or intramuscular injection in a dose of 1 mg per kg body-weight daily, but not exceeding 60 mg daily, generally for up to 5 days; courses should not be longer than 10 days or repeated at intervals of less than 6 weeks. Children may be given 500 µg per kg body-weight twice daily (up to a maximum of 60 mg daily) for up to 5 days. Dosage should be reduced in elderly or debilitated patients. It is advisable for the patient to remain in bed during the emetine treatment and a careful watch should be kept on cardiac function with ECG monitoring; strenuous exercise should be avoided for several weeks.

Emetine was formerly administered by mouth as emetine and bismuth iodide.

Preparations

Emetine Hydrochloride Injection *(U.S.P.)*

Emetine Injection *(B.P.)*. Contains emetine hydrochloride. When prepared from the pentahydrate the strength is stated as the equivalent amount of the heptahydrate.

Proprietary Names and Manufacturers

Hemometina *(Cusi, Spain)*;
Manufacturers also include—*Lilly, USA.*

The following names have been used for multi-ingredient preparations containing emetine hydrochloride— Cophylac Expectorant *(Hoechst, Canad.)*.

12705-w

Ethopabate *(BAN).*

Methyl 4-acetamido-2-ethoxybenzoate.
$C_{12}H_{15}NO_4=237.3$.

CAS — 59-06-3.

Pharmacopoeias. In *B.P. Vet.*

A white or pinkish-white, odourless or almost odourless powder. Very slightly **soluble** in water; soluble 1 in 30 of alcohol, 1 in 10 of chloroform, and 1 in 15 of methyl alcohol; slightly soluble in ether.

Ethopabate is an antiprotozoal agent used in veterinary practice, usually in conjunction with other agents such as amprolium, pyrimethamine, or sulfaquinoxaline, for the control of coccidiosis in poultry.

Proprietary Veterinary Names and Manufacturers
Merck Sharp & Dohme, UK.

4783-n

Etofamide *(rINN).*

Ethychlordiphene; K-430. 2,2-Dichloro-*N*-(2-ethoxyethyl)-*N*-[4-(4-nitrophenoxy)benzyl]acetamide.
$C_{19}H_{20}Cl_2N_2O_5=427.3$.

CAS — 25287-60-9.

Etofamide, a dichloroacetamide derivative, is a luminal amoebicide with actions and uses similar to those of diloxanide furoate (see p.663). It is available in some countries as tablets of 200 mg for use in the treatment of intestinal amoebiasis.

Proprietary Names and Manufacturers
Kitnos *(Carlo Erba, Ital.)*.

4784-h

Furazolidone *(BAN, USAN, rINN).*

Nifurazolidonum. 3-(5-Nitrofurfurylideneamino)-2-oxazolidone.
$C_8H_7N_3O_5=225.2$.

CAS — 67-45-8.

Pharmacopoeias. In *Br., Braz., Cz., Egypt., Fr., Ind., It., Nord., Roum., Rus.,* and *U.S.* Also in *B.P. Vet.*

A yellow odourless or almost odourless crystalline powder. Very slightly **soluble** in water and alcohol; slightly soluble in chloroform; practically insoluble in ether. The filtrate from a 1% suspension in water has a pH of 4.5 to 7.0. **Store** in airtight containers. Protect from light.

Adverse Effects

The most common adverse effects of furazolidone involve the gastro-intestinal tract and include nausea and vomiting. Dizziness, drowsiness, headache, and a general malaise have also been reported.

Allergic reactions, most commonly skin reactions such as rashes or angioedema, may occur. There have been instances of acute pulmonary reactions, similar to those seen with the structurally related drug nitrofurantoin, and of hepatotoxicity. Agranulocytosis has been reported rarely. Haemolytic anaemia may occur in patients with a deficiency of glucose-6-phosphate dehydrogenase given furazolidone.

Darkening of the urine has been attributed to the presence of metabolites.

Precautions

Furazolidone is contra-indicated in patients known to be hypersensitive to it. Because of the risk of haemolytic anaemia it should be used with caution in those with glucose-6-phosphate dehydrogenase deficiency and should not be given to infants under one month of age since their enzyme systems are immature.

Interactions. A disulfiram-like reaction has been reported in patients taking alcohol while on furazolidone therapy; alcohol should be avoided during and for a short period after treatment with furazolidone.

Furazolidone is a monoamine oxidase inhibitor and the cautions advised for these inhibitors regarding the concomitant administration of other drugs, especially indirect acting sympathomimetic amines, and the consumption of food and drink containing tyramine should be observed (see Phenelzine Sulphate, p.378). However, there have been no reports of hypertensive crises in patients receiving furazolidone and it has been suggested (W.A. Pettinger *et al.*, *Clin. Pharmac. Ther.*, 1968, *9*, 442) that, since furazolidone inhibits monoamine oxidase gradually over several days, the risks are small if treatment is limited to a 5-day course. Toxic psychosis has been reported in a patient receiving furazolidone and amitriptyline (R.M. Aderhold and C.E. Muniz, *J. Am. med. Ass.*, 1970, *213*, 2080).

Absorption and Fate

Most of a dose of furazolidone passes through the intestinal tract without being absorbed, although coloured metabolites have been noted in the urine.

Uses and Administration

Furazolidone is a nitrofuran derivative with antiprotozoal and antibacterial activity. It is active against the protozoan *Giardia intestinalis* (*Giardia lamblia*) and against a range of enteric bacteria *in vitro*, including staphylococci, enterococci, *Escherichia coli*, *Salmonella* spp., *Shigella* spp., and *Vibrio cholerae*. Furazolidone is bactericidal and appears to act by interfering with bacterial enzyme systems. Resistance is reported to be limited.

Furazolidone is used in the treatment of giardiasis and is given by mouth in a dose of 100 mg four times daily for 7 to 10 days; children may be given 1.25 mg per kg body-weight four times daily. It has also been given in diarrhoea and gastro-enteritis of bacterial origin in similar doses, but treatment is generally restricted to a period of 2 to 5 days.

Reviews of the actions and uses of furazolidone.— R. E. Chamberlain, *J. antimicrob. Chemother.*, 1976, *2*, 325; K. F. Phillips and F. J. Hailey, *J. int. med. Res.*, 1986, *14*, 19.

ENTERIC BACTERIAL INFECTIONS. Furazolidone had a broad spectrum of activity *in vitro* against bacterial pathogens associated with acute diarrhoea. Minimum inhibitory concentrations for 90% of strains of *Salmonella* spp., *Shigella* spp., enterotoxigenic *Escherichia coli*, *Campylobacter jejuni*, *Aeromonas hydrophila*, *Plesiomonas shigelloides*, and *Vibrio parahaemolyticus* ranged from about 0.5 to 2 µg per mL; it was much less active against *Yersinia enterocolitica*, the MIC being 128 µg per mL.— J. R. Carlson *et al.*, *Antimicrob. Ag. Chemother.*, 1983, *24*, 509.

Of 232 strains of enteropathogenic *Escherichia coli* only 1 was resistant to furazolidone at a concentration of 20 µg per mL.— R. J. Gross *et al.*, *Br. med. J.*, 1982, *285*, 472. Of 2753 strains of *Shigella dysenteriae*, *S. flexneri*, and *S. boydii* only 1 was resistant to furazolidone at a concentration of 20 µg per mL.— R. J. Gross *et al.*, *ibid.*, 1984, *288*, 784. See also S. C. Pal (letter), *Lancet*, 1984, *1*, 1462.

In a double-blind study furazolidone 100 mg four times daily for 5 days was more effective than ampicillin 500 mg four times daily for 5 days in the treatment of acute traveller's diarrhoea, but not dramatically so.— H. L. DuPont *et al.*, *Antimicrob. Ag. Chemother.*, 1984, *26*, 160. In a review of the prophylaxis and treatment of traveller's diarrhoea it was noted that furazolidone has the advantage of a broad spectrum of activity including *Campylobacter* and *Giardia*. An antimicrobial agent should probably be given to patients with moderate to severe diarrhoea and other disabling symptoms. Although not as effective, furazolidone can be used as an alternative to treatment with co-trimoxazole.— H. L. DuPont *et al.*, *Ann. intern. Med.*, 1985, *102*, 260.

ENTERIC PROTOZOAL INFECTIONS. In a study of AIDS patients with enteric coccidiosis, 1 of 2 patients with isosporiasis responded to treatment with furazolidone 100 mg four times daily for 10 days, but subsequently relapsed and was successfully treated with a prolonged course of co-trimoxazole. None of 3 patients with cryptosporidiosis responded to furazolidone.— M. E. Whiteside *et al.*, *Am. J. trop. Med. Hyg.*, 1984, *33*, 1065.

Giardiasis. The view that furazolidone should be tried if metronidazole fails to eradicate giardiasis.—D. R. Bell, *Br. med. J.*, 1985, *291*, 815.

In a study of 22 children with giardiasis, 11 of 12 were cured when given furazolidone 8 mg per kg body-weight daily (as a suspension) in 3 divided doses for 10 days compared to only 2 of 10 who received similar treatment for 5 days. The authors conclude that furazolidone treatment for less than 7 to 10 days cannot be recommended for children with giardiasis.— T. V. Murphy and J. D. Nelson, *Am. J. Dis. Child.*, 1983, *137*, 267.

For a brief description of giardiasis and its treatment, see p.659.

For a comparative study *in vitro* of the activity of various drugs, including furazolidone, against *Giardia intestinalis*, see Metronidazole, p.671.

LEISHMANIASIS. Furazolidone has been reported to be active *in vitro* against *Leishmania tropica* (J.D. Berman and L.S. Lees, *Am. J. trop. Med. Hyg.*, 1983, *32*, 947), but 7 of 8 patients with cutaneous leishmaniasis attributed to *Leishmania braziliensis braziliensis* failed to respond to treatment with furazolidone 8 mg per kg body-weight daily for 10 days.—J. M. L. Costa *et al.*, *Trans. R. Soc. trop. Med. Hyg.*, 1985, *79*, 274.

PEPTIC ULCER. Beneficial results with furazolidone in the treatment of peptic ulcer.— Z. -T. Zheng *et al.* (letter), *Lancet*, 1985, *1*, 1048; H. -Y. Zhao *et al.* (letter), *ibid.*, *2*, 276. *Campylobacter pylori* (*C. pyloridis*) was very sensitive to furazolidone in a study *in vitro*, supporting the possibility that its effect on peptic ulcer healing could be related to this antibacterial activity.— A. Howden *et al.* (letter), *ibid.*, 1986, *2*, 1035.

For further reference to the possible association between *Campylobacter pylori* and peptic ulcer, see Metronidazole, p.671.

Preparations

Furazolidone Oral Suspension *(U.S.P.)*

Furazolidone Tablets *(U.S.P.)*

Proprietary Names and Manufacturers

Dialidene *(Ital.)*; Enterar *(Arnaldi, Ital.)*; Furoxane *(Oberval, Fr.)*; Furoxona *(Arg.)*; Furoxone *(Norwich-Eaton, Austral.*; *Belg.*; *Formenti, Ital.*; *Neth.*; *Eaton, S.Afr.*; *Norwich-Eaton, UK*; *Norwich Eaton, USA)*; Giardil *(Arg.)*; Intefuran *(Crosara, Ital.)*; Sirben *(Arg.)*; Tricofuron *(Fr.)*; Trifurox *(Norw.)*.

The following names have been used for multi-ingredient preparations containing furazolidone— Tricofuron *(Norwich Eaton, USA)*.

NOTE. The name Tricofuron has also been used to denote preparations containing only furazolidone.

12813-j

Halofuginone Hydrobromide *(BANM, USAN, rINNM).*
RU-19110. (±)-*trans*-7-Bromo-6-chloro-3-[3-(3-hydroxy-2-piperidyl)acetonyl]quinazolin-4(3*H*)-one hydrobromide.
$C_{16}H_{17}BrClN_3O_3$, HBr=495.6.

CAS — 55837-20-2 (halofuginone); 64924-67-0 (hydrobromide).

Halofuginone hydrobromide is an antiprotozoal agent used in veterinary practice for the prevention of coccidiosis in poultry.

Proprietary Veterinary Names and Manufacturers
Stenorol *(Hoechst Animal Health, UK)*.

4785-m

Halquinol *(BAN).*
Chlorhydroxyquinoline; Chlorquinol; Halquinols *(USAN)*; SQ-16401. A mixture of the chlorinated products of quinolin-8-ol containing 57 to 74% of 5,7-dichloroquinolin-8-ol (chloroxine), 23 to 40% of 5-chloroquinolin-8-ol (cloxyquin), and not more than 4% of 7-chloroquinolin-8-ol.

CAS — 8067-69-4 (halquinol); 773-76-2 (5,7-dichloroquinolin-8-ol).

Pharmacopoeias. Cz. has Chlorchinolinolum, a mixture of 5-chloro-and 5,7-dichloroquinolin-8-ol.

Halquinol is a halogenated hydroxyquinoline with properties similar to those of clioquinol (p.661). It was formerly given in the treatment of intestinal amoebiasis and other infective diarrhoeas.

Halquinol has been used topically in infected skin conditions and one of its constituents, 5,7-dichloroquinolin-8-ol (chloroxine), is applied as a cream in the treatment of dandruff and seborrhoeic dermatitis of the scalp.

Proprietary Names and Manufacturers
Capitrol *(Westwood, USA)*; Quixalin *(Squibb, S.Afr.*; *Squibb, UK)*; Quixaline *(Squibb, Belg.*; *Squibb, Fr.)*.

The following names have been used for multi-ingredient preparations containing halquinol— Remiderm *(Squibb, UK)*; Remotic *(Squibb, UK)*; Tardrox *(Carlton Laboratories, UK)*; Tarquinor *(Squibb, Austral.)*.

12826-t

Homidium Bromide *(BAN, rINN).*
Ethidium Bromide; RD-1572. 3,8-Diamino-5-ethyl-6-phenylphenanthridinium bromide.
$C_{21}H_{20}BrN_3$=394.3.

CAS — 1239-45-8.

Pharmacopoeias. In *B.P. Vet.*

A dark purple, odourless or almost odourless, crystalline or amorphous powder. **Soluble** 1 in 20 of water; slightly soluble in chloroform. A 2% solution in water has a pH of 4.0 to 7.0.

Homidium bromide is a trypanocide used in veterinary medicine.

12844-r

Imidocarb Hydrochloride *(BANM, USAN, rINNM).*
4A65. 3,3′-Di(2-imidazolin-2-yl)carbanilide dihydrochloride; 1,3-Bis[3-(2-imidazolin-2-yl)phenyl]urea dihydrochloride.
$C_{19}H_{20}N_6O$,2HCl=421.3.

CAS — 27885-92-3 (imidocarb); 5318-76-3 (hydrochloride).

Imidocarb hydrochloride is an antiprotozoal agent used in veterinary practice in the treatment of babesiosis. Imidocarb dipropionate has also been used.

Proprietary Veterinary Names and Manufacturers
Wellcome, USA.

12863-n

Ipronidazole *(BAN, USAN, rINN).*
M&B-16905; NSC-109212; Ro-7-1554. 2-Isopropyl-1-methyl-5-nitroimidazole.
$C_7H_{11}N_3O_2$=169.2.

CAS — 14885-29-1.

Ipronidazole is a 5-nitroimidazole derivative similar to metronidazole. It has been used in veterinary practice in the management of blackhead (histomoniasis) in turkeys.

Proprietary Veterinary Names and Manufacturers
Ipropran *(Roche, USA).*

12890-b

Lasalocid Sodium *(BANM, rINNM).*
Ro-02-2985 (lasalocid). An antibiotic produced by *Streptomyces lasaliensis.* Sodium 6-[(3*R*,4*S*,5*S*,7*R*)-7-{(2*S*,3*S*,5*S*)-5-ethyl-5-[(2*R*,5*R*,6*S*)-5-ethyltetrahydro-5-hydroxy-6-methyl-2*H*-pyran-2-yl]tetrahydro-3-methyl-2-furyl}-4-hydroxy-3,5-dimethyl-6-oxononyl]-2-hydroxy-*m*-toluate.
$C_{34}H_{53}NaO_8$=612.8.

CAS — 11054-70-9 (lasalocid); 25999-31-9 (lasalocid); 25999-20-6 (lasalocid sodium).

NOTE. Lasalocid is *USAN.*

Lasalocid sodium is an antiprotozoal agent used in veterinary practice for the prevention of coccidiosis in poultry.

Proprietary Veterinary Names and Manufacturers
Avatec *(Roche, UK).*

792-c

Meglumine Antimonate
Antimony Meglumine; Meglumine Antimoniate; Protostib; RP-2168. 1-Deoxy-1-methylamino-D-glucitol antimonate.
$C_7H_{18}NO_8Sb$=366.0.

CAS — 6284-40-8 (meglumine); 133-51-7 (antimonate).

Meglumine antimonate is a pentavalent antimony compound with the properties of sodium stibogluconate (p.677) and is used similarly in the treatment of leishmaniasis. It is administered by deep intramuscular injection as a solution containing the equivalent of 85 mg of pentavalent antimony per mL. Doses are expressed in terms of pentavalent antimony and are generally as described under sodium stibogluconate.

A report of agranulocytosis occurring in a 23-month-old child during treatment of visceral leishmaniasis with meglumine antimonate. The child had received intramuscularly 20 mg per kg body-weight for 2 days, 40 mg per kg for 2 days, and 60 mg per kg for 3 days.— P. Bourée and O. Dulac, *Archs fr. Pédiat.*, 1977, *34*, 659.

Proprietary Names and Manufacturers
Glucantim *(Farmitalia, Ital.)*; Glucantime *(Specia, Fr.; Spain).*

4787-v

Melarsonyl Potassium *(BAN, rINN).*
Mel W; Melarsenoxide Potassium Dimercaptosuccinate; Pentylthiarsphenylmelamine; RP-9955. Dipotassium 2-[4-(4,6-diamino-1,3,5-triazin-2-ylamino)phenyl]-1,3,2-dithiarsolan-4,5-dicarboxylate.
$C_{13}H_{11}AsK_2N_6O_4S_2$=532.5.

CAS — 37526-80-0 (melarsonyl); 13355-00-5 (potassium salt).

Melarsonyl potassium is a water-soluble derivative of melarsoprol and may be administered by subcutaneous or intramuscular injection. It was formerly used in the treatment of African trypanosomiasis as an alternative to melarsoprol, but was probably more toxic and less effective.

Proprietary Names and Manufacturers
Trimélarsan *(Specia, Fr.).*

4788-g

Melarsoprol *(BAN, rINN).*
Mel B; Melarsen Oxide-BAL; RP-3854. 2-[4-(4,6-Diamino-1,3,5-triazin-2-ylamino)phenyl]-1,3,2-dithiarsolan-4-ylmethanol.
$C_{12}H_{15}AsN_6OS_2$=398.3.

CAS — 494-79-1.

Adverse Effects
Adverse effects are common and may be severe during the treatment of African trypanosomiasis with melarsoprol. It may be difficult to distinguish between effects of the disease, Herxheimer-type reactions resulting from the trypanocidal activity of melarsoprol, and adverse effects of the drug itself attributed to its arsenic content or to hypersensitivity. For the adverse effects of arsenic and their treatment, see Arsenic Trioxide, p.1544.

A severe febrile reaction may occur after the first injection of melarsoprol, especially in patients with large numbers of trypanosomes in their blood. It is therefore common practice to give one or two injections of suramin prior to starting melarsoprol therapy.

The greatest risk is from reactive encephalopathy which occurs in about 10% of patients treated with melarsoprol and is usually seen between the end of the first 3- or 4-day course of injections and the start of the second course. Some have attributed it to a toxic effect of melarsoprol and others to a Herxheimer-type reaction resulting from the release of antigen from trypanosomes killed in the brain; a combination of drug toxicity and host immune responses may be responsible. Encephalopathy may be sudden in onset or develop slowly. Symptoms include fever, headache, tremor, slurring of speech, convulsions, and coma; death has occurred in up to 5% of patients treated with melarsoprol. Less commonly, haemorrhagic encephalopathy may occur. The prophylactic use of corticosteroids has been suggested during treatment courses of melarsoprol, but is of no proven benefit. Treatment of reactive encephalopathy has included the use of corticosteroids, hypertonic solutions to combat cerebral oedema, anticonvulsants such as diazepam, and subcutaneous adrenaline; dimercaprol has been given on the assumption that encephalopathy resulted from arsenic poisoning, but has not generally been of benefit.

Hypersensitivity reactions to melarsoprol may occur during the second and subsequent courses of treatment. Desensitisation has been attempted by recommencing treatment with smaller and gradually increasing doses of melarsoprol; the concomitant administration of corticosteroids may help to control symptoms during this procedure. Some authorities consider that the use of small doses of melarsoprol may increase the risk of resistance.

Melarsoprol injection is very irritant and extravasation during intravenous administration should be avoided. Vomiting and abdominal colic may occur if it is injected too rapidly. Other adverse effects reported include peripheral neuropathy, albuminuria, severe diarrhoea, cardiac arrhythmias, exfoliative dermatitis, and hepatic disturbances.

Experience over the past 25 years indicates that reactive encephalopathy is an unpredictable risk of melarsoprol treatment for African trypanosomiasis and is not related to the dose. The associated use of corticosteroids did not reduce the incidence of this complication.—J. O. L. Arroz, *Trans R. Soc. trop. Med. Hyg.*, 1987, *81*, 192.

Precautions
Melarsoprol should not be administered during epidemics of influenza. Severe haemolytic reactions have been reported in patients with glucose-6-phosphate dehydrogenase deficiency. It may precipitate erythema nodosum when administered to patients with leprosy.

Patients should be in hospital when they are treated with melarsoprol and dosage decided after taking into account their general condition.

Absorption and Fate
Melarsoprol is reported to be fairly well absorbed if given by mouth but is usually given by intravenous injection. A small amount penetrates to the CSF where it has local trypanocidal action. It is rapidly excreted so any prophylactic effect is short-lived.

Uses and Administration
Melarsoprol, a trivalent arsenical derivative, is a trypanocide which appears to act by inhibiting trypanosomal pyruvate kinase. It is effective in the treatment of all stages of African trypanosomiasis due to *Trypanosoma brucei gambiense* or *T. brucei rhodesiense*, but because of its toxicity its use is usually reserved for later stages of the disease involving the central nervous system. Resistance has been reported to develop.

Patients undergoing therapy with melarsoprol should be treated in hospital. Melarsoprol is administered by intravenous injection as a 3.6% solution in propylene glycol. The injection should be given slowly, care being taken to prevent leakage into the surrounding tissues, and the patient should remain supine and fasting for at least 5 hours after the injection.

Treatment protocols vary, but in general melarsoprol is given in low doses initially, especially in children and debilitated patients, increased gradually to the maximum daily dose of 3.6 mg per kg body-weight. Doses are given daily for 3 or 4 days and the course repeated 2 or 3 times with an interval of at least 7 days between courses.

TRYPANOSOMIASIS. For a brief description of African trypanosomiasis and WHO guidelines for its treatment, including the use of melarsoprol, see p.658.

Proprietary Names and Manufacturers
Arsobal *(May & Baker, S.Afr.)*; Arsorbal *(Fr.).*

12946-b

Methyl Benzoquate *(BAN).*
AY-20385; ICI-55052; Nequinate *(USAN, pINN).*
Methyl 7-benzyloxy-6-butyl-1,4-dihydro-4-oxoquinoline-3-carboxylate.
$C_{22}H_{23}NO_4$=365.4.

CAS — 13997-19-8.

Methyl benzoquate is an antiprotozoal agent used in veterinary practice, in association with clopidol, for the prevention of coccidiosis in poultry.

16893-c

Metronidazole *(BAN, USAN, rINN).*
Bayer-5360; Metronidaz.; NSC-50364; RP-8823; SC-10295. 2-(2-Methyl-5-nitroimidazol-1-yl)ethanol.
$C_6H_9N_3O_3$=171.2.

CAS — 443-48-1.

Pharmacopoeias. In *Br., Braz., Chin., Cz., Egypt., Ind., Int., It., Jpn., Jug., Nord., Roum., and U.S.*
Also in *B.P. Vet.*

A white to pale yellow crystalline powder or crystals, odourless or with a slight odour. It darkens on exposure to light.

Slightly **soluble** in water, alcohol, chloroform, and in ether. The *U.S.P.* injection has a pH of 4.5 to 7.0. **Protect** from light.
See below for **incompatibilities**.

4757-f

Metronidazole Benzoate *(BAN)*.

Benzoyl Metronidazole; RP-9712. 2-(2-Methyl-5-nitroimidazol-1-yl)ethyl benzoate.
$C_{13}H_{13}N_3O_4$=275.3.
CAS — 13182-89-3.
Pharmacopoeias. In *Ind.*

4751-c

Metronidazole Hydrochloride *(USAN)*.

SC-32642.
$C_6H_9N_3O_3$,HCl=207.6.
CAS — 69198-10-3.

INCOMPATIBILITY. Metronidazole hydrochloride for intravenous infusion has a low pH of 0.5 to 2.0 when reconstituted and reacts with aluminium in equipment such as needles to produce a reddish-brown discoloration. Although occurring less readily with the diluted and neutralised infusion solution or with solutions of metronidazole base, precipitation and discoloration have been reported after contact with aluminium for 6 hours or more (K.H. Schell and J.R. Copeland, *Am. J. Hosp. Pharm.*, 1985, *42*, 1040; B.J. Struthers and R.J. Parr, *ibid.*, 2660).

Several studies have assessed the compatibility of antibiotic injections and other drugs when added to metronidazole solution for intravenous infusion. Results have varied according to the criteria applied and the conditions used. Because of shifts in pH benzylpenicillin potassium, cefoxitin sodium, and cephamandole nafate were considered to be physically incompatible with metronidazole and ampicillin sodium, cephalothin sodium, and hydrocortisone sodium succinate to be conditionally compatible (S. Bisaillon and R. Sarrazin, *J. parent. Sci. Technol.*, 1983, *37*, 129). However, when chemical stability was assessed benzylpenicillin potassium, cefoxitin sodium, and hydrocortisone sodium succinate were compatible with metronidazole, whereas ampicillin sodium and cephalothin sodium were incompatible (V.D. Gupta and K.R. Stewart, *ibid.*, 1985, *39*, 145); in a further study (V.D. Gupta *et al.*, *J. clin. Hosp. Pharm.*, 1985, *10*, 379) cephamandole nafate was also chemically incompatible.

Regardless of these studies, it is generally recommended that other drugs should not be added to intravenous solutions of metronidazole or its hydrochloride.

Adverse Effects

The adverse effects of metronidazole are generally dose-related. The most common are gastro-intestinal disturbances, especially nausea and an unpleasant metallic taste; nausea is sometimes accompanied by headache, anorexia, and vomiting. Diarrhoea, dry mouth, a furred tongue, glossitis, and stomatitis may also occur. There have been rare reports of pseudomembranous colitis associated with metronidazole.

Peripheral neuropathy, usually presenting as numbness or tingling in the extremities, and epileptiform seizures are serious adverse effects on the nervous system that have been associated especially with high doses of metronidazole or prolonged treatment. Weakness, dizziness, ataxia, drowsiness, insomnia, and changes in mood or mental state such as depression or confusion have also been reported.

Temporary moderate leucopenia may occur in some patients receiving metronidazole. Skin rashes and pruritus occur occasionally and anaphylaxis has been reported rarely. Other side-effects include urethral discomfort and darkening of the urine. Raised liver enzyme values have occasionally been reported. Thrombophlebitis may follow the intravenous administration of metronidazole.

Studies have shown metronidazole to be mutagenic in bacteria and carcinogenic in some *animals*.

A study involving 37 cancer patients given high oral doses of metronidazole in conjunction with radiation. Doses of 6 g per m^2 body-surface three times a week for 3 weeks were associated with a 50% incidence of gastro-intestinal toxicity, a 25% incidence of central nervous system toxicity, including dizziness, tremors, ataxia, and confusion, and a 6% incidence of neuropathies.— R. C. Urtasun *et al.*, *Surgery, St Louis*, 1983, *93*, 145.

ALLERGY. A serum-sickness-like syndrome, with arthralgias, myalgias, and malaise followed by fever, chills, and a pruritic rash, developed in a 32-year-old woman about 5 days after starting treatment with metronidazole; leucopenia and neutropenia also occurred. Symptoms resolved on the withdrawal of metronidazole.— C. W. Weart and L. C. Hyman, *Sth. med. J.*, 1983, *76*, 410.

CARCINOGENICITY AND MUTAGENICITY. Metronidazole is mutagenic in some strains of bacteria (C.E. Voogd *et al.*, *Mutat. Res.*, 1974, *26*, 483) and the urine of patients treated with metronidazole was found to be mutagenic in bacteria (W.T. Speck *et al.*, *J. natn. Cancer Inst.*, 1976, *56*, 283). However, although increased chromosome aberrations were noted in patients following prolonged treatment with relatively high doses of metronidazole (F. Mitelman *et al.*, *Lancet*, 1976, *2*, 802) no evidence of a cytogenic effect was found in a subsequent controlled study (F. Mitelman *et al.*, *ibid.*, 1980, *1* 1249). Tumours have been induced in *rats* and *mice* given metronidazole in chronic studies, but there was no appreciable increase in the incidence of cancer in a retrospective study of 771 patients given metronidazole for vaginal trichomoniasis (C.M. Beard *et al.*, *New Engl. J. Med.*, 1979, *301*, 519) nor in a similar study of 2460 patients (G.D. Friedman, *ibid.*, 1980, *302*, 519); longer term surveillance was considered necessary before the risk of carcinogenicity could, be excluded (F.E. Mirer and M.A. Silverstein, *ibid.*). Small amounts of acetamide, a weak carcinogen in *rats*, was found in the urine of 5 patients taking metronidazole (R.L. Koch *et al.*, *Science*, 1981, *211*, 398), but the authors stress that this should not be interpreted as evidence that metronidazole is carcinogenic in man.

From a review of the available evidence, Roe (*Surgery, St Louis*, 1983, *93*, 158) concluded that metronidazole can be used without fear of carcinogenic or mutagenic risk and is apparently free of teratogenic potential. Nevertheless, metronidazole is mutagenic in bacteria and carcinogenic in rodents and the long-term risks in man have not been evaluated completely. Metronidazole crosses the placenta and, in a summary of risk to the foetus (*Drugs in Pregnancy and Lactation*, 2nd Edn, G.C. Briggs *et al.* (Ed.), Baltimore, Williams & Wilkins, 1986, p. 292/m) it is noted that available reports on the safety of metronidazole in preganancy are conflicting and additional data is required before the risk can be assessed. See also under Pregnancy and the Neonate in Precautions (below).

EFFECTS ON THE BLOOD. A report of bone marrow aplasia, with leucopenia and markedly reduced erythropoiesis and granulopoiesis on examination of the bone marrow, in a 74-year-old man given metronidazole 200 mg three times daily for 7 days before and 10 days after operation.— C. M. White *et al.* (letter), *Br. med. J.*, 1980, *280*, 647.

Aplastic anaemia occurred in 2 patients who had previously received metronidazole.— R. Raman *et al.*, *Clinician*, 1982, *46*, 464.

EFFECTS ON THE GASTRO-INTESTINAL TRACT. Reports of pseudomembranous colitis associated with the administration of metronidazole.— G. Thomson *et al.*, *Br. med. J.*, 1981, *282*, 864; J. J. Daly and K. V. S. Chowdary, *Dig. Dis. Scis*, 1983, *28*, 573.

EFFECTS ON LIPID METABOLISM. A significant drop in serum concentrations of cholesterol and triglycerides was noted in a patient after 7 days of treatment with metronidazole 750 mg three times daily for giardiasis. The lipid-lowering effect was confirmed in 5 further patients receiving similar doses.— J. L. Davis *et al.*, *Ann. intern. Med.*, 1983, *99*, 43.

EFFECTS ON THE LIVER. Severely elevated liver enzyme values, consistent with a drug-induced hepatitis, occurred in a patient given metronidazole hydrochloride 500 mg every 6 hours intravenously for 4 days. He was also receiving cefapirin sodium and tobramycin sulphate.— D. H. Appleby and H. D. Vogtland, *Clin. Pharm.*, 1983, *2*, 373.

EFFECTS ON THE NERVOUS SYSTEM. On neurological examination, sensory peripheral neuropathy was found in 11 of 13 patients with Crohn's disease aged 12 to 22 years who had received metronidazole for 4 to 11 months to a total dose ranging from 92 to 257 g. At the time of the study daily doses ranged from 10 to 33 mg per kg body-weight. Five of the 11 with neuropathy complained of paraesthesias or hypoaesthesias in the lower extremities, 5 were asymptomatic, and one had reduced nerve conduction velocity but a normal neurological examination and no symptoms. The 11 patients with peripheral neuropathy were re-evaluated 6 to 12 months after metronidazole was either discontinued or the dose reduced. Of the 9 taken off metronidazole there was complete resolution of neuropathy in 5, improvement in 3, and no change in one. The 2 patients in whom dosage was reduced to 10 mg per kg daily were studied after 10 and 12 months respectively on the reduced dose; the neuropathy had worsened in one and resolved in the other.— L. F. Duffy *et al.*, *Gastroenterology*, 1985, *88*, 681.

Individual reports of neurological effects associated with metronidazole: A. J. Voth (letter), *Can. med. Ass. J.*, 1969, *100*, 1012 (agitated depression); A. J. Giannini (letter), *Am. J. Psychiat.*, 1977, *134*, 329 (depression); S. Frytak *et al.*, *Ann. intern. Med.*, 1978, *88*, 361 (major motor seizures associated with high-dose therapy); R. K. Kusumi *et al.*, *ibid.*, 1980, *93*, 59 (acute encephalopathy, cerebellar dysfunction with ataxia, and sensory neuropathy associated with high-dose therapy); J. J. Schentag *et al.*, *Pharmacotherapy*, 1982, *2*, 384 (confusion, hallucinations, and agitation associated with intravenous administration); T. J. Halloran, *Drug Intell. & clin. Pharm.*, 1982, *16*, 409 (convulsions associated with high cumulative doses); J. Bailes *et al.*, *Am. J. Dis. Child.*, 1983, *137*, 290 (grand mal seizures, mental changes, and neurophysiological abnormalities associated with intravenous administration); R. S. Alvarez *et al.*, *Am. J. Obstet. Gynec.*, 1983, *145*, 640 (toxic encephalopathy with agitation, confusion, and disorientation); A. D. Hibberd *et al.* (letter), *N.Z. med. J.*, 1984, *97*, 128 (temporary sensorineural deafness); M. Wienbren *et al.* (letter), *J. clin. Path.*, 1985, *38*, 1076 (epileptiform seizures, encephalopathy, and urinary retention, probably a result of sensory neuropathy, associated with a high cumulative dose); B. Kirkham and J. Gott, *Br. med. J.*, 1986, *292*, 174 (oculogyric crisis).

EFFECTS ON THE PANCREAS. A report of acute pancreatitis associated with the administration of metronidazole; there was no evidence of a hypersensitivity reaction.— B. H. Plotnick *et al.*, *Ann. intern. Med.*, 1985, *103*, 891.

GYNAECOMASTIA. Gynaecomastia occurred in a 36-year-old man with ulcerative colitis after taking metronidazole 250 mg three times daily for about a month.— T. C. Fagan *et al.*, *J. Am. med. Ass.*, 1985, *254*, 3217.

PREGNANCY AND THE NEONATE. See Carcinogenicity and Mutagenicity (above).

Precautions

Metronidazole should be used with great care in patients with blood dyscrasias or with active disease of the central nervous system. All patients receiving metronidazole for more than 10 days should be monitored and treatment discontinued if signs of peripheral neuropathy or CNS toxicity develop. Doses should be reduced in patients with severe liver disease.

It is suggested that the use of metronidazole should be avoided during pregnancy, especially the first trimester. Some authorities consider that women taking metronidazole should not breast-feed their babies.

Interactions. When given in conjunction with *alcohol*, metronidazole may provoke a disulfiram-like reaction in some individuals; reactions have occurred after the administration of pharmaceutical preparations formulated with alcohol, including injections (*Drug Interact. News.*, 1987, *7*, 19), as well as after drinking alcohol. Acute psychoses or confusion have been associated with the concomitant use of metronidazole and *disulfiram* (E. Rothstein and D.D. Clancy, *New Engl. J. Med.*, 1969, *280*, 1006).

Although metronidazole had no effect on the elimination of antipyrine in healthy subjects (C. Staiger *et al.*, *Br. J. clin. Pharmac.*, 1984, *17*, 627P; J.C. Jensen and R. Gugler, *Clin. Pharmac. Ther.*, 1985, *37*, 407) and, by inference, has little effect on hepatic drug-metabolising enzymes, it enhances the anticoagulant effect of *warfarin* (see p.346) and may impair the clearance of *phenytoin* (see p.409). There is some evidence that phenytoin might accelerate the metabolism of metronidazole (L.A. Wheeler *et al.*, *Antimicrob. Ag. Chemother.*, 1978, *13*, 205). Plasma concentrations of metronidazole are decreased by the concomitant administration of *phenobarbitone*, with a consequent reduction in the effectiveness of metronidazole (P.B. Mead *et al.*, *New Engl. J. Med.*, 1982, *306*, 1490; S. Gupte, *ibid.*, 1983, *308*, 529). *Cimetidine* has increased plasma concentrations of metronidazole and might increase the risk of neurological side-effects (R. Gugler and J.C. Jensen, *New Engl. J. Med.*, 1983, *309*, 1518).

Metronidazole may interfere with the measurement of liver enzymes in blood to produce abnormally low results (J.P. Rissing *et al.*, *Antimicrob. Ag. Chemother.*, 1978, *14*, 636) and may interfere with the hexokinase method of measuring blood-glucose concentrations. It has also been reported to interfere with assays for blood concentrations of procainamide (R.H. Gannon and L.R. Phillips, *Am. J. Hosp. Pharm.*, 1982, *39*, 1966) and theophylline (D. Garfinkel *et al.*, *Ann. intern. Med.*, 1987, *106*, 171).

Metronidazole has anti-treponemal activity and may mask the immunological response seen in untreated early syphilis (R.S. Pattman and M.S. Sprott, *Eur. J. sex. transm. Dis.*, 1985, *2*, 73); contacts of syphilis receiving metronidazole should probably be screened for an additional 4 to 8 weeks.

For incompatibilities between metronidazole and other drugs in solutions for injection, see above.

ADMINISTRATION. For administration of metronidazole in the elderly, in hepatic failure, and in renal failure, see under Uses (below).

PORPHYRIA. Metronidazole was considered to be unsafe in patients with acute porphyria because it has been shown to be porphyrinogenic in *animals* or *in vitro* systems.— M.R. Moore and K.E.L. McColl, *Porphyrias, Drug Lists*, Glasgow, Porphyria Research Unit, University of Glasgow, 1987.

PREGNANCY AND THE NEONATE. A summary of the use of metronidazole during pregnancy and lactation. Metronidazole is mutagenic in bacteria and carcinogenic in *rodents*. It crosses the placenta to the foetus and its use in pregnancy is controversial. Additional data needs to be collected before the risk to the foetus can be assessed. However, the manufacturer and the Center for Disease Control consider metronidazole to be contra-indicated during the first trimester in patients with trichomoniasis; use for trichomoniasis during the second and third trimesters may be acceptable if alternative therapies have failed, but single-dose therapy should be avoided. For other indications the risks and benefits of treatment with metronidazole should be weighed carefully, especially in the first trimester. Metronidazole is excreted in breast milk and, since unnecessary exposure to the drug should be avoided, a single 2-g oral dose has been recommended for the treatment of trichomoniasis in mothers who are breast-feeding; if this dose is given the American Academy of Pediatrics (*Pediatrics*, 1983, *72*, 375) recommends discontinuing breast-feeding for 12 to 24 hours to allow excretion of the drug.— *Drugs in Pregnancy and Lactation*, 2nd Edn, G.C. Briggs *et al.* (Ed.), Baltimore, Williams & Wilkins, 1986, p. 292/m.

The view that metronidazole, given to nursing mothers, appears to be safe for the baby but causes the milk to have a bitter taste which may impair feeding.— P. C. Rubin, *Br. med. J.*, 1986, *293*, 1415.

See also Carcinogenicity and Mutagenicity in Adverse Effects (above).

For reference to the pharmacokinetics of metronidazole in neonates, see under Administration in Infants and Children in Absorption and Fate (below).

Absorption and Fate

Metronidazole is readily absorbed following administration by mouth and bioavailability approaches 100%. Peak plasma concentrations of approximately 5 and 10 µg per mL are achieved an average of 1 hour after single doses of 250 and 500 mg respectively. Some accumulation and consequently higher concentrations occur when multiple doses are given. Concentrations may vary according to the type of assay used. Absorption may be delayed, but is not reduced overall by administration with food. Metronidazole benzoate is also given by mouth and is hydrolysed in the gastro-intestinal tract to release metronidazole, which is then absorbed.

Following the intravenous administration of metronidazole, peak steady-state plasma concentrations of about 25 µg per mL with trough concentrations of about 18 µg per mL have been reported in patients given a loading dose of 15 mg per kg body-weight followed by 7.5 mg per kg every 6 hours. The bioavailability of metronidazole from rectal suppositories is 60 to 80%; peak plasma concentrations are half those achieved with equivalent oral doses and occur after about 4 hours. Absorption from vaginal pessaries has been reported to be poor.

Metronidazole is widely distributed. It appears in most body tissues and fluids including bile, bone, breast milk, cerebral abscesses, cerebrospinal fluid, liver and liver abscesses, saliva, seminal fluid, and vaginal secretions, and achieves concentrations similar to those in plasma. It also crosses the placenta and rapidly enters the foetal circulation. No more than 20% is bound to plasma proteins.

Metronidazole is metabolised in the liver by side-chain oxidation and glucuronide formation. The principal oxidative metabolites are 1-(2-hydroxyethyl)-2-hydroxymethyl-5-nitroimidazole (the 'hydroxy' metabolite), which has antibacterial activity and is detected in plasma and urine, and 2-methyl-5-nitroimidazole-1-acetic acid (the 'acid' metabolite), which has virtually no antibacterial activity and is often not detected in plasma, but is excreted in urine. Small amounts of reduced metabolites, acetamide and *N*-(2-hydroxyethyl)oxamic acid (HOA), have also been detected in urine and are probably formed by the intestinal flora.

The plasma elimination half-life of metronidazole is about 8 hours; that of the hydroxy metabolite is slightly longer. The half-life of metronidazole is reported to be longer in neonates and in patients with severe liver disease; that of the hydroxy metabolite is prolonged in patients with renal failure.

The majority of a dose of metronidazole is excreted in the urine, mainly as metabolites; a small amount appears in the faeces. Depending on the assay method used, up to 80% of a dose has been recovered in the urine within 48 hours.

A detailed review of the pharmacokinetics of metronidazole, including a brief description of the assay methods used. Reported metronidazole concentrations can vary considerably depending on the type of assay used. There are three major types: non-specific chemical assays, such as polarographic, spectrophotometric, and absorptiometric assays, in which all compounds containing a nitro group, including metronidazole and its major oxidative metabolites are measured collectively; bioassays using *Trichomonas vaginalis* or anaerobic bacteria as the test organisms, but unable to distinguish between metronidazole and any bioactive metabolites; and specific chromatographic assay techniques in which metronidazole and its major metabolites can be measured separately. High pressure liquid chromatography (HPLC) has provided most of the recent data on the metabolites of metronidazole.— E. D. Ralph, *Clin. Pharmacokinet.*, 1983, *8*, 43.

References to studies on the pharmacokinetics of metronidazole: I. Amon *et al.*, *Int. J. clin. Pharmac.*, 1978, *16*, 384; G. W. Houghton *et al.*, *Br. J. clin. Pharmac.*, 1979, *8*, 337; J. C. Jensen and R. Gugler, *Clin. Pharmac. Ther.*, 1983, *34*, 481.

References to studies on the pharmacokinetics of metronidazole after administration as metronidazole benzoate: G. W. Houghton *et al.*, *Br. J. clin. Pharmac.*, 1982, *14*, 201 (in healthy adults); M. A. Homeida *et al.*, *J. antimicrob. Chemother.*, 1986, *18*, 213 (in children with giardiasis).

For comparative studies of the pharmacokinetics of metronidazole and tinidazole, see Tinidazole, p.681.

ADMINISTRATION IN THE ELDERLY. Serum concentrations of metronidazole following a single 500-mg oral dose were significantly higher in 20 elderly patients than in 15 healthy young subjects. The area under the plasma versus time curve was almost doubled in the elderly group; an important factor appeared to be a decrease in volume of distribution. Erythrocytes of the elderly patients bound significantly less metronidazole *in vitro* than those of the younger subjects which might contribute to the reduced volume of distribution. It is suggested that the standard dose of metronidazole should be reduced by 30 to 40% in the elderly.—E. Ludwig *et al.*, *Int. J. clin. Pharmac. Ther. Toxic.*, 1983, *21*, 87.

ADMINISTRATION IN HEPATIC FAILURE. For reference to pharmacokinetic studies of metronidazole elimination in patients with liver disease, see under Uses (below).

ADMINISTRATION IN INFANTS AND CHILDREN. The overall mean half-life of metronidazole was 23.4 hours in a study involving 24 neonates given 7.5 mg per kg body-weight every 8 hours by intravenous infusion for a mean of 5 days; half-life was inversely related to gestational age. In contrast to Jager-Roman *et al.* (*J. Pediat.*, 1982, *100*, 651) who found that a considerably extended half-life in neonates shortened as the infants matured, mean half-lives after the first and last doses of metronidazole did not differ appreciably. The highest mean blood concentration of metronidazole after the first dose was 9.6 µg per mL compared with 19.31 µg per mL after the final dose; mean peak concentrations for the hydroxy metabolite (20396-RP) were 0.7 and 5.2 µg per mL respectively. Since the half-life is about three times that reported in adults, it is suggested that less frequent dosage would be appropriate in neonates.— P. Hall *et al.*, *Archs Dis. Childh.*, 1983, *58*, 529.

The pharmacokinetics of metronidazole given by mouth to an infant of 6 weeks and 19 children aged from 4 to 14 years were similar to those seen in adults.— I. Amon *et al.*, *Eur. J. clin. Pharmac.*, 1983, *24*, 113.

ADMINISTRATION IN INFLAMMATORY BOWEL DISEASES. Absorption of metronidazole given by mouth was found to be slightly reduced in patients with Crohn's disease when compared with healthy subjects (A. Melander *et al.*, *Eur. J. clin. Pharmac.*, 1977, *12*, 69). In a subsequent study in which patients first received metronidazole intravenously to ensure that they were at a steady state for the oral study (J.L. Shaffer *et al.*, *Br. J. clin. Pharmac.*, 1986, *21*, 431), there was no evidence that Crohn's disease or ulcerative colitis impaired the absorption of metronidazole.

ADMINISTRATION IN RENAL FAILURE. The pharmacokinetics of metronidazole, given as a single intravenous infusion of 500 mg, were studied in 29 patients with varying degrees of renal failure. Results were compared with those previously reported from healthy subjects (G.W. Houghton *et al.*, *Br. J. clin. Pharmac.*, 1979, *8*, 337). None of the pharmacokinetic parameters of unchanged metronidazole, including elimination half-life, were significantly different in the patients with renal impairment from those seen in healthy subjects, except for renal clearance. However, the mean plasma elimination half-life of 1-(2-hydroxyethyl)-2-hydroxymethyl-5-nitroimidazole (metabolite I) was significantly increased with decreasing renal function from 9.2 hours in healthy subjects to 16 hours in those with moderate renal insufficiency (creatinine clearance between 10 and 50 mL per minute), 28 hours in those with severe renal insufficiency (creatinine clearance 2 to 10 mL per minute), and 34 hours in dialysis patients (creatinine clearance below 1 mL per minute). Metabolite I is eliminated by renal and hepatic routes and its urinary excretion was reduced in patients with severe renal insufficiency to only 25% of that in healthy subjects. 2-Methyl-5-nitroimidazole-1-acetic acid (metabolite II) appears to be excreted almost exclusively in urine and although not detected in the plasma of healthy subjects it accumulated in patients with renal impairment proportionately to the severity of renal failure. It was considered that the accumulation of metronidazole or its 2 major metabolites is unlikely to have any toxicological implications in patients with creatinine clearances greater than 10 mL per minute and that doses should not be altered. Those with creatinine clearances below 10 mL per minute will show marked accumulation of both metabolites on repeated dosing, but doses need not be changed unless therapeutically acceptable. Unchanged drug and its metabolites are removed during haemodialysis and a further dose of metronidazole should be given after haemodialysis to replace that lost.— G. W. Houghton *et al.*, *Br. J. clin. Pharmac.*, 1985, *19*, 203.

Further references: A. A. Somogyi *et al.*, *J. antimicrob. Chemother.*, 1984, *13*, 183.

METABOLISM. Metronidazole and its principal metabolites were measured using HPLC in plasma from 10 patients with anaerobic infections who received metronidazole 13.6 mg per kg body-weight by intravenous infusion over one hour followed by 1.43 mg per kg every hour for up to 12 days. Concentrations of metronidazole and its hydroxy metabolite ranged from 7.2 to 44.8 µg per mL and from 1.6 to 15.2 µg per mL respectively; concentrations of the acid metabolite ranged from 0 to 1.4 µg per mL. The ratio of metronidazole to hydroxy metabolite was 0.03 to 0.3 in 9 patients and 1.0 in a patient taking phenytoin.— L. A. Wheeler *et al.*, *Antimicrob. Ag. Chemother.*, 1978, *13*, 205.

Small amounts of acetamide and *N*-(2-hydroxyethyl)oxamic acid (HOA), representing about 1 to 2% of the daily dose of 750 mg, were found in the urine of 5 patients taking metronidazole.— R. L. Koch *et al.*, *Science*, 1981, *211*, 398.

PREGNANCY AND THE NEONATE. In 8 women given suppositories of metronidazole 1 g 8-hourly for 7 doses following caesarean section the mean concentration of metronidazole in breast milk 30 minutes after completing treatment was 10 µg per mL (maximum 25 µg per mL).— B. Moore and J. Collier (letter), *Br. med. J.*, 1979, *2*, 211.

No significant difference was found between mean maternal and arterial cord-blood concentrations following prophylactic intravenous infusion of metronidazole 500 mg to 16 women undergoing caesarean section. Mean elimination half-life was 6.9 hours, and pharmacokinetics were similar to those expected in non-pregnant subjects.— A. A. Visser and H. K. L. Hundt, *J. antimicrob. Chemother.*, 1984, *13*, 279.

For the pharmacokinetics of metronidazole in neonates, see Administration in Infants and Children, above.

Uses and Administration

Metronidazole is a 5-nitroimidazole derivative with activity against anaerobic protozoa and anaerobic bacteria; it also has a radiosensitising effect on hypoxic tumour cells. Its mechanism of action is thought to involve interference with DNA by a metabolite in which the nitro group of metronidazole has been reduced.

Metronidazole is active against several protozoa including *Balantidium coli*, *Blastocystis hominis*, *Entamoeba histolytica*, *Giardia intestinalis* (*Giardia lamblia*), and *Trichomonas vaginalis*. Most obligate anaerobic bacteria, including *Bacteroides* and *Clostridium* spp., are sensitive *in vitro* to metronidazole. It is bactericidal. Minimum inhibitory concentrations for susceptible anaerobic bacteria generally range from 0.1 to 8 µg per mL. It also has activity against the facultative anaerobes *Gardnerella vaginalis* and *Campylobacter* spp. and against some spirochaetes. Resistance to metronidazole appears to be rare; cross-resistance to other nitroimidazoles, such as tinidazole, has been demonstrated.

Metronidazole is used in the treatment of susceptible protozoal infections and in the treatment and prophylaxis of anaerobic bacterial infections. Specific bacterial infections treated with metronidazole include bacterial vaginosis (nonspecific vaginitis), acute necrotising ulcerative gingivitis (Vincent's infection), and pseudomembranous colitis. It is also used in the treatment of dracontiasis (guinea-worm infection) and has been given in inflammatory bowel disease and as an adjunct to the radiotherapy of malignant neoplasms.

Metronidazole is administered by mouth in tablets or, as metronidazole benzoate, in oral suspension; the tablets are taken with or after food and the suspension at least 1 hour before food. Metronidazole is also given rectally in suppositories or by intravenous infusion of metronidazole or metronidazole hydrochloride. Doses are expressed in terms of metronidazole base. Pharmacokinetic studies indicate that the frequency of dosage should be reduced in patients with severe liver disease and possibly in neonates and the elderly. Patients undergoing haemodialysis may require an additional dose after dialysis.

In amoebiasis, metronidazole acts as an amoebicide at all sites of infection with *Entamoeba histolytica*. Because of its rapid absorption it is probably less effective against parasites in the bowel lumen and is therefore used in conjunction with a luminal amoebicide such as diloxanide furoate or di-iodohydroxyquinoline in the treatment of amoebic dysentery and in extra-intestinal amoebiasis, including hepatic amoebiasis. Metronidazole may also be used in asymptomatic cyst-passers, but is less effective than a luminal amoebicide. Metronidazole is given in doses of 400 to 800 mg three times daily by mouth for 5 to 10 days. Children aged 1 to 3 years may be given one-quarter, those aged 3 to 7 years one-third, and those aged 7 to 10 years one-half the adult dose; alternatively 35 to 50 mg per kg body-weight daily in divided doses has been suggested.

In balantidiasis and *Blastocystis hominis* infection, metronidazole has been given in doses similar to those used in amoebiasis.

In giardiasis, the usual dose of metronidazole is 2 g daily by mouth as a single dose for 3 successive days. Dosage for children is proportional, as for amoebiasis (above). An alternative suggested schedule is 250 mg three times daily for 5 to 7 days for adults or 15 mg per kg daily in divided doses for children.

In trichomoniasis, metronidazole is given by mouth as a single 2-g dose or as a 7-day course of 200 or 250 mg three times daily or 400 mg twice daily; other regimens used include a 2-day course of 800 mg in the morning and 1.2 g in the evening. Sexual partners should be treated concomitantly. Treatment may need to be repeated; some advocate an interval of 7 days between courses whereas others advise an interval of 4 to 6 weeks. Vaginal preparations containing metronidazole are available for the treatment of vaginal trichomoniasis in some countries. Children with trichomoniasis may be given a 7-day course of metronidazole by mouth as follows: 1 to 3 years, 50 mg three times daily; 3 to 7 years, 100 mg twice daily, and 7 to 10 years, 100 mg three times daily. An alternative children's dose is 15 mg per kg daily in divided doses for 7 days.

Bacterial vaginosis is treated similarly to vaginal trichomoniasis with which it may co-exist; metronidazole is given by mouth as a single 2-g dose or as a 7-day course of 400 or 500 mg twice daily.

In acute necrotising ulcerative gingivitis, metronidazole 200 mg three times daily is given by mouth for 3 days; similar doses are used in acute dental infections.

For the treatment of most anaerobic bacterial infections, metronidazole is given by mouth in an initial dose of 800 mg followed by 400 mg every 8 hours, usually for about 7 days. When oral therapy is precluded metronidazole may be administered intravenously, 500 mg being infused as 100 mL of a 5 mg per mL solution at a rate of 5 mL per minute every 8 hours, or rectally as a 1-g suppository every 8 hours for 3 days, then every 12 hours; oral therapy should be substituted as soon as possible. Suppositories may be unsuitable for the initiation of therapy in serious infections because of the slower absorption of metronidazole. Children may be given 7.5 mg per kg every 8 hours by mouth or by intravenous infusion; rectal doses of 125 mg in children under 1 year, 250 mg in those aged 1 to 5 years, and 500 mg in those aged 5 to 10 years, given every 8 hours for 3 days then every 12 hours, have also been used. In the *US* recommended adult doses of metronidazole are 7.5 mg per kg every 6 hours by mouth or 15 mg per kg by intravenous infusion followed by 7.5 mg per kg every 6 hours, doses being infused over 1 hour; by either route a total dose of 4 g in 24 hours should not be exceeded. In mixed anaerobic and aerobic infections metronidazole is given in association with the appropriate antibiotics.

For the prevention of postoperative anaerobic bacterial infections, especially in patients undergoing abdominal or gynaecological surgery, metronidazole is administered orally, intravenously, or rectally in doses similar to those used for the treatment of established infections. Various schedules have been employed and other antibacterial agents have sometimes been given concomitantly. By mouth, 400 mg of metronidazole may be given every 8 hours for 3 to 4 days followed postoperatively by intravenous or rectal administration until oral therapy is possible; shorter pre-operative courses and oral doses of up to 1 g have also been used. By intravenous infusion, 500 mg may be given shortly before operation and repeated every 8 hours, oral doses of 400 mg every 8 hours being substituted as soon as possible. By rectum, 1 g may be administered every 8 hours. Children's prophylactic doses are as for treatment (above). In the *US* the recommended schedule for adults undergoing colorectal surgery is metronidazole 15 mg per kg by intravenous infusion over 30 to 60 minutes, completed about 1 hour before surgery, followed by two further intravenous doses of 7.5 mg per kg infused at 6 and 12 hours after the initial dose.

Reviews of the actions and uses of metronidazole.— S. M. Finegold, *Ann. intern. Med.*, 1980, *93*, 585; P. Goldman, *New Engl. J. Med.*, 1980, *303*, 1212; *idem*, 1981, *304*, 547 (correction); *Lancet*, 1981, *1*, 818; J. E. Rosenblatt and R. S. Edson, *Mayo Clin. Proc.*, 1983, *58*, 154.

A discussion on the mechanism of antimicrobial action of metronidazole.— D. I. Edwards, *J. antimicrob. Chemother.*, 1979, *5*, 499.

ADMINISTRATION IN THE ELDERLY. The view that the daily dosage of metronidazole should be reduced in patients of 60 years or more.— A. J. McLean *et al.*, *Med. J. Aust.*, 1984, *141*, 163.

See also under Absorption and Fate (above).

ADMINISTRATION IN HEPATIC FAILURE. There have been differing results from pharmacokinetic studies of the elimination of metronidazole in patients with liver disease. Daneshmend *et al.* (*Gut*, 1982, *23*, 807) reported no marked difference between patients with cirrhosis or hepatosplenic schistosomiasis given a single 500-mg oral dose of metronidazole when compared with healthy subjects and suggested that, in the absence of renal impairment, dosage adjustment was not needed in patients with liver disease. However, Farrell *et al.* (*Br. med. J.*, 1983, *287*, 1845) found that elimination of metronidazole, administered intravenously, was considerably impaired in a study of 10 patients with alcoholic liver disease or chronic active hepatitis, 7 of whom had reduced creatinine clearance. Daneshmend and Roberts (*ibid.*, 1984, *288*, 405) commented that these differing results were probably due to impaired renal elimination, whereas Farrell *et al.* (*ibid.*, 1009) suggested that impaired elimination of metronidazole was due to impaired hepatic metabolism rather than decreased renal clearance; other studies have shown metronidazole clearance to be normal in renal failure. Farrell *et al.* nevertheless agreed that reduction in the dosage of metronidazole is required only when liver function is very poor, particularly when renal function is impaired. A study in 10 severely ill patients with or without impaired hepatic and/or renal function (B. Ljungberg *et al.*, *J. antimicrob. Chemother.*, 1984, *14*, 275) also suggested that liver function is a very important determinant of metronidazole elimination.

ADMINISTRATION IN INFANTS AND CHILDREN. For reference to the pharmacokinetics and dosage of metronidazole in neonates, see under Absorption and Fate (above).

ADMINISTRATION IN RENAL FAILURE. Pharmacokinetic studies have indicated that doses of metronidazole need not be altered in patients with renal insufficiency although an additional dose after haemodialysis is recommended to replace that lost during haemodialysis (see Absorption and Fate, above).

Routine adjustment of dosage was not considered necessary in patients undergoing peritoneal dialysis (J.G. Cassey *et al.*, *Antimicrob. Ag. Chemother.*, 1983, *24*, 950). However, the potential for metabolites to accumulate was noted in patients on continuous ambulatory peritoneal dialysis (D.R. Guay *et al.*, *ibid.*, 1984, *25*, 306) and it was suggested that dosage reduction may be necessary if excessive concentrations of metabolites are found to be toxic.

Metronidazole and its hydroxy metabolite were efficiently cleared and extensively removed in patients undergoing haemodialysis (A. Somogyi *et al.*, *Eur. J. clin. Pharmac.*, 1983, *25*, 683) and adjustments in dosage and timing of dosage were considered essential in such patients. In a further study (A.H. Lau *et al.*, *Antimicrob. Ag. Chemother.*, 1986, *29*, 235) the amount of metronidazole and its hydroxy metabolite cleared was found to depend on the type of dialysis membrane used; the authors concluded that dosage supplementation may be needed only for seriously ill patients undergoing haemodialysis with a membrane having high metronidazole clearance.

AMOEBIC INFECTIONS. *Entamoeba polecki* is almost exclusively a parasite of the large intestine of pigs and monkeys. Most infections in man have been found in Papua New Guinea. The infection is rather refractory to therapy with amoebicidal drugs but diloxanide furoate in combination with metronidazole has been used successfully.— Report of a WHO Scientific Group on Intestinal Protozoan and Helminthic Infections, *Tech. Rep. Ser. Wld Hlth Org. No. 666*, 1981, p. 56. Metronidazole, given in doses similar to those used for *Entamoeba histolytica* infections, was successful in the treatment of 6 of 8 Southeast Asian refugees with *Entamoeba polecki* infection. Further courses of metronidazole eradicated the infection in the remaining 2 patients.— J. D. Gay *et al.*, *Mayo Clin. Proc.*, 1985, *60*, 523. See also J. M. Boles and O. Masure (letter), *ibid.*, 1986, *61*, 226.

Beneficial results with metronidazole 500 or 750 mg three times daily by mouth for 10 days in 11 homosexual men with AIDS and severe diarrhoea. The diarrhoea appeared to be associated with the presence of intestinal protozoa such as *Entamoeba hartmanni*, *Entamoeba coli*, *Endolimax nana*, and *Iodamoeba buetschlii*, previously considered to be nonpathogenic. Cryptosporidia were also present in the stools of 6 patients, but persisted after treatment.— K. V. I. Rolston *et al.* (letter), *New Engl. J. Med.*, 1986, *315*, 192.

Amoebiasis. For a description of amoebiasis (*Entamoeba histolytica* infection) and reference to the use of metronidazole in its treatment, see p.658.

ANAEROBIC BACTERIAL INFECTIONS. Metronidazole has well-established bactericidal activity against obligate anaerobic bacteria *in vitro*, including the Gram-negative organisms *Bacteroides fragilis* and other *Bacteroides* spp., *Fusobacterium* spp., and *Veillonella* spp. and the Gram-positive organisms *Clostridium difficile*, *Cl. perfringens*, and other *Clostridium* spp., *Eubacterium* spp., *Peptococcus* spp., and *Peptostreptococcus* spp.; *Propionibacterium* and *Actinomyces* spp. are often resistant (J. Wüst, *Antimicrob. Ag. Chemother.*, 1977, *11*, 631; L. Dubreuil *et al.*, *ibid.*, 1984, *25*, 764; G.B. Hill and O.M. Ayers, *ibid.*, 1985, *27*, 324; A.W. Chow *et al.*, *ibid.*, *28*, 842; J.S. Brazier *et al.*, *J. antimicrob. Chemother.*, 1985, *15*, 181; P. Van der Auwera *et al.*, *ibid.*, 1987, *19*, 205). It also has activity against the facultative anaerobe *Gardnerella vaginalis*, although its bactericidal effect is reported to be much slower than against obligate anaerobes (E.D. Ralph and Y.E. Amatnieks, *Antimicrob. Ag. Chemother.*, 1980, *18*, 101), and against some strains of *Campylobacter* spp. including *C. fetus* subsp. *jejuni* (H. Hof *et al.*, *Antimicrob. Ag. Chemother.*, 1982, *22*, 332; A.M. Freydiere *et al.*, *ibid.*, 1984, *25*, 145) and *C. pylori* (*C. pyloridis*) (B.J. Marshall *et al.*, *Med. J. Aust.*, 1985, *142*, 439; A. Howden *et al.*, *Lancet*, 1986, *2*, 1035).

The oxidative metabolites of metronidazole have antibacterial activity; MICs of the 'hydroxy' metabolite against anaerobic bacteria are reported to be generally within one dilution of the parent compound whereas the 'acid' metabolite is much less active (I. Haller, *Antimicrob. Ag. Chemother.*, 1982, *22*, 165; J.P. O'Keefe *et al.*, *ibid.*, 426). The hydroxy metabolite has been reported to be consistently more active than metronidazole against strains of *G. vaginalis* (E.D. Ralph and Y.E. Amatnieks, *Sex. transm. Dis.*, 1980, *7*, 157; S. Shanker and R. Munro, *Lancet*, 1982, *1*, 167).

The mode of action of metronidazole is not entirely clear, but is thought to involve reduction by bacterial 'nitroreductases' to an unstable intermediate which interacts with DNA, effectively preventing further replication. A number of factors affect the sensitivity of micro-organisms to metronidazole *in vitro* (H.R. Ingham *et al.*, *J. antimicrob. Chemother.*, 1982, *10*, 84). Anaerobic conditions are important for optimal activity. Interactions between micro-organisms and metronidazole have been described, including inhibition of *Escherichia coli* by metronidazole in the presence of *B. fragilis* and enhancement of the rate of killing of *B. fragilis* by metronidazole in the presence of *E. coli*.

Resistance to metronidazole is rare in sensitive species. In a study on the susceptibility of the *B. fragilis* group in the *US* in 1981 (F.P. Tally *et al.*, *Antimicrob. Ag. Chemother.*, 1983, *23*, 536) two threshold concentrations (breakpoints) of 8 μg per mL and 16 μg per mL, above which strains were considered resistant to metronidazole, were selected on the basis of achievable blood concentrations; none of 753 isolates were resistant at either concentration and MICs ranged from 0.25 or less to 2 μg per mL. On continuation of the study (F.P. Tally *et al.*, *ibid.*, 1985, *28*, 675) no resistance was found over a 3-year period; in 1983 MICs for 543 isolates ranged from 0.12 or less to 8 μg per mL. There have however been occasional reports of metronidazole-resistant strains of *Bacteroides* spp. isolated from patients, including *B. fragilis* (H.R. Ingham *et al.*, *Lancet*, 1978, *1*, 214; V.O. Rotimi *et al.*, *ibid.*, 1979, *1*, 833; M.A. Eme *et al.*, *J. antimicrob. Chemother.*, 1983, *12*, 523; F. Lamothe *et al.*, *ibid.*, 1986, *18*, 642), *B. melaninogenicus* (M.S. Sprott *et al.*, *Lancet*, 1983, *1*, 1220), and *B. bivius* (P.W. McWalter and D.R. Baird, *ibid.*). The mechanism of resistance to metronidazole is uncertain. Although some have considered the lack of pyruvate dehydrogenase in resistant strains of *B. fragilis* to be responsible (M.L. Britz and R.G. Wilkinson, *Antimicrob. Ag. Chemother.*, 1979, *16*, 19; *idem*, *J. antimicrob. Chemother.*, 1984, *13*, 393), others (S. Tabaqchali *et al.*, *J. antimicrob. Chemother.*, 1983, *11*, 393; *idem*, 1984, *13*, 394) disagree.

The activity *in vitro* of metronidazole and other nitroimidazoles, such as tinidazole and ornidazole, against *Bacteroides fragilis* and *Fusobacterium* spp. has been considered broadly comparable (A.A. Carmine *et al.*, *Drugs*, 1982, *24*, 85). Results from individual studies have varied. Reynolds *et al.* (*J. clin. Path.*, 1975, *28*, 775) found nimorazole to have about three-fold less activity than metronidazole or tinidazole against *Bacteroides* and *Fusobacterium* spp. with geometric mean MICs of 1.05, 0.34, and 0.28 μg per mL respectively, whereas Wise *et al.* (*Chemotherapy, Basle*, 1977, *23*, 19) reported median MICs of 0.25 μg per mL for metronidazole and nimorazole, compared with 0.12 μg per mL for tinidazole against *B. fragilis*. More recently, Jokipii and Jokipii (*Antimicrob. Ag. Chemother.*, 1985, *28*, 561) found 7 nitroimidazole compounds to be very active against *B. fragilis*; tinidazole was the most active, followed in decreasing order of activity by panidazole, ornidazole, metronidazole and secnidazole (similar activity), carnidazole, and dimetridazole.

Anaerobic bacteria are important pathogens at nearly all anatomical sites. Their importance in intra-abdominal sepsis, non-venereal infections of the female genital tract, aspiration pneumonia, and lung abscess is well-established and high isolation-rates have been reported more recently in cutaneous, breast, and non-traumatic cerebral abscesses, chronic sinusitis, chronic otitis media, suppurative infections of the male genitourinary tract, pelvic inflammatory disease, peritonsillar abscesses, perimandibular space infections, dental infections, diabetic foot ulcers, and decubitus ulcers. Tissue necrosis or abscess formation is characteristic of infections due to anaerobic bacteria and debridement or drainage is often paramount in treatment. Metronidazole is active *in vitro* against virtually all anaerobic Gram-negative bacilli and also clostridia. It is reported to be effective against anaerobic infections at a variety of sites and is used, especially in the *UK* for surgical infection prophylaxis.— J. G. Bartlett, *Lancet*, 1982, *2*, 478.

Guidelines from the *US* on the choice of drugs for treating anaerobic infections. Useful drugs include benzylpenicillin, metronidazole, clindamycin, chloramphenicol, and cefoxitin, but the best antimicrobial regimen varies according to the site of infection. Metronidazole is generally not active against aerotolerant bacteria, including aerobic and microaerophilic streptococci commonly found in oral, pulmonary, and cerebral infections, and is usually given in association with penicillin in infections at these sites. In intra-abdominal infections *Escherichia coli* and *B. fragilis* tend to predominate and an aminoglycoside plus metronidazole may be given. Mixed infections are also common in the female genital tract; in pelvic inflammatory disease cefoxitin or metronidazole plus a tetracycline or other agent active against gonococci and *Chlamydia trachomatis* has been advised.— *Med. Lett.*, 1984, *26*, 87.

A report of the successful substitution of rectal for intravenous metronidazole in the majority of patients undergoing surgery.— A. McLean *et al.*, *Lancet*, 1983, *1*, 41. Therapeutic serum concentrations were achieved in 10 severely ill patients given metronidazole rectally in suppositories, although to achieve these concentrations rapidly an intravenous loading dose was given initially.— E. M. Barker *et al.*, *Br. med. J.*, 1983, *287*, 311. The view that, since metronidazole is as effective when given rectally as intravenously and is much cheaper, there is no reason to use the intravenous infusion except in emergencies and in patients with severe anaerobic infection for whom the oral or rectal route is contra-indicated.— *Drug & Ther. Bull.*, 1983, *21*, 53.

References to the use of metronidazole in various anaerobic infections: G. E. Cree *et al.*, *Br. med. J.*, 1982, *284*, 859 (balanoposthitis); P. Van der Auwera *et al.*, *J. antimicrob. Chemother.*, 1982, *10*, 57 (similar efficacy to clindamycin in intra-abdominal infection); D. G. Kelly *et al.*, *Gut*, 1983, *24*, 193 (ileostomy dysfunction); J.-P. Capron *et al.*, *Lancet*, 1983, *1*, 446 (prevention of cholestasis associated with total parenteral nutrition, possibly related to intestinal overgrowth of anaerobic bacteria); J. S. Dooley *et al.*, *Gut*, 1984, *25*, 988 (acute cholecystitis and acute cholangitis); I. Ahmadsyah and A. Salim, *Br. med. J.*, 1985, *291*, 648 (tetanus).

See also under Bacterial Vaginosis, Mouth Infections, Pseudomembranous Colitis, and Skin Disorders (below).

Surgical infection prophylaxis. A review of the use of metronidazole and related nitroimidazoles in surgical applications. Many studies have established that these drugs are effective in lowering the rate of wound infection in particular types of surgery. Benefit has been shown or can be expected when the surgical procedure broaches a viscus, a body cavity, or a space which normally harbours a flora of anaerobic organisms; *B. fragilis* has been implicated as the most common anaerobic pathogen. A marked fall in wound infection has been reported after bowel, biliary, gynaecological, and otolaryngological surgery in patients given metronidazole. It is widely accepted that metronidazole concentrations in plasma should be at least 6.25 μg per mL at the time of surgery and during recovery although data from single-dose studies and knowledge of the pharmacokinetics of metronidazole suggest that lower concentrations may be effective. There is no firm statement on how long these concentrations should be maintained after surgery and recommendations range from allowing the drug to be eliminated without further administration to the earlier regimens which involved therapy for approximately 1 week. Peak blood concentrations of metronidazole occur about 1 or 4 hours after oral or rectal administration respectively and administration by these routes is generally indicated rather than by the intravenous route, on the basis of efficacy, safety, and cost. Intravenous administration should be restricted to emergency pre-operative loading, to patients with proven anaerobic infections or serious sepsis associated with an unidentified organism, and to those unable to receive oral or rectal administration.— A. J. McLean *et al.*, *Med. J. Aust.*, 1984, *141*, 163.

Administration of metronidazole orally, parenterally, or rectally together with an antibiotic active against aerobic Gram-negative rods has become the mainstay of colorectal surgical prophylaxis in Great Britain although there is no convincing data allowing recommendation of this regimen over the pre-operative use of oral erythromycin and neomycin. Metronidazole has been found effective prophylactically in general and gynaecological surgery in which anaerobes constitute a large part of the colonising bacterial flora. However, it has not proved superior to the cephalosporins and in the *US* metronidazole will probably continue to serve as an alternative prophylactic agent in gynaecological surgery, colon surgery, and appendectomy when the more popular cephalosporin regimens cannot be used.— A. B. Kaiser, *New Engl. J. Med.*, 1986, *315*, 1129.

BACTERIAL VAGINOSIS. A brief review of anaerobic vaginosis (nonspecific vaginitis, bacterial vaginosis), a common and often distressing vaginal condition associated with a fishy-smelling vaginal discharge and an abnormal vaginal flora. The abnormal flora comprises *Gardnerella vaginalis* (*Haemophilus vaginalis*, *Corynebacterium vaginale*) and mixed anaerobes, with *Mobiluncus* spp. in up to 50% of cases. Many of these bacteria adhere to vaginal epithelial cells forming 'clue cells'. Since the full clinical syndrome is invariably associated with the presence of anaerobic bacteria, as well as *G. vaginalis*, and responds to treatment with metronidazole, the term anaerobic vaginosis is suggested to describe clue-cell-associated vaginal infections (in the absence of *Trichomonas vaginalis*) where the vaginal pH is greater than 5.0 and amine testing is positive. Other workers favour the broader term bacterial vaginosis. Topical treatment with a variety of drugs including sulphonamide vaginal cream and povidone-iodine pessaries has not been effective. Systemic treatment is effective; ampicillin was the preferred drug from 1972 to 1978, but since then metronidazole or other nitroimidazoles have become the treatment of choice. Most studies suggest that anaerobic vaginosis is a sexually-transmitted disease and it seems prudent to treat the sexual partners of infected women.— A. Blackwell, *J. antimicrob. Chemother.*, 1984, *14*, 445. The view that bacterial vaginosis is a preferable term to 'anaerobic vaginosis'. Several bacterial species are associated with this infection, including anaerobic *Bacteroides* spp., but *G. vaginalis* and *Mobiluncus* spp. are not obligate anaerobes.— B. M. Jones *et al.*, *J. antimicrob. Chemother.*, 1985, *16*, 189.

Several studies have demonstrated the efficacy of metronidazole 400 or 500 mg twice daily by mouth for 7 days in the treatment of bacterial vaginosis (T.A. Pheifer *et al.*, *New Engl. J. Med.*, 1978, *298*, 1429; M.J. Balsdon *et al.*, *Lancet*, 1980, *1*, 501; A.L. Blackwell *et al.*, *ibid.*, 1983, *2*, 1379). Single-dose therapy has potential advantages, including patient compliance. A single 2-g dose of metronidazole was found to be less effective than a 7-day regimen by some workers (A.L. Blackwell *et al.*; J. Swedberg *et al.*, *J. Am. med. Ass.*, 1985, *254*, 1046), but others have found single-dose and 5- or 7-day regimens to be equally effective (B.M. Jones *et al.*, *J. antimicrob. Chemother.*, 1985, *16*, 189; K.C. Mohanty and R. Deighton, *ibid.*, 799) and have recommended a 2-g dose of metronidazole as the preferred initial treatment for bacterial vaginosis; trichomoniasis was also diagnosed in 18.6% of Mohanty and Deighton's patients and was also cured by the single-dose regimen. In a study of several different dosage regimens (F. Jerve *et al.*, *Br. J. vener. Dis.*, 1984, *60*, 171), the best treatment schedule for bacterial vaginosis was considered to be metronidazole 2 g given on days 1 and 3. Single 2-g doses of metronidazole and the nitroimidazole derivatives nimorazole and tinidazole were equally effective in a comparative study (K.C. Mohanty and R. Deighton, *J. antimicrob. Chemother.*, 1987, *19*, 393).

Metronidazole has also been administered vaginally and 500 mg in a vaginal pessary each evening for 7 days was as effective as 400 mg twice daily by mouth for 7 days in a randomised open study in women with bacterial vaginosis (P. Bistoletti *et al.*, *Gynec. Obstet. Invest.*, 1986, *21*, 144).

BALANTIDIASIS. For a brief description of balantidiasis and its treatment, see p.659.

BLASTOCYSTIS HOMINIS INFECTION. Reports of the successful use of metronidazole in the treatment of diarrhoea associated with *Blastocystis hominis*, a protozoan parasite usually considered to be a harmless commensal of the intestinal tract.— N. Ricci *et al.* (letter), *Lancet*, 1984, *1*, 966 (2 g daily for 5 days); J. B. Vannatta *et al.*, *Ann. intern. Med.*, 1985, *102*, 495 (500 mg three times daily for 7 days).

DRACONTIASIS. Despite some contradictory results (D.R. Kulkarni and S.J. Nagalotimath, *Trans. R. Soc. trop. Med. Hyg.*, 1975, *69*, 169) metronidazole has been of benefit in the management of dracontiasis (dracunculiasis; guinea-worm infection). Like niridazole and thiabendazole it has marked anti-inflammatory properties and is thought to act probably be lessening the intense host tissue reaction, thus allowing the emerging worms to be removed more quickly, rather than by a direct anthelmintic effect (R. Muller, *Bull. Wld Hlth Org.*, 1979, *57*, 683). In a field study in Nigeria (O.O. Kale *et al.*, *Ann. trop. Med. Parasit.*, 1983, *77*, 151), metronidazole and thiabendazole were both significantly better than placebo in relieving symptoms and healing guinea-worm ulcers, although elimination of worms and parasitological relapses were not significantly improved. Kale *et al.* conclude that metronidazole, niridazole, and thiabendazole are each better than placebo and have a place in the treatment of dracontiasis.

Metronidazole has been given in a variety of dosage regimens including: 400 mg three times daily for 5 days (K.O. Padonu, *Am. J. trop. Med. Hyg.*, 1973, *22*, 42); 40 mg per kg body-weight daily in three divided doses, to a maximum daily dose of 2.4 g, for 3 days (O.O. Kale, *Ann. trop. Med. Parasit.*, 1974, *68*, 91); 400 mg daily for 10 to 20 days (R. Muller, 1979). A dose of 250 mg three times daily for 10 days has also been recommended (*Med. Lett.*, 1986, *28*, 9) as an alternative to treatment with niridazole.

GIARDIASIS. A comparison of the activity *in vitro* of 11 nitroimidazoles, including metronidazole, nimorazole, ornidazole, secnidazole, and tinidazole, and a range of other compounds, including furazolidone and mepacrine, against *Giardia intestinalis*. With the exception of panidazole and fexinidazole, the nitroimidazoles were equipotent to, or more active than metronidazole; most active were S-750400A, flunidazole, satranidazole, and ronidazole. Of the non-nitroimidazole compounds, the anthelmintic niridazole was the most active of all the compounds tested, being at least 10 times more active than metronidazole. Furazolidone and mepacrine had relative activities of 1.18 and 0.74 respectively compared to metronidazole. Paromomycin sulphate, erythromycin, and sulphasalazine, all of which have been reported effective in the treatment of giardiasis, had no activity in this study.— P. F. L. Boreham *et al.*, *J. antimicrob. Chemother.*, 1985, *16*, 589.

Mention of controversy over treating symptomless carriers of *Giardia intestinalis* and a report of a child who had 3 episodes of infection over 10 months. The first 2 episodes responded favourably to treatment based on metronidazole, but cysts persisted in the faeces despite identical treatment in the third episode. Her family were all found to be symptomless carriers and were treated and cured; the child's symptoms disappeared.— J. M. C. Pancorbo *et al.* (letter), *Lancet*, 1985, *2*, 951.

For a brief description of giardiasis and its treatment, see p.659.

HEPATIC ENCEPHALOPATHY. Treatment of hepatic encephalopathy includes the administration of an antibacterial agent to reduce excessive endogenous ammonia formation by the intestinal flora. Gram-negative anaerobes are thought to make a major contribution to the generation of this ammonia and metronidazole 200 mg four times daily for 1 week was as effective as neomycin, a well-recognised form of treatment, in a study in 18 patients with acute or chronic hepatic encephalopathy (M.H. Morgan *et al.*, *Gut*, 1982, *23*, 1). In a review of therapy for chronic encephalopathy (I.R. Crossley and R. Williams, *ibid.*, 1984, *25*, 85) it is suggested that substitution of metronidazole for neomycin, or a combination of the 2, be tried if there is no improvement with moderate dietary protein restriction, neomycin, and lactulose. However, in view of the CNS toxicity of metronidazole caution is advised with long courses, especially in patients with liver disease.

INFECTIOUS MONONUCLEOSIS. Following a favourable report of the use of metronidazole in anginose infectious mononucleosis and the suggestion that anaerobic bacteria may be involved in the pathogenesis of the disease (S.Å. Hedström *et al.*, *Scand. J. infect. Dis.*, 1978, *10*, 7), conflicting results have been described. There was no significant improvement with metronidazole 400 mg three times daily for up to 5 days in a double-blind placebo-controlled study in 40 patients over the age of 15 years (D.W. Spelman and H.F. Newton-John, *ibid.*, 1982, *14*, 99) whereas 5 patients, aged 3 to 13 years, with anginose infectious mononucleosis responded to treatment with metronidazole 750 mg daily in 3 divided doses for 5 days (S. Davidson *et al.*, *ibid.*, 103). More recently (G. Marklund *et al.*, *Scand. J. infect. Dis.*, 1986, *18*, 503), clinical improvement was noted in 13 patients with acute infectious mononucleosis after 5 days of treatment with tinidazole 2 g by mouth, followed by 1 g on 4 successive days, when compared with 11 patients who received no treatment.

INFLAMMATORY BOWEL DISEASES. A discussion on the treatment of inflammatory bowel disease. In ulcerative colitis, corticosteroids are the mainstay of treatment of acute attacks. Oral or intravenous metronidazole may be added to the treatment of severely ill patients although its efficacy is dubious. Corticosteroids also relieve the symptoms of Crohn's disease, although metronidazole 400 mg twice daily by mouth for 1 to 3 months is worth trying in colonic Crohn's disease not responding to corticosteroid enemas. Corticosteroids are generally ineffective in perianal Crohn's disease; much of the damage probably results from secondary infection and oral metronidazole may sometimes be very effective.— J. M. Rhodes, *Prescribers' J.*, 1986, *26*, 1.

Of 21 patients with chronic unremitting perineal Crohn's disease given metronidazole 20 mg per kg body-weight daily by mouth in divided doses, 17 were maintained on metronidazole for 5 to 21 months and 15 of these had complete or advanced healing. Five patients on metronidazole for 3 to 7 months developed peripheral neuropathy; treatment was discontinued in one, dosage reduced in 3, and the fifth patient who had minimal numbness was maintained on the same dosage.— L. H. Bernstein *et al.*, *Gastroenterology*, 1980, *79*, 357. The continued efficacy of metronidazole over longer treatment periods was established in a follow-up study of these 17 and 9 further patients with perineal Crohn's disease; 16 patients received metronidazole for 12 to 36 months and 8 of these, 4 off and 4 on the drug, healed completely and remain healed whereas the other 8 have advanced but incomplete healing. Attempts to reduce the dose or stop treatment with metronidazole indicated that this will be successful in only a minority of patients although the resulting exacerbation of the disease should respond to reinstitution of therapy. The major limiting factor of long-term therapy with metronidazole remains paraesthesias, which developed in 50% of patients 1 to 14 months after the onset of treatment; they appear to be dose-related and nonprogressive but tend to persist for prolonged periods even after metronidazole is discontinued.— L. J. Brandt *et al.*, *ibid.*, 1982, *83*, 383.

Metronidazole 400 mg twice daily for 4 months was considered to be slightly more effective than sulphasalazine 1.5 g twice daily in a multicentre double-blind crossover study (the Cooperative Crohn's Disease Study in Sweden) in 78 patients with active Crohn's disease. Nonresponders to sulphasalazine responded more favourably to metronidazole than did metronidazole nonresponders to sulphasalazine. Both drugs were less effective in small intestine disease than in colonic disease.— B. Ursing *et al.*, *Gastroenterology*, 1982, *83*, 550.

Metronidazole 500 mg administered intravenously every 8 hours for 5 days was of no benefit when given as an adjunct to intravenous corticosteroid therapy in a double-blind placebo-controlled study in 39 patients with severe ulcerative colitis.— R. W. Chapman *et al.*, *Gut*, 1986, *27*, 1210.

For the effect of inflammatory bowel diseases on the absorption of metronidazole, see under Absorption and Fate (above).

For an overview of the management of inflammatory bowel diseases, see the section on Corticosteroids.

LEISHMANIASIS. There have been variable results with metronidazole in the treatment of leishmaniasis. Favourable responses have been reported in individual patients with cutaneous leishmaniasis (P.I. Long, *J. Am. med. Ass.*, 1973, *223*, 1378) and, together with co-trimoxazole, kala-azar (K.J. Murphy and A.C.W. Bong, *Lancet*, 1981, *1*, 323); 6 of 10 patients with Indian kala-azar responded to treatment with metronidazole 25 mg per kg body-weight daily by intravenous infusion for 5 days followed by 40 mg per kg daily by mouth, in 4 divided doses, for 7 days (M. Mishra *et al.*, *Br. med. J.*, 1985, *291*, 1611). However, metronidazole was not effective in 5 of 6 patients with American cutaneous leishmaniasis due to *Leishmania brasiliensis* (B.C. Walton *et al.*, *J. Am. med. Ass.*, 1974, *228*, 1256) nor in 5 patients with Ethiopian mucocutaneous leishmaniasis (A. Belehu *et al.*, *Br. J. Derm.*, 1978, *99*, 421).

MALARIA. Beneficial results with metronidazole in 5 patients with vivax malaria.— R. F. James (letter), *Lancet*, 1985, *2*, 498. Criticism; metronidazole is not indicated for *Plasmodium vivax* infections.— R. Esposito (letter), *ibid.*, 784. Metronidazole failed to clear the parasites in symptomless children with *Plasmodium falciparum* and is unlikely to have a role in the treatment of *P. falciparum* malaria.— K. J. Pallangyo *et al.* (letter), *ibid.*, 1986, *1*, 922.

MALIGNANT NEOPLASMS. A review of the use of hypoxic sensitisers such as metronidazole and misonidazole as adjuncts to radiotherapy in patients with solid tumours.— J. D. Chapman, *New Engl. J. Med.*, 1979, *301*, 1429.

An apparently enhanced tumour response to radiotherapy in some of 36 patients with advanced head and neck tumours and 12 with alimentary metastatic adenocarcinoma, given metronidazole, might represent radiosensitisation, precision radiotherapy, or a direct cytotoxic effect of metronidazole, or a combined effect. Metronidazole was given in doses of 2.5 g daily in 3 divided doses for 5 days a week, to a total of up to 94 g.— A. B. M. F. Karim, *Br. J. Cancer*, 1978, *37*, *Suppl.* 3, 299.

See also Malodorous Tumours under Skin Disorders (below).

MOUTH INFECTIONS. *Dry socket*. Beneficial results with metronidazole applied topically in a double-blind placebo-controlled study in 55 patients with dry socket (a painful tooth socket following recent extraction and accompanied by partial or total loss of the blood clot). After irrigation of the affected socket with warm sterile saline, metronidazole 10% in carmellose gelatin paste (Orabase) flavoured with peppermint or the paste alone was inserted using a 2-mL syringe. Patients were reviewed after 2 or 3 days, the dressing re-applied, and further reviews made until a cure was achieved. The treatment period was significantly shorter with metronidazole than with paste thus implicating anaerobic bacteria in the pathogenesis of dry socket.— L. Mitchell, *Br. dent. J.*, 1984, *156*, 132. Query as to the amount of metronidazole administered. The effect of metronidazole might have been partly or wholly systemic.— A. I. McAughtry (letter), *ibid.*, 240. About 0.25 mL of paste, providing 25 mg of metronidazole, was required to treat one dry socket and applications were repeated only once every 2 to 3 days. The amount available for systemic absorption was thus unlikely to significantly inhibit pathogenic anaerobes.— L. Mitchell (letter), *ibid.*, 348.

Gingivitis. A review of the diagnosis, aetiology, and treatment of acute necrotising ulcerative gingivitis. Over the years the disease has been assigned a multitude of names including trench mouth; Vincent's gingivitis, infection, stomatitis, or angina; and fuso-spirochaetal gingivitis. Vincent originally described a spirochaete, *Borrelia vincentii*, and a fusiform bacterium as being linked with this clinical syndrome. The fusiform-spirochaete character of acute necrotising ulcerative gingivitis is still valid although more recently other species, including *Bacteroides melalinogenicus*, have also been implicated. Treatment includes reduction of the bacterial burden mechanically, and by the administration of penicillin or metronidazole in advanced cases, together with attempts to control precipitating factors.— B. D. Johnson and D. Engel, *J. Periodontol.*, 1986, *57*, 141.

PEPTIC ULCER. A close association between active gastritis and the presence of *Campylobacter pylori* (*Campylobacter pyloridis*) has been reported and convincing arguments for the probable causal significance of *C. pylori* in gastritis and peptic ulceration have been presented. Metronidazole is active against *C. pylori* and has been reported to heal peptic ulcers.— C. S. Goodwin and J. A. Armstrong, *J. antimicrob. Chemother.*, 1986, *17*, 1.

Beneficial results with metronidazole in the treatment of peptic ulcer.— M. Q. Diaz and A. S. Escobar (letter),

Lancet, 1986, *1*, 907.

PREGNANCY AND THE NEONATE. A review of the use of metronidazole in obstetrics and gynaecology.— M. O. Robbie and R. L. Sweet, *Am. J. Obstet. Gynec.*, 1983, *145*, 865.

For recommendations regarding the use of metronidazole during pregnancy and lactation, see under Pregnancy and the Neonate in Precautions (above).

For reference to dosage in neonates, see under Administration in Infants and Children in Absorption and Fate (above).

PSEUDOMEMBRANOUS COLITIS. Anecdotal reports suggest that oral metronidazole is an alternative to vancomycin in the treatment of pseudomembranous colitis caused by *Clostridium difficile* and commonly associated with antibiotic treatment. In a randomised comparative study in 101 patients treated for *Cl. difficile*-associated diarrhoea and colitis (D.G. Teasley *et al.*, *Lancet*, 1983, *2*, 1043), metronidazole 250 mg four times daily for 10 days was considered to be as effective as vancomycin, although the statistical conclusions of the study were criticised (R.S. Gordon, *ibid.*, 1417). Treatment of *Cl. difficile* carriers with metronidazole, along with other control measures, failed to eradicate infection in a chronic hospital ward (B.S. Bender *et al.*, *ibid.*, 1986, *2*, 11); the use of metronidazole was criticised (R.A. O'Connor *et al.*, *ibid.*, 751) since it was considered less reliable than vancomycin and had itself been implicated in the induction of colitis (see Effects on the Gastro-intestinal Tract in Adverse Effects, above). Doubt as to the efficacy of metronidazole has also been expressed on the grounds that it is rapidly and usually completely absorbed from the upper gastro-intestinal tract after administration by mouth, whereas effective therapy requires bactericidal concentrations in the colon. Metronidazole was not detected in the faeces of most healthy subjects following oral administration (Y. Arabi *et al.*, *J. antimicrob. Chemother.*, 1979, *5*, 531). However, bactericidal faecal concentrations of metronidazole and its hydroxy metabolite were measured in 9 patients during successful oral and intravenous therapy for antibiotic-associated colitis due to *Cl. difficile* (R.P. Bolton and M.A. Culshaw, *Gut*, 1986, *27*, 1169); these workers conclude that metronidazole 400 mg every 8 hours by mouth should be the first alternative to treatment with vancomycin and that metronidazole 500 mg every 8 hours given intravenously is also effective.

RHEUMATOID ARTHRITIS. Beneficial results have been achieved with metronidazole 2 g at night for 2 successive nights each week for 6 weeks in patients with rheumatoid arthritis. A proper controlled study is advocated.— P. K. Pybus (letter), *S. Afr. med. J.*, 1985, *67*, 1039.

SKIN DISORDERS. *Malodorous tumours.* The smell of some fungating tumours is identical to that associated with anaerobic infection, suggesting that it may be caused by colonisation of the tumour with anaerobes. Metronidazole 200 mg three times daily successfully reduced the smell of an ulcerating tumour in a woman with breast cancer.— R. F. U. Ashford *et al.* (letter), *Lancet*, 1980, *1*, 874. This result was confirmed in a double-blind crossover study completed by 6 patients with breast cancer in whom the smell of fungating tumours was troublesome. Metronidazole 200 mg three times daily for 14 days significantly reduced the smell compared with placebo; anaerobes or anaerobic products could no longer be isolated.— R. Ashford *et al.* (letter), *ibid.*, 1984, *1*, 1232.

A topical gel formulation of metronidazole has been developed which can be applied directly to fungating tumours and other severe skin lesions to control offensive odour. Once-daily application has proved effective. Treatment is supplemented by metronidazole irrigation for wound cleansing of large or deep cavities.— M. C. Allwood *et al.* (letter), *Pharm. J.*, 1986, *1*, 158.

Pressure sores and ulcers. Metronidazole, as a sterile 1% topical solution in 0.6% saline (P.H. Jones *et al.*, *Lancet*, 1978, *1*, 214) or by mouth in a dose of 400 mg three times daily (P.G. Baker and G. Haig, *Practitioner*, 1981, *225*, 569), has been used successfully to treat foul-smelling anaerobically infected pressure sores and leg ulcers. However, Baker and Haig's study has been criticised as have the *UK* manufacturers' recommendations for use in these conditions which are said to be based on this study (*Drug & Ther. Bull.*, 1982, *20*, 9). A more recent review on pressure sores also concludes that the efficacy of metronidazole still remains to be proven (R.L. Longe, *Clin. Pharm.*, 1986, *5*, 669).

Rosacea. Several double-blind studies have indicated that metronidazole is effective in the treatment of rosacea. Metronidazole 200 mg twice daily by mouth was significantly better than placebo (R.J. Pye and J.L. Burton, *Lancet*, 1976, *1*, 1211) and as effective as oxytetracycline by mouth (E.M. Saihan and J.L. Burton, *Br. J. Derm.*, 1980, *102*, 443). Similarly, topical application of a 1% metronidazole cream was found to be better than placebo (P.G. Nielsen, *Br. J. Derm.*, 1983, *108*, 327) and as effective as oxytetracycline by mouth (*idem*, *109*, 63). A 0.75% metronidazole gel also proved effective when compared with placebo in patients with acne rosacea, although the telangiectatic component of the disease was not altered (I.K. Aronson *et al.*, *Drug Intell. & clin. Pharm.*, 1987, *21*, 346). It has been suggested that the beneficial effect of metronidazole in rosacea may be due to its antiparasitic activity on *Demodex folliculorum* (N. Kurkcuoglu and N. Atakan, *Archs Derm.*, 1984, *120*, 837), but others (Y. Miyachi *et al.*, *Br. J. Derm.*, 1986, *114*, 231) propose an anti-inflammatory effect as a result of anti-oxidant action affecting neutrophil cell functions.

TRICHOMONIASIS. Trichomoniasis is caused by invasion of the genito-urinary tract with the protozoan *Trichomonas vaginalis.* It is a common cause of vaginitis and vaginal discharge; some infected women are asymptomatic but should still be treated. Men are usually asymptomatic although it may cause urethritis. Transmission is primarily sexual and sexual partners should be treated concomitantly. The treatment of choice is metronidazole given by mouth or other nitroimidazoles such as nimorazole or tinidazole. Metronidazole is trichomonicidal and is reported to be active at concentrations of 1.0 to 2.5 μg per mL; resistant strains of *T. vaginalis* have occasionally been reported. It has no effect on *Candida* spp. and mixed vaginal infections should be treated with metronidazole and an antifungal drug such as nystatin.

Resistance of *Trichomonas vaginalis* to metronidazole has been controversial because of the inability to confirm conclusively the resistance of strains isolated from patients with refractory vaginal trichomoniasis. Treatment failure has thus been attributed to re-infection by the sexual partner, noncompliance, and poor absorption of metronidazole or its inactivation by the vaginal flora. However, a resistant strain has been identified in a woman resistant to standard courses of treatment (J. Thurner and J.G. Meingassner, *Lancet*, 1978, *2*, 738); the isolate was found to be unequivocally resistant to metronidazole, tinidazole, and nimorazole, but only under aerobic testing conditions (J.G. Meingassner and J. Thurner, *Antimicrob. Ag. Chemother.*, 1979, *15*, 254). There have since been similar reports of resistant strains associated with treatment failure; infection in one patient proved totally refractory to repeated treatment with high doses of metronidazole (up to 6 g daily for 5 days, in hospital) (J.G. Lossick, *New Engl. J. Med.*, 1981, *304*, 735) whereas another was eventually treated successfully with a high-dose regimen of 750 mg four times daily by mouth for 14 days, together with 500 mg nightly by vaginal pessary (S. Krajden *et al.*, *Can. med. Ass. J.*, 1986, *134*, 1373).

In a comparison of the 2 recommended regimens for the treatment of vaginal trichomoniasis, metronidazole was given by mouth as a single 2-g dose to 96 women or as a 7-day course of 250 mg three times daily to 74 women. The same regimens were prescribed for sexual partners in 90% of cases and women were requested to avoid sexual intercourse during treatment. Cure-rates of 93.8% for the single-dose regimen and 97.3% for the 7-day regimen were achieved and were not significantly different. The only side-effects reported were nausea and/or vomiting in 4 women taking the single 2-g dose. The use of a single 2-g dose of metronidazole is therefore recommended for the treatment of vaginal trichomoniasis; it has the advantages of easy administration, better patient compliance, and lower cost.— J. M. Aubert and H. J. Sesta, *J. reprod. Med.*, 1982, *27*, 743.

A cure-rate of 94% was achieved in a series of 79 patients with vaginal trichomoniasis given a single 2-g dose of metronidazole in rectal suppositories.— S. K. Panja, *Br. J. vener. Dis.*, 1982, *58*, 257.

Preparations

Metronidazole Injection *(U.S.P.)*

Metronidazole Suppositories *(B.P.)*

Metronidazole Tablets *(B.P.)*

Metronidazole Tablets *(U.S.P.)*

Proprietary Preparations

Elyzol *(CP Pharmaceuticals, UK). Suppositories*, metronidazole 0.5 and 1 g.

Flagyl *(May & Baker, UK). Tablets*, metronidazole 200 and 400 mg.
Intravenous infusion, metronidazole 5 mg/mL, in ampoules of 20 mL and bottles and plastic bags of 100 mL.
Suppositories, metronidazole 0.5 and 1 g.

Flagyl Compak *(May & Baker, UK). Combination pack*, 21 metronidazole 200 mg tablets and 14 nystatin 100 000 units pessaries.

Flagyl-S *(May & Baker, UK). Suspension*, metronidazole 200 mg (as benzoate)/5mL.

Metrolyl *(Lagap, UK). Tablets*, metronidazole 200 and 400 mg.
Intravenous infusion, metronidazole 5 mg/mL, in bottles and plastic bags of 100 mL.
Suppositories, metronidazole 0.5 and 1 g.

Nidazol *(Steinhard, UK). Tablets*, scored, metronidazole 200 mg.

Vaginyl *(DDSA Pharmaceuticals, UK). Tablets*, scored, metronidazole 200 and 400 mg.

Zadstat *(Lederle, UK). Tablets*, scored, metronidazole 200 mg.
Intravenous infusion, metronidazole 5 mg/mL, in plastic bags of 100 mL.
Suppositories, metronidazole 0.5 and 1 g.

Proprietary Names and Manufacturers of Metronidazole and its Salts

Anaerobyl *(Searle, S.Afr.)*; Arilin *(Wolff, Ger.; Cimex, Switz.)*; Clont *(Bayer, Ger.)*; Debetrol *(Arg.)*; Deflamon *(SPA, Ital.)*; Elyzol *(Dumex, Denm.; Dumex, Norw.; Dumex, Swed.; Dumex, Switz.; CP Pharmaceuticals, UK)*; Entizol *(Pol.)*; Flagyl *(Arg.; May & Baker, Austral.; Belg.; Rhône-Poulenc, Canad.; Rhone-Poulenc, Denm.; Specia, Fr.; Rhône-Poulenc, Ger.; Farmitalia, Ital.; Neth.; Rhône-Poulenc, Norw.; NZ; May & Baker, S.Afr.; Rhone, Spain; Leo Rhodia, Swed.; Rhone-Poulenc, Switz.; May & Baker, UK; Searle, USA)*; Flagyl-S *(May & Baker, UK)*; Fossyol *(Merckle, Ger.)*; Gineflavir *(Crosara, Ital.)*; Klion *(Hung.)*; Kreucosan *(Kreussler, Ger.)*; Meronidal *(Jpn)*; Metazol *(Wilson, Pakistan)*; Metizol *(Glenwood, USA)*; Metric 21 *(Fielding, USA)*; Metrolag *(Lagap, Switz.)*; Metrolyl *(Lagap, UK)*; Metroni *(Casen Fisons, Spain)*; Metrozine *(Searle, Austral.)*; Metryl *(Lagamed, S. Afri.; Lemmon, USA)*; Nalox *(Arg.)*; Narobic *(Schwulst, S.Afr.)*; Neo-Metric *(Neolab, Canad.)*; Neo-Tric *(Canad.)*; Nida *(Jpn)*; Nidazol *(Steinhard, UK)*; Novonidazol *(Novopharm, Canad.)*; Protostat *(Ortho Pharmaceutical, USA)*; Rathimed N *(Pfleger, Ger.)*; Salandol *(Jpn)*; Sanatrichom *(Ger.)*; Satric *(Savage, USA)*; SK-Metronidazole *(Smith Kline & French, USA)*; Tranoxa *(Arg.)*; Trichazole *(Lennon, S.Afr.)*; Tricho Cordes *(Ichthyol, Ger.)*; Trichocide *(Jpn)*; Tricho-Gynaedron oral *(Ger.)*; Trichomol *(GEA, Denm.)*; Trichozole *(Protea, Austral.)*; Tricocet *(Lusofarmaco, Ital.)*; Tricofin Oral *(Arg.)*; Tricowas B *(Wasserman, Spain)*; Trikacide *(Canad.)*; Trivazol *(Ital.)*; Vagilen *(Farmigea, Ital.)*; Vaginyl *(DDSA Pharmaceuticals, UK)*; Zadstat *(Lederle, UK)*; Zolerol *(Rolab, S.Afr.)*.

The following names have been used for multi-ingredient preparations containing metronidazole and its salts— Entamizole *(Boots, UK)*; Flagyl Compak *(May & Baker, UK)*; Flagystatin *(Rhône-Poulenc, Canad.)*.

12973-q

Monensin Sodium *(BANM, rINNM)*.

Lilly-67314 *(monensin)*. An antibiotic produced by *Streptomyces cinnamonensis*. Sodium 4-{2-[2-ethyl-3′-methyl-5′-(tetrahydro-6-hydroxy-6-hydroxymethyl-3,5-dimethyl-2*H*-pyran-2-yl)perhydro-2,2′-bifuran-5-yl]-9-hydroxy-2,8-dimethyl-1,6-dioxaspiro[4.5]dec-7-yl}-3-methoxy-2-methylvalerate.

$C_{36}H_{61}NaO_{11}$=692.9.

CAS — 17090-79-8 (monensin); 22373-78-0 (sodium salt).

NOTE. Monensin is *USAN*.

Monensin sodium is an antiprotozoal agent used in veterinary practice for the prevention of coccidiosis in poultry and as a growth promoter for cattle.

Proprietary Veterinary Names and Manufacturers
Elancoban *(Elanco, UK)*; Romensin *(Elanco, UK)*.

12016-p

Narasin *(BAN, USAN, rINN)*.

Lilly-79891. An antibiotic produced by *Streptomyces aureofaciens*. 2-(6-{5-[2-(5-Ethyltetrahydro-5-hydroxy-6-methylpyran-2-yl)-15-hydroxy-2,10,12-trimethyl-1,6,8-trioxadispiro[4.1.5.3]pentadec-13-en-9-yl]-2-

hydroxy-1,3-dimethyl-4-oxoheptyl}tetrahydro-3,5-dimethylpyran-2-yl)butyric acid.
$C_{43}H_{72}O_{11}$=765.0.

CAS — 55134-13-9.

Narasin is an antiprotozoal agent used in veterinary practice for the prevention of coccidiosis in poultry.

Proprietary Veterinary Names and Manufacturers
Monteban *(Elanco, UK).*

13007-z

Nicarbazin *(BAN).*

An equimolecular complex of 1,3-bis(4-nitrophenyl)urea ($C_{13}H_{10}N_4O_5$) and 4,6-dimethylpyrimidin-2-ol ($C_6H_8N_2O$).
$C_{19}H_{18}N_6O_6$=426.4.

CAS — 330-95-0.

Nicarbazin is an antiprotozoal agent used in veterinary practice for the prevention of coccidiosis in poultry.

Proprietary Veterinary Names and Manufacturers
Nicrazin *(Merck Sharp & Dohme, UK).*

4789-q

Nifuratel *(BAN, USAN, rINN).*

Methylmercadone. 5-Methylthiomethyl-3-(5-nitrofurfurylideneamino)-2-oxazolidone.
$C_{10}H_{11}N_3O_5S$=285.3.

CAS — 4936-47-4.

Pharmacopoeias. In *Nord.*

Adverse Effects

Gastro-intestinal discomfort and skin rashes occasionally occur with nifuratel.

ALLERGY. A report of contact dermatitis after only one application of nifuratel ointment in a man whose wife was undergoing treatment with nifuratel vaginal pessaries.— P. G. Bedello *et al., Contact Dermatitis,* 1983, *9,* 166.

Precautions

Nausea and flushing of the skin may occur if large quantities of alcohol are taken during treatment with nifuratel.

Absorption and Fate

When taken by mouth nifuratel is absorbed from the gastro-intestinal tract. A metabolite, with activity against bacteria but not against trichomonads, is excreted in the urine.

Uses and Administration

Nifuratel is a nitrofuran derivative with a broad antimicrobial spectrum. It is active against the protozoan *Trichomonas vaginalis,* has an antibacterial spectrum similar to that of nitrofurantoin, and some activity against *Candida albicans.* Nifuratel has been used in the treatment of susceptible infections of the genito-urinary tract in doses of 200 to 400 mg three times daily by mouth. It has also been administered vaginally.

Proprietary Names and Manufacturers
Inimur *(Rorer, Ger.);* Macmiror *(Beta, Arg.; Poli, Ital.; Neth.; Adcock Ingram, S.Afr.; Farma-Lepori, Spain; Poli, Switz.);* Magmilor *(Calmic, UK);* Omnes *(Belg.; Fumouze, Fr.);* Polmiror *(Astra, Denm.; Astra, Swed.).*

13015-z

Nifursol *(BAN, USAN, pINN).*

3,5-Dinitro-2′-(5-nitrofurfurylidene)salicylohydrazide.
$C_{12}H_7N_5O_9$=365.2.

CAS — 16915-70-1.

Nifursol is an antiprotozoal agent used in veterinary practice for the management of blackhead (histomoniasis) in turkeys.

Proprietary Veterinary Names and Manufacturers
Salfuride *(Salsbury, UK).*

4790-d

Nifurtimox *(BAN, rINN).*

Bayer-2502. Tetrahydro-3-methyl-4-(5-nitrofurfurylideneamino)-1,4-thiazine 1,1-dioxide.
$C_{10}H_{13}N_3O_5S$=287.3.

CAS — 23256-30-6.

Adverse Effects

Adverse effects are common with nifurtimox and include gastro-intestinal effects such as anorexia with loss of weight, abdominal pain, nausea, and vomiting and effects on the nervous system, especially peripheral neuropathy. Psychoses, CNS excitement, insomnia, drowsiness, headache, dizziness, and convulsions have also been reported. Skin rashes and other allergic reactions may occur.

Absorption and Fate

Nifurtimox is well absorbed and rapidly metabolised following administration by mouth.

Uses and Administration

Nifurtimox is a nitrofuran derivative with antiprotozoal activity. It is of value in the treatment of South American trypanosomiasis (Chagas' disease) due to infection by *Trypanosoma cruzi,* especially the early acute stage of the disease.

Nifurtimox is given by mouth in divided doses. It is better tolerated by children than by adults. Recommended doses are: adults, 8 to 10 mg per kg body-weight daily for 60 to 120 days; children of 1 to 10 years, 15 to 20 mg per kg daily; of 11 to 16 years, 12.5 to 15 mg per kg daily.

LEISHMANIASIS. Pentavalent antimony, usually meglumine antimonate, is considered the treatment of choice for mucocutaneous leishmaniasis of the New World. Nifurtimox 10 mg per kg body-weight daily for a minimum of 4 weeks has been shown to be effective in a large proportion of cases of cutaneous leishmaniasis and in a smaller proportion of mucocutaneous leishmaniasis in Colombia and Brazil. However, toxic effects with nifurtimox are common and its role as a second-line drug or in combination with pentavalent antimony has not yet been established.— Report of a WHO Expert Committee on the Leishmaniases, *Tech. Rep. Ser. Wld Hlth Org. No. 701,* 1984.

Nifurtimox has been tried as an adjunct or alternative to antimonial therapy in mucosal leishmaniasis, but is weak in cutaneous disease in comparison to the antimonials and relatively ineffective in mucosal disease.— P. D. Marsden, *Trans. R. Soc. trop. Med. Hyg.,* 1986, *80,* 859.

For further information on leishmaniasis and its treatment, see Leishmaniasis, p.659.

TRYPANOSOMIASIS. *African trypanosomiasis.* Nifurtimox has recently been found suitable for curing African trypanosomiasis due to *Trypanosoma brucei gambiense,* including late-stage disease refractory to melarsoprol. However, few data are available at present and further studies are needed.— Report of a WHO Expert Committee on Epidemiology and Control of African Trypanosomiasis, *Tech. Rep. Ser. Wld Hlth Org. No. 739,* 1986.

References: F. Moens *et al., Annls Soc. belge Med. trop.,* 1984, *64,* 37.

American trypanosomiasis. The acute stage of South American trypanosomiasis is controlled effectively by nifurtimox. However, there has been controversy over its ability to cure completely, that is eradicate all parasites, in chronic disease. Cure-rates appear to decrease going from south to north in Latin America and this is probably due in part to variation in the sensitivity of different strains of *Trypanosoma cruzi.* Nifurtimox is not well tolerated and few patients complete the full 120-day treatment period that has been recommended for the cure of chronic cases. Two hypotheses have been advanced to explain the mode of action of nifurtimox. One involves interaction of a nitro-anion radical metabolite with nucleic acids, especially DNA, and is similar to the mechanism proposed for the antibacterial action of other nitrofuran drugs. The other involves the production of superoxide anions; the ability of *T. cruzi* to generate free radical metabolites from nifurtimox has been demonstrated. Both proposed mechanisms might have a role.— W. E. Gutteridge, *Br. med. Bull.,* 1985, *41,* 162.

Success-rates of 90% (xenodiagnosis) and 80% (immunological response) had been achieved in 550 patients with acute Chagas' disease treated with nifurtimox. Of 89 patients with chronic Chagas' disease treated with nifurtimox 8 to 10 mg per kg body-weight daily for short (30 to 60 days) or long (90 to 120 days) periods 76 were considered to be free of infection (xenodiagnosis) after follow-up for at least 11 months. Results from treatment for short or long periods were comparable. The cure-rate was about 92% in Argentina, Chile, and Southern Brazil, and about 53% in central Brazil.— J. A. Cerisola, in *Chagas' Disease,* Proceedings of an International Symposium, New York City, 27 June 1977, Washington, Pan American Health Organization, Scientific Publication No. 347,, p. 35.

For a brief description of South American trypanosomiasis, see p.658.

Proprietary Names and Manufacturers
Lampit *(Bayer, Ger.).*

4791-n

Nimorazole *(BAN, rINN).*

Nitrimidazine. 4-[2-(5-Nitroimidazol-1-yl)ethyl]-morpholine.
$C_9H_{14}N_4O_3$=226.2.

CAS — 6506-37-2.

Pharmacopoeias. In *It.*

Adverse Effects and Precautions

As for Metronidazole, p.667.

Absorption and Fate

Nimorazole is readily absorbed from the gastro-intestinal tract. Peak blood concentrations are achieved within 2 hours, and high concentrations are reported to occur in salivary and vaginal secretions. It is excreted in the urine together with 2 active metabolites.

Uses and Administration

Nimorazole is a 5-nitroimidazole derivative. It has antimicrobial actions and uses similar to those of metronidazole (see p.669) and is used similarly in the treatment of protozoal infections. It is also used in the treatment of acute necrotising ulcerative gingivitis (Vincent's infection) and has been given in the treatment of bacterial vaginosis (nonspecific vaginitis).

In the treatment of trichomoniasis, the usual dose of nimorazole is 2 g by mouth as a single dose with a main meal. Sexual partners should be treated concomitantly. In giardiasis, nimorazole 500 mg is given twice daily for 5 days; a suggested dose for children is 500 mg daily for those over 10 kg body-weight and 250 mg daily for those under 10 kg, both for 5 days. Similar dosage regimens are suggested for the treatment of amoebiasis.

In the treatment of acute necrotising ulcerative gingivitis, nimorazole 500 mg is given twice daily for 2 days.

ANAEROBIC BACTERIAL INFECTIONS. For reports indicating that nimorazole is less active than metronidazole or of similar activity against anaerobic bacteria *in vitro,* see Metronidazole, p.670.

BACTERIAL VAGINOSIS. Single 2-g oral doses of metronidazole, nimorazole, or tinidazole were equally effective in the treatment of vaginitis associated with *Gardnerella vaginalis* in a study involving 280 patients, although tinidazole proved more active *in vitro.*— K. C. Mohanty and R. Deighton, *J. antimicrob. Chemother.,* 1987, *19,* 393.

Proprietary Preparations

Naxogin 500 *(Farmitalia Carlo Erba, UK). Tablets,* scored, nimorazole 500 mg.

Proprietary Names and Manufacturers
Acterol Forte *(Ger.);* Esclama *(Farmitalia, Ger.);* Naxogin *(Arg.; Belg.; Carlo Erba, Ital.; Neth.; Farmitalia Carlo Erba, S.Afr.; Spain; Farmitalia Carlo Erba, UK);* Naxogyn *(Farmitalia Carlo Erba, Fr.);* Sirledi *(Inverni della Beffa, Ital.).*

1626-w

Nitrofurazone *(BAN, USAN).*

Furacilinum; Nitrofural *(pINN).* 5-Nitro-2-furaldehyde semicarbazone.

$C_6H_6N_4O_4$=198.1.

CAS — 59-87-0.

Pharmacopoeias. In *Aust., Br., Braz., Cz., Ind., It., Pol., Port., Rus.,* and *U.S.* Also in *B.P. Vet.*

A lemon to brownish-yellow odourless or almost odourless, crystalline powder. It slowly darkens on exposure to light and discolours on contact with alkalis.

Soluble 1 in 4200 of water, 1 in 590 of alcohol, and 1 in 350 of propylene glycol; soluble in dimethylformamide; practically insoluble in chloroform and ether. The filtrate from a 1% suspension in water has a pH of 5.0 to 7.5. **Store** at a temperature not exceeding 40° in airtight containers. Protect from light.

Adverse Effects

Sensitisation and generalised allergic skin reactions may be produced by the topical application of nitrofurazone.

Nitrofurazone is a toxic drug when given by mouth and serious adverse effects include severe peripheral neuropathy; haemolysis may occur in patients with a deficiency of glucose-6-phosphate dehydrogenase. Nitrofurazone in high oral doses is carcinogenic in *rats.*

Precautions

Topical preparations of nitrofurazone are contra-indicated in patients with known hypersensitivity. Those preparations containing macrogols should be used with caution in patients with renal dysfunction since macrogols can be absorbed through denuded skin and their accumulation in such patients may result in symptoms of progressive renal impairment.

Because of the risk of haemolysis nitrofurazone by mouth should be used with caution in patients with glucose-6-phosphate dehydrogenase deficiency.

Uses and Administration

Nitrofurazone is a nitrofuran derivative and has an antibacterial action against a number of Gram-negative and Gram-positive bacteria. *Pseudomonas* spp. are not generally susceptible. It is used as a local application for wounds, burns, ulcers, and skin infections, and for the preparation of surfaces before skin grafting. It is usually applied in a concentration of 0.2% in a water-soluble or water-miscible basis. A solution of nitrofurazone was formerly used for bladder irrigation.

Nitrofurazone also has antiprotozoal activity and, despite its toxicity when administered systemically, has been given in the treatment of late-stage African trypanosomiasis refractory to melarsoprol.

A review of the use of nitrofurazone as a topical antibacterial agent in the treatment of wounds, dermatological conditions, and burns.— G. Hooper and J. Covarrubias, *J. int. med. Res.,* 1983, *11,* 289.

TRYPANOSOMIASIS. Nitrofurazone can be employed in African trypanosomiasis resistant to melarsoprol, but its toxicity makes it unsuitable for regular use. Nitrofurazone is given by mouth in an adult dosage of 500 mg three or four times daily for 5 to 7 days. Its use is restricted to hospitals where haematocrit and glucose-6-phosphate dehydrogenase estimations can be done.— Report of a Joint WHO Expert Committee and FAO Expert Consultation on The African Trypanosomiases, *Tech. Rep. Ser. Wld Hlth Org. No. 635,* 1979. Nitrofurazone has been the only compound available with proven activity against late-stage African trypanosomiasis refractory to melarsoprol. More recently nifurtimox and eflornithine have shown promise although further studies are needed.— Report of a WHO Expert Committee on Epidemiology and Control of African Trypanosomiasis, *Tech. Rep. Ser. Wld Hlth Org. No. 739,* 1986.

Preparations

Nitrofurazone Cream *(U.S.P.)*
Nitrofurazone Ointment *(U.S.P.)*
Nitrofurazone Topical Solution *(U.S.P.)*

Proprietary Preparations

Furacin *(Norwich-Eaton, UK). Soluble ointment,* nitrofurazone 0.2%, in a water-soluble macrogol basis.

Proprietary Names and Manufacturers

Acutol *(Switz.)*; Becafurazona *(Carol, Spain)*; Furacin *(Arg.; Norwich-Eaton, Austral.; Canad.; Röhm, Ger.; Formenti, Ital.; Eaton, S.Afr.; Seid, Spain; Switz.; Norwich-Eaton, UK; Norwich Eaton, USA)*; Furacine *(Belg.; Neth.)*; Furesol *(Norw.)*; Germex *(Lennon, S.Afr.)*; Rivafurazon *(Carol, Spain).*

4792-h

Ornidazole *(USAN, rINN).*

Ro-7-0207. 1-Chloro-3-(2-methyl-5-nitroimidazol-1-yl)propan-2-ol.

$C_7H_{10}ClN_3O_3$=219.6.

CAS — 16773-42-5.

Adverse Effects and Precautions

As for Metronidazole, p.667.

Absorption and Fate

Ornidazole is readily absorbed from the gastro-intestinal tract and peak plasma concentrations of about 30 µg per mL have been achieved within 2 hours of a single dose of 1.5 g, falling to about 9 µg per mL after 24 hours and 2.5 µg per mL after 48 hours. Ornidazole is also absorbed from the vagina and peak plasma concentrations of about 5 µg per mL have been reported 12 hours after the insertion of a 500-mg vaginal pessary.

The plasma elimination half-life of ornidazole is 12 to 14 hours. Less than 15% is bound to plasma proteins. It is widely distributed in body tissues and fluids, including the cerebrospinal fluid.

Ornidazole is metabolised in the liver and is excreted in the urine, mainly as conjugates and metabolites, and to a lesser extent in the faeces; 85% of a single oral dose has been reported to be eliminated within 5 days, 63% in the urine and 22% in the faeces. Biliary excretion may be important in the elimination of ornidazole and its metabolites.

References to pharmacokinetic studies of ornidazole: D. E. Schwartz and F. Jeunet, *Chemotherapy, Basle,* 1976, *22,* 19 (comparison with metronidazole); I. Matheson *et al., Br. J. vener. Dis.,* 1977, *53,* 236 (plasma concentrations); D. E. Schwartz *et al., Xenobiotica,* 1979, *9,* 571 (metabolism); H. Merdjan *et al., Br. J. clin. Pharmac.,* 1985, *19,* 211 (in renal failure); A. M. Taburet *et al., Clin. Pharmac. Ther.,* 1986, *40,* 359 (in liver disease); A. Turcant *et al., Eur. J. clin. Pharmac.,* 1987, *32,* 111 (in neonates and infants).

Uses and Administration

Ornidazole is a 5-nitroimidazole derivative. It has the antimicrobial actions of metronidazole and is used similarly (see p.669) in the treatment of susceptible protozoal infections and in the treatment and prophylaxis of anaerobic bacterial infections.

It is administered by mouth in tablets after food, by vaginal pessary, or intravenously. When given intravenously, solutions of ornidazole should be diluted to 5 mg or less per mL and 100 or 200 mL infused over 15 to 30 minutes.

In amoebiasis, 500 mg of ornidazole is given twice daily by mouth for 5 to 10 days; children are given 25 mg per kg body-weight daily as a single dose. Patients with amoebic dysentery may be given 1.5 g as a single daily dose for 3 days; the children's dose is 40 mg per kg daily. In severe amoebic dysentery and amoebic liver abscess ornidazole may be given by intravenous infusion in a dose of 0.5 to 1 g initially, followed by 500 mg every 12 hours for 3 to 6 days; the children's dose is 20 to 30 mg per kg daily.

In giardiasis, 1.5 g of ornidazole is given by mouth as a single dose for 1 or 2 days; the children's dose is 40 mg per kg.

In trichomoniasis, a single dose of 1.5 g by mouth or 1 g by mouth together with 500 mg vaginally is given; 5-day courses of ornidazole 500 mg twice daily, with or without 500 mg vaginally, are also used. Sexual partners should be treated concomitantly. The children's dose is 25 mg per kg daily.

For the treatment of anaerobic bacterial infections, ornidazole is given by intravenous infusion in an initial dose of 0.5 to 1 g, followed by 500 mg every 12 hours for 5 to 10 days; oral therapy with 500 mg every 12 hours should be substituted as soon as possible. Children are given 10 mg per kg every 12 hours.

For the prevention of postoperative anaerobic bacterial infections, 1 g is given by intravenous infusion about 30 minutes before surgery.

Toxicological and clinical evaluation of ornidazole.— R. Richle *et al., Arzneimittel-Forsch.,* 1978, *28,* 612.

ADMINISTRATION IN HEPATIC FAILURE. The elimination of ornidazole following a single intravenous dose of 500 mg was impaired in 10 patients with severe liver cirrhosis when compared with 10 healthy subjects; mean half-lives were 21.9 hours and 14.1 hours respectively. It is suggested that the interval between doses of ornidazole should be doubled in patients with marked hepatic impairment.— A. M. Taburet *et al., Clin. Pharmac. Ther.,* 1986, *40,* 359.

ADMINISTRATION IN INFANTS AND CHILDREN. The pharmacokinetics of ornidazole in infants aged 1 to 42 weeks given 20 mg per kg body-weight by intravenous infusion over 20 minutes, before surgery, were similar to those reported in adults. Such a dose daily appears adequate for the therapy of anaerobic bacterial infections in neonates and infants.— A. Turcant *et al., Eur. J. clin. Pharmac.,* 1987, *32,* 111.

ADMINISTRATION IN RENAL FAILURE. The half-life of ornidazole administered intravenously was not prolonged in a study in patients with advanced chronic renal failure, including those on continuous ambulatory peritoneal dialysis, and modification of the usual dosage is not necessary in such patients. However, ornidazole was removed by haemodialysis and ornidazole should be given after the dialysis session rather than before.— H. Merdjan *et al., Br. J. clin. Pharmac.,* 1985, *19,* 211.

AMOEBIASIS. For the successful use of treatment with ornidazole for a single day in amoebic liver abscess, see Tinidazole, p.681.

ANAEROBIC BACTERIAL INFECTIONS. Mixed aerobic-anaerobic infections, in which *Escherichia coli* and *Bacteroides fragilis* were the predominant isolates, were cured in 15 of 16 patients given ornidazole 500 mg by intravenous infusion over 30 minutes every 12 hours after an initial dose of 1 g. Oral administration at the same dose was substituted when possible. Duration of treatment ranged from 5 to 60 days (mean 21 days).— H. Giamarellou *et al., J. antimicrob. Chemother.,* 1981, *7,* 569.

For comparison of the activity *in vitro* of nitroimidazole compounds against anaerobic bacteria, including a report that ornidazole was more active than metronidazole and less active than tinidazole against *Bacteroides fragilis,* see Metronidazole, p.670.

BACTERIAL VAGINOSIS. In a pilot study all of 39 women with vaginal infection associated with *Gardnerella vaginalis* had complete resolution of their symptoms, although *G. vaginalis* was not always eradicated, after treatment with one of the following 7-day regimens: ornidazole 500 mg vaginally each night; ornidazole 500 mg twice daily by mouth, with or without 500 mg vaginally each night; or metronidazole 400 mg three times daily by mouth. No one regimen was clearly superior to another, but it was considered that topical therapy with ornidazole might have some advantage over oral therapy.— R. J. Meech and J. Loutit, *N.Z. med. J.,* 1985, *98,* 389.

Vaginal infection with *Gardnerella vaginalis* had been eradicated in 119 of 129 women (92%) at follow-up 7 to 14 days after single-dose treatment with ornidazole 1 g by mouth and intravaginally. In most cases, including 9 of the 10 treatment failures, the regular sexual partner received a single oral dose of ornidazole 1.5 g.— K. Haukka *et al., Eur. J. sex. transm. Dis.,* 1985, *2,* 129.

GIARDIASIS. Single oral 1.5-g doses of ornidazole or tinidazole were equally effective against giardiasis in a study in 100 symptomatic patients.— L. Jokipii and A.

M. M. Jokipii, *Gastroenterology*, 1982, *83*, 399.

TRICHOMONIASIS. In a double-blind study all of 45 women with vaginal trichomoniasis were cleared of infection after a single dose of ornidazole 1.5 g by mouth; of 43 given tinidazole 2 g as a single dose 43 were cleared. Sexual partners were treated concomitantly.— L. Hillström *et al.*, *Br. J. vener. Dis.*, 1977, *53*, 193.

Proprietary Names and Manufacturers
Kolpicid *(Roche, Swed.)*; Ornidal *(Selvi, Ital.)*; Tiberal *(Roche, Arg.; Roche, Austral.; Roche, Fr.; Roche, Ger.; Roche, Ital.; Roche, S.Afr.; Roche, Switz.)*.

18671-a

Parvaquone *(BAN, rINN)*.
2-Cyclohexyl-3-hydroxy-1,4-naphthoquinone.
$C_{16}H_{16}O_3$=256.3.

CAS — 4042-30-2.

Parvaquone is an antiprotozoal agent used in veterinary practice in the treatment of theileriosis.

Proprietary Veterinary Names and Manufacturers
Wellcome, UK.

4794-b

Pentamidine Isethionate *(BANM)*.

M & B-800; Pentamidine Isetionate *(rINNM)*; Pentamidini Isethionas. 4,4′-(Pentamethylenedioxy)dibenzamidine bis(2-hydroxyethanesulphonate).
$C_{19}H_{24}N_4O_2,2C_2H_6O_4S$=592.7.

CAS — 100-33-4 (pentamidine); 140-64-7 (isethionate).

Pharmacopoeias. In *Br., Egypt., Ind., Int., It.,* and *Turk.*

White or almost white, odourless or almost odourless hygroscopic crystals or powder. Pentamidine isethionate 1.74 mg is approximately equivalent to 1 mg of pentamidine.

Soluble 1 in 10 of water; slightly soluble in alcohol; practically insoluble in chloroform and ether. A 5% solution in water has a pH of 4.5 to 6.5. Aqueous solutions deteriorate on storage and should be used immediately after preparation; solutions for injection are prepared aseptically. **Store** in well-closed containers.

4793-m

Pentamidine Mesylate *(BANM)*.

Pentamidine Dimethylsulphonate; Pentamidine Mesilate *(rINNM)*; Pentamidine Methanesulphonate; RP-2512. Pentamidine dimethanesulphonate.
$C_{19}H_{24}N_4O_2,2CH_3SO_3H$=532.6.

CAS — 6823-79-6.

Pharmacopoeias. In *Fr.*

A white or very faintly pink, almost odourless, granular powder. Pentamidine mesylate 1.56 mg is approximately equivalent to 1 mg of pentamidine. Slightly **soluble** in water and alcohol; practically insoluble in acetone, chloroform, and ether. A 5% solution in water has a pH of 4.5 to 6.5.

Adverse Effects

Pentamidine is a toxic drug and adverse effects are frequent and sometimes severe. Impaired renal function is common, but is usually manifest as mild and reversible raised blood urea nitrogen and serum creatinine concentrations. Raised liver enzyme values and haematological disturbances such as leucopenia, and occasionally thrombocytopenia, may occur. Hypoglycaemia, sometimes followed by hyperglycaemia and insulin-dependent diabetes mellitus, is well documented; there have been occasional reports of acute pancreatitis.

The rapid intravenous injection of pentamidine has resulted in sudden hypotension and immediate reactions such as dizziness, headache, vomiting, breathlessness, tachycardia, and fainting. Hypotension may also occur when pentamidine is administered intramuscularly or by slow intravenous infusion. The intramuscular administration of pentamidine often causes pain, swelling, and sterile abscess formation at the site of injection. Thrombophlebitis has occasionally followed intravenous administration.

Other adverse effects reported include hypocalcaemia, hyperkalaemia, skin rashes, the Stevens-Johnson syndrome, fever, flushing, gastro-intestinal effects such as nausea, vomiting, and taste disturbances, confusion, hallucinations, and cardiac arrhythmias.

In an analysis from the Center for Disease Control, 189 of 404 patients (46.8%) given pentamidine for the treatment of *Pneumocystis carinii* pneumonia experienced a total of 347 adverse reactions to the drug. These included impaired renal function (23.5% of patients), abnormal liver function (9.6%), hypoglycaemia (6.2%), haematological disturbances (4.2%), skin rashes (1.5%), and hypocalcaemia (1.2%). Local reactions at injection sites such as pain and abscess occurred in 18.3% and immediate side-effects such as hypotension in 9.6%. Nephrotoxicity was often the most serious adverse reaction although it was impossible to attribute it solely to pentamidine. Severe renal impairment occurred in 15 patients and contributed materially to 12 of 14 ensuing deaths. However elevation of blood urea nitrogen was usually relatively mild and reversible in those patients who had normal pretreatment renal function and had received no other nephrotoxic agents.— P. D. Walzer *et al.*, *Ann. intern. Med.*, 1974, *80*, 83.

Cardiotoxicity and metabolic disturbance were found to be limiting factors in the use of pentamidine in a study of 82 patients with visceral leishmaniasis resistant to treatment with sodium stibogluconate. The majority were given pentamidine intramuscularly, but in 9 patients it was given intravenously and in one patient both routes were used. Cardiotoxicity, manifested by tachycardia, hypotension, and ECG changes of nonspecific myocarditis, occurred in about 23% of patients. No hypoglycaemic reaction was noted, but 4 patients developed diabetes mellitus and 3 of them were found to be insulin-dependent. Other adverse reactions included gastro-intestinal effects (anorexia, nausea, vomiting, abdominal pain, or diarrhoea) in about 78%; CNS effects (headache associated with flushing, delirium, or sensory disturbances resembling pins and needles) in about 24%; mild reversible albuminuria in about 7%; and allergic manifestations (generalised urticaria, itching, and conjunctival congestion) in about 5%. One patient had severe anaphylaxis with shock, hypotension, abdominal and chest pain, breathlessness, and vomiting.— T. K. Jha, *Trans. R. Soc. trop. Med. Hyg.*, 1983, *77*, 167.

Contrary to previous experience with pentamidine and co-trimoxazole in the treatment of *Pneumocystis carinii* pneumonia, pentamidine was less toxic than co-trimoxazole in a retrospective review of AIDS patients treated for *Pn. carinii* pneumonia. Toxicity was seen in 13 of 30 patients (43%) given pentamidine intramuscularly, an incidence similar to that previously reported in patients without AIDS, but in 29 of 37 given co-trimoxazole, a substantially higher incidence than that seen in patients without AIDS. Adverse reactions to pentamidine occurred a median of 9.5 days after beginning treatment and were severe in 7 patients. Overall they included renal and hepatic abnormalities in 6 and 9 patients, respectively; leucopenia in 3; fever, rash, and thrombocytopenia in 1; and symptomatic hypoglycaemia requiring glucose infusion in 2.— F. M. Gordin *et al.*, *Ann. intern. Med.*, 1984, *100*, 495. In a further retrospective review of similar patients the incidence of toxicity with pentamidine was much higher. Adverse effects were experienced by 20 of 24 patients (83%) given pentamidine intramuscularly for the treatment of *Pn. carinii* pneumonia; 23 patients had AIDS and one had leukaemia. The most frequent were elevations in liver function tests, nausea and vomiting, hypoglycaemia, elevations in serum creatinine, and pain and induration at the site of injection. Other adverse effects noted included anaemia, leucopenia, and fever.— R. Andersen *et al.*, *Drug Intell. & clin. Pharm.*, 1986, *20*, 862.

A comparison of the toxicity of pentamidine given intramuscularly or intravenously. Severe hypotension has been reported following the intravenous injection of pentamidine over 5 to 10 minutes and the Centers for Disease Control (CDC) have recommended that the intramuscular route be used. However, analysis of reports to the CDC on 74 patients given pentamidine intramuscularly (52 patients) or by intravenous infusion over at least 60 minutes (22 patients) revealed a similar frequency of adverse reactions for both routes of administration and, in contrast to previous experience, hypotension was reported only with intramuscular administration. It is suggested that the previous high risk of hypotension associated with intravenous pentamidine was related to more rapid infusion rates and that the intravenous route is acceptable provided the drug is infused over at least 60 minutes under close medical supervision.— T. R. Navin and R. E. Fontaine (letter), *New Engl. J. Med.*, 1984, *311*, 1701. Hypotension occurred frequently in 167 patients given pentamidine, but the incidence was similar whether it was given intramuscularly or infused intravenously over 60 minutes or more.— C. G. Helmick and J. K. Green (letter), *Ann. intern. Med.*, 1985, *103*, 480. In patients with diarrhoea, renal toxicity occurred more frequently with intramuscular than with intravenous pentamidine and it is suggested that fluid status may have an important role in renal toxicity attributed to pentamidine.— J. K. Stehr-Green and C. G. Helmick (letter), *New Engl. J. Med.*, 1985, *313*, 694.

References to severe reactions associated with pentamidine: J. J. Wang *et al.*, *J. Pediat.*, 1970, *77*, 311 (toxic epidermal necrolysis, nephrotoxicity, and death); F. R. Stark *et al.* (letter), *Lancet*, 1976, *1*, 1193 (fatal Herxheimer-like reaction).

EFFECTS ON THE BLOOD. Pentamidine isethionate inhibited platelet adhesiveness, platelet aggregation, and clot retraction *in vitro* in a dose-dependent manner. The thrombin clotting time was prolonged at concentrations of pentamidine of 5 µg per mL and above and the prothrombin time at concentrations above 10 µg per mL.— S. J. Kempin *et al.*, *Antimicrob. Ag. Chemother.*, 1977, *12*, 451.

Severe reversible neutropenia developed in 3 patients with AIDS and *Pneumocystis carinii* pneumonia during treatment with pentamidine; in 2 of them neutropenia also developed or worsened during the administration of other anti-infective drugs. Earlier reports to the Centers for Disease Control on 179 similar patients noted that 26 had developed leucopenia and of these treatment with pentamidine had been withdrawn in 12; neutropenia or granulocytopenia was mentioned specifically in 6 of the 12.— *Morb. Mortal.*, 1984, *33*, 65.

EFFECTS ON CARBOHYDRATE METABOLISM. Severe fasting hypoglycaemia in 4 patients receiving pentamidine isethionate for *Pneumocystis carinii* pneumonia was followed later by hyperglycaemia and insulin-dependent diabetes mellitus. Following metabolic studies in 2 of the patients, studies *in vitro*, and an analysis of 90 published cases of pentamidine-induced hypoglycaemia, it was suggested that pentamidine, like streptozocin, has a toxic effect on the β-cells of the pancreatic islets and can induce an early cytolytic release of insulin and hypoglycaemia, followed by β-cell destruction, insulin deficiency, and diabetes mellitus.— P. Bouchard *et al.*, *Diabetes*, 1982, *31*, 40. A study *in vitro* using human insulinoma tissue supported this hypothesis, but *in vivo* pentamidine had no demonstrable effect when given to a patient with malignant insulinoma in an attempt to induce hyperglycaemia.— K. Osei *et al.*, *Am. J. Med.*, 1984, *77*, 41.

Pentamidine-induced hypoglycaemia and the associated inappropriate elevation of serum-insulin concentrations were successfully reversed in 2 patients by treatment with diazoxide by mouth.— D. B. Fitzgerald and I. S. Young, *J. trop. Med. Hyg.*, 1984, *87*, 15.

A retrospective study indicating that pentamidine-induced hypoglycaemia is more frequent and severe in AIDS patients. Hypoglycaemia developed in 10 (27%) of 37 AIDS patients during or shortly after treatment with pentamidine for *Pneumocystis carinii* pneumonia, an incidence at least 3-fold higher than that previously reported in patients with immunosuppression but not AIDS. Hypoglycaemia was symptomatic in all 9 evaluable patients and most developed CNS symptoms including dizziness, lightheadedness, agitation, lethargy, or altered mental status such as delirium or psychotic reactions; one patient developed permanent brain damage. Milder symptoms included anxiety, tremulousness, nausea, or vomiting. All of those with hypoglycaemia required therapy with 50% glucose intravenously. Insulin concentrations were normal in the 2 hypoglycaemic patients tested and no patient subsequently developed diabetes, although follow-up was relatively short. All those who developed hypoglycaemia also developed nephrotoxicity.— C. M. Stahl-Bayliss *et al.*, *Clin. Pharmac. Ther.*, 1986, *39*, 271.

Fatal acute pancreatitis occurred in 2 patients with

AIDS given pentamidine for *Pneumocystis carinii* pneumonia. Before the onset of clinical symptoms of pancreatitis, both had progressive renal impairment associated with hypoglycaemia that occurred after a week of therapy; in these circumstances pentamidine therapy should be interrupted.— S. Salmeron *et al.* (letter), *Ann. intern. Med.*, 1986, *105*, 140. A report of hyperglycaemia and fatal acute pancreatitis associated with pentamidine in a patient with AIDS.— A. Zuger *et al.*, *J. Am. med. Ass.*, 1986, *256*, 2383.

Further references: A. Belehu and B. Naafs (letter), *Lancet*, 1982, *1*, 1463 (diabetogenic effect associated with pentamidine mesylate but not the isethionate); T. K. Jha and V. K. Sharma, *Trans. R. Soc. trop. Med. Hyg.*, 1984, *78*, 252 (diabetogenic effect).

EFFECTS ON THE KIDNEY. Reports of uncommon forms of nephrotoxicity associated with the administration of pentamidine to AIDS patients: J. W. Sensakovic *et al.*, *Archs intern. Med.*, 1985, *145*, 2247 (myoglobinuria and acute renal failure); M. Shuster and M. Dunn (letter), *Ann. intern. Med.*, 1986, *105*, 146 (acute renal dysfunction and gross haematuria).

For reference to the relatively mild and reversible nephrotoxicity commonly associated with pentamidine therapy and also to the role of fluid status, see above.

EFFECTS ON THE PANCREAS. See under Effects on Carbohydrate Metabolism (above).

Precautions

Pentamidine should be used under close supervision. Patients should remain supine during administration and their blood pressure should be monitored. Kidney and liver function, blood-glucose concentrations, blood counts, and other parameters indicative of developing toxicity, such as serum-calcium concentrations and the ECG, should also be assessed regularly during courses of treatment with pentamidine.

The dosage of pentamidine may need to be reduced in patients with renal failure. The concomitant use of other nephrotoxic drugs should preferably be avoided.

Absorption and Fate

Pentamidine disappears rapidly from the blood following intramuscular or intravenous administration of the isethionate. It is deposited in tissues and excreted slowly in the urine.

Using fluorescence spectrophotometry, average low plasma-pentamidine concentrations of 400 ng per mL at 0.5 hour, 500 ng per mL at 1 hour, and 300 ng per mL at 3, 6, and 24 hours were observed in 7 patients following the daily intramuscular injection of pentamidine isethionate 4 mg per kg body-weight. The highest plasma concentrations of pentamidine were found in patients with an elevated blood urea nitrogen. Measurement in 5 patients showed that half to two-thirds of the urinary excretion took place in the first 6 hours and after treatment was stopped decreasing amounts were found in the urine up to 8 weeks later.— T. P. Waalkes *et al.*, *Clin. Pharmac. Ther.*, 1970, *11*, 505.

Using a newly developed bioassay for pentamidine, peak serum concentrations ranged from 0.5 to 3.2 μg per mL in 3 patients at the end of intravenous infusion over 1 to 2 hours of pentamidine [isethionate] 4 mg per kg body-weight. Concentrations declined rapidly and the mean half-life of elimination from serum was 17 minutes. Urinary excretion of pentamidine continued long after completion of treatment in 2 patients, with half-lives of about 5 and 9 days respectively. High tissue concentrations were found at autopsy in 4 patients who had received pentamidine intravenously and increased with the duration of therapy. The highest concentrations were in spleen and liver, followed by kidneys and adrenals; concentrations in lung were markedly lower.— E. M. Bernard *et al.*, *J. infect. Dis.*, 1985, *152*, 750.

Uses and Administration

Pentamidine, an aromatic diamidine derivative, is an antiprotozoal agent used in the treatment of the early stages of African trypanosomiasis, especially *Trypanosoma brucei gambiense* infections, and in *Pneumocystis carinii* pneumonia and some forms of leishmaniasis. It may act by several mechanisms including interference with protozoal DNA and folate transformation, and by inhibition of RNA and protein synthesis.

It has been given as the isethionate or mesylate salt, but pentamidine isethionate is the only form now available in the *UK* and *USA* and the manufacturers intend the isethionate to replace pentamidine mesylate worldwide. There is considerable confusion in the literature regarding the dosage of pentamidine since it is often not clear whether doses are being expressed in terms of pentamidine base, the isethionate salt, or the mesylate salt. In the treatment of *Pneumocystis carinii* pneumonia individual doses are clearly expressed as pentamidine isethionate 4 mg per kg body-weight. However, there is uncertainty as to whether the doses for African trypanosomiasis and leishmaniasis quoted in the literature are in terms of base or salt; in the 1986 WHO report on African trypanosomiasis a dose of pentamidine base 4 mg per kg (as the isethionate or mesylate) is specified whereas other guidelines for treatment specify pentamidine isethionate 4 mg per kg. In general it would appear that when the isethionate is used doses are expressed in terms of pentamidine isethionate, individual doses usually being up to 4 mg per kg, whereas when the mesylate is used doses are expressed in terms of pentamidine base. Pentamidine isethionate 4 mg per kg is approximately equivalent to pentamidine base 2.3 mg per kg; pentamidine mesylate 3.6 mg per kg is approximately equivalent to pentamidine base 2.3 mg per kg.

Pentamidine isethionate is administered by deep intramuscular injection or by slow intravenous infusion over at least 60 minutes; direct intravenous injection must be avoided. Patients should be lying down during administration. The mesylate has usually been given intramuscularly.

In the treatment of early African trypanosomiasis due to *T.b. gambiense*, pentamidine isethionate 4 mg per kg may be given daily or on alternate days by intramuscular injection or intravenous infusion to a total of 7 to 10 doses (WHO has specified a dose of pentamidine base 4 mg per kg). Pentamidine is not effective in trypanosomiasis with central nervous system involvement, but 1 or 2 injections of pentamidine may be given in late-stage *T.b. gambiense* infection before starting treatment with melarsoprol. Prophylaxis with single doses of pentamidine has been used in areas where trypanosomiasis is endemic, but in general is no longer recommended.

In the treatment of *Pneumocystis carinii* pneumonia, pentamidine isethionate 4 mg per kg is given once daily for 14 days, or longer in patients with AIDS, by intramuscular injection or preferably slow intravenous infusion.

In the treatment of visceral leishmaniasis, pentamidine isethionate 3 to 4 mg per kg may be given intramuscularly on alternate days to a maximum of 10 injections; the course may need to be repeated. In cutaneous leishmaniasis, pentamidine isethionate 3 to 4 mg per kg may be given intramuscularly once or twice a week until the condition resolves.

Reviews of the actions and uses of pentamidine: R. D. Pearson and E. L. Hewlett, *Ann. intern. Med.*, 1985, *103*, 782; M. Sands *et al.*, *Rev. infect. Dis.*, 1985, *7*, 625.

ADMINISTRATION. For comparison of the toxicity of pentamidine when given intramuscularly or intravenously, see Adverse Effects (above).

BABESIOSIS. In 3 nonsplenectomised patients infected with *Babesia microti* and presenting with severe symptoms, clinical improvement occurred 2 to 4 days after starting treatment with pentamidine [isethionate] 4 mg per kg body-weight daily by deep intramuscular injection. Treatment was continued for 2 weeks in 2 patients but was stopped after 7 days in the third because of raised creatinine concentrations. Pain at the injection site occurred in all 3 patients. Parasitaemia declined and in 2 patients organisms were no longer seen in blood smears 5 days after starting therapy; in the remaining patient, given pentamidine for 2 weeks, parasitaemia persisted and was still evident 5 weeks after treatment.— P. B. Francioli *et al.*, *Ann. intern. Med.*, 1981, *94*, 326. Comment. Although symptoms improved after pentamidine therapy the evidence for its efficacy against *B. microti* is not convincing. As previously seen in an asplenic patient with a much higher parasitaemia rate, a decreasing trend in parasitaemia may have already begun before treatment was started. Less toxic drugs such as chloroquine have provided similar symptomatic relief and pentamidine should be reserved for severe cases of babesiosis unresponsive to more conservative therapy.— S. M. Teutsch and D. D. Juranek (letter), *ibid.*, *95*, 241.

LEISHMANIASIS. In *visceral leishmaniasis* pentamidine is used, more commonly in the Old World, in patients who are unresponsive to the pentavalent antimonials sodium stibogluconate or meglumine antimonate. Pentamidine should be given in doses of 4 mg per kg body-weight three times a week for 5 to 25 weeks or longer, depending on the response [salt used and route of administration not stated]. *Cutaneous leishmaniasis of the Old World* due to *Leishmania aethiopica* is unresponsive to antimonials at conventional doses and most sores should be left to heal spontaneously. Mucocutaneous lesions are, however, extremely chronic and disfiguring and justify the use of pentamidine 3 to 4 mg per kg once or twice a week until resolution is complete, usually in a few weeks; relapse is unusual. In *diffuse cutaneous leishmaniasis* due to *L. aethiopica*, pentamidine 3 to 4 mg per kg is given once a week for 4 months longer than it takes to eliminate the parasites from slit-skin smears. Relapses may occur up to 7 months after remission and are treated in the same way. *Cutaneous leishmaniasis of the New World* due to *L. braziliensis* is treated with pentavalent antimonials. Lesions due to *L. braziliensis guyanensis* are particularly slow to respond and liable to relapse, but these lesions respond well to pentamidine. In *mucocutaneous leishmaniasis of the New World* failure to respond to pentavalent antimony is an indication for the use of amphotericin or pentamidine.— Report of a WHO Expert Committee on the Leishmaniases, *Tech. Rep. Ser. Wld Hlth Org. No. 701*, 1984.

References to the use of pentamidine in patients with visceral leishmaniasis unresponsive to sodium stibogluconate: C. P. Thakur *et al.*, *Br. med. J.*, 1984, *288*, 895; A. D. M. Bryceson *et al.*, *Trans. R. Soc. trop. Med. Hyg.*, 1985, *79*, 705.

For further information on leishmaniasis and its treatment, see Leishmaniasis, p.659.

PNEUMOCYSTIS CARINII PNEUMONIA. The protozoan *Pneumocystis carinii* is an opportunistic organism. It is probably acquired in childhood following subclinical infection by the airborne route and is then thought to become latent in the lungs, kept in check by T lymphocytes (*Lancet*, 1985, *1*, 676). In immunocompromised individuals such as premature or malnourished infants and patients of all ages with inherited or acquired immunodeficiency it causes pneumonia which is generally fatal if untreated.

Before the introduction of co-trimoxazole, pentamidine was the standard treatment for *Pneumocystis carinii* pneumonia. In an analysis of data submitted to the Center for Disease Control (P.D. Walzer *et al.*, *Ann. intern. Med.*, 1974, *80*, 83) the highest incidence of *Pn. carinii* pneumonia was in children less than 1 year old and the commonest underlying disease was leukaemia; 69 (42%) of 163 patients with confirmed *Pn. carinii* pneumonia treated with pentamidine recovered and 59 (63%) of 93 treated for 9 or more days recovered. Pentamidine, however, is toxic and almost half of the patients experienced side-effects. Subsequently, a comparative study in children with acute leukaemia or other malignancies found co-trimoxazole to be as effective as pentamidine in the treatment of *Pn. carinii* pneumonia, but to be less toxic (W.T. Hughes *et al.*, *J. Pediat.*, 1978, *92*, 285); co-trimoxazole can also be given by mouth. For further information on co-trimoxazole, see p.206.

Since the advent of the acquired immune deficiency syndrome (AIDS) the incidence of opportunistic infections with *Pn. carinii* has increased dramatically. At a National Institutes of Health workshop serious pulmonary disorders were reported in 441 (41%) of 1067 AIDS patients and of these 373 were *Pn. carinii* pneumonia (J.F. Murray *et al.*, *New Engl. J. Med.*, 1984, *310*, 1682); co-trimoxazole was recommended as the treatment of choice for first episodes of *Pn. carinii* pneumonia in patients with AIDS, although pentamidine should be given to those with hypersensitivity to co-trimoxazole or other sulphonamides and substitution of pentamidine should be considered on day 4 or 5 of treatment with co-trimoxazole if there has been continued progression of disease. There is no evidence that simultaneous treatment with co-trimoxazole and pentamidine is beneficial and the drug toxicities could be additive. Many patients treated for second episodes of *Pn. carinii* pneumonia did not respond to co-trimoxazole and in these circumstances the more frequent initial use of pentamidine may be justified. Patients with AIDS appear to have an increased incidence of adverse reactions to co-trimoxazole and it had to be withdrawn in about 20% of patients. In a retrospective study (J.A. Kovacs *et al.*, *Ann. intern. Med.*, 1984, *100*, 663) a much higher incidence of adverse reactions to co-trimoxazole was noted in AIDs patients than in those with other immunosuppressive diseases; *Pn. carinii* pneumonia was also found to present as a more insidious disease process in those with AIDS. The necessity for more prolonged therapy and a higher relapse-rate was noted in AIDS patients (H.W. Haverkos, *Am. J. Med.*, 1984, *76*, 501). In another retrospective study (F.M. Gordin *et al.*, *Ann. intern. Med.*, 1984, *100*, 495; see also Adverse Effects, above) co-trimoxazole was found to be more toxic than pentamidine in AIDS patients, contrary to earlier experience in patients without AIDS. However, in a small prospective study in 40 AIDS patients with *Pn. carinii* pneumonia (J.M. Wharton *et al.*, *Ann. intern. Med.*, 1986, *105*, 37) there was no significant difference in the incidence of adverse reactions to pentamidine or co-trimoxazole; efficacy was not considered by Wharton *et al.* to be significantly different either although in the short term 5 of 20 patients given co-trimoxazole died compared with only 1 of 20 given pentamidine. Others commenting on these results felt that pentamidine might indeed be more effective than co-trimoxazole for the initial treatment of *Pn. carinii* pneumonia in AIDS patients and that a larger study is needed to clarify the issue (T. Dennis, *Ann. intern. Med.*, 1986, *105*, 629; P.R. Marantz, *ibid.*, 630; P. Bégin and J. Hanley, *ibid.*, 1987, *106*, 474; M.A. Polis and W.C. Blackwelder, *ibid.*, 475; J.K. Erban, *ibid.*). Meanwhile, guidelines for the treatment of *Pn. carinii* pneumonia in AIDS patients continue to recommend co-trimoxazole as the treatment of first choice and pentamidine isethionate 4 mg per kg body-weight daily for 14 to 21 days by intramuscular injection or slow intravenous infusion, in 250 mL of 5% glucose over 2 hours, as alternative therapy when side-effects with co-trimoxazole are severe (A. Millar, *Br. med. J.*, 1987, *294*, 1334; I.V.D. Weller, *ibid.*, *295*, 200). In a recent review of pentamidine in the treatment of *Pn. carinii* pneumonia (K.L. Goa and D.M. Campoli-Richards, *Drugs*, 1987, *33*, 242) it was concluded that co-trimoxazole is more appropriate as initial therapy in patients without AIDS, but that pentamidine should be considered the treatment of first choice for those with AIDS. Improved outcome will probably depend on the development of new antipneumocystis drugs or the ability to reverse or prevent immunodeficiency rather than manipulation of the two available drugs, pentamidine and co-trimoxazole (C.U. Tuazon and A.M. Labriola, *Drugs*, 1987, *33*, 66); alternative drugs under study include dapsone, eflornithine, and trimetrexate.

There have been encouraging results with pentamidine administered by aerosol. In a preliminary study 13 of 15 AIDS patients with first episodes of *Pn. carinii* pneumonia responded to therapy solely with pentamidine inhaled for 20 minutes daily for 21 days (A.B. Montgomery *et al.*, *Lancet*, 1987, *2*, 480); there were no adverse systemic reactions and the only local adverse effect was coughing in 12 patients. Further beneficial results have also been reported in individual patients given pentamidine by inhalation for the treatment or prophylaxis of *Pn. carinii* pneumonia (A.J. Jesuthasan *et al.*, *Lancet*, 1987, *2*, 971; A. Heley, *ibid.*, 1092); pretreatment with nebulised terbutaline or ipratropium prevented the bronchospasm or cough associated with pentamidine inhalation.

Reviews of pentamidine isethionate and its use in the treatment of *Pneumocystis carinii* pneumonia.— S. Drake *et al.*, *Clin. Pharm.*, 1985, *4*, 507; *Med. Lett.*, 1985, *27*, 6; K. L. Goa and D. M. Campoli-Richards, *Drugs*, 1987, *33*, 242.

TRYPANOSOMIASIS. For a brief description of African trypanosomiasis and WHO guidelines for its treatment, including the use of pentamidine, see p.658.

Preparations

Pentamidine Injection *(B.P.)*. Contains pentamidine isethionate.

Proprietary Preparations

Pentamidine Isethionate *(May & Baker, UK)*. *Injection*, powder for reconstitution, pentamidine isethionate 200 mg and 300 mg. Also known as Pentacarinat.

Proprietary Names and Manufacturers
Lomidine *(Specia, Fr.; Rhône-Poulenc, Ger.)*; Pentam *(Lyphomed, USA)*; Pentacarinat *(May & Baker, UK)*.

13099-l

Phenamidine Isethionate

4,4′-Oxydibenzamidine bis(2-hydroxyethanesulphonate).
$C_{14}H_{14}N_4O, 2C_2H_6O_4S = 506.6$.

CAS — 101-62-2 (phenamidine); 620-90-6 (isethionate).

Phenamidine isethionate, an aromatic diamidine derivative, is an antiprotozoal agent which has been used in veterinary practice in the treatment of babesiosis.

13193-w

Pyrithidium Bromide *(BAN)*.

Pyritidium Bromide *(pINN)*; RD-2801. 3-Amino-8-(2-amino-1,6-dimethylpyrimidinium-4-ylamino)-6-(4-aminophenyl)-5-methylphenanthridinium dibromide.
$C_{26}H_{27}Br_2N_7 = 597.4$.

CAS — 3616-05-5 (pyrithidium); 14222-46-9 (bromide).

Pharmacopoeias. In *B.P. Vet.*

A brick-red to reddish-purple, odourless or almost odourless, hygroscopic powder. **Soluble** 1 in 40 of water; very slightly soluble in alcohol. A 2% suspension in water has a pH of 4.0 to 7.0. **Store** in airtight containers.

Pyrithidium bromide is an antiprotozoal agent used in veterinary practice as a trypanocide.

18609-l

Quinfamide *(USAN, rINN)*.

Win-40014. 1-(Dichloroacetyl)-1,2,3,4-tetrahydroquinolin-6-ol 2-furoic acid ester.
$C_{16}H_{13}Cl_2NO_4 = 354.2$.

CAS — 62265-68-3.

Quinfamide is a luminal amoebicide (see Amoebiasis, p.658) which has been given by mouth in the treatment of chronic intestinal amoebiasis.

References: L. Guevara *et al.*, *Clin. Ther.*, 1983, *6*, 43; F. A. Rojas *et al.*, *ibid.*, 47.

Proprietary Names and Manufacturers
Amenox *(Winthrop-Breon, USA)*.

13205-r

Quinuronium Sulphate

Quinolyl Urea. 6,6′-Ureylenebis(1-methylquinolinium) bis(methyl sulphate).
$C_{23}H_{26}N_4O_9S_2 = 566.6$.

CAS — 135-14-8.

Quinuronium sulphate is an antiprotozoal agent used in veterinary practice for the treatment of babesiosis.

Proprietary Veterinary Names and Manufacturers
Ludobal *(Bayer Agrochem, UK)*; Pirevan V *(Evans Medical, UK)*.

13216-n

Robenidine Hydrochloride *(BANM, USAN, rINNM)*.

CL-78116; Robenzidene Hydrochloride. 1,3-Bis(4-chlorobenzylideneamino)guanidine hydrochloride.
$C_{15}H_{13}Cl_2N_5,HCl = 370.7$.

CAS — 25875-51-8 (robenidine); 25875-50-7 (hydrochloride).

Robenidine hydrochloride is an antiprotozoal agent used in veterinary practice for the prevention of coccidiosis in poultry and rabbits.

Proprietary Veterinary Names and Manufacturers
Cycostat *(Cyanamid, UK)*.

13219-b

Ronidazole *(BAN, USAN, pINN)*.

(1-Methyl-5-nitroimidazol-2-yl)methyl carbamate.
$C_6H_8N_4O_4 = 200.2$.

CAS — 7681-76-7.

Pharmacopoeias. In *B.P. Vet.*

A white to yellowish-brown, odourless or almost odourless powder. Slightly **soluble** in water, alcohol, and chloroform; very slightly soluble in ether. **Protect** from light.

Ronidazole is a 5-nitroimidazole derivative similar to metronidazole. It is used in veterinary practice for the treatment and control of swine dysentery in pigs and has also been added to turkey feeding stuffs.

References to the activity of ronidazole against *Giardia intestinalis*: P. F. L. Boreham *et al.*, *J. antimicrob. Chemother.*, 1985, *16*, 589; *idem*, 1986, *18*, 393.

Proprietary Veterinary Names and Manufacturers
Ridzol *(Merck Sharp & Dohme, UK)*.

12017-s

Salinomycin Sodium *(BANM, rINNM)*.

AHR-3096 (salinomycin); K-364 (salinomycin); K-748364A (salinomycin). An antibiotic produced by *Streptomyces albus*. Sodium (2*R*)-2-{(2*R*,5*S*,6*R*)-6-[(1*S*,2*S*,3*S*,5*R*)-5-{(2*S*,5*S*,7*R*,9*S*,10*S*,12*R*,15*R*)-2-[(2*R*,5*R*,6*S*)-5-ethyltetrahydro-5-hydroxy-6-methylpyran-2-yl]-15-hydroxy-2,10,12-trimethyl-1,6,8-trioxadispiro[4.1.5.3]pentadec-13-en-9-yl}-2-hydroxy-1,3-dimethyl-4-oxoheptyl]tetrahydro-5-methylpyran-2-yl}butyrate.
$C_{42}H_{69}NaO_{11} = 773.0$.

CAS — 53003-10-4 (salinomycin); 55721-31-8 (salinomycin sodium).

Salinomycin is an antiprotozoal agent used in veterinary practice for the prevention of coccidiosis in poultry.

Proprietary Veterinary Names and Manufacturers
Sacox *(Hoechst Animal Health, UK)*.

13227-b

Secnidazole *(BAN, rINN)*.

14539-RP; PM-185184; RP-14539. 1-(2-Methyl-5-nitroimidazol-1-yl)propan-2-ol.
$C_7H_{11}N_3O_3 = 185.2$.

CAS — 3366-95-8.

Secnidazole is a 5-nitroimidazole derivative with properties similar to those of metronidazole, apart from a much longer plasma half-life. It is used in the treatment of amoebiasis and has also been tried in trichomoniasis.

In 10 healthy subjects, 5 men and 5 women, given single oral 2-g doses, the elimination serum half-life of secnidazole was 20 hours in men and 14 hours in women compared with 13 and 12 hours respectively for tinidazole.— D. Videau *et al.*, *Br. J. vener. Dis.*, 1978, *54*, 77.

AMOEBIASIS. Beneficial results with a single oral dose of secnidazole 2 g in the treatment of acute intestinal amoebiasis.— K. Soedin *et al.*, *Pharmatherapeutica*, 1985, *4*, 251.

A single 2-g oral dose of secnidazole had cured 136 of 140 male and female patients with urogenital trichomoniasis 48 hours later.— D. Videau *et al.*, *Br. J. vener. Dis.*, 1978, *54*, 77.

Proprietary Names and Manufacturers
Flagentyl *(Specia, Fr.)*.

809-s

Sodium Stibogluconate *(BAN, rINN)*.

Sod. Stibogluc.; Sodium Antimony Gluconate; Stibogluconat-Natrium.

CAS — 16037-91-5.

Pharmacopoeias. In *Br.*, *Ind.*, and *It.*

A pentavalent antimony compound of indefinite composition containing, when dried, 30 to 34% of pentavalent antimony. It has been represented by the formula $C_6H_9Na_2O_9Sb$ but usually there are less than 2 atoms of Na for each atom of Sb.

It is a colourless, odourless or almost odourless, mostly amorphous powder.

Very **soluble** in water; practically insoluble in alcohol and ether. A solution containing 10% of pentavalent antimony has a pH of 5.0 to 5.6 after autoclaving. Solutions may be **sterilised** by autoclaving. **Store** in well-closed containers. The *B.P.* injection should be protected from light.

Adverse Effects, Treatment, and Precautions

As for Antimony Sodium Tartrate, p.49.

Adverse effects are generally less frequent and less severe with the pentavalent antimony compounds sodium stibogluconate and meglumine antimonate than with trivalent compounds such as antimony sodium tartrate. Nevertheless, similar precautions should be observed, especially in patients on high-dose therapy.

Intramuscular injections of sodium stibogluconate can be painful and intravenous administration has been associated with thrombophlebitis.

On a weight-for-weight basis children require more pentavalent antimony than adults and tolerate it better, but in both adults and children tolerance is adversely affected by impaired renal function. Doses of 10 mg of pentavalent antimony per kg body-weight every 8 hours for 10 days have been shown not to be toxic; single doses of 30 mg per kg are associated with toxicity. Common side-effects are anorexia, vomiting, nausea, malaise, myalgia, headache, and lethargy. ECG changes are dose-dependent and most commonly T-wave inversion and prolonged QT interval. Renal damage is a rarely reported toxic effect. The rapid excretion of pentavalent antimony and its limited accumulation, in contrast to trivalent antimony, make interruption of treatment with rest periods for fear of cumulative toxicity unnecessary.— Report of a WHO Expert Committee on the Leishmaniases, *Tech. Rep. Ser. Wld Hlth Org. No. 701*, 1984.

See under Leishmaniasis in Uses, (below) for adverse effects reported in clinical studies with high-dose sodium stibogluconate therapy.

EFFECTS ON THE HEART. A detailed evaluation of the cardiac effects of a standard 10-day regimen of intravenous sodium stibogluconate in 22 soldiers with cutaneous leishmaniasis, but otherwise healthy. No serious cardiac effects were noted, though T-wave amplitude fell in every case and such minor ECG changes should be expected.— A. Henderson and D. Jolliffe, *Br. J. clin. Pharmac.*, 1985, *19*, 73. The ECG was monitored during 65 courses of treatment with sodium stibogluconate in 59 Kenyan patients with leishmaniasis. ECG abnormalities developed during 35 treatment courses. They were qualitatively similar to those previously described during treatment with trivalent antimonial drugs, but occurred less frequently and later during the course of treatment. The most common abnormality was inversion and/or decreased amplitude of T waves. Incidence was related to total daily dose and duration of treatment. One patient died suddenly during the 4th week of treatment with 60 mg of antimony per kg body-weight daily. Guidelines for monitoring during treatment with sodium stibogluconate include the recommendation that ECGs be obtained every 3 to 4 days in patients receiving 20 mg of antimony per kg daily for more than 20 days or a higher dose for more than 10 days. If Stokes-Adams attacks or ventricular tachyarrhythmias develop, sodium stibogluconate should be stopped and treatment with atropine started. If this is unsuccessful isoprenaline or atrial pacing should be considered.— J. D. Chulay *et al.*, *Am. J. trop. Med. Hyg.*, 1985, *34*, 702.

EFFECTS ON THE KIDNEY. Evidence of renal tubular dysfunction in patients with mucocutaneous leishmaniasis given meglumine antimonate or sodium stibogluconate in a dose of 20 mg of pentavalent antimony per kg body-weight daily for 30 days or more.— J. P. R. Veiga *et al.* (letter), *Lancet*, 1983, *2*, 569. Sodium stibogluconate given to 16 young men with cutaneous leishmaniasis, but otherwise healthy, in a standard dose of 600 mg of pentavalent antimony daily intravenously for 10 days had no apparent adverse effect on glomerular or tubular renal function. Larger doses of pentavalent antimonial drugs given to sick, elderly, or malnourished patients may have more serious effects on renal function.— D. S. Jolliffe (letter), *ibid.*, 1985, *1*, 584.

Absorption and Fate

In common with other pentavalent antimony compounds sodium stibogluconate is not bound by red blood cells but remains in the plasma and is rapidly excreted by the kidney. Small amounts may be reduced to trivalent antimony in the liver.

A study of the renal excretion of sodium stibogluconate in healthy subjects and in patients with kala-azar. Preliminary observations failed to demonstrate antimony in the faeces during a course of sodium stibogluconate. Following intravenous administration sodium stibogluconate appeared to be confined to the extracellular fluid compartment, and was rapidly excreted in a manner similar to that of inulin (over 95% being excreted in the urine in the first 6 hours), hence it is probably not metabolised. Following intramuscular injection blood concentrations were lower and more sustained, but over 80% was excreted in the first 6 hours. It thus appears that the fears of cumulative toxicity following sodium stibogluconate administration may be unfounded.— P. H. Rees *et al.*, *Lancet*, 1980, *2*, 226.

Uses and Administration

Sodium stibogluconate is a pentavalent antimony compound used in the treatment of leishmaniasis. It is administered by intravenous or intramuscular injection as a solution containing the equivalent of 100 mg of pentavalent antimony per mL. Intravenous injections must be administered very slowly (over at least 5 minutes) and preferably through a fine needle to avoid thrombophlebitis; they should be discontinued immediately if coughing, vomiting, or substernal pain occurs (see Adverse Effects on Antimony Sodium Tartrate, p.49).

Doses are expressed in terms of the equivalent amount of pentavalent antimony. In general, the doses now used are higher and the duration of treatment longer than in earlier standard regimens. Treatment schedules depend on the type of leishmaniasis, the severity of the disease, and the endemic area. Doses of 10 to 20 mg of pentavalent antimony per kg body-weight daily for 30 consecutive days or more are now usual in the treatment of visceral leishmaniasis (kala-azar) and mucocutaneous leishmaniasis (espundia). In cutaneous leishmaniasis of the Old World (oriental sore) doses of 10 mg of pentavalent antimony per kg daily for up to 10 days have been recommended, but again higher dosage may be necessary; in early disease the solution may be infiltrated around the edges of the lesions rather than being given systemically.

For further details on dosage in the treatment of leishmaniasis, see below.

LEISHMANIASIS. After many years the pentavalent antimony compounds, sodium stibogluconate and meglumine antimonate, remain the drugs of choice for all forms of leishmaniasis, but dosage schedules have been revised. Standard regimens were based on a course of 600 mg (10 mg per kg body-weight) of pentavalent antimony daily for 6 to 10 days with 10-day rest periods between courses. More recent studies, especially in visceral leishmaniasis, with higher doses for longer periods have indicated that fears of toxicity may have been exaggerated and because of rapid urinary excretion rest periods appear to be unnecessary.

These changes are reflected in the WHO recommendations (*Tech. Rep. Ser. Wld Hlth Org. No. 701*, 1984), which are summarised as follows. In *visceral leishmaniasis* initial treatment should be based on a daily intravenous or intramuscular injection of 10 mg of pentavalent antimony per kg body-weight [according to A.D.M Bryceson *et al.* (*Trans. R. Soc. trop. Med. Hyg.*, 1985, *79*, 700) this is a misprint and the dose should be 20 mg per kg] to a maximum of 850 mg for at least 20 days. The length of treatment varies from one endemic area to another, but should be continued for at least 2 weeks after anticipated parasitological cure, the exact length being determined for each country. Most patients seem to respond rapidly to treatment, but relapse rates differ in various parts of the world. Patients should be examined after 3 and 12 months to detect any relapse. Those relapsing after the initial recommended course of pentavalent antimony should be re-treated with the same drug at the same daily dose of 20 mg per kg to a maximum of 850 mg daily for twice the initial treatment period.

Early non-inflamed lesions of *cutaneous leishmaniasis* due to *Leishmania tropica, L. major, L. mexicana*, or *L. peruviana* may be treated by infiltration with intralesional injections of 1 to 3 mL of sodium stibogluconate or meglumine antimonate, repeated once or twice if necessary at intervals of 1 to 2 days. Systemic therapy with 10 to 20 mg of pentavalent antimony per kg daily should be given if the lesions are more severe and continued until a few days after clinical and parasitological cure is achieved.

Cutaneous leishmaniasis due to *L. aethiopica* is not responsive to antimonials at conventional doses.

In *cutaneous leishmaniasis* due to *L. braziliensis*, prolonged systemic treatment with 10 to 20 mg of pentavalent antimony per kg daily for a minimum of 3 weeks is indicated to prevent the later development of mucocutaneous leishmaniasis.

New patients with parasitologically confirmed *diffuse cutaneous leishmaniasis in the New World*, usually due to *L. mexicana amazonensis*, should be treated with 10 to 20 mg of pentavalent antimony per kg every 24 or 12 hours, continuing for several months longer than it takes to achieve clinical and parasitological cure.

In *mucocutaneous leishmaniasis*, usually occurring in areas where *L. braziliensis* is endemic, pentavalent antimony, usually meglumine antimonate, is considered the drug of choice, and is used in widely differing regimens. Single daily doses of 20 mg of pentavalent antimony per kg are given for a minimum of 4 weeks; if toxic effects develop or the response is poor, 10 to 15 mg per kg may be given every 12 hours.

For further information on leishmaniasis and its treatment, see p.659.

A study of the biochemical mechanisms contributing to the activity of sodium stibogluconate against *Leishmania*.— J. D. Berman *et al.*, *Antimicrob. Ag. Chemother.*, 1985, *27*, 916.

Cutaneous leishmaniasis. Cutaneous leishmaniasis caused by *Leishmania aethiopica* usually responds poorly to conventional doses of pentavalent antimonial drugs. High-dose treatment with sodium stibogluconate intravenously in a dose of 20 mg of antimony per kg body-weight twice daily for 30 days was found to be effective in 3 Kenyan patients. Toxicity was not a problem, although mild transient increases in liver enzymes and ECG changes occurred in all 3 and local venous thrombosis at the injection site was common. In one patient, dosage was reduced to 18 mg per kg because of anorexia.— J. D. Chulay *et al.*, *Trans. R. Soc. trop. Med. Hyg.*, 1983, *77*, 717.

In a comparison of 3 treatment schedules in 36 patients with American cutaneous leishmaniasis, sodium stibogluconate given intravenously for 10 days at a dose of 600 mg of antimony daily was most effective and better tolerated when administered once daily by rapid intravenous infusion rather than by continuous infusion over 24 hours or in divided doses every 8 hours by rapid infusion. When infused rapidly the dose was dissolved in 50 mL of glucose 5% and given over 10 minutes. For continuous infusion the daily dose was given in 1 litre of glucose 5% at a constant rate.— C. N. Oster *et al.*, *Am. J. trop. Med. Hyg.*, 1985, *34*, 856.

High-dose therapy with sodium stibogluconate was assessed in 40 patients with American cutaneous leishmaniasis caused primarily by *Leishmania braziliensis panamensis*. Patients received either 10 or 20 mg of antimony per kg body-weight daily for 20 consecutive days administered intravenously in 50 mL of 5% glucose over 5 to 10 minutes. No upper limit for total daily dose of antimony was specified and doses ranged from 620 to 850 mg in those given 10 mg per kg and from 1220 to 1850 mg in those given 20 mg per kg. At 9 weeks after starting treatment all 19 patients given 20 mg per kg daily were cured, but 5 of 21 given the lower dose had persistent active disease. Both treatment regimens were generally well tolerated and there was a similar incidence of reversible side-effects. Mild to moderate muscle and joint stiffness occurred in more than half of the patients. Laboratory abnormalities included increases in liver enzymes, mild leucopenia, and ECG changes. It was concluded that existing guidelines for treatment of cutaneous leishmaniasis, established as 10 to 20 mg of antimony per kg up to a maximum of 850 mg daily for 10 to 20 days were inadequate and should be revised to reflect the safety and efficacy of sodium stibogluconate administered at a dose of 20 mg of antimony per kg daily for 20 days.— W. R. Ballou *et al.*, *Lancet*, 1987, *2*, 13.

Post-kala-azar dermal leishmaniasis in 108 Indian patients was treated with sodium stibogluconate in doses of 10, 15, or 20 mg [of antimony] per kg body-weight daily by intramuscular injection for 120 days. The cure-rate was significantly higher with the 20 mg per kg regimen.— C. P. Thakur *et al.*, *Br. med. J.*, 1987, *295*, 886.

Further references to the use of pentavalent antimonial drugs in the treatment of cutaneous leishmaniasis: S. Belazzoug and R. A. Neal (letter), *Trans. R. Soc. trop.*

Med. Hyg., 1986, *80*, 670 (failure of meglumine antimonate to cure cutaneous lesions of *Leishmania major* in Algeria).

Visceral leishmaniasis. A comparison of 2 dosage schedules of sodium stibogluconate in the treatment of visceral leishmaniasis in Kenya, where the disease is particularly difficult to treat. A dose of 10 or 20 mg of antimony per kg body-weight daily was given intramuscularly for up to 9 weeks. The higher dose was found to be safe and well tolerated; in children, but not in adults, 20 mg per kg was more effective than 10 mg per kg.— G. M. Anabwani *et al.*, *Lancet*, 1983, *1*, 210.

In a study involving 126 Indian patients with visceral leishmaniasis, sodium stibogluconate given in a dose of 600 mg of antimony daily (20 mg per kg body-weight daily in those under 12 years of age) by intramuscular injection for 20 days, or for a further 10 or 20 days if necessary, was well tolerated and effective. Side-effects were restricted to pain at the injection site (14 patients), a feeling of warmth (23), and swelling, without abscess, at the injection site (3).— C. P. Thakur *et al.*, *Br. med. J.*, 1984, *288*, 895.

Ten Kenyan children with visceral leishmaniasis unresponsive to sodium stibogluconate, most recently in doses of 16 to 25 mg of antimony per kg body-weight daily for 30 to 98 days, were given high-dose therapy with 20 mg of antimony per kg every 8 hours, by intravenous injection when possible, otherwise intramuscularly. Treatment for 30 days at this dosage was achieved in only 4, and was abandoned or modified in the remaining 6 because of toxicity or suspected toxicity; in 2 patients the dose was reduced to 20 mg per kg every 12 hours and in one to 18 mg per kg every 8 hours. One patient died; cardiac arrest probably resulted from a tachyarrhythmia caused by sodium stibogluconate. ECG changes were noted in 3 further patients examined. Other toxic effects during treatment were malaise and anorexia (6 patients), vomiting (6), fever (2), cough (2), fall in haemoglobin (2), elevation of transaminases (3), elevation of blood urea (1), and albuminuria (1). Malaise was commonly profound. Toxic effects generally appeared within 3 to 10 days of starting treatment. Injections of large volumes of sodium stibogluconate were painful when given intramuscularly and often caused superficial venous thrombosis when given intravenously.

Only 2 patients responded fully to treatment and one of these died suddenly. Pentamidine was given to 8 patients; in 7 after high-dose treatment with sodium stibogluconate was stopped and in one before sodium stibogluconate treatment. Three patients were given allopurinol in addition to pentamidine. Stepwise development of resistance to both sodium stibogluconate and pentamidine was observed. Overall 9 patients were cured parasitologically with the following treatment regimens: high-dose sodium stibogluconate alone (2 patients), prolonged pentamidine alone (2), sodium stibogluconate plus pentamidine (2), pentamidine plus allopurinol (2), and sodium stibogluconate plus allopurinol (1). Of the original 10 patients, one died of apparent drug toxicity, one was transferred to another unit, and the other 8 have remained well without relapse for at least a year. The authors currently treat relapsed patients with sodium stibogluconate in a dose of 20 mg of antimony per kg daily for 60 days. In patients unresponsive to this dosage or who subsequently relapse, 20 mg per kg every 12 hours is usually well tolerated and may be effective. Long-term low-frequency pentamidine therapy may also be effective and both drugs can be used together, although toxicity may be increased. The place of allopurinol remains uncertain.— A. D. M. Bryceson *et al.*, *Trans. R. Soc. trop. Med. Hyg.*, 1985, *79*, 705. In 5 Kenyan patients, visceral leishmaniasis unresponsive to sodium stibogluconate in a dose of 20 mg of antimony per kg body-weight once or twice daily intavenously or intramuscularly for at least 50 days was treated successfully with sodium stibogluconate at the same dosage for 14 to 54 days together with allopurinol in a dose of about 20 mg per kg daily by mouth in 3 divided doses. Parasites had disappeared from splenic aspirate smears in all patients within 19 days and none had relapsed in at least 12 months of follow-up. Treatment was well tolerated. Optimum dosage remains to be established, but at least 30 days of treatment with sodium stibogluconate in a dose of 20 mg of antimony per kg once or possibly twice daily, with allopurinol 6 to 8 mg per kg three times daily, is currently recommended for Kenyan patients with visceral leishmaniasis unresponsive to antimonials.— C. N. Chunge *et al.*, *ibid.*, 715.

Further references to the use of pentavalent antimonial drugs in the treatment of visceral leishmaniasis: A. S. Khot and M. H. Thompson, *Archs Dis. Childh.*, 1983, *58*, 930 (contracted in the Mediterranean by 2 infants; successful treatment with sodium stibogluconate).

Preparations

Sodium Stibogluconate Injection *(B.P.)*

Proprietary Preparations

Pentostam *(Wellcome, UK)*. *Injection*, sodium stibogluconate equivalent to pentavalent antimony 100 mg/mL in bottles of 100 mL.

13279-c

Sulfanitran *(BAN, USAN, rINN)*.

NSC-77120; Sulphanitran. 4′-(4-Nitrophenylsulphamoyl)acetanilide.

$C_{14}H_{13}N_3O_5S$=335.3.

CAS — 122-16-7.

Sulfanitran, a sulphonamide, is an antiprotozoal agent which has been used in veterinary practice for the control of coccidiosis in poultry.

Proprietary Veterinary Names and Manufacturers

Salsbury, UK.

4797-q

Suramin

Antrypol; Bayer-205; Fourneau-309; Naganinum; Naganol. The symmetrical 3″-urea of the sodium salt of 8-(3-benzamido-4-methylbenzamido)naphthalene-1,3,5-trisulphonic acid.

$C_{51}H_{34}N_6Na_6O_{23}S_6$=1429.2.

CAS — 145-63-1 (acid); 129-46-4 (sodium salt).

NOTE. Suramin Sodium is *rINN*.

Pharmacopoeias. In *Egypt.*, *Fr.*, *Int.*, *It.*, and *Rus.* Also in *B.P.C. 1973.*

A white, pinkish-white, or slightly cream-coloured, odourless or almost odourless, hygroscopic powder. **Soluble** 1 in less than 1 of water; very slightly soluble in alcohol; practically insoluble in chloroform and ether. Solutions deteriorate on storage and should be used immediately after preparation; solutions for injection are prepared aseptically. **Store** in a cool place in airtight containers. Protect from light.

Adverse Effects

An immediate reaction, with nausea, vomiting, shock, and loss of consciousness, may follow the injection of suramin in some patients and thus it is usual practice to give a small test dose before initiating treatment. Abdominal pain and skin reactions such as urticaria and pruritus may also occur. The risk of hypersensitivity reactions is reported to be greater when onchocerciasis is present.

Later adverse effects include paraesthesia, hyperaesthesia of the palms and soles, skin eruptions, fever, raised liver enzyme values, and effects on the eye including photophobia and lachrymation. Albuminuria is common; haematuria and casts in the urine may also occur. There have been occasional reports of adrenal insufficiency. Agranulocytosis and haemolytic anaemia are rare.

Suramin was associated with significant toxicity in a study in 12 patients with AIDS given 1 g weekly by intravenous infusion for up to 36 weeks. Adverse effects included: hepatic enzyme elevations (9 patients), usually relatively mild and transient but requiring discontinuation of suramin in one and dosage reduction in another; fever (9), most commonly within the first 4 weeks of treatment; malaise (11), especially on the day of drug administration; proteinuria (10); mild transient renal dysfunction (2); reversible neutropenia (4); reversible thrombocytopenia (2); increasing anaemia (8); clinical evidence of adrenal insufficiency (2) after the 25th and 29th weeks of therapy, respectively, and abnormal adrenocorticotrophic hormone stimulation tests (5) after many months of treatment; transient skin rash (10), including an intensely pruritic erythematous maculopapular eruption (2); metallic or salty taste in the mouth (6); sensory paraesthesias in the feet and hands (8) with depressed deep tendon reflexes in one; and constipation (2).— A. M. Levine *et al.*, *Ann. intern. Med.*, 1986, *105*, 32.

EFFECTS OF THE EYE. The incidence of optic atrophy increased from 1 in 25 to 5 in 25 three years after patients had been treated with suramin 5.2 g (total dose) for ocular onchocerciasis. There was no change in the incidence (1 in 23) in 23 patients not given suramin.— B. Thylefors and A. Rolland, *Bull. Wld Hlth Org.*, 1979, *57*, 479.

A report of toxic keratopathy in AIDS patients treated with suramin.— S. A. Teich *et al.* (letter), *New Engl. J. Med.*, 1986, *314*, 1455.

PREGNANCY AND THE NEONATE. See under Precautions (below).

Precautions

Suramin should be administered under close medical supervision, especially when patients are in poor condition, and treatment discontinued if initial doses are not tolerated. It should not be used in the presence of renal disease. The urine should be tested before each dose; mild albuminuria may be acceptable but treatment should be interrupted if it increases or casts appear in the urine.

PREGNANCY AND THE NEONATE. Suramin has been reported to be teratogenic in *mice* but not in *rats* (L. Mercier-Parot and H. Tuchmann-Duplessis, *C.r.Séanc. Soc. Biol.*, 1973, *167*, 1518) and some authorities (*Med. Lett.*, 1987, *29*, 61) have advised that it should only be used during pregnancy when there is no suitable alternative. Pregnancy is stated by the manufacturers to be a contra-indication to the use of suramin for the treatment of onchocerciasis.

Absorption and Fate

Following intravenous injection, suramin becomes bound to plasma proteins and a low concentration in plasma is maintained for months. Unbound suramin is excreted in the urine. Penetration of suramin into the cerebrospinal fluid appears to be poor.

The clinical pharmacokinetics of suramin were studied in 4 patients with AIDS given 6.2 g intravenously over 5 weeks. Suramin accumulated during treatment and plasma concentrations exceeded 100 µg per mL for several weeks. After the last dose the terminal half-life of suramin ranged from 44 to 54 days. At least 99.7% was bound to plasma proteins. Renal clearance accounted for most of the elimination of suramin from the body. There appeared to be little or no metabolism of suramin.— J. M. Collins *et al*, *J. clin. Pharmac.*, 1986, *26*, 22.

Uses and Administration

Suramin is a trypanocide used in the treatment of the early stages of African trypanosomiasis and is effective as an anthelmintic in the treatment of onchocerciasis. It also has activity *in vitro* against human immunodeficiency virus (HIV) and has been tried in patients with AIDS.

Suramin is administered by slow intravenous injection, usually as a 10% solution. Because of the danger of severe reations it is advisable to give a test dose of 100 to 200 mg before initiating treatment.

In African trypanosomiasis suramin is used mainly for the early stages of *Trypanosoma brucei rhodesiense* infection; pentamidine is generally preferred for early-stage treatment of *T.b. gambiense* infection. Suramin is not used as sole therapy for late-stage infections with central nervous system involvement since its penetration into the cerebrospinal fluid is not considered to be adequate. Provided the test dose is well tolerated, early-stage trypanosomiasis is treated with a dose of 20 mg per kg body-weight of suramin (up to a maximum of 1 g in adults) given every 5 to 7 days, usually to a total of 5 injections and not exceeding 7 injections. In late-stage *T.b. rhodesiense* infection 2 or 3 injections of suramin are often given before starting treatment with melarsoprol; combined therapy with suramin and tryparsamide has been used in late-stage *T.b. gambiense* infection.

In onchocerciasis, suramin is effective in clearing the adult worms and also has microfilaricidal activity. The standard dosage of suramin has been 1 g (after an initial test dose) weekly for 5 or 6 weeks, often given after a course of diethylcarbamazine which is active only against microfilariae. However, weekly doses of suramin starting at 200 mg and gradually increasing to 1 g may be tolerated better. More recently (see below) a total dose of 4 g given over 6 weeks has been recommended.

AIDS. In studies *in vitro* suramin was found to inhibit the reverse transcriptase of human immunodeficiency virus (HIV) (S. Broder and R.C. Gallo, *New Engl. J. Med.*, 1984, *311*, 1292) and to inhibit the infectivity of HIV and its cytopathic effect on helper-inducer T cells at concentrations of 100 µg or more per mL (H. Mitsuya *et al.*, *Science*, 1984, *226*, 172). However, pilot studies with suramin in patients with AIDS have been disappointing. In 10 patients with HIV infection suramin had a virustatic effect but did not produce clinical or immunological improvement (S. Broder *et al.*, *Lancet*, 1985, *2*, 627); most patients received a total dose of 6.2 g, a test dose of 200 mg on day 0 being followed by 1 g intravenously over 20 minutes on days 3, 7, 14, 21, 28, and 35. Broder *et al.* suggested that longer courses of treatment with suramin or the concomitant use of other antiviral agents or a T-cell stimulating agent such as interleukin-2 might be of benefit. Longer term treatment proved no more successful in a study in 12 patients with AIDS given suramin for up to 36 weeks (A.M. Levine *et al.*, *Ann. intern. Med.*, 1986, *105*, 32). Following induction therapy with suramin 1 g weekly for 6 weeks, maintenance doses of 500 mg weekly were given but were subsequently increased to 1 g weekly when it was recognised that the antiviral effect of suramin was dose-dependent and nadir serum concentrations of above 100 µg per mL were sought. HIV reverse transcriptase levels were suppressed for at least 18 weeks in 3 of 11 evaluable patients, but clinical improvement occurred in only one patient and none had improved immune function. There was also significant toxicity associated with suramin.
Following analysis of results in 98 patients with AIDS or AIDS-related complex treated between April 1985 and April 1986 at various centres, the *US* Suramin Working Group has concluded that suramin as currently administered cannot be recommended as effective therapy for AIDS (*J. Am. med. Ass.*, 1987, *258*, 1347). Dosage regimens used were either 0.5, 1, or 1.5 g of suramin intravenously weekly for 6 weeks, followed by 0.5 or 1 g weekly for up to 1 year. Although virus suppression was confirmed this did not appear to be associated with clinical response or immunological improvement. As a result there are no ongoing trials in the *US* testing suramin in patients with AIDS. Nevertheless, at least additive activity against HIV *in vitro* has been reported between suramin and either zidovudine or acyclovir and there may be a role in the future for combination therapies using suramin analogues that are less toxic and penetrate the cns better.

ONCHOCERCIASIS. Diethylcarbamazine and suramin have been used in the treatment of the filarial infection onchocerciasis for more than 30 years, but their serious and long-lasting side-effects have only recently been understood and efforts are now being made to find improved chemotherapeutic regimens. Suramin kills both microfilariae and adult worms, but is an inherently dangerous drug because of its high protein-binding affinity with alteration of enzyme function. The risk of optic neuropathy, nephrotoxicity, and the occasional death severely limit its usefulness especially for mass treatment. When used in a reduced dosage suramin appears to be safer and to have a lower frequency of side-effects although it does not necessarily kill all the adult worms.— H. R. Taylor, *Bull. Wld Hlth Org.*, 1984, *62*, 509.
Suramin is the only macrofilaricide available for use against *Onchocerca volvulus*. Knowledge of its complications, especially those associated with the eye, has advanced but little is known about its mode of action. A total of at least 6 g of suramin must be given over 6 weeks to kill all adult worms, but can produce significant and dangerous side-effects in 10 to 30% of patients and cannot be recommended for general use. A total dose of 4 g given over 6 weeks is now recommended for an adult weighing 60 kg or more. It should be given as follows: 0.2 g (or 3.3 mg per kg body-weight) in the first week, followed by 0.4, 0.6, 0.8, 1, and 1 g in the following 5 weeks. In patients showing no signs of toxicity, macrofilaricidal action can be improved by a final injection of 1 g, raising the total dose to 5 g. Anterior uveitis may develop, but can usually be controlled by topical corticosteroid therapy. Treatment with suramin has long-term effects on ocular onchocerciasis. Lesions of the anterior segment usually improve or stabilise, but advanced sclerosing keratitis does not respond and new lesions may also appear. Conditions affecting the posterior segment and optic nerve rarely improve; optic neuritis and optic atrophy have been observed during and after treatment with a regimen of 6 g of suramin. A Mazzotti skin reaction may appear during the first few weeks of treatment with suramin and, together with the ocular changes, is presently attributed to the microfilaricidal effect of suramin. Adverse effects specifically due to suramin also occur.
Thus, the use of suramin is restricted because of the frequency of associated complications and because it is intrinsically toxic and relatively difficult to handle. In the treatment of onchocerciasis suramin is given following a course of diethylcarbamazine, the major indication for such treatment being onchocerciasis severe enough to threaten sight; severe onchodermatitis may also justify treatment.— Third Report of the WHO Expert Committee on Onchocerciasis, *Tech. Rep. Ser. Wld Hlth Org. No. 752*, 1987.
For further information on onchocerciasis and its treatment, see under Diethylcarbamazine Citrate, p.53.
Investigations of the suitability of suramin, given in small gradually increasing doses, for the mass treatment of onchocerciasis in hyperendemic communities in West Africa. Adults without major contra-indications, such as blindness, advanced age, poor general condition, or pregnancy, and living in a region where transmission had not been interrupted were given weekly doses increasing from 0.2 to 1 g. In most of those who had received a total dose of 45 to 50 mg per kg body-weight or more the parasite load in the skin and eyes fell by over 75% of the initial load. There was an almost complete absence of disturbing side-effects.— A. Rougemont *et al.*, *Bull. Wld Hlth Org.*, 1980, *58*, 917. In a region where transmission was controlled, tolerance was generally good and the worm burden was reduced by 90% within 3 months of starting treatment in 78 patients with onchocerciasis given suramin in small gradually increasing doses. Weekly injections corresponded to 0.2, 0.4, 0.6, 0.8, and 1 g, with a further 1 g for patients weighing more than 60 kg; doses were proportionately reduced for lighter patients and, depending on individual tolerance the last dose was either halved or dispensed with. It was concluded that such flexible use of suramin may continue until a new drug without its disadvantages becomes available.— A. Rougemont *et al.*, *ibid.*, 1984, *62*, 261.

TRYPANOSOMIASIS. For a brief description of African trypanosomiasis and WHO guidelines for its treatment, including the use of suramin, see p.658.

Preparations

Suramin Injection *(B.P.C. 1973).* A sterile solution of suramin in Water for Injections, prepared immediately before use.

Proprietary Names and Manufacturers

Germanin *(Bayer, Ger.)*; Moranyl *(Specia, Fr.)*.

4798-p

Teclozan *(USAN, pINN).*

NSC-107433; Win-13146. *NN'*-*p*-Phenylenedimethylenebis[2,2-dichloro-*N*-(2-ethoxyethyl)acetamide].
$C_{20}H_{28}Cl_4N_2O_4$=502.3.

CAS — 5560-78-1.

Teclozan, a dichloroacetamide derivative, is a luminal amoebicide with actions and uses similar to those of diloxanide furoate (see p. 663). It may be given by mouth in the treatment of intestinal amoebiasis in one of the following dosage schedules, all supplying a total dose of 1.5 g: 500 mg every 12 hours for 3 doses; or 500 mg daily in divided doses for 3 days; or 100 mg three times daily for 5 days.

Proprietary Names and Manufacturers
Falmonox *(Winthrop-Breon, USA).*

13318-q

Tenonitrozole *(rINN).*

TC-109; Thenitrazole. *N*-(5-Nitrothiazol-2-yl)thiophene-2-carboxamide.
$C_8H_5N_3O_3S_2$=255.3.

CAS — 3810-35-3.

Tenonitrozole is a trichomonacide and is given by mouth or vaginally in the treatment of trichomoniasis. It is also said to be active against *Candida albicans.*

Proprietary Names and Manufacturers
Atrican *(Innothéra, Fr.; Bouty, Ital.).*

17008-h

Tilbroquinol *(pINN).*

7-Bromo-5-methylquinolin-8-ol.
$C_{10}H_8BrNO$=238.1.

CAS — 7175-09-9.

Tilbroquinol is a halogenated hydroxyquinoline with properties similar to those of clioquinol (p.661). It has been used together with tiliquinol (see below) in the treatment of intestinal infections including amoebiasis.
A report of neurotoxicity, considered to be subacute myelo-opticoneuropathy, in a patient who had taken tilbroquinol together with tiliquinol for 4 years.— M. Soffer *et al.* (letter), *Lancet*, 1983, *1*, 709.

Proprietary Names and Manufacturers
The following names have been used for multi-ingredient preparations containing tilbroquinol— Intetrix *(Beaufour, Fr.).*

17009-m

Tiliquinol *(rINN).*

5-Methylquinolin-8-ol.
$C_{10}H_9NO$=159.2.

CAS — 5541-67-3.

Tiliquinol has been used in conjunction with tilbroquinol in the treatment of intestinal infections (see above).

Proprietary Names and Manufacturers
The following names have been used for multi-ingredient preparations containing tiliquinol— Intetrix *(Beaufour, Fr.).*

4799-s

Tinidazole *(BAN, USAN, rINN).*

CP-12574. 1-[2-(Ethylsulphonyl)ethyl]-2-methyl-5-nitroimidazole.
$C_8H_{13}N_3O_4S$=247.3.

CAS — 19387-91-8.

Adverse Effects and Precautions

As for Metronidazole, p.667.

ADMINISTRATION IN RENAL FAILURE. See under Uses (below).

PREGNANCY AND THE NEONATE. For a recommendation regarding the initiation of breast-feeding after the use of tinidazole, see under Pregnancy and the Neonate in Absorption and Fate (below).

SHOCK. An acute severe toxic reaction occurred in a healthy subject shortly after the intravenous infusion of tinidazole 1.6 g over 80 minutes. He fainted for about 10 seconds and low blood pressure, nausea, and tiredness persisted for several hours. Spasms in the left arm were also experienced but no generalised convulsions. The reaction was not considered to be allergic.— S. Aase *et al.*, *Eur. J. clin. Pharmac.*, 1983, *24*, 425.

Absorption and Fate

The pharmacokinetics of tinidazole resemble those of metronidazole although the half-life is longer.
Tinidazole is almost completely absorbed following administration by mouth and, typically, a peak plasma concentration of about 40 µg per mL is achieved 2 hours after a single 2-g dose, falling to 10 µg per mL at 24 hours and 2.5 µg

per mL at 48 hours; concentrations above 8 μg per mL are maintained by daily maintenance doses of 1 g. Comparable concentrations are achieved with equivalent intravenous doses. The plasma elimination half-life of tinidazole is 12 to 14 hours.

Tinidazole is widely distributed and concentrations similar to those in plasma have been achieved in bile, breast milk, cerebrospinal fluid, saliva, and a variety of body tissues; it crosses the placenta readily. Only 12% is reported to be bound to plasma proteins.

Unchanged drug and metabolites are excreted in the urine and, to a lesser extent, in the faeces.

A review of the pharmacokinetics, metabolism, and tissue distribution of tinidazole.— B. A. Wood *et al.*, *J. antimicrob. Chemother.*, 1982, *10, Suppl.* A, 43.

Comparative studies of the pharmacokinetics of tinidazole and metronidazole.— J. Mattila *et al.*, *Antimicrob. Ag. Chemother.*, 1983, *23,* 721 (intravenous, rectal, and intravaginal administration); J. Viitanen *et al.*, *Chemotherapy, Basle,* 1984, *30,* 211 (serum and abdominal tissue concentrations); J. Viitanen *et al.*, *Antimicrob. Ag. Chemother.*, 1985, *28,* 812 (concentrations in male genital tissues).

See also under Pregnancy and the Neonate (below).

ADMINISTRATION IN RENAL FAILURE. For reference to pharmacokinetic studies with tinidazole in patients with renal failure, see under Uses (below).

METABOLISM AND EXCRETION. The pharmacokinetics and metabolism of ^{14}C-tinidazole were studied in 2 healthy subjects following the intravenous infusion of 800 mg. Excretion of ^{14}C was predominantly in the urine but was fairly slow; a mean of 44% of the dose was excreted during the first 24 hours, increasing to a total of 63% after 5 days. About 12% was excreted in the faeces over 5 days. Biliary excretion and enterohepatic circulation might be partly responsible for the delayed excretion. On HPLC analysis, unchanged tinidazole accounted for a mean of 32% of the total drug-related material excreted in the urine at 5 days, equivalent to about 20% of the dose. Ethyl 2-(5-hydroxy-2-methyl-4-nitro-1-imidazolyl)-ethyl sulphone, a product of the hepatic biotransformation of tinidazole involving hydroxylation and nitro-group migration, was the major metabolite in urine collected between 0 and 12 hours (about 30% urinary ^{14}C); 2-hydroxymethyltinidazole was a minor metabolite (about 9% urinary ^{14}C). Unchanged drug and the major urinary metabolite were present in faeces. In plasma, ^{14}C was associated mainly with unchanged drug; the minor metabolite 2-hydroxymethyltinidazole was also present, but not the major urinary metabolite.— S. G. Wood *et al.*, *J. antimicrob. Chemother.*, 1986, *17,* 801.

PREGNANCY AND THE NEONATE. Placental transfer of metronidazole and tinidazole into foetal and placental tissues did not differ significantly after a single intravenous infusion over 20 minutes of 500 mg of either drug in 21 patients undergoing first trimester abortion. Using high-performance liquid chromatography, mean concentrations of tinidazole in serum, foetal tissue, and placental tissue were 13.2 μg per mL, 7.6 μg per mg, and 4.9 μg per mg compared with metronidazole concentrations of 13.5 μg per mL, 9.0 μg per mg, and 3.5 μg per mg respectively, 1 hour after the start of the infusion.— M. Karhunen, *Br. J. clin. Pharmac.*, 1984, *18,* 254.

The excretion of tinidazole in breast milk was highly related to serum concentration in 5 women given 1.6 g intravenously for prophylaxis before Caesarean section. The average milk/serum concentration ratio varied between 0.62 and 1.39. Low concentrations in milk were reached 53 to 84 hours after the dose of tinidazole and exceeded the lowest detectable limit of 0.5 μg per mL in only one woman 72 hours after administration. It was considered that breast-feeding should not be initiated until 3 days after such prophylactic treatment.— G. R. Evaldson *et al.*, *Br. J. clin. Pharmac.*, 1985, *19,* 503.

Uses and Administration

Tinidazole is a 5-nitroimidazole derivative. It has the antimicrobial actions of metronidazole and is used similarly (see p.669) in the treatment of susceptible protozoal infections and in the treatment and prophylaxis of anaerobic bacterial infections.

Tinidazole is usually administered as a single daily dose by mouth with or after food; it is also given by intravenous infusion.

In amoebiasis, tinidazole is administered, usually in conjunction with a luminal amoebicide such as diloxanide furoate or di-iodohydroxyquinoline, in a dose of 2 g daily by mouth for 2 or 3 days; in hepatic amoebiasis 1.5 to 2 g daily may be given for up to 5 days. Children are given 50 to 60 mg per kg body-weight daily.

A single dose of tinidazole 2 g is given by mouth in the treatment of giardiasis, trichomoniasis, and acute necrotising ulcerative gingivitis (Vincent's infection); 50 to 75 mg per kg as a single dose is suggested for children with giardiasis or trichomoniasis, although it may sometimes be necessary to repeat this dose once. In trichomoniasis sexual partners should be treated concomitantly. In bacterial vaginosis (nonspecific vaginitis) a single 2-g dose is usually given, although higher cure-rates have been achieved with a 2-g dose on 2 successive days.

For the treatment of most anaerobic bacterial infections tinidazole is given by mouth, usually for 5 or 6 days, in an initial dose of 2 g followed on subsequent days by 1 g daily or 500 mg twice daily. If oral therapy is not possible tinidazole may be administered intravenously, 800 mg being infused as 400mL of a 2 mg per mL solution at a rate of 10 mL per minute; this initial dose is followed by 800 mg daily or 400 mg twice daily until oral therapy can be substituted. For the prevention of postoperative anaerobic bacterial infections 2 g is given by mouth about 12 hours before surgery. Alternatively 1.6 g is given as a single intravenous infusion before surgery or in two divided doses, one just before surgery and the other during surgery or no later than 12 hours postoperatively.

Proceedings of a symposium on the use of tinidazole in the treatment of amoebiasis, giardiasis, and trichomoniasis.— *Drugs*, 1978, *15, Suppl.* 1, 1–60.

A brief comparison of the actions and uses of tinidazole and metronidazole demonstrating the similarities between the two drugs apart from a reduction in dosage frequency with tinidazole.— *Drug & Ther. Bull.*, 1983, *21,* 90.

ADMINISTRATION IN RENAL FAILURE. Single-dose studies indicate that the pharmacokinetics of tinidazole in patients with chronic renal failure are not significantly different from those in healthy subjects and that no modification of tinidazole dosage is necessary. However, tinidazole is rapidly removed by haemodialysis and it is recommended that patients on regular dialysis are given an additional half-dose infusion of tinidazole after the end of haemodialysis if treatment precedes dialysis (B.L. Flouvat *et al*, *Br. J. clin. Pharmac.*, 1983, *15,* 735) or that tinidazole is administered in full dosage after each dialysis (R. A. Robson *et al.*, *Clin. Pharmacokinet.*, 1984, *9,* 88).

AMOEBIASIS. A parasite cure-rate of only 44% was achieved in 18 patients with non-invasive amoebiasis given tinidazole 40 mg per kg body-weight in one daily dose for 5 days compared with 91% in 23 similar patients given tinidazole for 5 days together with diloxanide furoate 20 mg per kg daily in three divided doses for 10 days.— P. Pehrson and E. Bengtsson, *Trans. R. Soc. trop. Med. Hyg.*, 1983, *77,* 845.

Treatment of amoebic liver abscess for a single day with 2 g of tinidazole or ornidazole in 2 divided doses by mouth was equally effective in a double-blind study in 72 patients; overall cure-rates of 94.3 and 94.6%, respectively, were achieved. The abscess cavity was aspirated in 56 patients.— R. Lasserre *et al.*, *Am. J. trop. Med. Hyg.*, 1983, *32,* 723.

ANAEROBIC BACTERIAL INFECTIONS. A review of the antibacterial activity of tinidazole and its use in the treatment and prophylaxis of anaerobic infections.— A. A. Carmine *et al.*, *Drugs*, 1982, *24,* 85.

A series of papers on the role of tinidazole in the treatment and prophylaxis of anaerobic infections.—*J. antimicrob. Chemother.*, 1982, *10, Suppl.* A, 1-187.

A review of the antibacterial activity of tinidazole. Studies *in vitro* have shown minimum inhibitory concentrations to be less than 4 μg per mL for more than 90% of strains of anaerobic bacteria such as *Bacteroides*, *Fusobacterium*, and *Clostridium* spp.— C. E. Nord, *J. antimicrob. Chemother.*, 1982, *10, Suppl.* A, 35.

The hydroxy metabolite of tinidazole was more active *in vitro* than tinidazole itself and significantly more active than the hydroxy metabolite of metronidazole against *Gardnerella vaginalis*.— S. Shanker and R. Munro (letter), *Lancet*, 1982, *1,* 167.

For comparisons of the activity *in vitro* of tinidazole against anaerobic bacteria with that of other nitroimidazoles, see Metronidazole, p.670.

BACTERIAL VAGINOSIS. Single 2-g oral doses of metronidazole, nimorazole, or tinidazole were equally effective in the treatment of vaginitis associated with *Gardnerella vaginalis* in a study involving 280 patients, although tinidazole proved more active *in vitro*.— K. C. Mohanty and R. Deighton, *J. antimicrob. Chemother.*, 1987, *19,* 393.

GIARDIASIS. Results indicating that a single oral dose of tinidazole 50 mg per kg body-weight to a maximum of 2 g is effective in the treatment of giardiasis. The single dose of tinidazole was more effective than a single dose of metronidazole 60 mg per kg (maximum 2.4 g) and as effective as metronidazole 50 mg per kg (maximum 2 g) on three successive days in studies in 63 patients.— P. Speelman, *Antimicrob. Ag. Chemother.*, 1985, *27,* 227.

For a study demonstrating the effectiveness of a 1.5-g oral dose of tinidazole in giardiasis, see Ornidazole, p.674.

For a comparative study *in vitro* of the activity of various drugs, including tinidazole, against *Giardia intestinalis*, see Metronidazole, p.671.

INFECTIOUS MONONUCLEOSIS. For a report of the use of tinidazole in infectious mononucleosis, see Metronidazole, p.671.

TRICHOMONIASIS. Single 2-g oral doses of tinidazole or metronidazole were equally effective in a single-blind study in 82 women with vaginal trichomoniasis.— G. Gabriel *et al.*, *J. int. med. Res.*, 1982, *10,* 129.

Proprietary Preparations

Fasigyn *(Pfizer, UK). Tablets*, tinidazole 500 mg.

Proprietary Names and Manufacturers

Fasigin *(Pfizer, Ital.)*; Fasigyn *(Pfizer, Arg.; Pfizer, Austral.; Roerig, Belg.; Pfizer, Denm.; Pfizer, Neth.; Pfizer, Norw.; Pfizer, S.Afr.; Pfizer, Swed.; Pfizer, UK)*; Fasigyne *(Pfizer, Fr.; Pfizer, Switz.)*; Simplotan *(Pfizer, Ger.)*; Sorquetan *(Basotherm, Ger.)*; Tiniba *(Cadila, Ind.)*; Trichogin *(Chiesi, Ital.)*; Tricolam *(Pfizer, Spain)*; Trimonase *(Tosi-Novara, Ital.)*.

6000-c

Tryparsamide *(rINN).*

Glyphenarsine; Tryparsam.; Tryparsone. Sodium hydrogen 4-(carbamoylmethylamino)phenylarsonate hemihydrate.

$C_8H_{10}AsN_2NaO_4,\frac{1}{2}H_2O$=305.1.

CAS — 554-72-3 (anhydrous); 6159-29-1 (hemihydrate).

Pharmacopoeias. In *Int.*, *Mex.*, and *Turk.*

Tryparsamide, a pentavalent arsenical compound, is a trypanocide which penetrates into the cerebrospinal fluid and has been used in the treatment of late-stage African trypanosomiasis due to *Trypanosoma brucei gambiense*. However, because of its toxicity, especially the risk of blindness resulting from damage to the optic nerve, tryparsamide has generally been replaced by melarsoprol.

TRYPANOSOMIASIS. In African trypanosomiasis the drug of choice in late disease with CNS involvement is melarsoprol. Alternative treatment is with tryparsamide plus suramin. The adult dosage is one injection of tryparsamide 30 mg per kg body-weight and one injection of suramin 10 mg per kg, both given intravenously every 5 days to a total of 12 injections; the course may be repeated after 1 month.— *Med. Lett.*, 1986, *28,* 9.

Antithyroid Agents

830-g

The main antithyroid agents included in this section are the thioureylenes (or thiourea or thiocarbamide derivatives); this group comprises the imidazole derivatives (carbimazole and methimazole), the thiouracils (benzylthiouracil, iodothiouracil sodium, methylthiouracil, propylthiouracil, and thiouracil), and thibenzazoline. Also included in this section are perchlorates (potassium and sodium perchlorate), tyrosine derivatives (dibromotyrosine and di-iodotyrosine), and some miscellaneous agents (aminomethiazole tartrate, isobutiacilic acid, and mercaptothiazoline).

Antithyroid agents have also sometimes been termed thyrostatic substances.

Other agents, not included in this section but described elsewhere, used in the management of hyperthyroidism are iodine and iodides, iodine radiopharmaceuticals, and propranolol.

Adverse Effects

Side-effects due to the thioureylene antithyroid agents, such as carbimazole, methimazole, and propylthiouracil, occur most commonly during the first 2 months of treatment. Those most frequently encountered include nausea, vomiting, gastric distress, headache, and skin rashes including maculopapular eruptions, urticaria, and pruritus. Among other adverse effects that have occurred are fever, arthralgia, a lupus-like illness, vasculitis, hepatitis, and alopecia.

Agranulocytosis is the most serious adverse reaction, and patients should be instructed to report the development of mouth ulcers or sore throat, fever, or rashes, since these may sometimes precede abnormal findings in the blood by several days. Thrombocytopenia, leucopenia, and aplastic anaemia have also been reported.

Cross-sensitivity between antithyroid agents may occur.

Antithyroid agents cross the placenta and may cause foetal or neonatal hypothyroidism or goitre.

There is national favouritism for different thioureylene antithyroid agents. Propylthiouracil is used widely in the United States where carbimazole is difficult to obtain, yet carbimazole is the drug of choice in the United Kingdom. These differences have, in part, been fostered by the belief that one is less toxic than the other. In comparable doses, there is probably little or no difference in side-effects. Skin rashes, usually maculopapular eruptions, occur in about 5% of patients. Drug fever, arthralgia, jaundice, nephrotic syndrome, and lupus-like syndrome are rare complications. The most important problems, because of their potential seriousness and incidence, are granulocytopenia and agranulocytosis. Serious agranulocytosis occurs in about 1 in 200 patients. The problem usually occurs within 3 months of starting therapy, is rapid in onset, and usually will not be diagnosed by differential white counts at clinic visits. Marrow aplasia has been noted on rare occasions after carbimazole. Side-effects occur most frequently in the first four to eight weeks of treatment and are somewhat dose related.— I. R. McDougall, *J. clin. Pharmac.*, 1981, *21*, 365.

Serious adverse reactions to antithyroid drugs are sufficiently infrequent in adults so that concern about them does not usually affect the choice of therapy.— D. V. Becker, *New Engl. J. Med.*, 1984, *311*, 464.

A review of antithyroid drugs, specifically propylthiouracil and methimazole. Side-effects are encountered in only 1 to 5% of patients given antithyroid agents. The important side-effects include fever, rash, urticaria, and arthralgias or frank arthritis, and all seem to occur more frequently with higher drug doses. Perhaps the most common side-effect is transient leucopenia, occurring in up to 12% of adults and 25% of children; it is not ordinarily a reason to discontinue therapy. If a minor adverse reaction occurs with one antithyroid agent, therapy can be switched to the other, but cross-sensitivity is seen in about 50% of patients. Mild dermatologic reactions often disappear, despite continued therapy with the same drug.

Both propylthiouracil and methimazole can cause agranulocytosis which has been shown to be an auto-immune rather than a toxic phenomenon. Rates in various series have ranged from 0.1 to 1%, and the generally accepted figure is 0.5%. It almost always develops within the first 3 months of therapy; because of the sudden onset routine monitoring of the white-cell-count is fruitless. If the drugs are discontinued there is gradual improvement, although deaths have been reported. All patients taking antithyroid drugs should be advised to stop taking the drug immediately if fever, pharyngitis, mouth sores, or other symptoms of infection develop. Low doses of methimazole have been reported to be safer with respect to agranulocytosis than either high doses of methimazole or standard doses of propylthiouracil. If agranulocytosis occurs with one antithyroid drug, the other should not be given, to obviate cross-reactivity. Agranulocytosis can develop upon re-institution of therapy after an uncomplicated course of antithyroid treatment, when its onset is often more rapid, suggesting that sensitisation has taken place. The risk of agranulocytosis does not appear to be greater in patients who are re-exposed to antithyroid agents than in those receiving the drugs for the first time.

Toxic hepatitis may occur during antithyroid therapy. Drug-related hepatotoxicity has been reported almost exclusively with propylthiouracil, whereas cholestatic jaundice, without evidence of hepatic necrosis, has been typically associated with methimazole. Propylthiouracil-related hepatitis can be severe and has been fatal. Vasculitis and a lupus-like syndrome have also been reported, again much more frequently with propylthiouracil than with methiomazole, and may occur within weeks or sometimes months or years of starting antithyroid therapy.

Other very rare complications include aplastic anaemia, thrombocytopenia, nephrotic syndrome (with methimazole), and loss of taste (with methimazole). Hypoprothrombinaemia is a rare adverse effect with propylthiouracil and potentially disastrous in the surgical patient. Its cause is unknown but may be related to a warfarin-like effect of propylthiouracil, since it can be partially reversed with large doses of vitamin K or fresh plasma.— D. S. Cooper, *New Engl. J. Med.*, 1984, *311*, 1353.

Pruritus and a maculopapular rash or a sensitivity reaction with arthralgia, jaundice, lymphadenopathy, vomiting, and pyrexia may occur with both carbimazole and propylthiouracil (2 to 3%). Cross-sensitivity between carbimazole and propylthiouracil is seldom seen so patients with side-effects may be given the alternative drug. The rare but serious adverse effect of both drugs is agranulocytosis (0.05 to 0.3%).— R. Wilkinson, *Prescribers' J.*, 1984, *24*, 97.

EFFECTS ON THE BLOOD. An analysis of drug-induced blood dyscrasias reported to the Swedish Adverse Drug Reaction Committee for the 10-year period 1966-75 showed that agranulocytosis attributable to antithyroid agents had been reported on 29 occasions and had caused 5 deaths. The relative risk of dyscrasias appeared to be the same for the 3 commonly used drugs (carbimazole, methimazole, and propylthiouracil).— L. E. Böttiger *et al.*, *Acta med. scand.*, 1979, *205*, 457.

Results of a retrospective survey regarding the incidence and causes of neutropenia in hospitalised patients during 1973-78 in the Stockholm County region revealed a total of 84 episodes of drug-induced neutropenia; patients with neutropenia induced by antineoplastic agents were excluded. When the patient had taken only one drug, carbimazole, methimazole, and propylthiouracil were involved in 4, 1, and 4 episodes respectively and carbimazole was also implicated in one episode when more than one drug had been taken. Calculations of the estimated risk of drug-induced neutropenia per million tablets sold was 1.52 for carbimazole, 0.94 for methimazole, and 4.35 for propylthiouracil. Only 29 of the total 84 episodes of neutropenia had been reported to the Swedish Adverse Drug Reaction Committee.— P. Arneborn and J. Palmblad, *Acta med. scand.*, 1982, *212*, 289.

Comparison of 14 patients with methimazole- or propylthiouracil-induced agranulocytosis, and a further 36 patients with antithyroid-induced agranulocytosis reported in the literature, with 50 similar patients who did not develop agranulocytosis in association with antithyroid therapy. Those developing agranulocytosis had a significantly higher mean age than those who did not and, whereas agranulocytosis was associated with all dose levels of propylthiouracil, it was only associated with doses of methimazole greater than 30 mg daily. Moreover, those developing agranulocytosis usually did so within the first 2 months of treatment. Based on these findings the following guidelines were formulated for therapy: warnings about symptoms of malaise, chills, and pharyngitis are particularly important during the earliest phases of treatment; antithyroid drugs should be administered cautiously to older patients; low doses of methimazole may be associated with a lower incidence of agranulocytosis than higher doses or than conventional doses of propylthiouracil.— D. S. Cooper *et al.*, *Ann. intern. Med.*, 1983, *98*, 26. Comment that the omission of a 1981 Japanese study concerning 10 patients (N. Hamada *et al.*, *Endocrinol. Jpn*, 1981, *28*, 823) from this short literature review casts serious doubts on several of the paper's conclusions.— B. A. Warner (letter), *ibid.*, 562. Reply that none of the conclusions should be altered.— D. S. Cooper and E. C. Ridgeway (letter), *ibid.* Since the original publication the authors have heard the results interpreted by others to mean that methimazole in daily doses of 30 mg or less does not cause agranulocytosis; this was clearly not the intention. It is emphasized that agranulocytosis can occur at any methimazole dose, but that the likelihood is diminished at doses less than 30 mg daily. A daily dose of 30 mg or less does not, however, protect the patient from agranulocytosis.— D. S. Cooper *et al.* (letter), *ibid.*, 1984, *101*, 283.

The International Agranulocytosis and Aplastic Anaemia Study carried out in Israel and Europe indicated that there was an estimated excess risk of agranulocytosis with antithyroid drugs of 6.3 per million users in a one-week period. Aplastic anaemia was associated with these drugs; the excess risk could not be estimated, but was considered to be very low.—*Br. med. J.*, 1988, *297*, 262.

PREGNANCY AND THE NEONATE. Of 417 reported cases where the mother received antithyroid drugs alone, neonatal goitre occurred in 18 (4.3%), cretinism in 9 (2.2%), and congenital abnormalities in 6 (1.4%). Foetal losses occurred in 58 (13.9%) and neonatal thyrotoxicosis in 4 (1%). In 165 cases where the mother received antithyroid drugs plus thyroxine, neonatal goitre occurred in 1 (0.6%), cretinism in none and congenital abnormalities in 9 (5.5%). Foetal losses occurred in 15 (9.1%) and neonatal thyrotoxicosis in 5 (3.0%).—I. Ramsay *et al.*, *Clin. Endocr.*, 1983, *18*, 73. For a discussion regarding the controversial nature of the combined use of antithyroid agents and thyroxine in pregnancy, see under Uses (below).

Treatment of Adverse Effects

If blood disorders, such as agranulocytosis or bone-marrow depression, occur antithyroid agents should be immediately withdrawn and, if necessary, antibiotics and blood transfusions may be given.

Precautions

Patients should be warned to report the development of mouth ulcers or sore throat, fever, or skin rashes that occur during therapy with antithyroid agents since these may be indicative of abnormalities in the blood.

PREGNANCY AND THE NEONATE. Since the recommendation that women taking antithyroid agents should not breast-feed appeared to be based on one report of high concentrations of thiouracil in 2 samples of milk (R.H. Williams *et al.*, *J. clin. Invest.*, 1944, *23*, 613), L.C.K. Low *et al.* (*Lancet*, 1979, *2*, 1011) investigated the excretion in milk of agents in current use. They found in 2 patients given a single dose of radio-labelled carbimazole 10 mg or propylthiouracil 100 mg the milk-to-serum ratio for non-protein bound radioactivity was 1.05 and 0.55 respectively. They felt that antithyroid therapy should not be an absolute contra-indication to breast-feeding provided that the mother was on a small dose and that the circulating thyroid hormones of the baby were closely monitored. They also suggested that if mothers did breast-feed, propylthiouracil should be preferred to carbimazole or methimazole. In a study on the excretion of propylthiouracil in the milk of lactating women following the administration of propylthiouracil 400 mg, J.P. Kampmann *et al.* (*Lancet*, 1980, *1*, 736) found that the concentration in milk was only about 10% of the maximum concentration in serum. They also failed to note any changes in the thyroid parameters of a suckling infant whose mother received propylthiouracil 200 to 300 mg daily and who was studied over a period of 5 months. They concluded that lactating mothers receiving propylthiouracil could continue nursing, if they wished, with close supervision of the infant. In response to these 2 studies L. Tegler and B. Lindström (*Lancet*, 1980, *2*, 591) suggested that the revision of the dogma that antithyroid agents were contra-indicated in lactating mothers should be restricted to propylthiouracil until further studies of the metabolism of other antithyroid drugs, particularly methimazole, were available. Studying the excretion of methimazole following administration of carbimazole 40 mg to 5 lactating women K. Johansen *et al.* (*Eur. J. clin. Pharmac.*, 1982, *23*, 339) found that the milk-to-serum ratio was 0.98. This was accounted for by the fact that methimazole is unionised and not bound to proteins in serum. Similarly D.S. Cooper *et al.* (*J. clin. Endocr. Metab.*, 1984, *58*, 473) found a milk-to-serum ratio of 1.03 for methimazole, following administration of methimazole, and concluded that propylthiouracil, because it was reported to cross into milk only one-tenth as well as methimazole, should probably be used if breast-feeding was considered in patients requiring antithyroid drug therapy. Lamberg *et al.* (*Clin. Endocr.*, 1984, *21*, 81) concluded from the study of 12 mother-infant pairs that breast-feeding could be carried out if the daily dose of antithyroid agent did not exceed 15 mg of carbimazole or 150 mg of propylthiouracil and if the thyroid function of the infants was monitored. However, based on their own data from 2 infants and the results of a long-term study by other workers involving 7 children, Rylance *et al.* (*Lancet*, 1987, *1*, 928) suggested that carbimazole could be given in doses of up to 30 mg daily. They also considered that discarding breast-milk produced 2 to 4 hours after a dose of carbimazole could be expected to reduce an infant's daily intake of methimazole considerably.

For reviews and discussions on the use of antithyroid agents in the management of hyperthyroidism in pregnancy, and precautions to be observed, see below under Pregnancy and the Neonate.

Uses and Administration

The antithyroid agents are used in the treatment of hyperthyroidism, a common form of which is Graves' disease. Those most commonly employed are carbimazole, methimazole, and propylthiouracil; carbimazole is the drug most widely used in the UK whereas methimazole and propylthiouracil are those most used in the USA.

Unlike thyroidectomy or therapy with radio-iodine, the antithyroid agents have a reversible effect on the thyroid gland. High doses are given initially, usually for 1 to 3 months, until the patient becomes euthyroid. The dose is then reduced to the minimum necessary to maintain euthyroidism. Treatment is normally continued for 1 to 2 years. Alternatively, treatment with antithyroid agents has been continued at the initial dosage and thyroid hormones, such as thyroxine or liothyronine, given additionally to prevent the development of hypothyroidism. Following withdrawal of therapy some patients enter remission and remain euthyroid for long periods, although many, however, will relapse, usually shortly after the discontinuation of treatment.

If hyperthyroidism is to be treated by subtotal thyroidectomy, the patient may first be treated with antithyroid agents such as carbimazole, methimazole, or propylthiouracil, until euthyroid and then given iodine (as Aqueous Iodine Solution) or iodides (such as potassium iodide) for about 1 to 2 weeks before operation in order to reduce the vascularity of the thyroid.

Antithyroid agents, such as carbimazole, methimazole, and propylthiouracil, are used in the treatment of thyroid storm in conjunction with other measures which usually include propranolol and iodine or iodides.

Antithyroid agents have been used as growth promoters in animal feeds when they are known as thyrostats or thyrostatic substances. Because of the dangers of residues of these substances being present in foods for human consumption, the administration of antithyroid agents, by any means to animals intended for human consumption in order to increase body-weight, or the import of animals or the meat from animals treated with antithyroid agents, is now prohibited within Great Britain and other EEC countries. In addition, the sale and supply of thyrostatic substances for use in any animal is now prohibited within the EEC.

Discussions on auto-immune thyroid disorders including Graves' disease and Hashimoto's thyroiditis and the possible mode of action of antithyroid agents as immunomodulators.— P. Kendall-Taylor, *Br. med. J.*, 1984, *288*, 509; R. Volpé, *New Engl. J. Med.*, 1987, *316*, 44.

HYPERTHYROIDISM. A review and discussion on the treatment of thyroid disorders, including hyperthyroidism. There is no doubt that antithyroid drugs will render hyperthyroid patients euthyroid. In addition, a proportion of patients with Graves' disease (30 to 50%) will have a lasting remission when antithyroid drugs are discontinued. In practice patients should be observed for relapse after treatment is stopped since tests to predict relapse are not absolutely reliable. Most physicians treat hyperthyroid children with antithyroid drugs, and this is certainly the treatment of choice for pregnant hyperthyroid patients. The cut-off age for using radio-iodine therapy instead of antithyroid drugs varies. In the USA patients above 30 years are usually advised to have radio-iodine whereas in the UK the arbitrary age is 40 years. Loading doses [for adults] given daily are usually carbimazole 30 to 60 mg, methimazole 30 to 60 mg, and propylthiouracil 300 to 600 mg. Improvement is noted in 10 to 20 days but euthyroidism is often delayed for 6 to 10 weeks. As the patient improves the dose is titrated to produce euthyroidism and maintenance doses given daily are usually carbimazole 5 to 30 mg, methimazole 5 to 30 mg, and propylthiouracil 50 to 150 mg. The maintenance therapy is continued for 12 to 18 months. There are several variations on this theme. Some believe that it is easier to prescribe thyroid replacement with antithyroid drugs, since the dose of antithyroid drug need not be altered and hypothyroidism will be prevented. If this approach is adopted the thyroid replacement should not be prescribed until the patient has been rendered euthyroid with antithyroid drugs. Severe hyperthyroidism or hyperthyroidism causing complications can be treated with larger doses of thioureylenes or by combining propranolol with the antithyroid drug. When the clinical features come under control, the propranolol can be discontinued and at the same time the dose of the antithyroid agent titrated downward.— I. R. McDougall, *J. clin. Pharmac.*, 1981, *21*, 365.

A brief review and discussion on the choice of therapy for Graves' hyperthyroidism. Surgery, antithyroid drugs, and radio-iodine are all effective for the treatment of adult Graves' hyperthyroidism. However, reports present widely varying and often conflicting data with regard to cure, relapse, frequency of side-effects, cost, and convenience. Antithyroid drugs, such as propylthiouracil and methimazole, if taken regularly in adequate doses, almost always control the symptoms of hyperthyroidism. However, permanent remission occurs in only 10 to 40% of patients with Graves' hyperthyroidism. Antithyroid drugs are a reasonable first choice for many patients with hyperthyroidism and are particularly useful as ancillary therapy. Patterns of use and preferences vary widely. The use of antithyroid drugs requires a prolonged period of close medical supervision. Permanent remission is seldom achieved within the first year of therapy. Since the relapse rate is high, patients should be closely observed for 2 or 3 years after cessation of therapy. During this period the eventual resolution of the illness remains unknown. The ability to predict the long-term outcome of antithyroid drug therapy could substantially alter management strategy, but to date various tests have not proved to be reliable indicators. No single form of therapy is suitable for or acceptable to all patients. Surgery appears to be less advantageous than previously. Antithyroid drugs may be an acceptable initial therapy for selected patients, but radio-iodine is currently the preferred therapy for the majority of adults with Graves' hyperthyroidism.— D. V. Becker, *New Engl. J. Med.*, 1984, *311*, 464.

A review of antithyroid drugs, specifically propylthiouracil and methimazole. Antithyroid agents are most frequently employed to treat children, young adults, and pregnant women with hyperthyroidism due to Graves' disease. Other treatment is preferred for hyperthyroidism due to toxic nodular goitre, a single autonomously functioning nodule, or subacute or lymphocytic thyroiditis. The choice of antithyroid drug is usually based on personal experience. However, there are situations in which one drug may be preferred over the other. Propylthiouracil may be preferred to methimazole in severe hyperthyroidism, since it acutely lowers serum concentrations of tri-iodothyronine, but no studies have compared the 2 drugs in this situation. Propylthiouracil is also preferred over methimazole for pregnant patients. Generally, therapy begins [in adults] with propylthiouracil 300 mg [daily] or methimazole 30 mg [daily]. Occasionally, doses have to be increased to 600 to 1000 mg of propylthiouracil or 60 to 90 mg of methimazole before thyroid function becomes normal. The majority of patients may be given methimazole or carbimazole as a single daily dose; a single daily dose of propylthiouracil may be less satisfactory. There have been anecdotal reports of propylthiouracil-resistance, but such resistance appears to be almost always due to poor compliance. Patients are usually euthyroid after 2 to 4 months of treatment, when the dose can often be reduced by 50 to 75%. Some clinicians do not reduce the dose but continue with full blocking doses and supplement with thyroxine replacement if drug-induced hypothyroidism develops. It is the author's practice to titrate the dose to maintain biochemical euthyroidism. Many patients with Graves' disease enter remission after drug therapy. The duration of therapy, drug dose, and other clinical factors all influence the remission rate. Studies on the optimum duration of treatment provide conflicting results and most clinicians continue to treat patients for 12 to 24 months rather than withdraw therapy as soon as the patient is euthyroid. Unfortunately there is no consistently reliable method of predicting which patients will obtain a remission or relapse when therapy is withdrawn, so it is best to follow patients closely. If remission occurs, the patient should be re-evaluated every 6 to 12 months for life; if relapse occurs a second course of antithyroid drugs or preferably radio-iodine may be given. Controversies still surround the use of these agents.— D. S. Cooper, *New Engl. J. Med.*, 1984, *311*, 1353.

A discussion on the clinical management of thyroid diseases. The choice of medical treatment, surgery, or radio-iodine for Graves' disease is often arbitrary. In children and young adults it is usual to try antithyroid agents initially. Carbimazole and propylthiouracil are the most commonly used drugs to control the disease until remission occurs. Treatment [in adults] is usually started with carbimazole 30 to 60 mg daily or propylthiouracil 300 to 450 mg daily. It takes on average 4 to 8 weeks to attain clinical and biochemical euthyroidism; if a good response is not obtained by 3 months the patient should be suspected of failing to comply with treatment. When control is achieved either the dose may be gradually reduced to the lowest level required to maintain the patient euthyroid, usually carbimazole 5 to 15 mg daily or propylthiouracil 50 to 150 mg daily, or secondly the initial blocking dose of antithyroid drugs is continued and a replacement dose of thyroxine added to maintain euthyroidism. Treatment is continued for at least 12 months. The major disadvantage of antithyroid drug treatment is a 40 to 70% incidence of recurrent disease. There is no satisfactory way of predicting which patients will relapse.— R. Wilkinson, *Prescribers' J.*, 1984, *24*, 97.

Evidence from studies in 4 patients to suggest that in some patients an initial daily dose of carbimazole 10 mg may be as effective as 40 mg in the treatment of thyrotoxicosis.— L. C. K. Low *et al.* (letter), *Lancet*, 1979, *1*, 493. Similar observations with methimazole.— N. Riccioni *et al.* (letter), *ibid.*, 1087. A further study again suggesting that carbimazole 10 mg daily may be an effective starting dose in many patients.— L. C. K. Low *et al.*, *Br. J. clin. Pharmac.*, 1981, *12*, 315.

A comparison of the effects of high and low dosage regimens of antithyroid agents in the management of Graves' hyperthyroidism. Remission occurred in 75.4% of 65 patients after withdrawal of high-dose maintenance therapy with either methimazole 40 to 100 mg daily or propylthiouracil 0.5 to 1.2 g daily in association with supplementary liothyronine. In a similar group of 48 patients who received only antithyroid agents in conventional low maintenance doses (methimazole 5 to 25 mg daily or propylthiouracil 100 to 300 mg daily) remission occurred in 41.6% after discontinuation of therapy.— J. H. Romaldini *et al.*, *J. clin. Endocr. Metab.*, 1983, *57*, 563.

Patients apparently resistant to carbimazole are a rare but important group, and, although poor compliance is often blamed, evidence of high dietary-iodine intake should also be considered. Iodine may affect the response of the thyroid to antithyroid agents by increasing the thyroidal stores of preformed hormone and by altering the thyroid's metabolism of carbimazole. Studies are required to assess the effect of iodine state on the response to antithyroid agents.— R. Hall and J. H. Lazarus, *Br. med. J.*, 1987, *294*, 721.

Early surveys had shown that the continuing decline in the rates of remission in patients treated with antithyroid agents for Graves disease in the *USA* was associated with an increase in the intake of dietary-iodine in the general population. Furthermore, the improvement found in rates of remission since the end of these studies appears to be in line with a recent decline in dietary-iodine intake.— B. L. Solomon *et al.*, *Ann. intern. Med.*, 1987, *107*, 510. Remission-rates in Japan were much higher than would be expected considering the high dietary-iodine intake in the population. This difference between remission-rates may be related to the longer duration of antithyroid therapy in Japan when compared with the *USA*.— S. Sakata, *ibid.*, 1988, *108*, 308.

Further reviews.— D. S. Cooper, *Am. J. Med.*, 1986, *80*, 1165; J. R. Stockigt and D. J. Topliss, *Med. J. Aust.*, 1986, *145*, 278.

Adjunct to radio-iodine. Most patients who are younger than 55 years and who are candidates for radio-iodine therapy can be treated with radio-iodine without using antithyroid drugs. There is, however, a role for adjuvant antithyroid therapy, especially in older patients, in those with large multinodular glands, and in those in whom the clinical features of the disease are severe or where slight worsening might precipitate complications such as cardiac failure. Pretreatment of patients with antithyroid drugs usually requires 2 or 3 months of therapy, stoppage of antithyroids for 3 or 4 days, measurement of radio-iodine uptake, and then prescription of the radio-iodine therapy dose. If the clinical situation warrants it, the antithyroid drug can be re-introduced 2 days after radiotherapy and continued for several weeks. Some physicians prescribe antithyroid drugs only after radio-iodine but this author prefers to pretreat as well.— I. R. McDougall, *J. clin. Pharmac.*, 1981, *21*, 365.

Pregnancy and the neonate. In a detailed review of methimazole and propylthiouracil D.S. Cooper (*New Engl. J. Med.*, 1984, *311*, 1353) considered that these compounds had supplanted surgery in the treatment of the pregnant hyperthyroid patient although they could affect the foetal thyroid. Both crossed the placenta, but transfer was 4 times greater with methimazole (explained by propylthiouracil being heavily protein bound, poorly soluble in aqueous solution, and ionised at pH 7.4); because of this and reports of congenital scalp defects reported with methimazole, propylthiouracil was preferred. Methimazole might reasonably be used in patients allergic to propylthiouracil. Typical starting doses of 300 mg of propylthiouracil daily in divided doses could usually be reduced to 50 to 150 mg daily after 4 to 6 weeks. In another review, I. Ramsay (in *Medical Disorders in Obstetric Practice*, M. de Swiet (Ed.) London, Blackwell Scientific Publications, 1984, p.385) considered that thyrotoxicosis diagnosed during pregnancy should be controlled as quickly as possible and could usually be achieved within 4 or 5 weeks by carbimazole 15 mg or propylthiouracil 150 mg both every 8 hours. These doses should be progressively lowered to a maintenance dose of 15 mg or less daily for carbimazole or 150 mg or less daily for propylthiouracil. Similar doses were recommended by Z.M. van der Spuy and H.S. Jacobs (*Postgrad. med. J.*, 1984, *60*, 245). Although it appears that the lowest possible dose should be used to maintain the maternal free-thyroxine concentration in the high-normal to mildly thyrotoxic range thyrotoxicosis should be controlled even if daily doses of more than 450 mg of propylthiouracil are necessary. Failure to control symptoms at a dose of 600 mg daily may indicate the need for surgery. (G.N. Burrow, *New Engl. J. Med.*, 1985, *313*, 562; W.M. Hague, *Br. med. J.*, 1987, *294*, 297). Diffusion of antithyroid agents across the placenta and foetal goitre formation does not appear to be a purely dose-related phenomenon and women have given birth to healthy children even after receiving large amounts of anti-thyroid agents. Some physicians try to withdraw therapy during the last trimester because of a possible diminution of thyroid activity at this time and Ramsay considered that this might avoid effects on the foetal thyroid but required careful supervision of the mother in case she became toxic again. However, some (P.E. Belchetz, *Br. med. J.*, 1987, *294*, 264) still consider that the optimal treatment of thyrotoxicosis in pregnancy remains open to debate and that mid-trimester partial thyroidectomy in patients rendered euthyroid by treatment, is safe and effective when conducted by an experienced surgeon.

Carbimazole has been given to mothers to control foetal thyrotoxicosis. D.H. Cove and P. Johnston (*Lancet*, 1985, *1*, 430) reported that the foetus of a mother whose hyperthyroidism has been controlled by ablative treatment might be exposed to thyroid-stimulating immunoglobulins. In such an instance the foetus and not the mother might require antithyroid therapy. In a study to determine the optimal therapy for maintaining normal foetal thyroid function Momotani *et al.* (*New Engl. J. Med.*, 1986, *315*, 24) found that high concentrations of maternal thyroid stimulating hormone binding antibodies and free thyroxine concentrations were an indication of the foetal need for antithyroid treatment. They concluded that in order to maintain euthyroid status in the foetus, thionamide dosage should be adjusted to keep maternal free-thyroxine concentrations in a mildly thyrotoxic range.

The treatment of hyperthyroidism in pregnancy with antithyroid agents plus supplementary thyroxine remains controversial. The addition of thyroxine to the antithyroid drug regimen in pregnant hyperthyroid women has been suggested in an attempt to protect both the mother and the foetus from antithyroid-induced hypothyroidism and its complications. A preliminary report by R. Fraser and M. Wilkinson (*Br. med. J.*, 1953, *1*, 481) and later studies, including those of A.L. Herbst and H.A. Selenkow (*Obstet. Gynec.*, 1963, *21*, 543 and *New Engl. J. Med.*, 1965, *273*, 627), indicated that this was a successful form of therapy. A more recent study by I. Ramsay *et al.* (*Clin. Endocr.*, 1983, *18*, 73) again reported favourable results using antithyroid agents in combination with thyroxine whereas R.G. Cheron *et al.* (*New Engl. J. Med.*, 1981, *304*, 525) found that supplementation with thyroxine in combination with liothyronine did not appear to prevent neonatal hypothyroxinaemia. Despite the favourable reports the block-replacement regimen has still not been generally accepted and many critics and reviewers (J.I. Hamburger, *Obstet. Gynec.*, 1972, *40*, 114; D.S. Cooper, *New Engl. J. Med.*, 1984, *311*, 1353; Z.M. van der Spuy and H.S. Jacobs, *Postgrad. med. J.*, 1984, *60*, 245; R. Wilkinson, *Prescribers' J.*, 1984, *24*, 97) have objected to it, mainly on the grounds that higher doses of antithyroid agents are used in combination than when used alone, and also that the placental transfer of thyroxine is very limited, thus being unlikely to be able to afford any protection to the foetus.

The value of antithyroid agents in the treatment of transient hyperthyroidism associated with hyperemesis gravidarum has not been confirmed (R. Bouillon *et al.*, *Am. J. Obstet. Gynec.*, 1982, *143*, 922) although some consider that they may be of use if the abnormality worsens or persists into the later stages of pregnancy (T.T.H. Lao *et al.*, *J. R. Soc. Med.*, 1986, *79*, 613).

If treatment of the hyperthyroid phase of postpartum thyroiditis is necessary, a beta-adrenoceptor blocking agent such as propranolol should be used and not an antithyroid agent.— *Lancet*, 1987, *1*, 962.

Thyroid storm. Thyroid storm is a medical emergency. Treatment includes antithyroid agents (propylthiouracil 300 mg three times daily) to prevent more formation of thyroid hormones and to reduce conversion of thyroxine to tri-iodothyronine, propranolol, and iodine to prevent release of formed hormones from the thyroid.— I. R. McDougall, *J. clin. Pharmac.*, 1981, *21*, 365.

The treatment of thyroid storm, a life-threatening acceleration of hyperthyroidism, has been revolutionised by the use of beta blockers, given as propranolol 5 to 10 mg intravenously, slowly at intervals, titrated to relieve the signs. Large doses of carbimazole or propylthiouracil are given orally or via a nasogastric tube and iodine is given orally or intravenously as potassium iodide.— R. Wilkinson, *Prescribers' J.*, 1984, *24*, 97.

12361-h

Aminomethiazole Tartrate

2-Amino-4-methylthiazole hydrogen tartrate.

$C_4H_6N_2S,C_4H_6O_6$=264.3.

CAS — 1603-91-4 (aminomethiazole).

Aminomethiazole tartrate is an antithyroid agent which was formerly used in the treatment of hyperthyroidism.

Proprietary Names and Manufacturers

Normotiroide *(Vita, Ital.)*.

832-p

Benzylthiouracil

6-Benzyl-2,3-dihydro-2-thioxopyrimidin-4(1*H*)-one; 6-Benzyl-2-mercaptopyrimidin-4-ol; 6-Benzyl-2-thiouracil.

$C_{11}H_{10}N_2OS$=218.3.

CAS — 33086-27-0; 6336-50-1.

Benzylthiouracil is an antithyroid agent which has been used in the treatment of hyperthyroidism.

Proprietary Names and Manufacturers

Basdène *(Théraplix, Fr.)*.

831-q

Carbimazole *(BAN, rINN)*.

Ethyl 3-methyl-2-thioxo-4-imidazoline-1-carboxylate.

$C_7H_{10}N_2O_2S$=186.2.

CAS — 22232-54-8.

Pharmacopoeias. In *Br.*, *Chin.*, *Cz.*, *Egypt.*, *Fr.*, *Ind.*, *Int.*, and *Turk.*

A white or creamy-white crystalline powder with a characteristic odour. Slightly **soluble** in water and ether; soluble 1 in 50 of alcohol, 1 in 17 of acetone, and 1 in 3 of chloroform. **Store** in well-closed containers.

Adverse Effects and Treatment

As for Antithyroid Agents, p.682.

For reviews and discussions regarding the nature and incidence of the adverse effects of antithyroid agents, including carbimazole, see under Antithyroid Agents, p.682.

EFFECTS ON THE BLOOD. For studies comparing the incidence of antithyroid-induced blood disorders, including agranulocytosis and neutropenia associated with carbimazole, see under Antithyroid Agents, p.682.

EFFECTS ON THE IMMUNE SYSTEM. For reports of the insulin autoimmune syndrome in patients receiving carbimazole or methimazole, see under Methimazole, p.686.

EFFECTS ON THE LIVER. Jaundice in a young woman receiving carbimazole appeared immediately after an operation and also re-appeared later on challenge with carbimazole. It was suggested that the anaesthetic agents might have produced an alteration in the liver-cell membranes making them susceptible to carbimazole injury, possibly through an immunological step.— W. W. Dinsmore *et al.* (letter), *New Engl. J. Med.*, 1983, *309*, 438.

Further reports of cholestatic jaundice in patients treated with carbimazole.— D. C. Wheeler *et al.*, *J. R. Soc. Med.*, 1985, *78*, 75; H. Blom *et al.*, *Archs intern. Med.*, 1985, *145*, 1513.

PREGNANCY AND THE NEONATE. Of 25 children whose mothers had taken carbimazole during pregnancy 5 to 16 years earlier, one had partial adactyly of one foot and the other bilateral congenital cataracts. A third child had a small goitre but was euthyroid, as were all the others.— A. M. McCarroll *et al.*, *Archs Dis. Childh.*, 1976, *51*, 532.

For a review of antithyroid agents in pregnancy, see under Antithyroid Agents, p.682 and p.684.

Precautions

As for Antithyroid Agents, p.682.

PREGNANCY AND THE NEONATE. For discussions of precautions to be observed during the administration of antithyroid agents, including carbimazole, to pregnant and nursing mothers, see under the Precautions and Uses of Antithyroid Agents, p.682 and p.684.

Absorption and Fate

Carbimazole and methimazole are rapidly absorbed from the gastro-intestinal tract. Carbimazole is considered to be totally metabolised to methimazole which is widely distributed throughout the body, although it is concentrated in the thyroid gland. Methimazole is not bound to proteins in blood and although the elimination half-life from blood is relatively short, the biological effects are much longer lasting. Methimazole is excreted in the urine.

Methimazole readily crosses the placenta and is excreted in breast milk.

A review of the clinical pharmacokinetics of antithyroid drugs, including carbimazole and methimazole.— J. P. Kampmann and J. M. Hansen, *Clin. Pharmacokinet.*, 1981, *6*, 401.

A study of the pharmacokinetics of methimazole after the oral administration of single doses of carbimazole 60 mg or methimazole 60 mg to 15 previously untreated hyperthyroid patients. In 10 given carbimazole maximum plasma-methimazole concentrations occurred between 30 minutes and 1 hour after the dose with what appeared to be a second smaller peak or inflection at 4 hours; similar plasma concentration-time curves were observed in the 5 given methimazole. The large differences in the area-under-the-curves for both groups would seem to indicate large interindividual differences in the amount of the dose absorbed, particularly within the carbimazole group. It was possible in one patient to measure the concentration of 3-methyl-2-thiohydantoin, a metabolite of methimazole. The mean half-life of methimazole after administration of carbimazole and methimazole was 3.18 and 2.96 hours respectively. These half-lives were less than half those observed in the majority of other reports, and are due to the more specific assay for methimazole which is possible by HPLC. The observed protein binding of methimazole reported in an earlier study (G.G. Skellern *et al.*, *Br. J. clin. Pharmac.*, 1974, *1*, 265) has since been shown to be artefactual owing to the procedure used.— G. G. Skellern *et al.*, *Br. J. clin. Pharmac.*, 1980, *9*, 137. Studies of the pharmacokinetics of methimazole using a radio-immunoassay. In 6 healthy subjects given a single dose of methimazole 30 or 60 mg by mouth mean peak serum-methimazole concentrations of 0.65 and 1.54 μg per mL respectively occurred after 2 hours. In 5 patients with Graves' disease, also given the 2 doses, mean peak concentrations were similar, being 0.78 and 1.35 μg per mL respectively, but occurred after only 1 hour. Considerable interindividual variation was found, however, which could have been due to differences in drug absorption, although previously published data had indicated almost complete absorption of methimazole from the gastro-intestinal tract. In 4 patients with hepatic cirrhosis a mean peak serum-methimazole concentration of 1.3 μg per mL occurred 40 minutes after the administration of methimazole 60 mg. The mean half-life of disappearance from the plasma was 6.0 hours in the controls, and 6.8 hours in the hyperthyroid patients; the difference was not significant. In contrast patients with cirrhosis had a markedly prolonged mean half-life of 21.2 hours. This difference suggested a major role for the liver in the metabolism of methimazole although the possibility of delayed absorption could not be excluded. It was suggested that patients with liver disease might benefit from a less frequent methimazole dosing schedule, but further studies were needed before specific recommendations could be made.— D. S. Cooper *et al.*, *J. clin. Endocr. Metab.*, 1984, *58*, 473.

A study using gas chromatography-mass spectrometry of the intrathyroidal concentrations of methimazole in 20 patients with hyperthyroidism due to Graves' disease undergoing subtotal thyroidectomy. All patients had received carbimazole 15 to 45 mg daily for at least 2 months before surgery and all were euthyroid. The results strongly indicated that the elimination time for methimazole from the thyroid gland is much longer than that from the blood. Previous clinical trials have provided evidence of a much longer antithyroid effect than could be expected from blood elimination time, and thus this study supports the recommendation of a single daily dose of methimazole for the treatment of Graves' disease in most instances.— R. Jansson *et al.*, *J. clin. Endocr. Metab.*, 1983, *57*, 129.

Further references.— R. Jansson *et al.*, *Clin. Pharmacokinet.*, 1985, *10*, 443.

PREGNANCY AND THE NEONATE. Studies in 9 women undergoing therapeutic abortion given single doses of carbimazole, methimazole, or propylthiouracil indicated that the placenta appeared to be more permeable to methimazole than to propylthiouracil.— B. Marchant *et al.*, *J. clin. Endocr. Metab.*, 1977, *45*, 1187.

A study of the pharmacokinetics of methimazole in hyperthyroid women at various stages of pregnancy following the administration of a single dose of carbimazole.— G. G. Skellern *et al.*, *Br. J. clin. Pharmac.*, 1980, *9*, 145.

For references to the excretion of antithyroid agents, including methimazole (a metabolite of carbimazole), in breast milk, and precautions to be observed in nursing mothers, see under Antithyroid Agents, p.682.

Uses and Administration

Carbimazole, which is metabolised to methimazole, is an antithyroid agent which depresses the formation of thyroid hormones. The main effect, within the thyroid gland, is the reduction of formation of iodotyrosines by inhibition of the iodination of thyroglobulin and reduction of the synthesis of tri-iodothyronine and thyroxine by inhibition of the coupling reaction between iodotyrosines. The release of any preformed thyroid hormones is not affected. Unlike the perchlorates carbimazole does not reduce the uptake of iodide by the thyroid gland. It is considered that the clinical antithyroid activity of carbimazole is attributable entirely to methimazole. Carbimazole and methimazole also possess some immunosuppressant activity.

Carbimazole is used to control hyperthyroidism such as Graves' disease and is given by mouth usually in an initial dosage of 30 to 60 mg daily in divided doses, at 8-hourly intervals, according to the severity of the disorder. Improvement is usually seen in 1 to 3 weeks and control of symptoms is achieved in 1 to 3 months. The dose is then gradually reduced to the smallest amount that will control the disease. Usual maintenance doses are 5 to 15 mg daily. A suggested initial dose for children is 0.75 to 1 mg per kg bodyweight daily in divided doses.

HYPERTHYROIDISM. For reviews, discussions, and reports on the use of antithyroid agents, including carbimazole, in the management of hyperthyroidism, see under Antithyroid Agents, p.683.

Pregnancy and the neonate. A report of the outcome of four pregnancies in a woman previously made hypothyroid (which was controlled by thyroxine) after partial thyroidectomy for hyperthyroidism. During the first 2 pregnancies she received no antithyroid therapy; the first resulted in a late intra-uterine death of a foetus with features compatible with foetal hyperthyroidism and the second in a child with skull deformities probably due to uncontrolled foetal hyperthyroidism. During the third pregnancy carbimazole 10 mg four times daily was started at 25 weeks because of foetal tachycardia. A normal infant was delivered but hyperthyroidism developed at 4 days which was treated with propranolol 3 mg three times daily and from day 21 with carbimazole 1 mg twice daily. Again during the fourth pregnancy, because of foetal tachycardia, the mother received carbimazole 5 mg three times daily at 23 weeks, reduced to 5 mg twice daily at 31 weeks. Initially the baby was clinically and biochemically euthyroid but clinical features of hyperthyroidism appeared 7 days after delivery. Propranolol 3 mg four times daily and carbimazole 0.75 mg daily rapidly controlled the features of hyperthyroidism and treatment was continued for 8 weeks. These findings supported the hypothesis that the morbidity and mortality associated with foetal and neonatal hyperthyroidism are preventable by treatment during pregnancy. Probably at greatest risk are the infants of mothers who have had previous ablative thyroid treatment, since the foetus may be exposed to thyroid-stimulating immunoglobulins throughout pregnancy without the modifying effect of carbimazole given for maternal hyperthyroidism.— D. H. Cove and P. Johnston, *Lancet*, 1985, *1*, 430. Similar reports of the use of carbimazole to treat foetal and neonatal hyperthyroidism in infants whose mothers had previously undergone partial thyroidectomy.— I. Ramsay, *Br. med. J.*, 1976, *2*, 1110; P. L. Robinson *et al.*, *Br. med. J.*, 1979, *1*, 383.

For reviews and discussions concerning the use of antithyroid agents, including carbimazole, in the management of hyperthyroidism in pregnancy, see under Antithyroid Agents, p.684.

Preparations

Carbimazole Tablets *(B.P.)*

Proprietary Preparations

Neo-Mercazole *(Nicholas, UK)*. *Tablets* (Neo-Mercazole 5), scored, carbimazole 5 mg.
Tablets (Neo-Mercazole 20), carbimazole 20 mg.

Proprietary Names and Manufacturers

Basolest *(Neth.)*; Carbazole *(Austral.)*; Carbotiroid *(Borromeo, Ital.)*; Neo-Carbimazole *(Spain)*; Neo-Mercazol *(Belg.)*; Neo-Mercazole *(Nicholas, Austral.; Canad.; Nicholas, Denm.; Nicholas, Fr.; Nicholas, Norw.; MPS Lab., S.Afr.; Nicholas, Swed.; Nicholas, Switz.; Nicholas, UK)*; Neo-Morphazole *(Nicholas, Ger.)*; Neo-Thyreostat *(Herbrand, Ger.)*; Neo-Tireol *(Ital.)*; Neo-Tomizol *(Robert, Spain)*.

12643-l

Dibromotyrosine

3,5-Dibromo-L-tyrosine.
$C_9H_9Br_2NO_3$=339.0.

CAS — 300-38-9.

Dibromotyrosine is an antithyroid agent which has been used in the treatment of hyperthyroidism.

Symptoms of restlessness, anxiety, and insomnia associated with anginal syndrome were significantly reduced when dibromotyrosine was added to therapy with diltiazem.— R. C. Merchan *et al.*, *Clin. Trials J.*, 1987, *24*, 227.

Proprietary Names and Manufacturers

Biotiren *(Benvegna, Ital.)*; Bromotiren *(Baldacci, Ital.; Spain)*.

9005-f

Diiodotyrosine

Diotyrosine; Iodogorgoic Acid. 3,5-Di-iodo-L-tyrosine dihydrate.
$C_9H_9I_2NO_3,2H_2O$=469.0.

CAS — 66-02-4 (anhydrous); 300-39-0 (L, anhydrous).

Pharmacopoeias. In *Aust.*, *Cz.*, and *Rus.*

A white to slightly brownish powder. Very slightly **soluble** in water; slightly soluble in alcohol; practically insoluble in chloroform and ether; freely soluble in solutions of alkali hydroxides and dilute mineral acids. **Protect** from light.

Diiodotyrosine has been used in the treatment of hyperthyroidism.

Proprietary Names and Manufacturers

Itir *(Boniscontro & Gazzone, Ital.)*; Normotiroides Fuerte *(Inexfa, Spain)*.

833-s

Iodothiouracil Sodium *(BANM, rINNM)*.

Athyriodacil Sodique; Iothiouracil Sodium. The dihydrate of the sodium salt of 2,3-dihydro-5-iodo-2-thioxopyrimidin-4(1*H*)-one; the dihydrate of the sodium salt of 5-iodo-2-mercaptopyrimidin-4-ol; the dihydrate of the sodium salt of 5-iodo-2-thiouracil.
$C_4H_2IN_2NaOS,2H_2O$=312.1.

CAS — 5984-97-4 (iodothiouracil); 3565-15-9 (sodium salt, anhydrous).

Iodothiouracil sodium is an antithyroid agent which was formerly used in the treatment of hyperthyroidism.

12867-v

Isobutiacilic Acid

2-(4-Hydroxy-6-methylpyrimidin-2-yl)-2-(methyl)thiopropionic acid.
$C_9H_{12}N_2O_2S$=212.3.

Isobutiacilic acid is an antithyroid agent which has been used in the treatment of hyperthyroidism.

Proprietary Names and Manufacturers

Isotiran *(Zilliken, Ital.)*.

834-w

Mercaptothiazoline

2-Thiazoline-2-thiol.
$C_3H_5NS_2$=119.2.

CAS — 96-53-7; 12758-33-7; 25377-76-8.

Mercaptothiazoline is an antithyroid agent which was formerly used in the treatment of hyperthyroidism.

835-e

Methimazole *(BAN, USAN)*.

Mercazolylum; Thiamazole *(rINN)*; Tiamazol. 1-Methylimidazole-2-thiol.
$C_4H_6N_2S$=114.2.

CAS — 60-56-0.

Pharmacopoeias. In *Arg.*, *Braz.*, *Chin.*, *Hung.*, *It.*, *Jpn*, *Jug.*, *Nord.*, *Rus.*, and *U.S.*

A white to pale buff crystalline powder with a faint characteristic odour. M.p. 144° to 147°.**Soluble**1 in 5 of water, 1 in 5 of alcohol, 1 in 4.5 of chloroform, and 1 in 125 of ether. Solutions in water are practically neutral to litmus. **Protect** from light.

Methimazole, like phenylthiourea and propylthiouracil, had a dualistic taste response and was bitter to nearly 30% of persons tested.— G. H. Hamor and A. Lafdjian, *J. pharm. Sci.*, 1967, *56*, 777.

Adverse Effects and Treatment

As for Antithyroid Agents, p.682.

For reviews and discussions regarding the nature and incidence of the adverse effects of antithyroid agents, including methimazole, see under Antithyroid Agents, p.682.

EFFECTS ON THE BLOOD. Aplastic anaemia in 1 patient induced by methimazole. Failure to recognise the initial complaints as indicators of drug toxicity in the patient and a 2-week delay in discontinuing methimazole may have been responsible for the unusually severe bone marrow suppression.— J. Moreb *et al.*, *Acta haemat.*, 1983, *69*, 127.

For studies comparing the incidence of antithyroid-induced blood disorders, including agranulocytosis and neutropenia associated with methimazole, see under Antithyroid Agents, p.682.

EFFECTS ON THE IMMUNE SYSTEM. A report of the insulin autoimmune syndrome in 85 patients in Japan covering the period 1970-82; 15 of the patients had received methimazole. It appeared that some drugs containing sulphydryl groups could induce the formation of insulin autoantibodies in predisposed individuals, especially among Japanese people.— Y. Hirata (letter), *Lancet*, 1983, *2*, 1037. Mention of the syndrome in 2 patients receiving carbimazole.— A. C. Burden and F. D. Rosenthal (letter), *ibid.*, 1311.

Methimazole-induced serum sickness, comprising sore throat, pruritus, arthralgias, facial oedema, and fever, in 1 patient.— M. Van Kuyk *et al.*, *Acta clin. belg.*, 1983, *38*, 68.

EFFECTS ON THE KIDNEYS. A report of the nephrotic syndrome in 1 patient associated with methimazole therapy.— L. R. Reynolds and D. Bhathena, *Archs intern. Med.*, 1979, *139*, 236.

EFFECTS ON THE LIVER. Jaundice was attributed to methimazole in one patient. Symptoms cleared on substituting propylthiouracil for methimazole.— C. E. Becker *et al.*, *J. Am. med. Ass.*, 1968, *206*, 1787. Another case of jaundice associated with methimazole.— M. G. Fischer *et al.*, *ibid.*, 1973, *223*, 1028.

PREGNANCY AND THE NEONATE. Mention of scalp defects in 3 infants of 2 mothers who had received methimazole during pregnancy.— S. Milham and W. Elledge (letter), *Teratology*, 1972, *5*, 125. A further report mentioning scalp defects in 2 infants whose mother had received methimazole.— Q. Mujtaba and G. N. Burrow, *Obstet. Gynec.*, 1975, *46*, 282. Besides the 5 published cases of aplasia cutis congenita associated with methimazole 5 verbally reported cases are known. Because of this association propylthiouracil may be the preferred drug for the management of thyrotoxicosis in pregnant women.— L. K. Bachrach and G. N. Burrow (letter), *Can. med. Ass. J.*, 1984, *130*, 1264. A further similar report of congenital scalp defects. Although examination of the records of over 49 000 infants born in a Dutch hospital between 1959 and 1986 failed to exclude a causal relationship between maternal usage of carbimazole or methimazole during pregnancy and congenital skin defects it appeared that this association was not as strong as earlier reports had suggested.— C. P. Van Dijke *et al.*, *Ann. intern. Med.*, 1987, *106*, 60.

For further reports of the effect of methimazole on the foetus, see Propylthiouracil, p.687.

For a review of antithyroid agents in pregnancy, see under Antithyroid Agents, p.682 and p.684.

Precautions

As for Antithyroid Agents, p.682.

PREGNANCY AND THE NEONATE. For discussions of precautions to be observed during the administration of antithyroid agents, including methimazole, to pregnant and nursing mothers, see under Precautions and Uses of Antithyroid Agents, p.682 and p.684.

Absorption and Fate

Methimazole is a metabolite of carbimazole and the absorption and fate of both compounds is described under Carbimazole, p.684.

Uses and Administration

Methimazole is an antithyroid agent whose action is described under its parent, carbimazole (see p.685). Methimazole is used similarly to carbimazole to control hyperthyroidism and is given by mouth usually in an initial dosage of 15 to 60 mg daily in divided doses, at 8-hourly intervals, according to the severity of the disorder. When the condition is controlled, probably in 1 to 3 months, the dose is reduced to a maintenance dose, usually 5 to 15 mg daily. A suggested initial dose for children is 400 µg per kg body-weight daily in divided doses; for maintenance this dose may be halved.

Reference to the possible use of topical methimazole as a radioprotectant during radiotherapy.— M. M. Ferguson *et al.* (letter), *Lancet*, 1985, *2*, 325.

HYPERTHYROIDISM. For reviews, discussions, and reports on the use of antithyroid agents, including methimazole, in the management of hyperthyroidism, see under Antithyroid Agents, p.683.

Preparations

Methimazole Tablets *(U.S.P.)*

Proprietary Names and Manufacturers

Antitiroide GW *(Panthox & Burck, Ital.)*; Danantizol *(Gador, Arg.)*; Favistan *(Asta Pharma, Ger.)*; Mercaptol *(Nessa, Spain)*; Metazolo *(Ital.)*; Strumazol *(Christiaens, Belg.; Neth.)*; Tapazole *(Lilly, Canad.; Lilly, Ital.; Lilly, Norw.; Lilly, S.Afr.; Lilly, Switz.; Lilly, USA)*; Thacapzol *(Kabi, Swed.)*; Thycapzol *(GEA, Denm.)*; Tirodril *(Estedi, Spain)*; Tomizol *(Spain)*.

836-l

Methylthiouracil *(USAN, rINN)*.

2,3-Dihydro-2-thioxo-6-methylpyrimidin-4(1*H*)-one; 2-Mercapto-6-methylpyrimidin-4-ol; 6-Methyl-2-thiouracil.

$C_5H_6N_2OS$=142.2.

CAS — 56-04-2.

Pharmacopoeias. In *Arg., Aust., Braz., Int., It., Nord., Pol., Rus.*, and *U.S.*

A white odourless crystalline powder. M.p. about 330° with decomposition. **Soluble** 1 in 150 of boiling water; very slightly soluble in water; sparingly soluble in alcohol; slightly soluble in chloroform and ether; freely soluble in ammonium hydroxide and in solutions of alkali hydroxides. **Protect** from light.

Methylthiouracil is an antithyroid agent which has been used in the treatment of hyperthyroidism.

Proprietary Names and Manufacturers

Atiroid *(Spain)*; Methiocil *(Helvepharm, Switz.)*; Thyreostat *(Herbrand, Ger.)*; Thyrostabil *(Streuli, Switz.)*; Tiouracil *(Spain)*.

837-y

Potassium Perchlorate

$KClO_4$=138.5.

CAS — 7778-74-7.

Pharmacopoeias. In *Cz.* and *Hung.*

Odourless colourless crystals or white crystalline powder. It decrepitates on heating and evolves oxygen. Each g represents 7.2 mmol of potassium. **Soluble** 1 in 65 of water and 1 in 15 of boiling water; practically insoluble in alcohol.

WARNING. *Potassium perchlorate has been used for the illicit preparation of explosives or fireworks; care is required with its supply.*

Adverse Effects

Fatal aplastic anaemia has occurred in a small proportion of patients. Other blood disorders including agranulocytosis, thrombocytopenia, and leucopenia have been reported. Signs of intolerance may precede changes in the blood by several days. The nephrotic syndrome occurs rarely. Nausea and vomiting and hypersensitivity reactions such as maculopapular rashes, fever, and lymphadenopathies may occur, but are reported to be infrequent if the daily dosage is kept below 1 g.

Treatment of Adverse Effects and Precautions

As for Antithyroid Agents, p.682.

Uses and Administration

Potassium perchlorate is an antithyroid agent which reduces the uptake of iodide by the thyroid gland and also releases inorganic iodide already taken up by the gland. However, because of toxicity its use is generally limited to patients who cannot tolerate other forms of antithyroid therapy.

To control hyperthyroidism potassium perchlorate has been given by mouth in an initial dose of 200 mg three or four times daily, reduced after 2 to 4 weeks to 100 mg three or four times daily. More than 1 g daily should not be given. Thyroid function may remain depressed for some weeks after withdrawal of the drug. Potassium perchlorate has been used to prepare patients for partial thyroidectomy when the goitre was small and nodular.

Potassium perchlorate may also be used in thyroid function studies because it releases inorganic iodide already taken up by the gland. Radio-iodine is given initially and decreased counts of radioactivity over the thyroid gland following the administration of potassium perchlorate demonstrate that the perchlorate has caused the release of inorganic iodide from the gland; this is termed a positive discharge test. The test is usually considered to provide an abnormal result if more than about 10% of the radioactivity is discharged. This indicates a defect in the binding of iodide involved in the synthesis of thyroid hormones and a cause of thyroid dysfunction. The test has also been used to investigate the action and efficacy of antithyroid agents such as carbimazole and propylthiouracil.

Potassium perchlorate is also used in nuclear medicine to reduce unwanted uptake of radiopharmaceuticals such as radio-iodine or pertechnetate (^{99m}Tc) by the choroid plexus, salivary glands, and thyroid gland, thus enhancing the visibility of scans of the head and neck.

Proprietary Names and Manufacturers

Peroidin *(Protea, Austral.; Purdue Frederick, Canad.; Larkhall Laboratories, UK)*; Pertiroid *(Piam, Ital.)*.

838-j

Propylthiouracil *(BAN, USAN, rINN)*.

Propylthiouracilum. 2,3-Dihydro-6-propyl-2-thioxopyrimidin-4(1*H*)-one; 2-Mercapto-6-propylpyrimidin-4-ol; 6-Propyl-2-thiouracil.

$C_7H_{10}N_2OS$=170.2.

CAS — 51-52-5.

Pharmacopoeias. In *Aust., Br., Braz., Chin., Egypt., Eur., Ger., Ind., Int., It., Jpn, Jug., Mex., Nord., Swiss, Turk.*, and *U.S.*

White or practically white crystals or crystalline powder. *B.P.* **solubilities** are: very slightly soluble in water and ether; sparingly soluble in alcohol; dissolves in aqueous solutions of alkali hydroxides. *U.S.P.* solubilities are: slightly soluble in water, chloroform, and ether; sparingly soluble in alcohol; soluble in ammonium hydroxide and solutions of alkali hydroxides. **Store** in well-closed containers. Protect from light.

Propylthiouracil had a dualistic taste response and was bitter to nearly 30% of persons tested.— G. H. Hamor and A. Lafdjian, *J. pharm. Sci.*, 1967, *56*, 777.

Adverse Effects and Treatment

As for Antithyroid Agents, p.682. A rare complication of therapy with propylthiouracil is a tendency to haemorrhage; it may be controlled by the administration of phytomenadione.

For reviews and discussions regarding the nature and incidence of the adverse effects of antithyroid agents, including propylthiouracil, see under Antithyroid Agents, p.682.

EFFECTS ON THE BLOOD. Severe hypoprothrombinaemia developed in a 60-year-old diabetic, hypertensive, hyperthyroid woman after administration of propylthiouracil 300 mg daily for 2 weeks.— G. D'Angelo and L. P. Le Gresley, *Can. med. Ass. J.*, 1959, *81*, 479.

In 1 patient with propylthiouracil-induced agranulocytosis, cytotoxicity was shown to be complement-dependent and mediated by an IgM antibody thus demonstrating an immunologic basis for the development of the agranulocytosis. Cytotoxic activity of the patient's serum could be demonstrated against the granulocytes of only 2 of 8 normal subjects suggesting the possibility that only a subset of patients receiving propylthiouracil may be susceptible to induced agranulocytosis.— M. M. Guffy *et al.*, *Archs intern. Med.*, 1984, *144*, 1687.

For studies comparing the incidence of antithyroid-induced blood disorders, including agranulocytosis and neutropenia associated with propylthiouracil, see under Antithyroid Agents, p.682.

EFFECTS ON THE IMMUNE SYSTEM. Cutaneous vasculitis, leucocytopenia, and arthralgia in 3 patients associated with propylthiouracil therapy; all patients had received propylthiouracil for at least 1 year before developing the symptoms. Histologic examination revealed the usual features of an allergic vasculitis, and immunofluorescence-staining suggested immune complex deposition.— M. Gammeltoft and J. K. Kristensen, *Acta derm.-vener., Stockh.*, 1982, *62*, 171.

Fatal agranulocytosis with cutaneous hypersensitivity vasculitis in 1 patient after propylthiouracil therapy.— T. J. Reidy *et al.*, *Sth. med. J.*, 1982, *75*, 1297.

The suggestion that in 1 patient propylthiouracil precipitated a lupus-like syndrome in which, besides cutaneous vasculitis, leucopenia, positive antinuclear factor and lupus erythematosus cells, polyarthritis was a prominent feature. The cutaneous eruption was considered to be a typical "allergic" leucocytoclastic vasculitis.— B. K. Oh *et al.*, *Br. J. Rheumatol.*, 1983, *22*, 106.

EFFECTS ON THE LIVER. A report of 2 cases of propylthiouracil-induced hepatitis, one of which was fatal. There have been reports of at least 8 cases in which it is reasonable to implicate propylthiouracil as causing hepatic injury. However, all cases before this report lack sufficient serologic evidence to exclude hepatitis A, cytomegalovirus, or Epstein-Barr virus. The mechanism of the injury is most likely to be host idiosyncrasy given the small number of cases and the frequency of drug use. The diagnosis of a hepatotoxic effect should always be suspected in the patient receiving propylthiouracil therapy in whom clinical or biochemical evidence of acute hepatitis develops; this should lead to prompt discontinuation of the drug therapy while appropriate testing for viral hepatitis is performed.— J. S. Hanson, *Archs intern. Med.*, 1984, *144*, 994.

Individual reports of liver disorders associated with propylthiouracil.— M. S. Fedotin and L. G. Lefer, *Archs intern. Med.*, 1975, *135*, 319 (liver disease similar to chronic active hepatitis); L. N. Parker (letter), *Ann. intern. Med.*, 1975, *82*, 228 (jaundice and hepatitis in a child); A. A. Mihas *et al.*, *Gastroenterology*, 1976, *70*, 770 (hepatic necrosis); M. Weiss *et al.*, *Archs intern. Med.*, 1980, *140*, 1184 (increased liver function test values); M. M. Safani *et al.* (letter), *Archs intern. Med.*, 1982, *142*, 838 (fatal fulminant hepatitis).

EFFECTS ON THE LUNGS. A report of a diffuse interstitial pneumonitis in 2 patients who had received propylthiouracil.— K. Miyazono *et al.*, *Archs intern. med.*, 1984, *144*, 1764.

OVERDOSAGE. Ingestion of an amount of propylthiouracil considered to be at least 5 g produced no acute effects in a 12-year-old girl.— G. L. Jackson *et al.*, *Ann. intern. Med.*, 1979, *91*, 418.

PREGNANCY AND THE NEONATE. Goitre in 5 neonates was recorded in infants born to 30 patients given propylthiouracil in 41 pregnancies. The dosage of propylthiouracil appeared to be an important but not the only factor.— G. N. Burrow, *J. clin. Endocr. Metab.*, 1965, *25*, 403.

Long-term follow-up of 15 children born to thyrotoxic mothers treated with propylthiouracil during pregnancy suggested that exposure to propylthiouracil *in utero* did not appear to have an adverse effect on subsequent intellectual and physical development.— G. N. Burrow *et al.*, *Am. J. Dis. Child.*, 1968, *116*, 161.

Transient neonatal goitre occurred in 2 infants, 1 in each of 2 sets of twins, born to mothers who had taken propylthiouracil or methimazole during pregnancy.— S. Refetoff *et al.*, *J. Pediat.*, 1974, *85*, 240.

Propylthiouracil or methimazole was administered to 21 women during 26 pregnancies. Three infants had goitre at birth and of these 2 had neonatal thyrotoxicosis. There were congenital defects in 5 children of 3 mothers (developmental retardation, aortic atresia, and hypospadias with propylthiouracil and scalp defects and imperforate anus with methimazole).— Q. Mujtaba and G. N. Burrow, *Obstet. Gynec.*, 1975, *46*, 282.

For a review of antithyroid agents in pregnancy, see under Antithyroid Agents, p.682 and p.684.

Precautions

As for Antithyroid Agents, p.682.

INTERACTIONS. Studies *in vitro* showed that the addition of aspirin, phenylbutazone, or warfarin to serum containing propylthiouracil significantly increased the free fraction of propylthiouracil. No effect was observed after the addition of nortriptyline, phenazone, phenytoin, or propranolol.— J. P. Kampmann and J. E. M. Hansen, *Br. J. clin. Pharmac.*, 1983, *16*, 549.

PREGNANCY AND THE NEONATE. For discussions of precautions to be observed during the administration of antithyroid agents, including propylthiouracil, to pregnant and nursing mothers, see under the Precautions and Uses of Antithyroid Agents, p.682 and p.684.

Absorption and Fate

Propylthiouracil is rapidly absorbed from the gastro-intestinal tract. It undergoes metabolism and is widely distributed throughout the body, although it is concentrated in the thyroid gland. Propylthiouracil is appreciably bound to proteins in blood and although the elimination half-life from blood is short, the biological effects are much longer lasting. Propylthiouracil and metabolites are excreted in the urine.

Propylthiouracil crosses the placenta and is excreted in breast milk.

A review of the clinical pharmacokinetics of antithyroid agents, including propylthiouracil.— J. P. Kampmann and J. M. Hansen, *Clin. Pharmacokinet.*, 1981, *6*, 401.

A study using high pressure liquid chromatography on the disposition of propylthiouracil following administration by intravenous infusion to 10 healthy subjects. Distribution of propylthiouracil was rapid and after distribution equilibrium had been achieved the median apparent elimination half-life was calculated as 1.28 hours. The extensive metabolism of propylthiouracil was demonstrated by no more than about 2% of the administered dose being excreted in the urine of any subject. The median free fraction of propylthiouracil in plasma was 18.2%. The hepatic extraction ratio was calculated to be 0.33; thus first pass biotransformation would reduce the systemic availability by about 33% after oral administration. The results suggested that renal clearance of propylthiouracil was not a simple process and that there was passive tubular reabsorption back into the circulation. The data also in part explained the reported variable efficacy of single daily dose regimens; the clearance of propylthiouracil was sufficiently rapid so that many patients failed to sustain a therapeutic concentration after a single large dose, although some patients who absorb the drug comparatively slowly might sustain effective drug concentrations.— H. G. Giles *et al.*, *J. clin. Pharmac.*, 1981, *21*, 466.

A study in 17 hyperthyroid patients given propylthiouracil 200 mg three times daily for 3 weeks showed a significant correlation between serum-propylthiouracil concentrations and the percentage decrease in serum concentrations of thyroid hormones. Concentrations of propylthiouracil were measured spectrophotometrically. It was suggested that serum-propylthiouracil concentrations above 4 to 5 µg per mL one hour after an oral dose of 400 mg would secure a sufficient and rapid antithyroid effect during continuous therapy.— J. P. Kampmann and J. E. M. Hansen, *Br. J. clin. Pharmac.*, 1981, *12*, 681.

A study of the pharmacokinetics of propylthiouracil using a radio-immunoassay. In 5 healthy subjects and 4 patients with untreated Graves' disease given single doses of propylthiouracil 50, 200, or 300 mg, mean peak serum-propylthiouracil concentrations were 0.91, 2.9, and 4.0 µg per mL respectively in the controls and 1.04, 4.5, and 7.1 µg per mL respectively in the patients; statistical difference was achieved only at the 300-mg dose. Although the explanation for higher concentrations in patients than controls was uncertain, the most plausible reason was heightened absorption of propylthiouracil from the gut in hyperthyroidism. The effects of propylthiouracil on thyroidal iodide organification [the process of thyroid hormone biosynthesis from inorganic iodide] was assessed by perchlorate discharge testing. Both groups had normal basal results but after propylthiouracil the hyperthyroid patients had a greater percentage of perchlorate-dischargable radio-iodine than the controls. In both groups there was a highly significant correlation between serum-propylthiouracil concentrations and perchlorate-dischargeable iodide. This striking positive correlation led to the suggestion that determination of serum-propylthiouracil concentrations might be of benefit in estimating propylthiouracil efficacy more precisely in individual patients; the data suggested that concentrations of 3 µg per mL or more 4 hours after ingestion of propylthiouracil would be associated with a perchlorate-dischargeable iodide level of 50% or more in a hyperthyroid patient. Although it was not possible to demonstrate an unequivocal dose-response relationship between changes in serum concentrations of tri-iodothyronine or reverse tri-iodothyronine and propylthiouracil dosage, a greater and more long-lasting response was clearly observed with higher doses.—D. S. Cooper *et al.*, *J. clin. Endocr. Metab.*, 1982, *54*, 101.

Studies indicating that the mean serum protein binding of propylthiouracil of 76.2% in 12 euthyroid subjects was not significantly different from that of 76.6% in 10 hyperthyroid patients.— J. P. Kampmann and J. E. M. Hansen, *Br. J. clin. Pharmac.*, 1983, *16*, 549.

In 6 children or adolescents with Graves' disease pharmacokinetic studies after the administration of a single dose of propylthiouracil by mouth showed that intake of food before drug ingestion was associated with a lower and delayed peak plasma-propylthiouracil concentration and variable area-under-the-curve values compared to intake of food after drug administration. It was suggested that administration of propylthiouracil in the fasting state is more advisable for obtaining a consistent bioavailability.— A. Okuno *et al.*, *Pediat. Pharmacol.*, 1983, *3*, 43.

PREGNANCY AND THE NEONATE. Studies in 9 women undergoing therapeutic abortion given single doses of carbimazole, methimazole, or propylthiouracil indicated that the placenta appeared to be more permeable to methimazole than to propylthiouracil.— B. Marchant *et al.*, *J. clin. Endocr. Metab.*, 1977, *45*, 1187.

Evidence from studies in 3 hyperthyroid women during pregnancy and post partum suggesting that pregnancy does not have a major effect on the pharmacokinetics of propylthiouracil.— D. S. Sitar *et al.*, *Pharmacology*, 1982, *25*, 57.

For references to the excretion of antithyroid agents, including propylthiouracil, into breast milk, and precautions to be observed in nursing mothers, see under Antithyroid Agents, p.682.

Uses and Administration

Propylthiouracil is an antithyroid agent with actions similar to those of carbimazole (see p.685) but additionally it inhibits the peripheral de-iodination of thyroxine to tri-iodothyronine. Propylthiouracil, like carbimazole and methimazole, also possesses some immunosuppressant activity.

Propylthiouracil is used to control hyperthyroidism and is given by mouth usually in an initial dosage of 300 to 600 mg daily in divided doses, at 8-hourly intervals, according to the severity of the disorder. When the condition is controlled, probably in 1 to 3 months, the dose is reduced to a maintenance dose, usually 50 to 200 mg daily. A suggested initial dose for children aged 6 to 10 years is 50 to 150 mg daily in divided doses, and for children over 10 years 150 to 300 mg daily.

Following an earlier study indicating that propylthiouracil hastened clinical improvement in patients with alcoholic liver disease, Orrego *et al.* (*New Engl. J. Med.*, 1987, *317*, 1421) conducted a double-blind study to determine the effect of long-term treatment on survival. In contrast to Hallé *et al.* (*Gastroenterology*, 1982, *82*, 925) who had failed to find any beneficial effect, Orrego *et al.* found that during their 2-year study the 13% mortality-rate in patients receiving propylthiouracil 300 mg daily was significantly lower than the 25% mortality-rate in patients receiving placebo. The main effect of propylthiouracil appeared to be on acute alcoholic hepatitis as the difference in mortality-rate was greatest during the first 12 weeks. Although subgroup analysis indicated that the effect was greater in severely ill patients, the validity of this result is considered to be uncertain as the patients had not been randomised according to the severity of their disease on entry to the study (*Lancet*, 1988, *1*, 450).

ADMINISTRATION IN GASTRO-INTESTINAL DISORDERS. A study indicating that propylthiouracil could be administered in usual doses to patients with intestinal shunts.— J. P. Kampmann *et al.*, *Clin. Pharmacokinet.*, 1984, *9*, 168.

ADMINISTRATION IN RENAL FAILURE. Propylthiouracil could be given in usual doses in renal failure.— W. M. Bennett *et al.*, *Am. J. Kidney Dis.*, 1983, *3*, 155.

HYPERTHYROIDISM. For reviews, discussions, and reports on the use of antithyroid agents, including propylthiouracil, in the management of hyperthyroidism, see under Antithyroid Agents, p.683.

Pregnancy and the neonate. Thyrotoxicosis in a neonate was treated with propylthiouracil 6 mg at 8-hourly intervals for 2 weeks. Thyrotoxic symptoms reappeared after 2 weeks and were treated with propylthiouracil 6.25 mg twice daily for 8 weeks. The infant then remained euthyroid.— G. J. Robards and J. R. Davis, *Med. J. Aust.*, 1973, *2*, 432.

A report of the use of propylthiouracil to manage foetal hyperthyroidism in a woman with a genetic predisposition to hyperthyroidism. At 26 weeks of gestation the foetus was noted to have become hyperactive with tachycardia and propylthiouracil 300 mg daily was given to the mother; dosage was reduced to 150 mg daily at 28 weeks, reduced again at 37 weeks to 62.5 mg daily, and finally discontinued at birth. A euthyroid boy was born at 37 weeks, with slight signs of neonatal thyrotoxicosis that did not require treatment. The mother had no symptoms of hyperthyroidism or hypothyroidism during the pregnancy.— J. Serup (letter), *Lancet*, 1978, *2*, 896.

For reviews and discussions concerning the use of antithyroid agents, including propylthiouracil, in the management of hyperthyroidism in pregnancy, see under Antithyroid Agents, p.684.

Preparations

Propylthiouracil Tablets *(B.P.)*

Propylthiouracil Tablets *(U.S.P.)*

Proprietary Names and Manufacturers

Propycil *(Kali-Chemie, Ger.; Farmades, Ital.)*; Propyl-Thyracil *(Frosst, Canad.)*; Thyreostat II *(Herbrand, Ger.)*; Tiotil *(Pharmacia, Swed.)*.

13255-p

Sodium Perchlorate

$NaClO_4,H_2O$=140.5.

CAS — 7601-89-0 (anhydrous); 7791-07-3 (monohydrate).

WARNING. *Sodium perchlorate has been used for the illicit preparation of explosives or fireworks; care is required with its supply.*

Sodium perchlorate is an antithyroid agent with actions similar to those of potassium perchlorate (see p.686). Like potassium perchlorate it has been used in the treatment of hyperthyroidism, in perchlorate discharge tests, and to reduce unwanted uptake of radiopharmaceuticals.

Proprietary Names and Manufacturers

Irenat *(Tropon, Ger.; Medichemie, Switz.)*.

839-z

Thibenzazoline

2-Mercaptobenzimidazole-1,3-dimethylol. 1,3-Bis(hydroxymethyl)benzimidazolin-2-thione.

$C_9H_{10}N_2O_2S$=210.3.

CAS — 6028-35-9.

M.p. 160° to 162°. **Soluble** in dilute alkalis.

Thibenzazoline is an antithyroid agent which was formerly used in the treatment of hyperthyroidism.

840-p

Thiouracil

2,3-Dihydro-2-thioxopyrimidin-4(1*H*)-one; 2-Mercaptopyrimidin-4-ol; 2-Thiouracil.

$C_4H_4N_2OS$=128.2.

CAS — 141-90-2.

Pharmacopoeias. In *Span.*

Thiouracil is an antithyroid agent which was formerly used in the treatment of hyperthyroidism.

Thiouracil was the first widely used antithyroid drug but it had a rather high rate of side-effects and its use was soon abandoned.— D. S. Cooper, *New Engl. J. Med.*, 1984, *311*, 1353.

Antiviral Agents

1680-c

The drugs described in this section are used in the treatment of a number of viral infections or for providing protection, usually for a brief period only, against infection. Treatment has to be started early in the infection for the antiviral agent to be effective and inhibit the replicating virus. There is little evidence that these compounds affect latent or nonreplicating viruses.

They do not provide an alternative to available immunisation for the long-term prophylaxis of infection—for details of such treatment see the section on vaccines and other immunological products, p.1155. Other drugs used in the treatment of viral infection discussed elsewhere include amantadine hydrochloride (p.1009), cytarabine (p.620), and levamisole (p.56). Immunoglobulins are also used in the treatment of viral infections. While this section includes several new antiviral agents there are many more under development and they include:

the phospholipid, AL-721;

the mismatched double-stranded RNA compound, ampligen;

the dideoxynucleosides, dideoxycytidine and dideoxyadenosine;

the antipicornaviral, disoxaril (Win-51711); and

the ammonium tungsto-antimoniate, HPA-23.

Reviews of antiviral agents and their use in viral infections: G. J. Galasso, *Bull. Wld Hlth Org.*, 1981, *59*, 503; M. S. Hirsch and R. T. Schooley, *New Engl. J. Med.*, 1983, *309*, 963 and 1034; P. E. Hermans and F. R. Cockerill, *Mayo Clin. Proc.*, 1983, *58*, 217; G. J. Galasso, *J. antimicrob. Chemother.*, 1984, *14, Suppl. A*, 127; D. O. White, *Med. J. Aust.*, 1984, *140*, 715; K. G. Nicholson, *Lancet*, 1984, *2*, 617, 677, and 736; C. Stuart-Harris, *J. antimicrob. Chemother.*, 1985, *15*, 387; D. A. J. Tyrrell and J. S. Oxford (Ed.), *Br. med. Bull.*, 1985, *41*, 307; Progress in the Development and Use of Antiviral Drugs and Interferon, *Tech. Rep. Ser. Wld Hlth Org. No. 754*, 1987; M. J. Wood and A. M. Geddes, *Lancet*, 1987, *2*, 1189.

1682-a

Acyclovir *(BAN, USAN)*.

Aciclovir *(rINN)*; Acycloguanosine; BW-248U. 9-(2-Hydroxyethoxymethyl)guanine; 2-Amino-1,9-dihydro-9-(2-hydroxyethoxymethyl)purin-6-one.

$C_8H_{11}N_5O_3$=225.2.

CAS — 59277-89-3.

A white crystalline powder. Slightly **soluble** in water.

Oleic acid and oleyl alcohol each enhanced the penetration of acyclovir in propylene glycol across human skin *in vitro*.— E. R. Cooper *et al.*, *J. pharm. Sci.*, 1985, *74*, 688.

16177-e

Acyclovir Sodium *(BANM, USAN)*.

Aciclovir Sodium *(rINNM)*. 9-(2-Hydroxyethoxymethyl)guanine sodium.

$C_8H_{10}N_5NaO_3$=247.2.

CAS — 69657-51-8.

A white crystalline powder. **Soluble** 1 in 10 of water.

Each g of acyclovir sodium represents 4.05 mmol of sodium. Acyclovir sodium 1.1 g is approximately equivalent to 1 g of acyclovir.

Adverse Effects

Acyclovir when administered intravenously as acyclovir sodium may cause local reactions at the injection site with inflammation, pain, and phlebitis; these reactions may be associated with extravasation that leads to ulceration. Some patients experience rapid increases in blood concentrations of urea and creatinine. In a few patients renal impairment may occur and may progress to acute renal failure. The rate of administration influences renal toxicity since acyclovir crystals can be precipitated in the tubules following bolus injection. The patient's state of hydration also affects renal toxicity.

Occasional adverse effects include increased values for liver enzymes, haematological and encephalopathic changes, and skin rashes.

Topical application of acyclovir may sometimes produce burning or erythema. Eye ointments may occasionally produce stinging and superficial punctate keratopathy.

There have been reports of skin rashes and gastro-intestinal effects with acyclovir given by mouth, but it is usually well tolerated.

A possible drug-related necrotising vasculitis; acyclovir was one of many drugs used in this patient.— G. K. von Schulthess (letter), *New Engl. J. Med.*, 1981, *305*, 1349. A vasculitic rash in an immunocompromised child given acyclovir by infusion as part of the treatment for chickenpox.— M. P. W. Platt and O. B. Eden (letter), *Lancet*, 1982, *2*, 763. Erythema leading to maculopapular eruption in a patient given acyclovir by mouth.— C. E. H. Grattan and J. Boyle, *Br. med. J.*, 1984, *289*, 1424.

Transient renal impairment associated with acyclovir in 2 patients. The dose in each patient was 10 mg per kg body-weight infused over 1 hour and given every 8 hours; hydration was reported to be good. Both patients experienced transient lymphopenia and one thrombocytopenia.— M. G. Harrington *et al.* (letter), *Lancet*, 1981, *2*, 1281.

Raised serum-creatinine concentrations occurred in 11 of a group of 19 patients with herpes zoster given acyclovir 500 mg per m^2 body-surface intravenously three times daily for 5 days. Ten of these 11 patients experienced nausea or vomiting, 3 abdominal pain, and 2 thirst. Out of the 8 patients whose creatinine concentrations were unaltered, 3 experienced nausea or vomiting and 1 light-headedness. Of the 10 patients in the control group given placebo 3 experienced nausea or vomiting and 1 light-headedness.—B. Bean *et al.*, *Lancet*, 1982, *2*, 118.

Acyclovir was given to 143 patients in doses ranging from 0.75 to 3.6 g per m^2 body-surface daily by intravenous infusion for the treatment of herpesvirus infections following bone-marrow transplantation. Six of the 143 developed reversible neurological symptoms including tremor, agitation, nausea, lethargy, mild disorientation, autonomic instability, hemiparaesthesia, and slurred speech. EEGs were diffusely abnormal in all 6. Symptoms improved in all patients on withdrawing acyclovir; reinstituting acyclovir in 2 produced a recurrence of symptoms. Concomitant therapy included irradiation and methotrexate intrathecally for all 6, interferon alfa for 3, and cyclosporin for 1.— J. C. Wade and J. D. Meyers, *Ann. intern. Med.*, 1983, *98*, 921. Individual case reports of neurological adverse effects in patients given acyclovir.— C. V. Vartian and D. M. Shlaes (letter), *ibid.*, *99*, 568; J. Auwerx *et al.* (letter), *ibid.*, 882; S. M. Z. Cohen *et al.* (letter), *ibid.*, 1984, *100*, 920.

EFFECTS ON BLOOD. No evidence of bone-marrow toxicity in three patients given acyclovir following bone-marrow transplantation.— F. T. Serota *et al.*, *J. Am. med. Ass.*, 1982, *247*, 2132. See also E. Gluckman *et al.*, *J. antimicrob. Chemother.*, 1983, *12, Suppl. B*, 161.

The bone marrow of 3 patients showed evidence of megaloblastic haemopoiesis during therapy with acyclovir for suspected or proven herpes simplex encephalitis.— R. J. Amos and J. A. L. Amess (letter), *Lancet*, 1983, *1*, 242.

Inhibition of human peripheral blood lymphocytes in samples taken from subjects given acyclovir.— P. Tauris *et al.*, *J. antimicrob. Chemother.*, 1984, *13*, 71.

Treatment of Adverse Effects

Renal impairment is reported to respond rapidly to hydration and/or dosage reduction or withdrawal. Overdosage has not been reported to be a problem; single doses of up to 80 mg per kg body-weight of acyclovir injected accidentally did not produce any adverse consequences. However, should acyclovir need to be removed then haemodialysis would be effective.

Precautions

Acyclovir should be administered with caution to patients with renal impairment and doses should be adjusted according to creatinine clearance. Parenteral administration should be by slow intravenous infusion over one hour to avoid precipitation of acyclovir in the kidney. The risk of renal impairment is increased by dehydration and by the concomitant use of other nephrotoxic drugs.

Probenecid is reported to block the renal clearance of acyclovir.

Hypersensitivity does not appear to be a problem, although the manufacturer states that acyclovir is contra-indicated in patients known to be hypersensitive to it.

Bolus injections of 10 mg of acyclovir per kg body-weight increased creatinine values in two patients. Although the authors had found no adverse renal effects on giving 5 mg per kg by bolus injection to 27 patients every 8 hours (*Lancet*, 1982, *2*, 827) this could not be used as evidence that bolus injections were suitable for higher doses. For doses greater than 5 mg per kg acyclovir should be dissolved in 100 mL of glucose injection and infused over one hour as recommended by the manufacturer.— N. A. Peterslund *et al.* (letter), *Lancet*, 1983, *1*, 243.

Reversible psychiatric adverse effects occurred within 12 to 24 hours in 3 patients with chronic renal failure given acyclovir in large intravenous doses of 7.8 to 9.5 mg per kg body-weight daily.— C. R. Tomson *et al.* (letter), *Lancet*, 1985, *2*, 385. See also P. Bataille *et al.* (letter), *ibid.*, 724.

Overwhelming fatigue associated with the use of acyclovir and zidovudine. When each agent was given alone there was no such effect.— M. C. Bach (letter), *New Engl. J. Med.*, 1987, *316*, 547.

Antiviral Action

Acyclovir is active against herpes simplex virus type 1 and type 2 and against varicella zoster virus. This activity is due to intracellular conversion of acyclovir by viral thymidine kinase to the monophosphate with subsequent conversion to the diphosphate and the active triphosphate. This active form inhibits the herpesvirus DNA polymerase enzyme as well as being incorporated into viral DNA. This process is highly selective for infected cells. Studies in *animals* and *in vitro* show various sensitivities but demonstrate that these viruses are inhibited by concentrations of acyclovir that are readily achieved clinically. Herpes simplex virus type 1 appears to be the most susceptible, then type 2, followed by varicella zoster virus.

The Epstein-Barr virus is also susceptible to acyclovir, although for this virus it does not appear to be activated by thymidine kinase.

Acyclovir has no activity against latent viruses, but there is some evidence that it inhibits latent herpes simplex virus at an early stage of reactivation.

A review of the spectrum of activity of acyclovir *in vitro* and *in vivo*. Herpes simplex virus types 1 and 2 are both sensitive, with type 2 being perhaps slightly less sensitive. Sensitivity also varies with different cell lines. Various studies have demonstrated acyclovir's activity against herpes simplex infections in *animals*. Acyclovir can prevent the establishment of latent infections but an established latent infection becomes unresponsive. Recurrent episodes of acute disease are reported to respond to treatment with acyclovir and prophylaxis is reported to prevent recurrence. Varicella zoster virus is susceptible to acyclovir but to a lesser extent than herpes simplex because of poorer phosphorylation. Human cytomegalovirus is relatively insensitive in cell cultures, probably due to the virus being deficient in a specific thymidine kinase. The Epstein-Barr virus is inhibited by acyclovir despite the apparent absence of a specific thymidine kinase; the latent state is unaffected. Activity *in vivo* has been demonstrated against *Herpesvirus simiae* and equine rhinotracheitis virus. There is some evidence for activity against hepatitis B virus.— P. Collins, *J. antimicrob. Chemother.*, 1983, *12, Suppl. B*, 19.

A detailed review of the biochemistry and mechanism of action of acyclovir.— G. B. Elion, *J. antimicrob.*

Chemother., 1983, *12, Suppl. B*, 9. See also *idem, Am. J. Med.*, 1982, *73, Suppl. 1A*, 7.

The potentiation *in vitro* of the activity of acyclovir on pseudorabies virus [a herpes virus] by amphotericin.— B. Malewicz *et al.*, *Antimicrob. Ag. Chemother.*, 1983, *23*, 119. See also *idem*, 1984, *25*, 772.

CYTOMEGALOVIRUS. Antiviral synergy *in vitro* with acyclovir and interferon alfa when tested against human cytomegalovirus. This contrasts with earlier reports that showed an additive not a synergistic effect.— C. A. Smith *et al.*, *Antimicrob. Ag. Chemother.*, 1983, *24*, 325. Synergy *in vitro* with acyclovir and vidarabine.— S. A. Spector and E. Kelley, *ibid.*, 1985, *27*, 600.

EPSTEIN-BARR VIRUS. Studies on the activity of acyclovir *in vitro* against the Epstein-Barr virus indicated that here the phosphorylation of acyclovir was not carried out by thymidine kinase.— A. K. Datta and J. S. Pagano, *Antimicrob. Ag. Chemother.*, 1983, *24*, 10.

HERPES SIMPLEX VIRUS. The activity of acyclovir against herpes simplex virus types 1 and 2 was compared *in vitro* using Vero cells with that of idoxuridine, cytarabine, trifluridine, and vidarabine. Acyclovir was found to be the most active.— P. Collins and D. J. Bauer, *J. antimicrob. Chemother.*, 1979, *5*, 431. Different sensitivities of herpes simplex virus type 1 were observed for acyclovir and other antiviral agents when tested on various cell lines. For acyclovir the ID_{50} ranged between 0.01 and 2.00 μg per mL; for bromovinyldeoxyuridine and for fluoroiodoaracytosine the ID_{50} ranged between 0.004 and 0.200 μg per mL. For most cell lines tested the order of decreasing potency was bromovinyldeoxyuridine followed by fluoroiodoaracytosine and then acyclovir. For murine cell lines the order was bromovinyldeoxyuridine followed by acyclovir then fluoroiodoaracytosine.— E. De Clercq, *Antimicrob. Ag. Chemother.*, 1982, *21*, 661.

Enhanced activity was observed with human interferon and acyclovir against herpes simplex virus types 1 and 2 in Vero cells.— T. L. Stanwick *et al.*, *Antimicrob. Ag. Chemother.*, 1981, *19*, 672. See also S. M. Hammer *et al.*, *ibid.*, 1982, *21*, 634.

An additive effect with acyclovir and vidarabine against herpes simplex viruses in Vero cells and in *mice*.— R. F. Schinazi *et al.*, *Antimicrob. Ag. Chemother.*, 1982, *22*, 499.

Acyclovir alteration of lymphocyte transformation response to herpes simplex virus infection.— W. E. Lafferty *et al.*, *Antimicrob. Ag. Chemother.*, 1984, *26*, 887.

Latent infection. Acyclovir inhibited herpes simplex virus reactivation in an *in vitro* model using human trigeminal ganglia. It did not eradicate latent virus; when acyclovir was withdrawn herpes simplex virus was obtained from 3 of 18 cultures.— M. E. Lewis *et al.*, *Antimicrob. Ag. Chemother.*, 1983, *23*, 487.

Acyclovir does not affect latent infections but could affect the latent virus during early stages of reactivation. Intermittent exposure *in vitro* of latently infected ganglia to acyclovir reduced the proportion of ganglia containing reactivatable herpes simplex virus.— R. J. Klein *et al.*, *Antimicrob. Ag. Chemother.*, 1983, *24*, 129. There was no evidence in *rabbits* that acyclovir or bromovinyldeoxyuridine given by mouth prevented the recurrence of viral shedding or clinical corneal disease in experimental herpes simplex keratitis. Resistant viruses were not found in tears.— H. E. Kaufman *et al.*, *Antimicrob. Ag. Chemother.*, 1983, *24*, 888.

The development of acyclovir-resistant strains of herpes simplex virus type 1.— J. Christophers and R. N. P. Sutton, *J. antimicrob. Chemother.*, 1987, *20*, 389.

VARICELLA ZOSTER VIRUS. Acyclovir and interferon alfa showed synergistic activity *in vitro* against varicella zoster virus. An additive to synergistic activity was also observed between interferon alfa and bromovinyldeoxyuridine, vidarabine, or foscarnet.— M. Baba *et al.*, *Antimicrob. Ag. Chemother.*, 1984, *25*, 515.

Resistance

Herpes simplex virus develops resistance to acyclovir *in vitro* and *in vivo* due to the selection of mutants deficient in thymidine kinase. Other mechanisms of resistance include altered specificity of thymidine kinase and reduced sensitivity of viral DNA polymerase.

Resistance has not yet emerged as a problem in treating herpes simplex infections partly because of the low incidence of resistant mutants *in vivo* and because viruses deficient in thymidine kinase appear to be of altered if not low virulence. Patients with a suppressed immune response appear to be most susceptible to developing resistance.

Cross-resistance occurs with other antiviral agents that require activation by thymidine kinase. Resistance to bromovinyldeoxyuridine and idoxuridine may develop because of the deficiency in thymidine kinase or in the case of bromovinyldeoxyuridine because of altered thymidine kinase specificity. Mutants with altered DNA polymerase may show cross-resistance to bromovinyldeoxyuridine, fosfonet, and vidarabine.

Resistance has also been reported with varicella zoster virus.

A review of resistance to acyclovir in herpes simplex virus. Thymidine-kinase-defective strains occur frequently but have reduced pathogenicity *in vivo*, although this may not be so when the immune system is impaired. Defective strains cannot readily be reactivated from latent infections, but mixtures of defective strains and normal or sensitive strains will establish latent infections and on reactivation yield further resistant viruses. Resistance may be mediated through routes other than the recognised modification of thymidine kinase or DNA polymerase; the thymidine-kinase-defective phenotype probably disguises a heterogeneous series of mutants.— H. J. Field, *J. antimicrob. Chemother.*, 1983, *12, Suppl. B*, 129. See also C. Crumpacker, *Drugs*, 1983, *26*, 373; H. H. Balfour, *Ann. intern. Med.*, 1983, *98*, 404.

Acyclovir-resistant mutants of herpes simplex virus in 2 bone-marrow transplant patients. The mutants were deficient in thymidine kinase.— W. H. Burns *et al.*, *Lancet*, 1982, *1*, 421.

Development of clinical resistance to suboptimal doses of acyclovir in *mice* infected with herpes simplex virus.— H. J. Field, *Antimicrob. Ag. Chemother.*, 1982, *21*, 744 (for correction to figures see *ibid.*, *22*, 719).

Herpes simplex virus type 1 resistance to acyclovir developed in one patient during the third course of treatment with acyclovir. Resistance had also developed to bromovinyldeoxyuridine but not to vidarabine or to fosfonet.— C. S. Crumpacker *et al.*, *New Engl. J. Med.*, 1982, *306*, 343. Various explanations for the mechanism of resistance.— D. M. Coen (letter), *ibid.*, *307*, 681. It has been reported that acyclovir-resistant mutants are latency-negative and protect against reinfection. Thus it is possible that the spread of resistant mutants in susceptible persons would lead only to a mild infection and might induce a refractory state against infections with wild, virulent virus populations. Also, strains of herpes simplex virus resistant to acyclovir are sensitive to other antiviral agents.— R. J. Klein (letter), *ibid.* See also D. W. Barry (letter), *ibid.*, 1209. In reply it was accepted that resistance could have been due to an altered DNA polymerase that remained sensitive to fosfonet and vidarabine. However, the large majority of viruses in the resistant isolate exhibited little viral thymidine kinase activity.— C. Crumpacker *et al.* (letter), *ibid.*, 682.

Resistance patterns in isolates of herpes simplex virus from 301 patients, 149 of whom had received acyclovir. Initial sensitivity varied widely but most of the isolates were sensitive to 1 to 2 μg per mL. Acyclovir did not significantly affect sensitivity with the exception of severely immunocompromised patients.— C. Dekker *et al.*, *J. antimicrob. Chemother.*, 1983, *12, Suppl. B.*, 137.

Pathogenic acyclovir-resistant viruses that are thymidine-kinase-deficient mutants have been observed and it is probable that pathogenic DNA polymerase mutants will emerge. It is proposed that resistance will occur predominantly among patients being treated for active disease rather than in those being treated prophylactically since the likelihood of mutation to resistance is proportional to the number of replicating virions. Experience in the authors' hospital supports this hypothesis which could be tested in a multicentre study.— R. F. Ambinder *et al.*, *Lancet*, 1984, *1*, 1154. Criticism. Resistance patterns could change when exposing an increased population to prophylaxis. Selectivity for the infected cell is not absolute and there may be risks from resistant mutants.— J. H. Abeles (letter), *ibid.*, *2*, 95.

Further references to acyclovir resistance: S. M. Hammer *et al.*, *Antimicrob. Ag. Chemother.*, 1982, *21*, 634 (herpes simplex virus); K. K. Biron *et al.*, *Am. J. Med.*, 1982, *73, Suppl. 1A*, 383 (varicella zoster virus); D. S. Parris and J. E. Harrington, *Antimicrob. Ag. Chemother.*, 1982, *22*, 71 (herpes simplex virus).

Absorption and Fate

The intravenous infusion of acyclovir as the sodium salt produces plasma-acyclovir concentrations that demonstrate a biphasic pattern. The infusion of a dose equivalent to 5 mg of acyclovir per kg body-weight has produced steady-state plasma concentrations with a peak of 9.8 μg per mL and a trough of 0.7 μg per mL.

Acyclovir is excreted through the kidney by both glomerular filtration and tubular secretion. The terminal or beta-phase half-life is reported to be about 2.5 to 2.9 hours for adults without renal impairment and 18 hours, reduced to 5.7 hours during haemodialysis, for those with chronic renal failure. Most of a dose by intravenous infusion is excreted unchanged with only up to 14% appearing in the urine as the inactive metabolite 9-carboxymethoxymethylguanine. Faecal excretion may account for about 2% of a dose. There is wide distribution to various tissues, including the cerebrospinal fluid where concentrations achieved are about 50% of those achieved in plasma. Protein binding is reported to range from 9 to 33%.

Up to 20% of a dose of acyclovir given by mouth is considered to be absorbed from the gastro-intestinal tract. Administration of a prodrug, desciclovir, is being investigated to overcome this poor absorption. Absorption of acyclovir is usually slight following topical application although it may be increased by changes in formulation.

A detailed review of the pharmacokinetics of acyclovir given intravenously and by mouth.— P. de Miranda and M. R. Blum, *J. antimicrob. Chemother.*, 1983, *12, Suppl. B.*, 29. See also O. L. Laskin, *Clin. Pharmacokinet.*, 1983, *8*, 187.

The pharmacokinetics of acyclovir given intravenously as the sodium salt in single doses of 2.5, 5, 10, and 15 mg per kg body-weight as an infusion over 1 hour to 13 patients with various malignant disorders. The declining plasma concentration was considered to be well described by a two-compartment open model. At the end of the infusion the mean plasma-acyclovir concentrations were 4.52, 8.28, 14.6, and 22.7 μg per mL respectively. The mean terminal (beta) half-lives were 2.9, 2.8, 3.3, and 2.4 hours respectively. Total clearance was 239, 268, 321, and 394 mL per minute and the volumes of distribution at steady state were 44.1, 43.1, 55.9, and 53.4 litres per 1.73 m^2 body-surface respectively. Renal clearance amounted to 77.4% of total clearance and was about three times greater than the estimated creatinine clearance; 70.2% of total acyclovir was excreted in the urine over 72 hours. It was considered that elimination involved both tubular secretion and glomerular filtration. Local reactions due to extravasation occurred in 2 patients.— O. L. Laskin *et al.*, *Antimicrob. Ag. Chemother.*, 1982, *21*, 393.

Probenecid 1 g given one hour before infusion of acyclovir enhanced the plasma concentrations of acyclovir in 3 patients given 5 mg per kg body-weight by intravenous infusion over one hour. Probenecid increased the mean terminal plasma half-life by 18% from 2.3 to 2.7 hours and the area under the plasma concentration-time curve by 40%. The mean 25-hour urinary excretion declined by 12.4% from 79.0 to 69.2% of the dose. Total body clearance declined by 29% from 300 to 213 mL/min per 1.73 m^2 body-surface; renal clearance declined by 32% but was still about two-fold greater than the estimated creatinine clearance. It was considered that the clinical significance of probenecid's inhibitory effect was probably limited.— O. L. Laskin *et al.*, *Antimicrob. Ag. Chemother.*, 1982, *21*, 804.

Good intra-ocular penetration was achieved after the administration of acyclovir by mouth to 16 patients undergoing cataract extraction. Patients received 5 doses of acyclovir 400 mg in the 24 hours before surgery and a mean concentration of acyclovir 3.26 μmol per litre (0.73 μg per mL) was found in aqueous humour removed during surgery. The mean concentration in plasma obtained at the same time was 8.74 μmol per litre (1.97 μg per mL). There was a significant correlation between plasma and aqueous humour concentrations.— S. O. Hung *et al.*, *Br. J. Ophthal.*, 1984, *68*, 192.

Further references to the pharmacokinetics of acyclovir: P. de Miranda *et al.*, *Clin. Pharmac. Ther.*, 1979, *26*, 718; P. J. Selby *et al.*, *Lancet*, 1979, *2*, 1267; P. de Miranda *et al.*, *Clin. Pharmac. Ther.*, 1981, *30*, 662; S. A. Spector *et al.*, *Antimicrob. Ag. Chemother.*, 1981, *19*, 608; W. M. Sullender *et al.*, *ibid.*, 1987, *31*, 1722.

PREGNANCY AND THE NEONATE. Acyclovir has been reported to cross the placenta (B.S. Greffe *et al.*, *J. Pediat.*, 1986, *108*, 1020). The manufacturers have also reported that acyclovir has been detected in breast milk.

Uses and Administration

Acyclovir is used for the treatment of viral infections due to herpes simplex virus (types 1 and 2) and varicella zoster virus (herpes zoster and chickenpox).

Herpes simplex infections including herpes keratitis, herpes labialis, and genital herpes respond to acyclovir given by intravenous, oral, or topical routes as soon as possible after symptoms appear. Both initial and recurrent infections can be successfully treated. Prolonged treatment can reduce the incidence of recurrence which is important in immunocompromised patients. However, when prolonged treatment is withdrawn infections may recur.

Acyclovir also improves the healing of herpes zoster lesions when given intravenously or by mouth, although studies indicate that it has little effect on pain.

Acyclovir is administered by intravenous infusion as the sodium salt over a period of 1 hour. Solutions for infusion are usually prepared to give a concentration of 25 mg of acyclovir per mL; this may then be further diluted. The dose by this route is 5 mg per kg body-weight administered every 8 hours and recommended periods of treatment range from 5 to 7 days. A higher dose of 10 mg per kg every 8 hours may be required in varicella zoster infections in patients whose immune response is impaired.

The usual dose by mouth in herpes simplex is 200 mg of acyclovir five times daily every 4 hours for 5 days; prolonged treatment may consist of 200 or 400 mg four times daily every 6 hours. An ointment or cream containing acyclovir 5% may be applied 5 or 6 times daily every 3 or 4 hours for periods of 5 to 10 days. In herpes simplex keratitis a 3% eye ointment may be applied 5 times daily every 4 hours until 3 days after healing.

Doses should be reduced in renal failure. This may be done by increasing the interval between infusions to 12 hours when the creatinine clearance is between 25 and 50 mL per minute or to 24 hours for 10 to 25 mL per minute. When the creatinine clearance is less than 10 mL per minute, 2.5 mg per kg may be given every 24 hours. Patients on haemodialysis require a dose after each dialysis. The oral dose should be reduced to 200 mg every 12 hours for patients with a creatinine clearance of less than 10 mL per minute.

Dosage reduction might be required in elderly patients. In children the intravenous dose is best calculated by body-surface using 250 mg per m^2 as an equivalent of 5 mg per kg and 500 mg per m^2 for 10 mg per kg.

Reviews on the actions and uses of acyclovir: D. M. Richards *et al.*, *Drugs*, 1983, *26*, 378; A. W. Hopefl, *Drug Intell. & clin. Pharm.*, 1983, *17*, 623; *Can. med. Ass. J.*, 1984, *131*, 1045; *Drug & Ther. Bull.*, 1984, *22*, 85; D. J. Jeffries, *Br. med. J.*, 1985, *290*, 177; C. Fletcher and B. Bean, *Drug Intell. & clin. Pharm.*, 1985, *19*, 518; D. J. Jeffries, *Br. med. J.*, 1986, *293*, 1523.

The recommended treatment for infections with monkey B virus (*Herpesvirus simiae*) is acyclovir 10 mg per kg body-weight given by intravenous infusion over one hour every 8 hours for 14 days. Treatment should be started if a monkey that has caused an injury however trivial develops any signs of infection or if the injured person shows any signs or symptoms.— C. C. Baker *et al.* (letter), *Br. med. J.*, 1982, *285*, 1350.

AIDS. Improvement in generalised lymphadenopathy in one patient given acyclovir. It was suggested that acyclovir may block the progression to the acquired immune deficiency syndrome (AIDS).— L. Resnick *et al.* (letter), *Lancet*, 1984, *1*, 798. In 2 patients given acyclovir there was, over a prolonged period, no change in persistent lymphadenopathy despite short-term improvement.— J. Weber and D. Jeffries (letter), *ibid.*, 1236. Spontaneous regression of lymphadenopathy.— J. Goudsmit (letter), *ibid.*

APLASTIC ANAEMIA. A beneficial response to acyclovir 15 mg per kg body-weight daily for 10 days given intravenously to one patient with refractory aplastic anaemia. A similar case had previously been reported. Treatment was based on the possible viral aetiology of severe aplastic anaemia.— A. Bacigalupo *et al.* (letter), *New Engl. J. Med.*, 1984, *310*, 1606. See also D. Gomez-Almaguer *et al.* (letter), *ibid.*, 1986, *314*, 584.

BEHÇET'S SYNDROME. Individual reports of acyclovir producing a beneficial response in Behçet's syndrome: L. Resegotti and M. Pistone (letter), *Ann. intern. Med.*, 1984, *100*, 319; J. Prieto *et al.* (letter), *ibid.*, *101*, 565. A disappointing response.— T. Sözen and B. Ateş (letter), *ibid.*, 406.

CHICKENPOX. Acyclovir 500 mg per m^2 body-surface given intravenously every 8 hours for 7 days was compared with placebo in 20 immunocompromised children with chickenpox recruited from 9 centres. Acyclovir produced no significant increase in healing or reduction in the period of virus shedding. However, fewer children in the acyclovir group developed pneumonitis.— C. G. Prober *et al.*, *J. Pediat.*, 1982, *101*, 622.

Reduction in the duration of vesicles and of fever in adults with chickenpox treated with acyclovir 10 mg per kg body-weight infused every 8 hours for 5 days in a double-blind study involving 34 adults in the treatment group and 34 in the placebo group. Pain and itching were not affected. Virus particles in the vesicles were reduced on day 1 in the treatment group but not on day 2.— W. Al-Nakib *et al.*, *J. Infect.*, 1983, *6*, *Suppl. 1*, 49.

Further references: J. W. M. van der Meer *et al.* (letter), *Lancet*, 1980, *2*, 473 (favourable report on the treatment of 1 patient with very severe chickenpox); M. H. van Weel-Sipman *et al.* (letter), *ibid.*, 1981, *1*, 147 (recurrent atypical varicella in 2 leukaemic children previously treated with acyclovir for early chickenpox); H. H. Balfour, *J. Pediat.*, 1984, *104*, 134 (rapid resolution in 4 children with chickenpox given early treatment but no benefit in 4 treated at least 5 days after onset of rash).

Pregnancy and the neonate. Acyclovir has been given, usually in conjunction with immunoglobulin therapy, to neonates with congenital varicella infection (B. Bose *et al.*, *Lancet*, 1986, *1*, 449; J. Haddad *et al.*, *ibid.*, 1494; P.E. Carter *et al.*, *ibid.*, *2*, 1460; J.A. Sills *et al.*, *ibid.*, 1987, *1*, 161). Holland has recommended a dose of 10 mg per kg body-weight intravenously every 8 hours (*Lancet*, 1986, *2*, 1156). However doses, where mentioned in the above reports, were usually 15 mg per kg every 8 hours. Haddad *et al.* (*Lancet*, 1987, *1*, 161) have also recommended prophylactic acyclovir before delivery where there is high risk to the neonate.

CREUTZFELDT-JAKOB DISEASE. Individual reports of acyclovir failing to produce a response in Creutzfeldt-Jakob disease: A. S. David *et al.* (letter), *Lancet*, 1984, *1*, 512; P. K. Newman (letter), *ibid.*, 793.

CYTOMEGALOVIRUS INFECTIONS. Acyclovir 500 mg per m^2 body-surface given intravenously three times a day for 7 days to 9 immunocompromised patients with cytomegalovirus disease produced a faster rate of improvement and defervescence than placebo given to 7 similar patients (H.H. Balfour *et al.*, *Am. J. Med.*, 1982, *73*, *Suppl. 1A*, 241). A beneficial result was also obtained with acyclovir in a cardiac transplant patient with cytomegalovirus pneumonia (M.H. Ashraf *et al.* (letter), *Lancet*, 1982, *1*, 173). Other reports have failed to show a beneficial response. In one study 7 of 8 transplant patients with cytomegalovirus pneumonia died despite acyclovir treatment with doses of up to 1.2 g per m^2 daily infused intravenously over 2 hours (J.C. Wade *et al.*, *Am. J. Med.*, 1982, *73*, *Suppl. 1A*, 249). In another study 4 infants with congenital cytomegalovirus infections failed to show improvement with acyclovir (S.A. Plotkin *et al.*, *Am. J. Med.*, 1982, *73*, *Suppl. 1A*, 257).

When acyclovir was given for the prophylaxis of infections with herpes simplex viruses, Saral *et al.* (*New Engl. J. Med.*, 1981, *305*, 63) found that during treatment cytomegalovirus was cultured from 1 of 10 bone-marrow transplant patients receiving acyclovir compared with none of 10 receiving placebo; after cessation of treatment the virus was cultured from 4 and 2 patients respectively. Acyclovir was started 3 days before transplantation and continued for a total of 18 days, a dose of 250 mg per m^2 being given by intravenous infusion every 8 hours. In contrast, in another controlled study involving 39 transplant patients, acyclovir was considered to provide protection against cytomegalovirus infection (E. Gluckman *et al.*, *Lancet*, 1983, *2*, 706). In this study acyclovir was given by mouth to 20 of the patients in a dose of 200 mg every 6 hours for a period starting 8 days before to 35 days after marrow transplantation; 19 patients received a placebo. No patient given acyclovir developed cytomegalovirus infection during treatment but 7 given placebo did. After treatment 7 of the acyclovir group and 11 of the placebo group had developed cytomegalovirus infections; none in the acyclovir group had pneumonitis, but 3 of the 11 placebo-group patients died of cytomegalovirus interstitial pneumonitis. The results of Gluckman *et al.* could not be reproduced in another study (P. Selby *et al.* (letter), *Br. med. J.*, 1984, *289*, 253) that used larger doses in marrow transplant patients so leaving uncertainty as to the value of acyclovir in the prophylaxis of cytomegalovirus infections.

DOSAGE IN RENAL FAILURE. The pharmacokinetics of acyclovir in 6 patients with end-stage renal disease showed markedly reduced elimination of a dose of 2.5 mg per kg body-weight given by intravenous infusion over one hour. Haemodialysis carried out 48 hours after the start of infusion removed 60% of the drug.— O. L. Laskin *et al.*, *Clin. Pharmac. Ther.*, 1982, *31*, 594.

Acyclovir could be administered to patients with renal failure by adjusting the dosage interval. A dosage interval of 8 hours is suitable for patients whose glomerular filtration-rates exceed 50 mL per minute; an interval of 24 hours between doses is advisable for rates of between 10 and 50 mL per minute. Where the rate is less than 10 mL per minute the dosage interval should be 48 hours. A dose supplement should be given to patients undergoing haemodialysis.— W. M. Bennett *et al.*, *Am. J. Kidney Dis.*, 1983, *3*, 155.

Individual dosing of acyclovir based on measured plasma concentrations might be required in patients with a creatinine clearance of 25 mL or less per minute for a body-surface area of 1.73 m^2.— D. M. Brundage *et al.*, *Drug Intell. & clin. Pharm.*, 1984, *18*, 501.

For reversible psychiatric effects in patients with chronic renal failure given acyclovir, see under Precautions, p.689.

EPSTEIN-BARR INFECTIONS. Acyclovir produced a response on 2 occasions in a transplant patient with a lymphoproliferative disease associated with Epstein-Barr virus. No response was obtained when the condition occurred for a third time when the lymphoproliferation appeared to have changed from polyclonal to monoclonal B-cell proliferation.— D. W. Hanto *et al.*, *New Engl. J. Med.*, 1982, *306*, 913. Successful treatment in 2 patients with polyclonal lymphoproliferation. When the lymphoproliferation becomes monoclonal, conventional cancer chemotherapy with or without radiotherapy is indicated.— *idem* (letter), *307*, 896. See also J. L. Sullivan *et al.*, *ibid.*, 1984, *311*, 1163.

A beneficial response with acyclovir in infectious mononucleosis.— J. Andersson *et al.*, *J. infect. Dis.*, 1986, *153*, 283.

HEPATITIS. Poor results in treating 3 patients with chronic hepatitis B with acyclovir.— C. I. Smith *et al.*, *Am. J. Med.*, 1982, *73*, *Suppl. 1A*, 267.

Antiviral activity against hepatitis B virus in 2 patients given acyclovir 10 and 15 mg per kg body-weight respectively by intravenous infusion every 8 hours for 5 to 7 days. No response was seen with doses of 5 or 7.5 mg per kg.— I. V. D. Weller *et al.* (letter), *Lancet*, 1982, *1*, 273.

Enhanced antiviral activity in patients with chronic hepatitis B given acyclovir in association with interferon alfa, when compared with either drug alone.— S. W. Schalm *et al.*, *Lancet*, 1985, *2*, 358.

Further references: G. J. M. Alexander *et al.*, *Gut*, 1984, *25*, A1134 (partial inhibition of viral replication).

HERPES SIMPLEX. Acyclovir given by mouth or injection has been shown to be effective in the treatment of patients with mucocutaneous herpes simplex including those who are immunosuppressed (C.D. Mitchell *et al.*, *Lancet*, 1981, *1*, 1389; S. Chou *et al.*, *ibid.*, 1392; J.C. Wade *et al.*, *Ann. intern. Med.*, 1982, *96*, 265; S.E. Straus *et al.*, *ibid.*, 270; D.H. Shepp *et al.*, *ibid.*, 1985, *102*, 783). Topical treatment of infections with herpes simplex virus, with the exception of keratitis, has produced conflicting results which may in part be due to poor penetration of acyclovir. Spruance *et al.* (*Antimicrob. Ag. Chemother.*, 1984, *25*, 553) found in a study involving 352 patients that an ointment of acyclovir 10% in a macrogol basis was ineffective in the treatment of herpes labialis whereas Whitley *et al.* (*J. infect. Dis.*, 1984, *150*, 323) found a similar 5% ointment to be of benefit. Van Vloten *et al.*, (*J. antimicrob. Chemother.*, 1983, *12*, *Suppl. B.*, 89) found that a cream of acyclovir 5% in propylene glycol produced a beneficial effect in a study involving 30 patients; Fiddian *et al.* (*Br. med. J.*, 1983, *286*, 1699) also showed some response with such a cream. However, Shaw *et al.* (*Br. med. J.*, 1985, *291*, 7) could not demonstrate any advantage of acyclovir over propylene glycol in 45 patients with recurrent herpes labialis.

A short review of acyclovir prophylaxis for herpes simplex virus infection.— D. Gold and L. Corey, *Antimicrob. Ag. Chemother.*, 1987, *31*, 361.

Encephalitis. Acyclovir 10 mg per kg body-weight infused intravenously over 1 hour every 8 hours was compared with vidarabine 15 mg per kg infused intravenously over 12 hours each day in 127 patients with suspected herpes simplex encephalitis in a multicentre study. Infection was confirmed in 53 patients who received treatment for 10 days; analysis was possible in 51 patients, 27 on acyclovir and 24 on vidarabine. There were 5 deaths in the acyclovir group and 12 in the vidarabine group. Follow-up was until death or for 6 months or more. After acyclovir therapy, 15 of the 22 survivors returned to normal compared with 3 of the 12 vidarabine survivors.— B. Sköldenberg *et al.*, *Lancet*, 1984, *2*, 707. In an interim summary of progress in the studies being carried out by the *US* National Institute of Allergy and Infectious Diseases it was considered that there was no evidence pointing to acyclovir being superior to vidarabine in neonatal herpes simplex virus infection or herpes simplex encephalitis (R.J. Whitley *et al.*, *J. antimicrob. Chemother.*, 1983, *12*, *Suppl. B*, 105). Also Whitley *et al.* criticised Sköldenberg *et al.*'s, study, mainly on the diagnosis of herpes simplex encephalitis. However, Whitley *et al.*, in a more recent study (*New Engl. J. Med.*, 1986, *314*, 144) have produced results similar to those of Sköldenberg *et al.* and they consider acyclovir to be the treatment of choice for biopsy-proved herpes simplex encephalitis in non-neonates.

Herpes genitalis. Reviews of genital herpes simplex virus infections and treatment including acyclovir: A. Mindel and S. Sutherland, *J. antimicrob. Chemother.*, 1983, *12*, *Suppl. B*, 51; L. Corey and K. K. Holmes, *Ann. intern. Med.*, 1983, *98*, 973.

Reviews on the use of acyclovir in the management of initial and recurrent episodes of herpes simplex genital infection: Y. J. Bryson, *J. antimicrob. Chemother.*, 1983, *12*, *Suppl. B*, 61 (oral route); A. Mindel, *J. antimicrob. Chemother.*, 1984, *14*, *Suppl. A*, 75 (oral, intravenous, and topical routes); *Med. Lett.*, 1985, *27*, 41 (oral route); M. E. Guinan, *J. Am. med. Ass.*, 1986, *255*, 1747 (oral route); S. L. Sacks, *Can. med. Ass. J.*, 1987, *136*, 701 (oral route).

Acyclovir has been shown to be effective in the treatment of primary episodes of herpes genitalis. Mindel *et al.* (*Lancet*, 1982, *1*, 697 and 976) showed that acyclovir given intravenously in doses of 5 mg per kg body-weight every 8 hours for 15 doses in a study involving 30 patients reduced viral shedding time and the healing time of some lesions as well as the duration of vesicles, new lesion formation, and symptoms. Corey *et al.* (*Ann. intern. Med.*, 1983, *98*, 914) obtained similar results with the same intravenous regimen.

Treatment by mouth with a dose of 200 mg five times daily for 5 days (A.E. Nilsen *et al.*, *Lancet*, 1982, *2*, 571 and 834) or 10 days (Y.J. Bryson *et al.*, *New Engl. J. Med.*, 1983, *308*, 916) produced results similar to those achieved with the intravenous route. Corey *et al.* (*J. antimicrob. Chemother.*, 1983, *12*, *Suppl. B*, 79) also found oral therapy with acyclovir to be effective in treating primary first-episode infections except that unlike intravenous therapy it did not reduce the duration of vaginal discharge. In a subsequent study (G.J. Mertz *et al.*, *J. Am. med. Ass.*, 1984, *252*, 1147) there was a beneficial response to oral therapy in primary first-episode genital herpes but in nonprimary first-episode infection the duration of lesions and the symptoms were not affected although the duration of viral shedding was reduced. Mindel *et al.* (*Lancet*, 1987, *1*, 1171) have also shown that acyclovir 200 mg four times daily for 7 days produced a more rapid response than inosine pranobex 1 g four times daily for 7 days.

Topical therapy with acyclovir as a 5% cream in propylene glycol has also proved effective in initial infection (A.P. Fiddian *et al.*, *J. antimicrob. Chemother.*, 1983, *12*, *Suppl. B.*, 67). In another study the effects of topical acyclovir were less marked than with systemic acyclovir therapy and there was no effect on vaginal discharge (L. Corey *et al.*, *J. antimicrob. Chemother.*, 1983, *12*, *Suppl. B*, 79), although in this study acyclovir was applied in a polyethylene glycol basis (see p.691).

Acyclovir has also been assessed in the treatment of recurrent episodes of genital herpes. A dose of 200 mg five times daily for 5 days given by mouth reduced viral shedding and healing time (A.E. Nilsen *et al.*, *Lancet*, 1982, *2*, 571 and 834). However, the reduction in new lesion formation was less marked than in the treatment of initial episodes. Another multicentre study (R.C. Reichman *et al.*, *J. Am. med. Ass.*, 1984, *251*, 2103) employing the same dose showed that acyclovir reduced viral shedding and healing time. Also starting self-treatment as soon as symptoms appeared proved more effective than treatment which started within 48 hours of symptoms emerging. Topical treatment has also been found effective in recurrent episodes (A.P. Fiddian *et al.*, *J. antimicrob. Chemother.*, 1983, *12*, *Suppl. B*, 67). However, in another multicentre study (J.P. Luby *et al.*, *J. infect. Dis.*, 1984, *150*, 1) topical treatment with acyclovir 5% in a macrogol basis provided no beneficial effect on recurrent infection or its prevention, apart from a reduction in the duration of virus excretion.

The recurrence rate of genital herpes was not affected by acyclovir given systemically or topically for a treatment period of 5 to 10 days (L. Corey *et al.*, *J. antimicrob. Chemother.*, 1983, *12*, *Suppl. B*, 79) and this was confirmed in subsequent studies when acyclovir was given by mouth for 10 days (G.J. Mertz *et al.*, *J. Am. med. Ass.*, 1984, *252*, 1147) or for 7 days (A. Mindel *et al*, *Lancet*, 1987, *1*, 1171). However, treatment for periods of 84 to 125 days reduced the number of recurrent infections during the period of treatment; when treatment was stopped all patients had recurrences (S.E. Straus *et al.*, *New Engl. J. Med.*, 1984, *310*, 1545; J.M. Douglas *et al.*, *ibid.*, 1551; A. Mindel *et al.*, *Lancet*, 1984, *2*, 57, R.N. Thin *et al.*, *J. antimicrob. Chemother.*, 1985, *16*, 219). Doses ranged from 200 mg twice daily to 200 mg five times daily; in one study the initial dose was 200 mg five times daily for the first 5 days thereafter reduced to 200 mg three times daily.

Keratitis. Reviews of acyclovir in the treatment of herpes simplex virus infections of the eye: M. G. Falcon, *J. antimicrob. Chemother.*, 1983, *12*, *Suppl.* B, 39; *idem*, *Br. J. Ophthal.*, 1987, *71*, 102.

In a double-blind study 12 patients with dendritic corneal ulcers were treated by minimal wiping debridement followed by application of 3% acyclovir eye ointment 5 times daily for 7 days; 12 similar patients received debridement followed by application of a placebo ointment. Within 7 days of debridement there were 7 recurrences in the placebo group and none in the acyclovir group. Brisk healing rates occurred in a further 4 patients with dendritic ulcers treated with 3% acyclovir ointment alone. No side-effects associated with acyclovir topical therapy were noted in any of the 16 patients treated.— B. R. Jones *et al.* (preliminary communication), *Lancet*, 1979, *1*, 243.

There was no difference in response to topical treatment with ophthalmic ointments containing acyclovir 3% or vidarabine 3% in a double-blind study involving 68 patients with dendritic keratitis. Treatment consisted of 5 applications daily for 14 days and good results with re-epithelialisation within 14 days occurred in 31 of 32 patients given acyclovir and 33 of 36 given vidarabine.— P. R. Laibson *et al.*, *Am. J. Med.*, 1982, *73*, *Suppl. 1A*, 281. Similar results.— J. McGill and P. Tormey, *ibid.*, 286. Acyclovir 3% applied as an eye ointment produced faster healing of herpetic corneal ulceration than vidarabine 3% in a study of 93 patients. Healing occurred in 45 of 48 given acyclovir and 37 of 45 given vidarabine.— B. J. Young *et al.*, *Br. J. Ophthal.*, 1982, *66*, 361.

Similar responses with acyclovir and trifluridine in a study of 59 patients with dendritic keratitis.— C. La Lau *et al.*, *Br. J. Ophthal.*, 1982, *66*, 506.

In a double-blind study treatment of disciform keratitis with acyclovir eye ointment 3% plus betamethasone eye-drops 0.01% was compared with acyclovir plus placebo. Healing occurred in all of 21 patients who received acyclovir and corticosteroid in a median time of 21 days; 11 of the 19 treated with acyclovir and placebo were withdrawn from the study because their condition remained static or worsened.— L. M. T. Collum *et al.*, *Br. J. Ophthal.*, 1983, *67*, 115.

Acyclovir 400 mg or placebo was given by mouth five times daily to patients with superficial dendritic herpetic corneal ulcers after a minimal wiping debridement of the ulcer. After 7 days 67% of ulcers had healed in 15 patients given acyclovir compared with 43% in 14 patients given placebo. This was a non-significant difference, but the rate of healing was significantly faster in the acyclovir-treated group.— S. O. Hung *et al.*, *Br. J. Ophthal.*, 1984, *68*, 398.

Effective treatment with acyclovir or vidarabine ointments in herpes simplex geographic corneal ulceration.— L. M. T. Collum *et al.*, *Br. J. Ophthal.*, 1985, *69*, 847.

Oral acyclovir produced a similar response to topical acyclovir in herpes simplex dendritic corneal ulceration.— L. M. T. Collum *et al.*, *Br. J. Ophthal.*, 1986, *70*, 435.

Pregnancy and the neonate. The effective use of acyclovir in the treatment of a pregnant patient with disseminated herpes simplex.— D. C. Lagrew *et al.*, *J. Am. med. Ass.*, 1984, *252*, 2058.

For neonatal herpes simplex, see Encephalitis, above.

Prophylaxis. None of 10 marrow transplant patients developed herpes simplex when receiving acyclovir 250 mg per m^2 body-surface every 8 hours for 18 days by intravenous infusion; 7 of 10 similar patients given placebo did develop herpes simplex. After acyclovir prophylaxis was stopped 7 patients showed evidence of infection. Two patients in the acyclovir group developed delirium.— R. Saral *et al.*, *New Engl. J. Med.*, 1981, *305*, 63.

In 20 patients undergoing allogenic bone-marrow transplantation, the incidence of oropharyngeal herpes simplex virus infection was reduced by acyclovir 5 mg per kg body-weight intravenously every 12 hours during the period of granulocytopenia — from 5 of 10 given placebo to none of 10 given acyclovir. In patients undergoing chemotherapy for the induction of remission of leukaemia the incidence of infection was similarly reduced. There was a high incidence of herpes infections in both groups after the study, but recurrences were often clinically mild.— I. M. Hann *et al.*, *Br. med. J.*, 1983, *287*, 384.

In a 32-week double-blind crossover study in 16 patients acyclovir 5% cream (propylene glycol basis) applied twice daily was no more effective than placebo in preventing the recurrence of herpes simplex infection or associated erythema multiforme.— H. A. Fawcett *et al.*, *Br. med. J.*, 1983, *287*, 798. Individual reports of herpetic erythema multiforme being prevented by acyclovir: C. T. C. Kennedy *et al.*, *ibid.*, 1981, *283*, 1360 (topical application); J. A. Green *et al.*, *Ann. intern. Med.*, 1985, *102*, 632 (oral route).

In a double-blind placebo-controlled study involving 39 patients, acyclovir 200 mg every 6 hours by mouth for 8 days before to 35 days after bone-marrow transplantation, gave complete protection against herpes simplex infections. After cessation of treatment the frequency of infection was the same in the placebo and the active groups. Although the incidence and severity of graft-versus-host disease was not significantly reduced by acyclovir this might be worth investigating in a larger study.— E. Gluckman *et al.*, *Lancet*, 1983, *2*, 706. In a similar study, 24 transplant patients received 400 mg of acyclovir five times daily by mouth starting 1 week before transplantation and continuing for a total of 35 days; 5 developed active herpes simplex during that period compared with 17 of 25 given placebo. Two of the five remained asymptomatic and as prophylaxis continued viral shedding ceased. Drug compliance was erratic because of oral mucosal damage and the 3 patients who developed herpes simplex lesions during prophylaxis with acyclovir had stopped taking the study drug at least 6 days before the occurrence of their first positive cultures. When prophylaxis was withdrawn another 9 patients in the acyclovir group developed infection after a median period of 8 weeks; another 2 patients in the placebo group developed infection. There was no prophylactic effect on other herpesvirus infections. Acyclovir prophylaxis significantly increased the rate of marrow engraftment in those patients receiving methotrexate but not those receiving cyclosporin. The occurrence of graft-versus-host disease was not affected by acyclovir.— J. C. Wade *et al.*, *Ann. intern. Med.*, 1984, *100*, 823.

Acyclovir given by mouth in a dose of 0.4 to 1 g daily for up to 180 days to 4 immunodeficient patients reduced the incidence of recurrence of herpes simplex. All 4 patients had previously responded to treatment for culture-proven herpes simplex with acyclovir, but consistently had new outbreaks within one month of completing treatment. During 23 suppressive treatment periods with acyclovir there were 6 episodes of herpes simplex. Infection always recurred when suppression was stopped.— S. E. Straus *et al.*, *Ann. intern. Med.*, 1984, *100*, 522.

Further references: H. G. Prentice, *J. antimicrob. Chemother.*, 1983, *12*, *Suppl. B*, 153; R. Saral *et al.*, *Ann. intern. Med.*, 1983, *99*, 773.

See also Herpes genitalis, above.

HERPES ZOSTER. Acyclovir 5 mg per kg body-weight intravenously every 8 hours for 5 days improved healing and also shortened the duration of pain in the acute phase in 20 patients with herpes zoster when compared with placebo given to 22 similar patients. At 1-month follow-up acyclovir had no effect on the persistence of pain.— N. A. Peterslund *et al.*, *Lancet*, 1981, *2*, 827. In a subsequent controlled study involving 40 elderly patients with severe herpes zoster, acyclovir 400 mg given by mouth five times daily for 5 days was as effective as 5 mg per kg given three times daily by intravenous infusion for 5 days. While the mean concentration of acyclovir in the vesicular fluid after oral dosage was approximately half that seen after intravenous administration it was still within the effective range for varicella zoster virus. The oral route should be preferred in uncomplicated herpes zoster.— *idem*, *J. antimicrob. Chemother.*, 1984, *14*, 185. A further study showing some benefit from this oral dose. A dose of 800 mg five times daily might produce a better response.— M. W. McKendrick *et al.*, *ibid.*, 661. A planned interim analysis of 41 patients showed that acyclovir 800 mg given by mouth five times daily for 7 days significantly reduced the duration of the vesicles, the time to crusting, and pain in the first week. Like the previous study, treatment was started within 72 hours of the onset of rash. The 800-mg dosage regimen was considerably more effective than that employing 400 mg. A 200-mg regimen as used by Finn and Smith (*Lancet*, 1984, *2*, 575) seemed unlikely to be ideal for herpes zoster.— *idem* (letter), *Lancet*, 1984, *2*, 925. The effectiveness of the 800-mg dose was confirmed in a placebo-controlled multicentre study of 205 patients. The benefit was most pronounced in patients who began treatment within 48 hours of the onset of rash.— *idem*, *Br. med. J.*, 1986, *293*, 1529.

Acyclovir reduced the duration of viral shedding, reduced pain during the treatment period, and accelerated healing of lesions in a controlled study involving 29 patients with acute herpes zoster. Acyclovir was given by intravenous infusion over 50 to 90 minutes to 19 of the patients within 72 hours of the rash appearing in a dose of 500 mg per m^2 body-surface three times daily for 5 days; 10 patients received placebo. However, pain recurred or worsened in 6 of the 17 patients who had shown improvement during treatment with acyclovir compared with 2 of 5 given placebo. Eleven of the patients given acyclovir developed raised serum concentrations of creatinine.— B. Bean *et al.*, *Lancet*, 1982, *2*, 118. See also *idem*, *J. antimicrob. Chemother.*, 1983, *12, Suppl. B*, 123.

A multicentre controlled study involving 94 immunocompromised patients with localised or disseminated cutaneous herpes zoster, demonstrated that acyclovir 500 mg per m^2 body-surface infused intravenously over 1 hour three times daily for 7 days halted progression of zoster. There was no difference in pain resolution between acyclovir and placebo.— H. H. Balfour *et al.*, *New Engl. J. Med.*, 1983, *308*, 1448. Responses to comments.— *idem* (letter), *309*, 1254; *idem* (letter), *310*, 988. See also H. H. Balfour *et al.*, *J. antimicrob. Chemother.*, 1983, *12, Suppl. B*, 169. Similar findings of improvement in healing but no significant resolution of pain with a dose of 5 mg per kg body-weight given intravenously every 8 hours for 5 days to 17 patients compared with 20 control patients.— J. McGill *et al.*, *J. Infect.*, 1983, *6*, 157. No significant effects on healing or acute pain with 10 mg per kg infused intravenously every 8 hours for 5 days in a double-blind study involving 40 patients.— B. E. Juel-Jensen *et al.*, *ibid.*, *Suppl. 1*, 31.

Acyclovir 500 mg per m^2 body-surface infused over 1 hour every 8 or 12 hours was more effective than vidarabine 10 mg per kg body-weight given daily as a 12-hour infusion in a study of 22 severely immunocompromised patients with varicella-zoster virus infection.— D. H. Shepp *et al.*, *New Engl. J. Med.*, 1986, *314*, 209.

Encephalitis. Case reports of herpes zoster encephalitis responding to treatment with acyclovir.— J. S. Cheesbrough *et al.*, *Postgrad. med. J.*, 1985, *61*, 145; D. V. Ehrensaft and M. M. Safani (letter), *Ann. intern. Med.*, 1985, *102*, 421; M. K. B. Whyte and P. W. Ind, *Br. med. J.*, 1986, *293*, 1536.

Keratitis. In a double-blind study acyclovir and betamethasone eye ointments applied 5 times daily were compared in the treatment of herpes zoster kerato-uveitis; treatment was continued until active ocular involvement ceased and was then tailed off over 4 to 6 weeks. In the acyclovir group healing occurred in 16 of 17 patients with a median treatment duration of 76 days. The median initial length of treatment for patients receiving betamethasone was 96.9 days but in 12 of 19 patients the kerato-uveitis recurred when treatment was tailed off or stopped; in these patients corticosteroids were restarted and thus the total median treatment time of 280 days for the whole of the corticosteroid group was significantly longer. Corneal lesions resolved significantly faster in acyclovir-treated eyes. The results supported the theory that if corticosteroids are to be used for the treatment of herpes zoster ophthalmicus low-dose maintenance therapy should be continued for a considerable time to prevent reactivation of the disease.— J. McGill and C. Chapman, *Br. J. Ophthal.*, 1983, *67*, 746.

MYCOSIS FUNGOIDES. Remission of mycosis fungoides in one patient given acyclovir.— L. Resnick *et al.*, *J. Am. med. Ass.*, 1984, *251*, 1571. There was no effect in 2 patients.— G. Mahrle *et al.* (letter), *ibid.*, 1985, *253*, 977. Preliminary results from a multicentre study point to benefit in some patients.— S. N. Horwitz and P. Frost (letter), *ibid.*

Proprietary Preparations

Zovirax *(Wellcome, UK)*. *Tablets*, acyclovir 200 mg and 400 mg.
Suspension, acyclovir 200 mg/5 mL.
Intravenous infusion, powder for reconstitution, acyclovir 250 mg (as sodium salt).
Cream, acyclovir 5% in an aqueous cream base.
Eye ointment, acyclovir 3%.

Zovirax tablets and suspension are free from azo dyes.— R. Smith, *Pharm. J.*, 1985, *1*, 15.

Proprietary Names and Manufacturers of Acyclovir and Acyclovir Sodium

Acyvir *(Isnardi, Ital.)*; Cusiviral *(Cusi, Spain)*; Cycloviran *(Sigmatau, Ital.)*; Maynar *(Novag, Spain)*; Milavir *(Frumtost, Spain)*; Sifiviral *(SIFI, Ital.)*; Viclovir *(Abello, Spain)*; Vipral *(Pharmainvesti, Spain)*; Virherpes *(Pensa, Spain)*; Virmen *(Menarini, Spain)*; Zovirax *(Wellcome, Austral.; Wellcome, Canad.; Wellcome, Denm.; Wellcome, Fr.; Wellcome, Ger.; Wellcome, Ital.; Wellcome, S.Afr.; Gayoso Wellcome, Spain; Wellcome, Swed.; Wellcome, Switz.; Wellcome, UK; Wellcome, USA)*.

12455-p

Bromovinyldeoxyuridine

BVDU. (*E*)-5-(2-Bromovinyl)-2′-deoxyuridine.
$C_{11}H_{13}BrN_2O_5$=333.1.

Bromovinyldeoxyuridine has antiviral activity and is effective *in vitro* against herpes simplex virus type 1 and varicella zoster virus; other viruses including herpes simplex virus type 2 have been reported to be sensitive, but only at relatively high concentrations. The activity appears to be due, at least in part, to selective phosphorylation of bromovinyldeoxyuridine by viral deoxythymidine kinase in preference to cellular kinases. There is the possibility of cross-resistance developing between bromovinyldeoxyuridine and acyclovir because of some similar features in their mode of action (see p.690). It has been tried in the treatment of herpes simplex and herpes zoster.

ANTIVIRAL ACTION. A review of the antiviral spectrum of bromovinyldeoxyuridine.— E. De Clercq, *J. antimicrob. Chemother.*, 1984, *14, Suppl. A*, 85.

Antiviral studies of bromovinyldeoxyuridine *in vitro*: E. De Clercq *et al.*, *Antimicrob. Ag. Chemother.*, 1982, *21*, 33 (varicella zoster virus); H. Machida *et al.*, *ibid.*, 358 (varicella zoster virus); J. -C. Lin *et al.*, *Science*, 1983, *221*, 578 (Epstein-Barr virus); S. R. Preblud *et al.*, *Antimicrob. Ag. Chemother.*, 1984, *25*, 417 (varicella zoster virus). See also under Acyclovir, Antiviral Action, p.690.

Antiviral studies of bromovinyldeoxyuridine in *animals*: P. C. Maudgal *et al.*, *Antimicrob. Ag. Chemother.*, 1980, *17*, 8 (herpes simplex type 1 in *rabbits*); E. De Clercq *et al.*, *ibid.*, 1982, *22*, 421 (herpes simplex virus in *mice*); E. De Clercq, *ibid.*, 1984, *26*, 155 (herpes simplex virus in *mice*); I. S. Sim, *J. antimicrob. Chemother.*, 1984, *14, Suppl. A*, 111 (genital herpes in *guinea pigs*).

EFFECTS ON BLOOD. Bromovinyldeoxyuridine demonstrated a variable suppressive effect on human cells grown *in vitro*. Granulocyte-monocyte colony-forming cells and peripheral-blood mononuclear cells were resistant to any suppressive effect except at very high concentrations of the drug; human fibroblasts were somewhat more sensitive. The results suggested that bromovinyldeoxyuridine compared favourably *in vitro* with currently used antiviral agents in terms of myelotoxicity and immunotoxicity.— A. E. Wittek *et al.*, *Antimicrob. Ag. Chemother.*, 1983, *24*, 803.

HERPES SIMPLEX. Beneficial results with bromovinyldeoxyuridine 0.1% eye-drops instilled 9 times daily, at hourly intervals during the day only, in herpes simplex keratitis. Patients who were clinically resistant to idoxuridine, trifluridine, or vidarabine responded promptly to topical bromovinyldeoxyuridine therapy. In patients with ophthalmic herpes zoster, bromovinyldeoxyuridine 375 mg daily by mouth in 3 divided doses in association with bromovinyldeoxyuridine 0.1% eye-drops led to prompt healing of skin lesions and kerato-uveitis.— P. C. Maudgal *et al.*, *Antiviral Res.*, 1984, *4*, 281.

HERPES ZOSTER. Beneficial results with bromovinyldeoxyuridine given by mouth to 4 patients with severe herpes zoster.— E. de Clercq *et al.*, *Br. med. J.*, 1980, *281*, 1178.

In a study of 20 immunocompromised patients with severe localised or disseminated herpes zoster, bromovinyldeoxyuridine in an oral dose of approximately 7.5 mg per kg body-weight daily in 3 or 4 divided doses for 5 days produced rapid clearance of infection in 19 patients; appearance of new lesions ceased within one day in 12 patients.— J. Wildiers and E. De Clercq, *Eur. J. Cancer clin. Oncol.*, 1984, *20*, 471.

16807-h

Desciclovir *(USAN, rINN)*.

BW-515U; BW-A515U; Deoxyacyclovir. 6-Deoxyacyclovir.
$C_8H_{11}N_5O_2$=209.2.
CAS — 84408-37-7.

Desciclovir is an acyclovir prodrug reported to provide higher plasma-acyclovir concentrations than acyclovir following oral administration.

References: P. Selby *et al.*, *Lancet*, 1984, *2*, 1428; P. D. Whiteman *et al.*, *Eur. J. clin. Pharmac.*, 1984, *27*, 471; *idem*, *Br. J. clin. Pharmac.*, 1985, *19*, 149P; B. G. Petty *et al*, *Antimicrob. Ag. Chemother.*, 1987, *31*, 1317.

Proprietary Names and Manufacturers
Wellcome, UK.

12706-e

Edoxudine *(USAN, rINN)*.

Ethyl Deoxyuridine; ORF-15817. 5-Ethyl-2′-deoxyuridine.
$C_{11}H_{16}N_2O_5$=256.3.
CAS — 15176-29-1.

Edoxudine has been used in herpes infections especially affecting the eye.

Edoxudine preferentially inhibited herpes simplex virus type 2 *in vitro* compared with type 1.— C. -Z. Teh and S. L. Sacks, *Antimicrob. Ag. Chemother.*, 1983, *23*, 637.

Edoxudine in an aqueous cream basis or in dimethyl sulphoxide was found to be comparable or superior to acyclovir ointment in the treatment of herpes simplex virus type 1 infection in *guinea-pigs*.— S. L. Spruance *et al.*, *Antimicrob. Ag. Chemother.*, 1985, *28*, 103.

Proprietary Names and Manufacturers
Aedurid *(Robugen, Ger.)*; Edurid *(Medipharm, Switz.)*.

12692-r

Enviroxime *(USAN, rINN)*.

LY-122772; Viroxime Component B. (*E*)-2-Amino-6-benzoyl-1-(isopropylsulphonyl)-1*H*-benzimidazole oxime.
$C_{17}H_{18}N_4O_3S$=358.4.
CAS — 72301-79-2.

Enviroxime has antiviral activity *in vitro* against a wide range of rhinoviruses. Clinical results have not been encouraging.

A mixture of enviroxime and its isomer zinviroxime known as viroxime has been investigated.

Preliminary findings indicated a beneficial effect with enviroxime administered intranasally and orally against rhinovirus infection. Enviroxime by mouth was poorly tolerated and therefore nasal administration should be studied further.— R. J. Phillpotts *et al.*, *Lancet*, 1981, *1*, 1342. Enviroxime administered to healthy subjects as a nasal spray before or after rhinovirus challenge neither prevented nor eliminated infection. Although statistically insignificant, some reduction of symptoms and diminished viral shedding were seen when enviroxime concentrations in nasal washings exceeded 100 ng per mL. It was suggested that attempts to improve the formulation of the nasal spray should be made.— R. A. Levandowski *et al.*, *Antimicrob. Ag. Chemother.*, 1982, *22*, 1004. In a double-blind placebo-controlled study, enviroxime administered intranasally had no consistent significant therapeutic effect against natural rhinovirus infections.— F. D. Miller *et al.*, *ibid.*, 1985, *27*, 102.

Further references: F. G. Hayden and J. M. Gwaltney, *Antimicrob. Ag. Chemother.*, 1982, *21*, 892; R. J. Phillpotts *et al.*, *ibid.*, 1983, *23*, 671.

Proprietary Names and Manufacturers
Lilly, USA.

10251-m

Fluoroiodoaracytosine
1-(2′-Deoxy-2′-fluoro-β-D-arabinofuranosyl)-5-iodocytosine; 2′-Fluoro-5-iodo-aracytosine; FIAC.
$C_9H_{11}FIN_3O_4$=371.1.

CAS — 69123-90-6; 69124-05-6 (hydrochloride).

Fluoroiodoaracytosine is reported to be active against various herpesviruses including herpes simplex viruses.

A brief review of fluoroiodoaracytosine.— A. L. Donner and B. Leyland-Jones, *Drug Intell. & clin. Pharm.*, 1984, *18*, 885.

Phase 1 evaluation of fluoroiodoaracytosine in immunosuppressed patients with herpesvirus infections.—C. W. Young *et al.*, *Cancer Res.*, 1983, *43*, 5006.

The pharmacokinetics of fluoroiodoaracytosine, given intravenously and by mouth to immunosuppressed patients with herpesvirus infections.—A. Feinberg *et al.*, *Antimicrob. Ag. Chemother.*, 1985, *27*, 733.

Antiviral activity of fluoroiodoaracytosine against human cytomegalovirus.— J. M. Colacino and C. Lopez, *Antimicrob. Ag. Chemother.*, 1983, *24*, 505.

Antiviral activity of fluoroiodoaracytosine against Epstein-Barr virus.— J. -F. Chiou and Y. -C. Cheng, *Antimicrob. Ag. Chemother.*, 1985, *27*, 416; J. -C. Lin *et al.*, *ibid.*, 971.

Antiviral activity of fluoroiodoaracytosine against herpes simplex viruses.— Y. -C. Cheng *et al.*, *Antimicrob. Ag. Chemother.*, 1981, *20*, 420; D. R. Mayo and G. D. Hsiung, *ibid.*, 1984, *26*, 354; R. F. Schinazi *et al.*, *ibid.*, 1986, *29*, 77; J. Colacino *et al.*, *ibid.*, 877.

Antiviral activity of fluoroiodoaracytosine against varicella zoster virus.— S. R. Preblud *et al.*, *Antimicrob. Ag. Chemother.*, 1984, *25*, 417.

Proprietary Names and Manufacturers
Bristol-Myers Products, USA.

16817-b

Foscarnet Sodium *(USAN, rINN).*
A-29622; EHB-776; Phosphonoformate Trisodium.
CNa_3O_5P=192.

CAS — 63585-09-1; 34156-56-4 (hexahydrate).

Foscarnet sodium is active against herpes simplex viruses and human cytomegalovirus. It has also shown some activity against the HIV virus. It is being investigated in the treatment of cytomegalovirus infections especially in patients with AIDS. Administration has been by continuous intravenous infusion and doses have ranged from about 50 to 160 µg per kg body-weight per minute.

A brief discussion on the actions and uses of foscarnet, an inhibitor of reverse transcriptase activity: *Lancet*, 1985, *2*, 648.

ADVERSE EFFECTS. Acute renal failure with foscarnet. Haemodialysis reduced plasma-foscarnet concentrations.— G. Deray *et al.*, *Lancet*, 1987, *2*, 216.

AIDS AND CYTOMEGALOVIRUS INFECTIONS. References to foscarnet in the management of AIDS often with associated cytomegalovirus infections: D. R. J. Singer *et al.* (letter), *Ann. intern. Med.*, 1985, *103*, 962; J. N. Weber *et al.*, *Gut*, 1987, *28*, 482; C. F. Farthing *et al.*, *AIDS*, 1987, *1*, 21; J. Gaub *et al.*, *AIDS*, 1987, *1*, 27.

For activity against the HIV virus, see also E. G. Sandstrom *et al.*, *Lancet*, 1985, *1*, 1480; K. L. Hartshorn *et al.*, *Antimicrob. Ag. Chemother.*, 1986, *30*, 189.

References to foscarnet being used in cytomegalovirus infections in transplant patients: J. F. Apperley *et al.* (letter), *Lancet*, 1985, *1*, 1151; O. Ringden *et al.* (letter), *ibid.*, 1503; *idem*, *J. antimicrob. Chemother.*, 1986, *17*, 373.

HEPATITIS B. Effective treatment with foscarnet in a patient with fulminant hepatitis B.— J. S. Price *et al.* (letter), *Lancet*, 1986, *2*, 1273.

Proprietary Names and Manufacturers
Astra, Swed.

10273-s

Fosfonet Sodium *(USAN, rINN).*
Abbott-38642; Phosphonoacetate Disodium Monohydrate.
$C_2H_3Na_2O_5P,H_2O$=202.

CAS — 54870-27-8; 36983-81-0 (anhydrous); 4408-78-0 (acid).

Fosfonet sodium is reported to be active against various herpesviruses including herpes simplex viruses.

Proprietary Names and Manufacturers
Abbott, USA.

19084-q

Ganciclovir *(BAN, pINN).*
2′-NDG; 2′-Nor-2′-deoxyguanosine; 9-(1,3-Dihydroxy-2-propoxymethyl)guanine; BIOLF-62; BN-B759V; BW-759; BW-759U; BWB-759U; DHPG; Dihydroxypropoxymethylguanine; RS-21592. 9-[2-Hydroxy-1-(hydroxymethyl)ethoxymethyl]guanine.
$C_9H_{13}N_5O_4$=364.3.

CAS — 82410-32-0.

The stability of ganciclovir sodium in glucose 5% or sodium chloride 0.9% injections. G. C. Visor *et al.*, *Am. J. Hosp. Pharm.*, 1986, *43*, 2810.

Ganciclovir is an antiviral agent similar to acyclovir but with greater activity against cytomegalovirus.
It has been given usually in doses of 2.5 or 5 mg per kg body-weight by intravenous infusion every 8 or 12 hours for the treatment of cytomegalovirus infections in patients with AIDS or in immunosuppressed states. The most common infections have been pneumonia, colitis, and retinitis. Intravitreal injections have been tried in retinitis. Improvement has been reported with ganciclovir, but usually only for as long as treatment is continued.
Adverse effects have included bone marrow suppression. *Animal* studies suggest that there might be a risk of adverse testicular effects. Absorption from the gastro-intestinal tract is poor.
Some studies have indicated that ganciclovir sodium was used.

The pharmacokinetics of ganciclovir.— C. Fletcher *et al.*, *Clin. Pharmac. Ther.*, 1986, *40*, 281.

References to ganciclovir in cytomegalovirus infections: D. Felsenstein *et al.*, *Ann. intern. Med.*, 1985, *103*, 377 (retinitis); D. H. Shepp *et al.*, *Ann. intern. Med.*, 1985, *103*, 368 (pneumonia); Collaborative DHPG Treatment Study Group, *New Engl. J. Med.*, 1986, *314*, 801 (pneumonia, retinitis, and gastro-intestinal infection); M. L. Harris and M. B. R. Mathalone, *Br. med. J.*, 1987, *294*, 92 (retinitis); A. Erice *et al.*, *J. Am. med. Ass.*, 1987, *257*, 3082 (pneumonitis, retinitis, hepatitis, and gastro-intestinal infection); A. Chachoua *et al.*, *Ann. intern. Med.*, 1987, *107*, 133 (gastro-intestinal infection).

Proprietary Preparations
Cymevene *(Syntex, UK). Intravenous infusion*, powder for reconstitution, ganciclovir 500 mg (as sodium salt).

12854-d

Ibacitabine *(rINN).*
Iododesoxycytidine. 2′-Deoxy-5-iodocytidine.
$C_9H_{12}IN_3O_4$=353.1.

CAS — 611-53-0.

Ibacitabine has been used via ocular and topical routes in the treatment of herpes infections.

Proprietary Names and Manufacturers
Cébévir *(Chauvin-Blache, Fr.; Novopharma, Switz.)*; Cuterpès *(Chauvin-Blache, Fr.)*.

1681-k

Idoxuridine *(BAN, USAN, rINN).*
5-IDUR; IDU; SKF-14287. 2′-Deoxy-5-iodouridine.
$C_9H_{11}IN_2O_5$=354.1.

CAS — 54-42-2.

Pharmacopoeias. In *Br.*, *Chin.*, *Egypt.*, *Ind.*, *Jpn*, and *U.S.*

Odourless or almost odourless, colourless crystals or a white crystalline powder from which iodine vapour is liberated on heating.
Slightly **soluble** in water and in alcohol; practically insoluble in chloroform and in ether. It has been reported that some decomposition products such as iodouracil are more toxic than idoxuridine and reduce its antiviral activity. **Store** in airtight containers. Protect from light.

STABILITY. References to the stability of solutions of idoxuridine and their decomposition due to heating or autoclaving: L. J. Ravin and J. J. Gulesich, *J. Am. pharm. Ass.*, 1964, *NS4*, 122; E. T. Backer and J. van de Langerijt, *Pharm. Weekbl. Ned.*, 1966, *101*, 489.

Adverse Effects
Adverse effects, which occur occasionally when idoxuridine is applied to the eyes, include irritation, pain, conjunctivitis, oedema of the eyelids, photophobia, and occlusion of the lachrymal duct. Allergic reactions may occur. Prolonged use may damage the cornea.
Idoxuridine applied to the skin may produce irritation and allergic reactions. Adverse effects after intravenous administration of idoxuridine may be severe; bone marrow depression and liver damage have been reported. Other systemic adverse effects include glossitis, stomatitis, alopecia, and gastro-intestinal disturbances.

Adverse effects on the cornea from ophthalmic use of idoxuridine.— J. H. Lass *et al.*, *Archs Ophthal.*, *N.Y.*, 1983, *101*, 747.

Squamous carcinoma in one patient associated with topical idoxuridine treatment. Reference is made to one earlier similar case.— H. S. Koppang and E. Aas, *Br. J. Derm.*, 1983, *108*, 501.

ALLERGY. Reports of allergic reactions to idoxuridine applied to the eye or to the skin: P. E. Osmundsen, *Contact Dermatitis*, 1975, *1*, 251; R. B. Amon *et al.*, *Archs Derm.*, 1975, *111*, 1581.

PREGNANCY AND THE NEONATE. Idoxuridine applied topically to the eye in doses similar to those used clinically was teratogenic to *rabbits*, causing exophthalmic-like deformities and malformed forelegs.— M. Itoi *et al.*, *Archs Ophthal.*, *N.Y.*, 1975, *93*, 46.

Precautions
Idoxuridine should be used with caution in conditions where there is also deep ulceration involving the stromal layers of the cornea, as delayed healing has resulted in corneal perforation. Prolonged topical use should be avoided. Corticosteroids should be applied with caution in patients also receiving idoxuridine. Boric acid preparations should not be applied to the eye in patients also receiving ocular preparations of idoxuridine as irritation ensues.
Idoxuridine is no longer given parenterally.

Antiviral Action
Following intracellular phosphorylation, idoxuridine is incorporated into viral DNA instead of thymidine so inhibiting replication of the virus. Idoxuridine is also incorporated into mammalian DNA. Idoxuridine is active against herpes simplex and varicella zoster viruses. It has also been shown to inhibit vaccinia virus and cytomegalovirus.
Resistance to idoxuridine occurs *in vitro* and *in vivo*. Viruses have been observed that are deficient in thymidine kinase activity.

Absorption and Fate
Following systemic administration idoxuridine is rapidly metabolised to iodouracil, uracil and iodide which are excreted in the urine and have no antiviral activity. Idoxuridine is not bound to plasma proteins. Penetration of the cornea is reported to be poor.

Uses and Administration
Idoxuridine is used topically in the treatment of herpes simplex keratitis with best results being achieved in superficial ulcers. Treatment may also involve the cautious use of corticosteroids if

there is deep ulceration. Solutions of idoxuridine in dimethyl sulphoxide are used for the topical treatment of cutaneous forms of herpes simplex and herpes zoster. Idoxuridine is no longer given parenterally.

In the treatment of herpes simplex keratitis idoxuridine may be applied as an 0.1% ophthalmic solution, one drop being instilled every hour during the day and every 2 hours at night until the corneal ulcers have healed. Treatment should then be continued generally for about 5 days with one drop every 2 hours during the day and one drop every 4 hours at night. An ophthalmic ointment containing 0.5% idoxuridine is also available and is administered five times daily every 4 hours.

Idoxuridine 5% in dimethyl sulphoxide to aid absorption can be painted onto the lesions of cutaneous herpes simplex and herpes zoster four times daily for 4 days. In severe cutaneous herpes zoster a 40% solution in dimethyl sulphoxide may be applied on a dressing once daily for 4 days. It is recommended that the dressing be retained over the dermatome for 24 hours. This treatment should not be continued for longer than 4 days.

The development and therapeutic uses of topical preparations of idoxuridine 5%.— R. P. R. Dawber, *Scott. med. J.*, 1977, *22*, 310.

A short review on the actions and uses of idoxuridine.— D. J. Jeffries, *Prescribers' J.*, 1981, *21*, 159.

In a double-blind study in 11 women with widespread condyloma acuminatum, idoxuridine 0.25% in Vaseline and lanolin applied twice daily was compared with placebo. The condylomata in those treated with the idoxuridine ointment disappeared macroscopically and microscopically whereas in the placebo group there was progression or no change.— K. Hasumi *et al.* (letter), *Lancet*, 1984, *1*, 968.

HERPES GENITALIS. In a double-blind study 53 patients with recurrent genital herpes were treated with topical applications of idoxuridine 20% in dimethyl sulphoxide, idoxuridine 5% in dimethyl sulphoxide, or dimethyl sulphoxide alone. Both treatments with idoxuridine were superior to dimethyl sulphoxide alone and lesions treated with idoxuridine 20% healed more rapidly and shed virus for a shorter period than those treated with idoxuridine 5%. There was no significant difference in the recurrence-rate of lesions for the different groups in 34 patients who were followed up for up to 2 years.— J. D. Parker, *J. antimicrob. Chemother.*, 1977, *3*, *Suppl. A*, 131. Following an open study to select an appropriate concentration of idoxuridine, a preparation of idoxuridine 30% in dimethyl sulphoxide was compared with dimethyl sulphoxide and sodium chloride solution 0.9% in the topical treatment of 96 episodes of recurrent genital herpes in a group of 88 patients. Each preparation was applied four times daily for 7 days. Idoxuridine had no effect on symptoms and signs or on recurrence although it did shorten the duration of virus shedding. However there was no significant effect on virus shedding in a group of patients with primary infection.— D. L. Silvestri *et al.*, *J. Am. med. Ass.*, 1982, *248*, 953.

HERPES SIMPLEX ENCEPHALITIS. The termination of studies on idoxuridine being used parenterally to treat herpes simplex encephalitis because of the high mortality-rate and severe toxicity in patients receiving the drug.— Boston Interhospital Virus Study Group and the NIAID-Sponsored Cooperative Antiviral Clinical Study, *New Engl. J. Med.*, 1975, *292*, 599.

HERPES SIMPLEX KERATITIS. For a comparative study of the efficacy of idoxuridine and trifluridine in herpes simplex keratitis, see Trifluridine, p.701.

For comparative studies of the efficacy of idoxuridine and vidarabine in herpes simplex keratitis, see Vidarabine, p.703.

HERPES ZOSTER. In a double-blind study 100 patients with acute herpes zoster received treatment with idoxuridine 40% in dimethyl sulphoxide or one of the following ointments: a basis of macrogol; a basis with dimethyl sulphoxide 60%; a basis with idoxuridine 5% and dimethyl sulphoxide 60%; or a basis with idoxuridine 40% and dimethyl sulphoxide 60%. Treatment with any of the ointments was without any positive effect and although the effect of idoxuridine in solution was statistically significant, it was only slightly better than the ointments with respect to healing and there was no apparent effect on pain and sensitivity. However, analysis revealed that the age of the patient correlated with the duration of pain and with delayed healing, that rapid healing was influenced by the duration of pain, and that herpes zoster in the trigeminal area healed more quickly than in other areas. It was suggested that treatment with idoxuridine should be re-evaluated and these variables taken into account.— K. E. Wildenhoff *et al.*, *Scand. J. infect. Dis.*, 1979, *11*, 1. Results of a double-blind randomised study comparing idoxuridine in dimethyl sulphoxide with dimethyl sulphoxide alone and with saline, again showed that trigeminal zoster (in 42 patients) healed faster than thoracic zoster (in 80 patients). Patients with thoracic zoster, however, experienced pain significantly longer before the eruption of the skin lesions, which might explain the apparent therapeutic failure of idoxuridine in thoracic zoster.— V. Esmann and K. E. Wildenhoff (letter), *Lancet*, 1980, *2*, 474.

Further references to idoxuridine in herpes zoster: R. Dawber, *Br. med. J.*, 1974, *2*, 526; B. E. Juel-Jensen and F. O. MacCallum (letter), *ibid.*, 1974, *3*, 41; J. R. Simpson, *Practitioner*, 1975, *215*, 226.

ORF. Idoxuridine 35% in dimethyl sulphoxide applied as a wet dressing for 4 to 5 days cleared lesions of orf, the DNA virus becoming undetectable on electron microscopy.— B. E. Juel-Jensen (letter), *J. R. Coll. gen. Pract.*, 1977, *27*, 57.

Preparations

Idoxuridine Eye Drops *(B.P.)*

Idoxuridine Ophthalmic Ointment *(U.S.P.)*. A sterile ointment containing 0.45 to 0.55% of idoxuridine in a soft paraffin (petrolatum) basis.

Idoxuridine Ophthalmic Solution *(U.S.P.)*. A sterile aqueous solution containing 0.09 to 0.11% of idoxuridine; it may contain suitable buffers, stabilisers, and antimicrobial agents. pH 4.5 to 7.0.

Proprietary Preparations

Herpid *(Boehringer Ingelheim, UK)*. *Application*, idoxuridine 5% in dimethyl sulphoxide.

Idoxene *(Spodefell, UK)*. *Eye ointment*, idoxuridine 0.5%.

Iduridin *(Ferring, UK)*. *Application*, idoxuridine 5% and 40% in dimethyl sulphoxide.

Kerecid *(Allergan, UK)*. *Ophthalmic ointment*, idoxuridine 0.5%.
Ophthalmic solution, idoxuridine 0.1%.

Ophthalmadine *(Sas, UK)*. *Eye-drops*, idoxuridine 0.1%.
Eye ointment, idoxuridine 0.5%.

Proprietary Names and Manufacturers

Cheratil *(Francia Farm., Ital.)*; Col Cusi Virucida *(Cusi, Spain)*; Collyre 'V' P.O.S. *(Switz.)*; Dendrid *(Arg.; Alcon, Switz.; Alcon, UK; Farillon, UK)*; Gel V P.O.S. *(P.O.S., Fr.)*; Herpetil *(Ital.)*; Herpid *(Boehringer Ingelheim, UK)*; Herpidu *(Norw.; Dispersa, Switz.)*; Herplex *(Arg.; Allergan, Austral.; Belg.; Allergan, Canad.; Neth.; S.Afr.; Allergan, UK; Allergan, USA)*; Idoxene *(Spodefell, UK)*; Iducher 2% *(Farmigea, Ital.)*; Iducutit *(Ferring, Ger.)*; Idulea *(Arg.)*; Iduridin *(Ferring, Denm.; Ger.; Ayerst, Ital.; Neth.; Ferring, Norw.; Ferring, Swed.; Ferring, UK)*; Idustatin *(Isnardi, Ital.)*; Iduviran *(Chauvin-Blache, Fr.; Switz.)*; Kerecid *(Allergan, UK)*; Oftalmolosa Cusi Virucida *(Cusi, Spain)*; Ophthalmadine *(Sas, UK)*; Spectanefran *(Allergan, Ger.)*; Stoxil *(Allergan, Austral.; Smith Kline & French, Austral.; Smith Kline & French, Canad.; Smith Kline & French, S.Afr.; Smith Kline & French, USA)*; Synmiol *(Winzer, Ger.)*; Virexen *(Vinas, Spain; Sapos, Switz.)*; Virucida *(Spain)*; Virunguent *(Hermal, Ger.)*; Vistaspectran *(Ger.)*; Zostrum *(Eire; Basotherm, Ger.)*.

12941-f

Inosine Pranobex *(BAN)*.

Inosiplex; Methisoprinol; NPT-10381. Inosine 2-hydroxypropyldimethylammonium 4-acetamidobenzoate (1:3).

$C_{10}H_{12}N_4O_5{:}C_{14}H_{22}N_2O_4$ (1:3)=1115.2.

CAS — 36703-88-5.

NOTE. Inosine pranobex has sometimes been described as inosine with dimepranol and acedoben. Dimepranol is the pINN name for (±)-1-(dimethylamino)-2-propanol and acedoben is the pINN name for *p*-acetamidobenzoic acid.

Adverse Effects and Precautions

Some patients have experienced transient nausea and vomiting. Metabolism of the inosine content of inosine pranobex leads to increased serum and urine concentrations of uric acid; caution is therefore recommended in treating patients with impaired renal function, gout, or hyperuricaemia.

Antiviral Action

Inosine pranobex appears to owe its activity in viral infections more to its capacity to modify or stimulate cell-mediated immune processes than to a direct action on the virus.

Slight activity of inosine pranobex against some viruses *in vitro*; some activity in *animals* infected with herpes simplex virus type 2 and influenza virus.— T. -W. Chang and L. Weinstein, *Am. J. med. Sci.*, 1973, *265*, 143. Lack of activity in experimental model infections.— L. A. Glasgow and G. J. Galasso, *J. infect. Dis.*, 1972, *126*, 162.

Absorption and Fate

Inosine pranobex is reported to be rapidly absorbed following administration by mouth. It is also rapidly metabolised, the inosine portion of the complex yielding uric acid; the other part of the complex undergoes oxidation and glucuronidation. The metabolites are excreted in the urine.

The metabolism and excretion of *NN*-dimethylaminoisopropanol and *p*-acetamidobenzoic acid in 2 subjects given inosine pranobex.— P. Nielsen and A. H. Beckett, *J. Pharm. Pharmac.*, 1981, *33*, 549.

Uses and Administration

Inosine pranobex is used in the treatment of various viral infections. Preparations are available for use in herpes simplex and in genital warts. It has been tried in subacute sclerosing panencephalitis and in immunodeficiency disorders including AIDS. The recommended dose in herpes simplex is 1 g four times daily by mouth for 7 to 14 days. A dose of 1 g three times daily is given for 14 to 28 days as an adjunct to traditional topical treatment for genital warts.

Reviews of the actions and uses of inosine pranobex: D. M. Campoli-Richards *et al.*, *Drugs*, 1986, *32*, 383; *Drug & Ther. Bull.*, 1986, *24*, 93.

AIDS. References to immunomodulatory effects of inosine pranobex in AIDS: K. Y. Tsang *et al.* (letter), *New Engl. J. Med.*, 1984, *310*, 987; M. H. Grieco *et al.*, *Ann. intern. Med.*, 1984, *101*, 206; *Pharm. J.*, 1984, *2*, 385.

CONDYLOMAS. A brief report of inosine pranobex with conventional treatment producing improvement in genital warts. Inosine pranobex given alone was considered to be no more effective than conventional therapy.— *Pharm. J.*, 1985, *2*, 187.

A report of improvement in genital warts with inosine pranobex alone or with conventional treatment.— K. C. Mohanty and C. S. Scott, *Genitourinary Med.*, 1986, *62*, 352.

DIABETES MELLITUS. Since inosine pranobex had been shown to diminish islet B-cell destruction in *mice* with induced diabetes, it was tested in a controlled study involving 19 patients with newly diagnosed insulin-dependent diabetes. No clinically important effect was seen on the endogenous insulin reserve.— B. Greulich *et al.*, *Diabetologia*, 1983, *25*, 158.

ENCEPHALITIS. Twenty-three of 27 patients with acute viral encephalitis (due to herpes viruses in 7) treated with inosine pranobex recovered; 19 of these did so without sequelae. The usual dose of inosine pranobex was 100 mg per kg body-weight daily by mouth or intravenously, in courses of 8 to 10 days, with 8 days between courses; 1 to 3 courses were given for benign forms, and 2 to 6 or 9 courses for severe forms. In general, therapy was well tolerated; vomiting sometimes occurred at the beginning of oral therapy. Discontinuous therapy at moderate doses yields the best results for all forms of the disorder. Immunostimulants given continuously or in high doses may enhance proliferation of suppressor T-lymphocytes yielding results opposite to those sought.— A. Buge *et al.* (letter), *Lancet*, 1979, *2*, 691.

Subacute sclerosing panencephalitis. Various early reports indicated that some patients with subacute sclerosing panencephalitis might benefit from inosine pranobex (L.J. Streletz and J. Cracco, *Ann. Neurol.*, 1977, *1*, 183; P.R. Huttenlocher and R.H. Mattson, *Neurology*, 1979, *29*, 763) while other reports indicated that it offered no benefit (R. Silverberg *et al.*, *Archs Neurol.*, 1979, *36*, 374; F.S. Haddad and W.S. Risk, *Ann. Neu-*

rol., 1980, *7*, 185). However, a large multicentre non-randomised study covering 98 patients found that inosine pranobex seemed to be able to prolong life in patients with this condition (C.E. Jones *et al.*, *Lancet*, 1982, *1*, 1034). The 98 patients were treated with inosine pranobex 100 mg per kg body-weight daily by mouth for periods ranging from less than one month to 9.5 years. The organisation of the study, which involved comparing survival in the treated group with 3 control groups, produced criticism and doubts on the validity of the findings (*Lancet*, 1982, *1*, 1052; T.C. Chalmers and H. Smith, *ibid.*, 1475; C. Jones, *ibid.*, *2*, 495). The study also prompted a reminder that subacute sclerosing panencephalitis can be successfully prevented by efficient measles vaccination. Further investigations of patients treated with inosine pranobex indicated that responses were greater in patients with slowly developing or chronic disease than in those with rapidly developing subacute sclerosing panencephalitis (R.H. DuRant *et al.*, *J. Pediat.*, 1982, *101*, 288; R.H. DuRant and P.R. Dyken, *Neurology*, 1983, *33*, 1053).

HEPATITIS. A report of no benefit with inosine pranobex in patients with acute viral hepatitis.— K. C. Lam *et al.*, *Am. J. dig. Dis.*, 1978, *23*, 893.

Inosine pranobex 1.5 g four times daily for a mean period of 28 days produced significant improvement in some symptoms and liver signs in 28 patients with hepatitis B when compared with 29 controls. The treated group also showed greater reduction in HBsAg values.— A. Scasso *et al.*, *Curr. ther. Res.*, 1983, *34*, 423.

References to responses to inosine pranobex in viral hepatitis: F. Di Blasi *et al.*, *Arch. Med. intern.*, 1981, *33*, 457; C. E. Zanda, *Riv. Patol. clin.*, 1981, *36*, 95.

HERPES SIMPLEX. The number of recurrences of herpes labialis and herpes genitalis was significantly reduced in 70 patients in a year of study in which they were given either placebo or inosine pranobex 70 mg per kg body-weight daily for a week and during the subsequent 5th, 9th, and 12th weeks; comparison was made with the incidence of infections that had been observed the previous year. During the year of the study the number of recurrences of herpes labialis but not of herpes genitalis was significantly lower in the treatment group than in the controls. An intermittent schedule was selected in part because of the reluctance of a previous group to take tablets for more than 20 to 30 consecutive days.— M. Galli *et al.* (letter), *Lancet*, 1982, *2*, 331 and 926.

There was no difference between inosine pranobex and placebo in reducing the incidence of recurrent attacks of herpes simplex or the duration of symptoms in a double-blind study involving 18 patients. The study was intended to be crossover in design but only 10 patients received both placebo and inosine pranobex; also 5 patients received 2 courses of inosine pranobex. The dose of inosine pranobex was 1 g by mouth four times a day for 7 days starting within 3 days of the first visible signs of an attack. Thirty-three attacks were observed before treatment, 18 during treatment with inosine pranobex, 18 during placebo treatment, and 32 after the treatment period.— K. O. K. Kalimo *et al.*, *Archs Derm.*, 1983, *119*, 463.

Although reports on inosine pranobex in herpes simplex are somewhat lacking in detail the effects look clinically useful. However published work allows no conclusions about which is the best agent for mucocutaneous herpes and inosine pranobex needs to be compared with other therapies for both therapeutic and prophylactic efficiency (*Lancet*, 1985, *1*, 200). This judgement was endorsed by Mindel (*ibid.*, 631). Saurat, who had collaborated on some of the early work, responded with doubts about the dose (*ibid.*, 877). Most studies employed 3 to 4 g daily for 4 to 7 days and at this dose Saurat has observed a biphasic effect, the initial improvement being followed by a relapse. The best regimen might be 1 day's treatment with 3 g. Mindel *et al.* (*ibid.*, 1987, *1*, 1171) subsequently compared inosine pranobex 1 g four times daily with acyclovir 200 mg four times daily or with a combination of both drugs in first-attack genital herpes. Treatment was for 7 days and showed acyclovir or both drugs producing a more rapid healing and a shorter duration of viral shedding than inosine pranobex alone.

Further references to inosine pranobex in herpes simplex: O. Salo and A. Lassas, *Eur. J. sex. transm. Dis.*, 1983, *1*, 101 (genital herpes); *Pharm. J.*, 1984, *2*, 385 (genital herpes); D. J. Talbot and A. P. Menday (letter), *Lancet*, 1985, *1*, 877 (preliminary report of multicentre study in herpes labialis).

HERPES ZOSTER. Inosine pranobex had no important influence on the course of infection in a comparative study involving 6 children with cancer and herpes zoster given 1.8 to 2.7 g per m^2 body-surface daily for at least 5 days and 7 similar patients given a placebo. Lymphocytes from the treated children were no more responsive to varicella-zoster antigen than those from controls.— S. Feldman *et al.*, *Antimicrob. Ag. Chemother.*, 1978, *14*, 495.

References to inosine pranobex being tried with good results in herpes zoster: F. Torregrossa, *Acta Gerontol.*, 1978, *28*, 105; S. Bunta and Z. Peris, *Z. Hautkrankheiten*, 1981, *56*, 1457; B. Lesourd *et al.*, *Nouv. Presse méd.*, 1982, *11*, 191; D. Tanphaichitra and S. Srimuang, *J. antimicrob. Chemother.*, 1987, *19*, 255.

INFLUENZA AND THE COMMON COLD. Inosine pranobex 2.5 g twice daily for 10 days by mouth was no more effective than a placebo in a double-blind study in 30 subjects infected, 48 hours after starting treatment, with an intranasal instillation of Hong Kong influenza virus.— S. Longley *et al.*, *Antimicrob. Ag. Chemother.*, 1973, *3*, 506. Inosine pranobex 4 g daily, taken by mouth in divided doses, reduced symptoms when compared with placebo in a double-blind study of healthy subjects infected experimentally with influenza A virus either before or after inosine pranobex was started.— R. A. Khakoo *et al.*, *J. antimicrob. Chemother.*, 1981, *7*, 389. Similar mixed results had been achieved in studies on rhinovirus infection.— D. M. Pachuta *et al.*, *Antimicrob. Ag. Chemother.*, 1974, *5*, 403; R. H. Waldman and R. Ganguly, *Ann. N.Y. Acad. Sci.*, 1977, *284*, 153.

RHEUMATOID ARTHRITIS. References to inosine pranobex being tried in rheumatoid arthritis: J. Wybran *et al.*, *J. Rheumatol.*, 1981, *8*, 643.

Proprietary Preparations

Imunovir *(Leo, UK). Tablets*, inosine pranobex 500 mg.

Proprietary Names and Manufacturers

Anavir *(Errekappa, Ital.)*; Aviral *(Medici Domus, Ital.)*; Bodaril *(Elmu, Spain)*; Delimmun *(Delalande, Ger.)*; Immunoviral *(Port.)*; Imunovir *(Leo, UK)*; Isoprinosin *(Andreu, Spain)*; Isoprinosina *(Delalande, Ital.)*; Isoprinosine *(Organon, Canad.*; *Fisons, Ger.*; *Newport, USA)*; Isoviral *(Janus, Ital.)*; Modimmunal *(Ravizza, Ital.)*; Modimunal *(Jug.)*; Prinosine *(Kor.)*; Virac *(Crosara, Ital.)*; Viral-Os *(Berenguer-Beneyto, Spain)*; Virustop *(Pulitzer, Ital.)*; Viruxan *(Gramon, Arg.*; *Sigmatau, Ital.)*; Viruxprine *(Faes, Spain)*.

1683-t

Interferons

Proteins or glycoproteins produced in human or animal cells following exposure chiefly to viruses. They may also be produced through recombinant DNA technology.

CAS — 9008-11-1; 76543-88-9 (alfa-2a); 99210-65-8 (alfa-2b); 98059-18-8 (gamma-1a); 98059-61-1 (gamma-2a or 1b).

The 3 main types of interferon (IFN) are now generally known as interferon alfa, interferon beta, and interferon gamma.

Interferon alfa (*BAN, rINN*) (interferon-α; IFN-α) was also known as leucocyte interferon or lymphoblastoid interferon as it can be derived from those cells as well as through recombinant DNA technology. Protein variants from the human alfa gene may be designated by a number as in interferon alfa-2, and in the case of interferon alfa-2 the number may be qualified by a letter to indicate the peptide sequence at positions 23 and 34. Interferon alfa-2a (*USAN*) has lysine at 23 and histidine at 34, interferon alfa-2b (*USAN*) has arginine at 23 and histidine at 34, while interferon alfa-2c has arginine at both 23 and 34. Interferon alfa may consist of a mixture of proteins and be described as multicomponent; this may be indicated by a letter and then a number as interferon alfa-n1 (*USAN*). The name may be further elaborated on the label by approved sets of initials in parentheses to indicate the method of production: (rbe) indicates production from bacteria (*Escherichia coli*) genetically modified by recombinant DNA technology; (lns) indicates production from cultured lymphoblasts from the Namalwa cell line that have been stimulated by a Sendai virus; (bls) indicates production from leucocytes from human blood that have been stimulated by a Sendai virus. In *Martindale* interferon alfa may be described as leucocyte or lymphoblastoid interferon alfa or as recombinant interferon alfa since the precise method of production was not always clear.

Interferon beta (*BAN, rINN*) (interferon-β; IFN-β) was also known as fibroblast interferon after the cell type used for production.

Interferon gamma (*BAN, rINN*) (interferon-γ; IFN-γ) was also known as immune interferon since it was derived from immunologically stimulated T-lymphocytes. Like interferon alfa, protein variants of interferon gamma have been produced and are designated by a number and letter to indicate the sequences at position 1 and terminal position 139. Interferon gamma-1a has at position 1, hydrogen, cysteine, tyrosine, and cysteine and at terminal position 139, arginine, alanine, serine, glutamine, and hydroxyl. Interferon gamma-1b (*USAN*) has at position 1, hydrogen and methionine, and at position 139, hydroxyl; in the *BAN* description of interferon gamma, this form is given as interferon gamma-2a. This type of interferon may also be produced through recombinant DNA technology when the letters (rbe) may be used as with interferon alfa.

Units

25 000 units of human lymphoblastoid interferon alfa are contained in one ampoule of the first International Standard Preparation (1984).

12 000 units of human leucocyte interferon alfa are contained in one ampoule of the first International Standard Preparation (1984).

9000 units of human recombinant interferon alfa-2a are contained in one ampoule of the first International Standard Preparation (1984).

17 000 units of human recombinant interferon alfa-2b are contained in one ampoule of the first International Standard Preparation (1987).

8000 units of human recombinant interferon alfa-1 (alpha D) are contained in one ampoule of the first International Standard Preparation (1987).

15 000 units of human fibroblast interferon beta are contained in one ampoule of the second International Standard Preparation (1987).

6000 units of human recombinant interferon beta (Ser 17) are contained in one ampoule of the first International Standard Preparation (1987).

4000 units of human interferon gamma are contained in one ampoule of the first International Standard Preparation (1984).

There are also International Standard Preparations (1987) for murine interferon alfa, beta, and gamma as well as International Reference Preparations (1978) for chick and rabbit interferon.

Adverse Effects and Precautions

Most of the reports of the adverse effects of interferons have involved interferon alfa given intramuscularly or sometimes intravenously. Some of the effects have been observed with interferon beta. It is considered that interferon alfa produced by recombinant DNA technology has similar adverse effects to interferon alfa from cultured human cells that contains a mixture of subtypes.

Interferon alfa produces 'flu-like symptoms with fever, chills, and myalgia that may respond to paracetamol. Anorexia with weight loss and alopecia occur as does bone marrow depression. There may be nausea and vomiting, headache, and signs of altered liver function; liver necrosis has been reported. Renal failure has occurred as has the nephrotic syndrome. Cardiovascular effects include hypo- or hypertension, myocardial infarction, and strokes. Fatigue and mental depression may be severe. EEG abnormalities and neurological symptoms including convulsions, ataxia, and coma have been reported.

Nasal administration may produce mucosal irritation.

Because of the range of potentially serious

adverse effects that can occur with interferons, they should be used with caution in patients with conditions that might be exacerbated. It is felt by some that interferons are contra-indicated in patients with severe cardiac, renal, hepatic, or CNS disorders.

Interferons can inhibit hepatic oxidising activity and so block the metabolism of drugs subject to that process.

Human leucocyte interferon alfa was given intrathecally in increasing doses to 5 patients severely disabled with multiple sclerosis. The aim was to give 4 individual doses in 5 mL of sodium chloride injection at weekly intervals starting with 0.1 million units then 0.3, 1.0, and finally 3.0 million units. Three patients dropped out before the fourth dose. All patients experienced fever that did not respond to conventional antipyretics. Extreme fatigue occurred in all patients increasing their need for help and was considered to be unbearable with doses greater than 0.3 million units. Recovery from the fatigue occurred in the 24 hours after the temperature fell to below 37°. Respiratory difficulties occurred in 2 patients when given the fourth dose. Four patients experienced an increase in lymphocytes.— J. Ruutiainen *et al.*, *Br. med. J.*, 1983, *286*, 940.

The effects of increasing doses of recombinant interferon alfa-2 were studied in 6 subjects. No adverse effects were experienced with a dose of 0.3 million units given intramuscularly. A dose of 1 million units produced mild transient headache, malaise, myalgia, and a slight increase in temperature in 5 subjects. When the dose was increased to 3 million units all 6 subjects developed, within 2 to 4 hours, headache, malaise, myalgia, chills and then fevers. Other effects experienced by some of the subjects included nausea, vomiting, somnolence, confusion, photophobia, and herpes labialis. Indomethacin given with the 3 million units dose suppressed the fever. Subjects experienced significant increases in plasma concentrations of 11-hydroxycorticosteroids and significant decreases in concentrations of zinc with the 3 million units dose.— G. M. Scott *et al.*, *Antimicrob. Ag. Chemother.*, 1983, *23*, 589. Indomethacin 50 mg every 6 hours for 3 doses and ibuprofen 400 mg every 6 hours each blocked fever and myalgias and attenuated fatigue in patients given interferon alfa intrathecally.— J. S. Mora *et al.* (letter), *New Engl. J. Med.*, 1984, *310*, 126.

Lack of response to interferon alfa-2b in chronic myelogenous leukaemia associated with the emergence of interferon antibodies. It is considered that the effect of these antibodies is underestimated and that patients treated with interferons should be monitored for antibodies using blood samples taken at a time when the antibodies can be measured.— P. von Wussow *et al.* (letter), *Lancet*, 1987, *2*, 635.

EFFECTS ON BLOOD. Restoration of bone-marrow function following marrow transplantation was delayed in 3 patients given a human interferon alfa preparation. In a 4th patient also given interferon alfa the transplant failed to take. Laboratory results showed an inhibition of granulocyte colony growth by human leucocyte interferon alfa. It was considered that interferon alfa was contra-indicated in patients with severe bone-marrow insufficiency and should not be given to marrow transplant patients before the graft was fully functional.— C. Nissen *et al.* (letter), *Lancet*, 1977, *1*, 203. Bone-marrow transplants were not affected by recombinant interferon alfa given to 5 patients with interstitial pneumonia 3 of whom had cytomegalovirus infections. Two of the patients recovered; one was given 36 million units daily for 18 days and the other 50 million units daily for 15 days. Three patients experienced fever and chills, 4 experienced more than a 60% reduction in the absolute peripheral granulocyte counts, and 4 had a 37 to 80% reduction in absolute platelet counts. All experienced an increase in lymphocytes. Peripheral blood counts returned to normal after interferon therapy was completed.— D. J. Winston *et al.*, *Antimicrob. Ag. Chemother.*, 1983, *23*, 846.

Immune thrombocytopenia in 5 cancer patients given interferon alfa.— P. McLaughlin *et al.*, *J. Am. med. Ass.*, 1985, *254*, 1353.

Immune haemolytic anaemia in 2 patients given interferon alfa-2.— L. P. Akard *et al.*, *Ann. intern. Med.*, 1986, *105*, 306.

EFFECTS ON THE KIDNEY. In a double-blind parallel-group study all of 8 renal transplant patients given, in addition to routine immunosuppression, high doses of recombinant interferon alfa (36 million units intramuscularly three times a week for 6 weeks followed by twice weekly for a further 6 weeks) had early rejection episodes which were corticosteroid resistant; 3 also had transient nephrotic syndrome. All of 8 control patients, given human albumin and saline solution, also had early rejection episodes but only one was corticosteroid resistant. These adverse effects on the transplant contrasted with the absence of adverse effect on kidney transplants reported by Hirsch *et al.* (*New Engl. J. Med.*, 1983, *308*, 1489) who gave lower doses of leucocyte interferon alfa for the prophylaxis of cytomegalovirus infections.— P. Kramer *et al.*, *Lancet*, 1984, *1*, 989.

Case reports of the nephrotic syndrome associated with interferon alfa: S. D. Averbuch *et al.*, *New Engl. J. Med.*, 1984, *310*, 32; P. Selby *et al.*, *Br. med. J.*, 1985, *290*, 1180.

In a toxicity study of recombinant interferon gamma involving 18 patients, doses of 22 and 110 million units by intravenous infusion led to mild proteinuria. No increases in urea or creatinine concentrations were observed. There was no proteinuria with smaller doses.— K. Sriskandan *et al.* (letter), *Br. med. J.*, 1985, *290*, 1590.

Nephrotic syndrome secondary to membranoproliferative glomerulonephritis in a patient given interferon alfa-2.— J. Herrman *et al.* (letter), *New Engl. J. Med.*, 1987, *316*, 112.

EFFECTS ON THE NERVOUS SYSTEM. Adverse effects reported in 10 women with advanced breast cancer treated for up to 12 weeks with recombinant interferon alfa in doses of 20 million units daily or 50 million units three times a week included fever, anorexia, nausea, and transient leucopenia. All patients showed an abnormal EEG pattern and neurological adverse effects included profound lethargy and somnolence in 6 patients, confusion and dysphasia in 5, paraesthesia in 2, and an upper motor-neurone lesion of the legs in 1. These effects resolved when interferon alfa was withdrawn and all patients tolerated its reintroduction at a lower dose.— H. Smedley *et al.*, *Br. med. J.*, 1983, *286*, 262. Changes in the EEG occurred in one patient given human lymphoblastoid interferon alfa 4 million units per m^2 body-surface daily before neurological symptoms developed.— L. Honigsberger *et al.* (letter), *ibid.*, 719.

A prospective study involving 8 cancer patients given interferon alfa prepared either via cell culture or recombinant DNA technology showed that all experienced severe reversible EEG abnormalities; 3 patients studied retrospectively also experienced the same effects. The dose was usually 100 million units per m^2 body-surface daily administered by continuous intravenous infusion for 7 days. All patients showed signs of hepatic dysfunction and 2 patients became hypocalcaemic, one of them developing signs of renal failure.— A. Z. S. Rohatiner *et al.*, *Br. J. Cancer*, 1983, *47*, 419.

Further references: C. C. Suter *et al.*, *Mayo Clin. Proc.*, 1984, *59*, 847 (EEG abnormalities); F. Adams, *J. Am. med. Ass.*, 1984, *252*, 938 (neuropsychiatric changes); P. L. J. A. Bernsen *et al.* (letter), *Lancet*, 1985, *1*, 50 (neuralgic amyotrophy and polyradiculopathy).

EFFECTS ON THE SKIN. Exacerbation or stimulation of psoriasis in 3 patients given recombinant interferon alfa.— J. R. Quesada and J. U. Gutterman, *Lancet*, 1986, *1*, 1466. Interferon gamma might produce a more marked exacerbation.— B. S. Baker *et al.* (letter), *ibid.*, *2*, 342. No exacerbation was seen in 7 patients given interferon gamma.— H. -J. Schulze and G. Mahrle (letter), *ibid.*, 926.

EFFECTS ON THE THYROID. Three women complaining of hair loss during treatment with leucocyte interferon alfa for breast cancer were found to have clinical hypothyroidism.— I. S. Fentiman *et al.* (letter), *Lancet*, 1985, *1*, 1166. Hypothyroidism was observed in 4 and hyperthyroidism in 2 of 41 patients with carcinoid tumour and liver metastases given leucocyte interferon alfa for an average of 8 months. The thyroid activity might have been due to interferon gamma which might be present in some preparations of interferon alfa.— P. Burman *et al.* (letter), *ibid.*, *2*, 100. Recombinant interferon gamma did not produce alopecia or hypothyroidism in 18 patients given 3 infusions a week for 4 weeks.— H. Bhakri *et al.* (letter), *ibid.*, 457.

INTERACTIONS. Combining vidarabine and human leucocyte interferon alfa was reported to increase toxicity in an uncontrolled study involving 29 patients with chronic hepatitis B. The combination led to accumulation and increased plasma concentrations of vidarabine.— S. L. Sacks *et al.*, *Antimicrob. Ag. Chemother.*, 1982, *21*, 93. See also G. Garcia *et al.*, *Ann. intern. Med.*, 1987, *107*, 278.

Inhibition of theophylline metabolism by interferon.— S. J. Williams *et al.*, *Lancet*, 1987, *2*, 939.

Antiviral Action

Interferons are produced by virus-infected cells and confer protection on uninfected cells. They affect many cell functions demonstrating, in addition to their antiviral activity, antiproliferative and immunoregulatory properties. These activities are considered to be interrelated and several enzyme systems appear to be activated by interferons to block viral and possibly cellular RNA development. Antimicrobial activity has been observed against chlamydia, plasmodium, and toxoplasma.

Studies *in vitro* have not shown that interferons inhibit all viruses and clinically their use is limited to a number of infections where studies have shown benefit and these involve hepatitis B virus, herpes simplex viruses, varicella zoster virus, human cytomegalovirus, and rhinoviruses.

Reviews of the actions of interferons: E. R. Stiehm *et al.*, *Ann. intern. Med.*, 1982, *96*, 80; B. Rager-Zisman and B. R. Bloom, *Br. med. Bull.*, 1985, *41*, 22.

Some references to the activity of interferons against individual viruses: T. L. Stanwick *et al.*, *Antimicrob. Ag. Chemother.*, 1981, *19*, 672 (herpes simplex virus; enhanced activity with acyclovir); S. M. Hammer *et al.*, *ibid.*, 1982, *21*, 634 (herpes simplex virus; enhanced activity with acyclovir); J. A. Armstrong *et al.*, *ibid.*, 1983, *24*, 137 (herpes simplex virus); C. A. Smith *et al.*, *ibid.*, 325 (human cytomegalovirus; enhanced activity with acyclovir); F. G. Hayden *et al.*, *ibid.*, 1984, *25*, 53 and 787 (influenza viruses; enhanced activity with rimantadine or tribavirin); M. Baba *et al.*, *ibid.*, 515 (varicella zoster virus; enhanced activity with vidarabine); L. E. Rasmussen *et al.*, *ibid.*, *26*, 599 (herpes simplex virus and human cytomegalovirus; comparison of cloned and native alfa and beta forms); D. D. Ho *et al.*, *Lancet*, 1985, *1*, 602 (HIV); S. W. Schalm *et al.*, *ibid.*, *2*, 358 (hepatitis B virus; enhanced activity with acyclovir); K. L. Hartshorn *et al.*, *Antimicrob. Ag. Chemother.*, 1986, *30*, 189 (HIV; Enhanced activity with fosfonet).

Absorption and Fate

Following intramuscular injection interferon alfa produced by recombinant techniques and from cultured leucocytes produce similar plasma concentrations; half-lives of up to 8 hours have been reported. Intravenous administration produces more rapid distribution and elimination. Interferon alfa does not cross the blood-brain barrier.

Interferon beta is less well absorbed than interferon alfa following intramuscular injection and is therefore usually given intravenously.

Some references to the pharmacokinetics of interferon alfa: J. U. Gutterman *et al.*, *Ann. intern. Med.*, 1982, *96*, 549; R. J. Wills *et al.*, *Clin. Pharmac. Ther.*, 1984, *35*, 283; L. D. Bornemann *et al.*, *Eur. J. clin. Pharmac.*, 1985, *28*, 469; R. J. Wills and H. E. Spiegel, *J. clin. Pharmac.*, 1985, *25*, 616.

Uses and Administration

Interferons are used for their antiviral activity as well as for their effect on certain tumours. Most of the studies on the application of this group of compounds have involved interferon alfa derived from relevant human cells or produced through recombinant DNA technology.

Interferons provide effective prophylaxis against rhinoviruses and may be useful for patients at serious risk from colds. Some studies have shown a prophylactic effect against cytomegalovirus infections in transplant patients. Herpetic infections have been treated with interferon alfa and it has formed part of effective treatment for herpetic keratitis. Condylomas and laryngeal papillomas have responded to treatment as has Kaposi's sarcoma. Malignant neoplasms reported to be responsive to interferons include hairy-cell leukaemia, chronic myeloid leukaemia, and non-Hodgkin's lymphoma.

There are now several preparations of interferons readily available with approved uses and recommended doses. Within the interferon alfa group there is interferon alfa-2a (rbe), interferon alfa-2b (rbe), and alfa-n1 (lns). In hairy cell leukaemia the dose of interferon alfa-2a or alfa-n1 is 3 million units daily by deep intramuscular or subcutaneous injection until there is improvement or for up to 24 weeks, then reduced to a maintenance dose of 3 million units three times a week. The recommended dose for interferon alfa-2b is 2 million units per m² body-surface subcutaneously three times a week. Interferon alfa-2a and alfa-2b are recommended for AIDS-related Kaposi's sarcoma; the dose of the former is 36 million units daily by intramuscular injection for 4 to 10 weeks then three times weekly for maintenance. Doses of interferon alfa-2b in chronic myelogenous leukaemia are 4 to 5 million units per m² body-surface daily by subcutaneous injection, reduced for maintenance to an alternate day schedule. Condyloma acuminata are treated by the intralesional injection of 1 million units of interferon alfa-2b on alternate days for 3 weeks; the maximum weekly dose should not exceed 15 million units. Up to 5 million units may be injected daily into multiple sites of large lesions.

Reviews and discussions on interferons: M. S. Hirsch and M. N. Swartz, *New Engl. J. Med.*, 1980, *302*, 949; G. M. Scott and D. A. J. Tyrrell, *Br. med. J.*, 1980, *280*, 1558. Correction.— *ibid.*, *281*, 695; R. B. Pollard, *Drugs*, 1982, *23*, 37; Interferon Therapy, *Tech. Rep. Ser. Wld Hlth Org. No. 676*, 1982 (see also Technical Report No. 754); J. E. Houglum, *Clin. Pharm.*, 1983, *2*, 20; T. C. Merigan, *New Engl. J. Med.*, 1983, *308*, 1530; P. G. Higgins, *J. clin. Path.*, 1984, *37*, 109; D. C. Burke, *Br. med. Bull.*, 1985, *41*, 333; G. P. Sarna, *Ann. intern. Med.*, 1987, *106*, 260.

Some references to interferons being used in a variety of disorders: D. Ikic *et al.*, *Int. J. clin. Pharmac.*, 1981, *19*, 450 (burns and ulcers); A. M. Arvin *et al.*, *Antimicrob. Ag. Chemother.*, 1982, *21*, 259 (rubella); A. Bomholt, *Archs Otolar.*, 1983, *109*, 550 (laryngeal papilloma); W. A. Hendrickse *et al.*, *Br. med. J.*, 1984, *289*, 290 (laryngeal papilloma); K. Öberg *et al.*, *Lancet*, 1985, *1*, 725 (pancreatic cholera); C. F. Nathan *et al.*, *New Engl. J. Med.*, 1986, *315*, 6 (leprosy).

AIDS. Preliminary observations in 12 homosexual men with Kaposi's sarcoma who were immunosuppressed indicated that recombinant interferon alfa might prove to be a useful treatment.— S. E. Krown *et al.*, *New Engl. J. Med.*, 1983, *308*, 1071.

Recombinant interferon alfa-2 produced a complete response in 2 and a partial response in 6 of 20 men with Kaposi's sarcoma and AIDS. The number of patients was too small to prove the superiority of a high-dose regimen over a low-dose one.— J. E. Groopman *et al.*, *Ann. intern. Med.*, 1984, *100*, 671.

A study of 16 patients with AIDS, 15 of whom also had opportunistic infections, and of corresponding controls, showed that mononuclear cells from patients in the AIDS group did not properly secrete activating lymphokines nor produce interferon gamma in response to antigen stimulation. However, macrophages from the AIDS patients were activated *in vitro* by interferon gamma. These findings suggest a rationale for using interferon gamma in the treatment of AIDS.— H. W. Murray *et al.*, *New Engl. J. Med.*, 1984, *310*, 883. The impairment of synthesis of interferon gamma by lymphocytes can also be detected in persons at risk of AIDS.— E. Buimovici-Klein *et al.* (letter), *ibid.*, *311*, 328; H. W. Murray *et al.* (letter), *ibid.*, 329. Different results were achieved in a study involving 12 patients with the lymphadenopathy syndrome and 6 with AIDS. Mononuclear cells from the majority of these patients were able to proliferate *in vitro* and generate interferon gamma.— J. L. Moore *et al.* (letter), *ibid.*, 1985, *312*, 442.

Recombinant interferon gamma produced improvement in atopic manifestations in 2 adults with AIDS.— J. M. Parkin *et al.*, *Br. med. J.*, 1987, *294*, 1185.

Reports of improvement in HIV associated thrombocytopenia with interferon alfa-2a (rbe) or interferon alfa-n1 (lns). Thrombocytopenia associated with hepatitis B also improved.— M. E. Ellis *et al.*, *Br. med. J.*, 1987, *295*, 1519; A. M. L. Lever *et al.*, *ibid.*

Further reports of interferon alfa being used to treat AIDS-related Kaposi's sarcoma: J. N. Weber *et al.*, *Gut*, 1985, *26*, 295; W. R. Frederick *et al.*, *J. infect. Dis.*, 1985, *152*, 162.

COMMON COLD. Various studies demonstrating that interferon alfa given intranasally could provide effective prophylaxis against the common cold, although there may be problems of local irritation: S. B. Greenberg *et al.*, *J. infect. Dis.*, 1982, *145*, 542; G. M. Scott *et al.*, *Br. med. J.*, 1982, *284*, 1822; G. M. Scott *et al.*, *Lancet*, 1982, *2*, 186; C. Herzog *et al.* (letter), *ibid.*, 1983, *2*, 962; P. G. Higgins *et al.*, *Antimicrob. Ag. Chemother.*, 1983, *24*, 713; B. M. Farr *et al.*, *ibid.*, 1984, *26*, 31; D. A. J. Tyrrell, *J. antimicrob. Chemother.*, 1986, *18*, *Suppl. B*, 153; R. M. Douglas *et al.*, *New Engl. J. Med.*, 1986, *314*, 65; F. G. Hayden *et al.*, *ibid.*, 71.

CONDYLOMAS. Beneficial results, but not complete cures, with interferon alfa in the topical treatment of widespread vaginal flat condylomata.— E. Vesterinen *et al.* (letter), *Lancet*, 1984, *1*, 157.

In an open study in women with condylomata acuminata intramuscular administration of interferon beta was found to be a more suitable route than topical application of a cream or subcutaneous intralesional injections. In a subsequent double-blind study 9 women and 2 men with condylomata acuminata were given interferon beta 2 million units by intramuscular (intragluteal) injection daily for 10 consecutive days and 11 women were given placebo. Lesions disappeared from about 5 weeks after completion of the course of injections in 9 of the 11 treated patients (82%) and only 2 of the 11 control patients (18%). After 3 months the two non-responders in the treated group and 6 in the placebo group were given another course of 10 injections of interferon beta and all responded to treatment. None of the treated patients who responded had had a recurrence in 10 to 12 months. Side-effects were mild fever, myalgia, "flu-like" syndrome, and headaches (lasting for 3 to 4 hours).— A. Schonfeld *et al.*, *Lancet*, 1984, *1*, 1038. Resolution of vaginal warts was also achieved in 12 women by intramuscular injections of interferon alfa in doses of 4 to 6 million units three times weekly for 6 weeks; cervical and vulval warts also responded to this treatment.— A. B. Alawattegama and G. R. Kinghorn (letter), *ibid.*, 1468. A note of caution.— G. Gross *et al.* (letter), *ibid.*, 1467.

Intralesional injection of interferon alfa-2b produced significantly better improvement in genital warts than placebo in a multicentre study.— L. J. Eron *et al.*, *New Engl. J. Med.*, 1986, *315*, 1059.

Further references to interferons in the treatment of warts: J. R. Gibson *et al.*, *Br. J. Derm.*, 1986, *115*, *Suppl.* 31, 76.

CYTOMEGALOVIRUS INFECTION. Preliminary results of a double-blind controlled study in 41 patients undergoing renal transplantation suggested that a prophylactic course of interferon alfa delayed the shedding of cytomegalovirus and decreased the incidence of viraemia after transplantation when compared with placebo, whereas treatment with antithymocyte immunoglobulin was associated with an increase in the severity of cytomegalovirus infection. Effects on herpes simplex infection were less striking but the trend was similar.— S. H. Cheeseman *et al.*, *New Engl. J. Med.*, 1979, *300*, 1345. Study of these patients also indicated that increasing immunosuppression with antithymocyte immunoglobulin increased excretion of Epstein-Barr virus but this was partially reversed in patients also receiving interferon.— S. H. Cheeseman *et al.*, *Ann. intern. Med.*, 1980, *93*, 39.

Interferon alfa was given to 20 renal transplant patients by intramuscular injection in a dose of 3 million units three times a week for 6 weeks reduced to twice a week for a further 8 weeks. Treatment was started just before transplantation. One of these patients developed the cytomegalovirus syndrome during a period when he missed some doses. Seven of 22 similar patients given a placebo under double-blind conditions developed the syndrome. Cytomegalovirus was isolated from 12 of 20 interferon-alfa recipients and 17 of 22 placebo recipients; urinary excretion of cytomegalovirus was delayed in interferon-alfa recipients who also received antithymocyte immunoglobulin.— M. S. Hirsch *et al.*, *New Engl. J. Med.*, 1983, *308*, 1489.

Lack of benefit with interferon alfa in the treatment of cytomegalovirus retinitis in 4 patients, 3 of them with AIDS.— S. Chou *et al.*, *Antimicrob. Ag. Chemother.*, 1984, *25*, 25.

Further studies and reports of the use of interferon in patients receiving organ and tissue transplants.— W. Weimar *et al.*, *Eur. J. clin. Invest.*, 1978, *8*, 255; J. D. Meyers *et al.*, *J. infect. Dis.*, 1980, *141*, 555.

See also under Effects on Blood in Adverse Effects, above.

HEPATITIS. In a double-blind study administration of interferon alfa did not appear to have any beneficial effect in 8 patients with chronic HBsAg-positive hepatitis when compared with 8 similarly affected control patients who received albumin as placebo. The interferon was given in a dose of 12 million units daily by intramuscular injection in the first week, this dose being subsequently halved each week until discontinuation after the sixth week. The only effect on the hepatitis was a transient reduction in DNA-polymerase activity, without apparent clinical significance. Side-effects included chills and/or fever in all of the 8 patients after the first injection and one patient had increasing hair loss. Leucocytes decreased significantly during the first 3 weeks of treatment and 6 patients developed leucopenia; thrombocytes also decreased significantly after the first week of treatment.— W. Weimar *et al.*, *Lancet*, 1980, *1*, 336. Better results have been obtained with much higher doses (400 to 900 million units) and patients must be treated for 4 to 6 months and followed up for 6 to 12 months.— T. C. Merigan *et al.* (letter), *ibid.*, 422. Comment.— W. Weimar and H. Schellekens (letter), *ibid.*, 590.

A more recent report of loss of HBsAg with lymphoblastoid interferon given in a dose of 10 million units per m² body-surface daily then adjusted to 3 times a week for 6 months or until HBeAg was not detectable.— G. J. M. Alexander *et al.*, *Lancet*, 1987, *2*, 66. There was no difference in response to placebo or similar doses of recombinant interferon alfa-2 given for 12 weeks to Chinese children positive for HBsAg.—C. -L Lai *et al.*, *Ibid.*, 877.

Combinations of interferons are also being tried.— W. H. Caselmann *et al.* (letter), *ibid.*, 454; V. Carreno and I. Mora (letter), *ibid.*, 1086.

A discussion on corticosteroid with interferon treatment for hepatitis B.— T. F. Kirn, *J. Am. med. Ass.*, 1987, *258*, 427.

Further references to interferon alfa in hepatitis B: D. M. Novick *et al.*, *Gut*, 1984, *25*, A541 (comparison with vidarabine); M. G. Anderson *et al.*, *ibid.*, A570 (effect on natural killer activity); M. Mondelli *et al.*, *ibid.*, A1178 (susceptibility of hepatocytes *in vitro*); K. G. Nicholson, *Lancet*, 1984, *2*, 736 (short review with reference to combined therapy with vidarabine); S. W. Schalm *et al.*, *ibid.*, 1985, *2*, 358 (enhanced activity with acyclovir in chronic hepatitis B); M. G. Anderson *et al.*, *Gut*, 1987, *28*, 619 (improvement in chronic active hepatitis B limited to treatment period); E. M. McDonald *et al.*, *Lancet*, 1987, *2*, 1175 (increase in psychiatric morbidity with interferon treatment of hepatitis B); F. La Banda *et al.* (letter), *ibid.*, 1988, *1*, 250 (response in children).

Reports of patients with non-A, non-B hepatitis improving on treatment with interferon alfa.— J. H. Hoofnagle *et al.*, *New Engl. J. Med.*, 1986, *315*, 1575; B. J. Thomson *et al.*, *Lancet*, 1987, *1*, 539.

See also under Adverse Effects, above.

HERPES SIMPLEX. Interferon alfa significantly reduced the reactivation of latent herpes simplex infection when compared with placebo in a double-blind study in 37 patients, with a history of herpes infection, who underwent an operation on the trigeminal root, a procedure associated with reactivation. Interferon alfa 70 000 units per kg body-weight daily was given intramuscularly morning and evening for 5 days starting on the day before operation. Total reactivation occurred in 9 of 19 patients given interferon compared with 15 of 18 given placebo.— G. J. Pazin *et al.*, *New Engl. J. Med.*, 1979, *301*, 225. Follow-up 3 weeks after surgery revealed recurrence in some patients who had remained asymptomatic throughout the initial period of observation. A subsequent survey of patients involved in the study suggested that a single course of treatment of a recurrent herpes simplex infection, with interferon, does not itself cure latency in the neural ganglions.— H. W. Haverkos *et al.* (letter), *ibid.*, 1980, *303*, 699.

Significant improvement in labial and genital herpes with topical interferon beta.— M. Glezerman *et al.*, *Lancet*, 1988, *1*, 150.

Keratitis. Eleven patients with dendritic keratitis obtained a beneficial response (mean healing time: 2.9 days) to daily application of 5 drops of trifluridine 1% in association with 2 drops of a preparation containing 30 million units of interferon alfa per mL. There was no significant difference between 15 patients who received the trifluridine with albumin (mean healing time: 5.7 days) and those who received it with an interferon-alfa preparation containing only 1 million units per mL (mean healing time: 5.3 days).— R. Sundmacher *et al.* (letter), *Lancet*, 1978, *2*, 687. A further study involving 38 patients with keratitis did not demonstrate any difference in effectiveness between interferon alfa 100 million units per mL and 30 million units per mL when one drop was given daily in conjunction with one drop of trifluridine 1% five times daily.— *idem*, *Archs Ophthal.*, *N.Y.*, 1984, *102*, 554. Another controlled study involving 53 patients with dendritic keratitis and confirmed infection with herpes simplex virus. The combination treatment of 2 drops daily of interferon alfa 10 million units per mL with 5 drops daily of trifluridine 1% reduced partial and complete healing times to a significantly greater extent than trifluridine and placebo; the partial healing times were 3.3 and 6.5 days while the complete healing times were 6.6 and 11.3 days. All healing times were considered to be better than those achieved with no treatment. Interferon alfa and placebo were each given until the third day of partial healing. Trifluridine was continued until complete healing occurred.— E. W. J.

de Koning *et al.*, *Br. J. Ophthal.*, 1982, *66*, 509.

HERPES ZOSTER. Three double-blind controlled studies in 90 patients with cancer assessed the effect of interferon alfa given intramuscularly at doses between 42 000 and 510 000 units per kg body-weight daily in the treatment of early localised herpes zoster infections. At the highest dose early treatment prevented cutaneous dissemination completely and reduced the spread of infection within the primary dermatome. Visceral complications were also reduced among interferon recipients. Post-herpetic neuralgia was less severe at the higher doses.— T. C. Merigan *et al.*, *New Engl. J. Med.*, 1978, *298*, 981. Comments and criticisms.— M. S. Hirsch, *ibid.*, 1022; W. Weimar and H. Schellekens (letter), *ibid.*, 1979, *300*, 923. A reply.— T. C. Merigan (letter), *ibid.*, 924. A later series of 2 multicentre double-blind controlled studies involving 44 children being treated for cancer showed that interferon alfa started within 72 hours of the appearance of the varicella exanthem reduced the number of days of new lesion formation. Doses in the first study ranged from 42 000 to 250 000 units per kg body-weight daily by intramuscular injection until no new vesicles had appeared for 24 hours; in the second study 350 000 units per kg were given daily for 2 days then 175 000 units per kg daily for 3 days.— A. M. Arvin *et al.*, *ibid.*, 1982, *306*, 761. See also T. C. Merigan *et al.*, *Antimicrob. Ag. Chemother.*, 1981, *19*, 193.

Encephalitis. Three patients with viral encephalitis were treated with interferon beta 0.5 to 1.2 million units intrathecally daily for 8 to 10 days. The 2 patients in whom the virus was not identified improved dramatically. The third patient whose encephalitis was due to varicella zoster virus relapsed and required a second course within 3 weeks; this produced further improvement until another relapse 6 months later. Problems associated with this treatment were transient fever, a slight increase in liver enzyme concentrations, and, in 2 patients, an occasional fall in blood pressure.— H. Prange and H. Wismann (letter), *New Engl. J. Med.*, 1981, *305*, 1283.

MALIGNANT NEOPLASMS. Many reports have been published on the effects of interferons on various neoplasms; many have involved human interferon alfa and some recombinant interferon alfa. Some deal with interferon beta and interferon gamma is being assessed.

Large doses of interferon alfa have been tried although there is a limit to what patients may tolerate because of adverse effects (S.A. Sherwin *et al.*, *J. Am. med. Ass.*, 1982, *248*, 2461; K. Sikora and H. Smedley, *Br. med. J.*, 1983, *286*, 739).

Tumours that have shown benefit from human interferon alfa include malignant neoplasms of the breast (J. Gutterman *et al.*, *Ann. intern. Med.*, 1980, *93*, 399; E.C. Borden *et al.*, *ibid.*, 1982, *97*, 1) although Sherwin *et al.* (*ibid.*, 1983, *98*, 598) did not obtain any benefit with recombinant interferon alfa. Metastatic carcinoid tumours improved in some patients given human interferon alfa (K. Öberg *et al.*, *New Engl. J. Med.*, 1983, *309*, 129) and in one patient given interferon beta (D.R. Strayer *et al.*, *J. Am. med. Ass.*, 1984, *251*, 1682).

Patients with hairy-cell leukaemia have obtained remissions with human or recombinant interferon alfa (J.R. Quesada *et al.*, *New Engl. J. Med.*, 1984, *310*, 15; J.T.P. Janssen *et al.*, *Lancet*, 1984, *1*, 1025; M.J. Ratain *et al.*, *Blood*, 1985, *65*, 644; B.D. Cheson and A. Martin, *Ann. intern. Med.*, 1987, *106*, 871) and preparations of interferon alfa are available for this condition. Chronic myelogenous leukaemia has also responded to interferon alfa, usually recombinant (M. Talpaz *et al.*, *New Engl. J. Med.*, 1986, *314*, 1065; *idem*, *Blood*, 1987, *69*, 1280).

Non-Hodgkin's lymphomas have responded to recombinant interferon alfa (K.A. Foon *et al.*, *New Engl. J. Med.*, 1984, *311*, 1148; P.A. Bunn *et al.*, *Ann. intern. Med.*, 1984, *101*, 484). Responses have been observed in patients with malignant melanoma given human interferon alfa with cimetidine (S. Borgström *et al.*, *New Engl. J. Med.*, 1982, *307*, 1080) as well as in patients given recombinant interferon alfa (J.M. Kirkwood *et al.*, *Ann. intern. Med.*, 1985, *103*, 32; J.R. Quesada *et al.*, *Blood*, 1986, *67*, 275).

Some further references to the use of interferon alfa in various neoplasms: H. Mellstedt *et al.*, *Lancet*, 1979, *1*, 245 (myeloma); J. U. Gutterman *et al.*, *Ann. intern. Med.*, 1980, *93*, 399 (myeloma and lymphoma as well as breast cancer); T. J. Priestman, *Lancet*, 1980, *2*, 113 (tolerance in advanced malignant disease); D. Ikič *et al.*, *ibid.*, 1981, *1*, 1022 (breast cancer; bladder cancer; melanoma); *idem*, 1025 (cancer of the head and neck); *idem*, 1027 (cervical carcinoma); S. J. Horning *et al.*, *J. Am. med. Ass.*, 1982, *247*, 1718 (tolerance in advanced malignant neoplasms); J. B. deKernion *et al.*, *J. Urol., Baltimore*, 1983, *130*, 1063 (renal carcinoma); J. M. Kirkwood *et al.*, *Cancer Res.*, 1985, *45*, 863 (renal carcinoma); J. S. Berek *et al.*, *ibid.*, 4447 (ovarian cancer); R. Ohno *et al.*, *Cancer Chemother. Pharmac.*, 1985, *14*, 34 (multiple myeloma, plasma cell leukaemia, and primary macroglobulinaemia); B. Eriksson *et al.*, *Lancet*, 1986, *2*, 1307 (malignant endocrine pancreatic tumours); R. G. Steis *et al.*, *New Engl. J. Med.*, 1988, *318*, 1409 (resistance in hairy-cell leukaemia).

MULTIPLE SCLEROSIS. Interferon is reported to stabilise or improve exacerbations of multiple sclerosis. Both interferon alfa (R.L. Knobler *et al.*, *Neurology*, 1984, *34*, 1273; H.S. Panitch, *Archs Neurol.*, 1987, *44*, 61) and interferon beta (L. Jacobs *et al.*, *Lancet*, 1986, *2*, 1411) have been used and administration has been by the intrathecal route for interferon beta and sometimes for interferon alfa (see p.697 under Adverse Effects). Interferon gamma exacerbates multiple sclerosis (H.S. Panitch *et al.*, *Lancet*, 1987, *1*, 893; M.A. Armstrong *et al.*, *ibid.*, 1369).

Proprietary Preparations

Intron A *(Kirkby-Warwick, UK)*. *Injection*, powder for reconstitution, interferon alfa-2b (rbe) 3, 5, 10, and 30 million units per vial.

Roferon-A *(Roche, UK)*. *Injection*, powder for reconstitution, interferon alfa-2a (rbe) 3, 9, and 18 million units per vial.

Wellferon *(Wellcome, UK)*. *Injection*, interferon alfa-n1 (lns) 3 or 10 million units per vial.

Proprietary Names and Manufacturers

Berofor *(Basotherm, Ger.)*; Exovir-HZ *(Exovir, USA)*; Fiblaferon *(Rentschler, Ger.)*; Frone *(Serono, Hong Kong; Inter-Yeda, Israel; Serono, Ital.)*; Immuneron; Intron A *(Essex, Austral.; Schering, Canad.; Kirby-Warrick, Eire; Essex, Ger.; Scherag, S.Afr.; Essex, Switz.; Kirby-Warrick, UK; Schering, USA)*; Introna *(Schering Corp., Denm.; Schering, Swed.)*; Roferon-A *(Roche, Fr.; Roche, Ger.; Roche, UK; Roche, USA)*; Wellferon *(Pacific, Canad.; Wellcome, UK)*.

1684-x

Methisazone *(BAN, USAN)*.

33-T-57; AN-5051; *N*-Methylisatin β-Thiosemicarbazone; Metisazone *(rINN)*. 1-Methylindoline-2,3-dione 3-thiosemicarbazone.

$C_{10}H_{10}N_4OS = 234.3$.

CAS — 1910-68-5.

An orange-yellow powder. Practically **insoluble** in water and in dilute mineral acids; soluble 1 in 800 of chloroform, and 1 in 2000 of methyl alcohol; soluble in warm dilute solutions of alkali hydroxides and in hot glacial acetic acid. **Protect** from light.

Freshly prepared methisazone occurred as orange-yellow fluffy microneedles. On standing, the milled powder slowly developed outgrowths or 'whiskers', which showed that the powder was unsuitable for pharmaceutical use. In solution, a short exposure to light caused a reversible change, but irreversible decomposition occurred on prolonged exposure.— J. C. Deavin and D. H. Mitchell, *J. Pharm. Pharmac.*, 1965, *17*, 56S.

The properties of methisazone and the problems of formulating suspensions and tablets.— A. Axon, *J. mond. Pharm.*, 1972, *15*, 221.

A study of the crystal modification of methisazone by grinding; there appeared to be at least 2 polymorphic forms of methisazone.— K. C. Lee and J. A. Hersey, *J. Pharm. Pharmac.*, 1977, *29*, 249.

Adverse Effects

Nausea and vomiting are common side-effects during treatment with methisazone. Anorexia, diarrhoea, skin rashes, and alopecia may also occur.

Precautions

Methisazone is contra-indicated in patients with impaired liver function except in vaccination complications and in subjects accidentally exposed to laboratory specimens of smallpox virus.

Alcohol taken concomitantly may enhance the side-effects.

Antiviral Action

Methisazone is active against pox viruses and RNA viruses probably through inhibition of viral protein synthesis.

Absorption and Fate

Methisazone is irregularly absorbed from the gastro-intestinal tract. It is extensively metabolised in the body and is excreted in the urine as metabolites and unchanged drug.

Uses and Administration

Methisazone was formerly used in the prophylaxis of smallpox when adults were given two doses each of 3 g. It was also used in the treatment of eczema vaccinatum and vaccinia gangrenosa when an initial dose of 200 mg per kg body-weight was given followed by 50 mg per kg every 6 hours for 8 doses, repeated, if necessary, after 7 days.

For reports on the use of methisazone, see Martindale 28th Edn, p. 823.

Proprietary Names and Manufacturers

Marboran *(Wellcome, Switz.; Wellcome, UK)*.

12979-y

Moroxydine Hydrochloride *(BANM, rINNM)*.

ABOB. 1-(Morpholinoformimidoyl)guanidine hydrochloride.

$C_6H_{13}N_5O,HCl = 207.7$.

CAS — 3731-59-7 (moroxydine); 3160-91-6 (hydrochloride).

Moroxydine hydrochloride has been used in the prophylaxis and treatment of various herpes infections. Usual doses range from 200 to 400 mg by mouth three or four times daily.

Proprietary Names and Manufacturers

Biguan *(Septa, Spain)*; Flumadon *(Globopharm, Switz.)*; Flumidin *(Kabi, Ger.)*; Virustat *(Delagrange, Belg.; Delagrange, Fr.)*.

1686-f

Rimantadine Hydrochloride *(USAN, rINNM)*.

α-Methyl-1-adamantanemethylamine Hydrochloride; EXP-126. 1-(1-Adamantyl)ethylamine hydrochloride; 1-(Tricyclo[3.3.1.1^{3,7}]dec-1-yl)ethylamine hydrochloride.

$C_{12}H_{21}N,HCl = 215.8$.

CAS — 13392-28-4 (rimantadine); 1501-84-4 (hydrochloride).

Adverse Effects

The incidence and severity of adverse effects associated with rimantadine appear to be low. Those reported include gastro-intestinal disturbances such as nausea and vomiting, and central nervous system effects such as insomnia, nightmares, anxiety or nervousness, and concentration difficulties.

A double-blind placebo-controlled study in healthy subjects to compare the relative toxicities of equal doses of rimantadine hydrochloride and amantadine hydrochloride. Both drugs were well tolerated at doses of 200 mg daily for 4.5 days, but rimantadine was significantly better tolerated than amantadine at a dosage of 300 mg daily. At the higher dosage the amantadine recipients reported significantly more frequent and prominent side-effects related to the central nervous system (nervousness, lightheadedness, difficulty concentrating and sleep disturbance) than did rimantadine or placebo recipients; performance was also significantly decreased. Both amantadine and rimantadine recipients reported gastro-intestinal complaints (loss of appetite, nausea) significantly more frequently than did the placebo group. Rimantadine appeared to offer more promise than amantadine because of better tolerance at increased dosage.— F. G. Hayden *et al.*, *Antimicrob. Ag. Chemother.*, 1981, *19*, 226. The differences in adverse effects between the 2 drugs might be related to differences in pharmacokinetics.— F. G. Hayden *et al.*, *ibid.*, 1983, *23*, 458.

Comparable and minimal central nervous system adverse effects with rimantadine, amantadine, or chlorpheniramine.— V. M. Millet *et al.*, *Antimicrob. Ag. Chemother.*, 1982, *21*, 1.

A double-blind placebo-controlled study to evaluate the safety of rimantadine hydrochloride for elderly, chronically ill individuals during an influenza A epidemic. Rimantadine hydrochloride 100 mg twice daily was administered to 18 patients of whom 11 completed the study and received rimantadine for a mean of 80 days; 17 similar patients received placebo. A significantly greater proportion of the rimantadine group developed anxiety and/or nausea compared with the placebo group; there was also a significantly greater number of days in which anxiety, nausea, confusion, depression, or vomiting were reported. Most of these side-effects lasted less than 9 days and were seldom severe except in 2 patients who withdrew after days 5 and 9 because of insomnia, anxiety, or both. Plasma concentrations of rimantadine obtained 3 to 4 hours after the last dose ranged from 0.634 to 2.602 μg per mL. Additional pharmacokinetic studies should be carried out to determine whether lower dosages should be prescribed in the elderly.— P. A. Patriarca *et al., Antimicrob. Ag. Chemother.*, 1984, *26*, 101.

Antiviral Action

Rimantadine hydrochloride inhibits influenza A viruses.

Studies of the action of rimantadine *in vitro* against influenza type A virus: G. A. Galegov *et al.* (letter), *Lancet*, 1979, *1*, 269; W. C. Koff and V. Knight, *Proc. Soc. exp. Biol. Med.*, 1979, *160*, 246.

Rimantadine, at concentrations ranging from 0.5 to 2 μg per mL, was found to be more effective *in vitro* against influenza A viruses than amantadine at the same concentrations; these concentrations were comparable to those achieved in the plasma after administration of amantadine 200 mg daily by mouth. Both drugs showed increasing antiviral acitvity as concentrations were increased, however, at concentrations of 16 and 32 μg per mL rimantadine was found to be toxic to ferret tracheal ciliated epithelium during weeks 2 to 3 whereas amantadine appeared to be nontoxic.— D. B. Burlington *et al., Antimicrob. Ag. Chemother.*, 1982, *21*, 794.

The combination of rimantadine hydrochloride and tribavirin resulted in an enhanced antiviral effect *in vitro* against influenza A viruses compared with the effects of either drug alone.— F. G. Hayden *et al., Antimicrob. Ag. Chemother.*, 1980, *18*, 536.

Interferon alfa-2 interacted additively or synergistically *in vitro* with rimantadine hydrochloride or tribavirin in the inhibition of influenza virus replication.— F. G. Hayden *et al., Antimicrob. Ag. Chemother.*, 1984, *25*, 53 and 787.

Absorption and Fate

Rimantadine hydrochloride is absorbed from the gastro-intestinal tract. It has a long plasma half-life; reported figures ranging from 24 to 33 hours.

References to the pharmacokinetics of rimantadine: R. J. Wills *et al., Antimicrob. Ag. Chemother.*, 1987, *31*, 826; E. L. Anderson *et al., ibid.*, 1140.

Uses and Administration

Rimantadine hydrochloride is used similarly to amantadine hydrochloride (see p.1009) in the prophylaxis and treatment of influenza A infections. It has been given in usual doses of 200 mg daily by mouth in single or divided doses.

INFLUENZA. Reviews and discussions on the use of rimantadine in the prophylaxis and treatment of influenza infections: D. M. Zlydnikov *et al., Rev. infect. Dis.*, 1981, *3*, 408.

Rimantadine hydrochloride 150 mg, amantadine hydrochloride 100 mg, or a placebo, was given twice daily for 10 days to 95 patients with influenza due to type A virus. The duration of fever in the 3 groups was 19 hours, 23 hours, and 45 hours respectively, and overall clinical improvement was more rapid in those taking the drugs than the placebo. Serological conversion occurred in 35 of 48 taking the placebo, 21 of 24 taking rimantadine, and 19 of 23 taking amantadine.— W. L. Wingfield *et al., New Engl. J. Med.*, 1969, *281*, 579.

Both amantadine and rimantadine in doses of 100 mg twice daily by mouth produced faster resolution of symptoms and signs of influenza in naturally infected subjects than placebo. In addition, both frequency and quantity of virus shed were diminished in drug recipients. Although minor central side-effects were noted with amantadine there was a slight, but not striking, therapeutic advantage with amantadine when compared with rimantadine.— L. P. Van Voris *et al., J. Am. med. Ass.*, 1981, *245*, 1128. In a double-blind placebo-controlled study of 450 healthy subjects both rimantadine and amantadine, given in doses of 100 mg twice daily by mouth for 6 weeks, were highly effective in preventing influenza-like illness; compared with placebo, reductions in the rates of illness of 65% and 78%, respectively, were found. However, significant differences in the rates of side-effects were observed. Rimantadine was not associated with side-effects any more frequently than placebo, but amantadine recipients had a higher rate of side-effects, largely central symptoms, than either placebo or rimantadine recipients. On the basis of this study, rimantadine appeared to be the drug of choice for the chemoprophylaxis of influenza A.— R. Dolin *et al., New Engl. J. Med.*, 1982, *307*, 580. There is little evidence that current dosage regimens are equivalent for amantadine and rimantadine. Further clinical studies based on pharmacokinetic data are necessary to decide which drug is superior.— R. G. Douglas, *ibid.*, 617.

In a study involving 36 healthy subjects rimantadine by inhalation had a therapeutic effect comparable to that found with larger doses of rimantadine by mouth in experimental influenza type A infection.— F. G. Hayden *et al., Antiviral Res.*, 1982, *2*, 147.

Rimantadine, generally in a single daily dose of 200 mg for 5 days produced a rapid reduction in virus titre and oral temperature in 7 patients with influenza A (H3N2) than did placebo given to 7 other patients. Rimantadine also tended to produce a more rapid resolution of respiratory and systemic symptoms.— F. G. Hayden and A. S. Monto, *Antimicrob. Ag. Chemother.*, 1986, *29*, 339.

Proprietary Names and Manufacturers

Roflual *(Roche, Fr.)*;

Manufacturers also include—*Du Pont, USA*.

1687-d

Stallimycin Hydrochloride *(USAN, pINNM)*.

Distamycin A Hydrochloride; FI-6426. *N*″-(2-Amidinoethyl)-4-formamido-1,1′,1″-trimethyl-*N*,4′:*N*′,4″-ter-[pyrrole-2-carboxamide] hydrochloride.

$C_{22}H_{27}N_9O_4,HCl=518$.

CAS — 636-47-5 (stallimycin); 6576-51-8 (hydrochloride).

Stallimycin hydrochloride is an antibiotic derived from *Streptomyces distallicus*. A yellowish white crystalline powder. M.p. 184° to 187°.

Adverse Effects and Precautions

Hypersensitivity reactions may occur after topical application of stallimycin hydrochloride. It should be applied with care to patients with kidney or liver impairment. Preparations containing stallimycin hydrochloride should not be applied to the conjunctiva.

Uses and Administration

Stallimycin hydrochloride is an antibiotic which has been reported to have antiviral activity against DNA viruses such as herpesviruses and vaccinia. It has been used in the form of a 1% ointment or paste for cutaneous or mucocutaneous infections produced by herpes simplex, herpes zoster, and vaccinia viruses.

References to the clinical use of stallimycin hydrochloride: D. Bassetti, *G. Mal. infett. parassit.*, 1968, *20*, 827 (varicella); D. Bassetti, *G. Mal. infett. parassit.*, 1969, *21*, 849 (severe herpes zoster); A. De Vriendt and I. Weemaes, *G. Mal. infett. parassit.*, 1972, *24*, 63 (chickenpox, herpes zoster, and vaccinia).

Proprietary Names and Manufacturers

Herperal *(Farmitalia, Ital.)*.

1685-r

Tribavirin *(BAN)*.

ICN-1229; Ribavirin *(USAN, pINN)*. 1-β-D-Ribofuranosyl-1*H*-1,2,4-triazole-3-carboxamide.

$C_8H_{12}N_4O_5=244.2$.

CAS — 36791-04-5.

Adverse Effects and Precautions

Patients have experienced increased serum-bilirubin concentrations when given tribavirin by mouth. Other effects that have been reported include headache, abdominal cramps, fatigue, and reversible anaemia.

When given by inhalation tribavirin has sometimes caused deterioration in pulmonary function and adverse effects on the cardiovascular system including a fall in blood pressure and cardiac arrest. Tribavirin given by this route may adversely affect any ventilation equipment being used coincidentally.

Tribavirin has been reported to be teratogenic in *animals*.

Animal toxicity of tribavirin, including teratogenicity.— L. H. Kilham and V. H. Ferm, *Science*, 1977, *195*, 413; D. M. Kochhar *et al., Toxic. appl. Pharmac.*, 1980, *52*, 99.

Tribavirin and zidovudine inhibited each others' antiviral activity *in vitro*.— M. W. Vogt *et al., Science*, 1987, *235*, 1376.

Antiviral Action

Tribavirin inhibits a wide variety of viruses. However, activity *in vitro* and in *animal* models has not necessarily correlated with activity against human infections. Tribavirin is phosphorylated but its mode of action is still unclear. Susceptible DNA viruses include herpes viruses. Susceptible RNA viruses include lassa virus, members of the bunyaviridae group, influenza, parainfluenza, measles, mumps, and respiratory syncytial viruses, togaviridae, and human immunodeficiency virus (HIV).

The combination of rimantadine hydrochloride and tribavirin resulted in an enhanced antiviral effect *in vitro* against influenza A viruses compared with the effects of either drug alone.— F. G. Hayden *et al., Antimicrob. Ag. Chemother.*, 1980, *18*, 536.

Interferon alfa-2 interacted additively or synergistically *in vitro* with rimantadine hydrochloride or tribavirin in the inhibition of influenza virus replication.— F. G. Hayden *et al., Antimicrob. Ag. Chemother.*, 1984, *25*, 53 and 787.

Absorption and Fate

Tribavirin is rapidly absorbed following oral administration and peak blood concentrations have been reported within 60 to 90 minutes. It is phosphorylated to produce active metabolites and is excreted chiefly in the urine. However, there is some faecal excretion and retention in tissues, chiefly the red blood cells.

Tribavirin is also absorbed from the respiratory tract following inhalation.

Radio-immunoassay of serum samples from 4 subjects given tribavirin 1 g daily in divided doses for 10 days by mouth showed a mean concentration of 3.1 μmol. The mean serum concentration in 5 subjects given 4 g of tribavirin daily in divided doses intravenously was 32.1 μmol. The mean plasma concentration in 4 children given tribavirin by aerosol for several hours a day for 3 days at a dose of 820 μg per kg body-weight per hour was 0.8 μmol.— R. K. Austin *et al., Antimicrob. Ag. Chemother.*, 1983, *24*, 696.

Distribution of tribavirin into the CSF in man.— C. Crampacker *et al.* (letter), *Lancet*, 1986, *2*, 45.

Uses and Administration

Tribavirin is effective against several viral infections. Influenza A and B have been reported to respond to tribavirin administered by aerosol as have respiratory syncytial viral infections; this route appears to give better results than the oral route. Other infections being studied include lassa fever.

Up to 1 g daily has been given in divided doses by mouth. The aerosol form of tribavirin has been delivered at a constant rate for periods ranging from several hours a day to almost continuous administration.

Preparations of tribavirin have recently become available for administration to infants and children with severe respiratory syncytial infections via a small particle aerosol generator. Solutions containing 20 mg per mL are used; over a 12-hour period 300 mL, representing 6 g of tribavirin, are delivered by aerosol at an average concentration of 190 μg per litre of air. Treatment is for 3 to 7 days and may be extended to 18 hours a day. The triacetate is also under study.

AIDS. No benefit from tribavirin in 7 children with HIV infection.— S. Blanche *et al.* (letter), *Lancet*, 1986, *1*, 863.

HEPATITIS. In a double-blind placebo-controlled study tribavirin 100 mg given by mouth every 6 hours for 10 days produced beneficial signs in the treatment of acute hepatitis B.— P. A. Ayrosa-Galvão and I. O. Castro, *Ann. N.Y. Acad. Sci.*, 1977, *284*, 278. In 13 patients with chronic hepatitis B virus infection, given tribavirin usually 800 mg daily for 21 days, the failure of treatment to cause disappearance of surface antigen from the serum suggested that treatment was not likely to be effective. One patient, and a 14th patient, developed transient mild intravascular haemolysis.— M. C. Kew and H. C. Seftel (letter), *Br. med. J.*, 1977, *1*, 904. Another report showing lack of benefit from tribavirin in chronic hepatitis B.— S. Jain *et al.*, *J. antimicrob. Chemother.*, 1978, *4*, 367. Improvement in hepatitis A with tribavirin.— S. A. Patki and P. Gupta, *Chemotherapy, Basle*, 1982, *28*, 298.

INFLUENZA. Conflicting results have been obtained in studies of tribavirin being given to treat influenza. Cohen *et al.* (*J. infect. Dis.*, 1976, *133*, *Suppl.*, A144) showed little benefit from tribavirin given by mouth in artificially induced influenza type A although Salido-Rengell *et al.* (*Ann. N.Y. Acad. Sci.*, 1977, *284*, 272) and Magnussen *et al.* (*Antimicrob. Ag. Chemother.*, 1977, *12*, 498) demonstrated activity. Influenza type B also failed to respond to tribavirin given by mouth in a study by Togo and McCracken (*J. infect. Dis.*, 1976, *133*, *Suppl.*, A109). More recent studies have shown that tribavirin administered by aerosol was effective in both types of influenza (V. Knight *et al.*, *Lancet*, 1981, *2*, 945; H.W. McClung *et al.*, *J. Am. med. Ass.*, 1983, *249*, 2671; B.E. Gilbert *et al.*, *Antimicrob. Ag. Chemother.*, 1985, *27*, 309).

LASSA FEVER. Lassa fever in *monkeys* responded to tribavirin given intramuscularly.— E. L. Stephen and P. B. Jahrling (letter), *Lancet*, 1979, *1*, 268. An enhanced response was obtained when *monkeys* were given tribavirin with lassa virus antiserum.— P. B. Jahrling *et al.*, *J. infect. Dis.*, 1984, *149*, 420.

A reduction in the fatality-rate of lassa fever in patients given tribavirin, especially within 6 days of the onset of fever. Tribavirin was given intravenously in a loading dose of 2 g then 1 g every six hours for 4 days then, 500 mg every eight hours for 6 days.— J. B. McCormick *et al.*, *New Engl. J. Med.*, 1986, *314*, 20.

PNEUMONIA. Following a preliminary study in which volunteers with experimental respiratory syncytial viral infection showed a beneficial response to tribavirin given by aerosol (C.B. Hall *et al.*, *J. Am. med. Ass.*, 1983, *249*, 2666), a double-blind study was set up involving 33 infants with pneumonia due to the virus. Tribavirin was given to 16 of the infants by aerosol for a minimum of 3 days. The particles in the aerosol were about 1.3 micrometre in diameter and were administered at a rate of 12.5 litres per minute. The reservoir contained 20 mg of tribavirin per mL. When compared with placebo, tribavirin produced significant improvement in lower respiratory-tract signs and in arterial oxygen saturation and diminished viral shedding.— C. B. Hall *et al.*, *New Engl. J. Med.*, 1983, *308*, 1443. See also *idem*, *J. Am. med. Ass.*, 1985, *254*, 3047.

Further references to tribavirin in respiratory syncytial viral pneumonia in children: E. W. Gelfland *et al.* (letter), *Lancet*, 1983, *2*, 732; L. H. Taber *et al.*, *Pediatrics*, 1983, *72*, 613; *Lancet*, 1986, *1*, 362; W. Barry *et al.*, *Archs Dis. Childh.*, 1986, *61*, 593.

Two children with adenovirus pneumonia improved with tribavirin given by inhalation.—R. M. Buchdahl *et al.* (letter), *Lancet*, 1985, *2*, 1070.

Proprietary Preparations

Virazid *(Britannia Pharmaceuticals, UK)*. *Inhalation*, tribavirin 6 g for reconstitution.

Proprietary Names and Manufacturers

Virazid *(Britannia Pharmaceuticals, UK)*; Virazole *(ICN, Canad.; ICN, USA)*.

1688-n

Trifluridine *(USAN, rINN).*

F_3T; F_3TDR; Trifluorothymidine. ααα-Trifluorothymidine; 2′-Deoxy-5-trifluoromethyluridine.
$C_{10}H_{11}F_3N_2O_5$=296.2.

CAS — 70-00-8.

The assessment in an *animal* model of the effect of different formulations on the penetration of trifluridine following topical application.— S. L. Spruance, *Antimicrob. Ag. Chemother.*, 1984, *26*, 819.

Adverse Effects

Adverse effects occurring after the use of trifluridine in the eyes are similar to those for idoxuridine (p.694) but have been reported to occur less frequently.

Trifluridine injected into the yolk sac was shown to be teratogenic in *chicken* embryos.— G. Kury and R. J. Crosby, *Toxic. appl. Pharmac.*, 1967, *11*, 72. Trifluridine applied topically to the eye in doses similar to those used clinically was not teratogenic to *rabbits*.— M. Itoi *et al.*, *Archs Ophthal., N.Y.*, 1975, *93*, 46.

Conjunctival cicatrisation associated in one patient with trifluridine.— I. J. Udell (letter), *Am. J. Ophthal.*, 1985, *99*, 363.

Antiviral Action

Trifluridine is structurally similar to idoxuridine and following phosphorylation it acts similarly against herpes simplex virus. It is also reported to be active against adenoviruses, varicella zoster and vaccinia viruses, and cytomegalovirus. Like idoxuridine it is incorporated into mammalian DNA.

Absorption and Fate

Trifluridine is absorbed through the cornea following ocular administration and absorption may be increased in the presence of damage or inflammation. There is no evidence of metabolism in man when trifluridine is administered by this route nor is there any evidence of systemic absorption.

Uses and Administration

Trifluridine is used in the treatment of primary keratoconjunctivitis and recurrent epithelial keratitis due to herpes simplex viruses. Some studies show it to be more effective than idoxuridine and as effective as vidarabine. Patients who have not responded to either of these two antiviral agents might respond to trifluridine; it might also be useful in patients unable to tolerate idoxuridine.

One drop of a 1% ophthalmic solution is instilled into the eye every 2 hours up to a maximum of 9 times daily until complete re-epithelialisation has occurred. Treatment is then reduced to one drop every 4 hours to a maximum of 5 drops a day for a further 7 days. It has also been used as a 1 or 2% ophthalmic ointment.

Reviews on the actions and uses of trifluridine: C. Heidelberger and D. H. King, *Pharmac. Ther.*, 1979, *6*, 427; A. A. Carmine *et al.*, *Drugs*, 1982, *23*, 329.

Trifluridine as 1% drops produced improvement in 6 eyes of 4 patients with Thygeson's superficial punctate keratitis and might be an alternative to corticosteroid therapy.— A. Nesburn *et al.*, *Ophthalmology*, 1984, *91*, 1188.

HERPES SIMPLEX KERATITIS. In a double-blind two-centre study in 40 patients with herpes simplex virus ulcers of the cornea, treatment failures were significantly lower after the use of trifluridine 1% than after the use of idoxuridine 0.1%. The mean time to healing was significantly less with trifluridine (6.3 compared with 8.2 days).— P. C. Wellings *et al.*, *Am. J. Ophthal.*, 1972, *73*, 932.

In a single-blind study, 40 patients with active herpes simplex corneal ulcers were treated with either 1% trifluridine or 0.1% idoxuridine eye-drops. There was no significant difference between the rates of healing in the 2 groups but significantly more eyes healed successfully within 14 days with trifluridine (96%) compared with idoxuridine (75%). Three patients treated with trifluridine and corticosteroids together healed, but one treated with idoxuridine and corticosteroids failed to heal; numbers were too small for statistical analysis. Of a further 15 similar patients considered to be treatment failures with idoxuridine or vidarabine, 87% healed when given trifluridine.— D. Pavan-Langston and C. S. Foster, *Am. J. Ophthal.*, 1977, *84*, 818. For another report of trifluridine being effective in herpetic keratitis resistant to other therapy, see R. A. Hyndiuk *et al.*, *Archs Ophthal., N.Y.*, 1978, *96*, 1839.

A multicentre double-blind study involving 59 patients with herpetic keratitis showed that ointments containing acyclovir 3% or trifluridine 2% applied 5 times daily for up to 16 days were equally effective. Healing occurred within an average of 6.3 days with acyclovir and 7.1 days with trifluridine. After 2 weeks' treatment 27 of 31 in the acyclovir group and 23 of 28 in the trifluridine group were healed.— C. La Lau *et al.*, *Br. J. Ophthal.*, 1982, *66*, 506.

For studies of interferon alfa being used with trifluridine in herpes keratitis, see under Interferons, p.698.

For studies indicating that trifluridine is as effective as vidarabine in the treatment of herpes simplex keratitis, see under Vidarabine, p.703.

Proprietary Names and Manufacturers

Aflomin *(Frumtost, Spain)*; Bephen *(Thilo, Ger.)*; TFT *(Thilo, Ger.; Mann, Neth.)*; Triherpin *(Dispersa, Norw.)*; Triherpine *(Dispersa, Switz.)*; Viromidin *(Cusi, Spain)*; Virophta *(Dulcis, Mon.)*; Viroptic *(Wellcome, Canad.; Wellcome, USA)*.

1689-h

Tromantadine Hydrochloride *(rINNM).*

D-41. *N*-1-Adamantyl-2-(2-dimethylaminoethoxy)acetamide hydrochloride; 2-(2-Dimethylaminoethoxy)-*N*-(tricyclo[3.3.1.1^{3,7}]dec-1-yl)acetamide hydrochloride.
$C_{16}H_{28}N_2O_2$,HCl=316.9.

CAS — 53783-83-8 (tromantadine); 41544-24-5 (hydrochloride).

Adverse Effects

Contact dermatitis has been reported following the topical use of tromantadine hydrochloride.

Of 240 patients with herpes simplex treated with a gel containing tromantadine hydrochloride 1%, 20 showed local irritation. Patch testing confirmed that this was due to contact dermatitis to tromantadine in 12 of the patients. None of the patients tested was sensitive to the gel basis.— D. Fanta and P. Mischer, *Contact Dermatitis*, 1976, *2*, 282.

Contact dermatitis after application of tromantadine hydrochloride in one patient.— G. Lembo *et al.*, *Contact Dermatitis*, 1984, *10*, 317.

Uses and Administration

Tromantadine hydrochloride is a derivative of amantadine (see p.1008) used for its antiviral activity. It is applied as a 1% ointment in the treatment of herpes simplex infections of the skin and eye.

ANTIVIRAL ACTION. Synthesis of tromantadine and its activity against herpes simplex virus. Results *in vitro* suggested that tromantadine inhibited an early event and also a late event in herpes simplex virus replication.— K. S. Rosenthal *et al.*, *Antimicrob. Ag. Chemother.*, 1982, *22*, 1031.

HERPES SIMPLEX. In a double-blind study of 20 patients with herpes simplex lesions (on the lips, skin, or genitals) tromantadine hydrochloride 1% ointment applied 6 times daily significantly reduced the frequency of all symptoms compared with placebo; the healing time was also significantly reduced. In a further open study 19 similar patients with recurrent herpes simplex applied tromantadine hydrochloride 1% ointment prophylactically at least twice daily for periods varying from 2 months to 3 years; the symptom-free intervals were significantly extended and the rate of recurrence reduced. However, 2 patients with genital herpes simplex developed eczematous reactions after several months' treatment.— L. Hellgren and L. S. Hermann, *Dermatologica*, 1983, *167*, 267.

Proprietary Names and Manufacturers

Viru-Merz *(Merz, Ger.; Merz, Neth.; Merz, Switz.)*; Virumerz *(Merz, Denm.)*; Viru-Serol *(Lacer, Spain)*; Viruserol *(Zyma, Ital.)*.

17027-v

Vidarabine *(BAN, USAN, rINN).*

Adenine Arabinoside; Ara-A; CI-673. 9-β-D-Arabinofuranosyladenine monohydrate.
$C_{10}H_{13}N_5O_4,H_2O$=285.3.

CAS — 5536-17-4 (anhydrous); 24356-66-9 (monohydrate).

Pharmacopoeias. U.S. includes Sterile Vidarabine.

A purine nucleoside obtained from *Streptomyces*

antibioticus. It is a white to off-white powder. **Soluble** 1 in about 2220 of water; slightly soluble in dimethylformamide. **Store** in airtight containers.

1690-a

Vidarabine Phosphate *(BANM, USAN, rINNM)*.

Ara-AMP; Arabinosyladenine Monophosphate; Cl-808; Vidarabine 5′-Monophosphate. 9-β-D-Arabinofuranosyladenine 5′-(dihydrogen phosphate).

$C_{10}H_{14}N_5O_7P$=347.2.

CAS — 29984-33-6; 71002-10-3 (vidarabine sodium phosphate).

Stability of vidarabine phosphate in aqueous solutions.— W. -H. Hong and D. H. Szulczewski, *J. parent. Sci. Technol.*, 1984, *38*, 60.

Formulation of a stable vidarabine phosphate injection.— M. S. L. Kwee and L. M. L. Stolk, *Pharm. Weekbl. Ned., scient. Edn*, 1984, *6*, 101. See also S. D. Patel and S. H. Yalkowsky, *J. parent. Sci. Technol.*, 1987, *41*, 15.

Adverse Effects

Adverse effects which may occur when vidarabine is applied to the eyes include irritation, pain, superficial punctate keratitis, photophobia, lachrymation, and occlusion of the lachrymal duct.

Following intravenous administration of vidarabine the most common adverse effects are gastro-intestinal disturbances including nausea, vomiting, diarrhoea, anorexia, and weight loss. Encephalopathic changes have also occurred. Haematological changes induced by vidarabine have included decreases in haemoglobin concentrations or haematocrit, leucopenia, and thrombocytopenia.

Other side-effects occurring occasionally after intravenous administration of vidarabine have included malaise, pruritus, rash, haematemesis, thrombophlebitis and pain at the site of injection, elevation in bilirubin concentrations, and abnormal liver enzyme values.

Vidarabine has been reported to be teratogenic, carcinogenic, and mutagenic in some species of *animals*.

Forty-two patients with compromised immunity and complications of infections due to herpesviruses were evaluated for adverse effects to intravenous treatment with vidarabine. Patients received either a placebo or vidarabine in a daily dosage of 10, 15, or 20 mg per kg body-weight for 4 to 10 days; one patient received vidarabine 30 mg per kg. Six forms of reversible adverse effects were observed: nausea and vomiting, weight loss, weakness (often with impaired ambulation), megaloblastosis in erythroid series in bone marrow, tremors 5 to 7 days after the start of therapy (including tremors in one patient with an abnormal EEG that was consistent with toxic metabolic encephalopathy), and thrombophlebitis at the site of injection. The incidence of side-effects was generally greater in patients who received 20 mg per kg daily.— A. H. Ross *et al.*, *J. infect. Dis.*, 1976, *133, Suppl.*, A192.

Adverse effects in 15 patients with chronic hepatitis B treated with vidarabine (12 also received interferon alfa concomitantly) included gastro-intestinal symptoms, weakness or fatigue, myalgia, reversible granulocytopenia and thrombocytopenia, jaw pain, tremor, ataxia, difficulty in walking, and neurological effects with EEG changes mimicking metabolic encephalopathy. The patient with the most severe neurological effects also had a transient compromise in renal function. Close monitoring of liver function, renal function, neurological status, and haematologic values should be undertaken during treatment with vidarabine.— S. L. Sacks *et al.* (letter), *J. Am. med. Ass.*, 1979, *241*, 28. See also under Interferons, Interactions, p.697.

A patient with disseminated herpes zoster developed a syndrome of inappropriate secretion of antidiuretic hormone and hyponatraemia secondary to the administration of vidarabine.— E. Ramos *et al.*, *Antimicrob. Ag. Chemother.*, 1979, *15*, 142.

EFFECTS ON THE BLOOD. Seven patients with herpesvirus infections were given intravenous infusions of vidarabine 10 or 20 mg per kg body-weight daily. Haematologic changes occurred most often in patients with concomitant underlying chronic diseases, were most frequent with the higher dose, and were limited to patients who also had decreases in haemoglobin concentrations. All 5 patients receiving 20 mg per kg daily had decreases in haemoglobin of more than 2 g per 100 mL, whereas only 1 of 3 patients who received 10 mg per kg had a similar reduction. The number of neutrophils, white blood cells, and platelets did not decrease during treatment, even in patients who had low counts before treatment. Two patients, who had received the same chemotherapy for Hodgkin's disease and were treated with vidarabine 20 mg per kg daily for disseminated herpes zoster infection, developed a transient motor aphasia resembling akinetic mutism. The condition resolved on cessation of therapy with vidarabine.— C. B. Lauter *et al.*, *J. infect. Dis.*, 1976, *134*, 75.

Further references: B. Hafkin *et al.*, *Antimicrob. Ag. Chemother.*, 1979, *16*, 781 (lymphopenia).

EFFECTS ON THE NERVOUS SYSTEM. A report of fatal neurological toxicity associated with vidarabine sodium phosphate therapy in a cancer patient with normal renal function.— L. Van Etta *et al.*, *J. Am. med. Ass.*, 1981, *246*, 1703.

In a study of 31 patients with chronic hepatitis B treated with vidarabine phosphate, 6 patients experienced myalgia and 7 developed peripheral neuropathy. The neurological toxicity was associated with the duration of treatment. It was suggested that the total dose should not exceed 300 mg per kg body-weight in any one course.— A. S. F. Lok *et al.*, *J. antimicrob. Chemother.*, 1984, *14*, 93.

A discussion on the neurological toxicity of vidarabine and a report of 2 such cases. Tremor or any other mild presentation of neurotoxicity should be considered an indication for withdrawal of the drug as more serious, even life-threatening, neurotoxic effects may rapidly follow.— D. R. Burdge *et al.*, *Can. med. Ass. J.*, 1985, *132*, 392.

Further references to neurotoxicity with vidarabine: R. W. Vilter, *Antimicrob. Ag. Chemother.*, 1986, *29*, 933 (one case); J. P. Quinn *et al.*, *Curr., ther. Res.*, 1987, *41*, 706 (seven cases, 5 fatal). See also under Hepatitis, below.

Precautions

Vidarabine when injected should be given intravenously but rapid administration is not advised. Vidarabine phosphate has been injected by other routes. Caution is recommended in all patients at risk from fluid overload such as those with cerebral oedema or impaired renal function; the dose may also need to be reduced in renal impairment because of the slower rate of excretion of the metabolite hypoxanthine arabinoside. Blood counts should be carried out during treatment.

INTERACTIONS. Two patients with chronic lymphocytic leukaemia who were receiving allopurinol daily developed severe neurotoxicity on the fourth day of treatment with vidarabine. Xanthine oxidase has a role in the degradation of vidarabine and inhibition of this enzyme by allopurinol could increase concentrations of hypoxanthine arabinoside, the major metabolite of vidarabine.— H. M. Friedman and T. Grasela (letter), *New Engl. J. Med.*, 1981, *304*, 423.

Vidarabine could produce homocysteine deficiency resulting in possible risks when vidarabine is given with methotrexate.— G. L. Cantoni *et al.* (letter), *New Engl. J. Med.*, 1982, *307*, 1079.

For a possible interaction between vidarabine and theophylline, resulting in increased serum concentrations of theophylline, see R. Gannon *et al.* (letter), *Ann. intern. Med.*, 1984, *101*, 148.

For a report of increased toxicity of vidarabine in patients also receiving interferon alfa, see p.697. See also Hepatitis under Uses, below.

Antiviral Action

Vidarabine appears to act by interfering in the early stages of viral DNA synthesis, but several mechanisms may be involved. It is phosphorylated intracellularly to the triphosphate which inhibits among other enzymes viral DNA polymerase; it may also be incorporated into the viral DNA.

Following administration, vidarabine is rapidly converted to hypoxanthine arabinoside which also appears to interfere with viral DNA synthesis but is reported to have less antiviral activity than the parent compound.

The activity of vidarabine *in vitro* is limited to DNA viruses such as herpes simplex virus type 1 and type 2, and varicella zoster virus; with few exceptions it does not inhibit RNA viruses.

Vidarabine's metabolite hypoxanthine arabinoside appeared to be involved in the susceptibility and resistance of herpes simplex viruses to vidarabine.— K. F. Bastow *et al.*, *Antimicrob. Ag. Chemother.*, 1983, *23*, 914. Herpes simplex virus mutants resistant to vidarabine were found to retain their resistance in the presence of the adenosine deaminase inhibitor deoxycoformycin (pentostatin; covidarabine). Herpes simplex virus polymerase appeared to govern the susceptibility to vidarabine.— H. E. Fleming and D. M. Coen, *ibid.*, 1984, *26*, 382.

Combinations of vidarabine or vidarabine phosphate with acyclovir produced an additive effect *in vitro* against herpes simplex virus type 1 and type 2 without increasing drug toxicity. These results were further substantiated in *mice*, however some adverse effects were noted at high dosages particularly for combinations with vidarabine.— R. F. Schinazi *et al.*, *Antimicrob. Ag. Chemother.*, 1982, *22*, 499. Vidarabine and acyclovir were found to be synergistic *in vitro* against most human cytomegalovirus isolates studied.— S. A. Spector and E. Kelley, *Antimicrob. Ag. Chemother.*, 1985, *27*, 600.

Synergistic antiviral effect *in vitro* of vidarabine and interferon alfa against varicella zoster virus.— M. Baba *et al.*, *Antimicrob. Ag. Chemother.*, 1984, *25*, 515.

Absorption and Fate

Following intravenous administration vidarabine is rapidly metabolised, principally by deamination to hypoxanthine arabinoside (arabinosyl hypoxanthine). Peak plasma concentrations of 6 μg and 0.4 μg per mL have been obtained for hypoxanthine arabinoside and vidarabine respectively at the end of a 12-hour infusion of vidarabine 10 mg per kg body-weight. The plasma half-life for hypoxanthine arabinoside appears to be about 3.5 hours.

Hypoxanthine arabinoside is widely distributed in tissues, with the highest concentrations being detected in kidney, liver, and spleen and lower concentrations in brain and skeletal muscle. It diffuses into the cerebrospinal fluid to give concentrations about one-third to one-half of those in plasma.

Excretion is principally through the kidney with about 40 to 50% of a dose appearing in the urine as hypoxanthine arabinoside within 24 hours and 1 to 3% as unchanged drug.

Twenty-five samples of aqueous humour were obtained from 21 patients during routine cataract surgery. Each patient had used a 3% vidarabine ointment pre-operatively every 6 hours for a total of 8 doses. Vidarabine could not be detected in any of the samples but varying concentrations of hypoxanthine arabinoside from 0.02 μg per mL (the lower limit of sensitivity of the assay) to 0.28 μg per mL were found.— R. H. Poirier *et al.*, in *Adenine Arabinoside: An Antiviral Agent*, D. Pavan-Langston *et al.* (Ed.), New York, Raven Press, 1975, p.307.

Vidarabine was given for 5 days in a daily dose of 10 mg per kg body-weight by slow intravenous infusion over 12 hours to 5 immunosuppressed patients with herpes zoster. Vidarabine appeared to be rapidly deaminated since virtually all of the drug present in plasma and urine was in the form of hypoxanthine arabinoside with a peak mean plasma concentration of about 3 μg per mL occurring at the end of each infusion. There was no indication of drug accumulation. Mean urinary excretion in 24 hours ranged from 1.94 to 2.39% for vidarabine and from 40.8 to 49.5% for hypoxanthine arabinoside.— R. A. Buchanan *et al.*, *Clin. Pharmac. Ther.*, 1980, *27*, 690.

The infusion kinetics and haemodialysis clearance of hypoxanthine arabinoside following vidarabine administration to a patient with renal failure. Due to the increased half-life of hypoxanthine arabinoside it was recommended that the dose of vidarabine be reduced by 25% in patients with severe renal insufficiency. It was also recommended that the dose be given after dialysis because of the estimated removal of as much as 50% of the hypoxanthine arabinoside in the body during a 6-hour haemodialysis at a plasma flow-rate of 200 mL per minute.— G. R. Aronoff *et al.*, *Antimicrob. Ag. Chemother.*, 1980, *18*, 212.

In a study of 29 patients the pharmacokinetics and metabolism of vidarabine phosphate were found to be similar to those of vidarabine.— R. J. Whitley *et al.*, *Antimicrob. Ag. Chemother.*, 1980, *18*, 709.

Further references: A. J. Glazko *et al.*, in *Adenine Arabinoside: An Antiviral Agent*, D. Pavan-Langston *et al.* (Ed.), New York, Raven Press, 1975, p.111; T. C. Shope *et al.*, *J. infect. Dis.*, 1983, *148*, 721.

Uses and Administration

Vidarabine is used topically in the treatment of herpes simplex keratitis in the form of a 3% ophthalmic ointment and can be used when there has been no response to treatment with antiviral agents such as idoxuridine or when ocular toxicity or hypersensitivity to other agents has occurred. The ointment is applied 5 times daily every 3 hours until corneal re-epithelialisation has occurred then twice daily for a further 7 days to prevent recurrence. If there is no improvement within 7 days or if complete healing has not occurred within 21 days, other forms of therapy should be considered. Severe conditions or conditions which have not healed with idoxuridine treatment may take longer to respond.

Vidarabine is also used intravenously in the treatment of encephalitis due to herpes simplex. A suggested dose is 15 mg per kg body-weight daily for 10 days; this is infused at a constant rate over a period of 12 to 24 hours. As each mg of vidarabine requires 2.22 mL of intravenous fluid for complete solubilisation large quantities of fluids have to be infused in order to administer the daily dose. The more soluble vidarabine phosphate has been used to try and overcome this problem and has also been given intramuscularly.

Vidarabine has also been given by intravenous infusion in a dose of 10 mg per kg daily for at least 5 days in the treatment of varicella zoster infections in immunosuppressed patients.

Vidarabine sodium phosphate has also been used. The valerate is under study.

Reviews and discussions covering the use of vidarabine in the treatment of viral infections: *Lancet*, 1980, *1*, 1337; R. J. Whitley *et al.*, *Drugs*, 1980, *20*, 267; R. J. Whitley, *J. antimicrob. Chemother.*, 1984, *14*, *Suppl. A.*, 57.

For the proceedings of a symposium on vidarabine, see *Adenine Arabinoside: An Antiviral Agent*, D. Pavan-Langston *et al.* (Ed.), New York, Raven Press, 1975.

CHICKENPOX. Results of a double-blind placebo-controlled study of 34 immunosuppressed patients indicated that vidarabine 10 mg per kg body-weight daily infused over 12 hours was useful for the treatment of chickenpox.— R. Whitley *et al.*, *J. Pediat.*, 1982, *101*, 125.

CREUTZFELDT-JAKOB DISEASE. A report of a woman with pathologically-proven Creutzfeldt-Jakob disease that was repeatedly suppressed for more than 6 months with vidarabine.— T. W. Furlow *et al.* (letter), *Lancet*, 1982, *2*, 564.

CYTOMEGALOVIRUS INFECTIONS. Two patients with acute cytomegalovirus encephalitis were successfully treated with vidarabine 15 mg per kg body-weight daily for 10 days given intravenously. One patient also received dexamethasone 4 mg every 6 hours by intravenous injection. No serious toxic reactions to vidarabine were reported at this dosage.— C. A. Phillips *et al.*, *J. Am. med. Ass.*, 1977, *238*, 2299.

In 5 of 6 immunocompromised patients with cytomegalovirus retinitis vidarabine 15 mg or more per kg body-weight daily by intravenous infusion was associated with some improvement in the course of the disease. However, significant gastro-intestinal and haematological toxicity occurred.— R. B. Pollard *et al.*, *Ann. intern. Med.*, 1980, *93*, 655.

Vidarabine showed no therapeutic effect against cytomegalovirus infection in renal transplant patients.— S. C. Marker *et al.*, *Archs intern. Med.*, 1980, *140*, 1441.

Further references: J. V. Baublis *et al.*, in *Adenine Arabinoside: An Antiviral Agent*, D. Pavan-Langston *et al.* (Ed.), New York, Raven Press, 1975, p.247 (improvement in some infants and adults).

DOSAGE IN RENAL FAILURE. Vidarabine could be administered to patients with renal failure by adjusting the dose. Usual doses are suitable for patients whose glomerular filtration-rates exceed 10 mL per minute; a reduction to 75% of the normal dose is advisable for rates below this. A dose supplement should be given to patients undergoing haemodialysis.— W. M. Bennett *et al.*, *Am. J. Kidney Dis.*, 1983, *3*, 155.

See also above under Absorption and Fate.

EPSTEIN-BARR INFECTIONS. Possible therapeutic effect of vidarabine in infectious mononucleosis encephalitis.— S. F. Berkovic *et al.*, *Med. J. Aust.*, 1982, *2*, 343.

HEPATITIS. For a brief discussion on the use of vidarabine in the treatment of viral hepatitis, see V. Damjanovic and W. Brumfitt, *J. antimicrob. Chemother.*, 1980, *6*, 11.

In 5 patients positive for hepatitis B surface antigen, vidarabine phosphate 10 or 15 mg per kg body-weight daily administered as intermittent intravenous or intramuscular bolus injections produced transient inhibition of viral replication. Reversible thrombocytopenia occurred in 2 patients when treatment was continued beyond 10 days. In 3 similar patients reduction of the dosage after 5 days to 5 mg per kg daily, or treatment with this lower dose throughout, allowed therapy for up to 34 days without serious adverse effects. Long-term inhibition of viral replication occurred in these 3 patients and they developed antibodies to hepatitis B antigen. The results indicated that a long course of vidarabine phosphate was successful in reducing the concentration of viral particles in the blood and therefore in reducing the level of infectivity of the patients.— I. V. D. Weller *et al.*, *Gut*, 1982, *23*, 717.

In a controlled study involving 64 patients with chronic hepatitis B, no benefit was achieved with vidarabine phosphate 5 mg per kg body-weight daily in 2 divided doses in months 1, 3, and 5 when compared with placebo. Nor was there any benefit when leucocyte interferon was also used in the intervening months; on the contrary there was an increase in neurotoxicity. Side-effects of vidarabine occurred both during treatment and after the drug was discontinued, and were considered responsible for treated patients remaining significantly more symptomatic than controls 6 months after therapy was discontinued.— G. Garcia *et al.*, *Ann. intern. Med.*, 1987, *107*, 278.

See also under Precautions for Interferons, p.697 for another study showing increased toxicity with vidarabine used with interferon alfa in chronic hepatitis B.

Further references to the use of vidarabine in the treatment of viral hepatitis: R. G. Chadwick *et al.*, *Br. med. J.*, 1978, *2*, 531; R. B. Pollard *et al.*, *J. Am. med. Ass.*, 1978, *239*, 1648; M. F. Bassendine *et al.*, *Gastroenterology*, 1981, *80*, 1016; D. M. Novick *et al.*, *Gut*, 1984, *25*, A541.

HERPES SIMPLEX. The application of vidarabine 3% in a basis of soft paraffin 60% and liquid paraffin 40% did not modify the clinical course or viral titre of herpes progenitalis in 15 episodes when compared with a placebo in a double-blind study. Possibly this lack of effect was due to limited diffusion into the lesion which might be improved by use of a more soluble form or a different vehicle.— E. L. Goodman *et al.*, *Antimicrob. Ag. Chemother.*, 1976, *8*, 693. Similar results.— H. G. Adams *et al.*, *J. infect. Dis.*, 1976, *133*, *Suppl.*, A151; A. L. Hilton *et al.*, *Br. J. vener. Dis.*, 1978, *54*, 50.

Vidarabine phosphate, used topically as a 10% cream, was found to be ineffective when compared with placebo in the treatment of recurrent herpes simplex labialis in a collaborative double-blind study of 233 patients. Inadequate penetration of the skin might be responsible for this failure.— S. L. Spruance *et al.*, *New Engl. J. Med.*, 1979, *300*, 1180.

Vidarabine 3% in a water-miscible gel basis applied 6 times daily for 7 days was significantly more effective than placebo in reducing lesion size in 70 patients with recurrent herpes simplex labialis who were evaluated over 12 months, but there was no statistical difference between the vidarabine and placebo groups in episode frequency or lesion duration. Treatment during the tingling stage accelerated development of the lesion.— N. H. Rowe *et al.*, *Oral Path.*, 1979, *47*, 142.

A report of radiculomyelopathy associated with herpes simplex genitalis in a 20-year-old woman. The patient responded to treatment with vidarabine 600 mg per 24 hours intravenously for 5 days together with idoxuridine applied topically.— C. E. Handler *et al.*, *Postgrad. med. J.*, 1983, *59*, 388.

In a randomised crossover study by the US National Institute of Allergy and Infectious Diseases Collaborative Antiviral Study Group 39 immunocompromised patients with progressive mucocutaneous (oral and/or genital) herpes simplex virus infections received vidarabine intravenously for 7 days followed by placebo for an additional 7 days; 46 similar patients received the reverse regimen. Therapy did not significantly accelerate healing for the total population, but there was accelerated loss of pain and temperatures became normal sooner in the group who received vidarabine first. Furthermore, therapy accelerated the clearance of virus from lesions for patients over 40 years of age as well as for those who had herpes simplex virus type 1 infections. Vidarabine could be used as a therapeutic agent in older immunocompromised patients with herpes simplex virus type 1 infections, but its value may be limited by the mandatory fluid load and consequent hospitalisation.— R. J. Whitley *et al.*, *J. infect. Dis.*, 1984, *149*, 1.

Encephalitis and neonatal herpes simplex. A report of beneficial results with vidarabine in neonatal herpes simplex infections, from a double-blind study carried out by the US National Institute of Allergy and Infectious Diseases. Vidarabine 15 mg per kg body-weight daily, given intravenously over 12 hours, was administered for 10 days to 28 neonates; a further 28 received placebo. The type of neonatal herpetic disease was the major determinant of outcome. In the most severe forms, namely disseminated herpes simplex and localised central nervous system disease, vidarabine significantly reduced mortality from 74 to 38%; of the survivors, 29% of treated patients were without demonstrable neurological defects at 1-year follow-up compared with only 11% of untreated patients. However, those with localised CNS infection had a much better prognosis than those with disseminated infection. Neonates with apparent localised infections of the skin, eye, or mouth had a far better prognosis than other forms of infection.— R. J. Whitley *et al.*, *Pediatrics*, 1980, *66*, 495. In a follow-up study in 39 similar neonates vidarabine 30 mg per kg body-weight daily was of no more benefit than 15 mg per kg daily.— R. J. Whitley *et al.*, *ibid.*, 1983, *72*, 778.

Whitley *et al.* have also shown vidarabine to be of benefit in adults with herpes simplex encephalitis (*New Engl. J. Med.*, 1977, *297*, 289; *ibid.*, 1981, *304*, 313). However, others have shown acyclovir to be superior (B. Sköldenberg *et al.*, *Lancet*, 1984, *2*, 707) and in a more recent study Whitley *et al.* (*New Engl. J. Med.*, 1986, *314*, 144) also found acyclovir to be superior to vidarabine in biopsy-proved herpes simplex encephalitis in non-neonates. According to Whitley *et al.* there is as yet no evidence of acyclovir being superior to vidarabine in neonatal herpes simplex infection.

Further references to vidarabine in herpes simplex encephalitis: M. L. Landry *et al.*, *J. Am. med. Ass.*, 1982, *247*, 332; W. M. Wenman *et al.*, *Can. med. Ass. J.*, 1982, *126*, 819.

Keratitis. Discussions and reviews on the use of vidarabine in the treatment of herpetic keratitis: J. I. McGill *et al.*, *Trans. ophthal. Soc. U.K.*, 1975, *95*, 246; *Drug & Ther. Bull.*, 1979, *17*, 43.

In a study of 54 patients with ocular herpes simplex, there was no significant difference between the healing time of ulcers of 27 eyes treated with vidarabine 3% ointment (12.4 days) and 24 eyes treated with idoxuridine 0.5% ointment (11.5 days). Visual acuity was improved in more patients treated with vidarabine and was considered to be due to smoother epithelial healing rather than to any differences in stromal scarring. In a further study vidarabine was used successfully in 49 of 57 patients who had had severe allergy or toxic reaction to idoxuridine, or had no improvement or deterioration of herpetic ulcers while receiving idoxuridine therapy; the mean healing time was 10.6 days. Except for one patient, who had redness and irritation and punctate keratitis, there were no adverse reactions in these patients during therapy lasting up to 192 days.— D. Pavan-Langston, *Am. J. Ophthal.*, 1975, *80*, 495. See also D. Pavan-Langston and R. A. Buchanan, *Trans. Am. Acad. Ophthal. Oto-lar.*, 1976, *81*, 813; D. M. O'Day *et al.*, *Am. J. Ophthal.*, 1976, *81*, 642.

In a double-blind study vidarabine 3.3% ointment or trifluridine 1% eye-drops were used 5 times daily to treat 102 patients with dendritic or amoeboid ulcers of the cornea due to herpes simplex. The frequency of treatment was reduced to three times daily when the epithelial defect healed and the total treatment was given for a maximum of 14 days. The dendritic ulcers of only 1 of 87 patients failed to heal and this was in a patient treated with vidarabine. The mean time required to heal was not significantly different for the 2 groups being 5.13 days for vidarabine and 5.75 days for trifluridine. Recurrence or recrudescence of epithelial herpetic disease occurred in 10 patients treated with vidarabine and in 4 treated with trifluridine, but was considered to be due to the arbitrary choice of the length of treatment after initial healing. In the 15 patients with amoeboid ulcers, trifluridine appeared to be more effective than vidarabine.— D. J. Coster *et al.*, *J. infect. Dis.*, 1976, *133*, *Suppl.*, A173. See also J. P. Travers and A. Patterson, *J. int. med. Res.*, 1978, *6*, 102. Similar results were obtained in 63 patients treated with 2% trifluridine ointment or 3% vidarabine ointment but the mean healing times were 11.14 days and 10.54 days respectively. The difference in the healing times between this study and that of D.J. Coster *et al.* may have been due to the criteria used to decide healing.— O. P. Van Bijsterveld and H. Post, *Br. J. Ophthal.*, 1980, *64*, 33.

For comparison of vidarabine and acyclovir in the treatment of herpes simplex virus infections of the eye, see Acyclovir, p.692.

HERPES ZOSTER. Discussions on the use of vidarabine in the treatment of disseminated herpes zoster particularly in immunosuppressed patients.— R. Dolin *et al.*, *Ann. intern. Med.*, 1978, *89*, 375; A. W. Hopefl, *Drug Intell. & clin. Pharm.*, 1979, *13*, 255.

From a randomised controlled crossover collaborative study by the US National Institute of Allergy and Infectious Diseases of a total of 87 immunosuppressed patients with active herpes zoster, it was reported that although there was rapid healing with a placebo, the clearance of virus from vesicles, the cessation of new vesicle formation, and the time to total pustulation were significantly improved when vidarabine 10 mg per kg body-weight was given daily, by slow intravenous infusion over 12 hours, for the first 5 days of treatment. The treatment was of particular value when given within the first 6 days of the disease to young patients with reticuloendothelial neoplasms.— R. J. Whitley *et al.*, *New Engl. J. Med.*, 1976, *294*, 1193.

A report of herpes-zoster myelitis which rapidly improved after treatment with vidarabine.— R. N. Corston *et al.*, *Br. med. J.*, 1981, *283*, 698 and 1156.

A study indicating that intravenous vidarabine therapy reduces the complications of herpes zoster when instituted within 72 hours of the onset of localised infection in immunocompromised patients.— R. J. Whitley *et al.*, *New Engl. J. Med.*, 1982, *307*, 971. Comment on the concomitant administration of corticosteroids in many of the patients and the possible benefit in reducing the frequency of post-herpetic neuralgia.— M. S. Topiel and G. L. Simon (letter), *ibid.*, 1983, *308*, 526. In the patients evaluated a beneficial corticosteroid effect could not be substantiated.— R. J. Whitley *et al.* (letter), *ibid.*

In a double-blind study of 20 immunosuppressed patients with varicella or disseminated zoster vidarabine phosphate was found to be as clinically effective as vidarabine. In both treatment groups, all patients survived, no new vesicles were observed after the third day of treatment, and, in those patients with a fever, a sudden and sharp drop in temperature was observed a mean of 3.8 days after admission to hospital. Both drugs were given in a usual dose of 15 mg per kg body-weight daily for 5 days, but vidarabine phosphate had the advantage that it could be infused over shorter periods (30 minutes) every 12 hours.— J. L. Vilde *et al.*, *J. med. Virol.*, 1983, *12*, 149.

For a study showing acyclovir producing better results than vidarabine in severely immunocompromised patients with varicella-zoster virus infection, see acyclovir, p.693.

Further references: B. Juel-Jensen, *J. antimicrob. Chemother.*, 1976, *2*, 261.

Encephalitis. A 3-year-old child with viral encephalitis associated with increased titres of antibodies to varicella zoster virus improved dramatically within 2 days of receiving vidarabine phosphate 15 mg per kg body-weight. Another child with severe encephalitis associated with cytomegalovirus made a slow recovery under treatment with vidarabine phosphate.— G. T. Werner and O. Sauer (letter), *Lancet*, 1979, *1*, 1040.

LARYNGEAL PAPILLOMA. Three of 6 children with frequently recurring human laryngeal papillomatosis had a beneficial response to courses of vidarabine. One of the 3 had needed a tracheostomy for 7 years.— J. Pritchard *et al.* (letter), *Lancet*, 1980, *2*, 1383. Vidarabine was not considered to have been useful in the treatment of respiratory papillomatosis in 9 children.— W. A. Hendrickse *et al.*, *Archs Dis. Childh.*, 1985, *60*, 374.

VACCINIA. Rapid resolution of a vaccinial lesion of the eye of a 5-year-old boy was felt to be largely due to topical application of 3% vidarabine eye ointment.— P. Gatenby (letter), *Lancet*, 1979, *1*, 676. See also D. Pavan-Langston and C. H. Dohlman, *Am. J. Ophthal.*, 1972, *74*, 81.

Preparations

Vidarabine Concentrate for Injection *(U.S.P.)*
Vidarabine Ophthalmic Ointment *(U.S.P.)*

Proprietary Preparations

Vira-A *(Parke, Davis, UK). Injection*, vidarabine 200 mg/mL, in vials of 5 mL. To be diluted before use. *Eye ointment*, vidarabine 3%.

Proprietary Names and Manufacturers of Vidarabine and its Salts

Vira-A *(Parke, Davis, Austral.; Parke, Davis, Canad.; Substantia, Fr.; Parke, Davis, S.Afr.; Parke, Davis, Spain; Parke, Davis, UK; Parke, Davis, USA).*

1691-t

Xenazoic Acid *(rINN).*
Xenalamine; Xenalmine. 4-[2-(Biphenyl-4-yl)-1-ethoxy-2-oxoethylamino]benzoic acid.
$C_{23}H_{21}NO_4$=375.4.

CAS — 1174-11-4.

Xenazoic acid has been reported to have antiviral properties.

18797-s

Zidovudine *(BAN, USAN, pINN).*

Azidodeoxythymidine; Azidothymidine; AZT; BW-509U; BW-A509U; BWA-509U; Compound-S. 3′-Azido-3′-deoxythymidine.
$C_{10}H_{13}N_5O_4$=267.2.

CAS — 30516-87-1.

Adverse Effects and Treatment

The commonest adverse effects reported with zidovudine are anaemia and leucopenia, mainly neutropenia, which have been reported to affect about half the patients being treated depending on their existing blood picture. This haematological toxicity can be severe enough to require blood transfusion.

Other significant adverse effects reported with zidovudine include nausea, headache, insomnia, and myalgia.

Other adverse effects have occurred in patients treated with zidovudine but their incidence is no greater than that observed in placebo groups.

CNS toxicity contributing to death in an AIDS patient being treated with zidovudine.— D. N. Hagler and P. T. Frame (letter), *Lancet*, 1986, *2*, 1392. Wernicke's encephalopathy might have been brought on by zidovudine in one patient.— D. G. Davtyan and H. V. Vinters (letter), *ibid.*, 1987, *1*, 919.

An analysis of the adverse reactions observed in a placebo-controlled study of zidovudine involving 282 patients with AIDS or AIDS-related complex. Nausea, myalgia, and insomnia were reported with significantly greater frequency by the zidovudine recipients compared with the placebo group. Anaemia and leucopenia (mainly neutropenia) occurred in the majority of patients given zidovudine; erythrocyte transfusions were required by 31% of the zidovudine group and 11% of the placebo group. Decreases in platelets occurred in 12% of the zidovudine group and 31% of the placebo group; however, there was a significantly greater increase in platelet count in those given zidovudine. Patients at risk of haematological adverse effects were those with more advanced disease, with low initial serum-vitamin B_{12} concentrations, or those taking paracetamol.— D. D. Richman *et al.*, *New Engl. J. Med.*, 1987, *317*, 192.

Severe depression of white cells and platelets as well as haemoglobin in an AIDS patient receiving zidovudine.— G. Forester (letter), *New Engl. J. Med.*, 1987, *317*, 772. Four further cases of pancytopenia and bone-marrow aplasia with zidovudine.— P. S. Gill *et al.*, *Ann. intern. Med.*, 1987, *107*, 502.

Progressive pigmentation of all fingernails in 2 patients receiving zidovudine.— P. A. Furth and A. M. Kazakis (letter), *Ann. intern. Med.*, 1987, *107*, 350.

Abnormal liver-function values associated with zidovudine in 3 patients necessitating its withdrawal. Zidovudine was reinstated in 2 patients without further liver changes.— A. J. Melamed *et al.* (letter), *J. Am. med. Ass.*, 1987, *258*, 2063.

Precautions

Zidovudine should be used with care in patients with anaemia or bone-marrow suppression. It has been recommended that it should not be used if the neutrophil count or haemoglobin count is abnormally low. Care is also required in the elderly and in patients with reduced kidney or liver function.

Because of the haematological toxicity of zidovudine it is recommended that blood tests should be carried out every 2 weeks for the first 3 months of treatment, thereafter tests should be carried out at least monthly.

Paracetamol has been reported to increase zidovudine's toxicity on the blood. Probenecid delays its excretion.

Overwhelming fatigue associated with the use of acyclovir and zidovudine. When each agent was given alone there was no such effect.— M. C. Bach (letter), *New Engl. J. Med.*, 1987, *316*, 547.

Tribavirin and zidovudine inhibited each others' antiviral activity *in vitro*.— M. W. Vogt *et al.*, *Science*, 1987, *235*, 1376.

Acute meningo-encephalitis on dose reduction of zidovudive probably as a result of an increase in HIV replication.— M. Helbert *et al.*, *Lancet*, 1988, *1*, 1249.

Antiviral activity

Zidovudine halts the DNA synthesis of HIV through competitive inhibition of its reverse transcriptase following its staged conversion to the triphosphate via thymidine kinase and other kinases. It also possesses some antibacterial activity.

Ampligen, a mismatched polymer of double-stranded RNA, reduced the concentration of zidovudine required for the inhibition of HIV *in vitro*.— W. M. Mitchell *et al.*, *Lancet*, 1987, *1*, 890.

Synergy between dextran sulphate and zidovudine against HIV *in vitro*.— R. Ueno and S. Kuno (letter), *Lancet*, 1987, *1*, 1379; M. C. Berenbaum (letter), *ibid.*, *2*, 461; R. Ueno and S. Kuno (letter), *ibid.*, 796.

Absorption and Fate

Zidovudine is rapidly absorbed from the gastro-intestinal tract with a bioavailability of about 50 to 70%. It crosses the blood-brain barrier. The plasma half-life is about 1 hour.

Zidovudine is metabolised intracellularly to the antiviral triphosphate. It is also metabolised in the liver to the glucuronide and is excreted in the urine as unchanged drug and metabolite. As there is some tubular secretion, probenecid can delay excretion.

Uses and Administration

Zidovudine is used in the management of AIDS and the AIDS-related complex, and at present is generally restricted to patients who have recovered recently from *Pneumocystis carinii* pneumonia or have multiple symptoms of HIV infection.

It is given by mouth in doses of 200 to 300 mg every four hours day and night based on 3.5 mg per kg body-weight every 4 hours. Blood tests should be carried out regularly as described under Precautions. Should the white-cell count or haemoglobin level fall the dose interval can be reduced to 8 hours. Should the effects on the blood be severe, zidovudine may need to be suspended.

Other nucleoside antiviral agents under investigation include dideoxycytidine and dideoxyadenosine.

Zidovudine has been reported to produce improvement in patients with AIDS or AIDS-related complex (R. Yarchoan *et al.*, *Lancet*, 1986, *1*, 575) including patients with neurological involvement (R. Yarchoan *et al.*, *Lancet*, 1987, *1*, 132). A multicentre, double-blind, placebo-controlled study was set up to investigate zidovudine's safety and effectiveness initially in 282 patients with AIDS manifested by a recent history of first-episode *Pneumocystis carinii* pneumonia or with multiple symptoms of AIDS-related complex (M.A. Fischl *et al.*, *New Engl. J. Med.*, 1987, *317*, 185). However, it was decided to halt the study prematurely when a significant difference in mortality was detected between the zidovudine and placebo groups; there was also a reduced frequency of opportunistic infection in the treatment group. When given to patients with HIV antigen but no symptoms zidovudine was found to reduce the antigen levels (F. De Wolf *et al.*, *Lancet*, 1988, *1*, 373). It has also been reported to be of benefit in a few patients with AIDS associated psoriasis (M. Duvic *et al.*, *Lancet*, 1987, *2*, 627; T. Ruzicka *et al.*, *ibid.*, 1469), but there are conflicting reports of benefit in another few with lymphocytic interstitial pneumonia associated with AIDS

(M.C. Bach, *Lancet*, 1987, *2*, 796; M. Helbert *et al.*, *ibid.*, 1333). Recent investigations have also involved alternating zidovudine with dideoxycytidine (R. Yarchoan *et al.*, *Lancet*, 1988, *1*, 76).

Some reviews on zidovudine: R. Yarchoan and S. Broder, *New Engl. J. Med.*, 1987, *316*, 557; *Lancet*, 1987, *1*, 957.

Proprietary Preparations

Retrovir *(Wellcome, UK)*. *Capsules*, zidovudine 100 and 250 mg.

Proprietary Names and Manufacturers

Retrovir *(Gayoso Wellcome, Spain; Wellcome, UK; Wellcome, USA)*.

14030-f

Zinviroxime *(USAN, rINN)*.

LY-122771; Viroxime Component A. (*Z*)-2-Amino-6-benzoyl-1-(isopropylsulphonyl)-1*H*-benzimidazole oxime. $C_{17}H_{18}N_4O_3S = 358.4$.

CAS — 72301-78-1.

Zinviroxime is an isomer of enviroxime and is reported to have antiviral activity. Viroxime which is a mixture of the 2 isomers has been investigated.

Proprietary Names and Manufacturers

Lilly, USA.

Anxiolytic Sedatives Hypnotics and Neuroleptics

7000-n

The drugs in this chapter include sedative agents used in the management of anxiety and neurosis (anxiolytic sedatives), as well as those used to produce sleep (hypnotics), and agents used in the treatment of psychoses (neuroleptics or major tranquillisers).

For agents used in disorders of affect, such as mental depression, see Antidepressants, p.350.

Many other drugs have sedative and hypnotic effects or side-effects: these include alcohol (p.950), antihistamines (p.443), general anaesthetics (p.1113), hyoscine (p.534), and opioid analgesics (p.1294).

Dependence

Dependence is liable to occur in susceptible patients given any of the sedatives in this section although the potential of the benzodiazepines for evoking dependence is less than that of, for example, the barbiturates. Dependence is characterised by a strong need to continue taking the drug, a tendency to increase the dose, a psychic dependence on the effects of the drug, and a physical dependence on the effects of the drug for the maintenance of homoeostasis, with a characteristic abstinence syndrome on withdrawal.

The detrimental effects of hypnotic dependence arise particularly from the persistence of effects such as ataxia, dysarthria, mental impairment and confusion, and poor judgement.

Withdrawal symptoms are similar to those of alcohol abstinence and are characterised after several hours by apprehension and weakness, followed by anxiety, headache, dizziness, tremors, and vomiting and then by nausea, abdominal cramps, insomnia, and tachycardia. Orthostatic hypotension and convulsions may develop after a day or two, sometimes leading to status epilepticus. Hallucinations and delirium tremens may develop after several days followed by a deep sleep before the symptoms disappear.

The time at which symptoms develop varies with the duration of action of the drug used. Symptoms may be dramatically reversed by the administration of almost any sedative and this should be followed by the slow withdrawal of the sedative over a period of days or weeks.

The neuroleptic agents have not been reported to cause dependence of this type; however, mild symptoms resembling the withdrawal symptoms of dependence have been seen following the abrupt withdrawal of phenothiazines from patients receiving prolonged maintenance therapy.

A review of dependence on psychotropic drugs. Of prescribed drugs, the anxiolytic sedatives are by far the major drugs of dependence, and no drug of this category is free from addictive potential. Many former barbiturate addicts have become dependent on benzodiazepines following reduced prescribing of the former due to concern over their toxicity and potential for abuse. In contrast, reports of dependence on antidepressants and neuroleptics are rare.— J. G. Edwards *et al.*, *Postgrad. med. J.*, 1984, *60, Suppl.* 2, 29.

Discussions of benzodiazepine abuse and dependence: WHO Review Group, *Bull. Wld Hlth Org.*, 1983, *61*, 551; P. J. Tyrer, *Br. med. J.*, 1984, *288*, 1101; P. Grantham, *Br. J. Hosp. Med.*, 1987, *37*, 292.

A review of the management of benzodiazepine dependence. Withdrawal symptoms have been reported after treatment for as little as 4 to 6 weeks, and may be wide-ranging: increased sensory perception is frequent, but gastro-intestinal disturbances, headaches, muscle spasms, vertigo, and sleep disturbances are frequent. The proportion of long-term users in whom dependence develops has been variably estimated as between 15 and 44%. The withdrawal syndrome was previously reported as lasting up to 3 months but patients have been seen in whom symptoms have persisted for a year or more. Withdrawal is, in general, best tackled in the outpatient setting. Stopping the drug abruptly is more likely to lead to severe withdrawal symptoms but no consensus exists on the optimum length for the withdrawal process or the size of each dosage reduction. Four weeks is probably the minimum period but up to 16 weeks has been recommended; over the withdrawal period dosage should be tapered off in steps ranging from 0.5 to 2.5 mg diazepam or its equivalent. Rough equivalents to 2.5 mg of diazepam are 5 mg of chlordiazepoxide, 0.5 mg of lorazepam, 5 mg of nitrazepam, 7.5 mg of oxazepam, 5 mg of temazepam, or 0.125 mg of triazolam. In the authors' view the rate of reduction of dosage should not be fixed at the outset but should be adjusted according to the appearance and severity of withdrawal symptoms. Generally symptoms emerge 4 or 5 days after reduction in dosage, but they may not become evident until several steps in the withdrawal programme have been completed. Reduction can thus be in weekly steps until the first withdrawal symptoms emerge, at which stage the rate of reduction should be reduced. A further reduction should be made once the initial symptoms have waned sufficiently for the patient to be willing to contemplate a further consequent accentuation of symptoms. This procedure should be followed until the last few milligrams, at which stage the psychological aspects of dependence are likely to intensify and may require judicious use of placebo. Reduction of the usual dosage frequency from daily to alternate days, or even less frequently, before finally withdrawing the drug, may also be useful. Other drugs may be used to assist withdrawal; long-acting benzodiazepines, which are associated with less pronounced withdrawal symptoms than short-acting drugs have been recommended for substitution of the latter prior to withdrawal. Clonidine is moderately but not dramatically helpful, and propranolol attenuates some features of withdrawal syndromes but does not decrease their frequency or subjective aspects. Antidepressants may be needed for frank depressive episodes. Patients should be seen frequently by the treating physician; formal psychological help has not yet been shown to be of particular help but recent developments, especially in cognitive treatments, may prove most valuable. It is difficult to obtain an accurate estimate of the likelihood of recovery: 88 to 100% of volunteers succeed in stopping benzodiazepine intake with gradual withdrawal, but only one-third of these are free of subsequent problems. The optimum strategy remains prevention of dependence through thoughtful prescribing.— A. C. Higgitt *et al.*, *Br. med. J.*, 1985, *291*, 688.

A statement on benzodiazepines and dependence from a consensus meeting of the Royal College of Psychiatrists. Benzodiazepines should be prescribed primarily for the short-term relief of anxiety or insomnia which is disabling, severe, or subjecting the patient to extreme or unacceptable distress. Ideally benzodiazepines should be prescribed for no more than 1 month, at as low a dose as possible, and given only intermittently for sleep induction. Patients should be encouraged to withdraw gradually from long-term use; high-dose dependence is common, but dependence at therapeutic doses is also common. Even after short-term benzodiazepine use, a tapering-off regime is recommended to minimise rebound; the longer the period of use, the longer the reduction period indicated. Certain benzodiazepines are associated with dependence and some have more severe withdrawal reactions than others. In general, compounds of higher potency incur a greater level of dependence and the use of benzodiazepines of low potency may reduce the risk of long-term dependence.— R. G. Priest *et al.*, *Bull. R. Coll. Psychiat.*, 1988, *12*, 107.

Further references to the management of benzodiazepine dependence and withdrawal: P. J. Tyrer and N. Seivewright, *Postgrad. med. J.*, 1984, *60, Suppl.* 2, 41; P. Tyrer *et al.* (letter), *Lancet*, 1985, *1*, 1042; *Lancet*, 1987, *1*, 78.

Adverse Effects

All the drugs in this chapter possess varying degrees of depressant action on the central nervous system, and may produce undesirable sedation and drowsiness during the day. Many of them also produce varying degrees of dependence (see above).

The adverse effects of the **barbiturates** include respiratory depression, allergic reactions, particularly skin rashes, hepatitis, cholestasis, and photosensitivity. Erythema multiforme (Stevens-Johnson syndrome) and exfoliative dermatitis, sometimes fatal, have been reported. Folate deficiency has occurred following chronic administration, and hypoprothrombinaemia has been reported in infants born to mothers who have received a barbiturate during pregnancy. As with other sedatives paradoxical excitement and irritability may occur, particularly in children, the elderly, and patients in acute pain.

Nystagmus and ataxia may occur with excessive doses. The toxic effects of overdosage result from profound central depression and include coma, respiratory and cardiovascular depression, with hypotension and shock leading to renal failure. Hypothermia may occur with subsequent pyrexia on recovery. Characteristic erythematous or haemorrhagic blisters reportedly occur in about 6% of patients.

The barbiturates are extremely alkaline, and necrosis has followed subcutaneous injection of the sodium salts. Intravenous injection may be hazardous, and has resulted in hypotension, shock, laryngospasm and apnoea. Gangrene has resulted from intra-arterial injection into an extremity.

In contrast to the barbiturates the incidence of adverse effects with the **benzodiazepines** is lower, and the effects usually less severe. Nonetheless, dizziness, vertigo, light-headedness, headache, confusion, mental depression, slurred speech or dysarthria, changes in libido, ataxia, tremor, blurred vision, urinary retention or incontinence, gastro-intestinal disturbances, changes in salivation, jaundice, and occasional blood disorders have been reported. The benzodiazepines can cause amnesia, and like the barbiturates, may produce paradoxical excitation. Respiratory depression and hypotension are rare or absent at usual doses but may occasionally occur with high dosage and parenteral administration.

Overdosage can produce central nervous system depression and coma.

Pain and thrombophlebitis have been associated with the intravenous administration of a benzodiazepine.

The **phenothiazines** and related neuroleptics produce in general a lesser degree of central depression than the barbiturates or benzodiazepines, and tolerance to their initial sedative effects develops fairly quickly in most patients. Adverse effects of phenothiazine therapy may include antimuscarinic effects such as dry mouth, constipation, urinary retention, and mydriasis, as well as agitation, insomnia, depression, convulsions, nasal congestion, tachycardia, electrocardiographic changes, postural hypotension, miosis, blurred vision, and inhibition of ejaculation.

Allergic reactions include urticaria, exfoliative dermatitis, and contact sensitivity. Jaundice has occurred, and is probably allergic in origin. Prolonged therapy may lead to deposition of pigment in the skin, or more frequently the eyes; corneal and lens opacities have been observed. Photosensitivity reactions also occur.

Various haematological disorders, including a potentially fatal agranulocytosis have occurred in patients receiving phenothiazines. Most cases of agranulocytosis have occurred within 4 to 10 weeks of starting treatment, and symptoms such as sore throat or fever should be watched for and white cell counts instituted should they appear.

The phenothiazines produce extrapyramidal dysfunction due to their effects on central dopaminergic transmission. Resultant disorders include acute dystonia, a parkinsonism-like syndrome, akathisia, and the neuroleptic malignant syndrome; tardive dyskinesia and perioral tremor may subsequently develop.

The phenothiazines alter endocrine and metabolic functions. Patients have experienced amenorrhoea, galactorrhoea, gynaecomastia, weight gain, hyperglycaemia and altered glucose tolerance, and increased serum-cholesterol concentrations. Body temperature regulation is impaired and may result in both hypo- or hyperthermia depending on environment.

Pain and irritation at the injection site have been reported with some phenothiazines given by injection.

The relative incidence of different adverse effects varies between the different groups of phenothiazines. The more potent group with a piperazine side-chain reportedly provoke a higher incidence of extrapyramidal effects, particularly dystonia, whereas hypotension may be more likely with phenothiazines having an aliphatic (dimethylaminopropyl) side-chain.

EFFECTS ON THE BLOOD. An incidence of neutropenia of 0.8 per 1000 treated individuals, which has been reported with the phenothiazines, is high, and is only acceptable because the effect is usually reversible on the cessation of the agent, and because of the serious nature of psychotic illness. The long-term use of these drugs for less serious psychiatric disorders is hard to justify.— H. P. Roeser, *Med. J. Aust.*, 1987, *146*, 145.

Benzodiazepines had been alleged to cause both leucopenia and leucocytosis in addition to eosinophilia.— J. G. Edwards, *Practitioner*, 1977, *219*, 117.

EFFECTS ON CARBOHYDRATE METABOLISM. Studies in healthy subjects and patients with latent diabetes mellitus suggested that administration of low doses (50 or 75 mg daily by mouth) of chlorpromazine would not significantly modify glucose tolerance or plasma insulin concentrations. However a chlorpromazine infusion (50 mg over 1 hour) could induce hyperglycaemia and inhibit insulin secretion in both groups.— G. Erle *et al.*, *Eur. J. clin. Pharmac.*, 1977, *11*, 15.

EFFECTS ON THE CARDIOVASCULAR SYSTEM. ECG abnormalities, including sinus tachycardia, T-wave abnormality, S-T depression, Q-T prolongation, and right bundle branch block, were found in 59 of 140 schizophrenic patients (135 men, 5 women) taking phenothiazines including chlorpromazine, thioridazine, trifluoperazine, and fluphenazine. None of the patients had shown evidence of heart disease. Exercise increased S-T depression but the abnormalities were all reversible in 48 patients. There was no significant difference between drugs.— M. V. J. Raj and R. Benson, *Postgrad. med. J.*, 1975, *51*, 65.

Cardiac arrest in a hypothyroid woman may have been due to phenothiazine sensitivity.— J. Gomez and G. Scott, *Br. J. Psychiat.*, 1980, *136*, 89.

A report of a Stokes-Adams attack with complete heart block in a patient receiving a phenothiazine and pimozide with orphenadrine.— M. A. Chughtai, *Br. med. J.*, 1984, *289*, 162.

Cardiac arrest occurred following apparent recovery in a patient who had taken an overdose of chlorpromazine and flurazepam. Re-entrant ventricular arrhythmias may be precipitated by overdosage of a phenothiazine and electrocardiography on admission is strongly recommended in such cases.— W. Reid and A. D. B. Harrower, *Br. med. J.*, 1984, *288*, 1880.

EFFECTS ON THE ENDOCRINE SYSTEM. A discussion of the potential danger of using phenothiazines in patients with breast cancer when the increase in serum-prolactin concentrations might have some effect on the tumour.— P. Ettigi *et al.* (letter), *Lancet*, 1973, *2*, 266. An epidemiological study demonstrating no association between neuroleptic use and breast cancer.— S. Wagner and N. Mantel, *Cancer Res.*, 1978, *38*, 2703.

Over a threefold increase in plasma-prolactin concentrations in men and women schizophrenics treated with chlorpromazine or thioridazine.— H. Y. Meltzer and V. S. Fang, *Archs gen. Psychiat.*, 1976, *33*, 279.

The majority of patients receiving chronic phenothiazine therapy have only moderately raised serum-prolactin concentrations. Of 9 patients with galactorrhoea associated with phenothiazine therapy, 6 had prolactin concentrations towards the upper end of normal and 3 had elevated concentrations ranging from 75 to 100 ng per mL.— D. L. Kleinberg *et al.*, *New Engl. J. Med.*, 1977, *296*, 589.

Hyperprolactinaemia in alcoholic patients might be exacerbated if they are treated with phenothiazines. In 5 alcoholic patients serum-prolactin concentrations were raised after treatment with promazine (to above the normal range in 3).— S. K. Majumdar (letter), *Lancet*, 1978, *2*, 101.

A study in 21 males receiving long-term phenothiazine therapy indicated no increase in pituitary size despite the theoretical risk associated with phenothiazine therapy.— S. Rosenblatt *et al.* (letter), *Lancet*, 1978, *2*, 319. A report of 2 patients who developed pituitary tumours while on long-term therapy with phenothiazine neuroleptics. A further 2 patients who had been on phenothiazine therapy were found to have sellar enlargement and the empty sellar syndrome which is recognised to be related to the development of pituitary tumours. In 10 further patients measurements of the sellar volume indicated that this was within normal limits, although above the normal mean in 9.— K. Asplund *et al.* (letter), *Ann. intern. Med.*, 1982, *96*, 533. There was no evidence of an increased incidence of pituitary abnormalities on examination of skull X-rays in 69 patients receiving long-term phenothiazine therapy. Earlier X-rays were available for 41 patients and there was no evidence of changes in the pituitary despite the high prolactin concentrations in the blood of these patients.— V. A. Lilford *et al.*, *Br. J. Psychiat.*, 1984, *144*, 421.

Four patients with galactorrhoea taking benzodiazepines all had normal serum-prolactin concentrations. A causal relationship between benzodiazepines and either galactorrhoea or abnormalities of prolactin secretion has yet to be established.— D. L. Kleinberg *et al.*, *New Engl. J. Med.*, 1977, *296*, 589. A 55-year-old man who had increased his diazepam intake to 80 to 140 mg daily developed bilateral gynaecomastia. The gynaecomastia resolved on withdrawal of the diazepam.— H. J. Moerck and G. Magelund (letter), *Lancet*, 1979, *1*, 1344. Diazepam does not affect plasma-prolactin concentrations.— J. D. Wilson *et al.* (letter), *Br. med. J.*, 1979, *1*, 123. Raised serum-oestradiol concentrations in 5 men with diazepam-associated gynaecomastia.— D. Bergman *et al.* (letter), *Lancet*, 1981, *2*, 1225.

Benzodiazepines may affect the central control of endocrine function by an action on the hypothalamus or anterior pituitary. Temazepam and oxazepam have been shown to increase plasma cortisol and prolactin concentrations, and diazepam to raise growth hormone secretion in healthy subjects. Endocrine symptoms occurring in long-term benzodiazepine users include menstrual irregularities, premenstrual tension, breast engorgement, gynaecomastia, and galactorrhoea, but the mechanisms are not understood.— H. Ashton, *Adverse Drug React. Bull.*, 1986, (Jun.), 440.

EFFECTS ON THE EYES. Those phenothiazine derivatives with piperidine side-chains such as thioridazine have a higher risk of inducing retinal toxicity than other phenothiazine derivatives, with relatively few cases reported for those with aliphatic side-chains, while the piperazine group do not appear to exert direct ocular toxicity. The phenothiazines as a group can also cause cataract formation, mainly of an anterior polar variety.— A. L. Crombie, *Prescribers' J.*, 1981, *21*, 222.

Phenothiazines may induce a retinopathy related both to the dose and its duration. The critical dose in phenothiazine-induced retinopathy is 800 mg daily. Interestingly, the retinopathy may present either acutely, with sudden loss of vision associated with retinal oedema and hyperaemia of the optic disc, or chronically, with a fine pigment scatter appearing in the central area of the fundus, extending peripherally but sparing the macula. Chronic paracentral and pericentral scotomas may be found.— M. A. Spiteri and D. G. James, *Postgrad. med. J.*, 1983, *59*, 343.

EFFECTS ON THE LIVER. Chlorpromazine and other phenothiazines may cause hepatocanalicular cholestasis in which cholestasis is associated with features of hepatocyte damage, often suggesting immunological liver injury. Only a small number of patients taking the drug are affected and the onset is usually in the first 4 weeks of therapy. The phenothiazine or one of its metabolites may induce alteration in the liver-cell membrane so that it becomes antigenic; there is also good evidence that direct hepatotoxicity may also be related to the production of free drug radical.— S. Sherlock, *Lancet*, 1986, *2*, 440. Results suggesting patients with a genetically-determined low capacity for sulphoxide formation may be predisposed to the development of jaundice following chlorpromazine therapy.— E. Elias *et al.*, *Gut*, 1984, *25*, A1130. See also A. Olomu *et al.* (letter), *Lancet*, 1985, *1*, 1504.

EFFECTS ON MENTAL FUNCTION. *Catatonia*. Neuroleptic-associated catatonia in 2 patients. One patient, who had received chlorpromazine, died of pneumonia and the other, who had received haloperidol, and was subsequently given chlorpromazine after the development of catatonia, was still comatose after 7 months.— Q. R. Regestein *et al.*, *J. Am. med. Ass.*, 1977, *238*, 618. Comments. When catatonic stupor arises or substantially worsens after the beginning of treatment with neuroleptic agents a reaction to treatment should be suspected and a period of drug withdrawal should follow.— D. R. Weinberger and R. J. Wyatt (letter), *ibid.*, 1978, *239*, 1846.

Depression. A brief discussion of the role of phenothiazines and butyrophenones in causing depression.— F. A. Whitlock and L. E. J. Evans, *Drugs*, 1978, *15*, 53.

EFFECTS ON SEXUAL FUNCTION. A discussion on the impairment of male sexual function by psychotropic drugs, including mention that thioridazine appears to be the worst offender.— *Br. med. J.*, 1979, *2*, 883.

Phenothiazines, particularly thioridazine, have been reported to inhibit female orgasm.— W. W. Shen and L. S. Sata, *J. reprod. Med.*, 1983, *28*, 497.

A review of drug-induced sexual dysfunction and infertility. The phenothiazines can cause both impotence and ejaculatory dysfunction, and from the limited evidence available the incidence appears to be higher than with antidepressants. Priapism has been described particularly with the phenothiazines and is attributed to their alpha-antagonist effects which prevent constriction of the blood vessels supplying erectile tissue. Other neuroleptics such as the butyrophenones and diphenylbutylpiperidines lack the peripheral autonomic effects of the phenothiazines and rarely cause sexual dysfunction. Benzodiazepines and other sedative-hypnotic drugs have no direct effects on erection or ejaculation but their sedative effect may reduce sexual arousal and lead to impotence in some patients. Conversely sexual performance may be improved where it is impaired by anxiety.— L. Beeley, *Adverse Drug React. Ac. Pois. Rev.*, 1984, *3*, 23.

A report of increased libido and orgasmic function on withdrawal of long-term benzodiazepine therapy in 2 women.— D. Nutt *et al.* (letter), *Lancet*, 1986, *2*, 1101.

EFFECTS ON THE SKIN. Chlorpromazine caused both phototoxic and photoallergic skin reactions. In a sensitised patient a photoallergic response will be achieved with a concentration of drug that will not produce a phototoxic reaction. The two reactions can be distinguished histologically if skin tests are biopsied within 24 hours after the reaction becomes apparent. There is evidence of the reaction in the first 24 hours in phototoxicity and in 24 to 96 hours in photoallergy.— S. Epstein, *Archs Derm.*, 1968, *98*, 354.

Phototoxicity. Several experiments were made on about 100 patients with schizophrenia to test their sensitivity to light after varying dosage treatments with chlorpromazine. The critical dosage of chlorpromazine hydrochloride required to produce a phototoxic reaction appeared to be about 600 mg daily.— A. Satanove and J. S. McIntosh, *J. Am. med. Ass.*, 1967, *200*, 209.

Testing in 7 subjects taking chlorpromazine revealed that photosensitivity reactions manifested primarily as immediate erythema and that sensitivity was primarily to light in the long ultraviolet (UV-A) and visible wavebands (335 to 400 nm). Sensitivity to UV-B was normal.— J. Ferguson *et al.*, *Br. J. Derm.*, 1986, *115*, *Suppl.* 30, 35.

Pigmentation. The pigment found in the skin of patients treated with chlorpromazine was considered to be formed in a light-catalysed anaerobic reaction in which chlorpromazine was polymerised and deposited with melanin and hydrogen chloride liberated. The acid could account for the skin irritation. The polymer was prepared and produced a bluish-purple discoloration which faded in 3 days when injected intracutaneously into 2 volunteers.— C. L. Huang and F. L. Sands, *J. pharm. Sci.*, 1967, *56*, 259.

EXTRAPYRAMIDAL DISORDERS. *Akathisia*. A discussion of akathisia. The condition is characterised by an inability to sit still, and is the most common motor side-effect of treatment with neuroleptics, with an overall incidence reported to be around 20%. It may be caused by phenothiazines, thioxanthenes, and butyrophenones: more potent neuroleptics such as trifluoperazine and haloperidol are more likely to cause the syndrome than less potent ones such as chlorpromazine or thioridazine. Although akathisia may occur in isolation it is often combined with other drug-induced extrapyramidal syndromes such as parkinsonism or dyskinesia. Acute akathisia usually develops within a few days of beginning treatment, is dose-dependent, and disappears if the drug is stopped or the dose reduced. It often responds to antimuscarinics and if treatment with the neuroleptic is continued commonly subsides after 2 to 3 months. In contrast, the tardive form, like tardive dyskinesia appears after several months of treatment, is not dose-dependent, does not respond to antimuscarinics, and is made worse by stopping treatment.— E. Szabadi, *Br. med. J.*, 1986, *292*, 1034. A further review.— *Lancet*, 1986, *2*, 1131.

Comments on the theory that neuroleptic chelation of iron, which is essential to the D_2 dopamine receptor, may be implicated in akathisia induced by neuroleptics: H. S. Pall *et al.* (letter), *Lancet*, 1986, *2*, 1469; J. De Keyser *et al.* (letter), *ibid.*, 1987, *2*, 336.

Parkinsonism. A reminder of the fact that neuroleptics may cause parkinsonism, and of the need to exclude neuroleptic-induced extrapyramidal effects when making this diagnosis.— P. S. Murdoch and J. Williamson, *Lancet*, 1982, *1*, 1212. The typical 4 to 5 Hz resting tremor of idiopathic Parkinson's disease is rarely encountered in the drug-induced parkinsonian syndrome.— R. J. M. Lane and P. A. Routledge, *Drugs*, 1983, *26*, 124. In a study of 95 cases of parkinsonism referred to a hospital geriatric department, 48 were judged to have drug-induced parkinsonism. Clinical findings in the 2 groups were surprisingly similar, including the incidence of tremor. Drug-induced parkinsonism resolved in 66% of cases but in a further 11% resolution was followed by development of idiopathic Parkinson's disease.— P. J. Stephen and J. Williamson, *Lancet*, 1984, *2*, 1082. Corrections.— *ibid.*, 1410. and *ibid.*, 1985, *1*, 113. Contrary results.— R. Rozzini *et al.* (letter), *ibid.* Drug-induced cases can make a considerable contribution to the prevalence of parkinsonism. In a survey of 393 patients with Parkinson's disease 71 had drug-induced disease and thioridazine and prochlorperazine were the principal drugs involved.— W. J. Mutch (letter), *ibid.* The prognosis of drug-induced parkinsonism, and the risk of subsequent development of idiopathic Parkinson's disease: J. A. Wilson *et al.* (letter), *ibid.*, 1987, *1*, 443; J. S. Bamrah and S. D. Soni (letter), *ibid.*, 1031.

Tardive dyskinesia. Tardive, or delayed, dyskinesia generally occurs only in patients treated with neuroleptics for longer than a year, although much shorter exposures have been implicated. It occurs in between 5 and 40% of patients on long-term neuroleptic medication and is believed to result from proliferation of central post-synaptic dopamine receptors causing imbalance between dopaminergic and cholinergic activity. Increasing the neuroleptic dose improves the dyskinesia but only temporarily; conversely, stopping the drug usually worsens the condition at first, or it may appear after treatment is stopped for other causes. Such withdrawal dyskinesia usually settles after a further 6 months abstinence from neuroleptics. No satisfactory drug treatment exists, and the only proven way of avoiding tardive dyskinesia is to lower the dose of neuroleptic when symptoms first appear.— *Drug & Ther. Bull.*, 1986, *24*, 27.

A report of tardive dyskinesia in 6 patients receiving benzodiazepines, 3 of whom had previously received neuroleptics; benzodiazepines might worsen or even induce dyskinesia-like symptoms, and their use to treat tardive dyskinesia is controversial at best.— A. H. Rosenbaum and J. R. de la Fuente (letter), *Lancet*, 1979, *2*, 900.

NEUROLEPTIC MALIGNANT SYNDROME. A review of the neuroleptic malignant syndrome. The symptoms include catatonia, clouded consciousness, extrapyramidal disorders (akinesia, rigidity, and opisthotonos), and autonomic disturbances, most importantly hyperpyrexia. The syndrome always develops in close association with neuroleptic treatment, often early on but sometimes only after several months. The syndrome develops rapidly, usually in 24 to 72 hours and has a high mortality. There is no specific treatment other than to stop the offending neuroleptic immediately; symptomatic management may include cooling, correction of fluid imbalance, benzodiazepines for muscle rigidity, and dantrolene.— E. Szabadi, *Br. med. J.*, 1984, *288*, 1399. Further reviews of the neuroleptic malignant syndrome: *Lancet*, 1984, *1*, 545; B. H. Guzé and L. R. Baxter, *New Engl. J. Med.*, 1985, *313*, 163; R. J. Abbott and L. A. Loizou, *Br. J. Psychiat.*, 1986, *148*, 47; T. J. Ingall and C. Tennant, *Med. J. Aust.*, 1986, *145*, 454; C. Harpe and A. Stoudemire, *Med. Toxicol.*, 1987, *2*, 166.

For the use of dantrolene in the treatment of neuroleptic malignant syndrome, see under Dantrolene Sodium, p.1233.

OEDEMA. A report of severe persistent oedema and fluid retention in a patient receiving long-term chlorpromazine therapy, which resolved following withdrawal of the drug and recurred on re-introduction. Peripheral oedema occurs in 1 to 3% of patients taking phenothiazines and may be due to the antidopaminergic activity of these compounds.— L. Witz *et al.*, *Br. med. J.*, 1987, *294*, 807.

PREGNANCY AND THE NEONATE. Psychotropic drugs have been suspected of teratogenesis but their teratogenic potential at therapeutic dosage is small, if present at all.— H. Ashton, *Adverse Drug React. Bull.*, 1983, (Aug.), 372.

In a study of the maternal drug histories of the mothers of 764 infants born with CNS anomalies, and 764 controls, benzodiazepine use up to the end of the first trimester was not associated with central nervous system defects despite an earlier report (C. Greenberg *et al.*, *Br. med. J.*, 1977, *2*, 853) of such an association.— K. A. Winship *et al.*, *Archs Dis. Childh.*, 1984, *59*, 1052.

SUDDEN DEATH. A report of the sudden death of a 37-year-old manic-depressive woman who had received high doses of chlorpromazine over the previous 2 days. Her death was believed to have been due to phenothiazine-induced depression of the medullary respiratory centres of the brain stem.— A. Whyman, *J. nerv. ment. Dis.*, 1976, *163*, 214. A suggestion that occasional reports of sudden death due to aspiration or asphyxiation in patients receiving phenothiazines may be due to a syndrome similar to bulbar palsy. It is not reversed by antiparkinsonian medication.— K. Solomon, *Am. J. Psychiat.*, 1977, *134*, 308.

Treatment of Adverse Effects

Following recent ingestion of an overdose the stomach may be emptied by gastric lavage and aspiration. Patients should be managed with intensive symptomatic and supportive therapy, with particular attention being paid to the maintenance of cardiovascular, respiratory, and renal functions, and to the maintenance of the electrolyte balance.

Various measures aimed at the active removal of drug have been employed in poisoning by those barbiturates with long half-lives but with the possible exception of charcoal haemoperfusion their value is questionable. Dialysis is of little or no value in poisoning by benzodiazepines or phenothiazines.

In the management of phenothiazine-induced hypotension the use of adrenaline or other sympathomimetics with beta-adrenergic agonist properties should be avoided; since the alpha-blocking effects of phenothiazines impair the usual alpha-mediated vasoconstriction these agents may exacerbate hypotension in such cases.

The management of poisoning with sedatives or hypnotics. The airway will become obstructed unless the patient is nursed in the coma position until alert enough to maintain his own airway. Central respiratory depression occurs less often with benzodiazepines than with barbiturates but combination with other CNS depressants has an additive if not synergistic effect. If there is a respiratory depression the patient should be mechanically ventilated. Primary respiratory acidosis may be compounded by secondary metabolic acidosis, resulting in an acidaemia the correction of which will tend to cause hypokalaemia. Aspiration pneumonitis is the other main respiratory complication, and should be prevented if possible. Hypotension should be managed initially with fluids or, if persistent, a positive inotrope such as dobutamine. In barbiturate poisoning prediction of the depth and duration of symptoms is notoriously difficult: plasma concentrations can only act as an approximate guide and the overriding factor must be the patient's condition. Active elimination may be considered in the minority of severely poisoned patients who do not respond adequately to supportive measures or who develop life-threatening complications. The most effective form is haemoperfusion; haemodialysis and forced alkaline diuresis are ineffective for short-acting barbiturates and should be considered only for barbitone or phenobarbitone. However, forced diuresis may prejudice an already compromised haemodynamic equilibrium. The general principles of barbiturate overdosage apply equally well to the benzodiazepines; however, active elimination is of no benefit. The clinical usefulness of benzodiazepine antagonists has yet to be established. Chloral derivatives are all metabolised within minutes to trichloroethanol, and apart from irritation of the gastro-oesophageal mucosa the principal effects resemble those of alcohol. Profound respiratory and cardiac depression may occur, and cardiac arrhythmias are not uncommon, although usually not sustained. If treatment is needed, such arrhythmias respond well to propranolol. Haemodialysis and haemoperfusion can both increase clearance of the drug. Following poisoning with glutethimide a characteristic fluctuating level of consciousness is seen; cerebral oedema, convulsions, and sudden apnoea may complicate severe poisoning. Forced diuresis and haemodialysis are not useful and the former may be harmful; haemoperfusion is the treatment of choice where supportive care fails. In overdosage with chlormethiazole the half-life may be significantly prolonged. Since the drug is often prescribed to alcoholics it is prudent to assume that alcohol may also be present in chlormethiazole overdose and that alcohol withdrawal syndrome may complicate the later stages of recovery.— C. Byatt and G. Volans, *Br. med. J.*, 1984, *289*, 1214.

The management of poisoning with neuroleptics. Gastric lavage should be performed up to 6 hours after ingestion, and be followed with activated charcoal. The mainstay of treatment is supportive care; if dystonic reactions occur they normally respond rapidly to procyclidine 5 to 10 mg or orphenadrine 20 to 40 mg given intramuscularly or intravenously. Dantrolene is the drug of choice in the neuroleptic malignant syndrome.— J. Henry and G. Volans, *Br. med. J.*, 1984, *289*, 1291.

There is no place for forced diuresis in poisoning due to one of the shorter-acting barbiturates since these drugs are largely eliminated by hepatic metabolism. Diuresis does increase the urinary excretion of long-acting barbiturates such as phenobarbitone but should now be regarded as obsolete since it is potentially hazardous and less efficient than haemoperfusion or haemodialysis. It has been superceded by conservative management, while oral charcoal is becoming the preferred method of treatment. Haemoperfusion is most effective, often dramatically so, in the treatment of barbiturate poisoning. It is now rarely performed, however, in the *UK* since serious barbiturate poisoning has become less common, and because there is an increasing tendency to use conservative measures in managing the poisoned patient where possible.— J. A. Henry, *Br. J. Anaesth.*, 1986, *58*, 223.

Discussion of the value of specific benzodiazepine antagonists in benzodiazepine overdose.— C. H. Ashton, *Br. med. J.*, 1985, *290*, 805.

For the use of a specific benzodiazepine antagonist in benzodiazepine poisoning see under Flumazenil, p.841. For discussion of the treatment of neuroleptic-induced extrapyramidal disorders, see Levodopa, p.1019. For the management of neuroleptic malignant syndrome see Bromocriptine Mesylate p.1014 and Dantrolene p.1233.

Precautions

Sedatives and neuroleptics should be given with care in elderly or debilitated patients who may be more prone to adverse effects. Caution is required in patients with impaired liver, kidney, or respiratory function, and in patients receiving other central nervous system depressant drugs in whom CNS depression may be potentiated: pre-existing CNS depression or coma is normally a contra-indication. Because of the drowsiness and impaired concentration that may ensue, affected patients should not drive or operate machinery where loss of attention might be hazardous.

The **barbiturates** are contra-indicated in patients with acute intermittent porphyria, in whom they may provoke an attack, and in patients whose hepatic, renal, or respiratory impairment is severe. Like other sedatives they should be given with care to patients in pain, in whom they may provoke a paradoxical reaction, unless an analgesic is given concomitantly.

With continued administration, tolerance develops to the sedative or hypnotic effects of the barbiturates but not to their lethal effects, and the therapeutic index thus decreases with time.

The barbiturates induce liver enzymes, and thus increase the rate of metabolism, and decrease the activity, of many other drugs.

Sedative anxiolytics, such as the **benzodiazepines** should be avoided in general in psychotic patients, and in those suffering from mental depression or suicidal tendencies (this applies also to the barbiturates) unless there is a marked component of anxiety in their illness. Care may be needed in epileptic patients, in whom the initiation or abrupt withdrawal of benzodiazepine therapy has occasionally provoked seizures.

The **phenothiazines** should be avoided in patients with bone-marrow depression, and should not be given with other drugs that may induce leucopenia and blood dyscrasias such as phenylbutazone or the thiouracil derivatives. They should be given with caution to patients in whom a sudden drop in blood pressure would be undesirable, in phaeochromocytoma, and cardiovascular disorders. When given with other drugs that produce postural hypotension dosage adjustments may be necessary; however, it should be noted that phenothiazines have been reported to reduce the antihypertensive action of guanethidine and other adrenergic neurone blockers.

Phenothiazines should be given with care in patients with parkinsonism. They inhibit the actions of levodopa. As many phenothiazines possess antimuscarinic actions they may potentiate the adverse effects of other antimuscarinics, including the antimuscarinic antiparkinsonian agents which may be given to treat phenothiazine-induced extrapyramidal effects. Phenothiazine effects on the vomiting centre may mask the symptoms of overdosage of other agents, or of disorders such as gastro-intestinal obstruction. Care may be required in patients with diabetes because of their effects on metabolism, and administration at extremes of temperature may be hazardous since body temperature regulation is impaired by these agents.

Care is required in epileptic patients receiving anticonvulsant therapy as phenothiazines may lower the seizure threshold; they should be avoided if possible in untreated epileptics.

Patients receiving phenothiazine therapy should receive regular examinations for abnormal pigmentation or ocular changes; those agents with antimuscarinic side-effects should be avoided in closed-angle glaucoma.

Withdrawal. All the drugs in this chapter may produce withdrawal symptoms if therapy is abruptly terminated: these are most likely to be severe on withdrawal of barbiturate therapy. When long-term therapy with a barbiturate or a benzodiazepine is to be withdrawn the dose should be reduced gradually over 2 to 3 weeks. Although gradual withdrawal has been suggested following therapy with a phenothiazine some sources suggest that it may be adequate simply to continue concomitant antimuscarinic antiparkinsonian therapy for several weeks after discontinuing the neuroleptic. See Dependence on p.706.

Concentrations of folate in serum and erythrocytes were lower than normal in 16 patients who took anticonvulsants, in 15 who took phenothiazines and in 7 who took tricyclic antidepressants with a benzodiazepine. All the patients showed significant induction of hepatic microsomal enzymes. Folate deficiency occurred in patients after 2 to 5 years' treatment and was greater in those treated for longer periods. It was suggested that folate deficiency due to the induction of microsomal enzymes might subsequently limit enzyme induction and hence reduce drug metabolism and could thereby lead to symptoms of toxicity in patients apparently stabilised for a number of years. The dietary intake of patients on long-term treatment with enzyme-inducing drugs might be inadequate.— D. Labadarios *et al.*, *Br. J. clin. Pharmac.*, 1978, *5*, 167. An investigation in 28 schizophrenic patients receiving long-term neuroleptic treatment with fluphenazine or flupenthixol, in some cases with chlorpromazine, showed no biochemical evidence of hepatic microsomal enzyme induction.— S. K. Majumdar and P. P. Kakad, *Postgrad. med. J.*, 1978, *54*, 789.

A study showing that the rate of non-trivial accidents in patients taking benzodiazepines was significantly increased compared with controls; there was no such increase for those taking phenothiazines or antidepressants.— G. A. C. Binnie, *Br. med. J.*, 1983, *287*, 1349.

A review of the likelihood of drug-induced heat-stroke. Patients receiving neuroleptics may be at serious risk in hot weather (most reported cases have occurred when the ambient temperature was greater than 30°, often combined with high humidity), particularly when also given antimuscarinics. Exertion and dehydration should be avoided and patients should stay in cooler areas as much as possible. One should also remember that patients receiving neuroleptics are far more susceptible to hypothermia in cold weather due to their impaired thermoregulation.— *Drug Interact. News.*, 1985, *5*, 23.

ADMINISTRATION IN CHILDREN. A report of phenothiazine intoxication in 30 children as a complication of phenothiazine treatment. It was considered that a large number had received excessive doses.— B. Duffy, *Med. J. Aust.*, 1971, *1*, 676. Data suggesting that impaired gut absorption or accelerated metabolism of chlorpromazine may occur in children.— L. Rivera-Calimlim *et al.*, *Clin. Pharmac. Ther.*, 1977, *21*, 115.

ADMINISTRATION IN THE ELDERLY. A review of the use of psychotropic drugs, including hypnotics, sedatives, and neuroleptics, in the elderly. There is now little place for the use of barbiturates, particularly in the elderly. Benzodiazepines are widely prescribed both as anxiolytics and hypnotics, but may also produce excessive effects on the central nervous system in the elderly. Those benzodiazepines with longer half-lives such as chlordiazepoxide, flurazepam, and diazepam should be prescribed for the elderly in smaller doses and at more widely spaced intervals than in younger patients. Those with shorter half-lives such as lorazepam, oxazepam, or temazepam should also be given in reduced dose, but in a dosage schedule similar to that in younger patients. Chloral hydrate may be a useful hypnotic in the elderly but the benzodiazepines are usually a wiser choice since its metabolites may displace drugs such as warfarin and phenytoin from plasma proteins. Neuroleptics should also be given in the smallest effective dose to elderly patients, in whom parkinsonian effects and tardive dyskinesia are more common than in younger patients. Rare side-effects such as photosensitivity, retinopathy, and agranulocytosis are also more likely in elderly patients.— T. L. Thompson *et al.*, *New Engl. J. Med.*, 1983, *308*, 134 and 194. Comment.— S. H. Zavaro (letter), *ibid.*, 1985, *312*, 652. Reply and correction.— T. L. Thompson *et al.* (letter), *ibid.*

Further references to the administration of psychotropic agents in the elderly: J. C. A. Morrant, *Can. med. Ass. J.*, 1983, *129*, 245; *Drugs for the Elderly*, F.I. Caird (Ed.), Copenhagen, WHO, 1985, pp. 118 and 121; G. J. Fancourt and C. M. Castleden, *Br. J. Hosp. Med.*, 1986, *35*, 321.

AIDS. Acute extrapyramidal syndromes developed in 2 patients with AIDS given prochlorperazine 10 mg by mouth every 6 hours. Persons with AIDS may be more susceptible to the neurological effects of phenothiazines perhaps because of the neurotropism of the HIV virus.— H. Edelstein and R. T. Knight (letter), *Lancet*, 1987, *2*, 341.

For a further report of a possibly increased incidence of extrapyramidal effects following low doses of a phenothiazine in patients with the acquired immune deficiency syndrome see Metoclopramide, p.1098.

HYPOPARATHYROIDISM. Five patients with untreated hypoparathyroidism suffered a severe dystonic reaction within 5 to 31 hours of an intramuscular injection of prochlorperazine in a dose of 10 mg for adults and 130 to 160 μg per kg body-weight for children. After being given vitamin D_2 to establish normocalcaemia, 2 of 3 patients challenged with prochlorperazine suffered milder reactions than before. One patient with idiopathic latent tetany suffered a severe reaction when given perphenazine. Caution was recommended in giving phenothiazine derivatives to patients with hypoparathyroidism and it was suggested that any acute reaction to such a drug should prompt investigation for some form of latent tetany.— M. Schaaf and C. A. Payne, *New Engl. J. Med.*, 1966, *275*, 991.

INTERFERENCE WITH DIAGNOSTIC TESTS. Phenothiazines are the drugs most commonly implicated in reports of interference with pregnancy tests, probably by causing increased secretion of luteinising hormone. Barbiturates have also been stated as causes of false-positive results in pregnancy tests.— S. Yosselson-Superstine (letter), *Am. J. Hosp. Pharm.*, 1984, *41*, 1098.

Phenothiazines may produce false-negative results in assays for urinary 5-hydroxyindoleacetic acid (5-HIAA) used in the diagnosis of carcinoid syndrome.— B. Clarke and H. J. F. Hodgson, *Br. J. Hosp. Med.*, 1986, *35*, 146.

LUPUS ERYTHEMATOSUS. Patients with systemic lupus erythematosus or those taking prednisone were more susceptible to extrapyramidal symptoms produced by phenothiazines or tricyclic antidepressants.— Boston Collaborative Drug Surveillance Program, *J. Am. med. Ass.*, 1973, *224*, 889.

MOUNTAIN SICKNESS. A plea that sedatives should not be given at altitude. Since diazepam, and possibly other sedatives blunt the hypoxic ventilatory response, sleep hypoxaemia might be exacerbated.— J. R. Sutton *et al.* (letter), *Lancet*, 1979, *1*, 165.

PORPHYRIA. Acute attacks of porphyria have been reported after the use of diazepam, chlordiazepoxide, oxazepam, flunitrazepam, and nitrazepam, and there is experimental confirmation for the first two. The quoted data must be put in perspective, however, as the reports of clinical exacerbations are few in relation to the widespread use of these agents in clinical practice. With the possible exception of chlordiazepoxide they could be used cautiously, if necessary, as tranquillisers or hypnotics, although for the latter indication chloral hydrate is perhaps the drug of choice. Among the neuroleptics, chlorpromazine has been reported to be safe in porphyric patients.— M. R. Moore and P. B. Disler, *Adverse Drug React. Ac. Pois. Rev.*, 1983, *2*, 149.

PREGNANCY AND THE NEONATE. If an anxiolytic or hypnotic is given during pregnancy it should be a benzodiazepine; barbiturates and older drugs such as meprobamate are obsolete. Although early reports suggested an association between maternal benzodiazepine use and defects of the palate in the offspring this has not been substantiated, and abrupt withdrawal of diazepam from an anxious woman in early pregnancy is not justified. There is no evidence that benzodiazepines are harmful later in pregnancy but the need for the drug has to be clear to justify its use. During labour a single bolus dose of diazepam up to 30 mg has no effect on Apgar score; however, a larger dose, or sustained prenatal benzodiazepine ingestion, can lead to the floppy infant syndrome. There is also good evidence for a withdrawal syndrome in infants whose mothers have taken benzodiazepines regularly during pregnancy. Many benzodiazepines are present in breast milk in amounts sufficient to cause problems. Assessment of the dangers of neuroleptic drugs is more difficult because of the already increased risk of neonatal mortality in schizophrenic mothers. Several studies have failed to show a teratogenic effect of neuroleptics; however, the phenothiazine prochlorperazine, used as an antiemetic, has been shown to be teratogenic between the 6th and 10th weeks of gestation. Neuroleptics enter breast milk in clinically insignificant amounts.— J. B. Loudon, *Br. med. J.*, 1987, *294*, 167.

See also under Adverse Effects, above.

Uses and Administration

The drugs in this chapter may be classed as psychotropic agents; that is drugs acting on psychic function, behaviour, or experience which alter the mental state by affecting the neurophysiological and biochemical activity of the functional units of the CNS, or, in the pharmacological sense, as narcotics, i.e. CNS-depressants capable of producing a state of insensibility.

The **anxiolytic sedatives**, also known as anti-anxiety sedatives or minor tranquillisers include the benzodiazepines, the carbamates, and a number of chemically unrelated compounds such as chlormezanone. They are used in the management of psychoneuroses to reduce pathological anxiety, agitation, and tension; a benzodiazepine is usually the drug of choice for this purpose although concern about the risks of dependence (see above) has led to some falling-off in their use. Some benzodiazepines are also employed in anaesthetic premedication.

There is no sharp distinction between sedatives and the **hypnotics**, which are used to induce sleep: the difference in action is mainly one of degree and the same drug or group of drugs can have both effects, larger doses being necessary to produce a state of sleep. Hypnotics produce a state similar to, but distinguishable from normal sleep, with characteristic alterations in the EEG; most hypnotics reduce the duration and intensity of the rapid-eye-movement (REM) phase of sleep, during which most dreaming takes place, at the expense of the non-dreaming, orthodox or 'slow-wave' phase. When the hypnotic is withdrawn there is a rebound increase in the proportion of REM sleep. Since insomnia arises from a variety of causes it may require other treatment than hypnotics; where a hypnotic is required, short-term use is preferable. The choice of a suitable hypnotic depends upon the onset and duration of action required, as well as the period of treatment and the age and personality of the patient; again, a benzodiazepine is frequently the drug of first choice.

The **neuroleptics** or major tranquillisers are also known as antipsychotic agents as their major use is in the symptomatic management of psychoses, including schizophrenia and mania. They include the butyrophenones, the phenothiazines, and the thioxanthenes. They are believed to owe their action to competitive antagonist properties at dopaminergic receptors in the brain. Some neuroleptics have also been employed in anaesthetic procedures, and in certain neuropsychiatric disorders such as Gilles de la Tourette syndrome.

ADMINISTRATION. For precautions to be observed when administering sedatives and neuroleptics to children and the elderly see under Precautions, above.

ANALGESIA. Analgesic effects have been suggested with some neuroleptics, such as chlorpromazine, and analgesic-potentiating effects with others such as haloperidol, but these have not been substantiated by studies in clinical practice.— G. W. Hanks, *Postgrad. med. J.*, 1984, *60*, 881. The patient in pain may be unable to sleep and combined therapy with a hypnotic and an anti-inflammatory at night can be helpful in rheumatoid arthritis. However the use of psychotropic drugs to enhance the analgesic effect of painkillers is more contentious. Neuroleptic drugs have analgesic effects in their own right and can be used as analgesic-sparing agents in the treatment of chronic severe pain. However, partners must be matched with care as side-effects may be unacceptable in combination.— *Lancet*, 1984, *2*, 793.

As part of the pain equation consists of mental distress it seems logical that some attempts should be made to relieve this. Anxiolytics may be of considerable value in some cases, and the author has found chlordiazepoxide in a dose of 5 to 25 mg by mouth every 6 to 8 hours of particular value. Diazepam is also valuable and may be used intravenously in severe pain to produce a state of extreme drowsiness in which minor surgical and other procedures may be carried out.— S. G. F. Matts, *Br. J. clin. Pract.*, 1984, *38*, 337.

ANXIETY AND NEUROSIS. The classification of neuroses.— P. Tyrer, *Lancet*, 1985, *1*, 685; M. G. Gelder, *Br. med. J.*, 1986, *292*, 972.

The presentation of the anxious patient.— K. Granville-Grossman, *Postgrad. med. J.*, 1984, *60*, 7.

Comment on the use of psychotropic drugs to alleviate stress, with particular reference to the nationwide survey in the USA by G.D. Mellinger *et al.* (*Archs gen. Psychiat.*, 1978, *35*, 1045). Among other findings it appears that men with high levels of distress tend to increase their alcohol consumption rather than take drugs, whereas the opposite trend was evident in women. It is not known whether patients with psychic distress turn to alcohol if denied drugs, therefore caution should be exercised in exhorting doctors to cut down their prescribing of psychotropic drugs, since the problems of alcohol abuse are far greater.— *Lancet*, 1978, *2*, 1347. See also G. D. Mellinger *et al.*, *J. Am. med. Ass.*, 1984, *251*, 375 (characteristics of long-term anxiolytic users).

With a reasoned approach to treatment, acute and chronic anxiety can be diminished by medications, particularly the benzodiazepines. Patients should expect that treatment will be of limited duration and will diminish but not eradicate the disorder. For situational or phobic anxiety, occasional use is indicated. For persistent symptoms, the use of anxiolytics for periods of exacerbation may be effective, although patients often report sustained improvement with maintenance treatment.— J. F. Rosenbaum, *New Engl. J. Med.*, 1982, *306*, 401.

Anxiety is a normal reaction but when severe and disabling it becomes pathological. Patients should be carefully assessed to detect associated problems in their lives and for the presence of underlying physical or mental illness. Drugs are often unnecessary in treating neurotic anxiety and psychotherapy or behaviour therapy may be successful. Where an anxiolytic is prescribed it is commonly one of those benzodiazepines with a longer duration of action. Diazepam and chlordiazepoxide have been used for many years and are cheaper than newer alternatives such as medazepam. Oxazepam and lorazepam have a shorter duration of action and may be useful in acute attacks of anxiety, while clobazam is claimed to produce less impairment of psychomotor function than other benzodiazepines in equivalent doses. The decision to give anxiolytic therapy should not be taken lightly. The risk of dependence increases if the duration of treatment exceeds about 2 months, and so patients should be told at the outset that treatment is for a limited period only. Some patients with chronic anxiety will need more prolonged treatment but to justify continued prescription there must be regular review and assessment of response.— N. Hockings and B. R. Ballinger, *Br. med. J.*, 1983, *286*, 1949.

A discussion on the rational use of anxiolytics. Neuroleptics such as chlorpromazine, thioridazine, and trifluoperazine have been advocated for the treatment of anxiety. The suggested dose is quite low, typically half or less of the usual dose in psychosis, but even at low doses autonomic side-effects such as dry mouth and dizziness may lead to poor tolerance in anxious patients because such symptoms mimic those of their disorder. Concern over the development of more serious effects, notably tardive dyskinesia has also led to a decrease in the use of neuroleptics for anxiety. The chief indication for such use is in patients with a history of dependence on other drugs, since dependence on neuroleptic drugs is virtually unknown. Dosage should be cautious and reviewed periodically and extrapyramidal symptoms should be monitored for carefully. However, the main, and most widely used anxiolytics have become benzodiazepines. There is little to choose among these drugs in terms of effectiveness, so the choice of drug is likely to be based on pharmacokinetic factors. A benzodiazepine with a long half-life, such as diazepam or clorazepate, is appropriate if the anxiety is sustained, whereas for episodic anxiety, shorter-acting compounds such as lorazepam can be used, taken 30 minutes or so before entering an anxiety-provoking situation, or even once the panic attack has already started. In patients with chronic disabling anxiety, which is usually alleviated by anxiolytics but which recrudesces on stopping medication, long-term usage becomes inevitable, with the risk of dependence; nonetheless, the risk is worth taking if the patient is handicapped by his or her anxiety, and if the response to medication is unequivocal. The recommendations made by the American Medical Association in 1974 remain relevant and cogent:

anxiolytics should be reserved for the relief of severe symptoms.

any underlying disorder should be diagnosed and treated before settling for symptomatic relief.

drugs should be avoided in patients with a history of drug or alcohol abuse.

doses should be kept modest to avoid psychological impairment.

be familiar with the need for gradual withdrawal, with support and encouragement, if abuse occurs or when discontinuing after long-term use.

dependence should be watched for during long courses of treatment, the risk becoming appreciable after 4 to 6 months.

the amount prescribed should be limited to that appropriate to the interval between visits.

patients should be warned that sedation may occur, especially initially, and that interactions with alcohol and other central depressants may be hazardous.

it should be emphasised that drugs are only part of an overall strategy for the management and treatment of anxiety.— M. Lader and H. Petursson, *Drugs*, 1983, *25*, 514.

A discussion of panic attacks and phobias and their management. Although benzodiazepines have been tried in most patients with these disorders there is no evidence of their effectiveness, whereas antidepressants have been shown to be uniquely effective.— D. V. Sheehan, *New Engl. J. Med.*, 1982, *307*, 156.

CEREBRAL ISCHAEMIA. The barbiturates have been used to protect the brain from neurological damage resulting from inadequate oxygenation following cerebral ischaemia, the rationale for their use being to reduce cellular metabolism, and hence oxygen requirement, in the CNS. However, studies with thiopentone and pentobarbitone have failed to demonstrate benefit.— A. Aitkenhead, *Br. J. Hosp. Med.*, 1986, *35*, 290. See also N. M. Dearden, *ibid.*, 1986, *36*, 94.

CONVULSIONS. A review of the management of persistent epileptic seizures. If the patient fails to respond to modification of conventional dosage regimens then oral benzodiazepines such as clobazam and lorazepam may be useful in small doses, given at night, in addition to conventional anti-epileptics. Where psychosis associates with epilepsy, phenothiazines in association with adequate anticonvulsants are usually effective, and there are usually no great problems despite the convulsant actions of the former.— D. F. Scott, *Br. J. Hosp. Med.*, 1984, *32*, 306.

Oral benzodiazepines may sometimes be a useful adjunct to conventional anticonvulsants for seizure prophylaxis in epilepsy. They are most effective at the beginning of therapy since tolerance often develops, and long-term therapy has proved disappointing; they seem most appropriate for short-term prophylaxis, for example to cover changes in anti-epileptic medication. Clobazam and clonazepam are the best studied; diazepam and clorazepate are seldom used alone for seizure prevention because of unwanted effects. Nitrazepam has been widely used in the treatment of infantile spasms with hypsarrhythmia, and in myoclonic epilepsy of childhood, but there is no evidence that it has a specific role in these conditions or is superior to other benzodiazepines.— *Drug & Ther. Bull.*, 1986, *24*, 45.

The treatment of convulsions in children. Immediate treatment must be effective and safe and a rectal solution of diazepam in a dose of 250 to 500 µg per kg, or 5 mg for children of 1 to 3 years and 10 mg for older children may be easily and conveniently administered. Absorption is rapid and bioavailability almost complete. Doctors may prefer to give diazepam intravenously. In those children who do not respond to diazepam, clonazepam may have some benefit but intramuscular or rectal paraldehyde is the more common alternative. If these and other drugs such as intravenous phenytoin do not produce a response chlormethiazole [edisylate] may prove helpful, an initial infusion of a 0.8% solution at a rate of 2 mL per minute (or 1 mL per minute in children under 3) for 5 to 10 minutes usually being adequate, followed by a reduced rate appropriate to response. Careful monitoring is required because of the risk of additive respiratory depression from previous therapy. If all the above measures fail induction of anaesthesia and continued anticonvulsant therapy is necessary.— G. Rylance, *Prescribers' J.*, 1986, *26*, 9.

Febrile convulsions. For a view on the management of febrile convulsions see Phenobarbitone, p.405.

Status epilepticus. For a review of the treatment of status epilepticus, including the role of diazepam, see under Phenytoin Sodium, p.411.

DEMENTIA. A discussion of the definition, differential diagnosis, and subtypes of dementia.— M. -M. Mesulam, *J. Am. med. Ass.*, 1985, *253*, 2559.

The prevailing opinion is that on the whole neuroleptics should be avoided in early dementia and should be used cautiously when behavioural symptoms, especially when associated with paranoid states, make sedative treatment necessary. Anxiolytic sedatives such as the benzodiazepines are often to be preferred to neuroleptics for treatment of anxiety and agitation in deteriorated elderly patients; however, if the patient's condition worsens and moderate doses of these agents no longer suffice it may be preferable to switch to neuroleptics rather than use high doses of an anxiolytic sedative which might induce ataxia or somnolence.— J. M. Orgogozo and R. Spiegel, *Postgrad. med. J.*, 1987, *63*, 337.

Reviews and discussions of dementia including the role of hypnotics, anxiolytics, and neuroleptics in its management: K. Davison, *Br. J. Hosp. Med.*, 1985, *34*, 112; *J. Am. med. Ass.*, 1986, *256*, 2234.

A review of Alzheimer's disease and its management.— L. E. Hollister, *Drugs*, 1985, *29*, 483.

DEPRESSION. A critical review of the use of benzodiazepines in depression. The benzodiazepines are extensively prescribed as a primary treatment for depression in clinical practice, particularly to women, despite a lack of evidence for any antidepressant effect. With the possible exception of alprazolam they are clearly inferior to the tricyclic antidepressants in relieving depressive symptoms, nor is there any evidence that a combination of such an antidepressant with a benzodiazepine is more effective than a tricyclic alone, even though individual anxiety symptoms may benefit in the first 2 or 3 weeks.— D. A. W. Johnson, *Br. J. clin. Pharmac.*, 1985, *19*, 31S.

EXTRAPYRAMIDAL DISORDERS. A discussion of the management of dystonias. The word is usually taken to mean an abnormal movement, or dyskinesia, in a group with tremor, chorea, myoclonus, and tic. The abnormal posturing is usually intermittent. The commonest cause is perhaps drug therapy, particularly acute dystonic reactions to phenothiazines, butyrophenones, or metoclopramide; such reactions respond well to intravenous diazepam or antimuscarinic drugs, which may need to be repeated over 24 to 48 hours. However, treatment for the primary dystonias is generally disappointing. Many drugs, including diazepam, the phenothiazines, and haloperidol have been tried, and have seemed beneficial in a small proportion of cases, but the results are unpredictable, and side-effects may limit their use.— *Lancet*, 1985, *1*, 321.

See also under Adverse Effects, above.

MANIA. A review of drug treatment for bipolar depression and mania. Moderate or severe acute mania is usually most rapidly controlled by a neuroleptic. Phenothiazines and thioxanthenes are effective but the butyrophenone haloperidol, in doses of 10 to 60 mg daily, is often particularly useful. The more disturbed patient may be given haloperidol 10 mg intramuscularly at half-hourly intervals until calmed. Larger intramuscular doses are to be discouraged as they may be excessive in some patients and their prolonged effects may make subsequent diagnosis and management difficult. In some patients chlorpromazine may be useful because of its greater sedative effects, if the patient will accept them. After an initial improvement when medication is commenced the manic state tends to improve further over the next 2 weeks; there is no evidence that increasing the dose of haloperidol further achieves faster improvement. In some patients failure to improve is due to poor compliance and here depot neuroleptics can be used satisfactorily. For manic patients who are not adequately sedated by neuroleptic medication, or to avoid prescribing such medication, sedation can be achieved with diazepam 10 to 20 mg intravenously or 30 mg by mouth, or else with intramuscular amylobarbitone. The anticonvulsant benzodiazepine clonazepam has also been reported to improve mania.— J. C. Cookson, *Br. J. Hosp. Med.*, 1985, *34*, 172.

NAUSEA AND VOMITING. A review of anti-emetics, including phenothiazines, butyrophenones, and sedatives such as the benzodiazepines.— J. Stonham and S. Ross, *Br. J. Hosp. Med.*, 1984, *31*, 354.

A review of the optimum management of nausea and vomiting in cancer chemotherapy. The phenothiazines are effective anti-emetics of approximately equal therapeutic value; choice of a particular drug must be guided by side-effects. They remain the standard treatment for drugs that produce mild or moderate emesis but are of little if any value against more severly emetogenic programmes. Prochlorperazine 10 mg by mouth or intramuscularly, or 25 mg rectally, given every 4 to 6 hours has been found to be effective and well tolerated for chemotherapy regimens that are mildly or moderately emetogenic. Butyrophenones such as haloperidol or droperidol are also effective anti-emetics; haloperidol in doses of 1 to 2 mg has been reported to offer more protection against severely emetogenic compounds than prochlorperazine and tetrahydrocannabinol. Benzodiazepines such as diazepam and lorazepam have been reported to decrease the incidence of chemotherapy-induced nausea and vomiting, although the mechanism is unknown; the capacity of lorazepam to induce amnesia has also been of benefit in improving compliance and has been investigated in the prevention of conditioned or anticipatory nausea and vomiting. Sedation with short-acting barbiturates has also been tried. There remains no single ideal anti-emetic; combination anti-emetic regimens are an attractive, if still largely empirical, approach.— P. L. Triozzi and J. Laszlo, *Drugs*, 1987, *34*, 136. See also J. H. Kearsley and M. H. N. Tattersall, *Med. J. Aust.*, 1985, *143*, 341.

See also Treatment of Adverse Effects of Antineoplastic Agents, p.583, and under Anti-emetics, p.1073.

PREMENSTRUAL SYNDROME. Diazepam and other benzodiazepines are frequently employed in general practice to treat patients with premenstrual syndrome where anxiety and tension are dominant. However, there are no studies to evaluate such therapy and it is probable that these drugs exaggerate depression and lethargy.— P. M. S. O'Brien, *Drugs*, 1982, *24*, 140. A discussion on the premenstrual syndrome.— *Lancet*, 1983, *2*, 950.

PSYCHOSIS. *Schizophrenia*. A review of biological aspects of schizophrenia.— S. Snyder, *Lancet*, 1982, *2*, 970.

An aetiological classification of schizophrenia.— R. M. Murray *et al.*,, *Lancet*, 1985, *1*, 1023. Further comments on the classification of schizophrenia.— L. E. DeLisi *et al.*, (letter), *ibid.*, 1502; J. L. Waddington (letter), *ibid;* M. A. Reveley and B. Chitkara (letter), *ibid.*, 1503; A. M. Reveley *et al.*, (letter), *ibid.*, *2*, 216.

A discussion of calcium-channel blockers, and the hypothesis that the calcium-channel blocking action of diphenylbutylpiperidine neuroleptics such as pimozide may possibly be associated with improvement of emotional withdrawal in schizophrenic patients.— S. H. Snyder and I. J. Reynolds, *New Engl. J. Med.*, 1985, *313*, 995.

A detailed discussion of the action, uses, and adverse effects of neuroleptics in the management of schizophrenia. It has become clear that dopamine interacts with more than one type of receptor in the brain, the D_1 receptor being linked to adenylate cyclase activation, whereas the D_2 receptor is not. Established drugs such as chlorpromazine appear to show little specificity, although the butyrophenones show preferential affinity for the D_2 receptor and the substituted benzamides such as sulpiride are highly D_2-selective. Although it is not yet possible to say for certain, the therapeutic effects of the neuroleptics appear to be mediated through an interaction with the D_2 receptor.— A.V.P. Mackay, Antischizophrenic Drugs, in **Drugs in psychiatric practice**, P.J. Tyrer (Ed.), London, Butterworths, 1982,, p.42.

Reviews of the use of neuroleptic agents: J. L. Black *et al.*,, *Mayo Clin. Proc.*, 1985, *60*, 777; M. G. Livingston, *Prescribers' J.*, 1985, *25*, 134.

The use of neuroleptics in acute schizophrenia. Neuroleptics are the mainstay of treatment; however, they are not a cure, and the long-term outcome in schizophrenic patients is often poor.— E. C. Johnstone, *Br. J. Hosp. Med.*, 1985, *34*, 198.

The management of chronic schizophrenia. Finding the best drug for a patient remains a matter of trial and error, and choice may be guided by knowledge of adverse effects, avoiding, for example sedative drugs in torpid patients. All authorities recommend the use of only one neuroleptic at a time, and dosage can often be simplified to twice or even once daily in view of the long half-lives of many of these agents. An adequate dose should be given, as failure to prescribe a big enough dose is the commonest reason for treatment failure; the highest doses are needed in patients who are agitated, more psychotic, younger, heavier, and male. If even a high dose is ineffective there are excellent pharmacokinetic reasons for trying a different route of administration, or a different drug. The ideal dose is the lowest one that is effective, which may be determined by stepwise reduction, but it is important to remember that the patient's current behaviour reflects changes that were made days, weeks, or even months ago. The question of when to stop maintenance treatment of chronic schizophrenia is difficult. Some evidence suggests a need to continue treatment indefinitely but many practitioners agree that it is difficult to justify not having a trial withdrawal of drugs every few years in most hospitalised chronic schizophrenics. However enthusiasm for regular drug holidays has waned for fear of causing enhanced receptor sensitivity. It is impossible as yet to generalise, and at the end, as well as the beginning, of drug treatment trial and error seems necessary.— R. Morgan, *Br. J. Hosp. Med.*, 1985, *34*, 202.

Criticism of the administration of high doses of antipsychotic therapy early in treatment. A double-blind study comparing loading against standard doses of haloperidol has demonstrated that for the average decompensated schizophrenic patient a moderate dose is sufficient to start the reintegrative process, which cannot be accelerated by loading doses. A patient can be started on a sufficient but moderate dose with therapeutic response and side-effects being carefully monitored. If there was no progress after 3 or 4 days a gradual increase in dosage would be indicated. The completely refractory patient, however, deserves a trial on high doses of potent phenothiazines or haloperidol.— S. E. Ericksen *et al.* (letter), *New Engl. J. Med.*, 1976, *294*, 1296.

The use of depot injections of neuroleptics in the maintenance therapy of schizophrenia.— D. Ginestet and L. Julon, *Trends pharmacol. Sci.*, 1982, *3*, 62.

Discussion of low-dose maintenance therapy for schizophrenia. Evidence suggests that a substantial proportion of patients who are presently maintained on fluphenazine decanoate at up to 25 mg every 2 weeks may do just as well on as little as 5 mg (but not less), with the added advantage of fewer side-effects. The approach should now be tried in the outpatient management of patients with chronic schizophrenia.— R. Manchanda and S. R. Hirsch, *Br. med. J.*, 1986, *293*, 515. Criticism. Such a conclusion is premature and incautious; many studies suggest an increased relapse-rate with low-dose therapy. As yet there are no clear indications that the standard practices of the last few years can be abandoned.— D. A. W. Johnson (letter), *ibid.*, 1099. Reply.— S. R. Hirsch and R. Manchanda (letter), *ibid.*

RESTLESS LEG SYNDROME. A review of the restless leg syndrome. The syndrome is characterised by aching discomfort in the calves associated with restlessness of the legs and an irresistible urge to move them. The disorder is intermittent but characteristically begins during relaxation in the evenings or in bed; it should be distinguished from neuroleptic-induced akathisia which is accompanied by inner restlessness of the mind and body and which is often eased rather than aggravated by lying down. Many drugs have been advocated for the treatment of restless leg syndrome, reflecting the high placebo response and spontaneous remission rates. Although the phenothiazines have been reported to exacerbate symptoms, chlorpromazine 50 to 100 mg at night has been recommended; however the safest and most effective drug therapy is a benzodiazepine such as clonazepam 0.5 mg in the evening.— W. R. G. Gibb and A. J. Lees, *Postgrad. med. J.*, 1986, *62*, 329. See also E. M. R. Critchley, *Br. med. J.*, 1986, *292*, 1729. Most patients do not require treatment, but in those that do levodopa should be tried first; then clonazepam, carbamazepine, and for resistant cases chlorpromazine.— C. Clough, *ibid.*, 1987, *294*, 262.

SLEEP DISORDERS. A review of the parasomnias. Parasomnias are motor or autonomic disturbances during sleep that result from disturbed sleep mechanisms. The main parasomnias include hypnic jerks, fragmentary sleep myoclonus, restless legs syndrome, periodic movements in sleep (PMS), bruxism (tooth grinding), head banging, sleepwalking, aggression during sleep, sleep dystonia, sleep paralysis, nocturnal enuresis, night terrors and nightmares, and sleep pain.— J. D. Parkes, *Lancet*, 1986, *2*, 1021.

A review of some sleep disorders. Insomnia is the most commonly encountered and requires multidimensional treatment: a hypnotic drug should be prescribed only as an adjunct to improvements in lifestyle, sleep-wake routines and sleeping environments. Sleepwalking or night terrors are more likely to be encountered in children, who usually outgrow them; when they occur in adults emotional disturbance is often present and psychiatric evaluation and treatment is generally indicated. Certain drugs that markedly suppress stage 3 and 4 sleep, primarily benzodiazepines such as diazepam and flurazepam may be given as adjunctive therapy in adults but are not recommended in children. Nightmares, which should be distinguished from night terrors in that the former occur in REM sleep, and are vividly recalled, may result in sleep disturbance if recurrent. Psychotherapy is often indicated and in patients in whom psychotic behaviour is associated with nightmares neuroleptic drugs are indicated.— A. Kales *et al.*, *Ann. intern. Med.*, 1987, *106*, 582.

A discussion of the treatment of insomnia. Insomnia is a symptom of various conditions and is best considered as being transient, short-term, or long-term. Transient insomnia occurs in those who usually sleep well and is usually due to an alteration in sleeping conditions e.g. noise, or an unusual pattern of rest, as in shiftwork. A hypnotic may not be needed, but when treatment is given a rapidly eliminated hypnotic is appropriate and it should be needed on only a couple of occasions. Short-term insomnia is usually related to an emotional problem or serious illness. A hypnotic is likely to be useful but should be given preferably for only about a week, and not for more than three weeks. Intermittent rather than nightly use is desirable, and a rapidly-eliminated drug is usually appropriate to avoid impaired daytime alertness, though in more anxious patients a longer-lasting drug may be preferred. There has been some controversy over the use of hypnotics in the third category of patients, those with chronic or long-term insomnia. Possibly one-third to half such patients have an underlying psychiatric disorder such as depression and it is this that should be treated. Others may be chronic abusers of alcohol or other drugs, while some may have specific sleep disorders. The most important of the latter is probably sleep apnoea and in such patients sedatives are contra-indicated. Nonetheless in many patients with chronic insomnia no apparent cause can be found. In such patients the essentials are exercise, controlled curtailment of sleep, reduction in stress, restriction of caffeine and alcohol, and the intermittent use of a hypnotic for 1 night in 3 for up to a month. In these patients longer-acting benzodiazepines may be more appropriate. If, after about a month, such treatment is unsuccessful a trial of a sedative antidepressant has been suggested, even in the absence of overt depression, although this approach is controversial. In general the benzodiazepines are to be preferred as hypnotics for their safety and usefulness but it is emphasised that patients should always receive the smallest possible dose for the shortest clinically necessary time; drug dosage has often been unnecessarily high, particularly in patients with transient and short-term insomnia.— J. Marks and A. N. Nicholson, *Br. med. J.*, 1984, *288*, 261.

Further reviews and discussions of the use of hypnotics for insomnia: N. Hockings and B. R. Ballinger, *Br. med. J.*, 1983, *286*, 1949; C. Hallstrom, *Br. J. Hosp. Med.*, 1983, *30*, 188; I. Oswald, *ibid.*, 1984, *31*, 219; *Lancet*, 1985, *2*, 253; A. Clift, *J. R. Coll. gen. Pract.*, 1985, *35*, 365; M. Lader, *Br. med. J.*, 1986, *293*, 1048; A. N. Nicholson, *Drugs*, 1986, *31*, 164.

The management of sleep disturbance in the elderly. Prescription of hypnotics should be the exception rather than the rule, and there should be regular review and discontinuation after a short course. Chlormethiazole is generally a safe drug in the elderly, although it may make some frail old people very drowsy. Dichloralphenazone is also used and causes fewer gastro-intestinal side-effects than chloral hydrate. Promazine is useful in demented patients with nocturnal confusion and agitation unresponsive to the other 2 drugs. Of the benzodiazepines longer-acting drugs such as nitrazepam or flurazepam are no longer considered suitable in the elderly due to adverse sedative effects and impairment of psychomotor performance. However a medium-acting drug such as lormetazepam may be of benefit and seems to lack the rebound anxiety sometimes seen with short-acting drugs such as temazepam and triazolam.— M. J. Bendall, *Prescribers' J.*, 1985, *25*, 99.

7001-h

Acepromazine Maleate *(BANM, USAN, rINNM).* Acetylpromazine Maleate; ACP *(base)*. 10-(3-Dimethylaminopropyl)phenothiazin-2-yl methyl ketone hydrogen maleate.

$C_{19}H_{22}N_2OS,C_4H_4O_4$=442.5.

CAS — 61-00-7 (acepromazine); 3598-37-6 (maleate).

Pharmacopoeias. In *Fr.* Also in *B.P. Vet.*

A yellow odourless crystalline powder. Acepromazine maleate 13.5 mg is approximately equivalent to 10 mg of acepromazine.

Soluble 1 in 27 of water, 1 in 13 of alcohol, and 1 in 3 of chloroform; slightly soluble in ether. A 1% solution in water has a pH of 4 to 4.5. **Store** in well-closed containers.

Acepromazine is a phenothiazine with general properties resembling those of the other phenothiazines (see p.706) which has been given in doses of 2 to 3 mg of the base by mouth three times daily. It has also been used as the maleate in conjunction with etorphine hydrochloride (see p.1304), for the immobilisation of large *animals*.

Proprietary Names and Manufacturers
Plegicil *(Pharmacia, Denm.; Clin Midy, Fr.; Seid, Spain).*

7002-m

Acetophenazine Maleate *(USAN, rINNM).*

Acephenazine Maleate; Acetophenazine Dimaleate; NSC-70600; Sch-6673. 10-{3-[4-(2-Hydroxyethyl)piperazin-1-yl]propyl}phenothiazin-2-yl methyl ketone dimaleate.
$C_{23}H_{29}N_3O_2S,2C_4H_4O_4$=643.7.

CAS — 2751-68-0 (acetophenazine); 5714-00-1 (maleate).

Pharmacopoeias. In *U.S.*

A fine yellow powder. **Soluble** 1 in 10 of water, 1 in 260 of alcohol, 1 in 370 of acetone, 1 in 2850 of chloroform, 1 in 6000 of ether, and 1 in 11 of propylene glycol. **Store** in airtight containers.

Adverse Effects, Treatment, and Precautions
As for other phenothiazines, p.706.

Absorption and Fate
For an account of the absorption and fate of a phenothiazine, see Chlorpromazine, p.723.

Uses and Administration
Acetophenazine maleate is a phenothiazine with general properties similar to those of chlorpromazine (p.724). It has a piperazine side-chain.
The usual initial dose for the treatment of psychoses is 20 mg three times daily, with a range of 40 to 120 mg daily. In severe schizophrenia doses of up to 400 to 600 mg daily have been given.

Preparations
Acetophenazine Maleate Tablets *(U.S.P.)*

Proprietary Names and Manufacturers
Tindal *(Schering, Denm.; Schering, Swed.; Schering, USA).*

4002-h

Acetylglycinamide-Chloral Hydrate

AGAC; AGAK.
$C_6H_{11}Cl_3N_2O_4$=281.5.

A complex of chloral hydrate and *N*-acetylglycinamide.

Acetylglycinamide-chloral hydrate is a derivative of chloral hydrate (p.717) used as a hypnotic, in doses of 1.7 g at night (equivalent to 1 g of chloral hydrate). It is also used as a sedative.

Proprietary Names and Manufacturers
Ansopal *(Gobbi-Novag, Arg.; Ferrosan, Swed.).*

12327-d

Adinazolam *(USAN, rINN).*

U-41123. 8-Chloro-1-(dimethylaminomethyl)-6-phenyl-4*H*-1,2,4-triazolo[4,3-*a*][1,4]benzodiazepine.
$C_{19}H_{18}ClN_5$=351.8.

CAS — 37115-32-5 (base); 57938-82-6 (mesylate).

NOTE. *USAN* also includes the mesylate.

Adinazolam is a triazolobenzodiazepine structurally related to alprazolam (below) and which is reported to have similar properties.

Studies *in vitro* indicated that the metabolites of adinazolam, U-40125, U-41128, U-42352, and U-33737 (estazolam) might be more active than the parent compound.— V. H. Sethy *et al., J. Pharm. Pharmac.*, 1984, *36*, 546.

Proprietary Names and Manufacturers
Upjohn, USA.

1676-x

Alpidem *(BAN, rINN).*

SL-800342-00. 2-(6-Chloro-2-*p*-chlorophenylimidazo-[1,2-*a*]pyridin-3-yl)-*N,N*-dipropylacetamide.
$C_{21}H_{23}Cl_2N_3O$=404.3.

CAS — 82626-01-5.

Alpidem is an imidazopyridine derivative that has been investigated for its sedative and anxiolytic properties.

Reference: B. Saletu *et al., Curr. ther. Res.*, 1986, *40*, 769.

Proprietary Names and Manufacturers
Ananxyl *(Synthelabo, Fr.).*

7003-b

Alprazolam *(BAN, USAN, rINN).*

U-31889. 8-Chloro-1-methyl-6-phenyl-4*H*-1,2,4-triazolo[4,3-*a*][1,4]benzodiazepine.
$C_{17}H_{13}ClN_4$=308.8.

CAS — 28981-97-7.

Pharmacopoeias. In *U.S.*

A white to off-white crystalline powder. **Insoluble** in water; soluble in alcohol; freely soluble in chloroform; slightly soluble in ethyl acetate and sparingly soluble in acetone. **Store** in well-closed containers. The *U.S.P.* directs that the tablets should be stored in airtight containers and protected from light.

Dependence, Adverse Effects, Treatment, and Precautions
As for the benzodiazepines in general, p.706.

ABUSE. Report of the abuse of alprazolam by patients receiving methadone maintenance therapy for opiate dependence. Ingestion of high doses of alprazolam following the taking of methadone produces a 'high' without pronounced sedation. Alprazolam is also being reportedly abused by other nonopiate-drug abusers, and the usual urine toxicology screens for benzodiazepines often give false-negative results for alprazolam because of the extremely low concentrations of metabolites excreted, making abuse difficult to detect.— W. W. Weddington and A. C. Carney (letter), *J. Am. med. Ass.*, 1987, *257*, 3363.

EFFECTS ON THE LIVER. Abnormal liver enzyme values occurred on 2 occasions when alprazolam was added to the treatment regimen of a patient receiving phenelzine for depression. Clinicians should be alert to a possible hepatotoxic effect, especially if alprazolam is used in combination with a monoamine oxidase inhibitor.— P. Roy-Byrne *et al.* (letter), *Lancet*, 1983, *2*, 787.

EFFECTS ON MENTAL FUNCTION. A report of the emergence of anger and hostility in patients given alprazolam.— J. F. Rosenbaum *et al., Am. J. Psychiat.*, 1984, *141*, 792.

A report of mania in two patients taking alprazolam; both recovered following withdrawal of alprazolam and treatment with lithium.— G. W. Arana *et al., Am. J. Psychiat.*, 1985, *142*, 368.

Stuttering developed on treatment with alprazolam in a 22-year-old woman. The condition regressed following withdrawal of the drug, and recurred on rechallenge with alprazolam but not with diazepam, lorazepam, or placebo.— R. L. Elliott and B. J. Thomas, *J. clin. Psychopharmacol.*, 1985, *5*, 159.

INTERACTIONS. *Cimetidine.* For the interactions of benzodiazepines with cimetidine see under Diazepam, p.729.

Dextropropoxyphene. In a study in healthy subjects dextropropoxyphene 65 mg every 6 hours significantly prolonged the half-life of alprazolam from 12 to 18 hours, and reduced total alprazolam clearance; there was no significant effect on half-life or clearance of diazepam or lorazepam.— D. R. Abernethy *et al., Br. J. clin. Pharmac.*, 1985, *19*, 51.

Digoxin. For the effect of alprazolam on serum-digoxin concentrations, see under Digoxin, p.828.

Oral contraceptives. For reference to interactions between benzodiazepines, including alprazolam, and oral contraceptives, see under Diazepam, p.730.

PREGNANCY AND THE NEONATE. Comment by the manufacturers (Upjohn) on cases of congenital abnormalities in children exposed to alprazolam and triazolam. Over half the cases of reported exposure completed their pregnancy and were delivered of a normal child without complications but benzodiazepines in general may be capable of increasing the risk of congenital abnormalities, and therapy or abuse during pregnancy may produce withdrawal symptoms in the neonate after birth.— W. S. Barry and S. M. St Clair (letter), *Lancet*, 1987, *1*, 1436.

WITHDRAWAL. Confusion, agitation, and visual hallucinations in an elderly patient, following abrupt withdrawal of alprazolam, were followed by unconsciousness and grand mal seizures. Benzodiazepines with short half-lives, such as alprazolam, may present a greater risk of withdrawal symptoms than those with longer half-lives such as diazepam.— A. B. Levy, *J. clin. Psychiat.*, 1984, *45*, 38. An earlier study suggesting that withdrawal symptoms are minimal after alprazolam or lorazepam. Seventeen of 40 patients given alprazolam, in doses up to 4.5 mg daily, for 6 months, subsequently experienced symptoms when placebo was substituted for active drug; 16 of 29 who had been receiving lorazepam up to 9 mg daily for the same period also reported symptoms. Of the patients with symptoms, 12 from each group dropped out of the study because of them, but only 4 of the 24 required benzodiazepines to alleviate their symptoms.— J. B. Cohn and E. P. Noble, *Psychopharmac. Bull.*, 1983, *19*, 751.

A review of 8 reported cases of severe withdrawal symptoms following discontinuation of alprazolam, including grand mal seizures, rebound anxiety, and psychotic symptoms.— J. L. Browne and K. J. Hauge, *Drug Intell. & clin. Pharm.*, 1986, *20*, 837.

Reference to the use of carbamazepine in attenuating alprazolam withdrawal symptoms.— E. Klein *et al., Am. J. Psychiat.*, 1986, *143*, 235.

Absorption and Fate
Alprazolam is well absorbed from the gastro-intestinal tract following oral administration, with peak plasma concentrations being achieved within 1 to 2 hours of a dose. The half-life in plasma is 12 to 15 hours. Alprazolam is extensively bound to plasma protein. It is metabolised in the liver, primarily by hydroxylation to α-hydroxy-alprazolam which is reported to be approximately half as active as the parent compound; plasma concentrations of metabolites are very low. It is excreted in urine as unchanged drug and metabolites.

References: D. J. Greenblatt *et al., Clin. Pharmacokinet.*, 1983, *8*, 233; R. B. Smith and P. D. Kroboth, *Drug Intell. & clin. Pharm.*, 1985, *19*, 450; D. A. Ciraulo *et al., J. clin. Pharmac.*, 1986, *26*, 292.

The pharmacokinetics of alprazolam in obese patients.— D. R. Abernethy *et al., Clin. Pharmacokinet.*, 1984, *9*, 177.

For the pharmacokinetics of alprazolam in patients with cirrhosis of the liver, see Administration in Hepatic Failure, under Uses, below.

Uses and Administration
Alprazolam is a benzodiazepine with general properties similar to those of diazepam p.731. It is used in the treatment of anxiety in doses of 0.25 to 0.5 mg three times daily by mouth, increased where necessary up to a total daily dose of 4 mg. In elderly or debilitated patients an initial dose of 0.25 mg twice or three times daily has been suggested.

A review of alprazolam. The basic pharmacology of alprazolam is similar to that of other benzodiazepines, such as diazepam, although it is about 10 times more potent than the latter. However, it appears to possess, unlike other benzodiazepines, some antidepressant activity. Clinical experience indicates that alprazolam 1.5 to 2 mg daily is comparable in efficacy to diazepam 15 to 20 mg daily in outpatients with anxiety, while initial studies in patients with both depression and anxiety suggest that alprazolam is comparable to imipramine in this group. Further studies will be required to determine the extent of alprazolam's antidepressant action in patients with depression alone. Alprazolam has also been investigated in the management of agoraphobia and panic attacks. Treatment of depression or panic disorders may require doses of up to 10 mg daily, although optimum dosages have yet to be determined in these disorders; if clinical response is not observed after 4 to 7 days of treatment with usual maximum doses, therapy should be gradually discontinued.— G. W. Dawson *et al.*, *Drugs*, 1984, *27*, 132.

Further reviews: *Med. Lett.*, 1982, *24*, 41; *Drug & Ther. Bull.*, 1983, *21*, 63; R. N. Straw, *Br. J. clin. Pharmac.*, 1985, *19*, 57S.

ADMINISTRATION IN HEPATIC FAILURE. A study of the effect of alcoholic liver disease on alprazolam pharmacokinetics. Alprazolam 1 mg by mouth was absorbed more slowly in 17 patients with alcoholic cirrhosis but no ascites than in 17 healthy subjects; the peak alprazolam concentrations in the 2 groups were achieved at a mean of 3.34 hours and 1.47 hours respectively, and the mean elimination half-lives were 19.7 hours and 11.4 hours. However, there were no significant differences in the maximum plasma concentrations achieved. The results indicate that alprazolam, in common with other benzodiazepines which undergo oxidative metabolism, would accumulate to a greater extent in patients with alcoholic liver disease than in healthy subjects; alprazolam may need to have the daily dose reduced by half in this population.— R. P. Juhl *et al.*, *J. clin. Pharmac.*, 1984, *24*, 113.

ANXIETY. A placebo-controlled multicentre study involving 976 outpatients with moderate to severe anxiety of at least one month's duration found that alprazolam 0.5 to 3 mg daily for 4 weeks tended to be more effective than diazepam 10 to 60 mg daily in relieving symptoms of anxiety. Doses were adjusted to minimise side-effects; drowsiness, the major side-effect, was seen more frequently with diazepam. The percentage of patients who were considered to respond to treatment was 80% among those receiving alprazolam, 73% among those taking diazepam, and 45% among those given placebo.— J. B. Cohn, *J. clin. Psychiat.*, 1981, *42*, 347. Alprazolam 1.5 to 3 mg daily was equivalent in its anxiolytic effect to diazepam 15 to 30 mg daily in a multicentre placebo-controlled study involving 46 patients, but there was also some evidence for an antidepressant effect of the former.— K. Davison *et al.*, *Br. J. clin. Pharmac.*, 1985, *19*, 37S.

Some further studies of the use and efficacy of alprazolam in anxiety: J. B. Cohn, *Curr. ther. Res.*, 1984, *35*, 100 (in geriatric patients); J. B. Cohn and C. S. Wilcox, *Pharmacotherapy*, 1984, *4*, 93 (comparison with lorazepam); M. A. Morphy, *Curr. ther. Res.*, 1986, *40*, 551 (in anxious schizophrenics); E. Väisänen and E. Jalkanen, *Acta psychiat. scand.*, 1987, *75*, 536 (comparison with oxazepam).

DEPRESSION. In a multicentre study involving 723 patients with unipolar depression of at least a month's duration, treatment with alprazolam in doses up to 1.5 mg three times daily, or with imipramine hydrochloride in doses up to 75 mg three times daily was more effective than placebo in relieving depression. Alprazolam was at least as effective as imipramine in relieving symptoms of depression, and was considered more effective on somatic symptoms during the 6-week period of study. At the mean doses taken (alprazolam 2.87 mg daily and imipramine 131.75 mg daily), which are equivalent therapeutically, there was evidence for a faster onset of antidepressant action with alprazolam. The results appear to confirm earlier reports of alprazolam's effect on depressive symptoms.— J. P. Feighner *et al.*, *J. Am. med. Ass.*, 1983, *249*, 3057. Criticism. The mean doses of the two drugs are not, as stated, equivalent. Most experts believe that a minimum of 150 mg of imipramine hydrochloride daily is necessary for an adequate therapeutic trial in most patients, whereas the mean dose given in this study was consistently below this. If adequate doses of imipramine had been given the results might have been different.— K. Jaffe (letter), *ibid.*, 1984, *251*, 215.

In a double-blind study alprazolam, in doses up to 6 mg daily in 9 patients was compared with imipramine hydrochloride up to 300 mg daily in a further 7 for the treatment of endogenous depression. A further 5 patients received electroconvulsive therapy (ECT). All patients showed an improvement in the first 10 days of therapy; however, after this there was no further response to alprazolam, whereas patients receiving imipramine or ECT continued to improve. After 24 days patients receiving imipramine showed an overall mean reduction of 71% in ratings of depression (Hamilton Scale), compared with 67% for ECT and 29% for alprazolam; improvement with alprazolam was mainly related to vegetative features of the illness rather than the cognitive symptoms of depression.— R. H. Lenox, *Psychopharmac. Bull.*, 1984, *20*, 79.

Further studies of alprazolam in depression: W. M. Pitts *et al.*, *J. clin. Psychiat.*, 1983, *44*, 213 (in geriatrics); M. Ansseau *et al.*, *J. Affect. Dis.*, 1984, *7*, 287 (compared with doxepin); K. Rickels *et al.*, *Archs gen. Psychiat.*, 1985, *42*, 134 (compared with amitriptyline and doxepin); N. W. Imlah, *Br. J. Psychiat.*, 1985, *146*, 515 (compared with amitriptyline).

PANIC. Mention of excellent response of panic attacks to alprazolam 750 µg four times daily by mouth in a patient with a Raynaud-like syndrome.— R. Pies (letter), *J. Am. med. Ass.*, 1985, *253*, 2833.

A 12-week open study of the effects of alprazolam in panic was completed by 30 patients, 19 with panic disorder and 11 suffering from agoraphobia with panic attacks. Patients received alprazolam in an initial dose of 0.5 mg three times daily increased gradually as required to a maximum of 10 mg daily. Fourteen of the 30 were considered to have responded by the third week of treatment, and 22 of the 30 by the 12th week; of this 22, 15 were completely panic free, while the remainder had occasional milder or less frequent attacks. The mean dose at the end of the study was 4.5 mg daily. Alprazolam was generally well tolerated, the chief side-effect being sedation, which was transient in most patients. Alprazolam appears to be a rapidly-acting and effective treatment for panic disorder or agoraphobia-associated panic attacks, but placebo-controlled comparisons with other therapies are needed before its place can be established.— M. R. Liebowitz *et al.*, *J. clin. Psychopharmacol.*, 1986, *6*, 13.

PREMENSTRUAL SYNDROME. Results of a crossover study in 19 women with severe premenstrual syndrome suggested that alprazolam 250 µg three times daily was superior to placebo in reducing symptoms.— S. Smith *et al.*, *Obstet. Gynec.*, 1987, *70*, 37.

Preparations

Alprazolam Tablets *(U.S.P.)*

Proprietary Preparations

Xanax *(Upjohn, UK)*. *Tablets*, scored, alprazolam 250 and 500 µg.

Proprietary Names and Manufacturers

Tafil *(Upjohn, Denm.; Upjohn, Ger.)*; Trankimazin *(Upjohn, Spain)*; Valeans *(Valeas, Ital.)*; Xanax *(Upjohn, Austral.; Upjohn, Canad.; Upjohn, Fr.; Upjohn, Ital.; Upjohn, Switz.; Upjohn, UK; Upjohn, USA)*; Xanor *(Upjohn, S.Afr.; Upjohn, Swed.)*.

1759-d

Amisulpride *(rINN)*.

4-Amino-*N*-[(1-ethyl-2-pyrrolidinyl)methyl]-5-(ethylsulphonyl)-2-methoxybenzamide.

$C_{17}H_{27}N_3O_4S = 369.5$.

CAS — 71675-85-9.

Amisulpride is a substituted benzamide related to sulpiride (p.766). It is used as a neuroleptic in the management of schizophrenia and acute psychoses.

Proprietary Names and Manufacturers

Solian *(Delagrange, Fr.)*.

18810-y

Amperozide *(BAN, rINN)*.

FG-5606. 4-[4,4-Bis(4-fluorophenyl)butyl]-*N*-ethylpiperazine-1-carboxamide.

$C_{23}H_{29}F_2N_3O = 401.5$.

CAS — 75558-90-6.

Amperozide is a neuroleptic that has been used in the treatment of animals.

Proprietary Veterinary Names and Manufacturers

Hogpax *(Ferrosan, Norw.; Ferrosan, Swed.)*.

4005-v

Amylobarbitone *(BAN)*.

Amobarbital *(USAN, rINN)*; Amobarbitalum; Pentymalum. 5-Ethyl-5-isopentylbarbituric acid.

$C_{11}H_{18}N_2O_3 = 226.3$.

CAS — 57-43-2.

Pharmacopoeias. In *Arg., Br., Chin., Cz., Egypt., Fr., Hung., Ind., Int., It., Jpn, Nord., Port.,* and *U.S.*

A white odourless crystalline powder. At 25° it absorbs insignificant amounts of moisture at relative humidities up to about 90%.

Very slightly **soluble** in water; soluble 1 in 5 of alcohol, 1 in 20 of chloroform, and 1 in 6 of ether; soluble in aqueous solutions of alkali hydroxides and carbonates. A saturated solution in water has a pH of about 5.6. **Store** in well-closed containers.

4006-g

Amylobarbitone Sodium *(BANM)*.

Amobarbital Sodium *(USAN, rINNM)*; Amobarbitalum Natricum; Barbamylum; Pentymalnatrium; Sodium Amobarbital; Soluble Amylobarbitone. Sodium 5-ethyl-5-isopentylbarbiturate.

$C_{11}H_{17}N_2NaO_3 = 248.3$.

CAS — 64-43-7.

Pharmacopoeias. In *Arg., Aust., Br., Braz., Chin., Egypt., Eur., Fr., Ger., Ind., Int., It., Jpn, Neth., Roum., Rus., Swiss,* and *U.S.*

A white, odourless, hygroscopic, granular powder. The *B.P.* specifies that it loses not more than 3% of its weight on drying, whereas the *U.S.P.* requires that the loss should not be more than 1%. Very **soluble** in water free of dissolved carbon dioxide, sometimes leaving a small insoluble residue; freely soluble in alcohol; practically insoluble in chloroform and in ether. Solutions decompose on standing; decomposition is accelerated by heat. The *B.P.* specifies that a 10% solution in water has a pH of not more than 11.0; the *U.S.P.* specifies a pH between 9.6 and 10.4

Incompatible with acids, acidic salts such as ammonium bromide, acidic syrups such as lemon syrup, and with chloral hydrate. Amylobarbitone may be precipitated from mixtures containing amylobarbitone sodium. This precipitation is dependent upon the concentration and the pH. **Store** in airtight containers.

INCOMPATIBILITY. There was loss of clarity when intravenous solutions of amylobarbitone sodium were mixed with dimenhydrinate, diphenhydramine hydrochloride, hydrocortisone sodium succinate, hydroxyzine hydrochloride, insulin, opioid analgesics, noradrenaline acid tartrate, procaine hydrochloride, streptomycin sulphate, tetracycline hydrochloride, or vancomycin hydrochloride.— J. A. Patel and G. L. Phillips, *Am. J. Hosp. Pharm.*, 1966, *23*, 409.

STABILITY OF SOLUTIONS. A 10% solution of amylobarbitone sodium in water lost 1.8% of its strength in 5 days at 20°, 3.7% in 14 days, 5.6% in 32 days, and 15.1% in 90 days. When heated at 100°, a 10% solution lost 4.2% of its strength in 10 minutes, 6.2% in 20 minutes, and 17.9% in 1 hour.— H. Nuppenau, *Dansk Tidsskr. Farm.*, 1954, *28*, 261.

Dependence, Adverse Effects, Treatment, and Precautions

As for the barbiturates in general, p.706.

Absorption and Fate

Amylobarbitone is readily absorbed from the gastro-intestinal tract and following absorption some 60% is bound to plasma proteins. It has a half-life of about 20 to 25 hours which is considerably extended in neonates. It is metabolised in the liver; up to about 50% is excreted in the urine as 3′-hydroxyamylobarbitone and up to about 30% as *N*-hydroxyamylobarbitone, less than 1% appearing unchanged; up to about 5% is excreted in the faeces.

METABOLISM AND EXCRETION. Following administration of radioactively labelled amylobarbitone to 2 healthy subjects 79 to 92% was recovered in the urine in 6 days, and only 4 to 5% in the faeces. Unchanged drug was practically absent from both urine and faeces, and less than 50% of the dose was identified as 3′-hydroxyamylobarbitone. A second main metabolite was identified as *N*-hydroxyamylobarbitone and found to account for up to 30% of the dose.— B. K. Tang *et al.*, *Drug Metab. & Disposit.*, 1975, *3*, 479.

5-(3′-Carboxybutyl)-5-ethylbarbituric acid appeared to be a significant urinary metabolite of amylobarbitone.— W. Baldeo *et al.* (letter), *J. Pharm. Pharmac.*, 1977, *29*, 254.

PREGNANCY AND THE NEONATE. Following intramuscular injection of amylobarbitone sodium 200 mg to mildly hypertensive women in labour 0.7 to 3.5 hours before delivery, the plasma half-life of amylobarbitone was 2.5

times as long in the neonates as in the mothers.— B. Krauer *et al.*, *Clin. Pharmac. Ther.*, 1973, *14*, 442. A similar distribution of half-lives was noted in 7 of 10 neonates whose mothers had also received amylobarbitone or phenobarbitone chronically for hypertension during pregnancy. There was no evidence of induction of amylobarbitone hydroxylation possibly because the foetal liver microsomes were not inducible by barbiturates in the doses used or because they had already been induced by other substances such as maternal hormones. Two apparently healthy children had very considerably longer half-lives (about 86 and 118 hours) and in one initially lethargic child the plasma-amylobarbitone concentration did not change significantly throughout the study-period.— G. H. Draffan *et al.*, *Clin. Pharmac. Ther.*, 1976, *19*, 271.

Uses and Administration

Amylobarbitone is a barbiturate that is used as a hypnotic and sedative. As a hypnotic it is usually given in doses of 65 to 200 mg at night. As a sedative it may be given in doses of 15 to 50 or 60 mg two to four times daily; higher doses have been given to patients under supervision in hospitals. A more rapid onset of effect is obtained with similar doses of the sodium salt.

Amylobarbitone sodium may also be given by deep intramuscular injection, when oral administration is not possible or for the emergency control of status epilepticus (it is not suitable for the routine control of grand mal epilepsy); no more than 500 mg should be given intramuscularly and no more than 5 mL should be injected at any one site. Under close hospital supervision, in emergency, it may also be given by intravenous injection as a 10% solution at a rate not exceeding 1 mL per minute in usual doses of 65 to 500 mg; the dose should not exceed 1 g. Subcutaneous injections may cause tissue necrosis.

ADMINISTRATION. *In the elderly.* Investigations in 2 groups of healthy adult male subjects indicated that the rate of hydroxylation of amylobarbitone sodium decreased with age.— R. E. Irvine *et al.*, *Br. J. clin. Pharmac.*, 1974, *1*, 41.

ADMINISTRATION IN HEPATIC FAILURE. Metabolism of amylobarbitone, after intravenous injection of 3.23 mg per kg body-weight, was compared in 10 healthy subjects and 10 patients with chronic liver disease. Of the patients with hepatic disorders, 5 had low serum-albumin concentrations and showed reduced serum binding of amylobarbitone and impaired metabolism: the other 5 had normal serum-albumin concentrations and showed no abnormality in amylobarbitone metabolism. No differences in clinical response were observed between the groups.— G. E. Mawer *et al.*, *Br. J. Pharmac.*, 1972, *44*, 549.

TINNITUS. A study demonstrating the beneficial effect of amylobarbitone in tinnitus.— I. Donaldson, *J. Lar. Otol.*, 1978, *92*, 123.

Preparations of Amylobarbitone and Amylobarbitone Sodium

Amobarbital Elixir *(U.S.P.)*. An elixir containing amylobarbitone with alcohol 26 to 32%. Store in airtight containers.

Amobarbital Sodium Capsules *(U.S.P.)*. Capsules containing amylobarbitone sodium.

Amobarbital Tablets *(U.S.P.)*. Tablets containing amylobarbitone.

Sterile Amobarbital Sodium *(U.S.P.)*. Amylobarbitone sodium suitable for parenteral use.

Proprietary Preparations of Amylobarbitone and Amylobarbitone Sodium

Amytal *(Lilly, UK)*. *Tablets*, amylobarbitone 15, 30, 50, and 100 mg.
Tablets, scored, amylobarbitone 200 mg.

Sodium Amytal *(Lilly, UK)*. *Capsules*, amylobarbitone sodium 60 and 200 mg.
Tablets, amylobarbitone sodium 60 and 200 mg.
Injection, powder for reconstitution, amylobarbitone sodium 250 and 500 mg.

Proprietary Names and Manufacturers

Amal *(Austral.)*; Amycal *(Norw.)*; Amylbarb *(Austral.)*; Amylobeta *(Austral.)*; Amytal *(Lilly, Austral.; Belg.; Lilly, Canad.; Ital.; Neth.; Lilly, UK; Lilly, USA)*; Amytal Sodium *(Lilly, Austral.; Lilly, Canad.; Lilly, S.Afr.; Lilly, USA)*; Etamyl *(Ital.)*; Eunoctal *(Fr.)*; Isoamitil Sedante *(Hosbon, Spain)*; Neur-Amyl *(Fawns & McAllan, Austral.)*; Neur-Amyl Sodium *(Fawns & McAllan, Austral.)*; Placidel *(Miquel, Spain)*; Sodium Amytal *(Lilly, UK)*; Stadadorm *(Ger.)*.

The following names have been used for multi-ingredient preparations containing amylobarbitone and amylobarbitone sodium—Amesec *(Lilly, Austral.; Lilly, Canad.)*; Amylomet *(Woodward, UK)*; Amylozine *(Smith Kline & French, UK)*; Drinamyl *(Smith Kline & French, UK)*; Ephedrine and Amytal *(Lilly, USA)*; Gerisom *(Winthrop, UK)*; Hypercal-B *(Carlton Laboratories, UK)*; Hypertane Compound *(Medo, UK)*; Neutradonna Sed *(Nicholas, UK)*; Placitate *(Faulding, Austral.)*; Potensan *(Medo, UK)*; Salimed Compound *(Medo, UK)*; Tuinal *(Lilly, Austral.; Lilly, Canad.; Lilly, UK; Lilly, USA)*; Vitaphen *(Faulding, Austral.)*.

4007-q

Aprobarbitone

Allylisopropylmalonylurea; Allypropymal; Aprobarbital *(rINN)*. 5-Allyl-5-isopropylbarbituric acid.
$C_{10}H_{14}N_2O_3$=210.2.

CAS — 77-02-1.

Pharmacopoeias. In *Nord.*

Aprobarbitone is a barbiturate and shares the general properties of the group (see p.706). It has been used as a hypnotic in doses of 40 to 160 mg at night and as a sedative in usual doses of 40 mg three times daily.

Proprietary Names and Manufacturers

Alurate *(Roche, USA)*.

7004-v

Azacyclonol Hydrochloride *(BANM, rINNM)*.

Azacyclonolium Chloride; MER-17. α-Phenyl-α-4-piperidylbenzyl alcohol hydrochloride.
$C_{18}H_{21}NO,HCl$=303.8.

CAS — 115-46-8 (azacyclonol); 1798-50-1 (hydrochloride).

Azacyclonol is an isomer of pipradrol (see p.1448) but lacks the latter's central stimulant properties. It has been given as the hydrochloride in the treatment of anxiety in doses of 100 to 800 mg daily.

Proprietary Names and Manufacturers

Frenquel *(Merrell, Fr.)*.

12412-x

Azaperone *(BAN, USAN, rINN)*.

R-1929. 4′-Fluoro-4-[4-(2-pyridyl)piperazin-1-yl]butyrophenone.
$C_{19}H_{22}FN_3O$=327.4.

CAS — 1649-18-9.

Pharmacopoeias. In *B.P. Vet.*

A white to yellowish-white microcrystalline powder. M.p. 90° to 95°. Practically **insoluble** in water; soluble 1 in 29 of alcohol, 1 in 4 of chloroform, and 1 in 31 of ether. Solutions are **sterilised** by filtration. **Store** in well-closed containers. Protect from light.

Azaperone is a tranquilliser used in veterinary practice.

Proprietary Veterinary Names and Manufacturers

Suicalm *(Crown, UK)*.

4009-s

Barbitone

Barbital *(rINN)*; Barbitalum; Diemalum; Diethylmalonylurea; Malonal. 5,5-Diethylbarbituric acid.
$C_8H_{12}N_2O_3$=184.2.

CAS — 57-44-3.

Pharmacopoeias. In *Arg., Aust., Belg., Br., Eur., Fr., Ger., Hung., It., Jpn, Jug., Mex., Neth., Nord., Pol., Port., Roum., Rus., Span., Swiss,* and *Turk.*

A white, odourless, crystalline powder or colourless crystals. Slightly soluble in water and chloroform; soluble in boiling water, alcohol, and ether. Dissolves in aqueous solutions of alkali hydroxides and carbonates and in aqueous ammonia.

4010-h

Barbitone Sodium

Barbital Sodium *(rINN)*; Barbitalum Natricum; Diemalnatrium; Soluble Barbitone. Sodium 5,5-diethylbarbiturate.
$C_8H_{11}N_2NaO_3$=206.2.

CAS — 144-02-5.

Pharmacopoeias. In *Arg., Aust., Egypt., Fr., Hung., Int., It., Pol., Roum., Rus., Span., Swiss,* and *Turk.* Also in *B.P.C. 1973.*

STABILITY IN SOLUTION. A 10% solution in water lost 2% of its strength in 10 days at 20°, 3.2% in 20 days, 8.1% in 40 days, and 15.1% in 80 days. When heated at 100°, a 10% solution lost 11% of its strength in 30 minutes and 34.7% in 2 hours.— H. Nuppenau, *Dansk Tidsskr. Farm.*, 1954, *28*, 261.

Dependence, Adverse Effects, Treatment, and Precautions

As for the barbiturates in general, p.706.

Mention of severe barbitone poisoning in a laboratory technician. Barbitone was widely used as an electrophoresis buffer and in the preparation of reagents to determine the kaolin-cephalin clotting time, and was therefore available in clinical chemistry and haematology laboratories.— M. Pye and D. J. Dawson (letter), *Br. med. J.*, 1984, *289*, 1625.

PREGNANCY AND THE NEONATE. Barbitone sodium appeared in foetal blood within 2 or 3 minutes of administration to the mother; blood concentrations comparable with those of the mother persisted for up to 15 hours.— C. E. Flowers, *Obstet. Gynec.*, 1957, *9*, 332.

Quantities of barbitone excreted in breast milk were enough to produce marked sedation in the infant.— T. E. O'Brien, *Am. J. Hosp. Pharm.*, 1974, *31*, 844.

Uses and Administration

Barbitone is a barbiturate that has been used as a hypnotic in doses of 300 to 600 mg about an hour before bedtime. Owing to its slow rate of excretion there is a special risk of a cumulative action. Barbitone sodium has been preferred for its more rapid onset of action following administration by mouth; it was also formerly given by intramuscular injection as a 10% solution and rectally as a 5% solution.

Proprietary Names and Manufacturers

Diemal *(DAK, Denm.)*; Dormileno *(Faes, Spain)*.

The following names have been used for multi-ingredient preparations containing barbitone sodium— Plexonal *(Sandoz, Canad.)*; Somnytic Tablets *(Philip Harris, UK)*.

7005-g

Benactyzine Hydrochloride *(BANM, rINNM)*.

2-Diethylaminoethyl benzilate hydrochloride.
$C_{20}H_{25}NO_3,HCl$=363.9.

CAS — 302-40-9 (benactyzine); 57-37-4 (hydrochloride).

Pharmacopoeias. In *Cz.* and *Pol.*

Benactyzine has been used as the hydrochloride in the management of psychoneurotic disorders in doses of 1 to 2 mg three times daily.

Proprietary Names and Manufacturers

Alin *(Lazar, Arg.)*; Lucidex *(Arg.)*.

The following names have been used for multi-ingredient preparations containing benactyzine hydrochloride—Deprol *(Wallace, USA)*.

7006-q

Benperidol *(BAN, USAN, rINN)*.

Benperidol; CB-8089; R-4584. 1-{1-[3-(4-Fluorobenzoyl)propyl]-4-piperidyl}benzimidazolin-2-one.
$C_{22}H_{24}FN_3O_2$=381.4.

CAS — 2062-84-2.

Benperidol is a butyrophenone with general properties similar to those of haloperidol (p.743).

Doses of 0.25 to 1.5 mg daily have been given in the management of aberrant sexual behaviour.

EFFECTS ON SEXUAL FUNCTION. Results of a double-blind placebo-controlled crossover study demonstrated no significant difference between the effect of benperidol 1.25 mg daily, chlorpromazine 125 mg daily, or placebo, on sexual drive and arousal in 12 paedophilic sexual offenders. The only significant difference was that self-rating of frequency of sexual thoughts was lower with benperidol. The effects of benperidol are unlikely to be sufficient to control severe forms of antisocial sexually deviant behaviour.— G. Tennent *et al.*, *Archs sex. Behav.*, 1974, *3*, 261. Current evidence is insufficient to substantiate the claim that benperidol has a specific action on sexual disorders.— *Drug & Ther. Bull.*, 1974, *12*, 12.

Proprietary Preparations

Anquil *(Janssen, UK)*. *Tablets*, benperidol 0.25 mg.

Proprietary Names and Manufacturers

Anquil *(S.Afr.; Janssen, UK)*; Frenactil *(Belg.; Clin Midy, Fr.; Neth.)*; Glianimon *(Tropon, Ger.)*; Psicoben *(Ravizza, Ital.)*.

12429-g

Bentazepam *(USAN, rINN).*

CI-718; QM-6008. 1,3,6,7,8,9-Hexahydro-5-phenyl-2*H*-[1]benzothieno[2,3-*e*]-1,4-diazepin-2-one.

$C_{17}H_{16}N_2OS$=296.4.

CAS — 29462-18-8.

Bentazepam is a benzodiazepine derivative with general properties similar to those of diazepam (p.728). It has been used in the treatment of anxiety states in usual doses of 25 mg three times daily by mouth.

Proprietary Names and Manufacturers

Tiadipona *(Knoll-Made, Spain)*.

7007-p

Benzoctamine Hydrochloride *(BANM, USAN, rINNM).*

Ba-30803. *N*-(9,10-Dihydro-9,10-ethanoanthracen-9-ylmethyl)methylamine hydrochloride.

$C_{18}H_{19}N,HCl$=285.8.

CAS — 17243-39-9 (benzoctamine); 10085-81-1 (hydrochloride).

Adverse Effects

Sedation and dryness of the mouth appear to be the most common effects. It is reported not to depress the respiratory centre.

Precautions

Benzoctamine should be used with caution in patients with renal or hepatic impairment. It may impair the patient's ability to drive vehicles or take charge of other machinery.

Absorption and Fate

Benzoctamine is readily absorbed from the gastro-intestinal tract and has been reported to have a plasma half-life of 2 to 3 hours. It is metabolised in the liver and rapidly excreted mainly as glucuronide conjugates in the urine.

Uses and Administration

Benzoctamine hydrochloride is used in the treatment of anxiety and tension states in usual doses of 10 mg three times daily. Benzoctamine has also been used as the mesylate for intramuscular or slow intravenous injection.

In a double-blind comparison of benzoctamine and chlordiazepoxide in patients with anxiety neurosis, both drugs produced a similar therapeutic response. With both drugs, doses of 10 to 30 mg were given and 26 patients received benzoctamine compared with 29 who received chlordiazepoxide. Side-effects were more frequent in the benzoctamine group.— W. H. Lo and T. Lo, *J. clin. Pharmac.*, 1973, *13*, 48.

Benzoctamine 10 mg three times daily was not significantly more effective than placebo in a double-blind study of 25 anxious patients.— J. S. Teja *et al.*, *Curr. ther. Res.*, 1975, *18*, 354.

Proprietary Names and Manufacturers

Tacitin *(Denm.; Ger.; Neth.; Ciba, Norw.; S.Afr.; Ciba, UK)*; Tacitine *(Ciba, Fr.; Ciba, Switz.)*.

7008-s

Bromazepam *(BAN, USAN, rINN).*

Ro-5-3350. 7-Bromo-1,3-dihydro-5-(2-pyridyl)-1,4-benzodiazepin-2-one.

$C_{14}H_{10}BrN_3O$=316.2.

CAS — 1812-30-2.

Dependence, Adverse Effects, Treatment, and Precautions

As for the benzodiazepines in general, p.706.

Absorption and Fate

For an account of the absorption and fate of a benzodiazepine, see Diazepam, p.730.

A study of the clinical pharmacokinetics of bromazepam in healthy subjects. Following administration of 12 mg by mouth to 10 subjects bromazepam appeared to be completely absorbed from the gastro-intestinal tract and peak plasma concentrations were obtained within 1 to 4 hours of administration. The plasma elimination half-life ranged from 7.9 to 19.3 hours (mean 11.9 hours). It was excreted in the urine almost entirely as the glucuronide conjugates of 3-hydroxybromazepam and the 3-hydroxybenzoylpyridine derivative (a mean of 27% and 40% of the dose, respectively), with a mean of only 2.3% as intact bromazepam and only 0.66% as the intact benzoylpyridine derivative. Studies of multiple daily dosing in 6 of the 10 subjects revealed similar pharmacokinetic findings.— S. A. Kaplan *et al.*, *J. Pharmacokinet. Biopharm.*, 1976, *4*, 1.

METABOLISM. The major metabolites excreted in the urine of 3 women after a single 12-mg oral dose of bromazepam were conjugated 3-hydroxylated derivatives [3-hydroxybromazepam and 2-(2-amino-5-bromo-3-hydroxybenzoyl)pyridine].— M. A. Schwartz *et al.*, *J. pharm. Sci.*, 1973, *62*, 1776.

Uses and Administration

Bromazepam is a benzodiazepine with actions and uses similar to those of diazepam (p.731). The usual dose for the treatment of anxiety is between 3 and 18 mg daily in divided doses by mouth, depending on the patient's response and the severity of the condition. Higher doses have occasionally been given. Doses should be reduced by half in elderly patients.

Proprietary Preparations

Lexotan *(Roche, UK)*. *Tablets*, scored, bromazepam 1.5 and 3 mg.

Proprietary Names and Manufacturers

Bartul *(Mepha, Switz.)*; Brozam *(Rolab, S.Afr.)*; Compendium *(Polifarma, Ital.)*; Durazanil *(Durachemie, Ger.)*; Gityl *(Krewel, Ger.)*; Lectopam *(Roche, Canad.)*; Lexatin *(Roche, Spain)*; Lexomil *(Roche, Fr.)*; Lexotan *(Roche, Austral.; Roche, Belg.; Roche, Denm.; Roche, Ital.; Jpn; Roche, S.Afr.; Roche, UK)*; Lexotanil *(Roche, Arg.; Roche, Ger.; Roche, Neth.; Roche, Switz.)*; Neo-Opt *(Braun & Herberg, Ger.)*; Normoc *(Merckle, Ger.)*.

7009-w

Bromperidol *(BAN, USAN, rINN).*

R-11333 (bromperidol); R-46541 (decanoate). 4-[4-(*p*-Bromophenyl)-4-hydroxypiperidino]-4′-fluorobutyrophenone.

$C_{21}H_{23}BrFNO_2$=420.3.

CAS — 10457-90-6.

Bromperidol is a butyrophenone with general properties similar to those of haloperidol (p.743). It has been given in doses of about 6 to 8 mg daily in the treatment of psychosis; higher doses have also been used. The decanoate has been given by intramuscular injection as a depot preparation.

Proprietary Names and Manufacturers

Azuren *(Janssen, Belg.)*; Bromidol *(Janssen, Denm.)*; Impromen *(Janssen, Ger.; Janssen, Ital.)*; Tesoprel *(Organon, Ger.)*.

4013-v

Bromvaletone

Bromisoval *(rINN)*; Bromisovalerylurea; Bromisovalum; Bromvalerylurea; Bromylum. *N*-(2-Bromo-3-methylbutyryl)urea.

$C_6H_{11}BrN_2O_2$=223.1.

CAS — 496-67-3.

Pharmacopoeias. In *Aust., Cz., Hung., Jpn, Neth., Nord., Pol., Roum., Rus.,* and *Span.*

Bromvaletone has actions and uses similar to those of carbromal (see p.717).

Proprietary Names and Manufacturers

Bromural *(Knoll, Austral.; Knoll, Ger.; Knoll, Neth.)*.

The following names have been used for multi-ingredient preparations containing bromvaletone— Menopax *(Nicholas, UK)*; Menopax Forte *(Nicholas, UK)*.

12458-e

Brotizolam *(BAN, USAN, rINN).*

We-941. 2-Bromo-4-(2-chlorophenyl)-9-methyl-6*H*-thieno[3,2-*f*][1,2,4]triazolo[4,3-*a*][1,4]diazepine.

$C_{15}H_{10}BrClN_4S$=393.7.

CAS — 57801-81-7.

Dependence, Adverse Effects, Treatment, and Precautions

As for the benzodiazepines in general, p.706.

INTERACTIONS. *Alcohol.* The clearance of brotizolam was slightly impaired in 13 healthy subjects when it was given with *alcohol*; co-administration enhanced subjective feelings of sedation but had no significant effect on measurements of psychomotor performance.— J. M. Scavone *et al.*, *Br. J. clin. Pharmac.*, 1986, *21*, 197.

Hypoglycaemics. Brotizolam did not appear to interfere with the hypoglycaemic response to *tolbutamide* or *phenformin*.— C. Rodriguez *et al.*, *Curr. ther. Res.*, 1982, *31*, 185.

Absorption and Fate

For an account of the absorption and fate of a benzodiazepine see Diazepam, p.730.

The pharmacokinetics of oral brotizolam. The drug is rapidly absorbed from the gastro-intestinal tract and almost completely metabolised; less than 1% of a dose being excreted unchanged in urine. The two major hydroxylated metabolites, WE-964 and WE-1061, are excreted in urine as glucuronide or sulphate conjugates. The elimination half-life of the parent drug is reported to range from 3.6 to 7.9 hours and the major metabolites probably have similar half-lives to brotizolam itself. Following administration of radiolabelled brotizolam approximately 65% of the radioactivity was excreted in urine, and 22% in faeces.— W. D. Bechtel, *Br. J. clin. Pharmac.*, 1983, *16*, 279S.

The mean oral bioavailability of brotizolam was 70% in a study in 8 healthy subjects.— R. Jochemsen *et al.*, *Br. J. clin. Pharmac.*, 1983, *16*, 285S.

Uses and Administration

Brotizolam is a benzodiazepine derivative with general properties similar to those of diazepam (p.731). It is used as a hypnotic in usual doses of 125 or 250 µg at night.

A review of the pharmacodynamic properties of brotizolam.— M. S. Langley and S. P. Clissold, *Drugs*, 1988, *35*, 104.

For a series of papers on brotizolam, see *Br. J. clin. Pharmac.*, 1983, *16*, *Suppl.* 2, 200S-440S.

JET LAG. A study of the use of brotizolam in the management of sleep disturbances following change of time zone after transatlantic flights.— A. N. Nicholson *et al.*, *Lancet*, 1986, *2*, 1205.

Proprietary Names and Manufacturers

Lendormin *(Boehringer Ingelheim, Ger.)*.

12471-p

Buspirone Hydrochloride *(BANM, USAN, rINNM).*

MJ-9022-1. 8-[4-(4-Pyrimidin-2-ylpiperazin-1-yl)butyl]-8-azaspiro[4.5]decane-7,9-dione hydro-

chloride.
$C_{21}H_{31}N_5O_2,HCl=422.0$.

CAS — 36505-84-7 (buspirone); 33386-08-2 (hydrochloride).

Dependence, Adverse Effects, Treatment, and Precautions

Dizziness, nausea, headache, nervousness, light-headedness, excitement, paraesthesias, sleep disturbances, chest pain, tinnitus, and nasal congestion have been reported following the use of buspirone. It is reported to produce less sedation, and have a lower potential for dependence, than other anxiolytics such as the benzodiazepines (see p.706).

Uses and Administration

Buspirone is an anxiolytic agent with dopaminergic and antiserotonergic properties but which is reported to be largely lacking in sedative, anticonvulsant, and muscle relaxant actions. It is given, in initial doses of 5 mg of the hydrochloride three times daily, in the management of anxiety and tension states; the dose may be increased if necessary to a maximum of 60 mg daily in divided doses.

Reviews of buspirone: K. V. Kastenholz and M. L. Crismon, *Clin. Pharm.*, 1984, *3*, 600; H. L. Goldberg, *Pharmacotherapy*, 1984, *4*, 315; C. S. Dommisse and C. L. DeVane, *Drug Intell. & clin. Pharm.*, 1985, *19*, 624; K. L. Goa and A. Ward, *Drugs*, 1986, *32*, 114; *Med. Lett.*, 1986, *28*, 117; *Lancet*, 1988, *1*, 804.

ACTION. Evidence from a study in 8 subjects that buspirone may have both agonist and antagonist properties at central dopamine receptors, resulting in stimulation of both growth hormone and prolactin secretion.— H. Y. Meltzer *et al.*, *Archs gen. Psychiat.*, 1983, *40*, 1099.

In a study in patients with generalised anxiety disorder 43 were assigned to treatment with buspirone and 13 were given diazepam, the mean daily doses being 16.5 and 13 mg respectively. Diazepam gave significantly greater improvement overall and in symptom scores during the first 3 weeks; however, at 4 weeks there was no significant difference between the treatments in terms of efficacy. More patients taking diazepam had CNS-related adverse effects such as drowsiness and nightmares, but the frequency of gastro-intestinal disturbances was greater with buspirone. Although buspirone appears to be as effective as the benzodiazepine after 4 weeks of treatment, diazepam appears to have a significantly earlier onset of action.— A. F. Jacobson *et al.*, *Pharmacotherapy*, 1985, *5*, 290.

In a multicentre study involving 293 patients with moderate to severe anxiety patients received either buspirone in doses of up to 60 mg daily or clorazepate in doses up to 90 mg daily, and treatment was continued for up to 4 weeks. The mean daily dose of buspirone ranged from 16 to 20.5 mg and that of clorazepate from 21 to 30.8 mg. There was no significant difference in the overall effectiveness of the 2 treatments, although fatigue was improved by buspirone, whereas clorazepate significantly improved sleep duration. Buspirone also reduced depression in patients with anxiety with depression. Sedation occurred more frequently in patients given clorazepate, who were significantly more likely to suffer a drug-related adverse effect. Buspirone appears to be a promising agent for the treatment of anxiety, alone or with associated depression, which causes less sedation than the benzodiazepines.— J. B. Cohn *et al.*, *Am. J. Med.*, 1986, *80, Suppl.* 3B, 10. Similar results from a comparison of buspirone with diazepam.— L. F. Fabre, *Curr. ther. Res.*, 1987, *41*, 751.

Retrospective analysis of data indicated that patients treated with buspirone who had previously used benzodiazepines had significantly less improvement than those without a history of past use. Prior benzodiazepine use did not alter the outcome of treatment with diazepam.— E. Schweizer *et al.* (letter), *New Engl. J. Med.*, 1986, *314*, 719. Similar results.— D. Olajide and M. Lader, *J. clin. Psychopharmacol.*, 1987, *7*, 148.

Beneficial effects of buspirone in the management of an elderly, agitated, demented patient.— C. C. Colenda (letter), *Lancet*, 1988, *1*, 1169.

Proprietary Preparations

Buspar *(Bristol-Myers Pharmaceuticals, UK). Tablets*, buspirone hydrochloride 5 mg.

Proprietary Names and Manufacturers

Bespar *(Bristol, Ger.)*; Buspar *(Astra, Austral.; Bristol-Myers Pharmaceuticals, UK; Mead Johnson Pharmaceutical, USA).*

4014-g

Butalbital *(USAN, rINN).*

Alisobumalum; Allylbarbital; Allylbarbituric Acid; Itobarbital; Tetrallobarbital. 5-Allyl-5-isobutylbarbituric acid.
$C_{11}H_{16}N_2O_3=224.3$.

CAS — 77-26-9.

NOTE. The name Butalbital has also been applied to talbutal (p.768), the s-butyl analogue.

Pharmacopoeias. In *U.S.*

A white odourless crystalline powder. Slightly **soluble** in cold water; soluble in boiling water; freely soluble in alcohol, chloroform, and ether; soluble in aqueous solutions of alkali hydroxides and carbonates. A saturated solution is acid to litmus.
Store in well-closed containers.

Butalbital is a barbiturate and shares the general properties of the group (see p.706). It has been used as a hypnotic and sedative.

Proprietary Names and Manufacturers

Sandoptal *(Sandoz, USA).*

The following names have been used for multi-ingredient preparations containing butalbital— Amaphen *(Trimen, USA)*; Amaphen with Codeine *(Trimen, USA)*; Anoquan *(Mallard, USA)*; Axotal *(Adria, USA)*; B-A-C *(Mayrand, USA)*; B-A-C 3 *(Mayrand, USA)*; Bancap *(Forest Pharmaceuticals, USA)*; Bancap with Codeine *(Forest Pharmaceuticals, USA)*; Bucet *(UAD, USA)*; Cafergot-PB *(Sandoz, Austral.)*; Esgic *(Forest Pharmaceuticals, USA)*; Fioricet *(Sandoz, USA)*; Fiorinal *(Sandoz, Canad.; Sandoz, USA)*; Fiorinal with Codeine *(Sandoz, USA)*; Fiorinal-C *(Sandoz, Canad.)*; G-1/G-2/G-3 Capsules *(Hauck, USA)*; Medigesic Plus *(US Pharmaceutical, USA)*; Neo-HS *(Neolab, Canad.)*; Pacaps *(Lasalle, USA)*; Phrenilin *(Carnrick, USA)*; Phrenilin with Codeine *(Carnrick, USA)*; Plexonal *(Sandoz, Canad.)*; Repan *(Everett, USA)*; Sedapap *(Mayrand, USA)*; Tecnal *(Technilab, Canad.)*; Tecnal C *(Technilab, Canad.)*; T-Gesic *(T.E. Williams, USA)*; Triad *(UAD, USA)*; Two-Dyne *(Hyrex, USA).*

7010-m

Butaperazine Maleate *(USAN, rINNM).*

AHR-3000 (butaperazine); Bayer-1362 (butaperazine); Butaperazine Dimaleate; Riker-595 (butaperazine). 1-{10-[3-(4-Methylpiperazin-1-yl)propyl]phenothiazin-2-yl}butan-1-one dimaleate.
$C_{24}H_{31}N_3OS,2C_4H_4O_4=641.7$.

CAS — 653-03-2 (butaperazine); 1063-55-4 (maleate).

Pharmacopoeias. In *Jug.*

7011-b

Butaperazine Phosphate *(rINNM).*

$C_{24}H_{31}N_3OS,2H_3PO_4=605.6$.

CAS — 7389-45-9.

Adverse Effects, Treatment, and Precautions

As for the phenothiazines in general, p.706.

Absorption and Fate

For an account of the absorption and fate of a phenothiazine, see Chlorpromazine, p.723.

Uses and Administration

Butaperazine is a phenothiazine with general properties similar to those of chlorpromazine (p.724). It has a piperazine side-chain.
Butaperazine has been administered by mouth as the maleate and has been given by injection as the phosphate.
The usual dose for the treatment of psychoses is 5 to 10 mg of butaperazine three times daily, given by mouth as the maleate, to a maximum of 100 mg daily, in divided doses. It has also been given by deep intramuscular injection as the phosphate.

Proprietary Names and Manufacturers

Randolectil *(Bayer, Arg.)*; Repoise *(Robins, USA).*

4015-q

Butobarbitone *(BAN).*

Butethal; Butobarbital (distinguish from Butabarbital, which is secbutobarbitone); Butobarbitalum. 5-Butyl-5-ethylbarbituric acid.
$C_{10}H_{16}N_2O_3=212.2$.

CAS — 77-28-1.

Pharmacopoeias. In *Aust., Br., Eur., Fr., Ger., Hung., It., Neth.,* and *Swiss.*

Colourless crystals or white crystalline, almost odourless, powder. Slightly **soluble** in water; freely soluble in alcohol and in chloroform; soluble in ether; soluble in aqueous solutions of alkali hydroxides and carbonates and ammonia, forming salts.

Dependence, Adverse Effects, Treatment, and Precautions

As for the barbiturates in general, p.706.

A 28-year-old conscious woman, who later stated that she had taken butobarbitone 6 g in the 3 previous days, had vertical gaze paralysis suggestive of brain lesions. Recognition of such paralysis in barbiturate poisoning might obviate unnecessary neurological investigation.— R. H. Edis and F. L. Mastaglia, *Br. med. J.*, 1977, *1*, 144.

INTERACTIONS. Results suggesting that metronidazole alters the metabolism of butobarbitone when taken concomitantly.— M. A. Al Sharifi *et al.*, *J. Pharm. Pharmac.*, 1982, *34*, 126.

Absorption and Fate

Butobarbitone is inactivated in the liver mainly by hydroxylation; small amounts are excreted in the urine as unchanged drug. It has been reported to have a half-life of about 40 to 55 hours and to be about 26% bound to plasma proteins.

A kinetic study of urinary excretion in 2 healthy subjects; results for butobarbitone and its 3′-hydroxyl, 3′-oxo, and 3-acid metabolites. The half-life of butobarbitone was estimated as 50.2 hours in one subject and 55.5 hours in the other.— J. N. T. Gilbert *et al.*, *J. Pharm. Pharmac.*, 1974, *26, Suppl.*, 16P.

Following administration of butobarbitone 200 mg to 5 healthy subjects, half-lives of 33.6 to 41.5 hours were measured. Nightly administration of 50 to 200 mg for several days to 4 of the subjects led to substantial accumulation; the half-lives decreased by about 20 to 25% probably due to enzyme induction. Repeated administration of butobarbitone should be avoided, and occasional use restricted to hospital in-patients in whom daytime sedation is required.— D. D. Breimer, *Eur. J. clin. Pharmac.*, 1976, *10*, 263.

See also under Interactions, above.

Uses and Administration

Butobarbitone is a barbiturate that has been used as a hypnotic and sedative. As a hypnotic it is usually given by mouth in doses of 100 to 200 mg at night.

A report of the use of butobarbitone to alleviate attacks of paroxysmal atrial fibrillation.— H. Yarrow (letter), *Br. med. J.*, 1983, *286*, 1980.

Proprietary Preparations

Soneryl *(May & Baker, UK). Tablets*, scored, butobarbitone 100 mg.

Proprietary Names and Manufacturers

Sonabarb *(Protea, Austral.)*; Soneryl *(May & Baker, Austral.; Belg.; Rhône-Poulenc, Canad.; Denm.; Fr.; Neth.; May & Baker, S.Afr.; Switz.; May & Baker, UK).*

The following names have been used for multi-ingredient preparations containing butobarbitone— Butomet *(Woodward, UK)*; Dolalgin *(May & Baker, UK)*; Sonalgin *(May & Baker, Austral.; May & Baker, UK)*; Sonergan *(May & Baker, UK).*

18886-w

Butoctamide Hemisuccinate *(rINNM).*
Butoctamide Semisuccinate. *N*-(2-Ethylhexyl)-3-hydroxybutyramide hydrogen succinate.
$C_{16}H_{29}NO_5$=315.4.

CAS — 32838-26-9.

Butoctamide is a hypnotic that has been used in the short-term management of insomnia in doses of 200 mg of the hemisuccinate at night.

Proprietary Names and Manufacturers
Listomin *(Lion, Jpn).*

3901-g

Calcium Carbamoylaspartate
Calcium *N*-Carbamoylaspartate; Calcium Ureidosuccinate.
$C_5H_6CaN_2O_5$=214.2.

CAS — 16649-79-9.

Calcium carbamoylaspartate is reported to possess sedative properties and has been given in the treatment of insomnia and behavioural disorders in children.

Proprietary Names and Manufacturers
Sedalin *(Rocador, Spain).*

7012-v

Camazepam *(rINN).*
SB-5833. 7-Chloro-2,3-dihydro-1-methyl-2-oxo-5-phenyl-1*H*-1,4-benzodiazepin-3-yl dimethylcarbamate.
$C_{19}H_{18}ClN_3O_3$=371.8.

CAS — 36104-80-0.

Camazepam is a benzodiazepine and shares the general properties of the group (see p.706). The usual dose for the treatment of anxiety is 10 mg twice or three times daily; in severe conditions up to 20 mg three times daily has been given.

Proprietary Names and Manufacturers
Albego *(Sintesa, Belg.; Boehringer Ingelheim, Ger.; Simes, Ital.; ICN, Neth.; Farmasimes, Spain; Inpharzam, Switz.)*; Limpidon *(Crinos, Ital.)*; Paxor *(Bristol, Belg.).*

7013-g

Captodiame Hydrochloride *(BANM, rINNM).*
Captodiamine Hydrochloride. 2-(4-Butylthiobenzhydrylthio)ethyldimethylamine hydrochloride.
$C_{21}H_{29}NS_2$,HCl=396.0.

CAS — 486-17-9 (captodiame); 904-04-1 (hydrochloride).

Captodiame hydrochloride has been given in doses of 50 mg three times daily for the treatment of anxiety and tension.

Proprietary Names and Manufacturers
Covatine *(Bailly, Fr.).*

4018-w

Carbromal *(BAN, rINN).*
Bromodiethylacetylurea; Karbromal. *N*-(2-Bromo-2-ethylbutyryl)urea.
$C_7H_{13}BrN_2O_2$=237.1.

CAS — 77-65-6.

Pharmacopoeias. In *Arg., Aust., Belg., Br., Ger., Hung., Mex., Nord., Pol., Port., Rus.,* and *Span.*

A white, odourless or almost odourless, crystalline powder. Slightly **soluble** in water; soluble 1 in 18 of alcohol, 1 in 2 of chloroform, and 1 in 25 of ether.

Dependence, Adverse Effects, Treatment, and Precautions
As for the barbiturates, p.706.
Continuous use of carbromal over long periods may give rise to symptoms of chronic toxicity resembling bromism, including CNS depression, irritability, and slurring of speech. Skin eruptions including non-thrombocytopenic purpura, have been reported. Deaths have occurred following excessive dosage.

Reversible cataracts were seen in a man who had taken half or one Carbrital capsule every night continuously for 5 years. The condition appeared to have been due to the carbromal and cleared up on stopping administration of the drug.— R. Crawford, *Br. med. J.*, 1959, *2*, 1231.

OVERDOSAGE. Six of 7 patients who had ingested an estimated 26 to 60 g of carbromal and in whom routine gastric lavage had been unsuccessful survived after gastroscopic lavage had been performed until the stomach appeared free of tablet mass.— H. -J. Marsteller and R. Gugler (letter), *New Engl. J. Med.*, 1977, *296*, 1003.

Absorption and Fate
Carbromal is readily absorbed from the gastro-intestinal tract and is partly metabolised to 2-ethylbutyrylurea and bromide ion.

Excretion of bromine in the urine after therapeutic and suicidal doses of carbromal.— H. Schütz and Y. D. Ha, *Arzneimittel-Forsch.*, 1975, *25*, 432.

Uses and Administration
Carbromal is a bromureide which has been used as a hypnotic, in doses of 0.5 to 1 g at night, and as a sedative in doses of 0.25 to 0.5 g two or three times daily.

Proprietary Names and Manufacturers
Adalin *(Bayer, Ger.)*; Diacid *(Neth.)*; Mirfudorm *(Merckle, Ger.)*; Neo-diacid *(Neth.).*

The following names have been used for multi-ingredient preparations containing carbromal— Carbrital *(Parke, Davis, Austral.; Parke, Davis, Canad.; Parke, Davis, UK*; Menopax *(Nicholas, UK)*; Menopax Forte *(Nicholas, UK).*

7014-q

Carphenazine Maleate *(BANM, USAN).*
Carfenazine Maleate *(rINNM)*; NSC-71755; Wy-2445. 1-(10-{3-[4-(2-Hydroxyethyl)piperazin-1-yl]propyl-}phenothiazin-2-yl)propan-1-one dimaleate.
$C_{24}H_{31}N_3O_2S,2C_4H_4O_4$=657.7.

CAS — 2622-30-2 (carphenazine); 2975-34-0 (maleate).

Pharmacopoeias. In *U.S.*

A fine yellow powder, odourless or with a slight odour. **Soluble** 1 in 600 of water and 1 in 400 of alcohol; practically insoluble in chloroform and ether. A 1% suspension in water has a pH of 2.5 to 3.5; the *U.S.P.* Oral Solution has a pH of between 5.8 and 6.8. **Store** in airtight containers. Protect from light.

Adverse Effects, Treatment, and Precautions
As for the phenothiazines in general, p.706.

Absorption and Fate
For an account of the absorption and fate of a phenothiazine, see Chlorpromazine, p.723.

Uses and Administration
Carphenazine is a phenothiazine with general properties similar to those of chlorpromazine (p.724). It has a piperazine side-chain.
Carphenazine has been given in psychoses as the maleate in usual doses of 25 to 50 mg three times daily, to a maximum of 400 mg daily in divided doses.

Preparations
Carphenazine Maleate Oral Solution *(U.S.P.)*

Proprietary Names and Manufacturers
Proketazine *(Wyeth, USA).*

7015-p

Carpipramine Hydrochloride *(rINNM).*
PZ-1511. 1-[3-(10,11-Dihydro-5*H*-dibenz[*b,f*]azepin-5-yl)propyl]-4-piperidinopiperidine-4-carboxamide dihydrochloride monohydrate.
$C_{28}H_{38}N_4O$,2HCl,H_2O=537.6.

CAS — 5942-95-0 (carpipramine); 7075-03-8 (hydrochloride, anhydrous).

Carpipramine is structurally related both to imipramine (p.362) and to butyrophenones like haloperidol (p.743). It has been used in the management of psychoses, particularly in withdrawn or apathetic patients. It is given as the hydrochloride in a usual dose equivalent to 50 mg of the base three times daily, with a range of 50 to 400 mg daily.

Proprietary Names and Manufacturers
Defekton *(Jpn)*; Prazinil *(Fournier Frères, Fr.).*

4020-b

Chloral Hydrate *(BAN, USAN).*
Chloral; Chloral Hydr.; Chlorali Hydras; Kloralhydrat. 2,2,2-Trichloroethane-1,1-diol.
$C_2H_3Cl_3O_2$=165.4.

CAS — 302-17-0.

Pharmacopoeias. In *Arg., Aust., Belg., Br., Braz., Chin., Cz., Egypt., Eur., Fr., Ger., Hung., Ind., Int., It., Jpn, Jug., Mex., Neth., Nord., Pol., Port., Roum., Rus., Span., Swiss, Turk.,* and *U.S.* Also in *B.P. Vet.*

Colourless or white crystals with a pungent odour. It volatilises slowly on exposure to air and melts at about 55°.
The *B.P.* states that it is **soluble** 1 in 0.3 of water, 1 in 0.2 of alcohol, and 1 in 3 of chloroform; freely soluble in ether. *U.S.P.* solubilities are: 1 in 0.25 of water, 1 in 1.3 of alcohol, 1 in 2 of chloroform, and 1 in 1.5 of ether; very soluble in olive oil. A 10% solution in carbon dioxide-free water has a pH of 3.5 to 5.5.
Incompatible with alkalis, alkaline earths, alkali carbonates, soluble barbiturates, borax, tannin, iodides, oxidising agents, permanganates, and alcohol (chloral alcoholate may crystallise out). It forms a liquid mixture when triturated with many organic compounds, such as camphor, menthol, phenazone, phenol, thymol, and quinine salts. **Store** in airtight containers.
The *U.S.P.* directs that the syrup should be protected from light.
NOTE. Aqueous solutions are liable to develop mould growth.

STABILITY OF SOLUTIONS. Aqueous solutions of chloral hydrate decomposed rapidly when exposed to ultraviolet light, with the formation of hydrochloric acid, trichloroacetic acid, and formic acid. Under ordinary storage conditions decomposition was slow; a 1% solution lost about 5% of its strength after storage at room temperature for 20 weeks.— P. W. Dankwortt, *Arch. Pharm., Berl.*, 1942, *280*, 197.

Adverse Effects
Chloral hydrate has an unpleasant taste and is corrosive to skin and mucous membranes unless well diluted. In therapeutic doses side-effects include gastric irritation, light-headedness, ataxia, nightmares, excitement, and confusion (sometimes with paranoia). Hangover is less common than with barbiturates. Allergic reactions include skin rashes and eosinophilia. Leucopenia may occur. The effects of acute overdosage resemble acute barbiturate intoxication (see p.706). In addition the irritant effect may cause initial vomiting, and gastric necrosis leading to strictures. Cardiac arrhythmias have been reported. Jaundice may follow liver damage, and kidney damage is associated with albuminuria.
Chronic ingestion of high doses may be associated with gastritis, skin rashes, peripheral vasodilatation, hypotension, and myocardial depression. Renal damage may occur.
Tolerance may develop with high or prolonged dosage and dependence may occur (see p.706). Sudden withdrawal of chloral hydrate from a dependent patient may result in symptoms similar to delirium tremens.

In a drug surveillance programme, 1618 patients received chloral hydrate as a hypnotic, usually in doses of 0.5 to 1 g. In 1130 patients evaluated the response was considered good in 70.9%. Side-effects, which were reversible, occurred in 2.3% of patients and included gastro-intestinal symptoms (10 patients), CNS depression (20), and skin rash (5). In 1 patient the prothrombin time was increased; in 1 patient hepatic encephalopathy seemed to worsen; and bradycardia developed in 1 patient.— S. Shapiro *et al.*, *J. Am. med. Ass.*, 1969, *209*, 2016. In a Boston Collaborative Drug Surveillance

Program side-effects occurred in approximately 2% of 5435 patients who received chloral hydrate. Three reactions were described as life-threatening.— R. R. Miller and D. J. Greenblatt, *J. clin. Pharmac.*, 1979, *19*, 669.

OVERDOSAGE. A 6-year-old boy awoke from a deep sleep 18 hours after taking 8 g of chloral hydrate and was subsequently well.— R. H. S. Mindham (letter), *Br. med. J.*, 1968, *3*, 187.

Cardiac and respiratory arrest occurred in a 22-month-old boy immediately after aspiration of a dose of chloral hydrate elixir. The child recovered after receiving immediate cardiac massage and oxygen.— D. M. Granoff *et al.*, *Am. J. Dis. Child.*, 1971, *122*, 170.

A 25-year-old woman who ingested 20 g of chloral hydrate developed initial respiratory failure, hypotension, hypothermia, and pulmonary oedema, and was deeply unconscious. Massive gastric necrosis with generalised peritonitis was found, followed by complete obstruction at the oesophago-gastric junction.— I. D. A. Vellar *et al.*, *Br. J. Surg.*, 1972, *59*, 317.

Of 76 cases of chloral hydrate poisoning reported to the National Poisons Information Service 47 were severe. Of 39 adults 12 had cardiac arrhythmias including 5 with cardiac arrest. Anti-arrhythmic drugs such as lignocaine were recommended unless obviously contra-indicated. In prolonged coma haemoperfusion through charcoal, or haemodialysis, was recommended.— H. M. Wiseman and G. Hampel (letter), *Br. med. J.*, 1978, *2*, 960.

WITHDRAWAL. A 45-year-old woman with a history of barbiturate dependence became dependent upon chloral hydrate, taking doses of up to 10 g daily. She was admitted to hospital and suffered no ill effects on abrupt withdrawal, but to minimise the risk of symptoms such as delirium tremens it would probably be better to treat such a patient with low doses of chloral hydrate for at least a week.— C. B. Stone and R. Okun, *Clin. Toxicol.*, 1978, *12*, 377.

Treatment of Adverse Effects

Treatment is essentially supportive. Demulcents such as liquid paraffin may be given to relieve gastric and oesophageal irritation. Haemoperfusion or dialysis may be beneficial in severe poisoning.

A 38-year-old woman who had taken about 38 g of chloral hydrate was successfully treated with haemodialysis; lignocaine was used initially to control arrhythmias, and dopamine to maintain blood pressure.— N. E. Stalker *et al.*, *J. clin. Pharmac.*, 1978, *18*, 136.

Precautions

Chloral hydrate should not be used in patients with marked hepatic or renal impairment or severe cardiac disease and oral administration is best avoided in the presence of gastritis. It should be used with caution in patients susceptible to porphyria.

Chloral hydrate and similar sedatives cause drowsiness and patients receiving them should not take charge of vehicles or machinery where loss of attention could lead to accidents. These effects are enhanced by the simultaneous administration of depressants of the central nervous system such as alcohol (the 'Mickey Finn' of detective fiction), barbiturates, and other sedatives. A vasodilator reaction has also occurred after concomitant administration with alcohol.

It has been suggested on theoretical grounds that its effects may be enhanced if monoamine oxidase inhibitors are given concurrently but the validity of any reported interactions has been questioned. Chloral hydrate has been reported both to decrease and to enhance the effects of coumarin anticoagulants. Chloral hydrate is reported not to induce liver enzymes. A hypermetabolic state, apparently due to displacement of thyroid hormones from their binding proteins, has been reported following concomitant administration of chloral hydrate and frusemide.

INTERACTIONS. *Alcohol.* In a controlled study of 5 healthy subjects, alcohol 500 mg per kg body-weight, given after chloral hydrate 15 mg per kg, increased and prolonged the plasma-trichloroethanol concentrations and reduced plasma concentrations of trichloroacetic acid. In turn chloral hydrate increased the absorption of alcohol leading to more rapidly achieved and higher blood concentrations in the first 30 minutes.— E. M. Sellers *et al.*, *Clin. Pharmac. Ther.*, 1972, *13*, 37. The heart-rate of these subjects was increased when given alcohol after having received chloral hydrate 15 mg per kg daily for 7 days, the last dose being given 12 hours before the alcohol. Systolic pressure was increased at 1 hour and decreased at 3 hours, motor performance was reduced when alcohol was taken after chloral hydrate, and auditory vigilance impaired. One subject had a vasodilator reaction with palpitations, anxiety, and flushing; although similar to the 'acetaldehyde syndrome' the blood-alcohol concentration was only half that found after alcohol alone, which had caused no reaction.— *idem*, 50.

INTERFERENCE WITH DIAGNOSTIC TESTS. *Glucose.* Chloral hydrate may produce false positive results in some tests for glucose.— M. Lubran, *Med. Clins N. Am.*, 1969, *53*, 211.

Steroids. The administration of chloral hydrate could interfere with measurements of urinary 17-hydroxycorticosteroids.— J. M. Rosenberg and I. S. Kampa, *Drug Intell. & clin. Pharm.*, 1973, *7*, 33.

Urea. Chloral hydrate could interfere technically with chemical estimations for urea in the blood to produce erroneous raised results.— *Drug & Ther. Bull.*, 1972, *10*, 69.

PREGNANCY AND THE NEONATE. Maternally administered chloral hydrate lowers the bilirubin concentrations of the infants.— J. H. Drew and W. H. Kitchen, *J. Pediat.*, 1976, *89*, 657.

Chloral hydrate was reported to enter breast milk in amounts sufficient to cause minimal sedation after large feeds.— R. L. Savage, *Adverse Drug React. Bull.*, 1976, Dec., 212. See also J. B. Bernstine, *J. Obstet. Gynaec. Br. Commonw.*, 1956, *63*, 228; J. B. Bernstine *et al.*, *Am. J. Obstet. Gynec.*, 1957, *73*, 801; J. H. Lacey, *Br. med. J.*, 1971, *4*, 684; M. S. Meskin and E. J. Lien, *J. clin. Hosp. Pharm.*, 1985, *10*, 269.

Absorption and Fate

Chloral hydrate is rapidly absorbed from the stomach and starts to act within 30 minutes. It is widely distributed throughout the body. It is metabolised to trichloroethanol and trichloroacetic acid in the erythrocytes, liver, and other tissues and excreted partly in the urine as trichloroethanol and its glucuronide (urochloralic acid) and as trichloroacetic acid. Significant amounts are also excreted in the bile.

Trichloroethanol is the active metabolite, and passes into the cerebrospinal fluid, into milk, and through the placenta to the foetus. The half-life of trichloroethanol in plasma is reported to range from about 7 to 11 hours.

Studies on the absorption of chloral hydrate and chloral betaine following oral and rectal administration.— M. Simpson and E. L. Parrott, *J. pharm. Sci.*, 1980, *69*, 227.

METABOLISM AND EXCRETION. In a comparative study 7 healthy subjects were given chloral hydrate 15 mg per kg body-weight and triclofos 22.5 mg per kg. Peak plasma concentrations of trichloroethanol were 8.5 µg per mL after a single dose of chloral hydrate and 8.2 µg per mL after a single dose of triclofos, no unchanged chloral hydrate or triclofos being detected. The plasma half-lives of trichloroacetic acid and trichloroethanol were 67.2 and 8.2 hours, and the plasma protein binding was 94% and 35% respectively. The pattern of urinary metabolites was similar for both drugs with 7.1% of the chloral hydrate dose and 4.6% of the triclofos dose being recovered as trichloroethanol glucuronide, trichloroethanol, and trichloroacetic acid. After 24 hours less than 12% of each drug was recovered in the urine and it was considered that biliary excretion is probably an important elimination route. Following administration of either drug for 7 days, plasma concentrations of trichloroacetic acid greater than 80 µg per mL were obtained.— E. M. Sellers *et al.*, *Clin. Pharmac. Ther.*, 1973, *14*, 147.

Uses and Administration

Chloral hydrate is a hypnotic and sedative with properties similar to those of the barbiturates; therapeutic doses have little effect on respiration and blood pressure.

Externally, chloral hydrate has a rubefacient action and was formerly employed as a counter-irritant.

Chloral hydrate is administered by mouth as an oral liquid or as gelatin capsules with chloral hydrate dissolved in a suitable vehicle. It has also been dissolved in a bland fixed oil and given by enema or as suppositories. It should not be given as tablets or pills as these concentrated forms may damage the mucous membrane of the alimentary tract.

The usual hypnotic dose is 0.5 to 2 g at night and as a sedative 250 mg may be given three times daily, up to a maximum single or daily dose of 2 g. It should be taken well diluted with water or milk. Children usually tolerate chloral hydrate well and 50 mg per kg body-weight daily may be given to a maximum single dose of 1 g as a hypnotic. A suggested sedative dose in children is 8 mg per kg three times daily.

Derivatives of chloral hydrate, such as butylchloral hydrate, chloral betaine, chloralformamide, chloralose, chlorhexadol, and dichloralphenazone, which break down in the body to yield chloral hydrate, have been used similarly.

ADMINISTRATION IN THE ELDERLY. No relationship between clinical toxicity and age had been noted for chloral hydrate.— D. J. Greenblatt *et al.*, *Clin. Pharmac. Ther.*, 1977, *21*, 355.

ADMINISTRATION IN RENAL FAILURE. Chloral hydrate could be given in usual doses to patients with a glomerular filtration-rate greater than 50 mL per minute, but should be avoided in those with a glomerular filtration-rate less than this.— W. M. Bennett *et al.*, *Am. J. Kidney Dis.*, 1983, *3*, 55.

Preparations

Chloral Hydrate Capsules *(U.S.P.)*

Chloral Hydrate Syrup *(U.S.P.)*

Chloral Mixture *(A.P.F.).* Mist. Chloral.; Chloral Hydrate Mixture. Chloral hydrate 1 g, orange syrup 1 mL, concentrated chloroform water 0.25 mL or compound hydroxybenzoate solution 0.1 mL, water to 10 mL.

Chloral Mixture CF *(A.P.F.).* Chloral Hydrate Mixture for Children. Chloral hydrate 250 mg, orange syrup 2 mL, concentrated chloroform water 0.1 mL or compound hydroxybenzoate solution 0.05 mL, water to 5 mL.

Chloral Mixture *(B.P.).* Chloral Hydrate Mixture; Chloral Oral Solution. Contains chloral hydrate 10% in a suitable vehicle. An extemporaneous preparation may be prepared containing chloral hydrate 1 g, syrup 2 mL, water to 10 mL. It should be recently prepared. To be well diluted with water before use.

When protected from light Chloral Mixture was stable for at least 12 weeks at room temperature. Benzoic acid was a suitable preservative.— Pharm. Soc. Lab. Rep. P/77/15, 1977. Chloral Mixture preserved with benzoic acid and protected from light was stable for 48 weeks at 25°.— Pharm. Soc. Lab. Rep. P/78/6, 1978. Microbiological studies indicated that unpreserved Chloral Mixture was very rapidly bactericidal and sporicidal, and the inclusion of benzoic acid as an additional preservative appeared to be unnecessary.— Pharm. Soc. Lab. Rep. P/78/3, 1978.

Paediatric Chloral Elixir *(B.P.).* Paediatric Chloral Oral Solution. Contains chloral hydrate 4% in a suitable vehicle with a blackcurrant flavour. An extemporaneous preparation may be prepared containing chloral hydrate 200 mg, black currant syrup 1 mL, water 0.1 mL, syrup to 5 mL; it should be recently prepared.

Proprietary Preparations

Noctec *(Squibb, UK). Capsules,* chloral hydrate 500 mg.

Proprietary Names and Manufacturers

Aquachloral *(Webcon, USA)*; Chloradorm *(Austral.)*; Chloraldurat *(Pohl, Ger.; Neth.; Pohl-Boskamp, Switz.)*; Chloralex *(Canad.)*; Chloralix *(Riker, Austral.)*; Chloralvan *(Canad.)*; Dormel *(Drug Houses Austral., Austral.)*; Elix-Nocte *(Nelson, Austral.)*; Kloral *(DAK, Denm.)*; Médianox *(Grossmann, Switz.)*; Noctec *(Squibb, Austral.; Squibb, Canad.; Squibb, UK; Squibb, USA)*; Novochlorhydrate *(Novopharm, Canad.)*; Rectules *(USA)*; SK-Chloral Hydrate *(Smith Kline & French, USA)*; Somnox *(Belg.)*.

4022-g

Chloralose *(rINN)*.

Alphachloralose; α-Chloralose; Chloralosane; Glucochloral. 1,2-*O*-(2,2,2-Trichloroethylidene)-α-D-glucofuranose.

$C_8H_{11}Cl_3O_6$=309.5.

CAS — 15879-93-3.

Chloralose was formerly employed as a hypnotic with actions similar to those of chloral hydrate (p.717), of which it is a derivative; it is now chiefly used as a pesticide.

Proprietary Names and Manufacturers

Somio *(Dergo, Belg.)*.

7017-w

Chlordiazepoxide *(BAN, USAN, rINN)*.

Methaminodiazepoxide. 7-Chloro-2-methylamino-5-phenyl-3*H*-1,4-benzodiazepine 4-oxide.

$C_{16}H_{14}ClN_3O$=299.8.

CAS — 58-25-3.

Pharmacopoeias. In *Br., Braz., Chin., Cz., Ind., Jpn, Jug., Nord., Roum.,* and *U.S.*

A yellow, odourless or almost odourless, crystalline powder, sensitive to sunlight. Chlordiazepoxide 1 mg is approximately equivalent to 1.1 mg of chlordiazepoxide hydrochloride. Practically **insoluble** in water; soluble 1 in 50 of alcohol and 1 in 130 of ether; sparingly soluble in chloroform. **Store** in airtight containers. Protect from light.

7018-e

Chlordiazepoxide Hydrochloride *(BANM, USAN, rINNM)*.

Chlordiazepoxidi Hydrochloridum; Methaminodiazepoxide Hydrochloride; NSC-115748; Ro-5-0690.

$C_{16}H_{14}ClN_3O,HCl$=336.2.

CAS — 438-41-5.

Pharmacopoeias. In *Belg., Br., Egypt., Eur., Fr., Ger., It., Neth., Swiss, Turk.,* and *U.S.*

An odourless white or slightly yellowish crystalline powder.

Soluble 1 in 10 of water and 1 in 40 of alcohol; practically insoluble in chloroform, ether, and petroleum spirit. **Store** in airtight containers. Protect from light.

Dependence, Adverse Effects, Treatment, and Precautions

As for the benzodiazepines in general, p.706.

EFFECTS ON THE BLOOD. Aplastic anaemia was an established clinical reaction ocurring in some patients as an idiosyncratic response to chlordiazepoxide. Chlordiazepoxide has also been reported as being associated with cases of agranulocytosis.— P. C. Vincent, *Drugs*, 1986, *31*, 52.

Purpura. Non-thrombocytopenic purpura occurred in a 65-year-old woman following administration of chlordiazepoxide for at least 12 months in irregular courses of 10 mg twice daily for about 1 week at approximately monthly intervals. The purpura reappeared within 48 hours of restarting chlordiazepoxide in a dosage of 30 mg daily.— I. J. Copperman (letter), *Br. med. J.*, 1967, *4*, 485.

INTERACTIONS. *Alcohol.* A study in 5 healthy subjects demonstrating that moderate doses of alcohol impair the elimination of chlordiazepoxide, accounting in part for the increased sedation when the two are taken together.— P. V. Desmond *et al.*, *Eur. J. clin. Pharmac.*, 1980, *18*, 275.

Antacids. A study in 10 healthy subjects indicated that although concurrent administration of antacid (magnesium and aluminium hydroxide) delayed absorption of chlordiazepoxide it did not affect the completeness of absorption or the apparent rate of elimination.— D. J. Greenblatt *et al.*, *Clin. Pharmac. Ther.*, 1976, *19*, 234. See also *idem*, *Clin. Pharmac. Ther.*, 1977, *21*, 105.

Cimetidine. For mention of interactions between the benzodiazepines and cimetidine see under Diazepam, p.729.

Disulfiram. For an interaction between chlordiazepoxide and disulfiram see under Diazepam, p.730.

Ketoconazole. Ketoconazole impaired the clearance of chlordiazepoxide, apparently due to an effect on hepatic metabolism; clinically significant interactions might occur if the two drugs were given concurrently.— M. W. Brown *et al.*, *Clin. Pharmac. Ther.*, 1985, *37*, 290.

Levodopa. For the effects of benzodiazepines on levodopa, see Levodopa, p.1016.

Oral contraceptives. For the effect of oral contraceptives on chlordiazepoxide metabolism see under Diazepam, p.730.

INTERFERENCE WITH DIAGNOSTIC TESTS. In 14 euthyroid patients and 6 mildly thyrotoxic patients, administration of chlordiazepoxide in a dosage of 10 mg thrice daily for 4 weeks did not significantly affect the results of tests of thyroid iodide trapping or of thyroid hormone release. Chlordiazepoxide did not alter the commonly used tests of thyroid function.— F. Clark and R. Hall, *Br. med. J.*, 1970, *2*, 266. Similar findings.— S. D. Slater, *Br. J. clin. Pract.*, 1972, *26*, 463.

PREGNANCY AND THE NEONATE. *Early pregnancy.* Results of a prospective study of 19 044 live births indicated an increased incidence of defects in children of mothers exposed to chlordiazepoxide during the first 42 days of pregnancy.— L. Milkovich and B. J. van den Berg, *New Engl. J. Med.*, 1974, *291*, 1268.

Of 50 282 children born to mothers monitored by the Collaborative Perinatal Project 257 were found to have been exposed to chlordiazepoxide, and possibly other drugs, at some time during the first 4 months of the pregnancy. No association between chlordiazepoxide exposure and any type of malformation could be detected.— O. P. Heinonen *et al.*, *Birth Defects and Drugs in Pregnancy*, Littleton MA, Publishing Sciences Group, 1977, p. 335.

See also p.709.

Late pregnancy. In a double-blind study in 166 women in early labour, the effect of chlordiazepoxide was compared with a placebo. Chlordiazepoxide was found to cross the placenta but no foetal or neonatal depression occurred. No significant difference between the 2 treatments was detected.— P. M. Mark and J. Hamel, *Obstet. Gynec.*, 1968, *32*, 188.

Concentrations of chlordiazepoxide in cord blood were as high as those of maternal blood in 3 of 4 infants born to mothers given chlordiazepoxide for pre-eclampsia or eclampsia; in the fourth infant the concentration was about 40% of that in maternal blood.— G. M. Stirrat *et al.* (letter), *Br. med. J.*, 1974, *2*, 729.

Absorption and Fate

For an account of the absorption and fate of a benzodiazepine, see Diazepam, p.730.

Chlordiazepoxide has been reported to have an elimination half-life ranging from about 5 to 30 hours. Pharmacologically active metabolites include desmethylchlordiazepoxide, demoxepam, desmethyldiazepam, and oxazepam.

A detailed review of the clinical pharmacokinetics of chlordiazepoxide.— D. J. Greenblatt *et al.*, *Clin. Pharmacokinet.*, 1978, *3*, 381.

ABSORPTION AND PLASMA CONCENTRATIONS. In 8 volunteers the average peak blood concentration of chlordiazepoxide after administration of 50 mg by mouth was 1.75 µg per mL and occurred in 1 to 1.5 hours. However after intramuscular injection the average peak concentration of 1 µg per mL was delayed.— D. J. Greenblatt *et al.*, *New Engl. J. Med.*, 1974, *291*, 1116.

The biological half-life of chlordiazepoxide was found to be shorter than previously reported, and also more variable, ranging from 6.6 to 28 hours. Most of a dose was eliminated as the intermediate desmethylchlordiazepoxide. The metabolite demoxepam was not found in the plasma of any of 6 volunteers after the administration of single doses of chlordiazepoxide.— M. A. Schwartz *et al.*, *J. pharm. Sci.*, 1971, *60*, 1500.

Studies in 14 healthy subjects (7 male and 7 female) given chlordiazepoxide by intravenous infusion indicated that the apparent half-lives of distribution and elimination and the total blood clearance did not differ significantly between the sexes but that the apparent volumes of the central compartment and of the total distribution space were significantly larger in the female group. A further study in 3 subjects indicated a limited uptake of chlordiazepoxide by red blood cells.— D. J. Greenblatt *et al.*, *Clin. Pharmac. Ther.*, 1977, *22*, 893. See also: K. Wilson, *Clin. Pharmacokinet.*, 1984, *9*, 189.

PLASMA PROTEIN BINDING. A study of the CSF of 30 patients who received chlordiazepoxide hydrochloride 100 mg by mouth prior to surgical procedures indicated that simultaneous CSF concentrations of chlordiazepoxide were considerably lower than those in the plasma. Since only the unbound chlordiazepoxide in plasma has been reported to be available for diffusion into CSF (J. Koch-Weser and E.M. Sellers, *New Engl. J. Med.*, 1976, *294*, 311 and 526; W.H. Oldendorf, *A. Rev. Pharmac.*, 1974, *14*, 239), the ratio of the concentration in CSF and plasma was used to calculate that chlordiazepoxide is about 90 to 97% protein bound. The data suggested that variations in protein binding might be responsible for differences in clinical response.— D. R. Stanski *et al.*, *Clin. Pharmac. Ther.*, 1976, *20*, 571.

Uses and Administration

Chlordiazepoxide is a benzodiazepine with actions and uses similar to those of diazepam (p.731).

Chlordiazepoxide is administered by mouth as the hydrochloride and sometimes as the base. It may also be administered by intramuscular injection where the dose may be expressed in terms of the base or the hydrochloride.

The usual dose of either the base or the hydrochloride for the treatment of anxiety is 30 mg daily in divided doses; in severe conditions the dose is 40 to 100 mg daily; for elderly and debilitated patients the usual initial dose is 10 mg daily. A suggested dose for children is 5 mg two to four times daily; another suggested dose for children is 500 µg per kg body-weight daily, in 3 or 4 divided doses.

For the control of the acute symptoms of alcohol withdrawal chlordiazepoxide hydrochloride may be given by deep intramuscular or slow intravenous injection; the usual dose is 50 to 100 mg calculated as the base or as the hydrochloride, repeated if required within 2 to 4 hours; doses should be reduced by half in elderly or debilitated patients. Preparations formulated for intramuscular use are stated to be unsuitable for intravenous administration due to the formation of air bubbles in the solvent; intravenous injections should be dissolved in Water for Injections or sodium chloride injection.

ADMINISTRATION. Studies showing that the absorption of chlordiazepoxide after intramuscular injection is much slower than the same dose given by mouth.— D. J. Greenblatt *et al.*, *Eur. J. clin. Pharmac.*, 1978, *13*, 267.

In the elderly. A study on the absorption and disposition of chlordiazepoxide in young and elderly men.— R. I. Shader *et al.*, *J. clin. Pharmac.*, 1977, *17*, 709.

ADMINISTRATION IN RENAL FAILURE. Chlordiazepoxide could be given in usual doses to patients with renal failure. Concentrations of chlordiazepoxide were not affected by haemodialysis.— W. M. Bennett *et al.*, *Am. J. Kidney Dis.*, 1983, *3*, 155.

ALCOHOL AND DRUG WITHDRAWAL. For a discussion of the management of alcohol withdrawal, including the role of chlordiazepoxide, see under Diazepam, p.732.

Preparations

Chlordiazepoxide Capsules *(B.P.)*. Contain chlordiazepoxide hydrochloride.

Chlordiazepoxide Tablets *(B.P.)*. Store at a temperature not exceeding 25°.

Chlordiazepoxide Tablets *(U.S.P.)*

Chlordiazepoxide Hydrochloride Capsules *(U.S.P.)*

Chlordiazepoxide Hydrochloride Tablets *(B.P.)*. Store at a temperature not exceeding 25°.

Sterile Chlordiazepoxide Hydrochloride *(U.S.P.)*. Chlordiazepoxide hydrochloride suitable for parenteral use. pH of a 1% solution 2.5 to 3.5.

Proprietary Preparations of Chlordiazepoxide and its Salts

Librium *(Roche, UK)*. *Capsules*, chlordiazepoxide hydrochloride 5 and 10 mg.
Tablets, chlordiazepoxide 5, 10, and 25 mg.
Injection, powder for reconstitution, chlordiazepoxide 100 mg (as hydrochloride), supplied with diluent.

Tropium *(DDSA Pharmaceuticals, UK)*. *Capsules*, chlordiazepoxide hydrochloride 5 and 10 mg.
Tablets, chlordiazepoxide hydrochloride 5, 10, and 25 mg.

Proprietary Names and Manufacturers of Chlordiazepoxide and its Salts
Ansiacal *(Ital.)*; A-Poxide *(Abbott, USA)*; Benzodiapin *(Lisapharma, Ital.)*; Binomil *(Spain)*; Calmoden *(Berk Pharmaceuticals, UK)*; Cebrum *(Ital.)*; Chlortran *(S.Afr.)*; Corax *(Canad.)*; C-Tran *(Canad.)*; Diazebrum *(Arg.)*; Diazepina *(Arg.)*; Elenium *(Pol.)*; Endequil *(Ital.)*; Equibral *(Ravizza, Ital.)*; Helogaphen *(Ger.)*; Huberplex *(Hubber, Spain)*; Karmoplex *(Lennon, S.Afr.)*; Klopoxid *(DAK, Denm.)*; Labican *(Boniscontro & Gazzone, Ital.)*; Liberans *(Ital.)*; Libritabs *(Roche, USA)*; Librium *(Roche, Austral.; Belg.; Roche, Canad.; Roche, Denm.; Roche, Fr.; Roche, Ger.; Roche, Ital.; Neth.; Roche, Norw.; Roche, S.Afr.; Roche, Spain; Roche, Swed.; Roche, Switz.; Roche, UK; Roche, USA)*; Lixin *(Ital.)*; Medilium *(Medic, Canad.)*; Multum *(Chephasaar, Ger.)*; Nack *(Canad.)*; Normide *(Inibsa, Spain)*; Novopoxide *(Novopharm, Canad.)*; O.C.M. *(Arg.)*; Omnalio *(Estedi, Spain)*; Paliatin *(Lasa, Spain)*; Philcorium *(Ital.)*; Psicofar *(Terapeutico M.R., Ital.)*; Psicoterina *(Francia Farm., Ital.)*; Raysedan *(Arg.)*; Relaxedans *(Salvat, Spain)*; Relaxil *(Canad.)*; Reliberan *(Geymonat, Ital.)*; Reposal *(Arg.)*; Risachief *(Jpn)*; Risolid *(Dumex, Denm.; Dumex, Norw.; Swed.)*; Seren *(Vita, Ital.)*; Sintesedan *(Arg.)*; SK-Lygen *(Smith Kline & French, USA)*; Smail *(Edmond Pharma, Ital.)*; Solium *(Horner, Canad.)*; Trilium *(Canad.)*; Tropium *(DDSA Pharmaceuticals, UK)*; Viansin *(Ital.)*; Zeisin *(Ger.)*.

The following names have been used for multi-ingredient preparations containing chlordiazepoxide and its salts—Apo-Chlorax *(Apotex, Canad.)*; Clipoxide *(Schein, USA)*; Corium *(ICN, Canad.)*; Librax *(Roche, Austral.; Roche, Canad.; Roche, USA)*; Libraxin *(Roche, UK)*; Limbatril; Limbitrol *(Roche, UK; Roche, USA)*; Menrium *(Roche, Canad.; Roche, USA)*; Pentrium *(Roche, Canad.; Roche, UK)*.

4023-q

Chlorhexadol *(BAN)*.
Chloralodol *(rINN)*; Chloralodolum. 2-Methyl-4-(2,2,2-trichloro-1-hydroxyethoxy)pentan-2-ol.
$C_8H_{15}Cl_3O_3$=265.6.

CAS — 3563-58-4.

Pharmacopoeias. In *Nord.*

Chlorhexadol has the actions of Chloral Hydrate, p.717. It has been given as a hypnotic in doses of 0.8 to 1.6 g at night and as a sedative in doses of 400 mg three times daily.

Proprietary Names and Manufacturers
Mechloral *(Dumex, Denm.)*; Mecoral *(Dumex, Norw.)*; Medodorm *(Medo, UK)*.

18200-w

Chlormethiazole *(BAN)*

Clomethiazole *(rINN)*. 5-(2-Chloroethyl)-4-methylthiazole.
C_6H_8ClNS=161.6.

CAS — 533-45-9.

Pharmacopoeias. In *Br.*

A colourless to slightly yellowish-brown liquid with a characteristic odour. Slightly **soluble** in water; miscible with alcohol, with chloroform, and with ether. A 0.5% solution in water has a pH of 5.5 to 7.0.
Store in well-closed containers at a temperature of 2° to 8°.

4024-p

Chlormethiazole Edisylate *(BANM)*.

Chlormethiazole Ethanedisulphonate; Clomethiazole Edisilate *(rINNM)*; SCTZ. 5-(2-Chloroethyl)-4-methylthiazole ethane-1,2-disulphonate.

$(C_6H_8ClNS)_2,C_2H_6O_6S_2$=513.5.

CAS — 1867-58-9.

Pharmacopoeias. In *Br.*

A white crystalline powder with a characteristic odour. Freely **soluble** in water; soluble in alcohol; practically insoluble in ether. **Store** in well-closed containers.

INCOMPATIBILITY. Chlormethiazole 8 g per litre in glucose 4% injection reacted with plastic giving sets.— S. Lingam *et al., Br. med. J.*, 1980, *280*, 155.

Further references to the sorption of chlormethiazole by plastic giving sets: S. E. Tsuei *et al., Eur. J. clin. Pharmac.*, 1980, *18*, 333; E. A. Kowaluk *et al., Am. J. Hosp. Pharm.*, 1982, *39*, 460; *idem*, 1983, *40*, 118; *idem, J. pharm. Sci.*, 1984, *73*, 43; M. G. Lee, *Am. J. Hosp. Pharm.*, 1986, *43*, 1945.

STABILITY. A commercial infusion formulation of chlormethiazole edisylate (Heminevrin) was reported to be stable for 18 months when stored at the recommended temperature of 5 to 8°. The breakdown of active substance was increased by approximately 1% per month per 10° increase in storage temperature above this range, and a shelf-life of 2 weeks had been reported at room temperature, assuming that a maximum loss of 0.5% was acceptable.— *Pharm. J.*, 1987, *1*, 148. See also K. Gustavii and K. Ekstrand-Asker, *Acta pharm. suec.*, 1986, *23*, 21 (stability of chlormethiazole solution at differing ph and temperature).

Dependence

Dependence (see p.706) may develop, particularly with prolonged use.

A man who had been given chlormethiazole for the treatment of alcoholism appeared to have transferred his dependence to chlormethiazole; he was taking 40 to 50 tablets daily.— A. Foster (letter), *Br. med. J.*, 1977, *1*, 1355.

Warnings on the risk of using chlormethiazole in ambulant alcoholic patients are timely but should not be taken out of context. Experience over 15 years at the St Bernard's Hospital Alcoholic Unit has not only confirmed the findings of many observers that chlormethiazole is an extremely valuable drug in the treatment and prophylaxis of severe alcohol withdrawal syndromes (including delirium tremens) but has also indicated that when used in patients for a limited period only (usually no more than 6 or 7 days) the risk of dependence is extremely low. It should be stressed that the risk of chlormethiazole dependence is a real one when it is given indiscriminately for lengthy use in unstable alcoholics treated as outpatients but seems very low when it is used in the withdrawal phase of alcoholism in the correct way, and equally so when used in sections of the population not prone to dependence.— M. M. Glatt (letter), *Br. med. J.*, 1978, *2*, 894. See also *idem*, 1976, *2*, 582; *idem*, 1977, *2*, 1088.

A report on 5 patients who were considered to have become physically dependent on chlormethiazole, taken by 4 of them in doses of up to about 5 to 10 g daily. Withdrawal symptoms included suicidal depression and an acute psychotic state.— M. A. Hession *et al., Lancet*, 1979, *1*, 953. The doses prescribed in the first patients were far in excess of the recommended dosage. The criticisms made should more appropriately be levelled at other hypnotics rather than chlormethiazole which is rarely associated with withdrawal symptoms when used in the correct dosage.— A. N. Exton-Smith and A. E. McLean (letter), *ibid.*, 1093. Similar severe criticisms.— S. K. Majundar (letter), *ibid.*, 1093 and 1254; M. M. Glatt (letter), *ibid.*, 1093; C. J. Scott (letter), *ibid.*, 1094.

Adverse Effects

Chlormethiazole may produce nasal irritation and sneezing on administration; conjunctival irritation, headache, and, following oral administration, gastro-intestinal disturbances including nausea and vomiting, have occurred. A transient fall in blood pressure, related to the rate of infusion, may follow intravenous dosage, and rapid infusion has resulted in hypotension and apnoea. Phlebitis or thrombophlebitis may occur after intravenous infusion. Other adverse effects that have been reported with chlormethiazole include fever, cough, increased bronchial secretion, tachycardia and cardiac arrhythmias, and, rarely, anaphylaxis.
Excessive doses may produce coma, respiratory depression, hypotension, and hypothermia; pneumonia may follow increased respiratory secretion.

EFFECTS ON THE GASTRO-INTESTINAL TRACT. Long-standing dysphagia and a gross motility disorder of the oesophagus in a patient receiving chlormethiazole improved gradually once the drug was withdrawn. Six weeks after the drug was stopped oesophageal motility had returned almost to normal, and the patient remained free of dysphagia during the succeeding months.— P. Dewis *et al., Br. med. J.*, 1982, *284*, 705.

EFFECTS ON THE HEART. Cardiac arrest in 2 chronic alcoholics might have been associated with chlormethiazole infusion.— G. T. McInnes *et al., Postgrad. med. J.*, 1980, *56*, 742.

EFFECTS ON MENTAL STATE. Alpha coma (normally associated with a poor prognosis in structural brain damage) was noted in 3 patients given chlormethiazole for alcohol-withdrawal states. Withdrawal of the chlormethiazole was accompanied by complete recovery, indicating that such a finding in association with drug intoxication need not imply that secondary hypoxic brain damage has occurred.— W. M. Carroll and F. L. Mastaglia, *Br. med. J.*, 1977, *2*, 1518.

OVERDOSAGE. A report of suicide by chlormethiazole poisoning in 5 alcoholic men being treated for depression with chlormethiazole; at least 2 of the men had also ingested alcohol.— J. M. Horder, *Br. med. J.*, 1978, *1*, 693.

A report of chlormethiazole poisoning on 16 occasions in 13 patients, some of whom had also taken other drugs and alcohol. There was increased salivation on 7 occasions; otherwise the clinical features were those of barbiturate poisoning. The highest plasma-chlormethiazole concentration was 36 μg per mL, with the highest value in a conscious patient 11.5 μg per mL. All the patients survived following intensive supportive treatment as for barbiturate poisoning.— R. N. Illingworth *et al., Br. med. J.*, 1979, *2*, 902.

PREGNANCY AND THE NEONATE. Severe depression with hypotonia, hypoventilation, or apnoea was reported to have occurred in the immediate neonatal period in 13 infants among 21 born to mothers treated for toxaemia of pregnancy. All the mothers had received chlormethiazole edisylate 4 to 24 g by intravenous infusion, and 12 of the affected infants came from a group of 14 mothers who also received diazoxide as intravenous boluses of 75 to 150 mg to control hypertension. Adverse reactions were not considered to be related to the doses used.— R. A. Johnson, *Br. med. J.*, 1976, *1*, 943.

Ten of 16 babies whose mothers were given chlormethiazole for pre-eclampsia were sleepy compared with only one of 15 whose mothers were given hydralazine. Nine of the chlormethiazole infants required forced feeding compared with 4 in the hydralazine group.— C. Wood and P. Renou (letter), *Med. J. Aust.*, 1978, *2*, 73.

Treatment of Adverse Effects, and Precautions

Treatment of the adverse effects of chlormethiazole is supportive, as for hypnotics and sedatives in general (see p.708).
Chlormethiazole is contra-indicated in patients with acute pulmonary insufficiency, and should be given with care to patients with chronic pulmonary insufficiency, renal failure, or liver disease. When given parenterally, means to maintain the airway should be at hand.
Chlormethiazole causes drowsiness and patients receiving it should not take charge of vehicles or machinery where loss of attention could lead to accidents. These effects are enhanced by the simultaneous administration of depressants of the central nervous system such as alcohol, barbiturates, and other sedatives and by neuroleptics.

INTERACTIONS. *Alcohol.* Comment on the dangers of concomitant ingestion of chlormethiazole and alcohol. Although chlormethiazole is a popular choice for the treatment of alcohol withdrawal symptoms, if it is given long-term, alcoholics readily transfer dependency to it, often while continuing to abuse alcohol. The outcome of such combined abuse is often severe self-poisoning with deep coma and potentially fatal respiratory depression.— G. T. McInnes, *Br. med. J.*, 1987, *294*, 592.

Beta blockers. Sinus bradycardia developed in an 84-year-old woman taking *propranolol* for hypertension 3 hours after she took a second dose of chlormethiazole 192 mg. Her pulse-rate increased on discontinuation of propranolol and chlormethiazole and later stabilised when she took propranolol with haloperidol.— *Med. J.*

Aust., 1979, *2*, 553.

H_2-antagonist antihistamines. A study of the pharmacokinetics of chlormethiazole edisylate 1 g by mouth in 8 healthy subjects, before and after administration of *cimetidine* 1 g daily for 1 week, demonstrated that mean clearance of chlormethiazole was reduced to 69% of its original value by cimetidine therapy. This was associated with an increase in the mean peak plasma concentration of the hypnotic from 2.664 to 4.507 μg per mL and an increase in the mean elimination half-life from 2.33 to 3.63 hours. The pharmacokinetic alterations were accompanied by an increase in clinical response. After the original dose of chlormethiazole subjects slept for 30 to 60 minutes, whereas following cimetidine treatment, most slept for at least 2 hours.— G. Shaw *et al.*, *Eur. J. clin. Pharmac.*, 1981, *21*, 83. *Ranitidine* did not significantly affect the pharmacokinetics of chlormethiazole in a study in 7 healthy subjects.— M. L. Mashford *et al.*, *Clin. Pharmac. Ther.*, 1983, *34*, 231.

Absorption and Fate

Chlormethiazole is rapidly absorbed from the gastro-intestinal tract, peak plasma concentrations appearing about 15 to 45 minutes after oral administration. It is widely distributed in the body, and extensively metabolised, probably by first-pass metabolism in the liver with only small amounts appearing unchanged in the urine. It crosses the placenta.

ABSORPTION. A study in 10 healthy subjects indicated more rapid and complete absorption of chlormethiazole after capsules than after tablets. Degree and speed of absorption increased even further after the oral solution.— M. Fischler *et al.*, *Acta pharm. suec.*, 1973, *10*, 483. See also E. P. Frisch and B. Ortengren, *Acta psychiat. scand.*, 1966, *42*, *Suppl.* 192, 35.

METABOLISM AND EXCRETION. A study of the pharmacokinetics of chlormethiazole following intravenous infusion in 6 healthy subjects. Unlike earlier workers a biphasic decay was found for the plasma concentrations, with half-lives of 0.54 and 4.05 hours. Hepatic metabolism is probably the main process of elimination of chlormethiazole and in 3 subjects studied less than 5% was found unchanged in the urine. A significant first-pass effect of chlormethiazole was predicted with the systemic availability of an orally administered dose being about 15%.— R. G. Moore *et al.*, *Eur. J. clin. Pharmac.*, 1975, *8*, 353.

A study of the pharmacokinetics of chlormethiazole and 2 metabolites after administration by mouth to young adult and old subjects. Reduced plasma binding and higher plasma concentrations were noted in the elderly.— R. L. Nation *et al.*, *Eur. J. clin. Pharmac.*, 1977, *12*, 137. See also *idem*, 1976, *10*, 407.

Urinary metabolites of chlormethiazole.— M. Ende *et al.*, *Arzneimittel-Forsch.*, 1979, *29*, 1655.

PREGNANCY AND THE NEONATE. Intravenous administration of a 0.8% solution of chlormethiazole edisylate at a rate of 20 mL per minute was found in 19 pregnant women at term to give plasma concentrations in maternal blood of 4.7 to 22.4 μg per mL of chlormethiazole and concentrations of 4.5 to 16.9 μg in the umbilical vein.— G. M. Duffus *et al.* (preliminary communication), *Lancet*, 1968, *1*, 335.

A study of maternal and neonatal concentrations of chlormethiazole following the use of chlormethiazole edisylate in the treatment of 4 patients with pre-eclampsia. After breast-feeding started, chlormethiazole was detectable in only 3 of 27 serial blood samples from babies and the concentrations were 18, 9, and 6 ng per g. The highest calculated amount of chlormethiazole ingested at a single breast feed was 37.2μg.— M. E. Tunstall *et al.*, *Br. J. Obstet. Gynaec.*, 1979, *86*, 793.

See also Adverse Effects.

Uses and Administration

Chlormethiazole edisylate is a hypnotic and sedative with anticonvulsant effects. It is used in confusion, agitation, and restlessness, particularly of geriatric patients, in sleep disorders in the elderly, and in the treatment of acute alcohol and drug withdrawal symptoms. It is also used in status epilepticus and toxaemia of pregnancy, and as a sedative in regional anaesthesia.

Chlormethiazole as Heminevrin (*Astra*) has been used as tablets containing 500 mg of edisylate, as well as capsules containing 192 mg of chlormethiazole base and as syrup containing 250 mg of edisylate in 5 mL, or as a 0.8% intravenous infusion of the edisylate. As a result of differences in the bioavailability of these different preparations, 500 mg of the edisylate in the tablets is equivalent to 192 mg of the base in the capsules, but it is also equivalent to only 250 mg (5 mL) of the edisylate in the syrup, ie. one tablet or one capsule or 5 mL of syrup are all equivalent in their effects. For further details see under Preparations, below.

The usual hypnotic dose of chlormethiazole is 1 or 2 capsules (192 or 384 mg of the base) or the equivalent. For daytime sedation 1 capsule (192 mg of the base), or the equivalent dose as one of the other dosage forms, may be given three times daily.

Various regimens have been suggested for the treatment of drug and alcohol withdrawal, usually starting with 9 to 12 capsules, or the equivalent, divided into 4 doses, on the first day, and gradually reducing the dosage over the following 5 days. Treatment should be carried out in hospital, and administration for longer than 9 days is not recommended because of the risk of dependence (see above).

For pre-eclamptic toxaemia an initial infusion of 30 to 50 mL of a 0.8% solution of the edisylate is given at the rate of 60 drops (4 mL) per minute until the patient is drowsy, then reduced to a rate of about 10 to 15 drops per minute. An infusion of 40 to 100 mL of the 0.8% solution may be given over 5 to 10 minutes to control convulsions in status epilepticus. Thereafter an intravenous infusion may be required according to the patient's response. Either of these 2 regimens may also be used for acute alcohol withdrawal symptoms and delirium tremens but, owing to the short half-life of chlormethiazole, the rapid infusion method must be followed either by a further intravenous infusion of 0.8% solution or by oral therapy with the capsules. Close supervision is essential during intravenous infusions to avoid the risk of overdose.

In the management of status epilepticus in children a suggested initial infusion rate is 0.01 mL of the 0.8% solution per kg body-weight per minute, adjusted according to response until seizures are abolished or drowsiness occurs.

ADMINISTRATION IN THE ELDERLY. Chlormethiazole was less safe than a benzodiazepine as a hypnotic in elderly patients, because of the risk of overdosage.— *Drugs for the Elderly*, F.I. Caird (Ed.), Copenhagen, WHO, 1985.

For a study indicating an increased response to chlormethiazole in elderly patients, see N. Hockings *et al.*, *Br. J. clin. Pharmac.*, 1982, *14*, 143P.

ADMINISTRATION IN HEPATIC FAILURE. Studies in 8 patients with advanced cirrhosis of the liver and in 6 healthy men showed that the amount of unmetabolised chlormethiazole reaching the circulation after an oral dose was about 10 times higher in the patients than in the controls. Low concentrations in the controls were related to extensive first-pass metabolism in the liver.— P. J. Pentikäinen *et al.*, *Br. med. J.*, 1978, *2*, 861. See also *idem*, *Eur. J. clin. Pharmac.*, 1980, *17*, 275.

ALCOHOL AND DRUG WITHDRAWAL. In a double-blind study in 97 alcoholic patients with symptoms from the recent withdrawal of alcohol, chlormethiazole [edisylate as tablets] in a dosage of respectively 2, 5, 3.5, 2.5, 1.5, 1, and 0.5 g on each of the 7 days after admission, was compared with placebo. During the trial period almost all of the individual symptoms, particularly psychiatric symptoms, improved more rapidly in the treated group. The incidence of sedation was 53% in the treated group compared with 25% in the placebo group. Overall assessment on the first, second, and third days showed an improvement in respectively 50, 67, and 71% of the patients given chlormethiazole, and respectively 22, 27, and 41% of patients given the placebo. There was no evidence that chlormethiazole was contra-indicated in depression. Side-effects included a sneezing reflex in 11 given chlormethiazole. In view of the possible risk of dependence, chlormethiazole should not be continued beyond 6 days.— M. M. Glatt *et al.*, *Br. med. J.*, 1965, *2*, 401.

For discussion of the management of alcohol withdrawal, including the role of chlormethiazole, see Diazepam, p.732.

ANAESTHESIA. In 5 healthy adults, 1 to 2 g of chlormethiazole [edisylate] was infused over about 8 minutes (a rate 2 to 3 times greater than recommended) to produce unconsciousness. Cardiac output, mean arterial pressure, central venous pressure, and respiration showed no significant changes; heart-rate increased by an average of about 48%. Chlormethiazole might be of value to produce sedation in patients undergoing intensive care.— J. Wilson *et al.*, *Br. J. Anaesth.*, 1969, *41*, 840.

Chlormethiazole [edisylate] as a 0.8% solution, caused local pain when given by rapid infusion (20 mL per minute) prior to fibre-endoscopic examination of the upper gastro-intestinal tract. It was ineffective as a sedative in 5 of 25 patients compared with only 1 of 50 given diazepam 5 mg per minute intravenously.— E. J. Galizia *et al.*, *Br. J. Anaesth.*, 1975, *47*, 402.

The use of chlormethiazole edisylate 0.8% infusion to provide prolonged sedation in 4 intensive care patients. Initially the infusion was given at a rate of 8 mL per minute for 5 minutes, which produced unconsciousness in all patients in 2 to 4 minutes. The infusion was then stopped and the patients began to recover in 1 to 3 minutes. Subsequently, prolonged infusion at a rate of 1.5 or 2 mL per minute was commenced and maintained at more or less this rate for 48 hours. The prolonged infusion took 15 to 30 minutes to produce unconsciousness but once established the patients responded only to gross stimulation, and were easily managed. There was a slight tachycardia and an increase in mucous secretions in the upper airway during infusion but no other changes in vital signs. Opioid analgesics were given where necessary during painful procedures. At the end of the prolonged infusion recovery of consciousness was slow, taking from 4 to 12 hours. Chlormethiazole is extremely useful in the management of seriously-ill patients requiring artificial ventilation, provided that administration is discontinued every few hours to avoid excessive accumulation and thus excessively delayed recovery. Care should be taken to avoid fluid overload, and suction is necessary to clear increased nasal and pharyngeal secretion. Infusion should be given via a large central vein to avoid thrombosis.— D. B. Scott *et al.*, *Br. J. Anaesth.*, 1980, *52*, 541.

In contrast to etomidate, which causes adrenocortical suppression and increases the fatality rate in severely-injured patients, chlormethiazole infusion given for 7 days to an accident victim had no adverse effect on adrenal function. Chlormethiazole may have a role in the treatment of intensive care patients who are difficult to sedate.— P. M. Pfeifer and M. Marshall (letter), *Lancet*, 1985, *1*, 460.

CONVULSIONS. In 9 episodes of status epilepticus, unresponsive to diazepam, in 8 patients the condition responded on 7 occasions to the infusion of chlormethiazole [edisylate] 500 to 700 mg per hour, without serious impairment of consciousness or depression of respiration.— P. K. P. Harvey *et al.*, *Br. med. J.*, 1975, *2*, 603.

A report of the long-term use of oral chlormethiazole to treat 3 children with epilepsy refractory to other anticonvulsants. One was subsequently withdrawn from chlormethiazole therapy after 4 months without evidence of any withdrawal reactions. Oral chlormethiazole may be a useful adjunct in the management of difficult cases of childhood epilepsy.— T. V. Stanley (letter), *Archs Dis. Childh.*, 1982, *57*, 242.

A preterm neonate with status epilepticus that had not responded to other treatment, including phenobarbitone, diazepam, and paraldehyde, was successfully managed with a chlormethiazole [edisylate] infusion of 10 mg per kg body-weight per hour. Convulsions returned when attempts were made to reduce the chlormethiazole dosage over the next 10 days; the drug was stopped after 19 days and replaced with phenytoin by mouth.— P. Miller and I. Kovar, *Postgrad. med. J.*, 1983, *59*, 801.

For further discussion of the treatment of convulsions in children, including the role of chlormethiazole, see p.710.

Proprietary Preparations of Chlormethiazole and Chlormethiazole Edisylate

Heminevrin *(Astra, UK). Capsules,* chlormethiazole 192 mg.
Syrup, chlormethiazole edisylate 250 mg/5 mL.
Intravenous infusion, chlormethiazole edisylate 8 mg/mL, in bottles of 500 mL.

Based on plasma levels of chlormethiazole in man, one Heminevrin tablet containing 500 mg chlormethiazole edisylate is considered to be clinically equivalent to one Heminevrin capsule containing 192 mg chlormethiazole base in arachis oil or 5 mL Heminevrin syrup containing 250 mg chlormethiazole edisylate.— A. K. Watson, *Astra, Personal Communication*, 1979.

Proprietary Names and Manufacturers of Chlormethiazole and Chlormethiazole Edisylate
Distraneurin *(Astra, Ger.; Astra, Switz.)*; Distraneurine *(Belg.; Spain)*; Hemineurin *(Arg.; Astra, Austral.)*; Hémineurine *(Debat, Fr.; Debat, Switz.)*; Heminevrin *(Astra, Denm.; Astra, Norw.; Astra, S.Afr.; Astra, Swed.; Astra, UK)*.

7019-l

Chlormezanone *(BAN, rINN)*.

Chlormethazanone; Chlormezanonum. 2-(4-Chlorophenyl)-3-methylperhydro-1,3-thiazin-4-one 1,1-dioxide.
$C_{11}H_{12}ClNO_3S$=273.7.

CAS — 80-77-3.

Pharmacopoeias. In *Cz.*

Adverse Effects

Drowsiness, weakness, nausea, dizziness, skin rash, flushing of the skin, confusion, excitement, depression, and dryness of the mouth have been reported. There may be difficulty in micturition. Cholestatic jaundice has occasionally occurred.

EFFECTS ON THE BLOOD. A brief report of immune thrombocytopenia in a patient receiving chlormezanone.— R. D. Finney and J. Apps, *Br. med. J.*, 1985, *290*, 1112.

EFFECTS ON THE SKIN. In a retrospective study of fixed eruptions in 86 patients, confirmed by a positive challenge test in 84, chlormezanone was the agent responsible in 5 cases.— K. Kauppinen and S. Stubb, *Br. J. Derm.*, 1985, *112*, 575.

OVERDOSAGE. A patient who had ingested 7 g of chlormezanone became comatose and hypotensive with flaccid muscle tone and diminished reflexes. The patient recovered without treatment.— D. Armstrong *et al.*, *Br. med. J.*, 1983, *286*, 845.

Following ingestion of 11 g of chlormezanone a patient was initially comatose, with hot, dry skin, dilated pupils, flaccidity, and absent reflexes, but subsequently developed hypertonicity and periods of excitement provoked by minor disturbances. The predominance of antimuscarinic symptoms may have been due to the high dose ingested.— B. W. Kirkham and J. B. Edelman, *Br. med. J.*, 1986, *292*, 732.

Treatment of Adverse Effects

For general guidelines to the symptomatic therapy of overdosage with hypnotics, sedatives, and neuroleptics, see p.708.

Precautions

For guidelines to the precautions to be observed with hypnotics, sedatives, and neuroleptics, see p.708.

Uses and Administration

Chlormezanone is used in the treatment of anxiety and tension states. It has been claimed to be of benefit in conditions associated with muscle spasm but has not been shown to have a direct action on muscle. The usual dose for the treatment of anxiety is 200 mg three or four times daily, with a range of 300 to 800 mg daily in divided doses.

As a hypnotic a dose of 400 mg at night is recommended.

ANXIETY. In a 4-week general practice multicentre study chlormezanone 400 mg by mouth at night, in 22 patients, appeared to be as effective as diazepam 5 mg three times daily, in a further 22, in relieving anxiety. A further patient in each group was withdrawn due to excessive daytime drowsiness; drowsiness was the most common side-effect, reported in 4 of those taking chlormezanone and 7 of those receiving diazepam.— D. M. Allin, *Curr. med. Res. Opinion*, 1982, *8*, 33.

INSOMNIA. In a multicentre crossover study in general practice, completed by 76 patients with sleep disturbances and mild anxiety, both the quality and duration of sleep were significantly improved by treatment at night with chlormezanone. Doses of 400 mg were considered more effective than 200 mg, and were preferred by the majority of patients, although side-effects, including daytime sedation, were more common with the higher dose. There was no evidence of a specific anxiolytic effect but reduction of anxiety might result from improved sleep.— G. M. Hunter, *Curr. med. Res. Opinion*, 1982, *8*, 22.

Further studies of the hypnotic effect of chlormezanone: K. Adam and I. Oswald, *Br. J. clin. Pharmac.*, 1982, *14*, 57 (comparison with nitrazepam); D. Van Steenis, *Curr. med. Res. Opinion*, 1982, *8*, 28 (comparison with temazepam).

Chlormezanone has no advantages over currently available hypnotics, and its long plasma half-life seems undesirable. Its potential for dependence and safety in overdosage have not been established with any certainty, and it cannot be recommended as a hypnotic.— *Drug & Ther. Bull.*, 1983, *21*, 32.

Proprietary Preparations

Trancopal *(Winthrop, UK)*. *Tablets*, chlormezanone 200 mg.

Proprietary Names and Manufacturers

Alinam *(Lucien, Fr.)*; Chlomedinon *(Jpn)*; Muskel Trancopal *(Winthrop, Ger.)*; Myolespen *(Jpn)*; Relizon *(Jpn)*; Rexan *(Ital.)*; Rilaquil *(Ital.)*; Supotran *(Fr.)*; Tanafol *(Ital.)*; Toyomezanon *(Jpn)*; Trancopal *(Aust.; Belg.; Winthrop, Canad.; Winthrop, Denm.; Laakefarmos, Fin.; Winthrop, Fr.; Iceland; Maggioni-Winthrop, Ital.; Neth.; Winthrop, Norw.; S.Afr.; Sterling-Winthrop, Swed.; Winthrop, Switz.; Winthrop, UK; Winthrop-Breon, USA)*; Trancote *(Jpn)*; Transanate *(Jpn)*.

The following names have been used for multi-ingredient preparations containing chlormezanone.— Lobak *(Sterling Research, UK)*; Trancoprin *(Winthrop, UK)*.

7020-v

Chlorproethazine Hydrochloride *(rINNM)*.

RP-4909 *(base)*. 3-(2-Chlorophenothiazin-10-yl)-*NN*-diethylpropylamine hydrochloride.
$C_{19}H_{23}ClN_2S,HCl$=383.4.

CAS — 84-01-5 (chlorproethazine); 4611-02-3 (hydrochloride).

Chlorproethazine is a phenothiazine derivative differing chemically from chlorpromazine by the substitution of a diethyl for a dimethyl group. It has general properties similar to those of chlorpromazine (below) but has been used mainly as a muscle relaxant. A recommended dosage of chlorproethazine hydrochloride by mouth is 25 to 100 mg daily (in divided portions); it has also been given by injection. Although exposure of the skin to phenothiazines has been associated with sensitivity reactions, chlorproethazine hydrochloride has also been applied topically in an ointment, with the warning to avoid direct exposure to sunlight.

Proprietary Names and Manufacturers

Neuriplège *(Génévrier, Fr.)*.

7021-g

Chlorpromazine *(BAN, USAN, rINN)*.

3(2-Chlorophenothiazin-10-yl)propyldimethylamine.
$C_{17}H_{19}ClN_2S$=318.9.

CAS — 50-53-3.

Pharmacopoeias. In *Br.* and *U.S.*

A white to creamy-white powder or waxy solid, odourless or with an amine-like odour. It darkens on prolonged exposure to light. M.p. 56° to 58°. Chlorpromazine 100 mg is approximately equivalent to 111 mg of chlorpromazine hydrochloride.

The *B.P.* states that it is practically **insoluble** in water; soluble 1 in 2 of alcohol, 1 in less than 1 of chloroform, and 1 in 1 of ether. *U.S.P.* solubilities are: 1 in 3 of alcohol, 1 in 2 of chloroform, and 1 in 3 of ether; freely soluble in dilute mineral acids; practically insoluble in dilute alkali hydroxides. **Store** in airtight containers. Protect from light.

7022-q

Chlorpromazine Embonate *(BANM, rINNM)*.

Chlorpromazine Pamoate. Chlorpromazine 4,4′-methylenebis(3-hydroxy-2-naphthoate).
$(C_{17}H_{19}ClN_2S)_2,C_{23}H_{16}O_6$=1026.1.

7023-p

Chlorpromazine Hydrochloride *(BANM, USAN, rINNM)*.

Aminazine; Chlorpromazini Hydrochloridum; Cloridrato de Clorpromazina.
$C_{17}H_{19}ClN_2S,HCl$=355.3.

CAS — 69-09-0.

Pharmacopoeias. In *Arg., Aust., Belg., Br., Braz., Chin., Cz., Egypt., Eur., Fr., Ger., Hung., Ind., Int., It., Jpn, Jug., Neth., Nord., Pol., Port., Rus., Swiss, Turk.*, and *U.S.* Also in *B.P. Vet.*

An odourless white or creamy-white crystalline powder. It decomposes on exposure to air and light becoming yellow, pink, and finally violet. The *B.P.* states that it is **soluble** 1 in 0.4 of water, 1 in 1.3 of alcohol, and 1 in 1 of chloroform; practically insoluble in ether. *U.S.P.* solubilities are: 1 in 1 of water, 1 in 1.5 of alcohol and of chloroform. A freshly prepared 10% solution in water has a pH of 4 to 5. The *B.P.* injection is **sterilised** by autoclaving after distribution into containers in which the air has been replaced by nitrogen or other suitable gas and has a pH of 5.0 to 6.5. **Store** in airtight containers. Protect from light.

CAUTION. *Chlorpromazine may cause severe dermatitis in sensitised persons. Pharmacists, nurses, and others who handle the drug frequently should wear masks and rubber gloves.*

When a solution of chlorpromazine was shaken for 1 hour with a number of synthetic materials, soft plastic materials such as silicone, latex, and thin polyvinyl chloride tubing adsorbed 99, 84, and 86% of chlorpromazine respectively. Adsorption occurred with hard plastic materials, cotton wool, filter paper, and glass wool but to a lesser extent. Other lipophilic phenothiazines and thiopentone were shaken with latex and polyvinyl chloride tubing and found to be adsorbed whereas hydrophilic compounds were not. A positive relationship between temperature and adsorption was demonstrated.— G. Krieglstein *et al.*, *Arzneimittel-Forsch.*, 1972, *22*, 1538.

A study of drug loss from intravenous delivery systems. There was a 41% loss of chlorpromazine hydrochloride from solution when infused for 7 hours via a plastic infusion set, and a 79% loss after infusion for 1 hour from a glass syringe through silastic tubing; however, loss was negligible from a system comprising a glass syringe with polythene tubing.— E. A. Kowaluk *et al.*, *Am. J. Hosp. Pharm.*, 1982, *39*, 460. See also *idem*, 1983, *40*, 118.

INCOMPATIBILITY. An immediate precipitate occurred when chlorpromazine hydrochloride 200 mg per litre was mixed with aminophylline 1 g per litre, ampicillin sodium 2 g per litre, chlorothiazide 2 g per litre, ethamivan 2 g per litre, methohexitone sodium 2 g per litre, phenobarbitone sodium 800 mg per litre, sulphadiazine sodium 4 g per litre, and sulphadimidine sodium 4 g per litre in 5% glucose solution and 0.9% sodium chloride solution. An immediate precipitate occurred with amphotericin 200 mg per litre in 5% glucose solution, and a haze developed over 3 hours with chloramphenicol 4 g per litre in 0.9% sodium chloride solution, but an immediate precipitate was formed in 5% glucose solution. A haze developed over 3 hours when chlorpromazine hydrochloride was mixed with benzylpenicillin 6 g per litre, cloxacillin sodium 1 g per litre, or methicillin sodium 4 g per litre in 0.9% sodium chloride solution.— B. B. Riley, *J. Hosp. Pharm.*, 1970, *28*, 228.

Solutions containing 2.5% of chlorpromazine hydrochloride could be diluted to 100 mL with 0.9% sodium chloride solution provided the pH of the saline solution was such that the pH of the dilution did not exceed the critical range of pH 6.7 to 6.8. With saline of pH 7 or

7.2, the final solution had a pH of 6.4.— P. F. D'Arcy and K. M. Thompson (letter), *Pharm. J.*, 1973, *1*, 28.

Morphine sulphate injection containing chlorocresol 0.2% was incompatible with chlorpromazine hydrochloride injection. Morphine injection without chlorocresol should be compatible.— J. B. Crapper, *Br. med. J.*, 1975, *1*, 33.

Chlorpromazine hydrochloride 25 mg in 1 mL produced an immediate haze when mixed with 2 mL of a solution containing cimetidine hydrochloride 150 mg per mL.— P. F. Souney *et al.*, *Am. J. Hosp. Pharm.*, 1984, *41*, 1840.

A proprietary oral solution containing chlorpromazine hydrochloride 5 mg per mL was physically compatible for 30 minutes, but not for 1 hour, with a solution containing thioridazine hydrochloride 30 mg per mL.— W. A. Parker, *Can. J. Hosp. Pharm.*, 1984, *37*, 133.

Adverse Effects

As for the phenothiazines in general, p.706.

In 556 patients who received chlorpromazine, adverse reactions attributed to the drug occurred in 68 (12.2%). Reactions were life-threatening in 1.3%. Drowsiness or disorientation (30) and hypotension (12) were the most common adverse effects.— C. Swett, *Curr. ther. Res.*, 1975, *18*, 199.

EFFECTS ON THE BLOOD. Chlorpromazine has been reported to cause aplastic anaemia. Agranulocytosis is also associated with its use and an incidence of 1 in 1300 has been reported.— P. C. Vincent, *Drugs*, 1986, *31*, 52.

Treatment of Adverse Effects

As for the phenothiazines in general, p.708.

Precautions

As for the phenothiazines in general p.708.

For precautions in administering chlorpromazine to patients with AIDS see Metoclopramide, p.1098. See also p.709.

INTERACTIONS. *Alcohol.* Akathisia and dystonia occurred after consumption of alcohol in patients taking phenothiazines. Alcohol might lower the threshold of resistance to neurotoxic side-effects.— E. G. Lutz, *J. Am. med. Ass.*, 1976, *236*, 2422.

Antacids. Studies in 6 patients showed that chlorpromazine plasma concentrations were significantly lower after administration of chlorpromazine with an aluminium hydroxide and magnesium trisilicate antacid gel (Gelusil) than after chlorpromazine alone. *In vitro* studies indicated that chlorpromazine was highly bound to the gel.— W. E. Fann *et al.*, *J. clin. Pharmac.*, 1973, *13*, 388.

Aspirin and other anti-inflammatory analgesics. In 4 of 5 psychiatric patients taking chlorpromazine, serum concentrations of 'free' chlorpromazine increased when acetanilide 3 g daily was given concomitantly. The amounts of unchanged chlorpromazine excreted in the urine increased in all the patients. Salicylamide 3 g daily produced a qualitatively similar but lesser effect, but aspirin in the same dose had a negligible effect. Acetanilide, and to a lesser extent salicylamide, competed with chlorpromazine in forming hydroxy derivatives and glucuronides.— C. L. Huang and K. Hirano, *Biochem. Pharmac.*, 1967, *16*, 2023.

Benzhexol and other antiparkinsonian agents. A study of plasma-chlorpromazine concentrations in relation to clinical response. Concurrent administration of benzhexol appeared to lower chlorpromazine concentrations.— L. Rivera-Calimlim *et al.*, *Clin. Pharmac. Ther.*, 1973, *14*, 978. A placebo-controlled study indicating that benzhexol had no effect on plasma-chlorpromazine concentration.— G. M. Simpson *et al.*, *Archs gen. Psychiat.*, 1980, *37*, 205.

Beverages. In vitro findings of an interaction between the antipsychotic drugs, fluphenazine and haloperidol, and coffee or tea.— F. Kulhanek *et al.* (letter), *Lancet*, 1979, *2*, 1130. Agreement. The interaction might account for variations in blood concentrations.— S. R. Hirsch (letter), *ibid.* A study in patients receiving chlorpromazine, haloperidol, fluphenazine, or trifluoperazine indicated that limitations on coffee and tea intake in psychiatric hospitals cannot be justified on the grounds that such beverages might lower the efficacy of antipsychotic drugs.— S. Bowen *et al.* (letter), *Lancet*, 1981, *1*, 1217. Results supporting the view that coffee or tea alter the pharmacokinetics of neuroleptics by reducing the overall effect and by producing a retard drug out of the short-acting one.— F. Kulhanek and O. K. Linde (letter), *ibid.*, *2*, 359. Despite the interaction *in vitro* a study in 12 healthy subjects indicated no significant reduction in plasma concentrations of fluphenazine on concomitant ingestion of the hydrochloride with tea or coffee.— S. M. Wallace *et al.* (letter), *Lancet*, 1981, *2*, 691.

Cimetidine. Despite evidence that cimetidine reduced the metabolism of chlorpromazine, mean steady-state plasma concentrations of chlorpromazine fell rather than rose in 8 patients given cimetidine for 7 days in addition to regular chlorpromazine therapy. The explanation was probably that cimetidine interfered with chlorpromazine absorption.— C. A. Howes *et al.*, *Eur. J. clin. Pharmac.*, 1983, *24*, 99.

Desferrioxamine. The combination of phenothiazines with desferrioxamine should be strictly avoided: loss of consciousness lasting 48 to 72 hours has been reported in patients given a phenothiazine during desferrioxamine therapy, possibly because this combination of drugs removes essential iron from the nervous system.— *Lancet*, 1985, *1*, 143.

Phenobarbitone and other barbiturates. Phenobarbitone increased the rate of urinary chlorpromazine excretion by 10 to 81%. When epileptic patients normally receiving barbiturates and chlorpromazine had their barbiturate withdrawn for 7 days there was a 17 to 55% decrease in urinary chlorpromazine excretion. A preparation of aluminium hydroxide with magnesium hydroxide adsorbed chlorpromazine when administered simultaneously and reduced the chlorpromazine urinary excretion-rate by 10 to 45%. This effect could be reduced by giving the medications 2 hours apart.— F. M. Forrest *et al.*, *Biol. Psychiat.*, 1970, *2*, 53.

Phenytoin and other anticonvulsants. A 55-year-old man who had been receiving phenytoin 300 mg daily for over 3 years and who was suffering from stable tardive dyskinesia which had been induced by haloperidol (discontinued 2 years previously) obtained amelioration of his symptoms on discontinuation of phenytoin for a week. On reintroduction of phenytoin the dyskinesia relapsed to its original severity. Phenytoin might exacerbate neuroleptic-induced dyskinesia.— J. DeVeaugh-Geiss (letter), *New Engl. J. Med.*, 1978, *298*, 457. Criticism.— P. A. Nausieda (letter), *ibid.*, 1093.

Piperazine. A child who had received piperazine for worms convulsed when given chlorpromazine several days later. Experiments in *dogs* and *goats* demonstrated that though piperazine or chlorpromazine given separately produced no ataxia, severe clonic convulsions, sometimes fatal, occurred when they were given together.— B. M. Boulos and L. E. Davis (letter), *New Engl. J. Med.*, 1969, *280*, 1245.

For references to further studies of the interaction between piperazine and chlorpromazine in *animals*, see under Piperazine, p.63.

Propranolol and other beta-blockers. Caution is essential when giving propranolol for hypertension to patients already stabilised on phenothiazines or tricyclic antidepressants.— R. Galinsky (letter), *New Engl. J. Med.*, 1976, *295*, 281. There was little reported evidence of trouble with this association.— N. M. Kaplan (letter), *ibid.*

A study completed by 6 chronic schizophrenic patients in good general health indicated that addition of propranolol to chlorpromazine therapy raises plasma concentrations of chlorpromazine.— M. Peet *et al.* , *I.C.I. Pharmaceuticals* (letter), *Lancet*, 1980, *2*, 978.

Tetracyclines. Black galactorrhoea occurred in a patient receiving concomitant therapy with minocycline and a phenothiazine.— R. S. W. Basler and P. J. Lynch, *Archs Derm.*, 1985, *121*, 417.

Tricyclic antidepressants. Since phenothiazines, tricyclic antidepressants, and antiparkinsonian agents had antimuscarinic properties the use of combinations of any of these drugs could produce confusion, impaired memory, hallucinations, and disorientation.— D. S. Janowsky *et al.*, *Am. J. Psychiat.*, 1972, *129*, 360.

Raised concentrations of phenothiazines caused by concomitant amitriptyline therapy.— A. Jus *et al.*, *Neuropsychobiology*, 1978, *4*, 305. See also R. S. Lott, *Drug Interact. News.*, 1985, *5*, 31.

In 7 psychotic patients who received chlorpromazine 100 mg by mouth every 8 hours for 9 weeks, addition of nortriptyline 50 mg 8-hourly by mouth during weeks 4, 5, and 6 resulted in a significant increase in plasma chlorpromazine concentrations and a profound worsening of the clinical state; these changes were reversed when nortriptyline was withdrawn. Addition of nortriptyline in full antidepressant doses to chlorpromazine therapy for psychosis should be avoided, and the same may hold true for other antidepressants and neuroleptics.— S. Loga *et al.*, *Clin. Pharmacokinet.*, 1981, *6*, 454.

INTERFERENCE WITH DIAGNOSTIC TESTS. Chlorpromazine is reported to interfere with pregnancy tests, thyroid-function tests, the Coombs' test where a false-positive result can be achieved, and with adrenal medullary tests. It is also reported to interfere with estimations for serum 5-hydroxyindole-acetic acid, blood urea, urinary ketones and steroids, urinary porphobilinogen, and vitamin B_{12}.

PREGNANCY AND THE NEONATE. *Diffusion across the placenta.* Chlorpromazine and its metabolites were found in the maternal plasma and urine, in the foetal plasma and amniotic fluid, and in neonatal urine after doses of 50 to 100 mg of chlorpromazine were given intramuscularly to pregnant women shortly before delivery.— S. E. F. O'Donoghue (letter), *Nature*, 1971, *229*, 124.

If given in high doses over a long period during pregnancy, chlorpromazine might cause damage to the retina of the foetus.— G. M. Stirrat, *Prescribers' J.*, 1973, *13*, 135. *Animal* studies on accumulation of chorio-retinotoxic drugs in the foetal eye.— N. G. Lindquist *et al.*, *Acta pharmac. tox.*, 1970, *28*, *Suppl.* 1, 64.

Excretion in breast milk. Preliminary data suggesting that in mothers taking chlorpromazine, concentrations can be higher in milk than in maternal plasma and might be associated with drowsiness and lethargy in the infant.— D. H. Wiles *et al.* (letter), *Br. J. clin. Pharmac.*, 1978, *5*, 272.

Absorption and Fate

Chlorpromazine is readily absorbed from the gastro-intestinal tract but is subject to considerable first-pass metabolism in the gut wall. It is also extensively metabolised in the liver and is excreted in the urine and bile in the form of numerous active and inactive metabolites; there is evidence of enterohepatic recycling. Owing to the first-pass effect, plasma concentrations following oral administration are much lower than those following intramuscular administration. Moreover, there is very wide intersubject variation in plasma concentrations of chlorpromazine; no simple correlation has been found between plasma concentrations of chlorpromazine and its metabolites, and their therapeutic effect. Paths of metabolism of chlorpromazine include hydroxylation and conjugation with glucuronic acid, *N*-oxidation, oxidation of a sulphur atom, and dealkylation. Although the plasma half-life of chlorpromazine itself has been reported to be only a few hours, elimination of the metabolites may be very prolonged.

Chlorpromazine is very extensively bound to plasma proteins. It is widely distributed in the body and crosses the blood-brain barrier to achieve higher concentrations in the brain than in the plasma. Chlorpromazine and its metabolites also cross the placental barrier and are excreted in milk (see under Precautions).

A review of the literature on the absorption and fate of chlorpromazine. Blood and urinary studies by and large favour a fairly short sojourn of the bulk of chlorpromazine in the body. For the blood studies this is in the range of 2 to 3 days and for the urinary studies up to about 18 days. There is no doubt, however, that chlorpromazine brings about changes that can persist much longer than this after drug discontinuation. The exact relationship of persisting therapeutic effects to administered chlorpromazine is uncertain. There is the possibility that minute amounts of chlorpromazine and-or metabolites persist at active sites in slowly reversible or relatively irreversible ways. It also seems that some chlorpromazine is stored in adipose tissue and slowly mobilised after stopping chlorpromazine administration.— R. B. Lacoursiere and H. E. Spohn, *J. nerv. ment. Dis.*, 1976, *163*, 267.

PLASMA PROTEIN BINDING. Chlorpromazine is highly bound to plasma protein, varying from 91.8 to 97% over the range of clinical blood concentrations (0.01 to 1 μg per mL). Binding is easily reversed.— S. H. Curry, *J. Pharm. Pharmac.*, 1970, *22*, 193.

Studies on the protein binding of phenothiazines, using bovine serum albumin, indicated that chlorpromazine has the highest affinity, followed in order by trifluoperazine, perphenazine, fluphenazine, and promazine. These results indicated that the order of binding affinity was based on the hydrophobicity of the phenothiazine, with the more hydrophobic molecules being more strongly bound.— H. Zia and J. C. Price, *J. pharm. Sci.*, 1975, *64*, 1177.

Uses and Administration

Chlorpromazine has a wide range of activity arising from its depressant actions on the central nervous system and its alpha-adrenergic blocking and weaker antimuscarinic activities. It is a dopamine inhibitor; it inhibits prolactin-release-inhibitory factor, considered to be dopamine, thus stimulating the release of prolactin. The turnover of dopamine in the brain is also increased. There is some evidence that the antagonism of central dopaminergic function, especially at the postulated D_2-dopaminergic receptor, is related to therapeutic effect in psychotic conditions.

Chlorpromazine possesses sedative properties but patients usually develop tolerance rapidly to the sedation. It has anti-emetic, antipruritic, serotonin-blocking, and weak antihistaminic properties and slight ganglion-blocking activity. It inhibits the heat regulating centre so that the patient tends to acquire the temperature of his surroundings (poikilothermy). Chlorpromazine can relax skeletal muscle. It has membrane-stabilising and hence local anaesthetic properties. Its actions on the autonomic system produce vasodilatation, hypotension, and tachycardia. Salivary and gastric secretions are reduced.

Chlorpromazine is widely used in the management of psychotic conditions. It controls excitement, agitation, and other psychomotor disturbances in schizophrenic patients and reduces the manic phase of manic-depressive conditions. It is used to control hyperkinetic states and aggression and is sometimes given in other psychiatric conditions for the control of anxiety and tension.

Chlorpromazine is anti-emetic and is used to control the nausea and vomiting of a variety of diseases and that caused by various drugs. It does not appear to be of benefit in motion sickness.

Chlorpromazine is effective in the alleviation of intractable hiccup. It has been used for the management of alcohol withdrawal symptoms but compounds such as diazepam are now preferred.

Chlorpromazine was formerly given in conjunction with pethidine and sometimes promethazine in a form of neuroleptanalgesia; however, such a combination was associated with considerable adverse effects and a combination of haloperidol with fentanyl is now usually preferred for this procedure. Chlorpromazine may be given to reduce pre-operative anxiety. Postoperative nausea and vomiting is reduced by chlorpromazine.

Since analgesic requirements are reduced by chlorpromazine it is used as an adjunct in the management of severe pain especially in malignant disease. It has also been used as an adjunct in the treatment of tetanus and is given to control acute intermittent porphyria.

Chlorpromazine is administered as the hydrochloride by mouth or injection, and as the embonate by mouth as a concentrated suspension in doses equivalent to those of the hydrochloride, and as the base rectally by suppository.

Dosage varies both with the individual and with the purpose for which the drug is being used. In most patients oral treatment may be used from the start, commencing with a dosage of 25 to 50 mg of the hydrochloride, or its equivalent as the embonate, three times daily and increasing as necessary; the usual daily maintenance dose ranges from 25 to 100 mg three times daily. Psychotic patients may require daily doses of up to 1 g or more.

For parenteral use, deep intramuscular injection is preferable. Subcutaneous injection is contra-indicated and intravenous injection is usually limited to severe hiccups; the injection must be diluted before intravenous administration. After injection of chlorpromazine, patients should remain in the supine position for at least 30 minutes. It is fairly well tolerated for short periods and is especially useful during the initial stages of treatment in psychiatric cases. The usual dose by injection is 25 to 50 mg repeated as required.

As an adjunct to the treatment of tetanus, 25 to 50 mg has been given intramuscularly 3 or 4 times daily.

If intractable hiccup does not respond to 25 to 50 mg three or four times daily by mouth for 2 to 3 days then 25 to 50 mg should be administered intramuscularly and if this fails 25 to 50 mg in 500 to 1000 mL of sodium chloride injection should be infused slowly, with the patient supine, and careful monitoring of the blood pressure.

If the oral and parenteral routes are not suitable chlorpromazine is administered rectally and suppositories containing 100 mg of chlorpromazine base may be employed; this is stated to have an effect comparable with 40 mg of the hydrochloride by mouth or 20 mg intramuscularly. Up to 4 suppositories may be given in 24 hours.

During the first few days of treatment, patients taking chlorpromazine should be advised not to drive vehicles or to use machinery.

For children over 5 years of age, one-third to one-half the adult dose may be given, and below this age a dose of 500 µg per kg body-weight may be given 4 times daily.

ADMINISTRATION IN HEPATIC FAILURE. There was no difference in the plasma clearance and cerebral effects of chlorpromazine in 24 patients with cirrhosis compared with matched controls. The susceptibility to chlorpromazine of some patients with cirrhosis was probably due to increased sensitivity of cerebral neurones and not to impaired liver metabolism.— J. D. Maxwell *et al.*, *Clin. Sci.*, 1972, *43*, 143. Further references.— A. E. Read *et al.*, *Br. med. J.*, 1969, *3*, 497.

ADMINISTRATION IN RENAL FAILURE. Chlorpromazine could be given in usual doses to patients in renal failure.— W. M. Bennett *et al.*, *Am. J. Kidney Dis.*, 1983, *3*, 155.

Chlorpromazine in total doses of 0.1 to 1 g given over periods of 2 to 7 days induced toxic psychoses in 4 patients with chronic renal failure requiring haemodialysis. In a fifth patient toxic psychosis was associated with administration of promethazine.— C. J. McAllister *et al.*, *Clin. Nephrol.*, 1978, *10*, 191.

ALCOHOL AND DRUG WITHDRAWAL. *Alcohol.* Chlorpromazine and mesoridazine each produced improvement which was most marked in the first week, in a controlled study of 40 patients in alcohol withdrawal states. Agitation, tremor, anxiety, and hallucinations were relieved or reduced.— J. B. Frost, *Can. psychiat. Ass. J.*, 1973, *18*, 385.

Although alcoholic hallucinosis may accompany withdrawal symptoms it may also present during a spell of sustained drinking, or more rarely during periods of sustained abstinence; for persistent or predominant hallucinosis which does not respond to withdrawal regimens, phenothiazines are indicated in antipsychotic dosage. However, in the management of withdrawal phenothiazines are generally contra-indicated as they may precipitate convulsions and are associated with liver damage.— A.P. Thorley, Alcohol, in *Drugs in Psychiatric Practice*, P.J. Tyrer (Ed.), London, Butterworths, 1982,, p.352.

Opioid analgesics. Chlorpromazine in a daily dose of 2.2 mg per kg body-weight in divided doses at 6-hourly intervals by mouth or injection was effective in relieving all the symptoms of diamorphine withdrawal in 178 infants born to diamorphine-addicted mothers. The dose of chlorpromazine was gradually reduced over 10 to 40 days.— C. Zelson *et al.*, *Pediatrics*, 1971, *48*, 178. See also *Med. Lett.*, 1973, *15*, 47. A discussion of neonatal opiate withdrawal. In the *USA* opiates, diazepam, and phenobarbitone are widely used in the management of this condition; however, in the *UK* chlorpromazine has tended to be the preferred treatment. Where drug treatment is needed to control withdrawal chlorpromazine is begun with a loading dose of 3 mg per kg body-weight, followed by a total maintenance dose of 3 mg per kg by mouth daily, divided into 4 or 6 doses. This dose is increased by 3 mg per kg daily if withdrawal is becoming increasingly severe, until control is achieved; occasionally as much as 15 mg per kg daily is required. Once the baby's condition is stable reduction in chlorpromazine dosage by 2 mg per kg every third day is attempted. Complications of phenothiazine usage have been notably absent, although rarely seizures may occur.— R. P. A. Rivers, *Archs Dis. Childh.*, 1986, *61*, 1236.

For a comparison of chlorpromazine with haloperidol in the management of phencyclidine-induced psychosis see Haloperidol, p.745.

ANALGESIA. For debate as to the analgesic and analgesic-potentiating effects of neuroleptics, see p.709.

BREATHLESSNESS. Preliminary results in healthy subjects indicated that chlorpromazine reduced the sensation of breathlessness evoked by exercise without altering the drive to breathe. It is conceivable that chlorpromazine, a constituent of the Brompton Cocktail, might offer relief for distressing breathlessness in terminally-ill patients.— P. A. O'Neill *et al.*, *Br. J. clin. Pharmac.*, 1985, *19*, 793.

See also under Respiratory distress syndrome, below.

CARDIOVASCULAR DISORDERS. Beneficial effect of chlorpromazine in heart failure in patients with myocardial infarction.— U. Elkayam *et al.*, *Chest*, 1977, *72*, 623. Intravenous injection of chlorpromazine, diluted to 2.5 mg per mL with saline, at a rate of 2.5 mg every 5 minutes until recovery was complete or a total dose of 25 mg had been reached, was used to treat 5 patients with pulmonary oedema who did not respond to conventional treatment. As soon as vasodilatation was apparent a bolus dose of frusemide 40 mg was given intravenously. Four of the 5 patients recovered fully.— E. Romano and A. Gullo, *Lancet*, 1980, *1*, 1000.

In 9 patients with severe hypertension a single dose of chlorpromazine 50 mg intramuscularly and frusemide 50 mg intravenously with bedrest resulted in a gradual and adequate reduction in blood pressure and pulse-rate. Maintenance therapy, by mouth, with a diuretic and beta-blocker was started 4 to 8 hours after parenteral treatment.— R. J. Young *et al.*, *Br. med. J.*, 1980, *280*, 1579. Comment.— P. E. Nielsen *et al.* (letter), *ibid.*, *281*, 873. In a 5-year prospective study, 27 of 30 patients presenting as hypertensive emergencies were satisfactorily treated by administration of chlorpromazine 50 mg intramuscularly combined with intravenous injection of frusemide 50 mg. The resultant decrease in blood pressure was gradual and progressive and reduced diastolic blood pressure to 100 mmHg or less in 4 hours. A further 2 patients required a second course at 4 hours, which produced a satisfactory response in both, and 1 patient died before response to treatment could be assessed. One of the 30 who experienced an acute fall in blood pressure had taken metoprolol shortly before treatment; none of the other patients experienced any adverse effects from the treatment regimen. The combination of frusemide and chlorpromazine appears to be a simple, safe, and predictable method of treatment for severe hypertension.— G. R. Nimmo and A. A. H. Lawson, *Curr. med. Res. Opinion*, 1986, *10*, 203.

A report of complete remission of a case of severe thrombotic thrombocytopenic purpura following administration of chlorpromazine 1 g daily for 6 weeks. Relapse did not occur when chlorpromazine was withdrawn.— R. T. Wensley and A. C. Cuthbert, *Br. med. J.*, 1982, *284*, 1446.

CHOLERA. Administration of chlorpromazine to 11 cholera patients with severe purging significantly reduced loss of fluid over 4 successive 8-hour periods compared with 20 similar control patients. Four of the patients received chlorpromazine 1 mg per kg body-weight intramuscularly, 4 received 4 mg per kg intramuscularly, and 3 received 1 mg per kg by mouth. After 32 hours, purging virtually stopped in those given the higher dose of chlorpromazine. In a few of the lower-dose patients a rebound purging occurred after the initial effect but was controlled by a second dose. Patients receiving chlorpromazine were mildly sedated, more comfortable, and had no nausea or vomiting. No hypotension occurred in these well-hydrated patients but this risk needs evaluation before the widespread use of chlorpromazine in cholera can be recommended.— G. H. Rabbani *et al.* (preliminary communication), *Lancet*, 1979, *1*, 410. In a subsequent controlled study patients with cholera and persistent diarrhoea despite intravenous rehydration therapy were given chlorpromazine 1 or 4 mg per kg body-weight, either intramuscularly or by mouth; 34 received chlorpromazine therapy while a further 12 acted as controls. Chlorpromazine significantly reduced the purging-rate compared with controls. Although differences between treatment groups were not significant there was a tendency for a better effect with the higher dose, given by either route. Duration of diarrhoea, frequency of vomiting, and mean requirement for intravenous fluids were all reduced in treated patients compared with controls. The antisecretory effects of the drug appeared to be biphasic with an initial effect followed by a second peak 24 to 32 hours after administration. Use of chlorpromazine might obviate the need for much intravenous hydration and simplify rehydration procedures; however, sedation, particularly in children, may prove a limitation. The standard treatment for cholera remains rehydration fluid and tetracycline and it remains to be seen whether adjunctive use of chlorpromazine is of practical benefit.— G. H. Rabbani *et al.*, *Br. med. J.*, 1982, *284*, 1361. In a placebo-controlled study in 410 patients with diarrhoea, 316 of whom had cholera, addition of chlorpromazine 1 mg per kg body-weight by mouth to standard therapy (rehydration and tetracycline) was no more effective than placebo overall in improving failure rates, purging rates, intravenous fluid requirements, or length of hospital stay. In children with severe cholera chlorpromazine significantly improved the failure rate of oral therapy but this effect was not seen in children with less severe cholera, adults with cholera, or patients of all ages with noncholera diarrhoea. Failure to detect any benefit may be attributable in part to the strikingly low failure rate of standard therapy. On the basis of these results chlorpromazine cannot be recommended as an adjunct to standard therapy in watery diarrhoea, except possibly in children with severe disease.— M. R. Islam *et al.*, *Gastroenterology*, 1982, *82*, 1335.

DEMENTIA. For discussion of the role of neuroleptics in the management of dementia see p.710.

DIAGNOSTIC USE. *Huntington's chorea.* There were impaired prolactin responses to chlorpromazine and protirelin in patients with Huntington's chorea when compared with controls. This might be of value in early detection of the disorder and suggested that there was a dopaminergic influence.— M. R. Hayden *et al.*, *Lancet*, 1977, *2*, 423. Experience with bromocriptine (a dopaminergic agonist) in patients with Huntington's chorea did not show any evidence of dopaminergic hypersensitivity.— R. J. Chalmers *et al.* (letter), *ibid.*, 824.

Pituitary reserve. A comparison of the functional evaluation of pituitary reserve in patients with the amenorrhoea-galactorrhoea syndrome utilising gonadorelin, levodopa, or chlorpromazine.— A. Zárate *et al.*, *J. clin. Endocr. Metab.*, 1973, *37*, 855. Testing with chlorpromazine and protirelin could be of diagnostic value in distinguishing between those patients with galactorrhoea and amenorrhoea produced by pituitary tumours, idiopathic disease or other causes.— A. E. Boyd *et al.*, *Ann. intern. Med.*, 1977, *87*, 165. Chlorpromazine 25 mg intramuscularly, or 0.4 mg per kg body-weight intramuscularly in children, administered after an overnight fast could be used as an alternative to the protirelin test. In general, serum prolactin should at least double; absence of response implies impairment in hypothalamic-pituitary prolactin control.— C. F. Abboud, *Mayo Clin. Proc.*, 1986, *61*, 35.

GILLES DE LA TOURETTE'S SYNDROME. Chlorpromazine 500 to 700 mg daily controlled Gilles de la Tourette's syndrome in a 14-year-old boy, unable to tolerate haloperidol owing to the development of paranoid ideation and depersonalisation.— J. Feldman (letter), *Am. J. Psychiat.*, 1977, *134*, 99.

HEADACHE. Comment on the beneficial response of cluster headache to chlorpromazine therapy.— V. S. Caviness and P. O'Brien, *New Engl. J. Med.*, 1980, *302*, 446.

Chlorpromazine 1 mg per kg intramuscularly produced complete resolution of migraine symptoms within 20 to 55 minutes in 96 of 100 patients.— K. V. Iserson, *Ann. emerg. Med.*, 1983, *12*, 756. A similar report. Intravenous chlorpromazine 5 to 50 mg provided complete relief in 38 of 52 migraine attacks in 40 patients; relief was incomplete in 3 cases and on 11 occasions there was a mild residual headache. A randomised trial of chlorpromazine in acute migraine should be considered.— P. L. Lane and R. Ross, *Headache*, 1985, *25*, 302.

A brief discussion of the use of chlorpromazine in the prophylaxis and treatment of migraine and cluster headache.— B. A. Atkinson and C. B. Tuttle, *Can. J. Hosp. Pharm.*, 1985, *38*, 130.

HICCUP. Details of a protocol for treating hiccups. Any metabolic abnormality should be corrected, then granulated sugar should be swallowed dry; if this is successful the sugar should be repeated if hiccups recur. If the sugar is not successful, pass nasogastric tube, decompress stomach, then irritate pharynx; if successful, repeat if hiccups recur. If not successful, give chlorpromazine 25 to 50 mg intravenously, and if succcessful maintain on chlorpromazine by mouth for 10 days. If the intravenous chlorpromazine is not successful initially, repeat up to 3 times, and if eventually successful, maintain on chlorpromazine by mouth for 10 days. If chlorpromazine is not successful, give metoclopramide 10 mg intravenously every 4 hours, and if this is successful maintain on metoclopramide by mouth for 10 days. If metoclopramide is not successful, give quinidine 200 mg by mouth 4 times daily, and if this is not successful, carry out left phrenic nerve-block then crush.— B. W. A. Williamson and I. M. C. Macintyre, *Br. med. J.*, 1977, *2*, 501.

LEISHMANIASIS. Preliminary results in 3 patients suggested that chlorpromazine as a 2% ointment, applied 3 times daily for a month, might be of benefit in the management of diffuse cutaneous leishmaniasis.— T. -H. Henriksen and S. Lende (letter), *Lancet*, 1983, *1*, 126.

PHANTOM LIMB PAIN. Chlorpromazine 500 mg daily by mouth abolished severe phantom limb pain in a patient who had suffered for more than 30 years following a leg amputation.— T. P. Logan, *Sth. med. J.*, 1983, *76*, 1585.

RESPIRATORY DISTRESS SYNDROME. A report of beneficial results with chlorpromazine in the respiratory distress syndrome.— E. F. Diamond and V. R. DeYoung, *J. Am. med. Ass.*, 1966, *196*, 584.

SCORPION STING. Three children with scorpion stings were successfully sedated with chlorpromazine, in 1 patient administered intravenously and in the other 2 patients intramuscularly [no doses stated]. All 3 children responded dramatically within minutes, though the first patient had failed to respond to a total of 160 mg of phenobarbitone.— H. L. Masco (letter), *J. Am. med. Ass.*, 1970, *212*, 2122.

TEMPERATURE DISORDERS. *Heat stroke.* The main aim of treatment in heat stroke is to reduce body temperature rapidly. The patient should be placed in a cool air-conditioned room, clothing removed, and ice-packs applied. Convulsions and shivering were prevented by the intravenous infusion of 200 mL of glucose injection containing 100 mg each of chlorpromazine, pethidine, and promethazine. A double dose was sometimes used and occasionally hypnotic drugs were necessary.— S. Shibolet *et al.*, *Q. J. Med.*, 1967, *36*, 525.

Hypothermia. A treatment regimen, including chlorpromazine, for the prevention of brain damage in submersion hypothermia.— A. W. Conn, *Can. med. Ass. J.*, 1979, *120*, 397.

Preparations

Chlorpromazine Oral Solution *(B.P.).* Chlorpromazine Elixir. A solution of chlorpromazine hydrochloride in a suitable flavoured vehicle. Dilutions must be freshly prepared.

Chlorpromazine Hydrochloride Injection *(U.S.P.).* A sterile solution of chlorpromazine hydrochloride, 23.75 to 26.25 mg per mL, in Water for Injections. pH 3 to 5.

Chlorpromazine Hydrochloride Syrup *(U.S.P.).* A syrup containing chlorpromazine hydrochloride 190 to 210 mg in each 100 mL.

Chlorpromazine Hydrochloride Tablets *(U.S.P.)*

Chlorpromazine Injection *(B.P.).* A sterile solution containing chlorpromazine hydrochloride in Water for Injections free from dissolved air.

Chlorpromazine Suppositories *(B.P.).* Contain chlorpromazine in a suitable basis.

Chlorpromazine Suppositories *(U.S.P.).* Suppositories containing chlorpromazine.

Chlorpromazine Tablets *(B.P.).* Tablets containing chlorpromazine hydrochloride.

Proprietary Preparations

Chloractil *(DDSA Pharmaceuticals, UK). Tablets*, chlorpromazine hydrochloride 25 and 50 mg.

Largactil *(May & Baker, UK). Tablets*, chlorpromazine hydrochloride 10, 25, 50, and 100 mg.
Syrup, chlorpromazine hydrochloride 25 mg/5 mL.
Forte Suspension, chlorpromazine hydrochloride 100 mg (as embonate)/5 mL.
Injection, chlorpromazine hydrochloride 25 mg/mL, in ampoules of 1 and 2 mL.
Suppositories, chlorpromazine 100 mg.

Proprietary Names and Manufacturers of Chlorpromazine and its Salts

Amazin *(SCS, S.Afr.)*; Ampliactil *(Arg.)*; Aspersinal *(Arg.)*; BayClor *(Bay, USA)*; Chloractil *(DDSA Pharmaceuticals, UK)*; Chlorazine *(Streuli, Switz.)*; Chlorprom *(Canad.)*; Chlorpromanyl *(Technilab, Canad.)*; Clopratets *(Pharmadrug, Ger.)*; Cloracin *(Nessa, Spain)*; Dozine *(R.P. Drugs, UK)*; Hibanil *(Mekos, Norw.)*; Hibernal *(Leo Rhodia, Swed.)*; Klorazin *(Vernleigh, S.Afr.)*; Klorpromex *(Swed.)*; Largactil *(May & Baker, Austral.; Belg.; Rhône-Poulenc, Canad.; Rhone-Poulenc, Denm.; Specia, Fr.; Carlo Erba, Ital.; Neth.; Rhône-Poulenc, Norw.; May & Baker, S.Afr.; Rhone, Spain; Rhone-Poulenc, Switz.; May & Baker, UK)*; Megaphen *(Bayer, Ger.)*; Novochlorpromazine *(Novopharm, Canad.)*; Procalm *(Austral.)*; Promachlor *(USA)*; Promacid *(USV, Austral.)*; Promapar *(Parke, Davis, USA)*; Protran *(Protea, Austral.)*; Prozil *(Dumex, Denm.)*; Prozin *(Lusofarmaco, Ital.)*; Repazine *(Lennon, S.Afr.)*; Thorazine *(Smith Kline & French, USA)*.

The following names have been used for multi-ingredient preparations containing chlorpromazine and its salts— Amargyl *(May & Baker, UK)*.

7024-s

Chlorprothixene *(BAN, USAN, rINN).*

N-714; Ro-4-0403. (*Z*)-3-(2-Chlorothioxanthen-9-ylidene)-*NN*-dimethylpropylamine.
$C_{18}H_{18}ClNS = 315.9$.

CAS — 113-59-7.

Pharmacopoeias. In *Cz.* (as the hydrochloride, and as the mesylate), in *Nord.*, which also includes the hydrochloride, and in *U.S.*

A yellow, crystalline powder with a slight amine-like odour.
Soluble 1 in 1700 of water, 1 in 29 of alcohol, 1 in 2 of chloroform, 1 in 14 of ether, and 1 in 18 of acetone. The *U.S.P.* Oral Suspension has a pH of between 3.5 and 4.5. **Store** in airtight containers. Protect from light.

Adverse Effects, Treatment, and Precautions

As for the phenothiazines, p.706.

EFFECTS ON THE LIVER. A 59-year-old man receiving chlorprothixene (for the second time) for acute mania developed severe obstructive jaundice within a few days; he was also taking chlorpropamide, digoxin, and diuretics; chlorprothixene was considered the most likely cause of the jaundice, though chlorpropamide could not be excluded.— D. G. S. Ruddock and J. Hoenig (letter), *Br. med. J.*, 1973, *1*, 231.

WITHDRAWAL. A 9-year-old boy with mild choreoathetotic cerebral palsy, mild mental retardation, and a severe behaviour problem, who had been taking chlorprothixene 150 mg daily for about a year developed restlessness and insomnia the day after its abrupt withdrawal. Nausea and vomiting occurred on the fourth day, followed on the sixth day by severe extrapyramidal disorders. The vomiting, which occurred after meals, persisted until the twentieth day after withdrawal, and the extrapyramidal movements were still present on the twenty-eighth day, when neuroleptic therapy was resumed owing to the severity of his behaviour problem. Control of the abnormal involuntary movements was attained within 24 hours of resuming neuroleptic therapy.— L. E. Yepes and B. G. Winsberg, *Am. J. Psychiat.*, 1977, *134*, 574.

Absorption and Fate

For an account of the absorption and fate of a thioxanthene, see Flupenthixol, p.738.

Chlorprothixene and its sulphoxide metabolite were concentrated in the breast milk of 2 mothers receiving chlorprothixene 200 mg daily but it was calculated that the amount supplied to the nursing infant was only 0.1% of the maternal dose per kg body-weight.— I. Matheson *et al.*, *Eur. J. clin. Pharmac.*, 1984, *27*, 611.

METABOLISM. Studies on the metabolism of chlorprothixene in *animals* and man. In addition to the major metabolite chlorprothixene-sulphoxide, 2 further urinary metabolites were identified, namely *N*-desmethylchlorprothixene-sulphoxide and chlorprothixene-sulphoxide-*N*-oxide.— J. Raaflaub, *Arzneimittel-Forsch.*, 1967, *17*, 1393.

Uses and Administration

Chlorprothixene is a thioxanthene with general properties similar to those of the phenothiazine, chlorpromazine (p.724). The usual dose for the treatment of psychoses is 25 to 50 mg three or four times daily; in acute psychoses doses of up to 600 mg daily have been given. It may also be given intramuscularly in doses of 25 to 50 mg three or four times daily.
Doses of 10 to 25 mg three or four times daily have been suggested for children over 6 years of age.
Chlorprothixene has also been advocated for non-psychotic emotional disturbances in adults,

such as anxiety and tension, but safer and more appropriate agents such as the benzodiazepines are generally to be preferred.

Chlorprothixene should be given in reduced dosage to elderly patients.

PAIN. Of 30 patients with postherpetic neuralgia 25 were given chlorprothixene 50 mg by mouth every 6 hours and 5 with severe neuralgia were given an additional 100 mg initially by intramuscular injection. Complete pain relief was experienced within 72 hours by 27 patients (within 24 hours by 11).— G. A. Farber and J. W. Burks, *Sth. med. J.*, 1974, *67*, 808.

Only 4 of 13 patients with postherpetic neuralgia reported pain relief when given chlorprothixene 50 mg daily by mouth for 1 week, followed by 50 mg twice daily for a further week. Two of these 4 were subsequently forced to discontinue further therapy due to adverse effects, and the remaining 2 found that the effectiveness of maintenance treatment diminished after several months. In a second study, chlorprothixene 50 mg every 6 hours produced lasting pain relief only in 1 of 19 patients.— P. W. Nathan, *Pain*, 1978, *5*, 367.

Preparations

Chlorprothixene Injection *(U.S.P.)*. A sterile solution in Water for Injections, prepared with the aid of hydrochloric acid. pH 3 to 4.

Chlorprothixene Oral Suspension *(U.S.P.)*

Chlorprothixene Tablets *(U.S.P.)*

Proprietary Names and Manufacturers

Taractan *(Austral.; Belg.; Roche, Denm.; Fr.; Roche, Ger.; Roche, Ital.; Neth.; Roche, Switz.; Roche, UK; Roche, USA)*; Tarasan *(Roche, Canad.)*; Truxal *(Belg., Lundbeck, Denm.; Tropon, Ger.; Neth.; Lundbeck, Norw.; S.Afr.; Lundbeck, Swed.; Lundbeck, Switz.)*; Truxaletten *(Tropon, Ger.; Lundbeck, Switz.)*; Truxaletter *(Norw.)*; Truxalettes *(Belg.)*.

7025-w

Clobazam *(BAN, USAN, rINN)*.

HR-376; HR-4723; LM-2717. 7-Chloro-1,5-dihydro-1-methyl-5-phenyl-1,5-benzodiazepine-2,4(3*H*)-dione.

$C_{16}H_{13}ClN_2O_2$=300.7.

CAS — 22316-47-8.

Dependence, Adverse Effects, Treatment, and Precautions

As for the benzodiazepines in general, p.706.

INTERACTIONS. *Alcohol*. A study demonstrating interaction between clobazam and alcohol.— K. Taeuber *et al.*, *Br. J. clin. Pharmac.*, 1979, *7, Suppl.* 1, 91S.

Antiepileptics. For the effect of clobazam on blood concentrations of carbamazepine, see under Carbamazepine, p.401.

Cimetidine. Cimetidine reduced the rate of elimination of clobazam and its metabolite *N*-desmethylclobazam in a study involving 10 healthy subjects; the effect seemed to be greater on the metabolite than the parent drug. There was also some evidence that cimetidine increased the bioavailability of clobazam. The results of this single-dose study suggested that an interaction of clinical significance might occur if cimetidine were given to patients receiving clobazam.— T. Pullar *et al.*, *Br. J. clin. Pharmac.*, 1987, *23*, 317. See also H. -G. Grigoleit *et al.*, *Eur. J. clin. Pharmac.*, 1983, *25*, 139.

For further discussion of the interactions between the benzodiazepines and cimetidine see under Diazepam, p.729.

WITHDRAWAL. Withdrawal symptoms in 2 patients on withdrawal of clobazam.— H. Petursson and M. H. Lader, *Br. med. J.*, 1981, *282*, 1931.

Absorption and Fate

It has been reported that unlike the 1,4-benzodiazepines such as diazepam (see p.730), clobazam, a 1,5-benzodiazepine, is not hydroxylated at the 3-position.

A review of the clinical pharmacokinetics of some newer benzodiazepines, including clobazam. Clobazam is reasonably rapidly absorbed following single oral doses, with peak concentrations generally reached within 2 hours after administration in the fasting state. After the distribution phase elimination proceeds with a usual half-life ranging from 10 to 50 hours in young healthy subjects. Total clearance is reduced in elderly compared to young men, but such a difference with age has not been demonstrated in women. Clobazam is extensively protein bound, the free fraction in plasma being about 10 to 13%. The major metabolic pathway in humans involves removal of the N-1 methyl group to yield the active metabolite desmethylclobazam. Metabolism of clobazam involves hepatic microsomal oxidation, and clearance is likely to be impaired in patients with cirrhosis and in those receiving enzyme-inhibiting drugs.— D. J. Greenblatt *et al.*, *Clin. Pharmacokinet.*, 1983, *8*, 233.

A study of the disposition kinetics of clobazam. Peak serum concentrations were achieved a mean of 1.28 hours after a single dose of 20 mg by mouth in 16 healthy fasting subjects. The mean elimination half-life was 24 hours. Following administration of clobazam 5 mg twice daily by mouth to 13 of the subjects for 22 days there was significant accumulation of the drug and of its major metabolite desmethylclobazam. The mean accumulation half-lives of drug and metabolite were 24 hours and 106 hours respectively. The subjects reported an increase in daytime sedation during the study; this was maximal during the first week of dosage despite continued accumulation of the drug thereafter.— H. R. Ochs *et al.*, *Eur. J. clin. Pharmac.*, 1984, *26*, 499. See also W. Rupp *et al.*, *Br. J. clin. Pharmac.*, 1979, *7, Suppl.* 1, 51S.

The pharmacokinetics of clobazam in epileptics. Plasma concentrations of *N*-desmethylclobazam were much higher in 6 epileptic patients given clobazam 30 mg by mouth than in 6 healthy controls given the same dose. The results were probably due to enzyme induction in epileptics by concomitant antiepileptic medication.— S. Jawad *et al.*, *Br. J. clin. Pharmac.*, 1984, *18*, 873.

Uses and Administration

Clobazam is a benzodiazepine with actions and uses similar to those of diazepam (p.731). The usual dose for the treatment of anxiety is 20 to 30 mg daily given in divided doses or as a single dose at night; in severe conditions up to 60 mg daily has been given. Similar daily doses have been given as adjunctive therapy in the management of epilepsy.

Doses of 20 mg daily have been suggested in elderly patients; in children aged 3 years or over not more than half the recommended adult dose may be given.

ACTION. A view that the pharmacological profile of clobazam, which is a 1,5-benzodiazepine, differs from that of the 1,4-benzodiazepines, such as chlordiazepoxide and diazepam, in that it displays a wide separation of psychosedative or 'tranquillising' properties, from impairment of motor coordination, and that this is associated with a relative lack of muscle relaxant activity.— G. W. Hanks, *Hoechst*, *Br. J. clin. Pharmac.*, 1979, *7, Suppl.* 1, 151S. A review of some clinical studies on clobazam. In 15 studies comparing it with diazepam there was an equal incidence of drowsiness in 2, more drowsiness with clobazam in 5, and more drowsiness with diazepam in 8.— D. Koeppen, *Br. J. clin. Pharmac.*, 1979, *7, Suppl.* 1, 139S.

ALCOHOL AND DRUG WITHDRAWAL. Evidence from a study in 40 alcoholic patients that clobazam is of benefit in the management of alcohol withdrawal.— P. K. Mukherjee, *J. int. med. Res.*, 1983, *11*, 205.

CONVULSIONS. Like other benzodiazepines clobazam is a highly effective anticonvulsant. It appears to have a greater therapeutic potential, and a lower incidence of side-effects, than the 1,4-benzodiazepines. The development of tolerance to its effects is a problem, but as it is usually prescribed for patients with intractable seizures it is clearly worth a trial as adjunctive treatment, even if a small number of patients derive lasting benefit. It seems wise to start the drug on 10 or 20 mg; a single dose at night is preferable to minimise daytime sedation. Fixed doses of 20 mg daily and intermittent treatment, with re-prescribing of clobazam after clobazam-free intervals, are the regimes of choice in patients who exhibit tolerance.— M. R. Trimble and M. M. Robertson, Clobazam, in *New Anticonvulsant Drugs*, B.S. Meldrum and R.J. Porter (Eds), London, John Libbey, 1986, p.65. See also *Drug & Ther. Bull.*, 1986, *24*, 45.

For further reference to the use of the benzodiazepines in convulsive disorders see p.710.

PAIN. Mention of the complete relief of phantom limb pain refractory to other therapy in an elderly patient given clobazam 10 mg three times daily.— C. P. Rice-Oxley (letter), *Br. med. J.*, 1986, *293*, 1309.

Proprietary Preparations

Frisium *(Hoechst, UK)*. *Capsules*, clobazam 10 mg.

Proprietary Names and Manufacturers

Castilium *(Port.)*; Clarmyl *(Roussel, Spain)*; Clopax *(Funk, Spain)*; Frisin *(Chile)*; Frisium *(Hoechst, Austral.; Belg.; Hoechst, Denm.; Hoechst, Ger.; Hoechst, Ital.; Hoechst, UK)*; Karidium *(Arg.)*; Noiafren *(Hoechst, Spain)*; Sederlona *(Andreu, Spain)*; Sentil *(Kor.)*; Urbadan *(Arg.; Braz.; Col.; Ecuad.; Guat.; Mex.; Peru; Port.; Urug.)*; Urbanol *(Cassenne, S.Afr.)*; Urbanyl *(Diamant, Fr.; Roussel, Switz.)*.

12582-z

Clocapramine Hydrochloride *(rINNM)*.

Chlorcarpipramine Hydrochloride; Y-4153. 1′-[3-(3-Chloro-10,11-dihydro-5*H*-dibenz[*b,f*]azepin-5-yl)propyl]-[1,4′-bipiperidine]-4′-carboxamide dihydrochloride monohydrate.

$C_{28}H_{37}ClN_4O,2HCl,H_2O$=572.0.

CAS — 47739-98-0 (clocapramine).

Clocapramine is a chlorinated derivative of carpipramine (p.717) and has been used in the treatment of schizophrenia.

Reference: S. Yamagami, *J. int. med. Res.*, 1985, *13*, 301 (comparison with haloperidol).

Proprietary Names and Manufacturers

Clofekton *(Yoshitomi, Jpn)*.

7029-j

Clorazepate Monopotassium *(USAN)*.

Abbott-39083; CB-4311. Potassium 7-chloro-2,3-dihydro-2-oxo-5-phenyl-1*H*-1,4-benzodiazepine-3-carboxylate.

$C_{16}H_{10}ClKN_2O_3$=352.8.

CAS — 5991-71-9.

7030-q

Potassium Clorazepate *(BANM)*.

Abbott-35616; AH-3232; CB-4306; Clorazepate Dipotassium *(USAN)*; Dipotassium Clorazepate *(rINN)*. Compound of potassium 7-chloro-2,3-dihydro-2-oxo-5-phenyl-1*H*-1,4-benzodiazepine-3-carboxylate with potassium hydroxide.

$C_{16}H_{11}ClK_2N_2O_4$=408.9.

CAS — 20432-69-3 (clorazepic acid); 57109-90-7 (potassium clorazepate).

Dependence, Adverse Effects, Treatment, and Precautions

As for the benzodiazepines in general, p.706.

EFFECTS ON THE LIVER. A report of jaundice and hepatic necrosis associated with clorazepate administration.— J. L. W. Parker, *Postgrad. med. J.*, 1979, *55*, 908.

EFFECTS ON MENTAL STATE. *Paradoxical response*. A paradoxical rage reaction occurred in a 24-year-old man with mild anxiety symptoms who had taken 75 mg of clorazepate dipotassium in 8 hours. This reaction did not occur when intermittent low doses of diazepam were given.— F. E. Karch, *Ann. intern. Med.*, 1979, *91*, 61.

INTERACTIONS. *Alcohol*. Interactions between clorazepate and alcohol.— M. Staak *et al.*, *Int. J. clin. Pharmac. Biopharm.*, 1979, *17*, 205. See also M. Staak *et al.*, *Int. J. clin. Pharmac.*, 1980, *18*, 283.

Antacids. A study in 15 healthy subjects indicated that concurrent administration of clorazepate dipotassium with a magnesium and aluminium antacid tended to retard clorazepate absorption producing lower peak plasma concentrations of desmethyldiazepam; overall absorption and the elimination half-lives of clorazepate and desmethyldiazepam were unaffected.— A. H. C. Chun *et al.*, *Clin. Pharmac. Ther.*, 1977, *22*, 329.

Further references: R. I. Shader *et al.*, *Clin. Pharmac. Ther.*, 1978, *24*, 308.

Oral contraceptives. The discussion of the interactions between oral contraceptives and benzodiazepines, including clorazepate, see under Diazepam, p.730.

PREGNANCY AND THE NEONATE. Malformations in the infant of a mother who had taken clorazepate during the first trimester of pregnancy.— D. A. Patel and A. R. Patel (letter), *J. Am. med. Ass.*, 1980, *244*, 135.

See also under Absorption and Fate.

WITHDRAWAL. For reference to convulsions following withdrawal of clorazepate see under Lorazepam, p.747.

Absorption and Fate

For an account of the absorption and fate of a benzodiazepine, see Diazepam, p.730.

Clorazepate is decarboxylated rapidly at the low pH in the stomach to form desmethyldiazepam, which is quickly absorbed.

A peak plasma-desmethyldiazepam concentration of 379 ng per mL occurred 45 minutes after administration of clorazepate dipotassium 15 mg to a healthy subject.— D. J. Greenblatt, *J. pharm. Sci.*, 1978, *67*, 427.

For a comparison of the pharmacokinetics of oxazolam, prazepam, and clorazepate, see under Oxazolam, p.757.

BIOAVAILABILITY. A study of the bioavailability of potassium clorazepate following intramuscular injection in 6 healthy subjects. Comparison of plasma concentrations following intravenous and intramuscular injection of potassium clorazepate 20 mg revealed that the mean bioavailability co-efficient was 1.04, indicating it to be completely bioavailable on intramuscular administration; this compared with a bioavailability co-efficient of 0.85 for diazepam in the same subjects, but the clinical relevance of this difference was unknown.— Å. Bertler *et al.*, *Eur. J. clin. Pharmac.*, 1985, *28*, 229.

PREGNANCY AND THE NEONATE. *Diffusion across the placenta.* The mean transport fraction across the placenta of diazepam was 40% and of desmethyldiazepam 38%, but only 11% for clorazepate.— M. Guerre-Millo *et al.*, *Eur. J. clin. Pharmac.*, 1979, *15*, 171.

Excretion in breast milk. Desmethyldiazepam was found in small amounts in milk and in the blood of breast-fed infants when clorazepate was given to women who were breast-feeding.— E. Rey *et al.*, *Eur. J. clin. Pharmac.*, 1979, *15*, 181.

Uses and Administration

Clorazepate is a benzodiazepine with actions and uses similar to those of diazepam (p.731). In the *UK*, a usual dose of 15 mg of potassium clorazepate (the dipotassium salt) has been given as a single dose at night for the treatment of anxiety; alternatively a dose of 7.5 mg may be given up to three times daily.

In the *USA* rather higher doses have been recommended; 15 to 60 mg of potassium clorazepate may be given daily, as 2 to 4 divided doses or as a single dose at night. Doses of up to 90 mg have been given in the management of convulsive disorders or alcohol withdrawal syndrome.

Reduced doses should be given in elderly or debilitated patients.

The monopotassium salt has also been used similarly, in equivalent doses.

Proprietary Preparations

Tranxene *(Boehringer Ingelheim, UK). Capsules*, potassium clorazepate 7.5 and 15 mg.

Proprietary Names and Manufacturers

Azene *(Endo, USA)*; Belseren *(Belg.)*; Covengar *(Arg.)*; Enadine *(Arg.)*; Justum *(Arg.)*; Moderane *(Arg.)*; Nansius *(Berenguer-Beneyto, Spain)*; Novoclopate *(Novopharm, Canad.)*; Tencilan *(Arg.)*; Transene *(Midy, Ital.)*; Tranxen *(Searle, Denm.)*; Tranxene *(Glaxo, Austral.; Belg.; Abbott, Canad.; Clin Midy, Fr.; Boehringer Ingelheim, S.Afr.; Boehringer Ingelheim, UK; Abbott, USA)*; Tranxilen *(Ferrosan, Norw.; Ferrosan, Swed.)*; Tranxilium *(Arg.; Midy, Ger.; Labaz, Spain; Clin-Midy, Switz.)*; Uni-tranxene *(Belg.)*.

7031-p

Clothiapine *(BAN, USAN).*

Clotiapine *(rINN)*; HF-2159. 2-Chloro-11-(4-methylpiperazin-1-yl)dibenzo[*b,f*][1,4]thiazepine.

$C_{18}H_{18}ClN_3S$=343.9.

CAS — 2058-52-8.

Clothiapine has actions similar to those of the phenothiazines (see p.706) and has been given in doses of 40 to 120 mg daily for the treatment of psychoses. It may also be given by slow intravenous or deep intramuscular injection.

Proprietary Names and Manufacturers

Entumin *(Sandoz, Ital.)*; Entumine *(Wander, Switz.)*; Etomine *(Sandoz, S.Afr.)*; Etumina *(Sandoz, Arg.; Sandoz, Spain)*; Etumine *(Wander, Belg.; Sandoz, Fr.)*.

12592-k

Clotiazepam *(rINN).*

Y-6047. 5-(2-Chlorophenyl)-7-ethyl-1,3-dihydro-1-methyl-2*H*-thieno[2,3-*e*]-1,4-diazepin-2-one.

$C_{16}H_{15}ClN_2OS$=318.8.

CAS — 33671-46-4.

Pharmacopoeias. In *Jpn.*

Clotiazepam is a benzodiazepine and shows the general properties of the group, see p.706. It is used in the management of anxiety and tension states in usual doses of 10 to 15 mg daily, in divided doses by mouth. In more severe cases up to 30 mg daily may be given.

Proprietary Names and Manufacturers

Clozan *(Pfizer, Belg.)*; Distensan *(Esteve, Spain)*; Rize *(Jpn)*; Rizen *(Puropharma, Ital.)*; Tienor *(Farmaka, Ital.)*; Trecalmo *(Tropon, Ger.)*; Veratran *(Latéma, Fr.)*.

7032-s

Cloxazolam *(rINN).*

CS-370. 10-Chloro-11b-(2-chlorophenyl)-2,3,7,11b-tetrahydro-oxazolo[3,2-*d*][1,4]benzodiazepin-6(5*H*)-one.

$C_{17}H_{14}Cl_2N_2O_2$=349.2.

CAS — 24166-13-0.

Pharmacopoeias. In *Jpn.*

Cloxazolam is a benzodiazepine and shares the actions and uses of the group (see p.706). It has been given in doses of 3 to 12 mg daily for the treatment of anxiety.

Results of a double-blind placebo-controlled study in 8 healthy subjects comparing diazepam and cloxazolam. Cloxazolam 2 mg was approximately equivalent to diazepam 5 mg. The effect of cloxazolam could still be observed after 8 hours and it was considered that a dosage regimen of cloxazolam 2 mg twice daily should suffice.— B. Saletu *et al.*, *Curr. ther. Res.*, 1976, *20*, 510.

Proprietary Names and Manufacturers

Betavel *(Pharmainvesti, Spain)*; Enadel *(Jpn)*; Lubalix *(Lubapharm, Switz.)*; Sepazon *(Jpn)*; Tolestan *(Roemmers, Arg.)*.

12595-x

Clozapine *(BAN, USAN, rINN).*

HF-1854. 8-Chloro-11-(4-methylpiperazin-1-yl)-5*H*-dibenzo[*b,e*][1,4]diazepine.

$C_{18}H_{19}ClN_4$=326.8.

CAS — 5786-21-0.

Adverse Effects

For the adverse effects associated with neuroleptic therapy see p.706.

Agranulocytosis has been reported during clozapine treatment. Antimuscarinic side-effects, such as dry mouth and accommodation difficulties may be noted; orthostatic hypotension, tachycardia, hyperthermia, and delirium may occur. Extrapyramidal effects are reported to be rare or absent.

Clozapine caused hyperthermia associated with influenza-like symptoms in 4 of 16 patients.— E. Guirguis *et al.*, *Curr. ther. Res.*, 1977, *21*, 707.

EFFECTS ON BLOOD. During a 2-month period in Finland there were 18 reports of severe blood disorders (9 fatal) associated with clozapine. Agranulocytosis accounted for 8 of the deaths and leukaemia probably for the ninth. The sale and use of clozapine was stopped in Finland until further notice.— J. Idänpään-Heikkilä *et al.* (letter), *Lancet*, 1975, *2*, 611. See also *idem*, *Eur. J. clin. Pharmac.*, 1977, *11*, 193. Experience in 22 other countries outside Finland where clozapine had been marketed indicated an incidence of agranulocytosis of 0.3 per 1000 compared with an incidence almost 20 times as high in Finland and with 0.1 to 0.8 per 1000 for other tricyclic neuroleptics. A local factor or factors were possibly responsible for the higher incidence in Finland.— R. W. Griffith and K. Saameli, *Sandoz, Switz.* (letter), *Lancet*, 1975, *2*, 657. It was suggested that the frequency of agranulocytosis associated with clozapine was no higher than with phenothiazines. Weekly blood counts during the first 4 months of treatment would detect incipient granulocytopenia, and so reduce the mortality rate.— B. Anderman and R. W. Griffith, *Sandoz, Switz.*, *Eur. J. clin. Pharmac.*, 1977, *11*, 199.

Precautions

For general precautions to be observed with hypnotics, sedatives, and neuroleptics, see p.708.

Clozapine has antimuscarinic actions and its use should be avoided in patients with closed-angle glaucoma; care is also necessary in patients with ileus or prostatic hypertrophy. Clozapine should be given with caution in patients with epilepsy.

Clozapine is contra-indicated in patients with pre-existing bone marrow depression; patients receiving clozapine therapy require regular blood monitoring.

Uses and Administration

Clozapine is a neuroleptic agent used in the management of schizophrenia. Because of the risk of agranulocytosis it is generally reserved for patients who do not respond satisfactorily to other neuroleptic agents, or in whom there is a risk of provoking or exacerbating tardive dyskinesia with conventional neuroleptic therapy. It is given by mouth or intramuscular injection in usual doses of 25 to 200 mg daily; doses of up to 600 mg daily have been given in severe cases.

Patients receiving clozapine should undergo regular monitoring of white cell counts.

Proprietary Names and Manufacturers

Leponex *(Sandoz, Denm.; Sandoz, S.Afr.; Sandoz, Spain; Wander, Switz.)*.

7033-w

Cyamemazine *(rINN).*

Cyamepromazine; RP-7204. 10-(3-Dimethylamino-2-methylpropyl)phenothiazine-2-carbonitrile.

$C_{19}H_{21}N_3S$=323.5.

CAS — 3546-03-0.

Cyamemazine is a phenothiazine with general properties similar to those of the other phenothiazines (p.706). It has been used in the management of neuropsychiatric disorders and as an adjunct in the treatment of psychoses. The usual dose is 200 to 300 mg daily, with a range of 50 to 600 mg daily; the recommended daily dosage is given in 2 portions with the larger amount at night. It may also be given by intramuscular injection in doses of 25 to 200 mg daily.

Cyamemazine should be given in reduced dosage to elderly patients; the parenteral route is not recommended for the elderly.

Proprietary Names and Manufacturers

Tercian *(Théraplix, Fr.)*.

4025-s

Cyclobarbitone *(BAN).*

Cyclobarbital *(rINN)*; Ethylhexabital; Hexemalum. 5-(Cyclohex-1-enyl)-5-ethylbarbituric acid.

$C_{12}H_{16}N_2O_3$=236.3.

CAS — 52-31-3.

NOTE. The name ciclobarbital has been applied to hexobarbitone.

Pharmacopoeias. In *Aust., Braz., Hung., It., Jug., Pol.,* and *Roum.*

STABILITY. Samples 4 years old showed more than 20% decomposition (bromometric titration) and cyclobarbitone tablets showed considerable loss in strength after 1 to 4 years' storage. The decomposition was in the cyclohexene ring and was accompanied by the formation of peroxides. Cyclobarbitone calcium and hexobarbitone did not decompose on storage.— S. Åhlander, *Svensk farm. Tidskr.*, 1956, *60*, 249.

4026-w

Cyclobarbitone Calcium *(BANM)*.

Cyclobarbital Calcium *(rINNM)*; Cyclobarbitalum Calcicum; Hexemalcalcium. Calcium 5-(cyclohex-1-enyl)-5-ethylbarbiturate.
$(C_{12}H_{15}N_2O_3)_2Ca$=510.6.

CAS — 5897-20-1.

Pharmacopoeias. In *Aust., Br., Cz., Egypt., Eur., Fr., Ger., Ind., Int., It., Neth., Nord.,* and *Swiss.*

A white or slightly yellowish, crystalline powder. Slightly **soluble** in water; very slightly soluble in alcohol; practically insoluble in chloroform and in ether. **Store** in airtight containers.

Dependence, Adverse Effects, Treatment, and Precautions

As for the barbiturates in general, p.706.

Absorption and Fate

Cyclobarbitone is rapidly absorbed after oral administration and metabolised in the liver. It is reported to have a half-life ranging from 8 to 17 hours. It is excreted mainly in urine as metabolites; about 2 to 7% of a dose is reported to be excreted unchanged.

In a crossover study of the pharmacokinetics of cyclobarbitone calcium in 6 healthy subjects, 2 tablet formulations and an aqueous solution were compared. After oral administration of a 300-mg dose of the tablets peak plasma concentrations were obtained in 20 to 180 minutes. Absorption was most rapid with the aqueous solution but, contrary to expectations, bioavailability was lowest. In 4 of the subjects the half-lives of 8 to 11 hours were sufficiently short for a hypnotic agent, but in the other 2 subjects the half-lives of 15 to 17 hours were too long for its rational use in the treatment of insomnia.— D. D. Breimer and M. A. C. M. Winten, *Eur. J. clin. Pharmac.*, 1976, *9*, 443. See also D. D. Breimer (letter), *J. pharm. Sci.*, 1975, *64*, 1576.

A ketonic oxidation product (corresponding to 3-oxocyclobarbitone) was detected in the urine of subjects given cyclobarbitone by mouth.— R. Bouche *et al.*, *J. pharm. Sci.*, 1978, *67*, 1019.

Uses and Administration

Cyclobarbitone is a barbiturate that has been used as a hypnotic and sedative. As a hypnotic it is usually given in doses of 100 to 400 mg at night.

Proprietary Preparations

Phanodorm *(Winthrop, UK). Tablets*, cyclobarbitone calcium 200 mg.

Proprietary Names and Manufacturers

Ami-nal *(Belg.)*; Cyclosedal *(Belg.)*; Fanodormo Calcico *(Igoda, Spain)*; Panodorm-Calcium *(Ital.)*; Phanodorm *(Denm.; Bayer, Ger.; Neth.; Swed.; Winthrop, UK)*; Phanodorme Calcium *(Belg.)*; Prodorm *(Norw.)*; Rapidal *(Medo, UK)*; Somnupan *(Merckle, Ger.)*.

The following names have been used for multi-ingredient preparations containing cyclobarbitone calcium— Cyclomet *(Woodward, UK)*; Evidorm *(Winthrop, UK)*.

12552-s

Delorazepam *(rINN)*.

Chlordesmethyldiazepam; Clordesmethyldiazepam. 7-Chloro-5-(2-chlorophenyl)-1,3-dihydro-2*H*-1,4-benzodiazepin-2-one.
$C_{15}H_{10}Cl_2N_2O$=305.2.

CAS — 2894-67-9.

Delorazepam is a derivative of diazepam (p.728) and has similar general properties. It has been used in the treatment of anxiety states and psychoneurotic disorders in doses of 0.5 to 2 mg given 2 or 3 times daily by mouth; it has also been given by intramuscular or intravenous injection.

Proprietary Names and Manufacturers
En *(Ravizza, Ital.)*.

7036-y

Diazepam *(BAN, USAN, rINN)*.

Diazepamum; LA-111; NSC-77518; Ro-5-2807; Wy-3467. 7-Chloro-1,3-dihydro-1-methyl-5-phenyl-2*H*-1,4-benzodiazepin-2-one.
$C_{16}H_{13}ClN_2O$=284.7.

CAS — 439-14-5.

Pharmacopoeias. In *Belg., Br., Braz., Chin., Cz., Egypt., Eur., Fr., Ind., Int., It., Jpn, Jug., Neth., Nord.,* and *U.S.* Also in *B.P. Vet.*

A white or yellow, odourless or almost odourless, crystalline powder.

The *B.P.* states that it is very slightly **soluble** in water, soluble in alcohol and freely soluble in chloroform; *U.S.P.* solubilities are 1 in 16 of alcohol; 1 in 2 of chloroform, and 1 in 39 of ether; practically insoluble in water. The *B.P.* injection has a pH of 6.2 to 7.0, and is sterilised by filtration; the *U.S.P.* injection has a pH between 6.2 and 6.9.

Store in airtight containers. Protect from light.

SORPTION. A review of drug interactions with medical plastics and other surfaces. Continuous intravenous infusion of diazepam requires admixture with intravenous fluids raising both the problem of incompatibility and the more important one that diazepam is substantially sorbed by plastics in the apparatus used for administration; in some reports only a small fraction of the drug remained in the infused solution. It seems clear that the use of polyvinyl chloride bags and cellulose propionate volume-control chambers is contra-indicated; polyvinyl chloride lines also seem to be unsuitable but it is largely a question of having to put up with these until more suitable tubing becomes available. Diazepam solutions are stable in glass, and lack of sorption to polyolefin semi-rigid containers also makes these suitable alternatives.— P. F. D'Arcy, *Drug Intell. & clin. Pharm.*, 1983, *17*, 726.

Reports and studies of the adsorption of diazepam in various intravenous administration apparatuses: J. MacKichan *et al.* (letter), *New Engl. J. Med.*, 1979, *301*, 332 (extensive sorption to plastic tubing); A. Smith and G. Bird, *J. clin. Hosp. Pharm.*, 1982, *7*, 181 (in polyethylene, polyvinyl chloride, and glass containers); J. K. Yliruusi *et al.*, *Am. J. Hosp. Pharm.*, 1982, *39*, 1018 (a similar study); F. M. Smith and N. O. Nuessle, *ibid.*, 1687 (stability in glass unit-dose syringes); E. A. Kowaluk *et al.*, *ibid.*, 1983, *40*, 118 (negligible sorption from a polyolefin infusion system); *idem* (factors affecting diazepam loss to polyvinyl chloride bags and various infusion sets); F. Mathot *et al.* (letter), *Am. J. Hosp. Pharm.*, 1983, *40*, 948 (minimal loss from a polypropylene syringe, polyethylene tubing and a teflon catheter); B. G. Hancock and C. D. Black, *ibid.*, 1985, *42*, 335 (comparison of polyethylene-lined and polyvinyl chloride administration sets).

Dependence

As for the benzodiazepines in general, p.706.

Adverse Effects

For the adverse effects of the benzodiazepines, see p.706.

There have been reports of an association between infant cleft lip and palate, and maternal use of diazepam, but other studies have found no significant association between congenital malformations and maternal ingestion of benzodiazepines. Administration of diazepam in late pregnancy has been associated with intoxication of the neonate.

Intravenous injections of diazepam may be painful and can cause thrombophlebitis.

ALLERGY. A 9-year-old boy developed slight wheezing 18 hours after an intravenous injection of diazepam 5 mg. After an intramuscular injection of diazepam 5 mg 3 days later he became cyanotic within an hour, with wheezing, increased respiratory-rate, and abnormal blood gases. This was considered to be an immediate allergic reaction.— M. Z. Blumberg and S. Young, *Pediatrics*, 1974, *54*, 811.

A 28-year-old woman with a history of allergy to various substances, including chlordiazepoxide, developed an allergic reaction after a 10-mg intramuscular dose of diazepam.— L. Milner, *Br. med. J.*, 1977, *1*, 144. A similar report.— R. H. Falk (letter), *ibid.*, 287. The solvent, Cremophor EL, might have caused the allergy.— D. Blatchley (letter), *ibid.* A suggestion that solubilisation with Cremophor EL might promote hypersensitivity reactions to previously safe drugs.— A. Padfield and J. Watkins (letter), *ibid.*, 575. Of 1500 patients given intravenous injections of diazepam in soya oil only one allergic reaction had been noted, and the cause had been doubtful.— O. von Dardel *et al.* (letter), *ibid.*, 773.

A report of complement-mediated reactions attributed to the Cremophor EL solvent in 2 patients given intravenous injections of diazepam.— M. S. Hüttel *et al.*, *Br. J. Anaesth.*, 1980, *52*, 77.

An acute (type 1) hypersensitivity reaction in a patient given diazepam intravenously appeared on subsequent skin testing to be due to the lipid emulsion used as a carrier. Hypersensitivity to this formulation (Diazemuls) does not appear to have been previously reported.— D. J. Deardon and G. L. A. Bird (letter), *Br. J. Anaesth.*, 1987, *59*, 391.

CYTOGENETIC EFFECTS. Chromosome analysis performed on peripheral blood of 20 healthy young adults before and after a single 12- to 20-mg intravenous dose of diazepam revealed no significant increase in chromosomal aberrations due to diazepam.— B. J. White *et al.*, *J. Am. med. Ass.*, 1974, *230*, 414.

A report of preliminary animal studies suggesting that diazepam may have a tumour-growth-promoting effect.— D. F. Horrobin *et al.* (letter), *Lancet*, 1979, *1*, 978. Severe criticism; the reported effects have not been confirmed in another laboratory.— J. Genest, *Clinical Research Institute of Montreal*, *ibid.*, 1306. Oxazepam was found to have no significant influence on the tumour growth, or the survival-time, of tumour-bearing *rats*.— A. Guaitani *et al.* (letter), *ibid.*, 1147. Results of a 2-year study on substantial numbers of *animals* do not support the suggestion that diazepam may either cause or promote tumour growth.— M. R. Jackson and P. A. Harris, *Roche* (letter), *ibid.*, 1981, *1*, 104. Evaluation of diazepam from data previously collected during a multicentre breast cancer screening programme, the Breast Cancer Detection Demonstration Project, failed to demonstrate a relation between diazepam use and breast cancer.— R. A. Kleinerman *et al.* (letter), *ibid.*, 1153. A case control study involving 1236 women with breast cancer and 728 controls with other malignancies also failed to find any evidence that diazepam increased the risk of breast cancer relative to other cancers.— D. W. Kaufman *et al.*, *ibid.*, 1982, *1*, 537. Comment.— D. F. Horrobin (letter), *ibid.*, *2*, 223.

EFFECTS ON THE BLOOD. Diazepam has been reported to cause agranulocytosis.— P. C. Vincent, *Drugs*, 1986, *31*, 52.

EFFECTS ON BODY TEMPERATURE. After a single dose of diazepam 10 mg by mouth in 11 subjects body temperature on exposure to cold fell to a mean of 36.93°, compared with 37.08° on exposure to the same environmental temperature (approximately 12°) without the drug. Exposure to cold was less uncomfortable when diazepam had been taken.— S. M. Martin, *J. clin. Pharmac.*, 1985, *25*, 611.

EFFECTS ON THE ENDOCRINE SYSTEM. Plasma-testosterone concentrations were significantly increased in men taking diazepam 10 to 20 mg daily for 2 weeks.— A. E. Argüelles and J. Rosner (letter), *Lancet*, 1975, *2*, 607.

EFFECTS ON THE LIVER. Raised liver-enzyme values in a patient receiving diazepam fell when the drug was discontinued and rose again on rechallenge. Liver biopsy revealed focal necrosis and intracellular cholestasis.— F. Tedesco and L. R. Mills, *Dig. Dis. Scis*, 1982, *27*, 470. See also H. Jick *et al.*, *J. clin. Pharmac.*, 1981, *21*, 359 (cholestatic jaundice).

EFFECTS ON THE SKIN. Analysis by the Boston Collaborative Drug Surveillance Program of data on 15 438 patients hospitalised between 1975 and 1982 detected 2 allergic skin reactions attributed to diazepam among 4707 recipients of the drug. A reaction-rate of 0.4 per 1000 recipients was calculated from these figures.— M. Bigby *et al.*, *J. Am. med. Ass.*, 1986, *256*, 3358.

PORPHYRIA. Studies in *animals* indicating that diazepam had no porphyrinogenic effect.— R. K. Parikh and M. R. Moore, *Br. J. Anaesth.*, 1978, *50*, 1099. Acute intermittent porphyria in a 62-year-old man with alcoholic cirrhosis associated with the administration of diazepam.— D. R. Stone and E. S. Munson (letter), *ibid.*, 1979, *51*, 809.

See also p.709.

PREGNANCY AND THE NEONATE. *Early pregnancy.* Analysis of 278 mothers of children with various malformations carried out at the Center for Disease Control, Atlanta, demonstrated a significant fourfold risk of cleft lip with or without cleft palate in infants whose mothers had taken diazepam during the first trimester of pregnancy.— M. J. Safra and G. P. Oakley, *Lancet*, 1975, *2*,

478. A similar analysis in Finland of 599 children with oral clefts compared with 590 controls produced a significant association between oral clefts and intake of benzodiazepines during the first trimester.— I. Saxén and L. Saxén (letter), *ibid.*, 498. Of 836 mothers of congenitally malformed infants 33 had used benzodiazepines during the first trimester of pregnancy, compared with 21 in 836 controls. The case: control incidence ratio of 1.57 was not significant.— G. Greenberg *et al.*, *Br. med. J.*, 1977, *2*, 853.

A case-control study based on data collected from the mothers of 3109 children with birth defects between March 1976 and April 1982 suggested that diazepam use during the first trimester of pregnancy does not increase the risk of oral cleft anomalies. A possible risk of inguinal hernia related to diazepam use requires further evaluation.— L. Rosenburg *et al.*, *New Engl. J. Med.*, 1983, *309*, 1282. Criticism of the design of the study.— S. S. Entman and W. K. Vaughan (letter), *ibid.*, 1984, *310*, 1121. Reply.— L. Rosenberg and A. A. Mitchell (letter), *ibid.*, 1122. Prospective data from 33 249 pregnant women, 854 of whom had taken diazepam during the first trimester, also did not support an association between the diazepam use and the development of oral clefts.— P. H. Shiono and J. L. Mills (letter), *New Engl. J. Med.*, 1984, *311*, 919.

A further report of abnormalities in children exposed to benzodiazepines *in utero*.— L. Laegreid *et al.* (letter), *Lancet*, 1987, *1*, 108. Comments.— R. M. Winter (letter), *ibid.*, 627; W. S. Barry and S. M. St Clair (letter), *ibid.*, 1436. See also p.709.

Late pregnancy and labour. In a study in 18 infants born to mothers who had received 30 mg or less of diazepam (low-dose) in the 15 hours before delivery, none had low Apgar scores attributable to diazepam, 1 had a rectal temperature below 35°, 2 were reluctant to feed, and 1 had hypotonia. By contrast, in 14 infants whose mothers had received more than 30 mg of diazepam (high-dose) in the 15 hours before delivery, 10 had low Apgar scores, 8 had a low rectal temperature, 10 needed tube-feeding, and 12 had hypotonia. In 1 low-dose infant and 7 high-dose infants subjected to cold stress, the metabolic response was less than in 6 control infants whose mothers had not received diazepam. Cord-blood concentrations of diazepam and desmethyldiazepam were generally higher than maternal values. In 2 high-dose infants concentrations of diazepam rose after delivery possibly due to release from body stores. In 5 high-dose infants, concentrations of desmethyldiazepam rose after delivery and in many cases scarcely fell after 7 days. Care was necessary when diazepam was given in pre-eclampsia.— J. E. Cree *et al.*, *Br. med. J.*, 1973, *4*, 251.

In view of the wide variation in metabolism and excretion of diazepam in the neonate doses higher than 10 to 20 mg were not recommended for the mother during labour. Competitive inhibition of the conjugation of bilirubin might lead to hyperbilirubinaemia.— J. Kanto *et al.* (letter), *Br. med. J.*, 1974, *1*, 641. In 93 infants born to mothers who received diazepam during labour, the mean serum bilirubin concentration was increased by 6.3 μg per mL at 48 hours of age and 7.2 μg per mL at 72 hours. This effect would probably only be of importance in small premature infants.— J. H. Drew and W. H. Kitchen, *J. Pediat.*, 1976, *89*, 657. The concentration of sodium benzoate in Valium injection was not considered high enough to cause neonatal hyperbilirubinaemia following administration of 10 to 20 mg diazepam (with 100 to 200 mg sodium benzoate contained in the solvent) by intramuscular injection to the mother during labour.— R. Stockmann *et al.*, *J. int. med. Res.*, 1978, *6*, 468.

Hypotonia, difficulty in sucking, and hypothermia characteristic of the floppy-infant syndrome occurred in a newborn infant whose mother had taken diazepam 2 mg thrice daily on and off for the last 3 months of pregnancy to a total dose of 110 mg. An additional dose of 10 mg had been given rectally at delivery. The infant improved as the high serum concentrations of diazepam (about 550 nmol per litre on day 12) and desmethyldiazepam (about 700 nmol per litre on day 12) fell. Neonatal disturbances had been observed in other children whose mothers had taken diazepam late in pregnancy.— C. Gillberg (letter), *Lancet*, 1977, *2*, 244. No such effect on 2 infants whose mother had taken large doses of diazepam throughout pregnancy and during labour.— K. Haram (letter), *ibid.*, 612. Criticism. Two similar cases (of the floppy-infant syndrome), one involving diazepam and nitrazepam and the other nitrazepam alone.— A. N. P. Speight (letter), *ibid.*, 878. The floppy infant syndrome had not occurred in 30 pregnancies where the mothers had received oxazepam in doses of up to 75 mg daily.— K. A. D. Drury *et al.* (letter), *ibid.*, 1126.

Comment on the hazards of diazepam in labour which include loss of the beat-to-beat variation of the foetal heart. This may reflect a loss of adaptive ability of the foetal heart and circulatory system, or possibly a depression of the cardiac reflex centres in the brain.— J. M. B. Burn (letter), *Br. med. J.*, 1978, *1*, 1216.
See also p.709.

THROMBO-EMBOLIC EFFECTS. Skin pallor occurred within half an hour and discoloration and oedema of the forearm and hand rapidly followed in an 11-month-old child after the accidental intra-arterial injection of diazepam into the brachial artery. Pallor of the legs followed by oedema and cyanosis of the legs occurred in a 2-day-old infant given diazepam by umbilical artery catheter.— J. D. M. Gould and S. Lingan, *Br. med. J.*, 1977, *2*, 298.

A report of the accidental intra-arterial injection of diazepam in 2 patients with suggestions for the management of such accidents. Experience suggested that the clinical signs of ischaemia and gangrene may not occur until days after the event.— M. Rees and J. Dormandy, *Br. med. J.*, 1980, *281*, 289.

A comparison of local venous reactions following intravenous injection of diazepam in 3 different formulations - as a solution in propylene glycol (Stesolid), as a solution in Cremophor EL (Stesolid MR), and as an emulsion in soya oil and water (Diazemuls). The incidence of pain on injection and of subsequent thrombophlebitis was greatest in those given the propylene glycol solution, occurring in 50 and 31 of 64 patients respectively. These figures compared with 25 and 6 of 66 patients given the injection in Cremophor EL and 1 and 4 of 67 given the diazepam emulsion. On the basis of these results the frequency of local vascular side-effects would appear to be significantly decreased by using diazepam formulated in a lipid emulsion.— A. S. Olesen and M. S. Hüttel, *Br. J. Anaesth.*, 1980, *52*, 609. See also M. A. K. Mattila *et al.*, *Br. J. Anaesth.*, 1981, *53*, 1265; D. W. Bullimore, *Clin. Ther.*, 1982, *4*, 367; N. L. Rosenbaum, *Br. dent. J.*, 1982, *153*, 192.

Treatment of Adverse Effects

For general guidelines, see p.708.

Precautions

For precautions to be observed with the benzodiazepines, see p.708.

INTERACTIONS. Drowsiness as a side-effect of diazepam or chlordiazepoxide, was less frequent in smokers than in non-smokers. Nicotine, a hepatic enzyme inducer, might increase the metabolism of diazepam and chlordiazepoxide.—Report from the Boston Collaborative Drug Surveillance Program, *New Engl. J. Med.*, 1973, *288*, 277. No difference between smokers and non-smokers in plasma elimination half-lives or steady-state concentrations of diazepam.— U. Klotz *et al.*, *J. clin. Invest.*, 1975, *55*, 347. Tobacco smoking has no significant effect on the metabolism of chlordiazepoxide and therefore the smaller incidence of excessive sedation in smokers cannot be explained in terms of increased metabolism.— P. V. Desmond *et al.* (letter), *New Engl. J. Med.*, 1979, *300*, 199. A contrary study suggesting that smoking raised diazepam clearance, particularly among younger subjects.— D. J. Greenblatt *et al.*, *Clin. Pharmac. Ther.*, 1980, *27*, 301. See also R. W. Downing and K. Rickels, *Acta psychiat. scand.*, 1981, *64*, 398 (interaction of benzodiazepines, smoking, and coffee or tea drinking).

In groups of 10 or 12 patients, the absorption of a 10-mg oral dose of diazepam was significantly hastened when metoclopramide 10 mg was given intravenously at the same time; absorption was significantly reduced when morphine 10 mg was given intramuscularly 1 hour earlier; pethidine 100 mg intramuscularly 1 hour earlier had a similar, but lesser, effect; absorption was significantly reduced by atropine 600 μg intravenously given at the same time and, to a lesser degree, by atropine 600 μg intramuscularly.— J. A. S. Gamble *et al.*, *Br. J. Anaesth.*, 1976, *48*, 1181.

Alcohol. Reviews and comments on interactions between alcohol and diazepam: E. M. Sellers and M. R. Holloway, *Clin. Pharmacokinet.*, 1978, *3*, 440; M. Linnoila *et al.*, *Drugs*, 1979, *18*, 299.

In a double-blind crossover study in 40 healthy students diazepam 5 mg thrice daily increased choice reaction and attention and slightly increased coordination, but subjects drove faster and made more mistakes. When alcohol 500 mg per kg body-weight was added reaction was reduced, but subjects drove more slowly and made fewer mistakes.— M. Linnoila *et al.*, *Br. J. clin. Pharmac.*, 1974, *1*, 176P. A further study suggested that the impairment of skills associated with driving was due to an interaction between alcohol and diazepam itself, rather than its metabolites.— E. S. Palva and M. Linnoila, *Eur. J. clin. Pharmac.*, 1978, *13*, 345.

Conflicting views on the effect of alcohol on diazepam: S. L. Hayes *et al.*, *New Engl. J. Med.*, 1977, *296*, 186; R. Bernstein and J. S. Holcenberg (letter), *ibid.*, 1006; W. E. Boden (letter), *ibid;* S. L. Hayes *et al.* (letter), *ibid;* S. M. MacLeod *et al.*, *Eur. J. clin. Pharmac.*, 1977, *11*, 345; D. J. Greenblatt *et al.*, *Psychopharmacology*, 1978, *57*, 199; U. Laisi *et al.*, *Eur. J. clin. Pharmac.*, 1979, *16*, 263; E. M. Sellers *et al.*, *Clin. Pharmac. Ther.*, 1980, *27*, 286; *idem*, *28*, 638; E. H. Ellinwood *et al.*, *Clin. Pharmac. Ther.*, 1981, *30*, 534; E. M. Sellers and U. Busto, *J. clin. Psychopharmacol.*, 1982, *4*, 249; K. Aranko *et al.*, *Eur. J. clin. Pharmac.*, 1985, *28*, 559.

Antacids. In a study in 4 groups of 50 women undergoing minor gynaecological surgery the sedative effect of a single 10-mg oral dose of diazepam appeared to be enhanced by Aluminium Hydroxide Mixture 40 mL or 0.3M sodium citrate 30 mL, and reduced by Magnesium Trisilicate Mixture 30 mL. In 67 patients in whom plasma-diazepam concentrations were measured Aluminium Hydroxide Mixture appeared to promote early absorption.— S. G. Nair *et al.*, *Br. J. Anaesth.*, 1976, *48*, 1175.

Evidence to suggest that co-administration of diazepam with antacids reduces the rate of absorption of diazepam but does not reduce the extent of absorption.— D. J. Greenblatt *et al.*, *Clin. Pharmac. Ther.*, 1978, *24*, 600.

Anticoagulants. Reduced plasma binding of diazepam and desmethyldiazepam and increases in the free concentrations without changes in the total blood or plasma concentrations occurred immediately following heparin intravenously. Further studies were needed to assess the clinical relevance.— P. A. Routledge *et al.*, *Clin. Pharmac. Ther.*, 1980, *27*, 528.

Anti-epileptics. Valproic acid displaces diazepam from binding and decreases its metabolism; caution should be exercised when diazepam is given intravenously to patients receiving valproic acid.— *Med. Lett.*, 1983, *25*, 81. See also S. Dhillon and A. Richens, *Br. J. clin. Pharmac.*, 1981, *12*, 841.

Beta-blockers. The elimination half-life of single intravenous doses of diazepam was significantly prolonged, and clearance reduced, in patients receiving a propranolol regimen compared with values in the same patients when not receiving the beta-blocker. Propranolol did not affect the elimination half-life or clearance of intravenous lorazepam or alprazolam by mouth, although there was some evidence for a slower rate of absorption of alprazolam after propranolol. The clinical significance of the propranolol-diazepam interaction, if any, is unknown.— H. R. Ochs *et al.*, *Clin. Pharmac. Ther.*, 1984, *36*, 451. A study in 12 healthy subjects indicated that the metabolism of diazepam was inhibited by co-administration of the lipophilic beta-blockers propranolol and metoprolol, but not by the hydrophilic non-metabolised beta-blocker atenolol.— *Br. J. clin. Pharmac.*, 1984, *17*, 69S.

Cimetidine. Cimetidine has been reported to affect the hepatic metabolism of a wide range of drugs, and a number of studies have shown an alteration in the pharmacokinetics of benzodiazepines given concurrently. Klotz and Reimann (*New. Engl. J. Med.*, 1980, *302*, 1012) reported a reduced plasma clearance and increased elimination half-life of intravenous diazepam given after treatment for 1 day with cimetidine; similarly, cimetidine pretreatment has been reported to increase the elimination half-life and plasma concentration of diazepam by mouth (P. Gough *et al.*, *Br. J. clin. Pharmac.*, 1982, *14*, 739; J.W. Dundee, *ibid.*, 618P); the latter study suggested that this effect was more marked when diazepam was given as tablets rather than capsules.

Similar impairment of metabolism by cimetidine has been reported for chlordiazepoxide (P.V. Desmond *et al.*, *Ann. intern. Med.*, 1980, *93*, 266); alprazolam and triazolam (D.R. Abernethy *et al.*, *Psychopharmacology*, 1983, *80*, 275; S. Pourbaix *et al.*, *Int. J. clin. Pharmac. Ther. Toxic.*, 1985, *23*, 447); and midazolam (U. Klotz *et al.*, *Clin. Pharmac. Ther.*, 1985, *38*, 652). Cimetidine has been reported not to have a significant effect on the pharmacokinetics of oxazepam and lorazepam (D.J. Greenblatt *et al.*, *J. clin. Pharmac.*, 1984, *24*, 187) although other reports have purported to show a significant effect on both benzodiazepines by cimetidine (W.A.W. McGowan and J.W. Dundee, *Br. J. clin. Pharmac.*, 1982, *14*, 207; A.M. Lam and J.A. Parkin, *Can. Anaesth. Soc. J.*, 1981, *28*, 450). Lack of interaction has also been reported for temazepam (D.J. Greenblatt *et al.*, *J. pharm. Sci.*, 1984, *73*, 399). Benzodiazepines can be crudely divided into those metabolised primarily by oxidation, such as diazepam and chlordiazepoxide, and those metabolised primarily by

glucuronidation, such as temazepam, oxazepam, and lorazepam: it would appear that cimetidine is unlikely significantly to impair the metabolism of those benzodiazepines primarily metabolised by glucuronidation, whereas those cleared primarily by oxidation may undergo inhibition of metabolism by cimetidine (G.J. Dobb *et al.*, *Med. J. Aust.*, 1986, *145*, 58). However, it should be noted that cimetidine has also been reported to impair the clearance of nitrazepam (H.R. Ochs *et al.*, *Clin. Pharmac. Ther.*, 1983, *34*, 227), a drug stated to be metabolised primarily by nitroreduction.
The clinical significance of such interactions remains dubious. Greenblatt *et al.*, (*New Engl. J. Med.*, 1984, *310*, 1639) found that while standard doses of cimetidine given to patients on long-term diazepam therapy resulted in a marked increase in plasma concentrations of diazepam there was no evidence of increased daytime sedation, fatigue, or drowsiness. However, it was noted that the interaction might be of more significance in the elderly, in patients who had recently begun diazepam therapy and who had had less time to develop tolerance, and in those already receiving high doses of diazepam. A lack of clinically significant effects was also reported by Gough *et al.* (1982) for diazepam; Klotz *et al.* (*Clin. Pharmac. Ther.*, 1985, *38*, 652) likewise failed to note increased reaction times or sedation in patients given midazolam and cimetidine, despite a significant increase in midazolam steady-state plasma concentration.

Digoxin. For the effects of diazepam on digoxin pharmacokinetics see Digoxin, p.828.

Disulfiram. A study suggesting that concurrent administration of disulfiram inhibits chlordiazepoxide biotransformation. It is thought that diazepam disposition will be similarly affected, but that benzodiazepines metabolised by conjugation, such as oxazepam, may be less susceptible to inhibition of biotransformation.— E. M. Sellers *et al.*, *Clin. Pharmac. Ther.*, 1977, *21*, 117.

See also under Disulfiram, p.1566.

Levodopa. For reference to the effects of benzodiazepines on levodopa see Levodopa, p.1017.

Omeprazole. Following repeated daily administration of omeprazole to 8 healthy subjects the mean elimination half-life of diazepam was more than doubled, and the clearance decreased by 54%.— R. Gugler and J. C. Jensen (letter), *Lancet*, 1984, *1*, 969.

Oral contraceptives. A study demonstrating that long-term use of low-dose oestrogen oral contraceptives significantly impaired clearance of intravenous diazepam and prolonged its elimination half-life. Patients receiving both diazepam and oral contraceptives should be monitored for the possibility of increased clinical effects.— D. R. Abernethy, *New Engl. J. Med.*, 1982, *306*, 791. Results suggesting that in fact psychomotor impairment due to oral diazepam was greater during the menstrual pause than during the 21-day oral contraceptive cycle, perhaps due to an effect of oral contraceptives on diazepam absorption.— E. H. Ellinwood *et al.*, *Clin. Pharmac. Ther.*, 1984, *35*, 360. A study of the pharmacokinetics and clinical effects of alprazolam, lorazepam, temazepam, and triazolam in women using oral contraceptives and in controls. Results showed that women taking oral contraceptives appeared to be more sensitive to psychomotor impairment following single oral doses of alprazolam, lorazepam, and triazolam; the effects of temazepam were minimal in both groups. However, differences between the groups in terms of sedative or amnestic effect could not be established with any certainty. Differences in pharmacokinetics did not seem to explain the differences in psychomotor effects of benzodiazepines in women taking oral contraceptives.— P. D. Kroboth *et al.*, *ibid.*, 1985, *38*, 525.
Oral contraceptives appear to inhibit the metabolism of some benzodiazepines, such as chlordiazepoxide and diazepam, and increase the metabolism of others such as lorazepam and oxazepam. One would theoretically expect decreased metabolism of benzodiazepines that undergo oxidative metabolism in the liver, including alprazolam, halazepam, prazepam, clorazepate, and flurazepam. Conversely one might expect increased metabolism of those, like temazepam, that undergo glucuronide conjugation.— *Drug Interact. News.*, 1982, *2*, 41.

Penicillamine. Exacerbation of intravenous diazepam-induced phlebitis by oral penicillamine.— R. D. Brandstetter *et al.*, *Br. med. J.*, 1981, *283*, 525.

Ranitidine. In contrast to the results with cimetidine, most studies examining the effects of ranitidine on benzodiazepine metabolism have failed to show any significant effect; Klotz *et al.* (*Eur. J. clin. Pharmac.*, 1983, *24*, 357) found that the absorption of oral diazepam appeared to be slightly diminished by ranitidine but that there was no significant effect on diazepam metabolism, and similar results were reported by Abernethy *et al.* (*Clin. Pharmac. Ther.*, 1984, *35*, 188) and Fee *et al.* (*Br. J. clin. Pharmac.*, 1984, *17*, 617P).
Klotz *et al.* also reported a lack of any significant effect of ranitidine on the steady-state plasma concentration of midazolam (*Clin. Pharmac. Ther.*, 1985, *38*, 652); however, a number of other studies have reported that ranitidine and midazolam may interact in a clinically significant fashion. Elwood *et al.* (*Br. J. clin. Pharmac.*, 1983, *15*, 743) found that pretreatment for 24 hours with ranitidine resulted in increased bioavailability of midazolam, with higher plasma concentrations of the benzodiazepine for 6 hours after the dose; these pharmacokinetic changes were accompanied by an increased soporific effect. Similarly, Wilson *et al.* (*Br. J. Anaesth.*, 1986, *58*, 483) found that ranitidine resulted in a greater degree of drowsiness after single premedicant doses of midazolam than placebo; however, ranitidine did not affect the degree of drowsiness after temazepam.

Tuberculostatics. Prolongation of diazepam half-life by *isoniazid* and marked reduction of diazepam half-life by *rifampicin*.— H. R. Ochs *et al.*, *Clin. Pharmac. Ther.*, 1981, *29*, 671.

Xanthines. Deep sedation induced by intravenous injections of diazepam in patients undergoing surgical or diagnostic procedures was rapidly reversed by injection of aminophylline. Aminophylline 60 mg was given intravenously to 9 patients, repeated after 5 minutes in those not fully alert; a further 9 patients received placebo. After 20 minutes all but one of those given aminophylline were able to conduct a conversation, while none of the controls had regained this ability. The interaction seems important and offers the prospect that aminophylline in comparatively low doses could be used as an antagonist of diazepam.— S. B. Arvidsson (letter), *Lancet*, 1982, *2*, 1467. Aminophylline 2 mg per kg body-weight did not completely antagonise the sedative effect of diazepam in a healthy subject. After the injection of aminophylline the subject felt almost as alert as before diazepam administration and performance improved but did not reach baseline in tests of psychomotor function. About 20 minutes after injection of aminophylline the sedation and impaired performance returned and persisted until about 4 hours after administration of diazepam. This pattern of events corresponds well with the differing half-lives of the 2 drugs.— G. Kleindienst and P. Usinger (letter), *ibid.*, 1984, *1*, 113. Evidence that aminophylline antagonises diazepam sedation by blocking adenosine receptors.— D. Niemand *et al.* (letter), *ibid.*, 463.

A similar antagonism of diazepam-induced psychomotor impairment by infusion of aminophylline.— S. A. Henauer *et al.*, *Eur. J. clin. Pharmac.*, 1983, *25*, 743.

An investigation of the interaction between diazepam and caffeine.— M. M. Ghoneim *et al.*, *J. clin. Psychopharmacol.*, 1986, *6*, 75.

INTERFERENCE WITH DIAGNOSTIC TESTS. A number of drugs, including diazepam, can inhibit binding of thyroxine and liothyronine to their binding proteins, resulting in erroneously abnormal values from thyroid function tests.— I. Ramsay, *Postgrad. med. J.*, 1985, *61*, 375.

PREGNANCY AND THE NEONATE. See under Adverse Effects, above, and Absorption and Fate, and Uses and Administration, below.

Absorption and Fate

Diazepam is readily and completely absorbed from the gastro-intestinal tract, peak plasma concentrations occurring within about 30 to 90 minutes of oral administration. Absorption is erratic following intramuscular administration and lower peak plasma concentrations may be obtained compared with those following oral administration. Diazepam crosses the blood-brain barrier and is highly lipid soluble; these properties qualify it for intravenous use in short-term anaesthetic procedures, since it acts promptly on the brain, and its initial effects decrease rapidly as it is redistributed into fat depots and tissues.
Diazepam has a biphasic half-life with an initial rapid distribution phase followed by a prolonged terminal elimination phase of 1 or 2 days; its action is further prolonged by the even longer half-life of 2 to 5 days of its principal active metabolite, desmethyldiazepam (nordazepam), the relative proportion of which increases in the body on long-term administration. No simple correlation has been found between plasma concentrations of diazepam and its metabolites, and their therapeutic effect.
Diazepam is extensively metabolised in the liver and, in addition to desmethyldiazepam, its active metabolites include oxazepam, and temazepam. It is excreted in the urine, mainly in the form of its metabolites, either free or in conjugated form. Diazepam is very extensively bound to plasma proteins.
The plasma half-life of diazepam is prolonged in neonates, in the elderly, and in patients with kidney or liver disease. In addition to crossing the blood-brain barrier, diazepam and its metabolites also cross the placental barrier and are excreted in breast milk.

A detailed account of the clinical pharmacokinetics of diazepam.— M. Mandelli *et al.*, *Clin. Pharmacokinet.*, 1978, *3*, 72.

ABSORPTION AND PLASMA CONCENTRATIONS. In a double-blind study 14 of 29 patients admitted to hospital for acute anxiety were treated with diazepam 20 mg daily for at least 5 days. The minimal effective steady-state plasma concentration was found to be about 400 ng per mL and the degree of diazepam effect was directly proportional to plasma concentrations and reciprocal clearance values of diazepam and its metabolite desmethyldiazepam.— H. H. Dasberg *et al.*, *Clin. Pharmac. Ther.*, 1974, *15*, 473.

Mean peak serum-diazepam concentrations in 6 healthy subjects given single doses of diazepam 20 mg intravenously, intramuscularly, and by mouth were 1600, 290, and 490 ng per mL respectively, 15, 60, and 30 minutes after administration. Clinical effects were related to serum concentrations. Significant amounts of the metabolite, desmethyldiazepam, were not produced.— L. Hillestad *et al.*, *Clin. Pharmac. Ther.*, 1974, *16*, 479. Studies in 7 healthy subjects showed cumulation in the serum of diazepam and desmethyldiazepam when diazepam was given daily by mouth for up to 2 weeks. The mean biological half-life of diazepam in 3 subjects was 54 hours.— L. Hillestad *et al.*, *ibid.*, 485.

In 4 subjects given a single 5 mg dose of diazepam, peak plasma concentrations occurred between 0.5 and 1.5 hours after administration and ranged from 64 to 160 ng per mL.— R. C. Bourne *et al.*, *Br. J. Pharmac.*, 1978, *63*, 371P.

In a study of 36 patients who had received diazepam 2 to 30 mg daily for periods from one month to 10 years, plasma-diazepam concentrations were directly related to dose and inversely related to age. Most of the patients were also receiving other drugs. There was a close association between the plasma concentrations of diazepam and its metabolite desmethyldiazepam and both concentrations were independent of the duration of therapy. Plasma-diazepam concentration ranges were 0.02 to 1.01 μg per mL, and plasma-desmethyldiazepam concentration ranges were 0.055 to 1.765 μg per mL.— D. M. Rutherford *et al.*, *Br. J. clin. Pharmac.*, 1978, *6*, 69.

Nine patients requiring artificial ventilation were given diazepam 10 mg intravenously every 4 hours for up to 22 days; their plasma-diazepam concentrations rose over the first 6 days and reached a mean plateau value of 700 ng per mL in 8 to 10 days. The concentration of the metabolite desmethyldiazepam rose progressively throughout administration. Similar results occurred in 3 patients given 5-mg doses, with a mean plateau value of 400 ng per mL. When diazepam was discontinued plasma concentrations fell with a half-life of 2 to 4 days for diazepam and 4 to 8 days for the metabolite.— J. A. S. Gamble *et al.*, *Br. J. Anaesth.*, 1976, *48*, 1087.

Concentrations of diazepam and desmethyldiazepam in the plasma during long-term diazepam therapy.— D. J. Greenblatt *et al.*, *Br. J. clin. Pharmac.*, 1981, *11*, 35.

A study of the pharmacokinetics of rectal diazepam. In 6 subjects given diazepam 10 mg by mouth or as a solution (Valium injection) by rectum, mean bioavailability was 76 and 81% respectively compared with the same dose by intravenous injection. Mean peak serum concentrations were 331 and 309 ng per mL respectively, achieved after 48 and 37 minutes. Three patients were also given diazepam 20 mg as rectal solution and in these peak serum concentrations were between 335 and 510 ng per mL but were achieved more slowly than with the lower dose, after 1 to 2 hours. In a further study, pharmacokinetics of diazepam 10 mg formulated as a commercially-available suppository were compared with the same dose in a macrogol suppository basis. Mean peak serum concentrations of 131 ng per mL were obtained only after 185 minutes with the commercial suppository whereas the macrogol suppository gave a mean peak of 212 ng per mL after 75 minutes. Bioavailability from the 2 suppositories was 70 and 67% respectively and was not as great as from rectal solution. In view of the peak concentrations achieved and the delay in achieving them it is uncertain whether the rectal route would be a useful alternative to intravenous administration in the emergency management of adult patients, as distinct from children.— S. Dhillon *et al.*, *Br. J. clin. Pharmac.*, 1982, *13*, 427. In a study involving 13 children, administration of diazepam as a rectal solution to 9, in doses of 200 to 700 µg per kg body-weight, produced peak serum concentrations within 30 minutes in all but one case. In contrast, doses of 300 to 600 µg per kg as suppositories resulted in peaks only after 60 to 120 minutes or more in another group of 9 children. Although the mean dose was higher in the group given suppositories, mean serum concentration 10 minutes after administration was higher in the group given the rectal solution. Because of the slow rate of absorption currently available suppositories are unsatisfactory for use in an emergency, but the use of a rectal solution is a realistic alternative to intravenous administration in treating seizures in children.— S. Dhillon *et al.*, *Archs Dis. Childh.*, 1982, *57*, 264. See also H. Sonander *et al.*, *Br. J. Anaesth.*, 1985, *57*, 578.

In a crossover study in 8 subjects plasma-diazepam concentrations were significantly higher when diazepam was injected intravenously as a solution (Valium) than when injected in an emulsion formulation (Diazemuls); mean plasma concentrations 15 minutes after injection were 514 ng per mL after the solution and 380 ng per mL after the emulsion. Clinical effects may be less pronounced after injection of diazepam in the emulsion formulation.— J. P. H. Fee *et al.* (letter), *Lancet*, 1984, *2*, 813. Contrary results from a further study in 8 healthy subjects. There was no significant difference in mean plasma concentrations following the intravenous injection of diazepam as Valium or Diazemuls.— H. C. Naylor and A. N. Burlingham (letter), *ibid.*, 1985, *1*, 518.

BILIARY EXCRETION. In a study in 4 patients, who had undergone biliary surgery, biliary excretion of diazepam was insufficient to account for an enterohepatic circulation of the drug.— P. W. Eustace *et al.*, *Br. J. Anaesth.*, 1975, *47*, 983.

PLASMA PROTEIN BINDING. A study in which the amount of diazepam estimated as being bound to plasma proteins was 98%.— H. G. Giles (letter), *Br. J. clin. Pharmac.*, 1977, *4*, 711.

A study of the protein binding of diazepam and desmethyldiazepam in 62 healthy subjects. The mean free fractions for the drug and its metabolite were 1.48% and 2.97% respectively. Diazepam binding was significantly reduced by age, whereas sex had little or no effect; however, even taking into account variations due to age and plasma albumin there was considerable variation between subjects in the degree of binding, with the free fraction of diazepam ranging from 0.85% to 2.30%. The plasma albumin concentration, which decreased with age, was the primary determinant of desmethyldiazepam binding. The amount of unbound and active desmethyldiazepam present for a given total concentration is consistently greater than that for diazepam at the same total concentration, and this differential binding complicates attempts to relate plasma concentrations of diazepam and its active metabolites to their clinical effects.— M. D. Allen and D. J. Greenblatt, *J. clin. Pharmac.*, 1981, *21*, 219.

The percentage of diazepam unbound in 6 patients in need of liver transplantation ranged from 2.4% to 10.9%, with a mean of 5.1%; in 3 controls, the percentage unbound was 1.1%. Following orthotopic liver transplantation the mean percentage unbound improved significantly to 2.4% but did not reach control values despite normal albumin concentrations.— M. L. Huang *et al.*, *Clin. Pharmac. Ther.*, 1984, *35*, 247.

See also under Pregnancy and the Neonate, below.

PREGNANCY AND THE NEONATE. Clinical pharmacokinetics of benzodiazepines in neonates and infants: age-related differences and therapeutic implications.— P. L. Morselli *et al.*, *Clin. Pharmacokinet.*, 1980, *5*, 485.

Diffusion across the placenta. Diazepam 5 mg labelled with carbon-14 was given intramuscularly to 8 healthy pregnant women about to undergo abortions. The 12- to 16-week-old foetuses were removed at 1, 2, or 6 hours after injection. Concentrations in the cord blood were twice those of the maternal blood. The highest concentrations at 1 hour were: cord blood, 47.5 ng per mL; placenta, 39 ng per g; foetal liver, 31 ng per g; foetal brain, 29 ng per g. Low enzyme activity was detected in the liver which was capable of metabolising about 3% of added diazepam.— J. Idänpään-Heikkilä *et al.*, *Clin. Pharmac. Ther.*, 1971, *12*, 293.

Studies of the concentrations of diazepam and its metabolites (desmethyldiazepam, oxazepam, and its glucuronide) in the plasma of 5 infants whose mothers had received 10 to 15 mg of diazepam daily for 6 to 21 days before delivery indicated that the metabolism and excretion of diazepam in the newborn was subject to wide variation; concentrations might be high enough to be active for 10 days.— J. Kanto *et al.* (letter), *Br. med. J.*, 1974, *1*, 641.

In vitro studies indicated that foetal liver microsomes could metabolise diazepam from the 13th week of gestation, forming desmethyldiazepam and *N*-methyloxazepam. It was suggested that metabolites might accumulate in the foetal liver, as the placenta would be less permeable to them than to diazepam.— E. Ackermann and K. Richter, *Eur. J. clin. Pharmac.*, 1977, *11*, 43.

Excretion in breast milk. After 4 days' treatment with diazepam, 10 mg thrice daily given for 6 days to 3 nursing mothers immediately after childbirth, concentrations of 491 ng per mL were found in the mothers' plasma, 51 ng per mL in the milk, and 172 ng per mL in the children's plasma; concentrations of the metabolite, *N*-desmethyldiazepam were 340 ng, 28 ng, and 243 ng per mL respectively. On the 6th day concentrations of diazepam and *N*-desmethyldiazepam had increased in the mothers' plasma to 601 ng and 483 ng per mL and in the milk to 78 ng and 52 ng per mL, but had decreased in the children to 74 ng and 31 ng per mL. Because of possible competition for conjugation causing hyperbilirubinaemia, babies should not be breast fed if the mother was receiving diazepam.— R. Erkkola and J. Kanto (letter), *Lancet*, 1972, *1*, 1235. A similar study. Diazepam 10 mg daily may safely be given to a mother who is breast-feeding, but if large doses are needed breast-feeding should be discontinued.— R. Brandt, *Arzneimittel-Forsch.*, 1976, *26*, 454.

Plasma protein binding. The free fraction of diazepam was elevated in 54 women in the second and third trimesters of pregnancy compared with 15 healthy non-pregnant controls, and seemed to have a linear relationship with the stage of gestation. Diazepam binding in umbilical cord blood from 15 neonates was similar to that in the mother.— J. N. Lee *et al.*, *Br. J. clin. Pharmac.*, 1982, *14*, 551.

Studies indicating that the percentage of unbound diazepam is greater in maternal than in foetal plasma and that this may be related to higher concetrations of free fatty acids in maternal blood: W. Kuhnz and H. Nau, *Clin. Pharmac. Ther.*, 1983, *34*, 220; M. J. Ridd *et al.*, *Eur. J. clin. Pharmac.*, 1983, *24*, 595. The free fractions of diazepam and desmethyldiazepam were lower in foetal cord serum than in maternal serum but subsequently rose sharply in all the infants, paralleling a rise in neonatal plasma concentrations of free fatty acids, and remained above foetal values for up to 1 week. The results suggest strongly that displacement of diazepam and its metabolite from their binding sites by free fatty acids was responsible for the effect which may account for the adverse effects of diazepam observed in some neonates.— H. Nau *et al.*, *Br. J. clin. Pharmac.*, 1984, *17*, 92.

Uses and Administration

Diazepam is a benzodiazepine with anticonvulsant, anxiolytic, sedative, muscle relaxant, and amnestic properties. It is used in the treatment of anxiety and tension states, as a sedative and premedicant, in the control of muscle spasm, as in tetanus, and in the management of alcohol withdrawal symptoms.

It is of value in patients undergoing minor surgical procedures, endoscopy, and cardioversion. Diazepam may be beneficial in the treatment of some patients with epilepsy and it is the recommended treatment, when given by slow intravenous injection, for the control of status epilepticus. Diazepam is used in dentistry either to calm the patient or it is given parenterally to sedate the patient during the dental procedure.

The usual dose by mouth for mild anxiety states is 2 mg three times daily increasing in severe states to 15 to 30 mg daily in divided doses. It has been suggested that the prolonged duration of action of diazepam and its major metabolite, desmethyldiazepam, may qualify it for a 24-hour anxiolytic regimen given as a single dose at night. In muscle spasm 2 to 15 mg may be given daily in divided doses increased in severe spastic disorders, such as cerebral palsy, to up to 60 mg daily.

Diazepam may also be given rectally as suppositories or rectal solution in doses similar to those by mouth.

Diazepam is also given by deep intramuscular or slow intravenous injection; it is advisable to keep the patient in the supine position for at least an hour after administration. Intravenous injection should be carried out slowly at a recommended rate of no more than 1 mL of a 0.5% solution (5 mg) per minute. Solutions for intravenous infusion may be prepared by adding not more than 8 mL (40 mg) of diazepam as a 0.5% solution to 500 mL of sodium chloride injection or glucose injection; such solutions should be freshly prepared and used within 6 hours. Absorption following intramuscular injection is erratic and provides lower blood concentrations than those following oral administration.

In severe anxiety or acute muscle spasm diazepam 10 mg may be given intramuscularly or intravenously and repeated after 4 hours. Patients with tetanus may be given 100 to 300 µg per kg body-weight intravenously and repeated every 1 to 4 hours; alternatively, a continuous infusion of 3 to 10 mg per kg every 24 hours may be used or similar doses may be given by nasoduodenal tube. Considerably higher doses have also been used for tetanus. In status epilepticus 150 to 250 µg per kg is given by intramuscular or intravenous injection and repeated if required after 30 to 60 minutes. Once the patient is controlled recurrence of seizures may be prevented with intravenous phenytoin sodium or by a slow infusion (maximum total of 3 mg per kg over 24 hours) of diazepam. Facilities for respiratory assistance must be available. The usual dose in minor surgical procedures and dentistry is 200 µg per kg by injection adjusted to the patient's requirements.

A suggested sedative dose for children is 40 to 200 µg per kg body-weight up to 3 or 4 times daily. Dosage recommendations are not generally given for infants since they may be unable to metabolise diazepam, but a parenteral dose of 40 to 200 µg per kg given once only has been used. A suggested parenteral regimen for children with status epilepticus or severe recurrent seizures is 200 to 300 µg per kg body-weight or 1 mg per year of age; if necessary these doses may be repeated 30 minutes or 1 hour later; they may be followed by appropriate maintenance therapy if necessary. Facilities for respiratory assistance must be available.

Elderly and debilitated patients should be given one-half the usual adult dose.

The metabolite desmethyldiazepam is also used (see p.756).

A systematic review of the benzodiazepines and some guidelines for their use in anxiety, insomnia, and some other conditions. The usual division of benzodiazepines into rigid treatment categories of anti-anxiety agents and hypnotics did not appear to have a pharmacological basis; however, there were differences between the long-acting benzodiazepines, with a half-life exceeding 10 hours, such as diazepam, chlordiazepoxide, clorazepate, and medazepam, and the short-acting, rapidly cleared compounds such as triazolam, temazepam, oxazepam, and lorazepam. The latter group might have advantages over longer-acting benzodiazepines in the elderly, in patients with renal or hepatic impairment, and where daytime alertness is required. The benzodiazepines were not considered to have antidepressant or analgesic properties, and were thought unsuitable for use in depression, tension headaches, and dysmenorrhoea occurring in the absence of anxiety, and it was recommended that they should not be used in the treatment of anxiety or insomnia in children. It was noted that there was no firm evidence for the long-term, as distinct from short-term, efficacy of benzodiazepines in insomnia and anxiety.— Committee on the Review of Medicines, *Br. med. J.*, 1980, *29*, 910. Comment on the classification of benzodiazepines by half-life and the suggestion that classification should be based directly on the changes in plasma concentration.— D. M. Pierce and R. A. Franklin, *Br. J. clin. Pharmac.*, 1983, *16*, 345.

A review of the benzodiazepines: D. J. Greenblatt *et al.*, *New Engl. J. Med.*, 1983, *309*, 354 and 410.

ACTION. A review of drug and neurotransmitter receptors in the brain. In pharmacological studies the anxiolytic benzodiazepines seem to act by facilitating the synaptic actions of aminobutyric acid. Aminobutyric acid (GABA) does not act at the same receptor binding site as the benzodiazepines but at a presumably allosterically-linked site. The benzodiazepine receptors themselves appear to exist as at least 2 subtypes; although some evidence has suggested that the apparent subtypes may represent varying temperature-sensitive conformations of a single protein, other results favour distinct receptor proteins. The discrimination of type I from type II receptors offers the possibility of developing selective drugs. If one type of receptor were shown to mediate the anxiolytic effects of benzodiazepines, while the other accounted for their sedative actions, therapeutic advances might become possible but at present the relative behavioural roles of these receptor subtypes is unclear.— S. H. Snyder, *Science*, 1984, *224*, 22. See also L. Spero, *Lancet*, 1982, *2*, 1319.

A discussion of diazepam-binding inhibitor (DBI), a neuropeptide which may be the endogenous ligand for the benzodiazepine receptor.— *Lancet*, 1987, *1*, 307. Further references: A. Guidotti *et al.*, *Proc. natn. Acad. Sci. U.S.A.*, 1983, *80*, 3531; H. Alho *et al.*, *Science*, 1985, *229*, 179.

ADMINISTRATION. Significantly greater plasma-diazepam concentrations were found when the same dose of diazepam was administered intramuscularly into the buttock by doctors than by nurses. This might have been due to shallow injection into fat by the nurses, with little absorption from the organic solvent.— J. W. Dundee *et al.* (letter), *Lancet*, 1974, *2*, 1461. Comment on the poor, erratic, and incomplete absorption of diazepam and chlordiazepoxide following intramuscular injection.— C. B. Tuttle, *Am. J. Hosp. Pharm.*, 1977, *34*, 965.

The pharmacokinetics of diazepam following multiple-dose oral administration in healthy subjects. Single daily administration of the total daily dose at bedtime may represent a satisfactory dosage regimen.— F. B. Eatman *et al.*, *J. Pharmacokinet. Biopharm.*, 1977, *5*, 481. Evidence from a double-blind, placebo-controlled study that a long-acting benzodiazepine is more effective and better tolerated in divided doses. Of 20 patients with anxiety treated with prazepam, a long-acting benzodiazepine that is metabolised to desmethyldiazepam, 10 were given prazepam 10 mg twice daily and 20 mg at night, while the remainder received 40 mg as a single dose at night. The anxiolytic effect obtained with divided doses was significantly better and steadier than that with a single dose, and tolerance was also clearly better.— M. Ansseau *et al.* (letter), *New Engl. J. Med.*, 1984, *310*, 526.

A review of the choice of treatment for anxiety. Preparations containing an antidepressant and a sedative could not be recommended on pharmacological grounds since the dosage schedule for depression consisted of regular dosage until relief of depression followed by regular maintenance dosage whereas that for anxiety consisted of intermittent dosage, according to symptoms, for as brief a period as possible.— P. Tyrer, *Practitioner*, 1977, *219*, 479. See also J. Prutting (letter), *New Engl. J. Med.*, 1979, *300*, 372. A defence of the combined use of amitriptyline and chlordiazepoxide.— J. Cohen (letter), *ibid.*, 1164.

A review of endotracheal drug therapy, including reference to studies of endotracheal diazepam administration in *dogs*.— C. L. Raehl, *Clin. Pharm.*, 1986, *5*, 572.

For references to the rectal administration of diazepam in adults and children, including comparisons of suppositories and rectal solutions, see under Absorption and Fate, above. For precautions in the administration of benzodiazepines to the elderly see p.709.

ADMINISTRATION IN HEPATIC FAILURE. A study in 17 patients with chronic liver disease indicated that they required doses of diazepam about one-third lower than healthy subjects for premedication.— R. A. Branch *et al.*, *Gut*, 1976, *17*, 975. Comment.— *Br. med. J.*, 1977, *1*, 1241.

A study of the disposition of diazepam and its major metabolite desmethyldiazepam in 9 patients with cirrhosis, 5 with hepatic fibrosis and 1 with chronic hepatitis indicated that at least 2 steps in the metabolism of diazepam are impaired in patients with liver disease. The last step in the metabolism (glucuronidation of oxazepam) appeared to be unchanged since H.J. Shull *et al.*(*Ann. intern. Med.*, 1976, *84*, 420) had reported a normal disposition of oxazepam in patients with viral hepatitis and cirrhosis.— U. Klotz *et al.*, *Clin. Pharmac. Ther.*, 1977, *21*, 430. Based on pharmacokinetic findings in 5 patients with cirrhosis and 4 controls, diazepam could be given safely to cirrhotic patients provided the daily dosage was reduced to approximately half that in healthy subjects.— H. R. Ochs *et al.*, *ibid.*, 1983, *33*, 471.

ADMINISTRATION IN RENAL FAILURE. Diazepam could be given in usual doses to patients with renal failure although protein binding reduced to 90% in end-stage renal disease. Concentrations of diazepam were not affected by haemodialysis.— W. M. Bennett *et al.*, *Am. J. Kidney Dis.*, 1983, *3*, 155; H. R. Ochs *et al.*, *Br. J. clin. Pharmac.*, 1981, *12*, 829 (kinetics in renal insufficiency or hyperthyroidism).

ADMINISTRATION IN RESPIRATORY INSUFFICIENCY. A study in 8 healthy subjects indicated significantly depressed ventilatory response 15 and 30 minutes after intramuscular injection of diazepam 10 mg; a tendency to return towards control values at 60 minutes might be attributable to acute tolerance. In situations where diazepam is administered and hypoxia might be anticipated supplementary oxygen might be advisable. No significant effect was noted on hypercapnic ventilatory response after 70 to 130 minutes possibly owing to the time that had elapsed.— S. Lakshminarayan *et al.*, *Clin. Pharmac. Ther.*, 1976, *20*, 178.

A discussion on the effects of diazepam on ventilatory function, and its use for the symptomatic relief of breathlessness in the 'pink and puffing' type of patient with chronic bronchitis and emphysema, who unlike the 'blue and bloated' type, often keep their arterial blood gases near normal for many years. In view of the hazards to patients with carbon dioxide retention, diazepam should not be prescribed for the breathless patient with chronic bronchitis and emphysema, without a preliminary check on the arterial blood gases.— *Lancet*, 1980, *2*, 242.

ALCOHOL AND DRUG WITHDRAWAL. *Alcohol*. A discussion of alcohol and the management of alcohol withdrawal. Many drugs with tranquillising and anticonvulsant activity have been used for the management of alcohol withdrawal but it should be remembered that many cases of physical dependence do not require hospitalisation or drug treatment. In the *USA* chlordiazepoxide has emerged as the drug of choice; diazepam and chlormethiazole, despite real risks of dependence with the latter, are widely used in the *UK*. Abrupt abstinence usually requires treatment dispensed daily to avoid risk of overdose or misuse. The author's experience favours diazepam as drug of first choice; a practical regimen, which may be modified as needed, comprises 10 mg four times daily for 3 days, reduced to three times daily for a further three days, then 5 mg three and two times daily, each for 2 days. Ideally, after 10 days no further tranquillisers or hypnotics should be prescribed; most authorities agree that long-term replacement medication should be avoided, as most problem drinkers rapidly develop some degree of dependence on the new drug. Many physicians favour chlormethiazole in spite of mounting evidence of dependence problems, notably at regular doses above 3 g daily; the author has also noted withdrawal convulsions in otherwise uncomplicated cases, and the drug is contra-indicated in patients with respiratory disease. Where it is used, a suitable regimen is 1.5 g [of the edisylate, as tablets (see p.721)] three times daily for 2 days, reduced to 1 and then 0.5 g, for 2 days and 1 day respectively. Both the diazepam and chlormethiazole regimens should be sufficient to prevent withdrawal convulsions but may be complemented, where the patient is found to be seizure-prone or to exhibit myoclonic twitching, with an anti-epileptic such as phenytoin or sodium valproate; magnesium sulphate may be needed where serum magnesium concentrations are low. Should full-blown seizures occur, intravenous diazepam should provide adequate control. In the management of delirium tremens, which is relatively uncommon, large oral doses of diazepam or chlordiazepoxide, such as 100 to 400 mg over 24 hours, may be required initially; intravenous administration may be required in some cases. Chlormethiazole has been used similarly.— A.P. Thorley, Alcohol, in *Drugs in Psychiatric Practice*, P.J. Tyrer (Ed.), London, Butterworths, 1982,, p.352. A further review of the treatment of alcohol withdrawal. A benzodiazepine such as chlordiazepoxide or diazepam is the drug of choice, but beta-blockers or other adrenergic-blocking agents may also help relieve some symptoms of withdrawal.— *Med. Lett.*, 1986, *28*, 75.

Comment on the problems associated with the intramuscular route for diazepam in the treatment of alcohol withdrawal.— A. A. Wartenberg (letter), *J. Am. med. Ass.*, 1983, *250*, 1271.

A simplified diazepam loading regimen in the management of alcohol withdrawal. A placebo-controlled study in 25 patients given diazepam 20 mg by mouth every 1 to 2 hours, together with supportive care, including phenytoin in those with a history of seizures, indicated that 18 required no further therapy, compared with 14 of 25 controls who received placebo and supportive care. Patients treated with diazepam had faster and greater improvement than those given placebo. All patients who failed to respond by the sixth dose were withdrawn from the study and given standard diazepam therapy: 4 patients who had initially received placebo developed withdrawal symptoms (seizures, hallucinations, or arrhythmias), suggesting that delay in giving active drug may result in a higher rate of complications. On the basis of these observations it is recommended that inpatients with moderate to severe alcohol withdrawal should be given diazepam 20 mg every 1 to 2 hours within 1 hour of admission.— E. M. Sellers *et al.*, *Clin. Pharmac. Ther.*, 1983, *34*, 822. See also P. Devenyi and M. L. Harrison, *Can. med. Ass. J.*, 1985, *132*, 798.

A study of the effect of patient recognition of anxiolytic sedatives among medication in 120 patients undergoing alcohol withdrawal. Of 60 patients assigned to receive diazepam 10 mg, half were given a commercially-available form and half, masked in opaque capsules. A further 60 patients assigned to hydroxyzine embonate 50 mg were similarly divided. The sedatives were administered on patient request, and it was found that patients receiving the opaque capsules made significantly fewer requests, regardless of the drug. It was suggested that patients with a tendency to abuse drugs should be given non-indentifiable dosage forms.— D. A. Francis and A. A. Nelson, *Am. J. Hosp. Pharm.*, 1984, *41*, 488.

Opioid analgesics. Diazepam given to 85 adolescents dependent on diamorphine reduced the duration and severity of physiological withdrawal symptoms.— I. F. Litt *et al.*, *J. Pediat.*, 1971, *78*, 692. Diazepam was only moderately effective in reducing the withdrawal symptoms in patients dependent on methadone.— P. E. Rubin *et al.*, *Drug Intell. & clin. Pharm.*, 1973, *7*, 129.

Diazepam 1 to 2 mg was given intramuscularly every 8 hours to infants born to diamorphine-dependent mothers. Neonatal withdrawal symptoms were controlled within 24 to 72 hours when diazepam was gradually withdrawn.— G. Nathenson *et al.*, *Pediatrics*, 1971, *48*, 523.

For the suggestion that chlorpromazine is the drug of choice in the management of neonatal opioid withdrawal, see Chlorpromazine, p.724.

Diazepam 10 mg, given four times a day for 3 days has proved successful in the management of withdrawal among abusers of methadone, diamorphine, and alcohol, and is particularly useful in cases of multiple drug abuse. Experience has shown that preventing withdrawal seizures in diazepam addicts, however, is difficult; some of these patients may be consuming up to 200 mg per day, and seizures may occur 2 or 3 weeks after withdrawal. Tapered withdrawal over 3 weeks is usually adequate.— J. M. Sehmer (letter), *Can. med. Ass. J.*, 1985, *133*, 358.

ANAESTHESIA. A favourable review of the use of diazepam for minor procedures such as bronchoscopy, gastro-intestinal endoscopy, angiography, cardioversion, and some forms of dental treatment. Dose requirements usually lie between 10 to 40 mg and the margin between sedation and general anaesthesia is very narrow. Although it has a good safety record, respiratory depression may follow intravenous use, especially in debilitated patients and those with hypoxaemia, therefore resuscitation facilities should be at hand. Diazepam has a long duration of action and out-patients should be escorted home after the procedure, and warned not to drive or drink alcohol during the ensuing day; doses greater than 25 mg should not be given to out-patients. Because of its anti-analgesic properties it should not be given alone for painful procedures and when a procedure is likely to be painful adequate doses of an analgesic must be given before giving diazepam.— *Drug & Ther. Bull.*, 1976, *14*, 19. The limitations of sedatives for sedation and analgesia in minor painful procedures.— *Med. Lett.*, 1977, *19*, 26. In a comparative study involving 316 consecutive patients requiring endoscopy, 98 were randomly allocated to no preparation, 93 to throat analgesia with 10% lignocaine, and 125 were given diazepam 10 mg. Acceptability scores were highest in those given no preparation; those given local anaesthesia had a longer introduction time. It is concluded that proper instruction and a personal approach in the endoscopy room remain the best preparation for upper gastrointestinal endoscopy and that sedation is not usually beneficial.— G. F. Nelis (letter), *Lancet*, 1980, *2*, 861. The fact that some patients describe the discomfort of endoscopy as intolerable means that the procedure should not be attempted 'in cold blood'.— *Lancet*, 1980, *2*, 1064.

Diazepam is a sedative with amnestic action, not an anaesthetic and the usual intravenous dose of 200 µg per kg body-weight has a variable and unpredictable effect on the level of consciousness; even doses of 800 µg per kg may prove ineffective. This unpredictability, together with a slow onset and long duration of action are disadvantages in short procedures.— *Drug & Ther. Bull.*, 1983, *21*, 58.

Anaesthetic premedication. In a study in 240 patients, premedication with a combination of droperidol 2.5 mg with diazepam 5 mg produced better relief of anxiety, sedation, amnesia, and acceptance by patient and physician than either droperidol 10 mg or diazepam 10 mg alone. Larger doses of droperidol with diazepam increased the frequency of anxiety and larger doses of diazepam with droperidol might increase sedation.— G. P. Herr *et al.*, *Br. J. Anaesth.*, 1979, *51*, 537.

Pethidine 1 mg per kg body-weight, diazepam 250 µg per kg, and flunitrazepam 20 µg per kg intramuscularly were compared as premedicants in a double-blind study in 145 children, aged up to 15 years, undergoing otolaryngological surgery. All drugs were anxiolytic in the children 5 years and older, but diazepam was less effective in children under 5 years.— L. Lindgren *et al.*, *Br. J. Anaesth.*, 1979, *51*, 321.

In a double-blind crossover study in 18 healthy subjects, diazepam 70 or 140 µg per kg body-weight (a total dose of about 5 or 10 mg) given intravenously had no effect on lower oesophageal sphincter pressure; after 280 µg per kg pressure was increased. Diazepam does not therefore appear to increase the risk of regurgitation and pulmonary aspiration when used pre- or postoperatively.— T. R. Weihrauch *et al.*, *Gut*, 1979, *20*, 64.

In a study involving 101 children aged between 2 and 12 years and undergoing elective surgery diazepam 250 µg per kg body-weight was administered by mouth 90 minutes before surgery to 53, while 48 were given 500 µg per kg. There was no significant difference in premedication scores between the 2 groups 1 hour after taking the drug or at induction of anaesthesia. Although analysis by age suggested that when the lower dose was given younger patients (less than 5 years of age) were less sedated than older children this did not appear to affect recall. The results show that in children of this age range no advantage accrues to an increase in the dose of diazepam premedication from 250 to 500 µg per kg.— D. Fell *et al.*, *Anaesthesia*, 1985, *40*, 12.

Results of a study completed by 58 patients undergoing minor gynaecological surgery indicated that diazepam 10 mg given as a sustained-release tablet the night before surgery was effective in producing overnight sedation and reducing the frequency of awakening, but had no advantages as pre-operative medication compared with diazepam 10 mg as a conventional tablet on the morning of surgery.— R. J. Eastley *et al.*, *Curr. med. Res. Opinion*, 1986, *10*, 235.

Cardiac catheterisation. An intravenous infusion of diazepam (27 µg per kg body-weight per minute for 15 minutes) to 7 patients undergoing cardiac catheterisation produced a decrease in systemic and pulmonary arterial pressures; effects on cardiac output, vascular resistance, and oxygen consumption were variable.— G. D'Amelio *et al.*, *Eur. J. clin. Pharmac.*, 1973, *6*, 61. See also W. Markiewicz *et al.*, *J. clin. Pharmac.*, 1976, *16*, 637.

Cardiac pacemaker implantation. Pacemaker implantation is generally a straightforward procedure lasting less than 1 hour and carried out under local anaesthesia. Premedication is mild, e.g. pethidine 50 to 100 mg and prochlorperazine 12.5 mg one hour beforehand. Once the patient is prepared, with an intravenous cannula inserted into a forearm vein on the opposite side to the implant, a connection to the ECG monitor, and the operative site painted with antiseptic then diazepam 5 to 10 mg, as an emulsion, may be given via the intravenous cannula. The surgery may then be carried out under lignocaine local anaesthesia.— J. C. P. Crick, *Br. J. Hosp. Med.*, 1984, *31*, 116.

Cardioversion. Three groups, each of 50 patients, were given anaesthetics prior to DC cardioversion; the agents used were: diazepam in a mean dose of 320 µg per kg body-weight, thiopentone 3.7 mg per kg, and propanidid 4.6 mg per kg. Diazepam had minimal effects on blood pressure and might be of value in patients with cardiac disease; apnoea was infrequent but amnesia was poor. Thiopentone caused a transient fall in blood pressure; periods of apnoea exceeding 30 seconds occurred in 25 patients; thiopentone was preferable to diazepam in patients in good physical condition. Propanidid caused greater hypotension which was unlikely to be dangerous but this and a high incidence of excitation rendered it less suitable.— R. Orko, *Br. J. Anaesth.*, 1976, *48*, 257.

Dentistry. Diazepam 120 to 320 µg per kg body-weight, in doses up to 20 mg, was given intravenously in solutions containing 5 mg per mL at the rate of 1 mL per minute and induced suitable sedation prior to local analgesia in 105 patients undergoing dental treatment. Cavity preparation time was decreased in these patients but post-operative recovery was slow.— R. A. Dixon *et al.*, *Br. J. Anaesth.*, 1973, *45*, 202.

A study of intravenous diazepam, formulated as an emulsion to reduce pain on injection and thrombophlebitis, in providing sedation for dental procedures in 200 patients.— N. L. Rosenbaum, *Br. dent. J.*, 1982, *153*, 192.

Comparisons of diazepam with other benzodiazepines with a more rapid onset and shorter duration of action in dental patients: C. A. O'Boyle *et al.*, *Br. J. Anaesth.*, 1986, *58*, 378 (intravenous diazepam or oral temazepam); I. Barker *et al.*, *ibid.*, 371 (intravenous diazepam or midazolam); C. A. O'Boyle *et al.*, *ibid.*, 1987, *59*, 746 (midazolam by mouth or intravenous diazepam); H. E. Hosie *et al.*, *Br. dent. J.*, 1987, *162*, 190 (temazepam by mouth or intravenous diazepam).

Endoscopy. When given with atropine for premedication, diazepam was as effective as morphine for endoscopy. The only significant difference in response was that the conscious level was lower in those given diazepam.— R. Ludlam and J. R. Bennett, *Lancet*, 1971, *2*, 1397.

In 100 patients undergoing cystoscopy and related procedures good operating conditions were achieved in 45 by premedication with diazepam 10 mg by mouth 2 hours before surgery and induction of anaesthesia with pentazocine 1 mg per kg body-weight and diazepam 20 to 40 mg intravenously; 34 patients required supplements of nitrous oxide, and 21 required nitrous oxide and alphadolone with alphaxalone.— T. G. C. Smith *et al.*, *Br. J. Anaesth.*, 1977, *49*, 509.

A study of the effect of personality traits on the reaction to upper gastro-intestinal endoscopy. Diazepam increased the readiness of patients to accept further endoscopy because of its amnestic effect.— M. J. Webberley and A. Cuschieri, *Br. med. J.*, 1982, *285*, 251. Criticism of the study. It is important to distinguish clearly between premedication, which is given some minutes or hours before the procedure, and sedation, which is achieved by the use of intravenous diazepam given at the time of endoscopy. In 80 consecutive endoscopies carried out in a general practitioner endoscopy unit, premedication was lorazepam 2.5 to 5 mg given 90 minutes before the procedure, while sedation was achieved with intravenous diazepam emulsion 10 to 60 mg; 3 patients could not tolerate the endoscope despite large doses of diazepam, but of the remaining 77 only 2 had any accurate recollection of the procedure, and all 77 indicated that they would not object to its repetition.— R. Jones (letter), *ibid.*, 512.

A study suggesting that midazolam was as effective as diazepam for intravenous sedation during endoscopy, and was preferred by patients.— K. D. Bardhan *et al.*, *Br. med. J.*, 1984, *288*, 1046. Comment, and further results suggesting that recovery from the effects of midazolam may be more delayed than with diazepam.— J. R. B. Green *et al.* (letter), *ibid.*, 1383. Further comment. Midazolam may prove to be the drug of choice for endoscopy, but the benefits can be lost by giving too large a dose.— J. W. Dundee and J. P. H. Fee (letter), *ibid.*, 1614. Equipotent doses of midazolam offered no advantage over diazepam in terms of speed of recovery when given intravenously to patients undergoing bronchoscopy.— K. Korttila and J. Tarkkanen, *Br. J. Anaesth.*, 1985, *57*, 581. Comment. With larger doses (midazolam 300 µg per kg body-weight and diazepam 500 µg per kg) there is a marked difference in recovery time between the two drugs.— J. W. Dundee and J. P. H. Fee (letter), *ibid.*, 1986, *58*, 466. Reply. As with diazepam ambulatory patients given midazolam sedation must have an escort when discharged from hospital and patients should refrain from driving or operating machinery for at least 12 to 24 hours.— K. Korttila and J. Tarkkanen (letter), *ibid.*

Gynaecology. Diazepam, 10 mg given by intravenous injection 5 minutes before the intravenous injection of pethidine and promethazine, allowed minor gynaecological operations to be performed under excellent conditions in 1132 out of 1200 patients aged 16 to 78 years. No adverse reactions or complications were reported and patients slept for 4 to 5 hours.— J. A. Goldman *et al.*, *Br. J. Anaesth.*, 1972, *44*, 381.

Further studies of diazepam-containing regimens in gynaecological surgery: J. I. M. Lawson and M. K. Milne, *Br. dent. J.*, 1981, *151*, 379 (diazepam and pentazocine prior to general anaesthesia); P. Clyburn *et al.*, *Br. J. Anaesth.*, 1986, *58*, 872 (diazepam or midazolam with fentanyl and etomidate).

Intensive care. A review of sedation for anxiety, pain, and to assist ventilatory control in the intensive care unit. Diazepam is widely used and has an excellent safety record but its effects can be long-lasting. Midazolam is more potent and onset of action is more rapid but recovery from its effects can be prolonged in some critically ill patients. Lorazepam has similar properties to diazepam and has given satisfactory sedation in intensive care. Until controlled trials of newer drugs are complete the most acceptable regimen seems to be an infusion of morphine or pethidine, supplemented where necessary by small doses of a benzodiazepine.— *Lancet*, 1984, *1*, 1388. Comment. In an analysis of sedative techniques in 34 intensive therapy units in the *UK*, H.M. Merriman (*Intensive Care Med.*, 1981, *7*, 217) reported that the commonest first-line drugs were benzodiazepines or opioids alone or in combination. Diazepam was used in 64% of the units and lorazepam in 32%; nitrous oxide was employed in 26% of units to provide short-term sedation. Since the withdrawal of alphadalone-alphaxalone and doubts about the use of etomidate in the intensive therapy unit the authors carried out a further review of practice in 24 units. Opioids were used in the first-line regimens in 81% of units and benzodiazepines only in 29%; midazolam had now become the most frequently used benzodiazepine.— P. H. Gast *et al.* (letter), *ibid.*, *2*, 863. A further review.— S. M. Willatts, *Br. J. parent. Ther.*, 1985, *6*, 13.

Labour. In a small study in multiparous women diazepam 300 µg per kg body-weight intramuscularly did not reduce the requirement for pethidine during labour but was considered to have improved the quality of pain relief without affecting the neonate. A dose of 200 µg per kg had no effect on pain relief.— J. M. Davies and M. Rosen, *Br. J. Anaesth.*, 1977, *49*, 601.

ANXIETY. For discussion of the use of benzodiazepines in anxiety see p.710.

BREATHLESSNESS. Results suggesting that diazepam might be of benefit in giving symptomatic relief of breathlessness, and improving exercise tolerance in 'pink and puffing' patients.— P. Mitchell-Heggs *et al.*, *Q. J. Med.*, 1980, *49*, 9. In a crossover study of the effects of diazepam and promethazine in 15 'pink and puffing' patients diazepam had no effect on breathlessness and caused a significant deterioration in exercise tolerance. Not only does diazepam not seem to be of benefit in these patients, it may be positively harmful and is contra-indicated in patients with airways obstruction unless there is severe anxiety and a low arterial carbon dioxide pressure.— A. A. Woodcock *et al.*, *Br. med. J.*, 1981, *283*, 343. See also *Lancet*, 1986, *1*, 891.

CARDIAC DISORDERS. *Myocardial infarction.* Administration of diazepam 10 mg intravenously followed an hour later by 15 mg by mouth this dose being repeated every 8 hours for 3 days, produced safe, pleasant sedation in patients with myocardial infarction, and reduced the need for analgesics. Catecholamine excretion was reduced, suggesting that diazepam causes a lower stress reaction.— M. Melsom *et al.*, *Br. Heart J.*, 1976, *38*, 804.

Further references: A. Formanek *et al.*, *Radiology*, 1976, *121*, 541; R. A. Dixon *et al.*, *Br. Heart J.*, 1980, *43*, 535; B. W. Johansson, *Acta med. scand.*, 1980, *207*, 47.

CONVULSIONS. For the use of diazepam in the management of convulsions, see p.710.

A review of the use of diazepam by continuous intravenous infusion in the management of status epilepticus. Following intravenous injection of diazepam for initial control of seizures, subsequent therapy is usually with agents such as phenytoin, but where other agents are ineffective, intravenous infusion of diazepam may be considered. There is no data from controlled studies, and the administration rates and duration of infusion have varied widely in published reports. Both pharmacokinetic modelling and clinical experience seem to dictate that an initial loading dose of diazepam, of sufficient size to control the seizures, should be followed by intravenous infusion of 1 to 4 mg of diazepam per kg body-weight per day, adjusted if necessary. There has been some concern as to the stability of diazepam diluted in intravenous fluids; dilutions of 40 µg or less per mL seem to offer the greatest assurance of redissolution of diazepam and 24-hour stability.— H. E. Bell and J. S. Bertino, *Drug Intell. & clin. Pharm.*, 1984, *18*, 965.

EXTRAPYRAMIDAL DISORDERS. Results of a crossover study in 13 patients suggested that low-dose diazepam was not effective in the management of neuroleptic-induced tardive dyskinesia.— S. S. Weber *et al.*, *Drug Intell. & clin. Pharm.*, 1983, *17*, 523.

For the view that benzodiazepines should be avoided in tardive dyskinesia, see p.708. See also p.710.

MUSCULAR AND RHEUMATIC DISORDERS. In a double-blind crossover study in 24 patients with rheumatoid arthritis, 1 week's treatment with diazepam 5 mg thrice daily in addition to standard anti-inflammatory therapy was no more effective in relief of pain or other symptoms than placebo. Seven patients failed to complete the study.— J. D. Vince and D. Kremer, *Practitioner*, 1973, *210*, 264. Reduced morning stiffness on addition of diazepam to indomethacin at night.— D. Hobkirk *et al.*,

Rheumatol. Rehabil., 1977, *16*, 125.

References to the use of diazepam in muscle spasm: G. J. Dobb (letter), *Med. J. Aust.*, 1986, *144*, 112 (with pancuronium following sea-snake bite); J. A. Henry, *Br. J. Anaesth.*, 1986, *58*, 223 (in strychnine poisoning); R. G. Twycross, *Br. J. Hosp. Med.*, 1986, *36*, 244 (in muscle spasm associated with malignant disease).

For the use of diazepam to prevent suxamethonium-induced muscle pain, see Suxamethonium Chloride, p.1238.

See also Spasticity (below).

PREGNANCY AND THE NEONATE. *Eclampsia.* A brief discussion of the use of diazepam in pre-eclampsia and eclampsia.— B. M. Hibbard and M. Rosen, *Br. J. Anaesth.*, 1977, *49*, 3.

Sixteen women with eclampsia were treated with diazepam; all had convulsions and were unconscious. Convulsions ceased within 30 minutes in 13 patients and in all within 4 hours. There was one maternal death but no other maternal complications. Two mothers had been delivered before admission; there were 2 stillbirths (1 macerated) and 12 live births (by caesarean section if not delivered within 12 hours). Of the 12 live births 11 had Apgar scores of 7 to 8. Diazepam 40 mg was given intravenously followed by an infusion of 40 mg in 540 mL of 5% glucose at a rate of 30 to 40 drops per minute, increased if necessary; 20 to 40 mg was given intravenously every 4 to 6 hours for 24 hours after delivery, followed by 10 mg by mouth every 6 hours for a week.— P. Kawathekar *et al.*, *Curr. ther. Res.*, 1973, *15*, 845.

Criticism of low-dose long-term use of diazepam in mild pre-eclampsia. Not only is enough known about the harmful effects of benzodiazepines on the foetus to contra-indicate their use in this context, but there is no rationale for their use in the first place. It is irrational to assume that because diazepam is a useful anticonvulsant in fulminating pre-eclampsia and eclampsia, that smaller, tranquillising, doses might be useful in pre-eclampsia. Moreover, doses of diazepam far in excess of a reasonable anticonvulsant dose are often prescribed in fulminating pre-eclampsia, presumably in the false belief that diazepam is an antihypertensive agent.— A. N. P. Speight (letter), *Br. med. J.*, 1978, *1*, 1420.

Labour. For the use of diazepam during labour, see Anaesthesia (above).

Neonatal drug withdrawal. For the administration of diazepam to infants born to diamorphine-dependent mothers see Alcohol and Drug Withdrawal (above).

Tetanus neonatorum. For the use of diazepam in neonatal tetanus, see Tetanus (below).

PSYCHOSIS. *Schizophrenia.* In at least 25 schizophrenic patients, diazepam 5 mg three times daily greatly relieved auditory hallucinations which were uncontrolled by phenothiazines alone or in conjunction with antidepressants.— B. M. Irvine and F. Schaechter (letter), *Med. J. Aust.*, 1969, *1*, 1387.

Diazepam 10 to 20 mg intravenously relieved catatonic immobility in 2 schizophrenic patients. Subsequent administration of 40 mg daily by mouth maintained the improvement.— J. P. McEvoy and J. B. Lohr, *Am. J. Psychiat.*, 1984, *141*, 284.

In patients with schizophrenia resistant to adequate doses of neuroleptics addition of another drug from a different class may be tried, and diazepam has been suggested on the grounds that it may exert a specific antipsychotic effect via γ-aminobutyric acid as well as its general antianxiety effect.— R. Morgan, *Br. J. Hosp. Med.*, 1985, *34*, 202. See also M. Trabucchi and G. Ba (letter), *Lancet*, 1975, *2*, 868.

The use of diazepam in schizophrenic patients has been only poorly researched, but indications for its long-term use are likely to be rare, as the risks almost certainly outweigh the benefits.— D. A. W. Johnson, *Br. med. J.*, 1987, *294*, 302.

SPASTICITY. A review of drug therapy in the treatment of spasticity. Diazepam is useful alone or as adjunct therapy for spasticity, especially in patients with lesions affecting the spinal cord and occasionally in patients with cerebral palsy. It is particularly useful in patients who have painful or disabling, more-or-less continuous, muscle spasms, and who are able to cope with the drowsiness it sometimes produces. It is thought to be roughly equivalent to dantrolene in its therapeutic efficacy, although this has not been demonstrated; there are few demonstrable differences between diazepam and baclofen, although the former is probably less effective in patients with intermittent painful flexor spasms. Neither is particularly helpful in most patients with cerebral lesions. Diazepam, however, is also useful for the treatment of various nonspastic types of involuntary muscular activity, such as in tetanus, the stiff-man syndrome, or local muscle spasms of various traumatic causes.— R. R. Young and P. J. Delwaide, *New Engl. J. Med.*, 1981, *304*, 96.

A further brief review of the treatment of spasticity. Diazepam has been used for nearly 20 years in patients with spasticity and is the drug against which newer agents have been compared. Because of its sedative effect it is particularly useful in anxious patients or in those who have muscle spasms at night. The usual initial dose is 6 mg daily, increased as necessary up to 40 mg daily. The average dose is 15 mg daily, taken at bedtime to minimise sedation.— *Drug & Ther. Bull.*, 1983, *21*, 1.

Spasmodic torticollis. Spasmodic torticollis in 2 patients responded promptly to the intravenous injection of diazepam 5 to 10 mg.— S. Ahmad and M. K. Meeran (letter), *Br. med. J.*, 1979, *1*, 127.

Stroke. Reference to the use of diazepam in the management of spasticity after stroke.— *Drug & Ther. Bull.*, 1985, *23*, 9.

TETANUS. Eight children with tetanus recovered when given diazepam 9 mg per kg body-weight daily in addition to standard treatment.— G. Gedioğlu *et al.* (letter), *Lancet*, 1973, *2*, 454.

Five patients with severe tetanus were treated with diazepam and phenobarbitone. Large doses of diazepam were used, at times 480 mg daily, and all 5 patients became comatose for periods of 13 to 21 days. Treatment continued during the coma. All 5 patients recovered. Prolonged coma was considered to be a side effect of diazepam rather than a toxic effect and should not contra-indicate its use in the management of tetanus.— K. A. Odusote *et al.*, *Trop. geogr. Med.*, 1976, *28*, 194.

High-dose diazepam as a continuous intravenous infusion of 20 to 40 mg per kg body-weight daily and intragastric phenobarbitone 10 to 15 mg per kg daily in 4 divided doses were given to 19 neonates with tetanus; 7 infants also required intermittent positive-pressure ventilation, of whom 2 died. The main side-effects were severe drowsiness, coma, and apnoeic episodes which were reversed by reduction of diazepam dosage. At follow-up 2 of the 17 survivors were mentally retarded, probably due to cerebral hypoxia during severe tetanic spasms.— B. H. Khoo *et al.*, *Archs Dis. Childh.*, 1978, *53*, 737. A further study of the use of diazepam in the treatment of 10 infants with tetanus neonatorum.— S. Singhi and P. Singhi (letter), *Archs Dis. Childh.*, 1979, *54*, 650. Comment.— B. H. Khoo *et al.* (letter), *ibid.*, 651.

Preparations

Diazepam Capsules *(B.P.)*

Diazepam Capsules *(U.S.P.)*

Diazepam Extended-release Capsules *(U.S.P.)*

Diazepam Injection *(B.P.)*. A sterile solution of diazepam in Water for Injections or other suitable solvent.

Diazepam Injection *(U.S.P.)*. A sterile solution of diazepam in a suitable vehicle.

Diazepam Oral Solution *(B.P.)*

Diazepam Tablets *(B.P.)*

Diazepam Tablets *(U.S.P.)*

Proprietary Preparations

Alupram *(Steinhard, UK). Tablets*, diazepam 2, 5, and 10 mg.

Atensine *(Berk Pharmaceuticals, UK). Tablets*, scored, diazepam 2, 5, and 10 mg.

Diazemuls *(KabiVitrum, UK). Injection*, emulsion, diazepam 5 mg/mL, in ampoules of 2 mL.

Evacalm *(Unimed, UK). Tablets*, diazepam 2 and 5 mg.

Solis *(Galen, UK). Capsules*, diazepam 2 and 5 mg.

Stesolid *(CP Pharmaceuticals, UK). Injection*, diazepam 5 mg/mL, in ampoules of 2 and 4 mL.
Rectal tubes, rectal solution, diazepam 2 and 4 mg/mL, in tubes of 2.5 mL.

Tensium *(DDSA Pharmaceuticals, UK). Tablets*, diazepam 2, 5, and 10 mg.

Valium *(Roche, UK).*
Tablets, scored, diazepam 2, 5, and 10 mg.
Syrup, diazepam 2 mg/5mL.
Injection, diazepam 5 mg/mL, in ampoules of 2 mL.

Proprietary Names and Manufacturers

Aliseum *(Zoja, Ital.)*; Alupram *(Steinhard, UK)*; Amiprol *(Arg.)*; Ansiolin *(Scharper, Ital.)*; Antenex *(Alphapharm, Austral.)*; Apozepam *(A.L., Denm.; A.L., Swed.)*; Armonil *(Arg.)*; Atensine *(Berk Pharmaceuticals, UK)*; Avex *(Lipha, Ital.)*; Benzopin *(Schwulst, S.Afr.)*; Best *(Arg.)*; Betapam *(Be-Tabs, S.Afr.)*; Calmpose *(Ind.)*; Cuadel *(Arg.)*; Cyclopam *(S.Afr.)*; Diaceplex *(Salvat, Spain)*; Dialar *(Lagap, UK)*; Diapam *(Fin.)*; Diaquel *(Rolab, S.Afr.)*; Diatran *(GMP, S.Afr.)*; Diazemuls *(Pharmacia, Canad.; KabiVitrum, Denm.; Kabi, Ger.; KabiVitrum, Norw.; Kabi, Swed.; KabiVitrum, UK)*; Diazepan *(High Noon, Pakistan)*; Dipam *(S.Afr.)*; Dipezona *(Arg.)*; Dizam *(Pharmador, S.Afr.)*; Domalium *(Cronofar, Spain)*; Doval *(Ormed, S.Afr.)*; Drenian *(Ern, Spain)*; D-Tran *(Canad.)*; Ducene *(Sauter, Austral.)*; E-Pam *(ICN, Canad.)*; Eridan *(SIT, Ital.)*; Ethipam *(SCS, S.Afr.)*; Euphorin *(Jpn)*; Evacalm *(Unimed, UK)*; Gradual *(Arg.)*; Gubex *(Arg.)*; Lamra *(Merckle, Ger.)*; Lorinon *(Austral.)*; Mandro-Zep *(Henk, Ger.)*; Meval *(Medic, Canad.)*; Neo-Calme *(Canad.)*; Neosorex *(Rocador, Spain)*; Neurolytril *(Dorsch, Ger.)*; Noan *(Ravizza, Ital.)*; Notense *(Adcock Ingram, S.Afr.)*; Novazam *(Génévrier, Fr.)*; Novodipam *(Novopharm, Canad.)*; Paceum *(Orion, Switz.)*; Pax *(Lennon, S.Afr.)*; Paxel *(Canad.)*; Plidan *(Arg.)*; Pro-Pam *(Protea, Austral.)*; Quetinil *(Ital.)*; Quievita *(Vita, Ital.)*; Relanium *(Pol.)*; Relivan X *(S.Afr.)*; Rival *(Riva, Canad.)*; Saromet *(Arg.)*; Scriptopam *(Propan, S.Afr.)*; Sedapam *(Duncan, Flockhart, UK)*; Sedaril *(Jpn)*; Serenack *(Canad.)*; Solis *(Galen, UK)*; Somasedan *(Arg.)*; Sonacon *(Jpn)*; Stesolid *(Dumex, Denm.; Neth.; Dumex, Norw.; Dumex, Swed.; Dumex, Switz.; CP Pharmaceuticals, UK)*; Stress-Pam *(Canad.)*; Tensium *(DDSA Pharmaceuticals, UK)*; T-Quil *(Legere, USA)*; Tranquase *(Azuchemie, Ger.)*; Tranquirit *(Rorer, Ital.)*; Tranquo-Tablinen *(Beiersdorf, Ger.)*; Valaxona *(Schabru, Denm.; Schaper & Brümmer, Ger.)*; Valiquid *(Roche, Ger.)*; Valitran *(FIRMA, Ital.)*; Valium *(Arg.; Roche, Austral.; Belg.; Roche, Canad.; Roche, Denm.; Roche, Fr.; Roche, Ger.; Roche, Ital.; Neth.; Roche, Norw.; Roche, S.Afr.; Roche, Spain; Roche, Swed.; Roche, Switz.; Roche, UK; Roche, USA)*; Valrelease *(Roche, S.Afr.; Roche, UK; Roche, USA)*; Vatran *(Valeas, Ital.)*; Vival *(Apothekernes Laboratorium, Norw.)*; Vivol *(Horner, Canad.)*.

4028-l

Dichloralphenazone *(BAN)*.

A complex of chloral hydrate and phenazone.
$C_{15}H_{18}Cl_6N_2O_5$=519.0.

CAS — 480-30-8.

Pharmacopoeias. In *Br.*

A white microcrystalline powder with a slight odour characteristic of chloral hydrate. M.p. 64° to 67°.

Soluble 1 in 10 of water, 1 in 1 of alcohol, and 1 in 2 of chloroform; soluble in dilute acids. It is decomposed by dilute alkalis. **Store** in well-closed containers. The *B.P.* directs that the Oral Solution should be stored in a well-filled, well-closed container at a temperature not exceeding 25°, and protected from light.

In aqueous solution it dissociates into chloral hydrate and phenazone.

Dependence

Prolonged use of dichloralphenazone may lead to dependence (see p.706).

Adverse Effects, Treatment, and Precautions

As for Chloral Hydrate, p.717.

It is less likely than chloral hydrate to cause gastric irritation but phenazone-induced skin eruptions may occur (see p.35).

Dichloralphenazone is contra-indicated in patients with acute intermittent porphyria.

ALLERGY. A 66-year-old man suffered anaphylaxis 15 minutes after taking one tablet of dichloralphenazone; symptoms included pruritus, rash, peri-orbital oedema, chest pain, atrial fibrillation, and absence of recordable blood pressure; he recovered after treatment with hydrocortisone, promethazine, and oxygen. He had suffered a similar occurrence after taking dichloralphenazone about 14 years earlier; it had then been considered vasovagal syncope.— S. Perl, *Br. med. J.*, 1977, *2*, 1187.

A 55-year-old man given 2 tablets of dichloralphenazone developed severe bronchospasm and a widespread bullous skin eruption.— D. G. Limb (letter), *Br. med. J.*, 1977, *2*, 1480.

EFFECTS ON THE SKIN. A report of a fixed drug eruption to dichloralphenazone.— J. Verbov (letter), *Br. J.*

Derm., 1972, *86*, 438.

INTERACTIONS. For a report of the effect of dichloralphenazone on plasma concentrations of warfarin, see Warfarin Sodium, p.347.

OVERDOSAGE. Ventricular tachycardia on 2 occasions following severe overdosage with diazepam and dichloralphenazone was probably due to the dichloralphenazone.— J. A. Lockton, *Br. med. J.*, 1987, *294*, 1233. A similar report of life-threatening arrhythmia following ingestion of dichloralphenazone 6.5 g and lorazepam 25 mg together with alcohol.— R. J. I. Bain, *ibid.*, 1616.

PORPHYRIA. Dichloralphenazone was considered to be unsafe in patients with acute porphyria as it has been associated with acute attacks.— M.R. Moore and K.E.L. McColl, *Porphyrias, Drug Lists*, Glasgow, Porphyria Research Unit, University of Glasgow, 1987.

Absorption and Fate

Dichloralphenazone dissociates to form phenazone (see p.35) and chloral hydrate (see p.717).

PREGNANCY AND THE NEONATE. The concentration of the active metabolite, trichloroethanol, in the milk of a lactating mother taking 1.3 g of dichloralphenazone at night was 60 to 80% of that in the plasma.— J. H. Lacey (letter), *Br. med. J.*, 1971, *4*, 684.

Uses and Administration

Dichloralphenazone has the actions of chloral and phenazone and is used similarly to chloral hydrate (see p.718) as a hypnotic and sedative.

The usual hypnotic dose is 0.65 to 1.95 g at night. A suggested hypnotic dose for children is: up to 1 year of age 112 to 225 mg, 1 to 5 years 225 to 450 mg, 6 to 12 years 450 to 900 mg; this dose may be halved for a sedative dose.

Preparations

Dichloralphenazone Oral Solution *(B.P.)*. Dichloralphenazone Elixir

Dichloralphenazone Tablets *(B.P.)*. The tablets have a peppermint flavour.

Proprietary Preparations

Welldorm *(Smith & Nephew Pharmaceuticals, UK)*. *Tablets*, dichloralphenazone 650 mg. *Elixir*, dichloralphenazone 225 mg/5 mL.

Proprietary Names and Manufacturers

Bonadorm *(Austral.)*; Chloralol *(Horner, Canad.)*; Restwel *(S.Afr.)*; Welldorm *(Smith & Nephew Pharmaceuticals, UK)*.

The following names have been used for multi-ingredient preparations containing dichloralphenazone—Midrin *(Carnrick, USA)*; Paedo-Sed *(Pharmax, UK)*.

NOTE. Midrid *(Carnrick, UK)* has been reformulated to exclude dichloralphenazone.

7037-j

Dixyrazine

UCB-3412. 2-(2-{4-[2-Methyl-3-(phenothiazin-10-yl)propyl]piperazin-1-yl}ethoxy)ethanol.

$C_{24}H_{33}N_3O_2S$=427.6.

CAS — 2470-73-7.

Dixyrazine is a phenothiazine and shares the general properties of the group (see p.706). It has a piperazine side-chain. Various doses have been advocated for psychiatric disorders usually ranging from 12.5 to 75 mg daily.

Dixyrazine was considered to be unsafe in patients with acute porphyria because it has been shown to be porphyrinogenic in *animals* or *in vitro* systems.— M.R. Moore and K.E.L. McColl, *Porphyrias, Drug Lists*, Glasgow, Porphyria Research Unit, University of Glasgow, 1987.

Proprietary Names and Manufacturers

Esucos *(UCB, Arg.; UCB, Belg.; UCB, Denm.; UCB, Fr.; UCB, Ger.; SIT, Ital.; UCB, Neth.; UCB, Norw.; UCB, S.Afr.; UCB, Swed.; UCB, Switz.)*; Roscal *(Rosco, Denm.)*.

16612-j

Doxefazepam *(rINN)*.

SAS-643. 7-Chloro-5-(2-fluorophenyl)-1,3-dihydro-3-hydroxy-1-(2-hydroxyethyl)-2*H*-1,4-benzodiazepin-2-one.

$C_{17}H_{14}ClFN_2O_3$=348.8.

CAS — 40762-15-0.

Doxefazepam is a benzodiazepine derivative with general properties similar to those of diazepam (p.731). It is used as a hypnotic in the short-term management of insomnia in doses of 10 to 20 mg at night.

Proprietary Names and Manufacturers

Doxans *(Schiapparelli, Ital.)*.

7038-z

Droperidol *(BAN, USAN, rINN)*.

R-4749. 1-{1-[3-(4-Fluorobenzoyl)propyl]-1,2,3,6-tetrahydro-4-pyridyl} benzimidazolin-2-one.

$C_{22}H_{22}FN_3O_2$=379.4.

CAS — 548-73-2.

Pharmacopoeias. In *U.S.*

A white to light tan-coloured amorphous or microcrystalline powder. Practically **insoluble** in water; soluble 1 in 140 of alcohol, 1 in 4 of chloroform, and 1 in 500 of ether. The *U.S.P.* injection has a pH between 3.0 and 3.8. **Store** at 8° to 15° under an atmosphere of nitrogen in airtight containers. Protect from light.

A study of the stability of droperidol in glucose injection, sodium chloride injection, and lactated Ringer's injection. Although droperidol appeared to be stable for 7 days in mixtures stored in glass bottles there was some loss due to sorption when mixtures in lactated Ringer's injection were stored in polyvinyl chloride bags.— J. B. Ray *et al.*, *Am. J. Hosp. Pharm.*, 1983, *40*, 94.

Adverse Effects and Treatment

As for the phenothiazines, p.706.

EXTRAPYRAMIDAL EFFECTS. In a double-blind trial involving 100 healthy women undergoing gynaecological procedures, droperidol 5 mg used as premedicant caused an increase in tremor and no significant decrease in nausea. Postoperative anxiety appeared to increase.— F. R. Ellis and J. Wilson, *Br. J. Anaesth.*, 1972, *44*, 1288.

Extrapyramidal symptoms were reported in a 10-year-old boy 3 hours after an intravenous injection of droperidol 10 mg.— K. L. De Silva *et al.*, *Practitioner*, 1973, *211*, 316.

A 41-year-old man developed an acute dystonic reaction following intravenous administration of droperidol 10 mg in divided doses over 10 minutes. He developed severe perioral spasms, protruded his tongue and grimaced markedly; his eyes rotated upwards and to the right and seemed fixed in that position; his neck became rigid, his mandible protruded forward, and he bit his tongue; his entire face seemed to be in spasm and he became plethoric; he remained fully conscious, could breath deeply and move his unanaesthetised extremities on command, but was unable to speak. Within a minute of intravenous administration of diphenhydramine 75 mg all signs of the extrapyramidal reaction resolved.— C. M. Patton, *Anesthesiology*, 1975, *43*, 126.

Akathisia developed in 3 of 14 patients undergoing eye surgery within 90 minutes of administration of droperidol 20 mg and metoclopramide 10 mg by mouth for premedication.— T. R. E. Barnes *et al.* (letter), *Lancet*, 1982, *2*, 48.

Precautions

As for the phenothiazines, p.708.

Droperidol has a longer duration of action than opioid analgesics such as fentanyl and phenoperidine, therefore, during concurrent use, repeat doses of droperidol must not be given when only the opioid analgesic is required, since this would lead to accumulation of droperidol and overdosage.

Severely impaired psychomotor performance for at least 10 hours after droperidol administration. Droperidol is probably not suitable as an anaesthetic for outpatients.— K. Korttila and M. Linnoila, *Br. J. Anaesth.*, 1974, *46*, 961.

In 8 healthy subjects droperidol 5 mg intravenously appeared to increase the incidence of gastro-oesophageal reflux and might therefore increase the risk of regurgitation and aspiration of gastric contents during induction and recovery from anaesthesia.— J. G. Brock-Utne *et al.*, *Br. J. Anaesth.*, 1978, *50*, 295.

INTERACTIONS. *Antimuscarinic agents.* Droperidol appeared to have a mild atropinic action and enhanced the effect of atropine on heart-rate.— P. Parmentier and P. Dagnelie, *Br. J. Anaesth.*, 1979, *51*, 775.

MYASTHENIA GRAVIS. Although droperidol has not been implicated clinically, it has been shown experimentally to interfere with neuromuscular transmission, and should be used with caution in patients with myasthenia.— Z. Argov and F. L. Mastaglia, *New Engl. J. Med.*, 1979, *301*, 409.

PHAEOCHROMOCYTOMA. Intravenous administration of droperidol 1.25 mg to a 13-year-old boy with phaeochromocytoma caused severe hypertension which was easily controlled by phenoxybenzamine.— K. Sumikawa and Y. Amakata, *Anesthesiology*, 1977, *46*, 359. Further cases of droperidol-induced hypertension in patients with phaeochromocytoma.— D. A. Bittar, *ibid.*, 1979, *50*, 366. See also C. J. Hull, *Br. J. Anaesth.*, 1986, *58*, 1453.

Absorption and Fate

For a detailed account of the absorption and fate of a butyrophenone, see Haloperidol, p.744.

Droperidol has been reported to have an initial plasma half-life of 10 minutes and a terminal plasma half-life of about 2 hours. It is extensively bound to plasma proteins.

A study of the absorption, metabolism, and excretion of droperidol in healthy subjects following intramuscular and intravenous administration. Droperidol was so rapidly absorbed from the intramuscular site that a response almost equivalent to that following intravenous administration could be expected. Droperidol was extensively metabolised and of 75% excreted in the urine less than 1% was unchanged. About 22% was recovered in the faeces, about 50% of this as unchanged droperidol; this high faecal recovery suggests biliary excretion of a portion of the dose. Droperidol had an initial half-life of about 10 minutes and terminal half-life of an average of 2.2 hours (range 120 to 163 minutes).— W. A. Cressman *et al.*, *Anesthesiology*, 1973, *38*, 363. See also M. M. Ghoneim and K. Korttila, *Clin. Pharmacokinet.*, 1977, *2*, 344.

Uses and Administration

Droperidol is a butyrophenone with actions similar to those of haloperidol (p.744). The duration of action of droperidol has been variously reported to last from about 2 to 4 hours to up to as long as 6 hours; alteration of consciousness may last 12 hours or longer. It is used in conjunction with an analgesic such as fentanyl citrate (p.1305) to maintain the patient in a state of neuroleptanalgesia in which he is calm and indifferent to his surroundings and able to cooperate with the surgeon. The longer duration of action of droperidol must be kept in mind when using it in association with such opioid analgesics. Droperidol is also used as a premedicant, as an anti-emetic, and for the control of agitated patients in acute psychoses.

Droperidol is administered by mouth or by injection. The recommended dose in psychosis is 5 to 20 mg by mouth, repeated every 4 to 8 hours if necessary. For premedication 2.5 to 10 mg may be administered intramuscularly 30 to 60 minutes pre-operatively. As an adjunct to general anaesthesia 5 to 15 mg may be administered intravenously, followed by 1.25 to 2.5 mg, usually intravenously, if required for maintenance.

For the prevention of postoperative nausea and vomiting a dose of 5 mg intramuscularly or intravenously may be given. In cancer chemotherapy, a suggested regimen is 1 to 10 mg 30 minutes before commencement of antineoplastic therapy, followed by a continuous intravenous infusion of 1 to 3 mg per hour or 1 to 5 mg by intramuscular or intravenous injection every 1 to 6 hours as required.

In the *UK* droperidol 200 to 300 µg per kg body-weight intravenously has been suggested for anaesthetic use in children; in the *USA*, doses of

88 to 165 μg per kg have been recommended. Lower doses have been given. As an anti-emetic, children may be given doses between 20 and 75 μg per kg intramuscularly or intravenously. Droperidol should be used in reduced dosage in the elderly.

Preparations

Droperidol Injection *(U.S.P.)*. A sterile solution in Water for Injections prepared with the aid of lactic acid.

Proprietary Preparations

Droleptan *(Janssen, UK)*. *Tablets*, scored, droperidol 10 mg.
Oral liquid, droperidol 1 mg/mL.
Injection, droperidol 5 mg/mL, in ampoules of 2 mL.

Proprietary Names and Manufacturers

Dehydrobenzperidol *(Arg.; Belg.; Janssen, Denm.; Janssen, Ger.; Neth.; Janssen, Switz.)*; Dridol *(Janssen, Norw.; Janssen Pharmaceutica, Swed.)*; Droleptan *(Janssen, Austral.; Janssen, Fr.; Janssen, UK)*; Inapsin *(Janssen, S.Afr.)*; Inapsine *(Janssen, Canad.; Janssen, USA)*; Sintodian *(Carlo Erba, Ital.)*.

The following names have been used for multi-ingredient preparations containing droperidol— Innovar *(Janssen, Canad.; Janssen, USA)*; Thalamonal *(Janssen, UK)*.

4030-g

Estazolam *(rINN)*.

D-40TA. 8-Chloro-6-phenyl-4*H*-1,2,4-triazolo[4,3-*a*]-1,4-benzodiazepine.
$C_{16}H_{11}ClN_4$=294.7.

CAS — 29975-16-4.

Pharmacopoeias. In *Jpn*.

Estazolam is a benzodiazepine derivative with general properties similar to those of diazepam (p.728). It has been used as a hypnotic in the short-term management of insomnia in doses of 1 to 2 mg at night.

Proprietary Names and Manufacturers

Domnamid *(Lundbeck, Denm.)*; Esilgan *(Cyanamid, Ital.)*; Eurodin *(Takeda, Jpn)*; Nuctalon *(Takeda, Fr.)*.

4031-q

Ethchlorvynol *(BAN, USAN, rINN)*.

β-Chlorovinyl Ethyl Ethynyl Carbinol. 1-Chloro-3-ethylpent-1-en-4-yn-3-ol.
C_7H_9ClO=144.6.

CAS — 113-18-8.

Pharmacopoeias. In *U.S.*

A colourless to yellow, slightly viscous liquid with a characteristic pungent odour. Wt per mL about 1.072 g. It darkens on exposure to air and light.
Practically **insoluble** in water; miscible with most organic solvents. **Store** in airtight containers of glass or polyethylene, using polyethylene-lined closures. The *U.S.P.* directs that the capsules should be protected from light.

Dependence

Prolonged use of ethchlorvynol may lead to dependence (see p.706).

Ethchlorvynol withdrawal symptoms (including convulsions, hypertonicity, and hyperreflexia) occurred in a 67-year-old man who had taken the drug in a dose increased from 1 to at least 1.25 g daily over about 5 months.— H. T. Abuzahra and M. Rossdale (letter), *Br. med. J.*, 1968, *2*, 433.

Withdrawal symptoms in a neonate.— B. H. Rumack and P. A. Walravens, *Pediatrics*, 1973, *52*, 714.

Further reference to withdrawal.— M. W. Schottstaedt *et al., Crit. Care Med.*, 1981, *9*, 677.

Reports of abuse by intravenous injection: F. L. Glauser *et al., Ann. intern. Med.*, 1976, *84*, 46; P. Van Swearingen (letter), *ibid.*, 614.

See also under Adverse Effects (below).

Adverse Effects

Side-effects include gastro-intestinal disturbances including unpleasant after-taste, dizziness, headache, hangover, blurred vision, facial numbness, and hypotension. Skin rashes, urticaria, and occasionally, thrombocytopenia and cholestatic jaundice have also been reported as has toxic amblyopia. Idiosyncratic reactions include excitement, prolonged hypnosis, severe muscular weakness, and syncope without marked hypotension.
Acute overdosage is characterised by prolonged deep coma, respiratory depression, hypothermia, hypotension, and relative bradycardia. Pancytopenia has occurred.
Chronic intoxication causes incoordination, tremors, ataxia, confusion, slurred speech, hyperreflexia, diplopia, nystagmus, optic and peripheral neuropathy, and generalised muscle weakness. Pulmonary oedema has followed abuse by intravenous injection.

EFFECTS ON THE BLOOD. A report of fatal thrombocytopenia associated with ethchlorvynol.— E. S. Jacobson, *Ann. intern. Med.*, 1972, *77*, 73.

EFFECTS ON THE EYES. Toxic amblyopia occurred in a patient who received ethchlorvynol 0.5 to 1 g at night for about 3 months. Treatment consisted of cyanocobalamin injections of 1 mg daily for 10 days. Recovery was complete 6 months after withdrawal of ethchlorvynol.— W. M. Haining and G. W. Beveridge, *Br. J. Ophthal.*, 1964, *48*, 598.

A report of unusual nystagmus occurring after ethchlorvynol use.— A. H. Ropper (letter), *J. Am. med. Ass.*, 1975, *232*, 907.

EFFECTS ON THE LUNGS. A report of 2 subjects with rapid-onset severe non-haemodynamic pulmonary oedema following intravenous injection of the contents of ethchlorvynol capsules. This effect was reproduced in *dogs* and it was established that the polyethylene glycol vehicle was not responsible. Pulmonary oedema might be secondary to the direct effects of ethchlorvynol on the alveolar capillary membrane.— F. L. Glauser *et al., Ann. intern. Med.*, 1976, *84*, 46. See also P. Van Swearingen (letter), *ibid.*, 614; T. H. Self *et al., Drug Intell. & clin. Pharm.*, 1979, *13*, 96.

OVERDOSAGE. Six patients took ethchlorvynol with suicidal intent. Overdosage was characterised by deep, often prolonged coma, hypothermia, marked respiratory depression, and hypotension without compensatory tachycardia. Complications included peripheral neuropathy and severe pneumonia. Haemodialysis was more effective than peritoneal dialysis or forced diuresis.— B. P. Teehan *et al., Ann. intern. Med.*, 1970, *72*, 875. Recovery after taking 200 to 250 capsules of ethchlorvynol 500 mg. Haemodialysis for 14 hours removed 14 g of ethchlorvynol. Severe pancytopenia developed on the 15th day but there was no bleeding or infection.— J. C. Klock (letter), *ibid.*, 1974, *81*, 131.

Treatment of Adverse Effects

As for the barbiturates, p.708.
Haemoperfusion may be of value in the treatment of severe poisoning with ethchlorvynol.

The slow removal of ethchlorvynol from the body seen after therapeutic doses and overdosage may reflect localisation in adipose and other tissues rather than a slow rate of biotransformation.— P. F. Gibson and N. Wright, *J. pharm. Sci.*, 1972, *61*, 169.

A review of studies and reports on the removal of ethchlorvynol.— J. F. Winchester *et al., Trans. Am. Soc. artif. internal Organs*, 1977, *23*, 762. See also T. N. Tozer *et al., Am. J. Hosp. Pharm.*, 1974, *31*, 986.

DIALYSIS. A patient who had taken approximately 40 g of ethchlorvynol was treated successfully by haemodialysis using an oil dialysant.— L. T. Welch *et al., Clin. Pharmac. Ther.*, 1972, *13*, 745.

Other reports: J. S. Hyde *et al., Clin. Pediat.*, 1968, *7*, 739 (peritoneal dialysis); A. Hume *et al., Clin. Res.*, 1970, *18*, 62 (lipid haemodialysis).

HAEMOPERFUSION. Beneficial results with charcoal haemoperfusion in ethchlorvynol poisoning.— M. C. Gelfand *et al., Trans. Am. Soc. artif. internal Organs*, 1977, *23*, 599.

Three patients, who had ingested 12 to 22 g of ethchlorvynol, were successfully treated by haemoperfusion utilising Amberlite XAD-4 resin.— R. I. Lynn *et al., Ann. intern. Med.*, 1979, *91*, 549.

Further references to the use of resin haemoperfusion: S. L. Dua *et al.* (letter), *Ann. intern. Med.*, 1980, *92*, 436; N. Benowitz *et al., Clin. Pharmac. Ther.*, 1980, *27*, 236.

Precautions

Ethchlorvynol is contra-indicated in patients with porphyria, and caution is needed in hepatic or renal failure and in patients in severe uncontrolled pain. It may cause drowsiness and patients receiving ethchlorvynol should not drive or take charge of machinery where loss of attention could lead to accidents. The effect of ethchlorvynol may be enhanced by alcohol, barbiturates, and other central nervous system depressants. It has been reported to decrease the effects of coumarin anticoagulants, and delirium has followed concomitant use with tricyclic antidepressants.
Ethchlorvynol should be given with food, as excessively rapid absorption in some patients has been reported to produce giddiness and ataxia.

Absorption and Fate

Ethchlorvynol is readily absorbed from the gastro-intestinal tract and extensively metabolised in the liver, and possibly to some extent in the kidneys. It has a biphasic plasma half-life with a rapid initial phase and a terminal phase reported to last from 10 to 25 hours.

Studies in healthy subjects indicated that ethchlorvynol is rapidly absorbed following oral administration, and extensively metabolised with only traces of unchanged drug appearing in the urine. The metabolic half-life is a rather rapid 5.6 hours, but it disappears from plasma with a rapid α-phase and a much slower β-phase owing to extensive tissue redistribution.— L. M. Cummins *et al., J. pharm. Sci.*, 1971, *60*, 261. See also P. F. Gibson and N. Wright, *ibid.*, 1972, *61*, 169.

Ethchlorvynol is 35 to 50% bound to plasma proteins.— W. M. Bennett *et al., Ann. intern. Med.*, 1980, *93*, 286.

See also under Uses.

Uses and Administration

Ethchlorvynol has hypnotic effects which are manifest within 15 to 30 minutes of ingestion. It also has some anticonvulsant and muscle relaxant properties. The usual hypnotic dose is 500 mg at night but doses ranging from 0.2 to 1 g have been given. It has also been employed as a sedative in doses of 100 or 200 mg two or three times daily. Administration with food or milk has been recommended—see Precautions, above.

Following a study of ethchlorvynol as a hypnotic in 4 young insomniac patients it was concluded that side-effects militate against its use. One subject suffered severe headache, another experienced confusion and stuttering; the other 2 had feelings of tiredness, occasional headache, loss of concentration, and dizziness. There were also significant withdrawal effects.— D. F. Kripke *et al., Psychopharmacology*, 1978, *56*, 221.

ADMINISTRATION IN RENAL FAILURE. A single dose of ethchlorvynol 500 mg given to 9 normal subjects produced a rapid rise in plasma-ethchlorvynol concentration to about 4.2 μg per mL in 2 hours, followed by a fall to about 2.4 and 1.6 μg per mL at 4 and 6 hours after administration respectively. In 8 anephric patients on maintenance dialysis, the peak plasma concentration of about 3.9 μg per mL at 2 hours was maintained with little fall and was about 3.7 μg per mL 6 hours after administration.— J. K. Dawborn *et al., Med. J. Aust.*, 1972, *2*, 702.

Ethchlorvynol could be given in usual doses to patients with a glomerular filtration-rate greater than 50 mL per minute, but should be avoided in those with a glomerular filtration-rate less than this.— W. M. Bennett *et al., Am. J. Kidney Dis.*, 1983, *3*, 155.

Preparations

Ethchlorvynol Capsules *(U.S.P.)*

Proprietary Names and Manufacturers

Arvynol *(Pfizer, UK)*; Placidyl *(Abbott, Canad.; Abbott, USA)*; Serenesil *(Abbott, UK)*.

4032-p

Ethinamate *(BAN, USAN, rINN)*.

1-Ethynylcyclohexyl carbamate.
$C_9H_{13}NO_2$=167.2.

CAS — 126-52-3.

Pharmacopoeias. In *U.S.*

A white almost odourless powder. M.p. between 94° and 98°. **Soluble** 1 in 400 of water, 1 in about 3 of alcohol, 1 in 50 of petroleum spirit, 1 in 4.6 of propylene glycol, and 1 in 140 of sesame oil; freely soluble in chloroform and ether. A saturated solution in water has a pH of about 6.5. **Store** in airtight containers.

Dependence

As for the barbiturates, p.706.

Withdrawal of ethinamate had been followed by agitation, syncopal episodes, tremulousness, and hyperactive reflexes. Major convulsions, disorientation, delusions, and hallucinations had also been reported.— C. F. Essig, *J. Am. med. Ass.*, 1966, *196*, 714.

Adverse Effects

Gastro-intestinal discomfort, excitement in children, and skin rashes have been reported. Rarely, thrombocytopenic purpura and hypersensitivity with fever have occurred.

Treatment of Adverse Effects
As for the barbiturates, p.708.
Dialysis may be of value in the treatment of severe poisoning with ethinamate.

Precautions
Ethinamate causes drowsiness and patients receiving it should not take charge of vehicles or machinery where loss of attention could lead to accidents. These effects are enhanced by the simultaneous administration of other depressants of the central nervous system such as alcohol, or barbiturates.

PORPHYRIA. Ethinamate was considered to be unsafe in patients with acute porphyria because it has been shown to be porphyrinogenic in *animals* or *in vitro* systems.— M.R. Moore and K.E.L. McColl, *Porphyrias, Drug Lists*, Porphyria Research Unit, University of Glasgow, 1987.

Absorption and Fate
Ethinamate is rapidly absorbed from the gastro-intestinal tract and extensively metabolised in the body, partly by hydroxylation in the liver. It is excreted in the urine, almost entirely as metabolites; 36% of an oral dose is reported to be excreted in urine within 24 hours. It has a short half-life.

After administration of ethinamate 1 g by mouth to 8 healthy subjects the maximum blood concentrations occurred in 6 after about 60 minutes. The biological half-life was 135 minutes.— J. M. Clifford *et al.*, *Clin. Pharmac. Ther.*, 1974, *16*, 376.

Ethinamate 1 g was administered as tablets to 12 subjects. The mean peak plasma concentration was about 9.6 µg per mL. The biological half-life in plasma was calculated to be about 2 hours. Excluding one subject with a very low value mean 24-hour recovery from urine for the major metabolite *trans*-4-hydroxyethinamate was about 35%.— J. W. Kleber *et al.*, *J. pharm. Sci.*, 1977, *66*, 992.

Uses and Administration
Ethinamate has mild sedative and hypnotic properties and is used mainly as a hypnotic. It has been reported to induce sleep in about 20 minutes and to have an effect lasting about 4 hours. The usual dose is 0.5 to 1 g at night.

Preparations

Ethinamate Capsules *(U.S.P.)*

Proprietary Names and Manufacturers
Valamin *(Asche, Ger.)*; Valmid *(Dista, USA)*.

15319-n

Ethyl Loflazepate *(rINN)*.

CM-6912. Ethyl 7-chloro-5-(2-fluorophenyl)-2,3-dihydro-2-oxo-1*H*-1,4-benzodiazepine-3-carboxylate.
$C_{18}H_{14}ClFN_2O_3$=360.8.

CAS — 29177-84-2.

Ethyl loflazepate is a benzodiazepine with general properties similar to those of diazepam (p.728). It is used in the treatment of anxiety and tension states in usual doses of 1 to 3 mg daily by mouth.

Proprietary Names and Manufacturers
Victan *(Midy, Fr.)*.

16639-h

Etizolam *(rINN)*.

Y-7131. 4-(2-Chlorophenyl)-2-ethyl-9-methyl-6*H*-thieno[3,2-*f*]-*s*-triazolo[4,3-*a*][1,4]diazepine.
$C_{17}H_{15}ClN_4S$=342.9.

CAS — 40054-69-1.

Etizolam is a benzodiazepine derivative with general properties similar to those of diazepam (p.731). It has been used for its sedative and anxiolytic properties in doses of 0.5 to 1 mg three times daily.

Proprietary Names and Manufacturers
Depas *(Yoshitomi, Jpn)*.

12718-z

Etodroxizine *(rINN)*.

2-{2-[2-(4-*p*-Chlorobenzhydrylpiperazin-1-yl)ethoxy]-ethoxy}ethanol.
$C_{23}H_{31}ClN_2O_3$=419.0.

CAS — 17692-34-1.

Etodroxizine has been used as a sedative and for the relief of allergies.

Proprietary Names and Manufacturers
Indunox *(UCB, Belg.; UCB, Neth.; Vesta, S. Afr.)*.

12728-k

Febarbamate *(rINN)*.

Go-560. 1-(3-Butoxy-2-carbamoyloxypropyl)-5-ethyl-5-phenylbarbituric acid.
$C_{20}H_{27}N_3O_6$=405.4.

CAS — 13246-02-1.

Dependence, Adverse Effects, Treatment, and Precautions
As for the barbiturates in general, p.706.

Uses and Administration
Febarbamate is a barbiturate that has been used for its reported anxiolytic properties in the management of anxiety and insomnia. Doses of 100 to 200 mg daily have been given.

Proprietary Names and Manufacturers
G-Tril *(Sapos, Neth.; Vinas, Spain)*; Solium *(Lirca, Ital.)*; Tymium *(Sapos, Switz.)*.

7040-s

Fluanisone *(BAN, rINN)*.

Haloanisone; MD-2028; R-2028; R-2167. 4′-Fluoro-4-[4-(2-methoxyphenyl)piperazin-1-yl]butyrophenone.
$C_{21}H_{25}FN_2O_2$=356.4.

CAS — 1480-19-9.

Pharmacopoeias. In *B.P. Vet.*

An almost white to buff-coloured, odourless or almost odourless, crystalline powder. M.p. 72° to 76°. Practically **insoluble** in water; soluble 1 in 12 of alcohol, 1 in 1 of chloroform, and 1 in 22 of ether; freely soluble in dilute solutions of organic acids. **Store** in well-closed containers. Protect from light.

Fluanisone is a butyrophenone with general properties similar to those of haloperidol (p.743). It has been given in psychiatric disorders in doses of 2.5 mg twice or three times daily; higher doses have been given. Fluanisone may also be given intramuscularly.
Fluanisone is also used in veterinary medicine as a tranquilliser and for anaesthetic premedication.

Proprietary Names and Manufacturers
Sedalande *(Delalande, Belg.; Delalande, Fr.; Delalande, Ger.; Delalande, Switz.)*.

4034-w

Flunitrazepam *(BAN, USAN, rINN)*.

Ro-5-4200. 5-(2-Fluorophenyl)-1,3-dihydro-1-methyl-7-nitro-1,4-benzodiazepin-2-one.
$C_{16}H_{12}FN_3O_3$=313.3.

CAS — 1622-62-4.

Dependence, Adverse Effects, Treatment, and Precautions
As for the benzodiazepines in general, p.706.

INTERACTIONS. The effects of combined flunitrazepam and *alcohol* on performance.— M. Linnoila *et al.*, *J. clin. Pharmac.*, 1981, *21*, 430.

PORPHYRIA. Flunitrazepam was considered to be unsafe in patients with acute porphyria because it has been shown to be porphyrinogenic in *animals* or *in-vitro* systems.— M.R. Moore and K.E.L. McColl, *Porphyrias, Drug Lists*, Glasgow, Porphyria Research Unit, University of Glasgow, 1987.

THROMBO-EMBOLIC EFFECTS. Of 43 patients given a single intravenous dose of flunitrazepam 1 to 2 mg two had thrombosis 7 to 10 days later. The incidence was lower than in those given diazepam.— J. E. Hegarty and J. W. Dundee, *Br. med. J.*, 1977, *2*, 1384. See also H. Mikkelsen *et al.*, *Br. J. Anaesth.*, 1980, *52*, 817.

Absorption and Fate
Flunitrazepam is readily absorbed from the gastro-intestinal tract. About 77 to 80% is bound to plasma proteins. It is extensively metabolised in the liver and excreted mainly in the urine as metabolites. The elimination half-life is reported to be about 19 to 22 hours. Flunitrazepam crosses the placental barrier and is excreted in breast milk.

The mean terminal exponential half-life of flunitrazepam following administration of a single 2-mg dose to 8 healthy subjects was 13.5 hours; a half-life of 19.2 hours was obtained in a further 6 subjects following variable repeated doses.— H. G. Boxenbaum *et al.*, *J. Pharmacokinet. Biopharm.*, 1978, *6*, 283.

A terminal half-life of between 20 and 36 hours on prolonged administration of flunitrazepam.— E. Wickstrøm *et al.*, *Eur. J. clin. Pharmac.*, 1980, *17*, 189.

Concentrations of flunitrazepam in umbilical-vein and -artery plasma were lower than those in maternal venous plasma about 11 to 15 hours after administration of flunitrazepam 1 mg to 14 pregnant women; concentrations in amniotic fluid were lower still. Concentrations in breast milk after a single 2-mg dose were considered to be too low to produce clinical effects in breast-feeding infants but accumulation in the milk might occur after repeated administration.— J. Kanto *et al.*, *Curr. ther. Res.*, 1979, *26*, 539.

Further references: J. P. Cano *et al.*, *Arzneimittel-Forsch.*, 1977, *27*, 2383; P. J. Davis and D. R. Cook, *Clin. Pharmacokinet.*, 1986, *11*, 18.

Uses and Administration
Flunitrazepam is a benzodiazepine derivative with general properties similar to those of diazepam (p.731). It is given by mouth in the short-term management of insomnia, in doses of 0.5 to 2 mg at night. It has also been used for premedication, and, by intravenous injection, for the induction of general anaesthesia.

Reviews: M. A. K. Mattila and H. M. Larni, *Drugs*, 1980, *20*, 353. See also *Aust. J. Pharm.*, 1979, *60*, 246.

ANAESTHESIA. In 3 studies in a total of 220 subjects or patients flunitrazepam, in doses of 2 to 6 mg intravenously, exerted its maximum effect 1 to 1.5 minutes after injection; some patients were not asleep after doses equivalent to 100 µg per kg body-weight. Tremor, hypertonus, or involuntary muscle movements occurred in 11 patients; cough, hiccup, or laryngospasm occurred in 61 patients, and transient marked respiratory depression in 5; arterial hypotension in many patients did not cause concern; all these effects were more common in those who did not receive opiates as premedication. Prolonged drowsiness was not uncommon. Venous sequelae (in 21% of subjects) were similar to those observed after diazepam. Although flunitrazepam was considered to be 10 times more potent than diazepam it was too unreliable to be used as a routine induction agent.— J. W. Dundee *et al.*, *Br. J. Anaesth.*, 1976, *48*, 551.

In a double-blind study the induction of anaesthesia by flunitrazepam in 48 patients was comparable with the effect of alphaxalone and alphadolone in 49 patients. The maintenance of anaesthesia was considered superior in the flunitrazepam group. Transient erythema occurred in 4 patients given flunitrazepam, postoperative respiratory depression in 8, and laryngospasm on extubation in 2. The dose of flunitrazepam was 50 µg per kg body-weight with a supplementary dose of 10 µg per kg if needed and an additional dose of 10 µg per kg at incision.— M. A. K. Mattila *et al.*, *Br. J. Anaesth.*, 1977, *49*, 1041.

In 20 women undergoing total abdominal hysterectomy, anaesthesia was induced by flunitrazepam 30 µg per kg body-weight given intravenously and maintained using ketamine. No patients experienced emergence phenomena associated with ketamine and no patients had retrograde amnesia. Only 2 patients reported dreaming.— P. J. C. Houlton and J. W. Downing, *S. Afr. med. J.*, 1978, *54*, 1048.

In a study of 92 patients undergoing bronchoscopy flunitrazepam 10 µg per kg body-weight intravenously had a greater amnesic effect than diazepam 125 µg per kg. When the doses were doubled the effects of the 2 drugs were comparable. Mean serum-concentrations of flunitrazepam 2 hours after injection were 25 and 58 ng per mL respectively for the 2 doses.— K. Korttila *et al.*, *Br.*

J. Anaesth., 1978, *50*, 281.

In a double-blind study in 142 children undergoing routine surgery, flunitrazepam was compared with diazepam as premedication. The drugs were given by mouth 90 minutes before operation and atropine was not given. Flunitrazepam was associated with greater sedation before operation and less vomiting after operation and a greater frequency of amnesia before and immediately after operation. Flunitrazepam, 1, 1.5, or 2 mg, or diazepam, 10, 15, or 20 mg, was given, according to body-weight, to children weighing 31 to 40 kg, 41 to 50 kg, or more than 50 kg respectively.— F. J. Richardson and M. L. M. Manford, *Br. J. Anaesth.*, 1979, *51*, 313.

Flunitrazepam 1 mg or diazepam 10 mg intravenously was given, as an adjunct to general anaesthesia, immediately before operation to 90 female patients undergoing abdominal surgery. The quality of anaesthesia was better and the need for supplementary doses of pethidine lower in the flunitrazepam group. Flunitrazepam appeared to have a greater amnesic action than diazepam. Recovery was equally good in both groups.— M. A. K. Mattila *et al.*, *Br. J. Anaesth.*, 1979, *51*, 329.

The use of flunitrazepam 20 µg per kg body-weight as a premedicant in children undergoing otolaryngological surgery.— L. Lindgren *et al.*, *Br. J. Anaesth.*, 1980, *52*, 283.

Flunitrazepam 1 to 2 mg was used to induce sedation in 50 patients undergoing dental surgery. Further doses of 0.25 to 1 mg were given as required to maintain an adequate degree of sedation, and ensured satisfactory conditions in the majority of patients throughout the operations, which lasted up to 3 hours. In only 9 patients was it necessary to give a local anaesthetic. The majority of patients remained slightly drowsy the next morning but patient acceptability of the technique was high.— T. F. Breen, *J. int. med. Res.*, 1985, *13*, 74.

Proprietary Preparations

Rohypnol *(Roche, UK). Tablets*, scored, flunitrazepam 1 mg.

Proprietary Names and Manufacturers

Darkene *(Sigurtà, Ital.)*; Flunipam *(A.L., Denm.; Apothekernes Laboratorium, Norw.)*; Libelius *(Chiesi, Ital.)*; Narcozep *(Roche, Fr.)*; Noriel *(Biogalenique, Fr.)*; Primun *(Labinca, Arg.)*; Rohipnol *(Roche, Spain)*; Rohypnol *(Roche, Arg.; Roche, Austral.; Roche, Belg.; Roche, Denm.; Roche, Fr.; Roche, Ger.; Roche, Neth.; Roche, Norw.; Roche, S.Afr.; Roche, Swed.; Roche, Switz.; Roche, UK)*; Roipnol *(Roche, Ital.)*; Valsera *(Polifarma, Ital.)*.

7041-w

Fluopromazine *(BAN)*.

Triflupromazine *(USAN, rINN)*. *NN*-Dimethyl-3-(2-trifluoromethylphenothiazin-10-yl)propylamine.

$C_{18}H_{19}F_3N_2S$=352.4.

CAS — 146-54-3.

Pharmacopoeias. In *U.S.*

A pale amber viscous oily liquid which forms into large irregular crystals during prolonged storage. Practically **insoluble** in water. **Store** in airtight containers. Protect from light.

7042-e

Fluopromazine Hydrochloride *(BANM)*.

Triflupromazine Hydrochloride *(USAN, rINNM)*.

$C_{18}H_{19}F_3N_2S,HCl$=388.9.

CAS — 1098-60-8.

Pharmacopoeias. In *Ind.* and *U.S.*

A white to pale tan crystalline powder with a slight characteristic odour.

Soluble 1 in less than 1 of water and of alcohol and 1 in 1.7 of chloroform; soluble in acetone; practically insoluble in ether. The *U.S.P.* injection has a pH of between 3.5 and 5.2. **Store** in well-closed containers. Protect from light.

Adverse Effects, Treatment, and Precautions

As for the phenothiazines in general, p.706.

Absorption and Fate

For an account of the absorption and fate of a phenothiazine, see Chlorpromazine, p.723.

Uses and Administration

Fluopromazine hydrochloride is a phenothiazine with actions and uses similar to those of chlorpromazine (p.724). In the management of psychosis, 60 to 150 mg may be given daily by intramuscular injection; it has also been given by mouth in doses of 100 to 150 mg daily.

For the control of nausea and vomiting 5 to 15 mg may be given intramuscularly and repeated after 4 hours if necessary; a dose of 1 mg to a maximum total daily dose of 3 mg may be given intravenously. Elderly or debilitated patients may be given 2.5 mg intramuscularly. A suggested intramuscular dose for children is 200 µg per kg body-weight daily up to a maximum of 10 mg daily.

Preparations of Fluopromazine and Fluopromazine Hydrochloride

Triflupromazine Hydrochloride Injection *(U.S.P.)*. A sterile solution of fluopromazine hydrochloride in Water for Injections.

Triflupromazine Hydrochloride Tablets *(U.S.P.)*. Tablets containing fluopromazine hydrochloride.

Triflupromazine Oral Suspension *(U.S.P.)*. A suspension containing fluopromazine. Potency is expressed in terms of the equivalent amount of fluopromazine hydrochloride.

Proprietary Names and Manufacturers of Fluopromazine and Fluopromazine Hydrochloride

Psyquil *(Squibb, Fr.; Heyden, Ger.; Squibb, Switz.)*; Siquil *(Squibb, Belg.; Squibb, Neth.; Squibb, NZ; Squibb, Switz.)*; Vesprin *(Squibb, Canad.; Squibb, USA)*.

7043-l

Fluoresone *(rINN)*.

ANP-215; Floretione. Ethyl 4-fluorophenyl sulphone.

$C_8H_9FO_2S$=188.2.

CAS — 2924-67-6.

Fluoresone has been used in neuropsychiatric disorders in doses of up to 2 g daily.

Proprietary Names and Manufacturers

Caducid *(IFI, Ital.)*.

7044-y

Flupenthixol Decanoate *(BANM)*.

Flupentixol Decanoate *(rINNM)*. 2-{4-[3-(2-Trifluoromethylthioxanthen-9-ylidene)propyl]piperazin-1-yl}ethyl decanoate.

$C_{33}H_{43}F_3N_2O_2S$=588.8.

CAS — 2709-56-0 (flupenthixol); 30909-51-4 (decanoate).

7045-j

Flupenthixol Hydrochloride *(BANM)*.

Flupenthixol Dihydrochloride; Flupentixol Hydrochloride *(rINNM)*; LC-44 *(flupenthixol)*; N-7009 *(flupenthixol)*. 2-{4-[3-(2-Trifluoromethylthioxanthen-9-ylidene)propyl]piperazin-1-yl}ethanol dihydrochloride.

$C_{23}H_{25}F_3N_2OS,2HCl$=507.4.

CAS — 2413-38-9.

STABILITY. Studies on the decomposition of flupenthixol hydrochloride in aqueous solution.— R. P. Enever *et al.*, *J. pharm. Sci.*, 1979, *68*, 169. See also A. Li Wan Po and W. J. Irwin (letter), *Pharm. J.*, 1978, *2*, 430; *J. Pharm. Pharmac.*, 1980, *32*, 25.

Adverse Effects and Treatment

As for the phenothiazines, p.706.

OVERDOSAGE. Experience with 28 cases of flupenthixol poisoning failed to show serious toxicity.— P. Crome *et al.* (letter), *Br. med. J.*, 1978, *1*, 859.

SUDDEN DEATH. A report of sudden death in 3 patients who had received depot injections of flupenthixol decanoate.— J. Turbott and W. M. I. Smeeton, *Aust. N.Z. J. Psychiatry*, 1984, *18*, 91.

URINARY INCONTINENCE. Nocturnal enuresis in 4 young women was associated with depot injections of antipsychotic agents. One was receiving flupenthixol.— A. Shaikh (letter), *Br. med. J.*, 1978, *1*, 1698.

Precautions

As for the phenothiazines, p.708.

Flupenthixol is not recommended for excitable or overactive patients.

INTERACTIONS. A report of sudden cardiorespiratory arrest and death in an apparently healthy subject given an intravenous infusion of a class I anti-arrhythmic, eproxindine, during a clinical study. The subject was subsequently found to have received a depot injection of flupenthixol the previous day. Displacement of flupenthixol from its plasma binding sites by the anti-arrhythmic may have been responsible.— A. Darragh *et al.*, *Lancet*, 1985, *1*, 93. Comment by the *UK* and Danish manufacturers. The suggested interaction is speculative and idiosyncrasy to eproxindine seems a more likely cause of the fatal cardiotoxicity in this patient.— J. M. Simister and A. Jorgensen (letter), *ibid.*, 343. Reply, and a reminder that sudden death is not unknown in patients receiving depot neuroleptics, including flupenthixol.— A. Darragh *et al.* (letter), *ibid.*, 756.

See also under Adverse Effects, above.

Absorption and Fate

Flupenthixol is readily absorbed from the gastro-intestinal tract and is probably subject to first-pass metabolism in the gut wall. It is also extensively metabolised in the liver and is excreted in the urine and faeces in the form of numerous metabolites; there is evidence of enterohepatic recycling. Owing to the first-pass effect, plasma concentrations following oral administration are much lower than those following estimated equivalent doses of the intramuscular depot preparation. Moreover, there is very wide intersubject variation in plasma concentrations of flupenthixol, but in practice, no simple correlation has been found between plasma concentrations of flupenthixol and its metabolites, and the therapeutic effect. Paths of metabolism of flupenthixol include sulphoxidation, side-chain *N*-dealkylation, and glucuronic acid conjugation. It is widely distributed in the body, and crosses the blood-brain barrier.

The decanoate ester of flupenthixol is very slowly absorbed from the site of intramuscular injection and is therefore suitable for depot injection. It is gradually released into the blood stream where it is rapidly hydrolysed to flupenthixol.

A detailed account of pharmacokinetic studies on flupenthixol and flupenthixol decanoate.— A. Jørgensen, *Drug Metab. Rev.*, 1978, *8*, 235.

ABSORPTION AND DISTRIBUTION. A study of the pharmacokinetics of flupenthixol and flupenthixol decanoate in 10 schizophrenic women who had been receiving either the oral or the depot preparation for at least 6 months. Peak values of radioactivity were obtained 3 to 8 hours after oral administration of radioactively labelled flupenthixol 1 mg to 5 of the women but secondary peaks were seen in all cases. In 3 of the subjects the serum concentration subsequently fell very slowly, while in 2 the fall was rather steep; the half-life of total radioactivity was several days. Following intramuscular administration of flupenthixol decanoate 28 or 40 mg in the other 5 women, the serum concentrations were noted to build up rather slowly with maximum values seen 11 to 17 days after injection, indicating a very slow release of the radioactive substance from the site of injection. A plateau was reached around and just after the time of maximum concentration, and was estimated to last within 20% of the maximum, for about 2 weeks. Concentrations in the CSF 11 days after injection were 29 to 55% of the corresponding serum concentrations.— A. Jørgensen and C. G. Gottfries, *Psychopharmacologia*, 1972, *27*, 1.

Small, but not unimportant, amounts of flupenthixol reached the foetuses of 5 women treated with oral or intramuscular forms of flupenthixol during pregnancy. Amounts in the mothers' milk were about 30% higher than those in their serum and were considered to be of no importance unless the neonate differs considerably from the adult in metabolism of, or sensitivity to, flupenthixol.— L. Kirk and A. Jørgensen, *Psychopharmacology*, 1980, *72*, 107.

Uses and Administration

Flupenthixol is a thioxanthene with general properties similar to those of the phenothiazine, chlorpromazine (p.724). Unlike chlorpromazine, a certain activating effect has been ascribed to flupenthixol and, accordingly, it is not indicated in overactive patients. Flupenthixol is administered as the hydrochloride by mouth or as the longer-acting decanoate ester by deep intramuscular injection.

The usual dose of the hydrochloride for the treatment of psychoses is 3 to 9 mg twice daily; the maximum recommended dose is a total of 18 mg daily. The long-acting decanoate should be given by deep intramuscular injection in an initial test dose of 20 mg, as 1 mL of a 2% oily solution. According to the patient's response over the following 5 to 10 days, this may be followed by doses of 20 to 40 mg at intervals of 2 to 4 weeks. Shorter dosage intervals or greater amounts may be required according to the patient's response. If doses greater than 40 mg are considered necessary they should be divided between 2 separate injection sites; patients requiring high-dose therapy with flupenthixol decanoate in single doses of 100 mg or more may be given an injection containing 100 mg of the decanoate per mL (10%).

In patients already taking antipsychotic agents by mouth, the dosage should be gradually reduced on starting flupenthixol decanoate injections. In those being transferred from depot injections of phenothiazines, flupenthixol decanoate 40 mg is considered to be equivalent to fluphenazine decanoate 25 mg.

Flupenthixol has also been given as the hydrochloride by mouth, for the treatment of depression, with or without anxiety. The usual initial dose is 1 mg daily, increased to a maximum of 3 mg daily in divided doses. The last dose should be given no later than 4 p.m. and if no effect has been noted within 1 week of administration of the maximum dose, the treatment should be withdrawn.

Flupenthixol should be given in reduced dosage to elderly patients.

ACTION. Patients taking α-flupenthixol [(*Z*)-flupenthixol] showed a significantly greater improvement after three weeks than patients who were taking equal doses of β-flupenthixol [(*E*)-flupenthixol] or a placebo, in a study of 45 patients suffering from acute schizophrenic illnesses. The α-isomer had more effect on the positive symptoms of the disease (hallucinations, delusions and thought disorder) but this difference was less apparent for the negative symptoms (psychomotor retardation, poverty of speech and disturbances of affect).— T. J. Crow *et al.*, *Br. J. clin. Pharmac.*, 1977, *4*, 648P. See also P. M. Cotes *et al.*, *ibid.*, 651P. There is evidence that distribution of the 2 isomers across the blood-brain barrier is similar.— T. J. Crow and E. C. Johnstone (letter), *Lancet*, 1978, *1*, 1050.

A comment that flupenthixol is a D_1 receptor antagonist.— P. Jenner and C. D. Marsden (letter), *Lancet*, 1979, *2*, 900.

ADMINISTRATION. Results of a 12-week double-blind study involving 23 female schizophrenic patients who had been resistant to previous therapy, demonstrated no significant difference between those given flupenthixol decanoate 40 mg every 2 weeks, and those given 200 mg every 2 weeks. Those in the high-dose group experienced significantly more extrapyramidal side-effects compared with scores before the trial, and 3 of 4 who experienced excessive salivation were in the high-dose group. Although plasma concentrations varied considerably, they were consistently higher in the high-dose group, and there was improvement in the mental state of a sub-group of patients in the high-dose group, who may have been resistant for pharmacokinetic reasons.— R. G. McCreadie *et al.*, *Br. J. Psychiat.*, 1979, *135*, 175.

It must be clearly remembered that increase in the dose of flupenthixol decanoate to more than 40 mg twice weekly nullifies those antidepressant and activating properties which are of benefit in schizo-affective psychoses.— A. N. Singh, *J. int. med. Res.*, 1984, *12*, 17.

Proprietary Preparations

Depixol *(Lundbeck, UK). Tablets*, flupenthixol 3 mg (as hydrochloride).

Injection, oily, flupenthixol decanoate 20 mg (as *cis*-(*Z*)-isomer)/mL, in ampoules and disposable syringes of 1 and 2 mL, and vials of 10 mL.

Injection (Depixol-Conc.), oily, flupenthixol decanoate 100 mg (as *cis*-(*Z*)-isomer)/mL, in ampoules of 0.5 mL and 1 mL and vials of 5 mL.

Fluanxol *(Lundbeck, UK). Tablets*, flupenthixol 0.5 and 1 mg (as hydrochloride).

Proprietary Names and Manufacturers of Flupenthixol Salts and Esters

Depixol *(Lundbeck, UK)*; Émergil *(Fr.)*; Fluanxol *(Belg.; Merrell Dow, Canad.; Lundbeck, Denm.; Labaz, Fr.; Tropon, Ger.; Neth.; Lundbeck, Norw.; Lundbeck, S.Afr.; Lundbeck, Swed.; Lundbeck, Switz.; Lundbeck, UK)*; Fluanxol Depot *(Belg.; Merrell Dow, Canad.; Lundbeck, Denm.; Tropon, Ger.; Neth.; Lundbeck, Norw.; Lundbeck, S.Afr.; Lundbeck, Swed.; Lundbeck, Switz.)*.

7046-z

Fluphenazine Decanoate *(BANM, rINNM)*.

2-{4-[3-(2-Trifluoromethylphenothiazin-10-yl)propyl]piperazin-1-yl}ethyl decanoate.

$C_{32}H_{44}F_3N_3O_2S$=591.8.

CAS — 69-23-8 (fluphenazine); 5002-47-1 (decanoate).

Pharmacopoeias. In *Br.*, *Cz.*, and *Int.*

A pale yellow viscous liquid or a yellow crystalline oily solid with a faint ester-like odour. Fluphenazine decanoate 12.5 mg is approximately equivalent to 10.75 mg of fluphenazine hydrochloride. Practically **insoluble** in water; miscible with dehydrated alcohol, chloroform, and ether; soluble in fixed oils. The *B.P.* injection is **sterilised** by filtration. **Protect** from light.

7047-c

Fluphenazine Enanthate *(BANM, USAN)*.

Fluphenazine Enantate *(rINNM)*.

Fluphenazine Heptanoate. 2-{4-[3-(2-Trifluoromethylphenothiazin-10-yl)propyl]piperazin-1-yl}ethyl heptanoate.

$C_{29}H_{38}F_3N_3O_2S$=549.7.

CAS — 2746-81-8.

Pharmacopoeias. In *Br.*, *Int.*, and *U.S.*

A pale yellow to yellow-orange, clear to slightly turbid, viscous liquid or a yellow crystalline oily solid with a faint ester-like odour. Fluphenazine enanthate 12.5 mg is approximately equivalent to 11.6 mg of fluphenazine hydrochloride.

Practically **insoluble** in water; soluble 1 in less than 1 of alcohol and of chloroform and 1 in 2 of ether; soluble in fixed oils. The *B.P.* injection is **sterilised** by filtration. **Stable** in air at room temperature but unstable in strong light. **Store** in airtight containers. Protect from light.

7048-k

Fluphenazine Hydrochloride *(BANM, USAN, rINNM)*.

2-{4-[3-(2-Trifluoromethylphenothiazin-10-yl)propyl]piperazin-1-yl}ethanol dihydrochloride.

$C_{22}H_{26}F_3N_3OS,2HCl$=510.4.

CAS — 146-56-5.

Pharmacopoeias. In *Br.*, *Braz.*, *Chin.*, *Fr.*, *Ind.*, *Int.*, *Jug.*, and *U.S.*

A white or almost white, odourless, crystalline powder.

The *B.P.* states that it is **soluble** 1 in 10 of water; sparingly soluble in alcohol, and in ether. *U.S.P.* solubilities are: 1 in 1.4 of water and 1 in 6.7 of alcohol; slightly soluble in chloroform and in acetone; practically insoluble in ether. A 5% solution in water has a pH of 1.9 to 2.3. The *U.S.P.* injection has a pH between 4.8 and 5.2, the elixir a pH between 5.3 and 5.8, and the oral solution a pH between 4 and 5. **Store** in airtight containers. Protect from light.

Adverse Effects and Treatment

As for the phenothiazines in general, p.706.

Results of a double-blind crossover study in 7 evaluable patients indicated an important incidence of akinesia, involuntary movement, autonomic disturbances, and drowsiness in the first few hours following injection of fluphenazine decanoate and in the first 2 days following injection of fluphenazine enanthate.— S. H. Curry *et al.* (letter), *Lancet*, 1979, *1*, 331.

EFFECTS ON THE BLOOD. Fluphenazine has been associated with agranulocytosis.— P. C. Vincent, *Drugs*, 1986, *31*, 52.

EFFECTS ON BODY TEMPERATURE. For reference to fatal heat stroke in a patient receiving fluphenazine together with an antimuscarinic agent and methotrimeprazine see under Benztropine Mesylate, p.528.

EFFECTS ON THE ENDOCRINE SYSTEM. A 33-year-old schizophrenic man developed inappropriate secretion of antidiuretic hormone 2 days after the intramuscular injection of fluphenazine enanthate 50 mg.— J. L. G. de Rivera (letter), *Ann. intern. Med.*, 1975, *82*, 811.

EFFECTS ON THE LIVER. A patient given 3 injections of a depot neuroleptic containing fluphenazine decanoate over a 2-week period subsequently developed jaundice, beginning 17 days after the first dose. The patient subsequently developed indicators of severe liver toxicity, with extreme hyperbilirubinaemia and raised liver enzyme values, and remained very ill for the next 4 months. The patient was subsequently found to exhibit cross-sensitivity to haloperidol but not to flupenthixol. The case illustrates the necessity to treat patients for at least 2 weeks with a short-acting preparation of any new neuroleptic before transferring to a longer-acting depot preparation.— P. Kennedy (letter), *Br. J. Psychiat.*, 1983, *143*, 312.

EFFECTS ON MENTAL FUNCTION. *Depression.* Sixteen patients, initially diagnosed as schizophrenics, developed severe depression after an injection of fluphenazine enanthate or decanoate. Five suicides were attributed to the depression. Careful supervision in the follow-up period was essential after treatment with these drugs.— R. de Alarcon and M. W. P. Carney, *Br. med. J.*, 1969, *3*, 564. Comment. In the author's experience mild depressive psychosis is not uncommon during the convalescent period in schizophrenics treated with oral phenothiazines also, particularly those of high potency.— J. Johnson (letter), *ibid.*, 718. Mood disturbance is a common feature of schizophrenia, and suicide not an uncommon outcome: the risks of not treating the condition are greater than those of treatment.— N. W. Imlah (letter), *ibid.*, 1969, *4*, 49.

EFFECTS ON THE SKIN. Fluphenazine has been reported to cause photosensitivity reactions.— *Med. Lett.*, 1986, *28*, 51.

EXTRAPYRAMIDAL EFFECTS. Severe unpredictable extrapyramidal symptoms, which were not fully responsive to antiparkinsonian drugs, were an additional reaction in schizophrenics who were treated with fluphenazine enanthate or fluphenazine decanoate.— M. Segal and D. H. Ropschitz, *Br. med. J.*, 1969, *4*, 169.

Acute dystonia affecting the face occurred in 2 patients taking fluphenazine hydrochloride 5 mg at night.— X. G. Okojie (letter), *Br. med. J.*, 1972, *4*, 796.

Studies in 6 patients receiving fluphenazine decanoate every 4 weeks for control of schizophrenia indicated that signs of parkinsonism were most severe in the third week after the injection; this was at variance with suggestions of 3 to 5 days after injection as the peak period.— P. Lamb *et al.* (letter), *Lancet*, 1976, *1*, 484.

A suggestion that more extrapyramidal side-effects are associated with fluphenazine enanthate than with the decanoate.— J. Kane *et al.*, *Am. J. Psychiat.*, 1978, *135*, 1539.

Neuroleptic malignant syndrome. A discussion of the neuroleptic malignant syndrome. Fluphenazine and haloperidol are the most commonly implicated drugs, although it has been reported with several other neuroleptics.— *Lancet*, 1984, *1*, 545.

NAUSEA AND VOMITING. Severe nausea and vomiting associated with fluphenazine therapy was successfully treated with benztropine.— C. E. McDanal and R. A. Markoff, *Hawaii med. J.*, 1978, *37*, 268.

OVERDOSAGE. A patient who took about 30 fluphenazine 2.5 mg tablets was treated by gastric lavage. Twenty hours after hospital admission he experienced difficulty in breathing due to spasm of the respiratory muscles; other very severe extrapyramidal side-effects were also present. Muscle spasm was controlled by diazepam.— F. M. Ladhani (letter), *Med. J. Aust.*, 1974, *2*, 26.

There were few ill effects in a patient given fluphenazine decanoate 50 mg every 4 hours, instead of the intended 4 weeks, to a total of 1050 mg. Three weeks after the period of overdosage the patient had some degree of hypothermia and tachycardia, and after a further week parkinsonian signs appeared. No specific treatment was given.— H. K. Cheung and E. C. S. Yu, *Br. med. J.*, 1983, *286*, 1016.

PREGNANCY AND THE NEONATE. Four weeks after delivery, an infant born to a schizophrenic woman who had received fluphenazine decanoate intramuscularly every 3 weeks throughout pregnancy, developed mild extrapyramidal symptoms. He had been breast fed for 5 days. The extrapyramidal symptoms responded readily to administration of diphenhydramine by mouth.— M. F. Cleary, *Am. J. Psychiat.*, 1977, *134*, 815.

A report of multiple congenital abnormalities in a child born to a mother who was receiving intramuscular injections of fluphenazine enanthate during pregnancy. The mother had also received other drugs, including dicyclomine and doxylamine, paracetamol, and amylobarbitone sodium while pregnant.— G. L. Donaldson and R. G. Bury, *Acta paediat. scand.*, 1982, *71*, 335.

SUDDEN DEATH. A 49-year-old man developed a syndrome similar to bulbar palsy, with absent gag reflexes, following treatment with fluphenazine enanthate. Such a syndrome could be responsible for occasional reports of sudden death due to aspiration or asphyxiation in patients receiving phenothiazines. It is not reversed by antiparkinsonian medication.— K. Solomon, *Am. J. Psychiat.*, 1977, *134*, 308.

URINARY INCONTINENCE. Nocturnal enuresis in 3 young women was associated with fluphenazine decanoate therapy.— A. Shaikh (letter), *Br. med. J.*, 1978, *1*, 1698.

TREATMENT OF ADVERSE EFFECTS. In 8 patients who were receiving fluphenazine enanthate injections every 2 or 3 weeks, an attempt was made, under double-blind conditions, to replace benzhexol (given to reduce extrapyramidal side-effects of fluphenazine) with a placebo. Four patients developed severe reactions which indicated their continued need of benzhexol. Periodic review of the need for and dose of benzhexol was however justified.— L. Grove and J. L. Crammer, *Br. med. J.*, 1972, *1*, 276.

A 49-year-old man suffered a very severe parkinsonian syndrome associated with depression after receiving (in addition to amitriptyline and diazepam) fluphenazine decanoate 150 mg over 5 weeks with no antiparkinsonian medication. Both his parkinsonian symptoms and his depression responded remarkably to treatment with antiparkinsonian drugs.— A. H. Fry and A. W. Beard, *Practitioner*, 1977, *218*, 874.

A report of the beneficial effect of propranolol in preventing akathisia and tremor following injections of fluphenazine decanoate in an elderly patient. Propranolol was also effective in preventing these symptoms when the patient was given thiothixene.— R. Wilbur and A. V. Kulik (letter), *Lancet*, 1983, *2*, 917.

Precautions

As for the phenothiazines in general, p.708.

A report of dystonic reaction to fluphenazine causing risk to a patient while swimming.— M. W. Dysken and J. M. Davis (letter), *Br. med. J.*, 1978, *2*, 1164.

INTERACTIONS. *Clonidine*. Delirium in a 33-year-old man, was considered to have been caused by concomitant administration of clonidine and fluphenazine decanoate.— R. M. Allen and A. Flemenbaum, *J. clin. Psychiat.*, 1979, *40*, 236.

Lithium. A report of an acute neurotoxic reaction, manifest as tremor, confusion, ataxia, and severe dysarthria, in a patient receiving intramuscular fluphenazine decanoate injection and oral lithium carbonate.— S. V. Singh (letter), *Lancet*, 1982, *2*, 278.

Vitamins. Increase in manic behaviour necessitating increase in dosage with fluphenazine followed treatment with ascorbic acid to reduce vitamin C deficiency in a patient with steady-state fluphenazine plasma-concentrations.— M. W. Dysken *et al.* (letter), *J. Am. med. Ass.*, 1979, *241*, 2008.

Absorption and Fate

For an account of the absorption and fate of a phenothiazine, see Chlorpromazine, p.723.

Fluphenazine decanoate and fluphenazine enanthate are very slowly absorbed from the site of subcutaneous or intramuscular injection. They both gradually release fluphenazine into the body and are therefore suitable for use as depot injections.

The plasma half-life of fluphenazine after a single dose was 14.7 hours in 1 patient given the hydrochloride by mouth and 14.9 and 15.3 hours in 2 patients given the hydrochloride by intramuscular injection. The half-life was 3.6 and 3.7 days in 2 patients given the enanthate intramuscularly and 9.6 and 6.8 days in 2 patients given the decanoate intramuscularly. Fluphenazine sulphoxide and 7-hydroxyfluphenazine were identified in the urine and faeces.— S. H. Curry *et al.*, *Br. J. clin. Pharmac.*, 1979, *7*, 325. See also *idem* (letter), *Lancet*, 1978, *1*, 1217; K. K. Midha *et al.*, *Eur. J. clin. Pharmac.*, 1983, *25*, 709.

Slow decline, over a period of several months, of plasma drug and prolactin concentrations after discontinuation of chronic treatment with fluphenazine decanoate.— B. Wistedt *et al.* (letter), *Lancet*, 1981, *1*, 1163.

PLASMA PROTEIN BINDING. For the comparative protein binding of fluphenazine and other phenothiazines, see Chlorpromazine, p.723.

Uses and Administration

Fluphenazine is a potent phenothiazine with actions and uses similar to those of chlorpromazine (p.724). It has a piperazine side-chain. Fluphenazine is administered as the hydrochloride usually by mouth or as the longer-acting decanoate or enanthate esters by intramuscular or sometimes subcutaneous injection.

The usual initial dose of the hydrochloride for the treatment of psychoses is 2.5 to 10 mg daily in two to three divided doses; in severe schizophrenia up to 20 mg daily has been given. Dosage may subsequently be reduced to a usual maintenance dose of 1 to 5 mg daily. Treatment is sometimes started with intramuscular injections of 1.25 mg of the hydrochloride.

The long-acting decanoate or enanthate esters of fluphenazine are usually given by deep intramuscular injection. The onset of action is usually within 1 to 3 days of injection and significant effects on psychosis are usually evident within 2 to 4 days. The initial dose of fluphenazine decanoate or enanthate is 12.5 mg intramuscularly given to patients in hospital to assess the extrapyramidal effects. A dose of 25 mg may then be given every 2 weeks with subsequent adjustments in the amounts and the dosage interval according to the patient's response; the amounts required may range from 12.5 to 100 mg and the intervals required may range from 1 or 2 weeks to 5 or 6 weeks. If doses greater than 50 mg are considered necessary cautious increments should be made in steps of 12.5 mg.

Fluphenazine hydrochloride has also been given in doses of 1 to 2 mg daily, increased if necessary to 2 to 4 mg daily, for non-psychotic emotional disturbances, such as anxiety and tension. In general, however, neuroleptics are only suitable for such purposes in resistant conditions where more appropriate agents, such as the benzodiazepines (see Diazepam, p.731) have proved ineffective. If neuroleptic use is judged to be necessary, treatment should be directed at low dosages given on a short-term basis.

Fluphenazine should be given in reduced dosage to elderly patients.

ADMINISTRATION. A study substantiating earlier findings of a higher incidence of side-effects in patients receiving long-term intramuscular fluphenazine decanoate therapy than in those receiving fluphenazine by mouth.— A. Rifkin *et al.*, *Archs gen. Psychiat.*, 1977, *34*, 1215.

A study of the plasma concentrations of fluphenazine following intramuscular injection of 25 mg of the decanoate in 2 subjects and intramuscular injection of 25 mg of the enanthate in a further 2 subjects. The decanoate gave an early peak in keeping with its use in acute psychotic states whereas the enanthate gave its highest concentrations after 2 to 5 days.— S. H. Curry *et al.* (letter), *Lancet*, 1978, *1*, 1217.

High-dose therapy. A review of megadose therapy with fluphenazine using dosage regimens ranging from 0.8 to 1.2 g daily (equivalent to chlorpromazine 40 to 60 g daily). Three studies in chronic schizophrenics who were long-term hospital in-patients showed some improvement with megadose therapy. In acute patients, however, who had not responded to at least 6 weeks of standard treatment but who had been in hospital for less than 2 months, a better response was obtained in those given 30 mg daily than in those given 1.2 g daily, indicating that schizophrenics should not be considered refractory after only 6 weeks of treatment. The value of megadose therapy in long-term patients remains problematic since a limited degree of improvement may not be worth the increased risk of tardive dyskinesia. One remarkable finding in all studies is that such enormous doses are relatively well tolerated; the increase in extrapyramidal side-effects, typically seen as the dose approaches 30 mg daily, reaches a plateau or diminishes.— A. Rifkin and F. Quitkin, *Bull. N.Y. Acad. Med.*, 1978, *54*, 869.

BEHAVIOUR DISORDERS. Ten adolescent girls, disturbed, violent, and aggressive, had been treated for up to a year with fluphenazine decanoate 12.5 to 25 mg or flupenthixol decanoate 20 to 40 mg with benefit both at weekly to monthly intervals; 3 had been able to cease treatment.— M. S. Perinpanayagam and R. A. Haig (letter), *Br. med. J.*, 1977, *1*, 835. See also H. G. Kinnell (letter), *ibid.*, 1977, *2*, 578.

CHOREA. In a double-blind study in 9 patients, fluphenazine decanoate injection was more effective than a placebo in reducing chorea.— C. F. Terrence, *Curr. ther. Res.*, 1976, *20*, 177.

LESCH-NYHAN SYNDROME. Reference to a possible beneficial effect of fluphenazine in preventing self-mutilation in patients with Lesch-Nyhan syndrome.— M. Goldstein *et al.* (letter), *Lancet*, 1985, *1*, 338.

PAIN. For references to the use of fluphenazine in neurological pain, see Amitriptyline Hydrochloride, p.356.

Preparations of Fluphenazine Salts and Esters

Fluphenazine Decanoate Injection *(B.P.)*. A sterile solution of fluphenazine decanoate in sesame oil. For intramuscular use only.

Fluphenazine Enanthate Injection *(B.P.)*. A sterile solution of fluphenazine enanthate in sesame oil. For intramuscular use only.

Fluphenazine Enanthate Injection *(U.S.P.)*

Fluphenazine Hydrochloride Elixir *(U.S.P.)*. An elixir containing fluphenazine hydrochloride and alcohol 13.5 to 15%.

Fluphenazine Hydrochloride Injection *(U.S.P.)*

Fluphenazine Hydrochloride Tablets *(U.S.P.)*

Fluphenazine Hydrochloride Oral Solution *(U.S.P.)*. An aqueous solution of fluphenazine hydrochloride and not more than 15% alcohol. To be diluted before use.

Fluphenazine Tablets *(B.P.)*. Tablets containing fluphenazine hydrochloride.

Proprietary Preparations of Fluphenazine Salts and Esters

Modecate *(Squibb, UK)*. *Injection*, oily, fluphenazine decanoate 25 mg/mL, in ampoules of 0.5, 1, and 2 mL, disposable syringes of 1 and 2 mL, and vials of 10 mL. *Injection* (Modecate Concentrate), oily, fluphenazine decanoate 100 mg/mL, in ampoules of 0.5 and 1 mL.

Moditen *(Squibb, UK)*. *Tablets*, fluphenazine hydrochloride 1, 2.5, and 5 mg.
Injection (Moditen Enanthate), oily, fluphenazine enanthate 25 mg/mL, in ampoules of 1 mL.

Proprietary Names and Manufacturers of Fluphenazine Salts and Esters

Anatenazine *(Jpn)*; Anatensol *(Squibb, Austral.; Belg.; Squibb, Ital.; Neth.; Squibb, S.Afr.)*; Dapotum *(Heyden, Ger.; Squibb, Switz.)*; Eutimox *(Spain)*; Lyogen *(Promonta, Ger.; Byk Gulden, Switz.)*; Modecate *(Squibb, Austral.; Squibb, Canad.; Squibb, Fr.; Squibb, S.Afr.; Squibb, Spain; Squibb, UK)*; Moditen *(Belg.; Squibb, Canad.; Squibb, Fr.; Squibb, Ital.; Neth.; Switz.; Squibb, UK)*; Omca *(Heyden, Ger.)*; Pacinol *(Schering Corp., Denm.; Schering, Norw.; Schering, Swed.)*; Permitil *(Belg.; Schering, Canad.; Schering, USA)*; Prolixin *(Princeton, USA)*; Sevinol *(Belg.)*; Siqualone *(Novo, Norw.; Squibb, Swed.)*.

4035-e

Flurazepam Monohydrochloride *(BANM, rINNM)*.

7-Chloro-1-(2-diethylaminoethyl)-5-(2-fluorophenyl)-1,3-dihydro-1,4-benzodiazepin-2-one hydrochloride.

$C_{21}H_{23}ClFN_3O,HCl = 424.4$.

CAS — 17617-23-1 (flurazepam); 36105-20-1 (monohydrochloride).

Pharmacopoeias. In *Br.*

A white or almost white, odourless or almost odourless crystalline powder. Very **soluble** in water; freely soluble in alcohol; practically insoluble in ether. A 5% solution has a pH of 5 to 6. Flurazepam monohydrochloride 32.8 mg is

approximately equivalent to 30 mg of flurazepam.
Store in well-closed containers at a temperature of 8° to 15°.

4036-l

Flurazepam Hydrochloride *(USAN, rINNM).*

Flurazepam Dihydrochloride *(BANM)*; NSC-78559; Ro-5-6901.
$C_{21}H_{23}ClFN_3O,2HCl=460.8$.
CAS — 1172-18-5.

Pharmacopoeias. In *U.S.*

An off-white to yellow, odourless or almost odourless, crystalline powder. Flurazepam hydrochloride 30 mg is approximately equivalent to 25.3 mg of flurazepam. **Soluble** 1 in 2 of water, 1 in 4 of alcohol, 1 in 90 of chloroform, 1 in 3 of methyl alcohol, and 1 in 69 of isopropyl alcohol; very slightly soluble in ether and petroleum spirit. A solution in water is acid to litmus. **Store** in airtight containers. Protect from light.

Dependence, Adverse Effects, Treatment, and Precautions

As for the benzodiazepines in general, p.706.

DEPENDENCE. A report of 2 cases of flurazepam dependence. Both patients experienced marked withdrawal symptoms on discontinuation.— *Clin. Pharm.*, 1984, *3*, 316.

See also under Effects on Sexual Function, below.

Drug abuse. Reference to the intravenous abuse of flurazepam in order to relieve symptoms of opiate withdrawal.— J. Strang, *Br. med. J.*, 1984, *289*, 964.

EFFECTS ON THE LIVER. Reports of cholestatic jaundice following the use of flurazepam: M. H. Fang *et al.*, *Ann. intern. Med.*, 1978, *89*, 363; R. Reynolds *et al.*, *Can. med. Ass. J.*, 1981, *124*, 893.

EFFECTS ON SEXUAL FUNCTION. In 2 women in whom long-term flurazepam treatment was abruptly stopped severe withdrawal symptoms were accompanied by a marked increase in libido, in one case amounting to feelings of intense and almost constant sexual arousal which were only slightly abated by sexual intercourse. This increased sexual function was suppressed in both cases when the patients were restarted on an alternative benzodiazepine.— D. Nutt *et al.* (letter), *Lancet*, 1986, *2*, 1101.

PORPHYRIA. Flurazepam was considered to be unsafe in patients with acute porphyria because it has been shown to be porphyrinogenic in *animals* or *in vitro* systems.— M.R. Moore and K.E.L. McColl, *Porphyrias, Drug Lists*, Glasgow, Porphyria Research Unit, University of Glasgow, 1987.

TASTE DISTURBANCES. Flurazepam had been reported to cause dysgeusia.— J. M. T. Willoughby, *Adverse Drug React. Bull.*, 1983, Jun., 368.

Absorption and Fate

Flurazepam is fairly readily absorbed from the gastro-intestinal tract. It is rapidly metabolised and the metabolites and very little unchanged drug are excreted in the urine. The major active metabolite is *N*-desalkylflurazepam, which is reported to have a half-life ranging from 47 to 100 hours or more.

The metabolism of flurazepam was studied in 4 healthy male volunteers given 30 mg daily for 2 weeks. A hydroxyethyl metabolite was present in the blood shortly after administration. The *N*-desalkyl metabolite, the major metabolite in the blood, had a half-life ranging from 47 to 100 hours. Steady-state concentrations were reached after 7 to 10 days and were approximately 5 to 6 times greater than those observed on day 1.— S. A. Kaplan *et al.*, *J. pharm. Sci.*, 1973, *62*, 1932.

A review of the therapeutic activity of drug metabolites including those of flurazepam.— D. E. Drayer, *Clin. Pharmacokinet.*, 1976, *1*, 426.

A study in 3 patients indicating that following administration by mouth some metabolism of flurazepam occurred in the small bowel mucosa.— W. A. Mahon *et al.*, *Clin. Pharmac. Ther.*, 1977, *22*, 228.

Kinetics and clinical effects of flurazepam in young and elderly non-insomniac adults.— D. J. Greenblatt *et al.*, *Clin. Pharmac. Ther.*, 1981, *30*, 475.

Uses and Administration

Flurazepam is a benzodiazepine derivative with general properties similar to those of diazepam (see p.731). It is used as a hypnotic in the short-term management of insomnia. In the *USA* flurazepam is given in doses of 15 to 30 mg of the dihydrochloride (flurazepam hydrochloride) at night. In the *UK* it is given as the monohydrochloride in doses equivalent to 15 to 30 mg of flurazepam at night.

ADMINISTRATION IN THE ELDERLY. The frequency of reported toxicity due to flurazepam increased with age in a study from the Boston Collaborative Drug Surveillance Program involving 2542 patients in hospital for medical treatment, more than 40% of whom were over 60 years of age. None of the side-effects was serious and most related to residual drowsiness. Of patients aged under 60 years, 1.9% experienced unwanted effects whereas of those aged 80 or over toxicity reached 7.1%. Higher doses increased the frequency of adverse reactions this effect being most marked in the elderly; of patients aged 70 years or more who received an average dose of 30 mg or more, 39% experienced side-effects whereas at doses under 15 mg daily side-effects occurred in no more than 2% regardless of age.— D. J. Greenblatt *et al.*, *Clin. Pharmac. Ther.*, 1977, *21*, 355.

ADMINISTRATION IN RENAL FAILURE. Five patients on maintenance haemodialysis developed encephalopathy attributed to flurazepam and diazepam.— L. Taclob and M. Needle, *Lancet*, 1976, *2*, 704.

Flurazepam could be given in usual doses to patients with renal failure.— W. M. Bennett *et al.*, *Am. J. Kidney Dis.*, 1983, *3*, 155.

Preparations of Flurazepam Salts

Flurazepam Capsules *(B.P.).* Flurazepam Monohydrochloride Capsules. Contain flurazepam monohydrochloride. Potency is stated in terms of the equivalent amount of flurazepam.

Flurazepam Hydrochloride Capsules *(U.S.P.).* Contain flurazepam hydrochloride (dihydrochloride).

Proprietary Preparations

Dalmane *(Roche, UK). Capsules*, flurazepam monohydrochloride 16.4 and 32.8 mg (equivalent to flurazepam 15 and 30 mg).

Proprietary Names and Manufacturers of Flurazepam Salts

Benozil *(Jpn)*; Dalmadorm *(Roche, Denm.; Roche, Ger.; Roche, Ital.; Neth.; Roche, Norw.; Roche, S.Afr.; Sauter, Switz.)*; Dalmane *(Roche, Austral.; Roche, Canad.; Roche, UK; Roche, USA)*; Dalmate *(Jpn)*; Dormodor *(Roche, Spain)*; Felison *(Sigurtà, Ital.)*; Felmane *(Steinhard, UK)*; Flunox *(Boehringer Biochemia, Ital.)*; Fordrim *(Arg.)*; Insumin *(Jpn)*; Midorm A.R. *(Piam, Ital.)*; Natam *(Arg.)*; Niotal *(Belg.)*; Novoflupam *(Novopharm, Canad.)*; Paxane *(Steinhard, UK)*; Remdue *(Biomedica Foscama, Ital.)*; Somlan *(Arg.)*; Somnol *(Horner, Canad.)*; Som-Pam *(ICN, Canad.)*; Staurodorm *(Dolorgiet, Ger.)*; Valdorm *(Valeas, Ital.)*.

7049-a

Fluspirilene *(BAN, USAN, rINN).*

R-6218. 8-[4,4-Bis(4-fluorophenyl)butyl]-1-phenyl-1,3,8-triazaspiro[4.5]decan-4-one.
$C_{29}H_{31}F_2N_3O=475.6$.
CAS — 1841-19-6.

Adverse Effects, Treatment, and Precautions

As for the phenothiazines, p.706.

Of 24 patients who had been given fluspirilene injections weekly, 8 had deep subcutaneous lumps at the injection site; in a further 4 patients increased pressure was necessary to give the injection. Biopsy in one patient showed necrosis probably caused by precipitation of crystalline fluspirilene.— R. G. McCreadie *et al.*, *Br. med. J.*, 1979, *1*, 523.

Absorption and Fate

Fluspirilene is slowly absorbed after intramuscular injection of a microcrystalline aqueous suspension, detectable blood concentrations being reached within 4 hours of injection. It is rapidly metabolised on release from the injection site and the main metabolite, which is 4,4-bis(4-fluorophenyl)butyric acid obtained by *N*-dealkylation, is excreted in the urine.

Uses and Administration

Fluspirilene is a member of the diphenylbutylpiperidine group of antipsychotic agents which are structurally similar to the butyrophenones (see Haloperidol, p.743). When given by deep intramuscular injection it has a prolonged duration of action which lasts for about a week, with a range of 5 to 15 days.

The usual dose of fluspirilene for the treatment of schizophrenia is 2 mg weekly by deep intramuscular injection, increased by 2 mg weekly according to the patient's response. The usual maintenance dose is 2 to 8 mg weekly but in resistant conditions up to 12 mg weekly may be required. The maximum recommended dose is 20 mg weekly. Accumulation of fluspirilene, with signs of overdosage, may be managed by omission of one in 4 or 5 weekly injections.

ANXIETY. Fluspirilene 2 to 4 mg weekly given intramuscularly to 8 resistant neurotic patients was reported to be of value in patients with paranoid, depressive, or phobic symptoms associated with behavioural irritability, but not for patients whose symptoms were entirely subjective.— E. H. Bennie (letter), *Br. med. J.*, 1976, *1*, 1404.

Four patients with anxiety neurosis, anxiety state, or anorexia nervosa responded favourably to fluspirilene.— M. Trimble (letter), *Br. med. J.*, 1977, *2*, 1541.

Proprietary Preparations

Redeptin *(Smith Kline & French, UK). Injection*, fluspirilene 2 mg/mL, in ampoules of 1 and 3 mL, and vials of 6 mL.

Proprietary Names and Manufacturers

Imap *(Arg.; Belg.; McNeil, Canad.; Denm.; Janssen, Ger.; Neth.; Janssen, Norw.; Janssen, Switz.)*; Redeptin *(Smith Kline & French, UK)*.

16815-h

Flutazolam *(rINN).*

10-Chloro-11b-(2-fluorophenyl)-2,3,7,11b-tetrahydro-7-(2-hydroxyethyl)-oxazolo[3,2-*d*][1,4]benzodiazepin-6(5*H*)-one.
$C_{19}H_{18}ClFN_2O_3=376.8$.
CAS — 27060-91-9.

Flutazolam is a benzodiazepine derivative with general properties similar to those of diazepam (p.728). It has been used for its anxiolytic and sedative properties in doses of 4 mg three times daily.

Proprietary Names and Manufacturers

Coleminal *(Mitsui, Jpn)*.

12767-n

Flutroline *(USAN, rINN).*

CP-36584. (±)-8-Fluoro-α,5-bis(4-fluorophenyl)-1,3,4,5-tetrahydro-2*H*-pyrido[4,3-*b*]indol-2-ylbutan-1-ol.
$C_{27}H_{25}F_3N_2O=450.5$.
CAS — 70801-02-4.

Flutroline has been tried in the management of schizophrenia.

Results of a preliminary study involving 48 schizophrenic patients given flutroline indicated that doses of 20 mg or above, given once daily by mouth, were likely to be required for a beneficial effect.— A. A. Kurland *et al.*, *J. clin. Pharmac.*, 1982, *22*, 441. See also A. A. Kurland *et al.*, *ibid.*, 1983, *23*, 505.

Proprietary Names and Manufacturers

Pfizer, USA.

4037-y

Glutethimide *(BAN, USAN, rINN).*

Glutethimidum; Glutetimide. 2-Ethyl-2-phenylglutarimide; 3-Ethyl-3-phenylpiperidine-2,6-dione.
$C_{13}H_{15}NO_2$=217.3.

CAS — 77-21-4.

Pharmacopoeias. In *Belg., Br., Chin., Cz., Int., Jug., Pol.* (which also includes the monohydrate), and *U.S.*

Odourless or almost odourless colourless crystals or white crystalline powder.

Practically **insoluble** in water; soluble 1 in 5 of alcohol, 1 in less than 1 of chloroform, and 1 in 12 of ether; freely soluble in acetone and ethyl acetate; soluble in methyl alcohol. A saturated solution in water is acid to litmus. **Store** in well-closed containers. Protect from light.

STABILITY. Hydrolysis of glutethimide was a base-catalysed first-order reaction. At pH 5 the chemical half-life was 28.3 years at 25° and 1.02 months at pH 8, with decreasing stability at higher pH. Hydrolysis to 4-ethyl-4-phenylglutaramic acid occurred, and the use of the water-soluble glutethimide hydrochloride was suggested.— J. W. Wesolowski *et al., J. pharm. Sci.*, 1968, *57,* 811.

Dependence

As for the barbiturates, p.706.

ABUSE. A warning of the hazards associated with the abuse of glutethimide in a combination termed 'loads'.— J. J. Sramek and A. Khajawall (letter), *New Engl. J. Med.*, 1981, *305,* 231.

A report of chronic glutethimide abuse over 8 or 9 years culminating in severe tremor and incoordination rendering the patient unable to walk, faecal incontinence, and dysarthria. These symptoms resolved following withdrawal of the drug over 2 weeks.— A. H. Jones and J. F. Mayberry, *Br. J. clin. Pract.*, 1986, *40,* 213.

DEPENDENCE. Manifestations of glutethimide withdrawal had been reported to include nausea, vomiting, abdominal cramping, tachycardia, sweating, fever, agitation, and tremulousness. Major reactions included convulsions, or delirium, or both, characterised by confusion, disorientation, and hallucinations. The lowest dosages reported to have been followed by abstinence convulsions were 2.5 g and 5 g daily in 2 patients who had taken the drug for 3 months and 'several weeks' respectively.— C. F. Essig, *J. Am. med. Ass.*, 1966, *196,* 714.

Facial grimacing and a catatonia-like psychosis in a 37-year-old woman might have been due to glutethimide withdrawal in association with antihistamine administration.— M. I. Good, *Am. J. Psychiat.*, 1976, *133,* 1454.

A further report of catatonia associated with glutethimide withdrawal.— R. Campbell *et al., J. clin. Psychiat.*, 1983, *44,* 32.

NEONATAL DEPENDENCE. Neonatal withdrawal symptoms in an infant born to a mother addicted to diamorphine and glutethimide initially responded to chlorpromazine. Recurrence on the tenth day might have been due to glutethimide withdrawal.— M. Reveri *et al., Clin. Pediat.*, 1977, *16,* 424.

Adverse Effects

In therapeutic doses side-effects include nausea, headache, excitement, hang-over, blurred vision, and occasional skin rashes. Acute hypersensitivity reactions, blood disorders and exfoliative dermatitis have been reported in rare instances.

Overdosage with glutethimide produces symptoms similar to those of barbiturate overdosage; respiratory depression is usually less, and circulatory failure more severe than with the barbiturates (see p.706). There are considerable fluctuations in the depth of coma and wakefulness. Sudden apnoea, possibly linked to cerebral oedema, and convulsions may occur; severe hypotension may be unresponsive to volume expansion. Antimuscarinic effects such as mydriasis, dryness of the mouth, paralytic ileus, and urinary bladder atony often occur. Irregular absorption and storage in fat depots may complicate treatment.

Chronic ingestion of high doses of glutethimide is associated with impaired memory, inability to concentrate, impaired gait, ataxia, tremors, hyporeflexia, and slurring of speech; convulsions may also occur. Sudden withdrawal may produce symptoms ranging from nervousness and anxiety to grand mal convulsions.

EFFECTS ON THE BLOOD. A man aged 47, estimated to have taken 100 to 400 mg daily of glutethimide for 5 years, had megaloblastic anaemia and a haemoglobin value of 41%. Following drug withdrawal, he was given 20 mg of folic acid thrice daily. Within 7 days the haemoglobin rose to 80% and subsequently the dosage of folic acid was reduced to 15 mg daily. Haematological and other examinations indicated that the anaemia was probably due to glutethimide.— D. Pearson (letter), *Lancet*, 1965, *1,* 110.

EFFECTS ON THE BONES. For a report of osteomalacia following long-term glutethimide therapy see under Precautions, below.

EFFECTS ON THE NERVOUS SYSTEM. A woman who had taken increasingly large doses of glutethimide (up to 5 g daily) for about 5 years developed peripheral neuropathy and cerebral impairment, which persisted after the drug had been withdrawn.— R. Nover, *Clin. Pharmac. Ther.*, 1967, *8,* 283.

Three patients developed peripheral neuritis and cerebellar ataxia following prolonged glutethimide ingestion in doses varying from 0.75 to 4 g daily.— D. C. Haas and A. Marasigan, *J. Neurol. Neurosurg. Psychiat.*, 1968, *31,* 561.

A patient who took glutethimide about 15 to 22.5 g by mouth in a suicide attempt recovered with conventional support therapy. In the absence of cerebral ischaemia or hypoxaemia secondary to cardiopulmonary depression, complete clinical recovery from glutethimide-induced coma appeared to be possible no matter how severe the presenting neurological and EEG signs.— R. R. Myers and J. J. Stockard, *Clin. Pharmac. Ther.*, 1975, *17,* 212.

See also under Dependence, above.

Treatment of Adverse Effects

As for the barbiturates, p.708.

Forced diuresis is of no value in the management of glutethimide poisoning and is potentially hazardous, while haemodialysis, even with a lipid dialysate such as soya oil, has not been conclusively shown to offer any advantage over intensive supportive care. Where measures to enhance elimination are appropriate, haemoperfusion is the treatment of choice.

Precautions

Glutethimide is contra-indicated in patients with porphyria. Because of its antimuscarinic actions it should be given with great care to patients with conditions such as closed-angle glaucoma, prostatic hypertrophy or urinary tract obstruction, or cardiac arrhythmias, which may be exacerbated by such action.

Glutethimide causes drowsiness and patients receiving it should not take charge of vehicles or machinery where loss of attention could lead to accidents. These effects are enhanced by the simultaneous administration of depressants of the central nervous system such as alcohol, barbiturates, and other sedatives. Absorption of glutethimide is also markedly enhanced by concomitant administration of alcohol. Like the barbiturates glutethimide induces microsomal hepatic enzymes, and it can thus cause increased metabolism of coumarin anticoagulants and other drugs, with reduced effect. Chronic administration of glutethimide may also enhance vitamin D metabolism.

INTERACTIONS. *Calcium and vitamin D.* An elderly woman who ingested 18.75 g of glutethimide developed prolonged hypocalcaemia with an isolated episode of severe hypocalcaemia. She eventually recovered after about 7 weeks.— J. A. Crawshaw, *Practitioner*, 1968, *200,* 739.

A 53-year-old woman whose diet contained marginally adequate amounts of vitamin D and who had taken glutethimide 500 mg at night for 10 years developed osteomalacia. Study showed that this was due to increased enzymatic metabolism of cholecalciferol caused by glutethimide. Nitrazepam did not appear to have this effect.— R. H. Greenwood *et al., Br. med. J.*, 1973, *1,* 643.

Absorption and Fate

Glutethimide is irregularly absorbed from the gastro-intestinal tract and extensively metabolised in the liver. It has a biphasic plasma half-life. Glutethimide is excreted in urine, almost entirely as metabolites, with less than 2% of unchanged drug. Up to 2% of a dose has been reported to be present in the faeces. Glutethimide is reported to be about 50% bound to plasma proteins. It is highly lipid-soluble and may be stored in adipose tissue. It crosses the placental barrier and traces are found in breast milk.

ABSORPTION AND EXCRETION. Following oral administration of glutethimide 500 mg to 6 healthy subjects absorption was irregular with peak plasma-glutethimide concentrations of 2.85 to 7.05 µg per mL being achieved after 1 to 6 hours. In 4 of the 6 subjects decline after the peak was biphasic with initial half-lives of 2.7 to 4.3 hours and subsequent half-lives of 5.1 to 22 hours. Plasma protein binding of glutethimide was about 50%; little unmetabolised drug was excreted in the urine of 3 subjects studied. Mean glutethimide concentrations in the breast milk of 13 nursing mothers given 500 mg were 0.27, 0.27, 0.22, 0.12, and 0.04 µg per mL at 8, 12, 16, 20, and 23 hours respectively but in 32 of the 90 samples analysed no glutethimide was detected. Maternal and neonatal plasma concentrations were found to be similar when 4 women were given 1 g of glutethimide about 2 hours before parturition.— S. H. Curry *et al., Clin. Pharmac. Ther.*, 1971, *12,* 849. See also *idem, Br. J. clin. Pharmac.*, 1977, *4,* 109.

METABOLISM. Glutethimide was completely metabolised in the body and excreted mainly in the bile; there was considerable intestinal reabsorption, which consequently prolonged its action.— L. E. Hollister, *Clin. Pharmac. Ther.*, 1966, *7,* 142. Little unmetabolised glutethimide was detected in the bile of *dogs* and 5 patients undergoing biliary drainage who were given glutethimide. It was considered that the enterohepatic circulation had no significant effect on the absorption or excretion of glutethimide.— C. Charytan, *ibid.*, 1970, *11,* 816.

Two young women who went into coma after ingesting glutethimide woke after 24 hours, went back into a coma 12 hours later, and woke again about 40 hours after ingesting the drug. Concentrations of glutethimide in the serum rose and fell in correlation with the patients' states of consciousness; with a serum concentration of over 20 µg per mL the patients were asleep. Enterohepatic recirculation and other causes were suggested in explanation of the second peak concentration of glutethimide in the serum.— W. J. Decker *et al.* (letter), *Lancet*, 1970, *1,* 778.

The active metabolite of glutethimide, 4-hydroxy-2-ethyl-2-phenylglutarimide, was possibly a major contributory factor in the coma induced by glutethimide overdosage. The long duration of coma, which appeared to be unrelated to the half-life of glutethimide, might be due to the accumulation of this metabolite.— A. R. Hansen *et al., New Engl. J. Med.*, 1975, *292,* 250. The plasma concentrations of glutethimide and of 4-hydroxyglutethimide (4-hydroxy-2-ethyl-2-phenylglutarimide) did not correlate with the severity of coma in a patient who had taken an overdose of glutethimide.— S. C. Curry *et al., Med. Toxicol.*, 1987, *2,* 309.

Uses and Administration

Glutethimide is a piperidinedione hypnotic and sedative. It has been reported to act in about 30 minutes to induce sleep lasting 4 to 8 hours. The usual dose is 250 to 500 mg at night; some sources have recommended one repeat dose during the night if necessary.

ADMINISTRATION IN RENAL FAILURE. Glutethimide could be given in usual doses to patients with renal failure, but should be avoided in patients with a glomerular filtration-rate of less than 50 mL per minute.— W. M. Bennett *et al., Am. J. Kidney Dis.*, 1983, *3,* 155.

Preparations

Glutethimide Capsules *(U.S.P.)*
Glutethimide Tablets *(U.S.P.)*

Proprietary Names and Manufacturers

Doridène *(Belg.; Fr.; Ciba, Switz.)*; Doriden *(Ciba, Austral.; Canad.; Denm.; Ger.; Ital.; Neth.; Norw.; Spain; Ciba, UK; USV Pharmaceutical Corp., USA)*; Dorimide *(USA)*; Glimid *(Pol.)*.

7050-e

Halazepam *(BAN, USAN, rINN).*
Sch-12041. 7-Chloro-1,3-dihydro-5-phenyl-1-(2,2,2-trifluoroethyl)-1,4-benzodiazepin-2-one.
$C_{17}H_{12}ClF_3N_2O$=352.7.

CAS — 23092-17-3.

Dependence, Adverse Effects, Treatment, and Precautions
As for the benzodiazepines in general, p.706.

Absorption and Fate
For an account of the absorption and fate of a benzodiazepine see Diazepam, p.730.
Halazepam is well absorbed from the gastro-intestinal tract and is metabolised primarily to the long-acting metabolite *N*-desmethyldiazepam (nordazepam). It is extensively bound to plasma protein. Less than 1% is excreted unchanged in urine.

Comment on the pharmacokinetics of halazepam. Intact halazepam appears transiently in plasma, then is rapidly eliminated and is indetectable by 12 hours after a single dose. However, levels of desmethyldiazepam are much higher and persist in plasma for 14 days after the dose due to the long half-life of elimination. Such a profile indicates that desmethyldiazepam will be by far the most important active substance in blood during long-term therapy with halazepam, and it is therefore very unlikely that halazepam would provide a meaningful clinical advantage over other benzodiazepines that are transformed to desmethyldiazepam.— D. J. Greenblatt *et al.* (letter), *Lancet*, 1982, *1*, 1358.

A review of the clinical pharmacokinetics of some newer benzodiazepines including halazepam.— D. J. Greenblatt *et al.*, *Clin. Pharmacokinet.*, 1983, *8*, 233.

Uses and Administration
Halazepam is a benzodiazepine with actions and uses similar to those of diazepam (p.731). It has been given in doses of 20 to 40 mg three to four times daily for the treatment of anxiety. Dosage should be adjusted according to response. In elderly or debilitated patients a suggested initial dose is 20 mg once or twice daily, adjusted according to response.

For the view that halazepam is unlikely to have significant clinical advantages over similar existing benzodiazepines see under Absorption and Fate, above.

ADMINISTRATION. *High-dose therapy.* There was no significant difference in effectiveness between high doses of halazepam, escalating to 600 mg daily by mouth, and high-dose diazepam, up to 75 mg daily, in the management of 20 patients hospitalised for severe anxiety.— W. E. Fann *et al.*, *J. clin. Pharmac.*, 1983, *23*, 100.

Proprietary Names and Manufacturers
Alapryl *(Menarini, Spain)*; Paxipam *(Schering, USA)*.

18332-f

Haloperidol *(BAN, USAN, rINN).*

Aloperidolo; R-1625. 4-[4-(4-Chlorophenyl)-4-hydroxypiperidino]-4′-fluorobutyrophenone.
$C_{21}H_{23}ClFNO_2$=375.9.

CAS — 52-86-8.

Pharmacopoeias. In *Br.*, *Braz.*, *Chin.*, *Cz.*, *Fr.*, *Int.*, *It.*, *Jpn*, *Jug.*, *Nord.*, and *U.S.*

A white to faintly yellowish, odourless, amorphous or microcrystalline powder.
Practically **insoluble** in water; the *B.P.* has: soluble 1 in 50 of alcohol, 1 in 20 of chloroform, and slightly soluble in ether; the *U.S.P.* has: soluble 1 in 60 of alcohol, and 1 in 15 of chloroform. A saturated solution is neutral to litmus. The *B.P.* injection has a pH of 2.8 to 3.6, and the solution a pH of 2.5 to 3.5; the pH of the *U.S.P.* injection is between 3.0 and 3.8, and of the oral solution, between 2.75 and 3.75. The *B.P.* injection is **sterilised** by autoclaving. **Store** in airtight containers. Protect from light.

7051-l

Haloperidol Decanoate *(BANM, USAN, rINNM).*

R-13672.

$C_{31}H_{41}ClFNO_3$=530.1.

CAS — 74050-97-8.

Haloperidol was a weak monovalent base which formed a stable hydrochloride. In the presence of 1% lactic acid or tartaric acid, stable solutions in water could be prepared containing up to 20 mg per mL. Solutions for oral administration containing 2 mg of haloperidol per mL could be prepared by dissolving in purified water with a slight excess of lactic acid. The solution should be protected from sunlight or bright daylight and could be preserved with methyl hydroxybenzoate 0.19%. Solutions for intramuscular or intravenous injections containing 5 mg per mL could be prepared by dissolving in Water for Injections containing 0.5% of lactic acid. Methyl hydroxybenzoate 500 µg and propyl hydroxybenzoate 50 µg per mL could be added as preservative. The solution should be sterilised by filtration and stored in 1-mL amber glass ampoules. The solution had a pH of about 3.2 and was slightly hypo-osmotic. Haloperidol preparations were stable except that when exposed to light, solutions became discoloured after a few hours of exposure and deposited a greyish-red precipitate after several weeks.— P. J. A. W. Demoen, *J. pharm. Sci.*, 1961, *50*, 350.

INCOMPATIBILITY. Solutions of haloperidol (as the lactate) were incompatible with heparin sodium in glucose or sodium chloride injection; on injection of the haloperidol a precipitate formed immediately probably due to an acid-base reaction (mean pH of haloperidol lactate was 3.21 compared with 6.58 for heparin sodium).— D. A. Solomon and K. K. Nasinnyk, *Am. J. Hosp. Pharm.*, 1982, *39*, 843.

SOLUBILISATION. A study of haloperidol solubilisation in oils by aliphatic acids, and an evaluation *in vitro* of haloperidol release from solutions including oleic or linoleic acid.— B. L. Radd *et al.*, *J. parent. Sci. Technol.*, 1985, *39*, 48.

Adverse Effects

As for the phenothiazines, p.706. The effects of the butyrophenones most closely resemble those of phenothiazines with a piperazine side chain.

EFFECTS ON THE BLOOD. Although severe haematological effects are rare, agranulocytosis has been reported in association with haloperidol.— *Med. Lett.*, 1975, *17*, 11.
Further references: N. R. Cutler and J. F. Heiser, *J. Am. med. Ass.*, 1979, *242*, 2872.

EFFECTS ON BODY TEMPERATURE. A 30-year-old man receiving high-dose parenteral haloperidol therapy for withdrawal symptoms following barbiturate and methaqualone abuse, developed fatal hyperthermia.— D. J. Greenblatt *et al.*, *J. clin. Psychiat.*, 1978, *39*, 673.

A report of severe hyperthermia in a patient receiving haloperidol and benztropine during a period when ambient temperatures were high.— D. S. Bach and M. J. Rybak (letter), *Drug Intell. & clin. Pharm.*, 1985, *19*, 211.

For similar reports see under Benztropine Mesylate, p.528.

EFFECTS ON THE ENDOCRINE SYSTEM. Galactorrhoea has been reported in patients taking haloperidol.— G. M. Besser and C. R. W. Edwards, *Br. med. J.*, 1972, *2*, 280.

Inappropriate secretion of antidiuretic hormone in a woman taking haloperidol.— F. Matuk and K. Kalyanaraman, *Archs Neurol., Chicago*, 1977, *34*, 374. See also V. Peck and L. Shenkman, *Clin. Pharmac. Ther.*, 1979, *26*, 442.

EFFECTS ON THE HEART. Aside from occasionally causing some mild hypotension, haloperidol does not cause adverse cardiovascular effects. Unlike many phenothiazine neuroleptics, it rarely produces ECG changes.— F. Ayd, *J. clin. Psychiat.*, 1978, *39*, 807.

A study in 25 schizophrenic patients in good physical health, demonstrated a high degree of cardiovascular safety for healthy subjects who require treatment with moderate doses of haloperidol intramuscularly at intervals of 30 minutes. Nevertheless, it is prudent to assume that the risk of cardiovascular effects may be greater in elderly psychotic patients, and all patients who are medically ill, particularly with cardiovascular disease.— P. T. Donlan *et al.*, *Am. J. Psychiat.*, 1979, *136*, 233.

Cardiac arrhythmias in a 21-year-old man following rapid tranquillisation with haloperidol.— D. Mehta *et al.*, *Am. J. Psychiat.*, 1979, *136*, 1468.

A report of ventricular tachycardia and fibrillation in a patient who had received haloperidol 60 to 100 mg daily for 10 days.— J. H. N. Bett and G. W. Holt, *Br. med. J.*, 1983, *287*, 1264.

Two patients developed torsades de pointes after ingesting overdoses of haloperidol of 0.42 and 1 g respectively.— C. -S. Zee-Cheng *et al.* (letter), *Ann. intern. Med.*, 1985, *102*, 418.

EFFECTS ON THE LIVER. Cholestatic hepatitis has occurred in patients taking haloperidol.— *Med. Lett.*, 1975, *17*, 11. See also H. P. Dincsoy and D. A. Saelinger, *Gastroenterology*, 1982, *83*, 694.

Raised serum alkaline phosphatase concentrations in 7 of 10 patients receiving very high doses of haloperidol.— R. G. McCreadie and I. M. MacDonald, *Br. J. Psychiat.*, 1977, *131*, 310.

EFFECTS ON MENTAL STATE. Akathisia (a desire to keep moving), dysphoria, and anxiety in healthy subjects given single doses of haloperidol 5 mg.— B. G. Anderson *et al.* (letter), *New Engl. J. Med.*, 1981, *305*, 643.

Depression. Three patients given haloperidol for Gilles de la Tourette's syndrome suffered severe dysphoria, with symptoms which included sadness, crying, loss of energy, depression, despondency, drowsiness, lack of motivation, and substantial weight gain. Among a group of 72 patients treated, 3 others experienced similar, though less well documented responses to haloperidol.— E. D. Caine and R. J. Polinsky, *Am. J. Psychiat.*, 1979, *136*, 1216.

EFFECTS ON THE NERVOUS SYSTEM. Neurological symptoms of drug intoxication were attributed to haloperidol in 3 patients suffering from renal failure.— G. Richet *et al.*, *Br. med. J.*, 1970, *2*, 394.

A severe neurotoxic reaction occurred in a 74-year-old thyrotoxic patient given haloperidol.— K. Hamadah and A. F. Teggin (letter), *Lancet*, 1974, *2*, 1019. A similar report.— S. Yosselson and A. Kaplan (letter), *New Engl. J. Med.*, 1975, *293*, 201.

See also Interactions with lithium, under Precautions.

EFFECTS ON SEXUAL FUNCTION. Comment on the possible impairment of male sexual function by butyrophenones.— J. D. Horowitz and A. J. Goble, *Drugs*, 1979, *18*, 206.

Reports of male sexual dysfunction with haloperidol: S. H. Berger, *Am. J. Psychiat.*, 1979, *136*, 350; J. E. Mitchell and M. K. Popkin, *ibid.*, 1982, *139*, 633.

For comment that the butyrophenones rarely cause sexual dysfunction, see p.707.

EXTRAPYRAMIDAL EFFECTS. The Boston Collaborative Drug Surveillance Program monitored consecutively 32 812 medical in-patients. Drug-induced extrapyramidal symptoms occurred in 2 of 154 patients given a butyrophenone.— J. Porter and H. Jick, *Lancet*, 1977, *1*, 587.

A study of the incidence of extrapyramidal effects in patients receiving haloperidol by mouth in a median initial dose of 6 mg daily, increased to a maximum of 15 mg daily as required. Of 98 patients studied, 55 developed extrapyramidal symptoms, including parkinsonism in 38, dystonia in 12 and akathisia in 23. The risk of developing parkinsonism was greater in patients under 35 and in those given higher maximum doses, but a similar relationship was not demonstrated for other extrapyramidal symptoms. Of 43 patients who were receiving prophylactic anti-parkinsonian therapy 16 still developed parkinsonism; prophylactic therapy appeared to decrease the likelihood of parkinsonism in younger patients but to slightly increase the risk in older patients. In contrast only 1 of 19 patients given anti-parkinsonian therapy after developing symptoms failed to respond to it. Treatment with lorazepam 3 mg daily in divided doses was effective in controlling akathisia in 14 of 16 patients.— P. Moleman *et al.*, *J. clin. Psychiat.*, 1982, *43*, 492.

For further discussion of neuroleptic-induced extrapyramidal disorders see p.707.

See also under Uses (Administration in Children).

Tardive dyskinesia. Tardive dyskinesia developed in a 57-year-old woman after receiving haloperidol at a dose never exceeding 10 mg daily for 30 weeks. The symptoms disappeared within 12 weeks of withdrawal of haloperidol.— G. L. Stimmel, *Am. J. Hosp. Pharm.*,

1976, *33*, 961.

HYPOTENSION. For a comment on the mild degree of hypotension associated with haloperidol therapy, see under Effects on the Heart (above).

OVERDOSAGE. Symptoms in 2 young siblings who took an overdose of haloperidol included hypothermia; unexpected bradycardia was considered to be associated with the hypothermia.— J. V. K. Scialli and W. E. Thornton, *J. Am. med. Ass.*, 1978, *239*, 48.

Three children admitted to hospital with haloperidol overdosage had become drowsy, restless, and confused. They had marked extrapyramidal symptoms which included slurred speech, difficulty in swallowing, parkinsonian face, contracted masseter muscles, opisthotonus, hand tremors, and akathisia. The symptoms subsided within a few hours of biperiden administration.— C. A. Sinaniotis *et al.*, *J. Pediat.*, 1978, *93*, 1038.

About 36 hours after taking an estimated 15 to 20 mg of haloperidol a 22-month-old child suffered a severe hypertensive episode that required 5 days' therapy with hydralazine. Because of the delayed onset and the severity of the hypertension children should be observed in the hospital for at least 2 days after taking an overdose of haloperidol.— D. G. Cummingham, *J. Pediat.*, 1979, *95*, 489.

For torsades de pointes following massive overdosage of haloperidol, see under Effects on the Heart, above.

For another report mentioning hypertension in a child following haloperidol administration, see under Uses (Administration in Children).

SUDDEN DEATH. A woman admitted to hospital with acute psychosis died suddenly following attempts at rapid tranquillisation with high doses of haloperidol. She received 50 mg on the first day, 70 mg on the second, and 140 mg on the third. On the fourth day she was given 80 mg over 4 hours; 2 hours later she died.— R. Ketai *et al.*, *Am. J. Psychiat.*, 1979, *136*, 112. A further report.— J. Modestin *et al.*, *Am. J. Psychiat.*, 1981, *138*, 1616.

TARDIVE DYSKINESIA. See under Extrapyramidal Effects (above).

Treatment of Adverse Effects

As for the phenothiazines, p.708.

Precautions

As for the phenothiazines, p.708.

Severe dystonic reactions have followed the use of haloperidol, particularly in children and adolescents. It should therefore be used with extreme care in children. Haloperidol may also cause severe neurotoxic reactions in patients with hyperthyroidism. Haloperidol must be used with extreme caution in patients receiving lithium.

Evidence suggesting that cocaine addicts may be at increased risk of acute dystonic reactions following administration of haloperidol.— K. Kumor *et al.*, (letter), *Lancet*, 1986, *2*, 1341.

HYPERTHYROIDISM. A 43-year-old woman with hyperthyroidism and an acute psychosis developed a severe dystonic reaction to haloperidol therapy. She was salivating and tremulous and complained of difficulty in swallowing fluids and solid foods and subsequently died of aspiration asphyxia. Several reports in the literature suggest that hyperthyroidism enhances the neurotoxic effects of haloperidol. Moreover, the development of a severe extrapyramidal reaction to haloperidol may suggest undiagnosed hyperthyroidism.— M. F. Weiner, *Am. J. Psychiat.*, 1979, *136*, 717.

INTERACTIONS. *Anti-epileptic agents.* A 55-year-old man who had been receiving *phenytoin* 300 mg daily for over 3 years and who was suffering from stable tardive dyskinesia which had been induced by haloperidol (discontinued 2 years previously) obtained amelioration of his symptoms on discontinuation of phenytoin for a week. On reintroduction of phenytoin the dyskinesia relapsed to its original severity. Phenytoin might exacerbate neuroleptic-induced dyskinesia.— J. DeVaugh-Geiss (letter), *New Engl. J. Med.*, 1978, *298*, 457. Criticism.— P. A. Nausieda *et al.* (letter), *ibid.*, 1093.

Evidence to suggest that concomitant anticonvulsant medication (phenobarbitone and phenytoin) significantly reduces plasma-haloperidol concentrations. Plasma concentrations of the anticonvulsants were not affected.— M. Linnoila *et al.*, *Am. J. Psychiat.*, 1980, *137*, 819.

A report of delirium in a patient given *carbamazepine* while receiving haloperidol. The effect was postulated to be due to an interaction at the level of the CNS between carbamazepine and either haloperidol or the thioridazine which she had previously been given.— G. L. Kanter *et al.*, *Am. J. Psychiat.*, 1984, *141*, 1101. Concomitant administration of carbamazepine in 3 patients receiving long-term haloperidol therapy resulted in a decrease of 59 to 61% in plasma-haloperidol concentrations. There was no loss of psychiatric control, and 2 patients showed marked behavioural improvement when carbamazepine was added.— M. W. Jann *et al.*, *J. clin. Psychopharmacol.*, 1985, *5*, 106.

Beta blockers. Severe hypotension or cardiopulmonary arrest occurred on 3 occasions following administration of haloperidol and propranolol concurrently in a schizophrenic patient. The patient had received both drugs singly at different times without apparent ill effects.— H. A. Alexander *et al.*,, *J. Am. med. Ass.*, 1984, *252*, 87. Criticism of the proposed mechanism of interaction.— T. G. Burnakis (letter), *ibid.*, 1985, *253*, 1557.

Central stimulants. For an interaction between haloperidol decanoate and fenfluramine, see under Fenfluramine, p.1443.

Lithium. A report of encephalopathy in a 19-year-old man in association with high-dose haloperidol therapy and lithium. Similar forms of encephalopathy have also been noted in patients receiving high-dose haloperidol alone.— H. R. Veits, *Milit. Med.*, 1978, *143*, 201.

See also under Lithium Carbonate, p.368.

Methyldopa. For a report of dementia in 2 patients receiving methyldopa following concurrent administration of haloperidol, see Methyldopa, p.489.

Non-steroidal anti-inflammatory agents. A report of severe drowsiness and confusion in patients given haloperidol in combination with *indomethacin*.— H. A. Bird *et al.*, (letter), *Lancet*, 1983, *1*, 830.

PREGNANCY AND THE NEONATE. Administration of haloperidol to pregnant or lactating *rats* impaired the masculine sex behaviour of their male offspring.— E. M. Hull *et al.*,, *Science*, 1984, *224*, 1011.

Excretion in breast milk. Concentrations of haloperidol in the expressed breast milk of a woman receiving haloperidol were similar to observed therapeutic plasma concentrations in pharmacokinetic studies.— R. B. Stewart *et al.*, *Am. J. Psychiat.*, 1980, *137*, 849. See also L. J. Whalley *et al.* (letter), *Br. med. J.*, 1981, *282*, 1746.

Absorption and Fate

Haloperidol is readily absorbed from the gastro-intestinal tract. It is metabolised in the liver and is excreted in the urine and, via the bile, the faeces; there is evidence of enterohepatic recycling. Owing to the first-pass effect of metabolism in the liver, plasma concentrations following oral administration are lower than those following intramuscular administration. Moreover, there is wide intersubject variation in plasma concentrations of haloperidol, but in practice, no simple correlation has been found between plasma concentrations of haloperidol and its therapeutic effect. Paths of metabolism of haloperidol include oxidative *N*-dealkylation. Haloperidol has been reported to have a plasma half-life ranging from about 13 to nearly 40 hours. Haloperidol is very extensively bound to plasma proteins. It is widely distributed in the body and crosses the blood-brain barrier.

The decanoate ester of haloperidol is very slowly absorbed from the site of injection and is therefore suitable for depot injection. It is gradually released into the bloodstream where it is rapidly hydrolysed to haloperidol.

Peak plasma-haloperidol concentrations of up to 1.5% of a 2-mg tritiated dose were detected at 3 to 6 hours in 4 healthy subjects and 4 schizophrenic patients. About 26% was excreted in the urine by the healthy subjects and 20% by the patients in the first 5 days; by the third day about 15% had been excreted in the faeces. The amount excreted in the urine increased to 29% in the schizophrenic patients after 29 days treatment with haloperidol.— P. C. Johnson *et al.* (preliminary report), *Int. J. Neuropsychiat.*, 1967, *3*, *Suppl.* 1, S24.

Studies in 36 healthy men using radioactive haloperidol showed that after a 2-mg intramuscular injection, peak plasma concentrations were reached within 20 minutes. The half-life was 20.7 hours (range 12.8 to 35.5 hours).— W. A. Cressman *et al.*, *Eur. J. clin. Pharmac.*, 1974, *7*, 99.

A study in 10 healthy subjects demonstrated that haloperidol has a serum half-life ranging from about 10 to 19 hours following intravenous administration, and 12 to 36 hours following oral administration. It had an oral bioavailability of about 60%. In addition to evidence of enterohepatic recycling of the drug, there was some evidence of extrahepatic metabolism.— A. Forsman and R. Öhman, *Curr. ther. Res.*, 1976, *20*, 319. A study in psychiatric in-patients demonstrated that the biological half-life of haloperidol was of the same order as in healthy subjects; elimination was slower during the night. Bioavailability may have been as high as 70%. Measurement of plasma concentrations suggested that a therapeutic concentration in serum could be 3 to 10 ng per mL for many patients, but for some, considerably higher concentrations could be required, possibly due to pharmacodynamic variations.— *idem*, 1977, *21*, 396.

A further study of haloperidol kinetics after oral and intravenous doses.— F. O. Holley *et al.*,, *Clin. Pharmac. Ther.*, 1983, *33*, 477.

A multicentre study of the pharmacokinetics of haloperidol decanoate injection given at 4-week intervals.— A. J. M. Reyntjens *et al.*, *Int. Pharmacopsychiat.*, 1982, *17*, 238.

PLASMA PROTEIN BINDING. Haloperidol was about 92% bound to plasma proteins.— A. Forsman and R. Öhman, *Curr. ther. Res.*, 1977, *21*, 245.

Haloperidol protein binding was significantly increased in children of 4 to 11 years of age, and significantly decreased in cirrhotic patients, when compared with healthy adult subjects.— G. Tedeschi *et al.*,, *Br. J. clin. Pharmac.*, 1981, *11*, 430P.

No significant correlation was found between age and percentage haloperidol unbound in serum in a study involving 22 patients receiving long-term haloperidol therapy.— F. J. Rowell *et al.*,, *Br. J. clin. Pharmac.*, 1981, *11*, 377.

Uses and Administration

Haloperidol is a butyrophenone with actions and uses similar to those of the phenothiazine, chlorpromazine (p.724).

The usual dose for the treatment of psychoses is 0.5 to 5 mg twice or three times daily. In severe psychoses or resistant patients doses of up to 100 mg daily may be required; in very high dose therapy doses of 200 mg daily have been used. A suggested dose in children over 3 years of age is 50 µg per kg body-weight daily in divided doses, increased cautiously, if necessary, up to 150 µg per kg daily.

For the control of acute psychotic conditions haloperidol may be given intramuscularly in doses of 2 to 10 mg, subsequent doses of 5 mg may be given up to every hour until symptoms are controlled; dosage intervals of 4 to 8 hours may be adequate. Up to 30 mg intramuscularly may be required for the emergency control of very severely disturbed patients.

In patients already stabilised on an oral dose of haloperidol and requiring long-term therapy the long-acting decanoate ester may be given by deep intramuscular injection. The usual initial dose is the equivalent of 10 to 15 times the total daily dose of haloperidol by mouth, up to a maximum of 100 mg. Subsequent doses, usually given every 4 weeks, may be up to 300 mg or more, according to the patient's requirements, both dose and dose interval being adjusted as required.

Haloperidol may be used for its sedative and potent anti-emetic effects as premedication before surgery, in usual doses of 1 to 5 mg by intramuscular injection prior to anaesthetic induction. It has also been given intravenously.

Haloperidol is used in the management of Gilles de la Tourette's syndrome; a suitable dosage is reported to be up to about 10 mg daily, but requirements vary considerably and the dose must be very carefully adjusted to obtain the optimum response.

Doses of 500 µg twice daily have also been used for non-psychotic emotional disturbances, such as anxiety and tension. In general, however, like phenothiazines, the butyrophenones are only suitable for such purposes in resistant conditions, where more appropriate agents, such as the benzodiazepines (see Diazepam, p.731) have proved ineffective. If their use is judged to be necessary, treatment should be directed at low dosages given on a short-term basis.

A suggested dose of haloperidol for the management of behaviour disorders in disturbed and schizophrenic children is 50 μg per kg body-weight daily (in 2 divided doses), increased cautiously, if necessary, to up to 75 μg per kg daily. Haloperidol should be used in reduced dosage in the elderly; doses on the lower end of the scale are also advised for adolescents.

ACTION. A detailed review of the actions and uses of haloperidol. On a weight for weight basis, haloperidol is more potent than chlorpromazine; chlorpromazine has a greater propensity than haloperidol to cause sedation, antimuscarinic, and cardiovascular effects, and to alter the convulsive threshold, but haloperidol has a greater propensity than chlorpromazine to cause extrapyramidal reactions. Single daily doses of haloperidol seldom cause more side-effects than the same amount of drug taken in divided doses daily.— F. J. Ayd, *J. clin. Psychiat.*, 1978, *39*, 807. See also E. C. Settle and F. J. Ayd, *ibid.*, 1983, *44*, 440.

Results in *rats* suggested that ascorbic acid modulated the behavioural effects of haloperidol: as ascorbic acid concentrations increase, the response to haloperidol is enhanced.— G. V. Rebec *et al.*, *Science*, 1985, *227*, 438.

Controversy over the antimuscarinic effects of haloperidol: A. MacKay (letter), *Br. J. Hosp. Med.*, 1986, *35*, 132; K. Davison (letter), *ibid.*

ADMINISTRATION. A study suggesting a 'therapeutic window' of haloperidol concentrations in the treatment of psychosis.— J. R. Magliozzi *et al.*, *Am. J. Psychiat.*, 1981, *138*, 365. Similar results.— I. Extein *et al.*, *Psychopharmac. Bull.*, 1982, *18*, 156. See also I. Extein *et al.* (letter), *Lancet*, 1983, *1*, 1048. Contrary results.— J. M. Davis *et al.*, *Psychopharmac. Bull.*, 1985, *21*, 48. Inconsistent findings in studies of plasma haloperidol and clinical response may be at least partly due to failure to assess the ratio of haloperidol to the less active metabolite, reduced haloperidol.— A. C. Altamura *et al.* (letter), *Lancet*, 1987, *1*, 814.

A detailed preliminary review of haloperidol decanoate. Haloperidol decanoate is a depot form of haloperidol, given as an intramuscular injection in sesame oil. After injection it is released gradually from muscle tissue and hydrolysed into haloperidol and decanoic acid. Advantages of such a depot preparation include improved compliance and more stable plasma concentrations and haloperidol decanoate has been shown to be of value in the long-term management of psychotic conditions. The data available suggest that it is at least as effective as oral haloperidol or as other depot neuroleptics, although these results remain to be confirmed, and there is some evidence that the incidence and severity of extrapyramidal effects may be reduced compared with oral haloperidol. Although early studies mostly used a dose of the decanoate equivalent to 20 times the daily oral dosage, given monthly, current practice has tended to be more conservative. Patients are generally given 50 to 100 mg, and titrated upwards as required to up to 15 times the previous oral dose. Monthly injection appears to be convenient and satisfactory.— R. Beresford and A. Ward, *Drugs*, 1987, *33*, 31. See also *Drug & Ther. Bull.*, 1983, *21*, 39.

In children. Irreversible dystonia occurred in a 5-year-old hyperactive girl given treatment for 7 weeks with haloperidol 2 mg to 2.8 mg daily in divided doses; the dangers of giving haloperidol to children with self-limiting disease were discussed.— W. Shields and P. F. Bray, *J. Pediat.*, 1976, *88*, 301. Severe extrapyramidal and hypothalamic reactions developed in 2 adolescents given high doses of haloperidol. Symptoms included hyperthermia, semicoma, raised blood pressure and tachycardia, and generalised rigidity with cogwheeling and drooling.— B. Geller and D. E. Greydanus, *J. clin. Psychiat.*, 1979, *40*, 102.

In the elderly. Haloperidol is especially useful in the treatment of the older aggressive patient.— D. J. Williams, *Prescribers' J.*, 1978, *18*, 34.

ADMINISTRATION IN RENAL FAILURE. Haloperidol could be given in usual doses to patients with renal failure.— W. M. Bennett *et al.*, *Am. J. Kidney Dis.*, 1983, *3*, 155.

ADMINISTRATION IN RESPIRATORY INSUFFICIENCY. Comment on the advantage of haloperidol as an antipsychotic agent in patients with compromised pulmonary function but a warning that the dosage is often much lower than for patients with normal respiratory function.— J. A. Davis (letter), *J. Am. med. Ass.*, 1979, *241*, 1575.

ALCOHOL AND DRUG WITHDRAWAL. *Alcoholism.* A study of haloperidol for the control of alcohol withdrawal symptoms.— M. L. Palestine and E. Alatorre, *Curr. ther. Res.*, 1976, *20*, 289.

Barbiturates. Beneficial results were obtained with haloperidol in the management of barbiturate withdrawal.— R. Snyder, *Milit. Med.*, 1977, *142*, 885.

Phencyclidine. Haloperidol 5 mg was significantly more effective than chlorpromazine 50 mg in improving the effects of phencyclidine in a study involving 20 patients with phencyclidine-induced psychosis.— A. J. Giannini *et al.*,, *J. clin. Pharmac.*, 1984, *24*, 202.

BEHAVIOUR DISORDERS. The use of low doses of haloperidol (0.25 to 6 mg daily) to decrease sterotypical self-injurious behaviour in mentally retarded patients.— E. J. Mikkelsen (letter), *New Engl. J. Med.*, 1986, *315*, 398.

For reference to a study comparing haloperidol with lithium in children with aggressive behaviour disorder see under Lithium Carbonate, p.370.

CHOREA. Chorea associated with systemic lupus erythematosus in an 11-year-old boy responded rapidly to haloperidol 500 μg twice daily.— L. F. Kukla *et al.*, *Archs Dis. Childh.*, 1978, *53*, 345.

The treatment of chorea gravidarum in a pregnant woman with haloperidol 1 mg four times daily. The dosage was subsequently halved and then withdrawn without problems; there were no apparent adverse effects on the child, and both mother and offspring remained well 3 years later.— J. O. Donaldson, *Obstet. Gynec.*, 1982, *59*, 381.

GILLES DE LA TOURETTE'S SYNDROME. A review of Gilles de la Tourette's syndrome. The syndrome begins between 2 and 15 years of age, and is marked by rapid recurrent, involuntary movements of various muscle groups, and involuntary vocalisation (sounds, words, or profanities). Movements can be suppressed voluntarily for short periods, and the intensity of symptoms varies over weeks or months. Coprolalia is present in only 53% of patients, and the syndrome is often wrongly diagnosed. The most widely used treatment is haloperidol, which has proved beneficial in about 75% of cases tried, but its potentially severe side-effects are a cause for concern. Treatment with pimozide is equally effective and may have fewer side-effects. Clonidine is also reported to be effective in a minority of patients, although the mechanism is unclear. Treatment with methylphenidate is widely considered to be contra-indicated. Patients with mild symptoms may not need drug therapy, but psychotherapy and counselling remain necessary adjuncts to medical treatment.— R. D. Freeman *et al.*, *Can. med. Ass. J.*, 1984, *130*, 1554.

Experience in treating over 250 patients with Gilles de la Tourette's syndrome has indicated that some can only tolerate very gradual dosage increments of haloperidol. Whereas increments of 250 μg per day every 4 days are generally successful in most patients, this sub-group of patients should receive very gradual dosage increments such as 250 μg per day every 3 to 4 weeks.— A. K. Shapiro and E. Shapiro (letter), *J. Am. med. Ass.*, 1977, *238*, 29.

In a study of children and adolescents with Gilles de la Tourette's syndrome, a positive response to haloperidol was generally associated with plasma concentrations of 1 to 4 ng per mL. No relationship could be demonstrated for those with psychoses. Plasma concentrations of haloperidol bore no apparent relationship to the dose given.— P. L. Morselli *et al.*, *Ther. Drug Monit.*, 1979, *1*, 35.

GLAUCOMA. Topical application of haloperidol 0.125% or 1% eye-drops produced only a modest fall in intraocular pressure compared to placebo in a study involving 20 healthy subjects. The effect, which was maximal after 2 hours, was not significant, and haloperidol is unlikely to be of value in the treatment of glaucoma, despite previous results in *animals* suggesting an ocular hypotensive effect.— M. J. Lavin and V. Andrews, *Br. J. Ophthal.*, 1986, *70*, 448.

HEMIPLEGIA. See under Migraine, below.

HICCUP. In several patients haloperidol 5 mg given thrice daily by mouth or parenterally was successful in promptly halting persistent hiccup.— A. D. Korczyn (letter), *Br. med. J.*, 1971, *2*, 590. See also T. J. Ives *et al.*, *Am. J. Psychiat.*, 1986, *142*, 1368.

MANIA. A patient in the manic stage of manic-depressive psychosis was given haloperidol 100 mg and benzhexol 15 mg daily. Haloperidol dosage was increased to 500 mg daily and held for 8 weeks. Although the patient did not respond adequately to treatment he suffered no apparent side-effects, having received 27 g of haloperidol.— N. James (letter), *Med. J. Aust.*, 1973, *2*, 518.

Haloperidol has established itself as a rapidly acting mood corrective for acute mania, and the decanoate may prove appropriate as maintenance treatment for hypomania and in the management of the hospitalised manic patient.— J. Pollitt, *Br. J. Hosp. Med.*, 1983, *29*, 340.

For the risks pertaining to concomitant administration of haloperidol and lithium see under Precautions, above.

MIGRAINE. Haloperidol in doses of 50 to 100 μg per kg body-weight almost completely abolished attacks of alternating hemiplegic migraine in 3 of 6 children aged 3 to 15 years; in a further child the frequency of attacks was at least halved, while in 2 there was no obvious benefit. The results would appear to justify further trial.— M. A. Salmon and J. Wilson (letter), *Lancet*, 1984, *2*, 980.

NAUSEA AND VOMITING. A study in 65 postoperative patients demonstrated that haloperidol 2 mg intramuscularly has a rapid onset of action in postoperative vomiting (within 30 minutes of injection) but its activity decays over the following 4 hours at this dosage. Droperidol 5 mg intramuscularly had a slow onset of action, only reaching peak effectiveness 3 or 4 hours after administration, but had a prolonged anti-emetic action during the interval of 4 to 24 hours after administration. Prochlorperazine 10 mg intramuscularly had an onset and duration of action intermediate between the other two drugs. Use of haloperidol in association with droperidol might be more effective than any one compound alone.— E. A. Loeser *et al.*, *Can. Anaesth. Soc. J.*, 1979, *26*, 125.

In 17 patients with nausea and-or vomiting due to their antineoplastic treatment, marked relief was obtained in 5 and moderate relief in 7 after treatment with haloperidol, usually 1 mg thrice daily. The effect of haloperidol lasted about 5 hours.— D. A. Plotkin *et al.*, *Curr. ther. Res.*, 1973, *15*, 599.

Haloperidol 1 mg per m^2 body-surface intramuscularly, droperidol (in the same dosage), and prochlorperazine 6 mg per m^2 were equally effective as antiemetics in a double-blind crossover study in 27 patients receiving cisplatin chemotherapy.— N. J. Owens *et al.*, *Clin. Pharm.*, 1984, *3*, 167.

A review of the care of the terminally ill. For drug-induced vomiting haloperidol is used in a dose of 1.5 mg at once and nightly thereafter. If the patient is experiencing radiation-induced vomiting a higher dose, e.g. 5 mg, is indicated. If vomiting is associated with chemotherapy then 5 to 10 mg nightly may be necessary. Uraemic patients may also need higher doses: often 5 mg nightly, and sometimes 10 or 15 mg. Parkinsonian side-effects are more likely at doses over 3 mg and can be treated by dose reduction where possible or else an antiparkinsonian agent such as orphenadrine.— R. G. Twycross, *Br. J. Hosp. Med.*, 1986, *36*, 244.

RHEUMATOID ARTHRITIS. Evidence for an antirheumatic action of haloperidol 1.5 mg daily.— M. G. Grimaldi (letter), *Br. J. clin. Pharmac.*, 1981, *12*, 579.

SNEEZING. A patient with intractable sneezing that had continued every 4 to 5 seconds for 139 days, except during sleep and while talking, responded to treatment with haloperidol by mouth. With a dose of 1.5 mg twice daily the sneezing rate fell after a week to once every 30 seconds, and subsequent increase to 5 mg twice daily completely abolished symptoms. The patient stopped taking the medicine after 4 weeks, and symptoms recurred 6 weeks later, but responded to 5 mg three times daily. On gradual reduction of dosage over 6 months the patient experienced no recurrence of the sneezing and had remained symptom free after 6 months without medication.— K. Davison, *Br. med. J.*, 1982, *284*, 1163.

STUTTERING. In a controlled study of 36 patients with a stuttering impediment, haloperidol in an average dose of 0.75 to 1.5 mg thrice daily and orphenadrine 50 mg thrice daily, to reduce the side-effects of haloperidol, led to a significant improvement after 4 weeks in 10 of 12 patients. No further improvement was noted in the patients treated for a further 4 weeks although the initial improvement was maintained. Side-effects which included dry mouth, blurred vision, drowsiness, and depression occurred in patients given either the active medication or a placebo.— P. G. Wells and M. T. Malcolm, *Br. J. Psychiat.*, 1971, *119*, 603.

Haloperidol was given to 18 stutterers for 3 weeks. Of these, 4 patients showed a substantial improvement, 6 showed a lesser improvement, and 8 deteriorated. The mean dose of haloperidol was 2.5 mg daily. Side-effects occurring were drowsiness, poor concentration, restlessness, visual and eye disturbances, other extrapyramidal symptoms, and depression.— P. T. Quinn and C. Peachey, *Med. J. Aust.*, 1973, *2*, 809.

Preparations

Haloperidol Injection *(B.P.)*. A sterile solution of haloperidol in lactic acid diluted with Water for Injections.

Haloperidol Injection *(U.S.P.)*. A sterile solution of haloperidol in Water for Injections, prepared with the aid of lactic acid.

Haloperidol Oral Solution *(B.P.)*. Haloperidol Solution; Haloperidol Oral Drops. An aqueous solution containing not more than haloperidol 0.2%. Store at a temperature between 15° and 25°.

Haloperidol Oral Solution *(U.S.P.)*. Haloperidol Solution. A solution of haloperidol in water prepared with the aid of lactic acid.

Haloperidol Tablets *(B.P.)*

Haloperidol Tablets *(U.S.P.)*

Strong Haloperidol Oral Solution *(B.P.)*. Strong Haloperidol Oral Drops. An aqueous solution containing haloperidol 1%. It is intended to be diluted before use. Store at a temperature between 15° and 25°.

Proprietary Preparations

Dozic *(R.P. Drugs, UK)*. *Oral liquid*, haloperidol 1 and 2 mg/mL.

Fortunan *(Steinhard, UK)*. *Tablets*, haloperidol 500 µg. *Tablets* , scored, haloperidol 1.5, 5, 10 and 20 mg.

Haldol *(Janssen, UK)*. *Tablets*, scored, haloperidol 5 and 10 mg.
Oral liquid, haloperidol 2 mg/mL.
Oral liquid concentrate, haloperidol 10 mg/mL.
Injection, haloperidol 5 mg/mL, in ampoules of 1 and 2 mL.

Haldol Decanoate *(Janssen, UK)*. *Injection*, oily, haloperidol 50 and 100 mg (as decanoate)/mL, in ampoules of 1 mL.

Serenace *(Searle, UK)*. *Capsules*, haloperidol 500 µg.
Tablets, scored, haloperidol 1.5, 5, 10, and 20 mg.
Oral liquid, haloperidol 2 mg/mL.
Injection, haloperidol 5 mg/mL, in ampoules of 1 mL.
Injection, haloperidol 10 mg/mL, in ampoules of 2 mL.

Proprietary Names and Manufacturers

Bioperidolo *(FIRMA, Ital.)*; Brotopon *(Jpn)*; Dozic *(R.P. Drugs, UK)*; Duraperidol *(Durachemie, Ger.)*; Einalon S *(Jpn)*; Fortunan *(Steinhard, UK)*; Haldol *(Belg.; McNeil, Canad.; Janssen, Fr.; Janssen, Ger.; Janssen, Ital.; Neth.; Janssen, Norw.; Janssen Pharmaceutica, Swed.; Janssen, Switz.; Janssen, UK; McNeil Pharmaceutical, USA)*; Halopidol *(Arg.)*; Halosten *(Jpn)*; Linton *(Jpn)*; Novoperidol *(Novopharm, Canad.)*; Pacedol *(Protea, Austral.)*; Peluces *(Jpn)*; Peridol *(Technilab, Canad.)*; Serenace *(Searle, Austral.; Jpn; Searle, S.Afr.; Searle, UK)*; Serenase *(Janssen, Denm.; Lusofarmaco, Ital.)*; Sigaperidol *(Siegfried, Ger.; Sigamed, Switz.)*; Sylador *(Dumex, Denm.)*; Tamide *(Lennon, S.Afr.)*.

19283-j

Haloxazolam *(rINN)*.

10-Bromo-11b-(2-fluorophenyl)-2,3,7,11b-tetrahydrooxazolo[3,2-*d*][1,4]benzodiazepin-6(5*H*)-one.
$C_{17}H_{14}BrFN_2O_2$=377.2.

CAS — 59128-97-1.

Haloxazolam is a benzodiazepine derivative with general properties similar to those of diazepam (p.728). It has been used as a hypnotic in the short-term management of insomnia in doses of 5 to 10 mg at night.

Proprietary Names and Manufacturers

Somelin *(Sankyo, Jpn)*.

4039-z

Hexapropymate *(BAN, rINN)*.

L-2103; Propinylcyclohexanol Carbamate. 1-(Prop-2-ynyl)cyclohexyl carbamate.
$C_{10}H_{15}NO_2$=181.2.

CAS — 358-52-1.

Hexapropymate is a carbamate derivative with general properties similar to those of ethinamate (p.736), which has been used as a hypnotic in the short-term management of insomnia in usual doses of 400 mg at night. It has also been given rectally as suppositories.

Proprietary Names and Manufacturers

Biradon *(Osiris, Arg.)*; Merinax *(Labaz, Belg.; Labaz, Fr.; Sigmatau, Ital.; Labaz, Neth.; Labaz, Spain; Labaz, Switz.)*; Modirax *(Ferrosan, Swed.)*.

4040-p

Hexobarbitone *(BAN)*.

Ciclobarbital; Enhexymalum; Enimal; Hexobarbital *(USAN, rINN)*; Hexobarbitalum; Methexenyl; Methylcyclohexenylmethyl-barbitursäure; Methylhexabarbital. 5-(Cyclohex-1-enyl)-1,5-dimethylbarbituric acid.
$C_{12}H_{16}N_2O_3$=236.3.

CAS — 56-29-1.

Pharmacopoeias. In *Aust., Br., Cz., Eur., Fr., Ger., Hung., Int., It., Jug., Neth., Nord., Pol., Rus., Swiss, Turk.*, and *U.S.*

Odourless colourless crystals or a white crystalline powder. Very slightly **soluble** in water; slightly soluble in boiling water; sparingly soluble in alcohol; freely soluble in chloroform. Very soluble in solutions of alkali hydroxides but not in solutions of alkali carbonates. The *B.P.* states that it is freely soluble and the *U.S.P.* soluble, in ether. **Store** in airtight containers.

4041-s

Hexobarbitone Sodium

Enhexymalnatrium; Hexenalum; Hexobarbitalum Natricum; Narcosanum Solubile; Sodium Hexobarbital; Soluble Hexobarbitone. Sodium 5-(cyclohex-1-enyl)-1,5-dimethylbarbiturate.
$C_{12}H_{15}N_2NaO_3$=258.3.

CAS — 50-09-9.

Pharmacopoeias. In *Aust., Belg., Hung., Int., Jug., Nord., Pol., Rus.*, and *Turk.*

STABILITY OF SOLUTIONS. A 10% solution of hexobarbitone sodium in water lost 4.2% of its strength in 1 day at 20°, 7.3% in 2 days, 13.2% in 4 days, and 21.3% in 8 days.— H. Nuppenau, *Dansk Tidsskr. Farm.*, 1954, *28*, 261.

Hexobarbitone is a barbiturate and shares the general properties of the group (see p.706). It has been used as a hypnotic and sedative. Hexobarbitone sodium was formerly used intravenously for the induction of anaesthesia.

Preparations

Hexobarbital Tablets *(U.S.P.)*. Tablets containing hexobarbitone.

Proprietary Names and Manufacturers

Citopan *(Norw.)*; Cyclonal Sodium *(May & Baker, UK)*; Evipan *(Bayer, Ger.)*; Noctivane *(Fr.)*; Sombulex *(USA)*.

The following names have been used for multi-ingredient preparations containing hexobarbitone— Evidorm *(Winthrop, UK)*.

7052-y

Homofenazine Hydrochloride *(rINNM)*.

D-775 *(base)*. 2-{Hexahydro-4-[3-(2-trifluoromethylphenothiazin-10-yl)propyl]-1,4-diazepin-1-yl}ethanol dihydrochloride.
$C_{23}H_{28}F_3N_3OS,2HCl$=524.5.

CAS — 3833-99-6 (homofenazine); 1256-01-5 (hydrochloride).

Homofenazine hydrochloride is a phenothiazine and shares the general properties of the group (see p.706). It has been used in the management of neuropsychiatric disorders in doses of 3 mg twice or three times daily.

Proprietary Names and Manufacturers

Pasaden *(Homburg, Belg.; Homburg, Ger.; Farmades, Ital.)*.

4042-w

Ibomal

Bromoaprobarbitone; Isopropyl-bromallyl-barbitursäure; Propallylonal. 5-(2-Bromoallyl)-5-isopropylbarbituric acid.
$C_{10}H_{13}BrN_2O_3$=289.1.

CAS — 545-93-7.

Ibomal is a barbiturate and shares the general properties of the group (see p.706). It has been used as a hypnotic in the short-term management of insomnia in doses of 100 to 400 mg at night.

Proprietary Names and Manufacturers

Noctal *(UCB, Ger.)*.

7055-c

Ketazolam *(BAN, USAN, rINN)*.

U-28774. 11-Chloro-8,12b-dihydro-2,8-dimethyl-12b-phenyl-4*H*-[1,3]oxazino[3,2-*d*][1,4]benzodiazepine-4,7(6*H*)-dione.
$C_{20}H_{17}ClN_2O_3$=368.8.

CAS — 27223-35-4.

Dependence, Adverse Effects, Treatment, and Precautions

As for the benzodiazepines in general, p.706.

Absorption and Fate

For an account of the absorption and fate of a benzodiazepine, see Diazepam, p.730.

Following administration of ketazolam to *rats* metabolites included: oxazepam, 3-hydroxydiazepam, desmethyldiazepam, diazepam, and 4′-hydroxydiazepam.— F. S. Eberts *et al., Pharmacologist*, 1976, *18*, 153.

See also D. J. Greenblatt *et al., Clin. Pharmacokinet.*, 1983, *8*, 233.

Uses and Administration

Ketazolam is a benzodiazepine with general properties similar to those of diazepam (p.731). In the treatment of anxiety it is given in a usual dose of 30 mg daily, at night, with a range of 15 to 60 mg daily, either in divided doses or a single dose at night.

Ketazolam is also used in the management of spasticity associated with conditions such as stroke or spinal cord trauma.

A brief discussion on the actions and uses of ketazolam.— *Drug & Ther. Bull.*, 1980, *18*, 94.

Proprietary Preparations

Anxon *(Beecham Research, UK)*. *Capsules*, ketazolam 15 and 30 mg.

Proprietary Names and Manufacturers

Anxon *(Beecham Research, UK)*; Contamex *(Beecham-Wülfing, Ger.)*; Loftran *(Beecham, Canad.)*; Marcen *(Antibioticos, Spain)*; Sedotime *(Beecham, Spain)*; Solatran *(Belg.; Bencard, S.Afr.; Beecham, Switz.)*; Unakalm *(Belg.)*.

12903-c

Loprazolam *(BAN, rINN)*.

6-(2-Chlorophenyl)-2,4-dihydro-2-(4-methylpiperazin-1-ylmethylene)-8-nitroimidazo[1,2-*a*][1,4]benzodiazepin-1-one.
$C_{23}H_{21}ClN_6O_3$=464.9.

CAS — 61197-73-7.

18341-d

Loprazolam Mesylate *(BANM)*.

HR-158; Loprazolam Mesilate *(rINNM)*; Loprazolam Methanesulphonate; RU-31158.
$C_{23}H_{21}ClN_6O_3, CH_4O_3S$=561.0.

Dependence, Adverse Effects, Treatment, and Precautions

As for the benzodiazepines in general, p.706.

INTERACTIONS. A study of the effects of loprazolam and alcohol on performance.— I. C. McManus *et al., Br. J. clin. Pharmac.*, 1983, *16*, 291.

Absorption and Fate

For an account of the absorption and fate of a benzodiazepine, see Diazepam, p.730. The elimination half-life of loprazolam has been reported to range from 7 to 15 hours.

References: L. A. Stevens *et al., Eur. J. clin. Pharmac.*, 1983, *25*, 651; G. T. McInnes *et al., Br. J. clin. Pharmac.*, 1985, *19*, 649.

See also under Administration, below.

Uses and Administration

Loprazolam is an intermediate-acting benzodiazepine with general properties similar to those of diazepam (p.731).

It is used for its hypnotic properties in the management of insomnia, in usual doses of the equivalent of 1 mg of loprazolam, as the mesylate, at night. Dosage may be increased to 2 mg if necessary.

Reviews and discussions: G. Beaumont, *Br. J. clin. Pract.*, 1983, *37*, 307; *Drug & Ther. Bull.*, 1984, *22*, 48; B. G. Clark *et al.*, *Drugs*, 1986, *31*, 500.

ADMINISTRATION. *In the elderly*. There was a significant prolongation of the mean elimination half-life of loprazolam to 19.77 hours in 9 patients with a mean age of 72 given 1 mg by the mouth; this compared with a mean elimination half-life of 11.22 hours among 10 younger patients (mean age 28.8 years). In a further study there was an enhanced sedative response to loprazolam 1 mg in elderly compared with younger subjects; elderly subjects also showed sedative effects from a dose of 0.5 mg, whereas in younger subjects this had negligible effects. The results suggest that 0.5 mg may be an appropriate starting dose in elderly patients.— C. G. Swift *et al.*, *Br. J. clin. Pharmac.*, 1985, *20*, 119. See also A. J. Bayer and M. S. J. Pathy, *Curr. med. Res. Opinion*, 1986, *10*, 17.

Proprietary Names and Manufacturers

Dormonoct *(Cassenne, S.Afr.*; *Roussel, UK)*; Havlane *(Diamant, Fr.)*; Sonin *(Lipha, Ger.)*.

7060-y

Lorazepam *(BAN, USAN, rINN)*.

Wy-4036. 7-Chloro-5-(2-chlorophenyl)-1,3-dihydro-3-hydroxy-1,4-benzodiazepin-2-one. $C_{15}H_{10}Cl_2N_2O_2$=321.2.

CAS — 846-49-1.

Pharmacopoeias. In *Br.* and *U.S.*

A white or almost white, odourless or almost odourless crystalline powder. Practically **insoluble** in water; sparingly soluble in alcohol; slightly soluble in chloroform. **Store** in airtight containers. Protect from light.

A study of the solubility of lorazepam in fluids for intravenous administration (water, glucose injection, lactated Ringer's injection, and sodium chloride injection) and the potential drug loss due to sorption from mixtures to polyvinyl chloride bags and tubing. Solubility was greatest in glucose injection at 62 µg per mL and lowest in sodium chloride injection (27 µg per mL); these differences in solubility appeared to be pH related. Sorption was much slower than has been reported for diazepam, and it was concluded that reliable dose delivery could be maintained from intravenous admixtures of lorazepam in glucose injection infused over intervals up to 5 hours.— D. W. Newton *et al.*, *Am. J. Hosp. Pharm.*, 1983, *40*, 424.

Dependence

As for the benzodiazepines in general, p.706.

A brief review of lorazepam, including the comment that lorazepam is widely believed to carry a greater risk of dependence than other benzodiazepines.— *Drug & Ther. Bull.*, 1985, *23*, 61. See also M. Ross (letter), *J. R. Coll. gen. Pract.*, 1986, *36*, 86.

WITHDRAWAL. A report of withdrawal convulsions from benzodiazepines in 4 patients, involving clorazepate (1), oxazepam (1), and lorazepam (2).— T. R. Einarson (letter), *Lancet*, 1980, *1*, 151. A comment that 2 of these patients were also taking trifluoperazine, which has known epileptogenic potential. A patient has been seen, however, who suffered a grand-mal seizure 4 days after stopping lorazepam 5 mg daily alone; lorazepam had been taken for 2 years in a daily dose of 5 to 15 mg.— P. Tyrer (letter), *ibid*.

Adverse Effects, Treatment, and Precautions

As for the benzodiazepines in general, p.706.

EXTRAPYRAMIDAL DISORDERS. A report of orofacial dyskinesias in a patient receiving lorazepam.— R. Sandyk, *Clin. Pharm.*, 1986, *5*, 419.

Severe exacerbation of idiopathic parkinsonism occurred on 2 occasions in an elderly patient following administration of lorazepam. The patient had previously received triazolam without apparent ill-effect.— J. Rafferty and J. Williamson, *Br. med. J.*, 1983, *287*, 1596.

INTERACTIONS. *Alcohol*. Studies of the interactions between lorazepam and alcohol: A. K. Aucamp *et al.*, *S. Afr. med. J.*, 1984, *66*, 445; K. Aranko *et al.*, *Eur. J. clin. Pharmac.*, 1985, *28*, 559.

Beta-blockers. For the interactions of benzodiazepines, including lorazepam, with a beta-blocker, see under Diazepam, p.729.

Cimetidine. For the interactions of benzodiazepines, including lorazepam, with cimetidine, see under Diazepam, p.729.

Oral contraceptives. For the interaction of benzodiazepines, including lorazepam, with oral contraceptives, see under Diazepam, p.730.

Probenecid. The mean half-life of lorazepam following intravenous injection of 2 mg in 9 healthy subjects was increased from 14.3 to 33.0 hours following concurrent administration of probenecid. Probenecid selectively impairs glucuronide formation and thus the clearance of drugs like lorazepam.— D. R. Abernethy *et al.*, *Clin. Pharmac. Ther.*, 1984, *35*, 224.

OVERDOSAGE. A 6-year-old boy who had ingested not more than 30 mg (probably considerably less) of lorazepam was drowsy and ataxic and developed marked hallucinations persisting intermittently for 9 hours.— D. I. Jeffrey and M. F. Whitfield (letter), *Br. med. J.*, 1974, *4*, 719.

PREGNANCY AND THE NEONATE. Concentrations of lorazepam in cord plasma in 26 neonates were slightly lower than in maternal plasma. Lorazepam was slowly excreted by infants. In a study of 53 infants born to 51 mothers with hypertension treated with lorazepam and antihypertensives, oral treatment with lorazepam had little effect on the neonate other than delay in establishment of breast feeding. Lorazepam intravenously reduced the Apgar score at birth, increased the necessity for assisted respiration, and increased neonatal hypothermia and poor suckling. Premature infants had a very high incidence of depressed respiration, hypothermia, and feeding problems, regardless of route of administration. The use of lorazepam intravenously, and before 37 weeks of gestation, should be limited to hospitals with facilities for intensive neonatal care.— A. G. L. Whitelaw *et al.*, *Br. med. J.*, 1981, *282*, 1106. Comment.— M. Johnstone (letter), *ibid.*, 1973. Reply.— A. Whitelaw (letter), *ibid.*

THROMBO-EMBOLIC EFFECTS. Of 40 patients given a single intravenous dose of lorazepam 4 mg three had thrombosis 2 to 3 days later and 6 had thrombosis 7 to 10 days later. The incidence was lower than in those given diazepam.— J. E. Hegarty and J. W. Dundee, *Br. med. J.*, 1977, *2*, 1384. See also *Drug & Ther. Bull.*, 1981, *19*, 11.

Absorption and Fate

For an account of the absorption and fate of a benzodiazepine, see Diazepam, p.730.

Lorazepam is readily absorbed from the gastro-intestinal tract following oral administration, with a bioavailability of about 90%; peak plasma concentrations are reported to occur about 2 hours after an oral dose. Unlike other benzodiazepines such as diazepam it is also well absorbed when given intramuscularly.

The half-life has been reported to range from about 10 to 20 hours. Lorazepam is metabolised in the liver to the inactive glucuronide, and excreted in urine. It is about 85% bound to plasma protein.

ABSORPTION AND PLASMA CONCENTRATIONS. Studies in 4 healthy subjects given a single intravenous injection of lorazepam 5 mg suggested that the elimination half-life was about 13 hours; 69% of the dose was recovered from urine as the glucuronide.— D. J. Greenblatt *et al.*, *J. clin. Pharmac.*, 1977, *17*, 490. Further studies in 15 healthy subjects given lorazepam up to 10 mg daily by mouth for 26 weeks. With a dose of 6 mg daily, the mean steady-state plasma concentration was 88 ng per mL of lorazepam, and 170 ng per mL of the glucuronide; and with a daily dose of 10 mg the respective plasma concentrations were 164 and 266 ng per mL.— *idem*, 495. Following administration of lorazepam 4 mg into the deltoid muscles of 6 healthy subjects rapid absorption occurred (mean apparent absorption half-life of about 20 minutes) with peak plasma concentrations ranging from 49.6 to 82.7 ng per mL after 1 to 3 hours. An average of nearly 50% of the dose was recovered from the urine as the glucuronide during the first 24 hours and only about 0.3% as free lorazepam. The mean elimination half-life of 13.6 hours was similar to reported values following oral administration.— *idem*, *Clin. Pharmac. Ther.*, 1977, *21*, 222. In 6 and 7 healthy subjects given lorazepam 2 and 4 mg respectively by intravenous, intramuscular, or oral administration apparent elimination half-life was about 14 to 16 hours and about 65 to 79% of the administered dose was excreted in the urine within 72 hours as the glucuronide.— *idem*, *J. pharm. Sci.*, 1979, *68*, 57.

There were secondary peaks in plasma lorazepam concentrations on 12 of 18 occasions following ingestion of lorazepam by 6 healthy subjects; these secondary peaks occurred 1 to 5 hours after the initial peak and were occasionally higher. The plasma decay curve of lorazepam after oral administration cannot be represented by a smooth curve.— M. E. Dodson and M. Young, *Br. J. clin. Pharmac.*, 1982, *14*, 141P.

METABOLISM. Following administration of lorazepam 2 mg to 8 healthy subjects peak pooled plasma-lorazepam concentrations of 16.9 ng per mL were obtained after 2 hours at which time the clinical effects appeared to be maximum. Urinary excretion accounted for an average of about 88% of the dose, 86% (75% of the total dose) being as the major metabolite, lorazepam glucuronide; minor metabolites included a hydroxylated derivative, a quinazolinone derivative, and a quinazoline carboxylic acid. About 7% of the dose was recovered from the faeces but it was not established whether this was unabsorbed lorazepam or metabolites.— D. J. Greenblatt *et al.*, *Clin. Pharmac. Ther.*, 1976, *20*, 329.

PLASMA PROTEIN BINDING. In a study in 15 elderly and 15 younger subjects, of whom 6 and 9 respectively were female, there was a slight but significant increase in the mean free fraction of drug in the elderly; the volume of distribution was 18% less, and the clearance of free plus bound drug reduced by 28% compared with the younger group. These age-related differences were more apparent in female subjects.— M. Divoll and D. J. Greenblatt, *J. Pharm. Pharmac.*, 1982, *34*, 122.

PREGNANCY AND THE NEONATE. *Diffusion across the placenta*. Evidence to suggest that lorazepam does not appear to cross the placental barrier as readily as diazepam. Foetal concentration of lorazepam rarely exceeded that of the mother and following delivery the neonates were able to metabolise lorazepam at the same rate as the mother.— R. J. McBride *et al.*, *Br. J. Anaesth.*, 1979, *51*, 971.

Slow conjugation and elimination of lorazepam by the neonate.— A. J. Cummings and A. G. L. Whitelaw, *Br. J. clin. Pharmac.*, 1981, *12*, 511.

See also under Precautions.

Excretion in breast milk. Free lorazepam concentrations in the breast milk of 4 lactating mothers who had received lorazepam 3.5 mg by mouth as premedication, ranged from 8 to 9 ng per mL four hours after the dose. This represented approximately 15 to 26% of the concentration in plasma, and was probably sufficiently low to cause no adverse effects in breast-fed infants.— R. J. Summerfield and M. S. Nielsen (letter), *Br. J. Anaesth.*, 1985, *57*, 1042.

Uses and Administration

Lorazepam is a benzodiazepine with actions and uses similar to those of diazepam (p.731). The usual dose by mouth or sublingually for the treatment of anxiety is 2 to 6 mg daily in 2 to 3 divided doses with the largest dose taken at night; in severe conditions up to 8 to 10 mg daily has been given. A single dose of 1 to 4 mg at bedtime has been given for its hypnotic effect in insomnia.

Lorazepam may also be given intramuscularly or preferably intravenously as a sedative or for premedication. Recommended parenteral doses of lorazepam are: for anxiety, 25 to 30 µg per kg body-weight; for premedication, 50 µg per kg. The injection should be diluted before administration; intravenous injections should be given at a rate of not more than 2 mg per minute.

In the management of status epilepticus 4 mg may be given as a single intravenous dose; half this amount has been suggested as a dose in children.

Lorazepam should be given in reduced dosage to elderly or debilitated patients.

ADMINISTRATION. Despite poor water solubility intramuscular injection of lorazepam in 6 healthy subjects was found to be painless.— D. J. Greenblatt *et al.*, *Clin. Pharmac. Ther.*, 1977, *21*, 222.

Serum concentrations of lorazepam were similar whether the drug was given intramuscularly or by mouth preoperatively.— M. J. Diamond (letter), *Br. J. Anaesth.*, 1978, *50*, 730.

A study of the efficacy of sublingual lorazepam in the management of moderate to severe acute anxiety in 15 patients. A dose of 3 mg sublingually appeared optimal in providing relief from the symptoms without excessive side-effects.— A. N. Singh *et al.*, *Curr. ther. Res.*, 1983, *34*, 227.

An open study of a fast-dissolving wafer formulation of lorazepam as premedication in children undergoing elective surgery. Of 14 children who received a dose of 26 to 50 µg per kg body-weight, results in terms of efficacy and lack of side-effects were considered satisfactory in 4.— S. Underhill *et al.*, *Anaesthesia*, 1987, *42*, 319.

ADMINISTRATION IN HEPATIC FAILURE. A study indicating that both cirrhosis and hepatitis decrease the plasma binding of lorazepam and tend to depress its clearance but the latter effect was not statistically significant.— J. W. Kraus *et al.*, *Gastroenterology*, 1977, *73*, 1228. See also J. W. Kraus *et al.*, *Clin. Pharmac. Ther.*, 1978, *24*, 411.

If sedatives are required in patients with liver failure oxazepam or lorazepam seem to be safer than compounds such as diazepam; patients should be given a low dose and the therapeutic effects observed.— I. Corall and R. Williams, *Br. J. Anaesth.*, 1986, *58*, 234.

ADMINISTRATION IN RENAL FAILURE. The half-life of lorazepam was prolonged from a range of 9 to 16 hours to 32 to 70 hours in end-stage renal disease. Doses should be reduced by 50% in patients with a glomerular filtration-rate less than 10 mL per minute.— W. M. Bennett *et al.*, *Am. J. Kidney Dis.*, 1983, *3*, 155. See also R. K. Verbeeck *et al.* (letter), *Br. J. clin. Pharmac.*, 1981, *12*, 749.

ALCOHOL AND DRUG WITHDRAWAL. Withdrawal symptoms of 21 chronic alcoholic patients were successfully controlled by an initial intramuscular injection of lorazepam, usually 5 mg, followed by an average daily dose of 7 mg by mouth.— I. N. Hosein *et al.*, *Curr. med. Res. Opinion*, 1978, *5*, 632.

In a study in 52 patients experiencing symptoms from acute alcohol withdrawal, lorazepam in daily doses of 6 mg by mouth, reduced gradually to 2 mg over 4 days then withdrawn, was as effective as diazepam 30 mg, tapered to 10 mg over the same period, in reducing symptoms. Six of the 26 patients given lorazepam and 5 of 26 given diazepam failed to complete the study, but 19 of the 20 remaining in the lorazepam group and all of those remaining in the diazepam-treated group were considered to show improvement after treatment.— J. E. O'Brien *et al.*, *Curr. ther. Res.*, 1983, *34*, 825.

ANAESTHESIA. A summary of the important differences between diazepam and lorazepam in anaesthesia. As a premedicant diazepam 10 mg produces a degree of sedation comparable to lorazepam 2 to 2.5 mg; lorazepam has a duration of action 3 to 4 times greater than that of equivalent doses of diazepam; although diazepam by mouth has an earlier onset of action than following intramuscular injection this does not apply to lorazepam. These effects occur in parallel with plasma concentrations of the drugs. Both drugs are slowly excreted from the body, plasma concentrations remaining increased for 24 to 48 hours. Whereas desmethyldiazepam, the main metabolite of diazepam has an appreciable hypnotic action and accumulates following repeated administrations, this does not apply to lorazepam. A second peak concentration of both drugs may occur 5 to 8 hours after administration. In equivalent intravenous doses both drugs commonly produce anterograde amnesia which is not wholly dependent on sedation. Premedication with lorazepam will consistently reduce the undesirable emergence effect of ketamine, while diazepam is unreliable in this respect; in contrast, intravenous injection of diazepam near the end of a ketamine anaesthesia will reduce emergence sequelae, whereas lorazepam is not suitable for this purpose.— J. W. Dundee *et al.*, *Br. J. Anaesth.*, 1979, *51*, 439. A comparison of various injectable formulations of benzodiazepines and a reminder that lorazepam injection, while useful for prolonged procedures, is unsuitable as premedication in short procedures such as endoscopy since it may take up to 20 minutes to act after intravenous injection, whereas diazepam takes only 1 to 3 minutes. Furthermore, lorazepam has a much more prolonged action than diazepam.— *Drug & Ther. Bull.*, 1983, *21*, 45.

For further reference to the use of benzodiazepines in anaesthetic procedures, see Diazepam, p.732.

CONVULSIONS. A randomised double-blind study comparing lorazepam and diazepam in the treatment of status epilepticus. Of 70 episodes studied, 37 were treated with lorazepam and 33 with diazepam; most patients also received a loading dose of phenytoin, even if seizures had not recurred, after 30 minutes. Seizure activity was terminated by a single slow intravenous injection of diazepam 10 mg in 19 cases, and by lorazepam 4 mg in 29 episodes. A second dose was given to 13 of 14 cases not initially responding to diazepam, and seizures ceased in 6; similarly 4 of 8 patients given a second dose of lorazepam responded. The median time for the drug to take effect was 2 minutes with diazepam and 3 minutes with lorazepam. When seizures were analysed by type the two drugs appeared almost equally effective in treating generalised status epilepticus, whereas lorazepam was more frequently effective for other seizure types; however, these differences were not significant, and there was no significant difference in efficacy overall. The results indicate that lorazepam is at least as effective as diazepam in the initial treatment of status.— I. E. Leppik, *J. Am. med. Ass.*, 1983, *249*, 1452.

Lorazepam 50 µg per kg body-weight intravenously, abolished seizure activity within 5 minutes in 7 neonates with severe seizures refractory to conventional therapy. Symptoms recurred in 2 after 8 hours, but were less severe. Lorazepam did not appear to depress respiratory function further, even in 3 who were receiving ventilatory assistance. In view of the apparent efficacy and lack of severe adverse effects the use of intravenous lorazepam may be justifiable in severely ill neonates with refractory seizures.— A. Deshmukh *et al.*, *Am. J. Dis. Child.*, 1986, *140*, 1042.

A single intravenous injection of lorazepam 4 mg abolished seizure activity, on average after 4 minutes, in 6 patients who developed generalised myoclonic status epilepticus after cardiac arrest. Seizures did not recur, and no adverse effects were noted. Control of seizures did not result in improved survival in these patients, all of whom died, but was universally comforting to patients' families.— F. M. Vincent and T. Vincent (letter), *Ann. intern. Med.*, 1986, *104*, 586.

HYPNOTIC EFFECT. In a double-blind crossover study of 15 chronic insomniacs lorazepam 2 to 4 mg was approximately equivalent in hypnotic activity to flurazepam 30 mg. Side-effects were relatively frequent after the 4-mg dose and consisted of headache, drowsiness, lack of drive, dizziness, and tinnitus.— R. I. H. Wang *et al.*, *Clin. Pharmac. Ther.*, 1976, *19*, 191.

MANIA. A report of an encouraging response to lorazepam in severe manic-depressive illness unresponsive to conventional therapy. The patient, who had a 30-year history of manic depression, was given lorazepam 5 mg four times daily for a manic attack, and the illness settled within a few days. Subsequent maintenance was with lorazepam 7.5 mg daily; when the patient felt premonitory symptoms of mania increasing the dose to 20 mg daily for a few days would prevent a full-blown manic illness. This regimen had resulted in only 1 brief hospital admission during the past 2 years, compared with 17 over the 5 years before starting lorazepam, during much of which the patient was an inpatient or day-patient. The effects of lorazepam in mania deserve further exploration, especially in patients resistant to, or intolerant of, conventional therapy.— M. Jobling and G. Stein, *Lancet*, 1986, *1*, 510.

NAUSEA AND VOMITING. Lorazepam 4 to 5 mg given intravenously immediately before cancer chemotherapy had a beneficial effect as an adjunct to standard antiemetic therapy with perphenazine 5 mg given an hour beforehand, in 7 patients who had established a pattern of distressing vomiting at the time of their 3- or 4-weekly treatments; 4 of the patients had developed anticipatory vomiting. Although sleepy, they were awake enough to use a bowl if they did vomit. Lorazepam 2 mg by mouth up to every 4 hours was prescribed to keep patients asleep, but was rarely needed; standard parenteral anti-emetics were prescribed as required. Vomiting was reduced to a maximum of twice, in all but one patient, and anticipatory vomiting was abolished in 3 of 4.— J. Maher (letter), *Lancet*, 1981, *1*, 91.

Lorazepam and high-dose metoclopramide were comparably effective in reducing emesis induced by cisplatin and dacarbazine in a crossover study involving 19 patients. Lorazepam was given in doses of 2.5 mg per m^2 body-surface intravenously 30 minutes before the antineoplastic, or metoclopramide in 5 separate aliquots of 2 mg per kg body-weight, each infused over 15 minutes, and beginning 30 minutes before the antineoplastic. Although no difference was observed in efficacy lorazepam was preferred because of its simpler administration and its amnestic and anxiolytic effects.— S. J. Bowcock *et al.*, *Br. med. J.*, 1984, *288*, 1879. See also J. B. Craig *et al.*, *Oncology*, 1987, *44*, 90 (metoclopramide alone and with lorazepam in chemotherapy-induced emesis).

Addition of lorazepam 3 mg intravenously to standard antiemetic doses of haloperidol 5 mg did not reduce nausea and vomiting in all patients in a crossover study in 27 patients receiving cisplatin based chemotherapy. However, the combined regimen was preferred by 17 patients compared to 7 preferring haloperidol alone and 3 with no preference. There was a significant preference for the lorazepam-containing regimen among those patients in whom the amnestic effect of the benzodiazepine was greatest. Impairment of recall improves tolerance and acceptance of chemotherapy, and lorazepam plus haloperidol has since become the standard antiemetic treatment in the authors' institution for inpatients receiving cytotoxic chemotherapy.— M. L. Friedlander *et al.* (letter), *Lancet*, 1983, *2*, 686. See also *Drug & Ther. Bull.*, 1986, *24*, 46.

PSYCHOSIS. A suggestion that lorazepam 2 mg intramuscularly may be as effective as a neuroleptic such as haloperidol in restraining aggressive or violent psychotic patients.— P. A. Bick and A. L. Hannah (letter), *Lancet*, 1986, *1*, 206.

Preparations

Lorazepam Injection *(U.S.P.)*. A sterile solution of lorazepam in a suitable medium.

Lorazepam Tablets *(B.P.)*. Contain lorazepam. Store at a temperature not exceeding 25°.

Lorazepam Tablets *(U.S.P.)*

Proprietary Preparations

Almazine *(Steinhard, UK)*. *Tablets*, scored, lorazepam 1 and 2.5 mg.

Ativan *(Wyeth, UK)*. *Tablets*, scored, lorazepam 0.5, 1, and 2.5 mg.

Injection, lorazepam 4 mg/mL, in ampoules of 1 mL.

Proprietary Names and Manufacturers

Almazine *(Steinhard, UK)*; Alzapam *(Ultra, USA)*; Aplacasse *(Arg.)*; Ativan *(Wyeth, Austral.*; *Wyeth, Canad.*; *Wyeth, S.Afr.*; *Wyeth, UK*; *Wyeth, USA)*; Control *(Sigurtà, Ital.)*; Donix *(Llorens, Spain)*; Emotival *(Arg.)*; Idalprem *(Frumtost, Spain)*; Kalmalin *(Arg.)*; Laubeel *(Desitin, Ger.)*; Lorans *(Schiapparelli, Ital.)*; Lorax *(Braz.)*; Lorenin *(Port.)*; NIC *(Arg.)*; Novolorazem *(Novopharm, Canad.)*; Orfidal *(Orfi, Spain)*; Piralone *(Ferrer, Spain)*; Placidia *(Spain)*; Placinoral *(Robert, Spain)*; Pro Dorm *(Schürholz, Ger.)*; Punktyl *(Krewel, Ger.)*; Quait *(SIT, Ital.)*; Securit *(Ital.)*; Sedarkey *(Spain)*; Sedatival *(Arg.)*; Sedicepan *(Septa, Spain)*; Sidenar *(Arg.)*; Tavor *(Wyeth, Ger.)*; Temesta *(Wyeth, Denm.*; *Wyeth-Byla, Fr.*; *Kabi, Swed.*; *Wyeth, Switz.)*; Tolid *(Dolorgiet, Ger.)*; Tran-qil *(Rolab, S.Afr.)*; Tranqipam *(Lennon, S.Afr.)*; Trapax *(Arg.)*; Wypax *(Jpn)*.

4077-r

Lormetazepam *(BAN, USAN, rINN)*.

Wy-4082. 7-Chloro-5-(2-chlorophenyl)-1,3-dihydro-3-hydroxy-1-methyl-1,4-benzodiazepin-2-one.

$C_{16}H_{12}Cl_2N_2O_2$=335.2.

CAS — 848-75-9.

Dependence, Adverse Effects, Treatment, and Precautions

As for the benzodiazepines in general, p.706.

Absorption and Fate

Lormetazepam is rapidly absorbed from the gastro-intestinal tract and metabolised to the inactive glucuronide. The terminal half-life is reported to be about 12 hours.

References: D. J. Greenblatt *et al.*, *Clin. Pharmacokinet.*, 1983, *8*, 233; D. M. Pierce *et al.*, *Br. J. clin. Pharmac.*, 1984, *18*, 31.

Uses and Administration

Lormetazepam is a benzodiazepine derivative with general properties similar to those of diazepam (p.731). It has been used as a hypnotic in the short-term management of insomnia in usual doses of 0.5 to 2 mg at night.

Proprietary Names and Manufacturers

Loramet *(Orfi, Spain*; *Wyeth, Switz.*; *Wyeth, UK)*; Minias *(Farmades, Ital.)*; Noctamid *(Schering, Ger.*; *Schering, Ital.*; *Schering, S.Afr.*; *Schering, Spain*; *Schering, Switz.*; *Schering, UK)*; Pronoctan *(Schering, Denm.)*.

7061-j

Loxapine *(BAN, USAN, rINN).*
CL-62362; Oxilapine; SUM-3170. 2-Chloro-11-(4-methylpiperazin-1-yl)dibenz[*b,f*][1,4]oxazepine.
$C_{18}H_{18}ClN_3O$=327.8.

CAS — 1977-10-2.

3843-l

Loxapine Hydrochloride *(BANM, rINNM).*

$C_{18}H_{18}ClN_3O,HCl$=364.3.

Loxapine hydrochloride 28 mg is approximately equivalent to 25 mg of loxapine.

7062-z

Loxapine Succinate *(BANM, USAN, rINNM).*
CL-71563.
$C_{18}H_{18}ClN_3O,C_4H_6O_4$=445.9.

CAS — 27833-64-3.

Loxapine succinate 34 mg is equivalent to 25 mg of loxapine.

Adverse Effects, Treatment, and Precautions

As for the phenothiazines, p.706.

Extrapyramidal symptoms may be more common than those associated with chlorpromazine but less common than with those phenothiazines that have a piperazine side chain.

Other side-effects reported include nausea and vomiting, weight gain and loss, dyspnoea, ptosis, hyperpyrexia, headache, paraesthesia, flush, and polydipsia.

Loxapine succinate was given for 4 weeks to 13 patients with acute schizophrenia or acute exacerbations of chronic schizophrenia. The average daily dose of loxapine was 23.2 mg in week 1 and 26.8 mg daily in week 4. Side-effects occurred in all patients and included drowsiness in 10 and extrapyramidal symptoms in 2. Other side-effects included headache, dry mouth, dizziness, fatigue, tingling, nausea, agitation, lactation, palpitations, and inhibition of ejaculation.— E. Ucer and P. Casey, *Curr. ther. Res.*, 1979, *25*, 144.

ABUSE. A report of 3 cases of loxapine succinate abuse.— L. Sperry *et al.* (letter), *New Engl. J. Med.*, 1984, *310*, 598.

EFFECTS ON CARBOHYDRATE METABOLISM. Reversible nonketotic hyperglycaemia, coma, and delirium, developed in a patient receiving loxapine 150 mg daily in addition to lithium therapy. Symptoms improved following discontinuation of loxapine, but subsequently recurred when the patient was given amoxapine. The causative agent may have been 7-hydroxyamoxapine, a common metabolite of both amoxapine and loxapine.— G. Tollefson and T. Lesar, *J. clin. Psychiat.*, 1983, *44*, 347.

EXTRAPYRAMIDAL EFFECTS. A report on the successful use of loxapine by intramuscular injection in 12 acutely psychotic patients. Episodes of acute dystonia occurred in 3 patients.— K. Fruensgaard and K. Jensen, *Curr. ther. Res.*, 1976, *19*, 164.

Loxapine succinate in capsules, or hydrochloride as liquid concentrate, was effective in the treatment of 17 young adult patients with acute schizophrenia in an open 4-week study. Doses varied from 10 to 250 mg daily. Dystonia and constipation were the most frequent side-effects occurring in 13 and 7 patients respectively.— J. L. Thomas, *Curr. ther. Res.*, 1979, *25*, 371.

OVERDOSAGE. Rhabdomyolysis and acute renal failure in a young man following overdosage with loxapine succinate.— C. W. Tam *et al.*, *Archs intern. Med.*, 1980, *140*, 975.

Absorption and Fate

Loxapine is readily absorbed from the gastro-intestinal tract. It is very rapidly and extensively metabolised. It is mainly excreted in the urine, in the form of its conjugated metabolites, with smaller amounts appearing in the faeces as unconjugated metabolites; most of a dose is excreted in the first 24 hours. The major metabolites of loxapine are the active 7- and 8-hydroxyloxapine, which are conjugated to the glucuronide or sulphate; other metabolites include hydroxyloxapine-*N*-oxide, loxapine-*N*-oxide, and hydroxydesmethylloxapine (hydroxyamoxapine). Loxapine is widely distributed and *animal* studies have indicated that it crosses the placenta.

A comparative study of oral and intramuscular forms of loxapine in 10 schizophrenic patients. There was no difference in clinical action or side-effects between the 2 routes. Higher plasma concentrations were achieved following intramuscular administration indicating that bioavailability following oral administration is reduced by a first-pass effect.— G. M. Simpson *et al.*, *Psychopharmacology*, 1978, *56*, 225.

Further references: T. B. Cooper and R. G. Kelly, *J. pharm. Sci.*, 1979, *68*, 216.

Uses and Administration

Loxapine is a dibenzoxazepine with antipsychotic actions similar to those of chlorpromazine (p.724). It is given by mouth as the hydrochloride or the succinate and by intramuscular injection as the hydrochloride, but the doses are expressed in terms of the base.

The usual dose by mouth for the treatment of psychoses is 20 to 50 mg daily initially, in 2 to 4 divided doses, increased over the next 7 to 10 days to 60 to 100 mg daily or more; the maximum recommended dose is 250 mg daily. For the control of acute conditions it is given by intramuscular injection in doses of 12.5 to 50 mg at intervals of 4 to 6 hours or longer.

Loxapine should be given in reduced dosage to elderly patients.

ADMINISTRATION. Loxapine 12.5 to 50 mg administered intramuscularly twice or thrice daily as the hydrochloride for 5 days was considered to be an effective method of initiating treatment in 20 patients with acute schizophrenia. Patients were also given loxapine by mouth after 3 days and by the sixth day of treatment, loxapine was given by mouth only. Side-effects experienced only during parenteral administration of loxapine were hypotension, nausea, vomiting, dizziness, light headedness, muscle twitches, vertigo, fatigue, anorexia and headache. Other side-effects were similar to those produced after administration by mouth.— C. D. Van Der Velde, *Curr. ther. Res.*, 1978, *23*, 367.

Proprietary Names and Manufacturers of Loxapine and its Salts

Daxolin *(Dome, USA)*; Desconex *(Lafarquim, Spain)*; Loxapac *(Lederle, Arg.; Lederle, Austral.; Lederle, Belg.; Lederle, Canad.; Lederle, Denm.; Lederle, Fr.; Cyanamid, Ital.; Lederle, Neth.; Lederle, S.Afr.; Cyanamid, Spain)*; Loxitane *(Lederle, USA)*.

7063-c

Mebutamate *(BAN, USAN, rINN).*
W-583. 2-*sec*-Butyl-2-methyltrimethylene dicarbamate.
$C_{10}H_{20}N_2O_4$=232.3.

CAS — 64-55-1.

Mebutamate is a carbamate with general properties similar to those of meprobamate (p.750). It has been suggested for use as an adjunct in the treatment of hypertension in doses of 300 mg three or four times daily.

Proprietary Names and Manufacturers

Axiten *(Zambon, Ital.)*; Butatensin *(Benvegna, Ital.)*; Capla *(Inibsa, Spain)*; Ipotensivo Vita *(Vita, Ital.)*; Mebutina *(Formenti, Ital.)*; No-Press *(Janus, Ital.)*; Prean *(Chemil, Ital.)*; Sigmafon *(Lafare, Ital.)*; Vallene *(Simes, Ital.; Farmasimes, Spain)*.

7064-k

Medazepam *(BAN, rINN).*
Ro-5-4556 (hydrochloride). 7-Chloro-2,3-dihydro-1-methyl-5-phenyl-1*H*-1,4-benzodiazepine.
$C_{16}H_{15}ClN_2$=270.8.

CAS — 2898-12-6 (base); 2898-11-5 (hydrochloride).

NOTE. *USAN* includes the hydrochloride.

Pharmacopoeias. In *Br.*, *Jpn*, and *Nord.*

A yellowish, odourless or almost odourless crystalline powder. Practically **insoluble** in water; soluble 1 in 8 of alcohol, 1 in 1 of chloroform, and 1 in 5 of ether.

Dependence, Adverse Effects, Treatment, and Precautions

As for the benzodiazepines in general, p.706.

Absorption and Fate

For an account of the absorption and fate of a benzodiazepine, see Diazepam, p.730.

Medazepam is rapidly absorbed from the gastro-intestinal tract following oral administration. It is metabolised to a number of active metabolites including normedazepam, diazepam, and desmethyldiazepam which are present at higher concentrations than the parent drug following multiple doses.

A review of the pharmacokinetics of medazepam.— D. M. Hailey and E. S. Baird, *Br. J. Anaesth.*, 1979, *51*, 493.

ABSORPTION AND PLASMA CONCENTRATIONS. Mean plasma concentrations of 63 ng per mL of medazepam were measured in 20 patients given medazepam in a mean dose of 27 mg a day for 2 to 4 weeks. Mean diazepam concentrations were 28 ng per mL and desmethyldiazepam concentrations were 706 ng per mL.— A. J. Bond *et al.*, *Br. J. clin. Pharmac.*, 1977, *4*, 51.

Uses and Administration

Medazepam is a benzodiazepine with actions and uses similar to those of diazepam (p.731).

The usual dose for the treatment of anxiety is 15 to 30 mg daily in divided doses; in severe conditions up to 40 mg daily has been given.

ANAESTHESIA. *Anaesthetic premedication.* In a double-blind study of premedication in 150 women, medazepam 10 mg produced less drowsiness than diazepam 10 mg but the latter was preferred by patients. Nausea and vomiting were more frequent during the first hour postoperatively in patients given medazepam.— R. A. E. Assaf *et al.*, *Br. J. Anaesth.*, 1975, *47*, 464.

Preparations

Medazepam Capsules *(B.P.)*

Proprietary Preparations

Nobrium *(Roche, UK). Capsules,* medazepam 5 and 10 mg.

Proprietary Names and Manufacturers

Anxitol *(Denm.)*; Azepamid *(Jpn)*; Benson *(Ital.)*; Elbrus *(Arg.)*; Lasazepam *(Lasa, Spain)*; Lerisum *(Poli, Ital.)*; Medacepan *(Vinsi, Spain)*; Megasedan *(Andreu, Spain)*; Metonas *(Jpn)*; Narsis *(Jpn)*; Navizil *(Arg.)*; Nivelton *(Arg.)*; Nobrium *(Arg.; Belg.; Roche, Denm.; Roche, Fr.; Roche, Ger.; Roche, Ital.; Neth.; Roche, Norw.; Roche, S.Afr.; Roche, Spain; Roche, Switz.; Roche, UK)*; Raporan *(Austral.)*; Resmit *(Jpn)*; Serenium; Siman *(Arg.)*; Templane *(Arg.)*; Tranquilax *(Jpn)*.

7150-z

Melperone Hydrochloride *(BANM, rINNM).*
FG-5111; Flubuperone Hydrochloride; Methylperone Hydrochloride. 4′-Fluoro-4-(4-methylpiperidino)butyrophenone hydrochloride.
$C_{16}H_{22}FNO,HCl$=299.8.

CAS — 3575-80-2 (melperone); 1622-79-3 (hydrochloride).

Melperone is a butyrophenone with general properties similar to those of haloperidol (p.743). For the treatment of psychoses it is given as the hydrochloride in doses of up to 100 mg three or four times daily. In acute conditions it may be given intramuscularly in doses of 50 mg up to 4 times daily.

ACTION. Studies of the anti-arrhythmic properties of melperone: J. C. Mogelvang *et al.*, *Acta med. scand.*, 1980, *208*, 61; J. S. Millar and E. M. V. Williams, *Br. J. Pharmac.*, 1982, *75*, 109.

Proprietary Names and Manufacturers

Buronil *(Knoll, Belg.; Ferrosan, Denm.; Neth.; Ferrosan, Norw.; Ferrosan, Swed.)*; Eunerpan *(Nordmark, Ger.)*.

7065-a

Mephenoxalone *(rINN).*
AHR-233; Methoxadone; OM-518. 5-(2-Methoxyphenoxymethyl)oxazolidin-2-one.
$C_{11}H_{13}NO_4$=223.2.

CAS — 70-07-5.

Mephenoxalone has actions similar to those of meprobamate (see below). It has been used in usual doses of

400 mg three times daily in the treatment of anxiety or to relieve muscle spasm.

Proprietary Names and Manufacturers
Control-OM *(Om, Switz.)*; Dorsiflex *(Neth.; Syntex, Switz.)*; Riself *(Gibipharma, Ital.)*; Xérène *(Martinet, Fr.)*.

7066-t

Meprobamate *(BAN, USAN, rINN)*.

Meprobamatum; Meprotanum. 2-Methyl-2-propyltrimethylene dicarbamate.
$C_9H_{18}N_2O_4$=218.3.
CAS — 57-53-4.

Pharmacopoeias. In *Arg., Aust., Belg., Br., Braz., Chin., Cz., Egypt., Eur., Fr., Ger., Ind., Int., It., Jug., Neth., Pol., Port., Roum., Rus., Swiss, Turk.,* and *U.S.*

Odourless or almost odourless, colourless crystals or white crystalline powder.

***B.P.* solubilities** are: slightly soluble in water and in ether; soluble 1 in 7 of alcohol. *U.S.P.* solubilities are: slightly soluble in water; freely soluble in acetone and in alcohol; sparingly soluble in ether. **Store** in airtight containers.

Dependence

For discussion of dependence upon sedatives and hypnotics see p.706.

Adverse Effects

Drowsiness is the most frequent side-effect of meprobamate. Other effects include nausea, vomiting, diarrhoea, paraesthesia, weakness, and central effects such as headache, paradoxical excitement, dizziness, ataxia, and disturbances of vision. There may be hypotension, tachycardia, and cardiac arrhythmias. Hypersensitivity reactions occur occasionally. These may be limited to skin rashes, urticaria, and purpura or may be more severe with angioedema, bronchospasm, or anuria. Erythema multiforme and exfoliative or bullous dermatitis have been reported.

Blood disorders including agranulocytosis, eosinophilia, leucopenia, thrombocytopenia, and aplastic anaemia have occasionally been reported. Symptoms of porphyria may be exacerbated.

OVERDOSAGE. Of 773 admissions to Massachusetts General Hospital between 1962 and 1975 for psychotropic drug overdosage, meprobamate was implicated in 50. Serious intoxication was common and 2 patients died, one of whom had ingested an estimated 12 to 20 g, apparently with no other drugs. Hypotension was common and not always correlated with the depth of coma, indicating that it is not necessarily a consequence of CNS depression. Patients with meprobamate overdosage appear to be susceptible to cardiac failure and pulmonary oedema therefore care must be taken to avoid overhydration. The questionable efficacy and the potential for life-threatening intoxication are important drawbacks to the clinical use of this drug.— M. D. Allen *et al., Clin. Toxicol.,* 1977, *11,* 501.

Further reference S. Sato *et al., Hum. Toxicol.,* 1986, *5,* 243.

See also under Treatment of Adverse Effects, below.

PREGNANCY AND THE NEONATE. In a prospective study of 19 044 live births the incidence of severe congenital defects was compared in mothers who had presented with anxiety, tension, or mild depression, and who had received meprobamate, chlordiazepoxide, other drugs, or no drugs during or just before the pregnancy. Considering the first 42 days of pregnancy the rates of defects were: when meprobamate was prescribed 12.1 per 100 live births, chlordiazepoxide 11.4, other drugs 4.6, and no drug 2.6. Considering the later stages of pregnancy there was no significant difference in the rate of defects between the 4 groups. In the meprobamate group 5 of the children with abnormalities had congenital heart disease.— L. Milkovich and B. J. van den Berg, *New Engl. J. Med.,* 1974, *291,* 1268. In prospective English and French studies of 63 and 239 women respectively who had received meprobamate, chlordiazepoxide, and other anxiolytics during the first 13 weeks of pregnancy, there were significantly more malformed children (4 of 71) born to French mothers who had received meprobamate than to those who had not. None of these were cardiac abnormalities. However 3 of the mothers had had previous unsuccessful pregnancies. The incidence of malformations in the English group was not significant. In these studies malformations were defined as those present at birth or seen within the first 6 weeks of life compared with the L. Milkovich and B.J. van den Berg study which covered the first 5 years. Congenital heart disease would therefore not be so easily detected.— D. L. Crombie *et al.* (letter), *ibid.,* 1975, *293,* 198.

Of 50 282 children born to mothers monitored by the Collaborative Perinatal Project, 356 were found to have been exposed to meprobamate, and possibly other drugs, at some time during the first 4 months of the pregnancy. Although a slight association between hypospadias and meprobamate exposure was noted no relationship to other types of malformation could be detected.— O. P. Heinonen *et al., Birth Defects and Drugs in Pregnancy,* Littleton MA, Publishing Sciences Group, 1977, p. 335. See also S. C. Hartz *et al., New Engl. J. Med.,* 1975, *292,* 726.

WITHDRAWAL. Abstinence symptoms reported after the abrupt withdrawal of high doses of meprobamate included insomnia, vomiting, tremors, muscle twitches, anxiety, headache, ataxia, convulsions, and psychotic behaviour at times resembling delirium tremens.— C. F. Essig, *J. Am. med. Ass.,* 1966, *196,* 714.

Treatment of Adverse Effects

For general guidelines on the management of overdosage with sedatives and hypnotics, see p.708.

Meprobamate is rapidly metabolised, and intensive measures to reduce drug concentrations in overdosage are normally unecessary; however, in severe overdosage, charcoal haemoperfusion may be considered. Forced diuresis or haemodialysis have also been employed.

The stomach of a woman who died of meprobamate overdosage was found to contain about 25 g of meprobamate despite gastric lavage. Treatment should include gastric lavage through a wide calibre tube.— E. H. Jenis *et al., J. Am. med. Ass.,* 1969, *207,* 361. A 56-year-old woman was still deeply comatose 40 hours after ingestion of 36 g of meprobamate, despite gastric lavage, haemodialysis, and supportive therapy. Upon surgical operation a tarry mass weighing 140 g was removed from the stomach; it contained 24.9 g of meprobamate. She recovered following further haemodialysis.— H. S. Schwartz, *New Engl. J. Med.,* 1976, *295,* 1177.

A warning that expansion of plasma volume in hypotension due to meprobamate poisoning may cause pulmonary oedema.— F. Lhoste *et al.* (letter), *New Engl. J. Med.,* 1977, *296,* 1004.

Forced diuresis with physiological saline precipitated pulmonary oedema in a 23-year-old woman who had taken an overdose of meprobamate.— J. A. Axelson and J. F. Hagaman (letter), *New Engl. J. Med.,* 1977, *296,* 1481.

A review of some specific problems of drug intoxication. In severe meprobamate poisoning with plasma concentrations of 100 µg per mL or more the preferred elimination procedure would be haemoperfusion, although haemodialysis may also be used.— J. A. Henry, *Br. J. Anaesth.,* 1986, *58,* 223. Two children aged 2 and 2.5 years recovered with conservative management alone following overdosage of meprobamate with bendrofluazide despite measured plasma-meprobamate concentrations of 158 and 170 µg per mL respectively. Despite previous recommendations that haemoperfusion should be considered at plasma-meprobamate concentrations above 100 µg per mL these cases suggest that children may tolerate higher blood concentrations than adults, and recent experience with adults has suggested that haemoperfusion should normally only be considered at plasma concentrations above 200 µg per mL.— J. Dennison *et al., Hum. Toxicol.,* 1985, *4,* 215.

The treatment of meprobamate overdose with repeated oral doses of activated charcoal.— E. Hassan, *Ann. emerg. Med.,* 1986, *15,* 73.

Precautions

Meprobamate should not be given to patients with acute intermittent porphyria. Meprobamate may induce convulsions in patients with a history of epilepsy.

It may lower the tolerance to alcohol and other depressants of the central nervous system. Meprobamate is capable of inducing hepatic microsomal enzyme systems involved in drug metabolism: the metabolism of agents such as oral contraceptives, corticosteroids, phenytoin, phenothiazines, and tricyclic antidepressants may be enhanced if given concurrently.

Meprobamate may cause drowsiness and patients if affected should not drive vehicles or operate machinery where loss of attention could lead to accidents.

Because of the potential for the development of dependence (see above) withdrawal of meprobamate from patients who have received high or prolonged dosage should be gradual.

A study of the metabolism of meprobamate in human subjects suggested that chronic administration stimulates its own metabolism.— J. F. Douglas *et al., Proc. Soc. exp. Biol. Med.,* 1963, *112,* 436. Two patients receiving large doses of meprobamate for prolonged periods of time excreted meprobamate more slowly than subjects given single doses. This did not exclude the possibility of meprobamate enhancing its own metabolism.— L. E. Hollister and G. Levy, *Chemotherapia,* 1964, *9,* 20.

Absorption and Fate

Meprobamate is readily absorbed from the gastro-intestinal tract and peak concentrations in the plasma occur after 1 to 3 hours. Meprobamate is widely distributed. It is extensively metabolised in the liver and is excreted in the urine mainly as a hydroxylated metabolite and its glucuronide conjugate. Less than 10% of a dose is excreted unchanged. Meprobamate has a half-life reported to range from about 6 to 16 hours.

It diffuses across the placenta and appears in the milk of nursing mothers at concentrations of up to 4 times those in the maternal plasma.

The elimination of meprobamate was found to be variable following administration of 800 mg to 12 healthy subjects, the half-life ranging from 6.4 to 16.6 hours (mean 11.3 hours). Considerably longer half-lives of 24 and 48 hours respectively were found following abrupt discontinuation in 2 subjects who had been receiving high doses for prolonged periods of time.— L. E. Hollister and G. Levy, *Chemotherapia,* 1964, *9,* 20.

Uses and Administration

Meprobamate belongs to the carbamate group of anxiolytics. It has some muscle relaxant properties and has been reported to have anticonvulsant actions against petit mal seizures, but not against grand mal seizures (which may be exacerbated—see Precautions). It is used in the treatment of anxiety and tension but has largely been superseded by the benzodiazepines.

Meprobamate has sometimes been used as a muscle relaxant, alone or in combination with an analgesic, in the management of muscle spasm.

The usual anxiolytic dose is 400 mg three or four times daily to a maximum of 2.4 g daily. Children have been given 25 mg per kg body-weight daily in divided doses; alternatively children aged 6 to 12 years may be given 100 to 200 mg two or three times daily.

ADMINISTRATION IN HEPATIC FAILURE. Meprobamate elimination is reported to be prolonged in patients with chronic liver disease.— R. K. Roberts *et al., Drugs,* 1979, *17,* 198.

ADMINISTRATION IN RENAL FAILURE. The interval between doses of meprobamate should be extended from 6 hours to 9 to 12 hours in patients with a glomerular filtration-rate of 10 to 50 mL per minute, and to 12 to 18 hours in those with a glomerular filtration-rate of less than 10 mL per minute. Concentrations of meprobamate are affected by haemodialysis and peritoneal dialysis.— W. M. Bennett *et al., Am. J. Kidney Dis.,* 1983, *3,* 155.

Preparations

Meprobamate Oral Suspension *(U.S.P.)*

Meprobamate Tablets *(U.S.P.)*

Proprietary Preparations

Equanil *(Wyeth, UK). Tablets,* meprobamate 200 mg. *Tablets,* scored, meprobamate 400 mg.

Meprate *(DDSA Pharmaceuticals, UK). Tablets,* meprobamate 400 mg.

Tenavoid *(Leo, UK). Tablets,* meprobamate 200 mg, bendrofluazide 3 mg. *Dose.* For the premenstrual syndrome: 1 tablet 3 times daily for 5 to 7 days before each period.

Proprietary Names and Manufacturers

Aneural *(Ger.)*; Ansiowas *(Wasserman, Spain)*; Cyrpon *(Tropon, Ger.)*; Dapaz *(Alter, Spain)*; Distoncur *(Arg.)*;

Dystoid forte *(Ger.)*; Ecuanil *(Spain)*; Equanil *(Wyeth, Austral.; Wyeth, Canad.; Denm.; Clin Midy, Fr.; Wyeth, S.Afr.; Wyeth, UK; Wyeth, USA)*; Lan-Dol *(Canad.)*; Meditran *(Medic, Canad.)*; Mepavlon *(Spain; ICI Pharmaceuticals, UK)*; Mep-E *(Canad.)*; Meposed *(Vernleigh, S.Afr.)*; Meprate *(DDSA Pharmaceuticals, UK)*; Meprepose *(SCS, S.Afr.)*; Mepriam *(USA)*; Meprin *(Arg.)*; Meproban *(Norw.)*; Meprobil *(Nessa, Spain)*; Meprocompren *(Ger.)*; Meprodil *(Streuli, Switz.)*; Meprodiol *(Ital.)*; Mepron *(Hamilton, Austral.)*; Meprosa *(Ger.)*; Meprospan *(Horner, Canad.; Inibsa, Spain; Wallace, USA)*; Milonorm *(Wallace Mfg Chem., UK)*; Miltaun *(Ger.; Ital.)*; Miltaunetten *(Ger.)*; Miltown *(Horner, Canad.; Inibsa, Spain; Switz.; Pharmax, UK; Wallace, USA)*;
Neo-Tran *(Neolab, Canad.)*; Novomepro *(Novopharm, Canad.)*; Oasil *(Belg.; Ital.; Farmasimes, Spain; Switz.)*; Pantranquil *(S.Afr.)*; Perequil *(Ital.)*; Pertranquil *(Belg.; Switz.)*; Placidon *(Arg.)*; Probamyl *(Belg.; Switz.)*; Procalmadiol *(Belg.; Adrian-Marinier, Fr.)*; Quaname *(Belg.; Switz.)*; Quanil *(Wyeth, Ital.)*; Quietal *(Canad.)*; Restenil *(GEA, Denm.; Weiders, Norw.; Kabi, Swed.)*; Sedans *(Orravan, Spain)*; Sedoquil *(Ital.)*; Selene *(Ital.)*; SK-Bamate *(Smith Kline & French, USA)*; Stensolo *(Salfa, Ital.)*; Sycropaz *(Arg.)*; Tised *(Ticen, Eire)*; Urbilat *(Hermes, Ger.)*.

The following names have been used for multi-ingredient preparations containing meprobamate—282 Mep *(Frosst, Canad.)*; Deprol *(Wallace, USA)*; Ecuagesico; Equagesic *(Wyeth, Canad.; Wyeth, UK; Wyeth, USA)*; Mepogen *(Faulding, Austral.)*; Mepro Compound *(Schein, USA)*; Meprogesic *(Quantum, USA)*; Neo-HS *(Neolab, Canad.)*; Pathibamate *(Lederle, USA)*; Paxidal *(Wallace Mfg Chem., UK)*; Placitate *(Faulding, Austral.)*; PMB *(Ayerst, USA)*; Tenavoid *(Leo, UK)*.

7067-x

Mesoridazine Besylate *(BANM, USAN)*.

Mesoridazine Benzenesulphonate; Mesoridazine Besilate *(rINN)*; Mesoridazine Benzenesulphonate; NC-123 *(base)*; TPS-23 *(base)*. 10-[2-(1-Methyl-2-piperidyl)ethyl]-2-(methylsulphinyl)phenothiazine benzenesulphonate.

$C_{21}H_{26}N_2OS_2,C_6H_6O_3S=544.7$.

CAS — 5588-33-0 (mesoridazine); 32672-69-8(benzenesulphonate).

Pharmacopoeias. In *U.S.*

A white to pale yellow, almost odourless powder. **Soluble** 1 in 1 of water, 1 in 11 of alcohol, 1 in 3 of chloroform, and 1 in 6300 of ether; freely soluble in methyl alcohol. A freshly prepared 1% solution in water has a pH of between 4.2 and 5.7; the *U.S.P.* injection has a pH between 4 and 5.
Store in airtight containers. Protect from light.

INCOMPATIBILITY. A commercial formulation of mesoridazine besylate oral solution was incompatible on mixing with an oral solution of haloperidol (as the lactate). Mesoridazine was also incompatible with a solution of thioridazine hydrochloride.— W. A. Parker, *Can. J. Hosp. Pharm.*, 1984, *37*, 133.

Adverse Effects, Treatment, and Precautions
As for the phenothiazines in general, p.706.

INTERACTIONS. *Phenytoin and other anticonvulsants.* For the effect of phenytoin and phenobarbitone on plasma-mesoridazine concentrations in patients receiving thioridazine, see under Thioridazine, p.770.

Absorption and Fate
For an account of the absorption and fate of a phenothiazine, see Chlorpromazine, p.723.
Mesoridazine is a metabolite of thioridazine (p.770).

Uses and Administration
Mesoridazine is a phenothiazine with actions and uses similar to those of chlorpromazine (p.724). It has a piperidine side-chain and is a metabolite of thioridazine (p.770). Mesoridazine is usually given as the besylate but the doses are expressed in terms of the base. The usual dose for the treatment of psychoses is 50 mg three times daily; doses of up to 400 mg daily have been given. It may also be given intramuscularly in an initial dose of 25 mg repeated after 30 to 60 minutes if necessary; up to 200 mg daily has been given.
Doses of 10 mg three times daily have also been used for non-psychotic emotional disturbances, such as anxiety and tension. In general, however, phenothiazines are only suitable for such purposes in resistant conditions, where more appropriate agents, such as the benzodiazepines (see Diazepam, p.731), have proved ineffective. If their use is judged to be necessary, treatment should be directed at low dosages on a short-term basis. Mesoridazine should be given in reduced dosage to elderly patients.

A review of mesoridazine.— S. Gershon *et al.*, *J. clin. Psychiat.*, 1981, *42*, 463.

ALCOHOL AND DRUG WITHDRAWAL. Studies of mesoridazine in the treatment of alcoholism: J. B. Frost, *Can. psychiat. Ass. J.*, 1973, *18*, 385; I. Lowenstam, *J. chron. Dis.*, 1975, *28*, 431.

PSYCHOSES. There is no evidence that mesoridazine offers any advantage over other phenothiazines.— *Med. Lett.*, 1975, *17*, 68. In a double-blind study in 7 patients with schizophrenia considered refractory to neuroleptics, substitution of previous neuroleptic therapy (mesoridazine, haloperidol, or molindone) by mesoridazine 200 mg with amantadine 100 mg both twice daily by mouth, for 4 weeks, resulted in a significant improvement in mental state. Therapeutic progress appeared to be achieved by the third or fourth week of the combined therapy and was sustained during two subsequent weeks despite resumption of baseline neuroleptic therapy. The results support the hypothesis that combined mesoridazine and amantadine treatment is efficacious in a subgroup of neuroleptic-resistant schizophrenics and are consistent with the proposition that lack of response to neuroleptics may reflect in part a drug-induced catatonia-parkinsonism syndrome.— L. A. Opler *et al.*, *Curr. ther. Res.*, 1985, *37*, 318.

Preparations

Mesoridazine Besylate Injection *(U.S.P.)*. Potency is expressed in terms of the equivalent amount of mesoridazine.

Mesoridazine Besylate Oral Solution *(U.S.P.)*. Potency is expressed in terms of the equivalent amount of mesoridazine. To be diluted before use. Store at a temperature not exceeding 25°.

Mesoridazine Besylate Tablets *(U.S.P.)*. Potency is expressed in terms of the equivalent amount of mesoridazine.

Proprietary Names and Manufacturers
Imagotan *(Sandoz, Spain)*; Serentil *(Sandoz, Canad.; Boehringer Ingelheim, USA)*.

19474-r

Metaclazepam *(rINN)*.

Brometazepam; Ka-2547; KC-2547. 7-Bromo-5-(2-chlorophenyl)-2,3-dihydro-2-(methoxymethyl)-1-methyl-1*H*-1,4-benzodiazepine.

$C_{18}H_{18}BrClN_2O=393.7$.

CAS — 65517-27-3.

Metaclazepam is a benzodiazepine derivative with general properties similar to those of diazepam (p.731). It is used as the hydrochloride for its anxiolytic and sedative properties, in doses ranging from 5 to 30 mg daily in divided doses.

Reference K. -H. Molz *et al.*, *Eur. J. clin. Pharmac.*, 1985, *29*, 247 (pharmacokinetics).

Proprietary Names and Manufacturers
Talis *(Kali-Chemie, Switz.)*.

4045-y

Methaqualone *(BAN, USAN, rINN)*.

CI-705; CN-38703; Methachalonum; QZ-2; R-148; TR-495. 2-Methyl-3-*o*-tolylquinazolin-4(3*H*)-one.

$C_{16}H_{14}N_2O=250.3$.

CAS — 72-44-6.

Pharmacopoeias. In *Br., Cz., Eur., Nord., Swiss,* and *U.S.*

An odourless, white or almost white, crystalline powder. Very slightly **soluble** in water; the *B.P.* states that it is soluble 1 in 12 of alcohol, 1 in 1 of chloroform, and 1 in 50 of ether. *U.S.P.* solubilities are: 1 in 8 of alcohol, 1 in 2.2 of chloroform, 1 in 27 of ether, and 1 in 21 of isopropyl alcohol. **Store** in well-closed containers. Protect from light.

4046-j

Methaqualone Hydrochloride *(BANM, rINNM)*.

Methaqualoni Chloridum.

$C_{16}H_{14}N_2O,HCl=286.8$.

CAS — 340-56-7.

Pharmacopoeias. In *Nord.*

Methaqualone hydrochloride 200 mg is approximately equivalent to 175 mg of methaqualone.

Dependence
As for the barbiturates, p.706.

Addiction to methaqualone was recorded in a 47-year-old man who had taken increasing doses over a period of 4 years until he reached a dose of sixty 150-mg tablets daily. Delirium tremens was noted on withdrawal of methaqualone and dramatic improvement resulted from administration of thioridazine in doses up to 800 mg daily.— R. B. L. Ewart and R. G. Priest, *Br. med. J.*, 1967, *3*, 92.

In 3 subjects who had taken 1.5 to 2 g of methaqualone daily for several months abrupt cessation of the drug resulted in severe withdrawal symptoms, including grand mal seizure in 1 patient. Methaqualone was used when diamorphine was not available.— M. Swartzburg *et al.*, *Archs gen. Psychiat.*, 1973, *29*, 46.

In contrast to the generally declining trend in sedative abuse among young people in the *USA* there was an increase in methaqualone abuse from 1976 to 1981; this might be related to the increase in cocaine abuse since methaqualone is frequently used to counteract the stimulant effects of cocaine.— A. M. Nicholi, *New Engl. J. Med.*, 1983, *308*, 925.

Reviews of the misuse of methaqualone: F. A. Whitlock, *Drugs*, 1973, *6*, 167; D. S. Inaba *et al.*, *J. Am. med. Ass.*, 1973, *224*, 1505; E. F. Pascarelli, *ibid.*, 1512 and 1521; C. V. Wetli, *ibid.*, 1983, *249*, 621.

Adverse Effects
Side-effects of treatment with methaqualone or its hydrochloride in therapeutic doses include headache, 'hangover', dizziness, drowsiness, anorexia, nausea and gastro-intestinal discomfort, dry mouth, restlessness, and sweating. Skin reactions have also been reported. Aplastic anaemia may occur rarely but the association is not proven. Paraesthesia may occur, which is usually transient but may be a symptom of peripheral neuropathy and persist for months or even years.
The symptoms of mild acute poisoning are the same as those of the barbiturates and most other hypnotics (see p.706). Severe overdosage results in delirium, coma, restlessness, tachycardia, and hypertonia, hyperreflexia, and myoclonus, which may progress to convulsions. Cardiac and respiratory depression occurs less frequently than with acute barbiturate poisoning. Pulmonary and cutaneous oedema, cardiac and hepatic damage, renal insufficiency, and bleeding may occur with severe poisoning. Spontaneous vomiting and increased secretions are common and may lead to pneumonitis or respiratory obstruction.

EFFECTS ON THE EYES. Keratitis occurred in 2 subjects dependent on methaqualone.— F. C. Rodger (letter), *Br. J. Ophthal.*, 1973, *57*, 712.

OVERDOSAGE. Of 28 cases of poisoning due to tablets containing methaqualone 250 mg and diphenhydramine hydrochloride 25 mg (Mandrax) admitted to the Edinburgh Poisoning Treatment Centre, 19 were mildly poisoned and 9 more severely poisoned. All were treated by intensive supportive therapy and subsequently recovered. The most striking clinical features in the severe cases were pyramidal signs (marked hypertonia, increased tendon reflexes, and myoclonia). Four of the 9 showed impairment of cardiovascular function. Plasma-methaqualone concentrations on admission ranged from 2 to 20 µg per mL, in all except 1 case in which the concentration was below the limit of detection. It was considered that plasma concentrations greater than 30 µg per mL, corresponding to 20 tablets ingested, were indicative of dangerous poisoning in patients who had not become habituated. The diphenhydramine component of Mandrax did not appear to contribute significantly to its toxicity.— A. A. H. Lawson and S. S. Brown (letter), *Br. med. J.*, 1966, *2*, 1455.

A 38-year-old woman became deeply unconscious, hypotensive, and required mechanically assisted respiration after taking about 180 tablets of Mandrax. An ECG showed flat T-waves and a prolonged Q-T interval. Hypotension responded to treatment with metaraminol, and spontaneous respiration and tendon-reflexes returned after haemodialysis. An EEG taken 2 days after the drug was ingested was flat except for irregular bilateral spike complexes appearing at intervals of 1 to 8 seconds. Though the woman had many fits during the first few days, she made a slow recovery and 13 days after admission to hospital the EEG record was almost normal.— M. R. Wallace and E. Allen (letter), *Lancet*, 1968, *2*, 1247.

Although lack of respiratory depression has been proposed as characteristic of methaqualone poisoning, respiratory arrest and 36 hours of apnoea developed in a 21-year-old woman following overdosage with methaqualone.— R. E. Johnstone *et al.*, *Ohio St. med. J.*, 1971, *67*, 1018.

A woman who was a frequent drug abuser took a single dose of 9 g of methaqualone. She had no response to painful stimuli, exaggerated deep tendon reflexes, shivering and muscle twitching, and bilateral ankle clonus. After 16 hours muscle overactivity increased and could not be controlled by diazepam. She was given tubocurarine 12 mg, followed by 2 further doses at hourly intervals. Response to painful stimuli returned after 26 hours and the patient was conscious after 40 hours.— R. T. Abboud *et al.*, *Chest*, 1974, *65*, 204.

A 73-year-old man who had taken about 7 g of methaqualone (as Mandrax) and who was unconscious for 7 days developed severe peripheral motor and sensory neuropathy with numbness, tingling, and weakness of the legs.— K. Constantinidis, *Br. med. J.*, 1975, *2*, 370.

Treatment of Adverse Effects

As for the barbiturates, p.708.

Forced diuresis is of no value and may be harmful. In the management of severely poisoned patients haemoperfusion may be of value.

Precautions

Methaqualone should be used with caution in patients with impaired hepatic function. Its use should be avoided during pregnancy and in patients with epilepsy. It causes drowsiness and patients being treated with it should not take charge of vehicles or machinery where loss of attention could lead to accidents. These effects are enhanced by the simultaneous administration of depressants of the central nervous system such as alcohol, barbiturates, and other sedatives. Methaqualone may moderately induce microsomal hepatic enzymes.

INTERACTIONS. *Alcohol.* In a study on 12 subjects who received methaqualone 500 mg with diphenhydramine hydrochloride 50 mg at night followed by 3 single doses of alcohol 500 mg per kg body-weight at 24, 48, and 72 hours it was shown that residual levels of methaqualone reacted with alcohol 72 hours later. This resulted in greater subjective mental and physical sedation and impairment of cognitive tasks.— S. Roden *et al.* (letter), *Br. J. clin. Pharmac.*, 1977, *4*, 245.

Diphenhydramine. Studies *in vitro* demonstrated that diphenhydramine inhibited the metabolism of methaqualone by *rat* liver homogenate. This inhibition of conversion of methaqualone to an inactive metabolite may account for the enhanced effect claimed by drug abusers when the two drugs are taken together.— K. W. Hindmarsh *et al.*, *J. pharm. Sci.*, 1978, *67*, 1547.

PREGNANCY AND LACTATION. As the administration of methaqualone to pregnant *rats* had increased the incidence of cleft palate in the offspring, it was suggested that the use of methaqualone in women of child-bearing age should be avoided.— CanadaFood and Drug Directorate, *Pharm. J.*, 1970, *2*, 720.

See also under Absorption and Fate.

Absorption and Fate

Methaqualone is readily absorbed from the gastro-intestinal tract and extensively metabolised, mainly by hydroxylation, in the liver. Clearance from the plasma is biphasic, with a terminal half-life reported to range from 10 to 40 hours; it is extensively bound to plasma protein. It is excreted in the urine and faeces; about 2% is excreted in the urine unchanged.

In normal fasting subjects absorption of methaqualone base was rapid and peak plasma concentrations were reached within 2 hours; absorption of the hydrochloride was significantly faster. The drug was strongly protein bound at plasma concentrations up to those in severe acute overdosage and was largely excluded from red cells. The major route of metabolism in man involved relatively non-specific hydroxylation of the tolyl substituent and little unchanged drug was excreted either after therapeutic doses or after overdosage.— S. S. Brown and S. Goenechea, *Clin. Pharmac. Ther.*, 1973, *14*, 314. Methaqualone hydrochloride 300 mg was given by mouth to 7 healthy subjects. The maximum blood concentration occurred after an average of 3 hours and the concentration diminished in a biphasic manner. The biological half-lives were calculated to be about 50 minutes for the first component and 16 hours for the second. Methaqualone was detected in the plasma after 34 hours but not after 40 hours.— J. M. Clifford *et al.*, *ibid.*, 1974, *16*, 376.

Methaqualone was still detected in the blood of a healthy subject 17 days after the commencement of a 5-day administration period of methaqualone 250 mg and diphenhydramine hydrochloride 25 mg each night. The study had been terminated prematurely after 5 days because the subject had become too confused and drowsy.— M. E. Williams *et al.*, *J. clin. Pharm.*, 1976, *1*, 63.

Estimation of a 74-hour terminal half-life for methaqualone.— H. d'A. Heck *et al.*, *J. Pharmacokinet. Biopharm.*, 1978, *6*, 111.

Studies in women indicated that the metabolism of methaqualone to its hydroxylated metabolites was affected by the menstrual cycle, with significantly increased excretion of hydroxylated metabolites on day 15 of the cycle compared with day 1. No such significant difference could be demonstrated for the formation of the *N*-oxide metabolite.— K. Wilson *et al.*, *Br. J. clin. Pharmac.*, 1982, *14*, 333. See also M. Oram *et al.*, *ibid.*, 341.

PREGNANCY AND LACTATION. Inactive metabolites of methaqualone were possibly excreted in the milk of lactating mothers.— J. J. Rowan (letter), *Pharm. J.*, 1976, *2*, 184.

Studies in *mice* established that methaqualone crossed the placenta.— N. S. Shah *et al.*, *Toxic. appl. Pharmac.*, 1977, *40*, 497.

See also under Precautions.

Uses and Administration

Methaqualone is a quinazoline derivative that has been used as a hypnotic in the short-term management of insomnia in doses of 150 to 300 mg at night. It has sometimes been given in conjunction with diphenhydramine for an enhanced effect. Methaqualone has also been used as a sedative in usual doses of 75 mg given up to 4 times daily.

The hydrochloride, which is more rapidly absorbed has been used similarly to the base, in usual hypnotic doses of 200 to 400 mg at night, or 100 mg up to 4 times daily as a sedative.

Methaqualone has been withdrawn from the market in a number of countries because of problems with abuse.

ADMINISTRATION IN RENAL FAILURE. Methaqualone could be given in usual doses to patients with renal failure who had a glomerular filtration-rate greater than 50 mL per minute, but it should be avoided in those with a glomerular filtration-rate less than this.— W. M. Bennett *et al.*, *Am. J. Kidney Dis.*, 1983, *3*, 155.

Preparations

Methaqualone Tablets *(U.S.P.)*

Proprietary Names and Manufacturers

Cateudyl *(Belg.)*; Dormogen *(Cz.)*; Melsed *(Boots, UK)*; Melsedin *(Boots, UK)*; Mequelon *(Frosst, Canad.)*; Mequin *(Lemmon, USA)*; Metakvalon *(DAK, Denm.)*; Methasedil *(Cooper, Switz.)*; Nobadorm *(Streuli, Switz.)*; Normi-Nox *(Herbrand, Ger.; Herbrand, Switz.)*; Pallidan *(Berna, Spain)*; Parest *(Parke, Davis, USA)*; Quaalude *(Lemmon, USA)*; Rebuso *(Montpellier, Arg.)*; Revonal *(Merck, Belg.; Cascan, Ger.; E. Merck, Neth.; E. Merck, Swed.; E. Merck, UK)*; Rouqualone *(Rougier, Canad.)*; Sedalone *(Nordic, Canad.)*; Sindesvel *(York, Arg.)*; Sleepinal *(Austral.)*; Sopor *(American Critical Care, USA)*; Sovelin *(Weiders, Norw.)*; Sovinal *(ND & K, Denm.)*; Toquilone *(Belg.; Medichemie, Switz.)*; Torinal *(Med. y Prod. Quím., Spain)*; Triador *(Trianon, Canad.)*; Tualone *(ICN, Canad.)*; Vitalone *(Sabex, Canad.)*.

The following names have been used for multi-ingredient preparations containing methaqualone or methaqualone hydrochloride— Durophet-M *(Riker, UK)*; Mandrax *(Roussel, Canad.; Roussel, UK)*.

7068-r

Methotrimeprazine *(BAN, USAN).*

CL-36467; CL-39743; Levomepromazine *(rINN)*; RP-7044; SKF-5116. (−)-*NN*-Dimethyl-3-(2-methoxyphenothiazin-10-yl)-2-methylpropylamine; 3-(2-Methoxyphenothiazin-10-yl)-2-methylpropylimethylamine.

$C_{19}H_{24}N_2OS$=328.5.

CAS — 60-99-1.

Pharmacopoeias. In *Braz.* and *U.S.* Also in *B.P. Vet.*

A fine white almost odourless crystalline powder. Practically **insoluble** in water; soluble 1 in 2 of chloroform; sparingly soluble in alcohol and in methyl alcohol, but freely soluble in boiling alcohol; freely soluble in ether. **Protect** from light.

7069-f

Methotrimeprazine Hydrochloride *(BANM).*

Levomepromazine Hydrochloride *(rINNM)*; Levomepromazini Hydrochloridum.

$C_{19}H_{24}N_2OS,HCl$=364.9.

CAS — 4185-80-2.

Pharmacopoeias. In *Br.*, *Eur.*, and *Swiss.*

Methotrimeprazine hydrochloride 1.11 g is approximately equivalent to 1 g of methotrimeprazine. A white or slightly yellow, slightly hygroscopic crystalline powder. It deteriorates on exposure to air and light. Freely **soluble** in water, in alcohol, and in chloroform; practically insoluble in ether. **Store** in airtight containers. Protect from light.

7070-z

Methotrimeprazine Maleate *(BANM).*

Levomepromazine Maleate *(rINNM)*; Methotrimeprazine Hydrogen Maleate.

$C_{19}H_{24}N_2OS,C_4H_4O_4$=444.5.

CAS — 7104-38-3.

Pharmacopoeias. In *Cz.*, *It.*, *Jpn*, *Jug.*, and *Roum.*

Methotrimeprazine maleate 1.35 g is approximately equivalent to 1 g of methotrimeprazine.

Adverse Effects, Treatment, and Precautions

As for the phenothiazines in general, p.706. See also Antihistamines, p.443.

Methotrimeprazine may cause severe postural hypotension therefore patients receiving large initial doses or those receiving injections should be kept lying down. It should not be given to patients being treated with antihypertensive agents.

For a report of fatal heat stroke in a patient receiving methotrimeprazine concurrently with benztropine and fluphenazine, see Benztropine Mesylate, p.528.

Absorption and Fate

For an account of the absorption and fate of a phenothiazine, see Chlorpromazine, p.723.

In a study involving a total of 5 psychiatric patients peak plasma concentrations of methotrimeprazine were noted 1 to 4 hours after administration by mouth and 30 to 90 minutes after injection into the gluteal muscle. About 50% of orally administered drug reached the systemic circulation. Although the metabolite methotrimeprazine sulphoxide could not be detected after a single intramuscular injection it was found in concentrations higher than unmetabolised methotrimeprazine after single and multiple oral dosage, both substances reaching a steady state in the plasma within 7 days of starting multiple dose oral therapy. Fluctuations in plasma concentration during multiple dose oral therapy indicated that until the correlation between acute side-effects and peak plasma concentration of methotrimeprazine had been further studied the total daily dose should be divided into 2 or 3 portions when larger doses of methotrimeprazine were given by mouth.— S. G. Dahl, *Clin. Pharmac. Ther.*, 1976, *19*, 435.

In 8 psychiatric patients given methotrimeprazine 50 to 350 mg daily the plasma half-life showed wide variation, from 16.5 to 77.8 hours, and did not correlate with the dose given.— S. G. Dahl *et al.*, *Eur. J. clin. Pharmac.*, 1977, *11*, 305.

METABOLISM. Identification of metabolites of methotrimeprazine in plasma and urine of psychiatric patients.— S. G. Dahl and M. Garle, *J. pharm. Sci.*, 1977, *66*, 190.

Further references A. De Leenheer and A. Heyndrickx, *J. pharm. Sci.*, 1972, *61*, 914; S. G. Dahl and H. Refsum, *Eur. J. Pharmac.*, 1976, *37*, 241.

Uses and Administration

Methotrimeprazine is a phenothiazine with pharmacological activity similar to that of both chlorpromazine (p.724) and promethazine (p.460). It has the histamine-antagonist properties of the antihistamines together with central nervous system effects resembling those of chlorpromazine.

Methotrimeprazine may be given by mouth as the maleate in usual doses of 25 to 50 mg daily for the treatment of psychoses or as an adjunct to analgesics in the management of severe chronic pain; the daily dosage is usually divided into 3 portions with a larger portion taken at night. Doses of 100 to 200 mg have been given to patients in bed; gradual increase to doses of up to 1 g daily has been reported for severe psychoses.

Although the parenteral route is poorly tolerated, methotrimeprazine is also given by intramuscular injection as the hydrochloride in the management of acute terminal pain. The usual dose is 12.5 to 25 mg intramuscularly every 6 to 8 hours and patients should remain in bed for at least the first few doses; doses of up to 50 mg have been given. It may also be given in similar doses by intravenous infusion following dilution with an equal volume of sodium chloride injection. Alternatively it may be given, suitably diluted, by continuous subcutaneous infusion, via a syringe driver, in doses ranging from a total of 25 to 200 mg daily.

Care is required in elderly patients because of the risk of severe hypotension; if methotrimeprazine is given to such patients reduced doses may be necessary. Children are also susceptible to the hypotensive effects of methotrimeprazine: a suggested dose is 15 to 20 mg of the maleate daily in divided doses by mouth, and doses of 40 mg daily should not be exceeded.

Methotrimeprazine has also been given as the embonate.

ANALGESIA. Evidence of analgesic activity following oral administration of methotrimeprazine is unconvincing, and side-effects, particularly sedation, are common. There have been no reliable controlled studies which show a useful analgesic effect following oral administration of methotrimeprazine although analgesia has been reported after parenteral dosage.— G. W. Hanks, *Postgrad. med. J.*, 1984, *60*, 881. Methotrimeprazine was successfully used in the management of severe pain and anxiety in 4 patients with extensive burns. Favourable responses were generally achieved with a dose of 12.5 mg three times daily by mouth, or half this amount parenterally; methotrimeprazine did not appear to be less effective as an analgesic by mouth in these patients.— W. J. Peters and J. Friedman, *Can. med. Ass. J.*, 1983, *128*, 896.

The use of methotrimeprazine in terminal care. Methotrimeprazine has been suggested for symptomatic control in patients dying of advanced cancer, and particularly to control restlessness and severe vomiting and as an adjuvant to opioid analgesics in pain control. In a retrospective survey in 675 patients admitted to a hospice methotrimeprazine was given to 80; to 49 for restlessness, agitation, and confusion, to 16 for the control of pain, and to 15 patients for vomiting. The dose range was 12.5 to 50 mg every 4 to 8 hours in the majority of patients, although 9 required 75 mg, and 3 needed 100 mg doses. The drug's effect was rated as good in 33 of the 49 patients with agitation and restlessness, in 15 of the 16 in pain, and in 13 of the 15 receiving the treatment for vomiting. The most common side-effect was sedation; postural hypotension did not appear to a problem in these patients.— D. J. Oliver, *Br. J. clin. Pract.*, 1985, *39*, 339.

Reference to the use of an isotonic formulation of methotrimeprazine hydrochloride as a continuous subcutaneous infusion in terminal care; the use of an isotonic preparation in a syringe driver appears to reduce skin reactions and hence the number of site changes required.— N. P. Sykes and D. J. Oliver (letter), *Lancet*, 1987, *1*, 393. Correction.— *ibid.*, 522.

Preparations

Methotrimeprazine Injection *(U.S.P.)*. A sterile solution in Water for Injections prepared with the aid of hydrochloric acid. pH 3 to 5.

Proprietary Preparations

Nozinan *(May & Baker, UK). Injection,* methotrimeprazine hydrochloride 25 mg/mL, in ampoules of 1 mL.

Veractil *(May & Baker, UK). Tablets,* scored, methotrimeprazine maleate 25 mg.

Proprietary Names and Manufacturers

Levonormal *(Jpn)*; Levoprome *(Lederle, USA)*; Minozinan *(Rhone-Poulenc, Belg.; Specia, Neth.; Rhone-Poulenc, Switz.)*; Neurocil *(Tropon, Ger.)*; Nozinan *(Rhodia, Arg.; Rhone-Poulenc, Belg.; Rhône-Poulenc, Canad.; Rhone-Poulenc, Denm.; Specia, Fr.; Carlo Erba, Ital.; Specia, Neth.; Mekos, Norw.; Leo Rhodia, Swed.; Rhone-Poulenc, Switz.; May & Baker, UK)*; Procrazine *(Jpn)*; Sinogan *(Rhone, Spain)*; Sofmin *(Jpn)*; Tisercin *(EGIS, Hung.)*; Veractil *(Rhône-Poulenc, Norw.; May & Baker, UK)*.

4048-c

Methylpentynol *(BAN, rINN)*.

Meparfynol; Methylparafynol. 3-Methylpent-1-yn-3-ol. $C_6H_{10}O$=98.14.

CAS — 77-75-8.

4049-k

Methylpentynol Carbamate *(BANM, rINNM)*.

Mepentamate. 3-Methylpent-1-ynyl carbamate. $C_7H_{11}NO_2$=141.2.

CAS — 302-66-9.

Methylpentynol is a hypnotic and sedative. It has been used as a hypnotic in the short-term management of insomnia in usual doses of 0.5 to 1 g at night. It has also been given as a sedative.

The carbamate has been used similarly; the usual sedative dose is 400 to 600 mg daily in divided doses, but up to 1.2 g daily has been given in severe psychoneurotic disorders.

Proprietary Names and Manufacturers of Methylpentynol and Methylpentynol Carbamate

Allotropal *(Heyl, Ger.)*; Insomnol Elixir *(Medo, UK)*; N-Oblivon *(Latema, Belg.; Latéma, Fr.)*; Oblivon *(Doetsch, Grether, Switz.; Nicholas, UK)*; Oblivon-C *(Nicholas, UK)*; Olosed *(Ital.)*; Psicoland *(Landerlan, Spain)*; Vereden *(Ital.)*.

4052-l

Methyprylone *(BAN)*.

Methyprylon *(USAN, rINN)*; Ro-1-6463. 3,3-Diethyl-5-methylpiperidine-2,4-dione. $C_{10}H_{17}NO_2$=183.2.

CAS — 125-64-4.

Pharmacopoeias. In *Br.* and *U.S.*

A white or almost white crystalline powder with a slight characteristic odour. M.p. 74° to 77.5°. The *B.P.* states that it is **soluble** 1 in 14 of water, 1 in 0.7 of alcohol, 1 in 0.6 of chloroform, and 1 in 3.5 of ether. *U.S.P.* solubilities are: 1 in 11 of water, 1 in 2 of alcohol, chloroform and ether. **Store** in well-closed containers. Protect from light. The *U.S.P.* requires that the tablets or capsules be stored in airtight containers.

Dependence

As for the barbiturates, p.706.

Methyprylone withdrawal had been reported to cause confusion, restlessness, excitement, sweating, and polyuria. Generalised convulsions and auditory and visual hallucinations had also occurred. Psychotic behaviour was precipitated in a patient who had discontinued the daily use of 4.8 g of methyprylone, and death had been reported after withdrawal of methyprylone in a patient who had been taking 7.5 to 12 g daily for about 18 months.— C. F. Essig, *J. Am. med. Ass.*, 1966, *196*, 714. See also *idem*, *Clin. Pharmac. Ther.*, 1964, *5*, 334.

Adverse Effects, Treatment, and Precautions

As for glutethimide, p.742.

Dialysis or haemoperfusion may be of benefit in the management of severe poisoning.

Absorption and Fate

Methyprylone is absorbed from the gastro-intestinal tract and extensively metabolised in the liver. It is reported to be about 60% bound to plasma proteins. It is excreted in the urine, mostly as metabolites with small amounts of unchanged drug. A short half-life has been reported but it may be considerably prolonged in overdosage.

The pharmacokinetics of methyprylone following a single oral dose in 10 healthy subjects.— P. R. Gwilt *et al.*, *J. pharm. Sci.*, 1985, *74*, 1001.

Uses and Administration

Methyprylone, which like glutethimide is a piperidinedione derivative, is a hypnotic and sedative. It has been reported to act within an hour to induce sleep lasting 5 to 8 hours. The usual dose is 200 to 400 mg at night. It has been used as a sedative in doses of 50 to 100 mg up to 4 times daily.

Preparations

Methyprylon Capsules *(U.S.P.)*. Capsules containing methyprylone.

Methyprylon Tablets *(U.S.P.)*. Tablets containing methyprylone.

Methyprylone Tablets *(B.P.)*. Tablets containing methyprylone. The tablets may be sugar-coated. If not sugar-coated protect from light.

Proprietary Preparations

Noludar *(Roche, UK). Tablets,* scored, methyprylone 200 mg.

Proprietary Names and Manufacturers

Noludar *(Belg.; Roche, Canad.; Roche, Denm.; Roche, Ger.; S.Afr.; Roche, Swed.; Switz.; Roche, UK; Roche, USA)*.

16895-a

Mexazolam *(rINN)*.

CS-386. 10-Chloro-11b-(2-chlorophenyl)-2,3,7,11b-tetrahydro-3-methyloxazolo[3,2-*d*][1,4]benzodiazepin-6(5*H*)-one. $C_{18}H_{16}Cl_2N_2O_2$=363.2.

CAS — 31868-18-5.

Mexazolam is a benzodiazepine derivative with general properties similar to those of diazepam (p.731). It has been used for its anxiolytic and sedative properties in doses of 0.5 to 1 mg three times daily.

Proprietary Names and Manufacturers

Melex *(Sankyo, Jpn)*.

12958-p

Midazolam Hydrochloride *(BANM, USAN, rINNM)*.

Ro-21-3981/003. 8-Chloro-6-(2-fluorophenyl)-1-methyl-4*H*-imidazo[1,5-*a*][1,4]benzodiazepine hydrochloride. $C_{18}H_{13}ClFN_3$,HCl=362.2.

CAS — 59467-70-8 (midazolam); 59467-96-8 (hydrochloride); 59467-94-6 (maleate).

NOTE. *USAN* also includes Midazolam Maleate.

Dependence, Adverse Effects, Treatment, and Precautions

As for the benzodiazepines in general, p.706.

Pain and tenderness have been reported to occur at the site of injection. Headache, dizziness, and hiccoughs may occasionally occur. For a comment on the susceptibility of the elderly to midazolam, see below.

A discussion of the risks of using midazolam for conscious sedation. Higher doses were used initially in the *USA* than in the *UK*. Within about 6 months of its introduction in the *USA* in May 1986, 13 fatalities due to cardiorespiratory depression had been reported. By January 1988, 66 deaths had been reported, although in November 1987 the adult dosage recommendation had been reduced to 70 µg per kg body-weight and to 50 µg per kg for elderly patients. Fatalities have also occurred in the *UK* [where the dose is 70 µg per kg, reduced in the elderly]; 4 deaths having been reported to the CSM by November 1987. While it is agreed that midazolam can be used safely for conscious sedation, appropriate precautions must be taken to ensure that the correct dose is used and that allowances are made for age. The availability of flumazenil as an antagonist should not be an encouragement to use larger doses of midazolam. If the antagonist is used, due regard should be paid to the differences in the pharmacokinetics of the 2 compounds.— *Lancet*, 1988, *2*, 140. Details of 3 *UK* fatalities in elderly patients given doses of midazolam adjusted for age.— T. K. Daneshmend and R. F. A. Logan (letter), *ibid.*, 389.

Absorption and Fate

For an account of the absorption and fate of a benzodiazepine, see Diazepam, p.730.

Midazolam has a rapid onset of action and a relatively short duration. Sleep may be induced in 30 to 90 seconds following an intravenous injection. Midazolam is metabolised in the liver and less than 1% is excreted unchanged in the urine. Midazolam is extensively (about 96%) bound to plasma protein.

A review of the pharmacokinetics of newer intravenous anaesthetic agents including midazolam.— P. J. Davis and R. D. Cook, *Clin. Pharmacokinet.*, 1986, *11*, 18.

A brief review of the pharmacokinetic and pharmacodynamic properties of midazolam.— B. N. Swerdlow and F. O. Holley, *Clin. Pharmacokinet.*, 1987, *12*, 79.

Half-lives of midazolam of 19.4, 15.8, and 8.9 hours occurred in 3 patients, aged 68 years, 56 years, and 46 months respectively, who had been given repeated intravenous doses of midazolam for sedation; consciousness was recovered 6 days, the next day, and 48 hours respectively after the last dose of midazolam.— C. M. Byatt *et al.*, *Br. med. J.*, 1984, *289*, 799 and 1350. A similar report.— A. J. Byrne *et al.* (letter), *ibid.*, 1309. Comments: C. A. L. Moon (letter), *ibid.*, J. Dundee *et al.* (letter), *ibid.*, 1540.

Metabolism of midazolam was significantly impaired in 7 patients with alcoholic cirrhosis.— A. J. Macgilchrist *et al.*, *Gut*, 1986, *27*, 190.

Uses and Administration

Midazolam is a benzodiazepine derivative with general properties similar to those of diazepam (p.731). It is used as a sedative and premedicant in minor surgical, and anaesthetic procedures. It is used as the hydrochloride but doses are given in terms of the base. The maleate has also been used. The usual sedative dose ranges from 2.5 to 7.5 mg intravenously; an initial dose of 3.75 mg over 30 seconds has been suggested, with further doses if required. When used for the induction of anaesthesia, usual doses range from 0.1 to 0.2 mg per kg body-weight in premedicated patients and 0.2 to 0.3 mg per kg in those who have not received a premedicant.

Midazolam is also given intramuscularly as a premedicant. The usual dose is about 5 mg; doses range from 0.07 to 0.1 mg per kg.

Midazolam should be given in reduced doses to elderly and debilitated patients.

ADMINISTRATION. In a study of 14 patients undergoing abdominal surgery, 8 received intrathecal midazolam 2 mg and 6 were controls. None of the midazolam group required peroperative opiates, while all the control patients did. It was concluded that intrathecal midazolam provides a measure of analgesia similar to that of intravenous diamorphine.— T. P. Cripps and C. S. Goodchild, *Br. J. Anaesth.*, 1986, *58*, 1324P.

ANAESTHESIA. Induction by midazolam (0.2 mg per kg body-weight) or thiopentone (4 mg per kg) administered intravenously was compared in 33 women undergoing uterine curettage. Anaesthesia was maintained with nitrous oxide in oxygen (3:2). Supplementary doses of midazolam (0.15 mg per kg) or thiopentone (2 mg per kg) were given during anaesthesia. Induction was significantly more rapid after thiopentone, but the frequency of apnoea was greater than after midazolam. The recovery time after midazolam was significantly longer than after thiopentone but the duration of amnesia was much greater.— I. Freuchen *et al.*, *Curr. ther. Res.*, 1983, *34*, 269.

Midazolam was found to be suitable for the induction of anaesthesia for day-case surgery when compared with thiopentone in 100 patients undergoing termination of pregnancy as outpatients. Patients were randomly assigned to anaesthesia with midazolam, fentanyl, and nitrous oxide or thiopentone, fentanyl, and nitrous oxide. Midazolam 200 µg per kg body-weight was injected intravenously over 30 seconds followed by a further injection of 100 µg per kg if the eyelash reflex was present 3 minutes after the initial dose. The induction time for midazolam of about 40 seconds was significantly longer than the 31 seconds for thiopentone but significantly more patients required maintenance doses of thiopentone than of midazolam. Recovery was slower after midazolam but there were fewer unwanted side-effects than with thiopentone.— M. E. Crawford *et al.*, *Br. J. Anaesth.*, 1984, *56*, 165.

A placebo-controlled study of oral midazolam and temazepam as premedication for day-case patients. Ninety short-stay patients received midazolam 15 mg or temazepam 20 mg followed by anaesthesia with thiopentone and an inhalation agent. Midazolam and temazepam were both found to be superior to placebo regarding preoperative anxiolysis and sedation. Patients who received midazolam required a significantly smaller dose of thiopentone than the other groups. Midazolam patients showed a significant degree of anterograde amnesia compared with temazepam and placebo patients. Midazolam was considered to be the superior premedicant, although the delay in immediate and late recovery compared with temazepam would suggest that it is more suitable for inpatients.— J. Hargreaves, *Br. J. Anaesth.*, 1986, *58*, 1338P.

Successful use of midazolam 15 mg, by mouth, as a nocturnal sedative before caesarean section. Virtually no detectable levels of drug were found in the foetomaternal entity the following morning.— J. Kanto *et al.*, *Clin. Pharmac. Ther.*, 1983, *33*, 786.

A comparison of the effects of diazepam and midazolam on recovery from anaesthesia in 60 female patients scheduled for minor surgery. Patients received either intravenous bolus injections of midazolam 70 µg per kg and fentanyl 1.5 µg per kg or diazepam 150 µg per kg (as an emulsion) and fentanyl 1.5 µg per kg. Anaesthesia was then induced with etomidate 300 µg per kg and maintained with nitrous oxide 66% in oxygen with intermittent bolus injections of etomidate. The excitatory effects of etomidate were controlled by the benzodiazepine-fentanyl combination in both groups. No significant difference in the quality of recovery, amnesia, incidence of recall of pain on injection of etomidate, or nausea and vomiting could be demonstrated between the groups.— P. Clyburn *et al.*, *Br. J. Anaesth.*, 1986, *58*, 872.

Midazolam administered by a bolus dose of 2 mg followed immediately by an infusion at 2 mg per hour was found to be a safe and simple method of providing sedation during short-term ventilatory support after open-heart surgery H. M. L. Mathews *et al.*, *Br. J. Anaesth.*, 1987, *59*, 557.

Successful use of midazolam as an induction agent in a patient with Huntington's chorea.— M. R. C. Rodrigo (letter), *Br. J. Anaesth.*, 1987, *59*, 388.

DENTISTRY. A study comparing the clinical efficacy of midazolam with diazepam in 40 patients as a sedative-hypnotic in dentistry, followed by a more extensive study of midazolam in 80 patients. When used in dosages of midazolam 0.1 mg per kg body-weight or diazepam 0.2 mg per kg the degree of sedation was excellent for both drugs, while midazolam produced more complete amnesia and fewer side-effects.— J. G. McGimpsey *et al.*, *Br. dent. J.*, 1983, *155*, 47. Comment concerning difficulties in titration to patient response with a relatively concentrated formulation.— C. M. Hill (letter), *ibid.*, 1984, *156*, 240.

A study of 50 administrations of a dilution of midazolam hydrochloride (10 mg/5 mL) for dental sedation. An initial intravenous infusion of 3.5 mg over 30 seconds was followed by a pause of 90 seconds. Further increments of 1 mg were given every 30 seconds until sedation was deemed adequate. The dilute formulation provided easy assessment of dosage requirements and a reduced risk of oversedation.— A. M. Skelly and I. A. Nelson, *Br. dent. J.*, 1986, *160*, 99.

ENDOSCOPY. In a randomised study in 149 patients undergoing upper gastro-intestinal endoscopy midazolam (mean dose 10.3 mg) intravenously was as effective as diazepam [Valium] (mean dose 12.5 mg) for the induction of sedation. Endoscopists rated each drug highly satisfactory; patient assessment favoured midazolam.— K. D. Bardhan *et al.*, *Br. med. J.*, 1984, *288*, 1046. A similar study in 146 adults who received either diazepam [in lipid solution as Diazemuls] (mean dose 15.1 mg) or midazolam (mean dose 8.03 mg). Sedation was found to be adequate in both groups, although the rapidity of recovery was impaired in those patients receiving midazolam.— J. R. B. Green *et al.* (letter), *ibid.*, 1383. A critical comment. The age of the patients and concomitant administration of drugs should be taken into consideration in studies on the recovery from benzodiazepines.— J. W. Dundee and J. P. H. Fee (letter), *ibid.*, 1614.

Bronchoscopy was performed in 76 outpatients using local anaesthesia plus diazepam (Diapam) 0.2 mg per kg body-weight or midazolam (Dormicum) 0.05 or 0.1 mg per kg. The results showed that midazolam did not give a faster rate of recovery compared with diazepam at doses of comparable potency.— K. Korttila and J. Tarkkanen, *Br. J. Anaesth.*, 1985, *57*, 581. Comment that the preparation of diazepam used should be stated.— J. W. Dundee and J. P. H. Fee (letter), *ibid.*, 1986, *58*, 466. Reply that the two benzodiazepines were studied in doses of comparable potency. The half-lives for the initial distribution phase of both compounds are reported to be similar and hence recovery after administration of either drug would be expected to be similar.— K. Korttila and J. Tarkkanen (letter), *ibid.*

Proprietary Preparations

Hypnovel *(Roche, UK). Injection*, midazolam 2 mg (as hydrochloride)/mL, in ampoules of 5 mL and 5 mg (as hydrochloride)/mL, in ampoules of 2 mL.

Proprietary Names and Manufacturers

Dormicum *(Roche, Denm.; Roche, Ger.; Roche, Norw.; Roche, S.Afr.; Roche, Swed.; Roche, Switz.)*; Hypnovel *(Roche, UK)*; Versed *(Roche, USA)*.

12961-m

Milenperone *(BAN, USAN, rINN).*

R-34009. 5-Chloro-1-{3-[4-(4-fluorobenzoyl)piperidino]-propyl}-1,3-dihydrobenzimidazol-2-one.

$C_{22}H_{23}ClFN_3O_2$=415.9.

CAS — 59831-64-0.

Milenperone is reported to have neuroleptic activity.

Proprietary Names and Manufacturers

Janssen, Belg.

7072-k

Molindone Hydrochloride *(BANM, USAN, rINNM).*

EN-1733A. 3-Ethyl-1,5,6,7-tetrahydro-2-methyl-5-(morpholinomethyl)indol-4-one hydrochloride.

$C_{16}H_{24}N_2O_2$,HCl=312.8.

CAS — 7416-34-4 (molindone); 15622-65-8 (hydrochloride).

Adverse Effects, Treatment, and Precautions

As for the phenothiazines, p.706.

Leucopenia and leucocytosis have occasionally been reported and transient ECG changes have been noted.

For a suggestion that molindone may be less likely than haloperidol to induce tardive dyskinesia see W. M. Glazer *et al.*, *J. clin. Psychiat.*, 1985, *46*, 4.

EFFECTS ON THE LIVER. A report of hepatotoxicity, associated with a flu-like syndrome, in a patient given molindone. Symptoms and liver-enzyme values returned to normal on discontinuation of the drug and recurred on rechallenge with low doses. The effect was probably due to a hypersensitivity reaction.— S. C. Bhatia *et al.*, *Drug Intell. & clin. Pharm.*, 1985, *19*, 744.

Absorption and Fate

Molindone is readily absorbed from the gastro-intestinal tract, peak concentrations of unchanged molindone being obtained within about 1 to 2 hours of administration. It is rapidly and extensively metabolised and a large number of metabolites have been identified. It is excreted in the urine and faeces almost entirely in the form of its metabolites. The pharmacological effect from a single dose by mouth is reported to last for 24 to 36 hours.

The bioavailability of molindone following oral and intramuscular administration.— M. Zetin *et al.*, *Clin. Ther.*, 1985, *7*, 169.

Uses and Administration

Molindone is an indole derivative with antipsychotic actions similar to those of chlorpromazine (p.724). It is given as the hydrochloride by mouth.

The usual dose of molindone hydrochloride by mouth for the treatment of psychoses is 50 to 75 mg daily initially, increased within 3 or 4 days to 100 mg daily; in severe conditions doses of up to 225 mg daily may be required. The maintenance dosage can range from 15 to 225 mg daily. The recommended daily dosage is usually divided into 3 to 4 portions. For the control of acute conditions it has been given by intramuscular injection.

Molindone should be given in reduced dosage to elderly patients.

DEPRESSION. A comparison of molindone with tranylcypromine in the treatment of refractory depression.— J. G. Small *et al.*, *J. clin. Pharmac.*, 1981, *21*, 351.

SCHIZOPHRENIA. A long-term study of molindone hydrochloride given in doses of up to 200 mg daily to 23 chronic schizophrenic in-patients. The duration of the study ranged from 6 to 19 months. The general response was similar to that with the patients' previous and subsequent antipsychotic medication but some patients responded worse and others better. Although 5 patients gained weight another 5 lost substantial amounts indicating that molindone could be of benefit in overweight patients.— R. Kellner *et al.*, *Curr. ther. Res.*, 1976, *20*, 686.

Beneficial results with intramuscular injection of molindone in doses of up to 50 mg twice daily. It seemed reasonable to assume that higher daily doses would be tolerated if a suitable preparation were available.— D. H. Mielke and D. M. Gallant, *Curr. ther. Res.*, 1977, *22*, 356.

In a study involving 35 acutely ill schizophrenics patients were assigned to receive molindone in doses up to 225 mg daily by intramuscular injection or were given injections of haloperidol in doses up to 45 mg daily; treatment was continued for 12 to 72 hours until patients were able to receive drugs by mouth. The mean length of treatment by injection was 18.8 hours in those given molindone and 21.8 hours in those given haloperidol. There was a greater decrease in symptom intensity after the first 2 injections of molindone than after haloperidol. Thirty patients went on to complete more than one week of oral treatment with mean maximum doses of molindone 160 mg daily or haloperidol 32.4 mg daily. Improvement was seen with both drugs and there were no significant differences between the groups.— J. I. Escobar *et al.*, *J. clin. Psychiat.*, 1985, *46*, 15.

Proprietary Names and Manufacturers

Lidone *(Abbott, USA)*; Moban *(Endo, S.Afr.; Du Pont, USA)*.

7073-a

Moperone Hydrochloride *(rINNM)*.

Methylperidol Hydrochloride; R-1658 *(base)*. 4′-Fluoro-4-(4-hydroxy-4-*p*-tolylpiperidino)butyrophenone hydrochloride.

$C_{22}H_{26}FNO_2,HCl=391.9$.

CAS — 1050-79-9 (moperone); 3871-82-7 (hydrochloride).

Moperone is a butyrophenone with general properties similar to those of haloperidol (p.743). For the treatment of psychoses it has been given as the hydrochloride in doses of 10 to 60 mg daily.

Proprietary Names and Manufacturers

Luvatren *(Cilag-Chemie, Denm.; Cilag, Ital.; Yamanouchi, Jpn; Cilag-Chemie, Neth.; Cilag-Chemie, Norw.; Cilag, Swed.; Cilag, Switz.)*; Luvatrena *(Cilag, Ger.)*; Luvatrene *(Cilag-Chemie, Belg.; Cilag, Switz.)*.

13018-a

Nimetazepam *(rINN)*.

Menifazepam; S-1530. 1,3-Dihydro-1-methyl-7-nitro-5-phenyl-1,4-benzodiazepin-2-one.

$C_{16}H_{13}N_3O_3=295.3$.

CAS — 2011-67-8.

Nimetazepam is a benzodiazepine (see Diazepam, p.728) with sedative and hypnotic properties that has been given in doses of 3 to 5 mg.

Proprietary Names and Manufacturers

Erimin *(Sumitomo, Jpn)*.

4054-j

Nitrazepam *(BAN, USAN, rINN)*.

NSC-58775; Ro-4-5360; Ro-5-3059. 1,3-Dihydro-7-nitro-5-phenyl-1,4-benzodiazepin-2-one.

$C_{15}H_{11}N_3O_3=281.3$.

CAS — 146-22-5.

Pharmacopoeias. In *Aust., Br., Braz., Chin., Cz., Eur., Fr., Ger., It., Jpn, Neth., Nord.,* and *Swiss.*

A yellow, crystalline powder. Practically **insoluble** in water; slightly soluble in alcohol and in ether; sparingly soluble in chloroform. **Store** in well-closed containers. Protect from light.

Dependence, Adverse Effects, Treatment, and Precautions

As for the benzodiazepines in general, p.706.

Adverse reactions to nitrazepam were studied by the Boston Collaborative Drug Surveillance Program in 2111 hospital in-patients who received nitrazepam mainly for insomnia. Central nervous system (CNS) depression (drowsiness, fatigue, confusion, and ataxia) occurred in 49 patients, CNS stimulation (nightmares, hallucinations, insomnia and agitation) in 15, cutaneous reactions (rash and pruritus) in 5, and headache and gastro-intestinal disturbances in 3. The frequency of side-effects caused by CNS depression or stimulation were generally greater at higher doses of nitrazepam and those caused by CNS depression were also more frequent in elderly patients.— D. J. Greenblatt and M. D. Allen, *Br. J. clin. Pharmac.*, 1978, *5*, 407.

DEPENDENCE. Analysis of data from sleep laboratory evaluations of flunitrazepam, nitrazepam, and triazolam, and presentation of a hypothesis of benzodiazepine receptors to explain rebound withdrawal. Abrupt withdrawal of benzodiazepines with a relatively short duration of action may result in an intense form of rebound insomnia owing to a lag in the production and replacement of endogenous benzodiazepine-like compounds.— A. Kales *et al.*, *Science*, 1978, *201*, 1039. Comment.— A. N. Nicholson, *Br. J. clin. Pharmac.*, 1980, *9*, 223. See also R. T. Owen and P. Tyrer, *Drugs*, 1983, *25*, 385.

DROOLING. Two children given nitrazepam as part of their antiepileptic therapy developed drooling, eating difficulty, and aspiration pneumonia; symptoms improved in 1 patient when the dosage of nitrazepam was reduced. Manometric studies indicated that the onset of normal cricopharyngeal relaxation in swallowing was delayed in these patients until after hypopharyngeal contraction, resulting in impaired swallowing and spillover of material into the trachea. Manometry should be considered in the evaluation of patients taking nitrazepam who have eating difficulties or aspiration pneumonia.— E. Wyllie *et al.*, *New Engl. J. Med.*, 1986, *314*, 35.

EFFECTS ON THE NERVOUS SYSTEM. In a 55-year-old woman tingling and numbness of the hands was correlated with the ingestion of nitrazepam.— H. MacLean (letter), *Br. med. J.*, 1973, *1*, 488.

GOUT. A 40-year-old Chinese man with a history of gout had acute attacks on 5 occasions after taking nitrazepam 10 mg; attacks were also precipitated by diazepam 5 mg, chlordiazepoxide 15 mg, and Mandrax.— C. O. Leng (letter), *Br. med. J.*, 1975, *2*, 561.

HYPOTHERMIA. An 86-year-old woman developed hypothermia after administration of nitrazepam 5 mg. After recovery she was mistakenly given another 5-mg dose of nitrazepam and again developed hypothermia.— M. Impallomeni and R. Ezzat (letter), *Br. med. J.*, 1976, *1*, 223.

PORPHYRIA. Nitrazepam was considered to be unsafe in patients with acute porphyria because it has been shown to be porphyrinogenic in *animals* or *in vitro* systems.— M.R. Moore and K.E.L. McColl, *Porphyrias, Drug Lists*, Glasgow, Porphyria Research Unit, University of Glasgow, 1987.

PREGNANCY AND THE NEONATE. The floppy-infant syndrome in one neonate and sedation in another were associated with the maternal use of nitrazepam. The mother of the first child also took diazepam and this too was implicated.— A. N. P. Speight (letter), *Lancet*, 1977, *2*, 878. See also under Absorption and Fate.

RESPIRATORY IMPAIRMENT. Normal doses of nitrazepam could be fatal in patients with raised carbon dioxide concentrations due to chronic obstructive lung disease.— D. G. Model (letter), *Lancet*, 1974, *1*, 224.

A report of death by suicide of a 55-year-old man following ingestion of alcohol and nitrazepam; chronic bronchitis was considered to have been a major contributory factor in the death.— J. M. Torry, *Practitioner*, 1977, *217*, 648.

Absorption and Fate

Nitrazepam is fairly readily absorbed from the gastro-intestinal tract, although there is some individual variation. It is extensively bound to plasma proteins. It is metabolised in the liver, mainly by nitroreduction and acetylation (which is reported to be subject to genetic polymorphism). It is excreted in the urine in the form of its metabolites with only small amounts of a dose appearing unchanged. Up to about 20% of an oral dose is found in the faeces. It crosses the placental barrier and traces are found in breast milk.

ABSORPTION AND METABOLISM. After administration of nitrazepam 10 mg by mouth to volunteers, absorption varied from 53 to 94%. Maximum plasma concentrations were reached within 2 hours.— J. Rieder, *Arzneimittel-Forsch.*, 1973, *23*, 212.

When 9 healthy subjects took nitrazepam 5 mg, absorption was usually fairly rapid, but with some intersubject variation. A mean initial peak plasma concentration of 37.1 ng per mL (range 28.2 to 45.0 ng per mL) was obtained after a mean of 81 minutes (range 30 to 240 minutes). In most subjects there was a subsequent rapid decrease in plasma-nitrazepam concentration until 4 hours after taking the dose, followed by a slight increase to produce a second peak after 6 to 8 hours. The mean elimination half-life was 30 hours (range 18 to 36 hours).— D. D. Breimer *et al.* (letter), *Br. J. clin. Pharmac.*, 1977, *4*, 709.

Acetylation. The polymorphic acetylation of nitrazepam.— A. K. M. Karim and D. A. P. Evans, *J. med. Genet.*, 1976, *13*, 17.

Distribution. A study in 38 neurological patients indicated that nitrazepam is eliminated considerably more slowly from the CSF than from the plasma. Its β-phase half-life was found to be about 68 hours in the CSF compared with 27 hours in plasma. Whereas the CSF concentration after 2 hours was only 8% of that in plasma, after 36 hours it was nearly 16%.— L. Kangas *et al.*, *Acta pharmac. tox.*, 1977, *41*, 74.

ADMINISTRATION IN THE ELDERLY. The serum half-life (β-phase) of nitrazepam was 24.2 and 39.6 hours respectively in 25 healthy subjects aged 21 to 38 years who took nitrazepam 5 mg daily for 14 days and 12 hospitalised elderly patients aged 66 to 89 years who took nitrazepam 5 mg daily for 2 months. Peak serum-nitrazepam concentrations were 39.9 and 21.8 ng per mL respectively in the young and the old group, and the volumes of distribution were 2.4 and 4.8 litres per kg body-weight respectively. The immobility of the older patients and their diseases were considered to be responsible for the differences.— E. Iisalo *et al.*, *Br. J. clin. Pharmac.*, 1977, *4*, 646P. See also D. J. Greenblatt *et al.*, *Clin. Pharmac. Ther.*, 1985, *38*, 697 (effects of age and sex on nitrazepam kinetics).

See also under Uses, below.

PREGNANCY AND THE NEONATE. In early pregnancy a lower concentration of nitrazepam was found in foetal plasma than in maternal plasma, but as pregnancy progressed placental transfer of nitrazepam increased so that in late pregnancy foetal and maternal concentrations were not significantly different.— L. Kangas *et al.*, *Eur. J. clin. Pharmac.*, 1977, *12*, 355.

Uses and Administration

Nitrazepam is a benzodiazepine with actions similar to those of diazepam (see p.731). It is used as a hypnotic in the short-term management of insomnia and is reported to act in 30 to 60 minutes to produce sleep lasting for 6 to 8 hours. As a hypnotic the usual dose is 5 to 10 mg at night. Doses of 2.5 to 5 mg at night have been suggested for children, and these may also be more suitable for elderly patients.

Nitrazepam has also been used in epilepsy, notably for infantile spasms.

ADMINISTRATION IN HEPATIC FAILURE. A study of the pharmacokinetics of intravenous nitrazepam in 12 patients with cirrhosis of the liver compared with 9 healthy subjects aged 22 to 49 years and 8 healthy elderly subjects aged 67 to 76 years. The mean elimination half-life of nitrazepam was 26 hours in young and 38 hours in elderly subjects, the difference, which was not significant, being chiefly due to the greater volume of distribution in elderly subjects. Although there was also no significant difference between young and elderly subjects in percentage unbound nitrazepam (13.0 and 13.9% respectively) there was a substantially higher unbound fraction in the patients with cirrhosis, the mean value being 18.9%, and clearance of unbound nitrazepam was thus reduced relative to healthy subjects. When patients with liver cirrhosis take nitrazepam every night their levels of unbound nitrazepam will be higher than in healthy subjects.— R. Jochemsen *et al.*, *Br. J. clin. Pharmac.*, 1983, *15*, 295.

CONVULSIONS. Nitrazepam was given as an anticonvulsant to 24 infants, aged 1 to 18 months, with infantile spasms, including 22 with hypsarrhythmia. In 13 there was complete control of spasms with a dose of 0.6 to 1 mg per kg body-weight daily, in 6 there was temporary improvement followed by relapse, and in 5 there was no effect. Side-effects in 14 infants included hypersecretion of mucus and saliva in 7, drowsiness in 6, and difficulty in swallowing in 4. Hypersecretion occurred with doses as low as 700 µg per kg daily.— E. Völzke *et al.*, *Epilepsia*, 1967, *8*, 64.

In a double-blind crossover study comparing the anticonvulsant effects of nitrazepam and diazepam in 9 children with myoclonic seizure disorders, initial doses of 5 to 10 mg and 10 to 20 mg respectively were given daily in addition to phenobarbitone 30 to 60 mg and adjusted over periods of 6 months to an average of 18 and 40 mg respectively. Assessed by incidence of seizures and by EEG, the drugs were equally effective in producing at least 50% improvement in 5 patients, transient improvement in 2, and no improvement in 2. Side-effects included occasional drowsiness, hypotonia, and drooling with both drugs and bronchopneumonia in 3 while on high doses of diazepam.— J. M. Killian and G. H. Fromm, *Develop. Med. Child Neurol.*, 1971, *13*, 32.

A study of the use of nitrazepam for infantile spasms, childhood myoclonic epilepsy, or both in 56 children with tuberous sclerosis. Nitrazepam reduced or stopped seizures, for at least a few months, in 26 patients. The drug was subsequently withdrawn in 38 children after a median of 1.1 years, but the remainder were still receiving the drug after a median of 8 years, despite the fact that 9 were among those who had shown no benefit when the drug was introduced. In addition, there was evidence of impairment of motor and cognitive development associated with nitrazepam treatment. Although nitrazepam is undoubtedly effective in achieving initial control of refractory myoclonic seizures among some children its long-term efficacy is less clear, and its prescription to children needs to be evaluated.— J. Dennis and A. Hunt, *Br. med. J.*, 1985, *291*, 692. Comment. It would be unfortunate if nitrazepam fell into disrepute as a specific anticonvulsant for myoclonic epilepsy.— B. G. R. Neville (letter), *ibid.*, 1050. Reply.— J. Dennis and A. Hunt (letter), *ibid.*, 1421.

Further reference F. Dreifuss *et al.*, *Archs Neurol., Chicago*, 1986, *43*, 1107 (comparison with corticotrophin for infantile spasms).

See also p.710.

Preparations

Nitrazepam Capsules *(B.P.)*

Nitrazepam Tablets *(B.P.)*

Proprietary Preparations

Mogadon *(Roche, UK). Capsules*, nitrazepam 5 mg. *Tablets*, scored, nitrazepam 5 mg.

Remnos *(DDSA Pharmaceuticals, UK). Tablets*, scored, nitrazepam 5 and 10 mg.

Somnite *(Norgine, UK). Suspension*, nitrazepam 2.5 mg/5 mL.

Surem *(Galen, UK). Capsules*, nitrazepam 5 mg.

Proprietary Names and Manufacturers

Alodorm *(Alphapharm, Austral.)*; Apodorm *(A.L., Denm.; Apothekernes Laboratorium, Norw.; A.L., Swed.)*; Arem *(Lennon, S.Afr.)*; Dormicum *(Protea, Austral.)*; Dormo-Puren *(Klinge-Nattermann, Ger.)*; Dumolid *(Dumex, Denm.; Swed.; Dumex, Switz.)*; Eatan *(Desitin, Ger.)*; Hipsal *(Salvat, Spain)*; Hypnotin *(S.Afr.)*; Imeson *(Desitin, Ger.; Cimex, Switz.)*; Insomin *(Orion, Switz.)*; Ipersed *(Salus, Ital.)*; Lyladorm *(MPS Lab., S.Afr.)*; Mitidin *(Savoma, Ital.)*; Mogadan *(Roche, Ger.)*; Mogadon *(Arg.; Roche, Austral.; Belg.; Roche, Canad.; Roche, Denm.; Fr.; Roche, Ital.; Neth.; Roche, Norw.; Roche, S.Afr.; Roche, Spain; Roche, Swed.; Roche, Switz.; Roche, UK)*; Nitepam *(USV, Austral.)*; Nitrados *(Berk Pharmaceuticals, UK)*; Noctene *(Adcock Ingram, S.Afr.)*; Noctesed *(Unimed, UK)*; Novanox *(Pfleger, Ger.)*; Ormodon *(Ormed, S.Afr.)*; Pacisyn *(Syntetic, Denm.)*; Paxadorm *(Schwulst, S.Afr.)*; Paxisyn *(Norw.)*; Pelson *(Infale, Spain)*; Persopir *(Biopharma, Ital.)*; Prosonno *(Ital.)*; Quill *(Ital.)*; Relact *(Arg.)*; Remnos *(DDSA Pharmaceuticals, UK)*; Sindepres *(Arg.)*; Somnased *(Duncan, Flockhart, UK)*; Somnibel *(UCB, Ger.)*; Somnipar *(Rolab, S.Afr.)*; Somnite *(Norgine, UK)*; Sonnolin *(Ital.)*; Surem *(Galen, UK)*; Tri *(Vita, Ital.)*; Unisomnia *(Unigreg, UK)*.

7035-l

Nordazepam *(rINN)*.

A-101; Demethyldiazepam; Desmethyldiazepam; *N*-Desmethyldiazepam; Nordiazepam; Ro-5-2180. 7-Chloro-1,3-dihydro-5-phenyl-2*H*-1,4-benzodiazepin-2-one.

$C_{15}H_{11}ClN_2O$=270.7.

CAS — 1088-11-5.

Nordazepam is the principal metabolite of diazepam (p.728). It has been given in doses of 7.5 to 15 mg daily for the treatment of anxiety.

Proprietary Names and Manufacturers

Calmday; Demadar *(Volpino, Arg.)*; Madar *(Ravizza, Ital.)*; Nordaz *(Bouchara, Fr.)*; Praxadium *(Bottu, Fr.)*; Stilny; Tranxilium N *(Midy, Ger.)*; Vegesan *(Mack, Switz.)*.

7076-r

Oxazepam *(BAN, USAN, rINN)*.

Wy-3498. 7-Chloro-1,3-dihydro-3-hydroxy-5-phenyl-1,4-benzodiazepin-2-one.

$C_{15}H_{11}ClN_2O_2$=286.7.

CAS — 604-75-1.

Pharmacopoeias. In *Br., Braz., Cz., It., Nord.,* and *U.S.*

A white to pale yellow, odourless or almost odourless powder. Practically **insoluble** in water; soluble 1 in 220 of alcohol, 1 in 270 of chloroform, and 1 in 2200 of ether.

Store in well-closed containers. Protect from light.

Dependence, Adverse Effects, Treatment, and Precautions

As for the benzodiazepines in general, p.706.

INTERACTIONS. *Alcohol.* Alcohol-induced delay in oxazepam absorption.— H. J. Mallach *et al.*, *Arzneimittel-Forsch.*, 1975, *25*, 1840.

Analgesics. The peak plasma concentration of oxazepam was significantly decreased during treatment with diflunisal in 6 healthy subjects, while the clearance of the glucuronide metabolite was reduced and its mean elimination half-life increased from 10 to 13 hours. Diflunisal also displaced oxazepam from plasma protein binding sites *in vitro*.— A. M. Van Hecken *et al.*, *Br. J. clin. Pharmac.*, 1985, *20*, 225.

Anti-epileptics. The mean elimination half-life of oxazepam was 3.31 hours in 9 epileptics receiving long-term therapy with phenytoin alone or in combination with phenobarbitone, compared with 6.99 hours in 9 healthy subjects. The apparent oral clearance of oxazepam was almost twice as great in the group receiving anti-epileptic therapy as in the controls. The results were most probably due to enzyme induction by phenytoin and phenobarbitone; larger or more frequent doses of oxazepam may be needed for adequate therapeutic response in similar patients.— A. K. Scott *et al.*, *Br. J. clin. Pharmac.*, 1983, *16*, 441.

For further interactions with benzodiazepines, including oxazepam, see under Diazepam, p.729.

OVERDOSAGE. A 2-year-old girl was admitted to hospital 18 hours after taking 90 mg of oxazepam. She was apathetic and lethargic, though she showed paradoxical excitation. Reflexes were depressed and her face was oedematous. Her gait was ataxic. By the third hospital day the deep-tendon reflexes had returned to normal, and the ataxia disappeared slowly over 8 days, but at discharge, 2 weeks later, there was still slight facial puffiness.— P. M. Shimkin, *J. Am. med. Ass.*, 1966, *196*, 662.

A 45-year-old man, who ingested large doses [not stated] of oxazepam in an attempted suicide, went into a deep coma and had an apparent blood-glucose concentration of 1.68 g per 100 mL and an electrolyte imbalance. It was later discovered that oxazepam gave a positive reaction for glucose. The patient's condition did not improve until the fourth day when exchange transfusion was carried out. The importance of diagnosis of this pseudohyperglycaemic non-ketoacidotic coma and the dangers of insulin administration were emphasised.— M. S. Zileli *et al.* (letter), *J. Am. med. Ass.*, 1971, *215*, 1986. Tests indicated that lactose present as a filler in oxazepam preparations could have accounted for the false high blood-glucose concentration.— H. E. Spiegel and D. Enthoven (letter), *ibid.*, 1972, *220*, 1499. The effect of lactose could not be corroborated.— J. D. Teller (letter), *ibid.*, *222*, 209.

A 24-year-old man remained in a light sleep for 24 hours after drinking heavily over 40 hours then swallowing an estimated 2.4 g of oxazepam. A review of the literature confirms the belief that benzodiazepines are relatively safe drugs when taken in high doses.— K. Solomon, *N.Y. St. J. Med.*, 1978, *78*, 91.

PORPHYRIA. Oxazepam was considered to be unsafe in patients with acute porphyria although there is conflicting experimental evidence on porphyrinogenicity.— M. R. Moore and K.E.L. McColl, *Porphyrias, Drug Lists*, Glasgow, Porphyria Research Unit, University of Glasgow, 1987.

WITHDRAWAL. A 24-year-old man who had taken oxazepam 15 mg every 4 hours and 30 mg at night, for 2 years had withdrawal reactions when he suddenly stopped taking the drug. The symptoms which included increasing restlessness, rigidity of the limbs, stiffness of the joints, and a feeling of having great energy with impaired concentration resolved when he resumed taking oxazepam. He later stopped taking oxazepam by gradually reducing the dose without withdrawal symptoms.— G. Mendelson (letter), *Lancet*, 1978, *1*, 565 and 888.

Absorption and Fate

For an account of the absorption and fate of a benzodiazepine, see Diazepam, p.730.

Oxazepam has been reported to have a half-life ranging from about 6 to 20 hours. It is the ultimate pharmacologically active metabolite of diazepam and is itself largely metabolised to the inactive glucuronide.

ABSORPTION AND PLASMA CONCENTRATIONS. An account of the pharmacokinetics of oxazepam. Absorption of oxazepam is probably complete and in healthy subjects half-lives ranging from about 6 to 25 hours have been obtained.— G. Alván and I. Odar-Cederlöf, *Acta psychiat. scand.*, 1978, *Suppl.* 274, 47.

BILIARY EXCRETION. Following administration of oxazepam 45 mg to 2 subjects who had undergone cholecystectomy less than 0.1% of a dose was found in the bile.— H. J. Shull *et al.*, *Ann. intern. Med.*, 1976, *84*, 420. Increased biliary excretion and possible enterohepatic recycling in uraemic subjects.— G. Alván and I. Odar-Cederlöf, *Acta psychiat. scand.*, 1978, *Suppl.* 274, 47.

PREGNANCY AND THE NEONATE. *Diffusion across the placenta.* A study on the placental passage of oxazepam and its metabolism in 12 women given a single dose of oxazepam 25 mg during labour. Oxazepam was readily absorbed and peak plasma concentrations were in the same range as those reported in healthy males and non-pregnant females given the same dose although the plasma half-life (range 5.3 to 7.8 hours in 8 subjects studied) was shorter than that reported for non-pregnant subjects. Oxazepam was detected in the umbilical vein of all 12 patients with the ratio between umbilical to maternal vein concentration of oxazepam reaching a value of about 1.35 and remaining constant beyond a dose-delivery time of 3 hours. All of the babies had a normal Apgar score value. The oxazepam plasma half-life in the newborns was about 3 to 4 times that in the mothers although in 3 the plasma concentration of oxazepam conjugate rose during the first 6 to 10 hours after delivery indicating the ability of the neonate to conjugate oxazepam.— G. Tomson *et al.*, *Clin. Pharmac. Ther.*, 1979, *25*, 74.

Uses and Administration

Oxazepam is a benzodiazepine with actions and uses similar to those of diazepam (p.731). The usual dose for the treatment of anxiety is 15 to 30 mg three or four times daily. A suggested initial dose for elderly or debilitated patients is 10 mg three times daily.

Oxazepam has also been used as the hemisuccinate.

ADMINISTRATION. Neither the rate nor the extent of oxazepam absorption was reduced by food intake.— A. Melander, *Clin. Pharmacokinet.*, 1978, *3*, 337.

Further references: A. Melander *et al.*, *Acta pharmac. tox.*, 1977, *40*, 584.

In children. Numerous authors have employed oxazepam in paediatric psychiatry. Dosage varied according to age, indication, and individual response but normally a dose of about 1 mg per kg body-weight daily in divided doses proved adequate.— R. Deberdt, *Acta psychiat. scand.*, 1978, *Suppl.* 274, 104.

In the elderly. Oxazepam elimination appears to be unaffected by age.— R. E. Vestal, *Drugs*, 1978, *16*, 358.

ADMINISTRATION IN HEPATIC FAILURE. Seven patients with acute viral hepatitis, 6 with cirrhosis of the liver, and 16 age-matched healthy control subjects received oxazepam 15 or 45 mg by mouth. Urinary excretion rates and plasma elimination patterns were unaltered in patients with acute and chronic parenchymal liver disease. In a chronic study, oxazepam 15 mg was administered thrice daily by mouth for 2 weeks to 2 healthy subjects and to 2 patients with cirrhosis and did not appear to accumulate in any of the four.— H. J. Shull *et al.*, *Ann. intern. Med.*, 1976, *84*, 420.

ADMINISTRATION IN RENAL FAILURE. The half-life of oxazepam was increased from 6 to 25 hours to up to 90 hours in end-stage renal disease. Doses should be reduced to 75% in patients with a glomerular filtration-rate less than 10 mL per minute.— W. M. Bennett *et al.*, *Am. J. Kidney Dis.*, 1983, *3*, 155. Further references: U. Busch *et al.*, *Arzneimittel-Forsch.*, 1981, *31*, 1507; T. G. Murray *et al.*, *Clin. Pharmac. Ther.*, 1981, *30*, 805.

ADMINISTRATION IN THYROID DISORDERS. There was a reduction in half-life and an increase in the apparent oral clearance of oxazepam in 7 hyperthyroid patients. In 6 hypothyroid patients there was no overall change in oxazepam elimination, but the 2 most severely affected patients did show a reduction in half-life after treatment, and 5 of the 6 complained of drowsiness despite a relatively low dose of oxazepam (15 mg).— A. K. Scott *et al.*, *Br. J. clin. Pharmac.*, 1984, *17*, 49.

ANXIETY. Oxazepam in a dosage of 15 mg thrice daily was given to 48 patients suffering from anxiety states. Patients received plain uncoated tablets which were coloured green, red, and yellow, each for a period of 1 week. Though the differences in responses to treatment with the 3 colours of tablets were not significant, green tablets appeared to be the most effective for symptoms of anxiety, and yellow the most effective for depressive symptoms.— K. Schapira *et al.*, *Br. med. J.*, 1970, *2*, 446.

TINNITUS. For a study demonstrating beneficial results from oxazepam in patients with chronic subjective tinnitus, see under Clonazepam, p.402.

Preparations

Oxazepam Capsules *(B.P.)*. Store at a temperature not exceeding 25°.

Oxazepam Capsules *(U.S.P.)*

Oxazepam Tablets *(B.P.)*. Store at a temperature not exceeding 25°.

Oxazepam Tablets *(U.S.P.)*

Proprietary Preparations

Oxanid *(Steinhard, UK)*. *Tablets*, oxazepam 10, 15, and 30 mg.

Proprietary Names and Manufacturers

Adumbran *(Arg.; Austral.; Thomae, Ger.; Boehringer Ingelheim, Ital.; Boehringer Ingelheim, S.Afr.; Boehringer Ingelheim, Spain)*; Alepam *(Alphapharm, Austral.)*; Alopam *(A.L., Denm.; Apothekernes Laboratorium, Norw.; A.L., Swed.)*; Anxiolit *(Medichemie, Switz.)*; Aplakil *(Aristegui, Spain)*; Azutranquil *(Azuchemie, Ger.)*; Benzotran *(Protea, Austral.)*; Durazepam *(Durachemie, Ger.)*; Enidrel *(Arg.)*; Isodin *(Ital.)*; Limbial *(Chiesi, Ital.)*; Murelax *(Ayerst, Austral.)*; Nesontil *(Arg.)*; Neurofren *(Orfi, Spain)*; Noctazepam *(Brenner, Ger.)*; Novoxapam *(Novopharm, Canad.)*; Nulans *(Ital.)*; Oxaline *(Rolab, S.Afr.)*; Oxanid *(Steinhard, UK)*; Oxa-Puren *(Klinge-Nattermann, Ger.)*; Oxepam *(Fin.)*; Oxpam *(ICN, Canad.)*; Praxiten *(Arg.; Aust.; Wyeth, Ger.)*; Psiquiwas *(Wasserman, Spain)*; Purata *(Lennon, S.Afr.)*; Quen *(Ravizza, Ital.)*; Quilibrex *(Isnardi, Ital.)*; Sedokin *(Ital.)*; Serax *(Wyeth, Canad.; Wyeth, USA)*; Serenal; Serenid Forte *(Wyeth, UK)*; Serenid-D *(Wyeth, UK)*; Serepax *(Wyeth, Austral.; Wyeth, Denm.; Ferrosan, Norw.; Wyeth, S.Afr.; Kabi, Swed.)*; Seresta *(Wyeth-Byla, Fr.; Wyeth, Switz.)*; Serpax *(Wyeth, Ital.)*; Sigacalm *(Siegfried, Ger.)*; Sobile *(Lafarquim, Spain)*; Sobril *(KabiVitrum, Norw.; Kabi, Swed.)*; Uskan *(Desitin, Ger.; Cimex, Switz.)*; Wakazepam *(Jpn)*; Zapex *(Riva, Canad.)*.

The following names have been used for multi-ingredient preparations containing oxazepam— Fenprinax *(RBS Pharma, Ital.)*.

7077-f

Oxazolam *(rINN)*.

Oxazolazepam. 10-Chloro-2,3,7,11b-tetrahydro-2-methyl-11b-phenyloxazolo[3,2-*d*][1,4]benzodiazepin-6(5*H*)-one.
$C_{18}H_{17}ClN_2O_2=328.8$.

CAS — 24143-17-7.

Pharmacopoeias. In *Jpn.*

Oxazolam is a benzodiazepine with actions and uses similar to those of diazepam (p.728). It has been given in doses of 10 to 20 mg up to three times daily for the treatment of anxiety.

The pharmacokinetics of oxazolam in 12 healthy subjects. Following a 40-mg dose by mouth oxazolam was converted to desmethyldiazepam; mean peak serum concentrations of the latter were 115 ng per mL, achieved 8.6 hours after administration. The mean elimination half-life of desmethyldiazepam in these subjects was 61 hours. Three subjects also received single doses of prazepam and clorazepate which are also precursors of desmethyldiazepam, the latter being completely converted. The serum concentrations of desmethyldiazepam were greatest after clorazepate; the ratio of available desmethyldiazepam after equivalent doses of oxazolam and clorazepate was 0.22 to 1.00. The extent of desmethyldiazepam formation from oxazolam is either incomplete, or the drug is incompletely absorbed.— H. R. Ochs *et al.*, *J. clin. Pharmac.*, 1984, *24*, 446.

Proprietary Names and Manufacturers

Convertal *(Roemmers, Arg.)*; Hializan *(Pharmainvesti, Spain)*; Serenal *(Sankyo, Jpn)*; Tranquit *(Promonta, Ger.)*.

13064-n

Oxiperomide *(USAN, rINN)*.

Foxamide; Peromide; R-4714. 1-[1-(2-Phenoxyethyl)-4-piperidyl]benzimidazolin-2-one.
$C_{20}H_{23}N_3O_2=337.4$.

CAS — 5322-53-2.

Oxiperomide has been tried for the control of dyskinesias.

Proprietary Names and Manufacturers

Janssen, Belg.

7078-d

Oxypertine *(BAN, USAN, rINN)*.

Win-18501-2. 5,6-Dimethoxy-2-methyl-3-[2-(4-phenylpiperazin-1-yl)ethyl]indole.
$C_{23}H_{29}N_3O_2=379.5$.

CAS — 153-87-7.

Adverse Effects, Treatment, and Precautions

As for the phenothiazines, p.706.

Some sources have recommended that since oxypertine has been observed in *animal* studies to release small amounts of catecholamines it should be avoided in patients taking monoamine oxidase inhibitors.

Marked reduction in blood pressure in one patient and paralytic ileus in another, following administration of oxypertine.— *Jpn med. Gaz.*, 1978, *15*, (May 20), 12.

Uses and Administration

Oxypertine is a neuroleptic that has been used in the treatment of psychoses in doses of 80 to 120 mg daily in divided doses. The maximum recommended dose is 300 mg daily although higher doses have been used. Doses of 10 mg three or four times daily have also been used for non-psychotic emotional disturbances such as anxiety and tension. In general, however, neuroleptics are only suitable for such purposes in resistant conditions, where more appropriate agents, such as the benzodiazepines (see Diazepam, p.731) have proved ineffective. If their use is judged to be necessary treatment should be directed at low dosages given on a short-term basis.

Proprietary Preparations

Integrin *(Sterling Research, UK)*. *Capsules*, oxypertine 10 mg.
Tablets, scored, oxypertine 40 mg.

Proprietary Names and Manufacturers

Equipertine *(Belg.; Fr.; Neth.)*; Forit *(Winthrop, Ger.; Switz.)*; Integrin *(Sterling Research, UK)*; Opertil *(Denm.; Fin.; Neth.; Norw.)*.

4055-z

Paraldehyde *(BAN, USAN)*.

Paracetaldehyde; Paraldehydum. The trimer of acetaldehyde; 2,4,6-Trimethyl-1,3,5-trioxane.
$(C_2H_4O)_3=132.2$.

CAS — 123-63-7.

Pharmacopoeias. In *Arg., Aust., Br., Egypt., Eur., Fr., Ger., Hung., Ind., It., Neth., Nord., Span., Swiss, Turk.*, and *U.S.*

A clear colourless or pale yellow liquid with a strong characteristic odour. The *B.P.* specifies that it contains a suitable amount of an antoxidant; the *U.S.P.* permits a suitable stabiliser. Relative density 0.991 to 0.996. The *B.P.* gives the f.p. as 10° to 13°, and requires that not more than 10% distils below 123° and not less than 95% below 126°. The *U.S.P.* gives a congealing temperature of not lower than 11° and states that it distils completely between 120° and 126°.

Soluble 1 in 9 or 10 of water, but only 1 in 17 in boiling water; miscible with alcohol, chloroform, ether, and volatile oils. The *B.P.* injection is **sterilised** by filtration; contact with rubber should be avoided. **Store** at a temperature of 8° to 15° in small well-filled airtight containers. Protect from light. The *U.S.P.* specifies that it must not be used more than 24 hours after opening the container.

Because of its solvent action upon rubber, polystyrene, and styrene-acrylonitrile copolymer, paraldehyde should not be administered in plastic syringes made with these materials. The use of cork closures should be avoided.

At low temperature it solidifies to form a crystalline mass. If it solidifies, the whole should be liquefied before use.

CAUTION. *Paraldehyde decomposes on storage, particularly after the container has been opened. The administration of partly decomposed paraldehyde is dangerous. It must not be used if it has a brownish colour or a sharp penetrating odour of acetic acid.*

INCOMPATIBILITY. On re-evaluation of the compatibility of paraldehyde with plastic syringes and needle hubs it was recommended that, if possible, all-glass syringes should be used for the injection of paraldehyde or for the measurement of oral doses. Needles with plastic hubs could be used. The use of polypropylene syringes with rubber-tipped plastic plungers (Plastipak), or glass syringes with natural rubber-tipped plastic plungers (Glaspak) was acceptable only for the immediate administration or measurement of paraldehyde doses.— C. E. Johnson and J. A. Vigoreaux, *Am. J. Hosp. Pharm.*, 1984, *41*, 306.

SOLUBILITY IN WATER AND SALINE. In water: at 20°, 1 in 9; at 30°, 1 in 10; and at 37° 1 in 11.5. In 0.9% sodium chloride solution: at 20°, 1 in 9.5; at 30°, 1 in 11; and at 37°, 1 in 12.5.— Pharm. Soc. Lab. Rep. No. 856, 1962.

Dependence

Prolonged use of paraldehyde may lead to dependence (see p.706), especially in alcoholics.

Adverse Effects

Paraldehyde decomposes on storage and deaths

from corrosive poisoning have followed the use of such material. Paraldehyde has an unpleasant taste and imparts a smell to the breath; it may cause skin rashes.

Oral and rectal administration of paraldehyde may cause gastric or rectal irritation. Intramuscular administration is painful and associated with tissue necrosis, sterile abscesses, and nerve damage. Intravenous administration is extremely hazardous since it may cause pulmonary oedema and haemorrhage, hypotension and cardiac dilatation, and circulatory collapse; thrombophlebitis is also associated with intravenous administration.

Overdosage results in rapid laboured breathing owing to damage to the lungs and to acidosis. Nausea and vomiting may follow an overdose by mouth. Hepatic and renal damage may occur.

A patient with chronic tuberculosis died from corrosion of the upper air passages and subsequent bronchopneumonia 2 days after taking paraldehyde in water. The paraldehyde was old stock and contained 40% glacial acetic acid and excess oxidants.— *Br. med. J.*, 1954, *2*, 1114; A. S. Curry, *ibid.*, 1962, *1*, 687.

Pulmonary oedema was associated with paraldehyde given intravenously to a 2-year-old child with aplastic anaemia.— S. H. Sinal and J. E. Crowe, *Pediatrics*, 1976, *57*, 158.

Severe proctitis with stricture, and an excoriating rash affecting the buttocks and peri-anal area, were judged to have resulted from a paraldehyde enema given 4 days previously.— J. H. Stanley, *J. Am. med. Ass.*, 1980, *243*, 1749.

Pulmonary oedema followed intramuscular and intravenous administration of paraldehyde to an alcoholic patient.— R. Mountain *et al.*, *Chest*, 1982, *82*, 371.

Treatment of Adverse Effects

For general guidelines to the treatment of the acute adverse effects of hypnotics and sedatives, see p.708.

Precautions

Paraldehyde should not be given to patients with gastric disorders and it should be used with caution, if at all, in patients with bronchopulmonary disease or hepatic impairment. It should not be given rectally in the presence of colitis. Old paraldehyde must never be used.

Paraldehyde must be well diluted before oral or rectal administration; if it is deemed essential to give paraldehyde intravenously it must be well diluted and given very slowly with extreme caution (see also Adverse Effects and Uses). Intramuscular injections may be given undiluted but care should be taken to avoid nerve damage. Plastic syringes should be avoided (see Incompatibility, above).

Paraldehyde causes drowsiness and persons receiving it should not take charge of vehicles or machinery where loss of attention could lead to accidents. These effects are enhanced by simultaneous administration of depressants of the central nervous system such as alcohol, barbiturates, and other sedatives. Paraldehyde should not be administered to patients receiving disulfiram.

INTERACTIONS. *Alcohol*. A report on the deaths of 9 patients following administration of paraldehyde to treat acute alcohol intoxication. Preliminary *animal* studies confirmed a synergistic action between alcohol and paraldehyde.— S. Kaye and H. B. Haag, *Toxic. appl. Pharmac.*, 1964, *6*, 316.

Disulfiram. A study in *animals* of the enhancing effect of disulfiram on paraldehyde-induced sedation.— M. L. Keplinger and J. A. Wells, *Fedn Proc. Fedn. Am. Socs. exp. Biol.*, 1956, *15*, 445.

Absorption and Fate

Paraldehyde is reported to be readily absorbed when given by mouth, rectally, or intramuscularly and is distributed throughout the tissues. About 80% of a dose is metabolised in the liver probably to acetaldehyde, which is oxidised to acetic acid. Unmetabolised drug is largely excreted unchanged through the lungs; only small amounts appear in the urine. It crosses the placental barrier.

A constant proportion of about 7% of an oral dose was exhaled within 4 hours as unchanged paraldehyde and no metabolites were detected.— D. W. Lang and H. H. Borgstedt, *Toxic. appl. Pharmac.*, 1969, *15*, 269.

PREGNANCY AND LACTATION. Many hours after an initial dose of paraldehyde, the average concentration in the foetal circulation was almost equal to that in the maternal blood. The odour of paraldehyde was detectable in the breath of the newborn for 2 or 3 days after birth. It was considered that when given in sufficient dosage to cause amnesia, paraldehyde would cause neonatal depression in a large percentage of infants.— F. Moya and V. Thorndike, *Am. J. Obstet. Gynec.*, 1962, *84*, 1778.

Uses and Administration

Paraldehyde is a hypnotic and sedative with anticonvulsant effects. Following oral administration it is reported to act in 10 to 15 minutes to induce sleep lasting 4 to 8 hours but it has largely been superseded for that purpose by other agents.

The usual hypnotic dose by mouth or intramuscularly was 10 mL at night, while a dose of 5 mL has been given for its sedative effect. Oral doses must be well diluted to avoid gastric irritation and not more than 5 mL of an intramuscular dose should be injected into any one site. Similar doses have also been given rectally diluted with oil or water; higher doses were formerly given rectally as a basal anaesthetic.

Paraldehyde has also been used intramuscularly in doses up to 10 mL for the emergency treatment of epilepsy but the pain associated with its use, its tendency to react with plastic syringes, and the risk associated with deterioration, militate against its use. A suggested dose for children is 0.1 to 0.15 mL per kg body-weight.

Paraldehyde has also been given by intravenous infusion, diluted with several volumes of sodium chloride injection but severe untoward effects have been associated with its use by this route (see under Adverse Effects).

Preparations

Paraldehyde Injection *(B.P.)*. Sterile paraldehyde containing no added antimicrobial preservatives. Store at a temperature not exceeding 25° in complete darkness in ampoules sealed by fusion of the glass. Plastic syringes should not be used for administering this injection.

Sterile Paraldehyde *(U.S.P.)*. Paraldehyde suitable for parenteral use. Store at a temperature not exceeding 25°.

Proprietary Names and Manufacturers

Hypnotets *(Pharmadrug, Ger.)*; Paral *(Forest Pharmaceuticals, USA)*.

7080-k

Penfluridol *(BAN, USAN, rINN)*.

R-16341. 4-(4-Chloro-3-trifluoromethylphenyl)-1-[3-(*p,p'*-difluorobenzhydryl)propyl]piperidin-4-ol.
$C_{28}H_{27}ClF_5NO=524.0$.

CAS — 26864-56-2.

Pharmacopoeias. In *Cz.*

Adverse Effects, Treatment, and Precautions

As for the phenothiazines, p.706.

EFFECTS ON THE ENDOCRINE SYSTEM. Penfluridol 100 mg weekly for 6 weeks raised plasma-prolactin concentrations in 7 chronic schizophrenic males, but had no significant effect on plasma-testosterone concentrations. There were no correlations between individual changes in prolactin and testosterone concentrations. None of the patients complained of sexual difficulties.— R. S. Nathan *et al.* (letter), *Lancet*, 1980, *2*, 94. Comment.— R. T. Rubin (letter), *ibid.*, 370.

Absorption and Fate

Although penfluridol is absorbed from the gastro-intestinal tract, peak plasma concentrations are not achieved until about 12 to 24 hours after a dose by mouth. The initial peak plasma concentration is followed by a rapid decrease over the next 36 hours, probably due to tissue redistribution, followed by a slower decline over the next 120 hours. Penfluridol, accordingly, has a very long duration of action, and *animal* studies have indicated that this is partly related to its storage in, and slow release from, adipose tissue.

There is evidence of enterohepatic recycling, and penfluridol is mainly excreted unchanged in the faeces, with small amounts appearing in the urine as the metabolite 4,4-bis(4-fluorophenyl)butyric acid, which is obtained by *N*-dealkylation.

Uses and Administration

Penfluridol is a member of the diphenylbutylpiperidine group of neuroleptic agents, which are structurally similar to the butyrophenones (see haloperidol, p.743). Following administration by mouth it has a prolonged duration of action which lasts for about a week.

The usual dose of penfluridol for the treatment of psychoses is 20 to 60 mg weekly. Doses of up to 120 mg weekly may be required in resistant conditions.

SCHIZOPHRENIA. A brief review of the merits of a once-weekly oral preparation for schizophrenia.— *Lancet*, 1978, *2*, 879. Comment.— A. A. Schiff (letter), *ibid.*, 1101.

Results of a 3-week double-blind study completed by 29 of 33 schizophrenic patients requiring in-patient therapy, indicated that penfluridol is as effective as chlorpromazine in the treatment of schizophrenia, except for patients with very acute symptoms. Twenty-one of the 29 patients completed a 10-week follow-up study as outpatients. The mean dose of penfluridol was 102 mg weekly (range 80 to 120 mg weekly), and chlorpromazine 650 mg daily (range 100 to 900 mg daily). Five penfluridol patients required reduction of dose because of drowsiness (2), extrapyramidal effects (2), and weakness (1); 5 chlorpromazine patients also required dose reduction because of drowsiness. Two penfluridol patients were readmitted to hospital because of depression. Four chlorpromazine patients and 1 penfluridol patient left the study because of drowsiness. Supplementary chlorpromazine was required by 3 patients receiving penfluridol. Penfluridol was considered to be of similar efficacy as chlorpromazine, and to cause less drowsiness but more extrapyramidal effects.— G. Chouinard *et al.*, *J. clin. Pharmac.*, 1977, *17*, 162. A similar study involving 59 schizophrenics.— R. I. H. Wang *et al.*, *ibid.*, 1982, *22*, 236.

Proprietary Names and Manufacturers

Cyperon *(Esteve, Spain)*; Semap *(Johnson, Arg.; Janssen, Belg.; Janssen, Denm.; Janssen, Fr.; Janssen, Ger.; Janssen, Neth.; Janssen, Switz.)*.

4056-c

Pentobarbitone *(BAN)*.

Aethaminalum; Mébubarbital; Mebumal; Pentobarbital *(USAN, rINN)*; Pentobarbitalum. 5-Ethyl-5-(1-methylbutyl)barbituric acid.
$C_{11}H_{18}N_2O_3=226.3$.

CAS — 76-74-4.

Pharmacopoeias. In *Aust.*, *Br.*, *Eur.*, *Fr.*, *Ger.*, *It.*, *Neth.*, *Nord.*, *Span.*, *Swiss*, and *U.S.*

Odourless or almost odourless, colourless crystals or a white or almost white crystalline powder. Very slightly **soluble** in water and in carbon tetrachloride; soluble 1 in 4.5 of alcohol, 1 in 4 of chloroform, and 1 in 10 of ether; very soluble in acetone and in methyl alcohol. It dissolves in aqueous solutions of alkali hydroxides or carbonates, and in aqueous ammonia. **Store** in airtight containers.

4057-k

Pentobarbitone Calcium *(BANM)*.

Pentobarbital Calcium *(rINNM)*. Calcium 5-ethyl-5-(1-methylbutyl)barbiturate.
$(C_{11}H_{17}N_2O_3)_2Ca=490.6$.

4058-a

Pentobarbitone Sodium *(BANM)*.

Aethaminalum-Natrium; Ethaminal Sodium; Mebumalnatrium; Pentobarbital Sodium *(USAN, rINNM)*; Pentobarbitalum Natricum; Sodium Pentobarbital; Soluble Pentobarbitone. Sodium 5-ethyl-5-(1-methylbutyl)barbiturate.

$C_{11}H_{17}N_2NaO_3$=248.3.

CAS — 57-33-0.

Pharmacopoeias. In *Arg., Aust., Br., Braz., Cz., Egypt., Eur., Fr., Ger., Ind., It., Mex., Neth., Rus., Swiss,* and *U.S.* Also in *B.P. Vet.*

A white, hygroscopic, crystalline powder or granules, odourless or with a slight characteristic odour. The *B.P.* states that it is very **soluble** in water and in alcohol; practically insoluble in ether. The *U.S.P.* has it freely soluble in alcohol. The *B.P.* requires that a 10% solution in water has a pH of 9.6 to 11.0 when freshly prepared while the *U.S.P.* states that such a solution has a pH between 9.8 and 11.0 and that solutions for parenteral use have a pH between 10.0 and 10.5; however, the *U.S.P.* injection is stated to have a pH between 9.0 and 10.5, pentobarbitone base being added to adjust the pH. Solutions decompose on standing, the decomposition being accelerated at higher temperatures.

Incompatible with acids and acidic salts, and with chloral hydrate. Incompatibility has been reported with cephaloridine, cephazolin sodium, clindamycin phosphate, and pentazocine lactate. **Store** in airtight containers.

INCOMPATIBILITY. Fluopromazine hydrochloride injection was incompatible with pentobarbitone sodium.— C. Riffkin, *Am. J. Hosp. Pharm.*, 1963, *20*, 19.

There was loss of clarity when intravenous solutions of pentobarbitone sodium were mixed with those of chlorpheniramine maleate, dimenhydrinate, diphenhydramine hydrochloride, ephedrine sulphate, erythromycin gluceptate, hydrocortisone sodium succinate, hydroxyzine hydrochloride, insulin, opioid salts, noradrenaline acid tartrate, oxytetracycline hydrochloride, phenytoin sodium, prochlorperazine maleate, promazine hydrochloride (in glucose injection), promethazine hydrochloride, protein hydrolysate, sodium bicarbonate, streptomycin sulphate, suxamethonium chloride, tetracycline hydrochloride, or vancomycin hydrochloride.— J. A. Patel and G. L. Phillips, *Am. J. Hosp. Pharm.*, 1966, *23*, 409.

Pentobarbitone sodium was reported to be incompatible with cephalothin sodium, chlorpromazine hydrochloride, diphenhydramine hydrochloride, and prochlorperazine hydrochloride.— J. M. Meisler and M. W. Skolaut, *Am. J. Hosp. Pharm.*, 1966, *23*, 557.

Dependence, Adverse Effects, Treatment, and Precautions

As for the barbiturates in general, p.706.

EFFECTS ON THE NERVOUS SYSTEM. A report of toxic encephalopathy noted in 7 children, over a period of several years, following administration of suppositories containing pentobarbitone sodium and mepyramine maleate. In 3 children the dose was within the manufacturer's recommendations.— J. F. Schwartz and J. H. Patterson, *Am. J. Dis. Child.*, 1978, *132*, 37.

INTERACTIONS. *Beta blockers.* Mean plasma concentrations of *alprenolol* were reduced by 59% in 6 hypertensive patients given pentobarbitone, and this was associated with a significant reduction of the beneficial effects of the beta blocker on blood pressure and heart-rate.— P. Seideman *et al.*, *Br. J. clin. Pharmac.*, 1987, *23*, 267. See also R. A. Branch and R. J. Herman, *ibid.*, 1984, *17*, 77S.

Corynebacterium parvum. During evaluations of a vaccine of killed suspensions of *Corynebacterium parvum*, intravenous injections of *C. parvum* into *mice* rendered them lethally sensitive to normal safe anaesthetic doses of pentobarbitone. Caution was recommended when both preparations might be used in man.— B. Mosedale and M. A. Smith (letter), *Lancet*, 1975, *1*, 168.

OVERDOSAGE. Muscle necrosis and calcification occurred in a 35-year-old man during the course of severe acute renal failure due to intoxication with pentobarbitone. The calcification virtually disappeared by the end of 3 months.— J. G. Clark and M. D. Sumerling, *Br. med. J.*, 1966, *2*, 214.

PREGNANCY AND THE NEONATE. Doses of up to 300 mg of pentobarbitone administered intravenously to the mother before delivery had no appreciable effect upon the clinical condition of the infants at birth. By contrast doses of 600 to 750 mg had been followed by moderate to severe neonatal depression in 40% of the infants, with delay in the establishment of normal respiration.— F. Moya and V. Thorndike, *Clin. Pharmac. Ther.*, 1963, *4*, 628.

Absorption and Fate

Following oral or rectal administration pentobarbitone is well absorbed from the gastro-intestinal tract, and is reported to be approximately 50% bound to plasma protein. Clearance from the plasma is biphasic, and the terminal half-life is reported to range from 35 to 50 hours. It is metabolised in the liver, mainly by hydroxylation, and excreted in the urine mainly as metabolites.

Following intravenous administration of pentobarbitone sodium 50 mg to 5 healthy subjects pentobarbitone was noted to have a distribution phase (α phase) of about 4 hours, and elimination occurred with a harmonic mean β-phase half-life of about 50 hours. This suggested that for pentobarbitone the body has a central plasma compartment and one or more extravascular compartments. Following oral administration of pentobarbitone, absorption was found to be considerably delayed, but not reduced, by food.— R. B. Smith *et al.*, *J. Pharmacokinet. Biopharm.*, 1973, *1*, 5. Findings in 7 healthy subjects of an average β-phase half-life of only 22.3 hours following intravenous administration of pentobarbitone sodium 100 mg. After oral administration the half-life was about the same. A more detailed knowledge of pentobarbitone pharmacokinetics was needed to explain the deviation from the findings of R.B. Smith *et al.* (above). Of pentobarbitone in the central compartment of the body only about 13% was present in the blood, where about 4% was in the plasma water, 5% was bound to plasma protein, and 4% was distributed to blood cells. Pentobarbitone appeared to undergo extensive tissue binding in both the central and peripheral compartments.— M. Ehrnebo, *J. pharm. Sci.*, 1974, *63*, 1114.

Following oral administration to healthy subjects, capsules containing pentobarbitone sodium 100 mg were totally absorbed, with an absorption half-life of 0.35 hours. Absorption was slower following rectal administration of suppositories, and varied considerably according to the suppository basis.— J. T. Doluisio *et al.*, *J. pharm. Sci.*, 1978, *67*, 1586.

The pharmacokinetics of high-dose intravenous pentobarbitone in patients with severe head injury.— D. P. Wermeling *et al.*, *Drug Intell. & clin. Pharm.*, 1987, *21*, 459.

Uses and Administration

Pentobarbitone is a barbiturate that has been used as a hypnotic and sedative. Following an oral dose it is reported to act in 15 to 60 minutes to produce sleep lasting 1 to 4 hours. As a hypnotic it is usually given in doses of 100 to 200 mg at night, and about 30 mg has been given 3 or 4 times daily as a sedative. Similar doses may be given of the sodium or calcium salt.

Pentobarbitone has been used for premedication in anaesthetic procedures but its use for these purposes has largely been superseded by other agents, such as the benzodiazepines. It has also been used as an anticonvulsant by slow intravenous injection.

Intravenous pentobarbitone has also been tried in the management of cerebral ischaemia and raised intracranial pressure such as may result from traumatic injury to the head or from a stroke.

A technique for the management of patients with intracranial hypertension, using intravenous pentobarbitone as a sedative.— L. F. Marshall *et al.*, *Neurosurgery*, 1978, *2*, 100.

A report of the use of pentobarbitone in the treatment of submersion hypothermia.— A. W. Conn, *Can. med. Ass. J.*, 1979, *120*, 397.

ADMINISTRATION IN HEPATIC FAILURE. Prolongation of the half-life of pentobarbitone in patients with cirrhosis.— F. W. Ossenberg *et al.*, *Digestion*, 1973, *8*, 448.

ADMINISTRATION IN RENAL FAILURE. Pentobarbitone could be given in usual doses to patients with renal failure.— W. M. Bennett *et al.*, *Am. J. Kidney Dis.*, 1983, *3*, 155.

Preparations of Pentobarbitone and its Salts

Pentobarbital Elixir *(U.S.P.).* Contains pentobarbitone, with alcohol 16 to 20%.

Pentobarbital Sodium Capsules *(U.S.P.).* Contain pentobarbitone sodium.

Pentobarbital Sodium Elixir *(U.S.P.).* Pentobarbitone sodium 400 mg, glycerol 45 mL, alcohol 15 mL, orange oil 0.075 mL, caramel 200 mg, syrup 15 mL, dilute hydrochloric acid 0.6 mL, water to 100 mL.

Pentobarbital Sodium Injection *(U.S.P.).* A sterile solution of pentobarbitone sodium (or an equivalent amount of pentobarbitone for adjustment of the pH) in a suitable solvent. Dosage is given in terms of pentobarbitone sodium.

Pentobarbitone Capsules *(B.P.).* Pentobarbitone Sodium Capsules. Contain pentobarbitone sodium.

Pentobarbitone Tablets *(B.P.).* Pentobarbitone Sodium Tablets. Contain pentobarbitone sodium.

Proprietary Names and Manufacturers of Pentobarbitone Sodium and its Salts

Embutal *(Arg.)*; Insom Rapido *(Spain)*; Nembutal *(Abbott, Austral.*; *Belg.*; *Abbott, Canad.*; *Denm.*; *Fr.*; *Ger.*; *Ital.*; *Neth.*; *Switz.*; *Abbott, UK*; *Abbott, USA)*; Neodorm *(Nordmark, Ger.)*; Nova-Rectal *(Canad.)*; Penbon *(Nelson, Austral.)*; Pentogen *(Canad.)*; Pentone *(Faulding, Austral.)*; Petab *(Austral.)*; Praecicalm *(Molimin, Ger.)*; Repocal *(Desitin, Ger.)*; Schlafen *(Jpn)*; Sopental *(Continental Ethicals, S.Afr.)*.

The following names have been used for multi-ingredient preparations containing pentobarbitone sodium and its salts—Cafergot P-B *(Sandoz, Canad.*; *Sandoz, USA)*; Carbrital *(Parke, Davis, Austral.*; *Parke, Davis, Canad.*; *Parke, Davis, UK)*; Nembudeine *(Abbott, Austral.)*; Pentalgin *(Fawns & McAllan, Austral.)*; Wans *(Webcon, USA)*; Wigraine-PB *(Organon, USA)*.

7081-a

Perazine Dimalonate

P-725 *(perazine)*; Pemazine Dimalonate. 10-[3-(4-Methylpiperazin-1-yl)propyl]phenothiazine dimalonate.

$C_{20}H_{25}N_3S,2C_3H_4O_4$=547.6.

CAS — 84-97-9 (perazine); 14777-25-4 (dimalonate).

Perazine dimalonate is a phenothiazine with general properties similar to those of chlorpromazine (p.722). It has a piperazine side-chain. It has been given in usual doses equivalent to 75 to 600 mg of the base daily. It has also been given intramuscularly.

Proprietary Names and Manufacturers

Taxilan *(Promonta, Belg.*; *Promonta, Ger.*; *Byk, Neth.)*.

7082-t

Pericyazine *(BAN).*

Periciazine *(rINN)*; Propericiazine; RP-8909; SKF-20716. 10-[3-(4-Hydroxypiperidino)propyl]-phenothiazine-2-carbonitrile; 1-[3-(2-Cyanophenothiazin-10-yl)propyl]piperidin-4-ol.

$C_{21}H_{23}N_3OS$=365.5.

CAS — 2622-26-6.

Adverse Effects, Treatment, and Precautions

As for the phenothiazines in general, p.706.

Sedation and postural hypotension may be marked.

Absorption and Fate

For an account of the absorption and fate of a phenothiazine, see Chlorpromazine, p.723.

Uses and Administration

Pericyazine is a phenothiazine with actions and uses similar to those of chlorpromazine (p.724). It has a piperidine side-chain.

The usual dose for the treatment of psychoses is 15 to 30 mg daily; the daily dosage may be given in 2 portions, the larger amount in the evening. In severe psychoses initial doses of 75 mg daily have been given, increased if necessary, at weekly intervals, to up to 300 mg daily. It has also been given by intramuscular injection.

A suggested initial daily dose by mouth for children is 500 μg for a child of 10 kg, increased by 1 mg per 5 kg, to a maximum of 10 mg daily. Elderly subjects should be given reduced doses.

Proprietary Preparations

Neulactil *(May & Baker, UK). Tablets*, scored, pericyazine 2.5, 10, or 25 mg.
Forte syrup, pericyazine 10 mg/5 mL.

Proprietary Names and Manufacturers
Aolept *(Bayer, Ger.)*; Apamin *(Jpn)*; Nemactil *(Rhone, Spain)*; Neulactil *(May & Baker, Austral.; Rhone-Poulenc, Denm.; Rhône-Poulenc, Norw.; May & Baker, S.Afr.; Leo Rhodia, Swed.; May & Baker, UK)*; Neuleptil *(Arg.; Belg.; Rhône-Poulenc, Canad.; Specia, Fr.; Carlo Erba, Ital.; Neth.; Rhone-Poulenc, Switz.)*.

NOTE. The name Apamin has also been used to denote a neurotoxic polypeptide constituent of bee venom.

4059-t

Perlapine *(BAN, USAN, rINN).*
AW-142333; HF-2333. 6-(4-Methylpiperazin-1-yl)morphanthridine; 6-(4-Methylpiperazin-1-yl)-11*H*-dibenz-[*b,e*]azepine.
$C_{19}H_{21}N_3$=291.4.
CAS — 1977-11-3.

Perlapine is a hypnotic that has been used in the short-term management of insomnia in doses of 2.5 to 10 mg at night.

Proprietary Names and Manufacturers
Hypnodin *(Takeda, Jpn)*.

7084-r

Perphenazine *(BAN, USAN, rINN).*

Perphenazinum. 2-{4-[3-(2-Chlorophenothiazin-10-yl)propyl]piperazin-1-yl}ethanol.
$C_{21}H_{26}ClN_3OS$=404.0.
CAS — 58-39-9.

Pharmacopoeias. In *Br., Chin., Cz., Jpn,* and *U.S. Jpn* also includes the maleate.

A white or creamy-white odourless or almost odourless powder.
Practically **insoluble** in water; the *B.P.* states that it is soluble 1 in 20 of alcohol, 1 in 1 of chloroform, 1 in 80 of ether; soluble in dilute hydrochloric acid. *U.S.P.* solubilities are: 1 in 7 of alcohol, and 1 in 13 of acetone. The *B.P.* injection has a pH of 4.5 to 5.5; the *U.S.P.* injection has a pH of between 4.2 and 5.6. The *B.P.* injection is **sterilised** by autoclaving in an atmosphere of nitrogen.
Store in airtight containers. Protect from light.

Adverse Effects, Treatment, and Precautions
As for the phenothiazines in general, p.706.

EFFECTS ON THE HEART. The incidence (about 24% in the fasting state) of depolarisation abnormalities on the ECG in patients taking perphenazine or perphenazine with amitriptyline was increased after a glucose load.— G. Chouinard and L. Annable, *Archs gen. Psychiat.*, 1977, *34*, 951.

EFFECTS ON THE SKIN. Perphenazine had been reported to cause photosensitivity reactions.— *Med. Lett.*, 1986, *28*, 51.

EXTRAPYRAMIDAL EFFECTS. In a young woman with oculogyric crisis due to perphenazine 10 mg, the administration of atropine 600 µg and pethidine 50 mg produced complete remission of symptoms within 10 minutes.— J. J. Kimerling and S. R. Patel (letter), *Br. med. J.*, 1967, *4*, 554.

Severe spontaneous bucco-oro-lingual dyskinesia due to 2.5 mg of perphenazine given by intramuscular injection before and after an eye operation in a 17-year-old girl, was relieved within seconds by an intravenous injection of 5 mg of diazepam. No further attacks were seen after a further 5 mg of diazepam given intramuscularly.— D. M. Davies (letter), *Lancet*, 1970, *1*, 567.

Three patients developed acute extrapyramidal symptoms after treatment for nausea by a single dose of perphenazine. Benztropine mesylate intravenously gave complete relief of symptoms.— P. D. Ramsden and D. L. Froggatt (letter), *Br. med. J.*, 1972, *1*, 246.

Severe torticollis developed in a 19-year-old girl given perphenazine syrup in the early stages of jaundice. Severe extrapyramidal side-effects were also seen in a jaundiced boy given normal doses of prochlorperazine. Patients with liver disease were considered to be at special risk.— A. Paton (letter), *Br. med. J.*, 1974, *3*, 344.

An acute dystonic reaction, with symptoms of tetany and tetanus, but without extrapyramidal symptoms, occurred in an 8-year-old boy who had received four 5-mg doses of perphenazine in about 36 hours. The condition responded to diazepam.— W. D. Smith and M. A. Tobias, *Br. J. Anaesth.*, 1976, *48*, 703.

INTERACTIONS. A psychotic patient, previously maintained with plasma-perphenazine concentrations of 2 to 3 nmol per mL on a dose of 8 mg twice daily by mouth was readmitted with subtherapeutic plasma-perphenazine concentrations of less than 1 nmol per mL, despite unchanged dosage, following concomitant disulfiram therapy. The concentration of the sulphoxide metabolite of perphenazine was much increased. Following a change from oral to intramuscular perphenazine therapy there was a substantial clinical improvement associated with a return to therapeutic plasma concentrations of perphenazine and a fall in concentration of the metabolite. Disulfiram appears to greatly enhance biotransformation of perphenazine given by mouth to inactive metabolites, but parenteral administration avoids the 'first-pass' effect in the liver.— L. B. Hansen and N. -E. Larsen (letter), *Lancet*, 1982, *2*, 1472.

Absorption and Fate
For an account of the absorption and fate of a phenothiazine, see Chlorpromazine, p.723.

Perphenazine 5 or 6 mg administered intravenously had a plasma half-life from 8.4 to 12.3 hours in a study of 4 schizophrenic patients and 4 healthy subjects. Considerable fluctuations in plasma-perphenazine concentrations were observed 3 to 5 hours after administration before the exponential elimination phase. A dose of 6 mg by mouth in 4 healthy subjects failed to produce a detectable plasma concentration and only low plasma concentrations of its sulphoxide metabolite could be detected; this was attributed to a marked first-pass effect. Systemic availability was variable and poor in 4 schizophrenic patients given perphenazine 12 mg thrice daily. However, it was considered that oral therapy should be on an 8-hour dosage regimen. Intramuscular injection of perphenazine enanthate 50 or 100 mg every 2 weeks gave plasma-perphenazine concentrations similar to those after continuous oral administration but with a high initial absorption within 2 to 3 days associated with the most serious neurological and sedative side-effects.— C. E. Hansen *et al.*, *Br. J. clin. Pharmac.*, 1976, *3*, 915. See also J. R. Magliozzi, *Curr. ther. Res.*, 1986, *40*, 871.

Details of perphenazine enanthate, a long-acting ester of perphenazine, suitable for depot injection.— *Drugs Today*, 1978, *14*, 120.

Uses and Administration
Perphenazine is a phenothiazine with actions and uses similar to those of chlorpromazine (p.724). It has a piperazine side-chain. The usual dose for the treatment of psychoses is 4 to 8 mg three times daily; in severe psychoses doses of up to 64 mg daily have been permitted. It may be given by intramuscular injection for the immediate relief of acute psychotic symptoms in an initial dose of 5 to 10 mg and 5-mg doses may be given if necessary at 6-hourly intervals to a maximum of 15 to 30 mg daily.
For the control of nausea and vomiting the usual dose by mouth is 4 mg three times daily but up to 8 mg three times daily may be required. The usual intramuscular dose is 5 mg; occasionally 10 mg may be required.
Elderly subjects should be given reduced doses.
Perphenazine has also been used as the enanthate and as the decanoate.

Preparations
Perphenazine Injection *(B.P.)*
Perphenazine Injection *(U.S.P.)*. A sterile solution in Water for Injections prepared with the aid of citric acid.
Perphenazine Oral Solution *(U.S.P.)*. Perphenazine Solution
Perphenazine Syrup *(U.S.P.)*
Perphenazine Tablets *(B.P.)*
Perphenazine Tablets *(U.S.P.)*

Proprietary Preparations
Fentazin *(Allen & Hanburys, UK). Tablets*, perphenazine 2, 4, and 8 mg.
Injection, perphenazine 5 mg/mL, in ampoules of 1 mL.

Proprietary Names and Manufacturers
Decentan *(E. Merck, Ger.; Ital.; Igoda, Spain)*; Fentazin *(Allen & Hanburys, UK)*; F-Mon *(Jpn)*; Perfenil *(Ital.)*; Phenazine *(ICN, Canad.)*; Trilafon *(Essex, Austral.; Belg.; Schering, Canad.; Schering Corp., Denm.; Essex, Ital.; Neth.; Schering, Norw.; Scherag, S.Afr.; Spain; Schering, Swed.; Essex, Switz.; Schering, USA)*; Trilifan *(Unicet, Fr.)*.

The following names have been used for multi-ingredient preparations containing perphenazine— Elavil Plus *(Merck Sharp & Dohme, Canad.)*; Etrafon *(Schering, Canad.; Schering, USA)*; Mutabon *(Essex, Austral.)*; Proavil *(Pro Doc, Canad.)*; Triamed *(Medic, Canad.)*; Triavil *(Merck Sharp & Dohme, Canad.; Merck Sharp & Dohme, USA)*; Triptafen *(Allen & Hanburys, UK)*; Triptafen-DA *(Allen & Hanburys, UK)*; Triptafen-Forte *(Allen & Hanburys, UK)*; Triptafen-M *(Allen & Hanburys, UK)*; Triptafen-Minor *(Allen & Hanburys, UK)*.

7086-d

Phenprobamate *(BAN, rINN).*
MH-532; Proformiphen. 3-Phenylpropyl carbamate.
$C_{10}H_{13}NO_2$=179.2.
CAS — 673-31-4.

Phenprobamate is a carbamate with general properties similar to those of meprobamate (p.750). It has been given as an anxiolytic and muscle relaxant in doses of 400 to 800 mg three times daily.

Proprietary Names and Manufacturers
Actiphan *(Jpn)*; Gamaquil *(Pharmacia, Denm.; Siegfried, Ger.; Mekos, Norw.; Siegfried, Switz.)*; Nelaxan *(Jpn)*; Palmita *(Jpn)*; Paraquick *(Jpn)*.

13113-k

Picobenzide *(rINN).*
M-14012-4. 3,5-Dimethyl-*N*-(4-pyridylmethyl)benzamide.
$C_{15}H_{16}N_2O$=240.3.
CAS — 51832-87-2.

Picobenzide is reported to have neuroleptic activity.

Reference: M. V. Calvo *et al.*, *Int. J. clin. Pharmac. Ther. Toxic.*, 1985, *23*, 233 (pharmacokinetics).

Proprietary Names and Manufacturers
Made, Spain.

7087-n

Pimozide *(BAN, USAN, rINN).*

R-6238. 1-{1-[4,4-Bis(4-fluorophenyl)butyl]-4-piperidyl}benzimidazolin-2-one; 1-{1-[3-(4,4′-Difluorobenzhydryl)propyl]-4-piperidyl}benzimidazolin-2-one.
$C_{28}H_{29}F_2N_3O$=461.6.
CAS — 2062-78-4.

Adverse Effects, Treatment, and Precautions
As for the phenothiazines, p.706.
Extrapyramidal symptoms may be more common than those associated with chlorpromazine, whereas it may be less likely to cause sedation.

WITHDRAWAL. Three patients who had been taking pimozide had epileptiform fits 13 to 31 days after the dose of pimozide had been reduced or treatment stopped. In the absence of any other obvious reason a possible connection with pimozide has to be considered.— E. A. Burkitt and M. Faulkner (letter), *Br. med. J.*, 1972, *3*, 643.

Absorption and Fate
Following oral administration, about half of a dose of pimozide is reported to be absorbed. It undergoes significant first-pass metabolism. Peak plasma concentrations have been reported after 4 to 12 hours and there is a considerable interindividual variation in the concentrations achieved. Pimozide has a long terminal half-life of approximately 55 hours.
Pimozide is metabolised in the liver and excreted in the urine and faeces, both unchanged and in

the form of metabolites. The major path of metabolism of pimozide is *N*-dealkylation. *Animal* studies have indicated that it is widely distributed in the body, but with a large proportion of the dose stored in the liver and considerably lower concentrations elsewhere, including the brain.

In a crossover study in 14 schizophrenic patients given pimozide 2 to 10 mg daily it was estimated that the bioavailability was 79% when pimozide was given as tablets, and 84% when given as oral solution.— M. Larsson and A. Forsman, *Curr. ther. Res.*, 1984, *35*, 220.

Uses and Administration

Pimozide is a member of the diphenylbutylpiperidine group of antipsychotic agents, which are structurally similar to the butyrophenones (see Haloperidol, p.743). It is used in the management of psychoses, in a usual initial dose of 4 mg daily by mouth; in severe cases up to 20 mg or more daily may be given. Maintenance doses vary between 2 and 20 mg daily.

Pimozide has also been used in the management of Gilles de la Tourette's syndrome. The usual initial dose is 1 to 2 mg daily, increased if necessary to a maximum of 20 mg, or 300 µg per kg body-weight, daily. Most patients are maintained at about 10 mg daily.

Pimozide has also been given in doses of 2 to 4 mg daily for non-psychotic emotional disturbances, such as anxiety and tension. In general, however, neuroleptics are only suitable for such purposes in resistant conditions where more appropriate agents, such as the benzodiazepines (see Diazepam, p.731) have proved ineffective. If their use is judged to be necessary, treatment should be directed at low dosages given on a short-term basis.

Pimozide should be given in reduced dosage to elderly patients.

ADMINISTRATION. Pimozide had a mean plasma half-life of 55 hours after a multiple-dose regimen of 6 mg daily for 4 days and 53 hours after a single dose of 24 mg. The incidence of extrapyramidal effects was similar with both dose schedules. It was suggested that a single weekly dose might be useful.— R. G. McCreadie *et al.* (letter), *Br. J. clin. Pharmac.*, 1979, *7*, 533.

In a double-blind study in chronic schizophrenics, 13 were given pimozide by mouth (initially in daily doses, but adjusted gradually to weekly dosage after the first month), while 15 were assigned to treatment with fluphenazine decanoate injection fortnightly. At the end of the 10-month study the weekly dose of pimozide ranged from 10 to 60 mg, with an average of 40 mg, while the dose of fluphenazine ranged from the equivalent of 2 to 25 mg weekly, with an average of 14 mg. The study was completed by 8 of the 13 receiving pimozide and 9 of the 15 receiving fluphenazine and there were no significant differences between the 2 groups in mental state. The results show that weekly doses of pimozide were as effective as depot fluphenazine in preventing relapse in chronic schizophrenics.— R. McCreadie *et al.*, *Br. J. Psychiat.*, 1982, *140*, 280.

ANOREXIA NERVOSA. Since it had been suggested that anorexia could be related to a dopaminergic-receptor hyperactivity, pimozide 4 mg thrice daily for a month was used to treat an anorexic youth. Dramatic improvement occurred within 3 weeks. He gained 9 kg in weight and lost his obsession with his weight. Signs such as bradycardia and overactivity also disappeared.— F. Plantey (letter), *Lancet*, 1977, *1*, 1105.

BEHAVIOUR DISORDERS. A double-blind study on 30 disturbed male adolescents indicated that pimozide was more effective than placebo in alleviating anxiety and improving social behaviour. The initial dose of 2 mg pimozide daily was gradually increased by 1 mg until a satisfactory response was obtained or limiting side-effects occurred, the maximum used being 8 mg. Two subjects on pimozide became lethargic and were withdrawn from the study.— J. B. Goldberg and A. A. Kurland, *J. clin. Pharmac.*, 1974, *14*, 134.

DEMENTIA. Beneficial results with pimozide 2 to 12 mg daily in a placebo-controlled double-blind study in 40 patients with senile dementia.— A. Kodjian *et al.*, *Curr. ther. Res.*, 1986, *40*, 694.

GILLES DE LA TOURETTE'S SYNDROME. Pimozide in doses of up to 12 mg daily was as effective as haloperidol in a small controlled study of 5 patients with Gilles de la Tourette's syndrome and had fewer side-effects.— M. S. Ross and H. Moldofsky (letter), *Lancet*, 1977, *1*, 103.

Reviews of the use of pimozide in the management of Tourette's syndrome: C. L. Colvin and R. M. Tankanow, *Drug Intell. & clin. Pharm.*, 1985, *19*, 421; *Med. Lett.*, 1985, *27*, 3.

See also under Haloperidol, p.745.

MALIGNANT MELANOMA. Administration of pimozide appeared to induce a partial remission in a postmenopausal woman with metastatic malignant melanoma. It was given in a dose of 4 mg daily for the first week, 8 mg daily for the second, and 12 mg daily subsequently. Side-effects included lethargy, and dry mouth and eyes.— R. N. Taub and M. A. Baker (letter), *Lancet*, 1979, *1*, 605.

PSYCHOSES. Five patients with monosymptomatic psychosis, each having a single hypochondriacal complaint of delusional intensity, rapidly gained a remission when treated with pimozide 2 to 6 mg each morning. There was no improvement in a sixth patient who was considered to have a personality disorder.— B. E. J. Riding and A. Munro (letter), *Lancet*, 1975, *1*, 400. See also T. M. Reilly (letter), *ibid.*, 1385.

A discussion of delusions of parasitic infestation, and the use of pimozide. Retrospective study of 282 patients revealed that 66 had been treated with pimozide in doses of 2 to 12 mg: 44 of these responded and 16 did not; 6 were lost to follow-up. The response varied from total disappearance of the delusion to some improvement. Three patients were reported as developing drug-induced parkinsonism which limited use of the drug. Weight gain and drowsiness also occurred. As a rule relapse occurred on stopping treatment but control could be re-established on starting again. A few patients have had prolonged remissions.— A. Lyell, *Br. J. Derm.*, 1983, *108*, 485. See also *Lancet*, 1983, *2*, 261.

Pimozide 4 to 10 mg at night often reduces or abolishes symptoms in patients with delusions of venereal disease.— D. Goldmeier, *Br. med. J.*, 1984, *288*, 704.

A report of the response of a case of pathological jealousy to pimozide treatment.— A. Munro (letter), *Can. med. Ass. J.*, 1984, *131*, 852.

Mania. Improvement without sedation was obtained during a classical manic episode in 5 patients with recurrent manic-depressive psychoses given pimozide 8, 6 and 4 mg daily on successive days. There was a tendency to relapse on a fixed daily dose of 4 mg but 2 patients were controlled by increasing the dose to 8 mg twice daily. The response was considered to be better than that achieved with fenfluramine.— J. Cookson and T. Silverstone (letter), *Br. J. clin. Pharmac.*, 1976, *3*, 942.

The use of pimozide in post-partum mania.— J. C. Cookson *et al.*, *Acta psychiat. scand.*, 1981, *64*, 381.

Schizophrenia. Of 20 patients with chronic schizophrenia stabilised on neuroleptic medication and transferred under double-blind conditions to once-daily dosage with pimozide 17 maintained their status or improved, compared with 10 of 20 transferred to trifluoperazine and 7 of 20 transferred to a placebo. The dose of pimozide was 2 to 12 mg (mean 6.3 mg) and that of trifluoperazine 5 to 30 mg (mean 17.5 mg).— H. S. Gross, *Curr. ther. Res.*, 1974, *16*, 696. In a similar double-blind study, 12 of 22 patients remained the same or improved when transferred to pimozide compared to 16 of 22 given trifluoperazine. Side-effects occurred more frequently with pimozide, leading to withdrawal of 4 patients.— F. Kline *et al.*, *ibid.*, 1977, *21*, 768.

In a long-term study comparing pimozide and fluphenazine those on fluphenazine showed the largest improvement up to 6 months but for those remaining in the study for longer than a year there was a trend in favour of pimozide.— F. S. Abuzzahab, *Psychopharmac. Bull.*, 1977, *13*, 72.

Pimozide up to 60 mg daily was given to 16 acutely schizophrenic patients. Only 5 patients were suitable for discharge after 28 days' treatment, and the treatment was ineffective in a further 5. Extrapyramidal symptoms in 8 patients responded to antiparkinsonian therapy.— B. Shopsin and G. Selzer, *Curr. ther. Res.*, 1977, *21*, 755. In a study on the use of high-dose pimozide in 16 acutely agitated chronic schizophrenic patients, an initial single dose of 20 mg daily was rapidly increased to the maximum tolerated, but no more than 60 mg daily. In 3 patients, additional doses of pimozide 5 or 10 mg were given every hour until a calming effect developed or a maximum of 60 mg had been given. The treatment was effective in 14 patients, and 13 completed the 4-week study. The mean daily dose was 35 mg; side-effects were mainly extrapyramidal.— S. Piyakulmala *et al.*, *ibid.*, 1977, *22*, 453.

In a double-blind study of 18 chronic institutionalised patients no significant difference was found in the degree of increased socialisation between placebo and pimozide-treated groups.— E. J. McInnes *et al.*, *N.Z. med. J.*, 1978, *87*, 170.

In an uncontrolled study, 12 patients with schizophrenia of long duration took a placebo for 1 week, then up to 16 mg of pimozide daily followed by a mean maintenance dose of 6 mg for up to 9 weeks. Improvement occurred in 6 patients during the second week of the study with progressive improvement thereafter. The 4 patients who failed to improve during the first 2 weeks remained unchanged at the end of the study or in the case of 2 patients deteriorated with treatment. The main symptoms that improved were apathy, social withdrawal, thought disorders, depression and motor retardation. Side-effects experienced were dryness of the mouth, nausea, somnolence, weakness and parkinsonism.— C. S. Stier *et al.*, *Curr. ther. Res.*, 1978, *23*, 632.

A double-blind study comparing oral pimozide with injected fluphenazine in schizophrenic patients indicated that initially side-effects were similar but after 1 year they were considerably less in the group receiving oral therapy. There was evidence that reduction in side-effects on the oral preparation was due to the patients' adjustment of their own tablet dosage.— D. C. Watt (letter), *Lancet*, 1978, *2*, 1045.

Proprietary Preparations

Orap *(Janssen, UK). Tablets*, scored, pimozide 2, 4, and 10 mg.

Proprietary Names and Manufacturers

Opiran *(Cassenne, Fr.)*; Orap *(Arg.; Janssen, Austral.; Belg.; McNeil, Canad.; Janssen, Denm.; Janssen, Fr.; Janssen, Ger.; Janssen, Ital.; Neth.; Janssen, Norw.; Janssen, S.Afr.; Janssen, Spain; Janssen Pharmaceutica, Swed.; Janssen, Switz.; Janssen, UK; McNeil Pharmaceutical, USA)*.

7088-h

Pinazepam *(rINN)*.

7-Chloro-1,3-dihydro-5-phenyl-1-(prop-2-ynyl)-2*H*-1,4-benzodiazepin-2-one.

$C_{18}H_{13}ClN_2O$=308.8.

CAS — 52463-83-9.

Pinazepam is a benzodiazepine with actions and uses similar to those of diazepam (p.728). It is reported to be metabolised to desmethyldiazepam. It has been given in doses of 2.5 to 10 mg twice daily for the treatment of anxiety.

Proprietary Names and Manufacturers

Domar *(Zambeletti, Ital.)*; Duna *(Zambeletti, Spain)*.

7089-m

Pipamazine *(BAN, rINN)*.

1-[3-(2-Chlorophenothiazin-10-yl)propyl]piperidine-4-carboxamide.

$C_{21}H_{24}ClN_3OS$=402.0.

CAS — 84-04-8.

Pharmacopoeias. In *Fr.*

Adverse Effects, Treatment, and Precautions

As for the phenothiazines in general, p.706.

Uses and Administration

Pipamazine has general properties similar to those of chlorpromazine, p.724. It has a piperidine side-chain. It has been used as an anti-emetic in doses of 5 mg in the morning and 10 mg at night.

7090-t

Pipamperone Hydrochloride *(BANM, rINNM)*.

Floropipamide Hydrochloride; R-3345 *(pipamperone)*.

1-[3-(4-Fluorobenzoyl)propyl]-4-piperidinopiperidine-4-carboxamide dihydrochloride.

$C_{21}H_{30}FN_3O_2,2HCl$=448.4.

CAS — 1893-33-0 (pipamperone); 2448-68-2 (hydro-

chloride).

NOTE. Pipamperone is *USAN.*

Pipamperone hydrochloride 1.2 mg is approximately equivalent to 1 mg of pipamperone.

Pipamperone is a butyrophenone with general properties similar to those of haloperidol (p.743). It is given as the hydrochloride for the treatment of psychoses in doses equivalent to 40 to 120 mg of the base three times daily.

SKIN DISORDERS. Epidermolysis bullosa herpetiformis unresponsive to other treatment markedly improved when the patient was prescribed pipamperone 40 mg daily for psychological disturbance. The disease was found to be well controlled by 70 mg daily and partly controlled by 40 mg daily. Two attempts at drug withdrawal were followed by major bullous eruptions which responded to re-introduction of the drug.— J. M. Bonnetblanc and J. J. Bouquier (letter), *Lancet*, 1986, *1*, 1327.

Proprietary Names and Manufacturers

Dipiperon *(Janssen, Belg.; Janssen, Denm.; Janssen, Fr.; Janssen, Ger.; Janssen, Neth.; Janssen, Switz.)*; Piperonil *(Lusofarmaco, Ital.)*; Propitan *(Jpn).*

7091-x

Piperacetazine *(USAN, rINN).*

PC-1421. 10-{3-[4-(2-Hydroxyethyl)piperidino]propyl}-phenothiazin-2-yl methyl ketone.

$C_{24}H_{30}N_2O_2S=410.6.$

CAS — 3819-00-9.

Pharmacopoeias. In *U.S.*

A yellow granular powder. Practically **insoluble** in water; soluble 1 in 11 of alcohol, 1 in 1.3 of chloroform, 1 in 1200 of ether, and 1 in 25 of dilute hydrochloric acid. **Store** in airtight containers. Protect from light.

Adverse Effects, Treatment, and Precautions

As for the phenothiazines in general, p.706.

Extrapyramidal side-effects are reported to occur more frequently with piperacetazine than with other piperidine phenothiazines.

Absorption and Fate

For an account of the absorption and fate of a phenothiazine, see Chlorpromazine, p.723.

Uses and Administration

Piperacetazine is a phenothiazine with actions and uses similar to those of chlorpromazine (p.724). It has a piperidine side-chain.

It has been given in doses of up to 160 mg daily by mouth in the treatment of psychoses.

Preparations

Piperacetazine Tablets *(U.S.P.)*

Proprietary Names and Manufacturers

Quide *(Dow, Canad.; Merrell Dow, USA).*

7092-r

Pipothiazine *(BAN).*

Pipotiazine *(rINN)*; RP-19366. 10-{3-[4-(2-Hydroxyethyl)piperidino]propyl}-*NN*-dimethylphenothiazine-2-sulphonamide; 2-{4-[3-(2-Dimethylsulphamoylphenothiazin-10-yl)propyl]piperidin-1-yl}ethanol.

$C_{24}H_{33}N_3O_3S_2=475.7.$

CAS — 39860-99-6.

7093-f

Pipothiazine Palmitate *(BANM)*

IL-19552; Pipotiazine Palmitate *(USAN, rINNM)*; RP-19552.

$C_{40}H_{63}N_3O_4S_2=714.1.$

CAS — 37517-26-3.

7094-d

Pipothiazine Undecenoate *(BANM)*

Pipothiazine Undecylenate; Pipotiazine Undecenoate *(rINNM)*, RP-19551.

$C_{35}H_{51}N_3O_4S_2=641.9.$

CAS — 22178-11-6; 42573-55-7.

Adverse Effects, Treatment, and Precautions

As for the phenothiazines in general, p.706.

Manic symptoms developed in a schizophrenic patient following administration of pipothiazine palmitate. Symptoms recurred on subsequent rechallenge. The possible mania-inducing or antidepressant effects of pipothiazine should be investigated further.— A. N. Singh and J. Maguire, *Br. med. J.*, 1984, *289*, 734.

Absorption and Fate

For an account of the absorption and fate of a phenothiazine, see Chlorpromazine, p.723.

Pipothiazine palmitate and undecenoate are very slowly absorbed from the site of intramuscular injection. They both gradually release pipothiazine into the body and are therefore suitable for use as depot injections.

Pharmacokinetics of pipothiazine in patients with schizophrenia: P. J. De Schepper *et al.*, *Arzneimittel-Forsch.*, 1979, *29*, 1056; M. Blanc *et al.*, *Thérapie*, 1986, *41*, 27.

Uses and Administration

Pipothiazine is a phenothiazine with general properties similar to those of chlorpromazine (p.724). It has a piperidine side-chain. Pipothiazine itself is usually administered by mouth; the longer-acting palmitate and undecenoate esters are given by intramuscular injection.

The usual dose of pipothiazine for the treatment of psychoses is 10 to 20 mg daily in a single dose; in severe psychoses higher doses have been given for brief periods. In acute conditions treatment is sometimes started with intramuscular injections of 10 to 20 mg daily in one or two injections.

The long-acting palmitate and undecenoate esters of pipothiazine are given by deep intramuscular injection. The usual dose of both the palmitate and the undecenoate is 75 mg intramuscularly, given at average intervals of 4 weeks for the palmitate and 2 weeks for the undecenoate; in the case of both esters the amounts required may range from 25 to 200 mg.

Pipothiazine should be given in reduced dosage to elderly patients.

Proprietary Preparations

Piportil Depot *(May & Baker, UK). Injection*, oily, pipothiazine palmitate 50 mg/mL, in ampoules of 1 and 2 mL.

Proprietary Names and Manufacturers

Lonseren *(Rhone, Spain)*; Mi-Lonseren *(Spain)*; Piportil *(Rhone-Poulenc, Belg.; Rhône-Poulenc, Canad.; Specia, Fr.; Specia, Neth.; Rhone, Spain; Rhone-Poulenc, Switz.)*; Piportil Depot *(May & Baker, UK)*; Piportyl *(Rhodia, Arg.; Rhone-Poulenc, Denm.; Rhône-Poulenc, Norw.).*

13128-n

Pirenperone *(BAN, USAN, rINN).*

R-47465. 3-{2-[4-(4-Fluorobenzoyl)piperidino]ethyl}-2-methylpyrido[1,2-*a*]pyrimidin-4-one.

$C_{23}H_{24}FN_3O_2=393.5.$

CAS — 75444-65-4.

Pirenperone is reported to have neuroleptic activity.

Proprietary Names and Manufacturers

Janssen, Belg.

7095-n

Prazepam *(BAN, USAN, rINN).*

W-4020. 7-Chloro-1-(cyclopropylmethyl)-1,3-dihydro-5-phenyl-1,4-benzodiazepin-2-one.

$C_{19}H_{17}ClN_2O=324.8.$

CAS — 2955-38-6.

Pharmacopoeias. In *U.S.*

A white to off-white crystalline powder. **Soluble** in alcohol, chloroform, and dilute mineral acids; freely soluble in acetone. **Store** in airtight containers. Protect from light.

Dependence, Adverse Effects, Treatment, and Precautions

As for the benzodiazepines in general, p.706.

Absorption and Fate

For an account of the absorption and fate of a benzodiazepine, see Diazepam, p.730.

Prazepam is a precursor of desmethyldiazepam.

In 5 healthy men given a single dose of 25 mg of ^{14}C-labelled prazepam, peak radioactivity in the blood was reached in about 6 hours and fell gradually over the next 18 hours. The concentration of unconjugated material in the blood was about twice that of glucuronides. About 22% of the dose was excreted in the urine in 48 hours and about 7% in the faeces. Of the material excreted in the urine 4% was unconjugated (1.2% was desalkylprazepam), 83.7% was present as glucuronides (3-hydroxyprazepam glucuronide 40.7%, oxazepam glucuronide 29.7%), and 5.2% as sulphates. Unchanged prazepam was not detected.— F. J. DiCarlo *et al.*, *Ann. N.Y. Acad. Sci.*, 1971, *179*, 487. See also *idem*, *Clin. Pharmac. Ther.*, 1970, *11*, 890.

Following administration of prazepam 20 mg to 12 healthy subjects, considerable variation was noted in the plasma concentrations of desmethyldiazepam, which appears to be responsible for the pharmacological activity of prazepam. The appearance of desmethyldiazepam was not always first order and peak plasma-desmethyldiazepam concentrations were noted as little as 2.5 hours and as long as 72 hours after administration. If the clinical response to prazepam is dependent on the plasma concentration of desmethyldiazepam, the rate of onset of clinical effects could vary considerably after a single dose of prazepam. The elimination half-life in the 12 subjects was similarly very variable, ranging from 29 to 193 hours, with a mean of 69 hours.— M. D. Allen *et al.*, *J. clin. Pharmac.*, 1979, *19*, 445.

Further references: M. T. Smith *et al.*, *Eur. J. clin. Pharmac.*, 1979, *16*, 141; H. R. Ochs *et al.*, *J. clin. Pharmac.*, 1984, *24*, 446.

Uses and Administration

Prazepam is a benzodiazepine with actions and uses similar to those of diazepam (p.731). The usual dose for the treatment of anxiety is 10 mg three times daily; in severe conditions up to 60 mg daily has been given.

ADMINISTRATION. *In the elderly.* A study on the pharmacokinetics of prazepam in young and elderly subjects.— M. D. Allen *et al.*, *Clin. Pharmac. Ther.*, 1980, *28*, 196.

Preparations

Prazepam Capsules *(U.S.P.)*

Prazepam Tablets *(U.S.P.)*

Proprietary Names and Manufacturers

Centrax *(Parke, Davis, UK; Parke, Davis, USA)*; Demetrin *(Gödecke, Ger.; Warner, S.Afr.; Parke, Davis, Spain; Parke, Davis, Switz.)*; Equipaz *(Arg.)*; Lysanxia *(Substantia, Fr.)*; Prazene *(Parke, Davis, Ital.)*; Reapam *(Neth.)*; Trepidan *(Sigmatau, Ital.)*; Verstran *(USA).*

7096-h

Prochlorperazine *(BAN, USAN, rINN).*

Chlormeprazine; Prochlorpemazine. 2-Chloro-10-[3-(4-methylpiperazin-1-yl)propyl]phenothiazine.

$C_{20}H_{24}ClN_3S$=373.9.

CAS — 58-38-8.

Pharmacopoeias. In *Braz., Cz.,* and *U.S.*

A clear, pale yellow, viscous liquid, sensitive to light. Very slightly **soluble** in water; freely soluble in alcohol, chloroform, and in ether. **Store** in airtight containers. Protect from light.

7097-m

Prochlorperazine Edisylate *(BANM, USAN).*

Prochlorperazine Edisilate *(rINNM)*; Prochlorperazine Ethanedisulphonate. Prochlorperazine ethane-1,2-disulphonate.

$C_{20}H_{24}ClN_3S,C_2H_6O_6S_2$=564.1.

CAS — 1257-78-9.

Pharmacopoeias. In *U.S.*

A white to very light yellow odourless crystalline powder. Prochlorperazine edisylate 7.5 mg is approximately equivalent to 5 mg of prochlorperazine.

Soluble 1 in 2 of water and 1 in 1500 of alcohol; practically insoluble in chloroform and ether. Solutions in water are acid to litmus. The *U.S.P.* injection has a pH between 4.2 and 6.2. **Store** in airtight containers. Protect from light.

7098-b

Prochlorperazine Maleate *(BANM, USAN, rINNM).*

Prochlorperazine Dihydrogen Maleate; Prochlorperazine Dimaleate; Prochlorperazini Maleas.

$C_{20}H_{24}ClN_3S,2C_4H_4O_4$=606.1.

CAS — 84-02-6.

Pharmacopoeias. In *Br., Braz., Cz., Egypt., Eur., Fr., Ind., Int., It., Jpn, Jug., Neth., Roum., Swiss,* and *U.S.*

A white or pale yellow, almost odourless, crystalline powder. Prochlorperazine maleate 8 mg is approximately equivalent to 5 mg of prochlorperazine.

The *B.P.* states that it is very slightly **soluble** in water and in alcohol, and practically insoluble in chloroform and in ether. The *U.S.P.* states that it is practically insoluble in water; soluble 1 in 1200 of alcohol; slightly soluble in warm chloroform. A saturated solution in water has a pH of 3 to 4. **Store** in airtight containers. Protect from light.

7099-v

Prochlorperazine Mesylate *(BANM).*

Prochlorperazine Dimethanesulphonate; Prochlorperazine Mesilate *(rINNM)*; Prochlorperazine Methanesulphonate; Prochlorperazini Mesylas.

$C_{20}H_{24}ClN_3S,2CH_3SO_3H$=566.1.

CAS — 5132-55-8.

Pharmacopoeias. In *Br., Egypt., Ind.,* and *Int.*

A white or almost white odourless powder. Prochlorperazine mesylate 7.6 mg is approximately equivalent to 5 mg of prochlorperazine.

Soluble 1 in less than 0.5 of water and 1 in 40 of alcohol; slightly soluble in chloroform; practically insoluble in ether. A 2% solution in water has a pH of 2 to 3. The *B.P.* injection has a pH of 5.5 to 6.5 and is **sterilised** by autoclaving in containers in which the air has been replaced by nitrogen or other suitable gas.

Protect from light.

INCOMPATIBILITY. Particulate matter was observed within 2 hours when 1 mL of commercial prochlorperazine edisylate injection was mixed with sterile water 5 mL and 1 mL of any of the following commercial injection solutions: aminophylline, benzylpenicillin potassium, chloramphenicol sodium succinate, dexamethasone phosphate, dimenhydrinate, heparin, methicillin sodium, phenobarbitone sodium, phenytoin sodium, prednisolone sodium phosphate, and sulphafurazole diethanolamine.— R. Misgen, *Am. J. Hosp. Pharm.*, 1965, *22,* 92. Prochlorperazine edisylate 10 mg per litre was compatible with buffered benzylpenicillin for 24 hours.— E. A. Parker, *Am. J. Hosp. Pharm.*, 1969, *26,* 543.

Loss of clarity when solutions of prochlorperazine were mixed with those of calcium gluconate, chlorothiazide sodium, heparin, hydrocortisone sodium succinate, nitrofurantoin sodium, pentobarbitone sodium, and thiopentone sodium.— J. A. Patel and G. L. Phillips, *Am. J. Hosp. Pharm.*, 1966, *23,* 409.

Prochlorperazine hydrochloride was reported to be incompatible with benzylpenicillin, pentobarbitone sodium, and phenobarbitone sodium.— J. M. Meisler and M. W. Skolaut, *Am. J. Hosp. Pharm.*, 1966, *23,* 557.

An immediate precipitate occurred when prochlorperazine mesylate 100 mg per litre was mixed with aminophylline 1 g per litre or with ampicillin sodium 2 g per litre in glucose injection and sodium chloride injection, or with ethamivan 2 g per litre in sodium chloride injection. An immediate precipitate also occurred with phenobarbitone sodium 800 mg per litre, sulphadiazine sodium 4 g per litre, or sulphadimidine sodium 4 g per litre in sodium chloride injection, but when they were mixed in glucose injection a haze developed over 3 hours. A haze developed over 3 hours when prochlorperazine mesylate was mixed with amphotericin 200 mg per litre or methohexitone sodium 2 g per litre in glucose injection, or with benzylpenicillin 6 g per litre, chloramphenicol 4 g per litre, or chlorothiazide 2 g per litre in sodium chloride injection.— B. B. Riley, *J. Hosp. Pharm.*, 1970, *28,* 228.

A report of incompatibility, resulting in a cloudy solution, when prochlorperazine edisylate was diluted with sodium chloride injection containing methylparabens and propylparabens as preservatives. The problem was not encountered when sodium chloride injection without preservatives or using benzyl alcohol as preservative was used.— S. Jett *et al.* (letter), *Am. J. Hosp. Pharm.*, 1983, *40,* 210.

A precipitate formed immediately when a brand of morphine sulphate was mixed with either of 2 brands of prochlorperazine edisylate. Pharmacists should be aware of this potential incompatibility.— J. G. Stevenson and C. Patriarca (letter), *Am. J. Hosp. Pharm.*, 1985, *42,* 2651.

A statement by the manufacturers that prochlorperazine (Stemetil) syrup was incompatible with magnesium trisilicate mixture following a reformulation.— J. R. Greig (letter), *Pharm. J.*, 1986, *2,* 504.

Adverse Effects, Treatment, and Precautions

As for the phenothiazines in general, p.706.

Severe dystonic reactions have followed the use of prochlorperazine, particularly in children and adolescents. It should therefore be used with extreme care in children. Pain may occur at the site of injection.

EFFECTS ON THE BLOOD. Prochlorperazine has been reported to cause agranulocytosis.— P. C. Vincent, *Drugs*, 1986, *31,* 52.

EFFECTS ON THE CARDIOVASCULAR SYSTEM. For a report of episodes of hypertension associated with intravenous administration of prochlorperazine see under Alizapride, p.1074.

EFFECTS ON MENTAL STATE. *Catatonia.* Twenty-four hours after she had received the last of 3 injections of prochlorperazine given over a period of 6 days, a 34-year-old woman lapsed into a catatonic-like stupor. This was reversed within minutes of intravenous injection of diphenhydramine hydrochloride 50 mg. A relapse 4 hours later was again reversed within minutes of intravenous diphenhydramine hydrochloride in a dose of 25 mg. Five such recurrences over the next 36 hours were relieved in each instance by diphenhydramine hydrochloride 10 mg intravenously. Permanent relief was obtained after administration of benztropine mesylate 2 mg twice daily for several days.— T. Riley *et al., Postgrad. Med.*, 1976, *60,* 171.

EFFECTS ON THE MOUTH. A report of ulceration and soreness of the lip and tongue associated with administration of prochlorperazine maleate tablets. The erosive cheilitis resolved following withdrawal of prochlorperazine and recurred when it was reintroduced.— A. J. Duxbury *et al., Br. dent. J.*, 1982, *153,* 271. See also G. D. Reilly and M. L. Wood, *Acta derm.-vener., Stockh.*, 1984, *64,* 270.

EFFECTS ON THE SKIN. Prochlorperazine has been reported to cause photosensitivity reactions.— *Med. Lett.*, 1986, *28,* 51.

EXTRAPYRAMIDAL EFFECTS. Spasm of the muscles of the neck, extensor rigidity of the back, and carpopedal spasms occurred in a 14-year-old girl after taking 30 mg of prochlorperazine and in a 12-year-old boy after 100 mg administered over 12 hours as suppositories. Symptoms were abolished in 1 patient within a few minutes of an injection of 10 mg of diphenhydramine hydrochloride.— B. Z. Berk (letter), *Lancet*, 1969, *1,* 776.

A 20-year-old woman who had received oral prochlorperazine for 2 days for the treatment of postoperative nausea, developed stiffness and spasms of jaw, neck, arm, and pectoral muscles, which were relieved by an intravenous injection of benztropine mesylate 2 mg.— A. H. Qizilbash, *Can. med. Ass. J.*, 1973, *108,* 171.

Dyskinesia with involuntary jaw movements, similar to lockjaw, occurred in a 26-year-old pilot the day after he had used prochlorperazine suppositories for the treatment of gastroenteritis.— J. B. Lorenzo and E. A. Nisonger, *U.S. Navy Med.*, 1975, *66,* 6.

The Boston Collaborative Drug Surveillance Program monitored consecutively 32 812 medical inpatients. Drug-induced extrapyramidal symptoms occurred in 9 of 3013 patients given prochlorperazine. Also 1 patient out of 198 given prochlorperazine and chlorpromazine experienced extrapyramidal symptoms.— J. Porter and H. Jick, *Lancet*, 1977, *1,* 587.

Of 95 new cases of parkinsonism referred to a hospital department of geriatric medicine, 48 were associated with prescribed drugs; the most common cause was prochlorperazine which was associated with 21 cases.— P. J. Stephen and J. Williamson, *Lancet*, 1984, *2,* 1082.

Study of dystonic and dyskinetic reactions to prochlorperazine reported to the *UK* Committee on the Safety of Medicines revealed a total of 99 reports between 1967 and 1982, of whom 28 were male and 71 female. An estimated 36.96 million prescriptions were written for prochlorperazine (Stemetil) in this period. Eighteen of the male and 42 of the female patients were young adults (12 to 40 years). There was a highly significant effect of age on reporting rates, the highest incidence being in patients up to 19 years, in whom estimated rates were 15.7 and 16.9 per million prescriptions for males and females respectively. In comparison, rates fell to 0.24 and 0.40 respectively in patients aged over 40 years.— D. N. Bateman *et al., Br. J. clin. Pharmac.*, 1985, *20,* 258P.

Dysphagia was associated with cricopharyngeal dyskinesia in an elderly patient receiving prochlorperazine; swallowing returned to normal following withdrawal of prochlorperazine therapy, although there was a persistent orofacial dyskinesia.— A. J. Lobo and R. J. Dickinson, *Br. med. J.*, 1987, *295,* 333.

IMMUNE DEFICIENCY. For a report suggesting that persons with AIDS may be at increased risk of extrapyramidal disorders when taking phenothiazines, see p.709.

INTERACTIONS. *Desferrioxamine.* The combination of phenothiazines with desferrioxamine should be strictly avoided: loss of consciousness lasting 48 to 72 hours has been reported in patients given prochlorperazine during desferrioxamine therapy, possibly because this combination of drugs removes essential iron from the nervous system.— *Lancet*, 1985, *1,* 143.

PREGNANCY AND THE NEONATE. *Early pregnancy.* Evaluation of a number of antinauseant drugs, including prochlorperazine prescribed during the years 1959 to 66 for about 2000 pregnant women in the first 84 days of pregnancy, provided no evidence that prochlorperazine is associated with teratogenicity.— L. Milkovich and B. J. van den Berg, *Am. J. Obstet. Gynec.*, 1976, *125,* 244. See also M. M. Nelson and J. O. Forfar, *Br. med. J.*, 1971, *1,* 523.

The percentage of malformed children among 1309 children born to mothers who had taken phenothiazines during the first 4 months of pregnancy was comparable to that in 48 973 children not so exposed. When analysed for specific malformations there was some evidence of an association with cardiovascular and possibly respiratory malformations but the finding was of doubtful import. IQ scores at 4 years were not affected.— D. Slone *et al.*, *Am. J. Obstet. Gynec.*, 1977, *128*, 486. Of 50 282 children born to mothers monitored by the Collaborative Perinatal Project 1309 were found to have been exposed to phenothiazines, and possibly other drugs, at some time during the first 4 months of the pregnancy. A slight association between cardiovascular deformities and the phenothiazine group as a whole was noted with ventricular septal defects in particular being associated with prochlorperazine (877 exposures).— O. P. Heinonen *et al.*, *Birth Defects and Drugs in Pregnancy*, Littleton MA, Publishing Sciences Group, 1977, p. 322.

A reference to prochlorperazine having been shown to be teratogenic when the foetus was exposed between the 6th and 10th week.— J. B. Loudon, *Br. med. J.*, 1987, *294*, 167.

Absorption and Fate

For an account of the absorption and fate of a phenothiazine, see Chlorpromazine, p.723.

A study of the pharmacokinetics of prochlorperazine in 8 healthy subjects following doses of 6.25 and 12.5 mg intravenously, and 25 mg by mouth. There was a marked interindividual variation in pharmacokinetics following intravenous administration but no evidence of dose-dependent pharmacokinetics; mean terminal half-lives were 6.8 hours for the higher and 6.9 hours for the lower dose. The apparent volume of distribution was very high and plasma clearance values were apparently greater than liver plasma flow, suggesting that the liver may not be the only site of metabolism. After oral administration prochlorperazine concentrations were detectable in only 4 of the 8 subjects due in part to a low bioavailability but also due to the lack of sensitivity of the high-pressure liquid chromatographic assay used. The time to peak plasma concentration varied from 1.5 to 5 hours, and the peak concentrations varied from 1.6 to 7.6 ng per mL. Bioavailability was estimated to range from 0 to 16%. A low bioavailability due to high first-pass metabolism would be expected due to the high plasma clearance of prochlorperazine.— W. B. Taylor and D. N. Bateman, *Br. J. clin. Pharmac.*, 1987, *23*, 137.

Uses and Administration

Prochlorperazine is a phenothiazine with actions and uses similar to those of chlorpromazine (p.724). It has a piperazine side-chain.

Depending on the country or the manufacturer, doses of prochlorperazine are expressed either as the base or the salt. Most doses in the *UK*, including the rectal doses, are expressed in terms of the salt, while most doses in the *USA* are apparently expressed in terms of the base. As a result there is a disparity in the dosage recommendations for these countries, with the doses in the *USA* apparently tending to be higher.

In the *UK* the usual dose for the treatment of psychoses is 50 to 100 mg of the maleate daily in divided doses; when intramuscular injection is necessary, prochlorperazine may be given by deep intramuscular injection in a dose of 12.5 to 25 mg of the mesylate two or three times daily. In the *USA* prochlorperazine is given as the maleate or edisylate in doses equivalent to up to 150 mg of base daily by mouth. In severe disturbances it may be given by deep intramuscular injection as the edisylate in doses equivalent to 10 to 20 mg of base and repeated every 2 to 6 hours if necessary.

For the prevention of nausea and vomiting, in the *UK* the usual dose by mouth is 5 to 10 mg of the maleate three times daily. The usual intramuscular dose for nausea and vomiting is 12.5 mg of the mesylate; the rectal dose is given in suppositories as the base, but in a dose equivalent to 25 mg of the maleate. In the *USA* the dose by mouth for the control of nausea and vomiting is the equivalent of 5 to 10 mg of the base (as edisylate or maleate) given 3 or 4 times daily; alternatively the equivalent of 10 mg twice daily or 15 mg daily may be taken as controlled-release capsules. The recommended intramuscular dosage is the equivalent of 5 to 10 mg of the base, as the edisylate, given every 3 to 4 hours if necessary, up to a total of 40 mg of the base daily. The rectal dose is 25 mg of the base given twice daily. In the management of severe nausea and vomiting associated with anaesthetic and surgical procedures slow intravenous injection or intravenous infusion of prochlorperazine has been suggested, with the warning that hypotension may follow.

There are similar discrepancies with children's doses and owing to the risk of severe extrapyramidal reactions, prochlorperazine should be administered with extreme caution in children: in particular it is not recommended for those weighing less than 10 kg. Where the use of prochlorperazine in children is unavoidable, *UK* sources have suggested 250 µg of the mesylate (contained in the syrup) per kg body-weight, given two or three times daily; the intramuscular route is considered unsuitable. In contrast in the *USA* oral, rectal, and intramuscular routes have all been advocated. The usual oral or rectal anti-emetic dose ranges up to 7.5 mg of the base or its equivalent daily in children weighing 10 to 13 kg; in children 14 to 17 kg, up to 10 mg daily; from 18 to 39 kg, up to 15 mg daily. Higher doses have been given for psychoses. Special care should be taken not to supply or administer one 25-mg suppository in mistake for half a 5-mg suppository (i.e. 2.5 mg). The suggested intramuscular dose for children in the *USA* is the equivalent of about 130 µg of base given as a single deep intramuscular injection of the edisylate.

Prochlorperazine is also used in the *UK* in the treatment of vertigo including that due to Ménière's disease in doses of 15 to 30 mg of the maleate daily. It may also be used in the management of migraine.

Doses of 5 to 10 mg of the maleate (or, in the *USA*, the equivalent of 5 mg of the base) up to 3 or 4 times daily have also been used for non-psychotic emotional disturbances, such as anxiety and tension. In general, however, neuroleptics are only suitable for such purposes in resistant conditions, where more appropriate agents, such as the benzodiazepines (see Diazepam, p.731) have proved ineffective. If their use is judged to be necessary, treatment should be directed at low dosages given on a short-term basis.

Prochlorperazine should be given in reduced dosage to elderly patients.

Preparations

Prochlorperazine Edisylate Injection *(U.S.P.)*. A sterile solution of prochlorperazine edisylate in Water for Injections, containing the equivalent of 4.75 to 5.25 mg of prochlorperazine in each mL.

Prochlorperazine Edisylate Oral Solution *(U.S.P.)*. A solution containing prochlorperazine edisylate. Potency is expressed in terms of the equivalent amount of prochlorperazine. To be diluted before use.

Prochlorperazine Edisylate Syrup *(U.S.P.)*. A syrup containing, in each 100 mL, prochlorperazine edisylate equivalent to 92 to 108 mg of prochlorperazine.

Prochlorperazine Injection *(B.P.)*. Prochlorperazine Mesylate Injection. A sterile solution containing prochlorperazine mesylate in Water for Injections free from dissolved air.

Prochlorperazine Maleate Tablets *(U.S.P.)*. Tablets containing prochlorperazine maleate. Potency is expressed in terms of the equivalent amount of prochlorperazine.

Prochlorperazine Suppositories *(U.S.P.)*. Suppositories containing prochlorperazine. Store at a temperature not exceeding 37° in airtight containers; protect unwrapped suppositories from exposure to sunlight.

Prochlorperazine Tablets *(B.P.)*. Tablets containing prochlorperazine maleate.

Proprietary Preparations

Buccastem *(Reckitt & Colman Pharmaceuticals, UK)*. *Buccal tablets*, prochlorperazine maleate 3 mg.

Stemetil *(May & Baker, UK)*. *Tablets*, prochlorperazine maleate 5 mg.
Tablets, scored, prochlorperazine maleate 25 mg.
Effervescent powder, sachets, prochlorperazine mesylate 5 mg.
Syrup, prochlorperazine mesylate 5 mg/5 mL.
Injection, prochlorperazine mesylate 12.5 mg/mL, in ampoules of 1 and 2 mL.
Suppositories, prochlorperazine maleate 5 and 25 mg (as base).

Vertigon *(Smith Kline & French, UK)*. *Spansules*, controlled-release capsules, prochlorperazine 10 and 15 mg (as maleate).

Proprietary Names and Manufacturers of Prochlorperazine and its Salts

Anti-Naus *(Protea, Austral.)*; Buccastem *(Reckitt & Colman Pharmaceuticals, UK)*; Compazine *(Smith Kline & French, Austral.; Smith Kline & French, USA)*; Mitil *(Lennon, S.Afr.)*; Nibromin-A *(Jpn)*; Scripto-metic *(Bovit, S.Afr.)*; Stemetil *(May & Baker, Austral.; Belg.; Rhône-Poulenc, Canad.; Rhone-Poulenc, Denm.; Zambeletti, Ital.; Neth.; Rhône-Poulenc, Norw.; May & Baker, S.Afr.; Leo Rhodia, Swed.; Switz.; May & Baker, UK)*; Témentil *(Specia, Fr.)*; Vertigon *(Smith Kline & French, UK)*.

The following names have been used for multi-ingredient preparations containing prochlorperazine and its salts—Combid *(Smith Kline & French, Canad.; Smith Kline & French, USA)*; Prochlor-Iso *(Schein, USA)*; Pro-Iso *(Geneva, USA)*.

7100-v

Promazine Embonate *(BANM, rINNM)*.

Promazine Pamoate.

$(C_{17}H_{20}N_2S)_2,C_{23}H_{16}O_6$=957.2.

CAS — 58-40-2 (promazine).

Promazine embonate 1.5 g is approximately equivalent to 1 g of promazine hydrochloride.

7101-g

Promazine Hydrochloride *(BANM, USAN, rINNM)*.

Propazinum. *NN*-Dimethyl-3-phenothiazin-10-ylpropylammonium chloride.

$C_{17}H_{20}N_2S,HCl$=320.9.

CAS — 53-60-1.

Pharmacopoeias. In *Br.*, *Rus.*, and *U.S.* Also in *B.P. Vet.*

A white or slightly yellow, odourless or almost odourless, slightly hygroscopic, crystalline powder. It oxidises upon prolonged exposure to air and acquires a pink or blue colour.

The *B.P.* states that it is **soluble** 1 in 1 of water, 1 in 2 of alcohol, and 1 in 2 of chloroform; the *U.S.P.* specifies a solubility of 1 in 3 of water. The *B.P.* states that a 5% solution in water has a pH of 4.2 to 5.4; the *U.S.P.* gives 4.2 to 5.2. The pH of the *U.S.P.* injection is between 4.0 and 5.5, and that of the oral solution between 5.0 and 5.5. The *B.P.* injection has a pH of 4.4 to 5.2 and is **sterilised** by autoclaving and distributed in ampoules in which the air is replaced by nitrogen or other suitable gas. **Store** in airtight containers. Protect from light.

INCOMPATIBILITY. Particulate matter was observed within 2 hours when 1 mL of commercial promazine hydrochloride injection was mixed with sterile water 5 mL and 1 mL of any of the following commercial injection solutions: *aminophylline, benzylpenicillin potassium, chloramphenicol sodium succinate, dimenhydrinate, heparin, hydrocortisone sodium succinate, menaphthone sodium bisulphite, phenobarbitone sodium, phenytoin sodium, prednisolone sodium phosphate,* and *sulphafurazole diethanolamine*.— R. Misgen, *Am. J. Hosp. Pharm.*, 1965, *22*, 92.

Promazine 100 mg was 'physically incompatible' with *chlortetracycline* 50 mg, *fibrinogen* 200 mg, *plasmin* 200 mg, *penicillin* 1.2 g, *pentobarbitone sodium* 20 mg, *sodium bicarbonate* 375 mg, *sulphafurazole* 400 mg, *thiopentone sodium* 250 mg, or *warfarin sodium* 10 mg, in 100 mL of dextrose 5% injection.— R. D. Dunworth and F. R. Kenna, *Am. J. Hosp. Pharm.*, 1965, *22*, 190.

An immediate precipitate occurred when promazine hydrochloride 200 mg per litre was mixed with *aminophylline* 1 g per litre, *chlorothiazide* 2 g per litre, *ethamivan* 2 g per litre, *methohexitone sodium* 2 g per litre, or *sulphadimidine sodium* 4 g per litre in dextrose 5% injection or sodium chloride 0.9% injection, or with *phenobarbitone sodium* 800 mg per litre in sodium chloride 0.9% injection.— B. B. Riley, *J. Hosp. Pharm.*,

1970, *28*, 228.

STABILITY. A study of the stability of promazine diluted to a 0.1% infusion in sodium chloride solution (0.9%) or glucose (5%) found that solutions in glucose (5%) remained stable for up to 6 days at 4°, and at room temperature, provided they were stored in the dark. However, with saline as the diluent deterioration of the promazine was observed 24 hours after preparation, even when stored in the dark, and after 8 hours when exposed to light. Temperature had no effect on degradation rate.— I. R. Tebbett *et al.*, *Pharm. J.*, 1986, *2*, 172.

Adverse Effects, Treatment, and Precautions

As for the phenothiazines in general, p.706.

EFFECTS ON THE BLOOD. Promazine has been associated with agranulocytosis.— P. C. Vincent, *Drugs*, 1986, *31*, 52.

EFFECTS ON THE RESPIRATORY TRACT. Promazine has been reported to cause postoperative respiratory depression.— R. J. M. Lane and P. A. Routledge, *Drugs*, 1983, *26*, 124.

INTERACTIONS. *Adsorbents.* Absorption of promazine hydrochloride was delayed and reduced when its administration was preceded by a dose of an antidiarrhoeal mixture containing activated attapulgite 3 g, colloidal activated attapulgite 900 mg, and citrus pectin 300 mg in 30 mL.— D. L. Sorby and G. Liu, *J. pharm. Sci.*, 1966, *55*, 504. When promazine hydrochloride solution and activated attapulgite or charcoal suspensions were given simultaneously without prior equilibration, the effect of the adsorbents on absorption of promazine was negligible.— D. L. Sorby, *ibid.*, 1968, *57*, 1604.

PREGNANCY AND THE NEONATE. An increased incidence of neonatal jaundice coincided with the increased use of promazine. A decrease in the incidence of jaundice was noted 3 months after the total withdrawal of the drug from the hospital.— E. John, *Med. J. Aust.*, 1975, *2*, 342.

Absorption and Fate

For an account of the absorption and fate of a phenothiazine, see Chlorpromazine, p.723.

PLASMA PROTEIN BINDING. For the comparative protein binding of promazine and other phenothiazines, see Chlorpromazine, p.723.

Uses and Administration

Promazine is a phenothiazine with actions and uses similar to those of chlorpromazine (p.724). It is given by mouth, or in similar doses intramuscularly, as the hydrochloride. It has also been given as the embonate by mouth, in doses equivalent to those of the hydrochloride. Promazine hydrochloride has also been given by slow intravenous injection, in concentrations not exceeding 25 mg per mL.

Promazine has been given in usual doses of 100 to 200 mg of the hydrochloride up to four times daily for the treatment of psychoses; a maximum daily dose of 1 g has been specified. For the control of nausea and vomiting it has been given in doses of 25 to 50 mg up to four times daily.

Promazine should be given in reduced dosage to elderly subjects.

Preparations

Promazine Hydrochloride Injection *(U.S.P.)*

Promazine Hydrochloride Oral Solution *(U.S.P.)*. Promazine Hydrochloride Solution

Promazine Hydrochloride Syrup *(U.S.P.)*

Promazine Hydrochloride Tablets *(U.S.P.)*

Promazine Injection *(B.P.)*. A sterile solution containing promazine hydrochloride in Water for Injections free from dissolved air.

Promazine Tablets *(B.P.)*

Proprietary Preparations

Sparine (known in some countries as Liranol) *(Wyeth, UK)*. *Tablets*, promazine hydrochloride 25, 50, and 100 mg.
Suspension, promazine hydrochloride 50 mg (as embonate)/5 mL.
Injection, promazine hydrochloride 50 mg/mL, in ampoules of 1 or 2 mL.

Proprietary Names and Manufacturers

Calmotal *(Ital.)*; Liranol; Neuroplegil *(Ital.)*; Prazine *(Belg.; Neth.; Wyeth, Switz.)*; Promabec *(Canad.)*; Promanyl *(Canad.)*; Protactyl *(Wyeth, Ger.; Norw.)*; Sparine *(Wyeth, Austral.; Wyeth, Canad.; Wyeth, Denm.; Wyeth, S.Afr.; Wyeth, UK; Wyeth, USA)*; Talofen *(Pierrel, Ital.)*.

7102-q

Prothipendyl Hydrochloride *(BANM, rINNM)*.

D-206; Phrenotropin. *NN*-Dimethyl-3-(pyrido[3,2-*b*]-[1,4]benzothiazin-10-yl)propylamine hydrochloride monohydrate.
$C_{16}H_{19}N_3S,HCl,H_2O=339.9$.

CAS — 303-69-5 (prothipendyl); 1225-65-6 (hydrochloride, anhydrous).

Adverse Effects, Treatment, and Precautions

As for the phenothiazines, p.706.

Uses and Administration

Prothipendyl is an azaphenothiazine with general properties similar to those of chlorpromazine (p.724). It has been given by mouth as the hydrochloride in doses of 20 to 40 mg up to four times daily in psychoneuroses, and up to 240 mg or more daily in psychoses. Prothipendyl may also be given by injection.

Proprietary Names and Manufacturers

Dominal *(Asta Pharma, Ger.; Homburg, Neth.)*; Tolnate *(Smith Kline & French, UK)*.

4064-c

Proxibarbal *(rINN)*.

HH184; Proxibarbital. 5-Allyl-5-(2-hydroxypropyl)barbituric acid.
$C_{10}H_{14}N_2O_4=226.2$.

CAS — 2537-29-3.

Proxibarbal is a barbiturate and shares the general properties of the group (see p.706). It has been used as a sedative in doses of 300 to 600 mg daily.

Proprietary Names and Manufacturers

Axeen *(Hommel, Ger.; Zyma, Ital.; Frumtost, Spain; Zyma, Switz.)*; Centralgol *(Zyma, Fr.)*; Ipronal *(Biosedra, Arg.)*.

4065-k

Pyrithyldione *(rINN)*.

Didropyridinium; Nu 903. 3,3-Diethylpyridine-2,4(1*H*,3*H*)-dione.
$C_9H_{13}NO_2=167.2$.

CAS — 77-04-3.

Pyrithyldione is a hypnotic that has been given in doses of 200 to 400 mg at night in the short-term management of insomnia. It has also been used as a sedative.

Proprietary Names and Manufacturers

Persedon *(Roche, Belg.; Roche, Denm.; Roche, Ger.; Roche, Swed.; Roche, Switz.)*.

13196-y

Quazepam *(BAN, USAN, rINN)*.

Sch-16134. 7-Chloro-5-(2-fluorophenyl)-1,3-dihydro-1-(2,2,2-trifluoroethyl)-1,4-benzodiazepine-2-thione.
$C_{17}H_{11}ClF_4N_2S=386.8$.

CAS — 36735-22-5.

Dependence, Adverse Effects, Treatment, and Precautions

As for the benzodiazepines in general, p.706.

Absorption and Fate

For an account of the absorption and fate of a benzodiazepine see Diazepam, p.730.

Quazepam has been reported to have an elimination half-life of 39 hours and its two active metabolites, 2-oxoquazepam and *N*-desalkyl-2-oxoquazepam, to have half-lives of 39 and 73 hours respectively.

A study by the manufacturers of the single-dose pharmacokinetics of radiolabelled quazepam in 6 healthy subjects. Quazepam was well absorbed with a mean peak plasma concentration of 148 ng per mL 1.5 hours after a 25-mg dose. The major metabolites were found to be 2-oxoquazepam, *N*-desalkyl-2-oxoquazepam (which is identical to *N*-desalkylflurazepam), and 3-hydroxy-2-oxoquazepam glucuronide; the former 2 were active, and had mean plasma elimination half-lives of 40.2 and 69.5 hours, compared with 39.3 hours for the parent drug. Over a 5-day period, 31.3% of the total radioactivity was excreted in the urine, and 22.7% in the faeces. The metabolic profile and pharmaceutical characteristics of quazepam probably account for its pharmacodynamic behaviour; the rapidly appearing quazepam and 2-oxoquazepam may be chiefly responsible for induction of sleep while the desalkyl metabolite, with its long half-life, may account for the reported lack of rebound insommia.— N. Zampaglione *et al.*, *Drug Metab. & Disposit.*, 1985, *13*, 25.

PREGNANCY AND THE NEONATE. *Lactation.* A study in 4 lactating women indicated that quazepam was present in breast milk at approximately 4 times the plasma concentration for 48 hours following a dose of 15 mg by mouth; 2-oxoquazepam was also present in milk at about twice the plasma concentration, but only very small amounts of *N*-desalkyl-2-oxoquazepam were present, at less than one-tenth of the corresponding plasma concentrations. However, although quazepam and its metabolite were present in breast milk at relatively higher concentrations than in plasma the absolute amount of drug and metabolites excreted into milk was minimal, comprising about 0.11% of the administered dose over 48 hours. This was calculated to represent a dose of 4.9 µg per kg body-weight for a 3.5 kg infant, or about 2.3% of the adult dose.— J. M. Hilbert *et al.*, *J. clin. Pharmac.*, 1984, *24*, 457.

Uses and Administration

Quazepam is a long-acting benzodiazepine with general properties similar to those of diazepam (p.731). It has been used as a hypnotic in the short-term management of insomnia, in doses of 15 mg at night.

Studies of the use of quazepam as a hypnotic: J. W. Goethe and G. Kader, *Curr. ther. Res.*, 1982, *32*, 150; W. F. Powell, *ibid.*, 590; E. Wickstrøm and C. Allgulander, *Eur. J. clin. Pharmac.*, 1983, *24*, 67; H. J. Winsauer *et al.*, *Curr. ther. Res.*, 1984, *35*, 228; M. Mamelak *et al.*, *J. clin. Pharmac.*, 1984, *24*, 65; A. Kales *et al.*, *Clin. Pharmac. Ther.*, 1986, *39*, 345; A. Kales *et al.*, *ibid.*, 378; S. I. Ankier and K. L. Goa, *Drugs*, 1988, *35*, 42.

Proprietary Names and Manufacturers

Temodal *(Scherag, S. Afr.)*.

4066-a

Quinalbarbitone

Meballymal; Secobarbital *(USAN, rINN)*. 5-Allyl-5-(1-methylbutyl)barbituric acid.
$C_{12}H_{18}N_2O_3=238.3$.

CAS — 76-73-3.

Pharmacopoeias. In *Braz.* and *U.S.*

A white odourless amorphous or crystalline powder. Very slightly **soluble** in water; freely soluble in alcohol, ether, and solutions of fixed alkali hydroxides and carbonates; soluble in chloroform. A saturated solution in water has a pH of about 5.6. **Store** in airtight containers.

4067-t

Quinalbarbitone Sodium *(BAN)*.

Meballymalnatrium; Secobarbital Sodium *(USAN, rINNM)*; Secobarbitalum Natricum; Secobarbitone Sodium. Sodium 5-allyl-5-(1-methylbutyl)barbiturate.
$C_{12}H_{17}N_2NaO_3=260.3$.

CAS — 309-43-3.

Pharmacopoeias. In *Arg.*, *Aust.*, *Br.*, *Braz.*, *Chin.*, *Egypt.*, *Eur.*, *Fr.*, *Ger.*, *Ind.*, *Int.*, *It.*, *Neth.*, *Swiss*, and *U.S.*

A white odourless hygroscopic powder. **Soluble** 1 in 3 of water and 1 in 5 of alcohol; practically insoluble in chloroform and in ether. The *B.P.* states that a 10% solution in water has a pH of not more than 11; The *U.S.P.* gives the pH of a freshly prepared 10% solution as between 9.7 and 10.5, and the pH of the injection as between 9.0 and 10.5. Solutions decompose on standing, the process being accelerated at higher temperatures; the *U.S.P.* directs that the injection should be stored at 2° to 8°.

Incompatible with acids and acidic salts, and with chloral hydrate. **Store** in airtight containers.

INCOMPATIBILITY. There was loss of clarity when intravenous solutions of quinalbarbitone sodium were mixed with those of diphenhydramine hydrochloride, ephedrine sulphate, erythromycin gluceptate, hydrocortisone sodium succinate, insulin, opioid salts, noradrenaline acid tartrate, phenytoin sodium, procaine hydrochloride, streptomycin sulphate, tetracycline hydrochloride, or vancomycin hydrochloride.— J. A. Patel and G. L. Phillips, *Am. J. Hosp. Pharm.*, 1966, *23*, 409.

There was an immediate precipitate when a solution of cimetidine hydrochloride was mixed with one of quinalbarbitone sodium.— P. F. Souney *et al., Am. J. Hosp. Pharm.*, 1984, *41*, 1840.

Dependence, Adverse Effects, Treatment, and Precautions

As for the barbiturates in general, p.706.

Exposure to quinalbarbitone sodium among 6 workers in the pharmaceutical industry resulted in absorption of substantial amounts of the drug, with blood concentrations approaching those expected after a therapeutic dose. There continued to be evidence of absorption, despite protective masks to reduce inhalation, and it appeared that substantial absorption was taking place through the skin.— P. J. Baxter *et al., Br. med. J.*, 1986, *292*, 661.

Absorption and Fate

Quinalbarbitone is well absorbed from the gastro-intestinal tract following oral doses and has been reported to be extensively bound to plasma and tissue proteins. The elimination half-life is reported to be about 30 hours. It is metabolised in the liver, mainly by hydroxylation, and excreted in urine as metabolites and a small amount of unchanged drug.

Quinalbarbitone (as free acid) 3.3 mg per kg bodyweight was given by mouth to 6 healthy subjects. The maximum blood concentration was obtained after an average of 3 hours and in all 6 quinalbarbitone was detected in the blood after 108 hours; the calculated biological half-life was 28.9 hours.— J. M. Clifford *et al., Clin. Pharmac. Ther.*, 1974, *16*, 376.

A study of the metabolism of quinalbarbitone following administration of quinalbarbitone sodium 200 or 300 mg to 6 healthy subjects. No unchanged drug was detected in the urine.— J. N. T. Gilbert *et al., J. Pharm. Pharmac.*, 1975, *27*, 343.

PREGNANCY AND THE NEONATE. Quinalbarbitone sodium was detected in foetal cord blood within 1 minute of intravenous administration to the mother of 200 to 300 mg; equilibrium was reached within 3 to 5 minutes with the foetal concentration 70% of that of the mother. Of 76 infants, 90% showed little or no depression at birth.— F. Moya and V. Thorndike, *Clin. Pharmac. Ther.*, 1963, *4*, 628.

Uses and Administration

Quinalbarbitone is a barbiturate that is used as a hypnotic and sedative. As a hypnotic it is usually given in doses of 50 to 100 mg at night but occasionally 200 mg may be required; 30 to 50 mg has been given 3 or 4 times daily as a sedative. Similar doses may be given of the sodium salt.

Quinalbarbitone has been used for premedication in anaesthetic procedures but its use for these purposes has largely been superseded by other agents, such as the benzodiazepines.

ADMINISTRATION IN RENAL FAILURE. Quinalbarbitone could be given in usual doses to patients with renal failure. Concentrations of quinalbarbitone were not affected by haemodialysis or peritoneal dialysis.— W. M. Bennett *et al., Ann. intern. Med.*, 1980, *93*, 286.

Preparations

Secobarbital Elixir *(U.S.P.)*. Contains quinalbarbitone 0.417 to 0.461% w/v in a suitable flavoured vehicle containing 10 to 14% of alcohol.

Secobarbital Sodium and Amobarbital Sodium Capsules *(U.S.P.)*. Contain quinalbarbitone sodium and amylobarbitone sodium.

Secobarbital Sodium Capsules *(U.S.P.)*. Contain quinalbarbitone sodium.

Secobarbital Sodium Injection *(U.S.P.)*. A sterile solution of quinalbarbitone sodium in a suitable solvent.

Sterile Secobarbital Sodium *(U.S.P.)*. Quinalbarbitone sodium suitable for parenteral use.

Proprietary Preparations

Seconal Sodium *(Lilly, UK)*. *Capsules*, quinalbarbitone sodium 50 and 100 mg.

Tuinal *(Lilly, UK)*. *Capsules*, quinalbarbitone sodium 50 mg, amylobarbitone sodium 50 mg. For insomnia. *Dose*. 1 to 2 capsules at bedtime.

Proprietary Names and Manufacturers

Dormona *(Switz.)*; Imménoctal *(Houdé, Fr.)*; Immenox *(Ital.)*; Proquinal *(Austral.)*; Quinbar *(Austral.)*; Secogen *(Canad.)*; Seconal *(Lilly, USA)*; Seconal Sodium *(Lilly, Austral.; Belg.; Lilly, Canad.; Neth.; Lilly, S.Afr.; Switz.; Lilly, UK; Lilly, USA)*; Seconal-Natrium *(Norw.)*; Sedonal Natrium *(Denm.)*; Seral *(Canad.)*.

The following names have been used for multi-ingredient preparations containing quinalbarbitone sodium— Ephedrine and Seconal Sodium *(Lilly, USA)*; Tuinal *(Lilly, Austral.; Lilly, Canad.; Lilly, UK; Lilly, USA)*.

4068-x

Secbutobarbitone *(BAN)*.

Butabarbital *(USAN)*; Butabarbitone (distinguish from Butobarbitone); Secbutabarbital *(rINN)*. 5-*sec*-Butyl-5-ethylbarbituric acid.

$C_{10}H_{16}N_2O_3$=212.2.

CAS — 125-40-6.

Pharmacopoeias. In *U.S.*

A white, odourless, crystalline powder.

Very slightly**soluble** in water; soluble in alcohol, in chloroform, in ether, and in aqueous solutions of alkali hydroxides and carbonates. **Store** in airtight containers.

4069-r

Secbutobarbitone Sodium *(BANM)*.

Butabarbital Sodium *(USAN)*; Secbutabarbital Sodium *(rINNM)*; Secumalnatrium; Sodium Butabarbital. Sodium 5-*sec*-butyl-5-ethylbarbiturate.

$C_{10}H_{15}N_2NaO_3$=234.2.

CAS — 143-81-7.

Pharmacopoeias. In *U.S.*

A white powder. **Soluble** 1 in 2 of water, and 1 in 7 of alcohol; very slightly soluble in chloroform; practically insoluble in ether. A 10% solution in water free of carbon dioxide has a pH of between 10.0 and 11.2. **Store** in airtight containers.

Dependence, Adverse Effects, Treatment, and Precautions

As for the barbiturates in general, p.706.

Absorption and Fate

A study of the urinary excretion of secbutobarbitone in 3 male volunteers. From 5 to 9% of the drug was excreted unchanged and 24 to 34% was excreted as a terminal carboxylic acid; small amounts of 2 other metabolites were also found.— J. N. T. Gilbert *et al., J. Pharm. Pharmac.*, 1975, *27*, 923.

Uses and Administration

Secbutobarbitone is a barbiturate that is used as a hypnotic and sedative. As a hypnotic it is usually given in doses of 50 to 100 mg at night, as a sedative 15 to 30 mg has been given 3 or 4 times daily. Similar doses may be given of the sodium salt.

Preparations

Butabarbital Sodium Capsules *(U.S.P.)*. Contain secbutobarbitone sodium.

Butabarbital Sodium Elixir *(U.S.P.)*. An elixir containing secbutobarbitone sodium.

Butabarbital Sodium Tablets *(U.S.P.)*. Contain secbutobarbitone sodium.

Proprietary Names and Manufacturers

Buticaps *(Wallace, USA)*; Butisol Sodium *(Ethnor, Austral.; Horner, Canad.; Wallace, USA)*; Day-Barb *(Anca, Canad.)*; Neo-Barb *(Canad.)*.

The following names have been used for multi-ingredient preparations containing secbutobarbitone or secbutobarbitone sodium— Ancatropine Infant Drops *(Anca, Canad.)*; Butabell *(Saron, USA)*; Pyridium Plus *(Parke, Davis, USA)*; Quibron Plus *(Mead Johnson Laboratories, USA)*; Tedral-25 *(Parke, Davis, USA)*.

13261-g

Sodium Succinate

363 (succinic acid).

$C_4H_4Na_2O_4,6H_2O$=270.1.

CAS — 150-90-3 (anhydrous); 6106-21-4 (hexahydrate).

Sodium succinate has been used experimentally in the treatment of various psychotic disorders.

Succinic dinitrile ($C_4H_4N_2$ = 80.09) has been used in the treatment of exhaustion and depression.

7104-s

Spiclomazine Hydrochloride *(rINNM)*.

APY-606; Clospirazine Hydrochloride. 8-[3-(2-Chlorophenothiazin-10-yl)propyl]-4-thia-1,8-diazaspiro[4.5]-decan-2-one hydrochloride.

$C_{22}H_{24}ClN_3OS_2,HCl$=482.5.

CAS — 24527-27-3 (spiclomazine); 27007-85-8 (hydrochloride).

Spiclomazine hydrochloride is a phenothiazine with general properties similar to those of chlorpromazine (p.722). It has a piperidine side-chain. It has been given in doses of 50 to 150 mg three times daily in the treatment of psychoses.

Proprietary Names and Manufacturers

Diceplon *(Jpn)*.

7105-w

Spiperone *(BAN, USAN, rINN)*.

R-5147; Spiroperidol. 8-[3-(4-Fluorobenzoyl)propyl]-1-phenyl-1,3,8-triazaspiro[4.5]decan-4-one.

$C_{23}H_{26}FN_3O_2$=395.5.

CAS — 749-02-0.

Spiperone is a butyrophenone with general properties similar to those of haloperidol (p.743). Doses of 0.5 to 4.5 mg daily have been recommended in the treatment of schizophrenia.

Proprietary Names and Manufacturers

Spiropitan *(Jpn)*.

7106-e

Sulforidazine *(rINN)*.

Sulphoridazine; TPN-12. 10-[2-(1-Methyl-2-piperidyl)ethyl]-2-methylsulphonylphenothiazine.

$C_{21}H_{26}N_2O_2S_2$=402.6.

CAS — 14759-06-9.

Sulforidazine is a metabolite of thioridazine (p.770). It has been given in doses of 50 to 100 mg three times daily for the treatment of psychoses.

Proprietary Names and Manufacturers

Inofal *(Sandoz, Ger.)*.

7107-l

Sulpiride *(BAN, USAN, rINN)*.

N-(1-Ethylpyrrolidin-2-ylmethyl)-2-methoxy-5-sulphamoylbenzamide.

$C_{15}H_{23}N_3O_4S$=341.4.

CAS — 15676-16-1.

Pharmacopoeias. In *Jpn.*

Adverse Effects, Treatment, and Precautions

As for the phenothiazines, p.706.

Sleep disturbances, overstimulation, and agitation may occur.

Sulpiride is contra-indicated in patients with phaeochromocytoma (see under Hypertension, below). It should be given with care to manic or hypomanic patients in whom it may exacerbate symptoms.

EXTRAPYRAMIDAL DISORDERS. Although it has been suggested that sulpiride, with its more specific dopamine-blocking action, is less likely than other neuroleptics to cause tardive dyskinesia the evidence for this is unconvincing. Sulpiride has been advocated as a treatment for tardive dyskinesia but all neuroleptics will treat tardive dyskinesia in the short term.— F. Winton (letter), *Br. med. J.*, 1985, *291*, 1127. Disagreement (by the manufacturers).— A. A. Schiff (letter), *ibid.*, 1424. A report of tardive dyskinesia induced by sulpiride.— R. Sandyk, *Clin. Neuropharmacol.*, 1986, *9*, 100.

HYPERTENSION. Sulpiride 100 mg by mouth caused an attack of hypertension in 6 of 26 hypertensive patients; in 4 it induced a rise in urinary excretion of vanillylmandelic acid and catecholamines. A transient rise in blood pressure and catecholamines after administration of sulpiride occurred in 3 patients who were found to have a phaeochromocytoma; another patient probably had a phaeochromocytoma. The means by which sulpiride provoked hypertension were not known but appeared to be due to a noradrenergic effect. Sulpiride should be avoided during the treatment of phaeochromocytoma, and prescribed with great care in hypertensive patients.— P. Corvol *et al.*, *Sem. Hôp. Paris*, 1974, *50*, 1265.

INTERACTIONS. When sulpiride was given concomitantly with therapeutic doses of *sucralfate*, or of an *antacid* containing aluminium and magnesium hydroxides, in 6 healthy subjects the mean oral bioavailability of sulpiride was reduced by 40 and 32% respectively. When sulpiride was given 2 hours after the antacid or sulcralfate (each in 2 subjects) the reduction in bioavailability was about 25%. This interaction was expected to be clinically significant and it was recommended that if used concurrently sulpiride should be given before, rather than with or after, sucralfate or antacids.— M. W. Gouda *et al.*, *Int. J. Pharmaceut.*, 1984, *22*, 257.

Absorption and Fate

Sulpiride is absorbed from the gastro-intestinal tract and excreted in the urine and faeces. It is reported to have a plasma half-life of about 8 or 9 hours.

The pharmacokinetics of intravenous and oral sulpiride in healthy subjects.— F. -A. Wiesel *et al.*, *Eur. J. clin. Pharmac.*, 1980, *17*, 385.

A study of the pharmacokinetics of sulpiride in healthy subjects following intramuscular administration at doses of 50, 100, and 200 mg.— F. Bressolle *et al.*, *J. pharm. Sci.*, 1984, *73*, 1128.

Uses and Administration

Sulpiride is a substituted benzamide which is claimed to exert its antipsychotic action via a selective blockade of central dopamine D_2 receptors. It is also claimed to have mood elevating properties, and has anti-emetic actions and an effect on gastrin secretion.

In the treatment of schizophrenia initial doses of 200 to 400 mg twice daily by mouth may be given, increased if necessary up to a maximum of 1.2 g twice daily. Sulpiride may also be given initially by intramuscular injection, in doses of 600 to 800 mg daily. Usual maintenance doses are 400 to 800 mg daily by mouth. A dose of 3 to 5 mg per kg body-weight has been suggested in children.

Sulpiride has also been given in the management of neuroses, migraine, and vertigo; 150 to 300 mg daily has been given for gastric and duodenal ulcers.

Sulpiride should be given in reduced doses to elderly patients.

A brief review of sulpiride.— *Drug & Ther. Bull.*, 1984, *22*, 31.

ACTION. A study in *animals* suggesting that the central pharmacological activity of sulpiride and sultopride resides in the (−)-enantiomers and that this activity occurs at central dopamine receptors not dependent on adenylate cyclase for functional activity.— P. Jenner *et al.*, *J. Pharm. Pharmac.*, 1980, *32*, 39.

For discussion of the selective action of sulpiride at brain dopamine receptors see P. Jenner *et al.*, in *Schizophrenia: new pharmacological and clinical developments*, A.A. Schiff *et al.* (Eds), Royal Society of Medicine International Congress and Symposium Series No.94, London, Royal Society of Medicine, 1985, p.51.

Results of a study in *rats* given haloperidol or sulpiride continuously for 1 year showed that haloperidol produced changes in striatal dopamine function reflecting the development of postsynaptic dopamine receptor supersensitivity, which is believed to be related to the development of tardive dyskinesias. In contrast, the changes in function produced by sulpiride did not suggest postsynaptic receptor supersensitivity. These differences in effect may relate to the differing propensities of the two agents to produce tardive dyskinesias.— N. M. J. Rupniak *et al.*, *Psychopharmacology*, 1984, *84*, 503.

For a report that sulpiride can induce tardive dyskinesias see under Adverse Effects, above.

ALCOHOL AND DRUG WITHDRAWAL. Nalorphine-induced withdrawal symptoms in *monkeys* treated with morphine for 15 days were controlled by intramuscular administration of sulpiride 30 mg per kg body-weight. Sulpiride was not a pharmacological replacement for morphine.— J. Mercier and P. Etzensperger, *Thérapie*, 1975, *30*, 221. Studies in *dogs* have indicated that sulpiride can suppress the morphine-withdrawal syndrome.— A. De Permentier (letter), *Med. J. Aust.*, 1976, *1*, 98.

Relatively low doses of sulpiride induced extrapyramidal syndromes in heroin addicts.— D. De Maio *et al.*, *Neuropsychobiology*, 1978, *4*, 36.

A diamorphine addict given cyamemazine 1.8 g and sulpiride 4.8 g intravenously, over 48 hours for detoxification, developed hypertonia and malignant hyperthermia and died.— G. Bleichner *et al.* (letter), *Lancet*, 1981, *1*, 386.

ANOREXIA. Sulpiride 300 or 400 mg daily was no more effective than placebo in improving behavioural parameters or weight gain in a crossover study in 18 women with anorexia nervosa.— W. Vandereycken, *Br. J. Psychiat.*, 1984, *144*, 288.

CONTRACEPTION. A study suggesting that combination of a progestogen, norethisterone, with sulpiride, a dopamine antagonist, would provide improved contraception compared with either agent given alone.— M. R. Payne *et al.*, *Br. med. J.*, 1985, *291*, 559. Similar results might be achieved simply by increasing the dose of progestogen, and without the increase in prolactin concentrations which is a potential cause of concern. Furthermore the incidence of side-effects with the combination is quite high.— Y. Tayob and J. Guillebaud, *ibid.*, 1206.

DEPRESSION. In a single-blind study in 20 patients, sulpiride 0.4 to 1 g daily was shown to be slightly more effective than amitriptyline 75 to 200 mg daily in the treatment of psychotic and neurotic depression.— P. Niskanen *et al.*, *Curr. ther. Res.*, 1975, *17*, 281.

Further references: J. K. Salminen *et al.*, *Curr. ther. Res.*, 1980, *27*, 109.

EXTRAPYRAMIDAL DISORDERS. Sulpiride 100 mg three times daily was effective in relieving idiopathic torsion dystonia unresponsive to other treatment. Sulpiride therapy was stopped after 3 weeks due to galactorrhoea and weight gain.— R. Sandyk, *Br. med. J.*, 1984, *289*, 964.

GASTRO-INTESTINAL DISORDERS. Serum-gastrin concentrations following protein stimulation were reduced in 8 of 10 patients with duodenal ulcers after receiving sulpiride 300 mg daily by mouth for 8 days.— C. A. Dinelli *et al.*, *Arzneimittel-Forsch.*, 1976, *26*, 421. See also S. K. Lam and C. L. Lai, *Scand. J. Gastroenterol.*, 1976, *11*, 27. and R. Caldara *et al.*, *Gastroenterology*, 1978, *74*, 221.

Sulpiride reduced the stimulation of colonic motility caused by a standard meal in 12 patients with irritable bowel syndrome.— G. A. Lanfranchi *et al.*, *Eur. J. clin. Pharmac.*, 1983, *24*, 769.

In a study involving 42 healthy subjects intramuscular administration of sulpiride (the racemic substance) or its L-isomer decreased serum-gastrin concentration resulting from a food stimulus but had no effect on basal or stimulated gastric acidity. In contrast, the D-isomer significantly decreased gastric acid secretion without affecting serum-gastrin concentrations. The paradoxical response observed after D-sulpiride is similar to the action of dopamine and it is possible that the D-isomer has partial agonist actions. In view of the contradictory responses that have been reported following sulpiride treatment of peptic ulcer studies of the isomers may be of interest.— *Eur. J. clin. Pharmac.*, 1983, *25*, 319. See also A. Zanoboni *et al.*, *Curr. ther. Res.*, 1987, *41*, 903 (anti-emetic efficacy of L-sulpiride in digestive disorders).

In a double-blind study involving 73 patients with duodenal ulcers there was no significant difference in ulcer healing at 3 months between those treated with cimetidine 800 mg daily and those given in addition sulpiride 200 mg daily. However, on follow-up for up to 6 months ulcers recurred in 18 of 25 patients treated with cimetidine alone but in significantly fewer (11 of 29) of those given the combined regimen.— M. Tatsuta *et al.*, *Gut.*, 1986, *27*, 1512. See also S. K. Lam *et al.*, *Gastroenterology*, 1979, *76*, 315 (sulpiride and antacid treatment of duodenal ulcer).

LACTATION. In a double-blind study in women with inadequate lactation, daily milk yields rose (by 90 to 730 mL) in 13 of 14 given sulpiride 50 mg three times daily for 4 weeks, compared with a rise in only 3 of 12 given placebo. Mean serum-prolactin concentrations were elevated in women given sulpiride.— O. Ylikorkala *et al.*, *Br. med. J.*, 1982, *285*, 249. The best stimulus to inadequate lactation is to increase the frequency of nursing.— R. M. O'Leary (letter), *ibid.*, 807; D. P. Davies (letter), *ibid.*

Further references to the use of sulpiride in lactation promotion: T. Aono *et al.*, *Am. J. Obstet. Gynec.*, 1982, *143*, 927; O. Ylikorkala *et al.*, *Obstet. Gynec.*, 1984, *63*, 57.

Proprietary Preparations

Dolmatil *(Squibb, UK). Tablets*, scored, sulpiride 200 mg.

Sulpitil *(Tillotts, UK). Tablets*, scored, sulpiride 200 mg..

Proprietary Names and Manufacturers

Abilit *(Jpn)*; Aiglonyl *(Fumouze, Fr.)*; Arminol *(Krewel, Ger.)*; Biomaride *(Cheminova, Spain)*; Championyl *(Vita, Ital.)*; Confidan *(Bouty, Ital.)*; Coolspan *(Jpn)*; Co-Sulpir *(Smaller, Spain)*; Digton *(Areu, Spain)*; Dixibon *(Sandoz, Spain)*; Dobren *(Ravizza, Ital.)*; Dogmatil *(Delagrange, Belg.; Delagrange, Denm.; Delagrange, Fr.; Schürholz, Ger.; Delagrange, Neth.; Delagrange, Spain; Delagrange, Switz.)*; Dolmatil *(Squibb, UK)*; Drominetas *(Spain)*; Eglonyl *(Noristan, S.Afr.)*; Equilid *(Lepetit, Ital.)*; Eusulpid *(CT, Ital.)*; Guastil *(Uriach, Spain)*; Isnamide *(Isnardi, Ital.)*; Kapiride *(Spain)*; Lavodina *(IBE, Spain)*; Lebopride *(Spyfarma, Spain)*; Lusedan *(Spain)*; Meresa *(Dolorgiet, Ger.)*; Miradol *(Jpn)*; Mirbanil *(Boehringer Ingelheim, Spain)*; Misulvan *(Bernabó, Arg.)*; Neogama *(Hormosan, Ger.)*; Neoride *(Hosbon, Spain)*; Neuromyfar *(Valles Mestre, Spain)*; Normum *(Serpero, Ital.)*; Omperan *(Jpn)*; Psicocen *(Centrum, Spain)*; Quiridil *(Zoja, Ital.)*; Sato *(Scharper, Ital.)*; Sernevin *(Jpn)*; Sicofrenol *(Spain)*; Sulpisedan *(Llano, Spain)*; Sulpitil *(Tillotts, UK)*; Sulpril *(Astra, Denm.)*; Suprium *(IBYS, Spain)*; Sursumid *(Ital.)*; Synedil *(Beytout, Fr.)*; Tepavil *(Prodes, Spain)*; Tonofit *(Spain)*; Ulpir *(Lesvi, Spain)*; Vipral *(Roemmers, Arg.)*.

7108-y

Sultopride *(rINN)*.

LIN-1418. *N*-(1-Ethylpyrrolidin-2-ylmethyl)-5-ethylsulphonyl-2-methoxybenzamide.

$C_{17}H_{26}N_2O_4S$=354.5.

CAS — 53583-79-2.

Sultopride is a substituted benzamide related to sulpiride (above). It has been used in the emergency management of acute psychoses in doses of 0.4 to 1.2 g daily by mouth or intramuscularly; up to 1.6 to 1.8 g daily may be given intramuscularly, and up to 2.4 g daily by mouth. On control of the acute symptoms alternate antipsychotic therapy may be introduced for maintenance, or, in chronically aggressive patients, maintenance doses of sultopride 0.4 to 0.6 g daily may be given.

Proprietary Names and Manufacturers

Barnetil *(Delagrange, Belg.; Delagrange, Fr.)*; Barnotil *(Vita, Ital.)*.

13291-l

Suriclone *(BAN, rINN)*.

31264-RP. (*RS*)-6-(7-Chloro-1,8-naphthyridin-2-yl)-2,3,6,7-tetrahydro-7-oxo-5*H*-[1,4]dithi-ino[2,3-*c*]pyrrol-5-yl 4-methylpiperazine-1-carboxylate.

$C_{20}H_{20}ClN_5O_3S_2$=478.0.

CAS — 53813-83-5.

Suriclone is a cyclopyrrolone structurally related to zopiclone (p.775) and reported to possess similar properties. It has been tried as an anxiolytic.

Proprietary Names and Manufacturers

May & Baker, UK.

4071-z

Talbutal *(USAN, rINN).*
5-Allyl-5-*sec*-butylbarbituric acid.
$C_{11}H_{16}N_2O_3$=224.3.

CAS — 115-44-6.

Pharmacopoeias. In *U.S.*

A white crystalline powder which may have a slight odour of caramel. It occurs in 2 polymorphic forms. **Soluble** 1 in 500 of water, 1 in 1 of alcohol, 1 in 2 of chloroform, and 1 in 40 of ether; soluble in glacial acetic acid, and aqueous solutions of sodium hydroxide or sodium carbonate. **Store** in airtight containers.

Talbutal is a barbiturate and shares the general properties of the group (see p.706). It has been used as a hypnotic in doses of 120 mg at night, and as a sedative in doses of 30 to 60 mg two or three times daily.

Preparations

Talbutal Tablets *(U.S.P.)*

Proprietary Names and Manufacturers

Lotusate *(Winthrop-Breon, USA).*

4072-c

Temazepam *(BAN, USAN, rINN).*

3-Hydroxydiazepam; ER-115; K-3917; Ro-5-5345; Wy-3917. 7-Chloro-1,3-dihydro-3-hydroxy-1-methyl-5-phenyl-1,4-benzodiazepin-2-one.
$C_{16}H_{13}ClN_2O_2$=300.7.

CAS — 846-50-4.

Pharmacopoeias. In *Br.*

A white or almost white odourless crystalline powder. Practically **insoluble** in water; sparingly soluble in alcohol; freely soluble in chloroform. **Store** in well-closed containers. Protect from light.

Dependence, Adverse Effects, Treatment, and Precautions

As for the benzodiazepines in general, p.706.

Comment on individual variations in effectiveness and adverse effects with differing generic formulations of temazepam capsules.— T. Maguire (letter), *Pharm. J.*, 1986, *1*, 822.

EFFECTS ON THE SKIN. Generalised lichenoid drug eruption that had persisted for 5 months in an elderly patient receiving therapy including temazepam resolved within 10 days of discontinuing the benzodiazepine.— P. Norris and T. S. Sounex, *Br. med. J.*, 1986, *293*, 510.

INTERACTIONS. *Antihistamines.* Unexpected stillbirth less than 8 hours after maternal ingestion of temazepam and *diphenhydramine* was possibly due to a synergistic action of the two drugs. Studies in pregnant *rabbits* showed that 51 of 63 foetuses were stillborn or died shortly after birth when the mothers were given this combination of drugs.— G. A. Kargas *et al.* (letter), *New Engl. J. Med.*, 1985, *313*, 1417.

For the interaction of benzodiazepines, including temazepam, with agents such as cimetidine, ranitidine, and oral contraceptives, see Diazepam, p.729.

OVERDOSAGE. Evidence from a study of 15 deaths due to overdosage of various drugs in combination with temazepam suggested that while temazepam might be comparatively safe when taken alone in overdose it might have a synergistic effect when taken in combination with other agents.— A. R. W. Forrest *et al.* (letter), *Lancet*, 1986, *2*, 226.

PREGNANCY AND THE NEONATE. See under Interactions, above.

Absorption and Fate

Temazepam is fairly readily absorbed from the gastro-intestinal tract, although there is some individual variation. It is reported to be 96% bound to plasma protein. It has a biphasic half-life probably owing to tissue redistribution. It is excreted in the urine in the form of its conjugate together with small amounts of the demethylated derivative, oxazepam, also in conjugated form.

Following administration of three 10-mg capsules [type unspecified] of temazepam to each of 4 healthy subjects, temazepam was rapidly absorbed with peak plasma concentrations obtained within 2 hours in all 4 subjects. On the basis of urinary excretion the amount absorbed varied considerably, ranging from 51.1% to 84.8%. The decline in plasma concentrations was at least biphasic, suggesting extensive distribution in tissues. The rapid phase had a half-life of 2 to 3 hours, reflecting distribution in the tissues and the slow phase had a half-life of 15 to 20 hours representing the apparent elimination of the drug from plasma. Following rectal administration of 30-mg suppositories absorption was slow with more inter-subject variation, and lower peak plasma concentrations were achieved. Following administration of the capsules, conjugates of temazepam and its demethylated metabolite, oxazepam, were detected in the urine in the ratio of twenty to one. No oxazepam could be detected in the plasma after administration of the suppositories.— L. M. Fuccella *et al.*, *Int. J. clin. Pharmac.*, 1972, *6*, 303.

Results of a crossover study in 6 healthy subjects demonstrated that temazepam is more rapidly absorbed from soft than from hard gelatin capsules. Following repeated administration of temazepam 20 mg each night for 7 days, the mean half-life of 5.87 hours was not significantly longer than that of 5.28 hours obtained after the first administration. Following morning administration, however, the mean half-life was significantly longer, being 8.35 hours, suggesting a possible circadian rhythm in the rate of metabolism of temazepam.— L. M. Fuccella *et al.*, *Eur. J. clin. Pharmac.*, 1977, *12*, 383.

A study of the effects of age and sex on the pharmacokinetics of temazepam. The elimination half-life was significantly longer at 16.8 hours among 17 female subjects given temazepam 30 mg compared to 12.3 hours among 15 men. The total clearance was also lower among women. The unbound fraction of temazepam was affected both by age and sex, being 2.54% among the 7 young men, 2.30% among 7 young women, 3.12% among the 8 elderly men, and 2.75% among the 10 elderly women. Time to peak plasma concentration and volume of distribution were not affected by the age or sex of the subjects.— M. Divoll *et al.*, *J. pharm. Sci.*, 1981, *70*, 1104. Another study on the accumulation of temazepam in young healthy subjects.— H. R. Ochs *et al.*, *J. clin. Pharmac.*, 1984, *24*, 58.

Fasting produced a reduction in the half-life of temazepam, probably due to its redistribution. The displacement of temazepam from protein binding sites by free fatty acids may have played some part.— P. J. Cook *et al.*, *Br. J. clin. Pharmac.*, 1985, *19*, 587P.

The manufacturer of liquid preparations of temazepam reported on the more rapid absorption of liquid temazepam from soft gelatin capsules compared with temazepam absorption from powder-filled hard capsules. Such hard capsules were more suited to anxiolytic than to hypnotic use (A.P. Launchbury, *Lancet*, 1988, *1*, 833). Replying on behalf of the manufacturer of the hard capsules, Godfrey (*ibid.*, 1113) reported that *in-vivo* studies had shown no difference in bioavailability between the two capsules. In response Launchbury (*ibid.*, 1113) pointed out that no evidence was provided on the rate of absorption being similar with the 2 forms. Others also referred to studies showing slower absorption with hard capsules and their unsuitability for hypnotic use (R.G. Priest, *ibid.*, 1114; I. Hindmarch, *ibid.*).

Uses and Administration

Temazepam is a benzodiazepine with general properties similar to those of diazepam (p.731). It is used as a hypnotic in the short-term management of insomnia, in doses of 10 to 30 mg by mouth at night; exceptionally, doses up to 60 mg may be required.

Temazepam may also be given for premedication before minor surgical or investigative procedures; the usual dose is 20 to 40 mg given half to one hour beforehand.

Proprietary Preparations

Normison *(Wyeth, UK). Capsules*, temazepam 10 and 20 mg.

Proprietary Names and Manufacturers

Cerepax *(Arg.)*; Euhypnos *(Sigma, Austral.; Farmitalia, Denm.; Farmitalia Carlo Erba, S.Afr.; Farmitalia Carlo Erba, UK)*; Lenal *(Arg.)*; Levanxene *(Arg.)*; Levanxol *(Belg.; Ital.; Neth.; Farmitalia Carlo Erba, S.Afr.; Spain)*; Maeva *(Ital.)*; Normison *(Wyeth, Austral.; Wyeth, Denm.; Wyeth-Byla, Fr.; Wyeth, S.Afr.; Wyeth, Switz.; Wyeth, UK)*; Planum *(Farmitalia, Ger.; Farmitalia Carlo Erba, Switz.)*; Remestan *(Wyeth, Ger.)*; Restoril *(Anca, Canad.; Sandoz, USA)*; Somaz *(Quantum, USA)*; Temaz *(Quantum, USA)*; Tenso *(Castejon, Spain).*

7109-j

Tetrabenazine *(BAN, rINN).*

Ro-1-9569; TBZ. 1,3,4,6,7,11b-Hexahydro-3-isobutyl-9,10-dimethoxy-benzo[*a*]quinolizin-2-one.
$C_{19}H_{27}NO_3$=317.4.

CAS — 58-46-8.

Adverse Effects

Drowsiness is the most frequent side-effect of tetrabenazine. Postural hypotension, symptoms of extrapyramidal dysfunction, gastro-intestinal disturbances, and depression may also occur. Overdosage has produced sedation, sweating, hypotension, and hypothermia.

Postural hypotension and dysphagia are the serious side-effects of tetrabenazine, which require careful supervision. Depression is common in Huntington's chorea and it is difficult to know whether it is caused by tetrabenazine; parkinsonism was not noted in a series of patients studied.— C. Y. Huang and C. Elliott (letter), *Br. med. J.*, 1977, *2*, 1416. See also C. Y. Huang *et al.*, *Med. J. Aust.*, 1976, *1*, 583.

EXTRAPYRAMIDAL EFFECTS. Dysphagia and choking were associated with tetrabenazine in the treatment of Huntington's chorea.— R. P. Snaith and H. de B. Warren (letter), *Lancet*, 1974, *1*, 413.

A report of neuroleptic malignant syndrome following the use of tetrabenazine and metirosine in a patient with Huntington's chorea.— R. E. Burke *et al.*, *Neurology*, 1981, *31*, 1022.

OVERDOSAGE. A patient being treated for involuntary movements who swallowed approximately 1 g (40 tablets) of tetrabenazine during a period of depression became drowsy 2 hours later and marked sweating occurred. Her state of consciousness improved after 24 hours and she talked rationally and gained full control of micturition after 72 hours.' Her involuntary movements were reduced when she was somnolent but returned when full consciousness was restored.— D. W. Kidd and D. L. McLellan, *Br. J. clin. Pract.*, 1972, *26*, 179.

Precautions

Tetrabenazine has been reported to block the action of reserpine. It may also diminish the effects of levodopa and exacerbate the symptoms of parkinsonism. Tetrabenazine may cause drowsiness and patients so affected should not take charge of vehicles or machinery where loss of attention could lead to accidents. Use of tetrabenazine immediately following a course of a monoamine oxidase inhibitor has been reported to lead to a state of confusion, restlessness and disorientation; tetrabenazine should probably not be given with, or within 14 days of discontinuation of, such therapy.

Uses and Administration

Tetrabenazine is used in the management of movement disorders including chorea and similar symptoms of central nervous system dysfunction. It was formerly tried in the management of psychoses and psychoneuroses.

The usual initial dose is 25 mg three times daily by mouth, increased if required by 25 mg every 3 or 4 days to a maximum daily dose of 200 mg. If the patient does not respond within 7 days of receiving the maximum dose further treatment with tetrabenazine will have no effect.

CHOREA. Tetrabenazine was given to 30 patients with extrapyramidal movement disorders in doses of 75 to 225 mg daily. At least 80 to 90% reduction in abnormal movements occurred in 18 patients and a complete cessation in 10. Patients with choreiform motor activity showed a gradual diminution in involuntary movement after 2 or 3 days' treatment with doses of 150 to 220 mg. Higher dosage produced sedation. Two of 3 patients with hemiballismus of arteriosclerotic aetiology showed marked improvement after 2 days' treatment with 300 mg the first day and 200 mg for the following day. Tetrabenazine was of no benefit in patients with cerebellar parkinsonian tremors; these conditions could be aggravated. Side-effects occurred in 8 patients, and included fatigue in 3, excessive sweating in 2, and confusion, photophobia, and amenorrhoea in 1 each. Side-effects disappeared on reducing the dose by 25 to 50 mg daily.— M. A. Dalby, *Br. med. J.*, 1969, *2*, 422.

In a double-blind controlled study of 10 patients with chorea there was greater improvement with tetrabenazine 200 mg daily than thiopropazate 30 mg daily, as assessed by observing films of the patients at different stages of treatment.— D. L. McLellan *et al.*, *Lancet*, 1974, *1*, 104. Of 26 patients with chorea given 50 to 150 mg of tetrabenazine daily, choreiform movements were abolished in 10, were improved in 14, and remained unchanged in 2. Treatment was stopped because of hallucinations in 1 and depression in 2 patients.— K. J. Astin and E. W. J. Gumpert (letter), *ibid.*, 512.

A 10-year-old girl and a 12-year-old boy with Sydenham's chorea responded rapidly to treatment with tetrabenazine 25 mg twice or thrice daily.— C. H. Hawkes and C. H. Nourse, *Br. med. J.*, 1977, *1*, 1391.

Following administration of tetrabenazine in doses of up to 200 mg daily to 5 patients with Huntington's chorea and a positive family history, one showed excellent response with complete cessation of involuntary movements, 3 showed moderate improvement, and one showed no improvement. Of 2 patients with Huntington's chorea and no positive family history, one showed moderate improvement and one no improvement. No improvement was noted in a further 7 patients with miscellaneous hyperkinetic movement disorders.— J. U. Toglia *et al.*, *J. clin. Psychiat.*, 1978, *39*, 81.

Proprietary Preparations

Nitoman *(Roche, UK). Tablets*, scored, tetrabenazine 25 mg.

Proprietary Names and Manufacturers

Nitoman *(Roche, Austral.; Roche, Denm.; Roche, Norw.; Roche, UK).*

13314-m

Tetrazepam *(pINN).*

CB-4261. 7-Chloro-5-(cyclohex-1-enyl)-1,3-dihydro-1-methyl-2*H*-1,4-benzodiazepin-2-one.

$C_{16}H_{17}ClN_2O$=288.8.

CAS — 10379-14-3.

Tetrazepam is a benzodiazepine with general properties similar to those of diazepam (p.728). It has been used for its muscle relaxant properties in usual initial doses of 25 to 50 mg, increased if necessary to 150 mg or more daily.

Proprietary Names and Manufacturers

Musaril *(Midy, Ger.)*; Myolastan *(Clin Midy, Fr.; Labaz, Spain).*

7110-q

Thiethylperazine Malate *(BANM, USAN, rINNM).*

2-Ethylthio-10-[3-(4-methylpiperazin-1-yl)propyl]phenothiazine di(hydrogen malate).

$C_{22}H_{29}N_3S_2,2C_4H_6O_5$=667.8.

CAS — 1420-55-9 (thiethylperazine); 52239-63-1 (malate).

Pharmacopoeias. In *U.S.*

A white to faintly yellow crystalline powder with not more than a slight odour. **Soluble** 1 in 40 of water, 1 in 90 of alcohol, 1 in 525 of chloroform, and 1 in 3400 of ether. A freshly prepared 1% solution in water has a pH of 2.8 to 3.8 and the *U.S.P.* injection has a pH between 3 and 4. **Store** in airtight containers. The *U.S.P.* specifies that the injection should be protected from light.

7111-p

Thiethylperazine Maleate *(BANM, USAN, rINNM).*

GS-95; NSC-130044.

$C_{22}H_{29}N_3S_2,2C_4H_4O_4$=631.8.

CAS — 1179-69-7.

Pharmacopoeias. In *Cz., Fr., Swiss*, and *U.S.*

A yellowish granular powder, odourless or with not more than a slight odour.

Soluble 1 in 1700 of water and 1 in 530 of alcohol; slightly soluble in methyl alcohol; practically insoluble in chloroform and ether. A 0.1% solution in water has a pH of 2.8 to 3.8. **Store** in airtight containers. Protect from light.

Adverse Effects, Treatment, and Precautions

As for the phenothiazines in general, p.706.

EXTRAPYRAMIDAL EFFECTS. Administration of thiethylperazine to a 14-year-old boy resulted in oculogyric crises after only 20 mg; these effects stopped within an hour of discontinuing the drug.— J. McIvor (letter), *Br. med. J.*, 1967, *3*, 438.

Extrapyramidal symptoms were reported in a woman within 60 hours of taking thiethylperazine 10 mg thrice daily.— K. L. De Silva *et al.*, *Practitioner*, 1973, *21*, 316. Extrapyramidal reactions occurred in 40 patients, including children, who had received thiethylperazine, usually as a single intramuscular injection. Akathisia was seen in 4 patients and dyskinesia in 36.— A. R. Ahmad *et al.*, *J. Pakistan med. Ass.*, 1975, *25*, 129. See also P. G. Lacouture *et al.*, *Pediatrics*, 1979, *64*, 954.

A report of three attacks of acute dystonia in a 19-year-old patient given rectal thiethylperazine; the second and third attacks occurred approximately 23 and 35 hours respectively after the drug had been discontinued. The attacks were relieved by intravenous injections of diphenhydramine.— U. Khanderia, *Drug Intell. & clin. Pharm.*, 1985, *19*, 550. Correction.— *ibid.*, 682.

Absorption and Fate

For an account of the absorption and fate of a phenothiazine, see Chlorpromazine, p.723.

Uses and Administration

Thiethylperazine is a phenothiazine with general properties similar to those of chlorpromazine (see p.724). It has a piperazine side-chain. Thiethylperazine is used for the control of nausea and vomiting, and has also been used in vertigo. It has been used for the treatment of motion sickness but is not considered effective by some sources.

Thiethylperazine is given in usual doses of 10 mg of the maleate up to three times daily by mouth or rectally; where oral administration is impractical similar doses of the malate may be given by deep intramuscular injection.

Elderly patients should be given reduced doses of phenothiazines. Thiethylperazine is not recommended for use in children.

NAUSEA AND VOMITING. A study in 250 out-patients showed that thiethylperazine 10 mg, chlorprothixene 50 mg, and thiopropazate 10 mg, given before meals, were equally effective in countering nausea and vomiting during treatment with fluorouracil.— C. G. Moertel and R. J. Reitemeier, *Gastroenterology*, 1969, *57*, 262.

Thiethylperazine was effective in the prophylaxis and treatment of seasickness in a double-blind study of 300 passengers.— G. Rubensohn, *Läkartidningen*, 1970, *67*, 619. Thiethylperazine did not reduce the incidence of motion sickness among 10 subjects exposed to coriolis stimulation in a rotating chair.— R. L. Kohl *et al.*, *Clin. Pharmac. Ther.*, 1984, *35*, 251.

Preparations

Thiethylperazine Malate Injection *(U.S.P.)*

Thiethylperazine Maleate Suppositories *(U.S.P.)*. Suppositories containing thiethylperazine maleate. Store below 25° in airtight containers. Protect unwrapped suppositories from exposure to sunlight.

Thiethylperazine Maleate Tablets *(U.S.P.)*

Proprietary Preparations

Torecan *(Sandoz, UK). Tablets*, thiethylperazine maleate 10 mg (equivalent to thiethylperazine 6.33 mg).
Injection, thiethylperazine malate 10.86 mg (equivalent to thiethylperazine 6.5 mg)/mL, in ampoules of 1 mL.
Suppositories, thiethylperazine maleate 10.28 mg (equivalent to thiethylperazine 6.5 mg).

Proprietary Names and Manufacturers

Torecan *(Arg.; Sandoz, Austral.; Belg.; Sandoz, Denm.; Sandoz, Fr.; Sandoz, Ger.; Sandoz, Ital.; Neth.; Sandoz, Norw.; Sandoz, Spain; Sandoz, Swed.; Sandoz, Switz.; Sandoz, UK; Boehringer Ingelheim, USA).*

7112-s

Thiopropazate Hydrochloride *(BANM, rINNM).*

2-{4-[3-(2-Chlorophenothiazin-10-yl)propyl]piperazin-1-yl}ethyl acetate dihydrochloride.

$C_{23}H_{28}ClN_3O_2S,2HCl$=518.9.

CAS — 84-06-0 (thiopropazate); 146-28-1 (hydrochloride).

A white or pale yellow crystalline powder with a faint odour.

Soluble 1 in 4 of water, 1 in 130 of alcohol, and 1 in 65 of chloroform; practically insoluble in ether. A 10% solution in water has a pH of 1.4 to 1.7.

CAUTION. *Thiopropazate may cause severe dermatitis in sensitised persons, and pharmacists, nurses, and others who handle the drug frequently should wear masks and rubber gloves.*

Adverse Effects, Treatment, and Precautions

As for the phenothiazines in general, p.706.

Absorption and Fate

For an account of the absorption and fate of a phenothiazine, see Chlorpromazine, p.723.

Uses and Administration

Thiopropazate hydrochloride is a phenothiazine with actions and uses similar to those of chlorpromazine (p.724). It has a piperazine side-chain. In the management of psychoses it has been given in doses of 10 mg three times daily, adjusted if necessary, with a maximum total dose of 100 mg daily.

Proprietary Names and Manufacturers

Dartal *(Searle, Canad.; Neth.; Switz.)*; Dartalan *(Searle, Austral.; Belg.; Searle, UK).*

The following names have been used for multi-ingredient preparations containing thiopropazate hydrochloride—Pro-Banthine with Dartalan *(Searle, UK).*

7113-w

Thioproperazine Mesylate *(BANM).*

RP-7843; SKF-5883; Thioproperazine Dimethanesulphonate; Thioproperazine Mesilate *(rINNM)*; Thioproperazine Methanesulphonate. *NN*-Dimethyl-10-[3-(4-methylpiperazin-1-yl)propyl]phenothiazine-2-sulphonamide dimethanesulphonate.

$C_{22}H_{30}N_4O_2S_2,2CH_4O_3S$=638.8.

CAS — 316-81-4 (thioproperazine); 2347-80-0 (mesylate).

Pharmacopoeias. In *Fr.*

Adverse Effects, Treatment, and Precautions

As for the phenothiazines in general, p.706.

Absorption and Fate

For an account of the absorption and fate of a phenothiazine, see Chlorpromazine, p.723.

Uses and Administration

Thioproperazine is a phenothiazine with actions and uses similar to those of chlorpromazine (p.724). It has a piperazine side-chain. In the management of psychoses it may be given as the mesylate in initial doses of the equivalent of 5 mg of thioproperazine daily, increased as necessary; the usual effective dosage is 30 to 40 mg daily. In severe or resistant cases doses of 90 mg or more daily have been given.

Proprietary Names and Manufacturers

Majeptil *(May & Baker, Austral.; Rhone-Poulenc, Belg.; Rhône-Poulenc, Canad.; Specia, Fr.; Specia, Neth.; May & Baker, S.Afr.; Rhone, Spain; Rhone-*

Poulenc, Switz.; *May & Baker, UK)*; Mayeptil *(Rhodia, Arg.)*.

7114-e

Thioridazine *(BAN, USAN, rINN)*.

TP-21. 10-[2-(1-Methyl-2-piperidyl)ethyl]-2-methylthiophenothiazine.

$C_{21}H_{26}N_2S_2$=370.6.

CAS — 50-52-2.

Pharmacopoeias. In *Fr.*, *Nord.*, *Swiss*, and *U.S.*

A white or slightly yellow crystalline or micronised powder. Thioridazine 100 mg is approximately equivalent to 110 mg of thioridazine hydrochloride. Practically **insoluble** in water; freely soluble in dehydrated alcohol and in ether; very soluble in chloroform. The *U.S.P.* oral suspension has a pH of between 8 and 10.

Store in well-closed containers. Protect from light.

7115-l

Thioridazine Hydrochloride *(BANM, USAN, rINNM)*.

$C_{21}H_{26}N_2S_2,HCl$=407.0.

CAS — 130-61-0.

Pharmacopoeias. In *Br.*, *Cz.*, *Fr.*, *It.*, *Jpn*, *Jug.*, *Nord.*, *Swiss*, and *U.S.*

A white to cream-coloured or slightly yellow crystalline powder with a slight odour.

Soluble 1 in 9 of water, 1 in 10 of alcohol, and 1 in 1.5 of chloroform; freely soluble in methyl alcohol; practically insoluble in ether. A 1% solution in water has a pH of 4.2 to 5.2. **Store** in airtight containers. Protect from light.

An oral liquid formulation of thioridazine hydrochloride (Mellaril) was incompatible when mixed with a preparation of mesoridazine besylate, and was compatible for 30 minutes but not for 1 hour when mixed with preparations of chlorpromazine hydrochloride, fluphenazine hydrochloride, haloperidol lactate, hydroxyzine hydrochloride, loxapine, methotrimeprazine hydrochloride, perphenazine, prochlorperazine mesylate, procyclidine hydrochloride, trifluoperazine hydrochloride, and benzhexol hydrochloride.— W. A. Parker, *Can. J. Hosp. Pharm.*, 1984, *37*, 133.

Adverse Effects and Treatment

As for the phenothiazines in general, p.706.

The incidence of extrapyramidal symptoms is reported to be low.

Pigmentary retinopathy characterised by diminution of visual acuity, brownish colouring of vision, and impairment of night vision has been observed particularly in patients taking large doses. Changes in the electrocardiogram have also occurred. Sexual dysfunction is common with thioridazine but it is reported to have little epileptogenic effect.

ALLERGY. Pruritus and erythematous rash on the genitals in a woman following sexual intercourse were found to be due to thioridazine present in the seminal fluid of her husband, who was receiving 100 mg daily.— M. B. Sell, *Am. J. Psychiat.*, 1985, *142*, 271.

EFFECTS ON THE BLOOD. Thioridazine has been associated with agranulocytosis.— P. C. Vincent, *Drugs*, 1986, *31*, 52.

EFFECTS ON THE CARDIOVASCULAR SYSTEM. In a study of 252 male patients receiving thioridazine, the incidence of T-wave abnormalities only increased with the dose while the severity was related only to age. It was considered that the T-wave abnormalities induced by thioridazine were neither harmful nor cumulative and that they did not necessarily call for a reduction in dose or discontinuation of therapy.— C. C. Thornton and M. H. Wendkos, *Clin. Pharmac. Ther.*, 1971, *12*, 303. See also R. Axelsson and G. Aspenstrom, *J. clin. Psychiat.*, 1982, *43*, 332 (potential use of T-wave changes to indicate serum concentrations).

A 41-year-old man given thioridazine hydrochloride 600 mg daily for alcohol withdrawal developed ventricular ectopic beats, tachycardia, and fibrillation, and died. A 41-year-old woman similarly treated had ventricular tachycardia and frequent episodes of fibrillation, which responded to DC shock. Both patients had acidosis and hypokalaemia.— M. A. Sydney, *Br. med. J.*, 1973, *4*, 467. There was little reason to conclude that thioridazine was responsible for the arrhythmias.— R. W. Newton (letter), *ibid.*, 738.

A 54-year-old woman developed ventricular tachycardia associated with administration of thioridazine 1.3 g daily for manic-depressive psychosis.— T. B. Tri and D. T. Combs, *West. J. Med.*, 1975, *123*, 412.

Abnormal ECG patterns occurring in 4 of 5 schizophrenic patients given thioridazine 4 mg per kg bodyweight daily by mouth appeared to be associated with elevated plasma concentrations of the thioridazine ring sulphoxide metabolite.— L. A. Gottschalk *et al.*, *J. pharm. Sci.*, 1978, *67*, 155.

A report of thioridazine-induced torsade de pointes.— A. J. Kemper *et al.*, *J. Am. med. Ass.*, 1983, *249*, 2931.

See also Thyroid Disorders, under Precautions, below.

Epistaxis. A report of episodes of nasal bleeding in 3 patients, associated with introduction of thioridazine therapy.— S. Idupuganti, *Am. J. Psychiat.*, 1982, *139*, 1083.

EFFECTS ON THE ENDOCRINE SYSTEM. On 3 occasions a 39-year-old man with chronic schizophrenia developed massive oedema on administration of thioridazine. Prompt diuresis and marked weight loss occurred each time the drug was stopped. On the third occasion the patient suddenly died from multiple pulmonary emboli. Previous authors have suggested that oedema associated with thioridazine may be due to an increase in antidiuretic hormone.— J. Margolis, *J. Am. Geriat. Soc.*, 1972, *20*, 593. Inappropriate secretion of antidiuretic hormone in a woman receiving thioridazine.— F. Matuk and K. Kalyanaraman, *Archs Neurol., Chicago*, 1977, *34*, 374.

Conflicting views on the role of thioridazine in inducing water intoxication: K. J. Rao *et al.* (letter), *Ann. intern. Med.*, 1975, *82*, 61; C. M. Fischman (letter), *ibid.*, 852; M. Miller *et al.* (letter), *ibid.*

A report of significantly lowered mean serum testosterone concentrations in men receiving thioridazine, compared to those taking other neuroleptics. Serum luteinising hormone concentrations were also lowest in the thioridazine group.— W. A. Brown *et al.*, *Archs gen. Psychiat.*, 1981, *38*, 1270.

EFFECTS ON THE EYES. A description of chorioretinopathy in 3 patients receiving high doses of thioridazine. Progressive changes were noted in 2 of the patients for years after thioridazine was discontinued.— T. A. Meredith *et al.*, *Archs Ophthal., N.Y.*, 1978, *96*, 1172. A report of pigmentary retinopathy in a patient receiving long-term thioridazine therapy, in whom the maximum daily dose did not exceed 400 mg; it is necessary to be aware that retinal effects may also occur with low-dose thioridazine.— R. W. Lam (letter), *Can. med. Ass. J.*, 1985, *132*, 737.

See also Effects on the Eyes, p.707.

EFFECTS ON THE GASTRO-INTESTINAL TRACT. After about 1 month a 68-year-old woman taking thioridazine 150 mg daily developed severe diarrhoea which necessitated withdrawal of the drug. Fluphenazine and trifluoperazine, previously used unsuccessfully, had no effect on bowel function.— A. B. S. Mitchell, *Postgrad. med. J.*, 1975, *51*, 182.

Abdominal distension and aortic obstruction associated with thioridazine treatment.— M. M. Kemeny *et al.*, *J. Am. med. Ass.*, 1980, *243*, 683.

EFFECTS ON SEXUAL FUNCTION. There was a 60% incidence of sexual dysfunction in 57 male patients taking thioridazine, compared with a 25% incidence in 64 male patients who had taken other neuroleptics. A striking finding in the thioridazine group was the incidence of ejaculatory failures due to retrograde ejaculation; this did not occur in the other group.— J. Kotin *et al.*, *Am. J. Psychiat.*, 1976, *133*, 82. Psychotropic drugs have an adverse effect on male sexual function and thioridazine appears to be the worst offender.— *Br. med. J.*, 1979, *2*, 883.

For the effects of thioridazine on serum-testosterone concentrations see under Effects on the Endocrine System, above. See also p.707.

Priapism. A 24-year-old man developed priapism after taking an overdose of thioridazine in a suicide attempt.— R. A. Appell *et al.*, *Br. J. Urol.*, 1977, *49*, 160.

EXTRAPYRAMIDAL EFFECTS. The incidence of extrapyramidal effects with thioridazine is low, probably as a result of its high antimuscarinic potency; antimuscarinic activity, however, has unwanted effects of its own.— *Drug & Ther. Bull.*, 1977, *15*, 57.

Of 48 cases of parkinsonism associated with prescribed drugs and seen by a hospital department of geriatric medicine, 13 were associated with thioridazine.— P. J. Stephen and J. Williamson, *Lancet*, 1984, *2*, 1082.

OVERDOSAGE. Episodic ventricular tachycardia and fibrillation occurred in a patient 36 hours after ingesting 2.5 g of thioridazine. Cardiac monitoring might need to be extended in some patients for at least 48 hours.— D. F. Levine and A. J. Marshall (letter), *Lancet*, 1975, *2*, 990.

Death of 3 patients from overdosage with thioridazine; in 1 patient the dose was about 2 g, death was apparently due to cardiac arrhythmias. Arrhythmias developed in a further patient who survived after a dose of 500 mg.— P. T. Donlon and J. P. Tupin, *Archs gen. Psychiat.*, 1977, *34*, 955. See also K. R. Burgess *et al.*, *Med. J. Aust.*, 1979, *2*, 177.

See also under Effects on Sexual Function (above).

Precautions

As for the phenothiazines in general, p.708.

The influence of antipsychotic therapy on performance of judgement tasks was evaluated in 26 schizophrenic patients. Thioridazine appeared to block use of feedback information, whereas haloperidol and trifluoperazine enhanced use of feedback.— J. S. Gillis, *Curr. ther. Res.*, 1977, *21*, 224.

INTERACTIONS. *Antidepressants, tricyclic.* A woman developed life-threatening ventricular arrhythmias a month after the chlorpromazine in her drug regimen of chlorpromazine 800 mg daily and imipramine 100 mg daily was substituted by thioridazine 800 mg. Another woman, who was taking amitriptyline 300 mg daily, developed ventricular arrhythmias after she reported ingesting about 1.2 g of thioridazine.— E. M. Heiman, *J. nerv. ment. Dis.*, 1977, *165*, 139.

Anti-epileptics. Evidence to suggest that concomitant anti-epileptic medication (phenobarbitone and phenytoin) significantly reduces plasma-mesoridazine concentrations in patients given thioridazine; plasma-thioridazine concentration was not significantly different. Plasma concentrations of the anti-epileptics were not affected.— M. Linnoila *et al.*, *Am. J. Psychiat.*, 1980, *137*, 819.

For the effect of thioridazine on phenytoin, see Phenytoin, p.409.

Antihistamines. For the effect of a preparation containing chlorpheniramine maleate and phenylpropanolamine hydrochloride, on thioridazine, see Sympathomimetics (below).

Beta blockers. A report of increased plasma concentrations of thioridazine, probably due to reduced metabolism, in 2 schizophrenic patients following the introduction of concomitant propranolol therapy.— *Drug Interact. News.*, 1987, *7* (4), 17.

Dopaminergic agents. For the interaction of thioridazine with bromocriptine see Bromocriptine Mesylate, p.1012.

Lithium. A severe neurological reaction comprising choreoathetoid movements, akathisia, orofacial dyskinesia, and bruxism developed in a manic-depressive patient maintained on lithium following additional thioridazine treatment. The patient had previously received lithium with thioridazine, with chlorpromazine, and with haloperidol, without ill effect. Treatment with procyclidine was introduced, and symptoms subsided after 6 days.— H. M. A. S. Standish-Barry and M. A. Shelly (letter), *Lancet*, 1983, *1*, 771.

A report of encephalopathy possibly associated with concomitant administration of thioridazine and lithium.— C. H. Cantor (letter), *Med. J. Aust.*, 1986, *144*, 164.

Sympathomimetics. A 27-year-old woman with schizophrenia and T-wave abnormality of the heart, who had responded to thioridazine 100 mg daily with procyclidine 2.5 mg twice daily, died from ventricular fibrillation within 2 hours of taking a single dose of a preparation reported to contain chlorpheniramine maleate 4 mg with phenylpropanolamine hydrochloride 50 mg (Contac C), concurrently with thioridazine.— G. Chouinard *et al.*, *Can. med. Ass. J.*, 1978, *119*, 729. Critical comment; similar combinations of these drugs have not provoked untoward effects in other patients.— M. H. Wendkos (letter), *ibid.*, 1979, *120*, 1058. Reply, stressing the need for caution in the use of other drugs when large doses of thioridazine are prescribed.— G. Chouinard and B. D. Jones (letter), *ibid.*, 1058.

THYROID DISORDERS. Hyperpyrexia and ventricular tachycardia developed in a hyperthyroid patient after taking thioridazine. Thioridazine toxicity might have been enhanced by the hyperthyroid state.— M. B. Murphy and M. X. FitzGerald, *Postgrad. med. J.*, 1984, *60*, 445.

Hypothermic coma developed following administration of a single dose of thioridazine to a patient with myxoedema. The patient, who was receiving concomitant desipramine, subsequently recovered on symptomatic treatment.— D. Lauska and H. H. Harsch, *J. clin. Psychiat.*, 1984, *45*, 188.

WITHDRAWAL. Thioridazine 125 mg daily, which he had been taking for about 18 months, was abruptly withdrawn from a 9-year-old boy with minimal brain dysfunction characterised by hyperactivity, impulsiveness, and learning disability. Irritability appeared the next day, on the tenth day he complained of stomach aches, dyskinetic movements appeared on the fourteenth day, and nausea and vomiting, which began on the twenty-first day was so severe that he required intravenous fluids from the twenty-third to the twenty-sixth day. The vomiting improved on treatment with trimethobenzamide hydrochloride, but persisted intermittently until the thirty-second day. The extrapyramidal disorder persisted up to 90 days after withdrawal.— L. E. Yepes and B. G. Winsberg, *Am. J. Psychiat.*, 1977, *134*, 574.

Symptoms of nausea and vomiting were noted in a number of patients when long-term use of thioridazine 100 to 800 mg daily was stopped abruptly. The symptoms occurred between 24 and 48 hours after the last dose.— B. B. Kumar (letter), *J. Am. med. Ass.*, 1978, *239*, 25.

Akinesia and somnolence occurred in a patient following withdrawal of thioridazine and reduction of concomitant chlorpromazine dosage.— F. Inoui and A. M. Janikowski, *J. Neurol. Neurosurg. Psychiat.*, 1981, *44*, 958.

Absorption and Fate

For an account of the absorption and fate of a phenothiazine, see Chlorpromazine, p.723.

The serum half-life of thioridazine has been estimated to range from about 6 to over 40 hours. Its active metabolites include mesoridazine (p.751) and sulforidazine (p.766).

In 10 healthy subjects given thioridazine hydrochloride 100 mg, peak serum concentrations of 130 to 520 ng per mL were reached 1¼ to 4 hours after the dose; no correlation was shown between the weight, sex, and serum concentrations. In 3 healthy subjects given thioridazine 200 mg (in divided doses over 7 hours) the serum half-life was about 9 to 10 hours.— E. Mårtensson and B. -E. Roos, *Eur. J. clin. Pharmac.*, 1973, *6*, 181.

A study on the serum concentration and elimination from serum of thioridazine in psychiatric patients. The serum half-life in 38 patients ranged from 6 to 42 hours, with a mean of 16.4 hours in 20 who received only thioridazine and 17.1 hours in those who also received other medication. Elimination was reduced at night and with increasing age.— R. Axelsson and E. Mårtensson, *Curr. ther. Res.*, 1976, *19*, 242.

In 10 psychiatric patients stabilised on thioridazine, therapy was replaced by equipotent doses of the side-chain sulphoxide (mesoridazine) and side-chain sulphone (sulforidazine) metabolites of thioridazine. Both metabolites were shown to have an antipsychotic effect, the dose of each required being about two-thirds that of thioridazine. The serum half-lives were thioridazine 21 hours, mesoridazine 16 hours, and sulforidazine 13 hours. Apathy, depression, and restlessness gradually developed during treatment with the 2 metabolites and they could not be used for any length of time. Extrapyramidal symptoms, hypersalivation, and drowsiness were more common with the metabolites; 2 patients had epileptic seizures, and one receiving sulforidazine developed probable cholestatic jaundice.— R. Axelsson, *Curr. ther. Res.*, 1977, *21*, 587.

METABOLISM. Gas-chromatographic studies on the serum and urine of psychiatric patients receiving thioridazine identified the main nonconjugated metabolites as side-chain sulphoxide of thioridazine (mesoridazine), side-chain sulphoxide of demethylthioridazine, side-chain sulphone of thioridazine (sulforidazine), thioridazine disulphoxide, and the ring sulphoxide of thioridazine. Other metabolites tentatively identified were demethylthioridazine, the side-chain sulphone and ring sulphoxide of demethylthioridazine, and the ring sulphone of thioridazine.— E. Mårtensson *et al.*, *Curr. ther. Res.*, 1975, *18*, 687.

PLASMA PROTEIN BINDING. In 48 patients taking thioridazine the mean amount not bound to serum proteins was 0.15%, that of the side-chain sulphoxide 1.66%, side-chain sulphone 1.17%, and ring sulphoxide 1.7%.— G. Nyberg *et al.*, *Eur. J. clin. Pharmac.*, 1978, *14*, 341.

Uses and Administration

Thioridazine is a phenothiazine with actions and uses similar to those of chlorpromazine (p.724). It has a piperidine side-chain and, unlike chlorpromazine, has little anti-emetic activity. Doses are normally given in terms of the hydrochloride; however, some preparations contain the same dose of the base, which is equivalent to a slightly higher dose of the hydrochloride.

The usual initial dose for the treatment of psychoses is 50 to 100 mg of the hydrochloride three times daily; in severe conditions up to 800 mg daily may be required.

Doses of 20 to 200 mg daily have also been used for non-psychotic emotional disturbances, such as anxiety and tension. In general, however, phenothiazines are only suitable for such purposes in resistant conditions, where more appropriate agents, such as the benzodiazepines (see Diazepam, p.731) have proved ineffective. If their use is judged to be necessary treatment should be directed at low dosages on a short-term basis.

A suggested dose of thioridazine for children with behaviour disorders is 1 mg per kg bodyweight daily, in divided doses. Thioridazine should be given in reduced dosage to elderly patients.

ACTION. Improvement in 3 of 6 schizophrenic patients given thioridazine was associated with a high plasma concentration of the active side-chain sulphoxide (mesoridazine) or sulphone of thioridazine, whereas non-responders had a higher plasma concentration of the inactive ring sulphoxide. Plasma concentrations of thioridazine did not distinguish between the two groups.— G. Sakalis *et al.*, *Curr. ther. Res.*, 1977, *21*, 720.

Mention of the theory that thioridazine has a selective effect on dopamine receptors in the limbic system of the brain, and that this may account for its relative lack of extrapyramidal effects.— R. L. Borison and A. J. Blowers (letter), *Lancet*, 1982, *2*, 162. Disagreement and contrary results. The antimuscarinic properties of thioridazine are probably an adequate explanation of the rarity of drug-induced parkinsonism associated with its use.— G. P. Reynolds *et al.* (letter), *ibid.*, 499. Reply, and a defence of the theory that site specificity best explains differences in extrapyramidal activity among neuroleptics.— R. L. Borison and A. J. Blowers (letter), *ibid.*, 883.

ADMINISTRATION. White plaque formation on the oral mucosa of 3 women receiving thioridazine hydrochloride was attributed to the fact that the patients allowed the tablets to dissolve in the mouth. The symptoms cleared when thioridazine in liquid form was substituted for the tablets.— L. N. Folkerts (letter), *Am. J. Hosp. Pharm.*, 1978, *35*, 384.

ANXIETY. In a double-blind study in 45 patients with acute neurotic anxiety, thioridazine 25 or 50 mg three times daily impaired psychomotor skills more than diazepam 5 or 10 mg three times daily. In subjective studies thioridazine was considered to be less effective than diazepam as an anxiolytic agent.— I. Saario *et al.*, *Br. J. clin. Pharmac.*, 1976, *3*, 843.

EFFECTS ON SEXUAL FUNCTION. The use of thioridazine to suppress inappropriate ejaculation.— L. Clein (letter), *Br. med. J.*, 1962, *2*, 548.

Further references: D. Wheatley, *Practitioner*, 1972, *209*, 585.

Resort to drug therapy for premature ejaculation is usually unjustified because the condition nearly always has a psychogenic basis and is very often amenable to behavioural methods of treatment. Drugs are likely to have unacceptable side-effects and the benefits of medication are unlikely to persist after it is stopped.— K. Hawton, *Br. J. Hosp. Med.*, 1985, *34*, 207.

EXTRAPYRAMIDAL DISORDERS. Mentions of the use of thioridazine in the treatment of psychiatric disturbances associated with parkinsonism: G. Stern, *Prescribers' J.*, 1982, *22*, 1; *Drug & Ther. Bull.*, 1984, *22*, 37; A. E. Lang and R. D. G. Blair, *Can. med. Ass. J.*, 1984, *131*, 1031.

Tardive dyskinesia. Criticism of the view that thioridazine may be the phenothiazine of choice for patients with tardive dyskinesia who still require antipsychotic medication. Although antimuscarinic agents reduce the frequency of early extrapyramidal side-effects, they may worsen tardive dyskinesia. Hence, thioridazine, with its antimuscarinic activity may be relatively contra-indicated.— R. Linden (letter), *New Engl. J. Med.*, 1977, *296*, 1004. Comment.— R. M. Kobayashi (letter), *ibid.*

PAIN. Chronic pain was successfully treated with amitriptyline and thioridazine but excessive weight gain occurred when treatment lasted several months.— A. K. Pfister (letter), *J. Am. med. Ass.*, 1978, *239*, 1959.

Preparations

Thioridazine Hydrochloride Oral Solution *(U.S.P.)*. A solution containing thioridazine hydrochloride. It contains 2.5 to 4.7% of alcohol. To be diluted before use. Store at 15° to 30° in airtight containers.

Thioridazine Hydrochloride Tablets *(U.S.P.)*. Contain thioridazine hydrochloride. Store in airtight containers.

Thioridazine Oral Suspension *(U.S.P.)*. A suspension containing thioridazine. Store at a temperature not exceeding 30° in airtight containers.

Thioridazine Tablets *(B.P.)*. Tablets containing thioridazine hydrochloride.

Proprietary Preparations

Melleril *(Sandoz, UK)*. *Tablets*, thioridazine hydrochloride 10, 25, 50, and 100 mg.

Suspension, thioridazine 25 mg (equivalent to thioridazine hydrochloride 27.5 mg)/5 mL and 100 mg (equivalent to thioridazine hydrochloride 110 mg)/5 mL.

Syrup, thioridazine 25 mg (equivalent to thioridazine hydrochloride 27.5 mg)/5 mL.

Proprietary Names and Manufacturers

Mallorol *(Sandoz, Swed.)*; Meleril *(Arg.; Sandoz, Spain)*; Mellaril *(Sandoz, Canad.; Sandoz, USA)*; Mellaril-S *(Sandoz, USA)*; Mellerette *(Sandoz, Ital.)*; Melleretten *(Sandoz, Ger.; Neth.; Switz.)*; Mellerettes *(Belg.; Sandoz, Switz.)*; Melleril *(Sandoz, Austral.; Belg.; Sandoz, Denm.; Sandoz, Fr.; Sandoz, Ger.; Sandoz, Ital.; Neth.; Sandoz, Norw.; Sandoz, S.Afr.; Sandoz, Switz.; Sandoz, UK)*; Novoridazine *(Novopharm, Canad.)*; Ridazine *(Rolab, S.Afr.)*; Thioril *(Canad.)*.

7116-y

Thiothixene *(BAN, USAN)*.

NSC-108165; P-4657B; Tiotixene *(rINN)*. (*Z*)-*NN*-Dimethyl-9-[3-(4-methylpiperazin-1-yl)propylidene]thioxanthene-2-sulphonamide.

$C_{23}H_{29}N_3O_2S_2$=443.6.

CAS — 5591-45-7; 3313-26-6 (Z).

Pharmacopoeias. In *U.S.*

A white to tan-coloured almost odourless crystalline powder. Thiothixene 1 mg is approximately equivalent to 1.25 mg of thiothixene hydrochloride (dihydrate) or to 1.16 mg of the anhydrous hydrochloride. Practically **insoluble** in water; soluble 1 in 110 of dehydrated alcohol, 1 in 2 of chloroform, and 1 in 120 of ether; slightly soluble in acetone and in methyl alcohol. **Store** in airtight containers. Protect from light.

7117-j

Thiothixene Hydrochloride *(BANM, USAN)*.

CP-12252-1; Tiotixene Hydrochloride *(rINNM)*.

$C_{23}H_{29}N_3O_2S_2$,2HCl,$2H_2O$=552.6.

CAS — 58513-59-0 (anhydrous); 49746-04-5 (anhydrous, Z); 22189-31-7 (dihydrate); 49746-09-0 (dihydrate, Z).

Pharmacopoeias. In *U.S.*, which permits both the dihydrate and the anhydrous form ($C_{23}H_{29}N_3O_2S_2$,2HCl = 516.6).

A white or almost white crystalline powder with a slight odour.It is affected by light. **Soluble** 1 in 8 of water, 1 in 270 of dehydrated alcohol, and 1 in 280 of chloroform; practically insoluble in acetone and ether. The *U.S.P.* injection has a pH between 2.5 and 3.5, whilst a reconstituted solution of Thiothixene Hydrochloride for Injection *(U.S.P.)* may have a pH between 2.3 and 3.7; the oral solution has a pH between 2 and 3. **Store** in airtight containers. Protect from light.

Adverse Effects, Treatment, and Precautions

As for the phenothiazines, p.706.

EFFECTS ON THE BLOOD. Leucopenia in a patient associated with thiothixene therapy.— N. R. Cutler and J. F. Heiser, *J. Am. med. Ass.*, 1979, *242*, 2872.

EFFECTS ON THE ENDOCRINE SYSTEM. A 55-year-old man developed hyponatraemia associated with inappropriate secretion of antidiuretic hormone following administration of thiothixene 30 mg daily for 4 months.— K. Ajlouni *et al.*, *Archs intern. Med.*, 1974, *134*, 1103.

EFFECTS ON THE SKIN. Thiothixene has been reported to cause photosensitivity reactions.— *Med. Lett.*, 1986, *28*, 51.

EXTRAPYRAMIDAL DISORDERS. In a study involving 67 patients treated with thiothixene, 20% experienced akathisia within 12 hours of a test dose of 220 µg per kg body-weight by mouth, and 7 experienced a dystonic reaction. After maintenance treatment for 4 weeks, 63% of patients experienced akathisia, but this could be suppressed in all but 3 by antiparkinsonian medication.— T. Van Putten *et al.*, *Psychopharmac. Bull.*, 1984, *20*, 114.

For the use of propranolol to treat thiothixene-induced akathisia and tremor, see under Fluphenazine Hydrochloride, p.740.

Tardive dyskinesia. After receiving thiothixene 10 mg daily for a year, a 27-year-old schizophrenic man developed symptoms of tardive dyskinesia.— J. Ananth and A. Costin, *Am. J. Psychiat.*, 1977, *134*, 689.

WITHDRAWAL. Replacement of thiothixene, which he had been taking for 57 days, by thioridazine, was associated with the development of an acute brain syndrome in a 46-year-old man with chronic schizophrenia. Reinstitution of the thiothixene after 7 days controlled the symptoms. The thiothixene was again withdrawn 12 days later, this time without incident; the reason for this was not fully understood.— J. B. Ferholt and W. N. Stone, *J. nerv. ment. Dis.*, 1970, *150*, 400.

Absorption and Fate

For an account of the absorption and fate of a thioxanthene, see Flupenthixol, p.738.

Plasma concentrations of thiothixene were studied in schizophrenic patients using a method of analysis with a sensitivity equivalent to less than 1 ng per mL of plasma. In 15 adequately controlled patients receiving thiothixene 15 to 60 mg daily in 2, 3, or 4 divided doses by mouth, plasma concentrations were found to be in the relatively narrow range of 10 to 22.5 ng per mL 126 to 150 minutes after the last daily dose despite the four-fold difference in dosage. Investigations in a further 5 patients indicated that peak plasma concentrations were obtained about 1 to 3 hours after a dose, indicating rapid absorption with an absorption half-time of about 30 minutes. There was an early plasma half-life of about 210 minutes and a late half-life of about 34 hours; resurgence of drug concentrations in some subjects might have been due to enterohepatic recycling. Appreciable blood concentrations obtained 24 hours after a single dose indicated that a once-daily dose might be adequate for long-term therapy.— D. C. Hobbs *et al.*, *Clin. Pharmac. Ther.*, 1974, *16*, 473.

In a double-blind study, 40 schizophrenics received either thiothixene or thioridazine hydrochloride, the doses being adjusted for optimal effect. After 3 weeks, plasma concentrations of both drugs were dose-related, but after 8 weeks the plasma concentration of thiothixene had fallen, indicating enzyme induction, whilst the correlation was maintained for thioridazine.— R. Bergling *et al.*, *J. clin. Pharmac.*, 1975, *15*, 178.

Uses and Administration

Thiothixene is a thioxanthene with general properties similar to those of the phenothiazine, chlorpromazine (p.724). The usual initial dose of the base or the hydrochloride (expressed in terms of the base) for the treatment of psychoses is 2 mg three times daily, or 5 mg twice daily, gradually increasing to 20 to 30 mg daily if necessary; once-daily dosage may be adequate. In severe psychoses doses of up to 60 mg daily may be given. It may also be given intramuscularly as the hydrochloride in doses equivalent to 4 mg of the base two to four times daily increased if necessary to a maximum of 30 mg daily.

Thiothixene should be given in reduced dosage to elderly patients.

ANXIETY WITH DEPRESSION. In a double-blind trial involving 76 depressed anxious patients, 18 given thiothixene 2 to 12 mg daily achieved moderate to marked improvement compared with 16 patients given a placebo. Side-effects due to thiothixene were stimulation and sedation, but stimulation was also reported by patients receiving the placebo.— B. J. Goldstein and B. Brauzer, *J. clin. Pharmac.*, 1973, *13*, 167.

Preparations

Thiothixene Capsules *(U.S.P.)*

Thiothixene Hydrochloride for Injection *(U.S.P.)*. A sterile dry powder containing thiothixene hydrochloride. Potency is expressed in terms of thiothixene.

Thiothixene Hydrochloride Injection *(U.S.P.)*. A sterile solution in Water for Injections. Potency is expressed in terms of the equivalent amount of thiothixene.

Thiothixene Hydrochloride Oral Solution *(U.S.P.)*. A solution containing thiothixene hydrochloride. Potency is expressed in terms of the equivalent amount of thiothixene.

Proprietary Names and Manufacturers of Thiothixene and Thiothixene Hydrochloride

Navane *(Pfizer, Austral.; Roerig, Belg.; Pfizer, Canad.; Pfizer, Denm.; Pfizer, Ital.; Roerig, Neth.; Pfizer, Norw.; Pfizer, S.Afr.; Pfizer, Spain; Roerig, Swed.; Pfizer, UK; Roerig, USA)*; Orbinamon *(Pfizer, Ger.)*.

13339-l

Tiapride *(BAN, rINN)*.

FLO-1347 *(hydrochloride)*. *N*-(2-Diethylaminoethyl)-2-methoxy-5-methylsulphonylbenzamide.
$C_{15}H_{24}N_2O_4S$=328.4.

CAS — 51012-32-9 (tiapride); 51012-33-0 (hydrochloride).

Adverse Effects, Treatment, and Precautions

As for the phenothiazines, p.706.

Drowsiness or sedation are common.

Absorption and Fate

Tiapride is rapidly absorbed following oral administration and excreted in the urine. The half-life is reported to range from 3 to 4 hours.

A study of the steady-state pharmacokinetics of tiapride in 5 elderly patients with tardive dyskinesia, and in 2 patients with Huntington's chorea. All patients received tiapride 100 mg three times daily for 7 days. The mean peak plasma concentration of tiapride was 1.47 µg per mL, achieved a mean of 1.4 hours after dosing, and the mean elimination half-life was 3.8 hours. These values did not differ significantly from those previously reported in younger healthy subjects, although renal clearance was slightly lower in these patients. About half of the dose of tiapride was excreted unchanged by the kidney; a metabolite, probably *N*-monodesethyltiapride was detected in the urine but its identity was not confirmed.— R. A. C. Roos *et al.*, *Eur. J. clin. Pharmac.*, 1986, *31*, 191.

Uses and Administration

Tiapride is a substituted benzamide with general properties similar to those of sulpiride (p.767).

It has been used as a neuroleptic in the management of various psychiatric disorders, and to treat dyskinesias. Doses of 200 to 400 mg daily by mouth have usually been given, although higher daily doses have been used, in particular in the management of dyskinesia. Tiapride has also been given by intramuscular or intravenous injection.

Tiapride hydrochloride has also been used.

ALCOHOL AND DRUG WITHDRAWAL. Tiapride appeared to be effective in relieving major symptoms of alcohol withdrawal in a comparison with chlordiazepoxide involving 50 patients; however, significantly more of those given chlordiazepoxide considered their treatment effective. Tiapride might be useful in treating alcohol withdrawal symptoms where benzodiazepine side-effects were likely to prove a problem, but the benzodiazepine should be given where there is a risk of convulsions.— U. Lepola *et al.*, *Int. J. clin. Pharmacol. Res.*, 1984, *6*, 321. See also G. K. Shaw *et al.*, *Br. J. Psychiat.*, 1987, *150*, 164.

ANALGESIA. A comparison of tiapride with glafenine in the management of acute rheumatic pain.— F. Ginsberg *et al.*, *Curr. med. Res. Opinion*, 1983, *8*, 562.

EXTRAPYRAMIDAL DISORDERS. References to the use of tiapride in patients with tardive dyskinesia: W. Greil *et al.*, *Neuropsychobiology*, 1985, *14*, 17; A. Perényi *et al.*, *J. clin. Psychiat.*, 1985, *46*, 229.

For reference to the use of tiapride in reducing levodopa-induced dyskinesias and in suppressing the adverse effects of levodopa on respiration see Levodopa, p.1016.

Chorea. Disappointing results in a crossover study of tiapride 100 mg three times daily, compared with placebo, in 22 patients with Huntington's chorea.— R. A. C. Roos *et al.*, *Acta neurol. scand.*, 1982, *65*, 45.

Tiapride in doses of 3 g daily was significantly superior to placebo in relieving the symptoms of Huntington's chorea in a crossover study completed by 23 patients. Treatment with high-dose tiapride was generally well-tolerated, although associated with a higher incidence of sedation and extrapyramidal signs than placebo.— J. Deroover *et al.*, *Curr. med. Res. Opinion*, 1984, *9*, 329.

RHEUMATIC DISORDERS. For reference to the use of tiapride in rheumatic pain see under Analgesia, above.

Proprietary Names and Manufacturers of Tiapride and Tiapride Hydrochloride

Equilium *(Fumouze, Fr.)*; Italprid *(Prophin, Ital.)*; Porfanil *(Prodes, Spain)*; Pridonal *(Antibioticos, Spain)*; Sereprile *(Vita, Ital.)*; Tiapridal *(Millet, Arg.; Delagrange, Belg.; Delagrange, Fr.; Delagrange, Switz.)*; Tiapridex *(Schürholz, Ger.)*; Tiaprizal *(Delagrange, Spain)*.

17010-t

Timiperone *(rINN)*.

DD-3480. 4-Fluoro-4-[4-(2-thioxo-1-benzimidazolinyl)piperidino]butyrophenone.
$C_{22}H_{24}FN_3OS$=397.5.

CAS — 57648-21-2.

Timiperone is a butyrophenone derivative which is structurally related to haloperidol (p.743). It is used as a neuroleptic in the treatment of schizophrenia in total doses ranging from 0.5 to 12 mg daily.

Proprietary Names and Manufacturers

Tolopelon *(Daiichi, Jpn)*.

7118-z

Tofisopam *(rINN)*.

Egyt-341; Tofizopam. 1-(3,4-Dimethoxyphenyl)-5-ethyl-7,8-dimethoxy-4-methyl-5*H*-2,3-benzodiazepine.
$C_{22}H_{26}N_2O_4$=382.5.

CAS — 22345-47-7.

Adverse Effects, Treatment, and Precautions

As for the benzodiazepines in general p.706.

Somnolence may be less frequent or less marked than with conventional benzodiazepines, but has been reported, particularly in elderly patients. Skin rashes have occurred.

Uses and Administration

Tofisopam is a 2,3-benzodiazepine related structurally to the 1,4-benzodiazepines such as diazepam (p.728) and sharing some of the same actions; however it is reported to be largely lacking in the sedative, anticonvulsant, and muscle relaxant properties of the conventional benzodiazepines.

In the treatment of anxiety it has been given in doses of 50 mg three times daily; in severe cases, up to 300 mg daily may be given.

Tofisopam should be given in reduced dosage to elderly patients.

ABSORPTION AND FATE. A study of the pharmacokinetics of tofisopam in healthy subjects. It was found to have a plasma half-life of about 6 hours.— S. Rónai *et al.*, *Therapia hung.*, 1975, *23*, 139.

ACTION. In a crossover study in 12 subjects the effects of tofisopam 100 and 200 mg by mouth were compared with diazepam and a placebo. Tofisopam produced no changes in the EEG or in tests of psychological function, nor did it display a sedative action. There was some evidence of a very mild stimulant effect occurring 3 to 5 hours after ingestion and it is possible that tofisopam is acting as a prodrug.— A. Bond and M. Lader, *Eur. J. clin. Pharmac.*, 1982, *22*, 137.

ANAESTHESIA. Tofisopam as oral premedication.— A. Pakkanen *et al.*, *Br. J. Anaesth.*, 1980, *52*, 1009.

Tofisopam 100 mg was given by mouth to 47 patients as premedication before minor surgery under local or regional anaesthesia, compared with placebo (in 50) or no premedication; there was no significant difference between the groups except for increased postoperative sedation in those given tofisopam or placebo. In a second study tofisopam 100 mg given 3 times over the 24 hours before inpatient gynaecological surgery to 49 patients, significantly reduced pre-operative anxiety compared with placebo in a further 49; however, it did not cause sedation, and in fact there was a significant stimulatory effect on the morning of surgery.— J. Kanto *et al.*, *Int. J. clin. Pharmac. Ther. Toxic.*, 1982, *20*, 309. See also M. Hovi-Viander *et al.*, *Br. J. clin. Pharmac.*, 1985, *20*, 492.

Proprietary Names and Manufacturers
Grandaxin *(EGIS, Hung.)*; Grandaxine *(Ozothine, Fr.)*; Sériel *(Biogalenique, Fr.)*.

4073-k

Triazolam *(BAN, USAN, rINN).*

Clorazolam; U-33030. 8-Chloro-6-(2-chlorophenyl)-1-methyl-4*H*-[1,2,4]triazolo[4,3-*a*][1,4]-benzodiazepine.
$C_{17}H_{12}Cl_2N_4$=343.2.

CAS — 28911-01-5.

Pharmacopoeias. In *U.S.*

Store in well-closed containers. The *U.S.P.* directs that the tablets should be protected from light.

Dependence

As for the benzodiazepines in general, p.706.

DEPENDENCE. A report of triazolam dependence and comment on the potential of short-acting benzodiazepines for abuse.— J. A. E. Fleming (letter), *Can. med. Ass. J.*, 1983, *129*, 324.

WITHDRAWAL. A report of daytime rebound anxiety in 21 patients receiving triazolam 500 µg at night for 3 weeks; anxiety was greatest by the third week. Patients also experienced rebound insomnia in the fourth week, when active drug was replaced by placebo. In contrast there was evidence of reduced daytime anxiety when the patients were given the longer-acting drug loprazolam 1 mg at night, although rebound insomnia and anxiety were noted during the withdrawal week. Rebound phenomena are common on withdrawal of hypnotic agents, and the more rapidly the drug is eliminated, the earlier the rebound. These doses of triazolam appear to be metabolised sufficiently rapidly to produce rebound phenomena the following day.— K. Morgan and I. Oswald, *Br. med. J.*, 1982, *284*, 942. Criticism of the study and of the high dose of triazolam given.— A. N. Nicholson *et al.* (letter), *ibid.*, 1785. Reply. Such a dose, although considered high in the *U.K.*, is in common use in a number of countries.— K. Morgan and I. Oswald (letter), *ibid.* Further comment on withdrawal phenomena associated with very-short-acting hypnotics such as triazolam.— I. Oswald (letter), *ibid.*, 1983, *287*, 289.

A study of the effects of dose on triazolam-induced rebound insomnia in 12 healthy subjects demonstrated that wake time and sleep latency were significantly increased on the night following discontinuation of triazolam 500 µg for 6 nights; however, there was no significant difference in these parameters compared to placebo on the night following withdrawal of triazolam 250 µg for 6 nights. Both doses of triazolam were superior to placebo in increasing sleep time. Rebound insomnia appeared to occur only at the higher dose, which had no additional hypnotic efficacy in these subjects.— T. A. Roehrs, *Br. J. clin. Pharmac.*, 1986, *22*, 143. Data from a comparative study of triazolam and quazepam demonstrated marked rebound insomnia and daytime anxiety following withdrawal of triazolam 250 µg nightly (given for 14 nights) in 6 insomniac patients. Furthermore although this dose of triazolam appeared to have only minimal effects on insomnia in these patients it was associated with side-effects including irritability, anxiety, inability to concentrate, paranoid ideation, memory impairment, and hyperexcitability. Tolerance to the hypnotic effect developed rapidly. The study indicates that the adverse effects of the lower dose of triazolam are similar to those previously reported with doses of 500 µg.— A. Kales *et al.*, *Clin. Pharmac. Ther.*, 1986, *40*, 378.

A study involving 60 insomniac patients indicated that rebound insomnia following withdrawal from triazolam 500 µg nightly could be attenuated if the withdrawal was carried out by a tapered reduction in dose over several nights.— D. J. Greenblatt *et al.*, *New Engl. J. Med.*, 1987, *317*, 722.

See also under Nitrazepam, p.755.

Adverse Effects, Treatment, and Precautions

As for the benzodiazepines in general, p.706.

A report of a syndrome (adverse mental effects) associated with triazolam administration, with special reference to a close study of 25 patients.— C. van der Kroef (letter), *Lancet*, 1979, *2*, 526. Criticism by the manufacturers.— N. MacLeod and C. H. Kratochvil (letter), *ibid.*, 638. Further severe criticism.— F. J. Ayd *et al.* (letter), *ibid.*, 1018.

See also under Dependence, above.

EFFECTS ON THE LIVER. Fatal intrahepatic cholestasis possibly associated with triazolam.— I. Cobden *et al.*, *Postgrad. med. J.*, 1981, *57*, 730.

Absorption and Fate

Triazolam is rapidly and nearly completely absorbed from the gastro-intestinal tract. It is reported to be extensively bound to plasma proteins. It is metabolised in the liver and excreted in the urine in the form of its metabolites with only small amounts appearing unchanged.

In a study of triazolam tablets and a liquid formulation in healthy subjects, the bioavailability of the tablets was rapid and, relative to the liquid formulation, complete. The average half-life for absorption was 8 minutes with peak concentrations being achieved an average of 42 minutes after dosing.— C. M. Metzler *et al.*, *Clin. Pharmac. Ther.*, 1977, *21*, 111. In a study in 8 healthy subjects the bioavailability of triazolam 500 µg as an oral tablet was greater on average by 28% when the dose was given sublingually rather than orally. This might be due to avoidance of hepatic first-pass metabolism.— J. M. Scavone *et al.*, *J. clin. Pharmac.*, 1986, *26*, 208.

In a study in 10 healthy subjects the mean elimination half-life was 3.77 hours when triazolam 500 µg was given in the evening and 2.94 hours when the dose was given in the morning. Absorption was also significantly slower in the evening.— R. B. Smith *et al.*, *J. clin. Pharmac.*, 1986, *26*, 120.

Further references: F. S. Eberts *et al.*, *Clin. Pharmac. Ther.*, 1981, *29*, 81; D. J. Greenblatt *et al.*, *Clin. Pharmacokinet.*, 1983, *8*, 233.

OBESITY. The clearance of triazolam was considerably impaired in obese subjects.— D. R. Abernethy *et al.*, *Clin. Pharmacokinet.*, 1984, *9*, 177.

Uses and Administration

Triazolam is a benzodiazepine derivative with general properties similar to those of diazepam (p.731). It has been used as a hypnotic in the short-term management of insomnia, in doses of 250 µg at night; initial doses of 125 µg at night have been suggested for elderly subjects, increased to 250 µg if necessary.

In some countries, doses of up to 500 µg at night have been recommended; however, these may be associated with an increased risk of severe adverse effects (see under Dependence, and Adverse Effects, above).

Reviews of triazolam: *Br. J. clin. Pharmac.*, 1981, *11*, 3S; G. E. Pakes *et al.*, *Drugs*, 1981, *22*, 81; *Med. Lett.*, 1983, *25*, 32; P. D. Kroboth and R. P. Juhl, *Drug Intell. & clin. Pharm.*, 1983, *17*, 495.

Proprietary Preparations

Halcion *(Upjohn, UK)*. *Tablets*, scored, triazolam 125 and 250 µg.

Proprietary Names and Manufacturers

Halcion *(Belg.; Upjohn, Canad.; Upjohn, Denm.; Upjohn, Fr.; Upjohn, Ger.; Upjohn, Ital.; Upjohn, Norw.; Upjohn, S.Afr.; Upjohn, Spain; Upjohn, Switz.; Upjohn, UK; Upjohn, USA)*; Novodorm *(Rubio, Spain)*; Songar *(Valeas, Ital.)*.

4074-a

Triclofos Sodium *(BANM, USAN, rINNM).*

Sch-10159; Sodium Triclofos. Sodium 2,2,2-trichloroethyl hydrogen orthophosphate.
$C_2H_3Cl_3NaO_4P$=251.4.

CAS — 306-52-5 (triclofos); 7246-20-0 (sodium salt).

Pharmacopoeias. In *Br.*

A white or almost white, odourless or almost odourless, hygroscopic powder. **Soluble** 1 in 2 of water; slightly soluble in alcohol; practically insoluble in ether. A 2% solution in water has a pH of 3.0 to 4.5. **Store** in well-closed containers.

Dependence, Adverse Effects, Treatment, and Precautions
As for Chloral Hydrate, p.717.

Triclofos sodium is not corrosive to skin and mucous membranes.

OVERDOSAGE. A 47-year-old woman who took 100 triclofos tablets (50 g) was deeply unconscious and hypothermic; reflexes were absent and she was hypotensive. After intravenous fluids she recovered consciousness on the third day.— J. M. Orwin and H. G. Schroeder (letter), *Br. med. J.*, 1968, *3*, 187.

Absorption and Fate
Triclofos sodium is rapidly hydrolysed to trichloroethanol. For the distribution and fate of trichloroethanol, see Chloral Hydrate, p.718.

Uses and Administration
Triclofos sodium has hypnotic and sedative actions similar to those of chloral hydrate (see p.718) but it is more palatable and relatively free from the tendency to cause gastric irritation.

The usual adult dose as a hypnotic is 1 g (equivalent to 600 mg of chloral hydrate) at night, but up to 2 g may be necessary in some patients, and the usual dose as a daytime sedative is 500 mg once or twice daily. A suggested hypnotic dose for children up to 1 year of age is 100 to 250 mg; children aged 1 to 5 years may be given single doses of 250 to 500 mg, and children aged 6 to 12 years may be given single doses of 0.5 to 1 g.

Preparations

Triclofos Oral Solution *(B.P.)*. Triclofos Elixir. A solution of triclofos sodium in a suitable flavoured vehicle. Store at a temperature not exceeding 25°. If diluted, such dilutions must be freshly prepared and not used more than 2 weeks after issue.

Proprietary Names and Manufacturers
Tricloryl *(Glaxo, S.Afr.; Glaxo, UK)*; Triclos *(Merrell-National, USA: Merrell Dow, USA)*.

13378-t

Trifluomeprazine Maleate *(BANM, rINNM).*
Dimethyl[2-methyl-3-(2-trifluoromethylphenothiazin-10-yl)propyl]amine hydrogen maleate; 10-(3-Dimethylamino-2-methylpropyl)-2-trifluoromethylphenothiazine hydrogen maleate.
$C_{19}H_{21}F_3N_2S,C_4H_4O_4$=482.5.

CAS — 2622-37-9 (trifluomeprazine).

Pharmacopoeias. In *B.P. Vet.*

A white or almost white, odourless or almost odourless, crystalline powder. Very slightly **soluble** in water; soluble 1 in 25 of alcohol and of chloroform; practically insoluble in ether. **Protect** from light.

Trifluomeprazine maleate is a sedative used in veterinary medicine.

7120-s

Trifluoperazine Hydrochloride *(BANM, USAN, rINNM).*

Trifluoperazini Hydrochloridum; Triphthazinum. 10-[3-(4-Methylpiperazin-1-yl)propyl]-2-trifluoromethylphenothiazine dihydrochloride.
$C_{21}H_{24}F_3N_3S,2HCl$=480.4.

CAS — 117-89-5 (trifluoperazine); 440-17-5 (hydrochloride).

Pharmacopoeias. In *Belg., Br., Egypt., Eur., Fr., Ind., It., Neth., Roum., Rus., Swiss,* and *U.S.*

A white to pale yellow, odourless or almost odourless, slightly hygroscopic, crystalline powder. Trifluoperazine 1 mg is approximately equivalent to 1.2 mg of trifluoperazine hydrochloride.

Soluble 1 in 2 of water (*B.P.*) or 1 in 3.5 of water (*U.S.P.*); 1 in 11 of alcohol, and 1 in 100 of chloroform; practically insoluble in ether. The *U.S.P.* states that a 5% solution in water has a pH between 1.7 and 2.6; the *U.S.P* injection has a pH between 4 and 5. The *B.P.* states that a 10% solution in water has a pH of 1.6 to 2.5. In aqueous solution it is readily oxidised by atmospheric oxygen. **Store** in airtight containers. Protect from light.

Adverse Effects, Treatment, and Precautions

As for the phenothiazines in general, p.706.

EFFECTS ON THE BLOOD. *Aplastic anaemia.* Trifluoperazine has been reported to cause aplastic anaemia.— R. H. Girdwood, *Drugs*, 1976, *11*, 394.

EFFECTS ON THE EYES. Lenticular opacities occurred in 8 out of 31 schizophrenics who were given a succession of phenothiazine derivatives, mainly trifluoperazine, for periods of 3 to 10 years.— L. H. Margolis and J. L. Goble, *J. Am. med. Ass.*, 1965, *193*, 7.

EFFECTS ON SEXUAL FUNCTION. A report of anorgasmia in a woman taking trifluoperazine.— *Psychosomatics*, 1984, *3*, 23.

EFFECTS ON THE SKIN. Trifluoperazine has been reported to cause photosensitivity reactions.— *Med. Lett.*, 1986, *28*, 51.

EXTRAPYRAMIDAL EFFECTS. Acute dystonia affecting the tongue occurred in 2 patients after a single dose of 10 mg of trifluoperazine.— X. G. Okojie (letter), *Br. med. J.*, 1972, *4*, 796.

Extrapyramidal symptoms were reported in a 17-year-old girl within 60 hours of taking trifluoperazine 1 mg twice daily.— K. L. De Silva *et al.*, *Practitioner*, 1973, *211*, 316.

The Boston Collaborative Drug Surveillance Program monitored consecutively 32 812 medical inpatients. Drug-induced extrapyramidal symptoms occurred in 7 of 73 patients given trifluoperazine hydrochloride. Also 3 patients out of 44 given trifluoperazine with prochlorperazine or chlorpromazine experienced extrapyramidal symptoms.— J. Porter and H. Jick, *Lancet*, 1977, *1*, 587.

Of 48 cases of parkinsonism associated with prescribed drugs referred to a hospital department of geriatric medicine, 3 were associated with the use of trifluoperazine.— P. J. Stephen and J. Williamson, *Lancet*, 1984, *2*, 1082.

Tardive dyskinesia. A placebo-controlled study of phenothiazine-induced tardive dyskinesia in patients given trifluoperazine 16 mg or 80 mg daily. An attempt was made to replicate previous findings with chlorpromazine. The most significant finding was the high incidence of dyskinesia in chronic schizophrenic patients receiving high doses of chlorpromazine or trifluoperazine.— G. E. Crane and C. Chase, *Archs Neurol., Chicago*, 1970, *22*, 176.

A 60-year-old patient with manic depression maintained for several years on lithium and intermittent trifluoperazine developed tardive dyskinesia when trifluoperazine was discontinued.— *J. Am. med. Ass.*, 1985, *253*, 1633.

OVERDOSAGE. Seven youths each ingested 60 mg of trifluoperazine. Six had dystonic syndromes which lasted for 24 to 72 hours and were followed by akathisia. One, who had taken chlordiazepoxide 60 mg simultaneously, had an attenuated reaction. Amylobarbitone sodium given intravenously to 2 patients stopped the extrapyramidal attacks instantly, but in 1 patient 3 further severe attacks followed at 8-hourly intervals.— M. X. FitzGerald and O. FitzGerald (letter), *Lancet*, 1969, *1*, 1100.

Absorption and Fate

For an account of the absorption and fate of a phenothiazine, see Chlorpromazine, p.723.

Plasma-trifluoperazine concentrations during high-dose therapy.— S. H. Curry *et al.* (letter), *Lancet*, 1981, *1*, 395.

A study of the pharmacokinetics of trifluoperazine as a single 5-mg dose by mouth in 5 healthy subjects. Peak plasma concentrations of trifluoperazine, which were measured by a sensitive gas chromatography-mass spectrometry technique, were reached from 1.5 to 4.5 hours after ingestion and varied widely between subjects, ranging from 0.53 to 3.09 ng per ml. Elimination of trifluoperazine was multiphasic; the mean elimination half-life was estimated to be 5.1 hours over the period from 4.5 to 12 hours after ingestion, while the mean apparent terminal elimination half-life was estimated to be 12.5 hours.— K. K. Midha *et al.*, *Br. J. clin. Pharmac.*, 1983, *15*, 380. See also K. K. Midha *et al.* (letter), *Can. med. Ass. J.*, 1983, *129*, 324.

Further references: K. K. Midha *et al.*, *J. pharm. Sci.*, 1984, *73*, 261; M. Aravagiri *et al.*, *ibid.*, 1985, *74*, 1196; *idem*, *J. Pharmac. exp. Ther.*, 1986, *237*, 615.

PLASMA PROTEIN BINDING. For the comparative protein binding of trifluoperazine and other phenothiazines, see Chlorpromazine, p.723.

Uses and Administration

Trifluoperazine is a phenothiazine with actions and uses similar to those of chlorpromazine (p.724). It has a piperazine side-chain. Trifluoperazine is given as the hydrochloride but its doses are expressed in terms of the base.

The usual initial dose for the treatment of psychoses is 2 to 5 mg twice daily, gradually increased to a usual range of 15 to 20 mg daily in divided doses; in severe psychoses daily doses of 40 mg or more have been given. For the relief of acute psychotic symptoms it may be given by deep intramuscular injection in a dosage of 1 to 3 mg daily in divided doses; up to 6 mg may be given intramuscularly daily in severe psychoses. A suggested initial dose for use in children is 1 mg by mouth once or twice daily.

For the control of nausea and vomiting the usual dose by mouth is 1 or 2 mg twice daily; up to 6 mg daily may be given in divided doses.

Doses of 1 or 2 mg twice daily have also been used for non-psychotic emotional disturbances, such as anxiety and tension. In general, however, phenothiazines are only suitable for such purposes in resistant conditions, where more appropriate agents, such as the benzodiazepines (see Diazepam, p.731) have proved ineffective. If their use is judged to be necessary treatment should be directed at low dosages given on a short-term basis.

Trifluoperazine should be given in reduced dosage to elderly patients.

ANXIETY. Trifluoperazine was less effective than chlordiazepoxide in the treatment of 126 nonpsychotic patients with anxiety in a placebo-controlled study. Failure of treatment with trifluoperazine was considered to be due to the large number of patients who withdrew from the study because of side-effects which included drowsiness, akathisia, excitement and diarrhoea.— B. L. Weiss *et al.*, *Curr. ther. Res.*, 1977, *22*, 635.

CHOLERA SYNDROME. The diarrhoea of a patient with pancreatic cholera syndrome responded dramatically to trifluoperazine.— M. Donowitz *et al.*, *Ann. intern. Med.*, 1980, *93*, 284.

Preparations

Trifluoperazine Hydrochloride Injection *(U.S.P.).* A sterile solution in Water for Injections. Potency is expressed in terms of the equivalent amount of trifluoperazine.

Trifluoperazine Hydrochloride Syrup *(U.S.P.).* A syrup containing trifluoperazine hydrochloride. Potency is expressed in terms of the equivalent amount of trifluoperazine. pH 2.0 to 3.2.

Trifluoperazine Hydrochloride Tablets *(U.S.P.).* Potency is expressed in terms of the equivalent amount of trifluoperazine.

Trifluoperazine Hydrochloride Tablets *(B.P.).* Trifluoperazine Tablets. Potency is expressed in terms of the equivalent amount of trifluoperazine.

Proprietary Preparations

Stelazine *(Smith Kline & French, UK). Spansules*, sustained-release capsules, trifluoperazine 2, 10, and 15 mg (as hydrochloride).
Tablets, trifluoperazine 1 and 5 mg.
Oral concentrate, trifluoperazine 10 mg (as hydrochloride)/mL, for dilution before use.
Syrup, trifluoperazine 1 mg (as hydrochloride)/5 mL.
Injection, trifluoperazine 1 mg (as hydrochloride)/mL.

Proprietary Names and Manufacturers

Calmazine *(Protea, Austral.)*; Clinazine *(Canad.)*; Eskazine *(Smith Kline & French, Spain)*; Eskazinyl *(Switz.)*; Flumatets *(Pharmadrug, Ger.)*; Jatroneural *(Röhm, Ger.)*; Modalina *(Maggioni-Winthrop, Ital.)*; Nerolet *(Arg.)*; Novoflurazine *(Novopharm, Canad.)*; Pentazine *(Canad.)*; Solazine *(Horner, Canad.)*; Stelazine *(Smith Kline & French, Austral.; Smith Kline & French, Canad.; Smith Kline & French, S.Afr.; Smith Kline & French, UK; Smith Kline & French, USA)*; Terfluzin *(Austral.; Rhone-Poulenc, Denm.; Rhône-Poulenc, Norw.; Leo Rhodia, Swed.)*; Terfluzine *(Belg.; ICN, Canad.; Théraplix, Fr.; Neth.; Rhone-Poulenc, Switz.)*; Triflurin *(Canad.)*; Tripazine *(Canad.)*.

The following names have been used for multi-ingredient preparations containing trifluoperazine hydrochloride— Amylozine *(Smith Kline & French, UK)*; Expansyl *(Smith Kline & French, UK)*; Parstelin *(Smith Kline & French, Austral.; Smith Kline & French, UK)*; Stelabid *(Smith Kline & French, Austral.; Smith Kline & French, Canad.; Smith Kline & French, UK)*; Steladex *(Smith Kline & French, UK)*.

7121-w

Trifluperidol *(BAN, USAN, rINN).*

McN-JR-2498. 4′-Fluoro-4-[4-hydroxy-4-(3-trifluoromethylphenyl)piperidino]butyrophenone.

$C_{22}H_{23}F_4NO_2$=409.4.

CAS — 749-13-3.

7122-e

Trifluperidol Hydrochloride *(BANM, rINNM).*

$C_{22}H_{23}F_4NO_2,HCl$=445.9.

CAS — 2062-77-3.

Adverse Effects, Treatment, and Precautions

As for the phenothiazines, p.706.

Uses and Administration

Trifluperidol is a butyrophenone with general properties similar to those of haloperidol (p.744), and is used in the treatment of mania and schizophrenia. It is given by mouth as both the base and the hydrochloride in similar doses.

The initial dose is 500 µg daily and the dose is increased at intervals of 3 to 4 days until improvement occurs or a total dose of 6 to 8 mg daily is reached.

Proprietary Preparations

Triperidol *(Lagap, UK). Tablets*, scored, trifluperidol 0.5 and 1 mg.

NOTE. This product was formerly marketed in the *UK* containing trifluperidol hydrochloride; preparations of the hydrochloride are available under this name in some countries.

Proprietary Names and Manufacturers

Psicoperidol *(Denm.; Lusofarmaco, Ital.; Janssen, S.Afr.)*; Triperidol *(Janssen, Belg.; Janssen, Fr.; Janssen, Ger.; Janssen, Neth.; Spain; Lagap, UK)*.

7123-l

Trimetozine *(USAN, rINN).*

Abbott-22370; NSC-62939; PS-2383. 4-(3,4,5-Trimethoxybenzoyl)morpholine.

$C_{14}H_{19}NO_5$=281.3.

CAS — 635-41-6.

Pharmacopoeias. In *Hung.* and *Jug.*

Trimetozine has been used as a sedative and tranquilliser in anxiety states, in usual doses of 0.9 to 1.8 g daily.

Proprietary Names and Manufacturers

Neuristan *(Casasco, Arg.)*; Opalene *(Rhone-Poulenc, Belg.; Théraplix, Fr.)*; Serenitas *(Rocador, Spain)*; Trioxazine *(EGIS, Hung.; Labatec-Pharma, Switz.)*.

7124-y

Tybamate *(BAN, USAN, rINN).*

W713. 2-Methyl-2-propyltrimethylene butylcarbamate carbamate.

$C_{13}H_{26}N_2O_4$=274.4.

CAS — 4268-36-4.

Tybamate is a carbamate with general properties similar to those of meprobamate (p.750) which has been used in the treatment of anxiety and tension states.

Proprietary Names and Manufacturers

Tybatran *(Robins, USA)*.

7125-j

Valnoctamide *(USAN, rINN).*
McN-X-181; NSC-32363. 2-Ethyl-3-methylvaleramide.
$C_8H_{17}NO=143.2$.

CAS — 4171-13-5.

Valnoctamide has been given in doses of 400 to 800 mg daily in 2 or 3 divided doses for anxiety and tension states.

Proprietary Names and Manufacturers
Nirvanil *(Clin Midy, Fr.; Midy, Ital.; Sanofi Midy, Neth.; Sodip, Switz.).*

17026-b

Veralipride *(rINN).*
N-[(1-Allyl-2-pyrrolidinyl)methyl]-5-sulphamoyl-2-veratramide.
$C_{17}H_{25}N_3O_5S=383.5$.

CAS — 66644-81-3.

Veralipride is reported to possess neuroleptic properties. It has been used in the treatment of cardiovascular and psychological symptoms associated with menopause.

Proprietary Names and Manufacturers
Accional *(Fides, Spain)*; Agradil *(Vita, Ital.)*; Agréal *(Delagrange, Fr.; Delagrange, Spain)*; Faltium *(Prodes, Spain)*; Veralipril *(Midy, Ital.).*

4076-x

Vinylbitone *(BAN).*
Butyvinal; Vinylbital *(rINN)*; Vinymalum. 5-(1-Methylbutyl)-5-vinylbarbituric acid.
$C_{11}H_{16}N_2O_3=224.3$.

CAS — 2430-49-1.

Vinylbitone is a barbiturate and shares the general properties of the group (see p.706). It has been used as a hypnotic in the short-term management of insomnia in doses of 100 to 200 mg at night. It has also been given rectally as suppositories.

Proprietary Names and Manufacturers
Bykonox *(Byk, Belg.; Byk, Neth.)*; Optanox *(Valpan, Fr.)*; Speda *(Byk Gulden, Ger.; Byk Gulden, Switz.)*; Suppoptanox *(Valpan, Fr.).*

14031-d

Zopiclone *(BAN, rINN).*

27267-RP. 6-(5-Chloro-2-pyridyl)-6,7-dihydro-7-oxo-5*H*-pyrrolo[3,4-*b*]pyrazin-5-yl 4-methylpiperazine-1-carboxylate.
$C_{17}H_{17}ClN_6O_3=388.8$.

CAS — 43200-80-2.

Dependence, Adverse Effects, Treatment, and Precautions

As for the benzodiazepines, p.706.
A bitter taste in the mouth has been reported.

Absorption and Fate

The pharmacokinetics of zopiclone in 11 healthy subjects given 7.5 mg daily for 14 days. Zopiclone was well absorbed with mean peak plasma concentrations of 68 μg per mL 1.4 hours after administration. The decline in plasma-zopiclone concentrations was biexponential, with a mean terminal elimination half-life of 6.5 hours. Approximately 36% of a dose was excreted in urine as the metabolites *N*-desmethylzopiclone and zopiclone *N*-oxide together with small amounts of unchanged zopiclone; the two metabolites had mean elimination half-lives of 11 and 5.8 hours respectively, and excretion of drug and metabolites was essentially complete 48 hours after the final dose.— G. W. Houghton *et al., Int. J. clin. Pharmac. Ther. Toxic.*, 1985, *23*, 97.

PREGNANCY AND THE NEONATE. *Lactation.* Zopiclone was distributed into breast milk in 12 lactating women in concentrations approximately half those in plasma. The calculated dose that would be received by a neonate was 3.3 μg, which in a 3- kg child was equivalent to about 1% of the adult dose.— I. Matheson *et al., Br. J. clin. Pharmac.*, 1985, *20*, 290P.

Uses and Administration

Zopiclone is a cyclopyrrolone which is reported to have similar sedative, anxiolytic, muscle relaxant, and anticonvulsant properties to those of the benzodiazepines (see Diazepam, p.731).
It is used as a hypnotic in the short-term management of insomnia, in usual doses of 7.5 mg by mouth.

A review of zopiclone. The usual dose for the acute treatment of insomnia in adults is 7.5 mg; greater doses cause increased side-effects without improved hypnotic effect, although 10 to 15 mg of zopiclone may be of benefit in some treatment groups such as psychiatric inpatients. No dose reduction is required in treating the elderly unless hepatic or renal function are impaired. In clinical studies zopiclone has proved generally as effective as the benzodiazepines in the short-term treatment of chronic insomnia, or for pre-operative sleeplessness. The drug is well-tolerated, and because of its short half-life causes less 'morning-after' drowsiness and fatigue than longer-acting hypnotics, and minimal residual psychomotor impairment. Rebound phenomena following withdrawal have not proved a serious problem although some evidence of sleep deterioration does exist. The liability for dependence and the likelihood of long-term tolerance remain to be established. Although zopiclone also has anxiolytic, anticonvulsant, and muscle relaxant properties these are less marked in comparison with the benzodiazepines, due in part to its short duration of action, and it appears to find better use as a hypnotic.— K. L. Goa and R. C. Heel, *Drugs*, 1986, *32*, 48.

ADMINISTRATION. Results in 9 healthy subjects given zopiclone indicated a significant delay in onset of action when the drug was taken in the supine, as opposed to the standing, position; this was associated with a prolongation of more than 20 minutes in the lag time before absorption began. In order to obtain a rapid and complete hypnotic effect from zopiclone the tablet should be swallowed in the standing position.— K. S. Channer *et al., Br. J. clin. Pharmac.*, 1984, *18*, 879.

ADMINISTRATION IN HEPATIC INSUFFICIENCY. A study of the pharmacokinetics of zopiclone in cirrhosis. Zopiclone was given in a dose of 7.5 mg to 7 cirrhotic patients and 8 healthy subjects; a further 2 cirrhotic patients received 3.75 mg. Mean peak plasma concentrations were similar in healthy subjects and those with liver failure following equivalent doses but time to peak plasma concentration was significantly delayed in cirrhotics at 4 hours as compared to 2 hours in the healthy subjects. Elimination was greatly prolonged in cirrhotic patients, in whom the mean plasma half-life was 8.53 compared to 3.50 hours. The CNS-depressant effects of zopiclone were also delayed in the cirrhotic patients in a way consistent with the pharmacokinetic changes. There was also some evidence of an increased response in these patients. Caution should be exercised in administering zopiclone to patients with severe hepatic disease.— G. Parker and C. J. C. Roberts, *Br. J. clin. Pharmac.*, 1983, *16*, 259.

HYPNOTIC EFFECT. Comparisons with triazolam: C. P. Venter *et al., Curr. ther. Res.*, 1986, *40*, 1062 (equivalent in 41 geriatric patients); E. Autret *et al., Eur. J. clin. Pharmac.*, 1987, *31*, 621 (superior to triazolam in a crossover study in 121 patients).

Proprietary Names and Manufacturers

Immovane *(Thèraplix, Fr.).*

2479-d

Zotepine *(rINN).*
2-[(8-Chlorodibenzo[*b,f*]-thiepin-10-yl)oxy]-*N,N*-dimethylethylamine.
$C_{18}H_{18}ClNOS=331.9$.

CAS — 26615-21-4.

Zotepine is a neuroleptic which is also reported to possess antidepressant properties. It has been given in doses of 75 to 150 mg daily.

Proprietary Names and Manufacturers
Lodopin *(Fujisawa, Jpn).*

12014-g

Zuclopenthixol *(BAN, rINN).*

AY-62021 (clopenthixol); *Z*-Clopenthixol; N-746 (clopenthixol); NSC-64087 (clopenthixol). (*Z*)-2-{4-[3-(2-Chloro-10*H*-dibenzo[*b,e*]thiin-10-ylidene)propyl]piperazin-1-yl}ethanol.
$C_{22}H_{25}ClN_2OS=401.0$.

CAS — 53772-83-1 (zuclopenthixol); 982-24-1 (clopenthixol).

NOTE. Clopenthixol (the racemic mixture) is *USAN.*

7027-l

Zuclopenthixol Decanoate *(BANM, rINNM).*

$C_{32}H_{43}ClN_2O_2S=555.2$.

7028-y

Zuclopenthixol Hydrochloride *(BANM, rINNM).*

Zuclopenthixol dihydrochloride.
$C_{22}H_{25}ClN_2OS,2HCl=473.9$.

CAS — 633-59-0.

Zuclopenthixol hydrochloride 11.8 mg is approximately equivalent to 10 mg of zuclopenthixol.

STABILITY. The photochemical stability of *cis* and *trans* isomers of tricyclic neuroleptic drugs, including clopenthixol.— A. Li Wan Po and W. J. Irwin, *J. Pharm. Pharmac.*, 1980, *32*, 25.

Adverse Effects, Treatment, and Precautions

As for the phenothiazines, p.706.

Absorption and Fate

For an account of the absorption and fate of a thioxanthene, see Flupenthixol, p.738.

Uses and Administration

Zuclopenthixol is a thioxanthene with general properties similar to the phenothiazine, chlorpromazine (p.724). Zuclopenthixol is adminstered as the hydrochloride usually by mouth or as the longer-acting decanoate by deep intramuscular injection. Doses of the hydrochloride are expressed in terms of the base, and of the decanoate in terms of the ester.
The usual dose of the hydrochloride for the treatment of psychoses is the equivalent of 20 to 50 mg of the base daily in divided doses; in severe schizophrenia up to 150 mg daily has been given. It has also been given intramuscularly.
The long-acting decanoate should be given by deep intramuscular injection in an initial test dose of 100 mg as 0.5 mL of a 20% oily solution. According to the patient's response over the following week, this may be followed by doses of 200 to 400 mg every 2 to 4 weeks. Shorter dosage intervals or greater amounts may be required according to the patient's response. If doses greater than 400 mg are considered necessary they should be divided between 2 separate injection sites or, alternatively, given as a 50% oily solution. In patients already taking antipsychotic agents by mouth, the dosage should be gradually reduced on starting zuclopenthixol decanoate injections. In those being transferred from depot injections of phenothiazines, zuclopenthixol decanoate 200 mg is considered to be equivalent to fluphenazine decanoate 25 mg. Patients displaying agitation or aggression during therapy with flupenthixol may be better controlled by zuclopenthixol; zuclopenthixol decanoate 200 mg is considered to be equivalent to flupenthixol decanoate 40 mg.

For a symposium on the actions and uses of zuclopenthixol, see A. Gravem and K. Elgen, *Acta psychiat. scand.*, 1981, *64, Suppl.* 294, pp.1-77.

Proprietary Preparations

Clopixol *(Lundbeck, UK)*. *Tablets*, zuclopenthixol 2, 10, and 25 mg (as hydrochloride).
Injection (oily), zuclopenthixol decanoate 200 mg/mL, in ampoules of 1 mL and vials of 10 mL.
Injection (Clopixol-Conc.), (oily), zuclopenthixol decanoate 500 mg/mL, in ampoules of 1 mL.

Proprietary Names and Manufacturers

Ciatyl *(Tropon, Ger.)*; Cisordinol *(Lundbeck, Denm.; Lundbeck, Norw.; Lundbeck, Swed.)*; Cisordinol-acutard *(Lundbeck, Denm.)*; Clopixol *(Lundbeck, Switz.; Lundbeck, UK)*; Clopixol Depot *(Lundbeck, S.Afr.; Lundbeck, Switz.)*; Sedanxol *(Tropon, Ger.)*; Sordinol *(Belg., Denm.; Bracco, Ital.; Neth.; Norw.; S.Afr.; Swed., Switz.)*.

Astringents

290-k

Astringents precipitate proteins and when applied to mucous membranes or to damaged skin they form a superficial protective layer and are not usually absorbed.
They are used to harden the skin, to check exudative secretions and minor haemorrhage, for mouth ulcers, hyperhidrosis, and for haemorrhoids. Some have been taken internally for diarrhoea.
Compounds that have astringent as well as other properties may be found under Dermatological Agents, p.916, Gastro-intestinal Agents, p.1073, and Haemostatics, p.1131.

293-x

Albumin Tannate
Albutannin; Tannin Albuminate.
A compound of tannin with albumin.

CAS — 9006-52-4.

Pharmacopoeias. In *Arg., Aust., Cz., Hung., Jpn, Nord., Pol., Port.,* and *Span. Rus. P.* includes Thealbin, a compound of tannins from tea leaves with protein.

Albumin tannate has been used as an astringent in the treatment of diarrhoea.

Proprietary Names and Manufacturers
Tannalbin *(Schering, Austral.; Nordmark, Ger.; Knoll, Switz.).*

294-r

Alum *(BAN).*
Alaun; Allume; Aluin; Alumbre; Alumen; Aluminium Kalium Sulfuricum; Aluminium Potassium Sulphate; Alun; Potash Alum; Potassium Alum *(USAN).* Potassium aluminium sulphate dodecahydrate.
$KAl(SO_4)_2,12H_2O=474.4$.

CAS — 7784-24-9.

Pharmacopoeias. In *Arg., Aust., Belg., Br., Chin., Cz., Egypt., Eur., Fr., Ger., Hung., It., Jpn, Jug., Mex., Neth., Nord., Pol., Port., Roum., Span., Swiss,* and *U.S. U.S.* also includes ammonia alum (Ammonium Alum). *Arg., Belg., Hung., Jpn,* and *Span.* also include dried alum.

Colourless, transparent, odourless, crystalline masses or a granular powder.
B.P. **solubilities** are: soluble 1 in 7.5 of water, 1 in 0.3 of boiling water, and 1 in 3 of glycerol; practically insoluble in alcohol. A 10% solution in water has a pH of 3.0 to 3.5. **Store** in well-closed containers.

Adverse Effects
Large doses of alum are irritant and may be corrosive; gum necrosis and gastro-intestinal haemorrhage have occurred. Adverse effects on muscle and kidneys have been reported.

For a report of ileus in 2 patients after treatment with alum for bladder haemorrhage, see under Uses, below.

Uses and Administration
Alum precipitates proteins and is a powerful astringent. Alum, either as a solid or as a solution, may be used as a haemostatic. Dilute solutions have been used as mouth-washes or gargles. Recent applications include bladder irrigations with a 1% solution.
A 2% solution of alum has been applied for hyperhydrosis. Stronger solutions (5 to 10%) may be used to harden the epidermis.
Alum is also used as a mordant in the dyeing industry.

The use of alum for water purification during a cholera outbreak. The acidity of the alum-treated water was considered to be responsible for its vibriocidal activity.— M. U. Khan *et al.* (letter), *Lancet,* 1984, *2,* 1032.

The use of alum solution 1% irrigation for the control of massive bladder haemorrhage was found to be simple, effective, and without discernible side-effects (E.B. Ostroff and O.W. Chenault, *J. Urol., Baltimore,* 1982, *128,* 929), although a later study noted side-effects of ileus, suprapubic discomfort, and pyrexia (C. Kennedy *et al., Br. J. Urol.,* 1984, *56,* 673). Benefit may only be transient (A.K. Goel *et al., J. Urol., Baltimore,* 1985, *133,* 956).

Proprietary Names and Manufacturers
The following names have been used for multi-ingredient preparations containing alum— Cordocel *(Wigglesworth, UK);* Cordocel-H *(Wigglesworth, UK).*

296-d

Aluminium Acetate
Aluminum Acetate.
$C_6H_9AlO_6=204.1$.

CAS — 139-12-8.

Aluminium acetate is prepared from aluminium sulphate and acetic acid. The *B.P.* includes Aluminium Acetate Ear Drops which correspond to a solution of aluminium acetotartrate in that they are prepared from aluminium sulphate with the aid of acetic acid and tartaric acid. The *U.S.P.* includes Aluminum Acetate Topical Solution which is prepared from Aluminum Subacetate Topical Solution and glacial acetic acid; it does not involve tartaric acid.

Aluminium acetate solution is astringent. The solution is used as ear-drops; it has been used in dressings and as an astringent lotion. Aluminium subacetate (basic aluminium acetate) is used similarly.

Preparations

Aluminium Acetate Cream Oily *(A.P.F.).* Burow's Cream. Aluminium acetate solution (*A.P.F.*) 5 mL, zinc oxide 20 g, wool fat 25 g, arachis oil 25 mL, freshly boiled and cooled water 27 mL. Makes 100 g.

Aluminium Acetate Ear Drops *(A.P.F.).* Aurist. Alumin. Acet. Aluminium acetate solution (*A.P.F.*) 60 mL, freshly boiled and cooled water to 100 mL. The ear-drops should be freshly prepared.

Aluminium Acetate Ear Drops *(B.P.).* Aluminium Acetate Solution; Burow's Solution. A solution prepared from aluminium sulphate 22.5 g, acetic acid (33 per cent) 25 mL, tartaric acid 4.5 g, calcium carbonate 10 g, and water 75 mL. Store at a temperature not exceeding 25° in well-filled containers.
Burow's. Solution is also used in some countries as a synonym for Aluminium Acetotartrate Solution and for aluminium subacetate solutions.
A.P.F. uses this formula for aluminium acetate solution; a diluted form is included as Aluminium Acetate Ear Drops (*A.P.F.*).

Aluminium Acetate Lotion Aqueous *(A.P.F.).* Burow's Lotion. Aluminium acetate solution (*A.P.F.*) 5 mL, freshly boiled and cooled water to 100 mL. It should be freshly prepared and used within 7 days.

Aluminium Acetate Lotion Oily *(A.P.F.).* Burow's Emulsion. Aluminium acetate solution (*A.P.F.*) 25 mL, arachis oil 25 mL, zinc cream oily, to 100 g.

Aluminum Acetate Topical Solution *(U.S.P.).* Aluminum subacetate topical solution (*U.S.P.*) 54.5, glacial acetic acid 1.5, water to 100, all by vol.; it may be stabilised by the addition of not more than 0.6% of boric acid. pH 3.6 to 4.4. Store in airtight containers.

Aluminum Subacetate Topical Solution *(U.S.P.).* Aluminium sulphate 14.5 g, acetic acid (36 to 37% w/w) 16 mL, calcium carbonate 7 g, water to 100 mL; it may be stabilised by the addition of not more than 0.9% of boric acid. pH 3.8 to 4.6. Store in airtight containers.

Proprietary Names and Manufacturers of Aluminium Acetates
Acid Mantle *(Miles, Canad.; Dorsey Laboratories, USA);* Alsol *(Athenstaedt, Ger.);* Borofair *(Pharmafair, USA);* Domeboro *(Miles Pharmaceuticals, USA);* Eddikesur lerjord *(DAK, Denm.);* Eucéta *(Wander, Switz.);* Euceta *(Neth.);* Osti-Derm *(Pedinol, USA);* Pedi-Boro *(Pedinol, USA).*

The following names have been used for multi-ingredient preparations containing aluminium acetates— Xyloproct *(Astra, Austral.; Astra, UK).*

297-n

Aluminium Chloride
Aluminium Chloratum; Aluminum Chloride *(USAN);* Cloreto de Aluminio; Cloruro de Aluminio.
$AlCl_3,6H_2O=241.4$.

CAS — 7446-70-0 (anhydrous); 7784-13-6 (hexahydrate).

Pharmacopoeias. In *Arg., Hung., Jug., Swiss,* and *U.S.*

Soluble 1 in about 1 of water and 1 in 4 of alcohol. **Store** in airtight containers.

Adverse Effects
Aluminium chloride may cause irritation especially if applied to damp skin; this is attributed to the formation of hydrochloric acid.

Axillary granulomata requiring excision in 2 patients, associated with the use, after axillary shaving, of an antiperspirant spray of talc coated with aluminium trichloride. Examination showed the presence of aluminium and of talc.— S. Williams and A. J. Freemont, *Br. med. J.,* 1984, *288,* 1651.

Uses and Administration
Aluminium chloride is used in a 20% alcoholic solution as an antiperspirant in the treatment of hyperhidrosis. It is applied to dry skin usually at bedtime and is washed off in the morning before the sweat glands are fully active. Its mode of action is not clear since it does have an astringent action and has been reported to have a direct action on eccrine sweat glands.

HYPERHIDROSIS. A review of aluminium chloride in hyperhidrosis.— J. W. White, *Mayo Clin. Proc.,* 1986, *61,* 951.

A solution of aluminium chloride 20% in dehydrated alcohol was effective in relieving axillary hyperhidrosis in 64 of 65 patients. The solution was applied at night to the dry axilla, the axilla being washed with soap and water in the morning. After a week, applications were made only when necessary, usually every 7 to 21 days. Irritation was the only side-effect. Occlusion was not necessary.— K. T. Scholes *et al., Br. med. J.,* 1978, *2,* 84. Disappointing results in 38 patients with axillary hyperhidrosis, waiting for plastic surgery, treated with aluminium chloride 20%; by the end of the sixth month of treatment 26 patients had requested surgery. The results indicated that there is a group of patients with axillary hyperhidrosis who either cannot tolerate aluminium chloride or will not respond to it.— C. R. W. Rayner *et al., ibid.,* 1980, *280,* 1168.

Axillary skin biopsy was performed on 15 patients with axillary hyperhidrosis who had been applying aluminium chloride 15 or 20% in 2% [aqueous] solution of methylcellulose for at least 6 months. The apocrine sweat glands were histologically normal but the eccrine sweat glands showed structural changes of varying severity; 6 patients showing marked disintegration of glandular structures.— E. Hölzle and O. Braun-Falco, *Br. J. Derm.,* 1984, *110,* 399.

Proprietary Preparations

Anhydrol Forte *(Dermal Laboratories, UK). Application,* aluminium chloride 20% in an alcoholic basis.

Driclor *(Stiefel, UK). Application,* aluminium chloride 20% in an alcoholic basis.

Proprietary Names and Manufacturers
Aluminiumklorid *(DAK, Denm.);* Aluwets *(Stiefel, USA);* Anhydrol Forte *(Dermal Laboratories, UK);* Basoklin *(Basoderm, Denm.);* Driclor *(Stiefel, Austral.; Stiefel, UK);* Drysol *(Person & Covey, USA);* Ercoderm *(Denm.);* Hidrosol *(Alcon, Austral.);* Xerac AC *(Person & Covey, USA).*

298-h

Aluminium Chlorohydrate
Aluminium Chlorhydrate; Aluminum Chlorhydroxide; Aluminum Chlorohydrate *(USAN);* Aluminum Hydroxychloride; Basic Aluminium Chloride.
$Al_2(OH)_5Cl(+xH_2O)$.

CAS — 12042-91-0 (anhydrous).

Aluminium chlorohydrate is used as an astringent and antiperspirant. It is used similarly to aluminium chloride in hyperhidrosis and may be less irritant.

Preparations

Aluminium Chlorohydrate and Salicylic Acid Dusting Powder *(A.P.F.)*. Aluminium chlorohydrate, of commerce, 5 g, salicylic acid 3 g, purified talc, sterilised, 92 g.

Aluminium Chlorohydrate Dusting Powder *(A.P.F.)*. Aluminium chlorohydrate, of commerce, 2.5 g, purified talc, sterilised, 97.5 g.

Aluminium Chlorohydrate Paste *(A.P.F.)*. Colostomy Paste. Aluminium chlorohydrate, of commerce, 4 g, zinc oxide 20 g, dimethicone '350' 10 g, compound benzoin tincture 12.5 mL, emulsifying ointment to 100 g.

Proprietary Preparations

Chiron Barrier Cream *(Simcare, UK)*. *Cream*, aluminium chlorohydrate 2%.

Hyperdrol *(BritCair, UK)*. *Cream*, aluminium chlorohydrate 19%.
Roll-on, aluminium chlorohydrate 19%.

Proprietary Names and Manufacturers

Chiron Barrier Cream *(Simcare, UK)*; Dermun *(Basoderm, Denm.)*; Gelsica *(Sauter, Switz.)*; Hiposudol *(Vinas, Spain)*; Hyperdrol *(BritCair, UK)*; Phosphonorm *(Nefro-Pharma, Ger.)*; Primamed *(Schulke & Mayr, Ger.)*; Ronati *(Basotherm, Switz.)*.

The following names have been used for multi-ingredient preparations containing aluminium chlorohydrate—Breezee *(Pedinol, USA)*; Medrol Acne Lotion *(Upjohn, Austral.; Upjohn, Canad.)*; Medrone Acne Lotion *(Upjohn, UK)*; Neo-Medrol *(Upjohn, Austral.)*; Neo-Medrone Acne Lotion *(Upjohn, UK)*; Pedi-Dri *(Pedinol, USA)*; Pedi-Pro *(Pedinol, USA)*.

301-b

Aluminium Sulphate *(BAN)*.

Aluminii Sulfas; Aluminium Sulfuricum; Aluminium Trisulphate; Aluminum Sulfate *(USAN)*.
$Al_2(SO_4)_3,xH_2O$=342.1 (anhydrous).

CAS — 10043-01-3 (anhydrous); 17927-65-0 (hydrate).

Pharmacopoeias. In *Aust., Belg., Br., Eur., Fr., Ger., Hung., Ind., It., Jug., Neth., Nord., Pol., Port., Roum., Span., Swiss, Turk.,* and *U.S.*

Colourless or white odourless lustrous crystals or crystalline masses. The *B.P.* specifies 51 to 59% of $Al_2(SO_4)_3$; the *U.S.P.* specifies 54 to 59% of $Al_2(SO_4)_3$.
B.P. **solubilities** are: soluble in water; freely soluble in hot water; practically insoluble in alcohol. *U.S.P.* solubilities are: soluble 1 in 1 of water. A 2% solution in water has a pH of 2.5 to 4.0. **Store** in airtight containers.

Aluminium sulphate has an action similar to that of alum (see p.777) but is more astringent. A saturated solution has been used as a mild caustic. Solutions containing 5 to 10% have been used as astringent applications to ulcers and to mucous surfaces.
Aluminium sulphate is also used in the preparation of aluminium acetate solutions.

No effect of aluminium sulphate (20%) (Stingose) topically in wasp stings.— L. J. McLeod *et al.* (letter), *Med. J. Aust.*, 1986, *144*, 220.

Proprietary Names and Manufacturers

Stingose *(Hamilton, Austral.)*.

302-v

Ammonium Alum *(USAN)*.

Ammonia Alum. Ammonium aluminium sulphate dodecahydrate.
$NH_4Al(SO_4)_2,12H_2O$=453.3.

CAS — 7784-25-0 (anhydrous); 7784-26-1 (dodecahydrate).

Pharmacopoeias. In *U.S. U.S.* also includes Potassium Alum.

Colourless, transparent, odourless, crystalline masses or a granular powder. **Soluble** 1 in 7 of water, 1 in 0.5 of boiling water.

Ammonium alum has the actions and uses of alum (p.777).

303-g

Arnica Flower

Arnica; Arnicae Flos; Wolfsbane.

NOTE. Wolfsbane is also used as a common name for aconite.

Pharmacopoeias. In *Aust., Belg., Braz., Fr., Ger., Pol., Port., Roum., Span.,* and *Swiss. Aust.* also includes arnica root.

The dried flowerheads of *Arnica montana* (Compositae).

Arnica flower is irritant to mucous membranes and when ingested has produced severe symptoms including gastro-intestinal and nervous system disturbances, both tachycardia and bradycardia, and collapse. Tincture of arnica may cause dermatitis when applied to the skin of sensitive persons. Preparations of arnica flower and arnica root have been used as astringents for topical application to unbroken skin; they were not considered suitable for internal use.
Arnica is used in homoeopathic medicine.

306-s

Catechu *(BAN)*.

Gambier; Gambir; Pale Catechu.

CAS — 8001-48-7; 8001-76-1 (black catechu); 154-23-4 [(+)-catechin].

Pharmacopoeias. In *Br.* and *Jpn. B.P.* also allows Powdered Catechu. Catechu of *Chin. P.* and *Port. P.* is Black Catechu from *Acacia catechu* (Leguminosae).

A dried aqueous extract of the leaves and young shoots of *Uncaria gambier* (Rubiaceae) usually occurring as dull pale greyish-brown to dark reddish-brown cubes or pale brown powder.

Catechu is an astringent and is given as an ingredient of Aromatic Chalk with Opium Mixture in the treatment of diarrhoea.

Preparations

Catechu Tincture *(B.P.)*. Tinctura Catechu. Catechu 1 in 5 with cinnamon 1 in 20; prepared by maceration with alcohol (45%).

307-w

Chromium Trioxide

Anhídrido Crómico; Chromic Acid; Chromic Anhydride.
CrO_3=99.99.

CAS — 1333-82-0.

Pharmacopoeias. In *Mex., Nord., Port.,* and *Span.*

CAUTION. *Chromium trioxide is a powerful oxidising agent and is liable to explode in contact with small quantities of alcohol, ether, glycerol, and other organic substances.*

Solutions of chromium trioxide are corrosive, acting by oxidation. Repeated contact with chromium and its salts may cause eczematous dermatitis with oedema, particularly in hypersensitive persons and can also cause deep perforating ulcers known as 'chrome holes'. If inhaled, chromic dusts cause rhinitis and painless ulcers which may perforate the nasal septum; inhalation may cause severe lung damage, liver injury, and inflammation of the eyes. There may also be involvement of the central nervous system and there is an increased risk of lung cancer. Hexavalent chromium compounds are more dangerous than di- or trivalent compounds.
Acute symptoms of poisoning from the ingestion of chromium salts include intense thirst, dizziness, abdominal pain with vomiting, anuria or oliguria, and peripheral vascular collapse. Kidney damage may lead to fatal uraemia.
Treatment is symptomatic; dimercaprol has been tried. Protective measures should be taken when handling or working with chromium and its salts.
In Great Britain the recommended exposure limit of chromium (VI) compounds (as Cr) is 0.05 mg per m^3 (long-term). In the *US* the permissible and recommended exposure limits are 0.1 mg of chromates per m^3 and 0.025 mg of noncarcinogenic Cr (VI) per m^3 respectively.
Chromium trioxide was formerly used as a caustic and astringent.

Fatal poisoning with sodium dichromate. Ineffective treatment included haemodialysis and dimercaprol.— E. N. Ellis *et al.*, *J. Toxicol. clin. Toxicol.*, 1982, *19*, 249.

308-e

Cowberry Leaf

Red Whortleberry Leaf; Vitis Idaeae Folium.

Pharmacopoeias. In *Aust., Pol.,* and *Roum.*

The dried leaves of the cowberry, *Vaccinium vitis-idaea* (Ericaceae).

Cowberry leaf has astringent properties and has been used as a domestic remedy for diarrhoea.

309-l

Ellagic Acid *(rINN)*.

Benzoaric Acid. 4,4′,5,5′,6,6′-Hexahydroxydiphenic acid dilactone dihydrate; 2,3,7,8-Tetrahydroxy[1]benzopyrano[5,4,3-*cde*][1]benzopyran-5,10-dione dihydrate.
$C_{14}H_6O_8,2H_2O$=338.2.

CAS — 476-66-4 (anhydrous).

A tannin derivative which occurs free or combined in galls; it has been isolated from the juice of species of *Eucalyptus* (Myrtaceae) or it may be prepared synthetically.

Ellagic acid is astringent and has been used topically as a haemostatic.

310-v

Gall

Aleppo Galls; Blue Galls; Galla; Galläpfel; Galls; Noix de Galle; Nutgall.

Pharmacopoeias. In *Aust., Cz., Egypt.,* and *Pol.*

Excrescences on the twigs of *Quercus infectoria* (Fagaceae), resulting from the stimulus given to the tissues of the young twigs by the development of the larvae of the gall-wasp, *Adleria gallae-tinctoriae*(=*Cynips gallae-tinctoriae*) (Cynipidae). It contains about 50 to 70% of gallotannic acid.

Gall is an astringent and has been used in ointments and suppositories for the treatment of haemorrhoids. It is a source of tannic acid.

311-g

Hamamelis

Amamelide; Hamamelidis Folia; Hamamelis Leaves; Witch Hazel Leaves.

Pharmacopoeias. In *Arg., Belg., Egypt., Fr., It., Port., Roum., Span.,* and *Swiss.* Also in *B.P.C. 1973.* Hamamelis Water *B.P.C. 1973* is prepared from the twigs of *Hamamelis virginiana.*

The dried leaves of *Hamamelis virginiana* (Hamamelidaceae) containing tannins, gallic acid, a bitter principle, and a trace of volatile oil.

Hamamelis has astringent properties. It is used in ointments and suppositories in the treatment of haemorrhoids. Hamamelis water is used as a cooling application and has been applied as a haemostatic.
Hamamelis bark has also been used in the form of a tincture as an astringent and haemostatic. It is used in homoeopathy under the name Hamamelis.

Preparations

Hamamelis and Zinc Oxide Suppositories *(B.P.C. 1973)*. Suppositories containing hamamelis dry extract and zinc oxide. They are prepared with theobroma oil or other suitable fatty basis. About 1.5 g of hamamelis dry extract and 5 g of zinc oxide each displace 1 g of theobroma oil. Store in a cool place.

Hamamelis Dry Extract *(B.P.C. 1973)*. Ext. Hamam. Sicc.; Hamamelis Extract. A dry extract prepared by percolation with alcohol (45%). Store in a cool place in airtight containers.

Hamamelis Liquid Extract *(B.P.C. 1973)*. 1 in 1; prepared by percolation with alcohol (45%).

Hamamelis Ointment *(B.P.C. 1973).* Hamamelis liquid extract 1 g, wool fat 5 g, and yellow soft paraffin 4 g. Store in containers which prevent evaporation.

Hamamelis Suppositories *(B.P.C. 1973).* Suppositories containing hamamelis dry extract. They are prepared with theobroma oil or other suitable fatty basis. About 1.5 g of hamamelis dry extract displaces 1 g of theobroma oil. Store in a cool place.

Hamamelis Water *(B.P.C. 1973).* A clear liquid prepared by macerating the twigs of *Hamamelis virginiana* in water, distilling, and adjusting the distillate with the appropriate amount of alcohol.

Proprietary Names and Manufacturers of Hamamelis or one of its preparations
Hamasana *(Robugen, Ger.)*; Tucks *(Parke, Davis, USA).*

The following names have been used for multi-ingredient preparations containing hamamelis or one of its preparations—Hemocane *(Key, Austral.)*

314-s

Hypericum

Millepertuis; St. John's Wort.

CAS — 548-04-9 (hypericin).

Pharmacopoeias. In *Cz., Pol., Roum.,* and *Rus.*

The flowering tops of the common St. John's wort, *Hypericum perforatum* (Hypericaceae).

An infusion of hypericum has been used as an astringent and diuretic.
The herb contains a red pigment, hypericin, which causes photosensitisation. *Animals* are also sensitive and hypericum poses problems in agriculture.
Hypericum is used in homoeopathic medicine.

317-l

Oak Bark

Écorce de Chêne; Eichenrinde; Quercus; Quercus Cortex.

Pharmacopoeias. In *Aust., Cz., Hung., Jug., Nord., Pol., Port., Rus.,*and *Swiss.*

The dried bark from the smaller branches and young stems of the common oak,*Quercus robur* (=*Q. pedunculata*), or the durmast oak, *Q. petraea* (=*Q. sessiliflora*) (Fagaceae).

Oak bark contains quercitannic acid. It has astringent properties and was formerly used for haemorrhoids and as a gargle.

318-y

Potassium Chlorate

Kalium Chloricum; Potassii Chloras.
$KClO_3$=122.5.

CAS — 3811-04-9.

Pharmacopoeias. In *Belg., Port., Span.,* and *Swiss.* Also in *B.P.C. 1973.*

Colourless, odourless or almost odourless, crystals or white powder. **Soluble** 1 in 14 of water, 1 in 2 of boiling water, and 1 in 30 of glycerol; practically insoluble in alcohol. A 5% solution in water has a pH of about 7.

CAUTION. *Potassium chlorate is unstable and, in contact with organic or readily oxidisable substances such as charcoal, phosphorus, or sulphur it is liable to explode especially if heated or subjected to friction or percussion. It should not be allowed to come into contact with matches or surface containing phosphorus compounds. Potassium chlorate has been used for the illicit preparation of explosives or fireworks; care is required with its supply.*

Potassium chlorate has been used as an astringent, usually as a mouth-wash or gargle. Concentrated solutions are irritant. Acute poisoning from ingestion requires prompt symptomatic treatment. Symptoms include nausea, vomiting, diarrhoea, abdominal pain, haemolytic anaemia, haemorrhage, methaemoglobinaemia (not responsive to methylene blue), and renal failure. There may be liver damage and central effects with convulsions and coma.

Preparations

Potassium Chlorate and Phenol Gargle *(B.P.C. 1973).* Contains in each 100 mL, potassium chlorate 3 g, liquefied phenol 1.5 mL, blue colouring, water to 100 mL. It should be diluted with 10 times its volume of warm water before use. Protect from light.

319-j

Rhatany Root *(BAN).*

Krameria; Krameria Root; Ratanhiae Radix.

Pharmacopoeias. In *Arg., Aust., Belg., Br., Cz., Egypt., Eur., Fr., Ger., Hung., Mex., Neth., Port., Roum., Span.,* and *Swiss.*
Arg. and *Mex.* allow both *K. triandra* and *K. argentea; Span.* allows *K. triandra* and other species.
Br. also describes Powdered Rhatany Root.

The dried root of *Krameria triandra* (Krameriaceae), containing not less than 10% tannins. It is known in commerce as Peruvian rhatany.
The powder is reddish brown. **Store** in well-closed containers. Protect from light.

Rhatany root has been used in a wide range of preparations for its astringent properties.

320-q

Sambucus

Elder Flowers; Fleurs de Sureau; Holunderblüten; Sabugueiro; Sambuc.

Pharmacopoeias. In *Aust., Cz., Hung., Pol., Port., Roum.,* and *Swiss.*
Pol. also includes sambucus fruit.

The dried corollas and stamens of the flowers of the elder, *Sambucus nigra* (Caprifoliaceae), together with a proportion of buds, pedicels, and ovaries. **Store** in airtight containers in a cool place. Protect from light.

Sambucus, in the form of elder-flower water, has been used as a vehicle for eye and skin lotions. Elder-flower ointment has been used as a basis for pomades and cosmetic ointments.

A Morbidity and Mortality weekly report on acute gastro-intestinal and neurological symptoms from drinking elderberry juice from the fruits of *Sambucus mexicana.*— *J. Am. med. Ass.,* 1984, *251,* 2075. A comment on gastro-intestinal symptoms from other *Sambucus* species.— *Pharm. J.,* 1984, *1,* 660.

321-p

Sodium Chlorate

Natrium Chloricum; Sodii Chloras.
$NaClO_3$=106.4.

CAS — 7775-09-9.

Store in airtight containers.

CAUTION. As for Potassium Chlorate, above.
Investigations had indicated that technically pure sodium chlorate could explode under intense heat in an enclosed place; it had previously been believed that the chemical had to be contaminated by other substances before it would explode.— *Pharm. J.,* 1979, *1,* 325.

Sodium chlorate closely resembles potassium chlorate above in its properties and was formerly used as an astringent. Its main use is as a weedkiller and it is therefore a common household chemical. Poor storage conditions can lead to explosions.

Storage and Use of Sodium Chlorate, *Guidance Note CS3,* Great Britain, Health and Safety Executive, 1983.

322-s

Tannic Acid *(USAN).*

Acidum Tannicum; Gallotannic Acid; Tanin; Tann. Acid; Tannin.

CAS — 1401-55-4.

Pharmacopoeias. In *Arg., Aust., Belg., Cz., Egypt., Fr., Hung., It., Jpn, Jug., Mex., Neth., Nord., Pol., Port., Rus., Span., Swiss,* and *U.S.*

A tannin usually obtained from nut-galls, the excrescences produced on the young twigs of *Quercus infectoria* and allied species of *Quercus,* from the seed pods of tara (*Caesalpinia spinosa*), or from the nut-galls or leaves of sumac (any of genus *Rhus*).
Commercial grades of tannic acid may contain gallic acid and being less soluble are not suitable for medicinal use.
Yellowish-white or light brown glistening scales, light masses, or an amorphous powder, odourless or with a characteristic odour.
Very **soluble** in water, alcohol, and in acetone; soluble 1 in 1 of warm glycerol; practically insoluble in chloroform, ether, and petroleum spirit. **Store** in airtight containers. Protect from light.

Tannic acid has been used as an astringent for the mucous membrane of the mouth and throat. Suppositories of tannic acid have been used in the treatment of haemorrhoids.
Former uses of tannic acid include its application to burns and its addition to barium sulphate enemas to improve the quality of the pictures in the radiological examination of the colon. Both of these uses were associated with liver toxicity, sometimes fatal. If ingested tannic acid may cause nausea, vomiting, and other gastro-intestinal disturbances. It is metabolised to gallic acid which may cause kidney damage.

Abolition of allergens by tannic acid.— W. F. Green (letter), *Lancet,* 1984, *2,* 160.

The possible role of tannin in oesophageal cancer.— J. F. Morton (letter), *Lancet,* 1987, *2,* 327.

Preparations

Tannic Acid Glycerin *(B.P.C. 1973).* Glycer. Acid. Tannic. Tannic acid 15% w/w in glycerol.

Proprietary Preparations

Phytex *(Pharmax, UK). Paint,* tannic acid 4.89% (as borotannic complex), boric acid 3.12% (as borotannic complex), salicylic acid 1.46%. For fungal infections of the skin and nails.

Proprietary Names and Manufacturers

Tannosynt *(Hermal, Ger.)*; Zilactin *(Zila, USA).*

The following names have been used for multi-ingredient preparations containing tannic acid—Dalidyne *(Dalin, USA)*; Pernomol *(Laboratories for Applied Biology, UK)*; Phytex *(Drug Houses Austral., Austral.; Pharmax, UK)*; SM-33 *(Nicholas, Austral.).*

323-w

Tilia

Fleurs de Tilleul; Flor de Tilo; Lime Flowers; Lindenblüten.

Pharmacopoeias. In *Arg., Aust., Belg., Cz., Egypt., Fr., Ger., Hung., Jug., Pol., Port., Roum., Rus., Span.,* and *Swiss.*

The dried inflorescences, with their attached bracts, of the common lime, *Tilia* × *europaea* (Tiliaceae) and certain other species of *Tilia.*

Tilia is mildly astringent and is reputed to have antispasmodic and diaphoretic properties. Lime-flower 'tea' is a traditional domestic remedy.

Proprietary Names and Manufacturers
Hepamig *(Welcker-Lyster, Canad.).*

324-e

Tormentil Rhizome
Consolda Vermelha; Erect Cinquefoil.

Pharmacopoeias. In *Aust., Cz., Jug., Pol.,* and *Port.*

The dried rhizome of the common tormentil, *Potentilla erecta* (Rosaceae).

Tormentil has been used both internally and externally as an astringent, usually as a tincture.

Beta-adrenoceptor Blocking Agents

6300-v

Beta blockers (beta-adrenoceptor blocking agents or antagonists) are competitive inhibitors of the effects of catecholamines at beta-adrenergic receptor sites (see Sympathomimetics, p.1453). The principal effect of beta blockade is to reduce cardiac activity by diminishing or preventing beta-adrenoceptor stimulation. By reducing the rate and force of contraction of the heart, and decreasing the rate of conduction of impulses through the conducting system, the response of the heart to stress and exercise is reduced. These properties are used in the treatment of angina pectoris to reduce the oxygen consumption and increase the exercise tolerance of the heart. They are used in the treatment of cardiac arrhythmias to block adrenergic stimulation of cardiac pacemaker potentials.

The results of controlled studies suggest that beta blockers reduce the incidence of reinfarction and death after myocardial infarction, and if given sufficiently early may reduce infarct size and development.

The beta blockers are also beneficial in the long-term treatment of hypertension but their mode of action has not yet been fully elucidated. They are often used with thiazide diuretics and do not usually give rise to postural hypotension.

Since beta blockers reduce the responses to the beta-adrenoceptor stimulating effects of adrenaline they are used (in conjunction with an alpha-adrenoceptor blocking agent) in the management of phaeochromocytoma, and they have also been used for the symptomatic relief of catecholamine-provoked tremor in conditions such as anxiety or hyperthyroidism. Some beta blockers have also been found to be effective in the prophylaxis of migraine.

Beta blockers have been shown to reduce intraocular pressure following topical application to the eye, possibly by reducing the production of aqueous humour, and a number of beta blockers have been used to treat open angle glaucoma.

The actions and uses of beta blockers are mainly described under Propranolol Hydrochloride.

An account of beta blockade. The reason that beta-adrenoceptor blocking drugs lower the blood pressure seems to be a property of their beta-receptor inhibitory action. Regardless of associated properties, the presence or absence of membrane-stabilising or sympathomimetic action, a hypotensive effect is seen. A number of suggestions have been made to explain their hypotensive effect, including an effect on the CNS, an adrenergic neurone-blocking action, an anti-renin effect, an effect secondary to the reduced cardiac output, and, finally, a mechanism consequent on resetting the baroreceptors. It may be that a drug with such wide actions as a beta-receptor inhibitory drug may act to lower blood pressure by more than one mechanism. Providing patients are selected properly (excluding those with heart failure and asthma), adverse effects to beta-adrenoceptor blocking drugs are uncommon; severe adverse reactions may occur soon after initiation of therapy, even with small doses, but once therapy has been started, gradual dosage increase is most unlikely to be associated with precipitate adverse reactions. There is evidence that beta-adrenoceptor blocking drugs are of similar potency to adrenergic neurone inhibitory drugs and methyldopa. The beta-adrenoceptor blocking drugs have the advantage of the absence of postural and exercise hypotension, and possible long-term benefits in reducing the manifestations of ischaemic heart disease.— B. N. C. Prichard, *Br. J. clin. Pharmac.*, 1978, *5*, 379.

Choice and Classification of a Beta Blocking Agent

Although the clinical action of beta-adrenoceptor blocking agents seems to be a property of their beta-receptor inhibitory activity, associated properties, such as the presence or absence of cardioselectivity, membrane-stabilising (or local anaesthetic; or quinidine-like) activity, and intrinsic sympathomimetic action (ISA; or partial agonist activity) have been used (initially by J.D. Fitzgerald, *Clin. Pharmac. Ther.*, 1969, *10*, 292, and *Acta Cardiol.*, 1972, *Suppl.* 25, 199) as a basis for their classification. Accordingly, they are divided into non-cardioselective drugs (Division I) and cardioselective drugs (Division II). Both groups are then sub-divided depending on the presence or absence of membrane-stabilising activity and intrinsic sympathomimetic activity. Thus:

Division I, Group I drugs are non-cardioselective and possess both membrane activity and intrinsic sympathomimetic activity, e.g. alprenolol, p.782, oxprenolol, p.795;

Division I, Group II drugs are non-cardioselective and possess membrane activity but no intrinsic sympathomimetic activity, e.g. propranolol, p.798;

Division I, Group III drugs are non-cardioselective, have no membrane activity but do possess intrinsic sympathomimetic activity, e.g. pindolol, p.796;

Division I, Group IV drugs are non-cardioselective, and possess neither membrane activity nor intrinsic sympathomimetic activity, e.g. sotalol, p.807, timolol, p.808; and:

Division II, Group I drugs are cardioselective and possess both membrane activity and intrinsic sympathomimetic activity, e.g. acebutolol, below.

Division II, Group II drugs are cardioselective and possess membrane activity but no intrinsic sympathomimetic activity;

Division II, Group III drugs are cardioselective, have no membrane activity but do possess intrinsic sympathomimetic activity, e.g. practolol, p.798;

Division II, Group IV drugs are cardioselective, but possess neither membrane activity nor intrinsic sympathomimetic activity, e.g. atenolol, p.783, metoprolol, p.791.

A third group, Division III, describes beta blocking agents which also possess alpha blocking activity, e.g. labetalol, p.788. The additional alpha blocking properties of labetalol confer upon it a much more rapid onset of action, some enhancement of antihypertensive effect, and a certain incidence of postural hypotension.

Since the therapeutic effectiveness of the beta blocking agents seems to depend on their beta blocking action and since most side-effects stem from this action there is in general, little to choose between them when given in equi-effective doses. The membrane-stabilising and intrinsic sympathomimetic activities associated with some beta blockers are largely of pharmacological interest only.

The cardioselective properties of some beta blockers may, however, confer upon them some advantages since in usual doses they have a greater effect on the $beta_1$ receptors of the heart than on the $beta_2$ receptors found in the bronchi and lungs. In consequence they may have a reduced incidence of side-effects such as bronchospasm. However, cardioselectivity is relative and dose-dependent, and some effects on airway patency and respiratory function have been demonstrated even with so-called 'cardioselective' beta blockers.

Beta Blocking Therapy during Anaesthesia

Beta blocking agents alter the response of the body to stress and depress the myocardium. Some authorities have advocated temporary withdrawal prior to anaesthesia in order to provide better control of the circulatory system, but sudden withdrawal may expose the patient to severe uncontrolled angina or cardiac arrhythmias. There are also operative risks associated with uncontrolled hypertension. Anaesthesia may proceed safely under beta-adrenoceptor blockade provided that the patient is well monitored and that atropine is available to treat any bradycardia; alternatively the patient may be protected against bradycardia by the prior intravenous administration of atropine 1 to 2 mg. Anaesthetic agents causing myocardial depression, such as ether, chloroform, cyclopropane, and trichloroethylene, are best avoided.

Awareness by the anaesthetist that beta blockers are being taken is of the greatest importance.

For the use of beta blockers to treat cardiac arrhythmias arising under anaesthesia see under the individual monographs.

6302-q

Acebutolol Hydrochloride *(BANM, rINNM).*

IL-17803A; M & B-17803A. (±)-3′-Acetyl-4′-(2-hydroxy-3-isopropylaminopropoxy)butyranilide hydrochloride.

$C_{18}H_{28}N_2O_4,HCl = 372.9$.

CAS — 37517-30-9 (acebutolol, ±); 34381-68-5 (hydrochloride, ±).

NOTE. Acebutolol is *USAN*.

Adverse Effects, Treatment, and Precautions

As for Propranolol Hydrochloride, p.798.

ALLERGY. Cutaneous vasculitis due to acebutolol occurred in one patient. Hypersensitivity was confirmed by sensitivity testing. Rechallenge at a later date produced no reaction to acebutolol or other beta-blockers.— R. Ashford *et al.* (letter), *Lancet*, 1977, *2*, 462.

EFFECTS ON THE CIRCULATION. A report of near-fatal shock occurring within 40 minutes of acebutolol 400 mg in an elderly patient with chronic bronchitis and angina pectoris.— V. G. Tirlapur *et al.*, *Br. J. clin. Pract.*, 1986, *40*, 33.

EFFECTS ON IMMUNE RESPONSE. Development of antinuclear antibodies during acebutolol therapy.— R. J. Cody *et al.*, *Clin. Pharmac. Ther.*, 1979, *25*, 800.

A report of a case of a lupus syndrome associated with acebutolol therapy; the patient's symptoms remitted on withdrawal of acebutolol with the exception of a high antinuclear antibody titre.— P. Hourdebaigt-Larrusse *et al.*, *Annls Cardiol, Angeiol*, 1985, *34*, 421.

Further references: M. A. Martin (letter), *Br. J. clin. Pharmac.*, 1980, *10*, 313; J. D. Wilson, *Drugs*, 1980, *19*, 292; H. Leblanc *et al.*, *Presse méd.*, 1984, *13*, 2747; O. Bletry *et al.*, *ibid.*, 2751.

EFFECTS ON RESPIRATORY FUNCTION. A report of pleurisy and pulmonary granulomas in a patient receiving acebutolol and a diuretic; acebutolol was considered to be responsible.— G. M. Wood *et al.*, *Br. med. J.*, 1982, *285*, 936. Comment, and a further case of pleurisy associated with acebutolol.— R. J. E. Leggett (letter), *Br. med. J.*, 1982, *285*, 1425.

A report of hypersensitivity pneumonitis in a patient taking acebutolol.— G. M. Akoun *et al.*, *Br. med. J.*, 1983, *286*, 266.

Cardioselectivity. Acebutolol is generally considered to be a cardioselective beta blocker but there has been considerable controversy as to the degree of its selectivity and the selectivity of its primary metabolite, diacetolol. Whitsett *et al.* (*Chest*, 1982, *82*, 668) found no significant difference between acebutolol 200 to 400 mg twice daily and propranolol 40 to 80 mg twice daily in terms of their ability to largely abolish the beneficial effects of terbutaline on respiration in 10 asthmatics, while Nair *et al.* (*Int. J. clin. Pharmac. Ther. Toxic.*, 1981, *19*, 519) noted increased airway resistance and decreased FEV_1 in asthmatics given acebutolol 300 mg daily for 2 days; however these changes were not great enough to affect arterial oxygen desaturation. In contrast, Leary *et al.* (*S. Afr. med. J.*, 1973, *47*, 1245) have reported minimal effects on the airways in asthmatics given intravenous acebutolol. In a review of beta blockers, Feely *et al.* (*Br. med. J.*, 1983, *286*, 1043) have stated that acebutolol is less cardioselective than other agents such as atenolol or metoprolol, and Feely and Maclean propose (*ibid.*, 1972) that this may be because the metabolite accumulates during chronic dosage to reach concentrations which affect both $beta_1$ and $beta_2$ receptors since cardioselectivity is only a relative phenomenon and is dose-related. This remains uncertain and there is some evidence (M.S. Thomas and A.E. Tattersfield, *Eur. J. clin. Pharmac.*, 1986, *29*, 679) that at least after single doses, diacetolol is actually more cardioselective than acebutolol itself, but it should be remembered that all beta blockers may cause broncho-constriction in asthmatic subjects and the safety of cardioselective beta blockers is not absolute.

HYPOGLYCAEMIA. In 11 healthy subjects insulin-induced hypoglycaemia was significantly enhanced and return to normoglycaemia significantly delayed by propranolol 40 mg twice daily or metoprolol 50 mg twice daily. Acebutolol 100 mg twice daily significantly enhanced hypoglycaemia but did not significantly delay return to normoglycaemia.— R. J. Newman, *Br. med. J.*, 1976, *2*, 447.

Further references: J. Birnbaum *et al.*, *Clin. Pharmac. Ther.*, 1983, *33*, 294; A. Grimaldi *et al.*, *Curr. ther. Res.*, 1984, *36*, 361.

There were no significant adverse effects and no deterioration in diabetic control in patients given acebutolol rather than placebo in a study involving 20 diabetics.— D. M. Fraser *et al.*, *Curr. med. Res. Opinion*, 1986, *10*, 122.

INTERACTIONS. A report of enhancement of the effects of acebutolol by concomitant nicergoline.— N. Moore *et al.*, *Thérapie*, 1984, *39*, 103.

Absorption and Fate

Acebutolol is well absorbed from the gastro-intestinal tract following a dose by mouth, but undergoes extensive first-pass metabolism in the liver; the overall bioavailability is reported to be about 40%. It is widely distributed in the body but penetration into the CSF is reported to be poor; it crosses the placenta and is secreted in breast milk. Acebutolol is extensively metabolised; the major metabolite, diacetolol, is active and has a more prolonged half-life than the parent drug, with the result that after chronic administration plasma concentrations of diacetolol may be more than twice those of acebutolol. Acebutolol and diacetolol are secreted in the bile and may undergo enterohepatic recycling; acebutolol is also reported to be excreted directly from the intestinal wall. Drug and metabolites are also excreted extensively in the urine.

In 10 patients given a single 300-mg dose of acebutolol the mean plasma concentrations of acebutolol and its acetyl metabolite at 2 hours were 389 and 402 ng per mL respectively; at 7 hours the concentrations were 136 and 445 ng per mL. The elimination half-life of acebutolol was about 2.5 hours; elimination of the metabolite proceeded more slowly.— A. H. Gradman *et al.*, *Circulation*, 1977, *55*, 785.

Steady-state plasma concentrations of the acetyl metabolite were 2.7 times greater than those of the unchanged drug in 7 patients with cardiac arrhythmias given acebutolol 300 or 500 mg every 6 or 8 hours. Peak plasma-acebutolol concentrations occurred at 60 to 90 minutes in 3 patients with a half-life of about 2.5 hours whilst 4 patients had irregular plasma concentration curves suggestive of erratic or delayed absorption of acebutolol from the hard gelatin capsules or from enterohepatic recycling.— R. A. Winkle *et al.*, *Br. J. clin. Pharmac.*, 1977, *4*, 519.

DIALYSIS. Unlike beta-blockers such as pindolol and propranolol, acebutolol is subject to relatively important dialysis yield.— P. Aubert *et al.*, *J. Urol. Néphrol.*, 1976, *82*, 799.

PREGNANCY AND THE NEONATE. The pharmacokinetics of acebutolol and diacetolol in 29 pregnant women who received acebutolol for at least one month before delivery. Concentrations of acebutolol and diacetolol in arterial cord plasma at birth were from 0 to 138 ng per mL and from 0 to 647 ng per mL respectively; this compared with plasma concentrations of 0 to 661 and 113 to 1128 ng per mL in the mothers. Both acebutolol and its active metabolite cross the placenta to give therapeutic concentrations in the neonate; there was evidence of bradycardia in 12 of the 31 offspring and tachypnoea in 6 and these were associated with higher plasma concentrations of acebutolol than in those not so affected.— M. J. Boutroy *et al.*, *Develop. Pharmac. Ther.*, 1982, *4*, *Suppl.* 1, 109.

Uses and Administration

Acebutolol is a hydrophilic beta blocker with general properties similar to those of propranolol (see p.803). Acebutolol is classified as cardioselective and has some intrinsic sympathomimetic activity and membrane stabilising properties. It is used as the hydrochloride, but in the *UK*, doses are given in terms of the base, whereas in some other countries the same dose of the hydrochloride is given, resulting in slightly lower amounts of the active substance being administered.

In the treatment of hypertension the usual initial dose is 400 mg daily (at breakfast) or 200 mg twice daily, increased if necessary after 2 weeks according to the patient's response, to 800 mg once daily or 400 mg twice daily; some patients may require 800 mg in the morning and 400 mg in the evening.

The usual dose for angina pectoris is 200 mg twice daily but up to 300 mg three times daily may be required and total daily doses of 1.2 g have been given. The usual initial dose for cardiac arrhythmias is also 200 mg twice daily but up to 1.2 g daily in divided doses has been required. Acebutolol hydrochloride by mouth may take about 3 hours to exert its full effect.

For the emergency treatment of cardiac arrhythmias acebutolol hydrochloride has also been given by slow intravenous injection; doses equivalent to 25 mg of the base have been given, followed if necessary by the same dose as an intravenous infusion over an hour or more.

Reduced doses may be required in patients with impaired renal function; it has also been recommended that doses greater than 800 mg daily should be avoided in elderly patients.

Reviews of acebutolol B. N. Singh *et al.*, *Drugs*, 1985, *29*, 531; *Med. Lett.*, 1985, *27*, 58.

ADMINISTRATION IN RENAL FAILURE. A study involving 6 healthy subjects and 6 patients with chronic renal failure indicated that patients with chronic renal failure might require smaller doses of acebutolol. Subjects with renal failure appeared to exhibit a greater degree of non-renal elimination of acebutolol.— C. M. Kaye and J. F. Dufton (letter), *Br. J. clin. Pharmac.*, 1976, *3*, 198.

Evidence of prolongation of the half-life of acebutolol in patients with renal failure. In those undergoing haemodialysis, however, the half-life was similar to that of subjects with normal renal function.— P. Aubert *et al.*, *J. Urol. Néphrol.*, 1976, *82*, 799.

Acebutolol 400 mg in the morning effectively controlled the blood pressure of 5 of 11 patients with renal hypertension. A further 3 patients were controlled with this dose at 4 weeks but not at 12 weeks, and in the remaining 3 patients control could not be obtained with 800 mg each morning, possibly owing to weight gain reflecting subclinical salt and water retention. In 2 men with the most severe renal impairment a sharp deterioration in glomerular filtration-rate followed the introduction of acebutolol.— E. Begg *et al.*, *N.Z. med. J.*, 1979, *89*, 293.

Proprietary Preparations

Secadrex *(May & Baker, UK)*. *Tablets*, acebutolol 200 mg (as hydrochloride), hydrochlorothiazide 12.5 mg. *Dose*. One or 2 tablets daily.

Sectral *(May & Baker, UK)*. *Capsules*, acebutol 100 and 200 mg (as hydrochloride).
Tablets, acebutolol 400 mg (as hydrochloride).

Proprietary Names and Manufacturers

Acecor *(SPA, Ital.)*; Alol *(SIT, Ital.)*; Diasectral *(Rhone-Poulenc, Denm.)*; Molson *(Bayer, Spain)*; Neptal *(Röhm, Ger.)*; Prent *(Bayer, Arg.; Bayer, Ger.; Bayropharm, Ital.; Bayer, Switz.)*; Rhodiasectral *(Rhodia, Arg.)*; Sectral *(Specia, Fr.; Rhone-Poulenc, Ital.; Neth.; NZ; May & Baker, S.Afr.; Rhone, Spain; Rhone-Poulenc, Switz.; May & Baker, UK; Ives, USA)*; Wesfalin *(Roemmers, Arg.)*.

6303-p

Alprenolol Hydrochloride *(BANM, USAN, rINNM)*.

H56/28. (±)-1-(2-Allylphenoxy)-3-isopropylaminopropan-2-ol hydrochloride.

$C_{15}H_{23}NO_2,HCl = 285.8$.

CAS — 13655-52-2 (alprenolol); 13707-88-5 (hydrochloride).

Pharmacopoeias. In *Nord.*

Adverse Effects, Treatment, and Precautions

As for Propranolol Hydrochloride, p.798.

ALLERGY. A report of contact eczema in workers exposed to alprenolol. Alprenolol must be considered a very strong contact allergen.— L. Ekenvall and M. Forsbeck, *Contact Dermatitis*, 1978, *4*, 190.

EFFECTS ON THE BLOOD. Alprenolol-induced thrombocytopenia in 1 patient.— B. Magnusson and S. Rödjer, *Acta med. scand.*, 1980, *207*, 231.

EFFECTS ON RESPIRATORY FUNCTION. A study suggesting that alprenolol affects specific airway conductance less than propranolol.— C. K. Connolly and J. C. Batten, *Br. med. J.*, 1970, *2*, 515.

HYPOGLYCAEMIA. Exercise-induced hypoglycaemia in a patient taking alprenolol and hydralazine—the hypoglycaemia was suspected on one occasion and confirmed on another.— G. Holm *et al.*, *Br. med. J.*, 1981, *282*, 1360.

INTERACTIONS. A study in 5 healthy subjects indicated that pentobarbitone administration induced the metabolism of alprenolol. The decrease in plasma concentration following intravenous administration of alprenolol was insignificant, but that following oral administration was marked owing to the increased first-pass elimination.— G. Alván *et al.*, *Clin. Pharmac. Ther.*, 1977, *22*, 316. Concomitant pentobarbitone therapy significantly reduced the antihypertensive and negative chronotropic action of alprenolol in a study of 6 patients.— P. Seideman *et al.*, *Br. J. clin. Pharmac.*, 1987, *23*, 267.

Absorption and Fate

Alprenolol is almost completely absorbed from the gastro-intestinal tract but is reportedly subject to considerable first-pass metabolism in the liver. Peak plasma concentrations are achieved about 1 hour after a dose. It is metabolised in the liver, primarily to 4-hydroxyalprenolol, which is active. It is excreted in the urine mainly in the form of its metabolites. It is highly protein bound.

FIRST-PASS EFFECT. Support for the hypothesis that alprenolol is subject to significant first-pass metabolism.— G. Alván *et al.*, *J. Pharmacokinet. Biopharm.*, 1977, *5*, 193.

PROTEIN BINDING. Studies *in vitro* showed that the mean free fraction of alprenolol in the plasma obtained from 23 healthy subjects was 15.8% and this correlated inversely with the α_1-acid glycoprotein concentration. No relationship was found between plasma-albumin concentration and binding.— K. M. Piafsky and O. Borgå, *Clin. Pharmac. Ther.*, 1977, *22*, 545.

Uses and Administration

Alprenolol hydrochloride is a hydrophilic beta blocker with general properties similar to those of propranolol (see p.803). Alprenolol is classified as non-cardioselective and has some intrinsic membrane stabilising and sympathomimetic activity.

In the treatment of hypertension alprenolol hydrochloride is usually given in an initial dose of 200 mg daily, in divided doses, increased weekly according to the response of the patient up to a total of 800 mg daily in divided doses. The usual dose for angina pectoris and other cardiac disorders is 50 to 100 mg four times daily. For the emergency treatment of cardiac arrhythmias alprenolol hydrochloride has also been given by slow intravenous injection.

ADMINISTRATION IN HEPATIC FAILURE. The response to alprenolol which was metabolised by the liver was altered in the presence of hepatic disease.— G. L. Sanders, *Adverse Drug React. Bull.*, 1978, Feb., 240.

ENURESIS. A report of a beneficial effect of alprenolol on nocturnal enuresis in a 24-year-old woman.— B. Lake (letter), *Med. J. Aust.*, 1975, *1*, 367.

Proprietary Names and Manufacturers

Apllobal *(Jpn)*; Aptin *(Astra, Arg.; Astra, Austral.; Hässle, Denm.; Astra, Ger.; Byk Gulden, Ital.; Hässle, Norw.; Adcock Ingram, S.Afr.; Hässle, Swed.)*; Aptine *(Belg.; Astra, Fr.; Astra, Neth.)*; Aptol *(Astra, Switz.)*; Betacard *(Beecham, Austral.)*; Gubernal *(Geigy, Belg.; Geigy, Fr.; Geigy, Switz.)*; Regletin *(Jpn)*; Sinalol *(Jpn)*; Vasoton *(Astra, Arg.)*.

18779-q

Arotinolol Hydrochloride *(rINNM)*.

S-596. (±)-5-[2-{[3-(*tert*-Butylamino)-2-hydroxypropyl]-thio}-4-thiazolyl]-2-thiophenecarboxamide hydrochloride. $C_{15}H_{21}N_3O_2S_3,HCl=408.0$.

CAS — 68377-92-4 (arotinolol).

Arotinolol is an agent with beta blocking properties similar to those of propranolol (see p.798). In addition it has a less marked alpha blocking action. It has been tried in the management of hypertension and cardiac disorders.

The effects of topical arotinolol 0.5% ophthalmic solution on intra-ocular pressure.— M. Nakashima *et al.*, *Eur. J. clin. Pharmac.*, 1985, *28*, 391.

6304-s

Atenolol *(BAN, USAN, pINN)*.

ICI-66082. 4-(2-Hydroxy-3-isopropylaminopropoxy)phenylacetamide.

$C_{14}H_{22}N_2O_3=266.3$.

CAS — 29122-68-7; 60966-51-0 (±).

Pharmacopoeias. In *Br.*

A white or almost white, odourless or almost odourless powder. Sparingly **soluble** in water; soluble in absolute alcohol; practically insoluble in ether.

Adverse Effects, Treatment, and Precautions

As for Propranolol Hydrochloride, p.798.

A mean daily dose of atenolol 174 (range 12.5 to 600) mg was taken by 262 patients with hypertension for a mean of 23.3 (range 2 to 52) months in a multicentre open study. Significant reductions in supine and erect blood pressures and in supine heart-rate were obtained in the majority of patients. Treatment was discontinued in 14 patients, due to side-effects in 8. Overall side-effects included cold extremities, fatigue, sinus bradycardia, dry skin and eyes and heartburn. Of 11 patients with chronic bronchitis or bronchial asthma 3 reported slight respiratory symptoms.— L. Hansson *et al.*, *Curr. ther. Res.*, 1977, *22*, 839.

During post-marketing evaluation of atenolol in 34 120 patients adverse effects were reported in 6134 (15.4%) but in only about 1.6% of these was the adverse effect considered serious. The most common side-effects were headache, dizziness and lightheadedness, tiredness or fatigue, weakness, nausea, bradycardia, oedema, diarrhoea, depression, impotence, dyspnoea, anxiety, chest pain, lethargy, drowsiness, and malaise.— R. L. Herman *et al.*, *Curr. ther. Res.*, 1983, *33*, 165.

EFFECTS ON THE GASTRO-INTESTINAL TRACT. Reports of sclerosing peritonitis in patients receiving atenolol: N. Grefberg *et al.* (letter), *Lancet*, 1983, *2*, 733; B. V. Nielsen and K. G. Pedersen, *Br. med. J.*, 1985, *290*, 518.

For reports of retroperitoneal fibrosis in patients taking atenolol see under Fibrosis, below.

EFFECTS ON THE HEART. Evidence that atenolol may induce atrial fibrillation in susceptible patients.— K. Rasmussen *et al.*, *Eur. Heart J.*, 1982, *3*, 276.

EFFECTS ON THE KIDNEYS. Unilateral renal artery thrombosis, anuria, and death occurred in an elderly patient following a single dose of atenolol 100 mg.— A. B. Shaw and S. K. Gopalka, *Br. med. J.*, 1982, *285*, 1617.

EFFECTS ON MENTAL FUNCTION. Of 27 patients receiving atenolol, 3 developed vivid dreams and 2 became unable to cope with work.— H. J. Waal-Manning, *Clin. Pharmac. Ther.*, 1979, *25*, 8.

Acute psychotic behaviour developed in a patient given atenolol 50 mg daily. Symptoms regressed on discontinuation of atenolol and treatment with haloperidol.— J. J. Viadero *et al.*, *Am. J. Psychiat.*, 1983, *140*, 1382.

Evidence, from a study in 6 healthy subjects, that atenolol has central effects on performance. The results are surprising since atenolol has relatively low lipid solubility and might be expected to have fewer central effects than those beta blockers, such as propranolol, which penetrate the CNS more readily.— S. A. Salem and D. G. McDevitt, *Clin. Pharmac. Ther.*, 1983, *33*, 52.

A crossover study in 17 patients who had previously experienced central side-effects such as insomnia, nightmare, anxiety, confusion and irritability whilst receiving lipophilic beta-blockers (mostly propranolol, but also oxprenolol and pindolol) showed that introduction of atenolol produced no significant central side-effects, whereas metoprolol, which is moderately lipophilic, did produce an increase in sleep disturbances, although not to the extent previously experienced.— C. A. Kirk and R. Cove-Smith, *Postgrad. med. J.*, 1983, *59*, *Suppl.* 3, 161. See also J. H. Silas and J. C. McGourty (letter), *Lancet*, 1987, *2*, 108.

EFFECTS ON RESPIRATORY FUNCTION. In 20 patients with chronic obstructive airway disease, airway resistance was increased less by atenolol 100 mg than by propranolol 80 mg.— M. Beil and W. T. Ulmer, *Arzneimittel-Forsch.*, 1977, *27*, 419.

In 6 healthy subjects given atenolol 100 mg daily for 3 days the FEV_1 was significantly lower than that following placebo.— R. W. Fuller and P. J. T. Vallance, *Br. J. clin. Pharmac.*, 1982, *14*, 445.

Discussion of the effects of beta blockers on airways resistance. Atenolol appeared to have the least broncho-constrictive effect of the beta blockers available at the time in the *UK*.— A. E. Tattersfield and R. N. Harrison, *Drugs*, 1983, *25*, *Suppl.* 2, 227.

EFFECTS ON SEXUAL FUNCTION. Erectile dysfunction experienced by a 44-year-old man who was receiving propranolol 40 mg twice daily was reversed by substitution with atenolol 50 mg daily which also satisfactorily controlled his tachycardia.— J. Bathen (letter), *Ann. intern. Med.*, 1978, *88*, 716.

EFFECTS ON THE SKIN. *Necrosis.* Multiple areas of skin necrosis on the feet of a 57-year-old man taking atenolol.— P. J. Rees (letter), *Br. med. J.*, 1979, *1*, 955.

FIBROSIS. Severe criticism, by a representative of the manufacturer (*Stuart*), of a report by C.C. Doherty *et al.* (*Br. med. J.*, 1978, *2*, 1786) that retroperitoneal fibrosis in a 68-year-old woman might have been associated with atenolol.— M. J. Asbury (letter), *Br. med. J.*, 1979, *1*, 492.

Another report of retroperitoneal fibrosis associated with atenolol.— J. N. Johnson and J. McFarland (letter), *Br. med. J.*, 1980, *280*, 864. Severe criticism and comments.— M. J. Gavin *et al.* (letter), *ibid.*, 1227; D. W. Bullimore (letter), *ibid.*, *281*, 59; W. M. Castle *et al.* (letter), *ibid.*, 311; F. L. Rose and F. Bergel (letter), *ibid;* D. W. Bullimore (letter), *ibid.*, 564; F. L. Rose and F. Bergel (letter), *ibid.*, 745.

INTERACTIONS. *Antibiotics.* Bioavailability of atenolol 100 mg by mouth in 6 healthy subjects was reduced from 60% to 36% following co-administration of ampicillin 1 g, and exercise tachycardia was increased compared to results following atenolol alone. Following long-term combined therapy in 6 hypertensives, there was a reduction in bioavailability of atenolol to 24% but this was not associated with significantly greater blood pressure values than with atenolol alone.— M. Schäfer-Korting *et al.*, *Clin. Pharmac. Ther.*, 1983, *33*, 283. Results indicating that the interaction was unlikely to be clinically significant unless high doses of ampicillin were prescribed, in which case the drugs should be administered separately with atenolol preceding ampicillin.— A. J. McLean *et al.* (letter), *Br. J. clin. Pharmac.*, 1984, *18*, 969.

Anticoagulants. Studies suggesting a lack of interaction between atenolol and coumarin anticoagulants: F. Mantero *et al.*, *Br. J. clin. Pharmac.*, 1984, *17*, 94S (nicoumalone); H. Spahn *et al.*, *ibid.*, 97S (phenprocoumon).

Calcium-channel blockers. A report of severe hypotension in a patient with hypertension and angina taking atenolol when nifedipine was added to his treatment. When atenolol was withdrawn he developed unstable angina. In such situations the nifedipine should be withdrawn.— L. H. Opie and D. A. White, *Br. med. J.*, 1980, *281*, 1462.

For a report of complete heart block following combined administration of atenolol and verapamil, see under Verapamil, p.90.

Disopyramide. For the effect of atenolol on disopyramide clearance see Disopyramide, p.76.

Diuretics. For hypokalaemia associated with the use of atenolol combined with a diuretic see under Chlorothiazide, p.982.

Non-steroidal anti-inflammatory agents. Indomethacin but not sulindac reduced the antihypertensive action of chronic atenolol therapy in studies in hypertensive patients. The result might be connected with the fact that sulindac inhibits systemic prostaglandin synthesis only whereas indomethacin inhibits renal synthesis in addition.— A. Salvetti *et al.*, *Br. J. clin. Pharmac.*, 1984, *17*, 108S. A further study of the interaction of atenolol and indomethacin.— P. Ylitalo *et al.*, *Clin. Pharmac. Ther.*, 1985, *38*, 443.

OVERDOSAGE. Prolonged severe bradycardia and hypotension, as well as marked hypoglycaemia, occurred in an adolescent following an overdosage of atenolol; repeated doses of atropine 500 µg were required to maintain heart-rate and blood pressure over the following 36 hours.— I. A. Abbasi and S. Sorsby, *Clin. Pharm.*, 1986, *5*, 836. Severe bradycardia and hypotension following overdosage with an unknown amount of atenolol did not respond well to treatment with atropine and glucagon but treatment with intravenous prenalterol (in a total dose of 95 mg over 24 hours) increased heart-rate and blood pressure.— S. Freestone *et al.*, *Hum. Toxicol.*, 1986, *5*, 343.

PREGNANCY AND THE NEONATE. A report of bradycardia, hypotension, hypothermia, poor peripheral perfusion and oliguria in an infant born to a mother who had received atenolol for 3 days before delivery.— D. L. Woods and D. F. Morrell, *Br. med. J.*, 1982, *285*, 691. Severe criticism. The mother in question was also receiving phenobarbitone which could well have accounted for the symptoms. Controlled prospective studies have not generally substantiated anecdotal reports of an adverse effect of beta blockers on the foetus or neonate.— P. C. Rubin (letter), *ibid.*, 972; K. J. Thorley (letter), *ibid.*, 1116.

A study in 13 pregnant patients with severe pre-eclampsia suggested that the effects of atenolol 100 mg daily on the foetus were minimal.— K. J. Thorley *et al.*, *Br. J. clin. Pharmac.*, 1981, *12*, 725.

There was no evidence of short-term or medium-term paediatric complications in 55 infants whose mothers had received atenolol during the third trimester and who were followed for 1 year.— B. Reynolds *et al.*, *Archs Dis. Childh.*, 1984, *59*, 1061.

Absorption and Fate

Atenolol appears to be incompletely absorbed from the gastro-intestinal tract and is not significantly metabolised. It is excreted in the urine and its biological half-life is longer than would be anticipated from its plasma half-life of about 6 to 7 hours. Atenolol diffuses across the placenta and is excreted in breast milk. Only small amounts are reported to cross the blood-brain barrier, and it is only about 5% bound to plasma proteins.

Following intravenous administration of atenolol 50 mg to healthy subjects 100% of unchanged drug appeared in the urine indicating that atenolol was not significantly metabolised. Following administration of 50 mg by mouth absorption did not appear to be complete; bioavailability was about 63%. Following administration of 200 mg by mouth a mean of about 43% of the dose was excreted in the urine within 72 hours. Repeated administration of 200 mg daily by mouth either as a single dose or in 2 divided doses did not result in accumulation, the plasma elimination half-life after the first and the eighth days being a mean of about 6.31 hours and 6.66 hours respectively.— H. C. Brown *et al.*, *Clin. Pharmac. Ther.*, 1976, *20*, 524.

Five healthy male subjects were given atenolol 25 to 200 mg or a placebo; the reduction in heart-rate was still significant after 27 hours with the 100- and 200-mg doses.— J. D. Harry and J. Young, *Br. J. clin. Pharmac.*, 1977, *4*, 387P.

Investigations in 4 healthy subjects indicated that urinary pH had no influence on the excretion of atenolol.— C. M. Kaye (letter), *Br. J. clin. Pharmac.*, 1974, *1*, 513.

Whereas the buccal absorption of propranolol increased from 3.2% at pH 5 to 55.8% at pH 8 and 89.0% at pH 10, that of atenolol was pH-independent and less than 5%. Atenolol is considerably more hydrophilic than propranolol.— W. Schürmann and P. Turner, *Br. J. clin. Pharmac.*, 1977, *4*, 655P. On the premise that the distribution co-efficient is the basis of tissue distribution *in vivo*, atenolol may be regarded as the most hydrophilic of the clinically available beta blockers.— P. J. Taylor and J. M. Cruickshank, *J. Pharm. Pharmac.*, 1984, *36*, 118.

Food-induced reduction in bioavailability of atenolol.— A. Melander *et al.*, *Eur. J. clin. Pharmac.*, 1979, *16*, 327.

PREGNANCY AND THE NEONATE. In 6 women who had taken atenolol for at least 6 days up to the time of delivery concentrations of atenolol in maternal and umbilical serum were approximately equal. In a further woman who had discontinued treatment one day before delivery atenolol was not found in maternal or umbilical serum.— A. Melander *et al.*, *Eur. J. clin. Pharmac.*, 1978, *14*, 93.

Evidence that the elimination of atenolol is prolonged in

the neonate; mean half-life of elimination in 35 neonates whose mothers had received atenolol was calculated at 16 hours.— P. C. Rubin, *et al., Br. J. clin. Pharmac.*, 1983, *16*, 659.

Lactation. In a study in 10 lactating women given atenolol 100 mg daily the concentration of atenolol in breast milk varied from 380 to 1040 ng per mL, and the mean ratio of the concentration in blood to that in milk was 1.3 to 1. When the same women were given propranolol 40 mg twice daily, concentrations in breast milk ranged from 14 to 36 ng per mL and the mean blood/breast milk ratio was 2.0 to 1. Unlike propranolol atenolol appears to be distributed almost evenly between blood and milk but neither drug appears to be present in breast milk in sufficient quantity to provide a significant dose to the neonate.— K. J. Thorley and J. McAinsh, *Biopharm. Drug Disposit.*, 1983, *4*, 299. See also W. B. White *et al., Obstet. Gynec.*, 1984, *63, Suppl.*, 42S.

Uses and Administration

Atenolol is a hydrophilic beta blocker with general properties similar to those of propranolol (see p.803). Atenolol is classified as cardioselective and is reported to lack intrinsic sympathomimetic activity and membrane stabilising properties.

In the treatment of hypertension atenolol is usually given by mouth in a dose of 100 mg daily, as a single dose, although some patients may respond to 50 mg daily. The usual dose for angina pectoris is also 50 to 100 mg daily, given as single or divided doses. Although up to 200 mg daily has been given for angina pectoris additional benefit is not usually obtained from higher doses of atenolol.

For the emergency treatment of cardiac arrhythmias atenolol may be given by intravenous injection in a dose of 2.5 mg injected at a rate of 1 mg per minute, repeated if necessary every 5 minutes to a maximum total dosage of 10 mg. Alternatively atenolol may be given by intravenous infusion, a dose of 150 µg per kg bodyweight being administered over 20 minutes. The injection or infusion procedure may be repeated every 12 hours if necessary. When control is achieved maintenance doses of 50 to 100 mg daily may be given by mouth.

Atenolol is also used as an adjunct in the early management of acute myocardial infarction to limit progression and myocardial damage and reduce morbidity. Treatment should be given within 12 hours of the onset of chest pain; atenolol 5 to 10 mg should be given by intravenous injection at a rate of 1 mg per minute and followed after 15 minutes with 50 mg by mouth, provided no adverse effects result. A further 50 mg may be given after 12 hours, and subsequent dosage maintained, after a further 12 hours, with 100 mg daily.

The dosage of atenolol should be reduced in renal failure (see under Administration in Renal Failure, below).

A review of atenolol.— W. H. Frishman, *New Engl. J. Med.*, 1982, *306*, 1456.

For a series of papers relating to the adverse effects, precautions, pharmacokinetics, actions, and uses of atenolol, see *Drugs*, 1983, *25, Suppl.* 2.

ADMINISTRATION. In a study of 59 hypertensive patients there was no significant difference in the reduction in blood pressure produced by 50 mg daily (in 29) and 100 mg daily (in 30), both given for 1 month. Mean diastolic pressure fell from 106.0 to 95.4 mmHg in the group receiving the lower dose and from 107.8 to 97.7 mmHg in those given the higher dose. The number of responders in the 2 groups was 13 and 10 respectively, which was also not significantly different, and there was no detectable difference in adverse effects between groups. Under these circumstances there appears no reason to begin atenolol therapy with the higher dose.— E. van de Veur *et al., Eur. J. clin. Pharmac.*, 1985, *28*, 351. See also A. K. Scott *et al., Br. med. J.*, 1982, *284*, 1514.

Once-daily administration. In a double-blind crossover study in 12 patients with hypertension there was comparable reduction in blood pressure after atenolol 50 mg twice daily, 100 mg twice daily, or 100 mg daily.— C. M. Castleden *et al., Postgrad. med. J.*, 1977, *53*, 679. Further references: J. R. Ryan *et al., Curr. ther. Res.*, 1983, *33*, 1035; M. H. Maxwell *et al., ibid.*, *34*, 613.

ADMINISTRATION IN RENAL FAILURE. Atenolol could be given in usual doses to patients with a glomerular filtration-rate (GFR) greater than 50 mL per minute but the dosage should be reduced to 50% in those with a GFR between 10 and 50 mL per minute, and to 25% of the usual dose in those with a GFR less than 10 mL per minute. Alternatively, the conventional dose can be given with an extended dosage interval; doses which can be given every 24 hours in those with a glomerular filtration-rate greater than 50 mL per minute should be given only once in 48 hours where the GFR is between 10 and 50 mL per minute, and every 96 hours where the GFR is less than 10 mL per minute. The half-life of atenolol is extended from between 6 and 9 hours in patients with normal renal function to 15 to 35 hours in end-stage renal disease. It is removed by haemodialysis.— W. M. Bennett *et al., Am. J. Kidney Dis.*, 1983, *3*, 155.

Reports that atenolol causes less deterioration in renal function than non-selective beta-adrenoceptor blocking agents, such as propranolol: R. Wilkinson (letter), *Br. med. J.*, 1979, *1*, 617; H. J. Waal-Manning and P. Bolli (letter), *ibid.*, 1082.

ADMINISTRATION IN RESPIRATORY INSUFFICIENCY. In a double-blind crossover study in patients with bronchial asthma, intravenous injection of atenolol 3 mg caused a slight increase in airways resistance when compared to a placebo. Bronchial constriction caused by atenolol was readily overcome by inhalation of salbutamol.— N. P. Boye and J. R. Vale, *Eur. J. clin. Pharmac.*, 1977, *11*, 11.

Further references: C. Carlson and K. A. Järvinen, *Allergy*, 1978, *33*, 147; I. N. Findlay *et al., Br. J. clin. Pharmac.*, 1985, *19*, 150P.

ALCOHOL AND DRUG WITHDRAWAL. Addition of atenolol 50 to 100 mg daily, according to heart-rate, to standard therapy in 61 patients with the alcohol withdrawal syndrome reduced benzodiazepine requirements and the length of hospital stay compared with placebo in a further 59. Atenolol has a useful role in the therapy of patients with mild to moderate alcohol withdrawal syndrome.— M. L. Kraus *et al., New Engl. J. Med.*, 1985, *313*, 905.

ANXIETY. Atenolol 100 mg daily by mouth for 3 weeks in 31 patients with anxiety was no more effective than was placebo in a further 32 in relieving symptoms. There was an insignificant trend for greater improvement with atenolol at 3 weeks but whether this trend would continue and achieve significance with more prolonged treatment was unknown.— K. Rickels *et al., Curr. ther. Res.*, 1986, *40*, 149.

CARDIAC DISORDERS. Comparison of the ability of pindolol (a non-selective beta blocker) and atenolol (a cardioselective beta blocker) to protect against adrenaline-induced stimulation of myocardial oxygen demand in patients with angina pectoris. In patients given atenolol 62.5 µg per kg body-weight intravenously infusion of adrenaline provoked a mean 39% increase in myocardial oxygen demand, with increases in heart-rate and cardiac venous flow. In contrast, in those given intravenous pindolol 7.5 µg per kg body-weight, adrenaline produced only a mean 11% increase in demand with no significant change in heart-rate and a much smaller increase in cardiac venous flow. Pindolol provides better protection than atenolol against the increase in myocardial oxygen demand induced by concentrations of adrenaline equivalent to those observed in acute myocardial infarction; dose-response studies are needed to determine if this is a genuine difference of action or is related to dose.— H. Ihlen *et al., Eur. J. clin. Pharmac.*, 1984, *27*, 29.

Atenolol 10 mg every 6 hours intravenously for 3 days, followed by 100 mg daily by mouth for 4 days, was more effective than placebo in reducing catecholamine-induced myocardial damage in patients with abnormally elevated noradrenaline concentrations following acute head injury. Among the 56 patients given atenolol the blood concentration of the myocardial isoenzyme of creatine kinase, CKMB (a marker of myocardial damage) was 80% lower than in the 58 given placebo. Changes in ST segment and T-wave of the ECG were significantly less likely in patients who received atenolol. The benefit was considered likely to be a result of beta-blockade, *per se* and may be akin to the benefit in limiting the size of myocardial infarction; a cardioselective beta blocker was used in this study because of the potential risk of hypertension due to unmasked alpha constrictor activity if a non-selective beta blocker is given in the presence of high concentrations of adrenaline.— J. M. Cruickshank *et al., Lancet*, 1987, *2*, 585.

Angina pectoris. The work capacity of 8 patients with angina pectoris before an attack occurred was increased by a mean of 19 and 37%, 24 hours after taking a single daily dose of atenolol 50 or 100 mg respectively and by a mean of 44% four hours after the 100-mg dose. The effect of the 100-mg dose on the heart-rate after 24 hours was about 78% of the maximum effect produced after 4 hours. It was considered that a once-daily regimen of atenolol would be effective for patients with angina pectoris starting with a 50-mg dose and increased to 100 mg if this was tolerated.— G. H. Noer and T. Ekeli, *Curr. ther. Res.*, 1978, *24*, 17.

Studies of atenolol in the management of angina: J. B. Schwartz, *Drugs*, 1983, *25, Suppl.* 2, 160 (once daily dosage in stable angina); J. P. Godenir *et al., ibid.*, 172 (use in unstable angina); R. M. Boyle *et al., ibid.*, 193 (up to 200 mg daily in stable angina); P. Gruppillo *et al., ibid.*, 194 (comparison with nifedipine in angina of effort).

A study in 16 men with stable angina pectoris and normal left-ventricular function indicated that atenolol 100 mg daily together with nifedipine 20 mg three times daily, both by mouth, were more effective than either drug alone; the combination had no adverse effects on cardiac function in these patients.— I. N. Findlay *et al., Br. Heart J.*, 1986, *55*, 240.

Cardiac arrhythmias. A study of atenolol in 28 subjects indicated that the anti-arrhythmic properties of atenolol were similar to those of other beta-adrenoceptor blocking agents.— R. Sirbulescu, *Acta ther.*, 1977, *3*, 109.

Comment on the use of atenolol to prevent early ventricular fibrillation after myocardial infarction.— R. M. Norris (letter), *Lancet*, 1986, *2*, 396.

In a single-blind study atenolol 50 mg daily was given for 2 weeks to 32 patients suffering from frequent ventricular ectopic depolarisations and who had previously been receiving placebo. Two were withdrawn due to adverse effects; the remaining 30 were given 100 mg daily for 2 weeks. Of these 8 failed to tolerate the higher dose, but 22 went on to receive 200 mg daily for 2 weeks and all but 2 of these completed the study. A reduction in ventricular ectopy of at least 75% occurred in 6 of 32 patients taking 50 mg, 5 of 30 taking 100 mg and 3 of 21 taking 200 mg but only 4 who failed to give this response to 50 mg did so at 100 mg and none of those who failed to respond to a lower dose responded to 200 mg daily. However abolition of ventricular tachycardia, or reduction by at least 75% occurred among 8 of 17 receiving 50 mg, 7 of 16 taking 100 mg, and 8 of 11 given 200 mg daily; overall, of the 17 patients who had originally had ventricular tachycardia, 12 showed an effect with some dose of atenolol, despite the fact that 7 of them were among those whose ventricular ectopy failed to respond. Adverse reactions were common; the effect most frequently requiring discontinuation of the drug was symptomatic bradycardia.— P. E. Fenster *et al., Clin. Pharmac. Ther.*, 1987, *41*, 118.

Hypertrophy. Evidence from an open study in 71 hypertensive patients suggested that lowering blood pressure with atenolol may reduce existing left ventricular hypertrophy or prevent its development:—R. Fogari *et al., Int. J. clin. Pharmac., Ther. Toxic.* 1987, *25*, 334.

Myocardial infarction. Evidence, from a placebo-controlled study involving 22 patients, that atenolol 100 mg daily facilitates the recovery of the ECG signs of myocardial infarction.— S. Yusuf *et al., Lancet*, 1979, *2*, 868. Results of a randomised study in 214 patients with myocardial infarction, using intravenous atenolol given within 12 hours of chest pain, indicated that early beta-blockade reduced infarct development and lowered subsequent morbidity. However, it was not possible to be certain from this study if early intravenous beta-blockade had genuinely produced a moderate but worthwhile reduction in mortality.— *idem*, 1980, *2*, 273. See also P. R. F. Rossi *et al., Br. med. J.*, 1983, *286*, 506.

Evidence that early intravenous administration of atenolol to patients with acute myocardial infarction results in a significant reduction in pain (associated with lessened cardiac work) and therefore a reduction in the need for administration of opioid analgesics.— D. R. Ramsdale *et al., Am. Heart J.*, 1982, *103*, 459.

A multicentre randomised study involving 16 027 patients with suspected myocardial infarction of recent onset examined the benefits of early beta blockade against the absence of such treatment. Patients assigned to atenolol received an immediate intravenous injection of 5 mg given over 5 minutes and stopped if the heart-rate fell below 40 beats per minute; a further injection of up to 5 mg was given after 10 minutes if heart-rate was 60 beats per minute or greater. Provided the heart-rate did not fall below 40 beats per minute atenolol 50 mg was given by mouth 10 minutes after the end of the intravenous doses, followed by a further 50 mg 12 hours later; atenolol was subsequently given in doses of 100 mg by mouth daily for 6 days, although this dose could be halved or omitted if felt necessary.

Patients in the control group did not receive beta blockers unless there was a clear indication for such treatment. Of the 8037 patients assigned to receive atenolol 37% received less than the full course, but only 6% failed to receive at least the first 5 mg of intravenous atenolol. Upon analysis of the results there were 313 vascular-related deaths during the 7-day treatment period among patients receiving atenolol, compared with 365 deaths among the 7990 controls, a 15% difference in favour of atenolol; when patients were followed for 1 year the life-table estimates of vascular mortality were 10.7% among the atenolol group and 12.0% among controls, although the trend to fewer vascular deaths among the atenolol group during this period was not significant when follow-up was extended further. If early mortality is reduced by about 10 to 15% and if there is no additional difference in later mortality then 1-year vascular mortality will be reduced by only about 5% which is somewhat less than is suggested by direct examination of the data. If beta blockade does reduce cardiac arrest, re-infarction and mortality by the amount suggested by this and other studies then it is considerably more cost-effective an intervention than, for example, treatment of mild hypertension in middle age.—ISIS-1 (First International Study of Infarct Survival) Collaborative Group, *Lancet*, 1986, *2*, 57. Comment. It appears that intravenous administration of a beta blocker during evolution of an infarct has a beneficial effect similar to that of long-term administration following recovery. The benefit is modest, but addition of beta blockade to other agents such as thrombolytics to achieve early reperfusion could lead to more effective protection of the acutely ischaemic myocardium. The choice of beta blocker and whether to opt for a cardioselective agent remains to be resolved.— *ibid.*, 79.

For a similar large study using metoprolol see Metoprolol Tartrate, p.793.

GLAUCOMA. In a double-blind crossover study in 16 patients with intra-ocular pressures of or above 22 mmHg the topical application of atenolol 1, 2, or 4% (with benzalkonium chloride 0.02% and pH adjusted to 6) produced a mean maximum fall in intra-ocular pressure of 4.9, 6.1, and 6.3 mmHg respectively. The effect was evident at 1 hour, reached its maximum at 2 to 3 hours, and had disappeared after 7 hours. In 10 patients treated thrice daily for 7 days there was a sustained reduction in intra-ocular pressure with a tendency for the effect to be less at the end of the period. Pupil size, corneal sensitivity, blood pressure, and heart-rate were not affected.— K. Wettrell and M. Pandolfi, *Br. J. Ophthal.*, 1977, *61*, 334.

In a double-blind study in 8 patients with glaucoma a single dose of acetazolamide 500 mg reduced intra-ocular pressure to an insignificant extent, atenolol 50 mg reduced intra-ocular pressure significantly, and the effect of giving both drugs concomitantly was significantly greater than that of atenolol alone.— M. J. Macdonald *et al.*, *Br. J. Ophthal.*, 1977, *61*, 345. See also M. J. Elliot *et al.*, *ibid.*, 1975, *59*, 296.

A comparison of the reduction of intra-ocular pressure produced by atenolol 4% and adrenaline 1% eye-drops in 12 patients with intra-ocular hypertension showed that atenolol was more effective than adrenaline. No additive effect was observed when the drugs were used together.— C. I. Phillips *et al.*, *Br. J. Ophthal.*, 1978, *62*, 296. Both atenolol and adrenaline produced a reduction in intra-ocular pressure, and combined treatment produced a fall in pressure which was greater than that observed for either drug alone.— A. Rushton, *Br. J. clin. Pharmac.*, 1979, *7*, 575.

Similar decreases in intra-ocular pressure were noted following topical application thrice daily of atenolol 2% or pilocarpine 2% in a double-blind crossover study involving 8 patients with ocular hypertension.— K. Wettrell *et al.*, *Br. J. Ophthal.*, 1978, *62*, 292.

A brief comment on the problems associated with tolerance to atenolol eye-drops in glaucoma.— *Br. med. J.*, 1978, *1*, 460.

Atenolol in doses of 25 mg twice daily by mouth, or 50 or 100 mg once daily, produced a significant fall in mean intra-ocular pressure up to 6 hours after administration in a crossover study in 22 patients with chronic simple glaucoma or ocular hypertension. There was still a small non-significant reduction in intra-ocular pressure 12 hours after a 25-mg dose and 24 hours after the higher doses. Patients continued to receive their usual antiglaucoma therapy throughout the study but none were taking other beta blockers. Three patients reported less ache than usual in their eyes in the morning whilst receiving atenolol, which might indicate that there was less of a swing in intra-ocular pressure during atenolol treatment.— M. K. Tutton and R. J. H. Smith, *Br. J. Ophthal.*, 1983, *67*, 664.

HEPATIC DISORDERS. For evidence suggesting that atenolol is of no value in reducing portal hypertension, see under Propranolol Hydrochloride, p.805.

HYPERTENSION. A brief review of the use of atenolol for hypertension.— *Med. Lett.*, 1982, *24*, 15.

Withdrawal of long-term therapy with atenolol in hypertensive patients.— J. Webster *et al.*, *Br. J. clin. Pharmac.*, 1981, *12*, 211.

A dose-equivalence study of propranolol, metoprolol, and atenolol in the treatment of hypertension. There was a significant patient preference for atenolol, which had the lowest incidence of side-effects but was the most expensive treatment; metoprolol was the least expensive.— R. J. Haley and J. H. Licht, *Curr. ther. Res.*, 1984, *36*, 993.

In a crossover study involving 150 patients with mild to moderate hypertension (diastolic blood pressure of 95 to 120 mmHg) the effects of metoprolol 200 mg daily, atenolol 100 mg daily, and propranolol and oxprenolol both in doses of 160 mg daily as a slow-release tablet, were compared with placebo following administration for 4 weeks. Atenolol and propranolol caused a fall in mean supine blood pressure of 24/21 and 19/17 mmHg respectively, but metoprolol or oxprenolol resulted in non-significant reductions of only 10/5 and 6/2 mmHg.— M. Ravid *et al.*, *Archs intern. Med.*, 1985, *145*, 1321.

Studies of the use of atenolol with chlorthalidone: *Curr. ther. Res.*, 1984, *35*, 31 (combination more effective than either alone); A. Emanueli *et al.*, *J. int. med. Res.*, 1984, *12*, 314 (postmarketing surveillance in 2449 patients); J. A. Tweed and K. G. Edwards, *Acta ther.*, 1984, *10*, 15 (benefit in 6016 previously uncontrolled hypertensives).

For reference to the use of atenolol in the management of hypertension of pregnancy see under Pregnancy and the Neonate, below.

HYPERTHYROIDISM. In a double-blind crossover study in 21 patients with hyperthyroidism, propranolol 40 mg, atenolol 50 mg, or placebo were given 4 times daily for one week in randomised order. Both atenolol and propranolol were considered to have a beneficial effect on the peripheral manifestations of hyperthyroidism and both significantly reduced heart-rate, by 29.8% and 27.1% respectively, with no significant difference between the 2 drugs.— D. G. McDevitt and J. K. Nelson, *Br. J. clin. Pharmac.*, 1978, *6*, 233.

Reference to the use of atenolol or nadolol as preparation for thyroidectomy in patients with Graves' disease.— P. H. Gerst *et al.*, *Archs Surg.*, 1986, *121*, 838.

MIGRAINE. The use of atenolol in migraine.— P. Stensrud and O. Sjaastad, *Headache*, 1980, *20*, 204.

See also under Propranolol Hydrochloride, p.806.

PREGNANCY AND THE NEONATE. A study of atenolol in 13 pregnant women with severe pre-eclampsia.— K. J. Thorley *et al.*, *Br. J. clin. Pharmac.*, 1981, *12*, 725.

In a study in 120 women with hypertension in the last trimester of pregnancy, 60 were assigned to treatment with atenolol 100 or 200 mg daily while the remainder were given placebo. Four patients from the atenolol group with withdrawn due to inadequate blood pressure control or adverse effects (nausea); 8 patients were similarly withdrawn from the placebo group. Final analysis was carried out in 46 women who had received atenolol and 39 given placebo. Of those taking atenolol, 17 were managed on 100 mg daily whilst the remainder received 200 mg a day. Blood pressure fell in the atenolol group but not in the placebo group and proteinuria developed in only 3 of the former but in 10 of the latter group. Furthermore, there were substantial differences between groups in the rate of hospital admission, with 30 of the atenolol group being managed as outpatients whereas only 6 of those taking placebo could be so managed. There were 2 intra-uterine deaths in the placebo group and 1 in the atenolol group. Among those neonates successfully delivered, bradycardia was commoner in those born to mothers receiving atenolol. When children born to mothers excluded from analysis were also included on the basis of intention to treat there was evidence for an effect of atenolol in reducing the incidence of respiratory distress syndrome, probably because loss of blood-pressure control in the early third trimester may damage the immature foetal lung.— P. C. Rubin *et al.*, *Lancet*, 1983, *1*, 431.

The suggestion that labetalol may be superior to atenolol in the management of hypertension in pregnancy.— H. Lardoux *et al.* (letter), *Lancet*, 1983, *2*, 1194.

TREMOR. Atenolol 100 mg daily for 1 week reduced the intensity of essential tremor by 37.3% in a study in 24 patients, which was more than the 4.9% reported with placebo but less than the 42.3% reduction with propranolol 80 mg three times daily. Atenolol was preferred only by 1 patient whereas propranolol was preferred by 12, Atenolol appears to be less potent than propranolol but the difference is slight and atenolol may provide an alternative for patients who cannot tolerate propranolol.— T. A. Larsen *et al.*, *Acta neurol. scand.*, 1982, *66*, 547.

Preparations

Atenolol Tablets *(B.P.)*

Proprietary Preparations

Beta-Adalat *(Bayer, UK). Capsules*, atenolol 50 mg, nifedipine 20 mg (sustained-release).

Kalten *(Stuart, UK). Capsules*, atenolol 50 mg, hydrochlorothiazide 25 mg, amiloride hydrochloride equivalent to anhydrous amiloride hydrochloride 2.5 mg.

Tenif *(Stuart, UK). Capsules*, atenolol 50 mg, nifedipine 20 mg (sustained-release).

Tenoret 50 *(Stuart, UK). Tablets*, atenolol 50 mg, chlorthalidone 12.5 mg

Tenoretic *(Stuart, UK). Tablets*, atenolol 100 mg, chlorthalidone 25 mg.

Tenormin *(Stuart, UK). Tablets* (Tenormin LS), scored, atenolol 50 mg. *Tablets*, atenolol 100 mg. *Syrup*, atenolol 25 mg/5 mL. *Injection*, atenolol, 500 µg/mL, in ampoules of 10 mL.

Proprietary Names and Manufacturers

Atenol *(CT, Ital.)*; Blokium *(High Noon, Pakistan; Prodes, Spain)*; Felobits *(Duncan, Arg.)*; Ibinolo *(Ibi, Ital.)*; Myocord *(Beta, Arg.)*; Neatenol *(Fides, Spain)*; Prenormine *(ICI-Farma, Arg.)*; Seles Beta *(Farmitalia, Ital.)*; Telvodin *(Syncro, Arg.)*; Tenormin *(ICI, Austral.; Belg.; ICI, Canad.; ICI, Denm.; ICI, Ger.; ICI-Pharma, Ital.; Neth.; ICI, Norw.; Stuart, S.Afr.; ICI, Spain; ICI, Swed.; ICI, Switz.; Stuart, UK; Stuart Pharmaceuticals, USA)*; Ténormine *(I.C.I.-Pharma, Fr.)*; Vericordin *(Lazar, Arg.)*

The following names have been used for multi-ingredient preparations containing atenolol—Beta-Adalat *(Bayer, UK)*; Kalten *(Stuart, UK)*; Nif-Ten *(ICI, Ger.)*; Tenif *(Stuart, UK)*; Tenoret 50 *(Stuart, UK)*; Tenoretic *(Stuart, UK; Stuart Pharmaceuticals, USA)*.

16528-a

Befunolol Hydrochloride *(rINNM)*.

BFE-60. 7-[2-Hydroxy-3-(isopropylamino)propoxy]-2-benzofuranyl methyl ketone hydrochloride.

$C_{16}H_{21}NO_4,HCl=327.8$.

CAS — 39552-01-7 (befunolol).

Befunolol is a beta blocker with general properties similar to those of propranolol (see p.798). It has been tried as the hydrochloride in the management of hypertension and cardiac disorders.

Eye-drops containing befunolol hydrochloride 0.25% and 0.5% are instilled twice daily in the treatment of open-angle glaucoma.

Proprietary Names and Manufacturers

Bentos *(Kaken, Jpn)*; Glauconex *(Thilo, Ger.)*.

12439-p

Betaxolol Hydrochloride *(BANM, USAN, rINNM)*.

ALO-1401-02; SL 75212-10. 1-{4-[2-(Cyclopropylmethoxy)ethyl]phenoxy}-3-isopropylaminopropan-2-ol hydrochloride.

$C_{18}H_{29}NO_3,HCl=343.9$.

CAS — 63659-18-7 (betaxolol); 63659-19-8 (hydrochloride).

Adverse Effects, Treatment, and Precautions

As for Propranolol Hydrochloride, p.798.

Systemic side-effects have occasionally followed topical use of the eye-drops; local irritation and photophobia have been reported.

EFFECTS ON RESPIRATORY FUNCTION. A study in 8 healthy subjects indicated that neither betaxolol 40 or 80 mg, or propranolol 160 or 320 mg had any significant effect on specific airways conductance; however, the response to an inhaled dose of salbutamol was reduced significantly more following propranolol than after betaxolol.— R. Palminteri and G. Kaik, *Eur. J. clin. Pharmac.*, 1983, *24*, 741.

Studies suggesting that betaxolol eye-drops did not cause bronchoconstriction or deterioration of pulmonary function in patients with obstructive airways disease: R.

B. Schoene *et al.*, *Am. J. Ophthal.*, 1984, *97*, 86; E. M. Van Buskirk *et al.*, *ibid.*, 1986, *101*, 531.

Absorption and Fate

Betaxolol is reported to be completely absorbed from the gastro-intestinal tract following oral administration and to undergo only mimimal first-pass metabolism, resulting in a high oral bioavailability of 80 to 90%. It is extensively metabolised, and excreted in urine as unchanged drug and metabolites. It crosses the placenta and is excreted in breast milk.

In a study in 8 healthy middle-aged subjects given betaxolol 10 mg intravenously and 20 mg by mouth mean absolute bioavailability was 75.8%. The mean peak plasma concentration after oral dosage was 42.6 ng per mL, achieved 4 to 6 hours after administration; mean elimination half-life was 16.8 hours after oral and 16.4 hours after intravenous administration. 12.5% of an oral dose and 18.4% of the intravenous dose was excreted unchanged in the urine.— G. Bianchetti *et al.*, *Eur. J. clin. Pharmac.*, 1986, *31*, 231.

Uses and Administration

Betaxolol hydrochloride is a lipophilic beta blocker with general properties similar to those of propranolol (see p.803). It is classified as cardioselective and is reported to lack intrinsic sympathomimetic and membrane stabilising properties.

It is used in the management of hypertension in usual doses of 20 mg as a single daily dose, increased to 40 mg daily if necessary.

Eye-drops containing the equivalent of 0.5% betaxolol as the hydrochloride are instilled twice daily in the treatment of elevated intraocular pressure and open-angle glaucoma.

A review of betaxolol. Betaxolol is a relatively cardioselective beta blocker, but nonetheless should be given with care to patients with respiratory disease since the cardioselectivity of all beta blockers is only relative. It has a long elimination half-life, permitting once daily dosage, and has been shown to be effective in the management of hypertension; most patients respond to a dose of 10 to 20 mg daily. In elderly patients and those with severe renal dysfunction requiring dialysis treatment the usual recommended initial dose is 10 mg daily. Although clinical experience is limited, the drug appears to be relatively well tolerated; fatigue and impotence have been reported as the most frequent side-effects.— R. Beresford and R. C. Heel, *Drugs*, 1986, *31*, 6.

GLAUCOMA. Reviews of the use of betaxolol eye-drops in glaucoma: *Med. Lett.*, 1986, *28*, 45; C. P. Robinson, *Drugs Today*, 1986, *22*, 213; *Drug & Ther. Bull.*, 1987, *25*, 63.

GROWTH-HORMONE DEFICIENCY TEST. Reference to the use of betaxolol with glucagon in tests of growth-hormone deficiency.— M. Colle *et al.*, *Archs Dis. Childh.*, 1984, *59*, 670.

HYPERTENSION. A multicentre open study, involving 4685 patients, of the benefits of once-daily betaxolol treatment in mild to moderate hypertension.— J. Djian, *Br. J. clin. Pract.*, 1985, *39*, 188.

Proprietary Preparations

Betoptic *(Alcon, UK)*. *Eye-drops*, betaxolol 0.5% (as hydrochloride).

Kerlone *(Lorex, UK)*. *Tablets*, scored, betaxolol hydrochloride 20 mg.

Proprietary Names and Manufacturers

Betoptic *(Alcon, Canad.; Alcon, Denm.; Alcon, Fr.; Alcon, Ital.; Alcon, Swed.; Alcon, UK; Alcon Laboratories, USA)*; Betoptima *(Alcon, Ger.)*; Kerlon *(Lorex, Denm.; Lirca, Ital.; Kramer-Synthelabo, Switz.)*; Kerlone *(Robert et Carrière, Fr.; Beiersdorf, Ger.; Lorex, UK)*.

12440-n

Bevantolol Hydrochloride *(BANM, USAN, rINNM)*.

CI-775; NC-1400. 1-(3,4-Dimethoxyphenethylamino)-3-*m*-tolyloxypropan-2-ol hydrochloride.
$C_{20}H_{27}NO_4,HCl=381.9$.

CAS — 59170-23-9 (bevantolol); 42864-78-8 (hydrochloride).

Bevantolol hydrochloride is a moderately lipophilic beta blocker with general properties similar to those of propranolol (p.798). It is classified as cardioselective and is reported to be lacking in significant intrinsic sympathomimetic and membrane stabilising properties.

It has been investigated in doses of 200 to 400 mg daily in the management of hypertension; doses of 150 to 300 mg daily have been tried in patients with angina pectoris.

A preliminary review of bevantolol. Bevantolol is a beta blocker with a relatively high degree of selectivity for $beta_1$ receptors. It is generally well-tolerated; the most commonly reported side-effects have been headache, fatigue and dizziness, and gastro-intestinal disturbances. It is reported to be virtually completely absorbed from the gastro-intestinal tract and to undergo moderate first-pass metabolism, resulting in a bioavailabilty of about 60%. It is extensively metabolised and excreted largely in urine as metabolites and small amounts of unchanged drug; the elimination half-life has been reported as 1.5 hours. Studies have indicated that it is effective in the management of mild to moderate hypertension, and in angina pectoris; there is some evidence of a favourable effect on serum lipids and peripheral vascular resistance but this remains to be confirmed.— W. H. Frishman *et al.*, *Drugs*, 1988, *35*, 1.

For evidence of the need for caution when giving bevantolol to patients with asthma, see under Metoprolol Tartrate, p.792.

Proprietary Names and Manufacturers

Parke, Davis, USA.

18615-w

Bisoprolol Fumarate *(BANM, USAN, rINNM)*.

CL-297939; EMD-33512. 1-[4-(2-Isopropoxyethoxymethyl)phenoxy]-3-isopropylaminopropan-2-ol fumarate.
$(C_{18}H_{31}NO_4)_2,C_4H_4O_4=767.0$.

CAS — 66722-44-9 (bisoprolol); 66722-45-0 (fumarate).

Adverse Effects, Treatment, and Precautions

As for Propranolol Hydrochloride, p.798.

Absorption and Fate

Following oral administration bisoprolol is reported to be almost completely absorbed from the gastro-intestinal tract and to undergo only minimal first-pass metabolism; oral bioavailability is reported to be about 90%. Approximately 50% of a dose is metabolised in the liver and it is excreted in urine as unchanged drug and metabolites.

Uses and Administration

Bisoprolol is a relatively lipophilic beta blocker with general properties similar to those of propranolol, p.803. It is classified as cardioselective and is reported to be effectively lacking in intrinsic sympathomimetic and membrane stabilising properties.

Bisoprolol is given as the fumarate in the management of hypertension and angina pectoris. The usual dose ranges from 5 to 20 mg of bisoprolol fumarate as a single daily dose; most patients respond to 10 mg daily.

ADMINISTRATION IN RENAL FAILURE. Steady-state plasma concentrations of bisoprolol were significantly greater in 11 patients with renal failure given bisoprolol 10 mg daily for 7 days than in 8 healthy subjects given the same dose. Mean terminal elimination half-life was also greater at 18.5 hours in patients with renal failure than the value of 10.0 hours in healthy subjects. Following a single dose of bisoprolol 10 mg in a further 3 patients with uraemia and glomerular filtration-rates less than 5 mL per minute the half-life was even further prolonged at 24.2 hours. Patients with renal failure, especially advanced cases, may require dosage adjustment of bisoprolol.— W. Kirch *et al.*, *Br. J. clin. Pharmac.*, 1987, *23*, 623P.

Proprietary Preparations

Emcor *(E. Merck, UK)*. *Tablets* (Emcor LS), scored, bisoprolol fumarate 5 mg.
Tablets, scored, bisoprolol fumarate 10 mg.

Monocor *(Lederle, UK)*. *Tablets*, bisoprolol fumarate 5 and 10 mg.

Proprietary Names and Manufacturers

Concor *(E. Merck, Ger.; E. Merck, Switz.)*; Detensiel *(Merck-Clévenot, Fr.)*; Emcor *(E. Merck, UK)*; Monocor *(Lederle, UK)*.

16544-a

Bopindolol *(rINN)*.

LT-31-200. (±)-1-(*tert*-Butylamino)-3-[(2-methylindol-4-yl)oxy]propan-2-ol benzoate.
$C_{23}H_{28}N_2O_3=380.5$.

CAS — 62658-63-3.

Bopindolol is a beta blocker with general properties similar to those of propranolol (see p. 798). It is classified as non-cardioselective and is reported to possess some intrinsic sympathomimetic activity.

It is used in the management of hypertension and cardiac disorders in usual doses of 1 to 4 mg by mouth.

Proprietary Names and Manufacturers

Sandonorm *(Sandoz, Switz.)*.

12462-q

Bucindolol Hydrochloride *(BANM, USAN, rINNM)*.

MJ-13105-1. 2-[2-Hydroxy-3-(2-indol-3-yl-1,1-dimethylethylamino)propoxy]benzonitrile hydrochloride.
$C_{22}H_{25}N_3O_2,HCl=399.9$.

CAS — 71119-11-4 (bucindolol); 70369-47-0 (hydrochloride).

Bucindolol hydrochloride is a beta blocker with general properties similar to those of propranolol (see p.798). It is classified as non-cardioselective and is reported to possess intrinsic sympathomimetic activity as well as a vasodilator action. It has been investigated in the management of hypertension in doses up to 200 mg twice daily.

References: J. S. Gill and D. G. Beevers, *Eur. J. clin. Pharmac.*, 1984, *27*, 265; M. Maury *et al.*, *ibid.*, 1985, *27*, 649; J. Webster *et al.*, *Br. J. clin. Pharmac.*, 1985, *20*, 393; P. C. O'Connor *et al.*, *Br. J. clin. Pharmac.*, 1985, *20*, 659; C. Rosendorff *et al.*, *J. clin. Pharmac.*, 1985, *25*, 223.

Proprietary Names and Manufacturers

Bristol-Myers, UK; Mead Johnson Pharmaceutical, USA.

6305-w

Bufetolol Hydrochloride *(rINNM)*.

Y-6124. 1-*tert*-Butylamino-3-(2-tetrahydrofurfuryloxyphenoxy)propan-2-ol hydrochloride.
$C_{18}H_{29}NO_4,HCl=359.9$.

CAS — 53684-49-4 (bufetolol); 35108-88-4 (hydrochloride).

Bufetolol is a beta blocker with general properties similar to those of propranolol hydrochloride (see p.798). It has been given in doses of 5 to 30 mg or more daily by mouth in the treatment of various cardiovascular disorders.

Proprietary Names and Manufacturers

Adobiol *(Menarini, Ital.; Jpn)*.

6306-e

Bufuralol Hydrochloride *(BANM, rINNM).*
Ro-03-4787. 2-*tert*-Butylamino-1-(7-ethylbenzofuran-2-yl)ethanol hydrochloride.
$C_{16}H_{23}NO_2,HCl=297.8$.

CAS — 54340-62-4 (bufuralol); 60398-91-6 (hydrochloride).

Adverse Effects, Treatment, and Precautions
As for Propranolol Hydrochloride, p.798.

Side-effects of pallor, nausea and vomiting, bradycardia, and hypotension seen in some subjects given bufuralol appear to be related to vagal stimulation rather than beta blockade and are associated with poor metabolism of the drug to its hydroxylated metabolite.— P. Dayer *et al.* (letter), *Br. J. clin. Pharmac.*, 1982, *13*, 750.

Absorption and Fate
Following absorption from the gastro-intestinal tract bufuralol is reported to undergo first-pass metabolism in the liver. There is considerable interindividual variation in the ability to metabolise bufuralol. The major hydroxylated metabolite is reported to possess beta blocking activity and to have a longer half-life than that of the parent compound. Bufuralol is excreted in the urine almost entirely in the form of metabolites.

Following oral administration of radioactively labelled bufuralol 20 mg to 2 healthy subjects elimination was essentially complete within 3 days. About 75% was excreted in the urine, almost entirely in the form of metabolites.— R. J. Francis *et al.*, *Eur. J. Drug Metab. Pharmacokinet.*, 1976, *1*, 113.

The pharmacokinetic and pharmacodynamic behaviour of tolamolol and bufuralol cannot be explained adequately without taking into account their active metabolites.— L. P. Balant and J. Fabre (letter), *Lancet*, 1978, *2*, 425.

In a study involving 10 hypertensive patients given bufuralol 30 mg by mouth, bufuralol appeared rapidly in the plasma after ingestion; there was a 5-fold variation between patients in speed of absorption but in all cases it was complete by 2 hours. The calculated maximum concentration ranged from 44.6 to 200.3 ng per mL. Elimination appeared to be by a first-order process with a mean elimination half-life of 2.75 hours. In contrast the major metabolite 1-hydroxybufuralol (Ro-3-7410) had a longer mean half-life of 7.19 hours. Peak plasma concentrations of the metabolite ranged from 36.1 to 91.5 ng per mL.— M. Eckert *et al.*, *Eur. J. clin. Pharmac.*, 1983, *24*, 479.

Studies of genetic polymorphism in the oxidative metabolism of bufuralol: P. Dayer *et al.*, *Eur. J. clin. Pharmac.*, 1983, *24*, 797; P. Dayer *et al.*, *ibid.*, 1985, *28*, 317.

Uses and Administration
Bufuralol is a beta blocker with general properties similar to those of propranolol (see p.803). It is classified as non-cardioselective and has some intrinsic sympathomimetic activity.

ACTION. The haemodynamic effects of bufuralol hydrochloride 20 mg intravenously were compared with those of pindolol 2 mg intravenously. Further studies are needed to determine whether bufuralol is a selective or non-selective beta-adrenoceptor blocking agent. In addition to its beta-adrenoceptor blocking effects it was considered that bufuralol may also have a direct effect on peripheral resistance.— D. Magometschnigg *et al.*, *Int. J. clin. Pharmac. Biopharm.*, 1978, *16*, 54.

Further references: T. H. Pringle *et al.*, *Br. J. clin. Pharmac.*, 1986, *22*, 527; G. D. Johnston *et al.*, *Eur. J. clin. Pharmac.*, 1986, *30*, 649.

Proprietary Names and Manufacturers
Roche, UK.

6307-l

Bunitrolol Hydrochloride *(rINNM).*
Ko-1366 (bunitrolol). 2-(3-*tert*-Butylamino-2-hydroxypropoxy)benzonitrile hydrochloride.
$C_{14}H_{20}N_2O_2,HCl=284.8$.

CAS — 34915-68-9 (bunitrolol).

Adverse Effects, Treatment, and Precautions
As for Propranolol Hydrochloride, p.798.

Uses and Administration
Bunitrolol is a beta blocker with general properties similar to those of propranolol (see p.803). It is given as the hydrochloride in usual doses of 10 mg up to 3 times daily in the management of cardiovascular disorders.

Proprietary Names and Manufacturers
Stresson *(Boehringer Ingelheim, Ger.).*

6309-j

Bupranolol Hydrochloride *(rINNM).*
B-1312; KL-255. 1-*tert*-Butylamino-3-(6-chloro-*m*-tolyloxy)propan-2-ol hydrochloride.
$C_{14}H_{22}ClNO_2,HCl=308.2$.

CAS — 14556-46-8 (bupranolol); 15148-80-8 (hydrochloride).

Adverse Effects, Treatment, and Precautions
As for Propranolol Hydrochloride, p.798.
Bupranolol has been reported to be metabolised in the liver under the influence of monoamine oxidase; concomitant administration with monoamine oxidase inhibitors has been contra-indicated.

Uses and Administration
Bupranolol hydrochloride is a beta blocker with general properties similar to those of propranolol (see p.803). It has been given in doses of 100 to 400 mg daily, usually in 2 or 3 divided doses, in the management of cardiovascular disorders.

Proprietary Names and Manufacturers
Bétadran *(Logeais, Fr.)*; Betadrenol *(Galenica, Switz.; Melusin, Ger.; Schwarz, Ital.; Pharma-Schwarz, Switz.)*; Looser *(Jpn)*; Monobeltin *(Arg.)*; Ophtorenin *(Winzer, Ger.)*; Panimit *(Natrapharm, Ger.).*

12479-c

Butofilolol *(rINN).*
CM-6805a. (±)-2′-(3-*tert*-Butylamino-2-hydroxypropoxy)-5′-fluorobutyrophenone.
$C_{17}H_{26}FNO_3=311.4$.

CAS — 64552-17-6.

Butofilolol is a beta blocker with general properties similar to those of propranolol (see p.798). It is classified as non-cardioselective and is reported to be effectively lacking in intrinsic sympathomimetic and membrane stabilising properties. It is used in the management of hypertension in usual doses of the equivalent of 100 mg twice daily as the maleate; up to 400 mg daily may be given in some cases.

Proprietary Names and Manufacturers
Cafide *(Labaz, Fr.).*

12521-h

Carazolol *(BAN, rINN).*
BM-51052. 1-(Carbazol-4-yloxy)-3-isopropylaminopropan-2-ol.
$C_{18}H_{22}N_2O_2=298.4$.

CAS — 57775-29-8.

Carazolol is a beta blocker with general properties similar to those of propranolol (see p.798). It has been used in the management of hypertension in doses of 5 to 10 mg daily; up to 30 mg daily in divided doses has been given to patients with cardiac disorders.

Proprietary Names and Manufacturers
Conducton *(Klinge, Ger.).*

12533-g

Carteolol Hydrochloride *(BANM, USAN, rINNM).*

Abbott-43326; OPC-1085. 5-(3-*tert*-Butylamino-2-hydroxypropoxy)-3,4-dihydroquinolin-2(1*H*)-one hydrochloride.
$C_{16}H_{24}N_2O_3,HCl=328.8$.

CAS — 51781-06-7 (carteolol); 51781-21-6 (hydrochloride).

Adverse Effects, Treatment, and Precautions
As for Propranolol Hydrochloride, p.798.
Systemic side-effects may follow topical use of the eye-drops; local irritation and blurred vision have also been reported.

Uses and Administration
Carteolol hydrochloride is a beta blocker with general properties similar or those of propranolol (see p. 803). It is classified as non-cardioselective and is reported to possess intrinsic sympathomimetic activity.
It is used in the management of hypertension and cardiac disorders; doses of 5 to 20 mg daily have been given.
Eye-drops containing carteolol hydrochloride 1% or 2% are instilled twice daily in the treatment of open-angle glaucoma and ocular hypertension.

References: T. Ishizaki *et al.*, *Eur. J. clin. Pharmac.*, 1983, *25*, 95 (pharmacokinetics); T. D. Giles *et al.*, *Clin. Pharmac. Ther.*, 1984, *35*, 301 (antihypertensive action); M. T. Velasquez *et al.*, *J. clin. Pharmac.*, 1985, *25*, 601 (use in hypertension); R. R. Luther *et al.*, *J. int. med. Res.*, 1986, *14*, 167 (use in angina pectoris); R. R. Luther *et al.*, *ibid.*, 175 (use in hypertension); *Drug & Ther. Bull.*, 1987, *25*, 63 (topical use in glaucoma).

Proprietary Preparations
Teoptic *(Dispersa, UK). Eye-drops*, carteolol hydrochloride 1 and 2%.

Proprietary Names and Manufacturers
Arteolol *(Lacer, Spain)*; Arteoptic *(Dispersa, Ger.)*; Carteol *(Chauvin-Blache, Fr.)*; Endak *(Madaus, Ger.)*; Mikelan *(Otsuka, Jpn; Miquel, Spain)*; Teoptic *(Dispersa, UK).*

16573-d

Celiprolol Hydrochloride *(BANM, USAN, rINNM).*
3-{3-Acetyl-4-[3-(*tert*-butylamino)-2-hydroxypropoxy]-phenyl}-1,1-diethylurea hydrochloride.
$C_{20}H_{33}N_3O_4,HCl=416.0$.

CAS — 56980-93-9 (celiprolol); 57470-78-7 (hydrochloride).

Celiprolol is a beta blocker with general properties similar to those of propranolol (see p.798). It is classified as cardioselective and is reported to possess intrinsic sympathomimetic activity. Celiprolol hydrochloride is used in the treatment of hypertension and angina pectoris in usual doses of 200 to 300 mg daily; up to 600 mg may be required in some cases.

Proceedings of a symposium on celiprolol.— *Br. J. clin. Pract.*, 1985, *39*, *Suppl.* 40, 1–100.

Studies *in vitro* indicated that as well as beta$_1$ blocking properties celiprolol possessed alpha$_2$ blocking actions and some intrinsic sympathomimetic activity at beta$_2$ receptors.— E. Marmo *et al.*, *Curr. ther. Res.*, 1986, *40*, 475.

Proprietary Names and Manufacturers
Selectol *(Chemie-Linz, Aust.).*

12591-c

Cloranolol *(rINN).*
GYKI-41099. 1-(*tert*-Butylamino)-3-(2,5-dichlorophenoxy)propan-2-ol.
$C_{13}H_{19}Cl_2NO_2=292.2$.

CAS — 39563-28-5.

Cloranolol is reported to be a beta blocker.

Proprietary Names and Manufacturers
Tobanum *(Gedeon Richter, Hung.).*

6310-q

Dexpropranolol Hydrochloride *(BANM, USAN, rINNM).*
AY-20694; ICI-47319. (*R*)-1-Isopropylamino-3-(1-naphthyloxy)propan-2-ol hydrochloride.
$C_{16}H_{21}NO_2,HCl=295.8$.

CAS — 5051-22-9 (dexpropranolol); 13071-11-9 (hydrochloride).

Dexpropranolol is the dextro-isomer of propranolol (see p.798) and has similar membrane-stabilising effects but has little beta blocking activity.

For reference to the potential role of dexpropranolol as a vaginal contraceptive see under Propranolol Hydrochloride, p.805.

Proprietary Names and Manufacturers
ICI Pharmaceuticals, UK.

12638-z

Diacetolol Hydrochloride *(BANM, USAN, rINNM).*
EU-4891; M&B-16942A. 3′-Acetyl-4′-(2-hydroxy-3-isopropylaminopropoxy)acetanilide hydrochloride.
$C_{16}H_{24}N_2O_4$,HCl=344.8.

CAS — 28197-69-5 (diacetolol); 69796-04-9 (hydrochloride).

Diacetolol is an active metabolite of acebutolol (p.781).

Proprietary Names and Manufacturers
May & Baker, UK; Norwich Eaton, USA.

16636-f

Esmolol Hydrochloride *(BANM, USAN, pINNM).*
ASL-8052. Methyl 3-[4-(2-hydroxy-3-isopropylaminopropoxy)phenyl]propionate hydrochloride.
$C_{16}H_{25}NO_4$,HCl=331.8.

CAS — 84057-94-3 (esmolol); 81161-17-3 (hydrochloride).

Adverse Effects, Treatment and Precautions
As for Propranolol Hydrochloride, p.798.
Local irritation at the site of infusion, inflammation, and occasionally thrombophlebitis have occurred. Because of the very short duration of action of esmolol most adverse effects resolve rapidly on terminating the infusion.

Absorption and Fate
Following intravenous administration of esmolol the drug is rapidly hydrolysed by blood and tissue esterases. Blood concentrations are reported to decline in a biphasic manner with a distribution half-life of about 2 minutes and an elimination half-life of approximately 9 minutes. It is excreted in urine, primarily as the de-esterified metabolite ASL-8123.

References: C. Y. Sum *et al., Clin. Pharmac. Ther.*, 1983, *34,* 427; R. Achari *et al., J. clin. Pharmac.*, 1986, *26,* 44.

Uses and Administration
Esmolol is a relatively hydrophilic short-acting beta blocker with general properties similar to those of propranolol (see p.803). It is classified as cardioselective and is reported to be effectively lacking in intrinsic sympathomimetic and membrane stabilising properties.
Esmolol hydrochloride is given by intravenous infusion in the emergency treatment of cardiac arrhythmias. A loading dose of 500 μg per kg body-weight over 1 minute is followed by an initial maintenance infusion of 50 μg per kg per minute for 4 minutes. If there is no response, further loading doses may be followed by increases of the rate of maintenance infusion, in increments of 50 μg per kg per minute, to a maximum of 200 μg per kg per minute. Little additional benefit is obtained from further increases in maintenance dosage. Once a satisfactory response is obtained infusion may be continued, if necessary, for up to 48 hours.

Reviews of esmolol: D. M. Angaran *et al., Clin. Pharm.*, 1986, *5,* 288; *Med. Lett.*, 1987, *29,* 57; P. Benfield and E. M. Sorkin, *Drugs*, 1987, *33,* 392.
Further references: C. S. Reilly *et al., Clin. Pharmac. Ther.*, 1985, *38,* 579 (comparison with propranolol-induced beta blockade); R. D. Reynolds *et al., J. clin. Pharmac.*, 1986, *26, Suppl.* A, A3 (pharmacology and pharmacokinetics); R. J. Sung *et al., ibid.*, A15 (use in cardiac arrhythmias and myocardial ischaemia).

Proprietary Names and Manufacturers
Brevibloc *(Du Pont, USA).*

12849-m

Indenolol Hydrochloride *(BANM).*
Sch-28316Z (indenolol); YB-2. A 2:1 tautomeric mixture of 1-(inden-7-yloxy)-3-isopropylaminopropan-2-ol hydrochloride and 1-(inden-4-yloxy)-3-isopropylaminopropan-2-ol hydrochloride.
$C_{15}H_{21}NO_2$,HCl=283.8.

CAS — 60607-68-3 (indenolol); 68906-88-7 (hydrochloride).

Indenolol hydrochloride is a beta blocker with general properties similar to those of propranolol (p.798). It is classified as non-cardioselective and is reported to possess potent membrane stabilising properties; reports of intrinsic sympathomimetic activity have not been confirmed.
It has been tried in the management of hypertension in doses of 60 to 120 mg daily; up to 90 mg daily in divided doses has been given in angina pectoris and cardiac disorders.

Proprietary Names and Manufacturers
Pulsan *(Jpn)*; Securpres *(Poli, Ital.).*

6311-p

Labetalol Hydrochloride *(BANM, USAN, rINNM).*

AH-5158A; Ibidomide Hydrochloride; Sch-15719W. 5-[1-Hydroxy-2-(1-methyl-3-phenylpropylamino)ethyl]salicylamide hydrochloride; 2-Hydroxy-5-[1-hydroxy-2-(1-methyl-3-phenylpropylamino)ethyl]benzamide hydrochloride.
$C_{19}H_{24}N_2O_3$,HCl=364.9.

CAS — 36894-69-6 (labetalol); 32780-64-6 (hydrochloride).

Pharmacopoeias. In *Br.*

A white or almost white powder or granules. **Soluble** 1 in 60 of water and of alcohol; practically insoluble in chloroform and in ether. A 1% solution in water has a pH of 4 to 5. The *B.P.* injection has a pH of 3.5 to 4.5 and is **sterilised** by autoclaving.
Store in well-closed containers; the injection should be protected from light.

A study of the compatibility of labetalol injection with solutions for intravenous infusion. A precipitate occurred within six hours of admixture with sodium bicarbonate 5% injection but labetalol was apparently stable for 72 hours when mixed with Ringer's and lactated Ringer's injections, glucose injection (5%), and various strengths of glucose and sodium chloride injection.— P. -H. C. Yuen *et al., Am. J. Hosp. Pharm.*, 1983, *40,* 1007. Comment.— A. S. Alam (letter), *ibid.*, 1984, *41,* 74.

Adverse Effects
Since labetalol has alpha blocking properties plus beta blocking effects, postural hypotension may be associated with labetalol, particularly with high doses or in the early stages of therapy. Other side-effects reported include scalp tingling and other forms of paraesthesia, gastro-intestinal disturbances, headache, tiredness and lethargy, muscular weakness and cramps, dyspnoea, failure of ejaculation, reduced libido, impotence, urinary retention, nasal stuffiness, insomnia, vivid dreams, skin rashes, and depression. A positive antinuclear factor test has occasionally been associated with labetalol, and hypersensitivity reactions including pruritus, angioedema, and fever have been reported.

Analysis by the manufacturers of the side-effects associated with the first 3 months of labetalol therapy, in doses of up to 400 mg, in 1061 hypertensive patients was: lethargy (3.9%), dizziness (4.5%), headache (1.9%), upper gastro-intestinal tract symptoms, including nausea (2.6%), postural hypotension (0.7%), depression (0.7%), dyspnoea (1.4%), tingling sensation in skin or scalp (1.0%).— D. Harris and D. A. Richards (letter), *Br. med. J.*, 1978, *2,* 894.
Side-effects were reported by 91 of 163 patients with hypertension who received up to 6 months' therapy with labetalol at a mean initial dose of 399 mg increased to 420 mg at 4 to 6 months. Symptoms which were of sufficient severity for 29 patients to withdraw from treatment included tingling of scalp, muzzy head, tiredness, limb weakness, headaches, dizziness, gastro-intestinal effects, insomnia, and bronchospasm.— W. S. Manderson, *Practitioner*, 1979, *222,* 131.

ALLERGY. A report of an anaphylactoid reaction to labetalol given by mouth.— C. E. Ferree (letter), *Ann. intern. Med.*, 1986, *104,* 729.

EFFECTS ON THE BLOOD. *Leucopenia.* Mention of leucopenia in a patient taking labetalol.— G. L. Sanders *et al., Eur. J. clin. Pharmac.*, 1978, *14,* 301.

EFFECTS ON THE CARDIOVASCULAR SYSTEM. Labetalol 1 to 2 mg per kg body-weight by intravenous bolus injection produced a poor response in 5 of 6 patients with severe hypertension but an adequate reduction in diastolic blood pressure was obtained by the additional administration of other antihypertensive drugs. In the sixth patient there was an immediate and profound depressor response following labetalol which necessitated the infusion of a pressor agent.— E. P. MacCarthy *et al., Med. J. Aust.*, 1978, *1,* 399.
A comment on the incidence of postural hypotension in association with labetalol therapy. Of 57 patients treated with labetalol and a thiazide diuretic for up to 16 months, 20 had very minor symptoms of postural hypotension occurring usually 1 or 2 hours after taking the tablets. In only 5 were the effects severe enough to require a reduction in labetalol dose. This low incidence of serious postural hypotension may have reflected careful adjustment of labetalol doses, and concurrent use of a thiazide diuretic. Division of the daily dosage into 3 rather than 2 doses also reduced or abolished postural symptoms. Two patients appeared to be hypersensitive, with weakness and tachycardia in one and profound weakness and faintness in the second; their hypersensitivity may have been due to enhanced bioavailability of labetalol. This first-dose effect was similar to that seen after prazosin excepting that the patients remained sensitive to labetalol and needed only very small doses for satisfactory blood pressure control.— W. J. Louis *et al.* (letter), *Lancet*, 1978, *1,* 452.

EFFECTS ON THE EYES. *Melanin binding.* Studies in *animals* indicated that labetalol binds to ocular melanin, but no evidence of oculotoxicity was found.— D. Poynter *et al., Br. J. clin. Pharmac.*, 1976, *3, Suppl.* 3, 711.

EFFECTS ON IMMUNE RESPONSE. A positive antinuclear factor test in association with labetalol therapy.— W. J. Louis *et al.* (letter), *Lancet*, 1978, *1,* 452.
A finding of anti-mitochondrial antibodies in 7 of 90 patients on labetalol. The patients had been on labetalol for many months and were usually taking a high dose, and the anti-mitochondrial antibodies have not yet posed a clinical problem. Nevertheless, screening for anti-mitochondrial antibodies and the search for possible clinical complications seems warranted.— J. D. Wilson *et al.* (letter), *Lancet*, 1980, *2,* 312.
See also under Allergy, above.

EFFECTS ON LIPID METABOLISM. No significant changes were noted in plasma lipid and plasma urate concentrations in 33 patients treated with labetalol for a year.— R. J. S. McGonigle *et al.* (letter), *Lancet*, 1981, *1,* 163. A similar report.— Y. Goto *et al., Br. J. clin. Pract.*, 1987, *41,* 957.

EFFECTS ON THE MUSCLES. Toxic myopathy associated with the use of labetalol.— A. Teicher *et al., Br. med. J.*, 1981, *282,* 1824.

EFFECTS ON THE NERVOUS SYSTEM. Scalp tingling occurred in 2 patients receiving labetalol. In 1 patient the effect was severe enough to cause withdrawal of the drug.— A. S. P. Hua *et al.* (letter), *Lancet*, 1977, *2,* 295. One similar case of scalp tingling associated with labetalol; this patient also experienced a severe visual aura suggestive of migraine. Another patient given labetalol experienced tingling over his body, dizziness, and the desire but inability to urinate. A similar effect on urination was observed in a young diabetic with end-stage chronic renal failure given one dose of labetalol 100 mg.— R. R. Bailey (letter), *ibid.*, 720. The Committee on Safety of Medicines had received similar reports. The scalp alone was usually involved but in some instances there was widespread paraesthesia.— E. Scowen (letter), *ibid.*, 1978, *1,* 98.
A 39-year-old man developed peri-oral numbness and then tingling while taking labetalol 600 mg twice daily.— R. Gabriel (letter), *Br. med. J.*, 1978, *1,* 580.

EFFECTS ON RESPIRATORY FUNCTION. In 10 patients with asthma both propranolol 5 mg intravenously and labetalol 20 mg intravenously significantly reduced exercise-induced tachycardia, compared with a placebo. Patients had bronchoconstriction (assessed by forced expiratory volume and forced vital capacity) after propranolol but not after labetalol. This was consistent with blockade by labetalol of alpha-adrenoceptors in the bronchi.— C. Skinner *et al., Br. med. J.*, 1975, *2,* 59.
An asthmatic woman in hospital died after receiving labetalol 400 mg which had been intended for another patient.— *Pharm. J.*, 1977, *2,* 139.

Further references: S. H. D. Jackson and D. G. Beevers, *Br. J. clin. Pharmac.*, 1983, *15*, 553 (labetalol and atenolol had comparable effects on FEV_1 in asthmatics).

EFFECTS ON SEXUAL FUNCTION. Priapism resulting in impotence in a patient undergoing dialysis may have been associated either with the administration of labetalol or with the uraemic condition.— M. R. Law *et al.* (letter), *Br. med. J.*, 1980, *280*, 115.

EFFECTS ON THE SKIN. *Lichen planus.* An eruption resembling lichen planus developed in a 67-year-old man after taking labetalol for 12 weeks; the eruption subsided when labetalol was withdrawn and recurred 15 days after labetalol was again given. Lichenoid reactions were possibly related to beta-adrenoceptor blockade.— R. W. Gange and E. W. Jones, *Br. med. J.*, 1978, *1*, 816.

A 68-year-old woman developed a lichenoid eruption similar to both pityriasis rubra pilaris and follicular lichen planus after taking labetalol 200 to 400 mg thrice daily for several months. The rash resolved on cessation of therapy.— W. A. Branford *et al.*, *Practitioner*, 1978, *221*, 765.

A report of a hypertensive woman with scleroderma in whom a severe lichenoid skin eruption developed when she took labetalol; she was positive for anti-mitochondrial antibodies.— R. Staughton *et al.* (letter), *Lancet*, 1980, *2*, 581. The anti-mitochondrial antibodies may have been related to the scleroderma, not the labetalol.— C. J. Stevenson (letter), *ibid.*, 924.

Psoriasiform eruption. A patient who had taken labetalol 400 mg twice daily for 3 months developed a widespread scaly erythematous rash similar to that previously described in connection with other beta-blockers; the rash recurred after challenge with pure labetalol thus excluding incrimination of other ingredients of the commercial product.— A. Y. Finlay and E. Waddington (letter), *Br. med. J.*, 1978, *1*, 987. A similar report of rash in a 66-year-old woman who had taken labetalol for 13 months.— R. L. Savage *et al.* (letter), *ibid.*

LUPUS ERYTHEMATOSUS. Lupus-like illness in a woman taking labetalol; the condition resolved when labetalol was withdrawn.— I. D. Griffiths and J. Richardson (letter), *Br. med. J.*, 1979, *2*, 497.

SLE syndrome probably induced by labetalol.— R. C. Brown *et al.*, *Postgrad. med. J.*, 1981, *57*, 189.

OVERDOSAGE. Acute oliguric renal failure developed after a short period of moderate hypotension in a patient who ingested labetalol 16 g. Renal function subsequently recovered.— A. J. Smit *et al.*, *Br. med. J.*, 1986, *293*, 1142.

Treatment of Adverse Effects

In the treatment of overdosage with labetalol, account must be taken not only of its beta blocking properties (see Propranolol, Treatment of Adverse Effects, p.800) but also of its alpha blocking properties.

Severe hypotension may respond to placing the patient in the supine position with the feet raised. Bradycardia should be treated immediately by the intravenous injection of atropine, in doses up to 3 mg. If further measures are required it has been suggested that noradrenaline may be preferable to isoprenaline in restoring circulation. The recommended starting dose of noradrenaline is 5 to 10 µg intravenously repeated as necessary according to the patient's response; alternatively it may be given by intravenous infusion at a rate of 5 µg per minute until a satisfactory response is achieved. However, in severe overdosage treatment with glucagon, in doses similar to those advocated for beta blocker overdosage (see p.800), may be preferred.

The stomach should be emptied by aspiration and lavage, if ingestion of an overdose is recent.

Precautions

As for Propranolol Hydrochloride, p.801.

Owing to the alpha blocking properties of labetalol, postural hypotension may occur, particularly after initial doses. The effect of halothane on blood pressure may be enhanced by labetalol.

Hemiparesis with persistent paresis of the left arm developed in a 48-year-old woman given labetalol 35 mg intravenously over 2 or 3 minutes for hypertensive encephalopathy; her blood pressure fell from 250/150 to 160/95 mmHg. Labetalol should be given to slow infusion in such circumstances.— R. Solomons (letter), *Br. med. J.*, 1979, *2*, 672.

INTERACTIONS. A patient who had undergone renal transplantation and was taking methyldopa, propranolol, guanethidine, amiloride with hydrochlorothiazide, prednisolone, and azathioprine experienced a rise in blood pressure after 2 of 3 intravenous doses of labetalol.— M. Crofton and R. Gabriel, *Br. med. J.*, 1977, *2*, 737. Labetalol 1 mg per kg body-weight intravenously produced a significant fall in supine blood pressure in 10 of 17 patients with severe hypertension. Of the 7 non-responders all were receiving antihypertensive agents concurrently compared to 2 of the 10 responders.— B. P. McGarth *et al.*, *Med. J. Aust.*, 1978, *2*, 410.

The bioavailability of oral labetalol was significantly reduced from 30.3 to 17.0% in 5 healthy subjects following a 3-week course of glutethimide 500 mg daily. In contrast, following cimetidine 1.6 g daily for 3 days in 6 subjects systemic bioavailability of labetalol increased from 25.1 to 39.0%. Both glutethimide and cimetidine alter the first-pass metabolism of labetalol and this should be borne in mind in clinical practice.— T. K. Daneshmend and C. J. C. Roberts, *Br. J. clin. Pharmac.*, 1984, *18*, 393.

For a study indicating that *food* increases the bioavailability of labetalol see under Administration, below.

Interference with diagnostic tests. In 10 hypertensive patients taking labetalol 1 to 4.8 g daily there was no evidence, when sensitive and specific radio-enzymatic methods were used, that labetalol increased plasma concentrations of noradrenaline or the urinary excretion of endogenous adrenaline or noradrenaline.— C. A. Hamilton *et al.*, *Br. med. J.*, 1978, *2*, 800.

No significant elevation of plasma concentrations of noradrenaline or adrenaline occurs after acute intravenous administration of labetalol, but it interferes with fluorimetric measurements of urinary catecholamines to cause falsely elevated values, which could lead to a misdiagnosis of phaeochromocytoma. No such interference occurs when high-pressure liquid chromatographic methods are used.— D. A. Richards *et al.* (letter), *Br. med. J.*, 1979, *1*, 685.

Absorption and Fate

Labetalol is readily absorbed from the gastro-intestinal tract, but is subject to considerable first-pass metabolism; relative bioavailability is reported to be about 25%. Peak plasma concentrations occur about 1 or 2 hours after a dose. It is metabolised in the liver, the metabolites being excreted in the urine together with only small amounts of unchanged labetalol; its major metabolite has not been found to have significant alpha- or beta-adrenoceptor blocking effects. Excretion also occurs in the faeces via the bile. Labetalol crosses the placenta and is excreted in breast milk. Only very small amounts appear to cross the blood-brain barrier in *animals*. It is about 50% protein bound.

Increasing bioavailability of labetalol with age.— J. G. Kelly *et al.*, *Br. J. clin. Pharmac.*, 1982, *14*, 304.

A review of the clinical pharmacokinetics of labetalol. Labetalol is rapidly absorbed but undergoes presystemic metabolism in the liver and possibly the gut wall. Bioavailability has been reported to vary considerably between individuals and values ranging from 11 to 86% have been reported; bioavailability is increased when the drug is given with food, and appears to increase with age. The drug is widely distributed in the body; studies in *animals* have indicated accumulation in lung, liver, and kidney but little present in brain tissue. It binds reversibly to melanin in the uveal tract of the eye. Elimination is largely by glucuronidation in the liver, metabolites being excreted both in urine and faeces. The decline in plasma concentrations is bi- or tri-exponential, and the terminal elimination half-life has been reported to range from 1.7 to 6.1 hours.— J. J. McNeil and W. J. Louis, *Clin. Pharmacokinet.*, 1984, *9*, 157.

Uses and Administration

Labetalol hydrochloride is an antihypertensive agent with beta blocking properties similar to those of propranolol hydrochloride (see p.803). Its beta blocking properties are classified as non-cardioselective, and it is reported to possess some intrinsic sympathomimetic activity. In addition, however, it has selective $alpha_1$ blocking properties which reduce blood pressure by decreasing peripheral vascular resistance and, in addition, confer upon labetalol a rapid onset of action.

In the treatment of hypertension labetalol hydrochloride is usually given in an initial dose of 100 mg twice daily with food, if necessary gradually increased after about two weeks, according to the response of the patient, to 200 to 400 mg twice daily; total daily doses of 2.4 g have occasionally been required. Hospital in-patients may be given dosage increases on a daily basis where reduction of blood pressure is urgent.

For the emergency treatment of hypertension labetalol hydrochloride may be given by slow intravenous injection. In the *UK* a dose of 50 mg, over a period of at least 1 minute, has been recommended; if necessary this dose may be repeated at intervals of 5 minutes until a total of 200 mg has been given. In the *USA* an initial dose of 20 mg is recommended, given over 2 minutes; subsequent doses of 40 to 80 mg may be given every 10 minutes if necessary up to a maximum of 300 mg. Blood pressure should be monitored, and the patient should remain supine during intravenous administration and for 3 hours afterwards, to avoid excessive postural hypotension. Following bolus intravenous injection a maximum effect is usually obtained within 5 minutes and usually lasts up to 6 hours, although it may extend as long as 18 hours.

Labetalol hydrochloride has also been given by intravenous infusion.

A recommended initial dose in hypotensive anaesthesia is 10 to 20 mg intravenously, with increments of 5 to 10 mg if satisfactory hypotension is not achieved after 5 minutes. A higher initial dose may be required if halothane anaesthesia is not used (see under Precautions, above).

For a series of papers on labetalol, see *Br. J. clin. Pharmac.*, 1982, *13*, *Suppl.* 1, 1S-141S.

Reviews of labetalol: J. D. Wallin and W.M. O'Neill, *Archs intern. Med.*, 1983, *143*, 485; E. L. Michelson and W. H. Frishman, *Ann. intern. Med.*, 1983, *99*, 553; C. S. Conner, *Drug Intell. & clin. Pharm.*, 1983, *17*, 543; B. L. Carter, *ibid.*, 704; *Med. Lett.*, 1984, *26*, 83.

ACTION. It was estimated that the alpha : beta component activity of labetalol was about 1 : 3, its action being competitive at both sites.— D. A. Richards *et al.*, *Br. J. clin. Pharmac.*, 1976, *3*, 849.

Labetalol contains 2 asymmetric centres and exists as a mixture of equal proportions of the 4 stereoisomers. In a study in *animals* given the individual stereoisomers it was concluded that most of the $alpha_1$ blocking activity of labetalol resided in the (*SR*)-stereoisomer, and most of the beta blocking activity in the (*RR*)-stereoisomer.— R. T. Brittain *et al.*, *Br. J. Pharmac.*, 1982, *77*, 105.

ADMINISTRATION. In a study in 6 healthy subjects administration of labetalol 200 mg by mouth after a standard breakfast resulted in a 38% increase in mean systemic bioavailability compared with ingestion after an overnight fast. Food appears to increase the bioavailability of labetalol by reducing first-pass metabolism; labetalol should be taken at a standard time in relation to meals in order to minimise variations in availability.— T. K. Daneshmend and C. J. C. Roberts, *Br. J. clin. Pharmac.*, 1982, *14*, 73.

In the elderly. The use of labetalol 50 mg twice daily as an initial dose in elderly patients minimised side-effects and allowed eventual hypertensive control on lower maintenance doses.— S. R. Datta, *Br. J. clin. Pract.*, 1986, *40*, 434.

ADMINISTRATION IN HEPATIC FAILURE. Plasma concentrations of labetalol were similar, after intravenous administration, in patients with liver disease and in controls. After oral administration concentrations were higher in patients than in controls, due to reduced first-pass metabolism. The plasma half-life was similar in each group.— M. Homeida *et al.*, *Br. med. J.*, 1978, *2*, 1048.

CARDIAC DISORDERS. *Angina pectoris.* The value of combined alpha and beta blockade with labetalol in angina pectoris.— K. D. Mulac, *Postgrad. med. J.*, 1983, *59*, *Suppl.* 3, 33. See also S. H. Taylor *et al.*, *Br. med. J.*, 1982, *285*, 325.

Cardiac arrhythmias. A study on the anti-arrhythmic effects of labetalol.— C. Mazzola *et al.*, *Curr. ther. Res.*, 1981, *29*, 613.

Alpha receptors appear to play a role in the pathogenesis of ventricular arrhythmias in mitral valve prolapse syndrome and labetalol offers an alternative treatment for management of this condition.— G. S. Butrous *et al.*, *Postgrad. med. J.*, 1986, *62*, 259.

Myocardial infarction. Infusion of labetalol intravenously reduced systemic hypertension in 11 patients with myocardial infarction; myocardial oxygen demand was also reduced, as determined by double product, and there was no evidence of any worsening of left-sided heart failure. Labetalol appears to be ideal for the management of hypertension associated with acute myocardial infarction.— M. Renard *et al.*, *Br. Heart J.*, 1983, *49*, 522.

Intravenous infusion of labetalol followed by oral administration for 5 days in 83 patients with suspected myocardial infarction did not appear to be of benefit in limiting myocardial necrosis compared with 83 controls. Both groups received conventional therapy concomitantly. Labetalol should not be used to limit infarction in normotensive patients.— M. E. Heber *et al.*, *Eur. Heart J.*, 1987, *8*, 11.

HYPERTENSION. In a multicentre study involving 145 hypertensive patients (untreated standing diastolic pressures of 90 to 115 mmHg) patients received titrated doses of labetalol 100 to 600 mg twice daily or propranolol 40 to 240 mg twice daily for 3 months; hydrochlorothiazide was added if the standing diastolic blood pressure was still greater than 100 mmHg. At the end of monotherapy the reduction in standing blood pressure in patients receiving labetalol was 10.8/10.9 mmHg which was significantly greater than the fall of 4.0/5.1 mmHg in those receiving propranolol. Analysis of the results indicated that while the reductions in blood pressure were not significantly different in white patients, in black patients propranolol produced a significantly lesser fall in blood pressure than in whites whereas the effects of labetalol were maintained at a similar level to those in whites. Unlike pure beta blockers such as propranolol, which appear to be less effective in black hypertensives, labetalol is an effective antihypertensive agent in both black and white patients.— W. Flamenbaum, *J. natn. med. Ass.*, 1985, *77*, *Suppl.*, 14. Further evidence from post-marketing surveillance in 427 patients that labetalol is an effective antihypertensive agent in both black and non-black patients.— D. L. Due *et al.*, *Curr. ther. Res.*, 1986, *40*, 181.

A multicentre study of labetalol with hydrochlorothiazide in essential hypertension. In 83 patients in whom hydrochlorothiazide 25 mg twice daily failed to reduce standing diastolic pressure below 95 mmHg, addition of labetalol 100 to 400 mg twice daily induced a small but significant dose-related decrease in blood pressure; the mean fall was 10/9 mmHg supine and 17/13 mmHg standing. This compared with a fall of 3/4 mmHg in supine and 5/5 mmHg in standing pressures in a further 91 patients who had placebo added to their hydrochlorothiazide therapy. The effects of adding labetalol were significantly greater than those of adding placebo, and this applied in both black and non-black subjects. Five patients receiving labetalol were withdrawn from the study due to adverse effects including bronchospasm and elevated creatine kinase values with chest pain. One patient receiving placebo was also withdrawn due to adverse effects; 11 patients taking placebo and 2 receiving labetalol were also withdrawn due to unacceptably high blood pressure. Labetalol appears to be a relatively safe and effective step II agent in patients whose hypertension is not controlled by a diuretic alone.— *Clin. Pharmac. Ther.*, 1985, *38*, 24.

Clonidine withdrawal. The use of labetalol to prevent hypertensive rebound after clonidine withdrawal.— T. Rosenthal *et al.*, *Eur. J. clin. Pharmac.*, 1981, *20*, 237.

Controlled hypotension. Labetalol was used to produce controlled hypotension in 50 patients undergoing major surgery.— D. H. P. Cope and M. C. Crawford, *Br. J. Anaesth.*, 1979, *51*, 359.

Gradual reduction of blood pressure using labetalol was successfully achieved in a 43-year-old man who required reduction in blood pressure and no undue variability, in order to carry out arch aortography to confirm a suspected dissecting aneurysm of the aorta. The desired effect was achieved by using incremental infusions of labetalol, titrating the dose against the blood pressure and increasing the infusion-rate before the injection of dye to prevent any consequent rise in blood pressure.— A. M. M. Cumming and D. L. Davies (letter), *Lancet*, 1979, *1*, 929. For the successful use of intravenous labetalol to treat acute aortic dissection see B. P. Grubb *et al.*, *J. Am. med. Ass.*, 1987, *258*, 78.

A discussion of the use of induced hypotension in surgery. The beta blocking effects of labetalol are longer lasting than the alpha blockade which tends to result in rising peripheral resistance accompanied by continuing beta blockade during the recovery period, which is rarely desirable.— W. R. MacRae, *Br. J. Hosp. Med.*, 1985, *33*, 341.

Hypertensive crisis. A discussion of hypertensive emergencies and hypertensive urgencies. Labetalol 40 to 80 mg repeated at 15 minute intervals to a maximum of 320 mg has been successfully employed in hypertensive emergency to produce a prompt reduction in blood pressure. Once the desired blood pressure has been achieved oral maintenance therapy can be initiated. Some patients will not respond to labetalol, while others experience postural hypotension, and for these reasons sodium nitroprusside may be preferred in most true emergencies; however, labetalol has proved useful in acute perioperative hypertension, and may be appropriate in situations where careful monitoring is not possible. Labetalol has also shown promise when given by mouth in the treatment of hypertensive urgencies—situations where elevated blood pressure should be controlled within 24 hours but where the risks associated with very rapid reduction of blood pressure are not justified.— R. K. Ferguson and P. H. Vlasses, *J. Am. med. Ass.*, 1986, *255*, 1607. See also *Med. Lett.*, 1987, *29*, 18; J. Y. Garcia and D. G. Vidt, *Drugs*, 1987, *34*, 263.

Eleven patients admitted to hospital with diastolic blood pressures in excess of 130 mmHg were treated with labetalol by mouth—an initial dose of 300 mg (or 400 mg if the blood pressure exceeded 140 mmHg); subsequent doses were given 8-hourly—200 mg if the blood pressure was 120 to 130 mmHg or 100 mg if 100 to 120 mmHg. Successful control of mean blood pressure was achieved in 6 hours if the patients were supine.— R. R. Ghose *et al.*, *Br. med. J.*, 1978, *2*, 96.

Hypertensive crisis following chicken teriyaki (containing aged soy sauce rich in tyramine) in a patient receiving a monoamine oxidase inhibitor was successfully treated by intravenous administration of labetalol 20 mg over 5 minutes.— J. H. Abrams *et al.* (letter), *New Engl. J. Med.*, 1985, *313*, 52.

Labetalol 20 mg intravenously, followed by 20 mg every 10 minutes to a total of 200 mg produced a prompt but smooth reduction in blood pressure in a patient with hypertensive crisis (blood pressure 270/160 mmHg on admission) unresponsive to sodium nitroprusside and clonidine or propranolol, hydralazine, and prazosin. Five minutes after discontinuing intravenous labetalol the patient's blood pressure gradually decreased to 155/90 mmHg. The patient was subsequently maintained on oral labetalol and hydrochlorothiazide; blood pressure at discharge (after 8 days) was 140/85 mmHg.— P. M. Ngole, *Drug Intell. & clin. Pharm.*, 1987, *21*, 512.

PAIN. Peridural injection of labetalol 50 mg gave almost immediate relief of pain in 20 patients with terminal gynaecological cancers who had abdominal or perineal pain radiating to the lower limbs. Administration was repeated every 4 hours for 2 days and every 8 to 12 hours thereafter. The analgesic effect lasted 3 to 6 hours; 2 patients required alcoholisation of the nerve roots because of inadequate response while another required similar treatment after a month when pain symptoms resumed. Labetalol treatment, coupled with a low dose of morphine at night offers a useful means of maintaining pain relief in patients with terminal cancer.— E. Margaria *et al.*, *Int. J. clin. Pharmac. Ther. Toxic.*, 1983, *21*, 47.

PHAEOCHROMOCYTOMA. A report of the successful use of labetalol to control symptoms in 4 of 5 patients with phaeochromocytoma.— E. A. Rosei *et al.*, *Br. J. clin. Pharmac.*, 1976, *3*, *Suppl.* 3, 809. Although labetalol has been advocated as a first-line drug in the management of phaeochromocytoma on the basis of having both alpha and beta blocking effects the beta effect predominates and there have been reports of pulmonary oedema following its use.— C. J. Hull, *Br. J. Anaesth.*, 1986, *58*, 1453.

PREGNANCY AND THE NEONATE. Labetalol appears to be safe and reasonably effective in the management of hypertension of pregnancy.— A. M. Smith (letter), *Br. med. J.*, 1982, *285*, 972.

Labetalol reversed thrombocytopenia in patients with pre-eclampsia, possibly by increased production of prostacyclin.— J. J. Walker *et al.* (letter), *Lancet*, 1982, *2*, 279.

Labetalol 200 mg by mouth compared favourably with hydralazine 10 mg intramuscularly in a study in patients with pregnancy-related hypertension.— J. J. Walker *et al.*, *Postgrad. med. J.*, 1983, *59*, *Suppl.* 3, 168.

For the view that labetalol may be superior to atenolol in the management of hypertension in pregnancy, see Atenolol, p.785.

TETANUS. The continuous infusion over 19 days of labetalol to control adrenoceptor stimulation in a patient with severe tetanus.— J. W. Dundee and W. F. K. Morrow, *Br. med. J.*, 1979, *1*, 1121. Intermittent injections of labetalol have been found to be effective in some tetanus patients developing very high blood pressure.— M. A. K. Omar *et al.* (letter), *ibid.*, 1979, *2*, 274.

Further references: W. Hanna and G. A. C. Grell (letter), *Br. med. J.*, 1978, *2*, 772; H. Connor *et al.* (letter), *ibid.*, 1979, *2*, 502; G. M. Domenighetti *et al.*, *Br. med. J.*, 1984, *288*, 1483.

Preparations

Labetalol Injection *(B.P.)*. Labetalol Hydrochloride Injection. A sterile solution of labetalol hydrochloride in Water for Injections.

Labetalol Tablets *(B.P.)*. Labetalol Hydrochloride Tablets. Contain labetalol hydrochloride.

Proprietary Preparations

Labrocol *(Lagap, UK)*. *Tablets*, labetalol hydrochloride 100, 200, and 400 mg.

Trandate *(Duncan, Flockhart, UK)*. *Tablets*, labetalol hydrochloride 50, 100, 200, and 400 mg.
Injection, labetalol hydrochloride 5 mg/mL, in ampoules of 20 mL.

Proprietary Names and Manufacturers

Abetol *(CT, Ital.)*; Alfabetal *(Mitim, Ital.)*; Amipress *(Dox-Al, Ital.)*; Ipolab *(Von Boch, Ital.)*; Labrocol *(Lagap, UK)*; Lolum *(Lifepharma, Ital.)*; Mitalolo *(Ellem, Ital.)*; Normodyne *(Schering, USA)*; Presdate *(Pierrel, Ital.)*; Pressalolo *(Locatelli, Ital.)*; Trandate *(Glaxo, Austral.; Allen & Hanburys, Canad.; Glaxo, Denm.; Glaxo, Fr.; Cascan, Ger.; Glaxo, Ital.; Neth.; Glaxo, Norw.; NZ; Allen & Hanburys, S.Afr.; Glaxo, Spain; Glaxo, Swed.; Glaxo, Switz.; Duncan, Flockhart, UK; Glaxo, USA)*.

The following names have been used for multi-ingredient preparations containing labetalol hydrochloride—Normozide *(Schering, USA)*; Trandate HCT *(Glaxo, USA)*.

6312-s

Levobunolol Hydrochloride *(BANM, USAN, rINNM)*.

l-Bunolol Hydrochloride; (−)-Bunolol Hydrochloride; W-7000A. (−)-5-(3-*tert*-Butylamino-2-hydroxypropoxy)-3,4-dihydronaphthalen-1(2*H*)-one hydrochloride; (−)-5-(3-*tert*-Butylamino-2-hydroxypropoxy)-1,2,3,4-tetrahydronaphthalen-1-one hydrochloride.
$C_{17}H_{25}NO_3,HCl=327.9$.

CAS — 47141-42-4 (levobunolol); 27912-14-7 (hydrochloride).

Adverse Effects, Treatment, and Precautions

As for Propranolol Hydrochloride, p.798.

Systemic effects have followed topical use of the eye-drops; local irritation and blurred vision have also occurred.

Absorption and Fate

Following oral administration levobunolol is rapidly and almost completely absorbed from the gastro-intestinal tract. Some systemic absorption is reported to occur following topical application to the eye. It is extensively metabolised in the liver; the principal metabolite, dihydrolevobunolol, is reported to possess beta blocking activity. The metabolites and a certain amount of unchanged drug are excreted in the urine.

Following administration of a single dose of radioactively labelled levobunolol 3 mg by mouth to 5 healthy subjects absorption from the gastro-intestinal tract was rapid and virtually complete. Mean plasma concentrations of bunolol and dihydrobunolol, an active metabolite, were 3.26 and 2.4 ng per mL 0.5 and 1 hour after dosage respectively with corresponding half-lives of 6.1 and 7.1 hours; these concentrations were maintained for at least 3 hours. Bunolol glucuronide, dihydrobunolol glucuronide, and bunolol sulphate were also detected in plasma with half-lives of 9.1, 7.7, and 17.4 hours respectively. After 96 hours a mean of 77.6 and 3.1% of the administered dose had been excreted in the urine and faeces respectively.— F. J. Di Carlo *et al.*, *Clin. Pharmac. Ther.*, 1977, *22*, 858. See also F. -J. Leinweber *et al.*, *Pharmacology*, 1978, *16*, 70.

Animal studies on the metabolism of bunolol and levobunolol: F. -J. Leinweber *et al.*, *J. pharm. Sci.*, 1977, *66*, 1570; *idem*, 1978, *67*, 129; H. R. Kaplan *et al.*, *ibid.*, 132.

Uses and Administration

Levobunolol is a beta blocker with general properties similar to those of propranolol (see p.803). It is classified as non-cardioselective and is reported to lack intrinsic sympathomimetic activity and membrane stabilising properties.

Levobunolol is used as the hydrochloride to reduce raised intra-ocular pressure in open-angle glaucoma or ocular hypertension. The usual dosage is one drop of a 0.5% solution applied once or twice daily.
Bunolol, the racemic form, has also been investigated but its beta blocking activity is reportedly less potent.

CARDIAC DISORDERS. *Cardiac arrhythmias.* Following administration of a single dose of levobunolol to 22 patients, ventricular premature beats of high frequency and grade were reduced by at least 50% in 17. Reduction was over 90% in 11, being total in 9. Ventricular premature beats were exacerbated in 2 patients.— P. J. Podrid *et al.*, *Circulation*, 1977, *56, Suppl.* 3, 8.

Further references: W. Shapiro and J. Park, *Am. Heart J.*, 1978, *96*, 417.

HYPERTENSION. Evaluation of the antihypertensive effect of levobunolol in doses of 1 to 5 mg thrice daily in 17 hypertensive subjects. Side-effects included insomnia (6), asthenia (1), anorexia (1), dyspnoea (1), ankle oedema (1).— E. Arce-Gomez *et al.*, *Curr. ther. Res.*, 1976, *19*, 386.

Effect on plasma renin. A study in 11 patients with essential hypertension and high, normal, or low plasma-renin activity showed that levobunolol significantly depressed plasma-renin activity.— H. Gavras *et al.*, *J. clin. Pharmac.*, 1977, *17*, 350.

GLAUCOMA. A brief review of levobunolol and betaxolol for the treatment of glaucoma.— *Med. Lett.*, 1986, *28*, 45.

A further review of levobunolol in glaucoma and ocular hypertension.— J. P. Gonzalez and S. P. Clissold, *Drugs*, 1987, *34*, 648.

In a multicentre study in 88 patients with chronic open-angle glaucoma or ocular hypertension, 31 were treated with levobunolol 0.5%, 31 with levobunolol 1.0%, and 26 with timolol 0.5%; all 3 drugs were instilled in a dose of one drop twice daily. After 12 months the mean reduction in intra-ocular pressure in the 3 groups was 7.2, 6.2, and 6.0 mmHg respectively. Five patients receiving levobunolol 0.5% and 6 of those receiving levobunolol 1.0% were withdrawn due to lack of control of intra-ocular pressure, compared with 2 of those receiving timolol; these figures were not significantly different. Three patients receiving levobunolol 0.5% and 2 receiving levobunolol 1.0% were withdrawn due to side-effects including ocular irritation, headache, and gastro-intestinal disturbances. The study confirms that levobunolol appears to be as effective as timolol in treating elevated intra-ocular pressure.— M. Ober *et al.*, *Br. J. Ophthal.*, 1985, *69*, 593.

Further comparisons with timolol: A. Cinotti *et al.*, *Am. J. Ophthal.*, 1985, *99*, 11; D. Long *et al.*, *ibid.*, 18; T. Wandel *et al.*, *ibid.*, 1986, *101*, 298.

For a study comparing levobunolol with metipranolol see under Metipranolol, below.

Proprietary Names and Manufacturers
Betagan *(Allergan, Canad.; Allergan, USA)*; Vistagan *(Allergan, Ger.)*.

19406-s

Levomoprolol Hydrochloride *(pINNM)*.

Levomoprolol is the (−)-*S*-isomer of moprolol.

CAS — 77164-20-6 (levomoprolol).

12976-w

Moprolol Hydrochloride *(rINNM)*.

SD-1601. 1-Isopropylamino-3-(2-methoxyphenoxy)propan-2-ol hydrochloride.
$C_{13}H_{21}NO_3,HCl = 275.8$.

CAS — 5741-22-0 (moprolol); 27058-84-0 (hydrochloride).

Moprolol is a beta blocker with general properties similar to those of propranolol (see p.798). Its beta blocking activity resides in the (−)-enantiomer, levomoprolol.
Both moprolol hydrochloride and levomoprolol hydrochloride have been given in the management of hypertension; daily doses of 150 mg of the former and 75 mg of the latter have been given.

A comparison of moprolol hydrochloride and levomoprolol hydrochloride in patients with mild to moderate hypertension.— M. Volpe *et al.*, *Curr. ther. Res.*, 1984, *35*, 23.

Proprietary Names and Manufacturers of Moprolol Hydrochloride and Levomoprolol Hydrochloride
Levotensin *(Simes, Ital.)*; Omeral *(Simes, Ital.)*.

12921-a

Medroxalol Hydrochloride *(BANM, USAN, rINNM)*.

MDL-81968A; RMI-81968A. 5-{1-Hydroxy-2-[1-methyl-3-(3,4-methylenedioxyphenyl)propylamino]ethyl-}salicylamide hydrochloride; 5-{2-[3-(1,3-Benzodioxol-5-yl)-1-methylpropylamino]-1-hydroxyethyl}salicylamide hydrochloride.
$C_{20}H_{24}N_2O_5,HCl = 408.9$.

CAS — 56290-94-9 (medroxalol); 70161-10-3 (hydrochloride).

Medroxalol hydrochloride is reported to have alpha and beta blocking activity.

Comparison of medroxalol and labetalol.— H. L. Elliott *et al.*, *Br. J. clin. Pharmac.*, 1984, *17*, 565 and 573.

The use of medroxalol in doses up to 300 mg three times daily, in combination with hydrochlorothiazide, in patients with hypertension.— N. D. Vlachakis *et al.*, *J. clin. Pharmac.*, 1983, *23*, 419.

Proprietary Names and Manufacturers
Merrell Dow, USA.

12928-h

Mepindolol *(BAN, rINN)*.

LF-17895; SHE-222 *(sulphate)*. 1-Isopropylamino-3-(2-methylindol-4-yloxy)propan-2-ol.
$C_{15}H_{22}N_2O_2 = 262.4$.

CAS — 23694-81-7 (mepindolol); 56396-94-2 (sulphate).

Mepindolol is the methyl analogue of pindolol (p.796). It is a beta blocker with general properties similar to those of propranolol (see p.798). Mepindolol is classified as non-cardioselective and is reported to possess intrinsic sympathomimetic activity.
Mepindolol is given as the sulphate. It is used in the management of hypertension and angina pectoris in doses of 2.5 to 10 mg of the sulphate daily.

Proprietary Names and Manufacturers
Betagon *(Schering, Ital.)*; Corindolan *(Schering, Ger.)*; Mepicor *(Corvi, Ital.)*.

6313-w

Metipranolol *(BAN, rINN)*.

1-(4-Acetoxy-2,3,5-trimethylphenoxy)-3-isopropylaminopropan-2-ol; 4-(2-Hydroxy-3-isopropylaminopropoxy)-2,3,6-trimethylphenyl acetate.
$C_{17}H_{27}NO_4 = 309.4$.

CAS — 22664-55-7.

Pharmacopoeias. In Cz.

Adverse Effects, Treatment, and Precautions
As for Propranolol Hydrochloride, p.798.

INTERACTIONS. *With diuretics.* Antagonism of the hypokalaemic effect of chlorthalidone by metipranolol.— P. J. Neuvonen *et al.*, *Br. J. clin. Pharmac.*, 1978, *6*, 363.

Uses and Administration
Metipranolol is a beta blocker with general properties similar to those of propranolol (see p.803). It is classified as non-cardioselective and is reported to be largely lacking in intrinsic sympathomimetic activity and membrane stabilising properties.
Metipranolol is used to reduce raised intra-ocular pressure associated with open-angle glaucoma and other ocular disorders. It is instilled in usual initial doses of one drop of a 0.1% solution twice daily, increased to a 0.3 or 0.6% solution as required for control.
Metipranolol has also been used in the management of cardiac disorders in doses of 5 to 10 mg by mouth twice or three times daily; in the treatment of hypertension, doses of 20 mg have been given twice or three times daily.

GLAUCOMA. A brief review of some new beta blockers, including metipranolol, in the treatment of glaucoma.— *Drug & Ther. Bull.*, 1987, *25*, 63.

In a crossover study in 10 patients with open-angle glaucoma metipranolol 0.3% was as effective in reducing intra-ocular pressure as timolol 0.25% when instilled twice daily for 1 month. Good control of intra-ocular pressure was achieved with both preparations in 8 patients; 2 showed a poor or absent response. Mean intra-ocular pressure for both eyes was 23.34 mmHg before treatment, and fell to 21.47 mmHg after treatment with timolol and 20.65 mmHg after treatment with metipranolol. Two patients experienced a burning sensation following instillation of metipranolol, but no systemic side-effects were noted in this short-term study.— K. B. Mills and G. Wright, *Br. J. Ophthal.*, 1986, *70*, 39.

In a study in patients with ocular hypertension or chronic open-angle glaucoma metipranolol 0.6% in 25 was as effective as levobunolol 0.5% in 21 in reducing intra-ocular pressure when given twice daily for 3 months. One patient assigned to metipranolol was withdrawn from the study due to inadequate control of intra-ocular pressure and one receiving levobunolol withdrew due to development of dyspnoea and chest cramps. Reports of local stinging or burning were more frequent in patients receiving metipranolol, although not significantly so; heart rate fell significantly more in patients receiving levobunolol, although this was not considered clinically significant.— G. K. Krieglstein *et al.*, *Br. J. Ophthal.*, 1987, *71*, 250.

HYPERTENSION. In a controlled crossover study in 18 patients with mild to moderate hypertension each patient received, in randomised order, a placebo, metipranolol 10 to 40 mg twice daily, chlorthalidone 50 mg on alternate days, and metipranolol in association with chlorthalidone, each treatment being continued for 6 weeks. Metipranolol and chlorthalidone had a similar and significant hypotensive effect which was increased when the drugs were given in association with one another. Heart-rate was decreased by metipranolol when compared with the effect of placebo or chlorthalidone. Metipranolol antagonised the hypokalaemic effect of chlorthalidone.— P. J. Neuvonen *et al.*, *Br. J. clin. Pharmac.*, 1978, *6*, 363.

Proprietary Preparations
Glauline *(Smith & Nephew Pharmaceuticals, UK)*. *Eye-drops*, metipranolol 0.1%, 0.3%, and 0.6%, in bottles of 5 mL.

Minims Metipranolol *(Smith & Nephew Pharmaceuticals, UK)*. *Eye-drops*, metipranolol 0.1%, 0.3%, and 0.6%, in single-use disposable applicators.

Proprietary Names and Manufacturers
Betamann *(Mann, Ger.)*; Betanol *(Dulcis, Mon.)*; Betaophthiole *(Restan, S.Afr.)*; Disorat *(Boehringer Mannheim, Ger.; Boehringer Mannheim, Switz.)*; Glauline *(Smith & Nephew Pharmaceuticals, UK)*; Minims Metipranolol *(Smith & Nephew Pharmaceuticals, UK)*; Turoptin *(Dispersa, Switz.)*.

6314-e

Metoprolol Tartrate *(BANM, USAN, rINNM)*.

CGP-2175E; H-93/26. (±)-1-Isopropylamino-3-[4-(2-methoxyethyl)phenoxy]propan-2-ol tartrate.
$(C_{15}H_{25}NO_3)_2,C_4H_6O_6 = 684.8$.

CAS — 54163-88-1 (metoprolol); 37350-58-6 (metoprolol, ±); 56392-17-7 (tartrate, ±).

Pharmacopoeias. In *U.S.*

A white crystalline powder. Very **soluble** in water; freely soluble in alcohol, in chloroform, and in methylene choride; slightly soluble in acetone; practically insoluble in ether. A 10% solution in water has a pH of between 6 and 7. **Store** in airtight containers. Protect from light.

Adverse Effects
As for Propranolol Hydrochloride, p.798.

For debate as to whether the polymorphic oxidation of metoprolol contributes to the incidence of adverse effects see under Absorption and Fate, below.

DEAFNESS. Loss of hearing in a patient receiving metoprolol appeared to vary in extent according to the dose of metoprolol; hearing gradually improved over several months once the drug was withdrawn.— R. Fäldt *et al.*, *Br. med. J.*, 1984, *289*, 1490.

EFFECTS ON BONES AND JOINTS. Five cases of arthralgia associated with the use of metoprolol had been reported to the FDA; 6 reports of similar symptoms associated with propranolol, and one with atenolol, had been reported.— J. M. Sills and L. Bosco (letter), *J. Am. med. Ass.*, 1986, *255*, 198.

EFFECTS ON THE CARDIOVASCULAR SYSTEM. In 10 healthy subjects a single dose of propranolol 80 mg reduced skin temperature by a mean of 1.3°. Skin blood flow and muscle blood flow before and after exercise were significantly reduced. Metoprolol 100 mg reduced muscle blood flow after exercise but to a lesser degree and had no significant effect on the other parameters. The effects of the 2 drugs were similar in normal subjects and patients with hypertension except that metoprolol reduced skin blood flow in the latter. Metoprolol had advantages over propranolol in patients with impaired peripheral circulation.— P. D. McSorley and D. J. Warren, *Br. med. J.*, 1978, *2*, 1598.

Intermittent claudication and gangrene in a 58-year-old woman was associated with metoprolol therapy. She responded to discontinuation of smoking and metoprolol, and infusion of dextran, alcohol, and phenoxybenzamine.— J. A. Vale and D. B. Jefferys (letter), *Lancet*, 1978, *1*, 1216.

Evidence that peak hyperaemic calf blood flow was reduced by both metoprolol and methyldopa treatment in patients with intermittent claudication, and a reminder that all antihypertensive therapy should be given with care to patients with this condition.— M. Lepäntalo, *Br. J. clin. Pharmac.*, 1984, *18*, 90.

EFFECTS ON THE EYES. A woman developed pain and soreness of the eyes while taking metoprolol 200 mg daily; symptoms abated when metoprolol was withdrawn and recurred within 2 or 3 days when metoprolol was again given.— D. Scott (letter), *Br. med. J.*, 1977, *2*, 1221.

EFFECTS ON LIPID METABOLISM. A study in 9 hypertensive subjects indicating that metoprolol does not increase blood-triglyceride concentrations.— A. Nilsson *et al.* (letter), *Br. med. J.*, 1977, *2*, 126.

Acute pancreatitis was provoked by severe hypertriglyceridaemia in a patient in whom beta blockers (atenolol and metoprolol) greatly impaired triglyceride clearance.— P. N. Durrington and S. A. Cairns, *Br. med. J.*, 1982, *284*, 1016.

In a study involving 50 patients with mild to moderate hypertension metoprolol 200 mg daily caused a rise in mean very-low-density lipoprotein cholesterol concentrations and a small fall in concentration of the high-density lipoprotein fraction; in contrast, atenolol 50 mg daily did not affect serum lipoproteins in these patients.— S. Rössner and L. Weiner, *Eur. J. clin. Pharmac.*, 1983, *24*, 573.

See also Y. Lacourciere *et al.*, *Curr. ther. Res.*, 1986, *39*, 1033; G. Olsson *et al.*, *Eur. J. clin. Pharmac.*, 1987, *32*, 245.

EFFECTS ON MENTAL FUNCTION. For comparison of the central effects of metoprolol and atenolol see p.783.

EFFECTS ON RESPIRATORY FUNCTION. Metoprolol-associated bronchospasm developed in a 67-year-old patient with no history of asthma.— Adverse Drug Reactions Advisory Committee, *Aust. Prescriber*, 1978, *2*, 116.

See also Obstructive Airways Disease, under Precautions, below.

EFFECTS ON SEXUAL FUNCTION. Four of 14 men receiving metoprolol experienced disturbance of potency.— E. Arnesen, *Curr. ther. Res.*, 1978, *24*, 889.

See also under Fibrosis.

EFFECTS ON THE SKIN. *Alopecia.* Alopecia developed in an 18-year-old man following the start of metoprolol treatment, and did not improve when propranolol with hydralazine were substituted for metoprolol; discontinuation of the second beta blocker was followed by slow regrowth of scalp hair.— C. W. Graeber and R. A. Lapkin, *Cutis*, 1981, *28*, 633.

Psoriasiform eruptions. A report of eczematous and/or psoriasiform eruptions in 5 patients receiving long-term metoprolol therapy. The skin eruptions disappeared slowly within weeks or months of withdrawal of the drug.— H. A. M. Neumann *et al.* (letter), *Lancet*, 1979, *2*, 745.

FIBROSIS. Peyronie's disease [penile fibrosis] in one patient was associated with metoprolol. Symptoms improved when metoprolol was withdrawn.— J. S. Yudkin (letter), *Lancet*, 1977, *2*, 1355.

A report of retroperitoneal fibrosis in a patient who had been taking metoprolol and nifedipine for 11 months.— J. Thompson and D. G. Julian, *Br. med. J.*, 1982, *284*, 83.

A report of sclerosing peritonitis in a patient receiving metoprolol.— C. V. Clark and R. Terris (letter), *Lancet*, 1983, *1*, 937. Correction.— *ibid.*, 1174. See also N. Grefberg *et al.* (letter), *ibid.*, *2*, 733.

Treatment of Adverse Effects

As for Propranolol Hydrochloride, p.800.

Following ingestion of about 200 tablets of metoprolol 50 mg, prescribed for his father, a 19-year-old man was admitted to hospital conscious, with peripheral cyanosis and weak heart sounds, the heart-rate was 60 to 70 beats per minute, and the blood pressure was unrecordable. He was treated with infusions of electrolytes, sodium bicarbonate to correct acidosis, metaraminol 7 mg and glucagon 6 mg intravenously to raise the blood pressure followed by another intravenous dose of metaraminol (3 mg) 1 hour later after which the blood pressure stabilised at the patient's usual level. Frusemide was given to counteract fluid retention which occurred during the first 6 hours. Twelve hours after admission the patient was comfortable with no signs of cardiovascular depression. Although initial treatment included gastric lavage, measurement of the plasma concentrations indicated that most of the dose had been absorbed.— B. H. J. Möller (letter), *Br. med. J.*, 1976, *1*, 222. A similar case.— S. Sire (letter), *Lancet*, 1976, *2*, 1137.

Precautions

As for Propranolol Hydrochloride, p.801.

INTERACTIONS. *Anti-arrhythmics.* Prior administration of quinidine 50 mg produced a three-fold increase in the plasma metoprolol concentrations resulting from metoprolol 100 mg by mouth in 5 extensive metabolisers but had no effect in 5 poor metabolisers in whom plasma concentrations following metoprolol alone were in any case higher than in extensive metabolisers. Preliminary results indicate that this metabolic inhibition in the extensive metabolisers, effectively converting them to the poor metaboliser phenotype, lasted at least 48 hours after this subtherapeutic dose of quinidine.— T. Leemann *et al.*, *Eur. J. clin. Pharmac.*, 1986, *29*, 739.

Calcium channel blockers. For a report of atrioventricular block associated with concomitant metoprolol and verapamil administration, see Verapamil, p.90.

Histamine H_2 antagonists. For reference to interactions of metoprolol with cimetidine and ranitidine see under Propranolol Hydrochloride, p.801.

Lignocaine. For the effects of beta blockers on lignocaine elimination see under Propranolol Hydrochloride, p.802.

Oral contraceptives. A report of increased plasma-metoprolol concentrations in women who were taking an oral contraceptive.— M. J. Kendall *et al.*, *Br. J. clin. Pharmac.*, 1982, *14*, 120.

Parasympathomimetics. For a report of bronchospasm following acetylcholine injection in a patient receiving metoprolol see Acetylcholine Chloride, p.1328.

OBSTRUCTIVE AIRWAYS DISEASE. In 17 patients with chronic bronchitis there was no significant change in peak expiratory flow rate after treatment with metoprolol 200 mg daily (as a slow-release preparation) for 1 week; mean FEV_1 dropped from 1264 mL to 1218 mL, a reduction of 3.6%. One patient experienced an increase in wheeze associated with a 10% drop in FEV_1; subsequent monitoring suggested the presence of asthma as well as chronic bronchitis. The effects of these doses of metoprolol on respiratory function appear to be clinically unimportant in patients with chronic bronchitis, except where there is underlying asthma.— E. T. Peel and G. Anderson, *Postgrad. med. J.*, 1983, *59, Suppl.* 3, 73. Results in 16 patients with obstructive airways disease (asthma, bronchitis, and emphysema) suggested that any potential benefits of 'cardioselective' beta blockade with metoprolol over propranolol were marginal and of little practical significance. Patients with anatomically and functionally fixed airways obstruction appeared to tolerate beta blockers provided ventilatory impairment was not severe but in patients with reversible airways obstruction the response was unpredictable and potentially hazardous; beta blockers would be best avoided in this latter group.— H. W. Clague *et al.*, *Eur. J. clin. Pharmac.*, 1984, *27*, 517. In a study of the effects of 2 cardioselective beta blockers, metoprolol and bevantolol, on pulmonary function in asthmatic subjects, 7 of 15 had to be withdrawn before receiving the maximum dose of either drug; the maximum mean tolerated doses in these patients were 26.8 mg of metoprolol and 45.5 mg of bevantolol, which are subtherapeutic doses. These results emphasise the unpredictability of response to even cardioselective beta blockers in asthmatic patients.— P. G. Wilcox *et al.*, *Clin. Pharmac. Ther.*, 1986, *39*, 29.

WITHDRAWAL. About 78 hours after withdrawal of metoprolol a 52-year-old man with 4 previous myocardial infarctions suffered a dramatic worsening of his angina pectoris, and subsequently suffered ventricular fibrillation and myocardial infarction.— T. Meinertz *et al.* (letter), *Lancet*, 1979, *1*, 270. The symptoms may have been caused by administration of nifedipine rather than by withdrawal of metoprolol.— L. Beeley and J. Talbot (letter), *ibid.*, 387. A further report.— L. C. Williams *et al.* (letter), *ibid.*, 494.

Evidence of withdrawal phenomena in patients who had been receiving metoprolol for essential hypertension.— R. E. Rangno *et al.*, *Clin. Pharmac. Ther.*, 1982, *31*, 8; G. Olsson *et al.*, *Am. Heart J.*, 1984, *108*, 454; K. Lindvall *et al.*, *Eur. Heart J.*, 1986, *7*, 1045.

Absorption and Fate

Metoprolol is readily and completely absorbed from the gastro-intestinal tract but is subject to considerable first-pass metabolism. Peak plasma concentrations occur about 1.5 hours after a single dose. It is extensively metabolised in the liver, the metabolites being excreted in the urine together with only small amounts of unchanged metoprolol. The metabolism of metoprolol is reported to exhibit genetic polymorphism; the half-life of metoprolol in fast metabolisers is stated to be 3 to 4 hours, whereas in poor metabolisers it is about 7 hours. Metoprolol crosses the blood-brain barrier. It also crosses the placenta and is excreted in breast milk. It is only slightly bound to plasma protein.

The mean ratio of the saliva concentration of oxprenolol to the plasma concentration was 0.42 in 6 healthy subjects who took oxprenolol 80 mg. The concentrations of metoprolol were greater in saliva than in plasma in a further 6 healthy subjects who took metoprolol 100 mg and there was no clear relationship between them. It was suggested that while oxprenolol diffused passively, metoprolol was actively secreted, into saliva.— C. P. Dawes *et al.*, *Br. J. clin. Pharmac.*, 1978, *5*, 217.

The effect of age on the pharmacokinetics of metoprolol.— C. P. Quarterman *et al.*, *Br. J. clin. Pharmac.*, 1981, *11*, 287. A further study. There were disparities between the pharmacokinetics of metoprolol in young and elderly subjects and, although these had a negligible effect on the plasma concentration of metoprolol resulting from a given dose, institution of metoprolol therapy with relatively low doses was recommended in elderly individuals.— M. Larsson *et al.*, *Eur. J. clin. Pharmac.*, 1984, *27*, 217.

DIFFUSION INTO THE CSF. A 64-year-old hypertensive woman who had been taking metoprolol 50 mg thrice daily for 2 months had a CSF-metoprolol concentration of 267 ng per mL and plasma metoprolol of 341 ng per mL. It was considered that the concentration in CSF was approximately equal to the concentration of unbound drug in plasma.— A. J. Wood (letter), *Br. J. clin. Pharmac.*, 1977, *4*, 240.

METABOLISM. There has been considerable, and acrimonious, debate as to the influence of genetic polymorphism on the metabolism of metoprolol, and the clinical consequences, if any, of such variation. Lennard *et al.* (*Br. J. clin. Pharmac.*, 1982, *14*, 301) originally reported that of 8 subjects given metoprolol 200 mg daily for a week, 2 exhibited a prolonged half-life and duration of beta blockade; subsequent testing of oxidation phenotype with oral debrisoquine (a drug known to exhibit genetic polymorphism) showed that the subjects with increased metoprolol availability were also poor metabolisers of debrisoquine. In a subsequent study in 6 poor and 6 extensive hydroxylators of debrisoquine (M.S. Lennard *et al.*, *New Engl. J. Med.*, 1982, *307*, 1558) poor hydroxylators had threefold prolongation of the elimination half-life of metoprolol compared with extensive hydroxylators; it was suggested that dosage might need amending in poor hydroxylators, and that they might be at increased risk of adverse effects. Further confirmation of the existence of genetic polymorphism in metoprolol metabolism was obtained in studies involving 143 unselected hypertensive patients (J.C. McGourty *et al.*, *Br. J. clin. Pharmac.*, 1985, *20*, 555). The population comprised 131 extensive metabolisers of debrisoquine and 12 poor metabolisers; a bimodal distribution of metoprolol metabolism was seen and all poor metabolisers of metoprolol were poor metabolisers of debrisoquine. Further study in the families of 10 patients indicated genetic inheritance of impaired ability to hydroxylate metoprolol.

These findings have been vigorously disputed by Jack *et al.* (*Br. J. clin. Pharmac.*, 1983, *16*, 188) who suggested that the linkage between debrisoquine metabolism and that of metoprolol was fallacious, and in a subsequent letter that it was important to distinguish between examples where polymorphism was the determining factor in the pharmacokinetics, and those where it made only a minor contribution to elimination and hence variability (D.B. Jack and M.R. Wilkins, *ibid.*, 1984, *17*, 488. Although the importance of genetic polymorphism has been defended both in general and with regard to metoprolol (M.S. Lennard *et al.*, *ibid.*, 489; J.R. Idle and R.L. Smith, *ibid.*, 492). Regårdh and Johnsson (*ibid.*, 495) have suggested that there is no evidence of any clinical problem with metoprolol, and that in any case dosage should be individually adjusted according to pharmacological effect. Similarly, Clarke *et al.* (*ibid.*, *18*, 965) in a retrospective study involving 37 patients who had suffered adverse effects with metoprolol sufficient to prompt withdrawal did not find an increased incidence of poor metaboliser status compared with 37 controls.

The subject may be further confused by variations in the phenotype between ethnic groups. Although the incidence of the poor metaboliser phenotype in whites of European origin is reported to be about 9%, a study in 138 Nigerians (A.O. Iyun *et al.*, *Clin. Pharmac. Ther.*, 1986, *40*, 387) failed to identify evidence of polymorphic metabolism, and the authors caution against extrapolation of data between different racial groups.

PREGNANCY AND THE NEONATE. The disposition of metoprolol in newborn infants of mothers treated with metoprolol.— P. Lundborg *et al.* (letter), *Br. J. clin. Pharmac.*, 1981, *12*, 598.

The clearance of metoprolol was increased four-fold in 5 pregnant women during the last trimester, compared with that some months after delivery; this was probably due to enhanced hepatic metabolism in the pregnant state.— S. Högstedt *et al.*, *Eur. J. clin. Pharmac.*, 1983, *24*, 217.

Uses and Administration

Metoprolol tartrate is a beta blocker with general properties similar to those of propranolol (see p.803). It is classified as cardioselective and is reported to lack intrinsic sympathomimetic and membrane stabilising activity.

In the treatment of hypertension metoprolol tartrate is usually given in an initial dose of 100 mg daily, increased weekly according to the response of the patient to 400 mg daily or 200 mg twice daily. Better control may be obtained with the more frequent dosage regimens. The usual dose for angina pectoris is 50 to 100 mg twice or three times daily. As an adjunct in the treatment of hyperthyroidism metoprolol tartrate may be given in doses of 50 mg four times daily. In the treatment of cardiac arrhythmias the usual dose is 50 mg twice or three times daily, increased if necessary up to 300 mg daily in divided doses.

For the emergency treatment of cardiac arrhythmias metoprolol tartrate may be given intravenously in an initial dose of up to 5 mg administered at a rate of 1 to 2 mg per minute; this may be repeated, if necessary, at intervals of 5 minutes to a total dose of 10 to 15 mg. When acute arrhythmias have been controlled, maintenance therapy with doses not exceeding 50 mg three times daily by mouth is recommended and should be started 4 to 6 hours after intravenous therapy.

Arrhythmias may be prevented on induction of anaesthesia or controlled during anaesthesia, by the slow intravenous injection of 2 to 4 mg; further injections of 2 mg may be repeated as necessary to a maximum total dose of 10 mg.

Metoprolol is also used as an adjunct in the early management of acute myocardial infarction to limit progression and myocardial damage and reduce morbidity. Treatment should be given within 12 hours of the onset of chest pain; metoprolol 5 mg should be given intravenously at 2-minute intervals to a total of 15 mg, where tolerated. This should be followed, after 15 minutes, by the commencement of oral treatment, in patients who have received the full intravenous dose, with 50 mg every 6 hours for 2 days. In patients who have failed to tolerate the full intravenous dose a reduced oral dose should be given as and when their condition permits. Subsequent maintenance dosage is 100 mg given twice daily by mouth.

Doses of 100 to 200 mg are given daily in divided doses for migraine prophylaxis.

ADMINISTRATION. Studies in healthy subjects indicated that more metoprolol entered the general circulation following administration with food than when it was taken on an empty stomach; administration should always be standardised relative to meals.— A. Melander *et al.*, *Clin. Pharmac. Ther.*, 1977, *22*, 108.

In the elderly. A suggestion that metoprolol might need to be given in reduced dosage or once daily to elderly patients.— M. J. Kendall *et al.* (letter), *Br. J. clin. Pharmac.*, 1977, *4*, 497.

See also under Absorption and Fate, above.

Once-daily administration. Although metoprolol once-daily might be adequate in hypertension it might not suffice for angina and cardiac arrhythmias.— A. Lehtonen and H. Sundquist, *Curr. ther. Res.*, 1978, *23*, 131.

See also under Hypertension.

Studies of controlled-release tablets of metoprolol intended for once-daily administration: H. Folgering and M. van Bussel, *Eur. J. clin. Pharmac.*, 1980, *18*, 225; S. Freestone *et al.*, *Br. J. clin. Pharmac.*, 1982, *14*, 713; G. I. Hackett *et al.*, *Eur. J. clin. Pharmac.*, 1983, *25*, 717.

For a series of references to osmotic delivery systems for controlled release of metoprolol, see *Br. J. clin. Pharmac.*, 1985, *19*, *Suppl.* 2.

ADMINISTRATION IN RESPIRATORY INSUFFICIENCY. For warnings regarding the administration of metoprolol in patients with obstructive airways disease see Obstructive Airways Disease, under Precautions, above.

CARDIAC DISORDERS. A review of the use of metoprolol in cardiovascular disorders.— P. Benfield *et al.*, *Drugs*, 1986, *31*, 376.

Angina pectoris. In a double-blind crossover study in 14 patients with stable angina pectoris exercise tolerance was significantly greater when taking metoprolol 50 mg four times daily than when taking propranolol 40 mg four times daily. In a long-term study completed by 13 patients extending over a further 58 weeks exercise tolerance was maintained and no significant change occurred when the dose was changed to 100 mg twice daily. Mean serum-metoprolol concentrations at the end of the crossover study were 55.6 ng per g (range 12 to 136 ng) and 120 ng per g (range 51 to 256 ng) at the end of the long-term study. Treatment was well tolerated.— M. B. Comerford and E. M. M. Besterman, *Postgrad. med. J.*, 1976, *52*, 481. There was no significant difference in the beneficial effect of metoprolol 200 mg and propranolol 160 mg, both given once daily as a sustained-release preparation, in a crossover study in 11 patients with stable angina pectoris.— J. B. Irving and R. E. Edwards, *Br. J. clin. Pract.*, 1987, *41*, 872.

In a study involving 100 patients with angina pectoris the majority responded to treatment with metoprolol 50 or 100 mg twice daily by mouth, but the remaining 29 required individualisation of the dose at 150 to 200 mg twice daily.— O. Hammershøy, *Curr. ther. Res.*, 1982, *31*, 1026.

The benefits of combined nifedipine and metoprolol in patients with unstable angina uncontrolled by beta blockade alone.— J. Lubsen *et al.*, *Br. Heart J.*, 1986, *56*, 400.

Myocardial infarction. In a double-blind randomised study of 1395 patients with definite or suspected acute myocardial infarction mortality was reduced by metoprolol when compared with placebo. Metoprolol 15 mg was given intravenously on arrival in hospital, followed by 100 mg twice daily by mouth for 90 days. The cumulative mortality-rate for the treatment period was 8.9% (62 deaths) in the placebo group and 5.7% (40 deaths) in the metoprolol group, a reduction in mortality of 36%.— Å. Hjalmarson *et al.*, *Lancet*, 1981, *2*, 823. Analysis of the effects of metoprolol on ventricular tachyarrhythmias in these patients demonstrated a prophylactic effect against ventricular fibrillation, which may be a major reason for the reduction in mortality.— L. Rydén *et al.*, *New Engl. J. Med.*, 1983, *308*, 614. Mortality rate was still significantly lower at 2 years in the metoprolol group (13.2%) than in the placebo group (17.2%), but the benefit was most marked in patients treated within 8 hours of the onset of symptoms.— J. Herlitz *et al.*, *Int. J. Cardiol.*, 1986, *10*, 291.

Results of the Metoprolol in Acute Myocardial Infarction (MIAMI) study, a multicentre study involving 5778 patients with suspected or confirmed acute myocardial infarction. After randomisation, 2877 patients were assigned to treatment with metoprolol, initially in 3 doses of 5 mg intravenously each over 2 minutes, followed by 25 to 50 mg four times daily by mouth, according to response, for 2 days, and then by 100 mg twice daily for 13 days. The remaining 2901 patients received matching placebo. The mean interval between onset of symptoms and the beginning of treatment was 6.6 hours. There were 123 deaths among those treated with metoprolol (4.3%) compared with 142 among the placebo group (4.9%), and this difference was not significant. However, subgroup analysis suggested a more marked reduction in mortality among those patients considered at high risk. Furthermore there was a reduction in morbidity in all metoprolol-treated patients, with a lower incidence of ventricular fibrillation and arrhythmias and a lesser requirement for cardiac glycosides.— MIAMI Trial Research Group, *Eur. Heart J.*, 1985, *6*, 199. Comment on the use of intravenous beta blockers in myocardial infarction. The benefits of such treatment do exist, but they are modest.— *Lancet*, 1986, *2*, 79.

Further studies, indicating the benefit of long-term oral metoprolol in preventing re-infarction and sudden death after myocardial infarction: G. Olsson *et al.*, *J. Am. Coll. Cardiol.*, 1985, *5*, 1428; G. Olsson *et al.*, *Br. med. J.*, 1986, *292*, 1491.

See also G. Olsson *et al.*, *Br. med. J.*, 1987, *294*, 339 (cost-effectiveness of post-infarction prophylaxis with metoprolol).

DIABETIC NEPHROPATHY. Results in 5 insulin-dependent diabetics given metoprolol 100 to 200 mg daily suggested that the drug reduced microalbuminuria, an early symptom of diabetic nephropathy, in 4. If these results are confirmed it remains to be seen whether reducing urinary albumin excretion will prevent overt diabetic nephropathy.— P. J. Friedman *et al.* (letter), *Lancet*, 1986, *2*, 1042.

EXPLOSIVE RAGE. Two patients with a history of frequent explosive outbursts of temper improved following metoprolol treatment. One, who had responded to previous propranolol treatment, was given 50 mg twice daily by mouth, subsequently gradually increased to 300 mg daily in divided doses; the other received 100 mg twice daily in combination with carbamazepine 800 mg. Metoprolol may be helpful for patients with intermittent explosive disorder.— J. A. Mattes, *Am. J. Psychiat.*, 1985, *142*, 1108.

HEPATIC DISORDERS. For reference to the use of metoprolol in the management of variceal bleeding in cirrhotic patients see under Propranolol Hydrochloride, p.806.

HYPERTENSION. A double-blind crossover study in 20 patients with mild hypertension showed that 4 weeks' treatment with metoprolol 200 or 400 mg daily (in 2 doses) or atenolol 200 or 400 mg daily (in 2 doses) had similar hypotensive effects.— T. A. Jeffers *et al.*, *Br. med. J.*, 1978, *2*, 1269.

For further comparisons of metoprolol with atenolol in the management of hypertension see Atenolol, p.785.

Whereas propranolol produced a sharp reduction in heart-rate and blood pressure within the first 2 weeks of a 24-week study in 28 patients with hypertension, and a further slight decrease thereafter, metoprolol produced a slower but more uniform reduction during the study. Propranolol was more effective in reducing diastolic blood pressure while metoprolol was more effective in reducing heart-rate and systolic blood pressure. It was considered that metoprolol showed greater β_1 cardioselective properties than propranolol.— A. N. Singh *et al.*, *Curr. ther. Res.*, 1978, *24*, 571.

Results of a double-blind crossover study in healthy subjects comparing doses of metoprolol and propranolol that had an equivalent effect on exercise-induced tachycardia indicated that metoprolol was slightly more potent than propranolol in reducing blood pressure with exercise. Neither drug affected vascular tone at rest or in exercising muscle.— W. R. Hiatt *et al.*, *Clin. Pharmac. Ther.*, 1984, *35*, 12.

In the elderly. Studies of metoprolol and hydrochlorothiazide in elderly hypertensives: A. Pollet *et al.*, *Acta ther.*, 1986, *12*, 81; J. Wikstrand *et al.*, *J. Am. med. Ass.*, 1986, *255*, 1304.

Once-daily administration. In a controlled study in 16 patients with hypertension metoprolol 300 mg daily as a single dose or in 3 divided doses had a comparable effect in reducing blood pressure; the variations in plasma-metoprolol concentrations were more variable after once-daily dosage and the degree of blockade (assessed by heart-rate during exercise) was more consistent after thrice-daily dosage.— T. Reybrouck *et al.*, *Br. med. J.*, 1978, *1*, 1386.

Results in healthy subjects indicating that metoprolol can attenuate the systolic blood pressure response to moderate to severe exercise over a 24-hour period provided it is given twice or possibly thrice daily with a unit dose of 100 mg.— J. D. Harry *et al.* (letter), *Lancet*, 1979, *2*, 250. In a double-blind study involving 55 hypertensive patients atenolol and metoprolol were found to be equipotent after once-daily administration.— O. Lyngstam and L. Rydén (letter), *ibid.*, 634.

Studies indicating that once daily dosage with sustained-release formulations of metoprolol is as effective as twice daily dosage with conventional preparations in the management of hypertension: A. Howe, *Practitioner*, 1982, *226*, 573; A. N. Singh *et al.*, *Curr. ther. Res.*, 1983, *33*, 601. Contrary results. Once daily treatment of hypertension with metoprolol, even in long-acting formulations cannot be recommended because of waning antihypertensive effect over the 24 hours. Metoprolol should be prescribed twice daily in hypertension.— J. H. Silas *et al.*, *Br. J. clin. Pharmac.*, 1985, *20*, 387.

HYPERTHYROIDISM. Comparison of propranolol and metoprolol in the management of hyperthyroidism.— L. E. Murchison *et al.*, *Br. J. clin. Pharmac.*, 1979, *8*, 581.

Further references: O. R. Nilsson *et al.*, *Eur. J. clin. Pharmac.*, 1980, *18*, 315; A. Adlerberth *et al.*, *Ann. Surg.*, 1987, *205*, 182.

MIGRAINE. A report of the beneficial effect of metoprolol in 3 patients with migraine.— O. Ljung (letter), *New Engl. J. Med.*, 1980, *303*, 156.

Further studies of the benefits of metoprolol in migraine: J. -E. Olsson *et al.*, *Acta neurol. scand.*, 1984, *70*, 160 (50 mg twice daily as effective as propranolol 40 mg twice daily); P. Kangasniemi and C. Hedman, *Cephalalgia*, 1984, *4*, 91 (200 mg daily controlled-release comparable with propranolol 80 mg twice daily).

For a comparison of metoprolol and pizotifen in the prophylaxis of migraine, see Pizotifen Malate, p. 459.

TREMOR. Metoprolol was as effective as propranolol in relieving the symptoms of a 37-year-old man with essential tremor and, unlike propranolol, did not aggravate his asthma.— T. Riley and A. B. Pleet (letter), *New Engl. J. Med.*, 1979, *301*, 663.

Metoprolol, gradually increased to 50 mg thrice daily, produced a favourable response in 19 of 22 patients with long-standing essential or familial tremor. The 3 non-responders did not respond to propranolol either.— O. Ljung (letter), *New Engl. J. Med.*, 1979, *301*, 1005.

Further references: D. M. Turnbull and D. A. Shaw (letter), *Lancet*, 1980, *1*, 95.

For a study suggesting that metoprolol is less effective than propranolol in the management of essential tremor, see Propranolol Hydrochloride, p.807.

Preparations

Metoprolol Tartrate Injection *(U.S.P.)*

Metoprolol Tartrate Tablets *(U.S.P.)*

Metoprolol Tartrate and Hydrochlorothiazide Tablets *(U.S.P.)*

Proprietary Preparations

Betaloc *(Astra, UK). Tablets*, metoprolol tartrate 50 or 100 mg.
Tablets (Betaloc-SA), sustained-release, metoprolol tartrate 200 mg.
Injection, metoprolol tartrate 1 mg/mL, in ampoules of 5 mL.

Co-Betaloc *(Astra, UK). Tablets*, scored, metoprolol tartrate 100 mg, hydrochlorothiazide 12.5 mg.
Tablets (Co-Betaloc SA), metoprolol tartrate 200 mg (for sustained release), hydrochlorothiazide 25 mg.

Lopresor *(Geigy, UK). Tablets*, scored, metoprolol tartrate 50 and 100 mg.
Tablets (Lopresor SR), sustained-release, metoprolol tartrate 200 mg.
Injection, metoprolol tartrate 1 mg/mL in ampoules of 5 mL.

Lopresoretic *(Geigy, UK). Tablets*, metoprolol tartrate 100 mg, chlorthalidone 12.5 mg.

Proprietary Names and Manufacturers

Beloc *(Pfizer, Arg.; Astra, Ger.)*; Beprolo *(Lusofarmaco, Ital.)*; Betaloc *(Astra, Austral.; Astra, Canad.; NZ; Astra, UK)*; Lopresor *(Ciba, Arg.; Ciba, Austral.; Belg.; Geigy, Canad.; Ciba, Ger.; Geigy, Ital.; Neth.; Geigy, S.Afr.; Ciba, Switz.; Geigy, UK)*; Lopressor *(Geigy, Fr.; Ciba, Spain; Geigy, USA)*; Metoros *(Geigy, UK)*; Novometoprol *(Novopharm, Canad.)*; Prelis *(Brunnengräber, Ger.)*; Selokeen *(Neth.)*; Seloken *(Belg.; Hässle, Denm.; Astra, Fr.; Essex, Ital.; Lux.; Hässle, Norw.; Essex, Spain; Hässle, Swed.)*; Selo-Zok *(Hässle, Denm.)*.

The following names have been used for multi-ingredient preparations containing metoprolol tartrate— Co-Betaloc *(Astra, Canad.; Astra, UK)*; Lopresoretic *(Geigy, UK)*; Lopressor HCT *(Geigy, USA)*.

6315-l

Nadolol *(BAN, USAN, rINN)*.

SQ-11725. (2*R*,3*S*)-5-(3-*tert*-Butylamino-2-hydroxypropoxy)-1,2,3,4-tetrahydronaphthalene-2,3-diol.

$C_{17}H_{27}NO_4$=309.4.

CAS — 42200-33-9.

Pharmacopoeias. In *U.S.*

Store in well-closed containers.

Adverse Effects, Treatment, and Precautions

As for Propranolol Hydrochloride, p.798.

EFFECTS ON LIPID METABOLISM. Administration of nadolol to 6 hypertensive patients was associated with increases in triglyceride concentrations and significant reductions in serum concentrations of high-density lipoprotein.— N. R. Peden *et al.*, *Br. med. J.*, 1984, *288*, 1788.

EFFECTS ON MENTAL FUNCTION. A report of severe depression apparently precipitated by nadolol. The patient was much improved 3 days after withdrawal of the beta blocker.— J. W. Russell and M. A. Schuckit (letter), *Lancet*, 1982, *2*, 1286.

EFFECTS ON THE NERVOUS SYSTEM. A report of organic brain syndrome in a patient given nadolol. The patient was found unconscious and had no memory of the previous 3 days on awakening.— T.M. Kanefsky (letter), *Archs intern. Med.*, 1981, *141*, 1846.

EFFECTS ON RESPIRATORY FUNCTION. Near-fatal bronchospasm occurred in a young patient with asthma when given nadolol.— J. M. Raine *et al.*, *Br. med. J.*, 1981, *282*, 548.

Hypersensitivity pneumonitis was associated with nadolol in a patient prescribed the drug for migraine. Symptoms improved when nadolol was withdrawn.— M. B. Levy *et al.* (letter), *Ann. intern. Med.*, 1986, *105*, 806.

Absorption and Fate

Nadolol is incompletely absorbed from the gastro-intestinal tract to give peak plasma concentrations about 3 or 4 hours after a dose. It does not appear to be metabolised and is excreted unchanged in the urine and the bile. The plasma half-life has been variously reported as ranging from about 6 to 24 hours. It is only about 30% bound to plasma proteins and is reported to be dialysable. Nadolol is excreted in breast milk.

In 4 patients with mild hypertension given nadolol 2 mg by mouth or intravenously, the elimination half-life from plasma was an average of 10 to 12 hours (a range of 5.9 to 12.2 hours following intravenous administration, and a range of 9.6 to 14.2 hours following oral administration). This was shorter than unpublished data reporting an average terminal half-life of 17 hours for 4 healthy subjects. Calculations based on urinary excretion and plasma concentration data suggested that about 33% was absorbed after oral administration. There was evidence of biliary as well as urinary excretion since after intravenous administration about 73% was excreted in urine and 23% in faeces. Nadolol did not appear to be metabolised.— J. Dreyfuss *et al.*, *J. clin. Pharmac.*, 1977, *17*, 300. A similar study of therapeutic oral doses.— J. Dreyfuss *et al.*, *J. clin. Pharmac.*, 1979, *19*, 712.

A study of the effect of various beta-adrenoceptor blocking agents on exercise-induced changes in 9 patients with mild hypertension and 16 healthy subjects. The pharmacodynamic half-life of nadolol was about 39 hours.— R. A. Vukovich *et al.*, *Br. J. clin. Pharmac.*, 1979, *7*, *Suppl.* 2, 167S.

A study of nadolol binding to serum protein in 95 healthy subjects indicated that the average amount of nadolol bound was 14%, with considerable variation between individuals from 3.5% to 27%.— L. Patel *et al.*, *J. Pharm. Pharmac.*, 1984, *36*, 414.

Uses and Administration

Nadolol is a hydrophilic beta blocker with general properties similar to those of propranolol (see p.803). It is classified as non-cardioselective and is reported to lack intrinsic sympathomimetic and membrane stabilising activity.

In the treatment of hypertension nadolol is usually given in an initial dose of 40 to 80 mg daily, increased weekly according to the response of the patient to 240 mg or more daily; some patients have required doses of 640 mg daily. In the management of angina pectoris the usual initial dose is 40 mg daily, increased weekly according to the response of the patient to usual doses of up to 160 mg daily. Doses of 40 to 160 mg daily have also been given for the management of cardiac arrhythmias.

Similar doses are used in migraine prophylaxis.

In the management of thyrotoxicosis, doses of 80 to 160 mg daily have been given; most patients are reported to require the higher dose.

Reduced doses may be required in renal impairment.

ADMINISTRATION IN RENAL FAILURE. Nadolol could be given in usual doses to patients with a glomerular filtration-rate greater than 50 mL per minute but the dose should be reduced by half in those with a glomerular filtration-rate between 10 and 50 mL per minute, and to 25% of normal dosage in those in whom glomerular filtration-rate was less than 10 mL per minute. The half-life of nadolol was extended to 45 hours in patients with end-stage renal disease.— W. M. Bennett *et al.*, *Am. J. Kidney Dis.*, 1983, *3*, 155.

A study involving 15 hypertensive patients given nadolol 80 and 160 mg indicated that despite a fall in cardiac output there was no fall in renal blood flow or glomerular filtration-rate indicating that an increased percentage of cardiac output was redistributed to the kidneys.— S. C. Textor *et al.*, *New Engl. J. Med.*, 1982, *307*, 601. See also D. T. O'Connor (letter), *ibid.*, 1983, *308*, 49; K. O'Malley and E. O'Brien (letter), *ibid.*

Following high intravenous doses of nadolol and propranolol in healthy subjects there was no evidence that the former drug conferred any advantage in its effects on renal function.— D. G. Waller *et al.*, *Br. J. clin. Pharmac.*, 1985, *19*, 37.

GLAUCOMA. In a comparison in patients with glaucoma instillation of nadolol 2% eye-drops provided no long-term ocular hypotensive effect compared with timolol 0.5%. Diacetylnadolol 0.5% and 2.0% had some effect in decreasing intra-ocular pressure but 2 of 8 patients given the higher strength developed periorbital dermatitis.— E. Duzman *et al.*, *Br. J. Ophthal.*, 1983, *67*, 668.

In an open study nadolol 20, 40, or 80 mg daily by mouth in 51 patients was compared with twice daily topical timolol 0.25% or 0.5%, in a further 17 patients, in the treatment of chronic simple glaucoma. Both therapies were effective at lowering intra-ocular pressure although 8 patients receiving nadolol discontinued therapy due to side-effects. Nadolol 20 or 40 mg daily by mouth may be preferred to topical therapy for chronic simple glaucoma in patients who are already receiving beta blockers or who are unable to instil eye-drops.— J. Williamson *et al.*, *Br. J. Ophthal.*, 1985, *69*, 41. See also G. R. Duff *et al.*, *ibid.*, 1987, *71*, 698.

Preparations

Nadolol Tablets *(U.S.P.)*

Proprietary Preparations

Corgard *(Squibb, UK). Tablets*, nadolol 40 mg.
Tablets, scored, nadolol 80 mg.

Corgaretic *(Squibb, UK). Tablets*, scored, nadolol 40 and 80 mg, bendrofluazide 5 mg.

Proprietary Names and Manufacturers

Corgard *(Byk Liprandi, Arg.; Squibb, Canad.; Squibb, Fr.; Squibb, Ital.; Squibb, S.Afr.; Squibb, Spain; Squibb, Swed.; Squibb, Switz.; Squibb, UK; Princeton, USA)*; Corgard HS *(Squibb, S.Afr.)*; Solgol *(Heyden, Ger.)*.

The following names have been used for multi-ingredient preparations containing nadolol— Corgaretic *(Squibb, UK)*; Corzide *(Princeton, USA)*.

6316-y

Nifenalol *(rINN)*.
(±)-2-Isopropylamino-1-(4-nitrophenyl)ethanol; (±)-α-[(Isopropylamino)methyl]-4-nitrobenzyl alcohol.
$C_{11}H_{16}N_2O_3$=224.3.

CAS — 7413-36-7.

Nifenalol is a beta blocker with general properties similar to those of propranolol (see p.798) that has been tried in angina pectoris and some cardiac arrhythmias in doses of 150 to 300 mg of the hydrochloride daily by mouth. It has also been given by injection.

Proprietary Names and Manufacturers
Impeasel *(Roux-Ocefa, Arg.)*; Inpea *(Selvi, Ital.; Liade, Spain)*.

6317-j

Oxprenolol Hydrochloride *(BANM, USAN, rINNM)*.

Ba-39089; Oxyprenolol Hydrochloride. (±)-1-(2-Allyloxyphenoxy)-3-isopropylaminopropan-2-ol hydrochloride.
$C_{15}H_{23}NO_3$,HCl=301.8.

CAS — 6452-71-7 (oxprenolol); 6452-73-9 (hydrochloride).

Pharmacopoeias. In *Br.*, *Ind.* and *It.*

A white to slightly cream-coloured, odourless or almost odourless crystalline powder. **Soluble** 1 in less than 1 of water and 1 in 1.5 of alcohol; very slightly soluble in ether. A 5% solution in water has a pH of 4 to 6.

Adverse Effects and Treatment

As for Propranolol Hydrochloride, p.798.

ALLERGY. A report of oxprenolol-induced drug fever in a patient which was confirmed by a challenge test.— K. Hasegawa *et al.*, *Br. med. J.*, 1980, *281*, 27.

EFFECTS ON THE BLOOD. *Thrombocytopenia.* A 57-year-old man taking 640 mg of a slow-release preparation of oxprenolol daily developed thrombocytopenia which resolved a week after withdrawing oxprenolol. His platelet count fell on rechallenge with a single dose of slow-release oxprenolol 320 mg. His blood pressure was subsequently controlled with propranolol with no adverse effects.— W. N. Dodds and R. J. L. Davidson (letter), *Lancet*, 1978, *2*, 683.

EFFECTS ON THE EYES. A patient who had taken oxprenolol for 18 months (with clonidine, bendrofluazide, frusemide, and digoxin) developed redness of the eyes with conjunctival oedema and congestion and corneal opacities; the symptoms regressed within a week when oxprenolol was withdrawn.— M. S. Knapp and N. R. Galloway (letter), *Br. med. J.*, 1975, *2*, 557.

A 72-year-old man who had taken oxprenolol for about 7 months developed dryness of the eyes.— J. R. Clayden (letter), *Br. med. J.*, 1975, *2*, 557.

EFFECTS ON THE GASTRO-INTESTINAL TRACT. Filmy abdominal adhesions were found at laparotomy in a 50-year-old woman who had taken oxprenolol for about 3 months 4 years earlier; she had not taken practolol.— S. C. Kennedy and M. Ducrow (letter), *Br. med. J.*, 1977, *1*, 1598.

Severe gastro-intestinal symptoms perhaps with obstruction of the small bowel might have been associated with oxprenolol in a patient who also had renal failure. Necropsy revealed a generalised ileus without local cause and no peritonitis.— D. W. Young *et al.* (letter), *Lancet*, 1977, *2*, 1133.

EFFECTS ON MENTAL STATE. In a 66-year-old woman, with no family or personal history of schizophrenia, schizophrenic symptoms, occurring when the dose of oxprenolol was increased, regressed when the dose was reduced.— J. Steinert and C. R. Pugh, *Br. med. J.*, 1979, *1*, 790.

EFFECTS ON THE MUSCLES. A report of a myasthenia-like syndrome with weakness of ocular and limb muscles, occurring in a 67-year-old woman in association with oxprenolol therapy.— Y. Herishanu and P. Rosenberg (letter), *Ann. intern. Med.*, 1975, *83*, 834.

See also under Overdosage, below.

EFFECTS ON RESPIRATORY FUNCTION. A 39-year-old man with extrinsic atopic asthma became acutely breathless and cyanosed after taking 40 mg of oxprenolol.— J. Gaddie and C. Skinner (letter), *Br. med. J.*, 1972, *1*, 749. See also A. Mithal (letter), *ibid.*, 1974, *2*, 503.

FIBROSIS. Retroperitoneal fibrosis in one patient associated with the use of oxprenolol.— D. R. McCluskey *et al.*, *Br. med. J.*, 1980, *281*, 1459.

OVERDOSAGE. A report of rhabdomyolysis and myoglobinuria complicating severe overdosage with oxprenolol.— P. M. Schofield *et al.*, *Hum. Toxicol.*, 1985, *4*, 57.

TOLERANCE. A report of 2 cases of tolerance developing to the effects of oxprenolol. Both patients responded to substitution of another beta blocker.— Z. Weiss *et al.* (letter), *J. Am. med. Ass.*, 1985, *254*, 1454.

Precautions

As for Propranolol Hydrochloride, p.801.

INTERACTIONS. *Antihypertensives.* The effects of hydralazine on the pharmacokinetics of oxprenolol.— A. M. Dart *et al.*, *Br. J. clin. Pharmac.*, 1982, *13*, 587P.

Ergotamine. For a report of arterial spasm in a patient receiving oxprenolol and ergotamine see under Ergotamine Tartrate, p.1056.

Sympathomimetics. A very severe hypertensive reaction occurred in a 31-year-old hypertensive patient receiving methyldopa and oxprenolol when he was prescribed tablets containing phenylpropanolamine for a cold. Methyldopa was known to increase the pressor effects of sympathomimetic amines and the association with oxprenolol might have led to a particularly severe reaction since beta-blockade might allow an unopposed alpha constrictor response to adrenergic stimulation.— E. H. McLaren, *Br. med. J.*, 1976, *2*, 283.

Propranolol enhanced the vasoconstrictor response to noradrenaline in 8 healthy subjects; the addition of oxprenolol reversed the enhancement. This might be due to an alpha-blocking effect of oxprenolol, to a beta-agonist effect, or to a membrane-stabilising effect.— J. O'Grady *et al.*, *Eur. J. clin. Pharmac.*, 1978, *14*, 83.

PERIPHERAL VASCULAR DISEASE. Oxprenolol reduced peripheral blood flow in 8 hypertensive patients, although less than propranolol; neither drug should be used in patients with severe peripheral vascular disease, but if a beta blocker had to be prescribed to patients with mild peripheral vascular disease cautious use of oxprenolol was preferable to propranolol.— M. J. Vandenburg, *Br. J. clin. Pharmac.*, 1982, *14*, 733.

See also under Propranolol Hydrochoride, p.799.

Absorption and Fate

Oxprenolol is almost completely absorbed from the gastro-intestinal tract but is subject to considerable first-pass metabolism. Peak plasma concentrations have been reported to occur about 1 or 2 hours after a dose. It is metabolised in the liver and almost entirely excreted in the urine. Oxprenolol diffuses across the placenta. It also crosses the blood-brain barrier.

In 7 healthy subjects given 40, 80, or 160 mg of oxprenolol the plasma half-life was approximately 80 minutes, irrespective of the dose administered.— L. Brunner *et al.*, *Eur. J. clin. Pharmac.*, 1975, *8*, 3. Following intravenous administration of oxprenolol to 6 healthy subjects a triexponential decrease in plasma concentration was noted. An initial half-life of 5 minutes, corresponding to the initial rapid-distribution phase, was followed by an intermediate half-life of about an hour; a third half-life of 4.5 hours was considered to reflect slow release from storage depots in the body. Following administration by mouth less than 30% reached the systemic circulation owing to metabolism by the liver and gut during the absorption process.— M. J. Kendall *et al.*, *Eur. J. Drug Metab. Pharmacokinet.*, 1976, *1*, 155.

FIRST-PASS EFFECT. A study in 6 healthy subjects suggesting significant pharmacokinetic differences between oxprenolol, and propranolol and other beta-adrenoceptor blocking agents. Following administration of oxprenolol by mouth peak plasma concentrations were reached after 30 to 90 minutes with wide variation in bioavailability, and the plasma half-life was about 1.94 hours; unlike propranolol the plasma half-life was not significantly different following intravenous administration, being about 2.3 hours. The first-pass effect of oxprenolol appeared to differ from that of propranolol.— W. D. Mason and N. Winer, *Clin. Pharmac. Ther.*, 1976, *20*, 401.

METABOLITES. In 6 healthy volunteers oxprenolol 100 to 200 μg per kg body-weight intravenously had no effect on heart-rate, but doses of 40 to 80 mg by mouth significantly reduced the heart-rate, the effect being most evident 4 hours after a dose; this could represent the formation of an active metabolite.— A. Hedges and P. Turner (letter), *Br. med. J.*, 1973, *1*, 422.

PREGNANCY AND THE NEONATE. A study of the placental transfer of oxprenolol and its passage into breast milk in 32 pregnant women receiving oxprenolol in association with dihydralazine (Trasipressol). The mean plasma concentration of oxprenolol before delivery was 0.631 nmol per mL (range 0 to 4.226 nmol per mL) while that in amniotic fluid was 0.087 nmol per mL (range 0 to 0.370 nmol per mL). At the end of delivery the mean maternal plasma concentration was 0.386 nmol per mL. compared with 0.071 and 0.081 nmol per mL in plasma from the umbilical artery and vein respectively. Protein binding in maternal blood was 85%, which was higher than the figure of 78.3% reported in non-pregnant subjects. The concentrations of oxprenolol in breast milk 3 to 6 days after delivery ranged from 0 to 1.342 nmol per mL, and the milk to plasma concentration ratio was 0.45:1, which was lower than has been reported for metoprolol, perhaps because of the high protein binding of oxprenolol. The maximum daily dose that would be supplied to the infant in breast milk was only 0.07 mg per kg body-weight, which was at least 60 times less than the normal dose in adults.— A. Sioufi *et al.*, *Br. J. clin. Pharmac.*, 1984, *18*, 453.

Uses and Administration

Oxprenolol hydrochloride is a moderately lipophilic beta blocker with general properties similar to those of propranolol (see p.803). It is classified as non-cardioselective and is reported to possess intrinsic sympathomimetic and membrane-stabilising activity.

In the treatment of hypertension oxprenolol hydrochloride is usually given initially in a dosage of 80 mg twice daily by mouth, increased at weekly or fortnightly intervals. In conjunction with diuretic therapy a dosage of 80 to 320 mg is usually adequate; when given alone a dose of 480 mg daily should not be exceeded. The dose may also be given once daily as sustained-release tablets.

The usual dose for angina pectoris is 40 to 160 mg three times daily. For cardiac arrhythmias the usual dose is 20 to 40 mg three times daily, increased if necessary according to the patient's response.

For the emergency treatment of cardiac arrhythmias oxprenolol hydrochloride may be given by slow intravenous injection in a dose of 2 mg repeated if necessary after 5 minutes; a maximum cumulative dose of up to 16 mg may be given. Oxprenolol hydrochloride can also be given by the intramuscular route.

Oxprenolol hydrochloride has been given in doses of 40 to 80 mg to relieve anxiety in stressful situations.

ADMINISTRATION IN HEPATIC FAILURE. The response to oxprenolol, which was metabolised by the liver, was altered in the presence of hepatic disease.— G. L. Sanders, *Adverse Drug React. Bull.*, 1978, Feb., 240.

ANXIETY. In a 3-week double-blind trial in 29 patients with anxiety states, diazepam 15 to 35 mg daily was more effective and reduced symptoms more rapidly than oxprenolol 240 to 480 mg daily. Oxprenolol took 2 to 3 weeks to become effective.— G. Johnson *et al.*, *Med. J. Aust.*, 1976, *1*, 909.

A single dose of oxprenolol 40 mg taken 90 minutes before a concert performance significantly reduced anxiety with a significant improvement in musical performance in a double-blind crossover study of 24 musicians. Oxprenolol caused a significant reduction in pulse-rate and a slight fall in systolic blood pressure.— I. M. James *et al.*, *Lancet*, 1977, *2*, 952. Administration of oxprenolol 40 mg to 8 surgeons 1 hour before operations reduced their average heart-rate from 121 beats per minute to an average of 84 beats per minute.— G. E. Foster *et al.*, *ibid.*, 1978, *1*, 1323.

Oxprenolol 40 mg given 45 minutes before a stressful event (viewing of a necropsy) reduced subjective anxiety in a study involving 68 police cadets.— A. A. Landauer and D. A. Pocock, *Br. med. J.*, 1984, *289*, 592.

CARDIAC DISORDERS. *Angina pectoris.* In a double-blind study in 18 patients oxprenolol 160 mg daily as a sustained-release tablet was as effective as propranolol 40 mg thrice daily in controlling the symptoms of angina pectoris.— P. A. Majid *et al.*, *J. int. med. Res.*, 1979, *7*, 194.

Beta blockers such as oxprenolol, acebutolol, or pindolol,

with intrinsic sympathomimetic activity, are the logical choice to treat angina in patients with resting bradycardia or impaired peripheral circulation.— L. H. Opie, *Lancet*, 1984, *1*, 496.

Cardiac arrhythmias. In 41 patients with cardiac disease treated with digitalis, diuretics, quinidine, and anticoagulants, oxprenolol, 40 to 240 mg daily, had a beneficial effect in sinus tachycardia (especially associated with emotion), paroxysmal supraventricular tachycardia, and established atrial fibrillation. In conjunction with quinidine, it effectively prevented recurrences of paroxysmal atrial fibrillation or prevented its return after counter-current. There was little effect on extrasystoles whatever the origin.— L. Scebat and J. Bensaid, *Postgrad. med. J.*, 1970, (Nov.), *Suppl.*, 86.

Oxprenolol was used to treat 63 episodes of cardiac arrhythmias in 43 patients with acute myocardial infarction or ischaemia. Single intravenous injections were given, initially in a dose of 2 mg followed after 10 minutes by a further 4 mg and then 6 mg if the previous dose was not effective. The effects of continuous infusions of oxprenolol in a dose of 250 µg per minute were also studied. Oxprenolol successfully suppressed ventricular ectopic beats in 13 of 18 episodes and satisfactorily controlled 13 of 27 episodes of supraventricular tachycardia. It was less effective in suppressing other supraventricular arrhythmias. The most effective methods of administration were continuous intravenous infusion followed by the single intravenous injection of 6 mg. Hypotension occurred in more than 50% of patients, and oxprenolol should be given with caution to patients with low blood pressure and to patients with ventricular tachycardia.— G. Sandler and A. C. Pistevos, *Br. med. J.*, 1971, *1*, 254.

In a multicentre study involving 736 patients who had experienced acute myocardial infarction, oxprenolol 160 mg daily (as a slow-release tablet) for 3 days, followed by the same dose twice daily for a year was given to 358 patients while 378 received placebo. There was no significant difference in the incidence and frequency of ventricular arrhythmias; 22 patients in the oxprenolol group and 17 receiving placebo died during the following year. It was concluded that slow-release oxprenolol failed to demonstrate an antiarrhythmic effect at these doses in patients with postinfarction arrhythmias.— K.-P. Bethge *et al.*, *J. Am. Coll. Cardiol.*, 1985, *6*, 963.

Myocardial infarction. In a multicentre study involving 1103 patients who had undergone a myocardial infarction 632 were assigned to treatment with oxprenolol 40 mg by mouth twice daily while 471 received placebo. All but 5 patients began treatment one month or more after myocardial infarction. Overall, over the 6 years of the study there were 102 cardiac events (deaths and nonfatal infarctions) and 48 deaths in the placebo group while there were 119 events and 60 deaths in the oxprenolol group; there was no significant difference in these figures. Although there was a trend towards increased survival in the oxprenolol group for 42 months after entry this was subsequently reversed so that cumulative survival at 6 years was 85.1% in the oxprenolol group and 85.2% in the placebo group. However, subgroup analysis revealed that survival-rate was increased in patients given the drug within four months of infarction (cumulative 6-year survival 95.1% as against 76.6% in the placebo group) whereas it was reduced in those given oxprenolol more that 1 year after infarction. If confirmed these results suggest that the benefits of beta blockade may be confined to relatively early intervention, at the latest within the first few weeks after myocardial infarction.— S. H. Taylor *et al.*, *New Engl. J. Med.*, 1982, *307*, 1293.

Further studies: *Eur. Heart J.*, 1984, *5*, 189 (lack of benefit in preventing re-infarction).

HYPERTENSION. Evidence that prolonged therapy (10 weeks or more) may be needed for an antihypertensive effect with oxprenolol.— M. W. Millar-Craig *et al.*, *Eur. J. clin. Pharmac.*, 1983, *24*, 713.

For a lack of effect of single daily doses of oxprenolol on blood pressure in hypertensive patients, see under Atenolol, p. 785.

A multicentre study (the International Prospective Primary Prevention Study in Hypertension; IPPPSH) involving 6357 patients with essential hypertension and indicating lower average blood pressure and easier control in patients receiving oxprenolol rather than placebo as part of their antihypertensive medication.—IPPPSH Collaborative Group, *J. Hypertens.*, 1985, *3*, 379.

Once- and twice-daily administration. In a study completed by 15 hypertensive patients satisfactory control of blood pressure was obtained with a twice-daily dosage regimen of oxprenolol (together with diuretic therapy) despite its relatively short half-life.— B. J. Materson *et al.*, *Clin. Pharmac. Ther.*, 1976, *19*, 325.

Oxprenolol as a single daily dose of a sustained-release preparation was effective in controlling blood pressure in hypertensive patients.— G. N. Volans *et al.* (letter), *Br. J. clin. Pharmac.*, 1979, *8*, 86. See also B. J. Materson *et al.*, *Drug Intell. & clin. Pharm.*, 1983, *17*, 51.

A double-blind crossover study involving 23 hypertensive patients compared the effects of atenolol 100 mg once daily, sustained-release oxprenolol 160 mg once daily, and long-acting propranolol 160 mg once daily. The findings confirmed the effectiveness of atenolol and the long-acting propranolol formulation and showed them to be superior to sustained-release oxprenolol in lowering blood pressure over 24 hours. It was suggested that the present formulation of sustained-release oxprenolol may need to be reconsidered.— J. C. Petrie *et al.*, *Br. med. J.*, 1980, *280*, 1573.

The effects of slow-release oxprenolol 160 mg, alone or with cyclopenthiazide, and the same dose of oxprenolol in a conventional formulation were not significantly different in terms of plasma concentrations of oxprenolol produced, with peak plasma concentrations occurring after 3 hours and no significant effect compared with placebo after 24 hours. Slow-release formulations of oxprenolol should be given twice daily in order to maintain beta blockade over a 24-hour period.— M. J. Kerr *et al.*, *Br. J. clin. Pharmac.*, 1981, *12*, 869.

HYPERTHYROIDISM. In a controlled double-blind crossover study of 16 patients with moderately severe thyrotoxicosis, oxprenolol 40 mg every 8 hours for 1 week was no better than placebo. The probable explanation for the failure was that oxprenolol had some inherent sympathomimetic activity.— M. G. Gibberd and J. S. Staffurth (letter), *Lancet*, 1973, *1*, 205.

PREGNANCY AND THE NEONATE. *Hypertension in pregnancy.* In a randomised study in 53 women with hypertension of pregnancy 26 were treated with oxprenolol and 27 with methyldopa in doses designed to reduce sitting diastolic blood pressure to or below 80 mmHg; hydralazine was added when necessary. Those given oxprenolol had greater plasma volume expansion, with improved placental weight and birth weight. Blood-glucose concentrations in the infants in the oxprenolol group were significantly higher than in the methyldopa group. Oxprenolol appeared to have advantages over methyldopa.— E. D. M. Gallery *et al.*, *Br. med. J.*, 1979, *1*, 1591. See also E. D. M. Gallery *et al.*, *ibid.*, 1985, *291*, 563. No significant difference in foetal outcome was found in a case-controlled study comparing 50 women given methyldopa for hypertension in pregnancy and 50 given oxprenolol.— J. Fidler *et al.*, *Br. med. J.*, 1983, *286*, 1927.

Preparations

Oxprenolol Tablets *(B.P.).* Contain oxprenolol hydrochloride.

Proprietary Preparations

Apsolox *(Approved Prescription Services, UK). Tablets*, oxprenolol hydrochloride 20, 40, 80 and 160 mg.

Slow-Pren *(Norton, UK). Tablets*, sustained-release, oxprenolol hydrochloride 160 mg.

Trasicor *(Ciba, UK). Tablets*, oxprenolol hydrochloride 20, 40, 80 and 160 mg.
Tablets (Slow-Trasicor), sustained-release, oxprenolol hydrochloride 160 mg.

Trasidrex *(Ciba, UK). Tablets*, oxprenolol hydrochloride 160 mg (for sustained release), cyclopenthiazide 250 µg. For hypertension. *Dose.* Usually, 1 or 2 tablets daily.

Proprietary Names and Manufacturers

Apsolox *(Approved Prescription Services, UK)*; Captol *(Protea, Austral.)*; Laracor *(Lagap, UK)*; Lo-Tone *(Rolab, S.Afr.)*; Oxanol *(Spain)*; Slow-Pren *(Norton, UK)*; Slow-Trasicor *(Ciba, Arg.; Ciba, Canad.; Ciba, S.Afr.; Ciba, Switz.; Ciba, UK)*; Trasacor *(Jpn)*; Trasicor *(Ciba, Arg.; Ciba, Austral.; Belg.; Ciba, Canad.; Ciba, Denm; Ciba, Fr.; Ciba, Ger.; Ciba., Ital; Neth.; Ciba, Norw.; Ciba, S.Afr.; Ciba, Spain; Ciba, Swed.; Ciba, Switz.; Ciba, UK)*; Trasicor Retard *(Ciba, Denm.)*.

6318-z

Penbutolol Sulphate *(BANM, rINNM).*

Hoe-39893d; Hoe-893d; Penbutolol Hemisulphate; Penbutolol Sulfate *(USAN)*. *(S)*-1-*tert*-Butylamino-3-(2-cyclopentylphenoxy)propan-2-ol hemisulphate.

$(C_{18}H_{29}NO_2)_2,H_2SO_4=680.9$.

CAS — 38363-40-5 (penbutolol); 38363-32-5 (sulphate).

Adverse Effects, Treatment, and Precautions

As for Propranolol Hydrochloride, p.798.

Absorption and Fate

Penbutolol is readily absorbed from the gastro-intestinal tract and peak plasma concentrations occur about 1 or 2 hours after a dose. It is extensively metabolised, the metabolites being excreted in the urine together with only small amounts of unchanged penbutolol; several of its metabolites are believed to be biologically active.

The beta-adrenoceptor blocking effects of penbutolol 20 mg were compared with those of propranolol 80 mg in a double-blind trial involving 6 healthy subjects. Penbutolol differed from propranolol in that it did not lower resting heart-rates during the 2 hours following its administration, and did not reduce systolic blood pressure at rest. The peak plasma concentration of penbutolol occurred 1 hour after oral administration and its half-life was 4.5 hours. Peak biological activity occurred at 2 hours. This might be due to an active metabolite.— J. F. Giudicelli *et al.*, *Br. J. clin. Pharmac.*, 1977, *4*, 135.

In 8 healthy subjects penbutolol 50 mg by mouth was rapidly absorbed, producing a mean peak serum concentration of 770 ng per mL after about 1 hour. The mean plasma half-lives of the fast and slow phases were 2.5 and 27 hours respectively. The apparent elimination half-life was about 27 hours, suggesting that less frequent doses would be required, compared to other beta-adrenoceptor blocking agents. About 3% of the dose was recovered unchanged from the urine over 72 hours in 7 subjects, and 9.8% in the eighth, suggesting extensive metabolism.— J. J. Vallner *et al.*, *J. clin. Pharmac.*, 1977, *17*, 231.

Uses and Administration

Penbutolol is a beta blocker with general properties similar to those of propranolol (see p.803). It is classified as non-cardioselective and is reported to possess membrane stabilising properties but to lack intrinsic sympathomimetic activity.

Penbutolol sulphate has been given in the treatment of hypertension and cardiac disorders in usual doses of 40 mg daily as a single dose, increased to 80 mg daily if necessary.

Proprietary Preparations

Lasipressin *(Hoechst, UK). Tablets*, scored, penbutolol sulphate 40 mg, frusemide 20 mg. For hypertension. *Dose.* 1 tablet each morning, increased if necessary to 1 twice daily.

Proprietary Names and Manufacturers

Betapressin *(Hoechst, Ger.; Hoechst, Ital.; Hoechst, S.Afr.)*; Betapressine *(Roussel, Fr.; Hoechst, Switz.)*; Blocotin *(Hoechst, Spain)*; Hostabloc *(Hoechst, Arg.)*; Ipobar *(Miba, Ital.)*.

6319-c

Pindolol *(BAN, USAN, rINN).*

LB46; Prindolol; Prinodolol. 1-(Indol-4-yloxy)-3-isopropylaminopropan-2-ol.

$C_{14}H_{20}N_2O_2=248.3$.

CAS — 13523-86-9.

Pharmacopoeias. In *Br.*, *It.*, *Jpn*, and *U.S.*

A white or almost white, odourless or almost odourless, crystalline powder. Practically **insoluble** in water; slightly soluble in dehydrated alcohol and in chloroform; sparingly soluble in methyl alcohol. **Store** in well-closed containers. Protect from light.

Adverse Effects, Treatment, and Precautions

As for Propranolol Hydrochloride, p.798.

Fine tremor in the extremities of 5 patients during pindolol therapy was considered to have been due to its partial agonist activity.— H. Hod *et al.*, *Postgrad. med. J.*, 1980, *56*, 346.

EFFECTS ON THE BLOOD. Pindolol had been associated

with the development of agranulocytosis.— P. C. Vincent, *Drugs*, 1986, *31*, 52.

EFFECTS ON CARBOHYDRATE METABOLISM. Severe hypoglycaemia during haemodialysis occurred after 18 hours of fasting, in a 34-year-old man taking pindolol. The addition of glucose to the dialysis fluid was recommended.— K. Samii *et al.* (letter), *Lancet*, 1976, *1*, 545. See also A. Grimaldi *et al.*, *Curr. ther. Res.*, 1984, *36*, 361.

EFFECTS ON THE CARDIOVASCULAR SYSTEM. *Hypertension*. Paradoxically, high doses of pindolol could cause hypertension. In 9 patients taking a mean of 48 mg daily diastolic and systolic pressure, lying and standing, was significantly higher than when taking a mean of 19 mg daily.— H. J. Waal-Manning and F. O. Simpson (letter), *Br. med. J.*, 1975, *3*, 155. There was no evidence of a paradoxical rise of blood pressure in 24 patients with essential hypertension who received pindolol in increasing doses up to 45 mg per day.— O. H. Koldsland, *Curr. ther. Res.*, 1977, *22*, 853.

For comments on paradoxical hypertension associated with administration of beta-adrenoceptor blocking agents, see Propranolol, p.799.

Peripheral circulatory disorders. For the suggestion that pindolol may have less effect on peripheral circulation than beta blockers lacking intrinsic sympathomimetic activity, see under Propranolol Hydrochloride, p.799.

EFFECTS ON LIPID METABOLISM. Evidence from a study involving 28 subjects that pindolol, perhaps because of its intrinsic sympathomimetic action, may lack the adverse effects on serum lipids and lipoproteins that have been observed with other beta blockers.— L. A. Simons *et al.*, *Curr. ther. Res.*, 1987, *41*, 525.

EFFECTS ON RESPIRATORY FUNCTION. In 4 patients recovering from exacerbation of asthma pindolol, 200 µg intravenously or 15 mg by mouth, caused chest tightness and there was objective evidence of airways obstruction unresponsive to sympathomimetic aerosols.— K. Mattson and H. Poppius, *Eur. J. clin. Pharmac.*, 1978, *14*, 87.

Further reference: J. W. J. Lammers *et al.*, *Br. J. clin. Pharmac.*, 1985, *20*, 205.

For a comparison of the adverse effects of pindolol and propranolol on respiratory function see under Propranolol Hydrochloride, p.800.

LUPUS ERYTHEMATOSUS. A report of systemic lupus erythematosus associated with the use of pindolol.— J. Bensaid *et al.*, *Br. med. J.*, 1979, *1*, 1603.

RESTLESS LEG SYNDROME. A report of 1 patient in whom the restless leg syndrome occurred after commencing therapy with pindolol.— L. K. Morgan (letter), *Med. J. Aust.*, 1975, *2*, 753.

Absorption and Fate

Pindolol is almost completely absorbed from the gastro-intestinal tract and peak plasma concentrations are obtained about 1 to 2 hours after a dose. It is only partially metabolised and is excreted in the urine both unchanged and in the form of metabolites; small amounts are reported to be excreted in bile. About 40 to 60% is reported to be bound to plasma proteins. Pindolol is excreted in breast milk.

A review of studies on 57 subjects indicated that the systemic bioavailability of pindolol is at least 87%. It may be concluded that in man the first-pass effect of pindolol is so low as to be negligible.— J. Meier and E. Nüesch (letter), *Br. J. clin. Pharmac.*, 1977, *4*, 371. See also M. Guerret *et al.*, *Eur. J. clin. Pharmac.*, 1983, *25*, 357.

The plasma half-life of pindolol after administration to healthy subjects by mouth was about 3.5 hours and after intravenous administration about 3 hours; the difference was not significant. About 57% was bound to plasma proteins.— R. Gugler *et al.*, *Eur. J. clin. Pharmac.*, 1974, *7*, 17.

DIFFUSION INTO THE CSF. CSF: plasma ratios of propranolol and pindolol.— E. A. Taylor *et al.*, *Br. J. clin. Pharmac.*, 1979, *8*, 381P.

Uses and Administration

Pindolol is a moderately lipophilic beta blocker with general properties similar to those of propranolol (see p.803). It is classified as non-cardioselective and has intrinsic sympathomimetic actions but little membrane stabilising activity.

In the treatment of hypertension pindolol is usually given initially in a dosage of 5 mg twice or three times daily, subsequently increased according to the patient's response; additional benefit is rarely obtained from doses higher than 45 mg daily, although doses up to 60 mg daily have been given. A once-daily dosage regimen has been reported to be adequate for some patients.

The usual dose for angina pectoris is 2.5 to 5 mg up to three times daily; however, doses of up to 10 mg four times daily have been suggested.

For a series of papers on pindolol, see *Br. J. clin. Pharmac.*, 1982, *13, Suppl.* 2, 143S–450S.

Short reviews of pindolol: W. H. Frishman, *New Engl. J. Med.*, 1983, *308*, 940; *Med. Lett.*, 1983, *25*, 13.

ADMINISTRATION IN THE ELDERLY. A study of the pharmacokinetics of pindolol in 10 young and 10 elderly hypertensive patients indicated that half-life was prolonged and clearance reduced in the elderly patients; a significantly greater degree of beta blockade persisted 24 hours after a dose in the elderly group.— I. Gretzer *et al.*, *Eur. J. clin. Pharmac.*, 1986, *31*, 415.

ADMINISTRATION IN HEPATIC FAILURE. A study of the elimination of pindolol in patients with various forms of liver disease. The metabolism of pindolol was enhanced in patients with acute hepatitis, possibly because of increased hepatic blood flow. In contrast, decreased metabolism was found in most of the patients with hepatic cirrhosis; interestingly, some patients with impaired hepatic metabolism but normal renal function appeared to be able to compensate by increased renal excretion of unchanged drug. However, in patients with severely impaired hepatic metabolism (phenazone clearance less than 10 mL per minute) the elimination of pindolol was severely reduced and dosage modification may be required in these patients to avoid accumulation of pindolol.— E. E. Ohnhaus *et al.*, *Eur. J. clin. Pharmac.*, 1982, *22*, 247.

ADMINISTRATION IN RENAL FAILURE. Following administration of pindolol 40 µg per kg body-weight intravenously to 18 hypertensive patients, 9 in chronic renal failure exhibited decreased total-body and renal clearance of pindolol compared with 9 patients with normal renal function. Transfer rate-constants, distribution volumes, and non-renal clearance did not differ significantly between the 2 groups. After a single dose of pindolol 10 mg by mouth it was found that the patients with renal failure, compared with the patients with normal renal activity, effectively absorbed a decreased fraction of the dose, with increased initial rate of absorption being inversely correlated with creatinine clearance.— N. P. Chau *et al.*, *Clin. Pharmac. Ther.*, 1977, *22*, 505.

A comparative study of the pharmacokinetics of pindolol in subjects with essential hypertension suggested that when patients also had impaired renal function, the absorption of pindolol was decreased. No evidence was found for increased metabolism of pindolol in patients with reduced renal function.— D. Lavene *et al.*, *J. clin. Pharmac.*, 1977, *17*, 501.

ANXIETY. The changes in the EEG after pindolol 5 mg were similar to those produced by imipramine. Pindolol might be of use in treatment of somatic anxiety and anxiety with depression.— J. Roubicek (letter), *Br. J. clin. Pharmac.*, 1976, *3*, 661.

Pindolol 5 mg reduced subjective anxiety more than placebo in a study involving 30 musicians.— I. M. James *et al.*, *J. R. Soc. Med.*, 1983, *76*, 194.

See also under Haemostasis, below.

CARDIAC DISORDERS. *Angina pectoris*. In 12 healthy men pindolol 15 mg reduced exercise-induced tachycardia by a mean maximum of 36 beats per minute; about 40% of its activity remained 24 hours after the dose. Pindolol should be suitable for once-daily dosage in angina pectoris.— W. H. Aellig, *Eur. J. clin. Pharmac.*, 1978, *14*, 167.

Benefit from pindolol 5 to 10 mg twice daily in exertional angina.— D. L. Johnston *et al.*, *Can. med. Ass. J.*, 1984, *130*, 1449.

Pindolol was used successfully in the management of a patient with angina complicated by resting bradycardia; in contrast to atenolol, which exacerbated the bradycardia, pindolol slightly improved resting bradycardia while preventing exercise tachycardia.— M. A. James *et al.*, *Br. med. J.*, 1986, *293*, 1476.

Cardiac arrhythmias. Pindolol 200 to 400 µg given intravenously for 1 to 3 doses to 30 patients with cardiac arrhythmias slowed the ventricular rate within 2 hours in 13 of 14 patients with atrial fibrillation or flutter and converted 4 of these patients and 4 others with tachycardia to sinus rhythm. Premature ventricular beats of 6 or more per minute were abolished or reduced in 10 of 14 patients and premature atrial beats of 6 or more per minute were abolished in all of 3 patients.— W. S. Aronow and R. R. Uyeyama, *Clin. Pharmac. Ther.*, 1972, *13*, 15.

Myocardial infarction. A study involving 529 patients following myocardial infarction suggested that subsequent treatment with oral pindolol in 263 had no significant effect on mortality or re-infarction compared with placebo in 266. However, there was a reduced mortality in patients who started pindolol therapy more than 5 days after their original infarction, and this was still more evident in the group who started treatment after 12 days. In order to benefit, patients should not start therapy with pindolol for one week or more after myocardial infarction.—Australian and Swedish Pindolol Study Group, *Eur. Heart J.*, 1983, *4*, 367.

GLAUCOMA. Pindolol 1% eye-drops significantly lowered intra-ocular pressure in normal and glaucomatous eyes and were well tolerated. There was an increase in outflow facility when treatment was continued for about 1 month.— L. Bonomi and P. Steindler, *Br. J. Ophthal.*, 1975, *59*, 301.

Further references: S. E. Smith *et al.*, *Br. J. Ophthal.*, 1979, *63*, 63; R. J. H. Smith *et al.*, *ibid.*, 1982, *66*, 102; S. Andréasson and K. M. Jensen, *ibid.*, 1983, *67*, 228; Q. A. Mekki *et al.*, *Br. J. clin. Pharmac.*, 1983, *15*, 112.

HAEMOSTASIS. Following evidence of reduced bleeding in a study of pindolol given as an anxiolytic to patients undergoing tonsillectomy, a double-blind study was carried out on 36 tonsillectomy patients. Pindolol 5 mg was given the evening before and one hour before surgery in 19 patients; 17 received placebo. Mean blood loss in the group given pindolol was 1.77 mL, compared with 7.30 mL in the placebo group, and this significant difference was correlated with differences in heart-rate but not in blood pressure between groups. The mechanism of the apparent haemostatic action was uncertain.— R. Basjrah *et al.*, *J. int. med. Res.*, 1983, *11*, 263.

HYPERTENSION. In the short term the plasma concentration of pindolol was the most important factor determining its antihypertensive effect; but in the long term the initial elevation of blood pressure above normal was the most important factor.— Y. A. Weiss *et al.*, *Curr. ther. Res.*, 1977, *21*, 644.

In a multicentre study, 7062 hypertensive patients aged between 12 and 89 years were treated with pindolol 7.5 to 45 mg daily, 91.6% of the patients initially receiving 15 mg as a single daily dose, for 3 to 9 weeks. Treatment was considered to be effective in 75% of the 5989 patients assessed, and satisfactory in a further 12%. Treatment was discontinued in 53 patients because of lack of effect, and 1822 (25.8%) of the patients reported side-effects which were severe enough to cause discontinuation of treatment in 507 (7.2%) patients. The most common side-effects were dizziness (8.1%), gastro-intestinal complaints (7.1%), headache (4.9%), insomnia (3.5%), lassitude (3.0%), and subjective cardiac complaints (2.6%).— J. Rosenthal *et al.*, *Br. J. clin. Pract.*, 1979, *33*, 165.

HYPERTHYROIDISM. Pindolol 15 and 30 mg daily given in a controlled study to 20 patients with hyperthyroidism had no effect on thyroid function. Blood pressure was not reduced but the heart-rate was decreased in a dose-dependent manner.— J. L. Schelling *et al.*, *Clin. Pharmac. Ther.*, 1973, *14*, 158.

Pindolol 15 mg daily in divided doses did not reduce tachycardia in 6 hyperthyroid patients.— E. Abadie *et al.* (letter), *New Engl. J. Med.*, 1983, *309*, 795.

ORTHOSTATIC HYPOTENSION. The successful treatment of 3 patients, with severe orthostatic hypotension because of chronic autonomic failure, with pindolol, because of its intrinsic sympathomimetic activity.— A. J. Man in't Veld and M. A. D. H. Schalekamp, *Br. med. J.*, 1981, *282*, 929. No benefit with pindolol in 1 patient.— A. C. Davidson and S. E. Smith (letter), *ibid.*, 1704. See also P. Goldstraw and D. G. Waller (letter), *ibid.*, *283*, 310. Further comments.— A. J. Man in't Veld and M. A. D. H. Schalekamp (letter), *ibid.*, 561; G. Nyberg (letter), *ibid.*, 861. Pindolol was of no benefit in 5 patients with postural hypotension due to autonomic failure associated with multiple system atrophy. In 2 of the patients it produced cardiac failure.— B. Davies *et al.* (letter), *Lancet*, 1981, *2*, 982. Comment.— A. J. Man in't Veld and M. A. D. H. Schalekamp (letter), *ibid.*, 1279.

Preparations

Pindolol Tablets *(B.P., U.S.P.)*

Proprietary Preparations

Betadren *(Lagap, UK). Tablets*, pindolol 5 and 15 mg.

Viskaldix *(Sandoz, UK). Tablets*, scored, pindolol 10 mg, clopamide 5 mg. For hypertension. *Dose.* 1 tablet daily, increased if required to 3 tablets daily.

Visken *(Sandoz, UK). Tablets*, scored, pindolol 5 and 15 mg.

Proprietary Names and Manufacturers
Barbloc *(Alphapharm, Austral.)*; Betadren *(Lagap, UK)*; Carvisken *(Jpn)*; Decreten *(Dumex, Switz.)*; Durapindol *(Durachemie, Ger.)*; Hexapindol *(Durascan, Denm.)*; Pectobloc *(Siegfried, Ger.)*; Pinbetol *(Dolorgiet, Ger.)*; Viskeen *(Neth.)*; Visken *(Sandoz, Arg.; Sandoz, Austral.; Belg.; Sandoz, Canad.; Sandoz, Denm.; Sandoz, Fr.; Wander, Ger.; Sandoz, Ital.; Lux.; Sandoz, Norw.; Wander, S.Afr.; Sandoz, Spain; Sandoz, Swed.; Sandoz, UK; Sandoz, USA)*; Viskene *(Sandoz, Switz.)*.

The following names have been used for multi-ingredient preparations containing pindolol—Viskaldix *(Sandoz, NZ; Sandoz, UK)*; Viskazide *(Sandoz, Canad.)*; Visken 10 + Brinaldix 5 *(Sandoz, Austral.)*.

6320-s

Practolol *(BAN, USAN, pINN).*

AY-21011; ICI-50172; Practololum. 4′-(2-Hydroxy-3-isopropylaminopropoxy)acetanilide.
$C_{14}H_{22}N_2O_3$=266.3.

CAS — 6673-35-4.

Pharmacopoeias. In *Braz.*, and *Nord.*

Adverse Effects, Treatment, and Precautions

As for Propranolol Hydrochloride, below.

The 'oculomucocutaneous syndrome' of serious adverse effects on the skin, eyes, and mucous membranes, deafness, systemic lupus erythematosus, and sclerosing peritonitis, which may be fatal, has been associated with the use of practolol. The fibrotic changes are associated with immunological disturbances and there is little evidence of such effects with other beta blockers.

By the end of 1974, 187 reports had been received of adverse effects on the eyes of patients who had been treated with practolol for periods of a few weeks to several years. Two-thirds of the reports involved diminished tear secretion and conjunctivitis; the rest involved corneal damage sometimes leading to impairment or loss of vision. There had also been several hundred reports of psoriasiform or hyperkeratotic skin reactions, and 25 complaints of deafness. Fourteen patients had developed a syndrome resembling systemic lupus erythematosus and 8 had developed an unusual form of sclerosing peritonitis. In some patients the adverse reactions were multiple and half the patients with eye changes had a rash; the mild eye changes and most of the skin reactions were reversible on withdrawal of practolol but the damage could be irreversible in the case of corneal involvement. On the basis of reports to the Committee over 10 years it seemed unlikely that similar changes would occur even after prolonged therapy with propranolol but it was too early to comment on other beta-adrenoceptor blocking agents. In addition it had been reported that abrupt cessation of practolol might lead to worsening of angina pectoris and to cardiac arrhythmia.—Committee on Safety of Medicines, *Adverse Reactions Series No. 11*, Jan. 1975.

During 1974 and 1975 ninety-five patients were reported to the Swedish Adverse Drug Reaction Committee as having had an adverse reaction to practolol involving the skin and eyes. Data on 86 of these indicated that 64 had also received at least one other beta-adrenoceptor blocking agent (alprenolol, metoprolol, oxprenolol, pindolol, or propranolol). Analysis of these 64 cases confirmed the impression that serious side-effects of the type induced by practolol were uncommon with other beta-adrenoceptor blocking agents even in patients who were unable to tolerate practolol.— A. -K. Furhoff *et al.* (letter), *Br. med. J.*, 1976, *1*, 831.

Patients who develop typical practolol-induced eye and/or skin reactions were considered to be at high risk of later developing peritonitis and should be carefully monitored. Of 11 patients with induced peritonitis, 9 had such reactions before their first abdominal symptoms and in 8 the time-lag between discontinuing practolol and the onset of these symptoms ranged from 1 to 12 months.— J. E. Idänpään-Heikkilä *et al.* (letter), *Lancet*, 1977, *2*, 1354.

Antibody specific for a practolol metabolite was present in serum from all of 24 patients who had experienced adverse reactions to practolol; it was not present in 10 patients taking other beta-blockers nor in 21 controls; it was present in some of 15 patients who had taken practolol without adverse effect. In 5 patients antibody activity was increased by challenge with practolol and one patient had an adverse reaction. Reactions to practolol might represent a hitherto unknown type of hypersensitivity reaction.— H. E. Amos *et al.*, *Br. med. J.*, 1978, *1*, 402.

The tear-lysozyme ratio (the ratio of the concentration present to the lower limit of normality) was low in 21 patients who had taken practolol and who had the oculomucocutaneous syndrome (OCMS) and low in 31 who had taken practolol and who had not OCMS. The lysozyme ratio was also low in 5 patients who had taken tolamolol for at least a year. No reduction in lysozyme was found in 23, 26, and 23 patients who had taken respectively timolol, labetalol, and propranolol for at least 6 months, usually longer. Any patient developing a dry eye while taking a beta-adrenoceptor blocking agent should have the tear-lysozyme ratio measured; a low value, indicative of impaired function of the lachrymal gland, might precede clinical signs of adverse ocular reactions, as might high titres of antinuclear antibody and antibodies to the intercellular cement substance.— I. A. Mackie *et al.*, *Br. J. Ophthal.*, 1977, *61*, 354.

INTERACTIONS. For a report of an interaction between practolol and disopyramide see Disopyramide, p.76.

Absorption and Fate

Practolol is absorbed from the gastro-intestinal tract when given by mouth. It is not metabolised and is excreted unchanged in the urine.

Comparisons of the reduction in exercise-induced tachycardia and plasma concentrations of practolol suggested that practolol has a plasma half-life of 10 to 11 hours and a pharmacological half-life of 40 to 50 hours.— S. G. Carruthers *et al.* (letter), *Br. med. J.*, 1973, *2*, 177. Criticisms.— C. R. Kumana and T. R. D. Shaw (letter), *ibid.*, 1973, *2*, 715; S. E. Smith (letter), *ibid.*

Following oral administration of incremental doses of practolol to 7 patients with essential hypertension, absorption was found to be complete and the plasma half-life was 13.2 hours. There was no detectable metabolic transformation. Excretion was entirely by the kidneys and was unaffected by changes in urinary pH from 5.4 to 8.0.— G. Bodem and C. A. Chidsey, *Clin. Pharmac. Ther.*, 1973, *14*, 26.

Uses and Administration

Practolol is a beta blocker with general properties similar to those of propranolol (see p.803). It is classified as cardioselective and is reported to possess intrinsic sympathomimetic activity. Because of the serious adverse effects associated with its use it should be reserved for the management of life-threatening arrhythmias where alternative treatment is of no benefit.

For the emergency treatment of cardiac arrhythmias practolol may be given by slow intravenous injection in a dose of 5 mg, repeated if necessary according to the patient's response. Total dosages of more than 20 mg are not usually required.

Proprietary Preparations

Eraldin *(ICI Pharmaceuticals, UK). Injection*, practolol 2 mg/mL, in ampoules of 5 mL.

Proprietary Names and Manufacturers
Dalzic; Eraldin *(ICI, Austral.; ICI, Denm.; ICI, Norw.; ICI, S.Afr.; ICI Pharmaceuticals, UK)*; Eraldina *(ICI, Swed.)*.

6301-g

Propranolol Hydrochloride *(BANM, USAN, rINNM).*

AY-64043; ICI-45520; NSC-91523. (±)-1-Isopropylamino-3-(1-naphthyloxy)propan-2-ol hydrochloride.
$C_{16}H_{21}NO_2$,HCl=295.8.

CAS — 525-66-6 (propranolol)[5051-22-9(+); 4199-09-1(−); 13013-17-7(±)]; 318-98-9 (hydrochloride)[13071-11-9(+); 4199-10-4(−); 3506-09-0(±)].

Pharmacopoeias. In *Br., Braz., Chin., Cz., Egypt., Ind., Int., It., Jpn, Jug., Nord.*, and *U.S.*

A white or off-white, odourless or almost odourless, crystalline powder.

Soluble 1 in 20 of water and of alcohol; slightly soluble in chloroform; practically insoluble in ether. A 1% solution in water has a pH of 5 to 6. The *B.P.* injection has a pH of 3.0 to 3.5 and is **sterilised** by autoclaving. The *U.S.P.* injection has a pH between 2.8 and 4.0.

In aqueous solutions propranolol decomposes with oxidation of the isopropylamine side-chain, accompanied by a reduction in pH and discoloration of the solution. Solutions are most stable at pH 3 and decompose rapidly when alkaline.

Store in well-closed containers. The *U.S.P.* requires preparations to be protected from light.

Adverse Effects

The most common side-effects of propranolol are nausea, vomiting, and other gastro-intestinal disturbances, fatigue, and dizziness. Cardiovascular effects include bradycardia, hypotension, or occasionally paradoxical hypertension, cold extremities and Raynaud's phenomenon; congestive heart failure or heart block may be precipitated. Central nervous system effects include depression, hallucinations, confusion, psychotic episodes, and disturbances of sleep and vision. Paraesthesia and transient loss of hearing have been reported. Bronchospasm may occur, particularly in susceptible individuals. Blood disorders and skin rashes may also occur. Other adverse effects reported include impaired sexual function, allergic reactions, metabolic disturbances, fluid retention and weight gain, alopecia, myopathies, dry eyes, and stomatitis.

Side-effects may be minimised by starting treatment with a small dose and gradually increasing, although serious reactions have been reported after small doses.

For the adverse effects that may be associated with abrupt withdrawal of propranolol, see under Precautions, below.

In a Boston collaborative drug survey the following adverse reactions to propranolol occurred among a total of 319 hospital in-patients: pulmonary oedema (3), bradycardia and shock (3), complete heart block (1), bradycardia and angina (1), asymptomatic bradycardia (5), hypotension and syncope (5), asymptomatic hypotension (3), gastro-intestinal disturbance (3), dizziness (2), fatigue (1), fluid retention (1), 2:1 heart block (1), blurring of vision (1). In a survey of 23 published reports in which propranolol was administered by mouth to a total of 797 out-patients treated for periods of a few weeks to 6 years, the following adverse reactions were noted: gastro-intestinal disturbances (11.2%), cold extremities or exacerbation of Raynaud's phenomenon (5.8%), congestive heart failure (5.4%), sleep disturbances (4.3%), dizziness (4.1%), fatigue (3.1%), bronchospasm (2.6%), mental depression (1.6%), paraesthesias (1.5%), bradycardia (0.8%), hallucinations (0.8%), skin rash (0.8%), hypotension (0.5%), muscle cramps (0.5%), dry mouth (0.4%), heart block (0.3%), and blurring of vision (0.1%).— D. J. Greenblatt and J. Koch-Weser, *Drugs*, 1974, *7*, 118.

Other reviews of the incidence and management of adverse effects associated with propranolol and other beta-adrenoceptor blocking agents: *Br. med. J.*, 1977, *1*, 529; M. A. Riddiough, *Am. J. Hosp. Pharm.*, 1977, *34*, 465; G. L. Sanders, *Adverse Drug React. Bull.*, 1978, Feb., 240; *idem*, Apr., 247; *Lancet*, 1981, *2*, 539 (Medical Research Council Working Party on Mild to Moderate Hypertension); S. H. Croog *et al.*, *New Engl. J. Med.*, 1986, *314*, 1657.

A report by the manufacturers (ICI) suggesting that a lower incidence of side-effects may be associated with branded propranolol (Inderal) compared with generic products of the drug.— J. H. Sanderson and J. A. Lewis (letter), *Lancet*, 1986, *1*, 967. Criticism, and a reminder of the linkage between the adverse effects and therapeutic effects of propranolol.— L. Garcia-Buñuel (letter), *ibid.*, 1443.

ALLERGY. For the suggestion that beta blockers may exacerbate anaphylactic reactions, see under Precautions, below.

DYSKINESIA. A 35-year-old woman with a history of dystonic reactions to neuroleptic drugs suffered a similar reaction when her dose of propranolol reached 600 mg twice daily. Symptoms included rolled-up eyes, clenched teeth, perspiration and salivation, distortion of body and limbs, and arching of the back.— J. P. Crawford (letter), *Br. med. J.*, 1977, *2*, 1156.

EFFECTS ON THE BLOOD. *Agranulocytosis.* A 64-year-old man with cardiac arrhythmia who received propranolol 40 mg daily with procainamide 4 g daily for 6 weeks then propranolol alone 40 mg every 4 hours for 6 days developed agranulocytosis. On cessation of propranolol therapy he recovered completely.— I. U. Nawabi and N. D. Ritz, *J. Am. med. Ass.*, 1973, *223*, 1376. See also P. C. Vincent, *Drugs*, 1986, *31*, 52.

Platelet adhesiveness. Increased platelet adhesiveness associated with abrupt withdrawal of propranolol.— W. H. Frishman *et al.*, *Am. Heart J.*, 1978, *95*, 169.

Thrombocytopenic purpura. One case of thrombocytopenic purpura had been reported following administration of propranolol and 2 cases of non-thrombocytopenic purpura.— S. A. Stephen, *Am. J. Cardiol.*, 1966, *18*, 463.

EFFECTS ON CARBOHYDRATE METABOLISM. Severe hypoglycaemic episodes occurred in 2 children while taking propranolol. Both recovered after glucose therapy. The children had been eating poorly prior to the episodes.— J. M. Feller (letter), *Med. J. Aust.*, 1973, *2*, 92.

Severe hypoglycaemia during haemodialysis occurred, after 24 hours of fasting, in a 20-year-old woman taking propranolol. The addition of glucose to the dialysis fluid was recommended.— K. Samii *et al.* (letter), *Lancet*, 1976, *1*, 545. The use of propranolol did not appear to cause hypoglycaemia in a study of 10 hypertensive patients on chronic haemodialysis compared with 12 similar patients not taking beta-blocking agents.— H. A. Jensen *et al.* (letter), *ibid.*, 1976, *2*, 368. Relatively selective beta-adrenoceptor blocking agents might be less likely to produce hypoglycaemia.— R. J. Newman, *Br. med. J.*, 1976, *2*, 447.

A patient taking propranolol 960 mg daily developed diabetes; the blood-sugar concentration returned to normal when propranolol was withdrawn and no further treatment was necessary.— R. J. Inglis (letter), *Br. med. J.*, 1979, *1*, 1795.

Fasting plasma-glucose concentrations and glucose tolerance test values were significantly increased in hypertensive patients given either propranolol or hydrochlorothiazide as part of a multicentre study. Both drugs appear to have diabetogenic properties.—Veterans Administration Cooperative Study Group on Antihypertensive Agents, *Hypertension*, 1985, 7, 1008. Contrary findings.— M. E. Molitch *et al.*, *Curr. ther. Res.*, 1986, *39*, 398. See also A. Dornhorst *et al.*, *Lancet*, 1985, *1*, 123; I. Gove and M. J. Kendall (letter), *idib.*, 515; S. O'Rahilly (letter), *idib.*

EFFECTS ON THE CARDIOVASCULAR SYSTEM. Intermittent claudication was reported in 4 patients who had been treated with propranolol or practolol in doses of 120 to 300 mg daily for 3 weeks to 6 months.— J. C. Rodger *et al.*, *Br. med. J.*, 1976, *1*, 1125. Comment.— A. F. Lant and D. O. Gibbons (letter), *ibid.*, 1469.

Of 117 patients, usually with hypertension or angina, treated with a single drug (propranolol 42, practolol 19, oxprenolol 56) 22 had cold extremities before treatment; 5 were made worse; 18 patients developed cold extremities for the first time.— D. Trash *et al.* (letter), *Br. med. J.*, 1976, *2*, 527.

Vascular symptoms in patients with primary Raynaud's phenomenon were not exacerbated by propranolol or labetalol taken by mouth.— J. A. Steiner *et al.* (letter), *Br. J. clin. Pharmac.*, 1979, *7*, 401.

Bilateral incipient gangrene of the feet in 2 patients associated with the use of beta-adrenoceptor blocking agents.— D. A. O'Rourke *et al.* (letter), *Med. J. Aust.*, 1979, *2*, 88.

Of 4494 patients receiving antihypertensive therapy, 99 reported cold extremities, and 93 of these were among the 2280 receiving beta blockers. Patients on beta blockers with intrinsic sympathomimetic activity, such as oxprenolol or pindolol, reported a significantly lower incidence of this symptom; it was also less frequent in females than in males. Those on cardioselective beta blockers had similar reporting rates to those on beta blockers without cardioselectivity. If a patient is experiencing cold extremities while receiving a beta blocker they should be transferred to another medication if possible; if beta blockade is essential, a beta blocker with intrinsic sympathomimetic activity may offer some protection.— M. J. VandenBurg *et al.*, *Eur. J. clin. Pharmac.*, 1984, *27*, 47.

Effects on the heart. In 7 patients with mitral stenosis, propranolol was given during exercise and at rest. The decrease in heart-rate could have increased total diastolic time and allowed more blood to pass the mitral valve, but in practice there was a further overall decrease in cardiac performance.— G. R. Cumming and W. Carr, *Can. med. Ass. J.*, 1966, *95*, 527.

Heart failure occurred in 4 patients with atrial fibrillation and chronic rheumatic valvular disease who were given propranolol to control the ventricle-rate when digitalis failed.— N. Conway *et al.*, *Br. med. J.*, 1968, *2*, 213.

Propranolol 40 mg daily for 1 week caused an intermittent atrioventricular block in a 38-year-old man with angina pectoris.— M. Ilyas (letter), *New Engl. J. Med.*, 1972, *286*, 376.

A patient receiving propranolol developed syncopal episodes while eating or drinking.— J. Schluger *et al.*, *Chest*, 1973, *64*, 651.

Thirty-five elderly patients with severe chest pain but no ECG evidence of myocardial infarction were noted to be receiving propranolol or oxprenolol.— M. S. Pathy, *Am. Heart J.*, 1979, *98*, 168. But see also under Effects on the Gastro-intestinal Tract, below.

Chronic beta-blocker treatment may sometimes paradoxically be the cause of abnormal T-wave inversion.— T. M. Griffith *et al.*, *Br. med. J.*, 1982, *284*, 19.

Hypertension. Of 44 mental patients receiving propranolol in doses of 0.6 to 5 g daily for the treatment of psychoses, 8 developed a paradoxical rise in blood pressure; in 2 this was abrupt but in most the increase was progressive over 3 to 24 hours. The skin became pale, cold and clammy and the patients exhibited pronounced tension and outbursts of psychomotor unrest. In all cases the hypertension responded immediately to a single dose of phentolamine 15 to 30 mg intravenously, with phenoxybenzamine 10 to 20 mg daily for 3 to 4 days reducing the blood pressure to the previous low levels without discontinuing the propranolol; the other symptoms subsided with the blood pressure reduction. Most of the hypertensive episodes occurred when the propranolol dosage was increased after a previous reduction. In a few further cases when symptoms appeared phentolamine and phenoxybenzamine given together prevented the blood pressure rise despite continuing the propranolol.— I. Blum *et al.*, *Br. med. J.*, 1975, *4*, 623.

Leaving aside the special cases of phaeochromocytoma and psychosis, the occasional fluid retention that occurs with beta-adrenoceptor blocking agents could explain the paradoxical rise in blood pressure sometimes occurring in patients receiving beta-adrenoceptor blocking drugs.— B. N. C. Prichard (letter), *Lancet*, 1977, *1*, 536.

EFFECTS ON THE EYES. When 483 hypertensive patients being treated with propranolol or other hypotensive drugs were questioned about symptoms of gritty feelings, sore or red eyes, photophobia, and the need to use eye-drops, between 12 and 30% gave positive answers. There was no indication that patients taking beta-adrenoceptor blocking drugs were more likely to complain of eye symptoms than patients on other antihypertensive therapy.— C. T. Dollery *et al.*, *Br. J. clin. Pharmac.*, 1977, *4*, 295.

Ocular symptoms were reported by 14 of 71 patients when taking practolol but only by 4 of the 71 before practolol treatment. Skin rash was reported by 16 during but 8 before treatment; both ocular symptoms and rash occurred in 7 during and 1 before treatment. A similar investigation of 246 patients who had taken propranolol showed a smaller insignificant difference in the incidence of eye complaints consisting of 42 patients during and 31 patients before propranolol treatment. The overall incidence of rash was not significantly greater during propranolol treatment but 14 patients had both an eye complaint and rash during treatment compared to 4 patients before treatment.— D. C. G. Skegg and R. Doll, *Lancet*, 1977, *2*, 475.

Eye symptoms, including early cataract in 1 eye, occurred in a 70-year-old man during treatment with propranolol, and abated at the end of each course of treatment.— T. J. Halloran (letter), *J. Am. med. Ass.*, 1979, *241*, 2784.

For a statement that serious side-effects of the type induced by practolol were uncommon with other beta-adrenoceptor blocking agents, see Practolol, p.798.

Visual disturbances. A report of diplopia following concomitant inadvertent ingestion of therapeutic doses of oxprenolol and propranolol; the patient did not experience diplopia following ingestion of either drug alone. The Committee on Safety of Medicines were aware of 32 reports of diplopia in patients taking beta blockers; 24 of these were considered to be probably drug-related, of which 4 each were associated with propranolol, practolol, and atenolol, 3 each with oxprenolol and pindolol, 2 with nadolol, 1 each with acebutolol, metoprolol, sotalol, and timolol. Beta blockers can exacerbate or precipitate myasthenia gravis and also produce a myasthenic symptom, diplopia, in patients who otherwise appear neurologically normal. Although diplopia constitutes only 0.25% of the total suspected adverse reactions to beta blockers reported to the CSM over 16 years, awareness of the possibility may prevent unnecessary clinical investigation.— J. C. P. Weber (letter), *Lancet*, 1982, *2*, 826.

EFFECTS ON THE GASTRO-INTESTINAL TRACT. Intermittent chest pain suggestive of angina in a hypertensive patient was exacerbated by propranolol treatment. The patient's condition was subsequently diagnosed as being due to nutcracker oesophagus. Propranolol in common with other beta blockers may increase the amplitude of oesophageal contractions in patients with nutcracker oesophagus, thereby increasing the sensation of pain. Patients with chest pain suggestive of angina should be investigated carefully before treatment with beta blockers is given.— G. Bassotti *et al.*, *Br. med. J.*, 1987, *294*, 1655.

EFFECTS ON LIPID METABOLISM. Of 379 men who had been regularly followed for at least 5 years as untreated controls in the Oslo study drug trial of mild hypertension, the effects of propranolol alone, prazosin alone, and propranolol in association with prazosin, were studied in 23 with a stable diastolic blood pressure of 100 mmHg or more; each patient was given each of the 3 treatments for 8-week periods in a randomised crossover trial design. Propranolol significantly reduced both high-density-lipoprotein cholesterol and the cholesterol ratio, and increased total triglycerides. Conversely, prazosin reduced total cholesterol by reducing the low-density-lipoprotein plus very-low-density-lipoprotein fraction, and had no significant effect on high-density-lipoprotein cholesterol, so that the cholesterol ratio was significantly increased; total triglycerides were also significantly reduced by prazosin. The effects on lipids of the association of propranolol and prazosin included features of both, but owing partly to opposite effects of the 2 drugs, the net effect was small and did not reach statistical significance; the only significant effect of the association was a reduced high-density-lipoprotein cholesterol value. Propranolol alone significantly raised the serum-uric-acid concentration; this was also raised after the association of propranolol and prazosin but remained within normal limits, although the propranolol-induced rise might achieve clinical importance if the association were to be given with a diuretic. The clinical importance of the observed effects of the antihypertensives on blood lipids is uncertain, but all pharmacological effects of antihypertensive drugs should be taken into consideration, particularly when embarking on life-long treatment for young people.— P. Leren *et al.*, *Lancet*, 1980, *2*, 4. Comment.— *ibid.*, 19.

Treatment with beta blockers had no effect on plasma lipid and urate concentrations in a study of 51 hypertensive patients who had received propranolol (47 patients), atenolol (2), or metoprolol (2) for an average of 54 (range 8 to 79) months.— B. Ø. Kristensen, *Br. med. J.*, 1981, *283*, 191.

In a study completed by 18 hypertensive patients on propranolol therapy and by 14 receiving methyldopa neither drug significantly affected plasma concentrations of total cholesterol but both reduced high-density lipoprotein (HDL) cholesterol concentrations by about 10%. Propranolol also increased plasma-triglyceride concentrations by about 28%. Both drugs appear to have unfavourable effects on the blood-lipid profile. If these changes have the same prognostic significance as in epidemiological studies (which is not certain) then such a change in HDL cholesterol would be associated with about a 35% increase in the risk of coronary heart disease over 5 years.— A. S. Leon *et al.*, *J. clin. Pharmac.*, 1984, *24*, 209.

EFFECTS ON THE LIVER. For reports that propranolol may precipitate hepatic encephalopathy in patients with cirrhosis see Liver Disorders, under Precautions, below.

EFFECTS ON MENTAL STATE. Depression occurred in 28 of 89 patients given propranolol for cardiac arrhythmias. The incidence was highest in patients treated for periods over 3 months with doses higher than 120 mg daily.— H. J. Waal (letter), *Br. med. J.*, 1967, *2*, 50. There was no indication that an important incidence of depression was associated with propranolol administration.— J. D. Fitzgerald (letter), *ibid.*, 372. A brief discussion of the role of beta-adrenoceptor blocking agents in causing depression.— F. A. Whitlock and L. E. J. Evans, *Drugs*, 1978, *15*, 53. A report of 2 cases of depression in elderly patients associated with low doses of propranolol (20 and 30 mg daily, respectively). Both patients had evidence of a tendency to depression.— A. Cremona-Barbaro (letter), *Lancet*, 1983, *1*, 185. An open study of depressive symptoms in 34 patients receiving propranolol therapy found no correlation between dosage and depression scale scores overall, but there was a significant correlation among the 20 patients with no personal or family history of depression. The 14 patients with a positive personal or family history of depression had significantly higher scores than those with a negative history. It was concluded that propranolol therapy was associated with depressive symptoms in a greater than expected number of patients.— S. J. Griffin and M. J. Friedman, *J. clin. Psychiat.*, 1986, *47*, 453.

Visual hallucinations or illusions occurred in 11 of 63 patients taking propranolol 80 to 320 mg daily, alone or with diuretics, for hypertension.— R. Fleminger, *Br. med. J.*, 1978, *1*, 1182. In a 53-year-old woman, with a family history of schizophrenia but no personal history, schizophrenic symptoms, occurring when the dose of propranolol was increased, regressed when propranolol was withdrawn.— J. Steinert and C. R. Pugh, *ibid.*, 1979, *1*, 790. Nightly hallucinations, most commonly of a large white rabbit but occasionally of a human figure such as a statue of a knight in armour followed a switch from metoprolol 300 mg daily to propranolol 240 mg daily in a hypertensive patient. Hallucinations recurred on rechallenge with propranolol and resolved when the patient was returned to metoprolol therapy. Visual hallucinations and illusions are a rare, dose-related adverse effect of beta blocker therapy; the more lipid-soluble beta blockers such as propranolol penetrate the CNS more readily than hydrophilic drugs such as metoprolol.— W. B. White and K. Riotte (letter), *New Engl. J. Med.*, 1982, *307*, 558. Severe psychotic symptoms including hallucinations, paranoia, and aggressiveness, coupled with depression, were resolved in a patient receiving propranolol when atenolol, a less lipophilic drug, was substituted.— D. J. McGahan *et al.*, *Drug Intell. & clin. Pharm.*, 1984, *18*, 601. Hallucinations, depression, nightmares, and personality change with odd behaviour and violent outbursts followed an increase in dosage of propranolol from 160 to 240 mg daily in a patient with migraine. Symptoms improved markedly on stopping propranolol therapy but there was an unprovoked recurrence of depression, suicidal ideation and hallucinations nine days later which resolved with a short course of haloperidol. The patient subsequently remained free of symptoms.— J. G. Cunnane and G. W. Blackwood, *Postgrad. med. J.*, 1987, *63*, 57.

Evidence of memory impairment in hypertensive patients receiving propranolol therapy.— S. Solomon *et al.*, Archs gen. Psychiat, 1983, *40*, 1109.

EFFECTS ON THE MUSCLES. Three patients who were taking conventional doses of propranolol or oxprenolol developed myasthenia gravis or a myasthenia-like syndrome. It was considered that beta-blocking agents were capable of enhancing a myasthenic condition.— Y. Herishanu and P. Rosenberg (letter), *Ann. intern. Med.*, 1975, *83*, 834.

Clinical myotonia occurred in a patient receiving propranolol and disappeared when treatment was stopped. Examination of biopsy material revealed a pre-existing mild dystrophia myotonica.— W. Blessing and J. C. Walsh (preliminary communication), *Lancet*, 1977, *1*, 73. See also S. Satya-Murti *et al.* (letter), *New Engl. J. Med.*, 1977, *297*, 223.

A study in 6 healthy subjects indicated that neither propranolol nor metoprolol reduced muscle strength, coordination, endurance, or perception of effort. So far, no direct explanation can be given for the clinical experience of muscle fatigue associated with beta-adrenoceptor blockade.— G. Grimby and U. Smith (letter), *Lancet*, 1978, *2*, 1318. See also P. E. Hall *et al.*, *J. clin. Hosp. Pharm.*, 1984, *9*, 283 (possible mechanisms of beta-blocker-induced fatigue).

Proximal myopathy in a 68-year-old woman who had taken sotalol for several months persisted when sotalol was replaced by propranolol, regressed when propranolol was withdrawn, and recurred when it was again given.— J. C. Forfar, *Br. med. J.*, 1979, *2*, 1331.

A report of muscle wasting in 3 patients with thyrotoxicosis taking beta-blockers.— M. Uusitupa *et al.* (letter), *Br. med. J.*, 1980, *280*, 183.

Comment on muscle fatigue as a side-effect of beta-adrenoceptor blockade.— *Lancet*, 1980, *1*, 1285.

A further report of muscle weakness associated with propranolol. In view of the potential of beta blockade to increase exercise-induced hyperkalaemia, episodes of muscular weakness or tiredness may be caused in part by increased hyperkalaemic responses to protracted moderate or major exertions.— D. Lehr (letter), *New Engl. J. Med.*, 1985, *312*, 860.

EFFECTS ON RESPIRATORY FUNCTION. Propranolol given by intravenous injection in doses of 10 mg to healthy persons and in doses of 5 mg to asthmatics resulted in significant mean rises in airway resistance. In healthy persons the rise was not accompanied by any respiratory upset. In asthmatics there was a much greater rise in airway resistance and it usually resulted in dyspnoea, and occasionally in wheezing. Atropine sulphate in a dose of 1.2 mg by intravenous injection almost completely abolished the rise in airway resistance in normal persons and markedly reduced the rise in asthmatics.— A. G. Macdonald *et al.*, *Br. J. Anaesth.*, 1967, *39*, 919.

A drop of about 35% in specific airway conductance occurred in 5 asthmatic patients after an injection of 10 mg of propranolol whilst there was no significant effect in 10 normal subjects.— P. S. Richardson and G. M. Sterling, *Br. med. J.*, 1969, *3*, 143.

Dyspnoea, wheezing and coughing occurred following administration of propranolol on 2 separate occasions in a patient with migraine. The symptoms, which gave the appearance of bronchitis, resolved when the drug was stopped.— B. G. Clark *et al.*, *Drug Intell. & clin. Pharm.*, 1982, *16*, 776.

A study of the effects of long-term oral beta blockade on respiratory function in patients with angina pectoris but without airways disease. Propranolol was given three times daily to 21 patients, initially in a dose of 40 mg increased after 2 weeks to 80 mg; a further 19 patients received pindolol three times daily in a dose of 2.5 mg, increased subsequently to 5 mg. Over 52 weeks the FEV_1 fell by a mean of 240 mL in patients taking propranolol (from 87.1% to 80.6% of predicted value); the fall was significant as early as 2 weeks after commencing treatment. In contrast, FEV_1 among patients taking pindolol had fallen only by 120 mL after 52 weeks (from 89.5 to 85.6%). There was also a significant fall in forced vital capacity (FVC) among the propranolol group. None of the patients reported increased breathlessness or wheezing, but it is not known whether the deterioration in respiratory function would continue to progress in a cumulative fashion, and in patients with chronic obstructive airways disease this effect of propranolol would probably result in symptomatic deterioration of pulmonary function in previously asymptomatic patients. Beta blockers with a degree of intrinsic sympathomimetic activity; such as pindolol, appear to have a less pronounced effect on pulmonary function than those without, such as propranolol; cardioselectivity is also reported to moderate the effects on respiration. In consequence, although no beta blocker is entirely safe in patients with chronic obstructive airways disease, if one must be used then a cardioselective agent or one with intrinsic sympathomimetic activity should be preferred.— R. J. Northcote and D. Ballantyne, *Br. med. J.*, 1986, *293*, 97.

EFFECTS ON SEXUAL FUNCTION. Of 95 men treated with propranolol, 5 developed erectile dysfunction with doses of 120 mg or more daily.— S. C. Warren and S. G. Warren (letter), *Ann. intern. Med.*, 1977, *86*, 112. A further report of probable propranolol-induced reversible impotence in one patient.— R. A. Miller (letter), *Ann. intern. Med.*, 1976, *85*, 682.

Impotence was reported in 13.2% of men receiving propranolol as part of the MRC trial for the treatment of mild hypertension, which was greater than the 10.1% among those receiving placebo but significantly less than the 22.6% reported among those taking bendrofluazide.—Report of MRC Working Party on Mild to Moderate Hypertension, *Lancet*, 1981, *2*, 539.

A retrospective study of male sexual dysfunction associated with propranolol therapy. Sexual function was affected in up to 47% of patients.— W. Burnett and R. Chahine, *Cardiovasc. Med.*, 1979, *4*, 811.

Impotence is more common in hypertensive than in healthy controls; the manufacturers [ICI] do not feel that inclusion of impotence or sexual dysfunction on the *UK* data sheet is justified.— J. M. Bell and J. H. Sanderson (letter), *Pharm. J.*, 1985, *2*, 774. Comments and criticism: M. A. Davies and A. D'Mello (letter), *ibid.*, 1986, *1*, 34; J. Goldman (letter), *ibid.*

For the effects of propranolol on sperm, see Contraception, under Uses and Administration, below.

EFFECTS ON THE SKIN. Analysis, by the Boston Collaborative Drug Surveillance Program, of data on 15 438 patients hospitalised between 1975 and 1982 detected no allergic skin reactions attributed to propranolol hydrochloride among 1051 recipients of the drug.— M. Bigby *et al.*, *J. Am. med. Ass.*, 1986, *256*, 3358.

Necrosis. Three patients developed foot pain, with multiple areas of skin necrosis, but with palpable foot pulses, while taking beta-adrenoceptor blocking agents. The necrosis resolved when medication was withdrawn.— R. Gokal *et al.*, *Br. med. J.*, 1978, *1*, 721. See also B. I. Hoffbrand (letter), *ibid.*, 1979, *1*, 1082.

Psoriasiform eruptions. Details of 6 patients who developed reversible psoriasiform cutaneous eruptions during long-term propranolol therapy, similar to those reported after practolol.— H. A. Jensen *et al.*, *Acta med. scand.*, 1976, *199*, 363.

Further reports: P. L. Padfield *et al.* (letter), *Br. med. J.*, 1975, *1*, 626; N. J. Farr (letter), *ibid.*, 1976, *1*, 961; N. Hardwick and N. Saxe, *Br. J. Derm.*, 1986, *115*, 167.

FIBROSIS. Fibrosing conditions developed in 2 patients during treatment with propranolol. Peyronie's disease [penile fibrosis] occurred in 1 and the other developed Dupuytren's contracture of both hands.— W. W. Coupland (letter), *Med. J. Aust.*, 1977, *2*, 137.

A report of retroperitoneal fibrosis associated with propranolol in one patient.— J. R. Pierce *et al.* (letter), *Ann. intern. Med.*, 1981, *95*, 244. Studies indicating a lack of association between beta blocker therapy and retroperitoneal fibrosis: J. H. Marigold *et al.*, *Br. med. J.*, 1982, *284*, 870; J. P. Pyror *et al.*, *ibid.*, 1983, *287*, 639.

Peyronie's disease. Two patients taking propranolol developed pain in the penis on erection. Examination revealed fibrous plaques on the dorsum of the penis (Peyronie's disease). There might be an association between beta-adrenoceptor blocking agents and abnormal fibrous tissue production.— D. R. Osborne (letter), *Lancet*, 1977, *1*, 1111.

Of 146 patients with Peyronie's disease seen between January 1975 and May 1978, 19 had been on beta-adrenoceptor blocking therapy with propranolol (12), practolol (6), or both (1). None of a matched group of control patients had been taking these drugs. There might be an association between Peyronie's disease and beta-adrenoceptor blocking therapy or it might be that atherosclerosis and hypertension are the common aetiological factors.— J. P. Pryor and O. Khan (letter), *Lancet*, 1979, *1*, 331. Investigation of the medical and drug history of 98 consecutive men with Peyronie's disease showed that only 5 had taken beta-adrenoceptor blocking agents before the onset of the disease. It is considered that chronic degenerative arterial disease rather than beta blockers is associated with Peyronie's disease.— J. P. Pryor and W. M. Castle (letter), *ibid.*, 1982, *1*, 917.

HYPERKALAEMIA. Paradoxical changes in serum-potassium concentrations have been noted during cardiopulmonary bypass in association with non-cardioselective beta-adrenoceptor blockade.— D. W. Bethune and R. McKay (letter), *Lancet*, 1978, *2*, 380. Results confirming that beta-adrenoceptors are involved in the regulation of plasma-potassium concentrations.— E. Carlsson *et al.* (letter), *Lancet*, 1978, *2*, 424.

See also under Effects on the Muscles, above.

OVERDOSAGE. A 45-year-old man who had taken about 2 g of propranolol in a suicide attempt showed no signs of cardiac disturbance during a 5-day stay in hospital.— W. Wermut and M. Wójcicki (letter), *Br. med. J.*, 1973, *3*, 591.

Severe cardiac disturbances occurred in a 24-year-old woman who ingested 1 g of propranolol, 100 mL of whisky, and some beer in a suicide attempt.— G. Frithz (letter), *Br. med. J.*, 1976, *1*, 769.

A report of generalised seizures and broadening of the QRS complex of the ECG in 2 patients following massive overdosage with propranolol. The possibility of drug-induced hypoglycaemia and other metabolic causes for the seizures was ruled out and although cerebral hypoperfusion may have contributed the second patient suffered convulsions despite an adequate blood pressure. It was suggested that the ECG changes may have been due to the membrane-stabilising effect of propranolol. Both patients recovered.— A. Buiumsohn *et al.*, *Ann. intern. Med.*, 1979, *91*, 860.

A report of 3 cases of convulsions following induction of emesis to treat propranolol overdosage. The vagal stimulus associated with vomiting may be detrimental in the presence of significant beta blockade, leading to a reduction in cerebral perfusion and consequent convulsive activity. Where emetics are used to treat overdosage of beta blockers the prior administration of atropine may help prevent cardiovascular collapse.— N. Soni *et al.*, *Med. J. Aust.*, 1983, *2*, 629.

Beta blockers cause approximately 20 deaths per year in England and Wales; of 208 fatal poisonings due to beta blockers between 1975 and 1984, 141 were due to propranolol. Death is preceded by a profound depression of cardiac output and it is thought that the membrane stabilising activity of propranolol contributes to the lethal effects of overdose. Those beta blockers which lack membrane stabilising properties, such as atenolol, are rarely associated with fatal poisoning.— J. A. Henry and S. L. Cassidy, *Lancet*, 1986, *1*, 1414.

PREGNANCY AND THE NEONATE. See under Precautions, below.

Treatment of Adverse Effects

Following recent overdosage with a beta blocker the stomach should be emptied by gastric lavage. Severe bradycardia and hypotension may respond to atropine 1 to 2 mg or more intravenously. Where response is inadequate, the treatment of choice is high-dose glucagon, initially as a bolus dose of 5 to 10 mg, followed if necessary by an intravenous infusion of 1 to 5 mg per hour or more according to response; the rate of infusion should be reduced as the patient improves. Dobutamine or isoprenaline have also been used in the management of hypotension; large doses of the latter may be required to overcome competitive blockade of beta-adrenoceptors. The use of adrenaline has also been suggested, but see Precautions including Interactions.

Intravenous aminophylline, or inhaled or intravenous salbutamol, may be of benefit where bronchospasm occurs.

For evidence that emetics should not be used to empty the stomach following propranolol overdose, see under Overdosage, above.

A comment on the role of beta-stimulants and glucagon in beta-blocking poisoning, and the suggestion that aminophylline may also be beneficial. Care should be taken to avoid exacerbation of hypotension during administration of aminophylline.— B. Jones (letter), *Lancet*, 1980, *1*, 1031. A case report illustrating the value of glucagon during beta-blocker poisoning (with alprenolol). Glucagon should be given in an intravenous dose of 8 to 10 mg repeated one hour later if necessary. Dopamine was used as a β_1-stimulant and a pacemaker was inserted; the use of isoprenaline is viewed with reserve.— D. Jacobsen *et al.* (letter), *ibid.* Mention of the successful use of glucagon to treat 2 patients with no recordable blood pressure due to beta-blocker poisoning, and agreement that it is the treatment of choice for beta-blocker poisoning. It is considered that 2 patients known to have died with propranolol poisoning while being treated with atropine and catecholamines, might have survived had they been given large amounts of glucagon.— R. N. Illingworth (letter), *ibid.*, *2*, 86.

Further reference: R. S. Weinstein, *Ann. emerg. Med.*, 1984, *13*, 1123.

Precautions

Propranolol should not be given to patients with bronchospasm or obstructive airways disease, metabolic acidosis, sinus bradycardia, or partial heart block. It should be given to patients with congestive heart failure only when they are fully digitalised and only then with great caution. It should never be given to patients with phaeochromocytoma without concomitant alpha-adrenoceptor blocking therapy.

Propranolol may mask the symptoms of hyperthyroidism. It may also mask the symptoms of hypoglycaemia, as well as enhancing the effects of hypoglycaemic agents in patients with diabetes mellitus.

Great care should be exercised in giving propranolol to patients undergoing anaesthesia (see p.781) and myocardial depressants such as halothane, cyclopropane, or ether should be avoided. The effects of other myocardial depressant agents, including anti-arrhythmics such as quinidine, procainamide, or lignocaine, phenytoin, and drugs which interfere with calcium transport, such as verapamil, may also be enhanced by propranolol.

The effects of propranolol are diminished by beta-adrenoceptor stimulating agents such as isoprenaline; the hypotensive effects of propranolol may be dangerously reversed and the peripheral vasoconstrictor effects enhanced by alpha-adrenoceptor stimulating agents such as noradrenaline or those with mixed alpha- and beta-adrenoceptor stimulating properties such as adrenaline; bradycardia may also occur.

The effects of propranolol may be enhanced by adrenergic neurone blocking agents such as guanethidine or bethanidine, or catecholamine-depleting agents such as reserpine, and the hypotensive effects by diuretics.

Propranolol may enhance some of the cardiac effects of digitalis and diminish others. It has been suggested that clonidine withdrawal symptoms may be exacerbated in patients who are concurrently taking a beta blocker.

For comments on the withdrawal of propranolol, see below.

ALLERGY. A report of severe refractory anaphylaxis in 2 patients, apparently potentiated by concomitant beta blockade with propranolol.— R. L. Jacobs *et al.*, *J. Allergy & clin. Immunol.*, 1981, *68*, 125. A similar report in 5 further patients.— P. J. Hannaway and G. D. K. Hopper (letter), *New Engl. J. Med.*, 1983, *308*, 1536.

CARDIAC DISORDERS. A study confirming that beta-blocking agents should be prescribed only with extreme caution in heart failure of ischaemic origin.— S. H. Taylor and B. Silke, *Lancet*, 1981, *2*, 835.

CONTACT LENSES. Beta blockers may reduce tear flow, leading to irritation of the eye in wearers of contact lenses and potentially to the dehydration of soft lenses.— *Aust. J. Hosp. Pharm.*, 1987, *17*, 55.

EFFECTS ON PERFORMANCE. Comment on the possibility that beta blockers may impair response when driving; it may be unwise to take propranolol to reduce anxiety before a driving test.— K. Fox, *Br. med. J.*, 1984, *289*, 42. See also H. Ashton, *Adverse Drug React. Bull.*, 1983, Feb., 360.

HYPOGLYCAEMIA AND DIABETES MELLITUS. Studies in 6 healthy persons demonstrated that propranolol reduced the blood-sugar response to exercise and to hypoglycaemia. The danger of prescribing beta-adrenoceptor blocking agents for patients during treatment with hypoglycaemic agents is emphasised.— P. D. Bewsher (letter), *Lancet*, 1967, *1*, 104. The dangers of the concurrent use of insulin and propranolol may have been overestimated. Increased sweating in insulin-dependent diabetics taking propranolol is an indication of hypoglycaemia.— L. Strom (letter), *New Engl. J. Med.*, 1978, *299*, 487. A cardioselective β_1-adrenoceptor blocking agent should be used in diabetics rather than propranolol.— U. Smith and I. Lager (letter), *ibid.*, 1467. See also A. H. Barnett *et al.*, *Br. med. J.*, 1980, *280*, 976; U. Smith *et al.* (letter), *ibid.*, *281*, 1143.

In 20 hypertensive patients with diabetes blood-sugar concentrations rose significantly while the patients were treated with propranolol 80 mg twice daily or metoprolol 100 mg twice daily. The actual increase was relatively small and not detectable clinically in most patients.— A. D. Wright *et al.*, *Br. med. J.*, 1979, *1*, 159.

In 6 hypertensive diabetic patients studied under double-blind conditions propranolol 80 or 160 mg twice daily or metoprolol 100 or 200 mg twice daily had no significant effect on fasting plasma-glucose concentrations, glucose tolerance, or insulin response.— K. L. Woods *et al.*, *Br. med. J.*, 1980, *281*, 1321.

INTERACTIONS. A review of pharmacokinetic drug interactions with propranolol.— A. J. J. Wood and J. Feely, *Clin. Pharmacokinet.*, 1983, *8*, 253. Further reviews and studies of drug interactions with beta blockers: *Br. J. clin. Pharmac.*, 1984, *17*, *Suppl.* 1, 1S–114S; *Drug Interact. News.*, 1986, *6*, 17.

Alcohol. Studies in 7 healthy subjects did not demonstrate decreased tolerance to alcoholic beverages after beta-adrenoceptor blockade. The elimination-rate of alcohol was not decreased after administration of therapeutic doses of propranolol for 14 days.— T. L. Svendsen *et al.*, *Eur. J. clin. Pharmac.*, 1978, *13*, 91.

In healthy subjects alcohol increased the plasma clearance-rate of propranolol and diminished its hypotensive effect.— E. A. Sotaniemi *et al.*, *Clin. Pharmac. Ther.*, 1981, *29*, 705. See also P. Dorian *et al.*, *Eur. J. clin. Pharmac.*, 1984, *27*, 209.

Antacids. In 4 of 5 healthy subjects concomitant administration of propranolol and aluminium hydroxide mixture decreased the plasma concentration of propranolol.— J. H. Dobbs *et al.*, *Curr. ther. Res.*, 1977, *21*, 887.

Although there is evidence of a possible interaction between antacids and some beta blockers, perhaps because the antacid affects the rate of gastric emptying and hence the bioavailability of the beta blocker, such an interaction has not been demonstrated to have a clinical effect.— P. F. D'Arcy and J. C. McElnay, *Drug Intell. & clin. Pharm.*, 1987, *21*, 607.

Anti-arrhythmic agents. Beta-adrenoceptor blocking agents may enhance the negative inotropic action of anti-arrhythmic agents. In particular, prenylamine and verapamil should probably not be used in association with beta blockers.— P. J. Lewis, *Prescribers' J.*, 1979, *19*, 94.

Reports of serious adverse reactions, including some deaths, in patients stabilised on beta-adrenoceptor blocking agents who were given an oral loading dose of disopyramide (400 mg).— *Aust. J. Pharm.*, 1980, *61*, 446.

See also under interactions relating to Calcium-channel Blockers, and to Lignocaine, (below).

For a beneficial interaction between mexiletine and propranolol, used together in the treatment of refractory ventricular tachycardia, see E. B. Leahey *et al.*, *Br. med. J.*, 1980, *281*, 357.

Antiepileptic agents. A study of the effects of phenytoin and phenobarbitone on the clearance of propranolol and of sotalol.— E. A. Sotaniemi *et al.*, *Clin. Pharmac. Ther.*, 1979, *26*, 153.

Antihypertensive agents. Ketanserin reduced the oral clearance of propranolol and increased peak serum concentrations of the beta blocker in a study in 8 healthy subjects.— H. R. Ochs *et al.*, *Clin. Pharmac. Ther.*, 1987, *41*, 55. An earlier study. The pharmacokinetics of propranolol elimination were not affected by concurrent administration of ketanserin, nor vice versa, and the clinical effects of the combination were similar to those of propranolol alone.— F. M. Williams *et al.*, *Br. J. clin. Pharmac.*, 1986, *22*, 301.

Calcium-channel blockers. Reports of enhanced cardiac depression following combined use of beta blockers and verapamil: M. Packer *et al.*, *Circulation*, 1982, *65*, 660 (high-dose propranolol); J. N. H. Eisenberg and G. D. G. Oakley, *Postgrad. med. J.*, 1984, *60*, 705 (metoprolol); H. Kumagai *et al.*, *Curr. ther. Res.*, 1986, *40*, 1 (propranolol; in patients on haemodialysis).

See also interactions with Anti-arrhythmic agents, above.

A warning that administration of nifedipine might exacerbate the symptoms of beta-adrenoceptor blockade withdrawal, since it causes significant peripheral vasodilatation with subsequent reflex increase in sympathetic activity.— Ø. L. Pedersen and E. Mikkelsen (letter), *Lancet*, 1979, *1*, 554. Two patients developed heart failure when nifedipine was given in addition to beta blockers.— C. J. Anastassiades, *Br. med. J.*, 1980, *281*, 1251. Further references: R. H. Robson and M. C. Vishwanath, *ibid.*, 1982, *284*, 104; C. Anastassiades (letter), *ibid.*, 506.

Chlormethiazole. Profound bradycardia in an 84-year-old woman receiving propranolol 40 mg twice daily following the second of 2 doses of chlormethiazole 192 mg.— *Med. J. Aust.*, 1979, *2*, 553.

Dantrolene. For reference to a possible interaction between beta-adrenoceptor blocking agents and dantrolene, see Dantrolene Sodium, p.1233.

Digoxin. Two men with digoxin intoxication each developed progressive bradycardia within 2 hours of a single dose of 10 mg of propranolol by mouth, and both died. Bradycardia was possibly due to a synergistic action between propranolol and digoxin and could be prevented by the use of a test dose of propranolol or possibly by the routine administration of atropine with propranolol.— D. A. L. Watt, *Br. med. J.*, 1968, *3*, 413. Comments.— K. Hazell (letter), *ibid.*, 619; D. A. L. Watt (letter), *ibid.*, 1968, *4*, 58. Further comment.— M. O'Reilly *et al.* (letter), *Lancet*, 1974, *1*, 138. No antagonism was found in 15 patients though when digitalis was given alone the frequency of attacks increased.— M. H. Crawford *et al.* (letter), *ibid.*, 457.

Diuretics. For hypokalaemia associated with the use of a beta blocker combined with a diuretic see under Chlorothiazide, p.982.

Ergotamine tartrate. For a report of a possible interaction in a patient taking ergotamine tartrate and propranolol for migraine prophylaxis, see Ergotamine Tartrate, p.1056.

Histamine H_2-antagonists. Cimetidine has been reported to alter the pharmacokinetics of those beta blockers which are metabolised in the liver ('lipophilic' beta blockers). Feely *et al.* (*New Engl. J. Med.*, 1981, *304*, 692) reported a reduction in the clearance of intravenous propranolol, due to a decrease in liver blood flow, in subjects given cimetidine. The metabolism of oral propranolol was also inhibited, and Donovan (*Lancet*, 1981, *1*, 164) noted a very considerable increase in bioavailability of oral propranolol when cimetidine was given concomitantly, which might be due to reduced first-pass hepatic metabolism (A.M. Hegarty *et al.*, *Br. med. J.*, 1981, *282*, 1917). The clinical significance of the interaction is uncertain. Donn *et al.* (*J. clin. Pharmac.*, 1984, *24*, 500) found no significant difference in the heart-rate of 12 healthy subjects given propranolol concomitantly with cimetidine compared with propranolol alone, despite the fact that mean steady-state plasma concentrations of propranolol were 57% higher in the former case; however Donovan (1981) noted significant bradycardia and hypotension associated with the combination, and Cunningham (*Can. med. Ass. J.*, 1983, *128*, 892) has reported vertigo, vomiting, and ophthalmoplegia in 2 patients stabilised on propranolol when cimetidine was added to their therapy.

Other beta blockers that have been reported to interact similarly with cimetidine include metoprolol (W. Kirch *et al.*, *Clin. Sci.*, 1982, *63*, *Suppl.* 8, 451S; E. Mutschler *et al.*, *Br. J. clin. Pharmac.*, 1984, *17*, 51S) and the combined alpha and beta blocker, labetalol (T.K. Daneshmend and C.T.C. Roberts, *Lancet*, 1981, *1*, 565). Pindolol, which is only partly metabolised in the liver interacts with cimetidine to a lesser extent (E. Mutschler *et al.*, 1984). In contrast, 'hydrophilic' beta blockers such as atenolol (W. Kirch *et al.*, *Drugs*, 1983, *25*, *Suppl.* 2, 127) or nadolol (K.L. Duchin *et al.*, *Br. J. clin. Pharmac.*, 1984, *17*, 486), which are excreted largely unchanged by the kidneys, do not appear to interact in this way with cimetidine.

In contrast to cimetidine, the potential for interactions between the beta blockers and ranitidine appears to be low. A number of studies have indicated that ranitidine had no effect on the pharmacokinetics of propranolol (A.M. Hegarty *et al.*, *Br. med. J.*, 1982, *284*, 1304; L. Patel and K. Weerasuriya, *Br. J. clin. Pharmac.*, 1983, *15*, 152P; K.H. Donn *et al.*, *J. clin. Pharmac.*, 1984, *24*, 500). Surprisingly, Spahn *et al.* (*Br. med. J.*, 1983, *286*, 1546) found that addition of ranitidine to metoprolol therapy resulted in a marked increase of metoprolol bioavailability. Although the results and methodology of this study have been severely criticised by the manufacturers [Glaxo] (D. Jack *et al.*, *ibid.*, 1983, *286*, 2064, and *287*, 1218), another group has also reported increased plasma-metoprolol concentrations following addition of ranitidine (J.G. Kelly *et al.*, *Br. med. J.*, 1983, *287*, 1218 and *Br. J. clin. Pharmac.*, 1985, *19*, 219). However, these latter results applied only to single-dose studies and there was no evidence of any inhibition of metoprolol metabolism following chronic administration of both drugs.

Hypoglycaemic agents. Both acebutolol and propranolol significantly modified the effects of glibenclamide on blood-glucose concentrations after an oral glucose load in type II diabetics.— R. Zaman *et al.*, *Br. J. clin. Pharmac.*, 1982, *13*, 507.

Lignocaine. An increase in plasma half-life of lignocaine of up to 50% has been observed in the presence of propranolol.— *Aust. J. Pharm.*, 1974, *55*, 521.

A study demonstrating that, in healthy subjects, both prolonged infusion of lignocaine and co-administration of propranolol reduce the plasma clearance of lignocaine. It may be necessary to reduce the dosage of lignocaine when propranolol is given concomitantly and to reduce the rate of infusion when lignocaine is given for prolonged periods.— H. R. Ochs *et al.*, *New Engl. J. Med.*, 1980, *303*, 373. Two reports of the concomitant administration of propranolol possibly enhancing the toxicity of lignocaine.— C. F. Graham *et al.* (letter), *ibid.*, 1981, *304*, 1301.

Further references: K. A. Conrad *et al.*, *Clin. Pharmac. Ther.*, 1983, *33*, 133 (metoprolol or propranolol); N. D. S. Bax *et al.*, *Br. J. clin. Pharmac.*, 1985, *19*, 597 (propranolol inhibition of lignocaine metabolism).

Lipid-regulating agents. Concurrent administration of halofenate with propranolol resulted in decreased plasma-propranolol concentrations which correlated with reduced beta-adrenoceptor blockade. The mechanism of the interaction was not determined.— D. H. Huffman *et al.*, *Clin. Pharmac. Ther.*, 1976, *19*, 807.

Prior administration of cholestyramine or colestipol considerably reduced plasma-propranolol concentrations obtained following ingestion of propranolol 120 mg in 12 healthy subjects.— D. M. Hibbard *et al.*, *Br. J. clin. Pharmac.*, 1984, *18*, 337.

Neuroleptics. Caution is needed when using propranolol with phenothiazines and tricyclic antidepressants.— R. Galinsky (letter), *New Engl. J. Med.*, 1976, *295*, 281. The need for caution is accepted but there is little reported evidence of trouble with the association.— N. M. Kaplan (letter), *ibid.*

In healthy subjects given propranolol, plasma-propranolol concentrations increased after the introduction of chlorpromazine to the treatment.— R. E. Vestal *et al.*, *Clin. Pharmac. Ther.*, 1979, *25*, 19.

For a report of hypotension and cardiopulmonary arrest associated with concurrent propranolol and haloperidol therapy see Haloperidol Decanoate, p.744.

Nicergoline. For a study indicating that nicergoline enhances the cardiac depressant action of propranolol, see Nicergoline, p.1058.

Non-steroidal anti-inflammatory agents. Inhibition of prostaglandin synthesis by indomethacin in 7 hypertensive patients receiving propranolol or pindolol increased diastolic blood pressure. It was considered that salicylate-like compounds and non-steroidal anti-inflammatory agents should be avoided in hypertensive patients taking beta-blocking agents.— V. Durão *et al.* (preliminary communication), *Lancet*, 1977, *2*, 1005 and 1242. Indomethacin can cause hypertension on its own; this might explain the results.— M. VandenBurg (letter), *ibid.*, 1184. Further comments: C. Davidson (letter), *ibid;* A. Barrientos *et al.* (letter), *ibid.*, 1978, *1*, 277.

Although indomethacin produced no net effect in 19 untreated patients with essential hypertension, it blunted or reversed the antihypertensive effect of diuretic and beta-adrenoceptor blockade in 9 patients who received chlorthalidone or hydrochlorothiazide, sometimes with frusemide, and 11 patients treated with propranolol.— J. A. Lopez-Ovejero *et al.*, *Clin. Sci. & mol. Med.*, 1978, *55*, 203S.

In 15 patients whose mild essential hypertension was controlled by either propranolol or thiazide diuretics the addition of indomethacin 50 mg twice daily for 3 weeks caused an increase in blood pressure and body-weight.— J. Watkins *et al.*, *Br. med. J.*, 1980, *281*, 702. Comment that the antacid (aluminium hydroxide) taken if necessary to alleviate gastro-intestinal distress may have caused a decrease in the bioavailability of propranolol.— R. J. Mangini (letter), *ibid.*, 1353.

Pretreatment with aspirin reduced or abolished the hypotensive effects of a dose of pindolol or propranolol in hypertensive patients but did not prevent the beta-blocker-induced changes in heart-rate or systolic time intervals. It was suggested that the hypotensive effects of beta blockers, but not their negative chronotropic or inotropic effects, are dependent on endogenous prostaglandins and can be reversed by a prostaglandin synthesis inhibitor such as aspirin.— W. Sziegoleit *et al.*, *Int. J. clin. Pharmac. Ther. Toxic.*, 1982, *20*, 423.

Flurbiprofen attenuated the hypotensive effects of single doses of propranolol, but not those of atenolol, in 10 hypertensive patients.— J. Webster *et al.*, *Br. J. clin. Pharmac.*, 1984, *18*, 861.

For further references to interactions between non-steroidal anti-inflammatory drugs and beta blockers, see *Drug Interact. News.*, 1986, *6*, 1.

Oral contraceptives. A review of the effect of oral contraceptives on drug response. There is evidence for reduced first-pass metabolism of metoprolol in women receiving low-dose oral contraceptives, and a similar reduction, leading to higher plasma concentrations and potentially increased effect, might be expected for propranolol. Beta blockers which are excreted primarily unchanged in the urine such as atenolol and nadolol probably would not be affected by concurrent oral contraceptive use.— *Drug Interact. News.*, 1982, *2*, 41.

Rifampicin. Rifampicin markedly increased the oral clearance of propranolol in a study in 6 healthy subjects. The reduction in plasma concentrations of propranolol that results from chronic administration of rifampicin would probably lead to a significant alteration in the effects of the beta blocker if given concurrently.— R. J. Herman *et al.*, *Br. J. clin. Pharmac.*, 1983, *16*, 565.

Sympathomimetics. Adrenaline and noradrenaline should not be given to patients being treated with propranolol; when the beta receptors which caused vasodilatation were blocked by propranolol, adrenaline and similar drugs could produce a powerful vasoconstrictor effect by acting on the alpha receptors.— J. Grayson (letter), *Lancet*, 1967, *1*, 788. Bradycardia and atrioventricular block occurred in a subject given adrenaline 1 hour after propranolol in a laboratory investigation.— J. Kram *et al.* (letter), *Ann. intern. Med.*, 1974, *80*, 282.

A report of a fatality occurring in a 49-year-old woman with asymptomatic hypertension on a regimen of hydrochlorothiazide 50 mg twice daily and propranolol hydrochloride 40 mg four times daily, following the instillation of one drop of 10% phenylephrine hydrochloride solution in each eye during an ophthalmological examination.— E. Cass *et al.*, *Can. med. Ass. J.*, 1979, *120*, 1261.

A patient receiving minoxidil and propranolol for hypertension developed anaphylactic symptoms following a blood transfusion and was given a subcutaneous injection of adrenaline. The patient rapidly developed headache, paraesthesia, and weakness of the right arm and leg associated with a blood pressure of 220/130 mmHg. The hypertensive crisis, presumably mediated by an unopposed alpha-stimulated vasoconstriction, resolved following treatment with nifedipine and hydralazine. It is imperative to be aware of this potentially lethal interaction between adrenaline and beta blockers. In patients with known allergic conditions for which adrenaline treatment may be necessary, beta blockers should be avoided in favour of a combined alpha and beta blocker such as labetalol.— T. V. Whelan (letter), *Ann. intern. Med.*, 1987, *106*, 327.

Tricyclic antidepressants. For comments on the possible interaction between propranolol and tricyclic antidepressants see under interactions relating to Neuroleptics (above).

Xanthines. For the effect of propranolol on theophylline, see Theophylline p.1529.

INTERFERENCE WITH DIAGNOSTIC TESTS. A study indicating that a metabolite of propranolol, a conjugate of 4-hydroxypropranolol that is normally excreted in the urine, accumulates in the plasma of patients with chronic renal failure not receiving dialysis and interferes with the diazo reaction for detecting serum bilirubin to produce false-positive results. The Bilirubinometer method was not affected by this metabolite.— S. Al-Damluji and J. H. Meek, *Br. med. J.*, 1980, *280*, 1414. See also R. Belsey *et al.* (letter), *J. Am. med. Ass.*, 1984, *251*, 38.

Propranolol could interfere with tests of thyroid function.— *Med. Lett.*, 1981, *23*, 30.

LIVER DISORDERS. Evidence that propranolol worsens hepatic encephalopathy in cirrhotic patients deprived of portal perfusion of the liver, probably by decreasing arterial liver blood flow. The effect was not seen in cirrhotics with good hepatic function. If these observations are confirmed, beta blockers should be used with caution in patients with poor or absent portal perfusion.— P. Reding (letter), *Lancet*, 1982, *2*, 550. Contrary results. Of 5 patients with evidence of encephalopathy one deteriorated, one improved, and 3 remained unchanged while receiving propranolol therapy.— M. J. P. Arthur *et al.* (letter), *ibid.*, 879. Propranolol given to prevent variceal bleeding precipitated hepatic encephalopathy in a cirrhotic patient; challenge on 2 occasions confirmed the reaction.— D. Tarver *et al.*, *Br. med. J.*, 1983, *287*, 585. The case reported by Tarver *et al.* may represent an idiosyncratic mechanism. No exacerbation or precipitation of encephalopathy was observed in 6 patients with cirrhosis and varying degrees of liver dysfunction who received therapeutic doses of propranolol.— P. Watson and J. R. Hayes, *Br. med. J.*, 1983, *287*, 1067.

MALNUTRITION. Results of protein-binding studies suggesting that the dose of propranolol may need to be adjusted in undernourished subjects.— V. Jagadeesan and K. Krishnaswamy, *Eur. J. clin. Pharmac.*, 1985, *27*, 657.

PREGNANCY AND THE NEONATE. There is doubt about the use of beta blockers in pregnancy. There have been isolated reports of intra-uterine growth retardation, acute foetal distress in labour, and hypoglycaemia in the neonate. Although these may all be complications of hypertension in pregnancy, because of these reports beta blockers are not recommended as first-line treatment for hypertension in pregnancy.— M. de Swiet, *Prescribers' J.*, 1979, *19*, 59.

A study on the neonatal effects of maternal administration of acebutolol or methyldopa suggested that beta blockers should be used with caution during pregnancy. Blood pressure was significantly lower in 10 infants born to mothers who had received acebutolol and remained so for the first 3 days of life; heart-rate was also lower.— Y. Dumez *et al.*, *Br. med. J.*, 1981, *283*, 1077.

On current evidence beta blocker treatment of hypertension in pregnancy appears to improve the likelihood that the foetus will be normal.— P. C. Rubin, *New Engl. J. Med.*, 1981, *305*, 1323. Agreement; however, studies of oxprenolol or atenolol for hypertension in pregnancy demonstrate them to be frequently inadequate when given alone. Addition of prazosin may be needed, and this does not appear to increase the risk to the foetus.— W. F. Lubbe (letter), *ibid.*, 1982, *307*, 753.

A report of a child born with a congenital defect possibly associated with maternal administration of propranolol.— J. W. Campbell (letter), *New Engl. J. Med.*, 1985, *313*, 518.

SMOKING. Reports of potentially significant enhancement of propranolol clearance in patients who smoke: R. E. Vestal *et al.*, *Clin. Pharmac. Ther.*, 1979, *26*, 8; S. K. Gardner *et al.*, *Int. J. clin. Pharmac. Ther. Toxic.*, 1980, *18*, 421. See also I. H. Benedek *et al.*, *J. Pharm. Pharmac.*, 1984, *36*, 214.

THYROID DISORDERS. Propranolol treatment has masked symptoms of thyrotoxicosis (G.F. Cohen, *Lancet*, 1968, 2, 1349 and L. Shenkman *et al.*, *J. Am. med. Ass.*, 1977, *238*, 237); it can cause errors in the Achilles reflex test for thyroid disease (H.J. Waal-Manning, *Clin. Pharmac. Ther.*, 1969, *10*, 199). A number of investigators including Theilade *et al.* (*Lancet*, 1977, *2*,

363), Heyma *et al.* (*Br. med. J.*, 1980, *281*, 24) and Chambers *et al.* (*J. clin. Pharmac.*, 1982, *22*, 110) have shown that propranolol is a potent inhibitor of the peripheral conversion of thyroxine to tri-iodothyronine, [probably by inhibition of the enzyme 5′-monodeiodinase (M.R. Wilkins *et al.*, *Postgrad. med. J.*, 1985, *61*, 391)] and that therefore interpretation of serum tri-iodothyronine measurements in patients treated with propranolol requires caution. Furthermore, beta blockers may precipitate myxoedemic coma in hypothyroid patients (K. Murukami *et al.*, *Br. med. J.*, 1982, *285*, 543), perhaps by reducing further already critical tissue concentrations of tri-iodothyronine (N.P. Rowell, *ibid.*, 1210).

Another adverse effect in hyperthyroid patients may be dangerous depression of serum-calcium concentrations (Y.K. Seedat *et al.*, *Br. med. J.*, 1970, *3*, 525). The fall in cardiac output and heart-rate associated with propranolol given intravenously has been reported by Ikram (*Br. med. J.*, 1977, *1*, 1505) to be insignificant in patients with uncomplicated thyrotoxicosis, but to be significant in those also suffering from heart failure, contra-indicating its use in such patients; the effect of oral propranolol was not studied. Subsequently Staffurth and Stott (*Br. med. J.*, 1977, *2*, 191) have reported fatalities in 2 patients with thyrotoxicosis and propranolol may have contributed to these deaths. The results of a study by Harrower *et al.* (*Postgrad. med. J.*, 1977, *53*, 687) have indicated that propranolol-induced impairment of glucose tolerance is unlikely to be a serious contra-indication to treatment unless the patient has diabetes in addition to hyperthyrodism.

The pharmacokinetics of propranolol may also be altered in patients with thyrotoxicosis; Wilkinson and Burr (*Am. Heart J.*, 1984, *108*, 1160) found that both trough and peak serum concentrations of propranolol were significantly lower in the same patients when in the thyrotoxic state than when euthyroid; nadolol was not so affected. However, other groups have reported that the metabolism of propranolol (J.M. Bell *et al.*, *Br. J. clin. Pharmac.*, 1977, *4*, 79) and its protein binding (J.G. Kelly and D.G. McDevitt, *ibid.*, 1978, *6*, 123) are not significantly affected by thyroid status.

See also under Uses.

WITHDRAWAL. Reviews and comments on the withdrawal syndrome associated with beta blockers: *Lancet*, 1975, *2*, 592; D. G. Shand, *New Engl. J. Med.*, 1975, *293*, 449; *J. Am. med. Ass.*, 1975, *231*, 125; P. J. Ross *et al.* (letter), *Lancet*, 1979, *1*, 875; J. H. Botting and A. Gibson (letter), *ibid.*

In a retrospective analysis of a double-blind crossover efficacy study of propranolol 160 to 320 mg daily in angina pectoris it was noted that within 2 weeks of abrupt withdrawal of propranolol untoward ischaemic events occurred in 10 patients. Six had serious withdrawal complications: intermediate coronary syndrome (3), ventricular tachycardia (1), fatal myocardial infarction (1), and sudden death (1), and 4 suffered increased anginal symptoms.— R. R. Miller *et al.*, *New Engl. J. Med.*, 1975, *293*, 416.

A syndrome similar to florid thyrotoxicosis occurred in 3 patients within a week of the sudden withdrawal of propranolol 0.96 to 2 g daily for hypertension.— E. T. O'Brien (letter), *Lancet*, 1975, *2*, 819.

The effects of infusions of isoprenaline 2 µg per minute administered for 10 minutes before and after withdrawal of propranolol 40 mg four times daily over a 2-day period were studied in 6 healthy subjects. Hypersensitivity to isoprenaline was found 24 to 48 hours after propranolol withdrawal. Discontinuation of propranolol therapy for 24 hours or more before surgery might not be without risks.— H. Boudoulas *et al.*, *Ann. intern. Med.*, 1977, *87*, 433. To prevent rebound phenomena propranolol may have to be administered at reduced dosage or tapered for at least 10 to 14 days before withdrawal.— S. Nattel *et al.* (letter), *ibid.*, 1978, *89*, 288.

A withdrawal syndrome occurs with both cardioselective and nonselective beta blockers, and in both angina and hypertension.— B. Ø. Kristensen (letter), *Lancet*, 1979, *1*, 554.

In 4 hypertensive patients who had been taking propranolol 240 to 640 mg daily for 18 to 60 months, blood pressure and heart-rate rose and plasma concentrations of noradrenaline fell when propranolol was withdrawn; 3 patients experienced a forceful heart beat on the 3rd and 4th days after withdrawal.— T. J. B. Maling and C. T. Dollery, *Br. med. J.*, 1979, *2*, 366.

Gastro-intestinal bleeding due to ruptured oesophageal varices recurred in 2 cirrhotic patients after propranolol therapy was abruptly discontinued.— D. Lebrec *et al.* (letter), *New Engl. J. Med.*, 1982, *307*, 560. Haemorrhage on withdrawal of propranolol in a cirrhotic patient who had not previously suffered from variceal bleeding.— S. L. Alabaster *et al.* (letter), *J. Am. med. Ass.*, 1983, *250*, 3047.

Symptoms following withdrawal of propranolol from 100 consecutive patients undergoing coronary arteriography did not support the view that there is a propranolol withdrawal syndrome. Symptoms occurred exclusively in patients with class IV symptoms and were possibly due to loss of protection of beta blockade. There is virtually no evidence to support the view that propranolol dosage should be tapered off and no data have been presented comparing the relative merits of gradual versus abrupt withdrawal.— M. G. Myers *et al.*, *Am. Heart J.*, 1979, *97*, 298.

In a double-blind crossover study in 12 healthy subjects abrupt withdrawal of propranolol 120 mg twice daily after 1 week's administration did not lead to any significant increase in beta-adrenergic sensitivity either at rest or during periods of increased sympathetic activity. If the beta blocker withdrawal syndrome exists, hypersensitivity to beta stimulation does not appear to be the mechanism.— K. S. Kiyingi and J. Shaw, *Eur. J. clin. Pharmac.*, 1984, *27*, 423.

Absorption and Fate

Propranolol is almost completely absorbed from the gastro-intestinal tract, but is subject to considerable hepatic tissue binding and first-pass metabolism. Peak plasma concentrations occur about 1 to 2 hours after a dose, but vary greatly between individuals. It is metabolised in the liver, the metabolites being excreted in the urine together with only small amounts of unchanged propranolol; at least one of its metabolites (4-hydroxypropranolol) is considered to be biologically active but the contribution of metabolites to its overall activity is uncertain. The biological half-life of propranolol is longer than would be anticipated from its plasma half-life of about 3 to 6 hours. Propranolol crosses the placenta and traces are found in milk. It also crosses the blood-brain barrier. It is highly protein bound and reported not to be significantly dialysable.

FIRST-PASS EFFECT. Individual variation in the bioavailability of propranolol was determined mainly by first-pass metabolism rather than differences in gastric emptying.— C. M. Castleden *et al.*, *Br. J. clin. Pharmac.*, 1978, *5*, 121. See also C. F. George and M. Castleden (letter), *Br. med. J.*, 1977, *1*, 47.

Propranolol in low doses blocked cardiac, vascular, and renal beta-adrenoceptors in 6 healthy subjects who received 5 doses of 5 mg every 8 hours. Blood concentrations of propranolol could not be detected satisfactorily by fluorometry; gas-liquid chromatography showed concentrations ranging from 2.3 to 8.5 ng per mL. These results confound suggestions of a threshold dose by mouth being required to overcome a first-pass effect.— R. Davies *et al.*, *Lancet*, 1978, *1*, 407. The first-pass effect of propranolol has been amply proved and has important clinical implications.— C. F. George (letter), *ibid.*, 715. The first-pass effect was accepted; it was the threshold for this effect that was being questioned.— R. Davies *et al.* (letter), *ibid.*, 827. The active metabolite must also be considered.— L. P. Balant and J. Fabre (letter), *ibid.*, 1978, *2*, 425.

A report of significant first-pass uptake of propranolol by the lungs.— D. M. Geddes *et al.*, *Br. J. clin. Pharmac.*, 1978, *5*, 354P.

Food reduced the first-pass hepatic clearance of propranolol.— A. J. McLean *et al.*, *Clin. Pharmac. Ther.*, 1981, *30*, 31.

Further references to enhanced bioavailability when propranolol is given with food: H. Liedholm and A. Melander, *Clin. Pharmac. Ther.*, 1986, *40*, 29 (reduced presystemic conjugation of oral doses); L. S. Olanoff *et al.*, *ibid.*, 408 (reduced oral and increased intravenous clearance).

PROTEIN BINDING. Studies *in vitro* demonstrated that there was an inverse relationship between α_1 acid glycoprotein concentration and the amount of unbound propranolol in plasma. The most extensive binding of propranolol was seen in plasma from patients with inflammatory diseases such as rheumatoid arthritis and Crohn's disease, all of whom had elevated plasma concentrations of α_1 acid glycoprotein. Similar results were seen with chlorpromazine. Plasma-protein binding of cationic drugs appeared to be increased in inflammatory disease because of increased concentrations of α_1 acid glycoprotein which was able to bind them.— K. M. Piafsky *et al.*, *New Engl. J. Med.*, 1978, *299*, 1435.

Comment on the significance of drug binding to α_1 acid glycoprotein.— *Lancet*, 1979, *1*, 368.

The (−)-isomer of propranolol was more extensively bound to α_1 acid glycoprotein than was the (+)-isomer.— F. Albani *et al.*, *Br. J. clin. Pharmac.*, 1984, *18*, 244.

SUSTAINED-RELEASE PREPARATIONS. A comparison of the pharmacokinetics and pharmacodynamics of a long-acting capsule formulation of propranolol 160 mg with standard 40, 80, and 160 mg tablets.— J. McAinsh *et al.*, *Br. J. clin. Pharmac.*, 1978, *6*, 115.

Further references: A. P. Douglas-Jones, *J. int. med. Res.*, 1979, *7*, 221; D. B. Barnett *et al.*, *Br. J. clin. Pharmac.*, 1981, *11*, 432P; D. P. Nicholls *et al.*, *ibid.*, 1982, *14*, 727; M. J. Serlin *et al.*, *ibid.*, 1983, *15*, 519; D. Dvornik *et al.*, *Curr. ther. Res.*, 1983, *34*, 595; E. Perucca *et al.*, *Br. J. clin. Pharmac.*, 1984, *18*, 37; B. Zain *et al.*, *Curr. ther. Res.*, 1984, *35*, 896; J. M. Dunn. *et al.* (letter); *Lancet*, 1985, *2*, 1183.

PREGNANCY AND THE NEONATE. References to the metabolism of propranolol in pregnancy: M. T. Smith *et al.*, *Eur. J. clin. Pharmac.*, 1983, *24*, 727; *idem*, *25*, 481.

The disposition of propranolol was not altered in pregnancy in a study in 6 healthy subjects.— M. F. O'Hare *et al.*, *Eur. J. clin. Pharmac.*, 1984, *27*, 583.

Uses and Administration

Propranolol reduces cardiac activity by diminishing or preventing sympathetic beta-adrenoceptor stimulation. It reduces the rate and force of contraction of the heart and decreases the rate of conduction of impulses through the conducting system.

Its principal effect is to reduce the response of the heart to stress and exercise and it reduces blood pressure in patients with hypertension. It inhibits the release of renin from the kidney, but the contribution that this makes to its antihypertensive action is debatable. It also reduces some of the responses of the body to the effects of adrenaline and isoprenaline. It has weak membrane-stabilising properties and does not possess intrinsic sympathomimetic activity (but see p.781). Propranolol is classified as non-cardioselective.

Propranolol is used in the treatment of hypertension, often in conjunction with a thiazide diuretic. It does not produce postural hypotension but the full benefit of the treatment may not be evident for 6 to 8 weeks.

Propranolol is also used in the treatment of cardiac arrhythmias. It is often effective in paroxysmal supraventricular tachycardia. It is used with digitalis to reduce the ventricle-rate in atrial fibrillation and flutter which are not effectively controlled by digitalis alone. It is usually effective in the control of arrhythmias associated with digoxin intoxication and, administered intravenously, in the control of arrhythmias occurring during anaesthesia. It is generally less effective in ventricular than supraventricular arrhythmias but has been used in ventricular fibrillation when counter-shock cannot be employed.

Propranolol is used to improve the tolerance to exercise in patients with angina pectoris. It has been given for the prevention of re-infarction in patients who have suffered an acute myocardial infarction.

In hyperthyroidism, propranolol is given to reduce the heart-rate and control other symptoms of sympathetic nervous hyperactivity.

In the surgical treatment of phaeochromocytoma, propranolol may be given pre-operatively as an adjunct to an alpha blocking agent such as phenoxybenzamine.

Propranolol hydrochloride is usually given by mouth. Dosage is largely determined by the response of the patient. In most conditions, treatment should begin with a small dose which should be gradually increased. Usually 10 to 40 mg is given by mouth three or four times a day, but the dose may be increased up to 400 mg or more daily in the treatment of angina pectoris or hypertension. In phaeochromocytoma, 60 mg daily should be given on 3 pre-operative days always in association with alpha blockade (see Precautions).

For the emergency treatment of cardiac arrhythmias, propranolol hydrochloride may be given by slow intravenous injection in a dose of 1 mg injected over a period of 1 minute, repeated if necessary every 2 minutes until a maximum total of 10 mg has been given in conscious patients and 5 mg in patients under anaesthesia. Similar doses have been used in thyrotoxic crisis. Atropine, 1 to 2 mg, given intravenously has been recommended before propranolol is injected, in order to prevent excessive bradycardia. Propranolol is *not* suitable for the emergency treatment of hypertension; it should not be given intravenously in hypertension.

Propranolol is also used for some symptoms of anxiety, for migraine prophylaxis, and for essential tremor.

ADMINISTRATION. Studies in healthy subjects indicated that more propranolol entered the general circulation following administration with food than when it was taken on an empty stomach; administration should always be standardised relative to meals.— A. Melander *et al.*, *Clin. Pharmac. Ther.*, 1977, *22*, 108. See also T. Walle *et al.*, *Clin. Pharmac; Ther.*, 1981, *30*, 790 and under Absorption and Fate, above.

Comments and studies on responses to therapy with beta blockers in hypertensive persons of different races: Y. K. Seedat and J. Reddy, *S. Afr. med. J.*, 1971, *45*, 284; K. Jennings and V. Parsons, *Br. J. clin. Pharmac.*, 1976, *3*, *Suppl.* 3, 773; A. Reyes *et al.*, *Curr. ther. Res.*, 1978, *23*, 715; L. A. Salako *et al.*, *Eur. J. clin. Pharmac.*, 1979, *15*, 299.

For reference to treatment considerations in hypertensive black patients see under Hypertension, below.

Seventeen patients with mild to moderate hypertension receiving propranolol 240 mg, metoprolol 200 mg, or acebutolol 400 mg as a single daily dose between 7 a.m. and 8 a.m. were studied throughout 24 hours under carefully standardised conditions. Results indicated that once-daily beta-adrenoceptor blocking therapy reduces blood pressure substantially during both sleep and physical activity throughout 24 hours. Variability in arterial pressure associated with physical activity was also reduced throughout the 24-hour period. It is not known whether the average pressure is the major factor causing damage to the arterial wall or whether peaks in pressure are important, but reduction in variability as well as reduction in pressure is a potential advantage that beta-adrenoceptor blocking agents have over diuretics and anti-adrenergic drugs which would be expected to increase variability.— R. D. S. Watson *et al.*, *Lancet*, 1979, *1*, 1210.

Evidence that twice-daily dosage of propranolol was as effective as dosage 3 times daily in providing sustained beta blockade in patients receiving 180 mg daily.— J. B. Coelho *et al.*, *Clin. Pharmac. Ther.*, 1983, *34*, 440.

Propranolol, as a 10-mg dose of the hydrochloride in 0.2 mL of 2% methylcellulose gel, was well and rapidly absorbed from the nasal mucosa to produce serum concentrations equivalent to those after the same dose intravenously. The nasal route appears to be superior to the oral route for propranolol administration.— A. Hussain *et al.*, (letter), *J. pharm. Sci.*, 1980, *69*, 1240. Propranolol was well absorbed in 2 healthy subjects following buccal administration.— J. A. Henry *et al.*, *Br. J. clin. Pharmac.*, 1980, *10*, 61.

Stable propranolol concentrations and a predictable degree of beta blockade could be obtained by continuous rectal delivery from a rectal osmotic delivery system in a study in 6 subjects; results were comparable to those with intravenous infusion and offered a suitable alternative to the latter.— L. G. J. de Leede *et al.*, *Clin. Pharmac. Ther.*, 1984, *35*, 148.

For a report of significant serum-propranolol concentrations following intravaginal administration of propranolol tablets see under Contraception, below.

Controlled-release preparations. A review of the use of long-acting preparations of propranolol to provide beta blockade.— R. G. Shanks, *Postgrad. med. J.*, 1984, *60*, *Suppl.* 2, 61. See also *Br. J. clin. Pharmac.*, 1985, *19*, *Suppl.* 2.

ADMINISTRATION IN GASTRO-INTESTINAL DISORDERS. The plasma-propranolol concentration in 8 patients with coeliac disease was significantly higher 1 hour after a 40-mg dose than in 12 controls. In 10 patients with Crohn's disease the concentration was significantly higher from half to 6 hours after the dose.— R. E. Schneider *et al.*, *Br. med. J.*, 1976, *2*, 794. See also R. L. Parsons *et al.* (letter), *ibid.*, 1977, *1*, 103. Results following intravenous administration in 7 patients with Crohn's disease and 4 with rheumatoid arthritis showed that propranolol concentrations are elevated in patients with active inflammation because of a reduction in the apparent volume of distribution, probably as a result of increased plasma-protein binding. Since it is the free drug which is active it would be inappropriate to reduce the dose, and in fact there is a possibility that drug effect will be reduced in patients with these inflammatory conditions.— D. G. Waller *et al.* (letter), *Br. J. clin. Pharmac.*, 1982, *13*, 577.

ADMINISTRATION IN HEPATIC FAILURE. A study of the effects of cirrhosis on the disposition of propranolol during steady-state oral administration in 9 normal subjects and 7 with cirrhosis. There was a mean 3-fold increase in unbound propranolol concentrations in the blood in patients with cirrhosis when compared with the controls. Mean half-lives for the 2 groups were 11.2 and 4 hours respectively. Changes in systemic availability, clearance, and protein binding were proportional to the severity of the liver disease.— A. J. J. Wood *et al.*, *Clin. Pharmacokinet.*, 1978, *3*, 478. Further references: R. A. Branch *et al.*, *Br. J. clin. Pharmac.*, 1977, *4*, 630P; R. A. Branch and D. G. Shand, *Clin. Pharmacokinet.*, 1976, *1*, 264.

Study of the pharmacokinetics of propranolol in 10 patients with cirrhosis and portal hypertension led to the conclusion that for the majority of patients with severe liver disease therapy should be initiated in hospital with low doses such as propranolol 20 mg and results carefully monitored; if sustained-release preparations were used 80 mg would be safer than 160 mg unless liver function was well preserved.— M. J. P. Arthur *et al.*, *Gut*, 1985, *26*, 14. Agreement on the need to begin therapy in hospital with regular monitoring of the heart-rate.— D. B. Jones (letter), *ibid.*, 865.

ADMINISTRATION IN RENAL FAILURE. In 3 patients with hypertension and impaired renal function, there was further deterioration of renal function after treatment with propranolol for 9 and 70 days respectively and with oxprenolol for 20 days; 2 patients needed dialysis. It was recommended that beta-adrenoceptor blocking agents should not be given to patients with moderately severe renal failure.— D. J. Warren *et al.*, *Br. med. J.*, 1974, *2*, 193. Criticism.— P. Kincaid-Smith and A. S. P. Hua (letter), *ibid.*, 1974, *3*, 520. In 69 patients treated for not less than 6 months with propranolol mean initial creatinine clearance was 72.3 mL per minute and final clearance 69.2 mL per minute. In no instance had there been a fall in renal function sufficient to affect the patient clinically.— F. D. Thompson and A. M. Joekes (letter), *ibid.*, 1974, *2*, 555. Two further reports of sudden deterioration in renal function after administration of propranolol to patients with chronic renal failure.— C. P. Swainson and R. J. Winney (letter), *ibid.*, 1976, *1*, 459.

Propranolol 40 to 80 mg daily rapidly reduced blood pressure to normal and reduced plasma-renin activity in 2 patients with chronic renal failure and hypertension which had been refractory in spite of regular haemodialysis. The need for nephrectomy was avoided.— S. B. Moore and F. J. Goodwin, *Lancet*, 1976, *2*, 67.

The pharmacokinetics and effects of propranolol in terminal uraemic patients. Preliminary data suggested that, because of the greater systemic availability of the drug and reduced hepatic clearance, lower doses of propranolol should be given to patients with renal failure not yet undergoing dialysis. Although haemodialysis itself does not appear to contribute to removal of propranolol, marked fluctuations were noted in blood concentrations owing to variations in the hepatic elimination capacity and the apparent volume of distribution; no alteration in plasma protein binding was noted. Propranolol should be used with great caution and in low doses in patients with chronic renal failure.— G. Bianchetti *et al.*, *Clin. Pharmacokinet.*, 1976, *1*, 373. A similar study.— D. T. Lowenthal *et al.*, *Clin. Pharmac. Ther.*, 1974, *16*, 761.

Massive retention of propranolol metabolites in patients undergoing maintenance haemodialysis.— W. J. Stone and T. Walle, *Clin. Pharmac. Ther.*, 1980, *28*, 449.

A study indicating that there is no pharmacokinetic reason to amend the dosage of propranolol in patients with renal failure.— A. J. J. Wood *et al.*, *Br. J. clin. Pharmac.*, 1980, *10*, 561. See also W. Bennett *et al.*, *Am. J. Kidney Dis.*, 1983, *3*, 155.

ADMINISTRATION IN RESPIRATORY INSUFFICIENCY. A study of propranolol and other beta-adrenoceptor blocking agents in asthma, and the warning that no beta-adrenoceptor blocking agent, even if claiming to be cardioselective, is absolutely safe for the asthmatic patient.— P. B. S. Decalmer *et al.*, *Br. Heart J.*, 1978, *40*, 184.

Further reports and comments: K. N. V. Palmer (letter), *Br. med. J.*, 1977, *1*, 841; V. M. S. Oh *et al.*, *Br. J. clin. Pharmac.*, 1978, *5*, 107.

See also under Effects on Respiratory Function, under Adverse Effects, above.

ALCOHOL AND DRUG WITHDRAWAL. A review of the use of beta blockers in withdrawal states. Propranolol should be regarded as an adjuvant to other treatments for alcohol withdrawal symptoms, and should be used alone only in otherwise healthy patients with mild withdrawal symptoms in whom tremor or tachycardia are particularly troublesome. In more severe cases it may be combined with a benzodiazepine. There is no clear indication for the use of beta blockers in opiate withdrawal, with the possible exception of reactions in which somatic anxiety is prominent, but there is some preliminary evidence that propranolol may moderate the symptoms of the benzodiazepine withdrawal syndrome.— N. Seivewright and P. J. Tyrer, *Postgrad. med. J.*, 1984, *60*, *Suppl.* 2, 47.

For a report on the benefit of propranolol treatment in acute cocaine intoxication, see Cocaine Hydrochloride, p.1214.

ANXIETY. The (+)-isomer of propranolol (dexpropranolol) which caused no β-blockade had no effect on anxiety in a double-blind crossover pilot study of 10 patients indicating that the anti-anxiety effect observed previously with (±)-propranolol was due to its beta-blocking activity and not to a central action.— J. A. Bonn and P. Turner (letter), *Lancet*, 1971, *1*, 1355.

Beta-adrenoceptor function, as measured by cyclic AMP responsiveness to isoprenaline, was significantly reduced in 14 patients with untreated anxiety, compared with controls. This reduced response, which may represent downregulation, appeared similar to that seen previously in hypertensive patients. Treatment with propranolol 160 mg daily for 4 weeks in 7 patients markedly improved receptor responsiveness, whereas diazepam 15 mg daily in the remaining 7 did not.— D. R. Lima and P. Turner (letter), *Lancet*, 1983, *2*, 1505.

A brief review of beta blockers in the treatment of anxiety. The efficacy of beta blockers, particularly propranolol and oxprenolol, in the management of anxiety states is now well established. Beta blockers are effective mainly in somatic anxiety symptoms rather than psychic anxiety, and are probably less effective overall than the benzodiazepines, although this remains debatable. Long-term administration does not appear to produce dependence but the efficacy of long-term treatment and the possibility of withdrawal symptoms remain to be determined.— M. Peet, *Postgrad. med. J.*, 1984, *60*, *Suppl.* 2, 16.

Further reviews: I. M. James, *Postgrad. med. J.*, 1984, *60*, *Suppl.* 2, 19 (situational anxiety); C. Hallstrom, *ibid.*, 26 (morbid anxiety). See also M. Peet and R. A. Yates, *J. clin. Hosp. Pharm.*, 1981, *6*, 155.

CARDIAC DISORDERS. *Angina pectoris.* Views on the management of angina of effort. First line therapy is still sublingual glyceryl trinitrate; where this proves ineffective, one may add either a beta blocker, preferably a cardioselective one such as atenolol, or a calcium antagonist such as diltiazem, verapamil, or nifedipine. The third step is the combination of a beta blocker with nifedipine, which is likely to be better tolerated than the combination of a beta blocker with isosorbide dinitrate; combination of all three is less effective than beta blocker plus nifedipine (with short-acting nitrates as needed), probably due to excessive vasodilatation. In the author's view beta blockade is contra-indicated in angina at rest unless there is reactive tachycardia or hypertension, or unless the patient is already receiving beta blockers and may be at risk of a withdrawal reaction.— L. H. Opie, *Lancet*, 1984, *1*, 496. See also P. A. Poole-Wilson, *Postgrad. med. J.*, 1983, *59*, *Suppl.* 3, 11; D. Patterson, *Br. J. Hosp. Med.*, 1985, *33*, 8.

Of 35 patients with angina 19 of 29 who were sexually active experienced anginal pain during intercourse. After basic advice all were given beta-blocking agents. Patients experiencing pain became free from pain (6 also needed isosorbide dinitrate) and 4 resumed sexual activity.— G. Jackson, *Br. med. J.*, 1978, *2*, 16.

In a comparative study involving 16 patients with stable angina pectoris, single doses of propranolol, oxprenolol, practolol, tolamolol, and metoprolol were generally equally effective in the treatment of exercise-induced angina. A beneficial effect occurred within one hour and persisted for at least 8 hours.— U. Thadani *et al.*, *New Engl. J. Med.*, 1979, *300*, 750.

In a double-blind study involving 16 patients with severe exertional angina pectoris the incidence of pain and consumption of glyceryl trinitrate were significantly decreased by nifedipine 30 or 60 mg daily compared with placebo, but a significantly greater reduction was produced by propranolol 240 or 480 mg daily. Although the higher dose of propranolol had no additional benefit over the lower dose, the higher dose of nifedipine was significantly more effective than the lower. Combination of the 2 drugs in the higher doses produced further significant improvement.— P. Lynch *et al.*, *Br. med. J.*, 1980, *281*, 184.

Studies of combined beta blocker and calcium-channel blocker therapy in angina pectoris: A. C. Tweddel *et al.*, *Br. J. clin. Pharmac.*, 1981, *12*, 229 (propranolol and nifedipine); M. Bassan *et al.*, *Br. med. J.*, 1982, *284*, 1067 (propranolol and verapamil); L. Harris *et al.*, *ibid.*, 1148 (propranolol and nifedipine); J. C. McGourty *et al.*, *Br. J. clin. Pharmac.*, 1984, *17*, 638P (propranolol, pindolol, or atenolol, and verapamil); D. P. Humen *et al.*, *J. Am. Coll. Cardiol.*, 1986, *7*, 329 (propranolol and diltiazem); M. J. O'Hara *et al.*, *Clin. Cardiol.*, 1987, *10*, 115 (propranolol and diltiazem).

Cardiomyopathy. A comparative study of 24 patients with congestive cardiomyopathy taking beta blockers (alprenolol, practolol, or metoprolol) in addition to digitalis and diuretics, with a similar group of 13 controls selected retrospectively who had not taken beta blockers. The survival-rate in those also receiving beta blockers was 83%, 66%, and 52% after 1, 2, and 3 years respectively, compared with only 46%, 19%, and 10% in those who had not received beta blockers.— K. Swedberg *et al.* (preliminary communication), *Lancet*, 1979, *1*, 1374.

Comment on the use and hazards of beta blockade in congestive cardiomyopathy, and the view that a controlled trial is needed before it can be recommended.— *Lancet*, 1981, *1*, 598.

Results of a double-blind controlled study of acebutolol in 15 patients argued against routine administration of beta blocking agents in congestive cardiomyopathy.— H. Ikram and D. Fitzpatrick, *Lancet*, 1981, *2*, 490.

Propranolol is standard therapy for hypertrophic obstructive cardiomyopathy.— L. H. Opie, *Lancet*, 1980, *1*, 693.

Non-cardioselective beta blockers are more effective at reducing outflow tract obstruction in hypertrophic cardiomyopathy than are the cardioselective ones.— M. M. Webb-Peploe, *Postgrad. med. J.*, 1985, *61*, 1120.

The use of beta blockers in the treatment of dilated cardiomyopathy remains controversial. Beta blockers or calcium antagonists may afford symptomatic relief in hypertrophic cardiomyopathy, without, however, changing the long-term prognosis.—Memorandum from a WHO Meeting, *Bull. Wld Hlth Org.*, 1986, *64*, 365.

Beta blockers have for many years been the mainstay of medical therapy in symptomatic patients with either obstructive or nonobstructive hypertrophic cardiomyopathy, and can relieve all the principal cardiac symptoms including angina, dyspnoea, lightheadedness and syncope. Approximately one third to one half of symptomatic patients improve after treatment with propranolol in doses of 160 to 320 mg by mouth daily. After initial improvement symptoms may recur in some patients, mandating treatment with doses up to 640 mg daily, or even more.— B. J. Maron *et al.*, *New Engl. J. Med.*, 1987, *316*, 844.

Fallot's tetralogy. Propranolol by mouth was often of value in milder dyspnoeic spells associated with Fallot's tetralogy and where there was less severe organic narrowing of the right-ventricular outflow tract. Propranolol intravenously was often of value during acute attacks.— G. R. Cumming (letter), *Lancet*, 1966, *2*, 1317.

Marfan syndrome. Prophylactic propranolol is given to patients with Marfan syndrome who are unsuitable for surgery or whose operations are delayed.— R. M. Donaldson *et al.*, *Lancet*, 1980, *2*, 1178.

Myocardial infarction. An overview of randomised trials of beta blockade after myocardial infarction. Long-term beta blockade for perhaps a year or so following discharge after a myocardial infarction is now of proven value and for many such patients mortality reduction of about 25% can be achieved. No important differences are apparent among the benefits of different beta blockers although those with intrinsic sympathomimetic activity may confer less benefit. In contrast, although very early intravenous short-term beta blockade can definitely limit infarct size reliable information about the effects of such treatment on mortality must await the reports of the ISIS trial.— S. Yusuf *et al.*, *Prog. cardiovasc. Dis.*, 1985, *27*, 335.

For the results of the ISIS trial, confirming the benefits of early intervention with a beta blocker in myocardial infarction see under Atenolol, p.784.

A preliminary report of the double-blind randomised β-Blocker Heart Attack Trial (BHAT) in 3837 patients who had suffered acute myocardial infarction, indicating that patients receiving propranolol experienced a 26% lower mortality from all causes than did the control group. Overall mortality in the treated group was 7% (135 deaths) compared with 9.5% (183 deaths) in the placebo group. The study has consequently been curtailed. Patients entered the trial 5 to 21 days (average 13.8) after the onset of acute myocardial infarction and received either propranolol hydrochloride 40 mg or placebo thrice daily. A maintenance dose of 60 or 80 mg three times daily was prescribed at follow-up 1 month later. Beneficial effects occurred primarily in the first year after infarction and were not affected by the size of infarct or the age or sex of the patient.—β-Blocker Heart Attack Study Group, *J. Am. med. Ass.*, 1981, *246*, 2073. Final results of the study. After an average follow-up period of 25.1 months 138 patients in the propranolol group and 188 in the placebo group had died. Cardiovascular mortality was significantly reduced in the propranolol group (6.6% compared with 8.9%); sudden death was also less common in the patients receiving propranolol. Subgroup analysis suggested a beneficial effect of propranolol in both patients with anterior infarction and those with inferior infarction. Although the beneficial effects of propranolol appeared to be greatest in the first 12 to 18 months after myocardial infarction the effects were sustained for the duration of the trial. Based on these results the use of propranolol for at least 3 years is recommended in patients who have suffered recent myocardial infarction and who have no contra-indications to beta blockade.— *idem*, 1982, *247*, 1707.

In a double-blind randomised study of 560 high-risk patients who had survived acute myocardial infarction, treatment for one year with propranolol significantly reduced the number of sudden cardiac deaths when compared with placebo. Treatment was started 4 to 6 days after infarction and patients received either propranolol 40 mg four times daily or placebo.— V. Hansteen *et al.*, *Br. med. J.*, 1982, *284*, 155.

CONTRACEPTION. Comparison *in vitro* of the ability of propranolol, its (+)-isomer, and of procaine, to inhibit sperm motility. A 50% inhibition of sperm motility was obtained with a 1.3 mmol concentration of (+)-propranolol, 0.8 mmol of racemic (±)-propranolol, and 18 mmol for procaine.— C. Y. Hong *et al.*, *Br. J. clin. Pharmac.*, 1982, *13*, 285P. The sperm immobilising effects of 5 beta blockers *in vitro* were related to their lipid solubility, supporting the theory that they inhibit sperm motility by stabilising the cellular membrane. The concentrations required to reduce motility by 50% of control values were 0.8, 4.2, 6.2, 11.0, and 33.0 mmol respectively for propranolol, oxprenolol, metoprolol, acebutolol, and sotalol.— C. Y. Hong and P. Turner, *ibid.*, *14*, 269.

In 198 women who had used intra-uterine devices for contraception insertion of propranolol 80 mg (as an oral tablet) into the vagina each evening, except during menstruation, provided an effective alternative. Over 127 woman-years, the pregnancy rate at one year was calculated as 3.4 per 100 women, compared to an expected rate of 88.2 per 100 in the absence of contraception. Over the period of the study 33 women discontinued treatment because of local itching or discomfort. Propranolol would appear to be an effective vaginal contraceptive with a failure rate comparing favourably with other methods of contraception.— J. Zipper *et al.*, *Br. med. J.*, 1983, *287*, 1245. Propranolol appeared in the blood within 1 hour of insertion of an 80-mg oral tablet into the vagina in 6 healthy women; mean peak concentration was 106 ng per mL, achieved at 4.5 hours after administration. In contrast, propranolol appeared in the blood within 30 minutes of the same dose by mouth in 4 of the women, but the mean peak concentration (at 1.6 hours) was only 52.2 ng per mL. Supine and erect systolic blood pressure, pulse-rate, and FEV_1 fell after vaginal application but none of the women experienced symptomatic side-effects. Further studies of the contraceptive effects of propranolol should probably be conducted with the (+)-isomer, dexpropranolol which is almost devoid of beta-blocking effects.— L. G. Patel *et al.*, *ibid.*, 1247. See also R. M. Pearson *et al.* (letter), *Lancet*, 1984, *2*, 1480 (oral dexpropranolol).

The concentrations of propranolol in seminal fluid and in saliva from 6 healthy males following a dose of 80 mg by mouth were much less than those required to inhibit sperm motility.— P. Mahajan *et al.*, *Br. J. clin. Pharmac.*, 1984, *18*, 849.

ERYTHROMELALGIA. A woman with long-standing and worsening erythromelalgia with severe and frequent burning of the lower legs, ankles, and feet and occasional desquamation failed to respond to clonidine. Since these symptoms were the opposite of those of Raynaud's phenomenon which could be induced by beta blockers, treatment was tried with propranolol 10 mg three times daily. There was a rapid and complete response which had been maintained for 3 months.— J. L. Bada (letter), *Lancet*, 1977, *2*, 412.

EXPLOSIVE RAGE. The form of explosive rage that often occurs as a patient emerges from coma following head injury can sometimes be controlled rather dramatically by large doses of propranolol (up to 80 mg four times daily).— F. A. Elliott, *Practitioner*, 1976, *217*, 51.

Of 8 patients with intermittent explosive disorder (episodic outbursts of inappropriate rage), 2 had complete remission and 3 had substantial behavioural improvement when treated with propranolol in doses of 80 to 300 mg daily.— S. C. Jenkins and T. Maruta, *Mayo Clin. Proc.*, 1987, *62*, 204.

EXTRAPYRAMIDAL DISORDERS. Propranolol had proved beneficial in 12 patients with neuroleptic-induced akathisia, 9 of whom experienced complete remission. The mean dose required was 30 mg.— J. F. Lipinski *et al* (letter), *Lancet*, 1983, *2*, 685. Comment. While propranolol may turn out to be a useful treatment it may obscure the safer and more practical treatment of reducing the dose of neuroleptic medication.— J. C. Kuehnle (letter), *ibid.*, 1254. See also under Fluphenazine. See also under Parkinsonism, below.

Tardive dyskinesia. A preliminary study in psychiatric patients suggested that propranolol may be of benefit in tardive dyskinesia.— N. M. Bacher and H. A. Lewis, *Am. J. Psychiat.*, 1980, *137*, 495.

Further references: P. W. Roberts (letter), *Can med. Ass. J.*, 1980, *123* 1106; R. Wilbur and F. A. Kulik, *Prog. Neuropsychopharmacol. biol. Psychiatry*, 1981, *4*, 627.

GLAUCOMA. A review of beta blockers in the management of open-angle glaucoma.— W. P. Boger, *Drugs*, 1979, *18*, 25.

Propranolol hydrochloride eye-drops 1% significantly reduced intra-ocular pressure in 7 of 10 patients with raised pressure.— J. Vale *et al.*, *Br. J. Ophthal.*, 1972, *56*, 770.

A single-blind study in 12 patients with ocular hypertension showed that propranolol 20, 40, or 80 mg significantly reduced intra-ocular pressure in a dose-related manner.— K. Wettrell and M. Pandolfi, *Br. J. Ophthal.*, 1976, *60*, 680.

In a multicentre crossover study involving 103 patients with glaucoma propranolol 40 to 60 mg twice daily by mouth was as effective as twice daily application of timolol 0.5% eye-drops in reducing intra-ocular pressure. Combination of the two treatments produced further additive reductions in intra-ocular pressure in over 50% of patients. A. Öhrström *et al.*, *Acta Ophthalmol.*, 1985, *62*, 681.

HEPATIC DISORDERS. Long-term treatment with propranolol, in a dosage which reduced the heart-rate by about 25% (dose range, 20 to 180 mg twice daily), prevented recurrent gastro-intestinal bleeding in a controlled study of 74 patients with cirrhosis. A year after inclusion in the study 96% of treated patients were free of re-bleeding compared with 50% of the placebo group.— D. Lebrec *et al.*, *New Engl. J. Med.*, 1981, *305*, 1371. In a controlled study in 48 patients with cirrhosis and demonstrated variceal bleeding, 26 failed to benefit from propranolol in doses of 80 to 800 mg daily, compared with placebo in 22. Despite a fall in hepatic venous pressure gradient with propranolol in all patients measured, 12 of the 26 patients in the propranolol group rebled from oesophageal varices; this was not significantly different from the figure of 11 among the 22 receiving placebo. Four patients in the propranolol group and 2 in the placebo group died from variceal rebleeding. These results contrast markedly with those of Lebrec *et al.*, which may possibly be due to differences in patient selection; whereas the former study included mostly patients with alcoholic cirrhosis who had good liver function, the present study included patients with cirrhosis from a variety of causes and with varying severity of liver disease. Such good results as previously reported cannot necessarily be expected in patients with non-alcoholic cirrhosis and more severe liver damage.— A. K. Burroughs *et al.*, *ibid.*, 1983, *309*, 1539. Surgical shunts remain the gold standard, despite the risks. Initial therapy of varices should probably be by sclerotherapy, with surgery if bleeding episodes continue after a few months, provided the patient's condition permits.— T. B. Reynolds, *ibid.*, 1575.

Further reports of beneficial results from prophylactic propranolol therapy in chronic liver disease: P. C. Hayes and I. A. D. Bouchier, *Gut*, 1985, *26*, A1103; L. Pagliaro *et al.* (letter), *New Engl. J. Med.*, 1986, *314*, 244.

Propranolol (a non-selective beta blocker) or prazosin (an alpha blocker), but not atenolol (a cardioselective beta blocker), produced sustained reductions in portal venous pressure in an 8-week study involving 24 patients with cirrhosis, portal hypertension, and oesophageal varices. After 8 weeks of therapy the reduction in mean porto-hepatic venous pressure was 25% in the 8 given propranolol and 18% in those taking prazosin. Atenolol produced an initial significant drop in pressure at 2 to 3 weeks but this was not sustained at 8 weeks. There may be a reasonable case for studying propranolol combined with prazosin in patients with portal hypertension.— P. R. Mills *et al.*, *Gut*, 1984, *25*, 73.

Propranolol produced a more marked reduction in portal pressure following intravenous administration to 18 cirrhotic patients than did a comparable intravenous dose of metoprolol, but this was associated with a marked fall in hepatic blood flow which was not seen with the selective beta blocker. Because of the potential adverse effects of a fall in blood flow on hepatic function, metoprolol may be preferable to propranolol in preventing recurrence of gastro-intestinal bleeding, especially in patients with severely impaired liver function.— D. Westaby *et al.*, *Gut*, 1984, *25*, 121.

Comparisons of beta blockers with sclerotherapy in the prevention of variceal rebleeding: D. Westaby *et al.*, *Gut*, 1985, *26*, 421 (sclerotherapy more effective than metoprolol); J. M. Dollet *et al.* (letter), *Lancet*, 1985, *2*, 97 (sclerotherapy as effective as propranolol); P. Alexandrino *et al.*, *Gut*, 1986, *27*, A597 (sclerotherapy superior to propranolol).

HYPERPARATHYROIDISM. Although normal parathyroid tissue can be stimulated by catecholamines clinical studies of beta blockers in primary hyperparathyroidism have shown nothing approaching a consistent beneficial effect.— *Lancet*, 1984, *2*, 727.

HYPERTENSION. Debate over the choice of a beta blocker or a thiazide diuretic as the initial 'first-step' agent in the management of hypertension. Both groups are effective in a proportion of patients when given alone, but both have adverse effects on cardiovascular risk factors such as cholesterol, triglyceride, and uric acid concentrations. It is the authors' practice to use diuretics first in the drug treatment of hypertension and to use beta blockers as second line drugs; however, in some circumstances, as in patients with gout or ischaemic heart disease, it is preferred to initiate treatment with beta blockers.— J. A. Whitworth and P. Kincaid-Smith, *Drugs*, 1982, *23*, 394. A double-blind controlled study in 683 patients with mild to moderate hypertension compared treatment with propranolol in 340 with hydrochlorothiazide in 343. Both drugs effectively lowered blood pressure; with a reduction to target blood pressure in 57% of those given propranolol and 64% of those given hydrochlorothiazide. Hydrochlorothiazide was more effective overall than propranolol because of its greater efficacy in black patients, who comprised just over half of the total study population. The results seem to support the general use of a diuretic as a first-line drug, especially for black patients.—Veterans Administration Cooperative Study Group on Antihypertensive Agents, *J. Am. med. Ass.*, 1982, *248*, 1996. See also *idem*, 2004. Because of reservations about the side-effects of thiazide diuretics, in particular metabolic side-effects, a beta blocker, or perhaps an alpha blocker, may increasingly be chosen over a diuretic for initial therapy of uncomplicated hypertension.— L. H. Opie, *Lancet*, 1984, *1*, 496. There is no scientific evidence to support the use of beta blockers in preference to diuretics either in terms of effectiveness or of adverse effects.— G. Berglund, *J. cardiovasc. Pharmac.*, 1984, *6*, *Suppl.* 1, S256. A review of 9 major controlled studies of the treatment of hypertension, involving over 50 000 patients, and some guidelines for clinical practice. There is no real evidence that any particular form of drug treatment is superior to any other, except for a suggestion that beta blockers are less effective in preventing the complications of high blood pressure in smokers. Based on side-effects and cost, initial treatment should be with low-dose bendrofluazide.— R. G. Wilcox *et al.*, *Br. med. J.*, 1986, *293*, 433. Concerns about the safety of the thiazides have now been dispelled; where drug treatment of hypertension is necessary a thiazide should be preferred to a beta blocker unless contra-indicated. There is insufficient evidence of the long-term safety of calcium-channel blockers or angiotensin-converting-enzyme inhibitors, and these should be reserved as third-line drugs after thiazides and then beta blockers.— L. E. Ramsay, *Prescribers' J.*, 1987, *27*, (2), 1. The view that beta blockers are suitable first-line agents for the treatment of mild to moderate hypertension in most patients under 65 who do not have specific contra-indications to them.— D. C. Harrison, *Am. J. Cardiol.*, 1987, *60*, 13E.

For an outline of the stepped care approach to the management of hypertension, including the role of beta blockers, see under Choice of Antihypertensive Agent, p.466.

In children. In 9 hypertensive children propranolol in doses of 0.6 to 6.4 mg per kg body-weight daily (average 2.5 mg per kg) reduced blood pressure and heart-rate, and was well tolerated. Five children also received a diuretic and methyldopa or hydralazine.— W. R. Griswold *et al.*, *Archs Dis. Childh.*, 1978, *53*, 594.

Further references: J. G. Mongeau *et al.* (letter), *Can. med. Ass. J.*, 1977, *116*, 589 (adolescents with essential hypertension); D. E. Potter *et al.*, *J. Pediat.*, 1977, *90*, 309 (renal transplantation).

HYPERTHYROIDISM. Discussion of beta blockers in the treatment of hyperthyroid Graves' disease. Pre-operative therapy with a beta blocker, preferably combined with iodide can be considered the equal of pre-operative treatment with an antithyroid agent and iodide in patients with moderate hyperthyroidism but it is not superior. Use of a beta blocker allows surgery to be undertaken after one to two weeks. Maintenance of adrenergic blockade throughout the operation is important and thus use of longer-acting beta blockers is probably preferable, but apart from this there is no evidence that any one of them is superior for this purpose. However there has been a continuing trend away from surgical therapy of hyperthyroidism. In the drug treatment of hyperthyroidism beta blockers are widely considered to give symptomatic relief but should not be used alone nor given routinely; radioactive iodine or antithyroid agents remain the treatments of choice until more specific treatments aimed at the factors initiating the hyperthyroid condition are developed.— R. D. Utiger, *New Engl. J. Med.*, 1984, *310*, 1597.

An early study. Following its use in 100 hyperthyroid patients undergoing subtotal thyroidectomy, propranolol alone was considered to be safe and effective in the pre-operative preparation of hyperthyroid patients, with the main advantage of increased flexibility of date of operation. The following dosage regimen was used: propranolol 40 mg every 6 hours, the patient being admitted to hospital on the fourth pre-operative day and the dose increased if necessary until the resting pulse-rate was less than 90 per minute; propranolol was continued throughout the day of operation and for 7 days subsequently. Compared with a carbimazole-treated series of patients, blood loss was less presumably because the carbimazole-treated patients had increased vascularity and size of thyroid glands owing to overtreatment. Thyroid storm was avoided by high-quality perioperative supervision with no patient undergoing the operation until the resting pulse-rate was below 90, meticulous attention being paid to the important pre-operative dose of propranolol, and prompt treatment of postoperative chest infections; if a high standard was not attainable substitution of propranolol for antithyroid drugs would be unwise.— A. D. Toft *et al.*, *New Engl. J. Med.*, 1978, *298*, 643.

For the use of propranolol with potassium iodide in the pre-operative management of patients with Graves' disease, see Potassium Iodide, p.1187.

Neonatal thyrotoxicosis. Thyrotoxicosis evident 7 days after birth in a premature child born to a thyrotoxic mother was successfully treated with propranolol, 500 μg three times daily gradually increased to 7 mg four times daily; it was discontinued 53 days after birth. Despite vomiting which developed at 38 days and continued until the day after propranolol was stopped, the infant continued to gain weight.— K. N. Pearl and T. L. Chambers, *Br. med. J.*, 1977, *2*, 738.

Thyroid storm. An 11-year-old boy with signs of thyroid storm responded dramatically to intravenous administration of propranolol 3 mg, followed by a further 3 mg two hours later. After another 2 hours he was given 30 mg by mouth and subsequently 20 mg every six hours which controlled his symptoms until propylthiouracil could take effect. Two attempts to discontinue propranolol during the first 3 weeks were unsuccessful but he was eventually withdrawn from propranolol 40 mg daily during the fifth treatment week.— M. Galaburda *et al.*, *Pediatrics*, 1974, *53*, 920.

A report of 2 patients in whom administration of propranolol failed to prevent thyroid storm.— M. Eriksson *et al.*, *New Engl. J. Med.*, 1977, *296*, 263. Criticism; the dose might have been too low.— J. J. Abrams and J. Sandler (letter), *ibid.*, 1120. Further criticisms.— S. G. Dorfman *et al.* (letter), *ibid;* T. A. Bowdle (letter), *ibid.*, 1121. Reply.— S. Rubenfeld (letter), *ibid.* The dosage of propranolol might have been inadequate. In a study of 11 thyrotoxic patients given propranolol 40 mg four times daily the plasma-propranolol concentrations were not maintained above 50 ng per mL throughout the 6-hour dosage interval in 8, and in 4 peak concentrations were below 30 ng per mL.— R. Hellman *et al.* (letter), *ibid.*, *297*, 671.

Thyrotoxic hypercalcaemia. Propranolol, initially by intravenous infusion in a dose of about 10 mg per hour for 12 hours, followed by 20 or 25 mg four times daily by mouth for 3 to 4 weeks decreased serum-calcium concentrations in 2 patients with hypercalcaemia associated with hyperthyroidism.— R. K. Rude *et al.*, *New Engl. J. Med.*, 1976, *294*, 431. See also L. E. Mallette *et al.*, *Metabolism*, 1985, *34*, 999.

See also under Precautions.

LEPROSY. A study into the immunostimulant effect of the addition of propranolol to the standard therapy of 12 patients with lepromatous leprosy.— R. Anderson *et al.*, *Lepr. Rev.*, 1980, *51*, 137. *In vitro* studies indicating that metoprolol, propranolol, and sotalol may be useful in the *in vivo* restoration of leucotaxis in patients with lepromatous leprosy.— R. Anderson and E. M. S. Gatner (letter), *ibid.*, 195.

MIGRAINE. A review of beta blockers in the prophylaxis of migraine.— K. Weerasuriya *et al.*, *Cephalalgia*, 1982, *2*, 33. A further review. Beta blockers which lack intrinsic sympathomimetic activity, such as propranolol, timolol, atenolol, nadolol, and metoprolol have been shown to be effective in the prophylaxis of migraine in some, but not all, patients, regardless of whether they possess cardioselective properties or not. In contrast, partial agonists with a degree of intrinsic sympathomimetic activity such as alprenolol, oxprenolol, pindolol, or acebutolol have been shown to be ineffective. The mechanism of action is unknown, reflecting uncertainty as to the pathogenesis of migraine itself.— P. Turner, *Postgrad. med. J.*, 1984, *60*, *Suppl.* 2, 51. Experience with beta blockers at a large migraine clinic. Propranolol is the drug of first choice in the prophylaxis of migraine. Starting doses may be 80 mg per day or less but large doses are sometimes required; the dose may be increased rapidly by repeated doubling. In the absence of side-effects, up to 480 mg daily can be tried within a relatively short time period. Once an adequate response is achieved reduction of the dose may be attempted for maintenance therapy. In some patients who fail to respond even to large doses of propranolol, addition of small doses of amitriptyline may produce remarkable benefit. It is uncertain how long treatment should be continued, since the cyclical nature of the disease may tend to improvement with passage of time, but very long-term therapy should probably not be encouraged; however there is some evidence for the value of continuing propranolol for 6 months or more.— T. J. Steiner and R. Joseph, *ibid.*, 56.

For further reference see under Ergotamine Tartrate, p.1057.

NARCOLEPSY. Four patients with long-standing narcolepsy treated with methylphenidate were changed to therapy with propranolol 240 to 480 mg daily and this was considered to be at least as effective as methylphenidate in controlling sleep attacks. The effect of propranolol on the cataplexy, however, was variable with 1 improving, 2 remaining the same, and 1 deteriorating. In the latter 3 patients addition of a tricyclic antidepressant to propranolol essentially eliminated the cataplexy.— A. Kales *et al.*, *Ann. intern. Med.*, 1979, *91*, 741. See also A. Kales *et al.*, *ibid.*, 1987, *106*, 434.

A study of long-term propranolol treatment in the management of narcoleptic and cataplectic symptoms.— K. Meier-Ewart *et al.*, *Sleep*, 1985, *8*, 95.

ORTHOSTATIC HYPOTENSION. Propranolol had a beneficial effect in 3 of 5 patients with an orthostatic syndrome characterised by raised plasma-bradykinin concentrations.— D. H. P. Streeten *et al.*, *Lancet*, 1972, *2*, 1048.

A patient with orthostatic hypotension due to autonomic dysfunction was treated successfully with: tightly fitting stockings, a head-up body tilt at night, volume expansion with salt tablets and fludrocortisone, dexamphetamine for alpha-adrenergic stimulation, and propranolol for blocking beta-agonist-mediated vasodilatation and dexamphetamine-induced tachycardia. Dihydroergotamine subsequently replaced the dexamphetamine. None of the measures used alone was adequate.— K. K. P. Hui and M. E. Conolly, *New Engl. J. Med.*, 1981, *304*, 1473.

For reference to the absence of a beneficial effect of propranolol with ephedrine in orthostatic hypotension, see Ephedrine, p.1463.

PARKINSONISM. Propranolol in doses of not less than 60 mg daily was compared with a placebo in 18 patients with parkinsonism who were also receiving levodopa. The only significant effect of propranolol was an improvement in handwriting and circle-drawing and this was not considered to be of clinical value.— C. D. Marsden *et al.* (letter), *Lancet*, 1974, *2*, 410. Beta blockers have never been extensively used in parkinsonism, probably because specific agents such as levodopa and carbidopa exist, and because beta blockade affects only tremor and not rigidity. However, it may be worth considering adding a beta blocker to antiparkinsonism therapy where refractory tremor is a major problem, especially when it is accentuated greatly by emotion.—

P. J. Tyrer, *Drugs*, 1980, *20*, 300.

PORPHYRIA. Four patients with acute intermittent porphyria were relieved of tachycardia and hypertension after the administration of propranolol 40 to 400 mg daily.— A. D. Beattie *et al.*, *Br. med. J.*, 1973, *3*, 257.

Further references: A. Atsmon and I. Blum (letter), *Lancet*, 1970, *1*, 196; L. M. Flacks (letter), *ibid.*, 363; A. Atsmon *et al.*, *S. Afr. med. J.*, 1972, *46*, 311; D. Douer *et al.*, *J. Am. med. Ass.*, 1978, *240*, 766; A. S. Menawat *et al.*, *Postgrad. med. J.*, 1979, *55*, 546; M. R. Moore and P. B. Disler, *Adverse Drug React. Ac. Pois. Rev.*, 1983, *2*, 149.

PREGNANCY AND THE NEONATE. A review of the use of beta blockers in pregnancy.— P. C. Rubin, *New Engl. J. Med.*, 1981, *305*, 1323.

For warnings concerning the use of propranolol in pregnancy see also under Precautions.

Foetal tachycardia. Administration of propranolol to a diabetic woman during the last 20 days of pregnancy controlled tachycardia in the infant. After birth the concentration of propranolol in the child's blood was 20% of that in the mother's.— A. Teuscher *et al.*, *Am. J. Cardiol.*, 1978, *42*, 304.

Hypertension in pregnancy. In a retrospective study the foetal outcome was considerably worse in 9 hypertensive women given propranolol and other antihypertensive agents, than in 15 given antihypertensive therapy which excluded propranolol.— B. A. Lieberman *et al.*, *Br. J. Obstet. Gynaec.*, 1978, *85*, 678.

The successful control of blood pressure by propranolol, with other agents, in 8 of 9 pregnant women; there was no effect on uterine contractions and no increased frequency of abortion or premature labour.— P. Tcherdakoff *et al.*, *Br. med. J.*, 1978, *2*, 670.

A hypertensive woman was treated with propranolol 40 mg daily throughout pregnancy without complications. Estimated intake of propranolol in breast milk by the infant was about 3 μg daily.— E. A. Taylor and P. Turner, *Postgrad. med. J.*, 1981, *57*, 427.

Discussion of the treatment of cardiovascular disease in pregnancy. Beta blockers or methyldopa are the drugs of choice in the treatment of hypertension in pregnancy. Anecdotal reports of foetal morbidity linked with maternal administration of beta blockers have not been confirmed by controlled studies. The benefits to the foetus of treating maternal hypertension remain controversial; results of controlled studies suggest that treatment of both chronic hypertension and pregnancy-induced hypertension is beneficial to the foetus, but the size of the studies limits the ability to draw definitive conclusions.— K. R. Lees and P. C. Rubin, *Br. med. J.*, 1987, *294*, 358.

Hyperthyroidism in pregnancy. Opposition to the use of propranolol for hyperthyroidism in pregnancy.— G. P. Redmond (letter), *New Engl. J. Med.*, 1978, *298*, 917. Propranolol is only indicated in thyroid storm which is particularly apt to occur during labour and delivery.— G. N. Burrow (letter), *ibid.*, 918.

A review of the management of hyperthyroidism and hypothyroidism during pregnancy.— O. M. Edwards, *Postgrad. med. J.*, 1979, *55*, 340.

A discussion of post-partum thyroiditis. If treatment of the hyperthyroid phase is necessary a beta blocker such as propranolol should be given rather than an antithyroid agent.— *Lancet*, 1987, *1*, 962.

SCHIZOPHRENIA. Results of clinical studies of the use of propranolol in schizophrenia have been equivocal. Although there have been reports of benefit from uncontrolled studies, often with very high doses of around 3 g daily, controlled studies have failed to show any advantage over a placebo. Other work has shown that propranolol is less effective than chlorpromazine in the treatment of acute schizophrenia. Propranolol has sometimes been given as an adjunct to neuroleptic therapy, but any resultant clinical improvement is likely to be due to a pharmacokinetic interaction leading to increased plasma concentrations of the neuroleptic. Although the evidence does not support the use of propranolol in schizophrenia there is some evidence from case studies of a beneficial effect in patients with mania.— M. Peet and R. A. Yates, *J. clin. Hosp. Pharm.*, 1981, *6*, 155.

Evidence for a favourable effect of propranolol on both positive and negative symptoms of chronic schizophrenia in 22 patients; in contrast, thioridazine given to a further 23 improved positive but not negative symptoms.— D. Eccleston *et al.*, *Br. J. Psychiat.*, 1985, *147*, 623.

SEXUALLY INDUCED HEADACHES. Propranolol 20 mg twice daily completely abolished severe sexually induced headaches in a 32-year-old man.— N. R. Nutt (letter), *Br. med. J.*, 1977, *1*, 1664.

SHIVERING. Postoperative shivering occurred in only 1 of 97 patients who were receiving propranolol therapy before their operation; among 1360 patients who did not receive propranolol the prevalence of shivering was 29.8%.— D. S. Lee and M. J. Shaffer (letter), *Lancet*, 1986, *1*, 500.

TREMOR. Beta blockers, and in particular propranolol, have become the drugs of first choice in control of essential tremor in patients needing regular medication. Many comparative studies have shown beta blockers to be effective in controlling essential tremor, and none has been found to be superior to that originally tried, propranolol. The beneficial effect appears to be predominantly due to blockade of peripheral $beta_2$ receptors on extrafusal muscle fibres and muscle spindles, although there may also be a CNS effect. Treatment with propranolol may be with single doses in specific situations; the effect reaches a maximum after 1 to 2 hours and may persist for several hours. More usually, however, propranolol is given in doses of 40 to 80 mg three times daily as a continuous regimen. Response is not correlated with serum drug concentrations and is variable and unpredictable; a mean reduction in tremor amplitude of 45% has been recorded, with lower frequency and larger amplitude tremors responding best. The efficacy of long-term treatment is unknown.— L. J. Findley, *Br. J. Hosp. Med.*, 1986, *35*, 388.

Propranolol 30 to 80 mg daily reduced the tremor due to lithium but did not do so in patients also receiving tricyclic antidepressants.— L. Kirk *et al.* (letter), *Lancet*, 1972, *1*, 839. See also *idem*, 1973, *2*, 1086. Results indicating that beta blockade is ineffective in lithium-induced tremor.— J. M. Kellett *et al.*, *J. Neurol. Neurosurg. Psychiat.*, 1975, *38*, 719. Propranolol 30 to 40 mg daily controlled the lithium-induced tremor in 5 patients who had been taking lithium carbonate for 1 to 5 years. Tremor recurred in 3 patients when they stopped taking propranolol.— Y. D. Lapierre, *Can. med. Ass. J.*, 1976, *114*, 619.

Evidence that metoprolol, a cardioselective beta blocker, is less effective than the non-selective beta blocker propranolol in the management of essential tremor: S. Calzetti *et al.*, *J. Neurol. Neurosurg. Psychiat.*, 1982, *45*, 893.

For a comparison of propranolol with primidone in essential tremor and details of a combination regimen, see under Primidone, p.412.

WATER DRINKING, COMPULSIVE. The use of propranolol 960 mg daily to treat compulsive water drinking in a psychiatric patient.— S. Shevitz *et al.*, *J. nerv. ment. Dis.*, 1980, *168*, 246.

Preparations

Propranolol Hydrochloride Injection *(U.S.P.)*

Propranolol Hydrochloride Tablets *(U.S.P.)*

Propranolol Injection *(B.P.)*. A sterile solution of propranolol hydrochloride in Water for Injections containing citric acid or citric acid monohydrate.

Propranolol Tablets *(B.P.)*. Tablets containing propranolol hydrochloride.

Proprietary Preparations

Angilol *(DDSA Pharmaceuticals, UK). Tablets*, propranolol hydrochloride, 10, 40, 80, and 160 mg.

Apsolol *(Approved Prescription Services, UK). Tablets*, scored, propranolol hydrochloride 10, 40, 80, and 160 mg.

Berkolol *(Berk Pharmaceuticals, UK). Tablets*, scored, propranolol hydrochloride 10, 40, 80, and 160 mg.

Inderal *(ICI Pharmaceuticals, UK). Capsules* (Inderal LA), sustained-release, propranolol hydrochloride 160 mg.
Capsules (Half-Inderal LA), sustained-release, propranolol hydrochloride 80 mg.
Tablets, propranolol hydrochloride 10, 40, 80, and 160 mg.
Injection, propranolol hydrochloride 1 mg/mL, in ampoules of 1 mL.

Inderetic *(ICI Pharmaceuticals, UK). Capsules*, propranolol hydrochloride 80 mg, bendrofluazide 2.5 mg.

Inderex *(ICI Pharmaceuticals, UK). Capsules*, propranolol hydrochloride 160 mg (for sustained-release), bendrofluazide 5 mg.

Proprietary Names and Manufacturers

Angilol *(DDSA Pharmaceuticals, UK)*; Apsolol *(Approved Prescription Services, UK)*; Avlocardyl *(I.C.I.-Pharma, Fr.)*; Bedranol *(Lagap, Switz.; Lagap, UK)*; Beprane *(Riker, Fr.)*; Berkolol *(Berk Pharmaceuticals, UK)*; Beta-Neg *(Ital.)*; Bétaryl *(Nativelle, Fr.)*; Beta-Tablinen *(Beiersdorf, Ger.)*; Beta-Timelets *(Temmler, Ger.)*; Blocardyl *(Arg.)*; Cardinol *(Protea, Austral.)*; Cardispare *(Rolab, S.Afr.)*; Caridolol *(Jpn)*; Deralin *(Alphapharm, Austral.)*; Detensol *(Desbergers, Canad.)*; Dociton *(Rhein-Pharma, Ger.)*; Efektolol *(Efeka, Ger.)*; Elbrol *(Pfleger, Ger.)*; Euprovasin *(Magis, Ital.)*; Frekven *(Ferrosan, Denm.; Norw.; Ferrosan, Swed.)*; Herzul *(Jpn)*; Inderal *(ICI-Farma, Arg.; ICI, Austral.; Belg.; Ayerst, Canad.; ICI, Denm.; ICI-Pharma, Ital.; Jpn; Neth.; ICI, Norw.; ICI, S.Afr.; ICI, Swed.; ICI, Switz.; ICI Pharmaceuticals, UK; Ayerst, USA)*; Inderalici; Indobloc *(Degussa, Ger.)*; Kemi *(Jpn)*; Noloten *(Beta, Arg.)*; Novopranol *(Novopharm, Canad.)*; Oposim *(Arg.)*; Pranolol *(Apothekernes Laboratorium, Norw.)*; Prano-Puren *(Klinge-Nattermann, Ger.)*; Prolol *(USV, Austral.)*; Pronovan *(Nyco, Norw.)*; Propabbloc; *(Azuchemie, Ger.)*; Propalong *(Merck, Arg.)*; Propayerst *(Ayerst, Arg.)*; Propranur *(Henning Berlin, Ger.)*; Pur-Bloka *(Lennon, S.Afr.)*; Pylapron *Jpn)*; Rexigen *(Pharmador, S.Afr.)*; Sagittol *(Sagitta, Ger.)*; Sumial *(ICI, Spain)*; Tensiflex *(Bago, Arg.)*; Tesnol *(Jpn)*; *Tonum (Allergan, Ital.)*.

The following names have been used for multi-ingredient preparations containing propranolol hydrochloride— Inderetic *(ICI Pharmaceuticals, UK)*; Inderex *(ICI Pharmaceuticals, UK)*; Inderide *(Ayerst, Canad.; Ayerst, USA)*; Spiroprop *(Searle, UK)*.

6322-e

Sotalol Hydrochloride *(BANM, USAN, rINNM)*.

MJ-1999. 4′-(1-Hydroxy-2-isopropylaminoethyl)methanesulphonanilide hydrochloride.
$C_{12}H_{20}N_2O_3S,HCl=308.8$.

CAS — 3930-20-9 (sotalol); 959-24-0 (hydrochloride).

Adverse Effects, Treatment, and Precautions

As for Propranolol Hydrochloride, p.798.

EFFECTS ON THE HEART. Atypical ventricular tachycardia 'torsade de pointes' in a patient with chronic renal failure and hypertension was associated with administration of sotalol.— A. Kontopoulos *et al.*, *Postgrad. med. J.*, 1981, *57*, 321.

Prolonged Q-T_c intervals were seen in 29 patients taking sotalol 160 to 640 mg daily and were correlated with serum-sotalol concentrations. Since a prolonged Q-T_c interval is a risk factor for cardiac arrhythmia, ECG monitoring is recommended if sotalol is given to patients with renal insufficiency or is administered in high doses.— P. J. Neuvonen *et al.* (letter), *Lancet*, 1981, *2*, 426. See also J. K. McKibbin *et al.*, *Br. Heart J.*, 1984, *51*, 157 (syncope, prolonged QT interval and torsades de pointes).

Sustained torsades de pointes and ventricular tachycardia developed in a patient with normal renal function given sotalol 160 mg twice daily. The arrhythmogenic properties of sotalol are related to the class III antiarrhythmic properties which result in prolongation of the QT interval.— R. Krapf and M. Gertsch, *Br. med. J.*, 1985, *290*, 1784.

Severe bradycardia in an elderly patient who had apparently taken sotalol hydrochloride 560 mg.— K. Gupta, *Br. J. clin. Pract.*, 1985, *39*, 116.

EFFECTS ON THE SKIN. Cutaneous thickening in 6 hyperthyroid patients treated with radioactive iodine and beta-blockade might have been associated with the beta-blocking therapy with special reference to sotalol.— J. P. Michel *et al.* (letter), *Lancet*, 1979, *1*, 54.

FIBROSIS. A report of retroperitoneal fibrosis associated with the use of sotalol.— M. Laakso *et al.*, *Br. med. J.*, 1982, *285*, 1085.

INTERACTIONS. *Alcohol.* In a study of healthy subjects alcohol reduced the plasma clearance-rate of sotalol. The hypotensive effect of sotalol was increased.— E. A. Sotaniemi *et al.*, *Clin. Pharmac. Ther.*, 1981, *29*, 705.

Absorption and Fate

Sotalol is completely absorbed from the gastrointestinal tract and peak plasma concentrations are obtained about 2 or 3 hours after a dose. It is not metabolised and is excreted unchanged in the urine. It is not bound to plasma proteins. It crosses the placenta and is found in breast milk; however, only small amounts are reported to cross the blood-brain barrier and enter the CSF.

For a review including the pharmacokinetics of sotalol see B. N. Singh *et al., Drugs,* 1987, *34,* 311.

PREGNANCY AND THE NEONATE. The pharmacokinetics of sotalol in 6 healthy pregnant subjects. The systemic clearance of sotalol following an intravenous dose was significantly higher during pregnancy than in the postnatal period, and the mean elimination half-life shorter (6.6 versus 9.3 hours) although the latter difference was not significant. Clearance following an oral dose was also higher during pregnancy than afterwards, but half-lives (10.9 versus 10.3 hours) and mean bioavailability were similar. The changes were probably due to alterations in renal function in the antenatal period.— M. F. O'Hare *et al., Eur. J. clin. Pharmac.,* 1983, *24,* 521.

Uses and Administration

Sotalol hydrochloride is a beta blocker with general properties similar to those of propranolol (see p.803). It is classified as non-cardioselective and is reported to lack both intrinsic sympathomimetic and membrane stabilising properties.

When sotalol is given by mouth doses may be taken as a single daily dose, preferably on rising in the morning, or in divided doses.

In the treatment of hypertension sotalol hydrochloride is usually given in an initial dose of 160 mg daily increased at fortnightly intervals according to the response of the patient, to 600 mg or more daily. Doses of 4 g or more daily have occasionally been recorded.

The optimum dose for angina pectoris is also about 160 to 600 mg daily. For cardiac arrhythmias it has been given in doses of 120 to 240 mg daily, and similar doses may be given to reduce symptoms of sympathetic overactivity in hyperthyroidism.

For the emergency treatment of cardiac arrhythmias sotalol hydrochloride may be given by slow intravenous injection in a dose of 20 to 60 mg over 2 or 3 minutes, repeated if necessary after 10 minutes.

A dose of 320 mg has been given daily following myocardial infarction to prevent re-infarction.

Reduced doses may be required in renal impairment.

A review of sotalol.— B. N. Singh *et al. Drugs,* 1987, *34,* 311.

ACTION. A review of the classes of antiarrhythmic drug actions. Sotalol has been shown to have a greater anti-arrhythmic effect than can be attributed to its beta blocking (class II) actions alone which would accord with earlier results indicating an ability to delay repolarisation on acute administration (a class III property).— E. M. V. Williams, *J. clin. Pharmac.,* 1984, *24,* 129.

A comparison of the effects of (+)-sotalol and (±)-sotalol in 6 healthy subjects demonstrated that the beta-blocking activity resided almost entirely on the (−)-isomer, while the effects on the Q-T interval, which are consistent with type III anti-arrhythmic activity, appear to be due to both isomers. This would suggest that the electrophysiological effects of sotalol are unrelated to its beta-blocking properties.— G. D. Johnston *et al., Br. J. clin. Pharmac.,* 1985, *20,* 507.

ADMINISTRATION IN RENAL FAILURE. The pharmacokinetics of sotalol were studied in 4 healthy subjects and in 6 patients with end-stage renal failure. It was considered that reduced doses of sotalol should be used during maintenance treatment in patients with advanced renal failure and that haemodialysis over 6 to 7 hours would reduce plasma-sotalol concentrations by about 20%.— T. B. Tjandramaga *et al., Br. J. clin. Pharmac.,* 1976, *3,* 259.

Further references: G. Berglund *et al., Eur. J. clin. Pharmac.,* 1980, *18,* 321; A. D. Blair *et al., Clin Pharmac. Ther.,* 1981, *29,* 457; A. Kher *et al., Eur. J. clin. Pharmac.,* 1984, *27,* 361.

CARDIAC DISORDERS. A study of the effect of intravenous administration of sotalol 20 mg, at a rate of 1 mg per minute, in 20 patients with cardiac arrhythmias; a maximum of 3 doses could be given at intervals of 20 minutes (maximum cumulative dose 60 mg). A beneficial effect was noted in 2 of 2 patients with sinus tachycardia and 4 of 7 with other supraventricular tachycardias. Although beta-adrenoceptor blocking agents are not generally considered to be very effective in the treatment of ventricular arrhythmias, good results were obtained in 9 of 11 patients with lignocaine-resistant ventricular arrhythmias. Life-threatening bradycardia occurred in 2 patients.— Y. Latour *et al., Int. J. clin. Pharmac. Biopharm.,* 1977, *15,* 275.

A view that an intravenous dose of 10 to 20 mg of sotalol hydrochloride is only the initial starting dose, and that the range is up to 100 mg intravenously.— A. Simon (letter), *Lancet,* 1980, *1,* 1356. Refusal to recommend an intravenous dose of sotalol going up to 100 mg. Bearing in mind that the dose of sotalol is likely to be somewhat similar to practolol and that practolol may be less cardiodepressant, the dose should not exceed 20 mg except in an expert coronary care unit with full haemodynamic monitoring and facilities for coping with any untoward bradycardia.— L. H. Opie (letter), *ibid.*

Results in 16 patients suggesting that sotalol may be the drug of choice for patients with the Wolff-Parkinson-White syndrome.— K. -P. Kunze *et al., Circulation,* 1987, *75,* 1050.

Intravenous administration of sotalol 40 mg terminated combined atrial flutter/fibrillation and recurrent ventricular tachycardia in an 82-year-old patient with acute myocardial infarction.— D. R. Ramsdale and C. Peterson, *Postgrad. med. J.,* 1987, *63,* 579.

Myocardial infarction. In a multicentre study in 1456 patients who had survived myocardial infarction 873 were assigned to treatment with sotalol 320 mg daily while 583 received placebo; patients entered the study 5 to 14 days after infarction. The cumulative mortality-rate on 1-year follow-up was 7.3% in the group receiving sotalol which was less than the 8.9% in the placebo group but not significantly so. The difference in rates of confirmed re-infarction (3.3% in the sotalol group and 5.7% in controls) could be considered significant but the level of significance fell when unconfirmed re-infarctions were included. 25% of the patients randomised to sotalol and 21% of those randomised to placebo were withdrawn from the study during the 1-year follow-up; the excess of withdrawals in the sotalol group was due to hypotension, bradycardia, and other side-effects. Despite the lack of a significant difference in mortality it was concluded that the trial supported the results of other studies indicating a modest benefit of a 20 to 25% reduction in mortality from post-infarction beta blockade.— D. G. Julian *et al., Lancet,* 1982, *1,* 1142.

Sotalol 500 µg per kg body-weight intravenously over 15 minutes, followed by 600 µg per kg over 1 hour and then 200 µg per kg by continuous infusion for up to 12 hours had beneficial haemodynamic effects in 10 patients in the early stages of acute myocardial infarction compared with placebo in a further 10.— M. Åström *et al., Eur. Heart J.,* 1986, *7,* 931.

Proprietary Preparations

Beta-Cardone *(Duncan, Flockhart, UK). Tablets,* scored, sotalol hydrochloride 40, 80, and 200 mg.

Sotacor *(Bristol-Myers Pharmaceuticals, UK). Tablets,* sotalol hydrochloride 80 and 160 mg.
Injection, sotalol hydrochloride 10 mg/mL, in ampoules of 4 mL.

Sotazide *(Bristol-Myers Pharmaceuticals, UK). Tablets,* sotalol hydrochloride 160 mg, hydrochlorothiazide 25 mg. For hypertension. *Dose.* One or two tablets daily.

Tolerzide *(Bristol-Myers Pharmaceuticals, UK). Tablets,* sotalol hydrochloride 80 mg, hydrochlorothiazide 12.5 mg. For hypertension. *Dose.* One tablet daily.

Proprietary Names and Manufacturers

Beta-Cardone *(Duncan, Flockhart, UK)*; Betacardone *(Glaxo, Arg.)*; Betades *(Farmades, Ital.)*; Sotacor *(Astra, Austral.; Bristol, Canad.; Bristol-Myers, Denm.; Neth.; Bristol, S.Afr.; Bristol, Swed.; Bristol-Myers Pharmaceuticals, UK)*; Sotalex *(Allard, Fr.; Bristol, Ger.; Bristol Italiana Sud, Ital.; Bristol, Switz.)*; Sotapor *(Bristol-Myers, Spain)*.

1143-j

Tertatolol *(rINN).*

(±)-1-(*tert*-Butylamino)-3-(thiochroman-8-yloxy)propan-2-ol.
$C_{16}H_{25}NO_2S$=295.4.

CAS — 34784-64-0.

Tertatolol is a beta blocker with general properties similar to those of propranolol (see p.798). It is classified as non-cardioselective and is reported to lack intrinsic sympathomimetic activity. It has been investigated in the management of hypertension in single doses of 5 mg daily.

Proprietary Names and Manufacturers
Artex *(Servier, Fr.)*.

6323-l

Timolol Maleate *(BANM, USAN, rINNM).*

MK-950; Timololi Maleas. (*S*)-1-*tert*-Butylamino-3-(4-morpholino-1,2,5-thiadiazol-3-yloxy)propan-2-ol maleate.
$C_{13}H_{24}N_4O_3S,C_4H_4O_4$=432.5.

CAS — 26839-75-8 (timolol); 26921-17-5 (maleate).

Pharmacopoeias. In *Br., Neth.,* and *U.S.*

A white or almost white, odourless or almost odourless powder. **Soluble** 1 in 15 of water, 1 in 21 of alcohol, and 1 in 40 of chloroform; soluble in methyl alcohol; sparingly soluble in propylene glycol; practically insoluble in ether and in cyclohexane. A 2% solution in water has a pH of 3.8 to 4.3; the *B.P.* and *U.S.P.* specify that the ophthalmic preparations have a pH of 6.5 to 7.5. **Store** in well-closed containers. The *U.S.P.* specifies that the ophthalmic solution should be protected from light.

Adverse Effects, Treatment, and Precautions

As for Propranolol Hydrochloride, p.798.

Systemic side-effects have followed topical use of the eye-drops; mild local irritation and blurred vision have also been reported.

Reviews of systemic side-effects resulting from the ophthalmic administration of timolol: W. P. Munroe *et al., Drug Intell. & clin. Pharm.,* 1985, *19,* 85; W. L. Nelson *et al., Am. J. Ophthal.,* 1986, *102,* 606; F. T. Fraunfelder and S. M. Meyer, *Med. Toxicol.,* 1987, *2,* 287.

EFFECTS ON CARBOHYDRATE METABOLISM. Increased incidence of hypoglycaemic episodes in a diabetic woman was possibly related to the use of timolol eye-drops for glaucoma.— K. Angelo-Nielsen (letter), *J. Am. med. Ass.,* 1980, *244,* 2263. See also T. M. Velde and F. E. Kaiser, *Archs intern. Med.,* 1983, *143,* 1627.

EFFECTS ON THE CARDIOVASCULAR SYSTEM. Chronic congestive heart failure became more severe and bradycardia developed in a 72-year-old woman with severe rheumatic heart disease and atrial fibrillation after eye-drops containing timolol maleate 0.25% were substituted for her pilocarpine eye-drops.— N. A. Britman (letter), *New Engl. J. Med.,* 1979, *300,* 566.

Sinus arrest and junctional extrasystoles developed in a patient on long-term ocular timolol therapy; symptoms responded to withdrawal of timolol.— A. S. Treseder and T. P. L. Thomas, *Br. J. clin. Pract.,* 1986, *40,* 256.

Results of a study in patients given intravenous timolol, followed by oral dosage, after myocardial infarction showed that they had a significantly greater likelihood of developing a left ventricular thrombus than patients given placebo, probably because of the reduction in heart-rate and left ventricular apical wall motion induced by the beta blocker.— K. -A. Johannessen *et al., Circulation,* 1987, *75,* 151.

EFFECTS ON THE EYES. A report of dryness of the eyes in a man receiving timolol in doses up to 75 mg daily. His symptoms improved immediately on withdrawal of timolol.— M. A. Frais and T. J. Bayley, *Postgrad. med. J.,* 1979, *55,* 884.

A report of corneal anaesthesia in a patient receiving timolol eye-drops.— B. Calissendorff, *Acta Ophthalmol.,* 1981, *59,* 347.

EFFECTS ON MENTAL STATE. Hallucinations associated with the use of timolol for glaucoma.— D. Yates (letter), *J. Am. med. Ass.,* 1980, *244,* 768.

EFFECTS ON RESPIRATORY FUNCTION. Chronic but stable asthma in a 73-year-old woman was exacerbated and became uncontrollable after she started using timolol 0.5% eye-drops. The drops were withdrawn and pilocarpine substituted and within one week she was free of respiratory symptoms.— F. L. Jones and N. L. Ekberg (letter), *New Engl. J. Med.,* 1979, *301,* 270.

A report of life-threatening bradycardia, cyanosis, and respiratory distress associated with the instillation of timolol 0.25% eye-drops in an 18-month-old child.— T. Williams and W. H. Ginther (letter), *New Engl. J. Med.,* 1982, *306,* 1485.

At the time of writing, 16 fatal cases of status asthmaticus following ocular application of timolol in patients with a prior history of asthma or chronic lung disease had been reported in the *US.*— F. T. Fraunfelder and A. F. Barker (letter), *New Engl. J. Med.,* 1984, *311,* 1441.

Further reports of the adverse effects of timolol eye-drops on respiratory function: P. McGonigle and A. E.

Tribe (letter), *Med. J. Aust.*, 1985, *142*, 425; C. Botet *et al.* (letter), *Ann. intern. Med.*, 1986, *105*, 306.

Long-term beta blockade with oral timolol significantly reduced FEV_1 and peak expiratory flow-rate on 2-year follow-up involving 19 patients assigned to timolol therapy after myocardial infarction compared with 16 receiving placebo. The changes were clinically significant only in one patient, who was withdrawn from the study due to bronchial obstruction.— S. Johansen, *Eur. J. clin. Pharmac.*, 1985, *28*, 23.

EFFECTS ON SEXUAL FUNCTION. The National Registry of Drug-induced Ocular Side Effects at Oregon University had received more than 1700 case reports of adverse reactions following the topical use of timolol in the eye; 63% of these concerned systemic effects and they included 28 instances of sexual dysfunction in 25 patients, 2 of them female. Impotence was reported by 18 patients, decreased libido by 9, and decreased ejaculate volume by one. In most cases the symptoms were promptly reversed after timolol was discontinued.— F. T. Fraunfelder and S. M. Meyer (letter), *J. Am. med. Ass.*, 1985, *253*, 3092. Comment. The association remained uncertain.— I. M. Katz (letter), *ibid.*, 1986, *255*, 37.

FIBROSIS. It was considered that sclerosing peritonitis in a 50-year-old man might be associated with timolol therapy.— D. C. Baxter-Smith *et al.* (letter), *Lancet*, 1978, *2*, 149. Severe criticism; it is not considered that there is any objective evidence that this is a case of sclerosing peritonitis of the practolol type.— J. F. Nancarrow (letter), *ibid.*, 525.

A report of retroperitoneal fibrosis in a patient receiving oral timolol.— E. Rimmer *et al.* (letter), *Lancet*, 1983, *1*, 300.

INTERACTIONS. *Anti-arrhythmics*. A report of sinus bradycardia resulting from concomitant quinidine and timolol therapy, the latter as eye-drops, in an elderly patient.— Y. Dinai *et al.*, *Ann. intern. Med.*, 1985, *103*, 890.

Calcium channel blockers. For a report of an interaction between verapamil and timolol eye-drops see Verapamil, p.90.

Diuretics. A study in 6 healthy subjects indicated that timolol slightly ameliorated bendrofluazide-induced hypokalaemia. The interaction should be studied over prolonged periods and in disease states to establish whether it had clinical significance.— J. Hettiarachchi *et al.*, *Clin. Pharmac. Ther.*, 1977, *22*, 58.

For a report of dilutional hyponatraemia in a patient taking hydrochlorothiazide, amiloride, and timolol see under Chlorothiazide, p.982.

Sympathomimetics. Systemic hypertension and phaeochromocytoma-like symptoms developed in a patient receiving adrenaline eye-drops and timolol eye-drops as part of the therapy of open-angle glaucoma. Symptoms regressed when both eye-drops were withheld and recurred on their re-introduction. The patient was subsequently maintained on adrenaline but not timolol, without further incident.— G. T. Griffing *et al.* (letter), *New Engl. J. Med.*, 1982, *307*, 1344.

MYASTHENIA GRAVIS. Immediate deterioration in a patient with myasthenia following topical use of timolol for glaucoma.— S. A. Shaivitz (letter), *J. Am. med. Ass.*, 1979, *242*, 1611.

Further references: J. R. Coppeto, *Am. J. Ophthal.*, 1984, *98*, 244; A. Verkijk, *Ann. Neurol.*, 1985, *17*, 211.

Absorption and Fate

Timolol is almost completely absorbed from the gastro-intestinal tract but is subject to moderate first-pass metabolism. Peak plasma concentrations occur about 1 to 2 hours after a dose. It is extensively metabolised in the liver, the metabolites being excreted in the urine together with some unchanged timolol. It crosses the placenta and appears in breast milk. Protein binding is reported to be low.

Some timolol is absorbed systemically following instillation of the eye-drops.

Differing estimations of the half-life of timolol: D. J. Tocco *et al.*, *J. pharm. Sci.*, 1975, *64*, 1879 (3 hours); *idem*, *Drug Metab. & Disposit.*, 1975, *3*, 361 (4.5 hours); P. Vermeij *et al.*, *J. Pharm. Pharmac.*, 1978, *30*, 53 (about 2.5 hours); O. F. Else *et al.*, *Eur. J. clin. Pharmac.*, 1978, *14*, 431 (about 4.5 to 5 hours); T. Ishizaki and K. Tawara, *Eur. J. clin. Pharmac.*, 1978, *14*, 7 (about 2.8 hours).

A study in 6 poor metabolisers and 6 extensive metabolisers of debrisoquine indicated that the metabolism of timolol also exhibited genetic polymorphism. Following single doses of 20 mg of timolol by mouth the mean peak plasma concentration in poor metabolisers was 113.8 ng per mL whereas in the extensive metabolisers it was 60.7 ng per mL; 24 hours after the dose the mean plasma concentration was still 11.3 ng per mL in poor metabolisers whereas in extensive metabolisers it was indetectable. The calculated half-lives in the 2 groups were 7.5 hours and 3.7 hours respectively. Oral clearance, a measure of drug metabolising ability, was four times lower in poor than in extensive metabolisers; there was no significant difference in renal clearance. Reduction in exercise tachycardia was similar in both groups at 4 hours but was significantly greater in the poor metabolisers at 12 and 24 hours, suggesting that in this group twice daily dosage may be unnecessary.— J. C. McGourty *et al.*, *Clin. Pharmac. Ther.*, 1985, *38*, 409. See also R. V. Lewis *et al.*, *Br. J. clin. Pharmac.*, 1985, *19*, 329.

Studies of the penetration of timolol eye-drops into aqueous humour: C. I. Phillips *et al.*, *Br. J. Ophthal.*, 1981, *65*, 593; C. I. Phillips *et al.*, *ibid.*, 1985, *69*, 217.

PREGNANCY AND THE NEONATE. *Lactation*. Concentrations of timolol in breast milk were approximately six times greater than those in serum, the values being 5.6 and 0.93 ng per mL respectively, following instillation of timolol 0.5% eye-drops twice daily in a lactating woman. In view of this active secretion into the milk timolol may be contra-indicated in breast-feeding mothers.— J. S. Lustgarten and S. M. Podos, *Archs Ophthal., N.Y.*, 1983, *101*, 1381.

Uses and Administration

Timolol maleate is a hydrophilic beta blocker with general properties similar to those of propranolol (see p.803). It is classified as non-cardioselective and is reported to be effectively lacking in intrinsic sympathomimetic and membrane stabilising activity.

In the treatment of hypertension timolol maleate is usually given in initial doses of 5 to 10 mg twice daily, increased according to response at intervals of 3 to 7 days; usual maintenance doses are 10 to 30 mg daily in single or divided doses, but doses up to 60 mg daily may be required in some patients.

In angina pectoris most patients respond to 35 to 45 mg daily in divided doses; an initial dose of 5 mg two or three times daily has been recommended, increased at intervals of 3 or more days by no more than 10 mg daily initially and 15 mg daily subsequently, in divided doses.

Timolol maleate is also used in patients who have had a myocardial infarction to reduce the risk of mortality and re-infarction. Dosage has been recommended to begin with 5 mg twice daily for 2 days, increased subsequently in the absence of any contra-indicating adverse effects, to 10 mg twice daily.

Eye-drops containing timolol maleate 0.25 and 0.5% are instilled twice daily in the treatment of open-angle glaucoma. Once-daily instillation may suffice when the glaucoma has been controlled.

Doses of 10 to 20 mg daily of timolol maleate are used in the prophylaxis of migraine.

Reduced doses may be required in renal impairment.

ADMINISTRATION IN RENAL FAILURE. The mean half-life of timolol in patients with chronic renal disease was not significantly different from that of control subjects. Timolol was not significantly dialysable in patients undergoing dialysis, but 2 experienced haemodynamic complications during the haemodialysis procedure.— J. M. Pitone *et al.*, *Clin. Pharmac. Ther.*, 1977, *21*, 114.

CARDIAC DISORDERS. *Cardiac arrhythmias*. The use of oral timolol in reducing the incidence of atrial arrhythmias after coronary bypass surgery.— R. J. Vecht *et al.*, *Int. J. Cardiol.*, 1986, *13*, 125.

Myocardial infarction. Results of a multicentre double-blind randomised study involving 1884 patients suggesting that long-term treatment with timolol 10 mg twice daily started 7 to 28 days after myocardial infarction reduces mortality and the rate of reinfarction.—The Norwegian Multicenter Study Group, *New Engl. J. Med.*, 1981, *304*, 801. Six-year follow-up of the original study. The cumulative mortality-rates 72 months after assignment were 26.4% among patients receiving timolol, compared with 32.3% in the placebo group, representing a significant relative difference in mortality of 18.3%. These results indicate that the benefits of beta blockade after myocardial infarction are maintained over long-term administration.— T. R. Pedersen, *ibid.*, 1985, *313*, 1055. Criticism of the conclusion.— E. Y. Bellin (letter), *ibid.*, 1986, *314*, 1052. Reply.— T. R. Pedersen (letter), *ibid.*

Beneficial results following the early administration of timolol in a double-blind multicentre study of 144 patients with suspected first myocardial infarction. Patients were randomly assigned to timolol or placebo and treatment started within 5 hours of the onset of symptoms. Timolol maleate 1 mg was given by intravenous injection, repeated after 10 minutes, and followed by a constant infusion of timolol 600 µg per hour for 24 hours. Treatment was then continued with timolol 10 mg twice daily by mouth for the duration of the hospital stay. There was a significant reduction in myocardial ischaemia and ultimate infarct size as assessed by continuous vectorcardiography and creatine kinase release in the timolol group; analgesic requirements were also reduced.—The International Collaborative Study Group, *New Engl. J. Med.*, 1984, *310*, 9.

GLAUCOMA. A discussion of beta blockers in the treatment of chronic simple glaucoma. The hypotensive effect of timolol 0.25% given twice daily compares favourably with that of pilocarpine or adrenaline, while addition to pilocarpine or acetazolamide therapy further lowers intra-ocular pressure. Long-term studies have shown that the hypotensive effect is maintained for years, although some patients develop tolerance with a reduction in effect of up to 25% after one or more months of use. The advent of timolol has represented a major advance in the management of chronic simple glaucoma.— R. A. Hitchings, *Br. med. J.*, 1982, *285*, 84.

Further discussions of the management of glaucoma including the role of timolol: *Drug & Ther. Bull.*, 1983, *21*, 85; R. A. Hitchings, *Prescribers' J.*, 1983, *23*, 106.

In a 12-month double-blind study of 30 patients with open-angle glaucoma topical timolol 0.25% and timolol 0.5% showed little difference in effectiveness at controlling intra-ocular pressure. In one patient the intra-ocular pressure rose immediately after instillation of timolol 0.25% so therapy was discontinued. Eight patients in whom intra-ocular pressure was initially controlled by timolol subsequently required further anti-glaucoma medication to maintain their intra-ocular pressure below 22 mmHg, thus confirming the existence of the long-term loss of control which can occur with continuous topical timolol. It was suggested that timolol 0.25% should be the initial treatment of choice and if this proves ineffective alternative or additive anti-glaucoma therapy should be considered in preference to increasing the concentration of timolol to 0.5%.— K. B. Mills, *Br. J. Ophthal.*, 1983, *67*, 216.

A 200-week multicentre study in 117 glaucomatous patients confirmed the long-term efficacy of topical timolol maleate. The drug maintained intra-ocular pressure below 22 mmHg in 137 of 227 eyes throughout the study.— R. P. LeBlanc *et al.*, *Can. J. Ophthal.*, 1985, *20*, 128.

Closed-angle glaucoma. Studies on the use of timolol eye-drops in closed-angle glaucoma.— P. J. Airaksinen *et al.*, *Br. J. Ophthal.*, 1979, *63*, 822; C. I. Phillips, *ibid.*, 1980, *64*, 240.

HYPERTENSION. A brief review of the use of timolol as an antihypertensive agent.— *Med. Lett.*, 1982, *24*, 44.

An open multicentre general practice study of the benefits of therapy with timolol 10 mg twice daily for 1 month. The study involved 5190 hypertensive patients; 1057 patients failed to complete the study, 28% of them because of adverse effects. The mean reduction in blood pressure after 1 month was 20/13 mmHg; reduction was greater in patients with moderate or severe hypertension than in those with mild hypertension. The hypotensive effects were less marked in black or elderly patients. The majority of patients continued to receive timolol alone or in combination with another agent after the study was completed. During the study 22% of all patients experienced adverse effects of which the most frequent were fatigue, dizziness, and nausea. It was concluded that timolol is a well-tolerated and effective antihypertensive agent in a broad range of patients.— J. A. Bannon *et al.*, *Archs intern. Med.*, 1986, *146*, 654.

Post-marketing surveillance by the manufacturers in 11 685 patients given a proprietary combination of timolol 10 mg with bendrofluazide 2.5 mg for mild to moderate hypertension indicated that adequate control of blood pressure could be achieved in 61% of patients with this dose once daily. A further 29% required 2 tablets daily. Of the patients enrolled, 3033 were withdrawn, 1805 because of adverse effects. The results show combined timolol and bendrofluazide to be a highly effective treatment for hypertension which offers the possibility of control with a single daily dose in 90% of patients.— B. T. Marsh *et al.*, *J. int. med. Res.*, 1987, *15*, 106.

MIGRAINE. In a double-blind crossover study in 94 patients timolol maleate 10 mg twice daily for 4 weeks, increased if necessary to 10 mg in the morning and 20 mg in the evening for a further 4 weeks, was compared with placebo in the prophylaxis of migraine attacks. All patients were experiencing at least 3 headaches per month on entry into the study (mean 6.8); there was a mean decrease of 2.5 attacks per month with timolol therapy compared with 1.8 with placebo, a significant difference. Overall, 65% of the patients were characterised as responding to timolol, whereas only 40% responded to placebo. An increase from the initial dosage was required in 49% of patients while receiving timolol.— S. Stellar *et al.*, *J. Am. med. Ass.*, 1984, *252*, 2576.

Preparations

Timolol Eye Drops *(B.P.)*. Timolol Maleate Eye Drops. A sterile aqueous solution of timolol maleate.

Timolol Tablets *(B.P.)*. Timolol Maleate Tablets

Timolol Maleate Ophthalmic Solution *(U.S.P.)*. A sterile aqueous solution of timolol maleate. The strength is expressed in terms of timolol.

Timolol Maleate Tablets *(U.S.P.)*

Timolol Maleate and Hydrochlorothiazide Tablets *(U.S.P.)*

Proprietary Preparations

Betim *(Leo, UK)*. *Tablets*, scored, timolol maleate 10 mg.

Blocadren *(Merck Sharp & Dohme, UK)*. *Tablets*, scored, timolol maleate 10 mg.

Moducren *(Morson, UK)*. *Tablets*, scored, timolol maleate 10 mg, hydrochlorothiazide 25 mg, amiloride hydrochloride 2.5 mg. For hypertension. *Dose*. 1 or 2 tablets daily.

Prestim *(Leo, UK)*. *Tablets*, scored, timolol maleate 10 mg, bendrofluazide 2.5 mg.
Tablets (Prestim Forte), scored, timolol maleate 20 mg, bendrofluazide 5 mg. For hypertension. *Dose*. One to four Prestim tablets, or half to 2 tablets of Prestim Forte, daily.

Timoptol *(Merck Sharp & Dohme, UK)*. *Eye-drops*, timolol 0.25 and 0.5% (as maleate).

Proprietary Names and Manufacturers

Betim *(Denm.; Neth.; Leo, Norw.; Lövens, Swed.; Leo, (UK)*; Blocadren *(Frosst, Austral.; Belg.; Frosst, Canad.; Merck Sharp & Dohme, Ital.; Neth.; Merck Sharp & Dohme, Norw.; Merck Sharp & Dohme, S.Afr.; Spain; MSD, Swed.; Merck Sharp & Dohme, Switz.; Merck Sharp & Dohme, UK; Merck Sharp & Dohme, USA)*; Blocanol *(Fin.)*; Cusimolol *(Cusi, Spain)*; Oftan-Timolol *(NAF, Norw.)*; Proflax *(Merck Sharp & Dohme, Arg.)*; Temserin *(Frosst, Ger.; Greece)*; Tenopt *(Sigma, Austral.)*; Timacor *(Denm.; Merck Sharp & Dohme-Chibret, Fr.)*; Timoptic *(Merck Sharp & Dohme, Canad.; Chibret, Switz.; Merck Sharp & Dohme, USA)*; Timoptol *(Frosst, Austral.; Merck Sharp & Dohme-Chibret, Fr.; Chibret, Ger.; Merck Sharp & Dohme, Ital.; Neth.; NZ; S.Afr.; Merck Sharp & Dohme, UK)*.

The following names have been used for multi-ingredient preparations containing timolol maleate— Moducren *(Morson, UK)*; Prestim *(Leo, UK)*; Prestim Forte *(Leo, UK)*; Timolide *(Frosst, Canad.; Merck Sharp & Dohme, USA)*.

Blood Products and Substitutes

1210-s

Blood is a complex fluid with many functions including the maintenance of hydration of the tissues, maintenance of body temperature, and the transport within the body of gases, ions, nutrients, hormones, enzymes, antibodies, waste products of metabolism, and drugs.
This section is chiefly concerned with the use of blood, or blood products, in the prevention or treatment of disease and also covers other agents used as substitutes for blood products.

Blood Groups
The chief blood group systems are the ABO system and the Rhesus system.
In simple terms red blood cells carry on their surface genetically determined antigens. A person with antigen A, B, A plus B, or neither is classified as group A, B, AB, or O respectively. Such persons will have, in their serum, antibodies to B, A, neither, or both respectively—anti-B(β), anti-A(α), or anti-B plus anti-A ($\alpha + \beta$). Administration of blood containing red cells from a person of group A to a person with anti-A results in agglutination or possibly haemolysis. For the determination of the ABO group the agglutinogens of the red cells and the agglutinins of the serum are determined by testing against known standards.
In the Rhesus system many persons carry an antigen (Rh-positive) which stimulates antibody formation in Rh-negative persons; subsequent exposure to Rh-positive blood causes haemolysis.
Many variants of these systems, and other systems, are recognised.

Blood-clotting Factors
Roman numerals are used for the designation of those factors which are sufficiently defined as distinct entities by physio-pathological, physical, biochemical, and chemical properties; if considered desirable, a synonymous descriptive term can be used in parentheses following the Roman numeral. The following are the principal terms used:
Factor I (Fibrinogen)
Factor II (Prothrombin)
Factor III (Thromboplastin)
Factor IV (Calcium)
Factor V (Ac-globulin; Labile factor)
Factor VI (Unassigned)
Factor VII (Proconvertin; SPCA)
Factor VIII (Antihaemophilic factor; AHF)
Factor IX (Plasma thromboplastin component; PTC; Christmas factor)
Factor X (Stuart factor)
Factor XI (Plasma thromboplastin antecedent; PTA)
Factor XII (Hageman factor)
Factor XIII (Fibrin stabilising factor; FSF)
The letter 'a' after a factor name denotes the activated form. A number of other factors are also involved in blood clotting.
Hereditary deficiency of all the clotting factors (other than calcium and thromboplastin) has been described; the most important are deficiency of factor VIII causing haemophilia A and von Willebrand's disease, and deficiency of factor IX causing haemophilia B or Christmas disease. Vitamin K deficiency, treatment with anticoagulants, or liver disease may reduce the concentrations of the vitamin K-dependent factors II, VII, IX, and X.

Transmission of Infections
The use of blood, blood components, or blood products has been associated with the transmission of viruses, most notably transmission of the hepatitis B virus and the human immunodeficiency virus (HIV), leading in some cases to the subsequent development of the acquired immunodeficiency syndrome (AIDS); other reports of transmission include cytomegalovirus, non-A non-B hepatitis, and malaria. In many countries strenuous efforts have been made and continue to be made to screen donor material and to employ improved manufacturing methods with the aim of inactivating any micro-organisms present.

1215-j

Albumin

Albumin Solution (*B.P.*) (Albumin; Human Albumin; Human Albumin Solution (*Eur. P.*); Albumini Humani Solutio) is an aqueous solution of protein obtained from plasma or serum or from normal placentae frozen immediately after collection. The plasma, serum, or placentae are obtained from healthy donors who must, as far as can be ascertained, be free from detectable agents of infection transmissable by transfusion of blood or blood derivatives. It is prepared as a concentrated solution containing 15 to 25% of total protein or as an isotonic solution containing 4 to 5% of total protein; not less than 95% of the total protein is albumin. A suitable stabiliser, such as sodium caprylate, may be added but no antimicrobial preservative is added. It contains not more than 160 mmol of sodium per litre. The solution is sterilised by filtration and distributed aseptically into containers which are sealed to exclude micro-organisms and maintained at 59.5° to 60.5° for 10 hours. Finally, the containers are incubated for not less than 14 days at 30° to 32° or for not less than 4 weeks at 20° to 25° and examined visually for signs of microbial contamination. It should be stored at 2° to 25° and be protected from light.
Albumin Human (*U.S.P.*) is a sterile preparation, suitable for intravenous use, of serum albumin obtained by fractionating material (blood, plasma, serum, or placentas) from healthy human donors. It contains 4, 5, 20, or 25% of serum albumin and not less than 96% of the total protein is albumin. It may contain sodium acetyltryptophanate with or without sodium caprylate as a stabilising agent; it contains no added antimicrobial agent. It contains 130 to 160 mmol of sodium per litre.

Adverse Effects and Precautions
Albumin is a normal constituent of the blood and toxic effects are rare; urticaria, chills, and fever may occur. However, injection solutions containing 15 to 25% of albumin are hyperosmotic and should not be given to dehydrated patients unless additional fluid is given by mouth or by parenteral infusion.
Concentrated solutions are contra-indicated in patients with severe heart failure and should be given with caution in patients with diminished cardiac reserve because of circulatory overload and pulmonary oedema.

ALLERGY. There were 7 anaphylactic reactions in 60 048 infusions of human albumin.— J. Ring and K. Messmer, *Lancet*, 1977, *1*, 466.

ALUMINIUM TOXICITY. Aluminium was present in concentrations ranging from 0.064 to 2.570 mg per litre in 59 samples of proprietary human albumin solutions, from 5 different manufacturers. Following administration of albumin solutions on 2 occasions to a patient with stable renal function undergoing plasma exchange, urinary aluminium excretion was markedly elevated on the day of the exchange and fell slowly thereafter, remaining substantially above normal on the third day after the exchange. In view of the potential for aluminium toxicity, caution is warranted when albumin is infused repeatedly, particularly in patients with renal insufficiency; in such patients, plasma-aluminium concentrations should be monitored regularly.— D. S. Milliner *et al.*, *New Engl. J. Med.*, 1985, *312*, 165. See also: E. R. Maher *et al.*, *Br. med. J.*, 1986, *292*, 306.
Aluminium bone disease in patients receiving plasma exchange with contaminated albumin.— D. Maharaj *et al.*, *Br. med. J.*, 1987, *295*, 693. Comment that manufacturing processes are to be modified with the prospect of reducing substantially the level of aluminium and other metal ion contaminants in albumin products.— B. Cuthbertson *et al.* (letter), *ibid.*, 1062.

Uses and Administration
Albumin forms about 55% of the plasma proteins and provides most of the osmotic pressure of plasma. It has a low molecular weight (about 69 000) and is small enough to be excreted in the urine in nephrosis.
Albumin is administered intravenously as a 20% to 25% solution to replace protein lost in conditions such as the nephrotic syndrome and to compensate for reduced protein synthesis in cirrhosis of the liver. Doses vary according to the type of hypoalbuminaemic state present but are generally in the range of 100 to 400 mL for adults.
A 5% solution is approximately iso-osmotic with serum and may be administered intravenously for volume replacement in hypovolaemic shock associated with injury, surgery, or burns. The usual dose for adults is in the range of 200 to 800 mL although doses of up to 1600 mL may be necessary in burns. The 20% or 25% solution may be diluted with a suitable solution. If shock is associated with a loss of fluid to the extravascular component the use of a 20% solution in doses of 50 to 200 mL is recommended.

Proprietary Preparations
Albuminar *(Armour, UK). Infusion* (Albuminar 5), albumin 5%.
Infusion (Albuminar 20), albumin 20%.
Infusion (Albuminar 25), albumin 25%.
Human Albumin 20% *(Immuno, UK). Infusion*, albumin 20%.

Albumin is also available from *Blood Products Laboratory, UK.*

Proprietary Names and Manufacturers
Albuconn *(Cryosan, USA)*; Albuman *(Berna, Ital.)*; Albuminar *(Rorer, Ital.; Armour, UK)*; Albumisol *(USA)*; Albuspan *(USA)*; Albutein *(Alpha Therapeutic, USA)*; Buminate *(Hyland, USA)*; Buminate 20% *(Travenol, UK)*; Endalbumin *(Ismunit, Ital.)*; Haimaserum *(Aima, Ital.)*; Plasbumin *(Cutter, USA)*; Rhodalbumin *(Institut Merieux, Ger.)*; Rhodialbumin *(Rhone-Poulenc, Denm.; Rhône-Poulenc, Norw.; Rhone-Poulenc, Swed.)*; Seralbuman *(ISI, Ital.)*.
Manufacturers also include—*Commonwealth Serum Laboratories, Austral.; Connaught, Canad.; Behringwerke, Denm.; Nordisk Gentofte, Denm.; Behringwerke, Ger.; Biagini, Ital.; Immuno, Ital.; ISM, Ital.; Istituto Behring, Ital.; Merieux, Ital.; Pierrel, Ital.; Sclavo, Ital.; Travenol, Ital.; Immuno, Switz.; Merieux, Switz.; Immuno, UK; KabiVitrum, UK.*

1234-k

Anti-D Immunoglobulins

Anti-D (Rh_o) Immunoglobulin (*B.P.*) (Anti-D (Rh_o) Immunoglobulin Injection; Human Anti-D Immunoglobulin (*Eur. P.*); Immunoglobulinum Humanum Anti-D) is a liquid or freeze-dried preparation containing immunoglobulins, mainly immunoglobulin G (IgG). It is obtained from plasma or serum from D-negative donors who have been immunised against the rhesus D-antigen. It contains specific antibodies against the rhesus D-antigen of human red blood cells and may also contain small quantities of other blood group antibodies, such as anti-C, anti-E, anti-A, and anti-B. Normal Immunoglobulin may be added. Anti-D (Rh_o) Immunoglobulin is prepared in the same manner as Normal Immunoglobulin (see p.1170) except that the pooled material may be from fewer than 1000 donors. The liquid preparation should be stored, protected from light, in a sealed, colourless, glass container at a temperature of 2° to 8°. Under these conditions it may be expected to retain its potency for 3 years. The freeze-dried preparation should be stored, protected from light, under vacuum or under an inert gas; the *B.P.* specifies storage at a temperature of 2° to 8° whereas the *Eur. P.* specifies a temperature not exceeding 25°. Under these conditions it may be expected to retain its potency for 5 years.

Rh_0 (D) Immune Globulin (*U.S.P.*) is a sterile solution of globulins derived from human plasma containing antibody to the erythrocyte factor Rh_0 (D). It contains 10 to 18% of protein of which not less than 90% is gamma globulin. It contains glycine as a stabilising agent, and a suitable preservative. It should be stored at 2° to 8°.

Units

300 units of anti-D immunoglobulin, human are contained in 14.76 mg of human immunoglobulin (60 μg of anti-D immunoglobulin) in one ampoule of the first International Reference Preparation (1976).

Adverse Effects and Precautions

As for immunoglobulins in general, p.1155.

Anti-D immunoglobulin should be administered with caution to rhesus-positive persons for the treatment of blood disorders as it may cause haemolysis.

Uses and Administration

Anti-D immunoglobulin is used to prevent a rhesus-negative mother actively forming antibodies to foetal rhesus-positive red blood cells that may pass into the maternal circulation during childbirth, abortion, or certain other sensitising events. In subsequent rhesus-positive pregnancies these antibodies could produce haemolytic disease of the newborn. The injection of anti-D immunoglobulin is not effective once the mother has formed anti-D antibodies.

Anti-D immunoglobulin should always be given to rhesus-negative mothers with no anti-D antibodies in their serum and who have delivered rhesus-positive infants. It should be given intramuscularly as soon as possible after delivery in a dose of 500 units (100 μg) although a higher dose may be required depending on the amount of transplacental bleeding as assessed by the Kleihauer test. The dose should be given within 72 hours of delivery.

Rhesus-negative women having spontaneous or induced abortions should be given 250 units (50 μg) if the duration of pregnancy is 20 weeks or less; if the pregnancy is more advanced 500 units (100 μg) should be given.

There is also a risk of sensitisation during pregnancy from threatened abortion, amniocentesis, or external version. Any rhesus-negative woman at risk of transplacental haemorrhage during pregnancy and not known to be sensitised should be given 250 to 500 units (50 to 100 μg) of anti-D immunoglobulin depending upon the stage of pregnancy.

Anti-D immunoglobulin is also given after the transfusion of Rh-incompatible blood.

APLASTIC ANAEMIA. Response on 2 occasions of a rhesus-positive woman with aplastic anaemia and haemorrhagic symptoms due to thrombocytopenia to infusion of anti-D immunoglobulin; 2 μg per kg body-weight in 60 mL of sodium chloride was infused over 2 hours and given at intervals of 8 days. Therapy with corticosteroids, oxymetholone, and blood products had not been successful.— E. Rewald (letter), *Lancet*, 1987, *2*, 795.

BLOOD TRANSFUSION. Anti-D immunoglobulin failed to prevent rhesus immunisation when 3 mg was administered to a 29-year-old Rh-negative woman 24 hours after she was transfused with 1000 mL of Rh-positive blood. Subsequently anti-D immunoglobulin 8.4 mg by intramuscular injection over days 5 to 7 brought the total dose administered to 22.8 μg per mL Rh-positive red blood cells. It was recommended that Rh-negative patients given Rh-positive blood should immediately be given intramuscular anti-D immunoglobulin in divided doses until the total exceeds 20 μg per mL Rh-positive red blood cells within 72 hours. Anti-D titres should be monitored and if the titre at 6 months or later is greater than that at 1 month, active immunisation has occurred.— D. W. Branch *et al.* (letter), *Lancet*, 1985, *1*, 393.

HAEMOLYTIC DISEASE OF THE NEWBORN. A review and discussion of anti-D immunoglobulin prophylaxis. When an Rh(D)-negative woman bears an Rh(D)-positive foetus, the foetal red cells leaking into the maternal circulation may stimulate the production of anti-D antibody by the mother (iso-immunisation). This leak is greatest during delivery, so that the first child of a susceptible woman is unlikely to be affected by rhesus haemolytic disease. However, if the mother is sensitised, the anti-D antibody will cross into the foetal circulation in subsequent pregnancies, destroying foetal Rh(D)-positive cells and causing haemolytic disease.

Postnatal prophylaxis with anti-D immunoglobulin is not controversial and should always be given to an Rh-negative mother after delivery of an Rh-positive child; prophylaxis should also be given in similar circumstances after abortion or stillbirth. Anti-D immunoglobulin should be given in a dose of 250 units if before 20 weeks of gestation or 500 units if after 20 weeks and as soon as possible after delivery, certainly within 72 hours; a Kleihauer test, which is a measure of the number of foetal red cells in the maternal circulation and thus an indicator of the severity of the foeto-maternal transfusion, should be performed, and if raised the dose of immunoglobulin may be increased to a maximum of 2000 units daily.

Significant foeto-maternal transfusion may also occur antenatally during procedures such as amniocentesis or external cephalic version and prophylaxis should also be given, if indicated, at these times.

Some Rh(D)-negative women develop antibody during their first Rh(D)-positive pregnancy well before delivery and sensitisation may be avoided by giving anti-D immunoglobulin at 28 and 34 weeks of the pregnancy. As the immunoglobulin is scarce and expensive antenatal prophylaxis is best reserved for Rh(D)-negative mothers with no living children.— *Drug & Ther. Bull.*, 1985, *23*, 93. See also: S. J. Urbaniak, *Br. med. J.*, 1985, *291*, 4.

A study indicating that an antenatal regimen of anti-D immunoglobulin administration results in significant reduction in the incidence of Rh sensitisation. A control group of 2000 Rh(D)-negative primigravidas who gave birth to Rh(D)-positive infants in 1978–79 and who, in accordance with standard practice, had each received 100 μg anti-D immunoglobulin after delivery if the Kleihauer count was normal and higher doses for high foetal bleeds, was compared with a trial group of 2069 similar women having their first pregnancy in 1980–81. The trial women were given doses of anti-D immunoglobulin 100 μg at 28 and 34 weeks' gestation, a further dose of anti-D was given at delivery if the infant was Rh(D)-positive by the same criteria as for the control group. Two women in the trial group became actively immunised during the first pregnancy compared with 18 in the control group. Of 325 women in the trial group who had a further Rh(D)-positive pregnancy anti-D antibodies developed in 2 compared with a further 11 (making a total of 29) in 582 subsequent pregnancies in the control group. The reduction in the incidence of sensitisation was significant.— L. A. D. Tovey *et al.*, *Lancet*, 1983, *2*, 244.

A study indicating that the risk of iso-immunisation in Rh-negative women undergoing amniocentesis is small and the opinion that antenatal administration of anti-D immunoglobulin at amniocentesis is not warranted.— A. Tabor *et al.*, *Br. med. J.*, 1986, *293*, 533.

Discussion of the incidence of sensitisation and the need for anti-D immunoglobulin after early spontaneous or therapeutic abortion: M. Contreras *et al.* (letter), *Br. med. J.*, 1986, *293*, 1373; R. M. Hussey (letter), *ibid.*, 1987, *294*, 119; L. A. D. Tovey (letter), *ibid.*, 508.

Results of a survey of the reported management of threatened miscarriage by general practitioners highlighting differing policies in the use of anti-D immunoglobulin and calling for authoritative guidelines advising whether anti-D immunoglobulin should be given to women threatening to miscarry or to those who have miscarried.— C. Everett *et al.*, *Br. med. J.*, 1987, *295*, 583. A comment that clear-cut authoritative guidelines have been published in Great Britain (*Haemolytic disease of the newborn*, London, HMSO, 1976; Addendum 1981). All Rh(D)-negative women should receive anti-D immunoglobulin in a dose of 500 units (100 μg) for deliveries after 20 weeks and 250 units (50 μg) for deliveries before 20 weeks and for sensitising episodes. The dose should be given within 72 hours of delivery (unless the baby is known to be Rh(D)-negative), after abortion at whatever stage of pregnancy, and after every sensitising episode during pregnancy. Sensitising episodes include threatened abortion, antepartum haemorrhage, version, amniocentesis, and abdominal injuries. It is also recommended that the Kleihauer test be used to estimate the size of foetal bleed and that larger doses of anti-D immunoglobulin be administered if the situation merits it. If these guidelines are overlooked, as the survey suggests, a further reduction in the incidence of haemolytic disease of the newborn cannot be expected.— C. C. Entwhistle *et al.*, *ibid.*, 998.

THROMBOCYTOPENIA. Although normal immunoglobulin is established as a mode of therapy for immune thrombocytopenic purpura, some workers have also reported beneficial results with anti-D immunoglobulin. Treatment of an Rh(D)-positive patient with a long history of severe immune thrombocytopenic purpura and an associated cephalic haematoma with a single dose of 500 units (100 μg) of anti-D immunoglobulin intravenously was reported to result in a steady rise in platelet count and rapid resolution of haematoma (T.P. Baglin *et al.*, *Lancet*, 1986, *1*, 1329) although other investigators (M. Contreras and P.L. Mollison, *Lancet*, 1986, *2*, 49) considered that the improvement observed in the patient was unlikely to have been due to the low dose of immunoglobulin used and further considered that the use of anti-D immunoglobulin, a scarce material, in such circumstances was not justified. Further beneficial results in both rhesus-positive and rhesus-negative patients were reported (J.M. Durand *et al.*, *Lancet*, 1986, *2*, 49; R. Biniek *et al.*, *ibid.*, 627; P. Bierling *et al.*, *Ann. intern. Med.*, 1987, *106*, 773) and in some of these patients the immune thrombocytopenic purpura was associated with HIV-infection or AIDS; in these reports, however, much higher doses in the order of 1 to 3 mg daily were given intravenously.

Proprietary Names and Manufacturers

Beriglobina Anti D *(Behring, Spain)*; Gamma-Men *(ISM, Ital.)*; Gamulin Rh *(Armour, USA)*; Haima-D *(Aima, Ital.)*; HypRho-D *(Tropon-Cutter, Ger.*; *Cutter, USA)*; Immunorho *(ISI, Ital.)*; Inmunogamma Anti-D *(Leti, Spain)*; MICRhoGAM *(Ortho Diagnostic, USA)*; Mini-Gamulin Rh *(Armour, USA)*; Partobulin *(Immuno, Ger.*; *Immuno, Ital.)*; Partobulina *(Landerlan, Spain)*; Partobuline *(Immuno, Switz.)*; Parto-gamma *(Biagini, Ital.)*; Rhesogam *(Behringwerke, Ger.)*; Rhesogamma *(Istituto Behring, Ital.)*; Rhesonativ *(Kabi, Ger.*; *Pierrel, Ital.*; *Kabivitrum, USA)*; Rhesuman *(Berna, Ital.*; *Berna, Spain*; *Berna, Switz.)*; RhoGam *(Johnson & Johnson, Spain, Ortho Diagnostic, USA)*; Venogamma *(Ismunit, Ital.)*; WinRho (Rh *Institute, Canada.)*.

1216-z

Antithrombin III

Heparin Cofactor.

Antithrombin III is an $alpha_2$ globulin with a molecular weight of about 60 000 to 65 000.

Units

0.9 unit of antithrombin III, plasma is contained in one ampoule (which contains the freeze-dried residue of 1 mL of human plasma) of the first International Reference Preparation (1978).

Uses and Administration

Antithrombin III is a protein in plasma; it is the major inhibitor of thrombin, it inhibits factor Xa and possibly other factors, and is the cofactor through which heparin (see p.340) exerts its effect. Genetic and acquired deficiency of antithrombin III occurs and is associated with susceptibility to thrombo-embolic disorders.

Antithrombin III is used in doses of up to 3000 units intravenously daily in the management of patients with antithrombin III deficiency.

Antithrombins are inhibitors of thrombin and other coagulation proteases and antithrombin III appears to be the most important. Antithrombin III inactivates thrombin, factor Xa, and other serine proteases generated during coagulation. Reduced plasma concentrations of antithrombin III are found in many conditions, including the nephrotic syndrome, chronic liver disease, disseminated intravascular coagulation, and also during a major thrombo-embolic event and after surgery. An inherited deficiency of antithrombin III also occurs and is associated with recurrent venous thrombosis. The long-term treatment of individuals with antithrombin III deficiency remains controversial although an acute episode of thrombo-embolism is treated with heparin and antithrombin III concentrate. Antithrombin III concentrate is a blood product obtained by plasma fractionation; although the plasma half-life of antithrombin III in normal individuals, and in deficient patients in the steady state, is 16 to 24 hours, during an acute thrombotic event it is much shorter and infusions may need to be given every 12 hours.— *Lancet*, 1983, *1*, 1021. See also: J. H. Winter and A. S. Douglas, *Postgrad. med. J.*, 1983, *59*, 677.

Some references to the use of antithrombin III in various clinical conditions: H. G. Schipper *et al.* (preliminary communication), *Lancet*, 1978, *1*, 854 (disseminated intravascular coagulation); P. Brandt *et al.*, *Br. med. J.*, 1980, *280*, 449 (postpartum haemolytic-uraemic syndrome); G. Leone *et al.* (letter), *New Engl. J. Med.*, 1982, *307*, 1710 (antithrombin III deficiency and thrombosis).

Proprietary Preparations

Antithrombin III is available from *Blood Products Laboratory, UK*.

Proprietary Names and Manufacturers

Antitrombin *(KabiVitrum, Denm.)*; Atenativ *(Kabi, Ger.)*; Kybernin *(Behringwerke, Ger.)*.

1212-e

Blood

Whole Blood (*B.P.*) (Human Blood (*Eur. P.*); Sanguis Humanus) is blood which has been withdrawn aseptically from human beings and mixed with a suitable anticoagulant; the amount of anticoagulant should not exceed 22% of the final volume of the mixture. It contains no added preservative. The blood is obtained from a healthy donor who must, as far as can be ascertained, be free from detectable agents of infection transmissible by transfusion of blood or blood components. The donor blood has a haemoglobin value, in terms of the International Standard for Haemiglobincyanide, of not less than 12.5% w/v. Whole Blood has a haemoglobin value of not less than 9.7% w/v (calculated from the value of donor blood and the dilution due to the anticoagulant solution). Whole Blood is stored, immediately after collection and admixture with the anticoagulant, in sterile containers, sealed to exclude micro-organisms, at a temperature of 2° to 8° and the containers are not opened until immediately before transfusion. The label states the ABO group, the Rh group and the nature of specific antisera used in testing, the total volume of fluid, the proportion of blood, and the nature and percentage of anticoagulant. In order that compatibility and other tests can be carried out, a small quantity of Whole Blood is supplied in a small container attached to each main container. Whole Blood should be administered with suitable equipment such as that described in Section 3 or Section 4 of *Transfusion Equipment for Medical Use*, BS 2463: 1962.

Whole Blood (*U.S.P.*) (ACD Whole Blood; CPD Whole Blood; CPDA-1 Whole Blood; Heparin Whole Blood) is blood which has been withdrawn aseptically from suitable human donors. It contains acid citrate dextrose, citrate phosphate dextrose, citrate phosphate dextrose with adenine, or heparin sodium as an anticoagulant. It may consist of blood from which the antihaemophilic factor has been removed, in which case it is termed 'Modified'. The label states among other things the ABO group, the Rh group, the volume of blood, and the quantity and kind of anticoagulant; the ABO group may also be indicated by the use of specified labelling colours. It should be stored in hermetically-sealed sterile containers at 1° to 6° (with a range of not more than 2°) except during transport when the temperature may be 1° to 10°. The expiration date is not later than 48 hours after withdrawal (heparin anticoagulant), not later than 21 days after withdrawal (acid citrate dextrose or citrate phosphate dextrose), or not later than 35 days after withdrawal (citrate phosphate dextrose with adenine). In order that various tests can be carried out, a small quantity of Whole Blood is supplied in at least one small container attached to each main container.

ANTICOAGULANT SOLUTIONS FOR BLOOD. Anticoagulant solutions suitable for addition to whole blood are described under heparin sodium (p.341) and sodium citrate (p.1028).

STORAGE OF BLOOD. During storage changes and decomposition occur to whole blood. Stored whole blood is a potentially dangerous fluid, the maintenance of sterility of which depends entirely upon meticulous attention to cleanliness, faultless asepsis, and accurate and constant refrigeration from the time of collection until use. Whole blood should therefore only be stored under the conditions specified on the label and should only be administered with the recommended transfusion equipment.

Units

The expression 'unit of blood' generally represents a volume of about 500 to 540 mL, including anticoagulant. For blood preparations a unit generally refers to the quantity of a blood component obtained from 1 unit of whole blood. Specific units of activity are used for some blood components.

Adverse Effects

Transmission of infections has been associated with the transfusion of blood (see p.811).

The transfusion of massive volumes of whole blood may overload the circulation and cause pulmonary oedema. Repeated transfusions of blood, as in thalassaemia, may lead to iron overload. Allergic reactions may occur.

The transfusion of incompatible blood causes haemolysis, possibly with renal failure and disseminated intravascular coagulation; haemolytic reactions may occasionally occur where the screening tests have failed to detect antibody.

A report of a specific syndrome in thalassaemic patients, involving hypertension, convulsions, and cerebral haemorrhage, following multiple blood transfusions before splenectomy. Of 8 patients who suffered this syndrome 4 developed definite intracranial haemorrhage and 3 died. Vasopressive substances introduced by or related to multiple blood transfusion were considered responsible; host factors might also contribute.— P. Wasi *et al.*, *Lancet*, 1978, *2*, 602.

Data from patients who received blood transfusions during surgery for cancer indicated an association between the transfusion and recurrence of cancer; recurrence was higher in these patients than in those who did not have transfusion.— N. Blumberg *et al.*, *Br. med. J.*, 1986, *293*, 530. Comment.— T. J. Hamblin, *ibid.*, 517.

ALLERGY. Analysis, by the Boston Collaborative Drug Surveillance Program, of data on 15 438 patients hospitalised between 1975 and 1982 detected 24 allergic skin reactions attributed to blood among 1112 recipients.— M. Bigby *et al.*, *J. Am. med. Ass.*, 1986, *256*, 3358.

HAEMOLYTIC REACTION. Acute haemolytic transfusion reactions.— D. Goldfinger, *Transfusion, Philad.*, 1977, *17*, 85.

A report of antiglobulin-positive haemolytic anaemia due to a delayed haemolytic transfusion reaction in a patient who had received multiple blood transfusions.— B. J. Boughton and P. R. Galbraith, *Br. med. J.*, 1975, *4*, 430.

Delayed haemolytic reactions, presenting as sickle-cell crisis, in patients with sickle-cell disease after partial exchange transfusion.— W. J. Diamond *et al.*, *Ann. intern. Med.*, 1980, *93*, 231.

Further references: S. Panzer *et al.*, *Lancet*, 1987, *1*, 474.

IRON OVERLOAD. A man with thalassaemia who had received 404 units of blood triggered a metal detector at an airport security point. His total body-iron concentration was estimated to be over 100 g.— R. T. S. Jim (letter), *Lancet*, 1979, *2*, 1028. Iron overload after transfusion of thalassaemic patients for less than 4 years.— A. I. Schafer *et al.*, *New Engl. J. Med.*, 1981, *304*, 319.

Precautions

Whole blood should generally not be transfused unless the ABO and Rh groups of the patient's and the donor's blood have been verified and a compatibility check made between the patient's serum and the donor's red cells.

The Rh group of the recipient should always be determined and ideally all patients should be transfused with blood of homologous Rh groups.

To reduce the possibility of cardiac arrest from cardiac hypothermia when large volumes are used or the blood is transfused rapidly, and to minimise postoperative shivering, stored blood should be carefully warmed to about 37° before transfusion.

Drugs should *not* be added to blood.

Uses and Administration

Whole blood is used as a source of red cell concentrates, clotting factors, platelets, plasma proteins, and immunoglobulins, each of which has specific indications for use. Because of the risks involved in transfusing whole blood and the need for economy in its use, the appropriate blood component should be used whenever possible.

Whole blood may be used following blood loss during surgery and severe haemorrhage. It may also be used to supplement the circulation during cardiac bypass surgery.

The amount of whole blood transfused and the rate at which it is given depend upon the patient's age and general condition, upon the state of his circulatory system, and upon the therapeutic indication for transfusion. The haemoglobin concentration of the blood of the average adult is raised by about 1 g per 100 mL by the transfusion of 540 mL of whole blood.

AUTOLOGOUS BLOOD TRANSFUSION. Reviews, discussions, and comments on autologous blood transfusion, the procedure of a patient acting as his own blood donor, the blood usually being collected shortly before elective surgery: M. A. Popovsky *et al.*, *Mayo Clin. Proc.*, 1985, *60*, 125; *J. Am. med. Ass.*, 1986, *256*, 2378; *J. Am. med. Ass.*, 1987, *257*, 1220; L. A. Kay, *Br. med. J.*, 1987, *294*, 137.

TRANSPLANT SURGERY. A review of blood transfusion before renal transplantation resulting in prolonged survival of the allograft.— *Lancet*, 1984, *1*, 830.

1219-a

Blood Group Specific Substances A, B, and AB

Blood Group Specific Substances A, B, and AB (*U.S.P.*) is a sterile non-anaphylactic isotonic solution of the polysaccharide-amino-acid complexes that are capable of neutralising the anti-A and the anti-B isoagglutinins of group O blood. Substance A is prepared from hog stomach (gastric mucin) and substances B and AB from horse stomach (gastric mucosa). The substances contain no added preservative. They should be stored in single-dose containers at 2° to 8°.

The substances are used for immunisation of plasma donors for production of *in vitro* diagnostic reagents. The *U.S.P.* directs that the substances should not be given intravenously nor to fertile women. Blood group specific substance B may contain immunogenic A activity.

1222-y

Bone Marrow

Bone-marrow transplantation involves the injection, usually after immunosuppression, of material from a suitable HLA-compatible donor and has been used in some immunological deficiencies, in aplastic anaemia, and in leukaemia. The principal risks are infection, graft rejection, and graft-versus-host disease. Autologous transplantation, with material derived from the patient while in remission, has also been used.

A brief review of the use of bone-marrow transplantation for non-malignant disorders. When techniques of human histocompatibility typing made it possible to select HLA-identical siblings as donors, marrow transplantations became recognised as the therapy of choice for two non-malignant disorders, namely severe combined immunologic deficiency and severe aplastic anaemia. Although some success has been reported with marrow grafts in thalassaemia major the risk of early death as a complication of transplantation must be weighed against the possibility of a cure and the procedure is likely to remain controversial. Two major developments promise a wider application of marrow grafting for non-malignant disorders. The first is the prevention or amelioration of graft-versus-host disease by the removal of T-cells from the donor marrow inoculum and the second is the use of phenotypically HLA-identical unrelated volunteers as donors. Although a marrow graft, with its potential complications, is less than an ideal option for patients with hereditary haematopoietic disease it presently offers the only hope of cure.— E. D. Thomas, *New Engl. J. Med.*, 1985, *312*, 46. A further discussion on marrow transplantation for thalassaemia. The clinician is faced with a choice of bone marrow transplantation, with the possibility of cure but with a 25% probability of killing the patient, or transfusion and chelation therapy with uncertainty about its long-term efficacy. In countries where regular transfusion or chelation therapy is not available there seems little doubt that bone-marrow transplantation should be offered as the only possible form of therapy for thalassaemia. In centres with adequate facilities it seems more reasonable to embark on a transfusion programme with adequate chelation because the patients can be offered at least 15 to 20 years of reasonable life and it is very likely that within this period there will be genuine advances in chelation therapy.— *Lancet*, 1987, *1*, 1246. See also: K. Atkinson and J. C. Biggs, *Med. J. Aust.*, 1986, *144*, 338.

A discussion of the use of bone-marrow transplantation for neurovisceral storage disorders. Displacement bone-marrow transplantation (total displacement of the abnormal host bone marrow thus achieving lifelong engraftment) has already enabled satisfactory correction of over 40 previously fatal inborn errors of metabolism some of which result in brain damage.— *Lancet*, 1986, *2*, 788.

The rationale for bone-marrow transplantation in the treatment of malignant disease rests on three principles: that the disease is curable by very intensive chemotherapy and radiotherapy; that supportive care can be provided to keep the patient alive during the ensuing period of prolonged pancytopenia; that the marrow will repopulate with normal cells. Acute leukaemia was the first malignant disease successfully treated in this manner with identical twins as marrow donors (syngeneic bone-marrow transplantation). The majority of transplants are now carried out with bone marrow from an HLA-identical sibling donor (allogeneic transplantation) but there is the risk of graft-versus-host disease. If the patient acts as his own marrow donor while in remission this process of autologous bone-marrow transplantation has advantages. Autologous transplantation is being increasingly applied to the treatment of acute leukaemias, lymphomas, and non-haematological malignancies and can produce long, disease-free remissions in some patients.— *Lancet*, 1987, *1*, 303.

310187-z

Dextran 1 *(BAN, rINN).*

Dextranum 1.

CAS — 9004-54-0 (dextran).

Dextran 1 consists of dextrans of weight average molecular weight about 1000 that are polymers of glucose and are derived from the dextrans produced by the fermentation of sucrose by means of a certain strain of *Leuconostoc mesenteroides* (NCTC No. 10817).

Dextran 1 has been used to prevent severe anaphylactic reactions to infusions of dextran. It is reported to occupy the binding sites of dextran-reactive antibodies and so prevent the formation of large immune complexes with higher molecular weight dextrans.

In a multicentre study by Ljungström *et al.* (*Acta chir. scand.*, 1983, *149*, 341) involving about 29 200 patients, 10 mL of 15% dextran 1 was given intravenously 2 minutes before the start of an infusion of dextran 40 or 70. Severe dextran-induced anaphylactic reactions occurred in 7 patients and dextran 1 was not considered to have prevented all reactions. However the authors considered that the severity of reactions was reduced although the onset of symptoms was not delayed. The same group (H. Renck *et al. ibid.*, 355) carried out a further study involving about 34 950 patients given an injection of 20 mL of dextran 1 before the dextran infusion. There was only one severe likely reaction. It was considered that dextran 1 prevented anaphylactic reactions by hapten inhibition in a dose-dependent way. It did not reduce the incidence of mild reactions, which are not generally mediated by antibodies. Another large study (H. Renck *et al.*, *ibid.*, 349) comparing the effects of giving 20 mL of dextran 1 either 2 minutes before injection of dextran 40 or 70 or mixed with the injection, was discontinued after the occurrence of 2 severe reactions in the admixture group. There were 21, 20, and 2 adverse reactions to dextran 1 in the 3 studies respectively, including nausea, skin reactions, bradycardia, and hypotension. Apart from one patient, reactions to dextran 1 were mild and were considered to be of minor clinical importance.

Proprietary Names and Manufacturers

Promit *(Schiwa, Ger.; Hausmann, Switz.)*; Promiten *(Pharmacia, Norw.; Pharmacia, Swed.)*.

251-w

Dextran 40 *(BAN, USAN, rINN).*

Dextranum 40; Low-Molecular-Weight Dextran.

CAS — 9004-54-0 (dextran).

Pharmacopoeias. In *Braz.*, *Chin.*, *Jpn*, *Nord.*, and *Roum. Br.* describes Dextran 40 Intravenous Infusion.

Dextran 40 consists of dextrans of weight average molecular weight about 40 000 that are polymers of glucose and are derived from the dextrans produced by the fermentation of sucrose by means of a certain strain of *Leuconostoc mesenteroides* (NCTC No. 10817).

Solutions are **sterilised** by autoclaving.

Solutions should be **stored** at an even temperature and should not be used if they are cloudy or if a deposit is present.

Adverse Effects, Treatment, and Precautions

As for dextran 70, p.815.

Rapid renal excretion of dextran 40 can result in high urinary concentrations which increase urinary viscosity and may cause oliguria or renal failure. Dextran 40 can cause capillary oozing of wound surfaces due to improved perfusion pressure. Infusions of dextran 40 are contra-indicated in renal disease with anuria; should anuria or oliguria occur during treatment dextran 40 should be withdrawn.

ALLERGY. For reports of anaphylactic reactions associated with administration of dextran 40, see dextran 70, below, and dextran 1, above.

EFFECTS ON THE KIDNEYS. Seven of 8 cases of drug-induced acute renal failure seen in 8 months were due to dextran 40 (6 cases) or dextran 70 (1). Dextran injections had not been withdrawn despite falling urine outputs; 5 patients developed anuria.— T. G. Feest, *Br. med. J.*, 1976, *2*, 1300.

A report of acute renal failure and anuria associated with the use of dextran 40 infusions; the renal insufficiency was rapidly reversed following the removal of the dextran by plasmaphaeresis.— M. Moran and C. Kapsner, *New Engl. J. Med.*, 1987, *317*, 150.

EFFECTS ON THE LUNGS. In a study of 45 women undergoing gynaecological surgery, 25 received 400 to 500 mL of a 10% solution of dextran 40 intraperitoneally for prevention of adhesions. After 5 to 7 days, 12 of the dextran group and none of the controls had a pleural effusion visible on chest X-ray. The effusions were small to moderate, asymptomatic, and resolved without treatment.— A. Adoni *et al.*, *Int. J. Gynaecol. Obstet.*, 1980, *18*, 243.

Absorption and Fate

After intravenous infusion of dextran 40, about 70% is excreted unchanged in the urine within 24 hours. The dextran not excreted is slowly metabolised to carbon dioxide and water. A small amount is excreted into the gastro-intestinal tract and eliminated in the faeces.

Uses and Administration

Dextran 40 as a 10% solution exerts a slightly higher colloidal osmotic pressure than plasma proteins. It thus produces a greater expansion of plasma volume than dextrans of a higher molecular weight, although the expansion may have a shorter duration because of more rapid renal excretion. Dextran 40 also inhibits sludging or aggregation of red blood-cells.

Dextran 40 is therefore used like dextran 70 or dextran 75 for short-term plasma expansion and the prophylaxis of postoperative thrombo-embolic disorders. Because of its activity on red blood-cells it is also used to improve blood flow and prevent intravascular aggregation in conditions or procedures associated with impaired circulation.

Dextran 40 is given by intravenous infusion as a 10% solution in sodium chloride 0.9% or glucose 5%. Initial doses are often 500 to 1000 mL given rapidly over 30 to 60 minutes or occasionally over 4 to 6 hours. Subsequently doses of 500 mL are given, sometimes starting on the same day as the initial dose, but usually given on the next day for 5 days or on alternate days for 2 weeks. In peripheral vascular disorders 500 mL may be given every 12 hours for 4 doses and repeated as required every 3 to 6 months.

Infants may be given 5 mL per kg body-weight and children 10 mL per kg.

A dose of 10 to 15 mL per kg has been given before angiography, while 10 to 20 mL per kg body-weight has been added to extracorporeal perfusion fluids.

A 5% solution with electrolytes has been used for the washing and perfusion of organs for transplantation.

PERIPHERAL VASCULAR DISORDERS. Despite reports of improvement of peripheral circulation in patients with systemic sclerosis given low molecular weight dextran, a double-blind study of 29 patients with systemic sclerosis or Raynaud's syndrome did not show that dextran 40 produced significant improvement in finger temperature.— B. Dodman and N. R. Rowell, *Acta derm.-vener., Stockh.*, 1982, *62*, 440.

THROMBO-EMBOLIC DISORDERS. Dextran 40 is recommended for the prophylaxis of thrombo-embolic disorders resulting from surgical operations. In hip replacement surgery, Harris *et al.* (*J. Am. med. Ass.*, 1972, *220*, 1319) showed that warfarin and dextran 40 gave similar protection. In general surgery, Gruber *et al.* (*Lancet*, 1977, *1*, 207) found that heparin was better than dextran 40 in preventing deep-vein thrombosis.

More up-to-date references on the use of dextrans in the prophylaxis of thrombo-embolism are provided under dextran 70 (below).

Preparations

Dextran 40 Intravenous Infusion *(B.P.)*. Dextran 40 Injection

Proprietary Preparations

Gentran 40 *(Travenol, UK)*. *Intravenous infusion*, dextran 40 10% in glucose 5% or sodium chloride 0.9%, in bottles of 500 mL.

Lomodex 40 *(CP Pharmaceuticals, UK)*. *Intravenous infusion*, dextran 40 10% in glucose 5% or sodium chloride 0.9%, in bags of 500 mL.

Rheomacrodex *(Pharmacia, UK)*. *Intravenous infusion*, dextran 40 10% in glucose 5% or sodium chloride 0.9%, in bottles of 500 mL.

Proprietary Names and Manufacturers

Eudextran *(Stholl, Ital.)*; Fisiodex 40 *(Grifols, Spain)*; Gentran 40 *(Travenol, UK; Travenol, USA)*; Isodex *(Neth.)*; LMD 10% *(Abbott, Canad.; Abbott, USA)*; Lomodex 40 *(Fisons, Austral.; CP Pharmaceuticals, UK)*; Longasteril *(Fresenius, Ger.)*; Macrohorm *(Hormonchemie, Ger.)*; Onkovertin *(Braun Melsungen, Ger.)*; Perfadex *(Pharmacia, Swed.)*; Perfudex *(Austral.; Belg.; Pharmacia, UK)*; Plander *(Pierrel Hospital, Ital.)*; Rheofusin *(Pfrimmer, Ger.)*; Rheomacrodex *(Pharmacia, Austral.; Belg.; Pharmacia, Canad.; Pharmacia, Denm.; Cernep Synthelabo, Fr.; Schiwa, Ger.; Ital.; Neth.; Pharmacia, Norw.; Pharmacia, Swed.; Pharmacia, UK; Pharmacia, USA)*; Solplex 40 *(SIFRA, Ital.)*; Soludex *(Ital.)*; Thomaedex *(Thomae, Ger.)*.

252-e

Dextran 70 *(BAN, USAN, rINN).*

Dextranum 70.

CAS — 9004-54-0 (dextran).

Pharmacopoeias. In *Braz., Chin., Jpn, Nord.,* and *Roum. Br.* describes Dextran 70 Intravenous Infusion.

Dextran 70 consists of dextrans of weight average molecular weight about 70 000 that are polymers of glucose and are derived from the dextrans produced by the fermentation of sucrose by means of a certain strain of *Leuconostoc mesenteroides* (NCTC No. 10817).

Solutions are **sterilised** by autoclaving.

Solutions should be **stored** at an even temperature and should not be used if they are cloudy or if a deposit is present.

Adverse Effects and Treatment

Infusions of dextrans may occasionally produce allergic reactions such as fever, flushing, joint pains, urticaria, hypotension, and bronchospasm. Severe anaphylactic reactions occur rarely and may be fatal. Nausea and vomiting have also been reported. These reactions are treated symptomatically after withdrawal of the dextran. Dextran 40 can cause renal impairment as a result of increased urinary viscosity; capillary oozing has also been associated with its use.

Severe anaphylactic reactions occur in patients with high levels of dextran-reactive antibodies which may arise in response to dietary or bacterial polysaccharides. Dextrans may combine with these antibodies to form large immune complexes. Dextran 1 has been used to block the formation of these complexes and hence the reactions, see above.

ALLERGY. In a retrospective study of allergic reactions to dextran 40 and dextran 70 reported in Sweden from 1970 to 1979, there were 478 reports of reactions, 458 of which were considered to be due to dextran, out of 1 365 266 infusions given. There was a male to female ratio of 1.5 to 1 for all reactions and a ratio of 3 to 1 for the most severe reactions. The mean age of the patients was higher in those with severe reactions. Of the 28 fatal reactions, 27 occurred within 5 minutes of the start of the infusion and 25 when less than 25 mL had been infused. Three of the fatal reactions occurred after a test dose of only 0.5 to 1.0 mL and it was strongly recommended that such test doses should not be used.— K. -G. Ljungström *et al., Acta chir. scand.,* 1983, *149,* 253.

See also under dextran 1, above.

EFFECTS ON THE KIDNEYS. For a report of renal failure associated with administration of dextran 70, see dextran 40, above.

Precautions

Dextran infusions are contra-indicated in patients with severe congestive heart failure, bleeding disorders such as hypofibrinogenaemia or thrombocytopenia, renal failure, or in those allergic to dextrans.

Infusions produce a progressive dilution of oxygen-carrying capacity, coagulation factors, and plasma proteins and may overload the circulation. They should therefore be administered with caution to patients with impaired renal function, haemorrhage, chronic liver disease, or those at risk of developing pulmonary oedema or congestive heart failure. The haematocrit should not be allowed to fall below 30% and all patients should be observed for early signs of bleeding complications. Deficiency of coagulation factors should be corrected and fluid and electrolyte balance maintained. Dehydration should be corrected before or at least during dextran infusions, in order to maintain an adequate urine flow. Patients should be watched closely during the early part of the infusion period, and the infusion stopped immediately if signs of anaphylactic reactions appear. Infusions should also be stopped if there are signs of oliguria or renal failure.

The anticoagulant effect of heparin may be enhanced by dextran.

The higher molecular weight dextrans may interfere with blood grouping and cross matching of blood, while the lower molecular weight dextrans may interfere with some methods. Therefore, whenever possible, a sample of blood should be collected before giving the dextran infusion and kept frozen in case such tests become necessary.

The presence of dextran may interfere with the determination of glucose, bilirubin, or protein in blood or urine.

Absorption and Fate

After intravenous infusion dextrans with a molecular weight of less than 50 000 are excreted unchanged by the kidney and the rate of urinary excretion increases as the molecular weight decreases. Dextrans with a molecular weight greater than 50 000 slowly diffuse across the capillary wall and are slowly metabolised to carbon dioxide and water. Some molecules may be held in the reticuloendothelial system for prolonged periods. Small amounts of dextrans are excreted into the gastro-intestinal tract and eliminated in the faeces.

About 50% of dextran 70 is excreted unchanged in the urine within 24 hours.

Uses and Administration

Dextran 70 as a 6% solution exerts a colloidal osmotic pressure similar to that of plasma proteins. It is therefore used for the short-term expansion of the plasma volume in conditions such as shock or impending shock resulting from burns, surgery, haemorrhage, or trauma. It is also used in the prevention of postoperative thrombo-embolic disorders. Dextran 75 is used similarly. Doses depend on the severity of the plasma loss and on the type of operation. Initial doses consist of 500 or 1000 mL infused rapidly after haemorrhage, or over 4 to 6 hours when used for the prophylaxis of thrombosis. Subsequent doses of 500 mL may be given once, as in the management of haemorrhage, or on alternate days for up to 2 weeks for the prophylaxis of thrombosis. Patients with burns may require 3 litres or more plus electrolytes in the first few days.

A 32% solution of dextran 70 has been instilled into the uterus in a dose of 50 to 100 mL as a rinsing and dilatation fluid to aid hysteroscopy.

PELVIC ADHESIONS. In a double-blind study of 44 women undergoing gynaecological surgery 200 mL of a 32% solution of dextran 70 instilled into the peritoneal cavity was shown to be effective in reducing both the formation and reformation of adhesions.— S. M. Rosenberg and J. A. Board, *Am. J. Obstet. Gynec.,* 1984, *148,* 380.

Further references: *Fert. Steril.,* 1983, *40,* 612 (beneficial results); D. M. Magyar *et al., Am. J. Obstet. Gynec.,* 1985, *152,* 198 (beneficial results); R. P. S. Jansen *et al., ibid., 153,* 363 (no benefit).

THROMBO-EMBOLIC DISORDERS. Infusions of dextran 70 have been shown to reduce the incidence of pulmonary embolism (A. Kline *et al., Br. med. J.,* 1975, *2,* 109; K.-G. Ljungström, *Acta chir. scand.,* 1983, *514, Suppl.,* 1) and deep-vein thrombosis following surgery (J. Bonnar and J. Walsh, *Lancet,* 1972, *1,* 614; R.C. Smith, *Br. med. J.,* 1978, *1,* 952), although results have not been consistently uniform.

A number of studies have compared dextran 70 with other drugs. Lambie (*Br. med. J.,* 1970, *2,* 144) found it to be superior to warfarin yet Barber (*Postgrad. med. J.,* 1977, *53,* 130) obtained similar results with dextran 70, heparin, and warfarin in preventing deep-vein thrombosis. Multicentre studies have shown that dextran 70 produces similar results to heparin alone or with dihydroergotamine in the prophylaxis of fatal pulmonary embolisms (U.F. Gruber *et al., Br. med. J.,* 1980, *1,* 69; U.F. Gruber, *Br. J. Surg.,* 1982, *69, Suppl.,* 554). However, the use of dihydroergotamine with dextran 70 improved the prophylaxis of thrombo-embolisms in patients undergoing hip surgery (D. Bergqvist *et al., Br. J. Surg.,* 1984, *71,* 516).

Preparations

Dextran 70 Intravenous Infusion *(B.P.).* Dextran 70 Injection

Proprietary Preparations

Gentran 70 *(Travenol, UK). Intravenous infusion,* dextran 70 6% in glucose 5% or sodium chloride 0.9%, in bottles of 500 mL.

Hyskon *(Pharmacia, UK). Solution,* dextran 70 32% in glucose 10%. For hysteroscopy.

Lomodex 70 *(CP Pharmaceuticals, UK). Intravenous infusion,* dextran 70 6% in glucose 5% or sodium chloride 0.9%, in bags of 500 mL.

Macrodex *(Pharmacia, UK). Intravenous infusion,* dextran 70 6% in glucose 5% or sodium chloride 0.9%, in bottles of 500 mL.

Proprietary Names and Manufacturers

Fisiodex 70 *(Grifols, Spain)*; Gentran 70 *(Travenol, UK)*; Hyskon *(Pharmacia, Austral.; Pharmacia, Canad.; Pharmacia, Swed.; Pharmacia, UK; Pharmacia, USA)*; Lomodex 70 *(CP Pharmaceuticals, UK)*; Macrodex *(Pharmacia, Austral.; Belg.; Pharmacia, Canad.; Neth.; Pharmacia, Norw.; Pharmacia, Swed.; Pharmacia, UK; Pharmacia, USA)*; Perfudex 70 *(Belg.)*; Plander *(Pierrel Hospital, Ital.)*; Solplex 70 *(SIFRA, Ital.)*; Soludex *(Ital.)*.

The following names have been used for multi-ingredient preparations containing dextran 70— Tears Naturale *(Alcon, Austral.; Alcon, Canad.; Alcon, UK; Alcon Laboratories, USA)*; Tears Renewed *(Akorn, USA)*.

310188-c

Dextran 75 *(BAN, USAN, rINN).*

Dextranum 75.

CAS — 9004-54-0 (dextran).

Dextran 75 consists of dextrans of weight average molecular weight about 75 000 that are polymers of glucose and are derived from the dextrans produced by the fermentation of sucrose by means of a certain strain of *Leuconostoc mesenteroides* (NCTC No. 10817).

Solutions should be **stored** at an even temperature and should not be used if they are cloudy or if a deposit is present.

Dextran 75 has the same actions and uses as dextran 70.

ALLERGY. An anaphylactic reaction occurred 75 minutes after the intraperitoneal instillation of 300 mL of a 6% solution of dextran 75 for the prevention of adhesions after gynaecological surgery. After successful symptomatic treatment the reaction returned 20 minutes later due to slow absorption of dextran from the peritoneal cavity. There was no further reaction after removal of 200 mL of intraperitoneal fluid by culdocentesis.— M. Borten *et al., Obstet. Gynec.,* 1983, *61,* 755.

Proprietary Names and Manufacturers

Gentran 75 (*Travenol, USA*).

253-l

Dextran 110 *(BAN, rINN).*

Dextranum 110.

CAS — 9004-54-0 (dextran).

Pharmacopoeias. Br. describes Dextran 110 Intravenous Infusion.

Dextran 110 consists of dextrans of weight average molecular weight about 110 000 that are polymers of glucose and are derived from the dextrans produced by the fermentation of sucrose by means of a certain strain of *Leuconostoc mesenteroides* (NCTC No. 10817).

Solutions are **sterilised** by autoclaving.

Solutions should be **stored** at an even temperature and should not be used if they are cloudy or if a deposit is present.

Adverse Effects, Treatment, and Precautions

As for dextran 70, above.

Dextran 110 may cause rouleaux formation and may therefore interfere with blood grouping, cross matching, and rhesus typing, and may increase the erythrocyte sedimentation-rate. Therefore, whenever possible, a sample of blood should be collected before giving the dextran infusion and kept frozen in case such tests become necessary.

Absorption and Fate

The absorption and fate of dextrans are described under dextran 70, p.815.

Uses and Administration

Dextran 110 is used similarly to dextran 70 (see p.815) as a 6% solution for short-term plasma volume expansion in the treatment and prevention of shock from blood loss, burns, and surgery.

Preparations

Dextran 110 Intravenous Infusion *(B.P.)*. Dextran 110 Injection

Proprietary Preparations

Dextraven 110 *(CP Pharmaceuticals, UK). Intravenous infusion*, dextran 110 6% in sodium chloride 0.9%, in bottles of 500 mL.

1225-c

Factor VIII

Dried Factor VIII Fraction (*B.P.*) (Dried Human Antihaemophilic Fraction; Freeze-dried Human Coagulation Factor VIII (*Eur.P.*); Factor VIII Coagulationis Sanguinis Humani Cryodesiccatus) is prepared from human plasma obtained from blood from more than ten healthy donors who must, as far as can be ascertained, be free from detectable agents of infection transmissible by transfusion of blood or blood derivatives. The method of preparation is designed in particular to avoid the transmission of or to inactivate known agents of infection. The antihaemophilic fraction is prepared by a suitable fractionation technique and dissolved in an appropriate liquid, distributed in sterile containers, and immediately frozen. The preparation is freeze-dried and the containers sealed under vacuum or filled with oxygen-free nitrogen or other suitable inert gas before sealing. No antimicrobial preservative is added but an antiviral agent may be added provided it can be demonstrated to have no deleterious effect on the final product and to cause no adverse reactions in the patient; heparin may be added. A wide range of preparations is available varying in respect of activity and degree of purification. When the contents of a sealed container are dissolved in a volume of water as stated on the label the resulting solution contains not less than 3 units per mL and not less than 0.1 unit per mg of protein. The dried product should be stored at a temperature below 8° and be protected from light. The reconstituted solution should be used as soon as possible after, and not more than 3 hours after, reconstitution. If a gel forms the fraction should not be used. It should be administered with equipment that includes a filter.

Antihemophilic Factor (*U.S.P.*) is a sterile freeze-dried powder containing factor VIII fraction prepared from units of human venous plasma that have been tested for the absence of hepatitis B surface antigen, obtained from whole-blood donors and pooled; it may contain heparin sodium or sodium citrate. It contains not less than 100 units per g of protein. Unless otherwise specified it should be stored at 2° to 8° in hermetically-sealed containers. It should be used within 4 hours of reconstitution and should be administered with equipment that includes a filter.

Cryoprecipitated Antihemophilic Factor (*U.S.P.*) is a sterile frozen concentrate of human antihemophilic factor prepared from the cryoprotein fraction, rich in factor VIII, of human venous plasma obtained from suitable whole-blood donors from a single unit of plasma derived from whole blood or by plasmaphaeresis, collected and processed in a closed system. It contains no preservative. It has an average potency of not less than 80 units per container. It should be stored at or below −18° in hermetically-sealed containers. It should be thawed to 20° to 37° before use; this liquid should be stored at room temperature and used within 6 hours of thawing; it should also be used within 4 hours of opening the container and administered with equipment that includes a filter.

Units

3.9 units of blood coagulation factor VIII:C, concentrate, human are contained in 15 mg of a freeze-dried concentrate of human blood coagulation factor VIII in one ampoule of the third International Standard Preparation (1982).

Adverse Effects and Precautions

Allergic reactions may sometimes follow the use of factor VIII preparations. There is the possibility of intravascular haemolysis in patients with blood groups A, B, or AB receiving high doses or frequently repeated doses of factor VIII preparations due to the content of blood group iso-agglutinins.

Factor VIII preparations have been associated with the transmission of some viral infections, including hepatitis B and more notably transmission of the human immunodeficiency virus (HIV) leading to the subsequent development of the acquired immunodeficiency syndrome (AIDS). Strenuous efforts are now undertaken to screen the donor material from which factor VIII material is obtained and new methods of manufacture have also been introduced with the aim of inactivating any viruses present.

ALLERGY. Adverse reactions occurred in 15 of 70 patients who received factor VIII preparations. Effects included anaphylactic or febrile reactions, urticaria, angioedema, nausea, headache, light-headedness and visual disturbances. Antihistamines, prednisone, and isoprenaline were routinely supplied to haemophiliacs receiving out-patient therapy.— M. E. Eyster *et al.* (letter), *Ann. intern. Med.*, 1977, *87*, 248. The use of antihistamines could lead to more severe bleeding.— W. G. Hocking, *ibid.*, *88*, 130.

EFFECTS ON THE CARDIOVASCULAR SYSTEM. Unstable angina in one patient associated with the use of factor VIII preparations for severe haemophilia A.— R. G. Kopitsky and E. M. Geltman, *Ann. intern. Med.*, 1986, *105*, 215.

EFFECTS ON THE NERVOUS SYSTEM. A young man with severe haemophilia who had frequently received factor VIII experienced a grand mal seizure 40 minutes after he had given himself factor VIII. Further convulsive episodes occurred on 2 subsequent occasions, each time after rapid administration of the injection. There was no relevant history and no evidence of underlying CNS abnormality was found on investigation.— M. Small *et al.*, *Br. med. J.*, 1983, *286*, 1106. Comment that the seizures may have been due to a gradual accummulation of a substantial amount of aluminium which had been found in some batches of factor VIII preparations.— H. L. Elliott and G. S. Fell (letter), *ibid.*, 1900.

EFFECTS ON THE THYROID. Raised serum thyroxine values in a 15-year-old boy with classical haemophilia were associated with a factor VIII preparation which he had been receiving for 5 years for the prevention and treatment of haemarthroses. Care should be taken to avoid a mistaken diagnosis of hyperthyroidism.— J. S. D. Winter and P. J. Smail (letter), *Lancet*, 1980, *2*, 652.

Uses and Administration

Patients with haemophilia A have a genetic deficiency of factor VIII and are particularly susceptible to bleeding, which is closely related to the concentration of factor VIII. There is also a deficiency of factor VIII in von Willebrand's disease.

Preparations of factor VIII are used as infusions during bleeding episodes in the treatment of patients with haemophilia A and in the preparation of such patients for dental and surgical procedures. The dosage of factor VIII should be determined for each patient and will vary with the circumstances involving bleeding or type of surgery to be performed. A dose of 1 unit per kg body-weight has been reported to raise the plasma concentration of factor VIII by up to 2% (of normal). A suggested formula to calculate, approximately, the dose required for a given effect is:

units required =
Weight (kg) × 0.5 × % desired increase (of normal).

It is suggested that for mild to moderate haemorrhage the plasma concentration of factor VIII should be raised to 20 to 30% of normal, for more serious haemorrhage or minor surgery it should be raised to 30 to 50% of normal, and that for severe haemorrhage or major surgery an increase to 80 to 100% of normal may be necessary; thus doses commonly used are in the range of 10 to 50 units per kg.

Some patients develop antibodies to factor VIII and although large doses of preparations of both factor VIII and factor IX and sometimes also immunosuppressants have been used in the management of such patients, preparations having factor VIII inhibitor bypassing activity are now available (see below).

Some reviews and discussions on the management of haemophilia: P. Jones, *Archs Dis. Childh.*, 1984, *59*, 1010; C. R. Rizza, *Prescribers' J.*, 1984, *24*, 71.

Proprietary Preparations

Hemofil HT *(Travenol, UK). Injection*, freeze-dried factor VIII (heat treated) in vials containing 250, 750, and 1050 units.

Koate-HT *(Cutter, UK). Injection*, freeze-dried factor VIII (heat treated) in vials containing 250, 500, 1000, and 1500 units.

Kryobulin Heat Treated *(Immuno, UK). Injection*, freeze-dried factor VIII (heat treated) in vials containing 250, 500, and 1000 units.

Profilate Heat-Treated *(Alpha Therapeutic, UK). Injection*, freeze-dried factor VIII (heat treated) in vials containing 250, 500, 750, and 1000 units.

Factor VIII is also available from *Blood Products Laboratory, UK*.

Proprietary Names and Manufacturers

Actif VIII-HT *(Merieux, Ital.)*; Crioprecipitato *(Pierrel, Spain)*; Criostat HT *(Grifols, Spain)*; Emoclot *(Aima, Ital.)*; Factorate *(Armour, Ger.; Rorer, Ital.; Armour, UK; Armour, USA)*; Haemate *(Behringwerke, Ger.; Behring, Spain)*; Hematrate *(Hyland, Denm.)*; Hemofil *(Hyland, Canad.; Travenol, Ital.; Travenol, UK; Hyland, USA)*; Humafac *(USA)*; Humanate *(Speywood, UK)*; Humate *(Armour, USA)*; Hyate:C *(Speywood, UK)*; Koate *(Cutter, Canad.; Tropon-Cutter, Ger.; Sclavo, Ital.; Cutter, UK; Cutter, USA)*; Kryobulin *(Immuno, Canad.; Immuno, Denm.; Immuno, Ital.; Immuno, Spain; Immuno, UK)*; Kryobuline *(Immuno, Switz.)*; Nordiocto *(Nordisk Gentofte, Denm.)*; Profilate *(Alpha, Ger.; Alfa Farmaceutici, Ital.; Alpha, Swed.; Alpha Therapeutic, UK; Alpha Therapeutic, USA)*; Ristofact *(Behringwerke, Ger.)*; Uman-Cry-VIII *(Biagini, Ital.)*.

19165-p

Factor VIII Inhibitor Bypassing Fraction

Activated Prothrombin Complex Concentrate.

Preparations with factor VIII inhibitor bypassing activity are prepared from human plasma.

Adverse Effects and Precautions

Allergic reactions may follow the administration of preparations having factor VIII inhibitor bypassing activity.

Uses and Administration

Preparations with factor VIII inhibitor bypassing activity are used in patients with haemophilia A who have antibodies to factor VIII. The strength and doses of such preparations are expressed in units, 1 unit being defined as the factor VIII inhibitor bypassing activity which shortens the activated partial thromboplastin time of a high titre factor VIII inhibitor reference plasma to 50% of the blank value.

A recommended dose for spontaneous bleeding episodes in haemophiliac patients is 50 to 100 units per kg body-weight administered intravenously at 8- to 12-hourly intervals until clear signs of improvement occur; if improvement does not occur combined treatment with factor VIII is recommended.

A discussion on factor VIII inhibitors in haemophilia. The inhibitors are circulating immunoglobulins with specificity for the procoagulant component (VIII:C) of the factor VIII complex and their presence renders conventional factor VIII replacement therapy ineffective in the bleeding patient. High-dose human factor VIII replacement, whereby the antibodies are overwhelmed and haemostasis established, has been used to control haemorrhage as has the use of porcine factor VIII material which has a lower cross-reactivity with the human inhibitor. Physical depletion of the circulating inhibitor may also be obtained by procedures such as exchange transfusion or plasmaphaeresis but the effects are transient. Another approach is the use of immunosuppressive agents which occasionally eradicate the inhibitor.
The advent of activated prothrombin complex concentrates with factor VIII inhibitor bypassing activity has added a new dimension to the symptomatic management of these patients. Although the mechanism of action is not fully understood activated prothrombin complex concentrates are known to contain the activated coagulation factors VIIa and IXa and conceivably exert their effect in a manner irrespective of antibody titre, at a lower level in the coagulation cascade than factor VIII itself.— *Lancet*, 1983, *1*, 742.

Further reviews: C. K. Kasper, *J. Am. med. Ass.*, 1984, *251*, 68; C. R. Rizza, *Prescribers' J.*, 1984, *24*, 71.

Proprietary Preparations

Feiba *(Immuno, UK). Injection*, factor VIII inhibitor bypassing fraction in vials containing 500 and 1000 units.

Proprietary Names and Manufacturers

Autoplex *(Baxter, Ger.; Travenol, Spain; Hyland, USA)*; Feiba *(Immuno, Canad.; Immuno, Ger.; Immuno, Ital.; Immuno, Spain; Immuno, Switz.; Immuno, UK)*.

1227-a

Factor IX

Prothrombin Complex Concentrate.

Dried Factor IX Fraction *(B.P.)* (Freeze-dried Human Coagulation Factor IX *(Eur.P.)*; Factor IX Coagulationis Sanguinis Humani Cryodesiccatus) is rich in clotting factors II, IX, and X and may also contain clotting factor VII. It is prepared from human plasma obtained from blood from healthy donors who must, as far as can be ascertained, be free from detectable agents of infection transmissible by transfusion of blood or blood derivatives. The method of preparation is designed in particular to minimise thrombogenicity and to avoid the transmission of or to inactivate known agents of infection. The factor IX fraction is prepared by a suitable fractionation technique and dissolved in an appropriate liquid, sterilised by filtration, distributed in sterile containers, and freeze-dried. The containers are sealed under vacuum or filled with oxygen-free nitrogen or other suitable inert gas before sealing. When the contents of a sealed container are dissolved in a volume of water as stated on the label the resulting solution contains not less than 20 units of factor IX per mL, not less than 0.2 unit per mg of protein, not more than 300 mmol of sodium ions per litre, not more than 60 mmol of citrate ions per litre, and not more than 50 mmol of phosphate ions per litre. It may contain heparin at a concentration not exceeding 0.15 unit per unit of factor IX. The dried product should be stored at a temperature below 8° and be protected from light. The reconstituted solution should be used as soon as possible after, and not more than 3 hours after, reconstitution. If a gel forms the fraction should not be used.

Factor IX Complex *(U.S.P.)* is a sterile freeze-dried powder consisting of partially purified factor IX fraction, as well as concentrated factor II, VII, and X fractions of venous plasma obtained from healthy human donors. It contains no preservatives. It should be stored at 2° to 8° in hermetically-sealed containers. It should be used within 4 hours after reconstitution and administered with equipment that includes a filter.

Units

5.62 units of blood coagulation factor IX, human are contained in 5.92 mg of a freeze-dried concentrate of human blood coagulation factor IX in one ampoule of the first International Standard Preparation (1976).

Adverse Effects and Precautions

Allergic reactions may follow the administration of factor IX preparations. Intravascular coagulation has been reported in patients with liver disease. Overdosage may cause factors II and X to accumulate.

Factor IX preparations should not be given to patients with disseminated intravascular coagulation without prior treatment with heparin, and should be used with care in patients with liver disease.

Reports of adverse effects in patients with underlying hepatic disorders treated with factor IX preparations: P. M. Blatt *et al.*, *Ann. intern. Med.*, 1974, *81*, 766 (fatal thrombo-embolism); B. G. Gazzard *et al.*, *Gut*, 1974, *15*, 993 (intravascular coagulation); A. I. Cederbaum *et al.*, *Ann. intern. Med.*, 1976, *84*, 683 (intravascular coagulation).

Postoperative factor IX administration was associated with deep-vein thrombosis in a 63-year-old man with severe Christmas disease.— S. J. Machin and B. R. Miller (letter), *Lancet*, 1978, *1*, 1367.

A report of fatal myocardial necrosis in a patient receiving factor IX preparations.— R. A. Gruppo *et al.* (letter), *New Engl. J. Med.*, 1983, *309*, 242. Comment that the patient was receiving large doses for haemophilia A associated with factor VIII inhibitors.— J. M. Lusher (letter), *ibid.*, 1984, *310*, 464.

Uses and Administration

Patients with haemophilia B (Christmas disease) have a genetic deficiency of factor IX and are particularly susceptible to bleeding.

Factor IX preparations, being rich in other factors as well as factor IX, may sometimes be useful for the treatment of bleeding due to deficiencies of factors II, VII, and X, as well as IX, and in the preparation of such patients for surgery.

In patients with factor IX deficiency factor IX is given intravenously. The dosage should be determined for each patient and will vary with the circumstances involving bleeding or type of surgery to be performed. A dose of 1 unit per kg body-weight has been reported to raise the plasma concentration of factor IX by 1%. It is suggested that for mild haemorrhage the plasma concentration of factor IX should be raised to 5 to 10% of normal, for more serious haemorrhage or minor surgery it should be raised to 15 to 30% of normal, and that for major surgery an increase to over 50% of normal may be necessary; initial doses commonly used are in the range of 15 to 75 units per kg with doses in the range of 7 to 75 units per kg being given every 6 to 12 hours for maintenance.

Factor IX preparations have been used in the management of patients with haemophilia A who have antibodies to factor VIII but preparations having factor VIII inhibitor bypassing activity are now available (see above).

The biological half-life of factor IX was 15 to 30 hours, for factor II 2 to 4 days, for factor VII 4 to 6 hours, and for factor X 30 to 70 hours.— Inherited Blood Clotting Disorders, *Tech. Rep. Ser. Wld Hlth Org. No. 504*, 1972.

Proprietary Preparations

Prothromplex *(Immuno, UK). Injection*, freeze-dried factors IX, II, and X in vials containing 200 and 500 units of each factor.

Factor IX is also available from *Blood Products Laboratory, UK.*

Proprietary Names and Manufacturers

Bebulin *(Immuno, Denm.; Immuno, Ital.; Immuno, Spain)*; Bebuline *(Immuno, Switz.)*; Haimaplex *(Aima, Ital.)*; Konyne *(Cutter, Canad.; Sclavo, Ital.; Cutter, USA)*; Preconativ *(Pierrel, Ital.)*; Profilnine *(Alpha Therapeutic, USA)*; Proplex *(Hyland, Canad.; Hyland, USA)*; Prothar *(Armour, USA)*; Prothrombinex *(Commonwealth Serum Laboratories, Austral.)*; Prothromplex *(Immuno, UK)*; Protromplex *(Immuno, Ital.)*; Uman-Complex-IX *(Biagini, Ital.)*.

1228-t

Factor XIII

Fibrin-stabilising Factor; FSF.

Uses and Administration

Factor XIII deficiency is a genetic disorder. In the *UK* a preparation containing in each 4 mL after reconstitution factor XIII activity equivalent to at least 250 mL of fresh pooled citrated plasma is used in patients with factor XIII deficiency. In replacement therapy for the prophylaxis of haemorrhage a quantity, for an adult, equivalent to about 500 to 750 mL of fresh plasma may be given every 4 weeks. For the treatment of severe bleeding a dose equivalent to about 500 to 1250 mL of fresh plasma may be given daily until bleeding ceases. In prophylaxis in surgery a dose equivalent to 2500 mL of fresh plasma may be given and followed by the equivalent of 500 to 750 mL of fresh plasma daily for 5 days.

A discussion of factor XIII deficiency.— *Lancet*, 1980, *1*, 522.

Some references to the use of factor XIII concentrate in the management of patients with factor XIII deficiency: J. Francis and P. Todd, *Br. med. J.*, 1978, *2*, 1532; P. Stenberg *et al.* (letter), *Lancet*, 1980, *1*, 1136; S. Stenbjerg (letter), *ibid.*, *2*, 257; P. Stenberg *et al.* (letter), *ibid*; F. Delbarre *et al.* (letter), *ibid.*, 1981, *2*, 204.

Proprietary Preparations

Fibrogammin P *(Hoechst, UK). Injection*, freeze-dried factor XIII (heat treated) in vials each containing activity equivalent to at least 250 mL of fresh pooled citrated plasma.

Factor XIII is also available from *Blood Products Laboratory, UK.*

Proprietary Names and Manufacturers

Fibrogammin *(Behringwerke, Ger.; Istituto Behring, Ital.; Hoechst, UK)*; Fibrogammine *(Hoechst, Fr.)*.

1229-x

Fibrin

CAS — 9001-31-4.

Human Fibrin Foam *(B.P.C. 1973)* is a dry artificial sterile sponge of human fibrin. It is prepared by clotting with human thrombin a foam of a solution of human fibrinogen. The clotted foam is dried from the frozen state, cut into strips, and sterilised by heating at 130° for 3 hours. It should be stored below 25° in sterile containers sealed to exclude micro-organisms and moisture and be protected from light.

Uses and Administration

Fibrin foam has been used in conjunction with thrombin as a haemostatic in surgery at sites where bleeding cannot easily be controlled by the commoner methods of haemostasis. A piece of the foam is saturated with a solution of thrombin in sodium chloride 0.9% and placed in contact with the bleeding points. Blood coagulates in contact with the thrombin in the interstices of the foam. Since all the clotting materials are of human origin, they may be left in place when the wound is closed.

Proprietary Preparations of Animal Fibrin

Absele Sterile Absorbable Bone Sealant *(Ethicon, UK). Paste*, stabilised bovine fibrin 17.5%, solubilised bovine collagen 17.5%, dextran '70' 8%, glycerol 30%. For controlling bleeding from bone during surgery.

Biethium Sterile Absorbable Ox Fibrin Prosthesis *(Ethicon, UK). Implant* (absorbable prosthesis), heat-treated bovine fibrin 65%, glycerol 35%.

Proprietary Names and Manufacturers
Zimospuma *(Baldacci, Ital.; Zambon, Spain).*

1230-y

Fibrinogen

Factor I.

Dried Human Fibrinogen (*Eur.P.*) (Fibrinogenum Human Cryodesiccatum) contains the soluble constituent of human plasma that is transformed to fibrin on the addition of thrombin. It is prepared from liquid human plasma obtained from donors who must, as far as can be ascertained, be free from detectable agents of infection transmissible by transfusion. No antimicrobial preservative is added. It should be stored under vacuum or under an atmosphere of nitrogen at a temperature of 2° to 8° and be protected from light. When dissolved in the volume of water for injections stated on the label, the resulting solution contains not less than 1% of fibrinogen, the fibrinogen content being not less than 60% of the total protein content.

Uses and Administration

Fibrinogen has been used to control haemorrhage associated with low blood-fibrinogen concentration in afibrinogenaemia or hypofibrinogenaemia but the use of plasma or cryoprecipitate is often preferred. It has also been used in disseminated intravascular coagulation (the defibrination syndrome).

Fibrinogen labelled with radionuclides has also been used in diagnostic procedures.

Preparations

Dried Fibrinogen for Isotopic Labelling *(B.P.).* Dried Human Fibrinogen for Isotopic Labelling

Proprietary Names and Manufacturers

Fibrinogene *(Immuno, Switz.,)*;
Fibrinomer *(ISI, Ital.)*; Haemocomplettan *(Behringwerke, Ger.)*; Uman-Fibrin *(Biagini, Ital.).*

17041-m

Fluorocarbon Blood Substitutes

A fluorocarbon emulsion consisting of two fluorocarbons, perfluorodecalin and perfluorotripropylamine, has been used as a synthetic blood substitute in a variety of conditions.

Reviews and discussions on fluorocarbons as potential blood substitutes: P. M. Jones, *Br. med. J.*, 1983, *286*, 246; G. P. Biro, *Can. med. Ass. J.*, 1983, *129*, 237; K. C. Lowe, *Br. J. Hosp. Med.*, 1985, *34*, 195.

Perfluorochemical emulsions, or fluorocarbons, are inert fluorinated hydrocarbons whose primary use is in industry as refrigeration fluids and aerosol propellents. Their ability to carry oxygen and carbon dioxide, together with their ability to replace blood entirely in *rats*, led to the production of an emulsion of 20% fluorocarbons with an average particle size of 100 nm in a glucose/glycerol/electrolyte/hetastarch solution. (Fluosol-DA). This solution has been used clinically in a variety of situations, including resuscitation, refusal of blood transfusion, pre-operative anaemia, postpartum haemorrhage, carbon monoxide inhalation, and cerebral hypoxia. Although in most instances infusion volumes were modest (up to 25 mL per kg body-weight), haemodynamic indices and arterial oxygenation improved. There are, however, two major difficulties associated with the use of fluorocarbons. Some adverse reactions may be related to their effect on the immune system and secondly, the linear oxygen dissociation curve means that high inspired oxygen concentrations must be achieved for clinically useful oxygen carriage. Whilst there is reason for optimism that acceptable blood substitutes may become available in the foreseeable future, extensive *animal* and human studies are necessary before they should be considered for widespread clinical use.— *Lancet*, 1986, *1*, 717.

Proprietary Names and Manufacturers
Fluosol-DA *(Green Cross Corp., Jpn).*

5425-w

Gelatin *(BAN, USAN).*

CAS — 9000-70-8.

Pharmacopoeias. In *Arg., Aust., Br., Braz., Chin., Cz., Egypt., Eur., Fr., Ger., Hung., Ind., It., Jpn, Jug., Mex., Neth., Nord., Pol., Port., Roum., Rus., Span., Swiss,* and *Turk.* Also in *U.S.N.F.*

Gelatin is a purified protein obtained either by partial acid hydrolysis (type A) or by partial alkaline hydrolysis (type B) of animal collagen.

Colourless or pale yellowish or amber-coloured translucent sheets, shreds, flakes, powder, or granules with a slight odour.

Gelatin swells and softens when immersed in cold water, gradually absorbing 5 to 10 times its weight of water; **soluble** in hot water, forming a jelly on cooling; practically insoluble in alcohol, chloroform, and ether; soluble in a hot mixture of glycerol and water and in 6N acetic acid; insoluble in fixed and volatile oils. **Store** in airtight containers. The moisture content of powdered or finely divided gelatin varies rapidly with the humidity of the atmosphere to which it is exposed.

Gelatins are usually graded by jelly strength, expressed as 'Bloom strength' or 'Bloom rating'.

The gelatin described in some pharmacopoeias is not necessarily suitable for preparations for parenteral use or for other special purposes.

STANDARD FOR GELATIN. A British Standard Specification for methods of sampling and testing gelatin (BS 757:1975) is published by the British Standards Institution.

Adverse Effects

Allergic and anaphylactic reactions have occurred after the infusion of gelatin or its derivatives.

ALLERGY. Ten severe anaphylactoid reactions to an infusion of a modified fluid gelatin were reported over a period of 3 years.— Y. Blanloeil *et al.*, *Thérapie*, 1983, *38*, 539.

Precautions

Precautions that should be observed with plasma expanders are described under dextran 70, p.815, and these should be considered when gelatin and gelatin derivatives are used for this purpose. There does not appear to be any interference with blood grouping and cross matching of blood.

Absorption and Fate

Following infusion, gelatin is rapidly excreted, mostly in the urine.

Uses and Administration

Gelatin is a protein that has both clinical and pharmaceutical uses.

Gelatin is used as a haemostatic in surgical procedures as an absorbable film or sponge and can absorb many times its weight of blood.

It is also employed as a plasma substitute similarly to the dextrans. A 4% solution of a modified fluid gelatin with electrolytes has been infused at various rates, usually in doses of up to 2 litres for adults or 30 mL per kg body-weight for children.

Gelatin is used in the preparation of pastes, pastilles, suppositories, tablets, and hard and soft capsule shells. It is also used for the microencapsulation of drugs and other industrial materials. It has been used as a vehicle for injections; Pitkin's Menstruum, which consists of gelatin, glucose, and acetic acid, has been used in a modified form for heparin while hydrolysed gelatin has been used for corticotrophin. Gelatin is an ingredient of preparations used for the protection of stoma and lesions.

The Science and Technology of Gelatin, A.G. Ward and A. Courts (Ed.), London, Academic Press, 1977.

A brief review of 20 years' experience in the use of modified fluid gelatin as a plasma substitute. It is used routinely in the treatment of surgical haemorrhage, and has been used in doses of up to 15 litres in massive haemorrhage.— P. Lundsgaard-Hansen and B. Tschirren, *Develop. biol. Stand.*, 1981, *48*, 251.

A report of the use of modified fluid gelatin in leucophaeresis procedures.— D. W. Huestis *et al.*, *Transfusion, Philad.*, 1985, *25*, 343.

Preparations

Absorbable Gelatin Film *(U.S.P.)*

Absorbable Gelatin Sponge *(B.P.).* Gelatin Sponge

Absorbable Gelatin Sponge *(U.S.P.)*

Proprietary Preparations

Gelofusine *(Consolidated Chemicals, UK). Intravenous infusion*, modified fluid gelatin 40 g, sodium 154 mmol, potassium less than 0.4 mmol, magnesium less than 0.4 mmol, calcium less than 0.4 mmol, chloride 125 mmol/litre, in bottles of 500 mL.

Sterispon *(Allen & Hanburys, UK).* Absorbable Gelatin Sponge (*B.P.*).

Proprietary Names and Manufacturers

Crodyne *(Croda, UK)*; Dextricea Papilla *(Francisco Durban, Spain)*; Espongostan Film *(Leo, Spain)*; Fibrospuma Esponja *(Spain)*; Gelafundin *(Braun Melsungen, Ger.)*; Gelfilm *(Upjohn, Austral.; Upjohn, Ger.; Upjohn, USA)*; Gelfoam *(Upjohn, Austral.; Belg.; Ger.; Upjohn, S.Afr.; Switz.; Upjohn, USA)*; Gelofusine *(Consolidated Chemicals, UK)*; Gel-Phan *(Pierre Fabre, Fr.)*; Hemoce *(Behring, Spain)*; Marbagelan *(Behringwerke, Ger.)*; Neo-Plasmagel *(Ger.)*; Pharmagel *(USA)*; Physiogel *(Ger.)*; Spongostan *(Belg.; Ferrosan, Denm.; Ferrosan, Norw.; Novo, S.Afr.)*; Sterispon *(Allen & Hanburys, UK)*; Tanagel Papeles *(Francisco Durban, Spain)*; Thomaegelin *(Thomae, Ger.).*

12812-y

Haemoglobin

Haemoglobin is the red pigment of red blood cells. It is a tetrameric compound, each of the 4 subunits consisting of an iron-protoporphyrin complex containing 1 atom of ferrous iron (haem), in association with a polypeptide (globin). It contains about 0.34% of iron.

Haemoglobin has the property of reversible oxygenation and is the respiratory pigment of blood. Solutions of haemoglobin or modified haemoglobin have been investigated as blood substitutes.

Reviews and discussions on haemoglobin solutions as potential blood substitutes: G. P. Biro, *Can. med. Ass. J.*, 1983, *129*, 237; K. C. Lowe, *Br. J. Hosp. Med.*, 1985, *34*, 195.

Because the structure of haemoglobin gives a non-linear oxygen dissociation curve, almost maximum oxygen saturation occurs in normal arterial blood without the need for oxygen-enriched air; thus the use of haemoglobin solutions for emergency resuscitation appears logical. Initial *animal* experiments with haemoglobin from haemolysed erythrocytes resulted in serious renal damage but the development of stroma-free haemoglobin solutions reduced this toxicity somewhat. Polymerisation of haemoglobin (by the addition of glutaraldehyde) to produce high molecular weight substances has been reported as has the development of pyridoxylated haemoglobin solutions. There are, however, reservations concerning haemoglobin solutions as blood substitutes; blood itself must be available for their production, although expired blood maybe employed and there is also concern about impairment of immune mechanisms. Whilst there is reason for optimism that acceptable blood substitutes may become available in the foreseeable future, extensive *animal* and human studies are necessary before they should be considered for widespread clinical use.— *Lancet*, 1986, *1*, 717.

Proprietary Names and Manufacturers
Harimex-Ligos, Neth.

255-j

Hetastarch *(BAN, USAN).*

HES; Hydroxyethyl Starch. 2-Hydroxyethyl ether starch.

CAS — 9005-27-0.

Hetastarch is a starch that is composed of more than 90% of amylopectin and that has been etherified to the extent that an average of 7 to 8 of the hydroxy groups in each 10 D-glucopyranose units of starch polymer have been converted into OCH_2CH_2OH groups. Hetastarch as normally used has weight average molecular weight of about 450 000.

Adverse Effects

Infusions of hetastarch may occasionally produce allergic and anaphylactic reactions. Effects that have been reported include fever, headache, skin reactions, muscle pains, salivary enlargement, bronchospasm, periorbital oedema, and vomiting.

ALLERGY. Lichen planus occurred in one subject who received hetastarch as a consequence of granulocyte donation.— U. Bode and A. B. Deisseroth, *Transfusion, Philad.*, 1981, *21*, 83. Severe pruritus occurred in 4 subjects given hetastarch for the same purpose.— N. E. Parker *et al.*, *Br. med. J.*, 1982, *284*, 385.

EFFECTS ON THE BLOOD. In a review of the reported effects of hetastarch on blood coagulation it was concluded that when used in moderate doses hetastarch's effect on coagulation was slight, transient, and probably clinically insignificant.— R. G. Strauss, *Transfusion, Philad.*, 1981, *21*, 299.

A report of coagulopathy with intracranial haemorrhage in a patient treated with hetastarch. Hetastarch should probably be avoided in neurosurgical patients, in whom the prevention of intracranial haemorrhage is critical.— L. Damon *et al.* (letter), *New Engl. J. Med.*, 1987, *317*, 964. See also: B. E. Symington (letter), *Ann. intern. Med.*, 1986, *105*, 627.

Precautions

Precautions that should be observed with plasma expanders are described under dextran 70, p.815 and these should be considered when hetastarch is used. There does not appear to be any interference with blood grouping and cross matching of blood.

Serum-amylase concentrations can be increased by administration of hetastarch and this may interfere with diagnostic tests.

Absorption and Fate

After intravenous infusion of hetastarch, the molecules with a molecular weight of less than 50 000 are readily excreted unchanged by the kidney. About 40% of a dose is excreted in the urine in 24 hours. Accumulation occurs after multiple doses and it has been shown to persist in the body for several weeks.

The pharmacokinetics of hetastarch in healthy subjects: J. M. Mishler *et al.*, *Br. J. clin. Pharmac.*, 1979, *7*, 505; *idem*, *J. clin. Path.*, 1980, *33*, 155; A. Yacobi *et al.*, *J. clin. Pharmac.*, 1982, *22*, 206.

Uses and Administration

As a 6% solution hetastarch exerts a similar colloidal osmotic pressure to human albumin. It is used for short-term expansion of the plasma volume in shock or impending shock resulting from burns, surgery, haemorrhage, or trauma. The dose and rate of infusion depends on the condition of the patient. The usual dose is 500 to 1000 mL; more than 20 mL per kg body-weight per day is not usually required. In acute haemorrhagic shock up to 20 mL per kg per hour has been given.

Hetastarch increases the erythrocyte sedimentation-rate when added to whole blood. It is therefore used in leucophaeresis procedures to increase the yield of granulocytes. Doses of 250 to 700 mL are infused to venous blood in such procedures. There may be 2 such procedures per week to a total 10.

Hetastarch has also been used in extracorporeal perfusion fluids.

Reviews of the actions and uses of hetastarch: S. K. Nakasato, *Clin. Pharm.*, 1982, *1*, 509; J. D. Hulse and A. Yacobi, *Drug Intell. & clin. Pharm.*, 1983, *17*, 334.

A study involving 6 healthy subjects showed that hetastarch with a weight average molecular weight of 125 000 produced similar plasma expansion to dextran 70.— K. Korttila *et al.*, *J. clin. Pharmac.*, 1984, *24*, 273.

ADMINISTRATION IN RENAL FAILURE. In a study of the pharmacokinetics of hetastarch in 8 patients with creatinine clearances ranging from 28 to 100 mL per minute, it was concluded that this degree of renal function was adequate for the elimination of hetastarch.— J. Hulse *et al.*, *Clin. Pharmac. Ther.*, 1983, *33*, 254.

Proprietary Preparations

Hespan *(Du Pont Pharmaceuticals, UK)*. *Intravenous infusion*, hetastarch 6% in sodium chloride 0.9%, in bags of 500 mL.

Proprietary Names and Manufacturers

Elohast *(Hormonchemie, Ger.)*; Expafusin *(Pfrimmer, Ger.; Pfrimmer, Spain)*; Hes Grifols *(Grifols, Spain)*; Hespan *(Baxter, Ital.; Du Pont Pharmaceuticals, UK; American Critical Care, USA)*; Onkohas *(Braun Melsungen, Ger.)*; Plasmasteril *(Fresenius, Ger.)*; Volex *(McGaw, USA)*.

1244-t

Leucocytes

Transfusions of leucocytes (granulocytes) have been used in a variety of disorders as part of the management of infections not responsive to other treatments.

A brief discussion of infection and host defences in neonates including the use of the transfusion of mature granulocytes for fulminating early-onset sepsis and infection caused by antibiotic-resistant organisms.— M. L. Chiswick, *Br. med. J.*, 1983, *286*, 1377.

A discussion on recent advances in chronic granulomatous disease, a group of disorders involving recurrent infections and chronic inflammation. Leucocyte transfusions have been used when conventional medical and surgical treatments fail to control the infection or inflammation and when there is rapidly progressive life-threatening infection, but experience with these techniques is limited.— *Ann. intern. Med.*, 1983, *99*, 657.

5446-z

Oxypolygelatin

CAS — 9005-91-8.

Oxypolygelatin is a polymer derived from gelatin.

Oxypolygelatin has been used as a plasma substitute. There have been reports of anaphylaxis.

Proprietary Names and Manufacturers

Gelifundol *(Biotest, Ger.)*.

1245-x

Plasma

Fresh Frozen Plasma (*B.P.*) (Fresh Frozen Plasma for Infusion) is prepared from the supernatant liquid which is separated by centrifuging from Whole Blood from a single donor. It contains not less than 50% of the factor VIII activity of the Whole Blood. It is distributed in sterile containers which are immediately sealed and cooled to −30° or below as rapidly as possible and, in any case, within 18 hours of collection. It should be stored at a temperature of −30° or below until required for use except for any period (not exceeding 30 minutes) necessary for transportation. The label states the ABO group and the Rh group of the Whole Blood from which it was obtained and the nature of the specific antisera used in testing. It should be used within 3 hours of thawing and should not be refrozen. It should be administered with suitable equipment such as that described in Section 3 or Section 4 of *Transfusion Equipment for Medical Use*, BS 2463: 1962.

Adverse Effects

As for blood, p.813.

ALLERGY. Allergic pulmonary oedema after transfusion with fresh frozen plasma.— P. C. O'Connor *et al.*, *Br. med. J.*, 1981, *282*, 379.

Uses and Administration

Fresh frozen plasma contains useful amounts of clotting factors and may be used as a source of these factors when specific concentrates are not available. It has also been used in the treatment of thrombotic thrombocytopenic purpura.

Plasma exchange or plasmaphaeresis (the terms are commonly used synonymously) which involves the removal of blood, anticoagulation, centrifugation, and the return to the patient of the cellular components suspended in a suitable vehicle such as fresh frozen plasma or plasma protein fraction is used in a wide variety of disorders.

Following a consensus development conference in the *USA* involving the National Heart, Lung, and Blood Institute, the Food and Drug Administration (FDA), and the Office of Medical Applications of Research the following were considered to be indications for the use of fresh frozen plasma: the treatment of deficiencies of factors II, V, VII, IX, X, and XI when specific component therapy is neither available nor appropriate; reversal of the effect of warfarin in patients who are actively bleeding or requiring emergency surgery; reversal of haemostatic disorders associated with massive blood transfusion only in patients in whom factor deficiencies are presumed to be the sole or principal derangement; treatment of antithrombin III deficiency in patients undergoing surgery or who require heparin for treatment of thrombosis; treatment of infants with secondary immunodeficiency associated with severe protein-losing enteropathy; treatment of thrombotic thrombocytopenic purpura. There was no justification for the use of fresh frozen plasma as a volume expander or as a nutritional source. The risks associated with the use of fresh frozen plasma include disease transmission, anaphylactoid reactions, allo-immunisation, and excessive intravascular volume.— *J. Am. med. Ass.*, 1985, *253*, 551. See also: H. A. Oberman, *ibid.*, 556.

Discussion on the misuse of fresh frozen plasma and concluding that the proper indications for its use are few but include: abnormal bleeding in which a clotting defect has been proved; treatment of patients with rare isolated factor deficiencies such as factor V and factor X for which specific concentrates are unavailable; emergency use in patients to reverse the anticoagulant action of coumarin type compounds; and thrombotic thrombocytopenic purpura.— J. Jones, *Br. med. J.*, 1987, *295*, 287.

PLASMA EXCHANGE. General reviews of the use of plasma exchange: E. A. E. Robinson, *Archs Dis. Childh.*, 1982, *57*, 301; K. H. Shumak and G. A. Rock, *New Engl. J. Med.*, 1984, *310*, 762.

Report of the American Medical Association Panel on the current status of therapeutic plasmaphaeresis and related techniques: *J. Am. med. Ass.*, 1985, *253*, 819.

Reviews and discussions on the use of plasma exchange for neurological disorders: *J. Am. med. Ass.*, 1986, *256*, 1333; *Lancet*, 1986, *2*, 1313; P. O. Behan and W. M. H. Behan, *Br. med. J.*, 1987, *295*, 283.

1248-d

Plasma Protein Fraction

Plasma Protein Solution (*B.P.*) (Plasma Protein Fraction; Human Plasma Protein Solution (*Eur. P.*); Proteinorum Plasmatis Humani Solutio) is a sterile isotonic aqueous solution of the proteins of plasma or serum containing albumin and globulins which retain their solubility on heating. The plasma or serum is obtained from healthy donors who must, as far as can be ascertained, be free from detectable agents of infection transmissible by transfusion of blood or blood derivatives. It is sterilised by filtration and distributed aseptically into containers which are sealed to exclude micro-organisms and maintained at 60° for 10 hours. Finally, the containers are incubated for not less than 14 days at 30° to 32° or for not less than 4 weeks at 20° to 25° and examined visually for signs of microbial contamination. It contains 4 to 5% w/v of total protein, of which not less than 85% is albumin; it contains not more than 160 mmol of sodium per litre. It should be stored at 2° to 25° and be protected from light. It must not be used if the solution is cloudy or contains a deposit.

Plasma Protein Fraction (*U.S.P.*) is a sterile preparation of serum albumin and globulin obtained by fractionating material (blood, plasma, or serum) from healthy human donors, the source material being tested for the absence of hepatitis B surface antigen. It contains 5% of protein; not less than 83% of the total protein is albumin; not more than 17% is alpha and beta globulins; not more than 1% has the electrophoretic properties of gamma globulin. It contains 130 to 160 mmol of sodium per litre, and not more than 2 mmol of potassium per litre. It must not be used if the solution is turbid.

Adverse Effects and Precautions

Adverse effects are uncommon but nausea, vomiting, urticaria, chills, fever, hypotension, and salivation have been reported. Patients should be watched for signs of circulatory overload such as pulmonary oedema or heart failure.

ALLERGY. A 26-year-old woman developed acute urticaria after receiving 40 mL of an infusion of a plasma protein preparation (Plasmanate).— R. D. McMillin *et al.*, *Am. J. Surg.*, 1978, *135*, 706.

EFFECTS ON ELECTROLYTES. Metabolic alkalosis developed in 4 patients with limited renal function when they were given preparations of plasma protein fraction.— G. T. Rahilly and T. Berl, *New Engl. J. Med.*, 1979, *301*, 824.

Uses and Administration

Plasma protein fraction consists mainly of albumin with a small proportion of globulins. It is administered intravenously as a solution containing 4 to 5% of total protein for volume replacement in hypovolaemic shock associated with injury, surgery, or burns. The usual dose for adults is in the range of 250 to 500 mL. A suggested dose in children for shock associated with dehydration or infection is 20 to 30 mL per kg body-weight.

Doses of 1500 to 2000 mL or more have been suggested for use in adults for the treatment of hypoproteinaemia.

It does not contain blood-clotting factors.

Proprietary Preparations

Human Albumin Solution 4.5% 'Immuno' (*Immuno, UK*). Plasma Protein Fraction (*B.P.*).

Proprietary Names and Manufacturers

Buminate 5% *(Travenol, UK)*; Plasmanate *(Cutter, Canad.; Cutter, USA)*; Plasma-Plex *(Armour, USA)*; Plasmatein *(Alpha Therapeutic, USA)*; Plasmaviral *(ISI, Ital.)*; Protenate *(Hyland, Canad.; Hyland, USA)*.

1221-l

Platelets

Platelet Concentrate (*U.S.P.*) contains the platelets taken from plasma obtained by whole-blood collection, plasmaphaeresis, or plateletphaeresis from a single suitable human donor. The platelets are suspended in a specified volume (20 to 30 mL, or 30 to 50 mL) of the original plasma. The suspension contains not less than 5.5×10^{10} platelets per unit in not less than 75% of the units tested. It should be stored in hermetically-sealed sterile containers at 20° to 24° (30 to 50 mL volume), or at 1° to 6° (20 to 30 mL volume) except during transport when the temperature may be 1° to 10°. The expiration time is not more than 72 hours from the time of collection of the source material. Continuous gentle agitation must be maintained if stored at 20° to 24°. The suspension must be used within 4 hours of opening the container.

Adverse Effects

Blood platelets are antigenic, and immunological and allergic reactions have occurred. Because platelet preparations contain a small quantity of red cells, Rh immunisation may occur if platelets from an Rh-positive donor are given to an Rh-negative recipient.

ALLERGY. Analysis, by the Boston Collaborative Drug Surveillance Program, of data on 15 438 patients hospitalised between 1975 and 1982 detected 13 allergic skin reactions attributed to platelets among 29 recipients.— M. Bigby *et al.*, *J. Am. med. Ass.*, 1986, *256*, 3358.

Uses and Administration

Blood platelets assist in the clotting process by aggregation to form a platelet thrombus and by participating in the formation of thromboplastin. Transfusions of platelet concentrates are given to patients with thrombocytopenic haemorrhage. They may also be given prophylactically to reduce the frequency of haemorrhage in thrombocytopenia associated with the chemotherapy of neoplastic disease.

A consensus development conference in the *USA* involving the National Heart, Lung, and Blood Institute, the Food and Drug Administration (FDA), and the Office of Medical Applications of Research considered the following to be appropriate indications for platelet transfusion therapy: significant bleeding in patients with thrombocytopenia or an abnormality of platelet function if the platelet disorder is likely to be the cause of, or a contributory factor to, the bleeding; and prophylaxis in some patients with severe thrombocytopenia. The risks associated with platelet transfusion therapy were alloimmunisation, possible transmission of infection, and rarely graft-versus-host disease.— *J. Am. med. Ass.*, 1987, *257*, 1777.

A further review and discussion concerning platelet transfusion therapy.— *Lancet*, 1987, *2*, 490.

5449-a

Polygeline *(BAN, pINN)*.

Polygelinum.

CAS — 9015-56-9.

Polygeline is a polymer prepared by cross-linking polypeptides derived from denatured gelatin with a di-isocyanate to form urea bridges.

Intravenous preparations of polygeline contain calcium ions and are incompatible with citrated blood.

Adverse Effects

Allergic and anaphylactic reactions have occurred after the infusion of polygeline.

ALLERGY. In a study of 450 patients undergoing surgery, premedication with a histamine H_1-receptor antagonist (chlorpheniramine or dimethindene) and cimetidine reduced the incidence of cutaneous reactions to polygeline infusions.— B. Schöning *et al.*, *Klin. Wschr.*, 1982, *60*, 1048.

Precautions

Precautions that should be observed with plasma expanders are described under dextran 70, p.815, and these should be considered when polygeline is used for this purpose.

Preparations containing calcium ions should be used with caution in patients being treated with cardiac glycosides.

Absorption and Fate

Like gelatin, polygeline is excreted mainly in the urine.

Uses and Administration

Polygeline is used as a 3.5% solution with electrolytes as a plasma substitute for the treatment of shock due to haemorrhage, burns, injuries, or water and electrolyte loss. The rate of infusion depends on the condition of the patient and does not normally exceed 500 mL in 60 minutes. Initial doses usually consist of 500 to 1000 mL; up to 1500 mL of blood loss can be replaced by polygeline alone.

Polygeline is also used in patients undergoing extracorporeal circulation, as a perfusion fluid for isolated organs, as fluid replacement in plasma exchange, and as a carrier solution for insulin.

ADMINISTRATION IN RENAL FAILURE. In a study in 52 patients with normal or impaired renal function given 500 mL of polygeline 3.5% about 50% of the dose was excreted in the urine within 48 hours in those with normal renal function. Excretion was not impaired in those with a glomerular filtration-rate (GFR) of 31 to 90 mL per minute, slightly reduced in those with a GFR of 11 to 30 mL, reduced to 27% in 48 hours in those with a GFR of 2 to 10 mL, and to 9.3% in 48 hours in those with a GFR of 0.5 to 2 mL. The mean half-life of the elimination phase was 505 minutes in those with adequate renal function, increasing to 985 minutes in those with end-stage renal failure. Polygeline 500 mL of 3.5% solution could be given twice weekly for 1 to 2 months even in patients with total anuria.— H. Köhler *et al.*, *Eur. J. clin. Pharmac.*, 1978, *14*, 405.

PLASMA EXCHANGE. Polygeline as the sole replacement fluid in plasma exchange.— A. J. Stellon and P. J. Moorhead, *Br. med. J.*, 1981, *282*, 696.

Proprietary Preparations

Haemaccel *(Hoechst, UK)*. *Intravenous infusion*, polygeline 35 g, sodium 145 mmol, potassium 5.1 mmol, calcium 6.25 mmol, chloride 145 mmol/litre, in bottles of 500 mL.

Proprietary Names and Manufacturers

Emagel *(Istituto Behring, Ital.)*; Haemaccel *(Aust.; Hoechst, Austral.; Belg.; Hoechst, Fr.; Behringwerke, Ger.; Neth.; Behring, Norw.; Pol.; Behring, Swed.; Switz.; Hoechst, UK)*.

1218-k

Red Blood Cells

Concentrated Red Blood Cells (*B.P.*) is Whole Blood from a single donor from which part of the plasma and anticoagulant solution has been removed. It has a packed cell volume greater than 70%. It is prepared from Whole Blood which is preferably not more than 14 days old. The ABO group and the Rh group of the Whole Blood from which it was made and the nature of the specific antisera used in testing are stated on the label. It should be stored at 2° to 8° in sterile containers sealed to exclude micro-organisms. It should be administered with suitable equipment as described in Section 3 or Section 4 of *Transfusion Equipment for Medical Use*, BS 2463: 1962.

Plasma-reduced Blood (*B.P.*) (Plasma-reduced Whole Blood) is Whole Blood from a single donor from which part of the plasma and anticoagulant solution has been removed. It has a packed cell volume of 60 to 65%. It is prepared from Whole Blood which is preferably not more than 14 days old. The ABO group and the Rh group of the Whole Blood from which it was made and the nature of the specific antisera used in testing are stated on the label. It should be stored at 2° to 8° in sterile containers sealed to exclude micro-organisms. It should be administered with suitable equipment such as described in Section 3 or Section 4 of *Transfusion Equipment for Medical Use*, BS 2463: 1962.

Red Blood Cells (*U.S.P.*) is the remaining red blood cells of whole human blood from suitable donors, from which plasma has been removed. It is prepared not later than 21 days after the blood has been withdrawn except that the period may be 35 days if the anticoagulant used was acid citrate dextrose adenine solution. If intended for extended manufacturer's storage at or below −65° it contains a portion of the plasma sufficient to ensure cell preservation, or a cryophylactic substance. If unfrozen it should be stored in hermetically-sealed sterile containers at 1° to 6° (with a range of not more than 2°) except during transport when the temperature may be 1° to 10°.

Adverse Effects

As for blood, p.813.

Post-transfusion thrombocytopenic purpura occurred in a 43-year-old woman after the infusion of red blood cells; she had earlier had blood transfusions uneventfully.— P.

M. Dainer and E. D. Canada, *Br. med. J.*, 1977, *2*, 999.

Hypertension in 2 patients with sickle-cell anaemia and cerebral haemorrhage in one after the infusion of red blood cells.— J. E. Royal and R. A. Seeler (letter), *Lancet*, 1978, *2*, 1207. A similar report in thalassaemia.— S. Yetgin and G. Hicsonmez (letter), *ibid.*, 1979, *1*, 610.

Uses and Administration

Transfusions of red blood cells are given for the treatment of severe anaemia without hypovolaemia. The haemoglobin concentration of the blood of the average adult is raised by about 1 g per 100 mL by the red blood cells obtained from 540 mL of whole blood.

Red blood cells are also used for exchange transfusion in babies with haemolytic disease of the newborn.

A review of frozen red blood cells commenting that their use has declined and a reduction in the number of well-established indications for their use in preference to liquid-stored red cells has occurred.— H. Chaplin, *New Engl. J. Med.*, 1984, *311*, 1696.

1250-k

Thrombin

CAS — 9002-04-4.

Thrombin is a preparation of the enzyme which converts fibrinogen into fibrin. The prothrombin fraction is prepared by a suitable fractionation technique; the prothrombin is converted into thrombin in solution by the addition of calcium ions and thromboplastin.

Units

100 units of thrombin, human are contained in 3.5 mg of partially purified, freeze-dried human thrombin and 5 mg of sucrose in one ampoule of the first International Standard Preparation (1975).

Uses and Administration

A solution of human thrombin in sodium chloride 0.9%, prepared by means of an aseptic technique, has been used locally as a haemostatic in conjunction with fibrinogen and fibrin foam.

A preparation of bovine thrombin is used topically to control haemorrhage from puncture sites or from capillary oozing in surgery.

Solutions of thrombin should not be injected.

Preparations

Thrombin *(U.S.P.)*. A sterile freeze-dried powder containing the protein substance obtained from bovine prothrombin; it contains calcium. Solutions should be used within a few hours after preparation; they must not be injected or allowed to enter large blood vessels. Store at 2° to 8°.

Proprietary Preparations

Thrombins are available on a named-patient basis from *Armour, UK* and *Blood Products Laboratory, UK.*

Proprietary Names and Manufacturers

Thrombinar *(Armour, USA)*; Thrombostat *(Parke, Davis, Austral.; Parke, Davis, Canad.; Parke, Davis, UK; Parke, Davis, USA)*; Topostasin *(Roche, Denm.; Roche, Ital.; Roche, Swed.)*; Topostasine *(Roche, Ger.; Roche, Switz.)*; Zimotrombina *(Baldacci, Ital.)*.

1251-a

Thromboplastin

Factor III; Thrombokinase.

Thromboplastin is a blood-clotting factor which initiates conversion of prothrombin to thrombin in the formation of the blood clot.

Units

The second International Reference Preparation (1983) for thromboplastin, human, plain consists of ampoules containing freeze-dried human brain thromboplastin (international sensitivity index, 1.1).

The second International Reference Preparation (1983) for thromboplastin, bovine, combined consists of ampoules containing freeze-dried bovine brain thromboplastin (international sensitivity index, 1.0).

The second International Reference Preparation (1982) for thromboplastin, rabbit, plain consists of ampoules containing freeze-dried rabbit brain suspension (international sensitivity index, 1.4).

Uses and Administration

Preparations of thromboplastin have been used as haemostatics.

A preparation of thromboplastin derived from rabbit brain is employed in the determination of the prothrombin time for the control of anticoagulant therapy (for further details see under warfarin sodium, p.348).

Proprietary Preparations

Tachostyptan *(Consolidated Chemicals, UK). Injection,* thromboplastin (derived from porcine brain tissue) 2%, in ampoules of 5 mL. For intravenous injection in the control of haemorrhage. Available only on a named-patient basis.

Proprietary Names and Manufacturers

Clauden *(Luitpold, Ger.)*; Fibraccel *(Behringwerke, Ger.)*; Tachostyptan *(Hormonchemie, Ger.; Consolidated Chemicals, UK)*; Tacostiptan *(Chinoin, Ital.)*.

Cardiac Inotropic Agents

5800-k

Positive cardiac inotropic agents increase the force of contraction of the myocardium ultimately by increasing the intracellular calcium ion concentration. The cardiac glycosides are the main group of drugs to possess this activity which is mediated by inhibition of sodium-potassium ATPase. Other compounds such as amrinone and milrinone are potent inotropic agents and act through inhibition of phosphodiesterase. A number of compounds possess positive inotropic activity; those described in other sections include the β_1 agonists, such as dobutamine p.1459 and dopamine p.1460, and the β_2 agonists, such as pirbuterol p.1447. The partial β_1 agonist, xamoterol, is described on p.1486.

The cardiac glycosides are used to slow the heart-rate in atrial arrhythmias, especially atrial fibrillation, and are also given in congestive heart failure although their role in the long-term treatment of patients with heart failure and sinus rhythm is now questioned. The traditional treatment of heart failure includes restriction of physical activity, restriction of salt intake, and the use of a diuretic. If this proves insufficient, a digitalis glycoside may be given, and a vasodilator may also be beneficial. The more potent inotropic agents such as dopamine, dobutamine, and milrinone, are reserved for more severe disease.

The cardiac glycosides have very similar pharmacological effects but differ considerably in their speed of onset and duration of action. When rapid digitalisation is necessary, digoxin or ouabain may be given by intravenous injection; medigoxin may also be used. Digoxin is also given by mouth; because it has an intermediate half-life plasma concentrations respond rapidly to changes in dosage. Digitoxin has a longer half-life; it produces less variation in plasma concentrations, which may be advantageous if compliance is poor, but resolution of toxic symptoms will be delayed.

For reviews of the use of the newer cardiac inotropic agents, see under Digoxin, p.830.

5802-t

Acetyldigitoxin *(rINN)*.
α-Acetyldigitoxin; α-Digitoxin Monoacetate; Digitoxin 3‴-Acetate. 3β-[(*O*-3-*O*-Acetyl-2,6-dideoxy-β-D-*ribo*-hexopyranosyl-(1→4)-*O*-2,6-dideoxy-β-D-*ribo*-hexopyranosyl-(1→4)-2,6-dideoxy-β-D-*ribo*-hexopyranosyl)oxy]-14-hydroxy-5β,14β-card-20(22)-enolide.
$C_{43}H_{66}O_{14}$=807.0.

CAS — 1111-39-3.

Pharmacopoeias. In *Cz.*, *Hung.*, and *Roum. Pol.* includes the monohydrate.

Acetyldigitoxin is derived from Lanatoside A. It has the general properties of digoxin (p.825) and has been used similarly in maintenance doses of 100 to 200 µg daily by mouth.

Acetyldigitoxin has a half-life of between 8.5 and 8.8 days. About 21% of a dose was excreted in the urine in 6 days.— G. Bodem *et al.*, *Arzneimittel-Forsch.*, 1975, *25*, 1448.

In a study of 8 healthy subjects, digoxin tended to produce respiratory depression, but acetyldigitoxin which is more lipid-soluble tended to produce respiratory stimulation. The clinical implications for the treatment of cor pulmonale are discussed.— P. H. Joubert *et al.*, *Eur. J. clin. Pharmac.*, 1985, *28*, 155.

Proprietary Names and Manufacturers
Acetil Digitoxina *(Sandoz, Spain)*; Acylanid *(Sandoz, Arg.; Sandoz, Denm.; Sandoz, S.Afr.; Sandoz, Swed.; Sandoz, Switz.)*; Acylanide *(Sandoz-Wander, Belg.; Sandoz, Fr.; Sandoz, Neth.)*.

5803-x

Acetyldigoxin
α-Acetyldigoxin; Desglucolanatoside C. 3β-[(*O*-3-*O*-Acetyl-2,6-dideoxy-β-D-*ribo*-hexopyranosyl-(1→4)-*O*-2,6-dideoxy-β-D-*ribo*-hexopyranosyl-(1→4)-2,6-dideoxy-β-D-*ribo*-hexopyranosyl)oxy]-12β,14-dihydroxy-5β,14β-card-20(22)-enolide.
$C_{43}H_{66}O_{15}$=823.0.

CAS — 5511-98-8.

Pharmacopoeias. In *Aust.*

Acetyldigoxin has the general properties of digoxin (p.825). Both the α- and β-isomers have been used in maintenance doses of 200 to 400 µg daily by mouth.

In 4 patients given tritiated β-acetyldigoxin by mouth 90% rapidly passed through the stomach unchanged and was absorbed in the duodenum. Deacetylation to digoxin occurred on passage through the intestinal wall.— H. Flasch *et al.*, *Arzneimittel-Forsch.*, 1977, *27*, 656.

For reference to a decrease in the absorption of acetyldigoxin due to antineoplastic therapy, see Digoxin, Precautions p.828.

For a report of the successful treatment of acetyldigoxin poisoning with cholestyramine, see Digoxin, Treatment of Adverse Effects p.826.

Proprietary Names and Manufacturers of Acetyldigoxin Isomers
Agolanid *(Sandoz, Spain)*; Allocor *(Natrapharm, Ger.)*; Cardioreg *(Nattermann, Ital.)*; Cedigocin *(Sandoz, Switz.)*; Cedigocina *(Sandoz, Arg.)*; Cedigocine *(Sandoz-Wander, Belg.; Sandoz, Switz.)*; Cedigossina *(Sandoz, Ital.)*; Ceverin *(Schwarz, Ger.)*; Decardil *(Trenker, Belg.)*; Digistabil *(Hormonchemie, Ger.)*; Digostada *(Stadapharm, Ger.)*; Digotab *(Asta Pharma, Ger.)*; Dioxanin *(Boehringer Ingelheim, Ger.)*; Kardiamed *(Medice, Ger.)*; Lanadigin *(Promonta, Ger.)*; Longdigox *(Trommsdorff, Ger.)*; Novodigal *(Homburg, Belg.; Beiersdorf, Ger.)*; Sandolanid *(Sandoz, Ger.)*; Stillacor *(Wolff, Ger.)*.

5804-r

Acetylstrophanthidin
3β-Acetoxy-5,14-dihydroxy-19-oxo-5β,14β-card-20(22)-enolide.
$C_{25}H_{34}O_7$=446.5.

CAS — 60-38-8.

A synthetic derivative of strophanthidin, the aglycone of strophanthin.

Acetylstrophanthidin has actions similar to those of digoxin (p.825) but is rarely used clinically.

References: B. Lown *et al.*, *New Engl. J. Med.*, 1977, *296*, 301.

Proprietary Names and Manufacturers
Lilly, UK.

5805-f

Adonis Vernalis
Adonide; Adonis; Adoniskraut; Herba Adonidis.

Pharmacopoeias. In *Fr.*, *Ger.*, *Pol.*, *Rus.*, and *Span. Rus.* also includes Adonisidum (Adoniside), an aqueous solution of the glycosides of *A. vernalis*. *Ger.* also includes a standardised powder.

The dried aerial roots of *Adonis vernalis* (Ranunculaceae), containing glycosides which resemble digoxin (p.829) in action.

Adonis vernalis is inferior to digitalis in its therapeutic effect. It has been administered as an infusion and as a tincture.

18809-x

Alifedrine *(rINN)*.
D-13625. 1-Cyclohexyl-3{[(αS,βR)-β-hydroxy-α-methylphenethyl]amino}-1-propanone.
$C_{18}H_{27}NO_2$=289.4.

CAS — 78756-61-3.

Alifedrine is reported to possess positive inotropic activity.

References: P. Schanzenbächer *et al.*, *Z. Kardiologie*, 1984, *73*, 95.

12373-g

Amrinone *(BAN, USAN, rINN)*.
Win-40680. 5-Amino-3,4′-bipyridyl-6(1*H*)-one.
$C_{10}H_9N_3O$=187.2.

CAS — 60719-84-8.

Amrinone has been reported to be physically **incompatible** with glucose-containing solutions and with frusemide.

Adverse Effects
Amrinone produces gastro-intestinal disturbances that may necessitate withdrawal of treatment. It produces dose-dependent thrombocytopenia. Hepatotoxicity may occur, particularly during long-term treatment. Hypotension and cardiac arrhythmias have been reported. Other adverse effects include headache, fever, chest pain, and hypersensitivity reactions.

Intravenous injections of amrinone can cause local pain and burning at the injection site and extravasation should be avoided. The adverse effects associated with oral administration have made this route generally unacceptable.

A review of the adverse effects of amrinone and other newer inotropic agents.— M. W. I. Webster and D. N. Sharpe, *Med. Toxicol.*, 1986, *1*, 335.

A report of nephrogenic diabetes insipidus occurring in 1 patient and fever in another patient during treatment with amrinone 2 to 4 mg per kg body-weight by mouth two to three times daily. Thrombocytopenia also occurred in both patients, and all adverse effects resolved after amrinone was discontinued.— J. Wynne *et al.*, *Am. J. Cardiol.*, 1980, *45*, 1245.

The adverse effects of amrinone were assessed in 41 patients in chronic left ventricular failure. Hypotension occurred in 36 of 40 patients who received amrinone 1.5 to 2.0 mg per kg body-weight by intravenous infusion and in one patient after oral administration. Platelet counts fell below 100 x 10^9 per litre in 10 patients receiving amrinone orally and to some extent in all 17 patients who received the drug by this route. Thrombocytopenia was reversible in all cases. Abdominal symptoms included abdominal pain in 1 patient, nausea and vomiting in 3, and jaundice in 1. Splenomegaly was reported in 3 patients and pulmonary infiltration with and without vasculitis occurred in 2 patients. Other adverse effects reported included dryness of the skin, discoloration of the nails, reduced tear secretion, headache, and myositis. The phosphodiesterase inhibiting activity of amrinone could be responsible for the effects on the gastro-intestinal tract and on tear secretion, but there was also evidence suggestive of a drug-induced immunological abnormality.— P. T. Wilmshurst and M. M. Webb-Peploe, *Br. Heart J.*, 1983, *49*, 447.

Oral administration of amrinone, in a usual dose of 100 mg every 8 hours in addition to their usual medication, to 16 patients with refractory cardiac failure was associated with a significant reduction in platelet count in all patients; the percentage reduction correlated with plasma-amrinone concentrations. There was also a significant reduction in platelet survival in the 10 patients in whom it was measured. Although no haemorrhagic symptoms were observed, it was suggested that mean plasma concentrations should not exceed 2.5 µg per mL.— P. T. Wilmshurst *et al.*, *Br. J. clin. Pharmac.*, 1984, *17*, 317.

Adverse effects occurred in 15 out of 24 patients during treatment with amrinone 300 to 600 mg daily. The principal adverse effects were nausea, diarrhoea, fever, thrombocytopenia, and raised values for liver enzymes. Cardiac arrhythmias were reported in 3 patients. Amrinone was discontinued in 8 patients due to adverse effects.— B. D. Silverman *et al.*, *Archs intern. Med.*, 1985, *145*, 825.

A further report of amrinone-induced thrombocytopenia.— J. Ansell *et al.*, *Archs intern. Med.*, 1984, *144*, 949.

Precautions
Blood pressure and heart-rate should be monitored during parenteral amrinone administration. The fluid and electrolyte balance should be maintained. Platelet counts and liver function should also be monitored.

Absorption and Fate
Amrinone is absorbed from the gastro-intestinal tract with peak plasma concentrations being achieved within 3 hours. The half-life is variable and has been reported to be from about 2.5 hours in healthy subjects to up to 12 hours in patients with heart failure. Binding to plasma proteins is generally low. Amrinone is conjugated in the liver and excreted in the urine as the unchanged drug and its metabolites. About 18% of the administered dose has been detected in the faeces over 72 hours.

A review of the pharmacokinetics and pharmacodynamics of newer inotropic agents including amrinone.— M. L. Rocci and H. Wilson, *Clin. Pharmacokinet.*, 1987, *13*, 91.

Uses and Administration
Amrinone is a phosphodiesterase inhibitor which has vasodilatory and positive inotropic properties and has been used in the treatment of congestive heart failure. The mode of action has not been fully determined, but differs from that of digoxin. Although amrinone is effective when administered orally this route has been associated with an unacceptable level of adverse effects, and the drug is generally given intravenously for the short-term management of congestive heart failure unresponsive to other forms of therapy.
Amrinone is administered as the lactate either by slow intravenous injection or by continuous infusion and doses are adjusted according to the clinical response of the patient. The recommended initial dose is 750 µg per kg body-weight of amrinone base by slow intravenous injection over 2 to 3 minutes repeated after 30 minutes if necessary. Maintenance doses are 5 to 10 µg per kg per minute by infusion to a maximum of 10 mg per kg in 24 hours. Doses of up to 18 mg per kg per day have been used in a limited number of patients.

A review of the pharmacodynamics, clinical and adverse effects of amrinone. Amrinone has vasodilatory and positive inotropic properties that are concentration dependent. Studies *in vitro* suggest that increased calcium entry is the most prominent but not the sole mechanism responsible for its positive inotropic activity. Although the relative contributions of vasodilatation and increased contractility to the observed improvement in the haemodynamic state in patients with heart failure are controversial, the available data suggest that a combination of the 2 effects is responsible. Amrinone has been reported to improve exercise performance, but long-term beneficial effects have not been confirmed in at least 1 placebo-controlled study. Despite haemodynamic and symptomatic improvement, there is evidence of continued disease progression during long-term therapy. The usefulness of long-term therapy has been limited by the substantial number of adverse effects which occur.— W. S. Colucci *et al.*, *New Engl. J. Med.*, 1986, *314*, 349. The mode of action, clinical effectiveness, and safety of amrinone have been the subject of considerable debate. In general it has been concluded that, whatever the merits of the drug, its usefulness will be limited by the high incidence of adverse effects.— J. A. Franciosa, *Ann. intern. Med.*, 1985, *102*, 399. A brief comment that despite the early experience with amrinone being encouraging, the high incidence of adverse effects will clearly limit the long-term usefulness.— G. D. Johnston, *Br. med. J.*, 1985, *290*, 803. Further agreement that amrinone will never achieve acceptance as an orally effective agent in the treatment of heart failure.— P. Wilmshurst (letter), *ibid.*, 1515.

Further reviews: A. Ward *et al.*, *Drugs*, 1983, *26*, 468. Corrections.— *ibid.*, 1984, *28*, No. 3; *ibid.*, 1985, *30*, No. 5.

Proprietary Names and Manufacturers of Amrinone and its Salts
Inocor *(Winthrop, Canad.; Winthrop, Fr.; Winthrop, S.Afr.; Winthrop-Breon, USA)*; Wincoram *(Winthrop, Ger.; Sterwin, Spain)*.

18881-v

Bucladesine *(rINN)*.

N-(9-β-D-Ribofuranosyl-9*H*-purin-6-yl)butyramide cyclic 3′,5′-(hydrogen phosphate) 2′-butyrate.
$C_{18}H_{24}N_5O_8P$=469.4.

CAS — 362-74-3.

Bucladesine has been reported to have positive inotropic activity; it may be used as the sodium salt.

A brief review of the synthesis and pharmacology of bucladesine.— *Drugs of the Future*, 1985, *10*, 106.

Proprietary Names and Manufacturers
Actocin *(Daiichi, Jpn)*.

12470-q

Buquineran *(BAN, rINN)*.

UK-14275. 1-Butyl-3-[1-(6,7-dimethoxyquinazolin-4-yl)-4-piperidyl]urea.
$C_{20}H_{29}N_5O_3$=387.5.

CAS — 59184-78-0.

Buquineran is a phosphodiesterase inhibitor with inotropic effects on the heart. An analogue, carbazeran (UK-31557) has also been reported to possess inotropic activity.

Buquineran was found to have a significant inotropic action in 12 patients with coronary heart disease with little or no effect on heart rate.— I. Hutton *et al.*, *Br. J. clin. Pharmac.*, 1977, *4*, 513. See also K. Jennings *et al.*, *ibid.*, 1978, *5*, 13.

Possible adverse effects due to prolongation of the QT interval.— *Lancet*, 1979, *2*, 777.

Proprietary Names and Manufacturers
Pfizer, UK.

5806-d

Convallaria

Lily of the Valley Flowers; Maiblume; Maiglöckchenkraut; May Lily; Muguet.

CAS — 3253-62-1 (convallatoxol); 13473-51-3 (convalloside); 13289-19-5 (convallatoxoloside); 508-75-8 (convallatoxin).

Pharmacopoeias. In *Aust.*, *Ger.*, (from *C. majalis* or closely related species); *Pol.*, and *Span. Rus.* specifies aerial parts of *C. majalis* and its varieties and also includes convallatoxin. *Ger.* also includes a standardised powder.

The dried inflorescence or the rhizomes and roots of lily of the valley, *Convallaria majalis* (Liliaceae). Several crystalline glycosides have been obtained from the plant including convallarin, convalloside, convallatoxoloside, and convallatoxin.

Convallaria has an action on the heart similar to that of digoxin (p.829).

Convallaria majalis has been designated unsafe for inclusion in foods, beverages, or drugs by the Food and Drug Administration in the *USA*.— T. Larkin, *FDA Consumer*, 1983, *17* (Oct.), 5.

5807-n

Crataegus

Aubépine; Crataegus Oxyacantha; English Hawthorn; Haw; Pirliteiro; Weissdornblätter mit Blüten; Weissdornblüten.

Pharmacopoeias. In *Belg.*, *Braz.*, *Chin.*, *Cz.*, *Fr.*, *Ger.*, *Pol.*, *Port.*, *Rus.*, *Span.*, and *Swiss.*

The dried flowers, fruit, or leaves, or mixtures of these parts of *Crataegus oxyacantha* (=*C. monogyna*) or other spp.

Crataegus contains flavonoid glycosides claimed to have cardiotonic properties and has been used similarly to digoxin (p.829) as an extract or tincture.

Proprietary Names and Manufacturers
Cardiplant Schwabe *(Also, Ital.)*; Crasted *(Jpn)*; Crataegitan *(Amino, Switz)*; Crataegol *(Vernin, Fr.)*; Crataegutt *(Schwabe, Neth.; Med. y Prod. Quim., Spain)*; Crataegysat Bürger *(Ysatfabrik, Ger.)*; Cratamed *(Redel, Ger.)*; Esbericard *(Schaper & Brümmer, Ger.)*; Eurhyton *(Hausmann, Switz.)*; Oxacant *(Klein, Ger.)*.

5808-h

Cymarin

K-Strophanthin-α. A glycoside extracted from the roots of *Apocynum cannabinum*. 3β-[(2,6-Dideoxy-3-*O*-methyl-β-D-*ribo*-hexopyranosyl)oxy]-5,14-dihydroxy-19-oxo-5β,14β-card-20(22)-enolide.
$C_{30}H_{44}O_9$=548.7.

CAS — 508-77-0.

Cymarin has actions similar to those of digoxin (p.825).

Proprietary Names and Manufacturers
Alvonal MR *(Gödecke, Ger.)*.

5809-m

Deslanoside *(BAN, USAN, rINN)*.

Deacetyl-lanatoside C; Desacetyl-lanatoside C. 3β-[(*O*-β-D-Glucopyranosyl-(1→4)-*O*-2,6-dideoxy-β-D-*ribo*-hexopyranosyl-(1→4)-*O*-2,6-dideoxy-β-D-*ribo*-hexopyranosyl-(1→4)-2,6-dideoxy-β-D-*ribo*-hexopyranosyl)-oxy]-12β,14-dihydroxy-5β,14β-card-20(22)-enolide.
$C_{47}H_{74}O_{19}$=943.1.

CAS — 17598-65-1.

Pharmacopoeias. In *Arg.*, *Br.*, *Braz.*, *Chin.*, *Cz.*, *Egypt.*, *Eur.*, *Ind.*, *Jpn*, *Nord.*, *Swiss*, and *U.S.*

Odourless hygroscopic white crystals or crystalline powder.
Practically **insoluble** in water, chloroform, and ether; very slightly soluble in alcohol and methyl alcohol. Solutions are **sterilised** by autoclaving. **Store** in airtight, glass containers at a temperature not exceeding 10°. Protect from light.

Deslanoside is a derivative of lanatoside C and has similar actions and uses to those of digoxin (p.825). It is usually reserved for the treatment of emergencies although digoxin is generally preferred. Its effects occur about 10 minutes after intravenous administration and the full action on the heart is exerted after about 2 hours. It has a half-life of about 33 hours and its effects persist for 2 to 5 days.
The suggested rapid digitalising dose of deslanoside is 1.6 mg given by intravenous injection as a single dose or in divided doses over 12 hours. It has also been given by intramuscular injection. For maintenance treatment a cardiac glycoside is then given by mouth; lanatoside C may be used. A suggested digitalising dose for children is 20 to 25 µg per kg body-weight given intravenously as a single dose or in divided doses.

Preparations

Deslanoside Injection *(U.S.P.)*

Proprietary Names and Manufacturers
Cedilanid *(Austral.; Sandoz, Canad.; Sandoz, Denm.; Ger.; Sandoz, Ital.; Sandoz, Norw.; Sandoz, S.Afr.; Sandoz, Spain; Sandoz, Swed.; Sandoz, UK; Sandoz, USA)*; Cedilanide *(Belg.; Sandoz, Fr.; Neth.; Sandoz, Switz.)*; Desace *(Belg.; Fr.; Switz.)*; Desaci *(Simes, Ital.)*; Verdiana *(Farmasimes, Spain)*.

5811-x

Digitalin

Amorphous Digitalin; Digitalinum Purum Germanicum. A standardised mixture of glycosides from *Digitalis purpurea*.

Digitalin has actions similar to those of digoxin (p.825). Because of its ready solubility in water it was formerly used for the preparations of solutions for injection. Digitalin must be distinguished from digitoxin (Digitaline Cristallisée) which is very much more potent.

5812-r

Digitalis Leaf *(BAN)*.

Dedaleira; Digit. Fol.; Digit. Leaf; Digitale Pourprée; Digitalis *(USAN)*; Digitalis Folium; Digitalis Purpurea Folium; Digitalis Purpureae Folium; Feuille de Digitale; Fingerhutblatt; Foxglove Leaf; Hoja de Digital.

Pharmacopoeias. In *Arg., Aust., Belg., Br., Braz., Chin., Egypt., Eur., Fr., Ger., Hung., Int., Jpn, Jug., Mex., Neth., Nord., Pol., Port., Rus., Span., Swiss, Turk.,* and *U.S. Br.* also describes Powdered Digitalis Leaf.

The dried leaves of *Digitalis purpurea* (Scrophulariaceae). Digitalis leaf contains a number of glycosides, including digitoxin, gitoxin, and gitaloxin. **Store** in airtight containers. Protect from light.

5813-f

Prepared Digitalis *(BAN)*.

Digitalis Folii Pulvis Standardisatus; Powdered Digitalis *(USAN)*.

Pharmacopoeias. Standardised powders are included in *Arg., Aust., Belg., Br., Fr., Ger., Hung., Int., Jpn, Jug., Nord., Port., Turk.,* and *U.S.*

Digitalis leaf reduced to powder, no part being rejected, and biologically assayed. The *B.P.* states that, for therapeutic purposes, it should contain between 0.36% and 0.44% of cardenolic glycosides, calculated as digitoxin. The *U.S.P.* specifies a potency of 1 *U.S.P.* unit in 100 mg. **Store** in airtight containers. Protect from light.

Units

One unit of digitalis is contained in 76 mg of the third International Standard Preparation (1949) which contains 0.01316 units per mg.

Adverse Effects, Treatment, and Precautions

As for Digoxin, p.825.

A report of poisoning associated with the drinking of herbal tea made from the leaves of the foxglove which were mistaken for comfrey.— R. J. I. Bain, *Br. med. J.*, 1985, *290*, 1624.

Further references to accidental poisoning by herbal preparations containing digitalis: E. S. Dickstein and F. W. Kunkel, *Am. J. Med.*, 1980, *69*, 167.

Absorption and Fate

Digitalis is incompletely absorbed from the gastro-intestinal tract; 20 to 40% of the dose administered has been reported to reach the circulation. Digitalis has a half-life of 4 to 6 days.

Uses and Administration

Digitalis has the properties described under digoxin (p.829) and has a similar onset and duration of action to that of digitoxin (p.825). When treatment with a cardiac glycoside is required digoxin or digitoxin is preferred.

Provided that cardiac glycosides have not been given in the previous 10 to 14 days, digitalis as Prepared Digitalis has been used for rapid digitalisation in doses of 1 to 1.8 g given by mouth over 24 to 48 hours. Alternatively digitalisation can be achieved more slowly over 3 to 7 days. Maintenance doses of 60 to 200 mg daily have been given. Elderly patients may require smaller doses.

Preparations

Digitalis Capsules *(U.S.P.)*. Capsules containing prepared digitalis.

Digitalis Tablets *(U.S.P.)*. Tablets containing prepared digitalis.

Digitalis Tablets *(B.P.)*. Prepared Digitalis Tablets

Proprietary Names and Manufacturers of Digitalis Preparations

Augentonicum *(Stulln, Switz.)*; Digifortis *(Parke, Davis, USA)*; Digiglusin *(Lilly, USA)*; Digiplex *(Servier, Fr.)*; Digitalysat *(Ysatfabrik, Ger.)*; Pil-Digis *(Key, USA)*.

5814-d

Digitalis Lanata Leaf

Austrian Digitalis; Austrian Foxglove; Digitalis Lanatae Folium; Woolly Foxglove Leaf.

CAS — 17575-20-1 (lanatoside A).

Pharmacopoeias. In *Arg., Aust., Ger.,* and *Pol.* Also in *B.P.C. 1973.*

The dried leaves of the woolly foxglove, *Digitalis lanata* (Scrophulariaceae), containing about 1 to 1.4% of a mixture of cardioactive glycosides, including digoxin, digitoxin, acetyldigoxin, acetyldigitoxin, lanatoside A, and deslanoside. **Store** in airtight containers. Protect from light.

Digitalis lanata leaf is used as a source for the manufacture of digoxin and other glycosides.

Proprietary Names and Manufacturers

Digilanid *(Sandoz, UK)*.

5815-n

Digitoxin *(BAN, USAN, rINN)*.

Digitaline Cristallisée; Digitoxinum; Digitoxoside. 3β-[(*O*-2,6-Dideoxy-β-D-*ribo*-hexopyranosyl-(1→4)-*O*-2,6-dideoxy-β-D-*ribo*-hexopyranosyl-(1→4)-2,6-dideoxy-β-D-*ribo*-hexopyranosyl)oxy]-14-hydroxy-5β,14β-card-20(22)-enolide.

$C_{41}H_{64}O_{13}$=764.9.

CAS — 71-63-6.

Pharmacopoeias. In *Arg., Aust., Belg., Br., Braz., Chin., Cz., Egypt., Eur., Fr., Ger., Hung., Ind., Int., It., Jpn, Jug., Mex., Neth., Nord., Port., Roum., Rus., Span., Swiss, Turk.,* and *U.S.* Also in *B.P. Vet.*

A crystalline glycoside obtained from suitable species of *Digitalis*.

It is a white or pale buff-coloured, odourless, microcrystalline powder. Practically **insoluble** in water; soluble 1 in 150 of alcohol and 1 in 40 of chloroform; slightly soluble in methyl alcohol; slightly or very slightly soluble in ether; freely soluble in a mixture of equal volumes of chloroform and methyl alcohol. **Store** in airtight containers at a temperature not exceeding 15°. Protect from light.

Binding to an inline intravenous filter containing a cellulose ester membrane accounted for a reduction in digitoxin concentration of up to 25% from solutions of digitoxin 200 μg in 50 mL of glucose 5% or sodium chloride 0.9%.— L. D. Butler *et al., Am. J. Hosp. Pharm.*, 1980, *37*, 935. Treatment of cellulose filter membranes with an unidentified proprietary substance reduced adsorbance of digitoxin by about half compared with untreated membranes.— M. Kanke *et al., ibid.*, 1983, *40*, 1323.

Digitoxin was found to be adsorbed onto glass and plastic in substantial amounts from simple aqueous solutions but not from solutions in 30% alcohol, or in plasma, or urine.— L. Molin *et al., Acta pharm. suec.*, 1983, *20*, 129.

Adverse Effects and Treatment

As for Digoxin, p.825. Toxicity may be more prolonged after withdrawal of digitoxin because of the longer half-life. Treatment of toxicity with activated charcoal or adsorbent resins such as cholestyramine may be effective in reducing blood concentrations by interrupting enterohepatic recirculation of digitoxin.

Digitalis intoxication occurred in 179 patients who took 1 to 3 tablets daily for 8 weeks or more, each containing digitoxin 200 μg and digoxin 50 μg, instead of tablets each containing digoxin 250 μg. Fatigue and visual disturbances occurred in 95% of the patients, muscular weakness in 82%, anorexia and nausea in 80%, psychic complaints and abdominal pains in 65%, and dizziness, headache, diarrhoea, and vomiting in about one-half of the patients. Hallucination-like effects occurred in 12 patients. In 48 patients, 105 separate disturbances in rhythm or in atrioventricular conduction occurred. The patients were usually symptom-free from 1 to 4 weeks after withdrawal of the tablets, but 24 patients still had symptoms after 4 weeks. Use of the tablets was believed to have contributed to the death of 6 of 47 patients treated in hospital.— A. H. Lely and C. H. J. van Enter, *Br. med. J.*, 1970, *3*, 737.

Severe digitalis intoxication occurred in a patient considered to have taken about 100 tablets of digitoxin 100 μg. Gastric lavage was performed 3 hours after ingestion. The plasma-digitoxin concentration 21 hours after ingestion was 125 ng per mL (150 ng per mL on admission) when charcoal haemoperfusion was carried out for 8 hours and 1.24 mg of drug was removed. After an interval of one hour a second haemoperfusion was started and removed 870 μg of digitoxin by which time the plasma-digitoxin concentration had fallen to 70 ng per mL and most of the symptoms of intoxication had disappeared. Cholestyramine 4 g was then given three times daily for 5 days and considered to have increased the elimination of digitoxin.— H. -J. Gilfrich *et al.* (letter), *Lancet*, 1978, *1*, 505.

Serum-digitoxin concentrations in 2 patients with digitoxin toxicity (serum concentrations of 43 and 42 ng per mL respectively) returned to within the therapeutic range (10 to 30 ng per mL) following withdrawal of the drug, correction of hypokalaemia and cardiac arrhythmias where necessary, and 3 doses of cholestyramine 4 g given over 24 hours.— W. J. Cady *et al., Am. J. Hosp. Pharm.*, 1979, *36*, 92.

Treatment with activated charcoal 50 or 60 g and magnesium citrate solution every 8 hours for 72 hours decreased the serum-digitoxin concentration from 264 ng per mL to 27 ng per mL after 80 hours in a patient who had taken about 10 mg of digitoxin and 0.6 mg reserpine. The digitoxin half-life was reduced to 18 hours, and cardiac arrhythmias improved with the declining serum concentrations of digitoxin— S. Pond *et al.* (letter), *Lancet*, 1981, *2*, 1177.

Precautions

As for Digoxin, p.827.

Digitoxin should be used with caution in patients with impaired hepatic function.

INTERACTIONS. *Aminoglutethimide.* A mean overall increase of 109% was seen in digitoxin clearance in 5 patients during concomitant treatment with aminoglutethimide. The interaction was attributed to the induction of hepatic enzymes by aminoglutethimide.— P. E. Lønning *et al., Clin. Pharmac. Ther.*, 1984, *36*, 796.

Antibiotics. Report of acute heart failure in a patient taking digitoxin when treatment with rifampicin and isoniazid was started. Plasma-digitoxin concentrations fell from a pretreatment steady-state value of 27 ng per mL to 10 ng per mL. The reduction in the digitoxin concentration was attributed to induction of digitoxin metabolism by rifampicin.— G. Boman *et al.* (letter), *Br. J. clin. Pharmac.*, 1980, *10*, 89.

In 2 patients dependent on dialysis, digitoxin requirements increased by up to 50% when rifampicin therapy was started.— H. Gault *et al., Clin. Pharmac. Ther.*, 1984, *35*, 750.

Calcium-channel blocking agents. Steady-state concentrations of digitoxin in the plasma increased by an average of 35% over 2 to 3 weeks in 8 of 10 patients when verapamil 240 mg daily was added to their therapy. Total body clearance and extra-renal clearance of digitoxin were reduced by 27% and 29% respectively although renal excretion was unchanged. Plasma-digitoxin concentrations increased by a mean of 21% in 5 of 10 patients treated with diltiazem but were not increased by concomitant treatment with nifedipine.— J. Kuhlman, *Clin. Pharmac. Ther.*, 1985, *38*, 667.

Diuretics. Spironolactone decreased the half-life and the urinary elimination of unchanged digitoxin when it was given for at least 10 days to 8 patients on oral maintenance digitoxin therapy. The interaction was judged to be of minor clinical importance.— K. E. Wirth *et al., Eur. J. clin. Pharmac.*, 1976, *9*, 345. The half-life of digitoxin was found to be increased by the subsequent administration of spironolactone to 3 healthy subjects.— S. G. Carruthers and C. A. Dujovne, *Clin. Pharmac. Ther.*, 1980, *27*, 184.

INTERFERENCE WITH LABORATORY ESTIMATIONS. The administration of digitoxin could interfere with measurements of urinary 17-hydroxycorticosteroids.— J. M. Rosenberg and I. S. Kampa, *Drug Intell. & clin. Pharm.*, 1973, *7*, 33.

Digitoxin has been shown to produce an apparent elevation of digoxin concentrations as measured by radioimmunoassay, enzyme immunoassay, and fluoroimmunoassay.— S. Yosselson-Superstine, *Clin. Pharmacokinet.*, 1984, *9*, 67.

Absorption and Fate

Digitoxin is readily and completely absorbed from the gastro-intestinal tract. Therapeutic plasma concentrations may range from 10 to

35 ng per mL but there is considerable interindividual variation. Digitoxin is extensively bound to plasma protein. It is very slowly eliminated from the body and is metabolised in the liver, the major active metabolite being digoxin. Enterohepatic recycling occurs and digitoxin is excreted in the urine, mainly as metabolites. It is also excreted in the faeces and this route becomes significant in renal failure. Digitoxin has an elimination half-life of up to 7 days or more. The half-life is generally unchanged in renal failure.

An account of the clinical pharmacokinetics of digitoxin. Biological half-lives for digitoxin ranging from 2.4 to 16.4 days with a mean half-life of 7.6 days have been reported. This wide variation may be attributed to individual differences in hepatic metabolism of digitoxin and to the use of different assay methods. The shortest mean half-life of 4.8 days was observed with the most specific assay method and the longest mean half-life of 9.8 days with the least specific method.— D. Perrier *et al., Clin. Pharmacokinet.*, 1977, *2,* 292.

The pharmacokinetics of digitoxin were changed significantly in 5 patients with the nephrotic syndrome. The apparent volume of distribution of digitoxin was increased and protein binding decreased. Such patients should be maintained at lower serum-digitoxin concentrations than other patients but will need larger doses because of the shortened serum half-life and the increased renal excretion of digitoxin and its cardioactive metabolites.— L. Storstein, *Clin. Pharmac. Ther.*, 1976, *20,* 158.

Digitoxin half-life, apparent volume of distribution, and clearance were not found to differ in elderly subjects compared with young adults following intravenous injection in a single-dose study. The long half-life may make once weekly dosing possible in poorly compliant patients.— M. A. Donovan *et al.* (letter), *Br. J. clin. Pharmac.*, 1981, *11,* 401.

Children were found to have a greater volume of distribution of digitoxin than adults and a shorter mean half-life, although individual variation was considerable. The increase in total clearance in children compared to adults was attributed to greater metabolic clearance.— A. Larsen and L. Storstein, *Clin. Pharmac. Ther.*, 1983, *33,* 717.

In a study in 6 healthy subjects given single doses of digitoxin 1 mg intravenously or by mouth the mean elimination half-life of digitoxin was 174.9 and 157.7 hours by the two routes respectively when measured using a non-specific radio-immunoassay. When a specific assay was used, that separates digitoxin from its metabolites, the half-life values were 156.0 and 138.0 hours and mean bioavailability was reduced from 98% to 81.5%. Previously reported values for digitoxin bioavailability may have been elevated by the use of non-specific determinations.— R. T. MacFarland *et al., Eur. J. clin. Pharmac.*, 1984, *27,* 85.

The effect of multiple plasma exchanges on the steady-state pharmacokinetics of digitoxin was found to be quite small and was related to the amount of unbound drug in the plasma; 5.5% of the estimated amount of digitoxin in the body was removed by a single plasma exchange. The equivalent figure for removal of digoxin was 1.2% of the estimated amount in the body. It was recommended that, in patients treated with repetitive plasma exchanges, no alteration in dose is required as long as the dose of digitoxin or digoxin is administered after the procedure, and hypoalbuminaemia is corrected.— F. Keller *et al., Clin. Pharmacokinet.*, 1985, *10,* 514.

DISTRIBUTION AND PROTEIN BINDING. In a study of digitoxin metabolites in the myocardium, the mean ratio of myocardial to serum concentrations of digitoxin and its cardioactive metabolites was found to be 5.4:1. When calculated in terms of free drug the ratio was 200:1 and, since digitoxin is extensively bound to protein, gave a better estimate of affinity to heart tissue.— L. Storstein, *Clin. Pharmac. Ther.*, 1977, *21,* 395.

Digitoxin has been reported to be more than 90% bound to serum albumin in healthy subjects. Binding has been slightly reduced in patients with chronic active hepatitis or nephrotic syndrome. Conflicting effects on binding have been noted in uraemic patients; it is reduced in those on haemodialysis and a heparin-induced release of free fatty acids appears to be responsible. Where serum protein binding of digitoxin or digoxin is significantly decreased, total serum concentrations should be maintained below usual therapeutic values.— L. Storstein, *Clin. Pharmacokinet.*, 1977, *2,* 220.

METABOLISM. A study of digitoxin metabolism in patients on oral maintenance therapy and after a single intravenous dose showed that in both cases digitoxin is the main cardioactive substance in serum and in urine. All known cardioactive metabolites were present but there were differences between the single-dose and steady-state groups. In the steady-state group there was more unchanged digitoxin (89.7% in serum and 87% in urine compared with 80.4% and 56.6% respectively), far less digoxin (less than 1% in the steady-state group compared with 12.5% in serum and 25.5% in urine in the single-dose group), and less hydroxylated metabolites than in the single-dose group. The results indicate that caution is necessary in using single-dose data as a basis for maintenance therapy.— L. Storstein, *Clin. Pharmac. Ther.*, 1977, *21,* 125. See also *idem*, 536 (digitoxin metabolites in patients with renal impairment); L. Storstein and J. Amlie, *ibid.*, 659 (digitoxin metabolism in patients with biliary fistulas).

PLASMA CONCENTRATIONS. Serum and plasma concentrations of digitoxin are equivalent.— T. W. Smith and E. Haber, *New Engl. J. Med.*, 1973, *289,* 1063.

Uses and Administration

Digitoxin has the actions and uses of digoxin (p.829), and is completely and readily absorbed when given by mouth. It is the most potent of the digitalis glycosides and is the most cumulative in action. The onset of its action is slower than that of the other cardiac glycosides; its effects may be evident in about 2 hours and its full effects in about 12 hours after oral administration and somewhat more rapidly after intravenous injection. Its effects persist for about 3 weeks.

As described under digoxin, dosage should be carefully adjusted to the needs of the individual patient. Steady-state therapeutic plasma concentrations of digitoxin may range from 10 to 35 ng per mL; higher values may be associated with toxicity. Digoxin may be more suitable for rapid digitalisation but digitoxin can be given to patients who have not received cardiac glycosides during the past 2 weeks. In adults an initial dose of 600 µg may be given, followed by 400 µg after 4 to 6 hours, then 200 µg every 6 hours as necessary until a maximum total dose of 1.6 mg has been given over one to two days. For slow digitalisation 200 µg has been given twice daily for 4 days. The maintenance dose varies from 50 to 200 µg daily. Digitoxin may also be given in similar doses by slow intravenous injection when vomiting or other conditions prevent administration by mouth. It has also been given intramuscularly but injections may be irritant.

Suggested doses of digitoxin for digitalisation in children, to be given in 3 or more divided doses daily by mouth or by injection, are: premature and full-term infants, 22 µg per kg body-weight; 2 weeks to 1 year, 45 µg per kg; 1 to 2 years, 40 µg per kg; and over 2 years, 30 µg per kg. For maintenance one-tenth of the digitalising dose may be given daily.

ADMINISTRATION IN RENAL FAILURE. Doses of digitoxin should be reduced to 50 to 75% in patients with a glomerular filtration-rate of less than 10 mL per minute. Concentrations of digitoxin are not affected by haemodialysis or peritoneal dialysis.— W. M. Bennett *et al., Am. J. Kidney Dis.*, 1983, *3,* 155.

See also Absorption and Fate (above).

Preparations

Digitoxin Injection *(U.S.P.)*. A sterile solution in 5 to 50% alcohol.

Digitoxin Tablets *(B.P.)*

Digitoxin Tablets *(U.S.P.)*

Proprietary Names and Manufacturers

Asthenthilo *(Ger.)*; Coramedan *(Medice, Ger.)*; Crystodigin *(Lilly, USA)*; Digicor *(Hennig, Ger.)*; Digilong *(Arg.)*; Digimed *(Trommsdorff, Ger.)*; Digimerck *(Arg.; E. Merck, Ger.; Ital.; Spain; E. Merck, Switz.)*; Digipural *(Schaper & Brümmer, Ger.)*; Digitalina Bescansa *(Spain)*; Digitalina Mialhe *(Arg.)*; Digitalina Nativelle *(Nativelle, Ital.; Pan Química Farmac., Spain)*; Digitaline Nativelle *(Gamaprod, Austral.; Nativelle, Fr.; Lipomed, UK; Neth.; Spain; Nativelle, Switz.)*; Digitasid *(Belg.)*; Digitox *(Austral.)*; Digitoxina Simes *(Spain)*; Digitoxine *(Belg.; Mepha, Switz.; Streuli, Switz.)*; Digitrin *(Draco, Norw.; Draco, Swed.)*; Ditaven *(Cascan, Ger.)*; Mono-Glycocard *(RAN, Ger.)*; Purodigin *(Arg.; Wyeth, USA)*; Tardigal *(Beiersdorf, Ger.)*.

5801-a

Digoxin *(BAN, USAN, rINN)*.

Digoxinum; Digoxosidum. 3β-[(O-2,6-Dideoxy-β-D-*ribo*-hexopyranosyl-(1→4)-O-2,6-dideoxy-β-D-*ribo*-hexopyranosyl-(1→4)-2,6-dideoxy-β-D-*ribo*-hexopyranosyl)oxy]-12β,14-dihydroxy-5β,14β-card-20(22)-enolide.

$C_{41}H_{64}O_{14}$=780.9.

CAS — 20830-75-5.

Pharmacopoeias. In *Arg., Aust., Belg., Br., Braz., Chin., Cz., Egypt., Eur., Fr., Ger., Hung., Ind., Int., It., Jpn, Jug., Neth., Nord., Roum., Swiss, Turk.*, and *U.S.* Also in *B.P. Vet.*

A cardiac glycoside obtained from the leaves of *Digitalis lanata*. It occurs as odourless, colourless or white crystals or a white or almost white powder.

B.P. **solubilities** are: practically insoluble in water, slightly soluble in chloroform and in alcohol, freely soluble in a mixture of equal volumes of chloroform and methyl alcohol. *U.S.P.* solubilities are: practically insoluble in water and in ether, freely soluble in pyridine, slightly soluble in diluted alcohol and in chloroform. The *B.P.* injection is **sterilised** by autoclaving. **Store** in airtight containers. Protect from light.

Complexing digoxin with cyclodextrins was found to reduce acid hydrolysis and hasten dissolution *in vitro*.— K. Uekama *et al., J. Pharm. Pharmac.*, 1982, *34,* 627.

The stability of digoxin in injectable solutions. Solutions of digoxin 0.00025% in glucose injection, sodium chloride injection, and 2 compound electrolyte injections were stored for up to 48 hours under refrigeration and at room temperature. Digoxin was found to be physically compatible with the solutions tested and no reduction in digoxin concentration could be detected.— W. A. Shank and J. J. Coupal, *Am. J. Hosp. Pharm.*, 1982, *39,* 844.

A brief review of the stability of digoxin in parenteral nutrition solutions recommending that, although there have been several reports indicating that digoxin is effective when administered in this way, further studies of stability and availability are needed.— P. W. Niemiec and T. W. Vanderveen, *Am. J. Hosp. Pharm.*, 1984, *41,* 893.

Adverse Effects

Digoxin and the other cardiac glycosides commonly produce side-effects because the margin between the therapeutic and toxic doses is small; plasma concentrations in excess of 2 ng per mL are considered to be an indication that the patient is at special risk. There have been many fatalities, particularly due to cardiac toxicity.

Nausea, vomiting, and anorexia may be among the earliest symptoms of digoxin overdosage; diarrhoea and abdominal pain may also occur. Certain neurological effects are also common symptoms of digoxin overdosage and include headache, facial pain, fatigue, weakness, dizziness, drowsiness, disorientation, mental confusion, bad dreams and more rarely delirium, acute psychoses, and hallucinations. Convulsions have also been reported.

The most serious adverse effects are those on the heart. Toxic doses may cause or aggravate heart failure. Atrial or ventricular arrhythmias and defects of conduction are common and may be an early indication of excessive dosage. In general the incidence and severity of arrhythmias is related to the severity of the underlying heart disease. Almost any arrhythmia may ensue, but particular note should be made of supraventricular tachycardia, especially atrioventricular (AV) junctional tachycardia and atrial tachycardia with block. Ventricular arrhythmias including extrasystoles, sinoatrial block, sinus bradycardia, and AV block may also occur.

Chronic digoxin toxicity is associated with hypokalaemia and adverse reactions to digoxin may be precipitated if there is potassium depletion such as may be caused by the prolonged administration of diuretics. Hyperkalaemia occurs in acute overdosage.

Visual disturbances including blurred or misted vision may occur; colour vision may be affected with objects appearing yellow or less frequently green, red, brown, blue, or white. Allergic and skin reactions are rare; thrombocytopenia has been reported. The cardiac glycosides may occasionally cause gynaecomastia at therapeutic doses and may have some oestrogenic activity.

As digoxin has a shorter half-life than digitalis or digitoxin its adverse effects tend to be easier to manage.

A review of digitalis toxicity, including predisposing factors, drug interactions, contra-indications and treatment of adverse effects and acute poisoning.— R. E. Bullock and R. J. C. Hall, *Adverse Drug React. Ac. Pois. Rev.*, 1982, *1*, 201.

Further reviews: J. K. Aronson, *Clin. Sci.*, 1983, *64*, 253; C. F. George, *Br. med. J.*, 1983, *286*, 1533; J. Henry and G. Volans, *ibid.*, 1984, *289*, 1062.

An account of an outbreak of digoxin intoxication owing to a change in Lanoxin tablets affecting bioavailability not announced by the manufacturer.— A. Danon *et al.*, *Clin. Pharmac. Ther.*, 1977, *21*, 643.

The incidence of toxicity in patients taking digitalis preparations has been investigated by several groups. The Boston Collaborative Drug Surveillance Program reported an overall toxicity of 12.4% of patients receiving digoxin, with cardiac toxicity occurring in 8.5% and gastro-intestinal disturbances in 3.1% (D.J. Greenblatt, Digitalis Glycosides, in *Drug Effects in Hospitalized Patients*, R.R. Miller and D.J. Greenblatt (Ed.), London, Wiley, 1976, p.37). Of the 327 patients with cardiac toxicity, the effects were life-threatening in 79 and fatal in 2. In a prospective study in 135 hospital in-patients in Boston, Beller *et al.* (*New Engl. J. Med.*, 1971, *284*, 989) reported toxicity in 23% of patients and possible toxicity in a further 6%. Henry *et al.* (*Postgrad. Med. J.*, 1981, *57*, 358), monitoring hospital in-patients in Glasgow, recorded an incidence of adverse reactions of 19.5%. Side-effects were considered as generally benign, although there was a high incidence of gastro-intestinal reactions in women. No deaths were attributable to digoxin. Aronson (*Clin. Sci.*, 1983, *64*, 253) found the incidence of toxicity in out-patients to be as high as 16% in the Oxford area.

DIAGNOSIS OF TOXICITY. In a controlled study of 46 children receiving digoxin for the treatment of congestive heart failure, digitilisation significantly increased sodium concentrations in the red blood cells whilst potassium concentrations were decreased. Similar, but more marked effects were seen in patients on maintenance therapy, who were diagnosed as suffering from digoxin toxicity, when compared with non-toxic children. The ratio of red cell-sodium to red cell-potassium concentrations was successfully used to identify 32 of 34 patients with digoxin toxicity compared with 30 of 34 who were diagnosed using plasma-digoxin concentrations as a guide to toxicity.— M. W. Loes *et al.*, *New Engl. J. Med.*, 1978, *299*, 501.

The monitoring of red blood cell electrolytes in adults as a guide to the efficacy and toxicity of digitalis therapy was as effective as the measurement of plasma-digoxin concentrations and saved time and effort.— F. Wessels and H. Losse (letter), *New Engl. J. Med.*, 1979, *300*, 433.

Guidelines for the diagnosis of digoxin toxicity in individual patients. Toxicity should be suspected if the plasma-digoxin concentration is greater than 3 ng per mL, or there is hypokalaemia, or there are any two of the following four features: plasma potassium greater than 5 mmol per litre, plasma creatinine greater than 150 µmol per litre, age more than 60 years, or daily maintenance dose at a steady state of more than 6 µg per kg body-weight. Using these guidelines the incidence of overdiagnosis of toxicity in non-toxic patients is 41%.— J. K. Aronson, *Clin. Pharmacokinet.*, 1980, *5*, 137.

A view that plasma concentrations of digitalis glycosides used together with plasma-potassium concentrations may be helpful in diagnosing digitalis toxicity. If plasma-potassium concentrations are normal, toxicity is unlikely with plasma digoxin concentrations below 2 ng per mL (2.5 nmol per litre), whereas toxicity is very likely with concentrations above 4 ng per mL (5 nmol per litre). In hypokalaemic patients, plasma-glycoside concentrations between 1.3 and 2.5 nmol per litre may be associated with toxicity. Assessment of colour vision may be helpful in some patients, but pharmacological tests with acetylstrophanthidin, edrophonium, or edetic acid were considered to be unreliable and potentially dangerous.— C. F. George, *Br. med. J.*, 1983, *286*, 1533.

It was considered that serum cardiac glycoside concentrations should be used as a supplement to, not as a substitute for, clinical judgement. An isolated value should rarely if ever be used as the sole criterion for assessment of efficacy or toxicity.— T. H. Lee and T. W. Smith, *Clin. Pharmacokinet.*, 1983, *8*, 279.

See also under p.830 Administration in Uses.

EFFECTS OF ELECTROLYTES. In a study of 478 patients, digitalis intoxication was found more frequently in patients with hypomagnesaemia than in those with normal concentrations of magnesium but there was no correlation between serum-magnesium and serum-digitalis concentrations. Nausea, anorexia, extreme fatigue, and flickering of vision were more common in the patients with hypomagnesaemia although nausea and anorexia may have been the cause and not necessarily the symptoms of low serum-magnesium concentrations.— O. Storstein *et al.*, *Acta med. scand.*, 1977, *202*, 445.

Favourable response of digoxin-induced AV nodal tachycardias to parenteral magnesium sulphate in 7 patients receiving long-term diuretic treatment. Cellular magnesium deficiency can co-exist with normal serum-magnesium concentrations, and can lead to secondary potassium deficiency. It was concluded that cellular magnesium depletion with or without hypomagnesaemia seemed to predispose to digitalis-induced arrhythmias.— L. Cohen and R. Kitzes, *J. Am. med. Ass.*, 1983, *249*, 2808. Comment urging caution in administering magnesium supplements to patients with potential renal impairment who may have an impaired capacity to excrete a magnesium load. Additionally the reliance on lymphocyte magnesium estimation as a reliable marker of intracellular magnesium deficiency was questioned.— J. P. Sheehan (letter), *ibid.*, 1985, *253*, 513.

A combination of mild hypokalaemia and mild hypercalcaemia, assessed by means of the calcium to potassium ratio, was shown to be a predisposing factor for digoxin-induced automaticity, manifested by ventricular extrasystoles. Patients with digoxin-induced automaticity had serum-digoxin concentrations in the therapeutic range but had appreciable alkalosis and a mean calcium-to-potassium ratio higher than in patients with gastro-intestinal symptoms. There was a good correlation between high serum-digoxin concentrations and the occurrence of gastro-intestinal symptoms, but the calcium-to-potassium ratio and arterial pH in these patients were normal. It was considered that these observations could partly explain the lack of correlation found between serum-digoxin concentrations and symptoms of digoxin toxicity.— M. Sonnenblick *et al.*, *Br. med. J.*, 1983, *286*, 1089.

EFFECTS ON THE MENTAL STATE. Formed visual hallucinations occurred in 3 elderly patients receiving digoxin. All had high serum-digoxin concentrations. On temporary withdrawal of the drug the concentrations decreased to within the therapeutic range and the hallucinations subsided and never returned.— B. T. Volpe and R. Soave, *Ann. intern. Med.*, 1979, *91*, 865.

A report of organic brain syndrome, presenting as confusion, disorientation, memory deficit, and anorexia occurred in a 74-year-old patient 4 days after the start of digoxin therapy. Symptoms disappeared when digoxin was withdrawn, although serum-digoxin concentrations had remained within the therapeutic range. There were no signs of cardiac toxicity.— S. J. Eisendrath *et al.*, *Am. Heart J.*, 1983, *106*, 419.

Further references to cardiac glycosides adversely affecting the mental state: V. A. Portnoi, *J. clin. Pharmac.*, 1979, *19*, 747 (delirium in the elderly); M. Brezis *et al.* (letter), *Ann. intern. Med.*, 1980, *93*, 639 (nightmares).

EFFECTS ON SEX HORMONES. Mean serum-oestrogen concentrations were increased in 20 postmenopausal women and 18 men who had been taking digoxin for more than 2 years. Mean serum concentrations of luteinising hormone were decreased in both groups and the mean plasma-testosterone concentrations were decreased in the male group.— S. S. Stoffer *et al.*, *J. Am. med. Ass.*, 1973, *225*, 1643.

OVERDOSAGE. A report of fatal overdosage with digoxin in a 54-year-old woman; the blood-digoxin concentration was 50.4 ng per mL.— D. P. Nicholls, *Postgrad. med. J.*, 1977, *53*, 280.

PREGNANCY AND THE NEONATE. Despite extensive antenatal exposure to digitalis preparations, no adverse effects of maternal treatment have been seen in the foetus or newborn, although adverse effects have been found in the foetus when the mother developed digitalis toxicity. Concern has also been raised that digitalis may have a role in low birth weights observed occasionally in infants of mothers with heart disease. Digoxin is preferred to other glycosides because experience with digoxin in pregnancy is extensive.— H. H. Rotmensch *et al.*, *Ann. intern. Med.*, 1983, *98*, 487.

Treatment of Adverse Effects

For the treatment of *chronic poisoning* temporary withdrawal of digoxin or other cardiac glycosides may be all that is necessary, with subsequent doses adjusted according to the needs of the patient. Serum electrolytes should be measured and the ECG monitored. Potassium supplements should be given to correct hypokalaemia.

In the early stages of *acute poisoning* the stomach should be emptied by emesis or aspiration and lavage. Activated charcoal may be given in an attempt to prevent the absorption of cardiac glycosides; cholestyramine or colestipol has also been used, particularly to increase the elimination of digitoxin. Attempts to remove cardiac glycosides by haemodialysis or peritoneal dialysis have generally been ineffective and the value of haemoperfusion is controversial. Forced diuresis with frusemide is generally ineffective and may be dangerous; serious electrolyte imbalance may result from the use of such potent diuretics.

Cardiac toxicity in acute or chronic poisoning should be treated under ECG control and serum electrolytes should be monitored. Anti-arrhythmic treatment may be necessary particularly if there is a risk of progression to ventricular fibrillation. Potassium chloride may be given in hypokalaemic patients providing that renal function is normal and heart block is not present. Potassium has also been given to normokalaemic patients. Other electrolyte imbalance should be corrected. Phenytoin or lignocaine are also used in the treatment of digoxin-induced arrhythmias. Propranolol may also be tried, but can cause bradycardia. Procainamide has also been used, but it is generally considered to be more hazardous than other treatment. Atropine is given intravenously to control bradycardia and in patients with heart block. Pacing may be necessary if atropine is not effective. Cardioversion is very hazardous and is used only when other methods fail.

In *massive overdosage* progressive hyperkalaemia occurs and is fatal unless reversed. Glucose infusions and injections of soluble insulin have been given and, if the hyperkalaemia is refractory, dialysis may be tried. Massive overdosage has been treated successfully with fragments of digoxin-specific antibodies (p.839).

A review and discussion on the management of acute and chronic digitalis poisoning.— D. A. R. Boldy *et al.*, *J. clin. Hosp. Pharm.*, 1984, *9*, 147.

ACTIVATED CHARCOAL. Repeated doses of activated charcoal 25 g by mouth increased the total body clearance and decreased the elimination half-life of digoxin in 10 healthy subjects after intravenous administration of digoxin.— R. L. Lalonde *et al.*, *Clin. Pharmac. Ther.*, 1985, *37*, 367.

Multiple doses of activated charcoal were administered to a patient who had taken 6.5 mg digoxin. The plasma-digoxin concentration 14.5 hours after the overdose was 8.3 ng per mL and fell to 1.0 ng per mL over the ensuing 48 hours with a terminal elimination half-life of 14 hours. Activated charcoal was considered to have been beneficial in increasing digoxin elimination.— D. A. R. Boldy *et al.* (letter), *Lancet*, 1985, *2*, 1076.

For reference to the successful use of charcoal haemoperfusion in digitoxin toxicity, see Digitoxin, p.824.

ANTI-ARRHYTHMIC THERAPY. A 26-year-old man who had ingested 25 mg of digoxin developed intractable ventricular fibrillation unresponsive to lignocaine; he recovered after treatment with amiodarone given intravenously for 36 hours.— R. Maheswaran *et al.*, *Br. med. J.*, 1983, *287*, 392.

ION-EXCHANGE RESINS. Cholestyramine 8 g every 6 hours by mouth enhanced the elimination of β-acetyldigoxin and medigoxin in 2 patients with intoxication following acute overdose. Although the decline in the half-life of either drug was not as great as that reported for digitoxin, cholestyramine was considered to be a useful treatment for managing patients intoxicated with either digitoxin or digoxin derivatives.— J. Kuhlman, *Int. J. clin. Pharmac. Ther. Toxic.*, 1984, *22,* 543.

For the use of cholestyramine in digitoxin toxicity, see Digitoxin, p.824.

Precautions

Digoxin is generally contra-indicated in ventricular fibrillation and in patients with hypertrophic obstructive cardiomyopathy unless there is severe cardiac failure. Digoxin is also contra-indicated in patients with the Wolff-Parkinson-White syndrome, especially if it is accompanied by atrial fibrillation, since digoxin may precipitate ventricular tachycardia or fibrillation.

It should be used with caution in heart block; complete heart block may be induced if cardiac glycosides are used in partial heart block. It should be used with caution in acute myocarditis such as rheumatic carditis and in patients with advanced heart failure or severe pulmonary disease. Almost any deterioration in the condition of the heart or circulation may increase the sensitivity to digoxin. The role of digoxin in myocardial infarction is debated. Digoxin should be given with care to patients who have received cardiac glycosides previously. It may enhance the occurrence of arrhythmias in patients undergoing cardioversion and should be withdrawn 1 to 2 days before such procedures if possible. If cardioversion is essential and digoxin has already been given, low energy shocks must be used.

Early signs of digoxin toxicity should be watched for and the heart-rate should generally be maintained above 60 beats per minute. Toxicity may result from administering loading doses too rapidly and from accumulation of maintenance doses as well as from acute poisoning.

Digoxin doses should generally be reduced and plasma-digoxin concentrations monitored in patients with impaired renal function, in the elderly, and in premature infants; they should be carefully controlled in patients with electrolyte imbalance, or thyroid dysfunction. The effects of digoxin are enhanced by hypokalaemia, hypomagnesaemia, hypercalcaemia, hypoxia, and hypothyroidism and doses may need to be reduced until these conditions are corrected.

Interactions. There may be interactions between digoxin and drugs which alter its absorption, interfere with its excretion, or have additive effects on the myocardium. Drugs which cause electrolyte disturbances increase the risk of toxicity from cardiac glycosides. Thiazides and loop *diuretics* cause potassium depletion and also hypomagnesaemia which may lead to cardiac arrhythmias. Other causes of hypokalaemia include treatment with *corticosteroids, amphotericin, sodium polystyrene sulphonate, carbenoxolone* and also dialysis. Hypercalcaemia may also increase toxicity and intravenous administration of *calcium salts* is best avoided in patients taking cardiac glycosides. Digoxin should be given cautiously to patients receiving *parathyroid extract* or large doses of *vitamin D.*

The absorption of digitalis glycosides may be affected by intestinal adsorptive agents and antacids. *Sulphasalazine, neomycin,* and certain *antineoplastic agents* may cause clinically significant malabsorption, but *metoclopramide* and *propantheline* probably only significantly affect absorption from the more slowly dissolving dosage forms that have reduced bioavailability. About 10% of patients appear to metabolise digoxin to some extent through gut flora to produce cardio-inactive metabolites; in these patients administration of *antibiotics* that inhibit the organisms responsible may result in unexpectedly elevated serum-digoxin concentrations.

Quinidine invariably interacts with digoxin and plasma-digoxin concentrations may be doubled. Quinidine appears primarily to reduce renal excretion, but may also reduce non-renal excretion and displace digoxin from tissue-binding sites. Patients should be monitored for clinical signs of toxicity and increased plasma concentrations. It has been recommended that the dose of digoxin be reduced by 50% when concomitant treatment with quinidine is started. There is some evidence of a similar interaction with digitoxin. *Spironolactone* has also been reported to reduce the renal excretion of digoxin, but results are difficult to interpret since spironolactone and its metabolites can interfere with digoxin assays. *Phenytoin* may induce the hepatic metabolism of digitalis glycosides, and particularly digitoxin which is more dependent on the liver for elimination, during long-term therapy. Digoxin and digitoxin plasma concentrations should be monitored if phenytoin is administered, and larger doses of digitalis than anticipated may be necessary in patients on long-term phenytoin therapy. A similar effect may occur with *phenobarbitone* or with *rifampicin.* Concurrent administration of *verapamil* and digoxin may increase plasma-digoxin concentrations and lead to atrioventricular block. Increased plasma-digoxin concentrations have also been reported with *nifedipine* and *amiodarone* in some patients. *Suxamethonium* may increase the risk of cardiac arrhythmias, and bradycardia may be anticipated in patients given *beta-blockers* with digoxin.

Recommendation that liquid dosage forms of digoxin should be used in patients with small bowel resections to improve absorption. Absorption from tablet formulations may be decreased in patients with malabsorption syndromes or small bowel resections due to inadequate dissolution of the tablet.— K. P. Kumer *et al., Drug Intell. & clin. Pharm.*, 1983, *17,* 121. A patient with short-bowel syndrome absorbed 40 to 60% of the administered dose of digoxin given as an elixir.— S. J. Vetticaden *et al., Clin. Pharm.*, 1986, *5,* 62.

EFFECTS OF ELECTROLYTE IMBALANCE. Results indicating that the active tubular secretion of digoxin is reduced in hypokalaemic patients.— E. Steiness, *Clin. Pharmac. Ther.*, 1978, *23,* 511.

Seven patients with congestive heart failure receiving long-term diuretic treatment experienced AV nodal tachycardia in the presence of plasma-digoxin concentrations within the normal therapeutic range. Symptoms responded to parenteral magnesium supplements and it was concluded that cellular magnesium depletion with or without hypomagnesaemia appeared to predispose to digitalis-induced arrhythmias.— L. Cohen and R. Kitzes, *J. Am. med. Ass.*, 1983, *249,* 2808. Results of a study of the effect of hypomagnesaemia in patients with atrial fibrillation suggested that magnesium replacement therapy may be beneficial in patients with symptomatic atrial fibrillation for whom digoxin therapy is being contemplated.— C. DeCarli *et al., Am. J. Cardiol.*, 1986, *57,* 956. For comment on the administration of magnesium supplements to patients taking digoxin, see under Adverse Effects, above.

INTERACTIONS. Reviews of drug interactions occurring with cardiac glycosides.— P. F. Binnion, *Drugs,* 1978, *15,* 369; D. D. Brown *et al., Drugs,* 1980, *20,* 198; C. F. George, *Br. med. J.*, 1982, *284,* 291; S. R. Kayser, *Drug Interact. News.*, 1985, *5,* 1.

In a study of the drug profiles of 1825 surgical inpatients, at least one potential drug interaction was found in 17% of patients; digoxin was involved in 46% of these potential interactions.— C. W. Durrence *et al., Am. J. Hosp. Pharm.*, 1985, *42,* 1553.

Antacids and other gastro-intestinal agents. In a study involving 12 healthy subjects concurrent administration of digoxin in capsule or tablet form with either *kaolin with pectin* or *magnesium hydroxide* with *aluminium hydroxide* reduced the peak plasma-digoxin concentrations. Urinary excretion studies indicated that digoxin absorption was impaired to a greater extent from tablets than from capsules.— M. D. Allen *et al., J. clin. Pharmac.*, 1981, *21,* 26. A single dose of *kaolin with pectin* given with the digoxin dose reduced the peak digoxin concentration by 36% in a study involving 7 patients, but there was only a slight decrease in digoxin bioavailability. When the times of administration were separated by 2 hours, there was no evidence of an interaction.— K. S. Albert *et al., ibid.*, 449.

Concurrent *metoclopramide* administration was found to reduce the absorption of digoxin from tablets but not from soft gelatin capsules in 16 healthy subjects.— B. F. Johnson *et al., Clin. Pharmac. Ther.*, 1984, *36,* 724.

Anti-arrhythmic agents. An interaction between digoxin and *amiodarone* resulting in increases in plasma concentrations of digoxin has been reported on several occasions. Moysey *et al.* (*Br. med. J.*, 1981, *282,* 272) observed a progressive increase in plasma-digoxin concentrations by an average of 69% when amiodarone was added to digoxin therapy in 7 patients, and increases in serum-digoxin concentrations of 68 to 800% were associated with amiodarone therapy in 6 children (G. Koren *et al., J. Pediat.*, 1984, *104,* 467). Douste-Blazy *et al.* (*Lancet,* 1984, *1,* 905) found that both plasma and urinary concentrations of digoxin were increased by amiodarone, suggesting that a reduction in urinary excretion was unlikely to be responsible for the interaction, and this was supported by the observation by Mingardi (*ibid.*, 1238) of increased plasma-digoxin concentrations in an anuric man given amiodarone. However, Achilli and Serra (*Br. med. J.*, 1981, *282,* 1630) found no increase in plasma-digoxin concentrations during concomitant administration for 30 days.

The co-administration of *disopyramide* and digoxin was shown to reduce the cardiovascular effects of digoxin but there was no evidence to suggest that these changes were attributable to disturbances of the pharmacokinetics of digoxin.— H. L. Elliott *et al., Br. J. clin. Pharmac.*, 1982, *14,* 141P. Reductions in the volume of distribution and elimination half-life of digoxin were seen when disopyramide was administered concurrently. There was no alteration in serum-digoxin concentrations and the clinical significance of this interaction was not clear.— T. Risler *et al., Clin. Pharmac. Ther.*, 1983, *34,* 176.

A discussion of the interaction between digoxin and *quinidine* and its management. An increase in serum-digoxin concentration has been reported in almost 90% of patients when quinidine was added. The increase may be by up to 500%, although on average serum-digoxin concentrations were doubled, and an increase in symptoms of digoxin toxicity has been reported. However there is uncertainty about the relationships between increased serum concentrations and toxic and inotropic effects of digoxin. It may be necessary to reduce the dose of digoxin, or replace quinidine with another anti-arrhythmic drug.— J. T. Bigger and E. B. Leahey, *Drugs,* 1982, *24,* 229.

In a review of data collected from 4418 patients during the Boston Collaborative Drug Surveillance Program the incidence of gastro-intestinal and cardiac adverse effects in patients taking both digoxin and quinidine was greater than in those taking either drug separately, but the difference could be accounted for by an additive effect and was not attributed to a clinical interaction.— A. M. Walker *et al., Am. Heart J.*, 1983, *105,* 1025.

Comments on the mechanism of the digoxin-quinidine interaction: K. Schenck-Gustafsson and R. Dahlqvist, *Br. J. clin. Pharmac.*, 1981, *11,* 181; K. E. Pedersen *et al., Eur. J. clin. Pharmac.*, 1983, *24,* 41; K. E. Pedersen, *Acta med. scand.*, 1985, *Suppl.* 697, 7.

Further references to the quinidine digoxin interaction: P. D. Hirsh *et al., Am. J. Cardiol.*, 1980, *46,* 863; *Lancet,* 1980, *2,* 1064; B. Fichtl and W. Daering, *Clin. Pharmacokinet.*, 1983, *8,* 137.

Administration of *flecainide* 200 mg twice daily, to 15 healthy subjects taking digoxin caused a mean increase of 24% in predose digoxin concentrations and of 13% in digoxin concentrations 6 hours after the digoxin dose. It was considered that in most cases these increases in plasma-digoxin concentrations would not present a clinical problem, but that patients with higher plasma-digoxin concentrations or atrioventricular nodal dysfunction should be monitored.— C. E. Weeks *et al., J. clin. Pharmac.*, 1986, *26,* 27.

Antibiotics. Studies *in vivo* and *in vitro* indicating that antibiotics could reduce the metabolism of digoxin by gut flora, which could result in increased plasma-digoxin concentrations in a minority of subjects.— J. Lindenbaum *et al., New Engl. J. Med.*, 1981, *305,* 789.

Approximately 10% of patients receiving digoxin may metabolise 40% or more of the drug to cardio-inactive compounds. Gut flora contribute greatly to this process, and the administration of antibiotics to these patients appears to reduce this metabolic process resulting in higher serum concentrations. The greatest increase in serum-digoxin concentration has been seen with digoxin tablets of limited bioavailability.— J. E. Doherty, *New Engl. J. Med.*, 1981, *305,* 827.

Report of 2 patients dependent on dialysis in whom digoxin-dose requirements increased substantially when *rifampicin* therapy was started and fell by about 50% when rifampicin was discontinued.— H. Gault *et al., Clin. Pharmac. Ther.*, 1984, *35,* 750. A further report.— C. Novi *et al.* (letter), *J. Am. med. Ass.*, 1980, *244,* 2521.

Anticoagulants. For reference to digoxin having no effect on plasma-*warfarin* concentrations, see warfarin sodium (p.346).

Anti-epileptics. Phenytoin caused a marked decrease in steady-state serum-digoxin concentrations when phenytoin was administered with digoxin and acetyldigoxin to 6 healthy subjects for 7 days. The interaction was probably due to an increase in hepatic clearance.— H. Rameis, *Eur. J. clin. Pharmac.*, 1985, *29*, 49.

Antihypertensive agents. In a double-blind placebo-controlled study, serum-digoxin concentrations increased during *captopril* therapy in patients with heart failure. There was a weak positive correlation between the rise in the digoxin concentration and a fall in glomerular filtration rate.— J. G. F. Cleland *et al.*, *Br. J. clin. Pharmac.*, 1984, *17*, 214P.

Antimalarial agents. In 6 subjects given *quinine sulphate,* total body clearance of digoxin after an intravenous dose was decreased by 26%, primarily through a reduction .in non-renal clearance. Increased urinary excretion of digoxin was consistent with alterations in the non-renal clearance of digoxin and might be due to changes in the metabolism or biliary secretion of digoxin. Quinine increased the mean elimination half-life of digoxin from 34.2 to 51.8 hours but did not consistently change the volume of distribution.— M. Wandell *et al.*, *Clin. Pharmac. Ther.*, 1980, *28*, 425.

Antineoplastic agents. Time to peak plasma concentration was delayed after single doses of both β-acetyldigoxin and digitoxin in patients undergoing antineoplastic drug therapy. Steady-state concentrations of digoxin but not digitoxin were reduced. The effect was considered to be due to reduced absorption of the digitalis glucosides caused by damage to the gastro-intestinal mucosa by cytostatic therapy. Digitoxin may be preferred in patients receiving cytostatic drug therapy.— J. Kuhlmann, *Arzneimittel-Forsch.*, 1982, *32*, 698.

Absorption of digoxin was reduced by an average of 45.6% when taken in tablet form by 6 patients undergoing cancer chemotherapy. The absorption of digoxin from liquid-filled capsules by 7 additional patients was reduced by about 14.9%.— T. D. Bjornsson *et al.*, *Clin. Pharmac. Ther.*, 1986, *39*, 25.

Benzodiazepines. Raised plasma-digoxin concentrations were found in 3 patients also taking *diazepam.* Co-administration of diazepam was subsequently found to produce moderate increases of digoxin half-life in plasma, in 5 of 7 healthy subjects, whereas urinary excretion of digoxin was substantially reduced in all 7. Plasma concentrations of digoxin should be carefully monitored in patients also receiving diazepam.— J. R. Castillo-Ferrando *et al.* (letter), *Lancet*, 1980, *2*, 368.

The serum-digoxin concentration increased by about 300% when *alprazolam* 1 mg daily was administered to a 72-year-old patient stabilised on digoxin. There was a reduction in the apparent oral clearance of digoxin to 39% of normal.— G. Tollefson *et al.*, *Am. J. Psychiat.*, 1984, *141*, 1612. Therapeutic doses of *alprazolam* did not significantly alter digoxin clearance in 8 healthy subjects following a single intravenous dose of digoxin.— H. R. Ochs *et al.*, *Clin. Pharmac. Ther.*, 1985, *38*, 595.

Beta-blockers. For interactions between digoxin and *propranolol,* see propranolol hydrochloride (p.801).

Calcium-channel blocking agents. Studies on interactions between digoxin and *calcium antagonists* appear to show that *verapamil* can increase plasma-digoxin concentrations (G.G. Belz *et al.*, *Clin. Pharmac. Ther.*, 1983, *33*, 410; K.E. Pedersen *et al.*., *Eur. J. clin. Pharmac.*, 1983, *25*, 199). The effect of *nifedipine* is not as clear. While Belz *et al.* showed that it produced a 45% increase in plasma-digoxin concentrations, Schwartz and Migliore (*Clin. Pharmac. Ther.*, 1984, *36*, 19) reported no increase and Kleinbloesem *et al.* (*Ther. Drug. Monit.*, 1985, *7*, 372) reported only a 15% increase and considered that the interaction would have no clinical significance for most patients. *Gallopamil* was also investigated by Belz *et al.* who observed a 16% increase in plasma-digoxin concentrations in subjects given both drugs. Studies on the interaction between digoxin and *diltiazem* have also produced conflicting results. Rameis *et al.* (*Clin. Pharmac. Ther.*, 1984, *36*, 183) reported an increase of 20% in plasma-digoxin concentrations and Oyama *et al.* (*Am. J. Cardiol.*, 1984, *15*, 1480) reported that diltiazem increased digoxin plasma concentrations by up to 59% and medigoxin concentrations by up to 51%. Several other studies however have shown no change in digoxin pharmacokinetics or plasma concentration (T.R. Beltrami *et al.*, *J. clin. Pharmac.*, 1985, *25*, 390; P.M Young *et al.*, *Clin. Pharmac. Ther.*, 1985, *37*, 239; U. Elkayam *et al.*, *Am. J. Cardiol.*, 1985, *55*, 1393).

Dietary factors. Variations in *dietary fat* have been reported to change digoxin dosage requirements, possibly due to increased elimination secondary to increased biliary flow. However, this interaction is unlikely to be of clinical importance.— K. R. Hunter, *Prescribers' J.*, 1981, *21*, 177.

Diuretics. Amiloride administration increased renal clearance of digoxin and reduced the extrarenal digoxin clearance in 6 healthy subjects after a single intravenous dose of digoxin. Amiloride also inhibited the digoxin-induced positive inotropic effect, but the clinical implications in cardiac patients are unknown.— S. Waldorff *et al.*, *Clin. Pharmac. Ther.*, 1981, *30*, 172.

A review of the effects of *spironolactone* on assays, pharmacokinetics, and pharmacodynamics of digoxin. Plasma-digoxin concentrations could be increased by about 25%. Any clinical effect from such an increase might be mitigated by spironolactone metabolites protecting against digitalis-induced arrhythmias.— J. M. Horn, *Drug Interact. News.*, 1982, *2*, 51. Increases in measured serum-digoxin concentrations in patients taking spironolactone may be due to interference with radio-immunoassay procedures by spironolactone or its metabolites and/or decreased digoxin clearance. Since interference with assays is neither consistent nor predictable, digoxin concentrations in patients taking spironolactone should be interpreted with caution. Dosage decisions should be based primarily on clinical findings.— J. A. Paladino *et al.* (letter), *J. Am. med. Ass.*, 1984, *251*, 470. See also under Interference with Laboratory Estimations (below).

In a study of serum-digoxin concentrations involving 661 patients on continuous digoxin therapy, the mean serum-digoxin concentration was higher in 81 receiving concomitant diuretic therapy with *triamterene* in association with a thiazide or loop diuretic, than in patients receiving no diuretic, or a thiazide or loop diuretic alone or in association with amiloride. An interaction between triamterene and digoxin should be considered, although it is probably not sufficiently marked to be clinically important, except perhaps in patients with renal failure.— O. Impivaara and E. Iisalo, *Eur. J. clin. Pharmac.*, 1985, *27*, 627.

Non-steroidal anti-inflammatory agents. Steady-state serum concentrations of digoxin increased in 12 patients after 7 days treatment with *ibuprofen.* There was considerable individual variation, and the increase was no longer detectable after 28 days treatment.— F. P. Quattrocchi *et al.*, *Drug Intell. & clin. Pharm.*, 1983, *17*, 286.

Administration of *indomethacin* 50 mg three times a day by mouth did not significantly affect digoxin pharmacokinetics and dynamics in 6 healthy subjects given single doses of digoxin 750 μg intravenously.— M. B. Finch *et al.*, *Br. J. clin. Pharmac.*, 1984, *17*, 353. Serum-digoxin concentrations were elevated to potentially toxic levels when indomethacin at a mean total dose of 0.32 mg per kg body-weight was administered to 11 preterm infants with patent ductus arteriosus on digoxin therapy. There was a corresponding decrease in urine output but no alteration in serum creatinine concentration.— G. Koren *et al.*, *Pediat. Pharmacol.*, 1984, *4*, 25.

Sulphonamides. Reduced serum-digoxin concentrations were found in a patient being treated with digoxin and sulphasalazine. A study in 10 healthy subjects indicated that concurrent administration of sulphasalazine with digoxin impaired absorption of digoxin.— R. P. Juhl *et al.*, *Clin. Pharmac. Ther.*, 1976, *20*, 387.

INTERFERENCE WITH LABORATORY ESTIMATIONS. The presence of endogenous digoxin-like substances in neonates, and in patients with liver or kidney dysfunction may be responsible for elevated values or false-positive results in plasma-digoxin assays.

Individual cases of uraemic patients with anomalously high digoxin assays have been reported (J.L. Craver and R. Valdes, *Ann. intern. Med.*, 1983, *98*, 483; P.E. Rolan *et al.*, *ibid.*, *99*, 280). It has also been shown that patients with renal impairment who were being treated with digoxin not only had plasma concentrations that differed widely over several immunoassay methods, but that more than 60% of patients with renal impairment not on digoxin therapy had false positive results from most assays studied (S.W. Graves *et al.*, *Ann. intern. Med.*, 1983, *99*, 604). Rosenkranz and Fröhlich (*Ther. Drug Monit.*, 1985, *7*, 202) attributed false positive results with radio-immunoassay in patients with hepatic failure to a digitalis-like immunoreactive substance rather than to nonspecific interference with the assay method. They detected false-positive values as great as 3.6 ng per mL in patients with concomitant hepatic and renal failure.

It was suggested by Gault *et al.* (*Ann. intern. Med.*, 1984, *101*, 567) that bile salts could be examples of a class of endogenous compounds that alter nonspecifically the reactivity of digoxin with its antibody, perhaps by a detergent effect. In a subsequent study, Gault *et al.* (*Clin. Pharmac. Ther.*, 1986, *39*, 530) also found that varying plasma-digoxin values were dependent on the method used. They suggested that fluorescence polarisation immunoassay and certain commercial immunoassays rarely gave clinically important false values in renal failure, except where renal failure was associated with concomitant hepatic failure, during pregnancy, or in the neonate. Heazlewood *et al.* (*Ann. intern. Med.*, 1984, *100*, 618) recommended that the fluorescence polarisation immunoassay should be used for plasma-digoxin measurement in patients with renal failure. Nanji and Greenway (*Br. med. J.*, 1985, *290*, 432) reported that this also seemed to be the method of choice for patients with liver disease since it did not measure the digoxin-like immunoreactive substance.

Digoxin-like immunoreactivity has also been detected in premature and full-term infants not receiving digoxin (M.R. Pudek *et al.*, *New Engl. J. Med.*, 1983, *308*, 904; R. Valdes *et al.*, *J. Pediat.*, 1983, *102*, 947). The radial partition immunoassay was found to be less subject to interference than either radio-immunoassay or fluorescence polarisation immunoassay in low birth-weight infants (P.K. Ng *et al.*, *Am. J. Hosp. Pharm.*, 1985, *42*, 1977).

The administration of digoxin could interfere with measurements of urinary 17-hydroxycorticosteroids.— J. M. Rosenberg and I. S. Kampa, *Drug Intell. & clin. Pharm.*, 1973, *7*, 33.

Digoxin might interfere with fluorimetric estimations of urinary catecholamines.— J. Millhouse, *Adverse Drug React. Bull.*, 1974, Dec., 164.

The use of F(ab) antibody fragments in 2 patients caused gross method-dependent anomalies in the results of plasma-digoxin measurement by radio-immunoassay due to *in vitro* interactions. Use of immunotherapy may invalidate data obtained by direct immunoassay techniques.— I. Gibb *et al.*, *Br. J. clin. Pharmac.*, 1983, *16*, 445.

A review of drugs which can interfere with plasma-digoxin assays concluded that interference by spironolactone and prednisolone could be clinically significant. Interference by prednisone, progesterone, and testosterone was of questionable significance, and amiloride, triamterene, and phenytoin were not found to interact with digoxin assays.— S. Yosselson-Superstine, *Clin. Pharmacokinet.*, 1984, *9*, 67.

MALIGNANT HYPERPYREXIA. Comment that malignant hyperpyrexia may be aggravated by cardiac glycosides.— P. G. Blain and M. D. Rawlins, *Prescribers' J.*, 1981, *21*, 204.

Absorption and Fate

The absorption of digoxin from the gastro-intestinal tract is variable depending upon the formulation used. About 70% of the administered dose is absorbed from tablets which comply with *B.P.* or *U.S.P.* specifications, 80% is absorbed from an elixir, and over 90% is absorbed from liquid-filled soft gelatin capsules. Therapeutic plasma concentrations may range from 0.5 to 2.0 ng per mL. Digoxin has a large volume of distribution and is widely distributed in tissues, including the heart, brain, erythrocytes, and skeletal muscle. The concentration of digoxin in the myocardium is considerably higher than in plasma. From 20 to 30% is bound to plasma protein. Digoxin has been detected in cerebrospinal fluid and breast milk; it also crosses the placenta. It has an elimination half-life of 1.5 to 2 days.

Digoxin is mainly excreted unchanged in the urine by glomerular filtration and tubular secretion; reabsorption also occurs. Excretion of digoxin is proportional to the glomerular filtration rate. After intravenous injection 50 to 70% of the dose is excreted unchanged. Digoxin is not removed from the body by dialysis, and only small amounts are removed by exchange transfusion and during cardiopulmonary bypass.

A review of the clinical pharmacokinetics of digoxin. Discussion of the effects of various pathological and physiological conditions included a brief review of the effects of thyroid dysfunction on digoxin pharmacokinetics. Plasma-digoxin concentrations have been reported to be lower when patients are thyrotoxic than when they are euthyroid, although pharmacokinetic considerations alone cannot account for the apparent 'resistance' to digoxin in hyperthyroidism. In hypothyroidism plasma-digoxin concentrations have been reported to be elevated by some investigators, but this has not been confirmed by others. It was concluded that no reliable interpretation may be placed on the plasma-digoxin concentration in patients with thyroid dysfunction.

Elderly patients, apart from impairment of digoxin excretion because of impaired renal function, may have a reduced apparent volume of distribution of digoxin and should therefore be given lower loading doses.— J. K. Aronson, *Clin. Pharmacokinet.*, 1980, *5*, 137. See also E. Iisalo, *ibid.*, 1977, *2*, 1.

ABSORPTION. Studies in 6 healthy subjects demonstrated that ingestion of food decreased the rate but not the extent of absorption of concurrently administered digoxin.— B. F. Johnson *et al.*, *Clin. Pharmac. Ther.*, 1978, *23*, 315.

BIOAVAILABILITY. Large variations in the content, disintegration, and dissolution of solid dosage forms of digoxin preparations have led to large variations in plasma concentrations from different proprietary preparations. Other factors involved in varying bioavailability include the pharmaceutical formulation and presentation (capsules, solution, or tablets), particle size, and biological factors. Serious problems occurred in the *UK* in 1972 following changes in the manufacturing procedure for Lanoxin.

In 20 patients given digoxin in their usual dose as tablets for 4 weeks or, in a crossover period, as soft gelatin capsules containing 80% of the tablet dose as a solution in macrogol, mean digoxin concentrations were approximately proportional to the doses given. It was considered that the use of capsules would probably not represent an advance in treatment.— E. M. Rodgers *et al.*, *Br. med. J.*, 1977, *2*, 234. The absolute bioavailability of digoxin was about 84% from 3 strengths of soft gelatin capsule, 71% from aqueous solution, and 57% from tablets based on area under the serum concentration-time curve after a 0.4 mg dose in healthy subjects, and 92%, 82%, and 78% respectively based on cumulative urinary excretion.— J. E. Doherty *et al.*, *Curr. ther. Res.*, 1984, *35*, 301.

Hydrolysis. Studies *in vitro* indicated that pH influenced the extent of hydrolysis of digoxin and it was suggested that this may account for the variable bioavailability when administered by mouth since gastric pH could modify the composition of digoxin species available for absorption.— L. A. Sternson and R. D. Shaffer, *J. pharm. Sci.*, 1978, *67*, 327. Intragastric hydrolysis of digoxin occurred at roughly the same rate as *in vitro*. The 2 main factors which influenced hydrolysis were time and pH.— H. Gault *et al.*, *Clin. Pharmac. Ther.*, 1980, *27*, 16. Significant reduction of the hydrolysis of digoxin was observed after administration of a slowly dissolving enteric-coated formulation. However, in 4 of 7 healthy subjects studied there was greatly increased metabolism to inactive dihydrodigoxin.— J. O. Magnusson *et al.*, *Eur. J. clin. Pharmac.*, 1984, *27*, 197.

DISTRIBUTION AND PROTEIN BINDING. Reported values for digoxin protein binding have varied from 5 to 60% depending on the methods used, although the figure is usually around 20%. In the present study digoxin was found to be 21.2% bound. Binding was normal in uraemic patients but decreased from 23.5 to 15.4% during haemodialysis.— L. Storstein, *Clin. Pharmac. Ther.*, 1976, *20*, 6. Changes in protein binding during haemodialysis closely resembled those after injection of heparin and it is considered that displacement of digoxin from albumin by free fatty acids is responsible.— L. Storstein and H. Janssen, *ibid.*, 15.

Plasma-digoxin concentrations increased by between 28 and 91% after 2 hours rest in 8 healthy subjects. This was presumed to be due to changes in binding to tissues such as skeletal muscle.— K. E. Pedersen *et al.*, *Clin. Pharmac. Ther.*, 1983, *34*, 303.

Further references to the effect of exercise on digoxin binding: T. Joreteg and T. Jogestrand, *Eur. J. clin. Pharmac.*, 1983, *25*, 585; idem., 1984, *27*, 567.

Digoxin and digitoxin erythrocyte uptake was increased at reduced plasma albumin concentrations but was not affected by gamma globulin concentration *in vitro*. The results demonstrated the buffer capacity of erythrocytes and their ability to equilibrate changes in serum-digoxin and digitoxin concentrations even at low albumin levels.— M. L. Goncalves, *Clin. Pharmac. Ther.*, 1983, *34*, 347.

METABOLISM AND EXCRETION. Although hepatic metabolism, biliary excretion, and subsequent intestinal reabsorption of digoxin have been regarded as insignificant, a mean of about 30% of an intravenous dose of tritiated digoxin appeared in the small intestine of 5 healthy subjects in 24 hours.— J. H. Caldwell and C. T. Cline, *Clin. Pharmac. Ther.*, 1976, *19*, 410.

Although digoxin is reported to be excreted mainly unchanged in the urine there is evidence to suggest that metabolism may sometimes be extensive. Metabolites that have been detected in the urine include digoxigenin, dihydrodigoxigenin, the mono- and bisdigitoxosides of digoxigenin, and dihydrodigoxin. Digoxigenin mono- and bisdigitoxosides are known to be cardioactive whereas dihydrodigoxin is probably much less active than digoxin.— E. Iisalo, *Clin. Pharmacokinet.*, 1977, *2*, 1. The different metabolites of digoxin cross-react to a different extent with the anti-digoxin antibody used in radio-immunoassay. If digitoxosides are present, plasma-digoxin concentrations will be under estimated whereas digoxigenin results in an overestimate of circulating cardioactivity. In some patients the presence of digitoxosides may account for the occurrence of toxicity at apparently low concentrations of digoxin.— J. K. Aronson, *ibid.*, 1980, *5*, 137.

Results of a study indicating that digoxin was extensively inactivated by gastro-intestinal organisms in a minority of subjects who excrete cardio-inactive reduced metabolites of digoxin, and this may be responsible for clinical digoxin resistance and increased drug requirements.— J. Lindenbaum *et al.*, *New Engl. J. Med.*, 1981, *305*, 789.

Metabolism of digoxin by gut flora was reduced by the use of liquid-filled capsules.— D. G. Rund *et al.*, *Clin. Pharmac. Ther.*, 1983, *34*, 738. Production of digoxin-reduced products in the gut was appreciable in only 2 out of 10 patients taking digoxin, accounting for 5.7% and 3.7% of total glycoside elimination with the standard tablet formulation, and 6.1% and 1.6% respectively with liquid-filled capsules. No clinical differences were seen, and it was concluded that gut metabolism was unlikely to complicate clinical management of digoxin therapy with formulations of high bioavailability.— F. Lofts *et al.*, *Br. J. clin. Pharmac.*, 1986, *21*, 600P.

Further references to the metabolism of digoxin in the gastro-intestinal tract.— J. O. Magnusson *et al.*, *Br. J. clin. Pharmac.*, 1982, *14*, 284; J. O. Magnusson, *ibid.*, 1983, *16*, 741.

Effects of impaired renal function. The majority of a dose of digoxin is excreted in the urine and impaired renal function leads to a decreased rate of elimination and accumulation of digoxin if dosage is not adjusted. Renal clearance of digoxin is very often similar to the creatinine clearance. The volume of distribution of digoxin is reduced in severe renal impairment.— E. Iisalo, *Clin. Pharmacokinet.*, 1977, *2*, 1. See also: J. K. Aronson, *ibid.*, 1983, *8*, 155.

See also under Distribution and Protein Binding above and under Administration in Renal Failure in Uses.

PREGNANCY AND THE NEONATE. For comments on the presence of endogenous immunoreactive digoxin-like substances in neonates and during pregnancy, see Interference with Laboratory Estimations in Precautions (p.828) and Administration in Infants and Children in Uses (p.830).

A review of the pharmacokinetics of digoxin in *neonates and infants*. In full-term neonates or infants, 80 to 90% of a dose of digoxin administered by mouth in liquid form is absorbed, with peak plasma concentrations occurring within 30 to 120 minutes. The rate of absorption may be slower in preterm and low birth-weight infants, with peak concentrations achieved at 90 to 180 minutes, and may be significantly reduced in severe heart failure and in malabsorption syndromes. The intramuscular route should be avoided since the absorption of digoxin is erratic and very slow and tissue necrosis may occur. After the intravenous administration of digoxin there is a rapid distribution phase with an apparent half-life of 20 to 40 minutes followed by a slower exponential decay of plasma concentrations. In full-term neonates, digoxin has an apparent volume of distribution of 6 to 10 litres per kg body-weight. Smaller volumes have been noted in premature infants, while in older infants the volume may range from 10 to 22 litres per kg which is 1.5 to 2 times reported adult values. The apparent plasma half-life in healthy and sick neonates is generally very long and may range from 20 to 70 hours in full-term neonates or from 40 to 180 hours in preterm neonates. Digoxin is eliminated at a considerably faster rate in infants than in neonates and, in parallel with maturation of kidney function, a marked increase in clearance-rate is usually observed between the second and third month of life. The large apparent volume of distribution, higher clearance values, and greater concentrations of digoxin in the myocardial tissue and red cells of infants might justify the traditional assumption that infants tolerate digoxin better than adults and that higher doses are consequently needed in infants. However, studies have shown that in infants, as in adults, toxic signs become evident at plasma-digoxin concentrations above 3 ng per mL and that the therapeutic range may be 1.5 to 2 ng per mL. It is considered that doses of digoxin used in the past have been too high and that lower doses should be used, especially in premature and full-term neonates.— P. L. Morselli *et al.*, *Clin. Pharmacokinet.*, 1980, *5*, 485.

A study of the milk of 5 women receiving maintenance digoxin therapy for rheumatic heart disease who wished to breast feed their children, indicated that the total daily excretion of digoxin in the milk of mothers with therapeutic serum-digoxin concentrations would not exceed 1 to 2 µg. These amounts were not sufficient to affect the infants.— M. Levy *et al.* (letter), *New Engl. J. Med.*, 1977, *297*, 789. Digoxin could not be detected in the plasma of 2 infants about 10 days after breast feeding had been established. Their mothers had taken digoxin 250 µg daily throughout pregnancy and continued treatment post partum. The estimated daily intake of digoxin in the milk was only 120 ng per kg body-weight for one infant and 60 ng per kg for the other infant.— P. M. Loughnan, *J. Pediat.*, 1978, *92*, 1019.

In *neonates* with congestive heart failure the mean half-life of the distribution phase of digoxin was 37 minutes, and 44 hours for the elimination phase; in similar infants the corresponding values were 28 minutes and 19 hours respectively.— G. Wettrell, *Eur. J. clin. Pharmac.*, 1977, *11*, 329.

Studies in 34 *infants* aged 1 week to 2 years given digoxin for congestive heart failure showed that serum concentrations were markedly higher in those aged under 3 months, despite giving weight-adjusted doses.— H. Halkin *et al.*, *Eur. J. clin. Pharmac.*, 1978, *13*, 113.

A study of digoxin receptor binding properties in neonates which supported the hypothesis that decreased sensitivity to digoxin in the very young is a result of differences in receptor characteristics to those in adults.— M. Kearin *et al.*, *Clin. Pharmac. Ther.*, 1980, *28*, 346.

Uses and Administration

The principal actions of digoxin are an increase in the force of myocardial contraction and a reduction in the conductivity of the heart, particularly in conduction through the atrioventricular (AV) node. Digoxin also has a direct action on vascular smooth muscle and indirect effects mediated primarily by the autonomic nervous system, and particularly by an increase in vagal activity. There are also reflex alterations in autonomic activity due to the effects on the circulation. Overall, these actions result in positive inotropic effects, negative chronotropic effects, and decreased AV nodal activity.

In cardiac failure, the increased force of myocardial contraction results in increased cardiac output, decreased end-systolic volume, decreased heart size, and decreased end-diastolic pressure and volume. The decrease in systemic pressure and the reduction in sympathetic tone increase the blood flow through the kidneys causing diuresis with a reduction in oedema and blood volume, and the decrease in pulmonary venous pressure relieves dyspnoea and orthopnoea. In atrial arrhythmias direct and indirect actions cause a decrease in the conduction velocity through the AV node and an increase in the effective refractory period thus reducing ventricular rate. In addition there is a decrease in the refractory period of the cardiac muscle and depression of the sinus node partly in response to the increase in vagal activity.

Digoxin is given to slow the ventricular-rate in the management of atrial fibrillation; treatment is usually long term. In atrial flutter, the ventricular rate is normally more difficult to control with digoxin. Cardioversion with DC countershock is the preferred method of treatment, but treatment with digoxin may restore sinus rhythm, or it may convert the flutter to fibrillation and sinus rhythm may then be induced by subsequent withdrawal of digoxin. In patients with the Wolff-Parkinson-White syndrome and atrial fibrillation, digoxin can cause rapid ventricular rates, and possibly ventricular fibrillation and should be avoided. It may be given to relieve an attack of paroxysmal supraventricular tachycardia and has also been given to prevent further attacks. The use of digoxin in paroxysmal ventricular tachycardia is dangerous.

Digoxin is used in the treatment of congestive heart failure with atrial fibrillation although the beneficial effect of long-term treatment in patients in sinus rhythm is questioned. Diuretics are often given concomitantly and may be preferred to digoxin as initial treatment in patients with mild congestive heart failure and sinus rhythm. Vasodilators and angiotensin-converting enzyme inhibitors may also be used. There is controversy over the use of digoxin in patients with acute myocardial infarction and over its prophylactic use.

When given by mouth, digoxin may take effect within about 2 hours and the maximum effect may be reached in about 6 hours.

Higher doses are necessary to provide a chronotropic effect in cardiac arrhythmias than to produce an inotropic effect in congestive heart failure. Dosage should be carefully adjusted to the needs of the individual patient. Factors which may be considered include the patient's age, lean body mass, renal status, thyroid status, electrolyte balance, degree of tissue oxygenation, and the nature of the underlying cardiac or pulmonary disease. Steady-state plasma-digoxin concentrations (in a specimen taken at least 6 hours after a dose) of 0.5 to 2 ng per mL are generally considered acceptable; concentrations in excess of 2 ng per mL may be associated with toxicity. Because of considerable overlap, plasma concentrations are considered inadequate as the sole guide to dosage.

If rapid digitalisation is required, 500 to 750 μg of digoxin may be given by mouth followed by 250 μg every 6 hours until the desired therapeutic effect is obtained. A total dose of 1 to 1.5 mg given over 24 hours is normally adequate. If there is no great urgency a loading dose is omitted and digitalisation is achieved slowly over a week with doses of 125 to 500 μg daily. Steady-state plasma concentrations are achieved in about 6 to 7 days in patients with normal renal function. The usual maintenance dose of digoxin is 250 μg by mouth once or twice daily. In elderly patients therapy should generally be initiated gradually and with smaller doses; maintenance doses of 125 to 250 μg daily are usually adequate.

In urgent cases, provided that the patient has not been treated with cardiac glycosides during the previous 2 weeks, digoxin may be given by slow intravenous injection over 5 to 10 minutes or by intravenous infusion. The dosage ranges from 0.5 to 1 mg and produces a definite effect on the heart-rate in about 10 minutes, reaching a maximum within 1 to 2 hours. Alternatively an initial intravenous dose of 250 to 500 μg may be given, followed by 250 μg every 4 to 6 hours to a maximum total dose of 1 mg. Maintenance treatment is then usually given by mouth but intravenous doses of 125 to 500 μg daily have been given if oral administration is not possible. Digoxin has also been given intramuscularly but this route is not generally recommended since such injections may be painful and tissue damage has been reported.

A suggested dose for infants and children is 10 to 35 μg per kg body-weight by mouth or by injection in 3 or 4 divided doses over 24 hours, then 4 to 10 μg per kg daily, and later adjusted to the optimum maintenance dose. Premature and immature neonates are particularly sensitive to digoxin whereas children between one month and 2 years may require relatively larger doses than older children.

Digoxin should not be given subcutaneously as it may give rise to intense local irritation, and when given intravenously it should be administered slowly, care being taken to prevent extravasation.

General reviews on the actions and uses of digoxin and the other cardiac glycosides: *Am. J. Hosp. Pharm.*, 1978, *35*, 1495; L. H. Opie, *Lancet*, 1980, *1*, 912; A. J. Taggart and D. G. McDevitt, *Drugs*, 1980, *20*, 398; *Lancet*, 1982, *1*, 891; D. A. Chamberlain, *Br. Heart J.*, 1985, *54*, 227; B. Levitt and D. L. Keefe, *J. clin. Pharmac.*, 1985, *25*, 507; M. R. Wilkins *et al.*, *Br. med. J.*, 1985, *290*, 7; M. R. Wilkins, *Prescribers' J.*, 1986, *26*, 58.

ACTION. The role of the nervous system in the cardiovascular effects of digoxin.— R. A. Gillis and J. A. Quest, *Pharmac. Rev.*, 1979, *31*, 19.

The current hypothesis concerning the cellular mechanisms of digitalis action suggests that digitalis specifically inhibits Na-K ATPase. This produces an elevation in the intracellular sodium concentration that in turn produces an increase in the intracellular calcium level. The increased quantities of calcium available to the contractile elements of cardiac muscle provide the observed increased inotropy.— D. S. Miura and S. Biedert, *J. clin. Pharmac.*, 1985, *25*, 490.

ADMINISTRATION. A discussion on pharmacokinetic, pharmacodynamic, and other factors affecting digoxin dosage, with therapeutic guidelines. There is little evidence that prescribing aids such as nomograms or computer programs result in more accurate dosage determination. If patient compliance can be ensured and a preparation of uniform bioavailability is chosen, more accurate initial intuitive prescribing of digoxin should be possible with the help of careful clinical observation, critical use of plasma-digoxin concentrations, and awareness of factors which may modify the individual response such as age, other disease states, and interactions with other drugs.— G. D. Johnston, *Drugs*, 1980, *20*, 494. See also M. E. Burton *et al.*, *Clin. Pharmacokinet.*, 1985, *10*, 1.

An evaluation of 12 published methods of digoxin dosing in 85 patients demonstrated a low correlation between predicted and measured serum concentrations. However, since the methods tended to overpredict serum concentrations, the methods would generally allow safe first approximations for digoxin dosing.— W. N. Jones et al., *J. clin. Pharmac.*, 1982, *22*, 543.

Compliance. Compliance with prescribed digoxin therapy was estimated by comparing plasma-digoxin concentrations before and after a 10-day period when digoxin consumption was measured. There was non-compliance in 23 of 50 patients studied in general practice.— G. D. Johnston and D. G. McDevitt, *Br. J. clin. Pharmac.*, 1978, *6*, 339. Further references to the problem of non-compliance with digoxin therapy: J. R. Gilbert *et al.*, *Can. med. Ass. J.*, 1980, *123*, 119 (predicting compliance); A. J. Taggart *et al.*, *Br. J. clin. Pharmac.*, 1981, *1*, 31 (dose frequency did not influence compliance).

In infants and children. Review of the pharmacokinetics, actions, clinical uses, and toxicology of the cardiac glycosides in infants and neonates. There is an apparent increase in the affinity of the neonatal myocardium for digoxin compared with that of the adult. The volume of distribution of digoxin appears to be age-dependent, having an average value of about 5 litres per kg in low birth-weight infants and in adults and 12 to 16 litres per kg in full-term neonates. This difference has been attributed to greater tissue binding, and changes in body composition may be an additional factor. Measurement of serum-digoxin concentrations is complicated by the presence of an endogenous substance that cross-reacts with conventional radio-immunoassay materials and has been found in the serum of premature and full-term infants at concentrations ranging from 0.3 to 4.1 ng per mL. Digoxin clearance increases with maturation of renal function, and tubular secretion appears to be significant in full-term and older infants. In pre-term infants, total body clearance is significantly less than in other age groups, while in full-term infants, digoxin clearance is higher than in older children and adults, possibly due to increased non-renal clearance.

In infants with diminished myocardial contractility dosage requirements for optimal inotropic action are unclear. Some reports suggest that high-dose digoxin therapy is often necessary while others suggest clinical effectiveness with much lower dosage. The wide range of diseases and clinical conditions represented in studies make comparisons and extrapolation to other patients difficult and sometimes hazardous. For the treatment of arrhythmias dosage recommendations depend on age-related differences in pharmacokinetics. Published dosage schedules based on pharmacokinetic data at steady state are probably the most valid, but are necessarily based on average values. Individual clinical response and serum-digoxin concentrations should be taken into consideration when establishing the optimal maintenance dose for a patient. Since renal function increases in the first few weeks of life, digoxin requirements will increase with postnatal age. There is evidence to suggest that many cases of intoxication in infants occur during or immediately after digitalisation, and it is recommended that loading doses should not be given except for the management of arrhythmias and in emergencies. A dosing interval of 12 hours is generally recommended to minimise the possibility of toxic peak concentrations and sub-therapeutic trough concentrations, although a 24-hourly interval would be adequate in premature infants, increasing to 12-hourly as renal function increases, probably at 1 month of age.— R. J. Roberts, *Drug Therapy in Infants : Pharmacologic Principles and Clinical Experience*, London, W.B. Saunders, 1984, 138. Further references: L. Nyberg and G. Wettrell, *Clin. Pharmacokinet.*, 1978, *3*, 453; W. W. Pinsky *et al.*, *J. Pediat.*, 1979, *96*, 639.

Ampoules of digoxin for adult use should never be supplied to children's hospital wards; use of the paediatric injection should ensure that a fatal overdose cannot be given.— H. B. Valman, *Br. med. J.*, 1980, *280*, 1588.

See also Absorption and Fate (above).

In the elderly. Both loading and maintenance doses of digoxin should be reduced empirically in the small elderly patient with reduced lean body mass and impaired renal function. Plasma-digoxin concentrations correlate with symptoms of toxicity and should be used to achieve optimal maintenance dosage. Patients should be monitored for extra-cardiac symptoms as well as more overt signs of toxicity such as arrhythmias. Not all patients taking digoxin need maintenance therapy and in one study J.L.C. Dall (*Br. med. J.*, 1970, *2*, 705) found that in almost 75% of elderly patients in sinus rhythm, digoxin could be withdrawn safely. B. Whiting *et al.* (*Br. Heart J.*, 1978, *40*, 8) have reported that only about one third of a group of elderly patients were receiving an ideal dose of digoxin and withdrawal of the drug or a revision of dosage was beneficial.— R. E. Vestal, *Drugs*, 1978, *16*, 358. A view that in general digoxin is only necessary when there is rapid atrial fibrillation causing heart failure or signs of incipient failure and in patients with supraventricular paroxysmal tachycardia. Congestive heart failure in elderly patients in sinus rhythm is usually treated with simple diuretic therapy.— J. Williamson, *Practitioner*, 1978, *220*, 749.

Further references to the administration of digoxin to the elderly: G. Tsujimoto *et al.*, *Br. J. clin. Pharmac.*, 1982, *13*, 493.

In renal failure. In most patients with advanced renal failure an appropriate intravenous loading dose of digoxin is 10 μg per kg body-weight.— M. H. Gault *et al.*, *Br. J. clin. Pharmac.*, 1980, *9*, 593.

Evidence of cumulation of digoxin metabolites in patients requiring maintenance dialysis for end-stage renal failure. The clinical significance is not known.— T. P. Gibson and H. A. Nelson, *Clin. Pharmac. Ther.*, 1980, *27*, 219.

The use of an equation for calculating maintenance digoxin regimens in patients with renal insufficiency proved impractical.— F. Keller *et al.*, *Eur. J. clin. Pharmac.*, 1980, *18*, 433.

The normal half-life of digoxin of 36 to 44 hours is increased to 80 to 120 hours in end-stage renal disease. Standard doses should be reduced to 25 to 75% in patients with a glomerular filtration rate (GFR) of 10 to 50 mL per minute, and to 10 to 25% in those with a GFR of less than 10 mL per minute. Alternatively, the dosage interval may be increased to 36 hours in those with a GFR of 10 to 50 mL per minute and to 48 hours in those with a GFR of less than 10 mL per minute. No supplement to the dosage is required for haemodialysis or peritoneal dialysis. Serum concentrations may be overestimated by radio-immunoassay; the serum concentration 12 hours after a maintenance dose is the best guide to dosage.— W. M. Bennett *et al.*, *Am. J. Kidney Dis.*, 1983, *3*, 155.

Further references to the administration of digoxin to patients with renal failure: J. K. Aronson and D. G. Grahame-Smith, *Br. J. clin. Pharmac.*, 1976, *3*, 1045; L. Storstein and H. Janssen, *Clin. Pharmac. Ther.*, 1976, *20*, 15; S. M. Dobbs *et al.*, *Br. med. J.*, 1977, *2*, 168; S. Pancorbo and C. Comty (letter), *Ann. intern. Med.*, 1980, *93*, 639; E. E. Ohnhaus *et al.*, *Eur. J. clin. Pharmac.*, 1980, *18*, 467.

See also under Distribution and Protein Binding in Absorption and Fate (p.829).

In respiratory insufficiency. A review on the use of digoxin in pulmonary heart disease (cor pulmonale). There has been controversy over the use of digoxin in the treatment of congestive heart failure in patients with cor pulmonale although atrial arrhythmias appear to be legitimate indications for digoxin therapy in such patients. Patients with cor pulmonale may be more susceptible to the adverse effects of cardiac glycosides, especially since they are often elderly, thin, and may have impaired renal function. In general reduced doses are recommended except in the control of atrial fibrillation.— J. E. Doherty *et al.*, *Drugs*, 1977, *13*, 142. The efficacy of digoxin in the treatment of cor pulmonale remains controversial.— L. H. Green and T. W. Smith,

Ann. intern. Med., 1977, *87*, 459. Digoxin was not considered to be useful in cor pulmonale unless there is co-existent atrial fibrillation.— J. Rees, *Br. med. J.*, 1984, *289*, 1398.

Therapeutic drug monitoring. The use of erythrocyte-digoxin concentrations in monitoring digoxin therapy.— S. Kawai *et al.*, *Clin. Pharmac. Ther.*, 1982, *31*, 541. See also A. H. L. From *et al.*, *Eur. J. clin. Pharmac.*, 1983, *24*, 807; C. J. van Boxtel *et al.*, *Ther. Drug Monit.*, 1985, *7*, 191.

Discussion of the indications for the measurement of plasma-digoxin concentrations. While digoxin fulfils many of the criteria which make therapeutic monitoring worthwhile, there are difficulties in establishing a relationship between plasma and myocardial digoxin concentrations, and between plasma concentrations and therapeutic effects. Factors which may affect the interpretation of plasma-digoxin concentrations include those which can alter the kinetics of digoxin such as renal impairment and drug interactions, and those which alter the therapeutic response such as electrolyte imbalance and thyroid dysfunction. Plasma-concentration monitoring may contribute to the tailoring of individual dosage requirements, the diagnosis of toxicity or suspected overdosage, and the determination of the need for long-term therapy.— J. K. Aronson, *Drugs*, 1983, *26*, 230. See also: A. Richens, *Prescribers' J.*, 1983, *23*, 1.

A discussion on the reliability of serum-digoxin assays. The use of different antibodies in commercial radioimmunoassay kits means that it is not possible to compare results from assays obtained with different systems. Variations also occur in cross-reactivity with metabolites and endogenous substances, particularly in patients with renal failure. Correlation between dose and eventual blood concentration has not been achieved. Interpretation of results in those with reduced renal function, the very young, and the elderly is difficult, and serum-digoxin concentration measurement is often performed for unjustifiable reasons and at inappropriate times.— M. L. Hyneck, *Clin. Pharm.*, 1985, *4*, 81.

Analysis of 1599 requests for digoxin assays in 886 patients suggested that alteration in digoxin dosage resulted from digoxin measurement in few patients.— M. J. Hallworth and M. J. Brodie (letter), *Lancet*, 1986, *1*, 95.

Further references: F. H. M. Derkx *et al.*, *Br. J. clin. Pharmac.*, 1982, *14*, 139P; B. Whiting *et al.*, *Br. med. J.*, 1984, *288*, 541; G. R. Bailie and D. M. Angaran, *Pharm. J.*, 1986, *1*, 392; J. F. Doran (letter), *Lancet*, 1986, *1*, 321.

For further data on plasma concentrations, see under Diagnosis of Toxicity in Adverse Effects (p.826).

CARDIAC DISORDERS. *Arrhythmias.* Digoxin should only be administered to patients for the treatment of paroxysmal supraventricular tachycardia if the diagnosis is not in doubt since digoxin is dangerous in patients with ventricular tachycardia.— D. A. Chamberlain, *Prescribers' J.*, 1981, *21*, 153.

In a controlled study of 12 patients with atrial fibrillation on maintenance digoxin therapy, it was concluded that control of the resting heart-rate, even in a patient with high serum-digoxin concentration, does not ensure adequate control of the heart-rate at work-rates equivalent to usual daily activity.— R. Beasley *et al.*, *Br. med. J.*, 1985, *290*, 9.

An intravenous cardiac glycoside, preferably ouabain, was considered to be indicated for the treatment of acute atrial tachycardias if treatment with verapamil was not appropriate.— W. T. Brownlee, *Br. J. Hosp. Med.*, 1985, *33*, 138.

Intravenous verapamil was preferred to digoxin in the treatment of acute atrial fibrillation with rapid ventricular rate and of atrial flutter.— H. O. Klein and E. Kaplinsky, *Drugs*, 1986, *31*, 185.

Further references to digoxin in the treatment of arrhythmias.— J. L. Wilkinson, *Archs Dis. Childh.*, 1983, *58*, 945 (treatment of paroxysmal tachycardias); M. -L. Ong and G. Jackson, *Br. J. clin. Pract.*, 1985, *39*, 219 (digoxin combined with quinidine in the treatment of supraventricular arrhythmias).

Heart failure. A discussion of the value of positive inotropic agents in heart failure. Symptomatic improvement depends on improvement of the peripheral circulation, but even this may not improve survival which is determined by the amount of myocardial damage. In the early stages of heart failure, therapy should be directed towards prevention of further myocardial cell loss rather than stimulation of pump function. In the late stages of heart failure, positive inotropic agents may be used to stimulate the severely depressed myocardium although the response may be limited by the contractile reserve.— T. H. LeJemtel and E. H. Sonnenblick, *New Engl. J. Med.*, 1984, *310*, 1384.

The use of digoxin in patients with congestive heart failure in sinus rhythm remains controversial. Diuretics and vasodilators are generally considered to be more appropriate for first-line treatment of mild heart failure in sinus rhythm. The long-term benefits of digoxin are also contentious, and several studies have demonstrated that digoxin can be successfully withdrawn from certain patients on maintenance therapy. For studies and reviews, see: B. E. Griffiths *et al.*, *Br. med. J.*, 1982, *284*, 1819; M. Gheorghiade and G. A. Beller, *Am. J. Cardiol.*, 1983, *51*, 1243; L. H. Opie, *Lancet*, 1984, *1*, 496; T. B. Levine, *Br. J. clin. Pharmac.*, 1984, *18*, *Suppl.* 2, 147S; P. A. Poole-Wilson, *ibid.*, 151S; C. D. Mulrow *et al.*, *Ann. intern. Med.*, 1984, *101*, 113; D. P. Lipkin and P. A. Poole-Wilson, *Br. med. J.*, 1985, *291*, 993; M. M. Applefeld and D. S. Roffman, *Am. J. Med.*, 1986, *80*, 40; M. Packer and C. V. Leier, *Circulation*, 1987, *75*, *Suppl. IV*, 55.

Discussion of the alternatives to digitalis glycosides for heart failure.— G. D. Johnston, *Br. med. J.*, 1985, *290*, 803.

Reviews of the use of the newer positive inotropic agents in the treatment of congestive heart failure.— W. S. Colucci *et al.*, *New Engl. J. Med.*, 1986, *314*, 290; K. T. Weber *et al.*, *Drugs*, 1987, *33*, 503.

Heart surgery. Cardiac surgery appeared to produce an increased sensitivity to digoxin. Of 50 patients undergoing cardiac surgery 37 had postoperative arrhythmias and 17 had arrhythmias compatible with digoxin intoxication although measurements of serum-digoxin concentrations ranged from 0 to 2.8 ng per mL.— M. R. Rose *et al.*, *Am. Heart J.*, 1975, *89*, 288.

Prophylactic digoxin administration following surgery for coronary-artery bypass did not reduce the incidence of postoperative arrhythmias in a study of 98 patients. Supraventricular arrhythmias in 2 patients receiving prophylactic digoxin responded to discontinuation of the drug.— B. Weiner *et al.*, *Clin. Pharm.*, 1986, *5*, 55. See also: O. J. Ormerod *et al.*, *Br. Heart J.*, 1984, *51*, 618.

Myocardial infarction. Controversy surrounds the influence of digoxin therapy on the survival of patients after myocardial infarction. Moss *et al.* studied 972 patients during the first 4 months after myocardial infarction (*Circulation*, 1981, *64*, 1150). Their results suggested that digitalis therapy increased the mortality of coronary patients with congestive heart failure and complex ventricular premature depolarisations in the early post-hospital phase. In another study, cumulative survival rates at an average of 23 months were 66% in patients discharged on digoxin therapy compared with 87% of those not treated. However when differences in age, previous history of acute myocardial infarction, and severity of underlying heart disease were taken into consideration, the association between digoxin and decreased survival was of borderline significance (J.T. Bigger *et al.*, *Am. J. Cardiol.*, 1985, *55*, 623). Muller *et al.* observed 903 patients for up to 36 months after hospital discharge and found a cumulative mortality of 28% in patients taking digoxin and 11% in those not taking digoxin (*New Engl. J. Med.*, 1986, *314*, 265). However, patients treated with digoxin tended to have a poorer overall prognosis, and when the data were adjusted for risk factors it was concluded that no major hazard was associated with digoxin therapy. Yusuf *et al.* (*Circulation*, 1986, *73*, 14) criticised the statistical treatment of data collected retrospectively, and the validity of statistical manipulation to account for clinical differences in patient populations. It is likely that only a large prospective randomised study will be able to ascertain whether increased mortality is associated with digoxin therapy or with the clinical circumstances which form the basis for such therapy.

MALIGNANT NEOPLASMS. Discussion of a possible protective effect of cardiac glycosides against cancer. In a 5-year follow-up study of patients with breast cancer, the risk of recurrence within 5 years of mastectomy in patients not taking digoxin was 9.6 times that in patients taking digoxin.— B. Stenkvist *et al.* (letter), *New Engl. J. Med.*, 1982, *306*, 484. See also A. G. Goldin and A. R. Safa (letter), *Lancet*, 1984, *1*, 1134; G. D. Friedman (letter), *ibid.*, *2*, 875.

OBESITY. The use of digoxin or other cardiac glycosides in the treatment of obesity is unwarranted and dangerous.— *FDA Drug Bull.*, 1978, *8*, 21.

PREGNANCY AND THE NEONATE. Clinical improvement was seen in 12 of 21 infants aged between 1 and 7 months with a congested circulatory state due to an isolated ventricular septal defect treated with digoxin. Clinical benefit was only associated with evidence of an inotropic effect in 6 of the 12 infants.— W. Berman *et al.*, *New Engl. J. Med.*, 1983, *308*, 363.

A view that although administration of digitalis to non-pregnant patients with mitral stenosis is not considered to be beneficial it is advisable during pregnancy since atrial fibrillation is common and leads to pulmonary oedema with an associated maternal mortality of 14 to 17%.— J. M. Sullivan and K. B. Ramanathan, *New Engl. J. Med.*, 1985, *313*, 304.

Foetal arrhythmias. Supraventricular tachycardia in a foetus of 29 to 30 weeks' gestation was managed by giving digoxin to the mother.— T. D. Kerenyi *et al.*, *Lancet*, 1980, *2*, 393 and 546.

Maternal digoxin therapy is generally considered the drug treatment of choice in foetal tachyarrhythmias. If this fails, a combination of digoxin and verapamil may be contemplated, and a combination of digoxin and propranolol, procainamide, or quinidine as the next step.— J. W. Wladimiroff and P. A. Stewart, *Br. J. Hosp. Med.*, 1985, *34*, 134. See also J. T. Harrigan *et al.*, *New Engl. J. Med.*, 1981, *304*, 1527; M. Nagashima *et al.*, *Archs Dis. Childh.*, 1986, *61*, 996.

Preparations

Digoxin Elixir *(U.S.P.).* Contains 4.5 to 5.25 mg of digoxin in each 100 mL.

Paediatric Digoxin Oral Solution *(B.P.).* Digoxin Elixir Paediatric; Paediatric Digoxin Elixir. An elixir containing digoxin 50 µg in 1 mL. pH 6.8 to 7.2. The elixir should not be diluted.

Digoxin Injection *(B.P.).* Contains digoxin 250 µg in 1 mL. pH 6.7 to 7.3.

Paediatric Digoxin Injection *(B.P.).* Digoxin Paediatric Injection. Contains digoxin 100 µg in 1 mL. pH 6.7 to 7.3.

Digoxin Injection *(U.S.P.)*

Digoxin Tablets *(B.P.)*

Digoxin Tablets *(U.S.P.)*

Proprietary Preparations

Digoxin Nativelle (also known as Diganox) *(Nativelle, Fr.: Lipomed, UK). Tablets*, scored, digoxin 250 µg.

Lanoxin *(Wellcome, UK). Tablets* (Lanoxin-125), digoxin 125 µg.
Tablets, scored, digoxin 250 µg.
Injection, digoxin 250 µg/mL, in ampoules of 2 mL.

Lanoxin-PG *(Wellcome, UK). Tablets*, digoxin 62.5 µg. *Elixir*, digoxin 50 µg/mL.

Proprietary Names and Manufacturers

Allocor *(Natrapharm, Ger.)*; Cardigox *(Belg.)*; Cardiogoxin *(Arg.)*; Cardioreg *(Nattermann, Ital.)*; Cardiox *(Austral.)*; Coragoxine *(Nativelle, Fr.)*; Digacin *(Beiersdorf, Ger.)*; Digazolan *(Switz.)*; Digivern *(Vernleigh, S.Afr.)*; Digomal *(Malesci, Ital.)*; Dixina *(Ital.)*; Eudigox *(Simes, Ital.; Switz.)*; Lanacordin *(Gayoso Wellcome, Spain)*; Lanacrist *(Draco, Swed.)*; Lanicor *(Arg.; Boehringer Mannheim, Ger.; Boehringer Biochemia, Ital.; Neth.; Switz.)*; Lanorale *(Ital.)*; Lanoxicaps *(Wellcome, USA)*; Lanoxin *(Arg.; Wellcome, Austral.; Belg.; Wellcome, Canad.; Wellcome, Denm.; Wellcome, Ital.; Neth.; Wellcome, Norw.; Wellcome, S.Afr.; Wellcome, Swed.; Wellcome, Switz.; Wellcome, UK; Wellcome, USA)*; Lanoxine *(Fr.)*; LenoxiCaps *(Wellcome, Ger.)*; Lenoxin *(Wellcome, Ger.)*; Natigoxin *(Gamaprod, Austral.)*; Novodigal *(Beiersdorf, Ger.)*; Prodigox *(Austral.)*; Purgoxin *(Lennon, S.Afr.)*; SK-Digoxin *(USA)*.

16805-d

Enoximone *(BAN, USAN, rINN).*

Fenoximone; MDL-17043; MDL-19438; RMI-17043; YMDL-17043. 4-Methyl-5-[4-(methylthio)benzoyl]-4-imidazolin-2-one.

$C_{12}H_{12}N_2O_2S = 248.3$.

CAS — 77671-31-9.

Enoximone is a phosphodiesterase inhibitor which has been reported to have positive inotropic activity, and has been tried in the treatment of congestive heart failure.

Enoximone is reported to have pharmacologic and haemodynamic effects very similar to those of amrinone and milrinone. Beneficial responses have been seen in patients with congestive heart failure, although some investigators have reported an increase in myocardial oxygen consumption. Long-term therapy has been accompanied by a high incidence of gastro-intestinal disturbances and fluid retention is not infrequent. Thrombocytopenia is uncommon. Oral therapy with enoximone may produce symptomatic improvement of heart failure but does not appear to improve survival.— W. S. Colucci *et al.*, *New Engl. J. Med.*, 1986, *314*, 349.

A review of the pharmacokinetics and pharmacodynamics of newer inotropic agents including enoximone.— M. L. Rocci and H. Wilson, *Clin. Pharmacokinet.*, 1987, *13*, 91.

Further references to enoximone: *Lancet*, 1988, *1*, 1085.

Proprietary Names and Manufacturers
Merrell, UK.

5817-m

Gitalin

Gitalin Amorphous *(pINN)*. A mixture of glycosides obtained from *Digitalis purpurea* (Scrophulariaceae), containing 14 to 20% of digitoxin, 13 to 19% of gitaloxin, and 13 to 19% of gitoxin.

CAS — 1405-76-1 (gitalin, amorphous); 3261-53-8 (gitaloxin); 4562-36-1 (gitoxin).

Gitalin has the general properties of digoxin (p.825) and has been used similarly. It has been given by mouth in average maintenance doses of 500 μg daily.

Proprietary Names and Manufacturers of Gitalin and Gitaloxin
Cristaloxine *(Christiaens, Belg.; Pharmuka, Fr.)*; Formigital *(Padro, Spain)*; Gitalide *(Padro, Spain)*; Gitaligin *(Schering, USA)*; Verodigeno *(Boehringer Mannheim, Spain)*.

5818-b

Gitoformate *(rINN)*.

Gitoxin Pentaformate; Pentaformylgitoxin. 3β-[(*O*-2,6-Dideoxy-3,4-di-*O*-formyl-β-D-*ribo*-hexopyranosyl-(1→4)-*O*-2,6-dideoxy-3-*O*-formyl-β-D-*ribo*-hexopyranosyl-(1→4)-2,6-dideoxy-3-*O*-formyl-β-D-*ribo*-hexopyranosyl)oxy]-16β-formyloxy-14-hydroxy-5β,14β-card-20(22)-enolide.
$C_{46}H_{64}O_{19}$=921.0.

CAS — 10176-39-3; 7685-23-6.

Gitoformate is a synthetic cardiac glycoside with the general properties of digoxin (p.825) and has been used similarly in maintenance doses of 60 to 120 μg daily by mouth.

Proprietary Names and Manufacturers
Dynocard *(Madaus, Ger.)*; Formiloxine *(Christiaens, Belg.; Menarini, Ital.)*.

18963-q

Imazodan *(rINN)*.

CI-914 *(base or hydrochloride)*. 4,5-Dihydro-6-(*p*-imidazol-1-ylphenyl)-3(2*H*)-pyridazinone.
$C_{13}H_{12}N_4O$=240.3.

CAS — 84243-58-3.

NOTE. Imazodan Hydrochloride is *USAN*.

Imazodan is a phosphodiesterase inhibitor which is reported to have positive inotropic and vasodilatory activity.

In a study involving 12 patients with moderate to severe left ventricular dysfunction the results suggested that imazodan 1.2 μg or more per kg body-weight per minute by intravenous infusion improved the haemodynamic state of patients with severe congestive heart failure primarily by reducing systemic vascular resistance. A better response was obtained in patients whose initial systemic vascular resistance was elevated than in patients in whom it was not elevated. The positive inotropic effect also contributed to the beneficial effect of imazodan, and there was evidence of a reduction in myocardial oxygen consumption.— S. Terris *et al.*, *Am. J. Cardiol.*, 1986, *58*, 596.

Proprietary Names and Manufacturers
Warner-Lambert, USA.

5819-v

Lanatoside C *(BAN, rINN)*.

Celanide; Celanidum; Lanatosidum C. 3β-[(*O*-β-D-Glucopyranosyl-(1→4)-*O*-3-acetyl-2,6-dideoxy-β-D-*ribo*-hexopyranosyl-(1→4)-*O*-2,6-dideoxy-β-D-*ribo*-hexopyranosyl-(1→4)-*O*-2,6-dideoxy-β-D-*ribo*-hexopyranosyl)oxy]-12β,14-dihydroxy-5β,14β-card-20(22)-enolide.
$C_{49}H_{76}O_{20}$=985.1.

CAS — 17575-22-3.

Pharmacopoeias. In *Arg., Aust., Br., Braz., Cz., Egypt., Eur., Hung., Ind., Int., Jpn, Jug., Mex., Nord., Pol., Roum., Rus., Swiss,* and *Turk.*

A glycoside obtained from digitalis lanata leaf. It occurs as odourless, white or yellowish, hygroscopic crystals or crystalline powder.

Practically **insoluble** in water, in chloroform, and in ether; soluble 1 in 20 of methyl alcohol. **Store** in airtight, glass containers at a temperature not exceeeding 10°. Protect from light.

Adverse Effects, Treatment, and Precautions
As for Digoxin, p.825.

Absorption and Fate
Lanatoside C is poorly absorbed from the gastro-intestinal tract. It is weakly bound to serum albumin and rapidly passes to other tissues. About 20% of the dose administered has been stated to be inactivated daily. Its effects disappear after 3 to 6 days. Digoxin is reported to be a metabolite of lanatoside C excreted in the urine.

Following oral administration of tritiated lanatoside C to 31 subjects, an average of 74% of radioactive material in the plasma was digoxin and its metabolites. The results indicated that lanatoside C is converted to digoxin in the gastro-intestinal tract before absorption. Oral administration of lanatoside C might produce lower and more variable concentrations of digoxin in the body.— S. Aldous and R. Thomas, *Clin. Pharmac. Ther.*, 1977, *21*, 647.

BIOAVAILABILITY. Reformulation of Cedilanid tablets in 1982 resulted in increased bioavailability.— *Pharm. J.*, 1982, *1*, 51.

Uses and Administration
Lanatoside C is employed for the same purposes as digoxin (p.829). A suggested digitalising dose of lanatoside C is 1.5 to 2 mg daily by mouth in divided doses for 3 to 5 days. The maintenance dose varies from 0.25 to 1.5 mg daily.

Mixtures of lanatosides A, B, and C have also been used.

Proprietary Preparations
Cedilanid Tablets *(Sandoz, UK)*. *Tablets*, scored, lanatoside C 250 μg.

Proprietary Names and Manufacturers
Cedilanid *(Austral.; Sandoz, Denm; Sandoz, Ger.; Sandoz, Ital.; Sandoz, Spain; Sandoz, UK; USA)*; Cedilanide *(Belg.; Fr.; Neth.; Sandor, Switz)*; Celadigal *(Beiersdorf, Ger.)*; Celanat *(Switz.)*; Celanate *(Streuli, Switz.)*; Dilanosid-C *(Switz.)*; Lanatosid *(Denm.; Ger.)*; Lanimerck *(Ger.)*; Lanocide *(Austral.)*.

The following names have been used for multi-ingredient preparations containing lanatoside C— Dilanat *(Switz.)*; Pandigal *(Beiersdorf, Ger.)*.

5820-r

Medigoxin *(BAN)*.

β-Methyl Digoxin; β-Methyldigoxin; Metildigoxin *(rINN)*. 3β-[(*O*-2,6-Dideoxy-4-*O*-methyl-β-D-*ribo*-hexopyranosyl-(1→4)-*O*-2,6-dideoxy-β-D-*ribo*-hexopyranosyl-(1→4)-2,6-dideoxy-β-D-*ribo*-hexopyranosyl)oxy]-12β,14-dihydroxy-5β,14β-card-20(22)-enolide.
$C_{42}H_{66}O_{14}$=795.0.

CAS — 30685-43-9.

Adverse Effects, Treatment, and Precautions
As for Digoxin, p.825.

In contrast to digoxin, the rate of decline of radioactivity after intravenous administration of tritiated medigoxin was significantly retarded in patients with acute hepatitis. Delayed demethylation of medigoxin might explain the higher plasma concentrations in patients with liver disease when compared with healthy subjects.— W. Zilly *et al.*, *Clin. Pharmac. Ther.*, 1975, *17*, 302. Hepatic demethylation of medigoxin was reduced in 12 patients with cirrhosis of the liver compared with 12 healthy subjects. This resulted in a reduction in medigoxin clearance and a smaller volume of distribution.— H. Rameis *et al.*, *Int. J. clin. Pharmac. Ther. Toxic.*, 1984, *22*, 145.

Fairly good non-linear correlation was found between creatinine clearance and medigoxin half-life in a study of 15 patients with chronic renal impairment including 8 undergoing haemodialysis and 4 patients with congestive heart failure and unimpaired renal function. It was recommended that patients undergoing dialysis should be given 30 to 50% of the usual dose initially.— G. M. Trovato *et al.*, *Curr. ther. Res.*, 1983, *33*, 158.

For a report of the successful treatment of medigoxin intoxication with cholestyramine, see Digoxin p.826.

INTERACTIONS. For a report of an interaction between medigoxin and diltiazem see p.828.

Absorption and Fate
Medigoxin is rapidly and almost completely absorbed from the gastro-intestinal tract and in the steady state a half-life of 54-60 hours has been reported. Demethylation to digoxin occurs. About 60% of an oral or intravenous dose is excreted in the urine as unchanged drug and metabolites over 7 days. About 22% of a dose is reported to be lost each day through inactivation or excretion.

Similar mean steady state serum concentrations of about 1.5 ng per mL of medigoxin and digoxin were obtained when 6 healthy subjects took a daily dose of medigoxin 300 μg or digoxin 500 μg respectively. Subjects had a lower medigoxin dose requirement since only 50 to 80% of the digoxin dose was absorbed compared with 70 to 80% of the medigoxin dose. Renal clearances from total serum for digoxin and medigoxin were 126 and 87 mL per minute respectively. Medigoxin was about 22% bound to plasma protein and digoxin about 26%.— G. W. M. Kongola *et al.*, *Br. J. clin. Pharmac.*, 1976, *3*, 954P. Medigoxin had a half-life of about 2.29 days compared to 1.54 days for digoxin.— F. Keller *et al.*, *Eur. J. clin. Pharmac.*, 1977, *12*, 387.

Uses and Administration
Medigoxin has the general properties and uses of digoxin (p.829) but its onset of action is more rapid. When medigoxin is given by mouth an effect may appear within 5 to 20 minutes and a maximum effect on the myocardium may be seen in 15 to 30 minutes. The duration of action is similar to or a little longer than that of digoxin; therapeutic plasma concentrations are also similar. In stabilised patients a dose of 300 μg of medigoxin is as effective as 500 μg of digoxin. For rapid digitalisation medigoxin 200 μg is given three times daily for 2 to 4 days. Slower digitalisation may be achieved with 200 μg twice daily for 3 to 5 days and maintenance therapy is continued with 200 or 300 μg daily in divided doses. Children have been given 10 μg per kg body-weight every 6 hours, usually for 2 to 4 doses, and then 10 μg per kg daily.

A study of the comparative pharmacodynamics of medigoxin and digoxin in 5 healthy subjects. Although the better gastro-intestinal absorption of medigoxin was reflected in higher blood concentrations of the glycoside this did not result in greater positive inotropic response.— G. Das *et al.*, *Clin. Pharmac. Ther.*, 1977, *22*, 280.

Proprietary Names and Manufacturers
Cardiolan *(Tosi-Novara, Ital.)*; Lanirapid *(Boehringer Mannheim, Spain)*; Lanitop *(Arg.; Belg.; Boehringer Mannheim, Ger.; Boehringer Biochemia, Ital.; Neth.;*

Boehringer Mannheim, Switz.; *Roussel, UK*); Metidi *(Ital.)*; Miopat *(Polifarma, Ital.)*.

5821-f

Meproscillarin *(BAN, rINN)*.

4′-*O*-Methylproscillaridin; Knoll 570; Ky-18. 14-Hydroxy-3β-[(4-*O*-methyl-α-L-rhamnopyranosyl)oxy]-14β-bufa-4,20,22-trienolide.

$C_{31}H_{44}O_8$=544.7.

CAS — 33396-37-1.

NOTE. The name rambufaside was formerly used for meproscillarin.

Meproscillarin is the methyl ether of proscillaridin (below) and is used similarly to digoxin (p.829). It has been given by mouth in maintenance doses of 500 to 750 µg daily in divided doses and has also been administered intravenously.

No significant difference in plasma concentration was observed between 26 patients with impaired renal function and 7 healthy subjects given meproscillarin 500 µg daily for 2 weeks. It was concluded that, unlike digoxin, dose reduction of meproscillarin in patients with chronic renal failure was unnecessary.— W. D. Twittenhoff *et al., Arzneimittel-Forsch.*, 1978, *28*, 562.

Proprietary Names and Manufacturers

Clift *(Knoll, Ger.*; *Knoll, Switz.)*.

16896-t

Milrinone *(BAN, rINN)*.

Win-47203-2. 1,6-Dihydro-2-methyl-6-oxo[3,4′-bipyridine]-5-carbonitrile.

$C_{12}H_9N_3O$=211.2.

CAS — 78415-72-2.

Milrinone is a phosphodiesterase inhibitor structurally related to amrinone. It is reported to have greater inotropic activity than amrinone and to be less toxic. It also has vasodilatory activity. It has been reported to be beneficial in the management of congestive heart failure.

Milrinone has been reported to be approximately 15 times more potent than amrinone and to have very similar pharmacologic and haemodynamic effects. Marked haemodynamic improvement in patients with severe heart failure has followed both oral and intravenous administration. These improvements appear to be due to both mycocardial and vascular actions. Milrinone is reported to be much better tolerated than amrinone: thrombocytopenia and fever have not occurred and gastro-intestinal intolerance is rare. Adverse effects have included fluid retention and arrhythmias. Milrinone has a half-life of approximately 2 hours and is excreted largely unchanged in the urine.— W. S. Colucci *et al., New Engl. J. Med.*, 1986, *314*, 349. In another review of milrinone it was concluded that clinical studies have shown that the short-term haemodynamic benefits produced by milrinone are not necessarily sustained in patients with severe refractory congestive heart failure. In addition, milrinone does not appear to arrest the natural progression of congestive heart failure. Milrinone is likely to be useful for providing temporary palliation of symptoms of heart failure without prolonging life expectancy.— G. R. Hasegawa, *Clin. Pharm.*, 1986, *5*, 201.

Beneficial haemodynamic effects were demonstrated when milrinone was administered by intravenous infusion to 20 patients with congestive heart failure refractory to standard medical therapy. It was concluded that the combined inotropic and afterload-reducing properties of milrinone may prove advantageous by allowing maximal improvement in haemodynamic performance without excessively increasing myocardial oxygen demand. Treatment was generally well tolerated and there was no evidence of fever, thrombocytopenia, or gastro-intestinal effects. One patient withdrew because of headaches, one because of worsening of pre-existing muscle weakness, and four patients, all with coronary artery disease, died during treatment.— D. S. Baim *et al., New Engl. J. Med.*, 1983, *309*, 748.

A review of the pharmacokinetics and pharmacodynamics of newer inotropic agents including milrinone.— M. L. Rocci and H. Wilson, *Clin. Pharmacokinet.*, 1987, *13*, 91.

Proprietary Names and Manufacturers

Winthrop, UK.

5823-n

Ouabain *(BAN)*.

Acocantherin; G-Strophanthin; Ouabainum; Strophanthin-G; Strophanthinum; Strophanthoside-G; Uabaína; Ubaína. 3β-(α-L-Rhamnopyranosyloxy)-1β,5,11α,14,19-pentahydroxy-5β,14β-card-20(22)-enolide octahydrate.

$C_{29}H_{44}O_{12},8H_2O$=728.8.

CAS — 630-60-4 (anhydrous); 11018-89-6 (octahydrate).

Pharmacopoeias. In *Arg., Aust., Belg., Cz., Egypt., Eur., Fr., Ger., Int., It., Jpn, Mex., Neth., Nord., Pol., Roum., Span., Swiss,* and *Turk.* (all $8H_2O$); in *Port.* ($9H_2O$).

A glycoside obtained from the seeds of *Strophanthus gratus* or from the wood of *Acokanthera schimperi* or *A. ouabaio* (Apocynaceae).

Odourless colourless crystals or white crystalline powder. **Protect** from light.

Adverse Effects, Treatment, and Precautions

As for Digoxin, p.825.

Absorption and Fate

Absorption of ouabain from the gastro-intestinal tract is unpredictable. The plasma half-life has been reported to be about 21 hours.

Serum and plasma concentrations of ouabain are equivalent.— T. W. Smith and E. Haber, *New Engl. J. Med.*, 1973, *289*, 1063.

Uses and Administration

Ouabain is a cardiac glycoside with actions similar to those of digoxin (p.829). It takes effect in 3 to 10 minutes following intravenous injection and exerts its full action on the heart within ½ to 2 hours; the effect persists for 1 to 3 days. It is used when rapid benefit is required, especially in emergency situations.

Ouabain is given by slow intravenous injection in a dose of 250 µg; further injections of 100 µg may be given hourly if needed up to a total dose of 1 mg in 24 hours. Maintenance may be continued with digoxin by mouth.

Proprietary Names and Manufacturers

g-Strofantin *(DAK, Denm.*; *Swed.)*; Ouabaïne Aguettant *(Fr.)*; Ouabaine Arnaud *(Gamaprod, Austral.*; *Nativelle, Fr.*: *Lipomed, UK*; *Neth.*; *Spain)*; Purostrophan *(Kali-Chemie, Ger.)*; Strodival *(Herbert, Ger.)*; Strophoperm *(Ger.)*.

5824-h

Pengitoxin *(rINN)*.

Pentaacetylgitoxin. 16β-Acetoxy-3β-[(*O*-3,4-di-*O*-acetyl-2,6-dideoxy-β-D-*ribo*-hexopyranosyl-(1→4)-*O*-3-*O*-acetyl-2,6-dideoxy-β-D-*ribo*-hexopyranosyl-(1→4)-3-*O*-acetyl-2,6-dideoxy-β-D-*ribo*-hexopyranosyl)oxy]-14-hydroxy-5β,14β-card-20(22)-enolide.

$C_{51}H_{74}O_{19}$=991.1.

CAS — 7242-04-8.

Pengitoxin is a cardiac glycoside with the general properties of digoxin (p.825) and has been used similarly in maintenance doses of 400 µg daily by mouth. It has also been given by injection.

The absorption of pengitoxin was reported to be 99% after oral administration in a study involving 28 healthy subjects. The major metabolite was 16-acetylgitoxin. The elimination half-life of pengitoxin was longer than that of digoxin and shorter than that of digitoxin. The distribution volume and clearance were found to be closer to those of digitoxin than digoxin.— K. -O. Haustein *et al., Eur. J. clin. Pharmac.*, 1983, *25*, 369.

Proprietary Names and Manufacturers

Carnacid-Cor *(TAD, Ger.)*; Cordoval *(Ger.)*.

18672-t

Piroximone *(BAN, pINN)*.

MDL-19205. 4-Ethyl-5-isonicotinoyl-4-imidazolin-2-one.

$C_{11}H_{11}N_3O_2$=217.2.

CAS — 84490-12-0.

Piroximone is a phosphodiesterase inhibitor which has positive inotropic activity and has been investigated in the treatment of heart failure.

Piroximone produces haemodynamic effects similar to those of enoximone. Beneficial responses have been reported in the short-term treatment of patients with severe heart failure. The inotropic potency after oral administration is 5 to 10 times greater than that of enoximone, although piroximone produces a weaker hypotensive effect than enoximone at equivalent inotropic dosage.— W. S. Colucci *et al., New Engl. J. Med.*, 1986, *314*, 349.

A review of the pharmacokinetics and pharmacodynamics of newer inotropic agents including piroximone.— M. L. Rocci and H. Wilson, *Clin. Pharmacokinet.*, 1987, *13*, 91.

Proprietary Names and Manufacturers

Merrell, UK.

5826-b

Proscillaridin *(BAN, USAN, rINN)*.

A-32686; Proscillaridin A; PSC-801. 14-Hydroxy-3β-(α-L-rhamnopyranosyloxy)-14β-bufa-4,20,22-trienolide.

$C_{30}H_{42}O_8$=530.7.

CAS — 466-06-8.

A glycoside obtained from *Drimia maritima* (Liliaceae).

Adverse Effects, Treatment, and Precautions

As for Digoxin, p.825.

Absorption and Fate

Proscillaridin is absorbed erratically from the gastro-intestinal tract.

Results of a study suggesting that proscillaridin undergoes first-pass inactivation in the gut wall and enterohepatic recirculation.— K. -E. Andersson *et al., Eur. J. clin. Pharmac.*, 1977, *11*, 277.

The half-life of proscillaridin varied between 19 and 209 hours in a study involving 24 elderly patients with congestive heart failure. It was concluded that there may be difficulty in obtaining adequate plasma concentrations of proscillaridin and that a rapid elimination of the glycoside cannot be presumed in elderly patients.— B. Bergdahl, *Arzneimittel-Forsch.*, 1979, *29*, 343.

Uses and Administration

Proscillaridin is a cardiac glycoside which is used similarly to digoxin (p.829). It is reported to have a rapid onset and a short duration of action. In patients not previously treated with cardiac glycosides proscillaridin has been given by mouth in initial doses of 1 to 2.5 mg daily, followed by maintenance doses of 0.5 to 2 mg daily.

Proprietary Names and Manufacturers

Caradrin *(Asta, Ger.*; *Boehringer Biochemia, Ital.*; *Boehringer Mannheim, Spain*; *Laevosan, Switz.)*; Proscillan *(Streuli, Switz.)*; Sandoscill *(Sandoz, Ger.)*; Stellarid *(Zambeletti, Ital.)*; Sucblorin *(Jpn)*; Talucard *(Knoll, Arg.)*; Talusin *(Schering, Austral.*; *Knoll, Belg.*; *Biosédra, Fr.*; *Knoll, Ger.*; *Knoll, Ital.*; *Knoll, Neth.*; *Knoll, Norw.*; *Knoll, S.Afr.*; *Knoll, Swed.*; *Knoll, Switz.)*; Tradenal *(Medinsa, Spain)*; Urgilan *(Sintesa, Belg.*; *Simes, Ital.)*; Wirnesin *(Inpharzam, Ger.)*.

5827-v

Strophanthin-K

Estrofantina; Kombé Strophanthin; Strophanthin; Strophanthoside-K.

CAS — 11005-63-3.

Pharmacopoeias. In *Arg., Aust., Braz., It., Port., Rus.,* and *Span.*

Arg., Belg., Egypt., Fr., Port., Rus., and *Span.* all include monographs for Strophanthus.

A mixture of glycosides from strophanthus, the seeds of

Strophanthus kombe (Apocynaceae) or other spp., adjusted by admixture with a suitable diluent such as lactose so as generally to possess 40% of the activity of anhydrous ouabain.

Strophanthin-K has the general properties of digoxin (p.825) and has been used similarly. It is poorly absorbed from the gastro-intestinal tract. Strophanthin-K has been given intravenously in doses of 125 to 500 μg daily.

Proprietary Names and Manufacturers
Estrofosid *(Sandoz, Spain)*; Kombetin *(Boehringer, Arg.; Boehringer Mannheim, Ger.; Boehringer Biochemia, Ital.; Boehringer Mannheim, Spain)*; Myokombin *(Boehringer, Arg.; Boehringer Biochemia, Ital.)*; Strofopan *(Simes, Ital.; Farmasimes, Spain)*; Strophosid *(Sandoz, S.Afr.)*; Trauphantin *(Eifelfango, Ger.)*.

12392-s

Sulmazole *(pINN)*.
AR-L-115-BS. 2-(2-Methoxy-4-methylsulphinylphenyl)-1*H*-imidazo[4,5-*b*]pyridine.
$C_{14}H_{13}N_3O_2S = 287.3$.
CAS — 73384-60-8.

Sulmazole is a phosphodiesterase inhibitor and is reported to have inotropic effects on the heart.

Review of studies of the use of sulmazole in heart failure and obstructive pulmonary disease.— *Drugs of the Future*, 1985, *10*, 604.

A brief review of sulmazole. Sulmazole has been shown to improve left ventricular function in patients with severe congestive heart failure. The long-term safety and efficacy of sulmazole have not been established, and serious gastro-intestinal disturbances and mild thrombocytopenia have been seen in a high percentage of patients given sulmazole by intravenous infusion over 3 days. Visual disturbances have also been reported. Clinical studies have been discontinued following the development of hepatic neoplasms in *rodents*.— W. S. Colucci *et al.*, *New Engl. J. Med.*, 1986, *314*, 349.

Proprietary Names and Manufacturers
Vardax *(Thomae, Ger.)*.

Chelating Agents Antidotes and Antagonists

1030-v

In the treatment of acute poisoning most patients require only supportive and symptomatic therapy. The active removal of poisons from the stomach by gastric lavage or emesis induction may be considered, as should the administration of substances like activated charcoal by mouth to reduce their absorption. These measures should not be considered as routine; emesis and charcoal are for instance inappropriate in corrosive poisoning, and aspiration should only be carried out with great care.

Techniques intended to promote the elimination of poisons from the body such as forced diuresis, haemodialysis, or haemoperfusion are only of value for a limited number of poisons in a few severely poisoned patients. There are some specific antidotes and although they are not often necessary, their use in appropriate circumstances can be life-saving. Such use, however, does not preclude relevant supportive and symptomatic treatment.

The drugs included in this section act in a variety of ways. There are the antagonists such as naloxone hydrochloride that compete with the poison for receptor sites. There are compounds that inhibit the poison by reacting with it to form less active or inactive complexes or by interfering with its metabolism; chelating agents are typical examples of the first group and methionine is an example of the second. There are also compounds in other sections of *Martindale* that have a number of uses including the treatment of specific types of poisoning. Such compounds include those like atropine (p.523) that block essential receptors mediating the toxic effects, or compounds that reduce the rate of conversion of the poison to a more toxic compound, as with alcohol (p.950) in methyl alcohol poisoning, or bypass the effect of the drug as happens with calcium folinate (p.1264) in methotrexate overdosage. Ipecacuanha (p.910) is widely used for emesis induction. Many other compounds spread throughout *Martindale* are used for symptomatic treatment.

It should be noted that drugs acting on opioid receptors often have both agonist and antagonist properties, those included in this chapter such as naloxone are used specifically for their antagonist properties, those used for their agonist properties may be found under Opioid Analgesics (p.1294).

1031-g

Acetylpenicillamine

Acetyl-D-penicillamine. *N*-Acetyl-3,3-dimethyl-D-cysteine; *N*-Acetyl-3-mercaptovaline.

$C_7H_{13}NO_3S$=191.3.

CAS — 15537-71-0.

Acetylpenicillamine is a derivative of penicillamine. It is a weaker chelating agent than penicillamine (p.847), but has been used similarly in the treatment of mercury poisoning.

686-j

Activated Charcoal *(BAN, USAN).*

Adsorbent Charcoal; Carbo Activatus; Charbon Activé; Decolorising Charcoal; Medicinal Charcoal.

CAS — 16291-96-6 (charcoal).

Pharmacopoeias. In *Arg., Aust., Belg., Br., Braz., Chin., Cz., Egypt., Eur., Fr., Ger., Hung., Int., It., Jpn, Jug., Mex., Neth., Nord., Pol., Port., Roum., Rus., Span., Swiss, Turk.*, and *U.S. Port.* and *Span.* also include Animal Charcoal. *It. P.* also includes Carbone Vegetale.

A fine, odourless, tasteless, black powder, free from grittiness. The *B.P.* describes material prepared from vegetable matter by carbonisation processes intended to confer a high adsorbing power. The *U.S.P.* describes the residue from the destructive distillation of various organic materials, treated to increase its adsorptive power.

The *B.P.* specifies that it adsorbs not less than 40% of its own weight of phenazone, calculated with reference to the dried substance. The *U.S.P.* has tests for adsorptive power in respect of alkaloids and dyes. Practically **insoluble** in all usual solvents. **Store** in airtight containers.

Adverse Effects

Activated charcoal is relatively nontoxic when given by mouth but gastro-intestinal disturbances such as vomiting and constipation have been reported. It may colour the faeces black.

Haemoperfusion with activated charcoal has produced various adverse effects including platelet aggregation, charcoal embolism, thrombocytopenia, haemorrhage, hypoglycaemia, hypocalcaemia, hypothermia, and hypotension.

Report of death due to aspiration of activated charcoal in a 29-year-old man being treated for an overdose of desipramine and thiothixene.— H. H. Harsch (letter), *New Engl. J. Med.*, 1986, *314*, 318. Aspiration of activated charcoal in an 8-month-old child.— J. R. Hoffman (letter), *ibid.*, 1983, *308*, 157. Another fatality.— D. G. Menzies *et al.*, *Br. med. J.*, 1988, *297*, 459.

In a report on the treatment of salicylate poisoning with repeated oral activated charcoal it was noted that there were observable differences between the adverse effects of two proprietary preparations; Carbomix appeared to produce marked constipation whereas repeated doses of Medicoal could cause diarrhoea.— D. Boldy and J. A. Vale (letter), *Br. med. J.*, 1986, *292*, 136. For a report of faecal impaction associated with the use of activated charcoal (Carbomix) in a 32-year-old man who had taken overdoses of amitriptyline and chlorpromazine, see Treatment of Adverse Effects in Amitriptyline Hydrochloride, p.352.

Precautions

Activated charcoal diminishes the action of ipecacuanha and other emetics when given concomitantly by mouth; if indicated, emesis should be induced before activated charcoal is administered. Activated charcoal has the potential to reduce the absorption of many drugs from the gastro-intestinal tract and simultaneous oral therapy should therefore be avoided. In the management of acute poisoning, concurrent medication should be administered parenterally and activated charcoal is contra-indicated when specific oral antidotes such as methionine are used.

Uses and Administration

Activated charcoal can adsorb a wide range of plant and inorganic poisons and many drugs including salicylates, paracctamol, barbituratcs, and tricyclic antidepressants; thus when administered by mouth it reduces their systemic absorption from the gastro-intestinal tract and is used in the treatment of acute oral poisoning. It is of no value in the treatment of poisoning by strong acids or alkalis and its adsorptive capacity is too low to be of use in poisoning with iron salts, cyanides, malathion, dicophane, and some organic solvents such as methyl alcohol or ethylene glycol.

Activated charcoal is given by mouth usually as a slurry in water. The usual dose is 50 g, but higher doses have been used. For maximum efficacy, activated charcoal should be administered as soon as possible after ingestion of the toxic compound, preferably after gastric lavage or emesis. However, it may be effective several hours after poisoning with certain drugs that slow gastric emptying or undergo enterohepatic or entero-enteric recycling; repeated doses of activated charcoal are of value in enhancing the faecal elimination of these drugs including cardiac glycosides, barbiturates, salicylates, and theophylline. With repeated doses 50 g may be given every 4 hours or 25 g every 2 hours.

Mixtures such as 'universal antidote' that contained activated charcoal, magnesium oxide, and tannic acid should not be used.

In the haemoperfusion treatment of poisoning, activated charcoal may be used as the adsorbent to remove drugs from the blood stream. Charcoal haemoperfusion may be of value in acute poisoning by drugs such as the barbiturates, glutethimide, or theophylline.

Activated charcoal is used in dressings for ulcers and suppurating wounds to reduce malodour and may improve the rate of healing. Activated charcoal has been used as an intestinal marker and has also been tried in the treatment of flatulence. Technical grades of activated charcoal have been used as purifying and decolorising agents, for the removal of residual gases in low-pressure apparatus, and in respirators as a protection against toxic gases.

Charcoal (Carbo vegetabilis; Carbo veg.) is used in homoeopathic medicine.

Activated charcoal is most commonly administered as a slurry in water but this is often found to be unpalatable because of the colour, gritty taste, lack of flavour, and difficulty in swallowing (E.C. Scholtz *et al.*, *Am. J. Hosp. Pharm.*, 1978, *35*, 1355). Efforts have therefore been made to improve its palatability but studies *in vitro* or in healthy subjects have indicated that some foods such as ice cream, milk, and cocoa might inhibit the adsorptive capacity of activated charcoal whereas starches and jams appeared to have no effect (G. Levy *et al.*, *ibid.*, 1975, *32*, 289; R. De Neve, *ibid.*, 1976, *33*, 965). Carmellose has been demonstrated to improve palatability though it might also reduce the adsorptive power of activated charcoal (L.K. Mathur *et al.*, *ibid.*, 717; M. Manes, *ibid.*, 1120; L.K. Mathur *et al.*, *ibid.*, 1122). Scholtz *et al.*, 1978 found that activated charcoal formulations containing sorbitol, carmellose sodium, or starch were more palatable and essentially equivalent to the aqueous slurry formulation in efficacy. When chocolate syrup was used as a sweet flavouring agent it had to be added just before administration as the sweetness and flavour disappeared after a few minutes contact with the activated charcoal. Results of a study by Cooney (*ibid.*, 1980, *37*, 237) also suggested that saccharin sodium, sucrose, or sorbitol might be suitable flavouring agents for activated charcoal formulations.

ACUTE POISONING. Review of the efficacy of oral activated charcoal in the management of acute poisoning. Studies *in vitro* have only a limited relevance when the efficacy of charcoal as an antidote is evaluated. Experimental studies in *animals* and in man, careful observation of intoxicated patients, and adequate sampling are necessary to determine the role of activated charcoal in the management of overdoses by individual drugs. The efficacy of charcoal in the treatment of various intoxications including analgesics (such as aspirin, paracetamol, and dextropropoxyphene), hypnosedatives and anticonvulsants (such as barbiturates, phenytoin, and carbamazepine), tricyclic antidepressants, digitalis glycosides, theophylline, tolbutamide, and dapsone are discussed.— P. J. Neuvonen, *Clin. Pharmacokinet.*, 1982, *7*, 465. Further reviews: G. D. Park *et al.*, *Archs intern. Med.*, 1986, *146*, 969.

The administration of a single dose of activated charcoal has become an accepted method of preventing the absorption of ingested compounds. However, recent studies have indicated that repeated doses of activated charcoal by mouth may enhance the elimination of some drugs. Mechanisms by which activated charcoal may increase drug elimination from the body include interruption of the enterohepatic circulation of drugs excreted into the bile, reduction of the reabsorption of drugs which diffuse or are actively secreted into the intestines, and increased elimination of the drug via the gastro-intestinal tract when co-administered with a laxative to decrease gastro-intestinal transit time. Repeated oral doses of activated charcoal may therefore be considered for compounds that undergo enterohepatic or enteroenteric circulation, have a small volume of distribution, are not extensively bound to plasma proteins, and have a low endogenous clearance; the precise role of repeat dosing in acute intoxications will have to be determined for each individual compound.— S. M.

Pond, *Med. Toxicol.*, 1986, *1*, 3. Further discussions on the role of repeated dosing with oral activated charcoal in acute poisoning: G. Levy, *New Engl. J. Med.*, 1982, *307*, 676; *Lancet*, 1987, *1*, 1013; P. J. Neuvonen and K. T. Olkkola, *Med. Toxicol.*, 1988, *3*, 33.

Saline laxatives have been used as an adjunct to activated charcoal to hasten the elimination of the charcoal-poison complex and hence possibly reduce intestinal desorption of the drug. However, the role of laxatives in combination with activated charcoal in the management of poisoned patients is controversial. A study in 7 healthy subjects found that the administration of activated charcoal with magnesium citrate or metoclopramide with bisacodyl did not significantly change the bioavailability of aspirin, atenolol, or phenylpropanolamine when compared with the administration of activated charcoal alone. These results did not support the routine use of laxatives in combination with activated charcoal but in some instances such as with depot formulations, a beneficial effect might be obtained.— P. J. Neuvonen and K. T. Olkkola, *Hum. Toxicol.*, 1986, *5*, 255.

Review of factors influencing the clinical efficacy of activated charcoal.— W. A. Watson, *Drug Intell. & clin. Pharm.*, 1987, *21*, 160. Further references: K. T. Olkkola and P. J. Neuvonen, *Br. J. clin. Pharmac.*, 1984, *18*, 663 (effect of food); P. J. Neuvonen and K. T. Olkkola, *Eur. J. clin. Pharmac.*, 1984, *26*, 761 (effect of the charcoal-drug ratio and pH); G. D. Park *et al.*, *J. clin. Pharmac.*, 1984, *24*, 289 (effect of surface area); K. T. Olkkola, *Br. J. clin. Pharmac.*, 1985, *19*, 767 (effect of the charcoal-drug ratio).

For references to studies and reports on the effectiveness of activated charcoal in the management of overdoses with particular drugs such as theophylline, aspirin, amitriptyline, chlorpropamide, and digoxin, see under the Treatment of Adverse Effects section of their individual monographs.

Haemoperfusion. Haemoperfusion involves the passage of blood through an adsorbent material such as activated charcoal or synthetic hydrophobic polystyrene resins which can retain certain drugs and toxic agents. Early problems with charcoal haemoperfusion such as charcoal embolism, marked thrombocytopenia, fibrinogen loss, and pyrogen reactions have been largely overcome by purification procedures and by coating the carbon with biocompatible polymers. However, transient falls in platelet count, leucocyte count, and circulatory concentrations of clotting factors, calcium, glucose, urea, creatinine, and urate have been reported during haemoperfusion. While there is no substitute for supportive measures, haemoperfusion can significantly reduce the body burden of certain compounds with a low volume of distribution within 4 to 6 hours in some severely poisoned patients; haemoperfusion is not effective for drugs or poisons with very large volumes of distribution.— B. Widdop and J. A. Vale, *Hum. Toxicol.*, 1985, *4*, 345. For further reviews of haemoperfusion and its role in the treatment of acute poisoning, see S. Pond *et al.*, *Clin. Pharmacokinet.*, 1979, *4*, 329; *Med. Lett.*, 1986, *28*, 80; M. E. De Broe *et al.*, *Hum. Toxicol.*, 1986, *5*, 11.

For the use of haemoperfusion in hepatic failure, see below.

DIARRHOEA. A study of 204 patients with acute non-specific diarrhoea indicated that treatment with kaolin and pectin, diphenoxylate and atropine, or activated charcoal was no more effective than a controlled diet in reducing the frequency or looseness of stools.— K. Alestig *et al.*, *Practitioner*, 1979, *222*, 859.

FLATULENCE. Activated charcoal has been used to reduce gas in the intestines but reports on its efficacy have been conflicting. In a study involving 10 healthy subjects, oral activated charcoal was found to be an effective anti-gas medication and significantly reduced symptoms of bloating and abdominal discomfort. In contrast, the study failed to show that simethicone was effective in reducing gas in the colon.—N. K. Jain *et al.*, *Ann. intern. Med.*, 1986, *105*, 61.

HEPATIC FAILURE. Promising results were obtained using activated charcoal haemoperfusion in conjunction with infusions of the platelet-protective agent epoprostenol to treat fulminant hepatic failure in 76 patients with grade-III (sleeping but rousable, incoherent speech, and confused) or grade-IV (non-rousable) encephalopathy. The frequency of cerebral oedema was significantly less when haemoperfusion was started earlier; patients without cerebral oedema had a significantly better survival rate.— A. E. S. Gimson *et al.*, *Lancet*, 1982, *2*, 681. More clinical research was required before earlier haemoperfusion could be considered for the routine treatment of fulminant hepatic failure.— M. J. Weston (letter), *ibid.*, 983; T. M. S. Chang (letter), *ibid.*, 1039.

HYPERCHOLESTEROLAEMIA. In a preliminary study, 7 patients with primary hypercholesterolaemia resistant to therapy with fibric acid derivatives or nicotinic acid were treated with activated charcoal 8 g three times daily for 4 weeks. The plasma concentrations of total cholesterol and low-density-lipoprotein cholesterol were reduced by a mean of 25% and 41% respectively and there was a slight rise in high-density-lipoprotein cholesterol. The role of activated charcoal as a lipid-modulating agent ought to be assessed.— P. Kuusisto *et al.*, *Lancet*, 1986, *2*, 366. In contrast, 12-weeks' treatment with activated charcoal was not found significantly to decrease the mean serum-cholesterol concentrations in a double-blind study involving 12 hyperlipidaemic patients.— J. B. L. Hoekstra and D. W. Erkelens (letter), *ibid.*, 1987, *2*, 455.

PORPHYRIA. The efficacy of activated charcoal as a sorbent to retard enteral absorption of endogenous porphyrins excreted into the gut lumen was investigated in a patient with photomutilation diagnosed as having congenital erythropoietic porphyria. Activated charcoal 30 g given by mouth every 3 hours for 36 hours reduced the plasma-porphyrin concentration to normal values by 20 hours and was more effective than cholestyramine or transfusional therapy. After discontinuation of activated charcoal, plasma-porphyrin concentrations rose rapidly to near pretreatment levels within 10 days. Long-term treatment with oral charcoal over a 9-month period effected a clinical remission with low concentrations of plasma and skin porphyrin and an absence of photocutaneous activity. The optimal dose was determined to be 60 g three times a day. Decreased concentrations of vitamin B_{12}, vitamin D, and folic acid were observed during long-term charcoal therapy but were corrected by vitamin supplementation.— N. R. Pimstone *et al.*, *New Engl. J. Med.*, 1987, *316*, 390.

PRURITUS. Intractable pruritus associated with cholestasis was alleviated in all of 8 patients after 2 plasma perfusions through glass beads coated with activated charcoal. The duration of relief lasted for 24 hours to 5 months and was not correlated with the amount of bile acids removed.— B. H. Lauterburg *et al.*, *Lancet*, 1980, *2*, 53.

In a double-blind crossover study, administration of activated charcoal 6 g daily by mouth for 8 weeks was more effective than placebo in relieving generalised pruritus in 11 patients undergoing maintenance haemodialysis.— J. A. Pederson *et al.*, *Ann. intern. Med.*, 1980, *93*, 446.

ULCERS. A preliminary assessment of charcoal cloth in the management of discharging, infected, and malodorous wounds. A noticeable reduction in wound odour occurred in 24 of 26 patients with chronic stasis leg ulcers and in all of 13 patients with suppurating postoperative wounds. There was no conclusive evidence that the material facilitated wound healing, but wound cleansing was noted in 31 patients. Studies *in vitro* indicated that charcoal cloth could also adsorb bacteria.— R. Beckett *et al.* (letter), *Lancet*, 1980, *2*, 594.

In a controlled comparative study in the community, activated charcoal cloth (Actisorb) significantly increased the epithelialisation, and reduced the exudate levels, odour, and oedema of venous ulcers. During the 6-week treatment period, the mean reduction in ulcer size was 28.7% for the 65 patients treated with activated charcoal dressings compared to 11.7% in the control group of 32 patients treated with conventional dressings. There was no difference between the two groups with regard to pain levels.— C. M. Mulligan *et al.*, *Br. J. clin. Pract.*, 1986, *40*, 145.

Proprietary Preparations

Actisorb *(Johnson & Johnson, UK)*. *Dressing*, activated charcoal cloth. *Dressing* (Actisorb Plus), activated charcoal cloth with silver.

Carbellon *(Torbet Laboratories, UK)*. *Tablets*, activated charcoal 100 mg, belladonna dry extract 6 mg, magnesium hydroxide 100 mg, peppermint oil 0.003 mL. For indigestion, flatulence, and dyspepsia. *Dose.* 2 to 4 tablets three times daily; children, 1 to 5 years, 1 1/2 tablets three times daily, 6 to 12 years, 2 tablets three times daily.

Carbomix *(Penn, UK)*. *Oral powder*, activated charcoal 50 g/bottle. To be dispersed in water before administration. For acute poisoning.

Carbonet *(Smith & Nephew, UK)*. *Dressing*, activated charcoal cloth with absorbent layer and non-adherent layer.

Haemocol *(Smith & Nephew, UK)*. *Haemoperfusion unit*, activated charcoal granules coated with an acrylic hydrogel.

Lyofoam C *(Ultra, UK)*. *Dressing*, polyurethane foam with a hydrophilic, hydrophobic, and activated charcoal layer.

Medicoal *(Lundbeck, UK)*. *Granules*, effervescent, activated charcoal 5 g/sachet. To be dispersed in water before administration. For acute poisoning.

A warning on the possible adverse effects of the sodium content of the excipients in preparations of activated charcoal such as Medicoal.— A. Gorchein *et al.* (letter), *Lancet*, 1988, *1*, 1220.

Norit *(English Grains, UK)*. *Capsules*, activated charcoal 200 mg. For diarrhoea, indigestion, and flatulence.

Proprietary Names and Manufacturers

Actidose *(Paddock, USA)*; Actidose-Aqua *(Paddock, USA)*; Actisorb *(Johnson & Johnson, UK)*; Aqueous Charcodote *(Pharmascience, Canad.)*; Arm-A-Char *(Armour, USA)*; Carbomix *(S.C.A.T., Fr.; Medica, Swed.; Penn, UK)*; Carbonet *(Smith & Nephew, UK)*; Carbosorb *(Seton, UK)*; Char-Bons *(Langly, Austral.)*; Charcocaps *(Requa, USA)*; Charcodote *(Pharmascience, Canad.)*; Charcotabs *(USA)*; Darco G-60 *(Atlas, UK)*; Haemocol *(Smith & Nephew, UK)*; Intosan *(Sauter, Switz.)*; Kohle-Compretten *(E. Merck, Norw.)*; Kolsuspension *(ACO, Swed.)*; Kullsuspensjon *(Norw.)*; Lyofoam C *(Ultra, UK)*; Medicoal *(Protea, Austral.; Lundbeck, UK)*; Medikol *(Ferrosan, Swed.)*; Norit *(English Grains, UK)*; Norit Medicinaal *(Neth.)*.

The following names have been used for multi-ingredient preparations containing activated charcoal— Actisorb Plus *(Johnson & Johnson, UK)*; Carbellon *(Torbet Laboratories, UK)*; Carbomucil *(Norgine, UK)*; Kalto-Carb *(BritCair, UK)*; Karbokoff *(Arlo, USA)*.

5004-l

Calcium Polystyrene Sulphonate

Calcium Polystyrene Sulfonate.

CAS — 37286-92-3.

Pharmacopoeias. In *Jpn.*

The calcium salt of sulphonated styrene polymer.

Adverse Effects and Precautions

As for sodium polystyrene sulphonate, p.854. Sodium overloading is not a problem with calcium polystyrene sulphonate, but calcium overloading and hypercalcaemia may occur. Patients should be monitored for electrolyte disturbances, especially hypokalaemia and hypercalcaemia. The released calcium can also reduce the activity of tetracycline given by mouth. Calcium polystyrene sulphonate should not be used in patients presenting with renal failure together with hypercalcaemia.

EFFECTS ON THE LUNGS. An elderly man who died from cardiac arrest was found at necropsy to have bronchopneumonia associated with inhalation of calcium polystyrene sulphonate; the resin had been given by mouth to treat hyperkalaemia.— A. J. Chaplin and P. R. Millard, *Br. med. J.*, 1975, *3*, 77.

INTERACTIONS. *Antacids.* For a report of systemic alkalosis associated with the concomitant administration of sodium polystyrene sulphonate and antacids and the lack of such an effect with calcium polystyrene sulphonate, see Sodium Polystyrene Sulphonate, p.854.

Uses and Administration

Calcium polystyrene sulphonate is a cation-exchange resin which exchanges calcium ions for potassium ions and other cations. It is used similarly to sodium polystyrene sulphonate (see p.854) to reduce potassium concentrations in the treatment of hyperkalaemia and may be preferred to the sodium resin in patients who cannot tolerate an increase in their sodium load.

It is administered by mouth, in a dose of 15 g up to three or four times daily, as a suspension in water or syrup. A suggested dose for children is up to 1 g per kg body-weight daily in divided doses, reduced to a maintenance dose of 500 mg per kg. It should not be given in fruit juices that have a high potassium content and may reduce the exchange-capacity of the resin.

When oral administration is difficult, calcium polystyrene sulphonate may be administered rectally as an enema. The usual daily dose is 30 g given as a suspension in 100 mL of 2% methylcellulose '450' and 100 mL of water and retained, if possible, for at least 9 hours. Initial therapy may constitute administration by both oral and rectal routes. Children may be given rectal doses similar to those suggested by mouth.

Proprietary Preparations

Calcium Resonium *(Winthrop, UK). Powder,* calcium polystyrene sulphonate.

Proprietary Names and Manufacturers

Calcium Resonium *(Winthrop, Ger.; Winthrop, UK)*; CPS Pulver *(Gry, Ger.)*; Kalimate *(Jpn)*; Kayexalate Calcium *(Belg.; Fr.; USA)*; Resincalcio *(Rubio, Spain)*; Resonium Calcium *(Winthrop, Canad.; Winthrop, Denm.; Winthrop, Norw.; Sterling-Winthrop, Swed.; Winthrop, Switz.)*; Sorbisterit *(Fresenius, Fr.; Neth.; Fresenius, Switz.)*.

1032-q

Calcium Trisodium Pentetate *(BAN, rINN)*.

Calcium Trisodium DTPA; NSC-34249; Pentetate Calcium Trisodium *(USAN)*; Trisodium Calcium Diethylenetriaminepentaacetate. Calcium trisodium nitrilodiethylenedinitrilopenta-acetate.

$C_{14}H_{18}CaN_3Na_3O_{10}$=497.4.

CAS — 12111-24-9 (calcium trisodium pentetate); 67-43-6 (pentetic acid).

Pentetic acid and its salts are chelating agents with the general properties of the edetates (see Sodium Calciumedetate, p.852). Calcium trisodium pentetate has been used in the treatment of poisoning by heavy metals and radioactive metals such as plutonium. Doses of 1 g daily have been administered by slow intravenous infusion.

Pentetates have been labelled with metallic radionuclides and used in nuclear medicine.

Proprietary Names and Manufacturers

Calcium Chel 330 *(UK)*; Ditripentat-Heyl *(Heyl, Ger.)*.

7301-j

Cyclazocine *(USAN, rINN)*.

Win-20740. 3-Cyclopropylmethyl-1,2,3,4,5,6-hexahydro-6,11-dimethyl-2,6-methano-3-benzazocin-8-ol.

$C_{18}H_{25}NO$=271.4.

CAS — 3572-80-3.

Cyclazocine is an opioid antagonist with actions similar to those of naloxone (p.845); in addition it also possesses some agonist properties. It has been given by mouth as an adjunct in the treatment of opioid dependence. Withdrawal effects have been reported after abrupt discontinuation.

References: M. Fink *et al.*, *Am. J. Nurs.*, 1971, *71*, 1359; R. Resnick *et al.*, *Am. J. Psychiat.*, 1974, *131*, 595.

1041-p

Cysteamine Hydrochloride *(BANM)*.

L-1573 (cysteamine); MEA (cysteamine); Mercamine Hydrochloride; Mercaptamine Hydrochloride *(rINNM)*. 2-Aminoethanethiol hydrochloride.

C_2H_7NS,HCl=113.6.

CAS — 60-23-1 (cysteamine); 156-57-0 (hydrochloride).

Adverse Effects and Precautions

Cysteamine, administered intravenously, causes nausea, vomiting, and drowsiness; other side-effects reported include malaise, anorexia, flushing, and ventricular tachycardia. Cysteamine may precipitate hepatic coma in patients with overt hepatic damage.

Three patients with nephropathic cystinosis developed fever, maculopapular eruption, leucopenia, or headache within 2 weeks of starting cysteamine at doses of 53, 67, and 75 mg per kg body-weight daily by mouth. These side-effects resolved within 48 hours of drug withdrawal and all 3 patients were able to tolerate cysteamine when restarted at a dose of 10 mg per kg daily, slowly increased to therapeutic levels over 2 to 3 months. Higher doses of cysteamine had been associated with lethargy and seizures.— J. A. Schneider *et al.* (letter), *New Engl. J. Med.*, 1981, *304*, 1172.

Uses and Administration

Cysteamine hydrochloride facilitates glutathione synthesis and has been used in the treatment of severe paracetamol poisoning to prevent hepatic damage. Other forms of treatment are generally preferred and it has been largely superseded by acetylcysteine (p.903) and methionine (p.843). It is not effective unless given within 10 hours of the overdose of paracetamol. A suggested regimen is to give the equivalent of 2 g of the base by intravenous infusion over 10 minutes, followed by 3 doses of 400 mg infused over 4, 8, and 8 hours.

Cysteamine has been used as a radioprotective agent. It is also used in the treatment of cystinosis.

CYSTINOSIS. Cysteamine has been reported to be of benefit in children with nephropathic cystinosis, a rare autosomal recessive metabolic disorder characterised by the intracellular accumulation of cystine. Treatment with cysteamine administered by mouth has resulted in a reduction in the concentrations of cystine in leucocytes (M. Yudkoff *et al.*, *New Engl. J. Med.*, 1981, *304*, 141) and some reports have suggested that it may also prevent growth retardation and the development of nephropathy (V.A. Da Silva *et al.*, *ibid.*, 1985, *313*, 1460) though results have been conflicting (M. Yudkoff *et al.*, 1981; D.B.-E. Gradus *et al.*, *New Engl. J. Med.*, 1986, *314*, 1319; M. Pococco, *ibid.*, 1320). In the multicentre National Collaborative Cysteamine Study (W.A. Gahl *et al. ibid.*, 1987, *316*, 971), 93 children with nephropathic cystinosis were given cysteamine in gradually increasing daily doses of up to 66.4 mg per kg body-weight as the hydrochloride salt (mean 51.3 mg per kg daily) and compared with 55 historical controls. The results indicated that treatment with cysteamine reduced cystine concentrations in leucocytes, maintained renal function, particularly in those without substantial pre-existing glomerular dysfunction, and improved growth in children under 6 years of age; there was no improvement in the symptoms of the Fanconi syndrome, as measured by renal tubular function, or discernible changes in corneal accumulation of cystine crystals. Most patients found the taste and odour of cysteamine offensive; side-effects included nausea and vomiting and one boy developed hepatic veno-occlusive disease with an episode of life-threatening gastric variceal bleeding.

Cysteamine eye-drops 0.11% markedly reduced the number of cystine crystals in the corneas of 2 young children (less than 2 years old) with nephropathic cystinosis within 4 to 5 months of starting treatment.— M. I. Kaiser-Kupfer *et al.*, *New Engl. J. Med.*, 1987, *316*, 775.

Proprietary Names and Manufacturers

Lambratene *(Bracco, Ital.)*.

1034-s

Desferrioxamine Mesylate *(BANM)*.

Ba-33112; Deferoxamine Mesilate *(pINNM)*; Deferoxamine Mesylate *(USAN)*; Desferrioxamine Methanesulphonate. 30-Amino-3,14,25-trihydroxy-3,9,14,20,25-penta-azatriacontane-2,10,13,21,24-pentaone methanesulphonate.

$C_{25}H_{48}N_6O_8,CH_3SO_3H$=656.8.

CAS — 70-51-9 (desferrioxamine); 138-14-7 (mesylate).

Pharmacopoeias. In *Br.* and *U.S.*

A white to cream-coloured odourless or almost odourless powder. **Soluble** 1 in 5 of water and 1 in 20 of alcohol; practically insoluble in dehydrated alcohol, chloroform, and ether; slightly soluble in methyl alcohol. The *B.P.* specifies that a 10% solution in water has a pH of 3.5 to 5.5. The *U.S.P.* specifies that a 1% solution in water has a pH of 4.0 to 6.0. **Store** at a temperature not exceeding 4° in airtight containers. Protect from light. Desferrioxamine injection deteriorates on storage and should be used immediately after preparation; cloudy solutions should be discarded.

Adverse Effects

Rapid intravenous injection of desferrioxamine may cause flushing, urticaria, hypotension, and shock. Local pain may occur with subcutaneous or intramuscular injections and pruritus, erythema, and swelling have occurred after prolonged subcutaneous administration. Gastrointestinal disorders, dysuria, fever, allergic skin rashes, tachycardia, and leg cramps have been reported. Cataract formation and visual disturbances have occurred and hearing loss has also been reported.

ALLERGY. Individual reports of anaphylactoid reactions to desferrioxamine and methods of rapid desensitisation: K. B. Miller *et al.* (letter), *Lancet*, 1981, *1*, 1059; J. Bousquet *et al.* (letter), *ibid.*, 1983, *2*, 859.

EFFECTS ON THE BLOOD. A patient with end-stage renal disease developed reversible thrombocytopenia on 3 separate occasions after intravenous infusions of desferrioxamine for dialysis osteomalacia.— J. A. Walker *et al.*, *Am. J. Kidney Dis.*, 1985, *6*, 254.

EFFECTS ON THE EAR AND EYE. Lens opacities, retinal pigmentary changes, and ocular disturbances including loss of colour vision, night blindness, decreased visual acuity, and field defects have been reported in patients receiving long-term or high-dose treatment with desferrioxamine (S.C. Davies *et al.*, *Lancet*, 1983, *2*, 181; P. Simon *et al.*, *ibid.*, 512; C. Borgna-Pignatti *et al.*, *ibid.*, 1984, *1*, 681; M. Rubinstein *et al.*, *ibid.*, 1985, *1*, 817; A.H.S. Rahi *et al.*, *Br. J. Ophthal.*, 1986, *70*, 373). In most patients the visual defects improved when the drug was withdrawn. Arden *et al.* (*Br. J. Ophthal.*, 1984, *68*, 873) found a number of minor changes in retinal function in a study of 43 thalassaemia patients receiving desferrioxamine therapy; there was a significant correlation between the presence of abnormal ocular tests and the patients' diabetic status, but the incidence of visual defects appeared not to be related to drug dosage or ferritin concentrations. In contrast, Olivieri *et al.*, (*New Engl. J. Med.*, 1986, *314*, 869) found that in a group of 89 patients on long-term treatment with subcutaneous desferrioxamine, doses were significantly higher in those who developed visual symptoms and auditory problems. Most of the affected patients were also younger and had lower ferritin concentrations than those in the unaffected group. Of the 89 patients studied by Olivieri *et al.*, 9 had abnormal findings on eye examination but 22 had audiometric abnormalities with high-frequency sensorineural hearing loss in 13. Acute hearing loss has also been reported in a patient with chronic renal failure on haemodialysis who received desferrioxamine intravenously to reduce acquired iron overload. Hearing returned to normal 5 weeks after the desferrioxamine was stopped (A. Guerin *et al.*, *Lancet*, 1985, *2*, 39). Marsh *et al.* (*Postgrad. med. J.*, 1981, *57*, 582) have reported tinnitus in one patient on subcutaneous desferrioxamine therapy. For serial monitoring of adverse neurological effects in patients receiving long-term desferrioxamine treatment, Olivieri *et al.*, 1986, recommended complete eye examinations, audiological testing, and studies of visual evoked potentials every 3 months.

Precautions

Desferrioxamine is contra-indicated in patients with severe renal disease or anuria and should be used with caution in patients with impaired renal function. Skeletal foetal anomalies have occurred in *animals*. The desferrioxamine-iron complex excreted by the kidney may colour the urine reddish-brown.

The urinary excretion of iron should be regularly monitored during treatment and eye examinations have been recommended periodically for patients on long-term therapy. Monitoring of cardiac function has also been recommended for patients receiving combined treatment with high doses of ascorbic acid.

INFECTION SUSCEPTIBILITY. *Yersinia enterocolitica* is one of the most iron-dependent of all microbes, but unlike most other aerobic bacteria, it produces no detectable iron-binding compounds, or siderophores (*Lancet*, 1984, *1*, 84). Exogenous siderophores, such as desferrioxamine, may enable *Y. enterocolitica* to overcome this handicap (R.M. Robins-Browne and J.K. Prpic, *ibid.* 1983, *2*, 1372) and the apparent increased susceptibility to yersiniosis in patients with severe iron overload may therefore be attributable to desferrioxamine therapy rather than just the increased availability of iron. Infections due to *Y. enterocolitica* have been reported in patients receiving desferrioxamine for acute iron overdosage (K. Melby *et al.*, *Br. med. J.*, 1982, *285*, 467) or for chronic iron overload (R.M. Robins-Browne and J.K. Prpic, *Lancet*, 1983, *2*, 1372; M. Scharnetzky *et al.*, *ibid.*, 1984, *1*, 791; H.Y. Chiu *et al.*, *Br. med. J.*, 1986, *292*, 97; D. Kelly *et al.*, *ibid.*, 413; T. Gallant *et al.*, *New Engl. J. Med.*, 1986, *314*, 1643). Severe infection with *Y. pseudotuberculosis* has also been reported in a thalassaemia patient on long-term desferrioxamine therapy (B. Gordts *et al.*, *Lancet*, 1984, *1*, 41). When patients with iron overload become febrile with enteritis or pharyngitis, it has been recommended that desferrioxamine should be discontinued and that co-trimoxazole should be administered as prophylaxis against systemic yersiniosis (M. Scharnetzky *et al.*, 1984).

Possible drug-induced susceptibility to mucormycosis in dialysis patients given desferrioxamine.— J. J. Goodill and J. G. Abuelo (letter), *New Engl. J. Med.*, 1987, *316*, 54.

INTERACTIONS. *Ascorbic Acid.* Studies have indicated that ascorbic acid saturation considerably enhances the urinary excretion of iron in some patients treated for iron overload with subcutaneous infusions of desferrioxamine (M.A.M. Hussain *et al.*, *Lancet*, 1977, *1*, 977; M.J. Pippard *et al.*, *Clin. Sci. & mol. Med.*, 1978, *54*, 99). However, the relationship between ascorbic acid and iron metabolism is complex and it has been suggested that vitamin C deficiency may actually confer protection from iron-induced organ damage (A. Cohen *et al.*, *New Engl J. Med.*, 1981, *304*, 158). Cardiac disorders associated with oral ascorbic acid supplementation have also been reported in thalassaemic patients and the administration of ascorbic acid may therefore be harmful in iron overload. It has been recommended that ascorbic acid be given with extreme caution to patients with excess tissue iron; when used with desferrioxamine the need for ascorbic acid should be clearly established by measuring iron excretion before and after supplementation and the oral dose of ascorbic acid should be administered an hour or two after the infusion has been started (A.W. Nienhuis, *ibid.*, 170).

Phenothiazines. Oxidative damage by decompartmentalised copper might be involved in the pathogenesis of desferrioxamine's neuro-ophthalmic toxicity. Widespread oxidative damage was more likely in the presence of phenothiazines; prochlorperazine had already been shown to potentiate desferrioxamine toxicity.— H. Pall *et al.* (letter), *Lancet*, 1986, *2*, 1279.

Absorption and Fate

Desferrioxamine mesylate is poorly absorbed from the gastro-intestinal tract.

Studies on desferrioxamine and ferrioxamine metabolism in 16 healthy subjects and 24 patients with transfusional iron overload. Three minutes after an intravenous injection of desferrioxamine 10 mg per kg body-weight the concentration in plasma was between 80 and 130 μmol per litre. There was rapid clearance from the blood with the desferrioxamine concentration falling to half the initial value in about 5 to 10 minutes. The resulting ferrioxamine concentrations in the plasma were maximal within 5 hours and were about 3 times higher in iron-loaded than in normal subjects. During a continuous 24-hour subcutaneous infusion of desferrioxamine 100 mg per kg, plasma concentrations rose at different rates but a plateau level was usually reached within 12 hours. The plateau concentration of desferrioxamine appeared to be directly related to the degree of iron loading; heavily loaded subjects had relatively low concentrations of desferrioxamine in the plasma.— M. R. Summers *et al.*, *Br. J. Haemat.*, 1979, *42*, 547.

Uses and Administration

Desferrioxamine is a chelating agent which has a high affinity for iron. When given by injection it forms a stable water-soluble iron-complex (ferrioxamine) which is readily excreted in the urine and in bile. Desferrioxamine appears to remove iron from the storage forms such as haemosiderin or ferritin rather than from haemoglobin or cytochromes.

Desferrioxamine, administered as the mesylate, is used to aid the excretion of iron from the body in conditions associated with excessive iron storage in the tissues, such as haemochromatosis and haemosiderosis, in iron overload following repeated transfusions as in thalassaemia, and in acute iron poisoning.

In the treatment of chronic iron overload that may for instance follow multiple blood transfusions in thalassaemia, desferrioxamine mesylate is usually most effective when administered by subcutaneous or intravenous infusion preferably with the aid of a small portable infusion pump; intravenous infusions often prove more effective than subcutaneous infusions. The usual dose of desferrioxamine mesylate is 1 to 4 g daily infused over 12 hours but before long-term medication is started the optimum dose, the method of administration, and the duration of the infusion should be determined for each patient by monitoring urinary iron excretion and constructing a dose response curve. Some dosage regimens have required desferrioxamine to be infused on only 5 or 6 nights of each week. Desferrioxamine mesylate may also be administered by intramuscular injection; the initial dose is 0.5 to 1 g daily, but again the maintenance dose is determined by response. It has been suggested that in addition to intramuscular treatment, up to 2 g of desferrioxamine mesylate should be given by intravenous infusion for each unit of blood transfused, at a rate not more than 15 mg per kg body-weight per hour at the time of each blood transfusion. The co-administration of ascorbic acid supplements may enhance the excretion of iron in some patients.

In the treatment of acute iron poisoning a recommended procedure is to wash out the stomach with a 1% solution of sodium bicarbonate as quickly as possible and then to give 5 to 10 g of desferrioxamine mesylate in 50 to 100 mL of water by mouth, or by stomach tube to chelate any iron left in the stomach and prevent further absorption. To eliminate iron already absorbed, 1 to 2 g of desferrioxamine mesylate may be given intramuscularly every 3 to 12 hours or alternatively, desferrioxamine mesylate may be administered intravenously by slow infusion. It is considered that 100 mg of desferrioxamine mesylate can chelate approximately 8.5 mg of iron. Thus, 5 g can chelate the iron contained in about 10 tablets of ferrous sulphate or ferrous gluconate. The administration of desferrioxamine by mouth or gastric lavage as an adjunct in the treatment of iron poisoning is controversial; some authorities consider that the effiacy and safety of oral desferrioxamine for this indication still needs to be fully established.

In the *US*, a recommended procedure is to give desferrioxamine mesylate 1 g initially by intramuscular injection followed by 0.5 g every 4 hours for 2 doses. Subsequent doses of 0.5 g may be administered every 4 to 12 hours to a maximum of 6 g in 24 hours. Alternatively, the same doses may be given by slow intravenous infusion at a rate of not more than 15 mg per kg per hour, but this route of administration is only recommended for patients in a state of cardiovascular collapse.

Solutions for intravenous infusion may be prepared with sodium chloride injection (0.9%), glucose injection (5%), or lactated Ringer's injection.

Desferrioxamine has been used as a diagnostic test for iron storage disease in patients with normal renal function by injecting 0.5 g of the mesylate intramuscularly and estimating the excretion of iron in the urine collected over the next 6 hours; an excretion of more than 1 mg of iron by the patient under test is suggestive of iron storage disease.

Eye-drops containing 10% have been administered for the treatment of ocular siderosis and corneal rust stains.

ADMINISTRATION. Administration of desferrioxamine in solution by mouth to 14 thalassaemic patients increased urinary iron excretion above baseline values in every case but was clearly less efficient than subcutaneous infusion. Oral desferrioxamine might be a useful adjunct when compliance with parenteral administration was poor. The taste could be disguised.— S. T. Callender and D. J. Weatherall (letter), *Lancet*, 1980, *2*, 689. Similar findings with oral desferrioxamine given as the mesylate; the fat-soluble desferrioxamine stearate, however, was found to be relatively ineffective when given by mouth.— A. Jacobs and W. C. Ting (letter), *ibid.*, 794. The amount of iron excreted after oral administration of desferrioxamine to 18 young thalassaemic children was generally too low to be considered effective for the prevention of iron loading; even intravenous administration of desferrioxamine 1 g was not very effective for all these children (mainly those with lower iron stores).— C. Kattamis *et al.* (letter), *ibid.*, 1981, *1*, 51.

Preliminary study of administering desferrioxamine entrapped in red cell ghosts by intravenous infusion to improve the efficacy of iron chelation.— R. Green *et al.*, *Lancet*, 1980, *2*, 327. Comments: G. N. Smith (letter), *ibid.*, 1363; R. Green *et al.* (letter), *ibid;* G. N. Smith (letter), *ibid.*, 1981, *1*, 222.

The net iron excretion achieved by using desferrioxamine suppositories in 2 patients with thalassaemia iron-overload was only about 10% of that obtained after administration of an equivalent dose subcutaneously or intravenously.— G. Kontoghiorghes *et al.* (letter), *Lancet*, 1983, *2*, 454.

DIALYSIS. In a study involving 17 patients with chronic renal failure, there was no significant removal of aluminium by adsorbent haemoperfusion or haemodialysis alone, but when carried out 48 hours after desferrioxamine administration the clearance of aluminium was greatly increased. Adsorbent haemoperfusion with collodion-coated activated charcoal appeared to be more efficient than haemodialysis in removing aluminium after desferrioxamine infusion and might be used in series with haemodialysis to enhance aluminium clearance.— T. M. S. Chang and P. Barre, *Lancet*, 1983, *2*, 1051. Results at variance.— P. Simon *et al.* (letter), *ibid.*, 1489.

Bone disorders. Desferrioxamine in doses of 6 g once a week during haemodialysis had beneficial effects in 2 patients with long-standing severe dialysis osteomalacia; both patients reported an increase in joint flexibility and a decrease in bone pain within 2 weeks of treatment and x-rays after 4 to 6 months revealed that many fractures had healed completely. However, the bone structure after treatment remained abnormal and there was little change in the bone aluminium content.— D. J. Brown *et al.*, *Lancet*, 1982, *2*, 343. Intermittent desferrioxamine infusions were administered intravenously to 7 patients with renal failure on long-term dialysis; all had evidence of uraemic osteodystrophy and aluminium accumulation in bone, and 6 had symptoms of muscle or bone pain causing impairment of physical activity. Symptomatic improvement was noted within the first 2 to 4 weeks of treatment and was associated with the effective removal of aluminium from bone.

The diagnostic value of rises in serum-aluminium concentrations after a single intravenous infusion of desferrioxamine 28.5 mg per kg body-weight at the beginning of dialysis was also studied in 22 patients and serum-aluminium concentrations were measured before and 5 hours after the start of the infusion. Although all patients with aluminium accumulation in bone had a consistent rise in serum concentrations of aluminium after this desferrioxamine test, rises were also observed in some of the patients without bone-aluminium accumulation. It was concluded that the desferrioxamine test could not be used to diagnose the accumulation of aluminium in bone.— H. H. Malluche *et al.*, *New Engl. J. Med.*, 1984, *311*, 140. Desferrioxamine 40 mg per kg body-weight was infused within 4 hours of haemodialysis over a 2-hour period in 54 patients; plasma samples for the determination of aluminium concentrations were obtained before and 24 and 40 hours after the infusion. Results using this method suggested that the desferrioxamine test might be of value in the assessment of patients with suspected aluminium-related osteodystrophy.— D. S. Milliner *et al.*, *Ann. intern. Med.*, 1984, *101*, 775.

Encephalopathy. Dialysis encephalopathy, which can be a major complication of long-term haemodialysis, is thought to be related to the accumulation in the brain of aluminium, usually originating from the dialysis water supply. De-ionised or reverse-osmosis treated water with reduced aluminium concentrations may be of value in these patients, but in addition, desferrioxamine has been reported to have beneficial effects by the mobilisation and removal of aluminium when administered in doses of up to 6 g once a week via the arterial line during the first 2 hours of haemodialysis (P. Ackrill *et al.*, *Lancet*, 1980, *2*, 692; R.S. Arze *et al.*, *ibid.*, 1981, *2*, 1116). Of 11 patients with dialysis encephalopathy studied by Milne *et al* (*ibid.*, 1982, *2*, 502), 5 were treated with de-ionised or reverse-osmosis water alone and all died. The other 6 were treated similarly but were also given desferrioxamine 6 to 10 g intravenously each week at dialysis; 4 of these patients improved but 2 died of progressive dementia.

Although the total amount of aluminium removed with desferrioxamine treatment during peritoneal dialysis may be small compared with the amounts removed during haemodialysis, substantial improvement in early aluminium encephalopathy has been achieved in a patient on continuous ambulatory peritoneal dialysis by using intraperitoneal desferrioxamine (C.D. Payton *et al.*, *ibid.*, 1984, *1*, 1132).

IRON OVERLOAD DISEASES. A review of the treatment of

iron storage disorders. In patients with iron-loading anaemias such as aplastic anaemia, thalassaemia major, and sideroblastic anaemia, desferrioxamine may be used to increase the excretion of iron. In patients with idiopathic haemochromatosis, phlebotomy is the treatment of choice but when contra-indicated by severe anaemia, hypoproteinaemia, or cardiac disease, chelation therapy with desferrioxamine may be considered.— J. W. Halliday and M. L. Bassett, *Drugs*, 1980, *20*, 207. Suggested guidelines for the initiation of chelation therapy in transfusion-dependent adults with acquired anaemias or sickle-cell anaemia.— T. J. Ley and A. W. Nienhuis (letter), *New Engl. J. Med.*, 1983, *308*, 1422.

Patients homozygous for β-thalassaemia have severe anaemia requiring regular blood transfusions. As a consequence of this treatment iron overload develops and the excessive deposition of iron in the myocardium usually results in these patients dying in their second or third decade from arrhythmias or cardiac failure. Whether iron chelation with desferrioxamine measurably altered the survival of patients with β-thalassaemia was investigated by reviewing the medical records up to the end of 1980 of 92 patients with thalassaemia major born in or before 1963. The data available indicated significantly better survival among children for whom an average weekly dose of at least 3 g of desferrioxamine had been established (B. Modell *et al.*, *Br. med. J.*, 1982, *284*, 1081). In the late-1970's, administration of desferrioxamine by continuous subcutaneous infusion over 12 to 24 hours was established as more effective in increasing iron excretion than administration by intramuscular bolus injections (M.A.M. Hussain *et al.*, *Lancet*, 1976, *2*, 1278; R.D. Propper *et al.*, *New Engl. J. Med.*, 1977, *297*, 418; M.J. Pippard *et al.*, *Lancet*, 1978, *1*, 1178). Studies also indicated that with careful assessment of individual patterns of urinary-iron excretion in response to desferrioxamine, a negative iron balance could be achieved in most patients with iron-loading anaemias (M.J. Pippard *et al.*, *Clin. Sci. & mol. Med.*, 1978, *54*, 99) and that long-term subcutaneous desferrioxamine infusions might result in stabilisation of iron stores at a normal or near-normal level despite the continued need for transfusion (A.V. Hoffbrand *et al.*, *Lancet*, 1979, *1*, 947). There has also been preliminary evidence that organ function might improve with intensive desferrioxamine therapy. A reduction in liver-iron concentrations and an improvement in liver function has been reported in some patients with transfusional iron overload treated with desferrioxamine 2 to 4 g by slow subcutaneous infusion over 12 hours on 6 nights a week in conjunction with oral ascorbic acid supplements (A.V. Hoffbrand *et al.*, *Lancet*, 1979, *1*, 947). Some studies have also indicated that desferrioxamine treatment might preserve or possibly improve cardiac function impaired by iron overload in thalassaemic patients (S.B. Kaye and M. Owen, *Br. med. J.*, 1978, *1*, 342 and 555; A.P. Freeman *et al.*, *Ann. intern. Med.*, 1983, *99*, 450; R.E. Marcus *et al.*, *Lancet*, 1984, *1*, 392; L. Wolfe *et al.*, *New Engl. J. Med.*, 1985, *312*, 1600). Further reviews discussing the role of desferrioxamine in the management of iron overloading in thalassaemia.— D. J. Weatherall *et al.*, *New Engl. J. Med.*, 1983, *308*, 456; *Lancet*, 1984, *1*, 373; *ibid.*, 1987, *1*, 1246.

Ascorbic acid has been administered to patients with iron overload in conjunction with desferrioxamine therapy to enhance the excretion of iron but caution has been recommended, see under Precautions, above.

IRON POISONING. Review of acute iron poisoning and its management. In the majority of patients treatment requires no more than decisions on gastric emptying and the need for desferrioxamine administration. The use of a lavage fluid containing 2 g of desferrioxamine in a litre of water has been recommended to reduce iron absorption but its efficacy for this purpose is far from established. Nevertheless, until the value of enteral desferrioxamine has been determined the usual practice of leaving 10 g in the stomach seems advisable. For severe iron poisoning parenteral desferrioxamine is widely regarded as the treatment of choice even though its mechanism of action is still uncertain; increasing the elimination of iron does not appear to be its major role. Shock or coma are indications for the immediate administration of desferrioxamine without waiting for the result of serum iron estimations. If the patient is normotensive it is traditional to give a single intramuscular dose though this is of little merit if an intravenous infusion can be established within a few minutes. Intramuscular doses may be invaluable if delays are likely. In hypotensive patients the intravenous route is recommended. The maximum recommended total dose of desferrioxamine by intravenous administration is 80 mg per kg body-weight in 24 hours but in the absence of adverse effects, much larger doses may be tolerated. Disappearance of the orange-red colour imparted to the urine by ferrioxamine indicates that iron is no longer available for chelation. In less serious iron poisoning the use of desferrioxamine is more controversial and a majority of patients would probably survive without chelation therapy. However, if free iron is present in plasma it would seem logical to give desferrioxamine.— A. T. Proudfoot *et al.*, *Med. Toxicol.*, 1986, *1*, 83.

Pregnancy and the neonate. Desferrioxamine was successfully used to treat acute iron overdosage in a 24-year-old woman who was 34 weeks' pregnant. Eight hours after the overdose the patient began spontaneous labour and delivered an appropriately sized male infant whose clinical course was unremarkable except for low serum concentrations of iron which required iron supplementation.— W. F. Rayburn *et al.*, *Am. J. Obstet. Gynec.*, 1983, *147*, 717.

PORPHYRIA. In a study of 25 patients with porphyria cutanea tarda, subcutaneous infusion of desferrioxamine was found to be as effective as repeated phlebotomies in normalising porphyrin excretion and iron storage. Phlebotomy, which was less expensive and easier to perform, remained the treatment of choice, but desferrioxamine might be a useful alternative if phlebotomy was contra-indicated.— E. Rocchi *et al.*, *Br. J. Derm.*, 1986, *114*, 621.

Desferrioxamine was successfully used to treat haemodialysis-related porphyria cutanea tarda in a 22-year-old man in whom venesection therapy was contra-indicated because of severe anaemia requiring multiple blood transfusion. Each course of intravenous desferrioxamine therapy after the end of 3 haemodialysis sessions was accompanied by a marked decrease in plasma porphyrins, a sharp increase in haematocrit values, and a simultaneous improvement in skin lesions.— M. Praga *et al.* (letter), *New Engl. J. Med.*, 1987, *316*, 547.

RHEUMATOID ARTHRITIS. The generation of free radicals catalysed by iron resulting in peroxidation of synovial membranes has been proposed as the first event in the inflammation of rheumatoid arthritis (D.R. Blake *et al.*, *Lancet*, 1981, *2*, 1142). Preliminary data has suggested a possible role for desferrioxamine in the treatment of rheumatoid arthritis by removing iron from synovial membranes, decreasing synovial inflammation, restoring stores in bone marrow, and lessening anaemia (N. Giordano *et al.*, *Br. med. J.*, 1984, *289*, 961). A study using subcutaneous desferrioxamine to treat 6 patients with active rheumatoid disease refractory to conventional drugs has been initiated (R.J. Polson *et al.*, *Br. med. J.*, 1985, *291*, 448). One patient developed blurred vision after 5 days and was withdrawn from the study; the other 5 were withdrawn from the drug temporarily after 4 to 12 days because of nausea and vomiting but restarted therapy within 7 days on a lower maintenance dose without recurrence of symptoms. There was a close correlation between the total dose of desferrioxamine administered before the onset of side-effects and the haemoglobin and serum iron concentrations before treatment.

Preparations

Desferrioxamine Injection *(B.P.)*. Contains desferrioxamine mesylate.

Sterile Deferoxamine Mesylate *(U.S.P.)*. Desferrioxamine mesylate suitable for parenteral use.

Proprietary Preparations

Desferal *(Ciba, UK)*. *Injection*, powder for reconstitution, desferrioxamine mesylate, in vials of 500 mg.

NOTE. To prepare desferrioxamine eye-drops, dissolve 500 mg of Desferal in a sterile vehicle containing methylcellulose '4000' 0.5%, benzyl alcohol 1%, Water for Injections to 5 mL, with aseptic precautions. Use immediately; discard after 1 week.

Proprietary Names and Manufacturers

Desféral *(Ciba, Switz.)*; Desferal *(Ciba, Austral.; Belg.; Ciba, Canad.; Ciba, Denm.; Ciba, Fr.; Ciba, Ger.; Ciba, Ital.; Neth.; Ciba, Norw.; Ciba, S.Afr.; Ciba, Swed.; Ciba, UK; Ciba, USA)*; Desferin *(Ciba, Spain)*.

1033-p

Dicobalt Edetate *(BAN, rINN)*.

Cobalt Edetate; Cobalt EDTA. Cobalt [ethylenediaminetetra-acetato(4—)-*N*,*N'*,*O*,*O'*]-cobalt(II).

$C_{10}H_{12}Co_2N_2O_8$=406.1.

CAS — 36499-65-7.

Adverse Effects and Precautions

Dicobalt edetate may cause hypotension, tachycardia, and vomiting. Anaphylactic reactions have occurred; oedema of the face and neck, sweating, chest pain, cardiac irregularities, and skin rashes have been reported. Dicobalt edetate should not be injected in conditions other than known cyanide poisoning.

A patient with cyanide toxicity developed severe facial and pulmonary oedema after treatment with dicobalt edetate. When dicobalt edetate is used, facilities for intubation and resuscitation should be immediately available.— C. Dodds and C. McKnight, *Br. med. J.*, 1985, *291*, 785.

For further references to the adverse effects of dicobalt edetate and precautions necessary for clinical use, see under Uses and Administration, below.

Uses and Administration

Dicobalt edetate is a chelating agent used in the treatment of severe cyanide poisoning (see p.1350). Its use arises from the property of cobalt salts to form a relatively nontoxic stable ion-complex with cyanide. Dicobalt edetate should be used only in confirmed cyanide poisoning and never as a precautionary measure. Cyanide poisoning must be treated as quickly as possible. A suggested dose is 300 mg administered by intravenous injection, over about 1 minute, repeated if the response is inadequate; a further dose of 300 mg of dicobalt edetate may be given 5 minutes later if required. For less severe poisoning the injection should be given over 5 minutes. Each injection of dicobalt edetate may be followed immediately by 50 mL of glucose injection 50% intravenously though the value of giving glucose has been questioned.

Dicobalt edetate, an effective antidote for cyanide poisoning, was not without toxic effects when given to patients wrongly suspected of being poisoned. Careful clinical assessment was essential. If patients exposed to cyanides had indications of drowsiness and were considered to require the antidote, 300 mg of dicobalt edetate could be given slowly and the injection discontinued if adverse effects were noted. The antidote could be repeated if a beneficial response was not obtained and sodium thiosulphate used as supportive therapy.— D. D. Bryson (letter), *Lancet*, 1978, *1*, 92.

Report on the use of dicobalt edetate to treat 3 men exposed to cyanide gas. The patients survived but the immediate side-effects of dicobalt edetate were alarming. It was considered that dicobalt edetate should be reserved for comatose patients not responsive to classical treatment and for patients becoming unconscious despite such treatment.— J. Nagler *et al.*, *J. occup. Med.*, 1978, *20*, 414.

Further reports on the use of dicobalt edetate in the treatment of cyanide poisoning.— B. Hillman *et al.*, *Postgrad. med. J.*, 1974, *50*, 171; M. J. McKiernan (letter), *Lancet*, 1980, *2*, 86.

Proprietary Preparations

Kelocyanor *(Lipha, UK)*. *Injection*, dicobalt edetate 15 mg/mL, in ampoules of 20 mL.

Proprietary Names and Manufacturers

Kelocyanor *(Riker, Austral.; L'Arguenon, Fr.; Script Intal, S.Afr.; Lipha, UK)*.

19076-q

Digoxin-specific Antibody Fragments

Digoxin Immune Fab (Ovine); F(ab).

Digoxin-specific antibody fragments [F(ab)] are derived from antibodies produced in sheep immunised to digoxin. Digoxin has greater affinity for the antibodies than for tissue-binding sites, and the digoxin-antibody complex is then rapidly excreted in the urine. Digoxin-specific antibody fragments are generally restricted to the treatment of life-threatening digoxin intoxication in which conventional treatment is ineffective. Successful treatment of digitoxin and lanatoside C poisoning has also been reported. The dose of antibody fragments is based on the body-load of digoxin which can be estimated from the amount ingested or from the steady-state plasma concentration; approximately 60 mg is required to bind 1 mg of digoxin or digitoxin. Administration is by intravenous infusion over a 20-minute period. In the case of incomplete reversal or recurrence of toxicity a further dose can be given.

In a brief review of digoxin-specific F(ab) antibody fragments, Proudfoot (*Br. med. J.*, 1986, *293*, 642) reported that reversal of digitalis toxicity has been shown to be successful in clinical studies and that disappearance of symptoms could be rapid, at least in some patients. Infusion of F(ab) fragments had been well tolerated with no evidence of immediate or delayed hypersensitivity, although further monitoring would be necessary. In clinical studies, Smith *et al.* (*New Engl. J. Med.*, 1982, *307*, 1357) reported successful treatment of 21 out of 26 patients with life-threatening digitalis poisoning, and the same researchers subsequently reported similar results in 53 out of 56 patients who received appropriate treatment with F(ab) (T.L. Wenger *et al.*, *J. Am. Coll. Cardiol.*, 1985, *5*, 118A). In both studies, the death of 1 patient was attributed to insufficient F(ab) being available since arrhythmias recurred several hours after an initially favourable response. It was suggested that deterioration of cardiovascular function in some patients could have been associated with the reduction in inotropic support caused by the removal of cardiac glycosides.

In an attempt to rationalise treatment, Schaumann *et al.* (*Eur. J. clin. Pharmac.*, 1986, *30*, 527) studied the kinetics of F(ab) antibody fragments and bound digoxin in 17 patients with severe digoxin intoxication. They calculated the half-life of F(ab) antibody fragments to be 14.3 hours, and their results indicated that if F(ab) was infused over a short period about half would be cleared before enough digoxin had diffused from the tissue to allow adequate binding. They obtained good results using 160 mg as a loading dose followed by an infusion of a further 160 mg over 7 hours. Gibb and Parnham (*Br. med. J.*, 1986, *293*, 1171) pointed out that the measurement of serum-digoxin concentrations could not be relied upon to assess the severity of digoxin toxicity. Additionally, interference by F(ab) antibody fragments with immunoassay techniques can produce erroneous results; this may be partly overcome by appropriate determination of free and total glycoside. Evidence of the clearance of the inactive antibody-bound digoxin was conflicting with reported half-lives of between 16 and 34 hours. Thus modified assay techniques will be required for prolonged periods in patients requiring repeated serum-digoxin measurements. See also *Med. Lett.*, 1986, *28*, 87.

For a report of F(ab) antibody fragments interacting with plasma-digoxin measurements, see p.828.

Proprietary Preparations

Digibind *(Wellcome, UK). Injection*, powder for reconstitution, digoxin-specific antibody fragments F(ab) 40 mg.

Proprietary Names and Manufacturers

Digibind *(Wellcome, UK; Wellcome, USA).*

1036-e

Dimercaprol *(BAN, USAN, rINN).*

BAL; British Anti-Lewisite. 2,3-Dimercaptopropan-1-ol.

$C_3H_8OS_2$=124.2.

CAS — 59-52-9.

Pharmacopoeias. In *Aust., Br., Braz., Chin., Cz., Egypt., Eur., Fr., Ger., Hung., Ind., Int., It., Jpn, Jug., Neth., Nord., Pol., Swiss, Turk.*, and *U.S.* Also in *B.P. Vet.*

A clear colourless or slightly yellow liquid with an alliaceous odour. **Soluble** 1 in 20 of water and 1 in 18 of arachis oil; miscible with alcohol, benzyl benzoate, and methyl alcohol. Solutions in oil are **sterilised** by maintaining at a minimum of 150° for not less than 1 hour, the air in the containers having been replaced by nitrogen or other suitable gas. **Store** at 2° to 8° in well-filled airtight containers. Protect from light.

Adverse Effects and Treatment

The most consistent side-effects produced by dimercaprol are hypertension and tachycardia. Other side-effects include nausea, vomiting, headache, burning sensation of the lips, mouth, throat, and eyes, lachrymation and salivation, tingling of the extremities, a sensation of constriction in the throat and chest, muscle pains and muscle spasm, rhinorrhoea, conjunctivitis, sweating, restlessness, and abdominal pain. Pain may occur at the injection site and sterile abscesses occasionally develop. In children, fever commonly occurs and persists during therapy. Very high doses may cause convulsions and coma.

Side-effects are dose-related, relatively frequent, and usually reversible. It has been suggested that oral administration of ephedrine sulphate 30 to 60 mg half an hour before each injection of dimercaprol may reduce side-effects; antihistamines may alleviate some of the symptoms.

Dimercaprol applied topically is a potent skin sensitiser.

A report of haemolysis during dimercaprol chelation therapy for high blood-lead concentrations in 2 children with a deficiency of glucose-6-phosphate dehydrogenase.— N. Janakiraman *et al.*, *Clin. Pediat.*, 1978, *17*, 485.

Precautions

Dimercaprol should be used with care in patients with hypertension or impaired renal function. Alkalinisation of the urine may protect the kidney during therapy by stabilising the dimercaprol-metal complex. Dimercaprol should not be used in patients with impaired hepatic function unless due to arsenic poisoning. It should not be used in the treatment of poisoning due to cadmium, iron, or selenium as the dimercaprol-metal complexes formed are more toxic than the metals themselves.

Absorption and Fate

After intramuscular injection, maximum blood concentrations of dimercaprol may be attained within 1 hour. Dimercaprol is metabolised and rapidly excreted in the urine and bile.

Uses and Administration

Dimercaprol is a chelating agent used in the treatment of acute poisoning by arsenic, gold, and mercury; its role in the treatment of poisoning by antimony, bismuth, and thallium is less well established.

The sulphydryl groups on dimercaprol compete with endogenous sulphydryl groups on proteins such as enzymes to combine with these metals; chelation by dimercaprol therefore prevents or reverses any inhibition of the sulphydryl enzymes by the metal and the dimercaprol-metal complex formed is readily excreted by the kidney. Since the complex may dissociate, particularly at acid pH, or be oxidised, the aim of treatment is to provide an excess of dimercaprol in body fluids until the excretion of the metal is complete.

Dimercaprol should be administered by deep intramuscular injection. Various dosage schedules are in use.

In the *UK* a recommended schedule is to give doses of 400 to 800 mg on the first day of treatment, 200 to 400 mg on the second and third days, and 100 to 200 mg on the fourth and subsequent days, all administered in divided doses. Within these dose ranges, the individual dose is determined by body-weight, severity of symptoms, and the causative agent. Single doses should not generally exceed 3 mg per kg body-weight but single doses of up to 5 mg per kg may be required initially in patients with severe acute poisoning. A minimum interval of 4 hours between doses appears to reduce side-effects.

In the *US* a recommended schedule for severe arsenical or gold poisoning is 3 mg per kg body-weight given at 4-hourly intervals throughout the first 2 days, 4 doses are given on the third day, and 2 on the next 10 days. In milder cases 2.5 mg per kg body-weight is given 4 times daily on each of the first 2 days, twice daily on the third day, and once daily on subsequent days for 10 days. For acute mercurial poisoning an initial injection of 5 mg per kg body-weight is followed by 1 or 2 injections of 2.5 mg per kg body-weight daily for 10 days.

Some authorities have suggested that doses of up to 5 mg per kg every 4 hours may be required during the first 1 or 2 days of treatment in severe poisoning with gold, mercury, or arsenic.

Dimercaprol is also used in conjunction with sodium calciumedetate (p.852) in the treatment of lead poisoning. It can be of particular value in the treatment of acute lead encephalopathy and a suggested procedure is to administer an initial dose of dimercaprol 4 mg per kg body-weight alone followed at 4-hourly intervals by dimercaprol 3 to 4 mg per kg with concomitant doses of sodium calciumedetate administered at a separate site; treatment may be maintained for 2 to 7 days depending on the clinical response.

LEAD POISONING. Evidence that combined chelation therapy with dimercaprol and sodium calciumedetate was superior to sodium calciumedetate alone in the treatment of severe acute toxic episodes of lead poisoning.— J. J. Chisolm, *J. Pediat.*, 1968, *73*, 1.

See also under sodium calciumedetate (p.852)..

Preparations

Dimercaprol Injection *(B.P.).* BAL Injection. A sterile 5% w/v solution in benzyl benzoate and arachis oil. pH adjusted to 6.8 to 7.0 with alcoholic ammonia solution.

Dimercaprol Injection *(U.S.P.).* A sterile 9 to 11% w/w solution of dimercaprol in a mixture of benzyl benzoate and vegetable oil.

Proprietary Preparations

Dimercaprol *(Boots, UK). Injection*, oily, dimercaprol 50 mg/mL, in ampoules of 2 mL.

Proprietary Names and Manufacturers

BAL *(Boots, Austral.; Hynson, Westcott & Dunning, Canad.; L'Arguenon, Fr.; Boots-Formenti, Ital.; Hynson, Westcott & Dunning, USA)*; Dimercaprol *(Boots, UK)*; Sulfactin *(Degussa, Ger.).*

12658-t

4-Dimethylaminophenol Hydrochloride

$C_8H_{11}NO,HCl$=173.6.

CAS — 619-60-3 (4-dimethylaminophenol).

4-Dimethylaminophenol hydrochloride is reported to oxidise haemoglobin to methaemoglobin and has been used as an alternative to sodium nitrite (p.854) in the treatment of cyanide poisoning in conjunction with sodium thiosulphate. Doses of 3 mg per kg body-weight have been given intravenously.

A review of the treatment of cyanide poisoning with 4-dimethylaminophenol.— N. P. Weger, *Fundam. appl. Toxicol.*, 1983, *3*, 387.

Proprietary Names and Manufacturers

4-DMAP *(Köhler, Ger.).*

1037-l

Diphenylthiocarbazone

Dithizone.

$C_{13}H_{12}N_4S$=256.3.

CAS — 60-10-6.

Diphenylthiocarbazone is a chelating agent which has been suggested for use in thallium poisoning.

For a report on the treatment of thallium poisoning including the use of diphenylthiocarbazone as an oral intestinal chelating agent, see under Sodium Diethyldithiocarbamate, p.854.

7302-z

Diprenorphine Hydrochloride *(BANM, rINNM).*

M5050. (6*R*,7*R*,14*S*)-17-Cyclopropylmethyl-7,8-dihydro-7-(1-hydroxy-1-methylethyl)-6-*O*-methyl-6,14-ethano-17-normorphine hydrochloride; 2-[(−)-(5*R*,6*R*,7*R*,14*S*)-9a-Cyclopropylmethyl-4,5-epoxy-3-hydroxy-6-methoxy-6,14-ethanomorphinan-7-yl]propan-2-ol hydrochloride.

$C_{26}H_{35}NO_4,HCl$=462.0.

CAS — 14357-78-9 (diprenorphine); 16808-86-9 (hydrochloride).

Pharmacopoeias. In *B.P. Vet.*

A white or almost white crystalline powder. **Soluble** 1 in

30 of water; slightly soluble in alcohol; very slightly soluble in chloroform; practically insoluble in ether. A 2% solution in water has a pH of 4.5 to 6.0. **Store** in well-closed containers. Protect from light.

Diprenorphine hydrochloride is an opioid antagonist used in veterinary medicine to reverse the effects of etorphine hydrochloride.

Proprietary Veterinary Names and Manufacturers
Revivon *(C-Vet, UK)*.

1038-y

Disodium Edetate *(BAN)*.

Disodium Edathamil; Disodium EDTA; Disodium Tetracemate; Edetate Disodium *(USAN)*; Natrii Edetas; Sodium Edetate. Disodium dihydrogen ethylenediaminetetra-acetate dihydrate.
$C_{10}H_{14}N_2Na_2O_8,2H_2O=372.2$.

CAS — 139-33-3 (anhydrous); 6381-92-6 (dihydrate).

NOTE. In the *USA* the title sodium edetate is used to describe the tetrasodium salt.

Pharmacopoeias. In *Br., Eur., Fr., Ind., It., Jpn, Jug., Neth., Nord., Swiss, Turk.*, and *U.S.*

A white odourless crystalline powder. **Soluble** 1 in 11 of water; slightly soluble in alcohol; practically insoluble in chloroform and ether. The *B.P.* specifies that a 5% solution in water has a pH of 4.0 to 5.5. The *U.S.P.* specifies that a 5% solution in water has a pH of 4.0 to 6.0.

Adverse Effects

Disodium edetate has similar adverse effects to sodium calciumedetate (p.852).

Hypocalcaemia can occur if disodium edetate is administered by intravenous infusion too rapidly or in too concentrated a solution and tetany, convulsions, respiratory arrest, and cardiac arrhythmias may result.

Precautions

Disodium edetate has similar precautions to sodium calciumedetate (p.852). In addition, it should be used with caution in patients with tuberculosis, impaired cardiac function, or a history of seizures, and is contra-indicated in renal disease. Plasma-electrolyte concentrations, particularly of ionised calcium, should be monitored.

Absorption and Fate

Disodium edetate is poorly absorbed from the gastro-intestinal tract.

Uses and Administration

Disodium edetate is a chelating agent which forms a stable, soluble complex with calcium that is readily excreted by the kidney. It has been administered intravenously in the emergency treatment of hypercalcaemia and has been used to control digitalis-induced cardiac arrhythmias.

It has also been used in the treatment of calcium deposits from lime burns of the eye and in the treatment of calcified corneal opacities, either by topical application after removing the appropriate area of corneal epithelium or by iontophoresis.

In the *UK*, disodium edetate is usually administered as the trisodium salt. For the treatment of hypercalcaemia, 5 g of trisodium edetate should be diluted with at least 500 mL of glucose injection (5%) or sodium chloride injection (0.9%) and given by slow intravenous infusion over 2 to 3 hours. The usual dose is up to 70 mg per kg body-weight daily for adults, and up to 60 mg per kg for children. For topical application to the eye a 0.4% solution has been used.

Disodium edetate is also used as an antoxidant synergist in cosmetic and pharmaceutical preparations.

Estimated acceptable daily intake: up to 2.5 mg per kg body-weight.— Seventeenth Report of Joint FAO/WHO Expert Committee on Food Additives, *Tech. Rep. Ser. Wld Hlth Org. No. 539,* 1974.

ATHEROSCLEROSIS. Reviews of the use of disodium edetate chelating therapy to decalcify atherosclerotic plaques. There was no acceptable evidence that disodium edetate was effective in the treatment of atherosclerosis and the adverse effects could be lethal: *Med. Lett.*, 1981, *23,* 51; K. L. Rathmann and L. K. Golightly, *Drug Intell. & clin. Pharm.*, 1984, *18,* 1000; R. Magee, *Med. J. Aust.*, 1985, *142,* 514.

SCLEROMALACIA. In a patient with scleromalacia perforans associated with Crohn's disease, disodium edetate 0.5% eye-drops instilled 4 times daily produced beneficial results. It was considered to act as a collagenase inhibitor.— P. J. Evans and P. Eustace, *Br. J. Ophthal.*, 1973, *57,* 330.

Preparations

Disodium Edetate Eye Lotion *(A.P.F.)*. Disodium edetate 400 mg, Water for Injections to 100 mL. Sterilised by autoclaving.

Edetate Disodium Injection *(U.S.P.)*. A sterile solution of disodium edetate in Water for Injections, containing varying amounts of the disodium and trisodium salts as a result of pH adjustment. Potency is expressed in terms of the equivalent amount of anhydrous disodium edetate. pH 6.5 to 7.5.

Trisodium Edetate Intravenous Infusion *(B.P.)*. Trisodium Edetate Injection. Prepared immediately before use by diluting Strong Sterile Trisodium Edetate Solution with a suitable diluent.

Strong Sterile Trisodium Edetate Solution *(B.P.)*. Contains the equivalent of 20% w/v (limits 18 to 22%) of anhydrous trisodium edetate ($C_{10}H_{13}N_2Na_3O_8$) made by the interaction of sodium hydroxide and disodium edetate. Store in lead-free glass containers and sterilise by autoclaving. pH 7.0 to 8.0. To be diluted with sodium chloride injection (0.9%) or glucose injection (5%) before administration.

NOTE. 1 g of disodium edetate dihydrate is equivalent to about 962 mg of anhydrous trisodium edetate.

Proprietary Preparations

Limclair *(Sinclair, UK)*. *Injection*, trisodium edetate 200 mg/mL, in ampoules of 5 mL.

Proprietary Names and Manufacturers of Disodium and Trisodium Edetate

Complecal *(IBYS, Spain)*; Disotate *(Forest Pharmaceuticals, USA)*; Endrate *(Abbott, USA)*; Limclair *(Sinclair, UK)*; Nervanaid BA2 *(ABM Chemicals, UK)*; Nervanaid BA3 *(ABM Chemicals, UK)*; Sequestrene NA 2 *(Ciba-Geigy, UK)*; Sequestrene NA 3 *(Ciba-Geigy, UK)*; Sodium Versenate *(Austral.; Riker, UK; Riker, USA)*.

1039-j

Edetic Acid *(BAN, USAN, rINN)*.

Edathamil; EDTA. Ethylenediaminetetra-acetic acid.
$C_{10}H_{16}N_2O_8=292.2$.

CAS — 60-00-4.

Pharmacopoeias. In *Roum.* Also in *U.S.N.F.*

A white crystalline powder. Very slightly **soluble** in water; soluble in solutions of alkali hydroxides.

Edetic acid is used in pharmaceutical manufacturing and as an anticoagulant for blood taken for haematological investigations. Edetic acid and its salts have many industrial applications as chelating agents; for the use of edetates in medicine see disodium edetate above and sodium calciumedetate (p.852).

BLOOD TESTING. Edetic acid may induce platelet clumping in some specimens collected for blood-cell counting leading to diagnostic errors. The recognition of pseudothrombocytopenia resulting from the use of edetic acid as the anticoagulant in blood samples was discussed.— B. A. Payne, *Postgrad. Med.*, 1985, *77,* 75.

PHARMACEUTICAL FORMULATION. Review on the use of edetic acid and related chelating agents as antoxidant synergists, stabilisers, and preservative enhancers in the formulation of cosmetics and toiletries.— J. R. Hart, *Cosmet. Toilet.*, 1983, *98* (Apr.), 54.

Inhalation of edetic acid produced dose-related bronchoconstriction which persisted for longer than 60 minutes. Nebuliser solutions for bronchodilation should be made available without edetic acid as a preservative.— C. R. W. Beasley *et al.*, *Br. med. J.*, 1987, *294,* 1197.

Edetic acid has been reported to enhance the antimicrobial efficacy of some disinfectants such as chloroxylenol (p.959). However, for a report of edetates reducing the antimicrobial efficacy of thiomersal, see Thiomersal, p.970.

Proprietary Names and Manufacturers
Nervanaid B acid *(ABM Chemicals, UK)*; Sequestrene AA *(Ciba-Geigy, UK)*; Tracemate *(Marcofina, Fr.)*.

13215-d

Flumazenil *(BAN, rINN)*.

Flumazepil; Ro-15-1788. Ethyl 8-fluoro-5,6-dihydro-5-methyl-6-oxo-4*H*-imidazo[1,5-*a*][1,4]benzodiazepine-3-carboxylate.
$C_{15}H_{14}FN_3O_3=303.3$.

CAS — 78755-81-4.

Adverse Effects and Precautions

Nausea, vomiting, and flushing may occur. There have been rare reports of convulsions, especially in epileptics. Caution is advised when liver function is impaired. Because of its short duration of action, patients given flumazenil to reverse benzodiazepine-induced sedation should be kept under close observation; further doses of flumazenil may be necessary.

For a warning that the availability of flumazenil as an antagonist should not be an encouragement to use larger doses of midazolam for sedation, see p.753.

Uses and Administration

Flumazenil is a benzodiazepine antagonist which acts competitively at CNS benzodiazepine receptors. It is used postoperatively to reverse the sedative effects of benzodiazepine-induced anaesthesia. It may also be used to diagnose and treat benzodiazepine overdosage.

The usual initial dose is 200 μg given intravenously over 15 seconds followed at intervals of 60 seconds by further doses of 100 μg if required to a maximum of 1 mg or occasionally 2 mg (usual dose range, 300 to 600 μg). If drowsiness recurs 100 to 400 μg per hour may be infused intravenously, the rate being adjusted according to response.

ABSORPTION AND FATE. The pharmacokinetics of flumazenil after administration of high intravenous doses of 20 and 40 mg or oral doses of 200 mg were studied in 6 healthy men. Following intravenous administration, flumazenil was extensively distributed in the body and rapidly cleared from the plasma by hepatic metabolism. The elimination half-lives observed were less than 1 hour and less than 0.1% of a dose was excreted unchanged in the urine. After oral administration, the drug was rapidly absorbed reaching peak concentrations in the plasma after 20 to 90 minutes. Due to the high hepatic extraction ratio, orally administered flumazenil underwent pronounced first-pass metabolism and only about 16% of the dose reached the systemic circulation unchanged.— G. Roncari *et al.*, *Br. J. clin. Pharmac.*, 1986, *22,* 421. Further studies: U. Klotz *et al.*, *Eur. J. clin. Pharmac.*, 1984, *27,* 115; U. Klotz *et al.*, *Br. J. clin. Pharmac.*, 1985, *19,* 95.

ACTION. Studies on the effects of flumazenil.— A. Darragh *et al.*, *Br. J. clin. Pharmac.*, 1982, *14,* 677 (antagonsim of the central effects of diazepam); A. Darragh *et al.* (letter), *ibid.*, 871 (antagonism of the central effects of 3-methylclonazepam); J. -M. Gaillard and R. Blois, *ibid.*, 1983, *15,* 529 (effects on flunitrazepam-induced sleep changes); I. Gath *et al.*, *ibid.*, 1984, *18,* 541 (electrophysiological effects); G. Ziegler *et al.* (letter), *Lancet*, 1985, *2,* 510 (effects on sleep); U. Klotz *et al.*, *J. clin. Pharmac.*, 1985, *25,* 400 (reversal of midazolam-induced sedation); U. Klotz *et al.*, *Br. J. clin. Pharmac.*, 1986, *22,* 513 (effects on alcohol-induced sedation).

USES AND ADMINISTRATION. Brief discussion on the potential uses of flumazenil as a benzodiazepine antagonist.— C. H. Ashton, *Br. med. J.*, 1985, *290,* 805. Further reviews on the actions and uses of flumazenil: R. Amrein *et al.*, *Med. Toxicol.*, 1987, *2,* 411; R. N. Brogden and K. L. Goa, *Drugs*, 1988, *35,* 448.

Intravenous injection of 500 μg of flumazenil to a 25-year-old heroin addict with hepatic coma resulted in a remarkable improvement in consciousness which lasted for an hour.— G. Scollo-Lavizzari and E. Steinmann (letter), *Lancet*, 1985, *1,* 1324. Two of 4 patients with alcoholic liver cirrhosis and hepatic encephalopathy responded to the intravenous administration of flumazenil in doses of 200 to 500 μg.— G. Bansky *et al.* (letter), *ibid.* See also D. A. Burke *et al* (letter), *ibid.*, 1988, *2,* 505.

In a preliminary study, 13 patients with suspected benzodiazepine overdosage were given flumazenil 1.5 to

10 mg by slow intravenous injection. All patients intoxicated with benzodiazepines alone were fully awake and alert within 1 to 2 minutes but in the majority CNS depression returned 1 to 4 hours after the injection reflecting the short elimination half-life of flumazenil. Benzodiazepine overdosage alone is rarely fatal and generally only supportive measures are required but flumazenil might be an effective diagnostic tool in the primary management of self-poisoning to determine the intoxicating agents.— P. Hofer and G. Scollo-Lavizzari, *Archs intern. Med.*, 1985, *145*, 663.

Effective reversal of midazolam-supplemented general anaesthesia with flumazenil in a study involving 60 patients undergoing laparoscopy.— E. Alon *et al.*, *Br. J. Anaesth.*, 1987, *59*, 455.

When compared with placebo in a study of 60 patients with acute drug overdosage, flumazenil improved the level of consciousness in those who had taken benzodiazepines as well as in those who had taken benzodiazepines and other sedatives including alcohol. There was no response in those who had taken barbiturates alone or tricyclic antidepressants. Three patients given flumazenil complained of mild withdrawal symptoms that lasted for 15 minutes.— G. F. O'Sullivan and D. N. Wade, *Clin. Pharmac. Ther.*, 1987, *42*, 254.

Proprietary Preparations

Anexate *(Roche, UK)*. *Injection*, flumazenil 100µg/mL, in ampoules of 5 ml.

Proprietary Names and Manufacturers

Anexate *(Roche, Switz.; Roche, UK)*.

1610-h

Fuller's Earth

Terra Fullonica.

CAS — 8031-18-3.

Consists largely of montmorillonite, a native hydrated aluminium silicate, with which very finely divided calcite (calcium carbonate) may be associated.

Fuller's earth is an adsorbent which is used in dusting-powders, toilet powders, and lotions. Fuller's earth of high adsorptive capacity is used in industry as a clarifying and filtering medium.

It is used in the treatment of paraquat poisoning (see p.1352).

Proprietary Names and Manufacturers

Fuller's Earth (Surrey Finest Grade)*(Laporte, UK)*.

588-l

Glutathione

GSH. *N*-(*N*-L-γ-Glutamyl-L-cysteinyl)glycine.

$C_{10}H_{17}N_3O_6S$=307.3.

CAS — 70-18-8.

Glutathione has been used in the treatment of poisoning with a number of compounds including heavy metals. It has also been used in hepatitis and some skin diseases such as eczema.

Proprietary Names and Manufacturers

Agifutol S *(Kyorin, Jpn)*; Atomolan *(Kyowa, Jpn)*; Beamthion *(Jpn)*; Detoxan *(Jpn)*; Estathion *(Jpn)*; Glutathin *(Mochida, Jpn)*; Glutathiol *(Fr.)*; Glutide *(Tanabe, Jpn)*; Grutinal *(Sankyo, Jpn)*; Hydrathion *(Toyo Jozo, Jpn)*; Isethion *(Jpn)*; Ledac *(Jpn)*; Mohathion *(Jpn)*; Orglone *(Jpn)*; Panaron *(Dainippon, Jpn)*; Reglution *(Spain)*; Resithion *(Jpn)*; Tathiclon *(Jpn)*; Tathion *(Yamanouchi, Jpn)*; Tition *(Jorba, Spain)*; Torichion *(Jpn)*.

7303-c

Levallorphan Tartrate *(BANM, USAN, rINNM)*.

(−)-9a-Allylmorphinan-3-ol hydrogen tartrate.

$C_{19}H_{25}NO,C_4H_6O_6$=433.5.

CAS — 152-02-3 (levallorphan); 71-82-9 (tartrate).

Pharmacopoeias. In *Egypt.*, *Turk.*, and *U.S.*

A white or almost white odourless crystalline powder. **Soluble** 1 in 17 of water, 1 in 38 of alcohol, 1 in 5000 of ether, 1 in 3300 of chloroform, 1 in 13 of methyl alcohol, 1 in 665 of isopropyl alcohol, and 1 in 33 000 of petroleum spirit. The *U.S.P.* injection has a pH between 4.0 and 4.5. **Store** in airtight containers. Protect from light.

Adverse Effects

Levallorphan may give rise to drowsiness, miosis, and sweating. Restlessness, bradycardia, hypotension, dizziness, nausea, pallor, lethargy, and dysphoria may occur. Levallorphan may also cause respiratory depression and induce psychotic effects.

Precautions

As for Naloxone Hydrochloride (p.845). Levallorphan may exacerbate respiratory depression induced by low doses of opioids and non-opioid central depressants.

Uses and Administration

Levallorphan is an opioid antagonist with actions and uses similar to those of naloxone (p.845); in addition it also possesses some agonist properties. It should be used cautiously; levallorphan reverses severe opioid-induced respiratory depression but may exacerbate respiratory depression such as that induced by alcohol or other non-opioid central depressants.

In the treatment of opioid overdosage, an initial dose of 1 to 2 mg of levallorphan tartrate has been given intravenously followed by 1 or 2 doses of 0.5 mg at intervals of 5 to 15 minutes, if necessary. It has also been used to reverse opioid central depression resulting from the use of opioids during surgery and to reverse neonatal respiratory depression following administration of opioid analgesics to the mother during labour. Levallorphan tartrate may also be given subcutaneously or intramuscularly.

Preparations

Levallorphan Tartrate Injection *(U.S.P.)*

Proprietary Names and Manufacturers

Lorfan *(Austral.; Canad.; Ger.; Switz.; Roche, UK; Roche, USA)*.

The following names have been used for multi-ingredient preparations containing levallorphan tartrate— Pethilorfan *(Roche, UK)*.

3726-q

Mesna *(BAN, rINN)*.

Mesnum; UCB-3983. Sodium 2-mercaptoethanesulphonate.

$C_2H_5NaO_3S_2$=164.2.

CAS — 19767-45-4.

Solutions of mesna should be **stored** below 30° and protected from light.

There was no decrease in the concentration of free thiol groups of mesna after storage for 7 hours at room temperature of mesna (1.6 mg per mL) and ifosfamide (2.6 mg per mL) in glucose-saline in a polyethylene infusion bag. This suggests that mesna and ifosfamide do not react in the infusion bag.— I. C. Shaw and J. W. P. Rose (letter), *Lancet*, 1984, *1*, 1353. Confirmation of these conclusions after storage of mesna (40 mg per mL) and ifosfamide (50 mg per mL) in polypropylene syringes for 4 weeks at room temperature and also at 4°. However, ifosfamide concentrations fell by about 3% after 7 days and 12% after 4 weeks for both storage conditions.— C. G. Rowland *et al.* (letter), *ibid.*, *2*, 468.

Adverse Effects and Precautions

Adverse effects which may occur after administration of mesna include gastro-intestinal effects, headache, malaise, and skin rash. Bronchospasm has been reported after administration by nebuliser.

Mesna may produce a false positive result in diagnostic tests for urinary ketones.

A false positive result for urinary ketones using N-Multistix was obtained in 6 patients who had been given cyclophosphamide in association with mesna. This did not occur in 5 patients who received cyclophosphamide alone. The false positive colour reaction caused by mesna will fade when one drop of glacial acetic acid is added to the test strip, whereas true positive reactions will not.— E. C. Gordon-Smith *et al.* (letter), *Lancet*, 1982, *1*, 563. Similar findings of false positive reactions for urinary ketones when using Labstix during the administration of mesna.— A. B. Yehuda *et al.* (letter), *Drug Intell. & clin. Pharm.*, 1987, *21*, 547.

Meanwell *et al.* (*Lancet*, 1985, *1*, 406) reported a characteristic and severe encephalopathy associated with the administration of ifosfamide with mesna in 5 of 31 women with cervical and endometrial carcinoma. Cantwell and Harris (*ibid.*, 752) reported a similar encephalopathy in one patient with sarcoma of the uterus out of 119 patients with various forms of cancer treated with the combination. This patient was also receiving doxorubicin. They suggested that the neurotoxicity may be due to a direct effect of ifosfamide or mesna, or one of their metabolites, and that the higher total dose of mesna per treatment course used by Meanwell *et al.* might have contributed to the greater incidence of toxicity they described. However, Osborne and Slevin (*ibid.*, 1398) found no case of encephalopathy in 17 patients with ovarian or lung cancer given cyclophosphamide in association with mesna in higher doses than used by Meanwell *et al.* and they suggested that ifosfamide was the cause of the reported adverse effects. Pinkerton *et al.* (*ibid.*, 1399) reported a generalised seizure in a child within half an hour of the start of mesna administration before the infusion of ifosfamide, but agreed with Cantwell and Harris that either agent or their metabolites may be responsible. Meanwell *et al.* (*ibid.*, 1986, *2*, 406) have devised a nomogram to determine the probability of development of severe CNS effects, taking into account indicators of impairment of hepatic and renal function. This was tested in 45 patients receiving ifosfamide with mesna, and the authors suggested that it be used to identify a group of patients who should not be given the combination. A modification of this nomogram to take into account the rate of infusion has been suggested (T.J. Perren *et al.*, *ibid.*, 1987, *1*, 390). However, while these methods of predicting ifosfamide-related encephalopathy might be useful in pelvic disease, McCallum (*ibid.*, 987) found them to have little application in the evaluation of patients with small cell carcinoma of the lung.

A report of a hypersensitivity reaction, including rash, nausea, fever, and vomiting, in one patient given mesna intravenously.— E. Lang and M. Goos (letter), *Lancet*, 1985, *2*, 329.

Absorption and Fate

Mesna is rapidly excreted in the urine after oral or intravenous administration as the unchanged drug and as the metabolite mesna disulphide (dimesna).

Studies of the pharmacokinetics of mesna after oral and intravenous administration.— H. Burkert *et al.*, *Arzneimittel-Forsch.*, 1984, *34*, 1597; C. A. James *et al.*, *Br. J. clin. Pharmac.*, 1987, *23*, 561.

Uses and Administration

Mesna is used for the prophylaxis of urothelial toxicity in patients being treated with ifosfamide or cyclophosphamide. Unchanged mesna in the urine has free thiol groups that react with the metabolites of ifosfamide and cyclophosphamide, including acrolein, considered to be responsible for the toxic effects on the bladder.

If ifosfamide or cyclophosphamide is given as an intravenous bolus, mesna as 20% of the dose of the antineoplastic on a weight for weight basis is given intravenously on 3 occasions over 15 to 30 minutes at 4-hourly intervals beginning at the same time as the antineoplastic injection. This regimen is repeated for each dose of the antineoplastic. The dose of mesna may be increased to 40% of the dose of the antineoplastic and given 4 times at 3-hourly intervals. If the antineoplastic is given as an intravenous infusion over 24 hours, mesna as 20% of the total antineoplastic dose is given by intravenous injection, followed by 100% of the total dose by intravenous infusion over 24 hours, then followed by 60% by infusion over a further 12 hours. The final 12-hour infusion may be replaced by 3 injections each of 20% of the antineoplastic dose at 4-hourly intervals, or by mesna given by mouth in 3 doses each of 40% of the antineoplastic dose at 4-hourly intervals.

Mesna is also used as a mucolytic agent in a usual dose of 0.6 to 1.2 g administered by a nebuliser; it may also be given by direct instillation.

CYCLOPHOSPHAMIDE AND IFOSFAMIDE UROTOXICITY. References to mesna being given by mouth or intravenously to prevent the urotoxic effects of cyclophosphamide or ifosfamide: B. M. Bryant *et al.*, *Lancet*,

1980, *2*, 657; M. E. Scheulen *et al.*, in *New Experience with the Oxazaphosphorines with Special Reference to the Uroprotector Uromitexan*, H. Burkert and G.A. Nagel (Ed.), Basel, S. Karger, 1981, p.40; M. Varine and S. Monfardini, *ibid.*, p.47; C. E. Araujo and J. Tessler, *Eur. J. Cancer clin. Oncol.*, 1983, *19*, 195.

Findings *in vitro* that mesna does not prevent the chromosomal changes and, hence, the cell-killing effects of radiation. Mesna may therefore be given to prevent the urotoxic effects of cyclophosphamide and ifosfamide in patients being prepared for bone-marrow transplantation by treatment with these antineoplastic agents and total-body irradiation.— R. Becher *et al.* (letter), *New Engl. J. Med.*, 1982, *307*, 1152. In contrast, a study in *mice* has indicated that mesna is a radioprotector; an interval of at least 12 hours between cessation of the mesna infusion and total body irradiation has been recommended.— P. N. Plowman and K. Trott (letter), *Lancet*, 1987, *1*, 167. Further comment.— I. C. Shaw and A. J. Searle (letter), *ibid.*, 516.

Results of a study in 17 patients treated with cyclophosphamide and mesna indicating that mesna is rapidly excreted in the urine, and that the concentration of mesna in the bladder is related to the frequency of micturition. To maintain adequate protection against urotoxicity mesna should be given at frequent intervals (every 3 hours was suggested), urine output should not exceed 2 litres per day, and the bladder should be emptied immediately before the first mesna dose. Increased dosage, or more frequent injection may be required if concomitant diuretic therapy is given.— G. P. Finn *et al.* (letter), *New Engl. J. Med.*, 1986, *314*, 61.

RESPIRATORY DISORDERS. The minimum inhibitory concentration of azlocillin for *Pseudomonas aeruginosa* was reduced by the addition of a 1% solution of mesna *in vitro*. This was considered to be due to an independent effect of mesna on pseudomonal growth and not to a potentiation of azlocillin activity. This postulated antipseudomonal action in association with the mucolytic action of mesna may be of benefit in patients with cystic fibrosis.— D. P. Heaf *et al.*, *Archs Dis. Childh.*, 1983, *58*, 824.

Proprietary Preparations

Uromitexan *(Boehringer Ingelheim, UK). Injection*, mesna 100 mg/mL, in ampoules of 4 and 10 mL.

Proprietary Names and Manufacturers

Ausobronc Mesna *(Biochimica Zanardi, Ital.)*; Mistabron *(UCB, Belg.; UCB, Neth.; UCB, S.Afr.; UCB, Switz.)*; Mistabronco *(UCB, Ger.)*; Mucofluid *(UCB, Belg.; UCB, Fr.; UCB, Ger.; UCB, Ital.; UCB, Spain)*; Mucolene *(Formenti, Ital.)*; Sinomist *(Vesta, S.Afr.)*; Uromitexan *(Lucien, Fr.; Degussa-Asta, Ger.; Schering, Ital.; Funk, Spain; Degussa, Switz.; Boehringer Ingelheim, UK)*.

605-x

Methionine *(USAN)*.

L-Methionine. L-2-Amino-4-(methylthio)butyric acid.

$C_5H_{11}NO_2S$=149.2.

CAS — 63-68-3.

Pharmacopoeias. In *Cz., Jpn,* and *U.S.*

White crystals with a characteristic odour and taste.

Soluble in water, in warm dilute alcohol, and in dilute mineral acids; practically insoluble in acetone, dehydrated alcohol, and ether. A 1% solution in water has a pH of 5.6 to 6.1.

606-r

Racemethionine *(USAN)*.

Methionine *(rINN)*; DL-Methionine. DL-2-Amino-4-(methylthio)butyric acid.

$C_5H_{11}NO_2S$=149.2.

CAS — 59-51-8.

NOTE. The name methionine is often applied to racemethionine.

Pharmacopoeias. In *Aust., Belg., Braz., Cz., Egypt., Fr., Ger., Pol., Port., Roum., Rus., Span.,* and *U.S.*

White crystalline platelets or powder with a characteristic odour. **Soluble** 1 in 30 of water; soluble in dilute acids and solutions of alkali hydroxides; very slightly soluble in alcohol; practically insoluble in ether. A 1% solution in water has a pH of 5.6 to 6.1. **Protect** from light.

Adverse Effects and Precautions

Methionine may cause nausea, vomiting, drowsiness, and irritability. Methionine may precipitate hepatic encephalopathy in patients with established liver damage; it should be used with caution in patients with severe liver disease and should not be used in paracetamol poisoning if more than 10 hours have elapsed since ingestion of the overdose.

Review of the effects of nitrous oxide on the plasma concentrations of methionine.— J. F. Nunn, *Br. J. Anaesth.*, 1987, *59*, 3.

For the antagonism of the antiparkinsonian effect of levodopa by methionine, see under the Precautions of levodopa (p.1017).

Uses and Administration

Methionine is an amino acid which is an essential constituent of the diet and is incorporated into amino-acid solutions for parenteral nutrition (see p.1251).

Methionine also enhances the synthesis of glutathione and is used in the treatment of paracetamol poisoning to prevent hepatic damage. The usual dose is 2.5 g by mouth every 4 hours for 4 doses starting less than 10 hours after ingestion of the paracetamol. It has also been given intravenously. The literature relating to the use of methionine in paracetamol poisoning is, in general, imprecise as to the form of methionine used. In the *UK* the doses quoted above refer to racemethionine. Preparations containing both methionine and paracetamol have been formulated for use in situations where overdosage may occur.

Methionine has also been given by mouth to lower urinary pH and reduce odour and irritation due to ammoniacal urine.

PARACETAMOL POISONING. Discussions on the efficacy of methionine in paracetamol poisoning in comparison with acetylcysteine: J. A. Vale *et al.* (letter), *Br. med. J.*, 1979, *2*, 1435; T. J. Meredith *et al.*, *ibid.*, 1986, *293*, 345; J. M. Tredger *et al.* (letter), *ibid.*, 756; L. G. B. Tee *et al.* (letter), *Lancet*, 1986, *1*, 331.

For further references to the treatment of paracetamol poisoning see under acetylcysteine (p.903) and paracetamol (p.32).

Preparations

Racemethionine Capsules *(U.S.P.)*. Methionine Capsules

Racemethionine Tablets *(U.S.P.)*. Methionine Tablets

Proprietary Preparations

Methionine Tablets *(Evans Medical, UK). Tablets*, racemethionine 250 mg.

For proprietary preparations for enteral and parenteral nutrition containing racemethionine, see p.1289.

Proprietary Names and Manufacturers of Methionine or Racemethionine

Acimethin *(Gry, Ger.)*; Antamon *(S.Afr.)*; Antamonped *(Pediatric, S.Afr.)*; Lobamine *(Fr.)*; Meonine *(Wyeth, UK)*; Methnine *(Medical Research, Austral.)*; Monile *(Cortunon, Canad.)*; Ninol *(Horner, Canad.)*; Pedameth *(Forest Pharmaceuticals, USA)*; Uracid *(Wesley, USA)*; Uranap *(Vortech, USA)*.

The following names have been used for multi-ingredient preparations containing methionine or racemethionine—Amino-Cerv *(Milex, USA)*; G500 *(Cox, UK)*; Lipotrope *(Rougier, Canad.)*; Pameton *(Winthrop, UK)*.

1042-s

Methylene Blue *(USAN)*.

Azul de Metileno; Blu di Metilene; CI Basic Blue 9; Colour Index No. 52015; Methylenum Caeruleum; Methylthionine Chloride; Methylthioninium Chloride *(rINN)*; Schultz No. 1038; Tetramethylthionine Chloride Trihydrate. 3,7-Bis(dimethylamino)phenazathionium chloride trihydrate.

$C_{16}H_{18}ClN_3S,3H_2O$=373.9.

CAS — 61-73-4 (anhydrous); 7220-79-3 (trihydrate).

Pharmacopoeias. In *Arg., Belg., Chin., Cz., Fr., Hung., Int., It., Mex., Pol., Port., Rus., Span.,* and *U.S.*; in *Aust., Jug., Nord.,* and *Roum.* (xH_2O); in *Braz.* (anhydrous or $3H_2O$).

Dark green, odourless or almost odourless, crystals or crystalline powder with a bronze-like lustre. Solutions in water or alcohol are deep blue in colour.

Soluble 1 in 25 of water, 1 in 65 of alcohol; soluble in chloroform. Methylene Blue Injection U.S.P. has a pH of 3.0 to 4.5.

NOTE. Commercial methylene blue may consist of the double chloride of tetramethylthionine and zinc, and is not suitable for medicinal use.

Adverse Effects and Precautions

After intravenous administration methylene blue may cause nausea, vomiting, abdominal and chest pain, headache, dizziness, mental confusion, profuse sweating, and hypertension; with very high doses methaemoglobinaemia and haemolysis may occur. Oral administration may cause gastro-intestinal disturbances and dysuria.

Methylene blue should not be injected subcutaneously as it may cause necrotic abscesses. It should not be given by intrathecal injection as neural damage has occurred. Methylene blue should be used with caution in patients with severe renal impairment or glucose-6-phosphate dehydrogenase deficiency (see below).

Methylene blue imparts a blue colour to urine and faeces.

Necrotic ulcers developed on the feet of a 62-year-old man at the sites of methylene blue injections.— P. M. Perry and E. Meinhard, *Br. J. clin. Pract.*, 1974, *28*, 289.

In a 59-year-old man, an injection of methylene blue into the lumbar subarachnoid space resulted in paraparesis progressing to total paraplegia after 3½ years. The intrathecal use of methylene blue should be abandoned.— M. M. Sharr *et al.*, *J. Neurol. Neurosurg. Psychiat.*, 1978, *41*, 384.

Methylene blue should be used with caution in the treatment of toxic methaemoglobinaemia; high doses could cause haemolytic anaemias and patients with glucose-6-phosphate dehydrogenase (G6PD) deficiency were particularly susceptible. A rapid disappearance of cyanosis in response to methylene blue would be expected within one hour but might not occur if the patient had erythrocyte G6PD or NADPH-diaphorase deficiency or if methaemoglobinaemia was due to the ingestion of compounds such as aniline or dapsone. A second dose had been recommended if cyanosis did not disappear within one hour of methylene blue administration but results of a study in *animals* and of a patient with aniline poisoning indicated that an increased dosage of methylene blue might be of no additional benefit and could be potentially dangerous in that it could enhance Heinz body formation.— J. W. Harvey and A. S. Keitt, *Br. J. Haemat.*, 1983, *54*, 29.

PREGNANCY AND THE NEONATE. Although intra-amniotic injection of methylene blue has been used to diagnose premature rupture of foetal membranes or to identify separate amniotic sacs in twin pregnancies, there have been several reports of haemolytic anaemia (Heinz-body anaemia) and hyperbilirubinaemia in neonates exposed to methylene blue in the amniotic cavity (R.M. Cowett *et al.*, *Obstet. Gynec.*, 1976, *48*, *Suppl.* 1, 74S; F.T. Serota *et al.*, *Lancet*, 1979, *2*, 1142; J. Crooks, *Archs Dis. Childh.*, 1982, *57*, 872; M.J. Vincer *et al.*, *Can. med. Ass. J.*, 1987, *136*, 503). In most cases, exchange transfusions and/or phototherapy were required to control the jaundice. Crooks (1982) considered that the use of methylene blue for detecting premature rupture of the membranes should be avoided and Vincer *et al.* (1987) recommended that a safer dye, such as Azovan Blue (Evans Blue), be used for diagnosis in obstetric and neonatal practice.

Absorption and Fate

Methylene blue is absorbed from the gastro-intestinal tract. It is believed to be reduced in the tissues to the leuco form which is slowly excreted, mainly in the urine, together with some unchanged drug.

Results of a study in 7 healthy subjects indicated that although methylene blue was completely ionised at the pH of the gastro-intestinal tract, it was well absorbed. A mean of 74% of a 10-mg dose was recovered in the urine as unchanged drug or leucomethylene blue.— A. R. DiSanto and J. G. Wagner, *J. pharm. Sci.*, 1972, *61*, 1086.

Uses and Administration

In patients with methaemoglobinaemia, therapeutic doses of methylene blue can lower the levels of methaemoglobin in the red blood cells. It activates a normally dormant reductase enzyme system which reduces the methylene blue to leucomethylene blue, which in turn is able to reduce methaemoglobin to haemoglobin. However, in large doses methylene blue can itself produce methaemoglobinaemia and methaemoglobin concentration should therefore be closely monitored during treatment. Methylene blue is not effective for the treatment of methaemoglobinaemia in patients with glucose-6-phosphate dehydrogenase deficiency as these patients have a diminished capacity to reduce methylene blue to leucomethylene blue; it is also potentially harmful as patients with glucose-6-phosphate dehydrogenase deficiency are particularly susceptible to the haemolytic anaemias induced by methylene blue.

When methylene blue is used in the treatment of drug-induced methaemoglobinaemia as in nitrite poisoning, it is administered intravenously as a 1% solution in doses of 1 to 2 mg per kg bodyweight injected over a period of several minutes. A repeat dose may be given after one hour if required. It may be of some value in idiopathic methaemoglobinaemia; doses of up to 300 mg daily by mouth have been given.

Methylene blue is also used as a bacteriological stain, as a dye in diagnostic procedures such as fistula detection, and for the delineation of certain body tissues during surgery. It was formerly used in a renal-function test, and also in the treatment of urinary-tract infections.

DIAGNOSIS AND TESTING. References to the use of methylene blue as a colorant in diagnostic procedures: J. C. O'Sullivan (letter), *Br. med. J.*, 1973, *4*, 490 and 564 (tubal patency in female infertility); M. Nakajima *et al.*, *Am. J. Gastroent*, 1975, *63*, 240 (endoscopic examination of the duodenum); G. Girardi *et al.*, *Lancet*, 1978, *1*, 1236 (gastro-oesophageal reflux); C. E. Pope, *ibid.*, 1983, *1*, 1450 (gastro-oesophageal reflux dosage correction); F. L. M. Pattison (letter), *Can. med. Ass. J.*, 1983, *128*, 508 (*Neisseria gonorrhoeae* staining); K. Makiyama *et al.*, *Gut*, 1984, *25*, 337 (magnifying colonoscopy in Crohn's disease).

GLUTARICACIDURIA. Methylene blue may be of benefit in neonatal glutaricaciduria type II unresponsive to riboflavine.— J. -P. Harpey *et al.* (letter), *Lancet*, 1986, *1*, 391.

MANIC-DEPRESSIVE PSYCHOSIS. A 2-year double-blind crossover study of the prophylactic effect of methylene blue in 31 patients with recurrent bipolar manic-depressive psychosis; all patients were also taking lithium. During treatment with methylene blue 300 mg daily by mouth, the 17 patients who completed the study were significantly less depressed than when treated similarily with a placebo dose of 15 mg daily; no significant difference in the severity of manic symptoms was observed.— G. J. Naylor *et al.*, *Biol. Psychiat.*, 1986, *21*, 915.

SURGERY. Dudley (*Br. med. J.*, 1971, *3*, 680) demonstrated that methylene blue could be used successfully to stain and identify the parathyroid glands. The pre-operative intravenous administration of methylene blue injection in a dose of 5 mg per kg body-weight diluted in 500 mL of glucose-saline infused over 1 hour resulted in the staining of both normal and abnormal parathyroid glands, but adenomas could be distinguished by colour. Maximum staining occurred about 1 hour after infusion and lasted for about 20 minutes. No troublesome side-effects occurred, though the blue pallor of the patient had to be distinguished from cyanosis. Rowntree (*J. R. Soc. Med.*, 1980, *73*, 14) commented that the dose had to be related to lean body-weight as methylene blue was taken up by skeletal muscle but not by fat. High doses, if not diluted adequately, could cause thrombophlebitis; not more than 350 mg of methylene blue should be diluted in each 500 mL of infusion fluid. Bainbridge and Barnes (*Ann. R. Coll. Surg.*, 1983, *65*, 67) considered the use of intravenous dyes to facilitate intra-operative identification of the parathyroids a somewhat unneccessary exercise, but Young (*Br. J. Hosp. Med.*, 1984, *31*, 198) found it a valuable adjunct to parathyroid surgery.

Intra-operative localisation of small-bowel-bleeding sites with combined use of angiographic methods and methylene blue injection.— C. A. Athanasoulis *et al.*, *Surgery, St Louis*, 1980, *87*, 77.

Preparations

Methylene Blue Injection *(U.S.P.)*

Proprietary Preparations

Methylene Blue *(Harvey, USA: Farillon, UK). Solution*, methylene blue 1%, in ampoules of 10 mL.

Panatone *(Paines & Byrne, UK). Solution*, leucomethylene blue 1 mg/mL, in ampoules of 5 mL. For topical application for the delineation of the vagus nerve during vagotomy.

Proprietary Names and Manufacturers

Desmoid piller *(Denm.)*; Desmoidpillen *(Pohl, Ger.)*; Methylene Blue *(Harvey, USA; Farillon, UK)*; Panatone *(Paines & Byrne, UK)*; Urolene Blue *(Star, USA)*; Vitableu *(Faure, Fr.)*.

The following names have been used for multi-ingredient preparations containing methylene blue— Trac Tabs *(Hyrex, USA)*; Urised *(Webcon, USA)*; Uroblue *(Geneva, USA)*.

19554-r

Nalmefene *(USAN, pINN)*.

JF-1; Nalmetrene; ORF-11676. 17-(Cyclopropylmethyl)-4,5α-epoxy-6-methylenemorphinan-3,14-diol.

$C_{21}H_{25}NO_3$=339.4.

CAS — 55096-26-9.

Nalmefene is a specific opioid antagonist with actions similar to those of naloxone (p.845), but it may have a longer duration of action.

References: R. Dixon *et al.*, *Clin. Pharmac. Ther.*, 1986, *39*, 49 (pharmacokinetics after intravenous administration); K. M. Konieczko *et al.*, *Br. J. Anaesth.*, 1986, *58*, 1333P (opioid blockade after intravenous administration); T. J. Gal *et al.*, *Clin. Pharmac. Ther.*, 1986, *40*, 537 (opioid blockade after oral administration); R. Dixon *et al.*, *J. clin. Pharmac.*, 1987, *27*, 233 (pharmacokinetics after oral administration).

Proprietary Names and Manufacturers

Key, USA.

7304-k

Nalorphine Hydrobromide *(BANM, rINNM)*.

17-Allyl-17-normorphine hydrobromide; (−)-(5*R*,6*S*)-9a-Allyl-4,5-epoxymorphin-7-en-3,6-diol hydrobromide.

$C_{19}H_{21}NO_3$,HBr=392.3.

CAS — 62-67-9 (nalorphine); 1041-90-3 (hydrobromide).

Pharmacopoeias. In *Braz.*, *Chin.*, *Hung.*, and *It.* Also in *B.P. Vet.*

7305-a

Nalorphine Hydrochloride *(BANM, USAN, rINNM)*.

Nalorphini Hydrochloridum; Nalorphinium Chloride.

$C_{19}H_{21}NO_3$,HCl=347.8.

CAS — 57-29-4.

Pharmacopoeias. In *Arg.*, *Fr.*, *Ind.*, *Int.*, *Jug.*, *Nord.*, *Turk.*, and *U.S.*

Store in airtight containers. Protect from light.

Adverse Effects

Nalorphine may give rise to drowsiness, miosis, dysphoria, and lethargy; it may sometimes cause euphoria. There may be nausea, postural hypotension, and sweating. Nalorphine may also cause respiratory depression and induce disturbing psychotic effects. Mild withdrawal effects have been reported following prolonged administration, but it has little liability to abuse.

Precautions

As for Naloxone Hydrochloride (p.845). Nalorphine may exacerbate respiratory depression induced by low doses of opioids and non-opioid central depressants.

Absorption and Fate

Nalorphine is probably subject to considerable first-pass metabolism. It is largely metabolised in the liver and excreted in the urine. It crosses the placenta.

Uses and Administration

Nalorphine is an opioid antagonist with actions and uses similar to those of naloxone (p.845); in addition it also possesses some agonist properties. It should be used cautiously; nalorphine reverses severe opioid-induced respiratory depression but may exacerbate respiratory depression such as that induced by alcohol or other central non-opioid depressants.

In the treatment of opioid overdosage, nalorphine hydrobromide has been given by intravenous injection in a dose of 5 to 10 mg, repeated every 10 to 15 minutes as necessary. A maximum total dosage of 40 mg has been recommended but larger doses have been given. It has also been given intramuscularly or subcutaneously. Nalorphine hydrobromide has also been used to reverse neonatal respiratory depression following administration of opioid analgesics to the mother during labour.

Nalorphine hydrochloride has been used similarly.

Preparations

Nalorphine Hydrochloride Injection *(U.S.P.)*

Proprietary Names and Manufacturers

Lethidrone *(Wellcome, Austral.*; *Wellcome, S.Afr.*; *Wellcome, Switz.*; *Wellcome, UK)*; Norfin *(Lusofarmaco, Ital.)*.

7306-t

Naloxone Hydrochloride *(BANM, USAN, rINNM)*.

Allylnoroxymorphone Hydrochloride; EN-15304. 17-Allyl-6-deoxy-7,8-dihydro-14-hydroxy-6-oxo-17-normorphine hydrochloride; (−)-(5*R*,14*S*)-9a-Allyl-4,5-epoxy-3,14-dihydroxymorphinan-6-one hydrochloride.

$C_{19}H_{21}NO_4$,HCl=363.8.

CAS — 465-65-6 (naloxone); 357-08-4 (hydrochloride, anhydrous); 51481-60-8 (hydrochloride, dihydrate).

Pharmacopoeias. In *Braz.*, *Egypt.*, *It.*, and *U.S.* (anhydrous or dihydrate).

A white to slightly off-white powder. **Soluble** in water, dilute acids, and strong alkalis; slightly soluble in alcohol; practically insoluble in chloroform and ether. Aqueous solutions are acidic. **Store** in airtight containers. Protect from light.

It is recommended that infusions of naloxone hydrochloride should not be mixed with preparations containing bisulphite, metabisulphite, long-chain or high molecular weight anions, or solutions with an alkaline pH.

Adverse Effects

Adverse effects tend not to be a problem with naloxone at therapeutic doses. Nausea and vomiting have occurred and there have been individual reports of hypertension, cardiac arrhythmias, and pulmonary oedema, generally in patients given naloxone postoperatively. Seizures have also been reported infrequently.

Intravenous administration of high doses of naloxone 2 and 4 mg per kg body-weight to healthy subjects impaired cognitive performance and produced behavioural symptoms which included irritability, anxiety, sadness, difficulty in concentrating, and lack of appetite. Nausea and stomach-ache occurred frequently; tingling or numbness of extremities, dizziness, and occasionally yawning or sweating were also reported. Lower doses of naloxone 0.3 and 1 mg per kg had little or no discernible side-effects.— M. R. Cohen *et al.* (letter), *Lancet*, 1981, *2*, 1110.

Hypertension (G.Y. Tanaka, *J. Am. med. Ass.*, 1974, *228*, 25; I. Azar and H. Turndorf, *Anesth. Analg.*, 1979, *58*, 524), pulmonary oedema (J.W. Flacke *et al.*, *Anesthesiology*, 1977, *47*, 376), and cardiac arrhythmias including ventricular tachycardia and fibrillation (L.L. Michaelis *et al.*, *Ann. thorac. Surg.*, 1974, *18*, 608) have been reported following the use of naloxone postoperatively, generally in patients with pre-existing heart disease undergoing cardiac surgery. However, Taff (*Anesthesiology*, 1983, *59*, 576) reported a case of pulmonary oedema after postoperative intravenous administration of naloxone in increments of 40 to 80 μg over 5 to 10 minutes to a total of 300 μg in a healthy young man with no previous history of heart disease. Taff considered this case to be particularly significant because the recommendations for smaller incremental doses to be given over a longer time period had been followed.

Ventricular fibrillation has been observed in an opioid addict after administration of naloxone to reverse the effects of diamorphine (F.M. Cuss *et al.*, *Br. med. J.*, 1984, *288*, 363). However, this patient was later shown to have hepatic cirrhosis and alcoholic cardiomyopathy and the National Poisons Information Service in London noted that it had never been informed of such a suspected adverse reaction despite being contacted in about 800 cases of opiate poisoning each year (L. Barret *et al.*, *Br. med. J.*, 1984, *288*, 936).

Precautions

Naloxone hydrochloride should be used with caution in patients physically dependent on opioids, or who have received large doses of opioids, as an acute withdrawal syndrome may be precipitated (see under Morphine, Dependence, p. 1310). A withdrawal syndrome may also be precipitated in newborn infants of opioid-dependent mothers.

The duration of action of some opioids exceeds that of naloxone; patients should therefore be carefully observed after administration in case of relapse.

Absorption and Fate

Naloxone is absorbed from the gastro-intestinal tract but it is subject to considerable first-pass metabolism. It is metabolised in the liver, mainly by glucuronide conjugation, and excreted in the urine. It has a short plasma half-life of approximately one hour after parenteral administration.

A study *in vitro* on the protein binding of naloxone in adult and foetal plasma. The percentages of free naloxone in samples of plasma from 18 adults, 3 parturient women, and 18 neonates were 54.1%, 53.2%, and 61.5% respectively.— L. A. Asali and K. F. Brown, *Eur. J. clin. Pharmac.*, 1984, *27*, 459.

Pregnancy and the neonate. In 12 newborn infants given naloxone hydrochloride 35 or 70 μg intravenously via the umbilical vein, the mean plasma half-lives of naloxone were 3.53 and 2.65 hours respectively. These half-lives were 2 to 3 times longer than those reported for adults, possibly due to a diminished ability of the newborn to metabolise drugs by conjugation with glucuronic acid. Mean peak plasma concentrations of 8.2 ng per mL in those given 35 μg, and 13.7 ng per mL in those given 70 μg, were reached within 40 minutes of administration but this time was very variable, and in 5 infants peak plasma concentrations were reached within 5 minutes. When naloxone hydrochloride 200 μg was administered intramuscularly to 17 further newborn infants, peak concentrations of 7.4 to 34.6 ng per mL occurred at 0.5 to 2 hours.— T. A. Moreland *et al.*, *Br. J. clin. Pharmac.*, 1980, *9*, 609.

A study in 30 mothers given a single intravenous dose of naloxone during the second stage of labour, indicated that naloxone rapidly crossed the placental barrier so that some therapeutic effect might be anticipated in most babies. Placental transfer in 7 further mothers given naloxone intramuscularly was considered to be too variable for therapeutic purposes.— B. M. Hibbard *et al.*, *Br. J. Anaesth.*, 1986, *58*, 45.

Uses and Administration

Naloxone is a specific opioid antagonist that acts competitively at opioid receptors. It is an effective antagonist of opioids with agonist or mixed agonist-antagonist activity though larger doses may be needed for compounds with the latter activity. It is used to reverse opioid central depression, including respiratory depression, induced by natural or synthetic opioids.

Naloxone hydrochloride is usually given intravenously for a rapid onset of action which occurs within 2 minutes. The onset of action is only slightly less rapid when it is administered intramuscularly or subcutaneously. The duration of action of naloxone is dependent on the dose and route of administration; it may be 1 to 4 hours but may also be much shorter.

In the treatment of known or suspected opioid overdosage, an initial dose of naloxone hydrochloride 0.4 to 2 mg may be given intravenously and repeated if necessary at intervals of 2 to 3 minutes. If no response has been observed after a total dose of 10 mg then the diagnosis of overdosage with drugs other than opioids should be considered. In children, the usual initial dose is 10 μg per kg body-weight intravenously followed, if necessary, by a larger dose of 100 μg per kg.

Naloxone hydrochloride may also be used postoperatively to reverse central depression resulting from the use of opioids during surgery. A dose of 100 to 200 μg (1.5 to 3 μg per kg) may be given intravenously at intervals of at least 2 minutes to obtain an optimum respiratory response while maintaining adequate analgesia.

All patients receiving naloxone should be closely observed as the duration of action of some opioids exceeds that of naloxone and repeated doses by intravenous, intramuscular, or subcutaneous injection may be required. Alternatively, to sustain opioid antagonism, an intravenous infusion of naloxone hydrochloride has been suggested. Naloxone hydrochloride 4 μg per mL in sodium chloride injection (0.9%) or glucose injection (5%) may be infused at a rate titrated in accordance with the patient's response both to the infusion and previous bolus injections. Naloxone should not be mixed with preparations containing bisulphite, metabisulphite, long-chain or high molecular weight anions, or solutions with an alkaline pH.

Opioid-induced depression in neonates resulting from the administration of opioid analgesics to the mother during labour may be reversed by administering naloxone hydrochloride 10 μg per kg body-weight to the infant by intramuscular, intravenous or subcutaneous injection, repeated at intervals of 2 to 3 minutes if necessary. Alternatively, a single intramuscular dose of about 60 μg per kg may be given at birth for a more prolonged action.

Naloxone hydrochloride has been used to produce opioid blockade for the maintenance of addicts after opioid withdrawal in doses of up to 3 g by mouth. Some opioid analgesics have been formulated in combination with naloxone hydrochloride to reduce their potential for parenteral abuse.

Naloxone hydrochloride has also been used cautiously in small doses to diagnose opioid dependence by precipitating the withdrawal syndrome (see under naltrexone hydrochloride, p.846).

Review of the pharmacology of naloxone with respect to its effects on blood pressure, central nervous system ischaemia, respiration, mental illness, and non-opioid depressant drugs.— L. F. McNicholas and W. R. Martin, *Drugs*, 1984, *27*, 81. Further references on the pharmacology of naloxone: J. W. Holaday, *Annu. Rev. Pharmacol. Toxicol.*, 1983, *23*, 541 (effects on the cardiovascular system); A. I. Faden, *J. Am. med. Ass.*, 1984, *252*, 1177 (effects on blood pressure and shock); *idem*, 1452 (effects on central nervous system ischaemia after stroke and spinal cord injury).

Adjunct to intraspinal opioid analgesia. Naloxone reversed respiratory depression without abolition of pain relief in a patient given intrathecal morphine.— R. D. M. Jones and J. G. Jones, *Br. med. J.*, 1980, *281*, 645.

Urinary retention after epidural morphine was reversed by naloxone without reversal of analgesia.— N. Rawal *et al.* (letter), *Lancet*, 1981, *2*, 1411.

Administration. To overcome some of the problems inherent in a multiple intermittent intravenous dosing regimen, continuous intravenous administration of naloxone has been suggested. Although there have been several reports of the successful treatment of prolonged opioid overdosage with naloxone infusions (J.C. Bradberry and M.A. Raebel, *Drug Intell. & clin. Pharm.*, 1981, *15*, 945; G.K. Gourlay and K. Coulthard, *Br. J. clin. Pharmac.*, 1983, *15*, 269; N. Redfern, *Br. med. J.*, 1983, *287*, 751; S.G. Parker and D.G. Thomas, *ibid.*, 1547), definitive dosing guidelines have not yet been established (D.R. Romac, *Clin. Pharm.*, 1986, *5*, 251). Vale and Buckley (*Br. med. J.*, 1984, *288*, 406) considered that an infusion of naloxone alone was hazardous unless preceded by an adequate intravenous bolus injection of naloxone of not less than 1.2 mg to resuscitate the patient; continuous infusion was no substitute for frequent observation and appropriate intervention.

Anorexia. Naloxone infusions of up to 6.4 mg daily for 1 to 11 weeks were associated with a significantly increased weight gain in 12 patients with anorexia nervosa also receiving antidepressants and psychotherapy. An antilipolytic action for naloxone was suggested.— R. Moore *et al.*, *J. R. Soc. Med.*, 1981, *74*, 129. See also under Obesity, below.

Cerebrovascular disorders. Naloxone reversal of neurological deficits in patients with cerebral ischaemia has been reported (D.S. Baskin and Y. Hosobuchi, *Lancet*, 1981, *2*, 272; J.-Y. Bousigue *et al.*, *ibid.*, 1982, *2*, 618). However, Fallis *et al.* (*Stroke*, 1984, *15*, 627) found naloxone to be ineffective in reversing the neurological deficits of 15 patients with acute stroke and Parraro *et al.* (*Lancet*, 1984, *1*, 915) were unable to demonstrate a significant effect of naloxone on neurological motor deficits of acute onset. In a study by Jabaily and Davis (*Stroke*, 1984, *15*, 36) naloxone 0.8 to 1.2 mg administered intravenously improved the neurological status in 3 of 13 patients with cerebral infarction or ischaemia, although in one of these patients reversal was permanent and could have been spontaneous resolution. Naloxone reversal of neurological deficits appeared to be a rare event; results did not support routine administration.

Dementia. In a double-blind study in 7 patients with senile dementia of the Alzheimer type, administration of naloxone 1, 5, or 10 mg intravenously resulted in significant clinical and psychometric improvement.— B. Reisberg *et al.* (letter), *New Engl. J. Med.*, 1983, *308*, 721. In contrast, results of preliminary open studies indicated no notable improvements in 35 patients with Alzheimer's disease given naloxone 1 to 5 mg intravenously.— J. P. Blass *et al.* (letter), *ibid.*, *309*, 556. No cognitive measures improved after intravenous naloxone administration at doses of 0.1 mg per kg body-weight or 2 mg per kg in a double-blind study involving 12 patients with dementia of the Alzheimer type. Global assessments of restlessness, drowsiness, and irritability were increased.— P. N. Tariot *et al.*, *Psychopharmac. Bull.*, 1985, *21*, 680.

Extrapyramidal disorders. Naloxone 400 μg intravenously significantly reduced orofacial dyskinetic movements in a schizophrenic woman but had no effect in a second similar patient.— I. Blum *et al.*, *Clin. Neuropharmacol.*, 1984, *7*, 265.

Gastro-intestinal disorders. In 4 healthy subjects naloxone reversed pentazocine-induced delay in gastric emptying. Naloxone might be useful to reverse opioid effects on gastric emptying before the induction of anaesthesia during labour or in recurrent vomiting.— W. S. Nimmo *et al.*, *Br. med. J.*, 1979, *2*, 1189. In a placebo-controlled study involving 30 women in labour who had been given pethidine for analgesia, naloxone 1.2 mg intravenously appeared at least transiently to increase the rate of gastric emptying.— W. T. Frame *et al.*, *Br. J. Anaesth.*, 1984, *56*, 263.

Naloxone was of benefit in two patients with severe chronic idiopathic constipation.— M. -J. Kreek *et al.*, *Lancet*, 1983, *1*, 261. Criticism.— D. M. Preston and P. R. H. Barnes (letter), *ibid.*, 758.

Mania. See under Schizophrenia.

Menopausal flushing. Naloxone significantly reduced the frequency of flushes paralleled by a decrease in the number of pulses of luteinising hormone secretion in 5 of 6 climacteric women.— S. L. Lightman *et al.*, *Br. J. Obstet. Gynaec.*, 1981, *88*, 919. In 7 postmenopausal women, naloxone had no effect on the occurrence of hot flushes, episodic skin temperature elevations, or luteinising hormone secretion.— T. Tulandi *et al.*, *Am. J. Obstet. Gynec.*, 1985, *151*, 277.

Obesity. Naloxone 0.8 and 1.6 mg administered subcutaneously reduced food intake over an 8 hour period in 2 of 3 patients with Prader-Willi syndrome characterised by hyperphagia and gross obesity.— M. Kyriakides *et al.* (letter), *Lancet*, 1980, *1*, 876. Naloxone may suppress calorie intake by delaying gastric emptying rather than by acting at a hypothalamic level.— S. N. Sullivan, *ibid.*, 1140.

In a double-blind study, administration of an intravenous bolus injection of naloxone 500 μg per kg body-weight reduced the day-long calorie intake in 5 of 6 obese subjects. These results indicated that endogenous opioids might have a role in human eating and further studies of opioid antagonists in the treatment of obesity were suggested.— O. M. Wolkowitz *et al.* (letter), *New Engl. J. Med.*, 1985, *313*, 327. See also under naltrexone hydrochloride (p.847).

For a report of naloxone increasing weight gain in patients with anorexia nervosa, see under Anorexia, above.

Pain insensitivity. Results suggesting that congenital insensitivity to pain was related to a tonic hyperactivity of a morphine-like pain-inhibitory system, antagonised by naloxone.— H. Dehen *et al.* (letter), *Lancet*, 1977, *2*, 293. Naloxone failed to elicit any sensitivity to painful stimuli in 2 patients with congenital insensitivity to pain. Two forms of this disorder might exist, one naloxone antagonisable and the other not.— A. Pasi *et al.* (letter), *ibid.*, 1982, *1*, 622.

PREGNANCY AND THE NEONATE. Review of the use of naloxone for opioid-induced respiratory depression in newborn infants of mothers given opioid analgesics during labour. Central and respiratory depression in neonates might be attributable to many factors, customary resuscitation efforts should therefore be initiated immediately. The American Academy of Pediatrics Committee on Drugs recommended that naloxone should be reserved for adjunctive therapy in selected infants who had not initiated or established independent respiration following ventilation, who were significantly depressed, and who had a high probability of being narcotised. There was no clear-cut evidence to support routine use in opioid-exposed neonates and it was recommended that naloxone should not be administered to the infants of opioid-dependent mothers as a withdrawal syndrome might be precipitated.— *Pediatrics*, 1980, *65*, 667.

For studies indicating that naloxone might be useful in reversing the effects of opioid analgesics on gastric emptying during labour, see under Gastro-intestinal Disorders, above.

PRURITUS. Sustained clinical improvement with naloxone in one patient with generalised itch of unknown origin and in a second with a history of asthma, chronic urticaria, and angioedema.— S. Smitz *et al.* (letter), *Ann. intern. Med.*, 1982, *97*, 788.

RESPIRATORY FAILURE. An intravenous infusion of naloxone 200 µg per minute increased tidal volume and oxygen saturation in a patient with acute on chronic respiratory failure; after recovery the patient showed no response to naloxone. There might be overproduction of, or increased sensitivity to, endorphins in acute respiratory failure.— J. Ayres *et al.*, *Br. med. J.*, 1982, *284*, 927. Further report of beneficial results with naloxone in acute respiratory failure.— A. J. Williams *et al.* (letter), *Lancet*, 1982, *2*, 1470.

SCHIZOPHRENIA. Results of double-blind studies examining the effects of naloxone on schizophrenia were conflicting; some reported a significant reduction in symptoms, while others found no difference from placebo. Similarly, although there had been reports of naloxone reducing manic symptoms in some patients, one study had found naloxone to have no overall effect in such patients. A World Health Organization collaborative project investigated the behavioural effects of a single subcutaneous dose of naloxone hydrochloride 300 µg per kg body-weight in 32 schizophrenic patients and 26 manic patients in a multicentre double-blind placebo-controlled study. Significant drug effects indicating naloxone-associated improvement were found in the schizophrenic patients receiving concurrent treatment with neuroleptics but not in those who were medication-free. There was a significant improvement in auditory hallucinations in the neuroleptic-treated patients as assessed by self-ratings, and for the schizophrenic group as a whole when assessed by physician-ratings. Caution was recommended in extrapolating these results to any overall effectiveness of naloxone in schizophrenia and further long-term studies were needed, possibly with oral, long-acting opioid antagonists such as naltrexone. Naloxone was of no apparent benefit in the manic patients.— D. Pickar *et al.*, *Archs gen. Psychiat.*, 1982, *39*, 313. Criticism; the value of earlier positive reports of naloxone-associated improvement in schizophrenia may have been overrated and biased the study.— P. Skrabanek (letter), *Lancet*, 1982, *2*, 1270.

SHOCK. Anecdotal clinical reports indicated beneficial effects with naloxone in the treatment of septic and cardiogenic shock refractory to conventional therapy (M. Tiengo, *Lancet*, 1980, *2*, 690; R. Dirksen *et al.*, *ibid.*, 1360; D.J.M. Wright *et al.*, *ibid.*, 1361; W.R. Swinburn and P. Phelan, *ibid.*, 1982, *1*, 167). Peters *et al.*, (*ibid.*, 1981, *1*, 529) reported an immediate and striking increase in blood pressure after naloxone administration in 8 of 9 patients with sustained hypotension; 3 similar patients taking high doses of corticosteroids and one with hypoadrenocorticotropism did not respond. Higgins *et al.* (*Ann. intern. Med.*, 1983, *98*, 47) obtained favourable results using naloxone administered by bolus injection and infusion in an 80-year-old man with profound hypotension unresponsive to conventional treatment. However, in a double-blind study of 22 patients with septic shock, there was no significant difference in blood-pressure response between patients given intravenous bolus injections of naloxone hydrochloride 0.4 to 1.2 mg and placebo (vehicle of the commercially available injection) (A. DeMaria *et al.*, *Lancet*, 1985, *1*, 1363). Soulioti (*ibid.*, *2*, 452) suggested that the vehicle itself might have inherent effects. Pending the results of further work in animals and controlled clinical studies on survival as well as haemodynamic function, the widespread use of naloxone to treat shock was to be discouraged (J. W. Holaday and A. I. Faden, *ibid.*, 1981, *2*, 201). Roberts *et al.*, (ibid., 1988, *2*, 699) gave naloxone by continuous intravenous infusion to patients with septic shock and found that a positive haemodynamic effect only occurred 4 hours or more after the initial bolus injection.

TREATMENT OF OVERDOSAGE. *Alcohol.* For a review of studies on naloxone in the treatment of alcohol intoxication and an opinion that in view of the conflicting results there was no justification for the routine use of naloxone for this indication, see under Alcohol, p.950.

Chlorpromazine. Naloxone was successfully used to treat a 4-year-old boy with severe central nervous system depression associated with chlorpromazine ingestion.— O. Chandavasu and S. Chatkupt, *J. Pediat.*, 1985, *106*, 515.

Diazepam. Results of a study suggested that a large dose of naloxone 15 mg might be effective in relieving respiratory depression following diazepam overdosage.— C. Jordan *et al.*, *Br. J. Anaesth.*, 1979, *51*, 570P. Results of a double-blind study failed to demonstrate any antagonising action of naloxone on diazepam-induced sedation.— K. N. Christensen and M. Hüttel (letter), *Anesthesiology*, 1979, *51*, 187.

Preparations

Naloxone Hydrochloride Injection *(U.S.P.)*. A sterile iso-osmotic solution of naloxone hydrochloride in Water for Injections. It may contain suitable preservatives. pH 3.0 to 4.5.

Pentazocine and Naloxone Hydrochlorides Tablets *(U.S.P.)*

Proprietary Preparations

Min-I-Jet Naloxone Hydrochloride *(IMS, UK)*. *Injection*, naloxone hydrochloride 400 µg/mL, in single-use pre-filled syringes of 1 and 2 mL.

Narcan *(Du Pont Pharmaceuticals, UK)*. *Injection*, naloxone hydrochloride 400 µg/mL, in ampoules of 1 mL and vials of 10 mL. *Injection* (Narcan Neonatal), naloxone hydrochloride 20 µg/mL, in ampoules of 2 mL.

Proprietary Names and Manufacturers

Min-I-Jet Naloxone Hydrochloride *(IMS, UK)*; Nalonee *(Denm.; Fin.; Iceland; Norw.; Swed.)*; Narcan *(Aust.; Du Pont, Austral.; Belg.; Du Pont, Canad.; Du Pont de Nemours, Fr.; Crinos, Ital.; Neth.; Boots, S.Afr.; Du Pont de Nemours, Switz.; Du Pont Pharmaceuticals, UK; Du Pont, USA)*; Narcanti *(Du Pont, Denm.; DuPont, Ger.; Du Pont, Norw.; Du Pont, Swed.)*.

The following names have been used for multi-ingredient preparations containing naloxone hydrochloride— Talwin Nx *(Winthrop-Breon, USA)*.

7307-x

Naltrexone Hydrochloride *(BANM, rINNM)*.

EN-1639A. (5*R*)-*N*-Cyclopropylmethyl-3,14-dihydroxy-4,5-epoxymorphinan-6-one hydrochloride.

$C_{20}H_{23}NO_4,HCl = 377.9$.

CAS — 16590-41-3 (naltrexone); 16676-29-2 (hydrochloride).

NOTE. Naltrexone is *USAN*.

Adverse Effects

The adverse effects of naltrexone are usually transient and mild; some may be associated with opioid withdrawal. Difficulty in sleeping, lethargy, anxiety, dysphoria, abdominal pain, nausea, vomiting, alterations of appetite, joint and muscle pain, and headache may occur. Other side-effects including dizziness, nasal congestion, skin rashes, thrombocytopenic purpura, genito-urinary problems, minor increases in blood pressure, and non-specific ECG changes have also been reported. High doses may cause hepatocellular injury.

EFFECTS ON APPETITE. Four detoxified opiate addicts taking naltrexone experienced a marked reduction of appetite and loss of weight which required discontinuation of the drug.— H. A. Sternbach *et al.* (letter), *Lancet*, 1982, *1*, 388.

EFFECTS ON THE LIVER. Raised transaminase levels were noted in 5 of 26 obese patients after 3 weeks' treatment with naltrexone 300 mg daily; transaminase activity returned to normal when treatment was stopped. In view of the dose-related hepatotoxicity of naltrexone, further studies should avoid using high dosages.— J. E. Mitchell (letter), *Lancet*, 1986, *1*, 1215.

Precautions

Naltrexone should be avoided in patients taking opioids for medication or abuse as an acute withdrawal syndrome may be precipitated (see under Naloxone Hydrochloride, Precautions, p.845). Naltrexone should be discontinued at least 48 hours before elective surgery involving opioid analgesia. For further precautions when administering naltrexone hydrochloride as an adjunct in the treatment of opioid dependence, see under Uses and Administration, below.

Naltrexone should be used with caution in patients with hepatic dysfunction and is contra-indicated in patients with acute hepatitis or liver failure. Regular monitoring of hepatic function has been recommended.

Absorption and Fate

Naltrexone is well absorbed from the gastro-intestinal tract but is subject to considerable first-pass metabolism. It is extensively metabolised in the liver and may be recycled by the enterohepatic circulation. Naltrexone and its metabolites are excreted in the urine. The major metabolite, 6-β-naltrexol may also possess opioid antagonist activity.

Studies on the pharmacokinetics of naltrexone: K. Verebey *et al.*, *Clin. Pharmac. Ther.*, 1976, *20*, 315; M. E. Wall *et al.*, *Drug Metab. & Disposit.*, 1981, *9*, 369; M. E. Wall *et al.*, *ibid.*, 1984, *12*, 677; M. C. Meyer *et al.*, *J. clin. Psychiat.*, 1984, *45*, 15.

Preliminary pharmacokinetic evaluation of the sustained release of naltrexone from subcutaneous implants in 3 healthy subjects. Plasma-naltrexone concentrations were maintained at a relatively constant level for approximately one month but 2 of the subjects had local irritation at the site of implantation.— C. N. Chiang *et al.*, *Clin. Pharmac. Ther.*, 1984, *36*, 704.

Uses and Administration

Naltrexone is a specific opioid antagonist with actions similar to those of naloxone (p.845), however, it is more potent than naloxone and has a longer duration of action. It reversibly blocks the pharmacological effects of opioids and is used in the treatment of opioid dependence as an aid to maintaining abstinence following opioid withdrawal.

Naltrexone treatment should not be started until the patient has been detoxified and abstinent from opioids for at least 7 to 10 days; abstinence should be verified by analysis of the patient's urine. A naloxone challenge test should then be administered to confirm the absence of opioid dependence. Naloxone hydrochloride 200 µg should be administered intravenously and the patient observed for 30 seconds for evidence of withdrawal symptoms; if none occur a further dose of 600 µg should be given and the patient observed for 20 minutes; alternatively, naloxone hydrochloride 800 µg may be administered subcutaneously and the patient observed for 45 minutes. A confirmatory rechallenge with naloxone hydrochloride 1.6 mg intravenously may be considered if results are ambiguous. The administration of naltrexone should be delayed until a negative naloxone challenge test has been obtained.

Naltrexone hydrochloride is given by mouth. Treatment may be initiated with a dose of 25 mg and the patient then observed for an hour; if no signs of opioid withdrawal occur the remainder of the daily dose may be given. Lower initial doses have been used and some alternative regimens have involved gradually increasing an initial daily dose over several days. The usual maintenance dose of naltrexone hydrochloride is 350 mg weekly administered as 50 mg daily by mouth but the dosing interval may be lengthened to improve compliance; doses of 100 mg on alternate days or 150 mg every third day may be effective and intermittent dosage regimens have been used. Patients should be carefully counselled and warned that attempts to overcome the opioid blockade with large doses of opioids could result in fatal opioid intoxication.

BULIMIA. Significant reductions in bulimic symptoms were noted in 5 women with normal-weight bulimia after 6-weeks treatment with naltrexone.— J. M. Jonas and M. S. Gold (letter), *Lancet*, 1986, *1*, 807. See also.— idem, *Int. J. Psychiatry Med.*, 1987, *16*, 305.

ERECTILE DYSFUNCTION. Naltrexone 25 to 50 mg daily was of benefit in 6 of 7 men with idiopathic erectile dysfunction.— J. A. Goldstein (letter), *Ann. intern. Med.*, 1986, *105*, 799.

OBESITY. In a double-blind study involving 20 obese men and 40 obese women, 8 weeks' treatment with naltrexone 50 or 100 mg daily by mouth in 35 patients had no significant effect on weight loss in the group as a whole but evaluation of the results by sex did indicate a small but significant effect in women. Elevations in liver enzyme values occurred in 6 patients while taking naltrexone.— R. L. Atkinson *et al.*, *Clin. Pharmac. Ther.*, 1985, *38*, 419. See also under Naloxone Hydrochloride Uses and Administration, p.845.

OPIOID WITHDRAWAL. Reviews of naltrexone and its use as an adjunct in the management of opioid dependence: B. L. Crabtree, *Clin. Pharm.*, 1984, *3*, 273; *Med. Lett.*, 1985, *27*, 11; H. M. Ginzburg and M. G. MacDonald, *Med. Toxicol.*, 1987, *2*, 83; J. P. Gonzalez and R. N. Brogden, *Drugs*, 1988, *35*, 192.

Combined treatment with clonidine and naltrexone enabled 38 of 40 opioid addicts to withdraw completely and rapidly from long-term methadone therapy.— D. S. Charney *et al.*, *Am. J. Psychiat.*, 1986, *143*, 831.

Proprietary Names and Manufacturers

Nalorex *(Du Pont de Nemours, Fr.; Du Pont Pharmaceuticals, UK)*; Trexan *(Du Pont, USA)*.

1043-w

Obidoxime Chloride *(USAN, rINN)*.

LüH6. 1,1′-(Oxydimethylene)bis(4-hydroxyiminomethylpyridinium) dichloride.
$C_{14}H_{16}Cl_2N_4O_3$=359.2.

CAS — 7683-36-5 (obidoxime); 114-90-9 (chloride).

Pharmacopoeias. In *Swiss*.

Obidoxime chloride is a cholinesterase reactivator with similar actions and uses to pralidoxime (p.851). It is usually given in doses of 3 to 6 mg per kg body-weight by intramuscular or slow intravenous injection.

Obidoxime chloride, 2.5 to 10 mg per kg body-weight, given intramuscularly to 10 healthy men produced dose-related peak plasma concentrations within 30 minutes. The average half-life was 82.8 minutes, 84% of the dose being excreted unchanged in the urine in 24 hours. Side-effects included pain at the site of the injection, mild to moderate tachycardia and hypertension, transient paraesthesia, numbness and a sensation of warmth in the facial area, and a taste of menthol.— F. R. Sidell and W. A. Groff, *J. pharm. Sci.*, 1970, *59*, 793. Further studies on the pharmacokinetics of obidoxime chloride: *idem*, 1971, *60*, 860 (oral administration); F. R. Sidell *et al.*, *ibid.*, 1972, *61*, 1765 (comparison with pralidoxime after intravenous administration).

For references to the actions and uses of oximes in the treatment of organophosphorus poisoning, see under Uses and Administration in Pralidoxime Methylsulphate, p.851.

Proprietary Names and Manufacturers

Toxogonin *(E. Merck, Denm.; E. Merck, Ger.; E. Merck, Neth.; Merck, S.Afr.; E. Merck, Swed.)*.

1045-l

Penicillamine *(BAN, USAN, rINN)*.

D-Penicillamine. D-3,3-Dimethylcysteine; D-3-Mercaptovaline.
$C_5H_{11}NO_2S$=149.2.

CAS — 52-67-5 (penicillamine); 2219-30-9 (hydrochloride).

Pharmacopoeias. In *Br.*, *Cz.*, *Eur.*, *It.*, *Jug.*, and *U.S.*

A white or almost white, finely crystalline powder with a slight characteristic odour. **Soluble** 1 in 9 of water; slightly soluble in alcohol; practically insoluble in chloroform and ether. A 1% solution in water has a pH of 4.5 to 5.5. **Store** in airtight containers.

Adverse Effects and Treatment

Side-effects of penicillamine are frequent but many are reversible when the drug is withdrawn. Gastro-intestinal disturbances including anorexia, nausea, and vomiting may occur; oral ulceration and stomatitis have been reported and impaired taste sensitivity is common.

Skin rashes occurring early in treatment are commonly allergic and may be associated with pruritus, urticaria, and fever; they are usually transient but temporary drug withdrawal and treatment with corticosteroids or antihistamines may be required. Lupus erythematosus and pemphigus have been reported. A Stevens-Johnson-like syndrome has been observed during penicillamine treatment. Prolonged use of high doses may affect skin collagen and elastin, resulting in increased skin friability, elastosis perforans serpiginosa, and acquired epidermolysis bullosa (penicillamine dermatopathy).

Haematological side-effects have included thrombocytopenia and less frequently leucopenia; these are usually reversible but agranulocytosis, aplastic anaemia, and haemolytic anaemia have occurred and fatalities have been reported.

Proteinuria occurs frequently and in some patients may progress to glomerulonephritis or nephrotic syndrome. Penicillamine-induced haematuria is rare but normally requires drug discontinuation.

Other side-effects associated with penicillamine include Goodpasture's syndrome, obliterative bronchiolitis, myasthenia gravis, polymyositis, intrahepatic cholestasis, and pancreatitis.

Comparison of penicillamine toxicity in rheumatoid disease between 34 patients aged 60 years or over and a group of 67 younger patients. Penicillamine was of a similar efficacy in both groups but severe toxicity overall was significantly greater in the elderly. The incidence of skin rashes and severe taste abnormalities was significantly increased in the elderly group but there was no difference between the two groups in the incidence of mouth ulcers, haematological side-effects, proteinuria, or gastro-intestinal symptoms; 4 patients (3 in the elderly group) developed the nephrotic syndrome.— W. F. Kean *et al.*, *J. Am. Geriat. Soc.*, 1982, *30*, 94.

A study of penicillamine toxicity in 259 patients with systemic sclerosis given penicillamine in doses of 125 to 2000 mg (mean 635 mg) daily for 0.1 to 7.5 years (mean 1.8 years). A total of 144 side-effects occurred in 123 (47%) patients; penicillamine was successfully re-instituted following temporary withdrawal in 69 (28%) patients, but adverse effects required permanent discontinuation of therapy in 75 (29%) patients. The rate of increase in dosage appeared to be closely associated with the risk of toxicity. The main side-effects encountered were: cutaneous reactions (in 41 patients), nausea (20), fever (7), altered taste (7), mouth ulcers (7), thrombocytopenia (10), leucopenia (6), proteinuria (24), haematuria (5), and myasthenia gravis (4). A comparison of these results with those reported in previous studies on penicillamine toxicity in patients with rheumatoid arthritis, indicated that the side-effects were of a similar type and frequency, except that patients with systemic sclerosis might have an increased risk of developing other auto-immune diseases such as pemphigus and myasthenia gravis.— V. D. Steen *et al.*, *Ann. intern. Med.*, 1986, *104*, 699.

Of 20 patients with rheumatoid arthritis taking comparable doses of penicillamine, 5 of 6 patients with a poor capacity for producing sulphoxides developed toxic complications compared with only one of 14 patients who were extensive sulphoxidisers.— G. S. Panayi *et al.* (letter), *Lancet*, 1983, *1*, 414. Further results suggesting that the sulphoxidation capacity of an individual, although not the only factor involved, might be a significant determinant of penicillamine toxicity in rheumatoid patients. Measurements of the sulphoxidation capacity before starting penicillamine therapy might help identify those patients most at risk.— P. Emery *et al.*, *Br. J. clin. Pharmac.*, 1984, *18*, 286P. The poor sulphoxidation capacity found in many patients with primary biliary cirrhosis might partly explain their high incidence of adverse reactions to penicillamine therapy.— A. Olomu *et al.* (letter), *Lancet*, 1985, *1*, 1504. Confirmation of a high prevalence of impaired sulphoxidation in patients with primary biliary cirrhosis but failure to show any strong association between poor sulphoxidisers and penicillamine toxicity.— H. C. Mitchison *et al.*, *Gut*, 1986, *27*, A622.

ALLERGY. A report of urticaria, bronchial spasm, and angioedema in a woman receiving penicillamine for rheumatoid arthritis.— K. Tanphaichitr, *Sth. med. J.*, 1980, *73*, 788.

For a review of penicillamine-induced skin lesions including acute sensitivity reactions, see under Effects on the Skin, below.

EFFECTS ON THE BLOOD. Of the 18 deaths ascribed to penicillamine reported to the Committee on Safety of Medicines between January 1964 and December 1977, fourteen were apparently due to blood disorders, at least 7 of them being marrow aplasias. The myelotoxicity of penicillamine was reviewed in 10 patients with confirmed or suspected marrow depression during penicillamine treatment for rheumatoid arthritis or scleroderma; 6 of those 10 patients died.— A. G. L. Kay, *Ann. rheum. Dis.*, 1979, *38*, 232.

A 56-year-old woman developed agranulocytosis and toxic epidermal necrolysis 7 weeks after starting therapy with penicillamine 250 mg daily for primary biliary cirrhosis.— K. Ward and D. G. Weir, *Ir. J. med. Sci.*, 1981, *150*, 252.

Penicillamine-induced thrombocytopenia had a reported incidence of 12 to 27% in patients with rheumatoid arthritis and appeared to be due to bone-marrow suppression and a reduced platelet-production rate.— D. Thomas *et al.*, *Ann. rheum. Dis.*, 1984, *43*, 402.

Further reports of blood dyscrasias associated with penicillamine: E. E. Harrison and J. W. Hickman (letter), *Lancet*, 1976, *1*, 38 (thrombocytopenia and haemolytic anaemia); W. A. C. McAllister and J. A. Vale (letter), *ibid.*, *2*, 631 (fatal aplastic anaemia); A. J. Barnett and M. G. Whiteside (letter), *ibid.*, 682 (aplastic anaemia); S. Jones *et al.*, *Postgrad. med. J.*, 1978, *54*, 834 (erythro-myeloid aplasia); J. M. Trice *et al.*, *Archs intern. Med.*, 1983, *143*, 1487 (thrombotic thrombocytopenic purpura).

For reports of leukaemia in patients treated with penicillamine, see under Malignant Neoplasms, below.

EFFECTS ON THE BREAST. Breast enlargement has been reported in women taking penicillamine and may be a rare complication of penicillamine therapy (C. Passas and A. Weinstein, *Arthritis Rheum.*, 1978, *21*, 167; D.C.N. Thew and I.M. Stewart, *Ann. rheum. Dis.*, 1980, *39*, 200). In some patients breast enlargement was prolonged with poor resolution and others required surgery. Danazol has been used successfully to treat penicillamine-induced breast gigantism (P.J. Taylor *et al.*, *Br. med. J.*, 1981, *282*, 362; P.J. Rooney and J. Cleland, *ibid.*, 1627).

Gynaecomastia developed in a 30-year-old man 7 months after starting penicillamine treatment for rheumatoid arthritis. Symptoms receded 2 months after the drug had been discontinued.— D. M. Reid *et al.*, *Br. med. J.*, 1982, *285*, 1083.

EFFECTS ON THE EYE. Retinal pigment epithelial changes in a patient on long-term penicillamine treatment for Wilson's disease.— J. Dingle and W. H. Havener, *Ann. Ophthal.*, 1978, *10*, 1227.

EFFECTS ON THE GASTRO-INTESTINAL TRACT. Acute colitis in a 61-year-old woman with rheumatoid arthritis was attributed to penicillamine which had been started about 4.5 months earlier; the condition recurred when penicillamine was again given.— P. Hickling and J. Fuller, *Br. med. J.*, 1979, *2*, 367. A further report.— G. B. Grant (letter), *ibid.*, 555.

Ileal ulceration and stenosis in a patient with Wilson's disease was considered to be related to elastosis probably resulting from long-term penicillamine therapy.— M. Wassef *et al.* (letter), *New Engl. J. Med.*, 1985, *313*, 49.

EFFECTS ON THE KIDNEY. A discussion on penicillamine-induced nephropathy. Proteinuria associated with penicillamine usually occurred within 4 to 18 months of starting therapy though onset could be later. The incidence was greater in patients with rheumatoid arthritis and cystinuria than in those with Wilson's disease and also appeared to be related to the dose and its rate of increase. Proteinuria of nephrotic proportions usually developed rapidly but resolved on drug cessation. Minimal change, mesangioproliferative, and membranous nephropathy had all been associated with penicillamine treatment and progressive glomerulonephritis had been observed in a few patients who had developed features of Goodpasture's syndrome.— *Br. med. J.*, 1981, *282*,

761.

Penicillamine was successfully re-introduced and administered for at least 13 months in 5 patients with rheumatoid arthritis who had developed proteinuria during the first course of therapy. Proteinuria did not recur. The initial dose was 50 mg, increased by monthly increments of 50 mg to a maintenance dose of 150 mg daily. After 4 months the dose was increased further if necessary by increments of 50 mg at intervals of 3 months to 250 mg daily.— H. Hill *et al.*, *Ann. rheum. Dis.*, 1979, *38*, 229.

Two patients with progressive systemic sclerosis developed diffuse crescentic proliferative glomerulonephritis while taking penicillamine. Both responded to pulse methylprednisolone treatment and subsequent daily steroids.— K. A. Ntoso *et al.*, *Am. J. Kidney Dis.*, 1986, *8*, 159.

Further reports: G. H. Neild *et al.* (letter), *Lancet*, 1975, *1*, 1201 (membranous glomerulonephritis); I. Sternlieb *et al.*, *Ann. intern. Med.*, 1975, *82*, 673 (fatal pulmonary haemorrhages and rapidly progressive glomerulonephritis); T. Gibson *et al.* (letter), *ibid.*, 1976, *84*, 100 (similar clinical features ascribed to Goodpasture's syndrome). See also under Effects on the Respiratory System, below.

EFFECTS ON THE LIVER. Case report and review of penicillamine-associated hepatotoxicity. Of the 9 patients reviewed, all had liver function profiles consistent with intrahepatic cholestasis; one patient died of acute renal failure but the others improved rapidly after drug withdrawal. Monitoring of liver function and eosinophil counts in the early weeks of penicillamine therapy was recommended.— J. R. Seibold *et al.*, *Arthritis Rheum.*, 1981, *24*, 554. A 72-year-old man with rheumatoid arthritis developed jaundice approximately 4 weeks after starting penicillamine therapy. Liver biopsy indicated a slight degree of cholangitis with eosinophils in the portal tracts and severe predominantly intrahepatocellular cholestasis. Jaundice cleared within 3 weeks of stopping penicillamine and liver enzyme values approached normal after 6 weeks.— J. P. Devogelaer *et al.*, *Int. J. clin. Pharmacol. Res.*, 1985, *5*, 35.

EFFECTS ON THE MUSCLES AND THE NEUROMUSCULAR SYSTEM. A report of neuromyotonia in a patient taking penicillamine.— J. Reeback *et al.*, *Br. med. J.*, 1979, *1*, 1464.

Report on a patient taking penicillamine who developed profound sensory and motor neuropathy which improved rapidly after the initiation of pyridoxine supplementation.— K. D. Pool *et al.*, *Ann. intern. Med.*, 1981, *95*, 458.

Myasthenia. A review of 18 patients with rheumatoid arthritis who developed penicillamine-induced myasthenia; all had initial symptoms of diplopia and/or ptosis which in 7 progressed to a more generalised involvement. Treatment involved discontinuation of penicillamine in 16 patients facilitated by the use of anticholinesterase agents in 12; myasthenic symptoms resolved completely within 15 months for the majority but were persistent in at least 3 patients. The genetic features suggested that a different genetic background characterised drug-induced as opposed to spontaneous-onset myasthenia.— J. P. Delamere *et al.*, *Ann. rheum. Dis.*, 1983, *42*, 500.

Immunological evidence supporting the role of penicillamine in the induction of myasthenia gravis. The association of penicillamine-induced myasthenia gravis with acetylcholine receptor antibodies and HLA antigens was investigated.— M. J. Garlepp *et al.*, *Br. med. J.*, 1983, *286*, 338.

Further references to myasthenia with penicillamine.— R. L. Dawkins *et al.*, *J. Rheumatol.*, 1981, *8*, *Suppl.* 7, 169; H. Carter *et al.*, *Thérapie*, 1984, *39*, 689; J. P. Devogelaer *et al.*, *Int. J. clin. Pharmacol. Res.*, 1985, *5*, 143.

Polymyositis. One month after starting treatment with penicillamine, a 59-year-old woman with rheumatoid arthritis developed profound weakness followed by progressively severe cardiac arrhythmias and renal failure. Despite vigorous medical treatment, the patient died of intractable ventricular tachycardia. Autopsy revealed a skeletal muscle lesion similar to that of polymyositis-dermatomyositis. Thirteen previous reports of polymyositis-dermatomyositis associated with penicillamine use were reviewed. Dysphagia was the initial symptom in 6 of these patients, 4 had the rash of dermatomyositis, and 10 had weakness. Onset occurred 3 days to 2 years after starting penicillamine and doses ranged from 250 to 1200 mg daily; 11 patients had rheumatoid arthritis, 1 had progressive systemic sclerosis, and 1 had Wilson's disease. One patient died of cardiac complications but the other 12 recovered 1.5 to 7 months after stopping penicillamine therapy.— D. R. Doyle *et al.*, *Ann. intern. Med.*, 1983, *98*, 327.

Further reports of dermatomyositis or polymyositis: F. Wojnarowska, *J. R. Soc. Med.*, 1980, *73*, 884 (dermatomyositis); J. C. Renier *et al.*, *Thérapie*, 1984, *39*, 697 (polymyositis).

EFFECTS ON THE RESPIRATORY SYSTEM. A discussion on the adverse effects of penicillamine on the lungs. Reports of pulmonary haemorrhage associated with progressive renal failure in individual patients treated with penicillamine had commonly been classified as Goodpasture's syndrome, however it was considered that the immunological evidence tended to support an immune complex syndrome. It was also suggested that some cases might develop on a basis of penicillamine-induced renal disease with a nonspecific trigger factor promoting pulmonary involvement. Obliterative bronchiolitis had been reported in patients with rheumatoid arthritis treated with penicillamine but had also occurred in similar patients who had never taken the drug; in view of the extreme rarity of this condition a specific association with penicillamine was unlikely ever to be fully established. Evidence of an association between penicillamine and pulmonary infiltrates was scanty.— M. Turner-Warwick, *J. Rheumatol.*, 1981, *8*, *Suppl.* 7, 166.

References to the possible relationship of obliterative bronchiolitis to penicillamine treatment: W. H. Lyle (letter), *Br. med. J.*, 1977, *1*, 105; G. R. Epler *et al.*, *J. Am. med. Ass.*, 1979, *242*, 528; K. C. Murphy *et al.*, *Arthritis Rheum.*, 1981, *24*, 557.

For references on the association of Goodpasture's syndrome with penicillamine therapy, see also under Effects on the Kidney, above.

EFFECTS ON THE SKIN. A review of penicillamine-induced skin lesions. The cutaneous manifestations observed during penicillamine therapy included those resulting from interference with collagen and elastin such as penicillamine dermatopathy, elastosis perforans serpiginosa, and cutis laxa; those associated with auto-immune mechanisms such as pemphigus, pemphigoid, lupus erythematosus, and dermatomyositis; and those classified as acute sensitivity reactions including macular or papular eruptions and urticaria. The effects on collagen and elastin tended to occur only after prolonged treatment with high doses of penicillamine as in patients with Wilson's disease or cystinuria, whereas patients with diseases characterised by altered immune systems, such as rheumatoid arthritis, were more prone to develop the antibody-related adverse skin reactions. Acute hypersensitivity reactions tended to occur early in penicillamine treatment, usually within the first 7 to 10 days, and appeared not to be dose-related. Lichenoid reactions, stomatitis, nail changes, and adverse effects on hair had also been reported.— R. S. Levy *et al.*, *J. Am. Acad. Derm.*, 1983, *8*, 548.

For a report of toxic epidermal necrolysis and agranulocytosis in a patient taking penicillamine for primary biliary cirrhosis, see under Effects on the Blood, above.

Lichen planus. Graham-Brown *et al.* (*Br. J. Derm.*, 1982, *106*, 699) considered penicillamine to be of no aetiological significance in the development of lichen planus in 5 patients with primary biliary cirrhosis as only one had received prior penicillamine therapy. However, penicillamine has been reported to exacerbate pre-existing lichen planus in patients with primary biliary cirrhosis (F.C. Powell and R.S. Rogers, *Lancet*, 1981, *2*, 525). In a review by Powell *et al.* (*Br. J. Derm.*, 1982, *107*, 616) of 24 patients with lichen planus and primary biliary cirrhosis, 17 developed the initial lesions of lichen planus following the initiation of penicillamine therapy; in some the severity of the skin eruption was dose-related and when the drug was withdrawn the skin lesions gradually faded. Powell *et al.* (1982) suggested that penicillamine might therefore unmask a lichen planus diathesis in some patients with primary biliary cirrhosis and regarded the presence of lichen planus as a relative contra-indication to penicillamine treatment.

Pemphigus. Reports of pemphigus and pemphigoid eruptions associated with the use of penicillamine: R. A. Marsden *et al.*, *Br. J. Derm.*, 1977, *97*, 451 (herpetiform pemphigus); M. C. J. M. de Jong *et al.*, *ibid.*, 1980, *102*, 333 (pemphigus erythematosus); J. Zone *et al.*, *J. Am. med. Ass.*, 1982, *247*, 2705 (pemphigus foliaceus); P. J. Velthuis *et al.*, *Br. J. Derm.*, 1985, *112*, 615 (combined pemphigus and pemphigoid features); L. R. Lever and F. Wojnarowska, *ibid.*, 1985, *113*, *Suppl.* 29, 88 (benign mucous membrane pemphigoid); D. Shuttleworth and R. A. C. Graham-Brown, *ibid.*, 89 (cicatricial pemphigoid).

Penicillamine dermatopathy. A 20-year-old man who had received high-dose penicillamine treatment since the age of 12 for Wilson's disease developed haemorrhagic plaques typical of penicillamine dermatopathy over the pressure areas on his elbows, knees, knuckles, and shoulders.— I. H. Coulson and R. A. Marsden, *Br. J. Derm.*, 1985, *113*, *Suppl.* 29, 87.

Pseudoxanthoma elasticum. Pseudoxanthoma elasticum-like skin changes in a patient with cystinuria who had been treated with penicillamine 2.4 to 3 g daily for 19 years.— R. H. M. Thomas *et al.*, *J. R. Soc. Med.*, 1984, *77*, 794. A further report.— B. Bentley-Phillips (letter), *ibid.*, 1985, *78*, 787.

Psoriasiform eruptions. Two patients with rheumatoid arthritis developed psoriasiform eruptions during penicillamine treatment. In one patient the eruption resolved when penicillamine was stopped but worsened when treatment was restarted.— J. C. Forgie and A. S. Highet (letter), *Br. med. J.*, 1987, *294*, 1101.

EFFECTS ON TASTE. Taste impairment induced by penicillamine is commonly transient and may be less frequent in patients with Wilson's disease. It has been associated with the chelating action of penicillamine and copper and zinc induced deficiencies but evidence is lacking.— J. M. T. Willoughby, *Adverse Drug React. Bull.*, 1983, June, 368.

MALIGNANT NEOPLASMS. A 58-year-old woman with rheumatoid arthritis developed chronic lymphocytic leukaemia after taking penicillamine for 5 years.— J. E. Clausen *et al.* (letter), *Lancet*, 1978, *2*, 152. Report of acute lymphoblastic leukaemia in a 15-year-old girl receiving high doses of penicillamine for Wilson's disease.— P. A. Gilman and N. A. Holtzman, *J. Am. med. Ass.*, 1982, *248*, 467.

PREGNANCY AND THE NEONATE. Review of penicillamine teratogenicity. Evidence of the embryotoxicity of maternal penicillamine exposure in *animal* studies had been confirmed in man by 5 reports of cutis laxa in neonates of mothers who had taken penicillamine during pregnancy; 3 further reports of intra-uterine brain injury were less characteristic. Nevertheless most pregnancy outcomes were normal. Unless a safer therapy could be confirmed, penicillamine management of women with Wilson's disease should be continued throughout pregnancy since the benefits outweighed the risks. However, for conditions for which there were safer alternatives it would be prudent to discontinue penicillamine during pregnancy.— F. W. Rosa, *Teratology*, 1986, *33*, 127.

References to some individual reports of cutis laxa in neonates exposed to maternal penicillamine: O. K. Mjølnerød *et al.*, *Lancet*, 1971, *1*, 673 (generalised connective-tissue defect including lax skin, hyperflexibility of joints, vein fragility, varicosities, and impaired wound healing); L. Solomon *et al.* (letter), *New Engl. J. Med.*, 1977, *296*, 54 (growth retardation, flattened face, lax and wrinkled skin, inguinal hernias, and possible bowel perforation); A. Linares *et al.* (letter), *Lancet*, 1979, *2*, 43 (reversible cutis laxa and inguinal hernia); J. -P. Harpey *et al.* (letter), *ibid.*, 1983, *2*, 858 (loose skin folds and inguinal hernia possibly associated with zinc deficiency).

SYSTEMIC LUPUS ERYTHEMATOSUS. A syndrome resembling lupus erythematosus developed in 6 women with long-standing severe rheumatoid arthritis while being treated with penicillamine; these patients represented an approximate frequency of penicillamine-induced lupus erythematosus of 2%. All 6 had developed previous cutaneous reactions to gold therapy. Clinical manifestations, including pleurisy, leucopenia, rashes, thrombocytopenia, proteinuria, and neurological disturbances, occurred between the sixth and twelfth month of treatment in 3 patients and after one or two years in the others. All had high titres of antinuclear factor and 5 had lupus erythematosus cells; anti-double-stranded deoxyribonucleic acid antibodies and hypocomplementaemia were also noted in some patients. Recommended treatment included dosage reduction or drug discontinuation; corticosteroids and immunosupressants should be used only if necessary.— A. Chalmers *et al.*, *Ann. intern. Med.*, 1982, *97*, 659.

Precautions

Penicillamine is contra-indicated in patients with lupus erythematosus or a history of penicillamine-induced agranulocytosis, aplastic anaemia, or severe thrombocytopenia. It should be used with care, if at all, in patients with renal insufficiency.In the treatment of primary biliary cirrhosis, penicillamine should not be given to patients with a history of hepatic encephalopathy or bleeding varices and should be used with caution in patients with portal hypertension.

Penicillamine should not be given with other drugs capable of causing similar serious haematological or renal adverse effects. Patients who are

allergic to penicillin may react similarly to penicillamine but cross-sensitivity appears to be rare.
Patients need to be carefully supervised and observed for side-effects. In particular, frequent urine tests to detect proteinuria or haematuria and full blood and platelet counts are required regularly, especially in the first few weeks of treatment. Liver function tests have also been recommended at 6-monthly intervals.
Pyridoxine 25 mg daily may be given to patients on long-term therapy, especially if they are on a restricted diet, since penicillamine increases the requirement for this vitamin. The absorption of penicillamine may be reduced in patients taking iron supplements simultaneously and an interval of at least 2 hours between the administration of a dose of penicillamine and iron has been recommended; other metals may have a similar effect as may antacids.
Because of the effect of penicillamine on collagen and elastin and a possible delay in wound healing, it has been suggested that the dose should be reduced to 250 mg daily prior to surgery.

Results of a study in 40 patients with penicillin allergy suggested that while cutaneous crossreactivity with penicillamine had been documented, the risk of a severe allergic reaction to penicillamine in penicillin-allergic patients was probably quite low.— C. L. Bell and F. M. Graziano, *Arthritis Rheum.*, 1983, *26*, 801.

A report of a 57-year-old woman in whom penicillamine-induced myasthenia led to prolonged postoperative apnoea necessitating artificial ventilation. The significance of this report in planning anaesthesia for patients with rheumatoid arthritis treated with penicillamine was discussed.— M. J. Fried and D. T. Protheroe, *Br. J. Anaesth.*, 1986, *58*, 1191.

INTERACTIONS. *Antacids.* In a single-dose study in 6 healthy subjects, administration of penicillamine by mouth immediately after food, an oral dose of ferrous sulphate, or a dose of an antacid mixture of aluminium hydroxide, magnesium hydroxide, and simethicone, reduced the plasma concentrations of penicillamine to 52%, 35%, and 66% respectively of those obtained after administration in a fasting state. Results suggested that the reduction in plasma-penicillamine concentrations was associated with decreased penicillamine absorption.— M. A. Osman *et al.*, *Clin. Pharmac. Ther.*, 1983, *33*, 465.
Administration of an antacid containing aluminium and magnesium hydroxides significantly reduced the absorption of penicillamine but sodium bicarbonate had little effect; the inhibition of penicillamine absorption was therefore probably a result of chelation rather than a pH effect.— A. Ifan and P. G. Welling, *Biopharm. Drug Disposit.*, 1986, *7*, 401.

Diazepam. For a report of exacerbation of intravenous diazepam-induced phlebitis by oral penicillamine, see under Diazepam, (p.730).

Gold. There have been conflicting reports on the effect of previous gold therapy on the subsequent development of penicillamine toxicity in patients with rheumatoid arthritis.
A multicentre trial group (*Postgrad. med. J.*, 1974, *50*, *Suppl.* 2, 77) found no evidence of any interaction between gold and penicillamine but Webley and Coomes (*Br. med. J.*, 1978, *2*, 91) found that although the overall incidence of side-effects with penicillamine appeared unaffected by prior gold therapy, bone-marrow depression and rashes were more common in those patients previously treated with gold. Hill (*ibid.*, 961) reported that patients who had to stop gold therapy because of adverse effects were more prone to develop major adverse effects to penicillamine and a study by Dodd *et al.* (*ibid.*, 1980, *280*, 1498) indicated that patients who reacted adversely to gold were more likely to develop side-effects to penicillamine. Dodd *et al.* (1980) also found that the mean interval between finishing gold and beginning penicillamine in patients who developed identical adverse reactions to both drugs was significantly shorter than in those who developed different side-effects or no side-effects; this supported the theory that some adverse reactions to penicillamine might result from the mobilisation of gold previously stored in the tissues during gold therapy. An interval of at least 6 months between gold and penicillamine therapy in patients who had adverse reactions to gold was recommended. In contrast, Smith *et al.* (*ibid.*, 1982, *285*, 595) found no evidence that the interval between gold and penicillamine therapy had any influence on the subsequent development of penicillamine toxicity. A genetic susceptibility in certain patients to react adversely to either drug was suggested. However, in a prospective study by Steven *et al.* (*ibid.*, *284*, 79), prior gold, penicillamine, or levamisole treatment had no influence on the subsequent efficacy or toxicity of any one of these alternative drugs.
There has been a report of gold therapy causing a recurrence of myasthenia that had previously occurred with penicillamine (A.P. Moore *et al.*, *ibid.*, 1984, *288*, 192).

Insulin. Unexplained hypoglycaemia in 2 insulin-dependent diabetics occurred 6 to 8 weeks after penicillamine treatment for rheumatoid arthritis was started. Both patients required a reduction in their insulin dose.— P. Elling and H. Elling (letter), *Ann. intern. Med.*, 1985, *103*, 644. Comment on a possible association with immune mechanisms.— R. C. Becker and R. G. Martin (letter), *ibid.*, 1986, *104*, 127.

Iron. Patients stabilised on penicillamine whilst on oral iron therapy were unlikely to respond fully to penicillamine and would be exposed to a large increase in penicillamine absorption with possible adverse reactions if the iron was stopped.— J. A. L. Harkness and D. R. Blake, *Lancet*, 1982, *2*, 1368.
See also under Antacids, above.

Probenecid. Probenecid reduced the beneficial effects of penicillamine in cystinuria; co-administration in hyperuricaemic cystinuric patients was contra-indicated.— T. -F. Yu *et al.*, *J. Rheumatol.*, 1984, *11*, 467.

PREGNANCY AND THE NEONATE. For precautions in pregnancy see under Adverse Effects, (above).

Absorption and Fate

Penicillamine is readily absorbed from the gastro-intestinal tract and reaches peak concentrations in the blood within 1 to 2 hours. It is metabolised in the liver and excreted in the urine and faeces mainly as metabolites.

Studies on the pharmacokinetics of penicillamine: R. F. Bergstrom *et al.*, *Clin. Pharmac. Ther.*, 1981, *30*, 404; L. J. Notarianni *et al.*, *Br. J. clin. Pharmac.*, 1984, *18*, 303P; A. O. Muijsers *et al.*, *Arthritis Rheum.*, 1984, *27*, 1362.
For references to the reduction of penicillamine bioavailability by food, iron compounds, and antacids, see under Precautions, above.

Uses and Administration

Penicillamine is a chelating agent which aids the elimination from the body of certain heavy-metal ions, including copper, lead, and mercury by forming stable soluble complexes with them that are readily excreted by the kidney.
It is used in the treatment of Wilson's disease (hepatolenticular degeneration) in conjunction with a low-copper diet to promote the excretion of copper and in the treatment of heavy-metal poisoning. It may be used to treat asymptomatic lead intoxication or in the convalescent management of lead poisoning following initial treatment with sodium calciumedetate. It has also been used in primary biliary cirrhosis to reduce copper concentrations in the liver.
Penicillamine is used as an adjunct to diet and urinary alkalinisation in the management of cystinuria. It reacts with cystine to form a more soluble sulphide compound which is more readily excreted. By reducing urinary concentrations of cystine, penicillamine prevents the formation of cystine calculi and promotes the gradual dissolution of existing calculi.
Penicillamine is also used to treat severe active rheumatoid arthritis not adequately controlled by non-steroidal anti-inflammatory agents or conventional therapy and has been tried in the maintenance treatment of chronic active hepatitis after the disease has been controlled with corticosteroids and azathioprine.
Penicillamine is administered by mouth and should be taken on an empty stomach. A low initial dose increased gradually to the minimum optimal maintenance dosage may reduce the incidence of side-effects as well as provide closer control of the condition being treated.
In the treatment of Wilson's disease, the usual dosage range is 1 to 2 g daily in divided doses. The optimal dosage to achieve a negative copper balance should be determined by regular analysis of 24-hour urinary copper excretion. A maintenance dose of 0.75 to 1 g daily may be adequate once remission is achieved and should be continued indefinitely; the *UK* manufacturers recommend that a maintenance dose of 2 g daily should not be continued for more than a year. In children, a suggested dose is up to 20 mg per kg body-weight daily in divided doses.
In the management of lead poisoning, penicillamine may be given in doses of 0.5 to 2 g daily in divided doses until the urinary lead concentration is stabilised at less than 0.5 mg per day. A recommended dose for children is 20 to 25 mg per kg body-weight daily in divided doses.
In primary biliary cirrhosis, a suggested initial dose is 250 mg of penicillamine daily, increased at weekly intervals to a maintenance dose of 0.75 to 1 g daily in divided doses; when copper concentrations in the liver have returned to normal it may be possible to reduce the dose.
In cystinuria, doses of penicillamine are adjusted according to cystine concentrations in the urine. For the treatment of cystinuria and cystine calculi, the usual dose is 2 g daily in divided doses but may range from 1 to 4 g daily; a suggested dose for children is up to 30 mg per kg body-weight daily in divided doses. For the prevention of cystine calculi, lower doses of 0.25 to 1 g at bedtime may be given. An adequate fluid intake is essential to maintain urine flow during penicillamine administration for cystinuria.
In the treatment of rheumatoid arthritis an initial dose of penicillamine 125 to 250 mg daily is increased gradually by the same amount at intervals of 4 to 12 weeks. Remission is often achieved with maintenance doses of 500 to 750 mg daily but doses of up to 1.5 g daily have been required. Doses in excess of 500 mg daily should be taken in divided doses. Improvement may not occur for several months; the *US* manufacturers suggest that penicillamine should be discontinued if there is no response after treatment for 3 to 4 months with 1 to 1.5 g daily. After remission has been sustained for 6 months an attempt may be made gradually to reduce the dose by 125 to 250 mg daily every 2 to 3 months but relapse may occur. Lower doses may be required in the elderly who may be more susceptible to developing adverse effects. Initial doses of 50 to 125 mg daily have been recommended gradually increased to a maximum of 1 g daily if necessary. In children the maintenance dose is 15 to 20 mg per kg body-weight daily; a suggested initial dose is 50 mg daily for one month increased gradually at 4-weekly intervals.
In the management of chronic active hepatitis, an initial dose of penicillamine 500 mg daily in divided doses may be given after liver function tests have indicated that the disease has been controlled by corticosteroids; the dose is gradually increased over 3 months to 1.25 g daily with a concurrent reduction in the corticosteroid dose.

ADMINISTRATION. A report from a manufacturer of penicillamine on a formula and method of preparing granules of penicillamine for reconstitution as an oral liquid dosage form.— D. A. Rawlins and J. M. Smith, *J. clin. Hosp. Pharm.*, 1982, *7*, 141.
For references to the reduction of penicillamine bioavailability by food, iron compounds, and antacids, see under Precautions, above.

AIDS. In a preliminary study in 13 asymptomatic HIV-infected men with generalised lymphadenopathy, penicillamine in gradually increasing doses of up to 2 g daily by mouth decreased lymph-node size and suppressed viral replication. These results supported the need for further studies to assess the antiviral activity of penicillamine in patients with AIDS and AIDS-related complex. However, as penicillamine depressed T-cell lymphoproliferative responses, it should be given with caution to patients with impaired T-cell function.— R. S. Schulof *et al.*, *Arzneimittel-Forsch.*, 1986, *36*, 1531.

CHRONIC ACTIVE HEPATITIS. In a controlled study, penicillamine and prednisone were compared as maintenance therapy in chronic active hepatitis after the disease had been brought under control by corticosteroids. Of 18 patients receiving penicillamine (up to 1.2 g daily) 9 patients were withdrawn—side-effects (7) and lack of disease control (2). In the 17 patients given prednisone (15 mg daily) 6 were withdrawn—lack of disease control (4), side-effects (1), and carcinomatosis (1). Liver function tests in the patients remaining in the study after 1 year showed no significant differences. Because of side-effects penicillamine was not the drug of choice for maintenance, but if corticosteroids were contra-indicated penicillamine would be a useful alternative.— R. B. Stern *et al.*, *Gut*, 1977, *18*, 19.

CYSTINURIA. Of 24 patients with cystinuria treated for at least a year (or until dissolution of calculi) with oral fluids, alkalinisation of the urine, and penicillamine in a dose sufficient to reduce the excretion of cystine in the urine to about 200 mg in 24 hours, 10 experienced complete dissolution of calculi, 3 remained stone-free after urolithotomy, 5 had partial dissolution, and 6 no change or growth of calculi. Because toxic reactions with penicillamine are frequent and sometimes severe, this drug should be used only when necessary and then as an adjunct to, rather than a substitute for, increased oral fluids and urinary alkalinisation.— P. J. Dahlberg *et al.*, *Mayo Clin. Proc.*, 1977, *52*, 533.

METAL POISONING. Convincing evidence of the efficacy of penicillamine in metal poisoning appeared only in instances when urinary excretion of the metal was consistently and greatly increased by the drug. This was true in poisoning by copper, lead, and possibly arsenic but penicillamine was of doubtful or no value for cadmium, mercury, or gold intoxication.— W. H. Lyle, *J. Rheumatol.*, 1981, *8*, *Suppl.* 7, 96.

PRIMARY BILIARY CIRRHOSIS. Copper accumulation in the liver has been noted in patients with long-lasting cholestatic liver disorders such as primary biliary cirrhosis and initial studies (T.B. Deering *et al.*, *Gastroenterology*, 1977, *72*, 1208; S. Jain *et al.*, *Lancet*, 1977, *1*, 831) indicated that penicillamine might be of benefit by increasing the urinary excretion of copper and reducing liver-copper concentrations. It was also suggested that the immunological action of penicillamine might influence the course of the disease (O. Epstein *et al.*, *New Engl. J. Med.*, 1979, *300*, 274). However, preliminary results indicating that penicillamine improved survival in patients with primary biliary cirrhosis (O. Epstein *et al.*, *Lancet*, 1981, *1*, 1275) were not supported by further studies (D.S. Matloff *et al.*, *New Engl. J. Med.*, 1982, *306*, 319; E.R. Dickson *et al.*, *ibid.*, 1985, *312*, 1011; J. Neuberger *et al.*, *Gut*, 1985, *26*, 114) in which penicillamine did not significantly affect the overall survival or prevent progression of the disease. A review by James (*Gut*, 1985, *26*, 109) concluded that the value of penicillamine in the treatment of primary biliary cirrhosis was not proven; there was possibly a marginal decrease in mortality in an intermediate symptomatic group of patients but the incidence of side-effects was probably too high to justify further long and elaborate clinical studies.

RHEUMATIC DISORDERS. Reviews on the use of penicillamine in rheumatic disease.— K. D. Muirden, *Med. J. Aust.*, 1986, *144*, 32; H. E. Howard-Lock *et al.*, *Semin. Arthritis Rheum.*, 1986, *15*, 261.

Juvenile chronic arthritis. The results of a 6-month double-blind multicentre study in 70 children with juvenile chronic arthritis indicated that penicillamine (5 to 15 mg per kg body-weight daily) had beneficial effects which included a decrease in pain and a reduction in the total number of stiff or painful joints. In the penicillamine group the mean daily consumption of aspirin was also significantly reduced but the mean prednisone dosage was unaltered.— A. M. Prieur *et al.*, *Arthritis Rheum.*, 1985, *28*, 376. A 12-month double-blind multicentre study involving 162 children with severe active juvenile rheumatoid arthritis in the *USA* and *USSR* failed to demonstrate that, in the presence of non-steroidal anti-inflammatory drugs, either penicillamine or hydroxychloroquine had any greater therapeutic efficacy than placebo.— E. J. Brewer *et al.*, *New Engl. J. Med.*, 1986, *314*, 1269.

Palindromic rheumatism. Four of 5 patients with palindromic rheumatism had no further attacks for 1 year after being given penicillamine 250 mg daily.— E. C. Huskisson, *Br. med. J.*, 1976, *2*, 979.

Psoriatic arthritis. In a 24-week double-blind study involving 20 patients with psoriatic arthritis, penicillamine in a dose gradually increased to 500 mg daily significantly improved morning stiffness, pain, grip strength, articular index, and erythrocyte sedimentation rate.— S. O. Daunt *et al.*, *Br. J. Rheumatol.*, 1986, *25*, 74.

Rheumatoid arthritis. The Multicentre Trial Group (*Lancet*, 1973, *1*, 275) established penicillamine as an effective form of treatment in severe active rheumatoid disease. In a 12-month double-blind study involving 105 patients with severe refractory rheumatoid arthritis, penicillamine 1.5 g daily by mouth (as base or hydrochloride) improved all measurements (pain, morning stiffness, grip strength, articular index, functional assessment, erythrocyte sedimentation rate, haemoglobin concentrations, and sheep red-blood-cell agglutination titre) except for radiographic changes in small joints. Of the 52 patients receiving penicillamine, 16 withdrew from the study because of adverse effects. Further studies indicated that lower daily doses of penicillamine were also therapeutically effective (A.T. Day *et al.*,*Br. med. J.*, 1974, *1*, 180; Y. Shiokawa *et al.*, *Arthritis Rheum.*, 1977, *20*, 1464) and preferable as the incidence of side-effects could be reduced. Doses as low as 125 mg daily have been claimed to be effective in some patients but a 36-week multicentre controlled double-blind study (H.J. Williams *et al.*, *ibid.*, 1983, *26*, 581) involving 225 patients concluded that a dose of penicillamine 500 mg daily was only slightly more effective than placebo; a dose of 125 mg daily was not significantly different from either the 500 mg dose or placebo.

The choice of drug therapy for severe refractory rheumatoid arthritis and the role of penicillamine has still to be fully determined. A review of the effect of drug therapy on radiographic deterioration in rheumatoid arthritis (L. Iannuzzi *et al.*, *New Engl. J. Med.*, 1983, *309*, 1023) found no evidence that penicillamine delayed X-ray progression of the disease though there was not enough information to permit the conclusion that it was of no value in preventing erosive damage. Results of a prospective study in 112 patients with severe rheumatoid arthritis (D.L. Scott, *et al.*, *Lancet*, 1987, *1*, 1108) suggested that the beneficial effects of active drug therapy with gold, chloroquine, steroids, penicillamine, or cytotoxics extended over only a few years and did not influence long-term outcome. Emphasis was now on starting 'slow-acting' (second-line) antirheumatic drugs as soon as possible but only a small minority of patients appeared to remain on 'slow-acting' drugs for long, therapy often being stopped because of adverse reactions or loss of efficacy.

SCLERODERMA. In a retrospective study, 73 patients with progressive systemic sclerosis and diffuse scleroderma of less than 3 years duration were treated for at least 6 months with penicillamine in maximum daily doses of 500 to 1500 mg (median 750 mg) and compared with 45 similar patients taking colchicine, immunosuppressive agents, or no drugs; 21 of the patients taking penicillamine also received concurrent colchicine. Significant skin improvement was first observed in patients treated with penicillamine 19 to 42 months after therapy was initiated, and was maintained during subsequent follow-up. Results were promising and warranted a prospective controlled study of penicillamine in progressive systemic sclerosis.— V. D. Steen *et al.*, *Ann. intern. Med.*, 1982, *97*, 652.

Further reports of beneficial effects with penicillamine in patients with scleroderma (systemic sclerosis).— C. M. Herbert *et al.*, *Lancet*, 1974, *1*, 187 (effects on skin collagen); H. Mellstedt *et al.*, *Scand. J. Rheumatol.*, 1977, *6*, 92 (effects on skin capillary circulation); V. D. Steen *et al.*, *Arthritis Rheum.*, 1985, *28*, 882 (effects on pulmonary function).

Systemic sclerosis-like lesions developed in a 14-year-old boy with Wilson's disease who had been treated with penicillamine for 11 years. These findings questioned the suitability of penicillamine for the treatment of scleroderma.— S. Miyagawa *et al.*, *Br. J. Derm.*, 1987, *116*, 95.

WILSON'S DISEASE. A brief review of Wilson's disease and its treatment.— D. Parkes, *Br. med. J.*, 1984, *288*, 1180.

Penicillamine reduced serum-copper concentrations in 4 children with Wilson's disease, but in addition also reduced the serum-zinc concentrations, which were initially high, to the low normal range. The urinary zinc/copper ratios increased with the duration of treatment and might be useful in determining the adequacy of the dosage. One child developed hair loss and parakeratosis but symptoms were alleviated by a reduction in the dose with a subsequent reduction in urinary excretion of zinc; some of the adverse effects of penicillamine might be due to zinc deficiency.— M. Van Caillie-Bertrand *et al.*, *Archs Dis. Childh.*, 1985, *60*, 652.

Report of a woman with Wilson's disease who died of hepatic failure as a consequence of abandoning her long-term penicillamine therapy. One of the greatest hazards in patients with Wilson's disease was non-compliance especially as symptoms might not recur for 2 to 3 years. At follow-up it was therefore necessary to pay at least as much attention to the copper status of the patient as to possible penicillamine toxicity.— J. M. Walshe and A. K. Dixon, *Lancet*, 1986, *1*, 845. A further report.— P. Emery and I. R. Mackay (letter), *ibid.*, 1388.

Eight of 11 patients with Wilson's disease, who had been successfully treated with penicillamine for 3 to 19 years, died of hepatic decompensation or fulminant hepatitis 9 months to 6 years after stopping therapy. The short mean survival time of 2.6 years in these 8 patients was surprising if penicillamine had effectively removed the excess copper. It was suggested that penicillamine might act by the formation of a non-toxic complex which released copper when drug treatment was stopped. Thirteen further patients who had to discontinue penicillamine because of adverse effects were successfully managed on trientine dihydrochloride.— I. H. Scheinberg *et al.*, *New Engl. J. Med.*, 1987, *317*, 209. See also I.H. Scheinberg *et al.* (letter), *Lancet*, 1987, *2*, 95; M.E. Elmes and B. Jasani (letter), *ibid.*, 866.

Preparations

Penicillamine Tablets *(B.P.)*. Store at a temperature not exceeding 25°.

Penicillamine Tablets *(U.S.P.)*

Proprietary Preparations

Distamine *(Dista, UK)*. *Tablets*, scored, penicillamine 50 mg.

Tablets, penicillamine 125 and 250 mg.

Pendramine *(E. Merck, UK)*. *Tablets*, scored, penicillamine 125 and 250 mg.

Proprietary Names and Manufacturers

Artamin *(Switz.)*; Atamir *(Sandoz, Denm.)*; Cuprenil *(Pol.)*; Cuprimine *(Austral.*; *Merck Sharp & Dohme, Canad.*; *Neth.*; *Merck Sharp & Dohme, Norw.*; *MSD, Swed.*; *Merck Sharp & Dohme, Switz.*; *Merck Sharp & Dohme, UK*; *Merck Sharp & Dohme, USA)*; Cupripen *(Rubio, Spain)*; Depamine *(Berk Pharmaceuticals, UK)*; Depen *(Horner, Canad.*; *Wallace, USA)*; Dimetylcystein *(Dista, Denm.)*; Distamine *(Neth.*; *Switz.*; *Dista, UK)*; D-Penamine *(Dista, Austral.)*; Kelatin *(Belg.*; *Neth.)*; Mercaptyl *(Knoll, Switz.)*; Metalcaptase *(Heyl, Ger.*; *Jpn*; *Knoll, S.Afr.)*; Pemine *(Lilly, Ital.)*; Pendramine *(E. Merck, UK)*; Perdolat *(Schering, Austral.)*; Rhumantin *(GEA, Denm.)*; Sufortan *(Farmades, Ital.)*; Sufortanon *(Lacer, Spain)*; Trolovol *(Bayer, Fr.*; *Degussa, Ger.)*; Vistamin *(Wilson, Pakistan)*.

13157-g

Potassium Polystyrene Sulphonate

Potassium Polystyrene Sulfonate.

CAS — 9011-99-8.

The potassium salt of sulphonated styrene polymer.

Potassium polystyrene sulphonate is a cation-exchange resin similar to sodium polystyrene sulphonate (p.854). It exchanges potassium ions for calcium ions and other cations and has been used in the management of hypercalciuria and renal calculi.

Proprietary Names and Manufacturers

Campanyl *(Temmler, Ger.*; *Temmler, Switz.)*.

1050-s

Pralidoxime Chloride *(BANM, USAN)*.

2-PAM Chloride; 2-PAMCl; 2-Pyridine Aldoxime Methochloride. 2-Hydroxyiminomethyl-1-methylpyridinium chloride.

$C_7H_9ClN_2O$=172.6.

CAS — 6735-59-7; 495-94-3 (both pralidoxime);

51-15-0 (chloride).

Pharmacopoeias. In *Jug.*, *Ind.*, and *U.S.*

A white or pale yellow odourless crystalline powder. Freely **soluble** in water.

1048-z

Pralidoxime Iodide *(BANM, USAN, rINN).*

2-PAM Iodide; 2-PAMI.

$C_7H_9IN_2O$=264.1.

CAS — 94-63-3.

Pharmacopoeias. In *Chin.* and *Int.*

1049-c

Pralidoxime Mesylate *(BANM, USAN).*

2-PAMM; P2S; Pralidoxime Methanesulphonate.

$C_8H_{12}N_2O_4S$=232.3.

CAS — 154-97-2.

Pharmacopoeias. In *Nord.* which also includes an injection grade.

1047-j

Pralidoxime Methylsulphate *(BANM).*

$C_8H_{12}N_2O_5S$=248.3.

CAS — 1200-55-1.

Pharmacopoeias. In *It.*

Stability of pralidoxime salts in solution: A. W. Boeke, *Pharm. Weekbl. Ned.*, 1978, *113*, 713; R. I. Ellin, *J. pharm. Sci.*, 1982, *71*, 1057; E. M. May and J. E. Pearse, *Anal. Proc.*, 1983, *20*, 179. Studies on decomposition of pralidoxime solutions: D. G. Prue *et al.*, *J. pharm. Sci.*, 1983, *72*, 751; P. Fyhr *et al.*, *ibid.*, 1986, *75*, 608.

Adverse Effects

The administration of pralidoxime may be associated with drowsiness, dizziness, disturbances of vision, nausea, tachycardia, headache, hyperventilation, and muscular weakness. Tachycardia, laryngospasm, and muscle rigidity have been attributed to administering pralidoxime intravenously at too rapid a rate. Large doses of pralidoxime may cause transient neuromuscular blockade.

When atropine and pralidoxime are given together, the signs of atropinisation may occur earlier than might be expected when atropine is used alone.

Precautions

Pralidoxime should be used cautiously in patients with impaired renal function; a reduction in dosage may be necessary. Caution is also required in administering pralidoxime to patients with myasthenia gravis as it may precipitate a myasthenic crisis. Pralidoxime should not be used to treat poisoning by carbamate pesticides.

For conflicting reports of the effects of pralidoxime and atropine when the 2 agents were given mixed in the same syringe, see Atropine, p.524.

Absorption and Fate

Pralidoxime chloride is somewhat slowly absorbed from the gastro-intestinal tract. Blood concentrations are more rapidly attained after intramuscular or intravenous injection. It is not bound to plasma proteins, does not readily pass into the central nervous system, and is rapidly excreted in the urine partly unchanged and partly as a metabolite. The elimination half-life is approximately 1 to 2 hours.

References on the pharmacokinetics of pralidoxime salts: F. R. Sidell and W. A. Groff, *J. pharm. Sci.*, 1971, *60*, 1224 (pralidoxime chloride administered parenterally); F. R. Sidell *et al.*, *J. pharm. Sci.*, 1972, *61*, 1136 (pralidoxime mesylate by mouth); R. D. Swartz *et al.*, *Clin. Pharmac. Ther.*, 1973, *14*, 83 (effects of heat and exercise on elimination).

In a study of 6 healthy subjects concomitant intravenous administration of thiamine hydrochloride prolonged the plasma half-life of pralidoxime chloride.— J. Josselson and F. R. Sidell, *Clin. Pharmac. Ther.*, 1978, *24*, 95.

Uses and Administration

Pralidoxime is a cholinesterase reactivator. It is used as an adjunct to but *not* as a substitute for atropine in the treatment of poisoning by certain cholinesterase inhibitors. Its main indication is in poisoning due to organophosphorus pesticides or related compounds when it acts principally by reactivating the enzyme cholinesterase after this enzyme has been inhibited by phosphorylation. It thus restores the enzymatic destruction of acetylcholine at the neuromuscular junction and relieves muscle paralysis but concomitant administration of atropine is required to counteract directly the adverse effects of acetylcholine accumulation, particularly at the respiratory centre.

Pralidoxime is not equally antagonistic to all organophosphorus anticholinesterases as reactivation is dependent on the nature of the phosphoryl group and the rate at which inhibition becomes irreversible. It is not effective in the treatment of poisoning due to phosphorus, inorganic phosphates, or organophosphates without anticholinesterase activity. It is relatively ineffective in the treatment of poisoning by carbamate pesticides and it should not be used in carbaryl poisoning as it may increase toxicity. The use of pralidoxime for the treatment of overdosage by anticholinesterase drugs including those used to treat myasthenia gravis such as neostigmine has been suggested; however it is only slightly effective and its use is not generally recommended.

Pralidoxime may be administered subcutaneously, intramuscularly, or intravenously by slow intravenous injection of a 5% to 10% solution in Water for Injections over 5 to 10 minutes or alternatively by infusion in 100 mL of sodium chloride injection (0.9%) over a period of 15 to 30 minutes. It is usually given as the chloride or mesylate but the iodide and methylsulphate salts have also been used.

In the treatment of organophosphorus poisoning, atropine sulphate 2 mg should be given by subcutaneous, intravenous, or intramuscular injection and repeated at intervals of 5 to 60 minutes until the patient shows signs of atropine toxicity; atropinisation should then be maintained throughout the course of pralidoxime treatment which may continue for 48 hours or more. Large amounts of atropine may be required. Concomitantly, 1 to 2 g of pralidoxime should be administered intramuscularly or intravenously and repeated if necessary according to the patient's condition; a maximum dose of 12 g in 24 hours has been suggested. In children, pralidoxime 20 to 60 mg per kg body-weight may be given depending on the severity of poisoning and response to treatment. The dose of pralidoxime may need to be reduced in patients with impaired renal function.

Treatment should preferably be monitored by the determination of blood-cholinesterase concentrations.

The *US* manufacturers have suggested that if gastro-intestinal symptoms are not severe pralidoxime chloride may be given by mouth in doses of 1 to 3 g of pralidoxime every 5 hours.

Pralidoxime must be given within 24 hours of poisoning to be fully effective as cholinesterase inactivation usually becomes irreversible after this time; however patients with severe poisoning may occasionally respond more than 48 hours after exposure.

Other oximes with cholinesterase reactivating properties that have been used similarly include obidoxime chloride (p.847), diacetyl monoxime, and trimedoxime bromide (TMB-4).

ACTION. Review of the inhibition of cholinesterase by organophosphorus compounds and the mechanisms of action of pyridinium oximes in the treatment of organophosphorus intoxication.— R. I. Ellin, *Gen. Pharmacol.*, 1982, *13*, 457.

ORGANOPHOSPHORUS POISONING. A dramatic response in EEG with concomitant restoring of consciousness was observed 2 minutes after the start of an infusion of pralidoxime chloride in a 3½-year-old child with severe parathion poisoning. Oximes were generally thought to be unable to cross the blood-brain barrier but it was suggested that this response represented a direct action of pralidoxime on the central nervous system.— M. Lotti and C. E. Becker, *J. Toxicol. clin. Toxicol.*, 1982, *19*, 121.

In the treatment of intoxication with organophosphorus compounds, patients with peripheral symptoms should be given 2 to 4 mg of atropine sulphate and 1 to 2 g of a soluble salt of pralidoxime or 250 mg of obidoxime chloride by slow intravenous injection. A higher initial dose of atropine sulphate may be necessary in severe intoxication and further doses may be needed to maintain full atropinisation. Whenever possible, this treatment should be performed concurrently with measures to alleviate life-threatening effects and remove non-absorbed material. Continuous intensive observation should be maintained for at least 72 hours after initial improvement and blood samples for cholinesterase determinations should be taken before and during treatment. Reactivators are excreted fairly rapidly if kidney function is normal (in the case of pralidoxime 80% in 2 to 3 hours) and repeated doses may be needed.

Oximes should not be given in carbamate poisoning.— Ninth Report of the WHO Expert Committee on Vector Biology and Control, *Tech. Rep. Ser. Wld Hlth Org. No. 720*, 1985.

A review of poisoning from domestic products. In the management of poisoning with domestic organophosphorus insecticides the patient should be washed after removal of contaminated clothing, kept in a quiet environment, and given atropine 2 mg intravenously every 15 to 30 minutes until full atropinisation occurs if the parasympathetic symptoms of sialorrhoea, bronchorrhoea, and incontinence are troublesome. Pralidoxime should be given in a dose of 30 mg per kg body-weight intravenously every 4 hours for 24 hours. Pralidoxime is only of use if administered within 12 hours of exposure.— G. N. Volans and C. M. Byatt, *Prescribers' J.*, 1986, *26*, 87.

For references to the use of high doses of atropine in the treatment of organophosphorus poisoning, see under Uses and Administration in Atropine Sulphate, p.525.

Preparations of Pralidoxime Salts

Pralidoxime Chloride Tablets *(U.S.P.)*

Sterile Pralidoxime Chloride *(U.S.P.).* Pralidoxime chloride suitable for parenteral use; it may contain a small amount of sodium hydroxide for the adjustment of the pH. A 5% solution has a pH of 3.5 to 4.5.

Proprietary Names and Manufacturers of Pralidoxime Salts

Contrathion *(Rhodia, Arg.; L'Arguenon, Fr.; Farmitalia, Ital.)*; PAM Injection *(Abbott, Austral.)*; Protopam Chloride *(Ayerst, Canad.; Ayerst, USA).*

1051-w

Protamine Sulphate *(BAN).*

Protamine Sulfate *(USAN, rINN).*

CAS — 9012-00-4 (protamine); 9009-65-8 (sulphate).

Pharmacopoeias. In *Br.*, *Chin.*, *Eur.*, *Jpn*, *Jug.*, *Nord.*, and *U.S. Egypt.* includes the injection.

A purified mixture of the sulphates of basic peptides prepared from the sperm or the mature testes of suitable species of fish; the *B.P.* specifies fish belonging to the family Clupeidae or Salmonidae. A white or almost white hygroscopic powder. Sparingly **soluble** in water; practically insoluble in alcohol, chloroform, and ether. Solutions are **sterilised** by filtration. **Store** at 2° to 8° in airtight containers. Protamine sulphate is **incompatible** with certain antibiotics including several cephalosporins and penicillins.

Adverse Effects

Intravenous injections of protamine sulphate, particularly if given rapidly, may cause hypotension, bradycardia, and dyspnoea. A sensation of warmth, transitory flushing, nausea and vomiting, and lassitude may also occur. Anaphylactoid reactions have been reported.

A report on 4 patients who developed severe adverse reactions including marked hypotension, vascular collapse, and pulmonary oedema following the administration of protamine sulphate after cardiac surgery to neutralise the effect of heparin. Previous reports of similar reactions to protamine were reviewed. A total of 17 patients had immediate anaphylactic reactions; in 1 patient a complement-dependent IgG antibody-mediated reaction had been demonstrated and 3 patients tested for allergy to protamine had positive skin tests. In 15 of these 17 patients there was evidence of previous exposure to protamine; those with a high risk of sensitisation included leucophaeresis donors who had received the drug, diabetics using insulin containing protamine, and patients with fish allergy. Suspected reactions to protamine occurred in a further 10 patients after cardiac surgery. However, these reactions were characterised by severe vascular damage manifested as noncardiogenic pulmonary oedema or persistent hypotension and onset was delayed for 30 minutes to several hours. Evidence suggested that these reactions were not antibody mediated; only 2 of 7 evaluable patients had previous exposure. All patients required aggressive therapy.— C. L. Holland *et al.*, *Clin. Cardiol.*, 1984, *7*, 157.

Adverse cardiovascular responses to protamine were considered to be of 3 types, transient hypotension related to rapid drug administration, occasional anaphylactoid responses, and rarely, catastrophic pulmonary vasoconstriction. *Animal* investigations, prospective human studies, and individual case reports were reviewed and the toxicity of protamine was discussed.— J. C. Horrow, *Anesth. Analg.*, 1985, *64*, 348.

For a survey indicating that patients receiving isophane insulin, which contains protamine, were subject to an increased risk of anaphylaxis when protamine was used to reverse systemic heparinisation after cardiac catheterisation, see under Precautions in Insulin, p.393.

Uses and Administration

Protamine is a basic protein which combines with heparin to form a stable inactive complex. Protamine sulphate is used to neutralise the anticoagulant action of heparin in the treatment of haemorrhage resulting from severe heparin overdosage.

Protamine sulphate is administered by slow intravenous injection over a period of about 10 minutes. The dose is dependent on the amount of heparin to be neutralised and ideally should be titrated against assessments of the coagulability of the patient's blood. Protamine sulphate has weak anticoagulating properties and if given in gross excess its anticoagulant action could be significant. As heparin is being continuously excreted the dose should be reduced if more than 15 minutes have elapsed since heparin administration; for example, if protamine sulphate is given 30 minutes after heparin the dose may be reduced to about one-half. Not more than 50 mg of protamine sulphate should be injected for any one dose; patients should be carefully monitored as further doses may be required. The *B.P. 1988* specifies that 1 mg of protamine sulphate precipitates not less than 100 units of heparin sodium, but adds that this potency is based on a specific reference batch of heparin sodium. The *UK* manufacturer has stated that each mg of protamine sulphate will usually neutralise the anticoagulant effect of at least 80 international units of heparin (lung) or at least 100 international units of heparin (mucous). The *US* manufacturer has stated that each mg of protamine sulphate neutralises approximately 90 *USP* units of heparin (lung) or about 115 *USP* units of heparin (mucous).

Protamine sulphate has also been used to neutralise the effect of heparin given during leucophaeresis procedures or during extracorporeal circulation as in dialysis or cardiac surgery.

Protamine is also used to prolong the effects of insulin.

Preparations

Protamine Sulfate for Injection *(U.S.P.)*. A sterile mixture of protamine sulphate with 1 or more suitable dry diluents. The injection is prepared by the addition of solvent before use. Its solution has a pH of 6.5 to 7.5.

Protamine Sulfate Injection *(U.S.P.)*. A sterile iso-osmotic solution of protamine sulphate. Store at 2° to 8°.

Protamine Sulphate Injection *(B.P.)*. pH 2.5 to 3.5.

Proprietary Preparations

Protamine Sulphate *(Boots, UK)*. *Injection*, protamine sulphate 10 mg/mL in sodium chloride injection 0.9%, in ampoules of 10 mL.

Protamine Sulphate *(CP Pharmaceuticals, UK)*. *Injection*, protamine sulphate 10 mg/mL in sodium chloride injection 0.9%, in ampoules of 5 mL.

Proprietary Names and Manufacturers

Boots, UK; CP Pharmaceuticals, UK; Lilly, USA.

13186-e

Prussian Blue

Berlin Blue; CI Pigment Blue 27; Colour Index No. 77510; Ferric Ferrocyanide; Ferric Hexacyanoferrate (II).

$Fe_4[Fe(CN)_6]_3$=859.2.

CAS — 14038-43-8; 12240-15-2.

NOTE. The name Prussian Blue (CI Pigment Blue 27; Colour Index No. 77520) is also applied to potassium ferric hexacyanoferrate(II), $KFe[Fe(CN)_6]$ = 306.9.

Prussian blue is used in the treatment of thallium poisoning. When administered by mouth it forms a non-absorbable complex with thallium in the gastro-intestinal tract which is excreted in the faeces. It has been used similarly for the removal of radiocaesium from the body.

The following treatment of acute thallium poisoning has been suggested: gastric lavage; intravenous fluid challenge with forced diuresis until the 24-hour urinary thallium excretion is below 1 mg; prussian blue 10 g in 100 mL of 15% mannitol twice daily via a duodenal tube until 24-hour urinary thallium excretion is below 0.5 mg; intermittent haemoperfusion or haemodialysis, if possible, especially within 48 hours of ingestion.— G. De Groot *et al.* (letter), *Lancet*, 1987, *1*, 1084. See also under Sodium Diethyldithiocarbamate, p.854.

Proprietary Names and Manufacturers

Antidotum Thallii Heyl *(Heyl, Ger.)*; Radiogardase-Cs *(Heyl, Ger.)*.

1052-e

Sodium Calciumedetate *(BAN)*.

385; Calcium Disodium Edathamil; Calcium Disodium Edetate; Calcium Disodium Ethylenediaminetetra-acetate; Calcium EDTA; Edetate Calcium Disodium *(USAN)*; Natrii Calcii Edetas; Sodium Calcium Edetate *(rINN)*. The calcium chelate of disodium ethylenediaminetetra-acetate.

$C_{10}H_{12}CaN_2Na_2O_8,xH_2O$.

CAS — 62-33-9 (anhydrous).

Pharmacopoeias. In *Br.*, *Egypt.*, *Eur.*, *Fr.*, *It.*, *Jug.*, *Neth.*, *Nord.*, *Swiss*, *Turk.*, and *U.S. Cz.* includes the anhydrous form. Also in *B.P. Vet. Fr.* and *U.S.* specify a mixture of the dihydrate and trihydrate but predominantly the dihydrate. *Egypt.*, *Jug.*, and *Turk.* specify the dihydrate.

A white or almost white, slightly hygroscopic, odourless, crystalline powder or granules. **Soluble** 1 in 2 of water; practically insoluble in alcohol, chloroform, and ether. A 20% solution in water has a pH of 6.5 to 8.0. Solutions are **sterilised** by autoclaving and kept in containers made from lead-free glass. **Store** in airtight containers.

INCOMPATIBILITY. A haze developed over 3 hours when sodium calciumedetate 4 g per litre was mixed with amphotericin 200 mg per litre in glucose injection (5%), and a yellow colour when mixed with hydralazine hydrochloride 80 mg per litre in glucose injection.— B. B. Riley, *J. Hosp. Pharm.*, 1970, *28*, 228.

Adverse Effects

Sodium calciumedetate is nephrotoxic and may cause renal tubular necrosis. Nausea and cramp may also occur. Thrombophlebitis has followed the intravenous infusion of solutions greater than 3%. Other side-effects that have been reported include fever, malaise, headache, myalgia, histamine-like responses such as sneezing, nasal congestion, and lachrymation, bone-marrow depression, skin eruptions, transient hypotension, and ecg abnormalities.

EFFECTS ON THE KIDNEY. Of 130 children with lead poisoning who received combined chelation therapy of sodium calciumedetate (25 mg per kg body-weight intramuscularly every 12 hours) and dimercaprol (3 mg per kg intramuscularly every 4 hours) for a total of 5 days, 21 developed clinical evidence of nephrotoxicity and in 4 severe oliguric acute renal failure began 1 or 2 days after chelation therapy was discontinued. Nephrotoxicity was probably attributable to the use of sodium calciumedetate.— D. I. Moel and K. Kumar, *Pediatrics*, 1982, *70*, 259.

Precautions

Sodium calciumedetate should be used with caution, if at all, in patients with impaired renal function. Daily urinalysis for proteinuria and haematuria and regular monitoring of renal function has been recommended.

Sodium calciumedetate can chelate with several endogenous metals, including zinc, and may increase their excretion.

For the precautions necessary during sodium calciumedetate administration, see below under Uses and Administration.

Sodium calciumedetate 500 mg per m^2 body-surface was administered by deep intramuscular injection every 12 hours for 5 days to 10 children with asymptomatic lead poisoning. Lead concentrations in blood decreased to about 58% of the pretreatment values after 5 days treatment and were essentially unchanged for up to 60 hours after the last dose. Sodium calciumedetate also produced a marked fall in the mean plasma concentration of zinc but this rebounded rapidly after cessation of treatment. Mean urinary-lead excretion increased about 21-fold during the first 24 hours of therapy and urinary-zinc excretion increased about 17-fold. Sodium calciumedetate had little effect on the plasma concentrations or urinary excretion of copper. The results suggested that careful monitoring of zinc was required during treatment with sodium calciumedetate.— D. J. Thomas and J. J. Chisolm, *J. Pharmac. exp. Ther.*, 1986, *239*, 829.

Absorption and Fate

Sodium calciumedetate is poorly absorbed from the gastro-intestinal tract. After intravenous injection about 50% of a dose is excreted in the urine in 1 hour and over 95% in 24 hours.

The pharmacokinetics of sodium calciumedetate administered intramuscularly in doses of 1 g were studied in 10 subjects with normal body burdens of lead but with varying degrees of renal function. The clearance of sodium calciumedetate correlated with serum-creatinine values and creatinine clearance but not with the decrease in the concentrations of lead in the blood or with urinary-lead excretion over 3 days. Maximum serum concentrations of sodium calciumedetate and volume of distribution were no different for subjects with normal or abnormal creatinine clearance. The decrease in lead concentrations in the blood correlated significantly with creatinine clearance and urine protein but not with urinary lead excretion.— J. Osterloh and C. E. Becker, *Clin. Pharmac. Ther.*, 1986, *40*, 686.

Uses and Administration

Sodium calciumedetate is a chelating agent used in the treatment of lead poisoning. It mobilises lead from bone and tissues and aids elimination from the body by forming a stable, water-soluble, lead complex which is readily excreted by the kidney.

For administration by intravenous infusion, 1 g of sodium calciumedetate should be diluted with 250 to 500 mL of glucose injection (5%) or sodium chloride injection (0.9%). The infusion may be administered over a period of at least one hour, to a maximum of 40 mg of anhydrous sodium calciumedetate per kg body-weight, twice daily for up to 5 days, repeated if necessary after an interval of at least 2 days. Any further treatment with sodium calciumedetate should then not be recommenced for at least 7 days. The concentration of sodium calciumedetate infused should never exceed 3%.

Alternatively, the daily dose of sodium calciumedetate may be given intramuscularly in 2 to 4 divided doses as a 20% solution to which the addition of preservative-free procaine hydrochloride to a concentration of 0.5 to 1.5% has been recommended to minimise pain at the injection site. In children or in patients with lead encephalopathy and increased intracranial pressure in whom excess fluids must be avoided, the intramuscular route may be preferable.

Various alternative dosage regimens have been suggested and the concomitant use of dimercaprol (p.840) has been found to be beneficial in certain patients, particularly in children with acute lead encephalopathy.

As excretion is predominantly renal, an adequate urinary flow must be established and maintained during treatment. In patients with impaired renal function, smaller and less frequent doses have been recommended.

Sodium calciumedetate should not be given by mouth in the treatment of lead poisoning as it has been suggested that absorption of lead may be increased as a result.

Sodium calciumedetate may be used as a diagnostic test for lead poisoning.

Sodium calciumedetate is also a chelator of other heavy-metal polyvalent ions, including chromium and a cream containing sodium calciumedetate 10% has been used in the treatment of chrome ulcers and skin sensitivity reactions due to contact with heavy metals.

In some countries, sodium calciumedetate has been permitted for use as an antoxidant synergist in specified foodstuffs

Edetates have been labelled with metallic radionuclides and used in nuclear medicine.

Estimated acceptable daily intake: up to 2.5 mg per kg body-weight.— Seventeenth Report of Joint FAO/WHO Expert Committee on Food Additives, *Tech. Rep. Ser. Wld Hlth Org. No. 539,* 1974.

ADMINISTRATION IN RENAL FAILURE. For the pharmacokinetics of sodium calciumedetate and chelation of lead in renal failure, see under Absorption and Fate, above.

ANTIMICROBIAL ACTION. Successful eradication of *Pseudomonas aeruginosa* from the respiratory tract of 4 patients in intensive care using nebulised sodium calciumedetate together with parenteral benzylpenicillin. The mode of action probably involved the magnesium ions necessary to maintain cell membrane integrity.— K. M. Hillman and A. Twigley (letter), *Lancet,* 1984, *2,* 99.

LEAD POISONING. *Diagnosis.* Measuring the urinary excretion of lead after administration of a standard dose of sodium calciumedetate was considered to be a sensitive method of determining the potentially toxic fraction of lead stored in the body and of assessing response to chelation therapy in chronic lead poisoning.— M. E. Markowitz and J. F. Rosen, *J. Pediat.,* 1984, *104,* 337.

Treatment. A review of lead poisoning. Treatment is aimed primarily at alleviating the acute symptoms, and then at reducing the body-lead stores. Several chelating agents such as sodium calciumedetate, dimercaprol, and penicillamine may be used. Although rare, acute lead encephalopathy in children requires urgent treatment with dimercaprol and sodium calciumedetate. Because lead encephalopathy is unusual, the use of dimercaprol in adults is uncommon. Transient aggravation of symptoms may occur with high doses of sodium calciumedetate, possibly because of mobilisation of lead stores, and treatment must therefore be titrated according to clinical response. Penicillamine may be used after completion of parenteral therapy if the total body lead is still elevated. Protocols for drug administration are discussed.— L. S. Ibels and C. A. Pollock, *Med. Toxicol.,* 1986, *1,* 387.

Further reviews: J. J. Chisolm and D. Barltrop, *Archs Dis. Childh.,* 1979, *54,* 249; S. Piomelli *et al., J. Pediat.,* 1984, *105,* 523.

Preparations

Edetate Calcium Disodium Injection *(U.S.P.).* Sodium calciumedetate injection.

Sodium Calciumedetate Intravenous Infusion *(B.P.).* Sodium Calciumedetate Injection. Prepared immediately before use by diluting Strong Sterile Sodium Calciumedetate Solution with a suitable diluent.

Strong Sterile Sodium Calciumedetate Solution *(B.P.).* Contains the equivalent of 20% (limits 18 to 22%) of anhydrous sodium calciumedetate. To be diluted with sodium chloride injection (0.9%) or glucose injection (5%) before administration.

Proprietary Preparations

Ledclair *(Sinclair, UK). Injection,* sodium calciumedetate 200 mg/mL, in ampoules of 5 mL.

Proprietary Names and Manufacturers

Calcium Disodium Versenate *(Riker, Austral.; Riker, Canad.; Riker, USA);* Calciumedetat *(Ger.);* Chelante Ipit *(IPIT, Ital.);* Ledclair *(Sinclair, UK);* Piomburene *(Ital.);* Sequestrene NA2Ca *(Ciba-Geigy, UK).*

1053-l

Sodium Cellulose Phosphate

Cellulose Sodium Phosphate (*USAN*).

CAS — 9038-41-9; 68444-58-6.

Pharmacopoeias. In *U.S.*

The sodium salt of the phosphate ester of cellulose. A free-flowing cream-coloured, odourless, powder. The inorganic bound phosphate content is not less than 31.0% and not more than 36.0%, the free phosphate content is not more than 3.5%, and the sodium content is not less than 9.5% and not more than 13.0%, calculated on the anhydrous basis. Each g exchanges not less than 1.8 mmol of calcium, calculated on the anhydrous basis. Practically **insoluble** in water, dilute acids, and most organic solvents.

Store in well-closed containers.

Adverse Effects and Precautions

Side-effects with sodium cellulose phosphate are generally rare but diarrhoea and other gastro-intestinal upsets have been reported.

Patients should be monitored for electrolyte disturbances. Uptake of sodium and phosphate may increase and sodium cellulose phosphate should not be given to patients with renal failure or conditions requiring a restricted sodium intake such as congestive heart failure. Theoretically, long-term treatment could result in calcium deficiency; regular monitoring of calcium and parathyroid hormone has therefore been recommended. Sodium cellulose phosphate is not a totally selective exchange resin and the intestinal absorption of other dietary cations may be reduced; magnesium deficiency has been reported but may be corrected by dosage reduction or oral magnesium supplements. Urinary excretion of oxalate may increase and dietary restriction of oxalate intake may be necessary.

Sodium cellulose phosphate may interact with oral medicines containing calcium or magnesium salts including cation-donating antacids and laxatives; magnesium supplements should be administered at least one hour before or after any dose of the resin.

In a study involving 27 patients with absorptive hypercalciuria, sodium cellulose phosphate 5 g three times daily by mouth significantly decreased the urinary excretion of calcium and reduced renal stone formation. However, the renal excretion of oxalate increased in all patients and 8 were withdrawn from therapy when their urinary oxalate exceeded 80 mg per day. A significant decrease in urinary magnesium was also observed in those patients not receiving magnesium supplements. Patients on prolonged treatment with sodium cellulose phosphate required at least periodic monitoring for hypomagnesiuria and hyperoxaluria.— R. Hautmann *et al., J. Urol., Baltimore,* 1978, *120,* 712.

Potential complications of long-term sodium cellulose phosphate therapy include secondary hyperparathyroidism and bone disease; deficiency of magnesium, copper, zinc, and iron; and hyperoxaluria. A study in 18 patients with absorptive hypercalciuria and recurrent renal stones indicated that these complications could largely be avoided if patient selection was confined to those with absorptive hypercalciuria (hypercalciuria, intestinal hyperabsorption of calcium, and normal or suppressed parathyroid function); if the dose was adjusted so as not to reduce intestinal calcium absorption or urinary calcium subnormally (the optimal maintenance dose in most patients was 10 g daily); if oral magnesium supplements were provided; and if a moderate dietary restriction of calcium and oxalate was imposed. There was no evidence of zinc, copper, or iron deficiency.— C. Y. C. Pak, *J. clin. Pharmac.,* 1979, *19,* 451.

Uses and Administration

Sodium cellulose phosphate is a cation-exchange resin that exchanges sodium ions for calcium and other divalent cations. When administered by mouth, it binds calcium ions within the stomach and intestine to form a non-absorbable complex which is excreted in the faeces. It is used in the treatment of absorptive hypercalciuria with recurrent formation of calcium-containing renal stones to reduce the absorption of intestinal calcium usually in conjunction with a low calcium diet. A possible role in the treatment of osteopetrosis, hypercalcaemic sarcoidosis, idiopathic hypercalcaemia of infancy, and vitamin D intoxication has also been suggested.

The usual initial dose is 15 g daily by mouth in 3 divided doses with meals. A suggested dose for children is 10 g daily. The powder may be taken dispersed in water or sprinkled onto food. Oral magnesium supplements of 58 or 87 mg (2.39 or 3.58 mmol) of elemental magnesium twice daily have been recommended for patients taking daily doses of sodium cellulose phosphate 10 or 15 g respectively. The magnesium supplements should not be administered simultaneously with sodium cellulose phosphate.

Sodium cellulose phosphate may also be used for the investigation of calcium absorption.

A review of sodium cellulose phosphate in the treatment of absorptive hypercalciuria.— *Med. Lett.,* 1983, *25,* 67.

Sodium cellulose phosphate has been shown to be effective in decreasing the urinary excretion of calcium and in reducing renal-stone formation in patients with absorptive hypercalciuria (C.Y.C. Pak *et al., New Engl. J. Med.,* 1974, *290,* 175; C.Y.C. Pak *et al., Am. J. Med.,* 1981, *71,* 615). However, Backman *et al.* (*J. Urol., Baltimore,* 1980, *123,* 9) found the prophylactic effects of sodium cellulose phosphate (administered without specific dietary instructions or magnesium supplements) to be poor and suggested that thiazides should be the preferred treatment. Backman *et al.* (1980) also noted that 2 of the 35 patients they treated with sodium cellulose phosphate developed arthralgia which required drug withdrawal.

Proprietary Preparations

Calcisorb *(Riker, UK). Oral powder,* sodium cellulose phosphate, in sachets of 5 g.

Proprietary Names and Manufacturers

Calcibind *(Mission Pharmacal, USA);* Calcisorb *(Riker, Austral.; Belg.; Riker, Denm.; Kettelhack Riker, Ger.; Neth.; Whatman, S.Afr.; Switz.; Riker, UK).*

1054-y

Sodium Diethyldithiocarbamate

DDTC; Dithiocarb Sodium; Ditiocarb Sodium (*pINN*); DTC.

$C_5H_{10}NNaS_2$=171.3.

CAS — 148-18-5.

Sodium diethyldithiocarbamate is a chelating agent that has been used in the treatment of thallium poisoning. It has also been suggested for use in nickel carbonyl poisoning.

The immunomodulating properties of sodium diethyldithiocarbamate are under investigation.

Disulfiram is rapidly metabolised to diethyldithiocarbamate; for its further metabolism see p.1566.

The immunopharmacology and pharmacology of sodium diethyldithiocarbamate.— G. Renoux, *J. Pharmacol.,* 1982, *13, Suppl.* 1, 95.

AIDS. A double-blind crossover study to assess the effects of sodium diethyldithiocarbamate (10 mg per kg body-weight weekly) versus placebo in 83 patients with HIV infection. Each treatment was given for 4 months. Sodium diethyldithiocarbamate produced significant immunological and clinical improvement. Although this compound is known to be a T-cell recruiting agent with a theoretical risk of increasing the number of those cells that harbour the retrovirus, no aggravation was observed with its use in this study.— J.-M. Lang *et al.*, *Lancet.*, 1988. *2*, 702.

SYSTEMIC LUPUS ERYTHEMATOSUS. Sodium diethyldithiocarbamate 5 mg per kg body-weight by mouth once a week induced long-lasting remission of systemic lupus erythematosus in a 14-year-old girl.— N. Delepine *et al.* (letter), *Lancet*, 1985, *2*, 1246.

THALLIUM POISONING. A report on the treatment of a 27-year-old man with severe thallium intoxication; the effectiveness of forced diuresis, haemodialysis, intravenous diethyldithiocarbamate, and oral intestinal chelating agents such as prussian blue, diphenylthiocarbazone, and diethyldithiocarbamate was evaluated. Haemodialysis appeared to be very effective and diethyldithiocarbamate intravenously increased enormously the amount of thallium eliminated in urine; urinary clearances of thallium during forced potassium diuresis were as much as 20 mL per minute, but diethyldithiocarbamate perfusion enhanced the clearances to 200 mL per minute.— S. Nogué *et al.*, *J. Toxicol. clin. Toxicol.*, 1982, *19*, 1015. Intravenous administration of chelating agents in thallium poisoning should be avoided as they may cause a redistribution of thallium over the body, resulting in higher thallium concentrations in the brain.— G. De Groot *et al.* (letter), *Lancet*, 1987, *1*, 1084.

Proprietary Names and Manufacturers
Imuthiol.

1055-j

Sodium Nitrite *(USAN)*.

E250; Natrii Nitris; Natrium Nitrosum.
$NaNO_2$=69.00.

CAS — 7632-00-0.

Pharmacopoeias. In *Arg., Aust., Belg., Chin., Cz., Hung., Mex., Nord., Pol., Roum., Rus., Span., Swiss, Turk.*, and *U.S.*

White or slightly yellow granular powder or white or almost white opaque fused masses or sticks; deliquescent.
Soluble 1 in 1.5 of water; sparingly soluble in alcohol. Solutions in water are alkaline to litmus. The *U.S.P.* injection has a pH of 7.0 to 9.0. **Store** in airtight containers.

Adverse Effects

Sodium nitrite may cause nausea and vomiting, abdominal pain, dizziness, headache, cyanosis, and dyspnoea; vasodilatation resulting in syncope, hypotension, and tachycardia may occur. Overdosage may result in cardiovascular collapse, coma, convulsions, and death. Ionised nitrites readily oxidise haemoglobin to methaemoglobin, causing methaemoglobinaemia.
Sodium nitrite is a precursor for the formation of nitrosamines many of which are carcinogenic in *animals*, but a relationship with human cancer has not been established.

Three cases of methaemoglobinaemia through consumption of nitrite-contaminated meat.— T. Walley and M. Flanagan, *Postgrad. med. J.*, 1987, *63*, 643.

NITROSAMINES. For a review of the chemistry of nitrosamine formation, inhibition, and destruction, see M. L. Douglass *et al.*, *J. Soc. cosmet. Chem.*, 1978, *29*, 581.

Nitrates, nitrites, and gastric cancer in Great Britain.— D. Forman *et al.*, *Nature*, 1985, *313*, 620.

For a report on the occurrence and distribution of nitrate and nitrite in the environment with consideration of the formation of *N*-nitroso compounds from nitrite and the extent of human exposure to these compounds from dietary and other sources, see Nitrate, Nitrite, and *N*-Nitroso Compounds in Food, *Food Surveillance Paper No. 20*, London, HM Stationery Office, 1987.

Treatment of Adverse Effects

When nitrites are ingested, treatment is supportive and symptomatic; oxygen and methylene blue may be required for methaemoglobinaemia. Exchange transfusion may be considered when methaemoglobinaemia is severe.

A 36-year-old man who had taken sodium nitrite tablets (1 g daily) for several weeks thinking they were salt tablets became ill after taking 2 g on one hot day. He was obviously cyanosed, perspiring, and quite distressed, but recovered after treatment with oxygen and methylene blue.— L. G. Wilson (letter), *Med. J. Aust.*, 1976, *1*, 505.

Uses and Administration

Sodium nitrite is used in the treatment of cyanide poisoning in conjunction with sodium thiosulphate (see p.1350). The sodium nitrite produces methaemoglobinaemia and the cyanide ions combine with the methaemoglobin to produce cyanmethaemoglobin, thus protecting cytochrome oxidase from the cyanide ions. As the cyanmethaemoglobin slowly dissociates, the cyanide is converted to relatively nontoxic thiocyanate by the sodium thiosulphate and is excreted in the urine. The usual dosage regimen in adults is 300 mg of sodium nitrite (10 mL of a 3% solution) administered by intravenous injection over 3 minutes followed by 12.5 g of sodium thiosulphate (50 mL of a 25% solution or 25 mL of a 50% solution) administered intravenously over a period of about 10 minutes.
Sodium nitrite has been used as a rust inhibitor. It is also used as a preservative in foods such as cured meats. Potassium nitrite is also used as a food preservative.

Estimated acceptable daily intake of nitrites: up to 20 µg per kg body-weight. No change was made from the acceptable daily intake provided in the Seventeenth Report [however, in that report an intake of up to *200 µg* per kg was given].— Twenty-third Report of the Joint FAO/WHO Expert Committee on Food Additives, *Tech. Rep. Ser. Wld Hlth Org. No. 648*, 1980.

Preparations

Sodium Nitrite Injection *(B.P.C. 1973)*. A sterile solution of sodium nitrite 3% in Water for Injections.
Sodium Nitrite Injection *(U.S.P.)*

Proprietary Names and Manufacturers
OAR (Anti-Rust)*(Orapharm, Austral.)*.

1056-z

Sodium Phytate

Phytate Sodium *(USAN)*; Sodium Fytate *(rINNM)*. The nonasodium salt of *myo*-inositol hexakis(dihydrogen phosphate).
$C_6H_9Na_9O_{24}P_6$=857.9.

CAS — 83-86-3 (phytic acid); 7205-52-9 (nonasodium salt).

Sodium phytate reacts with calcium in the gastro-intestinal tract to form non-absorbable calcium phytate which is excreted in the faeces. Sodium phytate has been used in a similar manner to sodium cellulose phosphate (p.853) to reduce the absorption of calcium from the gut in the treatment of hypercalciuria.

The effects of dietary phytic acid.— *Lancet*, 1987, *2*, 664.

Proprietary Names and Manufacturers of Phytic Acid and its Salts
Alkalovert *(Klein, Ger.)*; Iliso *(Made, Spain)*; Phytat *(Daniel-Brunet, Fr.)*.

5009-k

Sodium Polystyrene Sulphonate

Sodium Polystyrene Sulfonate *(USAN)*.

CAS — 9003-59-2; 9080-79-9; 25704-18-1.

Pharmacopoeias. In *U.S.*

The sodium salt of sulphonated styrene polymer. An odourless, tasteless, golden brown, fine powder containing not more than 10% of water. The sodium content is not less than 9.4% and not more than 11.0%, calculated on the anhydrous basis. Each g exchanges not less than 110 mg (2.81 mmol) and not more than 135 mg (3.45 mmol) of potassium, calculated on the anhydrous basis. Practically **insoluble** in water.

Adverse Effects

Anorexia, nausea, vomiting, and occasionally diarrhoea may develop during treatment with sodium polystyrene sulphonate. Constipation may occur and large doses in elderly patients may result in faecal impaction. A mild laxative such as sorbitol has been recommended to prevent or treat constipation; magnesium-containing laxatives should not be used (see Precautions, below). Serious potassium deficiency can occur with sodium polystyrene sulphonate and signs of severe hypokalaemia may include irritability, confusion, ECG abnormalities, cardiac arrhythmias, and severe muscle weakness. Like other cation-exchange resins, sodium polystyrene sulphonate is not totally selective and its use may result in other electrolyte disturbances such as hypocalcaemia. Significant sodium retention may also occur, especially in patients with impaired renal function, and may lead to congestive heart failure.

EFFECTS ON THE LUNGS. Particles of sodium polystyrene sulphonate were found at autopsy in the lungs of 3 patients who had taken the resin by mouth and were associated with acute bronchitis and bronchopneumonia in 2 and with early bronchitis in the third. It was suggested that rectal administration of sodium polystyrene sulphonate may be preferable, but if administration by mouth is necessary the patient should be positioned carefully to facilitate ingestion of the resin and avoid aspiration.— H. M. Haupt and G. M. Hutchins, *Archs intern. Med.*, 1982, *142*, 379.

Precautions

Patients receiving sodium polystyrene sulphonate should be monitored for electrolyte disturbances, especially hypokalaemia. Since serum concentrations may not always reflect intracellular potassium deficiency, symptoms of hypokalaemia should also be watched for and the decision to stop treatment assessed individually. Hypokalaemia may exacerbate the adverse effects of digoxin and sodium polystyrene sulphonate should be used with caution in patients receiving cardiac glycosides.
Administration of sodium polystyrene sulphonate can result in sodium overloading and it should be used cautiously in patients with renal failure and with conditions requiring a restricted sodium intake, such as congestive heart failure and severe hypertension.
Metabolic alkalosis has been reported in patients with renal disease after the concomitant oral administration of sodium polystyrene sulphonate and cation-donating antacids and laxatives such as magnesium hydroxide or calcium carbonate; the potassium-lowering effect will also be diminished.
The possible effects of sodium polystyrene sulphonate on serum electrolytes should be considered when diagnostic measurements are contemplated in patients receiving such treatment.

INTERACTIONS. *Antacids.* In a study involving 11 patients, all but 2 with relatively stable chronic renal disease, systemic alkalosis occurred when sodium polystyrene sulphonate was given by mouth in association with an antacid containing magnesium hydroxide and aluminium hydroxide or with calcium carbonate; there was no effect with sodium polystyrene sulphonate and aluminium hydroxide alone. Alkalosis did not occur when calcium polystyrene sulphonate was administered with magnesium hydroxide and aluminium hydroxide.— E. T. Schroeder, *Gastroenterology*, 1969, *56*, 868. Metabolic acidosis in a 43-year-old man with chronic renal failure was reversed by the administration of sodium polystyrene sulphonate in association with magnesium hydroxide mixture. The patient's hyperkalaemia was markedly resistant to the resin.— P. C. Fernandez and P. J. Kovnat, *New Engl. J. Med.*, 1972, *286*, 23. The administration of sodium polystyrene sulphonate in association with magnesium hydroxide to a 49-year-old man with chronic renal failure resulted in severe metabolic alkalosis which, in the presence of the patient's chronic hypocalcaemia, precipitated a grand mal seizure.— H. A. Ziessman, *Sth. med. J.*, 1976, *69*, 497.

Uses and Administration

Sodium polystyrene sulphonate is a cation-exchange resin which exchanges sodium ions for potassium ions and other cations following oral or rectal administration. The exchanged resin is then excreted in the faeces. Each gram of resin exchanges about 3 mmol of potassium *in vitro*, and about 1 mmol *in vivo*.

Sodium polystyrene sulphonate is used to reduce potassium concentrations in the treatment of hyperkalaemia, including that associated with anuria or severe oliguria when caution is demanded. An effect may not be evident for several hours or longer, and in severe hyperkalaemia it should be used only in association with other more rapid potassium-lowering measures such as dialysis (see p.1037).

Serum-electrolyte concentrations should be monitored throughout treatment and doses given according to the patient's response. The usual dose is 15 g up to four times daily by mouth, as a suspension in water or syrup; administration in sorbitol solution has been recommended to avoid constipation. A suggested dose for children is up to 1 g per kg body-weight daily by mouth in divided doses, reduced to 500 mg per kg. It should not be given in fruit juices that have a high potassium content and may reduce the exchange-capacity of the resin.

When oral administration is difficult, sodium polystyrene sulphonate may be administered rectally as an enema. A dose of 30 g daily may be given as a suspension in 100 mL of 2% methylcellulose '450' and 100 mL of water and retained, if possible, for at least 9 hours. Initial therapy may constitute administration by both oral and rectal routes. In the *US* a rectal dose of 30 to 50 g in 100 mL of an aqueous vehicle such as sorbitol solution, retained as long as possible and repeated every 6 hours, has been recommended. Children may be given similar rectal doses to those suggested by mouth; particular care is needed with rectal administration in children as excessive dosage or inadequate dilution could result in impaction of resin.

Other polystyrene sulphonate resins include calcium polystyrene sulphonate (p.836), which may be used as an alternative to the sodium resin when sodium intake must be restricted; potassium polystyrene sulphonate (p.850), which has been used in the treatment of hypercalciuria; aluminium polystyrene sulphonate, which was formerly used in the treatment of hyperkalaemia; and ammonium polystyrene sulphonate, which was formerly used to reduce the absorption of sodium ions.

Preparations

Sodium Polystyrene Sulfonate Suspension *(U.S.P.)*

Proprietary Preparations

Resonium A *(Winthrop, UK). Powder,* sodium polystyrene sulphonate.

Proprietary Names and Manufacturers

Kayexalate *(Belg.; Winthrop, Canad.; Sterling Winthrop, Fr.; Maggioni-Winthrop, Ital.; Winthrop, S.Afr.; Winthrop-Breon, USA)*; Resinsodio *(Rubio, Spain)*; Resonium *(Winthrop, Denm.; Iceland; Sterling-Winthrop, Swed.)*; Resonium A *(Aust.; Winthrop, Austral.; Fin.; Winthrop, Ger.; Neth.; Winthrop, Switz.; Winthrop, UK)*.

1057-c

Sodium Thiosulphate *(BAN)*.

Natrii Thiosulfas; Natrium Thiosulfuricum; Sodium Hyposulphite; Sodium Thiosulfate *(USAN)*.

$Na_2S_2O_3,5H_2O = 248.2$.

CAS — 7772-98-7 (anhydrous); 10102-17-7 (pentahydrate).

Pharmacopoeias. In *Arg., Aust., Belg., Br., Chin., Cz., Egypt., Eur., Fr., Ger., Hung., Ind., It., Jpn, Jug., Mex., Neth., Nord., Pol., Port., Roum., Rus., Span., Swiss,* and *U.S.* Also in *B.P. Vet.*

Colourless transparent crystals or a coarse crystalline powder; efflorescent in dry air; deliquescent in moist air. It dissolves in its own water of crystallisation at about 49°. **Soluble** 1 in 0.5 of water; practically insoluble in alcohol. A 10% solution in carbon-dioxide-free water has a pH of 6.0 to 8.4. The *U.S.P.* injection has a pH of 8.0 to 9.5. **Store** in airtight containers.

Solutions of sodium thiosulphate 50% stored in air developed cloudiness or a deposit after autoclaving. Addition of sodium phosphate 0.5% or 1.2% improved stability but solutions became cloudy or developed a deposit after 12 and 6 weeks respectively at 25°. Solutions containing sodium bicarbonate 0.5% became cloudy or developed a deposit after 12 weeks at 25°. No significant improvement in stability was obtained when the concentration of sodium thiosulphate was reduced to 30% or 15%, or when the injection was sealed under nitrogen.— Pharm. Soc. Lab. Rep., 1975, P/75/3..

Adverse Effects

Apart from osmotic disturbances sodium thiosulphate is relatively non-toxic. Large doses by mouth have a cathartic action.

Absorption and Fate

Sodium thiosulphate is poorly absorbed from the gastro-intestinal tract. After intravenous injection it is distributed throughout the extracellular fluid and rapidly excreted in the urine.

An intravenous infusion of sodium thiosulphate 12 g per m^2 body-surface was administered over 6 hours to 8 patients receiving intraperitoneal antineoplastic therapy; in 6 of the patients it was given in conjunction with cisplatin to protect against the adverse effects of cisplatin. The thiosulphate was rapidly eliminated, 95% being excreted within 4 hours of stopping the infusion; on average only 28.5% of the dose was recovered unchanged in the urine. The mean plasma elimination half-life was 80 minutes.— M. Shea *et al., Clin. Pharmac. Ther.,* 1984, *35,* 419.

Uses and Administration

Sodium thiosulphate is used in the treatment of cyanide poisoning (see p.1350) in conjunction with sodium nitrite. The sodium nitrite produces methaemoglobinaemia, and the cyanide ions combine with the methaemoglobin to produce cyanmethaemoglobin, thus protecting cytochrome oxidase from the cyanide ions. As the cyanmethaemoglobin slowly dissociates, the cyanide is converted to relatively nontoxic thiocyanate by the sodium thiosulphate and is excreted in the urine.

The usual dosage regimen in adults is 300 mg of sodium nitrite (10 mL of a 3% solution) administered by intravenous injection over 3 minutes followed by 12.5 g of sodium thiosulphate (50 mL of a 25% solution or 25 mL of a 50% solution) administered intravenously over a period of about 10 minutes.

Sodium thiosulphate has antifungal properties and has been used in the treatment of pityriasis versicolor as a 20% or 25% solution applied once or twice daily. To prevent relapse, treatment must be continued for weeks or months after infection appears to have been cleared.

Estimated acceptable daily intake of sodium thiosulphate as SO_2: up to 700 µg per kg body-weight.— Twenty-second Report of Joint FAO/WHO Expert Committee on Food Additives, *Tech. Rep. Ser. Wld Hlth Org. No. 631,* 1978. See also Twenty-seventh Report of the Joint FAO/WHO Expert Committee on Food Additives, *Tech. Rep. Ser. Wld Hlth Org. No. 696,* 1983.

For a report of sodium thiosulphate given by intravenous infusion reducing the incidence of nephrotoxicity associated with intraperitoneal cisplatin, see under Treatment of Adverse Effects in Cisplatin, p.608.

Preparations

Sodium Thiosulfate Injection *(U.S.P.)*

Sodium Thiosulphate Injection *(B.P.C. 1973).* A sterile solution of sodium thiosulphate 50% in Water for Injections.

Sodium Thiosulphate Lotion *(A.P.F.).* Sodium thiosulphate 20% in freshly boiled and cooled water.

Proprietary Names and Manufacturers

Hyposulfène *(Rosa-Phytopharma, Fr.)*; Oligosol S *(Labcatal, Switz.)*; S-Hydril *(Laves, Ger.)*; Soufre Oligosol *(Labcatal, Fr.)*.

The following names have been used for multi-ingredient preparations containing sodium thiosulphate— Adasept *(Odan, Canad.)*; Komed *(Barnes-Hind, Canad.; Barnes-Hind, USA)*; Tineasol *(Arlo, USA)*; Tinver *(Barnes-Hind, Canad.; Barnes-Hind, USA)*.

1058-k

Succimer *(USAN, rINN)*.

DIM-SA; DMSA. *meso*-2,3-Dimercaptosuccinic acid.

$C_4H_6O_4S_2 = 182.2$.

CAS — 304-55-2.

Pharmacopoeias. In *Chin.* as the sodium salt.

Succimer is an analogue of dimercaprol (p.840) under study for the treatment of arsenic, lead, and mercury poisoning. It may be administered by mouth.

Reviews on the role of succimer in the treatment of heavy-metal poisoning: H. V. Aposhian, *Annu. Rev. Pharmacol. Toxicol.,* 1983, *23,* 193; J. H. Graziano, *Med. Toxicol.,* 1986, *1,* 155.

ARSENIC POISONING. Report of promising results in a patient with acute arsenic poisoning treated with succimer 300 mg by mouth every 6 hours for 3 days.— K. Lenz *et al., Arch. Tox.,* 1981, *47,* 241.

LEAD POISONING. Succimer was administered to 18 patients with occupational lead intoxication in doses of 10, 20, or 30 mg per kg body-weight daily by mouth for 5 days. The drug was well tolerated and there was a linear dose-dependent decline in lead concentrations in the blood during treatment. Succimer appeared to be a promising drug in the treatment of lead poisoning.— J. H. Graziano *et al., Clin. Pharmac. Ther.,* 1985, *37,* 431.

Further references: E. Friedheim *et al., Lancet,* 1978, *2,* 1234.

13334-q

Thymidine

NSC-21548; Thymine 2-Desoxyriboside. 1-(2-Deoxy-β-D-ribofuranosyl)-5-methyluracil; 1-(2-Deoxy-β-D-ribofuranosyl)-1,2,3,4-tetrahydro-5-methylpyrimidine-2,4-dione.

$C_{10}H_{14}N_2O_5 = 242.2$.

CAS — 50-89-5.

Thymidine is a nucleoside constituent of cells. It has been given by intravenous infusion to modulate the toxicity of methotrexate; it may also have an antineoplastic action of its own. Thymidine is not considered to be a substitute for calcium folinate.

A study indicated that acute lymphoblastic leukaemic cells were highly sensitive to growth inhibition by thymidine. Thymidine might have a role in the management of certain acute lymphoblastic leukaemias or lymphomas.— R. M. Fox *et al., Lancet,* 1979, *2,* 391. The antileukaemic potential of thymidine administered at the maximum tolerable dose was assessed in 6 patients with relapsed leukaemia or lymphoma. The dose was gradually escalated every few days until infusions of 180 to 240 g per m^2 body-surface were given daily and administered until bone-marrow aplasia resulted or unacceptable toxicity developed (14 to 29 days). Side-effects included nausea, vomiting, diarrhoea, and alopecia; liver function abnormalities, central nervous system toxicity, and electrolyte disturbance were also observed in some patients. Although bone-marrow aplasia was achieved in all patients and one had complete remission, this therapy which required prolonged continuous infusion of massive fluid volumes was impractical except in exceptional circumstances. The cell kill rate was much slower than that of other antineoplastic agents but thymidine might be a useful modulating agent, by inducing either cytokinetic or nucleotide pool alterations.— M. S. Blumenreich *et al., Cancer Res.,* 1984, *44,* 2203.

For conflicting reports on the enhancing effects of thymidine on the antineoplastic activity of fluorouracil, see under Fluorouracil, Uses and Administration, p.629.

For comments on the use of thymidine in the prevention of methotrexate toxicity, see under Methotrexate, Treatment of Adverse Effects, p.637.

13377-a

Trientine Dihydrochloride *(BAN, rINNM)*.

Trien Hydrochloride; Trientine Hydrochloride *(USAN)*; Triethylenetetramine Dihydrochloride. 2,2′-Ethylenediiminobis(ethylamine) dihydrochloride.

$C_6H_{18}N_4,2HCl=219.2.$

CAS — 112-24-3 (trientine); 38260-01-4 (dihydrochloride).

The manufacturers recommend that capsules of trientine dihydrochloride be **stored** at 2° to 8° in airtight containers.

Trientine dihydrochloride is a copper chelating agent used in a similar way to penicillamine (p.849) in the treatment of Wilson's disease in conjunction with a low-copper diet. It tends to be used in patients intolerant to penicillamine although systemic lupus erythematosus in patients treated with penicillamine has recurred during treatment with trientine.

Trientine dihydrochloride is administered by mouth, preferably on an empty stomach before meals. The usual dose is 1.2 to 2.4 g daily in 2 to 4 divided doses. The dose should be adjusted according to response and lower doses may be used to initiate therapy. In children, doses of up to 1.5 g daily have been given.

Iron deficiency has been reported in patients taking trientine dihydrochloride and iron supplements may be required; doses of trientine dihydrochloride and iron should not be administered together.

PRIMARY BILIARY CIRRHOSIS. Trientine dihydrochloride was effective in increasing urinary copper excretion in 4 patients with primary biliary cirrhosis but all 4 discontinued treatment within 6 months because of serious side-effects including acute gastritis, skin rash, severe anorexia, and rhabdomyolysis.— O. Epstein and S. Sherlock, *Gastroenterology*, 1980, *78*, 1442.

WILSON'S DISEASE. A review of trientine in Wilson's disease.— *Med. Lett.*, 1986, *28*, 67.

Report on the effective treatment of Wilson's disease with trientine dihydrochloride in 20 patients who were intolerant of penicillamine. In 19 patients serum-iron concentrations fell significantly but iron deficiency was readily corrected with iron supplements given at least 4 hours apart from any dose of trientine.— J. M. Walshe, *Lancet*, 1982, *1*, 643.

Further references: J. M. Walshe, *Q. J. Med.*, 1986, *58*, 81 (use in pregnancy).

Proprietary Names and Manufacturers
Cuprid *(Merck Sharp & Dohme, USA)*;
Manufacturers also include—*K & K-Greeff, UK.*

1059-a

Unithiol

DMPS; Unitiol. Sodium 2,3-dimercaptopropanesulphonate.

$C_3H_7NaO_3S_3=210.3.$

CAS — 4076-02-2.

Unithiol is an analogue of dimercaprol (p.840) used in the treatment of poisoning by heavy metals. It has been administered subcutaneously or intramuscularly in doses of 5 mg per kg body-weight 3 or 4 times during the first 24 hours, 2 or 3 times on the second day, and once or twice on subsequent days. It has also been given by mouth.

Reviews of unithiol in the treatment of heavy-metal poisoning.— H. V. Aposhian, *Annu. Rev. Pharmacol. Toxicol.*, 1983, *23*, 193; K. Hruby and A. Donner, *Med. Toxicol.*, 1987, *2*, 317.

LEAD POISONING. Twelve children with chronic lead poisoning were treated with unithiol 200 or 400 mg per m^2 body-surface daily by mouth in 4 divided doses for 5 days. Both dosages significantly reduced lead concentrations in blood but did not affect the concentrations of copper or zinc in plasma. During treatment the urinary excretion of lead, copper, and zinc was increased.— J. J. Chisolm and D. J. Thomas, *J. Pharmac. exp. Ther.*, 1985, *235*, 665.

MERCURY POISONING. Administration of unithiol 100 mg twice daily by mouth for a maximum of 15 days enhanced urinary elimination of mercury in 7 patients with mercury poisoning. The urinary elimination of copper and zinc were also increased in most patients and two developed skin rashes.— T. G. K. Mant, *Hum. Toxicol.*, 1985, *4*, 346.

Further references to unithiol in mercury poisoning: T. W. Clarkson *et al.*, *J. Pharmac. exp. Ther.*, 1981, *218*, 74 (methylmercury poisoning); J. R. Campbell *et al.*, *J. Am. med. Ass.*, 1986, *256*, 3127 (industrial exposure to mercury vapours).

WILSON'S DISEASE. Unithiol 200 mg twice daily was used successfully to maintain cupriuresis in a 13-year-old boy with Wilson's disease after he developed systemic lupus during treatment with penicillamine and with trientine dihydrochloride. Unithiol was started in two similar patients but both withdrew from treatment, one because of fever and a fall in leucocyte count and the other because of intense nausea and taste impairment.— J. M. Walshe, *Br. med. J.*, 1985, *290*, 673.

Proprietary Names and Manufacturers
Dimaval *(Heyl, Ger.)*.

Colouring Agents

2370-w

Colouring agents have long been used in foods and cosmetics in an attempt to improve the appearance of the product or subject. They are also used in medicinal preparations with the aim of improving their acceptability to patients. Such uses are now widely controlled and this has resulted in restrictions on the extent to which colouring agents may be used. Matters of concern that have received considerable publicity include sensitivity reactions (see tartrazine, p.860) and behaviour disorders (see below).

This chapter includes agents whose main use is to provide colour. Colouring agents with additional uses may be found in the chapters on disinfectants (p.949) and on diagnostic agents (p.938).

BEHAVIOUR DISORDERS. Food additives are implicated in behaviour disorders (J. Egger *et al.*, *Lancet*, 1985, *1*, 540). However, the role of foods and food additives is not clear (*Lancet*, 1979, *2*, 617; M.H. Lessof, *J. R. Coll. Physns*, 1987, *21*, 237). Lessof in discussing the conflicting evidence makes the point that many studies have failed to identify the restlessness and irritability of children with extensive eczema, asthma, or rhinitis and to give separate consideration to those whose behaviour problems are unaccompanied by somatic symptoms.

2372-l

Allura Red AC

CI Food Red 17; Colour Index No. 16035; E129; F D & C Red No. 40. Disodium 6-hydroxy-5-(6-methoxy-4-sulphonato-*m*-tolylazo)naphthalene-2-sulphonate.
$C_{18}H_{14}N_2Na_2O_8S_2$=496.4.

CAS — 25956-17-6.

Allura red AC is employed as a colouring agent. Its use extends to foods, medicines, and cosmetics.

Estimated acceptable daily intake of allura red: up to 7 mg per kg body-weight.— Twenty-fifth Report of Joint FAO/WHO Expert Committee on Food Additives, *Tech. Rep. Ser. Wld Hlth Org. No. 669*, 1981.

Although some of the *animal* studies had been criticised, allura red AC was considered to be provisionally acceptable in food in the *UK*. However, there was concern about *para*-cresidine a potential carcinogen used in the production of allura red AC. While this compound could not be detected in the free state in food-grade allura red AC down to a limit of 1 ppm, reassurance was required that it was not formed as a metabolite.— FdAC/REP/4, London, HM Stationery Office, 1987.

2373-y

Amaranth

Bordeaux S; CI Acid Red 27; CI Food Red 9; Colour Index No. 16185; formerly F D & C Red No. 2; E123. It consists mainly of trisodium 3-hydroxy-4-(4-sulphonato-1-naphthylazo)naphthalene-2,7-disulphonate.
$C_{20}H_{11}N_2Na_3O_{10}S_3$=604.5.

CAS — 915-67-3.

incompatibility between amaranth and cetrimide.— B. W. Barry and G. F. J. Russell, *J. pharm. Sci.*, 1972, *61*, 502.

Amaranth is used as a colouring agent in medicines, foodstuffs, and cosmetics.

Estimated acceptable daily intake of amaranth: up to 500 μg per kg body-weight.— Twenty-eighth Report of the FAO/WHO Expert Committee on Food Additives, *Tech. Rep. Ser. Wld Hlth Org. No. 710*, 1984.

Studies carried out by the *US* FDA showed no evidence of carcinogenicity with amaranth, but a subsequent study did show an increased tumour incidence in *rats* given amaranth. As a result of this, the *UK* Food Advisory Committee requested that carcinogenicity and metabolic studies be carried out in the *rat*. A satisfactorily conducted long-term study in the *rat* which included *in utero* exposure did not demonstrate any carcinogenicity. The increased incidence of renal pelvic calcification and epithelial hyperplasia that was observed was associated with senile changes and considered to be of doubtful relevance to human safety. The use of amaranth in food was recommended as acceptable.— FdAC/REP/4, London, HM Stationery Office, 1987.

Preparations

Amaranth Solution *(B.P.)*. Amaranth *food grade of commerce* 1 g, chloroform spirit 20 mL, glycerol 25 mL, freshly boiled and cooled water to 100 mL.

Amaranth Solution *(A.P.F.)*. Red Solution. Amaranth *food grade of commerce* 1 g, compound hydroxybenzoate solution 1 mL, freshly boiled and cooled water to 100 mL.

Red Syrup *(A.P.F.)*. Syr. Rubr.; Elixir Rubrum. Amaranth solution 2.5 mL, orange tincture 5 mL, lemon spirit 0.5 mL, syrup to 100 mL.

2375-z

Black PN

Brilliant Black BN; CI Food Black 1; Colour Index No. 28440; E151; Noir Brilliant PN. It consists mainly of tetrasodium 4-acetamido-5-hydroxy-6-[7-sulphonato-4-(4-sulphonatophenylazo)-1-naphthylazo]naphthalene-1,7-disulphonate.
$C_{28}H_{17}N_5Na_4O_{14}S_4$=867.7.

CAS — 2519-30-4.

Pharmacopoeias. In *Fr.*

Black PN is used as a colouring agent in medicines, cosmetics, and foods.

Estimated acceptable daily intake of black PN: up to 1 mg per kg body-weight.— Twenty-fifth Report of the Joint FAO/WHO Expert Committee on Food Additives, *Tech. Rep. Ser. Wld Hlth Org. No. 669*, 1981.

Animal studies supporting the recommendation that the use of black PN in food is acceptable.— FdAC/REP/4, London, HM Stationery Office, 1987.

2376-c

Bordeaux B

Azorubrum; CI Acid Red 17; Colour Index No. 16180. Consists mainly of disodium 3-hydroxy-4-(1-naphthylazo)naphthalene-2,7-disulphonate.
$C_{20}H_{12}N_2Na_2O_7S_2$=502.4.

CAS — 5858-33-3.

Bordeaux B was formerly used as a colouring agent for medicines and foods but has been replaced by other colours.

2377-k

Brilliant Blue FCF

133; Blue EGS; CI Acid Blue 9; CI Food Blue 2; Colour Index No. 42090; F D & C Blue No. 1; Patent Blue AC. Disodium 4′,4″-bis(*N*-ethyl-3-sulphonatobenzylamino)triphenylmethylium-2-sulphonate.
$C_{37}H_{34}N_2Na_2O_9S_3$=792.8.

CAS — 3844-45-9.

Brilliant blue FCF is used as a colouring agent in medicines, cosmetics, and foodstuffs.

An estimated acceptable daily intake of 12.5 mg of brilliant blue FCF per kg body-weight had been established after repeated subcutaneous injections to *animals*.— Thirteenth Report of an FAO/WHO Expert Committee on Food Additives, *Tech. Rep. Ser. Wld Hlth Org. No. 445*, 1970.

2378-a

Brown FK

154; Chocolate Brown FK; CI Food Brown 1. A mixture of 6 azo dyes: sodium 2′,4′-diaminoazobenzene-4-sulphonate; sodium 2′,4′-diamino-5′-methylazobenzene-4-sulphonate; disodium 4,4′-(4,6-diamino-1,3-phenylenebisazo) dibenzenesulphonate; disodium 4,4′-(2,4-diamino-1,3-phenylenebisazo) dibenzenesulphonate; disodium 4,4′-(2,4-diamino-5-methyl-1,3-phenylenebisazo) dibenzenesulphonate; trisodium 4,4′,4″-(2,4-diaminobenzene-1,3,5-triazo)tribenzenesulphonate.

CAS — 8062-14-4.

Brown FK is used as a colouring agent for foodstuffs such as smoked fish.

A temporary estimated acceptable daily intake (ADI) of up to 75 μg per kg body-weight for brown FK had been allocated at the 29th meeting pending the results of further long-term studies in *rats*. Since no results were forthcoming at the time of the thirtieth meeting, the temporary ADI was withdrawn.— Thirtieth Report of an FAO/WHO Expert Committee on Food Additives, *Tech. Rep. Ser. Wld Hlth Org. No. 751*, 1987.

Animal toxicity studies with brown FK provided inconsistent results and their toxicological significance was doubtful. Brown FK and its major colour components are mutagenic to bacterial systems *in vitro*, but mutagenicity was not demonstrated in the host-mediated assay. Given the absence of effects in carcinogenicity and multigeneration studies, it was considered that the *in vitro* mutagenicity findings did not constitute evidence of a possible hazard. The former Food Additives and Contaminants Committee had recommended that brown FK be restricted to smoked and smoke-flavoured fish and to meat marking. Brown FK was still recommended as being acceptable for these food uses.— FdAC/REP/4, London, HM Stationery Office, 1987.

2386-a

Brown HT

155; Chocolate Brown HT; CI Food Brown 3; Colour Index No. 20285. Disodium 4,4′-(2,4-dihydroxy-5-hydroxymethyl-1,3-phenylenebisazo)di(naphthalene-1-sulphonate).
$C_{27}H_{18}N_4Na_2O_9S_2$=652.6.

CAS — 4553-89-3.

Brown HT is used as a colouring agent for foodstuffs.

Estimated acceptable daily intake for brown HT: up to 1.5 mg per kg body-weight. Brown HT was manufactured with a higher salt content than most other colouring agents in order to reduce the content of organic impurity.— Twenty-eighth Report of the Joint FAO/WHO Expert Committee on Food Additives, *Tech. Rep. Ser. Wld Hlth Org. No. 710*, 1984.

Results of *animal* studies with brown HT were such that the Committee recommended that its use in food is acceptable.— FdAC/REP/4, London, HM Stationery Office, 1987.

2380-l

Canthaxanthin

CI Food Orange 8; Colour Index No. 40850; E161(g). *β,β*-Carotene-4,4′-dione.
$C_{40}H_{52}O_2$=564.9.

CAS — 514-78-3.

Canthaxanthin is a carotenoid but unlike betacarotene or *β*-apo-8′-carotenal it possesses no vitamin A activity. It is used to colour the flesh of trout or salmon when it may be given to the fish with astaxanthin. It is also used in cosmetics.

Canthaxanthin has also been given by mouth to produce an artificial suntan. Such use has led to retinal deposits and in some cases to impairment of vision.

Because of reports of crystal deposition in the retina following doses within the previously allocated estimated acceptable daily intake (ADI) of 25 mg per kg body-weight, the ADI was made temporary and reduced to up to 50 μg per kg. Further studies were required by 1989.— Thirty-first Report of the Joint FAO/WHO Expert Committee on Food Additives, *Tech. Rep. Ser. Wld Hlth Org. No. 759*, 1987.

Canthaxanthin had been classified in a previous review as being acceptable for use in food. Since that time there had been reports of deposits in the retina, termed gold speck maculopathy, sometimes associated with altered function. When used to colour the flesh of trout and salmon the maximum human intake from eating farmed fish flesh might be 1 to 5 mg per day. The infrequent consumption of such an amount was not considered to be a hazard. However canthaxanthin has been used to colour biscuits, confectionery, pickles, sauces, and preserves and these sources could provide 1 to 3 mg a day. It was considered that canthaxanthin be restricted to incorporation in the feed of farmed salmon and trout.— FdAC/REP/4, London, HM Stationery Office, 1987.

Some references to canthaxanthin retinopathy: P. Cortin *et al., Can. J. Ophthal.*, 1984, *19*, 215; R. McGuinness and P. Beaumont, *Med. J. Aust.*, 1985, *143*, 622.

2381-y

Caramel *(USAN).*

Burnt Sugar; E150; Sacch. Ust.; Saccharum Ustum.

CAS — 8028-89-5.

Pharmacopoeias. In *U.S.N.F.* Also in *B.P.C. 1973*

A thick, but free-flowing, dark brown liquid, with a characteristic odour and a pleasant bitter taste. Caramel *U.S.N.F.* is prepared from sucrose or glucose, a small amount of alkali or alkali carbonate or a trace of mineral acid being added while heating. In Great Britain caramel permitted for use in food may be a product obtained exclusively by heating sucrose or other edible sugars, or a water-soluble amorphous brown product obtained by heating an edible sugar in the presence of (a) certain organic or mineral acids or sulphur dioxide, or (b) alkali hydroxides or ammonia, or (c) ammonium, sodium, or potassium carbonates, phosphates, sulphates, or sulphites.

Caramel of commerce is made from many raw materials, including sucrose, glucose, liquid glucose, molasses, and invert sugar. It is supplied in various qualities and strengths, with different colour intensities, to suit the various commodities in which it is used.

Caramel is used as a colouring agent to produce pale yellow to dark brown colours. It has no calorific value. Some caramels also have flavouring properties.

Four classes of caramel were considered.

Caramel colour I (plain caramel; caustic caramel; spirit caramel). Although some materials classified as caramel colour I may contain sulphur compounds, an acceptable daily intake of 'not specified' was allocated provided that it complied with revised specifications.

Caramel colour II (caustic sulphite process caramel). No acceptable daily intake was established.

Caramel colour III (ammonia caramel; beer caramel). Lymphocyte depression caused by caramel colour III was attributed to a minor component, 2-acetyl-4-(5)-tetrahydroxybutylimidazole (THI). An estimated acceptable daily intake for caramel colour III of up to 200 mg per kg body-weight was allocated.

Caramel colour IV (ammonia sulphite caramel; soft-drink caramel). An estimated acceptable daily intake of up to 200 mg per kg body-weight was allocated to class IV caramel colours. These caramel colours contain 4-methylimidazole as a contaminant and a limit of 1 g per kg caramel colour IV was established; it was hoped that a substantial reduction could be made in this limit.— Twenty-ninth Report of the Joint FAO/WHO Expert Committee on Food Additives, *Tech. Rep. Ser. Wld Hlth Org. No. 733*, 1986. See also Thirty-first Report of the Joint FAO/WHO Expert Committee on Food Additives, *Tech. Rep. Ser. Wld Hlth Org. No. 759*, 1987.

In an Interim Report on the Review of the Colouring Matter in Food Regulations 1973, the Food Additives and Contaminants Committee paid special attention to the safety of caramels used in food. Because of their colouring and flavouring function caramels accounted for about 98% by weight of all colouring matter used in food. There are numerous different caramels in use and not one of these products could be chemically defined. Though some toxicological studies had been carried out on certain caramel products those tested had not been chemically defined and it was therefore impossible to extrapolate from one product to another. The Committee suggested that caramels should be considered as 4 distinct types, categorised according to their method of preparation: (a) burnt sugar (principally used as flavourings); (b) caustic; (c) ammonia; (d) ammonium sulphite. It was also suggested that the permitted number of caramels should be limited and that in the absence of a chemical specification those products permitted should be adequately defined by a full process specification. The British Caramel Manufacturers' Association considered that the needs of the food industry for caramels for colouring could be met by a limited number of caramels and proposed 6 specifications. Since much of the previous toxicological data relates to caramels other than those in the 6 specifications the Committee recommended that the biological properties of the caramels in each specification should be determined.— FAC/REP/29, London, HM Stationery Office, 1979.

The Food Advisory Committee reconsidered caramel. In reviewing the *animal* studies they could not rule out the possibility that 2-acetyl-4(5)-tetrahydroxybutylimidazole (THI) is not the only agent with haematological effects present in ammonia caramels, though it may be a marker for such compounds. An ammonia caramel should have a THI level below 25 ppm. It was recommended that caramel should remain classified as provisionally acceptable for use in food but further information was required on the lymphocytopenic effect. Confirmation was also required that caramels other than ammonia caramel do not cause lymphocytopenia under conditions of low vitamin-B_6 intake.— FdAC/REP/4, London, HM Stationery Office, 1987.

2382-j

Carmine

CI Natural Red 4; Colour Index No. 75470; E120. The aluminium lake or aluminium-calcium lake of the colouring matter of cochineal. It contains about 50% of carminic acid, an anthraquinone glycoside.

CAS — 1390-65-4.

Pharmacopoeias. In *Arg., Belg., Fr., Port.,* and *Swiss* which specify the aluminium-calcium lake. Also in *B.P.C. 1973* which specifies the aluminium lake.

Unless precautions are taken during manufacture and transport to prevent contamination, carmine may be infected with salmonella micro-organisms.

Carmine and some of its salts are used as colouring agents in medicines, foodstuffs, cosmetics, and toilet preparations.

Carmine passes through the gastro-intestinal tract unchanged and has been used as a faecal 'marker' in a dose of 200 to 500 mg.

Temporary estimated acceptable daily intake of ammonium carmine or equivalent amounts of the calcium, potassium, or sodium salts (the lithium salt is not acceptable for food-additive use): up to 2.5 mg per kg body-weight. Results from a long-term study were requested.— Twenty-fifth Report of the Joint FAO/WHO Expert Committee on Food Additives, *Tech. Rep. Ser. Wld Hlth Org. No. 669*, 1981.

2384-c

Carmoisine

Azorubine; CI Food Red 3; Colour Index No. 14720; E122. It consists mainly of disodium 4-hydroxy-3-(4-sulphonato-1-naphthylazo)naphthalene-1-sulphonate. $C_{20}H_{12}N_2Na_2O_7S_2$=502.4.

CAS — 3567-69-9.

Pharmacopoeias. In *Fr.*

Carmoisine is used as a colouring agent in foods and cosmetics.

Temporary estimated acceptable daily intake of carmoisine: up to 1.25 μg per kg body-weight. Further studies are required, including metabolic studies in man.— Twenty-second Report of the Joint FAO/WHO Expert Committee on Food Additives, *Tech. Rep. Ser. Wld Hlth Org. No. 631*, 1978.

The results of *animal* studies with carmoisine were such that the Committee recommended that its use in food is acceptable.— FdAC/REP/4, London, HM Stationery Office, 1987.

2385-k

Chlorophyll

CI Natural Green 3; Colour Index No. 75810; E140; E141 *(copper complexes of chlorophyll/chlorophyllin).*

CAS — 479-61-8 (chlorophyll a); 519-62-0 (chlorophyll b).

Chlorophyll is a green colouring matter of plants. It is a mixture of 2 closely related substances, chlorophyll a and chlorophyll b. The only difference between the 2 chlorophylls is that a methyl side-chain in chlorophyll a is replaced by a formyl group in chlorophyll b.

Oil-soluble chlorophyll derivatives. Replacement of the magnesium atom in the chlorophylls by 2 hydrogen atoms using dilute mineral acids produces olive-green water-insoluble phaeophytins. Copper phaeophytins (sometimes called copper chlorophyll complex) can be formed; these are more stable to acids and to light than the chlorophylls.

Water-soluble chlorophyll derivatives. When the chlorophylls are hydrolysed with alkali, phytyl alcohol and methyl alcohol are split off and green water-soluble chlorophyllins are formed. If sodium hydroxide is used, a mixture of sodium magnesium chlorophyllins a and b is the product. Similar water-soluble compounds can be prepared in which the magnesium is replaced by copper to give copper chlorophyllin complex.

Chlorophyll is employed principally as a colouring agent, in foods, medicines, and cosmetics.

Chlorophyll has been used as an external application in the treatment of wounds and ulcers. There is no clear evidence that it does accelerate healing but it is considered to have a deodorant action.

Commercial claims for the deodorant effect of chlorophyll tablets or toothpaste on halitosis and other body odours lack scientific proof.

Estimated acceptable daily intake of chlorophyllin copper complex and the sodium or potassium salts: up to 15 mg per kg body-weight.— Twenty-first Report of the Joint FAO/WHO Expert Committee on Food Additives, *Tech. Rep. Ser. Wld Hlth Org. No. 617*, 1978. See also Twenty-second Report of Joint FAO/WHO Expert Committee on Food Additives, *Tech. Rep. Ser. Wld Hlth Org. No. 631*, 1978.

Chlorophyllin had no effect on the urine odour in incontinent patients.— M. C. Nahata *et al., Drug Intell. & clin. Pharm.*, 1983, *17*, 732.

Proprietary Names and Manufacturers of Chlorophyll or a Related Substance

Amplex C *(Ashe, UK)*; Chloresium *(Rystan, USA)*; Derifil *(Rystan, USA)*; Derofil *(Langly, Austral.)*; Exodor *(Rorer, Ger.)*; Melodin *(Spain)*; Melodyn *(Rocador, Spain)*; Oligon *(Ger.)*; Sudroma *(Frosst, Canad.)*; Vulnotox *(Ger.)*.

The following names have been used for multi-ingredient preparations containing chlorophyll or a related substance— Gomaxide *(Seaford, UK)*; Panafil *(Rystan, USA)*; Prophyllin *(Rystan, USA)*.

2387-t

Cochineal *(BAN).*

CI Natural Red 4; Coccionella; Coccus; Coccus Cacti; Colour Index No. 75470; E120.

CAS — 1343-78-8.

Pharmacopoeias. In *Br., Egypt.,* and *Port.*

The dried female insect, *Dactylopius coccus* (=*Coccus cacti*) (Coccidae), containing eggs and larvae. It complies with a test for contamination with *Escherichia coli* and salmonellae.

Cochineal which is a source of carmine is used as a red colouring agent in food, medicines, and cosmetics.

Results of *animal* studies with cochineal were such that the Committee recommended that its use in food is acceptable.— FdAC/REP/4, London, HM Stationery Office, 1987.

2391-z

Eosin

CI Acid Red 87; Colour Index No. 45380; D & C Red No. 22; Éosine Disodique; Eosin Y. The disodium salt of 2′,4′,5′,7′-tetrabromofluorescein. $C_{20}H_6Br_4Na_2O_5$=691.9.

CAS — 548-26-5; 17372-87-1.

Pharmacopoeias. In *Fr.*

Eosin has been incorporated in solution-tablets to give a distinctive colour to solutions prepared from them. It is also used in cosmetics and as a reagent.

The unreliability of the Dill-Glazko eosin urine colour test for chloroquine.— F. Verdier *et al.* (letter), *Lancet*, 1985, *1*, 1282; L. Rombo *et al.* (letter), *ibid.*, 1509.

2392-c

Erythrosine

CI Food Red 14; CI No. 45430; E127; Erythrosine BS; Erythrosine Sodium *(USAN)*; F D & C Red No. 3. The monohydrate of the disodium salt of 2′,4′,5′,7′-tetra-iodofluorescein.

$C_{20}H_6I_4Na_2O_5,H_2O$=897.9.

CAS — 568-63-8; 16423-68-0 (both anhydrous); 49746-10-3 (monohydrate).

Pharmacopoeias. In *Braz.* and *U.S. Fr.* permits disodium or dipotassium salts.

Red or brownish-red odourless hygroscopic powder containing not less than 87% of dye, calculated as $C_{20}H_6I_4$–Na_2O_5,H_2O, together with smaller amounts of lower iodinated fluoresceins. **Soluble** in water forming a bluish-red solution that shows no fluorescence in ordinary light; sparingly soluble in alcohol; soluble in glycerol and propylene glycol; practically insoluble in fats and oils. **Store** in airtight containers.

Erythrosine is used as a colouring agent for medicines and foods. It is also used in cosmetics and as a disclosing agent for plaque on teeth.

A comment that erythrosine was being reviewed by the FDA because of carcinogenicity in *rats*.— B. E. Jones, *Pharm. J.*, 1984, *2*, 116.

Temporary estimated acceptable daily intake: up to 600 µg per kg body-weight. Erythrosine was absorbed only to a small extent in *animals* and man. Thyroid studies indicated that erythrosine inhibits the deiodination of thyroxine to tri-iodothyronine and at high doses activates secretory mechanisms for thyrotrophin in the pituitary. Results of pharmacokinetic studies were required to relate concentrations of erythrosine to the thyroid effects.— Thirtieth Report of the Joint FAO/WHO Expert Committee on Food Additives, *Tech. Rep. Ser. Wld Hlth Org. No. 751*, 1987.

Animal studies indicated that erythrosine or a metabolite acted on the thyroid by inhibiting the conversion of thyroxine to tri-iodothyronine so stimulating thyrotrophin. These actions were not attributable to free iodide. It was recommended that the use of erythrosine in food is acceptable provided limits are set so that intake would not exceed 100 µg per kg body-weight daily.— FdAC/REP/4, London, HM Stationery Office, 1987.

Preparations

Erythrosine Sodium Topical Solution *(U.S.P.)*

Erythrosine Sodium Soluble Tablets *(U.S.P.)*

Proprietary Preparations

Ceplac *(Rorer, UK). Dental disclosing tablets*, erythrosine 6 mg.

Proprietary Names and Manufacturers

Ceplac *(Rorer, UK)*; Disclo *(Orapharm, Austral.)*; En-De-Kay C-Red *(Westone, UK)*.

2394-a

Green S

Acid Brilliant Green BS; Acid Green S; CI Food Green 4; Colour Index No. 44090; E142; Lissamine Green; Wool Green B. Sodium 1-[4-dimethylamino-α-(4-dimethyliminiocyclohexa-2,5-dienylidene)benzyl]-2-hydroxynaphthalene-3,6-disulphonate.

$C_{27}H_{25}N_2NaO_7S_2$=576.6.

CAS — 3087-16-9.

Green S is used as a colouring agent in medicines, cosmetics, and foodstuffs.

Staining of the conjunctiva with Green S was found to be a reasonably specific but inadequately sensitive test for diagnosing early xerophthalmia.— N. Emran and A. Sommer, *Archs Ophthal., N.Y.*, 1979, *97*, 2333.

Studies in *animals* indicated that there is some absorption of green S and caecal enlargement but it was considered that there is a very large margin of safety between the highest estimated intake of green S of 130 µg per person daily and the level at which changes were seen in *animal* studies (500 mg per kg body-weight daily). It was recommended that the use of green S in food is acceptable.— FdAC/REP/4, London, HM Stationery Office, 1987.

12817-a

Henna

Henna Leaf; Lawsonia.

The dried leaves of *Lawsonia inermis* (= *L. alba*) (Lythraceae), containing lawsone (see p.1451).

Powdered henna is used for dyeing the hair and skin.

13078-q

Paraphenylenediamine

$C_6H_4(NH_2)_2$=108.1.

CAS — 106-50-3.

NOTE. Commonly known in the hairdressing trade as '*para*'.

Adverse Effects

It is estimated that about 4% of apparently normal subjects are sensitive to 'para', and 1% acutely sensitive; oedema and severe dermatitis may follow application in such persons. Effects on the eye may include chemosis, lachrymation, exophthalmos, and sometimes permanent blindness.

Following ingestion severe angioedema-like symptoms with respiratory difficulty and dyspnoea may occur and may require emergency tracheostomy; vomiting, massive oedema, gastritis, rise in blood pressure, vertigo, tremors, convulsions, and coma have been reported.

Some studies have linked hair dyes with mutagenicity and carcinogenicity.

In many countries the permitted concentration of paraphenylenediamine in hair dyes is controlled by law.

Of 1205 persons with dermatitis or eczema submitted to patch testing with paraphenylenediamine 2% in yellow soft paraffin, 15.2% gave a positive reaction.— E. Rudzki and D. Kleniewska, *Br. J. Derm.*, 1970, *83*, 543.

Comment on the severe toxicity associated with ingestion of paraphenylenediamine, alone or with henna; of 24 cases seen in the Sudan over 1 year, 8 had died, mainly due to acute respiratory distress of rapid onset.— E. H. El-Ansary *et al.* (letter), *Lancet*, 1983, *1*, 1341. See also F. Baud *et al.* (letter), *ibid.*, *2*, 514.

Chronic renal failure in 2 patients apparently associated with long-term topical application of paraphenylenediamine-containing hair dyes.— J. H. Brown *et al.*, *Br. med. J.*, 1987, *294*, 155. Criticism; there was no evidence of any association.— J. S. Savill and A. J. Rees (letter), *ibid.*, 646. See also C. M. Burnett and J. F. Corbett, *ibid.*, 1163.

CARCINOGENICITY. In a study of chromosomal damage and hair dyes no excess of chromosomal damage was noted in 60 professional hair tinters compared with 36 control subjects, possibly owing to the protective effect of gloves and poor percutaneous absorption through the hands. A significant excess of chromosomal damage (mainly chromatid breaks), was, however, noted in women with dyed hair compared with matched controls. This latter finding warranted further study in view of the known mutagenicity and carcinogenicity of some hair-dye constituents.— D. J. Kirkland *et al.*, *Lancet*, 1978, *2*, 124. Severe criticisms and comments.— N. J. Van Abbé (letter), *ibid.*, 271; D. J. Kirkland *et al.* (letter), *ibid.*, 272; N. J. Van Abbé (letter), *ibid.*, 368; D. J. Price (letter), *ibid.*; A. R. Feinstein (letter), *ibid.*, 627; D. J. Kirkland *et al.* (letter), *ibid.*, 628; C. Burnett (letter), *ibid.*, 685.

Analysis of data from 120 557 married, female, registered US nurses did not indicate evidence of any material carcinogenic risk occurring during the initial 20 years following first use of permanent hair dyes.— C. H. Hennekens *et al.*, *Lancet*, 1979, *1*, 1390. Criticisms.— A. K. Bahn (letter), *ibid.*, *2*, 475; J. M. Davies (letter), *ibid.*, 536.

For references to the mutagenic activity in bacteria of paraphenylenediamine derivatives used as hair dyes and its relevance to carcinogenicity, see C. E. Searle *et al.*, *Nature*, 1975, *255*, 506; D. J. Kirkland and S. Venitt, *Mutat. Res.*, 1976, *40*, 37; C. Burnett (letter), *Lancet*, 1976, *1*, 482; S. Venitt *et al.* (letter), *ibid.*, 641.

Further references: D. G. MacPhee and D. M. Podger (letter), *Med. J. Aust.*, 1975, *2*, 32; M. Jain *et al.* (letter), *Can. med. Ass. J.*, 1977, *117*, 1132; K. M. Stavraky *et al.*, *J. natn. Cancer Inst.*, 1979, *63*, 941.

Uses and Administration

Paraphenylenediamine is used as a hair dye and for dyeing furs.

13080-n

Paratoluenediamine

2-Methyl-1,4-phenylenediamine.

$C_7H_{10}N_2$=122.2.

CAS — 95-70-5.

Paratoluenediamine is used as a hair dye.

Of 612 persons with dermatitis or eczema submitted to patch testing with paratoluenediamine 2% in yellow soft paraffin, 4.2% gave a positive reaction.— E. Rudzki and D. Kleniewska, *Br. J. Derm.*, 1970, *83*, 543.

A report of aplastic anaemia in a woman who used a hair dye containing paratoluenediamine.— P. J. Toghill and R. G. Wilcox, *Br. med. J.*, 1976, *1*, 502. For comments suggesting that the aplastic anaemia might be attributed to antibiotics taken by the patient, see A. J. Jouhar (letter), *ibid.*, 1074.

A further report of aplastic anaemia in 2 patients following use of hair dye containing paratoluenediamine.— J. E. Hopkins and A. Manoharan, *Postgrad. med. J.*, 1985, *61*, 1003.

For references to the potential mutagenicity and carcinogenicity of hair dyes, see Paraphenylenediamine (above).

2397-r

Ponceau 4R

Brilliant Ponceau 4RC; Brilliant Scarlet; CI Food Red 7; Coccine Nouvelle; Cochineal Red A; Colour Index No. 16255; E124; Rouge Cochenille A. Trisodium 7-hydroxy-8-(4-sulphonato-1-naphthylazo)naphthalene-1,3-disulphonate.

$C_{20}H_{11}N_2Na_3O_{10}S_3$=604.4.

CAS — 2611-82-7.

Pharmacopoeias. In *Fr.*

Ponceau 4R is used as a colouring agent in medicines and foods. Sensitivity reactions have been reported.

Estimated acceptable daily intake of ponceau 4R: up to 4 mg per kg body-weight.— Twenty-seventh Report of the Joint FAO/WHO Expert Committee on Food Additives, *Tech. Rep. Ser. Wld Hlth Org. No. 696*, 1983.

The results of *animal* studies with ponceau 4R were such that the Committee recommended that its use in food is acceptable.— FdAC/REP/4, London, HM Stationery Office, 1987.

2398-f

Quinoline Yellow

Canary Yellow; CI Acid Yellow 3; CI Food Yellow 13; CI No. 47005; Jaune De Quinoléine. The sodium salts of a mixture of the mono- and disulphonic acids of quinophthalone or 2-(2-quinolyl)indanedione.

CAS — 8004-92-0.

NOTE. D & C Yellow No.10 and E104 are both used as synonyms or codes for quinoline yellow, but D & C Yellow No.10 describes a mixture mainly of the monosulphonic acid of quinophthalone while E104 describes a mixture mainly of the disulphonic acid.

Pharmacopoeias. In *Fr.*

Quinoline yellow is used as a colouring agent in medicines, cosmetics, and foodstuffs.

Estimated acceptable daily intake of quinoline yellow: up to 10 mg per kg body-weight; this applied to both the methylated and the unmethylated varieties of quinoline yellow.— Twenty-eighth Report of the Joint FAO/WHO Expert Committee on Food Additives, *Tech. Rep. Ser. Wld Hlth Org. No. 710*, 1984.

The results of *animal* studies with quinoline yellow were such that the Committee recommended that its use in food is acceptable.— FdAC/REP/4, London, HM Stationery Office, 1987.

2399-d

Raspberry

Framboise; Fructus Rubi Idaei; Himbeer; Rubus Idaeus. The fresh ripe fruit of *Rubus idaeus* (Rosaceae).

CAS — 8027-46-1.

Pharmacopoeias. In *Arg. B.P.* includes Concentrated Raspberry Juice and Raspberry Syrup.

Raspberry is used as a colouring and flavouring agent in medicines and foodstuffs.

Preparations

Concentrated Raspberry Juice *(B.P.).* Prepared from raspberry juice from which the pectin has been removed by the action of pectinase and subsequent clarification, adding to it sufficient sucrose to adjust the wt per mL to 1.05 to 1.06 g, then concentrating the juice to one-sixth of its original volume and adding sodium metabisulphite or other suitable antimicrobial preservative. Store at a temperature not exceeding 25°. Protect from light.

Raspberry Syrup *(B.P.).* Prepared by diluting 1 vol. of Concentrated Raspberry Juice with 11 vol. of syrup. It may contain permitted food-grade colours. It should be freshly prepared, but if it is prepared with precautions which will prevent fermentation, it may be recently prepared when it should be used within 4 weeks of opening the container. Store at a temperature not exceeding 25°. Protect from light.

2400-d

Red 2G

128; Acid Red 1; CI Food Red 10; Colour Index No. 18050; Ext. D & C Red No. 11; Geranine 2G. Disodium 5-acetamido-4-hydroxy-3-phenylazonaphthalene-2,7-disulphonate.

$C_{18}H_{13}N_3Na_2O_8S_2$=509.4.

CAS — 3734-67-6.

Red 2G is used as a colouring agent in medicines, cosmetics, and foods.

Estimated acceptable daily intake for red 2G: up to 100 µg per kg body-weight.— Twenty-fifth Report of the Joint FAO/WHO Expert Committee on Food Additives, *Tech. Rep. Ser. Wld Hlth Org. No. 669*, 1981.

There was concern that red 2G might produce haemolysis in subjects deficient in glucose-6-phosphate dehydrogenase, but investigations did not confirm such a risk. However, there might be a risk from red 2G hydrolysing in acid solution to red 10B about which there was inadequate data. It was considered undesirable to use red 2G in foods of high acidity that are subjected to a high temperature during processing. It was understood that in the *UK* use of red 2G is largely confined to meat products and use in this type of product is considered acceptable.— FdAC/REP/4, London, HM Stationery Office, 1987.

2401-n

Red Cherry

Cerasus; Cerise Rouge; Ginja; Griottier.

Pharmacopoeias. In *Fr.* and *Port. U.S.N.F.* includes Cherry Juice and Cherry Syrup.

The fresh ripe fruit of varieties of the red or sour cherry, *Prunus cerasus* (Rosaceae).

Red cherry is used as a colouring and flavouring agent.

Preparations

Cherry Juice *(U.S.N.F.).* The juice expressed from the fresh ripe fruit of *P. cerasus*, and containing not less than 1% of malic acid. pH 3 to 4. Store at a temperature not exceeding 40° in airtight containers. Protect from light.

Cherry Syrup *(U.S.N.F.).* Cherry juice 47.5 mL, sucrose 80 g, alcohol 2 mL, water to 100 mL. Store at a temperature not exceeding 40° in airtight containers. Protect from light.

2402-h

Red-Poppy Petal

Coquelicot; Klatschrose; Petalos de Amapola; Rhoead. Pet.; Rhoeados Petalum.

Pharmacopoeias. In *Arg.*, *Belg.*, *Fr.*, *Port.*, and *Span.*

The dried petals of *Papaver rhoeas* (Papaveraceae).

Red-poppy petal has been used as a colouring agent usually in the form of a syrup.

2403-m

Red-Rose Petal

Fleur de Rose; Flos Rosae; Red Rose Petals; Ros. Pet.; Rosae Gallicae Petala; Rosae Petalum; Rosenblüte.

Pharmacopoeias. In *Arg.*, *Chin.*, *Fr.*, *Port.*, and *Span.*

The petals of the red or Provins rose, *Rosa gallica* (Rosaceae). Some of the pharmacopoeias allow other species.

Red-rose petal has been employed, usually as an acid infusion, for its mild astringent properties and as a colouring agent.

2407-q

Saffron

Açafrão; Azafrán; CI Natural Yellow 6; Colour Index No. 75100; Croci Stigma; Crocus; Estigmas de Azafrán; Safran.

Pharmacopoeias. In *Arg.*, *Aust.*, *Belg.*, *Chin.*, *Fr.*, *Jpn*, *Mex.*, *Neth.*, *Port.*, *Roum.*, and *Span.*

The dried stigmas and tops of the styles of *Crocus sativus* (Iridaceae), containing crocines, crocetins, and picrocrocine. **Protect** from light.

Saffron is used as a food and cosmetic dye and flavouring agent. In some circles it is considered to be a food. It was once widely used for colouring medicines. There have been early reports of poisoning with saffron.

2410-h

Sunset Yellow FCF

CI Food Yellow 3; Colour Index No. 15985; E110; FD & C Yellow No. 6; Jaune Orangé S; Jaune Soleil; Orange Yellow S. Disodium 6-hydroxy-5-(4-sulphonatophenylazo)naphthalene-2-sulphonate.

$C_{16}H_{10}N_2Na_2O_7S_2$=452.4.

CAS — 2783-94-0.

Pharmacopoeias. In *Fr.*

Sunset yellow FCF is used as a colouring agent in foods, medicines, and cosmetics. Sensitivity reactions have been reported.

Estimated acceptable daily intake of sunset yellow FCF: up to 2.5 mg per kg body-weight.— Twenty-sixth Report of the Joint FAO/WHO Expert Committee on Food Additives, *Tech. Rep. Ser. Wld Hlth Org. No. 683*, 1982.

Consideration of 2 reports of an increased incidence of adrenal medullary adenomas in *rats* given sunset yellow FCF for 2 years as well as other studies in which there were no effects led to the opinion that the findings in the 2 reports were not attributable to treatment with sunset yellow FCF. It was recommended that this colour still be considered acceptable for use in food.— FdAC/REP/4, London, HM Stationery Office, 1987.

2411-m

Tartrazine

CI Food Yellow 4; Colour Index No. 19140; E102; F D & C Yellow No. 5; Jaune Tartrique; Tartrazin.; Tartrazol Yellow. It consists mainly of trisodium 5-hydroxy-1-(4-sulphonatophenyl)-4-(4-sulphonatophenylazo)pyrazole-3-carboxylate.

$C_{16}H_9N_4Na_3O_9S_2$=534.4.

CAS — 1934-21-0.

Pharmacopoeias. In *Fr.*

Tartrazine is used as a colouring agent in foods, cosmetics, and medicines. Some patients may experience sensitivity reactions (see below).

There have been numerous reports of reactions to tartrazine (see *Martindale 28th Edn*, p. 431) and these cover angioedema, asthma, urticaria, thrombocytopenic purpura, and anaphylactic shock. Some of the reports have dealt with cross-sensitivity, especially with aspirin, although the connection with aspirin has recently been questioned by the Food Advisory Committee (FdAC/REP/4, London, HM Stationery Office, 1987). A suggested incidence of tartrazine sensitivity is 1 in 10 000 (*Drug & Ther. Bull.*, 1980, *18*, 53). The mechanism of the reactions may not necessarily be immunological (R.D. Murdoch *et al.*, *J. R. Coll. Physns*, 1987, *21*, 257).

In considering the reports of tartrazine sensitivity or intolerance the Food Advisory Committee (1987) reported that similar evidence of intolerance might well be obtained for a variety of natural food ingredients if as many studies were conducted on them as on tartrazine. The Committee considered that tartrazine posed no more problems than other colours or food ingredients and recommended that the continued use of tartrazine in food is acceptable. However, use of tartrazine in medicines appears to be diminishing and in some countries its presence is declared on the label.

2415-q

Turmeric

CI Natural Yellow 3; Colour Index No. 75300; Curcuma; Indian Saffron. The dried rhizome of *Curcuma longa* (Zingiberaceae).

CAS — 458-37-7.

Pharmacopoeias. In *Chin.* Témoé-Lawaq (*Fr. P.*) and Javanische Gelbwurz (*Ger. P.*) are the rhizome of *C. zanthorrhiza*, containing not less than 5% (*Fr.*) or 3.5% (*Ger.*) of volatile oil.

Turmeric contains curcumin Colour Index No. 75300; E100 [1,7-bis(4-hydroxy-3-methoxyphenyl)hepta-1,6-diene-3,5-dione, $C_{21}H_{20}O_6$ = 368.4]. A yellow pigment.

Turmeric is used principally as a constituent of curry powders and other condiments. Turmeric and its main ingredient curcumin are used as yellow colouring agents in foods.

Temporary estimated acceptable daily intake (ADI) of curcumin: up to 100 µg per kg body-weight. The results of a carcinogenicity study and a reproduction/teratogenicity study were awaited.

Temporary ADI of turmeric oleoresin: up to 300 µg/kg. Histopathological change had been observed in the liver, kidney, bladder, and thyroid of *animals* given turmeric oleoresin and further data was required.

Turmeric or ground turmeric powder was also considered but because it is often regarded as a food rather than a food additive, it was not appropriate to allocate an ADI.— Thirtieth Report of FAO/WHO Expert Committee on Food Additives, *Tech. Rep. Ser. Wld Hlth Org. No. 751*, 1987.

Turmeric was considered to be provisionally acceptable for use in food as a colouring agent when it was not being used as a spice. However, further *animal* studies were required, especially as thyroid changes had been observed in the *pig*.— FdAC/REP/4, London, HM Stationery Office, 1987.

2419-e

Yellow 2G

107; Acid Light Yellow 2G; Acid Yellow 17; CI Food Yellow 5; Colour Index No. 18965. Disodium 2,5-dichloro-4-[5-hydroxy-3-methyl-4-(4-sulphonatophenylazo)pyrazol-1-yl]benzenesulphonate.

$C_{16}H_{10}Cl_2N_4Na_2O_7S_2$=551.3.

CAS — 6359-98-4.

Yellow 2G is used as a colouring agent in foodstuffs and cosmetics.

Yellow 2G was classified as a substance for which inadequate or no toxicological data are available and on which it is not possible to express an opinion as to its acceptability for use in food.— FdAC/REP/4, London, HM Stationery Office, 1987.

Contrast Media

1550-g

Contrast media (radiopaques) increase the absorption of X-rays as they pass through the body and are used for delineating body structures.

The use of gas (air, oxygen, or carbon dioxide) for visualisation has been described as negative contrast; that of radiopaque agents, positive contrast; when the two are used concomitantly the procedure is called double contrast. Tomography is the procedure whereby a selected plane of the subject is visualised.

Barium sulphate, the principal contrast medium for gastro-intestinal radiography, is described below.

The other contrast media described in this section are iodinated organic compounds whose degree of opacity is directly proportional to their iodine content. Being iodinated compounds, these contrast media carry the risk of unwanted effects from the iodine.

The iodinated contrast media may be classified as ionic and nonionic, and additionally as monomeric and dimeric.

The currently used monomeric ionic compounds are salts of substituted tri-iodobenzoic acid; they are soluble in water with comparatively low viscosity in solution. The toxicity of such media can be mainly attributed to their hyperosmolality. The ionic monomeric compounds include the acetrizoate, diatrizoate, metrizoate, iothalamate, ioxitalamate, and ioglicate salts.

The development of nonionic monomeric and ionic dimeric contrast media with reduced osmolality has led to a reduction in vascular pain and other haemodynamic side-effects. The nonionic monomeric contrast media include iohexol, iopamidol, iopromide, and metrizamide. Ionic dimeric contrast media include iocarmate, iodipamide, iodoxamate, ioglycamate, ioxaglate, and iotroxate.

Iotasul is a nonionic dimeric contrast medium.

Modifications of the cations of ionic contrast media can also reduce their toxicity in certain circumstances.

Most intravascular iodine-based contrast media are readily excreted by the kidneys and are used for examination of urinary and blood systems (urographic and angiographic media). Those principally used are salts of diatrizoic acid (p.863), iodamide (p.865), iopamidol (p.867), iothalamic acid (p.868), and ioxaglic acid (p.869).

Contrast media that are excreted primarily by the liver are used for examination of the biliary tract (cholecystographic media). They are usually given by mouth and include calcium ipodate (p.863), iocetamic acid (p.865), iopanoic acid (p.867), and sodium ipodate (p.871). Salts of iodipamide (p.866), iodoxamic acid (p.866), and of ioglycamic acid (p.867) are given intravenously.

Intravascular contrast media — the past, the present, and the future.— R. G. Grainger, *Br. J. Radiol.*, 1982, *55*, 1.

Contrast Media in Urography, Angiography, and Computerized Tomography, V. Taenzer and E. Zeitler (Ed.), Stuttgart, Georg Thieme Verlag, 1983.

The advantages of low-osmolar contrast media.— R. G. Grainger, *Br. med. J.*, 1984, *289*, 144. Comment.— P. Davies (letter), *ibid.*, 379; G. Ansell (letter), *ibid.*, 380; R. J. West (letter), *ibid.*, 698; R. G. Grainger (letter), *ibid.*

The pharmacology of intravascular radiocontrast media.— T. W. Morris and H. W. Fischer, *Annu. Rev. Pharmacol. Toxicol.*, 1986, *26*, 143.

Organic radiopaques: a review of the development of newer contrast media, the improved techniques for their use, and the resulting clinical benefits.— A. Bentley and K. Piper, *Pharm. J.*, 1987, *1*, 338.

EFFECTS ON THE CARDIOVASCULAR SYSTEM. Cardiovascular side-effects of various conventional, low-osmolar and nonionic contrast media.— K. Wink and J. Wissert, in *Contrast Media in Urography, Angiography and Computerized Tomography*, V. Taenzer and E. Zeitler (Eds), Stuttgart, Georg Thieme Verlag, 1983, p. 120.

EFFECTS ON THE KIDNEY. For a discussion on the effects of contrast media on the kidney, see sodium diatrizoate (p.864).

1520-d

Acetrizoic Acid

Acetriz. Acid; Acidum Acetrizoicum. 3-Acetamido-2,4,6-tri-iodobenzoic acid.

$C_9H_6I_3NO_3$=556.9.

CAS — 85-36-9.

Pharmacopoeias. In *Int.* and *Turk.*

Acetrizoic acid contains approximately 68.4% of I.

1551-q

Sodium Acetrizoate *(BAN, rINN).*

$C_9H_5I_3NNaO_3$=578.8.

CAS — 129-63-5.

Sodium acetrizoate contains approximately 65.8% of I. Each g of monograph substance represents 1.73 mmol of sodium.

Acetrizoic acid is a high-osmolal ionic monomeric contrast medium that was formerly used as its sodium salt in diagnostic radiology for a variety of procedures including hysterosalpingography, but has been replaced by better tolerated compounds, Acetrizoic acid has actions similar to the diatrizoates (p. 863).

Proprietary Names and Manufacturers

Angiombrine *(Medinsa, Spain)*; Densopax *(Arg.)*; Diaginol Viscous *(Austral.*; *May & Baker, UK)*; Fortombrine *(Medinsa, Spain)*; Salpix *(Ortho, Canad.)*.

1552-p

Barium Sulphate *(BAN).*

Barii Sulfas; Barii Sulphas; Barium Sulfate *(USAN)*; Barium Sulfuricum; Baryum (Sulfate de).

$BaSO_4$=233.4.

CAS — 7727-43-7.

Pharmacopoeias. In *Arg., Aust., Belg., Br., Braz., Chin., Cz., Egypt., Eur., Fr., Ger., Hung., Ind., Int., It., Jpn, Jug., Mex., Neth., Nord., Pol., Port., Roum., Rus., Span., Swiss, Turk.,* and *U.S.*

A fine, heavy, white, odourless, powder, free from grittiness.

Practically **insoluble** in water and organic solvents; very slightly soluble in acids and alkali hydroxides.

CAUTION. *When Barium Sulphate is prescribed the title should always be written out in full to avoid confusion with the poisonous barium sulphide or sulphite.*

Adverse Effects

Constipation may occur after oral or rectal barium sulphate administration; impaction, obstruction, and appendicitis have occurred. Cramping or diarrhoea have also been reported. Intravasation has led to the formation of emboli; deaths have occurred. Perforation of the bowel has led to peritonitis, adhesions, granulomas, and death.

The use of barium sulphate for bronchography, or aspiration into the lungs, has led to pneumonitis or granuloma formation.

Cardiac arrhythmias have occurred during the use of barium sulphate enemas.

In Great Britain the recommended exposure limit of barium sulphate respirable dust is 2 mg per m^3(long-term).

A healthy 64-year-old man developed fever and pelvic tenderness following a barium enema. This was attributed to the development of sepsis due to increased intracolonic pressure during the enema. Recovery after treatment with antibiotics was uneventful.— E. Larsen (letter), *J. Am. med. Ass.*, 1974, *229*, 639.

Accidental venous intravasation of barium sulphate occurred in an elderly woman given a barium sulphate enema. She developed hypotension and disseminated intravascular coagulation. The barium sulphate had high levels of endotoxins and it was considered that the endotoxic shock was responsible for the reaction. A barium granuloma developed 8 months later in the rectovaginal septum.— H. Blom *et al.*, *Archs intern. Med.*, 1983, *143*, 1253.

CARDIAC ARRHYTHMIAS. Of 95 patients undergoing barium enema examination, 44 had ECG changes during the procedure; the changes were more frequent in elderly patients and in those with heart disease. In 16 patients the changes were potentially serious.— G. L. Eastwood, *J. Am. med. Ass.*, 1972, *219*, 719.

Precautions

Barium sulphate should be used with caution in patients with obstructing lesions of the gastro-intestinal tract or pyloric stenosis. It should also be used with caution in acute diverticulitis, acute ulcerative colitis, and tracheoesophageal fistula. Use is not advisable in patients at risk from gastro-intestinal perforation; other contrast media such as diatrizoate or iothalamate may be considered.

Uses and Administration

Barium sulphate is used as a contrast medium for X-ray examination of the gastro-intestinal tract. It is not absorbed and hence does not produce the systemic effects of soluble barium salts. It is given in the form of a suspension.

For X-ray examination of the upper gastro-intestinal tract it may be given by mouth in the dose range 40 to 450 g. For examination of the colon, barium sulphate may be given by enema in the dose range 150 to 750 g. Higher doses may be employed with either route. Gas can be introduced into the gastro-intestinal tract for double-contrast examination by using suspensions of barium sulphate containing carbon dioxide; separate gas-producing preparations based on sodium bicarbonate are also available.

A review of barium sulphate preparations.— A. Bentley and K. Piper, *Pharm. J.*, 1987, *1*, 138.

Studies in which barium radiography compared unfavourably with endoscopy: M. W. Dronfield *et al.*, *Br. med. J.*, 1982, *284*, 545; C. P. Dooley *et al.*, *Ann. intern. Med.*, 1984, *101*, 538; P. B. Boulos *et al.*, *Lancet*, 1984, *1*, 95.

An investigation of the quality of barium enema films of 1000 patients. Over half the films were the result of a bad technique (single contrast) or of a good technique (double contrast) badly executed.— C. B. Williams and T. Nishigami (letter), *Lancet*, 1983, *2*, 48.

A study comparing 2 high density barium sulphate preparations, Micropaque HD and E-Z-HD, in double contrast investigations of the upper gastro-intestinal tract in 93 patients. E-Z-HD gave significantly better mucosal coating and was less liable to bubble formation.— J. M. Bell *et al.*, *Clin. Radiol.*, 1984, *35*, 367.

A double contrast technique using orally administered Baritop 300 mL diluted to 50% w/v, followed 30 minutes later by 100 Baritop effervescent tablets given in divided doses. The tablets yielded 1 litre of gas which rapidly passed into the small bowel. Results suggested that the main criticism of the small bowel barium examination has been largely overcome by this technique which increased the amount of barium and air in the small bowel and reduced the density of the contrast medium, thus distending the small bowel and reducing the number of overlapping loops of small bowel filled with barium.— G. M. Fraser and P. G. Preston, *Gut*, 1984, *25*, A1162.

Double contrast barium enemas were carried out on 151 patients using either air or carbon dioxide. Significant pain was experienced in 30% of patients receiving air compared to 11% when carbon dioxide was used. There was no difference in enema quality between the two groups.— R. A. Frost *et al.*, *Gut*, 1985, *26*, A582.

A study of 1358 referrals for barium enemas; the overall diagnostic yield for colonic or distal ileal pathology was 33% with 75 (5.5%) cancers detected.— K. D. Vellacott and J. Virjee, *Gut*, 1986, *27*, 182.

INTUSSUSCEPTION. Barium enemas have been recommended in the investigation of children with suspected acute intussusception which can also be reduced by the enema (*Lancet*, 1985, *2*, 250). Several studies have been reported to show success-rates ranging from about 8 to 80% (H. Carstensen *et al.*, *ibid.*, 954; G.J. Poston and M.P. Singh, *ibid.*, 1118).

Preparations

Barium Sulfate for Suspension *(U.S.P.)*. A dry mixture of not less than 90% of barium sulphate and one or more suitable dispersing and/or suspending agents. It may contain one or more suitable colours, flavours, fluidising agents, and preservatives. pH of a 60% w/w aqueous suspension is 4 to 10.

Barium Sulphate for Suspension *(B.P.)*. A dry mixture of not less than 85% of barium sulphate with a suitable dispersing agent and suitable flavouring agents and preservatives. pH of a 75% w/v aqueous suspension 4.5 to 7.0.

Barium Sulphate Oral Suspension *(B.P.)*. Barium Sulphate Suspension. An aqueous suspension containing not less than 75% w/v of barium sulphate with a suitable dispersing agent and suitable flavouring agents and preservatives. pH 4.5 to 7.0.

Proprietary Preparations

Baritop 100 *(Concept Pharmaceuticals, UK)*. *Suspension*, barium sulphate 100%. It contains carbon dioxide under pressure.
Baritop Tablets used to produce carbon dioxide are described under sodium bicarbonate (p.1027).

Baritop Plus *(Concept Pharmaceuticals, UK)*. *Suspension*, barium sulphate, granules for reconstitution.

E-Z-Cat *(Henleys, UK)*. *Suspension*, barium sulphate 4.6%.

E-Z-HD *(Henleys, UK)*. *Suspension*, barium sulphate, powder for reconstitution.

E-Z-PAQUE *(Henleys, UK)*. *Suspension*, barium sulphate, powder for reconstitution.

Micropaque DC *(Nicholas, UK)*. *Suspension*, barium sulphate 100%.

Micropaque HD *(Nicholas, UK)*. *Suspension*, barium sulphate, powder for reconstitution.

Micropaque Powder *(Nicholas, UK)*. *Suspension*, barium sulphate, powder for reconstitution.

Micropaque Standard *(Nicholas, UK)*. *Suspension*, barium sulphate 100%.
Suspension, powder for reconstitution.

Microtrast *(Nicholas, UK)*. *Paste*, barium sulphate 70%.

Polibar ACB *(Henleys, UK)*. *Suspension*, barium sulphate, powder for reconstitution.

Proprietary Names and Manufacturers

Bariopacin *(Serra Pamies, Spain)*; Baritop *(Boehringer Ingelheim, Austral.; Schering, Fr.; Concept Pharmaceuticals, UK)*; Barium Andreu *(Neth.)*; Baro-CAT *(Mallinckrodt, Canad.)*; Barosperse *(Mallinckrodt, Austral.; Mallinckrodt, Canad.; Swed.; Mallinckrodt, Switz.; Mallinckrodt, USA : Camlab, UK)*; Barotrast *(Neth.; Barnes-Hind, Switz.)*; Barytgen *(Fushimi, Denm.; Fushimi, Swed.)*; Baryx Colloïdal *(Fr.)*; Baryxine *(Fr.)*; Colobar *(Therapex, Canad.)*; Danobaryt *(Medicoteknik, Denm.)*; Disperbarium *(Rovi, Spain)*; Epi-C *(Mallinckrodt, Canad.)*; Epi-Stat *(Mallinckrodt, Canad.)*; Esobar *(Therapex, Canad.)*; Espho-Cat *(E-Z-EM, Canad.)*; Esophotrast *(Neth.; USA)*; E-Z-CAT *(E-Z-EM, Canad.; Henleys, UK)*; E-Z-HD *(E-Z-EM, Canad.; Henleys, UK)*; E-Z-Jug *(E-Z-EM, Canad.)*; E-Z-Paque *(E-Z-EM, Canad.; Henleys, UK)*; Gastropaque-S *(Arg.)*; Gastrorradiol *(Mabo, Spain)*; Gel-Unix *(Therapex, Canad.)*; Justebarin *(Juste, Spain)*; Liqui-Jug *(E-Z-EM, Canad.)*; Medebar *(Medefield, Austral.)*; Medescan *(Medefield, Austral.)*; Microbar *(Neth.; Max Ritter, Switz.)*; Microfanox *(Spain)*; Micropaque *(Graesser, Denm.; Nicholas, Fr.; Nicholas, Ger.; Neth.; Pan Quimica Farmac., Spain; Nicholas, Switz.; Nicholas, UK)*; Microtrast *(Nicholas, Fr.; Nicholas, Ger.; Neth.; Nicholas, Switz.; Nicholas, UK)*; Mixobar *(Astra Meditec, Denm.; Neth.; Astra Meditec, Norw.; Astra-Meditec, Swed.; Switz.)*; Neobar *(Belg.; E. Merck, Ger.)*; Oesobar *(Switz.)*; Oratrast *(Switz.)*; Polibar *(E-Z-EM, Canad.; Max Ritter, Switz.)*; Polibar ACB *(Henleys, UK)*; Radimix Colon *(Swed.)*; Radiobaryt *(Switz.)*; Radio-Baryx *(Fr.)*; Radiopaque *(Schering, Fr.; Switz.)*; Readi-Cat *(E-Z-EM, Canad.)*; Recto Barium *(Therapex, Canad.)*; Rugar *(USA)*; Sol-O-Pake *(E-Z-EM, Canad.)*; Steripaque *(Nicholas, UK)*; Suspobar *(Belg.)*; Telebar *(Guerbet, Fr.)*; Tixobar *(Astra, Austral.)*; Topcontral *(Boehringer Ingelheim, Ger.; Norw.)*; Ultra-R *(E-Z-EM, Canad.)*; Unibar-60 *(Therapex, Canad.)*; Unibaryt *(Röhm, Ger.; Neth.)*; Unik-Pak *(Canad.)*; X-Opac *(Fr.)*.

1553-s

Calcium Ipodate

Calcii Jopodas; Ipodate Calcium *(USAN)*. The calcium salt of 3-(3-dimethylaminomethyleneamino-2,4,6-tri-iodophenyl)propionic acid.
$(C_{12}H_{12}I_3N_2O_2)_2Ca = 1234.0$.

CAS — 5587-89-3 (ipodic acid); 1151-11-7 (calcium ipodate).

Pharmacopoeias. In *Nord.* (dihydrate) and *U.S.*

A fine, white or off-white odourless crystalline powder; contains approximately 61.7% of I. Slightly **soluble** in water, alcohol, chloroform, and methyl alcohol. **Store** in airtight containers.

Adverse Effects and Precautions

As for Iopanoic Acid, p.867. The effects on the gastro-intestinal tract may be less with calcium ipodate than with iopanoic acid. Headache has been reported.

Absorption and Fate

Calcium ipodate is absorbed from the gastro-intestinal tract following oral or rectal administration, and it appears in the bile within about 30 minutes of a dose. It is reported to be more rapidly absorbed than sodium ipodate. Maximum concentrations are found in the gall-bladder about 10 hours after administration. It is excreted mainly in the urine.

Uses and Administration

Calcium ipodate is a high-osmolal ionic monomeric contrast medium which is used for the examination of the biliary tract. It is given by mouth as an aqueous suspension. For cholecystography, 3 g is given in the evening, about 10 to 12 hours before the examination; a further 3 g may be given early next day 3 hours before the examination. For cholangiography and rapid cholecystography up to 6 g may be given. Sodium ipodate (p.871) is used similarly.

In 73 patients, cholecystography with iopanoic acid 3 g was unsuccessful. Immediately following the X-ray they were given 3 g of calcium ipodate and visualisation of the gall-bladder 5 hours later was adequate in 30 patients and unsuccessful in 30; in 13 patients the gall-bladder was partially opacified.— T. Klepetar *et al.*, *J. Am. med. Ass.*, 1970, *211*, 2154.

Preparations

Ipodate Calcium for Oral Suspension *(U.S.P.)*

Proprietary Preparations

Solu-Biloptin *(Schering, UK)*. *Sachets*, calcium ipodate 3 g.

Proprietary Names and Manufacturers

Oragrafin Calcium *(Squibb, Canad.; USA)*; Solu-Biloptin *(Austral.; Schering, Ger.; Norw.; Schering, Spain; Swed.; Switz.; Schering, UK)*; Solu-Biloptine *(Belg.)*.

1554-w

Diatrizoic Acid *(BAN, USAN)*.

Amidotrizoic Acid. 3,5-Diacetamido-2,4,6-tri-iodobenzoic acid.
$C_{11}H_9I_3N_2O_4 = 613.9$.

CAS — 117-96-4 (anhydrous); 50978-11-5 (dihydrate).

Pharmacopoeias. In *Chin.*, *Fr.*, and *Jpn* (all $2H_2O$); *U.S.* has anhydrous or dihydrate.

An odourless white powder, containing approximately 62% of I, calculated on the anhydrous substance.
Very slightly **soluble** in water and alcohol; soluble in dimethylformamide and in solutions of alkali hydroxides. **Store** in well-closed containers.

1555-e

Meglumine Diatrizoate *(BANM)*.

Diatrizoate Meglumine *(USAN)*; Methylglucamine Diatrizoate. *N*-Methylglucamine 3,5-diacetamido-2,4,6-tri-iodobenzoate.
$C_{11}H_9I_3N_2O_4,C_7H_{17}NO_5 = 809.1$.

CAS — 131-49-7.

Pharmacopoeias. In *Braz.* and *U.S.*

An odourless white powder containing approximately 47.1% of I. Freely **soluble** in water. **Incompatibilities** with some antihistamines have been reported.

1556-l

Sodium Diatrizoate *(BANM)*.

Diatrizoate Sodium *(USAN)*; Sodium Amidotrizoate *(rINN)*. Sodium 3,5-diacetamido-2,4,6-tri-iodobenzoate.
$C_{11}H_8I_3N_2NaO_4 = 635.9$.

CAS — 737-31-5.

Pharmacopoeias. In *Br. Braz.* and *U.S.* permit up to 10% water. In *Jug.*, *Nord.*, and *Turk.* as tetrahydrate.

An odourless white powder, containing 4 to 7% of water. It contains approximately 59.9% of I and each g of monograph substance represents 1.57 mmol of sodium, both calculated on the anhydrous substance.
Soluble 1 in 2 of water; slightly soluble in alcohol; practically insoluble in acetone and ether. **Incompatibilities** with some antihistamines have been reported. **Store** in well-closed containers. Protect from light.

DISPOSABLE SYRINGES. An increase in the severity and incidence of adverse effects following injection of contrast media for intravenous pyelography was attributed to the use of disposable syringes. Constituents of the rubber stopper of the syringe, particularly a phenolic compound, were found to leach out and dissolve in the contrast medium. It was strongly recommended that only inert syringes (e.g. glass) be used for the intravenous injection of contrast agents.— G. Hamilton (letter), *Can. med. Ass. J.*, 1983, *129*, 405. Critical comment that no evidence was provided that could attribute the reactions to use of the disposable syringes.— W. B. Chodirker (letter), *ibid.*, 1984, *130*, 343.

Adverse Effects and Treatment

Sodium diatrizoate and other water-soluble iodinated contrast media, given by injection, may cause nausea, a metallic taste, vomiting, sensations of heat, weakness, dizziness, paraesthesia, headache, coughing, rhinitis, sweating, retching, lachrymation, visual disturbances, pruritus, salivary gland enlargement, pallor, tachycardia, and hypotension. Rarely, convulsions, rigors, ventricular fibrillations, pulmonary oedema, circulatory failure, and cardiac arrest have occurred. Many of its effects can be attributed to its high osmolality which is a feature of the ionic monomeric contrast media; reducing the osmolality through altering the ionic or molecular profile produces a reduced incidence of adverse effects.
Anaphylactic shock and hypersensitivity reactions, with symptoms including dyspnoea, bronchospasm, oedema of the face and glottis, and urticaria, occasionally occur. Fatalities have occurred.
Pain may occur at the injection site and has been followed by extravasation and tissue damage, intramural injection, phlebitis, thrombosis, venospasm, and embolism.
Other infrequent reactions include: cerebral haematomas, sinus bradycardia, transient ECG abnormalities, haemodynamic disturbances, paralysis, and coma.
Fibrinolysis and a possible depressant effect on blood coagulation factors has been reported.

Renal failure and osmotic nephrosis have occurred after the intravenous use of these media. Contributing factors may include renal vasoconstriction and multiple myeloma; predisposing factors may include hypotension and dehydration.

Toxic effects after meglumine salts are generally less severe than after equivalent doses of sodium salts. Meglumine salts may have a diuretic effect. Mild diarrhoea may follow the oral or rectal administration of sodium and meglumine diatrizoates for gastro-intestinal examinations. The inhalation of solutions of these salts has caused fatal pulmonary oedema.

An intravenous injection of 0.5 to 1 mL of medium has been given as a test for sensitivity before administration of the main dose but it does not predict hypersensitivity with certainty and severe reactions and fatalities have followed the test dose. Adverse effects are treated symptomatically and adequate resuscitative facilities should be available when radiographic procedures are to be employed.

In a prospective study of 3509 patients undergoing urography using sodium diatrizoate 25 or 45%, sodium and meglumine diatrizoates, or sodium iothalamate, 1287 had no side-effects. Reversible heart failure occurred in 4 patients with pre-existing heart disease given large doses. Allergic reactions, usually urticaria, occurred in 52 patients including 13 of 355 with a history of allergy; the incidence of allergic reactions was 3.7% in those with a history of allergy compared with 1.2% in those without. Prophylactic use of an antihistamine did not reduce the incidence or severity of allergic reactions but increased threefold the incidence of flushing. Major reactions occurred in 4 patients—hypotension, bronchospasm, severe vomiting, and dyspnoea with urticaria. Nausea occurred in 286 patients and 90 vomited. Other reactions included warmth (1726), metallic taste (379), visceral sensations, usually an unpleasant feeling in the epigastrium (206), tingling (199), flushing (191), coughing and sneezing (72), and a variety of other symptoms, chiefly sensations in the perineum. Arm pain was usually associated with perivenous injection. Apart from an increased incidence of warmth the speed of injection did not influence side-effects. Special care was needed for small infants, the elderly, patients with renal or hepatic failure, myeloma, heart disease, or a previous major reaction. Full resuscitation facilities should be available.— P. Davies *et al.*, *Br. med. J.*, 1975, *2*, 434.

Of 32 964 patients undergoing excretion urography 6.8% had some side-effects; 1.72% had clinically important side-effects, sometimes severe and life-threatening. Reported estimates of mortality ranged from 1 in 400 000 to 1 in 116 000. Reactions were more common in patients with known hypersensitivity, but the incidence of severe or fatal reactions did not appear to be increased. Of 150 patients who had shown a reaction on previous urography 26 had a clinically important reaction on re-examination. In about 33 000 patients intravenous pretesting failed to identify 559 of 568 who developed significant reactions. Treatment of severe reactions included provision of an adequate airway, oxygen, adrenaline, intravenous fluids, and corticosteroids.— D. M. Witten, *J. Am. med. Ass.*, 1975, *231*, 974.

The use of meglumine diatrizoate might have contributed to the death, with bowel necrosis, perforation, and peritonitis, of 2 infants with meconium ileus.— J. C. Leonidas *et al.*, *Radiology*, 1976, *121*, 693. See also T. F. Hogan (letter), *Ann. intern. Med.*, 1977, *87*, 382; S. E. Seltzer and B. Jones, *Am. J. Roentg.*, 1978, *130*, 977.

Chromosome damage in 20 infants and children after cardiac catheterisation and angiocardiography with diatrizoates (Renografin-76) was greater than that calculated from the X-ray exposure dose to the patient. Long-term follow-up studies were indicated to determine the long-term hazards of this type of examination.— F. H. Adams *et al.*, *Pediatrics*, 1978, *62*, 312.

Neuralgic amyotrophy, associated with meglumine diatrizoate and iohexol in one patient.— J. M. S. Pearce and A. Al Jishi (letter), *Lancet*, 1985, *1*, 1400.

For a study comparing the tolerance of various contrast media with diatrizoic acid and its salts, see ioglicic acid (p. 866).

For a discussion of syringe materials affecting contrast media, see above.

EFFECTS ON THE BLOOD. There was a 60 to 70% inhibition of platelet function in 2 patients within 20 minutes of an injection of a contrast medium containing meglumine and sodium diatrizoate [Renovist II]. After 3 days there was still a 45% inhibition. *In vitro* studies suggested that the initial effect was due to the chelating agent present in the dye but that the longer term effect was possibly due to the metabolic products of iodinated fatty acids.— L. M. Zir *et al.*, *New Engl. J. Med.*, 1974, *291*, 134.

A report of intravascular haemolysis and renal failure in a 58-year-old man after angiocardiography with diatrizoates (Urografin 370).— J. R. Catterall *et al.*, *Br. med. J.*, 1981, *282*, 779.

Two cases of acute thrombocytopenia following the use of diatrizoate.— A. M. Shojania, *Can. med. Ass. J.*, 1985, *133*, 123.

An elderly man with a successful cadaveric renal transplant developed thrombotic microangiopathy leading to acute renal failure following aortofemoral angiography using 70 mL of 65% meglumine diatrizoate.— S. Fairley and B. U. Ihle, *Br. med. J.*, 1986, *293*, 922.

EFFECTS ON THE CARDIOVASCULAR SYSTEM. Severe hypotension in 2 patients undergoing urography with diatrizoate while receiving nadolol or propranolol. Both patients recovered within 15 minutes of receiving hydrocortisone sodium succinate and subcutaneous adrenaline plus supportive measures.— G. Hamilton, *Can. med. Ass. J.*, 1985, *133*, 122.

A case report of a 35-year-old woman who developed bradycardia and cardiac arrest after receiving 10 mL of Sinografin (meglumine diatrizoate and meglumine iodipamide) into the cervical canal. The sudden onset and rapid death, despite resuscitative procedures, suggested a lethal effect on the heart by the contrast medium.— J. M. Edelstein, *J. forens. Sci.*, 1986, *31*, 1142.

For a study comparing the haemodynamic side-effects of sodium meglumine diatrizoate and sodium meglumine ioxaglate see p.869.

EFFECTS ON THE KIDNEY. Renal toxicity is associated with contrast media (J.A. D'Elia *et al.*, *Am. J. Med.*, 1982, *72*, 719; C.P. Taliercio *et al.*, *Ann. intern. Med.*, 1986, *104*, 501). Pre-existing renal impairment appears to be a risk factor, although Mason *et al.* (*J. Am. med. Ass.*, 1985, *253*, 1001) found that patients with renal insufficiency given diatrizoate were not at a higher risk of sustaining a fall in creatinine clearance than patients with normal renal function. They also considered that angiography should not be withheld from a patient with borderline renal function (R.A. Mason *et al.*, *J. Am. med. Ass.*, 1985, *254*, 234). The renal function in such cases should be monitored after angiography carried out before surgery or other invasive procedures.

See also above under Effects on Blood.

EFFECTS ON THE PANCREAS. Acute pancreatitis after translumbar aortography, using sodium iothalamate or meglumine diatrizoate, was probably due to direct damage to the pancreas.— C. W. Imrie *et al.*, *Br. med. J.*, 1977, *2*, 681.

TREATMENT OF ADVERSE EFFECTS. In a study of 800 patients, the administration of clemastine with cimetidine five minutes before the intravenous infusion of meglumine diatrizoate reduced the frequency of anaphylactoid reactions. There was no reduction when clemastine or prednisolone were given alone.— J. Ring and K. -H. Rothenberger, *Münch. med. Wschr.*, 1984, *126*, 657.

Eight hundred and fifty-seven radiocontrast media procedures were performed in 743 patients who had previously experienced an immediate generalised (anaphylactoid) reaction to radiocontrast media. Pretreatment with prednisone and diphenhydramine hydrochloride in 415 of 695 intravascular infusions of radiocontrast media resulted in 45 (10.8%) reactions during which transient hypotension occurred in 3 (0.7%) patients. Prednisone-diphenhydramine-ephedrine sulphate pretreatment of 180 procedures was associated with 9 reactions (5.0%). The addition of cimetidine hydrochloride was not useful in that 14 reactions occurred during 100 procedures (14.0%). The 21 patients who had been receiving β-adrenergic antagonist therapy were protected as well as those who were not, in that none of the 11 patients receiving the three-drug regimen had a repeated reaction and only one of ten patients receiving the four-drug regimen reacted.— P. A. Greenberger *et al.*, *Archs intern. Med.*, 1985, *145*, 2197.

Precautions

Sodium diatrizoate and similar water-soluble contrast media should be used with caution in the presence of severe hepatic and renal impairment, severe hypertension, active tuberculosis, advanced cardiac disease, hyperthyroidism, phaeochromocytoma, or other grave general illness, and in patients with asthma, hay fever, sickle-cell disease, or hypersensitivity to contrast media or iodine. The administration of iodine-containing contrast media may interfere with thyroid-function tests, blood coagulation tests, and certain urine tests.

Precipitation of protein in the renal tubules, leading to uraemia, renal failure, and death has occurred in patients with multiple myeloma undergoing urography, possibly due to the additive effect of dehydration; particular care is necessary in such patients.

These media should not be given for hysterosalpingography in the presence of acute inflammatory conditions of the pelvic cavity, immediately before or during menstruation, or in pregnancy. Diatrizoates should not be used for urography in patients with anuria nor should they be used for myelography or in patients with suspected cranial subarachnoid haemorrhage.

Absorption and Fate

Diatrizoates are very poorly absorbed from the gastro-intestinal tract. Diatrizoates in the circulation are not significantly bound to serum proteins. If renal function is not impaired, unchanged sodium diatrizoate is rapidly excreted by glomerular filtration, but traces have been reported to remain in the circulation for 4 days.

Uses and Administration

Diatrizoates are ionic monomeric contrast media and are used in diagnostic radiology as solutions of the sodium or meglumine salt or as a mixture of the two. The high viscosity of concentrated solutions of the meglumine salt makes them difficult to administer rapidly.

For urography they are given by intravenous injection or infusion, or by retrograde injection. Solutions of diatrizoates may be given by mouth or rectally for the examination of the gastro-intestinal tract. Tomographic procedures may be used concomitantly to yield additional diagnostic information.

Diatrizoates are not suitable for myelography.

The integrity of colonic resection was studied in 117 patients using meglumine diatrizoate (Urografin 150) or meglumine metrizoate (Isopaque 100) as contrast enemas. The diagnostic accuracy of the radiological examination was 85%. Risk of complications has led to the abandonment by the authors of use of water-soluble contrast enemas for this purpose.— I. G. Haynes *et al.* (letter), *Lancet*, 1986, *1*, 675.

The successful treatment of 12 of 13 patients with tapeworm infections caused by *Diphyllobothrium latum* and *Taenia saginata*, by intraduodenal injection of sodium and meglumine diatrizoates (Gastrografin).— K. Waki *et al.*, *Lancet*, 1986, *2*, 1124.

MECONIUM ILEUS. Review of the treatment of babies with meconium ileus, including discussion on the use of diatrizoate enemas.— *Lancet*, 1982, *1*, 1000 (see also under Adverse Effects, above).

Preparations of Diatrizoates

Diatrizoate Meglumine and Diatrizoate Sodium Injection *(U.S.P.)*. Meglumine Diatrizoate and Sodium Diatrizoate Injection. When intended for intravascular use it contains no antimicrobial agents. pH 6.0 to 7.7. Protect from light.

Diatrizoate Meglumine Injection *(U.S.P.)*. Meglumine Diatrizoate Injection. When intended for intravascular use it contains no antimicrobial agents. pH 6.0 to 7.7. Protect from light.

Diatrizoate Sodium Injection *(U.S.P.)*. Sodium Diatrizoate Injection. When intended for intravascular use it contains no antimicrobial agents. pH 6.0 to 7.7. Protect from light.

Meglumine Diatrizoate Injection *(B.P.)*. Sterilised by autoclaving. pH 6 to 7. Protect from light.

Sodium Diatrizoate Injection *(B.P.)*. Sterilised by autoclaving. pH 6.6 to 7.6. Protect from light.

Diatrizoate Meglumine and Diatrizoate Sodium Solution *(U.S.P.)*. Meglumine Diatrizoate and Sodium Diatrizoate Solution. Not for parenteral use. pH 6.0 to 7.6. Store in airtight containers. Protect from light.

Diatrizoate Sodium Solution *(U.S.P.)*. Sodium Diatrizoate Solution. Not for parenteral use. pH 4.5 to 7.5.

Proprietary Preparations of Diatrizoates

Gastrografin *(Schering, UK)*. *Solution*, sodium diatrizoate 10%, meglumine diatrizoate 66%.

Hypaque *(Sterling Research, UK)*. *Injection* (Hypaque 25%), sodium diatrizoate 25%, in ampoules of 20 mL, and bottles of 250 and 350 mL.
Injection (Hypaque 45%), sodium diatrizoate 45%, in ampoules of 20 and 30 mL.
Injection (Hypaque 65%), sodium diatrizoate 25.23%, meglumine diatrizoate 50.46%, in ampoules of 20 mL.
Injection (Hypaque 85%), sodium diatrizoate 28.33%, meglumine diatrizoate 56.67%, in ampoules of 20 mL.
Powder (Hypaque Sodium), sodium diatrizoate.

Urografin *(Schering, UK)*. *Injection* (Urografin 150), sodium diatrizoate 3.9%, meglumine diatrizoate 26.1%, in ampoules of 10 and 20 mL, and bottles of 250 and 500 mL.
Injection (Urografin 290), sodium diatrizoate 7.9%, meglumine diatrizoate 52.1%, in ampoules of 20 mL and vials of 50 mL.
Injection (Urografin 310M), meglumine diatrizoate 65%, in ampoules of 20 mL and vials of 50 mL.
Injection (Urografin 325), sodium diatrizoate 40%, meglumine diatrizoate 18%, in ampoules of 20 mL and vials of 50 mL.
Injection (Urografin 370), sodium diatrizoate 10%, meglumine diatrizoate 66%, in ampoules of 20 mL and vials of 50, 100, and 200 mL.

Proprietary Names and Manufacturers of Diatrizoates

Angiografin *(Austral.; Schering, Ger.; Schering, Ital.; Schering, Norw.; Schering, Swed.; Switz.)*; Angiografine *(Belg.; Schering, Fr.)*; Cardiografin *(Squibb, USA)*; Cystografin *(Squibb, USA)*; Ethibloc *(Ethicon, Ger.)*; Gastrografin *(Austral.; Squibb, Canad.; Schering Corp., Denm.; Schering, Ger.; Schering, Ital.; Schering AG, Norw.; Schering, Swed.; Schering, Switz.; Schering, UK; Squibb, USA)*; Gastrografine *(Schering, Fr.)*; Hypaque *(Austral.; Winthrop, Canad.; Sterling Research, UK; Winthrop-Breon, USA)*; Hypaque-Cysto *(Winthrop-Breon, USA)*; Hypaque-M *(Winthrop-Breon, USA)*; MD-76 *(Mallinckrodt, Canad.)*; Peritrast *(Köhler, Ger.)*; Radialar *(Juste, Spain)*; Radiosélectan *(Schering, Fr.)*; Renografin *(Squibb, Canad.; Squibb, USA)*; Reno-M *(Squibb, Canad.; Squibb, USA)*; Renovist *(Squibb, Canad.; Squibb, USA)*; Triyosom *(Arg.)*; Urografin *(Austral.; Schering, Denm.; Schering, Ger.; Schering AG, Norw.; Schering, Swed.; Schering, UK)*; Urografine *(Schering, Fr.)*; Uropolinum *(Pol.)*; Urotrast *(Protea, Austral.)*; Urovison *(Austral.; Denm.; Schering, Fr.; Schering, Ger.; Norw.; Schering, Swed.)*; Urovist *(Schering, Ger.; Switz.)*; Urovist S *(Austral.)*.

The following names have been used for multi-ingredient preparations containing diatrizoates— Retrografin *(Squibb, Canad.)*; Sinografin *(Squibb, Canad.)*.

1557-y

Diodone *(pINN)*.

Iodopyracet. The diethanolamine salt of α-(1,4-dihydro-3,5-di-iodo-4-oxo-1-pyridyl)acetic acid.
$C_4H_{11}NO_2,C_7H_5I_2NO_3=510.1$.

CAS — 300-37-8.

Pharmacopoeias. In *Jug. Nord.* includes Diodonum, the acid, $C_7H_5I_2NO_3$ = 404.9.

Diodone contains approximately 49.8% of I.

Diodone is a high-osmolal ionic monomeric contrast medium with actions similar to those of the diatrizoates (p.863). It has been used for a variety of diagnostic procedures, including urography, hysterosalpingography, and salpingography.

Proprietary Names and Manufacturers
Diodon *(DAK, Denm.)*; Diodrast *(Winthrop, Canad.)*; Joduron *(Bracco, Ital.)*; Perjodal *(Pharmacia, Norw.)*; Umbradil *(Astra, Austral.; Astra, UK)*.

1558-j

Ethyl Monoiodostearate

A mixture of ethyl 9-iodostearate and ethyl 10-iodostearate (1:1).
$C_{20}H_{39}IO_2=438.4$.

Ethyl monoiodostearate is an oily liquid and contains approximately 28.9% (w/w) of I.

Ethyl monoiodostearate has been used for myelography and cerebral ventriculography.

Proprietary Names and Manufacturers
Duroliopaque *(Temis-Lostalo, Arg.; Belg.; Guerbet, Fr.; Byk Gulden, Ger.; Guerbet, Neth.; Guerbet, Switz.)*.

1559-z

Iobenzamic Acid *(BAN, USAN, rINN)*.

N-(3-Amino-2,4,6-tri-iodobenzoyl)-*N*-phenyl-β-alanine; 3-(3-Amino-2,4,6-tri-iodo-*N*-phenylbenzamido)propionic acid.
$C_{16}H_{13}I_3N_2O_3=662.0$.

CAS — 3115-05-7.

Iobenzamic acid contains approximately 57.5% of I.

Iobenzamic acid is a high-osmolal ionic monomeric contrast medium which has been given by mouth for the examination of the biliary tract in a dose of 3 g; heavy patients have been given 4.5 g.

Proprietary Names and Manufacturers
Bilibyk *(Byk Gulden, Ger.; Byk Gulden, Ital.)*; Osbil *(Byk Gulden, Ital.; Chemie-Linz, Switz.; May & Baker, UK)*; Osbiland *(Landerlan, Spain)*; Tracebil *(Christiaens, Belg.)*.

1522-h

Iocarmic Acid *(BAN, USAN, rINN)*.

MP-2032. 5,5′-(Adipoyldiamino)bis(2,4,6-tri-iodo-*N*-methylisophthalamic acid).
$C_{24}H_{20}I_6N_4O_8=1253.9$.

CAS — 10397-75-8.

Iocarmic acid contains approximately 60.7% of I.

1560-p

Meglumine Iocarmate *(BANM)*.

Iocarmate Meglumine *(USAN)*. The di(*N*-methylglucamine) salt of iocarmic acid.
$C_{24}H_{20}I_6N_4O_8, (C_7H_{17}NO_5)_2=1644.3$.

CAS — 54605-45-7.

Meglumine iocarmate contains approximately 46.3% of I.

Adverse Effects
As for Metrizamide, p.870. Spasm of the lower limbs has led to serious fractures.

Uses and Administration
Iocarmic acid is a low-osmolal ionic dimeric contrast medium which has been used as a 60% solution of meglumine iocarmate in lumbo-sacral radiculography, in cerebral ventriculography, in knee arthrography, and in hysterosalpingography.

Proprietary Names and Manufacturers of Meglumine Iocarmate
Dimer X *(Temis-Lostalo, Arg.; Belg.; Guerbet, Fr.; Byk Gulden, Ger.; Guerbet, Neth.; Rovi, Spain; Guerbet, Switz.; May & Baker, UK)*; Dimer-X *(Rovi, Spain)*; Dirax *(Jpn)*.

1561-s

Iocetamic Acid *(BAN, USAN, pINN)*.

DRC-1201; MP-620. *N*-Acetyl-*N*-(3-amino-2,4,6-tri-iodophenyl)-2-methyl-β-alanine; 3-[*N*-(3-Amino-2,4,6-tri-iodophenyl)acetamido]-2-methylpropionic acid.
$C_{12}H_{13}I_3N_2O_3=614.0$.

CAS — 16034-77-8.

Pharmacopoeias. In *U.S.*

Iocetamic acid contains approximately 62% of I. Store in well-closed containers.

Adverse Effects and Precautions
As for Iopanoic Acid, p.867.

Absorption and Fate
Iocetamic acid is absorbed from the gastro-intestinal tract. It is conjugated in the liver with glucuronic acid, and is excreted in the bile and concentrated in the gall-bladder; about 62% of a dose is excreted in the urine within 48 hours.

Uses and Administration
Iocetamic acid is a high-osmolal ionic monomeric contrast medium and is used for the examination of the biliary tract. A dose of 3.0 or 4.5 g is given by mouth 10 to 15 hours before examination. If visualisation is unsuccessful a repeat dose may be given on the evening of the first examination, and the examination repeated on the following day.

For a comparative study showing the similarities between sodium ipodate, iopanoic acid, and iocetamic acid in oral cholecystography, see Iopanoic Acid (p.868).

Preparations

Iocetamic Acid Tablets *(U.S.P.)*

Proprietary Names and Manufacturers
Cholebrin *(Nyco, Denm.; Nyco, Norw.; Nycomed, Swed.; Napp, UK)*; Cholebrine *(Belg.; Canad.; Fr.; Mundipharma, Ger.; Neth.)*; Colebrin *(Schering, Ital.)*; Colebrina *(Arg.; Sarget, Spain)*.

1523-m

Iodamide *(BAN, USAN, rINN)*.

Ametriodinic Acid; SH-926. α,5-Diacetamido-2,4,6-tri-iodo-*m*-toluic acid; 3-Acetamido-5-acetamidomethyl-2,4,6-tri-iodobenzoic acid.
$C_{12}H_{11}I_3N_2O_4=627.9$.

CAS — 440-58-4.

Pharmacopoeias. In *Cz.* and *Jpn.*

Iodamide contains approximately 60.6% of I.

1524-b

Meglumine Iodamide

Iodamide Meglumine *(USAN)*. The *N*-methylglucamine salt of iodamide.
$C_{12}H_{11}I_3N_2O_4, C_7H_{17}NO_5=823.2$.

CAS — 18656-21-8.

Meglumine iodamide contains approximately 46.3% of I.

1562-w

Sodium Iodamide

Iodamide Sodium.
$C_{12}H_{10}I_3N_2NaO_4=649.9$.

CAS — 10098-82-5.

Sodium iodamide contains approximately 58.6% of I. Each g of monograph substance represents 1.54 mmol of sodium.

Iodamide is a high-osmolal ionic monomeric contrast medium used, as its meglumine and sodium salts, in diagnostic radiology and has properties similar to the diatrizoates (see p.863).
Solutions used contain 65% of meglumine iodamide, 52.66% of sodium iodamide, or mixtures of the meglumine and sodium salts, and are given intravenously or by local application for a wide range of diagnostic procedures.

After intravenous administration to 7 healthy subjects, iodamide was eliminated rapidly and almost completely in urine, with negligible formation of metabolites. In 15 patients with renal failure elimination was slower, but still mainly in urine.— L. T. DiFazio *et al.*, *J. clin. Pharmac.*, 1978, *18*, 35. See also A. C. Bollerup *et al.*, *Eur. J. clin. Pharmac.*, 1975, *9*, 63.

Proprietary Preparations

Sodium Uromiro 300 *(E. Merck, UK)*. *Injection*, sodium iodamide 52.66%, in bottles of 50 mL.

Uromiro *(E. Merck, UK)*. *Injection* (Uromiro 300), meglumine iodamide 65%, in bottles of 50 mL.
Injection (Uromiro 340), meglumine iodamide 18.3%, sodium iodamide 43.4%, in ampoules of 20 mL and bottles of 50 mL.
Injection (Uromiro 380), meglumine iodamide 70%, sodium iodamide 9.7%, in bottles of 50 mL.
Injection (Uromiro 420), meglumine iodamide 40.8%, sodium iodamide 39.4%, in bottles of 50 mL.

Proprietary Names and Manufacturers of Iodamides
Isteropac E.R. *(Bracco, Ital.)*; Jodomiron *(Swed.)*; Opacist E.R. *(Bracco, Ital.)*; Renovue *(Squibb, Austral.; Squibb, USA)*; Sodium Uromiro *(E. Merck, UK)*; Urombrine *(Neth.)*; Uromiro *(Heyden, Ger.; Bracco, Ital.; Neth.; Bracco, Switz.; E. Merck, UK)*.

1525-v

Iodipamide *(BAN, USAN).*

Adipiodone *(rINN)*; Bilignostum. 3,3′-Adipoyldiaminobis(2,4,6-tri-iodobenzoic acid).

$C_{20}H_{14}I_6N_2O_6$=1139.8.

CAS — 606-17-7.

Pharmacopoeias. In *Braz., Chin., Cz., Jpn, Jug., Nord., Rus.,* and *U.S.*

A white, almost odourless, crystalline powder. Very slightly **soluble** in water, chloroform, and ether; slightly soluble in alcohol. Iodipamide contains approximately 66.8% of I. **Store** in well-closed containers.

1563-e

Meglumine Iodipamide

Iodipamide Meglumine *(BANM, USAN)*. The di(*N*-methylglucamine) salt of iodipamide.

$C_{20}H_{14}I_6N_2O_6$, $(C_7H_{17}NO_5)_2$=1530.2.

CAS — 3521-84-4.

Meglumine iodipamide contains approximately 49.8% of I. **Incompatibilities** have been reported with some antihistamines.

Administration of iodipamide meglumine (Cholografin) via a Y-injection site of an administration set through which gentamicin sulphate had previously been administered resulted in the immediate formation of a white precipitate downstream of the Y-site.— J. R. Jansen, *Am. J. Hosp. Pharm.*, 1975, *32*, 1225.

Adverse Effects, Treatment, and Precautions

As for the diatrizoates (p. 863).

Iodipamide may show some uricosuric activity.

Iodipamide was considered to be about 6 times more toxic than other contrast media being used for urography.— G. Ansell, *Adverse Drug React. Bull.*, 1978, Aug., 252.

EFFECTS ON THE HEART. For a case report of fatal cardiac arrest following administration of meglumine iodipamide and meglumine diatrizoate see p.864.

EFFECTS ON THE LIVER. Of 149 patients who received the dose of iodipamide recommended by the manufacturer 13 developed elevated serum aspartate aminotransferase (SGOT) values; of 126 who received twice the dose 23 developed elevated values.— F. J. Scholz *et al.* (letter), *J. Am. med. Ass.*, 1974, *229*, 1724.

Further references to hepatotoxicity: A. E. Stillman, *J. Am. med. Ass.*, 1974, *228*, 1420; L. R. Sutherland *et al., Ann. intern. Med.*, 1977, *86*, 437; S. Imoto (letter), *ibid.*, 1978, *88*, 129; T. Motoki *et al., Am. J. Gastroent.*, 1979, *72*, 71.

Absorption and Fate

Within 10 to 15 minutes of an intravenous injection, meglumine iodipamide appears in the hepatic duct and the common bile duct, and within 1 hour of the injection it appears in the gall bladder. About 90% of the dose is excreted in the faeces and the remainder in the urine.

Uses and Administration

Iodipamide is a low-osmolal ionic dimeric contrast medium which is used mainly as its meglumine salt for the examination of the biliary tract when oral procedures are considered unsuitable.

It is administered by slow intravenous injection over an average of 10 minutes or by infusion. Doses of 10 g are usually employed.

Preparations of Iodipamides

Meglumine Iodipamide Injection *(B.P.)*. Iodipamide Meglumine Injection. pH 6.0 to 7.1. Sterilised by autoclaving.

Iodipamide Meglumine Injection *(U.S.P.)*. Meglumine Iodipamide Injection. pH 6.5 to 7.7.

Proprietary Names and Manufacturers of Iodipamides

Biligrafin *(Schering, Austral.; Schering, Denm.; Schering, Ger.; Schering, Ital.; Schering, Norw.; Schering, Swed.; Schering, Switz.; Schering, UK)*; Biligrafina *(Schering, Arg.)*; Biligrafine *(Schering, Belg.)*; Cholografin *(Squibb, Canad.; Squibb, USA)*; Endocistobil *(Bracco, Ital.)*; Endografin *(Schering, Austral.; Schering, Ger.; Schering, Swed.; Schering, Switz.; Schering, UK)*; Intrabilix *(Guerbet, Fr.)*; Transbilix *(Codali, Belg.; Canad.; Guerbet, Denm.; Guerbet, Fr.; Guerbet, Neth.)*.

The following names have been used for multi-ingredient preparations containing iodipamides— Sinografin *(Squibb, Canad.)*.

1564-l

Iodised Oil Fluid Injection

Ethiodized Oil; Ethiodized Oil Injection.

CAS — 8001-40-9 (iodised oil); 8008-53-5 (ethiodized oil injection).

Pharmacopoeias. In *Br., Fr.,* and *U.S.*

A sterile iodine addition product of the ethyl esters of the fatty acids obtained from poppy-seed oil. The *B.P.* specifies 37 to 39% w/w of combined iodine. *U.S.P.* specifies 35.2 to 38.9% of combined iodine.

A straw-coloured, yellow, or amber-coloured, oily liquid which has not more than a slight alliaceous odour.

Practically **insoluble** in water; soluble in chloroform, ether, and petroleum spirit. **Store** in an atmosphere of carbon dioxide or nitrogen. Protect from light.

Because of its solvent action on polystyrene, iodised oil injection should not be administered in plastic syringes made with polystyrene.

Adverse Effects and Precautions

The risk of hypersensitivity reactions is greater after the use of iodised oil than after water-soluble iodinated contrast media such as sodium diatrizoate. Foreign body reactions have occurred. Cases of iodism have also occurred and have been fatal. Great care should be taken to avoid vascular structures, because of the danger of oil embolism; it should not therefore be used in areas affected by haemorrhage or local trauma. Iodised oil should be used with care in patients with thyroid dysfunction or a history of allergic reactions. A sensitivity test has been recommended before its use, although reactions are not always predictable from a patient's history or sensitivity tests. The administration of iodine-containing contrast media may interfere with thyroid-function tests.

The use of oily contrast media for hysterosalpingography was dangerous and unnecessary. Oil embolism and pelvic adhesions had occurred, and violent reactions with pelvic abscess in the presence of unsuspected pelvic tuberculosis. Several patients had been seen with bilateral tubal occlusion following an original investigation, using iodised oil, which had shown tubal patency.— F. W. Wright and J. Stallworthy (letter), *Br. med. J.*, 1973, *3*, 632.

In 9 patients given 6 or 7 mL of iodised oil fluid injection into each foot for lymphography there was no fall in forced expiratory volume or vital capacity, though severe breathlessness had been reported by other workers. Gas transfer factor was reduced by a mean of 22%, with the greatest reduction 24 to 48 hours after lymphography. Patients undergoing lymphography should not be submitted to general anaesthesia or irradiation of the mediastinum or lungs until a week had elapsed, and lymphography should not be performed in patients who had had recent radiotherapy.— R. J. White *et al., Br. med. J.*, 1973, *4*, 775.

Hyperplasia of the thyroid glands observed in several infants who died from Rhesus sensitisation was attributed to the use of iodised oil fluid injection for amniography. It was considered that this contrast medium was contra-indicated in amniography.— D. M. O. Becroft *et al.* (letter), *Lancet*, 1976, *2*, 1191.

Absorption and Fate

Iodised oil fluid injection is relatively rapidly absorbed after hysterosalpingography but may persist for several weeks or months after lymphangiography, and it is only slowly absorbed from most other body sites.

Uses and Administration

Iodised oil fluid injection is a contrast medium which is used for lymphangiography and for the visualisation of nasal and other sinuses. It has been used for hysterosalpingography but water-soluble agents are preferred. The dose is dependent upon the procedure. It is unsuitable for use in bronchography; a viscous injection was used for that purpose.

A review of the use of an iodised oil emulsion given intravenously for computed tomographic (CT) scans.— *J. Am. med. Ass.*, 1984, *251*, 707. See also: T. Kanematsu *et al.* (letter), *ibid.*, *252*, 3130.

Proprietary Preparations

Lipiodol Ultra Fluid *(May & Baker, UK)*. *Injection*, iodised oil, in ampoules of 10 mL.

Proprietary Names and Manufacturers

Lipiodol *(May & Baker, Austral.; Therapex, Canad.; Guerbet, Denm.; Guerbet, Fr.; Byk Gulden, Ger.; Byk Gulden, Ital.; Guerbet, Norw.; Rovi, Spain; Guerbet, Switz.; May & Baker, UK)*.

1527-q

Iodoxamic Acid *(BAN, USAN, rINN).*

B-10610; SQ-21982. 3,3′-(4,7,10,13-Tetraoxahexadecanedioyldiamino)bis(2,4,6-tri-iodobenzoic acid).

$C_{26}H_{26}I_6N_2O_{10}$=1287.9.

CAS — 31127-82-9.

Iodoxamic acid contains approximately 59.1% of I.

1567-z

Meglumine Iodoxamate *(BANM).*

Iodoxamate Meglumine *(USAN)*. The di(*N*-methylglucamine) salt of iodoxamic acid.

$C_{26}H_{26}I_6N_2O_{10}$, $(C_7H_{17}NO_5)_2$=1678.4.

CAS — 51764-33-1.

Meglumine iodoxamate contains approximately 45.4% of I.

Meglumine iodoxamate is a low-osmolal ionic dimeric contrast medium with similar properties to the diatrizoates (p.863). It is used for cholecystography and cholangiography, by intravenous infusion.

Some references to the use of meglumine iodoxamate in cholecystography: E. N. Sargent *et al., Am. J. Roentg.*, 1975, *125*, 251; A. Robbins *et al., ibid.*, 1976, *126*, 70; *idem*, *127*, 257; A. Moss, *ibid.*, 1977, *128*, 931.

Proprietary Preparations of Meglumine Iodoxamate

Endobil *(E. Merck, UK)*. *Injection*, meglumine iodoxamate 9.91%, in bottles of 100 mL.

Proprietary Names and Manufacturers

Cholovue *(Squibb, Canad.; Neth.)*; Endobil *(Bracco, Ital.; Bracco, Switz.; E. Merck, UK)*; Endomirabil *(Byk Gulden, Ger.)*.

12855-n

Ioglicic Acid *(BAN, USAN, rINN).*

SH-H-200-AB. 5-Acetamido-2,4,6-tri-iodo-*N*-(methylcarbamoylmethyl)isophthalamic acid.

$C_{13}H_{12}I_3N_3O_5$=671.0.

CAS — 49755-67-1.

Ioglicic acid contains approximately 56.7% of I.

Ioglicic acid is a high-osmolal ionic monomeric contrast medium used, as the meglumine and sodium salts, for urography, angiography, and related procedures. Ioglicic acid has actions similar to the diatrizoates (p. 863).

Ioglicate administered by 40-mL rapid injection, or by 100-mL and 250-mL infusions was compared with iothalamic acid in three multicentre studies on 995 patients. Sodium-meglumine mixed salts were used for rapid injection and meglumine salts for the other two investigations. The best opacification and lowest rates of unsatisfactory radiographs were achieved with the highest doses of iodine. The incidence of side-effects varied between 6% (high dose) and 22% (rapid injection), this increase was caused by a more significant occurrence of vascular pain and heat sensation. In all three comparisons ioglicate was tolerated somewhat better than iothalamate.— T. Baitsch *et al.*, Double Blind Comparison of Ioglicate and Iothalamate in Intravenous Urography, in

Contrast Media in Urography, Angiography and Computerized Tomography, V. Taenzer and E. Zeitler (eds), Stuttgart, Georg Thieme Verlag, 1983, p.143.

For a comparison of the incidence of adverse effects after administration of Rayvist or iopromide, see under iopromide (p.868).

Proprietary Names and Manufacturers
Rayvist *(Schering, Ger.; Schering, Ital.; Schering, Switz.).*

1528-p

Ioglycamic Acid *(BAN, USAN, rINN).*

BE-419. αα′-Oxybis(3-acetamido-2,4,6-tri-iodobenzoic acid).
$C_{18}H_{10}I_6N_2O_7$=1127.7.

CAS — 2618-25-9.

Ioglycamic acid contains approximately 67.5% of I.

1529-s

Meglumine Ioglycamate *(BANM).*

Ioglycamate Meglumine. The di(*N*-methylglucamine) salt of ioglycamic acid.
$C_{18}H_{10}I_6N_2O_7,(C_7H_{17}NO_5)_2$=1518.1.

CAS — 14317-18-1.

Meglumine ioglycamate contains approximately 50.2% of I.

1569-k

Sodium Ioglycamate *(BANM).*

Ioglycamate Sodium.
$C_{18}H_8I_6N_2Na_2O_7$=1171.7.

CAS — 3737-71-1.

Sodium ioglycamate contains about 65% of I. Each g of monograph substance represents 1.71 mmol of sodium.

Adverse Effects, Treatment, and Precautions

As for the diatrizoates (p.863).

Ioglycamates should not be used in patients with immunoglobulin IgM disorders such as macroglobulinaemia.

Intravascular precipitation and sudden death occurred in a patient with Waldenström's macroglobulinaemia given an intravenous injection of ioglycamic acid. IgM from this patient produced similar effects in *mice.*— M. Harboe *et al., Lancet,* 1976, *2,* 285.

There were 10 episodes of raised aminotransferase concentrations with hepatic necrosis in 7 patients given meglumine ioglycamate for infusion cholangiography.— K. Winckler, *Dt. med. Wschr.,* 1978, *103,* 420.

The biliary excretion of ioglycamates was impaired in diabetic patients taking sulphonylureas, and in Scandinavian women taking oral contraceptives.— G. Ansell, *Adverse Drug React. Bull.,* 1978, Aug., 252.

Uses and Administration

Ioglycamic acid is an ionic dimeric contrast medium which is extensively bound to plasma albumin. It is used, usually as meglumine ioglycamate, for the examination of the biliary tract when there is strong evidence of disease. Meglumine ioglycamate is given intravenously as a 35% solution over at least 5 minutes or as a 17% solution by infusion over not less than 30 minutes. The infusion should always be started at a low rate, and then increased after 3 to 5 minutes. A mixture of the meglumine and sodium salts has also been used. It has been suggested that meglumine ioglycamate should not be injected immediately after negative oral cholecystography.

In 50 patients submitted to cholangiography using 30 mL of 35% solution of meglumine ioglycamate and 50 given half the dosage, statistically better results were obtained with the higher dosage. The injection was given over 5 minutes. In 97% of those with intact gall-bladders maximum information was provided by 2 films taken at 60 and 90 minutes respectively. Absence of opacification at 60 minutes was indicative of cystic duct obstruction. In postcholecystectomy patients films at 30 and 60 minutes provided maximum information. Side-effects were nausea (3 patients), a metallic taste (8), and urticaria (2) readily responsive to chlorpheniramine maleate, 10 mg intramuscularly.— G. J. S. Parkin and H. Herlinger, *Gut,* 1974, *15,* 268.

Biliary excretion of meglumine ioglycamate began 20 minutes after the start of its intravenous infusion in 11 patients and was associated with a significant increase in bile flow compared with 10 controls and independently of bile salt secretion which was not significantly affected. Phospholipid and cholesterol secretion were significantly lowered in the treated group. There was a rise in the cholesterol-solubilising capacity of bile during meglumine ioglycamate excretion which suggested the possible development of a drug for dissolving cholesterol gall-stones.— G. D. Bell *et al., Gut,* 1978, *19,* 300.

Plasma binding, renal and biliary excretion studies of meglumine ioglycamate in jaundiced and anicteric patients.— G. D. Bell *et al., Br. J. Radiol.,* 1978, *51,* 251.

Proprietary Preparations of Ioglycamates

Biligram *(Schering, UK). Injection,* meglumine ioglycamate 17%, in vials of 100 mL.
Injection, meglumine ioglycamate 35%, in ampoules of 30 mL.

Proprietary Names and Manufacturers of Ioglycamates

Biligram *(Belg.; Denm.; Fr.; Ger.; Schering, Ital.; Norw.; Schering, Swed.; Switz.; Schering, UK)*; Bilivison *(Schering, Ital.)*; Bilivistan *(Ger.; Ital.; Norw.; Swed.)*; Bilograma *(Arg.).*

12856-h

Iohexol *(BAN, USAN, rINN).*

Win-39424. *N,N′*-Bis(2,3-dihydroxypropyl)-5-[*N*-(2,3-dihydroxypropyl)acetamido]-2,4,6-tri-iodoisophthalamide.
$C_{19}H_{26}I_3N_3O_9$=821.1.

CAS — 66108-95-0.

Iohexol contains approximately 46.4% of I.

Adverse Effects

As for Metrizamide p.870.

Encephalopathy developed in a 48-year-old man with sciatica within 9 hours of iohexol administration for lumbar myelography; the dose was 10 mL. The encephalopathy had largely resolved 48 hours after the myelogram, with complete resolution by 4 days.— M. Donaghy *et al.* (letter), *Lancet,* 1985, *2,* 887.

Neuralgic amyotrophy in one patient associated with meglumine diatrizoate and iohexol.— J. M. S. Pearce and A. Al Jishi (letter), *Lancet,* 1985, *1,* 1400.

For a comparison of the tolerance of adverse effects of iohexol, iopramide, and ioxaglate in aortofemoral arteriography, see iopromide (p.868).

For a comparison of the incidence of nausea and vomiting in patients receiving iohexol or sodium ioxaglate with meglumine ioxaglate for digital subtraction angiography, see sodium ioxaglate (p.869).

Uses and Administration

Iohexol is a low-osmolal nonionic monomeric contrast medium which is used for myelography, angiography, urography, and related procedures.

A review of the nonionic contrast media iohexol and iopamidol.— T. K. Kawada, *Drug Intell. & clin. Pharm.,* 1985, *19,* 525.

Initial report of a new method for determining the glomerular filtration rate, using X-ray fluorescence to measure the disappearance from the plasma of injected iohexol.— P. H. O'Reilly *et al., Br. med. J.,* 1986, *293,* 234.

The proceedings of a symposium on iohexol.— *Investve Radiol.,* 1985, *20, Suppl.*

ABSORPTION AND FATE. A study of the pharmacokinetics of iohexol given intravenously to 16 volunteers. Iohexol appeared to be distributed into extracellular water. It was not metabolised appreciably, renal excretion accounted for 95% of the total body clearance. A sensation of heat was recorded in a few cases following injection of iohexol.— J. Edelson *et al., J. pharm. Sci.,* 1984, *73,* 993.

Proprietary Names and Manufacturers

Omnigraf *(Juste, Spain)*; Omnipaque *(Winthrop, Canad.; Nyco, Denm.; Schering, Ger.; Schering, Ital.; Nyco, Norw.; Nycomed, Swed.; Schering, Switz.; Nycomed, UK; Winthrop-Breon, USA)*; Omnitrast *(Schering, Spain).*

14037-g

Iopamidol *(BAN, USAN, rINN).*

B-15000; SQ-13396. *N,N′*-Bis[2-hydroxy-1-(hydroxymethyl)ethyl]-2,4,6-tri-iodo-5-lactamidoisophthalamide.
$C_{17}H_{22}I_3N_3O_8$=777.1.

CAS — 60166-93-0; 62883-00-5.

Pharmacopoeias. In *U.S.*

Iopamidol contains approximately 49% of I.

Iopamidol is a low-osmolal nonionic monomeric contrast medium with actions similar to metrizamide (p.870). It is used for a variety of angiographic procedures; it is also used in arthrography, myelography, and urography.

A review of the nonionic contrast media iohexol and iopamidol.— T. K. Kawada, *Drug Intell. & clin. Pharm.,* 1985, *19,* 525.

Further references: K.-J. Wolf *et al.,* Comparative Evaluation of Low Osmolar Contrast Media in (Femoral) Arteriography in *Contrast Media in Urography, Angiography and Computerized Tomography,* V. Taenzer and E. Zeitler (Eds), Stuttgart, Georg Thieme Verlag, 1983, p.102.

ADVERSE EFFECTS. Phlebographies were carried out in 20 patients with meglumine iothalamate being injected into one leg and iopamidol into the other. There was significantly less thrombophlebitis with iopamidol, and it was concluded that iopamidol is a safer contrast medium for phlebography.— M. L. Thomas *et al., Br. J. Radiol.,* 1984, *57,* 205.

A case report of a 62-year-old man who had undergone lumbar myelography with 10 mL iopamidol. After the procedure headache, nausea, and vomiting developed. Rapidly worsening confusion followed and the patient became uncommunicative and was taken to hospital urgently. On arrival he was febrile, had very marked neck stiffness, and was irritable and restless. There were no abnormal neurological signs or evidence of infection. After supportive treatment the patient was discharged after 5 days with no residual symptoms.— C. Robinson and G. Fon, *Med. J. Aust.,* 1986, *144,* 553. See also K. Wallers *et al., Br. med. J.,* 1985, *291,* 1688.

Preparations

Iopamidol Injection *(U.S.P.)*

Proprietary Preparations

Niopam *(E. Merck, UK). Injection* (Niopam 200), iopamidol 40.8%, in ampoules of 10 and 20 mL.
Injection (Niopam 300), iopamidol 61.2%, in ampoules of 10 and 20 mL and bottles of 50 and 100 mL.
Injection (Niopam 370), iopamidol 75.5%, in ampoules of 10 and 20 mL and bottles of 50, 100, and 200 mL.

Proprietary Names and Manufacturers

Iopamiro *(Astra Meditec, Denm.; Heyden, Ger.; Bracco, Ital.; Astra Meditec, Norw.; Astra-Meditec, Swed.; Bracco, Switz.)*; Isovue *(Squibb, Canad.; Squibb, USA)*; Isovue-M *(Squibb, USA)*; Niopam *(E. Merck, UK)*; Solutrast *(Byk Gulden, Ger.).*

1570-w

Iopanoic Acid *(BAN, USAN, rINN).*

Acidum Iopanoicum; Iodopanoic Acid. 2-(3-Amino-2,4,6-tri-iodobenzyl) butyric acid.

$C_{11}H_{12}I_3NO_2$=570.9.

CAS — 96-83-3.

Pharmacopoeias. In *Arg., Br., Braz., Chin., Cz., Egypt., Int., Jpn, Jug., Nord., Roum.,* and *U.S.*

A white to cream-coloured powder, odourless or with a faint characteristic odour. It contains approximately 66.7% of I. Practically **insoluble** in water; soluble 1 in 25 of alcohol; soluble in acetone and aqueous solutions of alkali hydroxides. **Protect** from light.

Adverse Effects

Iopanoic acid gives rise occasionally to nausea, vomiting, abdominal cramp, diarrhoea, and, more rarely, dysuria. Acute renal failure, thrombocytopenia, and hypersensitivity reactions have been

reported.
Iopanoic acid has a uricosuric effect.

Precautions

Iopanoic acid is contra-indicated in severe hepatic or renal disease, and in patients with hypersensitivity to iodine; doses as high as 6 g should not be given to patients with renal impairment. It should not be used in the presence of acute gastro-intestinal disorders since its absorption may be impaired. It should be used with caution in patients with coronary artery disease, severe hyperthyroidism, hyperuricaemia, or cholangitis. Premedication with atropine has been suggested for patients with recent coronary heart disease. The administration of iodine-containing contrast media may interfere with thyroid-function tests.

Small doses of aspirin blocked the uricosuric effect of iopanoic acid.— A. E. Postlethwaite and W. N. Kelley (letter), *J. Am. med. Ass.*, 1972, *219*, 1479.

Absorption and Fate

Iopanoic acid is variably absorbed from the gastro-intestinal tract and is strongly and extensively bound to plasma protein. It is conjugated in the liver to the glucuronide and about 65% is excreted in the bile and the remainder in the urine. It appears in the gall-bladder about 4 hours after a dose is taken and maximum concentrations occur after about 17 hours. About 50% of a dose is excreted in 24 hours, but elevated protein-bound iodine concentrations may persist for several months.

A review of the intestinal absorption, hepatic uptake, biliary excretion, and gall-bladder concentration of iopanoic acid.— R. N. Berk *et al.*, *New Engl. J. Med.*, 1974, *290*, 204.

PREGNANCY AND THE NEONATE. The amount of iopanoic acid excreted in the milk of lactating mothers was considered to be too small to affect the child.— T. E. O'Brien, *Am. J. Hosp. Pharm.*, 1974, *31*, 844.

Uses and Administration

Iopanoic acid is a high-osmolal ionic monomeric contrast medium used for the examination of the biliary tract. It is given by mouth with a light fat-free meal about 10 to 14 hours before X-ray examination, the usual dose being 3 g. For repeat examinations on the same day as the original procedure, an additional 3 g may be administered. No more than 6 g should be taken during a 24-hour period. Adequate fluid intake is desirable. An interval of 5 to 7 days should elapse if a repeat examination is to be carried out with double the dose of iopanoic acid. Double doses should not be given to patients with renal disease. Doses of up to 6 g may be given in two doses to obtain better visualisation of the extrahepatic ducts. Adequate visualisation may not occur in patients with substantial gall-bladder disease or advanced liver disease.
For the visualisation of biliary calculi 1 g is given three times daily after relatively fat-free meals for 4 days and X-ray examination carried out on the morning of the 5th day in the fasting patient.
Sodium iopanoate has been similarly used.

A study of 300 patients showed that Cholebrin (iocetamic acid) was about as effective as Telepaque (iopanoic acid) and Biloptin (sodium ipodate) in outlining the gall-bladder and common bile duct. The frequency of side-effects was similar with each oral cholecystographic medium.— G. M. Roberts and M. R. Jones, *J. clin. Hosp. Pharm.*, 1984, *9*, 225.

Preparations

Iopanoic Acid Tablets *(B.P., U.S.P.)*

Proprietary Preparations

Cistobil *(E. Merck, UK). Tablets*, iopanoic acid 500 mg.
Telepaque *(Sterling Research, UK). Tablets*, iopanoic acid 500 mg.

Proprietary Names and Manufacturers

Bilijodon-Natrium *(Neth.; Swed.; Switz.)*; Biliopaco *(Rovi, Spain)*; Cistobil *(Medefield, Austral.; Bracco, Ital.; Uquifa, Spain; Bracco, Switz.; E. Merck, UK)*; Colegraf *(Estedi, Spain)*; Felombrine *(Medinsa, Spain)*; Jopanonsyre *(DAK, Denm.)*; Neocontrast *(Bama, Spain)*; Nigrantil *(Spain)*; Panjopaque *(Denm.)*; Telepaque *(Arg.; Aust.; Winthrop, Austral.; Belg.; Winthrop, Canad.; Winthrop, Denm.; Fin.; Fr.; Winthrop, Ger.; Maggioni-Winthrop, Ital.; Neth.; Norw.; Spain; Swed.; Switz.; Sterling Research, UK; Winthrop, UK; Winthrop-Breon, USA)*; Teletrast *(Swed.)*.

1571-e

Iophendylate *(BAN, USAN).*

Ethyl Iodophenylundecanoate; Ethyl Iodophenylundecylate; Iofendylate *(rINN)*. A mixture of stereoisomers of ethyl 10-(4-iodophenyl)undecanoate.
$C_{19}H_{29}IO_2$=416.3.

CAS — 99-79-6.

Pharmacopoeias. In *Chin.*, *Jpn*, and *U.S.* The *B.P.* only includes the injection.

A colourless to pale yellow viscous liquid, odourless or with a faint ethereal odour, darkening on prolonged exposure to air, and containing about 30.5% of I. Very slightly **soluble** in water; freely soluble in alcohol, chloroform, and ether.
Store in airtight containers. Protect from light.

ACTION ON PLASTICS. Polystyrene was soluble in iophendylate and syringes made from polystyrene were rapidly attacked. Syringes made from polypropylene appeared to be unaffected.— J. D. Irving and P. V. Reynolds (letter), *Lancet*, 1966, *1*, 362.

Adverse Effects

Side-effects such as headache, backache, neck stiffness, nausea, vomiting, and fever are common, and more serious symptoms of allergy and arachnoiditis sometimes occur with iophendylate. Aseptic meningitis has occurred. All but small amounts of iophendylate are usually removed from the spinal column after examination; any retained contrast medium may lead to the effects of absorbed iodine.

Hyperthyroidism, twice previously suspected, was considered to have been precipitated in a 47-year-old man by the injection of 6 mL of Iophendylate Injection.— A. M. Silas and A. G. White (letter), *Br. med. J.*, 1975, *4*, 162.

Chronic urticaria and intermittent anaphylaxis in a man were due to iophendylate used in myelography 17 years previously. After removal of about 8 mL of iophendylate from the spinal canal the patient remained almost totally asymptomatic.— P. Lieberman *et al.*, *J. Am. med. Ass.*, 1976, *236*, 1495.

Focal seizures, which developed in a 30-year-old woman 4 months after a myelogram, were believed to be associated with retained Pantopaque.— M. K. Greenberg and S. C. Vance (letter), *Lancet*, 1980, *1*, 312.

Precautions

Iophendylate should not be employed when lumbar puncture is contra-indicated, and to avoid subdural and extra-arachnoid extravasation it should not be used within 10 to 14 days of a previous lumbar puncture. Iophendylate should not be emulsified with cerebrospinal fluid, as this may increase the frequency of toxic reactions. It is recommended that iophendylate be administered using all-glass syringes as it may dissolve substances from some plastic syringes and/or their rubber plungers.

Reactions to iophendylate injection used for myelography occurred in 7 of 57 patients; 5 of the 7 patients had definite multiple sclerosis. It was considered that myelography should not be performed if multiple sclerosis was suspected.— P. Kauffmann and W. D. Jeans, *Lancet*, 1976, *2*, 1000.

Absorption and Fate

Iophendylate is very slowly absorbed from the spinal canal; its rate of disappearance has been reported to be about 1 mL per year.

Uses and Administration

Iophendylate is a high-osmolal ionic monomeric contrast medium which is used mainly for myelography. It has a low viscosity which makes it easy to inject; it forms a discrete mass and as much as possible of the material should be removed by aspiration from the spinal column after the examination is complete.
Iophendylate has also been used for examination of the third and fourth ventricles, and to visualise the foetus in the amniotic sac prior to intra-uterine blood transfusion.

Preparations

Iophendylate Injection *(B.P., U.S.P.)*

Proprietary Preparations

Myodil *(Glaxo, UK). Injection*, iophendylate, in ampoules of 3 mL.

Proprietary Names and Manufacturers

Ethiodan *(Allen & Hanburys, Canad.)*; Myodil *(Glaxo, Austral.; Glaxo, Ital.; Glaxo, UK)*; Pantopaque *(USA)*.

18651-j

Iopromide *(BAN, rINN).*

SH-414E. *N,N'*-Bis(2,3-dihydroxypropyl)-2,4,6-tri-iodo-5-(2-methoxyacetamido)-*N*-methylisophthalamide.
$C_{18}H_{24}I_3N_3O_8$=791.1.

CAS — 73334-07-3.

Iopromide contains approximately 48.1% of I.

Iopromide is a low-osmolal nonionic monomeric contrast medium which is used for angiography and urography. Iopromide has actions similar to metrizamide (p.870).

Iopromide and iohexol were studied against ioxaglate in 98 patients scheduled for aortofemoral arteriography. Iohexol and iopromide displayed better tolerance to idiosyncratic side-effects than ioxaglate. However, symptoms such as pain and heat were better tolerated with ioxaglate than with iohexol or possibly iopromide.— B. Hagen, Iohexol and Iopromide - Two New Non-ionic Water-soluble Radiographic Contrast Media: Randomized, Intraindividual Double-blind Study Versus Ioxaglate in Peripheral Angiography, in *Contrast Media in Urography, Angiography and Computerized Tomography*, V. Taenzer and E. Zeitler (Eds), Stuttgart, Georg Thieme Verlag, 1983 p.107. For some other comparisons see also K.-J. Wolf *et al.*, Comparative Evaluation of Low Osmolar Contrast Media in (Femoral) Arteriography, *ibid.*, p.102; V. Taenzer *et al.*, Urography with Non-ionic Contrast Media: Diagnostic Quality and Tolerance of Iopromide in Comparison with Ioxaglate, *ibid.*, p.153; E. Zeitler *et al.*, Experiences with Rayvist and Iopromid in Head and Body CT, *ibid.*, p.162.

Proprietary Names and Manufacturers

Ultravist *(Schering, Denm.; Schering, Ger.; Schering, Swed.; Schering, Switz.; Schering, UK)*.

12858-b

Iotasul *(USAN, rINN).*

ZK-79112. 5,5'-[Thiobis(ethylenecarboxamido)]bis-[*NN'*-bis(2,3-dihydroxypropyl)-2,4,6-tri-iodo-*NN'*-dimethylisophthalamide].
$C_{38}H_{50}I_6N_6O_{14}S$=1608.3.

CAS — 71767-13-0.

Iotasul contains approximately 47.3% of I.

Iotasul is a low-osmolal nonionic dimeric contrast medium.

Investigation of lymphoedema by means of indirect lymphography using iotasul.— H. Partsch *et al.*, *Br. J. Derm.*, 1984, *110*, 431.

Proprietary Names and Manufacturers

Schering, Ger.

1530-h

Iothalamic Acid *(BAN, USAN).*

Iotalamic Acid *(rINN)*; Methalamic Acid. 5-Acetamido-2,4,6-tri-iodo-*N*-methylisophthalamic acid.
$C_{11}H_9I_3N_2O_4$=613.9.

CAS — 2276-90-6.

Pharmacopoeias. In *Br.*, *Jpn*, and *U.S.*

A white, odourless powder. *B.P.* **solubilities** are: slightly soluble in water and in alcohol; practically insoluble in chloroform; very soluble in solutions of sodium hydroxide. It contains approximately 62% of I.
Store in well-closed containers. Protect from light.

1531-m

Meglumine Iothalamate *(BANM).*

Iothalamate Meglumine *(USAN).* The *N*-methylglucamine salt of iothalamic acid.
$C_{11}H_9I_3N_2O_4.C_7H_{17}NO_5$=809.1.
CAS — 13087-53-1.

Meglumine iothalamate contains approximately 47.1% of I.

1575-z

Sodium Iothalamate *(BANM).*

Iothalamate Sodium *(USAN).*
$C_{11}H_8I_3N_2NaO_4$=635.9.
CAS — 1225-20-3.

Sodium iothalamate contains approximately 59.9% of I. Each g of monograph substance represents 1.57 mmol of sodium.

Adverse Effects, Treatment, and Precautions

As for the diatrizoates (p.863).

In 40 patients undergoing phlebography, usually with about 200 mL of 60% meglumine iothalamate, pain at the injection site and in the calf were common; foot swelling also occurred; skin necrosis occurred as a delayed effect in 1 patient. Retrospective study revealed necrosis of the foot in 3 further patients and gangrene in 2. At the end of examination, in which tourniquets were used above the knee and ankle, the veins were flushed with saline and clearance of the contrast medium encouraged by muscle contraction.— M. L. Thomas and L. M. MacDonald, *Br. med. J.*, 1978, *2*, 317. For a study comparing meglumine iothalamate and iopamidol with regard to the incidence of venous thrombophlebitis see Iopamidol (p.867).

For a report of ventricular tachycardia in a patient receiving sodium iothalamate and prenylamine, see p.1516.

EFFECTS ON THE IMMUNE SYSTEM. A report of 2 homosexual men with generalised lymphadenopathy who had acute sensitivity reactions to meglumine iothalamate.— D. C. Doll, *Lancet*, 1984, *1*, 798.

EFFECTS ON THE NERVOUS SYSTEM. A case report of myasthenic crisis precipitated by infusion of iothalamic acid (Conray 60%) in a 25-year-old woman. It was concluded that iothalamic acid caused the crisis by a reversible neuromuscular blockade.— N. Canal and M. Franceschi (letter), *Lancet*, 1983, *1*, 1288.

INTERACTIONS. Iothalamic acid reduced the optical extinction in the colorimetric test used in the urinary hydroxyproline excretion test. It was recommended that at least 6 days should elapse before urine is collected for hydroxyproline measurement after intravenous injection of iodinated contrast medium.— P. Scalella (letter), *Lancet*, 1982, *1*, 907.

Absorption and Fate

Iothalamic acid in the circulation is not significantly bound to serum proteins. If renal function is not impaired, unchanged medium is rapidly excreted, primarily by glomerular filtration. The excretion of the meglumine salt is accompanied by a greater diuresis than accompanies the sodium salt.

Uses and Administration

Iothalamic acid is a high-osmolal ionic monomeric contrast medium and is used as its meglumine and sodium salts in diagnostic radiology. It has actions similar to the diatrizoates (p.864). The meglumine salt of iothalamic acid is generally better tolerated than the sodium salt but the high viscosity of solutions of the meglumine salt makes them difficult to administer rapidly. Solutions used contain up to 70% of the sodium salt, up to 60% of the meglumine salt, or mixtures of the 2 salts.
Iothalamates are given intravenously or by local application for a wide range of diagnostic procedures, including angiography, cholangiography, venography, and hysterosalpingography.
For urography they are given by intravenous injection or infusion, or by retrograde injection.
Iothalamates are not suitable for injection into the subarachnoid space.

ADMINISTRATION IN RENAL FAILURE. There was no deterioration of renal function in 15 patients, with reduced renal function but free from myelomatosis or diabetes, when they were given large doses of iothalamates for urography or angiography. Avoidance of dehydration and of repeated doses in rapid succession was recommended.— A. Rahimi *et al., Br. med. J.*, 1981, *282*, 1194.

Preparations of Iothalamates

Iothalamate Meglumine and Iothalamate Sodium Injection *(U.S.P.).* A sterile solution of iothalamic acid in Water for Injections, prepared with the aid of meglumine and sodium hydroxide. When intended for intravascular use it contains no antimicrobial agents. pH 6.5 to 7.7. Protect from light.

Iothalamate Meglumine Injection *(U.S.P.).* A sterile solution of iothalamic acid in Water for Injections, prepared with the aid of meglumine. When intended for intravascular use it contains no antimicrobial agents. pH 6.5 to 7.7. Protect from light.

Iothalamate Sodium Injection *(U.S.P.).* A sterile solution of iothalamic acid in Water for Injections, prepared with the aid of sodium hydroxide. When intended for intravascular use it contains no antimicrobial agents. pH 6.5 to 7.7. Protect from light.

Meglumine Iothalamate Injection *(B.P.).* pH 7.0 to 7.5. Protect from light.

Sodium Iothalamate Injection *(B.P.).* pH 7.0 to 7.5. Protect from light.

Proprietary Preparations of Iothalamates

Conray 280 *(May & Baker, UK). Injection,* meglumine iothalamate 60%, in ampoules of 20 mL and bottles of 50 mL.

Conray 325 *(May & Baker, UK). Injection,* sodium iothalamate 54%, in bottles of 50 mL.

Conray 420 *(May & Baker, UK). Injection,* sodium iothalamate 70%, in ampoules of 20 mL and bottles of 50 mL.

Proprietary Names and Manufacturers of Iothalamates

Angio-Conray *(Mallinckrodt, Canad.; Bracco, Ital.)*; Cardio-Conray *(May & Baker, Austral.; May & Baker, UK)*; Conray *(May & Baker, Austral.; Mallinckrodt, Canad.; Astra Meditec, Denm.; Byk Gulden, Ger.; Bracco, Ital.; Jpn; Astra Meditec, Norw.; Astra-Meditec, Swed.; May & Baker, UK)*; Contrix 28 *(Belg.; Fr.)*; Cysto-Conray *(Mallinckrodt, Canad.; USA)*; Gastro-Conray *(May & Baker, Austral.; May & Baker, UK)*; Retro-Conray *(Austral.; May & Baker, UK)*; Sombril *(Rovi, Spain)*; Vascoray *(Mallinckrodt, Canad.; Astra Meditec, Denm.).*

12859-v

Iotroxic Acid *(BAN, USAN, rINN).*

SH-213AB. 3,3′-(3,6,9-Trioxaundecanedioyldi-imino)bis(2,4,6-tri-iodobenzoic acid).
$C_{22}H_{18}I_6N_2O_9$=1215.8.
CAS — 51022-74-3.

Iotroxic acid contains approximately 62.6% of I.

12860-r

Meglumine Iotroxate *(BANM).*

Iotroxamide; Meglumine Iotroxinate; SH-H-273. The *N*-methylglucamine salt of iotroxic acid.
$C_{22}H_{18}I_6N_2O_9,2C_7H_{17}NO_5$=1606.2.

Meglumine iotroxate contains approximately 47.4% of I.

Iotroxic acid is an ionic dimeric contrast medium used, as the meglumine salt, intravenously for visualisation of the bilitary tract. Iotroxic acid has actions similar to metrizamide (p.870).

Proprietary Preparations

Biliscopin *(Schering, UK) Injection,* iodine 50 mg/mL (as meglumine iotroxate) in bottles of 100mL.
Injection, iodine 180 mg/mL (as meglumine iotroxate) in ampoules of 30 mL.

Proprietary Names and Manufacturers

Biliscopin *(Schering, Denm.; Schering, Ger.; Schering AG, Norw.; Schering, Swed.; Schering, Switz.; Schering, UK)*; Bilisegrol *(Schering, Spain)*; Chologram *(Schering, Ital.).*

12861-f

Ioxaglic Acid *(BAN, USAN, rINN).*

P-286. *N*-(2-Hydroxyethyl)-2,4,6-tri-iodo-5-[2′,4′,6′-tri-iodo-3′-(*N*-methylacetamido)-5′-methylcarbamoylhippuramido]isophthalamic acid.
$C_{24}H_{21}I_6N_5O_8$=1268.9.
CAS — 59017-64-0.

Ioxaglic acid contains approximately 60% of I.

15337-m

Meglumine Ioxaglate *(BANM).*

Ioxaglate Meglumine *(USAN)*; MP-302 *(with sodium ioxaglate)*. The *N*-methylglucamine salt of ioxaglic acid.
$C_{24}H_{21}I_6N_5O_8,C_7H_{17}NO_5$=1464.1.
CAS — 59018-13-2.

Meglumine ioxaglate contains approximately 52% of I.

15338-b

Sodium Ioxaglate *(BANM).*

Ioxaglate Sodium *(USAN)*; MP-302 *(with meglumine ioxaglate)*.
$C_{24}H_{20}I_6N_5NaO_8$=1290.9.
CAS — 67992-58-9.

Sodium ioxaglate contains approximately 59% of I. Each g of monograph substance represents 0.77 mmol of sodium.

Adverse Effects, Treatment, and Precautions

As for diatrizoic acid (p.863).

In a study on 24 patients, ventriculography was carried out using meglumine ioxaglate with sodium ioxaglate (Hexabrix) or meglumine diatrizoate with sodium diatrizoate (Urografin 76). Subjective tolerance was better and haemodynamic side-effects were less with Hexabrix than with Urografin.— A. Theler and H. R. Baur, *Cathet. Cardiovasc. Diagn.*, 1983, *9*, 577.

In a study of 47 phlebographies, diatrizoate (Urografin) and ioxaglate (Hexabrix) were compared with regard to postphlebographic thrombosis. A significantly lower rate was registered when the low-osmolar ioxaglate was used.— B. Eliasen *et al., Eur. J. Radiol.*, 1983, *3*, 97.

In an investigation of 100 patients undergoing ventriculography using meglumine ioxaglate with sodium ioxaglate (Hexabrix 320) or meglumine iothalamate (Conray 420), 13 patients found Hexabrix unpleasant compared with 24 receiving Conray; overall feelings of warmth and discomfort were less with Hexabrix. The incidence of nausea, vomiting, and hypersensitivity was similar. Angiographic quality was better with Conray. The slight advantages of Hexabrix over Conray may be valuable in patients requiring multiple angiograms or in those with impaired cardiac function, but do not justify its use for routine angiography.— J. Lyons *et al., Br. J. Radiol.*, 1984, *57*, 209.

A study of 101 patients undergoing central venous injections for digital subtraction angiography using meglumine ioxaglate with sodium ioxaglate (Hexabrix 320) or iohexol (Omnipaque 300). Nausea and vomiting did not occur in the iohexol group, whereas the incidence in the ioxaglate group was highly significant at 24.5%.— A. R. Manhire *et al., Clin. Radiol.*, 1984, *35*, 369.

For a comparison of the tolerance of adverse effects of ioxaglate, iohexol, and iopromide in aortofemoral arteriography, see Iopromide (p.868).

Uses and Administration

Ioxaglic acid is a low-osmolal ionic dimeric contrast medium given as its meglumine and sodium salts intravenously or by local application for a wide range of diagnostic procedures, including angiography, hysterosalpingography, phlebography, urography, and venography.
It must never be injected by the subarachnoid or

epidural routes. It is not suitable for myelography.

Some comparisons of ioxaglate with other contrast media: K.-J. Wolf *et al.*, Comparative Evaluation of Low Osmolar Contrast Media in (Femoral) Arteriography in *Contrast Media in Urography, Angiography and Computerized Tomography*. V. Taenzer and E. Zeitler (Eds), Stuttgart, Georg Thieme Verlag, 1983, p.102, V. Taenzer *et al.*, Urography with Non-ionic Contrast Media: Diagnostic Quality and Tolerance of Iopromide, *ibid.*, 1983, p.153.

Proprietary Preparations

Hexabrix *(May & Baker, UK). Injection* (Hexabrix 200), meglumine ioxaglate 24.56%, sodium ioxaglate 12.28%, in bottles of 50 mL.
Injection (Hexabrix 320), meglumine ioxaglate 39.3%, sodium ioxaglate 19.65%, in ampoules of 20 mL and bottles of 50 and 100 mL.

Proprietary Names and Manufacturers of Ioxaglic Acid and its Salts

Hexabrix *(May & Baker, Austral.; Mallinckrodt, Canad.; Guerbet, Denm.; Byk Gulden, Ger.; Guerbet, Norw.; Guerbet, Swed.; Guerbet, Switz.; May & Baker, UK; Mallinckrodt, USA).*

1532-b

Ioxitalamic Acid *(rINN).*

AG-58107; Ioxithalamic Acid. 5-Acetamido-*N*-(2-hydroxyethyl)-2,4,6-tri-iodoisophthalamic acid.
$C_{12}H_{11}I_3N_2O_5$=643.9.

CAS — 28179-44-4.

Ioxitalamic acid contains approximately 59.1% of I.

1533-v

Meglumine Ioxitalamate

Ioxitalamate Meglumine. The *N*-methylglucamine salt of ioxitalamic acid.
$C_{12}H_{11}I_3N_2O_5, C_7H_{17}NO_5$=839.2.

CAS — 29288-99-1.

Meglumine ioxitalamate contains approximately 45.4% of I.

1576-c

Sodium Ioxitalamate

Ioxitalamate Sodium.
$C_{12}H_{10}I_3N_2NaO_5$=665.9.

CAS — 33954-26-6.

Sodium ioxitalamate contains approximately 57.2% of I. Each g of monograph substance represents 1.5 mmol of sodium.

Salts of ioxitalamic acid (meglumine, sodium, and ethanolamine) are high-osmolal ionic monomeric contrast media with actions similar to those of the diatrizoates (p.863). They are used for intravenous urography, angiography, and peripheral and selective arteriography; the meglumine salt is also used for hysterosalpingography.

Proprietary Names and Manufacturers of Ioxitalamates

Telebrix *(Temis-Lostalo, Arg.; Codali, Belg.; Guerbet, Denm.; Guerbet, Fr.; Byk Gulden, Ger.; Byk Gulden, Ital.; Guerbet, Neth.; Rovi, Spain; Guerbet, Switz.)*; Vasobrix *(Guerbet, Denm.; Guerbet, Fr.).*

1577-k

Methiodal Sodium *(BAN, USAN, rINN).*

Sergosin; Sodium Methiodal; Urombral. Sodium iodomethanesulphonate.
CH_2INaO_3S=244.0.

CAS — 143-47-5 (methiodal); 126-31-8 (methiodal sodium).

Pharmacopoeias. In *Nord., Rus.,* and *U.S.*

A white odourless crystalline powder containing approximately 52% of I. On exposure to light it decomposes and becomes yellow.
Soluble 1 in 0.8 of water and 1 in 200 of alcohol; practically insoluble in acetone, chloroform, and ether; very soluble in methyl alcohol. A solution in water has a pH of 5 to 8. **Store** in airtight containers. Protect from light.

Methiodal sodium is a contrast medium with actions similar to those of the diatrizoates (p.863) and has been used for the examination of the urinary tract.

Preparations

Methiodal Sodium Injection *(U.S.P.)*

1578-a

Metrizamide *(BAN, USAN, rINN).*

Win-39103. 2-[3-Acetamido-2,4,6-tri-iodo-5-(*N*-methylacetamido)benzamido]-2-deoxy-D-glucose.
$C_{18}H_{22}I_3N_3O_8$=789.1.

CAS — 31112-62-6.

Metrizamide contains approximately 48.2% of I.

Adverse Effects

After intrathecal administration metrizamide may cause headache, nausea, and vomiting. Backache, neck stiffness, numbness, and leg or sciatic-type pain occur less frequently. Chest pain, tachycardia, bradycardia, apnoea, dizziness, pyrexia, hypertension, hypotension, cardiac arrest, vasculitis, haemorrhage, collapse, and shock have also been reported. Grand mal seizures, aseptic meningitis, and mild and transitory perceptual aberrations may occur occasionally. Renal failure, polyuria, haematuria, allergic reactions, and urinary retention have also been reported. Metrizamide is claimed to cause fewer side-effects than meglumine iocarmate.

No muscle spasm had been reported in the first 100 000 lumbar myelography examinations using metrizamide.— R. G. Grainger (letter), *Br. med. J.*, 1978, *1*, 1488.

A report of a grand mal seizure after lumbar myelography using metrizamide.— A. R. Wray *et al.* (letter), *Br. med. J.*, 1978, *2*, 1787.

In 100 patients undergoing venography one leg was examined using 50 mL of meglumine iothalamate (280 mg I per mL) and the other leg with metrizamide of comparable iodine content. Immediate pain was experienced by 68 and 15 patients respectively and pain one week later (74 patients) by 37 and 7 patients respectively. Flushing, nausea, vomiting, and foot or calf swelling were also reduced with metrizamide.— M. L. Thomas and H. L. Walters, *Br. med. J.*, 1979, *2*, 1036.

Cervical myelopathy, with arm weakness persisting 6 months later, after lumbar myelography with metrizamide.— M. Bastow and R. B. Godwin-Austen, *Br. med. J.*, 1979, *2*, 1262.

Severe delayed headaches and sometimes distressing nausea and vomiting associated with metrizamide given intrathecally. As these effects were possibly associated with cerebral swelling, iophendylate should be used rather than metrizamide for patients in whom a rise in intracranial pressure due to swelling might be harmful.— L. A. Cala (letter), *Lancet*, 1981, *2*, 922.

A 36-year-old man underwent lumbar myelography with metrizamide (1540 mg). Two hours later the patient developed an occipital and bitemporal headache. Severe symmetrical acral asterixis and head bobbing began between 12 and 14 hours after the procedure. Three months later asterixis and head bobbing persisted.— C. E. Davis *et al.*, *Archs Neurol., Chicago*, 1982, *39*, 128.

Reports of neuropsychiatric adverse effects associated with metrizamide: J. A. Kwentus *et al.*, *Am. J. Psychiat.*, 1984, *141*, 700 (mania); R. L. Elliott *et al.*, *J. Am. med. Ass.*, 1984, *252*, 2057 (prolonged delirium); J. B. Wade *et al.* (letter), *Lancet*, 1986, *2*, 102 (organic personality syndrome).

An intracranial subdural haematoma in a 31-year-old woman after myelography using 6.76 g of metrizamide.— N. G. Dan, *Med. J. Aust.*, 1984, *140*, 289.

EFFECTS ON THE KIDNEY. Rapid intravenous injection of metrizamide induced diffuse or focal osmotic nephrosis in 6 of 13 normohydrated patients with various types of kidney disease and various degrees of renal impairment. Renal impairment was mild and transient. Metrizamide nephrotoxicity is comparable to that of ionic contrast media.— J. -F. Moreau *et al.* (letter), *Lancet*, 1978, *1*, 1201.

Precautions

As for the diatrizoates (p.864).

Absorption and Fate

Metrizamide is eliminated from the CSF within several hours. It is not significantly bound to plasma albumin.

The pharmacokinetics of metrizamide were investigated after intrathecal injection in the lumbar area of 8 volunteers. There was considerable individual variation. Metrizamide was detected in the blood about 15 minutes after injection with maximum serum concentration in about 2 hours. About half of the dose had disappeared from the CSF in 45 minutes and about 70% of the injected dose was excreted unchanged in the urine within 24 hours.— K. Golman, *J. pharm. Sci.*, 1975, *64*, 405.

Uses and Administration

Metrizamide is a low-osmolal nonionic monomeric contrast medium used in myelography, cisternograpy, and ventriculography.

Computerised tomographic myelography with metrizamide was used in 63 subjects aged 6 days to 21 years. There were no false-positives and one false-negative. Vomiting and headaches occurred in half the children and 10 had fever. Metrizamide was considered better than contrast agents such as iophendylate for the study of the sacral, lumbar, and midthoracic regions.— *J. Am. med. Ass.*, 1977, *237*, 757.

Pancreatic parenchymography using metrizamide was carried out on 50 cases, only 4.6% developed clinical pancreatitis.— B. Twomey *et al.*, *Gut*, 1982, *23*, A432.

Some references: *Acta radiol., Diagnosis*, 1973, *Suppl.*, 1–390; R. G. Grainger *et al.*, *Br. J. Radiol.*, 1976, *49*, 996; J. Sackett *et al.*, *Radiology*, 1977, *123*, 779; R. D. Strand *et al.*, *Radiology*, 1978, *128*, 405.

Proprietary Names and Manufacturers

Amipaque *(Winthrop, Austral.; Winthrop, Canad.; Nyco, Denm.; Schering, Ger.; Maggioni-Winthrop, Ital.; Nyco, Norw.; Alter, Spain; Swed.; Switz.; Nycomed, UK; Winthrop-Breon, USA).*

1534-g

Metrizoic Acid

3-Acetamido-2,4,6-tri-iodo-5-(*N*-methylacetamido)benzoic acid.
$C_{12}H_{11}I_3N_2O_4$=627.9.

CAS — 1949-45-7.

Pharmacopoeias. In *Nord.*

Metrizoic acid contains approximately 60.6% of I.

1535-q

Meglumine Metrizoate

Metrizoate Meglumine. The *N*-methylglucamine salt of metrizoic acid.
$C_{12}H_{11}I_3N_2O_4, C_7H_{17}NO_5$=823.2.

CAS — 7241-11-4.

Meglumine metrizoate contains approximately 46.2% of I.

1579-t

Sodium Metrizoate *(BAN, rINN).*

Metrizoate Sodium *(USAN).*
$C_{12}H_{10}I_3N_2NaO_4$=649.9.

CAS — 7225-61-8.

Sodium metrizoate contains approximately 58.6% of I. Each g of monograph substance represents 1.54 mmol of sodium.

Adverse Effects, Treatment, and Precautions

As for the diatrizoates (p.863).

Thrombosis associated with phlebography using meglumine metrizoate.— U. Albrechtsson and C. -G. Olsson, *Lancet*, 1976, *1*, 723. Anticoagulant cover appeared to reduce the risk of thrombosis associated with phlebography and such cover was recommended.— F. Laerum *et al.* (letter), *ibid.*, 1980, *1*, 1141.

Uses and Administration

Metrizoic acid is a high-osmolal ionic monomeric contrast medium which, as its meglumine and sodium salts, has properties and uses similar to those of the diatrizoates (see p.864). It has been used as these salts often together with calcium metrizoate and magnesium metrizoate for a variety of diagnostic procedures including angiography and pyelography.

Proprietary Names and Manufacturers of Metrizoates
Isopaque *(Canad.; Nyco, Denm.; Fr.; Nyco, Norw.; Nycomed, Swed.; Nycomed, UK; USA)*; Nitigraf *(Juste, Spain)*; Ronpacon; Triosil.

1582-j

Propyliodone *(BAN, USAN, rINN).*

Propyliodonum. Propyl 1,4-dihydro-3,5-di-iodo-4-oxo-1-pyridylacetate.
$C_{10}H_{11}I_2NO_3$=447.0.

CAS — 587-61-1.

Pharmacopoeias. In *Br., Egypt., Jug., Nord.,* and *U.S.*

A white or almost white, crystalline powder, odourless or with a slight odour, containing approximately 56.8% of I.

B.P. **solubilities** are: practically insoluble in water; slightly soluble in alcohol and in chloroform; very slightly soluble in ether. **Store** in airtight containers. Protect from light.

Adverse Effects

Propyliodone may give rise to transient pyrexia, sometimes associated with malaise and aching of the joints, especially with the aqueous suspension, lasting 48 hours and sometimes accompanied by coughing. In a few cases, dyspnoea has occurred and, very rarely, transient lobar collapse. Allergic reactions may occur rarely.

Precautions

Propyliodone should be used with great care where there is hypersensitivity to iodine. It should also be used with caution in patients with asthma, bronchiectasis, or pulmonary emphysema. If bilateral examination is necessary in such patients an interval of several days should elapse between the examinations. Use of an excessive volume may result in lobar collapse. The administration of iodine-containing contrast media may interfere with thyroid-function tests.

Absorption and Fate

After instillation into the lungs some propyliodone may be expectorated and swallowed but the remainder is hydrolysed in the lungs and absorbed. Approximately 50% of the administered dose is eliminated in the urine within 3 days as di-iodopyridone acetate.

Uses and Administration

Propyliodone is a contrast medium used for the examination of the bronchial tract. It is usually administered in the form of either a 50% aqueous suspension or a 60% oily suspension and gives well-defined bronchograms for at least 30 minutes.

Preparations

Propyliodone Oily Suspension *(B.P.).* Sterile Propyliodone Oil Suspension *(U.S.P.)*; Propyliodone Oily Injection. A sterile 60% w/v suspension of propyliodone in arachis oil. Store below 30°.

Propyliodone Suspension *(B.P.).* Propyliodone Injection. A sterile 50% w/v suspension of propyliodone in Water for Injections. pH 6.0 to 7.5. Store between 10° and 30°.

Proprietary Preparations

Dionosil *(Glaxo, UK). Aqueous suspension*, propyliodone 50%, in vials of 20 mL.
Oily suspension, propyliodone 60%, in vials of 20 mL.

Proprietary Names and Manufacturers

Dionosil *(Glaxo, Austral.; Glaxo, Canad.; Glaxo, Ger.; Neth.; Glaxo, Norw.; Glaxo, Swed.; Switz.; Glaxo, UK).*

1584-c

Sodium Iodohippurate

Sodium Ortho-iodohippurate. Sodium α-(2-iodobenzamido)acetate dihydrate.
$C_9H_7INNaO_3,2H_2O$=363.1.

CAS — 147-58-0 (o-iodohippuric acid); 133-17-5 (sodium iodohippurate, anhydrous).

Sodium iodohippurate contains approximately 35% of I.

Sodium iodohippurate is a high-osmolal ionic monomeric, contrast medium and has been used for intravenous retrograde, and oral pyelography. Sodium iodohippurate has actions similar to the diatrizoates (p.863).

1585-k

Sodium Ipodate *(BAN).*

Ipodate Sodium *(USAN)*; Sodium Iopodate *(rINN).* Sodium 3-(3-dimethylaminomethyleneamino-2,4,6-tri-iodophenyl)propionate.
$C_{12}H_{12}I_3N_2NaO_2$=619.9.

CAS — 1221-56-3.

Pharmacopoeias. In *Jpn, Nord.,* and *U.S.*

A fine white or off-white, odourless, crystalline powder, containing approximately 61.4% of I. **Soluble** 1 in less than 1 of water, 1 in 2 of alcohol, 1 in 2 of dimethylacetamide, and 1 in 3.5 of dimethylformamide and dimethyl sulphoxide; very slightly soluble in chloroform; freely soluble in methyl alcohol. **Store** in airtight containers.

Adverse Effects and Precautions

As for Iopanoic Acid, p.867. The effects on the gastro-intestinal tract may be less with sodium ipodate than with iopanoic acid.

Absorption and Fate

Sodium ipodate is absorbed from the gastro-intestinal tract following oral or rectal administration, and maximum concentrations are found in the gall-bladder about 10 hours after ingestion. It is excreted in the urine.

Uses and Administration

Sodium ipodate is a high-osmolal ionic monomeric contrast medium and is used for examination of the biliary tract. It is used similarly to calcium ipodate (p.863) and in the same doses.

In a study of 4 patients with hyperthyroidism, sodium ipodate 3 g as a single dose by mouth lowered serum concentrations of tri-iodothyronine and thyroxine. It was suggested that sodium ipodate might be useful in the treatment of patients with hyperthyroid Graves' disease.— S. -Y. Wu, *Ann. intern. Med.*, 1978, *88*, 379.

For a comparative study showing the similarities between sodium ipodate, iopanoic acid, and iocetamic acid in oral cholecystography, see iopanoic acid (p.868).

Preparations

Ipodate Sodium Capsules *(U.S.P.)*

Proprietary Preparations

Biloptin *(Schering, UK). Capsules*, sodium ipodate 500 mg.

Proprietary Names and Manufacturers

Biloptin *(Arg.; Austral.; Schering, Denm.; Schering, Ger.; Schering, Ital.; Schering AG, Norw.; Schering, Swed.; Schering, Switz.; Schering, UK)*; Biloptine *(Belg.; Fr.)*; Oragrafin Sodium *(Squibb, Canad.; Squibb, USA).*

1586-a

Sodium Tyropanoate *(BAN, rINN).*

Tyropanoate Sodium *(USAN)*; Win-8851-2. Sodium 2-(3-butyramido-2,4,6-tri-iodobenzyl)butyrate.
$C_{15}H_{17}I_3NNaO_3$=663.0.

CAS — 27293-82-9 (tyropanoic acid); 7246-21-1 (sodium tyropanoate).

Pharmacopoeias. In *U.S.*

A white odourless hygroscopic powder containing approximately 57.4% of I. **Soluble** in water, alcohol, and dimethylformamide; very slightly soluble in acetone and ether. **Store** in airtight containers. Protect from light.

Sodium tyropanoate is a high-osmolal ionic monomeric contrast medium, with similar actions to iopanoic acid (p.867) also used for examination of the biliary tract. It is given by mouth in a dose of 3 g.

Preparations

Tyropanoate Sodium Capsules *(U.S.P.)*

Proprietary Names and Manufacturers

Bilopaque *(Winthrop, Canad.; Winthrop, Switz.; Winthrop-Breon, USA)*; Lumopaque *(Winthrop, Arg.).*

Corticosteroids

1060-e

The adrenal cortex produces a number of steroids which may be divided into 3 classes; those whose principal pharmacological actions are upon gluconeogenesis, glycogen deposition, and protein and calcium metabolism, together with inhibition of corticotrophin secretion, and anti-inflammatory activity (glucocorticoid actions), namely, cortisone and hydrocortisone (endogenous hydrocortisone often being termed cortisol); those whose principal actions are upon electrolyte and water metabolism (mineralocorticoid actions), namely, deoxycortone and aldosterone; and the sex corticoids which include mainly androgens.

The naturally occurring corticosteroids in the first 2 classes, except aldosterone which is relatively independent, are secreted under the influence of the anterior pituitary corticotrophic hormone, corticotrophin (see p.1139); all 4 have mineralocorticoid actions to a varying degree and they all, with the possible exception of deoxycortone, have some glucocorticoid actions.

In addition to the naturally occurring corticosteroids, many synthetic steroids with similar properties have been introduced. In developing these synthetic analogues the aim has usually been firstly to produce enhanced potency generally and secondly to separate the 2 main pharmacological actions so that, for example, an increase in glucocorticoid actions is not accompanied by a parallel increase in mineralocorticoid effects.

It appears that a measure of a corticosteroid's potency as a glucocorticoid is the degree of inhibition of corticotrophin secretion it produces.

The chemical structures of the corticosteroids described in this section are all very similar and resemble those of androgens and oestrogens.

The main corticosteroids used systemically are hydroxy compounds (alcohols). They are relatively insoluble in water and the sodium salt of the phosphate or succinate ester is generally used to provide water-soluble forms for injections or solutions. Such esters are readily hydrolysed in the body.

Esterification of corticosteroids at the 17 or 21 positions with fatty acids generally increases the activity on the skin. The formation of cyclic acetonides at the 16 and 17 positions further increases topical anti-inflammatory activity, usually without increasing systemic glucocorticoid activity, and fluorinated corticosteroids also generally have increased topical activity.

Some corticosteroids esterified at the 17 position are much more potent topically than systemically, e.g. beclomethasone dipropionate and betamethasone valerate; they are used by inhalation where their potent anti-inflammatory effect on the lungs has little systemic effect.

In the medical and pharmacological literature the names of unesterified corticosteroids have frequently been used indiscriminately for both the unesterified and esterified forms and it is not always apparent to which form reference is being made. The unesterified form is sometimes qualified by the phrase 'free alcohol'.

Adverse Effects of Corticosteroids

The side-effects associated with the use of corticosteroids in the large doses often necessary to produce a therapeutic response result from excessive action on electrolyte balance, excessive action on other aspects of metabolism including gluconeogenesis, the action on tissue repair and healing, and an inhibitory effect on the secretion of corticotrophin by the anterior lobe of the pituitary gland.

Disturbance of electrolyte balance is manifest in the retention of sodium and water, with oedema and hypertension, and in the increased excretion of potassium with the possibility of hypokalaemic alkalosis. In extreme cases, cardiac failure may be induced. Disturbances of electrolyte balance are common with the naturally occurring corticotrophin, cortisone, deoxycortone, and hydrocortisone, but are less frequent with many synthetic derivatives, such as betamethasone, dexamethasone, methylprednisolone, prednisolone, prednisone, and triamcinolone which have little or no mineralocorticoid activity.

Other excessive metabolic effects lead to mobilisation of calcium and phosphorus, with osteoporosis and spontaneous fractures, nitrogen depletion, and hyperglycaemia with accentuation or precipitation of the diabetic state. The insulin requirements of diabetic patients are increased. Increased appetite is often reported.

The effect on tissue repair is manifest in delayed wound healing, and increased liability to infection; infections may also be masked since corticosteroids have marked anti-inflammatory properties with analgesic and antipyretic effects. Increased susceptibility to all kinds of infection, including sepsis, fungal infections, and viral infections, has been reported in patients on corticosteroid therapy; for example, *Candida* infections of the mouth in patients treated with corticosteroids, especially if these are given conjointly with antibiotics, are not uncommon.

The dose of corticosteroid required to diminish corticotrophin secretion with consequent atrophy of the adrenal cortex and the time required for its occurrence vary from patient to patient. Acute adrenal insufficiency may occur during prolonged treatment or on cessation of treatment and may be precipitated by an infection or trauma. Growth retardation in children has been reported.

Large doses of corticosteroids, or of corticotrophin, may produce symptoms typical of hyperactivity of the adrenal cortex, with moon-face, sometimes with hirsutism, buffalo hump, flushing, increased bruising, striae, and acne, sometimes leading to a fully developed Cushing's syndrome. If administration is discontinued these symptoms are usually reversed, but sudden cessation is dangerous (see Withdrawal, p.873).

Other adverse effects include amenorrhoea, hyperhidrosis, mental and neurological disturbances, intracranial hypertension, acute pancreatitis, and aseptic necrosis of bone. An increase in the coagulability of the blood may lead to thrombo-embolic complications. Peptic ulceration has been reported but reviews of the literature do not always agree that corticosteroids are responsible for an increased incidence. Muscular weakness is an occasional side-effect of most corticosteroids, particularly when they are taken in large doses, and it is most evident with triamcinolone.

Adverse effects occur, in general, fairly equally with all corticosteroid preparations and their incidence rises steeply if dosage increases much above 7.5 mg daily of prednisolone or its equivalent. Short courses at high dosage for emergencies appear to cause less side-effects than prolonged courses with lower doses.

Most topically applied corticosteroids may, under certain circumstances, be absorbed in sufficient amounts to produce systemic effects. The topical application of corticosteroid preparations to the eyes has produced corneal ulcers, raised intraocular pressure, and reduced visual function, and systemic administration has caused posterior subcapsular cataract. Application of corticosteroids to the skin has led to loss of skin collagen and subcutaneous atrophy; local hypopigmentation of deeply pigmented skins has been reported following both the intradermal injection and topical application of potent corticosteroids.

Reviews of the adverse effects associated with corticosteroid therapy: M. G. C. Dahl, *Adverse Drug React. Bull.*, 1985, (Dec.), 428 (following topical application); J. P. Seale and M. R. Compton, *Med. J. Aust.*, 1986, *144*, 139 (following systemic administration).

ADRENAL SUPPRESSION. A review of inhibition of hypothalamo-pituitary-adrenocortical function associated with corticosteroid administration. Inhibition may persist for 6 to 12 months after treatment is withdrawn and may cause acute adrenal insufficiency with circulatory collapse during stress. In general, suppression of secretion of adrenocorticotrophic hormone and atrophy of the adrenal gland become progressively more definite as doses of corticosteroid exceed physiological amounts, i.e. more than 7.5 mg of prednisolone daily, and as the duration of therapy is prolonged. It is less when the corticosteroid is given as a single dose in the morning, and even less if this morning dose is given on alternate days or less frequently. In patients taking high enough doses of corticosteroids to suppress the adrenals the dose should be increased during any form of stress, and those treated within the last 2 or 3 months should be restarted on therapy. Where the interval since treatment is 3 to 12 months resumption of treatment depends on clinical assessment of signs of adrenal insufficiency. According to the disease and the duration of therapy patients may be weaned from corticosteroids at a rate ranging from 2.5 to 5 mg of prednisolone daily every 2 or 3 days to 2.5 mg every 1 to 3 weeks and possibly less, decrements being made with tablets of 1 mg when the dose has been reduced to 10 mg daily. Suppression may also occur after very short courses of high-dose therapy and since many such patients will be under continuing stress when the drugs are stopped, gradual withdrawal of corticosteroids over 5 to 7 days is preferable.— *Br. med. J.*, 1980, *280*, 813.

Corticosteroid-induced adrenal suppression has been associated not only with oral, rectal, and parenteral therapy, but has also followed topical application of corticosteroid preparations, particularly those containing potent corticosteroids. Adrenal suppression has also been associated with the use of inhalants, and the topical application of eye-drops, eye ointments, and nasal preparations. For further details of the problems associated with adrenal suppression see under Withdrawal, below.

ALLERGY AND ANAPHYLAXIS. There have been occasional reports of allergy, and sometimes anaphylaxis, caused by corticosteroids. In some cases the reaction is due to an ingredient used in the manufacture of the corticosteroid preparation.

EFFECTS ON BONES AND JOINTS. *Aseptic necrosis.* A review of corticosteroid-induced avascular necrosis of bone together with its diagnosis and treatment. It is one of the most disabling complications of therapy and is found in patients with a variety of disease states; even short courses of high-dose corticosteroids may be associated with its development. Many theories have been advanced to explain why corticosteroids should predispose to avascular necrosis but the question remains unresolved.— J. E. Nixon, *Br. med. J.*, 1984, *288*, 741.
A further review focussing on the problem in transplant recipients.— *Lancet*, 1985, *1*, 965.

Osteoporosis. Although it has long been recognised that supraphysiological doses of corticosteroids are associated with excess bone loss, osteoporosis, and fractures most studies concerning this association have been in patients with rheumatoid arthritis and renal disease and there has been some controversy over whether patients with certain other diseases may be less susceptible. Mueller (*Am. J. Roentg.*, 1976, *12*, 1300) reported that glucocorticoid therapy resulted in loss of bone in patients with rheumatoid arthritis but not in patients with asthma whereas Adinoff and Hollister (*New Engl. J. Med.*, 1983, *309*, 265) concluded that long-term steroid therapy in asthmatic patients was, in fact, associated with bone changes and fractures. Discussing glucocorticoid-induced osteoporosis Baylink (*ibid.*, 306) considered that the conclusions of Adinoff and Hollister were entirely consistent with the findings of a number of previous studies showing that in patients with various primary disease states, and in laboratory animals, glucocorticoids produced osteoporosis and that these findings eliminated any reasonable doubt that corticosteroids, in any disease state, may have a deleterious effect on bone. Baylink also discussed the treatment and prophylaxis of corticosteroid-induced osteoporosis and suggested the use of vitamin D, calcium, sodium fluoride, and if hypercalciuria was present, hydrochlorothiazide for treatment and vitamin D with calcium for prophylaxis in the patient at risk.

There does however appear to remain some controversy about the dose and duration of treatment with corticosteroids necessary to induce osteoporosis. Reid and colleagues (*Br. med. J.*, 1986, *293*, 1463) have tentatively suggested that even asthmatic patients using inhaled corticosteroids may be at risk although this has been severely criticised by Crompton (*Br. med. J.*, 1987, *294*, 123) who stated that the present evidence gave no grounds for such concern regarding the use of inhaled corticosteroids in conventional doses.

EFFECTS ON THE CARDIOVASCULAR SYSTEM. A short review of the adverse effects on the cardiovascular system following the rapid intravenous administration of corticosteroids.— A. M. Leathem, *Can. J. Hosp. Pharm.*, 1984, *37*, 109.

EFFECTS ON THE EYE. A short review and discussion on eye damage following the topical administration of corticosteroids and how to avoid it.— *Drug & Ther. Bull.*, 1987, *25*, 29.

For further comments regarding the use of topical corticosteroids on the eye, see Ocular Disorders under Uses and Administration (below).

EFFECTS ON THE GASTRO-INTESTINAL TRACT. The idea that corticosteroids might lead to peptic ulcers was an expectation that stemmed from observations of the alarm reaction and how stress produced acute ulcers. In the late 1940's corticotrophin and compound F [hydrocortisone] seemed to be the physiologic mediators of the alarm reaction so that evidence of corticosteroid-induced increases in gastric secretion and ulcers was looked for, and found. Later, it appeared that only patients with certain diseases were more susceptible to the development of an ulcer during therapy and in 1960 Spiro and Milles (*New Engl. J. Med.*, 1960, *263*, 286) concluded that there was little doubt that steroid therapy increased the frequency of peptic ulcer in rheumatoid arthritis but that control studies would be needed to prove the point. Later still, doubts surfaced about steroid-stimulated gastric secretion and even about the incidence of steroid ulcer and culminated in the report by Conn and Blitzer (*ibid.*, 1976, *294*, 473) who did not confirm any excess in the number of reported cases of ulcer associated with steroids. Recently, Messer and associates (*ibid.*, 1983, *309*, 21) on the basis of a statistical analysis of controlled clinical trials have again concluded that corticosteroids do increase the likelihood of ulcer and haemorrhage. As a gastro-enterologist, it is the author's view that common sense is needed before the clinician again changes habits; since an ulcer develops in 1% of control patients not receiving steroids, the 2% incidence for patients receiving steroids does not warrant the prophylactic use of anti-ulcer drugs in all patients. Prophylaxis does not seem to be required for patients with inflammatory bowel disease although a stronger case can be made for ulcer prophylaxis in rheumatoid arthritis when aspirin or non-steroidal anti-inflammatory agents are also being taken, but it should be remembered that there is, as yet, no certain proof that such prophylaxis works. If an ulcer does develop and there is good reason to continue with steroid therapy then corticosteroids may be continued along with some form of ulcer therapy, as the available evidence suggests that such ulcers heal as readily in patients who take steroids as in those who do not.— H. M. Spiro, *New Engl. J. Med.*, 1983, *309*, 45.

Further reviews: *Drug & Ther. Bull.*, 1987, *25*, 41.

EFFECTS ON GLUCOSE TOLERANCE. Short comments on the effect of corticosteroids on glucose tolerance.— R. Taylor, *Adverse Drug React. Bull.*, 1986, (Dec.), 452.

EFFECTS ON GROWTH. A review of the effects of corticosteroids on the growth of children.— I. A. Hughes, *Br. med. J.*, 1987, *295*, 683.

EFFECTS ON IMMUNE RESPONSE. Owing to their immunosuppressant effect administration of corticosteroids in doses greater than those required for physiological replacement therapy is associated with increased susceptibility to infection, aggravation of existing infection, and activation of latent infection. An additional problem is that the anti-inflammatory effect of corticosteroids may mask symptoms until the infection has progressed to an advanced stage; the altered response of the body may also permit the bizarre spread of infections, frequently in aberrant forms, such as disseminated parasitic infections. The risk is greater in patients receiving high doses, or associated therapy with other immunosuppressants such as cytotoxic agents, and in those who are already debilitated. Children receiving high doses of corticosteroids are at special risk from childhood ailments, such as chicken-pox, but vaccination with living organisms is contra-indicated since infection may be induced (killed vaccines or toxoids may be given). This increased susceptibility to infection coupled with masking of symptoms may also be caused by topical or local corticosteroid therapy. Thus, topical application to the skin has led to unusual changes such as atypical ringworm infection. Fungal infections, generally restricted to the upper respiratory tract, are associated with corticosteroid inhalations. Severe damage to the eye has followed the ocular use of corticosteroids in herpetic infections, and a similar generalised spread of herpes infection may follow application to the mouth in the presence of herpes infection.

Conversely, the effect of corticosteroids on the symptoms and course of some infections may be life-saving (see Uses). Before embarking on a long-term course of corticosteroid therapy general measures for the reduction of risk of infection include a diligent search for active or quiescent infection and, where appropriate, prevention or eradication of the infection before starting, or concurrent administration of chemoprophylaxis during corticosteroid treatment.

EFFECTS ON MENTAL STATE. A review of the effects of corticosteroids on mental state. A very wide range of mental disturbances has been reported but the evidence that they really cause psychological change is thin and largely circumstantial. However, the available evidence does suggest that some cases of mental disturbance may indeed result from corticosteroid therapy, particularly if high doses are used. Of the wide range of changes reported, psychosis, euphoria, and depression are the commonest.— D. M. Mitchell and J. V. Collins, *Postgrad. med. J.*, 1984, *60*, 467.

EFFECTS ON MUSCLES. Muscle weakness may be caused by potassium loss in patients receiving corticosteroids with a pronounced mineralocorticoid action, such as fludrocortisone. Muscle wasting is caused by the glucocorticoid properties of corticosteroids; it has been particularly noted in patients receiving 9α-fluorinated corticosteroids, such as triamcinolone, but can be caused by any glucocorticoid.

EFFECTS ON THE NERVOUS SYSTEM. A report of epidural lipomatosis leading to serious neurological complications in a 47-year-old man treated with prolonged high-dose corticosteroid therapy for severe asthma.— D. L. Butcher and S. A. Sahn, *Ann. intern. Med.*, 1979, *90*, 60. A similar report with a brief review of other published cases.— W. E. George *et al.*, *New Engl. J. Med.*, 1983, *308*, 316.

EFFECTS ON THE PANCREAS. A review of drug-induced acute pancreatitis reported in the English, German, and Japanese literature. Fifty-one patients with corticosteroid-related acute pancreatitis have been identified prior to 1975; the disease occurred in both sexes and in all age groups but the incidence appeared higher in males and in children. No inter-relation between the duration or dose of corticosteroids administered and the initiation of pancreatitis is apparent; the specific drug and its dosage have varied widely and the duration before onset has ranged from 6 days to 3.5 years.— Y. Nakashima and J. M. Howard, *Surgery Gynec. Obstet.*, 1977, *145*, 105.

EFFECTS ON SEXUAL FUNCTION. A review of drugs and sexual function. Although glucocorticoids have antagonistic effects on androgens in certain respects, replacement doses should cause no problem. Patients requiring supra-physiological doses are often quite seriously ill and this may be the limiting factor.— J. G. B. Millar, *Practitioner*, 1979, *223*, 634.

EFFECTS ON THE SKIN. A short discussion on the problems of skin sensitisers (ingredients of the product basis, preservatives, fragrances) present in topical corticosteroid preparations.— *Drug & Ther. Bull.*, 1986, *24*, 57.

EFFECTS ON THE VOICE. A short review and discussion on the problem of dysphonia associated with inhaled corticosteroids.— *Lancet*, 1984, *1*, 375. Comments and correspondence: C. H. Dash and G. M. Pover (letter), *ibid.*, 458; I. A. Campbell (letter), *ibid.*, 744; J. A. Streaton (letter), *ibid.*, 963.

Treatment of Adverse Effects of Corticosteroids

The adverse effects of corticosteroids are nearly always due to their use in excess of normal physiological requirements. They should be treated symptomatically, where possible the dosage being reduced or the drug slowly withdrawn.

The treatment of acute adrenal insufficiency in corticosteroid-treated patients, whether it be due to accidental abrupt withdrawal of the corticosteroid or the inability of the patient's adrenals to cope with the increased stress of infection or accidental or surgical trauma, is described under Uses and Administration of hydrocortisone (p.894).

Withdrawal of Corticosteroids

The use of pharmacological doses of corticosteroids to treat disease suppresses the endogenous secretion of corticotrophin by the anterior pituitary, with the result that the adrenal cortex becomes atrophied. Sudden withdrawal or reduction in dosage, or an increase in corticosteroid requirements associated with the stress of infection or accidental or surgical trauma, may then precipitate acute adrenal insufficiency. Symptoms of adrenal insufficiency include malaise, muscle weakness, mental changes, muscle and joint pain, desquamation of the skin, dyspnoea, anorexia, nausea and vomiting, fever, hypoglycaemia, hypotension, and dehydration; deaths have followed the abrupt withdrawal of corticosteroids. For the emergency treatment of acute adrenal insufficiency caused by abrupt withdrawal of corticosteroids, see under Uses and Administration of hydrocortisone (p.894).

In some instances, withdrawal symptoms may simulate a clinical relapse of the disease for which the patient has been undergoing treatment. Other effects that may occur during withdrawal or change of corticosteroid therapy include benign intracranial hypertension with headache and vomiting and papilloedema caused by cerebral oedema. Latent rhinitis or eczema may be unmasked.

Duration of treatment and dosage appear to be important factors in determining suppression of the pituitary-adrenal response to stress on cessation of corticosteroid treatment, and individual liability to suppression is also important.

Corticosteroid withdrawal should therefore always be gradual, the rate depending upon the individual patient's response, the dose, the disease being treated, and the duration of therapy. Recommendations for initial reduction, stated in terms of prednisolone, have varied from as little as steps of 1 mg monthly to 2.5 to 5 mg every 3 to 7 days. Adrenal function should be monitored throughout withdrawal and symptoms attributable to over-rapid withdrawal should be countered by resuming a higher dose and continuing the reduction at a slower rate. The administration of corticotrophin does not help to re-establish adrenal responsiveness.

This gradual withdrawal of corticosteroid therapy permits a return of adrenal function adequate for daily needs, but a further one to two years may be required for the return of function necessary to meet the stress of infection, surgical operations, or trauma. On such occasions patients with a history of recent corticosteroid withdrawal should be protected by means of supplementary corticosteroid therapy as described under Precautions, p.873.

A discussion of the problems of corticosteroid withdrawal. Short courses of a corticosteroid (up to 40 mg of prednisolone daily for less than 7 days) can be stopped suddenly without risk of hypothalamo-pituitary-adrenal suppression. Long-term treatment may require withdrawal over many months (such as a reduction of 1 mg in the daily dose of prednisolone every 3 to 4 weeks). Although after shorter-term treatment a reduction in the dose of prednisolone of 2.5 to 5 mg every 3 to 7 days has been recommended a more rapid tapering of the dose to 7.5 mg daily can sometimes be achieved, followed by more cautious reduction below this dose.— *Drug & Ther. Bull.*, 1987, *25*, 73.

See also Adrenal Suppression under Adverse Effects, p.872.

Precautions for Corticosteroids

Unless considered life-saving, systemic administration of corticosteroids is contra-indicated in patients with peptic ulcer, osteoporosis, psychoses, or severe psychoneuroses, and they should be used only with great caution in the presence of congestive heart failure or hypertension, in patients with diabetes mellitus, infectious diseases, chronic renal failure, and uraemia, and in elderly persons. Patients with active or doubtfully quiescent tuberculosis should not be given corticosteroids except, very rarely, as adjuncts to treatment with antitubercular drugs. Patients with quiescent tuberculosis should be observed closely and should receive chemoprophylaxis if corticosteroid therapy is prolonged.

Because of interference with inflammatory and immunological response, corticosteroids are usually contra-indicated (but see under Uses and Administration) in the presence of acute infections. Similarly, patients already receiving corticosteroid therapy are more susceptible to infection, the symptoms of which, moreover, may be masked until an advanced stage has been reached. Live vaccines should not be given to patients receiving high-dose systemic corticosteroid therapy; killed vaccines or toxoids may be given although the response may be attenuated. Children are at special risk of infection and may require prophylaxis with immunoglobulin.

During long courses of corticosteroid therapy, patients should be seen regularly and, in particular, checked for hypertension, glycosuria, hypokalaemia, gastric discomfort, and mental changes. Sodium intake may need to be reduced and potassium supplements may be necessary. Monitoring of the fluid intake and output, and daily weight records may give early warning of fluid retention; back pain may signify osteoporosis; children are at special risk from raised intracranial pressure; infections should be treated as an emergency. Patients should carry cards (and preferably also wear bracelets) giving full details of their corticosteroid therapy; they and their relatives should be fully conversant with the implications of their therapy and the precautions to be taken.

Measures to compensate for the adrenals' inability to respond to stress (see Withdrawal, above) include increasing the dose to cover minor intercurrent illnesses or similar stresses (with intramuscular administration to cover vomiting). Intramuscular injection of hydrocortisone sodium succinate 100 mg with the premedication has been used in patients on long-term corticosteroid therapy undergoing minor surgical procedures and doses of 100 mg intramuscularly every 6 to 8 hours for 3 days have been used in major procedures. Some studies, however, have suggested that such routine supplementation may not always be necessary and that in some patients only postoperative supplements need to be given when clinical symptoms of insufficiency arise (see below, under Operative Coverage).

Rapid intravenous injection of massive doses of corticosteroids may sometimes cause cardiovascular collapse and injections should therefore be given slowly or by infusion. High doses should not be used for prolonged treatment.

Concurrent administration of barbiturates, phenytoin, or rifampicin may enhance the metabolism and reduce the effects of corticosteroids. Response to anticoagulants may be reduced and, on some occasions, enhanced by corticosteroids. Concurrent administration of corticosteroids with the potassium-depleting diuretics, such as the thiazides or frusemide, may cause excessive potassium loss.

Many drugs have been reported to interfere with certain assay procedures for corticosteroids in body fluids and corticosteroids themselves may interfere with or alter the results of assays for some endogenous substances or drugs.

Topical applications of corticosteroids should not be made with an occlusive dressing to large areas of the body because of the increased risk of systemic toxicity and should not, in general, be used in the presence of infection. Occasionally they may be used with the addition of a suitable antimicrobial substance in the treatment of infected skin but there is a risk of sensitivity reactions occurring. Corticosteroids should not be applied to ulcers of the leg and long-term topical use is best avoided, especially in children.

Before starting long-term therapy with corticosteroids the following should be undertaken: an evaluation of the patient's pituitary-adrenal status; appropriate tests of carbohydrate metabolism to avoid precipitation of latent diabetes or aggravation of existing diabetes; X-ray films of spine and chest, since osteoporosis was a serious contra-indication and in tuberculosis or other chronic infections corticosteroid therapy could have an unfavourable effect on host-parasite balance; an ECG; and evaluation of blood pressure and renal functions; X-ray films of the upper gastro-intestinal tract in patients with a history of peptic-ulcer diathesis; and evaluation of the patient's psychological predisposition. Severe potassium depletion could occur during the administration of corticosteroids with a diuretic that causes potassium loss. In order to minimise the undesirable side-effects of prolonged corticosteroid therapy, supplementary potassium should be administered and sodium intake restricted, with antacids and a diet containing increased vitamin D and non-irritating foods.— G. W. Thorn, *New Engl. J. Med.*, 1966, *274*, 775.

INTERACTIONS. There was an appreciable and consistent increase in plasma corticosteroids after cigarette smoking in man.— A. Kershbaum *et al.*, *J. Am. med. Ass.*, 1968, *203*, 275. A review concerning the clinical importance of smoking and drug interactions concluding that in the majority of examples, including corticosteroids, there is little evidence that there is a recognisable hazard from the interaction per se.— P. F. D'Arcy, *Drug Intell. & clin. Pharm.*, 1984, *18*, 302.

A short review and discussion concerning several case reports of contraceptive failure in women using intra-uterine devices and receiving corticosteroid therapy. Although the evidence is largely anecdotal the contraceptive efficacy of intra-uterine devices may be related to an inflammatory reaction and there has been concern that anti-inflammatory agents may somewhat increase the failure-rate.— *Drug Interact. News.*, 1983, *3*, 35.

Analgesics. For the effect of corticosteroids on various analgesics, see aspirin, p.5 and phenylbutazone, p.36.

Antacids. Concurrent administration of antacids had no effect on serum concentrations of prednisolone attained.— A. R. Tanner *et al.*, *Br. J. clin. Pharmac.*, 1979, *7*, 397. Magnesium trisilicate and aluminium hydroxide did not affect absorption of prednisolone administered concurrently. Absorption might be reduced if small doses of prednisolone were taken with large doses of antacids.— D. A. H. Lee *et al.* (letter), *ibid.*, *8*, 92.

Further references: V. F. Naggar *et al.*, *J. pharm. Sci.*, 1978, *67*, 1029 (reduced dexamethasone bioavailability with magnesium trisilicate).

A view that weakness and debility attributed to corticosteroids may in fact be due to phosphorus depletion caused by concomitant administration of antacids.— M. Goodman *et al.*, *Am. J. Med.*, 1978, *65*, 868.

Anticoagulants. For the various effects of corticosteroids on anticoagulants see under warfarin sodium, p.346.

Anti-epileptics. A review of interactions between corticosteroids and anti-epileptic agents. Reduced efficacy of corticosteroids has been noted in asthmatic, arthritic, renal transplant, and other patients who also received phenytoin or phenobarbitone. Induction of microsomal liver enzymes by phenytoin or phenobarbitone resulting in enhanced clearance of the corticosteroid is believed to be the underlying mechanism. Different corticosteroids appear to be affected to different degrees, but the disease state, doses, and other determinants such as diet, sex, and other drugs administered may also be contributory factors. An increase in the dosage of the corticosteroids may be necessary in order to maintain the desired therapeutic response.— J. G. Gambertoglio, *Drug Interact. News.*, 1983, *3*, 55.

Antineoplastics and immunosuppressants. A review of drug interactions involving cyclosporin concluding that preliminary evidence indicates that mutual inhibition of metabolism occurs between cyclosporin and corticosteroids, increasing the plasma concentrations of both drugs. Additional studies are necessary to determine the incidence and clinical significance of the interaction.— *Drug Interact. News.*, 1984, *4*, 29.

For the effect of corticosteroids on various antineoplastic agents, see cyclophosphamide, p.612.

Antituberculous agents. Increased doses of corticosteroids were required by a patient with Addison's disease when given rifampicin. When ethambutol was substituted for rifampicin the corticosteroid dose had to be reduced. Cortisol-production rates increased in 4 patients with pulmonary tuberculosis being given rifampicin and there were signs of hepatic microsomal enzyme induction.— O. M. Edwards *et al.*, *Lancet*, 1974, *2*, 549. See also D. N. Maisey *et al.* (letter), *ibid.*, 896; W. van Marle *et al.* (letter), *Br. med. J.*, 1979, *1*, 1020.

Contrary to expectations, the administration of corticosteroids with rifampicin aggravated neuritis in borderline leprosy and was contra-indicated.— G. J. Steenbergen and R. E. Pfaltzgraff, *Lepr. Rev.*, 1975, *46*, 115. A warning that since rifampicin speeds the metabolism of corticosteroids, leprosy workers may find a poor response to corticosteroid therapy for severe type 2 lepra reaction (ENL reaction), if rifampicin is being given at the same time.— W. H. Jopling and J. H. S. Pettit (letter), *Lepr. Rev.*, 1979, *50*, 331.

Further references to rifampicin diminishing corticosteroid activity: G. A. Buffington *et al.*, *J. Am. med. Ass.*, 1976, *236*, 1958; W. Hendrickse *et al.*, *Br. med. J.*, 1979, *1*, 306; W. A. C. McAllister *et al.*, *Br. med. J.*, 1983, *286*, 923.

For the effect of corticosteroids on isoniazid, see p.566.

Muscle relaxants. For the effect of corticosteroids on pancuronium, see p.1236.

Sex hormones. Reviews discussing several reports of an enhanced effect of corticosteroids in women also receiving oestrogens or oral contraceptives and commenting that the dose of corticosteroids in some cases may need to be reduced.— *Drug Interact. News.*, 1982, *2*, 41; *ibid.*, 1983, *3*, 48; G. M. Shenfield, *Med. J. Aust.*, 1986, *144*, 205.

Reports of altered pharmacokinetics of corticosteroids in women taking oral contraceptives: P. J. Meffin *et al.*, *Br. J. clin. Pharmac.*, 1984, *17*, 655; U. F. Legler and L. Z. Benet, *Clin. Pharmac. Ther.*, 1986, *39*, 425.

Sympathomimetics. Studies in 21 asthmatic patients suggested that the plasma half-life of dexamethasone was decreased when it was administered with ephedrine.— S. M. Brooks *et al.*, *J. clin. Pharmac.*, 1977, *17*, 308.

Thalidomide. In a double-blind crossover study of thalidomide in the treatment of severe chronic erythema nodosum leprosum, the dose of prednisolone necessary to suppress symptoms was considerably reduced in 9 of 10 patients while they were receiving thalidomide 300 mg daily.— M. F. R. Waters, *Lepr. Rev.*, 1971, *42*, 26. For a comment that prednisolone should not be given with thalidomide, see *Lepr. Rev.*, 1979, *50*, 326.

Xanthines. For the effect of corticosteroids on theophylline, see theophylline hydrate, p.1529.

INTERFERENCE WITH DIAGNOSTIC TESTS. Some references to drugs interfering with the determination and assay of corticosteroids in body fluids: S. Borushek and J. J. Gold, *Clin. Chem.*, 1964, *10*, 41; O. Llerena and O. H. Pearson, *New Engl. J. Med.*, 1968, *279*, 983; C. L. Cope, *Adrenal Steroids and Disease*, London, Pitman Medical, 1972, p.125; J. Millhouse, *Adverse Drug React. Bull.*, 1974, (Dec.), 164.

OCCUPATIONAL EXPOSURE. A report of facial plethora in 12 men engaged in manufacture of a potent glucocorticoid despite adherence to safety regulations; 3 had abnormal responses to tetracosactrin. Such persons should be monitored regularly and should have periods of work not involving corticosteroids.— R. W. Newton *et al.*, *Br. med. J.*, 1978, *1*, 73.

OPERATIVE COVERAGE. A study and discussion concerning the management of surgical patients receiving corticosteroids. Supplementary corticosteroids used to be given to all surgical patients who were, or had been, receiving systemic steroid therapy for at least one week in the previous 6 months. Investigations have shown, however, that patients whose steroid therapy has been discontinued for more than 2 months have a normal cortisol response to surgery and can be regarded as non-steroid patients. Even in patients on long-term therapy there is a variable cortisol response to surgical stress and many do not develop shock when given no perioperative supplements. As steroid therapy involves risks, supplementary treatment should only be given where necessary and in the minimal effective dose.

In a series of 61 patients with rheumatoid arthritis on long-term corticosteroid treatment, hydrocortisone hemisuccinate 100 mg was given intramuscularly with the premedication on 71 occasions involving orthopaedic procedures while on 36 occasions no supplementary steroid was given with the premedication; patients resumed their oral maintenance doses of corticosteroids immediately after the operation, unless prevented from doing so by factors such as nausea and vomiting, and although supplementary intramuscular doses were not given routinely postoperatively they were allowed if indicated. Of the operations managed without a premedication dose of steroids, postoperative intramuscular supplements were required in only 17% compared with 24% when a premedication dose had been given. The patients most likely to need postoperative supplements were those on high-dose prednisolone (7.5 to 15 mg daily), but there were no consistent factors which would enable a requirement for supplementary steroids to be predicted in any particular individual.

It was considered that this study supported the suggestion that the requirement of steroid supplementation to maintain peri-operative homoeostasis is low and the comment was made that the nursing staff had expressed a preference for the regimen omitting the premedication dose and just allowing postoperative supplements when needed. It was considered that this regimen would also be suitable for patients receiving local therapy to the respiratory tract, eyes, or skin, routes in which adrenal suppression should not normally occur.— E. L. Lloyd, *Ann. R. Coll. Surg.*, 1981, *63*, 54. Some comments and correspondence: M. R. Masser (letter), *ibid.*, 216; C. S. Jones (letter), *ibid.*

PHAEOCHROMOCYTOMA. A case report of a 69-year-old woman with phaeochromocytoma in whom episodes of hypertension were related to the administration of corticosteroids.— P. Daggett and S. Franks, *Br. med. J.*, 1977, *1*, 84.

PORPHYRIA. A review of drug-induced porphyrias and comments on the conflicting evidence concerning corticosteroids. A report suggesting that corticosteroids may have a role in treating the acute attack together with many reports attesting to their safety, contrasts with their repeated incrimination as the offending agent in producing such episodes. It was considered that as corticosteroids may be life-saving, they should be used if really indicated.— M. R. Moore and P. B. Disler, *Adverse Drug React. Ac. Pois. Rev.*, 1983, *2*, 149.

PREGNANCY AND THE NEONATE. *Early pregnancy. Animal* studies by F.C. Fraser *et al.* (*J. cell. comp. Physiol.* 1954, *43*, 237), T. Fainstat (*Endocrinology*, 1954, *55*, 502) and others demonstrated an increase in foetal cleft palate following maternal ingestion of high corticosteroid doses, and cortisone has been used widely as a tool for the investigation of mechanisms responsible for cleft lip and palate. With doses used in clinical practice, however, the risk appears to be low. In an analysis of several hundred cases reported in the literature, A.J. Popert (*Br. med. J.*, 1962, *1*, 967) concluded that the incidence of cleft palate in exposed children was slightly higher than in a random sample, but that in the small selected group studied, this higher incidence might be fallacious. Although D.W. Warrell and R. Taylor (*Lancet*, 1968, *1*, 117) found an increased incidence of malformations in the children of asthmatic mothers given prednisolone 2.5 to 30 mg daily during pregnancy, J.K. Scott (*Lancet*, 1968, *1*, 208) has suggested that the outcome might have been worse in untreated asthmatic mothers. Moreover, other workers, such as M. Schatz *et al.* (*J. Am. med. Ass.*, 1975, *233*, 804) found no significant increase in the risk of foetal or maternal complications in a study of asthmatic mothers given prednisolone 2.5 to 20 mg daily. More recently, K.A. Winship *et al.* (*Archs Dis. Childh.*, 1984, *59*, 1052) found no evidence of a teratogenic effect for corticosteroids when comparing the maternal drug histories of the mothers of 764 infants born with anomalies of the CNS and 764 controls, and R.C. Holmes and M.M. Black (*Br. J. Derm.*, 1984, *110*, 67) found no striking differences in birthweight and frequency of 'small for dates' infants born to mothers who received systemic corticosteroids during pregnancy for pemphigoid gestationis and those who did not.

Further studies and surveys on the risks to the foetus of maternal corticosteroid therapy: A. M. Bongiovanni and A. J. McPadden, *Fert. Steril.*, 1960, *11*, 181 (low incidence of cleft palate); D. B. Yackel *et al.*, *Am. J. Obstet. Gynec.*, 1966, *96*, 985 (no association); S. D. Walsh and F. R. Clark, *Scott. med. J.*, 1967, *12*, 302 (no association); H. Serment and H. Ruf, *Bull. Féd. Socs Gynéc. Obstét. Lang. fr.*, 1968, *20*, 69 (low incidence of cleft palate and other defects); A. F. Fleming and N. C. Allan, *Br. med. J.*, 1969, *4*, 461 (no harmful effect); J. M. Reinisch *et al.*, *Science*, 1978, *202*, 436 (offspring of women given prednisone throughout pregnancy, significantly lighter).

Late pregnancy. Fears concerning the administration of corticosteroids during late pregnancy relate to their direct adverse effects on the foetus rather than any dysmorphogenic risk. These involve the known side-effects of corticosteroids, such as increased risk of infection and adrenal insufficiency. No such adverse effects were noted by M. Schatz *et al.* (*J. Am. med. Ass.*, 1975, *233*, 804) in the infants of 70 exposed pregnancies, but subclinical adrenal insufficiency has been reported by L.A. Grajwer *et al.* (*J. Am. med. Ass.*, 1977, *238*, 1279) in the infant of a mother given prolonged high-dose dexamethasone therapy for pseudotumor cerebri. Similarly, congenital cytomegalovirus infection was reported by T. J. Evans *et al.* (*Lancet*, 1975, *1*, 1359) in the infant of a woman receiving azathioprine and prednisone for renal transplantation. The potential dangers of maternal diabetogenic effects have been demonstrated by A.S. Gündoğdu *et al.* (*Lancet*, 1979, *2*, 1317) in a study of metabolic changes induced in diabetic women by salbutamol (used in the prevention of premature labour) which could be exacerbated by concomitant administration of dexamethasone (used to promote maturation of the foetal lung) with consequent danger to the foetus.

For details concerning the management of the respiratory distress syndrome in infants, see betamethasone, p.884.

Lactation. For studies on the excretion of corticosteroids into breast milk, see prednisolone, p.899.

Absorption and Fate of Corticosteroids

Corticosteroids, with the exception of deoxycortone, are absorbed from the gastro-intestinal tract. When administered by topical application, particularly under an occlusive dressing or when the skin is broken, or as a pulmonary aerosol inhalation or a rectal enema, sufficient corticosteroid may be absorbed to give systemic effects. Administration by mouth may give a more rapid response than intramuscular injection of an insoluble corticosteroid. Water-soluble forms of corticosteroids giving a rapid response are used for intravenous injection.

Corticosteroids in the circulation are extensively bound to plasma proteins, mainly to globulin and less so to albumin. The corticosteroid-binding globulin has high affinity but low binding capacity, while the albumin has low affinity but large binding capacity. Only unbound corticosteroid has pharmacological effects or is metabolised. The synthetic corticosteroids are less extensively protein bound than hydrocortisone (cortisol). They also tend to have longer half-lives.

Corticosteroids are metabolised mainly in the liver but also in the kidney, and are excreted in the urine. The slower metabolism of the synthetic corticosteroids with their lower protein-binding affinity may account for their increased potency compared with the natural corticosteroids.

A detailed review of the pharmacokinetics of some corticosteroids.— E. J. Begg *et al.*, *Med. J. Aust.*, 1987, *146*, 37.

Uses and Administration of Corticosteroids

The corticosteroids are used in physiological doses for replacement therapy in adrenal insufficiency. In primary adrenal insufficiency, such as Addison's disease or after adrenalectomy, both mineralocorticoid and glucocorticoid replacement is needed. In secondary adrenal insufficiency, associated with inadequate corticotrophin secretion, glucocorticoid replacement is usually adequate. Thus, in the treatment of primary adrenal insufficiency hydrocortisone is given by mouth, usually in association with fludrocortisone to provide supplementary mineralocorticoid replacement, whereas in secondary adrenal insufficiency supplementary mineralocorticoid therapy is not generally given. The emergency treatment of adrenal insufficiency usually involves the intravenous administration of hydrocortisone sodium succinate, together with infusions of sodium chloride and glucose to correct electrolyte disturbances.

The corticosteroids are used in pharmacological doses for their anti-inflammatory and immunosuppressant glucocorticoid properties, which suppress the clinical manifestations of disease in a wide range of disorders. For these purposes, the synthetic analogues with their considerably reduced mineralocorticoid properties linked with enhanced glucocorticoid properties, are preferred to cortisone and hydrocortisone. Despite the existence of very powerful synthetic glucocorticoids with virtually no mineralocorticoid activity, the hazards of inappropriately high glucocorticoid therapy are such that the less powerful prednisolone and prednisone are the glucocorticoids of choice for most conditions, since they allow for a greater margin of safety. There is little to choose between prednisolone and prednisone; prednisolone may be preferred since, like hydrocortisone, it exists in a metabolically active form, whereas prednisone, like cortisone, is inactive and must be converted into its active form by the liver; hence, particularly in some liver disorders, prednisone's bioavailability is less reliable.

Doses of corticosteroids higher than those required for physiological replacement will eventually lead to some degree of adrenal suppression, the extent depending on the dose given, the route of administration, and its duration of administration. The adrenal glands have a daily output equivalent to approximately 20 mg of hydrocortisone (cortisol), but individual blood-cortisol (hydrocortisone) concentrations may vary widely, and can increase up to tenfold or more during stress. Therefore, during periods of stress, such as during and after surgery and when suffering from intercurrent infections, the corticosteroid dosage of patients must be increased. The effects of different corticosteroids vary qualitatively as well as quantitatively, and it may not be possible to substitute one for another in equal therapeutic amounts without provoking side-effects. Thus, whereas cortisone and hydrocortisone have very appreciable mineralocorticoid (or sodium-retaining) properties relative to their glucocorticoid (or anti-inflammatory) properties, prednisolone and prednisone have considerably less, and others, such as betamethasone and dexamethasone, have none or virtually none. As a rough guide, the approximate equivalent doses of the main corticosteroids in terms of their glucocorticoid (or anti-inflammatory) properties alone, are: cortisone acetate 25 mg, betamethasone 0.75 mg, dexamethasone 0.75 mg, hydrocortisone 20 mg, methylprednisolone 4 mg, prednisolone 5 mg, prednisone 5 mg, triamcinolone 4 mg.

Because the therapeutic effects of corticosteroids seem to be of longer duration than the metabolic effects, intermittent treatment with corticosteroids has been used to allow the metabolic rhythm of the body to become re-established while maintaining the therapeutic effects. Regimens of intermittent therapy have usually consisted of short courses of treatment or of the administration of 2 days' doses of corticosteroids as a single dose on alternate days; such alternate-day therapy, however, is only appropriate for corticosteroids with a relatively short duration of action, such as prednisolone, and only in certain disease states. Corticosteroids are also given in single daily doses at times coinciding with maximum or minimum function of the adrenal cortex in order to enhance or diminish respectively the depressant effects of corticosteroids on the adrenals.

Although the empirical use of a corticosteroid is appropriate in a life-threatening situation, generally it is advisable not to begin corticosteroid therapy until a definite diagnosis has been made, for otherwise symptoms may be masked to such an extent that a true diagnosis becomes extremely difficult to make.

Oral therapy is indicated in a wide variety of conditions and examples include:

some allergic disorders such as bronchial asthma; the onset of action of oral glucocorticoids is too slow for the primary treatment of life-threatening allergic reactions such as anaphylaxis or angioedema, but they may be used as adjuncts following initial emergency administration of adrenaline (see p.1455);

some blood disorders, including auto-immune haemolytic anaemia and idiopathic thrombocytopenic purpura;

selected connective tissue disorders, such as giant-cell arteritis, polyarteritis nodosa, polymyalgia rheumatica, polymyositis, and systemic lupus erythematosus;

inflammatory gastro-intestinal disorders, such as Crohn's disease and ulcerative colitis;

selected hepatic disorders including auto-immune chronic active hepatitis;

infections accompanied by a severe inflammatory component provided that appropriate anti-infective chemotherapy is also given and that the benefits of corticosteroid therapy outweigh the possible risk of disseminated infection; examples of conditions where corticosteroid may be considered include helminthic infections, the Herxheimer reaction, and tuberculous meningitis;

some neurological disorders such as infantile seizures and sub-acute demyelinating polyneuropathy;

some inflammatory ocular disorders;

selected renal disorders including lupus nephritis and the minimal change nephrotic syndrome;

selected non-allergic respiratory disorders, such as pulmonary fibrosis, pulmonary sarcoid, and some aspiration syndromes;

selected rheumatic and collagen disorders (but rarely rheumatoid arthritis);

severe skin disorders such as pemphigus and pemphigoid.

Glucocorticoids are also used in conjunction with antineoplastic agents in regimens for the management of malignant disease as described under Antineoplastic Agents and Immunosuppressants, p.580. They are also given to reduce immune responses after organ transplantations, often in conjunction with azathioprine or cyclosporin.

Parenteral therapy may also be used for many of the above conditions when the disease is severe or if an emergency arises. Intravenous therapy is generally employed for intensive emergency treatment as the onset of action is relatively fast although intramuscular injections, often formulated as longer-acting depot preparations, may also be used to provide cover.

Intra-articular injection in the absence of infection and with full aseptic precautions, may be used in the treatment of rheumatoid arthritis, and, sometimes, of osteoarthritis. Cortisone acetate is not suitable for this purpose and either hydrocortisone acetate or one of the esters of the synthetic corticosteroids (betamethasone, dexamethasone, methylprednisolone, prednisolone, triamcinolone) are used. It should be noted that there have been several reports of joint damage after the intra-articular injection of corticosteroids into load-bearing joints.

Topical application often produces dramatic suppression of skin diseases, such as eczema, infantile eczema, atopic dermatitis, dermatitis herpetiformis, contact dermatitis, seborrhoeic dermatitis, neurodermatitis, some forms of psoriasis, and intertrigo, in which inflammation is a prominent feature. However, the disease may return or be exacerbated when corticosteroids are withdrawn and this appears to be a particular problem in some of the forms of psoriasis. Occasionally, corticosteroids may be used with the addition of a suitable antimicrobial substance, such as neomycin, in the treatment of infected skin. For comments on the topical application of preparations containing a corticosteroid and neomycin, see neomycin, p.269.

Intralesional injection sometimes hastens the resolution of chronic skin lesions such as lichen planus, lichen simplex, and keloids.

Topical application to the eye in inflammatory and traumatic disorders has led to dramatic results, but the occurrence of herpetic and fungal infections of the cornea and other serious complications generally militate against their use; eye-drops containing corticosteroids, particularly betamethasone and dexamethasone, should not usually be used for more than a week except under strict ophthalmic supervision with regular checks of intra-ocular pressure.

Inhalational therapy, particularly with beclomethasone dipropionate, is widely used in the prophylaxis of asthma.

Nasal application is also used in the prophylaxis of allergic rhinitis.

Rectal administration, by either suppository or enema, may be employed for some corticosteroids.

ADMINISTRATION. The diurnal rhythm of the adrenal cortex led to about 70% of the daily secretion being made between midnight and 9 am. In the treatment of adrenal cortical hyperplasia a dose of hydrocortisone given at night would be nearly twice as suppressive as the same dose given during the day. However, in treating allergic or collagen disease when suppression of adrenal cortical activity was best avoided a dose of hydrocortisone at about 8 am was indicated. When reducing steroid dosage after treatment, a single dose given at 8 am would be most beneficial and would not inhibit corticotrophin secretion.— C. H. Demos *et al.*, *Clin. Pharmac. Ther.*, 1964, *5*, 721.

The 17-ketogenic steroid excretion resulting when metyrapone was given to block adrenal hydrocortisone production was used to compare the duration of suppression produced by equal anti-inflammatory doses of corticosteroids. Duration of suppression was 3.25 days for betamethasone 6 mg, 2.75 days for dexamethasone 5 mg, 1.25 to 1.5 days for hydrocortisone 250 mg, methylprednisolone 40 mg, prednisolone 50 mg, and prednisone 50 mg, 2 days for paramethasone 20 mg, and 2.25 days for triamcinolone 40 mg.— J. G. Harter *et al.*, *Arthritis Rheum.*, 1965, *8*, 445.

Epidural route. A detailed review and discussion concerning the epidural use of corticosteroids in sciatica. The current controversy revolves around two main issues, safety and efficacy. Analysis of the literature attests to the safety of the procedure and the reported clinical complications are uncommon and relate mainly to the technical aspects of the injection. The adverse effects of epidural use should not be confused with the known and more serious complications following intrathecal administration. With respect to efficacy the literature is less definitive. The indications for optimal use remain unresolved and appropriate clinical studies are needed.— N. Bogduk and D. Cherry, *Med. J. Aust.*, 1985, *143*, 402.

ADMINISTRATION IN HEPATIC INSUFFICIENCY. A review of the pharmacokinetics of corticosteroids in patients with liver disease.— M. Uribe and V. L. W. Go, *Clin. Pharmacokinet.*, 1979, *4*, 233.

See also prednisolone, p.899.

For details of corticosteroid therapy in patients with hepatic insufficiency, see Hepatic Disorders (below).

ADMINISTRATION IN RENAL INSUFFICIENCY. For details of corticosteroid therapy in patients with impaired renal function see under Organ and Tissue Transplantation and Renal Disorders (below).

ADRENAL INSUFFICIENCY. For the management of acute and chronic primary adrenal insufficiency, see hydrocortisone, p.895, and fludrocortisone, p.890. For the management of adrenal insufficiency secondary to corticosteroid therapy, see hydrocortisone, p.895.

ALLERGY AND ANAPHYLAXIS. For the use of corticosteroids in the management of anaphylactic shock, see adrenaline, p.1455.

ASPIRATION SYNDROMES. A short comment that although the evidence in favour of the use of corticosteroids in pulmonary aspiration is equivocal there remains a strong view that high doses are of benefit.— J. S. M. Zorab, *Br. med. J.*, 1984, *288*, 1631. A reply stating that in any discussion of aspiration it is important to identify patients who inhale non-toxic substances such as water or blood and in whom no specific treatment apart from relief of airways obstruction and hypoxia is required. High-dose corticosteroid treatment has become fashionable in the past decade not only for serious respiratory problems but for other conditions and the view is held that if corticosteroids did indeed produce a clinical benefit in pulmonary aspiration it would undoubtedly have appeared by now. It is recommended that the use of high-dose corticosteroids in pulmonary aspiration should be abandoned.— D. W. Ryan (letter), *ibid.*, *299*, 51.

ASTHMA. The practical aspects of the management of asthma. Current practice recommends the use of drugs for an acute attack, and long-term therapy to prevent frequent recurrent attacks. Aerosol therapy with a beta$_2$-agonist is the first choice for the treatment of episodic mild asthma. An alternative is theophylline by mouth. In patients whose symptoms continue, regular bronchodilator therapy is indicated either by inhalation or by mouth. Sodium cromoglycate should then be added if control of symptoms is still insufficient. If no response to cromoglycate occurs bronchodilators should be used in conjunction with inhaled corticosteroids and in patients in whom control is still poor corticosteroids by mouth should be tried.— J. W. Paterson and R. A. Tarala, *Med. J. Aust.*, 1985, *143*, 453.

A discussion on the drugs available for the treatment of asthma. The drug of choice for the treatment of occasional acute symptoms is an inhaled beta$_2$-agonist. For suppressing the symptoms of chronic asthma inhaled cromoglycate or inhaled beta$_2$-agonist can be used. Oral theophylline is also effective but some would use an inhaled corticosteroid together with an inhaled adrenergic first. Patients with recurrent bronchodilator-unresponsive symptoms may require either inhaled or oral corticosteroids.— *Med. Lett.*, 1987, *29*, 11.

Discussion on the problem of some children with asthma being deprived of corticosteroids because of the fear of side-effects. The underdiagnosis of asthma is now well-known but the problem of undertreatment is less well appreciated. There should be no hesitation in using inhaled steroids in patients with chronic asthma not controlled by bronchodilators or cromoglycate. Failure to respond promptly to bronchodilators in acute asthma is an absolute indication for a short course of oral steroids. It should be remembered that there are also a few children with severe intractable asthma who need maintenance therapy with oral steroids.— T. J. David, *Archs Dis. Childh.*, 1987, *62*, 876.

Further general reviews on asthma: J. W. Paterson and R. A. Tarala, *Med. J. Aust.*, 1985, *143*, 390 (pharmacology); H. B. Valman, *Br. med. J.*, 1987, *294*, 753 (children); *Drug & Ther. Bull.*, 1987, *25*, 61 (infants).

Acute asthma. A discussion on the management of acute asthma. Therapy consists essentially of oxygen, corticosteroids, and bronchodilators although there are considerable differences in the approach in different countries, particularly in the choice of bronchodilator and route of administration. In the *UK* most respiratory physicians would probably start treatment, in a patient admitted to hospital, with oxygen, hydrocortisone 200 mg intravenously every 4 to 6 hours, and a nebulised beta$_2$-agonist. The dose of steroids is arbitrary but side-effects are very unusual with such doses of hydrocortisone even when continued for several days; doses higher than 200 mg have not been shown to be more effective. The use of bronchodilators is slightly less straightforward since there is a choice of agents and routes of administration.— *Lancet*, 1986, *1*, 131.

Further reviews: M. A. Branthwaite, *Br. J. Hosp. Med.*, 1985, *34*, 331.

Clinical studies on the role and use of corticosteroids in acute asthma: B. Littenberg and E. H. Gluck, *New Engl. J. Med.*, 1986, *314*, 150 (benefit of methylprednisolone intravenously when added to bronchodilators in patients with acute severe asthma); B. D. W. Harrison *et al.*, *Lancet*, 1986, *1*, 181 (no benefit of hydrocortisone intravenously when added to oral prednisolone and bronchodilators in patients with acute severe asthma but without ventilatory failure); A. Deshpande and S. A. McKenzie, *Br. med. J.*, 1986, *293*, 169 (value of a short course of prednisolone by mouth in the early treatment of acute asthma in children); J. Storr *et al.*, *Lancet*, 1987, *1*, 879 (value of a single dose of prednisolone by mouth in the early treatment of acute asthma in children).

For further details concerning the management of acute asthma, see salbutamol, p.1482.

Inhalational therapy. A discussion on inhaled corticosteroids, particularly in high doses, in asthma therapy. Inhaled corticosteroid therapy is well-established as an effective form of maintenance treatment in asthma and in recent years interest has been shown in the use of higher doses to treat the more severe forms. Several workers have confirmed that improvement in asthma control can be achieved in patients with severe or chronic asthma when the dose is increased although there are still surprisingly few prospective long-term studies. In some patients dependent upon oral corticosteroids significant reductions in the oral dose can be made by increasing the inhaled dose. With regard to adverse effects on adrenal function the message from the majority of studies is clear; systemic absorption does occur but clinically significant adrenal suppression does not occur at doses of up to 1500 or 1600 µg daily of beclomethasone dipropionate. For inhaled corticosteroids to be effective in the prophylaxis of asthma they must be taken regularly and patient compliance is important. Several studies have demonstrated that twice-daily therapy is as effective as four-times daily and that twice-daily administration may also improve compliance. Efficient delivery to the bronchial tree is crucial and a number of different devices are available for administration. The pressurised aerosol inhaler remains the most convenient and acceptable if the patient's technique is satisfactory. In patients unable to use an aerosol inhaler satisfactorily a spacer device may be an alternative. A powder inhalation from capsules using a rotahaler system is particularly useful for children and elderly patients.— M. J. Smith, *Drugs*, 1987, *33*, 423.

Further reviews of inhalational therapy, including corticosteroids, for asthma: M. F. Muers, *Prescribers' J.*,

1983, *23*, 32; M. T. Newhouse and M. B. Dolovich, *New Engl. J. Med.*, 1986, *315*, 870.

Pregnancy and the neonate. Reviews of the management of asthma during pregnancy: P. A. Greenberger and R. Patterson, *New Engl. J. Med.*, 1985, *312*, 897; H. Mawhinney and S. L. Spector, *Drugs*, 1986, *32*, 178; K. F. Chung and P. J. Barnes, *Br. med. J.*, 1987, *294*, 103.

Systemic therapy. Since the introduction of potent topically active inhaled corticosteroids in the early 1970's the number of asthmatic patients prescribed systemic steroids has dropped. However, a few patients with severe chronic asthma still require both forms of therapy. Although there is a wide range of corticosteroids available for systemic administration prednisolone is the most suitable for oral use. The side-effects may be minimised by giving a single daily dose in the early morning. Some workers suggest that alternate-day single-morning dosing reduces the side-effects even further, but unfortunately the control of asthma may be less effective on the non-steroid day although this appears to be less of a problem in children. Thus, where necessary, the optimal drug regimen for maintenance treatment with systemic corticosteroids in chronic severe asthma appears to be prednisolone once-daily in the early morning for adults and on alternate days for children.— L. D. Lewis and G. M. Cochrane, *Br. med. J.*, 1986, *292*, 1289.

BLOOD DISORDERS. *Aplastic anaemia.* The value of corticosteroids in aplastic anaemia was not clear and although occasional cases might respond to prednisolone most haematologists believed that it should be avoided.— C. G. Geary, *Br. med. J.*, 1974, *2*, 432.

Cold-haemagglutinin disease. Despite previously disappointing reports in high-titre cold-haemagglutinin disease, beneficial results were obtained with administration of high doses of corticosteroids to 2 patients with low-titre cold-haemagglutinin disease.— A. D. Schreiber *et al.*, *New Engl. J. Med.*, 1977, *296*, 1490.

A study suggesting that in contrast to patients with typical cold agglutinin disease, there is a subset of patients with IgG cold-reactive antibodies responsive to corticosteroids and splenectomy.— L. E. Silberstein *et al.*, *Ann. intern. Med.*, 1987, *106*, 238.

Haemangioma. Two infants with giant haemangioma with thrombocytopenia responded satisfactorily to prednisone 20 mg daily, continued in 1 patient for 5 weeks and then tapered off over 2 weeks. Tumours regressed and there was sustained haematological improvement. Prednisone was the treatment of choice for complicated haemangiomas.— J. Evans *et al.*, *Archs Dis. Childh.*, 1975, *50*, 809. A report of 2 children with haemangioma and thrombocytopenia in whom corticosteroids produced little or no improvement. The comment was made that large haemangiomas without thrombocytopenia are reported to regress well with corticosteroids but that when thrombocytopenia is a complication, only 50% of cases respond to corticosteroids.— T. J. David *et al.*, *Archs Dis. Childh.*, 1983, *58*, 1022.

Haemolytic anaemia. A short comment that although corticosteroids have become the mainstay of treatment in auto-immune haemolytic anaemia they have not been shown conclusively to be effective in the treatment of severe rhesus iso-immunisation.— K. H. Nicolaides and C. H. Rodeck, *Br. J. Hosp. Med.*, 1985, *34*, 141.

Hypereosinophilia. In a study of 16 patients with hypereosinophilia and progressive organ-system involvement, prednisone 60 mg daily for 1 week then on alternate days for 3 months gave a good response in 6 of the patients; 5 continued to be controlled on alternate-day therapy. Three of 5 patients who had a partial response and all 5 who had not responded to corticosteroids received hydroxyurea 1 to 2 g daily. Of these patients, some of whom were the most critically ill, 6 had a good response and 2 a partial response. Hydroxyurea was considered to be the drug of choice for corticosteroid-unresponsive patients with the hypereosinophilic syndrome.— J. E. Parrillo *et al.*, *Ann. intern. Med.*, 1978, *89*, 167.

Hypoplastic anaemia. A 24-year-old woman with congenital hypoplastic anaemia (Blackfan-Diamond syndrome) responded favourably to treatment with prednisone.— G. E. Zito and E. C. Lynch, *J. Am. med. Ass.*, 1977, *237*, 991. Beneficial effects in 4 patients with pure red-cell aplasia not totally responsive to corticosteroid therapy following the addition of cyclosporin.— T. H. Tötterman *et al.* (letter), *Lancet*, 1984, *2*, 693.

Sickle-cell anaemia. For comment on the use of dexamethasone in sickle-cell anaemia, see dexamethasone, p.888.

Thrombocytopenic purpura. Debate surrounds the use of corticosteroids in the newly diagnosed patient with idiopathic thrombocytopenic purpura. Most, but not all, authors conclude that steroids should be given and some merely indicate that they provide no measurable benefit. It would seem reasonable to give a 2- to 4-week course but longer-term treatment is universally condemned irrespective of whether the condition resolves or progresses.— J. S. Lilleyman, *Archs Dis. Childh.*, 1984, *59*, 701. See also R. W. Walker and W. Walker, *ibid.*, 316.

A review and discussion on the management of the pregnant patient with idiopathic thrombocytopenic purpura with the comment that most clinicians give corticosteroid therapy.— J. G. Kelton, *Ann. intern. Med.*, 1983, *99*, 796.

BONE DISORDERS. *Juvenile osteopetrosis.* Report of the use of prednisone 1 mg per kg body-weight daily by mouth, together with phosphate supplements and a low calcium diet in 4 children with juvenile osteopetrosis, a disorder characterised by an increase in bone density and neurological and haematological abnormalities and usually resulting in early death. Two of the children who started treatment after the age of 2 years showed a good clinical and radiological response and have continued therapy for 6 years; the third child who started treatment at 6 months showed a good clinical response but no radiological response but died later after being lost to follow-up and stopping therapy; the last child who started treatment as a neonate achieved complete clinical and radiological remission and has remained free of signs of the disease for 2 years after stopping therapy.— L. M. Dorantes *et al.*, *Archs Dis. Childh.*, 1986, *61*, 666.

CANCER CHEMOTHERAPY. Recent advances in the prevention or reduction of cytotoxic-induced emesis including a short review of studies using corticosteroids in the anti-emetic drug regimens. On the hypothesis that prostaglandin release may be involved in the nausea and vomiting after cytotoxic therapy, glucocorticoids have been used in an attempt to inhibit hypothalamic prostaglandin release and several early but uncontrolled studies have demonstrated an impressive anti-emetic action for dexamethasone and methylprednisolone when used either alone or in combination with other standard agents. A number of randomised controlled studies have also recently demonstrated the anti-emetic benefit of glucocorticoids. It is suggested that because of their minimal toxicity glucocorticoids, with or without a benzodiazepine, may be the anti-emetics of choice in patients who are receiving highly emetogenic drugs and that methylprednisolone 250 mg intravenously 2 hours before and after the administration of cytotoxic therapy affords reliable, reproducible, and significant control of emetic episodes.— J. H. Kearsley and M. H. N. Tattersall, *Med. J. Aust.*, 1985, *143*, 341. See also S. Gervais, *Can. J. Hosp. Pharm.*, 1986, *39*, 164.

For reports on the role of corticosteroids in combination chemotherapy for neoplastic disorders, see Antineoplastic Agents and Immunosuppressants, p.584.

CARDIAC DISORDERS. *Myocarditis.* On the basis of the supposition that after an initial infective stage the pathogenesis of acute inflammatory myopericarditis may depend upon an immunologic mechanism several workers have given corticosteroids for several months to patients with persistent heart failure due to acute inflammatory myocarditis. Although the studies were uncontrolled, some patients appeared to have a favourable response; the treatment, however, does entail considerable risk, especially of potentially fatal superinfection. Clinicians may be expected to disagree over the advisability of immunosuppressive therapy and controlled studies are needed to either confirm or refute efficacy.— R. A. Johnson and I. Palacios, *New Engl. J. Med.*, 1982, *307*, 1119.

A short comment that although there is no controlled data concerning the use of corticosteroids in the treatment of myocarditis related to drug hypersensitivity it does seem logical to try them in severe or persistent cases.— *Lancet*, 1985, *2*, 1165.

Postmyocardial infarction syndrome. The postmyocardial infarction syndrome consists of fever and pleuropericardial pain occurring after a coronary occlusion. The peak incidence is during the first three months and although symptoms do not last longer than 4 to 6 weeks they do tend to recur. Because the syndrome is self-limiting, evaluation of treatment is difficult. Simple anti-inflammatory analgesics usually control the symptoms but do not appear to influence the course of the illness. In severe cases corticosteroids often result in a dramatic response with resolution of fever and relief of pain within 24 hours although relapse tends to occur when treatment is stopped.— A. D. Timmis, *Br. med. J.*, 1984, *289*, 636.

CONNECTIVE TISSUE DISORDERS. *Arteritis.* A serious manifestation of cranial (temporal or giant-cell) arteritis is blindness which can be prevented by early recognition of the disease and prompt treatment with a corticosteroid. Prednisolone should be started immediately with an initial daily dose of 60 mg and the dose can be reduced after a week. Treatment may often need to be continued for years and after a year the symptoms may be controlled in about 80% of patients with prednisolone 2 to 7.5 mg daily as a single dose; alternate-day therapy has proved ineffective.— Drug & Ther. Bull., 1984, *22*, 11.

Dermatomyositis. See under Skin Disorders (below).

Lupus erythematosus. A review and discussion on the causative factors and treatment of systemic lupus erythematosus. Most patients, at some stage during their disease, require corticosteroid therapy and with the exception of some with cerebral involvement have a gratifying response in the majority of features; corticosteroids may not be required to treat arthritis, rash, or fever when only these features are present. The authors' preference is for a single morning dose of corticosteroid and where possible (usually when below the equivalent of prednisolone 10 mg daily) on alternate days. Following an acute flare-up it is the authors' practice to try and reduce the dose quickly, for example from 40 to 15 mg daily within one month.— K. D. Morley and G. R. V. Hughes, *Drugs*, 1982, *23*, 481.

A study of the use of corticosteroids in 35 patients with lupus pernio. Thirty-one patients received oral therapy of whom 5 also received local intra-lesional injections. Shrinkage of the lesions was observed in more than 50% of the patients on starting systemic therapy but a flare-up occurred in 35% following reduction of the dose to below a critical level, which was usually about 7.5 mg daily of prednisolone. Local injections did reduce the size of the lesion but the overall effect was very short-term.— M. A. Spiteri *et al.*, *Br. J. Derm.*, 1985, *112*, 315.

A report of the use of prednisone in association with low-dose aspirin to improve outcome of pregnancy in 8 women with the lupus anticoagulant, an autoantibody acquired by some patients with systemic lupus erythematosus and which is a clinical marker for recurrent first-trimester spontaneous abortion, as well as for second- and early third-trimester foetal death.— D. W. Branch *et al.*, *New Engl. J. Med.*, 1985, *313*, 1322. Similar reports.— R. G. Farquharson *et al.* (letter), *Lancet*, 1984, *2*, 228; R. G. Farquharson *et al.* (letter), *ibid.*, 1985, *2*, 842; W. F. Lubbe *et al.* (letter), *New Engl. J. Med.*, 1985, *313*, 1350.

See also under Renal Disorders (below).

Panniculitis. A report of relapsing, febrile, nodular, non-suppurative panniculitis (Weber-Christian syndrome) in 2 infants responding to treatment with prednisone.— W. M. Hendricks *et al.*, *Br. J. Derm.*, 1978, *98*, 175.

Polymyalgia rheumatica. A review of the diagnosis and treatment of polymyalgia rheumatica. Corticosteroids are clearly indicated in polymyalgia rheumatica where there is any evidence of an active arteritis, the initial dosage being about 20 to 30 mg of prednisolone daily. If the symptoms are essentially those of a polymyalgia, prednisolone 10 to 15 mg daily initially is usually adequate but 50 to 60 mg daily may be necessary if ophthalmic symptoms are present in order to prevent blindness. The author generally advises that dosage reduction should be by 0.5 to 1 mg every 3 to 4 weeks at the lower dose levels (10 mg daily) or by 2.5 to 5 mg weekly at higher levels (40 to 50 mg daily), providing symptoms are fully controlled, and the subsequent reduction is 1 mg every 2 weeks when a dosage of 20 mg daily is reached; these are suggestions only and individual cases vary considerably. Although, in some patients, corticosteroid therapy can be withdrawn within 1 to 2 years of onset, it usually takes considerably longer ranging from around 5 to 8 years and sometimes up to 10 years.— F. D. Hart, *Drugs*, 1987, *33*, 280.

Further reviews: J. R. Sewell, *Br. J. Hosp. Med.*, 1986, *35*, 299.

Polymyositis. See under Muscular Disorders (below).

EPILEPSY. A review and discussion on the use of corticosteroids in childhood seizures. For over 40 years it has been known that some children with otherwise intractable fits improve with corticosteroids and for over 30 years that a similar response may be obtained with corticotrophin. Since that time a considerable amount of work has centered on infantile spasms and particularly on the relative efficacies of prednisone and corticotrophin. Despite conflicting published reports it has emerged that more patients respond to corticotrophin although there are a few who will respond to prednisone but not to corticotrophin. The recommended dose of corticotrophin varies between 20 and 120 units daily; the author's choice is to start with 40 units daily, increased to 80 units daily after 3 to 4 weeks if there has been no response and, if then effective, continued for 3 to 6 months. Prednisone is usually started at 2 mg per kg body-weight daily, and in the event of a response, reduced to a maintenance dose of 10 to 20 mg daily; alternate-day therapy does not appear to result in a loss of control.— R. O. Robinson, *Archs Dis. Childh.*, 1985, *60*, 94.

GASTRO-INTESTINAL DISORDERS. A review of the use of corticosteroids in Crohn's disease with special reference to various aspects of the National Cooperative Crohn's Disease Study in the USA. Impressions gained from 2 large uncontrolled studies that a good initial symptomatic response to prednisone 30 mg daily or its equivalent, is obtained in 75 to 90% of patients, were confirmed in a double-blind controlled trial carried out as part of the National Cooperative Crohn's Disease Study (J.W. Singleton, *Gastroenterology*, 1977, *72*, 1133). Active disease involving the small bowel was especially responsive to corticosteroids, but the extra-intestinal complications and peri-anal disease were as unresponsive to prednisone as to placebo. Previous sulphasalazine therapy seemed to blunt subsequent response to corticosteroids, and the toxicity of corticosteroids at doses high enough to suppress active Crohn's disease was appreciable. The role of prophylactic corticosteroid therapy in both quiescent disease and after complete surgical extirpation of Crohn's disease has been examined in 3 recent controlled studies (L. Bergman and U. Krause, *Scand. J. Gastroenterol.*, 1976, *11*, 651; J.W. Singleton, *Gastroenterology*, 1977, *72*, 1133; R.C. Smith *et al.*, *Gut*, 1978, *19*, 606). Those receiving prophylactic corticosteroid therapy fared no better than those taking placebo or nothing and, in fact, fared noticeably, but not significantly, worse. Thus, prophylactic therapy with corticosteroids is not indicated for Crohn's disease. Although uncontrolled studies indicated a recrudescence of symptoms on withdrawal of corticosteroids, placebo-controlled National Cooperative Crohn's Disease Studies have shown that withdrawal during a quiescent phase is associated with no more relapses than continuation.— J. W. Singleton, *Ann. intern. Med.*, 1979, *90*, 983. See also The National Cooperative Crohn's Disease Study, J. W. Singleton (Ed.), *Gastroenterology*, 1979, *77*, 825-944.

A detailed review and discussion on the optimal use of corticosteroids in ulcerative colitis and Crohn's disease. The rationale of corticosteroid therapy in these disorders remains unknown and until their predominant action is known it cannot be hoped to design specific treatments aimed at altering particular aspects of the inflammatory response. Prednisolone is often used in the outpatient treatment of small bowel Crohn's disease but so far there is no support from controlled therapeutic studies to justify the use of either prednisolone or prednisone, in relatively small doses over prolonged periods in patients with quiescent disease with the aim of preventing relapse. Clinicians therefore withdraw corticosteroids as soon as possible after the treatment of an acute attack but patients often report that symptoms become worse below a certain dosage, which is often about 10 mg daily of prednisolone. Similar considerations also apply in the treatment of ulcerative colitis. Little is known about the relative therapeutic merits in either disease of giving corticosteroids intermittently or near continuously; thus prednisolone 40 mg daily as a single dose appears to be as effective as the same dose divided throughout the day and alternate-day therapy has also given encouraging results in active chronic colitis. Few attempts have been made to establish by prospective trial a relationship between dose and response although there is some evidence in ulcerative colitis that doses of 40 to 60 mg daily of prednisone are more effective than 20 mg daily. Topical corticosteroids applied from the gut lumen are also frequently used in the treatment of inflammatory bowel disease with the aim of attaining high tissue concentrations in the involved mucosa; interest is currently being shown in those poorly absorbed into the systemic circulation.— J. E. Lennard-Jones, *Gut*, 1983, *24*, 177.

Further reviews and comments on the general management of inflammatory bowel diseases: J. B. Kirsner and R. G. Shorter, *New Engl. J. Med.*, 1982, *306*, 775 (ulcerative colitis and Crohn's disease); I. W. Booth and J. T. Harries, *Gut*, 1984, *25*, 188 (ulcerative colitis and Crohn's disease in children); J. E. Lennard-Jones, *Postgrad. med. J.*, 1984, *60*, 797 (ulcerative colitis); R. M. Donaldson, *New Engl. J. Med.*, 1985, *312*, 1616 (inflammatory bowel disorders during pregnancy); *Drug & Ther. Bull.*, 1986, *24*, 13 (Crohn's disease); J. M. Rhodes, *Prescribers' J.*, 1986, *26*, 1 (ulcerative colitis and Crohn's disease).

For further references to the management of inflammatory bowel disease, see sulphasalazine, p.1110.

HEPATIC DISORDERS. A detailed review of the use of corticosteroids in liver disease, possible mechanisms of action, pharmacology, and rational use. Corticosteroids are contra-indicated in uncomplicated viral hepatitis, although they have a limited role in prolonged cholestasis. There has been considerable controversy over the years concerning the place of corticosteroids in the management of fulminant hepatic failure, but the general consensus at present is firmly against the use of corticosteroids. A problem in relation to chronic active hepatitis is that the meaning of the term has evolved since the instigation of some of the major studies, and current criteria are still not universally accepted. There is an established place for corticosteroid therapy in the management of the symptomatic and histologically severe forms, but the use of corticosteroids in hepatitis-B-positive chronic active hepatitis is still controversial. In patients who do benefit from corticosteroid therapy it has been shown that daily administration of prednisone 10 mg in association with azathioprine 50 mg, after an initial month of higher prednisone dose, offers the best chance of disease control, together with the lowest incidence of major corticosteroid side-effects. Assessment of alternate-day therapy has indicated that daily therapy appears to have advantages, but prednisolone has been recommended rather than prednisone, as the serum concentrations are more predictable. There is general agreement that corticosteroid therapy is not indicated in patients with chronic persistent hepatitis, as the condition is virtually asymptomatic, non-progressive, and associated with a good prognosis. If corticosteroids have a role in the management of alcoholic liver disease, it will probably be confined to patients with alcoholic hepatitis who have encephalopathy or a severe coagulation disorder. Corticosteroids often have a dramatic effect on patients with granulomatous hepatitis, but in a large variety of other hepatic disorders, including Wilson's disease, Gilbert's disease, Dubin Johnson syndrome, and hepatic amyloidosis, they have been shown to be of no value. They are of benefit in multi-system diseases that occasionally involve the liver, such as polyarteritis nodosa or systemic lupus erythematosus.— A. R. Tanner and L. W. Powell, *Gut*, 1979, *20*, 1109.

A review and discussion concerning the management of chronic hepatitis. An important aspect is the clear cut separation of chronic hepatitis into chronic persistent hepatitis and chronic active hepatitis, diagnoses which have very different therapeutic and prognostic implications. Chronic persistent hepatitis is often idiopathic, but may also be due to persistent infection with hepatitis B or the non-A, non-B virus. It does not require specific treatment, although may, particularly when associated with hepatitis B infection, occasionally progress to chronic active hepatitis. Chronic active hepatitis has a poor prognosis and treatment with corticosteroids is of value. Several controlled clinical studies have established that treatment with corticosteroids, with or without azathioprine, improves the survival of patients with chronic active hepatitis negative for hepatitis B (the autoimmune and cryptogenic variants of chronic active hepatitis). Patients with milder forms of the disease may be given corticosteroids for 3 to 6 months if incapacitating symptoms or severe disturbances in liver function are present while those with severe disease require long-term therapy. In general, the prognosis of chronic active hepatitis associated with hepatitis B virus is poorer than the form not associated with infection and treatment with corticosteroids is reported to only potentiate viral replication and to either be of no benefit or even to have a deleterious effect. However, it has recently been suggested that corticosteroids may have a beneficial effect in those patients who are negative for hepatitis B e antigen or positive for hepatitis B e antibody indicating cessation of viral replication with continuing hepatic damage being due to an autoimmune process.— J. Hegarty and R. Williams, *Br. med. J.*, 1985, *290*, 877.

Further reviews and comments on the role of corticosteroids in various liver disorders: J. A. Summerfield, *Postgrad. med. J.*, 1983, *59*, *Suppl.* 4, 99 (conflicting evidence in primary sclerosing cholangitis); *Ann. intern. Med.*, 1983, *99*, 500 (possible use in early primary biliary cirrhosis); S. Sherlock and H. C. Thomas, *Lancet*, 1985, *2*, 1343 (certain cases of chronic hepatitis due to hepatitis B); I. R. Mackay, *Med. J. Aust.*, 1987, *146*, 370 (chronic active hepatitis).

HYPERCALCAEMIA. Despite their unpredictability and the trivial short-term reduction they produce, corticosteroids are still widely used to lower serum-calcium concentrations. Although the hypercalcaemia of sarcoidosis and of vitamin-D intoxication is usually steroid-sensitive and that due to hyperparathyroidism steroid-resistant, this is not invariable. Some authors have considered corticosteroids to be highly effective in the treatment of hypercalcaemia complicating malignant disease whereas others considered them to be ineffective when used alone. Furthermore, the calcium-lowering effect of corticosteroids may take a week to develop, and reductions of less than 0.25 mmol per litre may be all that is achieved.— *Br. med. J.*, 1980, *280*, 204.

INFECTIONS. Although long-term corticosteroid therapy has an adverse effect on the body's response to infection (see Effects on Immune Response, under Adverse Effects), the judicious use of corticosteroids, usually on a short-term basis, and in conjunction with appropriate chemotherapeutic agents, may have a beneficial effect on the symptoms of selected acute infections, and may on occasions be life-saving.

Infectious mononucleosis. A short discussion on the use of corticosteroids in infectious mononucleosis. Although all cases will respond promptly to 'burst' therapy the author only treats patients with an unduly prolonged infection and those with an exceptionally severe sore throat that interferes with either respiratory function or eating. Most experts would use corticosteroids in patients with severe thrombocytopenia, haemolytic anaemia, encephalitis, pericarditis, or myocarditis associated with infection by the Epstein-Barr virus. Burst doses of prednisone may be 80 mg initially decreasing gradually, and withdrawn after 14 days. Prednisone is very safe in infectious mononucleosis but the theoretical risk of impairing immunity is a concern.— J. N. Sheagren, *J. Am. med. Ass.*, 1986, *256*, 1051.

Leprosy. For the use of corticosteroids in the management of leprosy reactions, see p.552.

For the use of corticosteroids to treat nerve damage associated with leprosy, see under Neurological Disorders (below).

Ocular infections. See under Ocular Disorders (below).

Pneumocystis carinii pneumonia. Reports of a beneficial response to corticosteroids in addition to antibiotics in patients with *Pneumocystis carinii* pneumonia: D. K. MacFadden *et al.*, *Lancet*, 1987, *1*, 1477 (in AIDS); N. J. Shaw *et al.* (letter), *ibid.*, *2*, 518 (in leukaemia).

Septic shock. A study to elucidate the role of corticosteroids in septic shock, a controversial issue because of studies previously reporting both a beneficial and a detrimental effect. Of 59 patients, 21 received methylprednisolone sodium succinate 30 mg per kg body-weight intravenously over 10 to 15 minutes, 22 received dexamethasone sodium phosphate 6 mg per kg intravenously over a similar time, and 16 did not receive a corticosteroid; a second dose was given after 4 hours if shock persisted but no further corticosteroids were given after the second dose. Although administration of corticosteroids did result in short-term improvements and benefits in certain groups of patients, particularly producing a higher incidence of shock reversal when administered within 4 hours of the onset of shock, the ultimate mortality or reversal of the shock state was not improved; there was no significant difference between either dexamethasone or methylprednisolone. It was concluded that corticosteroids do not improve the overall survival of patients with severe, late septic shock but may be helpful early in the course and in certain subgroups of patients; further studies are needed to identify such subgroups.— C. L. Sprung *et al.*, *New Engl. J. Med.*, 1984, *311*, 1137. Comments and correspondence concerning the study and on the controversial issue of corticosteroids in septic shock generally: *ibid.*, 1178; *ibid.*, 1985, *312*, 509-512. Results of a randomised double-blind, placebo-controlled study involving 382 patients indicated that methylprednisolone sodium succinate 30 mg per kg body-weight administered as an intravenous infusion over 20 minutes every 6 hours for a total of 4 doses and given within 2 hours of a presumptive diagnosis of severe sepsis or septic shock had no significant effect on the prevention of shock, reversal of shock, or overall mortality. It was concluded that high-dose corticosteroids provide no benefit in the treatment of such disorders.— R. C. Bone *et al.*, *ibid.*, 1987, *317*, 653. A similar conclusion that early high-dose corticosteroid therapy has no beneficial effect in patients with systemic sepsis after a similar study in which methylprednisolone sodium succinate was given intravenously, initially in a dose of 30 mg per kg over a 15-minute period and then in a dose of 5 mg per kg per hour for 9 hours.— The Veterans Administration Systemic Sepsis Cooperative Study Group, *ibid.*, 659.

Tuberculosis. It must be emphasised that corticosteroids must never be given to patients with tuberculous disease without adequate protective chemotherapy cover. Routine administration of corticosteroids in pulmonary tuberculosis is to be avoided although it is sometimes recommended that steroids be administered to patients whose symptoms are very toxic and who have extensive lung disease. As an adjunct to antituberculous therapy and depending upon the judgement of the clinician, possible indications for corticosteroids include: the control of drug hypersensitivity; where patients are so seriously ill from any form of tuberculosis that they may become moribund and suppression of the inflammatory response results in an immediate clinical improvement (cortisone being preferred); some tuberculous conditions such as peritonitis, pleural effusion, iridocyclitis, and pericarditis where deposition of fibrous tissue can cause undesirable and potentially serious mechanical effects. The role of corticosteroids in tuberculous meningitis remains debatable but they are useful when cerebral oedema is present and where adhesions block the circulation of the cerebrospinal fluid; prednisolone may be given intrathecally in usual doses of 12.5 to 25 mg daily until the CSF is normal. It should be noted, however, that steroids may restore the blood-brain barrier which is lessened in meningitis thus reducing the CSF-streptomycin concentration and making concurrent streptomycin intrathecal administration desirable.— *Modern Drug Treatment in Tuberculosis*, J.D. Ross *et al.* (Ed.), 6th Edn, The Chest, Heart and Stroke Association, London, 1983, p.53 and 84-8.

The value of prednisolone as adjuvant treatment in tuberculous constrictive pericarditis and pericardial effusion.— J. I. G. Strang *et al.*, *Lancet*, 1987, *2*, 1418; *idem*, 1988, *2*, 759.

Viral encephalitis. A short comment that there is some data to support the use of corticosteroid therapy in patients with acute viral encephalitis where there is evidence of raised intracranial pressure.— M. Swash, *Br. J. Hosp. Med.*, 1984, *32*, 250.

MALE INFERTILITY. A report of 98 men with immunologic infertility treated with one or more courses of oral methylprednisolone 96 mg daily for 7 days (beginning on day 21 of the partner's menstrual cycle). Of 71 men for whom complete follow-up was obtained pregnancy occurred in 31 of their partners within 12 months.— J. F. Shulman and S. Shulman, *Fert. Steril.*, 1982, *38*, 591.

A short comment stating that until large controlled studies have established the efficacy of steroid treatment for immunological infertility in men their use, because of the risk of severe and debilitating side-effects, cannot be justified.— M. Elstein *et al.* (letter), *Br. med. J.*, 1987, *294*, 1550.

MUSCULAR DISORDERS. *Dermatomyositis.* See under Skin Disorders (below).

Myasthenia Gravis. For a detailed review of the treatment of myasthenia gravis, including the role of corticosteroids, see under neostigmine methylsulphate, p.1333.

Polymyositis. A recommended therapeutic regimen for severe polymyositis: prednisone 60 mg daily in a single dose; azathioprine 2.5 to 3 mg per kg body-weight daily in divided doses; slow potassium tablets 1.2 g thrice daily; antacids and calcium tablets according to needs. After major improvement or at 6 months, the prednisone should be slowly reduced over 3 months to a maintenance level of 15 to 30 mg on alternate days in a single dose; the other therapy should be continued as before. At 2 years the therapy should be slowly tailed off over 3 months, monitoring for relapse of polymyositis and for adrenocortical failure. Therapy should be re-established if relapse occurs, and every subsequent year attempted withdrawal of therapy should be repeated.— W. G. Bradley, *Br. J. Hosp. Med.*, 1977, *17*, 351.

NEUROLOGICAL DISORDERS. *Bell's palsy.* A review and discussion concerning the diagnosis and management of facial paralysis. Prednisone dramatically relieves the pain of Bell's palsy and although some physicians suggest that the benefit is still in doubt it has become the standard treatment in the largest facial-paralysis clinics throughout the world. The suggested dose for adults is 1 mg per kg body-weight daily in divided doses morning and evening; if the paralysis remains incomplete after 5 or 6 days the prednisone is gradually withdrawn over the next 5 days but if the paralysis is complete the initial dosage should be continued for another 10 days and then gradually withdrawn.— K. K. Adour, *New Engl. J. Med.*, 1982, *307*, 348. Criticisms of the statement that prednisone has become the standard treatment, a statement that is based on opinion rather than fact and published controlled studies: R. Karis (letter), *ibid.*, 1647; A. Staal *et al.* (letter), *ibid.*

Cluster headache. Results of a double-blind study in 19 patients indicated that a single dose of prednisone 30 mg for acute attacks of cluster headaches gave almost immediate relief, and freedom from symptoms for about 60 days.— J. L. Jammes, *Dis. nerv. Syst.*, 1975, *37*, 375. See also J. R. Couch and D. K. Ziegler, *Headache*, 1978, *18*, 219.

Epilepsy. See under Epilepsy (above).

Leprosy. Preliminary results of a study on the effect of corticosteroid treatment for neural damage due to reversal reaction in borderline leprosy patients. In 36 patients who received a course of prednisolone for recent nerve damage, starting at 40 mg daily for the first 2 weeks and gradually reduced over a 6-month period, nerve function improved in 32 of the 53 affected ulnar nerves and 27 of the 40 affected median nerves.— E. M. J. Touw-Langendijk *et al.*, *Lepr. Rev.*, 1984, *55*, 41. In an out-patient study a semi-standardised regimen of prednisolone starting with an average daily dose of 25 mg by mouth and normally reduced by 5 mg daily per month was administered to 33 borderline leprosy patients to treat recent nerve damage of less than 6 months duration; dosage was adjusted for body-weight and the severity and persistence of the neuritis. Prednisolone treatment produced a marked improvement in 38 of the 57 damaged nerves and none got worse. Side-effects were few.— K. U. Kiran *et al.*, *ibid.*, 1985, *56*, 127.

Multiple sclerosis. In reviews of the management of multiple sclerosis (B. Giesser, *Drugs*, 1985, *29*, 88; A. Compston, *Br. J. Hosp. Med.*, 1986, *36*, 200; *Drug & Ther. Bull.*, 1986, *24*, 41) it is stated that corticosteroids are often used to hasten the recovery from an acute exacerbation although they have no effect on the degree of recovery nor do they affect the overall course of the disease. Prednisone or prednisolone are the agents reported to be used, usually in an initial dose of 60 mg daily for about a week and then gradually withdrawn over the next few weeks. Giesser has also commented that intrathecally administered corticosteroids are occasionally useful to temporarily relieve spasticity in patients unresponsive to oral therapy but that such use is controversial as adverse effects such as arachnoiditis or aseptic meningitis have occurred; a short comment is also made that there is no unequivocal evidence that administration of systemic corticosteroids produces a better degree of functional visual recovery in retrobulbar neuritis, a symptom in many patients with multiple sclerosis. In a small preliminary study involving 25 patients in acute relapse (M.P. Barnes *et al.*, *J. Neurol. Neurosurg. Psychiat.*, 1985, *48*, 157) it was found that methylprednisolone 1 g intravenously daily for 7 days produced a more rapid clinical improvement than a standard corticotrophin regimen but again no long-term benefit from corticosteroids was noted after 3 months.

Pain syndromes. A short comment that the reports which appear periodically of the dramatic effect of large doses of corticosteroids in Sudeck's atrophy and the shoulder-hand syndrome do not stand up to critical analysis and most workers have abandoned their use.— C. B. W. Parry and R. H. Withrington, *Postgrad. med. J.*, 1984, *60*, 869.

Subacute demyelinating polyneuropathy. A report of 10 patients with subacute demyelinating polyneuropathy who obtained a beneficial response to corticosteroid therapy; in one patient the response was initially slight, but became dramatic when azathioprine was added. Prednisone was given in initial single daily doses of 40 to 150 mg, until definite clinical improvement was obtained, and followed by a single-dose alternate-day regimen. After a detailed review of different forms of polyneuropathy, including the Guillain-Barré syndrome, and their response to corticosteroid therapy, it was concluded that subacute demyelinating neuropathy appears to be a distinct and clinically identifiable entity in which corticosteroid therapy is indicated.— S. J. Oh, *Archs Neurol., Chicago*, 1978, *35*, 509.

OCULAR DISORDERS. Ocular disorders and their treatment, including details of those conditions in which topical or systemic corticosteroid therapy is appropriate.— R. A. Thoft, *New Engl. J. Med.*, 1978, *298*, 1239. See also S. I. Davidson, *Prescribers' J.*, 1978, *18*, 139.

A discussion on the use of corticosteroids and the eye. Topical corticosteroids have transformed the management of inflammatory disease of the anterior segment of the eye and it should be noted that their proper use may be sight-saving but that their inappropriate use is potentially blinding. The dangers include the conversion of a simple dendritic herpes simplex epithelial lesion into an extensive amoeboid ulcer with the likelihood of permanent corneal scarring and loss of vision and also the risk of potentiation of bacterial and fungal infections. Other dangers include the development of open-angle glaucoma and cataracts. Topical steroids are used by ophthalmologists in herpes simplex keratitis but always under appropriate antiviral cover and their use requires considerable experience. Topical corticosteroids should never be given for an undiagnosed red eye and many consultant ophthalmic surgeons believe that general practitioners should never initiate therapy without an ophthalmic opinion.— D. St. Clair Roberts, *Br. med. J.*, 1986, *292*, 1414. See also: M. J. Lavin and G. E. Rose, *ibid.*, 1448; C. M. P. Claoué and K. E. Stevenson, *ibid.*, 1450. For debate and correspondence concerning the suggestion that topical corticosteroids for the eye should only be prescribed by ophthalmologists and not by general practitioners, see *Br. med. J.*, 1986, *292*, 1737-8 and *ibid.*, *293*, 205.

A review with recommendations for the treatment of viral keratitis including the use of corticosteroids in selected cases.— J. McGill and G. M. Scott, *Br. med. Bull.*, 1985, *41*, 351. See also: J. McGill, *Br. J. Ophthal.*, 1987, *71*, 118.

A short comment that corticosteroid eye-drops are used to control the inflammatory response commonly observed following cataract surgery; prednisolone is usually used but dexamethasone may be necessary if the inflammation is severe.— B. A. Noble, *Br. med. J.*, 1986, *292*, 1578.

See also under Thyroid Disorders (below).

ORGAN AND TISSUE TRANSPLANTATION. A review and discussion of the use of corticosteroids in immunosuppression following transplant surgery. For many years an immunosuppressive protocol using high doses of corticosteroids was unchallenged despite the fact that rejection was seldom totally suppressed and side-effects were inevitable. In 1977 it was reported (M.G. McGeown *et al.*, *Lancet*, 1977, *2*, 648) that excellent survival of transplanted kidneys could be obtained with azathioprine and lower doses of corticosteroids, a daily maintenance dose of just 20 mg (300 μg per kg body-weight) of prednisolone being used. This approach has since been supported by experimental and clinical studies showing that lowering the dose of prednisolone from about 75 to 150 mg daily to about 20 to 30 mg daily did not jeopardise the survival of the graft. Another factor that may be important is the time of day when immunosuppressive treatment is taken because of the diurnal variations involved in the endogenous production of steroids. The unit with the best results in the *UK* is the only one using a single morning dose of azathioprine and prednisolone although there is little experimental evidence to indicate that this is the optimal regimen; the point needs clarification and a study is needed to compare single-daily and twice-daily administration. Alternate-day therapy has also been advocated and uncontrolled studies suggest it does provide adequate immunosuppression but whether such treatment yields fewer complications and side-effects is less certain. The apparently universal practice in kidney and heart transplant units of prescribing a large dose of corticosteroids at the time of the transplant operation is another aspect that requires examination since experimental justification for such a practice is difficult to find. Current evidence suggests that small doses of corticosteroids (at least prednisolone 7 mg daily) are needed indefinitely in patients with functioning transplants to prevent rejection although azathioprine may sometimes be discontinued. A rejection episode can often be halted and reversed by increasing the dose of corticosteroids but the optimal dose is not known; a dose of [prednisolone] 3 mg per kg daily by mouth is customarily used and is generally effective but the usual dose of methylprednisolone 16 mg per kg daily intravenously is probably excessive. Until recently it was believed that corticosteroids were the only agents that could reliably reverse rejection episodes but antilymphocyte globulin appears to be an alternative and at least one kidney transplant unit uses it routinely in preference to corticosteroids. Cyclosporin is now being used and investigated in transplant centres and a regimen involving its use with corticosteroids has been adopted by a number of renal units particularly in the *USA*. In Europe the emphasis has been on using cyclosporin alone but rejection has quite often been a problem with many patients requiring steroids additionally at some time. If corticosteroids are necessary with cyclosporin then the precise dose needs to be established to avoid some potentially toxic regimen being adopted as a world standard.— J. R. Salaman, *Br. med. J.*, 1983, *286*, 1373.

An overview prepared by the Council on Scientific Affairs of the American Medical Association of the major forms of immunosuppression, including corticosteroids, used in organ transplantation: *J. Am. med. Ass.*, 1987, *257*, 1781.

For some reports giving details of immunosuppressant regimens used in transplant patients, see Ortho Multicenter Transplant Study Group, *New Engl. J. Med.*, 1985, *313*, 337 (renal; monoclonal antibodies, azathioprine, and corticosteroids compared with azathioprine and corticosteroids); R. Y. Calne *et al.* (letter), *Lancet*, 1985, *1*, 1448 (renal; cyclosporin initially followed by alternate-day maintenance with azathioprine, corticosteroids, and cyclosporin); J. R. Salaman and P. J. A. Griffin (letter), *ibid.*, *2*, 1066 (renal; cyclosporin initially followed by maintenance with azathioprine and corticosteroids compared with cyclosporin alone throughout); B. Levin *et al., ibid.*, 1321 (renal; pre-operative total lymphoid irradiation, postoperative antithymocyte globulin, and maintenance corticosteroids); C. M. Burke *et al., ibid.*, 1986, *1*, 517 (heart-lung; azathioprine, corticosteroids, and cyclosporin initially followed by maintenance with corticosteroids and cyclosporin); A. J. Hoitsma *et al., ibid.*, 1987, *1*, 584 (renal; cyclosporin initially followed by maintenance with azathioprine and corticosteroids compared with azathioprine and corticosteroids throughout); P. J. Morris *et al., ibid.*, 586 (renal; cyclosporin initially followed by maintenance with azathioprine and corticosteroids compared with azathioprine and corticosteroids throughout).

For further details concerning immunosuppression following organ and tissue transplantation, see under cyclosporin, p.617.

PANCREATITIS. In 2 patients with acute episodes of pancreatitis caused by sarcoidosis a response to corticosteroids occurred; corticosteroids are generally contra-indicated for most other forms of pancreatitis.— P. A. McCormick *et al., Br. med. J.*, 1985, *290*, 1472.

PREGNANCY AND THE NEONATE. For a review of the effects of corticosteroids during pregnancy, see Pregnancy and the Neonate under Precautions.

For reference to the use of corticosteroids in various disorders during pregnancy, see Asthma (above), Haemolytic Anaemia and Thrombocytopenic Purpura both under Blood Disorders (above), Lupus Erythematosus under Connective Tissue Disorders (above), and Pemphigus and Pemphigoid under Skin Disorders (below).

For the prevention of the neonatal respiratory distress syndrome, see Betamethasone, p.884.

RENAL DISORDERS. A review of the drug therapy of glomerulonephritis, including a discussion on studies attempting to elucidate the role of corticosteroids, with or without other immunosuppressant therapy. Controlled studies carried out to date in *membranous nephropathy* and in *mixed proliferative glomerulonephritis*, employing anti-inflammatory corticosteroids and immunosuppressant drugs have shown no effect other than some short-term benefit from cyclophosphamide (which was not subsequently confirmed) and diminution of proteinuria of membranous patients treated with chlorambucil. Indeed, the mortality of the treated group in the Medical Research Council's trials [D.A.K. Black *et al., Br. med. J.*, 1970, *3*, 421] of corticosteroids alone and with azathioprine was higher than in the control group, which suggests that in some patients the glomerulonephritis was made worse. Few of these trials were ideal and some doubt remains in several directions, so that a further trial of corticosteroids with or without immunosuppressant drugs seems justified.
There also seems to be a case for further trial of indomethacin in *proliferative glomerulonephritis* in doses higher than those of the 100-mg daily dose given by the Medical Research Council to patients with predominantly normal renal function. Reports of successful restoration of declining renal function towards normal have been with higher doses of indomethacin, sometimes accompanied by small doses of cyclophosphamide.
Antithrombin and antiplatelet drugs have usually been given against a background of immunosuppression and this toxic association of drugs should not be given to those whose disease does not satisfy strict criteria for serious disease. Results in patients with *proliferative glomerulonephritis and extensive crescent formation* have been encouraging but it must be remembered that these are obtained in the absence of controlled trials, which will be difficult in these rare, extremely ill patients. In the absence of controlled studies it must be remembered that the prognosis for the patient now includes regular dialysis and transplantation with a reasonable prospect for survival.
Although a considerable improvement has occurred in the prognosis of *lupus nephritis*, several controlled clinical trials, all of them open to criticism, have failed to show any clear advantage of corticosteroid therapy alone, although there are indications that the addition of immunosuppressants, even for a relatively short period, reduces the number of patients subsequently going into renal failure. Our current policy is to use corticosteroids and azathioprine routinely in all patients with severe forms of *lupus nephritis*; some judged to have milder renal disease on histological examination, are managed with corticosteroid therapy alone. The corticosteroid doses are maintained at 10 to 25 mg of prednisone daily, usually at the lower end of this range, in association with azathioprine rather than cyclophosphamide. We have also used anticoagulants and antiplatelet agents and, rarely, pulses of methylprednisolone, in acutely ill patients with *severe crescentic glomerulonephritis*. Plasmaphaeresis has also been tried in acute severe *renal lupus*.
The form of glomerulonephritis described as *minimal-change disease*, which is of unknown aetiology, responds reliably to both corticosteroid and immunosuppressive drugs. Corticosteroids, purine antagonists, and mustard-like drugs considerably accelerate remission of minimal-change disease but, whereas those treated with corticosteroids or purine-antagonists may relapse persistently, cyclophosphamide, at doses of 2.5 to 3 mg per kg body-weight daily for 6 to 8 weeks or longer, induces permanent remission in about a third of these relapsing patients. Administration of corticosteroids at a dose of about 60 mg of prednisone daily will induce remission in over 90% of the patients, and since only half will subsequently relapse, cyclophosphamide or other drugs are not justified as primary treatment except possibly in the elderly where a nephrotic syndrome is more serious and subsequent gonadal function of less importance. Corticosteroids may also be used for subsequent relapses, cyclophosphamide only being introduced when they become unsafe or unsatisfactory. Chlorambucil is reserved for those who relapse after cyclophosphamide therapy, but such patients may respond to lower doses of corticosteroids as if the cyclophosphamide had 'softened' the disease. The impact of diuretics and antibiotics must not be forgotten in this condition which used to carry a mortality of about 50% over 5 years and now has a mortality of less than 5% over 10 years.— J. S. Cameron, *Br. med. J.*, 1977, *1*, 1457 and 1520.

Further reviews of the use of corticosteroids in renal disease. Corticosteroids remain the treatment of choice for minimal-change glomerulonephritis. Initial therapy is with prednisolone or prednisone 60 to 80 mg daily in adults and 60 mg per m^2 body-surface in children for 4 to 8 weeks and then withdrawn progressively over 4 to 8 weeks. Alternate-day prednisolone is also capable of inducing remission in a high proportion of patients. The role of corticosteroids in membranous glomerulonephritis remains controversial. The author's personal approach in this condition is not to use corticosteroids unless the nephrotic state is clinically severe. In rapidly-progressive crescentic glomerulonephritis there are several reports demonstrating an often dramatic improvement after methylprednisolone intravenously followed by prednisolone. Corticosteroid therapy has also improved dramatically the prognosis of glomerulonephritis associated with systemic lupus erythematosus and the concomitant use of immunosuppressive therapy reduces the doses of corticosteroids required.— N. M. Thomson, *Med. J. Aust.*, 1987, *146*, 530. See also: B. M. Hall, *ibid.*, 1984, *140*, 758 (lupus nephritis).

In an attempt to clarify the role of corticosteroids in lupus nephritis several workers have either conducted new studies or re-analysed the results of previously published work (N.W. Boyce *et al., Med. J. Aust.*, 1984, *140*, 775; D.T. Felson and J. Anderson, *New Engl. J. Med.*, 1984, *311*, 1528; J.E. Balow *et al., ibid.*, 491; H.A. Austin *et al., ibid.*, 1986, *314*, 614). In general it was concluded that corticosteroids together with immunosuppressive therapy such as azathioprine or cyclophosphamide were more effective than corticosteroids alone although debate arose over which particular immunosuppressive drug was the better (*New Engl. J. Med.*, 1986, *315*, 458-9).

Some references to corticosteroids in the minimal-change nephrotic syndrome: C. Pru *et al., Ann. intern. Med.*, 1984, *100*, 69 (response initially, and generally even after late relapse, to corticosteroids); R. S. Trompeter *et al., Lancet*, 1985, *1*, 368 (good long-term prognosis after corticosteroids); E. Imbasciati *et al., Br. med. J.*, 1985, *291*, 1305 (intravenous pulse methylprednisolone and low-dose or high-dose oral prednisone); P. F. Hoyer *et al.* (letter), *Lancet*, 1986, *2*, 335 (benefit of cyclosporin in steroid-relapsing patients); C. Lagrue *et al.* (letter), *ibid.*, 693 (benefit of cyclosporin after failure of steroids).

Renal transplants. For reference to the use of corticosteroids in the management of renal transplant patients, see Organ and Tissue Transplantation (above).

RESPIRATORY DISORDERS. Reviews and discussions on the adult respiratory distress syndrome with the general conclusions that, although corticosteroids have been used and been reported to be of benefit in some cases, no controlled clinical studies have yet been performed to prove efficacy and that their use remains controversial.— C. R. M. Boggis and R. Greene, *Br. J. Hosp. Med.*, 1983, *29*, 167; B. A. Boucher and T. S. Foster, *Drug Intell. & clin. Pharm.*, 1984, *18*, 862; M. R. Flick and J. F. Murray, *J. Am. med. Ass.*, 1984, *251*, 1054; *Lancet*, 1986, *1*, 301.

A review of the use of corticosteroid therapy in some respiratory disorders (allergic bronchopulmonary aspergillosis, cryptogenic fibrosing alveolitis, extrinsic allergic alveolitis, prolonged pulmonary eosinophilia, sarcoidosis, and Wegener's granulomatosis). Although the use of corticosteroids in the management of a variety of respiratory diseases has mostly not been clarified by controlled clinical studies, the understanding of the pathological processes does give some justification for the continued use of steroids in these frequently troublesome diseases.— P. W. Trembath, *Med. J. Aust.*, 1985, *143*, 607.

See also Aspiration Syndromes (above), Asthma (above), and Sarcoidosis (below).

RHEUMATOID DISEASE. A review and discussion concerning the current management of rheumatoid arthritis. Patients with rheumatoid arthritis, which is better called rheumatoid disease, should be given anti-inflammatory drugs and/or analgesics. If the rheumatoid disease remains localised, there is a case for local treatment and the judicious use of corticosteroids into the synovial tendon sheaths or the joint cavity often provides considerable relief of pain and inflammation. Several studies have shown that intra-articular triamcinolone is the most efficacious and longest-lasting drug for rheumatoid synovitis of the joint but, arguably, it also carries the highest risk of side-effects; prednisolone or even hydrocortisone may be the preparation of choice for tendon sheaths. In the treatment of established rheumatoid disease opinions differ on the time to commence treatment with disease-modifying drugs (antirheumatoid drugs or second-line agents). Most physicians feel that the resultant symptomatic improvement is greater than that provided by non-steroidal anti-inflammatory agents and analgesics alone and justifies the calculated risk in their use. Traditionally gold has been the first choice although some consider penicillamine is just as effective and has fewer side-effects. Chloroquine and hydroxychloroquine are thought to be less powerful perhaps for initial use. Immunosuppressive agents, of which azathioprine is most widely used in the *UK*, are reserved for older patients or those who have failed to respond to other agents. Systemic corticosteroids produce the supreme symptomatic response very quickly but probably have no subsequent effect on the disease process and have many side-effects; they are probably best kept for use in the problem 2 to 3% of patients needing immediate rescue from severe rheumatoid disease.— H. A. Bird, *Br. J. Hosp. Med.*, 1986, *35*, 374. A further review and discussion on the treatment of severe rheumatoid arthritis. A personal preference for the second-line agent is sulphasalazine, penicillamine or gold, chloroquine or hydroxychloroquine, combination treatment, and captopril. Pulsed corticosteroids may be used for acute exacerbations with a second-line agent and long-term oral corticosteroids may be used in the elderly.— V. Wright, *Br. med. J.*, 1986, *292*, 431.

Further references: *Prescribers' J.*, 1987, *27*, 13-35 (a symposium).

RHINITIS. Comments on the treatment of allergic rhinitis. Topical (intranasal) corticosteroids are of considerable value. The technique of administration, covering as much of the nasal mucosa as possible, is critical: it is important to explain to patients that nasal corticosteroids must be used prophylactically. In hay fever, symptoms of rhinitis are largely or completely controlled in the majority of patients whereas in perennial rhinitis, reduction rather than complete elimination of symptoms is the dominant effect. Systemic corticosteroids are rarely indicated and should be reserved for very special circumstances.— P. W. Ewan, *Prescribers' J.*, 1983, *23*, 40. See also *Drug & Ther. Bull.*, 1985, *23*, 25.

SARCOIDOSIS. A short comment that corticosteroids are widely used in sarcoidosis but without proof that they affect the natural history of the disease, alter prognosis, or even prevent the development of pulmonary fibrosis. Although studies have shown that treatment produces early clinical, physiological, and radiographic improvement, no benefit is seen at long-term follow-up when treated patients are compared with controls. The problem lies with the fact that conventional methods of assessing patients with sarcoidosis are too crude and unreliable to identify individual patients with active and aggressive disease who might benefit from early treatment with corticosteroids.— J. T. Macfarlane, *Br. med. J.*, 1984, *288*, 1557.

SKIN DISORDERS. A detailed review of the clinical pharmacology and therapeutic use of topical corticosteroids. Guidelines for the correct use of topical corticosteroids are: be prepared to apply an appropriately potent compound to bring the condition under control; continue treatment with a less potent preparation after control is obtained; reduce the frequency of application; if required, continue daily application with the weakest preparation that will control the condition; once healed, tail off treatment; be especially careful in children and in certain anatomical sites, such as the face and flexures. The following is a rough guide to the clinical potencies of topical corticosteroids: *very potent* (*group 1*): beclomethasone dipropionate 0.5%, clobetasol propionate 0.05%, diflucortolone valerate 0.3%, fluocinolone acetonide 0.2%; *potent* (*group 2*): beclomethasone dipropionate 0.025%, betamethasone benzoate 0.025%, betamethasone dipropionate 0.05%, betamethasone valerate 0.1%, desonide 0.05%, desoxymethasone 0.25%, diflorasone diacetate 0.05%, diflucortolone valerate 0.1%, fluclorolone acetonide 0.025%, fluocinolone acetonide 0.025%, fluocinonide 0.05%, fluocortolone 0.5%, fluprednidene acetate 0.1%, flurandrenolone 0.05%, halcinonide 0.1%, hydrocortisone butyrate 0.1%, triamcinolone acetonide 0.1%; *moderately potent* (*group 3*): clobetasone butyrate 0.05%, flumethasone pivalate 0.02%, fluocinolone acetonide 0.01%, fluocortin butylester 0.75%, fluocortolone 0.2%, flurandrenolone 0.0125 to 0.025%, hydrocortisone 1% with urea; *mild* (*group 4*): dexamethasone 0.01%, hydrocortisone or hydrocortisone acetate 0.1 to 1%, methylprednisolone 0.25%. While the borderline between groups 1 and 2 is quite well defined, distinction between those preparations in groups 2 and 3 is not always easy. Some are available in different concentrations, which may be presumed (often erroneously, and seldom on the basis of reliable evidence) to qualify them for inclusion in a different category of clinical potency. There is a several-fold difference in topical absorption of corticosteroids between those absorbed the most and those absorbed the least, and in addition to a large variation in absorption between individuals, there is also a large variation between various anatomical sites which explains the difference in response of different areas to the same corticosteroid formulations. Compared with 1% on the forearm, the scalp absorbs approximately 4%, the forehead 7%, and the scrotum 36%. The groin, axillae and face are also areas of higher penetrability and it is these sites which tend to develop local side-effects more easily.— J. A. Miller and D. D. Munro, *Drugs*, 1980, *19*, 119.

Some guidelines to the use of topical corticosteroids. It was once fashionable for a patient with severe eczema or psoriasis to be coated with a corticosteroid and then slipped into a polythene suit. Such procedures are now largely discredited as stronger preparations will achieve the same result without occlusion. Some patients have been so frightened by vague rumours about side-effects that they will not use topical corticosteroids at all, and some doctors are so unworried by side-effects that they prescribe corticosteroids in too large quantities or inappropriately high strengths. A sensible balance is needed which may usually be achieved by following some simple ground rules. Firstly, eczema of various types is the main indication for topical corticosteroid therapy; psoriasis is less responsive to steroids and often better treated with tar, dithranol, or ultraviolet light. Secondly, accept that special rules apply to the face; problems may be largely avoided by using only hydrocortisone 0.5 or 1%. Thirdly, preparations of the right potency should be chosen. The safest rule is to use the lowest potency which will achieve the purpose, although some like to use a more potent preparation initially before changing to a weaker one. Caution is necessary when prescribing for children but potent preparations may be needed briefly in older children. Reasonable amounts of preparation should be prescribed; the whole body of an adult may be covered once with between 12 and 26 g and an arm takes 2 to 3 g. Finally, patients should be told that topical corticosteroids work best after a bath, should be applied sparingly in thin layers, and be smoothed gently into the skin; little is gained by applications more frequent than twice daily or by vigorous rubbing.— J. A. Savin, *Br. med. J.*, 1985, *290*, 1607.

Results of a study in 16 adult patients with eczema treated with a variety of topical corticosteroids until substantial clearing had occurred (up to 10 days) indicated that the mean requirement of preparation was 6.86 g per m^2 body-surface area. Using this value the calculated quantities of topical corticosteroid (cream or ointment) to the nearest 5 g required for twice daily application for one week for the whole body, arms and legs only, and trunk only respectively were as follows: 6 months of age, 35 g, 20 g, and 15 g; 1 year, 45 g, 25 g, and 15 g; 4 years, 60 g, 35 g, and 20 g; 8 years, 90 g, 50 g, and 35 g; 12 years, 120 g, 65 g, and 45 g; 16 years, 155 g, 85 g, and 55 g; adult (70-kg male), 170 g, 90 g, and 60 g. Calculated quantities for the same application schedule for an adult (70-kg male) for individual portions of the body were: face and neck, 10 g; one arm, 15 g; one leg, 30 g; hands and feet, 10 g.— P. D. L. Maurice and E. M. Saihan, *Br. J. clin. Pract.*, 1985, *39*, 441.

Acne. A review of the treatment of acne mentioning that intralesional corticosteroids (triamcinolone acetonide or hexacetonide) may accelerate the resolution of inflammatory nodules, prevent re-accumulation after aspiration of inflammatory cysts, and help flatten keloidal or hypertrophic scars. Strengths greater than 10 mg per mL should not be used and skin atrophy is a problem following repeated injections into the same site.— *Drug & Ther. Bull.*, 1984, *22*, 93.

Alopecia. Corticosteroids, either injected locally or given systemically usually make the hair regrow. Unfortunately the regrowth is often only temporary and the hazards of long-term treatment with corticosteroids are not justified. Repeated local injections of triamcinolone often induce atrophy of the scalp.— *Br. med. J.*, 1979, *1*, 505.

In alopecia areata intralesional corticosteroids, most commonly triamcinolone, will induce hair growth. Regrowth is confined to the site of injection and therefore patchy, although soon concealed by spontaneous growth from uninjected regions. Some atrophy of the scalp is inevitable but of no great consequence. Topical corticosteroids, even under occlusion, are not effective.— S. Shuster, *Prescribers' J.*, 1985, *25*, 12.

Dermatomyositis. A review of the treatment of 29 children with dermatomyositis. In 10 children an initial dose of prednisolone 1 mg per kg body-weight daily suppressed the disease successfully and following dosage reduction and withdrawal 6 have remained off treatment for at least a year. In the other group of children the induction dose of prednisolone was generally higher, being 1 to 3 mg per kg daily and was usually given for a longer period. Compared to the low-dose group only one child did as well and of the 12 in the high-dose group who have had corticosteroid therapy totally withdrawn there have been more serious problems. The present data suggest that the method of management with prednisolone may be critical in determining the final outcome. The use of a high induction dose and maintaining it beyond the time that remission has started to occur will inevitably lead to a more prolonged course of treatment which may in itself induce a certain chronicity in the disease and lead to the development of complications.— G. Miller *et al.*, *Archs Dis. Childh.*, 1983, *58*, 445.

Further references: M. Yoshioka *et al.*, *Archs Dis. Childh.*, 1985, *60*, 236.

Eczema. A discussion of the treatment of atopic eczema in childhood. Topical corticosteroids are undoubtedly helpful but should not be overvalued. Applications containing hydrocortisone acetate 1% can be used in all but the very smallest infants, even on the face, and ointments are preferable to creams. In a few children with severe atopic eczema other standard dermatological and systemic treatments produce little benefit and the use of prednisolone by mouth may be considered but is associated with significant hazard; prednisolone should be avoided in children below the age of 2 years or above the age of 11 years because of its effect on growth. Successful therapy will usually involve relatively high doses of 1.5 mg per kg daily initially, thereafter reduced very gradually and continued for about a year; alternate-day dosage is rarely effective.— D. J. Atherton, *Prescribers' J.*, 1986, *26*, 140.

Further reviews: J. Verbov, *Archs Dis. Childh.*, 1986, *61*, 518; T. J. David, *ibid.*, 1987, *62*, 876.

Erythema multiforme. Dramatic symptomatic relief could sometimes be provided in erythema multiforme (the Stevens-Johnson syndrome) by systemic corticosteroids, with an initial dose of 60 mg of prednisone in severe cases.— *Br. med. J.*, 1972, *1*, 63.

From a study of 32 children aged 8 months to 14 years with severe erythema multiforme, recovery among the 17 given prednisone 40 to 80 mg per m^2 body-surface or an equivalent corticosteroid was considered to be less rapid than among the 15 patients given supportive treatment; there was also a significant incidence of medical complications among those given corticosteroids.— J. E. Rasmussen, *Br. J. Derm.*, 1976, *95*, 181.

Keloids. Fluorinated corticosteroids in high concentrations could be applied as creams with occlusive dressings or impregnated in occlusive adhesive tape for the treatment of keloids. Intralesional injections with 0.05 to 0.1 mL of triamcinolone acetonide 1% suspension were commonly used and subcutaneous injection of a local anaesthetic below the keloid would reduce pain associated with the procedure.— D. D. Munro, *Practitioner*, 1974, *212*, 773.

Pemphigus and pemphigoid. A discussion concerning the treatment of pemphigus. Systemic corticosteroids are the mainstay of management and high doses are often required with adjuvant therapy frequently being added also. Initially high doses are used although most dermatologists attempt to keep the dose below 120 mg of prednisolone daily. Adjuvant therapy with azathioprine, cyclophosphamide, or gold has been used to good effect. Maintenance treatment must be individualised to every patient but in general the dose of prednisolone should be reduced by 50% every 2 to 3 weeks. When the daily dose has been lowered to 80 mg daily it is desirable to convert gradually to alternate-day therapy. During this period topical therapy with potent corticosteroids is useful and is also a valuable first-line treatment for early relapses. A combined corticosteroid-antibiotic preparation also reduces the chance of infection. Therapy for mucous membranes is also based on the use of corticosteroids, applied topically, sucked as lozenges, or possibly inhaled.— J. H. Barth and V. A. Venning, *Br. J. Hosp. Med.*, 1987, *37*, 326.

Pemphigoid gestationis (herpes gestationis) is a very uncommon skin condition almost specific to pregnancy. The intense itching and severe constitutional effects may be successfully treated with oral corticosteroids, initially in high dosage.— M. de Swiet, *Archs Dis. Childh.*, 1985, *60*, 794.

Psoriasis. A review of psoriasis and its management. Topical corticosteroids are still widely used for psoriasis but with diminishing enthusiasm from those who look after the long-term interests of such patients. Atrophy and other side-effects compound the problem that corticosteroids seem to become less effective after continued therapy and may even make the disease worse if overused. Nevertheless, they may be valuable in patients with the not uncommon mixtures of psoriasis with eczema or seborrhoeic dermatitis and also on those sites (the face, flexures, genitalia, and hands) where it might be expected they would be contra-indicated. In theory, the combination of corticosteroids with dithranol or tar should be desirable, but the published evidence is confusing. A few patients with chronic plaque psoriasis may be greatly improved by just a few nights use of a really strong topical preparation perhaps even under polythene occlusion, but in general dermatologists now rarely prescribe strong steroids under occlusion.— R. H. Champion, *Br. med. J.*, 1986, *292*, 1693.

A further discussion on the treatment of psoriasis including brief comments concerning the choice of suitable topical corticosteroid preparations.— S. M. Going, *Br. med. J.*, 1987, *295*, 984.

Urticaria pigmentosa. The effect of topical corticosteroids on human dermis including mention of the successful use of corticosteroids either by topical application or by intralesional injection in urticaria pigmentosum.— R. M. Lavker *et al.*, *Br. J. Derm.*, 1986, *115*, *Suppl.* 31, 101.

THYROID DISORDERS. A review of the management of thyroid diseases noting that high dose corticosteroid therapy is the mainstay of medical treatment when severe congestive ophthalmopathy occurs in Graves' disease. A starting dose of 60 to 80 mg of prednisolone daily for 1 to 2 weeks usually produces an improvement and the dosage can be slowly reduced.— R. Wilkinson, *Prescribers' J.*, 1984, *24*, 97.

The various forms of thyroiditis and treatment. Corticosteroids are indicated in all severe cases of subacute granulomatous thyroiditis and should be considered in patients with subacute lymphocytic thyroiditis with severe clinical symptoms. In invasive fibrous thyroiditis treatment is usually surgical with corticosteroids having been used after the operation to relieve symptoms and to decrease the size of the goitre but in some instances their withdrawal has led to the recurrence of thyroiditis or to the appearance of a previously unrecognised extracervical fibrosclerosis.— I. D. Hay, *Mayo Clin. Proc.*, 1985, *60*, 836.

12338-m

Alclometasone Dipropionate *(BANM, USAN, rINNM)*.

Sch-22219. 7α-Chloro-11β,17α,21-trihydroxy-16α-methylpregna-1,4-diene-3,20-dione 17,21-dipropionate.

$C_{28}H_{37}ClO_7$=521.0.

CAS — 67452-97-5 (alclometasone); 66734-13-2 (dipropionate).

Pharmacopoeias. In *U.S.*

Store in airtight containers.

Adverse Effects, Treatment, Withdrawal, and Precautions

As for corticosteroids, p.872.

When applied topically, particularly to large areas, when the skin is broken, or under occlusive dressings, corticosteroids may be absorbed in sufficient amounts to cause systemic effects.

Absorption and Fate
For a brief outline of the absorption and fate of corticosteroids, see p.875.

Uses and Administration
Alclometasone dipropionate is a corticosteroid used topically in the treatment of various skin disorders, as described under corticosteroids (see p.875). It is usually employed as a cream or ointment containing 0.05%.

A brief review of alclometasone.— *Med. Lett.*, 1987, *29*, 42.

SKIN DISORDERS. For recommendations concerning the correct use of corticosteroids on the skin, see Corticosteroids, p.880.

Preparations
Alclometasone Dipropionate Cream *(U.S.P.)*
Alclometasone Dipropionate Ointment *(U.S.P.)*

Proprietary Preparations
Modrasone *(Kirby-Warrick, UK). Cream, Ointment,* alclometasone dipropionate 0.05%.

Proprietary Names and Manufacturers
Aclovate *(Glaxo, USA)*; Alclosone *(Scherag, S.Afr.)*; Delonal *(Essex, Ger.)*; Legederm *(Schering Corp., Denm.)*; Modrasone *(Kirby-Warrick, UK)*.

1061-l

Aldosterone *(BAN, rINN).*
Electrocortin. 11β,18-Epoxy-18,21-dihydroxypregn-4-ene-3,20-dione.
$C_{21}H_{28}O_5$=360.4.

CAS — 52-39-1(+).

Adverse Effects
As for corticosteroids, p.872. Aldosterone has very pronounced mineralocorticoid actions and little effect on carbohydrate metabolism.

Uses and Administration
Aldosterone is probably the main mineralocorticoid secreted by the adrenal cortex. It has no anti-inflammatory properties.
Aldosterone has been used in association with a glucocorticoid in the treatment of Addison's disease. Doses of 500 μg have been given by slow intravenous injection or by intramuscular injection.

Evidence that aldosterone has a half-life of 50 minutes after infusion of 1 mg. About 75% of aldosterone is bound to plasma proteins.— R. E. Peterson, *Ann. N.Y. Acad. Sci.*, 1959, *82*, 846.

Proprietary Names and Manufacturers
Aldocorten *(Ciba, Ger.; Ciba, UK)*.

12351-d

Amcinonide *(BAN, USAN, rINN).*

Amcinopol; CL-34699. 16α,17α-Cyclopentylidenedioxy-9α-fluoro-11β,21-dihydroxypregna-1,4-diene-3,20-dione 21-acetate.
$C_{28}H_{35}FO_7$=502.6.

CAS — 51022-69-6.

Pharmacopoeias. In *U.S.*

Adverse Effects, Treatment, Withdrawal, and Precautions
As for corticosteroids, p.872.
When applied topically, particularly to large areas, when the skin is broken, or under occlusive dressings, corticosteroids may be absorbed in sufficient amounts to cause systemic effects.

Absorption and Fate
For a brief outline of the absorption and fate of corticosteroids, see p.875.

Uses and Administration
Amcinonide is a corticosteroid used topically in the treatment of various skin disorders, as described under corticosteroids (see p.875). It is usually employed as a cream or ointment containing 0.1%.

SKIN DISORDERS. For recommendations concerning the correct use of corticosteroids on the skin, see Corticosteroids, p.880.

Preparations
Amcinonide Cream *(U.S.P.)*
Amcinonide Ointment *(U.S.P.)*

Proprietary Names and Manufacturers
Amciderm *(E. Merck, Ger.)*; Amicla *(Lederle, Neth.)*; Cyclocort *(Lederle, Canad.; Lederle, USA)*; Penticort *(Lederle, Fr.)*.

1062-y

Beclomethasone Dipropionate *(BANM, USAN).*

9α-Chloro-16β-methylprednisolone Dipropionate; Beclometasone Dipropionate *(rINNM)*; Sch-18020W. 9α-Chloro-11β,17α,21-trihydroxy-16β-methylpregna-1,4-diene-3,20-dione 17,21-dipropionate.
$C_{28}H_{37}ClO_7$=521.0.

CAS — 4419-39-0 (beclomethasone); 5534-09-8 (dipropionate).

Pharmacopoeias. In *Br.* and *It. U.S.* allows either the anhydrous or monohydrate form.

A white to creamy-white odourless or almost odourless powder. Practically **insoluble** in water; soluble 1 in 60 of alcohol and 1 in 8 of chloroform; freely soluble in acetone. **Protect** from light.

Adverse Effects, Treatment, Withdrawal, and Precautions
As for corticosteroids, p.872.
Adrenal suppression may occur in some patients treated with high-dose long-term inhalation therapy for asthma. It has been stated that in the majority of patients no significant suppression is likely to occur when total daily doses of less than 1.5 mg are employed.

ADRENAL SUPPRESSION. Some references and correspondence concerning the potential of high-dose beclomethasone inhalation therapy to cause adrenal suppression: I. W. B. Grant and G. K. Crompton (letter), *Br. med. J.*, 1983, *286*, 644; I. M. Slessor (letter), *ibid.*, 645; P. Ebden and B. H. Davies (letter), *Lancet*, 1984, *2*, 576; C. M. Law *et al.*, *ibid.*, 1986, *1*, 942; H. M. Brown (letter), *ibid.*, 1269; J. M. Littlewood *et al.* (letter), *ibid.*, 1988, *1*, 115.

ALLERGY. Blood blisters in the mouth of an elderly patient using beclomethasone dipropionate inhalers.— *Med. J. Aust.*, 1979, *1*, 460. Haemorrhagic ulceration of the nasal mucosa in a patient after using a beclomethasone nasal spray.— N. Doble, *Br. med. J.*, 1985, *290*, 518.

Reports of asthmatic responses to beclomethasone dipropionate inhalations, possibly associated with materials used in their formulation, or with the containers: P. J. Maddern *et al.* (letter), *Med. J. Aust.*, 1978, *1*, 274; J. Godin and J. L. Malo, *Clin. Allergy*, 1979, *9*, 585; R. J. Clark (letter), *Lancet*, 1986, *2*, 574; R. Beasley *et al.* (letter), *ibid.*, 1227.

CANDIDIASIS. Results of a study involving 229 asthmatic children indicated that the presence of a sore throat or a hoarse voice was not related to the presence of *Candida* or to treatment with inhaled corticosteroids (beclomethasone). The occurrence of only one clinical case of oral candidiasis in 129 of the children receiving corticosteroids confirmed previous observations that it is an uncommon finding in children compared with the reported incidence of between 4.5 and 13% in adults. The incidence of colonisation with *Candida* was greater in those children who received steroids than in those who did not but was not affected by either the dose used or type of inhaler employed.— N. J. Shaw and A. T. Edmunds, *Archs Dis. Childh.*, 1986, *61*, 788.

EFFECTS ON THE LUNGS. Pulmonary eosinophilia developed in 3 adults during the gradual withdrawal of systemic corticosteroid therapy following the introduction of beclomethasone dipropionate inhalations.— I. C. Paterson *et al.*, *Br. J. Dis. Chest*, 1975, *69*, 217. Pulmonary eosinophilia in a patient also taking oral corticosteroid therapy.— J. L. Mollura *et al.*, *Ann. Allergy*, 1979, *42*, 326.
Further references to pulmonary eosinophilia in patients inhaling beclomethasone dipropionate: D. W. Hudgel and S. L. Spector, *Chest*, 1977, *72*, 359; L. R. Klotz *et al.*, *Ann. Allergy*, 1977, *39*, 133.

Absorption and Fate
For a brief outline of the absorption and fate of corticosteroids, see p.875.
Beclomethasone dipropionate is readily absorbed after administration by mouth. It has been reported that about 25% of an inhaled dose reaches the lungs.
Beclomethasone dipropionate is considerably more active topically or by inhalation than by mouth.

Uses and Administration
Beclomethasone dipropionate is a glucocorticoid with the general properties described under corticosteroids (see p.875).
Beclomethasone dipropionate exerts a topical effect on the lungs without significant systemic activity at recommended doses and is used by inhalation, generally from a metered aerosol, for the prophylaxis of the symptoms of asthma. The adult dosage of the aerosol is usually 400 μg daily, inhaled in 2 to 4 divided doses for maintenance treatment; if necessary, 600 to 800 μg may be inhaled daily initially, subsequently adjusted according to the patient's response. In patients with severe asthma or in those showing only a partial response to standard inhalation doses, high-dose inhalation therapy may be considered; doses of 1 mg daily (250 μg four times daily or 500 μg twice daily) may be used and may be increased to 1.5 to 2 mg daily (500 μg three or four times daily) if necessary; a maximum of 2 mg daily should not be exceeded. In children, 50 or 100 μg may be inhaled 2 to 4 times daily according to the response. Although beclomethasone dipropionate is generally inhaled in aerosol form, inhalation capsules are available for patients who experience difficulty in using the aerosol. Owing to differences in the relative bioavailability to the lungs of the 2 preparations a 100-μg dose from an inhalation capsule is approximately equivalent in activity to a 50-μg dose from an aerosol. Recommended maintenance doses of beclomethasone dipropionate from inhalation capsules are therefore 200 μg inhaled 3 or 4 times daily for adults, and 100 μg inhaled 2 to 4 times daily for children.
Beclomethasone dipropionate is also used as a nasal spray in the prophylaxis and treatment of allergic rhinitis. Usual doses are 50 μg in each nostril 3 or 4 times daily or 100 μg in each nostril twice daily; a total of 400 μg daily should not generally be exceeded.
In the *UK* the doses of beclomethasone dipropionate for asthma and rhinitis are expressed in units of 50-μg or multiples thereof whereas in the *USA* the dose-unit is 42-μg or multiples thereof.
Beclomethasone dipropionate is also used topically in the treatment of various skin disorders. Concentrations of 0.025 or 0.5% are generally employed.

ASTHMA. A review of clinical studies of the efficacy of varying doses of beclomethasone dipropionate suggests that the high-dose metered aerosols may improve the control of asthma in patients incompletely controlled by the standard-dose aerosols, and in some patients may allow a reduction in the dose of oral corticosteroids or may even avoid their use.— *Drug & Ther. Bull.*, 1986, *24*, 1. See also: *Lancet*, 1984, *2*, 23.
A brief review of the advantages and disadvantages of proprietary inhaler preparations containing a combination of salbutamol and beclomethasone dipropionate. Such fixed combinations will not help most patients with asthma since the flexible use of the individual components required for optimal control is prevented; some patients who cannot cope satisfactorily using two individual inhalers might find such a product helpful however.— *Drug & Ther. Bull.*, 1986, *24*, 13.

In studies on the use of nebulised beclomethasone dipropionate in childhood asthma Storr *et al.* (*Archs Dis. Childh.*, 1986, *61*, 270) found that it was more effective than saline in preschool children but that the response was less than that usually observed with beclomethasone as an inhalation aerosol or inhalation capsules in older children. Webb *et al.* (*ibid.*, 1108) failed to find any clear benefit at all with the nebulised suspension. These two studies have been subject to a brief comment by Clarke (*ibid.*, 1110) who concluded that, in the study by Webb, beclomethasone somehow failed to reach the lungs.

SKIN DISORDERS. For recommendations concerning the correct use of corticosteroids on the skin, and a rough guide to the clinical potencies of topical corticosteroids, see corticosteroids, p.880.

Preparations

Beclomethasone Cream *(B.P.)*. Beclomethasone Dipropionate Cream

Beclomethasone Ointment *(B.P.)*. Beclomethasone Dipropionate Ointment

Proprietary Preparations

Becloforte *(Allen & Hanburys, UK)*. *Inhaler*, beclomethasone dipropionate 250 μg/metered dose.

Becodisks *(Allen & Hanburys, UK)*. *Discs*, beclomethasone dipropionate 100 and 200 μg/dose, for use in a specially designed inhaler (Diskhaler).

Beconase *(Allen & Hanburys, UK)*. *Nasal spray*, beclomethasone dipropionate 50 μg/metered dose.
Nasal spray (aqueous), beclomethasone dipropionate 50 μg/metered dose.

Becotide *(Allen & Hanburys, UK)*. *Inhaler* (Becotide 50), beclomethasone dipropionate 50 μg/metered dose.
Inhaler (Becotide 100), beclomethasone dipropionate 100 μg/metered dose.
Rotacaps (inhalation capsules), beclomethasone dipropionate 100, 200, and 400 μg. For use with a specially designed inhaler (Rotahaler).
Suspension for nebulisation, beclomethasone dipropionate 50 μg/mL.

Propaderm *(Allen & Hanburys, UK)*. *Cream*, *Ointment*, beclomethasone dipropionate 0.025%.
Cream (Propaderm-Forte), beclomethasone dipropionate 0.5%.

Propaderm-A *(Allen & Hanburys, UK)*. *Ointment*, beclomethasone dipropionate 0.025%, chlortetracycline hydrochloride 3%.

Proprietary Names and Manufacturers

Aldecin *(Essex, Austral.; Belg.; Merck Sharp & Dohme, Denm.; Schering Corp., Denm.; Jpn; Neth.; MSD, Swed.; Schering, Swed.; Essex, Switz.)*; Aldecine *(Unicet, Fr.)*; Anceron *(Arg.)*; Andion *(Roche, Denm.)*; Beclo-Asma *(Aldo, Spain)*; Becloforte *(Glaxo, Denm.; Glaxo, Switz.; Allen & Hanburys, UK)*; Beclorhinol *(Declimed, Ger.)*; Beclo-Rino *(Aldo, Spain)*; Beclosona *(Spyfarma, Spain)*; Beclovent *(Allen & Hanburys, Canad.; Glaxo, USA)*; Becocent *(Glaxo, Denm.)*; Becodisks *(Allen & Hanburys, UK)*; Beconase *(Glaxo, Austral.; Belg.; Allen & Hanburys, Canad.; Glaxo, Denm.; Glaxo, Ger.; Neth.; Allen & Hanburys, S.Afr.; Glaxo, Switz.; Allen & Hanburys, UK; Glaxo, USA)*; Beconasol *(Glaxo, Switz.)*; Becotide *(Glaxo, Austral.; Belg.; Glaxo, Denm.; Glaxo, Fr.; Bonomelli, Ital.; Jpn; Neth.; Glaxo, Norw.; Allen & Hanburys, S.Afr.; Glaxo, Spain; Glaxo, Swed.; Glaxo, Switz.; Allen & Hanburys, UK)*; Bronco-Turbinal *(Valeas, Ital.)*; Clenilderm *(Chiesi, Ital.)*; Clenil *(Chiesi, Ital.)*; Dermisone Beclo *(Frumtost, Spain)*; Entyderma *(Jpn)*; Hibisterin *(Jpn)*; Inalone *(Lampugnani, Ital.)*; Korbutone *(Jpn)*; Menaderm Simple *(Menarini, Spain)*; Menaderm Simplex *(Menarini, Ital.)*; Propaderm *(Allen & Hanburys, Canad.; Bonomelli, Ital.; Allen & Hanburys, S.Afr.; Allen & Hanburys, UK)*; Propavent *(Arg.)*; Rino-Clenil *(Chiesi, Ital.)*; Sanasthmax *(Glaxo, Ger.)*; Sanasthmyl *(Glaxo, Ger.)*; Turbinal *(Valeas, Ital.)*; Vancenase *(Schering, Canad.; Schering, USA)*; Vanceril *(Schering, Canad.; Schering, USA)*; Viarox *(Essex, Ger.; Schering, Norw.; Scherag, S.Afr.)*.

The following names have been used for multi-ingredient preparations containing beclomethasone dipropionate—Propaderm-A *(Allen & Hanburys, UK)*; Propaderm-C *(Allen & Hanburys, UK)*; Propaderm-N *(Allen & Hanburys, UK)*.

1063-j

Betamethasone *(BAN, USAN, rINN)*.

9α-Fluoro-16β-methylprednisolone; Betamethasonum; Flubenisolonum. 9α-Fluoro-11β,17α,21-trihydroxy-16β-methylpregna-1,4-diene-3,20-dione.
$C_{22}H_{29}FO_5$=392.5.

CAS — 378-44-9.

Pharmacopoeias. In *Aust., Br., Braz., Chin., Cz., Egypt., Eur., Fr., Ger., Ind., Int., It., Jpn, Neth., Swiss,* and *U.S.* Also in *B.P. Vet.*

A white to practically white, odourless, crystalline powder. *B.P.* **solubilities** are: practically insoluble in water; soluble 1 in 75 of alcohol; very slightly soluble in chloroform. *U.S.P.* solubilities are: soluble 1 in 5300 of water, 1 in 65 of alcohol, and 1 in 15 of warm alcohol, 1 in 325 of chloroform, and 1 in 3 of methyl alcohol; sparingly soluble in acetone; very slightly soluble in ether. **Store** in well-closed containers. Protect from light.

1064-z

Betamethasone Acetate *(BANM, USAN, rINNM)*.

Betamethasone 21-acetate.
$C_{24}H_{31}FO_6$=434.5.

CAS — 987-24-6.

Pharmacopoeias. In *U.S.*

A white to creamy-white odourless powder. Betamethasone acetate 1.1 mg is approximately equivalent to 1 mg of betamethasone. **Soluble** 1 in 2000 of water, 1 in 9 of alcohol, and 1 in 16 of chloroform; freely soluble in acetone. **Store** in airtight containers.

1065-c

Betamethasone Benzoate *(BANM, USAN, rINNM)*.

W-5975. Betamethasone 17α-benzoate.
$C_{29}H_{33}FO_6$=496.6.

CAS — 22298-29-9.

Pharmacopoeias. In *U.S.*

A white to practically white, practically odourless, powder. Betamethasone benzoate 1.3 mg is approximately equivalent to 1 mg of betamethasone. Practically **insoluble** in water; soluble in alcohol, chloroform, and methyl alcohol. **Store** in airtight containers.

1066-k

Betamethasone Dipropionate *(BANM, USAN, rINNM)*.

Sch-11460. Betamethasone 17α,21-dipropionate.
$C_{28}H_{37}FO_7$=504.6.

CAS — 5593-20-4.

Pharmacopoeias. In *It., and Jpn,* and *U.S.*

A white or creamy-white odourless powder. Betamethasone dipropionate 1.3 mg is approximately equivalent to 1 mg of betamethasone. Practically **insoluble** in water; sparingly soluble in alcohol; freely soluble in acetone and chloroform.

1067-a

Betamethasone Sodium Phosphate *(BANM, USAN, rINNM)*.

Betamethasone Disodium Phosphate. Betamethasone 21-(disodium phosphate).
$C_{22}H_{28}FNa_2O_8P$=516.4.

CAS — 360-63-4 (phosphate); 151-73-5 (sodium phosphate).

Pharmacopoeias. In *Br., Ind.,* and *U.S.* Also in *B.P.Vet.*

A white or almost white, odourless, hygroscopic powder. Betamethasone sodium phosphate 1.3 mg is approximately equivalent to 1 mg of betamethasone. **Soluble** 1 in 2 of water, 1 in 470 of alcohol; slightly soluble in dehydrated alcohol; freely soluble in methyl alcohol; practically insoluble in acetone, chloroform, and ether. A 0.5% solution in water has a pH of 7.5 to 9.0. **Store** in airtight containers. Protect from light.

1068-t

Betamethasone Valerate *(BANM, USAN, rINNM)*.

9α-Fluoro-16β-methylprednisolone 17-Valerate; Flubenisoloni Valeras. Betamethasone 17α-valerate.
$C_{27}H_{37}FO_6$=476.6.

CAS — 2152-44-5.

Pharmacopoeias. In *Br., Ind., Jpn,* and *U.S.*

A white to creamy-white, odourless powder. Betamethasone valerate 1.2 mg is approximately equivalent to 1 mg of betamethasone.

Practically **insoluble** in water; soluble 1 in 12 to 16 of alcohol, 1 in 2 of chloroform, and 1 in 400 of ether; freely soluble in acetone. **Store** in airtight containers. Protect from light.

Adverse Effects, Treatment, Withdrawal, and Precautions

As for corticosteroids, p.872.

The effects of betamethasone on sodium and water retention are less than those of prednisolone or prednisone and approximately equal to those of dexamethasone.

Absorption and Fate

For a brief outline of the absorption and fate of corticosteroids, see p.875.

Some references to studies on the pharmacokinetics of betamethasone and its esters: A. B. M. Anderson *et al.*, *Obstet. Gynec.*, 1977, *49*, 471 (in pregnancy); M. C. Petersen *et al.*, *Eur. J. clin. Pharmac.*, 1980, *18*, 245 (intramuscular or intravenous administration in pregnancy); M. C. Petersen *et al.*, *ibid.*, 1983, *25*, 643 (intravenous administration in healthy subjects); M. C. Petersen *et al.*, *ibid.*, 803 (intravenous administration in pregnancy); M. C. Petersen *et al.*, *Br. J. clin. Pharmac.*, 1984, *18*, 383 (intravenous or intramuscular administration in pregnancy); H. Derendorf *et al.*, *Clin. Pharmac. Ther.*, 1986, *39*, 313 (intra-articular administration).

Uses and Administration

Betamethasone is a glucocorticoid and has the general properties described under corticosteroids (see p.875); 750 μg of betamethasone is equivalent in anti-inflammatory activity to about 5 mg of prednisolone. It has been used, either in the form of the free alcohol or in one of the esterified forms, in the treatment of all conditions for which corticosteroid therapy is indicated, except adrenal-deficiency states for which its lack of sodium-retaining properties makes it less suitable than hydrocortisone with supplementary fludrocortisone.

For administration by mouth betamethasone or betamethasone sodium phosphate are used; the usual dose, expressed in terms of betamethasone, is 0.5 to 5 mg daily in divided doses.

For parenteral administration the sodium phosphate ester may be given intravenously by injection or infusion or intramuscularly by injection in doses equivalent to 4 to 20 mg of betamethasone. It may also be given by local injection into soft tissues in doses equivalent to 4 to 8 mg of betamethasone. The sodium phosphate ester is also sometimes used in conjunction with the acetate ester. Suggested doses for intramuscular injection of such a combination are up to 4.5 mg daily for each ester and for intra-articular injection up to 6 mg for each ester.

Betamethasone sodium phosphate is also used in the topical treatment of allergic and inflammatory conditions of the eyes, ears, or nose, usually as drops containing 0.1%.

For topical application in the treatment of various skin disorders the benzoate, dipropionate, and valerate esters of betamethasone are used; the usual concentrations available are 0.025% of betamethasone benzoate, 0.05% of betamethasone as the dipropionate, and 0.01 to 0.1% of betamethasone as the valerate.

Betamethasone valerate is also used by inhalation for the prophylaxis of the symptoms of asthma. The initial dose for both adults and children is 200 µg inhaled 4 times daily, slowly reduced according to the patient's response to the minimum amount necessary to control the asthma.

Other esters of betamethasone which have occasionally been used include the divalerate, hemisuccinate, and valero-acetate.

Betamethasone adamantoate has been used in veterinary practice.

NEONATAL RESPIRATORY DISTRESS SYNDROME. After work showing that the functional maturation of foetal *animal* lungs can be accelerated by stimulation of the foetal adrenal cortex or by administration of glucocorticoids, G.C. Liggins and R.N. Howie, (*Pediatrics*, 1972, *50*, 515) found that intramuscular injection of a preparation containing betamethasone acetate 6 mg and betamethasone phosphate 6 mg, to mothers, more than 24 hours before premature delivery of infants of less than 32 weeks' gestation, was associated with a significant reduction in the incidence of respiratory distress syndrome. In controlled studies using hydrocortisone M. Baden *et al.* (*Pediatrics*, 1972, *50*, 526) and H.W. Taeusch *et al.* (*Pediatrics*, 1973, *52*, 850), found that this benefit did not extend to post-natal administration, and found an increased incidence of ventricular haemorrhage in the treated infants. Other fears concerning prenatal corticosteroid therapy (including possible growth retardation and increased risk of infection) were also expressed, but these adverse effects appear to be outweighed by clinical benefit where corticosteroid therapy is clearly indicated.

This advantage of corticosteroid therapy does not apply to toxaemia of pregnancy where it has been associated with a high incidence of foetal death and is generally contra-indicated. Contrary to other reports, however, in an open study, D.J. Nochimson and R.H. Petrie (*Am. J. Obstet. Gynec.*, 1979, *133*, 449) concluded that pregnancy-related hypertension does not appear to be an absolute contra-indication to glucocorticoid therapy.

In an endeavour to delay the onset of premature labour for long enough to enable corticosteroid therapy to act, beta-receptor stimulants, such as salbutamol, have been given concomitantly.

Further references to corticosteroids and the neonatal respiratory distress syndrome: E. Caspi and P. Schreyer (letter), *Lancet*, 1976, *1*, 973 (dexamethasone; need for administration for up to 7 days before delivery); M. Panter-Brick (letter), *Lancet*, 1976, *2*, 421 (dexamethasone; prophylaxis for an infant with a family history of pulmonary insufficiency); M. F. Block *et al.*, *Obstet. Gynec.*, 1977, *50*, 186 (betamethasone; time factor not significant; methylprednisolone not beneficial); S. N. Caritis *et al.*, *Am. J. Obstet. Gynec.*, 1977, *127*, 529 (betamethasone; in rhesus-sensitised women); A. Kauppila *et al.*, *Br. J. Obstet. Gynaec.*, 1977, *84*, 124 (dexamethasone; no short-term effect on maternal or infant corticotrophin secretion); A. Lazzarin *et al.* (letter), *Lancet*, 1977, *2*, 1354 (betamethasone; reduced infant polymorphonuclear leucocyte function); W. Siebert *et al.*, *Geburtsh. Frauenheilk.*, 1977, *2*, 149 (betamethasone; similar incidence but reduced mortality); C. Sutton, *Br. med. J.*, 1977, *2*, 1069 (dexamethasone; in diabetic mothers); I. Szabó *et al.* (letter), *Lancet*, 1977, *2*, 243 (prednisolone sodium succinate; advantage of longer interval before delivery); S. Sybulski, *Am. J. Obstet. Gynec.*, 1977, *127*, 871 (betamethasone; rapid recovery of infant adrenal activity); F. P. Zuspan *et al.*, *Am. J. Obstet. Gynec.*, 1977, *128*, 571 (hydrocortisone; beneficial effect prenatally); D. Bielawski *et al.* (letter), *Lancet*, 1978, *1*, 218 (betamethasone; leukaemoid reaction in infant); K. D. Gunston and D. A. Davey, *S. Afr. med. J.*, 1978, *54*, 1141 (dexamethasone; with fenoterol); T. R. Johnson and J. Schneider (letter), *New Engl. J. Med.*, 1978, *298*, 56 (betamethasone; chorioamnionitis with foetal and maternal sepsis); A. Kauppila *et al.*, *Obstet. Gynec.*, 1978, *51*, 288 (dexamethasone; with ritodrine); A. M. Butterfill and D. R. Harvey, *Archs Dis. Childh.*, 1979, *54*, 725 (betamethasone; follow-up of treated infants); T. R. Eggers *et al.*, *Med. J. Aust.*, 1979, *1*, 213 (betamethasone; with salbutamol); A. N. Papageorgiou *et al.*, *Pediatrics*, 1979, *63*, 73 (betamethasone; beneficial effect but increased neonatal hypoglycaemia); H. W. Taeusch *et al.*, *Pediatrics*, 1979, *63*, 64 (dexamethasone; beneficial effect but increased incidence of infection); I. Szabo *et al.*, *Lancet*, 1980, *2*, 751 (prednisolone sodium succinate; no benefit below 25 weeks' gestation possibly owing to lack of cortisol receptors in foetal lung); Collaborative Group on Antenatal Steroid Therapy, *Am. J. Obstet. Gynec.*, 1981, *141*, 276 (dexamethasone; beneficial effect prenatally); D. E. Johnson *et al.*, *Pediatrics*, 1981, *68*, 633 (betamethasone,; beneficial effect prenatally); Y. C. Wong *et al.*, *Archs Dis. Childh.*, 1982, *57*, 536 (dexamethasone; no long-term adverse effects on the lungs); *J. Pediat.*, 1984, *104*, 259 (dexamethasone; no adverse effects after 3-year follow-up); W. J. Morales *et al.*, *Am. J. Obstet. Gynec.*, 1986, *154*, 591 (dexamethasone; beneficial effect prenatally).

SKIN DISORDERS. For recommendations concerning the correct use of corticosteroids on the skin, and a rough guide to the clinical potencies of topical corticosteroids, see corticosteroids, p.880.

Preparations of Betamethasone and its Esters

In addition to the preparations below, further official preparations containing betamethasone or its esters may be found listed under clotrimazole.

Injections

Betamethasone Injection *(B.P.)*. Betamethasone Sodium Phosphate Injection. Sterilised by filtration. pH 8.0 to 9.0.

Betamethasone Sodium Phosphate Injection *(U.S.P.)*

Sterile Betamethasone Sodium Phosphate and Betamethasone Acetate Suspension *(U.S.P.)*. A sterile preparation containing betamethasone sodium phosphate in solution, and betamethasone acetate in suspension in Water for Injections.

Ophthalmic Dosage Forms

Betamethasone Eye-drops *(B.P.C. 1973)*. Betamethasone Sodium Phosphate Eye-drops; BET. A solution of betamethasone sodium phosphate. Sterilised by filtration.

Oral Dosage Forms

Betamethasone Syrup *(U.S.P.)*

Betamethasone Tablets *(B.P.)*

Betamethasone Tablets *(U.S.P.)*

Betamethasone Sodium Phosphate Tablets *(B.P.)*

Topical Dosage Forms

Betamethasone Dipropionate Topical Aerosol *(U.S.P.)*

Betamethasone Valerate Topical Aerosol *(U.S.P.)*

Betamethasone Valerate Scalp Application *(B.P.)*

Betamethasone Cream *(U.S.P.)*

Betamethasone Dipropionate Cream *(U.S.P.)*

Betamethasone Valerate Cream *(B.P.)*

Betamethasone Valerate Cream *(U.S.P.)*

Betamethasone Benzoate Gel *(U.S.P.)*

Betamethasone Dipropionate Lotion *(U.S.P.)*

Betamethasone Valerate Lotion *(B.P.)*

Betamethasone Valerate Lotion *(U.S.P.)*

Betamethasone Dipropionate Ointment *(U.S.P.)*

Betamethasone Valerate Ointment *(B.P.)*

Betamethasone Valerate Ointment *(U.S.P.)*

Betamethasone Valerate with Chlortetracycline Ointment *(B.P.C. 1973)*. Betamethasone with Chlortetracycline Ointment. Contains betamethasone valerate equivalent to betamethasone 0.1% and chlortetracycline hydrochloride 3%. When a strength less than that specified above is prescribed, the ointment should be diluted with white soft paraffin or chlortetracycline ointment, as appropriate.

Proprietary Preparations of Betamethasone and its Esters

Betnelan *(Glaxo, UK)*. *Tablets*, scored, betamethasone 500 µg.

Betnesol *(Glaxo, UK)*. *Tablets*, soluble, scored, betamethasone 500 µg (as sodium phosphate).
Injection, betamethasone 4 mg (as sodium phosphate)/mL, in ampoules of 1 mL.
Drops, for eye, ear, or nose, betamethasone sodium phosphate 0.1%.
Eye ointment, betamethasone sodium phosphate 0.1%.

Betnesol-N *(Glaxo, UK)*. *Drops*, for eye, ear, or nose, betamethasone sodium phosphate 0.1%, neomycin sulphate 0.5%.
Eye ointment, betamethasone sodium phosphate 0.1%, neomycin sulphate 0.5%.

Betnovate *(Glaxo, UK)*. *Cream, Lotion, Ointment, Scalp application*, betamethasone 0.1% (as valerate).

Betnovate RD (Ready Diluted) *(Glaxo, UK)*. *Cream, Ointment*, betamethasone 0.025% (as valerate).

Betnovate Rectal Ointment *(Glaxo, UK)*. *Ointment*, betamethasone valerate 0.05%, lignocaine hydrochloride 2.5%, phenylephrine hydrochloride 0.1%.

Betnovate-C *(Glaxo, UK)*. *Cream, Ointment*, betamethasone 0.1% (as valerate), clioquinol 3%.

Betnovate-N *(Glaxo, UK)*. *Cream, Ointment*, betamethasone 0.1% (as valerate), neomycin sulphate 0.5%.

Bextasol Inhaler *(Glaxo, UK)*. *Inhaler*, aerosol, betamethasone valerate 100 µg/metered inhalation.

Diprosalic *(Kirby-Warrick, UK)*. *Ointment*, betamethasone 0.05% (as dipropionate), salicylic acid 3%.
Scalp application, betamethasone 0.05% (as dipropionate), salicylic acid 2%.

Diprosone *(Kirby-Warrick, UK)*. *Cream, Lotion, Ointment*, betamethasone 0.05% (as dipropionate).

Fucibet *(Leo, UK)*. *Cream*, betamethasone 0.1% (as valerate), fusidic acid 2%.

Lotriderm *(Kirby-Warrick, UK)*. *Cream*, betamethasone 0.05% (as dipropionate), clotrimazole 1%.

Vista-Methasone *(Richard Daniel, UK)*. *Drops*, for eye, ear, or nose, betamethasone sodium phosphate 0.1%.

Vista-Methasone N *(Richard Daniel, UK)*. *Drops*, for eye, ear, or nose, betamethasone sodium phosphate 0.1%, neomycin sulphate 0.5%.

Proprietary Names and Manufacturers of Betamethasone and its Esters

Alphatrex *(Savage, USA)*; Bebate *(Warner, UK)*; Beben *(Parke, Davis, Canad.; Parke, Davis, Ital.; Substantia, Neth.)*; Bedermin *(Damor, Ital.)*; Benisone *(Cooper Dermatology, USA)*; Bentelan *(Glaxo, Ital.)*; Beta 21 *(IDI, Ital.)*; Betacort *(ICN, Canad.)*; Betaderm *(Taro, Canad.)*; Betadival *(Ital.)*; Betafluorene *(Ital.)*; Betallorens *(Spain)*; Betamamallet *(Jpn)*; Betamatil *(Dibios, Spain)*; Betameson *(Ital.)*; Betapred *(Glaxo, Swed.)*; Betasona *(Venez.)*; Betatrex *(Savage, USA)*; Beta-Val *(Lemmon, USA)*; Betnasol *(Col.; Peru; Port.)*; Betnelan *(Belg.; Glaxo, Canad.; Neth.; Glaxo, S.Afr.; Spain; Glaxo, UK)*; Betnelan-V *(Belg.; Lux.; Neth.)*; Betnesol *(Glaxo, Canad.; Schering Corp., Denm.; Glaxo, Fr.; Glaxo, Ger.; Neth.; Glaxo, S.Afr.; Glaxo, Switz.; Glaxo, UK)*; Betnesol-V *(Glaxo, Ger.)*; Betneval *(Glaxo, Fr.)*; Betnevate *(Jpn)*; Betnovat *(Glaxo, Denm.; Glaxo, Norw.; Glaxo, Swed.; Turk.)*; Betnovate *(Glaxo, Austral.; Glaxo, Canad.; Glaxo, S.Afr.; Glaxo, Spain; Glaxo, Switz.; Glaxo, UK)*; Bextasol *(Glaxo, UK)*; Bifosona *(Arg.)*; Célestène *(Unicet, Fr.)*; Celestan *(Essex, Ger.)*; Celestan-V *(Essex, Ger.)*; Celestoderm *(Unicet, Fr.; Neth.; Schering, Norw.; Essex, Spain)*; Celestoderm-V *(Arg.; Belg.; Schering, Canad.; Essex, Ital.; Scherag, S.Afr.; Essex, Switz.)*; Celeston *(Schering Corp., Denm.; Schering, Norw.)*; Celestona *(Schering, Swed.)*; Celestone *(Arg.; Essex, Austral.; Belg.; Schering, Canad.; Essex, Ital.; Neth.; Scherag, S.Afr.; Essex, Spain; Essex, Switz.; Schering, USA)*; Corteroid *(Arg.)*; Cortico LG *(Aandersen, Ital.)*; Cuantin *(Spain)*; Cuantona *(Mabo, Spain)*; Dermizol *(Roux-Ocefa, Arg.)*; Dermosol *(Jpn)*; Dermovaleas *(Valeas, Ital.)*; Desacort-Beta *(Ital.)*; Diprocort *(Essex, Switz.)*; Diproderm *(Schering Corp., Denm.; Essex, Spain; Schering, Swed.)*; Diprolène *(Unicet, Fr.; Essex, Switz.)*; Diprolen *(Schering Corp., Denm.)*; Diprolene *(Schering, Canad.; Schering, S.Afr.; Schering, USA)*; Diprophos *(Essex, Switz.)*; Diprosis *(Essex, Ger.)*; Diprosone *(Essex, Arg.; Essex, Austral.; Schering, Belg.; Schering, Canad.; Unicet, Fr.; Essex, Ger.; Essex, Ital.; Essex, NZ; Scherag, S.Afr.; Essex, Switz.; Kirby-Warrick, UK; Schering, USA)*; Diprospan *(Schering Corp., Denm.)*; Durabetason *(Durachemie, Ger.)*; Ecoval *(Glaxo, Ital.)*; Ectosone *(Technilab, Canad.)*; Emilan *(Perkins, Ital.)*; Euvaderm *(Sasse, Ger.)*; Hormezon *(Jpn)*; Linolosal *(Jpn)*; Maxivate *(Westwood, USA)*; Metaderm *(Desbergers, Canad.)*; Minisone *(IDI, Ital.)*; Muhibeta-V *(Jpn)*; No-Reumar *(Ital.)*; Novobetamet *(Novopharm, Canad.)*; P 10 Pomata *(Pulitzer, Ital.)*; Parbetan *(Parke, Davis, Spain)*; Paucisone *(ITA, Ital.)*; Persivate *(Lennon, S.Afr.)*; Pertene *(Ital.)*; Rinderon *(Jpn)*; Rolazote *(Arg.)*; Sclane *(Llorente, Spain)*; Skincort *(Parke, Davis, S.Afr.)*; Solu-Celeston *(Schering Corp., Denm.)*; Uticort *(Parke, Davis, USA)*; Valisone *(Schering, Canad.; Schering, USA)*; Viobeta *(IDI, Ital.)*; Vista-Methasone *(Richard Daniel, UK)*; Visubeta *(Merck Sharp & Dohme, Spain)*.

The following names have been used for multi-ingredient preparations containing betamethasone or its esters—Betnesol-N *(Glaxo, UK)*; Betnovate Compound Suppositories *(Glaxo, UK)*; Betnovate Rectal Ointment *(Glaxo, UK)*; Betnovate-A *(Glaxo, Austral.; Glaxo, UK)*; Betnovate-C *(Glaxo, Austral.; Glaxo, UK)*; Betnovate-N *(Glaxo, Austral.; Glaxo, Canad.; Glaxo, UK)*; Celestone Chronodose *(Essex, Austral.)*; Celestone Soluspan *(Sch-*

ering, Canad.; *Schering, USA*); Celestone-S (*Schering, Canad.*); Celestone-VG (*Essex, Austral.*); Diprogen (*Schering, Canad.*); Diprosalic (*Schering, Canad.*; *Kirby-Warrick, UK*); Diprosone-F (*Essex, Austral.*); Fucibet (*Leo, UK*); Garasone (*Schering, Canad.*); Lotriderm (*Kirby-Warrick, UK*); Lotrisone (*Schering, USA*); Valisone-G (*Schering, Canad.*); Vista-Methasone N (*Richard Daniel, UK*).

12463-p

Budesonide (*BAN, USAN, rINN*).

S-1320. An epimeric mixture of the α- and β-propyl forms of 16α,17α-butylidenedioxy-11β,21-dihydroxypregna-1,4-diene-3,20-dione.
$C_{25}H_{34}O_6$=430.5.

CAS — 51333-22-3 (11β,16α); 51372-29-3 (11β,16α(R)); 51372-28-2 (11β,16α(S)).

Adverse Effects, Treatment, Withdrawal, and Precautions

As for corticosteroids, p.872.

Psychosis in a child inhaling budesonide.— L. D. Lewis and G. M. Cochrane (letter), *Lancet*, 1983, *2*, 634.

Absorption and Fate

For a brief outline of the absorption and fate of corticosteroids, see p.875.

Uses and Administration

Budesonide is a glucocorticoid used as a nasal spray for the prophylaxis and treatment of allergic rhinitis. It is used in a usual initial dose of 100 μg into each nostril twice daily, subsequently reduced to the lowest dose adequate to control symptoms which may be 50 μg into each nostril twice daily.
Budesonide is also used by inhalation from a metered aerosol in the management of asthma. The usual adult dosage is 200 μg inhaled twice daily; in severe asthma the dosage may be increased but should not exceed a total of 1.2 mg daily. A suggested dose for children is 50 to 200 μg inhaled twice daily.

Proprietary Preparations

Pulmicort (*Astra, UK*). *Inhaler*, aerosol, budesonide 200 μg/metered inhalation.

Pulmicort LS (*Astra, UK*). *Inhaler*, aerosol, budesonide 50 μg/metered inhalation.

Rhinocort (*Astra, UK*). *Nasal spray*, aerosol, budesonide 50 μg/metered dose.

Proprietary Names and Manufacturers

Preferid (*Gist-Brocades, Denm.*; *Gist-Brocades, Swed.*); Pulmicort (*Astra, Ger.*; *Draco, Swed.*; *Astra, Switz.*; *Astra, UK*); Rhinocort (*Draco, Denm.*; *Draco, Swed.*; *Astra, Switz.*; *Astra, UK*); Spirocort (*Draco, Denm.*).

1069-x

Clobetasol Propionate (*BANM, USAN, rINNM*).

CCI-4725; GR2/925. 21-Chloro-9α-fluoro-11β,17α-dihydroxy-16β-methylpregna-1,4-diene-3,20-dione 17-propionate.
$C_{25}H_{32}ClFO_5$=467.0.

CAS — 25122-41-2 (clobetasol); 25122-46-7 (propionate).

Adverse Effects, Treatment, Withdrawal, and Precautions

As for corticosteroids, p.872.
When applied topically, particularly to large areas, when the skin is broken, or under occlusive dressings, corticosteroids may be absorbed in sufficient amounts to cause systemic effects.

Absorption and Fate

For a brief outline of the absorption and fate of corticosteroids, see p.875.

Uses and Administration

Clobetasol propionate is a corticosteroid used topically in the treatment of various skin disorders, as described under corticosteroids (see p.876). It is usually employed as a cream, ointment, or scalp application containing 0.05%.

SKIN DISORDERS. For recommendations concerning the correct use of corticosteroids on the skin, and a rough guide to the clinical potencies of topical corticosteroids, see Corticosteroids, p.880.

Proprietary Preparations

Dermovate (*Glaxo, UK*). *Cream, Ointment, Scalp application*, clobetasol propionate 0.05%.

Dermovate-NN (*Glaxo, UK*). *Cream, Ointment*, clobetasol propionate 0.05%, neomycin sulphate 0.5%, nystatin 100 000 units/g.

Proprietary Names and Manufacturers

Butavat (*Greece*); Clobesol (*Glaxo, Ital.*); Clovate (*Glaxo, Spain*); Decloban (*Cusi, Spain*); Dermadex (*Arg.*); Dermatovate (*Mex.*); Dermoval (*Glaxo, Fr.*); Dermovat (*Glaxo, Denm.*; *Fin.*; *Glaxo, Norw.*; *Glaxo, Swed.*); Dermovate (*Belg.*; *Glaxo, Canad.*; *Jpn*; *Neth.*; *Glaxo, S.Afr.*; *Glaxo, Switz.*; *Glaxo, UK*); Dermoxin (*Glaxo, Ger.*); Dermoxinale (*Glaxo, Ger.*); Temovate (*Glaxo, USA*).

1070-y

Clobetasone Butyrate (*BANM, USAN, rINNM*).

CCI-5537; GR2/1214. 21-Chloro-9α-fluoro-17α-hydroxy-16β-methylpregna-1,4-diene-3,11,20-trione 17-butyrate.
$C_{26}H_{32}ClFO_5$=479.0.

CAS — 54063-32-0 (clobetasone); 25122-57-0 (butyrate).

Adverse Effects, Treatment, Withdrawal, and Precautions

As for corticosteroids, p.872.
When applied topically, particularly to large areas, when the skin is broken, or under occlusive dressings, corticosteroids may be absorbed in sufficient amounts to cause systemic effects.

Absorption and Fate

For a brief outline of the absorption and fate of corticosteroids, see p.875.

Uses and Administration

Clobetasone butyrate is a corticosteroid used topically in the treatment of various skin disorders, as described under corticosteroids (see p.876). It is usually employed as a cream or ointment containing 0.05% and is also used as eye-drops containing 0.1%.

SKIN DISORDERS. For recommendations concerning the correct use of corticosteroids on the skin, and a rough guide to the clinical potencies of topical corticosteroids, see Corticosteroids, p.880.

Proprietary Preparations

Eumovate (formerly known as Molivate) (*Glaxo, UK*). *Cream, Ointment*, clobetasone butyrate 0.05%. *Eye-drops*, clobetasone butyrate 0.1%.

Eumovate-N (*Glaxo, UK*). *Eye-drops*, clobetasone butyrate 0.1%, neomycin sulphate 0.5%.

Trimovate (*Glaxo, UK*). *Cream*, clobetasone butyrate 0.05%, oxytetracycline 3% (as calcium salt), nystatin 100 000 units/g.
Ointment, clobetasone butyrate 0.05%, chlortetracycline hydrochloride 3%, nystatin 100 000 units/g.

Proprietary Names and Manufacturers

Cloptison (*Chibret, Switz.*); Emovat (*Glaxo, Denm.*; *Glaxo, Swed.*); Emovate (*Glaxo, Ger.*; *Neth.*; *Glaxo, Spain*; *Glaxo, Switz.*); Eumovate (*Glaxo, Austral.*; *Glaxo, Canad.*; *Glaxo, Ital.*; *Glaxo, S.Afr.*; *Glaxo, UK*).

12584-k

Clocortolone Pivalate (*USAN, rINNM*).

SH-863. 9α-Chloro-6α-fluoro-11β,21-dihydroxy-16α-methylpregna-1,4-diene-3,20-dione 21-pivalate.
$C_{27}H_{36}ClFO_5$=495.0.

CAS — 4828-27-7 (clocortolone); 34097-16-0 (pivalate).

Pharmacopoeias. In *U.S.*

A white to yellowish-white odourless powder. **Soluble** in acetone; freely soluble in chloroform and dioxan; sparingly soluble in alcohol; slightly soluble in ether. **Store** in airtight containers. Protect from light.

Clocortolone pivalate is a corticosteroid with the general properties described under corticosteroids (see p.872). It has been used topically in the treatment of various skin disorders.
When applied topically, particularly to large areas, where the skin is broken, or under occlusive dressings, corticosteroids may be absorbed in sufficient amounts to cause systemic effects.
For recommendations concerning the correct use of corticosteroids on the skin, see Corticosteroids, p.880.

Preparations

Clocortolone Pivalate Cream (*U.S.P.*)

Proprietary Names and Manufacturers

Cloderm (*Ortho Dermatological, USA*); Kaban (*Asche, Ger.*); Kabanimat (*Asche, Ger.*); Purantix (*Schering, Ital.*; *Sandoz, Spain*; *Wander, Switz.*).

1072-z

Cortisone Acetate (*BANM, USAN, rINNM*).

11-Dehydro-17-hydroxycorticosterone Acetate; Compound E Acetate; Cortisoni Acetas.
17α,21-Dihydroxypregn-4-ene-3,11,20-trione 21-acetate.
$C_{23}H_{30}O_6$=402.5.

CAS — 53-06-5 (cortisone); 50-04-4 (acetate).

Pharmacopoeias. In *Arg., Aust., Belg., Br., Braz., Chin., Egypt., Eur., Fr., Ger., Ind., Int., It., Jpn, Jug., Neth., Nord., Pol., Port., Roum., Rus., Swiss, Turk.*, and *U.S.*

A white or almost white, odourless, crystalline powder. Practically **insoluble** in water; soluble 1 in 350 of alcohol, 1 in 75 of acetone, 1 in 4 of chloroform, and 1 in 30 of dioxan; slightly soluble in ether and methyl alcohol. **Store** in well-closed containers. Protect from light.

Adverse Effects, Treatment, Withdrawal, and Precautions

As for corticosteroids, p.872.

Absorption and Fate

For a brief outline of the absorption and fate of corticosteroids, see p.875.
Cortisone acetate is readily absorbed from the gastro-intestinal tract and the cortisone is rapidly converted in the liver to its active metabolite, hydrocortisone (cortisol). The biological half-life of cortisone itself is only about 30 minutes. Absorption of cortisone acetate from intramuscular sites is considerably slower than following oral administration.

Uses and Administration

Cortisone is a glucocorticoid secreted by the adrenal cortex and has the general properties described under corticosteroids (p.875).
Cortisone acetate is rapidly effective when given by mouth, and more slowly by intramuscular injection.
Cortisone acetate has appreciable mineralocorticoid properties and has been used mainly for replacement therapy in Addison's disease or chronic adrenocortical insufficiency secondary to hypopituitarism. The normal daily requirement has ranged from 10 to 50 mg of cortisone acetate by mouth in divided doses. Hydrocortisone (p.894) is now generally preferred since cortisone itself is inactive and must be converted by the liver to hydrocortisone, its active metabolite; hence, in some liver disorders its bioavailability is less reliable. Additional sodium chloride may be required if there is defective aldosterone secretion, but mineralocorticoid activity is usually supplemented by fludrocortisone acetate by mouth. Acute adrenal insufficiency should be treated with a glucocorticoid such as hydrocortisone given intravenously.
Cortisone acetate has been used in the treatment of many allergic and inflammatory disorders but

prednisolone or other synthetic glucocorticoids are generally preferred because of their reduced sodium-retaining properties. Doses of cortisone acetate employed have generally ranged from about 20 to 300 mg daily by mouth or by intramuscular injection. It is ineffective when injected into joint capsules or applied to the skin.

Preparations

Cortisone Injection *(B.P.)*. Cortisone Acetate Injection. A sterile suspension of cortisone acetate, in water for injections, prepared using aseptic technique. It must not be given intravenously. Store at a temperature not exceeding 25° and avoid freezing.

Cortisone Tablets *(B.P.)*. Tablets containing cortisone acetate in fine powder.

Cortisone Acetate Tablets *(U.S.P.)*

Sterile Cortisone Acetate Suspension *(U.S.P.)*

Proprietary Preparations

Cortelan *(Glaxo, UK)*. *Tablets*, scored, cortisone acetate 25 mg.

Cortisone Acetate *(Merck Sharp & Dohme, UK)*. *Tablets*, cortisone acetate 5 mg.
Tablets, scored, cortisone acetate 25 mg.

Cortistab *(Boots, UK)*. *Tablets*, cortisone acetate 5 and 25 mg.
Injection, cortisone acetate 25 mg/mL in ampoules of 10 mL.

Cortisyl *(Roussel, UK)*. *Tablets*, scored, cortisone acetate 25 mg.

Proprietary Names and Manufacturers

Acetisone *(Ital.)*; Adreson *(Belg.; Neth.)*; Altesona *(Alter, Spain)*; Corlin *(Ind.)*; Cortal *(Organon, Swed.)*; Cortate *(Protea, Austral.)*; Cortelan *(Glaxo, UK)*; Cortemel *(S.Afr.)*; Cortisol *(Ital.)*; Cortistab *(Boots, UK)*; Cortisyl *(Roussel, UK)*; Cortogen *(Scherag, S.Afr.)*; Cortone *(Austral.; Merck Sharp & Dohme, Canad.; Merck Sharp & Dohme, Norw.; MSD, Swed.; Merck Sharp & Dohme, USA)*; Cortone Acetat *(Denm.)*; Cortone Acetato *(Merck Sharp & Dohme, Ital.)*; Kortison *(Denm.)*; Sterop *(Austral.)*.

NOTE. The name cortisol is also applied to endogenous hydrocortisone.

1073-c

Cortivazol *(USAN, pINN)*.

H-3625; NSC-80998. 11β,17α,21-Trihydroxy-6,16α-dimethyl-2′-phenyl-2′*H*-pregna-2,4,6-trieno[3,2-*c*]-pyrazol-20-one 21-acetate.
$C_{32}H_{38}N_2O_5$=530.7.

CAS — 1110-40-3.

Cortivazol is a glucocorticoid with the general properties described under corticosteroids (see p.872). It has been given by mouth in doses of about 0.4 to 3.2 mg daily, and by intra-articular injection in doses of about 1.25 to 3.75 mg, according to the size of the joint, usually at intervals of one to three weeks.

Proprietary Names and Manufacturers

Altim *(Roussel, Fr.)*; Diaster *(Diamant, Fr.)*; Dilaster *(Roussel, Spain)*; Idaltim *(Roussel, Arg.)*.

12627-l

Deflazacort *(BAN, rINN)*.

Azacort; DL-458-IT; L-5458; MDL-458; Oxazacort. 11β,21-Dihydroxy-2′-methyl-5′βH-pregna-1,4-dieno-[17,16-*d*]oxazole-3,20-dione 21-acetate.
$C_{25}H_{31}NO_6$=441.5.

CAS — 14484-47-0.

Deflazacort is a glucocorticoid with the general properties described under corticosteroids (see p.872). It has been given by mouth in doses of about 6 to 60 mg daily.

Proprietary Names and Manufacturers

Deflan *(Guidotti, Ital.)*; Flantadin *(Lepetit, Ital.)*.

1075-a

Deoxycortone Acetate *(BANM)*.

Cortin; Decortone Acetate; Deoxycorticosterone Acetate; Desoxycorticosterone Acetate *(USAN)*; Desoxycortone Acetate *(rINNM)*; Desoxycortoni Acetas. 21-Hydroxypregn-4-ene-3,20-dione 21-acetate.
$C_{23}H_{32}O_4$=372.5.

CAS — 64-85-7 (deoxycortone); 56-47-3 (acetate).

Pharmacopoeias. In *Arg., Aust., Belg., Br., Braz., Cz., Eur., Egypt., Fr., Ger., Hung., Ind., Int., It., Jug., Mex., Neth., Nord., Pol., Port., Roum., Rus., Swiss, Turk.,* and *U.S.*

Odourless colourless crystals or white or creamy-white crystalline powder. Practically **insoluble** in water; soluble 1 in 50 of alcohol, 1 in 30 of acetone; freely soluble in chloroform; slightly soluble in vegetable oils. **Store** in well-closed containers. Protect from light.

1074-k

Deoxycortone Pivalate *(BANM)*.

Deoxycorticosterone Trimethylacetate; Deoxycortone Trimethylacetate; Desoxycorticosterone Pivalate *(USAN)*; Desoxycorticosterone Trimethylacetate; Desoxycortone Pivalate *(rINNM)*. 21-Hydroxypregn-4-ene-3,20-dione 21-pivalate.
$C_{26}H_{38}O_4$=414.6.

CAS — 808-48-0.

Pharmacopoeias. In *U.S.* Also in *B.P.C. 1973.*

A white or creamy-white, odourless crystalline powder. Practically **insoluble** in water; soluble 1 in 500 of alcohol, 1 in 3 of chloroform, and 1 in 640 of ether; sparingly soluble in acetone; slightly soluble in methyl alcohol and vegetable oils. **Protect** from light.

Adverse Effects and Precautions

As for corticosteroids, pp.872-3. Overdoses of deoxycortone acetate may produce excessive sodium and water retention, leading to hypertension, oedema, pulmonary congestion, and signs and symptoms of congestive heart failure. Salt restriction is advisable in such cases. Excessive loss of potassium may result in muscular weakness and paralysis.

EFFECTS ON BONES AND JOINTS. Reports of joint pains in patients given deoxycortone acetate alone: K. Kirkeby, *Acta med. scand.*, 1954, *149*, 43.

Uses and Administration

Deoxycortone is a mineralocorticoid secreted by the adrenal cortex and has the general properties of mineralocorticoids described under corticosteroids (see p.875). It has a pronounced effect on sodium retention and potassium excretion but no significant glucocorticoid action. It is destroyed in the gastro-intestinal tract and has only a feeble action when given by mouth.

Deoxycortone, as the acetate or pivalate, has been used in the treatment of Addison's disease and other adrenocortical deficiency states as an adjunct to cortisone or hydrocortisone when these substances alone did not prevent the development of sodium deficiency. For this purpose, however, fludrocortisone given by mouth is now usually preferred.

Deoxycortone acetate has usually been administered as a subcutaneous implant, containing about 125 mg; the duration of action is reported to be between 8 and 12 months. It has also been given as an oily intramuscular injection. Deoxycortone pivalate has usually been given as an intramuscular injection of 25 to 100 mg every 4 weeks.

Preparations of Deoxycortone Esters

Desoxycorticosterone Acetate Pellets *(U.S.P.)*. Sterile implants of compressed deoxycortone acetate.

Desoxycorticosterone Acetate Injection *(U.S.P.)*. A sterile solution of deoxycortone acetate in vegetable oil.

Sterile Desoxycorticosterone Pivalate Suspension *(U.S.P.)*. A sterile suspension of deoxycortone pivalate in an aqueous vehicle.

Proprietary Names and Manufacturers of Deoxycortone Esters

Cortexon *(Schering, Arg.)*; Corticosterone *(Mitim, Ital.)*; Cortiron *(Schering, Ger.; Schering, Ital.; Schering, Spain)*; Cortisteril *(Ital Suisse, Ital.)*; Cortisteron *(Streuli, Switz.)*; Cortitron *(Schering, Ital.)*; Deoxycortone Acetate Implants *(Organon, UK)*; Desoxykorton *(DAK, Denm.)*; Doca *(Organon, Neth.; Organon, Swed.; Organon, USA)*; Leocortex *(Leo, Spain)*; Neodin Depositum *(Lusofarmaco, Ital.)*; Ormossurenol *(Ital.)*; Percorten *(Ciba, Canad.; Ciba, Spain)*; Percorten Acetate *(Ciba, USA)*; Percorten Hidrosoluble *(Ciba, Spain)*; Percorten M *(Neth.; Spain)*; Percorten M Crystules *(Ciba, UK)*; Percorten Pivalate *(Ciba, USA)*; Percorten wasserlöslich *(Ciba, Ger.)*; Percortene *(Belg.; Ciba, Switz.)*; Percortene M *(Belg.; Ciba, Switz.)*; Syncorta *(Jpn)*; Syncortyl *(Roussel, Fr.)*.

The following names have been used for multi-ingredient preparations containing deoxycortone esters—Plex-Hormone Injection *(Consolidated Chemicals, UK)*; Plex-Hormone Tablets *(Consolidated Chemicals, UK)*.

1076-t

Desonide *(BAN, USAN, rINN)*.

16-Hydroxyprednisolone 16,17-Acetonide; D2083; Desfluorotriamcinolone Acetonide. 11β,21-Dihydroxy-16α,17α-isopropylidenedioxypregna-1,4-diene-3,20-dione.
$C_{24}H_{32}O_6$=416.5.

CAS — 638-94-8.

Adverse Effects, Treatment, Withdrawal, and Precautions

As for corticosteroids, p.872.

When applied topically, particularly to large areas, when the skin is broken, or under occlusive dressings, corticosteroids may be absorbed in sufficient amounts to cause systemic effects.

Absorption and Fate

For a brief outline of the absorption and fate of corticosteroids, see p.875.

Uses and Administration

Desonide is a corticosteroid used topically in the treatment of various skin disorders, as described under corticosteroids (see p.876). It is usually employed as a cream or ointment or ear-drops containing 0.05%.

The pivalate ester has also been used in dermatological preparations and the sodium phosphate in ophthalmological preparations.

SKIN DISORDERS. For recommendations concerning the correct use of corticosteroids on the skin, and a rough guide to the clinical potencies of topical corticosteroids, see corticosteroids, p.880.

Proprietary Preparations

Tridesilon *(Lagap, UK)*. *Cream*,, desonide 0.05%.

Proprietary Names and Manufacturers

Apolar *(Apothekernes Laboratorium, Norw.; A.L., Swed.)*; Desowen *(Owen, USA)*; Locapred *(Pierre Fabre, Fr.)*; PR 100 *(Farmacologico Milanese, Ital.)*; Prenacid *(SIFI, Ital.)*; Reticus *(Farmila, Ital.)*; Sine-Fluor *(Knoll-Made, Spain)*; Sterax *(Alcon, Ger.; Alcon, S.Afr.; Alcon, Switz.)*; Steroderm *(Ital.)*; Topifug *(Wolff, Ger.)*; Tridésonit *(Dome-Hollister-Stier, Fr.)*; Tridesilon *(Miles, Canad.; Klinge, Ger.; Lagap, UK; Miles Pharmaceuticals, USA)*.

The following names have been used for multi-ingredient preparations containing desonide— Tridesilon Otic *(Miles Pharmaceuticals, USA)*.

1077-x

Desoxymethasone *(BAN)*.

A41-304; Desoximetasone *(USAN, rINN)*; Hoe-304; R-2113. 9α-Fluoro-11β,21-dihydroxy-16α-methylpregna-1,4-diene-3,20-dione.

$C_{22}H_{29}FO_4$=376.5.

CAS — 382-67-2.

Pharmacopoeias. In *U.S.*

A white or almost white, odourless, crystalline powder. Practically **insoluble** in water; freely soluble in alcohol, acetone, and chloroform.

Adverse Effects, Treatment, Withdrawal, and Precautions

As for corticosteroids, p.872.

When applied topically, particularly to large areas, when the skin is broken, or under occlusive dressings, corticosteroids may be absorbed in sufficient amounts to cause systemic effects.

Absorption and Fate

For a brief outline of the absorption and fate of corticosteroids, see p.875.

Uses and Administration

Desoxymethasone is a corticosteroid used topically in the treatment of various skin disorders, as described under corticosteroids (see p.876). It is usually employed as a cream, gel, or ointment; concentrations used range from 0.05% to 0.25%.

SKIN DISORDERS. For recommendations concerning the correct use of corticosteroids on the skin, and a rough guide to the clinical potencies of topical corticosteroids, see corticosteroids, p.880.

Preparations

Desoximetasone Cream *(U.S.P.).* Contains desoxymethasone.

Desoximetasone Gel *(U.S.P.).* Contains desoxymethasone.

Desoximetasone Ointment *(U.S.P.).* Contains desoxymethasone.

Proprietary Preparations

Stiedex *(Stiefel, UK). Oily cream,* desoxymethasone 0.25%.

Stiedex LP *(Stiefel, UK). Oily cream,* desoxymethasone 0.05%.

Stiedex LPN *(Stiefel, UK). Oily cream,* desoxymethasone 0.05%, neomycin 0.5% (as sulphate).

Proprietary Names and Manufacturers

Actiderm *(Hoechst, Arg.)*; Flubason *(Albert-Farma, Ital.; Hoechst, Spain)*; Ibaril *(Hoechst, Belg.; Hoechst, Denm.; Hoechst, Neth.; Hoechst, Norw.; Hoechst, Swed.)*; Stiedex *(Stiefel, UK)*; Topicorete *(Roussel, Belg.)*; Topicort *(Hoechst, Canad.; Roussel Maestretti, Ital.; Hoechst, USA)*; Topicorte *(Roussel, Fr.; Roussel, Neth.)*; Topiderm *(Roussel, Spain)*; Topisolon *(Cassella-Riedel, Ger.; Hoechst, S.Afr.; Hoechst, Switz.)*.

1084-t

Dexamethasone *(BAN, USAN, rINN).*

9α-Fluoro-16α-methylprednisolone; Desamethasone; Dexametasona; Dexamethasonum. 9α-Fluoro-11β,17α,21-trihydroxy-16α-methylpregna-1,4-diene-3,20-dione.

$C_{22}H_{29}FO_5$=392.5.

CAS — 50-02-2.

Pharmacopoeias. In *Aust., Br., Braz., Cz., Egypt., Eur., Fr., Ger., Ind., Int., It., Jpn, Jug., Neth., Roum., Swiss, Turk.,* and *U.S.* Also in *B.P. Vet.*

A white or almost white odourless crystalline powder. Practically **insoluble** in water; sparingly soluble in alcohol, acetone, dioxan, and methyl alcohol; slightly soluble in chloroform; very slightly soluble in ether. **Store** in well-closed containers. Protect from light.

1079-f

Dexamethasone Acetate *(BANM, USAN, rINNM).*

Dexamethasone 21-acetate.

$C_{24}H_{31}FO_6$=434.5.

CAS — 1177-87-3 (anhydrous); 55812-90-3 (monohydrate).

Pharmacopoeias. In *Chin.* and *Eur. Int.* and *U.S.* allow the anhydrous form or the monohydrate.

A clear white to off-white odourless powder. Dexamethasone acetate 1.1 mg is approximately equivalent to 1 mg of dexamethasone. Practically **insoluble** in water; freely soluble in acetone, dioxan, and methyl alcohol.

1080-z

Dexamethasone Isonicotinate *(BANM).*

Dexamethasone 21-isonicotinate.

$C_{28}H_{32}FNO_6$=497.6.

CAS — 2265-64-7.

Dexamethasone isonicotinate 1.3 mg is approximately equivalent to 1 mg of dexamethasone.

1083-a

Dexamethasone Sodium Metasulphobenzoate *(BANM).*

Dexamethasone 21-(sodium *m*-sulphobenzoate).

$C_{29}H_{32}FNaO_9S$=598.6.

CAS — 3936-02-5.

Dexamethasone sodium metasulphobenzoate 1.5 mg is approximately equivalent to 1 mg of dexamethasone.

1078-r

Dexamethasone Sodium Phosphate *(BANM, USAN, rINNM).*

Dexamethasone Phosphate Sodium; Sodium Dexamethasone Phosphate. Dexamethasone 21-(disodium orthophosphate).

$C_{22}H_{28}FNa_2O_8P$=516.4.

CAS — 2392-39-4.

Pharmacopoeias. In *Br., Braz., Chin., Eur., Ind., Jug.,* and *U.S.* Also in *B.P. Vet.*

A white or slightly yellow, very hygroscopic, crystalline powder; odourless or with a slight odour of alcohol. Dexamethasone sodium phosphate 1.3 mg is approximately equivalent to 1 mg of dexamethasone and 1.1 mg of dexamethasone sodium phosphate is approximately equivalent to 1 mg of dexamethasone phosphate.

Soluble 1 in 2 of water; slightly soluble in alcohol; sparingly soluble in dehydrated alcohol; practically insoluble in chloroform and ether; very slightly soluble in dioxan. The *B.P.* states that a 1% solution in water has a pH of 7.5 to 9.5; the *U.S.P.* specifies a pH of between 7.5 and 10.5. **Store** in airtight containers. Protect from light.

Adverse Effects, Treatment, Withdrawal, and Precautions

As for corticosteroids, p.872.

It has little or no effect on sodium and water retention.

INTERACTIONS. Some comments on the interaction between dexamethasone and phenytoin which results in reduced dexamethasone activity: I. Stockley, *Pharm. J.*, 1982, *1*, 515; *Drug Interact. News.*, 1985, *5*, 51; D. D. Wong *et al.* (letter), *J. Am. med. Ass.*, 1985, *254*, 2062.

PARAESTHESIA. A single dose of dexamethasone sodium phosphate 2 mg per kg body-weight given by intravenous infusion at various rates to 30 healthy subjects in a double-blind controlled study produced temporary itching, burning, or tingling, which was most intense in the ano-genital region, in all subjects given the infusion over 2 minutes. This effect was less frequent when the duration of administration was prolonged. Laboratory studies showed no untoward results apart from the expected hyperglycaemic effect.— A. W. Czerwinski *et al.*, *Clin. Pharmac. Ther.*, 1972, *13*, 638. In a study of 42 healthy subjects, side-effects were more common in those given hydrocortisone sodium phosphate with 16 of 18 subjects experiencing ano-rectal itching or burning compared with none of 18 in the hydrocortisone sodium succinate group, and 1 of 6 in the placebo group. The effect was observed within 10 seconds to 6 minutes after the start of administration.— E. Novak *et al.*, *ibid.*, 1976, *20*, 109. Comment on paraesthesia associated with intravenous injection of hydrocortisone sodium phosphate; the phosphate ester should not be used.— *Drug & Ther. Bull.*, 1979, *17*, 71. Further comments on reports of paraesthesia or perineal irritation associated with corticosteroids administered intravenously. The cause of this unusual side-effect remains unclear and is unlikely to be related to the phosphate ion itself although the corticosteroid phosphate ester may be responsible.— V. L. Thomas (letter), *New Engl. J. Med.*, 1986, *314*, 1643. Mention that dilution of dexamethasone sodium phosphate in physiological saline and administration by slow intravenous infusion abolished this side-effect.— S. G. Allan and R. C. F. Leonard (letter), *Lancet*, 1986, *1*, 1035.

Further references to itching and paraesthesia associated with corticosteroids: D. Barltrop and Y. T. Diba (letter), *Lancet*, 1969, *1*, 529 (hydrocortisone sodium phosphate); E. S. Snell (letter), *ibid.*, 530 (hydrocortisone sodium phosphate); N. G. Kounis (letter), *Br. med. J.*, 1973, *2*, 663 (hydrocortisone sodium phosphate); E. Baharav *et al.* (letter), *New Engl. J. Med.*, 1986, *314*, 515 (dexamethasone sodium phosphate); G. P. Sartiano *et al.* (letter), *ibid.*, 1644 (dexamethasone sodium phosphate).

Absorption and Fate

For a brief outline of the absorption and fate of corticosteroids, see p.875.

Dexamethasone is readily absorbed from the gastro-intestinal tract. Its biological half-life in plasma is about 190 minutes. Binding of dexamethasone to plasma proteins is less than for most other corticosteroids.

References to the pharmacokinetics of dexamethasone and its esters: J. McCafferty *et al.* (letter), *Br. J. clin. Pharmac.*, 1981, *12*, 434; T. R. O'R. Brophy, *Eur. J. clin. Pharmac.*, 1983, *24*, 103.

Uses and Administration

Dexamethasone is a glucocorticoid and has the general properties described under corticosteroids (see p.875); 750 µg of dexamethasone is equivalent in anti-inflammatory activity to about 5 mg of prednisolone.

It has been used, either in the form of the free alcohol or in one of the esterified forms, in the treatment of all conditions for which corticosteroid therapy is indicated, except adrenal-deficiency states for which its lack of sodium-retaining properties make it less suitable than hydrocortisone with supplementary fludrocortisone.

For administration by mouth dexamethasone is used in usual doses of 0.5 to 9 mg daily in divided doses. Dexamethasone is also used by mouth in the dexamethasone suppression tests for the diagnosis of Cushing's syndrome (for further details see under Diagnosis and Testing, below).

For parenteral administration in intensive therapy or in emergencies, the sodium phosphate ester may be given intravenously by injection or infusion or intramuscularly by injection; doses are sometimes expressed in terms of the free alcohol, the phosphate, or the sodium phosphate. Doses used, expressed in terms of dexamethasone phosphate, range from about 0.5 to 20 mg daily. Intravenous doses of the equivalent of 2 to 6 mg of dexamethasone phosphate per kg body-weight given slowly over a minimum period of several minutes have been suggested for the treatment of severe shock in an attempt to promote rapid vasodilation. These high doses may be repeated within 2 to 6 hours and this treatment should be continued only until the patients' condition is stable and usually for no longer than 48 to 72 hours. Dexamethasone sodium phosphate is also used in the treatment of cerebral oedema caused by malignancy. An initial intravenous dose of the equivalent of 10 mg of the phosphate is usually given followed by 4 mg intramuscularly every 6 hours; a response is usually obtained after 12 to 24 hours and dosage may be reduced after 2 to 4 days, and gradually discontinued over 5 to 7 days. A much higher dosage schedule has also been suggested for use in cerebral oedema in patients with inoperable brain tumours; initial doses of 50 mg intravenously have been given on the first day together with 8 mg intravenously every 2 hours reduced gradually over several days to a maintenance dose of 2 mg two or three times daily.

The acetate and sodium phosphate esters are given by intra-articular, intralesional, intramuscular, or soft-tissue injection; for intra-articular injection doses equivalent to 0.8 to 4 mg of dexamethasone sodium phosphate are employed depending upon the size of the joint.

For ophthalmic disorders or for topical application in the treatment of various skin disorders, dexamethasone or the sodium phosphate ester are usually employed; concentrations are usually expressed in terms of dexamethasone or dexamethasone phosphate and are commonly 0.05 to 0.1% for eye-drops or ointments and 0.1% for topical skin preparations.

Dexamethasone sodium phosphate is also used by inhalation for the prophylaxis of the symptoms of asthma. The initial dose is equivalent to 300 µg of dexamethasone phosphate inhaled three or four times daily, slowly reduced according to the patients' response to the minimum amount necessary to control the asthma.

For allergic rhinitis and other allergic or inflammatory nasal conditions a nasal spray containing dexamethasone isonicotinate or dexamethasone sodium phosphate is available.

Other esters of dexamethasone which have occasionally been used include the linoleate, sodium hydrogen sulphate, tebutate, and valerate.

The phenpropionate, pivalate, and trioxa-undecanoate esters have been used in veterinary medicine.

BLOOD DISORDERS. *Sickle-cell anaemia.* Administration of dexamethasone 2 mg every 6 hours to 2 siblings with sickle-cell anaemia causes subsidence of symptoms of a crisis within 48 hours. The drug is then tapered off over 3 to 7 days depending on the symptoms. Dexamethasone appears not only to reverse the symptoms but also to decrease the number of crises. Experience with a third sibling, who requires periodic transfusions, has been less good.— B. Robinson (letter), *Lancet*, 1979, *1*, 1088. The use of steroid hormones has been associated with venous thrombosis and may be contra-indicated. Nevertheless, properly controlled studies are indicated.— A. J. Bennett and F. Rosner (letter), *ibid.*, *2*, 474. *In vitro* studies on the blood of 3 patients with homozygous sickle-cell disease indicated that dexamethasone has no effect at the red blood cell level.— I. M. Franklin and D. C. Linch (letter), *ibid.*, 645.

CEREBRAL MALARIA. Despite some reports of patients with cerebral malaria benefiting from dexamethasone, a double-blind study involving 100 comatose patients with cerebral malaria showed that dexamethasone provided no benefit, prolonged the coma, and increased the incidence of complications.— D. A. Warrell *et al.*, *New Engl. J. Med.*, 1982, *306*, 313.

CEREBRAL OEDEMA. A review of cerebral oedema covering the use of corticosteroids in its management. Corticosteroids are very effective in reducing cerebral oedema associated with brain tumours and although several hypotheses have been proposed their exact mechanism of action is unknown. There has also been extensive animal and human research using corticosteroids for head injury but the results have varied widely and the role of steroids in the management of traumatic cerebral oedema remains controversial. Dexamethasone is the corticosteroid used most frequently in the treatment of severe head injuries and the optimal dose and length of treatment have not been established. There is no conclusive evidence that high doses intravenously of 100 to 400 mg daily for the first 24 to 72 hours, decreased to 4 mg every six hours, significantly improve the outcome compared to the more traditional low doses intravenously of 10 mg initially followed by 4 mg every six hours. Methylprednisolone has also been used to treat head injury but there is no known therapeutic advantage of one steroid over another.— C. M. Quandt and R. A. de los Reyes, *Drug Intell. & clin. Pharm.*, 1984, *18*, 105.

Some references to the use of dexamethasone in various situations displaying cerebral oedema: J. D. Weinstein *et al.*, *Neurology*, 1973, *23*, 121 (benefit in metastatic brain tumours); B. M. Frier and J. B. McConnell, *Br. med. J.*, 1975, *3*, 208 (benefit in diabetic ketoacidosis); J. W. Fletcher *et al.*, *J. Am. med. Ass.*, 1975, *232*, 1261 (benefit in metastatic brain tumours); H. J. Ruelen, *Br. J. Anaesth.*, 1976, *48*, 741 (benefit in vasogenic brain oedema); G. Mulley *et al.*, *Br. med. J.*, 1978, *2*, 994 (no benefit in acute stroke); P. R. Cooper *et al.*, *J. Neurosurg.*, 1979, *51*, 307 (disappointing results in head injury); H. E. James *et al.*, *Acta neurochir.*, 1979, *45*, 225 (benefit in head injury); T. S. Johnson, *New Engl. J. Med.*, 1984, *310*, 683 (benefit in preventing experimental acute mountain sickness); P. Ferreira and P. Grundy (letter), *ibid.*, 1985, *312*, 1390 (benefit in treatment of symptoms of acute mountain sickness); D. R. Shlim (letter), *ibid.*, *313*, 891 (no clear-cut response in the treatment of acute mountain sickness); J. W. Norris and V. C. Hachinski, *Br. med. J.*, 1986, *292*, 21 (no benefit in acute cerebral infarction); G. Ferrazzini *et al.*, *Br. med. J.*, 1987, *294*, 1380 (benefit in the treatment of moderate to severe acute mountain sickness); N. Poungvarin *et al.*, *New Engl. J. Med.*, 1987, *316*, 1229 (no benefit in primary supratentorial intracerebral haemorrhage).

See also under Cerebral Malaria (above).

DELIRIUM TREMENS. A report of dexamethasone being effective in benzodiazepine-resistant delirium tremens.— D. K. Fischer *et al.* (letter), *Lancet*, 1988, *1*, 1340.

DIAGNOSIS AND TESTING. *Cushing's syndrome.* Dexamethasone has been used to differentiate Cushing's disease (adrenal hyperplasia caused by defects of pituitary origin) from other forms of Cushing's syndrome (caused by ectopic ACTH secretion from non-pituitary tumours or by cortisol secretion from adrenal tumours). The dexamethasone suppression test first proposed by Liddle (*J. clin. Endocr. Metab.*, 1960, *20*, 1539) involved the administration of dexamethasone in low doses of 500 µg four times daily for 8 doses followed by higher doses of 2 mg again four times daily for 8 doses. In the low-dose tests the urinary excretion of cortisol and 17-hydroxycorticosteroids is suppressed in healthy persons but not in patients and in the high-dose tests the excretion is still not suppressed in those with Cushing's syndrome but is partially suppressed in those with Cushing's disease. Because this test usually involves patients being admitted to hospital for urine collection over a number of days and because false-negative responses are reported to be fairly frequent, more rapid and reliable tests have been sought. Kennedy *et al.* (*Br. med. J.*, 1984, *289*, 1188) have used the low-dose test in conjunction with the measurement of serum-cortisol concentrations and the excretion of free cortisol in urine over 24 hours and considered it to be a reliable method for screening for Cushing's syndrome. Another variation of the test has been reported by Tyrrell *et al.* (*Ann. intern. Med.*, 1986, *104*, 180) who administered a single dose of dexamethasone 8 mg at night and measured plasma-cortisol concentrations the next day; again they also concluded this test to be a practical and reliable alternative for the differential diagnosis of Cushing's syndrome.

Depression. Comments by the Health and Public Policy Committee of the American College of Physicians concerning the dexamethasone suppression test for the detection, diagnosis, and management of mental depression. The test is based on the premise that endogenously depressed patients have shown pituitary-adrenal axis abnormalities but has been found to have a low sensitivity for detecting depression. It is not recommended as a screening test for endogenous depression and pending further investigation and evaluation should be considered a diagnostic test of unproven value.— M. Young and J. S. Schwartz, *Ann. intern. Med.*, 1984, *100*, 307.

HIRSUTISM. Unbound testosterone concentrations were consistently elevated in 32 hirsute women. When concentrations were suppressed to normal by dexamethasone 0.5 to 1 mg at night hirsutism was generally improved or ceased to progress after 8 to 10 months of treatment.— J. D. Paulson *et al.*, *Am. J. Obstet. Gynec.*, 1977, *128*, 851.

NEONATAL RESPIRATORY DISTRESS SYNDROME. For reference to the use of dexamethasone for the prophylaxis of the neonatal respiratory distress syndrome, see under betamethasone, p.884.

SKIN DISORDERS. For recommendations concerning the correct use of corticosteroids on the skin, and a rough guide to the clinical potencies of topical corticosteroids, see p.880.

Preparations of Dexamethasone and its Esters

In addition to the preparations below, further official preparations containing dexamethasone or its esters may be found listed under neomycin sulphate.

Injections

Sterile Dexamethasone Acetate Suspension *(U.S.P.)*

Dexamethasone Sodium Phosphate Injection *(U.S.P.)*

Ophthalmic Dosage Forms

Dexamethasone Ophthalmic Suspension *(U.S.P.)*

Dexamethasone Sodium Phosphate Ophthalmic Ointment *(U.S.P.)*

Dexamethasone Sodium Phosphate Ophthalmic Solution *(U.S.P.)*

Oral Dosage Forms

Dexamethasone Elixir *(U.S.P.)*

Dexamethasone Tablets *(B.P.)*

Dexamethasone Tablets *(U.S.P.)*

Respiratory Dosage Forms

Dexamethasone Sodium Phosphate Inhalation Aerosol *(U.S.P.)*

Topical Dosage Forms

Dexamethasone Topical Aerosol *(U.S.P.)*

Dexamethasone Sodium Phosphate Cream *(U.S.P.)*

Dexamethasone Gel *(U.S.P.)*

Proprietary Preparations of Dexamethasone and its Esters

In addition to those given below, details of further proprietary preparations containing dexamethasone or its esters may be found under framycetin sulphate, neomycin sulphate, and tramazoline hydrochloride.

Decadron *(Merck Sharp & Dohme, UK)*. *Tablets*, scored, dexamethasone 500 µg.
Injection, dexamethasone 3.33 mg (as sodium phosphate)/mL (equivalent to dexamethasone phosphate 4 mg/mL), in vials of 2 mL.
Shock-Pak, dexamethasone 20 mg (as sodium phosphate)/mL in vials of 5 mL.

Maxidex *(Alcon, UK)*. *Eye-drops*, dexamethasone 0.1%.

Oradexon-Organon *(Organon, UK)*. *Tablets*, dexamethasone 500 µg and 2 mg.
Injection, dexamethasone 4 mg (as sodium phosphate)/mL (equivalent to dexamethasone sodium phosphate 5 mg/mL), in ampoules of 1 mL or vials of 2 mL.

Proprietary Names and Manufacturers of Dexamethasone and its Esters

Aacidexam *(Belg.)*; Acidocort *(Fr.)*; Aeroseb-Dex *(Herbert, USA)*; Ak-Dex *(Akorn, Canad.)*; Artrosone *(Davur, Spain)*; Auxiloson *(Thomae, Ger.)*; Auxison *(Boehringer Sohn, Switz.)*; Auxisone *(Boehringer Ingelheim, Belg.; Boehringer Ingelheim, Fr.)*; Azoman *(Boehringer Sohn, Arg.)*; BayDex *(Bay, USA)*; Carulon *(Jpn)*; Cébédex *(Chauvin-Blache, Fr.)*; Chronocorte *(Streuli, Switz.)*; Corson *(Jpn)*; Corti-Attritin *(Atmos, Ger.)*; Corti-summan *(Winzer, Ger.)*;

Dalalone *(Forest Pharmaceuticals, USA)*; Dalaron *(USA)*; Decacort *(Swed.)*; Decadeltosona *(Spain)*; Decaderm *(Jpn; Merck Sharp & Dohme, USA)*; Decadran *(Merck Sharp & Dohme, Spain)*; Decadron *(Arg.; Merck Sharp & Dohme, Austral.; Belg.; Merck Sharp & Dohme, Canad.; Merck Sharp & Dohme, Denm.; Merck Sharp & Dohme-Chibret, Fr.; Chibret, Ger.; Merck Sharp & Dohme, Ger.; Merck Sharp & Dohme, Ital.; Jpn; Chibret, Neth.; Merck Sharp & Dohme, Norw.; Merck Sharp & Dohme, S.Afr.; MSD, Swed.; Chibret, Switz.; Merck Sharp & Dohme, UK; Merck Sharp & Dohme, USA)*; Decadrone *(Jpn)*; Decalix *(USA)*; Decasone *(Austral.)*; Decaspray *(Merck Sharp & Dohme, USA)*; Decasterolone *(Ital.; Spain)*; Decoderm *(Spain)*; Decofluor *(Salfa, Ital.)*; Dectan *(Jpn)*; Dectancyl *(Roussel, Fr.)*; Dekacort *(Farber-Ref, Ital.)*; Dermadex *(Zambeletti, Ital.)*; Dermax *(Ital.)*; Deronil *(Schering, Canad.; Spain)*; Desacort *(Ital.)*; Desacortone *(Neopharmed, Ital.)*; Desalark *(Farmacologico Milanese, Ital.)*; Desaval *(Lusofarmaco, Ital.)*; Deseronil *(SCA, Ital.)*; Dethamedin *(Jpn)*; Dexa-Aldon *(Spain)*; Dexabene *(Merckle, Ger.)*; Dexa-Brachialin *(Steigerwald, Ger.)*; Dexacen *(Central Pharmaceuticals, USA)*; Dexacortal *(Organon, Swed.)*; Dexacortin *(Streuli, Switz.)*; Dexacortisyl *(Austral.; Roussel, UK)*; Dexafarma *(Spain)*; Dexa-Life *(Spain)*; Dexalocal *(Fink, Ger.; Medinova, Switz.)*; Dexamamallett *(Jpn)*; Dexamecortin *(Switz.)*; Dexamed *(Medice, Ger.)*; Dexametaluy *(Spain)*; Dexametosona *(Arg.)*; Dexamiso *(Oftalmiso, Spain)*; Dexamonozon *(Medice, Ger.)*; Dexane *(P.O.S., Fr.)*; Dexanteric *(Spain)*; Dexaplast *(Llorens, Spain)*; Dexapos *(Ursapharm, Ger.)*; Dexa-Rhinosan *(Switz.)*; Dexasan *(Spain)*; Dexa-Scherosana *(Arg.; Spain)*; Dexasine *(Thilo, Ger.)*; Dexa-sol *(Roussel, Belg.)*; Dexasone *(ICN, Canad.; Legere, USA)*; Dexa-Wolner *(Kairon, Spain)*; Dexmethsone *(Protea, Austral.)*; Dexona *(Cadila, Ind.)*; Dexone *(Rowell, USA)*; Dinormon *(Ital.)*; Esacortene *(Ital.)*; Eta-Cortilen *(SIFI, Ital.)*; Exadion *(Ital.)*; Exosterol *(Zyma, Switz.)*; Falban *(Spain)*; Firmalone *(FIRMA, Ital.)*; Fluormone *(Ital.)*; Fluorocort *(Ital.)*; Fluorodelta *(Ital.)*; Fortecortin *(E. Merck, Ger.; Ital.; Igoda, Spain; E. Merck, Switz.)*; Fosfodexa *(Llorens, Spain)*; Grosodexon *(Switz.)*; Hemidexa *(Llorens,

Spain); Hexadrol *(Organon Teknika, Canad.; Organon, USA)*; Hubersona *(Hubber, Spain)*; Isopto-Dex *(Alcon, Ger.)*; Isopto-Maxidex *(Alcon, Norw.; Alcon, Swed.)*; Lapiz Labial Alesa *(Ale, Spain)*; Linoderm *(Sigma Tau, Spain)*; Lokalison *(Dorsch, Ger.)*; Luxazone *(Allergan, Ital.)*; Maxidex *(Alcon, Austral.; Belg.; Alcon, Canad.; Alcon, Denm.; Alcon, Fr.; Neth.; Alcon, S.Afr.; Alcon, Spain; Alcon, Switz.; Alcon, UK)*; Megacort *(Aandersen, Ital.)*; Mephamesone *(Mepha, Switz.)*; Metasolon *(Jpn)*; Methazon-Ion *(Ital.)*; Millicortène *(Ciba, Switz.)*; Millicorten *(Ger.; Spain; Switz.)*; Miral *(USA)*; Moco *(Jpn)*; Moderix *(Spain)*;
Novadex *(Canad.)*; Oradexon *(Organon, Austral.; Belg.; Neth.; Organon, S.Afr.; Spain; Organon, Switz.; Organon, UK)*; Orgadrone *(Jpn)*; Predni-F *(Beiersdorf, Ger.)*; Savacort-D *(Savage, USA)*; Sawasone *(Jpn)*; Selftison-F *(Jpn)*; Situalin *(Puropharma, Ital.)*; SK-Dexamethasone *(Smith Kline & French, USA)*; Sokaral *(Allergan, Ger.)*; Soldesam *(Farmacologico Milanese, Ital.)*; Solone *(Liade, Spain)*; Soludécadron *(Merck Sharp & Dohme-Chibret, Fr.)*; Spersadex *(Dispersa, Ger.; Dispersa, Norw.; S.Afr.; Dispersa, Switz.)*; Spondy *(Efeka, Ger.)*; Sunia Sol-D *(Jpn)*; Topolyn *(Ital.)*; Totocortin *(Winzer, Ger.)*; Visumetazone *(Merck Sharp & Dohme, Ital.)*.

The following names have been used for multi-ingredient preparations containing dexamethasone or its esters—Ak-Trol *(Akorn, USA)*; Decaspray *(Merck Sharp & Dohme, UK)*; Dexacidin *(Coopervision, USA)*; Dexa-Rhinaspray *(Boehringer Ingelheim, UK)*; Dexasporin *(Pharmafair, USA)*; Maxitrol *(Alcon, Canad.; Alcon, UK; Alcon Laboratories, USA)*; Neodecadron *(Merck Sharp & Dohme, USA)*; NeoDecadron *(Merck Sharp & Dohme, Canad.)*; Ocu-Trol *(Ocumed, USA)*; Sofracort *(Roussel, Canad.)*; Sofradex *(Roussel, Austral.; Roussel, UK)*; Tobispray *(Boehringer Ingelheim, Austral.)*.

12645-j

Dichlorisone Acetate *(rINNM)*.
Diclorisone Acetate. 9α,11β-Dichloro-17α,21-dihydroxypregna-1,4-diene-3,20-dione 21-acetate.
$C_{23}H_{28}Cl_2O_5$=455.4.

CAS — 7008-26-6 (dichlorisone); 79-61-8 (acetate).

Dichlorisone acetate is a corticosteroid with the general properties described under corticosteroids (see p.872) and is used topically in the treatment of various skin disorders. It is usually employed as a cream or ointment containing 0.05% to 1%.
When applied topically, particularly to large areas, when the skin is broken, or under occlusive dressings, corticosteroids may be absorbed in sufficient amounts to cause systemic effects.

For recommendations concerning the correct use of corticosteroids on the skin, see Corticosteroids p.880.

Proprietary Names and Manufacturers
Astroderm *(Lagap, Ital.)*; Dermaren *(Areu, Spain)*; Diclasone *(Liberman, Spain)*; Dicloderm *(Cruz, Spain)*.

12651-l

Diflorasone Diacetate *(BANM, USAN, rINNM)*.

U-34865. 6α,9α-Difluoro-11β,17α,21-trihydroxy-16β-methylpregna-1,4-diene-3,20-dione 17,21-diacetate.
$C_{26}H_{32}F_2O_7$=494.5.

CAS — 2557-49-5 (diflorasone); 33564-31-7 (diacetate).

Pharmacopoeias. In *U.S.*

A white to pale yellow, crystalline powder. Practically **insoluble** in water; soluble in acetone and methyl alcohol; sparingly soluble in ethyl acetate; slightly soluble in toluene; very slightly soluble in ether. **Store** in airtight containers.

Adverse Effects, Treatment, Withdrawal, and Precautions

As for corticosteroids, p.872.
When applied topically, particularly to large areas, when the skin is broken, or under occlusive dressings, corticosteroids may be absorbed in sufficient amounts to cause systemic effects.

Absorption and Fate

For a brief outline of the absorption and fate of corticosteroids, see p.875.

Uses and Administration

Diflorasone diacetate is a corticosteroid used topically in the treatment of various skin disorders, as described under corticosteroids (see p.876). It is usually employed as a cream or ointment containing 0.05%.

SKIN DISORDERS. For recommendations concerning the correct use of corticosteroids on the skin, and a rough guide to the clinical potencies of topical corticosteroids, see Corticosteroids, p.880.

Preparations

Diflorasone Diacetate Cream *(U.S.P.)*
Diflorasone Diacetate Ointment *(U.S.P.)*

Proprietary Names and Manufacturers

Bexilona *(Isdin, Spain)*; Dermonilo *(Aristegui, Spain)*; Florone *(Upjohn, Canad.; Basotherm, Ger.; Upjohn, Neth.; Dermik, USA)*; Flutone *(Rorer, Canad.)*; Fulixan *(Esteve, Spain)*; Maxiflor *(Herbert, USA)*; Murode *(Hubber, Spain)*; Psorcon *(Dermik, USA)*; Sterodelta *(Gibipharma, Ital.)*.

1087-f

Diflucortolone Valerate *(BANM, rINNM)*.

6α,9α-Difluoro-11β,21-dihydroxy-16α-methylpregna-1,4-diene-3,20-dione 21-valerate.
$C_{27}H_{36}F_2O_5$=478.6.

CAS — 2607-06-9 (diflucortolone); 59198-70-8 (valerate).

NOTE. Diflucortolone and Diflucortolone Pivalate are *USAN*.

Adverse Effects, Treatment, Withdrawal, and Precautions

As for corticosteroids, p.872.
When applied topically, particularly to large areas, when the skin is broken, or under occlusive dressings, corticosteroids may be absorbed in sufficient amounts to cause systemic effects.

Absorption and Fate

For a brief outline of the absorption and fate of corticosteroids, see p.875.

Uses and Administration

Diflucortolone valerate is a corticosteroid used topically in the treatment of various skin disorders, as described under corticosteroids (see p.876). It is usually employed as a cream or ointment containing 0.1% or 0.3%.

SKIN DISORDERS. For recommendations concerning the correct use of corticosteroids on the skin, and a rough guide to the clinical potencies of topical corticosteroids, see corticosteroids, p.880.

Proprietary Preparations

Nerisone *(Schering, UK)*. *Cream, Oily cream, Ointment,* diflucortolone valerate 0.1%.

Nerisone Forte *(Schering, UK)*. *Oily cream, Ointment,* diflucortolone valerate 0.3%.

Proprietary Names and Manufacturers

Claral *(Schering, Spain)*; Dermaval *(FIRMA, Ital.)*; Flu-Cortanest *(Piam, Ital.)*; Neriforte *(Schering, Switz.)*; Nerisona *(Arg.; Schering, Denm.; Scherax, Ger.; Schering, Ital.; Neth.; Schering, Switz.)*; Nerisone *(Stiefel, Canad.; Schering, Fr.; NZ; Schering, S.Afr.; Schering, UK)*; Talacort *(Bergamon, Ital.)*; Temetex *(Arg.; Roche, Ger.; Roche, Ital.; S.Afr.; Roche, Spain; Sauter, Switz.; Roche, UK)*.

12652-y

Difluprednate *(USAN, rINN)*.
CM-9155; W-6309. 6α,9α-Difluoro-11β,17α,21-trihydroxypregna-1,4-diene-3,20-dione 21-acetate 17-butyrate.
$C_{27}H_{34}F_2O_7$=508.6.

CAS — 23674-86-4.

Difluprednate is a corticosteroid with the general properties described under corticosteroids (see p.872) and is used topically in the treatment of various skin disorders. It is usually employed as a cream, gel, or ointment; concentrations used range from 0.02% to 0.05%.
When applied topically, particularly to large areas, when the skin is broken, or under occlusive dressings, corticosteroids may be absorbed in sufficient amounts to cause systemic effects.

For recommendations concerning the correct use of corticosteroids on the skin, see corticosteroids, p.880.

Proprietary Names and Manufacturers
Épitopic *(Clin Midy, Fr.)*.

19106-x

Domoprednate *(rINN)*.
Ro-12-7024. 11β-17a-Dihydroxy-*D*-homopregna-1,4-diene-3,20-dione 17a-butyrate.
$C_{26}H_{36}O_5$=428.6.

CAS — 66877-67-6.

Domoprednate is a corticosteroid with the general properties described under corticosteroids (see p.872) and is under investigation for use topically in the treatment of various skin disorders.
When applied topically, particularly to large areas, when the skin is broken, or under occlusive dressings, corticosteroids may be absorbed in sufficient amounts to cause systemic effects.

For recommendations concerning the correct use of corticosteroids on the skin, see corticosteroids, p.880.

12689-m

Endrysone *(USAN)*.
Endrisone *(rINN)*. 11β-Hydroxy-6α-methylpregna-1,4-diene-3,20-dione.
$C_{22}H_{30}O_3$=342.5.

CAS — 35100-44-8.

Endrysone is a corticosteroid with the general properties described under corticosteroids (see p.872). It is used in eye-drops and eye ointments usually at a concentration of 0.5%.

Proprietary Names and Manufacturers
Aldrisone *(SIFI, Ital.)*.

12755-x

Fluazacort *(USAN, rINN)*.
L-6400. 9α-Fluoro-11β,21-dihydroxy-2′-methyl-5′βH-pregna-1,4-dieno[17,16-*d*]oxazole-3,20-dione 21-acetate.
$C_{25}H_{30}FNO_6$=459.5.

CAS — 19888-56-3.

Fluazacort is a corticosteroid with the general properties described under corticosteroids (see p.872) and is used topically in the treatment of various skin disorders. It is usually employed as a cream containing 0.025%.
When applied topically, particularly to large areas, when the skin is broken, or under occlusive dressings, corticosteroids may be absorbed in sufficient amounts to cause systemic effects.

For recommendations concerning the correct use of corticosteroids on the skin, see corticosteroids, p.880.

Proprietary Names and Manufacturers
Azacortid *(Lepetit, Ital.)*.

1088-d

Fluclorolone Acetonide *(BAN, rINN).*

Flucloronide *(USAN)*; RS-2252. 9α,11β-Dichloro-6α-fluoro-21-hydroxy-16α,17α-isopropylidenedioxypregna-1,4-diene-3,20-dione.

$C_{24}H_{29}Cl_2FO_5$=487.4.

CAS — 3693-39-8.

Pharmacopoeias. In *Br.*

A white or creamy white odourless or almost odourless, crystalline powder. Practically **insoluble** in water; soluble in alcohol and chloroform; slightly soluble in ether. **Protect** from light.

Adverse Effects, Treatment, Withdrawal, and Precautions

As for corticosteroids, p.872.

When applied topically, particularly to large areas, when the skin is broken, or under occlusive dressings, corticosteroids may be absorbed in sufficient amounts to cause systemic effects.

Absorption and Fate

For a brief outline of the absorption and fate of corticosteroids, see p.875.

Uses and Administration

Fluclorolone acetonide is a corticosteroid used topically in the treatment of various skin disorders, as described under corticosteroids (see p.876). It is usually employed as a cream or ointment containing 0.025%.

SKIN DISORDERS. For recommendations concerning the correct use of corticosteroids on the skin, and a rough guide to the clinical potencies of topical corticosteroids, see corticosteroids, p.880.

Preparations

Fluclorolone Ointment *(B.P.).* Fluclorolone Acetonide Ointment

Proprietary Preparations

Topilar *(Syntex, UK). Cream, Ointment,* fluclorolone acetonide 0.025%.

Proprietary Names and Manufacturers

Cutanit *(Syntex-Latino, Spain)*; Topilar *(Syntex, Austral.; Denm.; Syntex, Fr.; Norw.; Syntex, UK).*

1089-n

Fludrocortisone Acetate *(BANM, USAN, rINNM).*

9α-Fluorohydrocortisone 21-Acetate. 9α-Fluoro-11β,17α,21-trihydroxypregn-4-ene-3,20-dione 21-acetate.

$C_{23}H_{31}FO_6$=422.5.

CAS — 127-31-1 (fludrocortisone); 514-36-3 (acetate).

Pharmacopoeias. In *Br., Braz., Chin., Cz., Egypt., Fr., Ind.,* and *U.S.*

A white to pale yellow, odourless or almost odourless, hygroscopic, crystalline powder. Practically **insoluble** in water; soluble 1 in 50 of alcohol, 1 in 50 of chloroform; slightly soluble in ether. **Store** in well-closed containers. Protect from light.

Adverse Effects, Treatment, Withdrawal, and Precautions

As for corticosteroids, p.872.

Fludrocortisone acetate has glucocorticoid actions about 15 times as potent as hydrocortisone and mineralocorticoid effects more than 100 times as potent.

EFFECTS ON THE ELECTROLYTE BALANCE. Muscular weakness associated with hypokalaemia and raised serum-creatine phosphokinase concentrations in a patient was attributed to fludrocortisone acetate which he had taken for 2½ years in doses of 100 μg three to six times daily for severe postural hypotension. The patient showed no muscular weakness after serum-potassium concentrations were raised by potassium chloride given intravenously and maintained with potassium supplements and a high salt diet.— V. M. Rivera (letter), *J. Am. med. Ass.*, 1973, *225*, 993.

Severe hypokalaemia which resulted in extreme metabolic alkalosis in a woman who had been taking fludrocortisone 200 μg daily over a period of 1 year for postural hypotension; she was successfully treated with diuretics and potassium supplements.— A. Burns *et al., Postgrad. med. J.*, 1983, *59*, 506.

Absorption and Fate

For a brief outline of the absorption and fate of corticosteroids, see p.875.

Fludrocortisone is readily absorbed from the gastro-intestinal tract.

Studies in 5 volunteers showed the absorption of fludrocortisone by mouth to be rapid and complete with maximum blood concentrations after 1.7 hours. After intravenous injection the elimination half-life was 30 minutes.— W. Vogt *et al., Arzneimittel-Forsch.*, 1971, *21*, 1133.

Uses and Administration

Fludrocortisone is a corticosteroid with both mineralocorticoid and glucocorticoid actions as described under corticosteroids (see p.875).

With a dose that is just sufficient to correct sodium loss in Addison's disease or following total adrenalectomy, the glucocorticoid actions are not sufficient to maintain the patient in normal health; it is therefore given as an adjunct in patients who become sodium deficient on hydrocortisone alone. The suggested dose range of fludrocortisone acetate is 50 to 300 μg daily.

Fludrocortisone acetate may also be given concomitantly with glucocorticoid therapy in the salt-losing form of congenital adrenal hyperplasia.

Fludrocortisone is also used in the management of severe orthostatic hypotension.

ADRENAL INSUFFICIENCY. A study of fludrocortisone requirements in 10 patients with Addison's disease. Nine were initially on fludrocortisone 50 to 100 μg daily in addition to cortisone or hydrocortisone; 5 were also taking thyroxine for an associated auto-immune thyroid disease; one, who had detectable levels of aldosterone, was not initially receiving fludrocortisone. All the patients had evidence of sodium and water depletion and initiation of fludrocortisone 300 μg daily, with downwards adjustments, demonstrated that most patients required 200 μg daily. Two patients elected to remain on 300 μg daily, but in most this dose caused pronounced sodium and water retention. The patient with detectable aldosterone levels required 50 μg daily. Eight of the 10 patients felt better on the higher fludrocortisone doses while 2 felt no change.— S. J. Smith *et al., Lancet*, 1984, *1*, 11.

CONGENITAL ADRENAL HYPERPLASIA. In 4 children with salt-losing congenital adrenal hyperplasia, receiving maintenance doses of hydrocortisone or cortisone acetate, raised plasma concentrations of 17-hydroxyprogesterone and increased plasma renin activity were restored to normal following treatment with fludrocortisone 100 μg daily. It was recommended that these patients should be given mineralocorticoid, in addition to glucocorticoid, therapy at least until adult life.— I. A. Hughes *et al., Archs Dis. Childh.*, 1979, *54*, 350.

In 6 children with congenital adrenal hyperplasia receiving glucocorticoids, and in whom clinical and biochemical control was inadequate, an increase in the dose of fludrocortisone in 5 and introduction of fludrocortisone in the sixth resulted in improvement. In the 5 who were salt-losers and already receiving fludrocortisone in doses of 25 to 100 μg daily, the dose after increase and adjustment was 100 to 150 μg daily; in the sixth child with no history of salt loss the dose of fludrocortisone after initial adjustment was 25 μg daily. It was stated that although it is recognised that mineralocorticoid therapy should be continued indefinitely (because the withdrawal of such therapy while not always provoking a salt-losing crisis may make control with even large doses of glucocorticoid more difficult) this study showed that the dose of fludrocortisone used may be as critical as the dose of glucocorticoid.— K. D. Griffiths *et al., Archs Dis. Childh.*, 1984, *59*, 360.

DIAGNOSIS AND TESTING. Mention of the use of fludrocortisone as part of the sweat test for the diagnosis of cystic fibrosis. The sweat test involves analysis of the electrolyte content of a patient's sweat and in cystic fibrosis the values for sodium and chloride are raised. If the result is marginal, fludrocortisone 3 mg per m^2 body-surface is given daily for 2 days and the sweat test repeated; persons whose values return to within the normal range after suppression with fludrocortisone do not have cystic fibrosis.— J. M. Littlewood, *Archs Dis. Childh.*, 1986, *61*, 1041.

HYPOALDOSTERONISM. A discussion on hyporeninaemic hypoaldosteronism. Traditionally a mineralocorticoid such as fludrocortisone acetate has been used to reduce the hyperkalaemia and acidosis. Unfortunately pharmacologic rather than physiologic doses are often needed and these may not always be effective.— *New Engl. J. Med.*, 1986, *314*, 1041.

The use of fludrocortisone acetate in a patient with hyperkalaemia due to aldosterone deficiency.— J. J. Brown *et al., Br. med. J.*, 1973, *1*, 650. Fludrocortisone in the amelioration of metabolic acidosis in 4 patients with hyporeninaemic hypoaldosteronism.— A. Sebastian *et al., New Engl. J. Med.*, 1977, *297*, 576.

ORTHOSTATIC HYPOTENSION. A review and discussion on the management of postural hypotension. Drug treatment may be necessary if the cornerstone of management consisting of tilting the patient's bed at night is ineffective; fludrocortisone is the drug of choice. It should be introduced at a low dosage of 100 μg daily and adjusted at intervals of 1 to 2 weeks. The efficacy is limited by the side-effects of fluid retention, supine hypertension, and hypokalaemia.— R. D. S. Watson, *Br. med. J.*, 1987, *294*, 390. See also *Lancet*, 1987, *1*, 197.

Fourteen diabetic patients with postural hypotension, usually with features of autonomic neuropathy, were treated for 6 to 30 months with fludrocortisone, 100 μg twice daily initially, adjusted as required to a final mean dose of 100 to 400 μg daily. Lying blood pressure was not significantly changed but standing systolic and diastolic pressures rose significantly; 13 patients had symptomatic improvement. Fludrocortisone should be used with care in patients with proteinuria.— I. W. Campbell *et al., Br. med. J.*, 1976, *1*, 872.

A study of the effects of treatment with fludrocortisone in 7 patients with severe orthostatic hypotension. Doses of 0.3 to 1 mg daily were given for one to 14 years; in some patients the dose was reduced when severe hypertension or hypokalaemia appeared whilst the patient was recumbent. Although blood pressure in the recumbent and standing positions was substantially increased in all patients there was incomplete symptomatic relief; clinical benefit was greatest during the first 6 months of treatment. Complications of treatment included recumbent hypertension, cardiomegaly, hypertensive retinopathy, and hypokalaemia; these risks should be borne in mind when long-term treatment with fludrocortisone is considered.— A. V. Chobanian *et al., New Engl. J. Med.*, 1979, *301*, 68.

Preparations

Fludrocortisone Tablets *(B.P.).* Tablets containing fludrocortisone acetate.

Fludrocortisone Acetate Tablets *(U.S.P.)*

Proprietary Preparations

Florinef *(Squibb, UK). Tablets,* scored, fludrocortisone acetate 0.1 mg.

Proprietary Names and Manufacturers

Alfa-Fluorone *(Ausonia, Ital.)*; Alfanonidrone *(Ital.)*; Astonin *(E. Merck, Ger.; Igoda, Spain)*; Astonin-H *(Ger.)*; Cortineff *(Pol.)*; Florinef *(Squibb, Austral.; Squibb, Canad.; Squibb, Denm.; Novo, Norw.; Squibb, S.Afr.; Squibb, Swed.; Squibb, Switz.; Squibb, UK)*; Florinef Acetate *(Squibb, USA)*; Scherofluron *(Schering, Ger.).*

1090-k

Flumethasone *(BAN, USAN).*

Flumetasone *(rINN)*. 6α,9α-Difluoro-11β,17α,21-trihydroxy-16α-methylpregna-1,4-diene-3,20-dione.

$C_{22}H_{28}F_2O_5$=410.5.

CAS — 2135-17-3.

1091-a

Flumethasone Pivalate *(BANM, USAN).*

Flumetasone Pivalate *(rINNM)*; Flumethasone Trimethylacetate. Flumethasone 21-pivalate.

$C_{27}H_{36}F_2O_6$=494.6.

CAS — 2002-29-1.

Pharmacopoeias. In *U.S.*

A white to off-white crystalline powder. Practically **insoluble** in water; soluble 1 in 89 of alcohol, 1 in 350 of chloroform, and 1 in 2800 of ether; slightly soluble in methyl alcohol; very slightly soluble in methylene chloride. **Store** in airtight containers. Protect from light.

Adverse Effects, Treatment, Withdrawal, and Precautions
As for corticosteroids, p.872.
when applied topically, particularly to large areas, when the skin is broken, or under occlusive dressings, corticosteroids may be absorbed in sufficient amounts to cause systemic effects.

Absorption and Fate
For a brief outline of the absorption and fate of corticosteroids, see p.875.

Uses and Administration
Flumethasone pivalate is a glucocorticoid used by topical application in the treatment of various skin disorders as described under corticosteroids (see p.876). It is usually employed as 0.02% cream or ointment.
Flumethasone pivalate is also used in ear-drops in a concentration of 0.02% with clioquinol 1%.

SKIN DISORDERS. For recommendations concerning the correct use of corticosteroids on the skin, and a rough guide to the clinical potencies of topical corticosteroids, see corticosteroids, p.880.

Preparations of Flumethasone and its Esters
Flumethasone Pivalate Cream *(U.S.P.)*

Proprietary Preparations of Flumethasone and its Esters
Locorten-Vioform *(Zyma, UK). Ear-drops,* flumethasone pivalate 0.02%, clioquinol 1%.

Proprietary Names and Manufacturers of Flumethasone and its Esters
Locacorten *(Ciba, Austral.; Ciba, Canad.; Ciba, Denm.; Zyma, Ger.; Neth.; Ciba, Norw.; Ciba, Swed.)*; Locacortene *(Belg.; Ciba, Switz.)*; Locorten *(Arg.; Ciba, Ital.; Ciba, UK; Ciba, USA)*; Locortene *(Frumtost, Spain)*.

The following names have been used for multi-ingredient preparations containing flumethasone or its esters—Locacorten-Vioform *(Ciba, Austral.; Ciba, Canad.)*; Locasalen *(Ciba, Canad.)*; Locorten-Vioform *(Zyma, UK)*.

1092-t

Flunisolide *(BAN, USAN, rINN).*

RS-3999. 6α-Fluoro-11β,21-dihydroxy-16α,17α-isopropylidenedioxypregna-1,4-diene-3,20-dione.
$C_{24}H_{31}FO_6$=434.5.

CAS — 3385-03-3 (flunisolide); 77326-96-6 (hemihydrate).

Pharmacopoeias. In *U.S.* which specifies the hemihydrate.

A white to creamy-white crystalline powder. Practically **insoluble** in water; soluble in acetone; sparingly soluble in chloroform; slightly soluble in methyl alcohol.

Adverse Effects, Treatment, Withdrawal, and Precautions
As for corticosteroids, p.872.

Absorption and Fate
For a brief outline of the absorption and fate of corticosteroids, see p.875.

A study suggesting that the lack of systemic effect of flunisolide is due to rapid and extensive first-pass metabolism in the liver.— M. D. Chaplin *et al., Clin. Pharmac. Ther.,* 1980, *27,* 402.

Uses and Administration
Flunisolide is a glucocorticoid used as a nasal spray for the prophylaxis and treatment of allergic rhinitis. It is used in a usual initial dose of 50 µg into each nostril two or three times daily, subsequently reduced to the lowest dose adequate to control symptoms which may be as little as 25 µg into each nostril daily. Children over 5 years of age may be given 25 µg into each nostril three times daily.
Flunisolide is also used by inhalation from a metered aerosol in the management of asthma. The usual adult dosage is 500 µg inhaled twice daily; in severe asthma the dosage may be increased but should not exceed a total of 2 mg daily. A suggested dose for children over 5 years of age is 500 µg inhaled twice daily.

Preparations
Flunisolide Nasal Solution *(U.S.P.)*

Proprietary Preparations
Syntaris *(Syntex, UK). Nasal spray,* flunisolide 25 µg/metered dose.

Proprietary Names and Manufacturers
Aerobid *(Forest Pharmaceuticals, USA)*; Bronalide *(Syncare, Canad.; Syntex, Ger.)*; Bronilide *(Syntex, Switz.)*; Gibiflu *(Gibipharma, Ital.)*; Locasyn *(Syntex, Denm.)*; Lokilan *(Astra-Syntex, Norw.; Astra-Syntex, Swed.)*; Nasalide *(Syntex, USA)*; Rhinalar *(Syntex, Austral.; Syncare, Canad.)*; Syntaris *(Syntex, Ger.; Recordati, Ital.; Syntex, S.Afr.; Syntex, Switz.; Syntex, UK)*.

1093-x

Fluocinolone Acetonide *(BANM, USAN, rINN).*

6α,9α-Difluoro-16α-hydroxyprednisolone Acetonide; Fluocinoloni Acetonidum. 6α,9α-Difluoro-11β,21-dihydroxy-16α,17α-isopropylidenedioxypregna-1,4-diene-3,20-dione.
$C_{24}H_{30}F_2O_6$=452.5.

CAS — 67-73-2.

Pharmacopoeias. In *Br., Braz., Cz., Eur., It., Jpn, Jug.,* and *Swiss.* Also in *B.P. Vet. U.S.* allows either the anhydrous form or the dihydrate.

A white or almost white, odourless, crystalline powder. Practically **insoluble** in water; soluble 1 in 10 of acetone, 1 in 45 of alcohol, 1 in 26 of dehydrated alcohol, 1 in 15 to 25 of chloroform, and 1 in 350 of ether; soluble in methyl alcohol. **Store** in well-closed containers. Protect from light.

Adverse Effects, Treatment, Withdrawal, and Precautions
As for corticosteroids, p.872.
When applied topically, particularly to large areas, when the skin is broken, or under occlusive dressings, corticosteroids may be absorbed in sufficient amounts to cause systemic effects.

Absorption and Fate
For a brief outline of the absorption and fate of corticosteroids, see p.875.

Uses and Administration
Fluocinolone acetonide is a corticosteroid used topically in the treatment of various skin disorders, as described under corticosteroids (see p.876). It is usually employed as a cream, gel, lotion, or ointment; concentrations used range from 0.0025% to 0.2%.

SKIN DISORDERS. For recommendations concerning the correct use of corticosteroids on the skin, and a rough guide to the clinical potencies of topical corticosteroids, see corticosteroids p.880.

Preparations
In addition to the preparations below, further official preparations containing fluocinolone acetonide may be found listed under neomycin sulphate.
Fluocinolone Cream *(B.P.).* Fluocinolone Acetonide Cream
Fluocinolone Acetonide Cream *(U.S.P.)*
Fluocinolone Ointment *(B.P.).* Fluocinolone Acetonide Ointment
Fluocinolone Acetonide Ointment *(U.S.P.)*
Fluocinolone Acetonide Topical Solution *(U.S.P.)*

Proprietary Preparations
Synalar *(ICI Pharmaceuticals, UK). Cream,Gel, Ointment,* fluocinolone acetonide 0.025%.
Synalar 1 in 4 *(ICI Pharmaceuticals, UK). Cream, Ointment,* fluocinolone acetonide 0.00625%.
Synalar 1 in 10 *(ICI Pharmaceuticals, UK). Cream,* fluocinolone acetonide 0.0025%.
Synalar C *(ICI Pharmaceuticals, UK). Cream, Ointment,* fluocinolone acetonide 0.025%, clioquinol 3%.
Synalar N *(ICI Pharmaceuticals, UK). Cream, Ointment,* fluocinolone acetonide 0.025%, neomycin sulphate 0.5%.

Proprietary Names and Manufacturers
Alfabios *(Ausonia, Ital.)*; Alvadermo *(Oftalmiso, Spain)*; Anatopic *(Spain)*; Boniderma *(Boniscontro & Gazzone, Ital.)*; Coderma *(Biotrading, Ital.)*; Co-Fluocin *(Smaller, Spain)*; Coriphate *(Jpn)*; Cortalar *(Bergamon, Ital.)*; Cortamide *(Ottolenghi, Ital.)*; Cortiderma *(Ital.)*; Cortiespec *(Centrum, Spain)*; Cortiplastol *(Medici Domus, Ital.)*; Cortoderm *(Lennon, S.Afr.)*; Dermacort *(Biochimici, Ital.)*; Dermaisom *(ISOM, Ital.)*; Dermalar *(Canad.)*; Dermaplus *(Ripari-Gero, Ital.)*; Derma-Smoothe *(Hill, USA)*; Dermatin *(Ital.)*; Dermil *(Ital.)*; Dermisone Fluocinolona *(Spain)*; Dermobeta *(Terapeutico M.R., Ital.)*; Dermobiomar *(Spain)*; Dermofil *(Nuovo, Ital.)*; Dermoframan *(Oftalmiso, Spain)*; Dermolin *(Lafare, Ital.)*; Dermomagis *(Ital.)*; Dermotergol *(Kairon, Spain)*; Doricum *(Farmila, Ital.)*;
Elasven *(Cheminova, Spain)*; Esacinone *(Lisapharma, Ital.)*; Esilon *(SIT, Ital.)*; Flucort *(Jpn)*; Flulone *(Arg.)*; Fluocid *(Bicther, Spain)*; Fluocinil *(Coli, Ital.; Spain)*; Fluocinone *(Ital.)*; Fluocit *(CT, Ital.)*; Fluocortan *(Unibios, Spain)*; Fluoderm *(Taro, Canad.)*; Fluodermo *(Valles Mestre, Spain)*; Fluodermol *(Medosan, Ital.)*; Fluogisol *(Ital.)*; Fluolar *(Riva, Canad.)*; Fluomix Same *(Savoma, Ital.)*; Fluonid *(Herbert, USA)*; Fluonide *(Technilab, Canad.)*; Fluonide Dermica *(Ital.)*; Fluordima *(Fisons, Ital.)*; Fluoskin *(Dessy, Ital.)*; Fluovitef *(Italfarmaco, Ital.)*; Flupollon *(Jpn)*; Fluvean *(Jpn)*; Fluzon *(Jpn)*;
Gelidina *(Syntex-Latino, Spain)*; Intradermo Cort *(Pental, Spain)*; Isnaderm *(Isnardi, Ital.)*; Isoderma *(Isola-Ibi, Ital.)*; Jellin *(Grünenthal, Ger.)*; Lenar *(Ital.)*; Leniderm *(Salus, Ital.)*; Localyn *(Recordati, Ital.)*; Monoderm *(Neth.)*; Neoderm *(Janus, Ital.)*; Omniderm *(Face, Ital.)*; Oxidermiol *(Mazuelos, Spain)*; Percutina *(Ital.)*; Prodermin *(IBIS, Ital.)*; Psoranide *(Elder, USA)*; Radiocin *(Radiumfarma, Ital.)*; Roliderm *(Neopharmed, Ital.)*; Sterolone *(Francia Farm., Ital.)*; Straderm *(ITA, Ital.)*; Supricort *(Ind.)*; Synalar *(Arg.; ICI, Austral.; Belg.; Syncare, Canad.; ICI, Denm.; Cassenne, Fr.; Neth.; ICI, Norw.; ICI, S.Afr.; Syntex-Latino, Spain; ICI, Swed.; Grünenthal, Switz.; ICI Pharmaceuticals, UK; Syntex, USA)*; Synamol *(Syncare, Canad.)*; Synandone *(ICI Pharmaceuticals, UK)*; Synemol *(Syntex, USA)*; Topifluor *(Tiber, Ital.)*; Ultraderm *(Ecobi, Ital.)*; Ungovac *(Spain)*.

The following names have been used for multi-ingredient preparations containing fluocinolone acetonide— Neo-Synalar *(Syntex, USA)*; Synalar Bi-otic *(Syncare, Canad.)*; Synalar C *(ICI Pharmaceuticals, UK)*; Synalar N *(ICI Pharmaceuticals, UK)*.

1094-r

Fluocinonide *(BAN, USAN, rINN).*

Fluocinolide; Fluocinolone Acetonide 21-Acetate; NSC-101791. 6α,9α-Difluoro-11β,21-dihydroxy-16α,17α-isopropylidenedioxypregna-1,4-diene-3,20-dione 21-acetate.
$C_{26}H_{32}F_2O_7$=494.5.

CAS — 356-12-7.

Pharmacopoeias. In *Chin.* and *U.S.*

A white to cream-coloured crystalline powder with not more than a slight odour. Practically **insoluble** in water; sparingly soluble in acetone and chloroform; slightly soluble in alcohol, methyl alcohol, and dioxan; very slightly soluble in ether.

Adverse Effects, Treatment, Withdrawal, and Precautions
As for corticosteroids, p.872.
When applied topically, particularly to large areas, when the skin is broken, or under occlusive

dressings, corticosteroids may be absorbed in sufficient amounts to cause systemic effects.

Absorption and Fate

For a brief outline of the absorption and fate of corticosteroids, see p.875.

Uses and Administration

Fluocinonide is a corticosteroid used topically in the treatment of various skin disorders, as described under corticosteroids (see p.876). It is usually employed as a cream, gel, lotion, ointment, or scalp application containing 0.05%.

SKIN DISORDERS. For recommendations concerning the correct use of corticosteroids on the skin, and a rough guide to the clinical potencies of topical corticosteroids, see corticosteroids, p.880.

Preparations

Fluocinonide Cream *(U.S.P.)*

Fluocinonide Gel *(U.S.P.)*

Fluocinonide Ointment *(U.S.P.)*

Fluocinonide Topical Solution *(U.S.P.)*

Proprietary Preparations

Metosyn *(Stuart, UK). Cream* (FAPG Cream), *Ointment, Scalp lotion,* fluocinonide 0.05%.

Proprietary Names and Manufacturers

Bestasone *(Jpn)*; Biscosal *(Jpn)*; Cusigel *(Cusi, Spain)*; Flu 21 *(Aandersen, Ital.)*; Fludex *(San Carlo, Ital.)*; Klariderm *(Clariana, Spain)*; Lidemol *(Syncare, Canad.)*; Lidex *(Syncare, Canad.; Syntex, USA)*; Lidex-E *(Syntex, USA)*; Lyderm *(Taro, Canad.)*; Metosyn *(ICI, Denm.; ICI, Norw.; Stuart, S.Afr.; ICI, Swed.; Stuart, UK)*; Novoter *(Cusi, Spain)*; Topsym *(Grünenthal, Ger.; Jpn; Grünenthal, Switz.)*; Topsymin *(Grünenthal, Ger.; Grünenthal, Switz.)*; Topsyn *(Syncare, Canad.; Recordati, Ital.)*; Topsyne *(Belg.; Cassenne, Fr.; Neth.)*.

The following names have been used for multi-ingredient preparations containing fluocinonide— Lidecomb *(Syncare, Canad.)*; Trisyn *(Syncare, Canad.)*.

12761-a

Fluocortin Butyl *(BAN, USAN, rINNM).*

SH-K-203. Butyl 6α-fluoro-11β-hydroxy-16α-methyl-3,20-dioxopregna-1,4-dien-21-oate.

$C_{26}H_{35}FO_5$=446.6.

CAS — 33124-50-4 (fluocortin); 41767-29-7 (butyl ester).

Fluocortin butyl is a corticosteroid with the general properties described under corticosteroids (see p.872) and is used topically in the treatment of various skin disorders. It is usually employed as a cream or ointment containing 0.75%.

When applied topically, particularly to large areas, when the skin is broken, or under occlusive dressings, corticosteroids may be absorbed in sufficient amounts to cause systemic effects.

For recommendations concerning the correct use of corticosteroids on the skin, and a rough guide to the clinical potencies of topical corticosteroids, see corticosteroids, p.880.

Proprietary Names and Manufacturers

Vaspid *(Schering, Austral.)*; Vaspit *(Scherax, Ger.; Schering, Ital.; Schering, Spain; Schering, Switz.)*.

1095-f

Fluocortolone *(BAN, USAN, rINN).*

6α-Fluoro-16α-methyldehydrocorticosterone; SH-742. 6α-Fluoro-11β,21-dihydroxy-16α-methylpregna-1,4-diene-3,20-dione.

$C_{22}H_{29}FO_4$=376.5.

CAS — 152-97-6.

1096-d

Fluocortolone Hexanoate *(BANM, rINNM).*

Fluocortolone Caproate *(USAN)*; SH-770. Fluocortolone 21-hexanoate.

$C_{28}H_{39}FO_5$=474.6.

CAS — 303-40-2.

Pharmacopoeias. In *Br.*

An odourless or almost odourless, white to creamy-white, crystalline powder. Practically **insoluble** in water and ether; very slightly soluble in alcohol and methyl alcohol; sparingly soluble in chloroform; slightly soluble in acetone and dioxan. **Protect** from light.

1097-n

Fluocortolone Pivalate *(BANM, rINNM).*

Fluocortolone Trimethylacetate. Fluocortolone 21-pivalate.

$C_{27}H_{37}FO_5$=460.6.

CAS — 29205-06-9.

Pharmacopoeias. In *Br.*

Odourless or almost odourless, white to creamy-white, crystalline powder. Practically **insoluble** in water; sparingly soluble in alcohol and methyl alcohol; freely soluble in chloroform and dioxan; slightly soluble in ether. **Protect** from light.

Adverse Effects, Treatment, Withdrawal, and Precautions

As for corticosteroids, p.872.

When applied topically, particularly to large areas, when the skin is broken, or under occlusive dressings, corticosteroids may be absorbed in sufficient amounts to cause systemic effects.

Absorption and Fate

For a brief outline of the absorption and fate of corticosteroids, see p.875.

Fluocortolone hexanoate has a longer duration of action than the free alcohol or pivalate ester.

Uses and Administration

Fluocortolone and its esters are corticosteroids used topically in the treatment of various skin disorders, as described under corticosteroids (see p.876). They are usually employed as a cream or ointment; concentrations usually used are 0.1% of the hexanoate with 0.1% of the pivalate and 0.25% of the hexanoate with 0.25% of either the free alcohol or pivalate ester.

SKIN DISORDERS. For recommendations concerning the correct use of corticosteroids on the skin, and a rough guide to the clinical potencies of topical corticosteroids, see corticosteroids, p.880.

Preparations of Fluocortolone and its Esters

Fluocortolone Cream *(B.P.).* Fluocortolone Pivalate and Fluocortolone Hexanoate Cream

Fluocortolone Ointment *(B.P.).* Fluocortolone Pivalate and Fluocortolone Hexanoate Ointment

Proprietary Preparations of Fluocortolone and its Esters

Ultradil Plain *(Schering, UK). Cream, Ointment,* fluocortolone hexanoate 0.1%, fluocortolone pivalate 0.1%.

Ultralanum Plain *(Schering, UK). Cream,* fluocortolone pivalate 0.25%, fluocortolone hexanoate 0.25%. *Ointment,* fluocortolone 0.25%, fluocortolone hexanoate 0.25%.

Ultraproct *(Schering, UK). Rectal ointment,* fluocortolone pivalate 920 µg, fluocortolone hexanoate 950 µg, cinchocaine hydrochloride 5 mg/g. *Suppositories,* fluocortolone pivalate 610 µg, fluocortolone hexanoate 630 µg, cinchocaine hydrochloride 1mg.

Proprietary Names and Manufacturers of Fluocortolone and its Esters

Ficoid *(Fisons, UK)*; Syracort *(Beiersdorf, Ger.)*; Topodil *(Schering, Austral.)*; Ultracur *(Scherax, Ger.)*; Ultradil *(Schering, Ital.)*; Ultradil Plain *(Schering, UK)*; Ultralan *(Schering, Austral.; Schering, Fr.; Schering, Ger.; Schering, Ital.; Neth.; Schering, Spain; Schering, Switz.)*; Ultralanum *(Norw.; Schering, S.Afr.)*; Ultralanum Plain *(Schering, UK)*.

1098-h

Fluorometholone *(BAN, USAN, rINN).*

9α-Fluoro-11β,17α-dihydroxy-6α-methylpregna-1,4-diene-3,20-dione.

$C_{22}H_{29}FO_4$=376.5.

CAS — 426-13-1.

Pharmacopoeias. In *U.S.*

A white to yellowish-white, odourless, crystalline powder. Practically **insoluble** in water; soluble 1 in 200 of alcohol and 1 in 2200 of chloroform; very slightly soluble in ether. **Store** in airtight containers. Protect from light.

Adverse Effects, Treatment, Withdrawal, and Precautions

As for corticosteroids, p.872.

Prolonged application to the eye of preparations containing corticosteroids has caused raised intra-ocular pressure and reduced visual function.

Absorption and Fate

For a brief outline of the absorption and fate of corticosteroids, see p.875.

Uses and Administration

Fluorometholone is a glucocorticoid employed, usually as eye-drops containing 0.1% or 0.25%, in the treatment of allergic and inflammatory conditions of the eye.

Fluorometholone has also been used topically in the treatment of various skin disorders.

Preparations

In addition to the preparations below, further official preparations containing fluorometholone may be found listed under neomycin sulphate.

Fluorometholone Cream *(U.S.P.)*

Fluorometholone Ophthalmic Suspension *(U.S.P.)*

Proprietary Preparations

FML *(Allergan, UK). Eye-drops,* fluorometholone 0.1%.

FML-Neo *(Allergan, UK). Eye-drops,* fluorometholone 0.1%, neomycin sulphate 0.5%.

Proprietary Names and Manufacturers

Cortilet *(Swed.)*; Cortisdin *(Spain)*; Delmeson *(Hoechst, Denm.; Switz.)*; Efflumidex *(Allergan, Ger.)*; Fluaton *(Allergan, Ital.)*; Flucon *(Alcon, Austral.; Alcon, Fr.; Alcon, S.Afr.; Alcon, Switz.)*; Flumetholon *(Jpn)*; Flumetol semplice *(Farmila, Ital.)*; FML *(Canad.; Neth.; Allergan, S.Afr.; Allergan, UK)*; FML Liquifilm *(Allergan, Austral.; Allergan, Canad.; Allergan, USA)*; FML TM *(Belg.)*; Isopto-Flucon *(Alcon, Ger.; Alcon, Spain)*; Lerna *(Jpn)*; Oxylone *(USA)*; Regresin Sine *(Spain)*; Ursnon *(Jpn)*.

The following names have been used for multi-ingredient preparations containing fluorometholone— FML-Neo *(Allergan, UK)*; FML-Neo Liquifilm *(Allergan, Canad.)*.

1099-m

Fluperolone Acetate *(BANM, USAN, rINNM).*
9α-Fluoro-21-methylprednisolone Acetate. (21*S*)-9α-Fluoro-11β,17α,21-trihydroxy-21-methylpregna-1,4-diene-3,20-dione 21-acetate.
$C_{24}H_{31}FO_6$=434.5.

CAS — 3841-11-0 (fluperolone); 2119-75-7 (acetate).

Fluperolone acetate is a corticosteroid with the general properties described under corticosteroids (see p.872). It has been used topically in the treatment of various skin disorders.
When applied topically, particularly to large areas, when the skin is broken, or under occlusive dressings, corticosteroids may be absorbed in sufficient amounts to cause systemic effects.

For recommendations concerning the correct use of corticosteroids on the skin, see corticosteroids, p.880.

1100-m

Fluprednidene Acetate *(BANM, rINNM).*
Fluprednylidene 21-Acetate. 9α-Fluoro-11β,17α,21-trihydroxy-16-methylenepregna-1,4-diene-3,20-dione 21-acetate.
$C_{24}H_{29}FO_6$=432.5.

CAS — 2193-87-5 (fluprednidene); 1255-35-2 (acetate).

Pharmacopoeias. In *Nord.*

Fluprednidene acetate is a corticosteroid with the general properties described under corticosteroids (see p.872) and is used topically in the treatment of various skin disorders. It is usually employed as a cream, lotion, or ointment containing 0.1%.
When applied topically, particularly to large areas, when the skin is broken, or under occlusive dressings, corticosteroids may be absorbed in sufficient amounts to cause systemic effects.

For recommendations concerning the correct use of corticosteroids on the skin, and a rough guide to the clinical potencies of topical corticosteroids, see corticosteroids, p.880.

Proprietary Names and Manufacturers
Corticoderm *(E. Merck, Denm.; E. Merck, Norw.; E. Merck, Swed.)*; Décoderme *(Merck-Clévenot, Fr.)*; Decoderm *(Merck, Aust.; Merck, Belg.; E. Merck, Ger.; E. Merck, Neth.; Merck, S.Afr.; Igoda, Spain; E. Merck, Switz.; E. Merck, UK)*; Emcortina *(Merck, Arg.)*; Etacortin *(Hermal, Ger.)*; Vobaderm *(Hermal, Ger.)*.

1101-b

Fluprednisolone *(BAN, USAN, rINN).*
6α-Fluoroprednisolone. 6α-Fluoro-11β,17α,21-trihydroxypregna-1,4-diene-3,20-dione.
$C_{21}H_{27}FO_5$=378.4.

CAS — 53-34-9.

Fluprednisolone is a glucocorticoid with the general properties and uses described under corticosteroids (see p.872); 1.5 mg of fluprednisolone has been reported to be equivalent in anti-inflammatory activity to about 5 mg of prednisolone. It has been used by mouth in the form of the free alcohol and as the acetate and by injection as the acetate. The sodium hemisuccinate has also been used.

Proprietary Names and Manufacturers of Fluprednisolone and its Esters
Alphadrol *(Upjohn, USA)*; Selectren *(Hoechst, Spain)*; Vladicort *(Spain)*.

1102-v

Flurandrenolone *(BAN).*
6α-Fluoro-16α-hydroxyhydrocortisone 16,17-Acetonide; Fludroxycortide *(rINN)*; Flurandrenolide *(USAN)*. 6α-Fluoro-11β,21-dihydroxy-16α,17α-isopropylidenedioxypregn-4-ene-3,20-dione.
$C_{24}H_{33}FO_6$=436.5.

CAS — 1524-88-5.

Pharmacopoeias. In *U.S.*

An odourless, white to off-white, fluffy, crystalline powder. Practically **insoluble** in water and ether; soluble 1 in 72 of alcohol, 1 in 10 of chloroform, and 1 in 25 of methyl alcohol. **Store** at a temperature not exceeding 8° in airtight containers. Protect from light.

Adverse Effects, Treatment, Withdrawal, and Precautions
As for corticosteroids, p.872.
When applied topically, particularly to large areas, when the skin is broken, or under occlusive dressings, corticosteroids may be absorbed in sufficient amounts to cause systemic effects.

Absorption and Fate
For a brief outline of the absorption and fate of corticosteroids, see p.875.

Uses and Administration
Flurandrenolone is a corticosteroid used topically in the treatment of various skin disorders, as described under corticosteroids (see p.876). It is usually employed as a cream, lotion, or ointment; concentrations used range from 0.0125 to 0.05%. It is also used as a polyethylene tape with an adhesive containing 4 μg of flurandrenolone per cm^2 of tape.

SKIN DISORDERS. For recommendations concerning the correct use of corticosteroids on the skin, and a rough guide to the clinical potencies of topical corticosteroids, see corticosteroids, p.880.

Preparations
In addition to the preparations below, further official preparations containing flurandrenolone may be found listed under neomycin sulphate.

Flurandrenolide Cream *(U.S.P.).* Contains flurandrenolone.

Flurandrenolide Lotion *(U.S.P.).* Contains flurandrenolone.

Flurandrenolide Ointment *(U.S.P.).* Contains flurandrenolone.

Flurandrenolide Tape *(U.S.P.).* Non-porous, pliable, adhesive tape having flurandrenolone impregnated in the adhesive material.

Proprietary Preparations
Haelan *(Dista, UK). Cream, Ointment,* flurandrenolone 0.0125%.
Impregnated tape, flurandrenolone 4 μg/cm^2.
Haelan-C *(Dista, UK). Cream, Ointment,* flurandrenolone 0.0125%, clioquinol 3%.
Haelan-X *(Dista, UK). Cream, Ointment,* flurandrenolone 0.05%.

Proprietary Names and Manufacturers
Cordran *(Dista, USA)*; Drenison *(Lilly, Canad.; Lilly, Ital.; Derly, Spain; Lilly, UK)*; Haelan *(Austral.; Dista, UK)*; Haelan-X *(Dista, UK)*; Sermaka *(Lilly, Ger.)*.

The following names have been used for multi-ingredient preparations containing flurandrenolone— Cordran-N *(Dista, USA)*; Haelan-C *(Dista, UK)*.

1103-g

Formocortal *(BAN, USAN, rINN).*
3-(2-Chloroethoxy)-9α-fluoro-11β,21-dihydroxy-16α,17α-isopropylidenedioxy-20-oxopregna-3,5-diene-6-carbaldehyde 21-acetate.
$C_{29}H_{38}ClFO_8$=569.1.

CAS — 2825-60-7.

Formocortal is a corticosteroid with the general properties described under corticosteroids (see p.872) and is used topically in the treatment of various skin disorders. It is used as eye-drops and eye ointments containing 0.05% and has been employed as a cream or ointment containing 0.025%.
When applied topically, particularly to large areas, when the skin is broken, or under occlusive dressings, corticosteroids may be absorbed in sufficient amounts to cause systemic effects.

For recommendations concerning the correct use of corticosteroids on the skin, see corticosteroids, p.880.

Proprietary Names and Manufacturers
Deflamene *(Montedison, Arg.; Spain; Farmitalia Carlo Erba, UK)*; Formoftil *(Farmigea, Ital.)*.

1104-q

Halcinonide *(BAN, USAN, rINN).*
SQ-18566. 21-Chloro-9α-fluoro-11β-hydroxy-16α,17α-isopropylidenedioxypregn-4-ene-3,20-dione.
$C_{24}H_{32}ClFO_5$=455.0.

CAS — 3093-35-4.

Pharmacopoeias. In *U.S.*

A white to off-white, odourless, crystalline powder. Practically **insoluble** in water; soluble in acetone and chloroform; slightly soluble in alcohol and ether.

Adverse Effects, Treatment, Withdrawal, and Precautions
As for corticosteroids, p.872.
When applied topically, particularly to large areas, when the skin is broken, or under occlusive dressings, corticosteroids may be absorbed in sufficient amounts to cause systemic effects.

Absorption and Fate
For a brief outline of the absorption and fate of corticosteroids, see p.875.

Uses and Administration
Halcinonide is a corticosteroid used topically in the treatment of various skin disorders, as described under corticosteroids (see p.876). It is usually employed as a cream, lotion, or ointment; concentrations used range from 0.025% to 0.1%.

SKIN DISORDERS. For recommendations concerning the correct use of corticosteroids on the skin, and a rough guide to the clinical potencies of topical corticosteroids, see corticosteroids, p.880.

Preparations
Halcinonide Cream *(U.S.P.)*
Halcinonide Ointment *(U.S.P.)*
Halcinonide Topical Solution *(U.S.P.)*

Proprietary Preparations
Halciderm *(Squibb, UK). Cream,* halcinonide 0.1%.

Proprietary Names and Manufacturers
Halciderm *(Arg.; Squibb, Austral.; Belg.; Squibb, Ital.; Neth.; Squibb, Switz.; Squibb, UK)*; Halcimat *(Heyden, Ger.)*; Halcort *(FAIR Laboratories, UK)*; Halog *(Squibb, Canad.; Squibb, Denm.; Squibb, Fr.; Heyden, Ger.; Novo, Norw.; S.Afr.; Squibb, Spain; Swed.; Princeton, USA)*; Halog-E *(Princeton, USA)*; Heyden-Dermol *(Med. y Prod. Quím., Spain)*.

The following names have been used for multi-ingredient preparations containing halcinonide— Halcicomb *(Squibb, Canad.; FAIR Laboratories, UK)*.

16830-n

Halometasone *(rINN).*
Halomethasone. 2-Chloro-6α,9-difluoro-11β,17,21-trihydroxy-16α-methylpregna-1,4-diene-3,20-dione.
$C_{22}H_{27}ClF_2O_5$=444.9.

CAS — 50629-82-8.

Halometasone is a corticosteroid with the general properties described under corticosteroids (see p.872) and is used topically in the treatment of various skin disorders. It is usually employed as a cream or ointment containing 0.05% of halometasone monohydrate.
When applied topically, particularly to large areas, when the skin is broken, or under occlusive dressings, corticosteroids may be absorbed in sufficient amounts to cause systemic effects.

For recommendations concerning the correct use of corticosteroids on the skin, see corticosteroids p.880.

Proprietary Names and Manufacturers
Sicortène *(Ciba, Switz.)*; Sicorten *(Zyma, Ger.; Ciba-Geigy, Malaysia; Ciba, Neth.; Ciba, S.Afr.; Ciba-Geigy, Singapore)*.

12814-z

Halopredone Acetate *(USAN, rINNM).*
2-Bromo-6β,9α-difluoro-11β,17α,21-trihydroxypregna-1,4-diene-3,20-dione 17,21-diacetate.
$C_{25}H_{29}BrF_2O_7$=559.4.

CAS — 57781-15-4 (halopredone); 57781-14-3 (acetate).

Halopredone acetate is a corticosteroid with the general properties described under corticosteroids (see p.872) and is used topically in the treatment of various skin disorders. It is usually employed as a cream, gel, or lotion containing 0.01%.
When applied topically, particularly to large areas, when the skin is broken, or under occlusive dressings, corticosteroids may be absorbed in sufficient amounts to cause systemic effects.

For recommendations concerning the correct use of corticosteroids on the skin, see corticosteroids, p.880.

Proprietary Names and Manufacturers
Topicon *(Pierrel, Ital.).*

1105-p

Hydrocortamate Hydrochloride *(rINNM).*
Ethamicort; Hydrocortisone Diethylaminoacetate Hydrochloride. 11β,17α,21-Trihydroxypregn-4-ene-3,20-dione 21-diethylaminoacetate hydrochloride.
$C_{27}H_{41}NO_6$,HCl=512.1.

CAS — 76-47-1 (hydrocortamate); 125-03-1 (hydrochloride).

Hydrocortamate hydrochloride is a corticosteroid with the general properties described under corticosteroids (see p.872) It has been used topically in the treatment of various skin disorders.
When applied topically, particularly to large areas, when the skin is broken, or under occlusive dressings, corticosteroids may be absorbed in sufficient amounts to cause systemic effects.

For recommendations concerning the correct use of corticosteroids on the skin, see corticosteroids, p.880.

1138-k

Hydrocortisone *(BAN, USAN, rINN).*

17-Hydroxycorticosterone; Compound F; Cortisol; Hydrocortisonum. 11β,17α,21-Trihydroxypregn-4-ene-3,20-dione.
$C_{21}H_{30}O_5$=362.5.

CAS — 50-23-7.

Pharmacopoeias. In *Arg., Aust., Br., Braz., Chin., Egypt., Eur., Fr., Ger., Hung., Ind., Int., It., Jpn, Jug., Neth., Nord., Pol., Roum., Swiss, Turk.,* and *U.S.*

A white or almost white, odourless, crystalline powder. *B.P.* **solubilities** are: practically insoluble in water; soluble 1 in 40 of alcohol and 1 in 80 of acetone; slightly soluble in chloroform; very slightly soluble in ether. *U.S.P.* solubilities are: very slightly soluble in water and ether; soluble 1 in 40 of alcohol and 1 in 80 of acetone; slightly soluble in chloroform. **Store** in well-closed containers. Protect from light.

1107-w

Hydrocortisone Acetate *(BANM, USAN, rINNM).*

Cortisol Acetate; Hydrocortisoni Acetas. Hydrocortisone 21-acetate.
$C_{23}H_{32}O_6$=404.5.

CAS — 50-03-3.

Pharmacopoeias. In *Arg., Aust., Belg., Br., Braz., Chin., Cz., Egypt., Eur., Fr., Ger., Hung., Ind., Int., It., Jpn, Jug., Neth., Nord., Pol., Port., Roum., Swiss, Turk.,* and *U.S.*

An odourless, white or almost white, crystalline powder. Hydrocortisone acetate 112 mg is approximately equivalent to 100 mg of hydrocortisone.
Practically **insoluble** in water; soluble 1 in 230 of alcohol and 1 in 200 of chloroform. **Store** in well-closed containers. Protect from light.

1108-e

Hydrocortisone Butyrate *(BANM, USAN, rINNM).*

Cortisol Butyrate. Hydrocortisone 17α-butyrate.
$C_{25}H_{36}O_6$=432.6.

CAS — 13609-67-1.

Pharmacopoeias. In *Jpn* and *U.S.*

A white to practically white practically odourless crystalline powder. Hydrocortisone butyrate 119 mg is approximately equivalent to 100 mg of hydrocortisone.
Practically **insoluble** in water; slightly soluble in ether; soluble in acetone, alcohol, and methyl alcohol; freely soluble in chloroform.

1109-l

Hydrocortisone Cypionate *(BANM, USAN).*

Cortisol Cypionate; Hydrocortisone Cipionate *(rINNM)*; Hydrocortisone Cyclopentylpropionate. Hydrocortisone 21-(3-cyclopentylpropionate).
$C_{29}H_{42}O_6$=486.6.

CAS — 508-99-6.

Pharmacopoeias. In *U.S.*

A white to practically white, crystalline powder, odourless or with a slight odour. Hydrocortisone cypionate 134 mg is approximately equivalent to 100 mg of hydrocortisone.
Practically **insoluble** in water; soluble in alcohol, very soluble in chloroform; slightly soluble in ether. **Store** at a temperature not exceeding 8° in airtight containers. Protect from light.

1110-v

Hydrocortisone Hemisuccinate *(USAN).*

Cortisol Hemisuccinate; Hydrocortisone Hydrogen Succinate *(BAN).* Hydrocortisone 21-(hydrogen succinate).
$C_{25}H_{34}O_8$=462.5.

CAS — 2203-97-6 (anhydrous); 83784-20-7 (monohydrate).

Pharmacopoeias. In *Br., Cz., Fr.,* and *Jpn. U.S.* allows the anhydrous form or the monohydrate.

A white or almost white odourless or almost odourless crystalline powder. Hydrocortisone hemisuccinate 128 mg is approximately equivalent to 100 mg of hydrocortisone.
Practically **insoluble** in water; soluble 1 in 40 of alcohol, 1 in 7 of dehydrated alcohol, and 1 in 25 of sodium bicarbonate solution; soluble, with decomposition, in sodium hydroxide solution. **Store** in airtight containers. Protect from light.

1111-g

Hydrocortisone Sodium Phosphate *(BANM, USAN, rINNM).*

Cortisol Sodium Phosphate. Hydrocortisone 21-(disodium orthophosphate).
$C_{21}H_{29}Na_2O_8P$=486.4.

CAS — 6000-74-4.

Pharmacopoeias. In *Br.* and *U.S.*

A white or light yellow, odourless or almost odourless, hygroscopic powder. Hydrocortisone sodium phosphate 134 mg is approximately equivalent to 100 mg of hydrocortisone.
B.P. **solubilities** are: soluble 1 in 4 of water; practically insoluble in dehydrated alcohol and chloroform; *U.S.P.* solubilities are: soluble 1 in 1.5 of water; slightly soluble in alcohol; practically insoluble in chloroform, dioxan, and ether. A 0.5% solution in water has a pH of 7.5 to 9.0. Solutions are **sterilised** by filtration. **Store** in airtight containers. Protect from light.

1112-q

Hydrocortisone Sodium Succinate *(BANM, USAN, rINNM).*

Cortisol Sodium Succinate. Hydrocortisone 21-(sodium succinate).
$C_{25}H_{33}NaO_8$=484.5.

CAS — 125-04-2.

Pharmacopoeias. In *Braz., Egypt., It., Jpn,* and *U.S.*

A white or almost white, odourless, hygroscopic, amorphous solid. Hydrocortisone sodium succinate 134 mg is approximately equivalent to 100 mg of hydrocortisone.
Very **soluble** in water and alcohol; very slightly soluble in acetone; practically insoluble in chloroform. **Store** in airtight containers. Protect from light.

1106-s

Hydrocortisone Valerate *(BANM, USAN, rINNM).*

Cortisol Valerate. Hydrocortisone 17-valerate.
$C_{26}H_{38}O_6$=446.6.

CAS — 57524-89-7.

Pharmacopoeias. In *U.S.*

Hydrocortisone valerate 123 mg is approximately equivalent to 100 mg of hydrocortisone.

Adverse Effects, Treatment, Withdrawal, and Precautions
As for corticosteroids, p.872.

ALLERGY. A short review and discussion concerning anaphylactoid reactions to hydrocortisone: J. P. Seale, *Med. J. Aust.,* 1984, *141,* 446.

Reports of allergic reactions following the intravenous administration of hydrocortisone: C. S. Chan *et al., Med. J. Aust.,* 1984, *141,* 444 (anaphylactic reaction; airflow obstruction); C. E. Corallo and M. Sosnin, *Aust. J. Hosp. Pharm.,* 1985, *15,* 103 (bronchospasm).

PARAESTHESIA. For reports and comments on paraesthesia or perineal irritation associated with the administration of hydrocortisone sodium phosphate intravenously, see under dexamethasone, p.887.

Absorption and Fate
For a brief account of the absorption and fate of corticosteroids, see p.875.
Hydrocortisone is readily absorbed from the gastro-intestinal tract and peak blood concentrations are attained in about an hour. The biological half-life is about 100 minutes. It is more than 90% bound to plasma proteins. It is absorbed more slowly following intramuscular injection and is no longer administered by this route. Hydrocortisone acetate given by mouth is less readily absorbed than hydrocortisone, and it is very poorly absorbed from intramuscular injections; it is also very poorly absorbed from intrasynovial and soft-tissue injections but may be used by these routes to produce a prolonged local effect.
Hydrocortisone is absorbed through the skin, particularly in denuded areas; the acetate is less well absorbed and has a more prolonged action.
Hydrocortisone is metabolised in the liver and most body tissues to hydrogenated and degraded forms such as tetrahydrocortisone and tetrahydrocortisol. These are excreted in the urine, mainly conjugated as glucuronides, together with a very small proportion of unchanged hydrocortisone.

For details of the metabolism of hydrocortisone, see C. L. Cope, *Adrenal Steroids and Disease,* London, Pitman Medical, 1972.. See also: E. J. Begg *et al., Med. J. Aust.,* 1987, *146,* 37.

Uses and Administration
Hydrocortisone (cortisol) is the main glucocorticoid secreted by the adrenal cortex and has the

properties described under corticosteroids (see p.875). It has been used, either in the form of the free alcohol, or in one of the esterified forms, in the treatment of all conditions for which corticosteroid therapy is indicated. Hydrocortisone is now preferred to cortisone since it is already pharmacologically active, whereas cortisone must be converted in the liver to hydrocortisone.

For administration by mouth hydrocortisone is usually used and sometimes the cypionate ester is also employed. The usual dose range, expressed in terms of hydrocortisone, is generally 10 to 40 mg daily in divided doses.

For replacement therapy in acute or chronic adrenocortical insufficiency the normal requirement is 10 to 20 or 30 mg daily (usually 20 mg is taken in the morning and 10 mg in the early evening, to mimic the circadian rhythm of the body). Additional sodium chloride may be required if there is defective aldosterone secretion, but mineralocorticoid activity is usually supplemented by fludrocortisone acetate (see p.890) by mouth. Similar doses of about 10 to 30 mg hydrocortisone are also given to correct glucocorticoid deficiency in the salt-losing form of congenital adrenal hyperplasia, again in association with fludrocortisone, and together with an adequate sodium intake.

Hydrocortisone may be given intravenously, by slow injection or infusion, in the form of a water-soluble derivative such as hydrocortisone sodium succinate or hydrocortisone sodium phosphate when a rapid effect is required in emergencies; such conditions are acute adrenal insufficiency caused by addisonian or post-adrenalectomy crises, by the abrupt accidental withdrawal of therapy in corticosteroid-treated patients, or by the inability of the adrenal glands to cope with increased stress in such patients; certain allergic emergencies; acute severe asthma (status asthmaticus); and shock. The usual dose is the equivalent of 100 to 500 mg of hydrocortisone, repeated 3 or 4 times in 24 hours, according to the severity of the condition and the patient's response. Children up to 1 year of age may be given 25 mg, those aged 1 to 5 years 50 mg, and those aged 6 to 12 years 100 mg. Fluids and electrolytes should be given as necessary to correct any associated metabolic disorder. Similar doses to those specified above may also be given intramuscularly but the response is likely to be less rapid than that observed following intravenous administration. In some forms of shock much higher initial doses in the order of 1 g have been given intravenously.

In patients with adrenal deficiency states supplementary corticosteroid therapy may be necessary during some surgical operations and hydrocortisone sodium succinate or sodium phosphate may be given intramuscularly or intravenously before surgery.

For local administration by injection into soft tissues hydrocortisone in the form of the sodium phosphate or sodium succinate esters is usually employed; doses in terms of hydrocortisone are usually up to 200 mg. For intra-articular injection hydrocortisone acetate is usually used in doses of 5 to 50 mg depending upon the size of the joint.

For topical application in the treatment of various skin disorders hydrocortisone and the acetate, butyrate, and valerate esters are normally employed. Concentrations usually used for hydrocortisone have ranged from 0.1 to 2.5%, for the acetate from 0.25 to 2.5%, for the butyrate 0.1%, and for the valerate 0.2%. Although it is considered that hydrocortisone has fewer side-effects on the skin and is less liable to cause adrenal suppression than the more potent topical corticosteroids, it should be borne in mind, especially in view of the availability of 'over-the-counter' hydrocortisone preparations in certain countries, that this property may be considerably modified both by the type of formulation or vehicle used and by the type of esterification present; other factors that may also influence absorption include the site of application and the degree of skin damage.

Hydrocortisone or its esters are also available in a variety of other dosage forms including ophthalmic and rectal forms, for use in allergic and inflammatory disorders.

Other esters of hydrocortisone which have occasionally been used include the aceponate and hexanoate.

CONGENITAL ADRENAL HYPERPLASIA. References to the successful use of corticosteroids, administered to the mother during pregnancy, for the prevention of genital virilisation of high-risk female foetuses with congenital adrenal hyperplasia: M. David and M. G. Forest, *J. Pediat.*, 1984, *105*, 799 (dexamethasone or hydrocortisone); M. I. Evans *et al.*, *J. Am. med. Ass.*, 1985, *253*, 1015 (dexamethasone).

NEONATAL RESPIRATORY DISTRESS SYNDROME. For reference to the use of hydrocortisone in the prophylaxis of the neonatal respiratory distress syndrome, see under betamethasone, p.884.

SKIN DISORDERS. For recommendations concerning the correct use of corticosteroids on the skin, and a rough guide to the clinical potencies of topical corticosteroids, see corticosteroids, p.880.

Preparations of Hydrocortisone and its Esters

In addition to the preparations below, further official preparations containing hydrocortisone or its esters may be found listed under chloramphenicol, colistin, neomycin, neomycin sulphate, oxytetracycline hydrochloride, and polymyxin B sulphate.

Aural Dosage Forms

Hydrocortisone Ear Drops *(A.P.F.)*. Hydrocortisone 500 mg, propylene glycol to 100 mL.

Hydrocortisone and Acetic Acid Otic Solution *(U.S.P.)*

Injections

Sterile Hydrocortisone Suspension *(U.S.P.)*

Hydrocortisone Acetate Injection *(B.P.)*. An aqueous suspension of hydrocortisone acetate intended for local injection only.

Sterile Hydrocortisone Acetate Suspension *(U.S.P.)*

Hydrocortisone Sodium Phosphate Injection *(B.P.)*

Hydrocortisone Sodium Phosphate Injection *(U.S.P.)*

Hydrocortisone Sodium Succinate Injection *(B.P.)*. It is prepared by dissolving, immediately before use, the sterile contents of a sealed container (Hydrocortisone Sodium Succinate for Injection) which are made from hydrocortisone hemisuccinate with the aid of a suitable alkali.

Hydrocortisone Sodium Succinate for Injection *(U.S.P.)*. It may be prepared from hydrocortisone sodium succinate or hydrocortisone hemisuccinate and sodium hydroxide or sodium carbonate.

Ophthalmic Dosage Forms

Hydrocortisone Eye-drops *(B.P.C. 1973)*. HCOR. A sterile suspension containing up to 1% of hydrocortisone acetate.

Hydrocortisone Eye Ointment *(B.P.C. 1973)*. Hydrocortisone Acetate Eye Ointment. A sterile eye ointment containing hydrocortisone acetate.

Hydrocortisone Acetate Ophthalmic Ointment *(U.S.P.)*

Hydrocortisone Eye Ointment *(A.P.F.)*. Hydrocortisone acetate 2.5% in Eye Ointment Base.

Hydrocortisone Acetate Ophthalmic Suspension *(U.S.P.)*

Oral Dosage Forms

Hydrocortisone Lozenges *(B.P.C. 1973)*. Hydrocortisone Sodium Succinate Lozenges. Lozenges containing hydrocortisone sodium succinate.

Hydrocortisone Tablets *(U.S.P.)*

Hydrocortisone Cypionate Oral Suspension *(U.S.P.)*

Rectal Dosage Forms

Hydrocortisone Enema *(U.S.P.)*

Hydrocortisone Suppositories *(B.P.C. 1973)*. Suppositories containing hydrocortisone or hydrocortisone acetate.

Hydrocortisone Suppositories *(A.P.F.)*. Each contains hydrocortisone 25 mg or an equivalent amount of hydrocortisone acetate.

Topical Dosage Forms

Hydrocortisone Cream *(B.P.)*

Hydrocortisone Cream *(U.S.P.)*

Hydrocortisone Cream Aqueous *(A.P.F.)*. Hydrocortisone 1%, or an equivalent amount of hydrocortisone acetate, in aqueous cetomacrogol cream.

Hydrocortisone Acetate Cream *(B.P.)*

Hydrocortisone Acetate Cream *(U.S.P.)*

Hydrocortisone Acetate and Clioquinol Cream *(B.P.)*

Hydrocortisone Butyrate Cream *(U.S.P.)*

Hydrocortisone Valerate Cream *(U.S.P.)*

Hydrocortisone Gel *(U.S.P.)*

Hydrocortisone Lotion *(B.P.C. 1973)*. Hydrocortisone 1 g, chlorocresol 50 mg, self-emulsifying glyceryl monostearate 4 g, glycerol 6.3 g, water to 100 g. Any other suitable basis may be used.

Hydrocortisone Lotion *(U.S.P.)*

Hydrocortisone Lotion *(A.P.F.)*. Hydrocortisone 1 g, chlorocresol 50 mg, self-emulsifying glyceryl monostearate 4 g, glycerol 5 g, water to 100 g.

Hydrocortisone Acetate Lotion *(U.S.P.)*

Hydrocortisone Ointment *(B.P.)*

Hydrocortisone Ointment *(U.S.P.)*

Hydrocortisone Ointment *(A.P.F.)*. Hydrocortisone 1 g, liquid paraffin 10 g, wool fat 10 g, and white soft paraffin 79 g.

Hydrocortisone Acetate Ointment *(B.P.)*

Hydrocortisone Acetate Ointment *(U.S.P.)*

Hydrocortisone and Clioquinol Ointment *(B.P.)*

Proprietary Preparations of Hydrocortisone and its Esters

In addition to those given below, details of further proprietary preparations containing hydrocortisone or its esters may be found under bismuth oxide, bismuth subgallate, calamine, chloramphenicol, clioquinol, clotrimazole, coal tar, crotamiton, econazole nitrate, framycetin sulphate, fusidic acid, gentamicin sulphate, lignocaine, miconazole nitrate, neomycin sulphate, nystatin, oxytetracycline hydrochloride, potassium hydroxyquinoline sulphate, sulphacetamide sodium, and urea.

Anflam *(Cox, UK)*. *Cream*, *Ointment*, hydrocortisone 1%.

Cobadex *(Cox, UK)*. *Cream*, hydrocortisone 0.5 and 1%.

Colifoam *(Stafford-Miller, UK)*. *Rectal foam*, hydrocortisone acetate 10%.

Corlan *(Glaxo, UK)*. *Pellets* (lozenges), hydrocortisone 2.5 mg (as sodium succinate).

Cortacream Bandage *(Smith & Nephew, UK)*. *Impregnated bandage*, hydrocortisone acetate 1%.

Cortenema *(Bengué, UK)*. *Retention enema*, hydrocortisone 100 mg/60 mL.

Dermacort *(Panpharma, UK)*. *Cream*, hydrocortisone 0.1%.

Dioderm *(Dermal Laboratories, UK)*. *Cream*, hydrocortisone 0.1%.

Efcortelan *(Glaxo, UK)*. *Cream*, *Ointment*, hydrocortisone 0.5, 1, and 2.5%.
Lotion, hydrocortisone 1%.

Efcortelan Soluble *(Glaxo, UK)*. *Injection*, powder for reconstitution, hydrocortisone 100 mg (as sodium succinate), supplied with solvent.

Efcortesol *(Glaxo, UK)*. *Injection*, hydrocortisone 100 mg (as sodium phosphate)/mL, in ampoules of 1 and 5 mL.

Epifoam *(Stafford-Miller, UK)*. *Foam*, hydrocortisone acetate 1%, pramoxine hydrochloride 1%.

Evacort *(Evans Medical, UK)*. *Cream*, hydrocortisone 1%.

Hc45 *(Crookes Healthcare, UK)*. *Cream*, hydrocortisone acetate 1%.

Hydrocortistab *(Boots, UK)*. *Tablets*, scored, hydrocortisone 20 mg.
Injection (aqueous suspension), hydrocortisone acetate 25 mg/mL.
Cream, hydrocortisone acetate 1%.
Ointment, hydrocortisone 1%.

Hydrocortisyl *(Roussel, UK)*. *Cream*, *Ointment*, hydrocortisone 1%.

Hydrocortone *(Merck Sharp & Dohme, UK)*. *Tablets*, scored, hydrocortisone 10 and 20 mg.

Hydroderm *(Merck Sharp & Dohme, UK)*. *Ointment*, hydrocortisone 10 mg, neomycin sulphate 5 mg, bacitracin zinc 1000 units/g.

Lanacort *(Combe, UK)*. *Cream*, *Ointment*, hydrocortisone acetate 1%.

Locoid *(Brocades, UK)*. *Cream*, *Ointment*, *Scalp lotion*, hydrocortisone butyrate 0.1%.

Locoid C *(Brocades, UK)*. *Cream*, *Ointment*, hydrocortisone butyrate 0.1%, chlorquinaldol 3%.

Locoid Lipocream *(Brocades, UK). Oily cream,* hydrocortisone butyrate 0.1%.

Medicort *(Care, UK). Cream,* hydrocortisone 1%.

Proctofoam HC *(Stafford-Miller, UK). Rectal foam,* hydrocortisone acetate 1%, pramoxine hydrochloride 1%.

Proctosedyl *(Roussel, UK). Rectal ointment,* hydrocortisone 0.5%, cinchocaine hydrochloride 0.5%. *Suppositories,* hydrocortisone 5 mg, cinchocaine hydrochloride 5 mg.

NOTE. Proctosedyl was reformulated to exclude aesculus and framycetin sulphate.

Quinocort *(Quinoderm, UK). Cream,* hydrocortisone 1%, potassium hydroxyquinoline sulphate 0.5%.

Solu-Cortef *(Upjohn, UK). Injection,* powder for reconstitution, hydrocortisone 100 mg (as sodium succinate).

Timocort *(Reckitt & Colman Pharmaceuticals, UK). Cream,* hydrocortisone 1%.

Uniroid *(Unigreg, UK). Rectal ointment,* hydrocortisone 5 mg, neomycin sulphate 5 mg, polymyxin B sulphate 6250 units, cinchocaine hydrochloride 5 mg/g. *Suppositories,* hydrocortisone 5 mg, neomycin sulphate 10 mg, polymyxin B sulphate 12 500 units, cinchocaine hydrochloride 5 mg.

Wasp-eze Hydrocortisone *(International Laboratories, UK). Cream,* hydrocortisone 1%.

Zenoxone *(Biorex, UK). Cream,* hydrocortisone 1%.

Proprietary Names and Manufacturers of Hydrocortisone and its Esters

Aacicortisol *(Belg.)*; Actocortin *(Erco, Denm.; Ger.; Cortec, Norw.; Swed.)*; Actocortina *(Leo, Spain)*; Adacor *(Nelson, Austral.)*; Aeroseb-HC *(Herbert, USA)*; A-Hydrocort *(Abbott, USA)*; Alfason *(Thomae, Ger.)*; Algicortis *(Vaillant, Ital.)*; Anflam *(Cox, UK)*; Bacid *(Farma-Lepori, Spain)*; Bactine Hydrocortisone *(Miles Laboratories, USA)*; Buccalsone *(Belg.)*;
CaldeCORT *(Pharmacraft, USA)*; Carmol HC *(Syntex, USA)*; Cetacort *(Owen, USA)*; Chemysone *(Ital.)*; Cleiton *(Jpn)*; Cobadex *(Cox, UK)*; Colifoam *(Stafford-Miller, Austral.; Stafford-Miller, Denm.; Trommsdorff, Ger.; Stafford-Miller, Norw.; Stafford-Miller, S.Afr.; Stafford-Miller, Switz.; Stafford-Miller, UK)*; Colofoam *(Stafford-Miller, Fr.)*; Cordes-H *(Ichthyol, Ger.)*; Corlan *(Glaxo, Austral.; Neth.; Glaxo, S.Afr.; Glaxo, UK)*; Cortacream Bandage *(Smith & Nephew, UK)*; Cortaid *(Upjohn, Austral.; Upjohn, USA)*; Cortamed *(Berlex, Canad.)*; Cortate *(Schering, Canad.)*; Cort-Dome *(Austral.; Canad.; Miles Pharmaceuticals, USA)*; Cortef *(Upjohn, Austral.; Upjohn, Canad.; Upjohn, USA)*; Cortenema *(Interfalk, Canad.; Bengué, UK; Rowell, USA)*; Cortes *(Jpn)*; Cortesal *(Pharmacia, Swed.)*; Corti-Basileos *(Spain)*; Cortic *(Sigma, Austral.)*; Corticaine *(Glaxo, USA)*; Corticare *(Essex, Austral.)*; Corticotets *(Pharmadrug, Ger.)*; Corticreme *(Rougier, Canad.)*; Cortidro *(Ital.)*; Cortifair *(Pharmafair, USA)*; Cortifoam *(Reed & Carnrick, Canad.; Reed & Carnrick, USA)*; Cortiment *(Nordic, Canad.; Ferring, Swed.)*; Cortioftal *(Cusi, Spain)*; Cortoderm *(Taro, Canad.)*; Cortomister *(Fr.)*; Cortoxide *(USA)*; Cortril *(Austral.; Belg.; Canad.; Ital.; S.Afr.; Pfizer, UK; Pfizer, USA)*; Cotacort *(USA)*; Crema Transcutanea Astier *(Semar, Spain)*; Cutaderm *(Scherag, S.Afr.)*; Cycort *(Lederle, Austral.)*;
Dermacort *(Parke, Davis, Austral.; Panpharma, UK; Rowell, USA)*; Derm-Aid *(Ego, Austral.)*; Dermolate *(Schering, USA)*; Dermolene *(Switz.)*; Dilucort *(Triomed, S.Afr.)*; Dioderm *(Dermal Laboratories, UK)*; Dome-Cort *(Bayer, UK : Lagap, UK)*; Ef-corlin *(Ital.)*; Efcorlin *(Ind.)*; Efcortelan *(Glaxo, UK)*; EF-Cortelan *(Glaxo, Austral.; Glaxo, S.Afr.)*; Efcortesol *(Glaxo, UK)*; Egocort *(Ego, Austral.)*; Eldecort *(Elder, USA)*; Emi-Corlin *(Ital.)*; Emo-Cort *(Trans Canaderm, Canad.)*; Evacort *(Evans Medical, UK)*; Excerate *(Jpn)*; Ficortril *(Pfizer, Ger.; Pfizer, Swed.)*; Flebocortid *(Lepetit, Ital.; Spain)*; Hc45 *(Crookes Healthcare, UK)*; Hidroaltesona *(Alter, Spain)*; Hidrotisona *(Arg.)*; Hycor *(Sigma, Austral.)*; Hycort *(ICN, Canad.)*; Hyderm *(Taro, Canad.)*; Hydro-Adreson *(Neth.; Switz.)*; Hydro-Adreson SSC *(Belg.)*; Hydrocortal *(Organon, Swed.)*; Hydrocortemel *(S.Afr.)*; Hydrocortifor *(Switz.)*; Hydro-Cortilean *(Canad.)*; Hydrocortisat *(Denm.)*; Hydrocortistab *(Boots, UK)*; Hydrocortisyl *(Austral.; S.Afr.; Roussel, UK)*; Hydrocortone *(Austral.; Canad.; Neth.; MSD, Swed.; Merck Sharp & Dohme, Switz.; Merck Sharp & Dohme, UK; Merck Sharp & Dohme, USA)*; Hydrosone *(USV, Austral.)*; Hysone *(Protea, Austral.)*; Hysone-A *(Protea, Austral.)*; Hytone *(Dermik, USA)*;
Idracemi *(Farmigea, Ital.)*; Idrocortigamma *(IBP, Ital.)*; Ivocort *(USA)*; Lanacort *(Combe, UK)*; Lenirit *(Bonomelli, Ital.)*; Litraderm *(Ger.)*; Locoid *(Astra, Austral.; Belg.; Gist-Brocades, Denm.; Beytout, Fr.; Neth.; Gist-Brocades, Norw.; Brocades, S.Afr.; Gist-Brocades, Swed.; Gist-Brocades, Switz.; Brocades, UK; Owen, USA)*; Locoidon *(Brocades, Ital.)*; Manticor *(Canad.)*; Medicort *(Care, UK)*; Microcort *(Canad.)*; Milliderm *(A.L., Denm.)*; Munitren *(Robugen, Ger.)*; Mylocort *(Triomed, S.Afr.)*; Nordicort *(Ascot, Austral.)*; Novohydrocort *(Novopharm, Canad.)*; Nutracort *(Canad.; Owen, USA)*; Odoncortex *(Besins-Iscovesco, Fr.)*; Ophticor H *(Belg.)*; Optef *(USA)*; Orabase HCA *(Colgate-Hoyt, USA)*; Oralsone *(Gramon, Arg.; Vinas, Spain)*; Pabracort *(Paines & Byrne, UK)*; Penecort *(Herbert, USA)*; Phiacort *(Austral.)*; Physiocortison *(Spain)*; Plancol *(Jpn)*; Pro-Cort *(Barnes-Hind, USA)*; Proctocort *(Biothérax, Fr.; Reid-Rowell, USA)*; Procutan *(Scherag, S.Afr.)*; Promecort *(Schering, Swed.)*;
Rectocort *(Welcker-Lyster, Canad.)*; Rectoid *(USA)*; Sarna-HC *(Stiefel, Canad.)*; Schericur *(Scherax, Ger.; Schering, Spain)*; Scheroson F *(Austral.; Scherax, Ger.; Schering, Ger.; Spain)*; S-Cortilean *(Canad.)*; Sigmacort *(Sigma, Austral.)*; Siguent Hycor *(Sigma, Austral.)*; Skincalm *(Glaxo, S.Afr.)*; Solu-Cortef *(Arg.; Upjohn, Austral.; Belg.; Upjohn, Canad.; Upjohn, Denm.; Upjohn, Ital.; Neth.; Upjohn, Norw.; Upjohn, S.Afr.; Upjohn, Swed.; Upjohn, Switz.; Upjohn, UK; Upjohn, USA)*; Solu-Cortril *(Arg.)*; Solu-Glyc *(Erco, Norw.; Erco, Swed.; Switz.)*; Squibb-HC *(Squibb, Austral.)*; Supralef *(Spain)*; Synacort *(Syntex, USA)*; Tega-cort *(USA)*; Texacort *(Genderm, USA)*; Timocort *(Reckitt & Colman Pharmaceuticals, UK)*; Ulcort *(USA)*; Unicort *(Allen & Hanburys, Canad.)*; Uniderm *(Schering, Denm.; Schering, Swed.)*; Urecortyn *(Scharper, Ital.)*; Venocort *(Austral.)*; Venocortin *(S.Afr.)*; Wasp-eze Hydrocortisone *(International Laboratories, UK)*; Westcort *(Westwood, Canad.; Westwood, USA)*.

The following names have been used for multi-ingredient preparations containing hydrocortisone or its esters—Acne-sol *(Fawns & McAllan, Austral.)*; Actinac *(Roussel, Canad.; Roussel, UK)*; Aerocortin *(Wellcome, Austral.)*; Allersone *(Mallard, USA)*; Alphaderm *(Norwich-Eaton, UK; Vivan, USA)*; Alphosyl HC *(Stafford-Miller, UK)*; Analpram-HC *(Ferndale, USA)*; Anucaine-HC *(Searle, Canad.)*; Anugesic-HC *(Parke, Davis, Canad.; Parke, Davis, UK)*; Anusol HC *(Warner, Austral.)*; Anusol-HC *(Parke, Davis, Canad.; Parke, Davis, UK; Parke, Davis, USA)*; Bacticort *(Rugby, USA)*; Barquinol HC *(Fisons, UK)*; Barriere-HC *(Allen & Hanburys, Canad.)*; Barseb HC *(Barnes-Hind, USA)*; Barseb Thera *(Barnes-Hind, USA)*; BaySporin *(Bay, USA)*;
Calmurid HC *(Pharmacia, Canad.; Pharmacia, UK)*; Canesten-HC *(Baypharm, UK)*; Carbo-Cort *(Lagap, UK)*; Chlorocort *(Parke, Davis, Austral.)*; Chloromycetin Hydrocortisone *(Parke, Davis, UK; Parke, Davis, USA)*; Chymacort Ointment *(Armour, UK)*; Cobadex-Nystatin *(Cox, UK)*; Coly-Mycin S Otic *(Parke, Davis, USA)*; Cortar *(Hamilton, Austral.)*; Cor-Tar-Quin *(Lagap, UK)*; Cortisporin Cream *(Wellcome, Canad.; Wellcome, USA)*; Cortisporin Ointment *(Wellcome, Canad.; Wellcome, USA)*; Cortucid *(Nicholas, UK)*; Daktacort *(Janssen, UK)*; Derma-Sone *(Hill, USA)*; Di-Hydrotic *(Legere, USA)*; Dioderm C *(Dermal Laboratories, UK)*; Drotic *(Ascher, USA)*; Econacort *(Squibb, UK)*; Eczederm with Hydrocortisone *(Quinoderm, UK)*; Epifoam *(Stafford-Miller, UK; Reed & Carnrick, USA)*; Eurax-Hydrocortisone *(Geigy, UK)*; F-E-P Creme *(Boots, USA)*; Fostril HC *(Bristol-Myers, Austral.)*; Framycort *(Fisons, UK)*; Fucidin H *(Leo, UK)*; Genticin HC *(Nicholas, UK)*; Gentisone HC *(Nicholas, UK)*; Gregoderm *(Unigreg, UK)*;
HCV Creme *(Saron, USA)*; Hedal HC *(Arlo, USA)*; Hemcort HC *(Technilab, Canad.)*; Hepacort Plus *(Lipha, UK)*; Hill Cortac *(Hill, USA)*; Hydroderm *(Merck Sharp & Dohme, UK)*; Hydroform *(Dermacare, Austral.)*; Hysone *(Mallard, USA)*; Iodo-Cortifair *(Pharmafair, USA)*; Komed HC *(Barnes-Hind, Canad.; Barnes-Hind, USA)*; Lacticare-HC *(Stiefel, USA)*; LazerSporin-C *(Pedinol, USA)*; Locoid C *(Brocades, UK)*; Mantadil *(Wellcome, USA)*; Medicone Derma-HC *(Medicone, USA)*; Neo Hycor *(Sigma, Austral.)*; Neo-Cortef *(Upjohn, Austral.; Upjohn, Canad.; Upjohn, UK; Upjohn, USA)*; Nystaform-HC *(Bayer, UK)*; Occicair *(Pharmafair, USA)*; Ocu-Cort *(Ocumed, USA)*; Ocutricin HC Ointment *(Pharmafair, USA)*; Ophthocort *(Parke, Davis, Canad.; Parke, Davis, USA)*; Otic-HC *(Hauck, USA)*; Oticol *(Arlo, USA)*; Otizol-HC *(Nadeau, Canad.)*; Otobiotic *(Schering, USA)*; Otocort *(Lemmon, USA)*; Otoseptil *(Napp, UK)*; Otosporin *(Calmic, UK)*; Pedi-Cort V *(Pedinol, USA)*; Pentamycetin-HC *(Berlex, Canad.)*; Pimafucort *(Astra, Austral.)*; Plegettes *(Hamilton, Austral.)*; Pramosone *(Ferndale, USA)*; Pricort Cream *(Arlo, USA)*; Pricort Lotion *(Arlo, USA)*; Proctofoam HC *(Stafford-Miller, UK)*; Proctofoam-HC *(Reed & Carnrick, Canad.; Reed & Carnrick, USA)*; Proctosedyl *(Roussel, Austral.; Roussel, Canad.; Roussel, UK)*; Proctosone *(Technilab, Canad.)*; Pyocidin-Otic *(Forest Pharmaceuticals, USA)*;
Quinocort *(Quinoderm, UK)*; Quinoderm with Hydrocortisone *(Quinoderm, UK)*; Rectal Medicone-HC *(Medicone, USA)*; Sential *(Pharmacia, UK)*; Steroxin-Hydrocortisone *(Geigy, UK)*; Tarcortin *(Stafford-Miller, UK)*; Terra-Cortril *(Roerig, USA)*; Terra-Cortril Ear Suspension *(Pfizer, UK)*; Terra-Cortril Nystatin *(Pfizer, UK)*; Terra-Cortril Spray *(Pfizer, UK)*; Terra-Cortril Topical Ointment *(Pfizer, UK)*; Timodine *(Lloyd-Hamol, Reckitt & Colman Pharm., UK)*; Uniroid *(Unigreg, UK)*; Uremol-HC *(Trans Canaderm, Canad.)*; Vanoxide-HC *(Rorer, Canad.; Dermik, USA)*; Vasocort *(Smith Kline & French, UK)*; Vioform-Hydrocortisone *(Ciba, Austral.; Ciba, Canad.; Ciba, UK; Ciba, USA)*; VoSoL HC *(Wallace, USA)*; Vytone *(Dermik, USA)*; Xyloproct *(Astra, Austral.; Astra, UK)*; Zone-A *(USA)*.

12869-q

Isoflupredone Acetate *(BANM, USAN, rINNM).*

9α-Fluoroprednisolone Acetate; U-6013. 9α-Fluoro-11β,17α,21-trihydroxypregna-1,4-diene-3,20-dione 21-acetate.

$C_{23}H_{29}FO_6$=420.5.

CAS — 338-95-4 (isoflupredone); 338-98-7 (acetate).

Isoflupredone acetate is a corticosteroid with the general properties described under corticosteroids (see p.872). It has been used topically in the treatment of various skin disorders.

When applied topically, particularly to large areas, when the skin is broken, or under occlusive dressings, corticosteroids may be absorbed in sufficient amounts to cause systemic effects. See also p.880.

2481-k

Mazipredone *(rINN).*

11β,17-Dihydroxy-21-(4-methyl-1-piperazinyl)pregna-1,4-diene-3,20-dione.

$C_{26}H_{38}N_2O_4$=442.6.

CAS — 13085-08-0.

Mazipredone is a corticosteroid with the general properties described under corticosteroids (see p.872) and is used topically in the treatment of various skin disorders. It is usually employed as an ointment containing 0.25% of mazipredone hydrochloride.

When applied topically, particularly to large areas, when the skin is broken, or under occlusive dressings, corticosteroids may be absorbed in sufficient amounts to cause systemic effects. See also p.880.

Proprietary Names and Manufacturers

Depersolon *(Gedeon Richter, Hung.)*.

1113-p

Medrysone *(USAN, pINN).*

11β-Hydroxy-6α-methylprogesterone; Medrisona; U-8471. 11β-Hydroxy-6α-methylpregn-4-ene-3,20-dione.

$C_{22}H_{32}O_3$=344.5.

CAS — 2668-66-8.

Pharmacopoeias. In *Braz.* and *U.S.*

Adverse Effects, Treatment, Withdrawal, and Precautions

As for corticosteroids, p.872.

Prolonged application to the eye of preparations containing corticosteroids has caused raised intra-ocular pressure and reduced visual function.

Absorption and Fate

For a brief outline of the absorption and fate of corticosteroids, see p.875.

Uses and Administration

Medrysone is a glucocorticoid employed, usually as eye-drops containing 1%, in the topical treatment of allergic and inflammatory conditions of the eye as described under corticosteroids (see p.875).

Preparations

Medrysone Ophthalmic Suspension *(U.S.P.)*

Proprietary Names and Manufacturers

HMS Liquifilm *(Allergan, Austral.; Allergan, Canad.; Allergan, Neth.; Allergan, USA)*; Ipoflogin *(Allergan, Ital.)*; Medrifar *(Farmila, Ital.)*; Medriusar *(Difa, Ital.)*; Ophtocortin *(Winzer, Ger.)*; Sedesterol *(Poen, Arg.)*; Spectramedryn *(Allergan, Ger.)*; Visudrisone *(LOA, Arg.)*.

1114-s

Meprednisone *(USAN, rINN).*
16β-Methylprednisone. 17α,21-Dihydroxy-16β-methylpregna-1,4-diene-3,11,20-trione.
$C_{22}H_{28}O_5$=372.5.

CAS — 1247-42-3.

Pharmacopoeias. In *U.S.*

Store at a temperature not exceeding 40° in airtight containers. Protect from light.

Adverse Effects, Treatment, Withdrawal, and Precautions

As for corticosteroids, p.872.

Absorption and Fate

For a brief outline of the absorption and fate of corticosteroids, see p.875.

Uses and Administration

Meprednisone is a glucocorticoid with the general properties described under corticosteroids (see p.875); 4 mg of meprednisone is reported to be equivalent in anti-inflammatory activity to 5 mg of prednisolone.

It has been used in the treatment of all conditions for which corticosteroid therapy is indicated except adrenal-deficiency states, for which its lack of sodium-retaining properties makes it less suitable than hydrocortisone with supplementary fludrocortisone. It has been given by mouth as either the free alcohol or the acetate and by injection as the sodium hemisuccinate.

Proprietary Names and Manufacturers

Betapar *(Parke, Davis, USA)*; Corti-Bi *(Ital.)*.

1115-w

Methylprednisolone *(BAN, USAN, rINN).*

6α-Methylprednisolone. 11β,17α,21-Trihydroxy-6α-methylpregna-1,4-diene-3,20-dione.
$C_{22}H_{30}O_5$=374.5.

CAS — 83-43-2.

Pharmacopoeias. In *Br., Eur., It., Jpn,* and *U.S.*

A white or almost white odourless or almost odourless crystalline powder.

Practically **insoluble** in water; soluble 1 in 100 of alcohol, 1 in 800 of chloroform, and 1 in 800 of ether; slightly soluble in dehydrated alcohol; sparingly soluble in dioxan and methyl alcohol; slightly soluble in acetone. **Store** in airtight containers. Protect from light.

1116-e

Methylprednisolone Acetate *(BANM, USAN, rINNM).*

Methylprednisolone 21-acetate.
$C_{24}H_{32}O_6$=416.5.

CAS — 53-36-1.

Pharmacopoeias. In *Br.* and *U.S.* Also in *B.P. Vet.*

A white or almost white, odourless or almost odourless, crystalline powder. Methylprednisolone acetate 44 mg is approximately equivalent to 40 mg of methylprednisolone. *B.P.* **solubilities** are: practically insoluble in water; slightly soluble in dehydrated alcohol; very slightly soluble in ether. *U.S.P.* solubilities are: soluble 1 in 1500 of water and ether, 1 in 400 of alcohol, and 1 in 250 of chloroform; sparingly soluble in acetone and methyl alcohol; soluble in dioxan. **Store** in airtight containers. Protect from light.

1117-l

Methylprednisolone Hemisuccinate *(USAN).*

Methylprednisolone 21-(hydrogen succinate).
$C_{26}H_{34}O_8$=474.5.

CAS — 2921-57-5.

Pharmacopoeias. In *U.S.*

A white or almost white, odourless or almost odourless, hygroscopic solid. Methylprednisolone hemisuccinate 51 mg is approximately equivalent to 40 mg of methylprednisolone.

Very slightly **soluble** in water; freely soluble in alcohol; soluble in acetone. **Store** in airtight containers.

1118-y

Methylprednisolone Sodium Succinate *(BANM, USAN, rINNM).*

Methylprednisolone 21-(sodium succinate).
$C_{26}H_{33}NaO_8$=496.5.

CAS — 2375-03-3.

Pharmacopoeias. In *U.S.*

A white or almost white, odourless, hygroscopic, amorphous powder. Methylprednisolone sodium succinate 53 mg is approximately equivalent to 40 mg of methylprednisolone.

Soluble 1 in 1.5 of water, and 1 in 12 of alcohol; very slightly soluble in acetone; practically insoluble in chloroform and ether. **Store** in airtight containers. Protect from light.

Adverse Effects, Treatment, Withdrawal, and Precautions

As for corticosteroids, p.872.

Methylprednisolone may be slightly less likely than prednisolone to cause sodium and water retention.

Methylprednisolone sodium succinate should not be injected into the deltoid muscle since it may cause subcutaneous atrophy.

Reports of various adverse effects associated with intravenous administration of methylprednisolone in high-dose pulse therapy: K. J. Newmark *et al.* (letter), *Lancet*, 1974, *2*, 229 (bilateral knee-pain); R. R. Bailey and P. Armour (letter), *ibid.*, 1014 (bilateral knee-pain); W. M. Bennett and D. Strong (letter), *ibid.*, 1975, *1*, 332 (bilateral knee-pain); R. E. Moses *et al.* (letter), *Ann. intern. Med.*, 1981, *95*, 781 (fatal cardiac arrhythmia); A. Oto *et al.* (letter), *ibid.*, 1983, *99*, 282 (acute noninfectious peritonitis); A. L. Suchman *et al.*, *Arthritis Rheum.*, 1983, *26*, 117 (tonic-clonic seizures); W. T. Ayoub *et al.*, *ibid.*, 809 (cns toxicity); A. J. Williams *et al.* (letter), *Lancet*, 1983, *1*, 1222 (disseminated aspergillosis); D. F. Barrett (letter), *ibid.*, *2*, 800 (cardiac arrest; left ventricular failure); B. A. Baethge and M. D. Lidsky, *Ann. intern. Med.*, 1986, *104*, 58 (intractable hiccups).

ALLERGY. An account of an anaphylactic reaction to methylprednisolone sodium succinate 40 mg intravenously in a 17-year-old male asthmatic patient.— L. M. Mendelson *et al.*, *J. Allergy & clin. Immunol.*, 1974, *54*, 125. Comment.— *Br. med. J.*, 1974, *4*, 551.

EFFECTS ON THE SKIN. A 30-year-old African woman developed a persistent area of complete depigmentation at the site of an intra-articular injection of methylprednisolone.— E. Bloomfield (letter), *Br. med. J.*, 1972, *3*, 766.

Absorption and Fate

For a brief outline of the absorption and fate of corticosteroids, see p.875.

The half-life of methylprednisolone has been reported to be slightly longer than that of prednisolone.

Methylprednisolone acetate is absorbed from joints in a few days but is more slowly absorbed following deep intramuscular injection. It is less soluble than methylprednisolone.

Uses and Administration

Methylprednisolone is a glucocorticoid with the general properties described under corticosteroids (see p.875); 4 mg of methylprednisolone is equivalent in anti-inflammatory activity to about 5 mg of prednisolone.

It has been used, either in the form of the free alcohol or in one of the esterified forms, in the treatment of all conditions for which corticosteroid therapy is indicated except adrenal-deficiency states, for which its lack of sodium-retaining properties makes it less suitable than hydrocortisone with supplementary fludrocortisone.

For administration by mouth, methylprednisolone is usually given in a dosage range of 4 to 48 mg daily; higher doses have been suggested in certain blood disorders.

For parenteral administration in intensive or emergency therapy, methylprednisolone sodium succinate may be administered by intramuscular or intravenous injection or by intravenous infusion. The usual intramuscular or intravenous dose is the equivalent of 10 to 40 mg of methylprednisolone, repeated as required.

The intramuscular route is less likely to produce a rapid effect in emergency therapy than the intravenous route. In some forms of emergency or intensive therapy much higher doses of the equivalent of up to 30 mg per kg body-weight of methylprednisolone have been given as bolus intravenous injections repeated after 4 hours if necessary. Large doses should be given slowly over 10 to 20 minutes and should generally not be given for prolonged periods. For slow intravenous infusion methylprednisolone is dissolved in an appropriate volume of glucose injection or sodium chloride injection or sodium chloride and glucose injection. The dose in children is determined by the severity of the condition rather than by age, but should generally not be less than 500 µg per kg body-weight daily.

For intra-articular injection and for injection into soft tissues methylprednisolone acetate as an aqueous suspension is employed. The dose by intra-articular injection varies from 4 to 80 mg according to the size of the affected joint. Methylprednisolone acetate may also be administered by intramuscular injection for a prolonged systemic effect, the dose varying from 40 mg every 2 weeks to 80 mg weekly; doses of up to 120 mg weekly have also been given.

For use in the treatment of various skin disorders methylprednisolone acetate may be applied topically usually in concentrations of 0.25 to 1%. The acetate may also be administered by intralesional injection in doses of 20 to 60 mg.

Other esters of methylprednisolone which have occasionally been used include the cypionate.

ADMINISTRATION. For short-term intensive therapy or in certain emergency situations a technique of corticosteroid administration known as 'pulse therapy' has been employed. Methylprednisolone has often been used in this manner and typically high doses of about 1 g intravenously have been given, usually daily or on alternate days, or weekly, for a limited number of doses.

BLOOD DISORDERS. Reports of the response of various blood disorders to methylprednisolone administered intravenously in relatively high doses for short periods; the disorders had been refractory to previous standard therapy including other corticosteroids, usually prednisolone or prednisone.— A. Menichelli *et al.*, *Archs Dis. Childh.*, 1984, *59*, 777 (chronic idiopathic thrombocytopenia); S. Özsoylu (letter), *Lancet*, 1984, *2*, 1033 (Blackfan-Diamond syndrome); S. Issaragrisil and A. Painkijagum (letter), *Ann. intern. Med.*, 1985, *103*, 964 (aplastic anaemia); D. Meytes *et al.* (letter), *New Engl. J. Med.*, 1985, *312*, 318 (acute immune cold haemolysis).

CEREBRAL OEDEMA. For reference to the use of methylprednisolone in cerebral oedema, see under dexamethasone, p.888.

SEPTIC SHOCK. For reference to the use of methylprednisolone in septic shock, see under corticosteroids, p.878.

SKIN DISORDERS. For recommendations concerning the correct use of corticosteroids on the skin, and a rough guide to the clinical potencies of topical corticosteroids, see p.880.

Preparations of Methylprednisolone and its Esters

In addition to the preparations below, further official preparations containing methylprednisolone or its esters may be found listed under neomycin sulphate.

Injections

Methylprednisolone Acetate Injection *(B.P.)*. An aqueous suspension of methylprednisolone acetate that should not be given intravenously.

Sterile Methylprednisolone Acetate Suspension *(U.S.P.)*

Methylprednisolone Sodium Succinate for Injection *(U.S.P.)*. It may be prepared from methylprednisolone sodium succinate or from methylprednisolone hemisuccinate with the aid of sodium carbonate or sodium hydroxide.

Oral Dosage Forms

Methylprednisolone Tablets *(B.P.)*

Methylprednisolone Tablets *(U.S.P.)*

Rectal Dosage Forms

Methylprednisolone Acetate for Enema *(U.S.P.)*

Topical Dosage Forms

Methylprednisolone Acetate Cream *(U.S.P.)*

Proprietary Preparations of Methylprednisolone and its Esters

Depo-Medrone *(Upjohn, UK)*. *Injection* (aqueous suspension), methylprednisolone acetate 40 mg/mL, in vials of 1, 2, and 5 mL, and in disposable syringes of 2 mL.

Depo-Medrone with Lidocaine *(Upjohn, UK)*. *Injection* (aqueous suspension), methylprednisolone acetate 40 mg, lignocaine hydrochloride 10 mg/mL, in vials of 1 and 2 mL.

Medrone *(Upjohn, UK)*. *Tablets*, scored, methylprednisolone 2, 4, and 16 mg.

Medrone Acne Lotion *(Upjohn, UK)*. *Lotion*, methylprednisolone acetate 0.25%, aluminium chlorohydroxide complex 10%, sulphur 5%.

Neo-Medrone Acne Lotion *(Upjohn, UK)*. *Lotion*, methylprednisolone acetate 0.25%, aluminium chlorohydroxide complex 10%, sulphur 5%, neomycin sulphate 0.25%.

Neo-Medrone Cream *(Upjohn, UK)*. *Cream*, methylprednisolone acetate 0.25%, neomycin sulphate 0.5%.

Min-I-Mix Methylprednisolone *(IMS, UK)*. *Injection*, powder for reconstitution, methylprednisolone 500 mg and 1 g (as sodium succinate), in Min-I-Mix Vials (two-part vials with solvent) of 8 and 16 mL respectively.

Solu-Medrone *(Upjohn, UK)*. *Injection*, powder for reconstitution, methylprednisolone 0.5, 1.0, and 2.0 g (as sodium succinate), supplied with solvent.

Injection, powder for reconstitution, methylprednisolone 40 and 125 mg (as sodium succinate), in Mix-O-Vials (two-part vials with solvent) of 1 and 2 mL respectively.

Proprietary Names and Manufacturers of Methylprednisolone and its Esters

A-Methapred *(Abbott, USA)*; Asmacortone *(Nuovo, Ital.)*; BayMep *(Bay, USA)*; Betalona *(Spain)*; Caberdelta-M *(Caber, Ital.)*; Cortalfa *(Ital.)*; depMedalone *(Forest Pharmaceuticals, USA)*; Depo-Medrate *(Upjohn, Ger.)*; Depo-Medrol *(Arg.; Upjohn, Austral.; Belg.; Upjohn, Canad.; Upjohn, Denm.; Upjohn, Fr.; Upjohn, Ital.; Neth.; Upjohn, Norw.; Upjohn, S.Afr.; Upjohn, Switz.; Upjohn, USA)*; Depo-Medrone *(Upjohn, Swed.; Upjohn, UK)*; Depo-Moderin *(Upjohn, Spain)*; Depo-Predate *(Legere, USA)*; D-Med *(USA)*; Dura-Meth *(Foy, USA)*; Emmetipi *(Ital.)*; Esametone *(Lisapharma, Ital.)*; Eutisone *(IBIS, Ital.)*; Firmacort *(FIRMA, Ital.)*; Horusona *(Spain)*;
Medesone *(Fargal-Pharmasint, Ital.)*; Medrate *(Upjohn, Ger.)*; Medrol *(Arg.; Upjohn, Austral.; Belg.; Upjohn, Canad.; Denm.; Upjohn, Fr.; Upjohn, Ital.; Upjohn, Norw.; Upjohn, S.Afr.; Upjohn, Switz.; Upjohn, USA)*; Medrone *(Upjohn, Swed.; Upjohn, UK)*; Mega-Star *(Ausonia, Ital.)*; Mepred *(Savage, USA)*; Metilbetasone *(Coli, Ital.)*; Metilcort *(Ital.)*; Metilprednilone *(Ital.)*; Metilstendiolo *(Ital.)*; Min-I-Mix Methylprednisolone *(IMS, UK)*; Moderin *(Spain)*; Nixolan *(Ital.)*; Prednilen *(Lenza, Ital.)*; Radiosone *(Ital.)*; Reactenol *(Lafare, Ital.)*; Rep-Pred *(Central Pharmaceuticals, USA)*; Sieropresol *(Sifarma, Ital.)*; Solu-Medrol *(Upjohn, Austral.; Belg.; Upjohn, Canad.; Upjohn, Denm.; Upjohn, Fr.; Upjohn, Ital.; Neth.; Upjohn, Norw.; Upjohn, S.Afr.; Upjohn, Switz.; Upjohn, USA)*; Solu-Medrone *(Upjohn, Swed.; Upjohn, UK)*; Solu-Moderin *(Upjohn, Spain)*; Summicort *(Benvegna, Ital.)*; Suprametil *(Switz.)*; Urbason *(Belg.; Denm.; Hoechst, Ger.; Hoechst, Ital.; Neth.; Norw.; Hoechst, Spain; Swed.; Hoechst, Switz.)*; Urbason Solubile *(Hoechst, Denm.; Hoechst, Ital.; Norw.; Hoechst, Spain; Swed.; Hoechst, Switz.)*; Urbason-Depot *(Belg.; Switz.)*; Vériderm Médrol *(Upjohn, Fr.)*.

The following names have been used for multi-ingredient preparations containing methylprednisolone or its esters—Cordex *(Upjohn, Canad.)*; Medro-Cordex *(Upjohn, UK)*; Medrol Acne Lotion *(Upjohn, Austral.; Upjohn, Canad.)*; Medrone Acne Lotion *(Upjohn, UK)*; Neo-Medrol *(Upjohn, Austral.; Upjohn, Canad.)*; Neo-Medrone Acne Lotion *(Upjohn, UK)*; Neo-Medrone Cream *(Upjohn, UK)*.

1119-j

Paramethasone Acetate *(BANM, USAN, rINNM)*.

6α-Fluoro-16α-methylprednisolone 21-Acetate. 6α-Fluoro-11β,17α,21-trihydroxy-16α-methylpregna-1,4-diene-3,20-dione 21-acetate.

$C_{24}H_{31}FO_6$=434.5.

CAS — 53-33-8 (paramethasone); 1597-82-6 (acetate).

Pharmacopoeias. In *Fr.*and*U.S.*

A white to creamy-white, fluffy, odourless, crystalline powder. Practically **insoluble** in water; soluble 1 in 50 of chloroform and 1 in 40 of methyl alcohol; soluble in ether. **Store** in airtight containers.

Adverse Effects, Treatment, Withdrawal, and Precautions

As for corticosteroids, p.872.

Absorption and Fate

For a brief outline of the absorption and fate of corticosteroids, see p.875.

Uses and Administration

Paramethasone acetate is a glucocorticoid and has the general properties described under corticosteroids (see p.875); 2 mg of paramethasone is equivalent in anti-inflammatory activity to about 5 mg of prednisolone. It has been suggested for use by mouth in the treatment of all conditions in which corticosteroid therapy is indicated except adrenal-deficiency states for which its lack of sodium-retaining properties makes it less suitable than hydrocortisone with supplementary fludrocortisone.

Preparations

Paramethasone Acetate Tablets *(U.S.P.)*

Proprietary Names and Manufacturers of Paramethasone and its Esters

Alfa 6 *(Ital.)*; Cortidene *(Syntex-Latino, Spain)*; Depodillar *(Syntex, Belg.; Sarva, Neth.)*; Dilar *(Cassenne, Fr.)*; Dillar *(Syntex, Belg.; Sarva, Neth.)*; Haldrate *(Lilly, UK)*; Haldrone *(Lilly, USA)*; Metilar *(Syntex, Austral.; Astra-Syntex, Norw.; Syntex, UK)*; Monocortin *(Grünenthal, Ger.; Grünenthal, Switz.)*; Paramesone *(Jpn)*; Paramezone *(Recordati, Ital.)*; Soludillar *(Syntex, Belg.)*; Triniol *(Syntex-Latino, Spain)*.

2367-z

Prednicarbate *(USAN, rINN)*.

HOE-777; S-770777. 11β,17,21-Trihydroxypregna-1,4-diene-3,20-dione 17-(ethyl carbonate) 21-propionate.

$C_{27}H_{36}O_8$=488.6.

CAS — 73771-04-7.

Prednicarbate is a corticosteroid with the general properties described under corticosteroids (see p.872) and is used topically in the treatment of various skin disorders. It is usually employed as a cream or ointment containing 0.25%.

When applied topically, particularly to large areas, when the skin is broken, or under occlusive dressings, corticosteroids may be absorbed in sufficient amounts to cause systemic effects.

For recommendations concerning the correct use of corticosteroids on the skin, see corticosteroids p.880.

Proprietary Names and Manufacturers

Dermatop *(Cassella-Riedel, Ger.)*.

1120-q

Prednisolamate Hydrochloride *(BANM, rINNM)*.

Prednisolone 21-Diethylaminoacetate Hydrochloride.

11β,17α,21-Trihydroxypregna-1,4-diene-3,20-dione 21-diethylaminoacetate hydrochloride.

$C_{27}H_{39}NO_6$,HCl=510.1.

CAS — 5626-34-6 (prednisolamate).

Prednisolamate hydrochloride has the general properties of prednisolone (below) and was formerly used in some countries as a water-soluble form of prednisolone for intravenous injection and as an ointment.

1129-c

Prednisolone *(BAN, USAN, rINN)*.

1,2-Dehydrohydrocortisone; Deltahydrocortisone; Metacortandralone; Prednisolonum.

11β,17α,21-Trihydroxypregna-1,4-diene-3,20-dione.

$C_{21}H_{28}O_5$=360.5.

CAS — 50-24-8 (anhydrous); 52438-85-4 (sesquihydrate).

Pharmacopoeias. In *Arg., Aust., Br., Braz., Chin., Cz., Egypt., Eur., Fr., Ger., Hung., Ind., Int., It., Jpn, Jug., Neth., Nord., Pol., Port., Roum., Rus., Swiss,* and *Turk.* Also in *B.P. Vet. Nord.* and *U.S.* allow the anhydrous form or the sesquihydrate.

An odourless, white or almost white, crystalline, hygroscopic powder. Very slightly **soluble** in water; soluble 1 in 27 of dehydrated alcohol, 1 in 30 of alcohol, 1 in 50 of acetone, and 1 in 180 of chloroform; soluble in dioxan and methyl alcohol. **Store** in well-closed containers. Protect from light.

1122-s

Prednisolone Acetate *(BANM, USAN, rINNM)*.

Prednisolone 21-acetate.

$C_{23}H_{30}O_6$=402.5.

CAS — 52-21-1.

Pharmacopoeias. In *Arg., Chin., Egypt., Fr., Ind., Jpn, Jug., Pol., Roum., Turk.,* and *U.S.*

An odourless, white or almost white, crystalline powder. Prednisolone acetate 11 mg is approximately equivalent to 10 mg of prednisolone.

Practically **insoluble** in water; soluble 1 in 120 of alcohol; slightly soluble in acetone and chloroform.

1128-z

Prednisolone Hemisuccinate *(USAN)*.

Prednisolone 21-(hydrogen succinate).

$C_{25}H_{32}O_8$=460.5.

CAS — 2920-86-7.

Pharmacopoeias. In *Jpn* and *U.S.*

A fine, creamy-white, almost odourless powder with friable lumps. Prednisolone hemisuccinate 128 mg is approximately equivalent to 100 mg of

prednisolone.
Soluble 1 in 4170 of water, 1 in 6.3 of alcohol, 1 in 1064 of chloroform, and 1 in 248 of ether; soluble in acetone. **Store** in airtight containers.

1123-w

Prednisolone Hexanoate *(BANM, rINNM).*

Prednisolone Caproate. Prednisolone 21-hexanoate.
$C_{27}H_{38}O_6$=458.6.

Prednisolone hexanoate 127 mg is approximately equivalent to 100 mg of prednisolone.

1124-e

Prednisolone Pivalate *(BANM, rINNM).*

Prednisolone Trimethylacetate. Prednisolone 21-pivalate.
$C_{26}H_{36}O_6$=444.6.

CAS — 1107-99-9.

Prednisolone pivalate 123 mg is approximately equivalent to 100 mg of prednisolone.

1125-l

Prednisolone Sodium Metasulphobenzoate

Prednisolone Metasulphobenzoate Sodium *(BANM)*; R-812. Prednisolone 21-(sodium *m*-sulphobenzoate).
$C_{28}H_{31}NaO_9S$=566.6.

CAS — 630-67-1.

Prednisolone sodium metasulphobenzoate 157 mg is approximately equivalent to 100 mg of prednisolone.

1126-y

Prednisolone Sodium Phosphate *(BANM, USAN, rINNM).*

Prednisolone 21-(disodium orthophosphate).
$C_{21}H_{27}Na_2O_8P$=484.4.

CAS — 125-02-0.

Pharmacopoeias. In *Br., Turk.*, and *U.S.*

A white or slightly yellow hygroscopic powder or granules, odourless or with a slight odour. Prednisolone sodium phosphate, 27 mg is approximately equivalent to 20 mg of prednisolone.
Soluble 1 in 3 or 4 of water and 1 in 13 of methyl alcohol; slightly soluble in alcohol and dehydrated alcohol; practically insoluble in chloroform; very slightly soluble in acetone and dioxan. The *B.P.* states that a 0.5% solution in water has a pH of 7.5 to 9.0; the *U.S.P.* specifies that a 1% solution has a pH of 7.5 to 10.5. Solutions are **sterilised** by filtration. **Store** in airtight containers. Protect from light.

1127-j

Prednisolone Steaglate *(rINN).*

Prednisolone Stearoylglycollate *(BANM)*. Prednisolone 21-stearoylglycolate.
$C_{41}H_{64}O_8$=685.0.

CAS — 5060-55-9.

Prednisolone steaglate 190 mg is approximately equivalent to 100 mg of prednisolone.

1121-p

Prednisolone Tebutate *(BANM, USAN, rINNM).*

Prednisolone Butylacetate; Prednisolone Tertiary-butylacetate. Prednisolone 21-(3,3-dimethylbutyrate).
$C_{27}H_{38}O_6,H_2O$=476.6.

CAS — 7681-14-3 (anhydrous).

Pharmacopoeias. In *U.S.*

A white to slightly yellow hygroscopic powder, odourless or with a characteristic odour. Prednisolone tebutate 132 mg is approximately equivalent to 100 mg of prednisolone.
Very slightly **soluble** in water; freely soluble in chloroform and dioxan; soluble in acetone; sparingly soluble in alcohol and methyl alcohol. **Store** at a temperature not exceeding 8° in an atmosphere of nitrogen in airtight containers.

Adverse Effects, Treatment, Withdrawal, and Precautions

As for corticosteroids, p.872.
Owing to its less pronounced mineralocorticoid activity prednisolone is less likely than cortisone or hydrocortisone to cause sodium retention, electrolyte imbalance, and oedema.

Absorption and Fate

For a brief outline of the absorption and fate of corticosteroids, see p.875.
Prednisolone and prednisone are both readily absorbed from the gastro-intestinal tract, but whereas prednisolone already exists in a metabolically active form, prednisone must be converted in the liver to its active metabolite, prednisolone. In general, this conversion is rapid so that prednisone has a preconversion biological half-life of only about 60 minutes. Hence, although prednisone has been estimated to have only about 80% the bioavailability of prednisolone, this difference is of little consequence when seen in the light of intersubject variation in the pharmacokinetics of prednisolone itself; bioavailability also depends on the dissolution-rates of the tablet formulations. Nevertheless, prednisolone is the more reliably absorbed of the 2 corticosteroids, particularly in some liver diseases where the conversion of prednisone may be diminished. Following intramuscular administration the sodium phosphate ester of prednisolone is rapidly absorbed whereas the acetate, in the suspension form, is only slowly absorbed.
Peak plasma concentrations of prednisolone are obtained 1 or 2 hours after administration by mouth, and it has a usual plasma half-life of 2 or 3 hours. Its initial absorption, but not its overall bioavailability, is affected by food.
Prednisolone is extensively bound to plasma proteins, although less so than hydrocortisone (cortisol).
Prednisolone is excreted in the urine as free and conjugated metabolites, together with an appreciable proportion of unchanged prednisolone. Prednisolone crosses the placenta and small amounts are excreted in breast milk.
Prednisolone has a biological half-life lasting several hours, intermediate between those of hydrocortisone (cortisol) and the longer-acting glucocorticoids, such as dexamethasone. It is this intermediate duration of action which makes it suitable for the alternate-day administration regimens which have been found to reduce the risk of adrenocortical insufficiency, yet provide adequate corticosteroid coverage in some disorders.

Reviews of the clinical pharmacokinetics of prednisone and prednisolone: M. E. Pickup, *Clin. Pharmacokinet.*, 1979, *4*, 111; J. G. Gambertoglio *et al., J. Pharmacokinet. Biopharm.*, 1980, *8*, 1; E. J. Begg *et al., Med. J. Aust.*, 1987, *146*, 37.

A study of the pharmacokinetics of prednisolone following oral and intravenous administration.— H. Bergrem *et al., Eur. J. clin. Pharmac.*, 1983, *24*, 415.

The pharmacokinetics of prednisolone in various disease states: L. M. Berghouse *et al., Gut*, 1982, *23*, 980 (acute colitis); J. S. Shaffer *et al., ibid.*, 1983, *24*, 182 (crohn's disease); P. A. Reece *et al., Br. J. clin. Pharmac.*, 1985, *20*, 159 (renal transplant patients).

Administration in children. Variability in plasma-prednisolone concentrations was observed from samples taken immediately prior to, and at hourly intervals from 4 to 7 hours, after ingestion of the usual prescribed doses of prednisone by mouth, taken before breakfast, in 29 children with various diseases. In 22 children, the half-life for prednisolone ranged from 84 to 210 minutes; in a further 4 it ranged from 264 to 360 minutes. In most patients, peak concentrations occurred 1 or 2 hours after the dose, but in 5 patients this took 3 to 4 hours, and 3 others had a progressive increase in plasma concentrations during the study period; half-lives could not be calculated for the last 3.— O. C. Green *et al., J. Pediat.*, 1978, *93*, 299.

Administration in hepatic insufficiency. Comparison of the metabolic effects of prednisolone and prednisone. Active chronic liver disease or acute viral hepatitis caused lower concentrations and a slower rise to peak concentrations of plasma prednisolone after administration of prednisone than after prednisolone. In patients with inactive chronic liver disease similar concentrations were reached 1 hour after administration of either drug. The amount of prednisolone bound to protein was lower in patients with active liver disease and there was positive correlation between bound prednisolone and serum albumin concentrations; protein binding was not affected by the presence of azathioprine *in vitro*.— L. W. Powell and E. Axelsen, *Gut*, 1972, *13*, 690. Although plasma-prednisolone concentrations were more predictable after administration of prednisolone than after prednisone in 10 healthy subjects, no difference was noted in 25 patients with chronic active hepatitis. In the patients with liver disease, impaired hepatic conversion of prednisone to prednisolone was counteracted by impaired elimination of the prednisolone.— M. Davis *et al., Br. J. clin. Pharmac.*, 1978, *5*, 501. Impaired conversion of prednisone to prednisolone in patients with liver cirrhosis.— S. Madsbad *et al., Gut*, 1980, *21*, 52.

Pregnancy and the neonate. Concentrations of prednisone and prednisolone in human milk 120 minutes after prednisone 10 mg by mouth were 26.7 ng and 1.6 ng per mL.— F. H. Katz and B. E. Duncan (letter), *New Engl. J. Med.*, 1975, *293*, 1154.

Seven lactating women volunteers were given a single 5-mg dose of tritium-labelled prednisolone by mouth. A mean of 0.14% of the radioactivity from the dose was recovered per litre of milk during the following 48 to 61 hours.— S. A. McKenzie *et al., Archs Dis. Childh.*, 1975, *50*, 894.

Uses and Administration

Prednisolone is a glucocorticoid with the general properties described under corticosteroids (see p.875); 5 mg of prednisolone is equivalent in anti-inflammatory activity to about 25 mg of cortisone acetate. In general, prednisolone, either in the form of the free alcohol or in one of the esterified forms, is the drug of choice for all conditions in which routine systemic corticosteroid therapy is indicated, except adrenal-deficiency states for which its lack of sodium-retaining properties usually makes it less suitable than hydrocortisone (cortisol) with supplementary fludrocortisone. The more potent pituitary-suppressant properties of a glucocorticoid such as dexamethasone may, however, be required for the diagnosis and management of conditions associated with adrenal hyperplasia.
For administration by mouth prednisolone is usually used although prednisolone sodium phosphate or prednisolone steaglate are also employed; the usual dose, expressed in terms of prednisolone, is about 5 to 60 mg daily in divided doses, as a single daily dose at 8 a.m., or as a double dose on alternate days. Alternate-day early-morning dosage regimens produce less suppression of the hypothalamic-pituitary axis and may provide satisfactory control of symptoms in certain conditions although they may not always provide adequate control. Enteric-coated tablets of prednisolone are also available.
For parenteral administration the sodium phosphate ester is normally employed and may be given intravenously by injection or infusion or intramuscularly by injection; doses appear to have been variously expressed in terms of prednisolone, prednisolone phosphate, or prednisolone sodium phosphate but are generally within the range of 4 to 60 mg daily. An aqueous suspension of prednisolone acetate is also used intramuscularly to give a prolonged effect with doses of 25 to 100 mg of the acetate being given once or twice weekly.
For intra-articular injection the acetate, sodium phosphate, and tebutate esters are used. Suggested doses are 5 to 25 mg of prednisolone acetate, 2 to 30 mg of prednisolone phosphate (for

the sodium phosphate ester), and 8 to 40 mg of prednisolone tebutate. The sodium phosphate and tebutate are also given by intralesional injection and by injection into soft tissue.

Prednisolone sodium phosphate is also used in the topical treatment of allergic and inflammatory conditions of the eyes or ears, usually as drops containing 0.5%.

For rectal use prednisolone sodium metasulphobenzoate or prednisolone sodium phosphate may be employed. Retention enemas containing the equivalent of 20 mg of prednisolone per 100 mL or suppositories containing the equivalent of 5 mg of prednisolone are available.

Other esters of prednisolone which have occasionally been used include the palmitate, sodium tetrahydrophthalate, and valeroacetate.

Preparations of Prednisolone and its Esters

In addition to the preparations below, further official preparations containing prednisolone or its esters may be found listed under chloramphenicol, neomycin, and neomycin sulphate.

Injections

Sterile Prednisolone Acetate Suspension *(U.S.P.)*

Prednisolone Sodium Phosphate Injection *(B.P.)*

Prednisolone Sodium Phosphate Injection *(U.S.P.)*

Prednisolone Sodium Succinate for Injection *(U.S.P.)*. It is prepared from prednisolone hemisuccinate with the aid of sodium hydroxide or sodium carbonate.

Sterile Prednisolone Tebutate Suspension *(U.S.P.)*

Ophthalmic Dosage Forms

Prednisolone Eye-drops *(B.P.C. 1973)*. Prednisolone Sodium Phosphate Eye-drops; PRED. Eye-drops containing prednisolone sodium phosphate 0.518%.

Prednisolone Sodium Phosphate Eye Drops *(A.P.F.)*. Prednisolone Eye Drops. Eye-drops containing prednisolone sodium phosphate 0.518%.

Prednisolone Sodium Phosphate Ophthalmic Solution *(U.S.P.)*

Oral Dosage Forms

Prednisolone Tablets *(B.P.)*

Prednisolone Tablets *(U.S.P.)*

Rectal Dosage Forms

Prednisolone Enema *(B.P.C. 1973)*. Prednisolone Sodium Phosphate Enema. An aqueous solution of prednisolone sodium phosphate.

Topical Dosage Forms

Prednisolone Cream *(U.S.P.)*

Proprietary Preparations of Prednisolone and its Esters

Deltacortril Enteric *(Pfizer, UK)*. *Tablets*, enteric-coated, prednisolone 2.5 and 5 mg.

Delta-Phoricol *(Wallace Mfg Chem., UK)*. *Tablets*, prednisolone 5 mg.

Deltastab *(Boots, UK)*. *Tablets*, scored, prednisolone 1 and 5 mg.
Injection (aqueous suspension), prednisolone acetate 25 mg/mL, in ampoules of 1mL.

Minims Prednisolone Sodium Phosphate *(Smith & Nephew Pharmaceuticals, UK)*. *Eye-drops*, prednisolone sodium phosphate 0.5%, in single-use disposable applicators.

Precortisyl *(Roussel, UK)*. *Tablets*, prednisolone 1 mg.
Tablets, scored, prednisolone 5 mg.

Precortisyl Forte *(Roussel, UK)*. *Tablets*, scored, prednisolone 25 mg.

Pred Forte *(Allergan, UK)*. *Eye-drops*, prednisolone acetate 1%.

Predenema *(Pharmax, UK)*. *Enema*, prednisolone 20 mg (as sodium metasulphobenzoate)/100 mL, in disposable containers of 100 mL.

Predfoam *(Pharmax, UK)*. *Rectal foam*, prednisolone 20 mg (as sodium metasulphobenzoate)/metered dose.

Prednesol *(Glaxo, UK)*. *Tablets*, soluble, scored, prednisolone 5 mg (as sodium phosphate).

Predsol *(Glaxo, UK)*. *Drops*, for eye or ear, prednisolone sodium phosphate 0.5%.
Retention enema, prednisolone 20 mg (as sodium phosphate)/100 mL, in disposable containers of 100 mL.
Suppositories, prednisolone 5 mg (as sodium phosphate).

Predsol-N *(Glaxo, UK)*. *Drops*, for eye or ear, prednisolone sodium phosphate 0.5%, neomycin sulphate 0.5%.

Scheriproct *(Schering, UK)*. *Rectal ointment*, prednisolone hexanoate 0.19%, cinchocaine hydrochloride 0.5%.
Suppositories, prednisolone hexanoate 1.3 mg, cinchocaine hydrochloride 1 mg.

Sintisone *(Farmitalia Carlo Erba, UK)*. *Tablets*, scored, prednisolone steaglate 6.65 mg (claimed to be therapeutically equivalent to 5 mg of prednisolone).

Proprietary Names and Manufacturers of Prednisolone and its Esters

Acepreval *(Ital.)*; Adnisolone *(Nelson, Austral.)*; Ak-Tate *(Akorn, Canad.)*; Alconisolone *(Ital.)*; Caberdelta *(Ital.)*; Codelcortone *(Merck Sharp & Dohme, UK)*; Codelcortone-TBA *(Merck Sharp & Dohme, Austral.; Merck Sharp & Dohme, Switz.; Merck Sharp & Dohme, UK)*; Codelsol *(Frosst, Austral.; Neth.; Swed.; Merck Sharp & Dohme, UK)*; Corti-Clyss *(Vifor, Switz.)*; Cortipred *(Ital.)*; Cortisolone *(SIT, Ital.)*; Cortomas *(Ital.)*; Dacortin *(Switz.)*; Dacortin-H *(Igoda, Spain)*; Désocort *(Fr.)*; Decaprednil *(Dorsch, Ger.)*; Decortin-H *(E. Merck, Ger.)*; Delcortol *(Leo, Denm.)*; Delta-Cortef *(Upjohn, Austral.; Upjohn, USA)*; Delta-Cortilen *(SIFI, Ital.)*; Deltacortril *(Belg.; Pfizer, Ger.; Norw.; Spain; Swed.; Pfizer, UK)*; Delta-Larma *(Spain)*; Deltalone *(DDSA Pharmaceuticals, UK)*; Delta-Phoricol *(Wallace Mfg Chem., UK)*; Deltasolone *(USV, Austral.)*; Deltastab *(Boots, UK)*; Deltidrosol *(Poli, Ital.)*; Deltolio *(Farmila, Ital.)*; Deltosona *(Spain)*; Derpo PD *(Jpn)*; Di-Adreson-F *(Organon, Belg.; Organon, Neth.)*; Domucortone *(Medici Domus, Ital.)*; Donisolone *(Jpn)*; Dulmicort *(Fr.)*; Dura Prednisolon *(Ger.)*; Econopred *(Alcon Laboratories, USA)*; Encortolone *(Pol.)*; Endoprenovis *(Vister, Ital.)*; Estilsona *(Ifesa, Spain)*; Fiasone Parenteral *(Orfi, Spain)*; Glitisone *(Vis, Ital.)*; Hemilagar *(Spain)*; Hexacortone *(Spirig, Switz.)*; Hostacortin *(Hoechst, Ger.)*; Hydeltrasol *(Merck Sharp & Dohme, USA)*; Hydeltra-TBA *(Merck Sharp & Dohme, USA)*; Hydrocortancyl *(Roussel, Fr.)*; Ibisterolon *(Ibi, Ital.)*; Inflamase *(Coopervision, Canad.; Ger.; Coopervision, USA)*; Inflanefran *(Allergan, Ger.)*; Klismacort *(Bene, Ger.)*; Lenisolone *(S.Afr.)*; Lentosone *(Arg.)*; Longiprednil *(Dorsch, Ger.)*; Marsolone *(Marshall's Pharmaceuticals, UK)*; Mecortolon *(Pol.)*; Meprisolon *(Switz.)*; Meticortelone *(Essex, Ital.; Scherag, S.Afr.; Schering, USA)*; Meti-Derm *(Schering, USA)*; Metreton *(Schering, USA)*; Minims Prednisolone *(Smith & Nephew, Austral.; Smith & Nephew Pharmaceuticals, UK)*; Nisolone *(Llorente, Spain)*; Normonsona *(Normon, Spain)*; Optocort *(Austral.)*; Panafcortelone *(Protea, Austral.)*; Pediapred *(Fisons, USA)*; Phortisolone *(Fr.)*; Precortalon *(Organon, Swed.)*; Precortilon *(Ger.)*; Precortisyl *(Austral.; Roussel, UK)*; Pred Forte *(Allergan, Canad.; Allergan, S.Afr.; Switz.; Allergan, UK; Allergan, USA)*; Pred Mild *(Allergan, Canad.; Allergan, S.Afr.; Switz.; Allergan, USA)*; Predartrina *(Ital.)*; Predate *(Legere, USA)*; Predate S *(Legere, USA)*; Predate TBA *(Legere, USA)*; Pred-Clysma *(KabiVitrum, Denm.; KabiVitrum, Norw.; ACO, Swed.)*; Predeltilone *(SCS, S.Afr.)*; Predenema *(Pharmax, UK)*; Predfoam *(Pharmax, UK)*; Prednabene *(Merckle, Ger.)*; Prednesol *(Glaxo, UK)*; Predni-Coelin *(Pfleger, Ger.)*; Prednicort *(Cortec, Swed.)*; Prednicortelone *(Belg.)*; Prednifor *(Switz.)*; Predni-H *(Beiersdorf, Ger.)*; Predni-Helvacort *(Switz.)*; Predniment *(Ferring, Denm.)*; Predniretard *(Boots-Dacour, Fr.)*; Prednis *(USA)*; Prednisolona Alonga *(Spain)*; Predonine *(Jpn)*; Predonine Water-soluble *(Jpn)*; Predsol *(Glaxo, Austral.; Glaxo, S.Afr.; Glaxo, UK)*; Prelone *(Austral.; Muro, USA)*; Prenesei *(Ital.)*; PSP-IV *(Reid-Provident, USA)*; Rolisone *(Farmitalia, Norw.)*; Ropredlone *(USA)*; Savacort *(Savage, USA)*; Savacort-S *(USA)*; Scherisolon *(Schering, Austral.; Schering, Ger.; Switz.)*; Scherisolona *(Spain)*; Sintisone *(Sigma, Austral.; Belg.; Ital.; Farmitalia Carlo Erba, Swed.; Farmitalia Carlo Erba, UK)*; Sodasone *(USA)*; Solone *(Fawns & McAllan, Austral.)*; Solucort *(Merck Sharp & Dohme-Chibret, Fr.)*; Solu-Dacortin *(Merck, Aust.; Austral.; Bracco, Ital.; Igoda, Spain; E. Merck, Switz.)*; Solu-Dacortine *(Merck, Belg.; E. Merck, Switz.)*; Solu-Decortin *(E. Merck, Ger.)*; Solupred *(Houdé, Fr.)*; Sterane *(Pfipharmecs, USA)*; Sterofrin *(Alcon, Austral.)*; Ulacort *(USA)*; Ultracorten-H *(Ciba, Ger.; Switz.)*; Ultracortene-H *(Belg.; Ciba, Switz.)*; Ultracortenol *(Austral.; Belg.; Schering, Denm.; Dispersa, Ger.; Neth.; Dispersa, Norw.; Dispersa, Swed.; Dispersa, Switz.; Ciba, UK)*; Verisone *(Ital.)*.

The following names have been used for multi-ingredient preparations containing prednisolone or its esters—Ak-Cide *(Akorn, Canad.; Akorn, USA)*; Anacal *(Panpharma, UK)*; Blephamide *(Allergan, Austral.; Allergan, Canad.; Allergan, USA)*; Cetapred *(Alcon, Canad.; Alcon Laboratories, USA)*; Cordex *(Upjohn, UK)*; Hydromycin-D *(Boots, UK)*; Isopto Cetapred *(Alcon, Canad.; Alcon Laboratories, USA)*; Metimyd *(Schering, Canad.; Schering, USA)*; Mydrapred *(Alcon, Canad.)*; Ocu-Lone-C *(Ocumed, USA)*; Optimyd *(Schering, USA)*; Poly-Pred *(Allergan, USA)*; Prednefrin *(Allergan, Austral.)*; Predsol-N *(Glaxo, UK)*; Predsulfair *(Pharmafair, USA)*; Scheriproct *(Schering, Austral.; Schering, UK)*; Sulfacort *(Rugby, USA)*; Sulphrin *(Bausch & Lomb, USA)*; Sulpred *(Pharmafair, USA)*; Vasocidin *(Coopervision, Canad.; Coopervision, USA)*.

1131-w

Prednisone *(BAN, USAN, rINN)*.

1,2-Dehydrocortisone; Deltacortisone; Deltadehydrocortisone; Metacortandracin; Prednisonum.
17α,21-Dihydroxypregna-1,4-diene-3,11,20-trione.
$C_{21}H_{26}O_5$=358.4.

CAS — 53-03-2.

Pharmacopoeias. In *Arg., Aust., Br., Braz., Cz., Egypt., Eur., Fr., Ger., Ind., Int., It., Jug., Neth., Nord., Pol., Port., Roum., Rus., Swiss, Turk.*, and *U.S.*

A white or almost white, odourless, crystalline powder. *B.P.* **solubilities** are: practically insoluble in water; slightly soluble in alcohol and chloroform. *U.S.P.* solubilities are: very slightly soluble in water; soluble 1 in 150 of alcohol and 1 in 200 of chloroform; slightly soluble in dioxan and methyl alcohol. **Store** in well-closed containers. Protect from light.

1130-s

Prednisone Acetate *(BANM, rINNM)*.

Prednisone 21-acetate.
$C_{23}H_{28}O_6$=400.5.

CAS — 125-10-0.

Pharmacopoeias. In *Arg., Chin., Egypt., Fr., Ind., Int., Jug., Pol., Roum.*, and *Turk.*

Prednisone acetate 11 mg is approximately equivalent to 10 mg of prednisone.

Prednisone is a biologically inert glucocorticoid which is converted to prednisolone in the liver. It has the same chemical relationship to prednisolone as cortisone has to hydrocortisone. The indications and dosage of prednisone for oral use are exactly the same as those for prednisolone but since its bioavailability may, under some circumstances, be less reliable, prednisolone is now the preferred drug. For further details, see prednisolone, p.899.

Preparations of Prednisone and its Esters

Prednisone Oral Solution *(U.S.P.)*

Prednisone Syrup *(U.S.P.)*

Prednisone Tablets *(B.P.)*

Prednisone Tablets *(U.S.P.)*

Proprietary Preparations of Prednisone and its Esters

Decortisyl *(Roussel, UK)*. *Tablets*, scored, prednisone 5 mg.

Econosone *(DDSA Pharmaceuticals, UK)*. *Tablets*, prednisone 1 and 5 mg.

Proprietary Names and Manufacturers of Prednisone and its Esters

Adasone *(Nelson, Austral.)*; Colisone *(Canad.)*; Cortancyl *(Roussel, Fr.)*; Cortialer *(Spain)*; Dacortin *(Igoda, Spain)*; Decortin *(E. Merck, Ger.)*; Decortisyl *(Austral.; Roussel, UK)*; Decorton *(Salfa, Ital.)*; Deidrocortisone *(Ital.)*; Delcortin *(Denm.)*; Delta Prenovis *(Ital.)*; Deltacortene *(Lepetit, Ital.)*; Deltacortone *(Merck Sharp & Dohme, UK)*; Delta-Dome *(USA)*; Delta-Scherosona *(Spain)*; Deltasone *(Austral.; Upjohn, Canad.; S.Afr.; Upjohn, USA)*; Deltison *(Ferring, Swed.)*; Deltison Clysma *(Norw.)*; Deltisona *(Arg.)*; Di-Adreson *(Organon, UK)*; Econosone *(DDSA Pharmaceuticals, UK)*; Encorton *(Pol.)*; Fiasone Oral *(Spain)*; Hostacortin *(Ger.)*; Itacortone *(Ghimas, Ital.)*; Liquid Pred *(Muro, USA)*; Lisacort *(USA)*; Marnisonal *(Spain)*; Marsone *(Marshall's Pharmaceuticals, UK)*; Marvidiene *(Ital.)*; Méprisone *(Mepha, Switz.)*; Meprison *(Switz.)*; Meticorten *(Arg.; Scherag, S.Afr.; Schering, USA)*; Nisone *(Llorente, Spain)*; Orasone *(Rowell, USA)*; Panafcort *(Protea, Austral.; Propan, S.Afr.)*; Paracort *(Canad.)*; Parmenison *(Aust.)*; Predeltin *(SCS, S.Afr.)*; Predniartrit *(Spain)*; Prednicen-M *(Central Pharmaceuticals, USA)*; Prednicort *(Belg.)*; Prednilonga *(Dorsch, Ger.)*; Predniment *(Ferring, Ger.)*; Predni-Tablinen *(Beiersdorf, Ger.)*; Predni-Wolner *(Spain)*; Prednovister *(Spain)*; Presone *(Austral.)*; Proped *(Austral.)*; Rectodelt *(Trommsdorff, Ger.)*; Servisone *(USA)*; SK-Prednisone *(Smith Kline & French, USA)*; Sone *(Fawns & McAllan, Austral.)*; Sterapred *(Mayrand, USA)*; Supopred *(Spain)*; Ultracorten *(Ciba, Ger.; Spain)*; Ultracortene *(Ciba, Switz.)*; Urtilone *(Fr.)*; Winpred *(ICN, Canad.)*.

The following names have been used for multi-ingredient preparations containing prednisone or its esters—Delta-Butazolidin *(Geigy, UK)*; Metreton *(Schering, Canad.)*.

1132-e

Prednylidene *(BAN, rINN)*.

16-Methylene Prednisolone. 11β,17α,21-Trihydroxy-16-methylenepregna-1,4-diene-3,20-dione.

$C_{22}H_{28}O_5$=372.5.

CAS — 599-33-7.

Prednylidene has the general properties of prednisolone (p.899) and has been used for similar purposes; 6 mg is equivalent in effect to about 5 mg of prednisolone. It has been given by mouth and by injection as the diethylaminoacetate hydrochloride.

Proprietary Names and Manufacturers of Prednylidene and its Salts

Dacorsol *(Igoda, Spain)*; Dacortilen *(Merck, Aust.; Bracco, Ital.; Igoda, Spain; E. Merck, Swed.)*; Décortilène *(Merck-Clévenot, Fr.)*; Decortilen *(E. Merck, Ger.)*.

1133-l

Suprarenal Cortex

Suprarenal cortex contains a number of steroid compounds the most active of which are corticosterone, dehydrocorticosterone, hydrocortisone, cortisone, and aldosterone. It has been prepared from the adrenal glands of oxen.

Suprarenal cortex was formerly used for the treatment of Addison's disease but it has been superseded by hydrocortisone and other corticosteroids.

Proprietary Names and Manufacturers

Alfacortex *(Alfa Farmaceutici, Ital.)*; Biocortone *(SIT, Ital.)*; Cortelan *(Aandersen, Ital.)*; Cortical *(Caber, Ital.)*; Corticopan *(Ist. Chim. Inter., Ital.)*; Cortidin *(Crinos, Ital.)*; Cortigen *(Richter, Ital.)*; Cortine *(Laroche Navarron, Fr.)*; Fluxalgin *(Baer, Ger.)*; Liocortex *(Radiumfarma, Ital.)*; Master Cortex *(Coli, Ital.)*; Maxicortex *(Manetti Roberts, Ital.)*; Mencortex *(Menarini, Ital.)*; Novacort *(Pulitzer, Ital.)*; Novocortex *(Besins-Iscovesco, Fr.)*; Opocortin *(Spain)*; Pleocortex *(Menarini, Spain)*; Pleocortin *(Menarini, Spain)*; Recortex *(Fellows, USA)*; Sicortex *(Sifarma, Ital.)*; Solcort *(Von Boch, Ital.)*; Supracort *(Samil, Ital.; Paines & Byrne, UK)*; Sustal *(FIRMA, Ital.)*; Tomcor *(Croce Bianca, Ital.)*; Ultracort *(Ripari-Gero, Ital.)*.

The following names have been used for multi-ingredient preparations containing suprarenal cortex—Movelat *(Luitpold, Austral.; Panpharma, UK)*.

13356-y

Tixocortol Pivalate *(BANM, rINNM)*.

JO-1016. 11β,17α-Dihydroxy-21-mercaptopregn-4-ene-3,20-dione 21-pivalate.

$C_{26}H_{38}O_5S$=462.7.

CAS — 61951-99-3 (tixocortol).

Tixocortol pivalate is a glucocorticoid with the general properties described under corticosteroids (see p.872). It is used as nasal, throat, and rectal preparations.

Proprietary Names and Manufacturers

Pivalone *(Jouveinal, Fr.; Uhlmann-Eyraud, Switz.)*; Rectovalone *(Jouveinal, Fr.)*; Tiovalon *(Intersan, Ger.)*; Tiovalone *(Juste, Spain)*.

1134-y

Triamcinolone *(BAN, USAN, rINN)*.

9α-Fluoro-16α-hydroxyprednisolone; Fluoxiprednisolonum. 9α-Fluoro-11β,16α,17α,21-tetrahydroxypregna-1,4-diene-3,20-dione.

$C_{21}H_{27}FO_6$=394.4.

CAS — 124-94-7.

Pharmacopoeias. In *Br., Cz., Ind., It., Jpn, Jug.,* and *U.S.*

A white or almost white, odourless or almost odourless, slightly hygroscopic, crystalline powder. Slightly **soluble** in water; very slightly soluble in chloroform and ether; soluble 1 in 40 of alcohol; slightly soluble in methyl alcohol. **Store** in well-closed containers.

1137-c

Triamcinolone Acetonide *(BANM, USAN, rINNM)*.

CL-61965, CL-106359 (both triamcinolone acetonide sodium phosphate); Triamcinoloni Acetonidum. 9α-Fluoro-11β,21-dihydroxy-16α,17α-isopropylidenedioxypregna-1,4-diene-3,20-dione.

$C_{24}H_{31}FO_6$=434.5.

CAS — 76-25-5.

Pharmacopoeias. In *Br., Braz., Cz., Eur., Ind., It., Jpn, Jug., Swiss, Turk.,* and *U.S.* Also in *B.P. Vet.*

A white or cream-coloured, almost odourless, crystalline powder. Triamcinolone acetonide 11 mg is approximately equivalent to 10 mg of triamcinolone.

B.P. **solubilities** are: practically insoluble in water; sparingly soluble in alcohol and chloroform; very slightly soluble in ether. *U.S.P.* solubilities are: practically insoluble in water; very soluble in dehydrated alcohol, chloroform, and methyl alcohol. **Store** in well-closed containers. Protect from light.

1136-z

Triamcinolone Diacetate *(BANM, USAN, rINNM)*.

Triamcinolone 16α,21-diacetate.

$C_{25}H_{31}FO_8$=478.5.

CAS — 67-78-7.

Pharmacopoeias. In *U.S.*

White to off-white, fine crystalline powder with a slight odour. Triamcinolone diacetate 12 mg is approximately equivalent to 10 mg of triamcinolone.

Practically **insoluble** in water; soluble 1 in 13 of alcohol, 1 in 80 of chloroform, and 1 in 40 of methyl alcohol; slightly soluble in ether.

1135-j

Triamcinolone Hexacetonide *(BAN, USAN, rINN)*.

Triamcinolone Acetonide 21-(3,3-Dimethylbutyrate). 9α-Fluoro-11β,21-dihydroxy-16α,17α-isopropylidenedioxypregna-1,4-diene-3,20-dione 21-(3,3-dimethylbutyrate).

$C_{30}H_{41}FO_7$=532.6.

CAS — 5611-51-8.

Pharmacopoeias. In *U.S.*

A white to cream-coloured powder. Triamcinolone hexacetonide 14 mg is approximately equivalent to 10 mg of triamcinolone.

Practically **insoluble** in water; soluble in chloroform; slightly soluble in methyl alcohol.

Adverse Effects, Treatment, Withdrawal, and Precautions

As for corticosteroids, p.872.

Its effects on sodium and water retention are less than those of prednisolone. Anorexia, weight loss, flushing, depression, and muscle wasting are reported to have been particularly associated with triamcinolone.

ALLERGY. References to allergic reactions to topical triamcinolone preparations caused by the content of ethylenediamine: S. Wright and R. R. M. Harman, *Br. med. J.*, 1983, *287*, 463; S. Freeman (letter), *Med. J. Aust.*, 1986, *145*, 361.

Absorption and Fate

For a brief outline of the absorption and fate of corticosteroids, see p.875.

Triamcinolone is reported to have a biological half-life in plasma of about 300 minutes. It is bound to plasma albumin to a much smaller extent than hydrocortisone.

The acetonide, diacetate, and hexacetonide esters of triamcinolone are only very slowly absorbed from injection sites.

References to the pharmacokinetics of triamcinolone and its esters: H. Möllmann *et al.*, *Eur. J. clin. Pharmac.*, 1985, *29*, 85; H. Derendorf *et al.*, *Clin. Pharmac. Ther.*, 1986, *39*, 313.

Uses and Administration

Triamcinolone is a glucocorticoid and has the general properties described under corticosteroids (see p.875); 4 mg of triamcinolone is equivalent in anti-inflammatory activity to about 5 mg of prednisolone. It has been used, either in the form of the free alcohol or in one of the esterified forms, in the treatment of all conditions for which corticosteroid therapy is indicated, except adrenal-deficiency states for which its lack of sodium-retaining properties makes it less suitable than hydrocortisone with supplementary fludrocortisone.

For administration by mouth triamcinolone is used in usual doses of 4 to 48 mg daily.

For parenteral administration the acetonide or diacetate esters are used in doses of about 40 mg by intramuscular injection. They are usually given as suspensions to provide a prolonged systemic effect.

For intra-articular injection triamcinolone acetonide, diacetate, and hexacetonide have all been used. Doses for these esters have been in the range of 2.5 to 40 mg, 5 to 40 mg, and 2 to 30 mg respectively depending upon the size of the joint injected.

For topical application in the treatment of various skin disorders triamcinolone acetonide is used, usually in a concentration of 0.1% although concentrations ranging from 0.025 to 0.5% have been employed. Triamcinolone esters are also commonly used by intralesional injection in the treatment of some inflammatory skin disorders such as keloids. Suggested doses for the various esters have been: acetonide, 1 mg per site; diacetate, a total of 5 mg in divided doses into small lesions or up to a total of 48 mg in divided doses into large lesions with no more than 12.5 mg injected into any one site; hexacetonide, up to 500 μg per square inch (approximately 80 μg per cm^2) of affected skin.

Triamcinolone acetonide is also used by inhalation for asthma.

Other esters of triamcinolone which have occasionally been used include the acetonide dipotassium phosphate, aminobenzal benzamidoisobutyrate, and benetonide. Another derivative of triamcinolone, flupamesone has also been used.

SKIN DISORDERS. For recommendations concerning the correct use of corticosteroids on the skin, and a rough guide to the clinical potencies of topical corticosteroids, see corticosteroids, p.880.

Preparations of Triamcinolone and its Esters

In addition to the preparations below, further official preparations containing triamcinolone or its esters may be found listed under neomycin sulphate and nystatin.

Dental Dosage Forms

Triamcinolone Dental Paste *(B.P.)*. Triamcinolone Acetonide Dental Paste

Triamcinolone Acetonide Dental Paste *(U.S.P.)*

Injections

Sterile Triamcinolone Acetonide Suspension *(U.S.P.)*

Sterile Triamcinolone Diacetate Suspension *(U.S.P.)*

Sterile Triamcinolone Hexacetonide Suspension *(U.S.P.)*

Oral Dosage Forms

Triamcinolone Tablets *(B.P.)*

Triamcinolone Tablets *(U.S.P.)*

Triamcinolone Diacetate Syrup *(U.S.P.)*

Topical Dosage Forms

Triamcinolone Acetonide Topical Aerosol *(U.S.P.)*

Triamcinolone Cream *(B.P.)*. Triamcinolone Acetonide Cream

Triamcinolone Acetonide Cream *(U.S.P.)*

Triamcinolone Lotion *(B.P.C. 1973)*. Triamcinolone Acetonide Lotion. A dispersion of triamcinolone acetonide.

Triamcinolone Acetonide Lotion *(U.S.P.)*

Triamcinolone Ointment *(B.P.)*. Triamcinolone Acetonide Ointment

Triamcinolone Acetonide Ointment *(U.S.P.)*

Proprietary Preparations of Triamcinolone and its Esters

In addition to those given below, details of further proprietary preparations containing triamcinolone or its esters may be found under neomycin and nystatin.

Adcortyl *(Squibb, UK)*. *Injection* (aqueous suspension), triamcinolone acetonide 10 mg/mL, in ampoules of 1 mL and vials of 5 mL.
Cream, Ointment, triamcinolone acetonide 0.1%.
Dental paste (Adcortyl in Orabase), triamcinolone acetonide 0.1%.

Adcortyl with Graneodin *(Squibb, UK)*. *Cream, Ointment*, triamcinolone acetonide 0.1%, neomycin 0.25% (as sulphate), gramicidin 0.025%.

Aureocort *(Lederle, UK)*. *Cream, Ointment*, triamcinolone acetonide 0.1%, chlortetracycline hydrochloride 3%.

Kenalog *(Squibb, UK)*. *Injection* (aqueous suspension), triamcinolone acetonide 40 mg/mL, in disposable syringes of 1 and 2 mL and vials of 1 mL.

Ledercort *(Lederle, UK)*. *Tablets*, triamcinolone 2 and 4 mg.
Cream, Ointment, triamcinolone acetonide 0.1%.

Ledermix *(Lederle, UK)*. *Paste*, triamcinolone acetonide 1%, demeclocycline hydrochloride 3% (as demeclocycline calcium). For application to exposed tooth pulp under temporary filling.
Cement, triamcinolone acetonide 0.67%, demeclocycline hydrochloride 2%, calcium hydroxide, zinc oxide, supplied with 2 types of hardening fluids. For use as a permanent lining cement for tooth cavities in cases of pulp exposure.

Lederspan *(Lederle, UK)*. *Injection* (aqueous suspension), triamcinolone hexacetonide 5 mg/mL, in vials of 5 mL.
Injection (aqueous suspension), triamcinolone hexacetonide 20 mg/mL, in vials of 1 and 5 mL.

Proprietary Names and Manufacturers of Triamcinolone and its Esters

Adcortyl *(Squibb, UK)*; Albacort *(Teknofarma, Ital.)*; Albicort *(Neth.)*; Alcorten *(Alcon, Spain)*; Aristocort *(Lederle, Austral.; Lederle, Canad.; Lederle, USA)*; Aristogel *(USA)*; Aristospan *(Lederle, Canad.; Lederle, USA)*; Azmacort *(Rorer, USA)*; BayTac *(Bay, USA)*; BayTac-D *(Bay, USA)*; Bucalsone *(Spain)*; Cenocort A *(Central Pharmaceuticals, USA)*; Cenocort Forte *(Central Pharmaceuticals, USA)*; Cinalone *(Legere, USA)*; Cino-40 *(Reid-Provident, USA)*; Cinolone *(Ital.)*; Cinonide *(Legere, USA)*; Corticothérapique *(Mepha, Switz.)*; Cortinovus *(Ital.)*; Cutinolone Simple *(Labaz, Fr.)*; Delphi *(Belg.)*; Delphicort *(Cyanamid-Lederle, Ger.)*; Delsolone *(Medosan, Ital.)*; Ditrizin *(Spain)*; Dolsolone *(Medosan, Ital.)*;
Eczil *(Ital.)*; Extracort *(Basotherm, Ger.)*; Flogicort *(Ital.)*; Fortcinolona *(Arg.)*; Ftorocort *(Hung.)*; Hexatrione *(Lederle, Fr.)*; Ipercortis *(AGIPS, Ital.)*; Kenacort *(Arg.; Squibb, Austral.; Belg.; Squibb, Canad.; Squibb, Fr.; Squibb, Ital.; Neth.; Novo, Norw.; Squibb, Swed.; Squibb, Switz.; Squibb, USA)*; Kenacort A *(Squibb, Austral.; Belg.; Fr.; Neth.; Squibb, Switz.)*; Kenacort Diacetate *(Squibb, USA)*; Kenacort-T *(Novo, Norw.; Squibb, Swed.)*; Kenalog *(Squibb, Austral.; Squibb, Canad.; Squibb, Denm.; Squibb, UK; Squibb, USA)*; Kenalone *(Squibb, Austral.)*; Kortikoid *(Ratiopharm, Ger.)*; Ledercort *(Arg.; Lederle, Denm.; Cyanamid, Ital.; Neth.; Lederle, Norw.; Lederle, S.Afr.; Cyanamid, Spain; Lederle, Swed.; Lederle, Switz.; Lederle, UK)*; Ledercort A *(Cyanamid, Ital.)*; Ledercort Depot *(Lederle, UK)*; Lederlon *(Cyanamid-Lederle, Ger.)*; Lederspan *(Arg.; Belg.; Lederle, Denm.; Ital.; Neth.; Lederle, Norw.; Lederle, S.Afr.; Lederle, Swed.; Switz.; Lederle, UK)*; Medicort *(Ital.)*; Paralen *(Switz.)*; Proctosteroid *(Aldo, Spain)*; Rineton *(Jpn)*; Sadocort *(Ital.)*; SK-Triamcinolone *(Smith Kline & French, USA)*; Solodelf *(Ger.)*; Tédarol *(Specia, Fr.)*; Taucorten *(Sigmatau, Ital.)*; Tibicorten *(Stiefel, Fr.; Sigmatau, Ital.)*; Tracilon *(Savage, USA)*; Tramacin *(USA)*; Triaceton *(Cusi, Spain)*; Triaderm *(Taro, Canad.)*; Triam *(Nattermann, Ger.)*; Triam-A *(USA)*; Triamcet *(Ger.)*; Triamcinair *(Pharmafair, USA)*; Triamcort *(Ital.; Switz.)*; Trianciterap *(Arg.)*; Tri-Anemul *(Pharmasal, Ger.)*; Trianide *(Technilab, Canad.)*; Tricinolon *(Jpn)*; Tricortale *(Bergamon, Ital.)*; Trigon *(Squibb, Spain)*; Trilon *(Ital.)*; Trimacort *(Canad.)*; Trymex *(Savage, USA)*; Volon *(Heyden, Ger.)*; Volonimat *(Heyden, Ger.)*; Voncort *(Ital.)*.

The following names have been used for multi-ingredient preparations containing triamcinolone or its esters—Adcortyl with Graneodin *(Squibb, UK)*; Aristoform *(Lederle, Canad.)*; Audicort *(Lederle, UK)*; Aureocort *(Lederle, Canad.; Lederle, UK)*; Kenacomb *(Squibb, Austral.; Squibb, Canad.)*; Kenalog-S *(USA)*; Ledermix *(Lederle, UK)*; Mycolog *(Squibb, USA)*; Mycolog-II *(Squibb, USA)*; Myco-Triacet *(Lemmon, USA)*; Myco-Triacet-II *(Lemmon, USA)*; Mytrex *(Savage, USA)*; Mytrex-F *(Savage, USA)*; Nystadermal *(Squibb, UK)*; Nyst-olone *(Schein, USA)*; Remiderm *(Squibb, UK)*; Remotic *(Squibb, UK)*; Silderm *(Lederle, UK)*; Tri-Adcortyl *(Squibb, UK)*; Triamalone *(Trans Canaderm, Canad.)*; Tricaderm *(Squibb, UK)*; Viaderm-KC *(Taro, Canad.)*.

Cough Suppressants Expectorants and Mucolytics

2000-q

Described in this section are drugs that are reported to have cough suppressant, expectorant, or mucolytic actions, and which are mainly used in various respiratory conditions.

Cough and cold preparations containing various combinations of cough suppressants, expectorants, sympathomimetics, antihistamines, or analgesics are available, but some of these combinations such as a cough suppressant and an expectorant are illogical and there is little evidence to support their efficacy. As with many combinations, doses of individual drugs may be inadequate or inappropriate, and the large number of ingredients may expose the patient to unnecessary adverse effects.

Other agents reported to be beneficial in respiratory tract conditions and described in other sections include demulcents such as Glycerol (p.1128) and decongestant inhalations of Menthol (p.1586) or volatile oils.

Cough Suppressants

The cough suppressants described in this section have either a central or peripheral action on the cough reflex or a combination of both. The centrally-acting agents described in this section include dextromethorphan and other morphinan or opium-alkaloid compounds or derivatives that have little or no analgesic properties. Those that also have an analgesic effect such as codeine, diamorphine, and methadone are described in the section on Opioid Analgesics. The centrally-acting cough suppressants generally have little sedative activity. Cough suppressants with a peripheral action, such as benzonatate, may act on the cough receptors present in the respiratory mucosa, or are reported to act by a bronchodilatory effect.

Cough suppressants are used to suppress irritant, unproductive coughs, but few have been shown to be effective by controlled clinical studies. The ideal cough suppressant should diminish the frequency and distress of coughing whilst not impairing reflex mechanisms allowing clearance of secretions. Their use in conditions characterised by the production of bronchial secretions, such as chronic bronchitis or cystic fibrosis may result in sputum retention and the development of pneumonia.

A long review of the analgesic and cough suppressant effects of codeine and its alternatives.— N. B. Eddy *et al.*, *Codeine and its Alternates for Pain and Cough Relief*, Geneva, World Health Organization, 1970; *idem*, *Bull. Wld Hlth Org.*, 1969, *40*, 639 and 721.

Further references: D. T. D. Hughes, *Br. med. J.*, 1978, *1*, 1202.

Expectorants

The expectorants described in this section are reported to increase the volume of secretions in the respiratory tract and therefore to facilitate their removal by ciliary action and coughing. Some, such as small doses of ipecacuanha and squill, ammonium salts, some volatile oils, and various compounds described in the section on Iodine Compounds (p.1184), are believed to achieve this by an irritant effect on the gastric mucosa, although there is no evidence to show that they are effective.

Other agents that have been used as expectorants include Acetic Acid (p.1537), Garlic (p.1573), Tar (p.933), and various plant products and extracts such as adhatoda, ammoniacum, angelica, euphorbia, euphorbium, galbanum, grindelia, primula rhizome, and saponaria.

Mucolytics

The mucolytics described in this section alter the structure of mucus to decrease its viscosity and therefore facilitate its removal by ciliary action or expectoration. Acetylcysteine, carbocisteine, methyl cysteine, mesna (p.842), and stepronin all have thiol groups; if this group is free as in acetylcysteine it may be substituted for disulphide bonds in mucus and therefore break the mucus chains. However, drugs such as carbocisteine with 'protected' thiol groups cannot act by this mechanism. Thiol groups are also involved in the mechanism of action of some of these agents when they are used in the treatment of poisoning.

Although mucolytics have been shown to affect sputum viscosity and structure, and patients have reported alleviation of their symptoms, no consistent improvement has been demonstrated in lung function.

Inhalation aerosols of water, sodium bicarbonate, sodium chloride, surfactants such as Tyloxapol (p.1248), and proteolytic enzymes such as Chymotrypsin (p.1043), and Trypsin (p.1050), have also been used for their reported hydrating or mucolytic effects on respiratory secretions. However, it should be remembered that water is not readily incorporated into mucus when administered by inhalation, and such inhalations may act more by an irritant action on the mucosa.

3701-r

Acetylcysteine *(BAN, USAN, rINN).*

5052; *N*-Acetylcysteine; NSC-111180. *N*-Acetyl-L-cysteine.

$C_5H_9NO_3S = 163.2$.

CAS — 616-91-1.

Pharmacopoeias. In *Br.*, *Braz.*, *Chin.*, and *U.S.*

A white crystalline powder with a slight acetic odour.

B.P. **solubilities** are: soluble 1 in 8 of water and 1 in 2 of alcohol; practically insoluble in chloroform and ether. *U.S.P.* solubilities are: 1 in 5 of water and 1 in 4 of alcohol; practically insoluble in chloroform and ether. A 1% solution in water has a pH of 2.0 to 2.8.

Incompatible with most metals, with rubber, and with oxygen and oxidising substances. Some antibiotics including amphotericin, ampicillin sodium, erythromycin lactobionate, and some tetracyclines are either physically incompatible with or may be inactivated on mixture with acetylcysteine.

A change in colour of solutions of acetylcysteine to light purple does not indicate significant impairment of safety or efficacy. **Store** in airtight containers at a temperature below 15°. Protect from light.

For a report of the effect *in vitro* of acetylcysteine on the antimicrobial activity of some antibiotics, see under Uses and Administration, below.

Adverse Effects

Adverse effects reported with acetylcysteine include bronchospasm, nausea, vomiting, stomatitis, rhinorrhoea, headache, tinnitus, urticaria, chills, fever, and haemoptysis. Anaphylactic reactions have been reported rarely.

In 38 patients identified by The National Poisons Information Service and the manufacturer as experiencing anaphylactoid reactions after the intravenous use of acetylcysteine the most common feature was rash or pruritus; other features included flushing, nausea or vomiting, angioedema, tachycardia, bronchospasm, and hypotension. Symptoms in 19 cases of overdosage (often due to misinterpretation of the label) were similar but more severe and included respiratory depression (1), haemolysis (1), disseminated intravascular coagulation (1), renal failure (3), and death (2); some of these effects could be attributable to paracetamol poisoning. Three further cases of overdosage had also been seen.— T. G. K. Mant *et al.*, *Br. med. J.*, 1984, *289*, 217.

For further reports of adverse reactions after intravenous administration of acetylcysteine for the treatment of paracetamol poisoning see J. A. Vale and D. C. Wheeler (letter), *Lancet*, 1982, *2*, 988 (allergy); S. W. -C. Ho and L. J. Beilin, *Br. med. J.*, 1983, *287*, 876 (bronchospasm); *Lancet*, 1984, *1*, 1421 (fatal cardiovascular collapse); D. N. Bateman *et al.*, *Hum. Toxicol.*, 1984, *3*, 393 (urticaria; responses suggest a pseudo-allergic rather than an immunological reaction).

Precautions

Acetylcysteine should be used with caution in asthmatic patients.

For a report of the effect *in vitro* of acetylcysteine on the antimicrobial activity of some antibiotics, see under Uses and Administration, below.

Absorption and Fate

Acetylcysteine is rapidly absorbed from the gastro-intestinal tract.

Single-dose studies using radioactively-labelled acetylcysteine demonstrating that it is distributed to the lungs and metabolised to cysteine, diacetylcysteine, and cystine.— D. Rodenstein *et al.*, *Clin. Pharmacokinet.*, 1978, *3*, 247. See also J. Maddock, *Eur. J. resp. Dis.*, 1980, *61*, *Suppl.* 111, 52.

Uses and Administration

Acetylcysteine is a mucolytic agent that reduces the viscosity of secretions probably by the splitting of disulphide bonds in mucoproteins. It is used in cystic fibrosis, respiratory conditions associated with the production of viscous mucus such as acute and chronic bronchitis, or asthma, and in the routine cleansing of tracheostomies.

It is most active in concentrations of 10 to 20% at a pH of 7 to 9 and the pH may have been adjusted in commercial preparations with sodium hydroxide. It is sometimes stated that acetylcysteine sodium is used, although the dose is expressed in terms of acetylcysteine. Administration can be by nebulisation of 2 to 5 mL of a 20% solution or 4 to 10 mL of a 10% solution through a face mask or mouthpiece 3 to 4 times daily. If necessary 1 to 10 mL of a 20% solution or 2 to 20 mL of a 10% solution may be given by nebulisation every 2 to 6 hours. It can also be given by direct instillation of 1 to 2 mL of a 10 to 20% solution every 1 to 4 hours. Mechanical suction of the liquefied secretions may be necessary, and nebulisers containing metal or rubber components should not be used.

Acetylcysteine may also be given by mouth in doses of 200 mg three times daily as granules dissolved in water. Children aged up to 2 years may be given 200 mg once daily, and those aged 2 to 6 years 200 mg twice daily.

In the treatment of dry eye syndromes associated with abnormal mucus production, acetylcysteine is administered topically usually as a 5% solution with hypromellose, 1 to 2 drops being given 3 to 4 times daily.

Acetylcysteine is also used in the treatment of paracetamol poisoning. An initial dose of 150 mg per kg body-weight of acetylcysteine in 200 mL of glucose injection is given intravenously over 15 minutes, followed by an intravenous infusion of 50 mg per kg in 500 mL of glucose injection over the next 4 hours and then 100 mg per kg in one litre over the next 16 hours. The volume of intravenous fluids should be modified for children. In the *US*, acetylcysteine has been given by mouth in an initial dose of 140 mg per kg as a 5% solution followed by 70 mg per kg every 4 hours for 17 doses. Acetylcysteine is reported to be very effective when administered within 8 hours of paracetamol overdosage, with the protective effect diminishing after this time and being ineffective when administered later than 15 hours.

At a concentration of 20 µg per mL, acetylcysteine inhibited the growth of 12 of 13 strains of *Pseudomonas aeruginosa*, 1 of 8 strains of *Staphylococcus aureus*, and none of 10 strains of *Klebsiella* and *Enterobacter* species. An additive effect was demonstrated against *Ps. aeruginosa* with combinations of acetylcysteine with carbenicillin or ticarcillin. Antagonism against this organism was demonstrated with combinations of acetylcysteine with gentamicin or tobramycin; antagonism against *Kl. pneumoniae* was also demonstrated with acetylcysteine and gentamicin. It was suggested that, although acetylcysteine and aminoglycoside antibiotics were chemically compatible, they should not be administered at the same time by aerosol in patients with cystic fibrosis because of the possibility of local inactivation of the antibiotic.— M. F. Parry and H. C. Neu, *J. clin. Microbiol.*, 1977, *5*, 58.

CARBON TETRACHLORIDE POISONING. In a report of acute carbon tetrachloride poisoning in 19 patients, 13 were given acetylcysteine intravenously according to the dosage regimen recommended for paracetamol poisoning. It was concluded that prompt intravenous therapy with acetylcysteine in addition to supportive treatment may minimise hepatorenal damage. However, due to the slow elimination of carbon tetrachloride, treatment may be required for longer than the 20 hours recommended for paracetamol poisoning.— M. Ruprah *et al.*, *Lancet*, 1985, *1*, 1027. See also P. W. Mathieson *et al.*, *Hum. Toxicol.*, 1985, *4*, 627.

COLPOSCOPY. Acetylcysteine had been used in association with a 2 to 3% solution of acetic acid in 1500 women to clean the cervix and remove cervical mucus prior to colposcopy.— A. D. Martins, *Eur. J. resp. Dis.*, 1980, *61*, *Suppl.* 111, 172.

CYSTIC FIBROSIS. A report of 8 patients with 'meconium ileus equivalent' secondary to cystic fibrosis; 7 were treated with 10 mL of acetylcysteine 20% four times a day by mouth and 100 mL of acetylcysteine 10% as an enema 1 to 4 times a day. There was symptomatic improvement in 24 hours.— J. G. Hanly and M. X. Fitzgerald, *Br. med. J.*, 1983, *286*, 1411.

There was no clinical or subjective benefit from acetylcysteine or ambroxol given by mouth for 12 weeks in a double-blind placebo-controlled study involving 32 patients with cystic fibrosis.— F. Ratjen *et al.*, *Eur. J. Pediat.*, 1985, *144*, 374.

CYSTINURIA. Complete dissolution of cystine stones was achieved after direct percutaneous infusion of a solution of acetylcysteine and sodium bicarbonate in 2 of 6 patients, and after infusion of trometamol in 3 of 5 patients. Dissolution with acetylcysteine required a longer period of treatment than with trometamol.— S. P. Dretler *et al.*, *J. Urol., Baltimore*, 1984, *131*, 216. See also W. P. Mulvaney *et al.*, *ibid.*, 1975, *114*, 107.

DOXORUBICIN CARDIOTOXICITY. It has been suggested that acetylcysteine may be useful in doxorubicin-induced cardiotoxicity due to its ability to act as a free-radical scavenger. However Dresdale *et al.* (*Am. J. clin. Oncol.*, 1982, *5*, 657) found it to be ineffective in reversing established cardiotoxicity and Unverferth *et al.* (*J. natn. Cancer Inst.*, 1983, *71*, 917) could demonstrate no preventative effect on acute toxicity.

IFOSFAMIDE UROTOXICITY. Results of a preliminary study indicating that acetylcysteine given by mouth may be effective in preventing the urotoxicity caused by ifosfamide.— J. H. Saiers and M. Slavik, *Vet. hum. Toxicol.*, 1981, *23*, *Suppl.* 1, 12.

OTITIS MEDIA. For references to the possible use of acetylcysteine in the treatment of secretory otitis media (glue ear), see under Carbocisteine, p.907.

PANCREATITIS. Beneficial response to acetylcysteine in a patient with acute pancreatitis complicated by adult respiratory distress syndrome and renal failure. Acetylcysteine was given at half the dosage recommended for paracetamol poisoning over a period of 56 hours.— J. M. Braganza *et al.* (letter), *Lancet*, 1986, *1*, 914.

PARACETAMOL POISONING. Intravenous acetylcysteine was considered to be the treatment of choice for paracetamol overdosage, and to be very effective in preventing the liver damage, renal failure, and death that may occur. Treatment with acetylcysteine should be initiated in all patients with plasma-paracetamol concentrations above the 'treatment line' (a line joining 200 µg per mL at 4 hours and 30 µg per mL at 15 hours on a semilogarithmic graph).If ingestion of paracetamol is within the last 4 hours, gastric lavage or induction of emesis should also be carried out. Acetylcysteine should be started as soon as possible and should not be delayed beyond 8 hours after ingestion while awaiting laboratory results. Treatment should be started immediately in patients admitted between 8 and 15 hours after ingestion; it can then be discontinued if found to be unnecessary after subsequent results of plasma-paracetamol concentrations. Treatment after 15 hours is of no value and may aggravate the risk of hepatic failure.

Although acetylcysteine by mouth has been used for paracetamol poisoning in the *USA*, even large doses were considered to be less effective than intravenous administration due to the slow and incomplete absorption in patients with nausea and vomiting. This more than outweighed the possible advantage of direct delivery to the liver after oral administration. Oral therapy would also be contra-indicated in patients who have been given emetics or activated charcoal.— L. F. Prescott, *Drugs*, 1983, *25*, 290. See also *idem.*, *Br. med. J.*, 1983, *287*, 274; K. J. Breen *et al.*, *Med. J. Aust.*, 1982, *1*, 77.

In an open study involving 662 patients with paracetamol poisoning, acetylcysteine by mouth was concluded to be effective if administered during the first 16 hours after ingestion.— B. H. Rumack *et al.*, *Archs intern. Med.*, 1981, *141*, 380.

For references to the role of glutathione in paracetamol poisoning and the possible mechanisms of action of acetylcysteine see G. J. Beckett *et al.*, *Gut*, 1985, *26*, 26; L. G. B. Tee *et al.* (letter), *Lancet*, 1986, *1*, 331.

RESPIRATORY DISORDERS. *Atelectasis.* Relief of severe atelectasis during mechanical ventilation after administration of nebulised acetylcysteine in 5 premature infants with pulmonary diseases.— J. Amir *et al.*, *Clin. Pharm.*, 1985, *4*, 255.

Chronic bronchitis. In 2 double-blind multicentre studies of 495 and 203 patients with chronic bronchitis (Multicentre Study Group, *Eur. J. resp. Dis.*, 1980, *61*, *Suppl.* 111, 93; G. Boman *et al.*, *ibid.*, 1983, *64*, 405) acetylcysteine 200 mg twice daily by mouth for 6 months was shown to be more effective than placebo in decreasing acute exacerbations; lung function tests however did not appear to be improved to a clinically significant extent.

In an open study, 1392 patients with chronic bronchitis received acetylcysteine 200 mg by mouth three times daily for 2 months. There was a general improvement in symptoms and in sputum viscosity and purulence. Adverse effects were reported in 230 patients: they included gastro-intestinal effects, dry mouth, headache or dizziness, rashes, bronchospasm, malaise, alteration of taste, skeletal muscle effects, frequency of micturition, flushing, sweating, and blurred vision.— A. B. Tattersall *et al.*, *J. int. med. Res.*, 1983, *11*, 279. Confirmation of results in a similar study of 248 patients; 27 patients reported similar adverse effects.— *idem.*, 1984, *12*, 96.

In a double-blind, multicentre study of 121 patients with chronic bronchitis receiving acetylcysteine 200 mg by mouth three times daily for 3 months, cough and ease of expectoration, but not sputum viscosity and purulence, improved to a greater extent than with placebo.— I. M. Jackson *et al.*, *ibid.*, 198.

Preparations

Acetylcysteine Solution *(U.S.P.)*

Proprietary Preparations

Fabrol *(Zyma, UK). Granules,* acetylcysteine 200 mg/sachet. To be dissolved in water before administration.

Ilube *(Duncan, Flockhart, UK). Eye-drops,* acetylcysteine 5%, hypromellose 0.35%.

Parvolex *(Duncan, Flockhart, UK). Concentrate for intravenous infusion,* acetylcysteine 200 mg/mL in ampoules of 10 mL.

Proprietary Names and Manufacturers

Airbron *(Allen & Hanburys, Canad.; Duncan, Flockhart, UK)*; Brunac *(Bruschettini, Ital.)*; Eurespiran *(Nicholas, Ger.)*; Exomuc *(Bouchara, Fr.)*; Fabrol *(Ciba, Denm.; Inpharzam, Swed.; Zyma, UK)*; Fluimucil *(Arsac, Fr.; Inpharzam, Ger.; Zambon, Ital.; Neth.; Zambon, Spain; Inpharzam, Switz.)*; Fluprowit *(Thiemann, Ger.)*; Granon *(DAK, Denm.)*; Ilube *(Duncan, Flockhart, UK)*; Inspir *(Swed.)*; L-Cimexyl *(Cimex, Switz.)*; Lysomucil *(Belg.)*; Mucisol *(Deca, Ital.)*; Muciteran *(Schwabe-Farmasan, Ger.)*; Muco Sanigen *(Beecham-Wülfing, Ger.)*; Mucocedyl *(Kettelhack Riker, Ger.)*; Mucofilin Sol *(Jpn)*; Mucolysin *(Durascan, Denm.)*; Mucolyticum *(Bristol, Ger.)*; Mucomist *(Bristol Italiana Sud, Ital.)*; Mucomyst *(Arg.; Astra, Austral.; Belg.; Bristol, Canad.; Astra, Denm.; Allard, Fr.; Neth.; Draco, Norw.; Tika, Norw.; Tika, Swed.; Switz.; Mead Johnson Pharmaceutical, USA)*; Mucosal *(Dey, USA)*; Mucothiol *(Ozothine, Fr.)*; Mucret *(Astra, Ger.)*; Nac *(Canad.)*; Parvolex *(Glaxo, Austral.; Allen & Hanburys, Canad.; Duncan, Flockhart, UK)*; Solmucol *(Ibsa, Switz)*; Tixair *(Valpan, Fr.)*.

1231l-z

Acetyldihydrocodeine Hydrochloride

4,5-Epoxy-3-methoxy-9a-methylmorphinan-6-yl acetate hydrochloride.

$C_{20}H_{25}NO_4,HCl = 379.9$.

CAS — 3861-72-1 (acetyldihydrocodeine).

Acetyldihydrocodeine hydrochloride is a centrally-acting cough suppressant.

Proprietary Names and Manufacturers

Acetylcodone *(Bios, Belg.)*.

3900-v

Adamexine *(rINN)*.

α-(1-Adamantylmethylamino)-4′,6′-dibromo-2-acetotoluidide.

$C_{20}H_{26}Br_2N_2O = 470.2$.

CAS — 54785-02-3.

Adamexine has been used as a mucolytic in the treatment of respiratory-tract disorders in doses of 20 to 25 mg three times daily.

Proprietary Names and Manufacturers

Adamucol *(Ferrer, Spain)*; Broncostyl *(Robert, Spain)*.

5603-l

Alloclamide Hydrochloride *(rINNM)*.

264-CE. 2-Allyloxy-4-chloro-*N*-(2-diethylaminoethyl)benzamide hydrochloride.

$C_{16}H_{23}ClN_2O_2,HCl = 347.3$.

CAS — 5486-77-1 (alloclamide); 5107-01-7 (hydrochloride).

Alloclamide hydrochloride is a cough suppressant; it is given by mouth in doses of 12.5 to 25 mg.

Proprietary Names and Manufacturers

Tuselin *(Liade, Spain)*.

2002-s

Ambroxol *(rINN)*.

NA-872. *trans*-4-(2-Amino-3,5-dibromobenzylamino)cyclohexanol.

$C_{13}H_{18}Br_2N_2O = 378.1$.

CAS — 18683-91-5.

Ambroxol is a metabolite of bromhexine and has similar actions and uses. It is given as the hydrochloride in doses of 15 to 30 mg two or three times daily by mouth, by inhalation, or by injection.

References to pharmacokinetic studies of ambroxol: R. Hammer *et al.*, *Arzneimittel-Forsch.*, 1978, *28*, 899; R. Jauch *et al.*, *ibid.*, 904; H. Vergin *et al.*, *ibid.*, 1985, *35*, 1591.

No adverse effect on gastric mucus was observed in a study of 10 patients with respiratory disorders given ambroxol 30 mg three times daily by mouth for 10 days.— M. Guslandi and M. E. Zanoni, *J. int. med. Res.*, 1985, *13*, 281.

ALVEOLAR PROTEINOSIS. A 39-year-old man who refused serial alveolar lavage for proteinosis had a beneficial response to inhalation of ambroxol aerosols, 3 mL every six hours, in association with ambroxol 30 mg by mouth every six hours. This was considered to be due to an activating effect on surfactant in the lung.— J. P. Diaz *et al.* (letter), *Lancet*, 1984, *1*, 1023.

BRONCHITIS. References to the use of ambroxol by mouth, by inhalation, or by intravenous injection in the treatment of bronchitis: K. J. Wiessmann and K. Niemeyer, *Arzneimittel-Forsch.*, 1978, *28*, 918; P. Göbel and H. Rensch, *ibid.*, 929; H. Hoffmann, *ibid.*, 931; R. Kranicke, *ibid.*, 934.

CYSTIC FIBROSIS. For a report of the use of ambroxol in cystic fibrosis, see Acetylcysteine, above.

HYALINE MEMBRANE DISEASE. Evidence to suggest that ambroxol given antenatally had some protective effect against hyaline membrane disease although the effect appeared to be dependent on the period of gestation.— R. R. Wauer *et al.*, *Int. J. biol. Res. Pregnancy*, 1982, *3*, 84. See also J. Henahan, *J. Am. med. Ass.*, 1983, *249*, 2425.

SILICOSIS. Ambroxol was considered to be more effective in patients with silicosis than in patients with chronic obstructive bronchitis. It was suggested that the twofold action of ambroxol as a secretolytic and surfactant stimulant would account for the increased activity in the silicosis patients.— P. C. Curti and H. D. Renovanz, *Arzneimittel-Forsch.*, 1978, *28*, 922.

SJÖGREN'S SYNDROME. In a double-blind crossover study of 36 patients with primary Sjögren's syndrome, ambroxol 60 mg twice daily by mouth for 3 weeks had no effect on lachrymal secretion as measured by objective ophthalmological tests. Three patients reported a subjective increase in tear and saliva production.— R. Manthorpe *et al.*, *Acta Ophthalmol.*, 1984, *62*, 537.

Proprietary Names and Manufacturers

Ambril *(Allergopharma, Ger.)*; Ambrolitic *(Wasserman, Spain)*; Bronchopront *(Mack, Illert., Ger.)*; Duramucal *(Durachemie, Ger.)*; Expit *(Jossa-Arznei, Ger.)*; Frenopect *(Hefa-Frenon, Ger.)*; Lindoxyl *(Lindopharm, Ger.)*; Lisopulm *(Esseti, Ital.)*; Motosol *(Castejon, Spain)*; Mucibron *(Hosbon, Spain)*; Muciclar *(Piam, Ital.)*; Muco-Aspecton *(Krewel, Ger.)*; Mucobron *(OFF, Ital.)*; Mucoclear *(Mundipharma, Ger.)*; Mucophlogat *(Azuchemie, Ger.)*; Mucosan *(Fher, Spain)*; Mucosolvan *(Thomae, Ger.*; *De Angeli, Ital.)*; Mucosolvon *(Boehringer Ingelheim, Switz.)*; Muco-Tablinen *(Beiersdorf, Ger.)*; Mucovent *(Byk Gulden, Ger.)*; Naxpa *(Novag, Spain)*; Pulmonal *(Schaper & Brümmer, Ger.)*; Secretil *(Caber, Ital.)*; Stas *(Stada, Ger.)*; Tauxolo *(Ibi Sud, Ital.)*; Tusso-Basan *(Sagitta, Ger.)*; Viscomucil *(ABC, Ital.)*.

5604-y

Aminothiazoline Camphorate

Camfazolinum. 2-Amino-2-thiazoline camphorate.
$(C_3H_6N_2S)_2,C_{10}H_{16}O_4=404.6$.

CAS — 1779-81-3 (aminothiazoline); 2387-58-8 (camphorate).

Aminothiazoline camphorate has been used as a cough suppressant in doses of 200 mg by mouth three or four times daily.

2003-w

Ammonium Acetate

$CH_3CO_2NH_4=77.08$

CAS — 631-61-8 (ammonium acetate); 8013-61-4 (ammonium acetate solution).

2004-e

Ammonium Bicarbonate *(BAN)*.

503. Ammonium hydrogen carbonate.
$NH_4HCO_3=79.06$.

CAS — 1066-33-7.

Pharmacopoeias. In *Br.* and *Egypt.*

A fine, white, slightly hygroscopic, crystalline powder, white crystals, or glassy colourless solid, with a slightly ammoniacal odour. It volatilises rapidly at 60° with dissociation into ammonia, carbon dioxide, and water; volatilisation takes place slowly at ordinary temperatures if slightly moist.

Soluble 1 in 5 of water; practically insoluble in alcohol. **Store** in a cool place in well-closed containers.

NOTE. The *B.P.* directs that when Ammonium Carbonate is prescribed or demanded Ammonium Bicarbonate be supplied.

2005-l

Ammonium Carbonate *(USAN)*.

503; Carbonato de Amonio.

CAS — 8000-73-5.

Pharmacopoeias. In *Arg., Fr., It., Mex., Port.,* and *Span.* Also in *U.S.N.F.*

A white powder or hard white or translucent masses with an ammoniacal odour, consisting of a variable mixture of ammonium bicarbonate and ammonium carbamate, $NH_2.CO_2.NH_4$. It yields 30 to 34% of NH_3. On exposure to air it loses ammonia and carbon dioxide, becoming opaque, and is finally converted into friable porous lumps or a white powder of ammonium bicarbonate. **Soluble** 1 in 4 of water. It is decomposed by hot water. A solution in water is alkaline to litmus. **Store** at a temperature not exceeding 30° in airtight containers. Protect from light.

NOTE. The *B.P.* directs that Ammonium Bicarbonate be supplied when Ammonium Carbonate is prescribed or demanded.

2006-y

Ammonium Chloride *(BAN, USAN)*.

510; Ammonii Chloridum; Ammonium Chloratum; Cloruro de Amonio; Muriate of Ammonia; Sal Ammoniac.
$NH_4Cl=53.49$.

CAS — 12125-02-9.

NOTE. The food additive number 380 is used for ammonium citrate.

Pharmacopoeias. In *Arg., Aust., Belg., Br., Braz., Chin., Egypt., Eur., Fr., Ger., Hung., Ind., It., Jug., Mex., Neth., Nord., Pol., Port., Roum., Span., Swiss,* and *U.S.*

White crystalline powder or colourless crystals with a cooling saline taste; somewhat hygroscopic. Each g represents 18.69 mmol of chloride. *B.P.* **solubilities** are: soluble 1 in 2.7 of water. *U.S.P.* solubilities are: freely soluble in water and glycerol, and more so in boiling water; sparingly soluble in alcohol. A 5% solution in water has a pH of 4.6 to 6.0. A 0.8% solution is iso-osmotic with serum. Solutions are **sterilised** by autoclaving or by filtration. **Store** in airtight containers.

Adverse Effects and Treatment

Ammonium salts are irritant to the gastric mucosa and may produce nausea and vomiting particularly in large doses. Large doses of ammonium chloride may cause a profound acidosis and hypokalaemia which should be treated symptomatically. Intravenous administration of ammonium chloride may cause pain and irritation at the site of injection, which may be decreased by slowing the rate of infusion.

Excessive doses of ammonium salts, particularly if administered by rapid intravenous injection, may give rise to hepatic encephalopathy. This results from the inability of the liver to convert the increased load of ammonium ions to urea, and is similar to the symptoms of terminal liver failure.

In Great Britain the recommended exposure limits of ammonium chloride fumes are 10 mg per m^3 (long term); 20 mg per m^3 (short term).

Precautions

Ammonium salts are contra-indicated in the presence of impaired hepatic or renal function.

Absorption and Fate

Ammonium chloride is effectively absorbed from the gastro-intestinal tract. The ammonium ion is converted into urea in the liver; the anion thus liberated into the blood stream and extracellular fluid causes a metabolic acidosis and decreases the pH of the urine; this is followed by transient diuresis.

Uses and Administration

The administration of ammonium chloride produces a transient diuresis and a mild acidosis. It may be used in the treatment of severe metabolic alkalosis, particularly that resulting from chloride loss following prolonged vomiting or excessive diuresis. It is administered usually as a 1 to 2% solution by slow intravenous infusion, in a dosage depending on the severity of the alkalosis. A concentrated solution of ammonium chloride may be diluted by sodium chloride or glucose injection.

Ammonium chloride may also be used to maintain the urine at an acid pH in the treatment of some urinary-tract disorders, or in forced acid diuresis procedures to aid the excretion of basic drugs, such as amphetamines, in severe cases of overdosage. It is usually given by mouth, often as enteric-coated tablets, in a dose of 1 to 2 g every four to six hours, although 4 g every two hours has been given in forced acid diuresis procedures.

Ammonium chloride was formerly used to increase the diuretic effect of mercurial diuretics.

Ammonium chloride is used as an expectorant.

Other ammonium salts used similarly include the acetate, benzoate, bicarbonate, carbonate, and citrate.

Report of a preliminary study of the use of an ammonia tolerance test to differentiate between ascites of cirrhotic and malignant origin. Plasma ammonia concentrations were measured before, and 15 and 30 minutes after the rectal instillation of 100 mL of a 5% ammonium acetate solution. The mean plasma-ammonia concentration rose significantly in the group of patients with cirrhosis but not in those with malignancies.— C. Felding *et al.*, *Scand. J. Gastroenterol.*, 1984, *19*, 365.

Preparations of Ammonium Salts

Strong Ammonium Acetate Solution *(B.P.)*. Ammonium bicarbonate 47.0 g, glacial acetic acid 45.3 g, a sufficient quantity of Strong Ammonia Solution to neutralise the acid, freshly boiled and cooled water to 100 mL. It contains 55% to 60% of ammonium acetate. A 10% v/v solution in water has a pH of 7 to 8. Wt per mL 1.085 to 1.095 g. Store in containers of lead-free glass.

The *B.P.* directs that when Ammonium Acetate Solution or Dilute Ammonium Acetate Solution is prescribed or demanded, Strong Ammonium Acetate Solution diluted to 8 times its volume with freshly boiled and cooled water be supplied.

Ammonium Chloride Tablets *(B.P.C. 1973)*. May be enteric-coated.

Ammonium Chloride Tablets *(U.S.P.)*. Enteric-coated tablets.

Ammonium Chloride Mixture *(A.P.F.)*. Mist. Ammon. Chlorid.; Expectorant Mixture; Mist. Expect. Ammonium chloride 1 g; ipecacuanha tincture 0.25 mL, aromatic ammonia solution (or aromatic ammonia spirit) 0.5 mL, liquorice liquid extract 0.5 mL, concentrated chloroform water 0.25 mL or methyl hydroxybenzoate solution 0.1 mL, water to 10 mL. *Dose.* 10 to 20 mL.

Ammonium Chloride Mixture *(B.P.)*. Ammonium Chloride Oral Solution. Ammonium chloride 1 g, aromatic ammonia solution 0.5 mL, liquorice liquid extract 1 mL, water to 10 mL. It should be recently prepared.

Ammonium Chloride Mixture *B.P.* was not adequately preserved against microbial spoilage as determined by the *B.P.* challenge test.— T. R. R. Kurup and L. S. C. Wan, *Pharm. J.*, 1986, *2*, 761.

Ammonia and Ipecacuanha Mixture *(B.P.)*. Ammonia and Ipecacuanha Oral Solution; Mistura Expectorans; Mist. Expect. Ammonium bicarbonate 200 mg, liquorice liquid extract 0.5 mL, ipecacuanha tincture 0.3 mL, concentrated camphor water 0.1 mL, concentrated anise water 0.05 mL, double-strength chloroform water 5 mL, water to 10 mL. It should be recently prepared.

Ammonia and Ipecacuanha Mixture *B.P.* was not adequately preserved against microbial spoilage as determined by the *B.P.* challenge test.— T. R. R. Kurup and L. S. C. Wan, *Pharm. J.*, 1986, *2*, 761.

Ammonium Chloride and Morphine Mixture *(B.P.)*. Ammonium Chloride and Morphine Oral Solution; Mist. Ammon. Chlorid. Co.; Mist. Ammon. Chlor. Sed.; Mistura Tussi Sedativa. Ammonium chloride 300 mg, ammonium bicarbonate 200 mg, chloroform and morphine tincture 0.3 mL, liquorice liquid extract 0.5 mL, water to 10 mL. It should be recently prepared. Contains about 500 µg of anhydrous morphine in 10 mL.

Various quantities of Ammonium Chloride and Morphine Mixture *B.P.* were stored in 300 mL bottles for 25 weeks in the dark under ambient temperature conditions. Bottles stored containing 300 mL, 200 mL, 100 mL, or 50 mL of the mixture retained 100%, 95%, 60%, and 30% of the original morphine content respectively. It was recommended that to minimise the storage of partially filled containers of the mixture a maximum of 100 mL in a single container should be supplied to the patient, and an expiry date of 2 months following the date of sale or dispensing should be given.— K. Helliwell and P. Jennings, *Pharm. J.*, 1982, *2*, 600.

Senega and Ammonia Mixture *(A.P.F.)*. Ammonium bicarbonate 250 mg, compound camphor spirit 1 mL, liquorice liquid extract 0.5 mL, concentrated senega infusion 0.5 mL, concentrated chloroform water 0.25 mL or compound hydroxybenzoate solution 0.1 mL, water to 10 mL. *Dose*. 10 to 20 mL.

Ammonium Chloride Injection *(U.S.P.)*. pH (of a 10% solution) 4 to 6.

Proprietary Names and Manufacturers of Ammonium Chloride and other Ammonium Salts

Chlorammonic *(Promedica, Fr.)*; Expigen *(Pharmacia, Denm.)*; Gen-Diur *(Leo, Spain)*; Hi-Amchlor *(High Noon, Pakistan)*; Nuseals Ammonium Chloride *(Lilly, UK)*.

The following names have been used for multi-ingredient preparations containing ammonium chloride and other ammonium salts—Ambenyl *(Parke, Davis, Canad.)*; Avil Decongestant *(Hoechst, Austral.)*; Benadryl Expectorant *(Parke, Davis, Austral.)*; Benafed *(Parke, Davis, UK)*; Benatuss *(Parke, Davis, Austral.)*; Benylets *(Parke, Davis, UK)*; Benylin Expectorant *(Parke, Davis, Canad.; Warner-Lambert, UK)*; Benylin-DM *(Parke, Davis, Canad.)*; Benyphed *(Parke, Davis, Austral.)*; Broncodeine *(Nadeau, Canad.)*; Calmylin with codeine *(Technilab, Canad.)*; Cheracol *(Upjohn, Canad.)*; Delixir *(Hamilton, Austral.)*; Drixine Cough Expectorant *(Essex, Austral.)*; Dytuss *(Lasalle, USA)*; Flavelix *(Pharmax, UK)*; Guanor *(R.P. Drugs, UK)*; Histadyl EC *(Lilly, UK)*; Histalix Expectorant *(Wallace Mfg Chem., UK)*; Hycomine *(Du Pont, Austral.; Du Pont, Canad.)*; Pectomed *(Medo, UK)*; P-V-Tussin Syrup *(Reid-Provident, USA)*; Pyramenso *(Nordic, Canad.)*; Quelidrine *(Abbott, USA)*; Senamon *(Drug Houses Austral., Austral.)*; Thenfacol *(Winthrop, Austral.)*; Ticipect *(Ticen, Eire)*; Twin-K-Cl *(Boots, USA)*; Unitussin *(Unimed, UK)*.

12427-b

Benproperine *(rINN)*.

ASA-158/5 (phosphate). 1-[2-(2-Benzylphenoxy)-1-methylethyl]piperidine.

$C_{21}H_{27}NO = 309.5$.

CAS — 2156-27-6.

Benproperine is a cough suppressant reported to have a peripheral and central action. It has been given by mouth as the embonate and the phosphate.

Proprietary Names and Manufacturers of Benproperine Salts

Blascorid *(Guidotti, Ital.)*; Cofrel; Pirexil *(Astra, Arg.)*; Pirexyl *(Pharmacia, Denm.; Pharmacia, Norw.; Pharmacia, Swed.)*; Tussafug *(Robugen, Ger.; Medipharm, Switz.)*.

5605-j

Benzonatate *(BAN, USAN, rINN)*.

Benzononatine; KM-65.

3,6,9,12,15,18,21,24,27-Nonaoxaoctacosyl 4-butylaminobenzoate.

$C_{13}H_{18}NO_2(OCH_2CH_2)_nOCH_3$, where *n* has an average value of 8.

CAS — 104-31-4 (where n = 8).

Pharmacopoeias. In *U.S.*

A clear, pale yellow, viscous liquid with a faint characteristic odour. **Soluble** 1 in less than 1 of water, alcohol, chloroform, and ether. **Store** in airtight containers. Protect from light.

Adverse Effects

Headache, dizziness, gastro-intestinal disturbances, nasal congestion, hypersensitivity, and skin rash have been reported. There may be drowsiness. Convulsions may occur in overdosage. Benzonatate has local anaesthetic properties and may produce numbness of the mouth, tongue, and pharynx.

Uses and Administration

Benzonatate is a cough suppressant stated to act both centrally and peripherally. It is given by mouth in a dose of 100 mg three to 6 times daily. Benzonatate is reported to act within 20 minutes and its effects are reported to last for 3 to 8 hours.

HICCUP. Intractable hiccup in 6 patients was relieved within 20 minutes following the administration of benzonatate.— C. M. Ayres, *Dis. nerv. Syst.*, 1966, *27*, 397.

Preparations

Benzonatate Capsules *(U.S.P.)*

Proprietary Names and Manufacturers

Tessalin *(Ciba, Norw.)*; Tessalon *(Ciba-Geigy, Canad.; Ciba, Neth.; Ciba, Swed.; Ciba, Switz.; Du Pont, USA)*.

5640-k

Bibenzonium Bromide *(BAN, rINN)*.

Diphenetholine Bromide; ES132. [2-(1,2-Diphenylethoxy)ethyl]trimethylammonium bromide.

$C_{19}H_{26}BrNO = 364.3$.

CAS — 59866-76-1 (bibenzonium); 15585-70-3 (bromide).

Bibenzonium bromide is a cough suppressant which is stated to have a central action. It is given by mouth in doses of 20 to 30 mg.

Proprietary Names and Manufacturers

Bractos *(Volpino, Arg.)*; Lysobex *(Bracco, Ital.)*; Rea-Tos Jarabe *(Rocador, Spain)*; Sedobex *(Continental Pharma, Belg.)*.

2008-z

Bromhexine Hydrochloride *(BANM, USAN, rINNM)*.

NA-274. 2-Amino-3,5-dibromo-*N*-cyclohexyl-*N*-methylbenzylamine hydrochloride.

$C_{14}H_{20}Br_2N_2,HCl = 412.6$.

CAS — 3572-43-8 (bromhexine); 611-75-6 (hydrochloride).

Pharmacopoeias. In *Br., Chin., Jpn*, and *Jug.*

A white or almost white, odourless or almost odourless, crystalline powder. Practically **insoluble** in water; sparingly soluble in alcohol and methyl alcohol; slightly soluble in chloroform. **Protect** from light.

Adverse Effects

Gastro-intestinal side-effects may occur occasionally with bromhexine and a transient rise in serum aminotransferase values has been reported.

Precautions

Since bromhexine may disrupt the gastric muscosal barrier it should be given cautiously to patients with gastric ulceration.

Absorption and Fate

Bromhexine hydrochloride is absorbed from the gastro-intestinal tract and is excreted in the urine mainly as metabolites. Ambroxol (p.904) is a metabolite of bromhexine.

In a study involving 10 healthy subjects bromhexine hydrochloride was absorbed from the gastro-intestinal tract, peak plasma concentrations occurring after about 1 hour. Only small amounts of the unchanged drug were excreted in the urine with a half-life of about 6.5 hours.— E. Bechgaard and A. Nielsen, *Biopharm. Drug Disposit.*, 1982, *3*, 337.

Uses and Administration

Bromhexine hydrochloride is a mucolytic agent used in the treatment of respiratory disorders associated with viscid mucus. The usual adult dose is 8 to 16 mg three or four times daily. Suggested dosage for children under 5 years is 4 mg twice daily, and for children aged 5 to 10 years, 4 mg four times daily.

It is also given by deep intramuscular or slow intravenous injection in doses of 8 to 24 mg daily; up to 20 mg in 500 mL of glucose injection or up to 40 mg in 500 mL of sodium chloride injection, may be given by slow intravenous infusion. It has also been used as the camsylate.

OTITIS MEDIA. In a study of 95 children with secretory otitis media, bromhexine 8 to 16 mg three times daily by mouth for 4 or 8 weeks was no more effective than placebo for the resolution of effusion. Five children being treated with bromhexine were withdrawn from the study because of rash, diarrhoea, or enuresis.— I. A. Stewart *et al.*, *Clin. Otolaryngol.*, 1985, *10*, 145.

USE WITH AN ANTIBIOTIC. Bromhexine was shown by Bergogne-Berezin *et al.* (*Therapie*, 1979, *34*, 705) in a preliminary study to enhance the penetration of erythromycin into bronchial secretions. In a study of 81 elderly patients with acute exacerbations of chronic bronchopulmonary diseases (F. Boraldi and B. Palmieri, *Curr. ther. Res.*, 1983, *33*, 686), 41 received cephalexin 1 g and bromhexine hydrochloride 8 mg both given by mouth three times daily for 10 days, and 40 received cephalexin only in the same dosage. Symptoms and ventilatory function were improved to a greater extent in the group treated with the antibiotic and mucolytic combination than with the antibiotic alone. Similar studies have shown a beneficial effect of treatment with a combination of cephalexin and bromhexine hydrochloride in post-surgical bronchial complications (G. Busca *et al.*, *Clin. Trials J.*, 1983, *20*, 115), acute and chronic bronchitis (R. Dattoli and A. Lechi, *ibid.*, 141), bronchopneumonia in children (M. Ramenghi and V. Angelozzi, *ibid.*, 177), and in women with lower respiratory tract infections (O. Ghidini and A. Tomba, *ibid.*, 248). However, in these studies the combination of cephalexin and bromhexine hydrochloride was not compared with cephalexin alone.

SJÖGREN'S SYNDROME. A group from Denmark (K. Frost-Larsen *et al.*, *Br. med. J.*, 1978, *1*, 1579; J.U. Prause *et al.*, *Acta Ophthalmol.*, 1984, *62*, 489) have shown that although bromhexine 16 mg three times daily by mouth for 2 and 3 weeks respectively appears to stimulate lachrymal secretion, as shown by objective ophthalmological tests, there was no subjective improvement in the feeling of dryness in the eyes; there was also no effect on dryness of the mouth. Tapper-Jones *et al.* (*Br. med. J.*, 1980, *280*, 1356) also found bromhexine 16 mg four times daily by mouth for 2 weeks no more effective than placebo. However, the results from both groups have been criticised in that not all the patients fulfilled the criteria for Sjögren's syndrome (I. Mackie and D.V. Seal, *Br. med. J.*, 1978, *2*, 638; R. Manthorpe *et al.*, *ibid.*, 1980, *281*, 1216).

Preparations

Bromhexine Tablets *(B.P.)*. Bromhexine Hydrochloride Tablets

Proprietary Names and Manufacturers

Aletor *(Spain)*; Auxit *(Heyden, Ger.)*; Bisolvon *(Boehringer Ingelheim, Austral.; Belg.; Boehringer Ingelheim, Denm.; Boehringer Ingelheim, Fr.; Thomae, Ger.; Boehringer Ingelheim, Ital.; Jpn; Lux.; Neth.; Boehringer Ingelheim, Norw.; Boehringer Ingelheim, S.Afr.; Fher, Spain; Boehringer Ingelheim, Swed.; Boehringer Ingelheim, Switz.; Boehringer Ingelheim, UK)*; Bromcilate *(Spain)*; Broncokin *(Geymonat, Ital.)*; Bronkese *(Lennon, S.Afr.)*; Dakryo *(Basotherm, Ger.)*; Ophtosol *(Winzer, Ger.)*; Viscolyt *(GEA, Denm.)*.

The following names have been used for multi-ingredient preparations containing bromhexine hydrochloride—Bisolvomycin *(Boehringer Ingelheim, UK)*.

5606-z

Butamyrate Citrate *(BANM).*
Abbott-36581; Butamirate Citrate *(USAN, rINNM)*; HH-197. 2-(2-Diethylaminoethoxy)ethyl 2-phenylbutyrate dihydrogen citrate.
$C_{18}H_{29}NO_3,C_6H_8O_7$=499.6.

CAS — 18109-80-3 (butamyrate); 18109-81-4 (citrate).

Butamyrate citrate is a cough suppressant stated to have a central action. It has been given by mouth in doses of 5 to 10 mg.

Proprietary Names and Manufacturers
Pertix *(Hommel, Ger.)*; Sincodix *(Beta, Arg.)*; Sinecod *(CCP, Belg.; Zyma, Ger.; Zyma, Ital.; Frumtost, Spain; Zyma, Switz.).*

12481-w

Butopiprine Hydrobromide *(rINNM).*
LD-2351. 2-Butoxyethyl α-phenyl-1-piperidineacetate hydrobromide.
$C_{19}H_{29}NO_3,HBr$=400.4.

CAS — 55837-15-5 (butopiprine); 60595-56-4 (hydrobromide).

Butopiprine hydrobromide has been used as a cough suppressant.

Proprietary Names and Manufacturers
Laucalon *(Castejon, Spain)*; Rutacel *(Promeco, Arg.).*

577-s

Carbocisteine *(BAN, rINN).*

AHR-3053; Carbocysteine *(USAN)*; LJ-206. *S*-Carboxymethyl-L-cysteine.
$C_5H_9NO_4S$=179.2.

CAS — 2387-59-9; 638-23-3 (L).

Carbocisteine is **incompatible** with Pholcodine Linctus, causing precipitation of carbocisteine from solution.

Adverse Effects

Nausea, headache, gastric discomfort, diarrhoea, gastro-intestinal bleeding, and skin rash have occasionally occurred with carbocisteine.

A report of transient hypothyroidism associated with the administration of carbocisteine in a patient with compromised thyroid function.— W. M. Wiersinga, *Br. med. J.*, 1986, *293*, 106.

Precautions

It is recommended that carbocisteine be used with caution in patients with a history of peptic ulcer and be avoided in patients with active ulceration.

Absorption and Fate

Carbocisteine is absorbed from the gastro-intestinal tract and excreted in the urine as unchanged drug and metabolites.

In a study of 200 healthy volunteers given a single dose of carbocisteine there was almost a 100-fold variation in the amount of sulphoxide metabolites detected in the urine. Family studies suggested that this may be due to a genetic effect.— S. C. Mitchell *et al.*, *Br. J. clin. Pharmac.*, 1984, *18*, 507.

Uses and Administration

Carbocisteine is used in the treatment of disorders of the respiratory tract associated with excessive mucus. It is given by mouth in a dose of 750 mg three times daily, reduced by one-third when a response is obtained. Children aged 2 to 5 years may be given 62.5 to 125 mg four times daily and those aged 6 to 12 years 250 mg three times daily.

In a study of 10 patients with gastro-intestinal phytobezoars, treatment of one patient with carbocisteine resulted in complete disappearance of the bezoar in 3 days.— C. M. Stein and M. Gelfand, *Trans. R. Soc. trop. Med. Hyg.*, 1985, *79*, 508.

BRONCHITIS. In a double-blind study involving 109 patients with chronic bronchitis, peak expiratory flow-rates improved to a greater extent in those patients given carbocisteine 750 mg by mouth three times daily for 6 months than in those given placebo. However, carbocisteine appeared to have no effect on the number of acute exacerbations.— M. Grillage and K. Barnard-Jones, *Br. J. clin. Pract.*, 1985, *39*, 395. Inconclusive effect on lung function tests and sputum viscosity in a similar study in 36 patients given carbocisteine for 6 weeks.— M. Aylward *et al.*, *Clin. Trials J.*, 1985, *22*, 36. See also R. Glosauer *et al.*, *Therapiewoche*, 1976, *26*, 6533.

OTITIS MEDIA. There have been several studies investigating the use of carbocisteine by mouth in secretory otitis media, however most of them have used small numbers of patients and the results have in general been inconclusive. Taylor and Dareshani (*Br. J. clin. Pract.*, 1975, *29*, 177), and McGuiness (*ibid.*, 1977, *31*, 105) found the response to carbocisteine to be favourable, however Ramsden *et al.* (*J. Lar. Otol.*, 1977, *91*, 847) found no evidence of efficacy.

A study *in vitro* of the effect of mucolytics on the rheological properties of mucus collected from patients with secretory otitis media. Although acetylcysteine produced a large decrease in viscosity of secretions, carbocisteine produced no such effect.— J. P. Pearson *et al.* (letter), *Lancet*, 1985, *2*, 674. Acetylcysteine is unlikely to achieve adequate concentrations in the ear to have this effect after oral administration. Studies are required to investigate the mucus secreted before and after oral administration of mucolytics.— C. Marriott (letter), *ibid.*, 1068. Reply that mucolytics could possibly be used topically for the treatment of blocked grommets.— J. P. Pearson *et al.* (letter), *ibid.*, 1300.

Proprietary Preparations

Mucodyne *(Berk Pharmaceuticals, UK). Capsules*, carbocisteine 375 mg.
Paediatric syrup, carbocisteine 125 mg/5 mL.
Syrup, carbocisteine 250 mg/5 mL.

Proprietary Names and Manufacturers

Anatac *(UCB, Spain)*; Betaphlem *(Be-Tabs, S.Afr.)*; Bronchathiol *(Martin, Fr.)*; Bronchette *(Continental Ethicals, S.Afr.)*; Bronchipect *(Neth.)*; Broncodeterge Simple *(Spain)*; Carbocit *(CT, Ital.)*; Corbar-M *(Vesta, S.Afr.)*; Flemex *(Parke, Davis, S.Afr.)*; Fluifort *(Dompè, Ital.)*; Lessmusec *(Beige, S.Afr.)*; Lisil *(Lenza, Ital.)*; Lisomucil *(Lirca, Ital.)*; Muciclar *(Substantia, Fr.)*; Mucocaps *(Fisons, S.Afr.)*; Mucocis *(Crosara, Ital.)*; Mucodyne *(Berk Pharmaceuticals, UK)*; Mucojet *(Polifarma, Ital.)*; Mucolase *(Lampugnani, Ital.)*; Mucolex *(Parke, Davis, UK)*; Mucolitic *(Arg.)*; Mucopront *(Mack, Illert., Ger.)*; Mucosirop *(Fisons, S.Afr.)*; Mucosol *(Tosi-Novara, Ital.)*; Mucospect *(Triomed, S.Afr.)*; Mucotreis *(Ecobi, Ital.)*; Pectox *(Nattermann, Ger.; Infar Nattermann, Spain; Degussa, Switz.)*; Pulmoclase *(UCB, Ger.)*; Reomucil *(Tosi, Ital.)*; Rhinathiol *(Synthelabo, Fr.; Neth.; Kramer-Synthelabo, Switz.)*; Rinatiol *(Difersa, Spain)*; Solfomucil *(Locatelli, Ital.)*; Solucis *(Magis, Ital.)*; Superthiol *(Crinos, Ital.)*; Transbronchin *(Degussa, Ger.)*; Visclair S *(Sinclair, UK)*; Viscoteina *(Iquinosa, Spain).*

5608-k

Chlophedianol Hydrochloride *(BANM, USAN).*
Clofedanol Hydrochloride *(rINNM)*; SL-501. 2-Chloro-α-(2-dimethylaminoethyl)-α-phenylbenzyl alcohol hydrochloride.
$C_{17}H_{20}ClNO,HCl$=326.3.

CAS — 791-35-5 (chlophedianol); 511-13-7 (hydrochloride).

Chlophedianol hydrochloride is a centrally-acting cough suppressant.

Proprietary Names and Manufacturers
Detigon *(Bayer, Arg.; Bayer, Ital.)*; Eletuss *(Serpero, Ital.)*; Eutus 24 *(IBIS, Ital.)*; Farmatox *(Ital.)*; Gentos *(Morgens, Spain)*; Pectolitan *(Kettelhack Riker, Ger.)*; Prontosed *(Francia Farm., Ital.)*; Tigonal *(IBP, Ital.)*; Tuxidin *(Ital.)*; Ulone *(Riker, Canad.)*; Ulotos *(Riker, Arg.).*

The following names have been used for multi-ingredient preparations containing chlophedianol hydrochloride— Quiactin *(Merrell Dow, Austral.).*

5609-a

Clobutinol Hydrochloride *(rINNM).*
KAT-256. 2-(4-Chlorobenzyl)-3-(dimethylaminomethyl)butan-2-ol hydrochloride.
$C_{14}H_{22}ClNO,HCl$=292.2.

CAS — 14860-49-2 (clobutinol); 1215-83-4 (hydrochloride).

Clobutinol hydrochloride is a centrally-acting cough suppressant given by mouth in doses of 40 to 80 mg three times daily; doses of 20 mg have been given by subcutaneous, intramuscular, or intravenous injection.

Proprietary Names and Manufacturers
Lomisat *(Boehringer Ingelheim, Spain)*; Silomat *(Boehringer, Arg.; Boehringer Ingelheim, Belg.; Boehringer Ingelheim, Denm.; Biothérax, Fr.; Thomae, Ger.; Boehringer Ingelheim, Ital.; Jpn; Boehringer Ingelheim, Norw.; Boehringer Ingelheim, S.Afr.; Boehringer Ingelheim, Swed.; Boehringer Sohn, Switz.).*

5610-e

Cloperastine Hydrochloride *(pINNM).*
1-[2-(4-Chlorobenzhydryloxy)ethyl]piperidine hydrochloride.
$C_{20}H_{24}ClNO,HCl$=366.3.

CAS — 3703-76-2 (cloperastine); 14984-68-0 (hydrochloride).

Cloperastine hydrochloride is a centrally-acting cough suppressant with some antihistaminic action. It is given by mouth in doses of 10 to 20 mg three times daily.
Cloperastine fendizoate ($C_{20}H_{24}ClNO,C_{20}H_{14}O_4$ = 648.2) is used similarly; 177 mg of cloperastine fendizoate is approximately equivalent to 100 mg of cloperastine hydrochloride.

Proprietary Names and Manufacturers
Hustazol *(Yoshitomi, Jpn)*; Nitossil *(Zyma, Ital.)*; Seki *(Simes, Ital.)*; Sekisan *(Farmasimes, Spain).*

2009-c

Cocillana *(BAN).*
Grape Bark; Guapi Bark; Huapi Bark.

CAS — 1398-77-2.

Pharmacopoeias. In *Br.* which also describes Powdered Cocillana.

The dried bark of *Guarea rusbyi* and closely related species (Meliaceae) containing not less than 3.5% of alcohol (60%)-soluble extractive.

Cocillana is used as an expectorant and, in large doses, as an emetic.

Preparations
Cocillana Liquid Extract *(B.P.C. 1973).* 1 in 1; prepared by percolation with alcohol (60%). *Dose.* 0.5 to 1 mL.

Proprietary Names and Manufacturers
The following names have been used for multi-ingredient preparations containing cocillana— Cosanyl *(Parke, Davis, Austral.).*

2010-s

Creosote
Creosote; Creosotal (carbonate); Wood Creosote.

CAS — 8021-39-4 (creosote); 8001-59-0 (carbonate).

Pharmacopoeias. In *Belg., Jpn, Pol., Port.*, and *Span.*. *Belg.* and *Port.* also include Creosote Carbonate.

A liquid consisting of a mixture of phenols obtained from wood tar. Commercial creosote used for timber preservation is obtained from coal tar.

Creosote possesses disinfectant properties and has been used as an expectorant. It has also been used as the carbonate.
Adverse effects are similar to those of Phenol, p.967.

5634-t

Dextromethorphan *(BAN, USAN, pINN).*

(+)-3-Methoxy-9a-methylmorphinan.
$C_{18}H_{25}NO$=271.4.

CAS — 125-71-3.

Pharmacopoeias. In *U.S.*

A practically white or slightly yellow odourless crystalline powder. Dextromethorphan 7.3 mg is approximately equivalent to 10 mg of dextromethorphan hydrobromide. Practically **insoluble** in water; freely soluble in chloroform. **Store** in airtight containers.

5613-j

Dextromethorphan Hydrobromide

(BANM, USAN, pINNM).

Dextromethorphani Hydrobromidum. Dextromethorphan hydrobromide monohydrate.
$C_{18}H_{25}NO,HBr,H_2O$=370.3.

CAS — 125-69-9 (anhydrous); 6700-34-1 (monohydrate).

Pharmacopoeias. In *Belg., Br., Braz., Eur., Fr., It., Jpn, Neth., Swiss,* and *U.S.*

A white or almost white crystalline powder, odourless or with a faint odour.

Soluble 1 in 60 to 65 of water and 1 in 10 of alcohol; freely soluble in chloroform with the separation of water; practically insoluble in ether. A 1% (*U.S.P.*) or 2% (*B.P.*) solution in water has a pH of 5.2 to 6.5. **Store** in airtight containers.

Adverse Effects

Adverse effects with dextromethorphan appear to be rare and may include dizziness and gastro-intestinal disturbances. Excitation, confusion, and respiratory depression may occur after overdosage. Dextromethorphan has been subject to abuse, but there does not appear to be any evidence of dependence of the morphine type.

ABUSE AND DEPENDENCE. Dextromethorphan was capable of producing very slight psychic dependence but not physical dependence of the morphine type.— Seventeenth Report of WHO Expert Committee on Drug Dependence, *Tech. Rep. Ser. Wld Hlth Org. No. 437,* 1970.

A report of the abuse of pure dextromethorphan hydrobromide powder by a 30-year-old man. Euphoria and restlessness occurred about 15 minutes after "snorting" the powder and lasted for up to 2 hours; this was then followed by depression, nausea, tiredness, and dizziness. The powder was used regularly 2 to 3 times daily for 2 to 3 months; sometimes he also smoked cannabis to enhance the effect. The patient experienced no particular symptoms after withdrawal but complained of a continued craving for the drug.— P. M. Fleming, *Br. med. J.*, 1986, *293*, 597. See also M. W. Orrell and P. G. Campbell (letter), *ibid.*, 1242.

OVERDOSAGE. For reports of overdosage of dextromethorphan hydrobromide in children and reversal of toxicity with intravenous naloxone see W. L. Shaul *et al.*, *Pediatrics*, 1977, *59*, 117; B. Katona and S. Wason, *New Engl. J. Med.*, 1986, *314*, 993.

INTERACTIONS. For a report of a possible interaction between dextromethorphan and phenelzine sulphate see under Phenelzine Sulphate p.379.

Absorption and Fate

Dextromethorphan is well absorbed from the gastro-intestinal tract. It is metabolised in the liver and excreted in the urine as unchanged dextromethorphan and demethylated metabolites including dextrorphan, which has some cough suppressant activity.

For evidence of a common genetic control of *O*-demethylation of dextromethorphan to dextrorphan, and debrisoquine hydroxylation, and the possible use of dextromethorphan in the phenotyping of oxidative drug metabolism see G. Pfaff *et al.*, *Int. J. Pharmaceut.*, 1983, *14*, 173; A. Küpfer *et al.* (letter), *Lancet*, 1984, *2*, 517; B. Schmid *et al.*, *Clin. Pharmac. Ther.*, 1985, *38*, 618; A. Küpfer *et al.*, *Xenobiotica*, 1986, *16*, 421.

Uses and Administration

Dextromethorphan hydrobromide is a cough suppressant which has a central action on the cough centre in the medulla. Although structurally related to morphine, dextromethorphan and other centrally-acting cough suppressants have no analgesic properties and in general they have little sedative activity.

Dextromethorphan hydrobromide is used for the relief of unproductive cough. It is reported to act within half an hour of administration by mouth and to exert an effect for up to 6 hours. It is given by mouth in doses of 10 to 30 mg every 4 to 8 hours to a usual maximum of 120 mg in 24 hours. Children aged 6 to 12 years may be given 5 to 15 mg every 4 to 8 hours to a maximum of 60 mg in 24 hours, and children aged 1 to 6 years 2.5 to 7.5 mg every 4 to 8 hours to a maximum of 30 mg in 24 hours.

Dextromethorphan polistirex (a dextromethorphan and sulphonated diethenylbenzene-ethenylbenzene copolymer complex) is also used. Dextrorphan, the *O*-demethylated metabolite of dextromethorphan also has cough suppressant properties, but does not have the analgesic properties of its isomer levorphanol, (see p.1307).

In a double-blind, crossover study of 16 patients with chronic stable cough, 2 doses of dextromethorphan hydrobromide or codeine phosphate 20 mg by mouth were given at night 4 hours apart. Both suppressed cough frequency and intensity to a greater extent than placebo as measured by a pressure transducer placed over the trachea. Dextromethorphan hydrobromide had a greater effect than codeine phosphate on cough intensity, but their effects on frequency were similar.— H. Matthys *et al.*, *J. int. med. Res.*, 1983, *11*, 92.

Preparations

Dextromethorphan Hydrobromide Syrup *(U.S.P.)*

Proprietary Preparations

Brontyl *(Reckitt & Colman Pharmaceuticals, UK). Capsules,* chewable, dextromethorphan hydrobromide 15 mg.

Cosylan *(Warner-Lambert, UK). Syrup,* dextromethorphan hydrobromide 13.5 mg/5 mL.

Paranorm *(Wallace Mfg Chem., UK). Paediatric syrup,* dextromethorphan hydrobromide 2.75 mg, ephedrine hydrochloride 2 mg, guaiphenesin 10 mg/5 mL.

Robitussin Cough Soother *(Robins, UK). Oral liquid,* dextromethorphan hydrobromide 7.5 mg/5 mL.

Robitussin Junior Cough Soother *(Robins, UK). Oral liquid,* dextromethorphan hydrobromide 3.75 mg/5 mL.

Tancolin *(Ashe, UK). Linctus,* dextromethorphan hydrobromide 2.62 mg, theophylline 15 mg, ascorbic acid 12.35 mg/5 mL.

Proprietary Names and Manufacturers of Dextromethorphan Salts

Akindex *(Fournier S.A., Fr.)*; Balminil D.M. *(Rougier, Canad.)*; Benylin DM *(Parke, Davis, USA)*; Bronchenolo Tosse *(Midy, Ital.)*; Broncho-Grippol-DM *(Charton, Canad.)*; Brontyl *(Reckitt & Colman Pharmaceuticals, UK)*; Calmerphan-L *(Siegfried, Switz.)*; Canfodion *(Gentili, Ital.)*; Congespirin Cough Syrup *(Bristol-Myers Products, USA)*; Cosylan *(Warner-Lambert, UK)*; Cremacoat 1 *(Richardson-Vicks, USA)*; Deca-Toux *(Canad.)*; Delsym *(Pennwalt, Canad.; McNeil Consumer, USA)*; Dexofan *(DAK, Denm.)*; Dextphan *(Jpn)*; DM Syrup *(Canad.)*; Extuson *(Leo, Swed.)*; Fluprim *(Roche, Ital.)*; Koffex *(Rougier, Canad.)*; Nodex *(Brothier, Fr.)*; Pectobron *(Arg.)*; Pediacare-1 *(McNeil Consumer, USA)*; Robidex *(Robins, Canad.)*; Robitussin Cough Soother *(Robins, UK)*; Romilar *(Arg.; Ital.; Roche, Spain)*; Sedatuss *(Trianon, Canad.)*; Sedotus *(Ital.)*; Tussidyl *(Tika, Swed.)*; Tussistop *(Ital.)*; Tussorphan *(Canad.)*; Valatux *(Farmacologico Milanese, Ital.)*.

The following names have been used for multi-ingredient preparations containing dextromethorphan salts—Actifed Compound Linctus *(Wellcome, UK)*; Actifed DM *(Wellcome, Canad.)*; Actifed-CC *(Wellcome, Austral.)*; Albatussin *(Bart, USA)*; Ambenyl-D *(Forest Pharmaceuticals, USA)*; Bayer Cough Syrup *(Glenbrook, USA)*; Benadryl Cold and Flu Tablets *(Parke, Davis, Austral.)*; Benafed *(Parke, Davis, UK)*; Benatuss *(Parke, Davis, Austral.)*; Benylin Fortified *(Warner-Lambert, UK)*; Benylin Mentholated *(Warner-Lambert, UK)*; Benylin-DM *(Parke, Davis, Canad.)*; Benylin-DM-D *(Parke, Davis, Canad.)*; Benylin-DME *(Parke, Davis, USA)*; Benyphed *(Parke, Davis, Austral.)*; Biohisdex DM *(Everest, Canad.)*; Biohisdine DM *(Everest, Canad.)*; Bromphen Expectorant *(Schein, USA)*; Cardec DM *(Schein, USA)*; Cepacol Cough and Sore Throat Lozenges *(Merrell Dow, Austral.)*; Cerose-DM *(Wyeth, USA)*; Chemhisdex-DM *(Clark, Canad.)*; Chemhisdine-DM *(Clark, Canad.)*; Chloraseptic DM *(Richardson-Vicks, Canad.)*; Codimal DM *(Central Pharmaceuticals, USA)*; Comtrex *(Bristol-Myers Products, USA)*; Coryban-D Cough Syrup *(Pfipharmecs, USA)*; Cotaminol *(Gen, Canad.)*; CoTylenol *(McNeil Consumer, USA)*; Cremacoat *(Richardson-Vicks, Canad.)*; Cremacoat 3 *(Richardson-Vicks, USA)*; Cremacoat 4 *(Richardson-Vicks, USA)*; Dexylets *(Parke, Davis, UK)*; Dimetane-DX *(Robins, USA)*; Dimetapp-DM *(Robins, Canad.)*; Dorcol *(Ancalab, Canad.)*; Dorcol Children's Cough Syrup *(Dorsey Laboratories, USA)*; Dorcol Paediatric *(Dorsey Laboratories, USA)*; Drixine Cough Suppressant *(Essex, Austral.)*; Guiatuss D-M *(Schein, USA)*; Histalet DM *(Reid-Rowell, USA)*; Lotussin *(Searle, UK)*; Muflin *(Concept Pharmaceuticals, UK)*; Naldecon-DX *(Bristol, USA)*; Neo-Diophen *(Hamilton, Austral.)*; Neo-Tuss *(Neolab, Canad.)*; Novahistex DM *(Dow, Canad.)*; Novahistine DM *(Dow, Canad.; Lakeside, USA)*; Nyquil *(Richardson-Vicks, Canad.)*; Ornade-DM *(Smith Kline & French, Canad.)*; Orthoxicol Cough Suppressant For Children *(Upjohn, Austral.)*; Orthoxicol Expectorant *(Upjohn, Austral.)*; Paranorm *(Wallace Mfg Chem., UK)*; Pediacare-3 *(McNeil Consumer, USA)*; Pharma-Col *(Rosken, Austral.)*; Phenergan with Dextromethorphan *(Wyeth, USA)*; Poly-Histine DM *(Bock, USA)*; Promatussin *(Wyeth, Canad.)*; Pulmorphan *(Riva, Canad.)*; Quelidrine *(Abbott, USA)*; Robitussin-CF *(Robins, Canad.; Robins, USA)*; Robitussin-DM *(Robins, Austral.; Robins, Canad.; Robins, USA)*; Rondec-DM *(Ross, USA)*; Ru-Tuss Expectorant *(Boots, USA)*; Scot-Tussin Cough & Cold *(Scot-Tussin, USA)*; Sigma Relief *(Sigma, Austral.)*; Sigma Relief Junior *(Sigma, Austral.)*; Sorbutuss *(Dalin, USA)*; Spec-T Orange *(Squibb, Canad.)*; Sudafed DM *(Wellcome, Canad.)*; Syrtussar *(Armour, UK)*; Tancolin *(Ashe, UK)*; Triaminic-DM *(Dorsey Laboratories, USA)*; Triaminic-DM Expectorant *(Ancalab, Canad.)*; Triaminicol *(Dorsey Laboratories, USA)*; Triaminicol DM *(Ancalab, Canad.)*; Triolix *(Drug Houses Austral., Austral.)*; Tusibron-DM *(Ram, USA)*; Tussafed *(Everett, USA)*; Tussar DM *(USV Pharmaceutical Corp., USA)*; Tusselix *(Key, Austral.)*; Tusselix Cough Silencers *(Key, Austral.)*; Tussi-Organidin DM *(Wallace, USA)*; Unitussin *(Unimed, UK)*; Vasofrinic Plus *(Trianon, Canad.)*; Vicks Formula 44 *(Richardson-Vicks, Canad.)*; Vicks Formula 44D *(Richardson-Vicks, Canad.)*.

5615-c

Dimemorfan Phosphate *(rINNM).*

AT-17. (+)-3,9a-Dimethylmorphinan phosphate.
$C_{18}H_{25}N,H_3PO_4$=353.4.

CAS — 36309-01-0 (dimemorfan); 36304-84-4 (phosphate).

Dimemorfan phosphate is a centrally-acting cough suppressant. It is given by mouth in doses of 10 to 20 mg.

Proprietary Names and Manufacturers

Astomin *(Yamanouchi, Jpn)*; Dastosin *(Morrith, Spain)*; Gentus *(Gentili, Ital.)*.

5616-k

Dimethoxanate Hydrochloride *(BANM, rINNM).*

2-(2-Dimethylaminoethoxy)ethyl phenothiazine-10-carboxylate hydrochloride.
$C_{19}H_{22}N_2O_3S,HCl$=394.9.

CAS — 477-93-0 (dimethoxanate); 518-63-8 (hydrochloride).

Dimethoxanate hydrochloride is a cough suppressant which is stated to have a central and some peripheral action. It is given by mouth in doses of 25 to 50 mg.

Proprietary Names and Manufacturers

Cothera *(Ayerst, Ital.; Inibsa, Spain)*; Cotrane *(Labaz, Belg.; Midyfarm, Fr.)*; Perlatos *(Farmacologico Milanese, Ital.)*; Tussizid *(Ital.)*.

12678-d

Domiodol *(USAN, pINN).*
MG-13608. 2-Iodomethyl-1,3-dioxolan-4-ylmethanol.
$C_5H_9IO_3$=244.0.

CAS — 61869-07-6.

Domiodol has been used for its mucolytic properties in the relief of respiratory disorders.

Proprietary Names and Manufacturers
Mucolitico *(Maggioni-Winthrop, Ital.).*

12680-k

Dropropizine *(BAN, rINN).*
UCB-1967. 3-(4-Phenylpiperazin-1-yl)propane-1,2-diol.
$C_{13}H_{20}N_2O_2$=236.3.

CAS — 17692-31-8.

Dropropizine is a cough suppressant reported to have a peripheral action. It is given by mouth in doses of 15 to 30 mg.

Proprietary Names and Manufacturers
Catabex *(Sarva, Belg.)*; Domutussina *(Medici Domus, Ital.)*; Ribex *(Formenti, Ital.)*; Tusofren *(Prodes, Spain).*

5617-a

Drotebanol *(BAN, rINN).*
Oxymethebanol. 3,4-Dimethoxy-9a-methylmorphinan-6β,14-diol.
$C_{19}H_{27}NO_4$=333.4.

CAS — 3176-03-2.

Drotebanol is an opioid, centrally-acting cough suppressant with actions similar to Morphine (see p.1310). It is given by mouth in doses of 2 mg three times daily. It has also been given subcutaneously or intramuscularly.

Proprietary Names and Manufacturers
Metebanyl *(Sankyo, Jpn).*

12696-h

Eprazinone Hydrochloride *(rINNM).*
CE-746. 3-[4-(β-Ethoxyphenethyl)piperazin-1-yl]-2-methylpropiophenone dihydrochloride.
$C_{24}H_{32}N_2O_2$,2HCl=453.5.

CAS — 10402-90-1 (eprazinone); 10402-53-6 (hydrochloride).

Eprazinone hydrochloride is a cough suppressant reported to have a peripheral action and also to have expectorant properties. It is given by mouth in doses of 50 to 100 mg three times daily.

Report of a skin eruption with subcorneal pustulation associated with the administration of eprazinone.— M. Faber *et al.*, *Hautarzt*, 1984, *35*, 200.

Proprietary Names and Manufacturers
Eftapan *(Merckle, Ger.)*; Mucitux *(Sanders-Probel, Belg.*; *Riom, Fr.*; *Recordati, Ital.*; *Liade, Spain)*; Resplene *(Chugai, Jpn).*

2012-e

Eriodictyon *(USAN).*
Mountain Balm; Yerba Santa.

CAS — 8013-08-9.

Pharmacopoeias. In *U.S.N.F.*

The dried leaves of *Eriodictyon californicum* (Hydrophyllaceae).

Eriodictyon has been used as an expectorant. It has also been used to mask the taste of bitter drugs.

Preparations

Aromatic Eriodictyon Syrup *(U.S.N.F.).* Eriodictyon fluidextract 3.2 mL, potassium hydroxide solution (1 in 20) 2.5 mL, compound cardamom tincture *U.S.N.F.* 6.5 mL, lemon oil 0.05 mL, clove oil 0.1 mL, alcohol 3.2 mL, sucrose 80 g, magnesium carbonate 500 mg, water to 100 mL. Store at a temperature not exceeding 40° in airtight containers. Protect from light.

Eriodictyon Fluidextract *(U.S.N.F.).* 1 in 1; prepared by percolation with a mixture of alcohol 4 vol. and water 1 vol. Store at a temperature not exceeding 40° in airtight containers. Protect from light.

5618-t

Ethyl Orthoformate
Ether de Kay; Triethoxymethane. Triethyl orthoformate.
$C_7H_{16}O_3$=148.2.

CAS — 122-51-0.

Pharmacopoeias. In *Fr.*

Ethyl orthoformate is a cough suppressant. It is reported to be a respiratory antispasmodic and is administered by mouth or rectally.

Proprietary Names and Manufacturers
Aethone *(Sopar, Belg.*; *Laboratoires Biologiques de l'Île-de-France, Fr.)*; Orthoformyl *(Belg.).*

5619-x

Fedrilate *(rINN).*
Fedrilatum; UCB-3928. 1-Methyl-3-morpholinopropyl perhydro-4-phenylpyran-4-carboxylate.
$C_{20}H_{29}NO_4$=347.5.

CAS — 23271-74-1.

Fedrilate is a cough suppressant which has been given by mouth as the maleate in doses of 50 mg three or four times daily.

Proprietary Names and Manufacturers
Corbar-S Linctus *(Vesta, S.Afr.)*; Tussapax *(Vesta, S.Afr.)*; Tussefan *(ICN, Neth.).*

5620-y

Fominoben Hydrochloride *(rINNM).*
PB-89. 3′-Chloro-2′-[*N*-methyl-*N*-(morpholinocarbonylmethyl)aminomethyl]benzanilide hydrochloride.
$C_{21}H_{24}ClN_3O_3$,HCl=438.4.

CAS — 18053-31-1 (fominoben); 24600-36-0 (hydrochloride).

Fominoben hydrochloride is a centrally-acting cough suppressant which is also reported to have respiratory stimulant properties. It is given in doses of 160 mg two or three times daily by mouth or 40 to 80 mg two or three times daily by slow intravenous injection.

ABSORPTION AND FATE. The biotransformation of fominoben hydrochloride.— A. Zimmer *et al.*, *Arzneimittel-Forsch.*, 1978, *28*, 688.

RESPIRATORY STIMULATION. The respiratory analeptic effect of fominoben hydrochloride after administration of pethidine and promethazine.— S. Völpel *et al.*, *Arzneimittel-Forsch.*, 1979, *29*, 334. Further studies on the respiratory effects of fominoben.— J. Scholtze, *ibid.*, 337; J. Patsch, *ibid.*, 340.

In a double-blind study of 60 patients with chronic obstructive lung disease, fominoben hydrochloride 160 mg three times daily be mouth for 15 days resulted in an increase in arterial oxygen pressure and a decrease in arterial carbon dioxide pressure. This effect was not observed with dextromethorphan hydrobromide and was considered to be due to a respiratory stimulant effect of fominoben.— T. Sasaki *et al.*, *J. int. med. Res.*, 1985, *13*, 96.

Proprietary Names and Manufacturers
Broncomenal *(Alacan, Spain)*; Finaten *(Finadiet, Arg.)*; Noleptan *(Thomae, Ger.)*; Tasadox *(Castejon, Spain)*; Terion *(Lusofarmaco, Ital.)*; Tosifar *(Aristegui, Spain)*; Tussirama *(Serpero, Ital.).*

19251-g

Glaucine
DL-832 (phosphate); *dl*-Glaucine; MDL-832 (phosphate). DL-1,2,9,10-Tetramethoxyaporphine.
$C_{21}H_{25}NO_4$=355.4.

CAS — 5630-11-5.

Glaucine is a centrally-acting cough suppressant under investigation. It has been used both as the phosphate and the hydrobromide.
D-Glaucine is an alkaloid obtained from *Glaucium flavum* (Papaveraceae) and has been used as a cough suppressant in Eastern Europe.

References: J. B. S. Redpath and B. J. Pleuvry, *Br. J. clin. Pharmac.*, 1982, *14*, 555; K. H. Rühle *et al.*, *ibid.*, 1984, *17*, 521; H. Gastpar *et al.*, *Curr. med. Res. Opinion*, 1984, *9*, 21.

Proprietary Names and Manufacturers of Glaucine or a Salt of Glaucine
Glauvent *(Pharmachim, Bulg.).*

2016-z

Guaiacol
Methyl Catechol.

CAS — 90-05-1 (guaiacol); 553-17-3 (guaiacol carbonate); 4112-89-4 (guaiacol phenylacetate).

Pharmacopoeias. In *Arg.*, *Fr.*, *Mex.*, *Port.*, *Roum.*, *Span.*, and *Swiss. Port.* and *Span.* also include Guaiacol Carbonate.

The main constituent of guaiacol is 2-methoxyphenol, $CH_3O.C_6H_4.OH$=124.1.

Guaiacol has disinfectant properties and has been used as an expectorant. It has also been used as the carbonate and the phenylacetate.
Adverse effects are similar to those of Phenol, p.967.

Results of a study in 8 healthy subjects and 20 patients with reflux oesophagitis indicating that guaiacol may prove useful in the treatment of this condition.— R. V. Heatley *et al.*, *Gut*, 1982, *23*, 1044.

Proprietary Preparations

Pulmo Bailly *(Bengué, UK). Oral liquid concentrate*, guaiacol 75 mg, codeine 7 mg, phosphoric acid 75 mg/5 mL.

Proprietary Names and Manufacturers of Guaiacol and its Salts
Gujaphenyl *(DDD, Ger.)*; Gunyl *(Galactina, Switz.).*
The following names have been used for multi-ingredient preparations containing guaiacol and its salts—Creo-Rectal *(Nadeau, Canad.)*; Dolodent *(Sabex, Canad.)*; Omni-Tuss *(Pennwalt, Canad.)*; Pulmo Bailly *(Bengué, UK).*

12803-l

Guaiapate *(USAN, rINN).*
MG-5454. 1-{2-[2-(2-*o*-Methoxyphenoxyethoxy)ethoxy]-ethyl}piperidine.
$C_{18}H_{29}NO_4$=323.4.

CAS — 852-42-6.

Guaiapate is reported to be a centrally-acting cough suppressant. It has been given by mouth in doses of 25 mg.

Proprietary Names and Manufacturers
Klamar *(Maggioni-Winthrop, Ital.).*

12795-v

Guaietolin *(rINN).*
Glycerylguethol; Glyguetol. 3-(2-Ethoxyphenoxy)propane-1,2-diol.
$C_{11}H_{16}O_4$=212.2.

CAS — 63834-83-3.

Guaietolin is an analogue of guaiphenesin which is used as an expectorant. It has been used in doses of 300 to 600 mg two to three times daily.

Proprietary Names and Manufacturers
Guéthural 300 *(Elerte, Fr.).*

2018-k

Guaiphenesin *(BAN).*

Glyceryl Guaiacolate; Glycerylguayacolum; Guaiacol Glycerol Ether; Guaiacyl Glyceryl Ether; Guaifenesin *(USAN, rINN)*; Guajacolum Glycerolatum. 3-(2-Methoxyphenoxy)propane-1,2-diol.

$C_{10}H_{14}O_4$=198.2.

CAS — 93-14-1.

Pharmacopoeias. In *Aust., Br., Cz., Jpn, Roum.,* and *U.S.*

White or slightly grey crystals or crystalline aggregates, odourless or with a slight characteristic odour.

B.P. **Solubilities** are: soluble 1 in 33 of water, 1 in 11 of alcohol and of chloroform; slightly soluble in ether; soluble 1 in 15 of glycerol with warming, and 1 in 15 of propylene glycol. *U.S.P.* has soluble 1 in 60 to 70 of water. A 1% (*U.S.P.*) or 2% (*B.P.*) solution in water has a pH of 5 to 7. **Store** in airtight containers.

Adverse Effects and Precautions

Gastro-intestinal discomfort has occasionally been reported. Very large doses cause nausea and vomiting. Guaiphenesin may interfere with diagnostic measurements of urinary 5-hydroxyindoleacetic acid or vanillylmandelic acid.

Ramsdell and Kelley (*Ann. intern. Med.*, 1973, *78*, 239) observed hypouricaemia (serum-urate concentrations of less than 20 μg per mL) in 6 patients who were being treated with guaiphenesin. Therapeutic doses for 3 days reduced serum urate by up to 30 μg per mL in 4 patients. In a study involving 10 healthy subjects, however, Matheson *et al.* (*Drug Intell. & clin. Pharm.*, 1982, *16*, 332) concluded that guaiphenesin 200, 400, or 600 mg given as a single dose or every 3 hours for up to 48 hours, does not decrease serum-urate concentrations to a statistically or clinically significant degree.

Absorption and Fate

Guaiphenesin is absorbed from the gastro-intestinal tract. It is metabolised and excreted in the urine.

Uses and Administration

Guaiphenesin is reported to reduce the viscosity of tenacious sputum and is used as an expectorant. It has been given by mouth in doses of 200 to 400 mg every 4 hours.

INFERTILITY. Results indicating that guaiphenesin may improve fertility, by increasing sperm motility through an effect on cervical mucus. In 10 women whose fertility problem seemed likely to be related to the cervical factor only, 8 conceived after treatment with guaiphenesin 200 mg three times daily by mouth given from day 5 of the cycle until a rise in temperature. Of 30 women who may have had other causes of infertility 8 also conceived.— J. H. Check *et al., Fert. Steril.*, 1982, *37*, 707.

RESPIRATORY DISEASE. While Yeates *et al.* (*Am. Rev. resp. Dis.*, 1977, *115*, *Suppl.* 4, 182) found guaiphenesin no better than placebo in aiding clearance of secretions from the lungs in 19 patients with chronic bronchitis, Robinson *et al.* (*Curr. ther. Res.*, 1977, *22*, 284) reported a sputum-thinning effect and reduced cough frequency and intensity in a study of 239 patients with dry or productive cough although sputum volume was increased only in patients with productive cough. In a double-blind study involving 65 patients (J.J. Kuhn *et al., Chest*, 1982, *82*, 713) the effect of guaiphenesin on cough frequency was no different to placebo when measured objectively. However, on subjective evaluation, guaiphenesin was associated with a decrease in sputum quantity and thickness. See also: *Drug & Ther. Bull.*, 1985, *23*, 63 and 86.

Preparations

Guaifenesin Capsules *(U.S.P.)*

Guaifenesin Syrup *(U.S.P.)*. A syrup containing guaiphenesin and alcohol 3 to 4%.

Guaifenesin Tablets *(U.S.P.)*

Proprietary Preparations

Noradran *(Norma, UK). Syrup*, guaiphenesin 25 mg, diphenhydramine hydrochloride 5 mg, diprophylline 50 mg, ephedrine hydrochloride 7.5 mg/5 mL.

Pholcomed Expectorant (formerly known as Pulmodrine Expectorant) *(Medo, UK). Syrup*, guaiphenesin 62.5 mg, methylephedrine hydrochloride 625 μg/5 mL.

Robitussin *(Robins, UK). Oral liquid*, guaiphenesin 100 mg/5 mL.

Robitussin Plus *(Robins, UK). Oral liquid*, guaiphenesin 100 mg, pseudoephedrine hydrochloride 30 mg/5 mL.

Proprietary Names and Manufacturers of Guaiphenesin or a related substance

2/G Expectorant *(Merrell Dow, USA)*; Anastil *(Eberth, Ger.)*; Balminil Expectorant *(Rougier, Canad.)*; Breonesin *(Winthrop-Breon, USA)*; Broncho-Grippex *(Canad.)*; Broncovanil *(Scharper, Ital.)*; Corutol Expectorant *(Canad.)*; Cremacoat 2 *(Richardson-Vicks, USA)*; Gaiapect *(Canad.)*; Globipen Balsamico Infantil *(Andromaco, Spain)*; Glycotuss *(Vale, USA)*; Glytuss *(Mayrand, USA)*; Guajasyl *(Mepha, Switz.)*; Guiatuss *(Schein, USA)*; Humibid *(Adams, USA)*; Hytuss *(Hyrex, USA)*; Idropulmina *(ISI, Ital.)*; Motussin *(Canad.)*; Myoscain 'E' *(Ger.)*; Reed's Croup Syrup *(Lagamed, S.Afr.)*; Reorganin *(Ger.)*; Resyl *(Belg.; Ciba-Geigy, Canad.; Ciba, Ital.; Spain; Ciba, Swed.; Ciba, Switz.)*; Robitussin *(Robins, Austral.; Robins, Canad.; Scheurich, Ger.; Ital.; Rovi, Spain; Robins, UK; Robins, USA)*; Scot-Tussin Expectorant *(Scot-Tussin, USA)*; Sedatuss Expectorant *(Canad.)*; S-T Expect *(USA)*; Tusibron *(Ram, USA)*; Tussanca *(Canad.)*.

The following names have been used for multi-ingredient preparations containing guaiphenesin or a related substance—Acet-Am *(Organon, Canad.)*; Actifed CC *(Wellcome, Austral.)*; Actifed Expectorant *(Wellcome, UK)*; Actifed-C *(Wellcome, USA)*; Adatuss *(Mastar, USA)*; Ambenyl-D *(Forest Pharmaceuticals, USA)*; Asbron *(Anca, Canad.)*; Asbron G *(Sandoz, USA)*; Benylin-DME *(Parke, Davis, USA)*; Brexin EX *(Savage, USA)*; Bricanyl Compound *(Astra, UK)*; Bricanyl Expectorant *(Astra, UK)*; Broncho-Grippol *(Charton, Canad.)*; Brondecon *(Parke, Davis, USA)*; Brondecon Expectorant *(Warner, Austral.)*; Bronkolixir *(Winthrop-Breon, USA)*; Bronkotabs *(Winthrop-Breon, USA)*; CAM Decongestant *(Rybar, UK)*; Chemhisdex-DHC-Expectorant *(Clark, Canad.)*; Chemhisdine-DHC-Expectorant *(Clark, Canad.)*; Cheracol *(Upjohn, Canad.)*; Choledyl Expectorant *(Parke, Davis, Canad.)*; CoActifed Expectorant *(Wellcome, Canad.)*; Codiclear DH *(Central Pharmaceuticals, USA)*; Codimal Expectorant *(Central Pharmaceuticals, USA)*; Cold War *(Key, Austral.)*; Conar-A *(Beecham Laboratories, USA)*; Conex *(Forest Pharmaceuticals, USA)*; Conex with Codeine *(Forest Pharmaceuticals, USA)*; Congess *(Fleming, USA)*; Congestac *(Menley & James, USA)*; Coryban-D Cough Syrup *(Pfipharmecs, USA)*; Cremacoat *(Richardson-Vicks, Canad.)*; Cremacoat 3 *(Richardson-Vicks, USA)*; Daribiol *(Cambridge Laboratories, Austral.)*; Deconsal *(Adams, USA)*; Deproist with Codeine *(Geneva, USA)*; Detussin Expectorant *(USA)*; Dilor-G *(Savage, USA)*; Dimetane Expectorant *(Robins, Canad.)*; Dimetane Expectorant-C *(Robins, Canad.)*; Dimetane Expectorant-DC *(Robins, Canad.)*; Dimotane Expectorant *(Robins, UK)*; Dimotane Expectorant DC *(Robins, UK)*; Donatussin DC *(Laser, USA)*; Donatussin Drops *(Laser, USA)*; Dorcol *(Ancalab, Canad.)*; Dorcol Children's Cough Syrup *(Dorsey Laboratories, USA)*; Dorcol Paediatric *(Dorsey Laboratories, USA)*; Drixine Cough Expectorant *(Essex, Austral.)*; Dura-Gest *(Dura, USA)*; Dura-Vent *(Dura, USA)*; Eclabron *(Wharton, USA)*; Elixophyllin-GG *(Forest Pharmaceuticals, USA)*; Emfaseem *(Saron, USA)*; Entair *(Duncan, Flockhart, UK)*; Entex *(Norwich Eaton, USA)*; Entex LA *(Norwich-Eaton, Canad.; Norwich Eaton, USA)*; Entuss Tablets *(Hauck, USA)*; Entuss-D *(Hauck, USA)*; Ex-Span *(Rotex, USA)*; Exyphen *(Norton, UK)*; Fedahist Expectorant *(Kremers-Urban, USA)*; Franol Expect *(Winthrop, UK)*; Guaifed *(Muro, USA)*; Guaifed-PD *(Muro, USA)*; Guiatuss A-C *(Schein, USA)*; Guiatuss D-M *(Schein, USA)*; Head & Chest *(Richardson-Vicks, USA)*; Histalet X *(Reid-Rowell, USA)*; Hycotuss *(Du Pont, USA)*; IDM-Expectorant *(Rougier, Canad.)*;
Kwelcof *(Ascher, USA)*; Linctifed *(Wellcome, UK)*; Lotussin *(Searle, UK)*; Lufyllin-GG *(Wallace, USA)*; Mudrane GG *(Poythress, USA)*; Mudrane GG-2 *(Poythress, USA)*; Mudrane GG Elixir *(Poythress, USA)*; Naldecon-CX *(Bristol, USA)*; Naldecon-DX *(Bristol, USA)*; Naldecon-EX *(Bristol, USA)*; Neo-Tuss *(Neolab, Canad.)*; Nethaprin Expectorant *(Merrell, UK)*; Nezcaam *(Rybar, UK)*; Noradran *(Norma, UK)*; Novahistex DH Expectorant *(Dow, Canad.)*; Novahistex DM Expectorant *(Dow, Canad.)*; Novahistex Expectorant *(Dow, Canad.)*; Novahistine DM Expectorant *(Dow, Canad.)*; Novahistine DMX *(Lakeside, USA)*; Novahistine Expectorant *(Lakeside, USA)*; Nucofed Expectorant *(Beecham Laboratories, USA)*; Ornade Expectorant *(Smith Kline & French, Canad.)*; Orthoxicol Expectorant *(Upjohn, Austral.)*; Oxycap *(Hyrex, USA)*; Paranorm *(Wallace Mfg Chem., UK)*; PEM *(Loveridge, UK)*; Phenephrin *(Nelson, Austral.)*; Pholcomed Expectorant *(Medo, UK)*; Poly-Histine Expectorant Plain *(Bock, USA)*; Promist LA *(Russ, USA)*; Pseudo-Bid *(Holloway, USA)*; Pseudo-Hist Expectorant *(Holloway, USA)*; Pulmodrine Expectorant *(Medo, UK)*; Pulmorphan *(Riva, Canad.)*; P-V-Tussin Tablets *(Reid-Provident, USA)*; Quiactin *(Merrell Dow, Austral.)*; Quibron *(Astra, Austral.; Bristol, USA)*; Quibron Plus *(Mead Johnson Laboratories, USA)*;
Respaire *(Laser, USA)*; Riddovydrin Elixir *(Riddell, UK)*; Robitussin A-C *(Robins, Canad.; Robins, USA)*; Robitussin AC *(Robins, UK)*; Robitussin Plus *(Robins, UK)*; Robitussin-CF *(Robins, Canad.; Robins, USA)*; Robitussin-DAC *(Robins, USA)*; Robitussin-DM *(Robins, Austral.; Robins, Canad.; Robins, USA)*; Robitussin-PE *(Robins, Canad.; Robins, USA)*; Robitussin-PS *(Robins, Austral.)*; Ru-Tuss Expectorant *(Boots, USA)*; Rymed *(Edwards, USA)*; Rymed-Jr. *(Edwards, USA)*; Rymed-TR *(Edwards, USA)*; Sigma Relief *(Sigma, Austral.)*; Sinufed *(Hauck, USA)*; Slo-phyllin GG *(Rorer, USA)*; Sorbutuss *(Dalin, USA)*; S-T Forte *(Scot-Tussin, USA)*; Sudafed Expectorant *(Wellcome, Canad.; Calmic, UK)*; Sudelix Junior *(Wellcome, Austral.)*; Synophylate-GG *(Central Pharmaceuticals, USA)*; Tedral Expectorant *(Warner, UK)*; Terpoin *(Hough, Hoseason, UK)*; Theolair-Plus *(Riker, USA)*; Thylline-GG *(Schein, USA)*; T-Moist *(T.E. Williams, USA)*; Totolin *(Galen, UK)*; Triafed-C *(Schein, USA)*; Triaminic Expectorant *(Ancalab, Canad.; Dorsey Laboratories, USA)*; Triaminic Expectorant DH *(Ancalab, Canad.)*; Triaminic Expectorant with Codeine *(Ancalab, Canad.)*; Triaminic-DM Expectorant *(Ancalab, Canad.)*; Trinex *(Mastar, USA)*; Tusibron-DM *(Ram, USA)*; Tussar *(USV Pharmaceutical Corp., USA)*; Tusselix *(Key, Austral.)*; Tussend Expectorant *(Merrell Dow, USA)*; Vasofrinic Plus *(Trianon, Canad.)*; Vicks Formula 44D *(Richardson-Vicks, Canad.)*; Zephrex *(Bock, USA)*; Zephrex-LA *(Bock, USA)*.

2020-e

Ipecacuanha *(BAN).*

Ipecac *(USAN)*; Ipecacuanha Root; Ipecacuanhae Radix.

CAS — 8012-96-2.

Pharmacopoeias. In *Arg., Aust., Belg., Br., Braz., Cz., Egypt., Eur., Fr., Ger., Hung., Int., It., Jpn, Jug., Mex., Neth., Nord., Pol., Port., Roum., Span., Swiss, Turk.,* and *U.S. Br.* also describes Powdered Ipecacuanha. Prepared Ipecacuanha is described in *Aust., Belg., Br., Eur.* (Ipecacuanhae Pulvis Normatus), *Fr., Ger., Int., It., Jpn, Mex., Neth., Turk.,* and *U.S.* (Powdered Ipecac).

The dried underground organs of *Cephaelis ipecacuanha* (= *Uragoga ipecacuanha*) (Rubiaceae), known in commerce as Matto Grosso ipecacuanha or of *C. acuminata*, (= *U. granatensis*), known in commerce as Costa Rica ipecacuanha, or of a mixture of both species. It contains not less than 2% of total alkaloids, calculated as emetine. *U.S.P.* specifies not less than 2% of ether-soluble alkaloids of which not less than 90% is emetine and cephaeline; the content of cephaeline is equal to, or not more than 2.5 times, that of emetine.

Prepared Ipecacuanha (*B.P.*) is finely powdered ipecacuanha adjusted with powdered ipecacuanha of lower alkaloidal strength or powdered lactose to contain 1.9 to 2.1% of total alkaloids, calculated as emetine. *U.S.P.* specifies 1.9 to 2.1% of ether-soluble alkaloids, with emetine and cephaeline content as for Ipecacuanha.

Store in airtight containers. Protect from light.

NOTE. The *B.P.* directs that when Ipecacuanha, Ipecacuanha Root, or Powdered Ipecacuanha is prescribed, Prepared Ipecacuanha shall be dispensed.

Adverse Effects

Large doses of ipecacuanha have an irritant effect on the gastro-intestinal tract, and persistent bloody vomiting or bloody diarrhoea may occur. Mucosal erosions of the entire gastrointestinal tract have been reported. The absorption of emetine, which is most likely if vomiting does not occur after the administration of emetic doses of ipecacuanha, may give rise to adverse effects on the heart, such as conduction abnormalities or myocardial infarction. These, combined with dehydration due to vomiting may cause vasomotor collapse followed by death.

There have been several reports of chronic abuse of ipecacuanha to induce vomiting in eating disorders; cardiotoxicity and myopathy have occurred and may be a result of accumulation of emetine.

There have also been several reports of ipecacuanha poisoning due to the unwitting substitution of ipecac fluidextract (*U.S.P. XVI*) for ipecac syrup (*U.S.P.*); the fluidextract was about 14 times the strength of the syrup.

ABUSE. In a review of bulimarexia and related eating disorders (R.T. Harris, *Ann. intern. Med.*, 1983, *99*, 800) attention was drawn to the abuse of ipecac syrup to induce vomiting. Adverse effects of repeated vomiting, such as metabolic complications, aspiration pneumonitis, parotid enlargement, dental abnormalities, oesophagitis or haematemesis due to mucosal lacerations, (the Mallory-Weiss syndrome) may be observed. Adler *et al.* (*J. Am. med. Ass.*, 1980, *243*, 1927) reported fatal cardiotoxicity in a patient who had ingested 90 to 120 mL of ipecac syrup daily for 3 months. Palmer and Guay (*New Engl. J. Med.*, 1985, *313*, 1457) reported the development of reversible myopathy in 2 patients; one had ingested ipecac syrup daily for 4 months, and less frequently previously, and the other had taken ipecac syrup at least twice a week for 4 years. Both patients also showed electrocardiogram abnormalities. These effects were considered to be due to the long-term accumulation of emetine, although Isner expressed doubt (*ibid.*, 1986, *314*, 1253). In a retrospective study of 100 patients with eating disorders by Pope *et al.* (*ibid.*, 245), symptomatic myopathy was reported in one patient who had ingested a total of 2000 doses but not in 3 patients who had ingested between 100 and 400 doses.

Treatment of Adverse Effects

After acute overdose of ipecacuanha, activated charcoal is given to delay absorption followed if necessary by gastric lavage. Prolonged vomiting can be controlled by the intramuscular injection of anti-emetics. Fluid and electrolyte imbalance should be corrected and facilities should be available to correct any cardiac effects and subsequent shock.

After the withdrawal of ipecacuanha following chronic abuse, recovery may be prolonged due to the slow elimination of emetine.

Precautions

Ipecacuanha should not be used as an emetic in patients whose condition increases the risk of aspiration or in patients who have taken substances, such as corrosive compounds, that might be especially dangerous if aspirated. Petroleum products are dangerous when aspirated, so those who consider it worthwhile using ipecacuanha in the management of such poisoning should give it with great care. Ipecacuanha should not be given to patients in shock or to those at risk from seizures either as a result of their condition or from the compound, such as strychnine, that has been ingested.

Its use should also be avoided in patients unlikely to respond to its emetic action, although it has successfully induced emesis in patients who have ingested anti-emetics. Patients with cardiovascular disorders are at risk if ipecacuanha is absorbed.

The action of ipecacuanha may be delayed or diminished if given with or after milk or charcoal.

Although MacLeod (*New Engl. J. Med.*, 1963, *268*, 146) reported the failure of ipecacuanha syrup to induce emesis after an overdose of pipamazine, a drug with a depressant action on the vomiting centre, 2 studies (M.E. Thoman and H.L. Verhulst, *J. Am. med. Ass.*, 1966, *196*, 147; A.S. Manoguerra and E.P. Krenzelok, *Am. J. Hosp. Pharm.*, 1978, *35*, 1360) have shown it to be as effective in inducing emesis after overdoses of anti-emetic drugs as after drugs without anti-emetic action. In a review of the management of ingestion of poisons Henry and Volans (*Br. med. J.*, 1984, *289*, 304) stated that although agents with anti-emetic effects are a theoretical contra-indication to the use of an emetic, few problems occur in practice, and emesis usually occurs satisfactorily.

Uses and Administration

Ipecacuanha is used as an expectorant in doses of 0.5 to 2 mg of total alkaloids represented by 0.025 to 0.1 mL of Ipecacuanha Liquid Extract (*B.P.*) or 0.4 to 1.4 mL of Ipecac Syrup (*U.S.P.*). It is also used in larger doses as an emetic for selected patients. Vomiting usually occurs within 30 minutes of administration by mouth of an emetic dose due to an irritant effect on the gastro-intestinal tract and a central action on the chemoreceptor trigger zone.

Doses are usually followed by a copious drink of water or fruit juice; in young children this may be given before the dose. Adults may be given doses of 21 to 42 mg of total alkaloids represented by 15 to 30 mL of Paediatric Ipecacuanha Emetic Mixture (*B.P.*) or of Ipecac Syrup (*U.S.P.*). Children aged 6 months to 1 year may be given 7 to 14 mg of total alkaloids, represented by 5 to 10 mL of Paediatric Ipecacuanha Emetic Mixture (*B.P.*) or of Ipecac Syrup (*U.S.P.*); older children may be given 21 mg, represented by 15 mL of Paediatric Ipecacuanha Emetic Mixture (*B.P.*) or of Ipecac Syrup (*U.S.P.*). Doses may be repeated once only after 20 to 30 minutes if emesis has not occurred.

Ipecacuanha is used in homoeopathic medicine.

EMESIS IN ACUTE POISONING. In a review of the management of drug overdosage and poisoning, gastric aspiration and lavage was considered to be the preferred method for removing unabsorbed drug or poison, but was recognised to be traumatic in young children. This had led to an increasing tendency to use emetics, ipecacuanha syrup [Ipecac Syrup *U.S.P.*, Ipecacuanha Syrup (Emetic) *A.P.F.*, or Paediatric Ipecacuanha Emetic Mixture *B.P.*] being the agent of choice. There is controversy over the relative efficacy of gastric lavage and induced emesis, however neither can be relied on to empty the stomach completely.— L. F. Prescott, *Br. med. J.*, 1983, *287*, 274. In a similar review ipecacuanha syrup was also considered to be the emetic of choice. Although originally advocated only in children it is equally effective in adults and, when correctly used, may be preferable to gastric lavage. The authors do not normally recommend its use outside hospital since it may occasionally produce prolonged vomiting, and there have been cases where parents have administered it inappropriately in a moment of panic, despite adequate instruction.— J. Henry and G. Volans, *ibid.*, 1984, *289*, 304. Like gastric lavage, ipecacuanha is sometimes thought to be ineffective more than 4 hours after ingestion of the poison, however lack of serious adverse effects from this treatment have led to its general acceptance up to 6 hours after ingestion.— *idem*, 486. Although ipecacuanha syrup is an efficient and rapidly acting emetic, there is no evidence that it prevents drug absorption or systemic toxicity. It only rarely produces serious adverse effects, but in large doses vomiting can be persistent. Ipecacuanha may also prevent the use of specific treatments such as methionine and charcoal. It was therefore considered that the use of ipecacuanha syrup in the management of poisoning should be reconsidered.— J. A. Vale *et al.*, *ibid.*, 1986, *293*, 1321. The basis for promoting emesis rests more on the occasional recovery of large quantities of drug than on verification of its efficacy in routine use.— G. Gordon (letter), *ibid.*, 1987, *294*, 247.

In a study of 24 306 cases of paediatric poisoning it was concluded that the risk of having ipecacuanha syrup in the home was outweighed by the saving in treatment time.— C. Chafee-Bahamon *et al.*, *Pediatrics*, 1985, *75*, 1105.

Preparations

Ipecac Syrup *(U.S.P.)*. Prepared by percolation from powdered ipecac *U.S.P.* 7 g, glycerol 10 mL, syrup to 100 mL. It contains 123 to 157 mg of ether-soluble alkaloids in each 100 mL.

Paediatric Ipecacuanha Emetic Mixture *(B.P.)*. Paediatric Ipecacuanha Emetic. Ipecacuanha liquid extract 0.7 mL, hydrochloric acid 0.025 mL, glycerol 1 mL, syrup to 10 mL.

Ipecacuanha Syrup (Emetic) *(A.P.F.)*. Ipecacuanha liquid extract 6 mL, dilute acetic acid 2.5 mL, glycerol 10 mL, syrup to 100 mL. *Dose*. 30 mL; children under 2 years, 15 mL; 2 to 3 years, 20 mL; 3 to 4 years, 25 mL.

Ammonia and Ipecacuanha Mixture *(B.P.)*. See p.905.

Paediatric Ipecacuanha and Ammonia Mixture *(B.P.C. 1973)*. Ipecacuanha tincture 0.1 mL, ammonium bicarbonate 30 mg, sodium bicarbonate 100 mg, tolu syrup 0.5 mL, double-strength chloroform water 2.5 mL, water to 5 mL. It should be recently prepared. *Dose*. Children, up to 1 year, 5 mL; 1 to 5 years, 10 mL.

Paediatric Ipecacuanha Mixture *(B.P.C. 1973)*. Ipecacuanha tincture 0.1 mL, sodium bicarbonate 100 mg, tolu syrup 1 mL, double-strength chloroform water 2.5 mL, water to 5 mL. It should be recently prepared. *Dose*. Children; up to 1 year, 5 mL; 1 to 5 years, 10 mL.

For a report of incompatibility when Paediatric Ipecacuanha Mixture was prepared with or diluted with syrup preserved with hydroxybenzoates, see under Sucrose, p.1276.

Ipecacuanha and Camphor Mixture CF *(A.P.F.)*. Expectorant Mixture for Children. Ipecacuanha tincture 0.1 mL, compound camphor spirit 0.25 mL, glycerol 1 mL, water to 5 mL. *Dose*. 5 mL.

Paediatric Ipecacuanha and Squill Linctus *(B.P.C. 1973)*. Ipecacuanha tincture 0.1 mL, squill tincture 0.15 mL, compound orange spirit 0.0075 mL, black currant syrup 2.5 mL, syrup to 5 mL. *Dose*. Children, 5 mL.

Ipecacuanha and Tolu Mixture *(A.P.F.)*. Cough Mixture. Ipecacuanha tincture 0.25 mL, compound camphor spirit 1 mL, tolu syrup 1 mL, concentrated chloroform water 0.15 mL or compound hydroxybenzoate solution 0.1 mL, concentrated anise water 0.15 mL, water to 10 mL. *Dose*. 10 mL.

Paediatric Opiate Ipecacuanha Mixture *(B.P.C. 1973)*. Ipecacuanha tincture 0.1 mL, camphorated opium tincture 0.15 mL, sodium bicarbonate 100 mg, tolu syrup 1 mL, double-strength chloroform water 2.5 mL, water to 5 mL. It should be recently prepared. *Dose*. Children, up to 1 year, 5 mL; 1 to 5 years, 10 mL.

For a report of incompatibility when Paediatric Opiate Ipecacuanha Mixture was prepared with or diluted with syrup preserved with hydroxybenzoates, see under Sucrose, p.1276.

Ipecacuanha Liquid Extract *(B.P.)*. Prepared by percolation with alcohol (80%) and adjusted to contain 1.9 to 2.1% w/v of total alkaloids calculated as emetine; about 2 mg in 0.1 mL.

Ipecacuanha Tincture *(B.P.)*. Ipecacuanha liquid extract 10 mL, dilute acetic acid 1.65 mL, alcohol (90%) 21 mL, glycerol 20 mL, water to 100 mL. It contains 0.19 to 0.21% w/v of total alkaloids, calculated as emetine; about 2 mg in 1 mL.

The *B.P.* directs that Ipecacuanha Tincture be dispensed when Ipecacuanha Wine is prescribed.

Ipecacuanha and Opium Powder *(B.P.C. 1973)*. Dover's Powder; Compound Ipecacuanha Powder. Prepared ipecacuanha 10 g, powdered opium 10 g, lactose 80 g. It contains 1% of anhydrous morphine; 6 mg in 600 mg. *Dose*. 300 to 600 mg.

Ipecacuanha and Opium Tablets *(B.P.C. 1973)*. Dover's Powder Tablets. Tablets containing ipecacuanha and opium powder. *Dose*. 300 to 600 mg.

Proprietary Names and Manufacturers

The following names have been used for multi-ingredient preparations containing ipecacuanha—Alophen *(Warner-Lambert, UK)*; Aperient Dellipsoids D9 *(Pilsworth, UK)*; Bronchial Dellipsoids D15 *(Pilsworth, UK)*; Dasin *(Beecham Laboratories, USA)*; Linituss *(Ayrton, Saunders, UK)*; Neo-Pectol *(Neolab, Canad.)*; Pectomed *(Medo, UK)*; Phenergan Compound Expectorant *(May & Baker, UK)*; Phenergan Expectorant *(May & Baker, Austral.)*; Quelidrine *(Abbott, USA)*; Terra-Bron *(Pfizer, UK)*; Tussifans *(Norton, UK)*; Unitussin *(Unimed, UK)*.

5622-z

Isoaminile Citrate *(BANM, rINNM).*
4-Dimethylamino-2-isopropyl-2-phenylvaleronitrile dihydrogen citrate.
$C_{16}H_{24}N_2,C_6H_8O_7$=436.5.

CAS — 77-51-0 (isoaminile); 126-10-3; 28416-66-2 (both citrate).

Isoaminile citrate is a cough suppressant which has actions and uses similar to Dextromethorphan Hydrobromide (see p.908). It is given by mouth in a dose of 40 mg three to five times daily. It has also been given as the cyclamate.

Isoaminile citrate was responsible for a fixed drug eruption in 1 patient.— J. A. Savin, *Br. J. Derm.*, 1970, *83*, 546.

Proprietary Preparations

Dimyril *(Fisons, UK). Linctus,* isoaminile citrate 40 mg/5 mL.

Proprietary Names and Manufacturers of Isoaminile and its Salts

Dimyril *(Fisons, UK)*; Peracan *(Belg.)*; Peracon *(Arg.; Denm.; Kali-Chemie, Ger.; Ital.; Neth.; Norw.; Ethimed, S.Afr.; Swed.; Switz.)*; Perogan *(Spain)*; Sedotosse *(Panthox & Burck, Ital.)*.

12893-q

Letosteine *(pINN).*
2-[2-(Ethoxycarbonylmethylthio)ethyl]thiazolidine-4-carboxylic acid.
$C_{10}H_{17}NO_4S_2$=279.4.

CAS — 53943-88-7.

Letosteine is a mucolytic agent which has been used in the treatment of respiratory disorders in a dose of 50 mg by mouth three times daily. Gastro-intestinal adverse effects have been reported.

Proprietary Names and Manufacturers

Letoclar *(Zyma, Ital.)*; Letofort *(Salus, Ital.)*; Soluidal *(Frumtost, Spain)*; Viscotiol *(Farmitalia Carlo Erba, Fr.; Searle, Ital.)*.

5623-c

Levopropoxyphene Napsylate *(BANM, USAN).*
Levopropoxyphene Napsilate *(rINNM)*. (−)-1-Benzyl-3-dimethylamino-2-methyl-1-phenylpropyl propionate naphthalene-2-sulphonate monohydrate.
$C_{22}H_{29}NO_2,C_{10}H_8O_3S,H_2O$=565.7.

CAS — 2338-37-6 (levopropoxyphene); 5714-90-9 (napsylate, anhydrous); 55557-30-7 (napsylate, monohydrate).

Pharmacopoeias. In *U.S.*

A white almost odourless powder. Levopropoxyphene napsylate 1.67 g is approximately equivalent to 1 g of levopropoxyphene. Very slightly **soluble** in water; soluble 1 in 17 of alcohol and 1 in 2 of chloroform; soluble in acetone and methyl alcohol. **Store** in airtight containers.

Levopropoxyphene napsylate, an isomer of dextropropoxyphene, is a centrally-acting cough suppressant. It has actions and uses similar to Dextromethorphan Hydrobromide (see p.908). It is given by mouth in doses of 50 to 100 mg. It has also been given as the dibudinate.

Preparations

Levopropoxyphene Napsylate Capsules *(U.S.P.)*

Levopropoxyphene Napsylate Oral Suspension *(U.S.P.)*. Avoid freezing. Protect from light.

Proprietary Names and Manufacturers

Novrad *(Lilly, USA)*; Sotorni *(Ravensberg, Ger.)*.

607-f

Methyl Cysteine Hydrochloride *(BANM).*

Mecysteine Hydrochloride *(rINNM)*; Methylcysteine Hydrochloride. Methyl L-2-amino-3-mercaptopropionate hydrochloride.
$C_4H_9NO_2S,HCl$=171.6.

CAS — 2485-62-3 (methyl cysteine); 18598-63-5 (hydrochloride).

Adverse Effects

Nausea and heartburn have occasionally been reported.

Uses and Administration

Methyl cysteine hydrochloride is used similarly to acetylcysteine in the treatment of disorders of the respiratory tract associated with excessive mucus. It is given by mouth in a dose of 100 to 200 mg three to four times daily. Children over 5 years of age may be given 100 mg three times daily. It has also been administered by inhalation.

In 2 double-blind studies in patients with chronic bronchitis (K.N.V. Palmer *et al.*, *Br. med. J.*, 1962, *1*, 280; M. Aylward *et al.*, *Curr. med. Res. Opinion*, 1978, *5*, 461), methyl cysteine hydrochloride given by mouth for 4 and 6 weeks respectively reduced symptoms of cough and had a beneficial effect on sputum. In a double-blind crossover study of 26 patients with a range of respiratory disorders (J.N. Sahay *et al.*, *Clin. Trials J.*, 1982, *19*, 137), there was a general reduction in sputum production, but a variable effect on symptoms and lung function after treatment with methyl cysteine hydrochloride 200 mg by mouth 4 times daily for 4 weeks.

A good clinical response was seen in only 2 of 15 patients with rheumatoid arthritis treated with methyl cysteine by mouth.— F. McKenna *et al.* (letter), *Br. J. Rheumatol.*, 1986, *25*, 132.

Proprietary Preparations

Visclair *(Sinclair, UK). Tablets,* enteric-coated, methyl cysteine hydrochloride 100 mg.

Proprietary Names and Manufacturers

Acthiol J *(Fr.; Switz.)*; Actiol *(SIT, Ital.)*; Actithiol *(Funk, Spain)*; Daiace *(Jpn)*; Ethitanin *(Jpn)*; Visclair *(Sinclair, UK)*.

5624-k

Morclofone Hydrochloride *(rINNM).*
Dimeclofenone Hydrochloride. 4′-Chloro-3,5-dimethoxy-4-(2-morpholinoethoxy)benzophenone hydrochloride.
$C_{21}H_{24}ClNO_5,HCl$=442.3.

CAS — 31848-01-8 (morclofone); 31848-02-9 (hydrochloride).

Morclofone hydrochloride is a centrally-acting cough suppressant given by mouth in doses of 100 mg four to six times daily.

Proprietary Names and Manufacturers

Medicil *(Medici, Ital.)*; Nitux *(Inpharzam, Switz.)*; Plausitin *(Montedison, Arg.; Carlo Erba, Ital.)*.

5625-a

Noscapine *(BAN, USAN, rINN).*

Narcotine; Noscapinum; L-α-Narcotine. (3*S*)-6,7-Dimethoxy-3-[(5*R*)-5,6,7,8-tetrahydro-4-methoxy-6-methyl-1,3-dioxolo[4,5-*g*]isoquinolin-5-yl]-phthalide.
$C_{22}H_{23}NO_7$=413.4.

CAS — 128-62-1.

NOTE. The name Camphoscapine has been used for noscapine camsylate.

Pharmacopoeias. In *Aust., Br., Egypt., Eur., Fr., Ger., Ind., Int., It., Jpn, Neth., Swiss, Turk.,* and *U.S.*

Noscapine is an alkaloid obtained from opium. It occurs as colourless crystals or as a fine white or practically white crystalline powder.
Practically **insoluble** in water at 20°, very slightly soluble at 100°; slightly soluble in alcohol and ether; soluble in acetone and chloroform; soluble in strong acids although the base may be precipitated on dilution with water. **Store** in well-closed containers. Protect from light.

5626-t

Noscapine Hydrochloride *(BANM, rINNM).*

Narcotine Hydrochloride; Noscapini Hydrochloridum; Noscapinium Chloride.
$C_{22}H_{23}NO_7,HCl,H_2O$=467.9.

CAS — 912-60-7 (anhydrous).

Pharmacopoeias. In *Aust., Br., Eur., Ger., It., Jug., Neth., Nord.,* and *Swiss* (all with H_2O); *Hung.* (with $2H_2O$); *Fr.* and *Jpn* (both with xH_2O).

Colourless crystals or a white crystalline powder; hygroscopic.
Freely **soluble** in water, alcohol, chloroform; practically insoluble in ether. A 2% solution in water has a pH not below 3.0. Aqueous solutions may deposit the base on standing.
Store in well-closed containers. Protect from light.

Noscapine is a centrally-acting cough suppressant that has actions and uses similar to Dextromethorphan Hydrobromide (see p.908). It is given by mouth in a dose of 15 to 30 mg every 4 to 6 hours. Children aged 6 to 12 years may be given half the adult dose, and those aged 2 to 6 years a quarter of the adult dose. It has also been given as the embonate and the camsylate.

Preparations of Noscapine and its Salts

Noscapine Linctus *(B.P.)*. Contains noscapine 0.3% and citric acid monohydrate 1%. Store at a temperature not exceeding 25°.

For a report of incompatibility when Noscapine Linctus was prepared with or diluted with syrup preserved with hydroxybenzoates, see under Sucrose, p.1276.

Proprietary Names and Manufacturers of Noscapine and its Salts

Bequitusin *(Spain)*; Capval *(Dreluso, Ger.)*; Coscopin *(Duncan, Flockhart, UK)*; Dru Tosse *(Ital.)*; Finipect *(Neth.)*; Longactin *(Dumex, Norw.)*; Longatin *(Dumex, Denm.; Dumex, Swed.)*; Lyobex retard *(Lappe, Ger.)*; Narcotos *(Searle, Arg.)*; Narcotussin *(Biologici Italia, Ital.)*; Nipaxon *(Mekos, Swed.)*; Nitepax *(MPS Lab., S.Afr.)*; Noscapect *(Belg.; Roter, Neth.)*; Noscatuss *(Fisons, Canad.)*; Rode Hoestsiroop *(Neth.)*; Tucotine *(Sanders-Probel, Belg.)*; Tulisan *(Logeais, Fr.)*; Tusscapine *(Fisons, USA)*; Tussicare *(Belg.)*; Tussinil *(Pental, Spain)*.

The following names have been used for multi-ingredient preparations containing noscapine and its salts—Conar-A *(Beecham Laboratories, USA)*; Extil Compound *(Evans Medical, UK)*; Theonar *(MCP Pharmaceuticals, UK)*.

NOTE. The *UK* preparation Triotussic had been reformulated to exclude noscapine hydrochloride prior to its withdrawal from the market.

5627-x

Oxeladin Citrate *(BANM, rINNM).*
2-(2-Diethylaminoethoxy)ethyl 2-ethyl-2-phenylbutyrate dihydrogen citrate.
$C_{20}H_{33}NO_3,C_6H_8O_7$=527.6.

CAS — 468-61-1 (oxeladin); 52432-72-1 (citrate).

Oxeladin citrate is a centrally-acting cough suppressant.

Proprietary Names and Manufacturers

Antusel *(Arg.)*; Dorex *(Woelm, Ger.)*; Frenotos *(Disprovent, Arg.)*; Neobex *(Lampugnani, Ital.)*; Paxeladine *(Beaufour, Belg.; Beaufour, Fr.)*; Pectamol *(Malesci, Ital.; Apothekernes Laboratorium, Norw.)*; Pectamon *(Hässle, Swed.)*; Tussilisin *(Ibirn, Ital.)*; Tussilong *(Restan, S.Afr.)*.

13067-b

Oxolamine Citrate *(rINNM).*
683M; AF-438; SKF-9976. 2-(3-Phenyl-1,2,4-oxadiazol-5-yl)triethylamine citrate.
$C_{14}H_{19}N_3O,C_6H_8O_7$=437.4.

CAS — 959-14-8 (oxolamine); 1949-20-8 (citrate).

Oxolamine citrate is a cough suppressant with a predominantly peripheral action, given by mouth in doses of 100 to 200 mg. It is also given as the phosphate.
Hallucinations in children have been reported after its use.

Proprietary Names and Manufacturers of Oxolamine Citrate and Phosphate
Bentox *(Ital.)*; Bredon *(Organon, Austral.; Organon, Belg.; Organon, Denm.; Organon, Neth.)*; Broncatar *(Pulitzer, Ital.)*; Encelad *(Ital.)*; Flogobron *(Fisons, Ital.)*; Oxolev *(Giusto, Ital.)*; Perebron *(Angelini, Ital.; Farma-Lepori, Spain)*; Tussibron *(Sella, Ital.)*.

5607-c

Pentoxyverine Citrate *(rINNM).*
Carbetapentane Citrate; UCB-2543. 2-(2-Diethylaminoethoxy)ethyl 1-phenylcyclopentane-1-carboxylate dihydrogen citrate.
$C_{20}H_{31}NO_3,C_6H_8O_7$=525.6.

CAS — 77-23-6 (pentoxyverine); 23142-01-0 (citrate).

Pharmacopoeias. In *Chin.*

Pentoxyverine citrate is a cough suppressant. It is given by mouth in doses of 25 to 50 mg. The hydrochloride and the tannate are also used.

Proprietary Names and Manufacturers of Pentoxyverine Salts
Atussil *(Delagrange, Fr.)*; Germapect *(UCB, Ger.)*; Sedotussin *(UCB, Ger.)*; Toclase *(UCB, Arg.; UCB, Denm.; UCB, Norw.; UCB, Swed.)*; Tuclase *(UCB, Belg.; UCB, Ital.; UCB, Neth.)*; Tussa-Tablinen *(Beiersdorf, Ger.)*.

The following names have been used for multi-ingredient preparations containing pentoxyverine salts— Rynatuss *(Wallace, USA)*; Tussar *(USV Pharmaceutical Corp., USA)*.

5602-e

Pholcodine *(BAN, rINN).*
Pholcodinum. 3-*O*-(2-Morpholinoethyl)morphine monohydrate.
$C_{23}H_{30}N_2O_4,H_2O$=416.5.

CAS — 509-67-1 (anhydrous).

Pharmacopoeias. In *Aust., Br., Egypt., Eur., Fr., Ger., Ind., Int., It., Jug., Neth.,* and *Swiss.*

Colourless crystals or a white or almost white crystalline powder.
Soluble 1 in 50 of water; freely soluble in alcohol and acetone; very soluble in chloroform; slightly soluble in ether; dissolves in dilute mineral acids.
Store in well-closed containers.

Pholcodine is a centrally-acting cough suppressant that has actions and uses similar to Dextromethorphan Hydrobromide, p.908. It is administered by mouth in a dose of 5 to 10 mg three or four times daily; children over 2 years of age may be given 5 mg four times daily and children under 2 years, 1 to 2.5 mg also four times daily. The tartrate and the citrate have also been used.

A comparative study of the pharmacokinetics of pholcodine and codeine in healthy subjects.— J. W. A. Findlay *et al., Br. J. clin. Pharmac.,* 1986, *22,* 61.

Preparations

Pholcodine Linctus *(A.P.F.).* Pholcodine 5 mg, citric acid monohydrate 50 mg, concentrated chloroform water 0.15 mL or methyl hydroxybenzoate solution 0.05 mL, glycerol 1.5 mL, water to 5 mL.

Pholcodine Linctus CF *(A.P.F.).* Pholcodine 2.5 mg, citric acid monohydrate 25 mg, concentrated chloroform water 0.1 mL or compound hydroxybenzoate solution 0.05 mL, glycerol 2 mL, water to 5 mL.

Pholcodine Linctus *(B.P.).* Contains pholcodine 0.1% and citric acid monohydrate 1%. Protect from light.

Strong Pholcodine Linctus *(B.P.).* Contains pholcodine 0.2% and citric acid monohydrate 2%. Protect from light.

Proprietary Preparations

Copholco *(Rorer, UK). Linctus,* pholcodine 5.63 mg, terpin hydrate 2.82 mg, menthol 1.41 mg, cineole 0.0026 mL/5 mL.

Copholcoids *(Rorer, UK). Pastilles,* pholcodine 4 mg, terpin hydrate 16 mg, menthol 2 mg, cineole 0.004 mL.

Dia-Tuss *(Lipha, UK). Oral liquid,* pholcodine 10 mg/5 mL.

Expulin *(Galen, UK). Linctus,* pholcodine 5 mg, pseudoephedrine hydrochloride 15 mg, chlorpheniramine maleate 2 mg, menthol 1.1 mg/5 mL.
Paediatric linctus, pholcodine 2 mg, chlorpheniramine maleate 1 mg, menthol 1.1 mg/5 mL.

Galenphol (formerly known as Galphol) *(Galen, UK). Linctus,* pholcodine 5 mg/5 mL.
Linctus, strong, pholcodine 10 mg/5 mL.
Paediatric linctus, pholcodine 2 mg/5 mL.

Pavacol-D *(Boehringer Ingelheim, UK). Mixture,* pholcodine 5 mg/5mL.

PEM *(Loveridge, UK). Linctus,* pholcodine 5 mg, ephedrine hydrochloride 10 mg, guaiphenesin 12.5 mg, menthol 1.25 mg/5 mL.

Pholcomed *(Medo, UK). Linctus,* pholcodine 5 mg, papaverine hydrochloride 1.25 mg/5 mL.
Pastilles, pholcodine 4 mg, papaverine hydrochloride 1 mg.

Pholcomed D (formerly known as Pholcomed Diabetic) *(Medo, UK). Diabetic linctus,* pholcodine 5 mg, papaverine hydrochloride 1.25 mg/5 mL.

Pholcomed Forte *(Medo, UK). Linctus* or *Diabetic linctus,* pholcodine 19 mg, papaverine hydrochloride 5 mg/5 mL.

Pholtex *(Riker, UK). Mixture,* pholcodine 15 mg, phenyltoloxamine 10 mg/5 mL.

Triolinctus *(Sandoz, UK). Syrup,* pholcodine 5 mg, pseudoephedrine hydrochloride 20 mg, chlorpheniramine maleate 2 mg/5 mL.

Proprietary Names and Manufacturers of Pholcodine and its Salts
Actuss *(Sigma, Austral.)*; Adaphol *(Nelson, Austral.)*; Cherry Bark Linctus *(Loveridge, UK)*; Codisol *(Denm.)*; Dia-Tuss *(Lipha, UK)*; Duro-Tuss *(Riker, Austral.)*; Galenphol *(Galen, UK)*; Galphol *(Galen, UK)*; Homocodeina Jarabe *(Boizot, Spain)*; Lantuss *(Austral.)*; Linctus Tussinol *(G.P. Laboratories, Austral.)*; Pavacol-D *(Boehringer Ingelheim, UK)*; Pectolin *(Faulding, Austral.)*; Pholcolin *(Drug Houses Austral., Austral.)*; Pholcolin Red *(Drug Houses Austral., Austral.)*; Pholtrate *(McGloin, Austral.)*; Pholtussin *(Austral.)*; Sancos *(Sandoz, UK)*; Sedlingtus *(Faulding, Austral.)*; Triopaed *(Sandoz, UK)*; Tussinol *(Austral.)*; Tussokon *(Pharmacia, Swed.)*; Tuxi *(Weiders, Norw.)*.

The following names have been used for multi-ingredient preparations containing pholcodine and its salts—Cold War *(Key, Austral.)*; Copholco *(Rorer, UK)*; Copholcoids *(Rorer, UK)*; Davenol *(Wyeth, UK)*; Expulin *(Galen, UK)*; Falcodyl *(Norton, UK)*; PEM *(Loveridge, UK)*; Phensedyl Linctus *(May & Baker, Austral.)*; Pholcolix *(Parke, Davis, UK)*; Pholcomed *(Medo, UK)*; Pholdrine *(Austral.)*; Pholtex *(Riker, UK)*; Rinurel *(Warner, UK)*; Rubelix *(Pharmax, UK)*; Sancos Co *(Sandoz, UK)*; Tixylix *(May & Baker, Austral.; May & Baker, UK)*; Triocos *(Sandoz, UK)*; Triolinctus *(Sandoz, UK)*; Valledrine *(May & Baker, Austral.; May & Baker, UK)*.

NOTE. The name Pavacol-D was formerly used to denote a preparation containing, in addition to pholcodine, papaverine hydrochloride.

5629-f

Pipazethate Hydrochloride *(BANM).*
Pipazetate Hydrochloride *(rINNM)*; Piperestazine Hydrochloride. 2-(2-Piperidinoethoxy)ethyl pyrido[3,2-*b*][1,4]benzothiazine-10-carboxylate hydrochloride.
$C_{21}H_{25}N_3O_3S,HCl$=436.0.

CAS — 2167-85-3 (pipazethate); 6056-11-7 (hydrochloride).

NOTE. Pipazethate is *USAN.*

Pipazethate hydrochloride is a cough suppressant which is stated to have a central and some peripheral action. It is given by mouth in doses of 20 to 40 mg up to three times daily.

A healthy 4-year-old child became somnolent and agitated, with convulsions, followed by coma, after swallowing an unknown number of tablets containing pipazethate; cardiac arrhythmias also developed.— O. A. da Silva and M. Lopez, *Clin. Toxicol.,* 1977, *11,* 455.

Proprietary Names and Manufacturers
Lenopect *(Draco, Swed.)*; Selvigon *(Homburg, Ger.; Smith Kline & French, UK)*; Selvjgon *(Rorer, Ital.)*; Toraxan *(Unifa, Arg.)*.

5630-z

Piperidione
NU-1510. 3,3-Diethylpiperidine-2,4-dione.
$C_9H_{15}NO_2$=169.2.

CAS — 77-03-2.

Piperidione is a centrally-acting cough suppressant with sedative properties.

Proprietary Names and Manufacturers
Sedulon *(Roche, Swed.)*.

2022-y

Potassium Guaiacolsulfonate *(USAN).*
Kalium Guajacolsulfonicum; Potassium Guaiacolsulphonate; Sulfogaiacol *(rINN)*. Potassium hydroxymethoxybenzenesulphonate hemihydrate.
$C_7H_7KO_5S,\frac{1}{2}H_2O$=251.3.

CAS — 1321-14-8 (anhydrous); 78247-49-1 (hemihydrate).

Pharmacopoeias. In *U.S.* Also in *Aust., Belg., Fr., Jpn, Neth., Pol., Port., Roum.,* and *Span.* none of which specify hemihydrate.

Potassium guaiacolsulfonate should be **protected** from light.

Potassium guaiacolsulfonate is used as an expectorant; it is given by mouth in doses of 500 mg two or three times daily.

Proprietary Names and Manufacturers
Bron *(Scharper, Ital.)*; Silborina *(Iema, Ital.)*.

The following names have been used for multi-ingredient preparations containing potassium guaiacolsulfonate—Albatussin *(Bart, USA)*; Ambenyl *(Parke, Davis, Canad.)*; Entuss Liquid *(Hauck, USA)*; Phenergan Compound Expectorant *(May & Baker, UK)*; Phenergan Expectorant *(May & Baker, Austral.; Rhône-Poulenc, Canad.)*; Phenergan Expectorant with Codeine *(Rhône-Poulenc, Canad.)*; Phenergan VC Expectorant *(Rhône-Poulenc, Canad.)*; Phenergan VC Expectorant with Codeine *(Rhône-Poulenc, Canad.)*; Poly-Histine Expectorant with Codeine *(Bock, USA)*; Thenfacol *(Winthrop, Austral.)*.

5631-c

Prenoxdiazine Hydrochloride *(rINNM).*
HK-256; Prenoxdiazin Hydrochloride. 3-(2,2-Diphenylethyl)-5-(2-piperidinoethyl)-1,2,4-oxadiazole hydrochloride.
$C_{23}H_{27}N_3O,HCl$=397.9.

CAS — 47543-65-7 (prenoxdiazine); 982-43-4 (hydrochloride).

Prenoxdiazine hydrochloride is a peripherally-acting cough suppressant given by mouth in doses of 100 mg three or four times daily. Prenoxdiazine benzhydrate is also used.

Proprietary Names and Manufacturers of Prenoxdiazine Salts
Libexin *(Chinoin, Hung.; Master Pharma, Ital.)*; Libexine *(Labatec-Pharma, Switz.)*; Lomapect *(TAD, Ger.)*; Tibexin *(Christiaens, Belg.)*; Varoxil *(Padro, Spain)*.

2025-c

Senega Root *(BAN).*
Polygalae Radix; Rattlesnake Root; Seneca Snakeroot; Senega.

CAS — 1260-04-4 (polygalic acid).

Pharmacopoeias. In *Arg., Aust., Belg., Br., Chin., Egypt., Eur., Fr., Jpn, Mex., Neth., Nord., Port., Span.*, and *Swiss. Br.* also describes Powdered Senega Root.

The dried root and root crown of *Polygala senega* or certain closely related species of *Polygala* or a mixture of these. **Protect** from light.

Senega root has been given by mouth as an expectorant in doses of 2.5 to 5 mL of a concentrated infusion, or 0.3 to 1 mL of a liquid extract.

Preparations

Senega Tincture *(B.P.C. 1973).* Senega liquid extract 1 mL, alcohol (60%) to 5 mL. *Dose.* 2.5 to 5 mL.

Senega and Ammonia Mixture *(A.P.F.).* See p.906.

Proprietary Names and Manufacturers

The following names have been used for multi-ingredient preparations containing senega root—Cosanyl *(Parke, Davis, Austral.)*; Senamon *(Drug Houses Austral., Austral.).*

13239-p

Sobrerol

Sobrerolo. *p*-Menth-6-ene-2,8-diol.
$C_{10}H_{18}O_2$=170.3.

CAS — 498-71-5.

Pharmacopoeias. In *It.*

Sobrerol is claimed to have expectorant and mucolytic activity and is used in respiratory disorders.

Report of a study of the pharmacokinetics of sobrerol after oral or intravenous administration to 2 groups of 4 patients with acute exacerbations of chronic bronchitis. Sobrerol was rapidly absorbed from the gastro-intestinal tract and rapidly distributed. Thirteen and 23% of the dose was excreted in the urine as unchanged drug, glucuronidated sobrerol, and hydrated carvone after intravenous and oral administration respectively. After both routes of administration it was shown to accumulate in bronchial mucus.— P. C. Braga *et al.*, *Eur. J. clin. Pharmac.*, 1983, *24*, 209.

Proprietary Names and Manufacturers

Ditifene *(Almirall, Spain)*; Lysmucol *(Essex, Switz.)*; Sobrepin *(Unifa, Arg.; Corvi, Ital.; Zambeletti, Spain).*

5632-k

Sodium Dibunate *(BAN, rINN).*

L-1633. Sodium 2,6-di-*tert*-butylnaphthalene-1-sulphonate.
$C_{18}H_{23}NaO_3S$=342.4.

CAS — 14992-58-6 (dibunate); 14992-59-7 (sodium dibunate).

NOTE. The name naftoclizine has been used for chlorcyclizine dibunate.

Sodium dibunate is a cough suppressant claimed to have central and peripheral actions. It is given by mouth in doses of 30 to 60 mg.

Ethyl dibunate and chlorcyclizine dibunate have also been used.

Proprietary Names and Manufacturers

Becantal *(Labaz, Spain)*; Becantex *(Labaz, Belg.; Labaz, Fr.; Labaz, Neth.)*; Bechisan *(Salus, Ital.)*; Bexedan *(UCB, Ital.)*; Licolen *(Molteni, Ital.).*

The following names have been used for multi-ingredient preparations containing sodium dibunate—Balminil *(Rougier, Canad.)*; Daribiol *(Cambridge Laboratories, Austral.).*

2027-a

Indian Squill *(BAN).*

Urginea.

Pharmacopoeias. In *Br.*

The bulb of *Drimia indica* (Liliaceae), with the outer membranous scales removed, usually sliced and dried. It contains cardiac glycosides similar to those in squill. **Store** at a temperature not exceeding 25° in a dry place. Powdered Indian squill is very hygroscopic and should be stored in a desiccated atmosphere.

2026-k

Squill *(BAN).*

Bulbo de Escila; Cebolla Albarrana; Cila; Meerzwiebel; Scilla; Scillae Bulbus; Scille; White Squill.

Pharmacopoeias. In *Arg., Br., Egypt., Ger., Port.*, and *Span. Br.* also describes Powdered Squill.

The dried sliced bulb of *Drimia maritima* (Liliaceae), with the membranous outer scales removed, and containing not less than 68% of alcohol (60%)-soluble extractive.

Store at a temperature not exceeding 25° in a dry place. Powdered squill is very hygroscopic and should be stored in a desiccated atmosphere.

Adverse Effects, Treatment, and Precautions

The adverse effects of squill and Indian squill include nausea, vomiting, and diarrhoea. As squill and Indian squill contain cardiac glycosides they can cause similar adverse effects to digoxin (p.825). The treatment of the adverse effects is similar and similar precautions should be considered.

For reports of cardiac glycoside toxicity and myopathy associated with the abuse of Codeine Linctus (*A.P.F.*), which used to contain squill oxymel, see: M. Kennedy, *Med. J. Aust.*, 1981, *2*, 686; C. Kilpatrick *et al.* (letter), *ibid.*, 1982, *2*, 410; S. S. W. Seow (letter), *ibid.*, 1984, *140*, 54.

For similar reports associated with the abuse of Opiate Squill Linctus (*B.P.*) see: D. Thurston and K. Taylor (letter), *Pharm. J.*, 1984, *2*, 63; W. Smith *et al.*, *Br. med. J.*, 1986, *292*, 868.

Uses and Administration

Squill and Indian squill are used as expectorants and have been given in doses of 30 to 250 mg, as the oxymel, elixir, tincture, or vinegar. Red squill has been used as a rodenticide (see p.1354).

It was recommended by the Food Additives and Contaminants Committee that squill be prohibited for use in foods as a flavouring agent.— *Report on the Review of Flavourings in Food*, FAC/REP/22, Minist. Agric. Fish. Fd, London, HM Stationery Office, 1976.

A history of the use of squill.— W. E. Court, *Pharm. J.*, 1985, *2*, 194.

Preparations

Squill Liquid Extract *(B.P.).* 1 in 1; prepared by percolation with alcohol (70%).

Squill Oxymel *(B.P.).* Contains squill or Indian squill in acetic acid, purified honey, and water.

Opiate squill preparations are listed under p.1315.

Proprietary Names and Manufacturers

The following names have been used for multi-ingredient preparations containing squill—Broncodeine *(Nadeau, Canad.)*; Cosanyl *(Parke, Davis, Austral.)*; Linituss *(Ayrton, Saunders, UK)*; Neo-Pectol *(Neolab, Canad.)*; Pectomed *(Medo, UK)*; Sedatussin *(Lilly, UK)*; Tussifans *(Norton, UK).*

980-x

Stepronin *(rINN).*

Tiofacic. *N*-(2-Mercaptopropionyl)glycine 2-thiophenecarboxylate.
$C_{10}H_{11}NO_4S_2$=273.3.

CAS — 72324-18-6.

Stepronin has been reported to have mucolytic actions, and has also been used in the treatment of acute and chronic hepatitis. It is also used as the sodium and lysinate salts.

Proprietary Names and Manufacturers of Stepronin or its Salts

Broncoplus *(Sigmatau, Ital.)*; Masor *(Formenti, Ital.)*; Mucodil *(Valeas, Ital.)*; Tiase *(Mediolanum, Ital.; Mediolanum, Switz.)*; Tioten *(Mediolanum, Ital.)*; Valase *(Logifarm, Ital.).*

2029-x

Terpin Hydrate *(USAN).*

Terpene Hydrate; Terpinol. *p*-Menthane-1,8-diol monohydrate; 4-Hydroxy-α,α,4-trimethylcyclohexanemethanol monohydrate.
$C_{10}H_{20}O_2,H_2O$=190.3.

CAS — 80-53-5 (anhydrous); 2451-01-6 (monohydrate).

Pharmacopoeias. In *Arg., Belg., Fr., Hung., Mex., Port., Roum., Rus., Span., Swiss,* and *U.S.*

Colourless lustrous crystals or white powder with a slight odour. It effloresces in dry air. **Soluble** 1 in 200 of water, 1 in 35 of boiling water, 1 in 13 of alcohol, 1 in 3 of boiling alcohol, 1 in 140 of chloroform, and 1 in 140 of ether. A 1% solution in hot water is neutral to litmus. **Store** in airtight containers.

Terpin hydrate has been stated to increase bronchial secretion directly and is used as an expectorant. It is given by mouth in doses of 170 to 200 mg every 4 to 6 hours.

Nausea, vomiting, or abdominal pain may follow the ingestion of terpin hydrate on an empty stomach.

Preparations

Terpin Hydrate Elixir *(U.S.P.).* Terpin hydrate 85 mg, glycerol 2 mL, syrup 0.5 mL, alcohol 2.15 mL, benzaldehyde 0.00025 mL, sweet orange peel tincture 0.1 mL (or orange oil 0.005 mL dissolved in alcohol 0.075 mL), water to 5 mL.

Terpin Hydrate and Codeine Elixir *(U.S.P.).* Codeine 10 mg, terpin hydrate elixir to 5 mL.

Terpin Hydrate and Dextromethorphan Hydrobromide Elixir *(U.S.P.).* Dextromethorphan hydrobromide 10 mg, terpin hydrate elixir to 5 mL.

Proprietary Preparations

Tercoda *(Sinclair, UK). Elixir,* terpin hydrate 8 mg, codeine phosphate 8 mg/5 mL.

Terpoin *(Hough, Hoseason, UK). Elixir,* terpin hydrate 9.15 mg, guaiphenesin 50 mg, cineole 4.15 mg, codeine phosphate 15 mg, menthol 18.3 mg/5 mL.

Proprietary Names and Manufacturers

The following names have been used for multi-ingredient preparations containing terpin hydrate— Copholco *(Rorer, UK)*; Copholcoids *(Rorer, UK)*; Coterpin *(Ayrton, Saunders, UK)*; SK-Terpin Hydrate and Codeine *(Smith Kline & French, USA)*; Tercoda *(Sinclair, UK)*; Tercolix *(Norton, UK)*; Terpalin *(Norton, UK)*; Terpo-Dionin *(Winthrop, Canad.)*; Terpoin *(Hough, Hoseason, UK).*

NOTE. The *UK* preparation Triotussic had been reformulated to exclude terpin hydrate prior to its withdrawal from the market.

6261-j

Thebacon Hydrochloride *(BANM, rINNM).*

Acethydrocodone Hydrochloride; Acetyldihydrocodeinone Hydrochloride; Dihydrocodeinone Enol Acetate Hydrochloride. 6-*O*-Acetyl-7,8-dihydro-3-*O*-methyl-6,7-didehydromorphine hydrochloride; (−)-(5*R*)-4,5-Epoxy-3-methoxy-9a-methylmorphin-6-en-6-yl acetate hydrochloride.
$C_{20}H_{23}NO_4,HCl$=377.9.

CAS — 466-90-0 (thebacon).

Thebacon hydrochloride is used for cough suppression in doses of 5 to 10 mg.

Proprietary Names and Manufacturers

Acedicon *(Boehringer Ingelheim, Ger.; Boehringer Ingelheim, Ital.)*; Acedicone *(Boehringer Ingelheim, Belg.)*; Thebacetyl *(Belg.).*

13352-s

Tipepidine Hybenzate

AT-327 *(tipepidine)*; CR-662 *(tipepidine)*; Tipepidine Hibenzate *(rINNM)*. 3-[Di(2-thienyl)methylene]-1-methylpiperidine 2-(4-hydroxybenzoyl)benzoate.
$C_{15}H_{17}NS_2,C_{14}H_{10}O_4$=517.7.

CAS — 5169-78-8 (tipepidine); 31139-87-4 (hybenzate).

Tipepidine hybenzate is a cough suppressant which is claimed also to have an expectorant action.

Report of generalised convulsions associated with the administration of tipepidine hybenzate by mouth in one patient.— R. M. Cuomo, *Acta neurol. Napoli*, 1982, *37*, 110.

Proprietary Names and Manufacturers
Asvelik *(Medinsa, Spain)*; Asverin *(Searle, Ital.; Tanabe, Jpn)*; Sotal *(Gramon, Arg.)*.

287-f

Tolu Balsam *(BAN, USAN)*.

Baume de Tolu.

CAS — 9000-64-0.

Pharmacopoeias. In *Arg., Belg., Egypt., Fr., It., Mex., Port., Roum., Span., Swiss,* and *U.S.*

A balsam obtained from *Myroxylon balsamum* (=*M. toluiferum*) (Leguminosae). It is a brownish-yellow or brown plastic solid when fresh, but it subsequently becomes harder and finally brittle. It has an aromatic and vanilla-like odour.

Practically **insoluble** in water and light petroleum; soluble in alcohol, chloroform, and ether, but sometimes leaving some insoluble residues. **Store** at a temperature not exceeding 40° in airtight containers.

Tolu balsam is considered to have very mild antiseptic properties and some expectorant action but is mainly used to flavour cough mixtures. However, it is generally used in the form of a syrup and Tolu Syrup (*B.P.*) no longer contains tolu balsam but is based on cinnamic acid, (see p.1359).

Preparations

Tolu Balsam Syrup *(U.S.N.F.)*. Tolu balsam tincture 5 mL, magnesium carbonate 1 g, sucrose 82 g, water to 100 mL.

Tolu Balsam Tincture *(U.S.N.F.)*. Tolu balsam 20 g, alcohol to 100 mL; prepared by maceration.

5633-a

Zipeprol Hydrochloride *(rINNM)*.

CERM-3024. 1-Methoxy-3-[4-(β-methoxyphenethyl)piperazin-1-yl]-1-phenylpropan-2-ol dihydrochloride.

$C_{23}H_{32}N_2O_3,2HCl=457.4$.

CAS — 34758-83-3 (zipeprol); 34758-84-4 (hydrochloride).

Zipeprol hydrochloride is a cough suppressant which is stated to have a peripheral action on bronchial spasm; 150 to 300 mg may be given daily by mouth in divided doses. There have been reports of abuse and overdosage producing neurological symptoms.

ABUSE AND OVERDOSAGE. A Milan Poison Control Centre report of 32 patients with severe neurological symptoms associated with zipeprol overdosage, most of whom were young adults whose history pointed to habitual use for euphoria. Eleven of these patients dealt with directly, presented with generalised seizures, followed by coma. Three further patients were children and their symptoms were restlessness (in keeping with a low overdose of 27 mg per kg body-weight), abnormalities of posture and gait, and generalised seizures followed by choreic movements and forced right deviation of the head and eyes.— C. Moroni *et al.* (letter), *Lancet*, 1984, *1*, 45. A report of convulsions in 2 teenagers associated with zipeprol overdoses of 750 mg and 975 mg. One had several opisthotonic crises during examination and also developed cerebral oedema.— F. Perraro and A. Beorchia (letter), *ibid.*

Proprietary Names and Manufacturers
Antituxil-Z *(Ghimas, Ital.)*; Balutox *(Baldacci, Ital.)*; Broncozina *(Mendelejeff, Ital.)*; Bronx *(Lisapharma, Ital.)*; Citizeta *(CT, Ital.)*; Mirsol *(Permamed, Switz.)*; Respilène *(Winthrop, Fr.)*; Respirase *(Gibipharma, Ital.)*; Respirex *(Inibsa, Spain)*; Talasa *(Andromaco, Arg.)*; Zitoxil *(Lifepharma, Ital.)*.

Dermatological Agents

1590-j

The skin is subject to a very wide range of disorders including pruritus, erythema, inflammation, purpura, vesicles and bullae, urticaria, photosensitivity, and disorders of pigmentation and of the scalp.
Some disorders are characteristic of specific diseases and fade as the disease regresses. Some are caused by specific local infections and are best treated by the appropriate antimicrobial agent. Many skin disorders are side-effects of therapeutic and other agents, ranging from mild hypersensitivity to the life-threatening Stevens-Johnson syndrome or toxic epidermal necrolysis. There remains a wide range of disorders the aetiology of many of which is poorly understood.
This section describes many of the agents that have been used, often over many years; their pharmacology is often poorly understood.
Agents that have a traditional place in the treatment of skin disorders include dithranol, ichthammol, resorcinol, sulphur, tar, and coal tar. More recent developments include the use of etretinate and methoxsalen in psoriasis and isotretinoin and tretinoin in acne.
Agents with primarily a protective function include calamine, starch, talc, titanium dioxide, and zinc oxide.
Agents used to increase pigmentation include dihydroxyacetone, methoxsalen, and trioxsalen. Agents used to reduce pigmentation include hydroquinone, mequinol, and monobenzone. Other agents used to protect against sunlight are described under Sunscreen Agents, p.1450.
For the use of corticosteroids in the treatment of skin disorders, see p.875.
For the use of immunosuppressants in the treatment of psoriasis, see p.639.

ACNE. A brief review of the treatment of acne vulgaris.— W. J. Cunliffe, *Archs Dis. Childh.*, 1982, *57*, 245.

DANDRUFF. A discussion of the aetiology of dandruff and the mode of action of therapeutic agents.— S. Shuster, *Br. J. Derm.*, 1984, *111*, 235.

ECZEMA. The treatment of atopic eczema in childhood.— D. J. Atherton, *Prescribers' J.*, 1986, *26*, 140; J. Verbov, *Archs Dis. Childh.*, 1986, *61*, 518.

LEUCODERMA. A brief discussion on the causes and treatment of leucoderma.— S. S. Bleehen, *Br. med. J.*, 1987, *294*, 360.

PSORIASIS. Reviews of psoriasis and its treatment.— E. M. Farber and L. Nall, *Drugs*, 1984, *28*, 324; M. Klaber, *Prescribers' J.*, 1986, *26*, 147; R. H. Champion, *Br. med. J.*, 1986, *292*, 1693. Comments: C. E. M. Griffiths *et al.* (letter), *ibid.*, *293*, 266; R. A. Wakeel and D. C. Dick (letter), *ibid.*

ULCERS. The current management of leg ulcers.— T. J. Ryan, *Drugs*, 1985, *30*, 461.

URTICARIA. Current concepts in the pathogenesis and treatment of urticarias.— K. P. Mathews, *Drugs*, 1985, *30*, 552.

19160-m

Acitretin *(pINN)*.
Etretin; Ro-10-1670. (*all-trans*)-9-(4-Methoxy-2,3,6-trimethylphenyl)-3,7-dimethyl-2,4,6,8-nonatetraenoic acid.
$C_{21}H_{26}O_3$=326.4.

CAS — 55079-83-9.

Acitretin is a metabolite of etretinate reported to have anti-psoriatic activity and a shorter biological half-life than etretinate.

For an *in vitro* study demonstrating that acitretin is potentially phototoxic, see Etretinate, p.921.

References to the use of acitretin in psoriasis: J. M. Geiger *et al.*, *Curr. ther. Res.*, 1984, *35*, 735; T. P. Kingston *et al.*, *Archs Derm.*, 1987, *123*, 55.

1591-z

Alcloxa *(USAN, rINN)*.
ALCA; Aluminium Chlorhydroxyallantoinate; RC-173. Chlorotetrahydroxy[(2-hydroxy-5-oxo-2-imidazolin-4-yl)ureato]dialuminium.
$C_4H_9Al_2ClN_4O_7$=314.6.

CAS — 1317-25-5.

Alcloxa is an astringent and keratolytic containing allantoin.

Proprietary Names and Manufacturers
The following names have been used for multi-ingredient preparations containing alcloxa—Acnederm *(Ego, Austral.)*; Miol (Formula M.I.) Cream *(BritCair, UK)*; Miol (Formula M.I.) Lotion *(BritCair, UK)*.

1592-c

Aldioxa *(USAN, rINN)*.
ALDA; Aluminium Dihydroxyallantoinate; RC-172. Dihydroxy[(2-hydroxy-5-oxo-2-imidazolin-4-yl)ureato]-aluminium.
$C_4H_7AlN_4O_5$=218.1.

CAS — 5579-81-7.

Aldioxa is an astringent and keratolytic containing allantoin. Aldioxa has been used for gastro-intestinal disorders.

Proprietary Preparations
ZeaSorb *(Stiefel, UK)*. *Dusting powder*, aldioxa 0.2%, chloroxylenol 0.5%, pulverised maize core 45%.

Proprietary Names and Manufacturers
Alanetorin *(Jpn)*; Alanta-SP *(Jpn)*; Arlanto *(Jpn)*; Ascomp *(Jpn)*.

The following names have been used for multi-ingredient preparations containing aldioxa—Cetanorm *(Norma, UK)*; Rikospray Silicone *(Riker, UK)*; Zeasorb *(Stiefel, Canad.)*; ZeaSorb *(Stiefel, UK)*.

1593-k

Allantoin *(BAN, USAN)*.
Glyoxyldiureide. 5-Ureidohydantoin; 5-Ureidoimidazolidine-2,4-dione.
$C_4H_6N_4O_3$=158.1.

CAS — 97-59-6.

Allantoin is used in psoriasis and other skin disorders.

Proprietary Names and Manufacturers
The following names have been used for multi-ingredient preparations containing allantoin—Acne-sol *(Fawns & McAllan, Austral.)*; Actinac *(Roussel, Canad.; Roussel, UK)*; Alphosyl *(Stafford-Miller, Austral.; Reed & Carnrick, Canad.; Stafford-Miller, UK; Reed & Carnrick, USA)*; Alphosyl HC *(Stafford-Miller, UK)*; AVC *(Merrell Dow, Canad.)*; Blistik Medicated Lip Balm *(Key, Austral.)*; Dermalex *(Labaz Sanofi, UK)*; Ego Antiseptic Cream *(Ego, Austral.)*; Egoderm Cream *(Ego, Austral.)*; Egoderm M *(Ego, Austral.)*; Egopsoryl *(Ego, Austral.)*; Epicare *(Rosken, Austral.)*; Hemocane *(Key, Austral.)*; Herpecin-L *(Campbell, USA)*; Medi Creme *(Rosken, Austral.)*; Medi Pulv *(Rosken, Austral.)*; Oticane *(Rosken, Austral.)*; Paxyl Cream *(Faulding, Austral.)*; Vagimide *(Legere, USA)*.

12348-v

Aluminium Oxide

Al_2O_3=102.0.

CAS — 1344-28-1.

Fused synthetic aluminium oxide, of graded particle size, is used as an abrasive paste as an adjunct in the treatment of acne.

Proprietary Preparations
Brasivol *(Stiefel, UK)*. *Cleansing paste*, fused synthetic graded particles of aluminium oxide 38% (No.1 fine), 52% (No.2 medium), or 65% (No.3 coarse) in a soap-detergent base.

Other Proprietary Abrasive Preparations
Ionax Scrub *(Alcon, UK)*. *Gel*, polyethylene granules in a detergent basis, with benzalkonium chloride. For the abrasive treatment of acne.

Proprietary Names and Manufacturers
Brasivil *(Stiefel, Ger.)*; Brasivol *(Stiefel, Austral.; Stiefel, Canad.; Stiefel, S.Afr.; Stiefel, UK)*.

12370-m

Ammonium Salicylate

$C_7H_9NO_3$=155.2.

CAS — 528-94-9.

Ammonium salicylate has been used topically as a keratolytic in skin disorders.

Proprietary Names and Manufacturers
Salicyl-Vasogen *(Pearson, Ger.)*.

The following names have been used for multi-ingredient preparations containing ammonium salicylate— Aspellin *(Rorer, UK)*.

5905-m

Benzoyl Peroxide *(BANM, USAN)*.

Dibenzoyl peroxide.
$C_{14}H_{10}O_4$=242.2.

CAS — 94-36-0.

Pharmacopoeias. In *Braz. Br.* and *U.S.* include Hydrous Benzoyl Peroxide which contains not less than 23% or 26% respectively of water.

A white amorphous or granular powder with a characteristic odour. Sparingly **soluble** in water and in alcohol; soluble in acetone, chloroform, and ether.
Store in original container, treated to reduce static charges, at room temperature. Unused material should not be returned to its original container but should be destroyed by the addition of sodium hydroxide solution (10%). Destruction can be considered to be complete if the addition of a crystal of potassium iodide does not result in the release of free iodine. Protect from light.

CAUTION. *Benzoyl peroxide may explode if subjected to grinding, percussion, or heat. Hydrous benzoyl peroxide containing water to reduce the risk of explosion may still explode if exposed to temperatures higher than 60° or cause fires in the presence of reducing substances.*

Adverse Effects and Precautions
Application of benzoyl peroxide may produce an initial stinging effect. Contact sensitisation has been reported in some patients using preparations containing benzoyl peroxide. Caution is required when applying it near mucous membranes. Patients should be alerted to benzoyl peroxide's bleaching property.
In Great Britain the recommended exposure limit of benzoyl peroxide is 5 mg per m^3 (long-term). In the *US* the permissible and recommended exposure limits are 5 mg per m^3.

Of 50 patients studied, 38 demonstrated sensitivity to gel preparations containing benzoyl peroxide 5%; patch tests using a 1% solution of benzoyl peroxide in acetone on 10 of the sensitive subjects showed the sensitivity to be retained for at least 3 months.— J. J. Leyden and A. M. Kligman, *Contact Dermatitis*, 1977, *3*, 273.

A report of an unusual unpleasant body odour in one patient attributed to the topical use of benzoyl peroxide.— P. Molberg (letter), *New Engl. J. Med.*, 1981, *304*, 1366.

Concern at the implications of some *animal* studies

showing benzoyl peroxide to possess some tumour-promoting activity G. R. N. Jones (letter), *Hum. Toxicol.*, 1985, *4*, 75.

Uses and Administration

Benzoyl peroxide has keratolytic properties. Antimicrobial activity has been reported against *Staphylococus epidermidis* and *Propionibacterium acnes*. It is used mainly in the treatment of acne, usually in topical preparations containing 2.5 to 10% often in conjunction with other antimicrobial agents. Strengths are expressed as anhydrous benzoyl peroxide although it is usually employed in a hydrous form for safety (see above).

Benzoyl peroxide is also used as a bleaching agent in the food industry and as a catalyst in the plastics industry.

ACNE. Reduction of inflamed acne lesions with 5 days' treatment with benzoyl peroxide 5%.— H. Schutte *et al.*, *Br. J. Derm.*, 1982, *106*, 91.

A rise in sebum excretion-rate with benzoyl peroxide.— W. J. Cunliffe *et al.*, *Br. J. Derm.*, 1983, *109*, 577.

Further references to benzoyl peroxide in acne: B. Burke *et al.*, *Br. J. Derm.*, 1983, *108*, 199 (comparable with erythromycin topically); S. B. Tucker *et al.*, *ibid.*, 1984, *110*, 487 (comparable with clindamycin topically).

Preparations

Benzoyl Peroxide Cream *(B.P.)*

Benzoyl Peroxide Gel *(B.P., U.S.P.)*

Benzoyl Peroxide Lotion *(B.P., U.S.P.)*

Erythromycin and Benzoyl Peroxide Topical Gel *(U.S.P.)*

Potassium Hydroxyquinoline Sulphate and Benzoyl Peroxide Cream *(B.P.)*

Proprietary Preparations

Acetoxyl *(Stiefel, UK)*. *Gel* (Acetoxyl 2.5), benzoyl peroxide 2.5% in an acetone basis.
Gel (Acetoxyl 5) benzoyl peroxide 5% in an acetone basis.

Acnegel *(Stiefel, UK)*. *Gel*, benzoyl peroxide 5%.
Gel (Acnegel Forte), benzoyl peroxide 10%.

Acnidazil *(Janssen, UK)*. *Cream*, benzoyl peroxide 5%, miconazole nitrate 2%.

Benoxyl *(Stiefel, UK)*. *Cream* and *lotion* (Benoxyl 5), benzoyl peroxide 5%.
Cream (Benoxyl 5 with Sulphur), benzoyl peroxide 5%, sulphur 2%.
Lotion (Benoxyl 10), benzoyl peroxide 10%.
Cream (Benoxyl 10 with Sulphur), benzoyl peroxide 10% sulphur 5%.
Lotion (Benoxyl 20), benzoyl peroxide 20%.

Benzagel *(Bioglan, UK)*. *Gel* (Benzagel 5), benzoyl peroxide 5%.
Gel (Benzagel 10), benzoyl peroxide 10%.

Clearasil Acne Treatment *(Richardson-Vicks, UK)*. *Cream*, benzoyl peroxide 10%.

Nericur *(Schering, UK)*. *Gel* (Nericur 5), benzoyl peroxide 5%.
Gel (Nericur 10), benzoyl peroxide 10%.

Oxy *(Beecham Proprietaries, UK)*. *Lotion* (Oxy 5), benzoyl peroxide 5%.
Lotion (Oxy 10), benzoyl peroxide 10%.

PanOxyl *(Stiefel, UK)*. *Gel*, aqueous (PanOxyl Aquagel 2.5), benzoyl peroxide 2.5%.
Gel (PanOxyl 5), benzoyl peroxide 5% in an ethanolic base.
Gel, aqueous (PanOxyl Aquagel 5) benzoyl peroxide 5%.
Gel (PanOxyl 10), benzoyl peroxide 10% in an ethanolic base.
Gel, aqueous (PanOxyl Aquagel 10) benzoyl peroxide 10%.
Lotion (PanOxyl Wash), benzoyl peroxide 10% in a detergent base.

Quinoderm *(Quinoderm, UK)*. *Cream*, benzoyl peroxide 10%, potassium hydroxyquinoline sulphate 0.5%.
Cream (Quinoderm Cream 5), benzoyl peroxide 5%, potassium hydroxyquinoline sulphate 0.5%.
Cream (Quinoderm Cream with Hydrocortisone), benzoyl peroxide 10%, potassium hydroxyquinoline sulphate 0.5%, hydrocortisone 1%.
Lotion (Quinoderm Lotio-Gel), benzoyl peroxide 10%, potassium hydroxyquinoline sulphate 0.5%.
Lotion (Quinoderm Lotio-Gel 5%), benzoyl peroxide 5%, potassium hydroxyquinoline sulphate 0.5%.

Quinoped *(Quinoderm, UK)*. *Cream*, benzoyl peroxide 5%, potassium hydroxyquinoline sulphate 0.5%.

Theraderm *(Bristol-Myers Pharmaceuticals, UK)*. *Gel* (Theraderm 5), benzoyl peroxide 5%.
Gel (Theraderm 10), benzoyl peroxide 10%.

Proprietary Names and Manufacturers

AcetOxyl *(Stiefel, Canad.; Stiefel, UK)*; Acnacyl *(Rosken, Austral.)*; Acnéfuge *(Spirig, Switz.)*; Acnegel *(Stiefel, UK)*; Acnomel BP5 *(Smith Kline & French, Canad.)*; Akne-Aid *(Stiefel, Ger.)*; Aknefug *(Wolff, Ger.)*; Akneroxid *(Hermal, Ger.; Hermal, Switz.)*; Alquam-X *(Westwood, Canad.)*; Basiron *(Basoderm, Denm.; Basotherm, Switz.)*; Benoxid *(Pharma-Medica, Denm.)*; Benoxyl *(Stiefel, Austral.; Stiefel, Canad.; Stiefel, Fr.; Stiefel, Ger.; Stiefel, UK)*; Benzac *(Alcon, Austral.; Alcon, Canad.; Alcon, Switz.; Owen, USA)*; Benzagel *(Rorer, Canad.; Rorer, Fr.; Rorer, Switz.; Bioglan, UK; Dermik, USA)*; Benzaknen *(Alcon, Ger.)*; Clearasil Acne Treatment *(Richardson-Vicks, Canad.; Richardson-Vicks, UK; Richardson-Vicks, USA)*; Conex *(Schering, Swed.)*; Curaderm *(Pharma-Medica, Denm.)*; Cutacnyl *(Galderma, Fr.)*; Debroxide *(Alcon, UK : Farillon, UK)*; Dermodex *(USA)*; Dermoxyl *(ICN, Canad.)*; Desanden *(Max Ritter, Switz.)*; Desquam-X *(Westwood, Canad.; Westwood, USA)*; Diafen *(Cilag, Fr.)*; Eclaran *(Pierre Fabre, Fr.)*; Effacne *(Roche, Fr.)*; Fostex BPO *(Westwood, USA)*; H_2Oxyl *(Stiefel, Canad.; Stiefel, Switz.)*; Kerolyte *(NZ)*; Loroxide *(Rorer, Canad.)*; Mytolac *(Richardson-Vicks, Swed.)*; Nericur *(Schering, UK)*; Oxy *(USV, Austral.; Fink, Ger.; Norcliff Thayer, Swed.; Beecham Proprietaries, UK)*; Oxyderm *(ICN, Canad.)*; Pannogel *(Schering, Fr.)*; PanOxyl *(Stiefel, Austral.; Stiefel, Canad.; Stiefel, Fr.; Stiefel, Ger.; Nyco, Norw.; Stiefel, Switz.; Stiefel, UK; Stiefel, USA)*; Persadox *(Owen, USA)*; Persa-Gel *(Canad.; Ortho Dermatological, USA)*; Persa-Gel W *(Ortho Dermatological, USA)*; Sanoxit *(Basotherm, Ger.)*; Scherogel *(Scherax, Ger.)*; Stioxyl *(Stiefel, Swed.)*; Teen *(USA)*; Theraderm *(Bristol-Myers Pharmaceuticals, UK)*; Topacil *(Cilag, Switz.)*; Topex *(Richardson-Vicks, Austral.; Richardson-Vicks, UK; Richardson-Vicks, USA)*; Xerac BP *(Person & Covey, USA)*.

The following names have been used for multi-ingredient preparations containing benzoyl peroxide— Acnidazil *(Janssen, UK)*; Benoxyl with Sulphur *(Stiefel, UK)*; Benzamycin *(Dermik, USA)*; Persol *(Horner, Canad.)*; Quinoderm *(Quinoderm, UK)*; Quinoderm with Hydrocortisone *(Quinoderm, UK)*; Quinoped *(Quinoderm, UK)*; Sulfoxyl *(Stiefel, Canad.)*; Vanair *(Carter-Wallace, UK)*; Vanoxide-HC *(Rorer, Canad.; Dermik, USA)*.

1595-t

Cade Oil

Alquitrán de Enebro; Goudron de Cade; Juniper Tar *(USAN)*; Juniper Tar Oil; Kadeöl; Oleum Cadinum; Oleum Juniperi Empyreumaticum; Pix Cadi; Pix Juniperi; Pix Oxycedri; Pyroleum Juniperi; Pyroleum Oxycedri; Wacholderteer.

CAS — 8013-10-3.

Pharmacopoeias. In *Arg., Hung., Mex., Port., Roum., Span., Swiss,* and *U.S.*

Cade oil is obtained by the destructive distillation of the branches and wood of *Juniperus oxycedrus* (Pinaceae). It is a dark, reddish-brown or nearly black, oily liquid with an empyreumatic odour. It contains guaiacol, ethylguaiacol, creosol, and cadinene. Very slightly **soluble** in water; soluble 1 in 3 of ether; soluble 1 in 9 of alcohol; miscible with amyl alcohol, chloroform, and glacial acetic acid. Avoid exposure to excessive heat. Protect from light.

Cade oil is used for its antipruritic and keratoplastic properties as an ingredient in topical preparations for psoriasis, eczema, and seborrhoea.

It was recommended that cade oil be prohibited for use in foods as a flavouring agent.— *Food Standards Committee Report on Flavouring Agents*, London, HM Stationery Office, 1965.

Proprietary Names and Manufacturers

Caditar *(I.P.R.A.D., Fr.)*.

The following names have been used for multi-ingredient preparations containing cade oil—Gelcotar Liquid *(Quinoderm, UK)*; Multi-Tar Plus *(ICN, Canad.)*; Polytar Emollient *(Stiefel, Austral.; Stiefel, UK)*; Polytar Liquid *(Stiefel, Austral.; Stiefel, UK)*; Polytar Plus *(Stiefel, UK)*.

1598-f

Calamine *(BAN, USAN)*.

Prepared Calamine.

CAS — 8011-96-9.

Pharmacopoeias. In *Arg., Br., Chin., Egypt., Ind.,* and *U.S.*

Calamine (*B.P.*) is a basic zinc carbonate coloured with ferric oxide, yielding on ignition 68 to 74% of oxides of zinc and iron. It is an amorphous, impalpable, pink or reddish-brown powder, the colour depending on the variety and amount of ferric oxide present and the process by which it is incorporated. Practically **insoluble** in water; soluble with effervescence in hydrochloric acid.

Calamine (*U.S.P.*) is zinc oxide with a small proportion of ferric oxide yielding on ignition not less than 98% of ZnO.

Calamine has a mild astringent action on the skin and is used as a dusting-powder, cream, lotion, or ointment in a variety of skin conditions.

Preparations

Aqueous Calamine Cream *(B.P.)*. Calamine Cream. Calamine 4 g, zinc oxide 3 g, liquid paraffin 20 g, self-emulsifying glyceryl monostearate 5 g, cetomacrogol emulsifying wax 5 g, phenoxyethanol 500 mg, and freshly boiled and cooled water 62.5 g.
A.P.F. (Calamine Cream Aqueous) has a similar preparation which may be tinted by the addition of up to 1% of caramel solution.

Evaluation of microbial preservation of reformulated calamine creams.— T. R. R. Kurup and L. S. C. Wan, *Pharm. J.*, 1983, *1*, 100.

Calamine and Coal Tar Ointment *(B.P.)*. Compound Calamine Ointment; sometimes known as Unguentum Sedativum. Calamine 12.5 g, zinc oxide 12.5 g, strong coal tar solution 2.5 g, hydrous wool fat 25 g, white soft paraffin 47.5 g.

Calamine Cream Oily *(A.P.F.)*. Calamine 32 g, oleic acid 0.5 mL, arachis oil 21.5 mL, wool fat 17.5 g, calcium hydroxide solution 30.5 mL. It may be tinted by the addition of up to 1% of caramel solution.

Calamine Lotion *(B.P.)*. Calam. Lot. Calamine 15 g, zinc oxide 5 g, bentonite 3 g, sodium citrate 500 mg, liquefied phenol 0.5 mL, glycerol 5 mL, freshly boiled and cooled water to 100 mL.
A.P.F. has a similar formula with sterilised bentonite.

Calamine Lotion *(U.S.P.)*. Calamine *U.S.P.* 8 g, zinc oxide 8 g, glycerol 2 mL, bentonite magma 25 mL, calcium hydroxide topical solution to 100 mL. If a more viscous consistency is desired, the quantity of bentonite magma may be increased to not more than 40 mL.

Calamine Lotion Oily *(A.P.F.)*. Lot. Calam. Oleos. Calamine 5 g, wool fat 1 g, oleic acid 0.5 mL, arachis oil 50 mL, calcium hydroxide solution to 100 mL. May be tinted by the addition of about 0.5% of caramel solution.

Calamine Ointment *(B.P.)*. Calamine 15 g and white soft paraffin 85 g.

Compound Calamine Application *(B.P.C. 1973)*. Compound Calamine Cream; Compound Calamine Liniment; Linimentum Calaminae Compositum. Calamine 10 g, zinc oxide 5 g, zinc stearate 2.5 g, wool fat 2.5 g, yellow soft paraffin 25 g, and liquid paraffin 55 g.

Phenolated Calamine Lotion *(U.S.P.)*. Liquefied phenol 1 mL, calamine lotion *U.S.P.* 99 mL.

Zinc Paste, Calamine and Clioquinol Bandage *(B.P.)*. See under Zinc Oxide, p.936.

Proprietary Preparations

Eczederm *(Quinoderm, UK)*. *Cream*, calamine 20.88% and arachis oil 12.5%.
Cream (Eczederm cream with hydrocortisone 0.5%), contains in addition hydrocortisone 0.5%.

Lacto-Calamine *(Kirby-Warrick, UK)*. *Lotion*, calamine 4%, hamamelis water 5%, phenol 0.2%.

Proprietary Names and Manufacturers

The following names have been used for multi-ingredient preparations containing calamine— Calaband *(Seton, UK)*; Caladryl *(Parke, Davis, Austral.; Parke, Davis, Canad.; Warner-Lambert, UK; Parke, Davis, USA)*; Calistaflex *(Glaxo, Austral.)*; Calmasol *(Ethipharm, Canad.)*; Calsept *(Norton, UK)*; Dome-Paste *(Miles Pharmaceuticals, USA)*; Eczederm with Hydrocortisone *(Quinoderm, UK)*; Globolotion *(R.P. Drugs, UK)*; Histofax *(Wellcome, UK)*; Lacto-Calamine *(Kirby-Warrick, UK)*; Quinaband *(Seton, UK)*; RBC *(Rybar, UK)*; Vasogen *(Pharmax, UK)*.

1599-d

Calcium Thioglycollate

Calcium Mercaptoacetate. Calcium mercaptoacetate trihydrate.

$C_2H_2CaO_2S,3H_2O=184.2$.

CAS — 814-71-1; 68-11-1 (thioglycollic acid).

Calcium thioglycollate is used as a depilatory, usually in concentrations of 2 to 4% in creams and lotions made alkaline by the addition of calcium hydroxide. It has been used pre-operatively to avoid shaving. Thioglycollates are used in home hair waving lotions together with potassium bromate as the neutraliser. There have been reports of skin reactions associated with the use of thioglycollate.

1600-d

Centella

Herba Centellae; Hydrocotyle; Indian Pennywort.

CAS — 18449-41-7 (madecassic acid); 464-92-6 (asiatic acid); 16830-15-2 (asiaticoside).

Pharmacopoeias. In *Chin.*

The fresh and dried leaves and stems of *Centella asiatica* (=*Hydrocotyle asiatica*) (Umbelliferae). It contains madecassic acid, asiatic acid, and asiaticoside.

Centella has mainly been used in the management of ulcers.

Proprietary Names and Manufacturers

Blastoestimulina *(Funk, Spain)*; Centelase *(Ital.)*; Madecassol *(Belg.; Syncare, Canad.; Laroche Navarron, Fr.; Neth.; Laroche Navarron, Switz.; Lipha, UK)*; Marticassol *(Martinet, Fr.)*.

1602-h

Chrysarobin

Araroba Depurata; commonly but erroneously called Chrysophanic Acid.

Pharmacopoeias. In *Arg., Aust., Jug., Mex., Nord., Port.,* and *Span.*

Chrysarobin is obtained from araroba, a substance obtained from *Andira araroba* (Leguminosae).

Chrysarobin has been used similarly to dithranol in psoriasis and in the treatment of skin infections. It should not be used on the face, genitalia, or scalp, owing to its irritant action, and should not be employed over a large area of skin. The ointment stains the skin and clothing a brownish-violet colour. Absorption of chrysarobin through the skin causes excretion of a yellow pigment which colours alkaline urine red.

Proprietary Names and Manufacturers

Chrysamone *(Andard-Mount, UK)*.

12610-m

Cosmetics

In the *UK* The Cosmetic Products (Safety) Regulations 1984 (SI 1984: No. 1260), as amended (SI 1985: No. 2045) define a 'cosmetic product' as 'any substance or preparation intended to be applied to any part of the external surfaces of the human body (that is to say, the epidermis, hair system, nails, lips and external genital organs) or to the teeth or buccal mucosa wholly or mainly for the purpose of cleaning, perfuming or protecting them or keeping them in good condition or changing their appearance or combating body odour or perspiration except where such cleaning, perfuming, protecting, keeping, changing, or combating is wholly for the purpose of treating or preventing disease'. A 'cosmetic product intended to come into contact with the mucous membranes' means 'a cosmetic product intended to be applied in the vicinity of the eyes, on the lips, in the oral cavity or to the external genital organs, and does not include any cosmetic product which is intended to come into only brief contact with the skin'.

The use of a large number of substances or groups of substances (generally with potent pharmacological activity or recognised toxicity) is prohibited in cosmetics.

The use of colouring agents for cosmetics is controlled. Some substances or groups of substances may be used only for specified purposes, with specified maximum concentrations, and subject to labelling and other requirements. In the *UK* these substances include alkali and alkaline earth sulphides, ammonia, benzoic acid, its salts and esters, benzyl alcohol, 1,3-bis(hydroxymethyl)imidazolidene-2-thione, boric acid, chlorates of alkali metals, chlorbutanol, dichloromethane, dichlorophen, fluorides, fluorosilicates, formaldehyde and paraformaldehyde, hexachlorophane, hydrogen peroxide, hydroquinone, 4-hydroxybenzoic acid and its salts and esters (except benzyl ester), inorganic sulphites and hydrogen sulphites, 6-methylcoumarin, monofluorophosphates, nicomethanol hydrofluoride, nitromethane, oxalic acid, its esters and alkaline salts, phenol and its alkali salts, *o*-phenylphenol and its salts, potassium and sodium hydroxide, propionic acid and its salts, pyrithione zinc, pyrogallol, quinine and its salts, resorcinol, salicylic acid and its salts, silver nitrate, sodium iodate, sodium nitrite, sorbic acid and its salts, thioglycollic acid, its salts and esters, tosylchloramide sodium, and water-soluble zinc salts. There have been a number of reports of contact allergy and photosensitivity reactions associated with cosmetics.

12614-q

Covering Creams

Covering creams usually contain opacifying agents and pigments in a suitable basis. They are used for the concealment of birth marks, scars, and disfiguring skin disease.

Proprietary Preparations

Boots Covering Cream *(Boots, UK). Cream,* opaque, pigmented, available in a range of shades.

Covermark *(Stiefel, UK). Cream,* opaque, based on beeswax and mineral oil, available in a variety of tints. A range of other covering and tinting products is also available.

Keromask *(Innoxa, UK). Creams,* for masking and shading, with finishing powder.

Veil *(Blake, UK). Cream,* available in a range of shades.

1603-m

Crotamiton *(BAN, USAN, rINN).*

Crotam. *N*-Ethyl-*N*-*o*-tolylcrotonamide; *N*-Ethylcrotono-*o*-toluidide; *N*-Ethyl-*N*-(2-methylphenyl)-2-butenamide.

$C_{13}H_{17}NO=203.3$.

CAS — 483-63-6.

Pharmacopoeias. In *Br., Egypt.,* and *U.S.*

A colourless or pale yellow oily liquid with a faint amine-like odour. It solidifies partly or completely at low temperatures and it must be completely liquefied by warming before use. The *B.P.* specifies that it is predominantly the (*E*)-isomer, with not more than 15% of the (*Z*)-isomer. *U.S.P.* specifies a mixture of (*E*)- and (*Z*)- isomers.

Slightly **soluble** in water; miscible with alcohol, methyl alcohol, and ether. **Store** in small airtight containers. Protect from light.

Adverse Effects and Precautions

Applied topically, crotamiton occasionally causes irritation. There have been reports of sensitivity reactions. Crotamiton should not be used in the presence of acute exudative dermatitis. It should not be applied near the eyes.

Uses and Administration

Crotamiton is an acaricide and in the treatment of scabies a 10% cream or lotion is applied, after first bathing and drying, to the whole of the body surface below the chin particular attention being paid to body folds and creases. A second application is advisable 24 hours later. Appropriate measures should be taken to avoid reinfection especially from contaminated clothing and bed-linen.

Crotamiton is also an antipruritic agent and local application gives rapid relief from itching. It is used for the relief of anogenital pruritus, senile pruritus, and pruritus associated with various disorders. One application is usually effective for 6 to 10 hours.

Preparations

Crotamiton Cream *(B.P.)*

Crotamiton Cream *(U.S.P.)*

Crotamiton Lotion *(B.P.)*

Proprietary Preparations

Eurax *(Ciba Consumer, UK). Ointment,* crotamiton 10%. *Lotion,* crotamiton 10%.

Eurax-Hydrocortisone *(Geigy, UK). Cream,* crotamiton 10%, hydrocortisone 0.25%.

Proprietary Names and Manufacturers

Bestloid *(Jpn)*; Crotamitex *(Stockhausen, Ger.)*; Eurax *(Geigy, Austral.; Belg.; Ciba-Geigy, Canad.; Geigy, Fr.; Geigy, Ital.; Neth.; Geigy, Norw.; Geigy, S.Afr.; Geigy, Swed.; Geigy, Switz.; Ciba Consumer, UK; Westwood, USA)*; Euraxil *(Zyma, Ger.; Padro, Spain)*.

The following names have been used for multi-ingredient preparations containing crotamiton— Eurax-Hydrocortisone *(Geigy, UK)*; Teevex *(Geigy, UK)*.

1604-b

Dextranomer *(BAN, rINN).*

Dextran cross-linked with epichlorohydrin (1-chloro-2,3-epoxypropane); Dextran 2,3-dihydroxypropyl 2-hydroxypropane-1,3-diyl ether.

CAS — 56087-11-7.

Practically **insoluble** in water.

Precautions

Dextranomer should not be used in deep wounds or cavities from which its removal cannot be assured, nor should it be used on dry wounds. Care should be exercised when paste formulations of dextranomer are used near the eyes. Spillage may render surfaces very slippery.

Uses and Administration

The action of dextranomer depends upon its ability to absorb up to 4 times its weight of fluid, including dissolved and suspended material of molecular weight up to about 5000.

Dextranomer is used for the cleansing of exudative and infected wounds, including burns and ulcers, and for preparation for skin grafting. The wound is cleansed with sterile water or saline and allowed to remain wet; dextranomer in the form of spherical beads is sprinkled on to a depth of at least 3 mm and covered with a sterile dressing. Occlusive dressings are not recommended as they may lead to maceration around the wound. The dextranomer can be renewed up to 5 times daily (usually once or twice daily), before the layer has become saturated with exudate; the old layer is washed off with a stream of sterile water or saline before renewal. All dextranomer must be removed before skin grafting. Dextranomer may also be applied as a paste or a paste-containing absorbent pad which need only be changed twice daily to every 2 days according to the rate of wound exudation.

Cadexomer-iodine (p.1184) has similar properties of absorption and releases iodine.

Correctly used on exudative venous ulcers, with daily or more frequent changes, dextranomer accelerates removal of pus and necrotic debris, and may help to relieve pain. It is better than saline dressings for infected wounds, but whether it improves the rate of healing compared with antiseptic dressings is still not clear. It does not influence hard eschar, is ineffective on avascular ulcers and is not needed on healthy granulation tissue.— *Drug & Ther. Bull.,* 1984, *22,* 15.

The treatment time of alveolar osteitis (painful tooth sockets, 'dry sockets') was reduced by the use of dextranomer compared with the use of zinc oxide and eugenol dressings.— R. W. Matthews, *Br. dent. J.,* 1982, *152,* 157. Criticism of the methods used.— B. Mitchell (letter), *ibid.,* 261. Reply.— R. W. Matthews (letter), *ibid.*, 335.

Some references to the use of dextranomer: S. Jacobsson *et al.*, *Scand. J. plast. reconstr. Surg.*, 1976, *10*, 65 (benefit in leg ulcers and miscellaneous wounds); P. Paavolainen and B. Sundell, *Annls Chir. Gynaec. Fenn.*, 1976, *65*, 313 (improvement in burns); A. Lassus *et al.*, *Acta derm.-vener., Stockh.*, 1977, *57*, 361 (improvement in penile ulcers); G. Arturson *et al.*, *Burns*, 1978, *4*, 225 (improvement in burns); G. Eriksson *et al.*, *Curr. ther. Res.*, 1984, *35*, 678 (no difference between dextranomer and saline dressings in leg ulcers).

Proprietary Preparations

Debrisan *(Pharmacia, UK)*. *Beads*, dextranomer, diameter 100 to 300 µm.

Absorbent pad, dextranomer 90%, polyethylene glycol and water 10%, in textile bag.

Paste, dextranomer 6.4 g, polyethylene glycol and water 3.6 g.

Proprietary Names and Manufacturers

Debrisan *(Pharmacia, Austral.; Pharmacia, Canad.; Pharmacia, Denm.; Schering, Fr.; Neth.; Pharmacia, Norw.; NZ; Keatings, S.Afr.; Pharmacia, Swed.; Pharmacia, Switz.; Pharmacia, UK; Johnson & Johnson, USA)*; Debrisorb *(Parke, Davis, Ger.)*.

1605-v

Dihydroxyacetone

DHA; Ketotriose. 1,3-Dihydroxypropan-2-one.

$C_3H_6O_3$=90.08.

CAS — 96-26-4.

Adverse Effects and Precautions

Skin irritation and rashes have occasionally been reported. Avoid contact with eyes and clothing.

Uses and Administration

Applied to the skin as a lotion or cream, dihydroxyacetone causes the slow development of a brown coloration similar to that caused by exposure to the sun. The coloration is considered to be due to a reaction with the amino acids of the skin.

A single application may give rise to a patchy appearance; progressive darkening of the skin results from repeated use until a point is reached when no further darkening takes place. If the treatment is stopped the colour starts to fade after about 2 days and disappears completely within 8 to 14 days as the external epidermal cells are lost by normal attrition.

Creams and lotions containing 0.2 to 5% of dihydroxyacetone have been used. The presence of at least 20% of water is recommended; the colour reaction is most rapid in acid media and is facilitated by the addition of a surfactant; no reaction occurs above pH 8. Some preparations have included compounds such as lawsone for sun-screening purposes, since dihydroxyacetone gives no protection against sunburn.

Proprietary Names and Manufacturers

Vitadye *(Elder, Canad.; Elder, USA)*.

1606-g

Dithranol *(BAN, rINN)*.

Anthralin *(USAN)*; Dioxyanthranol. 1,8-Dihydroxyanthrone; 1,8-Dihydroxy-9(10*H*)-anthracenone.

$C_{14}H_{10}O_3$=226.2.

CAS — 1143-38-0.

Pharmacopoeias. In *Belg., Br., Cz., Ind., Swiss,* and *U.S.*

A yellow to orange-yellow or yellowish-brown, odourless, crystalline powder. Practically **insoluble** in water; slightly soluble in alcohol, ether, and glacial acetic acid; soluble in acetone, chloroform, solutions of alkali hydroxides, and fixed oils. The filtrate from a suspension in water is neutral to litmus. **Store** in airtight containers. Protect from light.

CAUTION. *Dithranol is a powerful irritant and should be kept away from the eyes and tender parts of the skin.*

In dithranol pastes containing zinc oxide the presence of salicylic (or benzoic) acid was necessary to prevent the development of discoloration due to interaction between dithranol and zinc oxide; such discoloration was indicative of ineffectiveness. Zinc oxide and starch could be omitted without loss of effectiveness provided stiffness was maintained. The effect of dithranol 0.25 or 0.5% in yellow soft paraffin was not affected by the presence or absence of 0.5 or 2.0% of salicylic acid. If milling facilities were not available, dithranol could be dissolved in chloroform and then dispersed in Lassar's paste.— S. Comaish *et al.*, *Br. J. Derm.*, 1971, *84*, 282.

Studies on the discoloration of various dithranol pastes. It was suggested that the application of heat, even indirect, should be avoided in the manufacture of dithranol pastes, and that metal spatulas should not be used.— Pharm. Soc. Lab. Rep. P/79/1, 1979.

A study evaluating the stability of dithranol in various bases. Stability was found to vary with concentration; weaker preparations being less stable. Dithranol was found to be unstable in yellow soft paraffin and 'Unguentum Merck', although ascorbic and oxalic acids could be added to the latter to increase stability. Salicylic acid produced a destabilising effect on dithranol in 'Unguentum Merck' and yellow soft paraffin, a stabilising effect in Lassar's paste, but little effect in white soft paraffin. Dithranol is relatively stable in white soft paraffin which is the preferred base for short-contact therapy. The inclusion of salicylic acid in these preparations is questionable because it has a negligible effect as an anti-oxidant, is irritant to the skin, and percutaneous absorption can be significant.— P. G. Green *et al.*, *Br. J. Derm.*, 1985, *113*, *Suppl.* 29, 26.

Adverse Effects and Precautions

Dithranol may cause a burning sensation especially on perilesional skin. It is irritant to the eyes and mucous membranes. Hands should be washed after use.

Dithranol should not be used for acute or pustular psoriasis or on inflamed skin. It stains skin, hair, some fabrics, plastics, and enamel. Staining of bathroom ware may be less of a problem with creams than ointments. Stains on skin and hair disappear on cessation of treatment.

EFFECTS ON THE SKIN. Kingston and Marks (*Br. J. Derm.*, 1983, *108*, 307) and Maurice and Greaves (*ibid.*, *109*, 337) found that fair-skinned individuals (skin type I, Boston Classification) were more sensitive to the irritant and erythemal effects of dithranol than those of skin types II to IV. Roberts (*ibid.*, 1984, *110*, 247) felt that complete absence of pigmentation predisposed to a marked increase in sensitivity in 2 vitiliginous patients who developed a severe inflammatory reaction with marked worsening of psoriasis after dithranol application.

It has been suggested that dithranol irritancy is due to free radical formation (M.J. Finnen *et al.*, *Lancet*, 1984, *2*, 1129; M.W. Greaves, *Br. J. Derm.*, 1984, *110*, 247), although there has been dispute concerning this mechanism (M. Whitefield *et al.*, *Lancet*, 1985, *1*, 173; Y. Paramsothy *et al.*, *Br. J. Derm.*, 1986, *115*, 251). Barr *et al.* (*Br. J. clin. Pharmac.*, 1983, *16*, 715) suggested that irritancy was due, in the early stages, to prostaglandin E_2, but this mechanism has also been disputed (C.M. Lawrence and S. Shuster, *Br. J. Derm.*, 1985, *113*, 107). Systemic pretreatment with indomethacin partially blocked the irritant response to dithranol (T. Kingston and R. Marks, *ibid.*, 1983, *108*, 307), but prednisone (L. Juhlin, *ibid.*, 1981, *105*, *Suppl.* 20, 87) chlorpheniramine, and aspirin (K. Misch *et al.*, *ibid.*, 82) were without effect. Pretreatment of the skin with erythemogenic u.v.-B and oral PUVA (L. Juhlin, 1981), coal tar solution (C.M. Lawrence *et al.*, *Br. J. Derm.*, 1984, *110*, 671), free-radical scavengers (M.J. Finnen *et al.*, 1984), high potency topical corticosteroids (C.M. Lawrence and S. Shuster, *Br. J. Derm.*, 1985, *113*, 117), potassium hydroxide solution, or an anionic surfactant solution (Teepol) (C.M. Lawrence *et al.*, *ibid.*, 1987, *116*, 171) have all been tried with some success, although low concentrations of dithranol itself were ineffective (C.M. Lawrence and S. Shuster, *ibid.*, 1985, *113*, 117). Kingston and Lowe (*Br. J. Derm.*, 1986, *115*, *Suppl.* 31, 80) found that reducing dithranol contact time from 24 hours to one hour was significantly more effective in reducing irritancy than pretreatment with suberythemogenic u.v.-B or coal tar.

Uses and Administration

Dithranol is used in the treatment of psoriasis. Conventional treatment is commonly started with an ointment or paste containing 0.1% dithranol (0.05% in very fair patients) applied for 2 hours or longer; the strength is gradually increased as necessary to 0.5 or 0.6%, occasionally to 1%, and the duration of contact extended to overnight periods or longer. The preparation is sparingly and accurately applied to the lesions only. If, on initial treatment, lesions spread or excessive irritation occurs, the concentration of dithranol or the frequency of application should be reduced; if necessary, treatment should be stopped. The face, skin flexures, and genitals are particularly sensitive. After each treatment period the patient should bathe or shower to remove any residual dithranol.

With short contact therapy dithranol up to 2% in a soft base is applied to the lesions for 30 to 60 minutes daily, or occasionally longer, before being washed off. Surrounding unaffected skin may be protected by the prior use of white soft paraffin. If stick formulations are used, overnight treatment may be started with 1% dithranol and reduced to 0.5% or increased to 2% as necessary. The 2% concentration is more suitable for short contact therapy. Treatment should be continued until the skin is entirely clear. Intermittent courses may be needed to maintain the response. Treatment schedules often involve coal tar and u.v. irradiation (preferably u.v.-B) before the application of dithranol. An example is the Ingram regimen (see below). Salicylic acid is included in many topical preparations of dithranol as a stabiliser or antoxidant.

Dithranol has been reported to possess fungicidal properties.

Butantrone (10-butyryldithranol) has been used similarly to dithranol but is claimed to cause less staining and skin irritation.

The mechanism of action of dithranol is unknown in detail. Dithranol, its 10-acetyl analogue, and dimers completely inhibit cell growth and thymidine incorporation in human cultured cells, and inhibit both DNA replication and repair synthesis. The interference seems to be specific for mitochondrial DNA.— E. M. Farber and L. Nall, *Drugs*, 1984, *28*, 324.

In vitro experiments on isolated *rat* liver mitochondria showed that dithranol acted as an uncoupler of oxidative phosphorylation and suggested that it could inhibit the adenosine triphosphate supply in epidermal cells. This loss of energy supply in keratinocytes could explain, at least in part, the therapeutic efficiency of dithranol in psoriasis.— P. Morlière *et al.*, *Br. J. Derm.*, 1985, *112*, 509.

ALOPECIA. Dithranol applied at concentrations sufficient to maintain a mild contact dermatitis (0.1% to 0.5%) in 10 patients with alopecia areata failed to stimulate hair regrowth.— D. A. Nelson and R. L. Spielvogel, *Int. J. Derm.*, 1985, *24*, 606.

PSORIASIS. The larger and fewer the psoriatic plaques, the more feasible and appropriate is dithranol; the smaller and more numerous, the less appropriate is dithranol, leaving tar or corticosteroids as the options. If tar fails, dithranol should be tried; used skilfully, it is faster and more effective. Under in-patient conditions or in day-centre treatment, dithranol in a stiff vehicle e.g. dithranol paste *B.P.*, is highly effective and will clear most psoriasis within 3 weeks. Unlike tar, dithranol must be used carefully. Under out-patient domestic conditions, dithranol in a cream formulation may be found easier to handle, although response may be less satisfactory.— H. Baker, *Prescribers' J.*, 1982, *22*, 64.

Combination with etretinate. For the combined use of dithranol with etretinate in psoriasis, see p.922.

Combination with u.v. irradiation. In the complete form of the Ingram regimen, the patient was soaked in a warm tar bath, dried, and exposed to u.v. light to produce the slightest erythematous reaction. Each psoriatic lesion was then obscured with dithranol 0.4% in Lassar's paste, dressings applied, and left for 24 hours; the procedure was then repeated (J.T. Ingram, *Br. med. J.*, 1953, *2*, 591). A modification of this regimen, reported to be as effective, consisted of a daily hot tar bath followed by incremental u.v. irradiation and corticosteroid cream application to the lesions every 3 hours. Dithranol 0.1 to 0.4% in a stiff paste was applied overnight; irritation and staining were minimised (E.M. Farber and D.R. Harris, *Archs Derm.*, 1970, *101*, 381). Young (*Br. J. Derm.*, 1970, *82*, 516) found that a modification of the Ingram regimen in which the tar bath or u.v. irradiation were omitted was no less effective than the standard regimen, and this was confirmed by Seville (*ibid.*, 1975, *93*, 205). A possible explanation is that lamps with substantial u.v.-C emission, such as the mercury arc lamps most commonly used in the *UK* have little effect because delivery of therapeutic doses of u.v.-B is limited by erythema induced by u.v.-C (P.M. Farr *et al.*, *Br. med. J.*, 1987, *294*, 205). Hindson *et al.* (*Br. J. Derm.*, 1983, *108*, 457) investigated the effect of combining u.v.-A irradiation with short-contact dithranol therapy and reported a favourable clearance time for psoriasis, but Reshad *et al.* (*ibid.*, 1984, *111*, 155), in a study controlled for the beneficial effects of short-contact therapy alone, found no benefit from additional u.v.-A exposure.

In a study of 224 patients with chronic plaque psoriasis, treated with either a modified Ingram dithranol regimen or PUVA (see p.927), lesions in 91% of the PUVA group and 82% of the dithranol group cleared satisfactorily. Clearing took longer with PUVA treatment (mean 34.4 days) than with dithranol (mean 20.4 days), but took less patient and nurse time and was more convenient and acceptable to the patients. Twelve of 16 patients in whom dithranol failed responded to PUVA and 3 of 3 in whom PUVA failed responded to dithranol (S. Rogers *et al.*, *Lancet*, 1979, *1*, 455). Relapse rate in 53 patients with plaque psoriasis after clearing with PUVA was found to be the same as in 76 patients cleared with dithranol when no maintenance treatment was given. The estimated probability of remaining in remission at 16 months was about 13%. However, in 112 patients given maintenance PUVA either weekly or once every 3 weeks after initial clearing with PUVA, relapse rate was reduced such that the estimated probability of remaining in remission at 16 months was about 80%. There was no difference in relapse rate whichever maintenance PUVA schedule was used (D.V. Briffa *et al.*, *Br. med. J.*, 1981, *282*, 937). In 41 patients whose psoriasis had been cleared with dithranol and who were then given maintenance PUVA once weekly, the estimated probability of remaining in remission at 16 months was 42% (J.M. Marks *et al.*, *ibid.*, 1984, *288*, 95). Patients in remission who withdrew from PUVA maintenance had a low relapse rate; one year after withdrawal, half were still well (P.C.M. van de Kerkhof, *ibid.*, 939).

Continuous application at low dithranol concentration. Twenty-four patients with psoriasis were treated with continuous application of dithranol 0.01 to 0.05% with salicylic acid 4 to 10% in a soft base. Between 4½ to 14½ month's treatment was needed for a response of considerable improvement to complete clearing in 17 patients, including 1 with pustular psoriasis. There was no irritation of psoriatic or non-involved skin nor was there staining of skin, hair, nails, or clothing.— I. Brody and A. Johansson, *J. cutaneous Pathol.*, 1977, *4*, 233.

Short-contact and 'minutes' therapy. Following a preliminary study suggesting that a 1 hour application of dithranol may be effective in the treatment of psoriasis (H. Schaefer *et al.*, *Br. J. Derm.*, 1980, *102*, 571), two studies found that daily application for 1 to 3 hours (short-contact therapy) of dithranol 0.1% to 2% with salicylic acid as a stabiliser in soft bases was as effective as 24 hour application in clearing psoriasis (U. Runne and J. Kunze, *ibid.*, 1982, *106*, 135; J.R. Marsden *et al.*, *ibid.*, 1983, *109*, 209). Therapy for 10 to 30 minutes daily ('minutes' therapy) was also effective, although there was disagreement about the rate of improvement compared to 24 hour regimens (B.N. Statham *et al.*, *Br. J. Derm.*, 1984, *110*, 703). Jones *et al.* (*ibid.*, 1985, *113*, 331) found 30-minute and overnight therapy with dithranol concentrations of 1% to 3% to be equally effective in clearing plaque psoriasis in 30 patients. MacDonald and Marks (*ibid.*, 1986, *114*, 235), investigating dithranol 2% at contact times between immediate removal and 20 minutes in 18 patients with chronic plaque psoriasis, found clinical efficacy and side-effects to be independent of contact time. Ryatt *et al.* (*ibid.*, 1984, *111*, 455) used dithranol 0.5% to 3% in Lassar's paste due to the increased skin irritation reported with the softer bases by Marsden *et al.*, 1983 and Statham *et al.*, 1984. Application for 2 hours daily in 12 patients with plaque psoriasis was as effective as the standard Ingram regimen, whereas application for 30 minutes daily in 21 similar patients was less effective until day 20 of treatment.

Reports of the successful home management of psoriatic patients using short-contact therapy.— J. Donaldson and W. J. Cunliffe, *Br. med. J.*, 1983, *286*, 1939; R. H. Seville (letter), *ibid.*, *287*, 503.

Stick formulation. Reports of equal efficacy, but easier application and greater patient preference for dithranol in a paraffin-based stick formulation compared to paste or cream in the treatment of psoriasis: H. Gisslèn and P. Nordin, *J. int. med. Res.*, 1983, *11*, 46; G. Agrup and J. Agdell, *Br. J. clin. Pract.*, 1985, *39*, 185; U. Eilard and L. Edin, *ibid.*, 232.

Preparations

Anthralin Cream *(U.S.P.)*. Dithranol cream.

Anthralin Ointment *(U.S.P.)*. Dithranol ointment.

Dithranol and Salicylic Acid Ointment (Water-Washable) *(A.P.F.)*. Dithranol 100 mg, salicylic acid 500 mg, liquid paraffin 20 g, emulsifying ointment to 100 g.

Dithranol Ointment *(B.P., A.P.F.)*. Contains dithranol, in fine powder, in yellow soft paraffin.

Dithranol Paste *(B.P., A.P.F.)*. Dithranol and Zinc Paste. Dithranol 100 mg, zinc and salicylic acid paste to 100 g.

Proprietary Preparations

Anthranol *(Stiefel, UK)*. *Ointment*, dithranol 0.4%, 1.0%, and 2.0%.

Antraderm *(Brocades, UK)*. *Application stick*, dithranol 1%, in a solid wax basis.
Application stick (Antraderm Mild), dithranol 0.5%, in a solid wax basis.
Application stick (Antraderm Forte), dithranol 2%, in a solid wax basis.

Dithrocream *(Dermal Laboratories, UK)*. *Cream*, dithranol 0.1%, 0.25%, and 2.0%.
Cream (Dithrocream Forte), dithranol 0.5%.
Cream (Dithrocream HP), dithranol 1.0%.

Dithrolan *(Dermal Laboratories, UK)*. *Ointment*, dithranol 0.5%, salicylic acid 0.5%.

Psoradrate *(Norwich-Eaton, UK)*. *Cream*, dithranol 0.1%, 0.2%, and 0.4% with urea.

Psorin *(Thames, UK)*. *Ointment*, dithranol 0.11%, crude coal tar 1.1%, salicylic acid 1.6%.
Ointment (Psorin Forte), dithranol 0.32%, crude coal tar 1.0%, salicylic acid 3.2%.

Proprietary Names and Manufacturers

Amitase *(Schering Corp., Denm.; Schering, Norw.; Schering, Swed.)*; Anthra-Derm *(Canad.; Dermik, USA)*; Anthraderm *(Pharma-Medica, Denm.)*; Anthraforte *(Stiefel, Canad.)*; Anthranol *(Stiefel, Canad.; Stiefel, UK)*; Antraderm *(Protea, Austral.; Brocades, UK)*; Dicream *(Essex, Austral.)*; Dithrocream *(Dermal Laboratories, UK)*; Dithro-Crème *(Essex, Switz.)*; Dithroderm *(Wilson, Pakistan)*; Drithocreme *(American Dermal, USA)*; Dritho-Scalp *(American Dermal, USA)*; Lasan *(Canad.; Stiefel, USA)*; Lasan HP-1 *(Stiefel, USA)*; Psoralon *(Hermal, Switz.)*; Psorex *(Pharma-medica, Switz.)*.

The following names have been used for multi-ingredient preparations containing dithranol—Dithraderm *(Dermacare, Austral.)*; Dithrolan *(Dermal Laboratories, UK)*; Psoradrate *(Norwich-Eaton, Austral.; Norwich-Eaton, UK)*; Psorin *(Cambden, Austral.; Thames, UK)*; Stie-Lasan *(Stiefel, UK)*.

1607-q

Dithranol Triacetate *(BANM, rINNM)*.

Dithranol Acetate. 1,8,9-Triacetoxyanthracene.

$C_{20}H_{16}O_6$=352.3.

CAS — 16203-97-7.

Dithranol triacetate is hydrolysed in contact with water to form the active diacetyl compound, 1,8-diacetoxy-9-anthranol. It is claimed to be less staining and irritant to the skin than dithranol and is used similarly in the treatment of psoriasis as a 1% cream.

In a comparison of dithranol with dithranol triacetate in 20 patients with chronic psoriasis, the relative absence of inflammatory reactions and skin staining with the triacetate was confirmed. It was concluded that dithranol triacetate was less effective and slower to exert its therapeutic action than dithranol in the treatment of chronic psoriasis.— C. Hodgson and E. Hell, *Br. J. Derm.*, 1970, *83*, 397.

Proprietary Preparations

Exolan *(Dermal Laboratories, UK)*. *Cream*, dithranol triacetate 1%.

Proprietary Names and Manufacturers

The following names have been used for multi-ingredient preparations containing dithranol triacetate— Exolan Lotion *(Dermal Laboratories, UK)*.

1608-p

Enoxolone *(BAN, rINN)*.

Glycyrrhetic Acid; Glycyrrhetinic Acid. 3β-Hydroxy-11-oxo-olean-12-en-30-oic acid.

$C_{30}H_{46}O_4$=470.7.

CAS — 471-53-4.

A complex triterpene prepared from glycyrrhizinic acid.

Enoxolone is applied topically as ointment or suppositories in noninfective inflammatory skin or rectal disorders.

Proprietary Names and Manufacturers

PO 12 *(Biothérax, Fr.)*.

16638-n

Ethyl Lactate

$C_5H_{10}O_3$=118.1.

CAS — 97-64-3.

Ethyl lactate is applied topically in the treatment of acne vulgaris. It is reported to lower the pH within the skin thereby exerting a bactericidal effect.

Proprietary Preparations

Tri-ac *(Ciba Consumer, UK)*. *Lotion*, ethyl lactate 10%, zinc sulphate 0.3%.

1609-s

Etretinate *(BAN, USAN, rINN)*.

Ro-10-9359. Ethyl 3-methoxy-15-apo-φ-caroten-15-oate; Ethyl (*all-trans*)-9-(4-methoxy-2,3,6-trimethylphenyl)-3,7-dimethylnona-2,4,6,8-tetraenoate.

$C_{23}H_{30}O_3$=354.5.

CAS — 54350-48-0.

Adverse Effects

The adverse effects of etretinate are similar to those of vitamin A (p.1278) and isotretinoin (p.923) and are generally reversible and dose-related. Etretinate can cause dryness of the mucous membranes, sometimes with erosion, involving the lips (cheilitis), mouth, conjunctiva, sometimes causing conjunctivitis, and nasal mucosa, rarely causing epistaxis. Dryness of the skin may be associated with scaling, thinning, pruritus, exfoliation, and erythema. Hair thinning and alopecia may occur, usually 4 to 8 weeks after starting therapy. Skeletal hyperostosis, benign intracranial hypertension, musculo-skeletal pain, gastro-intestinal effects, and paronychia have been reported. Elevation of serum-hepatic-enzyme and triglyceride concentrations may occur.

Etretinate is teratogenic.

EFFECTS ON THE CARDIOVASCULAR SYSTEM. The Italian Ministry of Health was re-evaluating etretinate as a result of rare suspected cases of myocardial ischaemia and infarction reported in treated patients.— *WHO Drug Inf.*, 1987, *1*, 29.

EFFECTS ON THE EARS. Earache developed in 2 patients after receiving etretinate 50 to 75 mg daily for 2 to 3 weeks, but became less severe or disappeared on reduction of dosage or cessation of treatment.— L. Juhlin, *Acta derm.-vener., Stockh.*, 1983, *63*, 181.

EFFECTS ON THE EYES. Alterations in colour sense in 4 patients associated with prolonged etretinate therapy.— U. Weber (letter), *Lancet*, 1988, *1*, 236.

EFFECTS ON THE KIDNEY. A report of impaired renal function and hypercalcaemia associated with etretinate 25 mg daily for 36 months, given for prevention of recurrent superficial bladder tumours.— F. F. Horber *et al.* (letter), *Lancet*, 1984, *2*, 1093.

Oedema. Generalised oedema developed in a patient 14 days after commencing oral etretinate 1 mg per kg daily for psoriasis.— K. Moulopoulou-Karakitsou *et al.*, *Br. J. Derm.*, 1981, *104*, 709. A report of generalised oedema after etretinate 0.8 mg per kg daily for 3 weeks in a patient with pityriasis rubra pilaris.— J. Lauharanta (letter), *ibid.*, 1982, *106*, 251.

EFFECTS ON THE LIVER. Etretinate commonly causes transient slight elevations of serum concentrations of aminotransferases, lactate dehydrogenase, and alkaline phosphatase, but there have been few reports of acute hepatitis (E.K. Foged and F.K. Jacobsen, *Dermatologica*, 1982, *164*, 395; V.C. Weiss *et al.*, *Archs Derm.*, 1984, *120*, 104) or cholestatic jaundice (D. Gavish *et al.*, *J. Am. Acad. Derm.*, 1985, *13*, 669) after its administration. In one patient, acute hepatitis progressed to chronic active hepatitis, despite cessation of etretinate therapy (V.C. Weiss *et al.*, *Br. J. Derm.*, 1985, *112*, 591) but studies examining serial liver biopsies from patients receiving long-term etretinate have failed to show any significant chronic liver damage (S.D. Glazer *et al.*, *J. Am. Acad. Derm.*, 1984, *10*, 632; E. Foged *et al.*, *ibid.*, *11*, 580; H.H. Roenigk *et al.*, *Br. J. Derm.*, 1985, *112*, 77). The manufacturers have reported instances of hepatic fibrosis, necrosis, and/or cirrhosis.

EFFECTS ON THE MUSCULOSKELETAL SYSTEM. Diffuse hyperostosis in a 38-year-old man associated with long-term etretinate therapy.— S. Burge and T. Ryan (letter), *Lancet*, 1985, *2*, 397. A 4-year-old child with a major form of ichthyosis was treated with etretinate at doses of more than 1 mg per kg body-weight over a 7-year period. Laboratory results and radiological studies showed no evidence of adverse effects on growth or ossification.— P. Brun and R. Baran, *Curr. ther. Res.*, 1986, *40*, 657. Of 38 patients who had received an average etretinate dose of 0.8 mg per kg daily for an average of 60 months, 32 had radiographic evidence of extraspinal tendon and ligament calcification. The most commonly involved sites were the ankles (29 patients), pelvis (20), and knees (16) and involvement tended to be bilateral and multifocal. Spine involvement was uncommon. Fifteen of the 32 affected patients had no bone or joint symptoms at the sites of radiographic abnormality.— J. J. DiGiovanna *et al.*, *New Engl. J. Med.*, 1986, *315*, 1177. A report of spinal hyperostosis in 13 of 18 patients treated with etretinate 25 to 50 mg daily for 6 months to 4 years.— C. B. Archer *et al.* (letter), *Lancet*, 1987, *1*, 741. See also B. Melnick *et al.*, *Br. J. Derm.*, 1987, *116*, 207.

EFFECTS ON THE NAILS. Severe nail dystrophy in 2 patients associated with etretinate therapy.— M. M. Ferguson *et al.* (letter), *Lancet*, 1983, *2*, 974.

EFFECTS ON THE SERUM LIPIDS. After 16 weeks treatment with etretinate 0.5 to 1.5 mg per kg daily, the mean serum-triglyceride concentration in 21 psoriatic patients was significantly increased compared to the pre-treatment mean. The serum-triglyceride concentration exceeded the normal range in 10 of 13 patients starting therapy with normal values. The mean serum-cholesterol level for all patients was also significantly increased. The mean serum-triglyceride concentration had returned to its pre-treatment value by 8 weeks after cessation of therapy, but serum cholesterol was still increased in 6 patients. The mean high-density-lipoprotein (HDL) cholesterol concentration did not change significantly during the study. The benefits of prolonged etretinate therapy must be weighed against the risks of such treatment in patients whose serum-lipid concentrations increase over their pre-therapy values.— C. N. Ellis *et al.*, *Archs Derm.*, 1982, *118*, 559. The daily administration of 15 mL of an oil containing eicosapentaenoic acid (MaxEPA) by mouth for one month decreased raised serum-cholesterol values and significantly decreased raised serum-triglyceride values in 7 psoriatic patients receiving etretinate 50 or 75 mg daily.— J. R. Marsden, *Br. J. Derm.*, 1987, *116*, 450.

EFFECTS ON THE SKIN. Multiple pyogenic granulomata occurred in 2 patients during etretinate therapy.— D. M. Williamson and R. Greenwood (letter), *Br. J. Derm.*, 1983, *109*, 615. A report of erythroderma in a patient receiving etretinate 25 mg daily for psoriasis.— J. Levin and J. Almeyda (letter), *ibid.*, 1985, *112*, 373.

Five psoriatic patients developed papular lesions of the palms and soles shortly after beginning treatment with etretinate at an initial daily dose of 1 mg per kg body-weight. The lesions disappeared without tapering the dose.— M. David *et al.*, *Acta derm.-vener., Stockh.*, 1986, *66*, 87.

In vitro photohaemolysis studies demonstrated that tretinoin and isotretinoin have a phototoxic potential while etretinate has none. However, acitretin the major metabolite of etretinate had a phototoxic potential greater than that of tretinoin. The apparently low incidence of photosensitivity suggested that an idiosyncracy is responsible. Patients should use appropriate photoprotection against u.v.-B and u.v.-A wavebands.— J. Ferguson and B. E. Johnson, *Br. J. Derm.*, 1986, *115*, 275.

Nodular prurigo-like eruptions occurred in 2 patients during etretinate therapy.— J. Boer and G. Smeenk, *Br. J. Derm.*, 1987, *116*, 271.

INTRACRANIAL HYPERTENSION. A report of benign intracranial hypertension, due to acute hypervitaminosis A, in a patient receiving etretinate for Darier's disease in doses between 1.0 and 0.3 mg per kg body-weight.— J. M. Bonnetblanc *et al.* (letter), *Lancet*, 1983, *2*, 974.

MALIGNANT NEOPLASMS. A report of 2 patients developing lymphomas while receiving etretinate (P.J. Woll *et al.*, *Lancet*, 1987, *2*, 563) prompted a report of 3 other malignancies in patients taking etretinate (P.V. Harrison, *ibid.*, 801). However, Cunliffe *et al.* (*ibid.*, 1525) pointed to interest in etretinate being used to treat myelodysplastic disorders and to treat and prevent neoplasia.

PREGNANCY AND THE NEONATE. A report of skeletal deformations in a foetus conceived 4 months after the mother's last dose of etretinate.— W. Grote *et al.* (letter), *Lancet*, 1985, *1*, 1276.

Precautions

Etretinate is teratogenic and treatment should not be started in pregnant patients; also pregnancy should be avoided during treatment and for 2 years after treatment has been withdrawn. Etretinate is contra-indicated in hepatic and renal impairment, hypervitaminosis A, and in breast-feeding mothers.

Liver function and fasting blood lipids should be monitored at the start of therapy, 1 month after initiating therapy, and 3-monthly thereafter. Children receiving long-term therapy should be carefully monitored for any abnormalities of musculo-skeletal development. Patients receiving etretinate should avoid dietary supplements of vitamin A and should not donate blood during, or for 2 years after cessation of therapy.

Absorption and Fate

Following oral administration etretinate undergoes significant first pass metabolism and plasma concentrations of the active carboxyl-acid metabolite (acitretin) may be detected before those of the parent drug. Both etretinate and acitretin are extensively bound to plasma protein; on multiple dosing they have a prolonged half-life. Etretinate is excreted in the faeces mainly as unchanged drug and in the urine as metabolites.

References to the pharmacokinetics of etretinate: R. K. Brazzell and W. A. Colburn, *J. Am. Acad. Derm.*, 1982, *6*, 643; O. Rollman and A. Vahlquist, *Br. J. Derm.*, 1983, *109*, 439; W. A. Colburn *et al.*, *J. clin. Pharmac.*, 1985, *25*, 583; R. W. Lucek and W. A. Colburn, *Clin. Pharmacokinet.*, 1985, *10*, 38.

Data indicating that chronic dosing of etretinate with milk or a high fat meal compared to fasting conditions would result in higher concentrations of etretinate, which may ultimately lead to higher metabolite concentrations.— W. A. Colburn *et al.*, *J. clin. Pharmac.*, 1985, *25*, 583.

Uses and Administration

Etretinate is a derivative of tretinoin (p.935). It is given by mouth for the treatment of severe, extensive psoriasis that has not responded to other treatment. It is also used in palmo-plantar pustular psoriasis, severe congenital ichthyosis, and severe Darier's disease (keratosis follicularis) as well as other disorders of keratinisation.

The recommended initial daily dose of etretinate is up to 0.75 mg per kg body-weight, given by mouth in divided doses for 2 to 4 weeks. The dose may then be increased to 1 mg per kg daily if the therapeutic response is inadequate, but a total daily dose of 75 mg should not be exceeded. Once a response has been achieved, the dose should be reduced to 0.5 mg per kg daily, in divided doses and be given for a further 6 to 8 weeks. When patients, especially those with psoriasis or Darier's disease, obtain no further improvement, etretinate should normally be discontinued and patients may experience a worthwhile period of remission. Any subsequent exacerbations may be treated intermittently as necessary. Some patients, especially those with congenital ichthyosis, may experience such a short remission that maintenance therapy should be continued at the lowest dose that will prevent recurrences, usually 0.25 to 0.5 mg per kg daily. Children have been given the same dose as adults with the exception of long-term maintenance therapy which is not recommended.

The etretinate derivatives dichloroetretinate (Ro-12-7554), fenretinide (4-hydroxyphenylretinamide), and an arotinoid ethyl ester (Ro-13-6298; Ro-13-7410) are being investigated as dermatological and antineoplastic agents.

Reviews of etretinate: A. Ward *et al.*, *Drugs*, 1983, *26*, 9; *Med. Lett.*, 1987, *29*, 9; C. E. Orfanos *et al.*, *Drugs*, 1987, *34*, 459.

ACNE. Etretinate was given for 8 weeks at a daily dose of 1 mg per kg body-weight to 8 male patients with severe acne of 2 to 11 years' duration. Of 7 completing the study, 6 showed improvement and 5 had fewer acne lesions. Sebum excretion-rate was not measured because it has been reported that the dramatic reduction in sebaceous gland size, observed in patients receiving isotretinoin, is not seen with etretinate.— R. M. MacKie and D. C. Dick (letter), *Lancet*, 1980, *2*, 1300. A further report.— J. Wishart, *Aust. J. Derm.*, 1982, *23*, 24.

AMYLOIDOSIS. A report of apparent total regression of secondary amyloidosis in a psoriatic patient given etretinate.— E. af Ekenstam *et al.*, *Br. med. J.*, 1986, *293*, 733.

KERATINISATION DISORDERS. A report of the use of etretinate in several keratinisation disorders.— P. A. Viglioglia, *Br. J. Derm.*, 1980, *103*, 483.

A report of eruptive keratoacanthoma in a 63-year-old Japanese woman which responded well to etretinate by mouth. Treatment began with 40 mg daily reduced ultimately to a maintenance dose of 10 mg daily or on alternate days. Lesions reappeared when therapy was stopped.— K. Yoshikawa *et al.*, *Br. J. Derm.*, 1985, *112*, 579. See also.— E. Blitstein-Willinger *et al.*, *ibid.*, 1986, *114*, 109.

Etretinate controlled the skin symptoms and the pruritus of a patient with disseminated superficial actinic porokeratosis.— A. -L. Kariniemi *et al.*, *Br. J. Derm.*, 1980, *102*, 213.

In a double-blind study, 44 patients with actinic keratosis received oral etretinate 75 mg daily or placebo for 2 months, followed by the alternative therapy for a further 2 months. Thirty-seven of 44 patients had a complete or partial response with etretinate, compared to 2 of 42 receiving placebo. Response to treatment occurred within the first month and was maintained even when the dose was reduced because of toxicity.— M. Moriarty *et al.*, *Lancet*, 1982, *1*, 364. See also A. D. Pearse *et al.*, *ibid.*, 1987, *116*, 420.

Almost complete clinical clearance of Bazex paraneoplastic acrokeratosis with oral etretinate.— J. M. Wishart, *Br. J. Derm.*, 1986, *115*, 595.

Darier's disease. Seventeen patients with moderate to severe Darier's disease were given etretinate 25 mg twice daily for up to 10 weeks. Within 2 to 6 weeks, 6 patients demonstrated complete or nearly complete clearing, 5 stopped treatment because of side-effects (isomorphic reactions, pruritus, transient abdominal pain) and 6 continued for 10 weeks with progressive improvement. There was no initial worsening like that occasionally seen in psoriasis. The improvement of the trunk was slightly faster than of the head. Palms and soles showed slight improvement. Nails did not improve. Erythema, papules, and hyperkeratosis were reduced equivalently during the first 4 weeks; thereafter, erythema was reduced less favourably. All patients relapsed 6 days to 10 months after the end of the first treatment period; patients with severe disease had the shortest remissions and all patients with moderate disease had remissions exceeding 4 weeks. Patients retreated with mean doses of 0.41 to 0.61 mg per kg body-weight daily for 6.0 to 7.5 weeks showed similar improvement to that seen after the first course and side-effects were usually milder, although there was still a tendency to isomorphic reactions in some patients.— G. -B. Löwhagen *et al.*, *Dermatologica*, 1982, *165*, 123. See also S. M. Burge *et al.*, *Br. J. Derm.*, 1981, *104*, 675.

Ichthyosiform erythroderma. Marked improvement of ichthyosiform erythroderma with etretinate.— R. S. Matthews, *Br. J. Derm.*, 1984, *111*, *Suppl.* 26, 75. Another report.— D. Burrows, *ibid.*, 76. See also A. D. Pearse *et al.*, *ibid.*, 1986, *114*, 285.

Pityriasis rubra. Moderate to marked clinical improvement in 5 patients with pityriasis rubra pilaris treated with etretinate 0.5 to 1 mg per kg daily for up to 14 weeks.— L. Kanerva *et al.*, *Br. J. Derm.*, 1983, *108*, 653.

LICHEN PLANUS. A double-blind study of 28 patients with severe oral lichen planus showed that etretinate 75 mg daily by mouth had a marked beneficial effect, but the lesions did not usually disappear completely, relapses were common when medication had been discontinued and treatment probably did not shorten the natural course of the disease.— K. Hersle *et al.*, *Br. J. Derm.*, 1982, *106*, 77.

MALIGNANT NEOPLASMS. After 34 days treatment with etretinate 1 mg per kg body-weight daily, there was complete flattening of the lesions of mycosis fungoides in a 77-year-old woman and the mononuclear cell infiltrate decreased significantly. No clinical recurrences occurred after a 4-month follow-up, but discontinuation of etretinate led to a relapse in 3 weeks.— A. L. Claudy *et al.*, *Arch. dermatol. Res.*, 1982, *273*, 37.

The use of etretinate in 12 patients with various cutaneous lymphomas.— A. L. Claudy *et al.*, *Br. J. Derm.*, 1983, *109*, 49.

In a double-blind multicentre trial, 65 patients with recurrent superficial bladder tumours received etretinate 25 to 50 mg daily by mouth or placebo after tumour resection for 2 or more years. During the first year there was a decrease in the number of tumours and resections in the etretinate group, which was not significant. The incidence of recurrent bladder tumours after 3, 12, and 24 months was always lower in the etretinate group and the number of simultaneous multifocal recurrences was significantly lower.— U. E. Studer *et al.*, *J. Urol., Baltimore*, 1984, *131*, 47.

See also under Keratinisation Disorders.

PSORIASIS. Reviews of the use of etretinate in psoriasis: A. Ward *et al.*, *Drugs*, 1983, *26*, 9; *Med. Lett.*, 1987, *29*, 9.

In a 12 month double-blind crossover study, 74 patients with severe psoriasis of long duration received by mouth placebo or etretinate 100 mg daily, reduced after 2 weeks to 50 mg daily and, in some patients to 25 mg daily, for alternating 3-month periods. The severity of erythema, desquamation and infiltration were less, the extent of psoriasis was reduced and more patients were in complete remission after etretinate than placebo. Side-effects on uninvolved skin and mucous membranes seemed to be largely dose-dependent.— A. Lassus, *Br. J. Derm.*, 1980, *102*, 195.

After initial skin clearing, 36 psoriatic patients were given maintenance treatment of daily placebo or etretinate, at half of the maximal dose tolerated during the clearing phase, for 1 year. At the end of treatment relapses had occurred in 15 of 18 patients receiving placebo and 6 of 15 receiving etretinate.— L. Dubertret *et al.*, *Br. J. Derm.*, 1985, *113*, 323.

Twenty patients with palmoplantar pustular psoriasis were treated for 4 weeks with etretinate 70 mg daily by mouth, leading to clinical improvement and a significant fall in mean pustule count. Sixteen of these patients then received either placebo or etretinate 30 mg daily for 12 weeks. There was a rapid deterioration in the clinical condition and a rise in mean pustule count in the placebo group, but the etretinate group still showed moderate-to-good improvement in 6 of 8 patients and a significantly lower mean pustule count after 12 weeks. Only 1 patient withdrew from the study because of side-effects during the high-dose period. Adverse effects on liver function and serum lipids were not found.— S. I. White *et al.*, *Br. J. Derm.*, 1986, *115*, 577.

Combination therapy. Pustular types of psoriasis responded rather early in a few days and cleared in a few weeks after high doses of etretinate in the range of 75 mg daily. Erythrodermic types, or patients who tended to develop erythroderma, responded better to rather lower doses, 23 to 35 mg daily over a longer period (8 to 10 weeks). Plaque type of common psoriasis responds to etretinate if given alone or combined with dithranol, PUVA, u.v.-B, and with topical corticosteroids. These combinations produced earlier clearing and longer remissions.— E. M. Farber and L. Nall, *Drugs*, 1984, *28*, 324.

Combination therapy with dithranol. Twelve patients with widespread psoriasis were treated with oral etretinate 75 to 125 mg daily for 2 to 6 weeks. Six of these patients also received concomitant local treatment with salicylic acid 2% in petrolatum. Of these 1 had a very good response (full remission, nearly all lesions cleared), 2 had good responses (remission, over 75% of the lesions flattened), 1 had a moderate response (less than 75% of lesions improved), and in 2 response was deemed insufficient. The other 6 patients received local treatment with dithranol 0.1% and salicylic acid 2% in petrolatum. Very good responses were obtained in 4 and good responses in 2. The combined application of etretinate with low concentrations of dithranol seemed to increase the clinical response and to shorten the duration of the traditional local treatment.— C. E. Orfanos and U. Runne, *Br. J. Derm.*, 1976, *95*, 101.

Combination therapy with methotrexate. Two male patients with severe erythrodermic psoriasis and pustular episodes were successfully treated with etretinate 20 to 70 mg daily by mouth and methotrexate 10 to 20 mg weekly intravenously for 2½ years. Attempts to taper and then discontinue dosage of methotrexate resulted in loss of control of psoriasis. Caution must be exercised in the use of this combination regimen until it is determined whether the incidence of toxic hepatitis is increased with either short- or long-term treatment.— E. Tuyp and R. M. MacKie, *J. Am. Acad. Derm.*, 1986, *14*, 70 (see also under interactions with methotrexate, p.638).

Combination therapy with PUVA. Some studies have found that concurrent oral etretinate with PUVA therapy was more effective in producing complete remission in severe psoriasis than either treatment alone, and allowed a reduction in the total u.v.-A dose needed for clearing (K. Wolff and H. Hönigsmann, *Pharmac. Ther.*, 1981, *12*, 381; J. Lauharanta *et al.*, *Br. J. Derm.*, 1981, *104*, 325; R.A. Logan and W.A.D. Griffiths, *ibid.*, 1986, *115*, *Suppl.* 30, 11). Other studies have only shown significant benefit in the treatment of palmoplantar pustular psoriasis (C.M. Lawrence *et al.*, *ibid.*, 1984, *110*, 221) and not in chronic plaque psoriasis (S. Parker *et al.*, *ibid.*, 215). These disparate results have led to criticisms of study design (K. Wolff and H. Hönigsmann, *ibid.*, *111*, 247; M. Corbett, *ibid.*, 1985, *112*, 121; S. Shuster *et al.*, *ibid.*, 122).

For a further report of the beneficial use of etretinate with PUVA therapy, employing topical trioxsalen in psoriasis, see p.935.

For a study suggesting that etretinate and isotretinoin are equally effective when used in combination with PUVA for psoriasis, see p.925.

Combination therapy with topical corticosteroids. One hundred and eighteen psoriatic patients were treated for 8 weeks with daily oral etretinate (median initial dose 0.98 mg per kg body-weight), betamethasone valerate 0.1% cream applied twice daily, or both treatments combined. Improvement of erythema, desquamation, and infiltration was greatest with the combination treatment and least with betamethasone alone. Complete or satisfactory remission was achieved in significantly more patients on combined treatment (74.4%) than on etretinate alone (51.4%) or betamethasone alone (33.3%).— J. V. Christiansen *et al.*, *Dermatologica*, 1982, *165*, 204. Similar results using low-dose etretinate and triamcinolone acetonide cream, with markedly less retinoid side-effects.— H. J. van der Rhee *et al.*, *Br. J. Derm.*, 1980, *102*, 203.

Combination therapy with u.v.-B radiation. Sixty-three patients with extensive psoriasis were given either combined therapy with etretinate approximately 1 mg per kg body-weight daily, decreasing after therapeutic effects were obtained and u.v.-B irradiation 4 to 5 days per week, decreasing to once or twice weekly for maintenance, or u.v.-B irradiation alone. Very good or good improvement was achieved in 19 of 23 patients receiving combined therapy and 24 of 40 control patients. The effect of etretinate and u.v.-B radiation therapy was apparently additive.— C. E. Orfanos *et al.*, *Acta derm.-vener., Stockh.*, 1979, *59*, 241.

Comparison with isotretinoin. In a double-blind crossover study of 16 patients with recalcitrant hyperkeratotic or pustular disorders of the hands and feet (mainly palmoplantar pustulosis), equimolar doses of etretinate and isotretinoin were compared with respect to their clinical effects and changes in serum lipoprotein concentrations. The results suggested that, in the diseases studied, etretinate was preferable in both respects.— C. Vahlquist *et al.*, *Br. J. Derm.*, 1985, *112*, 69.

For a further study suggesting that etretinate is more effective than isotretinoin in psoriasis, see p.925.

Comparison with PUVA. Eighty-four patients with persistent palmoplantar pustulosis of long duration were treated with etretinate at a daily dose of 0.9 to 1.0 mg per kg body-weight for 2 weeks, then 0.6 to 0.7 mg per kg for maintenance or 1 of 3 PUVA regimens: u.v.-A with oral methoxsalen, 1% methoxsalen cream, or trioxsalen baths. After 12 weeks, 4 of 28 patients treated with local methoxsalen and 14 of 17 treated with etretinate had completely cleared, whereas none treated with local trioxsalen or oral methoxsalen showed complete clearance.— A. Lassus *et al.*, *Br. J. Derm.*, 1985, *112*, 455.

PSORIATIC ARTHRITIS. In a double-blind controlled study of 40 patients with psoriatic arthritis, etretinate 0.25 to 0.75 mg per kg daily was compared with ibuprofen 400 mg given four times daily. There was no significant advantage of one treatment over the other during the first 8 weeks. At 12 weeks, ibuprofen-treated patients showed a significant improvement in articular index and a trend towards improvement in early morning stiffness. In the etretinate-treated patients, there was a significant improvement in articular index at 16 weeks, but a gradual improvement in a majority of parameters over 24 weeks did not reach significance. There was a significant improvement in haemoglobin, ESR, C-reactive protein, and histidine over 24 weeks with etretinate, but only in histidine with ibuprofen. Almost all patients on etretinate noticed an improvement of the psoriatic skin lesions.— R. Hopkins *et al.*, *Ann. rheum. Dis.*, 1985, *44*, 189. See also.— J. Woo *et al.* (letter), *Postgrad. med. J.*, 1985, *61*, 843.

WARTS AND PAPULOSIS. Severe papillomavirus type 5-induced epidermodysplasia verruciformis in a 32-year-old man was treated successfully with etretinate 1 mg per kg body-weight daily by mouth. After 2 months most of his flat wart-like lesions had disappeared, plaques were repigmenting and no longer scaly, and 2 tumours at the inguinal-scrotal margin were much reduced in size. The patient appears to be almost free of causative virus.— M. A. Lutzner and C. Blanchet-Bardon (letter), *New Engl. J. Med.*, 1980, *302*, 1091.

Etretinate was used for the successful treatment of extensive bowenoid papulosis in 1 patient (F. de Mari *et al.*, *Lancet*, 1981, *2*, 936); however recurrence occurred 7 months after cessation of therapy (*idem.*, 1982, *1*, 1027). In 2 other patients etretinate resulted in slight flattening of lesions with no further improvement. It was concluded that etretinate treatment of bowenoid papulosis was not much help and that the benefits were temporary (C. Blanchet-Bardon *et al.*, *ibid.*, 1981, *2*, 1348).

Etretinate appreciably reduced the hyperkeratosis of resistant viral warts, but infection was not eradicated and the warts returned when the drug was stopped.— M. H. Bunney, *Br. med. J.*, 1986, *293*, 1045.

Proprietary Preparations

Tigason *(Roche, UK)*. *Capsules*, etretinate 10 and 25 mg.

Proprietary Names and Manufacturers

Tegison *(Roche, Canad.; Roche, USA)*; Tigason *(Roche, Austral.; Roche, Denm.; Roche, Fr.; Roche, Ger.; Roche, Ital.; Roche, Norw.; Roche, S.Afr.; Roche, Spain; Roche, Swed.; Sauter, Switz.; Roche, UK)*.

1612-b

Hydroquinone *(USAN)*.

Hydrochinonum; Quinol. Benzene-1,4-diol.

$C_6H_6O_2$=110.1.

CAS — 123-31-9.

Pharmacopoeias. In *Belg.*, *Braz.*, *Hung.*, and *U.S.*

Fine white crystals or white crystalline powder which darken on exposure to light and air. **Soluble** 1 in 17 of water, 1 in 4 of alcohol, 1 in 51 of chloroform, and 1 in about 16 of ether. **Store** in airtight containers. Protect from light.

Adverse Effects, Treatment, and Precautions

Hydroquinone may cause transient erythema and a mild burning sensation as well as undesirable pigmentation changes. Occasionally hypersensitivity has occurred and some sources recommend skin testing before use. Hydroquinone has caused conjunctival changes; contact with the eyes should be avoided. Systemic effects are similar to those of phenol (see p.967) and are treated similarly.

Hydroquinone should not be used for the prevention of sunburn or to bleach eyelashes or eyebrows.

In Great Britain the recommended exposure limits of hydroquinone are 2 mg per m^3 (long-term); 4 mg per m^3 (short-term); in the *US* the permissible and recommended exposure limits are 2 mg per m^3.

A report of patchy depigmentation of the palm, forefinger, and base of the neck in a West Indian woman after using a cosmetic cream containing hydroquinone.— C. M. Ridley *et al.* (letter), *Br. med. J.*, 1984, *288*, 1537.

Localised exogenous ochronosis (blue-black hyperpigmentation) of the face developed in a 50-year-old black woman who had used a proprietary bleaching cream containing 2% hydroquinone up to 6 times daily for about 2½ years. Eighteen months after discontinuing the use of the cream, there was clearing of the hyperpigmentation except for some residual changes in the periorbital areas.— D. Cullison *et al.*, *J. Am. Acad. Derm.*, 1983, *8*, 882.

Brown discoloration of the nails developed in 2 women after the use of hydroquinone-containing cosmetic skin-lightening creams for actinic lentigines of the hands.— R. J. Mann and R. R. M. Harman, *Br. J. Derm.*, 1983, *108*, 363.

Uses and Administration

Hydroquinone increases melanin excretion from melanocytes and may also prevent its production. Hydroquinone is used topically as a depigmenting agent for the skin in conditions such as chloasma, melasma, freckles, and lentigines. It should be applied only to intact skin which should be protected from sunlight to reduce repigmentation. It is also used as an antoxidant for ether and in photographic developers.

In the *UK* the maximum concentration of hydroquinone in hair dyes and cosmetic products for localised skin lightening is limited by law to 2%. Concentrations of 2 to 4% are used clinically.

A review of the actions and uses of bleaching creams containing hydroquinone.— P. G. Engasser and H. I. Maibach, *J. Am. Acad. Derm.*, 1981, *5*, 143.

The development of hydroquinone-containing skin lighteners.— W. R. Chapman and E. J. Shevlin, *Cosmet. Toilet.*, 1983, *98*, 69.

Two double-blind trials of the treatment of melasma with hydroquinone in 221 Hispanic patients revealed that epidermal-type melasma appeared to respond better than the dermal type; creams containing 2% hydroquinone with sunscreens were safe and better than 2% hydroquinone creams without sunscreens, but less effective than 4% hydroquinone formulations; 5% hydroquinone, with or without retinoic acid and corticosteroids, was highly irritant; alcoholic lotion containing 2% hydroquinone and retinoic acid 0.05 to 0.1% gave consistently good-to-excellent results provided patients avoided sun and used sunscreens; and for maintenance therapy, 2% hydroquinone-containing sunscreens were considered to be ideal.— M. A. Pathak *et al.*, *J. invest. Derm.*, 1981, *76*, 324.

Analysis of 41 skin lightening creams available over-the-counter in the *UK* revealed that 8 contained more than 2% hydroquinone.— J. Boyle and C. T. C. Kennedy, *Br. J. Derm.*, 1986, *114*, 501.

Preparations

Hydroquinone Cream *(U.S.P.)*

Hydroquinone Topical Solution *(U.S.P.)*

Proprietary Names and Manufacturers

Dermopaque *(Wilson, Pakistan)*; Dermoquin *(Wilson, Pakistan)*; Eldopaque *(Elder, Canad.; Elder, USA)*; Eldoquin *(Elder, Canad.; Elder, USA)*; Esoterica *(Lentheric Morny, UK; Norcliff Thayer, USA)*; Melanex *(Neutrogena Dermatologics, USA)*; Phiaquin *(Robins, Austral.)*; Ultraquin *(Canderm, Canad.)*.

The following names have been used for multi-ingredient preparations containing hydroquinone—Banquin *(Kramer, USA)*; Esoterica Facial *(Lentheric Morny, UK)*; Esoterica Fortified *(USV, Austral.; Lentheric Morny, UK)*; Solaquin Cream *(Elder, Canad.)*; Solaquin Forte Cream *(Elder, Canad.; Elder, USA)*; Solaquin Forte Gel *(Elder, USA)*.

1615-q

Ichthammol *(BAN, USAN)*.

Ammonii Sulfogyrodalas; Ammonio Sulfoittiolato; Ammonium Bithiolicum; Ammonium Bituminosulfonicum; Ammonium Ichthosulphonate; Ammonium Sulfobituminosum; Ammonium Sulpho-Ichthyolate; Bithiolate Ammonique; Bithyol; Bituminol; Ichthosulphol; Ichthyol; Ichthyolammonium; Sulphonated Bitumen.

CAS — 8029-68-3.

Pharmacopoeias. In *Arg., Aust., Belg., Br., Chin., Cz., Egypt., Fr., Ger., Hung., It., Jpn, Jug., Mex., Nord., Port., Roum., Span., Swiss, Turk.*, and *U.S.*

A reddish-brown to almost black viscous liquid with a strong characteristic empyreumatic odour. It consists mainly of the ammonium salts of the sulphonic acids of an oily substance prepared from the destructive distillation of a bituminous schist or shale, together with ammonium sulphate (about 5 to 7%). It contains not less than 10.5% of organically combined sulphur, calculated on the dried material, and not more than 25% of the total sulphur is in the form of sulphates.

B.P. **solubilities** are: soluble in water; partly soluble in alcohol and in ether; *U.S.P.* solubilities are: soluble 1 in 10 of water; miscible with glycerol, fixed oils, and fats; partially soluble in alcohol and in ether. **Store** in well-closed containers.

Ichthammol has slight bacteriostatic properties; it is slightly irritant to the skin and there have been rare reports of hypersensitivity. It is used in creams, ointments, and bandages often in combination with zinc oxide (see p.936), in the treatment of chronic skin diseases such as eczema and ulcers.

Preparations

Ichthammol Glycerin *(B.P.C. 1973)*. Glycerin of Ammonium Ichthosulphonate; Ichthammol Ear Drops *(A.P.F.)*; Ichthammol Paint *(A.P.F.)*. Ichthammol 10 g, glycerol 90 g. Used in inflammatory conditions.

Ichthammol Ointment *(U.S.P.)*. Ichthammol 10 g, wool fat 10 g, and yellow soft paraffin 80 g.

Ichthammol and Zinc Cream Oily *(A.P.F.)*. Oily Ichthammol Cream. Ichthammol 5 g, wool fat 15 g, and zinc cream oily 80 g.

Zinc and Ichthammol Preparations. For further preparations see under Zinc Oxide, p. 936.

Proprietary Names and Manufacturers of Ichthammol and Related Compounds

Adnexol *(Protina, Ger.; Bama, Spain)*; Bitamon *(Cooper, Switz.)*; Dermichthol *(Ichthyol, Ger.)*; Ichthalon *(Ichthyol, Switz.)*; Ichtho-Bad *(Ichthyol, Ger.; Ichthyol, Switz.)*; Ichtho-Cutan *(Ichthyol, Ger.)*; Ichtholan *(Ichthyol, Ger.; Ichthyol, Switz.)*; Ichthraletten *(Ichthyol, Ger.; Ichthyol, Switz.)*; Ichtopur *(Ichthyol, Ger.)*; Poudre Velours *(Alcon-Couvreur, Belg.)*.

The following names have been used for multi-ingredient preparations containing ichthammol and related compounds—Acnederm *(Ego, Austral.)*; Egoderm Cream and Ointment *(Ego, Austral.)*; Egoderm M *(Ego, Austral.)*; Ichthopaste *(Smith & Nephew, UK)*; Icthaband *(Seton, UK)*; Medicone Derma-HC *(Medicone, USA)*; Uraband *(Seton, UK)*.

1616-p

Isotretinoin *(BAN, USAN, rINN)*.

13-*cis*-Retinoic Acid; Ro-4-3780. (13*Z*)-15-Apo-β-caroten-15-oic acid; (2*Z*,4*E*,6*E*,8*E*)-3,7-dimethyl-9-(2,6,6-trimethylcyclohex-1-enyl)nona-2,4,6,8-tetraenoic acid.

$C_{20}H_{28}O_2$=300.4.

CAS — 4759-48-2.

Pharmacopoeias. In *U.S.*

Adverse Effects

The adverse effects of isotretinoin are similar to those of vitamin A (see p.1278) and are generally reversible and dose-related. Isotretinoin can cause dryness of the mucous membranes and of the skin with scaling, fragility, and erythema, especially of the face, cheilitis, pruritus, epistaxis, conjunctivitis, and dry sore mouth. There may be corneal opacities, skeletal hyperostosis, and premature epiphyseal closure, and musculoskeletal symptoms. Elevation of serum triglycerides, hepatic enzymes, erythrocyte sedimentation rate and, less often, serum creatine phosphokinase and blood glucose can occur. Less common effects include hair thinning, photosensitivity, gastro-intestinal symptoms, benign intracranial hypertension and an association with skin infections and an inflammatory bowel syndrome.

Isotretinoin is teratogenic.

EFFECTS ON CALCIUM HOMOEOSTASIS. A report of hypercalcaemia associated with oral isotretinoin in the treatment of severe acne.— J. P. Valentic, *J. Am. med. Ass.*, 1983, *250*, 1899.

EFFECTS ON THE EYES. A review of 261 adverse ocular reactions which occurred in 237 patients receiving isotretinoin. Blepharoconjunctivitis, subjective complaints of dry eyes, blurred vision, and contact lens intolerance were reversible side-effects. More serious ocular adverse reactions included papilloedema, pseudotumour cerebri, and white or grey subepithelial corneal opacities; all of these were reversible on discontinuation of isotretinoin.— F. T. Fraunfelder *et al.*, *Am. J. Ophthal.*, 1985, *100*, 534. Poor night vision and/or excessive glare sensitivity was reported by 3 patients treated with isotretinoin 1 mg per kg daily. It was suspected that isotretinoin may compete for normal retinol binding sites on cell surfaces or transport molecules.— R. G. Weleber *et al.*, *Archs Ophthal., N.Y.*, 1986, *104*, 831.

EFFECTS ON THE MUSCULOSKELETAL SYSTEM. Pittsley and Yoder (*New Engl. J. Med.*, 1983, *308*, 1012) observed an ossification disorder resembling diffuse idiopathic skeletal hyperostosis in 4 of 9 patients who had been taking isotretinoin 3 to 4 mg per kg daily for 2 to 6 years for refractory ichthyosis. It was not anticipated that the lower doses and much shorter period of treatment used in acne would cause any difficulties in this regard. However, small asymptomatic hyperostoses have been detected radiographically along 1 or more vertebrae in approximately 10% of isotretinoin-treated patients. In these prospective studies, the bony abnormalities were usually not seen until 8 months after the conclusion of treatment (P.E. Pochi, *ibid.*, 1985, *313*, 1013).

A florid case of osteoma cutis occurred in a 24-year-old woman following isotretinoin 100 mg daily for 20 weeks. A few scattered osteomata of the skin were observed prior to treatment.— R. H. Brodkin and A. A. Abbey, *Dermatologica*, 1985, *170*, 210.

A report of reversible skeletal muscle and myoneural junction damage induced by isotretinoin in 2 patients.— E. Hodack *et al.*, *Br. med. J.*, 1986, *293*, 425.

EFFECTS ON THE RESPIRATORY SYSTEM. A 20-year-old man noted the development of exercise-induced wheezing within 3 to 4 weeks of starting isotretinoin therapy. Wheezing was alleviated on stopping isotretinoin.— D. A. Fisher (letter), *J. Am. Acad. Derm.*, 1985, *13*, 524.

EFFECTS ON THE SERUM LIPIDS. In a study of 53 patients with severe nodulocystic acne, but otherwise healthy, given isotretinoin 1 mg per kg body-weight daily by mouth for 20 weeks, the mean plasma-triglyceride concentration increased and exceeded 200 mg per dL in 9 patients. The mean plasma-cholesterol concentration also increased, but mean plasma concentration of high-density-lipoprotein (HDL) cholesterol fell. Eight weeks after discontinuation of therapy, mean plasma lipid and lipoprotein concentrations had returned to pre-treatment values (S. Bershad *et al.*, *New Engl. J. Med.*, 1985, *313*, 981). Marsden *et al.* (*Lancet*, 1983, *1*, 134) had previously noted a rise in serum-triglyceride and cholesterol concentrations in 18 and 10 patients treated for 12 weeks with oral isotretinoin 0.8 and 0.05 mg per kg daily respectively; HDL cholesterol only fell with the higher dose. Kingston *et al.* (*ibid.*, 471) believed it would be correct to exclude the drug from subjects who are predisposed to vascular disease or have a pre-existing hyperlipidaemia.

For possible mechanisms and consequences of hyperlipidaemia due to isotretinoin, see J. Marsden, *Br. J. Derm.*, 1986, *114*, 401.

The daily administration of 15 mL of an oil containing eicosapentaenoic acid (MaxEPA) by mouth for one month significantly reduced raised serum-triglyceride and -cholesterol concentrations in 16 patients receiving isotretinoin 1 mg per kg body-weight daily by mouth for acne.— J. R. Marsden, *Br. J. Derm.*, 1987, *116*, 450.

EFFECTS ON THE SKIN. A 17-year-old man developed glistening, red, nodular granulomatous lesions in areas of healing acne cysts during therapy with isotretinoin which disappeared 4 weeks after cessation of treatment.— P. R. Lane and D. J. Hogan (letter), *Can. med. Ass. J.*, 1984, *130*, 550.

Acne fulminans has been reported as a complication of isotretinoin treatment (J.K. Kellett *et al.*, *Br. med. J.*, 1985, *290*, 820; N.R. Huston and R. Mules, *N.Z. med. J.*, 1985, *36*, 821) and treatment has included corticosteroids. However, there have been cases of acne fulminans being treated with isotretinoin (C.R. Darley *et al.*, *J. R. Soc. Med.*, 1984, *77*, 328).

A patient with plaque-stage mycosis fungoides developed a universal reddening of the skin, accompanied by exfoliation with a clinical pattern of severe seborrhoeic dermatitis after 2 days of treatment with isotretinoin 0.5 mg per kg body-weight. Treatment was discontinued after 4 days, but widespread dermatitis was still apparent 6 weeks later. This effect had previously been seen only in patients with Sézary syndrome.— G. L. Wantzin and K. Thomsen (letter), *J. Am. Acad. Derm.*, 1985, *13*, 665.

For an *in vitro* study demonstrating that isotretinoin is

potentially phototoxic, see Etretinate, p.921.

PREGNANCY AND THE NEONATE. Reports of intra-uterine exposure to isotretinoin causing spontaneous abortions or leading to the isotretinoin dysmorphic syndrome in the neonate. This syndrome is characterised by malformations of the head, CNS, heart, and thymus: F. W. Rosa (letter), *Lancet*, 1983, *2*, 513; J. T. Braun *et al.*, *ibid.*, 1984, *1*, 506; R. M. Hill (letter), *ibid.*, 1465; C. Marwick, *J. Am. med. Ass.*, 1984, *251*, 3208; P. J. Benke, *ibid.*, 3267; J. H. Hersh *et al.* (letter), *ibid.*, 1985, *254*, 909; E. J. Lammer *et al.*, *New Engl. J. Med.*, 1985, *313*, 837; M. Tremblay *et al.*, *Can. med. Ass. J.*, 1985, *133*, 208; R. Robertson and P. M. MacLeod, *ibid.*, 1147; F. Rosa (letter), *Lancet*, 1987, *2*, 1154.

Precautions

Isotretinoin is teratogenic and treatment should not be started in pregnant patients; also pregnancy should be avoided during treatment and for 1 month after treatment has been withdrawn. Isotretinoin is contra-indicated in patients with hepatic and renal impairment, hypervitaminosis A, and in breast-feeding mothers.

Liver-function and fasting blood lipids should be measured at the start of therapy, after the first month, and thereafter as appropriate. Blood glucose should be monitored throughout treatment in patients who either have, or are predisposed to, diabetes mellitus. Patients receiving isotretinoin should avoid dietary supplements of vitamin A and should not donate blood during, or for 1 month after cessation of therapy.

For reports that oral isotretinoin at a daily dose of 0.5 mg per kg did not interact adversely with oral contraceptives containing ethinyloestradiol and levonorgestrel, see: M. Orme *et al.* (letter), *Lancet*, 1984, *2*, 752; M. Orme *et al.*, *Br. J. clin. Pharmac.*, 1984, *17*, 227P.

Absorption and Fate

After oral administration isotretinoin is metabolised in the liver, without significant first-pass effect, to its major metabolite 4-oxo-isotretinoin; there is also some isomerisation of isotretinoin to tretinoin. Isotretinoin, tretinoin, and their metabolites undergo enterohepatic recycling. The elimination half-life of isotretinoin is 10 to 20 hours, much shorter than that of etretinate. Isotretinoin is highly bound to plasma proteins.

Isotretinoin is excreted in the faeces, largely as intact drug, and in the urine as metabolites.

References to the pharmacokinetics of isotretinoin: R. K. Brazzell and W. A. Colburn, *J. Am. Acad. Derm.*, 1982, *6*, 643; R. W. Lucek and W. A. Colburn, *Clin. Pharmacokinet.*, 1985, *10*, 38.

Following observations in 12 healthy subjects each given a single 100 mg oral dose of isotretinoin, it was suggested that steady-state blood concentrations should be observed within 1 week. Negligible amounts of unchanged drug were excreted in the urine, whereas 53.2 to 74.3% of the dose was recovered as intact isotretinoin in the faeces within 72 hours of administration.— K. -C. Khoo *et al.*, *J. clin. Pharmac.*, 1982, *22*, 395.

Isotretinoin was given as a suspension in a single oral dose of 80 mg to 15 healthy subjects. After rapid absorption, isotretinoin was distributed and eliminated with mean half-lives of 1.3 and 17.4 hours respectively. Maximum blood concentrations occurred at 1 to 4 hours after dosing. Maximum concentrations of 4-oxo-isotretinoin, the major blood metabolite, were approximately one-half those of isotretinoin and occurred at 6 to 16 hours after dosing. The ratio of areas under the curve for metabolite and parent drug suggests that their average steady-state ratios during a dosing interval would be approximately 2.5. Therefore, at steady state, the metabolite could contribute to the overall efficacy of the drug.— W. A. Colburn *et al.*, *Eur. J. clin. Pharmac.*, 1983, *24*, 689. Results suggesting that steady-state concentrations of isotretinoin could be predicted from single dose data, but that there were changes in the disposition of 4-oxo-isotretinoin during multiple dosing.— R. K. Brazzell *et al.*, *ibid.*, 695.

In a study of 20 healthy subjects given 80 mg isotretinoin orally as capsules, relative bioavailability was found to be approximately 1.5 to 2 times greater when the dose was administered 1 hour before, concomitantly with, or 1 hour after, a meal than when given during a complete fast. Co-administration of isotretinoin with, rather than 1 hour after, a meal may be the best method of administration as the maximum blood concentration which may be associated with increased side-effects, is then lower.— W. A. Colburn *et al.*, *J. clin. Pharmac.*, 1983, *23*, 534.

Uses and Administration

Isotretinoin is a derivative of tretinoin (p.935). It is given by mouth for the treatment of severe acne that has not responded to other measures. It is not indicated for uncomplicated adolescent acne.

The initial daily dose for acne is 0.5 to 1 mg per kg body-weight by mouth, given with food either as a single dose or in two divided doses and adjusted after 2 to 4 weeks according to response and side-effects. Acute exacerbation of acne is occasionally seen during the initial period, but usually subsides within 7 to 10 days on continued treatment. Patients intolerant to the initial dose may be able to continue treatment at 100 to 200 µg per kg daily. Patients whose disease is very severe or primarily on the body instead of the face may require up to 2 mg per kg daily.

Treatment should continue for 15 to 20 weeks or until the total cyst count has decreased by over 70%. Improvement may continue after cessation of treatment, therefore a period of 8 weeks should elapse before a subsequent course is considered. Prolonged remissions can occur.

Isotretinoin has been tried in a number of other skin disorders, including psoriasis, some keratinisation disorders, and some epithelial neoplasms.

For a review of the pharmacology and therapeutic uses of isotretinoin, see A. Ward *et al.*, *Drugs*, 1984, *28*, 6. See also C. E. Orfanos *et al.*, *Drugs*, 1987, *34*, 459.

ACNE. In a double-blind study, isotretinoin at doses of 0.1, 0.5, or 1.0 mg per kg body-weight daily by mouth for 16 weeks was used to treat 76 patients with previously unresponsive moderate to severe cystonodular acne. Sebum excretion-rate was reduced by 75%, 89%, and 91% in the 0.1, 0.5, and 1.0 mg per kg groups respectively, predominantly within the first 4 weeks. After 16 weeks, acne grade showed a 70% improvement in 0.1 mg per kg group and 65% in the other 2 groups, and the number of acne lesions was decreased by 80% in the 0.1 and 0.5 mg per kg groups and 89% in the 1.0 mg per kg group. Facial acne improved more than acne on the chest and back. A clinical improvement of greater than 50% was produced in 60 patients and a further 9 continued to improve to that level whilst off treatment. Seven patients, 1 in the 1.0 mg per kg group and 3 in each of the other groups failed to respond at all.

Sixteen weeks after stopping treatment, sebum excretion-rate in the 0.1 mg per kg group had returned to 95% of the pre-treatment level, whilst in the other 2 groups, rates had only returned to 60-66% of pre-treatment levels. Eleven patients relapsed, 5 in the 0.1 mg per kg group and 3 in each of the other 2 groups. Only 6 patients relapsed to 50% of their pre-treatment acne grade (D.H. Jones *et al.*, *Br. J. Derm.*, 1983, *108*, 333).

Sixty-nine patients were followed up. There was a considerably greater relapse-rate with the 0.1 mg per kg dose than with the other 2 doses, although the difference was not significant until 88 weeks post-therapy. Only in 8 patients did the acne return to within 50% of its pre-treatment level. A dose of 0.5 to 1.0 mg per kg was recommended as a balance between clinical effectiveness, toxicity, and prolonged remission of the acne. Although 0.1 mg per kg was effective in treating patients with severe resistant acne and was less toxic, it had a poor long-term effect and should not be used in such patients (D.H. Jones and W.J. Cunliffe, *ibid.*, 1984, *111*, 123). Similar results were achieved in a multicentre study involving 141 patients tested with the same 3 doses, (J.S. Strauss *et al.*, *J. Am. Acad. Derm.*, 1984, *10*, 490).

A 30-year-old patient with a renal transplant and a serum-creatinine concentration of 0.19 to 0.20 mmol/L, taking cyclosporin and prednisone, was successfully treated for severe cystic acne with isotretinoin 0.7 mg per kg body-weight daily by mouth.— M. Tam and A. Cooper (letter), *Br. J. Derm.*, 1987, *116*, 463.

Results indicating that isotretinoin is ineffective when applied topically in the treatment of acne.— M. Harms *et al.* (letter), *Lancet*, 1985, *1*, 398.

Combination therapy with cyproterone acetate. Twenty-seven male patients with severe acne were treated for 12 weeks with cyproterone acetate 5 mg daily, isotretinoin 0.05 mg per kg body-weight daily, or both drugs combined. Sebum excretion-rate and acne lesion count fell in all 3 groups, but the reduction was similar in those receiving isotretinoin alone and the combination and was not significant in those receiving cyproterone alone. Unwanted effects on serum-triglyceride concentrations were smaller with combined treatment than isotretinoin alone. Although no evidence of synergy was found, it was suggested that combination therapy might be useful in ameliorating isotretinoin side-effects on serum lipids.— J. R. Marsden *et al.*, *Br. J. Derm.*, 1984, *110*, 697.

Combination therapy with tetracycline. Twenty-nine patients with nodulocystic acne were treated for 16 weeks with isotretinoin 1 mg per kg body-weight daily or isotretinoin 0.25 mg per kg daily with tetracycline 250 mg twice daily. All patients receiving isotretinoin alone and 75% of those receiving the combination had marked improvement or complete clearing of acne, but side-effects were more frequent and severe in those receiving isotretinoin alone.— A. Langner *et al.*, *Dermatologica*, 1985, *170*, 185.

Comparison with minocycline. In an open study, 24 patients with severe nodular cystic acne were given isotretinoin 1 mg per kg body-weight daily for 10 weeks, followed by 0.5 mg per kg daily for 10 weeks, or minocycline 100 mg daily for 10 weeks, followed by 50 mg daily for 10 weeks. At the end of treatment, the number and mean diameter of the cysts were decreased in both groups, but the improvement was more striking in the isotretinoin-treated group. There was a significant remission in the acne of patients treated with isotretinoin, but not in that of the minocycline-treated patients.— P. D. Pigatto *et al.*, *Dermatologica*, 1986, *172*, 154.

Comparison with tetracycline. In a double-blind study, 30 patients with severe nodulocystic acne were treated with isotretinoin up to 2 mg per kg daily or tetracycline up to 1000 mg daily for 16 weeks. Both treatments which were given by mouth decreased the mean number of cysts, the sum of largest cyst diameters, and the number of comedones and pustules: isotretinoin was more effective than tetracycline only in reducing the number of comedones and pustules. Acne treated with isotretinoin continued to improve during the 8-week follow-up period whereas acne treated with tetracycline remained essentially unchanged. Isotretinoin also relieved acne-associated symptoms and improved healing time and the rate of development of new lesions to a greater extent than tetracycline. All isotretinoin-treated patients experienced side-effects compared with 7 of 15 tetracycline-treated patients.— R. S. Lester *et al.*, *Int. J. Derm.*, 1985, *24*, 252.

CELLULITIS. Isotretinoin at daily doses of 0.5 to 1.0 mg per kg body-weight for 12 weeks resulted in complete scalp healing and hair regrowth on 2 occasions in a 21-year-old man with dissecting cellulitis of the scalp. Improvement lasted for 3 months after discontinuing isotretinoin on both occasions. Previous antibiotic therapy had been ineffective.— A. E. M. Taylor (letter), *Lancet*, 1987, *2*, 225.

FOLLICULITIS. Thirty-two patients with gram-negative folliculitis were treated with isotretinoin 0.47 to 1.0 mg per kg daily. Facial pustules were completely cleared in all patients after 4 months of therapy and gram-negative organisms were eliminated from the skin in 31 patients and the nose in 30 after 5 months. There were no instances of recurrence in 11 patients assessed 6 months after stopping therapy.— W. D. James and J. J. Leyden, *J. Am. Acad. Derm.*, 1985, *12*, 319.

HIDRADENITIS. Four of 8 patients with extensive hidradenitis suppurativa experienced clinical improvement after 4 months of oral isotretinoin therapy at an average dose of 0.9 mg per kg.— C. H. Dicken *et al.*, *J. Am. Acad. Derm.*, 1984, *11*, 500.

KERATINISATION DISORDERS. *Darier's disease.* In an open multicentre study, 104 patients with Darier's disease (keratosis follicularis) were treated with isotretinoin. Mean daily dosage in short-term courses was 1.43 to 1.87 mg per kg body-weight and during long-term therapy 0.98 to 1.43 mg per kg. About 85% of patients had clearly improved by 5 to 8 weeks and this level was maintained through 16 weeks of treatment, with treatment failure in 5 patients. Similar improvement was seen in subsequent short- and long-term courses, indicating that in some patients after relapse of treatment, good clinical improvement could be maintained with either alternate-day or alternate-week medication schedules. Because prolonged remissions are not seen in patients with Darier's disease, chronic treatment would be necessary.— C. H. Dicken *et al.*, *J. Am. Acad. Derm.*, 1982, *6*, 721.

Ichthyosis. In an open multicentre study of 99 patients, the average effective daily dose of isotretinoin to treat lamellar ichthyosis and epidermolytic hyperkeratosis was approximately 2 mg per kg. By the end of each treatment course, over 90% of patients were clearly improved, but signs of involvement returned to pre-treatment levels on discontinuation. X-linked ichthyosis and congenital ichthyosiform erythroderma appeared to respond more satisfactorily than ichthyosis vulgaris. Total clearing was not the usual response and fewer of the patients with epidermolytic hyperkeratosis were found to be clear. Patients with the most severe disease cleared less completely.— H. P. Baden *et al.*, *J. Am. Acad. Derm.*, 1982, *6*, 716.

Keratosis. Of 6 patients with keratoderma palmaris et plantaris treated with isotretinoin at a mean daily dose of 1.95 mg per kg for a mean duration of 113 days, 3 showed definite to marked improvement and 2 demonstrated complete clearing. Relapses occurred when isotretinoin was discontinued and scaling and induration appeared to be significantly worsened, indicating that there was a rebound phenomenon.— W. F. Bergfeld *et al.*, *J. Am. Acad. Derm.*, 1982, *6*, 727.

Pityriasis rubra. Forty-five patients with pityriasis rubra pilaris were treated with oral isotretinoin at mean daily doses of 1.51 to 2.13 mg per kg in short- and long-term courses. Over 50% of patients were clearly improved by 4 weeks of therapy and in all but 1 course, over 90% of patients showed improvement. Erythema, scaling, and induration increased after stopping therapy, but did not return to pre-treatment levels and 6 patients experienced complete or almost complete remission at 6 months.— L. A. Goldsmith *et al.*, *J. Am. Acad. Derm.*, 1982, *6*, 710. See also.— J. A. Newton and M. M. Black, *Br. J. Derm.*, 1985, *113, Suppl.* 29, 69 (epidermal naevus).

LICHEN PLANUS. Twenty patients with oral lichen planus were treated in a double-blind study with either isotretinoin 0.1% gel or the vehicle alone twice daily for 2 months. Improvement was significantly greater in the patients receiving the isotretinoin gel. Side-effects were generally limited to transient burning with initial application of both the vehicle and active medication. Superficial desquamation and erythema were occasionally noted with the use of the isotretinoin gel. Serum concentrations of isotretinoin and its metabolites were undetectable.— T. A. Giustina *et al.*, *Archs Derm.*, 1986, *122*, 534.

LUPUS. Isotretinoin 80 mg daily by mouth clinically benefited 8 patients with chronic or subacute cutaneous (discoid) lupus erythematosus after 16 weeks. Peripheral blood B- and T-cell counts were unaffected by therapy, but there was resolution of routine histopathological abnormalities, normalisation of abnormal lesions on direct immunofluorescent microscopy and of the epidermis on electron microscopy, and reduction of all T-cells near the dermoepidermal junction without change in ratio of T-helper/inducer cells to T-suppressor/cytotoxic cells. The possibility that treated lesions would recur when therapy was discontinued should influence treatment decisions; isotretinoin may be most useful in establishing rapid control in treatment-resistant lesions and for intermittent treatment of acute flare-ups in selected patients.— R. C. Newton *et al.*, *Archs Derm.*, 1986, *122*, 170.

MALIGNANT NEOPLASMS. One-hundred-and-eight patients with advanced cancers or preneoplastic lesions were given isotretinoin at daily oral doses of 3 and 2 mg per kg body-weight respectively for at least 1 month. Considerable acitivity was seen in patients with squamous cell epithelial disease. Partial or mixed temporary responses were seen in 6 of 24 patients with advanced cancer (lung, head and neck) and 3 of 5 with preneoplastic lesions (keratoacanthomas, multiple basal carcinomas, and epidermal dysplasia verruciformis). All responses occurred in subcutaneous or skin disease sites. Of 45 patients with non-squamous cell epithelial malignancies, there was 1 partial (ovarian) and 2 minor (skin) responses. One of 13 patients with malignant melanoma had a partial response and no responses were seen in 21 patients with non-epithelial malignancies. The predominant limiting side-effects occurred in skin. Additionally, emotional lability and headaches were frequent, symptoms different from those seen in patients with dermatological conditions and probably reflecting the higher dose used.— F. L. Meyskens *et al.*, *Cancer Treat. Rep.*, 1982, *66*, 1315.

Beneficial responses in advanced squamous cell carcinoma of the skin with isotretinoin.— S. M. Lipman and F. L. Meyskens, *Ann. intern. Med.*, 1987, *107*, 499.

Kaposi's sarcoma. Six patients with cutaneous Kaposi's sarcoma associated with AIDS received isotretinoin by mouth in a daily dose of 2 mg per kg body-weight for four weeks. No patient showed tumour regression and new lesions developed.— J. L. Ziegler *et al.* (letter), *Lancet*, 1984, *2*, 641.

Malignant eccrine poroma. Isotretinoin produced remission in one case of malignant eccrine poroma (M. Roach, *Ann. intern. Med.*, 1983, *99*, 486), but no response in another case (M. Friedland *et al.*, *ibid.*, *100*, 614).

Mycosis fungoides. Four patients with refractory cutaneous T-cell lymphoma (mycosis fungoides) were treated with oral isotretinoin at a dose of 2 to 3 mg per kg body-weight daily, the dose being reduced after 4 weeks in 3 patients because of skin dryness and scaling. Near complete clearing of extensive tumours and plaques was seen in 1 patient, who remained in partial remission with continued improvement after 15 months. Two patients showed improvement in pruritus and 50% reduction in plaques by 4 and 6 weeks, respectively. The fourth patient had improvement in pruritus and clearing of plaques, but dryness and scaling necessitated further reduction and eventually withdrawal of the treatment.— J. F. Kessler *et al.*, *Lancet*, 1983, *1*, 1345. Similar results in a further 7 patients.— R. P. Warrell *et al.* (letter), *ibid.*, *2*, 629. See also M. Alexander (letter), *ibid.*, 463.

Oral leucoplakia. Forty-four patients with oral leucoplakia were treated with either isotretinoin 1 to 2 mg per kg body-weight daily by mouth or placebo for 3 months in a double-blind study and followed for 6 months. A complete or partial response, as classified by inspection, occurred in 16 of 24 patients receiving isotretinoin compared with 2 of 20 receiving placebo. Histologically, dysplasia was reversed in 13 patients receiving isotretinoin and in 2 receiving placebo. Intolerable conjunctivitis and hypertriglyceridaemia developed in 2 patients receiving isotretinoin 2 mg per kg, necessitating withdrawal of treatment. It was concluded that isotretinoin, even in short-term use, appears to be an effective treatment for oral leucoplakia and has an acceptable level of toxicity.— W. K. Hong *et al.*, *New Engl. J. Med.*, 1986, *315*, 1501.

Preleukaemia. Complete haematological and cytogenetic remission in a patient with a myelodysplastic syndrome (refractory anaemia with excess blast cells) and an abnormal karyotype after daily isotretinoin therapy for 10 months.— R. A. Larson, *Ann. intern. Med.*, 1985, *103*, 136.

Seventy patients with myelodysplastic syndrome having 5% or fewer marrow blast cells received either isotretinoin 10 to 20 mg daily for up to 145 weeks, or no treatment. Among non-sideroblastic patients the 1-year survival in the treated group was 77%, compared with 36% in the control group. There were too few deaths among patients with sideroblastic anaemia to allow any effect of therapy on survival to be evaluated. Larger trials were needed.— R. E. Clark *et al.*, *Lancet*, 1987, *1*, 763. Comment.— G. Tricot (letter), *ibid.*, 1271.

PSORIASIS. Sixty patients with severe, widespread psoriasis were treated with either isotretinoin or etretinate combined with PUVA therapy. Both retinoids were administered orally at a daily dose of 1 mg per kg body-weight 5 days before PUVA therapy was started and were continued until the psoriasis had cleared completely, at which time the retinoids were discontinued and patients were put on PUVA maintenance. There was no significant difference between the 2 regimens in respect of duration of the clearing phase, number of exposures, and, most importantly, cumulative u.v.-A dose. When the 2 patient groups were compared with an earlier series treated with PUVA alone (K. Wolff; H. Hönigsmann, *Pharmac. Ther.*, 1981, *12*, 381) both combinations were superior. The fact that isotretinoin could replace etretinate in retinoid-PUVA combination therapy meant that retinoid-PUVA treatment could be considered for women of childbearing age, provided they had severe psoriasis and took contraceptive precautions for a month after the psoriasis had cleared.— H. Hönigsmann and K. Wolff (letter), *Lancet*, 1983, *1*, 236.

A report of 4 patients with generalised pustular psoriasis, whose pustulation and other associated symptoms began resolving within 5 days after oral isotretinoin 1.2 to 1.75 mg per kg body-weight daily.— H. L. Sofen *et al.* (letter), *Lancet*, 1984, *1*, 40.

In an open study, 11 patients with generalised pustular psoriasis were treated with isotretinoin 1.5 to 2.0 mg per kg body-weight daily. Treatment was continued for 6 weeks after pustulation had ceased. Ten patients were successfully treated, with complete resolution of systemic symptoms and cessation of pustulation occurring after a mean of 3.4 days of therapy. Halving the isotretinoin dose after control of pustulation had been achieved resulted in recurrence. Follow-up for up to 24 months showed that the majority subsequently required an alternative agent to achieve satisfactory control of their psoriasis. Thus, while isotretinoin successfully aborted the attack of generalised pustulation, it was not effective in treating the residual psoriasis when used alone.

A further 29 patients with chronic plaque psoriasis were treated with isotretinoin 1.5 mg per kg daily or etretinate 0.75 mg per kg daily. In general, the etretinate group had more extensive psoriasis. After 8 weeks, 18 of 19 patients treated with etretinate had a complete or moderate response, compared with only 4 of 10 treated with isotretinoin. Etretinate was thus significantly more effective than isotretinoin in inducing a partial or complete clearing of chronic plaque psoriasis.— R. L. Moy *et al.*, *Archs Derm.*, 1985, *121*, 1297.

For a study suggesting that etretinate is preferable to isotretinoin in hyperkeratotic or pustular disorders of the hands and feet, see p.922.

ROSACEA. Nine patients with severe rosacea that had not responded to tetracycline improved when they were given isotretinoin 0.5 mg per kg body-weight daily for 6 weeks. All patients experienced side-effects.— R. Fulton *et al.*, *Br. J. Derm.*, 1983, *108*, 243. A further report of improvement in 12 of 13 patients. Ten patients were followed up for between 1 and 2 years after isotretinoin was stopped and 3 women and 2 men did not show any relapse.— J. B. Schmidt *et al.*, *Acta derm.-vener., Stockh.*, 1984, *64*, 15.

STEATOCYSTOMA. A report of marked improvement in 3 patients with steatocystoma multiplex suppurativum given isotretinoin 1 mg per kg daily for 6 months. Isotretinoin was recommended as the treatment of choice in cases with a severe inflammatory component.— B. N. Statham and W. J. Cunliffe (letter), *Br. J. Derm.*, 1984, *111*, 246. Despite the reported response in steatocystoma, treatment with isotretinoin 1 mg per kg body-weight by mouth daily for 20 weeks was of no benefit in a patient with eruptive vellus hair cysts.— F. Urbina-González *et al.* (letter), *Br. J. Derm.*, 1987, *116*, 465.

Proprietary Preparations

Roaccutane *(Roche, UK)*. *Capsules*, isotretinoin 5 mg and 20 mg.

Proprietary Names and Manufacturers

Accutane *(Roche, Canad.; Roche, USA)*; Roaccutan *(Roche, Denm.; Roche, Ger.)*; Roaccutane *(Roche, Austral.; Roche, Fr.; Roche, S.Afr.; Sauter, Switz.; Roche, UK)*; Roacutan *(Roche, Spain)*.

1619-e

Mequinol *(rINN)*.

Hydroquinone Monomethyl Ether. 4-Methoxyphenol.
$C_7H_8O_2$=124.1.

CAS — 150-76-5.

Mequinol is used similarly to monobenzone (see p.928), usually as a 10% cream, in the treatment of hyperpigmentation.

In Great Britain the recommended exposure limit of mequinol is 5 mg per m^3 (long-term).

A 19-year-old West Indian girl applied a bleaching wax containing mequinol for 2 to 3 months to lighten the colour of her skin. She subsequently developed severe irregular hypopigmentation of her hands, arms, neck, and legs. Despite discontinuing the use of the cream, hypopigmentation continued for some weeks.— J. Boyle and C. T. C. Kennedy (letter), *Br. med. J.*, 1984, *288*, 1998.

Proprietary Names and Manufacturers

Leucobasal *(Sodip, Switz.)*; Leucodinine B *(Promedica, Fr.)*; Novo-Dermoquinona *(Llorente, Spain)*.

1620-b

Ammoniated Mercury *(USAN)*.

Aminomercuric Chloride; Hydrargyri Aminochloridum; Hydrargyrum Amidochloratum; Hydrargyrum Ammoniatum; Hydrargyrum Praecipitatum Album; Mercuric Ammonium Chloride; Mercury Amide Chloride; Mercury Aminochloride; White Precipitate.
NH_2HgCl=252.1.

CAS — 10124-48-8.

Pharmacopoeias. In *Belg., Cz., Egypt., Hung., Int., Jug., Pol., Rus., Turk.*, and *U.S.*

Several pharmacopoeias assign the synonym 'White Precipitate' to Precipitated Mercurous Chloride.

A white odourless amorphous powder which is stable in

air, but darkens on exposure to light. Practically **insoluble** in water and alcohol; soluble in warm hydrochloric, nitric, and acetic acids. **Store** in well-closed containers. Protect from light.

Adverse Effects and Treatment

As for Mercury, p.1587. The topical application of preparations containing ammoniated mercury has resulted in allergic reactions, acrodynia, and mercury poisoning.

EFFECTS ON THE KIDNEY. Of 60 patients (16 men, 44 women) aged 15 to 56 with the nephrotic syndrome, 53% (70% of the women) were using skin-lightening creams containing 5 to 10% of ammoniated mercury or had used such creams. Concentrations of mercury in urine were 90 to 250 ng per mL (mean 150) for those using the creams and 0 to 90 ng per mL (mean 29) for those who had used them. The upper limit for normal was 80 ng per ml. Of 26 patients followed up for 6 months to 2 years, 10 had spontaneous remissions, 2 had remissions after treatment with corticosteroids, and 1 after treatment with cyclophosphamide; 13 did not respond to treatment.— R. D. Barr *et al.*, *Br. med. J.*, 1972, *2*, 131.

Precautions

Preparations of ammoniated mercury should not be applied to infants and young children as they may cause acrodynia (pink disease). They should not be applied to raw surfaces or the eyes.

Uses and Administration

Ammoniated mercury was formerly used topically in the treatment of impetigo and other staphylococcal skin infections, in dermatomycoses, and in psoriasis. The topical application of mercurial preparations is generally considered undesirable.

In the *UK* the use of ammoniated mercury in cosmetics is prohibited by law.

Preparations

Ammoniated Mercury and Coal Tar Ointment *(B.P.C. 1973).* Unguentum Hydrargyri Ammoniati et Picis Carbonis; Unguentum Picis Carbonis Compositum; Compound Ointment of Coal Tar. Ammoniated mercury 2.5 g, strong coal tar solution 2.5 g, and yellow soft paraffin 95 g.

Ammoniated Mercury, Coal Tar, and Salicylic Acid Ointment *(B.P.C. 1973).* Unguentum Hydrargyri Ammoniati et Picis Carbonis cum Acido Salicylico. Salicylic acid 2 g, ammoniated mercury and coal tar ointment to 100 g.

Ammoniated Mercury Ointment *(U.S.P.)*

Ammoniated Mercury Ophthalmic Ointment *(U.S.P.)*

1622-g

Mesulphen *(BAN).*

Dimethyldiphenylene Disulphide; Dimethylthianthrene; Mesulfen *(pINN)*. It consists mainly of 2,7-dimethylthianthrene.

$C_{14}H_{12}S_2$=244.4.

CAS — 135-58-0.

Pharmacopoeias. In *Aust.* and *Nord.* Thiantholum (*Jpn*) is a mixture of 2,7-dimethylthianthrene and ditolyl disulphide.

Mesulphen is a parasiticide and antipruritic agent and has been employed in the treatment of acne, pediculosis pubis, scabies, and seborrhoea. Sensitivity to mesulphen has occasionally been reported.

Proprietary Names and Manufacturers

Hispaderma *(Cidan, Spain)*; Mitigal *(Hermal, Ger.; Sigurtà, Ital.; Bayer, Norw.)*; Perozon *(Spitzner, Ger.)*; Soufrol *(Max Ritter, Switz.)*.

The following names have been used for multi-ingredient preparations containing mesulphen— Ringworm Ointment *(Wellcome, Austral.)*; Tineafax Ointment *(Wellcome, Austral.)*.

1623-q

Methoxsalen *(BAN, USAN).*

8-Methoxypsoralen; Ammoidin; Metoxaleno; Xanthotoxin. 9-Methoxy-7*H*-furo[3,2-*g*]-chromen-7-one.

$C_{12}H_8O_4$=216.2.

CAS — 298-81-7.

Pharmacopoeias. In *Braz.*, *Egypt.*, and *U.S.*

A constituent of the fruits of *Ammi majus*. It occurs as white to cream-coloured, odourless, fluffy, needle-like crystals.

Practically **insoluble** in water; sparingly soluble in boiling water and ether; freely soluble in chloroform; soluble in boiling alcohol, and in acetone, acetic acid, and propylene glycol. **Store** in well-closed containers. Protect from light.

Adverse Effects

Methoxsalen commonly causes nausea and less frequently mental effects including insomnia and mental depression.

Photochemotherapy or PUVA (see under Uses) may cause pruritus, mild transient erythema, oedema, dizziness, headache, vesiculation, bulla formation, onycholysis, acneiform eruption, and severe skin pain. Over-exposure to sunlight or u.v.-A radiation may produce severe burns.

The long-term risks of PUVA therapy include skin cancer in patients with pre-disposing factors, epidermal dystrophy, premature ageing of the skin, pigmentary changes, cataract formation, and alterations in the immune system. Numerous investigations indicate that PUVA is toxic to normal lymphocytes as well as to Langerhans' cells, which are important in antigen processing and presentation. It is possible that an immunosuppressive effect of PUVA is responsible for its carcinogenic potential, and it has been suggested that drugs that can bind to DNA are more likely to induce antinuclear antibody formation.— E. M. Farber *et al.*, *Archs Derm.*, 1983, *119*, 426.

EFFECTS ON THE BLOOD. After 1 year of PUVA treatment with oral methoxsalen, a 73-year-old psoriatic man developed a preleukaemic condition (haematopoietic dysplasia) characterised by a refractory anaemia, a slight thrombocytopenia, and leucopenia, and a bone marrow with an excess of myeloblasts.— J. Wagner *et al.*, *Scand. J. Haemat.*, 1978, *21*, 299. Acute myeloid leukaemia developed in a 73-year-old woman 2 years after the end of a course of 109 PUVA treatments, using oral methoxsalen, for psoriasis.— N. E. Hansen, *ibid.*, 1979, *22*, 57.

EFFECTS ON THE EYES. A 5-year study of 1299 psoriatic patients treated with PUVA using oral methoxsalen failed to demonstrate a significant dose-dependent increase in the risk of developing symptomatic cataracts, provided adequate eye protection was used. A small increase in the risk of development of nuclear sclerosis and posterior subcapsular opacities was observed among patients who had received at least 100 PUVA treatments compared with patients who had received fewer treatments, but these changes were not severe enough to impair vision.— R. S. Stern *et al.*, *J. invest. Derm.*, 1985, *85*, 269. See also: S. Lerman *et al.*, *ibid.*, 1980, *74*, 197; T. Y. Woo *et al.*, *Archs Derm.*, 1985, *121*, 1307.

Transient, apparently dose-related, visual-field defects in 3 patients during PUVA treatment.— D. A. Fenton and J. D. Wilkinson (letter), *Lancet*, 1983, *1*, 1106.

EFFECTS ON THE HAIR. Hypertrichosis was noticed in 15 of 23 female patients receiving PUVA therapy but only 2 of 14 patients treated with u.v.-A alone.— F. H. J. Rampen, *Br. J. Derm.*, 1983, *109*, 657.

EFFECTS ON THE IMMUNE SYSTEM. Compared to untreated controls, there was a decrease in circulating T-lymphocytes and a decreased response of lymphocytes to mitogens in 10 psoriatic patients who had received a high exposure to PUVA (more than 200 treatments over 2 to 6 years).— W. L. Morison *et al.*, *Br. J. Derm.*, 1983, *108*, 445.

For an *in-vitro* study of the effects of methoxsalen, u.v.-A irradiation, and PUVA on human leucocyte function, see: A. Bredberg and A. Forsgren, *Br. J. Derm.*, 1984, *111*, 159.

A 61-year-old psoriatic woman developed a drug fever after PUVA therapy on 2 occasions whereas neither oral methoxsalen nor u.v.-A irradiation alone caused a febrile reaction. The drug fever was felt to be an allergic phenomenon caused by a product of methoxsalen resulting from u.v.-A irradiation.— I. Tóth Kása and A. Dobozy, *Acta derm.-vener., Stockh.*, 1985, *65*, 557.

See also under Effects on the Kidney and Effects on the Skin, below.

EFFECTS ON THE KIDNEY. A report of nephrotic syndrome developing in a 38-year-old woman after 10 PUVA treatments.— L. T. K. Lam Thuon Mine *et al.*, *Br. med. J.*, 1983, *287*, 94.

EFFECTS ON THE LIVER. A 59-year-old woman with long-standing psoriasis, who had a damaged liver from methotrexate, twice developed a toxic hepatitis with fever and marked elevation of liver enzymes after taking methoxsalen 50 mg by mouth, during her fifteenth and sixteenth weekly PUVA treatments. On both occasions, there was spontaneous resolution within 5 days of the toxic hepatitis, which did not occur with topical methoxsalen.— D. M. Pariser and R. J. Wyles, *J. Am. Acad. Derm.*, 1980, *3*, 248.

EFFECTS ON THE NAILS. A report of nail pigmentation in 4 of 14 Indian patients with vitiligo after 2 months' treatment with methoxsalen.— R. P. C. Naik and G. Singh, *Br. J. Derm.*, 1979, *100*, 229.

EFFECTS ON THE SKIN. Squamous-cell carcinoma, basal cell carcinoma, nodular malignant melanoma, keratoacanthoma, actinic keratoses and Bowen's disease have all been recorded during or after cessation of PUVA therapy (R.S. Stern *et al.*, *New Engl. J. Med.*, 1984, *310*, 1156; D. Kemmett *et al.*, *Br. med. J.*, 1984, *289*, 1498; H. Reshad *et al.*, *Br. J. Derm.*, 1984, *110*, 299; D. Suurmond *et al.*, *ibid.*, 1985, *113*, 485). It was felt that previous skin carcinoma, arsenic therapy, or radiotherapy were strong risk factors for the development of cutaneous malignancies with PUVA and were relative contra-indications to its use in psoriasis (H. Reshad *et al.*, 1984; D. Suurmond *et al*, 1984). It was also suggested that methotrexate and PUVA might be synergistic in the induction of cutaneous malignancy (C.P. Fitzsimons *et al.*, *Lancet*, 1983, *1*, 235). However, Stern *et al.*, 1984, in a 5.7 year follow-up of 1380 patients treated with PUVA for psoriasis noted a significant increase in the relative risk of cutaneous squamous-cell carcinoma independent of prior exposure to cutaneous carcinogens, but related to cumulative u.v.-A exposure. Gibbs *et al.* (*Lancet*, 1986, *1*, 150) suggested that the increase in skin cancer risk noted in American surveys compared to European surveys might be explained by differences in therapeutic strategy; the American combination of a low u.v.-A dose and extended treatment times may increase tumour risk.

An 8-year follow-up study of cutaneous and ocular side-effects of PUVA therapy.— N. H. Cox *et al.*, *Br. J. Derm.*, 1987, *116*, 145.

Hyperpigmentation as freckles (PUVA lentigines) (S.S. Bleehen, *Br. J. Derm.*, 1978, *99*, *Suppl.* 16, 20) and hypopigmentation (G. Schuler *et al.*, *ibid.*, 1982, *107*, 173) have been reported after PUVA treatment and a mottled skin, consisting of irregular hyper- and depigmentation has been observed in PUVA-overdosed skin sites (F. Gschnait *et al.*, *ibid.*, 1980, *103*, 11).

Bullous pemphigoid developed in 2 patients during PUVA treatment; one had a history of bullous pemphigoid, and the other had taken co-trimoxazole which was not considered the precipitating factor.— K. Thomsen and H. Schmidt, *Br. J. Derm.*, 1976, *95*, 568. See also J. K. Robinson *et al.*, *ibid.*, 1978, *99*, 709.

Contact allergy to methoxsalen, confirmed by patch testing, in 2 patients treated with PUVA.— E. M. Saihan, *Br. med. J.*, 1979, *2*, 20. See also I. Weissmann *et al.*, *Br. J. Derm.*, 1980, *102*, 113.

Amongst 1380 patients with psoriasis treated with PUVA and followed for over 5 years, there was a significant, dose-dependent increase in the prevalence of clinical actinic degeneration (wrinkling, telangiectasia, and altered skin markings) of the skin of the buttocks and dorsa of the hands. However, the magnitude of the increase was small and, after 5 years, of little consequence to most patients.— R. S. Stern *et al.*, *J. invest. Derm.*, 1985, *84*, 135.

Precautions

Methoxsalen should not be given concomitantly with any drug known to cause photosensitisation nor to patients with diseases associated with light sensitivity such as porphyria, although it is used with care to decrease some patients' sensitivity to sunlight. Other contra-indications include aphakia, skin cancer, or a history of skin cancer. Methoxsalen should be used with caution in patients with hepatic insufficiency.

The skin should be protected from sunlight for at least 24 hours before and 8 hours after methoxsalen ingestion and patients should wear wrap-around u.v.-A absorbing glasses for 24 hours after ingestion. It is recommended that patients should undergo an ophthalmic examination, and that measurements of full blood count, anti-nuclear antibody titre, and hepatic and renal function be carried out before, and at intervals after, commencing therapy.

The Committee on Drugs of the American Academy of Pediatrics had recommended that PUVA should not be used for psoriasis in children except under investigational new drug protocols.— S. Segal *et al.*, *Pediatrics*, 1978, *62*, 253.

INTERACTIONS. PUVA treatment had no effect in a 48-year-old woman with psoriasis who was also receiving phenytoin 250 mg daily for epilepsy. PUVA treatment failure was due to abnormally low serum concentrations of methoxsalen, probably due to induction of hepatic enzymes by phenytoin.— B. Staberg and B. Hueg, *Acta derm.-vener., Stockh.*, 1985, *65*, 553.

Absorption and Fate

When taken by mouth methoxsalen is absorbed from the gastro-intestinal tract. Increased photosensitivity is present 1 hour after a dose, reaches a peak at about 2 hours, and disappears after about 8 hours. Up to 80% of a dose is excreted in the urine within 8 hours as the hydroxylated or glucuronide derivatives. Photosensitivity is more persistent after topical application.

A review of the clinical pharmacokinetics of the psoralens. The absorption of methoxsalen and hence clinical response, may be increased by concomitant food ingestion as well as by differences in drug formulation. A liquid preparation in soft gelatin capsules or a microenema gave higher serum concentrations more rapidly than did crystalline methoxsalen in tablets or capsules. Methoxsalen has a high, but variable, intrinsic metabolic clearance and is almost completely metabolised. There is a large interpatient variability in clearance. Individuals with a high clearance and low maximum serum concentration usually show reduced sensitivity to PUVA.— F. A. de Wolff and T. V. Thomas, *Clin. Pharmacokinet.*, 1986, *11*, 62.

Uses and Administration

Methoxsalen is a photosensitiser, markedly increasing skin reactivity to long-wavelength ultraviolet radiation, 320 to 400 nm, an effect used in photochemotherapy or PUVA [psoralen (P) and high- intensity long-wavelength (u.v.-A) irradiation]. In the presence of u.v.-A methoxsalen bonds with DNA inhibiting DNA synthesis and cell division, and can lead to cell injury. Recovery from the cell injury may be followed by increased melanisation of the epidermis. Methoxsalen may also increase pigmentation by an action on melanocytes.

PUVA is used to treat idiopathic vitiligo and severe, recalcitrant, disabling psoriasis not adequately responsive to other forms of therapy. PUVA has also been used to treat mycosis fungoides and under careful control to increase tolerance to sunlight.

To repigment vitiliginous areas, methoxsalen is given in a dose of 20 mg by mouth, with food or milk, 2 to 4 hours before measured periods of exposure to sunlight or u.v.-A two or three times a week, at least 48 hours apart. The length of exposure is adjusted according to the patient's skin type and response to therapy. An oral dose of 600 µg per kg body-weight should not be exceeded in vitiligo as severe burns may result. Methoxsalen is also used topically to repigment small, well-defined vitiliginous lesions. A 1% solution has been used, but this may need to be diluted 10-fold or 100-fold to avoid adverse cutaneous effects. The surrounding skin is protected by an opaque sunscreen, the lotion is applied to the lesion and after about 2 hours the treated area is exposed to sunlight or u.v.-A for measured periods once weekly or more often. Exposure time is adjusted according to skin type and response. The lesions are then washed and protected from light for 12 to 48 hours.

For the symptomatic treatment of psoriasis or mycosis fungoides, a similar schedule is used except that it employs high-intensity u.v.-A and that the initial oral methoxsalen dosage is based upon the patient's body-weight, ranging from 10 mg for a patient of less than 30 kg to 70 mg for a patient of over 115 kg. If there is no response or only minimal response after the fifteenth PUVA treatment dosage may be increased, once only, by 10 mg for the remainder of the course of treatment.

In the *UK* the use in cosmetics of *Ammi majus* and its galenical preparations, and methoxsalen, except for the natural content of essences, is prohibited by law.

For the mechanism of psoralen photosensitisation, see.— J. H. Epstein and B. U. Wintroub, *Drugs*, 1985, *30*, 42.

ALOPECIA. PUVA therapy has been used for alopecia areata with limited success. It has been recommended that it be used only after other approaches have been tried (O. Larkö and G. Swanbeck, *Acta derm.-vener., Stockh.*, 1983, *63*, 546; A.L. Claudy and D. Gagnaire, *Archs Derm.*, 1983, *119*, 975; M.A. Amer and A.E. Garf, *Int. J. Derm.*, 1983, *22*, 245).

KERATOSIS. A report of slow improvement in a patient with keratosis lichenoides chronica given PUVA therapy.— K. S. Ryatt *et al.*, *Br. J. Derm.*, 1982, *106*, 223. PUVA was effective in 5 patients with chronic hyperkeratotic dermatitis of the palms. Relapses occurred on cessation of therapy, but responded to re-treatment.— H. Mobacken *et al.*, *ibid.*, 1983, *109*, 205.

LICHEN. A report of good to excellent response to PUVA treatment by 6 of 7 patients with lichen planus, treated for an average of 10 weeks.— J. P. Ortonne *et al.*, *Br. J. Derm.*, 1978, *99*, 77.

A report of beneficial response to PUVA therapy in a 60-year-old woman with scleromyxoedema.— P. M. Farr and F. A. Ive, *Br. J. Derm.*, 1984, *110*, 347.

MALIGNANT NEOPLASMS. In 149 patients with mycosis fungoides treated with PUVA, some followed-up for 8 years from their first treatment, patients with macular disease were usually cleared by PUVA; some remissions of over 3 years followed discontinuation of treatment. Despite PUVA, plaque-stage patients may progress to tumour-stage disease, which required therapy additional to PUVA in most patients. Erythrodermic cases tolerated PUVA poorly. Irregular attendance was the most common reason for an apparent poor clinical response. The effect of PUVA on long-term prognosis remained to be determined.— R. A. Logan *et al.*, *Br. J. Derm.*, 1986, *115*, *Suppl.* 30, 17. Further references: D. V. Briffa *et al.*, *Lancet*, 1980, *2*, 49.

In a preliminary study, 27 of 37 patients with otherwise resistant cutaneous T-cell lymphoma responded to extracorporeal photochemotherapy. Treatment involved administration of methoxsalen 600 µg per kg body-weight. Two hours later 300 mL of the patient's plasma was removed. This was pooled with leukocyte-enriched blood and saline and exposed to u.v.-A before return to the patient.— R. Edelson *et al.*, *New Engl. J. Med.*, 1987, *316*, 297.

See also Effects on the skin under Adverse Effects.

PHOTODERMATOSES. Thirty-eight patients with polymorphic light eruption were treated with PUVA, low-dose u.v.-A with oral placebo (control), or u.v.-B with oral placebo 3 times weekly for 6 weeks. After completion of the treatment period, for each group itch, rash, and the proportion of patients with these symptoms increased with increasing u.v. exposure. However, compared with the control group, these effects were much less marked in the PUVA and u.v.-B groups for both itch and, to a lesser extent, rash.— G. M. Murphy *et al.*, *Br. J. Derm.*, 1984, *111*, *Suppl.* 26, 24.

Long-standing chronic actinic dermatitis in 4 patients was treated with a modified PUVA regime initially including generalised applications of topical steroids immediately after PUVA exposure. All patients were freed of rash, no longer needed protection from u.v. radiation, and were maintained on twice monthly PUVA therapy.— C. Hindson *et al.*, *Br. J. Derm.*, 1985, *113*, 157.

PITYRIASIS. In 3 patients with long-standing pityriasis lichenoides, which was resistant to other forms of therapy, there was complete clearing in 1 and marked improvement in 2 after PUVA therapy 3 times weekly for 3 to 12 months.— F. C. Powell and S. A. Muller, *J. Am. Acad. Derm.*, 1984, *10*, 59.

PSORIASIS. In the multicentre European PUVA Study a response better than marked improvement was obtained in 88.8% of 3136 patients with severe psoriasis treated with PUVA. The average number of treatments required was 20, clearing taking 37 days and the total cumulative u.v.-A dose was 96 J/cm^2. Within a follow-up period of 80 weeks, the chance that a patient would remain in remission was almost the same with or without maintenance therapy. Comparison of the clearing phase results with those reported for the *U.S.* Cooperative Clinical Trial (J.W. Melski *et al.*, *J. invest. Derm.*, 1977, *68*, 328) showed treatment duration to be twice as long in the *U.S.* study for a similar response even though the number of treatments was much the same; total u.v.-A requirements were also higher. In the *U.S.* study, treatments were given only 2 or 3 times a week and dose increments followed a predetermined rigid schedule. The European study protocol provided for 4 treatments per week and rapid dose increments adjusted to the patients' response, an approach that saved time and reduced the total u.v.-A dose.— T. Henseler *et al.*, *Lancet*, 1981, *1*, 853.

Twenty-two patients with bilaterally symmetrical persistent palmoplantar pustulosis were treated on one randomly selected side with PUVA using oral methoxsalen. After 30 treatments, the treated side had cleared completely in 12 patients, was much improved in 5, and improved in 4; one patient had improved on both sides. Fifteen of the 22 received a further 30 PUVA treatments employing topical methoxsalen on the control side. Seven patients cleared completely, 6 were much improved, and 2 improved. Frequent maintenance was needed, with early relapse if it was stopped.— D. Murray *et al.*, *Br. J. Derm.*, 1980, *102*, 659.

Plaque-type psoriasis cleared in 13 of 20 patients after PUVA treatment and improved but failed to clear in 4. Treatment failed in 3. Four patients with erythrodermic, pustular, or inflammatory psoriasis failed to respond. Factors to be considered in patient selection for PUVA are the type of psoriasis, the patient's skin type, and the proportion of body surface area involved.— J. -P. Des-Groseilliers *et al.*, *Can. med. Ass. J.*, 1981, *124*, 1016.

Symmetrical psoriatic lesions in 15 patients were treated with PUVA using topical methoxsalen 1%. One side was exposed to u.v.-A 2 hours after application, the other within 5 minutes (non-interval therapy). Both regimens were equally effective in 11 patients, the 2-hour interval therapy was preferred in 3, and the non-interval therapy was preferred in 1. With non-interval therapy, unfavourable side-effects were minimal and it was easy to treat patients as out-patients.— K. Danno *et al.*, *Br. J. Derm.*, 1983, *108*, 519.

In 5 patients with troublesome nail psoriasis, local PUVA treatment using topical methoxsalen 1% applied to the proximal nail fold followed by u.v.-A irradiation produced clearing in 2 and substantial improvement in a further 2. One failed to show sustained improvement.— S. E. Handfield-Jones *et al.* (letter), *Br. J. Derm.*, 1987, *116*, 280.

For a comparison of PUVA with dithranol in the treatment of psoriasis, see p.920 and with etretinate, see p.922.

For the combined use of PUVA with etretinate in psoriasis, see p.922.

For a comparison of the use of etretinate or isotretinoin combined with PUVA for psoriasis, see p.925.

Combination therapy with methotrexate. Two hundred and six patients with severe psoriasis were treated with the Ingram dithranol regime (see p.919). Sixty-one received no subsequent maintenance treatment, 37 received weekly to monthly PUVA, and 108 received methotrexate, cumulative dose 460 mg per year. After one year 24% of patients who had no maintenance therapy were in remission, compared with 82% of the PUVA maintenance group, and 96% of the methotrexate maintenance group. After 3 years, 83% of the methotrexate group were still in remission, but if methotrexate was discontinued a rapid relapse followed. After stopping PUVA maintenance, many patients remained in remission for many months.— P. C. M. Van de Kerkhof *et al.*, *Br. J. Derm.*, 1982, *106*, 605. See also P. C. M. Van de Kerkhof and J. W. H. Mali, *Br. J. Derm.*, 1982, *106*, 623.

Combination therapy with topical corticosteroids. In studies of 116 patients (W.L. Morison *et al.*, *Br. J. Derm.*, 1978, *98*, 125) and 90 patients (M. Schmoll *et al.*, *ibid.*, *99*, 693), PUVA with concurrent topical fluocinolone acetonide or triamcinolone acetonide cleared psoriasis more quickly than PUVA alone. Morison *et al.*, noted a greatly increased relapse rate immediately post-clearing whereas Schmoll *et al.* did not and attributed this to their more intensive PUVA regimen. Morison *et al.* also found that 6 weeks' pre-treatment with topical fluocinolone acetonide did not reduce the subsequent number of PUVA treatments needed to clear psoriasis whereas Gould and Wilson (*ibid.*, *98*, 133) found that one week's pre-treatment with topical clobetasol propionate did reduce the number in 8 of 16 patients. The beneficial effect was attributed to a shorter course, without occlusive dressings, and application only to symmetrical, equally affected plaques.

Combination therapy with u.v.-B radiation. A comparison of PUVA on its own and in combination with u.v.-B irradiation, both given twice weekly was carried out in 31 patients with chronic psoriasis. The addition of u.v.-B significantly decreased the number of PUVA treatments required to achieve clearance and in 3 cases, clearance was achieved where PUVA alone had failed.— K. M. Diette *et al.*, *Archs Derm.*, 1984, *120*, 1169.

WEALING DISORDERS. Reduced pruritus and wealing and partial to almost complete fading of macules in 7 of 8 patients with urticaria pigmentosa after an average of 27 PUVA exposures.— D. Vella Briffa *et al.*, *Br. J. Derm.*, 1983, *109*, 67.

Five of 14 patients with symptomatic dermographism reported worthwhile improvement of pruritus after 12 PUVA treatments.— R. A. Logan *et al.*, *Br. J. Derm.*, 1984, *111*, *Suppl.* 26, 41.

Preparations

Methoxsalen Capsules *(U.S.P.)*

Methoxsalen Topical Solution *(U.S.P.)*

Proprietary Preparations

Deltasoralen *(Delta Laboratories, Eire). Tablets*, methoxsalen 10 mg.
Paint, methoxsalen 1%.
Emulsion, methoxsalen 0.15%.

Oxysoralen *(Delta Laboratories, Eire). Capsules*, methoxsalen 10 mg.

Proprietary Names and Manufacturers

Deltasoralen *(Delta Laboratories, Eire)*; Geroxalen *(Aust.; Pharma-Medica, Denm.; Neth.)*; Meladinin *(Ger.; Switz.)*; Meladinine *(Promedica, Fr.; Basotherm, Ger.; Basotherm, Switz.)*; Mopsoralen *(Belg.)*; Novo Meladinina *(Llorente, Spain)*; Oxsoralen *(Aust.; Protea, Austral.; Belg.; Elder, Canad.; Lifepharma, Ital.; Neth.; Elder, S.Afr.; Alcon, Spain; Switz.; Elder, USA)*; Oxysoralen *(Delta Laboratories, Eire)*; Ultramop *(Canderm, Canad.)*.

The following names have been used for multi-ingredient preparations containing methoxsalen— Meladinine *(Delta Laboratories, Eire)*.

12944-h

5-Methoxypsoralen

Bergapten. 5-Methoxypsoralen is an ingredient of bergamot oil. 4-Methoxy-7*H*-furo[3,2-*g*]chromen-7-one.
$C_{12}H_8O_4$=216.2.

CAS — 484-20-8.

5-Methoxypsoralen has been used similarly to methoxsalen (p.927) in the PUVA treatment of psoriasis. Concern has been expressed at the possible risk of cancer, and the use of 5-methoxypsoralen in cosmetic suntan preparations is considered unwise by some authorities. Photosensitivity caused by 5-methoxypsoralen is sometimes known as Berloque dermatitis.

A discussion of the possible risk of cancer from sunlight, from the use of psoralens in the PUVA treatment of psoriasis, and from the use of 5-methoxypsoralen in suntan preparations.— *Br. med. J.*, 1981, *283*, 335.

A report of pruritus, pigmentation, and a tendency to sunburn in a 70-year-old woman with chronic liver disease after eating about 170 g of parsley, which contains 5-methoxypsoralen, daily for 30 years.— P. Cooles, *Br. med. J.*, 1982, *285*, 1719.

The absence of u.v.-A-induced erythema following the use of a commercial tablet preparation of 5-methoxypsoralen was probably due to the poor bioavailability of the preparation.— L. M. L. Stolk *et al.*, *Br. J. Derm.*, 1985, *112*, 469.

Proprietary Names and Manufacturers

Psoraderm *(Goupil, Fr.)*.

1624-p

Monobenzone *(USAN, rINN)*.

Monobenzyl Ether of Hydroquinone. 4-Benzyloxyphenol.
$C_{13}H_{12}O_2$=200.2.

CAS — 103-16-2.

Pharmacopoeias. In *U.S.*

A white odourless, crystalline powder. Practically **insoluble** in water; soluble 1 in about 15 of alcohol, 1 in 29 of chloroform, 1 in 14 of ether; soluble in acetone. **Store** at a temperature not exceeding 30° in airtight containers. Protect from light.

Adverse Effects

Monobenzone may cause skin irritation and sensitisation. In some patients, this may only be temporary and need not necessitate complete withdrawal of the drug. In other patients, an eczematous sensitisation may occur. Excessive depigmentation may occur even beyond the areas under treatment and may produce unsightly patches.

Uses and Administration

Monobenzone increases melanin excretion from melanocytes and may also prevent its production. It is used locally in the form of a cream containing up to 20% for final, permanent depigmentation of normal skin in extensive vitiligo. It is applied to the affected parts two or three times daily until a satisfactory response is obtained, and thereafter twice weekly. Excessive exposure to sunlight should be avoided. The results are variable. Depigmentation only becomes apparent when the preformed melanin pigments have been lost with the normal sloughing of the stratum corneum and this may take several months. If, however, no improvement is noted after 4 months treatment the use of the drug should be abandoned.

Monobenzone has no effect on melanomas or pigmented naevi and is not recommended for freckling, chloasma, or hyperpigmentation following skin inflammation or due to photosensitisation following the use of certain perfumes.

In the *UK* the use of monobenzone in cosmetics is prohibited by law.

Preparations

Monobenzone Cream *(U.S.P.)*

Proprietary Names and Manufacturers

Aloquin *(Prosana, Austral.)*; Benoquin *(Elder, Canad.; Switz.; Elder, USA)*; Depigman *(Hermal, Ger.; Hermal, Neth.; Hermal, Switz.)*; Dermochinona *(Chinoin, Ital.)*; Leucodinine *(Belg.)*.

12980-g

Motretinide *(USAN, rINN)*.

Ro-11-1430. (*all-trans*)-*N*-Ethyl-9-(4-methoxy-2,3,6-trimethylphenyl)-3,7-dimethylnona-2,4,6,8-tetraenamide.
$C_{23}H_{31}NO_2$=353.5.

CAS — 56281-36-8.

Motretinide is used topically, similarly to tretinoin, in the treatment of acne.

Fifty patients with mild-to-moderate acne vulgaris were treated once or twice daily for 1 to 6 months with motretinide cream or lotion 0.1% or pads impregnated with a solution containing motretinide 1 mg. Comedones, papules, and pustules were reduced by 58%, 53%, and 71% respectively and there was usually remission after 8 to 10 weeks. Good or very good results were recorded in 52% of patients. Mild erythema and burning of the skin occurred during the first 4 weeks; there was drying and desquamation in 16% of patients. It was concluded that although tretinoin is a more efficacious topical therapy in acne vulgaris, motretinide was to be preferred in moderate and mild cases, as well as in subjects who may be intolerant to tretinoin.— M. Papini, *Drugs exp. & clin. Res.*, 1982, *8*, 525.

In an 8-week open study, 30 patients with mild-to-moderate acne vulgaris were treated with motretinide cream 0.1% applied twice daily or benzoyl peroxide gel 5% applied once daily. Good results were obtained with both agents; there were no differences regarding the lesion count. Benzoyl peroxide caused local irritation in 11 of 15 patients, severe enough to warrant discontinuation in 2, whereas motretinide was well tolerated except in 1 case who experienced a severe flare-up reaction within the first week of treatment.— A. Lassus *et al.*, *Dermatologica*, 1984, *168*, 199.

Proprietary Names and Manufacturers

Tasmaderm *(Sauter, Switz.)*.

1627-e

Pentosalen *(BAN)*.

Ammidin; Imperatorin; Isoamylenoxypsoralen; Marmelosin. 9-(3-Methylbut-2-enyloxy)-7*H*-furo[3,2-*g*]-chromen-7-one.
$C_{16}H_{14}O_4$=270.3.

A constituent of the fruits of *Ammi majus* (Umbelliferae).

Pentosalen has been used with methoxsalen (see p. 927) in the treatment of alopecia and vitiligo.

In the *UK* the use of pentosalen in cosmetics is prohibited by law.

Proprietary Names and Manufacturers

The following names have been used for multi-ingredient preparations containing pentosalen— Meladinine *(Delta Laboratories, Eire)*.

7523-v

Podophyllum *(USAN)*.

American Mandrake; May Apple Root; Podoph.; Podophyllum Rhizome.

CAS — 9000-55-9 (podophyllum); 518-28-5 (podophyllotoxin); 568-53-6 (α-peltatin); 518-29-6 (β-peltatin).

Pharmacopoeias. In *Port., Span.*, and *U.S.*

The dried rhizome and roots of *Podophyllum peltatum* (Berberidaceae). The *U.S.P.* specifies not less than 5% of resin. The resin contains podophyllotoxin, α-peltatin, and β-peltatin.

7524-g

Indian Podophyllum

Ind. Podoph.; Indian Podophyllum Rhizome.

Pharmacopoeias. In *Chin.* Also in *B.P.C. 1973* .

The dried fruits of *Podophyllum emodi* (=*P. hexandrum*) (Berberidaceae).

7525-q

Podophyllum Resin *(BAN, USAN)*.

Podoph. Resin; Podophylli Resina; Podophyllin.

Pharmacopoeias. In *Arg., Aust., Belg., Egypt., Fr., Hung., Int., Nord., Port., Span., Swiss, Turk.*, and *U.S.* (all from podophyllum only). In *Br.* from Indian podophyllum or podophyllum.

A mixture of resins obtained from Indian podophyllum or from podophyllum; the *B.P.* specifies either, the *U.S.P.* specifies podophyllum. Resin from Indian podophyllum contains at least 40% podophyllotoxin, that from podophyllum only about 10%.

An amorphous powder, varying in colour from light brown to greenish-yellow or brownish-grey, with a characteristic odour. On exposure to light or to temperatures above 25° it becomes darker in colour.

Very slightly **soluble** in cold water; partly soluble in hot water but precipitated again on cooling; soluble completely or almost completely in alcohol; partly soluble in chloroform, ether, and dilute ammonia solution. A solution in alcohol is acid to litmus. **Store** in a cool place in airtight containers. Protect from light.

CAUTION. *Podophyllum resin is strongly irritant to the skin, eyes, and mucous membranes and requires careful handling.*

Adverse Effects

Podophyllum is very irritant. It can also cause severe systemic toxicity after ingestion or topical application, which is usually reversible but has been fatal. Symptoms of toxicity include nausea, vomiting, abdominal pain and diarrhoea; there may be thrombocytopenia, leucopenia, renal failure, and hepatotoxicity. Central effects include hallucinations, confusion, dizziness, stupor, ataxia, hypotonia, convulsions, and coma. EEG changes may persist for several days. Peripheral and autonomic neuropathies are delayed in onset and prolonged in duration and may result in paraesthesiae, reduced reflexes, muscle weakness, tachycardia, apnoea, orthostatic hypotension, paralytic ileus, and urinary retention.

A review of cases of podophyllum toxicity. Fatal poisoning in one patient following ingestion of about 10 to 11 g of podophyllum. Fourteen other cases of poisoning, some fatal, are reviewed.— D. E. Cassidy *et al.*, *J. Toxicol. clin. Toxicol.*, 1982, *19*, 35.

Coma and prolonged peripheral neuropathy after the ingestion of a large number of herbal laxative tablets containing podophyllin.— G. J. Dobb and R. H. Edis, *Med. J. Aust.*, 1984, *140*, 495.

A report of the transformation of a condyloma acuminatum into an invasive squamous cell carcinoma after treatment with podophyllin 25% in alcohol. It was noted that almost all reported cases of malignant transformation in condyloma acuminatum had occurred since the introduction of podophyllin for their treatment.— H. B. Svindland, *Eur. J. sex. transm. Dis.*, 1984, *1*, 165.

Precautions

Podophyllum resin should not be given by mouth or used topically during pregnancy.

The risk of systemic toxicity after topical application is increased by the treatment of large areas with excessive amounts for prolonged periods, by the treatment of friable, bleeding, or recently biopsied warts, and by inadvertent application to normal skin or mucous membranes.

Uses and Administration

Podophyllum resin has an antimitotic action and is used principally as a topical treatment for ano-genital warts (condylomata acuminata). It is applied as a 10 to 25% solution in alcohol or compound benzoin tincture, left on the warts for 1 to 6 hours, and then washed off. This procedure is carried out 1 to 3 times weekly and, if unsuccessful after about 4 applications, an alternative treatment should be tried. Podophyllum resin has been used on external genital, perianal, and intra-meatal warts, but should not be used on cervical or urethral warts. Care must be taken to avoid application to healthy tissue. Podophyllum resin is also used in an ointment for plantar warts.

When taken by mouth podophyllum resin has a drastic purging action and it is highly irritant to the intestinal mucosa and produces violent peristalsis. It has been superseded by less toxic laxatives.

Podophyllum peltatum has been designated as a herb unsafe for foods, beverages, and drugs by the Food and Drug Administration.— *Am. Pharm.*, 1984, *NS24*, (Mar.), 20.

ANO-GENITAL WARTS. One hundred and nine patients with ano-genital warts were treated weekly for 6 weeks in a double-blind study with either 10 or 25% podophyllin in tincture of benzoin compound. Three months after therapy ceased, 24 patients were free of warts, 12 each after treatment with 10 and 25% podophyllin. There was no significant difference in the number of applications needed with each treatment.— P. D. Simmons, *Br. J. vener. Dis.*, 1981, *57*, 208.

In a prospective, controlled study, 60 patients with first-episode perianal condylomata acuminata were treated by surgical excision or local application of a 25% podophyllin tincture of benzoin for 6 hours once weekly for up to 6 weeks. The median number of visits required to clear all warts was 5 in the podophyllin-treated group and 1 in the surgically-treated group. Of 23 patients whose warts were cured by podophyllin, 17 had recurrences requiring further treatment within 1 year, compared to 8 of 28 cured by surgical excision. There were significantly fewer recurrences among the surgically-treated than in the podophyllin-treated patients at each 3-monthly follow-up. Thus surgical excision produced faster clearance and lower recurrence rates than podophyllin application.— S. L. Jensen, *Lancet*, 1985, *2*, 1146. Similar results in a further 29 patients.— H. T. Khawaja (letter), *ibid.*, 1986, *1*, 208.

Comparison with fluorouracil. Thirty-seven patients with penile and urethral condylomata acuminata were treated with either podophyllin 25% alcoholic solution applied weekly for 4 weeks, or fluorouracil cream applied daily for 2 weeks. The 2 treatments gave the same results which were unrelated to distribution, type, and appearance of the warts. After 4 weeks of treatment, 56.7% of the patients were cured. By giving those who failed to respond to one drug the other, for 2 to 4 weeks, a total regression was seen in 64.9% after 4 to 9 months. Side-effects after podophyllin treatment were reported by only 1 of 22 patients, while the side-effects of the fluorouracil treatment were a problem for 11 of 20 patients within 10 to 14 days.— J. Wallin, *Br. J. vener. Dis.*, 1977, *53*, 240.

Comparison with podophyllotoxin. In a double-blind study, 77 patients with ano-genital warts were treated weekly with either podophyllin 20% or podophyllotoxin 5% in alcohol. After 6 weeks, 9 of 38 patients were cured with podophyllin and 8 of 39 with podophyllotoxin, and there was a 50% or more reduction in size and/or number of condylomata in 20 and 18 patients respectively. These differences were not significant. The low number of local adverse reactions with 5% podophyllotoxin compared to 20% podophyllin indicated that it may be used as drug of first choice.— C. S. Petersen *et al.*, *Eur. J. sex. transm. Dis.*, 1985, *2*, 155.

Comparison with trichloroacetic acid. Sixty patients with ano-genital warts were treated weekly with either podophyllin 25% and trichloroacetic acid 50% in industrial methylated spirits, or podophyllin 25% alone. There was no significant difference in the numbers of patients clear of warts at 6 and 12 weeks (32%) but of the patients without warts at 6 weeks, those treated with podophyllin alone had required a mean of 4.0 applications compared to 2.9 with the combination. Five of 31 patients experienced side-effects (superficial ulceration, excessive soreness) with the combination; no side-effects were reported with podophyllin alone.— G. Gabriel and R. N. T. Thin, *Br. J. vener. Dis.*, 1983, *59*, 124.

PLANTAR WARTS. Good results have been claimed in some plantar warts. After preliminary removal of callus, podophyllin 25% in liquid paraffin was applied under adhesive plaster and repeated at intervals of 1 to 2 weeks.— E. M. Saihan, *Br. J. Hosp. Med.*, 1983, *29*, 182.

Preparations

Compound Podophyllin Paint *(B.P., A.P.F.).* Pig. Podoph. Co.; Podophyllin Compound Paint. Podophyllum resin 15 g, compound benzoin tincture to 100 mL.

Podophyllum Resin Topical Solution *(U.S.P.).* A solution in alcohol containing podophyllum resin *U.S.P.* and an alcoholic extract of Siam or Sumatra benzoin.

Proprietary Preparations

Posalfilin *(Norgine, UK). Ointment*, podophyllum resin 20%, salicylic acid 25%.

Vericap *(Cuxson, Gerrard, UK). Dressing*, podophyllum resin 20%, linseed oil 20%.

Proprietary Names and Manufacturers of Podophyllum Resin and Related Compounds

Condofil *(Ital.)*; Condyline *(Gist-Brocades, Denm.)*; Pod-Ben-25 *(C & M, USA)*; Podofilm *(Pharmascience, Canad.)*; Vericap *(Cuxson, Gerrard, UK)*; Wartec *(Conpharm, Swed.)*; Warticon *(Cph, UK)*.

The following names have been used for multi-ingredient preparations containing podophyllum resin and related compounds—Boldolaxine *(Simes, Austral.)*; Canthacur-PS *(Pharmascience, Canad.)*; Cantharone Plus *(Dormer, Canad.*; *Seres, USA)*; Opobyl *(Bengué, UK)*; Posalfilin *(Norgine, Austral.*; *Norgine, UK)*; Salicylin-P *(Key, Austral.)*; Verban *(Welcker-Lyster, Canad.)*; Verrex *(C & M, USA)*; Verrusol *(C & M, USA)*; Wartkil *(Rosken, Austral.)*; Wart-Off *(Nelson, Austral.)*.

1663-z

Some Proprietary Protective Materials

Several types of dressing are available in addition to the traditional cotton or viscose dressings. Listed below are some proprietary protective materials that are aerosol polymer sprays, sleeved pads, semipermeable films, polymeric foams, hydrogels, or hydrocolloids.

Aerosol polymer sprays are used to provide flexible, protective films on the skin. These and semipermeable films are impermeable to wound exudate and reduce fluid loss from wounds.

Sleeved pads consist of absorbent pads covered with non-adherent polymeric wound contact material.

Polymeric polyurethane foams are permeable to water vapour and oxygen and maintain a moist wound surface whilst absorbing excess wound exudate.

Hydrogels and hydrocolloids consist of a matrix of polymeric material containing a high percentage of water. They are soft and conformable, and like the polymeric foams, are used to maintain optimum conditions for wound healing.

Some other proprietary protective materials are described under dimethicones (p. 1325), cadexomer-iodine (p. 1184), dextranomer (p. 919), and povidone-iodine (p. 1188).

References: T. D. Turner, *Pharm. J.*, 1984, *1*, 452 (semipermeable films); K. J. Harkiss, *ibid.*, 1985, *2*, 268 (dressings for leg ulcers); *Drug & Ther. Bull.*, 1986, *24*, 9 (dressings for leg ulcers); S. Thomas, *Pharm. J.*, 1988, *1*, 752.

Proprietary Preparations

Bioclusive *(Johnson & Johnson, UK). Dressing*, sterile, transparent semipermeable polyurethane film with adhesive edging.

Comfeel Ulcus *(Coloplast, UK). Dressing*, sterile, composite, hydrocolloid matrix backed by a polyurethane foam. Also available as a powder and paste.

Debrisan *(Pharmacia, UK).* See under Dextranomer, p.919.

Geliperm *(Geistlich, UK). Dressing*, sterile, hydrogel, polymerised acrylamide and agar matrix containing water. A Wet form, Dry form, and Granulate are available.

Description of a non-textile wound dressing (Geliperm) which is a gel polymer of agar and acrylamide.— J. A. Myers, *Pharm. J.*, 1983, *1*, 263.

Granuflex *(Squibb Surgicare, UK). Dressing*, sterile, composite, hydrocolloid matrix backed by a waterproof polyurethane foam. Also available as granules and paste.

Inadine *(Johnson & Johnson, UK).* See under Povidone-Iodine, p.1188.

Iodosorb *(Janssen, UK).* See under Cadexomer Iodine, p.1184.

Lyofoam *(Ultra, UK). Dressing*, sterile, polyurethane foam with a hydrophilic and a hydrophobic layer.

Melolin *(Smith & Nephew, UK). Dressing*, sterile, cotton and acrylic fibre pad sleeved with polyester film.

N-A Dressing *(Johnson & Johnson, UK). Dressing*, sterile, knitted viscose, acrylic coated.

Nobecutane *(Astra, UK). Dressing*, aerosol spray, acrylic resin equivalent to total solids 5.7%, ethyl acetate 27.3%.

NSB *(Geistlich, UK). Dressing*, aerosol spray, vinylpyrrolidone and vinyl acetate copolymer.

Opsite *(Smith & Nephew, UK). Dressing*, sterile, transparent semipermeable polyurethane film with adhesive edging.

Opsite Spray *(Smith & Nephew, UK). Dressing*, aerosol spray, ethoxyethyl methacrylate and methoxyethyl methacrylate copolymer (Hydron) 3%.

Scherisorb *(Smith & Nephew, UK). Dressing*, sterile, hydrogel, starch copolymer matrix containing water.

Silastic Foam Dressing *(Dow Corning, UK).* See under Dimethicones, p. 1325.

Sorbsan *(Steriseal, UK).* See under Calcium Alginate, p.1132.

Tegaderm *(3M Health Care, UK). Dressing*, sterile, transparent semipermeable polyurethane film with adhesive edging.

Vigilon *(Bard, UK). Dressing*, sterile, hydrogel.

Proprietary Names and Manufacturers

Aeroplast *(Parke, Davis, UK)*; Bioclusive *(Johnson & Johnson, UK)*; DuoDermflexible Hydroactive Dressings *(Squibb, Austral.)*; Hibispray No. 4 Clear Plastic Dressing *(Stuart, UK)*; Hollihesive Skin Barrier *(Abbott, Austral.)*; Lyofoam *(Ultra, UK)*; N-A Dressing *(Johnson & Johnson, UK)*; Nobecutane *(Astra, Austral.*; *Astra, UK)*; NSB *(Geistlich, UK)*; Nucopal *(Orapharm, Austral.)*; Opsite *(Smith & Nephew, Austral.*; *Smith & Nephew, UK)*; Scherisorb *(Smith & Nephew, UK)*; Skin Bond Cement *(Denyer, Austral.)*; Skin Gel *(Abbott, Austral.)*; Skin Prep *(Denyer, Austral.)*; Spray-on Bande *(Eagle, Austral.)*; Stomahesive *(Squibb, Austral.*; *Squibb Surgicare, UK)*; Synthaderm *(Armour, UK)*; Tegaderm *(3M Health Care, UK)*; Urihesive *(Squibb, Austral.*; *Squibb Surgicare, UK)*; Varihesive *(Squibb, Austral.*; *Squibb Surgicare, UK)*; Vigilon *(Bard, UK)*.

1631-q

Pumice *(USAN).*

Lapis Pumicis; Pierre Ponce Granulée; Pumex; Pumex Granulatus; Pumice Stone.

CAS — 1332-09-8.

Pharmacopoeias. In *Fr.* and *U.S.*

A substance of volcanic origin consisting chiefly of complex silicates of aluminium, potassium, and sodium. Odourless, very light, hard, rough, porous greyish masses or gritty, greyish powder. Practically **insoluble** in water and not attacked by acids.

The *U.S.P.* recognises 3 grades of powdered pumice: (1) superfine (=pumice flour)—not less than 97% passes through a No. 200 [US] sieve; (2) fine—not less than 95% passes through a No. 150 sieve and not more than 75% through a No. 200 sieve; (3) coarse—not less than 95% passes through a No. 60 sieve and not more than 5% through a No. 200 sieve.

Store in well-closed containers.

Powdered pumice is used as a dental and dermal abrasive and as a filtering medium.

Pneumoconiosis caused by pumice dust.— G. Babolini *et al.*, *Bull. int. Un. Tuberc.*, 1979, *54*, 425.

1633-s

Pyrithione Zinc *(BAN, USAN, rINN).*

Zinc 2-Pyridinethiol 1-Oxide; Zinc Pyridinethione. Bis-[1-hydroxypyridine-2(1*H*)-thionato]zinc.

$C_{10}H_8N_2O_2S_2Zn$=317.7.

CAS — 13463-41-7.

Pyrithione zinc has bacteriostatic and fungistatic properties. It is used similarly to selenium sulphide (p.932) in the control of seborrhoeic dermatitis and dandruff. It is an ingredient of some proprietary shampoos.

Pyrithione sodium has been used when a soluble form of pyrithione is required.

While less than 1% of pyrithione zinc was absorbed through the skin 13% of pyrithione sodium was absorbed.— C. K. Parekh (letter), *Lancet*, 1978, *1*, 940.

In 32 subjects, a shampoo containing zinc pyrithione 1% used twice weekly was more effective than a placebo shampoo in reducing dandruff, the relative difference becoming significant after a minimum of 3 washes.— R. Marks *et al.*, *Br. J. Derm.*, 1985, *112*, 415. See also N. J. Van Abbé *et al.*, *Int. J. cosmet. Sci.*, 1981, *3*, 233.

ADVERSE EFFECTS. Peripheral neuritis with paraesthesia and muscle weakness in one patient was associated with the prolonged use of a shampoo containing pyrithione zinc 2%. The muscle weakness had disappeared 3 months after stopping the shampoo and 2 years later the paraesthesia had improved by about 75%.— J. E. Beck (letter), *Lancet*, 1978, *1*, 444.

Proprietary Names and Manufacturers

Action Foam *(Upjohn, Austral.)*; Dan Gard *(Hoechst, Austral.; Stiefel, Canad.)*; Danex *(Herbert, USA)*; De-Squaman *(Hermal, Ger.)*; Desquaman *(Hermal, Switz.)*; DHS Zinc Dandruff Shampoo *(Person & Covey, USA)*; Hair Power *(Canad.)*; Sapoderm *(Austral.)*; Sebulon *(Westwood, Canad.; Westwood, USA)*; Skaelud *(ND & K, Denm.)*; Ultrex *(Pharmeurop, Fr.)*; Zinc Omadine *(Olin, USA: K & K-Greeff, UK)*; Zincon *(Lederle, USA)*; ZNP *(Stiefel, USA)*.

The following names have been used for multi-ingredient preparations containing pyrithione zinc— Multi-Tar Plus *(ICN, Canad.)*.

1634-w

Pyrogallol

Pyrogallic Acid. Benzene-1,2,3-triol.

$C_6H_6O_3$=126.1.

CAS — 87-66-1.

Pharmacopoeias. In *Aust., Fr., Jug., Pol., Port., Span.*, and *Swiss.*

Adverse Effects

Systemic effects of pyrogallol are similar to those of phenol (see p.967) and in addition include methaemoglobinaemia, haemolysis, and kidney damage; they are treated similarly.

Uses and Administration

Pyrogallol has been used as an ointment in psoriasis and parasitic skin diseases, but it is not suitable for application over large areas or denuded surfaces owing to the danger of toxic effects from absorption.

Pyrogallol stains the skin and hair black; skin stains are removed by ammonium persulphate or 10% oxalic acid solution.

In the *UK* the concentration of pyrogallol in hair dyes is limited to 5% by law.

Pyrogallol triacetate has been used for the same purposes as pyrogallol.

1636-l

Pyroxylin *(BAN, USAN, rINN).*

Algodão-Polvora; Cellulose Nitrate; Colloxylinum; Fulmicoton; Gossypium Collodium; Kollodiumwolle; Pyroxylinum; Soluble Guncotton.

CAS — 9004-70-0.

Pharmacopoeias. In *Arg., Aust., Belg., Br., Egypt., Jpn, Mex., Port., Span.*, and *U.S.*

A nitrated cellulose prepared, under carefully controlled conditions, by treating defatted wood pulp or cotton linters with a mixture of nitric and sulphuric acids. It occurs as white or almost white cuboid granules or fibrous material resembling cotton wool but harsher to the touch and more powdery. It is highly inflammable.

Soluble 1 in 25 of a mixture of 1 vol. of alcohol (90%) and 3 vol. of ether; soluble in acetone and glacial acetic acid. **Store** in well-closed containers, loosely packed, protected from light, and stored at a temperature not exceeding 15°, remote from fire. The container should be suitably designed to disrupt should the internal pressure reach or exceed 1400 kPa. The amount of damping fluid must not be allowed to fall below 25% w/w; should this happen, the material should be either rewetted or used immediately for the preparation of Collodion. It should be kept moistened with not less than 25% of industrial methylated spirit or isopropyl alcohol. When kept in well-closed bottles and exposed to light, it decomposes with the evolution of nitrous vapours, leaving a carbonaceous residue.

Uses and Administration

Pyroxylin is used in the preparation of collodions which are applied to the skin for the protection of small cuts and abrasions. Collodions have also been tried as vehicles for the application of drugs when prolonged local action is required.

Preparations

Collodion *(B.P.)*. A solution of pyroxylin (approximately 10%) in a mixture of alcohol (90%) (or industrial methylated spirit, suitably diluted) 1 volume and solvent ether 3 volumes, diluted with the same mixed solvent to a kinematic viscosity of 405 to 700 cSt.

NOTE. The *B.P.* directs that when Collodion is prescribed or demanded, Flexible Collodion be supplied.

Collodion *(U.S.P.)*. Pyroxylin 4 g, ether 75 mL, and alcohol 25 mL.

Flexible Collodion *(B.P.)*. Colophony 2.5 g, castor oil 2.5 g, collodion to 100 mL.

Flexible Collodion *(U.S.P.)*. Camphor 2 g, castor oil 3 g, collodion *U.S.P.* to 100 g.

Proprietary Names and Manufacturers

Collodion 33042 *(BDH Chemicals, UK)*; Necoloidine Solution *(BDH Chemicals, UK)*.

The following names have been used for multi-ingredient preparations containing pyroxylin— Syl *(Reckitt & Colman Pharmaceuticals, UK)*.

1637-y

Resorcinol *(BAN, USAN).*

Dioxybenzolum; *m*-Dihydroxybenzene; Resorcin. Benzene-1,3-diol.

$C_6H_6O_2$=110.1.

CAS — 108-46-3.

Pharmacopoeias. In *Arg., Aust., Belg., Br., Braz., Chin., Cz., Egypt., Eur., Fr., Ger., Hung., Jug., Mex., Neth., Nord., Pol., Port., Roum., Rus., Span., Swiss,* and *U.S.*

Colourless, white, practically white, or slightly pinkish-grey, acicular crystals or crystalline powder with a characteristic odour. M.p. 109° to 112°. It becomes red on exposure to air and light.

Soluble 1 in less than 1 of water, 1 in 1 of alcohol; freely soluble in ether, and glycerol; slightly soluble in chloroform. A 5% solution in water is neutral or acid to litmus.

Incompatible with Nitrous Ether Spirit, ferric salts, and caustic alkalis.**Store** in well-closed containers. Protect from light.

Adverse Effects, Treatment, and Precautions

Resorcinol is a mild irritant and may result in skin sensitisation. It may be absorbed through the skin or from ulcerated surfaces and prolonged use may lead to myxoedema due to the antithyroid action of the drug. Systemic effects are similar to those of phenol but convulsions may occur more frequently. Resorcinol toxicity is treated as for Phenol, p.967.

In Great Britain the recommended exposure limits of resorcinol are 10 ppm (long-term); 20 ppm (short-term).

A study of the percutaneous absorption of resorcinol from a hydro-alcoholic vehicle after repeated application in 3 subjects concluded that resorcinol 2% appeared safe for topical use.— D. Yeung *et al.*, *Int. J. Derm.*, 1983, *22*, 321.

Resorcinol could cause green discoloration of the urine.— J. Karlstrand, *J. Am. pharm. Ass.*, 1977, *NS17*, 735.

Uses and Administration

Externally, resorcinol has antipruritic, exfoliative, and keratolytic properties. It is used in the treatment of acne and seborrhoeic skin conditions.

Alcoholic hair lotions containing 2.5% have been employed in the treatment of dandruff but they should not be used on fair hair and before use it is important to free the hair from soap and alkali to avoid discoloration.

In the *UK* the concentration of resorcinol is limited by law to 5% in hair dyes and 0.5% in hair lotions and shampoos.

Preparations

Resorcinol and Sulfur Lotion *(U.S.P.)*

Compound Resorcinol Ointment *(B.P.C. 1973)*. Ung. Resorcin. Co. Resorcinol 4 g, bismuth subnitrate 8 g, zinc oxide 4 g, starch 10 g, cade oil 3 g, wool fat 10 g, sodium metabisulphite 200 mg, water 4 g, hard paraffin 2 g, yellow soft paraffin 54.8 g.

Compound Resorcinol Ointment *(U.S.P.)*. Resorcinol 6 g, zinc oxide 6 g, bismuth subnitrate 6 g, cade oil 2 g, yellow beeswax 10 g, yellow soft paraffin 29 g, wool fat 28 g, and glycerol 13 g.

Resorcinol and Sulphur Ointment Compound *(A.P.F.)*. Ung. Resorcin. et Sulphur. Co. Resorcinol 2 g, precipitated sulphur 3 g, salicylic acid 1 g, and white simple ointment 94 g.

Proprietary Preparations

Eskamel *(Smith Kline & French, UK)*. *Cream*, resorcinol 2%, precipitated sulphur 8%.

Proprietary Names and Manufacturers

Castel-Minus *(USA)*; Egosol R *(Ego, Austral.)*.

The following names have been used for multi-ingredient preparations containing resorcinol—Acne-aid *(Stiefel, Canad.)*; Acnil *(Fisons, UK)*; Acnomel *(Smith Kline & French, Canad.; Menley & James, USA)*; Anugesic-HC Cream *(Parke, Davis, UK)*; Anusol HC *(Warner, Austral.)*; Anusol-HC *(Parke, Davis, UK; Parke, Davis, USA)*; Clearasil Adult Care *(Richardson-Vicks, USA)*; Clearasil Cream *(Richardson-Vicks, UK)*; Derma Cas *(Hill, USA)*; Egomycol *(Ego, Austral.)*; Eskamel *(Smith Kline & French, Austral.; Smith Kline & French, UK)*; Fungi-Nail *(Kramer, USA)*; Hedal HC *(Arlo, USA)*; Nestosyl *(Bengué, UK)*; Night Cast S *(Dormer, Canad.; Seres, USA)*; pHorac *(Winthrop, Austral.)*; Resaltar *(Trans Canaderm, Canad.)*; Rezamid *(Rorer, Canad.)*; Seborrol *(Ego, Austral.)*.

1638-j

Resorcinol Monoacetate *(USAN).*

Resorcin Acetate. 3-Acetoxyphenol.

$C_8H_8O_3$=152.1.

CAS — 102-29-4.

Pharmacopoeias. In *U.S.*

A pale yellow or amber viscous liquid with a faint char-

acteristic odour.
Sparingly **soluble** in water; soluble in alcohol and most organic solvents. A saturated solution in water is acid to litmus. **Store** in airtight containers. Protect from light.

Resorcinol monoacetate is used for the same purposes as resorcinol; it liberates resorcinol slowly by hydrolysis so that the effects are milder and of longer duration than those of resorcinol. It is less likely than resorcinol to discolour fair hair.

Proprietary Names and Manufacturers
Euresol *(Knoll, Austral.)*.

The following names have been used for multi-ingredient preparations containing resorcinol monoacetate—Dome-Acne *(Lagap, UK)*; Salaphene *(Napp, UK)*.

2701-y

Salicylic Acid *(BAN, USAN)*.

Acido Ortóxibenzoico; Acidum Salicylicum; Salizylsäure. 2-Hydroxybenzoic acid.
$C_7H_6O_3$=138.1.

CAS — 69-72-7.

Pharmacopoeias. In Arg., Aust., Belg., Br., Braz., Chin., Cz., Egypt., Eur., Fr., Ger., Hung., Ind., Int., It., Jpn, Jug., Mex., Neth., Nord., Pol., Port., Roum., Rus., Span., Swiss, Turk., and *U.S.*

Colourless acicular crystals or a white crystalline powder with a sweetish acrid taste. The synthetic form is white and odourless but if prepared from natural methyl salicylate it may have a slightly yellow or pink tint, and a faint, mint-like odour. **Soluble** 1 in 460 to 550 of water, 1 in 15 of boiling water, 1 in 3 to 4 of alcohol, 1 in 3 of ether, and 1 in 45 of chloroform. **Store** in well-closed containers. Protect from light.

Adverse Effects

Salicylic acid is a mild irritant and application of salicylic acid preparations to the skin may cause dermatitis. Symptoms of acute systemic salicylate poisoning (see aspirin, p.3) have been reported after the application of salicylic acid to large areas of the body.

A review of the systemic risks resulting from topically-applied drugs, including salicylic acid.— A. Zesch, *Br. J. Derm.*, 1986, *115, Suppl.* 31, 63.

Symptoms of salicylism developed in 3 adults, with extensive psoriasis, between the second and fourth day of application 6 times daily of salicylic acid ointment (3 or 6%). The symptoms largely disappeared within 1 day after discontinuing the application of the ointment. Serum concentrations of salicylic acid ranged from 460 to 640 μg per mL. There were 13 deaths from salicylic acid poisoning following application of salicylic acid ointments reported in the literature. Ten of the 13 fatalities occurred in children.— J. F. von Weiss and W. F. Lever, *Archs Derm.*, 1964, *90,* 614.

Two patients died after more than 50% of their body areas had been painted twice with an alcoholic solution of salicylic acid 20.7% for tinea infection. The deaths were preceded by symptoms typical of salicylate poisoning.— C. P. Lindsey, *Med. J. Aust.*, 1968, *1,* 353.

Further reports of salicylate toxicity following topical application of preparations containing salicylic acid.— E. P. Cawley *et al.*, *J. Am. med. Ass.*, 1953, *151,* 372; L. V. Perlman (letter), *New Engl. J. Med.*, 1966, *274,* 164; J. B. Aspinall and K. M. Goel (letter), *Br. med. J.*, 1978, *2,* 1373; M. G. Davies *et al.*, *ibid.*, 1979, *1,* 661; P. A. Soyka and L. F. Soyka (letter), *J. Am. med. Ass.*, 1980, *244,* 660.

Uses and Administration

Salicylic acid has keratolytic properties and is applied topically in the treatment of hyperkeratotic and scaling skin conditions such as dandruff, ichthyosis, and psoriasis. Initially a concentration of about 2% is used, increased to about 6% if necessary. It is often used in conjunction with many other agents, such as benzoic acid, coal tar, resorcinol, and sulphur. Salicylic acid is also used in the form of a paint in a collodion basis (10 to 17%) or as a plaster (20 to 50%) to destroy warts or corns.

It also possesses fungicidal properties and is used topically in the treatment of such fungal skin infections as tinea.

ONYCHOMYCOSIS. The successful treatment of onychomycosis by boring holes in the affected nail plates, enlarging these with acid, then applying an ointment of precipitated sulphur 3% with salicylic acid 3% in soft paraffin.— J. Brem (letter), *Lancet*, 1977, *2,* 937.

SKIN DISORDERS. *Acne.* An opinion that salicylic acid, especially in a polar solvent, is an effective comedolytic agent.— H. P. Baden (letter), *New Engl. J. Med.*, 1980, *302,* 1419. There appear to be no controlled studies on the use of salicylic acid in acne.— J. W. Melski and K. A. Arndt (letter), *ibid.*

WARTS. In the course of studies assessing the value of treatments for viral warts in a total of 1807 patients, a study of 389 patients in 2 centres showed that against hand warts a mixture of salicylic acid 1 part and lactic acid 1 part in flexible collodion 4 parts (SAL paint) was as effective as liquid nitrogen or as a combination of both treatments, the percentage cures being 67, 69, and 78 respectively. No recurrences of hard warts were reported 6 months after treatment with SAL paints in 46 of 50 patients in a general practice. Other studies indicated that SAL paint cured 45% of patients with mosaic plantar warts and it was no less effective than preparations containing fluorouracil 5%, idoxuridine 5%, a 10% buffered solution of glutaraldehyde, or a paint prepared to contain 40% of an adduct of benzalkonium chloride and bromine (Callusolve 40).— M. H. Bunney *et al.*, *Br. J. Derm.*, 1976, *94,* 667.

A review of the treatment of warts including a short section on formulations of salicylic acid suitable for use.— F. E. Anderson, *Drugs*, 1985, *30,* 368.

Preparations

Collodions

Lactic and Salicylic Acid Paint *(A.P.F.)*. Lactic acid 20, salicylic acid 20, flexible collodion to 100.

Salicylic Acid Collodion *(B.P.)*. Salicylic acid 12 g, flexible collodion to 100 mL. Store at a temperature not exceeding 25°.

Salicylic Acid Collodion *(U.S.P.)*. Salicylic acid 10 g, flexible collodion *U.S.P.* to 100 mL. Store at 15° to 30° in airtight containers.

Salicylic Acid Paint *(A.P.F.)*. Corn Paint; Salicylic Acid Collodion. Salicylic acid 10 g, flexible collodion to 100 mL. Store in airtight containers below 25°.

Creams

Salicylic Acid and Resorcinol Cream Aqueous *(A.P.F.)*. Salicylic acid 2 g, resorcinol 2 g, aqueous cream to 100 g. Protect from light and avoid contact with metals.

Salicylic Acid and Sulphur Cream Aqueous *(A.P.F.)*. Crem. Acid. Salicyl. et Sulphur. Salicylic acid 2 g, precipitated sulphur 2 g, aqueous cream to 100 g. Avoid contact with metals.

Ear-drops

Salicylic Acid Ear Drops *(A.P.F.)*. Aurist. Acid. Salicyl. Salicylic acid 2 g, alcohol 90% 50 mL, freshly boiled and cooled water to 100 mL.

Foams

Salicylic Acid Topical Foam *(U.S.P.)*. Store in airtight containers.

Gels

Salicylic Acid Gel *(U.S.P.)*. Store at 15° to 30° in airtight containers.

Lotions

Salicylic Acid Lotion *(B.P.)*. Salicylic acid 2 g, castor oil 1 mL, alcohol (or industrial methylated spirit) to 100 mL. Keep away from an open flame.

Salicylic Acid Lotion *(A.P.F.)*. Lot. Acid. Salicyl.; Lotio Crinalis. Salicylic acid 2 g, castor oil 1 ml., alcohol 96% to 100 ml.

Salicylic Acid and Coal Tar Lotion *(A.P.F.)*. Salicylic acid 2 g, coal tar solution 5 mL, castor oil 1 mL, spike lavender oil 0.1 mL, alcohol 90% to 100 mL.

Salicylic Acid and Mercuric Chloride Lotion *(B.P.C. 1973)*. Lotio Acidi Salicylici et Hydrargyri Perchloridi. Salicylic acid 2 g, mercuric chloride 100 mg, castor oil 1 mL, acetone 12.5 mL, alcohol (or industrial methylated spirit) to 100 mL. Store in a cool place in airtight containers. Keep away from an open flame.

Ointments

Salicylic Acid Ointment *(B.P., A.P.F.)*. Salicylic acid 2% in wool alcohols ointment.

Salicylic Acid and Coal Tar Ointment *(A.P.F.)*. Salicylic acid 3 g, strong coal tar solution 3 mL, white soft paraffin 50 g, emulsifying ointment to 100 g.

Salicylic Acid and Sulphur Ointment *(B.P.C. 1973)*. Salicylic acid 3% and precipitated sulphur 3% in oily cream.

Plasters

Salicylic Acid Plaster *(U.S.P.)*. A uniform mixture of salicylic acid in a suitable base spread on paper, cotton cloth, or other suitable backing material. Store at 15° to 30°.

Proprietary Preparations

Cuplex *(Smith & Nephew Pharmaceuticals, UK)*. *Gel*, salicylic acid 11%, lactic acid 4%, copper acetate equivalent to copper 0.0011%.

Duofilm *(Stiefel, UK)*. *Paint*, salicylic acid 16.7% w/w, lactic acid 16.7% w/w in flexible collodion.

Keralyt *(Bristol-Myers Pharmaceuticals, UK)*. *Gel*, salicylic acid 6%.

Monphytol *(Laboratories for Applied Biology, UK)*. *Paint*, salicylic acid (free and methyl and propyl esters) 33%, chlobutol 3%, undecenoic acid (as methyl and propyl esters) 5.7%.

Pyralvex (formerly known as Peralvex) *(Norgine, UK)*. *Oral paint*, salicylic acid 1%, extract of anthraquinone glycosides 5%.

Salactol *(Dermal Laboratories, UK)*. *Paint*, salicylic acid 16.7% w/w, lactic acid 16.7% w/w in flexible collodion.

Verrugon *(Pickles, UK)*. *Ointment*, salicylic acid 50%.

Proprietary Names and Manufacturers

Clearasil Medicated Astringent *(Richardson-Vicks, USA)*; Compound-W *(Whitehall, UK; Whitehall, USA)*; Cornina *(Ger.)*; Coroplast *(Fournier, Spain)*; Egocappol *(Ego, Austral.)*; Fomac *(Dermik, USA)*; Gehwol *(Gerlach, Ger.)*; Guttaplast *(Beiersdorf, Ger.)*; Gyan *(Laves, Ger.)*; Hydrisalic *(Pedinol, USA)*; Ionil Plus *(Owen, USA)*; Keralyt *(Westwood, Canad.; Bristol-Myers Pharmaceuticals, UK; Westwood, USA)*; Occlusal *(Genderm, USA)*; Phytodermine *(May & Baker, UK)*; Salac *(Genderm, USA)*; Salicyl *(DAK, Denm.)*; Saligel *(Stiefel, Canad.; Stiefel, USA)*; SaSha *(Korn Pharma, Denm.)*; Sebcur *(Dermtek, Canad.)*; Sebucare *(Westwood, USA)*; Soluver *(Dermtek, Canad.)*; Squamasol *(Ichthyol, Ger.)*; Verrugon *(Pickles, UK)*; Viron *(Odan, Canad.)*; Wart-Off *(Leeming, USA)*; Xseb *(Dormer, Canad.; Baker/Cummins, USA)*.

The following names have been used for multi-ingredient preparations containing salicylic acid—Acnaveen *(Oral-B, Austral.; Oral-B, UK)*; Acnelab *(Austral.)*; Adasept *(Odan, Canad.)*; Antinea *(American Dermal, USA)*; Aserbine *(Bencard, UK)*; Aveenobar Medicated *(Cooper Dermatology, USA)*; Barseb HC *(Barnes-Hind, USA)*; Barseb Thera *(Barnes-Hind, USA)*; Canthacur-PS *(Pharmascience, Canad.)*; Cantharone Plus *(Dormer, Canad.; Seres, USA)*; Cornkil *(Rosken, Austral.)*; Cuplex *(Smith & Nephew Pharmaceuticals, UK)*; Dermacide *(Sabex, Canad.)*; Diprosalic *(Schering, Canad.; Kirby-Warrick, UK)*; Dithraderm *(Dermacare, Austral.)*; Dithrolan *(Dermal Laboratories, UK)*; Dome-Acne Medicated Cleanser *(Lagap, UK)*; Duofilm *(Stiefel, Austral.; Stiefel, Canad.; Stiefel, UK; Stiefel, USA)*; Duoplant *(Stiefel, Canad.)*; Egomycol *(Ego, Austral.)*; Egosol-BS *(Ego, Austral.)*; Egosulphyl *(Ego, Austral.)*; Fostex *(Bristol-Myers, Austral.; Westwood, Canad.; Westwood, USA)*; Fungi-Nail *(Kramer, USA)*; Gelcosal *(Quinoderm, UK)*; Ionil *(Alcon, Canad.; Owen, USA)*; Ionil T *(Alcon, Austral.; Alcon, Canad.; Alcon, UK; Owen, USA)*; Isophyl *(Ego, Austral.)*; Jadit *(Hoechst, UK)*; Komed *(Barnes-Hind, Canad.; Barnes-Hind, USA)*; Komed HC *(Barnes-Hind, Canad.; Barnes-Hind, USA)*; Locasalen *(Ciba, Canad.)*; Malatex *(Norton, UK)*; Monphytol *(Salmond & Spraggon, Austral.; Laboratories for Applied Biology, UK)*; Movelat *(Luitpold, Austral.; Panpharma, UK)*; Mycoderm Cream and Powder *(Ego, Austral.)*; Mycozol *(Parke, Davis, Austral.)*; Night Cast R *(Dormer, Canad.; Seres, USA)*; Oticane *(Rosken, Austral.)*; Peralvex *(Norgine, UK)*; Pernox *(Westwood, Canad.; Westwood, USA)*; Phytex *(Drug Houses Austral., Austral.; Pharmax, UK)*; Phytocil Cream *(Rorer, UK)*; Posalfilin *(Norgine, Austral.; Norgine, UK)*; Pragmatar *(Smith Kline & French, Austral.; Smith Kline & French, Canad.; Smith Kline & French, UK)*; P&S *(Baker/Cummins, USA)*; P&S Plus *(Dormer, Canad.)*; Psorin *(Cambden, Austral.; Thames, UK)*; Pyralvex *(Norgine, Austral.; Norgine, UK)*; Resaltar *(Trans Canaderm, Canad.)*; Salactic *(Pedinol, USA)*; Salactol *(Dermal Laboratories, UK)*; Salicylin-P *(Key, Austral.)*; Sastid *(Stiefel, Canad.)*; Sebaveen *(Knox, UK)*; Sebcur/T *(Dermtek, Canad.)*; Seborrol *(Ego, Austral.)*; Sebulan

(Bristol-Myers, Austral.); Sebulex *(Westwood, Canad.*; *Westwood, USA)*; Sebutone *(Westwood, Canad.*; *Westwood, USA)*; SLT *(C & M, USA)*; SM-33 *(Nicholas, Austral.)*; SSC Ointment *(Cambden, Austral.)*; Stie-Lasan *(Stiefel, UK)*; Sulsal *(Trans Canaderm, Canad.)*; Tardan *(Odan, Canad.)*; Tineasol *(Arlo, USA)*; Tinver *(Barnes-Hind, Canad.*; *Barnes-Hind, USA)*; Tricaderm *(Squibb, UK)*; Verrex *(C & M, USA)*; Verrusol *(C & M, USA)*; Viranol *(American Dermal, USA)*; Wartkil *(Rosken, Austral.)*; Wart-Off *(Nelson, Austral.)*.

1639-z

Selenium Sulphide *(BAN)*.

Selenium Disulphide; Selenium Sulfide *(USAN)*.
SeS_2=143.1.

CAS — 7488-56-4.

Pharmacopoeias. In *Br.* and *U.S.* Also in *B.P. Vet.*

A bright orange to reddish-brown powder with a faint odour of hydrogen sulphide. Practically **insoluble** in water; soluble 1 in about 160 of chloroform and 1 in about 1670 of ether; practically insoluble in most other organic solvents. Selenium sulphide may discolour metals. **Store** in well-closed containers.

Adverse Effects and Treatment

Topical application of selenium sulphide can produce irritation of the conjunctiva, scalp, and skin, especially in the genital area and skin folds. Scalp oiliness, hair discoloration and hair loss have been reported. Only traces of selenium sulphide are absorbed through intact skin.

When taken by mouth, selenium sulphide is highly toxic. Symptoms of poisoning include an odour of garlic in the breath, a metallic taste, anorexia, vomiting, anaemia, and fatty degeneration of the liver.

In Great Britain the recommended exposure limit of selenium compounds (as Se) is 0.2 mg per m^3 (long-term).

Treatment of poisoning is symptomatic. Dimercaprol should not be used.

Precautions

Selenium sulphide should not be applied to inflamed or exudative areas, or to extensive areas of the skin. It should not be allowed to enter the eyes.

Uses and Administration

Selenium sulphide has antifungal and anti-seborrhoeic properties. It is used as a shampoo in the treatment of dandruff (pityriasis capitis) and seborrhoeic dermatitis of the scalp. Five to 10 mL of a suspension containing 2.5% of selenium sulphide is applied to the wet scalp; the hair is rinsed and the application repeated; the suspension should remain in contact with the scalp for a total of 4 to 6 minutes. The hair should be well rinsed after the treatment and all traces of the suspension removed from the hands and nails. Applications are usually made twice weekly for 2 weeks, then once weekly for 2 weeks and then only when necessary. A 1% shampoo is also used.

Selenium sulphide is also used as a 2.5% lotion in the treatment of pityriasis versicolor. The lotion is applied to the affected areas with water and allowed to remain for 10 minutes before thorough rinsing. This procedure is repeated once daily for 7 days.

In the *UK* the use of selenium and its compounds in cosmetics is prohibited by law.

Some disorders have been attributed to selenium deficiency, however, dietary supplementation is not generally considered necessary. Trace elements are discussed under p.1250.

DANDRUFF. Selenium sulphide as a 2.5% suspension in a detergent vehicle can reduce scaling. In controlled trials, it reduced dandruff better than a non-medicated shampoo, and more quickly than zinc pyrithione, or a tar preparation.— *Drug & Ther. Bull.*, 1983, *21*, 41.

PITYRIASIS VERSICOLOR. Selenium sulphide is the treatment of choice for pityriasis versicolor.— D. T. Roberts, *Prescribers' J.*, 1985, *25*, 40.

TINEA CAPITIS. Forty-eight children with tinea capitis due to *Trichophyton tonsurans* were treated with griseofulvin 10 mg per kg daily by mouth alone (10 children) or with either topical clotrimazole lotion applied twice daily (12), or twice weekly shampooing with a non-medicated detergent shampoo (6) or selenium sulphide suspension 2% (16). Two weeks after starting treatment, only 1 child in the selenium sulphide group had viable spores recovered from the scalp surface whereas all of the children receiving the other treatments harboured viable spores. Selenium sulphide shampooing appears to offer an important adjunctive therapy for tinea capitis by suppressing viable spores on the scalp surface and minimising the chances for spread to occur.— H. B. Allen *et al.*, *Pediatrics*, 1982, *69*, 81.

Preparations

Selenium Sulfide Lotion *(U.S.P.)*. Selenium sulphide in an aqueous stabilised suspension containing a suitable dispersing agent, buffer, and depending on use, a detergent.

Selenium Sulphide Scalp Application *(B.P.)*. Selenium Sulphide Application. A suspension of selenium sulphide in a suitable liquid basis. pH 4.0 to 5.5.

Proprietary Preparations

Lenium *(Winthrop, UK)*. *Shampoo cream*, selenium sulphide 2.5%.

Selsun *(Abbott, UK)*. *Shampoo*, selenium sulphide 2.5%.

Proprietary Names and Manufacturers

Abbottselsun *(Abbott, Spain)*; Bioselenium *(Uriach, Spain)*; Caspiselenio *(Kin, Spain)*; Exsel *(Canad.*; *Herbert, USA)*; Iosel 250 *(USA)*; Lenium *(Winthrop, UK)*; Sébo-Lénium *(Winthrop, Switz.)*; Sebarex *(Austral.)*; Sebusan *(Canad.*; *Swed.)*; Selenol *(ND & K, Denm.*; *Switz.)*; Selgol *(Gohl, Switz.)*; Selsun *(Abbott, Austral.*; *Belg.*; *Abbott, Canad.*; *Abbott, Denm.*; *Abbott, Fr.*; *Abbott, Ger.*; *Abbott, Ital.*; *Abbott, Norw.*; *Abbott, S.Afr.*; *Abbott, Swed.*; *Abbott, Switz.*; *Abbott, UK*; *Abbott, USA)*; Selukos *(Kabi, Ger.*; *KabiVitrum, Norw.*; *ACO, Swed.*; *Switz.)*; Sul-Blue *(USA)*; Versel *(Trans Canaderm, Canad.)*.

1644-l

Precipitated Sulphur *(BAN)*.

Azufre Precipitado; Enxôfre Precipitado; Gefällter Schwefel; Lac Sulfuris; Magisterio de Azufre; Milk of Sulphur; Precipitated Sulfur *(USAN)*; Soufre Précipité.
S=32.07.

CAS — 7704-34-9.

Pharmacopoeias. In *Arg.*, *Aust.*, *Belg.*, *Braz.*, *Cz.*, *Egypt*, *Fr.*, *Ger.*, *Hung.*, *Jug.*, *Mex.*, *Nord.*, *Pol.*, *Port.*, *Roum.*, *Rus.*, *Span.*, *Turk.*, and *U.S. Jpn* and *Swiss* include Sulfur but do not specify precipitated or sublimed.

A pale yellow, odourless, amorphous or microcrystalline powder.

Practically **insoluble** in water; soluble 1 in 2 of carbon disulphide and 1 in 100 of olive oil; very slightly soluble in alcohol. Incompatible with topical mercurial compounds. **Store** in well-closed containers.

WARNING. *Sulphur has been used for the illicit preparation of explosives or fireworks; care is required with its supply.*

1643-e

Sublimed Sulphur

Azufre Sublimado; Enxôfre Sublimado; Fleur de Soufre; Flowers of Sulphur; Sublimed Sulfur *(USAN)*; Sublimierter Schwefel; Sulfur Sublimatum Depuratum; Sulphur Sublimatum.
S=32.07.

CAS — 7704-34-9.

Pharmacopoeias. In *Arg.*, *Aust.*, *Chin.*, *Egypt.*, *Fr.*, *Hung.*, *Jug.*, *Port.*, *Span.*, and *U.S.* Also in *B.P.C. 1973*. *Jpn* and *Swiss* include Sulfur but do not specify precipitated or sublimed.

In aqueous lotions containing precipitated sulphur, a few drops of a solution of a surfactant such as docusate sodium was recommended as a 'wetting' agent for the sulphur.— *Pharm. J. N.Z.*, 1957, *19*, No. 8, 21.

Sulphur is a keratolytic, a mild antiseptic, and a parasiticide and has been widely employed, in the form of lotions or ointments, in the treatment of acne, dandruff, seborrhoeic conditions, and scabies, though there are more convenient and effective preparations. Lotions of precipitated sulphur with lead acetate have been used to darken grey hair.

When taken by mouth, sulphur is converted in the small intestine into alkali sulphides which by their irritant action produce a mild laxative effect. However, sulphaemoglobinaemia may occur. Sublimed sulphur has been used similarly to precipitated sulphur.

Sulphur is used in homoeopathic medicine.

Comedone formation occurred when 2.5 or 5% suspensions of elemental sulphur were applied, under occlusive dressings, to the backs of 6 volunteers for 6 weeks. It was considered that, while the application of sulphur suspensions to acne vulgaris reduced the papulo-pustules, it promoted the formation of comedones and so established a vicious circle.— O. H. Mills and A. M. Kligman, *Br. J. Derm.*, 1972, *86*, 620.

Preparations

Compound Sulphur Lotion *(B.P.C. 1973)*. Sulphur Compound Lotion. Precipitated sulphur 4 g, alcohol (95%) (or industrial methylated spirit) 6 mL, glycerol 2 mL, quillaia tincture 0.5 mL, calcium hydroxide solution to 100 mL.

Resorcinol and Sulphur Preparations. See under Resorcinol, p. 930.

Sulfur Ointment *(U.S.P.)*. Precipitated sulphur 10%, liquid paraffin 10%, white ointment 80%.

Washed Sulphur. Sulphur Lotum; Sulfur Sublimatum Lotum; Purified Sulphur; Soufre Lavé; Gewaschener Schwefel; Azufre Lavado; Enxôfre Lavado. A fine, odourless, tasteless, yellow, crystalline powder prepared by washing sublimed sulphur with ammoniated water. It is included in many pharmacopoeias.

Proprietary Preparations

Dome-Acne *(Lagap, UK)*. *Cream*, colloidal sulphur 4%, resorcinol monoacetate 3%.

Proprietary Names and Manufacturers of Precipitated or Sublimed Sulphur

Aknaseb *(Prof. Pharm. Corp., Canad.)*; Bensulfoid Powder and Tablets *(Poythress, USA)*; Fostril *(Westwood, Canad.*; *Westwood, USA)*; Fostril T *(Bristol-Myers, Austral.)*; Lotio Alsulfa *(Trans Canaderm, Canad.)*; Postacne *(Rorer, Canad.*; *Dermik, USA)*; Schwefel-Diasporal *(Protina, Ger.)*; Sufrogel *(Weimer, Ger.)*; Sulfoïdal Robin *(Rosa-Phytopharma, Fr.)*; Svovl *(DAK, Denm.)*; Tetrazufre *(Quimica Medica, Spain)*; Transact *(Westwood, USA)*.

The following names have been used for multi-ingredient preparations containing precipitated or sublimed sulphur—Acnaveen *(Oral-B, Austral.*; *Oral-B, UK)*; Acne-aid *(Stiefel, Canad.)*; Acnederm *(Ego, Austral.)*; Acnelab *(Austral.)*; Acne-sol *(Fawns & McAllan, Austral.)*; Acnil *(Fisons, UK)*; Acnomel *(Smith Kline & French, Canad.*; *Menley & James, USA)*; Actinac *(Roussel, Canad.*; *Roussel, UK)*; Aveenobar Medicated *(Cooper Dermatology, USA)*; Benoxyl with Sulphur *(Stiefel, UK)*; Bensulfoid Lotion *(Poythress, USA)*; Clearasil Adult Care *(Richardson-Vicks, USA)*; Clearasil Cream *(Richardson-Vicks, UK)*; Dome-Acne *(Lagap, UK)*; Dome-Acne Medicated Cleanser *(Lagap, UK)*; Egopsoryl *(Ego, Austral.)*; Egosulphyl *(Ego, Austral.)*; Eskamel *(Smith Kline & French, Austral.*; *Smith Kline & French, UK)*; Fostex *(Bristol-Myers, Austral.*; *Westwood, Canad.*; *Westwood, USA)*; Fostril HC *(Bristol-Myers, Austral.)*; Hill Cortac *(Hill, USA)*; Medrol Acne Lotion *(Upjohn, Austral.*; *Upjohn, Canad.)*; Medrone Acne Lotion *(Upjohn, UK)*; Neo-Medrol *(Upjohn, Austral.)*; Neo-Medrone Acne Lotion *(Upjohn, UK)*; Night Cast R *(Dormer, Canad.*; *Seres, USA)*; Night Cast S *(Dormer, Canad.*; *Seres, USA)*; Pernox *(Westwood, Canad.*; *Westwood, USA)*; Persol *(Horner, Canad.)*; pHisoDan *(Sterling, Canad.)*; pHisodan *(Winthrop, Austral.)*; pHorac *(Winthrop, Austral.)*; Pragmatar *(Smith Kline & French, Austral.*; *Smith Kline & French, Canad.*; *Smith Kline & French, UK)*; Rezamid *(Rorer, Canad.)*; Sastid *(Stiefel, Canad.)*; Sebaveen *(Knox, UK)*; Sebulan *(Bristol-Myers, Austral.)*; Sebulex *(Westwood, Canad.*; *Westwood, USA)*;

Sebutone *(Westwood, Canad.; Westwood, USA)*; SSC Ointment *(Cambden, Austral.)*; Sulfacet-R *(Rorer, Canad.; Dermik, USA)*; Sulfoxyl *(Stiefel, Canad.)*; Sulsal *(Trans Canaderm, Canad.)*; Vanair *(Carter-Wallace, UK)*.

1645-y

Sulphurated Lime
Calcium Sulphide; Calx Sulphurata; Sulfurated Lime *(USAN)*.

CAS — 8028-82-8 (sulphurated lime solution).

A mixture containing calcium sulphate and not less than 50% of calcium sulphide, CaS.

Sulphurated lime is used topically as sulphurated lime solution for acne, scabies, seborrhoeic dermatitis, and boils. It was formerly given internally for the treatment of boils, carbuncles, and pustular acne. A solution containing calcium polysulphides and known as 'lime-sulphur' is used as a fungicide in horticulture.

An impure grade of calcium sulphide (Hepar Sulphuris; Hepar Sulph.) is used in homoeopathic medicine.

NOTE. The title Hepar Sulfuris is also applied to Sulphurated Potash—see below.

Preparations

Sulfurated Lime Topical Solution *(U.S.P.)*. The solution has sometimes been known as Sulfurated Lime Solution; Vleminckx's Solution or Lotion; Calcium Sulfuratum Solutum. Prepared by boiling together in water sublimed sulphur 25 g and calcium oxide 16.5 g to produce 100 ml. Store in completely-filled airtight containers.
Dilute 1 in 10 before use.

Proprietary Names and Manufacturers
Vlemasque *(Rorer, Canad.; Dermik, USA)*.

1646-j

Sulphurated Potash
Foie de Soufre; Hepar Sulfuris; Kalii Sulfidum; Liver of Sulphur; Potassa Sulphurata; Schwefelleber; Sulfurated Potash *(USAN)*.

CAS — 39365-88-3.

NOTE. The title Hepar Sulphuris is used in homoeopathic medicine for an impure grade of calcium sulphide—see Sulphurated Lime.

Pharmacopoeias. In *Nord., Port.,* and *U.S.* Also in *B.P.C. 1973.*

A mixture of potassium polysulphides and other potassium compounds, including sulphite and thiosulphate, containing 42 to 45% of sulphur. *U.S.P.* specifies not less than 12.8% of sulphur as sulphide. Greenish-yellow fragments, internally pale liver-brown rapidly changing to greenish-yellow on exposure to air and absorbing moisture and carbon dioxide. It has an odour of hydrogen sulphide.

Almost completely **soluble** 1 in 2 of water. Alcohol dissolves only the sulphides. A 10% solution in water is alkaline to litmus. **Incompatible** with acids. **Store** in small airtight containers.

Sulphurated potash is a mild counter-irritant and parasiticide. It is used in acne and scabies in the form of a lotion.

Sulphurated potash is used in homoeopathic medicine when it is known as hepar sulph.

Preparations

Sulphurated Lotion *(A.P.F.)*. Lot. Sulphurat. Sulphurated potash 5 g, zinc sulphate 5 g, acetone 5 mL, glycerol 5 mL, spike lavender oil 0.2 mL, freshly boiled and cooled water to 100mL. It should be freshly prepared, stored between 2° and 8°, and used within 7 days.

White Lotion *(U.S.P.)*. Lotio Alba. Sulphurated potash 4 g, zinc sulphate 4 g, water to 100 mL. It should be freshly prepared.

Zinc Sulphide Lotion *(B.P.C. 1973)*. Sulphurated Potash and Zinc Lotion; Sulphurated Potash Lotion. Sulphurated potash 5 g, zinc sulphate 5 g, concentrated camphor water 2.5 mL, water to 100 mL. It should be freshly prepared.

1647-z

Purified Talc *(BAN)*.
553(b); Powdered Talc; Purified French Chalk; Talc *(USAN)*; Talcum; Talcum Purificatum.

CAS — 14807-96-6.

Pharmacopoeias. In *Arg., Aust., Belg., Br., Chin., Cz., Egypt., Eur., Fr., Ger., Hung., Ind., It., Jpn, Jug., Mex., Neth., Nord., Pol., Port., Roum., Span., Swiss, Turk.,* and *U.S.* Also in *B.P. Vet.*

A purified native hydrated magnesium silicate, approximating to the formula $Mg_6(Si_2O_5)_4(OH)_4$; it may contain varying amounts of aluminium silicate and iron. A very fine, light, homogeneous, white, or greyish-white, odourless, impalpable, and unctuous powder, which adheres readily to the skin. Purified talc should be free from microscopic asbestos fibres.

Practically **insoluble** in water and in dilute mineral acids and dilute solutions of alkali hydroxides. It is **sterilised** by exposure to ethylene oxide or by heating so that the whole of the material is maintained at 160° for 1 hour.

Adverse Effects

Contamination of wounds or body cavities with talc is liable to cause granulomas.

Prolonged or intense aspiration of talc may produce pneumoconiosis.

Talc is liable to be heavily contaminated with bacteria, including *Clostridium tetani, Cl. welchii,* and *Bacillus anthracis.* When used in dusting-powders, it should be sterilised.

In Great Britain the recommended exposure limits of talc, total dust are 10 mg per m^3 (long-term) and talc, respirable dust 1 mg per m^3 (long-term).

A 4-month-old infant with a tracheotomy tube went into cardiorespiratory arrest and died when baby powder was spilled accidentally and a cloud of powder apparently blocked the child's airway. Talc acts as a pulmonary irritant if inhaled and this toxic inhalation is magnified by the bronchopulmonary dysplasia that such infants often have. The unneeded use of baby powder was discouraged.— W. H. Cotton and P. J. Davidson (letter), *New Engl. J. Med.,* 1985, *313,* 1662.

A report of pulmonary vascular talc granulomatosis in a 37-year-old man after the intravenous self-administration of pulverised pethidine hydrochloride tablets in suspension over a period of several months. Talc is a widely used filler substance in the manufacture of pharmaceutical tablets.— I. S. Schwartz and C. Bosken, *J. Am. med. Ass.,* 1986, *256,* 2584.

References to a possible association between ovarian cancer and exposure to cosmetic talc: W. J. Henderson *et al.* (letter), *Lancet,* 1979, *1,* 499; D. L. Longo and R. C. Young, *ibid.,* 1979, *2,* 349; M. L. Newhouse (letter), *ibid.,* 528; F. J. C. Roe (letter), *ibid.,* 744; D. L. Longo and R. C. Young (letter), *ibid.,* 1011; I. M. Phillipson (letter), *ibid.,* 1980, *1,* 48.

Uses and Administration

Purified talc is used in massage and as a dusting-powder to allay irritation and prevent chafing. It is usually mixed with starch to increase absorption of moisture, and zinc oxide. Talc used in dusting-powders should be sterilised. As purified talc is liable to cause foreign-body granulomas, it is not suitable for dusting surgical gloves. Purified talc is used as a lubricant in making tablets and to clarify liquids.

Talc poudrage has been used to treat recurrent spontaneous pneumothorax and pleural effusions.

The use of talc as a non-specific intracavitary sclerosing agent for malignant pleural effusion was effective, but caused severe local pain and required general anaesthesia.— D. P. Dhillon and S. G. Spiro, *Br. J. Hosp. Med.,* 1983, *29,* 506.

Preparations

Talc Dusting Powder *(B.P., A.P.F.)*. Purified talc, sterilised, 90 g and starch 10 g.

Zinc, Starch, and Talc Dusting-powder *(B.P.C. 1973)*. See under Zinc Oxide, p.936.

Proprietary Names and Manufacturers
The following names have been used for multi-ingredient preparations containing talc— Piz Buin (Factor 12) *(Greiter, Switz.: Ciba Consumer, UK)*.

1648-c

Tar *(BAN)*.
Alquitrán Vegetal; Brea de Pino; Goudron Végétal; Nadelholzteer; Pine Tar *(USAN)*; Pix Abietinarum; Pix Liquida; Pix Pini; Pyroleum Pini; Wood Tar.

CAS — 8007-45-2.

NOTE. It is known in commerce as Stockholm tar.

Pharmacopoeias. In *Arg., Aust., Belg., Br., Cz., Egypt., Mex., Nord., Port., Span.,* and *U.S. Aust.* and *Nord.* also include beech tar.

Tar is obtained by the destructive distillation of the wood of various trees of the family Pinaceae. It contains hydrocarbons and phenols. It is a dark brown or nearly black viscous semi-liquid with a characteristic empyreumatic odour; it is heavier than water. Tar has an acid reaction which it imparts to water when shaken with it, and it may thereby be distinguished from coal tar, which has an alkaline reaction.

B.P. solubilities are: **soluble** in alcohol, chloroform, ether, and in fixed and volatile oils. *U.S.P.* solubilities are: slightly soluble in water; miscible with alcohol, chloroform, ether, glacial acetic acid, and fixed and volatile oils.

When stored for some time tar separates into a layer which is granular in character due to minute crystallisation of catechol, resin acids, etc. and a surface layer of a syrupy consistence. **Store** in airtight containers.

Adverse Effects

Tar has similar adverse effects to coal tar (see p.934), but it is not reported to cause photosensitisation.

Uses and Administration

Tar is used in the treatment of chronic skin diseases, particularly eczema and psoriasis.

Tar has been given internally as an expectorant.

Proprietary Preparations

Polytar *(Stiefel, UK)*. *Bath additive*(Polytar Emollient), tar 7.5%, cade oil 7.5%, coal tar solution 2.5%, arachis oil extract of crude coal tar 7.5%, liquid paraffin 35%. *Shampoo*(Polytar Liquid), tar 0.3%, cade oil 0.3%, coal tar solution 0.1%, arachis oil extract of crude coal tar 0.3%, oleyl alcohol 1.0%.
Shampoo(Polytar Plus), ingredients as for Polytar Liquid, with hydrolysed animal protein 3.0%.

Tardrox *(Carlton Laboratories, UK)*. *Cream,* tar 1%, halquinol 1.5%.

Proprietary Names and Manufacturers
Lavatar *(Trans Canaderm, Canad.)*; Pinetarsol *(Ego, Austral.)*.

The following names have been used for multi-ingredient preparations containing tar—ESTP *(Martindale Pharmaceuticals, UK)*; Gelcosal *(Quinoderm, UK)*; Gelcotar *(Quinoderm, UK)*; Multi-Tar Plus *(ICN, Canad.)*; Polytar Emollient *(Stiefel, Austral.; Stiefel, UK)*; Polytar Liquid *(Stiefel, Austral.; Stiefel, UK)*; Polytar Plus *(Stiefel, UK)*; Resaltar *(Trans Canaderm, Canad.)*; Tardrox *(Carlton Laboratories, UK)*.

1650-w

Coal Tar *(BAN, USAN)*.
Alcatrão Mineral; Alquitrán de Hulla; Brea de Hulla; Crude Coal Tar; Goudron de Houille; Oleum Lithanthracis; Pix Carbon.; Pix Carbonis; Pix Lithanthracis; Pix Mineralis; Pyroleum Lithanthracis; Steinkohlenteer.

CAS — 8007-45-2.

NOTE. Pix Lithanthracis (*Arg. P.*) is Prepared Coal Tar.

Pharmacopoeias. In *Aust., Belg., Br., Cz., Fr., Jug., Nord., Port., Roum., Span.,* and *U.S.*

Coal tar is obtained by the destructive distillation of bituminous coal at about 1000°.

A thick, nearly black, viscous liquid with a strong characteristic penetrating odour. On exposure to air it gradually becomes more viscous. It burns in air with a luminous sooty flame. Wt per mL about 1.15 g.

Slightly **soluble** in water; partly soluble in alcohol, acetone, chloroform, ether, carbon disulphide, methyl alcohol, volatile oils, and petroleum spirit. A saturated solution in water is alkaline to litmus. **Store** in airtight containers. Prepared coal tar is commercial coal tar heated at 50° for 1 hour.

No significant therapeutic differences were noted during a study of 22 patients with stable symmetrical chronic psoriasis when the use of high-temperature tar from coke ovens was compared with low-temperature tar obtained during the manufacture of smokeless fuel.— R. S. Chapman and O. A. Finn, *Br. J. Derm.*, 1976, *94*, 71.

Adverse Effects

Coal tar may cause irritation and acne-like eruptions of the skin. It also has a photosensitising action, a property used in the treatment of psoriasis with coal tar and ultraviolet radiation. Hypersensitivity to coal tar has been reported.

In the *US* the permissible and recommended exposure limits of coal products are 0.2 mg per m^3 (benzene-soluble fraction) and 0.1 mg per m^3 (cyclohexane-extractable fraction) respectively.

Although Stern *et al.* (*Lancet*, 1980, *1*, 732) found an increased risk of skin carcinoma in 59 patients with psoriasis who had had very high exposures to tar and/or u.v. radiation, Pittelkow *et al.* (*Archs Derm.*, 1981, *117*, 465) found no such evidence in 260 patients followed for a mean of 20 years and Jones *et al.* (*Br. J. Derm.*, 1985, *113*, 97) noted that long-term topical tar therapy alone was not associated with an increase in malignancy in 719 patients.

Uses and Administration

Coal tar is antipruritic, keratoplastic, and a weak antiseptic. It is used in eczema, psoriasis, dandruff, and other skin affections. Prepared coal tar has been used similarly. Tar acids (see p.970) are used as disinfectants.

Daily epidermal application of 5% crude coal tar to 14 subjects caused an initial transient hyperplasia followed by a reduction in viable epidermal thickness, which reached 20% after 40 days, indicating that intensively applied crude coal tar could act as a cytostatic agent on normal human skin.— R. M. Lavker *et al.*, *Br. J. Derm.*, 1981, *105*, 77.

PSORIASIS. In a review of the treatment of psoriasis Baker (*Prescribers' J.*, 1982, *22*, 64) considered tar to be extremely safe although it may be messy and unpleasant for some patients. Allergic contact sensitisation is rare and primary irritation unusual, except in very inflamed unstable psoriasis. Response tends to be slow, but tar is the initial treatment of choice for the majority of mild to moderate cases. In another review, Farber and Nall (*Drugs*, 1984, *28*, 324) considered that crude coal tar which is a complex mixture of many hydrocarbons affects psoriasis by enzyme inhibition and antimitotic action. *Animal* studies (M.I. Foreman *et al.*, *Br. J. Derm.*, 1985, *112*, 323) suggest that isoquinoline and analogous ingredients of coal tar contribute to its anti-psoriatic activity.

Applications of coal tar, followed after 24 hours by u.v. irradiation (the Goeckerman regimen), gave good clinical results in psoriasis.— H. O. Perry *et al.*, *Archs Derm.*, 1968, *98*, 178.

A small, uncontrolled study examining the various components of the Goeckerman regimen noted that crude coal tar alone without u.v. radiation had definite antipsoriatic activity, that the addition of u.v.-B radiation greatly enhanced its effectiveness, that 1% crude coal tar was as effective as 5%, and 25%, that application 2 hours prior to irradiation was equivalent to overnight usage, and that there was little difference between hydrophilic ointment and petrolatum as vehicles.— J. W. Petrozzi *et al.*, *Br. J. Derm.*, 1978, *98*, 437.

In a review of 200 psoriatic patients treated with an ambulatory Goeckerman regimen consisting of the home application of a coal tar preparation at bedtime, followed the next day by exposure to u.v.-B radiation, psoriasis had cleared in 86% after treatment for 5 days a week for 1 month. Mean length of remission was 5.1 months.— J. -P. DesGroseilliers *et al.*, *Can. med. Ass. J.*, 1981, *124*, 1018.

Thirty-nine patients with stable plaque-type psoriasis were treated 3 times weekly with either a coal tar extract and suberythemogenic u.v.-B radiation or maximally erythemogenic u.v.-B radiation with emollients. The fraction of patients who cleared was not significantly different between groups, but in the coal tar group, patients who successfully cleared did so at a significantly lower mean number of treatments and mean total u.v.-B dose than patients in the control group. The coal tar and u.v.-B protocol provided an effective, inexpensive, and convenient outpatient treatment for patients with moderate psoriasis, but appeared less successful in patients with severe psoriasis.— A. Menkes *et al.*, *J. Am. Acad. Derm.*, 1985, *12*, 21.

Preparations

Ammoniated Mercury and Coal Tar Ointment *(B.P.C. 1973)*. See under Ammoniated Mercury, p.926.

Ammoniated Mercury, Coal Tar, and Salicylic Acid Ointment *(B.P.C. 1973)*. See under Ammoniated Mercury, p.926.

Calamine and Coal Tar Ointment *(B.P.)*. See under Calamine, p.917.

Coal Tar Ointment *(U.S.P.)*. Coal tar 1, polysorbate '80' 0.5, and zinc oxide paste 98.5.

Coal Tar Paint *(A.P.F.)*. Coal tar 10 g, acetone to 100 mL. Flammable. Keep away from an open flame.

Coal Tar Paste *(B.P.)*. Strong coal tar solution 7.5 g and compound zinc paste 92.5 g.

Coal Tar and Salicylic Acid Ointment *(B.P.)*. Coal tar 2 g, salicylic acid 2 g, emulsifying wax 11.4 g, polysorbate '80' 4 g, liquid paraffin 7.6 g, white soft paraffin 19 g, coconut oil 54 g.

NOTE. Coal Tar and Salicylic Acid Ointment *B.P.C. 1973* was prepared with prepared coal tar.

Coal Tar Solution *(B.P.)*. Coal tar 20 g, polysorbate '80' 5 g, alcohol (or industrial methylated spirit) to 100 mL. Store in well-closed containers.

Coal Tar Solution *(A.P.F.)*. Liquor Picis Carbonis; Liq. Pic. Carb. Prepared coal tar 20 g, polysorbate '80' 5 g, alcohol (96%) to 100 mL. A solution prepared from crude coal tar is included in the *B.P.* and *U.S.P.*

Coal Tar Solution Strong *(A.P.F.)*. Prepared coal tar 40 g, polysorbate '80' 5 g, alcohol (96%) to 100 mL.

Coal Tar Topical Solution *(U.S.P.)*. Coal tar 20 g, polysorbate '80' 5 g, alcohol, to 100 mL.

Coal Tar and Zinc Cream Oily *(A.P.F.)*. Coal tar 1 g, castor oil 1 g, and zinc cream oily *(A.P.F.)* 98 g.

Coal Tar and Zinc Ointment *(B.P.)*. Strong coal tar solution 10 g, zinc oxide 30 g, and yellow soft paraffin 60 g.

Coal Tar and Zinc Paste *(A.P.F.)*. Coal Tar Paste. Coal tar 1 g, castor oil 1 g, and compound zinc paste 98 g.

Strong Coal Tar Solution *(B.P.)*. Coal tar 40 g, polysorbate '80' 5 g, alcohol (or industrial methylated spirit) to 100 mL.

NOTE. Strong Coal Tar Solution *B.P.C. 1973* was prepared by maceration from Prepared Coal Tar *B.P.C. 1973*.

Zinc and Coal Tar Preparations. For further preparations see under Zinc Oxide, p.936.

Proprietary Preparations Containing Coal Tar and Mixtures of Coal Tar Fractions

Alphosyl *(Stafford-Miller, UK)*. *Cream* and *Lotion*, refined alcoholic extract of coal tar 5%, allantoin 2%. *Shampoo* (Application PC), refined alcoholic extract of coal tar 5%, allantoin 0.2%.

Alphosyl HC *(Stafford-Miller, UK)*. *Cream*, refined alcoholic extract of coal tar 5%, allantoin 2%, hydrocortisone 0.5%.

Baltar *(E. Merck, UK)*. *Shampoo*, coal tar distillate 1.5%.

Carbo-Dome *(Lagap, UK)*. *Cream*, coal tar solution 10%.

Clinitar *(Smith & Nephew, UK)*. *Cream*, standardised coal tar extract 1%.
Gel, standardised coal tar extract 2.5%.
Shampoo, standardised coal tar extract 2%.

Gelcosal *(Quinoderm, UK)*. *Gel*, strong coal tar solution 5%, tar 5%, salicylic acid 2%.

Gelcotar *(Quinoderm, UK)*. *Gel*, strong coal tar solution 5%, tar 5%.
Shampoo (Gelcotar Liquid), strong coal tar solution 1.25%, cade oil 0.5%.

Genisol *(Fisons, UK)*. *Shampoo application*, purified coal-tar fractions 0.25% equivalent to prepared coal tar 2%, sodium sulphosuccinated, undecylenic acid monoalkylolamide 1%.

Ionil T *(Alcon, UK)*. *Shampoo*, coal tar solution 5%, salicylic acid 2%, benzalkonium chloride 0.2%.

Meditar *(Brocades, UK)*. *Application stick*, coal tar 5%, in a solid wax basis.

Pragmatar *(Smith Kline & French, UK)*. *Ointment*, cetyl alcohol-coal tar distillate 4%, precipitated sulphur 3%, salicylic acid 3%.

Psoriderm *(Dermal Laboratories, UK)*. *Bath additive*, coal tar fraction 40%, in an emulsion.
Cream, coal tar fraction 6%, lecithin 0.4%.
Scalp lotion, coal tar fraction 2.5%, lecithin 0.3%.

Psorigel *(Alcon, UK)*. *Gel*, coal tar solution 7.5%.

Tarcortin *(Stafford-Miller, UK)*. *Cream*, alcoholic coal tar extract 5%, hydrocortisone 0.5%.

T/Gel *(Neutrogena, UK)*. *Shampoo*, coal tar extract 2%.

Proprietary Names and Manufacturers of Coal Tar and Mixtures of Coal Tar Fractions

Balnetar *(Bristol-Myers, Austral.; Westwood, Canad.)*; Baltar *(E. Merck, UK)*; Basotar *(Basoderm, Denm.)*; Carbo-Dome *(Dome-Hollister-Stier, Fr.; Lagap, UK)*; Clinitar *(Smith & Nephew, UK; Ulmer, USA)*; Denorex *(Whitehall, Canad.; Whitehall, USA)*; DHS Tar Shampoo *(Person & Covey, USA)*; Estar *(Westwood, Canad.; Westwood, USA)*; Exederm *(Austral.)*; Fototar *(Elder, USA)*; Meditar *(Brocades, UK)*; Pentrax *(Genderm, USA)*; Politar *(Arg.)*; Psoriderm *(Dermal Laboratories, UK)*; Psorigel *(Alcon, Austral.; Alcon, Canad.; Alcon, UK)*; Targel *(Odan, Canad.)*; Teerol *(Max Ritter, Switz.)*; T/Gel *(Prof. Pharm. Corp., Canad.; Neutrogena, UK)*; Waxtar *(Pharma-Medica, Denm.)*; Zetar *(Rorer, Canad.; Dermik, USA)*.

The following names have been used for multi-ingredient preparations containing coal tar and mixtures of coal tar fractions—Acnelab *(Austral.)*; Alphosyl *(Stafford-Miller, Austral.; Reed & Carnrick, Canad.; Stafford-Miller, UK; Reed & Carnrick, USA)*; Alphosyl-HC *(Stafford-Miller, UK)*; Balneum with Tar *(E. Merck, UK)*; Carbo-Cort *(Lagap, UK)*; Coltapaste *(Smith & Nephew, UK)*; Cor-Tar-Quin *(Lagap, UK)*; Eczema Cream *(Hamilton, Austral.)*; Egolotin *(Ego, Austral.)*; Egopsoryl *(Ego, Austral.)*; Exolan Lotion *(Dermal Laboratories, UK)*; Gelcosal *(Quinoderm, UK)*; Gelcotar *(Quinoderm, UK)*; Gelcotar Liquid *(Quinoderm, UK)*; Genisol *(Key, Austral.; Fisons, UK)*; Ionil T *(Alcon, Austral.; Alcon, Canad.; Alcon, UK; Owen, USA)*; Multi-Tar Plus *(ICN, Canad.)*; Polytar Emollient *(Stiefel, Austral.; Stiefel, UK)*; Polytar Liquid *(Stiefel, Austral.; Stiefel, UK)*; Polytar Plus *(Stiefel, UK)*; Pragmatar *(Smith Kline & French, Austral.; Smith Kline & French, Canad.; Smith Kline & French, UK)*; P&S Plus *(Dormer, Canad.)*; Psorin *(Cambden, Austral.; Thames, UK)*; Psorox *(Fisons, UK)*; Sebcur/T *(Dermtek, Canad.)*; Sebutone *(Westwood, Canad.; Westwood, USA)*; SLT *(C & M, USA)*; SSC Ointment *(Cambden, Austral.)*; Tar Doak *(Trans Canaderm, Canad.)*; Tarband *(Seton, UK)*; Tarcortin *(Stafford-Miller, UK)*; Tardan *(Odan, Canad.)*; Tarquinor *(Squibb, Austral.)*; Triamalone *(Trans Canaderm, Canad.)*.

1653-y

Tellurium Dioxide

TeO_2=159.6.

CAS — 7446-07-3.

A 2.5% suspension was formerly used similarly to selenium sulphide as a shampoo in the treatment of seborrhoeic dermatitis. In Great Britain the recommended exposure limit of tellurium and compounds, except the hexafluoride, (as Te) is 0.1 mg per m^3 (long-term); the use of tellurium and its compounds in cosmetics is prohibited by law.

1654-j

Thioxolone *(BAN)*.

OL-110; Tioxolone *(rINN)*. 6-Hydroxy-1,3-benzoxathiol-2-one.
$C_7H_4O_3S$=168.2.

CAS — 4991-65-5.

Thioxolone has been used topically in the treatment of acne.

Proprietary Names and Manufacturers

Camyna *(Boehringer Ingelheim, Denm.; Boehringer Ingelheim, Norw.; Boehringer Ingelheim, S.Afr.; Basoderm, Swed.)*; Gélacnine *(Furt, Fr.)*; Stepin *(Basotherm, Ger.)*; Vikura Salba *(Jpn)*; Wasacne *(IFI, Ital.)*.

1655-z

Titanium Dioxide *(BAN, USAN).*

CI Pigment White 6; Colour Index No. 77891; E171; Titanii Dioxidum; Titanium Oxide.
TiO_2=79.90.

CAS — 13463-67-7.

Pharmacopoeias. In *Aust., Br., Braz., Eur., Fr., Ind., It., Jpn, Jug., Neth., Swiss,* and *U.S.*

A white or almost white, infusible, odourless powder.
Practically **insoluble** in water, dilute mineral acids, and organic solvents; slowly soluble in hot sulphuric acid; soluble in hydrofluoric acid, and by fusion with potassium bisulphate and alkali hydroxides or carbonates. A 10% suspension in water is neutral to litmus.
Store in well-closed containers.

Titanium dioxide has an action on the skin similar to that of zinc oxide (p.936) and is employed for the relief of pruritus and in certain exudative dermatoses. Titanium peroxide, titanium salicylate, and titanium tannate are used in combination with titanium dioxide for the same indications. It reflects ultraviolet light and is used to prevent sunburn. It is an ingredient of certain face powders and other cosmetics. It is used to pigment and opacify hard gelatin capsules and tablet coatings and as a delustring agent for regenerated cellulose and other man-made fibres. Specially purified grades may be used in food colours.
In Great Britain the recommended exposure limits of titanium dioxide are, total dust 10 mg per m^3 (long-term), respirable dust 5 mg per m^3 (long-term).

Preparations

Titanium Dioxide Paste *(A.P.F.).* Titanium Dioxide Magma. Titanium dioxide 20 g, calamine 25 g, light kaolin or light kaolin (natural), sterilised, 10 g, bentonite, sterilised, 1 g, chlorocresol 100 mg, glycerol 15 g, freshly boiled and cooled purified water to 100 g.

Titanium Dioxide Paste *(B.P.).* Titanium dioxide 20 g, zinc oxide 25 g, sterilised light kaolin or light kaolin (natural) 10 g, red ferric oxide of commerce 2 g, chlorocresol 100 mg, glycerol 15 g, freshly boiled and cooled water to 100 g. Avoid contact with aluminium.

Proprietary Preparations

Metanium *(Bengué, UK). Ointment,* titanium dioxide 20%, titanium peroxide 5%, titanium salicylate 3%, titanium tannate 0.1%, in a silicone basis.

Proprietary Names and Manufacturers

Sun-Bar *(Odan, Canad.).*

The following names have been used for multi-ingredient preparations containing titanium dioxide— Acne-sol *(Fawns & McAllan, Austral.)*; Granugen *(Schering, Austral.)*; Herpecin-L *(Campbell, USA)*; Metanium *(Bengué, UK).*

1656-c

Tretinoin *(BAN, USAN, rINN).*

NSC-122758; Retinoic Acid; Vitamin A Acid. *all-trans*-Retinoic acid; 15-Apo-β-caroten-15-oic acid; 3,7-Dimethyl-9-(2,6,6-trimethylcyclohex-1-enyl)nona-2,4,6,8-*all-trans*-tetraenoic acid.
$C_{20}H_{28}O_2$=300.4.

CAS — 302-79-4.

Pharmacopoeias. In *Br.* and *U.S.*

A yellow to light-orange crystalline powder.
Practically **insoluble** in water; soluble in ether; slightly soluble in alcohol and chloroform. It is unstable in solution in the presence of strong oxidising agents. It is very sensitive to light and oxygen.
Store at −15° in well-closed containers. Protect from light.

Adverse Effects

The application of tretinoin may cause transitory stinging and a feeling of warmth. Correct application causes erythema and scaling similar to that of mild sunburn. Sensitivity to u.v. light may be increased. Temporary hypopigmentation and hyperpigmentation have been reported. Excessive application may cause marked redness, discomfort, and peeling without any increase of effect on the acne.

A discussion of the possible increased risk of sun-provoked cancer in patients using tretinoin.— *FDA Drug Bull.,* 1978, *8,* 26. See also H. P. Baden (letter), *New Engl. J. Med.,* 1980, *302,* 1419; J. W. Melski and K. A. Arndt (letter), *ibid.*

Critical comment on the advice (given by Health and Welfare, Canada) that tretinoin was potentially teratogenic and should not be used for the treatment of acne in young women.— F. W. Danby (letter), *Can. med. Ass. J.,* 1978, *119,* 854. Reply upholding the advice.— A. B. Morrison (letter), *ibid.*

For an *in vitro* study demonstrating that tretinoin is potentially phototoxic, see Etretinate, p.921.

Precautions

Tretinoin should not be applied to the eyes, mouth, or other mucous surfaces, nor to eczematous or abraded skin. Caution is needed when tretinoin is used concomitantly with other topical treatment, especially with keratolytic agents. Excessive exposure to sunlight and u.v. light should be avoided. Patients with sunburn should not use tretinoin until fully recovered.

Absorption and Fate

Tretinoin appears to be only slightly absorbed from the skin after topical application.

Uses and Administration

Tretinoin appears to stimulate the epithelium to produce horny cells at a faster rate and to reduce their cohesion, possibly by altering the synthesis or quality of the cement substance which binds horny layer cells into impactions.
Tretinoin is used primarily in the treatment of acne vulgaris in which comedones, papules, and pustules predominate. It is applied as a cream, gel, or alcoholic solution, usually containing 0.025% or 0.05%. The skin should be washed with soap and water to remove excessive oiliness and dried 15 to 20 minutes before applying tretinoin lightly, once or twice daily according to response and irritation. There may be apparent exacerbations of the acne during early treatment and a therapeutic response may not be evident for 6 to 8 weeks. When the condition has resolved application for maintenance should be less frequent.
Tretinoin has also been used in psoriasis and some disorders of keratinisation. Derivatives of tretinoin such as etretinate (see p.921) and isotretinoin (see p.924) are given by mouth, and other derivatives are also under study.
Tretinoin is vitamin A acid; for the actions and uses of vitamin A, see p.1278.

A brief review of tretinoin.— C. E. Orfanos *et al., Drugs,* 1987, *34,* 459.

A discussion of the prevention of cutaneous ageing with tretinoin.— *Lancet,* 1988, *1,* 977.

Tretinoin applied topically, was effective in hypertrophic lichen planus (usually permanently), autosomal dominant ichthyosis, keratoses of the palms or soles, and keratosis pilaris. Tretinoin was too irritating for use in ichthyosis associated with atopic eczema.— S. Gunther, *Cutis,* 1976, *17,* 287.

For the use of tretinoin with fluorouracil in the eradication of solar keratoses, especially those on the hands, see Fluorouracil, p.630.

ACNE VULGARIS. Tretinoin was considered to be most beneficial in patients with extensive comedones and can be usefully combined with benzoyl peroxide; tretinoin is used in the morning and benzoyl peroxide in the evening.— W. J. Cunliffe, *Prescribers' J.,* 1982, *22,* 7.

MALIGNANT NEOPLASMS. Two patients with cutaneous metastatic melanoma were treated daily for 12 weeks with topical tretinoin solution 0.05%. Complete regression of the treated lesions was noted in 1 patient and a partial response was seen in the other.— N. Levine and F. L. Meyskens, *Lancet,* 1980, *2,* 224.

Retinoic acid induced morphological maturation and markedly inhibited proliferation in cultured neuroblastoma cells and may be a useful therapy for metastatic neuroblastoma.— R. C. Seeger *et al., Ann. intern. Med.,* 1982, *97,* 873.

RHEUMATOID ARTHRITIS. Comment on possible retinoid therapy for rheumatoid arthritis.— E. D. Harris, *Ann. intern. Med.,* 1984, *100,* 146.

Preparations

Tretinoin Cream *(U.S.P.)*

Tretinoin Gel *(B.P.)*

Tretinoin Gel *(U.S.P.)*

Tretinoin Solution *(B.P.).* Contains tretinoin in a suitable alcoholic solvent. **Store** at a temperature between −5° and 0°.

Tretinoin Topical Solution *(U.S.P.).* Contains tretinoin in a suitable non-aqueous hydrophilic solvent.

Proprietary Preparations

Retin-A *(Ortho-Cilag, UK). Cream,* tretinoin 0.025 and 0.05%.
Gel, tretinoin 0.025%.
Lotion, tretinoin 0.025%.

Proprietary Names and Manufacturers

A-Acido *(Arg.)*; Aberel *(Cilag, Fr.; Neth.; Johnson & Johnson, Spain)*; Aberela *(Cilag-Chemie, Norw.; Cilag, Swed.)*; Acid A Vit *(Belg.; Neth.)*; Acnavit *(Denm.)*; Acretin *(Belg.)*; Airol *(Arg.; Roche, Austral.; Roche, Denm.; Roche, Ger.; Roche, Ital.; Roche, Norw.; Roche, S.Afr.; Sauter, Switz.)*; A-vitaminsyre *(DAK, Denm.)*; Avitoin *(Norw.)*; Cordes VAS *(Ichthyol, Ger.)*; Dermairol *(Roche, Swed.)*; Dermojuventus *(Juventus, Spain)*; Effederm *(Sauba, Fr.)*; Epi-Aberel *(Cilag, Ger.)*; Eudyna *(Nordmark, Ger.)*; Locacid *(Pierre Fabre, Fr.)*; Retiderma *(Cinfa, Spain)*; Retin-A *(Cilag, Austral.; Cilag, Ital.; NZ; Johnson & Johnson, S.Afr.; Cilag, Switz.; Ortho-Cilag, UK; Ortho Dermatological, USA)*; Stievaa *(Stiefel, Canad.).*

1657-k

Trioxsalen *(USAN).*

4,5′,8-Trimethylpsoralen; Trioxysalen *(rINN).* 2,5,9-Trimethyl-7*H*-furo[3,2-*g*]chromen-7-one.
$C_{14}H_{12}O_3$=228.2.

CAS — 3902-71-4.

Pharmacopoeias. In *U.S.*

A white to off-white or greyish, odourless, crystalline solid. Practically **insoluble** in water; soluble 1 in 1150 of alcohol, 1 in 84 of chloroform, 1 in 43 of methylene chloride, and 1 in 100 of methyl isobutyl ketone. **Protect** from light.

Trioxsalen has the actions of methoxsalen (see p.926) and is used similarly to enhance pigmentation or increase the tolerance to sunlight in selected patients in a dose of 5 to 10 mg daily by mouth 2 to 4 hours before exposure to sunlight or ultraviolet radiation. Treatment should generally not be continued for longer than 14 days and the total dosage should not exceed 140 mg on a continuous or interrupted regimen. However, patients with idiopathic vitiligo may require more prolonged therapy and higher doses.
Trioxsalen has also been used topically and by mouth in the PUVA treatment of psoriasis (see p.927).
In the *UK* the use of trioxsalen, except for the natural content of essences, in cosmetics is prohibited by law.

Nine patients with severe and extensive psoriasis were treated by immersion in a trioxsalen solution 0.33 mg per litre for 10 minutes, followed by u.v.-A irradiation (bath-PUVA). A further 25 similar patients were given etretinate 1 mg per kg body-weight daily by mouth accompanied after two weeks by daily bath-PUVA. Good-to-excellent results were obtained in 24 of 25 patients treated with bath-PUVA plus etretinate and in 8 of 9 receiving bath-PUVA alone. However, the addition of etretinate almost halved the total u.v.-A dose needed for clearing. After clearance of psoriasis 15 of the patients receiving the combined therapy were given maintenance therapy of only bath-PUVA once or twice weekly and 9 received only etretinate 25 to 50 mg daily. During maintenance, results in 14 of the 15 patients receiving bath-PUVA remained good-to-excellent during a mean follow-up of 10 weeks; in the etretinate group results remained good-to-excellent in 4 of 9 patients. Three additional patients with psoriasis resistant to bath-PUVA cleared in 4 to 8 weeks after the addition of etretinate.— N. Väätäinen *et al., J. Am. Acad. Derm.,* 1985, *12,* 52.

Preparations
Trioxsalen Tablets *(U.S.P.)*

Proprietary Names and Manufacturers
Levrison *(Rovi, Spain)*; Tripsor *(Orion, Fin.)*; Trisoralen *(Protea, Austral.; Belg.; Elder, Canad.; Delta Laboratories, Eire; Lifepharma, Ital.; Elder, S.Afr.; Elder, USA: Sas, UK)*.

1658-a

Xenysalate Hydrochloride *(BANM, rINNM)*.
Biphenamine Hydrochloride *(USAN)*. 2-Diethylaminoethyl 3-phenylsalicylate hydrochloride; 2-Diethylaminoethyl 2-hydroxy-3-phenylbenzoate hydrochloride.
$C_{19}H_{23}NO_3$, HCl=349.9.

CAS — 3572-52-9(xenysalate); 5560-62-3 (hydrochloride).

Xenysalate hydrochloride has been used for the control of seborrhoeic dermatitis of the scalp and dandruff.

Proprietary Names and Manufacturers
Salol *(DAK, Denm.)*; Sébaklen *(Fumouze, Fr.)*.

1659-t

Zinc Carbonate
Hydrated Zinc Carbonate; Zinci Subcarbonas.

CAS — 3486-35-9 ($ZnCO_3$).

Pharmacopoeias. In *Nord.*

Zinc carbonate is mildly astringent and protective to the skin and, in the form of calamine (see p.917), is used in creams, dusting-powders, lotions, and ointments.

1660-l

Zinc Oxide *(BAN, USAN)*.
Blanc de Zinc; Flores de Zinc; Zinci Oxidum; Zinci Oxydum; Zincum Oxydatum.
ZnO=81.39.

CAS — 1314-13-2.

NOTE. 'Zinc White' is a commercial form of zinc oxide for use as a pigment.

Pharmacopoeias. In *Arg., Aust., Belg., Br., Braz., Chin., Cz., Egypt., Eur., Fr., Ger., Hung., Ind., Int., It., Jpn, Jug., Mex., Neth., Nord., Pol., Port., Roum., Rus., Span., Swiss, Turk.,* and *U.S.*

A white or faintly yellowish-white, odourless, amorphous, soft powder, free from grittiness.
Practically **insoluble** in water and in alcohol; soluble in dilute mineral acids and in solutions of alkali hydroxides. **Store** in well-closed containers.

For a report of the impairment of the effectiveness of dithranol by Zinc Oxide, see p.919.

Zinc oxide is applied to the skin as a mild astringent, as a soothing and protective application in eczema, and as a protective to slight excoriations often with coal tar (see p.934). Zinc oxide reflects ultraviolet radiation and is used in sunscreens.

When zinc oxide is mixed with a strong solution of zinc chloride, an oxychloride is formed which sets into a hard mass; this forms the basis of some dental cements. A similar product is obtained by mixing zinc oxide with phosphoric acid to form an oxyphosphate. Mixed with clove oil or eugenol, zinc oxide is used as a temporary dental filling.

In Great Britain the recommended exposure limits of zinc oxide fume are 5 mg per m^3 (long-term); 10 mg per m^3 (short-term). In the *US* the permissible and recommended exposure limits are 5 mg per m^3. For further details of zinc and its salts see p.1287.

The treatment of uncomplicated superficial and plantar leprotic ulcers with adhesive zinc oxide tape.— A. Kumar and M. Lakshmanan, *Lepr. Rev.*, 1986, *57*, 45; R. T. Walton *et al.*, *ibid.*, 53.

COMPLICATIONS OF DENTAL USE. Solitary aspergillosis of the maxillary sinus in 29 of 30 patients was associated with zinc oxide from overfilled teeth. Treatment consists of removal of the fungal ball containing the zinc oxide; no antifungal treatment is necessary. Zinc oxide has been shown to accelerate the growth of *Aspergillus fumigatus*.— J. Beck-Mannagetta *et al.* (letter), *Lancet*, 1983, *2*, 1260.

Preparations

Compound Zinc Paste *(B.P.)*. Co. Zinc Paste; Zinc Compound Paste; Zinc Paste; Zinc Paste Compound *(A.P.F.)*; Compound Zinc Oxide Paste; Zinc Oxide Paste *(U.S.P.)*; Lassar's Plain Zinc Paste. Zinc oxide 25 g, starch 25 g, and white soft paraffin 50 g.

Ichthammol and Zinc Cream Oily *(A.P.F.)*. See under Ichthammol, p.923.

Zinc and Castor Oil Ointment *(B.P., A.P.F.)*. Zinc and Castor Oil Oint.; Zinc and Castor Oil Cream; Zinc Oxide and Castor Oil Ointment; Zinc and Castor Oil. Zinc oxide 7.5 g, castor oil 50 g, cetostearyl alcohol 2 g, white beeswax 10 g, and arachis oil 30.5 g.

Zinc and Coal Tar Ointment *(A.P.F.)*. Ung. Zinc. et Pic. Zinc oxide 20 g, coal tar 5 g, castor oil 3 g, and yellow soft paraffin 72 g.

Zinc and Coal Tar Paste *(B.P.)*. Zinc Oxide and Coal Tar Paste; White's Tar Paste. Coal tar 6 g, zinc oxide 6 g, starch 38 g, emulsifying wax 5 g, and yellow soft paraffin 45 g.
The title White's Tar Paste has also been used for: prepared coal tar 4, zinc oxide 25, soft paraffin to 100.

Zinc and Coal Tar Preparations. For further preparations see under Coal Tar, p.934.

Zinc Cream *(B.P.)*. Zinc Oxide Cream. Zinc oxide 32 g, oleic acid 0.5 mL, arachis oil 32 mL, wool fat 8 g, calcium hydroxide 45 mg, freshly boiled and cooled water to 100 g.

Zinc Cream Oily *(A.P.F.)*. Crem. Zinc. Oleos; Zinc Cream. Zinc oxide 32 g, oleic acid 0.5 mL, arachis oil 21.5 mL, wool fat 17.5 g, and calcium hydroxide solution 30.5 mL.

Zinc Gelatin *(U.S.P.)*. Zinc oxide 10 g, gelatin 15 g, glycerol 40 g, and water 35 g.

Zinc Gelatin Impregnated Gauze *(U.S.P.)*. Absorbent gauze impregnated with zinc gelatin that may contain a small amount of ferric oxide. Each 100 g contains 82.5 to 89.5 g of zinc gelatin *(U.S.P.)*, equivalent to 6.7 to 9.1% of zinc oxide.

Zinc and Ichthammol Cream *(B.P.)*. Zinc Oxide and Ichthammol Cream. Zinc Cream 82 g, wool fat 10 g, ichthammol 5 g, cetostearyl alcohol 3 g.

Zinc Ointment *(B.P.)*. Zinc Oint.; Ung. Zinc.; Zinc Oxide Ointment *(A.P.F.)*. Zinc oxide 15% in simple ointment.

Zinc Oxide Ointment *(U.S.P.)*. Zinc oxide 20 g, liquid paraffin 15 g, white ointment 65 g.

Zinc Oxide and Salicylic Acid Paste *(U.S.P.)*. Zinc Oxide Paste with Salicylic Acid; Lassar's Zinc Paste with Salicylic Acid. Salicylic acid 2% in zinc oxide paste.

Zinc Paste Bandage *(B.P.)*. A bandage of a white plain-weave cotton cloth impregnated with not less than 150 g per m^2 of a suitable paste containing not less than 6% of zinc oxide.

Zinc Paste, Calamine and Clioquinol Bandage *(B.P.)*. A bandage of a white plain-weave cotton cloth impregnated with not less than 175 g per m^2 of a paste containing zinc oxide 9.25%, clioquinol 1%, calamine 5.75%.

Zinc Paste and Coal Tar Bandage *(B.P.)*. A bandage of a white plain-weave cotton cloth impregnated with not less than 150 g per m^2 of a suitable paste containing coal tar 3.0% and not less than 6% of zinc oxide.

Zinc Paste and Ichthammol Bandage *(B.P.)*. A bandage of a white plain-weave cotton cloth impregnated with not less than 150 g per m^2 of a paste containing zinc oxide 6% and ichthammol 2%.

Zinc and Salicylic Acid Paste *(B.P.)*. Zinc Oxide and Salicylic Acid Paste; Lassar's Paste. Zinc oxide 24 g, salicylic acid 2 g, starch 24 g, and white soft paraffin 50 g.
A.P.F. has salicylic acid 2 g, liquid paraffin 2 g, compound zinc paste 96 g.

Zinc, Starch, and Talc Dusting-powder *(B.P.C. 1973)*. Conspersus Zinci, Amyli et Talci; Zinc Oxide and Starch Dusting-powder; Zinc Oxide, Starch, and Talc Dusting-powder; Zinc, Starch and Talc Dusting Powder *(A.P.F.)*. Zinc oxide 25 g, starch 25 g, and sterilised purified talc 50 g.

Zinc-Eugenol Cement *(U.S.P.)*. Zinc Compounds and Eugenol Cement. It consists of 2 preparations packed separately: (1) *The Powder.* Zinc oxide 70 g, zinc acetate 500 mg, zinc stearate 1 g, and colophony 28.5 g, (2) *The Liquid.* Eugenol 85 mL and cottonseed oil 15 mL; protect from light. To prepare the cement, mix 10 parts of the powder with 1 part of the liquid to a thick paste immediately before use. The amount of liquid may be varied to give any desired consistency.

Proprietary Preparations

Calaband *(Seton, UK)*. *Impregnated bandage*, white plain-weave cotton cloth, impregnated with not less than 175 g per m^2 of a paste containing zinc oxide 9.25%, calamine 5.75%.

Coltapaste *(Smith & Nephew, UK)*. *Impregnated bandage*, Zinc Paste and Coal Tar Bandage *(B.P.)*.

Ichthopaste *(Smith & Nephew, UK)*. *Impregnated bandage*, Zinc Paste and Ichthammol Bandage *(B.P.)*.

Icthaband *(Seton, UK)*. *Impregnated bandage*, Zinc Paste and Ichthammol Bandage *(B.P.)*.

Noratex *(Norton, UK)*. *Cream*, zinc oxide 21.8%, talc 7.4%, light kaolin 3.5%, cod-liver oil 2.15%, wool fat 1.075%.

Quinaband *(Seton, UK)*. *Impregnated bandage*, Zinc Paste, Calamine and Clioquinol Bandage *(B.P.)*.

Sudocrem *(Tosara, UK)*. *Cream*, zinc oxide 15.25%, hydrous wool fat 4%, benzyl benzoate 1.01%, benzyl cinnamate 0.15%, benzyl alcohol 0.39%.

Tarband *(Seton, UK)*. *Impregnated bandage*, Zinc Paste and Coal Tar Bandage *(B.P.)*.

Thovaline *(Ilon Laboratories, UK)*. *Ointment* and *Aerosol spray*, zinc oxide 19.8%, talc 3.3%, light kaolin 2.5%, cod-liver oil 1.5%, wool fat 2.5%.

Viscopaste PB7 *(Smith & Nephew, UK)*. *Impregnated bandage*, Zinc Paste Bandage *(B.P.)*.

Zincaband *(Seton, UK)*. *Impregnated bandage*, Zinc Paste Bandage *(B.P.)*.

Proprietary Names and Manufacturers

Amniolina *(Bama, Spain)*; Herisan *(Rougier, Canad.)*; Natusan ZINK-Barnesalve *(Benzon, Denm.)*; Oxyplastine *(Pharmeurop, Fr.; Wild, Switz.)*; Pangamma *(IBP, Ital.)*; Pharmakon *(Vine Chemicals, UK)*; Primer *(Glenwood, USA)*; Sénophile *(Bruneau, Fr.)*; Sudocrem *(Tosara, UK)*; Viscopaste PB7 *(Smith & Nephew, S.Afr.; Smith & Nephew, UK)*; Zincaband *(Seton, UK)*; Zincofax *(Wellcome, Canad.)*.

The following names have been used for multi-ingredient preparations containing zinc oxide—Allersone *(Mallard, USA)*; Anthical *(May & Baker, UK)*; Anugesic-HC *(Parke, Davis, UK)*; Anusol *(Warner, Austral.; Warner-Lambert, UK; Parke, Davis, USA)*; Anusol HC *(Warner, Austral.)*; Anusol-HC *(Parke, Davis, UK; Parke, Davis, USA)*; Bensulfoid Lotion *(Poythress, USA)*; Bismodyne *(Loveridge, UK)*; Calaband *(Seton, UK)*; Calmasol *(Ethipharm, Canad.)*; Coltapaste *(Smith & Nephew, UK)*; Cordocel *(Wigglesworth, UK)*; Cordocel-H *(Wigglesworth, UK)*; Dome-Paste *(Miles Pharmaceuticals, USA)*; Eczema Cream *(Hamilton, Austral.)*; Egoderm Ointment *(Ego, Austral.)*; Egolotin *(Ego, Austral.)*; Egozite *(Ego, Austral.)*; Esoban *(Southon-Horton, UK)*; ESTP *(Martindale Pharmaceuticals, UK)*; Granugen *(Schering, Austral.)*; Hemocane *(Key, Austral.; Intercare, UK)*; Hemorex *(Winthrop, Austral.)*; Hill Cortac *(Hill, USA)*; Ichthopaste *(Smith & Nephew, UK)*; Icthaband *(Seton, UK)*; Medicone Derma-HC *(Medicone, USA)*; Morhulin *(Napp, UK)*; Nestosyl *(Bengué, UK)*; Noratex *(Norton, UK)*; Nupercainal Suppositories *(Ciba, USA)*; Pazo *(Bristol-Myers Products, USA)*; Pedoz *(Hamilton, Austral.)*; Piz Buin (Factor 12) *(Greiter, Switz.: Ciba Consumer, UK)*; Quinaband *(Seton, UK)*; Rectal Medicone-HC *(Medicone, USA)*; Rectinol *(G.P. Laboratories, Austral.)*; RoC Total Sunblock *(Roc, UK)*; RVPaque *(Elder, USA)*; Septex Cream No. 1 *(Norton, UK)*; Septex Cream No. 2 *(Norton, UK)*; Silon *(Pharmacia, Canad.)*; Sprilon *(Pharmacia, UK)*; Tarband *(Seton, UK)*; Thovaline *(Ilon Laboratories, UK)*; Ung. Morrhuae Co *(Philip Harris, UK)*; Uraband *(Seton, UK)*; Vasogen *(Pharmax, UK)*; Wyanoids *(Wyeth, USA)*; Xyloproct *(Astra, Austral.; Astra, UK)*.

1662-j

Zirconium Dioxide
Zirconia; Zirconic Anhydride; Zirconium Oxide.
ZrO_2=123.2.

CAS — 1314-23-4.

Zirconium dioxide and salts, e.g. zirconium lactate and zirconium oxychloride, have been used in deodorant preparations. There have been reports of allergic reactions with granulomas.

Zirconium dioxide has also been used as a contrast medium. In Great Britain the recommended exposure limits of zirconium compounds (as Zr) are 5 mg per m^3 (long-term); 10 mg per m^3 (short-term).

Proprietary Names and Manufacturers
The following names have been used for multi-ingredient preparations containing Zirconium dioxide— Ziradryl (*Parke, Davis, Canad.; Parke, Davis, USA*).

Diagnostic Agents

2120-z

This section mainly describes compounds that are administered solely for diagnostic purposes. It does not include contrast media or radiopharmaceuticals as they are described in their own sections; nor does it include the many compounds with clinical as well as diagnostic uses, they are spread throughout *Martindale*.
No attempt has been made in this edition to describe the endogenous substances such as CEA (carcinoembryonic antigen) that are measured in various tests.
Tests carried out *in vitro* have generally been omitted with the exception of glucose tests and tests for pregnancy and ovulation.

2121-c

Ametazole Hydrochloride *(BANM).*
Betazole Hydrochloride *(pINNM)*; Betazoli Chloridum.
2-(Pyrazol-3-yl)ethylamine dihydrochloride.
$C_5H_9N_3,2HCl=184.1$.

CAS — 105-20-4 (ametazole); 138-92-1 (hydrochloride).

Pharmacopoeias. In *Nord.*

Ametazole hydrochloride is an analogue of histamine and was used as a diagnostic agent for testing gastric secretion when it was given in a dose of 500 µg per kg body-weight by subcutaneous or intramuscular injection.

Proprietary Names and Manufacturers
Betazol *(Lilly, Ger.)*; Histalog *(Lilly, Canad.; Lilly, UK; Lilly, USA)*; Testazid *(Apothekernes Laboratorium, Norw.)*.

2122-k

Aminohippuric Acid *(USAN).*
p-Aminobenzoylglycine; *p*-Aminohippuric Acid; PAHA; Para-aminohippuric Acid. *N*-4-Aminobenzoylaminoacetic acid.
$C_9H_{10}N_2O_3=194.2$.

CAS — 61-78-9 (aminohippuric acid); 94-16-6 (sodium salt).

Pharmacopoeias. In *Cz., Fr.,* and *U.S.*

A white crystalline powder which discolours on exposure to light. **Soluble** 1 in 45 of water, 1 in 50 of alcohol, and 1 in 5 (with decomposition) of dilute hydrochloric acid; very slightly soluble in carbon tetrachloride, chloroform, and ether; freely soluble, with decomposition, in alkaline solutions. **Store** in airtight containers. Protect from light.
The *U.S.P.* injection (Aminohippurate Sodium Injection) consists of an aqueous solution of aminohippuric acid prepared with the aid of sodium hydroxide. It has a pH between 6.7 and 7.6.

Adverse Effects
Sodium aminohippurate may cause nausea and vomiting, vasomotor disturbances, flushing, tingling, cramps, and a feeling of warmth. Patients may develop an urge to urinate or defaecate after infusion.

Precautions
The estimation of sodium aminohippurate may be affected in patients taking procaine, sulphonamides, or thiazosulphone. Probenecid diminishes the excretion of aminohippuric acid. Clearance is also affected by penicillins, salicylates, sulphinpyrazone, and other drugs that compete for the same excretory pathways.

Uses and Administration
Aminohippuric acid is given by intravenous infusion, as the sodium salt, as a diagnostic agent for the estimation of effective renal plasma flow. Doses are aimed at producing a plasma concentration of 10 to 20 µg per mL; at these concentrations plasma clearance of aminohippurate is considered to be equal to the effective renal plasma flow. As it is excreted by glomerular filtration as well as tubular secretion, sodium aminohippurate has also been used for the measurement of the renal tubular secretory mechanism. Doses for this purpose are infused slowly to achieve a plasma concentration of 400 to 600 µg per mL to saturate the tubular secretion.

Preparations
Aminohippurate Sodium Injection *(U.S.P.)*

Proprietary Preparations
Sodium Para-aminohippurate *(Merck Sharp & Dohme, UK). Injection,* sodium para-aminohippurate 200 mg/mL in vials of 10 mL.

Proprietary Names and Manufacturers
Nephrotest BAG *(Ger.)*
Manufacturers also include—*Merck Sharp & Dohme, Austral.; Merck Sharp & Dohme, UK; Merck Sharp & Dohme, USA* .

2123-a

Azovan Blue *(BAN).*
Azovanum Caeruleum; CI Direct Blue 53; Colour Index No. 23860; Evans Blue *(USAN)*; T-1824. Tetrasodium 6,6′-[3,3′-dimethylbiphenyl-4,4′-diylbis(azo)]bis[4-amino-5-hydroxynaphthalene-1,3-disulphonate].
$C_{34}H_{24}N_6Na_4O_{14}S_4=960.8$.

CAS — 314-13-6.

Pharmacopoeias. In *Arg.* and *U.S.*

A green, bluish-green, or brown, odourless powder. Very **soluble** in water; very slightly soluble in alcohol; practically insoluble in carbon tetrachloride, chloroform, and ether. The *U.S.P.* injection has a pH of 5.5 to 7.5. **Store** in airtight containers.

Azovan blue is a dye which has been used for the determination of blood volume. The uptake in the blood following the intravenous injection of up to 20 mg is used to calculate the blood volume. It is firmly bound to plasma proteins and is slow to leave the circulation. Some patients however, may experience staining of the skin.

Preparations
Evans Blue Injection *(U.S.P.).* Azovan Blue Injection

5003-e

Azuresin *(BAN).*
Azure A Carbacrylic Resin.

CAS — 8050-34-8 (azuresin); 531-53-3 (azure A).

Azuresin is a carbacrylic cation-exchange resin containing about 6% of 3-amino-7-dimethylaminophenothiazin-5-ium chloride (azure A). It was formerly given by mouth for the detection, without intubation, of free hydrochloric acid in the gastric juice. In the presence of free acid in the stomach the dye component of the resin is displaced by hydrogen ions and is subsequently excreted in the urine, to which it imparts a green or blue colour.

Proprietary Names and Manufacturers
Diagnex Blue *(Squibb, UK)*.

1957-g

Bentiromide *(BAN, USAN, rINN).*
BTPABA; E-2663; PFT; Ro-11-7891. 4-(*N*-Benzoyl-L-tyrosylamino)benzoic acid.
$C_{23}H_{20}N_2O_5=404.4$.

CAS — 37106-97-1.

Adverse Effects and Precautions
Reported adverse effects of bentiromide include headache, diarrhoea, and other gastro-intestinal effects. There may be hypersensitivity and transient increases in the values obtained in liver function studies.
Misleading results may be obtained in patients with gastro-intestinal, liver, or kidney disorders, or in patients receiving other drugs that are excreted as arylamines. Some of these drugs include benzocaine, chloramphenicol, lignocaine, procaine, procainamide, sulphonamides, and some diuretics.
Aminobenzoic acid can displace methotrexate from binding sites.

Absorption and Fate
Following administration by mouth, bentiromide is hydrolysed by chymotrypsin in the gut to release *p*-aminobenzoic acid and benzoyl-tyrosine. The aminobenzoic acid is absorbed, metabolised in the liver, and excreted in the urine as *p*-aminobenzoic acid and metabolites.

Uses and Administration
Bentiromide is used as a noninvasive test of pancreatic function, the amount of *p*-aminobenzoic acid and its metabolites being excreted in the urine being taken as a measure of the chymotrypsin-secreting activity of the pancreas. Some studies have questioned its reliability and led to modifications in the test.
The usual dose is 500 mg. Children aged 6 to 12 years may be given 14 mg per kg body-weight up to a maximum dose of 500 mg.

Some references to the assessment of bentiromide in the diagnosis of pancreatic disorders: C. Arvanitakis and N. J. Greenberger, *Lancet*, 1976, *1*, 663; M. Sacher *et al.*, *Archs Dis. Childh.*, 1978, *53*, 639; V. A. Tetlow *et al.*, *Clin. Trials J.*, 1980, *17*, 121; C. J. Mitchell *et al.*, *Br. med. J.*, 1981, *282*, 1751; G. Kay *et al. ibid.*, *283*, 382; P. G. Lankisch, *Gut*, 1982, *23*, 777; M. Okada *et al.*, *Postgrad. med. J.*, 1983, *59*, 79; P. N. Foster *et al.*, *Br. med. J.*, 1984, *289*, 13; J. Braganza (letter), *ibid.*, 562; I. Cobden *et al.* (letter), *ibid.*, 830; C. Lang *et al.*, *Gut*, 1984, *25*, 508; *Med. Lett.*, 1984, *26*, 50.

Proprietary Names and Manufacturers
Chymex (*Adria, Canad.; Adria, USA*).

2124-t

Ceruletide *(BAN, USAN, rINN).*
Caerulein.
$C_{58}H_{73}N_{13}O_{21}S_2=1352.4$.

CAS — 17650-98-5 (ceruletide); 71247-25-1 (ceruletide diethylamine).

NOTE. The name Ceruleinum has been applied to Indigo Carmine, p.941.

Ceruletide is a decapeptide amide originally isolated from the skin of the Australian frog, *Hyla caerulea*, and other amphibians. Ceruletide compound with diethylamine (ceruletide diethylamine) may exist as a salt with 1 to 3 moles of diethylamine.

Uses and Administration
Ceruletide has similar actions to pancreozymin. When administered by injection it stimulates gall-bladder contraction and relaxes the sphincter of Oddi; it also stimulates intestinal muscle.
As ceruletide diethylamine, it is used as an aid to cholecystography and in pancreatic function studies when it may be given intramuscularly in doses equivalent to 300 ng of ceruletide per kg body-weight. It has also been tried in paralytic ileus.

A review of the actions and uses of ceruletide.— M. E. Vincent *et al.*, *Pharmacotherapy*, 1982, *2*, 223.

Four patients with retained biliary calculi following cholecystectomy had their stones flushed out by large volumes of saline. The saline was administered via a T tube and this administration was made possible by the intravenous infusion of ceruletide 2 ng per kg body-weight per minute for 1 hour to produce relaxation of the sphincter. In 3 patients the biliary tree was clear of stones after one treatment; the fourth patient was clear after two treatments.— A. Cuschieri, *Br. med. J.*, 1984, *289*, 1582.

Ceruletide by intramuscular injection was considered superior to pentazocine intramuscularly in alleviating pain in a study involving 56 patients with biliary colic. Pentazocine was superior to ceruletide in patients with renal colic. Side-effects associated with ceruletide were profuse sweating (1 patient), dizziness (2), and vomiting (1).— M. Lishner *et al.*, *Drug Intell. & clin. Pharm.*, 1985, *19*, 433.

Further references to ceruletide: A. Agosti *et al.* (letter), *Lancet*, 1971, *1*, 395 (benefit in paralytic ileus); N. Basso *et al.*, *Eur. J. clin. Pharmac.*, 1982, *22*, 531 (ischaemic pain); G. Stacher *et al.*, *Gut*, 1984, *25*, 513 (increased jejunal motor activity and threshold as well as tolerance to pain); A. Cuschieri *et al.*, *ibid.*, A1140 (relaxant effect on choledochal sphincter).

Proprietary Names and Manufacturers of Ceruletide Diethylamine
Ceosunin *(Jpn)*; Takus *(Farmitalia, Ger.; Farmitalia Carlo Erba, Switz.)*.

7942-n

Coccidioidin

CAS — 12622-73-0.

Coccidioidin (*U.S.P.*) is a sterile solution containing the antigens obtained from the byproducts of mycelial growth or from the spherules of the fungus *Coccidioides immitis*; it contains a suitable antimicrobial agent. It should be stored at 2° to 8° and any dilutions should be used within 24 hours. The expiration date is not later than 3 years (mycelial product) or 18 months (spherule-derived product) after release from manufacturer's cold storage.

Coccidioidin is used as an aid to the diagnosis of coccidioidomycosis. The usual dose is 0.1 mL of a 1 in 100 dilution by intradermal (intracutaneous) injection.

Comments regarding skin testing for the detection of prior infection by *Coccidioides immitis*. Coccidioidin, prepared from mycelial culture filtrates, is commonly used in a dilution of 1 in 100 and provides good diagnostic accuracy. A dilution of 1 in 10 often cross-reacts with histoplasmin and can result in false-positive results in areas where histoplasmosis is endemic; even a 1 in 100 dilution may produce a false-positive result in persons with active histoplasmosis. A product (spherulin) prepared from the soluble fraction released by the spherules of *C. immitis* is also used, and this detects exposure to *C. immitis* in 35% more patients than does the mycelial product.— A. R. Ahmed and D. A. Blose, *Archs Derm.*, 1983, *119*, 934.

Proprietary Preparations

Coccidioidin may be available on a named-patient basis from *Cutter, USA*.

Proprietary Names and Manufacturers
Spherulin (*Berkeley, USA*).

2125-x

Congo Red

CI Direct Red 28; Colour Index No. 22120; Rubrum Congoensis. Disodium 3,3′-[biphenyl-4,4′-diylbis(azo)]-bis[4-aminonaphthalene-1-sulphonate].
$C_{32}H_{22}N_6Na_2O_6S_2$=696.7.

CAS — 573-58-0.

Pharmacopoeias. In *Hung.*, *Nord.*, and *Span.* Also in*B.P.C. 1973.*

A reddish-brown powder. **Soluble** in water. Solutions are **sterilised** by autoclaving or by filtration.

NOTE. The grade of congo red that is usually supplied as a microscopical stain is unsuitable for injection.

Congo red is used as a stain in the diagnosis of amyloid disease; deposits in tissue samples can be detected by congo red causing them to fluoresce under polarised light. Congo red was formerly given intravenously when the rate of removal from plasma was used in the diagnosis of amyloidosis. Injection was however not without danger especially from undissolved dye.

12666-t

2,4-Dinitrochlorobenzene

DNCB. 1-Chloro-2,4-dinitrobenzene.
$C_6H_3ClN_2O_4$=202.6.

CAS — 97-00-7.

Adverse Effects
Skin contact with 2,4-dinitrochlorobenzene usually produces hypersensitivity.

Not only was 2,4-dinitrochlorobenzene a potent sensitiser but it had been shown to cross-react with chloramphenicol.— R. J. Pye and J. L. Burton (letter), *Br. med. J.*, 1976, *2*, 1130.

2,4-Dinitrochlorobenzene had been shown to be mutagenic *in vitro*. It was best avoided in benign dermatoses.— R. Happle, *Archs Derm.*, 1985, *121*, 330.

Uses and Administration
2,4-Dinitrochlorobenzene is a potent sensitiser and the modification or absence of a hypersensitivity response to the application of 2,4-dinitrochlorobenzene has been used diagnostically in certain diseases. It has also been used as an immunostimulant in leprosy and some forms of cancer and was tried in the treatment of alopecia and warts.

A study and discussions of the sensitising action of 2,4-dinitrochlorobenzene.— M. M. Carr *et al.*, *Br. J. Derm.*, 1984, *110*, 637; A. R. Ahmed and D. A. Blose, *Archs Derm.*, 1983, *119*, 934. See also L. Millikan, *J. Am. Acad. Derm.*, 1982, *7*, 91A.

Some improvement has been reported in alopecia areata following the application of 2,4-dinitrochlorobenzene (R. Happle and K. Echternacht, *Lancet*, 1977, *2*, 1002) although patients may become tolerant to its sensitising effect (L.A. Daman and E.W. Rosenberg, *Lancet*, 1977, *2*, 1087). Experience in treating extensive alopecia has not been good (A.P. Warin, *Lancet*,, 1979, *1*, 927). There have been suggestions that warts might respond to 2,4-dinitrochlorobenzene (M. Goihman-Yahr *et al.*, *Lancet*, 1978, *1*, 447). However, in commenting on a report of its mutagenicity Happle (*Archs Derm.*, 1985, *121*, 330) considered that 2,4-dinitrochlorobenzene should not be used for benign dermatoses.

12714-e

Etiocholanolone

3α-Hydroxy-5β-androstan-17-one.
$C_{19}H_{30}O_2$=290.4.

CAS — 53-42-9.

Etiocholanolone is one of the 17-ketosteroids produced by the metabolism of steroid hormones and excreted in the urine. The rise in the number of blood granulocytes which follows an intramuscular injection of etiocholanolone has been used to assess bone-marrow granulocyte reserves.

Proprietary Names and Manufacturers
Etiolone *(Vister, Ital.)*.

2129-n

Fluorescein *(USAN).*

3′,6′-Dihydroxyspiro[isobenzofuran-1(3*H*),9′[9*H*]-xanthen]-3-one.
$C_{20}H_{12}O_5$=332.3.

CAS — 2321-07-5.

Pharmacopoeias. In *U.S.*

An odourless yellowish-red to red powder. Practically **insoluble** in water; soluble in dilute alkali hydroxides. **Store** in airtight containers.

1956-v

Fluorescein Dilaurate

$C_{44}H_{56}O_7$=696.9.

2130-k

Fluorescein Sodium *(BAN, USAN).*

CI Acid Yellow 73; Colour Index No. 45350; D & C Yellow No. 8; Fluoresc. Sod.; Fluorescein Natrium; Fluoresceinum Natricum; Obiturin; Resorcinolphthalein Sodium; Sodium Fluorescein; Soluble Fluorescein; Uranin. Disodium fluorescein.
$C_{20}H_{10}Na_2O_5$=376.3.

CAS — 518-47-8.

Pharmacopoeias. In *Aust.*, *Br.*, *Braz.*, *Chin.*, *Egypt.*, *Ind.*, *Int.*, *It.*, *Jpn*, *Jug.*, *Nord.*, *Swiss*, and *U.S.*

An orange-red, odourless, almost tasteless, hygroscopic powder. The *B.P.* **solubilities** are 1 in 1.5 of water and 1 in 10 of alcohol. The *B.P.* and *U.S.P.* injections have a pH of 8.0 to 9.8 and the *B.P.* specifies **sterilisation** by autoclaving. *B.P.* eye-drops have a pH of 7.0 to 9.0. **Store** in airtight containers. Protect from light.

Adverse Effects
The intravenous injection of fluorescein sodium may produce nausea and vomiting. Extravasation is painful. Allergic reactions may consist of urticaria; occasionally the reactions may be severe. There have been reports of cardiac arrests and fatalities. Concern that impurities or a defect in manufacturing processes might be responsible for the serious reactions led to a review of the *B.P.* specification and a reduction in the permitted level of impurities.

The skin and urine may be coloured yellow but this is transient. Patients may also experience an unpleasant taste.

Of 55 reported adverse reactions following the intravenous injection of fluorescein sodium, 37 were of an allergic type and most of these were characterised only by urticaria but 7 were severe and consisted of shock, respiratory obstruction and arrest, and hypotension. Serious non-allergic reactions occurred on 9 occasions and included cardiac arrest, and myocardial infarction. Reports from various institutions performing fluorescein angiography indicated a mean incidence for all types of reactions of 0.6% and for severe reactions 0.4%.— M. R. Stein and C. W. Parker, *Am. J. Ophthal.*, 1971, *72*, 861.

An increase in the total number of reactions to injections of fluorescein sodium prompted an analysis of the batch being used within the hospital. This showed that the batch contained a significant amount of dimethylformamide that might have accounted for the toxicity.— J. S. H. Jacob *et al.*, *Br. J. Ophthal.*, 1982, *66*, 567 (The *B.P.* introduced in the 1983 Addendum limits for dimethylformamide, resorcinol, and related substances).

Acute pancreatitis associated in one patient with an intravenous injection of fluorescein sodium.— L. H. Morgan and J. M. Martin, *Br. med. J.*, 1983, *287*, 1596.

Two patients with sickle cell disease experienced severe pain after fluorescein angiography.— R. Acheson and G. Serjeant (letter), *Lancet*, 1985, *1*, 1222.

Uses and Administration
A 1% or 2% solution of fluorescein sodium is applied to the eye as a diagnostic agent for detecting corneal lesions and foreign bodies. Special care should be taken to avoid microbial contamination. It is used as an aid to the fitting of hard contact lenses when it may be applied as eye-drops or as sterile papers impregnated with fluorescein; these papers are also used for diagnostic purposes. Fluorescein sodium may be given by rapid intravenous injection usually as a 10% to 25% solution in a dose of 500 mg for the

examination of the ophthalmic vasculature; the oral route has been tried for this purpose.
Other uses include the differentiation of healthy from diseased or damaged tissue.
Fluorescein dilaurate is given by mouth in a dose of 348.5 mg (0.5 mmol) to assess exocrine pancreatic function. The test relies on pancreatic enzymes hydrolysing the ester so that the amount of fluorescein excreted in the urine can be taken as a measure of pancreatic activity. A control dose of 188.14 mg (0.5 mmol) of fluorescein sodium forms part of the test.

Fluorescein mixed with sclerosant improves the accuracy of endoscopic injection of oesophageal varices.— K. R. Hine *et al.*, *Lancet*, 1984, *2*, 322.

In a series of 38 patients fluorescein sodium 1.25 g by mouth with single-frame photography was satisfactory for detecting cystoid macular oedema after cataract surgery. It was suggested that this technique was an adequate alternative to intravenous fluorescein angiography.— M. J. Noble *et al.*, *Br. J. Ophthal.*, 1984, *68*, 221.

DIABETIC RETINOPATHY. The retinal vessels were markedly impervious to fluorescein in the blood. In patients with diabetic retinopathy the blood-retinal barrier was reduced permitting escape of fluorescein into the vitreous. The presence of fluorescein, measured by fluorophotometry, in the vitreous of diabetic patients without apparent retinal involvement was an early sign of retinal degeneration.— J. Cunha-Vaz *et al.*, *Br. J. Ophthal.*, 1975, *59*, 649.

Fluorescein leakage could detect diabetic retinopathy before the development of microaneurysms. Angiofluorography should be carried out annually after the onset of diabetes by injecting 10 mL of fluorescein sodium 10% intravenously and taking photographs every second for 10 seconds with a further 2 photographs 15 and 30 minutes after the fluorescein injection.— H. Dorchy and D. Toussaint (letter), *Lancet*, 1978, *1*, 1200.

PANCREATIC FUNCTION TEST. Fluorescein dilaurate was reported by Barry *et al.* (*Lancet*, 1982, *2*, 742) to be a useful screening agent for the exclusion of pancreatic exocrine failure in outpatients. Cumming *et al.* (*Archs Dis. Childh.*, 1986, *61*, 573) found that results from the test correlated well with those from the faecal chymotrypsin test in cystic fibrosis. There have, however, been criticisms of the test's low specificity and of patients' difficulties in following the instructions (J.M. Braganza, *Lancet*, 1982, *2*, 927; A.J. MacGilchrist and B.M. Frier, *ibid.*, 1985, *1*, 1337). In response, Barry (*Lancet*, 1985, *2*, 96) reported that his false-positive response rate in over 200 outpatients (supplied with simple written instructions) was 10% and that this 10% consisted almost entirely of patients with hepatobiliary disease.

Preparations

Fluorescein Eye Drops *(A.P.F.)*. Gutt. Fluoresc. Fluorescein sodium 250 mg, phenylmercuric nitrate 4 mg, Water for Injections to 100 mL. Sterilised by autoclaving. These eye-drops are dispensed in single-dose containers to avoid contamination by cross-infection.

Fluorescein Eye Drops *(B.P.)*. Fluorescein Sodium Eye Drops. Contain fluorescein sodium.

Fluorescein Sodium Ophthalmic Strips *(U.S.P.)*

Fluorescein Injection *(B.P.)*. Fluorescein Sodium Injection. Contains fluorescein sodium.

Fluorescein Injection *(U.S.P.)*

Proprietary Preparations

Alcon Opulets Fluorescein Sodium 1% *(Alcon, UK)*. *Eye-drops*, fluorescein sodium 1%, in single-use disposable applicators.

Fluor-Amps *(Sas, UK)*. *Injection*, fluorescein sodium 5, 10, 15, 20, and 25%, in ampoules of 5 mL.

Fluorets *(Smith & Nephew Pharmaceuticals, UK)*. *Ophthalmic strips*, fluorescein sodium 1 mg.

Minims Fluorescein Sodium *(Smith & Nephew Pharmaceuticals, UK)*. *Eye-drops* fluorescein sodium 1 and 2%, in single-use disposable applicators.

Pancreolauryl Test *(International Laboratories, UK)*. *Capsules*, blue, fluorescein dilaurate 174.25 mg, and red, fluorescein sodium 188.14 mg.

Proprietary Names and Manufacturers of Fluorescein Compounds

Ak-Fluor *(Akorn, USA)*; Alcon Opulets Fluorescein Sodium *(Alcon, UK)*; Disclo-Plaque *(Orapharm, Austral.)*; Fluoflex *(Gelflex, Austral.)*; Fluor-Amps *(Sas, UK)*; Fluores IV *(Covan, S.Afr.)*; Fluoresceinnatrium Minims *(Smith & Nephew, Norw.; Smith & Nephew, Swed.)*; Fluorescite *(Arg.; Alcon, Austral.; Alcon, Canad.; Alcon, S.Afr.; Alcon Laboratories, USA)*; Fluorets *(Smith & Nephew, Denm.; Smith & Nephew, S.Afr.; Smith & Nephew Pharmaceuticals, UK)*; Fluor-I-Strip *(Ayerst, Austral.; Ayerst, Canad.; Ayerst, UK; Ayerst, USA)*; Ful-Glo *(Barnes-Hind, Austral.; Canad.; Barnes-Hind, USA)*; Funduscein *(Coopervision, Canad.; Coopervision, USA)*; Minims Fluorescein Sodium *(Smith & Nephew, Austral.; Smith & Nephew, Denm.; Smith & Nephew Pharmaceuticals, UK)*; Pancreolauryl Test *(Temmler, Ger.; Temmler, Switz.; International Laboratories, UK)*; Uranina *(Ferrer, Spain)*.

The following names have been used for multi-ingredient preparations containing fluorescein compounds— Fluorocaine *(Akorn, USA)*; Fluress *(Barnes-Hind, Austral.; Barnes-Hind, Canad.; Barnes-Hind, USA)*; Minims Fluorescein Sodium and Lignocaine *(Smith & Nephew, Austral.)*; Minims Lignocaine and Fluorescein *(Smith & Nephew Pharmaceuticals, UK)*.

12773-f

FST-Sawada Antigen

FST-Sawada antigen has been used in a skin test for filariasis where blood tests cannot be carried out.

FST-Sawada antigen is obtainable from Division of Malaria and Other Parasitic Diseases, World Health Organization, Geneva.— *Br. med. J.*, 1977, *2*, 170.

12778-b

Galactose

D-Galactose.

$C_6H_{12}O_6$=180.2.

CAS — 59-23-4.

Pharmacopoeias. In *Neth.* and *Swiss.*

Galactose has been used in liver-function tests.

1958-q

Glucose Tests

Several tests are available so that patients with diabetes mellitus can monitor their disease. Tests can be employed to detect the presence of glucose in the urine and some of the preparations are used to detect several substances in the urine. These tests are easy to carry out but are not considered reliable enough for insulin-dependent patients who should ideally check their blood-glucose concentrations using one of the blood tests now available. Newer methods of monitoring involve checking blood glycosylated haemoglobin values.
Urine tests generally employ either the copper-reduction method or the glucose-oxidase method and both methods produce a colour change in the presence of glucose. Blood tests generally employ the glucose-oxidase method and may require a reflectance meter to measure the reaction.
Patients should be aware that concomitant drug therapy might affect the result.

Preparations

Glucose Enzymatic Test Strip *(U.S.P.)*. Consists of glucose oxidase, horseradish peroxidase, a suitable substrate for the reaction of hydrogen peroxide catalysed by peroxidase, and other inactive ingredients impregnated and dried on filter paper. When tested in human urine containing known glucose concentrations it reacts in the specified times to produce colours corresponding to the colour chart provided. Store at 15° to 30°.

Proprietary Preparations

Bili-Labstix *(Ames, UK)*. *Reagent strips*, urine test for glucose and other substances.

BM-Test-BG *(Boehringer Corp., UK)*. *Reagent strips*, blood test for glucose. Use with a reflectance meter.

BM-Test-Glycemie 1-44 *(Boehringer Corp., UK)*. *Reagent strips*, blood test for glucose.

BM-Tests *(Boehringer Corp., UK)*. *Reagent strips*, urine tests for glucose and other substances.

Clinistix *(Ames, UK)*. *Reagent strips*, urine test for glucose.

Clinitest *(Ames, UK)*. *Reagent tablets*, urine test for glucose.
In the *UK* these are descibed in the Drug Tariff as Copper Solution Reagent Tablets.

Dextrostix *(Ames, UK)*. *Reagent strips*, blood test for glucose.

Diabur-Test 5000 *(Boehringer Corp., UK)*. *Reagent strips*, urine test for glucose.

Diastix *(Ames, UK)*. *Reagent strips*, urine test for glucose.

Fructosamine Test *(Roche, UK)*. *Reagent solution*, nitroblue tetazolium, supplied with a test kit. Laboratory test for the determination of blood glucose.

GA Blood Glucose *(Hypoguard, UK)*. *Reagent strips*, blood test for glucose.

Glucostix *(Ames, UK)*. *Reagent strips*, blood test for glucose.

Hema-Combistix *(Ames, UK)*. *Reagent strips*, urine test for glucose and other substances.

Keto-Diabur-Test 5000 *(Boehringer Corp., UK)*. *Reagent strips*, urine test for glucose and ketones.

Keto-Diastix *(Ames, UK)*. *Reagent strips*, urine test for glucose and ketones.

Labstix *(Ames, UK)*. *Reagent strips*, urine test for glucose and other substances.

Multistix *(Ames, UK)*. *Reagent strips*, urine test for glucose and other substances.

Nephur-Test + Leucocytes *(Boehringer Corp., UK)*. *Reagent strips*, urine test for glucose and other substances.

N-Labstix *(Ames, UK)*. *Reagent strips*, urine test for glucose and other substances.

N-Multistix *(Ames, UK)*. *Reagent strips*, urine test for glucose and other substances.

Reflotest *(Boehringer Corp., UK)*. *Reagent strips* (Reflotest-Glucose), blood test for glucose.
Reagent strips (Reflotest-Hypoglycemie), blood test for glucose.
Use with a reflectance meter.

Tes-Tape *(Lilly, UK)*. *Reagent tape*, urine test for glucose.

Uristix *(Ames, UK)*. *Reagent strips*, urine test for glucose and protein.

Visidex II *(Ames, UK)*. *Reagent strips*, blood test for glucose.

Proprietary Names and Manufacturers

Ames-BG *(Miles, Austral.)*; Autoclix *(Boehringer Mannheim, S.Afr.)*; Bili-Combur-6 *(Boehringer Mannheim, Austral.)*; Bili-Labstix *(Miles, Austral.; Ames, Canad.; Ames, S.Afr.; Ames, UK)*; BM-Test Glucose *(Boehringer Mannheim, S.Afr.)*; BM-Test-3 *(Boehringer Mannheim, S.Afr.)*; BM-Test-BG *(Boehringer Mannheim, Austral.; Boehringer Corp., UK)*; BM-Test-Glycemie 1-44 *(Boehringer Corp., UK)*; BM-Test-Glycemie 20-800 *(Boehringer Mannheim, Austral.)*; BM-Test-GP *(Boehringer Mannheim, S.Afr.)*; BM-Tests *(Boehringer Corp., UK)*; Chemstrip *(Boehringer Mannheim Diagnostics, USA)*; Chemstrip bG *(Boehringer Mannheim, Canad.; Boehringer Mannheim Diagnostics, USA)*; Chemstrip uG 5000 *(Boehringer Mannheim, Canad.)*; Clinistix *(Miles, Austral.; Ames, Canad.; Ames, S.Afr.; Ames, UK)*; Clinitest *(Miles, Austral.; Ames, S.Afr.; Ames, UK)*; Combistix *(Miles, Austral.; Ames, Canad.)*; Combur *(Boehringer Mannheim, Austral.; Boehringer Mannheim, S.Afr.)*; Dextrostix *(Ames, Canad.; Ames, S.Afr.; Ames, UK)*; Diabur-Test 5000 *(Boehringer Mannheim, Austral.; Boehringer Mannheim, S.Afr.; Boehringer Corp., UK)*; Diastix *(Miles, Austral.; Ames, Canad.; Ames, UK)*; Ecur 4-Test *(Boehringer Mannheim, S.Afr.)*; Ecur-Test *(Boehringer Mannheim, Austral.)*; Fructosamine Test *(Roche, UK)*; GA Blood Glucose *(Hypoguard, UK)*; Glucostix *(Ames, Canad.; Ames, S.Afr.; Ames, UK)*; Gluketur *(Boehringer Mannheim, Austral.)*; Haemo-Glukotest 20-800R *(Boehringer Mannheim, S.Afr.)*; Hema-Combistix *(Miles, Austral.; Ames, UK)*; Keto-Diabur-Test 5000 *(Boehringer Mannheim, Austral.; Boehringer Mannheim, S.Afr.; Boehringer Corp., UK)*; Keto-Diastix *(Miles, Austral.; Ames, Canad.; Ames, S.Afr.; Ames, UK)*; Labstix *(Miles, Austral.; Ames, Canad.; Ames, S.Afr.; Ames, UK)*; L-Combur-5-Test *(Boehringer Mannheim, Austral.; Boehringer Mannheim, S.Afr.)*; Medi-Test Combi *(Ascot, Austral.)*; Medi-Test Glucose *(Ascot, Austral.)*; Multistix *(Miles, Austral.; Ames, Canad.; Ames, UK)*; Multistix SG *(Miles, Austral.; Ames, S.Afr.)*; N-Combur Test *(Boehringer Mannheim, Austral.; Boehringer Mannheim, S.Afr.)*; Neostix-3 *(Miles, Austral.)*; Neostix-N *(Miles, Austral.)*; Nephur 7 Test *(Boehringer Mannheim, S.Afr.)*; Nephur-Test + Leucocytes *(Boehringer Mannheim, Austral.; Boehringer Corp., UK)*; N-Labstix *(Ames, Canad.; Ames, UK)*; N-Multistix *(Miles, Austral.; Ames, Canad.; Ames, UK)*; N-Multistix SG *(Miles, Austral.; Ames, Canad.; Ames, S.Afr.)*; N-Multistix-C *(Miles, Austral.)*; N-Uristix *(Ames, Canad.)*; Reflocheck *(Boehringer Mannheim, Canad.)*; Reflotest *(Boehringer*

Corp., UK); Reflotest-Glucose *(Boehringer Mannheim, S.Afr.)*; Reflotest-Hypoglycaemie *(Boehringer Mannheim, S.Afr.)*; Reflotest-Urea *(Boehringer Mannheim, S.Afr.)*; Tes-Tape *(Lilly, Austral.; Lilly, Canad.; Lilly, S.Afr.; Lilly, UK; Lilly, USA)*; Uristix *(Miles, Austral.; Ames, Canad.; Ames, S.Afr.; Ames, UK)*; Visidex II *(Miles, Austral.; Ames, Canad.; Ames, S.Afr.; Ames, UK)*.

278-r

Guaiacum Resin

Guaiac; Guaiacum; Guajakharz.

CAS — 9000-29-7.

The resin of guaiacum wood (lignum vitae; *Guaiacum officinale* or *G. sanctum*).

Guaiacum resin was formerly used in the treatment of rheumatism. It is now used in the detection of occult blood in the faeces. The accuracy of the guaicum test has been questioned and some drugs may interfere with the result.

Proprietary Preparations

Haemoccult *(Norwich-Eaton, UK). Test kit*, slides impregnated with guaiacum resin with a hydrogen peroxide reagent.

Okokit II *(Hughes & Hughes, UK). Test kit*, test-pads impregnated with guaiacum resin with reagents.

Proprietary Names and Manufacturers

Early Detector *(Warner-Lambert, USA)*; Fleet Detecatest *(Fleet, USA)*; Haemoccult *(Norwich-Eaton, UK)*; Hemoccult *(Menley & James, USA; SmithKline Diagnostics, USA)*; Okokit II *(Hughes & Hughes, UK)*.

2134-r

Histamine Acid Phosphate

Histam. Acid Phos.; Histamine Diphosphate; Histamine Phosphate *(USAN)*; Histamini Phosphas. 2-(Imidazol-4-yl)ethylamine diphosphate.

$C_5H_9N_3,2H_3PO_4$=307.1.

CAS — 51-74-1.

Pharmacopoeias. In *Arg., Aust., Br., Braz., Egypt., Eur., Fr., Ind., Int., It., Mex., Neth., Span., Swiss, Turk.*, and *U.S. Br., Eur.*, and *Ind.* specify 1 H_2O.

Colourless odourless crystals; stable in air but affected by light. Histamine acid phosphate (anhydrous) 2.76 mg or histamine acid phosphate monohydrate 2.93 mg is approximately equivalent to 1 mg of histamine.

Soluble 1 in 4 of water. The *B.P.* specifies that a 5% solution in water has a pH of 3.75 to 3.95; the pH of the *U.S.P.* injection ranges from 3.0 to 6.0. **Store** in airtight containers. Protect from light.

2133-x

Histamine Hydrochloride

Histamine Dihydrochloride; Histamini Dihydrochloridum. 2-(Imidazol-4-yl)ethylamine dihydrochloride.

$C_5H_9N_3,2HCl$=184.1.

CAS — 56-92-8.

Pharmacopoeias. In *Arg., Cz., Eur., Fr., Hung., It., Neth., Nord., Pol., Roum.*, and *Swiss.*

Odourless, hygroscopic, colourless crystals or white crystalline powder. Histamine hydrochloride 1.66 mg is approximately equivalent to 1 mg of histamine. Very **soluble** in water; soluble in alcohol; practically insoluble in chloroform and ether. A 5% solution in water has a pH of 2.85 to 3.60. **Store** in airtight containers. Protect from light.

Adverse Effects and Treatment

Injection of histamine as the acid phosphate or the hydrochloride can produce a range of adverse effects that includes headache, flushing of the skin, general vasodilatation with a fall in blood pressure, tachycardia, bronchial constriction and dyspnoea, visual disturbances, vomiting, diarrhoea, and other gastro-intestinal effects. These reactions may be serious and excessive dosage can produce collapse and shock, and may be fatal. Reactions may occur at the injection site. Some of these effects may be relieved by an antihistamine H_1 antagonist, but adrenaline may be required and should always be available.

Precautions

Histamine acid phosphate should be used with care in patients with asthma or other allergic conditions, in elderly patients, and in patients with cardiovascular disorders.

Absorption and Fate

Histamine acid phosphate is largely inactive when given by mouth. It exerts a rapid, though transient, effect when given by subcutaneous, intramuscular, or intravenous injection. It is metabolised by methylation and oxidation; the metabolites are excreted in the urine.

Uses and Administration

Histamine given parenterally causes stimulation of smooth muscle, especially of the bronchioles, and lowers blood pressure by dilating the arterioles and capillaries. It also stimulates many of the glands of internal secretion, especially the gastric glands.

Histamine has been given usually as the acid phosphate by subcutaneous injection to identify the causes of achlorhydria, but pentagastrin is considered to be safer. Doses equivalent to 10 or 14.5 µg of histamine per kg body-weight were employed.

Histamine has also been tried as a diagnostic test for phaeochromocytoma since it has a stimulant action on chromaffin cells, but this test is not without its dangers and is not considered definitive.

Other uses have included testing for histamine sensitivity.

Preparations

Histamine Phosphate Injection *(U.S.P.)*. A sterile solution of histamine acid phosphate in Water for Injection.

Proprietary Preparations

Akrotherm *(Napp, UK). Ointment*, histamine hydrochloride 0.034%, acetylcholine chloride 0.2%, cholesterol 1%. For chilblains and allied conditions.

Proprietary Names and Manufacturers of Histamine Salts

Alergenol *(Spain)*.

Manufacturers also include—*Bull, Austral.; DAK, Denm.; IBIS, Ital.*

The following names have been used for multi-ingredient preparations containing histamine salts— Akrotherm *(Napp, UK)*; Cremathurm *(Sinclair, UK)*.

NOTE. The names Algipan, Cremalgex, and Cremalgin were formerly used to denote preparations containing, in addition to other ingredients, histamine hydrochloride.

8040-k

Histoplasmin

CAS — 9008-05-3.

Histoplasmin *(U.S.P.)* is a sterile solution containing standardised culture filtrates of the fungus *Histoplasma capsulatum* grown on a synthetic liquid medium; it may contain a suitable antimicrobial agent. It should be stored at 2° to 8°.

Histoplasmin, in an intradermal (intracutaneous) dose of 0.1 mL of a 1 in 100 dilution, may be used as an aid to the diagnosis of histoplasmosis.

The histoplasmin skin test is relatively effective; lack of specificity is due to extensive cross-reactions in individuals sensitised to other fungi.— *FDA Drug Bull.*, 1978, *8*, 15. Further references: A. R. Ahmed and D. A. Blose, *Archs Derm.*, 1983, *119*, 934.

2135-f

Indigo Carmine

Blue X; Ceruleinum; CI Food Blue 1; Colour Index No. 73015; Disodium Indigotin-5,5′-disulphonate; E132; FD & C Blue No. 2; Indicarminum; Indigotindisulfonate Sodium *(USAN)*; Indigotine; Sodium Indigotindisulphonate. Disodium 3,3′-dioxo-2,2′-bi-indolinylidene-5,5′-disulphonate.

$C_{16}H_8N_2Na_2O_8S_2$=466.4.

CAS — 860-22-0.

NOTE. The name Caerulein has been applied to Ceruletide, p.938.

Pharmacopoeias. In *Arg., Belg., Fr., It., Jpn, Roum.*, and *U.S.*

A purplish-blue powder or blue granules with a coppery lustre.

Soluble 1 in 100 of water; slightly soluble in alcohol; practically insoluble in most other organic solvents. The *U.S.P.* injection has a pH of 3.0 to 6.5. **Store** in airtight containers. Protect from light.

Adverse Effects

Indigo carmine may cause nausea, vomiting, hypertension, and bradycardia, and occasionally, allergic reactions such as skin rash, pruritus, and bronchoconstriction.

A report of fatal cardiac arrest in 2 elderly patients following the administration of indigo carmine 80 mg intravenously. Both had a history of asthmatic bronchitis.— A. M. Voiry *et al.*, *Annls méd. Nancy*, 1976, *15*, 413.

Uses and Administration

The appearance of indigo carmine in the urine following injection has been used to test kidney function. It was usually injected intramuscularly or intravenously in a dose of 40 mg. It has also been used as a marker dye to aid urological and other procedures.

It has been used as a blue dye in medicinal preparations but it is relatively unstable. It is used as a food colour.

Estimated acceptable daily intake of indigo carmine: up to 2.5 mg per kg body-weight. Information from further studies was desirable.— Thirteenth Report of FAO/WHO Expert Committee on Food Additives, *Tech. Rep. Ser. Wld Hlth Org. No.* 445, 1971.

Preparations

Indigotindisulfonate Sodium Injection *(U.S.P.)*. A sterile solution of indigo carmine in Water for Injections.

Proprietary Preparations

Indigo Carmine *(Hynson, Westcott & Dunning, USA: Farillon, UK). Injection*, indigo carmine 0.8%, in ampoules of 5 mL.

Proprietary Names and Manufacturers

Bull, Austral.; Hynson, Westcott & Dunning Diagnostics, Canad.; Hynson, Westcott & Dunning, USA : Farillon, UK.

2136-d

Indocyanine Green *(USAN)*.

Sodium 2-{7-[1,1-dimethyl-3-(4-sulphobutyl)benz[*e*]indolin-2-ylidene]hepta-1,3,5-trienyl}-1,1-dimethyl-1*H*-benz[*e*]indolio-3-(butyl-4-sulphonate).

$C_{43}H_{47}N_2NaO_6S_2$=775.0.

CAS — 3599-32-4.

Pharmacopoeias. In *U.S.* which also includes Sterile Indocyanine Green.

An olive-brown, dark green, blue-green, dark blue, or black powder, odourless or with a slight odour. It contains not more than 5% of sodium iodide.

Soluble in water and methyl alcohol; practically insoluble in most other organic solvents. A 0.5% solution in water has a pH of about 6. Aqueous solutions are deep emerald green in colour and are stable for about 8 hours.

Adverse Effects and Precautions

Indocyanine green is reported to be well tolerated. Solutions contain a small amount of sodium iodide and should be used with caution in patients hypersensitive to iodine.

Two patients maintained on haemodialysis experienced headache, diaphoresis, and pruritus when given indocyanine green; a third patient had a severe anaphylactoid reaction.— D. D. Michie *et al.*, *J. Allergy & clin. Immunol.*, 1971, *48*, 235.

A report of allergic-type reactions, one fatal, in 4 patients following the administration of indocyanine green. Two of the patients had no previous history of allergy or asthma.— T. R. Carski *et al.* (letter), *J. Am. med. Ass.*, 1978, *240*, 635.

Absorption and Fate

After intravenous injection indocyanine green is bound to plasma protein. It is rapidly taken up by the liver and is excreted unchanged into the bile.

The mean half-life of indocyanine green, given in doses of 25 mg to 11 patients with normal liver function was 1.3 minutes, compared with 3.9 minutes in 38 patients with liver dysfunction. For 8 patients taking anticonvulsant drugs, 2 on phenylbutazone, 1 on haloperidol, 1 on nitrofurantoin, and 9 addicted to one or more of diamorphine, methadone, morphine, pethidine, or poppy heads the mean half-life was 0.65 minutes. The percentage disappearance-rate per minute from plasma in these 3 groups was 50.6, 24.8, and 115.8 respectively; the highest rates occurred in addicts and were elevated above normal even when liver dysfunction was present.— V. Melikian *et al.*, *Gut*, 1972, *13*, 755.

Uses and Administration

Indocyanine green is an indicator dye used for assessing cardiac output and liver function.

The usual dose for cardiac assessment is 5 mg injected via a cardiac catheter. A suggested dose for children is one-half, and for infants one-quarter, of the adult dose. Several doses need to be given to obtain a number of dilution curves. However, the total dose should not exceed 2 mg per kg body-weight.

The usual dose of indocyanine green for testing liver function is 500 µg per kg body-weight intravenously.

Preparations

Sterile Indocyanine Green *(U.S.P.)*

Proprietary Preparations

Cardio-green *(Hynson, Westcott & Dunning, USA: Farillon, UK)*. *Injection*, powder for reconstitution, indocyanine green 25 and 50 mg.

2137-n

Inulin *(BAN, USAN).*

Alant Starch.

CAS — 9005-80-5.

Pharmacopoeias. In *Br., Cz.,* and *U.S.*

The *B.P.* describes inulin as a polysaccharide obtained from the tubers of *Dahlia variabilis, Helianthus tuberosus,* and other genera of the family Compositae. It is a white, odourless or almost odourless, hygroscopic, amorphous, granular powder. Slightly **soluble** in cold water, but freely soluble in hot water; it is slightly soluble in organic solvents. A 10% solution has a pH of 4.5 to 7.0. The *B.P.* and the *U.S.P.* injections have a pH of 5.0 to 7.0 Inulin is hydrolysed to fructose. The *B.P.* injection is **sterilised** by filtration. **Store** in airtight containers.

Absorption and Fate

Inulin is rapidly removed from the circulation following intravenous administration. A trace may be found in the bile and may cross the placenta, but it is predominantly eliminated in the urine by glomerular filtration. It is not metabolised.

Uses and Administration

Inulin is used as a diagnostic agent to measure the glomerular filtration-rate. An initial dose of 50 mg per kg body-weight is given by slow intravenous injection and is followed by the intravenous infusion of a dose that has varied from about 1.6 to 7.0 g. The glomerular filtration-rate is calculated from the amount of inulin excreted in the urine and the concentration in the plasma.

Preparations

Inulin and Sodium Chloride Injection *(U.S.P.)*. Solid matter should be completely redissolved by heating.

Inulin Injection *(B.P.)*. A sterile solution containing inulin 10% and sodium chloride 0.8% in Water for Injections. Inulin Injection deposits on storage. Solid matter should be completely redissolved by heating for not more than 15 minutes and cooling before use. The solution should not be reheated.

12885-q

Kveim Antigen

A fine suspension in physiological saline of material from granulomatous lymph nodes taken from patients with active sarcoidosis.

Kveim antigen is used as an intradermal injection in the Kveim test for the diagnosis of sarcoidosis.

Kveim tests were carried out with 3 batches of material in 81 patients with various diseases and positive results were obtained in tuberculosis, lymphomas, inflammatory bowel diseases, and rheumatoid arthritis as well as sarcoidosis.— T. H. Hurley *et al.*, *Lancet*, 1975, *1*, 494.

12892-g

Lepromin

A suspension of killed *Mycobacterium leprae* prepared from the skin of heavily infected patients suffering from lepromatous leprosy (lepromin H) or from armadillo tissue infected with *M. leprae* (lepromin A).

CAS — 63163-81-5.

Lepromin is used in an intradermal skin test for the classification of leprosy and the assessment of immune responsiveness to *M. leprae*. The test is not diagnostic for leprosy.

Supplies of lepromin are available in Great Britain from Laboratories for Leprosy and Mycobacterial Research, National Institute for Medical Research, Mill Hill, London, NW7 1AA.

An account of the lepromin reaction. The original lepromin (of Mitsuda and Hayashi), a suspension of the whole autoclaved homogenised leproma including some tissue elements, was sometimes called integral lepromin, whereas purified bacillary suspensions were sometimes called bacillary lepromins. Leprolins were the soluble proteins of the bacilli with or without proteins of the lepra, not coagulated by heating, and did not elicit the early reaction. The Dharmendra antigen was neither a lepromin nor a leprolin and was used especially for testing the early reactions; it gave only a weak late reaction.— M. Abe *et al.*, *Lepr. Rev.*, 1974, *45*, 244.

A WHO memorandum on recommendations for the preparation of standard integral (Mitsuda-type) lepromin and its testing. The source material should be *M. leprae* from biopsy specimens of skin obtained from heavily infected patients suffering from lepromatous leprosy or from armadillo tissues infected with *M. leprae*.— *Bull. Wld Hlth Org.*, 1979, *57*, 921.

Some further references: S. G. Browne, *Lepr. Rev.*, 1983, *54*, 353; J. L. Stanford, *Tubercle*, 1984, *65*, 63; L. J. Reitan *et al.*, *Lepr. Rev.*, 1984, *55*, 33; E. González-Abreu *et al.*, *ibid.*, 337; K. Jesudasan *et al.*, *ibid.*, 1985, *56*, 303.

2138-h

Limulus Test

LAL Test; Limulus Amebocyte Lysate Test; Limulus Amoebocyte Lysate Test.

The limulus test is a test for the presence of bacterial endotoxins and is based on their ability to exhibit a protein coagulation reaction with limulus amoebocyte lysate prepared from the circulating blood cells of the horseshoe crab, *Limulus polyphemus*.

7970-v

Lymphogranuloma Venereum Antigen

Frei Antigen.

Lymphogranuloma Venereum Antigen *(U.S.P.)* is a sterile suspension of the inactivated agent of *Miyagawanella lymphogranulomatis*, prepared by growing the organism in the yolk-sac of embryonated chicken eggs. It contains an antimicrobial agent. It should be stored at 2° to 8°.

Lymphogranuloma venereum antigen was formerly used in the diagnosis of lymphogranuloma venereum.

Lymphogranuloma venereum antigen was not reactive in many patients with previous *Chlamydia trachomatis* infection and the test might be negative in confirmed cases of the disease. Removal from the market was recommended; it was so removed.— *FDA Drug Bull.*, 1978, *8*, 15.

2139-m

Metyrapone *(BAN, USAN, rINN).*

SU-4885. 2-Methyl-1,2-di(3-pyridyl)propan-1-one.

$C_{14}H_{14}N_2O = 226.3$.

CAS — 54-36-4.

Pharmacopoeias. In *Br., Jpn,* and *U.S.*

A white to light amber, fine, crystalline powder with a characteristic odour. M.p. 50° to 53°. It darkens on exposure to light.

Soluble 1 in 100 of water, 1 in 3 of alcohol and chloroform; soluble in methyl alcohol; soluble in dilute mineral acids forming water-soluble salts. **Store** in a cool place in airtight containers. Protect from light.

Adverse Effects

Metyrapone may give rise to nausea and vomiting, epigastric pain, headache, sedation, giddiness, and allergic rash.

Alopecia associated in one patient with metyrapone given for Cushing's syndrome.— P. L. Harris, *Clin. Pharm.*, 1986, *5*, 66.

Precautions

Metyrapone should be used with extreme caution, if at all, in patients with gross hypopituitarism or with reduced adrenal secretary activity because of the risk of precipitating acute adrenal failure.

Phenytoin is reported to increase the metabolism of metyrapone; doubling the dose of metyrapone may counteract the interaction. However, as many other drugs may interfere with the steroid assessment, medication is best avoided where possible during the metyrapone test.

PORPHYRIA. Metyrapone was considered to be unsafe in patients with acute porphyria because it has been shown to be porphyrinogenic in *animals* or *in vitro* systems.— M.R. Moore and K.E.L. McColl, *Porphyrias, Drug Lists*, Glasgow, Porphyria Research Unit, University of Glasgow, 1987.

Uses and Administration

Metyrapone inhibits the enzyme 11β-hydroxylase responsible for the synthesis of the glucocorticoids cortisone and hydrocortisone (cortisol) as well as aldosterone from their precursors. The consequent fall in the plasma concentrations of circulating glucocorticoids stimulates the anterior pituitary gland to produce more corticotrophin. This, in turn, stimulates the production of more 11-deoxycortisol and other precursors which are excreted in the urine where they can be measured. Metyrapone is therefore used as a test of the feedback hypothalamo-pituitary mechanism.

A prior test is performed, using 50 units of corticotrophin by infusion over 8 hours, to demonstrate the responsiveness of the adrenal cortex. If there is an adequate response, metyrapone is given after an interval of 2 days, usually in a dose of 750 mg by mouth every 4 hours for 6 doses. A suggested dose by mouth for children is 15 mg per kg body-weight, with a minimum dose of 250 mg every 4 hours for 6 doses. In patients with a normally functioning pituitary gland excretion of 17-hydroxycorticosteroids is increased 2- to 4-fold and that of 17-ketosteroids about 2-fold.

Since metyrapone inhibits the synthesis of aldosterone it has been used to treat some cases of resistant oedema in conjunction with a glucocorticoid to suppress the normal corticotrophin response to low plasma concentrations of glucocorticoids. The suggested dosage of metyrapone in resistant oedema is 2.5 to 4.5 g daily in divided doses.

Metyrapone is also used in the management of Cushing's syndrome when doses may range from 250 mg to 6 g daily.

Metyrapone tartrate has been given by injection.

CUSHING'S SYNDROME. Thirteen patients with Cushing's disease were treated for 2 to 66 months with metyrapone 0.25 g twice daily to 1 g four times daily ; 9 received pituitary irradiation. Clinical features improved rapidly, allowing time for pituitary irradiation to be effective, without worsening in oedema or hypertension or gastro-intestinal symptoms. Lightheadedness occurred in 4 patients for about 20 minutes after each dose; hirsutism was troublesome in some patients.— W. J. Jeffcoate *et al., Br. med. J.*, 1977, *2*, 215. Comment.— D. N. Orth, *Ann. intern. Med.*, 1978, *89*, 128. There have been several other reports on the use of metyrapone in Cushing's syndrome either with pituitary irradiation (S.R. Ahmed *et al., Br. med. J.*, 1984, *289*, 643) or, in one patient, as the primary treatment (G. Dickstein *et al., J. Am. med. Ass.*, 1986, *255*, 1167). It has been used sucessfully in the management of a pregnant patient (M.J.J. Gormley *et al., Clin. Endocrin.*, 1982, *16*, 283) and has been used in conjunction with sodium valproate (B. Glaser *et al., Lancet*, 1984, *2*, 640).

Preparations

Metyrapone Capsules *(B.P.)*
Metyrapone Tablets *(U.S.P.)*

Proprietary Preparations

Metopirone *(Ciba, UK). Capsules*, metyrapone 250 mg.

Proprietary Names and Manufacturers

Metopiron *(Ciba, Denm.; Ciba, Ger.; Ital.; Neth.; Ciba, Norw.; Ciba, Swed.)*; Metopirone *(Ciba, Austral.; Ciba, Canad.; Ciba, Switz.; Ciba, UK; Ciba, USA)*.

7980-q

Mumps Skin Test Antigen

Mumps Skin Test Antigen (*U.S.P.*) is a sterile aqueous suspension of formaldehyde-inactivated mumps virus prepared from the extra-embryonic fluid of virus-infected chick embryos, concentrated and purified by differential centrifugation, and diluted with isotonic sodium chloride solution. It contains a preservative and glycine as a stabilising agent. Each mL contains not less than 20 complement-fixing units. It should be stored at 2° to 8°.

Recovery from mumps produces skin hypersensitivity to mumps virus. A positive reaction to mumps skin test antigen, 0.1 mL intradermally (intracutaneously), may indicate previous infection with mumps virus but it is not considered to be very reliable. It should not be given to patients hypersensitive to egg protein.

Mumps skin test antigen is unreliable for identifying susceptible persons because of poor sensitivity and specificity and variable potency. It is now used as one of a number of tests to evaluate immunological (T-cell) competence.— *FDA Drug Bull.*, 1978, *8*, 15.

Preparations

A mumps skin test antigen is available on a named-patient basis from *Connaught, Canad.*

Proprietary Names and Manufacturers
MSTA *(Connaught, USA)*

2141-x

Pancreozymin *(BAN)*.

CCK; CCK-PZ. A hormone prepared from the duodenal mucosa of pigs. The endogenous hormone is known as cholecystokinin.

Store between 2° to 8°.

Units

The potency of pancreozymin may be expressed as Crick-Harper-Raper units based on the pancreatic secretion in *cats* or as Ivy *dog* units based on the increase in gall-bladder pressure. One Ivy dog unit is considered to be approximately equivalent to 1 Crick-Harper-Raper unit.

An *in vitro* bioassay of pancreozymin.— E. L. Giannoulis and R. E. Barry, *Gut*, 1982, *23*, 146 and 552.

Adverse Effects

Flushing of the skin and other vasomotor effects may occur, particularly after rapid intravenous injection of pancreozymin. Allergic reactions may occasionally occur.

Uses and Administration

Pancreozymin, administered by intravenous injection, causes an increase in the secretion of pancreatic enzymes, and also stimulates gall-bladder contraction.

Pancreozymin is used as a diagnostic agent in conjunction with secretin for testing the functional capacity of the pancreas and for testing gall-bladder function or bile-duct patency. It may also be used as an adjunct to cholecystography.

A procedure frequently used is to give secretin, 1 to 2 Crick-Harper-Raper units per kg body-weight, as a freshly prepared solution, by intravenous injection over about 2 minutes, followed by 1 to 2 units per kg of pancreozymin, as a freshly prepared solution, given by intravenous injection over about 5 minutes.

In 44 controls and 74 patients with possible gall-bladder disease, the gall-bladder, opacified with ipodate sodium, was observed following injection of pancreozymin. There was a high incidence of false positives in the control groups; it was concluded that pancreozymin cholecystography was not helpful in the diagnosis and management of patients with possible acalculous gall-bladder disease.— F. H. Dunn *et al., J. Am. med. Ass.*, 1974, *228*, 997. See also *idem*, *229*, 1283.

A 60-minute infusion of pancreozymin was a more efficient stimulus of gall-bladder contraction in 6 healthy subjects than a bolus injection. The contractions were stronger, more consistent, and more prolonged with the infusion. No untoward effects were observed with the infusion, but the bolus injection was associated with flushing, transient abdominal discomfort, cramp, and nausea.— W. P. M. Hopman *et al., Br. med. J.*, 1986, *292*, 375. In over 200 double-blind placebo-controlled infusions of pancreozymin in patients suspected of having acalculous biliary pain, about half the patients developed pain during the infusion. None of the healthy subjects developed pain.— T. W. J. Lennard *et al.* (letter), *ibid.*, 1138. Pain induced by pancreozymin may be colonic in origin and may not indicate gall-bladder dysfunction.— C. D. Johnson (letter), *ibid.*, 1398.

Some references to the pancreozymin-secretin test: J. Braganza *et al., Gut*, 1973, *14*, 383; E. A. Eikman *et al., Ann. intern. Med.*, 1975, *82*, 318; J. M. Braganza and J. J. Rao, *Br. med. J.*, 1978, *2*, 392; L. T. K. Wong *et al., Gut*, 1982, *23*, 744; P. G. Lankisch, *Gut*, 1982, *23*, 777.

Proprietary Names and Manufacturers

Pancreozymin *(Boots, UK)*.

The following names have been used for multi-ingredient preparations containing pancreozymin— Anorex-CCK *(Robertson/Taylor, USA)*.

2142-r

Patent Blue V

Acid Blue 3; CI Food Blue 5; Colour Index No. 42051; E131. Calcium α-(4-diethylaminophenyl)-α-(4-diethyliminiocyclohexa-2,5-dienylidene)-5-hydroxytoluene-2,4-disulphonate.

$(C_{27}H_{31}N_2O_7S_2)_2Ca = 1159.4$.

CAS — 3536-49-0.

NOTE. The name Patent Blue V is also used as a synonym for Sulphan Blue (CI No. 42045)—see p.946.

Pharmacopoeias. In *Fr.*

A dark blue-violet powder. Aqueous solutions are blue in colour.

Adverse Effects

Allergic reactions may occur immediately or after a few minutes; on rare occasions they may be severe and include shock, dyspnoea, laryngeal spasm, and oedema. Nausea, hypotension, and tremor have been reported.

Uses and Administration

Patent blue V is injected subcutaneously to colour the lymph vessels so that they can be injected with a contrast medium. The usual dose of 0.25 mL of the 2.5% solution diluted with an equal volume of sodium chloride injection or 1% lignocaine hydrochloride injection is injected subcutaneously in each interdigital web space. Additional injections may be required when the lower limbs are to be examined. The bluish skin colour which may develop after injection usually disappears after 24 to 48 hours.

Patent blue V is used as a food colour.

The temporary maximum acceptable daily intake (ADI) of patent blue V had been withdrawn in 1974 as the results of required studies had not been submitted. There was still insufficient data to allow for allocation of an ADI. Further studies were in progress.— Twenty-Sixth Report of the Joint FAO/WHO Expert Committee on Food Additives, *Tech. Rep. Ser. Wld Hlth Org. No. 683*, 1982.

Proprietary Preparations

Patent Blue V *(May & Baker, UK). Injection*, patent blue V 2.5%, in ampoules of 2 mL.

Proprietary Names and Manufacturers

May & Baker, Austral.; May & Baker, UK.

2143-f

Penicilloyl-polylysine

PO-PLL; PPL. A polypeptide compound formed by the interaction of a penicillanic acid and polylysine of an average degree of polymerisation of 20 lysine residues per molecule.

CAS — 53608-77-8.

Solutions should be **stored** between 2° and 8°.

Adverse Effects and Precautions

Severe allergic reactions have occasionally been reported following administration of penicilloyl-polylysine; a scratch test is recommended before intradermal administration.

Uses and Administration

Penicilloyl-polylysine is used as a diagnostic agent to detect penicillin hypersensitivity. After a preliminary scratch test it is given by intradermal injection. The development, usually within 15 minutes, of a wheal and of erythema is generally judged a positive reaction. The incidence of allergic reactions is stated to be less than 5% in patients showing a negative reaction. Pencilloyl-polylysine does not detect those liable to suffer late reactions or reactions due to minor antigen determinants; these reactions require other tests.

In an attempt to decrease the frequency of penicillin reactions in a hospital, 2 penicillin antigens, a minor determinant mixture of benzylpenicillin and its derivatives (MDM) and benzylpenicilloyl-polylysine were tested on the skin of each of 218 adults. Fifty of 66 patients with a history of penicillin allergy gave negative results to the tests and 37 of these were subsequently given penicillin without suffering any untoward effects. Ten of 152 patients with no history of penicillin hypersensitivity had positive skin-test reactions and were therefore not given penicillin. The remaining 142 patients had no history of penicillin reactions and a negative result to the skin tests and penicillin was administered without any adverse reactions.— N. F. Adkinson *et al., New Engl. J. Med.*, 1971, *285*, 22.

A survey of 14 000 tests recorded in the literature suggested that the use of penicilloyl-polylysine was safe, more reliable than a history of penicillin allergy, and would reveal sensitivity in patients with no previous history.— W. E. Herrell, *Clin. Med.*, 1972, *79* (Jan.), 12.

Proprietary Names and Manufacturers
Penkit *(Stallergenes, Switz.)*; Pre-Pen *(Kremers-Urban, USA)*.

2144-d

Pentagastrin *(BAN, USAN, rINN)*.

AY-6608; ICI-50123. *tert*-Butyloxycarbonyl-[β-Ala[13]]gastrin-(13-17)-pentapeptide amide.
$C_{37}H_{49}N_7O_9S$=767.9.

CAS — 5534-95-2.

Pharmacopoeias. In *Br.*, *Cz.*, and *Nord.*

A white or almost white odourless powder. Practically **insoluble** in water; slightly soluble in alcohol; soluble in dimethylformamide, and dilute ammonia solution. The *B.P.* injection is sterilised by filtration. **Protect** from light.

Adverse Effects
Pentagastrin may cause a number of gastro-intestinal effects including nausea and abdominal cramps. Cardiovascular effects include flushing of the skin and tachycardia. There may be headache, drowsiness, and dizziness. Allergic reactions are rare.

Some case reports of adverse reactions to pentagastrin: M. Aylward and J. B. Bourke (letter), *Lancet*, 1969, *2*, 267 (gastrointestinal effects and tachycardia); C. Wastell and J. MacNaughton (letter), *Br. med. J.*, 1975, *1*, 334 (rash, pruritus, and peri-orbital oedema); R. F. McCloy and J. H. Baron (letter), *Lancet*, 1977, *1*, 548 (severe bradycardia); D. Drucker (letter), *New Engl. J. Med.*, 1981, *304*, 1427 (atrial fibrillation with pentagastrin and calcium gluconate); M. Goldman, *Br. med. J.*, 1984, *289*, 470 (acute interstitial nephritis); J. Arnved *et al.*, *Lancet*, 1985, *2*, 1068 (thrombocytopenia associated with pentagastrin-induced release of serotonin from platelets).

Precautions
Pentagastrin should not be given to patients who have previously shown sensitivity to the drug. It should not be given to patients with acute peptic ulcer and should be given with care to patients with active pancreatic, hepatic, or biliary-tract disease.

Absorption and Fate
Pentagastrin is not active when given by mouth.

A study in 4 subjects indicated that pentagastrin might be absorbed intact from the gastro-intestinal tract.— M. T. Morrell and W. M. Keynes (letter), *Lancet*, 1975, *2*, 712.

Uses and Administration
Pentagastrin is a synthetic polypeptide which when given parenterally has effects similar to those of natural gastrin. Since it stimulates the secretion of gastric acid, pepsin, and intrinsic factor, it is used as a diagnostic agent to test the secretory action of the stomach. The usual dose is 6 µg per kg body-weight by subcutaneous injection; by intravenous infusion the dose is 0.6 µg per kg per hour, in sodium chloride injection. It has also been given intramuscularly and as a snuff. Because the response to pentagastrin is reduced after vagotomy it has been used as a test of the completeness of vagotomy.
Pentagastrin stimulates the secretion of pancreatic enzymes and thus has been used as a test for pancreatic function. It has also been tried in the diagnosis of medullary carcinoma of the thyroid.

DIAGNOSIS OF NEOPLASMS. Pentagastrin 5 µg per kg body-weight as an intravenous bolus injection was given to 10 brothers and sisters of 2 patients with proved medullary carcinoma of the thyroid. After pentagastrin the serum-calcitonin concentrations were sufficiently elevated in 4 members for diagnoses of thyroid carcinomas to be made; these were subsequently confirmed histologically.— H. Mulder and C. A. P. F. Su, *Dt. med. Wschr.*, 1977, *102*, 479.
A study in 3 patients with medullary thyroid neoplasms and in 36 asymptomatic relatives of these patients showed that pentagastrin 500 ng per kg body-weight given intravenously over 10 to 15 seconds provided more rapid and effective stimulation of immunoreactive calcitonin release into the blood, within 5 minutes, than did the slow infusion of a calcium salt. The release of calcitonin provided a diagnostic test for the presence of medullary thyroid neoplasm and was positive in 11 persons given pentagastrin and in 3 of them by the use of calcium.— M. Verdy *et al.*, *Can. med. Ass. J.*, 1978, *119*, 29.

DIAGNOSIS OF OESOPHAGEAL SPASM. Pentagastrin was given by intravenous infusion to 6 patients with idiopathic diffuse oesophageal spasm in doses of 1 to 10 µg per kg body-weight per hour and the response compared to that from sodium chloride injection. The differences between placebo and pentagastrin were very small and few were significant. It seemed unlikely that pentagastrin would be a useful provocative agent to assist in the diagnosis of diffuse oesophageal spasm.— R. M. Wexler and M. D. Kaye, *Gut*, 1981, *22*, 213.

EFFECTS ON THE GASTRO-INTESTINAL TRACT. Studies in 204 men showed that after an intramuscular injection of pentagastrin 6 µg per kg body-weight the output of gastric acid was similar to that following an injection of ametazole 2 mg per kg subcutaneously, histamine 40 µg per kg subcutaneously or 40 µg per kg per hour intravenously, or pentagastrin 6 µg per kg subcutaneously or 6 µg per kg per hour intravenously. Samples of gastric secretion were aspirated 10, 20, and 30 minutes after the intramuscular injection of pentagastrin. In 26% of the men given pentagastrin intramuscularly, peak acid output occurred 20 to 40 minutes after the injection so that collection up to 30 minutes after the injection underestimated the peak acid output of these men.—Report of a Multicentre Study, *Lancet*, 1969, *1*, 341.
Pentagastrin stimulated the uptake of pertechnetate labelled with technetium-99m by the gastric mucosa and aided the diagnosis of Meckel's diverticulum.— S. Treves *et al.*, *Radiology*, 1978, *128*, 711.

Preparations
Pentagastrin Injection *(B.P.)*. A sterile, isotonic solution of pentagastrin in Water for Injections. pH 7.0 to 8.5. Store at 2 to 8°. It should not be allowed to freeze. Protect from light.
The manufacturer recommends storage below 4°.

Proprietary Preparations
Peptavlon *(ICI Pharmaceuticals, UK)*. *Injection*, pentagastrin 250 µg/mL in ampoules of 2 mL.

Proprietary Names and Manufacturers
Gastrodiagnost *(E. Merck, Ger.)*; Peptavlon *(ICI, Austral.; Ayerst, Canad.; ICI, Denm.; I.C.I.-Pharma, Fr.; ICI, Norw.; ICI, Swed.; ICI, Switz.; ICI Pharmaceuticals, UK; Ayerst, USA)*.

2145-n

Phenolsulphonphthalein *(BAN)*.

Fenolsolfonftaleina; Phenol Red; Phenolsulfonphthalein *(USAN)*; Phenolsulfonphthaleinum; Phenolsulphonphthal.; PSP. 4,4′-(3*H*-2,1-Benzoxathiol-3-ylidene)diphenol *S,S*-dioxide.
$C_{19}H_{14}O_5S$=354.4.

CAS — 143-74-8.

Pharmacopoeias. In *Br.*, *Chin.*, *Eur.*, *Fr.*, *It.*, *Jpn*, *Mex.*, *Neth.*, *Nord.*, *Swiss*, and *U.S.*

A bright to dark red, odourless, crystalline powder. Very slightly **soluble** in water; slightly soluble in alcohol. The *U.S.P.* also has freely soluble in solutions of alkali hydroxides and carbonates (such solutions are violet-red to deep red in colour); practically insoluble in chloroform and in ether.

Adverse Effects
Allergic reactions may occasionally occur.

Precautions
Excretion of phenolsulphonphthalein may be affected in patients with gout or those taking aminohippuric acid, atropine, penicillin, probenecid, salicylates, sulphinpyrazone, some sulphonamides, diuretics, or contrast media. Phenolsulphonphthalein may interfere with a number of laboratory tests.

Absorption and Fate
After intravenous injection, phenolsulphonphthalein is in part bound to plasma proteins, and in a patient with normal kidney function is rapidly excreted, mainly in the urine; some is excreted by the liver. Renal clearance is predominantly by tubular secretion, only a small amount being eliminated by glomerular filtration.

Uses and Administration
Phenolsulphonphthalein has been used as a test of renal function by estimating the rate of excretion in the urine after the intravenous injection of 6 mg, after a water load of 0.5 to 1 litre. It has also been given intramuscularly.
Alkaline urine is coloured red to violet.
Phenolsulphonphthalein has also been used as a drug ingestion indicator, a marker in drug absorption studies and in a quantitative test of residual urine.

Preparations
Phenolsulfonphthalein Injection *(U.S.P.)*. A sterile solution of phenolsulphonphthalein, rendered soluble with sodium bicarbonate or sodium hydroxide, in Water for Injections and made iso-osmotic with sodium chloride. pH 6.0 to 7.5.

Proprietary Names and Manufacturers
PSP-Plasma-Test *(E. Merck, Ger.)*
Manufacturers also include—*DAK, Denm.; Hynson, Westcott & Dunning, USA : Farillon, UK.*

13103-z

Phenylthiourea
Phenylthiocarbamide; PTC. 1-Phenylthiourea.
$C_7H_8N_2S$=152.2.

CAS — 103-85-5.

Sensitivity to the bitter taste of phenylthiourea has been found to be genetically determined; weak solutions (about 1 in 100 000) usually taste bitter to 3 of 4 persons in the population. The possibility that some individuals or groups are predisposed genetically to certain diseases has been investigated by correlation of the occurrence of disease with taste sensitivity to phenylthiourea.

1959-p

Pregnancy and Fertility Tests

There are a number of kits available for simple pregnancy and fertility testing. Some of these are listed below. A common method of detecting pregnancy is to measure the increase in chorionic gonadotrophin in the urine with the aid of specific antibodies. The measurement may be carried out in different ways involving for instance immunoassays or agglutination. The period of ovulation can be detected by measuring luteinising hormone excretion in similar ways.
These tests can give false results. Those carrying out the tests should be aware of this and of problems such as contaminated specimens, concomitant drug therapy, or other factors that could affect the result.

Proprietary Preparations
Clearblue *(Unipath, UK)*. Home and professional pregnancy test kit.
Confirm *(Chefaro, UK)*. Home pregnancy test kit.
Directaclone CG *(Alpha Laboratories, UK)*. Professional pregnancy test kit.
Discover 2 *(Carter-Wallace, UK)*. Home pregnancy test kit.
Discover Colour *(Carter-Wallace, UK)*. Home pregnancy test kit.
Discretest *(Chefaro, UK)*. Home ovulation test kit.
Evatest *(Thames Genelink, UK)*. Home pregnancy test kit.

First Response *(Tambrands, UK)*. Home ovulation test kit.

Gravindex *(Ortho Diagnostics, UK)*. Professional pregnancy test kit.

β-HCG Slide Test *(Roche, UK)*. Professional pregnancy test kit.

β-HCG Tube Test *(Roche, UK)*. Professional pregnancy test kit.

Neo-Planotest Duoclon *(Organon Teknika, UK)*. Professional pregnancy test kit.

Neo-Pregnosticon 75 Duoclon *(Organon Teknika, UK)*. Professional pregnancy test kit.

Organon LH Color *(Organon, UK)*. Home ovulation test kit.

Ovustick *(MediMar, UK)*. Home ovulation test kit.

Predictor *(Chefaro, UK)*. Home pregnancy test kit.

Predictor Colour *(Chefaro, UK)*. Home pregnancy test kit.

Pregnospia Duoclon *(Organon Teknika, UK)*. Professional pregnancy test kit.

Pregnosticon All-In 1000 M *(Organon Teknika, UK)*. Professional pregnancy test kit.

Pregnosticon Planotest *(Organon Teknika, UK)*. Professional pregnancy test kit.

Prepurex *(Wellcome Diagnostics, UK)*. Professional pregnancy test kit.

Ramp *(MediMar, UK)*. Professional pregnancy test kit.

Tandem Icon *(Britpharm, UK)*. Professional pregnancy test kit.

Test Pack hCG-Urine *(Abbott, UK)*. Professional pregnancy test kit.

Proprietary Names and Manufacturers

Advance *(Ortho Pharmaceutical, USA)*; β-HCG Slide Test *(Roche, UK)*; β-HCG Tube Test *(Roche, UK)*; Beta-Placentex *(Roche, Canad.)*; Beta-Pregnosis *(Roche, Canad.)*; Clearblue *(Unipath, UK)*; Confirm *(Chefaro, UK)*; Daisy 2 *(Ortho Pharmaceutical, USA)*; Denco *(Carter-Wallace, Austral.; Horner, Canad.)*; Denco Beta-Preg *(Horner, Canad.)*; Directaclone CG *(Alpha Laboratories, UK)*; Discover 2 *(Carter-Wallace, Austral.; Carter-Wallace, UK)*; Discover Colour *(Carter-Wallace, UK)*; Discretest *(Chefaro, UK)*; EPT Plus *(Warner-Lambert, USA)*; Evatest *(Thames Genelink, UK)*; FACT *(Ortho Pharmaceutical, USA)*; First Response *(Tambrands, UK; Tambrands, USA)*; Gonavislide *(Sigma, Austral.; Ames, S.Afr.)*; Gravindex *(Ortho, Canad.; Ortho Diagnostics, UK)*; Neo-Planotest Duoclon *(Organon Teknika, Switz.; Organon Teknika, UK)*; Neo-Pregnosticon *(Organon, Austral.)*; Neo-Pregnosticon 75 Duoclon *(Organon Teknika, Switz.; Organon Teknika, UK)*; Organon LH Color *(Organon, UK)*; Oveia Dual Analyte *(Boots, UK)*; Ovustick *(MediMar, UK; Monoclonal Antibodies, USA)*; Placentex *(Roche, Canad.)*; Planosec *(Organon, Austral.; Organon, S.Afr.)*; Predictor *(British Pharmaceuticals, Austral.; Chefaro, UK)*; Predictor Colour *(Chefaro, UK)*; Pregcolor *(Organon, S.Afr.)*; Pregnancy Slide Test *(Roche, Austral.; Roche, S.Afr.)*; Pregnosis *(Roche, Canad.)*; Pregnospia Duoclon *(Organon Teknika, UK)*; Pregnosticon All-In *(Organon, Austral.; Organon Teknika, Switz.)*; Pregnosticon All-In 1000 M *(Organon Teknika, UK)*; Pregnosticon Planotest *(Organon, Austral.; Organon, S.Afr.; Organon Teknika, Switz.; Organon Teknika, UK)*; Pregtest *(Organon, Austral.)*; Prepurex *(Wellcome, Austral.; Wellcome, S.Afr.; Wellcome Diagnostics, UK)*; Ramp *(MediMar, UK)*; Tandem Icon *(Britpharm, UK)*; Test Pack hCG-Urine *(Abbott, UK)*; UCG-BETASlide *(Carter-Wallace, Austral.; Horner. Canad.)*; UCG-BETAStat *(Carter-Wallace, Austral.)*; UCG-Quiktube *(Horner, Canad.)*; UCG-Slide *(Carter-Wallace, Austral.; Horner, Canad.)*; UCG-Test *(Horner, Canad.; Carter-Wallace, Switz.)*.

2146-h

Rose Bengal Sodium

CI Acid Red 94; Colour Index No. 45440; ROS; Rose Bengal; Sodium Rose Bengal. The disodium salt of 4,5,6,7-tetrachloro-2′,4′,5′,7′-tetraiodofluorescein.
$C_{20}H_2Cl_4I_4Na_2O_5$=1017.6.

CAS — 11121-48-5 (rose bengal); 632-69-9 (disodium salt).

NOTE. Dichlorotetraiodofluorescein (CI Acid Red 93; Ext. D & C Reds Nos. 5 and 6; Colour Index No. 45435) has been used as its disodium or dipotassium salt, for colouring pharmaceutical and cosmetic preparations for external use and as a food colour. The name Rose Bengale has been applied to both CI Acid Red 93 and 94.

A brownish-red solid. Aqueous solutions are deep red in colour.

Rose bengal eye-drops prepared at University College Hospital, London were incompatible with phenylmercuric nitrate, benzalkonium chloride, and chlorhexidine, but were compatible with esters of hydroxybenzoic acid.— N. Harb, *J. Hosp. Pharm.*, 1968, *25*, 239 (Moorfields Eye Hospital have used phenylmercuric acetate successfully in similar eye-drops).

Uses and Administration

Rose bengal sodium is taken up by the liver and excreted in the bile; the iodine-131-labelled compound (see p.1380) is therefore used as a diagnostic aid in the determination of hepato-biliary function.

It is also used, as 1% eye-drops, to stain devitalised conjunctival and corneal cells and as an aid in the diagnosis of dry eye. It is reported to be of value in assessing Sjogren's syndrome and in detecting damage from ill-fitting contact lenses.

Instillation of this dye may be painful.

Proprietary Preparations

Minims Rose Bengal *(Smith & Nephew Pharmaceuticals, UK)*. *Eye-drops*, rose bengal sodium 1%, in single-use disposable applicators.

NOTE. The *B.P.* allows the synonym ROS to be used for single-dose eye-drops containing rose bengal sodium.

Proprietary Names and Manufacturers

Minims Rose Bengal *(Smith & Nephew, Austral.; Smith & Nephew Pharmaceuticals, UK)*.

8005-j

Schick Test

Schick Control (*B.P.*) is Schick Test Toxin (*B.P.*) which has been heated at 70° to 85° for not less than 5 minutes. It must be prepared from the same batch of Schick Test Toxin as that with which it is issued.

Schick Test Control (*U.S.P.*) is Diphtheria Toxin for Schick Test (*U.S.P.*) that has been inactivated by heat. It should be stored at 2° to 8°.

Schick Test Toxin (*B.P.*) is a preparation from sterile filtrate from a culture in a liquid medium of a toxigenic strain (a well-characterised PW-8 subculture is satisfactory) of *Corynebacterium diphtheriae*; the toxin may be purified; it is then diluted so that 0.1 or 0.2 mL contains the test dose. It contains a suitable antimicrobial preservative. It should be stored at 2° to 8°. If stored at 25° it retains its potency for 2 months.

Diphtheria Toxin for Schick Test (*U.S.P.*) is a sterile solution of the diluted standardised toxic products of growth of *Corynebacterium diphtheriae* prepared from toxin of specified minimum potency. It should be stored at 2° to 8°.

Units

900 units of diphtheria (Schick) test toxin are contained in 0.005 mg of purified diphtheria toxin with 1 mg of bovine albumin and 2.74 mg of phosphate buffer salts in one ampoule of the first International Standard Preparation (1954).

Uses and Administration

The Schick test is used for the diagnosis of susceptibility to diphtheria and to detect patients who might experience an adverse reaction to diphtheria vaccines. Young children up to the age of about 8 to 10 years are stated to rarely suffer from adverse reactions following vaccination and therefore the Schick test is not usually performed in this age group. In older children and adults the immunity to diphtheria may vary and therefore these patients usually undergo a Schick test before the use of certain diphtheria vaccines in order to detect either susceptibility to the disease or hypersensitivity to the vaccine. Some diphtheria vaccines are formulated with lesser amounts of toxoid especially for adult use so that the need for prior Schick testing is unnecessary; for further details see under diphtheria vaccines, p.1160.

A dose of 0.2 mL of the Schick toxin is administered intradermally (intracutaneously) into the flexor surface of the forearm. A similar dose of Schick control is injected into the other forearm. The reaction to the injections may be read after 24 to 48 hours, though 5 to 7 days may be necessary for late reactors and to confirm a reading taken earlier.

A *negative reaction*, indicating that the patient is immune to diphtheria, occurs when there is no redness at either injection site. A *positive reaction*, indicating susceptibility to diphtheria, occurs as a red flush about 10 mm or more in diameter at the site of injection of the test dose with no reaction to the control injection. A *negative-and-pseudo reaction*, also indicating immunity, is shown by a flush which develops rapidly at each injection site but the reaction fades more rapidly than a positive reaction; the reaction is due to non-specific constituents of the injection. A *combined* or *positive-and-pseudo reaction*, also indicating susceptibility, is shown by a flush which develops rapidly at each injection site, but as it fades a positive reaction develops at the site of the test dose.

A study in 39 healthy Swedish subjects suggesting that the Schick test was a poor predictor of both immunity to diphtheria and of side-effects likely to occur after immunisation with diphtheria-containing vaccines. The lack of correlation may indicate that the tetanus component of the combined diphtheria and tetanus vaccines employed caused the local reactions.— B. Settergren *et al.*, *Br. med. J.*, 1986, *292*, 524.

Preparations

Schick Test Toxin (*B.P.*) and Schick Control (*B.P.*) are available from *Wellcome, UK.*

2147-m

Secretin *(BAN, rINN)*.

A hormone, prepared from the duodenal mucosa of pigs.

CAS — 17034-35-4.

Store at 2° to 8°.

Secretin solutions in a range of strengths were pumped at a constant rate through a plastic infusion system, including syringe, tubing, and catheter, for 45 minutes. The amount of secretin, measured by radio-immunoassay, decreased on delivery through the system. The reductions in secretin concentrations after 45 minutes were similar in samples of solution from the syringe and catheter tip. The loss of secretin from solution might be due to its binding to plastic; the rate of loss was not related to the original concentration of a solution.— M. Miyata *et al.* (letter), *New Engl. J. Med.*, 1979, *300*, 95.

Units

Various units have been used; in the UK the potency of secretin is expressed as arbitrary Crick-Harper-Raper (CHR) units based on the volume of pancreatic juice secreted in cats; in Sweden potency is expressed as arbitrary Clinical units, the value of which was amended in the 1960s. The *UK* manufacturers state that 1 Clinical unit is approximately equivalent to 4 Crick-Harper-Raper units.

References.— L. V. Gutierrez and J. H. Baron, *Gut*, 1972, *13*, 721.

Adverse Effects

Allergic reactions may occasionally occur. Diarrhoea has occurred in patients given high doses by intravenous infusion.

Anaphylactoid local reactions after intradermal injection of secretin occurred in 8 of 8 patients with duodenal ulcer, 2 of 3 with gastric ulcer, 4 of 6 with ulcerative colitis or Crohn's disease, 13 of 23 with other gastrointestinal diseases, and possibly in 1 of 7 healthy subjects.— H. W. Baenkler *et al.* (letter), *Br. med. J.*, 1975, *2*, 747.

Precautions

The secretin test should be used with caution in patients with acute pancreatitis. An intradermal test for sensitivity has been suggested.

Uses and Administration

Since secretin administered by intravenous injection causes an increase in the secretion by the pancreas of water and bicarbonate into the duodenum, it is used in conjunction with pancreozymin (see p.943) as a diagnostic agent for testing the functional capacity of the pancreas. The usual dose in the *UK* is 1 to 2 Crick-Harper-Raper units per kg body-weight by slow intravenous injection over about 2 minutes. In the *USA* a recommended alternative dose is 1 Clinical unit per kg.

Patients with the Zollinger-Ellison syndrome show an increase in gastrin following the administration of secretin; this is used in the diagnosis of the syndrome.

Hyperparathyroid patients consistently produced very large insulin responses to secretin injection. This large insulin response in hyperparathyroid patients should be investigated as a safe, non-calcium-dependent diagnostic test for primary hyperparathyroidism.— D. J. Sanders *et al.* (letter), *Lancet*, 1980, *2*, 265.

DUODENAL ULCER. *Diagnosis.* Secretin in a dose of 20 Clinical units given intradermally to 7 patients with duodenal ulcer produced a definite skin reaction due to histamine release in 6. No reactions occurred in 6 control patients. Secretin might be of value in the diagnosis of duodenal ulcer.— H. W. Baenkler *et al.*, *Lancet*, 1977, *1*, 928.

See also under Adverse Effects.

Treatment. Studies in 7 patients with duodenal ulcer indicated that secretin given intravenously suppressed acid secretion in response to a meal or to pentagastrin. Serum-gastrin concentrations were reduced and bicarbonate secretions increased.— S. J. Konturek *et al.*, *Gut*, 1973, *14*, 842. Experience with 4 patients undergoing haemodialysis for terminal renal failure indicated that infusions of secretin might be useful in reducing the tendency to duodenal ulceration in such patients by inhibiting gastric hypersecretion of acid.— A. M. M. Shepherd *et al.*, *Br. med. J.*, 1974, *1*, 96. Three patients with a duodenal ulcer received 10 Clinical units per kg body-weight of a long-acting synthetic secretin preparation by subcutaneous injection twice daily for 1 week then once daily for 3 weeks. Improvement in epigastric pain occurred 2 to 8 days after the start of treatment and complete healing of the ulcer occurred after 2 to 3 weeks. Treatment did not result in a fall in basal serum-gastrin concentration nor in a reduced serum-gastrin response to a test meal nor was pancreatic-bicarbonate secretion enhanced.— L. Demling *et al.*, *Scand. J. Gastroenterol.*, 1976, *11*, *Suppl.* 42, 135. A study involving 14 patients with a duodenal ulcer given a placebo or synthetic porcine secretin 333 µg (approximately equivalent to 18 Clinical units per kg body-weight of natural porcine secretin) by subcutaneous injection every 4 hours was discontinued after 10 days because of transient, asymptomatic, hyperamylasaemia in secretin-treated patients. During the period of study it was considered that secretin was no more effective than a placebo in relieving pain or healing the ulcer.— R. M. Henn *et al.*, *Am. J. dig. Dis.*, 1976, *21*, 921.

PANCREOZYMIN-SECRETIN TEST. For some references to the pancreozymin-secretin test, see Pancreozymin, p.943.

ZOLLINGER-ELLISON SYNDROME. Secretin administered as an intravenous bolus injection was used to diagnose Zollinger-Ellison syndrome in 18 patients with a history of peptic ulcer disease and was preferred to calcium gluconate.— C. W. Deveney *et al.*, *Ann. intern. Med.*, 1977, *87*, 680. A report of a false-positive response of gastrin to a secretin test for diagnosis of the Zollinger-Ellison syndrome in a patient who had achlorhydria and hypergastrinaemia.— R. L. Wollmuth and J. B. Wagonfield (letter), *ibid.*, 1978, *88*, 718.

Proprietary Names and Manufacturers

Secrepan *(Jpn)*; Sekretolin *(Hoechst, Ger.)*

Manufacturers also include—*Boots, Austral.; KabiVitrum, Norw.; Ferring, Swed.; Boots, UK.*

2148-b

Sincalide *(BAN, USAN, rINN).*

CCK-OP; SQ-19844. De-1-(5-oxo-L-proline)-de-2-L-glutamine-5-methionine-ceruletide.

$C_{49}H_{62}N_{10}O_{16}S_3$=1143.3.

CAS — 25126-32-3.

Adverse Effects

In addition to the physiological effect of gall-bladder contraction, sincalide may produce dizziness and flushing.

Uses and Administration

Sincalide is the synthetic C-terminal octapeptide of pancreozymin and administered by intravenous injection it stimulates gall-bladder contraction.

Sincalide is used for testing gall-bladder function and as an adjunct to cholecystography. It is usually given in doses of 20 ng per kg body-weight by intravenous injection over ½ to 1 minute. It is also used as a diagnostic agent in conjunction with secretin for testing the functional capacity of the pancreas. A suggested procedure is to give secretin by intravenous infusion over 1 hour and 30 minutes after starting this infusion, sincalide 20 ng per kg is infused over a 30-minute period.

Maximum gall-bladder contraction occurred in 24 of 40 patients undergoing cholecystography given sincalide 20 ng per kg body-weight by intravenous injection over 1 minute. The remaining 16 patients required a second dose to achieve maximum contraction. Transient mild abdominal pain, cramps, or nausea occurred in 48% of the patients but these were considered to be manifestations of the physiologic actions of sincalide.— E. N. Sargent *et al.*, *Am. J. Roentg.*, 1976, *127*, 267.

Eight patients with chronic pancreatitis became symptom-free during treatment with sincalide given in a dose of 2 drops of a 0.1% solution intranasally thrice daily before meals for 3 weeks. There was also some evidence of improvement in exocrine pancreatic function. Three patients experienced borborygmi and loose stools which stopped when the dose was slightly decreased.— A. Pap and V. Varró (letter), *Lancet*, 1977, *2*, 294.

Proprietary Names and Manufacturers

Kinevac *(Squibb, Austral.; Squibb, Canad.; Heyden, Ger.; Squibb, USA).*

2150-r

Sulphan Blue *(BAN).*

Acid Blue 1; Alphazurine 2G; Blue VRS; Colour Index No. 42045; Isosulfan Blue *(USAN)*; Patent Blue V; Sulphanum Caeruleum. Sodium α-(4-diethylaminophenyl)-α-(4-diethyliminiocyclo-hexa-2,5-dienylidene)toluene-2,5-disulphonate.

$C_{27}H_{31}N_2NaO_6S_2$=566.7.

CAS — 68238-36-8; 129-17-9 (2,4 isomer).

NOTE. The name Patent Blue V is mainly used for CI No. 42051—see p.943. Sulphan blue was formerly described as the 2,4-disulphonate isomer.

A violet powder. Solutions are blue in colour.

Adverse Effects and Precautions

Sulphan blue occasionally causes nausea. Allergic reactions and attacks of asthma have occasionally been reported.

Sulphan blue should not be used during surgical shock. Sulphan blue has been reported to interfere with blood tests for protein and iron.

Fatal allergic shock in a burnt patient given 6 mL of a 10% solution of sulphan blue intravenously.— S. Hepps and M. Dollinger, *New Engl. J. Med.*, 1965, *272*, 1281. Another report of life-threatening anaphylaxis in a patient given sulphan blue 1% subcutaneously to visualise the lymphatics of the feet.— S. M. Longnecker *et al.*, *Clin. Pharm.*, 1985, *4*, 219.

Sulphan blue interfered with the laboratory determination of total protein, albumin, amylase, iron, and total iron binding capacity in one patient. It was considered that requests for these assays are inappropriate for up to 2.5 days after administration of the dye.— S. P. Halloran *et al.* (letter), *Lancet*, 1983, *1*, 188.

Absorption and Fate

Following intravenous injection, sulphan blue is widely distributed in the tissues and may appear in bile, bronchial secretions, faeces, gastro-intestinal secretions, and synovial fluid. It is mainly excreted in the urine, and skin staining should disappear within 48 hours.

Uses and Administration

Changes in skin colour occur 1 to 1½ minutes after an intravenous injection of sulphan blue and complete body staining is established in 3 to 5 minutes. This effect is used as a direct visual test of the state of the circulation in healthy and damaged tissues, particularly in assessing tissue viability in burns and soft-tissue trauma. The usual dose is 0.25 to 0.5 mL per kg body-weight of a 6.2% solution by slow intravenous injection.

Sulphan blue is also given subcutaneously in lymphangiography to outline lymph trunks; a 1% solution has been used.

Proprietary Preparations

Disulphine Blue *(ICI Pharmaceuticals, UK). Injection,* sulphan blue 6.2% in ampoules of 10 mL.

Proprietary Names and Manufacturers

Disulphine Blue *(Ger.; ICI Pharmaceuticals, UK)*; Lymphazurin *(Pharmascience, Canad.).*

2151-f

Sulphobromophthalein Sodium *(BAN).*

Bromsulfophthalein Sodium; BSP; SBP Sulphobromophthal. Sod; Sodium Sulfobromophthalein; Sulfobromophthalein Sodium *(USAN)*. Disodium 4,5,6,7-tetrabromophenolphthalein-3′,3″-disulphonate; Disodium 5,5′-(4,5,6,7-tetrabromophthalidylidene)bis(2-hydroxybenzenesulphonate).

$C_{20}H_8Br_4Na_2O_{10}S_2$=838.0.

CAS — 71-67-0.

Pharmacopoeias. In *Br., Chin., Cz., Egypt., Ind., It., Jpn,* and *U.S.*

A white, odourless, crystalline, hygroscopic powder. **Soluble** 1 in 12 of water; practically insoluble in alcohol and in acetone. The *U.S.P.* injection has a pH of 5.0 to 6.5. Solutions are **sterilised**by filtration. **Store** in airtight containers.

Adverse Effects

Allergic-type reactions, some fatal, have been reported in patients given sulphobromophthalein. Inadvertent subcutaneous infiltration may cause irritation and necrosis.

In view of the 15 deaths and 27 severe allergic reactions which had been reported in connection with the sulphobromophthalein test, the test was best reserved for cases not readily elucidated by other means.— C. Wierum (letter), *J. Am. med. Ass.*, 1969, *210*, 1102.

After the administration of sulphobromophthalein, severe reactions including cardiac arrest, cyanosis, dyspnoea, and imperceptible pulse, or loss of consciousness, occurred in 3 patients. Storage of sulphobromophthalein at too low a temperature was considered to be the cause of these reactions.— E. Juhl *et al.* (letter), *Lancet*, 1970, *2*, 424. See also T. W. Astin, *Br. med. J.*, 1965, *2*, 408.

A fixed drug eruption occurred in a patient 8 hours after she was given an injection of sulphobromophthalein; she responded similarly to phenolphthalein given by mouth.— E. L. Smith, *Br. J. Derm.*, 1977, *97*, 106.

Precautions

Because a 5% solution of sulphobromophthalein, on standing, may yield a deposit which is not readily visible, it has been recommended that ampoules of the solution should, immediately before use, be immersed for 20 minutes in boiling water, well shaken, and cooled to body temperature.

The clearance of sulphobromophthalein may be reduced by drugs which impair hepatic function and has been stated to be affected by a wide range of compounds including cholagogues, cholecystographic agents, opioid analgesics, probenecid, sex hormones, and drugs extensively excreted in bile.

Absorption and Fate

Sulphobromophthalein sodium, administered intravenously, is bound to plasma proteins. In patients with normal hepatic function it is rapidly excreted in the bile.

Uses and Administration

Sulphobromophthalein sodium is used as a diagnostic agent for testing the functional capacity of the liver.

The test is usually performed in the morning after the patient has had a fat-free breakfast; no food must be given during the test. A dose usually of 5 mg of sulphobromophthalein sodium per kg body-weight is given as a 5% solution by intravenous injection over a period of about 3 minutes. The dose may have to be adjusted if there is fluid retention. Forty-five minutes after the injection the amount of dye remaining in the serum is determined colorimetrically; less than 5 to 7% is considered to indicate normal liver function.

Preparations

Sulfobromophthalein Sodium Injection *(U.S.P.)*.

Proprietary Names and Manufacturers

Bromophthalein *(Abbott, Austral.)*; Bromotaleina *(Igoda, Spain)*; Bromsulphalein *(Hynson, Westcott & Dunning, Canad.)*; Bromthalein *(E. Merck, Ger.; E. Merck, Swed.; E. Merck, Switz.)*; Hepartest *(Ger.)*.

2152-d

Tolonium Chloride *(rINN)*.

CI Basic Blue 17; Colour Index No. 52040; Toluidine Blue O. 3-Amino-7-dimethylamino-2-methylphenazathionium chloride; 3-Amino-7-dimethylamino-2-methylphenothiazin-5-ium chloride.

$C_{15}H_{16}ClN_3S$=305.8.

CAS — 92-31-9.

NOTE. Distinguish from Toluidine Blue, Colour Index No. 63340.

A green crystalline powder with a bronze lustre. Aqueous solutions are blue-violet in colour.

Uses and Administration

Tolonium chloride has been used to stain oral and gastric neoplasms but its accuracy has been questioned. It was given intravenously to stain the parathyroid glands and has been given for menstrual disorders.

Proprietary Names and Manufacturers

Menodin *(Ital.)*.

8024-k

Tuberculins

Old Tuberculin (*B.P.*) (Old Tuberculin for Human Use (*Eur. P.*); Tuberculinum Pristinum ad Usum Humanum) is a sterile heat-concentrated filtrate from the soluble products of growth and lysis of one or more strains of mycobacteria. It contains a suitable preservative that does not give rise to false-positive reactions. It may be issued in concentrated or diluted form. It should be stored at 2° to 8°, not be allowed to freeze, and be protected from light. Under these conditions the undiluted form may be expected to retain its potency for at least 8 years. Diluted solutions are less stable depending on the degree of dilution and the nature of the diluent.

Tuberculin Purified Protein Derivative (*B.P.*) (Tuberculin P.P.D.; Tuberculin Purified Protein Derivative (*Eur. P.*); Tuberculin: Derivatum Proteinosum Purificatum ad Usum Humanum) is a sterile preparation made from the heat-treated products of growth and lysis of one or more strains of *Mycobacterium tuberculosis*. It may contain a suitable preservative that does not give rise to a false-positive reaction and a suitable stabiliser. It may be issued in concentrated or diluted form as a liquid and the diluted form may be freeze-dried. It should be stored at 2° to 8°, not be allowed to freeze, and be protected from light. Special care must be taken to avoid inhaling the powder.

Tuberculin (*U.S.P.*) is a sterile solution derived from the concentrated soluble products of growth of *Mycobacterium tuberculosis* or *M. bovis*. It is supplied as Old Tuberculin, a standardised culture filtrate or as Purified Protein Derivative (PPD), a further standardised purified protein fraction. It should be stored at 2° to 8°. Multiple-puncture devices may be stored at a temperature not exceeding 30°.

Units

500 000 units of mammalian tuberculin purified protein derivative are contained in 10 mg of purified protein derivative prepared from a human strain with 4 mg of salts in one ampoule of the first International Standard Preparation (1951).

500 000 units of avian tuberculin purified protein derivative are contained in 10 mg of purified protein derivative with 26.3 mg of salts in one ampoule of the first International Standard Preparation (1954).

The third International Standard Preparation (1965) of old tuberculin contains 90 000 units per mL.

Adverse Effects

Pain and pruritus may occur at the injection site, occasionally with vesiculation, ulceration, or necrosis in highly sensitive persons. If given to patients with tuberculosis a severe reaction may occur. Granuloma has been reported after Heaf tests.

Allergic reactions to tuberculin tine tests have been reported rarely and measures to deal with them should be available. For detailed recommendations concerning the management of anaphylaxis, see adrenaline, p.1455.

A 19-year-old youth collapsed and died shortly after receiving a Tuberculin Tine Test (old tuberculin intradermal test). He had also been given an oral poliomyelitis vaccine before the tine test. Death was considered probably to be due to an anaphylactic reaction to the tine test. No abnormality was found at autopsy.— V. J. M. DiMaio and R. C. Froede (letter), *J. Am. med. Ass.*, 1975, *233*, 769. A further report of a severe life-threatening anaphylactoid reaction to tuberculin in one patient.— M. A. Spiteri, *Br. med. J.*, 1986, *293*, 243.

A report of lymphangitis on 5 occasions after the Mantoux test and on 7 occasions after the Heaf test.— J. B. Morrison, *Br. med. J.*, 1984, *289*, 413. Comment that the tests were carried out unnecessarily on some patients with tuberculosis.— F. Festenstein (letter), *ibid.*, 625.

Precautions

Sensitivity to tuberculin may be diminished during virus infections, after ultraviolet light treatment, during corticosteroid therapy, and after virus vaccines.

Uses and Administration

Tuberculins are used as diagnostic agents for testing for hypersensitivity to tuberculoprotein. A person showing a specific sensitivity to tuberculin is considered to have been infected with tubercle bacillus, though the infection may be inactive. Sensitivity tests to tuberculin can be performed in different ways.

In the *UK* it is recommended that tuberculin testing should always be performed, except in neonates, when BCG vaccination is being considered; either the Mantoux test or the Heaf test is recommended.

For a routine Mantoux test, 0.1 mL of a diluted solution of tuberculin purified protein derivative, containing 100 units per mL, is injected intradermally. A positive and a strongly positive result are considered to consist of induration of at least 6 mm and 15 mm respectively in diameter; the results should be read after 72 hours but may, if necessary, be read for up to 96 hours after the test. If a patient is suspected of having tuberculosis a solution of tuberculin PPD containing 10 units per mL should be used.

For the Heaf test a solution of tuberculin purified protein derivative containing 100 000 units per mL is used. The solution is applied to the forearm and a multiple puncture gun is used; a puncture of 1 mm depth is recommended for children under 2 years of age and a puncture of 2 mm for older children and adults. Results may be read 3 to 10 days after the test and a positive result is considered to consist of a palpable induration around at least four puncture points. Positive results are also graded as follows: grade 1, at least 4 small indurated papules; grade 2, an indurated ring formed by confluent papules; grade 3, solid induration 5 to 10 mm wide; and grade 4, induration over 10 mm wide. In individuals with grade 1 reactions who have not previously received BCG vaccines, the reaction is not usually related to infection with *Mycobacterium tuberculosis* and these patients may be offered BCG vaccination. Grade 3 and 4 reactions are regarded as being strongly positive reactions and persons displaying such reactions along with those showing a strongly positive reaction to a Mantoux test should be investigated for the presence of active tuberculosis.

Disposable tine tests, coated with dried old tuberculin or moistened before use from an attached reservoir of tuberculin purified protein derivative are also available.

In some other countries the population tested, the procedures used, and grading of reactions may differ slightly from that outlined above.

Discussion on the need to isolate a specific tuberculin since it is now well established that a positive tuberculin skin test does not necessarily indicate infection with the typical tubercle bacillus, but rather emphasises that there is a group of closely-related acid-fast micro-organisms which may cause cross-skin sensitivity in man.— L. F. Affronti *et al.*, *Bull. int. Un. Tuberc.*, 1983, *58*, 233. See also: *Lancet*, 1984, *1*, 199.

Recommendations for the interpretation of positive tuberculin reactions in people with a history of BCG vaccination in the *USA*.— D. E. Snider, *J. Am. med. Ass.*, 1985, *253*, 3438.

Proprietary Preparations

Imotest-Tuberculin *(Servier, UK)*. A disposable plastic unit bearing 9 tines (prongs) which are wetted before application by 0.05 mL of tuberculin purified protein derivative contained in an attached removable reservoir; the amount of tuberculin injected is stated to be equivalent to 5 units. For intradermal tuberculin testing.

Tuberculin, Old, Tine Test (Rosenthal) *(Lederle, UK)*. A disposable plastic unit with a stainless steel disk bearing 4 tines (prongs) coated with old tuberculin; the amount of old tuberculin on the tines is stated to be equivalent to 5 units. For intradermal tuberculin testing.

Tuberculin Purified Protein Derivative (*B.P.*) is also available from *Evans Medical, UK*.

Proprietary Names and Manufacturers

Aplisol *(Parke, Davis, USA)*; Aplitest *(Parke, Davis, USA)*; Imotest-Tuberculin *(Servier, UK)*; Monotest *(Merieux, Ital.)*; Mono-Vacc *(Merieux, USA)*; Sclavo-Test *(Sclavo, Ital.; Sclavo, USA)*; Tubergen *(Behringwerke, Ger.; Berna, Switz.)*; Tubersol *(Connaught, USA)*;

Manufacturers also include—*Commonwealth Serum Laboratories, Austral.; Connaught, Canad.; Lederle, S.Afr.; Evans Medical, UK; Lederle, UK; Lederle, USA.*

2153-n

Tyramine Hydrochloride

p-Tyramine Hydrochloride; Tyrosamine Hydrochloride. 4-Hydroxyphenethylamine hydrochloride; 4-(2-Aminoethyl)phenol hydrochloride.

$C_8H_{11}NO,HCl$=173.6.

CAS — 51-67-2 (tyramine); 60-19-5 (hydrochloride).

Tyramine hydrochloride is a sympathomimetic agent which has indirect effects on adrenergic receptors. It has been given by mouth or injection in the tyramine pressor test in the investigation of monoamine oxidase inhibitory activity or of amine uptake blocking activity as well as of various physiological and diseased states.

It has also been tried in the diagnosis of migraine and phaeochromocytoma.
The hazards of taking foods rich in tyramine while under treatment with monoamine oxidase inhibitors are described in the antidepressants section.

ABSORPTION AND FATE. After intravenous administration tyramine was rapidly excreted; the equivalent of 70 to 90% of a dose appeared in the urine within 6 hours. It was not concentrated by the formed elements of the blood. About 85% of excreted material consisted of the main metabolite *p*-hydroxyphenylacetic acid and about 6% was free tyramine. Small amounts of 9 other metabolites were detected, 2 of which were probably *N*-acetyltyramine and *p*-hydroxyphenylacetaldehyde.— M. Tacker *et al.* (letter), *J. Pharm. Pharmac.*, 1972, *24*, 247.

MENTAL DEPRESSION. The amount of conjugated tyramine excreted in the urine following an oral dose was reduced in patients who were severely depressed, mildly depressed or who had recovered from depression when compared with controls.— W. M. Harrison *et al.*, *Archs gen. Psychiat.*, 1984, *41*, 681. Comment.— *Lancet*, 1984, *2*, 963.

ORTHOSTATIC HYPOTENSION. Tyramine on its own or with phenelzine produced severe supine hypertension in 4 patients with orthostatic hypotension but did not influence their hypotensive response to tilting. The addition of phenelzine merely prolonged the induced hypertension but did not affect its pattern. Phenylephrine and ephedrine controlled the postural symptoms but produced recumbent hypertension. Other therapy should be found.— B. Davies *et al.*, *Lancet*, 1978, *1*, 172. Good results were achieved in 3 patients with severe disabling orthostatic hypotension after treatment with tyramine and tranylcypromine. Treatment was continued for 5, 10, and 12 months.— P. M. Trust (letter), *Lancet*, 1978, *1*, 386. A favourable response in another patient given tyramine hydrochloride with phenelzine.— C. A. Wood *et al.* (letter), *Ann. intern. Med.*, 1985, *103*, 803.

PHAEOCHROMOCYTOMA. Some references to tyramine being used as a provocative test for phaeochromocytoma: K. Engelman and A. Sjoerdsma, *J. Am. med. Ass.*, 1964, *189*, 81; R. N. Thurm *et al.*, *ibid.*, 1966, *196*, 613; K. Engelman *et al.*, *New Engl. J. Med.*, 1968, *278*, 705.

Proprietary Names and Manufacturers
Mydrial *(Winzer, Ger.)*.

2154-h

Xylose *(BAN, USAN)*.

D-Xylose; Wood Sugar. α-D-Xylopyranose.
$C_5H_{10}O_5$=150.1.

CAS — 58-86-6; 6763-34-4.

Pharmacopoeias. In *Br.* and *U.S.*

Odourless colourless needles or white crystalline powder. **Soluble** 1 in less than 1 of water; slightly soluble in alcohol; soluble in hot alcohol. **Store** in airtight containers.

Adverse Effects and Precautions

Xylose may cause some gastro-intestinal discomfort with large doses. Other drugs may affect the absorption of xylose and interfere with the xylose test.

In the xylose test indomethacin reduced the intestinal absorption of xylose, possibly due to increased intestinal motility. Aspirin reduced the excretion of xylose, possibly by a renal effect.— M. J. Kendall *et al.*, *Br. med. J.*, 1971, *1*, 533.

Absorption and Fate

Xylose is incompletely absorbed from the gastro-intestinal tract. Part of the absorbed xylose is metabolised in the body mainly to carbon dioxide and water. Up to about 35% of a dose taken by mouth is reported to be excreted in the urine within 5 hours.

Uses and Administration

Xylose is used for the investigation of absorption from the gastro-intestinal tract. It is given by mouth, usually in a dose of either 5 or 25 g, with up to 500 mL of water. The amount recovered in the urine is estimated over a certain period and that figure can be used to assess any malabsorption. Adjustment may have to be made for renal impairment.

Xylan, a polymerisation product of xylose, is a possible filler and disintegrant for pharmaceutical tablets.— M. Juslin and P. Paronen, *J. Pharm. Pharmac.*, 1984, *36*, 256.

Results in 24 healthy men indicating no age-dependence in xylose absorption over the age range of 32 to 85 years. This finding is in contrast with the generally held belief that gastro-intestinal absorptive function decreases with age.— S. L. Johnson *et al.*, *Clin. Pharmac. Ther.*, 1985, *38*, 331.

Some references to the value or limitation of the xylose test in adults as well as children. Conditions being diagnosed include coeliac disease, Crohn's disease, gastroenteritis, and protein intolerance: H. Theile *et al.*, *Z. Kinderheilk.*, 1968, *103*, 247; G. E. Sladen and P. J. Kumar, *Br. med. J.*, 1973, *3*, 223; M. J. Kendall (letter), *ibid.*, 405; C. J. Rolles *et al.*, *Lancet*, 1973, *2*, 1043; S. P. Lamabadusuriya *et al.*, *Archs Dis. Childh.*, 1975, *50*, 34; C. J. Rolles *et al.*, *ibid.*, 259; F. M. Stevens *et al.*, *J. clin. Path.*, 1977, *30*, 76; C. L. Morin *et al.*, *Lancet*, 1979, *1*, 1102; M. E. Penny *et al.*, *Gut*, 1984, *25*, A1155.

Proprietary Preparations

Xylose-BMS (formerly known as Xylomed) *(Bio-Medical, UK)*. *Oral powder*, xylose 5 and 25 g, in unit dose packs.

Proprietary Names and Manufacturers

Xylomed *(Bio-Medical, UK)*; Xylo-Pfan *(Adria, Canad.; Adria, USA)*; Xylose-BMS *(Bio-Medical, UK)*.

Disinfectants

2200-z

Disinfectants and antiseptics are generally used to destroy or inhibit the growth of pathogenic micro-organisms in the non-sporing or vegetative state.

There is often confusion between the terms disinfectant and antiseptic. However, according to the British Standard Glossary of Terms Relating to Disinfectants (BS 5283: 1976) the term *disinfectant* is applied to a chemical agent which destroys micro-organisms, but not usually bacterial spores; it does not necessarily kill all micro-organisms, but reduces them to a level which is harmful neither to health nor the quality of perishable goods. The term is applicable to agents used to treat inanimate objects and materials and may also be applied to agents used to treat the skin and other body membranes and cavities. The term *antiseptic* is applied to a chemical agent which destroys or inhibits micro-organisms on living tissues having the effect of limiting or preventing the harmful results of infection.

Sterilisation is the total removal or destruction of all living micro-organisms; a few chemical agents are capable of producing sterility under suitable conditions but, in general, sterility is produced by heat or radiation methods.

Preservatives are used to prevent microbial spoilage of preparations; in pharmacy, preservatives should reduce pathogenic organisms to acceptable numbers or should maintain sterility during use of the preparation. Ideally they should destroy pathogenic organisms.

Some drugs can be used for disinfection and preservation, but those mainly used as preservatives are described in the section on Preservatives (p.1355).

The main types of disinfectants described in this section are alcohols, aldehydes, cationic surfactants, chlorhexidine salts, chlorine and its compounds, dyes, mercurials, phenols and related substances, and some gases and vapours.

Alcohols, suitably diluted, are used for the rapid disinfection of clean surfaces and skin, but not wounds. They are active against a wide range of bacteria, but are not reliably active against viruses or fungi. The alcohols described in this section are alcohol (p.950), isopropyl alcohol (p.964), and methylated spirits (p.965).

The *aldehydes* formaldehyde (p.961) and glutaraldehyde (p.963) are used for disinfection and sterilisation of clean surfaces but are too irritant for disinfection of the skin. Formaldehyde may be used as a vapour.

Cationic surfactants are quaternary ammonium or pyridinium compounds with activity against a wide range of Gram-positive organisms, some Gram-negative organisms, lipophilic viruses, and fungi. Resistant Gram-negative organisms include *Pseudomonas* spp. They may be used on the skin, where their detergent action is often useful in cleansing dirty wounds. They are also used for cleansing and disinfecting containers and equipment in the food and dairy industries. However, they are inactivated by soaps, anionic surfactants, and organic matter, and by adsorption onto cotton and some plastics. The quaternary compounds described include benzalkonium chloride (p.951), cetrimide (p.953), cetylpyridinium chloride (p.954), and domiphen bromide (p.960). Their general properties are described under Cetrimide.

Chlorhexidine (p.955) is a cationic bisbiguanide disinfectant, active against many Gram-positive and Gram-negative organisms, and some fungi and viruses. However, some Gram-negative organisms, particularly *Pseudomonas* spp. are resistant. It is used as a disinfectant for skin and mucous membranes and as a preservative for pharmaceutical preparations.

Chlorine and chlorine-releasing substances are bactericidal to most Gram-positive and Gram-negative bacteria, some bacterial spores, and some viruses. They also have a deodorant action. Their activity is reduced by organic matter and in alkaline conditions. The main chlorine-releasing compound is sodium hypochlorite (p.969); chloramine (p.955), chlorinated lime (p.957), dichlordimethylhydantoin (p.960), halazone (p.963), oxychlorosene (p.967), and sodium dichloroisocyanurate (p.969) also have the general properties described under chlorine (p.957). Some of the chlorine-releasing substances are used for cleansing foul wounds and ulcers, for disinfecting contaminated water, and since they have low toxicity, for disinfecting utensils in the food industry. Iodine has a similar action, see p.1184.

Two types of *dyes* are used for their antimicrobial action on the skin: the acridine derivatives acriflavine (p.950), aminacrine hydrochloride (p.951), and proflavine hemisulphate (p.969); and the triphenylmethane derivatives brilliant green (p.953), crystal violet (p.959), magenta (p.965), and malachite green (p.965). These dyes are bacteriostatic, particularly against Gram-positive organisms, and have some inhibitory activity against fungi and yeasts.

Gases and *vapours* are used for sterilising objects that cannot be satisfactorily sterilised by heat or chemical means and to sterilise the atmosphere. In general, only surface sterilisation occurs. Gases and vapours are used to sterilise metal or plastic surfaces of a variety of equipment as well as plastic catheters and syringes. Ethylene oxide (p.961) and propiolactone (p.969) are used for these purposes. Formaldehyde may also be used in vapour form.

Mercurials have antibacterial and antifungal activity but are affected by the presence of organic matter. The main mercurial disinfectant is thiomersal (p.970); others used include hydrargaphen (p.964), mercurochrome (p.965), and nitromersol (p.966). Phenylmercuric salts are used as preservatives.

Phenols and chlorinated phenols have a bactericidal action in appropriate concentrations but rapidly lose their effect on dilution or in the presence of organic matter, cationic surfactants, and some plastics. They are more active in acid conditions and more effective against Gram-positive organisms than against Gram-negative organisms. The more highly substituted phenolic derivatives are more selective in their action than the cruder mixed tar acids and some have antifungal activity. The more selective phenolics are used for skin disinfection and the less-refined products for disinfection of drains and floors and for contaminated bedding and instruments before heat sterilisation. Phenols are also used as preservatives in pharmaceutical preparations. The phenols described in this section include cresol (p.959), phenol (p.967), thymol (p.971), and tar acids and disinfectants (p.970). Chlorinated phenols include chlorocresol (p.958), chloroxylenol (p.959), hexachlorophane (p.963), and triclosan (p.971). Their general properties are described under phenol.

Substances used as disinfectants or antiseptics and described elsewhere include Ampholytic Surfactants, p.1416, Hydrogen Peroxide, p.1579, and Iodine, p.1184.

DISINFECTANT EVALUATION. The apparatus and reagents required, the standard techniques and the methods of calculating the various coefficients of disinfectants are fully described in British Standard (BS) Specifications:

The *Rideal-Walker Test*, in BS 541 (*Technique for Determining the Rideal-Walker Coefficient of Disinfectants*), requires distilled-water dilutions of the disinfectant to be tested against broth cultures of the specified micro-organisms.

The *Chick-Martin Test*, in BS 808 (*Modified Technique of the Chick-Martin Test for Disinfectants*), requires the disinfectant to be tested in the presence of a high concentration of organic matter, a yeast suspension being used for this purpose.

The *Crown Agents' Test*, in BS 2462 (*Specification for Black and White Disinfectant Fluids*), is for white fluids only and requires a sterile artificial sea-water dilution of the disinfectant to be tested in the presence of soluble and insoluble organic material.

The *Phenol Coefficient (Staphylococcus) Test*, in BS 2462, is designed to ensure that modified black and modified white fluids are not unduly selective in their bactericidal activity.

The method for the laboratory evaluation of disinfectant activity of quaternary ammonium compounds by suspension test procedure is given in BS 3286, and the determination of the antimicrobial value of quaternary ammonium compound disinfectant formulations is given in BS 6471.

An improved (1974) *Kelsey-Sykes test* for disinfectants.— J. C. Kelsey and I. M. Maurer, *Pharm. J.*, 1974, *2*, 528.

Methods of testing disinfectants.— A. Crémieux and J. Fleurette, in *Disinfection, Sterilization and Preservation*, S.S. Block (Ed.), Philadelphia, Lea and Febiger. 1983, 918.

RESISTANCE. Bacterial resistance to antiseptics and disinfectants.— A. D. Russell *et al.*, *J. Hosp. Infect.*, 1986, *7*, 213.

The minimum inhibitory concentrations (MIC) of cetrimide, propamidine, aminacrine, and chlorhexidine were increased in 30 strains of *Staphylococcus aureus* resistant to both methicillin and gentamicin (MGRSA), compared to 21 strains sensitive to the 2 antibiotics, but the MGRSA strains were not significantly more resistant to hexachlorophane. It was unclear whether such increased resistance would mean that certain antiseptics may be limited in their use against MGRSA, as antiseptic concentrations in clinical practice were much higher in most cases than the MIC's observed (W. Brumfitt *et al.*, *Lancet*, 1985, *1*, 1442). Ten epidemic strains of methicillin-resistant *Staphylococcus aureus* (MRSA) had greatly increased resistance to povidone-iodine, eusol, chlorhexidine acetate, and chlorhexidine gluconate. The relevance of this *in vitro* resistance to antiseptic efficacy *in vivo* was not known, especially since sub-lethal concentrations of chlorhexidine *in vitro* may reduce the infectivity of bacteria *in vivo*. It was felt that perhaps the use of povidone-iodine and eusol should be restricted in MRSA-infected patients until the *in vivo* effect of antiseptic resistance was known. If the antiseptic resistance was plasmid-mediated and inducible, then rotation or minimal use of the antiseptics may reduce selection pressure (G. Mycock, *ibid.*, *2*, 949). However, Lacey *et al.* (*ibid.*, 1307) in repeating the work of Mycock concluded that MRSA were as sensitive to povidone-iodine as were other cultures of *Staphylococcus aureus*.

USE OF DISINFECTANTS IN HOSPITALS. Guidance on disinfection in hospitals.— G. A. J. Ayliffe *et al.*, *Chemical Disinfection in Hospitals, Public Health Laboratory Service*, London 1984. See also Code of Practice for the Prevention of Infection in Clinical Laboratories and Post-mortem Rooms, London, Department of Health and Social Security, 1978; I. M. Maurer, *Hospital Hygiene*, London, Edward Arnold, 1985. and see below under Viral Disinfection.

Thorough physical cleaning of the endoscope and ancillary equipment is an essential prerequisite to any effective disinfection procedure and after disinfection, endoscopic equipment should be rinsed free of residual germicide and dried. Aqueous alkaline glutaraldehyde 2% is at present the liquid disinfectant of choice for fibre-endoscopes. In-use studies have shown that 2 minutes immersion adequately decontaminates fibre-endoscopes between patient procedures though some workers would advocate 10 to 30 minutes immersion in view of the risk of hepatitis B transmission and the disputed tuberculocidal efficacy of the solution. Ethylene oxide has no practical role in the routine disinfection of endoscopes between patient procedures, but remains the best available treatment for endoscopes used on patients known to have infectious diseases including hepatitis B, tuberculosis, and typhoid fever. Povidone-iodine has been shown adequately to decontaminate fibre-endoscopes with 2 to 4 minutes disinfection between patient procedures without causing yellowing of lenses. Properly manufactured povidone-iodine solution, assayed to ensure sterility was necessary. Succindialdehyde 10% adequately disinfected fibre-endoscopes in 30 minutes with no evidence of endoscope damage and is rapidly hepatovirucidal. Buffered hypochlorite solutions are rapidly germicidal and hepatovirucidal but could damage endoscope components. The following solutions do not reliably disinfect fibre-endoscopes: quaternary ammonium compounds, chlorhexidine, chlorhexidine-cetrimide mixtures, alcohol, isopropyl alcohol, hexachlorophane, and cresol.— H. J. O'Connor and A. T. R. Axon, *Gut*, 1983, *24*, 1067. See also G. L. Ridgway, *J. Hosp. Infect.*, 1985, *6*, 363; J. H. T. Wagenvoort *et al.*, *ibid.*, 1986, *7*, 78.

Recovered permanent cardiac pacemakers have been adequately sterilised for re-use in formaldehyde and glutaraldehyde. Some use a low-level disinfectant (dimethylbenzyl ammonium chloride) combined with ethylene oxide, formaldehyde, and glutaraldehyde. Resterilisation with ethylene oxide gas alone has also been reported.— M. D. Rosengarten *et al.*, *Can. med. Ass. J.*, 1985, *133*, 279.

USE OF DISINFECTANTS ON FARMS. For a list of disinfectants and their rate of dilution approved for use in Great Britain in foot-and-mouth disease, swine vesicular disease, fowl pest, and tuberculosis in animals, see The Diseases of Animals (Approved Disinfectants) Order 1978 (SI 1978: No. 32), as amended (SI 1986: No. 5).

VIRAL DISINFECTION. *Creutzfeldt-Jakob virus.* The virus causing Creutzfeldt-Jakob disease was resistant to inactivation by formaldehyde solutions. Hypochlorite 0.5% or povidone-iodine appeared to be most effective.— W. B. Patterson *et al.*, *Ann. intern. Med.*, 1985, *102*, 658.

See also under Chlorine, p.958.

Hepatitis B virus. Boiling for 1 minute, steam autoclaving, ethylene oxide gas sterilisation, glutaraldehyde 2%, formaldehyde 8%, and sodium hypochlorite 0.5% will inactivate hepatitis B virus. Phenolics, hexachlorophane, and quaternary ammonium compounds were not recommended.— W. B. Patterson *et al.*, *Ann. intern. Med.*, 1985, *102*, 658.

Human immunodeficiency virus. For spillage of LAV/HTLV III [HIV] positive blood, body fluid, and excreta onto surfaces, or when heat-sensitive articles were grossly contaminated, use should be made of either freshly activated glutaraldehyde 2%, or phenolic disinfectant 2%, or freshly-prepared hypochlorite solution containing 10 000 ppm 'available chlorine'. For the treatment of minor surface contamination, and as part of general good hygiene practice, hypochlorite solution containing 1000 ppm 'available chlorine' or phenolic disinfectant 1% were recommended, with alcohol 70%, isopropyl alcohol 70%, or glutaraldehyde 2% as alternatives.— Advisory Committee on Dangerous Pathogens, *LAV/HTLV III—The Causative Agent of AIDS and Related Conditions, Revised Guidelines*, London, Department of Health and Social Security, 1986.

Human immunodeficiency virus-contaminated bronchoscopes, gastroscopes, and other lensed instruments should be sterilised with ethylene oxide or receive high-level disinfection with an agent that was also mycobactericidal; a glutaraldehyde 2% soak for 45 minutes was sufficient.— J. E. Conte, *Ann. intern. Med.*, 1986, *105*, 730.

Viral haemorrhagic fevers. For the disinfection of materials in contact with viral haemorrhagic fever viruses, phenolic disinfectants are commonly used at working dilutions of between 1 and 5% according to the level of organic matter present. For disinfection of sites where there is no obvious or gross contamination, a final dilution of hypochlorite solution containing 1000 ppm 'available chlorine' was recommended. Where visible blood or vomit is encountered a final concentration of 10 000 ppm 'available chlorine' was indicated. Activated glutaraldehyde 2% was also suitable. Fumigation with formaldehyde vapour is recommended for the internal disinfection of isolators, ambulances, and residential premises.— *Memorandum on The Control of Viral Haemorrhagic Fevers* Department of Health and Social Security, London, HM Stationery Office, 1986.

2201-c

Acriflavine

Acriflavine Hydrochloride; Acriflavinium Chloride *(rINN)*. A mixture of 3,6-diamino-10-methylacridinium chloride hydrochloride and 3,6-diaminoacridine dihydrochloride.

CAS — 8063-24-9.

Pharmacopoeias. In *Aust.*, *Jug.* and *Swiss.*

Acriflavine has properties similar to other acridine derivatives (see p.969).

Proprietary Names and Manufacturers

Diacrid *(Siegfried, Switz.)*; Panflavin *(Chinosolfabrik, Ger.)*.

551-f

Alcohol *(USAN)*.

Aethanolum; Alcool; Ethanol; Ethanol (96 per cent) *(BAN)*; Ethyl Alcohol.

$C_2H_5OH=46.07$.

CAS — 64-17-5.

Pharmacopoeias. In *Arg.*, *Aust.*, *Belg.*, *Br.*, *Chin.*, *Cz.*, *Egypt.*, *Fr.*, *Ger.*, *Hung.*, *Ind.*, *Int.*, *It.*, *Jpn*, *Jug.*, *Mex.*, *Neth.*, *Nord.*, *Pol.*, *Port.*, *Roum.*, *Rus.*, *Span.*, *Swiss*, *Turk.*, and *U.S.* Also in *B.P. Vet.*

The *B.P.* specifies under Ethanol (96 per cent) not less than 96% and not more than 96.6% v/v; 93.8 to 94.7% w/w of C_2H_5OH. The *U.S.P.* specifies under Alcohol not less than 94.9% and not more than 96.0% v/v; 92.3 to 93.8% w/w of C_2H_5OH.

In *Martindale* the term alcohol is used for alcohol 95 or 96% v/v.

A mixture of ethyl alcohol and water. A clear, colourless, mobile, volatile, readily inflammable liquid with a characteristic spirituous odour and burning taste.

Miscible with water (with rise of temperature and contraction of volume), chloroform, ether, glycerol, and almost all other organic solvents. **Store** in a cool place in airtight containers.

Dehydrated alcohol (absolute alcohol) is also included in the *B.P.* under the title Ethanol (not less than 99.4% v/v or 99% w/w of C_2H_5OH; density 788.16 to 791.2 kg per m^3) and in the *U.S.P.* under the title Dehydrated Alcohol (not less than 99.5% v/v or 99.2% w/w of C_2H_5OH; sp. gr. not more than 0.7964 at 15.56°).

The *B.P.* also includes several **dilute alcohols** and one of these, alcohol(90%), is also known as rectified spirit. **Diluted Alcohol** *(U.S.N.F.)* contains 48.4 to 49.5% v/v or 41 to 42% w/w and is prepared by mixing equal volumes of Alcohol (*U.S.P.*) and water.

Alcoholic strength is expressed as a percentage by volume of alcohol. It was previously often expressed in terms of *proof spirit*. Proof spirit contained about 57.1% v/v or 49.2% w/w of C_2H_5OH, and was defined as 'that which at the temperature of 51° F weighs exactly twelve-thirteenths of an equal measure of distilled water'. Spirit of such a strength that 100 volumes contained as much ethyl alcohol as 160 volumes of proof spirit was described as '60 OP' (over proof). Spirit of which 100 volumes contained as much alcohol as 40 volumes of proof spirit was described as '60 UP' (under proof). An alternative method of indicating spirit strength was used on the labels of alcoholic beverages in the *UK* when the strength was given as a number of degrees, proof spirit being taken as 100°. In the *USA* alcoholic strength is expressed in degrees, the value of which is equal to twice the percentage by volume. Thus 70° proof (old *UK* system) is equivalent to 40% v/v, and therefore to 80° proof (*USA* system).

Adverse Effects

The concentration of alcohol in the blood producing a state of intoxication varies between individuals. Low to moderate concentrations of alcohol depress cortical function causing loss of judgement, emotional lability, muscle inco-ordination, visual impairment, slurred speech, and ataxia. Hangover effects may include nausea, headache, dizziness, and tremor. Higher concentrations of alcohol depress medullary action; lethargy, amnesia, hypothermia, hypoglycaemia (especially in children), stupor, coma, respiratory depression, and cardiovascular collapse may occur. The median lethal blood-alcohol concentration is generally estimated to be approximately 400 to 500 mg per 100 mL. Death may occur at lower blood-alcohol concentrations due to inhalation of vomit during unconsciousness.

It is an offence in many countries for motorists to drive when the blood-alcohol concentration is above a stated value. The alcohol concentration in expired air and urine can be used to estimate the blood-alcohol concentration.

Chronic intoxication with alcohol may cause damage to many organs, particularly the brain and the liver. Brain damage may lead to Korsakoff's syndrome and Wernicke's encephalopathy. Fat deposits may occur in the liver and there may be a reduction in various blood-cell counts. Nutritional diseases may occur due to inadequate diet.

Alcoholism is dependence of the barbiturate-alcohol type (see p.706) and usually involves tolerance to other sedatives and anaesthetics.

Frequent application of alcohol to the skin produces irritation and dry skin.

There are many references to alcohol and pregnancy. A foetal alcohol syndrome has been identified in which infants born to some alcoholic mothers have characteristic features and abnormalities. There have been some reports of the syndrome being associated with moderate alcohol intake in pregnancy.

In Great Britain the recommended exposure limit of alcohol is 1000 ppm (long-term).

DEPENDENCE. Adverse clinical and behavioural manifestations, including dependence and cirrhosis of the liver, tended to become apparent in persons with an average daily consumption of more than 150 mL of absolute alcohol for prolonged periods. Studies of selected groups of heavy drinkers (total about 12 500) showed that the death-rate from all causes was 2 to 4 times higher than in the general population.— Twentieth Report of the WHO Expert Committee on Drug Dependence, *Tech. Rep. Ser. Wld Hlth Org. No. 551*, 1974; Report of a WHO Expert Committee on Problems Related to Alcohol Consumption, *Tech. Rep. Ser. Wld Hlth Org. No. 650*, 1980.

Treatment of Adverse Effects

In acute poisoning the stomach may be emptied by aspiration and lavage if indicated. If respiration is depressed, assisted respiration may be necessary. It is important to provide good supportive treatment and to keep the patient warm. Fluid balance should be maintained by the use of suitable electrolyte solutions, and glucose may be needed for the treatment of hypoglycaemia. Intravenous infusions of fructose have been used to treat severe alcohol poisoning but as these may produce metabolic acidosis and other unpleasant side-effects their use is controversial. Haemodialysis or peritoneal dialysis is of value in severe alcoholic poisoning.

In chronic alcoholics withdrawal syndromes occurring in the presence of declining plasma concentrations of alcohol vary from mild to possibly fatal delirium tremens. Sedatives may be given to prevent or suppress withdrawal symptoms; chlormethiazole is one of the agents commonly used.

For the long-term treatment of alcoholics, see disulfiram (p.1566) and citrated calcium carbimide (p.1558).

Intravenous administration of glucose 25 g to 8 pregnant women did not reverse the suppression of foetal breathing movements produced by 0.25 g per kg body-weight of alcohol by mouth.— W. McLeod *et al.*, *Am. J. Obstet. Gynec.*, 1984, *148*, 634.

Jefferys and Volans of the British National Poisons Information Service reported that alcohol-induced coma was completely reversed within 10 minutes in patients given a dose of at least 1.2 mg of naloxone by the intravenous route (*Hum. Toxicol.*, 1983, *2*, 227). Cholewa *et al.* (*ibid.*, 217) reported that naloxone reduced the duration of alcohol-induced coma, but did not reverse it. Another study failed to show that naloxone effectively reverses alcohol intoxication (E. Nuotto *et al.*, *Lancet*, 1983, *2*, 167). In view of the lack of agreement between these studies, it has been suggested that there is no real justification for using naloxone to treat alcohol intoxication (*Lancet*, 1983, *2*, 145).

A brief discussion of propylthiouracil in alcoholic liver disease.— *Lancet*, 1988, *1*, 450.

Precautions

Alcohol may aggravate peptic ulcer, impaired liver or kidney function, diabetes mellitus, and epilepsy. Ingestion of alcohol during pregnancy or by nursing mothers is not advisable.

In chronic alcoholics there may be tolerance to the effects of other central nervous system depressants including general anaesthetics.

All processes requiring judgement and co-ordination are affected by alcohol and these include the driving of any form of transport and the operating of machinery.

Reports of interactions between alcohol and other drugs are not consistent, possibly because acute alcohol intake may inhibit drug metabolism while chronic alcohol intake may enhance the induction of drug-metabolising enzymes in the liver. Alcoholic beverages may cause reactions when taken by patients receiving monoamine oxidase inhibitors. Alcohol may enhance the acute effects of drugs which depress the central nervous system, such as hypnotics, antihistamines, muscle relaxants, opioid analgesics, antiepileptics, antidepressants, and tranquillisers. Unpleasant reactions, similar to those occurring with disulfiram (see p.1566), may occur when alcohol is taken concomitantly with chlorpropamide, metronidazole, and some cephalosporins.

Alcohol may cause hypoglycaemic reactions in patients receiving sulphonylurea antidiabetic agents or insulin, and may cause orthostatic hypotension in patients taking drugs with vasodilator action. It should be remembered that alcohol may be present in a number of pharmaceutical preparations such as elixirs and mouthwashes, and that children may be particularly susceptible to its hypoglycaemic effects.

INTERACTIONS. Reviews of interactions between alcohol and other drugs.— G. T. McInnes, *Prescribers' J.*, 1985, *25*, 87; E. A. Lane *et al.*, *Clin. Pharmacokinet.*, 1985, *10*, 228.

Absorption and Fate

Alcohol is rapidly absorbed from the gastro-intestinal tract and is distributed throughout the body fluids. It readily crosses the placenta. Alcohol vapour can be absorbed through the lungs.

Alcohol is mainly metabolised in the liver; it is converted by alcohol dehydrogenase to acetaldehyde and is then further oxidised to acetate. A hepatic microsomal oxidising system is also involved. About 90% to 98% of alcohol is oxidised and the remainder is excreted unchanged by the kidneys and the lungs and also in breast milk, saliva, sweat, and other secretions.

The rate of absorption of alcohol from the stomach may be modified by such factors as the presence of food and the period of time during which the alcohol is ingested; small volumes of alcohol are rapidly absorbed from an empty stomach.

The rate of metabolism may be accelerated following repeated excessive use and by certain substances including insulin and thyroxine. Rapid ingestion of alcohol may lead to accumulation and subsequent prolongation of its effects.

Absorption of alcohol through the intact skin is said to be negligible.

PREGNANCY AND THE NEONATE. A review of drug excretion in breast milk. Alcohol is freely secreted into milk in concentrations slightly below those in blood.— J. T. Wilson *et al.*, *Clin. Pharmacokinet.*, 1980, *5*, 1.

Uses and Administration

Alcohol has bactericidal activity and is used, often as methylated spirits, to disinfect skin prior to injection, venepuncture, or surgical procedures. A concentration of 70% is commonly employed. Alcohol should not be used for disinfection of surgical or dental instruments because of its low efficacy against bacterial spores.

Alcohol also has anhidrotic, astringent, and rubefacient properties. It is sometimes used to harden the skin in order to prevent bedsores.

Alcohol is widely used as a solvent and preservative in pharmaceutical preparations.

Severe and chronic pain including that caused by trigeminal neuralgia may be relieved by injection of alcohol close to the nerve. Intrathecal injection of alcohol has also been used in the treatment of spasticity. Alcohol is given intravenously in the treatment of acute poisoning from methyl alcohol (see p.1429).

Alcohol has been given in the suppression of essential tremor.

DIAGNOSTIC USE. Topical use of alcohol to aid detection of anaesthesia of the skin in patients with leprosy.— B. Rojas (letter), *Lepr. Rev.*, 1984, *55*, 182.

PAIN. It is doubtful whether alcohol or phenol have any place in peripheral nerve blocks as the analgesia is commonly patchy and there is a definite incidence of neuritis, but one exception is the injection of alcohol 40% into the muscle sheath of patients with painful muscular spasms in multiple sclerosis.— J. W. Lloyd, *Br. med. J.*, 1980, *281*, 432.

SCLEROTHERAPY. The use of alcohol as a sclerosant to produce infarction of the tumour veins of a 55-year-old woman with an aldosterone-producing adenoma.— C. J. Mathias *et al.*, *Br. med. J.*, 1984, *288*, 1416.

Beneficial results in 6 patients following treatment of hepatic cysts with aspiration and injection of alcohol.— W. J. Bean and B. A. Rodan, *Am. J. Roentg.*, 1985, *144*, 237.

Evidence of the efficacy and safety of absolute alcohol as a sclerosant in the treatment of patients with oesophageal varices using endoscopic sclerotherapy at weekly intervals.— S. K. Sarin *et al.*, *Gut*, 1985, *26*, 120. Of 17 patients with oesophageal varices treated every 2 weeks by endoscopic sclerotherapy using absolute alcohol as the sclerosant, 13 developed complications and 2 died. It was felt that its use as a sclerosant should be avoided.— D. K. Bhargava *et al.* (letter), *Gut*, 1986, *27*, 1518.

TREMOR. Intravenous administration of alcohol decreased essential tremor in all of 15 male patients, whereas only 11 of them responded to propranolol.— W. C. Koller and N. Biary, *Neurology*, 1984, *34*, 221.

VIRAL DISINFECTION. For the use of alcohol for the disinfection of surfaces contaminated with human immunodeficiency virus, see p.950.

Preparations

Alcohol and Dextrose Injection *(U.S.P.)*. A sterile solution of alcohol and glucose in Water for Injections.

Dehydrated Alcohol Injection *(U.S.P.)*

Rubbing Alcohol *(U.S.P.)*. Prepared from specially denatured alcohol and containing 68.5 to 71.5% v/v of dehydrated alcohol.

Spirit Ear-drops *(B.P.C. 1973)*. Auristillae Spiritus. Alcohol 50 mL, water to 100 mL. *A.P.F.* (Spirit Ear Drops) has alcohol (90%) 50 mL, freshly boiled and cooled water to 100 mL.

Proprietary Names and Manufacturers

Duonalc-E *(ICN, Canad.)*.

2203-a

Ambazone *(BAN, rINN)*.

Ambazonum. 4-Amidinohydrazonocyclohexa-2,5-dien-1-one thiosemicarbazone monohydrate.

$C_8H_{11}N_7S,H_2O$=255.3.

CAS — 539-21-9 (anhydrous); 6011-12-7 (monohydrate).

Pharmacopoeias. In *Roum.*

Ambazone is an antimicrobial agent which is used in the form of 10-mg lozenges for minor infections of the mouth and pharynx.

Proprietary Names and Manufacturers

Bridal *(Bayer, Neth.)*; Iversal *(Bayer, Fr.; Bayer, Ger.)*; Primal *(Bayer, Ital.; Bayer, Switz.)*; Primals *(Bayer, Norw.)*.

2204-t

Aminacrine Hydrochloride *(BANM, USAN)*.

Aminoacridine Hydrochloride *(rINNM)*; NSC-7571.

9-Aminoacridine hydrochloride monohydrate.

$C_{13}H_{10}N_2,HCl,H_2O$=248.7.

CAS — 90-45-9 (aminacrine); 134-50-9 (hydrochloride, anhydrous).

Pharmacopoeias. In *Arg.* and *Nord.*

Aminacrine has properties similar to those of other acridine derivatives (see p.969). It is applied locally for minor wounds and infections.

It is sometimes preferred to proflavine as it is non-staining.

Proprietary Names and Manufacturers

Aminopt *(Sigma, Austral.)*.

The following names have been used for multi-ingredient preparations containing aminacrine hydrochloride—AVC *(Merrell Dow, Canad.)*; Calistaflex *(Glaxo, Austral.)*; Medi Creme *(Rosken, Austral.)*; Medijel *(Key, Austral.; DDD, UK)*; Morrhuol Acridine Cream *(Hamilton, Austral.)*; Triva Jel *(Boyle, USA)*; Vagimide *(Legere, USA)*.

2205-x

Amylmetacresol *(BAN, rINN)*.

6-Pentyl-*m*-cresol; 5-Methyl-2-pentylphenol.

$C_{12}H_{18}O$=178.3.

CAS — 1300-94-3.

Pharmacopoeias. In *Br.*

A clear or almost clear liquid or a solid crystalline mass with a characteristic odour, colourless or slightly yellow when freshly prepared; it darkens on keeping. M.p. about 22°. Practically **insoluble** in water; soluble in alcohol, ether, and oils. **Store** in well-closed containers. Protect from light.

Amylmetacresol is a disinfectant used chiefly in minor infections of the mouth and throat.

Proprietary Preparations

Strepsils *(Crookes Healthcare, UK)*. *Lozenges*, amylmetacresol 600 µg, dichlorobenzyl alcohol 1.2 mg.

Lozenges, (Strepsils Honey and Lemon) contain the same active ingredients as Strepsils in a flavoured basis.

Lozenges, (Strepsils with vitamin C) contain the same active ingredients as Strepsils with ascorbic acid 100 mg.

Proprietary Names and Manufacturers

Mac *(Manetti Roberts, Ital.)*.

The following names have been used for multi-ingredient preparations containing amylmetacresol— Strepsils *(Boots, Austral.; Crookes Healthcare, UK)*.

2206-r

Benzalkonium Chloride *(BAN, USAN, rINN)*.

Benzalkonii Chloridum; Benzalkonium Chloratum; Cloreto de Benzalconio. A mixture of alkylbenzyldimethylammonium chlorides of the general formula $[C_6H_5.CH_2.N(CH_3)_2.R]Cl$, in which R represents a mixture of the alkyls from C_8H_{17} to $C_{18}H_{37}$. The *B.P.* specifies that it contains not less than 95% and not more than 104% of alkylbenzyldimethylammonium chlorides, calculated as $C_{22}H_{40}ClN$ with reference to the anhydrous substance. The *U.S.N.F.* specifies not less than 40% of the $C_{12}H_{25}$ compound, calculated on the dried substance, not less than 20% of the $C_{14}H_{29}$ compound, and not less than 70% of these 2 compounds. *Egypt.* specifies R from C_6H_{13} to $C_{18}H_{37}$.

CAS — 8001-54-5.

Pharmacopoeias. In *Arg., Aust., Belg., Braz., Br., Egypt., Eur., Fr., Hung., Int., It., Jpn, Jug., Neth., Port., Swiss,* and *Turk.* Also in *U.S.N.F. Chin.* includes benzalkonium bromide.

A white or yellowish-white powder, thick gel, or gelatinous pieces with a mild aromatic odour. It forms a clear molten mass on heating. The *B.P.* specifies that it contains not more than 10% of water; the *U.S.P.* specifies not more than 15%.

Very **soluble** in water and alcohol; the anhydrous form is slightly soluble in ether. A solution in water is usually slightly alkaline and foams strongly when shaken.

Incompatible with soaps and other anionic surfactants, citrates, iodides, nitrates, permanganates, salicylates, silver salts, and tartrates. Incompatibilities have been demonstrated with ingredients of some commercial rubber mixes or plastics. Incompatibilities have also been reported with other substances including aluminium, cotton dressings, fluorescein sodium, hydrogen peroxide, kaolin, hydrous wool fat, and some sulphonamides. **Store** in airtight containers.

Adverse Effects, Treatment, and Precautions

As for Cetrimide, p.953.

ALLERGY. An allergic reaction in one patient to benzalkonium chloride used as a preservative in nose drops and confirmed by challenge which produced nasal congestion and irritation of the eyes and throat lasting 48 hours.— G. Hillerdal, *J. Otorhinolaryngol. Borderl.*, 1985, *47*, 278.

The view that the production of bronchoconstriction in an asthmatic patient after nebulised beclomethasone dipropionate was due to benzalkonium chloride, present as a preservative. It was recommended that nebuliser solutions are formulated without benzalkonium chloride.— R. Beasley *et al.* (letter), *Lancet*, 1986, *2*, 1227. Six asthmatic patients developed bronchoconstriction after inhaling 4 mL of a nebulised isotonic ipratropium bromide formulation preserved with benzalkonium chloride and edetic acid (Atrovent), but showed bronchodilatation after inhaling 4 mL of a preservative-free formulation. Inhalation of the preservatives administered separately produced dose-related bronchoconstriction, persisting for over 60 minutes.— *idem, Br. med. J.*, 1987, *294*, 1197.

EFFECTS ON THE EAR. Benzalkonium chloride has been reported to be ototoxic.— J. L. Honigman (letter), *Pharm. J.*, 1975, *2*, 523.

EFFECTS ON THE EYE. Inflammation of the eye and deterioration of vision 3 days after change of soaking solution, for a soft contact lens, to one containing benzalkonium chloride.— A. R. Gasset, *Am. J. Ophthal.*, 1977, *84*, 169.

Uses and Administration

Benzalkonium chloride is a quaternary ammonium disinfectant with properties and uses similar to those of the other cationic surfactants as described under cetrimide (p.954).

Solutions of benzalkonium chloride 0.02 to 0.1% have been used for cleansing skin, mucous membranes, and wounds. A 0.02 to 0.05% solution has been used as a vaginal douche. An aqueous solution usually not stronger than 0.005% has been used for irrigation of the bladder and urethra and a 0.0025% solution for retention lavage of the bladder.

Creams containing benzalkonium chloride are used in the treatment of napkin rash.

A 0.2 to 0.5% solution is used as a shampoo in seborrhoeic dermatitis.

Benzalkonium lozenges are used for the treatment of superficial infections of the mouth and throat.

A 0.01% solution of benzalkonium chloride is used as a preservative for some eye-drops of the *B.P.* and *U.S.P.* It is not suitable for eye-drops containing local anaesthetics. Because some rubbers are incompatible with benzalkonium chloride the *B.P.C. 1973* recommended that, unless the suitability has been established, silicone rubber teats be used on eye-drop containers. Benzalkonium chloride is unsuitable as a preservative in solutions for washing and storing soft contact lenses of hydrophilic plastic.

Benzalkonium chloride is also used as a vaginal spermicide in the form of a 0.9 to 1.2% cream.

Benzalkonium chloride has also been used topically in herpes simplex infections.

Benzalkonium bromide has been similarly used.

The antibacterial effect of benzalkonium chloride (0.003%) was enhanced by 0.175% of benzyl alcohol, phenylpropanol, or phenethyl alcohol. The effect was more than additive, was most pronounced in respect of phenylpropanol, and least pronounced in respect of benzyl alcohol.— R. M. E. Richards and R. J. McBride, *J. pharm. Sci.*, 1973, *62*, 2035.

For the use of phenethyl alcohol with benzalkonium chloride as a preservative for ophthalmic solutions, see Phenethyl Alcohol, p.1361.

SPERMICIDE. In addition to inhibiting sperm motility there is evidence that benzalkonium chloride has been reported to disturb the electrolyte balance in the aqueous phase of cervical mucus, making it hostile to sperm.— R. M. Pearson, *Pharm. J.*, 1985, *1*, 686.

Preparations of Benzalkonium Salts

Benzalkonium Lozenges *(B.P.C. 1973).* Benzalkonium Chloride Lozenges. *Lozenges*, benzalkonium chloride solution 0.001 mL, menthol 600 µg, thymol 600 µg, eucalyptus oil 0.002 mL, and lemon oil 0.002 mL.

Benzalkonium Chloride Solution *(B.P., B.P. Vet.)*

Benzalkonium Chloride Solution *(U.S.N.F.)*

Benzalkonium Solution Compound *(A.P.F.).* Hard Contact Lens Solution. Benzalkonium chloride solution 0.02 mL, disodium edetate 50 mg, sodium chloride 900 mg, Water for Injections to 100 mL. Sterilised by autoclaving.

Proprietary Preparations of Benzalkonium Salts

Capitol *(Dermal Laboratories, UK). Gel*, benzalkonium chloride 0.5%.

Cetanorm *(Norma, UK). Cream*, benzalkonium chloride 0.1%, aldioxa 0.375%, chlorbutol 0.1%, cetrimide 0.4%, and nonoxinol '9' 2%.

Conotrane *(Boehringer Ingelheim, UK). Cream*, benzalkonium chloride 0.1%, dimethicone '350' 22%.

Drapolene *(Calmic, UK). Cream*, benzalkonium chloride 0.01%, cetrimide 0.2% in a water-miscible basis.

Roccal *(Winthrop, UK). Solution*, benzalkonium chloride 1%.

Solution (Roccal Concentrate 10X), benzalkonium chloride 10%.

Torbetol *(Torbet Laboratories, UK). Lotion*, benzalkonium chloride 0.05%, cetrimide 0.7%, hexachlorophane 0.75%. *Shampoo*, see p.954.

Proprietary Names and Manufacturers of Benzalkonium Salts

Alpagelle *(Pharmascience, Fr.)*; Armil *(Squibb, Spain)*; Baktonium *(Bode, Ger.)*; Benzalc *(Asens, Spain)*; Benzalchlor-50 *(Canad.)*; Benzalkon *(DAK, Denm.; NLH, Norw.)*; Benzaltex *(Atlantic, Switz.)*; Capitol *(Dermal Laboratories, UK)*; Cetal Conc. A and B *(Orapharm, Austral.)*; Cycloton B50 *(Witco, UK)*; Dermo-Sterol *(Bio-Chemical Laboratory, Canad.)*; Empigen BAC *(Albright & Wilson, Marchon Division, UK)*; Germiphene *(Stickley, Canad.)*; Hyamine 3500 *(Rohm & Haas, UK)*; Ice-O-Derm *(Wampole, Canad.)*; Laudamonium *(Henkel, Ger.)*; Lindemil *(Spain)*; Lysoform-Killavon *(Lysoform, Ger.)*; Morpan BC *(ABM Chemicals, UK)*; Oraldettes *(Parke, Davis, S.Afr.)*; Pameb *(Bio-Chemical Laboratory, Canad.)*; Pentalcol *(Pental, Spain)*; Pharmatex *(Interpharm, Canad.; Pharmelac, Fr.)*; Quartamon *(Schulke & Mayr, Ger.)*; Roccal *(Winthrop, UK)*; Rodalon *(Ferrosan, Denm.)*; Sabol *(Horner, Canad.)*; Silquat *(Tenneco, UK)*; Tearisol *(Inibsa, Spain)*; Vantoc CL *(ICI Organics, UK)*; Zephiran *(Winthrop, Austral.; Winthrop, Canad.; Winthrop-Breon, USA)*; Zephirol *(Bayer, Ger.)*.

The following names have been used for multi-ingredient preparations containing benzalkonium salts—Amino-Cerv *(Milex, USA)*; Bactine *(Miles, Canad.)*; Benzets *(Norton, UK)*; Callusolve *(Dermal Laboratories, UK)*; Cetanorm *(Norma, UK)*; Cetylcide *(Cetylite, USA)*; Conotrane *(Boehringer Ingelheim, UK)*; Drapolene *(Calmic, UK)*; Drapolex *(Wellcome, Canad.)*; Ionax Scrub *(Alcon, Canad.; Alcon, UK)*; Ionil *(Alcon, Canad.; Owen, USA)*; Ionil T *(Alcon, Canad.; Alcon, UK; Owen, USA)*; Polycide *(Cottrell, UK)*; Stomobar *(Thackray, UK)*; Stomogel *(Thackray, UK)*; Stomogol Concentrate *(Thackray, UK)*; Toracsol *(Torbet Laboratories, UK)*; Torbetol Lotion *(Torbet Laboratories, UK)*; Torbetol Shampoo *(Torbet Laboratories, UK)*.

NOTE. The name Conotrane was formerly used to denote a preparation containing hydrargaphen

---

2207-f

Benzethonium Chloride *(BAN, USAN, rINN).*

Benzethonii Chloridum. Benzyldimethyl(2-{2-[4-(1,1,3,3-tetramethylbutyl)phenoxy]ethoxy}ethyl)ammonium chloride.

$C_{27}H_{42}ClNO_2$=448.1.

CAS — 121-54-0.

Pharmacopoeias. In *Arg., Egypt., Int., Jpn, Nord.,* and *U.S.*

White crystals with a mild odour.

Soluble 1 in less than 1 of water, alcohol, and chloroform; slightly soluble in ether. A 1% solution in water is slightly alkaline to litmus and foams strongly when shaken. **Incompatible** with soaps and other anionic surfactants. **Store** in airtight containers. Protect from light.

Benzethonium chloride is a quaternary ammonium disinfectant with properties and uses similar to those of other cationic surfactants as described under cetrimide (p.953).

Benzethonium chloride produced mild skin irritation at a concentration of 5% but not lower, was not considered to be a sensitiser, and was considered to be safe at a concentration of 0.5% in cosmetics applied to the skin and at a maximum concentration of 0.02% in cosmetics used in the eye area.— The Expert Panel of the American College of Toxicology, *J. Am. Coll. Toxicol.*, 1985, *4*, 65.

Preparations

Benzethonium Chloride Tincture *(U.S.P.).* Benzethonium chloride 200 mg, alcohol 68.5 mL, acetone 10 mL, and water to 100 mL; it may be coloured. Inflammable.

Benzethonium Chloride Topical Solution *(U.S.P.)*

Proprietary Names and Manufacturers

Benzalcan *(Switz.)*; Desamon *(Switz.)*; Formula Magic *(Consolidated Chemical, USA)*; Hyamine 1622 *(Rohm & Haas, UK)*; Phemerol Chloride *(USA)*.

The following names have been used for multi-ingredient preparations containing benzethonium chloride—Buro-Sol *(Trans Canaderm, Canad.)*; Dermoplast *(Ayerst, Austral.; Ayerst, Canad.; Torbet Laboratories, UK)*.

2208-d

Benzododecinium Bromide

Benzyldodecyldimethylammonium bromide.

$C_{21}H_{38}BrN$=384.4.

CAS — 10328-35-5 (benzododecinium); 7281-04-1 (bromide).

NOTE. Benzododecinium Chloride is *rINN*.

Pharmacopoeias. In *Cz.*

Benzododecinium bromide is a quaternary ammonium disinfectant present in benzalkonium bromide. It is available in a variety of preparations for the local treatment of minor infections. It is also used as a spermicide. Benzododecinium chloride has also been used.

Proprietary Names and Manufacturers of Benzodocecinium and its Salts

Benzo-Davur *(Davur, Spain)*; Humex *(Fournier S.A., Fr.)*; Prorhinel *(Monal, Fr.; Interdelta, Switz.)*; Rewoquat B 50 *(Rewo, UK)*.

2209-n

Bisdequalinium Diacetate

R-199. 1,1′-Decamethylene-*NN*′-decamethylenebis(4-amino-2-methylquinolinium acetate).

$C_{44}H_{64}N_4O_4$=713.0.

Bisdequalinium diacetate is a bis-quaternary ammonium disinfectant applied topically in the treatment of a variety of minor infections.

Proprietary Names and Manufacturers

Alsol *(Also, Ital.)*; Salvizol *(Belg.; Ravensberg, Ger.; Vernleigh, S.Afr.; Grossmann, Switz.)*.

2211-a

Brilliant Green *(BAN)*.

CI Basic Green 1; Colour Index No. 42040; Viride Nitens. 4-(4-Diethylaminobenzhydrylidene)cyclohexa-2,5-dien-1-ylidenediethylammonium hydrogen sulphate.

$C_{27}H_{34}N_2O_4S$=482.6.

CAS — 633-03-4.

Pharmacopoeias. In *Hung*.

Viride Nitens (*Rus. P.*) is the oxalate.

Brilliant green is a disinfectant effective against vegetative Gram-positive bacteria but less effective against Gram-negative organisms and ineffective against acid-fast bacteria and bacterial spores. Its activity is greatly reduced in the presence of serum. A gel containing brilliant green 0.5% with lactic acid has been used in the treatment of ulcers.

A solution of brilliant green 0.5% and crystal violet 0.5% has been used for disinfecting the skin. However, concern at evidence of *animal* carcinogenicity with crystal violet has led to the decline of such paints. However, a paint consisting of this solution of the two disinfectants is still favoured by some surgeons for the marking of incisions, see p.960.

There have been occasional reports of sensitivity to brilliant green.

Proprietary Preparations

Variclene *(Dermal Laboratories, UK). Gel*, brilliant green 0.5% w/w, lactic acid 0.5% w/w.

The treatment of venous ulcers using Variclene.— C. F. Allenby *et al., Br. J. clin. Pract.*, 1983, *37*, 382.

2289-k

Bromsalans

A series of brominated salicylanilides which possess antimicrobial activity.

CAS — 55830-61-0.

2290-w

Dibromsalan *(USAN, pINN)*.

NSC-20527. 4′,5-Dibromosalicylanilide; 5-Bromo-*N*-(4-bromophenyl)-2-hydroxybenzamide.

$C_{13}H_9Br_2NO_2$=371.0.

CAS — 87-12-7.

2291-e

Metabromsalan *(USAN, pINN)*.

NSC-526280. 3,5-Dibromosalicylanilide; 3,5-Dibromo-2-hydroxy-*N*-phenylbenzamide.

$C_{13}H_9Br_2NO_2$=371.0.

CAS — 2577-72-2.

2213-x

Tribromsalan *(BAN, USAN, rINN)*.

ET-394; NSC-20526; TBS. 3,4′,5-Tribromosalicylanilide; 3,5-Dibromo-*N*-(4-bromophenyl)-2-hydroxybenzamide.

$C_{13}H_8Br_3NO_2$=449.9.

CAS — 87-10-5.

Bromsalans have antibacterial and antifungal activity and were used in medicated soaps, but there have been many reports of photosensitivity arising from this use. In the *UK* the maximum concentration of tribromsalan in soaps is restricted to 1% by law. The purity of the tribromsalan must not be less than 98.5%. Other bromsalans not to exceed 1.5%. 1′,5-Dibromosalan not to exceed 0.1%.

Proprietary Names and Manufacturers of Bromsalans

Diaphene *(Stecker, USA)*; Temasept I *(Hexcel, USA)*; Temasept IV *(Hexcel, USA)*.

2214-r

Cetalkonium Chloride *(BAN, USAN, rINN)*.

NSC-32942. Benzylhexadecyldimethylammonium chloride.

$C_{25}H_{46}ClN$=396.1.

CAS — 122-18-9.

Cetalkonium chloride is a quaternary ammonium disinfectant with properties and uses similar to those of other cationic surfactants as described under cetrimide (below).

Proprietary Names and Manufacturers

The following names have been used for multi-ingredient preparations containing cetalkonium chloride—AAA Mouth and Throat Spray *(Armour, UK)*; AAA Throat Spray *(USV, Austral.)*; Throsil *(Cox, UK)*.

2215-f

Cethexonium Bromide

Hexadecyl(2-hydroxycyclohexyl)dimethylammonium bromide.

$C_{24}H_{50}BrNO$=448.6.

CAS — 6810-42-0 (cethexonium); 1794-74-7 (bromide).

Pharmacopoeias. In *Fr.*

Cethexonium bromide is a quaternary ammonium disinfectant (see cetrimide, below). It is available in a variety of forms for the local treatment of minor infections.

Proprietary Names and Manufacturers

Biocidan *(Clin Midy, Fr.)*.

2216-d

Cetrimide *(BAN, rINN)*.

Cetrimide consists chiefly of trimethyltetradecylammonium bromide (= tetradonium bromide) together with smaller amounts of dodecyl- and hexadecyltrimethylammonium bromides. It contains not less than 96% of alkyltrimethylammonium bromides calculated as $C_{17}H_{38}BrN$ =336.4.

CAS — 505-86-2.

NOTE. The name cetrimonium bromide was often formerly applied to cetrimide. Cetrimonium bromide (CTAB; cetyltrimethylammonium bromide) is hexadecyltrimethylammonium bromide.

Pharmacopoeias. In *Aust., Belg., Br., Braz., Egypt., Eur., Fr., Ger., Ind., Int., It., Jug., Neth., Swiss,* and *Turk*. Also in *B.P. Vet.*

A white to almost white, voluminous, free-flowing powder with a faint characteristic odour.

Soluble 1 in 2 of water; freely soluble in alcohol and chloroform; practically insoluble in ether. **Incompatible** with soaps and other anionic surfactants, bentonite, iodine, phenylmercuric nitrate, and alkali hydroxides.

Strong Cetrimide Solution (*B.P.*) contains 20 to 40% cetrimide and up to 10% alcohol or isopropyl alcohol as a preservative; 1% aqueous solutions prepared from this may be sterilised by autoclaving.

For precautions to be taken in preparing and storing disinfectant and antiseptic solutions, see under Precautions, below.

Isolates from 63 hospital patients revealed *Pseudomonas maltophilia*, the source being deionised water used for making Savlon solutions.— M. M. Wishart and T. V. Riley, *Med. J. Aust.*, 1976, *2*, 710.

Adverse Effects and Treatment

When taken by mouth, cetrimide and other quaternary ammonium compounds cause nausea and vomiting; strong solutions may cause oesophageal damage and necrosis. They have depolarising muscle relaxant properties and toxic symptoms include dyspnoea and cyanosis due to paralysis of the respiratory muscles, possibly leading to asphyxia. Depression of the central nervous system (possibly preceded by excitement and with convulsions), hypotension, and coma may also occur. Intra-uterine or intravenous administration may cause haemolysis.

At the concentrations used on the skin, solutions of cetrimide and other quaternary compounds do not generally cause irritation, but some patients become hypersensitive to cetrimide after repeated applications. There have been rare reports of burns with concentrated solutions of cetrimide.

Treatment of poisoning is symptomatic; demulcents should be given if necessary but emesis and lavage avoided.

The fatal dose of quaternary ammonium detergents was estimated to be 1 to 3 g.— J. M. Arena, *J. Am. med. Ass.*, 1964, *190*, 56.

Chemical peritonitis associated with cetrimide washout after hydatid cyst surgery.— D. S. Gilchrist (letter), *Lancet*, 1979, *2*, 1374. Following liberal irrigation of multiple large hydatid cysts of the liver with cetrimide solution 0.1%, a 45-year-old woman developed methaemoglobinaemia with deep cyanosis. This was reversed by intravenous methylene blue 1 mg per kg body-weight. Whenever large amounts of cetrimide are used clinicians should be prepared to reverse the methaemoglobinaemia that may ensue.— A. Baraka *et al.* (letter), *Lancet*, 1980, *2*, 88. Metabolic acidosis developed in a 44-year-old man after the use of more than 1 litre of aqueous cetrimide solution 1% to sterilise hydatid cysts during surgery. Sustained alkalinisation and fluid loading led to rapid recovery. It was proposed that the acidosis was due to the large amount of cetrimide (pH 6) resorbed by cyst walls and peritoneum, and blood pH monitoring was suggested after operations on hydatid cysts, especially when large quantities of cetrimide had been used.— P. Momblano *et al.* (letter), *Lancet*, 1984, *2*, 1045.

Dilutions down to 1 in 1500 of an antiseptic preparation

containing cetrimide 15% and chlorhexidine gluconate 1.5% were found to be toxic to *mouse* connective tissue fibroblasts. Subsequent investigations revealed that that was due to the cetrimide present in the mixture. When dilutions of the individual components were examined, chlorhexidine failed to induce any detectable morphological changes when used in normal concentrations but cetrimide was found to be toxic at levels of 100 µg per mL. (The 2 dilutions most commonly used as antiseptics, 1 in 30 and 1 in 100, contain 5000 µg and 1500 µg of cetrimide respectively). It was suggested that in the absence of signs of clinical infection, basic wound toilet should consist of cleansing with an isotonic solution of saline. If an antimicrobial agent is required, a sterile solution of chlorhexidine should be considered, but the repeated application to an open wound of solutions containing cetrimide or other similar materials is likely to adversely affect granulation and hence delay wound healing.— S. Thomas and N. P. Hay (letter), *Pharm. J.*, 1985, *2*, 206.

Precautions

Prolonged and repeated applications of cetrimide to the skin are inadvisable as hypersensitivity may occur. Contact with the eyes, brain, meninges, and middle ear should be avoided. Cetrimide should not be used in body cavities or as an enema.

The antimicrobial activity of quaternary ammonium compounds may be diminished through incompatibility (see above), through adsorption, or through combination with protein. Thus soaps, blood, cotton, cellulose, and other organic matter will reduce the effectiveness of these agents.

Because of problems of contamination, many disinfectants and antiseptics are provided for clinical use in a sterile form in single application packs. If a bulk pack is employed, any unused contents are usually discarded immediately. The dilution of concentrated solutions should be carried out using appropriate measures to prevent contamination.

Uses and Administration

Cetrimide is a quaternary ammonium disinfectant with properties and uses typical of cationic surfactants. These surfactants dissociate in aqueous solution into a relatively large and complex cation, which is responsible for the surface activity, and a smaller inactive anion. In addition to the emulsifying and detergent properties usually associated with surfactants, the quaternary ammonium compounds have bactericidal activity against Gram-positive and, at a higher concentration, against some Gram-negative organisms. Some *Pseudomonas* spp. are particularly resistant as are strains of *Mycobacterium tuberculosis*. Bacterial spores are likely to survive even prolonged contact with solutions of these compounds. Some quaternary ammonium compounds have good activity against *Candida albicans*, but antifungal activity is variable. They are relatively ineffective against viruses.

Quaternary ammonium compounds are most effective in neutral or slightly alkaline solution and their bactericidal activity is appreciably reduced in acid media. They are compatible with each other. Alcohols enhance the activity of quaternary ammonium compounds.

Quaternary ammonium compounds, particularly cetrimide and benzalkonium chloride, have been employed as aqueous solutions or creams for cleansing skin and wounds. A mixture of cetrimide with chlorhexidine (see p.955) is now more commonly used for these purposes.

Quaternary ammonium compounds are not reliable agents for sterilising surgical instruments and heat-labile articles.

Solutions containing 1 to 3% of cetrimide are used as shampoos to remove the scales in seborrhoea. Cetrimide solution has been used as a scolicide to irrigate hydatid cysts during surgery to prevent spilled scolicides forming further cysts.

Cetrimide is also present in some emulsifying preparations.

For reference to the use of cetrimide for the disinfection of silicone-foam dressings, see Chlorhexidine Hydrochloride, p.956.

HYDATID DISEASE. The treatment of hydatid cysts by cetrimide.— G. J. Frayha *et al.*, *Trans. R. Soc. trop. Med. Hyg.*, 1981, *75*, 447 (See also under Adverse Effects).

MALIGNANT NEOPLASMS. In an *in vitro* test of cytocidal agents, cetrimide, eusol, mercuric perchloride, noxythiolin, povidone iodine, and water, for potential use in colorectal cancer operations to prevent live cell exfoliation and possible local recurrence, only cetrimide 30% and 100% achieved 100% kill-rate of cells at all exposure times from 2 to 15 minutes.— M. Crowson *et al.*, *Gut*, 1985, *26*, A570. Noxythiolin and to a lesser extent chlorhexidine showed some activity *in vitro* against neoplastic cells.— J. I. Blenkharn, *J. Pharm. Pharmac.*, 1987, *39*, 477.

Preparations

Cetrimide and Chlorhexidine Paint *(A.P.F.)*. Cetrimide 500 mg, chlorhexidine gluconate solution 2.5 mL, alcohol 90% 75 mL, freshly boiled and cooled water to 100 mL.

Cetrimide Cream *(B.P.)*. It may be prepared to the following formula: cetrimide 500 mg (or a suitable quantity), cetostearyl alcohol 5 g, liquid paraffin 50 g, freshly boiled and cooled water to 100 g.
A.P.F. (Cetrimide Cream Aqueous) has a similar preparation with chlorocresol 0.1%.

Cetrimide Emulsifying Ointment *(B.P.)*. Cetrimide 3 g, cetostearyl alcohol 27 g, liquid paraffin 20 g, and white soft paraffin 50 g.

Cetrimide Shampoo *(A.P.F.)*. Cetrimide 40, alcohol (90%) 30, water 30. Dilute 1 in 20 before use.

Cetrimide Solution *(B.P.)*. Strong Cetrimide Solution equivalent to cetrimide 1 g, freshly boiled and cooled water to 100 mL. It must be freshly prepared. The solution may be sterilised by autoclaving. Cetrimide solutions should not be used more than 7 days after first opening the container.

Strong Cetrimide Solution *(B.P., B.P. Vet.)*. A 20% to 40% aqueous solution of cetrimide, containing not more than 10% v/v of alcohol, isopropyl alcohol, or industrial methylated spirit. It may be perfumed and may contain colouring matter.

Proprietary Preparations

Ceanel Concentrate *(Quinoderm, UK)*. *Liquid*, cetrimide 10%, undecenoic acid 1%, phenethyl alcohol 7.5%.

Cetavlex *(Care, UK)*. *Cream*, cetrimide 0.5%.

Cetavlon *(ICI Pharmaceuticals, UK)*. *Solution*, cetrimide 40%.

Cetavlon PC *(Care, UK)*. *Shampoo*, cetrimide 17.5%.

Sensitivity of *Malassezia* sp. to commercial shampoos including Cetavlon PC.— W. Butterfield *et al.*, *Br. J. Derm.*, 1987, *116*, 233.

Cetriclens *(Smith & Nephew, UK)*. *Sterile solution*, cetrimide 0.15%, chlorhexidine gluconate 0.015%.
Sterile solution (Cetriclens Forte), cetrimide 0.5%, chlorhexidine gluconate 0.05%.

Savloclens *(ICI Pharmaceuticals, UK)*. *Sterile solution*, cetrimide 0.5%, chlorhexidine gluconate 0.05%.

Savlodil *(ICI Pharmaceuticals, UK)*. *Sterile solution*, cetrimide 0.15%, chlorhexidine gluconate 0.015%.

Savlon Hospital Concentrate *(ICI Pharmaceuticals, UK)*. *Solution*, cetrimide 15%, chlorhexidine gluconate 1.5%.

Tisept *(Seton, UK)*. *Sterile solution*, cetrimide 0.15%, chlorhexidine gluconate 0.015%.

Torbetol *(Torbet Laboratories, UK)*. *Shampoo*, cetrimide 17.5%, Benzalkonium Chloride Solution 5.0% v/v. *Lotion*, see p.952.

Travasept *(Travenol, UK)*. *Sterile solution* (Travasept 30), cetrimide 0.5%, chlorhexidine acetate 0.05%.
Sterile solution (Travasept 100), cetrimide 0.15%, chlorhexidine acetate 0.015%.

Vesagex *(Leo, UK)*. *Ointment*, cetrimide 1%.

Proprietary Names and Manufacturers

Cetavlex *(ICI, Austral.; Care, UK)*; Cetavlon *(ICI, Austral.; Denm.; I.C.I.-Pharma, Fr.; ICI, S.Afr.; ICI, Spain; ICI Pharmaceuticals, UK)*; Cetavlon PC *(Care, UK)*; Cetoderm *(Nelson, Austral.)*; Cetridal *(Arg.)*; Crodex C *(Croda, UK)*; Cycloton *(Witco, UK)*; Dermanatal *(Arg.)*; Empigen *(Albright & Wilson, Marchon Division, UK)*; Morpan CHSA *(ABM Chemicals, UK)*; Savlon *(ICI, Austral.; Ayerst, Canad.)*; Seboderm *(Napp, UK)*; Silquat C100 *(Tenneco, UK)*; Solufen *(Arg.)*; Vesagex *(Leo, UK)*; Xylonor *(Prats, Spain)*.

The following names have been used for multi-ingredient preparations containing cetrimide—Acnil *(Fisons, UK)*; Ceanel Concentrate *(Quinoderm, UK)*; Cetal Liquid *(Orapharm, Austral.)*; Cetanorm *(Norma, UK)*; Cetriclens *(Smith & Nephew, UK)*; Dermocaine *(Ego, Austral.)*; Drapolene *(Calmic, UK)*; Drapolex *(Wellcome, Canad.)*; Dri-Wash Medical Cleansing Towelette *(Linton, UK)*; Ego Antiseptic Cream *(Ego, Austral.)*; Ego Antiseptic Liquid *(Ego, Austral.)*; Gomaxine *(Seaford, UK)*; Medi Creme *(Rosken, Austral.)*; Medi-Prep *(Pharmax, UK)*; Medi-Sache *(Pharmax, UK)*; Pentaid *(Pennwalt, Canad.)*; RBC Cream *(Rybar, UK)*; Savloclens *(ICI Pharmaceuticals, UK)*; Savlodil *(Ayerst, Canad.; ICI Pharmaceuticals, UK)*; Savlon Antiseptic *(ICI, Austral.; Care, UK)*; Savlon Hospital Concentrate *(ICI, Austral.; Ayerst, Canad.; ICI Pharmaceuticals, UK)*; Septex Cream No. 1 *(Norton, UK)*; Tisept *(Seton, UK)*; Toracsol *(Torbet Laboratories, UK)*; Torbetol Lotion *(Torbet Laboratories, UK)*; Torbetol Shampoo *(Torbet Laboratories, UK)*; Travasept *(Travenol, UK)*.

2217-n

Cetylpyridinium Chloride *(BAN, USAN, rINN)*.

1-Hexadecylpyridinium chloride monohydrate.
$C_{21}H_{38}ClN,H_2O = 358.0$.

CAS — 7773-52-6 (cetylpyridinium); 123-03-5 (chloride, anhydrous); 6004-24-6 (chloride, monohydrate).

Pharmacopoeias. In *Br., Egypt., Eur., Fr., Hung., Int., It., Neth., Nord., Swiss,* and *U.S.*

A white unctuous powder with a slight characteristic odour.

B.P. **solubilities** are: soluble 1 in 20 of water; very soluble in alcohol and chloroform; very slightly soluble in ether. *U.S.P.* solubilities are: soluble 1 in 4.5 of water and of chloroform, and 1 in 2.5 of alcohol. A 1% solution in water has a pH of 5.0 to 5.4. **Incompatible** with soaps and other anionic surfactants. **Store** in well-closed containers.

Cetylpyridinium chloride is a cationic disinfectant with properties and uses similar to those of other cationic surfactants as described under cetrimide (p.953). It is available in a variety of preparations for the local treatment of minor infections.

In a double-blind crossover study in 100 subjects, use of a mouth-wash containing cetylpyridinium chloride 0.05% after meals reduced plaque accumulation in all subjects.— J. D. Holbeche *et al.*, *Aust. dent. J.*, 1975, *20*, 397. A double-blind study of 75 patients demonstrated that a mouth-wash containing cetylpyridinium chloride 0.1%, used twice daily for 6 weeks, reduced both the amount of plaque and the severity of gingivitis compared with a control mouth-wash. There was a reduction in thickness rather than surface coverage of plaque and this was accompanied by changes in the biochemical composition of plaque.— F. P. Ashley *et al.*, *Br. dent. J.*, 1984, *157*, 191.

Preparations

Cetylpyridinium Chloride Lozenges *(U.S.P.)*

Cetylpyridinium Chloride Topical Solution *(U.S.P.)*. Cetylpyridinium Chloride Solution

Proprietary Preparations

Merocet *(Merrell, UK)*. *Mouth-wash solution*, cetylpyridinium chloride 0.05%, alcohol 14%.

Merocets *(Merrell, UK)*. *Lozenges*, cetylpyridinium chloride 1.4 mg.

Merothol *(Merrell, UK)*. *Lozenges*, cetylpyridinium chloride 1.4 mg, menthol, and eucalyptus oil.

Proprietary Names and Manufacturers of Cetylpyridinium Chloride or another Salt

Benylin Sore Throat Lozenges *(Parke, Davis, Canad.)*; Cepacol Antibacterial Solution *(Merrell Dow, Austral.)*; Dobendan *(Merrell, Ger.; Merrell Dow, Switz.)*; Formamint *(Beecham-Wülfing, Ger.)*; Hiozon *(Denm.)*; Merocet *(Merrell, UK)*; Merocets *(Merrell, UK)*; Merothol *(Merrell, UK)*; Nedermin *(Spain)*; Neo Mentoformio *(Edmond Pharma, Ital.)*; Novoptine *(Dulcis, Mon.)*; Pyrisept *(Weiders, Norw.)*; Zepacole *(Merrell Dow, Spain)*.

The following names have been used for multi-ingredient preparations containing cetylpyridinium chloride or another salt—Balminil Pastilles *(Rougier, Canad.)*; Cepacaine *(Merrell Dow, Austral.)*; Cepacol *(Merrell Dow, Austral.; Dow, Canad.; Merrell Dow, USA)*; Codral Lozenges *(Wellcome, Austral.)*; Fungoid *(Pedinol, USA)*; Medilave Gel *(Martindale Pharmaceuticals, UK)*; Merocaine *(Merrell, UK)*; Seda-Gel Lotion *(Nelson, Austral.)*; Semets *(Beecham Laboratories, USA)*;

Toracsol *(Torbet Laboratories, UK)*; Tyrosolven *(Warner, UK)*.

2218-h

Chloramine *(BAN)*.
Chloramidum; Chloramine T; Chloraminum; Cloramina; Mianin; Natrium Sulfaminochloratum; Tosylchloramide Sodium *(rINN)*; Tosylchloramidum Natricum. Sodium *N*-chlorotoluene-*p*-sulphonimidate trihydrate.
$C_7H_7ClNNaO_2S, 3H_2O$=281.7.

CAS — 127-65-1 (anhydrous).

NOTE. The name Chloramin is applied to a preparation of chlorpheniramine maleate.

Pharmacopoeias. In *Aust., Belg., Br., Eur., Fr., Ger., Hung., It., Jug., Mex., Neth., Nord., Port., Span.,* and *Swiss.*

White or slightly yellow crystalline powder. It contains about 25% w/w of 'available chlorine' (see p.958).
Freely **soluble** in water; soluble in alcohol; practically insoluble in chloroform and ether. A 5% solution in water has a pH of 8 to 10. **Store** in airtight containers at a temperature of 8° to 15° Protect from light.

Adverse Effects

Vomiting, cyanosis, circulatory collapse, frothing at the mouth, and respiratory failure can occur within a few minutes of chloramine ingestion. Fatalities have occurred.
Chloramine in tap water has caused methaemoglobinaemia and haemolysis in patients undergoing dialysis.
Bronchospasm has occurred after inhalation.

Uses and Administration

Chloramine is an organic derivative of chlorine with the bactericidal actions and uses of chlorine (p.958).
It is stable at an alkaline pH but is much more active in acid media. It releases hypochlorous acid more slowly and is less active than hypochlorite solutions.
Chloramine has been employed as a wound disinfectant and general surgical antiseptic. It is less irritant than hypochlorites. It has also been used as a mouth-wash.
Chloramine is used for the treatment of drinking water containing little organic matter.
Chloramine was formerly used as a spermicide.
In the *UK* the maximum concentration of chloramine in cosmetics is limited to 0.2% by law.
Chloramine B (Chlorogenium; sodium *N*-chlorobenzenesulphonimidate sesquihydrate) has been used similarly to chloramine.

Proprietary Names and Manufacturers

Clonazone *(Promedica, Switz.)*; Clorina *(Med. y Prod. Qutm., Spain)*; Dercusan *(Cusi, Spain)*; Gineclorina *(Med. y Prod. Qutm., Spain)*; Gynomin *(Napp, UK)*; Hydroclonazone *(Promedica, Fr.; Promedica, Switz.)*; Kloramin *(DAK, Denm.)*; Klortee *(Protea, Austral.)*; Rendell Foam *(Rendell, UK)*; Santronex *(Rendell, UK)*.

2220-t

Chlorhexidine Acetate *(BANM, rINNM)*.

Chlorhexidine Diacetate. 1,1′-Hexamethylenebis-[5-(4-chlorophenyl)biguanide] diacetate.
$C_{22}H_{30}Cl_2N_{10},2C_2H_4O_2$=625.6.

CAS — 55-56-1 (chlorhexidine); 56-95-1 (acetate).

Pharmacopoeias. In *Br.* and *Chin.* Also in *B.P. Vet.*

A white to pale cream, odourless or almost odourless microcrystalline powder. **Soluble** 1 in 55 of water and 1 in 15 of alcohol; very slightly soluble in glycerol and propylene glycol. It is stable at ordinary temperatures but when heated it decomposes with the production of trace amounts of 4-chloroaniline. Aqueous solutions slowly decompose with the formation of trace amounts of 4-chloroaniline. **Store** in well-closed containers. Protect from light.

2221-x

Chlorhexidine Gluconate *(BANM, USAN, rINNM)*.

Chlorhexidine Digluconate. 1,1′-Hexamethylenebis[5-(4-chlorophenyl)biguanide] digluconate.
$C_{22}H_{30}Cl_2N_{10},2C_6H_{12}O_7$=897.8.

CAS — 18472-51-0 (chlorhexidine gluconate).

Pharmacopoeias. Br., Jpn, and *B.P. Vet.* include Chlorhexidine Gluconate Solution which contains 19 to 21% of chlorhexidine gluconate.

The solution is an almost colourless to pale straw-coloured, clear or slightly opalescent, odourless or almost odourless liquid.
Miscible with water, with up to 5 parts of alcohol, and with up to 3 parts of acetone. A 5% v/v dilution in water has a pH of 5.5 to 7.0.
Store the solution at a temperature not exceeding 25°. Protect from light.
NOTE. Commercial 5% concentrate contains a nonionic surfactant to prevent precipitation on dilution with hard water and is not suitable for use on mucous membranes; dilutions of the 20% concentrate should be used for this purpose.

2222-r

Chlorhexidine Hydrochloride *(BANM, USAN, rINNM)*.

AY-5312; Chlorhexidine Dihydrochloride. 1,1′-Hexamethylenebis[5-(4-chlorophenyl)biguanide] dihydrochloride.
$C_{22}H_{30}Cl_2N_{10},2HCl$=578.4.

CAS — 3697-42-5.

Pharmacopoeias. In *Br., Egypt.,* and *Jpn.* Also in *B.P. Vet.*

A white or almost white, odourless or almost odourless, crystalline powder.
Sparingly **soluble** in water; very slightly soluble in alcohol; soluble 1 in 50 of propylene glycol.
Chlorhexidine and its salts are stable at normal storage temperatures but when heated may decompose with the production of trace amounts of 4-chloroaniline. Chlorhexidine hydrochloride is less readily decomposed than chlorhexidine acetate and may be heated at 150° for 1 hour without appreciable production of 4-chloroaniline. Aqueous solutions of chlorhexidine salts decompose with the formation of trace amounts of 4-chloroaniline. This decomposition is increased by heating and alkaline pH. **Protect** from light.
Chlorhexidine Incompatibilities. Chlorhexidine is incompatible with soaps and other anionic materials. Chlorhexidine acetate is incompatible with potassium iodide. At a concentration of 0.05%, chlorhexidine is incompatible with borates, bicarbonates, carbonates, chlorides, citrates, phosphates, and sulphates, forming salts of low solubility which may precipitate from solution only after standing for 24 hours. At dilutions of 0.01% or more, these salts are generally soluble.
Chlorhexidine is inactivated by cork.
Fabrics which have been in contact with chlorhexidine solution may develop a brown stain if bleached with a hypochlorite. A perborate bleach may be used instead.

After storage for 72 hours, a decrease of more than 90% in the concentration of chlorhexidine acetate 0.05% occurred in aqueous suspensions containing insoluble magnesium compounds or starch; smaller losses occurred in the presence of insoluble zinc and calcium compounds.— T. J. McCarthy, *J. mond. Pharm.*, 1969, *12*, 321. The antibacterial activity of chlorhexidine acetate 0.005% against *Staphylococcus aureus* was reduced by between 70 and 100% by 1% of kaolin, magnesium trisilicate, aluminium magnesium silicate, or bentonite.— R. T. Yousef *et al., Can. J. pharm. Sci.*, 1973, *8*, 54. Binding of chlorhexidine to tragacanth reduced the antibacterial activity of chlorhexidine.— T. J. McCarthy and J. A. Myburgh, *Pharm. Weekbl. Ned.*, 1974, *109*, 265.

Adverse Effects and Treatment

Skin sensitivity to chlorhexidine has occasionally been reported. Strong solutions may cause irritation of the conjunctiva and other sensitive tissues. The use of chlorhexidine dental gel and mouth-wash has been associated with reversible discoloration of the tongue, teeth, and silicate or composite restorations. Transient taste disturbances and a burning sensation of the tongue may occur on initial use. Oral desquamation and occasional parotid gland swelling have been reported with the mouth-wash. If desquamation occurs, 50% dilution of the mouth-wash with water and less vigorous rinsing may allow continued use.
Chlorhexidine is poorly absorbed from the gastro-intestinal tract.
Toxic effects due to ingestion of chlorhexidine should be treated by gastric lavage.

ALLERGY. A severe allergic reaction with marked hypotension, generalised flushing, and impalpable peripheral pulses occurred in a 67-year-old man after application of a dressing containing chlorhexidine acetate 0.5% to the donor site of a skin graft.— J. Cheung and J. J. O'Leary, *Anaesth. & intensive Care*, 1985, *13*, 429.

EFFECTS ON THE LIVER. In a suicide attempt, a patient drank about 150 mL of chlorhexidine gluconate solution, corresponding to about 30 g of the pure substance. Besides pharyngeal oedema and necrotic oesophageal lesions, the patient had very high aminotransferase concentrations which rose to 30 times normal 5 days after ingestion and were still 8 times normal one week later. After one month the aspartate aminotransferase (SGOT) was returning to normal while the alanine aminotransferase (SGPT) was still 3 times normal. Six months after ingestion the aminotransferase levels were normal. A liver biopsy performed soon after the peak in aminotransferase levels showed diffuse fatty degeneration and lobular hepatitis suggesting that chlorhexidine was absorbed from the gastro-intestinal tract in a concentration high enough to produce liver necrosis.— G. Massano *et al.* (letter), *Lancet*, 1982, *1*, 289.

EFFECTS ON THE NOSE. Temporary hyposmia in some patients after transsphenoidal pituitary adenoma operation was assumed to be caused by preoperative disinfection of the nasal cavity with chlorhexidine gluconate solution.— M. Yamagishi *et al., Pract. Otol.*, 1985, *78*, 399.

EFFECTS ON THE TEETH. References to the mechanism of tooth discoloration associated with the oral use of chlorhexidine: M. Addy *et al., Br. dent. J.*, 1985, *159*, 281; M. Addy and J. Moran, *ibid.*, 331.

Precautions

Because it is irritant it is recommended that chlorhexidine should not be used on the brain, meninges, middle ear, or other sensitive tissues.
Chlorhexidine is sorbed on to contact lenses and may cause eye irritation. Syringes and needles that have been immersed in chlorhexidine solutions should be thoroughly rinsed with sterile water or saline before use.
The antimicrobial activity of chlorhexidine may be diminished through incompatibility or through adsorption (see above). Its activity may also be reduced in the presence of organic matter.
Chlorhexidine oral gel should not be used concomitantly with dentifrices.
Because of problems of contamination, many disinfectants and antiseptics are provided for clinical use in a sterile form in single application packs. If a bulk pack is employed, any unused contents are often discarded immediately. The dilution of concentrated solutions should be carried out using appropriate measures to prevent contamination.
Aqueous solutions of chlorhexidine used for instrument storage should contain sodium nitrite 0.1% to inhibit metal corrosion, and should be changed every 7 days.

Chlorhexidine was detected in low concentrations in the venous blood of 5 of 24 infants after bathing with a preparation containing chlorhexidine gluconate 4%

(Hibiscrub). No adverse effects due to percutaneous absorption of chlorhexidine were reported.— J. Cowen *et al.*, *Archs Dis. Childh.*, 1979, *54*, 379. Low or undetectable concentrations after the use of powder containing chlorhexidine 1%.— V. G. Alder *et al.*, *ibid.*, 1980, *55*, 277. Percutaneous absorption of chlorhexidine occurred in pre-term neonates but not in full-term infants treated with chlorhexidine 1% in alcohol for neonatal cord care. No absorption occurred when a dusting powder containing chlorhexidine 1% and zinc oxide 3% was used.— P. J. Aggett *et al.*, *ibid.*, 1981, *56*, 878.

Haemorrhagic skin necrosis associated with umbilical artery catheterisation in extremely pre-term infants was attributed to damage by the alcohol from the use of chlorhexidine 0.5% in spirit 70% as a disinfectant. The use of an aqueous solution was recommended.— N. Rutter (letter), *Archs Dis. Childh.*, 1983, *58*, 396.

A report of *Pseudomonas pickettii* septicaemia in 6 patients following the use of aqueous chlorhexidine 0.05%, prepared with contaminated twice-distilled water, for skin disinfection prior to venepuncture. This demonstrated again the danger of using unsterilised aqueous chlorhexidine solution. Aqueous chlorhexidine 0.05% alone, or with cetrimide 0.5% can be contaminated by pseudomonads, and several outbreaks of nosocomial infections caused by contaminated aqueous chlorhexidine solutions have been reported with *Ps. cepacia* being isolated in most cases. A 0.5% aqueous solution of chlorhexidine may be used for preoperative antisepsis, but 0.05% solutions should not be used to decontaminate skin before venepuncture.— A. Kahan *et al.* (letter), *Lancet*, 1984, *2*, 759.

Positive blood cultures of *Pseudomonas cepacia* in 2 patients were attributed to the inappropriate use of a chlorhexidine handwash (Hibiscrub) for the initial cleansing of venepuncture sites. Two containers of the handwash were shown to contain *Ps. cepacia* in numbers in excess of 10^5 colony forming units/mL (P.E. Gosden and P. Norman, *Lancet*, 1985, *2*, 671). Further studies showed that the handwash did not support the growth of the *Ps. cepacia* strain isolated unless diluted, and that dilution was the probable explanation for the contamination. The handwash contains isopropyl alcohol 4% as a preservative and dilution may leave it inadequately protected from contamination with certain micro-organisms (P. Norman *et al.*, *ibid.*, 1986, *1*, 209).

Uses and Administration

Chlorhexidine is a bisbiguanide disinfectant which is effective against a wide range of vegetative Gram-positive and Gram-negative bacteria. It is more effective against Gram-positive than Gram-negative bacteria, some species of *Pseudomonas* and *Proteus* being relatively less susceptible. Chlorhexidine is active against some viruses and some fungi. It is inactive against bacterial spores at room temperature. Chlorhexidine is most active at a neutral or slightly acid pH.

A 0.5% solution of chlorhexidine gluconate or acetate in alcohol (70%) is used for pre-operative skin disinfection and for the emergency disinfection of clean instruments (2 minutes immersion). A 0.05% aqueous solution is used as a wound disinfectant, as an eye irrigation, and for the storage and disinfection (30 minutes immersion) of clean instruments. A 0.05% solution in glycerol is used for urethral disinfection and catheter lubrication. A 0.02% aqueous solution is used for pleural, peritoneal, and bladder irrigation, and as a cystoscopy medium. A 0.01% concentration of chlorhexidine gluconate or acetate is used for eye-drop preservation. Tulle dressings impregnated with chlorhexidine acetate 0.5% are used for infected wounds.

For general disinfectant purposes, chlorhexidine gluconate is commonly used in combination with cetrimide (see p.954). Chlorhexidine gluconate is used in 1% creams for application to broken skin surfaces, as a barrier against bacterial hand infection, and in obstetrics; in a 4% detergent solution for pre-operative skin preparation and hand washing; in dusting powders; and in a 1% dental gel and 0.2% mouth-wash for the prevention of plaque and gingivitis. Chlorhexidine hydrochloride is also available in lozenges and has been used in the management of nasal staphylococcal infections.

The antibacterial effect of chlorhexidine acetate 0.002% was enhanced by benzyl alcohol, phenylpropanol, and phenethyl alcohol, all 0.175%.— R. M. E. Richards and R. J. McBride, *J. pharm. Sci.*, 1973, *62*, 2035.

Viable bacterial counts on the hands were reduced by a mean of 97.9% by the application to the hands of 0.5% chlorhexidine gluconate in 95% alcohol rubbed in until dry, by 65.1% by the application for 2 minutes of 0.5% chlorhexidine gluconate in water, by 86.7% by the application for 2 minutes of a 4% chlorhexidine gluconate detergent solution, and by 91.8% by a 0.1% solution of tetrabromo-*o*-cresol in 95.3% alcohol, rubbed in till dry. After 6 successive applications in 2 days the respective reductions were 99.7%, 91.8%, 99.2%, and 99.5%.— E. J. L. Lowbury *et al.*, *Br. med. J.*, 1974, *4*, 369.

A solution of chlorhexidine 0.5% is sporicidal after 5 minutes at 100°. Chlorhexidine could be used in an emergency when an autoclave breaks down or in countries or situations where steam pressure sterilisation was impossible.— A. W. Fowler (letter), *Lancet*, 1984, *2*, 760.

In an outbreak of epidemic methicillin resistant *Staphylococcus aureus* (EMRSA) chlorhexidine was used to try to ablate carriage in 6 subjects. It was used in daily washing and shampooing and as a 1% cream for nasal carriage. Despite these measures, it took from 3 to 20 days to clear the organism from the 6 subjects. Later, chlorhexidine cream was used in 15 nasal carriers. After 10 days' treatment all still carried the organism. They were all cleared within 2 days when treatment with nasal mupirocin was started and were still clear up to 14 days after the 5-day course of mupirocin.— G. Duckworth (letter), *Br. med. J.*, 1986, *293*, 885.

APHTHOUS STOMATITIS. Chlorhexidine gluconate mouth-wash 0.2% used 3 times daily for 6 weeks by 38 patients with minor aphthous ulceration significantly increased the number of days free of ulcers from 17 to 22 days and the interval between successive ulcers was almost doubled.— L. Hunter and M. Addy, *Br. dent. J.*, 1987, *162*, 106. Earlier studies: M. Addy *et al.*, *ibid.*, 1974, *136*, 452; idem, 1976, *141*, 118.

GINGIVAL HYPERPLASIA AND PLAQUE REDUCTION. A 66% reduction in plaque formation and a 24% reduction in gingival inflammation compared with controls was observed in 40 patients, aged 19 to 39 years, when they each used 10 mL of chlorhexidine acetate or gluconate 0.1 or 0.2% solution as a mouth-wash twice daily for 8 weeks. In the 2 months after the teeth were scaled and polished, the plaque reduction was 84% and the gingival index was reduced by 43%. There was no significant difference between the 0.2% and the 0.1% solution.— L. Flötra *et al.*, *Scand. J. dent. Res.*, 1972, *80*, 10.

In a double-blind study of 56 children with gingivitis, the use of a chlorhexidine gluconate gel (1%) as a toothpaste every night for 4 weeks was not more effective than placebo in improving the gingivitis. At the end of the 4-week period the gel produced a slightly greater reduction in plaque formation than placebo but 4 weeks later there was no difference. Tooth staining occurred in 75% of children given the gel, compared with 25% on placebo, and 4 weeks after stopping treatment 45% were still stained.— D. F. Hajos *et al.*, *Br. dent. J.*, 1977, *142*, 366.

In a study of 18 patients aged 25 years or less with gingival hyperplasia due to phenytoin therapy, chlorhexidine gluconate mouth-wash 0.1% used 3 times daily reduced plaque and the tendency for drug-induced hyperplasia to recur.— T. C. A. O'Neil and K. H. Figures, *Br. dent. J.*, 1982, *152*, 130 and 206.

Further references: T. C. A. O'Neil, *Br. dent. J.*, 1976, *141*, 276.

ORAL CANDIDIASIS. Chlorhexidine gluconate is an effective denture disinfectant for chronic atrophic candidiasis.— *Lancet*, 1986, *2*, 437.

PERITONEAL DIALYSIS. The addition of chlorhexidine to ambulatory dialysis fluid containing high concentrations of chloride ions was not recommended as precipitation of chlorhexidine was likely. In contrast, lavage with aqueous solutions of chlorhexidine had been shown to be both acceptable and very effective for controlling peritoneal sepsis.— G. W. Denton (letter), *Lancet*, 1984, *2*, 517.

PREGNANCY AND THE NEONATE. Chlorhexidine is as effective as hexachlorophane in preventing neonatal sepsis. Although chlorhexidine is absorbed percutaneously, its toxicity seems to be considerably lower than that of hexachlorophane.— *Lancet*, 1982, *1*, 87.

SILICONE-FOAM DRESSING DISINFECTION. Chlorhexidine, povidone iodine, cetrimide, and sodium hypochlorite were compared in the disinfection of silicone-foam dressing used in the management of open granulating wounds. Chlorhexidine 0.5% proved to be the most effective antiseptic, povidone iodine 1.0% and cetrimide 1.0% with isopropyl alcohol 0.4% were moderately successful, but sodium hypochlorite 0.2% gave poor results. A rinse of the dressing after disinfection prevented wound irritation by chlorhexidine due to carry-over, without compromising its antibacterial effect, but this procedure sometimes failed to prevent irritation when using the other antiseptics. It was noted that the chlorhexidine gluconate 5% concentrate (Hibitane 5% Concentrate) used contained non-ionic detergent and a stabilising agent and that pure preparations of chlorhexidine may not behave similarly.— B. K. Evans *et al.*, *J. clin. Hosp. Pharm.*, 1985, *10*, 289. See also: E. Thomas *et al.*, *Br. J. pharm. Pract.*, 1983, *5*, 12.

SPERMICIDE. Bisbiguanides of the chlorhexidine type are reported to have the ability to diffuse into mucus and render it impenetrable to sperm at concentrations as low as 1 mg per mL. Higher concentrations of chlorhexidine structurally modify the mucus, causing syneresis at the mucus/chlorhexidine interface which produces a barrier to both the entry of sperm and chlorhexidine. The potency of chlorhexidine in inhibiting sperm motility *in vitro* is identical to that of nonoxinol 9.— R. M. Pearson, *Pharm. J.*, 1985, *1*, 686.

URINARY-TRACT INFECTION. Although the Southampton Infection Control Team found that the addition of 10 mL of chlorhexidine gluconate 5% solution to catheter drainage bags, in conjunction with aseptic techniques, reduced the infection-rate and prevented cross-infection in patients undergoing urinary-tract catheterisation (*Lancet*, 1982, *1*, 89), it was suggested that the major pathway for bladder infections appears to be entry of bacteria colonising the periurethral zone (C.M. Kunin, *ibid.*, 626). A later prospective, controlled study in 58 post-prostatectomy patients found that the frequency of urinary infection in the chlorhexidine group (51%) did not differ significantly from that in the control group (45%) although chlorhexidine kept the contents of all drainage bags sterile (W.A. Gillespie *et al.*, *ibid.*, 1983, *1*, 1037).

Fifty-two geriatric patients with indwelling urinary catheters received twice daily bladder instillations for 3 weeks with either normal saline or chlorhexidine acetate solution 0.02%. Neither normal saline or chlorhexidine showed any significant decrease in urinary bacterial count, and there was an apparent overgrowth of *Proteus* spp. in 5 patients given chlorhexidine.— A. J. Davies *et al.*, *J. Hosp. Infect.*, 1987, *9*, 72.

WOUND DISINFECTION. Since cetrimide had been shown to be toxic to *mouse* cells, it was recommended that if an antimicrobial agent was required for wound disinfection, then chlorhexidine should be used without cetrimide.— S. Thomas and N. P. Hay (letter), *Pharm. J.*, 1985, *2*, 206.

Preparations

Chlorhexidine Gauze Dressing *(B.P.)*. Chlorhexidine Acetate Gauze Dressing. A sterile cotton and/or viscose dressing impregnated with a suitable ointment containing 0.4 to 0.6% chlorhexidine acetate.

Chlorhexidine Cream *(B.P.)*. Chlorhexidine gluconate solution in a suitable basis. For extemporaneous preparation the following formula may be used: chlorhexidine gluconate solution, a suitable quantity, liquid paraffin 10 g, cetomacrogol emulsifying wax 25 g, freshly boiled and cooled water to 100 g. *A.P.F.*(Chlorhexidine Cream Aqueous) specifies 1%.

Chlorhexidine Dusting Powder *(B.P.)*. Chlorhexidine hydrochloride 0.5% in sterilisable maize starch. Sterilised in quantities of not more than 30 g.

Chlorhexidine Ear Drops *(A.P.F.)*. Chlorhexidine acetate 50 mg, freshly boiled and cooled water to 100 mL.

Chlorhexidine Gel *(A.P.F.)*. Chlorhexidine gluconate solution 2.5 mL, tragacanth 2.5 g, glycerol 25 g, freshly boiled and cooled water to 100 g.

Chlorhexidine Irrigation *(A.P.F.)*. Chlorhexidine gluconate solution 0.1 mL, Water for Injections to 100 mL. Sterilised by autoclaving.

Chlorhexidine Mouth-wash *(D.P.F.)*. Chlorhexidine gluconate 0.2%.

Chlorhexidine Mouth-wash, Compound *(D.P.F.)*. Chlorhexidine gluconate 0.1%, chlorbutol 0.1%, chloroform 0.5%.

Proprietary Preparations of Chlorhexidine and its Salts

Bacticlens *(Smith & Nephew, UK)*. *Solution*, sterile, aqueous chlorhexidine gluconate 0.05%.

Bactigras *(Smith & Nephew, UK)*. *Dressing*, sterile, tulle, chlorhexidine acetate 0.5%.

Chlorasept 2000 *(Travenol, UK)*. *Solution*, sterile, aqueous chlorhexidine acetate 0.05%.

Corsodyl *(ICI Pharmaceuticals, UK). Dental gel*, chlorhexidine gluconate 1%.
Mouth-wash, chlorhexidine gluconate 0.2%.

CX Powder *(Bio-Medical, UK). Powder*, sterile, chlorhexidine acetate 1% in sterilisable maize starch.

Cyteal *(Concept Pharmaceuticals, UK). Solution*, chlorhexidine gluconate 0.5%, chlorocresol 0.3%, hexamidine di-isethionate 0.1%.

Dispray 1 Quick Prep *(Stuart, UK). Liquid aerosol spray*, industrial methylated spirit 70%, chlorhexidine gluconate 0.5%.

Elgydium *(Concept Pharmaceuticals, UK). Toothpaste*, chlorhexidine gluconate 0.004%.

Eludril *(Concept Pharmaceuticals, UK). Mouth-wash*, chlorhexidine gluconate 0.1%, chloroform 0.5%, chlorbutol 0.1%.
Spray, aerosol, chlorhexidine gluconate 0.05%, amethocaine hydrochloride 0.015%.

Hibidil *(ICI Pharmaceuticals, UK). Solution*, sterile, aqueous chlorhexidine gluconate 0.05%.

Hibiscrub *(ICI Pharmaceuticals, UK). Detergent solution*, chlorhexidine gluconate 4%.

Hibisol *(ICI Pharmaceuticals, UK). Solution*, chlorhexidine gluconate 0.5%, isopropyl alcohol 70%, and emollients.

Hibitane *(ICI Pharmaceuticals, UK). Cream* (Hibitane Antiseptic Cream), chlorhexidine gluconate 1%.
Cream (Hibitane Obstetric Cream), chlorhexidine gluconate 1%.
Powder (Hibitane Acetate), chlorhexidine acetate.
Solution (Hibitane 5% Concentrate), chlorhexidine gluconate 5% with surfactant.
Solution (Hibitane Gluconate 20% Solution), chlorhexidine gluconate 20%.

Hibitane Antiseptic Lozenges *(Care, UK). Lozenges*, chlorhexidine hydrochloride 5 mg, benzocaine 2 mg.

Instasept *(Bio-Medical, UK). Solution*, chlorhexidine acetate 0.5%, sodium nitrite 0.1%, industrial methylated spirit 70%.

Macrocide *(Macarthys, UK). Solution*, chlorhexidine gluconate 4%.

Medi-Wipe *(Smith & Nephew, UK). Swabs*, chlorhexidine gluconate solution 2.5%, alcohol 70%.

Naseptin *(ICI Pharmaceuticals, UK). Cream*, chlorhexidine hydrochloride 0.1%, neomycin sulphate 0.5%.

pHiso-MED *(Winthrop, UK). Solution*, chlorhexidine gluconate 4%.
NOTE. pHiso-MED previously contained hexachlorophane 3%.

Rotersept *(Roterpharma, UK). Aerosol spray*, chlorhexidine gluconate 0.2%.

Serotulle *(Johnson & Johnson, UK). Sterile tulle dressing*, chlorhexidine acetate 0.5%.

Unisept *(Seton, UK). Solution*, sterile, aqueous chlorhexidine gluconate 0.05%.

Uro-Tainer Chlorhexidine 1:5000 *(Vifor, Switz.: CliniMed, UK). Irrigation Solution*, sterile, chlorhexidine acetate 0.02%, in single-use packs of 100 mL.

Proprietary Names and Manufacturers of Chlorhexidine and its Salts

Bacticlens *(Smith & Nephew, UK)*; Bactigras *(Smith & Nephew, Austral.; Smith & Nephew, Canad.; Smith & Nephew, Denm.; Smith & Nephew, S.Afr.; Smith & Nephew, UK)*; Cetal Aerosols *(Orapharm, Austral.)*; Chlorasept 2000 *(Travenol, UK)*; Chlorhexamed *(Blend-a-med, Ger.)*; Chlorhex-a-myl *(Blend-a-pharm, Fr.)*; Chlorhexidine Acetate Irrigations *(Travenol, UK)*; Chlorohex *(Orapharm, Austral.; Geistlich, Switz.)*; Corsodyl *(ICI, Ger.; ICI, Switz.; ICI Pharmaceuticals, UK)*; CX Powder *(Bio-Medical, UK)*; Dispray 1 Quick Prep *(Stuart, UK)*; Dispray 2 Hard Surface Disinfectant *(Stuart, UK)*; Elgydium *(Concept Pharmaceuticals, UK)*; Exidine *(Xttrium, USA)*; Hansamed *(Beiersdorf, Ger.)*; Hexidin *(NAF, Norw.)*; Hexol *(Sigma, Austral.)*; Hexophene *(Ego, Austral.)*; Hibicare *(Canad.)*; Hibiclens *(ICI, Austral.; ICI, Ger.; Stuart Pharmaceuticals, USA)*; Hibicol *(ICI, Austral.)*; Hibident *(Belg.; ICI, S.Afr.)*; Hibidil *(Ayerst, Canad.; ICI, Denm.; ICI, S.Afr.; ICI Pharmaceuticals, UK)*; Hibigel *(Belg.)*; Hibiscrub *(Belg.; ICI, Denm.; Fr.; ICI, Norw.; S.Afr.; ICI, Spain; ICI, Swed.; ICI, Switz.; ICI Pharmaceuticals, UK)*; Hibisol *(ICI Pharmaceuticals, UK)*; Hibistat *(Stuart Pharmaceuticals, USA)*; Hibitane *(ICI, Austral.; Ayerst, Canad.; ICI, Denm.; I.C.I.-Pharma, Fr.; ICI, Norw.; ICI, S.Afr.; Spain; ICI, Swed.; ICI, Switz.; ICI Pharmaceuticals, UK; Stuart Pharmaceuticals, USA)*; Intasept *(Bio-Medical, UK)*; Larylin *(Beiersdorf, Ger.)*; Macrocide *(Macarthys, UK)*; Maskin *(Jpn)*; Medi-Swabs (H) *(Pharmax, UK)*; Medi-Wipe *(Smith & Nephew, UK)*; Peridex *(Procter & Gamble, USA)*; pHiso-MED *(Winthrop, UK)*; Plurexid *(Bottu, Fr.)*; Rhino-Blache *(Chauvin-Blache, Fr.)*; Rotersept *(Belg.; Maurer, Ger.; Neth.; Roterpharma, UK)*; Rouhex *(Rougier, Canad.)*; R(slashed o)dhex *(Denm.)*; Salvesept *(Spain)*; Savacol *(ICI, Austral.)*; Savlon Medicated Powder *(ICI, Austral.)*; Septeal *(Pierre Fabre, Fr.)*; Serotulle *(Johnson & Johnson, UK)*; Sterilon *(Belg.; Neth.; Roter, Switz.)*; Unisept *(Seton, UK)*; Uro-Tainer Chlorhexidine 1:5000 *(Vifor, Switz. : CliniMed, UK)*; Vitacontact *(Faure, Fr.)*.

The following names have been used for multi-ingredient preparations containing chlorhexidine and its salts—Cetal Liquid *(Orapharm, Austral.)*; Cetriclens *(Smith & Nephew, UK)*; Cyteal *(Concept Pharmaceuticals, UK)*; Dermocaine *(Ego, Austral.)*; Dermofax *(Hough, Hoseason, UK)*; Dri-Wash Medical Cleansing Towelette *(Linton, UK)*; Ego Antiseptic Cream and Liquid *(Ego, Austral.)*; Egomycol *(Ego, Austral.)*; Eludril Mouthwash and Spray *(Concept Pharmaceuticals, UK)*; Hexidin *(Barnes-Hind, Austral.)*; Hibitane Antiseptic Lozenges *(Care, UK)*; Instillagel *(Farco-Pharma, Ger.; CliniMed, UK)*; Medi Creme *(Rosken, Austral.)*; Medi Pulv *(Rosken, Austral.)*; Medi-Prep *(Pharmax, UK)*; Medi-Sache *(Pharmax, UK)*; Naseptin *(ICI, Austral.; ICI Pharmaceuticals, UK)*; Norgotin *(Norgine, UK)*; Nystaform *(Bayer, UK)*; Nystaform-HC *(Bayer, UK)*; Oticane *(Rosken, Austral.)*; Savloclens *(ICI Pharmaceuticals, UK)*; Savlodil *(Ayerst, Canad.; ICI Pharmaceuticals, UK)*; Savlon Antiseptic *(ICI, Austral.; Care, UK)*; Savlon Hospital Concentrate *(ICI, Austral.; Ayerst, Canad.; ICI Pharmaceuticals, UK)*; Seda-Gel Lotion *(Nelson, Austral.)*; Sterets H *(Seton, UK)*; Stomobar *(Thackray, UK)*; Stomogel *(Thackray, UK)*; Stomosol Concentrate *(Thackray, UK)*; Tisept *(Seton, UK)*; Travasept *(Travenol, UK)*; Tuscodin *(Schering, Austral.)*; Xylocaine Gel *(Astra, UK)*; Xylocaine with Hibitane *(Astra, Austral.)*.

2223-f

Chlorinated Lime *(BAN)*.

Bleaching Powder; Cal Clorada; Calcaria Chlorata; Calcii Hypochloris; Calcium Hypochlorosum; Calx Chlorata; Calx Chlorinata; Chloride of Lime; Chlorkalk; Chlorure de Chaux; Cloruro de Cal.
CAS — 7778-54-3.

Pharmacopoeias. In *Arg., Belg., Br., Chin., Fr., Jpn, Nord., Pol., Span.,* and *Swiss.*

A dull white powder with a characteristic odour, containing not less than 30% w/w of 'available chlorine' (see p.958). It becomes moist and gradually decomposes in air, carbon dioxide being absorbed and chlorine evolved.

Partly **soluble** in water and alcohol. Aqueous solutions are strongly alkaline. **Store** in well-closed containers.

For reference to the stability of Eusol, see below.

Adverse Effects, Treatment, and Precautions

As for Sodium Hypochlorite p.969.

Uses and Administration

Chlorinated lime has the actions and uses of chlorine (see below).

Its action is rapid but brief, the 'available chlorine' soon being exhausted by combination with organic material. It is used to disinfect faeces, urine, and other organic material, and as a cleansing agent for lavatories, drains, and effluents.

Chlorinated lime is used in the preparation of Surgical Chlorinated Soda Solution (Dakin's Solution) which has been employed as a wound disinfectant. The surrounding skin must be protected by smearing with soft paraffin to prevent irritation.

Chlorinated Lime and Boric Acid Solution (eusol) has been used as a disinfectant lotion and wet dressing, sometimes with equal parts of liquid paraffin.

Studies of the stability, skin irritancy, and uses of eusol (Chlorinated Lime and Boric Acid Solution) and other hypochlorite formulations used in hospitals.— S. F. Bloomfield and T. J. Sizer, *Pharm. J.*, 1985, *2*, 153.

A modified preparation of eusol (T-eusol) in which the borate buffer was replaced by acetate was considered to be as effective as eusol.— K. Greenblo *et al.*, *Pharm. J.*, 1985, *2*, 267.

For the use of eusol to prevent live cell exfoliation in colorectal cancer operations, see Cetrimide, p.954.

Preparations

Calcium Hypochlorite Solution *(A.P.F.)*. Eusol; Liq. Calc. Hypochlorit. Chlorinated lime 1.25 g, calcium hydroxide 0.5 g, water to 100 mL. Contains approximately 0.3% w/v (3000 ppm) of 'available chlorine'.

Chlorinated Lime and Boric Acid Solution *(B.P.)*. Eusol. Chlorinated lime 1.25 g, boric acid 1.25 g, water to 100 mL. It contains not less than 0.25% w/v (2500 ppm) of 'available chlorine'. Store at a temperature not exceeding 20° in well-filled, well-closed containers. Protect from light. It deteriorates on storage and should be used within 2 weeks.

Surgical Chlorinated Soda Solution *(B.P.C. 1973)*. Liq. Sod. Chlorinat. Chir.; Dakin's Solution. Prepared from chlorinated lime, sodium carbonate, boric acid, and freshly boiled and cooled water, the proportions varying with the amount of 'available chlorine' in the chlorinated lime. It contains 0.5 to 0.55% w/v (5000 to 5500 ppm) of 'available chlorine'. It should be recently prepared. Store in a cool place in well-filled airtight containers. Protect from light.

2224-d

Chlorine

925; 926 (chlorine dioxide).
Cl=35.45.
CAS — 7782-50-5 (Cl_2).

Adverse Effects

Chlorine gas is an irritant producing inflammation of the conjunctiva, burns and necrosis, and when inhaled causing pain, oedema, and spasm of the larynx and bronchi. The irritant effect of chlorine may produce extensive pulmonary oedema with cyanosis, venous engorgement, and rapid respiration. There may be vomiting, and acidosis may develop. Death may follow from either circulatory failure or pulmonary oedema.

In Great Britain the recommended exposure limits of chlorine are 1 ppm (long-term); 3 ppm (short-term). In the *US* the permissible and recommended exposure limits are 3 mg per m^3 and 1.45 mg per m^3 respectively.

A discussion on chlorine poisoning and its treatment.— *Lancet*, 1984, *1*, 321.

Repeated deliberate inhalation of chlorine in 1 patient.— P. Rafferty, *Br. med. J.*, 1980, *281*, 1178. A report of 2 further incidents of voluntary chlorine inhalation suggests that some individuals may be unusually insensitive to chlorine-induced irritation. Workers should be warned that concentrations of chlorine which can be tolerated for short periods without undue discomfort can still cause serious injury which may not be immediately apparent.— F. Dewhurst (letter), *Br. med. J.*, 1981, *282*, 565.

Eye examinations performed on 50 subjects immediately before and after swimming in a chlorinated pool (chlorine range 1.0 to 1.5 ppm) showed that 68% had symptoms of corneal oedema and 94% had corneal epithelial erosions. No subject experienced a measurable decrease in visual acuity.— J. R. Haag and R. G. Gieser, *J. Am. med. Ass.*, 1983, *249*, 2507.

Experience gained from 186 cases of acute chlorine exposure indicated that medical support was required for only a short time even when exposure was repeated. Late sequelae were not observed, even in patients with abnormal respiratory function tests or blood gases on admission.— L. Barret and J. Faure (letter), *Lancet*, 1984, *1*, 561.

The intoxication by chlorine gas of 76 children and their management.— J. Fleta *et al.*, *Hum. Toxicol.*, 1986, *5*, 99.

Treatment of Adverse Effects

Conjunctivitis may require frequent irrigations of water or saline. Respiratory distress should be treated with inhalations of humidified oxygen and bronchodilators. Corticosteroids may be required to minimise pulmonary damage. Acidosis may require the intravenous use of sodium bicarbonate or other suitable alkalising agent.

Precautions

The antimicrobial activity of chlorine disinfectants is diminished by the presence of organic material.

Uses and Administration

Chlorine has a rapid potent brief bactericidal action. It is used as liquid chlorine for the chlorination treatment of water, but for most other purposes it is used in the form of hypochlorites, organic chloramines, chlorinated hydantoins, chlorinated isocyanurates, and similar oxidising compounds capable of releasing chlorine.

In the presence of water these compounds produce hypochlorous acid and hypochlorite ion and it is generally considered that the lethal action on organisms is due to chlorination of cell protein or enzyme systems by nonionised hypochlorous acid. The activity of most of the compounds decreases with increase of pH, the activity of solutions of pH 4 to 7 being greater than those of higher pH values. However, stability is usually greater at an alkaline pH.

Chlorine is capable of killing most bacteria, and some fungi, yeasts, algae, viruses, and protozoa. It is relatively ineffective against spores.

The potency of chlorine disinfectants is expressed in terms of 'available chlorine'. This is based on the concept of chlorine gas (Cl_2) as the reference substance.

Two atoms of chlorine (2 × Cl) yield in water one molecule of hypochlorous acid (on which activity is based), while hypochlorites and chloramines yield one molecule of hypochlorous acid for each atom of chlorine. Thus the assayed chlorine in such compounds has to be multiplied by 2 to produce 'available chlorine'. The term 'active chlorine' has been used confusingly for either 'available chlorine' (Cl_2) or combined chlorine (Cl).

Because they have relatively low residual toxicity, chlorine compounds are useful for the disinfection of relatively clean impervious surfaces, such as babies' feeding bottles, baths, wash-basins, trolleys, and food and dairy equipment. A concentration of 200 to 250 ppm of 'available chlorine' is used, though lower concentrations may be adequate if a detergent is added to ensure wetting of the surface. Solutions containing 10 000 ppm 'available chlorine' are used to disinfect surfaces contaminated with spilled blood, body fluids, or excreta; this strength is effective against viruses including human immunodeficiency virus (HIV) and hepatitis B virus. These solutions are also used for grossly contaminated heat-sensitive articles. Solutions containing 1000 ppm 'available chlorine' are recommended for minor surface contamination and as part of general good hygiene practice.

In the *UK* the use of chlorine in cosmetics is prohibited by law.

Bromine (see p.1550) and Iodine (see p.1184) are also used as disinfectants.

On a large scale, chlorine gas is used to disinfect public water supplies. On a smaller scale, the use of chlorine compounds is more convenient and sodium hypochlorite, chloramine chlorine dioxide, and halazone are used. After satisfying the chlorine demand (the amount of chlorine needed to react with organic matter and other substances), a free-residual content of 0.2 to 0.4 ppm 'available chlorine' should be maintained for at least 15 minutes, though more is required for alkaline waters with a pH of 9 or more. For the disinfection of potentially contaminated water a concentration of 1 ppm for at least 30 minutes is recommended. The unpleasant taste of residual chlorine may be removed by adding a little citric acid or sodium thiosulphate.

For use in small swimming pools, sodium or calcium hypochlorite may be added daily to maintain a free-residual 'available chlorine' concentration of 1 to 3 ppm. Chloramine and the isocyanurates (see Sodium Dichloroisocyanurate, p.969) may also be used. To minimise irritation of the eyes, a pH of 7.2 to 7.8 should be maintained.

Potentiation of the sporicidal activity of hypochlorites has been achieved by the addition of low concentrations of ammonia, bromine, sodium hydroxide, and alcohols.— S. P. Gorman *et al.*, *Int. J. Pharmaceut.*, 1983, *17*, 291 (See sodium hypochlorite (p.969) for a note of caution on mixing hypochlorite with ammonia).

ORAL CANDIDIASIS. In denture stomatitis, fungi should be eliminated from the dentures by immersion each night in 2% sodium hypochlorite solution.— R. A. Cawson, *Prescribers' J.*, 1984, *24*, 124.

PERITONEAL DIALYSIS. The use of sodium hypochlorite solution containing 3000 to 6000 ppm of available free chlorine for flushing a Y-shaped dialysis solution transfer set reduced the incidence of peritonitis in patients receiving continuous ambulatory peritoneal dialysis.— R. Maiorca *et al.*, *Lancet*, 1983, *2*, 642.

SILICONE-FOAM DRESSING DISINFECTION. Sodium hypochlorite 0.2% solution gave poor results in the disinfection of silicone-foam dressings.— B. K. Evans *et al.*, *J. clin. Hosp. Pharm.*, 1985, *10*, 289.

SKIN GRAFTS. Exposure to a sodium hypochlorite 0.5% solution for 6 minutes effectively decontaminated skin infected with *Staphylococcus aureus*, *Pseudomonas aeruginosa*, and *Candida albicans* while leaving 66% of the basal cells viable, sufficient for subsequent growth and expansion in tissue culture, elements essential for grafting over wounds.— R. C. Fader *et al.*, *Antimicrob. Ag. Chemother.*, 1983, *24*, 181 (See also under Wound Disinfection, below).

VIRAL DISINFECTION. Autoclaving remained the method of choice for the sterilisation of material contaminated with Creutzfeldt-Jakob disease virus, but a one-hour exposure to 0.5% sodium hypochlorite solution should provide excellent disinfection when autoclaving was not possible.— P. Brown *et al.*, *New Engl. J. Med.*, 1982, *306*, 1279. In practice, the use of hypochlorite was limited by its variably corrosive effects on fabrics, metals, and skin. One-hour exposure to 1 N sodium hydroxide was recommended, which was less corrosive than hypochlorite for all materials except aluminium, and had nonvolatile properties especially desirable in the decontamination of work surfaces.— P. Brown *et al.* (letter), *ibid.*, 1984, *310*, 727.

In a study of 5 patients, twice daily topical application of dilute sodium hypochlorite solutions hastened the resolution of cutaneous and mucosal *Herpes simplex* virus lesions, ameliorated discomfort, and resulted in more rapid healing of vesicles. Sites treated during the prodrome stage failed to vesiculate.— D. T. Hunter, *Publ. Hlth, Lond.*, 1983, *97*, 218.

Sodium hypochlorite solution containing 500 ppm available chlorine killed adenovirus 8, herpes simplex virus type 1, and a strain of enterovirus 70 after exposure for 2 minutes. Phenylmercuric borate had no effect on adenovirus 8 or herpes simplex, and isopropyl alcohol killed only herpes simplex. The use of sodium hypochlorite solution for disinfection of tonometers with a 10-minute soaking was therefore recommended although care to avoid contact of the solution with metal must be taken.— J. Nagington *et al.*, *Br. J. Ophthal.*, 1983, *67*, 674.

WATER DISINFECTION. *Swimming Pool Disinfection Systems using Sodium Hypochlorite and Calcium Hypochlorite. A Survey of the Efficacy of Disinfection*, Department of the Environment, London, HM Stationery Office, 1981.

Swimming Pool Disinfection Systems using Electrolytically Generated Sodium Hypochlorite. Monitoring the Efficacy of Disinfection, Department of the Environment, London, HM Stationery Office, 1983.

The Treatment and Quality of Swimming Pool Water, Department of the Environment National Water Council, London, HM Stationery Office, 1985.

WOUND DISINFECTION. Solutions of sodium hypochlorite were highly toxic to *mouse* connective tissue fibroblasts when containing concentrations of hypochlorite as low as 0.005%, and some evidence of cell damage was still detectable at 0.0025%. It was suggested that in the absence of signs of clinical infection basic wound toilet should consist of cleansing with an isotonic saline solution. If an antimicrobial agent is required, a sterile solution of chlorhexidine should be considered, but the repeated application to an open wound of hypochlorites is likely adversely to affect granulation and hence delay wound healing.— S. Thomas and N. P. Hay (letter), *Pharm. J.*, 1985, *2*, 206. Comment. Eschar removal is an essential and primary stage in the mechanism of wound healing. The natural autolytic processes of the tissue are enhanced by the ability of sodium hypochlorite solution to hydrolyse tissue proteins and thereby aid in the dissolution of necrosed tissue. At the same time it serves as an antimicrobial agent, reducing the possibility of wound sepsis and septicaemia. These characteristics decrease the time interval between injury and the formation of granulation tissue, a major step in the process of wound healing, and reduce the time to the first tissue graft. It is at this point that hypochlorite solutions should be discontinued.— C. L. Gummer (letter), *ibid.*, 1986, *1*, 35. Further comment. The ability of hypochlorite solutions to hydrolyse and dissolve necrotic tissue was thought to be less important clinically than previously believed. An alternative explanation for the successful use of hypochlorite solutions to deslough wounds was probably eschar rehydration following the use of wet dressing packs, a process that could be achieved without the problems of cytotoxicity associated with the use of hypochlorite.— S. Thomas (letter), *ibid.*, 128.

2225-n

Chloroazodin

Azochloramid; Chlorazodin *(rINN)*. α,α′-Azobis(N^2-chloroformamidine).

$C_2H_4Cl_2N_6$=183.0.

CAS — 502-98-7.

Pharmacopoeias. In *Arg.*

Chloroazodin contains about 77% w/w of 'available chlorine' (see p.958). It explodes without melting at about 155°. All its solutions decompose on exposure to light. **Store** in airtight containers. Protect from light. Its decomposition is accelerated by contact with metals.

Chloroazodin aqueous solution liberates chlorine very slowly. It has been used as a wet dressing and for irrigating infected wounds.

2226-h

Chlorocresol *(BAN, USAN, rINN)*.

Chlorkresolum; Parachlorometacresol; PCMC. *p*-Chloro-*m*-cresol; 4-Chloro-3-methylphenol.

C_7H_7ClO=142.6.

CAS — 59-50-7.

Pharmacopoeias. In *Aust.*, *Belg.*, *Br.*, *Eur.*, *Fr.*, *Ind.*, *Int.*, *It.*, *Jug.*, *Neth.*, *Nord.*, *Swiss*, *Turk.*, and *U.S.N.F.*

Colourless or almost colourless crystals or white crystalline powder with a characteristic, odour; it is volatile in steam. M.p. 63° to 66°.

Slightly **soluble** in water; very slightly soluble in alcohol; freely soluble in ether and in fatty oils; dissolves in aqueous solutions of alkali hydroxides. Solutions in water acquire a yellowish colour on exposure to light and air. **Store** in airtight containers. Protect from light.

INCOMPATIBILITIES. Chlorocresol has long been recognised to be incompatible with a range of compounds including:

hydrated calcium chloride, codeine phosphate, diamorphine hydrochloride, papaveretum, quinine hydrochloride, methylcellulose, and nonionic surfactants.

References: J. S. McEwan and G. H. Macmorran, *Pharm. J.*, 1947, *1*, 260; W. E. Harris, *Australas. J. Pharm.*, 1961, *42*, 583; Pharm. Soc. Lab. Rep. P/70/15, 1970.; R. T. Yousef *et al.*, *Can. J. pharm. Sci.*, 1973, *8*, 54.

Adverse Effects, Treatment, and Precautions

As for Phenol, p.967.

Chlorocresol is much less toxic than phenol. Sensitisation reactions may follow application to the skin. The antimicrobial activity of chlorocresol may be diminished through incompatibility (see above), through adsorption, or through combination with organic matter. For comment on some measures that reduce the risk of contamination of disinfectants, see cetrimide (p.954).

Hypersensitivity occurred in a patient given heparin preserved with chlorocresol. Chlorocresol was considered to be responsible.— E. J. Ainley *et al.* (letter), *Lancet*, 1977, *1*, 705.

Uses and Administration

Chlorocresol is a potent disinfectant; it is more active in acid than in alkaline solution.

It was used in a concentration of 0.2% in the process of sterilisation by heating with a bactericide and is used, in a concentration of 0.1%, in aqueous injections issued in multidose containers to maintain sterility during the withdrawal of successive doses. It should not be employed for these purposes in solutions for use by intrathecal, intracisternal, or peridural injection, or in solutions for intravenous injections where the dose exceeds 15 mL.

It is also used as a preservative in creams and other preparations for external use which contain water but its effectiveness is reduced if oils, fats, or nonionic surfactants are present.

Proprietary Preparations

Wright's Vaporizing Fluid *(LRC Products, UK). Liquid,* chlorocresol 10%. For use in Wright's Vaporizer for congestion in whooping cough, the common cold, and catarrh.

A survey of poisoning by Wright's Vaporizing Fluid.— H. M. Wiseman *et al., Postgrad. med. J.,* 1980, *56,* 166.

Proprietary Names and Manufacturers

Wright's Vaporizing Fluid *(LRC Products, UK).*

The following names have been used for multi-ingredient preparations containing chlorocresol— Cyteal *(Concept Pharmaceuticals, UK)*; Gomaxine *(Seaford, UK)*; HEB 'A' (Anerythene) *(Waterhouse, UK)*; Hycolin *(Pearson, UK)*; Medol *(Austral.)*; Sterillium *(Pearson, UK).*

2228-b

Chloroxylenol *(BAN, USAN, rINN).*

Parachlorometaxylenol; PCMX. 4-Chloro-3,5-xylenol; 4-Chloro-3,5-dimethylphenol.

C_8H_9ClO=156.6.

CAS — 88-04-0.

Pharmacopoeias. In *Arg., Br.,* and *U.S.* Also in *B.P. Vet.*

White or cream-coloured crystals or crystalline powder with a characteristic odour; volatile in steam. Very slightly **soluble** in water; soluble 1 in 1 of alcohol; soluble in ether, terpenes, and fixed oils; dissolves in solutions of the alkali hydroxides. **Incompatible** with nonionic surfactants and methylcellulose.

Adverse Effects and Precautions

Chloroxylenol in the recommended dilutions is generally non-irritant but skin sensitivity has occurred. There have been isolated reports of poisoning.

The antimicrobial activity of chloroxylenol may be diminished through incompatibility (see above) or through combination with organic matter. For comment on some measures that reduce the risk of contamination of disinfectants, see cetrimide (p.954).

Reports of fatal or severe self-poisoning with chloroxylenol solution (Dettol): D. Meek *et al., Postgrad. med. J.,* 1977, *53,* 229; P. Joubert *et al., Br. med. J.,* 1978, *1,* 890.

Absorption and Fate

If chloroxylenol is ingested accidentally about one-third is excreted in the urine conjugated with glucuronic acid and sulphate.

Uses and Administration

Chloroxylenol is a disinfectant which is active against streptococci but less active against staphylococci and Gram-negative organisms, and is often inactive against *Pseudomonas* spp. Its activity against *Ps. aeruginosa* appears to be increased by the addition of edetic acid. It is inactive against bacterial spores.

It is used chiefly in the form of Chloroxylenol Solution for skin and wound disinfection.

Preparations

Chloroxylenol Solution *(B.P.).* Roxenol. Chloroxylenol 5 g, terpineol 10 mL, alcohol (or industrial methylated spirit) 20 mL, castor oil 6.3 g, potassium hydroxide 1.36 g, oleic acid 0.75 mL, freshly boiled and cooled water to 100 mL.

Proprietary Preparations

Dettol *(Reckitt & Colman Pharmaceuticals, UK). Liquid,* chloroxylenol 4.8%.
Lotion, chloroxylenol 1.3%, edetic acid 0.2%.
Cream, chloroxylenol 0.3%, triclosan 0.3%, edetic acid 0.2%.
Mouthwash, chloroxylenol 1.02%, with menthol, peppermint oil, anise oil, and other ingredients.

Proprietary Names and Manufacturers of Chloroxylenol and some other Chlorinated Phenols

Anti-Sept *(Seamless Hosp. Prod., USA)*; Bristol Pine Disinfectant *(Tenneco, UK)*; CX 140 *(BTP Cocker Chemicals, UK)*; CX 41 *(BTP Cocker Chemicals, UK)*; Dettol *(Reckitt & Colman, Austral.; Neth.; Reckitt & Colman Pharmaceuticals, UK)*; Espadol Quirúrgico *(Arg.)*; Iba-Cide *(Ingram & Bell, Canad.)*; Ibcol *(Jeyes, UK)*; Jeypine *(Jeyes, UK)*; Metasep *(Milance, USA)*; Prinsyl; Pynol *(Wellcome, UK).*

The following names have been used for multi-ingredient preparations containing chloroxylenol and some other chlorinated phenols—Acne-aid *(Stiefel, Canad.)*; Dettol Cream *(Reckitt & Colman, Austral.; Reckitt & Colman Pharmaceuticals, UK)*; Fungi-Nail *(Kramer, USA)*; Fungoid *(Pedinol, USA)*; Gomaxide *(Seaford, UK)*; Halocide 10 *(BTP Cocker Chemicals, UK)*; Hycolin *(Pearson, UK)*; Izal *(Sterling Health, UK)*; Medol *(Austral.)*; Otic-HC *(Hauck, USA)*; Oticol *(Arlo, USA)*; Steraskin *(G.P. Laboratories, Austral.)*; Sterillium *(Pearson, UK)*; Surgical Dettol *(Reckitt & Colman Pharmaceuticals, UK)*; Zal *(Sterling Health, UK)*; Zant *(Evans Medical, UK)*; ZeaSorb *(Stiefel, UK).*

2230-r

Clorophene *(USAN).*

Clorfene; Clorofene *(pINN)*; NSC-59989; Septiphene. 2-Benzyl-4-chlorophenol.

$C_{13}H_{11}ClO$=218.7.

CAS — 120-32-1.

Clorophene is stated to have a high phenol coefficient against a wide range of bacteria, fungi, protozoa, and viruses. It is used in disinfectant solutions and soaps.

Proprietary Names and Manufacturers

Manusept Emulsion *(Switz.)*; Santophen 1 *(Monsanto, UK).*

The following names have been used for multi-ingredient preparations containing clorophene— Hycolin *(Pearson, UK)*; Medol *(Austral.)*; Sterillium *(Pearson, UK).*

2231-f

Cresol *(BAN, USAN).*

Cresolum Crudum; Cresylic Acid; Kresolum Venale; Tricresol; Trikresolum. Methylphenol.

C_7H_8O=108.1.

CAS — 1319-77-3; 95-48-7 (o-cresol); 108-39-4 (m-cresol); 106-44-5 (p-cresol).

Pharmacopoeias. In *Arg., Aust., Belg., Br., Chin., Hung., Ind., Int., It., Jpn, Jug., Mex., Nord., Pol., Port., Roum., Span.,* and *Turk.* Also in *U.S.N.F.*

NOTE. Some grades of mixed cresols may be equivalent to Tar Acids, see p.970.

An almost colourless, or yellowish to pale brownish-yellow, or pinkish liquid, becoming darker with age or on exposure to light, with a characteristic odour resembling phenol, but more tarry, and consisting of a mixture of cresols and other phenols obtained from coal tar or petroleum.

Almost completely **soluble** 1 in 50 of water; freely soluble in alcohol, ether, chloroform, and in fixed and volatile oils; soluble in solutions of alkali hydroxides. A 2% solution in water is neutral to bromocresol purple. **Store** in airtight containers. Protect from light.

Cresol has a similar action to phenol (p.968). The majority of common pathogens are killed in about 10 minutes by solutions containing 0.3 to 0.6% of cresol but spores require higher concentrations for a much longer time.

It is used as Cresol and Soap Solution (Lysol) as a general disinfectant for hospital and domestic use but it has been largely superseded by less irritant phenolic disinfectants. In Great Britain the recommended exposure limit of cresols is 5 ppm (long-term); suitable precautions should be taken to prevent absorption through the skin. In the *US* the permissible and recommended exposure limits are 22 mg per m^3 and 10 mg per m^3. It is caustic to the skin and unsuitable for skin and wound disinfection. The cresols are widely used in commercial disinfectants.

A 52-year-old man who swallowed approximately 100 mL of a petroleum distillate containing cresol 12% suffered acute intravascular haemolytic anaemia with massive haemoglobinuria; this was attributed to haemoglobin denaturation and Heinz body formation, probably due to cresol intoxication. The patient was successfully treated with immediate erythrocytaphaeresis followed, over 5 days, by forced diuresis to prevent renal failure, and additional packed red cell transfusions.— M. A. Côté *et al., Can. med. Ass. J.,* 1984, *130,* 1319.

Preparations

See under Proprietary Names and Manufacturers of Preparations containing Cresols, Tar Acids, or other Phenols, p.970.

2232-d

Crystal Violet *(BAN).*

CI Basic Violet 3; Colour Index No. 42555; Gentian Violet *(USAN)*; Hexamethylpararosaniline Chloride; Methylrosanilinium Chloride *(rINN)*; Methylviolett; Pyoctaninum Caeruleum; Viola Crystallina. 4-[4,4′Bis(dimethylamino)benzhydrylidene]cyclohexa-2,5-dien-1-ylidenedimethylammonium chloride.

$C_{25}H_{30}ClN_3$=408.0.

CAS — 548-62-9.

Pharmacopoeias. In *Egypt., Fr., Ind., Nord.,* and *U.S. Arg., Aust., Braz., Hung., Jpn,* and *Jug.* include mixtures of hexamethylpararosaniline hydrochloride with the tetramethyl- and pentamethyl-compounds.

The name methyl violet—CI Basic Violet 1; Colour Index No. 42535—has been used as a synonym for crystal violet, but is applied to a mixture of the hydrochlorides of the higher methylated pararosanilines consisting principally of the tetramethyl-, pentamethyl-, and hexamethyl compounds.

Dark green powder or greenish, glistening crystals with a metallic luster; odourless or almost odourless. Sparingly **soluble** in water; soluble 1 in 10 of alcohol and 1 in 15 of glycerin; also soluble in chloroform; practically insoluble in ether. **Store** in well-closed containers. Aqueous solutions of greater strength than 0.5% can be prepared by the addition of alcohol, but are not suitable for use on mucous membranes.

The antibacterial activity of crystal violet was inhibited in suspension of bentonite with which it formed a stable complex.— W. A. Harris, *Australas. J. Pharm.,* 1961, *42,* 583.

REMOVAL OF STAINS. *From the skin.* Dilute hydrochloric acid was applied and rinsed immediately under running water; a second application and rinse might be necessary.—Pharm. Soc. Lab. Rep., *Pharm. J.,* 1961, *2,* 187.

Adverse Effects and Precautions

Crystal violet is usually well tolerated but may cause nausea, vomiting, diarrhoea, abdominal pain, and ulceration of mucous membranes. Avoid contact with the eyes.

The antimicrobial activity of crystal violet may be diminished through adsorption or through combination with organic matter.

Animal carcinogenicity has restricted its use.

In vitro, crystal violet was capable of interacting with DNA of living cells (indicating possible carcinogenicity); this suggested a need to re-evaluate its use clinically.— H. S. Rosenkranz and H. S. Carr (letter), *Br. med. J.,* 1971, *3,* 702. The Food Advisory Committee of the *UK* reported that crystal violet had demonstrated carcinogenicity in *mice.*— Fd AC/REP/4, London, HM Stationery Office, 1987..

A report of 3 patients who developed necrotic skin reactions after the topical application of a 1% aqueous solution of crystal violet. Other cases had been observed. The areas involved included the submammary folds, the genitalia, the gluteal fold, and the toe-webs. A similar reaction was produced in 2 subjects by the application of 1% crystal violet or brilliant green to stripped skin.— A. Björnberg and H. Mobacken, *Acta derm.-vener., Stockh.,* 1972, *52,* 55.

All of 6 neonates treated with aqueous crystal violet 0.5 or 1% for oral candidiasis developed oral ulceration not attributable to the candidiasis.— P. Horsfield *et al.* (letter), *Br. med. J.,* 1976, *2,* 529.

Severe haemorrhagic cystitis rapidly occurred in a 32-year-old woman after accidental injection through the urethra of a solution of crystal violet 1% and alcohol

2%. Her condition gradually improved with a high fluid intake.— C. Walsh and A. Walsh, *Br. med. J.*, 1986, *293*, 732. See also T. J. Christmas *et al.* (letter), *Lancet*, 1988, *2*, 459.

PORPHYRIA. Crystal violet was considered to be unsafe in patients with acute porphyria because it has been shown to be porphyrinogenic in *animals* or *in vitro* systems.— M.R. Moore and K.E.L. McColl, *Porphyrias, Drug Lists*, Glasgow, Porphyria Research Unit, University of Glasgow, 1987.

Uses and Administration

Crystal violet is a disinfectant effective against some vegetative Gram-positive bacteria, particularly *Staphylococcus* spp., and some pathogenic yeasts such as *Candida* spp. It is much less active against Gram-negative bacteria and ineffective against bacterial spores. Its activity increases as pH increases.

Crystal violet has been applied topically for the treatment of bacterial and fungal infections, but its use is now restricted to application to unbroken skin because of concern at *animal* carcinogenicity. This concern has also affected the use of crystal violet for food marking.

A plea that restricting the use of crystal violet to intact skin should not preclude its use as a skin marker for surgeons planning their incisions. A preparation of crystal violet [with brilliant green] known as Bonney's Blue does not permanently tattoo the skin, it withstands wetting with blood and saline, and it can be easily removed with spirit. Its use has not produced any reports of malignancy.— B. M. Jones and D. T. Gault (letter), *Lancet*, 1988, *1*, 949.

TRYPANOSOMIASIS. Crystal violet is used in some countries to prevent the transmission of Chagas' disease by blood transfusion. The recommended inclusion concentration is 1 mM; it appears to work for most but not all strains of *Trypanosoma cruzi in vitro*. No apparent side-effects have been reported from patients receiving treated blood.— W. E. Gutteridge, *Br. med. Bull.*, 1985, *41*, 162.

Preparations

Gentian Violet Cream *(U.S.P.)*. It contains gentian violet *U.S.P.* 1.2 to 1.6%, calculated as anhydrous hexamethylpararosaniline chloride in a suitable cream basis. Store at a temperature not exceeding 40° in airtight containers.

Gentian Violet Topical Solution *(U.S.P.)*. Gentian Violet Solution. Contains gentian violet (*U.S.P.*) equivalent to hexamethylpararosaniline chloride 0.95 to 1.05% with alcohol 8 to 10%. Store in airtight containers.

Proprietary Names and Manufacturers

Genapax *(Key, USA)*; Viogencianol *(Aprofa, Spain)*.

2234-h

Dequalinium Chloride *(BAN, rINN)*.

Decalinium Chloride; Decaminum. *N,N*-Decamethylenebis(4-amino-2-methylquinolinium chloride).

$C_{30}H_{40}Cl_2N_4$=527.6.

CAS — 6707-58-0 (dequalinium); 522-51-0 (chloride).

Pharmacopoeias. In *Br., Ind.,* and *Rus.*

A creamy-white odourless or almost odourless powder. Slightly **soluble** in water; soluble 1 in 30 of boiling water; slightly soluble in propylene glycol. **Incompatible** with soaps and other anionic surfactants, with phenol, and with chlorocresol.

Dequalinium is a bisquaternary ammonium antiseptic, active against many Gram-positive and Gram-negative bacteria, yeasts, and fungi. The action is little affected by the presence of serum. It is mainly used in the form of lozenges in the treatment of minor local infections.

Ulceration and necrosis have been reported following its topical use.

Proprietary Preparations

Dequadin *(Evans Medical, UK)*. *Lozenges*, dequalinium chloride 250 µg.

Labosept *(Laboratories for Applied Biology, UK)*. *Pastilles, dequalinium chloride 250 µg.*

Proprietary Names and Manufacturers of Dequalinium Salts

Angils *(Belg.)*; Danical *(Denm.)*; Decabis *(Gazzoni, Ital.)*; Dekadin *(Norw.)*; Dequadin *(Glaxo, Austral.; Glaxo, Canad.; Denm.; Eurospital Pharma, Ital.; Glaxo, S.Afr.; Inibsa, Spain; Switz.; Evans Medical, UK)*; Dequafungan *(Ger.)*; Dequavagyn *(Kreussler, Ger.)*; Dequin *(Inibsa, Spain)*; Eriosept *(Kreussler, Ger.)*; Evazol *(Ravensberg, Ger.)*; Faringina *(SIT, Ital.)*; Formocillina al Dequalinium *(Zyma, Ital.)*; Gargilon *(Neth.)*; Grocrème *(Grossmann, Switz.)*; Hexilin *(Evans Medical, UK)*; Labosept *(Laboratories for Applied Biology, UK)*; Leuco-Dibios *(Dibios, Spain)*; Maltyl *(Merckle, Ger.)*; Osangin *(Antonetto, Ital.)*; Phylletten *(Rorer, Ger.)*; Salvizol *(Norw.)*; Soor-Gel *(Engelhard, Ger.)*; Sorot *(Ravensberg, Ger.)*; SP *(Jpn)*.

The following names have been used for multi-ingredient preparations containing dequalinium chloride— Dequacaine (*Evans Medical, UK*); Dequadin Mouth Ulcer Paint (*Glaxo, Austral.*).

2235-m

Diacetylaminoazotoluene

Diacetazotol; Pellidol. 4-Diacetylamino-2′,3-dimethylazobenzene.

$C_{18}H_{19}N_3O_2$=309.4.

CAS — 83-63-6.

Pharmacopoeias. In *Aust.* and *Span.*

Diacetylaminoazotoluene is chemically related to scarlet red (see p.969) and has been used medicinally for similar purposes.

2236-b

Dibromopropamidine Isethionate *(BANM)*.

Dibromopropamidine Isetionate *(rINNM)*. 3,3′-Dibromo-4,4′-triethylenedioxydibenzamidine bis(2-hydroxyethanesulphonate).

$C_{17}H_{18}Br_2N_4O_2,2C_2H_6O_4S$=722.4.

CAS — 496-00-4 (dibromopropamidine); 614-87-9 (isethionate).

Pharmacopoeias. In *Br.*

A white or almost white, odourless, crystalline powder. **Soluble** 1 in 2 of water, 1 in 60 of alcohol, and 1 in 20 of glycerol; practically insoluble in chloroform, ether, fixed oils, and liquid paraffin. A 5% solution in water has a pH of 5 to 7. **Store** in well-closed containers.

Dibromopropamidine isethionate is an aromatic diamidine which is active against Gram-positive bacteria but is less active against Gram-negative bacteria and spore-forming organisms. It also has antifungal properties.

It is available as topical preparations for the local treatment of minor infections.

A report of the successful treatment of acanthamoeba keratitis with dibromopropamidine and propamidine isethionates, and neomycin.— P. Wright *et al.*, *Br. J. Ophthal.*, 1985, *69*, 778.

Proprietary Preparations

Brolene *(May & Baker, UK)*. *Eye ointment*, dibromopropamidine isethionate 0.15%.

Brulidine *(May & Baker, UK)*. *Cream*, dibromopropamidine isethionate 0.15%.

Proprietary Names and Manufacturers

Brolene *(May & Baker, Austral.; S.Afr.; May & Baker, UK)*; Brulidine *(May & Baker, Austral.; Rhône-Poulenc, Norw.; S.Afr.; May & Baker, UK)*.

The following names have been used for multi-ingredient preparations containing dibromopropamidine isethionate— Otamidyl *(May & Baker, UK)*; Phenergan Cream *(May & Baker, Austral.; May & Baker, UK)*.

2237-v

Dichlordimethylhydantoin

1,3-Dichloro-5,5-dimethylhydantoin; 1,3-Dichloro-5,5-dimethylimidazolidine-2,4-dione.

$C_5H_6Cl_2N_2O_2$=197.0.

It contains about 68% w/w of 'available chlorine'.

Dichlordimethylhydantoin is used as a source of chlorine, for sterilising babies' feeding bottles, and as a bleach.

In Great Britain the recommended exposure limits of dichlordimethylhydantoin are 0.2 mg per m^3 (long-term); 0.4 mg per m^3 (short-term).

Bromochlorodimethylhydantoin ($C_5H_6N_2O_2BrCl$=241.5) is a bromine-releasing compound used for the disinfection of swimming-pool water.

Proprietary Names and Manufacturers

Hydan *(ABM Chemicals, UK)*.

2238-g

Dichlorobenzyl Alcohol

2,4-Dichlorobenzyl alcohol.

$C_7H_6Cl_2O$=177.0.

CAS — 1777-82-8.

Dichlorobenzyl alcohol is an antiseptic used as an ingredient of throat lozenges.

Proprietary Names and Manufacturers

Dybenal; Myacide SP *(Boots, UK)*.

The following names have been used for multi-ingredient preparations containing dichlorobenzyl alcohol— Strepsils *(Boots, Austral.; Crookes Healthcare, UK)*.

2239-q

Dichloroxylenol *(BAN, rINN)*.

DCMX; Dichlorometaxylenol. 2,4-Dichloro-3,5-xylenol; 2,4-Dichloro-3,5-dimethylphenol.

$C_8H_8Cl_2O$=191.1.

CAS — 133-53-9.

Dichloroxylenol is a bactericide with actions similar to those of chloroxylenol (p.959) and may be used for the same purposes.

Proprietary Names and Manufacturers

Multiguard *(Sterling Industrial, UK)*.

The following names have been used for multi-ingredient preparations containing dichloroxylenol— Izal (*Sterling Industrial, UK*).

2242-h

Domiphen Bromide *(BAN, USAN, rINN)*.

NSC-39415; Phenododecinium Bromide. It consists chiefly of dodecyldimethyl-2-phenoxyethylammonium bromide.

$C_{22}H_{40}BrNO$=414.5.

CAS — 13900-14-6 (domiphen); 538-71-6 (bromide).

Pharmacopoeias. In *Br.* and *Chin.*

Colourless or faintly yellow crystalline flakes. **Soluble** 1 in less than 2 of water, 1 in less than 2 of alcohol, and 1 in 30 of acetone. A 10% solution in water is not more than slightly opalescent. A 1% solution in water has a pH of 6.4 to 7.6.

Incompatible with soaps and other anionic surfactants.

Domiphen bromide is a quaternary ammonium disinfectant with properties and uses similar to those of cetrimide (p.953).

Lozenges each containing 500 µg of domiphen bromide have been used in the treatment of minor local infections.

Proprietary Preparations

Bradosol *(Ciba Consumer, UK)*. *Lozenges*, domiphen bromide 500 µg. Bradosol Plus contains in addition lignocaine hydrochloride 5 mg.

Proprietary Names and Manufacturers

Bradoral *(Ciba, Ital.)*; Bradosol *(Ciba-Geigy, Canad.; Denm.; Ciba Consumer, UK)*; Neo-Bradoral *(Ciba, Switz.)*.

The following names have been used for multi-ingredient preparations containing domiphen bromide— Bradosol Plus (*Ciba Consumer, UK*); Oticol (*Arlo, USA*).

2243-m

Ethacridine Lactate *(rINNM)*.

Acrinol; Aethacridinium Lacticum; Lactoacridine. 6,9-Diamino-2-ethoxyacridine lactate.

$C_{15}H_{15}N_3O,C_3H_6O_3$=343.4.

CAS — 442-16-0 (ethacridine); 1837-57-6 (lactate).

Pharmacopoeias. In *Cz., Jug., Pol., Rus.,* and *Swiss*; in *Aust., Ger., Jpn, Port.,* and *Roum.* as monohydrate.

Ethacridine lactate has properties similar to other acridine derivatives (see p.969). It has been applied topically as a disinfectant; allergic reactions have occurred.

Ethacridine lactate has been given by extra-amniotic instillation for induction of abortion.

References to ethacridine being given by mouth: N. Madanagopalan *et al.*, *Curr. ther. Res.*, 1975, *18*, 546 (diarrhoea); T. J. Rising *et al.*, *Arzneimittel-Forsch.*, 1977, *27*, 872 (faecal elimination).

The intra-cervical introduction of 2 laminaria tents (see p.1582) 2 hours after extra-amniotic instillation of ethacridine decreased the mean induction-abortion interval from 32.7 to 19.7 hours in 80 women undergoing second trimester abortion compared to the instillation of ethacridine alone.— A. Jonasson *et al.*, *Curr. ther. Res.*, 1984, *35*, 793.

Proprietary Names and Manufacturers

Antidiar 200 *(Hoechst, Arg.)*; Gelastypt *(Hoechst, Ger.; Hoechst, Switz.)*; Hectalin *(Jpn)*; Metifex *(Cassella-med, Ger.)*; Rimaon *(Jpn)*; Rivanol *(Chinosolfabrik, Ger.)*.

2244-b

Ethylene Oxide

Oxirane.

C_2H_4O=44.05.

CAS — 75-21-8.

Mixtures of ethylene oxide with oxygen or air are explosive but the risk can be reduced by the addition of carbon dioxide or fluorocarbons.

Adverse Effects and Precautions

Ethylene oxide vapour irritates the nose and eyes and may also cause nausea and vomiting, diarrhoea, headache, vertigo, central nervous system depression, dyspnoea, and pulmonary oedema. Liver and kidney damage may occur. Fatalities have occurred. Excessive exposure of the skin to liquid or solution causes burns and blistering. There is some concern about the mutagenic and carcinogenic risk to man.

Many materials including plastics and rubber adsorb ethylene oxide. If such materials are being sterilised with ethylene oxide all traces of the gas must be removed before the materials can be used; removal may be by ventilation or more active means. Anaphylactic reactions have been associated with ethylene oxide-contaminated materials. Ethylene oxide may also react with materials being sterilised to produce substances such as ethylene chlorohydrin that may contribute to any toxicity.

In Great Britain the control exposure limit of ethylene oxide is 5 ppm (long-term). In the *US* the permissible and recommended exposure limits are 1.8 mg per m^3 and less than 0.18 mg per m^3 respectively.

Four men exposed to ethylene oxide at a concentration of greater than 700 ppm developed neurological disorders. One experienced headaches, nausea, vomiting, and lethargy followed by major motor seizures. The others experienced headaches, limb numbness and weakness, increased fatigue, trouble with memory and thought processes, and slurred speech. Three also developed cataracts, and one required bilateral cataract extractions.— W. M. Jay *et al.*, *Am. J. Ophthal.*, 1982, *93*, 727.

ALLERGY. Severe, sometimes fatal, anaphylactoid reactions occur very occasionally at the beginning of dialysis; almost universally a new dialyser sterilised with ethylene oxide has been implicated. Dyspnoea, wheezing, urticaria, flushing, headache, and hypotension are the most common adverse reactions, but acute severe bronchospasm, circulatory collapse, cardiac arrest, and death may occur. Allergy to ethylene oxide plays a part in these reactions, but exposure to cuprammonium cellulose (cuprophane) dialysis membranes may also be involved.— A. Nicholls, *Br. med. J.*, 1986, *292*, 1221. Some references to anaphylactoid reactions in dialysis patients resulting from the use of dialysis equipment sterilised with ethylene oxide: J. Bommer *et al.*, *Lancet*, 1985, *2*, 1382; K. W. Rumpf *et al.*, *ibid.*, 1385; A. Röckel *et al.* (letter), *ibid.*, 1986, *1*, 382; P. Piazolo and W. J. Brech (letter), *ibid.*, 918.

Allergic reactions in healthy plateletpheresis donors caused by sensitisation to ethylene oxide gas used to sterilise plastic components in disposable apheresis kits.— S. F. Leitman *et al.*, *New Engl. J. Med.*, 1986, *315*, 1192; L. Muylle *et al.* (letter), *Lancet*, 1986, *2*, 1225.

LEUKAEMIA. The recurrent finding of leukaemia in association with exposure to ethylene oxide is impressive, but the existence of a hazard cannot yet be regarded as established. The number of documented cases is small, the association has not been specific for any one type of leukaemia, and all of the workforces studied have been exposed to other chemicals.— *Lancet*, 1986, *2*, 201.

PREGNANCY AND THE NEONATE. A study of female hospital sterilising staff in all general hospitals in Finland showed that the incidence of spontaneous abortion (analysed according to employment at the time of conception and corrected for maternal age, parity, decade of pregnancy, smoking, and consumption of alcohol and coffee) was significantly increased in those exposed to ethylene oxide during pregnancy compared with those not so exposed.— K. Hemminki *et al.*, *Br. med. J.*, 1982, *285*, 1461. Criticisms: J. E. Gordon and T. J. Meinhardt (letter), *ibid.*, 1983, *286*, 1976; S. G. Austin (letter), *ibid.* Reply.— K. Hemminki *et al.* (letter), *ibid.*

Uses and Administration

Ethylene oxide is a bactericide and fungicide which is effective against most micro-organisms, including viruses. It is also sporicidal. It is used as a fumigant for foodstuffs and textiles and as an agent for the gaseous sterilisation of pharmaceutical and surgical materials.

The principal disadvantage of ethylene oxide is that it forms explosive mixtures with air, but this may be overcome by using mixtures containing 10% ethylene oxide in carbon dioxide or halogenated hydrocarbons, or by removing at least 95% of the air from the apparatus before admitting either ethylene oxide or a mixture of 90% ethylene oxide in carbon dioxide.

Certain fluorinated hydrocarbons form non-inflammable mixtures with ethylene oxide; mixtures of dichlorodifluoromethane and trichlorofluoromethane with 9 to 12% w/w of ethylene oxide are most commonly employed. The hydrocarbons permit a higher partial pressure of ethylene oxide in the exposure chamber at the same total pressure compared with that achieved with carbon dioxide.

Effective sterilisation by ethylene oxide depends on exposure time, temperature, humidity, the amount and type of microbial contamination, and the partial pressure of the ethylene oxide in the exposure chamber. The material being sterilised must be permeable to ethylene oxide if occluded micro-organisms are present. The bactericidal action is accelerated by increase of temperature; a temperature of about 55° can be used for most thermolabile materials.

Moisture is essential for sterilisation by ethylene oxide. In practice, dry micro-organisms need to be rehydrated before ethylene oxide can be effective, so a conditioning period in a suitable atmosphere should be used before sterilisation. Relative humidities of 40 to 60% are used. Control of physical factors does not assure sterility, and the process should be monitored usually by employing standardised suspensions of aerobic spores.

VIRAL DISINFECTION. For the use of ethylene oxide for the disinfection of articles contaminated with human immunodeficiency virus, see p.950.

Proprietary Names and Manufacturers

Cartox *(Rentokil, UK)*; Sterethox *(ICI Mond, UK)*.

2245-v

Euflavine

Neutral Acriflavine; Neutroflavin.

It consists of a mixture of 3,6-diamino-10-methylacridinium chloride and 3,6-diaminoacridine monohydrochloride. The latter is usually present to the extent of between 30 and 40%.

Euflavine has properties similar to other acridine derivatives (see p.969).

VASECTOMY. References to euflavine being used as a spermicide during vasectomy with some indication that it was not completely effective: D. Urquhart-Hay, *Br. med. J.*, 1973, *3*, 378; L. N. Jackson (letter), *ibid.*, 589; J. Slome (letter), *ibid.*, *4*, 233; I. S. Edwards, *Med. J. Aust.*, 1977, *1*, 847.

Preparations

Euflavine Lint *(B.P.C. 1973)*. Absorbent lint impregnated with 0.08 to 0.2% of euflavine.

2246-g

Formaldehyde *(BAN, USAN)*.

CH_2O=30.03.

CAS — 50-00-0.

NOTE. The names formalin and formol have been used for Formaldehyde Solution but in some countries Formalin is a trade mark.

Pharmacopoeias. Formaldehyde Solution is in *Arg., Aust., Belg., Br., Chin., Cz., Egypt., Fr., Ger., Hung., Int., It., Jpn, Jug., Mex., Nord., Pol., Port., Roum., Rus., Span., Swiss, Turk.*, and *U.S.* The specified content of formaldehyde varies slightly but is usually about the same as the *B.P.*

Formaldehyde is usually available as an aqueous solution containing as specified in the *B.P.* 34 to 38% w/w of CH_2O (= 30.03) with methyl alcohol as a stabilising agent to delay polymerisation of the formaldehyde to solid paraformaldehyde. The *U.S.P.* specifies not less than 36.5% or 37.0% (depending on the packaging) of CH_2O. It is a colourless liquid with a characteristic, pungent, irritating odour.

Miscible with water and alcohol. **Store** the solution at a temperature between 15° and 25° in airtight containers. A slight white deposit may form on keeping and develops more rapidly if the solution is kept in a cold place.

NOTE. There is often confusion about the terminology and strength of formaldehyde. In practice, the term formaldehyde is used to describe Formaldehyde Solution also known as formalin. Thus 1% formaldehyde is 1% of Formaldehyde Solution.

The Clinitest reaction fails to detect concentrations of formaldehyde below 50 ppm. Many dialysis units abandoned the use of Clinitest for this purpose in favour of the Schiff reagent (decolorised magenta solution) which, when used in ratios of 1 : 1 to 3 : 1 with the test sample, detects formaldehyde at a concentration of 3.6 to 5 ppm. A further advantage of the Schiff reagent is its insensitivity to glucose, making it usable in conjunction with a glucose-containing dialysate.— G. Zasuwa and N. W. Levin (letter), *New Engl. J. Med.*, 1982, *306*, 1550.

Adverse Effects and Precautions

Formaldehyde vapour is irritant to the eyes, nose, and respiratory tract, and may cause coughing, dysphagia, spasm and oedema of the larnyx, bronchitis, and pneumonia. Asthma has been reported after repeated exposure.

Concentrated solutions applied to the skin cause whitening and hardening. Contact dermatitis and sensitivity reactions have occurred after the use of conventional concentrations and after contact with residual formaldehyde in resins.

Ingestion of solutions of formaldehyde causes intense pain, with inflammation, ulceration, and necrosis of mucous membranes. There may be vomiting, haematemesis, blood-stained diarrhoea, haematuria, and anuria; metabolic acidosis, vertigo, convulsions, and circulatory failure may occur. Death has occurred after the ingestion of the equivalent of about 30mL of Formaldehyde Solution. If the patient survives 48 hours, recovery is probable.

In Great Britain the control exposure limit of formaldehyde is 2 ppm. In the *US* the permissible exposure limit is 3 ppm.

Formaldehyde reacts with protein and this may diminish its antimicrobial activity.

Toxicity Review 2, Formaldehyde, Health and Safety Executive, London, HMSO, 1981.

In reviews of the health risks in homes insulated with urea-formaldehyde foam, which releases formaldehyde, it was concluded that there was no good evidence that systemic and respiratory illness were directly attributable to exposure to the foam (J.R. Hoey *et al.*, *Can. med. Ass. J.*, 1984, *130*, 115; J.H. Day *et al.*, ibid., *131*, 1061; G.R. Norman *et al.*, *ibid.*, 1986, *134*, 1135).

ALLERGY. A report of acute exacerbation of eczema in a 24-year-old woman after injection of hepatitis B vaccine, containing formaldehyde up to 20 µg per mL. Patch-tests with formaldehyde were positive.— J. Ring (letter), *Lancet*, 1986, *2*, 522.

For a report of an allergic response to root canal paste containing paraformaldehyde, see Paraformaldehyde, p.967.

See also below under Effects on the Gingiva and Shock.

CARCINOGENICITY. From 1972 to 1979 the Ontario Cancer Registry recorded no deaths due to cancer of the nasal cavity among any of the following groups potentially exposed to formaldehyde in the course of their usual occupation: physicians, dentists, morticians, anatomists, and pathologists. If there is a risk of nasal cancer associated with inhalation of formaldehyde vapour, then it appears to be small.— N. Kreiger (letter), *Can. med. Ass. J.*, 1983, *128*, 248.

Examination of mortality statistics of 7680 men who had first been employed before 1965 in one of 6 factories in the British chemical or plastics industry where formaldehyde had been manufactured or used did not support the hypothesis that formaldehyde is a human carcinogen (E.D. Acheson *et al.*, *Lancet*, 1984, *1*, 611). Further analysis of the results was against the view that formaldehyde is a lung carcinogen in man, but did not exclude the possibility (*idem*, 1066). Sterling and Arundel (*ibid.*, 1985, *2*, 1366) felt that analysis of the data using proportional mortality rates indicated a substantial effect of formaldehyde on the respiratory system, but this method of analysis was deemed inappropriate (M.J. Gardner *et al.*, *ibid.*, 1366). Infante and Schneiderman (*ibid.*, 1986, *1*, 436) still felt that the data pointed to potential risks but Gardner *et al.* (*ibid.*, 437) thought that to detect such risks would require the follow-up of large cohorts exposed to high concentrations for long periods.

EFFECTS ON THE BLOOD. Haemolysis during chronic haemodialysis was due to formaldehyde eluted from filters.— E. P. Orringer and W. D. Mattern, *New Engl. J. Med.*, 1976, *294*, 1416.

EFFECTS ON THE GINGIVA. A report of painful, enlarged, and haemorrhagic gingival margins after the use of toothpaste containing a solution of formaldehyde.— I. M. Laws (letter), *Br. dent. J.*, 1984, *156*, 240.

EFFECTS ON THE RESPIRATORY SYSTEM. While asthma may occur after repeated exposure to formaldehyde, asthmatics may not experience an attack.— H. Harving *et al.*, *Br. med. J.*, 1986, *293*, 310; B. E. Heard (letter), *ibid.*, 821.

EFFECTS ON THE SKIN. A 78-year-old man developed formaldehyde photosensitivity, characterised by pruritus, burning, and redness within minutes of exposure to sunlight.— W. B. Shelley, *Archs Derm.*, 1982, *118*, 117.

See also under Allergy, above.

EFFECTS ON THE URINARY TRACT. Adverse effects of intravesical instillation of formaldehyde solutions have included dysuria, suprapubic pain, ureteric and bladder fibrosis, hydronephrosis, vesicoureteral reflux, and fatal acute renal failure (M. Melekos and J. Lalos, *Urology*, 1983, *21*, 331). Intraperitoneal spillage through a fistula, leading to adverse systemic effects, has also occurred (C.V. Capen *et al.*, *ibid.*, 1982, *19*, 599).

SHOCK. A report of 7 cases of shock, of possible toxic or anaphylactic aetiology, following the use of formaldehyde solutions during removal of hydatid cysts.— M. C. Galland *et al.*, *Thérapie*, 1980, *35*, 443.

Treatment of Adverse Effects

Contaminated skin should be washed with soap and water. After ingestion give water, milk, charcoal, and/or demulcents; avoid gastric lavage and emesis. Alleviate shock; acidosis, resulting from metabolism of formaldehyde to formic acid, may require the intravenous administration of sodium bicarbonate or sodium lactate. The use of haemodialysis has been suggested.

Uses and Administration

Formaldehyde is a disinfectant effective against vegetative bacteria, fungi, and many viruses, but it is only slowly effective against bacterial spores. Its sporicidal effect is greatly increased by increase in temperature. It has little penetrating power and readily polymerises and condenses on surfaces.

The effectiveness of formaldehyde gas depends on dissolving in a film of moisture before acting on micro-organisms, and in practice a relative humidity of 75% is necessary.

When applied to the unbroken skin, formaldehyde hardens the epidermis, renders it tough and whitish, and produces a local anaesthetic effect. A solution containing Formaldehyde Solution 3% has been used for the treatment of warts on the palms of the hands and soles of the feet. Sweating of the feet may be treated by the application of Formaldehyde Solution in glycerol or alcohol but such applications are liable to produce sensitisation reactions.

After surgical removal of hydatid cysts, diluted Formaldehyde Solution may be used for irrigating the cavities to destroy scolices. It is generally too irritant for use on mucous membranes but it has been used in mouthwashes as an antiseptic and hardening agent for the gums. In dentistry it has been used in endodontic treatment.

Formaldehyde gas is used for the disinfection of rooms and cabinets, when the gas may be produced by heating Formaldehyde Solution or by the reaction of the solution with potassium permanganate. Formaldehyde gas is used in combination with low-temperature steam for the sterilisation of heat-sensitive items. Formaldehyde Solution is used in the disinfection of blankets and bedding and in the disinfection of the membranes in dialysis equipment. It is important to ensure that there are no traces of formaldehyde on any equipment before it is used.

Formaldehyde Solution 10% in saline is used as a preservative for pathological specimens. It is not suitable for preserving urine for subsequent examination.

In applications where a solid form is required, paraformaldehyde is used (see p.967).

In the *UK* the use of formaldehyde in cosmetics is restricted to use in nail hardeners to a maximum concentration of 5%.

Taurolidine is a condensate of the amino acid taurine and formaldehyde which has a wide spectrum of antimicrobial activity.

HAEMORRHAGIC CYSTITIS. The Fair regimen (W.R. Fair, *Urology*, 1974, *3*, 573) for the intravesical administration of Formaldehyde Solution in haemorrhagic cystitis: instillation is carried out under general or regional anaesthesia, and patients with vesicoureteric reflux are treated with the head of the table raised. Formaldehyde Solution 1% 500 to 1 000 mL is passively run into the bladder until it is filled to capacity, and left in for 10 minutes. The bladder is then emptied and washed out with one litre of distilled water. Stronger concentrations of Formaldehyde Solution (up to 10%) and longer retention times (up to 30 minutes) can be used if bleeding does not stop (*Lancet*, 1987, *1*, 304). In a review of 118 patients treated with solutions of formaldehyde for intractable haematuria, the authors felt that this was probably the most effective treatment, but also probably the most dangerous (C.J. Godec and P. Gleich, *J. Urol., Baltimore*, 1983, *130*, 688). Bullock and Whitaker (*Br. med. J.*, 1985, *291*, 1522) noted that Formaldehyde Solution 5 to 10% controlled bladder haemorrhage in up to 80% of cases, but was absorbed systemically and so could cause toxicity, and could also cause severe mucosal damage. Ureteric fibrosis could be minimised by overhydration before treatment or by occluding the ureters during instillation. Murray *et al.* (*ibid.*, 1986, *292*, 57) felt that it was not necessary to use a concentration of 5 to 10% of Formaldehyde Solution. The incidence of side-effects such as urgency, dysuria, and suprapubic discomfort had been considerably reduced by the use of solutions of less than 4% with no loss of therapeutic effect, and retreatment was reliable and effective. However, of 4 patients treated with intravesical Formaldehyde Solution (two with a 10% solution and two with a 4% solution) by Smith *et al.* (*ibid.*, 412), 3 developed significant ureteral damage, presumed to be due to reflux of Formaldehyde Solution. A further 3 patients were treated with intravesical alum which successfully controlled bleeding without complications. Smith *et al.* concluded that alum was a safe and effective treatment for intractable bladder bleeding and should replace Formaldehyde Solution.

See also under Adverse Effects.

HYDATID DISEASE. Formaldehyde Solution 0.5% has been found to be a satisfactory scolicide for use during hydatid cyst surgery with minimal risk of systemic toxic effects or local damage, but in the event of biliary communication Formaldehyde Solution must not be injected into the cyst because a stenosing cholangitis may result.— D. L. Morris, *Br. J. Hosp. Med.*, 1981, *25*, 586.

URINARY-TRACT INFECTION. Twice daily instillation of 2 mL of Formaldehyde Solution into the urinary drainage bags of urology patients helped to control a hospital outbreak of *Klebsiella pneumoniae* urinary infection.— B. Suryaprakash *et al.* (letter), *Lancet*, 1984, *2*, 104.

USE OF DISINFECTANTS ON FARMS. In Great Britain, Formaldehyde Solution diluted 1 in 9 with water is an approved disinfectant for foot-and-mouth disease and swine vesicular disease under the Diseases of Animals (Approved Disinfectants) (Amendment) Order 1986 (SI 1986: No. 5).

VIRAL DISINFECTION. Formaldehyde Solution 0.1% was too slow in action to be recommended for the inactivation of human immunodeficiency virus (HIV) (B. Spire *et al.*, *Lancet*, 1984, *2*, 899) and the Creutzfeldt-Jakob virus was resistant to inactivation by Formaldehyde Solution (W.B. Patterson *et al.*, *Ann. intern. Med.*, 1985, *102*, 658). However Nye and Patou (*J. clin. Path.*, 1987, *40*, 119) have found a higher concentration of formaldehyde effective in inactivating HIV in CSF samples.

For the use of formaldehyde as a fumigant after exposure to viral haemorrhagic fever viruses, see p.950.

WARTS. Results of a retrospective survey of 446 children and a prospective survey of 200 children indicated that the advantages of formalin therapy for plantar warts are considerable, but it must be remembered that technique is all-important. In the initial stages of treatment 3% formalin solution was used. The patient was instructed to remove scale and dead tissue from the top of the wart by scraping with a nail-file or the side of the blade of a pair of scissors. The wart-bearing portion of the sole was then soaked in the 3% formalin solution for 15 to 20 minutes (stressing that the wart must not be placed in contact with the bottom of the receptacle). The whole process was repeated each night. To avoid the development of interdigital cracks due to hardening of the skin, if the warts were near toe clefts the patients were instructed to place a little soft paraffin between the toes before starting treatment. If there was little hardening of the skin after 3 weeks of treatment, the concentration of formalin was increased to 5%, 7% or even 10%. As a result of the survey in all 646 children, it was shown that formalin foot-soaks used each night for 6 to 8 weeks will cure 80% of all plantar warts up to 1 cm in diameter. Larger warts should be curetted after 3 weeks of treatment with formalin. By these means the recurrence and reinfection rates are reduced to extremely low levels; in addition the method is simple and painless.— C. F. H. Vickers, *Br. med. J.*, 1961, *2*, 743. Of 39 adults with plantar warts treated by soaking for 15 minutes daily in Formaldehyde Solution 3%, only 24 were cured after 8 weeks.— I. Anderson and E. Shirreffs, *Br. J. Derm.*, 1963, *75*, 29.

Preparations

Formaldehyde and Salicylic Acid Paint *(A.P.F.)*. Formaldehyde Solution 10 mL, salicylic acid 10 g, acetone 40 mL, alcohol (90%) to 100 mL.

Formaldehyde Lotion *(A.P.F.)*. Formalin Lotion. Formaldehyde Solution 3 mL, water to 100 mL. It must be freshly prepared.

Proprietary Preparations

Emoform *(Leo, UK)*. *Toothpaste*, Formaldehyde Solution 1.3%.

Veracur *(Typharm, UK)*. *Gel*, Formaldehyde Solution 1.5%.

Proprietary Names and Manufacturers

Emoform *(Leo, UK)*; Formitrol *(Ital.; Sandoz, Spain; Switz.)*; Formo-Cresol (*Orapharm, Austral.*); Lazer Formalyde (*Pedinol, USA*); Lysoform (*Lysoform, Ger.*; *Neth.*); Sporex (*Rougier, Canad.*); Veracur (*Typharm, UK*).

The following names have been used for multi-ingredient preparations containing formaldehyde— Duoplant (*Stiefel, Canad.*); Pedi-Dri (*Pedinol, USA*); Sterile Pack Fluid (*Ethicon, UK*).

2248-p

Glutaraldehyde *(BAN)*.

Glutaral *(USAN, rINN)*; Glutaric Dialdehyde. Pentane-1,5-dial.
$C_5H_8O_2$=100.1.
CAS — 111-30-8.

Adverse Effects

As for formaldehyde (p.961). Glutaraldehyde is less irritant to skin and mucous membranes than formaldehyde but it may cause dermatitis and sensitisation.

In Great Britain the recommended exposure limit of glutaraldehyde is 0.2 ppm.

Moderate chemical conjunctivitis followed accidental ocular contact with glutaraldehyde solution in a 57-year-old woman. Inflammation resolved after 3 days following saline irrigation and 6-hourly application of erythromycin ophthalmic ointment.— W. J. Murray and M. P. Ruddy, *Sth. med. J.*, 1985, *78*, 1012.

Asthma and rhinitis after exposure to glutaraldehyde in endoscopy units.— O. J. Corrado *et al.*, *Hum. Toxicol.*, 1986, *5*, 325.

Uses and Administration

Glutaraldehyde is a disinfectant which is rapidly effective against vegetative forms of Gram-positive and Gram-negative bacteria. It is also effective against acid-fast bacteria, bacterial spores, some fungi, and viruses, including hepatitis B virus and human immunodeficiency virus. Aqueous solutions show optimum activity between pH 7.5 and 8.5; such solutions are chemically stable for about 14 days. Solutions at acid pH values are more stable. The activity of glutaraldehyde is reported to be unaffected by up to 20% of serum.

A 2% aqueous solution buffered to a pH of about 8 (activated glutaraldehyde) is used for the sterilisation of endoscopic and dental instruments, thermometers, rubber or plastic equipment, and for other equipment which cannot be sterilised by heat. Glutaraldehyde is non-corrosive towards most materials. Complete immersion in the solution for 15 to 20 minutes is sufficient for rapid disinfection of thoroughly cleansed instruments but exposure for 10 hours is necessary for sterilisation as glutaraldehyde is only slowly effective against bacterial spores.

A 5 or 10% solution is used for the treatment of warts; it should not be used for facial or anogenital warts.

ENDOSCOPE DISINFECTION. For the use of glutaraldehyde for the disinfection of endoscopes, including endoscopes contaminated with human immunodeficiency virus, see Use of Disinfectants in Hospitals and Viral Disinfection, p.949.

HYPERHIDROSIS. Glutaraldehyde solution 10% applied on a swab to the soles has been recommended for idiopathic hyperhidrosis, but is no more effective than formaldehyde (which is not considered to be of much value) and has the disadvantage of staining the skin orange-brown.— W. A. D. Griffiths, *Prescribers' J.*, 1984, *24*, 38.

VIRAL DISINFECTION. For the use of glutaraldehyde for the disinfection of articles contaminated with human immunodeficiency virus, see p.950.

WARTS. Of 21 patients with plantar warts, 75% were cured in 8 weeks using twice daily applications of a stabilised gel containing activated glutaraldehyde 10%.— K. W. Scott, *Practitioner*, 1982, *226*, 1342.

Preparations

Glutaral Concentrate *(U.S.P.)*. A solution of glutaraldehyde 50% w/w in water. pH 3.7 to 4.5. Store at a temperature not exceeding 40° in airtight containers. Protect from light.

Glutaral Disinfectant Solution *(U.S.N.F.)*. A solution containing glutaraldehyde. pH 2.7 to 3.7. Store at a temperature not exceeding 40° in airtight containers. Protect from light.

Glutaraldehyde Solution *(B.P.)*. A dilution of Strong Glutaraldehyde Solution B.P. in a mixture of water and alcohol or industrial methylated spirits, containing 9.2 to 10.5% w/v of glutaraldehyde and 50.0 to 60.0% v/v of alcohol. Store at a temperature not exceeding 15° in well-closed containers.

Strong Glutaraldehyde Solution *(B.P.)*. An aqueous solution containing 47 to 53% w/w of glutaraldehyde. Store at a temperature not exceeding 15° in a well-closed container.

Proprietary Preparations

ASEP *(Galen, UK)*. *Solution*, activated glutaraldehyde 2%, stable for 14 days.

Cidex *(Surgikos, UK)*. *Solution*, activated glutaraldehyde 2%, stable for 14 days.
Solution (Cidex Long-Life), activated glutaraldehyde 2%, stable for 28 days.

Glutarol *(Dermal Laboratories, UK)*. *Solution*, glutaraldehyde 10%.

Verucasep *(Galen, UK)*. *Gel*, glutaraldehyde 10%.

Proprietary Names and Manufacturers

ASEP *(Galen, UK)*; Cidex *(Surgikos, UK)*; Diswart *(Essex, Austral.)*; Glutarol *(Panpharma, Switz.; Dermal Laboratories, UK)*; Pantasept *(Adroka, Switz.)*; Sonacide *(Ayerst, Canad.; USA)*; Sterihyde *(Jpn)*; Totacide 28 *(Tenneco, UK)*; Verucasep *(Galen, UK)*.

2249-s

Halazone *(USAN, pINN)*.

Pantocide. 4-(Dichlorosulphamoyl)benzoic acid.
$C_7H_5Cl_2NO_4S$=270.1.
CAS — 80-13-7.

Pharmacopoeias. In *Nord.*, *Rus.*, and *U.S.*

A white crystalline powder with a strong odour of chlorine, containing about 52% of 'available chlorine' (see p.958).

Very slightly **soluble** in water, chloroform, and ether; soluble 1 in 140 of alcohol; soluble in glacial acetic acid. It is soluble in aqueous solutions of alkali hydroxides and carbonates with the formation of a salt. Solutions are unstable and rapidly lose chlorine. **Store** in airtight containers. Protect from light.

Halazone has the properties of chlorine (see p.958) in aqueous solution and is used for the disinfection of drinking water. One tablet containing 4 mg of halazone, with sodium carbonate and sodium chloride, is sufficient to treat about a litre of water (500 mL for heavily contaminated water), in about 30 minutes to 1 hour. The taste of residual chlorine may be removed by adding sodium thiosulphate.

Preparations

Halazone Tablets for Solution *(U.S.P.)*

Proprietary Names and Manufacturers

Cloritines *(Torlan, Spain)*.

2250-h

Hexachlorophane *(BAN)*.

G-11; Hexachlorophene *(USAN, rINN)*. 2,2′-Methylenebis(3,4,6-trichlorophenol).
$C_{13}H_6Cl_6O_2$=406.9.
CAS — 70-30-4.

Pharmacopoeias. In *Arg.*, *Aust.*, *Br.*, *Braz.*, *Cz.*, *Hung.*, *Jug.*, *Nord.*, and *U.S.* Also in *B.P. Vet.*

A white or pale buff crystalline powder which is odourless or has a slight phenolic odour.

Practically **insoluble** in water; soluble 1 in 3.5 of alcohol, 1 in less than 1 of acetone, and 1 in less than 1 of ether; dissolves in dilute solutions of alkali hydroxides. **Store** in airtight containers. Protect from light.

Hexachlorophane was incompatible with benzalkonium chloride. The maximum loss of activity occurred at an approximate equimolar concentration of each component.— G. Walter and W. Gump, *J. pharm. Sci.*, 1962, *51*, 770.

The antibacterial activity of hexachlorophane was reduced in alkaline media. Products including hexachlorophane should have a pH between 5 and 6. Reduction in pH from 8 to 6 caused a fourfold increase in antibacterial activity. In addition, preparations should not contain large amounts of nonionic surfactants, which depressed or inactivated hexachlorophane completely.— G. Walter and W. Gump, *Soap chem. Spec.*, 1963, *39*, (July), 55.

DISCOLORATION OF DETERGENT SOLUTIONS. Hexachlorophane was extremely sensitive to iron, and to avoid discoloration due to traces of this metal in the detergent, it was advisable to incorporate a sequestrant such as disodium edetate (0.1 to 0.5%).— M. Bell, *Specialities*, 1965, *1*, 16.

Adverse Effects

Following ingestion, anorexia, nausea, vomiting, diarrhoea, abdominal pain, dehydration, shock, and confusion may occur. Convulsions and death may follow. Central nervous stimulation, convulsions, and death have also occurred after absorption of hexachlorophane from burns and damaged skin.

Photosensitivity and skin sensitisation have occurred occasionally after repeated use of hexachlorophane.

There have been reports showing that hexachlorophane can be absorbed through the skin of infants in amounts sufficient to produce spongy lesions of the brain, sometimes fatal.

EFFECTS ON THE CNS. Most reports of hexachlorophane toxicity relate to the 3% emulsion. In neonates washed regularly with this preparation a vacuolative myelinopathy has been seen at necropsy and the prevalence of these lesions correlates with the amount of exposure. The actively myelinating tracts of infants with a birth-weight of 1.4 kg or less are most susceptible, but Plueckhahn and Collins (*Med. J. Aust.*, 1976, *1*, 815) found no encephalopathy in babies weighing over 2.0 kg irrespective of their exposure to hexachlorophane, suggesting that this may be a safer limit for restricting hexachlorophane exposure in the newborn. The importance of the spongiform encephalopathy is questioned because there is no conclusive evidence relating any neurological features in the affected infants to the lesions in their brains; detection of such features affecting immature tracts would be difficult, however. A causal association between the myelinopathy and the death of infants has also been disputed. Furthermore, experimentally induced vacuolar lesions may be reversible and it has been proposed that many surviving children who were exposed in early life to hexachlorophane 3% emulsion may have acquired such changes but nonetheless progressed without physical or neurological sequelae.— *Lancet*, 1982, *1*, 87.

EFFECTS ON THE RESPIRATORY SYSTEM. Occupational asthma developed in a 43-year-old nurse after long-term exposure to hexachlorophane powder.— L. Nagy and M. Orosz, *Thorax*, 1984, *39*, 630.

PREGNANCY AND THE NEONATE. Halling (*Ann. N.Y. Acad. Sci.*, 1979, *320*, 426) reported a significant increase in congenital anomalies in infants born to nurses who had been exposed to hexachlorophane (15% compared with 3% in the general Swedish population). This study, however, has been critised on methodological grounds; most of the 'exposed' cases were selected because of a malformation rather than because of exposure to hexachlorophane. In a study by Baltzar *et al.* (*New Engl. J. Med.*, 1979, *300*, 627), infants born to women employed in hospital work in Sweden from 1973 to 1975 were compared with those born to women in the general population in Sweden during the same period. Although those investigators found a cluster of congenital malformations similar to those found by Halling, perinatal mortality and rates of occurrence of congenital malformations did not differ between the 2 groups. Reports on teratogenicity are controversial. Because hexachlorophane is rapidly absorbed from the skin and transplacental passage has been documented, restriction of the use of this product seems wise during pregnancy, at least during the first trimester.— L. M. Hill and F. Kleinberg, *Mayo Clin. Proc.*, 1984, *59*, 755.

See also above under Effects on the CNS.

Precautions

Hexachlorophane should not be applied to mucous membranes, large areas of skin, or to burnt or damaged skin and should not be used vaginally or applied under occlusive dressings. It should be used with caution on infants, especially premature and low birth-weight infants, and preferably only for the control of outbreaks of staphylococcal infection in nurseries. The antimicrobial activity of hexachlorophane may be diminished through incompatibility (see above), through adsorption, or through combination with protein. Blood reduces its effectiveness. Activity is also reduced at a pH that is not slightly acid. Some activity is retained in the presence of soap. Preparations of hexachlorophane are liable to contamination, especially with Gram-negative organisms.

Absorption and Fate

Hexachlorophane is absorbed from the gastro-intestinal tract and through intact and denuded skin. Percutaneous absorption may be significant in premature infants and through damaged skin. Hexachlorophane crosses the placenta.

Uses and Administration

Hexachlorophane is a chlorinated bisphenol disinfectant active against Gram-positive organisms, but much less active against Gram-negative organisms.

Hexachlorophane is mainly used in soaps and creams in a concentration of 0.23 to 3%. After repeated use of these preparations for several days there is a marked diminution of the bacterial flora due to accumulation of hexachlorophane in the skin. This residual effect is rapidly lost after washing with unmedicated soap or alcohol.

A preparation containing 3% is used for the disinfection of the hands of surgeons and others and, when other measures are not effective, for the control of staphylococcal infection in the newborn. Thorough rinsing is recommended before drying.

A 0.3% dusting powder has been applied to the cord stumps of the newborn.

The use of hexachlorophane in cosmetics and toiletries is restricted in Great Britain.

PREGNANCY AND THE NEONATE. In 1980, Plueckhahn (*Aust. paediat. J.*, 1980, *16*, 40) confirmed the prophylactic efficacy of a technique for antiseptic skin care in neonates using a 0.5% hexachlorophane powder instead of the 3% emulsion. The blood concentrations so attained were much lower than those associated with the emulsion. It thus appeared that the use of the 3% emulsion in infant skin care is no longer justifiable and that, if used at all, preparations containing a lower hexachlorophane concentration are preferable.— L. García-Buñuel (letter), *Lancet*, 1982, *1*, 1190. Powders containing chlorhexidine 1% or hexachlorophane 0.33% were equally effective in preventing colonisation and infection of the skin of newborn infants by ***Staphylococcus aureus*** but the skin became profusely colonised by coagulase-negative staphylococci, irrespective of the powder used.— V. G. Alder *et al.*, *Archs Dis. Childh.*, 1980, *55*, 277.

TINEA PEDIS. Treatment of tinea pedis with hexachlorophane produced a notable worsening of dermatophytosis simplex (itchy, scaly toe-web lesions), associated with proliferation of *Pseudomonas* spp.— *Lancet*, 1985, *2*, 81.

Preparations

Hexachlorophane Dusting Powder *(B.P.)*. Zinc and Hexachlorophane Dusting Powder. A mixture of hexachlorophane and zinc oxide with suitable inert diluents.

Hexachlorophene Cleansing Emulsion *(U.S.P.)*. Hexachlorophene Detergent Lotion

Hexachlorophene Liquid Soap *(U.S.P.)*. A 0.225 to 0.26% w/w solution of hexachlorophane in a 10 to 13% solution of a potassium soap. It may contain suitable water-hardness controls. The inclusion of nonionic detergents in amounts greater than 8% w/w may decrease the bacteriostatic activity of this preparation.

Proprietary Preparations

Ster-Zac DC Skin Cleanser *(Hough, Hoseason, UK)*. *Cream*, hexachlorophane 3%.

Ster-Zac Powder *(Hough, Hoseason, UK)*. *Dusting-powder*, hexachlorophane 0.33%.

Proprietary Names and Manufacturers

Fisohex *(Arg.)*; Gamophen Surgical Soap *(Switz.)*; Germibon *(Spain)*; Hexaphenyl *(Ingram & Bell, Canad.)*; Phaisohex *(Denm.; Iceland; Norw.)*; pHisoHex *(Winthrop, Austral.; Winthrop, Canad.; Winthrop-Breon, USA)*; pHisoScrub *(Winthrop-Breon, USA)*; Sapoderem *(Ingram & Bell, Canad.)*; Steridermis *(Sterling Industrial, UK)*; Ster-Zac *(Hough, Hoseason, UK)*; Sumasept *(Norw.)*; Zalpon *(Sterling Industrial, UK)*.

The following names have been used for multi-ingredient preparations containing hexachlorophane— Anacal *(Panpharma, UK)*; Aserbine Cream *(Bencard, UK)*; Bismodyne *(Loveridge, UK)*; Cordocel-H *(Wigglesworth, UK)*; Dermalex *(Labaz Sanofi, UK)*; Nestosyl *(Bengué, UK)*; pHisodan *(Winthrop, Austral.)*; Steraskin *(G.P. Laboratories, Austral.)*; Toracsol *(Torbet Laboratories, UK)*; Torbetol Lotion *(Torbet Laboratories, UK)*.

2251-m

Hexamidine Isethionate

Hexamidine Isetionate *(rINNM)*. 4,4′-(Hexamethylenedioxy)dibenzamidine bis(2-hydroxyethanesulphonate).
$C_{20}H_{26}N_4O_2,2C_2H_6O_4S=606.7$.

CAS — 3811-75-4 (hexamidine); 659-40-5 (isethionate).

NOTE. The name Hexamidinum has also been used for primidone.

Hexamidine isethionate has antibacterial and antifungal properties and is available in a variety of preparations for the local treatment of minor infections.

Proprietary Names and Manufacturers

Désomédine *(Chauvin-Blache, Fr.; Novopharma, Switz.)*; Hexomedine *(Rhone-Poulenc, Belg.; Théraplix, Fr.; Théraplix, Neth.; Rhone, Spain; Rhone-Poulenc, Switz.)*; Ophtamedine *(Bournonville, Neth.)*; Opthamedine *(de Bournonville, Belg.)*.

The following names have been used for multi-ingredient preparations containing hexamidine isethionate— Cyteal *(Concept Pharmaceuticals, UK)*; Medi Pulv *(Rosken, Austral.)*.

2587-b

Hexetidine *(BAN, rINN)*.

5-Amino-1,3-bis(2-ethylhexyl)perhydro-5-methylpyrimidine.
$C_{21}H_{45}N_3=339.6$.

CAS — 141-94-6.

Adverse effects

Allergic contact dermatitis and alterations in taste and smell have occasionally been reported.

Uses and Administration

Hexetidine is bactericidal and fungicidal.

It is used as a 0.1% mouthwash for local infections and oral hygiene.

References to the use of hexetidine in mouthwashes: T. H. Grenby and M. G. Saldanha, *Br. dent. J.*, 1984, *157*, 239; K. C. Ashley, *J. appl. Bact.*, 1984, *56*, 221; D. B. Wile *et al.*, *Curr. med. Res. Opinion*, 1986, *10*, 82.

Proprietary Preparations

Oraldene *(Warner-Lambert, UK)*. *Mouthwash*, hexetidine 0.1%.

Proprietary Names and Manufacturers

Buchex *(Arg.)*; Collu-Hextril *(Belg.; Substantia, Fr.)*; Drossadin *(Drossapharm, Switz.)*; Duranil *(Arg.)*; Glypesin *(Ger.)*; Hexoral *(Parke, Davis, Denm.; Gödecke, Ger.)*; Hextril *(Belg.; Substantia, Fr.; Neth.; Warner-Lambert, Switz.)*; Oraldene *(Warner-Lambert, UK)*; Oraldine *(Parke, Davis, S.Afr.; Parke, Davis, Spain)*; Oraseptic *(Parke, Davis, Ital.)*; Stas *(Stada, Ger.)*; Sterisil *(Ital.)*; Steri/Sol *(Parke, Davis, Canad.)*.

782-j

Hexylresorcinol *(BAN, USAN)*.

Esilresorcina; Hexylresorc. 4-Hexylbenzene-1,3-diol.
$C_{12}H_{18}O_2=194.3$.

CAS — 136-77-6.

Pharmacopoeias. In *Arg., Aust., Br., Braz., It., Mex., Nord., Swiss,* and *U.S.*

White or yellowish-white, acicular crystals, crystalline plates, or crystalline powder with a pungent odour and a sharp, astringent, numbing taste. It acquires a brownish-pink tint on exposure to light and air. M.p. 62° to 68°.

Soluble 1 in 2000 of water; freely soluble in alcohol, chloroform, ether, glycerol, methyl alcohol, and fixed oils; very slightly soluble in petroleum spirit. **Incompatible** with alkalis and oxidising agents.

Store in airtight containers. Protect from light.

CAUTION. *Hexylresorcinol is irritating to the oral mucosa, to the respiratory tract, and to the skin; alcoholic solutions have vesicant properties.*

Hexylresorcinol is a phenolic derivative which is used topically as an antiseptic in mouth-washes and throat lozenges and in solutions for cleansing skin wounds.

It also has anthelmintic activity, but has been superseded by newer drugs. It was given by mouth in the treatment of infections due to intestinal nematodes, dwarf tapeworm, and the intestinal fluke *Fasciolopsis buski* and by enema in severe trichuriasis.

High concentrations of hexylresorcinol are irritant and corrosive to skin and mucous membranes.

Preparations

Hexylresorcinol Pills *(U.S.P.)*. Pills with a rupture-resistant coating that is dispersible in the digestive tract.

Proprietary Names and Manufacturers

Oxana *(Biologici Italia, Ital.)*.

2252-b

Hydrargaphen *(BAN, rINN)*.

Hydraphen; Hygraphen. μ-[3,3′-Methylenebis(naphthalene-2-sulphonato)]-bis(phenylmercury).
$C_{33}H_{24}Hg_2O_6S_2=981.9$.

CAS — 14235-86-0.

Incompatible with metals, and sulphides.

Hydrargaphen is a mercurial disinfectant with antibacterial and antifungal properties. It was formerly used in the treatment of vaginitis, wounds, burns, and infections of the skin.

Proprietary Names and Manufacturers

Penotrane *(Boehringer Ingelheim, UK)*; Versotrane *(Austral.)*.

NOTE. The name Conotrane was formerly applied to a product containing hydrargaphen and dimethicone 350, but this product has now been reformulated to contain benzalkonium chloride instead of hydrargaphen.

555-m

Isopropyl Alcohol *(BAN, USAN)*.

2-Propanol; Alcohol Isopropylicus; Dimethyl Carbinol; Isopropanol; Secondary Propyl Alcohol. Propan-2-ol.
$(CH_3)_2CHOH=60.10$.

CAS — 67-63-0.

Pharmacopoeias. In *Aust., Belg., Br., Egypt., Jpn, Swiss,* and *U.S.*

A clear, colourless, mobile, volatile, inflammable liquid with a characteristic spirituous odour.

Very **soluble** in water, alcohol, chloroform, and ether. **Store** in a cool place in airtight containers.

Adverse Effects and Precautions

The toxicity of isopropyl alcohol is about twice that of ethyl alcohol (p.950), and the symptoms of intoxication appear to be similar, except that isopropyl alcohol has no initial euphoric action and gastritis, haemorrhage, pain, nausea, and vomiting are more prominent. The lethal dose by mouth is reported to be about 250 mL, however toxic symptoms may be produced by as little as 20 mL. Ketoacidosis and ketonuria commonly occur due to the presence of the major metabolite, acetone, in the circulation. Inhalation of isopropyl alcohol vapour has been reported to produce coma.

Application of isopropyl alcohol to the skin may cause dryness and irritation. Allergic eczema has also been reported.

In Great Britain the recommended exposure limits of isopropyl alcohol are 400 ppm (long-term);

500 ppm (short-term); suitable precautions should be taken to prevent absorption through the skin. In the *US* the permissible and recommended exposure limits are 980 mg per m^3 and 984 mg per m^3 respectively.

PREGNANCY AND THE NEONATE. A report of second- and third-degree chemical skin burns caused by isopropyl alcohol in 2 premature infants of very low birth-weight. In one infant isopropyl alcohol swabs had been used for conduction in electrocardiography; in the other it had been poured over the umbilical stump during surgical preparation for umbilical artery catheterisation.— J. B. Schick and J. M. Milstein, *Pediatrics*, 1981, *68*, 587. A similar report in 4 premature infants. It was recommended that the skin of small premature infants be dried immediately following the use of alcohols as part of the routine procedure of umbilical cord preparation for catheterisation.— Z. Weintraub and T. C. Iancu (letter), *ibid.*, 1982, *69*, 506.

Treatment of Adverse Effects

As for Alcohol, p.950.

Absorption and Fate

Isopropyl alcohol is readily absorbed from the gastro-intestinal tract but there appears to be little absorption through intact skin. Isopropyl alcohol is metabolised more slowly than ethyl alcohol and about 15% of an ingested dose is metabolised to acetone.

Uses and Administration

Isopropyl alcohol at a concentration of 70% has disinfectant properties similar to those of alcohol. It is used for pre-operative skin cleansing and as an ingredient of lotions but its marked degreasing properties may limit its usefulness in preparations used repeatedly. It is also used as a solvent, especially in cosmetics and perfumes, and as a vehicle for other germicidal compounds.

In a study involving 71 newborn infants, topical application of isopropyl alcohol to umbilical stumps was associated with a significantly shorter cord separation time than with triple dye (crystal violet, brilliant green, and proflavine hemisulphate) application.— A. J. Schuman and B. A. Oksol, *Milit. Med.*, 1985, *150*, 49 (See Adverse Effects, above).

VIRAL DISINFECTION. For the use of isopropyl alcohol for the disinfection of surfaces contaminated with human immunodeficiency virus, see p.950.

Preparations

Isopropyl Rubbing Alcohol *(U.S.P.)*. Contains 68 to 72% v/v of isopropyl alcohol.

Proprietary Names and Manufacturers

Alcojel *(Allen & Hanburys, Canad.)*; Avantine *(Laporte, UK)*; Duonalc *(ICN, Canad.)*; IPA/XG *(Shell Chemicals, UK)*; IPS *(Shell Chemicals, UK)*; IPS/C *(Shell Chemicals, UK)*; Medi-Swab *(Smith & Nephew, S.Afr.*; *Smith & Nephew, UK)*; Sterets *(Seton, UK)*.

The following names have been used for multi-ingredient preparations containing isopropyl alcohol— Cetylcide *(Cetylite, USA)*; Sterets H *(Seton, UK)*; Sterile Pack Fluid *(Ethicon, UK)*.

2253-v

Laurolinium Acetate *(BAN, rINN)*.

4-Amino-1-dodecyl-2-methylquinolinium acetate.
$C_{24}H_{38}N_2O_2$=386.6.

CAS — 6803-62-9 (laurolinium); 146-37-2 (acetate).

Laurolinium acetate is a cationic surfactant which has been used for skin disinfection.

2254-g

Magenta

Aniline Red; Basic Fuchsin *(USAN)*; Basic Magenta; CI Basic Violet 14; Colour Index No. 42510; Fuchsine; Rosaniline Hydrochloride.

CAS — 569-61-9 (pararosaniline hydrochloride); 632-99-5 (rosaniline hydrochloride).

Pharmacopoeias. In *Hung.* and *U.S.*

A mixture of the hydrochlorides of pararosaniline {4-[(4-aminophenyl)(4-iminocyclohexa-2,5-dien-1-ylidene)methyl]aniline} and rosaniline {4-[(4-aminophenyl)(4-iminocyclohexa-2,5-dien-1-ylidene)methyl]-2-methylaniline}. The dried material contains not less than 88% of dyestuff, calculated as rosaniline hydrochloride ($C_{20}H_{20}ClN_3$ = 337.9).

Odourless, iridescent green crystals, or a dark green, lustrous, crystalline powder. **Soluble** in water, alcohol, and amyl alcohol forming deep red solutions; practically insoluble in ether.

In Great Britain, the manufacture of magenta and auramine, and any process in the course of which these substances are formed, are controlled by the Carcinogenic Substances Regulations.

Magenta is a disinfectant effective against Gram-positive bacteria and some fungi. Magenta Paint (Castellani's paint) has been used in the treatment of superficial dermatophytoses, especially when moist eczematous dermatitis is present.

Decolorised magenta solution (Schiff reagent) is used as a test for the presence of aldehydes.

Magenta was considered unsafe for use in food.— Eighth Report of the Joint FAO/WHO Expert Committee on Food Additives, *Tech. Rep. Ser. Wld Hlth Org. No. 309*, 1965.

Methaemoglobinaemia in a 6-week-old child following topical use of a solution containing magenta, boric acid, phenol, and resorcinol.— E. Lundell and R. Nordman, *Ann. clin. Res.*, 1973, *5*, 404.

The handling of magenta was not thought to induce carcinogenesis but its actual manufacture may produce tumours.— R. W. Glashan, *Br. med. J.*, 1984, *288*, 1181.

Preparations

Carbol-Fuchsin Topical Solution *(U.S.P.)*. Magenta 300 mg, phenol 4.5 g, resorcinol 10 g, acetone 5 mL, alcohol 10 mL, water to 100 mL. Store in airtight containers. Protect from light.

Magenta Paint *(B.P.C. 1973)*. Castellani's Paint; Fuchsine Paint. Magenta 400 mg, boric acid 800 mg, phenol 4 g, resorcinol 8 g, acetone 4 mL, alcohol (90%) (or industrial methylated spirit, suitably diluted) 8.5 mL, water to 100 mL. Store in a cool place in airtight containers. Protect from light.

2255-q

Malachite Green

CI Basic Green 4; Colour Index No. 42000; Viride Malachitum. [4-(4-Dimethylaminobenzhydrylidene)cyclohexa-2,5-dienylidene]dimethylammonium chloride.

Malachite green is a disinfectant with actions and uses similar to those of brilliant green (see p.953).

Proprietary Names and Manufacturers

The following names have been used for multi-ingredient preparations containing malachite green— Mycozol *(Parke, Davis, Austral.)*.

2256-p

Mercurochrome

Chromargyre; Disodium 2,7-dibromo-4-hydroxymercurifluorescein; Merbromin *(rINN)*; Mercurescéine Sodique; Mercurodibromofluorescein. The disodium salt of [2,7-dibromo-9-(2-carboxyphenyl)-6-hydroxy-3-oxo-3*H*-xanthen-5-yl]hydroxymercury.
$C_{20}H_8Br_2HgNa_2O_6$=750.7.

CAS — 129-16-8.

NOTE. The use of the name Mercurochrome is limited; in some countries it is a trade-mark.

Pharmacopoeias. In *Braz., Egypt., Fr., It., Jpn, Port., Span.*, and *Swiss.*

Incompatible with acids, most alkaloidal salts, and many local anaesthetics, metals, and sulphides.

Adverse Effects, Treatment, and Precautions

As for Mercury, p.1587.

The antimicrobial activity of mercurochrome may be diminished through incompatibility (see above) and through the presence of organic material.

A report of contact dermatitis attributed to mercurochrome.— G. Camarasa, *Contact Dermatitis*, 1976, *2*, 120.

Mercurochrome used in topical antiseptic preparations was toxic to epidermal cells.— *Med. Lett.*, 1977, *19*, 83.

A report of fatal mercury poisoning from mercurochrome treatment of infected omphalocele. The high tissue concentrations of mercury might have contributed to cardiac arrest.— T. -F. Yeh *et al.* (letter), *Lancet*, 1978, *1*, 210. See also *idem, Clin. Toxicol.*, 1978, *13*, 463.

A 59-year-old woman had a 2% aqueous solution of mercurochrome applied to her surgical wounds and decubitus areas after surgery for an oesophageal stricture. By day 22 her blood contained 700 ng per mL of mercury and on day 23 she died in therapy-resistant shock. Aplastic anaemia, confirmed at autopsy, was tentatively ascribed to mercurochrome treatment.— P. H. T. J. Slee *et al.*, *Acta med. scand.*, 1979, *205*, 463.

Uses and Administration

Mercurochrome is a weak disinfectant that has been used for skin infections and for bladder and urethral irrigation.

Proprietary Names and Manufacturers

Cinfacromin *(Cinfa, Spain)*; Cromo Utin *(Deiters, Spain)*; Curichrome *(Goupil, Fr.)*; Glubel Cromo *(Spain)*; Mercromina *(Lainco, Spain)*; Mercrotona *(Orravan, Spain)*; Mercroverk *(Verkos, Spain)*; Mercuchrom *(Krewel, Ger.)*; Mercurasept *(Sauter, Switz.)*; Mercurin *(Monik, Spain)*; Mercuro Clinico *(Llano, Spain)*; Mercurocromo *(SIT, Ital.*; *Perez Jimenez, Spain)*; Pintacrom *(Sokatarg, Spain)*; Super Cromer Orto *(Normon, Spain)*; Veriscrom *(Cronofar, Spain)*; Yocrom *(Iquinosa, Spain)*.

557-v

Methylated Spirits

CAS — 8013-52-3 (ethyl alcohol-methyl alcohol mixture; industrial methylated spirit).

Three classes of methylated spirits are listed under the *UK* Methylated Spirits Regulations, 1983 (SI 1983: No. 252): industrial methylated spirits, mineralised methylated spirits, and denatured alcohol (denatured ethanol).

Industrial methylated spirits is defined as alcohol mixed with wood naphtha 5%. (See under Methyl Alcohol, p.1429, for a description of wood naphtha). Mineralised methylated spirits is alcohol mixed with wood naphtha 9.5 parts by volume and crude pyridine 0.5 parts by volume, and to every 2 000 litres of this mixture is added 7.5 litres of mineral naphtha (petroleum oil) and 3 g of synthetic organic dyestuff (methyl violet). This is the only variety that may be sold in Great Britain for general use. Denatured alcohol is alcohol (of a strength not less than 85%) mixed with *n*-propanol 2%, and to this mixture is added either Bitrex (denatonium benzoate) 10 mg per litre, solid quassin 120 mg per litre, or sucrose octa-acetate 4 g per litre.

Industrial Methylated Spirit *(B.P.)* (Industrial methylated spirits; IMS) is a mixture of 19 volumes of alcohol of an appropriate strength with 1 volume of approved wood naphtha, and is Industrial Methylated Spirit of the quality known as '66 OP' or '74 OP'. It is a colourless, clear, mobile, volatile, inflammable liquid with an odour which is spirituous and of wood naphtha.

Industrial Methylated Spirit (ketone-free) *(B.P.)* [Industrial Methylated Spirit (acetone-free)] is a mixture of the same strength as Industrial Methylated Spirit *B.P.*, but contains not more than the equivalent of 500 ppm of acetone.

Industrial Methylated Spirit may contain small amounts of acetone and should not then be used for the preparation of iodine solutions, since an irritating compound is formed by reaction between iodine and acetone; for such preparations Industrial Methylated Spirit (ketone-free) should be used.

Adverse Effects and Treatment

As for Methyl Alcohol, p.1428.

Bilateral abscesses of the thigh in a diabetic patient appeared to be associated with the use of surgical spirit instead of industrial methylated spirit for the storage of insulin syringes. It was considered that the additives such as castor oil, methyl salicylate, and diethyl phthalate in surgical spirit could produce oily residues on the inner surface of the syringe and that these residues would be sufficiently miscible with certain types of insulin to be deposited with the latter at the site of injection.— D. A. Leigh and G. W. Hough, *Br. med. J.*, 1980, *281*, 541.

Development of high blood-alcohol concentrations and severe haemorrhagic skin necrosis in an infant of 27 weeks gestational age which was attributed to skin cleansing with methylated spirits prior to umbilical arterial catheterisation.— V. Harpin and N. Rutter, *Archs Dis. Childh.*, 1982, *57*, 477.

Uses and Administration

Industrial methylated spirit, often in the form of surgical spirit, may be applied externally for its astringent action, but mucous membranes and excoriated skin surfaces must be protected. It may be used for skin preparation before injection.

Preparations

Surgical Spirit *(B.P.)*. Methyl salicylate 0.5 mL, diethyl phthalate 2 mL, castor oil 2.5 mL, Industrial Methylated Spirit to 100 mL.

2258-w

Methylbenzethonium Chloride *(BAN, USAN, rINN)*.

Benzyldimethyl-2-{2-[4-(1,1,3,3-tetramethylbutyl)-*o*-tolyloxy]ethoxy}ethylammonium chloride monohydrate.
$C_{28}H_{44}ClNO_2,H_2O$=480.1.

CAS — 25155-18-4 (anhydrous); 1320-44-1 (monohydrate).

Pharmacopoeias. In *U.S.*

White hygroscopic crystals with a mild odour. **Soluble** 1 in less than 1 of water, alcohol, and ether; practically insoluble in chloroform. **Store** in airtight containers.

Methylbenzethonium chloride is a quaternary ammonium disinfectant with properties and uses similar to those of other cationic surfactants, as described under Cetrimide, p.953.

It has been used principally to prevent ammoniacal dermatitis and skin irritation due to contact with urine, faeces, or perspiration; a 0.004 to 0.005% solution is used for rinsing babies' napkins and the undergarments and bedlinen of incontinent children and adults, or a cream, ointment, or dusting-powder (0.055 to 0.1%) may be applied locally.

Methylbenzethonium chloride was not considered to be a sensitiser, and was considered to be safe at a concentration of 0.5% in cosmetics applied to the skin and at a maximum concentration of 0.02% in cosmetics used in the eye area.— The Expert Panel of the American College of Toxicology, *J. Am. Coll. Toxicol.*, 1985, *4*, 65.

Sixty-seven patients with cutaneous leishmaniasis caused by *Leishmania major* were treated topically twice daily with an ointment comprising paromomycin sulphate 15% and methylbenzethonium chloride 12% in white soft paraffin (P ointment). After 10 days, 73% of patients had no parasites in their lesions; 14% became free within a further 20 days without further treatment; and 13% failed to respond. Clinical healing was generally completed 10 to 30 days after the end of treatment; 94% of the treated lesions healed with little or no scarring.— J. El-On *et al.* (letter), *Br. med. J.*, 1985, *291*, 1280. Reference to the successful use of P ointment for the treatment of recurrent cutaneous leishmaniasis caused by *Leishmania tropica*.— J. El-On *et al.*, *ibid.*, 704.

Preparations

Methylbenzethonium Chloride Lotion *(U.S.P.)*
Methylbenzethonium Chloride Ointment *(U.S.P.)*
Methylbenzethonium Chloride Powder *(U.S.P.)*

Proprietary Names and Manufacturers

Bedside-Care *(Sween, USA)*; Diaparene *(Glenbrook, USA)*; Hyamine 10-X *(Rohm & Haas, UK)*; Vi-Medin *(Sabex, Canad.)*.

The following names have been used for multi-ingredient preparations containing methylbenzethonium chloride— Dalidyne *(Dalin, USA)*.

2259-e

Miristalkonium Chloride *(BAN, rINN)*.

Myristylbenzalkonium Chloride. Benzyldimethyltetradecylammonium chloride.
$C_{23}H_{42}ClN$=368.0.

CAS — 139-08-2.

Miristalkonium chloride was used with other antimicrobial agents in lozenges for the treatment of throat infections.

12972-g

Monalazone Disodium *(rINN)*.

Disodium 4-(*N*-chlorosulphamoyl)benzoate.
$C_7H_4ClNNa_2O_4S$=279.6.

CAS — 61477-95-0.

Monalazone disodium is closely related structurally to halazone and was used as a vaginal disinfectant and spermicide.

Proprietary Names and Manufacturers

Speton *(Temmler, Ger.; Temmler, Switz.)*.

2261-v

Nitromersol *(USAN)*.

5-Methyl-2-nitro-7-oxa-8-mercurabicyclo[4.2.0]octa-1,3,5-triene.
$C_7H_5HgNO_3$=351.7.

CAS — 133-58-4.

Pharmacopoeias. In *U.S.*

A brownish-yellow to yellow odourless powder or granules. Very slightly **soluble** in water, alcohol, acetone, chloroform, and ether; soluble in solutions of alkalis and of ammonia with the formation of salts. **Store** in airtight containers. Protect from light.

Incompatible with metals and sulphides.

Adverse Effects, Treatment, and Precautions

As for Mercury, p.1587.

Nitromersol occasionally gives rise to hypersensitivity reactions. The antimicrobial activity of nitromersol may be diminished through incompatibility (see above) and through the presence of organic material.

Nitromersol had been reported to be ototoxic.— J. L. Honigman (letter), *Pharm. J.*, 1975, *2*, 523.

Nitromersol used in topical antiseptic preparations was toxic to epidermal cells.— *Med. Lett.*, 1977, *19*, 83.

Uses and Administration

Nitromersol is a disinfectant effective against some vegetative bacteria. It is not effective against spores. It is used as the sodium salt for disinfection of the skin prior to surgical treatment as a 0.5% alcohol-acetone-aqueous solution. A 0.2% solution is applied to the skin for the treatment of minor cuts.

Preparations

Nitromersol Tincture *(U.S.P.)*. Nitromersol 500 mg, sodium hydroxide 100 mg, acetone 10 mL, alcohol 52.5 mL, water to 100 mL; it may be coloured.

Nitromersol Topical Solution *(U.S.P.)*. Nitromersol Solution. Nitromersol 200 mg, sodium hydroxide 40 mg, sodium carbonate monohydrate 425 mg, water to 100 mL. Dilutions of this solution should be freshly prepared as they tend to precipitate on standing.

Proprietary Names and Manufacturers

Metaphen *(Abbott, Austral.)*.

The following names have been used for multi-ingredient preparations containing nitromersol— Butesin Picrate Ointment with Metaphen *(Abbott, Austral.)*.

2262-g

Noxythiolin *(BAN)*.

Noxytiolin *(rINN)*. 1-Hydroxymethyl-3-methyl-2-thiourea.
$C_3H_8N_2OS$=120.2.

CAS — 15599-39-0.

Noxythiolin solutions 1% and 2.5% could be stored in polypropylene containers. There was no adsorption of noxythiolin or of its degradation products (N-methylthiourea and formaldehyde).— D. F. McCafferty *et al.*, *J. clin. Hosp. Pharm.*, 1984, *9*, 241.

Adverse Effects

Noxythiolin 10 g per litre was added to the peritoneal dialysis fluid of 9 patients with continuous ambulatory peritoneal dialysis-associated peritonitis, immediately before instillation, in an attempt to sterilise the fluid. About 6 hours after this fluid had been drained, the breath of all 9 patients had acquired a pervasive sweetish odour of decaying vegetables, which persisted for 4 or 5 days.— W. K. Stewart and L. W. Fleming (letter), *Lancet*, 1983, *1*, 426.

Uses and Administration

Noxythiolin has wide antibacterial and antifungal actions. It probably acts in part by slowly releasing formaldehyde in solution. It has been used, usually as a 1 to 2.5% solution in water, for the irrigation of, or instillation into, body cavities and fistulas.

The normal total daily dosage in adults should not exceed 10 g.

In the treatment of bladder infections the intense burning sensation frequently experienced may be relieved by the addition of a local anaesthetic such as amethocaine hydrochloride. It has also been applied topically in gels and sprays.

In the management of surgical sepsis, noxythiolin was shown to be ineffective in 5 separate studies: 3 on appendicectomies and 2 on general surgical wounds.— O. J. A. Gilmore and R. G. Sprignall, *Br. J. Hosp. Med.*, 1983, *29*, 440.

Three patients with pleural empyema or pneumonectomy space infection were treated by irrigation of the cavity with noxythiolin 1% in normal saline for 3 hours, followed by drainage for 1 hour, the cycle being repeated 4-hourly. Infection was eradicated within 21 days in all 3 patients.— F. L. Rosenfeldt *et al.*, *Thorax*, 1984, *36*, 272.

Results indicated that much smaller amounts of formaldehyde are released from noxythiolin solutions than have previously been reported and that the antimicrobial effects of the solutions cannot be attributed solely to the presence of formaldehyde.— S. P. Gorman *et al.* (letter), *Pharm. J.*, 1984, *2*, 62.

The initial stage of infection may be associated with adherence of the organism to epithelial surfaces. Buccal or uroepithelial cells were incubated with *Candida albicans*, *Escherichia coli*, or *Staphylococcus saprophyticus* pretreated with noxythiolin 1% or 2.5%, or formaldehyde. Noxythiolin 1% and 2.5% significantly reduced adherence of the exponential phase blastospore of *C. albicans* while only the 2.5% solution significantly reduced the adherence of stationary phase cells. Similar results were obtained for noxythiolin 2.5% for the other 2 organisms. Formaldehyde solutions in equivalent concentrations to those found in noxythiolin solutions did not significantly reduce adherence.— L. Anderson *et al.*, *J. Pharm. Pharmac.*, 1985, *37*, *Suppl.*, 64P.

The susceptibility of 1000 recent pathogenic bacterial isolates to noxythiolin was determined by the disc susceptibility method. No Gram-positive strains were resistant to this method but 5.6% of Gram-negative strains were. The minimum inhibitory concentration (MIC) of the latter were determined; none had MIC values greater than 4.096 mg per mL (0.41%). Since concentrations of 50 mg per mL (5%) can be used for topical treatment, these organisms may be considered susceptible.— K. C. Ashley and D. L. Myerthall, *J. clin. Hosp. Pharm.*, 1986, *11*, 95.

MALIGNANT NEOPLASMS. For the use of noxythiolin to prevent live cell exfoliation in colorectal cancer operations, see under Malignant Neoplasms in Cetrimide, p.954.

Proprietary Preparations

Noxyflex *(Geistlich, UK)*. *Solution*, powder for reconstitution, noxythiolin 2.5 g, amethocaine hydrochloride 10 mg.
Solution, (Noxyflex 'S'), powder for reconstitution, noxythiolin 2.5 g.
Solutions are chemically stable for 7 days after preparation.

Proprietary Names and Manufacturers
Noxyflex *(Innothèra, Fr.)*; Noxyflex S *(Geistlich, UK)*.
The following names have been used for multi-ingredient preparations containing noxythiolin—Gynaflex *(Geistlich, UK)*; Noxyflex *(Geistlich, UK)*.

2263-q

Octaphonium Chloride *(BAN)*.

Octafonium Chloride *(rINN)*; Phenoctide. Benzyldiethyl-2-[4-(1,1,3,3-tetramethylbutyl)phenoxy]ethylammonium chloride monohydrate.
$C_{27}H_{42}ClNO,H_2O=450.1$.

CAS — 15687-40-8 (anhydrous).

Pharmacopoeias. In *Br.*

A white, odourless or almost odourless, crystalline powder. **Soluble** 1 in 5 of water; soluble in alcohol and chloroform. A 1% solution in water has a pH of 5 to 6.

Octaphonium chloride is a quaternary ammonium disinfectant with properties and uses similar to those of other cationic surfactants as described under Cetrimide, p.953.

2264-p

Oxychlorosene *(USAN)*.

Monoxychlorosene. The hypochlorous acid complex of a mixture of the phenyl sulphonate derivatives of aliphatic hydrocarbons.
$C_{20}H_{34}O_3S,HOCl=407.0$.

CAS — 8031-14-9.

Oxychlorosene is a chlorine disinfectant with the actions and uses described under Chlorine, p.957.
A 0.1 to 0.4% solution of the sodium salt of oxychlorosene is used for cleansing wounds.

CYSTITIS. Interstitial cystitis may respond to the instillation of the sodium salt of oxychlorosene.— A. L. Komaroff, *New Engl. J. Med.*, 1984, *310*, 368.

VIRAL DISINFECTION. At the concentration of virus likely to be found in clinical specimens, human immunodeficiency virus was inactivated by the sodium salt of oxychlorosene 4 mg per mL, the concentration recommended for clinical use.— R. J. Klein *et al.* (letter), *Lancet*, 1987, *1*, 281.

Proprietary Names and Manufacturers of Oxychlorosene and its Sodium Salt
Clorpactin WCS-90 *(Protea, Austral.; Guardian, Canad.; Guardian, USA: Farillon, UK)*; Clorpactin XCB *(Guardian, USA: Farillon, UK)*.

2265-s

Parachlorophenol *(USAN)*.

4-Chlorophenol.
$C_6H_5ClO=128.6$.

CAS — 106-48-9.

Pharmacopoeias. In *Aust., Braz., Jug., Nord., Pol., Swiss,* and *U.S.*

White or pink crystals with a characteristic phenolic odour. M.p. 42 to 44°.
Sparinglysoluble in water and liquid paraffin; very soluble in alcohol, chloroform, ether, glycerol, and fixed and volatile oils; soluble in melted soft paraffin. A 1% solution in water is acid to litmus. **Store** in airtight containers. Protect from light.

Parachlorophenol is a disinfectant with similar properties to phenol (see below).
Camphorated parachlorophenol is used in dentistry in the treatment of infected root canals.

Preparations

Camphorated Parachlorophenol *(U.S.P.)*. Parachlorophenol 35 g and camphor 65 g, triturated until the mixture liquefies.

2266-w

Paraformaldehyde

Paraform; Paraformic Aldehyde; Polymerised Formaldehyde; Polyoxymethylene; Trioxyméthylène.
$(CH_2O)_n$.

CAS — 30525-89-4.

Pharmacopoeias. In *Aust., Belg., Jpn, Jug., Nord., Pol., Port., Span.,* and *Swiss.* Also in *B.P.C. 1973.*

A solid polymer of formaldehyde.

Adverse Effects, Treatment, and Precautions
As for Formaldehyde, p.961. There have been reports of allergic and other reactions associated with the dental use of paraformaldehyde as a root canal sealant; it should not extrude beyond the apex.

Reports of nerve damage after the use of endodontic filling material containing paraformaldehyde: K. B. Fanibunda, *Br. dent. J.*, 1984, *157*, 231; J. D. Lilley and C. Russell (letter), *ibid.*, 340.
A type I allergic response followed deposition of a root canal paste containing paraformaldehyde into the periapical tissues of a 57-year-old man. The patient had a history of atopy and a previous allergic response to topical formaldehyde.— G. H. Forman and R. A. Ord, *Br. dent. J.*, 1986, *160*, 348.

Uses and Administration
Paraformaldehyde has the properties and uses of formaldehyde (see p.962) and is used as a source of formaldehyde. For disinfecting rooms it has been vapourised by heating. Tablets prepared for disinfecting rooms by vaporisation should be coloured by the addition of a suitable blue dye.
Paraformaldehyde is also used in lozenges. In dentistry, it has been used as an obtundent for sensitive dentine and as an antiseptic in mummifying pastes and for root canals.

Preparations

Formaldehyde Lozenges *(B.P.C. 1973)*. Formalin Throat Tablets; Formamint Tablets. Store in a cool place in airtight containers. These lozenges are liable to deteriorate on storage.
NOTE. The use of the names Formalin and Formamint is limited; in some countries they are trade-marks.

Proprietary Names and Manufacturers
Diformil *(Faes, Spain)*; Paraform *(Orapharm, Austral.)*.

13094-q

Peracetic Acid

Acetyl Hydroperoxide; Peroxyacetic Acid.
$C_2H_4O_3=76.05$.

CAS — 79-21-0.

Pharmacopoeias. In *Cz.*

Peracetic acid is a strong oxidising agent which is corrosive to the skin. It has been used as a spray for sterilisation of the air and interior of germ-free animal laboratories.

Proprietary Names and Manufacturers
Persteril *(Cz.)*.

2268-l

Phenol *(BAN, USAN)*.

Carbolic Acid; Fenol; Phenolum; Phenyl Hydrate. Hydroxybenzene.
$C_6H_5.OH=94.11$.

CAS — 108-95-2.

Pharmacopoeias. In *Arg., Aust., Belg., Br., Braz., Chin., Cz., Egypt., Fr., Ger., Hung., Ind., Int., It., Jpn, Jug., Mex., Neth., Nord., Pol., Port., Span., Swiss, Turk.,* and *U.S.*

Colourless or faintly pink deliquescent crystals or crystalline masses, becoming pink on keeping, with a characteristic, not tarry, odour. *U.S.P.* permits the addition of a suitable stabilising agent. F.p. 40° to 41°.
B.P. solubilities are: **soluble** 1 in 12 of water; freely soluble in alcohol, chloroform, ether, glycerol, and in fixed and volatile oils. *U.S.P.* solubilities are: soluble 1 in 15 of water; very soluble in alcohol, chloroform, ether, glycerol, and in fixed and volatile oils. A saturated solution in water at 20° is clear and is alkaline to methyl orange.
Incompatible with alkaline salts and nonionic surfactants. **Store** below 15° in airtight containers. Protect from light.
When phenol is to be mixed with collodion, fixed oils, or paraffins, melted phenol should be used, and not Liquefied Phenol.

CAUTION. *Phenol is caustic to the skin.*

Adverse Effects
When taken by mouth, phenol causes extensive local corrosion, with pain, nausea, vomiting, sweating, and diarrhoea. Initially fleeting excitation may occur but it is quickly followed by unconsciousness. There is depression of the central nervous system, with circulatory and respiratory failure. Acidosis may develop and occasionally there is haemolysis and methaemoglobinaemia with cyanosis. Pulmonary oedema may develop, and damage to the liver and kidneys may lead to organ failure. Death usually occurs from respiratory failure.
Severe or fatal poisoning may occur from the absorption of phenol from unbroken skin or wounds. Applied to skin, phenol causes blanching and corrosion, sometimes with little pain. Aqueous solutions as dilute as 10% may be corrosive.
In Great Britain the recommended exposure limits of phenol are 5 ppm (long-term); 10 ppm (short-term); suitable precautions should be taken to prevent absorption through the skin. In the *US* the permissible and recommended exposure limits are 19 mg per m^3 and 20 mg per m^3 respectively.

Cresols and other phenolic substances have similar, but often milder, effects.

A report of gastro-intestinal illness associated with contamination of drinking water supplies with phenol.— S. N. Jarvis *et al.*, *Br. med. J.*, 1985, *290*, 1800.
A 10-year-old boy developed life-threatening premature ventricular complexes during the application of a solution of phenol 40% and croton oil 0.8% in hexachlorophane soap and water for chemical peeling or exfoliation of a giant hairy naevus.— M. A. Warner and J. V. Harper, *Anesthesiology*, 1985, *62*, 366.

Treatment of Adverse Effects
If phenol has been swallowed, empty the stomach by aspiration and lavage, taking care to avoid perforation. Castor oil or olive oil may be added to the water to dissolve phenol and delay absorption; 50 mL of oil may be left in the stomach. Remove contaminated clothing and wash the skin with glycerol, vegetable oil, alcohol, or soap and water. Keep the patient warm and treat pulmonary oedema, systemic acidosis, respiratory failure, and circulatory failure symptomatically. Respiration may have to be assisted.

The following was recommended for skin contamination with phenol: remove all contaminated clothing immediately, flush excess phenol off the skin with water, then wash the affected area with macrogol 300 for at least 30 minutes, wearing protective gloves.— A. C. Houston (letter), *Chem. in Br.*, 1984, *20*, 116. A report of the use of eucalyptus oil to treat phenol burns.— H. R. C. Pratt (letter), *ibid.*, 1985, *21*, 149.

Precautions
Solutions should not be applied to large wounds since sufficient phenol may be absorbed to give rise to toxic symptoms.
The antimicrobial activity of phenol may be diminished through incompatibility (see above) or through combination with blood and other organic matter.
Appropriate measures should be taken to prevent contamination of phenol preparations during storage or dilution.

Absorption and Fate
Phenol is absorbed from the gastro-intestinal tract and through skin and mucous membranes. It is metabolised to phenylglucuronide and phenyl

sulphate, and small amounts are oxidised to catechol and quinol which are mainly conjugated. The metabolites are excreted in the urine; on oxidation to quinones they may tint the urine green.

Uses and Administration

Phenol is a disinfectant effective against vegetative Gram-positive and Gram-negative bacteria and some fungi, but only very slowly effective against spores. It is also active against certain viruses. Phenol is more active in acid solution.

Aqueous solutions up to 1% are bacteriostatic while stronger solutions are bactericidal.

A 0.5 to 1% solution has been used for its local anaesthetic effect to relieve itching. Weak solutions have also been used topically for disinfection. A 5% solution has been used as a disinfectant for excreta. Phenol has also been used as an obtundent and devitalising agent in dentistry.

Oily Phenol Injection is injected into the tissues around internal haemorrhoids as an analgesic sclerosing agent.

Phenol is administered intrathecally usually as a solution in glycerol for the alleviation of spasticity and severe intractable pain. Aqueous solutions of phenol have also been used for chemical sympathectomy.

In the *UK* the maximum concentration of phenol and its alkali salts in soaps and shampoos is limited by law to 1%, calculated as phenol.

Molluscum contagiosum could be treated by pricking liquefied phenol into each lesion with a sharpened stick.— F. A. Ive, *Br. med. J.*, 1973, *4*, 475.

A mixture of phenol, water, liquid soap, and croton oil containing approximately 50% of phenol was used for chemical face peeling in the treatment of facial wrinkling. The liquid was applied to the face after thorough cleansing and left for 24 hours under an occlusive dressing. In a group of about 1575 patients there was no evidence of systemic toxicity. Hypertrophic scarring occasionally occurred.— *J. Am. med. Ass.*, 1974, *228*, 898. See also R. P. Ariagno and D. R. Briggs, *Trans. Am. Acad. Ophthal. Oto-lar.*, 1975, *80*, 536. For a report of adverse cardiac effects associated with phenol being used for skin peeling, see under Adverse Effects, above.

ENLARGED PROSTATE. The intraprostatic injection of phenol and glacial acetic acid in 50 patients with benign enlargement of the prostate.— J. J. Shipman *et al.*, *Br. med. J.*, 1974, *3*, 734.

HAEMORRHOIDS. The technique most commonly used for preventing mucosal prolapse is to inject 2 to 5 mL of a 5% solution of phenol in arachis oil into the submucous space above each of the 3 principal haemorrhoids. Rather than causing the haemorrhoidal veins to thrombose, the injection works by producing submucosal fibrosis, fixing the mucosa to the underlying muscle. The injection may cause severe pain if it is too close to the anal verge. The treatment has proved quite effective in patients whose only symptom is bleeding and whose haemorrhoids do not prolapse; injection is less effective for prolapsing haemorrhoids.— J. Alexander-Williams, *Br. med. J.*, 1982, *285*, 1137. Rubber band ligation and photocoagulation were better long-term therapies for haemorrhoids than phenol injection (P.C. Gartell *et al.*, *Gut*, 1984, *25*, A563, N.S. Ambrose *et al.*, *ibid.*).

HYDROCELE. Five-year follow-up of 42 patients with 38 hydroceles and 10 epididymal cysts revealed recurrence of 4 hydroceles, only one of which was symptomatic and exceeded 20 mL. Phenol sclerotherapy should be considered for adults and is the treatment of choice for the elderly.— J. R. Nash, *Br. med. J.*, 1984, *288*, 1652.

INGROWING TOENAIL. Liquefied phenol applied to the nail-bed, nail-fold, and sulci was highly successful for destroying the matrix after removal of ingrowing nails.— A. Shepherdson, *Practitioner*, 1977, *219*, 725. A favourable report of cauterisation for 3 minutes with phenol 88% for onychogryphosis or ingrowing toenail.— T. Andrew and W. A. Wallace, *Br. med. J.*, 1979, *1*, 1539.

Further references: P. F. Cameron, *ibid.*, 1981, *283*, 821; P. J. Read (letter), *ibid.*, 1125; W. R. Murray and J. E. Robb (letter), *ibid;* P. A. G. Helmn (letter), *ibid;* A. J. Morkane *et al.*, *Br. J. Surg.*, 1984, *71*, 526.

PAIN. Neurolytic block of the splanchnic nerves or coeliac plexus achieved with 50% alcohol or 5 to 7% aqueous phenol is highly effective in relieving severe intractable pain caused by cancer of the pancreas, stomach, small intestine, gallbladder, or other abdominal viscera, and is most effective in patients in whom the cancer has not spread to the parietal peritoneum. Block of the splanchnic nerves or coeliac plexus first with local anaesthetic and subsequently with alcohol or phenol may also be indicated in patients with severe intractable pain of chronic pancreatitis, postcholecystectomy syndrome, or other chronic abdominal visceral diseases unrelieved by medical or surgical therapy.

Subarachnoid neurolysis achieved by injection of small amounts of alcohol or phenol into the subarachnoid space is one of the most effective methods for the relief of severe intractable pain below the neck. Pain relief lasts for several days to several months, and sometimes longer, although frequently it is necessary to do several blocks to effect prolonged relief. Numerous reports suggest that neurolytic subarachnoid block produces complete relief in 50 to 60% of cancer patients, partial relief in 20 to 25%, and no relief in the rest, comparing favourably with neurosurgery. With subarachnoid block of the roots supplying the upper limb, there is a 15 to 20% incidence of muscle weakness. If the block is done to relieve pain in the pelvis or lower limbs, there is a 20 to 25% incidence of bladder and/or rectal dysfunction and lower limb muscle weakness.— J. J. Bonica, *Postgrad. med. J.*, 1984, *60*, 897.

In the treatment of intractable postherpetic neuralgia, intrathecal phenol is not advocated nowadays as its effects on pain are temporary, it rarely affects dysaesthesia, and it can be dangerous.— S. Lipton, *Br. med. J.*, 1984, *289*, 98.

Jefferson (*J. Neurol. Neurosurg. Psychiat.*, 1963, *26*, 345) reported that of 37 patients with trigeminal neuralgia treated with phenol and glycerol injection of the trigeminal nerve, 7 did not obtain abatement of pain, or had recurrence within one week. Complications included weakness of the muscles of mastication on the side of the injection (present in about 40% of cases initially, but nearly always clearing within 3 months). Transient sixth nerve pareses are also relatively common.— R. D. Weeks, *Br. med. J.*, 1985, *291*, 190.

The lumbar sympathetic chain can be blocked for a period of up to a year using an aqueous solution of 6% phenol. The use of an X-ray image intensifier has made the placement of the needle tip onto the anterolateral surface of the body of the first or second lumbar vertebra relatively simple. An injection of the solution at this level will usually affect the whole length of the chain from the first to the fourth lumbar segment. The procedure can be performed after premedication with diazepam and insertion of local anaesthetic in the skin.— H. Ellis, *Br. J. Hosp. Med.*, 1986, *35*, 124.

The successful use of a glucose-glycerol-phenol solution injected into soft-tissue structures and spinal manipulation for chronic low back pain.— M. J. Ongley *et al.*, *Lancet*, 1987, *2*, 143.

SPASTICITY. In patients with multiple sclerosis unresponsive to medication, and in whom fibrous contractures have not set in, severe spasticity may be alleviated by chemical neurectomy, commonly by injection of the obturator nerves with phenol to relieve adductor spasm. Similarly, in cases of fixed paraplegia without the presence of contractures, chemical rhizotomy using intrathecal phenol or alcohol converts spastic paraplegia to a flaccid state, resulting in easier positioning of the patient with greater comfort. Adverse effects include complete loss of bladder and bowel control, and impotence.— B. Giesser, *Drugs*, 1985, *29*, 88.

URINARY INCONTINENCE. Twenty of 24 female patients with multiple sclerosis, with severe urge incontinence or leakage around an indwelling urethral catheter, were dry one week after subtrigonal injection of aqueous phenol 6.5%. All had previously failed to respond satisfactorily to drug therapy.— R. Ewing *et al.*, *Lancet*, 1983, *1*, 1304.

Preparations

Liquefied Phenol *(B.P.)*. Phenol 80 g, purified water to 100 g. Liquefied phenol may congeal or deposit crystals if stored below 4°. It should be completely melted before use. When phenol is to be mixed with collodion, fixed oils or paraffins, melted phenol should be used and not Liquefied Phenol.

Oily Phenol Injection *(B.P.)*. Contains phenol 5% in a suitable fixed oil. Sterilise by heating at 170° for 1 hour.

Phenol and Glycerol Injection *(B.P.)*. Phenol 5 g, glycerol, previously dried at 120° for 1 hour, to 100 g. Sterilise by heating at 170° for 1 hour.

Phenol Ear-drops *(B.P.C. 1973)*. Phenol glycerin 40 mL, glycerol to 100 mL. They contain 5.4 to 7.3% w/w of phenol.

CAUTION. *Dilution with water renders the ear-drops caustic; glycerol may be used as a diluent.*

Phenol Gargle *(B.P.C. 1973)*. Garg. Phenol.; Carbolic Acid Gargle. Phenol glycerin 5 mL, amaranth solution 1 mL, water to 100 mL; it contains 0.84 to 1.13% w/v of phenol. It should be diluted with an equal vol. of warm water before use.

Phenol Glycerin *(B.P.)*. Phenol 16 g, glycerol to 100 g.

CAUTION. *Dilution with water renders this preparation caustic; glycerol may be used as a diluent.*

Proprietary Preparations

Chloraseptic *(Norwich-Eaton, UK)*. *Liquid*, phenol and sodium phenolate equivalent to total phenol 1.4%, menthol, thymol, glycerol.

See also under Proprietary Names and Manufacturers of Preparations containing Cresols, Tar Acids, or other Phenols, p.970.

Proprietary Names and Manufacturers of Phenol and/or a Phenolate

Cepastat *(Dow, Canad.)*; Chloraseptic *(Norwich-Eaton, UK; Richardson-Vicks, USA)*; Fenicado *(Spain)*; Paoscle *(Jpn)*.

The following names have been used for multi-ingredient preparations containing phenol and/or a phenolate—Anbesol *(Whitehall, USA)*; Chloraseptic DM *(Richardson-Vicks, Canad.)*; Derma Cas *(Hill, USA)*; Egomycol *(Ego, Austral.)*; Egopsoryl *(Ego, Austral.)*; Merastat *(Merrell Dow, Austral.)*; Pernomol *(Laboratories for Applied Biology, UK)*; Sedaural *(Key, Austral.)*; URA *(Protea, Austral.)*.

2269-y

Picloxydine *(BAN, rINN)*.

1,1′-[Piperazine-1,4-diylbis(formimidoyl)]bis[3-(4-chlorophenyl)guanidine].

$C_{20}H_{24}Cl_2N_{10}$=475.4.

CAS — 5636-92-0.

Picloxydine is a biguanide disinfectant with actions similar to those of chlorhexidine gluconate (see p.955).

It has been used, as digluconate, with benzalkonium chloride, in a detergent basis for the cleansing and disinfection of surfaces.

Proprietary Names and Manufacturers

Vitabact *(Faure, Fr.)*.

The following names have been used for multi-ingredient preparations containing picloxydine— Resiguard *(Nicholas, UK)*.

2270-g

Polynoxylin *(BAN, rINN)*.

Poly{[bis(hydroxymethyl)ureylene]methylene}, a condensation product of formaldehyde and urea with the formula.

$(C_4H_8N_2O_3)_n$.

CAS — 9011-05-6.

Polynoxylin has antibacterial and antifungal actions and may act by the release of formaldehyde. It is available in a variety of preparations for the local treatment of minor infections.

The minimum inhibitory concentration (MIC) of polynoxylin for 1000 clinical isolates of bacteria and yeasts was in the range 1024 to 16 384 µg per mL. Cidal concentrations were within one dilution of the corresponding MIC values, suggesting a cumulative mode of antimicrobial activity. Formaldehyde was released into water from a 10% cream preparation giving a maximum yield of 1.56 mg within 6 hours.— J. I. Blenkharn, *J. clin. Hosp. Pharm.*, 1985, *10*, 367.

Proprietary Preparations

Anaflex *(Geistlich, UK)*. *Aerosol*, polynoxylin 2%. *Cream, Paste, and Powder*, polynoxylin 10%. *Lozenges*, polynoxylin 30 mg.

Ponoxylan *(Berk Pharmaceuticals, UK)*. *Gel*, polynoxylin 10%.

Proprietary Names and Manufacturers

Anaflex *(Gamaprod, Austral.; Denm.; Neth.; Geistlich, Switz.; Geistlich, UK)*; Larex *(Inibsa, Spain; Switz.)*; Noxylin *(Inibsa, Spain)*; Ponoxylan *(USV, Austral.; Fisons, S.Afr.; Berk Pharmaceuticals, UK)*.

2271-q

Proflavine Hemisulphate *(pINNM).*
Neutral Proflavine Sulphate; Proflavine. 3,6-Diaminoacridine sulphate dihydrate.
$(C_{13}H_{11}N_3)_2,H_2SO_4,2H_2O=552.6$.

CAS — 92-62-6 (proflavine).

Pharmacopoeias. In *Belg.* as the monohydrate. Also in *B.P.C. 1973* as the dihydrate.

The acridine derivatives, proflavine, acriflavine, aminacrine, ethacridine, and euflavine, are slow-acting disinfectants. They are bacteriostatic against many Gram-positive bacteria but less effective against Gram-negative organisms. They are ineffective against spores. Their activity is increased in alkaline solutions and is not reduced by tissue fluids.
The acridine derivatives have been used for the treatment of infected wounds or burns and for skin disinfection. Prolonged treatment may delay healing. They have also been used for the treatment of local infections of the ear, mouth, and throat.
Hypersensitivity has been reported.

Preparations

Proflavine Cream *(B.P.C. 1973).* Flavine Cream; Proflavine Emulsion. Proflavine hemisulphate 100 mg, chlorocresol 100 mg, yellow beeswax 2.5 g, wool fat 5 g, freshly boiled and cooled purified water 25 g, and liquid paraffin 67.3 g.

Proflavine Cream (*B.P.C.*) had little or no antibacterial activity when tested *in vitro* against 6 pathogenic organisms, as the proflavine hemisulphate was in the aqueous phase of a water-in-oil emulsion and was not released. Other salts of proflavine with a series of acids were tried in the same basis, and a water-in-oil cream containing 0.8% w/w of proflavine *n*-valerate, soluble in both oil and water, was found to be the most active. However, the hemisulphate was readily released from an oil-in-water cream and exhibited antibacterial activity. A suggested formula: proflavine hemisulphate 100 mg, cetomacrogol emulsifying wax 15 g, liquid paraffin 20 g, water to 100 g.— A. H. Fenton and M. Warren, *Pharm. J.*, 1962, *1*, 5.

2272-p

Propamidine Isethionate *(BANM).*
M&B-782; Propamidine Isetionate *(rINNM).* 4,4′-Trimethylenedioxydibenzamidine bis(2-hydroxyethanesulphonate).
$C_{17}H_{20}N_4O_2,2C_2H_6O_4S=564.6$.

CAS — 104-32-5 (propamidine); 140-63-6 (isethionate).

Propamidine isethionate is an aromatic diamidine which is active against Gram-positive, non-spore-forming organisms, but less active against Gram-negative bacteria and spore-forming organisms. It also has antifungal properties.
An ophthalmic solution containing 0.1% of propamidine isethionate is used for the treatment of conjunctivitis and blepharitis.

A report of the successful treatment of acanthamoeba keratitis with dibromopropamidine and propamidine isethionates, and neomycin.— P. Wright *et al.*, *Br. J. Ophthal.*, 1985, *69*, 778.

Proprietary Preparations

Brolene *(May & Baker, UK). Eye-drops,* propamidine isethionate 0.1%.

Proprietary Names and Manufacturers

Brolene Eye Drops *(May & Baker, Austral.; May & Baker, UK)*; M & B Antiseptic Cream *(May & Baker, Austral.; May & Baker, S.Afr.; May & Baker, UK).*

2273-s

Propiolactone *(BAN, USAN, rINN).*
β-Propiolactone; BPL; NSC-21626. Propiono-3-lactone.
$C_3H_4O_2=72.06$.

CAS — 57-57-8.

Propiolactone vapour is an irritant, mutagenic, possibly carcinogenic disinfectant which is very active against vegetative Gram-positive and Gram-negative bacteria, acid-fast bacteria, fungi, and viruses. It is rather less effective against bacterial spores.
Propiolactone vapour has been used for the gaseous sterilisation of pharmaceutical and surgical materials and for disinfecting large enclosed areas. It has low penetrating power.
Propiolactone has been used for the sterilisation of tissues for grafting. It is used for the sterilisation of rabies vaccine.

VIRAL DISINFECTION. Propiolactone 0.25% inactivates the reverse transcriptase activity of retrovirus HIV, but when added to whole blood it affected most biochemical determinations. When added to separated plasma, significant effects were limited to bicarbonate and some enzyme activities.— M. J. Ball and D. Griffiths (letter), *Lancet*, 1985, *1*, 1160. Propiolactone did not interfere with haemoglobin estimation, or total white cell or platelet counts. Coagulation studies were significantly affected and propiolactone should not be added to specimens taken for such purposes.— M. J. Ball and F. G. Bolton (letter), *ibid.*, *2*, 99.
A combined propiolactone and u.v. irradiation procedure was effective in the inactivation of non-A, non-B hepatitis virus.— A. M. Prince *et al.*, *J. med. Virol.*, 1985, *16*, 119.
For large-scale non-urgent work, HIV-infected specimens could be treated with propiolactone to inactivate the virus, but the procedure has hazards and is not recommended for routine use.— *Lancet*, 1986, *2*, 174.

Proprietary Names and Manufacturers

Betaprone *(Fellows, USA).*

2274-w

Scarlet Red
Biebrich Scarlet R Medicinal; CI Solvent Red 24; Colour Index No. 26105; Rubrum Scarlatinum; Scharlachrot; Sudan IV. 1-[4-(*o*-Tolylazo)-*o*-tolylazo]-naphth-2-ol.
$C_{24}H_{20}N_4O=380.4$.

CAS — 85-83-6.

Pharmacopoeias. In *Aust.*

Scarlet red has been used topically as a disinfectant. It can be irritant.

2276-l

Sodium Dichloroisocyanurate
Sodium Dichloro-*s*-triazinetrione; Sodium Troclosene. The sodium salt of 1,3-dichloro-1,3,5-triazine-2,4,6(1*H*,3*H*,5*H*)-trione.
$C_3Cl_2N_3NaO_3=219.9$.

CAS — 2893-78-9.

It contains about 62% of 'available chlorine' (see p.958).

Sodium dichloroisocyanurate has the actions and uses of chlorine (see p.957) and sodium hypochlorite (below) but its activity is only slightly affected by pH over the range 6 to 10. It is used for disinfecting babies' feeding bottles, for the treatment of water in swimming pools, and in various commercial bleach detergents and scouring powders as a relatively stable source of chlorine.
Dichloroisocyanuric acid ($C_3HCl_2N_3O_3$ = 198.0), potassium dichloroisocyanurate (potassium troclosene, troclosene potassium, $C_3Cl_2KN_3O_3$ = 236.1), and trichloroisocyanuric acid (symclosene, $C_3Cl_3N_3O_3$ = 232.4) are similarly used.

WATER DISINFECTION. The use of various biocides, including sodium dichloroisocyanurate, for the control of *Legionella pneumophila* in cooling water systems.— J. B. Kurtz *et al.*, *J. Hyg., Camb.*, 1982, *88*, 369.
Sodium dichloroisocyanurate 17 mg dissolved in 1 litre of water liberates 10 ppm of 'available chlorine' which kills viruses, bacteria, and encysted protozoa at around 20° at neutral pH after a contact time of 30 minutes. Organic matter in cloudy water reduces the available chlorine concentration, so turbidity should be allowed to settle and clear water decanted off for chlorination. Temperatures below 10° and increasing pH both reduce the cysticidal activity of halogens, and in those conditions water filtration is also necessary.— S. G. Wright, *Br. med. J.*, 1983, *287*, 741.
The Treatment and Quality of Swimming Pool Water, Department of the Environment, National Water Council, London, HM Stationery Office, 1985.

Proprietary Names and Manufacturers of Chlorinated Isocyanurates

ACL 56 *(Monsanto, UK)*; ACL 59 *(Monsanto, UK)*; ACL 60 *(Monsanto, UK)*; ACL 85 *(Monsanto, UK)*; Babysafe Tablets *(Kirby-Warrick, UK)*; Fi-Clor *(Chlor-Chem, UK)*; Fi-Clor Clearon *(Chlor-Chem, UK)*; Fi-Tab R/D *(Chlor-Chem, UK)*; Fi-Tab S/D *(Chlor-Chem, UK)*; Kirbychlor Tablets *(Kirby-Warrick, UK)*; Milton Tablets *(Richardson-Vicks, UK)*; Presept *(Surgikos, UK)*; Puritabs *(Essex, Austral.; Kirby-Warrick, UK)*; Simpla Tablets *(Ashe, UK)*; Softab *(Gelflex, Austral.)*; Tricidechlor *(Wingfield, UK).*

2277-y

Sodium Hypochlorite *(BAN, USAN).*

$NaOCl, 5H_2O=164.5$.

CAS — 7681-52-9.

Solutions of sodium hypochlorite should be **stored** in well-filled airtight containers at a temperature not exceeding 20°. Protect from light.

Sodium hypochlorite solutions providing 0.04 to 0.12% 'available chlorine' stored in amber glass bottles at room temperature could carry a 23-month expiry date based on chemical stability.— T. M. Fabian and S. E. Walker, *Am. J. Hosp. Pharm.*, 1982, *39*, 1016. See also S. F. Bloomfield and T. J. Sizer, *Pharm. J.*, 1985, *2*, 153.

Adverse Effects

Hypochlorite solutions release hypochlorous acid upon contact with gastric juice and acids, and ingestion causes irritation and corrosion of mucous membranes with pain and vomiting and, rarely, perforation of the oesophagus and stomach. A fall in blood pressure, delirium, and coma may occur. Inhalation of hypochlorous fumes causes coughing and choking and may cause severe respiratory tract irritation, pulmonary oedema, and oedema of the pharynx and larynx.

Treatment of Adverse Effects

If sodium hypochlorite solution is ingested, give water, milk, or other demulcents; antacids and sodium thiosulphate 1% to 2.5% solution may be of value.

Precautions

Topically applied hypochlorites may dissolve blood clots and cause bleeding.
Sodium hypochlorite solutions should not be mixed with solutions of strong acids or ammonia; the subsequent reactions release chlorine and chloramine.
The antimicrobial activity of hypochlorites is rapidly diminished in the presence of organic material; it is also pH dependent being greater in acid pH although they are more stable at alkaline pH.

Uses and Administration

Sodium hypochlorite solutions have the brief and rapid actions of chlorine (p.958). They are commonly used for the rapid disinfection of hard surfaces, food and dairy equipment, and babies' feeding bottles. Only diluted solutions containing up to 0.5% of 'available chlorine' are suitable for use on the skin and in wounds.
Labarraque's Solution is a solution of sodium hypochlorite with sodium chloride and an alkali and Eau de Javelle is a potassium hypochlorite solution.

For references to the uses of sodium hypochlorite, see chlorine (p.958).

Preparations

Dilute Sodium Hypochlorite Solution *(B.P.).* An aqueous solution containing 0.9 to 1.1% w/w of 'available chlorine'. It may contain stabilising agents and sodium chloride.

Sodium Hypochlorite Solution *(U.S.P.).* A solution containing 4 to 6% w/w of NaOCl.

Strong Sodium Hypochlorite Solution *(B.P.).* An aqueous solution containing not less than 8% w/w of 'available chlorine'. It may contain stabilising agents.

For other preparations containing hypochlorites, see under Chlorinated Lime, p.957.

Proprietary Preparations

Chlorasol *(Seton, UK). Solution,* sodium hypochlorite, 0.3 to 0.4% 'available chlorine'.

Milton *(Richardson-Vicks, UK). Solution,* stabilised sodium hypochlorite solution 1%.
Solution(Milton 2), sodium hypochlorite 2%.

Proprietary Names and Manufacturers

Bactot *(Arg.)*; Chlorasol *(Seton, UK)*; Chloros *(ICI Mond, UK)*; Deosan Green Label Steriliser *(Diversey, UK)*; Hygeol *(Wampole, Canad.)*; Hyposan *(Voxsan, UK)*; Milton *(Richardson-Vicks, UK)*; Parozone *(Jeyes, UK)*; Voxsan *(Voxsan, UK)*.

2278-j

Succinchlorimide

N-Chlorosuccinimide; 1-Chloropyrrolidine-2,5-dione.
$C_4H_4ClNO_2$=133.5.

CAS — 128-09-6.

It contains about 53% of 'available chlorine' (see p.958).

Succinchlorimide has been used for water disinfection.

13272-s

Succisulfone *(rINN).*

1500F; Fourneau-1500; Succinylsulphone. 4'-Sulphanilylsuccinanilic acid; 4-Amino-4'-(3-carboxypropionamido)diphenyl sulphone.
$C_{16}H_{16}N_2O_5S$=348.4.

CAS — 5934-14-5.

Succisulfone is a bacteriostatic agent applied topically as a 10% powder.

Proprietary Names and Manufacturers
Exosulfonyl *(Vaillant-Defresne, Fr.)*.

2279-z

Tar Acids

Tar acids are phenolic substances derived from the distillation of coal tar or, more recently, petroleum fractions. The lowest boiling fraction of coal tar, distilling at 188° to 205°, consists of mixed cresol isomers forming cresol *B.P.* The middle fraction, known as 'cresylic acids', distils at 205° to 230° and consists of cresols and xylenols. The 'high-boiling tar acids', distilling at 230° to 290°, consist mainly of alkyl homologues of phenol, with naphthalenes and other hydrocarbons.

Adverse Effects

As for Phenol, p.967.

Tar acids are generally very irritant and corrosive to the skin, even when diluted to concentrations used for disinfection.

A report of fatal self-poisoning in a 59-year-old man following the ingestion of approximately 250 mL of a xylenol-containing disinfectant (Stericol Hospital Disinfectant).— I. D. Watson *et al., Postgrad. med. J.*, 1986, *62*, 411.

Uses and Administration

Tar acids are used in the preparation of a range of disinfectant fluids used for household and general disinfection purposes.

The low-boiling range cresols produce fluids with low Rideal-Walker (RW) coefficients whose activity is not greatly reduced in the presence of organic matter but is reduced by some plastics. The cresylic acid fraction produces fluids with RW coefficients of 8 to 10 and the high-boiling fraction produces fluids with RW coefficients of 20 or more. This higher activity is greatly reduced by organic matter and is reflected in very much lower Chick-Martin coefficients. The higher boiling fractions are also more selective in action and less uniformly effective against Gram-positive organisms than the low-boiling range cresols.

The addition of chlorinated phenols to tar acids increases the RW coefficient but such mixtures are more selective and affected to a greater degree by organic matter. Hydrocarbons are often used to enhance the activity of the tar acids in disinfectant fluids; they also help to reduce crystallisation of phenols in cold weather.

Fluids based on tar acids are used similarly, but they must be used in adequate concentration as activity is markedly reduced by dilution.

Specifications for **disinfectants containing tar acids** are given in a British Standard Specification (BS 2462: 1961) and described as follows.

Black Fluids. Homogeneous solutions of coal-tar acids, or similar acids derived from petroleum, or any mixture of these, with or without hydrocarbons and with a suitable emulsifying agent.

White Fluids. Finely dispersed emulsions of coal-tar acids, or similar acids derived from petroleum, or any mixture of these, with or without hydrocarbons.

Modified Black Fluids and **Modified White Fluids** may contain, as an addition, any other active ingredients, but if these are used, the type and amount must be disclosed, if required, to the prospective buyer.

The fluids are required to be free from objectionable smell, to be packed in containers not liable to deleterious interaction with them, and to be labelled with certain particulars including directions for dilution.

VIRAL DISINFECTION. For the use of phenolic disinfectants for the disinfection of human immunodeficiency virus-contaminated articles, see p.950.

Proprietary Names and Manufacturers of Preparations containing Cresols, Tar Acids, or other Phenols

Clearsol *(Tenneco, UK)*; Creolin *(Pearson, UK)*; Cresolox *(Tenneco, UK)*; Desderman *(Sterling Industrial, UK)*; Jeyes' Fluid *(Jeyes, UK)*; Lubraseptic *(Guardian, USA)*; Lyseptol *(Philip Harris, UK)*; Novasapa *(Pharmaceutical Mfg, UK)*; Printol Hospital Disinfectant *(Tenneco, UK)*; Stericol Hospital Disinfectant *(Sterling Industrial, UK)*; Sterilite *(Tenneco, UK)*; Sudol *(Tenneco, UK)*.

The following names have been used for multi-ingredient preparations containing cresols, tar acids, or other phenols— Zal *(Sterling Health, UK)*; Zant *(Evans Medical, UK)*.

2281-s

Thiomersal *(BAN, pINN).*

Mercurothiolate; Mercurothiolate Sodique; Sodium Ethyl Mercurithiosalicylate; Thimerosal *(USAN)*; Thiomersalate. The sodium salt of (2-carboxyphenylthio)ethylmercury.
$C_9H_9HgNaO_2S$=404.8.

CAS — 54-64-8.

Pharmacopoeias. In *Arg., Br., Braz., Fr., Hung., Ind., It., Pol., Swiss,* and *U.S.*

A light cream-coloured crystalline powder with a slight characteristic odour.

B.P. solubilities are: **soluble** 1 in 1 of water and 1 in 8 of alcohol; practically insoluble in ether. *U.S.P.* solubilities are: soluble 1 in 1 of water and 1 in 12 of alcohol; practically insoluble in ether. A 1% solution in water has a pH of 6 to 8. **Store** in airtight containers. Protect from light.

The rate of oxidation of thiomersal in solution is greatly increased by traces of copper ions. In slightly acid solution thiomersal may be precipitated as the corresponding acid which undergoes slow decomposition with the formation of insoluble products.

Incompatible with metals and sulphides.

Propylene glycol, glycerol, and mannitol were suitable alternative isotonic agents to sodium chloride, which has been shown adversely to affect thiomersal stability.— M. J. Reader, *J. pharm. Sci.*, 1984, *73*, 840.

Adverse Effects, Treatment, and Precautions

As for Mercury, p.1587. Hypersensitivity reactions, usually with erythema and papular or vesicular eruptions, occasionally occur. Allergic conjunctivitis has been reported.

The antimicrobial activity of thiomersal may be diminished through incompatibility (see above) interaction, adsorption or combination with organic matter. Thus edetates, whole blood, plastics, and rubber will reduce its effectiveness. Appropriate measures should be taken to prevent contamination of thiomersal preparations during storage or dilution.

For a report of 6 cases of poisoning, 5 of them fatal, resulting from the presence of 1000 times the normal quantity of thiomersal in a preparation of chloramphenicol for intramuscular injection, see J. H. M. Axton, *Postgrad. med. J.*, 1972, *48*, 417.

Of 13 children with exomphalos (umbilical hernia) treated with a tincture of thiomersal, 10 had died. Tissue concentrations of mercury were above the minimum toxic concentrations in 6 examined. Neurological examination of 1 survivor showed no evidence of minimum mercury damage. It was recommended that organic mercurial disinfectants should be heavily restricted or withdrawn from hospital use as absorption occurred readily through intact membranes.— D. G. Fagan *et al., Archs Dis. Childh.*, 1977, *52*, 962.

Thiomersal used in topical antiseptic preparations was toxic to epidermal cells.— *Med. Lett.*, 1977, *19*, 83.

ALLERGY. False positive reactions to old tuberculin were attributed to the presence of thiomersal. In 63 subjects with positive thiomersal reactions, nearly all had positive reactions to old tuberculin but 23 had negative reactions to PPD, which contained no thiomersal.— H. Hansson and H. Möller, *Scand. J. infect. Dis.*, 1971, *3*, 169.

A vaccination reaction in a 5-year-old atopic girl was attributed to thiomersal allergy. Thiomersal was present in all brands of triple vaccine in the *UK* as a preservative and it was possible that many positive patch test reactions to thiomersal may be due to sensitisation at the time of vaccination.— N. H. Cox *et al.* (letter), *Br. med. J.*, 1987, *294*, 250.

EFFECTS ON THE EAR. Thiomersal had been reported to be ototoxic.— J. L. Honigman (letter), *Pharm. J.*, 1975, *2*, 523.

EFFECTS ON THE EYE. A study into the penetration of mercury (in thiomersal) from ophthalmic preservatives into the human eye. The study indicated that significant amounts of mercury may be found in the cornea and aqueous shortly after brief exposure of abnormal corneas to organic mercurials such as may occur in the course of normal ophthalmological procedures.— A. F. Winder *et al., Lancet*, 1980, *2*, 237.

INTERACTIONS. The antibacterial activity of thiomersal solutions was reduced by the addition of disodium edetate and also by the addition of sodium thiosulphate.— R. M. E. Richards and J. M. E. Reary, *J. Pharm. Pharmac.*, 1972, *24, Suppl.*, 84P. See also D. J. Morton, *Int. J. Pharmaceut.*, 1985, *23*, 357.

Nine patients using a contact lens solution containing 0.004% thiomersal developed varying degrees of ocular irritation after taking oral tetracyclines concurrently. Exposure to either the tetracyclines or thiomersal alone did not cause the response.— T. G. Crook and J. J. Freeman, *Am. J. Optom. physiol. Opt.*, 1983, *60*, 759.

Uses and Administration

Thiomersal is a bacteriostatic and fungistatic mercurial disinfectant that has been applied topically usually in a concentration of 0.1%.

Thiomersal, 0.01 to 0.02%, is used as a preservative in biological products.

In the *UK* the maximum concentration of thiomersal as a preservative in concentrated shampoos and hair creams is limited by law to 0.003%, and the maximum concentration in eye make-up and eye make-up remover to 0.007%. When mixed with other mercury compounds, the total mercury concentration must not exceed 0.007%.

Preparations

Thimerosal Tincture *(U.S.P.).* Thiomerosal Tincture. Contains thiomersal 0.09 to 0.11% w/v. Inflammable. Store at a temperature not exceeding 40°.

Thimerosal Topical Aerosol *(U.S.P.).* Thiomerosal Aerosol. An alcoholic solution of thiomersal mixed with suitable propellents in a pressurised container. Inflammable. Store at a temperature not exceeding 40°.

Thimerosal Topical Solution *(U.S.P.).* Thiomerosal Solution. Contains thiomersal 0.095 to 0.105% w/v. pH 9.6 to 10.2. Store at a temperature not exceeding 40°.

Proprietary Names and Manufacturers

Colluspray *(Belg.)*; Merseptyl *(Winthrop, Fr.)*; Merthiolate *(Austral.; Canad.; Lilly, S.Afr.; Lilly, UK; USA)*; Nutramersal *(S.Afr.)*; Topicaldermo *(Derly, Spain)*; Vitaseptol *(Fr.)*.

The following names have been used for multi-ingredient preparations containing thiomersal— Hexidin *(Barnes-Hind, Austral.)*.

13331-b

Thonzonium Bromide *(USAN).*

NC-1264; NSC-5648; Tonzonium Bromide *(rINN)*.
Hexadecyl[2-(*N-p*-methoxybenzyl-*N*-pyrimidin-2-ylamino)ethyl]dimethylammonium bromide.

$C_{32}H_{55}BrN_4O$=591.7.

CAS — 553-08-2.

Pharmacopoeias. In *U.S.*

Store in airtight containers.

Thonzonium bromide is a cationic detergent. As an additive in ear-drops and aerosol sprays it has been claimed to promote tissue contact by dispersion and penetration of cellular debris and exudate.

Proprietary Names and Manufacturers
Thonzide *(Parke, Davis, USA).*

2282-w

Thymol *(BAN, USAN).*

Acido Timico; Isopropylmetacresol; Timol. 2-Isopropyl-5-methylphenol.

$C_{10}H_{14}O$=150.2.

CAS — 89-83-8.

Pharmacopoeias. In *Arg., Aust., Belg., Br., Egypt., Fr., Ger., Hung., Ind., Int., It., Jpn, Mex., Pol., Port., Roum., Rus., Span., Swiss,* and *Turk.* Also in *U.S.N.F.*

Colourless crystals or white crystalline powder with a characteristic pungent aromatic thyme-like odour. M.p. 48° to 51°; when melted it remains liquid at a considerably lower temperature.
B.P. solubilities are: **soluble** 1 in 1000 of water, 1 in 0.3 of alcohol, 1 in 0.6 of chloroform, and 1 in 0.7 of ether. *U.S.N.F.* solubilities are: soluble 1 in 1000 of water, 1 in 1 of alcohol, 1 in 1 of chloroform, 1 in 1.5 of ether, and 1 in 2 of olive oil; soluble in glacial acetic acid and fixed and volatile oils. **Store** in airtight containers. Protect from light.

Adverse Effects, Treatment, and Precautions

As for Phenol, p.967.
When taken by mouth, thymol is less toxic than phenol. It is irritant to the gastric mucosa. Rashes may occur. Fats and alcohol increase absorption and aggravate the toxic symptoms.
The antimicrobial activity of thymol is diminished through combination with protein.
Appropriate measures should be taken to avoid contamination of thymol preparations during storage or dilution.

Thymol and other phenols could cause green or dark discoloration of the urine which could become black on standing.— R. B. Baran and B. Rowles, *J. Am. pharm. Ass.*, 1973, *NS13,* 139.

Contact allergy to a heparinoid cream (Hirudoid) was due to an allergen formed by the reaction between thymol and the degradation products of a triazine derivative, both present as preservatives.— G. Smeenk *et al.*, *Br. J. Derm.*, 1987, *116,* 223.

Absorption and Fate

Thymol is absorbed from the intestine. It is excreted in the urine as unchanged drug and as the glucuronide.

Uses and Administration

Thymol is a more powerful disinfectant than phenol but its use is limited by its low solubility in water, irritancy, and susceptibility to protein.
Thymol is used chiefly as a deodorant in mouth-washes and gargles and it has been used in dentistry. Externally, thymol has been used in dusting-powders for the treatment of fungous skin infections.
Thymol (0.01%) is added as an antoxidant to halothane, trichloroethylene, and tetrachloroethylene.

Preparations

Compound Thymol Glycerin *(B.P.).* Thymol 50 mg, sodium bicarbonate 1 g, borax 2 g, sodium benzoate 800 mg, sodium salicylate 520 mg, menthol 30 mg, cineole 0.13 mL, pumilio pine oil, of commerce 0.05 mL, methyl salicylate 0.03 mL, alcohol (90%) (or industrial methylated spirit, suitably diluted) 2.5 mL, glycerol 10 mL, sodium metabisulphite 35 mg, carmine, food grade of commerce, 30 mg, dilute ammonia solution 0.075 mL, water to 100 mL. pH 7.1 to 7.6. For use as a gargle or mouthwash dilute with about 3 times its vol. of warm water before use; diluted solutions should be prepared immediately before use.

Thymol Mouth-wash Compound *(A.P.F.).* Collut. Thymol. Alb.; Liq. Thymol. Co. Thymol 150 mg, menthol 10 mg, benzoic acid 800 mg, methyl salicylate 0.05 mL, cineole 0.05 mL, glycerol 2 mL, alcohol (90%) 20 mL, water to 100 mL. Dilute with 7 vol. of water for use as a gargle or mouth-wash.

Proprietary Names and Manufacturers

The following names have been used for multi-ingredient preparations containing thymol—Bensulfoid Lotion *(Poythress, USA).*

13361-w

Toloconium Methylsulphate

Toloconium Metilsulfate *(rINN).* Trimethyl[1-(*p*-tolyl)dodecyl]ammonium methylsulphate.

$C_{23}H_{43}NO_4S$=429.7.

CAS — 552-92-1.

Toloconium methylsulphate is a quaternary ammonium compound which has been used in infections of the mouth.

Proprietary Names and Manufacturers
Albert Crème *(Switz.)*; Désogène *(Geigy, Switz.)*; Desogen *(Geigy, Neth.)*; Stomatosan *(Ital.).*

2285-y

Triclobisonium Chloride *(rINN).*

Hexamethylenebis{dimethyl[1-methyl-3-(2,2,6-trimethylcyclohexyl)propyl]ammonium chloride}.

$C_{36}H_{74}Cl_2N_2$=605.9.

CAS — 7187-64-6 (triclobisonium); 79-90-3 (chloride).

Triclobisonium chloride is a quaternary ammonium compound with properties and uses similar to those of other cationic surfactants as described under Cetrimide, p.953. It has been applied topically in the treatment of skin infections and vaginitis.

2286-j

Triclocarban *(USAN, rINN).*

3,4,4′-Trichlorocarbanilide. 1-(4-Chlorophenyl)-3-(3,4-dichlorophenyl)urea.

$C_{13}H_9Cl_3N_2O$=315.6.

CAS — 101-20-2.

Adverse Effects and Precautions
When subjected to prolonged high temperatures triclocarban can decompose to form toxic chloroanilines, which can be absorbed through the skin and cause methaemoglobinaemia.
Mild photosensitivity has been seen in patch testing.

Uses and Administration
Triclocarban is an anilide disinfectant. It is bacteriostatic against Gram-positive organisms in high dilutions but is less effective against Gram-negative organisms and some fungi. It is used in soaps.

Proprietary Names and Manufacturers
Cutisan *(Innothéra, Fr.; Martindale Pharmaceuticals, UK)*; Genoface *(Genove, Spain)*; Nobacter; Procutene *(Bouty, Ital.)*; Septivon *(Midy, Fr.; Midysan, Switz.)*; Solubacter *(Belg.; Innothéra, Fr.)*; TCC *(Monsanto, UK)*; Ungel *(Arg.).*

The following names have been used for multi-ingredient preparations containing triclocarban— Crinagen *(Pharmax, UK).*

2287-z

Triclosan *(BAN, USAN, rINN).*

CH-3565; Cloxifenol. 5-Chloro-2-(2,4-dichlorophenoxy)phenol.

$C_{12}H_7Cl_3O_2$=289.5.

CAS — 3380-34-5.

Triclosan is a bis-phenol disinfectant, bacteriostatic against Gram-positive and most Gram-negative organisms. It has variable or poor activity against *Pseudomonas* spp. It is used in surgical scrubs, soaps, and deodorants in concentrations of 0.05 to 2%. There have been isolated reports of contact dermatitis.

The use of triclosan for washing and bathing in the control of methicillin-resistant *Staphylococcus aureus* infection on a surgical unit.— C. A. Bartzokas *et al.*, *New Engl. J. Med.*, 1984, *311,* 1422. Comment. Caution was necessary in attributing control to a single measure such as antiseptic bathing.— J. P. O'Keefe *et al.* (letter), *ibid.*, 1985, *312,* 858. Reply. Antiseptic bathing was the only specific measure adopted in addition to physical isolation and may prove an acceptable alternative to the use of systemic antibiotics.— C. A. Bartzokas (letter), *ibid.*

Proprietary Preparations
Gamophen *(Surgikos, UK). Soap,* triclosan 1.5%.
Manusept *(Hough, Hoseason, UK). Solution,* triclosan 0.5%, isopropyl alcohol 70%.
Ster-Zac Bath Concentrate *(Hough, Hoseason, UK). Solution,* triclosan 2%.

Proprietary Names and Manufacturers
Adasept Cleanser *(Odan, Canad.)*; Gamophen Antiseptic Soap *(Surgikos, UK)*; Hiozon *(Chemia, Denm.)*; Irgasan DP300 *(Ciba-Geigy, UK)*; Lipo-Sol *(Widmer, Switz.)*; Manusept *(Hough, Hoseason, UK)*; Pentaid *(Pennwalt, Canad.)*; Phisohex Reformulated *(Winthrop, Austral.)*; Procutol *(Spirig, Switz.)*; Sapoderm *(Reckitt & Colman, Austral.)*; Ster-Zac Bath Concentrate *(Hough, Hoseason, UK)*; Tersaseptic *(Trans Canaderm, Canad.)*; Zalclense Bactericidal Washing Cream

The following names have been used for multi-ingredient preparations containing triclosan—Adasept *(Odan, Canad.)*; Dettol Cream *(Reckitt & Colman, Austral.; Reckitt & Colman Pharmaceuticals, UK)*; Hycolin *(Pearson, UK)*; Tardan *(Odan, Canad.)*; Timoped *(Reckitt & Colman Pharmaceuticals, UK).*

2288-c

Trinitrophenol

Carbazotic Acid; Picric Acid; Picrinic Acid. 2,4,6-Trinitrophenol.

$C_6H_3N_3O_7$=229.1.

CAS — 88-89-1.

Pharmacopoeias. In *Arg., Fr., Port.,* and *Span.*

Trinitrophenol should be stored mixed with an equal weight of water; it must not be stored in glass-stoppered bottles.
Trinitrophenol burns readily and explodes when heated rapidly or when subjected to percussion. For safety in handling it is usually supplied mixed with not less than half its weight of water. It combines with metals to form salts, some of which are very explosive.

Adverse Effects
Dermatitis, skin eruptions, and severe itching may occur. Absorption through abraded skin or by ingestion has caused vomiting, pain, and diarrhoea, progressing to haemolysis, hepatitis, anuria, and convulsions. The metabolic-rate is increased, causing pyrexia.
In Great Britain the recommended exposure limits of trinitrophenol are 0.1 mg per m^3 (long-term); 0.3 mg per m^3 (short-term); suitable precautions should be taken to prevent absorption through the skin.

Uses and Administration
Trinitrophenol has disinfectant properties and was formerly used, mainly as a 1% aqueous solution, in the treatment of burns. Because of its toxic effects it is now rarely used in medicine.
In the *UK* the use of trinitrophenol in cosmetics is prohibited by law.

16330-b

Proprietary Preparations of Miscellaneous Cationic Surfactants

The main cationic surfactant disinfectant included in this section is cetrimide (p.953). However, there are a number of other cationic surfactant preparations used as disinfectants and the proprietary names of some of these are listed below.

Ambiteric D40 (*ABM Chemicals, UK*); Arquads (*Akzo, UK*); BTC (*Onyx Chemical Co., USA*); Contane (*Diversey, UK*); Deogen 3X (*Diversey, UK*); Dettol Endoscope Disinfectant (formerly known as Dettox ABC) (*Reckitt & Colman Pharmaceuticals, UK*); Dor (*Simpla, UK*); Emcol (*Witco, UK*); Ethoquads (*Akzo, UK*); Gloquat C (*ABM Chemicals, UK*); Hyamine 2389 (*Rohm & Haas, UK*); Morpan CHA (*ABM Chemicals, UK*); Resistone QD (*ABM Chemicals, UK*); Rewoquat B 41 (*Rewo, UK*); Rewoquat QA 100 (*Rewo, UK*); Task (*Brentchem, UK*); Tricidal (*Wingfield, UK*); Vantropol FHC (*ICI Organics, UK*).

Diuretics

2300-t

Diuretics promote the excretion of water and electrolytes by the kidneys. They are used in the treatment of patients with conditions such as congestive heart failure or hepatic, renal, or pulmonary disease when salt and water retention has resulted in oedema or ascites. The disease process in these conditions is not generally affected by the diuretic treatment.

Diuretics are also used, either alone, or in association with other antihypertensive agents, in the treatment of raised blood pressure (see p.466).

The principal groups of diuretics described in this section are:

1. Thiazides (benzothiadiazines), typified by chlorothiazide (p.981), and certain other compounds, often with structural similarities to the thiazides including: chlorthalidone, p.983, indapamide, p.993, mefruside, p.996, and metolazone, p.997. They inhibit sodium and chloride reabsorption in the kidney tubules and produce a corresponding increase in potassium excretion.
2. The "loop" or "high-ceiling" diuretics, which produce an intense, dose-dependent diuresis of relatively short duration. They include frusemide, p.987, bumetanide, p.980, and ethacrynic acid, p.986.
3. Potassium-sparing diuretics, which have a relatively weak diuretic effect and are normally used in conjunction with thiazide or loop diuretics, include amiloride, p.977, and triamterene, p.1003, and the aldosterone inhibitors such as spironolactone, p.1000.
4. Carbonic anhydrase inhibitors, including: acetazolamide, p.975, and dichlorphenamide, p.985. They are mainly used to reduce intra-ocular pressure in glaucoma.
5. Osmotic diuretics, such as mannitol (p.994) and urea (p.1005), which raise the osmolality of plasma and renal tubular fluid. They are used to reduce or prevent cerebral oedema and to reduce raised intra-ocular pressure.
6. Mercurial diuretics, typified by mersalyl (described under Mersalyl Acid, p.997), have largely been superseded by thiazide and loop diuretics.

The xanthines, (p.1521), are also used as diuretics and fructose (p.1264) is used as an osmotic diuretic.

A detailed review of the clinical pharmacology and therapeutic use of diuretics including discussion of the choice of diuretic in clinical practice.— A. Lant, *Drugs*, 1985, *29*, 57 and 162.

Further reviews and discussions on the use of diuretics: L. L. Francisco and T. F. Ferris, *Archs intern. Med.*, 1982, *142*, 28; D. Maclean and G. R. Tudhope, *Br. med. J.*, 1983, *286*, 1419.

A discussion of the factors affecting the choice of a diuretic including financial considerations. Bendrofluazide and frusemide were considered to be the thiazide and loop diuretics of choice respectively. Few patients were likely to need prophylaxis or treatment for hypokalaemia, and those who did should be given a potassium-sparing diuretic rather than potassium chloride.— L. E. Ramsay, *Prescribers' J.*, 1982, *22*, 49.

ADMINISTRATION. *In the elderly.* A discussion of the proper role of diuretics in the elderly.— *Br. med. J.*, 1978, *1*, 1092.

Comment on the safety of diuretics in the elderly.— W. J. MacLennan, *Br. med. J.*, 1988, *296*, 1551.

A double-blind placebo-controlled study was carried out on the effects of withdrawal of diuretic therapy from 106 elderly patients in whom its use was not deemed mandatory. During the following 12 weeks resumption of diuretic therapy was required in only 8 of the 54 patients receiving placebo. Overall, about 35% of the 141 patients initially considered for inclusion in the trial seemed to need the diuretic therapy they were receiving. These results indicated that many patients receive diuretics who do not need them. It was concluded that elderly people receiving long-term diuretic therapy without obvious current indication should have them withdrawn under careful supervision so that those who needed them can be identified.— M. L. Burr *et al.*, *Age & Ageing*, 1977, *6*, 38.

HEART FAILURE. A review of the treatment of heart failure. Despite the strong clinical impression that diuretics improve functional status in patients with heart failure, good evidence to either support or challenge this impression is not available. However, it was suggested that therapy with a diuretic was reasonable initial treatment for patients presenting with heart failure; digoxin and ACE-inhibitors could be added if diuretic therapy alone was ineffective.— G. H. Guyatt, *Drugs*, 1986, *32*, 538. See also I. Hutton and W. S. Hillis, *Br. J. Hosp. Med.*, 1986, *36*, 426.

HEPATIC DISORDERS. A review of the management of ascites in patients with liver disease. Spironolactone was generally the preferred diuretic: if diuresis was insufficient with spironolactone alone, the addition of a thiazide was indicated. A loop diuretic could be substituted for the thiazide in resistant cases but patients should be carefully monitored to ensure that diuresis was not too rapid. Rapid weight loss was considered acceptable when peripheral oedema was present but if ascites alone was present, weight loss should not exceed 1 kg per day.— E. Elias, *Prescribers' J.*, 1985, *25*, 26. See also J. S. Morris, *Br. med. J.*, 1984, *289*, 209; V. K. Rocco and A. J. Ware, *Ann. intern. Med.*, 1986, *105*, 573.

HYPERTENSION. A review of drugs used for the treatment of hypertension including diuretics. Thiazide diuretics are frequently used for the treatment of hypertension either alone or in conjunction with other antihypertensive agents. Loop diuretics may be useful in patients with fluid retention resistant to treatment with thiazides or in patients with impaired renal function. Potassium-sparing diuretics are used mainly with other diuretics to prevent or correct hypokalaemia.— *Med. Lett.*, 1987, *29*, 1.

Further references on the use of diuretics in hypertension: J. A. Whitworth and P. Kincaid-Smith, *Drugs*, 1982, *23*, 394; *Lancet*, 1982, *2*, 1316; J. H. Licht *et al.*, *Archs intern. Med.*, 1983, *143*, 1694; L. H. Opie, *Lancet*, 1984, *1*, 496.

For reference to the use of diuretics as part of the stepped-care approach to treating hypertension and general discussions on the treatment of hypertension, see Antihypertensives, p.466.

HYPERTENSION IN PREGNANCY. A discussion of the treatment of hypertension in pregnancy. Pre-eclampsia is a condition in which intravascular volume depletion occurs, and further depletion by diuretics may have a critical effect on the compromised uteroplacental blood flow. For this theoretical reason, diuretics are not generally used for controlling hypertension during pregnancy.— K. R. Lees and P. C. Rubin, *Br. med. J.*, 1987, *294*, 358. See also P. C. Rubin, *Prescribers' J.*, 1985, 25, 19; M. D. Lindheimer and A. I. Katz, *New Engl. J. Med.*, 1985, *313*, 675.

An overview of randomised studies of diuretics in pregnancy. Diuretics were found to have been effective in the treatment of pre-eclampsia, but this was to be expected since many studies included hypertension and oedema in their diagnostic criteria. The data on perinatal mortality suggested a reduction of roughly 10% in treated patients, but the incidence of perinatal mortality was small and much larger numbers of patients would be needed to confirm this result. However, there was no evidence of an increased risk of serious maternal or foetal side-effects due to diuretic therapy.— R. Collins *et al.*, *Br. med. J.*, 1985, *290*, 17. Comments that measures of outcome other than perinatal mortality would be more appropriate in assessing the success of treatment of pre-eclampsia: M. de Swiet and P. Fayers (letter), *ibid.*, 788; P. C. Rubin (letter), *ibid;* M. Ounsted and C. W. G. Redman (letter), *ibid.*, 1079.

For further references to the treatment of hypertension in pregnancy see under Antihypertensives, p.467.

LYMPHOSTATIC DISORDERS. Despite their widespread use, diuretics were considered to be ineffective in the management of lymphostatic disorders.— P. Mortimer and C. Regnard, *Br. med. J.*, 1986, *293*, 347.

MÉNIÈRE'S DISEASE. A review of the treatment of Ménière's disease including the use of diuretics. Thiazide diuretics have been shown to be effective in clinical studies. Although promising responses have also been reported with the loop diuretics, they are probably best avoided in view of their potential ototoxicity.— G. B. Brookes, *Drugs*, 1983, *25*, 77.

PREMENSTRUAL TENSION. A discussion of the premenstrual syndrome and its treatment. The effectiveness of drug treatment is difficult to evaluate. Results of studies have often given conflicting results but all agree that there is a very high placebo effect. Diuretics are frequently prescribed to relieve premenstrual bloating and symptoms attributed to fluid retention. Results of placebo-controlled studies support the use of diuretics only in cases where premenstrual weight gain can be demonstrated. Secondary hyperaldosteronism is a potential complication of long-term diuretic therapy, and treatment, if given, should be prescribed only during the symptomatic days and in the minimum effective dosage. Loop diuretics should be avoided. Spironolactone has the potential advantage that it does not cause secondary hyperaldosteronism.— C. P. West, *Prescribers' J.*, 1987, *27*, (Apr.), 9. See also H. Massil and P. M. S. O'Brien, *Br. med. J.*, 1986, *293*, 1289.

Adverse Effects and Precautions

There has been increasing concern about the known and suspected adverse effects of diuretics. Firstly, a high incidence of adverse effects has been shown by some, but not all, studies. Secondly, there was a possibility that diuretic-induced hypokalaemia, even when chronic and mild, could play a part in the genesis of ventricular arrhythmias and sudden death. Thirdly, despite the efficacy of thiazides in lowering blood pressure, there was no evidence that the risks of coronary artery disease were lessened in treated hypertensive patients and there was disquiet about adverse effects of diuretics on blood glucose, uric acid, and renin concentrations and on plasma lipids. There was some doubt as to whether diuretics would continue to be used as first-line treatment in hypertension.— J. G. Lewis, *Adverse Drug React. Bull.*, 1984, (Dec.), 404.

An analysis of data from the Multiple Risk Factor Intervention Trial and the Oslo Study in mild hypertension by Holme *et al.* (*J. Am. med. Ass.*, 1984, *251*, 1298) found a trend towards increased coronary heart disease mortality in patients with pre-existing ECG abnormalities taking diuretics. In a review of published reports, Kaplan (*Am. J. Nephrol.*, 1986, *6*, 1) also concluded that long-term treatment with diuretics could be hazardous. However, this conclusion was not supported by a number of large long-term studies in hypertension (Medical Research Council Working Party, *Br. med. J.*, 1985, *291*, 97; IPPPSH Collaborative Group, *J. Hypertension*, 1985, *3*, 379; J.D. Curb *et al.*, *J. Am. med. Ass.*, 1985, *253*, 3263; A. Amery *et al. Lancet*, 1985, *1*, 1349). Freis and Papademetriou (*Drugs*, 1985, *30*, 469) also concluded that the proposal that thiazide diuretics may increase cardiovascular risk was not supported by the data available.

Diuretics are one of the classes of drugs banned by the International Olympic Committee (IOC) for use by athletes in Olympic events. The Sports Council in the *UK* has issued guidelines based on IOC recommendations.— *Drug & Ther. Bull.*, 1987, *25*, 55.

EFFECTS ON THE ELECTROLYTE BALANCE. *Magnesium.* A discussion of the effects of diuretic therapy on the renal excretion of potassium and magnesium. Factors which affect potassium and magnesium depletion include the site and duration of action of the diuretic, the dose used, the duration of treatment, concomitant drug therapy, the underlying disease, and nutritional status. There was evidence to suggest that potassium and magnesium depletion may be related to an increased frequency of cardiac arrhythmias, especially in selected subgroups of patients. Electrolyte disturbances may have been responsible for some adverse effects found in large-scale multicentre studies of the treatment of hypertension; although the evidence linking diuretic administration to sudden death was circumstantial and inconclusive there was some cause for concern and diuretics should be administered at the lowest dosage necessary to achieve the desired antihypertensive effect. Potassium- and magnesium-sparing regimens should also be considered.— M. P. Ryan, *Am. J. Med.*, 1987, *82*, *Suppl.* 3A, 38.

The results of an open study by Dyckner and Wester (*Br. med. J.*, 1983, *286*, 1847) which indicated that magnesium supplementation in patients receiving long-term treatment with diuretics and a potassium supplement caused a further reduction in the blood pressure were not confirmed by Henderson *et al.* (*ibid.*, 1986, *293*, 664) in a double-blind randomised study in 41 hypertensive patients.

Potassium. The clinical consequences of diuretic-induced hypokalaemia remain controversial (L. Beeley, *Adverse Drug React. Bull.*, 1980, (Oct.), 304; F. Sandor *et al.*, *Br. med. J.*, 1982, *284*, 711; O.B. Holland, *Drugs*, 1984,

28, *Suppl.* 1, 86; N.M. Kaplan, *Am. J. Med.*, 1984, *77*, 1; B.J. Materson, *Archs intern. Med.*, 1985, *145*, 1966; N.M. Kaplan *et al.*, *New Engl. J. Med.*, 1985, *312*, 746; J.P. Kassirer and J.T. Harrington, *ibid.*, 785; M.J. Field and J.R. Lawrence, *Med. J. Aust.*, 1986, *144*, 641), although it is generally agreed that routine potassium supplementation in patients taking diuretics is unnecessary unless the serum-potassium concentration falls below 3.0 mmol per litre. However, potassium replacement is likely to be necessary in patients at risk from the cardiac effects of hypokalaemia (*Drug & Ther. Bull.*, 1985, *23*, 17) such as those with severe heart disease, those taking digitalis preparations or high doses of diuretics, and in patients with severe liver disease.

The amount of potassium in fixed combination diuretic and potassium preparations was considered to be insufficient to correct hypokalaemia (L. Beeley and S.P. Allison, *Br. J. Hosp. Med.*, 1984, *32*, 19), and the effectiveness of oral potassium supplements in increasing body stores of potassium has been questioned (P.R. Jackson *et al.*, *Br. J. clin. Pharmac.*, 1982, *14*, 257; G.M. Shenfield, *Drugs*, 1982, *23*, 462; V. Papademetriou *et al.*, *Archs intern. Med.*, 1985, *145*, 1986). Hypokalaemia may be overcome by adding a potassium-sparing diuretic to the regimen, but there is a danger of hyperkalaemia with indiscriminate use of these preparations (G.F.M. Whiting *et al.*, *Med. J. Aust.*, 1979, *1*, 409; L. Jaffey and A. Martin, *Lancet*, 1981, *1*, 1272). Potassium-sparing diuretics will not correct the potassium deficit unrelated to diuretic therapy in patients with severe heart failure (C. Davidson *et al.*, *Postgrad. med. J.*, 1978, *54*, 405).

Episodes of hypokalaemia occurred in 24 of 54 patients during treatment with a fixed-dose combination product containing amiloride 5 mg and hydrochlorothiazide 50 mg. The drop in plasma-potassium concentration usually occurred after 4 weeks of therapy, and most (74%) were seen during the first 12 months of therapy. Hyperkalaemia was found in 6 patients. The results demonstrate the necessity of monitoring plasma-potassium concentrations in patients on long-term diuretic therapy.— R. K. Penhall *et al.*, *Med. J. Aust.*, 1980, *1*, 376.

A correlation was seen between low serum-potassium concentrations and high counts of ventricular extrasystoles in patients treated with thiazide diuretics for mild to moderate hypertension, but there was no evidence of a simple causative relationship. The clinical significance of thiazide-induced ventricular extrasystoles was not clear.— Medical Research Council Working Party, *Br. med. J.*, 1983, *287*, 1249. Correction of diuretic-induced hypokalaemia with potassium chloride, triamterene, or both in 16 patients with uncomplicated hypertension did not significantly reduce the occurrence of spontaneous atrial or ventricular ectopic activity.— V. Papademetriou *et al.*, *Am. J. Cardiol.*, 1983, *52*, 1017.

In a crossover study in 16 hypertensive patients with diuretic-induced hypokalaemia, potassium (as potassium chloride) 24 to 96 mmol daily increased plasma-potassium concentrations to 3.5 mmol per litre or above in only 8 patients, and triamterene 50 to 200 mg daily increased potassium concentrations in 10 patients. Some patients who did not respond to potassium responded to triamterene and vice versa. Most of the administered potassium was excreted in the urine despite persisting hypokalaemia.— V. Papademetriou *et al.*, *Archs intern. Med.*, 1985, *145*, 1986.

Diuretics, primarily thiazides, remain the initial agents of choice in the treatment of hypertension in patients with chronic obstructive pulmonary disease (COPD), although calcium-channel blockers may provide an effective alternative. However, diuretic-induced hypokalaemia can be a particular problem in patients with COPD since hypokalaemia may exacerbate metabolic alkalosis and worsen hypoventilation in patients with chronic carbon dioxide retention. In addition, hypokalaemia may be potentiated by concurrent administration of corticosteroids or beta-agonists.— N. S. Hill, *Archs intern. Med.*, 1986, *146*, 129.

In an analysis of data from the Medical Research Council study of mild hypertension, potassium supplementation with potassium 16.8 or 33.6 mmol appeared to reduce the fall in serum-potassium concentration to some extent in patients taking bendrofluazide 5 or 10 mg respectively, but the change was not statistically significant. Potassium supplementation did not increase the antihypertensive effect of bendrofluazide.— Medical Research Council Working Party, *J. clin. Pharmac.*, 1987, *27*, 271.

The suggestion (B.R. Leslie, *Archs intern. Med.*, 1986, *146*, 1025; R. Whang, *ibid.*, 1026) that the failure of oral potassium chloride to correct diuretic-induced hypokalaemia could be explained by co-existent magnesium depletion was considered to be unlikely by Papademetriou (*ibid.*) in patients with uncomplicated hypertension on the basis of the available biochemical data.

Further references to diuretic-induced hypokalaemia and its prevention and treatment: J. G. Lewis, *Prescribers' J.*, 1982, *22*, 13; L. E. Ramsay *et al.*, *Br. J. clin. Pharmac.*, 1984, *17*, 605P; V. Papademetriou *et al.*, *Clin. Pharmac. Ther.*, 1984, *35*, 265; W. F. Stanaszek and J. A. Romankiewicz, *Drug Intell. & clin. Pharm.*, 1985, *19*, 176; J. R. E. Haalboom and A. Struyvenberg (letter), *New Engl. J. Med.*, 1985, *313*, 1021; T. G. Kelsey (letter), *ibid;* N. M. Kaplan (letter), *ibid;* R. D. Moore and G. D. Webb (letter), *ibid.*, 1022; J. P. Kassirer and J. T. Harrington (letter), *ibid;* P. Larochelle and A. G. Logan, *Can. med. Ass. J.*, 1985, *132*, 801; P. G. Cohen (letter), *ibid.*, *133*, 182; J. Lexchin (letter), *ibid.*, 183; A. G. Logan and P. Larochelle (letter), *ibid.*, 639.

Sodium. A review of reports of hyponatraemia associated with diuretic therapy published between 1966 and 1985. Hyponatraemia had been reported in 317 patients taking diuretics. The three diuretics most commonly associated with hyponatraemia were frusemide, 15.4%, amiloride plus hydrochlorothiazide, 13.6%, and hydrochlorothiazide alone, 13.6%. In 23.7% of patients the diuretic was not specified.— E. G. Walters *et al.*, *Br. J. clin. Pract.*, 1987, *41*, 841.

EFFECTS ON GLUCOSE TOLERANCE. A review of the effects of drugs including diuretics on glucose tolerance. Thiazide diuretics have been recognised as a cause of hyperglycaemia for many years, and it is now clear that all individuals taking thiazides for long periods may be at risk of developing hyperglycaemia, but the degree of risk depends on their pre-existing glucose tolerance. There is also evidence to suggest that concomitant administration of beta blockers can exacerbate the effect. It has been suggested that frusemide has an effect on glucose tolerance similar to that of the thiazide diuretics, but there is little evidence to support this.— R. Taylor, *Adverse Drug React. Bull.*, 1986, (Dec.), 452.

Glucose tolerance showed a progressive deterioration in 34 patients who had taken thiazide diuretics for 14 years. In 10 patients whose diuretic treatment was stopped an improvement in glucose tolerance was seen after 7 months.— M. B. Murphy *et al.*, *Lancet*, 1982, *2*, 1293.

A report of 12 cases of hyperosmolar non-ketotic diabetic syndrome. Treatment with diuretics was considered to have precipitated the syndrome in 9 of the patients. The syndrome is more common in elderly patients who should be monitored carefully during the first few months of diuretic therapy for the development of diabetes.— V. Fonseca and D. N. Phear, *Br. med. J.*, 1982, *284*, 36.

Results of a 12-year follow-up study on the association between the use of antihypertensive agents and the development of diabetes. A substantially increased risk of developing diabetes mellitus was observed for subjects with hypertension taking diuretics (895 women-years studied), those taking beta blockers (682 women-years), and those taking a combination of diuretics and beta blockers (281 women-years) compared with subjects not taking antihypertensive agents (13 855 control-years); those taking antihypertensive agents other than diuretics or beta blockers were too few to permit conclusions to be made. When the effects of diuretics and beta blockers were compared the relative risk was about the same.— C. Bengtsson *et al.*, *Br. med. J.*, 1984, *289*, 1495.

A double-blind study by the European Working Party on Hypertension in the Elderly in which 507 elderly hypertensive patients were followed up for 1 year, 371 for 2 years, and 270 for 3 years, indicated that those who received hydrochlorothiazide and triamterene (together with methyldopa if necessary) had impaired glucose tolerance compared with those who received placebo. The effects of diuretic therapy were established after one year and differences between treatment and placebo groups did not change further over the next 2 years. Overall there was an increase in fasting blood sugar of 5 mg per 100 mL in the active treatment group which occurred mainly in the first year. The hyperglycaemic effect of diuretics appeared to be related to potassium loss.— A. Amery *et al.*, *Postgrad. med. J.*, 1986, *62*, 919. See also A. Amery *et al.*, *Lancet*, 1978, *1*, 681.

EFFECTS ON LIPID METABOLISM. A review of the effect of diuretics on serum lipids and lipoproteins. Thiazide diuretics have been reported to increase blood-lipid and -lipoprotein concentrations in short-term studies, and there is evidence that frusemide produces a similar effect. There is little information about the effects of potassium-sparing diuretics. There is evidence to suggest that indapamide does not adversely affect blood lipids although raised blood lipids were found in one study. However, further comparative studies were considered necessary. In long-term studies total cholesterol has returned to baseline concentrations, suggesting that the hyperlipidaemic effect is transitory. However the long-term data were incomplete and convincing evidence of the long-term effects of diuretics on blood lipids was lacking.— R. P. Ames, *Drugs*, 1986, *32*, 260.

INTERACTIONS. *Non-steroidal anti-inflammatory drugs.* A review of the interaction between diuretics and non-steroidal anti-inflammatory drugs (NSAIDs). There have been a number of reports indicating that NSAIDs may antagonise the diuretic actions of loop and potassium-sparing diuretics and possibly also thiazides. The interaction is influenced by the age of the patient, the presence of renal disease and cardiac failure, and the dose, duration of treatment, and pharmacological profile of the drugs. Although there is evidence that indomethacin can alter the pharmacokinetics of frusemide, it is thought that inhibition of renal prostaglandin synthesis by NSAIDs has a greater bearing on the clinical interaction: inhibition of renal prostaglandin synthesis appears to inhibit activation of the renin-angiotensin-aldosterone system by all types of diuretic. The principal adverse clinical effect of the attenuated natriuretic response to diuretics by NSAIDs is worsening of cardiac failure. It is also possible that some NSAIDs may have deleterious effects on coronary perfusion. Clinicians should be aware of this important interaction and should exercise great care in the use of NSAIDs in patients with cardiac failure, especially if the failure is severe and associated with hyponatraemia, or if the patient is elderly and has renal impairment.

Indomethacin has also been shown to attenuate the antihypertensive effects of thiazides. Several actions of NSAIDs have been proposed as possible mechanisms for the interaction, including a possible pressor effect, fluid retention, and inhibition of renal and vasoactive prostaglandin synthesis. Sulindac, which has less effect on renal prostaglandin synthetase than indomethacin, does not inhibit the natriuretic response to frusemide and may enhance rather than attenuate the antihypertensive effect of thiazides. This suggests a major role for inhibition of renal prostaglandin synthesis in the attenuation of both diuretic and antihypertensive effects by non-selective NSAIDs, although there is other evidence which does not support the hypothesis for the effect on antihypertensive activity. Whatever the exact mechanism, the effect of NSAIDs is an important cause of inadequate blood pressure control in hypertensive patients. Patients in whom NSAIDs contribute to severe or refractory hypertension may be uncommon but are relatively easy to identify provided clinicians are aware of the possible interaction. More difficult to identify are the many patients whose blood-pressure control is marginally suboptimal but who may escape rigorous clinical audit. All hypertensive patients receiving NSAIDs should have their blood pressure monitored more frequently than usual.

It is increasingly recognised that NSAIDs produce a variety of toxic effects on the kidney. Patients receiving diuretic therapy may be at increased risk of NSAID-induced renal failure. Great care should be taken to avoid the combination of NSAIDs and diuretics in patients with renal disease, cirrhosis, or cardiac failure, as well as in elderly patients who usually have reduced renal function.— J. Webster, *Drugs*, 1985, *30*, 32.

Further reviews of the interaction between diuretics and NSAIDs: *Drug Interact. News.*, 1986, *6*, 27; *ibid.*, 1987, *7*, 7.

Other drugs. For reports of hyperkalaemia in patients receiving potassium-sparing diuretics or potassium supplements and ACE-inhibitors concurrently, see under Captopril (p.470).

For a discussion of the interaction between diuretics and lithium, see p.368.

For a discussion of the interaction between diuretics and anticoagulants, see p.346.

MISUSE. A discussion of bulimarexia and related eating disorders including the abuse of diuretics.— R. T. Harris, *Ann. intern. Med.*, 1983, *99*, 800.

PREGNANCY AND THE NEONATE. ***Breast feeding.*** A review of the excretion of antihypertensive agents including diuretics into human milk. The use of diuretics should probably be avoided during lactation. Although excessive amounts have not been reported in breast milk, a substantial decrease in milk volume may occur: thiazide diuretics have even been used to suppress lactation.— W. B. White, *Hypertension*, 1984, *6*, 297.

2301-x

Acetazolamide *(BAN, USAN, rINN).*

Acetazolam; Acetazolamidum. 5-Acetamido-1,3,4-thiadiazole-2-sulphonamide; *N*-(5-Sulphamoyl-1,3,4-thiadiazol-2-yl)acetamide.

$C_4H_6N_4O_3S_2$=222.2.

CAS — 59-66-5.

Pharmacopoeias. In *Br., Braz., Chin., Cz., Egypt., Eur., Fr., Hung., Ind., Int., It., Jpn, Jug., Nord., Roum., Swiss, Turk.,* and *U.S.*

A white to yellowish-white, odourless, crystalline powder.

Very slightly **soluble** in water; slightly soluble in alcohol and acetone; practically insoluble in carbon tetrachloride, chlorofom, and ether; dissolves in solutions of alkali hydroxides; sparingly soluble in practically boiling water.

2302-r

Acetazolamide Sodium *(USAN).*

Sodium Acetazolamide.

$C_4H_5N_4NaO_3S_2$=244.2.

CAS — 1424-27-7.

Pharmacopoeias. U.S. includes Sterile Acetazolamide Sodium.

Acetazolamide sodium 275 mg is approximately equivalent to 250 mg of acetazolamide. A freshly prepared 10% solution in water has a pH of 9 to 10.

Solutions of acetazolamide sodium in glucose 5% and sodium chloride 0.9% were stable for 5 days at 25° with a loss of potency of less than 7.2%. At 5° the loss of potency in both solutions was less than 6% after 44 days of storage. Small reductions in pH were recorded possibly due to the formation of acetic acid during the decomposition of acetazolamide. At −10° the loss in potency after 44 days of storage was less than 3% in both solutions. Results were similar in samples thawed in tap water and in a microwave oven.— J. Parasrampuria *et al., Am. J. Hosp. Pharm.,* 1987, *44,* 358.

Adverse Effects

Acetazolamide can commonly cause malaise, fatigue, depression, excitement, headache, weight loss, and gastro-intestinal disturbances. Drowsiness and paraesthesia involving numbness and tingling of the face and extremities are common particularly with high doses. Diuresis can be troublesome in patients being treated for glaucoma but generally abates after a few days of continuous therapy. Appreciable losses of potassium and sodium during prolonged therapy with acetazolamide may result in a tendency towards hypokalaemic acidosis. Severe metabolic acidosis has occasionally been reported, especially in elderly or diabetic patients or those with impaired renal function.

Blood dyscrasias occur rarely and may include aplastic anaemia, agranulocytosis, leucopenia, thrombocytopenia, and thrombocytopenic purpura. Acetazolamide therapy can give rise to crystalluria, renal calculi, and renal colic; renal lesions, possibly due to a hypersensitivity reaction, have also been reported. Other adverse reactions include allergic skin reactions, fever, thirst, dizziness, ataxia, transient myopia, tinnitus and hearing disturbances.

Intramuscular injections are painful owing to the alkalinity of the solution.

ALLERGY. A 54-year-old man with glaucoma who was treated with acetazolamide 500 mg daily for 26 days developed a generalised erythematous rash and became delirious, dehydrated, markedly jaundiced, with peripheral circulatory failure, and died from hepatic coma and anuria. Drug-induced hypersensitivity and hepatitis due to acetazolamide was suspected.— A. Kristinsson, *Br. J. Ophthal.,* 1967, *51,* 348.

EFFECTS ON THE BLOOD. *Agranulocytosis or aplastic anaemia.* Fatal bone-marrow depression, with anaemia, leucopenia, and thrombocytopenia, developed in a 66-year-old man after treatment with acetazolamide 500 mg twice daily for 3½ months.— G. W. Englund (letter), *J. Am. med. Ass.,* 1969, *210,* 2282.

Mention of 2 cases of fatal aplastic anaemia or agranulocytosis in one year probably due to acetazolamide.— W. H. W. Inman, *Br. med. J.,* 1977, *1,* 1500.

Severe aplastic anaemia in a 65-year-old woman was attributed to treatment with acetazolamide. The aplastic anaemia was treated successfully with antithymocyte immunoglobulin, oxymetholone, and corticosteroids.— B. I. Niven and A. Manoharan (letter), *Med. J. Aust.,* 1985, *142,* 120.

Thrombocytopenic purpura. Fatal thrombocytopenic purpura in a patient was associated with acetazolamide.— J. T. Corbett (letter), *Br. med. J.,* 1958, *1,* 1122.

EFFECTS ON THE ELECTROLYTE BALANCE. In a study of 27 elderly patients receiving acetazolamide for glaucoma, 4 patients had mild acidosis, 10 had moderate acidosis, and 1 had severe acidosis. Acidosis was not observed in 11 patients with glaucoma not receiving acetazolamide.— I. Heller *et al., Archs intern. Med.,* 1985, *145,* 1815.

Severe symptomatic metabolic acidosis was associated with acetazolamide therapy in a 93-year-old woman. A review of the published literature revealed 13 reports of severe metabolic acidosis induced by acetazolamide and references to a further 7 cases. Most severe cases of metabolic acidosis involved patients with renal disease or diabetes mellitus.— W. A. Parker and B. Atkinson, *Can. J. Hosp. Pharm.,* 1987, *40,* 31.

For further reports of severe metabolic acidosis associated with acetazolamide in patients with impaired renal function, see under Precautions, below.

EFFECTS ON ENDOCRINE FUNCTION. Hirsutism occurred in a 2½-year-old girl after treatment for 16 months with acetazolamide for congenital glaucoma. There was no evidence of virilisation.— I. S. Weiss, *Am. J. Ophthal.,* 1974, *78,* 327.

EFFECTS ON THE KIDNEYS. *Crystalluria.* Anuria preceded by backache and haematuria developed in 2 patients following short courses of acetazolamide. A high fluid intake was recommended for patients taking acetazolamide to reduce the risk of crystalluria.— T. Higenbottam *et al., Postgrad. med. J.,* 1978, *54,* 127.

Renal stones. A 21-year-old man with chronic glaucoma treated with acetazolamide 250 mg five times daily developed a calcium stone in the left ureter.— M. B. Pepys (letter), *Lancet,* 1970, *1,* 837.

EFFECTS ON THE LIVER. For a report of liver damage associated with acetazolamide administration, see Allergy (above).

EFFECTS ON MENTAL STATE. Apparent exacerbation of his chronic paranoid schizophrenia developed in a 69-year-old man given acetazolamide 250 mg three times daily for glaucoma. He returned to his previously adequate level of social behaviour on reduction of the dosage.— T. O. Rowe (letter), *Am. J. Psychiat.,* 1977, *134,* 587.

EFFECTS ON SEXUAL FUNCTION. A complex of malaise, fatigue, weight loss, anorexia, depression, and loss of libido occurred in 44 of 92 patients with chronic glaucoma during therapy with acetazolamide or methazolamide. These patients were found to be significantly more acidotic than those who did not experience such side-effects.— D. L. Epstein and W. M. Grant, *Archs Ophthal., N.Y.,* 1977, *95,* 1378.

Precautions

Acetazolamide is contra-indicated in the presence of sodium or potassium depletion, in idiopathic renal hyperchloraemic acidosis, in conditions such as Addison's disease and adrenal failure, and in marked hepatic or renal failure. It should not be used in chronic noncongested closed-angle glaucoma since it may mask deterioration of the condition. Its use is best avoided in the first trimester of pregnancy. It should be given with care to patients likely to develop acidosis or with diabetes mellitus; severe metabolic acidosis may occur in the elderly and in patients with impaired renal function.

By rendering the urine alkaline acetazolamide reduces the urinary excretion and so may enhance the effects of amphetamines, ephedrine, quinidine, quinine, and methadone, and reduces the effects of hexamine and its compounds. The diuretic effect of acetazolamide is diminished if ammonium chloride is taken concomitantly. Acetazolamide may enhance anticonvulsant-induced osteomalacia. Concurrent administration of acetazolamide and aspirin may result in severe acidosis.

For a contra-indication to the use of acetazolamide in the long-term management of chloridorrhoea, see Gastro-intestinal disorders under Uses.

Possible risks of cardiac arrhythmias during surgery in patients taking acetazolamide could be reduced by using positive pressure ventilation with muscle relaxation to prevent hypercapnia, and by correcting hypokalaemia pre-operatively.— R. Littlewood *et al.* (letter), *Med. J. Aust.,* 1984, *141,* 550.

ADMINISTRATION IN RENAL FAILURE. Acetazolamide has been reported to cause symptomatic metabolic acidosis in patients with mild renal failure (D.N. Maisey and R.D. Brown, *Br. med. J.,* 1981, *283,* 1527; M. Goodfield *et al., ibid.,* 1982, *284,* 422; W. Reid and A.D.B. Harrower, *ibid.,* 1114; see also under Adverse Effects, above). Many elderly patients have unrecognised mild renal failure, and these patients, and diabetic patients who are also susceptible to mild renal failure, should have urea and electrolyte concentrations measured before and during treatment with acetazolamide.

Large reductions in glomerular filtration-rate were observed during treatment with carbonic anhydrase inhibitors in 3 insulin-dependent diabetics with nephropathy and glaucoma. Kidney function improved when the carbonic anhydrase inhibitor was withdrawn.— P. Skøtt *et al., Br. med. J.,* 1987, *294,* 549.

INTERACTIONS. *Antacids.* The use of concurrent sodium bicarbonate therapy enhances the risk of calculus formation in patients taking acetazolamide.— M. A. Rubenstein and J. G. Bucy, *J. Urol., Baltimore,* 1975, *114,* 610.

Antiepileptics. For severe osteomalacia in patients taking acetazolamide with phenytoin and other antiepileptics, see Phenytoin, p.409.

For a suggestion that concurrent administration of acetazolamide impairs the absorption of primidone, see Primidone, p.412.

Aspirin. The acidosis caused by carbonic anhydrase inhibitors may increase the likelihood and severity of salicylate toxicity in patients taking salicylates, and conversely the acidosis caused by salicylates may increase the likelihood and severity of the acidotic syndrome complex in patients taking carbonic anhydrase inhibitors.— C. J. Anderson *et al., Am. J. Ophthal.,* 1978, *86,* 516.

A review of the interaction between acetazolamide and salicylate analgesics. Salicylate displaces acetazolamide from plasma protein binding sites and inhibits its renal excretion, whereas acetazolamide may enhance the penetration of salicylate into tissues by producing acidosis. Concurrent use of salicylates and acetazolamide should be avoided if possible, particularly if renal dysfunction is present. If the combination is used, patients should be carefully monitored for symptoms of central nervous system toxicity such as lethargy, confusion, somnolence, tinnitus, and anorexia.— *Drug Interact. News.,* 1987, *7,* 27.

Reports of severe metabolic acidosis in 2 patients with normal renal and hepatic function while taking salicylates (aloxiprin or salsalate) concomitantly with carbonic anhydrase inhibitors (dichlorphenamide or acetazolamide). R. A. Cowan *et al., Br. med. J.,* 1984, *289,* 347.

Further references: K. R. Sweeney *et al., Clin. Pharmac. Ther.,* 1986, *40,* 518.

Diuretics. For competition between acetazolamide and chlorthalidone for binding sites in blood cells, see Chlorthalidone, p.984.

Local anaesthetics. For the effect of acetazolamide on procaine, see Procaine Hydrochloride, p.1226.

INTERFERENCE WITH LABORATORY ESTIMATIONS. Reports of acetazolamide interfering with theophylline assays: I. K. Mecrow and B. P. Goldie (letter), *Lancet,* 1987, *1,* 558; H. C. Kelsey *et al.* (letter), *ibid.,* *2,* 403.

PREGNANCY AND THE NEONATE. A recommendation, based on results in *animals,* that carbonic anhydrase inhibitors should not be used in early pregnancy.— T. H. Maren, *Archs Ophthal., N.Y.,* 1971, *85,* 1.

Absorption and Fate

Acetazolamide is fairly rapidly absorbed from the gastro-intestinal tract with peak plasma concentrations occurring about 2 hours after administration by mouth. It has been estimated to have a plasma half-life of about 3 to 6 hours. It is tightly bound to carbonic anhydrase and high concentrations are present in tissues containing this enzyme, particularly red blood cells and the renal cortex; it is bound to plasma proteins. It is excreted unchanged in the urine.

The pharmacokinetics of acetazolamide in relation to its use in the treatment of glaucoma and its effects as an inhibitor of carbonic anhydrase.— B. Lehmann *et al.*, *Adv. Biosci.*, 1969, *5*, 197.

A single-dose study of acetazolamide in 4 elderly subjects indicating that the elderly have a reduced capacity to clear acetazolamide from plasma correlating with creatinine clearance; that they have reduced plasma protein binding which offsets the reduced unbound clearance; and that these factors predispose the elderly to enhanced accumulation of acetazolamide in erythrocytes. It was suggested that elderly patients may require reduced doses of acetazolamide.— D. J. Chapron *et al.*, *Br. J. clin. Pharmac.*, 1985, *19*, 363.

BIOAVAILABILITY. In 20 healthy subjects given acetazolamide 250 mg the mean peak plasma-acetazolamide concentration for 5 separate batches of tablets from a single manufacturer was 6.90, 8.55, 8.60, 11.28, and 11.44 μg per mL respectively. It was suggested that these results demonstrated bio-inequivalence.— G. J. Yakatan *et al.*, *J. pharm. Sci.*, 1978, *67*, 252.

A study comparing the bioavailability of acetazolamide from a sustained-release capsule and a conventional tablet following a single dose found that the extent of absorption from the capsule was less than half that from the tablet.— M. Ledger-Scott and J. Hurst, *Pharm. J.*, 1985, *2*, 451. The use of plasma concentrations rather than concentrations in whole blood was criticised. Using data from another study, calculations showed similar absorption of acetazolamide from tablets and controlled-release capsules.— R. G. Kelly (letter), *J. Pharm. Pharmac.*, 1986, *38*, 863.

PREGNANCY AND THE NEONATE. Following administration of acetazolamide 500 mg twice daily to a woman who was breast feeding, concentrations of acetazolamide in the breast milk were 1.3 to 2.1 μg per mL compared with maternal plasma concentrations of 5.2 to 6.4 μg per mL. Plasma concentrations of 0.2 to 0.6 μg per mL were found in the child 2 to 12 hours after breast feeding.— P. Söderman *et al.*, *Br. J. clin. Pharmac.*, 1984, *17*, 599.

RED CELL BINDING. Following administration of a single dose of acetazolamide 250 mg to 5 healthy subjects the range of peak plasma concentrations was 10 to 18 μg per mL over a period of 1 to 3 hours after dosage; this was about half those reported after a 500-mg dose. Red blood cell concentrations were higher and declined slowly; at 24 to 31 hours after dosage the ratio of red blood cell to plasma concentrations was greater than 4:1. Saliva concentrations were constant for each individual and were about 1% of those of plasma.— S. M. Wallace *et al.*, *J. pharm. Sci.*, 1977, *66*, 527.

Uses and Administration

Acetazolamide is an inhibitor of carbonic anhydrase. By inhibiting the reaction catalysed by carbonic anhydrase in the renal tubules, acetazolamide increases the excretion of bicarbonate and of cations, chiefly sodium and potassium, and so promotes an alkaline diuresis. Following oral administration, acetazolamide acts within 60 to 90 minutes and the effects last about 8 to 12 hours.

Continuous administration of acetazolamide is associated with metabolic acidosis and associated loss of diuretic activity. Therefore, although acetazolamide has been used as a diuretic, its effectiveness diminishes with continuous use and it has largely been superseded by agents such as the thiazides or frusemide. For diuresis the usual dose is 250 to 375 mg daily or on alternate days; intermittent therapy is required for a continued effect. A suggested dose for children is 5 mg per kg body-weight daily.

By inhibiting carbonic anhydrase in the eye acetazolamide decreases the formation of aqueous humour and so decreases intra-ocular pressure and is used in the pre-operative management of closed-angle glaucoma, or as an adjunct in the treatment of open-angle glaucoma. In the treatment of glaucoma the usual dose is 0.25 to 1 g daily, in divided doses for amounts over 250 mg daily.

Acetazolamide is also used, either alone or in association with other antiepileptics, for the treatment of various forms of epilepsy in doses of 0.25 to 1 g daily. A suggested dose for children for glaucoma or epilepsy is 8 to 30 mg per kg daily.

When oral administration is impracticable, similar doses of acetazolamide sodium may be given by intramuscular or preferably by intravenous injection.

Acetazolamide has also been used to prevent or ameliorate the symptoms of acute high-altitude (mountain) sickness when rapid ascent is necessary or in subjects who are particularly susceptible to altitude sickness despite gradual ascent. Acetazolamide shortens the time of acclimatisation but has little or no effect on established symptoms. Prompt descent will still be necessary if severe symptoms such as cerebral oedema or pulmonary oedema occur. For further details, see below.

When treatment is prolonged, or in susceptible patients, loss of potassium may be sufficient to produce hypokalaemia; potassium supplements should then be given as for Chlorothiazide (see p.983).

A detailed account of the chemistry, physiology, and inhibition of carbonic anhydrase.— T. H. Maren, *Physiol. Rev.*, 1967, *47*, 595–781.

A study of the effects of acetazolamide on renal and erythrocyte carbonic anhydrase. Acetazolamide 2.5 to 5 mg per kg body-weight intravenously effectively eliminates surplus water and bicarbonate in critically ill patients with metabolic alkalaemia. Concomitant transient inhibition of pulmonary carbon dioxide is small and of no clinical importance at this dose.— P. Berthelsen *et al.*, *Br. J. Anaesth.*, 1986, *58*, 512.

ADMINISTRATION AND POTASSIUM. In 16 patients with glaucoma who had taken acetazolamide and potassium supplements for more than 3 months serum-potassium concentrations remained in the normal range when potassium was withdrawn. Routine potassium supplementation is not indicated.— A. S. Critchlow *et al.*, *Br. med. J.*, 1984, *289*, 21.

ADMINISTRATION IN RENAL FAILURE. The interval between doses of acetazolamide should be extended from 6 hours to 12 hours in patients with a glomerular filtration-rate (GFR) of 10 to 50 mL per minute; it should be avoided in patients with a GFR of less than 10 mL per minute.— W. M. Bennett *et al.*, *Am. J. Kidney Dis.*, 1983, *3*, 155.

EPILEPSY. Acetazolamide was first used as an anticonvulsant in petit mal absences. It has been used in catamenial (menstrual) epilepsy because of its diuretic action. However, it is a poor diuretic but in practice may help to control a number of types of generalised epilepsy, especially myoclonic astatic epilepsy. It is essentially an adjuvant anticonvulsant.— P. M. Jeavons, *Practitioner*, 1977, *219*, 542.

Non-convulsive status epilepticus could be treated with intravenous diazepam, clonazepam, or acetazolamide.— *Lancet*, 1987, *1*, 958. Surprise at the recommendation of acetazolamide, whose usefulness is limited by the rapid development of tolerance and by adverse effects on prolonged use.— G. J. Hankey and E. G. Stewart-Wynne (letter), *ibid.*, 1427. Support for the use of acetazolamide as an antiepileptic agent, particularly in the management of petit mal (absence) seizures, in menstruation related seizures, and as an adjunct treatment in other refractory epilepsies of childhood. Acetazolamide has been shown to be as effective as ethosuximide and to have a lower incidence of side-effects. Acetazolamide toxicity was also considered mild compared with other antiepileptics. Acetazolamide is believed to have greater antiepileptic effectiveness in children than in adults, possibly due to differences in blood-brain barrier permeability.— J. G. Millichap (letter), *ibid.*, *2*, 163.

GASTRO-INTESTINAL DISORDERS. *Chloridorrhoea.* Administration of acetazolamide 125 mg every 8 hours to a 5-year-old child with congenital chloridorrhoea and metabolic alkalosis. Serum-bicarbonate concentrations were decreased but the underlying problem of chloride loss was exacerbated. Acetazolamide is therefore contra-indicated for the long-term management of this condition.— E. B. Clark and J. A. Vanderhoof, *J. Pediat.*, 1977, *91*, 148.

GLAUCOMA. Review of the treatment of glaucoma. Carbonic anhydrase inhibitors have an additive effect with miotics, timolol, adrenaline, and guanethidine.— R. A. Hitchings, *Prescribers' J.*, 1983, *23*, 106. See also: *Drug & Ther. Bull.*, 1983, *21*, 85.

In a short-term dose-response study completed by 9 patients with ocular hypertension, acetazolamide was given in single doses of 63, 125, 250, and 500 mg. Although plasma concentrations increased progressively with higher doses, the maximum fall in intra-ocular pressure exhibited a plateau effect with no difference between doses of 63 and 125 mg and very little average additional effect from 250 or 500 mg. A minor increase in the duration of response was observed with the 250-mg dose compared to lower doses, but 500 mg showed no further effect. A long-term study was now necessary.— B. R. Friedland *et al.*, *Archs Ophthal., N.Y.*, 1977, *95*, 1809.

A retrospective review of 222 patients with glaucoma indicating that those of 40 years or less tolerated treatment with carbonic anhydrase inhibitors much better than older patients.— C. E. Shrader *et al.*, *Am. J. Ophthal.*, 1983, *96*, 730.

MÉNIÈRE'S DISEASE. Acetazolamide 500 mg by intravenous injection might be useful diagnostically in patients with fluctuating Ménière's disease.— G. B. Brookes, *Drugs*, 1983, *25*, 77.

In a study of 14 patients with Ménière's disease (23 affected ears) treatment with acetazolamide 250 to 500 mg daily produced symptomatic improvement in only 4 patients (6 ears), which was only really significant in 2 patients. In 2 of the patients the improvement was not sustained, while another had to stop the drug due to the development of bilateral renal calculi. A deterioration in symptoms was seen in 3 cases. Significant adverse effects were encountered in 6 of 13 patients who had complied with dosage instructions. It was suggested that this high incidence of side-effects reflected a metabolic difference between patients with Ménière's disease and healthy subjects.— G. B. Brookes and J. B. Booth, *J. Lar. Otol.*, 1984, *98*, 1087.

MOUNTAIN SICKNESS. Symptoms of acute mountain sickness including headache, anorexia, nausea, insomnia, and lethargy often affect travellers to high altitudes and are most common above 10 000 feet (about 3000 metres): symptoms have been reported in over 50% of visitors to the Himalayas at 4243 metres, and were serious in 4%.

During acute exposure to high altitudes, hypoxia stimulates hyperventilation which leads to respiratory alkalosis. This alkalosis limits the ventilatory response to hypoxia. During acclimatisation, the bicarbonate concentration and the pH of extracellular fluid fall progressively. The falling pH increases the sensitivity of chemoreceptors to hypoxia and so permits greater ventilation, allowing acclimatisation. Acetazolamide accelerates the process of acclimatisation by causing bicarbonate diuresis and mild metabolic acidosis. Acetazolamide in doses of 250 mg to 1 g daily has been found to lower blood pH, improve blood gases, and improve symptom scores for acute mountain sickness. It produces striking improvements in sleep hypoxaemia and quality of sleep, reduces proteinuria, improves exercise performance, and reduces loss of muscle mass, probably by improving oxygen supplies to the tissues. It is not useful in treating established mountain sickness. The optimum dose and duration of treatment has yet to be established but 500 mg daily begun 24 to 72 hours before ascent has been suggested.

While the efficacy of acetazolamide in acute mountain sickness is not disputed, the desirability of its widespread use is still the subject of debate. It is generally agreed that gradual acclimatisation by slow ascent is preferable (A. Bradwell and J. Delamere, *Br. med. J.*, 1981, *283*, 1402; C. Clarke, *ibid.*, 1987, *294*, 1278; J.G. Dickinson, *ibid.*, *295*, 1161; *Drug & Ther. Bull.*, 1987, *25*, 45), but this is sometimes impractical due to constraints of time, for example in mountain rescue teams or in those engaged in mining or military operations. The use of acetazolamide on recreational visits to high altitudes was thought justifiable by Bradwell and Delamere and by the Drug & Therapeutics Bulletin, but Dickinson pointed out that severe and potentially fatal mountain sickness could still occur in those taking acetazolamide (A. Pines, *Lancet*, 1980, *2*, 807; M.K. Greene, *et al.*, *Br. med. J.*, 1981, *283*, 811; I. Wilson, *Postgrad. med. J.*, 1985, *61*, 472), and that freedom from minor symptoms could encourage people to go "too high too fast". It was suggested that prophylaxis with acetazolamide could be offered to those who make emergency ascents and those who have previously suffered acute mountain sickness at reasonable ascent rates. The use of acetazolamide does not obviate the need for prompt descent in severe forms of acute mountain sickness such as pulmonary or cerebral oedema.

Information sheets aimed at mountaineers and expedition doctors have been produced by the International Union of Alpinist Associations (IUAA) and are available in the *UK* from the Mountain Medicine Data Centre, St. Bartholomew's Hospital, 38 Little Britain, London EC1.

Further references to the use of acetazolamide in acute mountain sickness: P. H. Hackett *et al.*, *Lancet*, 1976, *2*, 1149; J. R. Sutton *et al.*, *New Engl. J. Med.*, 1979, *301*, 1329; Birmingham Medical Research Expeditionary Society Mountain Sickness Study Group, *Lancet*, 1981, *1*, 180; E. B. Larson *et al.*, *J. Am. med. Ass.*, 1982, *248*, 328; I. B. McIntosh and R. J. Prescott, *J. int. med. Res.*, 1986, *14*, 285; A. R. Bradwell *et al.*, *Lancet*, 1986, *1*, 1001.

A series of papers on the use of acetazolamide in acute mountain sickness from a symposium convened by the Birmingham Medical Research Expeditionary Society.— *Postgrad. med. J.*, 1987, *63*, 163-193.

MUSCULAR AND NEUROMUSCULAR DISORDERS. *Hypokalaemic periodic paralysis.* Acetazolamide 375 to 500 mg daily was an effective prophylactic agent in 2 patients with severe hypokalaemic periodic paralysis, and was well tolerated. Preliminary observations in 5 other patients given acetazolamide showed a striking improvement in 3.— J. S. Resnick *et al.*, *New Engl. J. Med.*, 1968, *278*, 582. In treating a further 12 patients, doses of 125 mg of acetazolamide were given three times daily to children and 250 mg two to six times daily to adults. There was dramatic improvement in 10 of the 12 and this lasted for up to 43 months. Chronic weakness between attacks in 10 patients was improved in 8.— R. C. Griggs *et al.*, *Ann. intern. Med.*, 1970, *73*, 39.

Paramyotonia congenita. Acetazolamide was tested on a patient with paramyotonia congenita, a condition marked by myotonia exacerbated by cold and exercise, and episodic weakness. Although acetazolamide had been used in the treatment of periodic paralysis, in this patient each administration of acetazolamide resulted in marked quadriparesis, although the myotonia was improved.— J. E. Riggs *et al.*, *Ann. intern. Med.*, 1977, *86*, 169.

RESPIRATORY DISORDERS. A review of the use of respiratory stimulants. Acetazolamide has been shown to produce chronic hyperventilation in healthy subjects. It has been used to improve hypoventilation in both acute and chronic metabolic alkalosis in patients with chronic obstructive pulmonary disease and decreases apnoeic awakenings and arousals in patients with central sleep apnoea. While acetazolamide appears to stimulate ventilation through its renal acid-base mechanism there is evidence that it might also have a direct but nonspecific effect on respiratory neurons.— B. M. Galko and A. S. Rebuck, *Drugs*, 1985, *30*, 475.

Studies in 8 patients with chronic obstructive lung disease who had chronic respiratory acidosis with superimposed metabolic alkalosis showed that correction of the alkalosis by the administration of acetazolamide, in 7 instances, or of ammonium chloride, in 3 instances, was followed by substantial improvement in clinical symptoms and in arterial oxygen pressures.— R. Bear *et al.*, *Can. med. Ass. J.*, 1977, *117*, 900.

Acetazolamide 500 mg by mouth induced bicarbonaturia and resulted in improved oxygenation in 2 patients with chronic obstructive pulmonary disease and congestive heart failure who had developed alkalosis following intravenous administration of frusemide 40 mg.— P. D. Miller and A. S. Berns, *J. Am. med. Ass.*, 1977, *238*, 2400.

Acetazolamide produced beneficial results in 6 patients with sleep apnoea, producing a 69% reduction in apnoeas after 1 week of therapy.— D. P. White *et al.*, *Archs intern. Med.*, 1982, *142*, 1816.

Preparations

Acetazolamide Tablets *(B.P.)*

Acetazolamide Tablets *(U.S.P.)*

Sterile Acetazolamide Sodium *(U.S.P.)*. A sterile powder suitable for parenteral use prepared from acetazolamide with the aid of sodium hydroxide. Potency is expressed in terms of the equivalent amount of acetazolamide.

Proprietary Preparations

Diamox *(Lederle, UK)*. *Tablets*, scored, acetazolamide 250 mg.

Sustets, sustained-release capsules, acetazolamide 500 mg.

Sodium Parenteral, injection, powder for reconstitution, acetazolamide 500 mg (as sodium salt).

Proprietary Names and Manufacturers

Acetamide *(Nessa, Spain)*; Atenezol *(Jpn)*; Défiltran *(Jouveinal, Fr.)*; Diamox *(Lederle, Austral.*; *Belg.*; *Lederle, Canad.*; *Lederle, Denm.*; *Théraplix, Fr.*; *Cyanamid-Novalis, Ger.*; *Cyanamid, Ital.*; *Neth.*; *Lederle, Norw.*; *Lederle, S.Afr.*; *Cyanamid, Spain*; *Lederle, Swed.*; *Lederle, Switz.*; *Lederle, UK*; *Lederle, USA)*; Didoc *(Jpn)*; Diuramid *(Pol.)*; Diuriwas *(IFI, Ital.)*; Edemox *(Wasserman, Spain)*; Glaucomide *(Austral.)*; Glauconox *(Spain)*; Glaupax *(Erco, Denm.*; *Dispersa, Ger.*; *Erco, Norw.*; *Erco, Swed.*; *Dispersa, Switz.)*; Inidrase *(Ital.)*; Oratrol *(Arg.)*.

12345-h

Althiazide *(USAN)*.

Altizide *(rINN)*; P-1779. 3-Allylthiomethyl-6-chloro-3,4-dihydro-2*H*-1,2,4-benzothiadiazine-7-sulphonamide 1,1-dioxide.

$C_{11}H_{14}ClN_3O_4S_3$=383.9.

CAS — 5588-16-9.

Althiazide is a thiazide diuretic (see p.981) that has been used in the treatment of hypertension.

References: D. Levitt, *Curr. med. Res. Opinion*, 1979, *6*, 136; E. N. Mngola, *J. int. med. Res.*, 1980, *8*, 199.

Proprietary Names and Manufacturers

Pfizer, USA.

2303-f

Ambuside *(BAN, USAN, rINN)*.

EX-4810; RMI-83047. 5-Allylsulphamoyl-2-chloro-4-(3-hydroxybut-2-enylideneamino)benzenesulphonamide; N^1-Allyl-4-chloro-6-(3-hydroxybut-2-enylideneamino)benzene-1,3-disulphonamide.

$C_{13}H_{16}ClN_3O_5S_2$=393.9.

CAS — 3754-19-6.

Ambuside is a diuretic which has certain structural similarities to the thiazides and has actions and uses similar to those of chlorothiazide (see p.983). It has been given in doses of 5 to 10 mg daily for hypertension and of up to 30 mg daily for oedema.

Proprietary Names and Manufacturers

Hydrion *(Robert et Carrière, Fr.)*;

Manufacturers also include—*Merrell Dow, USA.*

2304-d

Amiloride Hydrochloride *(BANM, USAN, rINNM)*.

Amipramizide; MK-870. *N*-Amidino-3,5-diamino-6-chloropyrazine-2-carboxamide hydrochloride dihydrate.

$C_6H_8ClN_7O,HCl,2H_2O$=302.1.

CAS — 2609-46-3 (amiloride); 2016-88-8 (hydrochloride, anhydrous); 17440-83-4 (hydrochloride, hydrous).

NOTE. Compounded preparations of amiloride hydrochloride and hydrochlorothiazide in the mass proportions of 1 part to 10 parts have the British Approved Name Co-amilozide.

Pharmacopoeias. In *Br.*, *Cz.*, *Egypt.*, *It.*, and *U.S.*

A yellow to yellowish-green, odourless or almost odourless powder. Slightly **soluble** in water and alcohol; practically insoluble in chloroform, ether, acetone, and ethyl acetate; freely soluble in dimethylsulphoxide; sparingly soluble in methyl alcohol. A 0.5% solution in water has a pH of 3.8 to 5.2. **Protect** from light.

Adverse Effects

Amiloride hydrochloride may cause nausea, vomiting, abdominal pain, diarrhoea or constipation, paraesthesia, thirst, dizziness, skin rash, pruritus, weakness, muscle cramps, and minor psychiatric or visual changes. Orthostatic hypotension and rises in blood-urea-nitrogen concentrations have been reported. Its potassium-sparing effect may lead to hyperkalaemia. Occasional abnormalities in liver-function tests have been reported.

EFFECTS ON THE ELECTROLYTE BALANCE. Metabolic acidosis was reported in 2 patients receiving total parenteral nutrition while taking either amiloride or triamterene. In both cases the acidosis resolved within a week of discontinuing the diuretic.— R. F. Kushner and M. D. Sitrin, *Archs intern. Med.*, 1986, *146*, 343.

For reports of severe hyponatraemia in patients taking amiloride with potassium-wasting diuretics, see Chlorothiazide, p.982 and Hydrochlorothiazide, p.992.

Potassium. Plasma-potassium concentrations rose above 5 mmol (5 mEq) per litre in 3 of 6 patients treated with amiloride. The plasma-potassium concentrations rose from 4.1 to 6.7 mmol (4.1 to 6.7 mEq) per litre after 3 days' treatment in a patient who received amiloride 40 mg daily, and a rise from 3.8 to 5.3 mmol (3.8 to 5.3 mEq) per litre followed 2 days' treatment with amiloride 10 mg daily in another patient. Treatment with amiloride increased the urinary sodium/potassium ratio.— I. Surveyor and R. A. Saunders (letter), *Lancet*, 1968, *2*, 516.

Precautions

Amiloride should not be given to patients with hyperkalaemia or progressive renal failure and should not be given with other potassium-sparing drugs or potassium supplements. Elderly patients, and patients with impaired renal function or diabetes mellitus are at particular risk of developing hyperkalaemia. It should be given with care to patients likely to develop acidosis, to patients with diabetes mellitus, and to those with impaired hepatic or renal function. Amiloride should be discontinued at least 3 days before glucose-tolerance tests are given to patients with diabetes mellitus because of the risks if patients are hyperkalaemic. Serum electrolytes and blood-urea-nitrogen should be estimated periodically.

INTERACTIONS. For the effects of amiloride on digoxin clearance, see under Digoxin (p.828).

For references on the antagonism of the action of potassium-sparing diuretics by non-steroidal anti-inflammatory drugs, see p.1.

Absorption and Fate

Amiloride is incompletely absorbed from the gastro-intestinal tract; bioavailability of about 50% is reported and is reduced by food. It is not bound to plasma proteins and has a half-life of 6 to 9 hours. It is excreted unchanged by the kidneys.

References to the pharmacokinetics of amiloride: P. Weiss *et al.*, *Clin. Pharmac. Ther.*, 1969, *10*, 401; E. Schmid and G. Fricke, *Pharmacol. Clin.*, 1969, *1*, 110; A. J. Smith and R. N. Smith, *Br. J. Pharmac.*, 1973, *48*, 646; J. E. Baer *et al.*, *J. Pharmac. exp. Ther.*, 1967, *157*, 472.

Uses and Administration

Amiloride is a mild diuretic which appears to act mainly on the distal renal tubules. It is described as potassium-sparing since, like spironolactone, it increases the excretion of sodium and chloride and reduces the excretion of potassium. Unlike spironolactone, however, it does not act by inhibiting aldosterone. Amiloride does not inhibit carbonic anhydrase. It takes effect about 2 hours after administration by mouth and its diuretic action has been reported to persist for about 24 hours. The full effect may be delayed until after several days of treatment.

Amiloride adds to the natriuretic but diminishes the kaliuretic effects of other diuretics, and is mainly used as an adjunct to the thiazides, frusemide, and similar diuretics, to conserve potassium and minimise the risk of alkalosis, in the treatment of refractory oedema associated with hepatic cirrhosis and congestive heart failure. It has also been used in combination with other diuretics in the treatment of hypertension. Amiloride hydrochloride is usually given in a dose of 5 to 10 mg daily which may be increased, if necessary, to a maximum of 20 mg daily. Once diuresis is established the dose should be reduced to a minimum effective level.

Compounded preparations of amiloride hydrochloride and hydrochlorothiazide in the mass proportions of 1 part to 10 parts have the British Approved Name Co-amilozide.

Potassium supplements should not be given.

Reviews of amiloride: *Med. Lett.*, 1981, *23*, 109.

A study of the metabolic effects of high-dose amiloride in healthy subjects.— J. A. Millar *et al.*, *Br. J. clin. Pharmac.*, 1984, *18*, 369.

Discussion of the actions of amiloride on the kidney.— J. E. Scoble *et al.*, *Lancet*, 1986, *2*, 326.

ADMINISTRATION IN RENAL FAILURE. In a study of amiloride in healthy subjects and patients with various degrees of renal failure, the natriuretic effect of amiloride was reduced in patients with creatinine clearance below 50 mL per minute. The terminal elimination half-life of amiloride was increased from 20 hours in healthy subjects to 100 hours in end-stage renal disease. The administration of amiloride in patients with severe renal impairment could aggravate potassium retention due to renal disease and amiloride should probably be avoided in patients with creatinine clearance of less than 50 mL per minute.— H. Knauf *et al.*, *Eur. J. clin. Pharmac.*, 1985, *28*, 61.

ADMINISTRATION WITH POTASSIUM-WASTING DIURETICS. Fixed dose combinations of a thiazide and a potassium-sparing diuretic did not significantly reduce the prevalence of hypokalaemia in 129 elderly patients compared with 68 patients taking a thiazide alone or with a potassium supplement. The co-amilozide combination was associated with a disproportionate number of cases of hyponatraemia. The desirability of the widespread use of fixed dose combination diuretics over less expensive single agents was questioned.— A. J. Bayer *et al.*, *Postgrad. med. J.*, 1986, *62*, 159.

In a study of 130 elderly hypertensive patients hypokalaemia occurred in 2 of 65 patients receiving co-amilozide compared with 10 of 65 receiving hydrochlorothiazide alone. Amiloride was well tolerated and maintained serum-potassium concentrations without causing hyperkalaemia.— M. G. Myers, *Archs intern. Med.*, 1987, *147*, 1026.

Further references on the potassium-sparing effects of amiloride used in combination with other diuretics: C. Venkata *et al.*, *J. clin. Pharmac.*, 1981, *21*, 484; U. G. Svendsen *et al.*, *Clin. Pharmac. Ther.*, 1983, *34*, 448; F. G. McMahon *et al.*, *Curr. ther. Res.*, 1983, *34*, 357.

For further references to the use of amiloride and other potassium-sparing diuretics to reduce hypokalaemia, and for comments on the use of potassium-sparing diuretics to prevent hypokalaemia during diuretic therapy, see p.973.

There was evidence to suggest that amiloride could prevent thiazide-induced magnesium losses (W.P. Leary *et al.*, *Curr. ther. Res.*, 1984, *35*, 293) but had no effect on magnesium excretion when given alone (*idem*, 1983, *34*, 205) in healthy subjects. A study of 66 patients with congestive heart failure treated with frusemide indicated that plasma-magnesium concentrations were raised by the addition of amiloride but not by spironolactone nor potassium supplements.— P. J. Robinson *et al.*, *Br. J. clin. Pharmac.*, 1984, *18*, 268P. Co-amilozide spared potassium and magnesium relatively more effectively than frusemide 40 mg with triamterene 50 mg and produced a longer and smoother diuresis.— A. Kohvakka and E. Hussi, *J. int. med. Res.*, 1986, *14*, 188.

HEPATIC DISORDERS. References on the use of amiloride and other potassium-sparing diuretics in ascites due to hepatic cirrhois: B. Senewiratne and S. Sherlock, *Lancet*, 1968, *1*, 120; S. Yamada and T. B. Reynolds, *Gastroenterology*, 1970, *59*, 833; P. Vesin, *Postgrad. med. J.*, 1975, *51*, 545; *Br. med. J.*, 1978, *1*, 66.

HYPERALDOSTERONISM. Amiloride therapy corrected hypokalaemia and ameliorated hypertension in a study of 12 patients with primary hyperaldosteronism.— G. T. Griffing *et al.*, *Clin. Pharmac. Ther.*, 1982, *31*, 56.

Amiloride increased plasma-potassium concentrations and plasma-aldosterone concentrations in patients with both primary hyperaldosteronism and Bartter's syndrome. Plasma renin activity was increased in primary hyperaldosteronism and decreased in Bartter's syndrome.— G. Griffing *et al.*, *J. clin. Pharmac.*, 1982, *22*, 505.

HYPERTENSION. The blood pressure of 10 hypertensive patients was reduced by the administration of amiloride 10 mg twice daily but the effect was less than that of hydrochlorothiazide 50 mg twice daily.— E. A. Gombos *et al.*, *New Engl. J. Med.*, 1966, *275*, 1215.

Amiloride, alone or in conjunction with hydrochlorothiazide, had little effect on blood pressure in 17 patients with hypertension.— H. Kampffmeyer and J. Conway, *Clin. Pharmac. Ther.*, 1968, *9*, 350.

A double-blind, multicentre study to compare the hypotensive effects of amiloride, hydrochlorothiazide, and co-amilozide in 179 patients with mild to moderate hypertension. Diastolic reductions were similar with all three treatments, but the systolic reductions were consistently greater with co-amilozide than with the two drugs separately. Hypokalaemia occurred in 14 of 62 patients receiving hydrochlorothiazide, in 1 of 57 patients receiving co-amilozide, and in none of 60 patients receiving amiloride. Transient elevations in plasma-potassium concentrations occurred in 6 patients receiving amiloride, in 1 patient receiving co-amilozide, and in 1 patient receiving hydrochlorothiazide.— Multicenter Diuretic Cooperative Study Group, *Archs intern. Med.*, 1981, *141*, 482.

Amiloride (mean dose 10 mg) with metoprolol (mean dose 125 mg) or hydrochlorothiazide (mean dose 15.6 mg) with metoprolol (mean dose 125 mg) were both effective in controlling hypertension in a study of 40 previously untreated hypertensive patients. In 38 previously treated patients the use of amiloride was associated with fewer biochemical abnormalities than thiazides.— J. P. Thomas and W. H. Thomson, *Br. med. J.*, 1983, *286*, 2015. Criticism of the study on the grounds of the doses used, concomitant administration of metoprolol, and the number of patients involved, and comment on the greater cost of amiloride compared with thiazides.— L. E. Ramsay (letter), *ibid.*, *287*, 614. Reply.— J. P. Thomas and W. H. Thomson (letter), *ibid.*

For further references to the use of amiloride with hydrochlorothiazide, see Hydrochlorothiazide, p.992.

LITHIUM-INDUCED POLYURIA. For references on the use of amiloride in patients with polyuria associated with long-term lithium therapy, see p.367.

RENAL DISORDERS. Results indicating that amiloride 5 mg daily, or hydrochlorothiazide 50 mg daily or both could correct an inherited cellular defect in oxalate transport thought to be a factor in calcium oxalate kidney stone formation.— B. Baggio *et al.*, *New Engl. J. Med.*, 1986, *314*, 599.

Preparations

Amiloride Tablets *(B.P.).* Amiloride Hydrochloride Tablets

Amiloride Hydrochloride Tablets *(U.S.P.)*

Amiloride Hydrochloride and Hydrochlorothiazide Tablets *(U.S.P.)*

Proprietary Preparations

Midamor *(Morson, UK). Tablets,* amiloride hydrochloride equivalent to anhydrous amiloride hydrochloride 5 mg.

Proprietary Names and Manufacturers

Arumil *(Merck Sharp & Dohme, Ger.)*; Midamor *(Merck Sharp & Dohme, Austral.; Merck Sharp & Dohme, Canad.; Neth.; Merck Sharp & Dohme, Norw.; S.Afr.; MSD, Swed.; Merck Sharp & Dohme, Switz.; Morson, UK; Merck Sharp & Dohme, USA)*; Modamide *(Merck Sharp & Dohme-Chibret, Fr.)*; Nirulid *(Merck Sharp & Dohme, Denm.)*; Pandiuren *(Arg.)*.

The following names have been used for multi-ingredient preparations containing amiloride hydrochloride— Amilco *(Norton, UK)*; Amizide *(Protea, Austral.)*; Frumil *(Rorer, UK)*; Hypertane *(Sanol Schwarz, UK)*; Kalten *(Stuart, UK)*; Lasoride *(Hoechst, UK)*; Moducren *(Morson, UK)*; Moduret *(Merck Sharp & Dohme, Canad.; Morson, UK)*; Moduretic *(Merck Sharp & Dohme, Austral.; Merck Sharp & Dohme, UK; Merck Sharp & Dohme, USA)*; Normetic *(Abbott, UK)*; Synuretic *(DDSA Pharmaceuticals, UK)*.

2305-n

Aminometradine *(BAN, rINN).*

Aminometramide. 1-Allyl-6-amino-3-ethylpyrimidine-2,4(1*H*,3*H*)-dione.

$C_9H_{13}N_3O_2$=195.2.

CAS — 642-44-4.

Aminometradine is a relatively weak diuretic which has been used to control oedema in patients with mild congestive heart failure.

12414-f

Azolimine *(USAN, rINN).*

CL-90748. 2-Imino-3-methyl-1-phenylimidazolidin-4-one.

$C_{10}H_{11}N_3O$=189.2.

CAS — 40828-45-3.

Azolimine is a potassium-sparing diuretic.

Pharmacology in *animals*.— R. Z. Gussin *et al.*, *J. Pharmac. exp. Ther.*, 1975, *195*, 8.

Proprietary Names and Manufacturers

Lederle, USA.

12415-d

Azosemide *(USAN, rINN).*

BM-02001; Ple-1053. 2-Chloro-5-(1*H*-tetrazol-5-yl)-4-(2-thenylamino)benzenesulphonamide.

$C_{12}H_{11}ClN_6O_2S_2$=370.8.

CAS — 27589-33-9.

Azosemide is a diuretic with actions similar to those of frusemide.

A brief review of the clinical pharmacokinetics of azosemide.— B. Beermann and M. Grind, *Clin. Pharmacokinet.*, 1987, *13*, 255.

Further references to azosemide: F. Krück *et al.*, *Eur. J. clin. Pharmac.*, 1978, *14*, 153; D. C. Brater, *Clin. Pharmac. Ther.*, 1979, *25*, 428; D. C. Brater *et al.*, *ibid.*, 435; C. Brater *et al.*, *ibid.*, 1979, *26*, 437; R. Seiwell and C. Brater, *ibid.*, 1980, *27*, 285; K. Horky *et al.*, *Eur. J. Pharmac.*, 1981, *69*, 439.

Proprietary Names and Manufacturers

Luret *(Boehringer Mannheim, Ger.)*.

12423-d

Bemetizide *(BAN, rINN).*

Diu-60. 6-Chloro-3,4-dihydro-3-(α-methylbenzyl)-2*H*-1,2,4-benzothiadiazine-7-sulphonamide 1,1-dioxide.

$C_{15}H_{16}ClN_3O_4S_2$=401.9.

CAS — 1824-52-8.

Bemetizide is a thiazide diuretic which has been used with triamterene in the treatment of hypertension in a usual dose of 25 mg daily or on alternate days.

Interaction of bemetizide and indomethacin in the kidney.— R. Düsing *et al.*, *Br. J. clin. Pharmac.*, 1983, *16*, 377.

Study of bemetizide with triamterene in patients with chronic liver disease and ascites.— I. R. Crossley *et al.*, *Clin. Trials J.*, 1983, *20*, 197.

References to the use of bemetizide in combination with triamterene in the treatment of hypertension: R. Hornung *et al.*, *Curr. med. Res. Opinion*, 1983, *8*, 425; R. Wray *et al.*, *ibid.*, 665.

Proprietary Names and Manufacturers

The following names have been used for multi-ingredient preparations containing bemetizide— Diucomb *(Melusin, Ger.)*; Tensigradyl *(Oberval, Fr.)*.

2306-h

Bendrofluazide *(BAN).*

Bendrofluaz.; Bendroflumethiazide *(USAN, rINN)*; Bendroflumethiazidum; Benzydroflumethiazide; FT-81. 3-Benzyl-3,4-dihydro-6-trifluoromethyl-2*H*-1,2,4-benzothiadiazine-7-sulphonamide 1,1-dioxide.

$C_{15}H_{14}F_3N_3O_4S_2$=421.4.

CAS — 73-48-3.

Pharmacopoeias. In *Br., Braz., Chin., Egypt., Eur., Fr., Ind., Int., It., Neth., Swiss,* and *U.S.* Also in *B.P. Vet.*

A white or cream-coloured, odourless or almost odourless, crystalline powder.

Practically **insoluble** in water; soluble 1 in 17 to 1 in 23 of alcohol, 1 in 1.5 of acetone, and 1 in 200 of ether; practically insoluble in chloroform. **Store** in airtight containers.

Adverse Effects, Treatment, and Precautions

As for Chlorothiazide, p.981.

Torsade de pointes occurred in a patient with a prolonged QT interval while taking bendrofluazide and diethylpropion. Diuretic-induced hypokalaemia was considered to be a contributory factor.— J. C. O'Keefe *et al.*, *Postgrad. med. J.*, 1985, *61*, 419.

OVERDOSAGE. Grand mal convulsions occurred in a previously healthy 14-year-old girl following ingestion of bendrofluazide 150 to 200 mg. The convulsions were not associated with any measurable disturbance of serum electrolytes.— K. R. Hine *et al.* (letter), *Lancet*, 1982, *1*, 564.

PORPHYRIA. Bendrofluazide was considered to be unsafe in patients with acute porphyria because it has been shown to be porphyrinogenic in *animals* or *in vitro* systems.— M.R. Moore and K.E.L. McColl, *Porphyrias, Drug Lists*, Glasgow, Porphyria Research Unit, University of Glasgow, 1987.

Absorption and Fate

Unlike chlorothiazide, bendrofluazide has been reported to be completely absorbed from the gastro-intestinal tract, and there are indications that it is fairly extensively metabolised; about 30% is excreted unchanged in the urine.

Following a dose of bendrofluazide 10 mg by mouth to 4 healthy subjects peak plasma concentrations ranged from 56 to 107 ng per mL at 2 to 2.5 hours after administration. The plasma half-life averaged 2.7 hours.— B. Beermann *et al.*, *Eur. J. clin. Pharmac.*, 1976, *10*, 293. A chronic placebo-controlled study in 8 hypertensive subjects. The plasma half-life averaged about 4 hours.— B. Beermann *et al.*, *ibid.*, 1978, *13*, 119.

A study of the pharmacokinetics of bendrofluazide in 9 healthy subjects. The mean half-life was 3 hours. About 30% of the dose was recovered in the urine within 48 hours, over 90% of this in the first 12 hours, but most of the drug was eliminated through non-renal mechanisms.— B. Beermann *et al.*, *Clin. Pharmac. Ther.*, 1977, *22*, 385.

Uses and Administration

Bendrofluazide is a thiazide diuretic with actions and uses similar to those of chlorothiazide (see p.983). Diuresis is initiated in about 2 hours and lasts for 12 to 18 hours or longer. In the treatment of oedema the usual initial dose is 5 to 10 mg daily or on alternate days; in some cases initial doses of up to 20 mg may be necessary. Maintenance doses have ranged from 2.5 to 10 mg taken daily or intermittently. In the treatment of hypertension the usual dose is 2.5 to 5 mg daily, either alone, or in conjunction with other antihypertensive agents; some sources have recommended initial doses of up to 20 mg daily.

A suggested initial dose for children is up to 400 µg per kg body-weight daily, reduced to 50 to 100 µg per kg for maintenance.

When treatment is prolonged, or in susceptible patients, loss of potassium may be sufficient to produce hypokalaemia; potassium supplements or a potassium-sparing diuretic should then be given as for chlorothiazide.

Bendrofluazide has also been used to suppress lactation.

HYPERKALAEMIA, FAMILIAL. Successful treatment of familial hyperkalaemia in a 9-year-old girl with bendrofluazide 2.5 mg twice daily. It is considered probable that she would eventually have developed significant hypertension and it is hoped to prevent this with long-term bendrofluazide therapy.— M. R. Lee and D. B. Morgan (letter), *Lancet*, 1980, *1*, 879.

HYPERTENSION. Results of a 6-year follow-up of previously untreated middle-aged men with mild to moderately severe essential hypertension. Bendrofluazide 2.5 to 5 mg daily or propranolol 80 to 160 mg daily produced similar reductions in blood pressure.— G. Berglund and O. Andersson, *Lancet*, 1981, *1*, 744.

Results of the Medical Research Council study of treatment of mild hypertension showed that treatment with either bendrofluazide or propranolol was associated with a reduction in the rate of strokes. Neither treatment had a clear advantage over the other, although bendrofluazide appeared somewhat better at preventing stroke, while propranolol may have prevented coronary events in non-smokers.— Medical Research Council Working Party, *Br. med. J.*, 1985, *291*, 97. See also p.806.

A study of the treatment of hypertension in 884 elderly patients found that active treatment reduced the rate of all strokes to 58% of that in the control group, and reduced the rate of fatal strokes to 30% of that in the control group. The principal antihypertensive agents were bendrofluazide and atenolol: 60% of patients treated took bendrofluazide and 70% took atenolol; 7% were on bendrofluazide alone. The incidence of myocardial infarction and total mortality was unaffected by treatment.— J. Coope and T. S. Warrender, *Br. med. J.*, 1986, *293*, 1145.

Further references to the use of bendrofluazide in hypertension: R. G. Wilcox and J. R. A. Mitchell, *Br. med. J.*, 1977, *2*, 547; D. A. van Staden *et al.*, *Curr. ther. Res.*, 1983, *34*, 620; A. C. Head, *Pharmatherapeutica*, 1984, *3*, 650; G. Berglund *et al.*, *Acta med. scand.*, 1986, *220*, 419; B. T. Marsh *et al.*, *J. int. med. Res.*, 1987, *15*, 106; R. L. Agrawal, *Br. J. clin. Pract.*, 1987, *41*, 916; A. C. Head *et al.*, *Curr. ther. Res.*, 1987, *10*, 562; P. F. Crowe *et al.*, *Br. J. clin. Pract.*, 1987, *41*, 967.

OSTEOPOROSIS. The use of bendrofluazide in regimens using ergocalciferol, dihydrotachysterol, and glucocorticoids to treat osteoporosis.— J. R. Condon *et al.*, *Postgrad. med. J.*, 1978, *54*, 249.

URINARY-TRACT DISORDERS. Beneficial response to prophylactic bendrofluazide for encrustation of bladder catheters.— I. Nielsen and P. Thorn, *Curr. ther. Res.*, 1986, *40*, 107.

Preparations

Bendrofluazide Tablets *(B.P.)*

Bendroflumethiazide Tablets *(U.S.P.)*. Tablets containing bendrofluazide.

Proprietary Preparations

Aprinox *(Boots, UK)*. *Tablets*, bendrofluazide 2.5 and 5 mg.

Berkozide *(Berk Pharmaceuticals, UK)*. *Tablets*, bendrofluazide 2.5 mg. *Tablets*, scored, bendrofluazide 5 mg.

Centyl *(Leo, UK)*. *Tablets*, bendrofluazide 2.5 mg. *Tablets*, scored, bendrofluazide 5 mg.

Centyl K *(Leo, UK)*. *Tablets*, bendrofluazide 2.5 mg, potassium chloride 573 mg (potassium 7.7 mmol) for sustained release.

Neo-NaClex *(Duncan, Flockhart, UK)*. *Tablets*, scored, bendrofluazide 5 mg.

Neo-NaClex-K *(Duncan, Flockhart, UK)*. *Tablets*, bendrofluazide 2.5 mg, potassium chloride 630 mg (potassium 8.4 mmol) for sustained release.

Owing to the risk of intestinal obstruction, sustained-release preparations such as Centyl K and Neo-NaClex-K, where the drug is released in transit, but the matrix ghost is often eliminated intact, should not be prescribed in patients with Crohn's disease or other intestinal disease in which strictures may form.— J. L. Shaffer *et al.* (letter), *Lancet*, 1980, *2*, 487.

Proprietary Names and Manufacturers

Aprinox *(Boots, Austral.; Boots, UK)*; Aprinox-M *(Austral.)*; Benuron *(Bristol-Myers Products, USA)*; Benzide *(Protea, Austral.)*; Berkozide *(Berk Pharmaceuticals, UK)*; Bristuron *(Bristol-Myers Products, USA)*; Centyl *(Leo, Denm.; Norw.; Lövens, Swed.; Leo, UK)*; Esberizid *(Schaper & Brümmer, Ger.)*; Naturetin *(Squibb, Canad.; Princeton, USA)*; Naturine *(Leo, Fr.)*; Neo-NaClex *(Austral.; Duncan, Flockhart, UK)*; Notens *(Farge, Ital.)*; Pluryl *(Austral.; Belg.; Neth.)*; Polidiuril *(Ital.)*; Salural *(Ital.)*; Salures *(Ferrosan, Swed.)*; Sinesalin *(ICI, Ger.; ICI, Switz.)*; Sodiuretic *(Squibb, Ital.)*; Tesical *(Arg.)*; Urinagen *(Arg.)*; Urizide *(DDSA Pharmaceuticals, UK)*.

The following names have been used for multi-ingredient preparations containing bendrofluazide— Abicol *(Boots, UK)*; Centyl K *(Leo, UK)*; Corgaretic *(Squibb, UK)*; Corzide *(Princeton, USA)*; Inderetic *(ICI Pharmaceuticals, UK)*; Inderex *(ICI Pharmaceuticals, UK)*; Naturetin-K *(Squibb, Canad.)*; Neo-NaClex-K *(Duncan, Flockhart, UK)*; Prestim *(Leo, UK)*; Prestim Forte *(Leo, UK)*; Rautractyl *(Squibb, Canad.)*; Rautrax-N *(Squibb, USA)*; Rauzide *(Princeton, USA)*; Tenavoid *(Leo, UK)*; Tensanyl *(Leo, UK)*.

2307-m

Benzthiazide *(BAN, USAN, rINN)*.

P-1393. 3-Benzylthiomethyl-6-chloro-2*H*-1,2,4-benzothiadiazine-7-sulphonamide 1,1-dioxide.

$C_{15}H_{14}ClN_3O_4S_3$=431.9.

CAS — 91-33-8.

Pharmacopoeias. In *U.S.*

A white crystalline powder with a characteristic odour. Practically **insoluble** in water and chloroform; slightly soluble in acetone; soluble 1 in 480 of alcohol; freely soluble in dimethylformamide and in solutions of alkali hydroxides; very slightly soluble or practically insoluble in ether. **Store** in airtight containers.

Benzthiazide is a thiazide diuretic with properties similar to those of chlorothiazide (see p.981). Diuresis is initiated in about 2 hours and lasts for about 12 hours. The initial dose in the treatment of oedema is 50 to 200 mg daily, followed by a maintenance dose of 25 to 150 mg daily. In the treatment of hypertension, the usual dose is 25 to 50 mg daily, either alone or in conjunction with other antihypertensive agents. Doses of up to 200 mg daily have been recommended. A suggested initial dose in children is 1 to 4 mg per kg body-weight daily in divided doses.

When treatment is prolonged, or in susceptible patients, loss of potassium may be sufficient to produce hypokalaemia; potassium supplements or a potassium-sparing diuretic should then be given as for chlorothiazide.

Preparations

Benzthiazide Tablets *(U.S.P.)*

Proprietary Preparations

Dytide *(Bridge, UK)*. *Capsules*, benzthiazide 25 mg, triamterene 50 mg.

Proprietary Names and Manufacturers

Aquatag *(Reid-Provident, USA)*; Diurin *(SCS, S.Afr.)*; Exna *(Robins, Canad.; Robins, USA)*; Fovane *(Pfizer, Belg.)*; Hydrex *(Trimen, USA)*; NaClex *(Robins, USA)*; Proaqua *(Reid-Provident, USA)*.

The following names have been used for multi-ingredient preparations containing benzthiazide— Decaserpyl Plus *(Roussel, UK)*; Dytide *(Bridge, UK)*.

2308-b

Benzylhydrochlorothiazide

Su-6227. 3-Benzyl-6-chloro-3,4-dihydro-2*H*-1,2,4-benzothiadiazine-7-sulphonamide 1,1-dioxide.

$C_{14}H_{14}ClN_3O_4S_2$=387.9.

CAS — 1824-50-6.

Benzylhydrochlorothiazide is a thiazide diuretic with properties similar to those of chlorothiazide (see p.981). It has been given in initial doses of 4 to 8 mg twice daily.

Proprietary Names and Manufacturers

3 BT *(Jpn)*; Behyd *(Jpn)*.

2309-v

Boldo

Boldo Leaves; Peumus.

CAS — 8022-81-9 (boldo leaf oil); 476-70-0 (boldine); 1398-22-7 (boldoglucin).

Pharmacopoeias. In *Arg.*, *Belg.*, *Cz.*, *Egypt.*, *Fr.*, *It.*, *Port.*, *Roum.*, *Span.*, and *Swiss.*

The dried leaves of *Peumus boldus* (Monimiaceae). It contains the alkaloid boldine (about 0.1%), the glycoside boldin or boldoglucin, and about 2% of volatile oil.

Boldo has been employed as a diuretic in the form of a tincture (1 in 10; in doses of 0.5 to 2 mL). It has also been used in herbal medicine in the treatment of gall-stones.

Proprietary Names and Manufacturers

The following names have been used for multi-ingredient preparations containing boldo— Bilogene *(Bio-Chemical Laboratory, Canad.)*; Boldolaxine *(Simes, Austral.)*; Hepax *(Sabex, Canad.)*; Opobyl *(Bengué, UK)*.

2310-r

Bumetanide *(BAN, USAN, rINN).*

Ro-10-6338. 3-Butylamino-4-phenoxy-5-sulphamoylbenzoic acid.

$C_{17}H_{20}N_2O_5S=364.4$.

CAS — 28395-03-1.

Pharmacopoeias. In *It.* and *U.S.*

An almost white powder. Slightly **soluble** in water; soluble in alkaline solutions. **Store** in airtight containers. Protect from light.

INCOMPATIBILITY. Bumetanide should not be added to infusion fluids with an acid reaction because of the risk of sedimentation.— R. N. Brogden *et al., Drugs,* 1975, *9,* 4.

Precipitation was noted when bumetanide injection was mixed with dobutamine injection.— G. R. Hasegawa and J. F. Eder, *Am. J. Hosp. Pharm.,* 1984, *41,* 949.

Adverse Effects

As for Frusemide, p.987. Bumetanide may cause muscle pain, particularly at high doses.

The 17 reports of adverse reactions to bumetanide received by the Committee on Safety of Medicines were: skin and muscle reactions (10), including 6 reports of muscular pain, thrombocytopenia (3), granulocytopenia or leucopenia (2), nausea and dizziness (1), and gynaecomastia (1). Two reactions proved fatal.— M. F. Cuthbert, *Committee on Safety of Medicines, Postgrad. med. J.,* 1975, *51, Suppl.* 6, 51.

A review of bumetanide. Adverse effects of bumetanide are similar to those of frusemide. Studies in *animals* have shown that bumetanide is less ototoxic than frusemide in equivalent diuretic doses, and there is evidence to suggest that this is also the case in humans. Bumetanide was associated with a higher incidence of hypochloraemia and hypokalaemia, and a lower incidence of hyperglycaemia than frusemide. Some controversy exists over the effects of bumetanide on carbohydrate metabolism.— A. Ward and R. C. Heel, *Drugs,* 1984, *28,* 426. See also I. H. Tuzel, *J. clin. Pharmac.,* 1981, *21,* 615.

EFFECTS ON THE EARS. Three patients with hearing loss associated with frusemide were able to tolerate bumetanide.— E. Bourke (letter), *Lancet,* 1976, *1,* 917.

EFFECTS ON THE MUSCLES. Mention of curious muscle stiffness, with tenderness to compression and pain on movement, in association with bumetanide therapy. The calf muscles were the first to be affected; shoulder girdle and thigh muscle tenderness also occurred in 2 patients, and one patient also had neck stiffness. The side-effect appeared to be dose-related for the individual patients.— J. E. Barclay and H. A. Lee, *Postgrad. med. J.,* 1975, *51, Suppl.* 6, 43.

EFFECTS ON THE PANCREAS. Increased serum-α-amylase values were observed in 4 of 11 patients with renal impairment and receiving bumetanide. In 3 of the patients the effect was dose-related. The cause was unknown; one possibility was a subclinical pancreatitis with some extrahepatic cholestasis.— F. Lynggaard and N. Bjørndal (letter), *Lancet,* 1977, *2,* 1355.

EFFECTS ON THE SKIN. *Erythema multiforme.* A skin reaction of the Stevens-Johnson type occurred in a patient with cirrhosis of the liver given bumetanide for 212 days.— H. Ring-Larsen, *Acta med. scand.,* 1974, *195,* 411.

Precautions

As for Chlorothiazide, p.982, Bumetanide may enhance the nephrotoxicity of cephalosporin antibiotics such as cephalothin and of the aminoglycoside antibiotics. Although the risk of ototoxicity may be less than with frusemide, bumetanide may enhance the ototoxic effects of aminoglycoside antibiotics in patients with renal impairment.

INTERACTIONS. For references to the lack of interaction between warfarin and bumetanide, see p.346.

Absorption and Fate

Bumetanide is almost completely and fairly rapidly absorbed from the gastro-intestinal tract; the bioavailability is reported to be about 95%. It has a plasma elimination half-life of about 1 to 1½ hours. It is about 95% bound to plasma proteins. About 80% of the dose is excreted in the urine, 50% as unchanged drug, and 10 to 20% in the faeces.

The pharmacokinetics of bumetanide in grossly oedematous patients was similar to that in non-oedematous subjects.— G. R. Bailie *et al., Clin. Pharmacokinet.,* 1987, *12,* 440.

References to the absorption and fate of bumetanide: S. C. Halladay *et al., Clin. Pharmac. Ther.,* 1977, *22,* 179; P. J. Pentikäinen *et al., Br. J. clin. Pharmac.,* 1977, *4,* 39; A. A. Holazo *et al., J. pharm. Sci.,* 1984, *73,* 1108.

Uses and Administration

Although chemically unrelated, bumetanide is a loop diuretic with actions and uses similar to those of frusemide (see p.989). Diuresis is initiated within about 30 minutes to an hour after a dose by mouth, and lasts for about 4 hours but may be prolonged to 6 hours after high doses; after intravenous injection its effects are evident within a few minutes and last for about 2 hours. As a general guide bumetanide 1 mg produces a diuretic effect similar to frusemide 40 mg.

In the treatment of oedema the usual initial dose is 0.5 to 2 mg by mouth in the morning or early evening; a second dose may be given 6 to 8 hours later if necessary. Most patients respond to doses of up to 10 mg, but higher doses may be needed in patients with severe renal or cardiac disease. In emergency or when oral therapy cannot be given 0.5 to 1 mg may be administered by intramuscular or intravenous injection, subsequently adjusted according to the patient's response. Intravenous injections should be given slowly over 1 to 2 minutes. A recommended dose for pulmonary oedema is 1 to 2 mg by intravenous injection, repeated 20 minutes later if necessary. Alternatively, 2 to 5 mg may be given over 30 to 60 minutes in 500 mL of a suitable infusion fluid (but see above under Incompatibility).

When treatment is prolonged, or in susceptible patients, loss of potassium may be sufficient to produce hypokalaemia; potassium supplements or potassium-sparing diuretics should then be given as for chlorothiazide (see p.983). When very high doses are used careful laboratory control is essential as described under the uses for frusemide (p.989; high-dose therapy).

Reviews and symposium reports on the actions, uses, and pharmacokinetics of bumetanide: *Drug & Ther. Bull.,* 1974, *12,* 49; *J. clin. Pharmac.,* 1981, *21,* 529–712; *Med. Lett.,* 1983, *25,* 61; A. Ward and R. C. Heel, *Drugs,* 1984, *28,* 426; C. E. Halstenson and G. R. Matzke, *Drug Intell. & clin. Pharm.,* 1983, *17,* 786.

References to the actions of bumetanide: M. J. Asbury *et al., Br. med. J.,* 1972, *1,* 211; R. A. Branch *et al., Clin. Pharmac. Ther.,* 1976, *19,* 538; S. Carrière and R. Dandavino, *Clin. Pharmac. Ther.,* 1976, *20,* 424; G. D. Johnston *et al., Br. J. clin. Pharmac.,* 1986, *21,* 359.

ADMINISTRATION. In 10 patients there was significantly increased diuresis and sodium excretion, but not potassium excretion, when their stabilised doses of bumetanide were taken in 2 divided doses at 8 am and 6 pm compared with a single stabilised dose taken in the morning.— K. R. Hunter and P. N. Underwood, *Postgrad. med. J.,* 1975, *51, Suppl.* 6, 91.

Studies have indicated that the rate of diuresis due to bumetanide is reduced and its onset delayed if given after food.— M. Homeida *et al., Br. J. clin. Pharmac.,* 1976, *3,* 969P.

Report of a synergistic response to bumetanide and metolazone given concurrently to healthy subjects.— D. C. Brater *et al., J. Pharmac. exp. Ther.,* 1985, *233,* 70. No synergistic effect was seen when bumetanide and metolazone were given concurrently to healthy subjects.— A. Greenberg *et al., J. clin. Pharmac.,* 1985, *25,* 369.

ADMINISTRATION IN RENAL FAILURE. Pharmacodynamic response to bumetanide and bumetanide excretion rate were reduced in a study of 6 patients with chronic renal failure. In 8 patients with chronic hepatic disease, diuretic response to bumetanide was impaired but bumetanide excretion rates were normal.— L. A. Marcantonio *et al., Br. J. clin. Pharmac.,* 1983, *15,* 245.

The bioavailability of bumetanide following a 5-mg dose was 66% in healthy subjects and 69% in patients with renal failure. The cumulative pharmacodynamic effects of oral and intravenous doses were essentially similar in both groups.— H. S. H. Lau *et al., Clin. Pharmac. Ther.,* 1986, *39,* 635.

CARDIAC DISORDERS. *Heart failure.* In 12 infants with heart failure a single oral dose of bumetanide 15 µg per kg body-weight produced significant diuresis and sodium excretion. In a long-term study in 13 similar infants, bumetanide, which was given with a potassium supplement, was considered to be an effective diuretic; doses ranged from 15 µg per kg on alternate days to 100 µg per kg daily. No significant side-effects occurred.— O. C. Ward and L. K. T. Lam, *Archs Dis. Childh.,* 1977, *52,* 877.

Bumetanide 1 mg was as effective as frusemide 40 mg in a study of 30 patients with congestive heart failure.— S. Sagar *et al., Int. J. clin. Pharmac. Ther. Toxic.,* 1984, *22,* 473.

HEPATIC DISORDERS. Bumetanide 0.5 to 4 mg daily appeared to be a satisfactory diuretic in the treatment of ascites in 15 of 17 patients with chronic liver disease.— P. J. A. Moult, *Gut,* 1974, *15,* 988.

Further references to the use of bumetanide in liver disease: R. F. Maronde and M. Quinn, *Clin. Pharmac. Ther.,* 1977, *21,* 110.

HYPERTENSION. No evidence of hypokalaemia was found in 12 mildly hypertensive patients given bumetanide 500 µg twice daily for a 6-month period, 6 of whom also received potassium supplements. Bumetanide did not have a sustained antihypertensive effect, it caused hyperuricaemia, and minor abnormalities of liver function were noted.— L. E. Murchison *et al., Br. J. clin. Pharmac.,* 1975, *2,* 87.

Preparations

Bumetanide Tablets *(U.S.P.)*

Proprietary Preparations

Burinex *(Leo, UK). Tablets,* scored, bumetanide 1 and 5 mg.

Liquid, bumetanide 1 mg/5 mL.

Injection, bumetanide 0.5 mg/mL, in ampoules of 2, 4, and 10mL.

Burinex K *(Leo, UK). Tablets,* bumetanide 500 µg, potassium chloride 573 mg (potassium 7.7 mmol) for sustained release.

Owing to the risk of intestinal obstruction, sustained-release preparations such as Burinex K, where the drug is released in transit, but the matrix ghost is often eliminated intact, should not be prescribed in patients with Crohn's disease or other intestinal disease in which strictures may form.— J. L. Shaffer *et al.* (letter), *Lancet,* 1980, *2,* 487.

Ulceration and perforation of a Meckel's diverticulum was attributed to administration of Burinex K in a 65-year-old patient.— G. T. Layer *et al., Postgrad. med. J.,* 1987, *63,* 211.

Proprietary Names and Manufacturers

Aquazone *(Prodes, Spain)*; Bonures *(Swed.)*; Bumex *(Roche, USA)*; Burinex *(Astra, Austral.; Belg.; Leo, Denm.; Leo, Fr.; Sigmatau, Ital.; Neth.; Leo, Norw.; Leo, S.Afr.; Lövens, Swed.; Leo Suede, Switz.; Leo, UK)*; Butinat *(Arg.; Mabo, Spain)*; Cambiex *(Arg.)*; Diurama *(Chiesi, Ital.)*; Farmadiuril *(Alter, Spain)*; Fontego *(Polifarma, Ital.)*; Fordiuran *(Thomae, Ger.; Boehringer Ingelheim, Spain)*; Lunetoron *(Jpn)*; Segurex *(Arg.)*.

2311-f

Buthiazide *(USAN).*

Butizide *(rINN)*; Thiabutazide. 6-Chloro-3,4-dihydro-3-isobutyl-2*H*-1,2,4-benzothiadiazine-7-sulphonamide 1,1-dioxide.

$C_{11}H_{16}ClN_3O_4S_2=353.8$.

CAS — 2043-38-1.

Pharmacopoeias. In *Roum.*

Buthiazide is a thiazide diuretic with properties similar to those of chlorothiazide (see p.981). It has been given in doses of 5 to 15 mg daily or on 2 or 3 days weekly for the treatment of oedema. It has also been given in doses of 5 to 10 mg daily for hypertension.

References: A. G. Dupont *et al., Curr. ther. Res.,* 1986, *40,* 990.

Proprietary Names and Manufacturers

Eunéphran *(Servier, Fr.)*; Saltucin *(Boehringer Mannheim, Ger.)*.

Manufacturers also include—*Searle, USA.*

2312-d

Canrenone *(USAN, pINN).*

Aldadiene; RP-11614; SC-9376. 3-Oxo-17α-pregna-4,6-diene-21,17β-carbolactone.

$C_{22}H_{28}O_3$=340.5.

CAS — 976-71-6.

STABILITY. For a study of the stability of canrenone and factors affecting its conversion to canrenoate potassium, see E. R. Garrett and C. M. Won, *J. pharm. Sci.*, 1971, *60*, 1801.

2313-n

Canrenoate Potassium *(BANM, USAN).*

Aldadiene Potassium; MF-465a; Potassium Canrenoate *(rINN)*; SC-14266. Potassium 17β-hydroxy-3-oxo-17α-pregna-4,6-diene-21-carboxylate.

$C_{22}H_{29}KO_4$=396.6.

CAS — 4138-96-9 (canrenoic acid); 2181-04-6 (canrenoate potassium).

Adverse Effects, Treatment, and Precautions

As for Spironolactone, p.1000. Irritation or pain may occur at the site of injection.

EFFECTS ON ENDOCRINE FUNCTION. Spironolactone-induced gynaecomastia in a 51-year old patient disappeared when treatment with canrenoate potassium was substituted.— A. Dupont (letter), *Lancet*, 1985, *2*, 731.

Gynaecomastia occurred in 16 of 30 patients taking canrenoate potassium and in all of 14 men treated with spironolactone for 6 months. It was suggested that canrenoate potassium may carry a reduced risk of gynaecomastia compared with spironolactone.— G. Bellati and G. Idéo (letter), *Lancet*, 1986, *1*, 626.

EFFECTS ON THE HEART. A report of a cardiac arrhythmia apparently associated with intravenous canrenoate potassium administration in one patient.— W. J. Mroczek *et al.*, *Clin. Pharmac. Ther.*, 1974, *16*, 336.

INTERACTIONS. *Fludrocortisone.* In 12 healthy subjects who were receiving fludrocortisone, single doses of canrenoate potassium 100, 150, or 200 mg caused a paradoxical dose-related increase in urinary potassium excretion 12 to 16 hours after administration; this was possibly related to increased urine volume. Similar results were obtained with spironolactone, but the dose-effect relationship was not clear.— L. E. Ramsay *et al.*, *Eur. J. clin. Pharmac.*, 1977, *11*, 101.

Uses and Administration

Canrenone has actions and uses similar to those of spironolactone (see p.1001) of which it is a metabolite. It has been given in doses of 50 to 200 mg daily or on alternate days, in one to three divided doses; up to 300 mg daily has been given.

Canrenoate potassium is a soluble form of canrenone suitable for parenteral administration. It may be given in doses of 200 to 400 mg daily, increasing to 800 mg daily in exceptional cases, by slow intravenous injection over a period of 2 to 3 minutes per 200 mg or by intravenous infusion in glucose 5% or sodium chloride 0.9%.

ANABOLISM. A study indicating improved nitrogen balance in patients receiving canrenoate potassium 600 to 800 mg daily in addition to total parenteral nutrition during the first 5 post-operative days following abdominal surgery. The effect was particularly marked in elderly subjects.— P. Guinot and Y. Metivier, *Clin. Ther.*, 1977, *1*, 56.

CARDIAC DISORDERS. An improvement in left ventricular function was reported following injection of a single dose of canrenoate potassium 400 mg into the right atrium of 13 patients with heart failure. The effect of canrenoate potassium was considered to be independent of its diuretic action.— O. De Divitiis *et al.*, *Curr. ther. Res.*, 1984, *35*, 40.

Beneficial response to canrenoate potassium given concurrently with digoxin and theophylline in 10 patients with chronic cor pulmonale.— L. Rufolo *et al.*, *Curr. ther. Res.*, 1985, *37*, 148

HEPATIC DISORDERS. In 12 patients with liver cirrhosis canrenoate potassium 200 mg intravenously significantly reduced the excretion of magnesium for up to 48 hours after the dose.— P. Lim and E. Jacob, *Br. med. J.*, 1978, *1*, 755.

Proprietary Preparations

Spiroctan-M *(MCP Pharmaceuticals, UK). Injection,* canrenoate potassium 20 mg/mL, in ampoules of 10 mL.

Proprietary Names and Manufacturers of Canrenone and Canrenoate Potassium

Aldactone *(Boehringer Mannheim, Ger.)*; Kanrenol *(SPA, Ital.)*; Luvion *(Simes, Ital.)*; Osiren *(Switz.)*; Osirenol *(Denm.; Hoechst, Norw.)*; Osyrol *(Hoechst, Ger.)*; Phanurane *(Théraplix, Fr.)*; Sincomen pro injectione *(Ger.)*; Soldactone *(Belg.; Searle, Denm.; Ital.; Neth.; Searle, Norw.; Searle, S.Afr.; Searle, Swed.; Searle, Switz.)*; Soludactone *(Searle, Fr.)*; Spiroctan *(Boehringer Mannheim, Switz.)*; Spiroctan-M *(MCP Pharmaceuticals, UK)*; Venactone (Lepetit, Ital.).

2314-h

Chlorazanil Hydrochloride *(rINNM).*

ASA-226. *N*-(4-Chlorophenyl)-1,3,5-triazine-2,4-diamine hydrochloride.

$C_9H_8ClN_5,HCl$=258.1.

CAS — 500-42-5 (chlorazanil); 2019-25-2 (hydrochloride).

Chlorazanil hydrochloride is a diuretic that has been given in usual doses of 150 mg. It is contra-indicated in patients with hepatic coma, hypokalaemia, or renal insufficiency with anuria.

Proprietary Names and Manufacturers

Daquin *(Riker, USA)*; Orpidan *(Heumann, Ger.)*.

2315-m

Chlormerodrin *(BAN, rINN).*

Chlormeroprin; Mercurylurée; Promeranum. (3-Chloromercuri-2-methoxypropyl)urea; Chloro(2-methoxy-3-ureidopropyl)mercury.

$C_5H_{11}ClHgN_2O_2$=367.2.

CAS — 62-37-3.

Pharmacopoeias. In *Rus.*

Chlormerodrin is a mercurial diuretic with actions and uses similar to those of mersalyl acid (see p.997), but which is suitable for oral administration.

Proprietary Names and Manufacturers

Mercloran *(Parke, Davis, USA)*; Neohydrin *(Merrell Dow, USA)*; Orimercur *(Reder, Spain)*.

2316-b

Chlorothiazide *(BAN, USAN, rINN).*

Chlorothiazidum; Clorotiazida. 6-Chloro-2*H*-1,2,4-benzothiadiazine-7-sulphonamide 1,1-dioxide.

$C_7H_6ClN_3O_4S_2$=295.7.

CAS — 58-94-6.

Pharmacopoeias. In *Arg., Br., Braz., Egypt., Eur., Fr., Int., It., Neth., Nord., Port., Swiss, Turk.,* and *U.S.*

A white or almost white, odourless, crystalline powder.

B.P. **solubilities** are: very slightly soluble in water; slightly soluble in alcohol; sparingly soluble in acetone; soluble in solutions of alkali hydroxides. *U.S.P.* solubilities are: very slightly soluble in water; freely soluble in dimethylformamide and dimethyl sulphoxide; slightly soluble in methyl alcohol and pyridine; practically insoluble in ether and chloroform. Alkaline solutions undergo decomposition, due to hydrolysis, upon standing or heating.

2317-v

Chlorothiazide Sodium *(USAN).*

Sodium Chlorothiazide.

$C_7H_5ClN_3NaO_4S_2$=317.7.

CAS — 7085-44-1.

Chlorothiazide sodium 537 mg is approximately equivalent to 500 mg of chlorothiazide.

INCOMPATIBILITY. There was loss of clarity when intravenous solutions of chlorothiazide sodium were mixed with those of insulin, some opioid analgesics, noradrenaline acid tartrate, procaine hydrochloride, prochlorperazine maleate, promazine hydrochloride, promethazine hydrochloride, streptomycin sulphate, tetracycline hydrochloride, or vancomycin hydrochloride.— J. A. Patel and G. L. Phillips, *Am. J. Hosp. Pharm.*, 1966, *23*, 409.

An immediate precipitate occurred when chlorothiazide 2 g per litre was mixed with chlorpromazine hydrochloride 200 mg per litre, promazine hydrochloride 200 mg per litre, or promethazine hydrochloride 100 mg per litre, and a yellow colour with a precipitate developed over 3 hours when chlorothiazide was mixed with hydralazine hydrochloride 80 mg per litre in glucose injection or sodium chloride injection. A yellow colour was produced when chlorothiazide was mixed with polymyxin B sulphate 2 mega units per litre in glucose injection. A haze developed over 3 hours when the drug was mixed with prochlorperazine mesylate 100 mg per litre in sodium chloride injection, but an immediate precipitate was formed when they were mixed in glucose injection.— B. B. Riley, *J. Hosp. Pharm.*, 1970, *28*, 228.

Chlorothiazide sodium was incompatible with amikacin sulphate.— B. C. Nunning and A. P. Granatek, *Curr. ther. Res.*, 1976, *20*, 417.

Adverse Effects

Chlorothiazide and other thiazide diuretics may cause a number of metabolic disturbances. They may provoke hyperglycaemia and glycosuria in diabetic and other susceptible patients. They may cause hyperuricaemia and precipitate attacks of gout in some patients. Administration of thiazide diuretics may be associated with electrolyte imbalances including hypochloraemic alkalosis, hyponatraemia, and hypokalaemia. Hypokalaemia intensifies the effect of digitalis on cardiac muscle and administration of digitalis or its glycosides may have to be temporarily suspended. Patients with severe coronary artery disease and cirrhosis of the liver are particularly at risk from hypokalaemia. Hyponatraemia may occur in patients with severe congestive heart failure who are very oedematous, particularly with large doses in conjunction with restricted salt in the diet. The urinary excretion of calcium is reduced. Hypomagnesaemia has also occurred. There is some evidence to suggest that electrolyte imbalances during long-term treatment with thiazides may be associated with an increased incidence of cardiac arrhythmias. Adverse changes in plasma lipids have also been noted but their clinical significance is unclear.

Signs of electrolyte imbalance include dry mouth, thirst, weakness, lethargy, drowsiness, restlessness, muscle pain and cramps, and gastro-intestinal disturbances.

Other side-effects include anorexia, gastric irritation, nausea, vomiting, constipation, diarrhoea, headache, dizziness, postural hypotension, paraesthesia, impotence, and yellow vision. Hypersensitivity reactions include skin rashes, photosensitivity, pulmonary oedema, and pneumonitis. Cholestatic jaundice, pancreatitis, and blood dyscrasias including thrombocytopenia and, more rarely, granulocytopenia, leucopenia, and aplastic and haemolytic anaemia have been reported.

Intestinal ulceration has occurred following the administration of tablets containing thiazides with an enteric-coated core of potassium chloride (see also under Potassium Chloride, p.1037).

The incidence of glucose intolerance in the Medical Research Council Study on Mild to Moderate Hypertension which led to withdrawal from the study was 9.38 per 1000 patient-years in men and 6.01 per 1000 patient-years in women taking bendrofluazide compared with 2.51 and 0.82 per 1000 patient-years respectively in patients taking placebo. Men also had higher incidences of gout (12.23 compared to 1.03 per 1000 patient-years) and impotence (19.58 compared to 0.89 per 1000 patient-years): overall 22.6% of men reported impotence after 2 years of treatment. Other adverse effects noted in patients taking bendrofluazide included lethargy, constipation, nausea, dizziness, headache, and paraesthesia. Serum concentrations of cholesterol were significantly higher in men taking bendrofluazide than in controls.— Medical Research Council Working Party, *Lancet*, 1981, *2*, 539. See also *idem*, *Br. med. J.*, 1985, *291*, 97.

An opinion that claims that diuretic-induced hypokalaemia and increased serum-cholesterol concentrations may be dangerous is not supported by the available evidence.— E. D. Freis, *Clin. Pharmac. Ther.*, 1986, *39*, 239.

In a discussion of the potential risks of hyperuricaemia during thiazide treatment for hypertension it was concluded that hyperuricaemia itself was not an important cause of renal failure. Increased serum-urate concentrations are observed in primary or secondary hypertension independently of drug treatment. It was concluded that symptomless hyperuricaemia in a hypertensive patient who is receiving diuretic treatment could be ignored.— *Lancet*, 1987, *1*, 1124.

For reference to the adverse effects of diuretics in general (including thiazides), especially effects on electrolyte balance, glucose tolerance, and lipid metabolism, see p.973.

ALLERGY. See under Effects on the Skin.

EFFECTS ON THE ELECTROLYTE BALANCE. *Calcium*. Thiazide diuretics reduced the urinary excretion of calcium by about 40% in patients with intact parathyroid glands but not in patients with hypoparathyroidism.— S. Middler *et al.*, *Metabolism*, 1973, *22*, 139.

Potassium. See diuretics in general, p.973.

Sodium. Symptoms of hyponatraemia with sodium deficit occurred in 4 patients without cardiac failure taking diuretics. Symptoms were lethargy, weakness, slowing of cerebration, anorexia, and nausea, possibly progressing to coma and convulsions; there was no peripheral oedema. The condition, which could easily be missed if plasma-electrolyte concentrations were not measured, responded to the administration of sodium and potassium and the withdrawal of diuretics.— C. J. C. Roberts *et al.*, *Br. med. J.*, 1977, *1*, 210. Of 44 patients with hyponatraemia (plasma-sodium concentration below 125 mmol per litre) 13 were taking diuretics; 5 were taking frusemide and 8 thiazides.— P. G. E. Kennedy *et al.*, *Br. med. J.*, 1978, *2*, 1251.

Severe dilutional hyponatraemia masquerading as subarachnoid haemorrhage occurred in a patient taking hydrochlorothiazide, amiloride, and timolol (G.F.A. Benfield *et al.*, *Lancet*, 1986, *2*, 341). A similar report (P.G. Bain *et al.*, *ibid.*, 634) in a patient taking hydrochlorothiazide and amiloride concomitantly, and later bendrofluazide alone suggested that thiazide diuretics could be responsible.

For further reports of severe hyponatraemia in patients taking thiazide diuretics and potassium-sparing diuretics concurrently see under Hydrochlorothiazide p.992.

EFFECTS ON THE GALL-BLADDER. Findings from a case-controlled drug surveillance programme of an association between the incidence of acute cholecystitis and the use of thiazide-containing drugs.— L. Rosenberg *et al.*, *New Engl. J. Med.*, 1980, *303*, 546.

A study of 91 patients with cholecystitis and 364 controls from the same population showed that the relative risk of developing cholecystitis was 2.1 in those who had taken thiazides during the past year; there was no association with earlier use of thiazides. Thiazides are not considered to cause cholelithiasis, but to increase the risk of cholecystitis in those with gall stones.— W. Van der Linden *et al.*, *Br. med. J.*, 1984, *289*, 654.

EFFECTS ON THE KIDNEYS. Thiazide diuretics can produce acute renal failure by over-enthusiastic use producing saline depletion and hypovolaemia and also, occasionally, by a hypersensitivity reaction. They can occasionally cause the formation of non-opaque urate calculi.— J. R. Curtis, *Br. med. J.*, 1977, *2*, 242 and 375.

For a report of a possible hypersensitivity reaction to thiazide diuretics or frusemide, resulting in reversible renal failure, see Frusemide, p.988.

EFFECTS ON THE SKIN. In Australia the preparation most commonly implicated in photosensitivity reactions was amiloride with hydrochlorothiazide (Moduretic). It was not known whether this reflected a high incidence of photosensitivity reactions to this product or its high usage. Other diuretics which had been reported to cause photosensitivity reactions included other thiazide diuretics alone or in combination, and frusemide.— K. Stone, *Aust. J. Pharm.*, 1985, *66*, 415.

A review of drug-induced photosensitivity. Photosensitivity reactions reported with thiazide diuretics include delayed erythema, eczematous reactions, lichenoid eruptions, and bullae.— J. H. Epstein and B. U. Wintroub, *Drugs*, 1985, *30*, 42.

Thiazide diuretics have been associated with lichen planus-like reactions which may be light-induced.— R. Graham-Brown, *Br. J. Hosp. Med.*, 1986, *36*, 281.

A report of 5 patients who developed photosensitive eruptions with clinical and histological features of subacute cutaneous lupus erythematosus while receiving thiazides.— S. K. Jones *et al.*, *Br. J. Derm.*, 1985, *113*, *Suppl.* 29, 25.

Eczema. Thiazide diuretics, which are sulphonamide derivatives, may produce eczematous eruptions if given to patients sensitised by topical use of sulphonamides.— J. Verbov, *Practitioner*, 1979, *222*, 400.

Vasculitis. In a series of 25 mostly elderly patients with necrotising vasculitis in the skin, 11 were on thiazides and 3 on chlorthalidone; 13 of the 25 had haematuria during the course of their vasculitis. In the 1 patient in whom provocative tests were tried there were reactions to hydrochlorothiazide and chlorthalidone.— A. Björnberg and H. Gisslén, *Lancet*, 1965, *2*, 982.

WITHDRAWAL. Serious oedema occurred in 8 patients within 2 weeks of abrupt withdrawal of thiazide diuretics. Thiazides were resumed and gradually tapered without recurrence of oedema.— K. Brandspigel (letter), *New Engl. J. Med.*, 1986, *314*, 515.

Treatment of Adverse Effects

Hypokalaemia in patients treated with thiazide diuretics may be avoided or treated by the administration of foods with a high potassium content, or by concurrent administration of potassium (but see the discussion on potassium supplements, p.973) or a potassium-sparing diuretic. With the exception of patients with conditions such as liver failure or kidney disease, chloride deficiency is usually mild and does not require specific treatment. Apart from the rare occasions when it is life-threatening, dilutional hyponatraemia is best treated with water restriction rather than salt therapy; in true hyponatraemia, appropriate replacement is the treatment of choice.

In massive overdosage, treatment should be symptomatic and directed at fluid and electrolyte replacement. In the case of recent ingestion gastric lavage should be carried out.

Precautions

Chlorothiazide and other thiazide diuretics should be used with caution in patients with impaired hepatic function since they may increase the risk of hepatic encephalopathy. They should also be given with caution in renal impairment since they can further reduce renal function. They may precipitate attacks of gout in susceptible patients. All patients should be carefully observed for signs of fluid and electrolyte imbalance, especially in the presence of vomiting or during parenteral fluid therapy. Thiazide diuretics may exacerbate or activate systemic lupus erythematosus in susceptible patients.

Chlorothiazide and other thiazide diuretics may enhance the toxicity of digitalis glycosides by depleting serum-potassium concentrations. They may enhance the neuromuscular blocking action of competitive muscle relaxants, such as tubocurarine. They may enhance the effect of antihypertensive agents, while postural hypotension associated with thiazide diuretic therapy may be enhanced by concomitant ingestion of alcohol, barbiturates, or opioids. The potassium-depleting effect of thiazide diuretics may be enhanced by corticosteroids, corticotrophin, or carbenoxolone. They have been reported to diminish the response to pressor amines, such as noradrenaline, but the clinical significance of this effect is uncertain.

Concomitant administration of thiazide diuretics and lithium is not generally recommended since the association may lead to toxic blood concentrations of lithium. Blood-glucose concentrations should be monitored in patients taking antidiabetic agents, since requirements may change.

Thiazide diuretics may interfere with a number of diagnostic tests, including tests for parathyroid function; serum concentrations of protein-bound iodine may increase without signs of thyroid disturbance.

Chlorothiazide crosses the placenta and there have been reports of neonatal jaundice, thrombocytopenia, and electrolyte imbalances following maternal treatment. Chlorothiazide is excreted in the breast milk. Treatment with thiazide diuretics can inhibit lactation.

INTERACTIONS. For references to the interaction between diuretics and nonsteroidal anti-inflammatory drugs, see p.974.

For the effect of thiazide diuretics on lithium, see p.368.

For the effect of thiazide diuretics on warfarin, see p.346.

Beta blockers. Hypokalaemia associated with the use of combined thiazide and beta blocker preparations has been reported by Skehan *et al.* (*Br. med. J.*, 1982, *284*, 83), Odugbesan *et al.* (*Lancet*, 1985, *1*, 1221), Williams (*ibid.*, 1395), Rodger *et al.* (*ibid.*), Scott (*ibid.*), Walters *et al.* (*ibid.*, *2*, 220), and Jacobs (*J. R. Coll. gen. Pract.*, 1986, *36*, 39). In the case reported by Odugbesan, hypokalaemia was complicated by ventricular fibrillation. The use of thiazides with beta blockers may also produce additive increases in serum triglyceride concentrations (*Drug Interact. News.*, 1986, *6*, 51).

In a randomised crossover study involving 14 hypertensive men with adult-onset (type II) diabetes, hydrochlorothiazide 50 mg twice daily for 3 weeks significantly raised fasting glucose concentrations and glycosylated haemoglobin. Propranolol 80 mg twice daily for 3 weeks had no significant effect on these parameters but significantly aggravated the effect of hydrochlorothiazide when the two drugs were given together. Hydrochlorothiazide in association with propranolol appeared to cause serious disturbances in glycaemic control in type II diabetics by mechanisms independent of insulin secretion.— A. Dornhorst *et al.*, *Lancet*, 1985, *1*, 123. Comments: I. Gove and M. J. Kendall (letter), *ibid.*, 515; S. O'Rahilly (letter), *ibid.*

Ion-exchange resins. Gastro-intestinal absorption of chlorothiazide in 10 patients was reduced by colestipol both when the drugs were ingested simultaneously (4 patients) and when chlorothiazide was ingested 1 hour prior to colestipol (6 patients).— R. E. Kauffman and D. L. Azarnoff, *Clin. Pharmac. Ther.*, 1973, *14*, 886.

In a study of 6 healthy subjects both cholestyramine and colestipol were found to reduce the absorption of hydrochlorothiazide. The total urinary excretion of hydrochlorothiazide was reduced by 85% by cholestyramine and 43% by colestipol.— D. B. Hunninghake *et al.*, *Int. J. clin. Pharmac. Ther. Toxic.*, 1982, *20*, 151.

Probenecid. Pretreatment with probenecid in 5 healthy subjects caused a significant increase in sodium excretion and urinary volume excretion after the intravenous administration of chlorothiazide 500 mg compared to values in the same subjects after only chlorothiazide. This increase was associated with a prolonged diuresis of chlorothiazide rather than an increase in intensity. No significant increase occurred when a dose of 1 g of chlorothiazide was employed.— D. C. Brater, *Clin. Pharmac. Ther.*, 1978, *23*, 259.

Propantheline. Gastro-intestinal absorption of chlorothiazide was increased by pretreatment with propantheline 30 mg. The effect was attributed to the reduction in stomach-emptying rate caused by propantheline.— M. A. Osman and P. G. Welling, *Curr. ther. Res.*, 1983, *34*, 404.

INTERFERENCE WITH DIAGNOSTIC TESTS. The administration of chlorothiazide could interfere with measurements of urinary 17-hydroxycorticosteroids.— J. M. Rosenberg and I. S. Kampa, *Drug Intell. & clin. Pharm.*, 1973, *7*, 33.

PREGNANCY AND THE NEONATE. Of 50 282 children born to mothers monitored by the Collaborative Perinatal Project 280 were found to have been exposed to diuretics, and possibly other drugs, at some time during the first 4 months of the pregnancy. In general exposure to diuretics was not associated with the production of malformations but a slight association with respiratory malformations was suggested.— O. P. Heinonen *et al.*, *Birth Defects and Drugs in Pregnancy*, Littleton MA,

Publishing Sciences Group, 1977, p. 371.

For a warning that chlorothiazide is an inappropriate diuretic for jaundiced infants, see Precautions for Frusemide, p.989.

Absorption and Fate

Chlorothiazide is incompletely and variably absorbed from the gastro-intestinal tract. It has been estimated to have a plasma half-life of 45 to 120 minutes although the clinical effects last for up to about 12 hours. It is excreted unchanged in the urine. Chlorothiazide crosses the placental barrier and small amounts are reported to be excreted in breast milk.

Interference by urinary constituents could cause appreciable errors in chlorothiazide bioavailability estimates based on colorimetric procedures. High-pressure liquid chromatography should be the analytical method of choice for urinary excretion-based bioavailability studies on chlorothiazide and, perhaps, other thiazide diuretics.— D. E. Resetarits and T. R. Bates, *J. pharm. Sci.*, 1979, *68*, 126.

Problems of bioavailability had been reported with 500-mg tablets of chlorothiazide.— *Pharm. J.*, 1981, *2*, 265.

PREGNANCY AND THE NEONATE. In 11 nursing mothers given chlorothiazide 500 mg the concentration in breast milk was less than an estimated 1 mg per litre. The risk to the infant was therefore remote.— M. W. Werthmann and S. V. Krees, *J. Pediat.*, 1972, *81*, 781.

Uses and Administration

Chlorothiazide and the other thiazides (which are chemically related to the sulphonamides) are diuretics which reduce the reabsorption of electrolytes from the renal tubules, thereby increasing the excretion of sodium and chloride ions, and consequently of water. The excretion of other electrolytes, notably potassium and magnesium, is also increased. The excretion of calcium is reduced. They also reduce carbonic-anhydrase activity so that bicarbonate excretion is increased, but this effect is generally small compared with the effect on chloride excretion and does not appreciably alter the acid-base balance or the pH of the urine. They may also reduce the glomerular filtration-rate.

The thiazides also have a hypotensive effect probably due to a reduction in peripheral resistance and enhance the effects of other antihypertensive agents. Paradoxically, they have an antidiuretic effect in patients with diabetes insipidus.

Chlorothiazide, like the other thiazide diuretics, is used in the treatment of oedema associated with congestive heart failure, and renal and hepatic disorders. It is also used in hypertension, either alone, or as an adjunct to other antihypertensive agents. However, thiazide diuretics are less effective in patients with impaired renal function.

Chlorothiazide and the other thiazide diuretics are no longer recommended for the routine treatment of toxaemia of pregnancy, although they have been used cautiously for some aspects of the management of pre-eclampsia, for example when there is cardiac failure (see under Hypertension in Pregnancy, p. 973).

The use of diuretic therapy has been advocated for the oedema accompanying premenstrual tension in otherwise healthy subjects although such use has little rationale unless there is evidence of fluid retention. Less common uses of chlorothiazide and other thiazide diuretics include the treatment of diabetes insipidus and the prevention of renal calculus formation in patients with hypercalciuria.

Following oral administration of chlorothiazide a response is usually obtained in about 2 hours and the diuresis is maintained for 6 to 12 hours. The onset of the hypotensive effect usually occurs within 3 to 4 days and the full effect may not be seen for up to 4 weeks.

Dosages of thiazide diuretics should be adjusted according to the response of individual patients. The usual dose of chlorothiazide for diuresis is 0.5 to 1 g once or twice daily; therapy on alternate days or on 3 to 5 days weekly may be adequate.

In the treatment of hypertension chlorothiazide may be given in an initial dose of 250 to 500 mg daily, given as a single or divided dose; doses of up to 2 g daily have been recommended. In general, doses given in hypertension are lower than those used for oedema since increasing the dose often produces an increase in adverse effects without an increase in hypotensive action. In patients who do not respond to a small dose of a thiazide diuretic the addition or substitution of a second antihypertensive agent is generally preferred to an increase in dosage.

The routine use of potassium supplements is no longer recommended in patients taking thiazide diuretics. However, prophylactic administration of a potassium supplement or a potassium-sparing diuretic may be necessary in patients at risk from hypokalaemia such as those taking digitalis preparations, those with cirrhosis of the liver, and those taking other potassium-depleting drugs concurrently.

A suggested dose of chlorothiazide in children is 25 mg per kg body-weight daily in two divided doses. Infants up to the age of 6 months may require up to 35 mg per kg daily in two divided doses.

Chlorothiazide has also been given intravenously as the sodium salt, in doses of 0.5 to 1 g once or twice daily; it is not suitable for subcutaneous or intramuscular injection and extravasation should be avoided. The diuretic effect lasts for up to 2 hours following intravenous injection.

For references to the choice of diuretics and their uses, and to prophylaxis and treatment of diuretic-induced hypokalaemia, see p.973.

ADMINISTRATION IN RENAL FAILURE. Thiazide diuretics are generally ineffective in patients with a glomerular filtration-rate below 30 mL per minute.— W. M. Bennett *et al.*, *Am. J. Kidney Dis.*, 1983, *3*, 155.

HYPERTENSION. Chlorothiazide 12.5, 25, or 50 mg with acebutolol 400 mg produced similar reductions in blood pressure in a study of 24 patients with mild to moderate essential hypertension. It was suggested that this represented a flat dose response and that use of larger doses of diuretic would be associated with increased adverse metabolic effects without improving control of the blood pressure.— G. A. MacGregor *et al.*, *Br. med. J.*, 1983, *286*, 1535. Comment that the range of doses used was inadequate to define the dose-response relationship.— L. E. Ramsay (letter), *ibid.*, *287*, 132. Reply.— N. D. Markandu and G. A. MacGregor, *ibid.*, 133.

Analysis of information from the Medical Research Council (MRC) trial of treatment of mild hypertension showed that bendrofluazide 5 and 10 mg daily produced similar reductions in blood pressure but that falls in serum-potassium concentrations and the incidence of adverse effects were dose-related. Potassium supplementation did not increase the antihypertensive effect. Data from the MRC study of the treatment of hypertension in the elderly showed that hydrochlorothiazide 25 mg with amiloride 2.5 mg and hydrochlorothiazide 50 mg with amiloride 5 mg daily also produced similar reductions in blood pressure but dose-related differences in the incidence of adverse effects.— Medical Research Council Working Party, *J. clin. Pharmac.*, 1987, *27*, 271.

HYPOPARATHYROIDISM. Administration of chlorthalidone 50 mg daily in association with a salt-restricted dietary regimen, given to 7 hypoparathyroid patients for periods of up to 25 months, effectively controlled the symptoms of hypoparathyroidism without incurring the hypercalcaemia or hypercalciuria associated with vitamin-D therapy. Neither the diuretic therapy nor the salt-restricted dietary regimen were as effective alone.— R. H. Porter *et al.*, *New Engl. J. Med.*, 1978, *298*, 577. Chlorothiazide 500 mg daily added to the regimen of a 14-year-old boy with hypoparathyroidism had no noticeable effect on plasma or urinary concentrations of calcium.— J. M. Gertner and M. Genel (letter), *ibid.*, 1478. Metabolic alkalosis was a common complication of treatment with thiazides and there was potential danger if they were used in hypoparathyroid patients with endogenous metabolic alkalosis.— U. S. Barzel (letter), *ibid.* Reply.— W. N. Suki (letter), *ibid.*, 1479. Further criticism.— D. A. McCarron (letter), *ibid.*, *299*, 900. Reply.— W. N. Suki (letter), *ibid.*

Bendrofluazide 10 mg daily was given to 9 patients with hypoparathyroidism in addition to their usual treatment with calcium and vitamin D. Bendrofluazide caused an increase in the renal threshold for calcium reabsorption and a modest increase in serum-calcium concentrations. The increase in renal threshold was due to a direct effect of the drug and was not caused by salt restriction or changes in glomerular filtration rate. Thiazide diuretics would not provide an alternative to vitamin D therapy except in patients with mild hypoparathyroidism but may reduce the oral calcium load required to maintain normocalcaemia.— G. H. Newman *et al.*, *Eur. J. clin. Pharmac.*, 1984, *27*, 41.

RENAL DISORDERS. Brocks *et al.* (*Lancet*, 1981, *2*, 124) found that the rate of renal stone formation was reduced to a similar extent by thiazide and by placebo in a study in 62 patients. However, urinary hypercalciuria was not used as a diagnostic criterion and no information was given about modifications to the diet that could have influenced the outcome (J.C. Birkenhäger *et al.*, *ibid.*, 578; G. Graziani *et al.*, *ibid.*; D.J. Sherrard, *ibid.*, 644). Birkenhäger and Graziani had shown beneficial responses to thiazides in patients with recurrent calcium stone formation. Although Graziani agreed that prolonged treatment with thiazides was not justified in patients with only a moderate rate of stone formation, it was generally considered that thiazides could be useful in patients with higher rates of calcium stone formation.

Preparations

Chlorothiazide Oral Suspension *(U.S.P.)*. pH 3.2 to 4.0. Store in airtight containers.

Chlorothiazide Sodium for Injection *(U.S.P.)*. A sterile mixture of chlorothiazide sodium, prepared from chlorothiazide with the aid of sodium hydroxide, and mannitol. Potency is expressed in terms of the equivalent amount of chlorothiazide. The solution has a pH of 9.2 to 10.

Chlorothiazide Tablets *(B.P., U.S.P.)*

Methyldopa and Chlorothiazide Tablets *(U.S.P.)*

Reserpine and Chlorothiazide Tablets *(U.S.P.)*

Proprietary Preparations

Saluric *(Merck Sharp & Dohme, UK)*. *Tablets*, scored, chlorothiazide 500 mg.

Proprietary Names and Manufacturers of Chlorothiazide and its Salts

Azide *(Fawns & McAllan, Austral.)*; Chlotride *(Frosst, Austral.; Merck Sharp & Dohme, Denm.; Neth.; Norw.; S.Afr.; Swed.)*; Clotride *(Ital.)*; Diuret *(Protea, Austral.)*; Diuril *(Merck Sharp & Dohme, USA)*; Diurilix *(Fr.)*; Diurone *(USV, Austral.)*; Saluretil *(Gayoso Wellcome, Spain)*; Saluric *(Merck Sharp & Dohme, UK)*; SK-Chlorothiazide *(Smith Kline & French, USA)*.

The following names have been used for multi-ingredient preparations containing chlorothiazide and its salts— Aldoclor *(Merck Sharp & Dohme, USA)*; Chloroserpine *(Schein, USA)*; Diupres *(Merck Sharp & Dohme, USA)*; Supres *(Frosst, Canad.)*.

2318-g

Chlorthalidone *(BAN, USAN)*.

Chlortalidone *(rINN)*; G-33182. 2-Chloro-5-(1-hydroxy-3-oxoisoindolin-1-yl)benzenesulphonamide.

$C_{14}H_{11}ClN_2O_4S$=338.8.

CAS — 77-36-1.

Pharmacopoeias. In *Br.*, *Braz.*, *Cz.*, *Egypt.*, *Eur.*, *Ind.*, *Int.*, *It.*, *Jug.*, and *U.S.*

A white or yellowish-white, odourless or almost odourless, crystalline powder.

Practically **insoluble** in water, in ether, and in chloroform; slightly soluble in alcohol; soluble 1 in 25 of methyl alcohol; soluble in solutions of alkali hydroxides.

Adverse Effects, Treatment, and Precautions

As for Chlorothiazide, p.981.

EFFECTS ON THE ELECTROLYTE BALANCE. Hypokalaemia was more marked in patients taking chlorthalidone than in those taking frusemide in a study of 25 patients.— F. Pupita *et al.*, *Pharmatherapeutica*, 1983, *3*, 475.

Depletion of magnesium and potassium was greater in

30 patients treated with chlorthalidone and beta blockers for a year than in 30 patients taking beta blockers alone.— G. Cocco *et al.*, *Eur. J. clin. Pharmac.*, 1987, *32*, 335.

EFFECTS ON THE KIDNEYS. *Inappropriate secretion of antidiuretic hormone.* Chlorthalidone 100 mg daily induced inappropriate secretion of antidiuretic hormone in a 60-year-old woman with mild hypertension and nephrolithiasis for which she had been instructed to increase her water intake.— R. Luboshitzky *et al.*, *J. clin. Pharmac.*, 1978, *18*, 336.

EFFECTS ON LIPID METABOLISM. Mean serum-cholesterol concentrations rose by 5.2% and serum-triglyceride concentrations by 25.7% in 32 hypertensive patients treated by diet and chlorthalidone 50 mg twice weekly to 100 mg daily for about 6 months. Only 15 of the 32 were significantly affected and the mean increases in these 15 were 13.9 and 51.9% respectively. In 31 similar patients with lower initial blood pressure treated by diet mean serum-cholesterol concentrations fell by 4.7% and triglyceride concentrations did not change.— R. P. Ames and P. Hill, *Lancet*, 1976, *1*, 721.

Serum concentrations of total cholesterol, low-density-lipoprotein cholesterol, and apoprotein B were increased significantly after 6 weeks chlorthalidone therapy in 18 postmenopausal women but not in 22 premenopausal women.— K. Boehringer *et al.*, *Ann. intern. Med.*, 1982, *97*, 206.

EFFECT ON THE MUSCLES. Hypokalaemic vacuolar myopathy developed in a 56-year-old woman following chlorthalidone therapy and laxative abuse.— S. J. Oh *et al.*, *J. Am. med. Ass.*, 1971, *216*, 1858.

EFFECTS ON SEXUAL FUNCTION. Sexual dysfunction, characterised by impotence or decreased libido, was associated with the administration of chlorthalidone in 5 men. In all patients sexual function improved on stopping, or reducing the dose of chlorthalidone.— J. Stessman and D. Ben-Ishay, *Br. med. J.*, 1980, *281*, 714.

In a survey of patients undergoing antihypertensive therapy sexual dysfunction was the most frequent side-effect in patients taking chlorthalidone or hydrochlorothiazide, with an incidence of 4.4%.— J. Lazar *et al.*, *Clin. Pharmac. Ther.*, 1984, *35*, 254.

INTERACTIONS. *Acetazolamide.* A study in 2 healthy subjects indicated that chlorthalidone and acetazolamide competed for the same binding sites in the blood cells. These showed greater affinity for acetazolamide which was able to inhibit the uptake of chlorthalidone into the red cells and also to displace chlorthalidone already attached to the binding sites.— B. Beermann *et al.*, *Clin. Pharmac. Ther.*, 1975, *17*, 424.

Warfarin. For references to the interaction between warfarin and chlorthalidone, see p.346.

PREGNANCY AND THE NEONATE. In the infants born to 9 women given chlorthalidone for toxaemia of pregnancy concentrations of 0.43 to 1.60 μg per mL were measured in cord blood of 8 at delivery. Treatment of the mothers was continued for 3 days after delivery, and concentrations of 90 to 860 ng per mL were found in milk on the third day. It was recommended that mothers receiving chlorthalidone should not breast-feed, as the infants might be less able than adults to eliminate it.— B. A. Mulley *et al.*, *Eur. J. clin. Pharmac.*, 1978, *13*, 129.

Absorption and Fate

Chlorthalidone is erratically absorbed from the gastro-intestinal tract. Its prolonged terminal half-life of 35 to 54 hours has been reported to be due to its strong binding to red blood cells. During long-term administration 30 to 60% has been reported to be excreted unchanged in the urine. It crosses the placental barrier and is excreted in breast milk.

References on the pharmacokinetics of chlorthalidone: W. Riess *et al.*, *Eur. J. clin. Pharmac.*, 1977, *12*, 375; H. L. J. Fleuren *et al.*, *Eur. J. clin. Pharmac.*, 1979, *15*, 35; H. L. J. Fleuren *et al.*, *Clin. Pharmac. Ther.*, 1979, *25*, 806; B. A. Mulley *et al.*, *Eur. J. clin. Pharmac.*, 1980, *17*, 203.

RED CELL BINDING. An *in vitro* study of the binding of chlorthalidone to human blood components. In the absence of red blood cells about 75% was bound to plasma proteins (mainly albumin) at a concentration range of 0.02 to 7.7 μg per mL. In whole blood, however, at concentrations of about 15 to 20 μg per mL, at least 98% was preferentially contained in the red blood cell fraction. Above this concentration the percentage of drug in the red blood cells decreased, and that in the plasma increased, indicating the presence of a saturable receptor in the red blood cells, which was identified as carbonic anhydrase. Chlorthalidone is much less strongly bound to albumin than carbonic anhydrase.— W. Dieterle *et al.*, *Eur. J. clin. Pharmac.*, 1976, *10*, 37. See also: G. D. Parr *et al.*, *J. Pharm. Pharmac.*, 1979, *31*, *Suppl.*, 42P.

Uses and Administration

Chlorthalidone is a diuretic which has certain structural similarities to the thiazides and has actions and uses similar to those of chlorothiazide (see p.983).

Diuresis is initiated in about 2 hours and lasts for 48 hours or longer. Its inhibitory action on carbonic anhydrase is only weak.

In the treatment of oedema the usual dose is 50 to 100 mg daily or 100 to 200 mg on alternate days; the maximum recommended dose is 400 mg, although some sources suggest that doses above 200 mg daily do not produce a greater response.

The usual dose in the treatment of hypertension is 25 to 50 mg daily, either alone, or in conjunction with other antihypertensive agents; in some cases doses of 100 mg may be necessary.

A suggested initial dose in children is 2 mg per kg body-weight 3 times a week.

In diabetes insipidus an initial dose of 100 mg twice daily has been recommended reduced to a maintenance dose of 50 mg daily.

When treatment is prolonged, or in susceptible patients, loss of potassium may be sufficient to produce hypokalaemia; potassium supplements or a potassium-sparing diuretic should then be given as for chlorothiazide.

ADMINISTRATION IN RENAL FAILURE. The interval between doses of chlorthalidone should be extended from 24 hours to 48 hours in patients with a glomerular filtration-rate of less than 10 mL per minute.— W. M. Bennett *et al.*, *Am. J. Kidney Dis.*, 1983, *3*, 155.

HYPERTENSION. In a crossover study in 33 hypertensive patients there was no significant difference between the antihypertensive effect of chlorthalidone 50 to 100 mg daily and frusemide 40 to 80 mg daily. Concomitant antihypertensive therapy remained the same throughout the study. Potassium supplements were required by 17 patients during the chlorthalidone period alone and by 2 patients during both drug periods.— M. E. Davidov *et al.*, *Curr. ther. Res.*, 1979, *25*, 1. See also F. Pupita *et al.*, *Pharmatherapeutica*, 1983, *3*, 475.

In a study involving 134 patients under 65 years old with previously untreated mild hypertension, chlorthalidone 25, 50, 75, or 100 mg produced similar reductions in blood pressure over 8 weeks. A decline in blood pressure was noted after 2 weeks of treatment and was maximal after 4 weeks. Diastolic pressure was reduced to below 95 mmHg in 70% of patients. Ten additional patients were withdrawn from the study due to adverse effects during chlorthalidone therapy. Metabolic effects tended to be greater with larger doses. The incidence of adverse effects was similar in the 4 groups.— J. G. Russell *et al.*, *Eur. J. clin. Pharmac.*, 1981, *20*, 407.

Chlorthalidone 15 mg daily was shown to be as effective as chlorthalidone 25 mg daily in reducing blood pressure in 222 patients with mild hypertension. The incidence of hypokalaemia was less with 15 mg than with 25 mg. Three patients taking chlorthalidone 15 mg withdrew from the study because of adverse reactions compared with 7 patients taking chlorthalidone 25 mg and 2 patients taking placebo.— S. Vardan *et al.*, *J. Am. med. Ass.*, 1987, *258*, 484. See also R. H. Grimm *et al.*, *Am. Heart J.*, 1985, *109*, 858.

Further references to chlorthalidone in hypertension: B. F. Robinson *et al.*, *Br. J. clin. Pharmac.*, 1983, *16*, 327; L. A. Ferrara *et al.*, *Eur. J. clin. Pharmac.*, 1984, *27*, 525; E. L. Webb *et al.*, *J. int. med. Res.*, 1984, *12*, 133; E. L. Webb *et al.*, *ibid.*, 140; H. Bachmann, *Helv. paediat. Acta*, 1984, *39*, 55; S. B. Hulley *et al.*, *Am. J. Cardiol.*, 1985, *56*, 913.

Effect on plasma renin. In a study of 50 patients with essential hypertension 10 of 13 patients with low-renin activity, 13 of 28 with normal-renin activity and 2 of 9 with high-renin activity responded to treatment with chlorthalidone 100 mg daily for 6 weeks. Increases in plasma-renin activity and particularly in the excretion-rate of aldosterone were higher in nonresponders than in responders. Factors governing the sensitivity of the aldosterone response to renin stimulation might determine the effectiveness of antihypertensive diuretics.— M. A. Weber *et al.*, *Ann. intern. Med.*, 1977, *87*, 558.

MÉNIÈRE'S DISEASE. Chlorthalidone could improve vertigo associated with Ménière's disease, but diuretics are not useful for dizziness of other origins.— L. M. Luxon, *Prescribers' J.*, 1985, *25*, 105.

Preparations

Chlorthalidone Tablets *(B.P.)*

Chlorthalidone Tablets *(U.S.P.)*

Proprietary Preparations

Hygroton *(Geigy, UK). Tablets*, scored, chlorthalidone 50 and 100 mg.

Hygroton-K *(Geigy, UK). Tablets*, chlorthalidone 25 mg, potassium chloride 500 mg (potassium 6.7 mmol) for sustained release.

Owing to the risk of intestinal obstruction, sustained-release preparations such as Hygroton-K, where the drug is released in transit, but the matrix ghost is often eliminated intact, should not be prescribed in patients with Crohn's disease or other intestinal disease in which strictures may form.— J. L. Shaffer *et al.* (letter), *Lancet*, 1980, *2*, 487.

Kalspare *(Rorer, UK). Tablets*, scored, chlorthalidone 50 mg, triamterene 50 mg.

Proprietary Names and Manufacturers

Axamin *(Lennon, S.Afr.)*; Higrotona *(Ciba, Spain)*; Hydro-long *(Beiersdorf, Ger.)*; Hygroton *(Arg.; Geigy, Austral.; Belg.; Geigy, Canad.; Geigy, Denm.; Geigy, Fr.; Ciba, Ger.; Neth.; Geigy, Norw.; Geigy, S.Afr.; Geigy, Swed.; Geigy, Switz.; Geigy, UK; USV Pharmaceutical Corp., USA)*; Igrolina *(Ital.)*; Igroton *(Geigy, Ital.)*; Novothalidone *(Novopharm, Canad.)*; Odemo-Genat *(Azuchemie, Ger.)*; Renidone *(Rolab, S.Afr.)*; Renon *(Ital.)*; Thalitone *(Boehringer Ingelheim, USA)*; Urid *(Protea, Austral.)*; Uridon *(ICN, Canad.)*; Urolin *(Salus, Ital.)*; Zambesil *(Lipha, Ital.)*.

The following names have been used for multi-ingredient preparations containing chlorthalidone—Combipres *(Boehringer Ingelheim, Canad.; Boehringer Ingelheim, USA)*; Demi-Regroton *(Rorer, USA)*; Hygroton-K *(Geigy, UK)*; Kalspare *(Rorer, UK)*; Lopresoretic *(Geigy, UK)*; Regroton *(USV Pharmaceutical Corp., USA)*; Tenoret 50 *(Stuart, UK)*; Tenoretic *(Stuart, UK; Stuart Pharmaceuticals, USA)*.

2843-b

Cicletanine *(rINN)*.

BN-1270; (±)-Cycletanide. (±)-3-(*p*-Chlorophenyl)-1,3-dihydro-6-methylfuro[3,4-*c*]pyridin-7-ol.

$C_{14}H_{12}ClNO_2$=261.7.

CAS — 89943-82-8.

Cicletanine is a diuretic which has been tried in the treatment of hypertension.

References: P. Braquet *et al.* (letter), *Lancet*, 1983, *1*, 1218.

Proprietary Names and Manufacturers Tenstatin (*IPSEN, Fr.*).

2320-d

Clopamide *(BAN, USAN, rINN)*.

DT-327. 4-Chloro-*N*-(2,6-dimethylpiperidino)-3-sulphamoylbenzamide.

$C_{14}H_{20}ClN_3O_3S$=345.8.

CAS — 636-54-4.

Clopamide is a diuretic which has certain structural similarities to the thiazides and has properties similar to those of chlorothiazide (see p.981). Diuresis is initiated in about 2 hours and lasts for up to 24 hours. In the treatment of oedema the usual initial dose is 40 to 60 mg daily; maintenance doses of 20 to 60 mg are given daily or intermittently. The usual dose in the treatment of hypertension is 20 to 40 mg daily, either alone, or in conjunction with other antihypertensive agents.

When treatment is prolonged, or in susceptible patients, loss of potassium may be sufficient to produce hypokalaemia; potassium supplements or a potassium-sparing diuretic should then be given as for chlorothiazide.

Proprietary Names and Manufacturers

Adurix *(Benzon, Denm.)*; Aquex *(Sandoz, USA)*; Brinaldix *(Sandoz, Austral.; Belg.; Denm.; Sandoz, Fr.; Sandoz, Ger.; Sandoz, Ital.; Neth.; Sandoz, Norw.; Spain; Sandoz, Swed.; Sandoz, Switz.; Sandoz, UK)*.

The following names have been used for multi-ingredient preparations containing clopamide— Brinaldix K *(Sandoz, UK)*; Viskaldix *(Sandoz, NZ; Sandoz, UK)*; Visken 10 + Brinaldix 5 *(Sandoz, Austral.)*.

2321-n

Clorexolone *(BAN, USAN, pINN).*
M&B-8430; RP-12833. 6-Chloro-2-cyclohexyl-3-oxoisoindoline-5-sulphonamide.
$C_{14}H_{17}ClN_2O_3S$=328.8.

CAS — 2127-01-7.

Clorexolone is a diuretic which has certain structural similarities to the thiazides and has actions and uses similar to those of chlorothiazide (see p.983). It has a diuretic action lasting 24 to 48 hours.
In the treatment of oedema, 25 to 100 mg may be given daily or on alternate days. In the treatment of hypertension, the usual dose is 10 to 25 mg daily, either alone, or in conjunction with other antihypertensive agents.
When treatment is prolonged, or in susceptible patients, loss of potassium may be sufficient to produce hypokalaemia; potassium supplements or a potassium-sparing diuretic should then be given as for chlorothiazide.

Proprietary Names and Manufacturers
Nefrolan *(May & Baker, Austral.; May & Baker, S.Afr.; May & Baker, UK)*;

2322-h

Couch-grass
Agropyrum; Graminis Rhizoma; Petit Chiendent; Twitch.

Pharmacopoeias. In *Fr.* and *Pol.*

The rhizome of *Agropyron repens*(=*Triticum repens*) (Gramineae). It contains glucose, mannitol, inositol, and triticin (a carbohydrate resembling inulin).

Couch-grass is a mild diuretic which has been used in the treatment of cystitis. It has usually been employed as a decoction or as a liquid extract.

2323-m

Cyclopenthiazide *(BAN, USAN, rINN).*
Cyclopenthiaz.; Su-8341. 6-Chloro-3-cyclopentylmethyl-3,4-dihydro-2*H*-1,2,4-benzothiadiazine-7-sulphonamide 1,1-dioxide.
$C_{13}H_{18}ClN_3O_4S_2$=379.9.

CAS — 742-20-1.

Pharmacopoeias. In *Br.*

A white, odourless or almost odourless powder. Practically **insoluble** in water; soluble 1 in 12 of alcohol; soluble in acetone and in ether; slightly soluble in chloroform.

Cyclopenthiazide is a thiazide diuretic with properties similar to those of chlorothiazide (see p.983). Diuresis is induced in 1 to 2 hours and lasts up to about 12 hours.
In the treatment of oedema the usual initial dose is 0.5 to 1 mg daily, reduced to a dose of 500 µg on alternate days. In the treatment of hypertension the usual dose is 250 to 500 µg daily either alone, or in conjunction with other antihypertensive agents. The maximum effective daily dose of cyclopenthiazide is reported to be 1.5 mg, and to be rarely required.
When treatment is prolonged, or in susceptible patients, loss of potassium may be sufficient to produce hypokalaemia; potassium supplements or a potassium-sparing diuretic should then be given as for chlorothiazide.
Cyclopenthiazide in a dose of 125 µg [daily] produced a similar hypotensive effect to the conventional dose of 500 µg in mild essential hypertension.— G. McVeigh *et al., Br. med. J.*, 1988, *297*, 95.

Preparations
Cyclopenthiazide Tablets *(B.P.)*
Navidrex *(Ciba, UK). Tablets*, scored, cyclopenthiazide 500 µg.
Navidrex-K *(Ciba, UK). Tablets*, cyclopenthiazide 250 µg, potassium chloride 600 mg (potassium 8.06 mmol) for sustained release.
Owing to the risk of intestinal obstruction, sustained-release preparations such as Navidrex-K, where the drug is released in transit, but the matrix ghost is often eliminated intact, should not be prescribed in patients with Crohn's disease or other intestinal disease in which strictures may form.— J. L. Shaffer *et al.* (letter), *Lancet*, 1980, *2*, 487.

Proprietary Names and Manufacturers
Navidrex *(Ciba, Austral.; Belg.; Denm.; Ger.; Neth.; S.Afr.; Ciba, Switz.; Ciba, UK)*.

The following names have been used for multi-ingredient preparations containing cyclopenthiazide— Navidrex-K *(Ciba, UK)*; Trasidrex *(Ciba, UK)*.

2324-b

Cyclothiazide *(BAN, USAN, rINN).*
MDi-193. 6-Chloro-3,4-dihydro-3-(norborn-5-en-2-yl)-2*H*-1,2,4-benzothiadiazine-7-sulphonamide 1,1-dioxide.
$C_{14}H_{16}ClN_3O_4S_2$=389.9.

CAS — 2259-96-3.

Pharmacopoeias. In *U.S.*

A white or almost white, practically odourless powder. Practically **insoluble** in water and chloroform; soluble 1 in 70 of alcohol and 1 in 30 of methyl alcohol; freely soluble in acetone.

Cyclothiazide is a thiazide diuretic with properties similar to those of chlorothiazide (see p.981). Diuresis is initiated within 6 hours and lasts for 18 to 24 hours.
In the treatment of oedema the usual initial dose is 1 to 2 mg daily, reduced to a dose of 1 or 2 mg on alternate days or twice or three times weekly. In the treatment of hypertension the usual dose is 2 mg daily, either alone, or in conjunction with other antihypertensive agents; in some cases doses of 2 mg up to three times daily may be required.
A suggested initial dose for children is 20 to 40 µg per kg body-weight daily.
When treatment is prolonged, or in susceptible patients, loss of potassium may be sufficient to produce hypokalaemia; potassium supplements or a potassium-sparing diuretic should then be given as for Chlorothiazide.

Preparations
Cyclothiazide Tablets *(U.S.P.)*

Proprietary Names and Manufacturers
Anhydron *(Lilly, USA)*; Doburil *(Boehringer Ingelheim, Austral.; Pharmacia, Denm.; Spain)*; Fluidil *(Adria, USA)*.

2325-v

Dichlorphenamide *(BAN, USAN).*
Diclofenamide *(rINN)*; Diclofenamidum. 4,5-Dichlorobenzene-1,3-disulphonamide.
$C_6H_6Cl_2N_2O_4S_2$=305.2.

CAS — 120-97-8.

Pharmacopoeias. In *Br., Chin.,* and *U.S.*

A white or almost white crystalline powder with a slight characteristic odour.
Practically **insoluble** or very slightly soluble in water; practically insoluble in chloroform; soluble 1 in 30 of alcohol; slightly soluble in ether; freely soluble in pyridine; soluble in solutions of alkali hydroxides and carbonates.

Dichlorphenamide is an inhibitor of carbonic anhydrase which has actions similar to those of acetazolamide (see p.976). When given by mouth, its effect begins within 1 hour and lasts for 6 to 12 hours.
Dichlorphenamide is used to reduce intra-ocular pressure in glaucoma. The usual initial adult dose is 100 to 200 mg, then 100 mg every 12 hours, followed by a maintenance dose of 25 to 50 mg onc to three times daily.
When treatment is prolonged, or in susceptible patients, loss of potassium may be sufficient to produce hypokalaemia; potassium supplements should then be given as for Chlorothiazide.

Preparations
Dichlorphenamide Tablets *(B.P., U.S.P.)*
Daranide *(Merck Sharp & Dohme, UK). Tablets*, scored, dichlorphenamide 50 mg.

Proprietary Names and Manufacturers
Antidrasi *(Arg.; ISF, Ital.; Merck Sharp & Dohme, Spain)*; Daranide *(Merck Sharp & Dohme, Austral.; Belg.; Canad.; Neth.; Swed.; Merck Sharp & Dohme, UK; Merck Sharp & Dohme, USA)*; Fenamide *(Farmigea, Ital.)*; Glauconide *(Llorens, Spain)*; Glaumid *(SIFI, Ital.)*; Hipotensor Oftalmico *(Spain)*; Oralcon *(Alcon, Denm.; Alcon, Swed.)*; Oratrol *(Austral.; Belg.; Fr.; Neth.; Alcon, Switz.; Alcon, UK; Alcon Laboratories, USA)*; Tensodilen *(Frumtost, Spain)*.

2326-g

Disulphamide *(BAN).*
Disulfamide *(pINN)*. 5-Chlorotoluene-2,4-disulphonamide.
$C_7H_9ClN_2O_4S_2$=284.7.

CAS — 671-88-5.

Disulphamide is an inhibitor of carbonic anhydrase with properties and uses similar to acetazolamide (see p.976). Potassium supplements should be given, where deemed necessary, as for chlorothiazide.
It has been given in doses of 100 to 400 mg daily.

Proprietary Names and Manufacturers
Diluen *(Ital.)*; Disamide *(BDH Chemicals, UK)*; Natirène *(Nativelle, Fr.)*; Toluidrin *(Radiumfarma, Ital.)*.

2327-q

Epithiazide *(BAN, USAN).*
Epitizide *(rINN)*; P-2105. 6-Chloro-3,4-dihydro-3-(2,2,2-trifluoroethylthiomethyl)-2*H*-1,2,4-benzothiadiazine-7-sulphonamide 1,1-dioxide.
$C_{10}H_{11}ClF_3N_3O_4S_3$=425.8.

CAS — 1764-85-8.

Epithiazide is a thiazide diuretic with properties similar to those of chlorothiazide (see p.981).

Proprietary Names and Manufacturers
Pfizer, USA.

The following names have been used for multi-ingredient preparations containing epithiazide— Thiaver *(Riker, UK)*.

2363-e

Ethacrynic Acid *(BAN, USAN).*
Acidum Etacrynicum; Etacrynic Acid *(rINN)*; Etacrynsäure; MK-595. [2,3-Dichloro-4-(2-ethylacryloyl)phenoxy]acetic acid.
$C_{13}H_{12}Cl_2O_4$=303.1.

CAS — 58-54-8.

Pharmacopoeias. In *Aust., Br., Chin., Cz., Eur., Fr., Ger., Ind., It., Neth., Nord., Swiss,* and *U.S.*

A white or almost white, odourless or almost odourless, crystalline powder. Very slightly **soluble** in water; soluble 1 in 1.6 of alcohol, 1 in 6 of chloroform, and 1 in 3.5 of ether; dissolves in ammonia and in dilute aqueous solutions of alkali hydroxides and carbonates. Solutions of the sodium salt containing the equivalent of ethacrynic acid 0.1% have a pH of 6.3 to 7.7. Solutions of the sodium salt are relatively stable at about pH 7 at room temperatures for short periods and less stable at higher pH values and temperatures. They are **incompatible** with solutions with a pH below 5. **Store** in well-closed containers. The injection should be protected from light and used immediately after preparation.

CAUTION. *Ethacrynic acid, especially in the form of dust, is irritating to the skin, eyes, and mucous membranes.*

2328-p

Sodium Ethacrynate *(BANM).*

Etacrynate Sodium; Ethacrynate Sodium *(USAN)*; Sodium Etacrynate.
$C_{13}H_{11}Cl_2NaO_4$=325.1.

CAS — 6500-81-8.

Pharmacopoeias. In *Chin. Br.* and *U.S.* include sodium ethacrynate for injection.

INCOMPATIBILITY. There were changes in the u.v. spectra indicating chemical change and possible incompatibility when sodium ethacrynate was added to sodium chloride injection containing hydralazine hydrochloride, procainamide hydrochloride, or tolazoline hydrochloride. A precipitate occurred with reserpine injection (Serpasil). Sodium ethacrynate appeared to be compatible with chlorpromazine hydrochloride, prochlorperazine edisylate, and promazine hydrochloride.— P. N. Catania and J. C. King, *Am. J. Hosp. Pharm.*, 1972, *29*, 141.

It has been recommended that ethacrynic acid may be dissolved in a 5% solution of glucose for infusion or slow injection, but if this has a pH below 5 the resulting solution may be cloudy and should not be used. In addition, ethacrynic acid should not be mixed with whole blood or blood derivatives; if it is desired to give ethacrynic acid at the same time as a blood transfusion it should be given independently.

Adverse Effects

As for Frusemide, p.987. Gastro-intestinal disturbances may be more common with ethacrynic acid; profuse watery diarrhoea is an indication for stopping ethacrynic acid therapy. Gastro-intestinal bleeding has been associated with ethacrynic acid and tinnitus and deafness may be more common. Other adverse effects include confusion, fatigue, nervousness, and apprehensiveness. Haematuria has been reported rarely.

Local irritation and pain may follow intravenous injection.

An account of the toxic effects of ethacrynic acid.— F. D. Schwartz *et al.*, *Am. Heart J.*, 1970, *79*, 427.

DIABETOGENIC EFFECT AND HYPOGLYCAEMIA. High doses of ethacrynic acid induced symptomatic hypoglycaemia with convulsions in 2 patients with uraemia.— J. F. Maher and G. E. Schreiner, *Ann. intern. Med.*, 1965, *62*, 15.

Ethacrynic acid 200 mg daily and hydrochlorothiazide 200 mg daily each reduced glucose tolerance when tested in 24 patients with essential hypertension. The effect was more pronounced with hydrochlorothiazide than with ethacrynic acid; the latter showed its most pronounced effect in diabetic subjects.— R. P. Russell *et al.*, *J. Am. med. Ass.*, 1968, *205*, 11.

One patient with heart failure developed hyperosmolar hyperglycaemic coma after 3 months' treatment with ethacrynic acid 200 to 400 mg daily in divided doses. Patients should be monitored for the development of hyperglycaemia.— A. J. Cowley and R. S. Elkeles (letter), *Lancet*, 1978, *1*, 154.

EFFECTS ON THE BLOOD. *Agranulocytosis.* A report of fatal agranulocytosis in association with ethacrynic acid.— J. G. Walker, *Ann. intern. Med.*, 1966, *64*, 1303.

Haemolysis. The addition of ethacrynic acid in concentrations greater than 2 mmol per litre caused immediate damage to red cells in whole blood. Frusemide did not have this effect.— J. Lieberman and W. Kaneshiro (letter), *Lancet*, 1971, *1*, 911.

Haemolytic anaemia. Suspected haemolytic anaemia in a patient receiving ethacrynic acid therapy.— M. Hanna, *Med. J. Aust.*, 1966, *1*, 534.

EFFECTS ON THE EARS. The Boston Collaborative Drug Surveillance Program monitored consecutively 32 812 medical inpatients. Drug-induced deafness occurred in 2 of 184 patients given ethacrynic acid.— J. Porter and H. Jick, *Lancet*, 1977, *1*, 587. See also Boston Collaborative Drug Surveillance Program, *J. Am. med. Ass.*, 1973, *224*, 515.

Deafness accompanied by nystagmus occurred in a patient following the slow intravenous infusion of 100 mg of ethacrynic acid; the side-effects resolved within 1 hour.— I. H. Gomolin and E. Garshick (letter), *New Engl. J. Med.*, 1980, *303*, 702.

EFFECTS ON THE GASTRO-INTESTINAL TRACT. Symptoms of gastro-intestinal intolerance, consisting of indigestion, nausea, vomiting, or occasional diarrhoea, occurred in 7 of 40 out-patients given ethacrynic acid therapy.— A. C. Newell, *Med. J. Aust.*, 1970, *1*, 320.

Of 26 294 hospital in-patients monitored by the Boston Collaborative Drug Surveillance Program, major gastro-intestinal bleeding occurred in only 57. Of these 57 patients, 37 had been receiving ethacrynic acid, heparin, warfarin, corticosteroids, or aspirin-containing drugs either alone or in different associations. The highest percentage of bleeds relative to patients exposed occurred in those receiving ethacrynic acid intravenously alone (4.5%) or by mouth in association with heparin or corticosteroids (6.3%).— H. Jick and J. Porter, *Lancet*, 1978, *2*, 87.

Further references to the incidence of gastro-intestinal bleeding with ethacrynic acid: D. Slone *et al.*, *J. Am. med. Ass.*, 1969, *209*, 1668.

EFFECTS ON THE KIDNEYS. Transient bilateral abdominal pain, radiating to the genitalia, occurred in a patient a few minutes after taking ethacrynic acid.— N. G. Kounis (letter), *Br. med. J.*, 1973, *3*, 641.

EFFECTS ON THE LIVER. A 25-year-old man developed hepatocellular damage on 3 occasions probably due to ethacrynic acid which he had taken in dosages varying from 50 to 200 mg daily for periods of 1 to 7 weeks. On 2 occasions the jaundice regressed when ethacrynic acid was discontinued, but on the third occasion the jaundice persisted and he died in congestive cardiac failure.— K. K. Datey *et al.*, *Br. med. J.*, 1967, *3*, 152.

EFFECTS ON THE SKIN. *Purpura.* A report of a patient in whom extensive purpuric and ecchymotic rashes might have been associated with ethacrynic acid administration. The patient subsequently died and among other post-mortem findings, there was extensive gastro-duodenal ulceration.— A. K. Pain (letter), *Br. med. J.*, 1967, *1*, 634.

Precautions

As for Chlorothiazide, p.982.

Ethacrynic acid may enhance the nephrotoxicity of cephalosporin antibiotics such as cephalothin and of the aminoglycoside antibiotics. It can also enhance the ototoxicity of aminoglycoside antibiotics. The risks of gastro-intestinal bleeding associated with ethacrynic acid administration may be enhanced by concurrent administration of anticoagulants.

INTERACTIONS. *Antibiotics.* For the effect of ethacrynic acid on the urinary elimination of chloramphenicol, see Chloramphenicol, p.188.

Anticoagulants. A study of haemolytic reactions and drug interactions in 500 warfarin-treated patients. Among interactions not previously noted clinically was one with ethacrynic acid.— J. Koch-Weser, *Clin. Pharmac. Ther.*, 1973, *14*, 139.

For further references to the interaction between warfarin and ethacrynic acid, see p.346.

Absorption and Fate

Ethacrynic acid is fairly rapidly absorbed from the gastro-intestinal tract. It is excreted both in the bile and the urine, partly unchanged and partly in the form of metabolites. It is extensively bound to plasma proteins.

Uses and Administration

Although chemically unrelated, ethacrynic acid is a diuretic with actions and uses similar to those of frusemide (see p.989). Diuresis is initiated within about 30 minutes after a dose by mouth, and lasts for about 6 to 8 hours; after intravenous injection of its sodium salt, the effects are evident within a few minutes and last for about 2 hours.

In the treatment of oedema, the usual initial dose is 50 mg in the morning, taken with or immediately after food; in some cases higher doses may be necessary, and severe cases have required gradual titration of the ethacrynic acid dosage up to a maximum of 400 mg daily, but the effective dose range is usually between 50 and 150 mg daily. Dosage of more than 50 mg daily should be given in divided doses, and it is preferable for all doses to be taken with food. Maintenance doses may be taken daily or intermittently and are usually less than the initial doses.

In emergency, such as acute pulmonary oedema, or when oral therapy cannot be given, ethacrynic acid may be given by slow intravenous injection either directly or into the tubing of a running infusion, as its salt, sodium ethacrynate, in a dose equivalent to 50 mg or 0.5 to 1 mg per kg body-weight of ethacrynic acid as a solution containing 1 mg per mL in glucose 5% (but see above under Incompatibility) or sodium chloride 0.9% solution; should a subsequent injection be required the site should be changed to avoid thrombophlebitis. Single doses of 100 mg have been given intravenously in critical situations. It is not suitable for subcutaneous or intramuscular injection.

For children over 2 years of age a suggested initial dose of ethacrynic acid is 25 mg daily by mouth, cautiously increased as necessary by 25 mg daily.

When treatment is prolonged, or in susceptible patients, loss of potassium may be sufficient to produce hypokalaemia; potassium supplements or potassium-sparing diuretics should then be given as for chlorothiazide (see p.983). If very high doses are used careful laboratory control is essential as described under the uses for frusemide (p.989; high-dose therapy).

A brief review of the clinical pharmacology of ethacrynic acid.— A. Lant, *Drugs*, 1985, *29*, 57.

ADMINISTRATION IN CHILDREN. In infants under 1 year of age with cardiac failure the dose of ethacrynic acid is 1 mg per kg body-weight intravenously repeated after 12 hours if necessary, or 3 mg per kg daily by mouth.— D. Goldring *et al.*, *Pediatrics*, 1971, *47*, 1056.

ADMINISTRATION IN RENAL FAILURE. Ethacrynic acid should be avoided in patients with a glomerular filtration-rate of less than 10 mL per minute.— W. M. Bennett *et al.*, *Am. J. Kidney Dis.*, 1983, *3*, 155.

CARDIAC DISORDERS. *Heart failure.* Reports of beneficial results with ethacrynic acid in patients with right or left heart failure: P. M. Buckfield and M. Hamilton, *J. Ther.*, 1966, *1*, (2), 5.

RENAL DISORDERS. Of 22 patients with oedema and severe chronic renal failure who received on average 150 mg of ethacrynic acid daily for 9 days, in only 3 did diuresis not occur.— K. D. G. Edwards *et al.*, *Med. J. Aust.*, 1967, *1*, 375.

Renal tubular acidosis. A patient with renal tubular acidosis, early renal insufficiency, and osteomalacia responded to treatment with ethacrynic acid 50 mg daily for 2 years. Urinary pH decreased and systemic acidosis disappeared. Osteomalacia receded and despite the hypercalciuric effect of ethacrynic acid, nephrocalcinosis did not get worse.— E. Heidbreder *et al.* (letter), *Lancet*, 1973, *1*, 52.

Preparations

Ethacrynate Sodium for Injection *(U.S.P.).* Potency is expressed in terms of the equivalent amount of ethacrynic acid.

Ethacrynic Acid Tablets *(B.P., U.S.P.)*

Sodium Ethacrynate Injection *(B.P.).* Potency is expressed in terms of the equivalent amount of ethacrynic acid.

Proprietary Preparations

Edecrin *(Merck Sharp & Dohme, UK). Tablets*, scored, ethacrynic acid 50 mg.

Injection, powder for reconstitution, ethacrynic acid 50 mg (as sodium ethacrynate).

Proprietary Names and Manufacturers of Ethacrynic Acid and its Sodium Salt

Crinuryl *(Israel)*; Edecril *(Merck Sharp & Dohme, Austral.; Jpn)*; Edecrin *(Belg.; Merck Sharp & Dohme, Canad.; Merck Sharp & Dohme, Denm.; Merck Sharp & Dohme, Ital.; Neth.; Merck Sharp & Dohme, Norw.; NZ; Merck Sharp & Dohme, Spain; Merck Sharp & Dohme, Switz.; Merck Sharp & Dohme, UK; Merck Sharp & Dohme, USA)*; Edecrina *(MSD, Swed.)*; Edecrine *(Merck Sharp & Dohme-Chibret, Fr.)*; Hydromedin *(Merck Sharp & Dohme, Ger.)*; Reomax *(Bioindustria, Ital.)*; Sodium Edecrin *(Merck Sharp & Dohme, Canad.; Merck Sharp & Dohme, USA)*; Taladren *(Malesci, Ital.)*; Uregyt *(Hung.)*.

2329-s

Ethiazide *(BAN, rINN).*
6-Chloro-3-ethyl-3,4-dihydro-2*H*-1,2,4-benzothiadiazine-7-sulphonamide 1,1-dioxide.
$C_9H_{12}ClN_3O_4S_2$=325.8.

CAS — 1824-58-4.

Ethiazide is a thiazide diuretic which has properties similar to those of chlorothiazide (see p.981). It has been given in doses of 2.5 to 5 mg twice daily or intermittently.

Proprietary Names and Manufacturers
The following names have been used for multi-ingredient preparations containing ethiazide— Hypertane Forte *(Medo, UK).*

2330-h

Ethoxzolamide
Ethoxyzolamide. 6-Ethoxybenzothiazole-2-sulphonamide.
$C_9H_{10}N_2O_3S_2$=258.3.

CAS — 452-35-7.

Ethoxzolamide is an inhibitor of carbonic anhydrase with actions and uses similar to those of acetazolamide (see p.976). Its effects last for about 10 hours.

In the treatment of glaucoma it is given in doses of 125 mg three times daily subsequently reduced to 62.5 mg three or four times daily if possible; an initial dose of 250 mg may be given.

Proprietary Names and Manufacturers
Cardrase *(Upjohn, Austral.; Upjohn, USA)*; Ethamide *(Allergan, USA)*; Glaucotensil *(Farmila, Ital.)*; Poenglausil *(Poen, Arg.)*; Redupresin *(Thilo, Ger.).*

12722-e

Etozolin *(USAN, rINN).*
Gö-687; W-2900A. Ethyl (3-methyl-4-oxo-5-piperidinothiazolidin-2-ylidene)acetate.
$C_{13}H_{20}N_2O_3S$=284.4.

CAS — 73-09-6.

Etozolin is a loop diuretic with properties similar to those of frusemide (see p.989). Etozolin is reported to be rapidly metabolised to ozolinone which also has diuretic activity. Etozolin is given in doses of 200 to 800 mg daily or intermittently.

For a series of papers on etozolin, see *Arzneimittel-Forsch.*, 1977, *27,* 1742–1817.

A study of the pharmacokinetics of etozolin and its active metabolite ozolinone in 6 hypertensive patients and 6 further hypertensive patients with chronic renal failure, following single doses of etozolin 400 mg by mouth. Etozolin had a prolonged diuretic effect lasting 12 to 18 hours, which was not significantly extended in chronic renal failure. In a further 15 hypertensive patients, of whom 11 had chronic renal failure, etozolin 400 mg daily for 14 days, alone or as part of an antihypertensive regimen, produced a decrease in blood pressure in 14, without any particular shift in electrolyte balance. All 15 patients lost weight during the study.— H. Knauf *et al., Eur. J. clin. Pharmac.*, 1984, *26,* 687.

Brief reviews of the properties of etozolin: A. Lant, *Drugs,* 1985, *29,* 57; B. Beermann and M. Grind, *Clin. Pharmacokinet.*, 1987, *13,* 254.

Proprietary Names and Manufacturers
Diuride *(Gibipharma, Ital.)*; Diuzolin *(Morgens, Spain)*; Elkapin *(Gödecke, Ger.; Parke, Davis, Ital.; Parke, Davis, Spain)*; Etopinil *(Wasserman, Spain).*

12745-a

Fenquizone Potassium *(rINNM).*
MG-13054. The potassium salt of 7-chloro-1,2,3,4-tetrahydro-4-oxo-2-phenylquinazoline-6-sulphonamide.
$C_{14}H_{11}ClKN_3O_3S$=375.9.

CAS — 20287-37-0 (fenquizone).

NOTE. Fenquizone is *USAN.*

Fenquizone potassium is a diuretic with properties similar to thiazides. It is given in usual doses of 10 to 20 mg daily.

References: R. Caldari *et al., Int. J. clin. Pharmacol. Res.*, 1982, *11,* 289; P. F. Angelino *et al., Int. J. clin. Pharmac. Ther. Toxic.*, 1985, *23,* 501; B. Beermann and M. Grind, *Clin. Pharmacokinet.*, 1987, *13,* 254.

Proprietary Names and Manufacturers
Idrolone *(Maggioni-Winthrop, Ital.).*

2331-m

Frusemide *(BAN).*
Furosemide *(USAN, rINN)*; Furosemidum; LB-502. 4-Chloro-*N*-furfuryl-5-sulphamoylanthranilic acid; 4-Chloro-2-furfurylamino-5-sulphamoylbenzoic acid.
$C_{12}H_{11}ClN_2O_5S$=330.7.

CAS — 54-31-9.

Pharmacopoeias. In *Aust., Br., Braz., Chin., Cz., Egypt., Eur., Fr., Ger., Ind., Int., It., Jpn, Jug., Neth., Nord., Swiss, Turk.*, and *U.S.* Also in *B.P. Vet.*

A white or slightly yellow, odourless, crystalline powder.

Practically **insoluble** in water; practically insoluble or very slightly soluble in chloroform; soluble 1 in 75 of alcohol; slightly soluble in ether; soluble or freely soluble in acetone; freely soluble in dimethylformamide; soluble in methyl alcohol and solutions of alkali hydroxides. **Protect** from light.

Solutions for injection are prepared with the aid of sodium hydroxide, giving solutions with a pH of 8.0 to 9.3 which can be **sterilised** by autoclaving. Such solutions should not be mixed or diluted with glucose injection or other acidic solutions.

INCOMPATIBILITY. Precipitation occurred when frusemide injection was mixed with dobutamine injection.— G. R. Hasegawa and J. F. Eder, *Am. J. Hosp. Pharm.*, 1984, *41,* 949.

Frusemide was precipitated when added to solutions containing either gentamicin or netilmicin in glucose 5% or sodium chloride 0.9%.— D. F. Thompson *et al., Am. J. Hosp. Pharm.*, 1985, *42,* 116.

STABILITY. Stability studies of frusemide in aqueous solutions.— A. G. Ghanekar *et al., J. pharm. Sci.*, 1978, *67,* 808. See also K. A. Shah *et al., ibid.*, 1980, *69,* 594.

Frusemide, 1 mg per mL in sodium chloride 0.9% in burette administration sets was found to be stable for up to 48 hours when exposed to diffuse daylight/fluorescent strip room lighting but decomposed rapidly on exposure to direct sunlight. Photodegradation could be overcome by the use of a burette protected with yellow PVC to protect the product from radiation in the 220 to 470 nm range (Amberset).— A. M. Yahya *et al., Int. J. Pharmaceut.*, 1986, *31,* 65.

Further references to the photodegradation of frusemide: D. E. Moore and V. Sithipitaks, *J. Pharm. Pharmac.*, 1983, *35,* 489; J. M. Neil *et al., Int. J. Pharmaceut.*, 1984, *22,* 105.

Adverse Effects
The most common side-effect associated with frusemide therapy is fluid and electrolyte imbalance including hyponatraemia, hypokalaemia, and hypochloraemic alkalosis, particularly after large doses or prolonged administration.

Other side-effects are relatively uncommon, and include allergy, nausea, diarrhoea, blurred vision, yellow vision, dizziness, headache, pancreatitis, photosensitivity, skin rashes, and hypotension. Bone marrow depression may occur rarely: agranulocytosis, thrombocytopenia, and leucopenia have been reported. Hepatic dysfunction, cholestatic jaundice, and paraesthesia have also been reported. Tinnitus and deafness may rarely occur in particular during rapid high-dose parenteral frusemide therapy. Rarely, deafness may be permanent particularly if frusemide has been given to patients taking other ototoxic drugs.

Frusemide may provoke hyperglycaemia and glycosuria, but probably to a lesser extent than the thiazide diuretics. It may cause hyperuricaemia and precipitate attacks of gout in some patients. Unlike the thiazide diuretics, it increases the urinary excretion of calcium. Renal stone formation has been reported when frusemide has been used to treat preterm infants.

A brief review of the clinical hazards of the powerful diuretics, frusemide and ethacrynic acid. By far the most frequently encountered problem is excessive depletion of blood volume, which can lead to profound shock, frequently complicated by hypokalaemia, and ending in death. Metabolic abnormalities comprise the second group of adverse effects from injudicious use of frusemide and ethacrynic acid; these include hypokalaemia, hyponatraemia, and metabolic or 'contraction' alkalosis. Less commonly, frusemide worsens carbohydrate tolerance; hyperuricaemia is frequent.— V. J. Plumb and T. N. James, *Mod. Concepts cardiovasc. Dis.*, 1978, *47,* 91.

Of 553 hospital in-patients receiving frusemide 220 experienced 480 adverse reactions. Considering only the most serious reactions, electrolyte disturbances occurred in 130 patients, extracellular volume depletion in 50, hepatic coma in 20, and other toxic effects in 20. Adverse reactions were more common in patients with cirrhosis of the liver.— C. A. Naranjo *et al., Am. J. Hosp. Pharm.*, 1978, *35,* 794.

The incidence of adverse effects attributed to frusemide in 585 hospital patients was: volume depletion (in 85), hyperuricaemia (54), hypokalaemia (21, equally in those with or without potassium supplements), hyponatraemia (6), gastro-intestinal effects (6), confusion (2), rash (1), thrombocytopenia (1), and glycosuria (1). Adverse effects were not related to renal function; in only 3 patients were adverse effects considered life-threatening (hypokalaemia in 2). Adverse effects were dose-related.— J. Lowe *et al., Br. med. J.*, 1979, *2,* 360.

Frusemide injection, which has a pH of about 9, would be expected to irritate tissues following extravasation.— R. Smith, *Br. J. parent. Ther.*, 1985, *6,* 30.

ALLERGY OR COLLAPSE. Death occurred in 2 elderly men almost immediately after they were given an injection of frusemide. Both patients had heart disease and mild diabetes.— I. Machtey (letter), *Lancet,* 1968, *2,* 1301.

Thirty seconds after an injection of frusemide a 7-year-old boy with the nephrotic syndrome collapsed with cardiac and circulatory arrest, and subsequently died. Although he had previously received frusemide both orally and intravenously, it was concluded that he had a cardiac arrest caused by hypersensitivity to frusemide.— C. P. Rance (letter), *ibid.*, 1969, *1,* 1265.

A report of cross allergy between glisoxepide, glibenclamide, frusemide, and probenecid in a 55-year-old diabetic man.— B. Ummenhofer and D. Djawari, *Dt. med. Wschr.*, 1979, *104,* 514.

See also under Effects on the Skin (below).

EFFECTS ON THE CIRCULATION. A report of leg ischaemia or superficial gangrene in 5 patients taking frusemide (plus amiloride in 3 patients). Dramatic improvement occurred on withdrawal of diuretics and rehydration.— D. A. O'Rourke and J. E. Hede, *Br. med. J.*, 1978, *1,* 1114.

In a study of 100 elderly patients with cerebral infarction or transient ischaemic attacks, a recent change in antihypertensive therapy was believed to have contributed to the pathogenesis of the stroke in 4 patients. Three of these 4 patients had been changed to frusemide therapy as had 3 other patients in whom the connection between treatment and stroke was less likely. It was considered that the use of powerful high-ceiling diuretics such as frusemide could cause cerebral ischaemia and should be avoided in the treatment of hypertension in the elderly.— P. A. F. Jansen *et al., Br. med. J.*, 1986, *293,* 914.

EFFECTS ON THE EARS. Reversible hearing loss in the medium- and high-frequency range occurred in 9 of 15 uraemic patients who were given intravenous infusions of 1 g of frusemide at the rate of 25 mg per minute. Very slight reversible impairment of hearing occurred in 4 of 10 patients given 600 mg at the rate of 15 mg per minute. There were no ototoxic effects in 10 patients who were given high doses of frusemide by slow infusion or by mouth for a prolonged period. Loss of hearing was considered to be a function of speed of infusion of frusemide.— A. Heidland and M. E. Wigand, *Klin. Wschr.*, 1970, *48,* 1052.

A report of permanent deafness in 6 patients following administration of frusemide during periods of impaired renal function. The onset of deafness was insidious and gradually progressive for up to 6 months after frusemide therapy.— C. A. Quick and W. Hoppe, *Ann. Otol. Rhinol. Lar.*, 1975, *84,* 94.

Further references to frusemide-induced ototoxicity: K. L. Gallagher and J. K. Jones, *Ann. intern. Med.*, 1979, *91,* 744.

EFFECTS ON THE ELECTROLYTE BALANCE. In 2 healthy subjects and 5 patients frusemide 80 mg caused no significant change in sodium, calcium, or magnesium concentrations in plasma; potassium and chloride fell; packed cell volume, protein, inorganic phosphorus, and urate rose; creatinine and urea rose after an initial fall. Frusemide causes acute changes in the concentrations of several plasma components and should be considered in any assessment of electrolyte disturbances.— T. O. Haug, *Br. med. J.*, 1976, *2*, 622.

Volume depletion and postural hypotension induced by diarrhoea in a patient taking frusemide and captopril.— P. R. Benett and S. A. Cairns (letter), *Lancet*, 1985, *1*, 1105.

Calcium. Despite the traditional view that frusemide administration lowers serum-calcium concentrations, they were raised in 11 of 13 male subjects by administration of 40 mg daily, for 3 weeks. It is suggested that low doses by mouth increase serum-calcium concentrations but that doses above 60 mg daily may depress them owing to urinary losses.— P. T. Chandler and S. A. Chandler, *Sth. med. J.*, 1977, *70*, 571.

Frusemide therapy in hypoparathyroid patients could result in hypocalcaemic tetany. In 6 hypoparathyroid patients the administration of frusemide 40 mg every 12 hours for 4 days produced a significant decrease in serum concentrations of ionised calcium. In 5 patients there was also an increase in urinary calcium excretion.— P. A. Gabow *et al.*, *Ann. intern. Med.*, 1977, *86*, 579. In a study of 36 patients with congestive heart failure, administration of frusemide or bumetanide produced an increase in serum concentrations of parathyroid hormone and a decrease in serum-calcium concentrations. An elevation in serum concentrations of alkaline phosphatase may have indicated accelerated bone remodelling as in primary hyperparathyroidism.— J. Elmgreen *et al.*, *Eur. J. clin. Pharmac.*, 1980, *18*, 363. Tetany was precipitated in a patient 18 years after thyroidectomy by administration of frusemide. The patient had asymptomatic hypocalcaemia before frusemide was given.— A. Bashey and W. MacNee, *Br. med. J.*, 1987, *295*, 960.

For reports of hypercalciuria, rickets, renal calculi, and hyperparathyroidism in neonates treated with frusemide, see under Pregnancy and the Neonate, below.

EFFECTS ON THE KIDNEY. Reversible renal failure associated with intestitial nephritis occurred in 4 patients with glomerulonephritis. It was considered that a hypersensitivity reaction to frusemide, taken by all 4, or a thiazide, taken by 3 could have been the cause, as renal function improved on cessation of the diuretics and administration of prednisone.— H. Lyons *et al.*, *New Engl. J. Med.*, 1973, *288*, 124. See also T. J. Fuller *et al.*, *J. Am. med. Ass.*, 1976, *235*, 1998.

EFFECTS ON LIPID METABOLISM. A study of the effects of frusemide on plasma lipoproteins in healthy subjects found that frusemide produced fewer changes in plasma lipids compared with thiazide diuretics, although increases in free palmitic and oleic acid concentrations were seen with all diuretics studied.— C. Joos *et al.*, *Eur. J. clin. Pharmac.*, 1980, *17*, 251.

EFFECTS ON THE NERVOUS SYSTEM. A report of severe generalised paraesthesia on 2 occasions in a cirrhotic patient following intravenous administration of frusemide. The mechanism was not understood and there were no clinical findings of anaphylaxis.— B. J. Materson, *J. Fla med. Assoc.*, 1971, *58*, 34.

EFFECTS ON THE PANCREAS. Brief case reports of 3 patients who developed pancreatitis after receiving frusemide intravenously.— N. Buchanan and R. D. Cane (letter), *Br. med. J.*, 1977, *2*, 1417.

EFFECTS ON THE SKIN. *Erythema multiforme.* A 65-year-old man developed erythema multiforme after treatment with a total dosage of 280 mg of frusemide by mouth. The rash and bullae resolved within 31 days.— T. P. Gibson and P. Blue (letter), *J. Am. med. Ass.*, 1970, *212*, 1709.

Further references to erythema multiforme in patients taking frusemide: C. Zugarman and E. J. La Voo (letter), *Archs Derm.*, 1980, *116*, 518.

Photosensitivity. Epidermolysis bullosa in 7 patients was attributed to frusemide which had been taken in doses of 0.5 to 2 g daily for 2 months to 3 years. The lesions persisted for 3 to 9 weeks and then regressed even when frusemide was continued.— A. C. Kennedy and A. Lyell, *Br. med. J.*, 1976, *1*, 1509.

Bullae and blistering of exposed areas of the skin occurred soon after the dose of frusemide was increased or high doses given in 4 patients with chronic renal failure. The reaction was considered to be phototoxic. There was no blistering following intermittent high intravenous doses of frusemide in 2 of these patients after the daily doses were discontinued and replaced by doses of ethacrynic acid, or in 1 patient when the high intermittent doses were given following a kidney transplant.— J. N. Burry and J. R. Lawrence, *Br. J. Derm.*, 1976, *94*, 495.

Frusemide had relatively high activity, similar to the phenothiazines, in an *in vitro* test for photosensitivity, and this might be the basis of reported skin reactions associated with its use.— D. E. Moore, *J. pharm. Sci.*, 1977, *66*, 1282.

Further references to photosensitivity reactions in patients taking frusemide: K. Keczkes and M. J. Farr (letter), *Br. med. J.*, 1976, *2*, 236.

Vasculitis. Cutaneous necrotising vasculitis in a 72-year-old man was presumably caused by an allergic reaction to frusemide.— W. H. Hendricks and R. S. Ader (letter), *Archs Derm.*, 1977, *113*, 375.

MISUSE. Deprecation of the use by jockeys of diuretics—usually frusemide 80 to 120 mg.— D. Price (letter), *Br. med. J.*, 1973, *1*, 804.

A woman had regularly taken frusemide 1.2 to 1.6 g daily for periods up to several weeks in an effort to lose weight. She had no evidence of renal dysfunction or other symptoms except malaise or fatigue and occasionally disturbances in potassium and chloride levels.— E. J. Howard (letter), *J. Am. med. Ass.*, 1976, *235*, 146.

PREGNANCY AND THE NEONATE. Administration of frusemide to 33 premature infants with respiratory distress syndrome was associated with a higher incidence of patent ductus arteriosus compared with infants treated with chlorothiazide. The mortality in the frusemide group was lower than in the chlorothiazide group. It was possible that the beneficial effects of frusemide could have balanced the harmful effects of patent ductus.— T. P. Green *et al.*, *New Engl. J. Med.*, 1983, *308*, 743.

Effects on calcium homoeostasis. Frusemide treatment was thought to have contributed to the development of rickets in 2 infants born prematurely, although it was not considered to have been a major factor.— A. E. Chudley *et al.*, *Archs Dis. Childh.*, 1980, *55*, 687.

Hypercalciuria was observed in 4 premature infants who were receiving long-term frusemide therapy. Parathyroid hormone concentration was elevated and bone mineral content depressed in 3 of the 4 infants, and 2 had ultrasound evidence of renal calcification. In one infant, autopsy showed evidence of calcium deposition in the kidney, and bone and parathyroid changes consistent with hyperparathyroidism.— P. S. Venkataraman *et al.*, *Am. J. Dis. Child.*, 1983, *137*, 1157.

Administration of frusemide to 2 premature infants with very low birth weights was associated with persistent disturbances in the calcium and phosphate balance. In one case this led to radiologically detectable osteopenia and fractures.— M. E. I. Morgan and S. E. Evans (letter), *Lancet*, 1986, *2*, 1399.

Renal calcification due to hypercalciuria during long-term treatment with frusemide has been reported in 10 premature infants (K.G. Hufnagle *et al.*, *Pediatrics*, 1982, *70*, 360). Report of a further case by Noe *et al.* (*J. Urol., Baltimore*, 1984, *132*, 93) also supported Hufnagle's observation that renal calcification could be reversed by the addition of a thiazide diuretic. Pearse *et al.* (*J. Ultrasound Med.*, 1984, *3*, 553) used renal ultrasound to diagnose renal calcification in 3 infants and recommended the use of ultrasound for regular examination of infants receiving frusemide to permit early diagnosis of calcification.

WITHDRAWAL. Apparent tolerance to the natriuretic action of frusemide in a patient following renal transplantation. When frusemide therapy was suddenly withdrawn, oedema rapidly recurrred. It was suggested that oedema could be perpetuated by secondary aldosteronism induced by the diuretic.— M. K. Chan *et al.*, *Br. med. J.*, 1979, *1*, 1604. Comment that the observed reduction in natriuresis was due to equilibration to a new steady state following the initiation of diuretic therapy and did not indicate that the diuretic response was reduced. The reaccumulation of oedema following withdrawal was to be expected since the underlying cause of the oedema had not been modified and it was not considered justifiable to suggest that withdrawal had led to rebound oedema or that diuretic therapy had perpetuated oedema.— L. E. Ramsay (letter), *ibid.*, *2*, 131. Reply.— M. K. Chan *et al.*, *ibid.*, 132.

Precautions

As for Chlorothiazide, p.982.

Frusemide is probably best avoided in pregnancy. It should be used with care in patients with prostatic hypertrophy or impairment of micturition. Frusemide may enhance the nephrotoxicity of cephalosporin antibiotics such as cephalothin and of aminoglycoside antibiotics. It can also enhance the ototoxicity of aminoglycoside antibiotics. Concurrent administration of phenytoin or indomethacin may reduce the clincal effects of frusemide.

INTERACTIONS. *Angiotensin-converting-enzyme inhibtors.* Although chronic therapy with frusemide and ACE inhibitors is generally effective and well tolerated, patients with volume depletion may develop an acute and severe hypotensive response following administration of ACE inhibitors.— *Drug Interact. News.*, 1987, *7*, 17.

Antibiotics. For the effect of frusemide on gentamicin, see Gentamicin Sulphate, p.238. For the effect of frusemide on chloramphenicol, see Chloramphenicol, p.188.

Antiepileptics. In 14 epileptic patients taking phenytoin and phenobarbitone (and in some cases other anti-epileptics) the mean diuretic effect of frusemide 20 mg was 68% of that in 10 healthy subjects and the peak effect was delayed from about 2 hours to about 4 hours. The diuretic effect of frusemide 40 mg in 17 epileptic patients was 51% of that in 10 healthy controls. The diuretic effect of frusemide 20 mg given intravenously to 12 epileptic patients was 50% of that in 5 healthy controls.— S. Ahmad, *Br. med. J.*, 1974, *3*, 657. In 5 healthy men absorption of frusemide and the maximum concentration in blood were reduced by about 50% when phenytoin 100 mg three times daily was taken for 10 days. Serum and renal clearance of frusemide were not changed. The mechanism was not clear but was not due to stimulation of microsomal enzymes.— A. Fine *et al.*, *ibid.*, 1977, *2*, 1061.

For the effect of frusemide on phenobarbitone, see Phenobarbitone, p.405.

Aspirin and other non-steroidal anti-inflammatory drugs. A review of the interactions between frusemide and non-steroidal anti-inflammatory drugs. Indomethacin, and other non-steroidal anti-inflammatory drugs including piroxicam, sulindac, naproxen, and ibuprofen have been reported to inhibit the diuretic and anti-hypertensive effects of frusemide. Sodium depletion due to frusemide may exacerbate the renal effects of non-steroidal anti-inflammatory drugs and result in a reduction in glomerular filtration. The interaction is probably due to the reduction of sodium excretion and inhibition of renal prostaglandins by non-steroidal anti-inflammatory drugs. The interaction is enhanced in patients who are sodium depleted including those with congestive heart failure, possibly because such patients exhibit greater renal vasodilatation in response to loop diuretics compared with patients with a normal sodium balance. However, frusemide-induced stimulation of renin release is suppressed by non-steroidal anti-inflammatory drugs independently of sodium balance and would appear to be mediated by prostaglandins.— *Drug Interact. News.*, 1986, *6*, 27.

Reports indicating that *aspirin* and other nonsteroidal anti-inflammatory agents can diminish the diuretic effect of frusemide: K. J. Berg, *Eur. J. clin. Pharmac.*, 1977, *11*, 111; *idem*, 117; H. Valette and E. Apoil (letter), *Br. J. clin. Pharmac.*, 1979, *8*, 592; E. Bartoli *et al.*, *J. clin. Pharmac.*, 1980, *20*, 452; A. C. Yeung Laiwah and R. A. Mactier, *Br. med. J.*, 1981, *283*, 714.

Results of a study suggesting that frusemide therapy may be ineffective in infants receiving *indomethacin* for patent ductus arteriosus.— Z. Friedman *et al.*, *J. Pediat.*, 1978, *93*, 512.

A pharmacokinetic evaluation of the attenuation of the diuretic effect of frusemide by indomethacin.— D. E. Smith *et al.*, *J. Pharmacokinet. Biopharm.*, 1979, *7*, 265.

For the effect of frusemide on indomethacin, see Indomethacin, p.23.

Chloral hydrate. Administration of frusemide intravenously to a patient who had been given chloral hydrate 8 and 12 hours previously on 2 occasions resulted in a sensation of heat, flushes, tachycardia, elevation of blood pressure to 160/90 mmHg, and severe diaphoresis. The reaction lasted 15 minutes. No adverse effects occurred after administration of frusemide alone.— M. Malach and N. Berman, *J. Am. med. Ass.*, 1975, *232*, 638. A retrospective study among 43 patients who had received both chloral hydrate and frusemide showed that 1 patient given frusemide 80 mg intravenously 8 hours after chloral hydrate had suffered a similar reaction; of 2 further patients who had possibly been affected, 1 had subsequently taken both drugs without side-effects.— M. P. Pevonka *et al.*, *Drug Intell. & clin. Pharm.*, 1977, *11*, 332.

Diuretics. For reference to severe electrolyte disturbances occurring in patients given metolazone concurrently with frusemide, see Metolazone, p.998.

Lithium. For comments on the use of diuretics including

frusemide in patients taking lithium, see Lithium Carbonate, p.368.

Probenecid. Reduction in the renal clearance of frusemide by concurrent administration of probenecid.— J. Honari *et al.*, *Clin. Pharmac. Ther.*, 1977, *22*, 395.

Further references to the effect of probenecid on frusemide: B. Odlind and B. Beermann, *Clin. Pharmac. Ther.*, 1980, *27*, 784; D. E. Smith *et al.*, *J. pharm. Sci.*, 1980, *69*, 571.

Theophylline. For the effect of frusemide on theophylline, see Theophylline, p.1529.

Warfarin. For reference to the lack of interaction between warfarin and frusemide, see p.346.

INTERFERENCE WITH DIAGNOSTIC TESTS. Frusemide, 20 mg intravenously, given to promote diuresis in tests for the localisation of urinary-tract infections, reduced the bacterial count in ureteric and bladder urine by a factor of 100 in a third of the patients. Thus it was impossible to distinguish renal from bladder infections.— K. F. Fairley (letter), *Lancet*, 1969, *1*, 1212.

Frusemide could interfere with the Schack and Waxler spectrophotometric assay for plasma-theophylline concentrations to give significantly false-positive elevations.— L. E. Matheson *et al.*, *Am. J. Hosp. Pharm.*, 1977, *34*, 496.

PORPHYRIA. A review of drug-induced porphyrias. Frusemide had been reported to be associated with clinical exacerbations of porphyria in isolated cases.— M. R. Moore and P. B. Disler, *Adverse Drug React. Ac. Pois. Rev.*, 1983, *2*, 149.

PREGNANCY AND THE NEONATE. A study indicating that frusemide is a potent displacer of bilirubin and should be used with caution in jaundiced infants.— S. Shankaran *et al.*, *J. Pediat.*, 1977, *90*, 642. A study indicating that on a molar basis, chlorothiazide, frusemide, and ethacrynic acid are at least as potent as sulphafurazole in displacing bilirubin from albumin. Frusemide and ethacrynic acid, when used in the recommended doses of 1 mg per kg body-weight, would probably not produce a significant increase in free bilirubin in most infants, but the weaker diuretic, chlorothiazide, in its recommended dose of 15 to 20 mg per kg, would result in substantially higher plasma concentrations, and hence would be an inappropriate alternative to frusemide for diuretic therapy in jaundiced infants.— R. P. Wennberg *et al.*, *ibid.*, 647. Confirmation that a single dose of frusemide 1 mg per kg body-weight does not displace bilirubin from the albumin binding site. Doses greater than 1.5 mg per kg or repeated doses could potentially do so.— J. V. Aranda *et al.*, *ibid.*, 1978, *93*, 507.

The use of frusemide in late pregnancy should be avoided if the adequacy of placental perfusion was suspect.— D. C. Dukes, *Practitioner*, 1978, *220*, 285.

Absorption and Fate

Frusemide is incompletely but fairly rapidly absorbed from the gastro-intestinal tract; bioavailability has been reported to be about 60 to 70% but is reduced in renal failure. It has a biphasic half-life in the plasma with a terminal elimination phase that has been estimated to range up to about 1½ hours although it is prolonged in renal and hepatic insufficiency. It is up to 99% bound to plasma proteins, and is mainly excreted in the urine, largely unchanged. Variable amounts are also excreted in the bile, non-renal elimination being considerably increased in renal failure. Frusemide crosses the placental barrier and is excreted in milk.

A detailed review of the clinical pharmacokinetics of frusemide. In healthy subjects the bioavailability from commercial tablets is 60 to 69% and is similar to that from an aqueous solution. In patients with end-stage renal disease, the absorption is reduced to 43 to 46%. Food delays the absorption but does not reduce the total amount absorbed. Plasma-protein binding in healthy subjects has been shown to be 91 to 99%. Frusemide binds almost exclusively to albumin and competes for binding sites with other acidic drugs. The proportion of bound frusemide is lower in patients with nephrotic syndrome and in acute and chronic renal failure. After intravenous administration intact frusemide is the major urinary product in the first 4 hours. After this time, frusemide glucuronide and the free amine metabolite are also found. Between 6 and 18% of an intravenous dose is found in the faeces in healthy subjects. In renal failure this is increased to 60%. The elimination half-life in neonates is prolonged, and a value of over 7 hours was reported in newborn infants with fluid overload. The elimination rate is also reduced in patients with end-stage renal disease, cardiac disease, hypertension, and liver disease.— R. E. Cutler and A. D. Blair, *Clin. Pharmacokinet.*, 1979, *4*, 279.

Further reviews of the pharmacokinetics of frusemide: L. Z. Benet, *J. Pharmacokinet. Biopharm.*, 1979, *7*, 1.

Confirmation in 6 healthy subjects that despite reduced bioavailability of frusemide given by mouth the total diuretic response is the same as after intravenous administration.— R. A. Branch *et al.*, *Br. J. Pharmac.*, 1976, *57*, 442P. The response to frusemide was determined by the concentration of drug in the tissue compartment rather than in plasma.— *idem*, *Br. J. clin. Pharmac.*, 1977, *4*, 121.

Evidence of reduced bioavailability of frusemide in oedema and suggestion that the intravenous route be tried before a diagnosis of diuretic resistance is made.— B. G. Odlind and B. Beermann, *Br. med. J.*, 1980, *280*, 1577.

References to altered kinetics of frusemide in some disease states: R. Fuller *et al.*, *Clin. Pharmac. Ther.*, 1981, *30*, 461 (in hepatic cirrhosis with ascites); D. E. Smith and L. Z. Benet, *Eur. J. clin. Pharmac.*, 1983, *24*, 787 (in kidney transplant patients); D. E. Smith *et al.*, *J. pharm. Sci.*, 1985, *74*, 603 (in nephrotic patients); M. R. Vasko *et al.*, *Ann. intern. Med.*, 1985, *102*, 314 (altered absorption in congestive heart failure); J. -P. Villeneuve *et al.*, *Clin. Pharmac. Ther.*, 1986, *40*, 14 (in cirrhosis); H. Nakahama *et al.*, *Eur. J. clin. Pharmac.*, 1987, *32*, 313 (in kidney transplant patients).

References to altered kinetics of frusemide in elderly patients: A. L. M. Kerremans *et al.*, *Clin. Pharmac. Ther.*, 1983, *34*, 181; F. Andreasen *et al.*, *Br. J. clin. Pharmac.*, 1983, *16*, 391.

Plasma protein binding was reduced in elderly patients.— G. M. Pacifici *et al.*, *Eur. J. clin. Pharmac.*, 1987, *32*, 199.

Uses and Administration

Frusemide is a potent diuretic with a rapid action. Its effects are evident within 30 minutes to 1 hour after a dose by mouth and last for about 4 to 6 hours; after intravenous injection its effects are evident in about 5 minutes and last for about 2 hours. Frusemide inhibits the reabsorption of electrolytes in the ascending limb of the loop of Henle and also in the distal renal tubules. It may also have a direct effect in the proximal tubules. Excretion of sodium, potassium, and chloride ions is increased and water excretion enhanced. It has no clinically significant effect on carbonic anhydrase.

Frusemide is used similarly to chlorothiazide (see p.983) and may be effective in patients unresponsive to thiazide diuretics. It is also used in the treatment of renal insufficiency.

Unlike the thiazide diuretics where, owing to their flat dose-response curve, very little is gained by increasing the dose, frusemide has a steep dose-response curve, which gives it a wide therapeutic range.

In the treatment of oedema, the usual initial dose is 40 mg once daily, adjusted as necessary according to response. Mild cases may respond to 20 mg daily or 40 mg on alternate days. Some patients may require doses of 80 mg or more daily given as one or two doses daily, or intermittently. Severe cases may require gradual titration of the frusemide dosage up to 600 mg daily. In emergency or when oral therapy cannot be given, 20 to 50 mg may be administered by intramuscular or slow intravenous (over 1 to 2 minutes) injection; if necessary further doses may be given, increasing by 20 mg increments and not given more often than every 2 hours. If doses greater than 50 mg are required it is recommended that they be given by slow intravenous infusion. For pulmonary oedema, sources in the *USA* have recommended that if an initial slow intravenous injection of 40 mg (over 1 to 2 minutes) does not produce a satisfactory response within one hour, the dose may be increased to 80 mg given slowly intravenously.

For children, the usual dose by mouth is 1 to 3 mg per kg body-weight daily or on alternate days; suggested doses by injection are 0.5 to 1.5 mg per kg although doses of up to 6 mg per kg have been given.

In the treatment of hypertension, frusemide is given in doses of 40 to 80 mg daily, either alone, or in conjunction with other antihypertensive agents. Doses of 40 to 80 mg have also been given by slow intravenous injection for hypertensive crises.

When treatment is prolonged, or in susceptible patients, loss of potassium may be sufficient to produce hypokalaemia; potassium supplements or potassium-sparing diuretics should then be given as for chlorothiazide (p.983).

High-dose therapy. In the management of oliguria in acute or chronic renal failure frusemide 250 mg diluted to 250 mL in a suitable diluent is infused over one hour. If urine output is insufficient within the next hour, this dose may be followed by 500 mg added to an appropriate infusion fluid, the total volume of which must be governed by the patient's state of hydration, and infused over 2 hours. If a satisfactory urine output has still not been achieved within one hour of the end of the second infusion then a third dose of 1 g may be infused over 4 hours. The rate of infusion should never exceed 4 mg per minute. In oliguric or anuric patients with significant fluid overload, the injection may be given without dilution directly into the vein, using a constant-rate infusion pump with a micrometer screw-gauge adjustment; the rate of administration should still never exceed 4 mg per minute. Patients who do not respond to a dose of 1 g probably require dialysis, although doses of up to 6 g daily have been tried. If the response to either method of administration is satisfactory, the effective dose (of up to 1 g) may then be given daily. Dosage adjustments should subsequently be made according to the patient's response. Alternatively, treatment may be maintained by mouth; 500 mg should be given by mouth for each 250 mg required by injection.

In the treatment of chronic renal insufficiency, an initial dose of 250 mg may be given by mouth, increased, if necessary in steps of 250 mg every 4 to 6 hours to a maximum of 2 g; dosage adjustments should subsequently be made according to the patient's response.

During treatment with these high-dose forms of frusemide therapy, careful laboratory control is essential. Fluid balance and electrolytes should be carefully controlled and, in particular, in patients with shock, measures should be taken to correct the blood pressure and circulating blood volume, before commencing this type of treatment. High-dose frusemide therapy is contra-indicated in renal failure caused by nephrotoxic or hepatotoxic agents, and in renal failure associated with hepatic coma.

For references to the choice of diuretics and their uses, and to prophylaxis and treatment of diuretic-induced hypokalaemia, see p.973.

A brief review of the actions of frusemide.— A. Lant, *Drugs*, 1985, *29*, 57.

A study suggesting that frusemide is eliminated predominantly by proximal tubular secretion, and that tubular, rather than plasma, concentration is the main determinant of its diuretic effect. The renal tubular site of action of frusemide is still debated, but most of the evidence points to the thick ascending limb of Henle's loop as the primary area of frusemide action, with somewhat conflicting results regarding its proximal tubular effect.— J. Honari *et al.*, *Clin. Pharmac. Ther.*, 1977, *22*, 395. See also M. Homeida *et al.*, *ibid.*, 402.

Contribution of prostaglandins to the systemic and renal vascular response to frusemide in normal man.— I. G. MacKay *et al.*, *Br. J. clin. Pharmac.*, 1984, *17*, 513.

The dose-response characteristics of the acute non-diuretic peripheral vascular effects of frusemide in healthy subjects.— G. D. Johnston *et al.*, *Br. J. clin. Pharmac.*, 1984, *18*, 75.

A review of the mechanisms and management of resistance to loop diuretics. In some cases sodium intake may be sufficient to overcome the diuretic effect, and limiting sodium intake could restore responsiveness. Often, however, the response to the diuretic is influenced by factors affecting the total amount of drug reaching the urine, the time course of its entry into the urine, and the pharmacodynamics of response to diuretic in the urine. Several clinical conditions can modify these factors leading to resistance: in patients with moderate renal insufficiency and the elderly insufficient drug may reach the urine; in nephrotic syndrome the diuretic may bind to proteins in urine; in hepatic cirrhosis an alteration in the pharmacodynamics appears to be responsible for resistance; and patients with congestive heart failure appear to have both an alteration in the dose-response curve and delayed absorption following oral administration. Strategies for overcoming resistance include increasing the size of the dose, increasing the frequency of administration or administering by continuous intravenous infusion, and concomitant administration of a diuretic with a different site of action such as hydrochlorothiazide or metolazone.— D. C. Brater, *Drugs*, 1985, *30*, 427.

Comment on the use of combined therapy with loop and thiazide-type diuretics in patients with resistant sodium retention. A synergistic effect has been reported with this combination and can be highly effective in refractory oedema. However the massive diuresis which results can lead to serious disturbances in fluid and electrolyte balance which have, on occasion, been fatal. The potential risk was considered justifiable in patients with marked resistant sodium retention and severe congestive heart failure or hypertension, particularly in the presence of renal insufficiency but therapy must be initiated cautiously and patients must be carefully monitored; hospitalisation may be indicated for the initiation of this therapy in some cases.— J. R. Oster *et al.*, *Ann. intern. Med.*, 1983, *99*, 405.

ADMINISTRATION IN RENAL FAILURE. Frusemide could be administered to patients with renal failure in normal doses. No dosage supplements were required in patients undergoing haemodialysis.— W. M. Bennett *et al.*, *Am. J. Kidney Dis.*, 1983, *3*, 155.

Study of the response to frusemide in chronic renal insufficiency. It was shown that the delivery of frusemide into the urine was prolonged in patients with chronic renal insufficiency, and this could account for the extended, low intensity diuresis found in such patients. It was also found that the nephrons remaining showed an exaggerated maximal response, and a dose of frusemide 160 mg intravenously was sufficient to reach the upper plateau of the dose-response curve in these patients, suggesting that the use of higher individual doses would not elicit a greater response in patients with chronic renal insufficiency.— D. C. Brater *et al.*, *Clin. Pharmac. Ther.*, 1986, *40*, 134.

CARDIAC DISORDERS. *Heart failure.* Indications that frusemide may have a beneficial haemodynamic effect on the heart, independent of its diuretic effect.— K. Dikshit *et al.*, *New Engl. J. Med.*, 1973, *288*, 1087.

The successful use of frusemide by infusion (4 to 16 mg per hour) in 10 patients with congestive heart failure unresponsive to single doses of 120 mg by mouth.— D. H. Lawson *et al.*, *Br. med. J.*, 1978, *2*, 476.

In patients with advanced cardiac failure a reduction in the excretion of frusemide into the urine compared with patients with moderate cardiac failure was correlated with the diuretic effect. Administration of hydralazine enhanced the diuretic effect of frusemide, possibly due to an improvement in renal blood flow.— A. Nomura *et al.*, *Clin. Pharmac. Ther.*, 1981, *30*, 177.

The successful use of frusemide 8 g daily intravenously for 9 days and 4 g daily for 4 days in a patient with severe cardiac failure secondary to primary hypertension which was unresponsive to digoxin, spironolactone, captopril, nifedipine, and frusemide, 2 g daily by mouth. Treatment was associated with no adverse effects, and specifically with no deterioration in renal or hepatic function and no signs of ototoxicity.— M. F. O'Rourke *et al.* (letter), *Archs intern. Med.*, 1984, *144*, 2429.

A study involving 14 patients with advanced congestive heart failure found that treatment with frusemide and captopril produced diuresis and correction of hyponatraemia not seen during treatment with captopril alone. It was suggested that captopril enhanced the renal effect of frusemide, either by increasing the distal delivery of solute or increasing the delivery of frusemide to the loop of Henle for its action.— V. J. Dzau and N. K. Hollenberg, *Ann. intern. Med.*, 1984, *100*, 777. Comment on the use of frusemide and captopril to correct hyponatraemia in patients with congestive heart failure.— R. W. Hamilton and V. M. Buckalew, *ibid.*, 902.

A study in 15 patients with chronic congestive heart failure indicating that intravenous frusemide could promote further clinical haemodynamic deterioration during the first 20 minutes. However, this was not considered to compromise the usefulness of frusemide in heart failure.— G. S. Francis *et al.*, *Ann. intern. Med.*, 1985, *103*, 1.

In a study of 10 patients with symptoms of heart failure despite treatment with frusemide 40 mg and amiloride 5 mg daily, greater symptomatic benefit was obtained by increasing the dose of frusemide than by adding captopril.— A. J. Cowley *et al.*, *Lancet*, 1986, *2*, 770. Although both increasing the dosage of frusemide and adding captopril produced symptomatic improvement in a study of 29 patients with heart failure, captopril produced a more favourable effect on the heart.— A. Boccanelli *et al.* (letter), *ibid.*, 1331.

Reports on sustained-release formulations of frusemide in the treatment of chronic heart failure: A. Vermeulen and D. R. Chadha, *J. clin. Pharmac.*, 1982, *22*, 513; idem, *Eur. J. clin. Pharmac.*, 1983, *24*, 449; S. K. Pehrsson, *ibid.*, 1985, *28*, 235.

Myocardial infarction. In a study of 73 patients with acute myocardial infarction, supraventricular tachyarrhythmias were more common in patients treated with frusemide 120 mg intravenously than in patients given frusemide 20 mg intravenously, while ventricular extrasystoles and ventricular tachycardia were more common with frusemide 20 mg. The study suggested that heart rate and the recurrence of both supraventricular and ventricular tachyarrhythmias were influenced by diuretic therapy, probably through mechanisms other than electrolyte disturbances.— F. F. Larsen and L. Mogensen, *Eur. Heart J.*, 1986, *7*, 210.

HEPATIC DISORDERS. Results of a controlled study (using spironolactone and/or frusemide in the active drug group) indicated that diuresis aiming at a modest rate of diuresis can be accomplished in patients with decompensated alcoholic liver disease and ascites of recent onset, without serious complications that can be attributed to diuretic therapy.— P. B. Gregory *et al.*, *Gastroenterology*, 1977, *73*, 534.

A review of the diagnosis and management of cirrhotic ascites. Frusemide had been found to be less effective than spironolactone in the management of ascites.— V. K. Rocco and A. J. Ware, *Ann. intern. Med.*, 1986, *105*, 573. Comment that frusemide could be effective in patients with cirrhotic ascites although there was the risk that frusemide-induced hypokalaemia could precipitate hepatic encephalopathy.— A. Spital (letter), *ibid.*, 1987, *106*, 169.

Frusemide may have synergistic actions with mannitol in the reduction of increased intracranial pressure and has also proved useful in the reduction of both cytotoxic and vasogenic cerebral oedema in patients with fulminant hepatic failure.— I. Corall and R. Williams, *Br. J. Anaesth.*, 1986, *58*, 234.

In children. Comment on the use of diuretic therapy for ascites and oedema associated with hepatic diseases in children. Hypokalaemia and dehydration are particular risks with frusemide and the thiazide diuretics. Spironolactone is the logical diuretic to use; it may be adequate used alone, or the addition of a small dose of frusemide or a thiazide diuretic may yield the desired diuresis.— D. M. Danks (letter), *J. Pediat.*, 1976, *88*, 695.

HYPERCALCAEMIA. Diuresis, resulting in a fall in serum-calcium concentrations of 23 to 38 μg per mL, occurred after a dose of frusemide of 80 to 100 mg intravenously in 8 patients with serum-calcium concentrations of 123 to 184 μg per mL due to various causes. Urinary losses of magnesium, potassium, sodium, and water were measured and replaced.— W. N. Suki *et al.*, *New Engl. J. Med.*, 1970, *283*, 836.

A discussion of the management of severe hypercalcaemia. Most patients with severe hypercalcaemia are profoundly salt and water depleted, often with renal impairment. Once the volume deficit has been corrected by infusion of sodium chloride 0.9%, the addition of frusemide 40 to 80 mg by intravenous infusion every 2 to 4 hours will further increase the urinary calcium excretion.— P. J. Altmann and J. Cunningham, *Postgrad. med. J.*, 1987, *63*, 77.

See also under Adverse Effects, Effects on the Electrolyte Balance.

HYPERTENSION. A review of the management of chronic hypertension. Frusemide has a shorter duration of action than the thiazide diuretics and may be less effective for treatment of hypertension. Use of frusemide in hypertension should be reserved for patients with fluid retention that cannot be controlled with thiazides or for patients with impaired renal function.— *Med. Lett.*, 1984, *26*, 107.

In 27 hypertensive patients whose blood pressure was not controlled by 3 or more drugs including a thiazide diuretic, a change in therapy, either by substituting frusemide for the thiazide or by adding spironolactone, resulted in a significant fall in blood pressure and loss of weight.— L. E. Ramsay *et al.*, *Br. med. J.*, 1980, *281*, 1101.

In patients with hypertension resistant to therapy with a thiazide diuretic, a beta blocker, and either prazosin, hydralazine, or methyldopa, the addition of frusemide produced a greater reduction in blood pressure than increasing the dose of thiazide, but at the expense of a decline in renal function, marked hypokalaemia, and an orthostatic effect.— S. Freestone *et al.*, *Br. J. clin. Pharmac.*, 1982, *14*, 137P.

Frusemide reversed hypertension, renal hypoprostaglandinism, and type IV renal tubular acidosis in a 13-year-old girl.— S. A. Sanjad *et al.*, *Ann. intern. Med.*, 1983, *99*, 624.

References to haemodynamic and endocrine responses to frusemide in hypertension: T. W. Wilson, *Clin. Pharmac. Ther.*, 1983, *34*, 590; I. G. MacKay *et al.*, *Clin. Sci.*, 1985, *68*, 159.

Once-daily administration. There was no significant difference between the mean arterial blood pressure obtained in 38 patients with hypertension when they took frusemide 80 mg as a once-daily dose for a mean of 191 days and in 2 divided doses for a mean of 173 days. Other antihypertensive therapy remained unchanged. Of 13 patients who had complained of nocturia during the twice-daily regimen, none reported this during the once-daily administration.— M. E. Davidov and W. J. Mroczek, *Curr. ther. Res.*, 1978, *23*, 300.

High-dose therapy. In 10 patients with severe hypertension (7 with essential arterial hypertension) frusemide in doses of 0.12 to 4 g daily produced a significantly greater reduction in blood pressure than previous conventional antihypertensive medication; maintenance doses were 40 mg to 2 g daily. Patients received dietary and/or supplementary sodium up to 680 mmol (680 mEq) daily and all received potassium 60 to 150 mmol (60 to 150 mEq) daily.— F. Cantarovich *et al.*, *Nephron*, 1974, *12*, 133.

Renin categorisation. A simple screening test for hypertension in outpatients was assessed in 40 hypertensive patients. Frusemide 60 mg was taken by mouth and plasma-renin activity measured 5 hours later. The results fell into 4 groups: extreme hyporeninaemia (primary aldosteronoma), suppressed renin (confirmed suppressed-renin hypertension), normal renin (essential hypertension), and elevated renin (renovascular hypertension). Identification of patients requiring further evaluation for remediable secondary causes was possible. All medication should be withheld for at least 1 week before testing because many drugs affected plasma-renin activity.— L. Wallach *et al.*, *Ann. intern. Med.*, 1975, *82*, 27.

INAPPROPRIATE SECRETION OF ANTIDIURETIC HORMONE. A review of the management of the syndrome of inappropriate secretion of diuretic hormone. Water restriction remains the mainstay of therapy. If acute water intoxication occurs, frusemide intravenously and hypertonic sodium chloride are effective but must be used cautiously to avoid adverse effects. Frusemide may also be helpful in long-term maintenance, and loop diuretics or demeclocycline appear to be the treatments of choice although further comparative studies are needed.— C. I. Miyagawa, *Drug Intell. & clin. Pharm.*, 1986, *20*, 527.

A patient with the syndrome of inappropriate secretion of antidiuretic hormone and symptomatic hyponatraemia was treated successfully with frusemide 40 mg daily together with a liberal sodium intake. A diet containing 100 mmol of salt was supplemented initially with sodium chloride tablets to give a total salt intake of 200 mmol.— G. Decaux *et al.*, *New Engl. J. Med.*, 1981, *304*, 329.

Seven out of 9 patients with chronic inappropriate secretion of antidiuretic hormone were successfully treated with frusemide 40 mg daily. One patient responded to frusemide 80 mg. The lack of response in the remaining patient could have been due to a relatively low creatinine clearance.— G. Decaux *et al.*, *Br. med. J.*, 1982, *285*, 89.

PREGNANCY AND THE NEONATE. *Diagnosis and testing.* Negative scanning for a foetal bladder following administration of frusemide to the mother to increase foetal urine production, strongly supports a diagnosis of renal agenesis (Potter syndrome).— R. P. Balfour and K. M. Laurence (letter), *Lancet*, 1980, *1*, 317. See also M. J. N. Keirse and R. H. Meerman, *Obstet. Gynec.*, 1978, *52*, 64.

Frusemide was used as a challenge test in assessing bilateral foetal hydronephrosis.— R. J. Barrett *et al.*, *Am. J. Obstet. Gynec.*, 1983, *147*, 846.

Lactation. Frusemide 40 mg each morning for 3 to 6 days was effective for the suppression of lactation.— R. G. H. Wade (letter), *Br. med. J.*, 1977, *1*, 442.

Patent ductus arteriosus. A discussion of delayed closure of ductus (DCD) in premature infants. The usual treatment for a haemodynamically significant ductus is reduction of fluid intake, correction of anaemia, and the administration of a diuretic. Frusemide is effective and widely used but there is some concern over a report that it may promote the development of DCD in infants with respiratory distress syndrome (see under Pregnancy and the Neonate in Adverse Effects, above). However, it is encouraging that the concurrent use of frusemide does not seem to inhibit duct closure during treatment with indomethacin.— *Lancet*, 1983, *2*, 436.

Respiratory distress syndrome. A brief discussion of the hazards of frusemide therapy in premature infants. Treatment with frusemide for bronchopulmonary dysplasia may produce both potential benefits and serious risks. Therapy should be undertaken cautiously with special attention to the risks to the kidneys.— L. Finberg, *Am. J. Dis. Child.*, 1983, *137*, 1145.

Study in 99 premature infants with severe respiratory distress syndrome indicating that frusemide administration is beneficial when spontaneous diuresis does not occur, and may be particularly effective if combined with early closure of the ductus arteriosus.— T. P. Green *et al.*, *J. Pediat.*, 1983, *103*, 618. Frusemide improved the pulmonary status in 29 infants with respiratory distress syndrome who required mechanical ventilation compared with 27 control infants, and was not associated with an increased incidence of patent ductus arteriosus. However, there was no difference in morbidity from bronchopulmonary dysplasia, or mortality between the two groups, and in consideration of potential adverse renal effects, routine use of frusemide could not be recommended.— T. F. Yeh *et al.*, *ibid.*, 1984, *105*, 603.

In a study of 85 premature babies with respiratory distress syndrome, 42 received three intravenous injections of frusemide 1 mg per kg body-weight at 24-hour intervals, and 43 received no diuretic treatment. The use of frusemide increased urine-sodium and chloride throughout the study period, but did not increase urine output until 24 hours after commencing treatment. Hypoxia, dehydration, and a low glomerular filtration-rate may contribute to the delay in diuretic response to frusemide.— T. F. Yeh *et al.*, *Archs Dis. Childh.*, 1985, *60*, 621.

Further references to the use of frusemide in respiratory distress syndrome: M. O. Savage *et al.*, *Archs Dis. Childh.*, 1975, *50*, 709.

See also under Precautions for Frusemide (Pregnancy and the Neonate) and Precautions for Chlorothiazide (Pregnancy and the Neonate).

PULMONARY OEDEMA. In a study involving 21 patients with pulmonary oedema, frusemide 40 or 80 mg intravenously did not deplete intravascular volume. It was suggested that the intravascular volume was replenished, possibly by reabsorption of oedematous fluid, at a rate equal to or greater than the volume removed by diuresis.— C. -J. Schuster *et al.*, *Am. J. Med.*, 1984, *76*, 585.

RAISED INTRACRANIAL PRESSURE. A study in 20 patients scheduled for craniotomy indicating that, while mannitol infusion could produce a transient increase in intracranial pressure, frusemide produced a decrease in intracranial pressure starting with the peak of diuresis. Frusemide may be preferred to mannitol in neurosurgery, especially when the patient already has increased intracranial pressure, an altered blood-brain barrier, or increased pulmonary water content, or in those with pre-existing cardiac and electrolyte abnormalities.— J. E. Cottrell *et al.*, *Anesthesiology*, 1977, *47*, 28.

The use of loop diuretics for the reduction of post-traumatic intracranial hypertension remains controversial. Concomitant administration of frusemide and mannitol has additive effects on the degree and duration of intracranial pressure. Osmotic therapy remains the treatment of choice for reduction of persistently elevated intracranial pressure. The authors' current practice was to administer mannitol 0.5 g per kg body-weight over 15 to 20 minutes combined with frusemide 300 to 600 µg per kg intravenously, followed by an infusion of plasma protein 1.5 mL per kg over the next hour. This regimen was repeated every 4 to 6 hours if needed, with close attention to serum-electrolyte concentrations and osmolality.— N. M. Dearden, *Br. J. Hosp. Med.*, 1986, *36*, 94.

Further references to the use of frusemide in cerebral oedema: S. G. F. Matts, *Br. J. clin. Pract.*, 1972, *26*, 361; J. Thilmann and H. Zeumer, *Dt. med. Wschr.*, 1974, *99*, 932.

Preparations

Frusemide Injection *(B.P.)*. Containing frusemide sodium, prepared from frusemide and sodium hydroxide. Potency is expressed in terms of the equivalent amount of frusemide.

Frusemide Tablets *(B.P.)*

Furosemide Injection *(U.S.P.)*. Containing frusemide and sodium hydroxide. Potency is expressed in terms of frusemide.

Furosemide Tablets *(U.S.P.)*. Tablets containing frusemide.

Proprietary Preparations

Aluzine *(Steinhard, UK)*. *Tablets*, scored, frusemide 20, 40, and 500 mg.

Diumide-K Continus *(Degussa, UK)*. *Tablets*, frusemide 40 mg, potassium chloride 600 mg (potassium 8 mmol) for sustained release.

Dryptal *(Berk Pharmaceuticals, UK)*. *Tablets*, scored, frusemide 40 and 500 mg.

Injection, frusemide 10 mg/mL, in ampoules of 2 and 5 mL.

Frumil *(Rorer, UK)*. *Tablets*, scored, frusemide 40 mg, anhydrous amiloride hydrochloride 5 mg.

Frusene *(Fisons, UK)*. *Tablets*, scored, frusemide 40 mg, triamterene 50 mg.

Frusetic *(Unimed, UK)*. *Tablets*, scored, frusemide 40 mg.

Frusid *(DDSA Pharmaceuticals, UK)*. *Tablets*, scored, frusemide 40 mg.

Lasikal *(Hoechst, UK)*. *Tablets*, frusemide 20 mg, potassium chloride 750 mg (potassium 10 mmol) for sustained release.

Owing to the risk of intestinal obstruction, sustained-release preparations such as Lasikal, where the drug is released in transit, but the matrix ghost is often eliminated intact, should not be prescribed in patients with Crohn's disease or other intestinal disease in which strictures may form.— J. L. Shaffer *et al.* (letter), *Lancet*, 1980, *2*, 487.

Lasilactone *(Hoechst, UK)*. *Capsules*, frusemide 20 mg, spironolactone 50 mg.

Lasix *(Hoechst, UK)*. *Tablets*, scored, frusemide 20, 40, and 500 mg.

Paediatric liquid, granules for reconstitution, frusemide 1 mg/mL when reconstituted with water.

Injection, frusemide 10 mg/mL, in ampoules of 2, 5, and 25 mL.

Lasix + K *(Hoechst, UK)*. *Tablets*, calendar pack; 30 tablets, scored, frusemide 40 mg; 60 tablets, potassium chloride 750 mg (potassium 10 mmol) for sustained release.

Lasoride *(Hoechst, UK)*. *Tablets*, frusemide 40 mg, amiloride hydrochloride 5 mg.

Min-I-Jet Frusemide Injection *(IMS, UK)*. *Injection*, frusemide 10 mg/mL, in single-use prefilled syringes of 4, 8, 10, 12, 25, and 50 mL.

Proprietary Names and Manufacturers

Aluzine *(Steinhard, UK)*; Aquamide *(Austral.)*; Aquasin *(Adcock Ingram, S.Afr.)*; Arasemide *(Jpn)*; Discoid *(Sagitta, Ger.)*; Diural *(A.L., Denm.*; *Apothekernes Laboratorium, Norw.*; *A.L., Swed.)*; Diuresal *(Lagap, Switz.*; *Lagap, UK)*; Diurolasa *(Lasa, Spain)*; Dryptal *(Berk Pharmaceuticals, UK)*; Durafurid *(Durachemie, Ger.)*; Errolon *(Arg.)*; Franyl *(Jpn)*; Frusetic *(Unimed, UK)*; Frusid *(Austral.*; *DDSA Pharmaceuticals, UK)*; Furetic *(Propan, S.Afr.)*; Furix *(Benzon, Denm.*; *Benzon, Norw.*; *Benzon, Swed.)*; Furo-basan *(Schönenberger, Switz.)*; Fur-O-Ims *(IMS, UK)*; Furo-Puren *(Klinge-Nattermann, Ger.)*; Furose *(Ascher, USA)*; Furoside *(ICN, Canad.)*; Fusid *(Schwarzhaupt, Ger.)*; Hydrex *(Rolab, S.Afr.)*; Hydro-rapid *(Beiersdorf, Ger.)*; Impugan *(Dumex, Denm.*; *Dumex, Norw.*; *Dumex, Swed.*; *Dumex, Switz.)*; Lasiletten *(Neth.)*; Lasilix *(Alg.*; *Hoechst, Fr.*; *Mor.*; *Tun.)*; Lasix *(Hoechst, Austral.*; *Belg.*; *Hoechst, Canad.*; *Hoechst, Denm.*; *Hoechst, Ger.*; *Hoechst, Ital.*; *Neth.*; *Hoechst, Norw.*; *Hoechst, S.Afr.*; *Hoechst, Swed.*; *Hoechst, Switz.*; *Hoechst, UK*; *Hoechst, USA)*; Laxur *(Chile)*; Min-I-Jet Frusemide *(IMS, UK)*; Moilarorin *(Jpn)*; Neo-Renal *(Canad.)*; Nicorol *(Denm.)*; Novosemide *(Novopharm, Canad.)*; Odemase *(Azupharma, Ger.)*; Oedemex *(Mepha, Switz.)*; Promedes *(Jpn)*; Puresis *(Lennon, S.Afr.)*; Seguril *(Hoechst, Spain)*; Sigasalur *(Siegfried, Ger.*; *Sigamed, Switz.)*; SK-Furosemide *(Smith Kline & French, USA)*; Uremide *(Protea, Austral.)*; Urex *(Fawns & McAllan, Austral.)*; Urex-M *(Fawns & McAllan, Austral.)*; Uritol *(Horner, Canad.)*.

The following names have been used for multi-ingredient preparations containing frusemide—Diumide-K *(Degussa, UK)*; Frumil *(Rorer, UK)*; Frusene *(Fisons, UK)*; Lasikal *(Hoechst, UK)*; Lasilactone *(Hoechst, UK)*; Lasipressin *(Hoechst, UK)*; Lasix + K *(Hoechst, UK)*; Lasoride *(Hoechst, UK)*.

2332-b

Hydrobentizide *(rINN)*.

Dihydrobenzthiazide. 3-Benzylthiomethyl-6-chloro-3,4-dihydro-2*H*-1,2,4-benzothiadiazine-7-sulphonamide 1,1-dioxide.

$C_{15}H_{16}ClN_3O_4S_3$=433.9.

CAS — 13957-38-5.

Hydrobentizide is a thiazide diuretic which has properties similar to those of chlorothiazide (see p.981). It has been given in doses of 20 to 30 mg daily, in conjunction with other antihypertensive agents.

2333-v

Hydrochlorothiazide *(BAN, USAN, rINN)*.

Hidroclorotiazida; Hydrochlorothiazidum. 6-Chloro-3,4-dihydro-2*H*-1,2,4-benzothiadiazine-7-sulphonamide 1,1-dioxide.

$C_7H_8ClN_3O_4S_2$=297.7.

CAS — 58-93-5.

NOTE. Compounded preparations of hydrochlorothiazide and amiloride hydrochloride in the mass proportions of 10 parts to 1 part have the British Approved Name Co-amilozide.

Pharmacopoeias. In *Br., Braz., Chin., Cz., Egypt., Eur., Hung., Ind., Int., It., Jpn, Jug., Neth., Nord., Pol., Roum., Swiss, Turk.*, and *U.S.* Also in *B.P. Vet.*

A white or almost white odourless or almost odourless crystalline powder.

Slightly or very slightly **soluble** in water; sparingly soluble in alcohol and in methyl alcohol; soluble in acetone; freely soluble in dimethylformamide, *n*-butylamine, and solutions of alkali hydroxides; insoluble in ether, chloroform, and dilute mineral acids. **Store** in well-closed containers.

Adverse Effects and Treatment

As for Chlorothiazide, p.981.

ALLERGY. Fatal intravascular immune haemolysis in a patient taking hydrochlorothiazide and methyldopa.— M. L. Beck *et al.*, *Am. J. clin. Path.*, 1984, *81*, 791.

Severe breathlessness believed to be duc to an idiosyncratic allergic pneumonitis occurred following a single dose of hydrochlorothiazide in a 56-year-old woman. The patient had taken hydrochlorothiazide for hypertension several months previously.— N. A. Parfrey and H. F. Herlong, *Br. med. J.*, 1984, *288*, 1880.

Further reports of pulmonary oedema associated with hydrochlorothiazide: A. D. Steinberg, *J. Am. med. Ass.*, 1968, *204*, 825; C. Beaudry and L. Laplante, *Ann. intern. Med.*, 1973, *78*, 251.

EFFECTS ON THE ELECTROLYTE BALANCE. For reports of hyponatraemia in patients taking hydrochlorothiazide with potassium-sparing diuretics, see below under Precautions.

EFFECTS ON THE KIDNEYS. A 43-year-old woman, who took hydrochlorothiazide 25 mg and triamterene 50 mg every second day for 10 days before menstruation for premenstrual oedema, suffered from renal colic following each dose of diuretic. Surgical investigation revealed a partial urinary-tract obstruction.— A. F. Delevett and M. Recalde (letter), *J. Am. med. Ass.*, 1973, *225*, 992.

Acute interstitial nephritis in 1 patient associated with the administration of hydrochlorothiazide.— A. L. Linton *et al.*, *Ann. intern. Med.*, 1980, *93*, 735.

Allergic interstitial nephritis associated with hydrochlorothiazide or triamterene in an 85-year-old man.— *New Engl. J. Med.*, 1983, *309*, 970.

EFFECTS ON THE SKIN. In a retrospective study of fixed eruptions in 86 patients, hydrochlorothiazide was identified as the agent responsible in 1 case.— K. Kauppinen and S. Stubb, *Br. J. Derm.*, 1985, *112*, 575.

Skin reactions identified in 5 patients taking hydrochlorothiazide and amiloride included vasculitis in 2, erythema multiforme in 1, and photosensitivity in 1. The type of reaction in the remaining patient was not described.— N. Hardwick and N. Saxe, *Br. J. Derm.*, 1986, *115*, 167.

Precautions

As for Chlorothiazide, p.982.

HYPONATRAEMIA. Hyponatraemia was reported in 8 patients taking chlorpropamide and hydrochlorothiazide with amiloride (Moduretic). It was possible that Moduretic alone could have been responsible for hyponatraemia in 6 patients, although the additive hyponatraemic effect of chlorpropamide was demonstrated in the remaining 2 patients.— A. M. Zalin *et al.*, *Br. med. J.*, 1984, *289*, 659. Comment: L. V. K. de Silva and W. S. Mula-Abed (letter), *ibid.*, 1081. Comment that the hyponatraemic effect of hydrochlorothiazide with amiloride deserves wider recognition, particularly in elderly patients in whom a thiazide alone may be more appropriate.— D. Millson *et al.* (letter), *ibid.*, 1308.

Further reports of hyponatraemia in patients taking hydrochlorothiazide and either amiloride or triamterene concomitantly: P. H. Strykers *et al.*, *J. Am. med. Ass.*, 1984, *252*, 389; C. J. C. Roberts *et al.*, *Br. med. J.*, 1984, *288*, 1962; R. Eastell and C. J. Edmonds, *ibid.*, *289*, 1658.

In a survey of 197 elderly patients taking thiazide diuretics, plasma-potassium concentrations were similar in patients taking thiazide alone, with a potassium supplement, or in combination with a potassium-sparing diuretic. Mean plasma-sodium concentration in patients taking amiloride-hydrochlorothiazide was significantly lower than in those taking triamterene-hydrochlorothiazide or a thiazide with or without potassium supplement: hyponatraemia (plasma sodium less than 130 mmol per litre) was present in 31% of patients taking amiloride-hydrochlorothiazide compared with 4% of those taking triamterene-hydrochlorothiazide and 9% of those taking thiazides alone. A contributory factor may have been the dose of hydrochlorothiazide (50 mg) in the amiloride-hydrochlorothiazide preparation commonly used which is twice that in the triamterene-hydrochlorothiazide preparation.— A. J. Bayer *et al.*, *Postgrad. med. J.*, 1986, *62*, 159.

INTERACTIONS. *Amantadine*. For a report of increased amantadine toxicity associated with hydrochlorothiazide and triamterene see p.1008.

Antibiotics. For the effect of hydrochlorothiazide on the urinary elimination of chloramphenicol, see Chloramphenicol, p.188.

Calcitonin. The addition of salcatonin to treat Paget's disease of bone in a patient receiving hydrochlorothiazide for idiopathic hypercalciuria reduced serum-potassium concentrations and these were not increased to usual values when potassium supplements were given.— W. C. Sturtridge *et al.*, *Can. med. Ass. J.*, 1977, *117*, 1031.

Cholestyramine. Results of a study suggesting that, in patients receiving both hydrochlorothiazide and cholestyramine, administration of cholestyramine 4 hours after hydrochlorothiazide would result in a 30 to 35% reduction in the absorption of hydrochlorothiazide.— D. B. Hunninghake and D. M. Hibbard, *Clin. Pharmac. Ther.*, 1986, *39*, 329.

Diuretics. See under Hyponatraemia (above).

Non-steroidal anti-inflammatory drugs. For the effect of non-steroidal anti-inflammatory drugs on the action of diuretics including hydrochlorothiazide, see p.974.

LUPUS ERYTHEMATOSUS. Photosensitivity reactions similar to subacute cutaneous lupus erythematosus associated with hydrochlorothiazide in 5 patients.— B. R. Reed *et al.*, *Ann. intern. Med.*, 1985, *103*, 49.

Absorption and Fate

Hydrochlorothiazide is variably but fairly rapidly absorbed from the gastro-intestinal tract. It has been estimated to have a plasma half-life of about 4 or 5 hours with a subsequent longer terminal phase; its biological half-life is up to about 15 hours. It is excreted unchanged in the urine. Hydrochlorothiazide crosses the placental barrier and is excreted in breast milk.

The gastro-intestinal absorption of hydrochlorothiazide was enhanced when it was given with food; this was probably due to delayed passage through the small intestine.— B. Beermann and M. Groschinsky-Grind, *Eur. J. clin. Pharmac.*, 1978, *13*, 125. The gastro-intestinal absorption of hydrochlorothiazide from oral tablets was reduced when it was taken after a meal. The discrepancy between this and other studies could be due to differences in fasting times.— R. H. Barbhaiya *et al.*, *J. pharm. Sci.*, 1982, *71*, 245.

A report of reduced absorption of hydrochlorothiazide in 5 patients who had previously undergone intestinal shunt surgery. The uptake of hydrochlorothiazide may depend on transit time through the small intestine.— L. Backman *et al.*, *Clin. Pharmacokinet.*, 1979, *4*, 63.

In a study of bioavailability of hydrochlorothiazide in 12 healthy subjects, absorption was rapid from all doses given, with peak plasma concentrations at 2 hours. The absorption of hydrochlorothiazide was proportional to the dose at doses of 25, 50, and 100 mg. Slightly higher plasma concentrations were obtained from suspensions than tablets immediately after dosing, but were not significantly different after half an hour.— R. B. Patel *et al.*, *J. pharm. Sci.*, 1984, *73*, 359.

Further references on the pharmacokinetics of hydrochlorothiazide: B. Beermann and M. Groschinsky-Grind, *Eur. J. clin. Pharmac.*, 1977, *12*, 297; B. Beermann *et al.*, *Clin. Pharmac. Ther.*, 1976, *19*, 531; E. Redalieu *et al.*, *J. pharm. Sci.*, 1985, *74*, 765.

RED CELL BINDING. In 2 healthy subjects given hydrochlorothiazide 50 mg by mouth, peak plasma concentrations of 428 and 450 ng per mL occurred 2.5 and 2 hours respectively after administration. Whole blood concentrations occurring after 3 hours were about 2.5 times the value of plasma concentrations.— E. Redalieu *et al.*, *J. pharm. Sci.*, 1978, *67*, 726.

Uses and Administration

Hydrochlorothiazide is a thiazide diuretic with actions and uses similar to those of chlorothiazide (see p.983). Diuresis is initiated in about 2 hours and lasts for 6 to 12 hours.

In the treatment of oedema the usual initial dose is 50 to 100 mg daily, reduced to a dose of 25 to 50 mg daily or intermittently; in some cases initial doses of up to 200 mg daily have been recommended. A suggested initial dose for children is 2.5 mg per kg body-weight daily in 2 divided doses. Infants under 6 months may need doses of up to 3.5 mg per kg daily.

In the treatment of hypertension the usual dose is 25 to 50 mg daily, either alone, or in conjunction with other antihypertensive agents. Doses of up to 100 mg have been recommended but are rarely necessary.

When treatment is prolonged or in susceptible patients, loss of potassium may be sufficient to produce hypokalaemia; potassium supplements or potassium-sparing diuretics should then be given as for chlorothiazide.

Compounded preparations of hydrochlorothiazide and amiloride hydrochloride in the mass proportions of 10 parts to 1 part have the British Approved Name Co-amilozide.

Comment that many fixed-dose combinations contain 25 or 50 mg of hydrochlorothiazide or equivalent doses of other diuretics and can result in alarmingly high daily doses being administered when several such combination tablets are given daily, as is frequent practice.— L. H. Opie, *Lancet*, 1984, *1*, 496.

Co-amilozide produced a longer and smoother diuresis than frusemide 40 mg with triamterene 50 mg which caused a short and somewhat unpleasant effect in a study in 10 healthy subjects. Co-amilozide also spared potassium and magnesium relatively more effectively than the frusemide-triamterene combination.— A. Kohvakka and E. Hussi, *J. int. med. Res.*, 1986, *14*, 188.

ADMINISTRATION IN RENAL FAILURE. The elimination half-life of hydrochlorothiazide increased from 6.4 hours in subjects with normal renal function to 11.5 hours in patients with mild renal impairment (endogenous creatinine clearance of between 30 and 90 mL per minute) and to 20.7 hours in patients with a creatinine clearance below 30 mL per minute.— C. Niemeyer *et al.*, *Eur. J. clin. Pharmac.*, 1983, *24*, 661.

HYPERTENSION. A double-blind study in 683 men with mild to moderate hypertension found that hydrochlorothiazide in doses of up to 200 mg daily was at least as effective as propranolol up to 640 mg daily in white patients, and more effective than propranolol in black patients.— Veterans Administration Cooperative Study Group, *J. Am. med. Ass.*, 1982, *248*, 1996. Long-term follow-up over 12 months of 394 patients from the previous study showed that hydrochlorothiazide was more effective in controlling blood pressure than propranolol. Fewer patients on hydrochlorothiazide were withdrawn from the study because of adverse effects than patients on propranolol although biochemical abnormalities were greater with hydrochlorothiazide.— idem, 2004.

In a study of 562 elderly patients (aged 60 to 75 years) treatment with hydrochlorothiazide 25 to 50 mg or metoprolol 100 mg with or without hydrochlorothiazide 12.5 mg were equally effective in reducing blood pressure. However, biochemical disturbances were greater in the hydrochlorothiazide group than in the metoprolol group. Adverse effects accounted for withdrawal from the study of 8 patients in the hydrochlorothiazide group and 5 patients from the metoprolol group, although overall there was no difference in the incidence of adverse effects.— J. Wikstrand *et al.*, *J. Am. med. Ass.*, 1986, *255*, 1304.

Further studies of hydrochlorothiazide in hypertension: E. D. Freis *et al.*, *Am. J. Med.*, 1983, *74*, 1029; F. Haimerl *et al.*, *Fortschr. Med.*, 1985, *103*, 812; I. G. Philip *et al.*, *Br. J. clin. Pract.*, 1987, *41*, 947.

MÉNIÈRE'S DISEASE. Hydrochlorothiazide could improve vertigo associated with Ménière's disease but diuretics are not useful for dizziness with other origins.— L. M. Luxon, *Prescribers' J.*, 1985, *25*, 105.

RENAL DISORDERS. Hydrochlorothiazide 50 mg twice daily appeared to be effective in preventing the formation of calcium stones in the urinary tract in a study of 67 patients with idiopathic hypercalciuria, urinary infection, or renal calculi with no apparent cause.— E. R. Yendt *et al.*, *Can. med. Ass. J.*, 1970, *102*, 614.

Treatment with hydrochlorothiazide 50 mg daily or amiloride 5 mg daily or both could be used to treat calcium oxalate stone formation in patients with an inherited cellular defect in oxalate transport.— B. Baggio *et al.*, *New Engl. J. Med.*, 1986, *314*, 599.

Preparations

Hydrochlorothiazide Tablets *(B.P.)*

Hydrochlorothiazide Tablets *(U.S.P.)*

Amiloride Hydrochloride and Hydrochlorothiazide Tablets *(U.S.P.)*

Methyldopa and Hydrochlorothiazide Tablets *(U.S.P.)*

Reserpine, Hydralazine Hydrochloride, and Hydrochlorothiazide Tablets *(U.S.P.)*

Reserpine and Hydrochlorothiazide Tablets *(U.S.P.)*

Timolol Maleate and Hydrochlorothiazide Tablets *(U.S.P.)*

Proprietary Preparations

Amilco *(Norton, UK)*. *Tablets*, scored, hydrochlorothiazide 50 mg, amiloride hydrochloride equivalent to anhydrous amiloride hydrochloride 5 mg.

Dyazide (known in some countries as Dytenzide) *(Bridge, UK)*. *Tablets*, scored, hydrochlorothiazide 25 mg, triamterene, 50 mg.

Esidrex *(Ciba, UK)*. *Tablets*, scored, hydrochlorothiazide 25 and 50 mg.

Esidrex-K *(Ciba, UK)*. *Tablets*, hydrochlorothiazide 12.5 mg, potassium chloride 600 mg (potassium 8.06 mmol) for sustained release.

Owing to the risk of intestinal obstruction, sustained-release preparations such as Esidrex-K, where the drug is released in transit, but the matrix ghost is often eliminated intact, should not be prescribed in patients with Crohn's disease or other intestinal disease in which strictures may form.— J. L. Shaffer *et al.* (letter), *Lancet*, 1980, *2*, 487.

HydroSaluric *(Merck Sharp & Dohme, UK)*. *Tablets*, scored, hydrochlorothiazide 25 and 50 mg.

Hypertane *(Sanol Schwarz, UK)*. *Tablets*, scored, hydrochlorothiazide 50 mg, amiloride hydrochloride 5 mg.

Moduret 25 *(Morson, UK)*. *Tablets*, hydrochlorothiazide 25 mg, amiloride hydrochloride equivalent to anhydrous amiloride hydrochloride 2.5 mg.

Moduretic *(Merck Sharp & Dohme, UK)*. *Tablets*, scored, hydrochlorothiazide 50 mg, amiloride hydrochloride equivalent to anhydrous amiloride hydrochloride 5 mg.
Oral solution, hydrochlorothiazide 50 mg, amiloride hydrochloride equivalent to anhydrous amiloride hydrochloride 5 mg/5 mL.

Normetic *(Abbott, UK)*. *Tablets*, scored, hydrochlorothiazide 50 mg, amiloride hydrochloride equivalent to anhydrous amiloride hydrochloride 5 mg.

Synuretic *(DDSA Pharmaceuticals, UK)*. *Tablets*, hydrochlorothiazide 50 mg, amiloride hydrochloride 5 mg.

Triamco *(Norton, UK)*. *Tablets*, scored, hydrochlorothiazide 25 mg, triamterene 50 mg.

Proprietary Names and Manufacturers

Apo-Hydro *(Apotex, Canad.)*; Atenadon *(Ital.)*; Catiazida *(Spain)*; Chlorzide *(Foy, USA)*; Chlothia *(Jpn)*; Cloredema H *(Cronofar, Spain)*; Delco-Retic *(USA)*; Di-Chlotride *(Merck Sharp & Dohme, Ger.)*; Dichlotride *(Merck Sharp & Dohme, Austral.*; *Belg.*; *Merck Sharp & Dohme, Denm.*; *Neth.*; *Merck Sharp & Dohme, Norw.*; *Merck Sharp & Dohme, S.Afr.*; *MSD, Swed.)*; Diclotride *(Ital.)*; Didral *(Ital.)*; Diidrotiazide *(Ital.)*; Direma *(Dista, UK)*; Diucen-H *(Central Pharmaceuticals, USA)*; Diuchlor H *(Medic, Canad.)*; Diu-Melusin *(Melusin, Ger.)*; Diurex *(Arg.)*; Diursana-H *(Spain)*; Dixidrasi *(Ital.)*; Edemex *(Adcock Ingram, S.Afr.)*; Esidrex *(Ciba, Austral.; Belg.; Canad.; Denm.; Ciba, Fr.; Ciba, Ital.; Neth.; Ciba, Norw.; Ciba, Spain; Ciba, Swed.; Ciba, Switz.; Ciba, UK)*; Esidrix *(Ciba, Ger.; Ciba, USA)*; Hidrenox *(Arg.)*; Hidrosaluretil *(Gayoso Wellcome, Spain)*; Hydro-Aquil *(Canad.)*; Hydro-DIURIL *(Merck Sharp & Dohme, Canad.; Merck Sharp & Dohme, USA)*; HydroSaluric *(Merck Sharp & Dohme, UK)*; Hydro-Z *(Mayrand, USA)*; Hydrozide *(USA)*; Idrodiuvis *(Vis, Ital.)*; Idrofluin *(Ital.)*; Idrolisin *(Ital.)*; Jen-Diril *(USA)*; Lexor *(Lemmon, USA)*; Loqua *(USA)*; Maschitt *(Jpn)*; Mictrin *(USA)*; Natrimax *(Trianon, Canad.)*; Neo Minzil *(Valeas, Ital.)*; Neo-Codema *(Neolab, Canad.)*; Neo-Flumen *(Austral.)*; Neoflumen *(Spain)*; Newtolide *(Jpn)*; Novohydrazide *(Novopharm, Canad.)*; Oretic *(Abbott, USA)*; Pantemon *(Jpn)*; Ridaq *(Lennon, S.Afr.)*; Ro-Hydrazide *(USA)*; SK-Hydrochlorothiazide *(Smith Kline & French, USA)*; Tandiur *(Arg.)*; Thiuretic *(Parke, Davis, USA)*; Urirex *(Pharmador, S.Afr.)*; Urozide *(ICN, Canad.)*.

The following names have been used for multi-ingredient preparations containing hydrochlorothiazide—Acezide *(Duncan, Flockhart, UK)*; Aldactazide *(Searle, Canad.; Searle, USA)*; Aldoril *(Merck Sharp & Dohme, Canad.; Merck Sharp & Dohme, USA)*; Amilco *(Norton, UK)*; Amizide *(Protea, Austral.)*; Apo-Methazide *(Apotex, Canad.)*; Apo-Triazide *(Apotex, Canad.)*; Apresazide *(Ciba, USA)*; Apresoline-Esidrix *(Ciba, USA)*; Capozide *(Squibb, UK; Squibb, USA)*; Co-Betaloc *(Astra, Canad.; Astra, UK)*; Dopazide *(Pharmascience, Canad.)*; Dyazide *(Smith Kline & French, Austral.; Smith Kline & French, Canad.; Bridge, UK; Smith Kline & French, USA)*; Dytenzide; Esidrex-K *(Ciba, UK)*; Esimil *(Ciba, USA)*; H-H-R *(Schein, USA)*; Hydral *(Reid-Provident, USA)*; Hydra-Zide *(Par, USA)*; Hydromet *(Merck Sharp & Dohme, UK)*; Hydropres *(Merck Sharp & Dohme, Canad.; Merck Sharp & Dohme, USA)*; HydroSaluric-K *(Merck Sharp & Dohme, UK)*; Hydroserpine *(Schein, USA)*; Hydrosine *(Major, USA)*; Hypertane *(Sanol Schwarz, UK)*; Hyserp *(Reid-Provident, USA)*; Inderide *(Ayerst, Canad.; Ayerst, USA)*; Kalten *(Stuart, UK)*; Lopressor HCT *(Geigy, USA)*; Maxzide *(Lederle, USA)*; Moducren *(Morson, UK)*; Moduret *(Merck Sharp & Dohme, Canad.; Morson, UK)*; Moduretic *(Merck Sharp & Dohme, Austral.; Merck Sharp & Dohme, UK; Merck Sharp & Dohme, USA)*; Normetic *(Abbott, UK)*; Normozide *(Schering, USA)*; Novodoparil *(Novopharm, Canad.)*; Novospirozine *(Novopharm, Canad.)*; Novotriamzide *(Novopharm, Canad.)*; Oreticyl *(Abbott, USA)*; Rezide *(Edwards, USA)*; Salupres *(Merck Sharp & Dohme, UK)*; Secadrex *(May & Baker, UK)*; Seragen *(Reid-Provident, USA)*; Ser-Ap-Es *(Ciba, Canad.; Ciba, USA)*; Serpasil-Esidrex *(Ciba, UK)*; Serpasil-Esidrex-K *(Ciba, UK)*; Serpasil-Esidrix *(Ciba, Canad.; Ciba, USA)*; Sotazide *(Bristol-Myers Pharmaceuticals, UK)*; Spironazide *(Schein, USA)*; Synuretic *(DDSA Pharmaceuticals, UK)*; Timolide *(Frosst, Canad.; Merck Sharp & Dohme, USA)*; Tolerzide *(Bristol-Myers Pharmaceuticals, UK)*; Trandate HCT *(Glaxo, USA)*; Triamco *(Norton, UK)*; Unipres *(Reid-Rowell, USA)*; Vaseretic *(Merck Sharp & Dohme, USA)*; Viskazide *(Sandoz, Canad.)*.

2334-g

Hydroflumethiazide *(BAN, USAN, rINN).*

Hydroflumethiazidum; Trifluoromethylhydrothiazide. 3,4-Dihydro-6-trifluoromethyl-2*H*-1,2,4-benzothiadiazine-7-sulphonamide 1,1-dioxide.

$C_8H_8F_3N_3O_4S_2$=331.3.

CAS — 135-09-1.

Pharmacopoeias. In *Br., Egypt., Int., Nord.,* and *U.S.*

White or cream-coloured, odourless or almost odourless, glistening crystals or crystalline powder. Practically **insoluble** or very slightly soluble in water, in chloroform, and in ether; soluble 1 in 39 of alcohol; freely soluble in acetone. **Store** in airtight containers.

A study of the effect of spray drying alone, or with excipients on physicochemical properties of hydroflumethiazide. A marked difference in apparent solubility of the spray dried form compared with that of the pure crystalline form was reported.— O. I. Corrigan *et al., Drug Dev. ind. Pharm.,* 1983, *9,* 1.

Adverse Effects, Treatment, and Precautions

As for Chlorothiazide, p.981.

Absorption and Fate

Hydroflumethiazide is incompletely but fairly rapidly absorbed from the gastro-intestinal tract. It has a metabolite which is reported to be extensively bound to the red blood cells. Hydroflumethiazide is excreted in the urine; its metabolite has also been detected in the urine.

References on the pharmacokinetics of hydroflumethiazide: G. J. Yakatan *et al., J. clin. Pharmac.,* 1977, *17,* 37; P. J. McNamara *et al., J. clin. Pharmac.,* 1978, *18,* 190; O. Brørs *et al., Eur. J. clin. Pharmac.,* 1978, *14,* 29; O. Brørs *et al., Eur. J. clin. Pharmac.,* 1979, *15,* 287; O. Brørs and S. Jacobsen, *Eur. J. clin. Pharmac.,* 1979, *16,* 125.

PROTEIN AND RED CELL BINDING. Hydroflumethiazide is 74% bound to human serum albumin *in vitro*.— A. Ågren and T. Bäck, *Acta pharm. suec.,* 1973, *10,* 223.

Evidence of extensive binding of 2,4-disulphamoyl-5-trifluoromethylaniline, a metabolite of hydroflumethiazide, to red blood cells.— O. Brørs and S. Jacobsen, *Eur. J. clin. Pharmac.,* 1979, *15,* 281.

Uses and Administration

Hydroflumethiazide is a thiazide diuretic with actions and uses similar to those of chlorothiazide (see p.983). Diuresis is initiated in about 2 hours and has been reported to last for up to 24 hours.

In the treatment of oedema the usual initial dose is 50 to 200 mg daily, in one or two divided doses, reduced to a dose of 25 to 50 mg on alternate days or intermittently. In the treatment of hypertension the usual dose is 25 to 50 mg daily in one or two divided doses, either alone, or in conjunction with other antihypertensive agents.

A suggested initial dose for children is 1 mg per kg body-weight daily, reduced for maintenance.

When treatment is prolonged, or in susceptible patients, loss of potassium may be sufficient to produce hypokalaemia; potassium supplements or a potassium-sparing diuretic should then be given as for chlorothiazide.

Preparations

Hydroflumethiazide Tablets *(B.P.)*

Hydroflumethiazide Tablets *(U.S.P.)*

Proprietary Preparations

Aldactide 25 *(Gold Cross, UK). Tablets,* spironolactone 25 mg, hydroflumethiazide 25 mg.

Aldactide 50 *(Gold Cross, UK). Tablets,* spironolactone 50 mg, hydroflumethiazide 50 mg.

Hydrenox *(Boots, UK). Tablets,* hydroflumethiazide 50 mg.

Proprietary Names and Manufacturers

Di-Ademil *(Austral.)*; Diucardin *(Canad.; Ayerst, USA)*; Enjit *(Jpn)*; Hydravern *(Vernleigh, S.Afr.)*; Hydrenox *(Austral.; Boots, UK)*; Leodrine *(Leo, Fr.)*; NaClex *(Glaxo, UK)*; Rivosil *(Benvegna, Ital.)*; Robezon *(Jpn)*; Rontyl *(Leo, Denm.; Neth.; Norw.)*; Saluron *(Bristol, USA)*; Salurona *(Spain)*.

The following names have been used for multi-ingredient preparations containing hydroflumethiazide—Aldactide *(Gold Cross, UK)*; Hydro-Fluserpine *(Schein, USA)*; Protensin; Rautrax *(Squibb, UK; Squibb, USA)*; Rautrax Sine K *(Squibb, UK)*; Salazide *(Major, USA)*; Salutensin *(Bristol, Canad.; Bristol, USA)*.

12847-n

Indacrinone *(USAN, rINN).*

Indacrinic Acid; MK-196. (±)-[(6,7-Dichloro-2-methyl-1-oxo-2-phenylindan-5-yl)oxy]acetic acid.

$C_{18}H_{14}Cl_2O_4$=365.2.

CAS — 57296-63-6.

Although chemically related to ethacrynic acid, indacrinone possesses both natriuretic and uricosuric properties. There is evidence to suggest that the (+) and (−) enantiomers have different modes of action.

Brief reviews of the clinical pharmacology and pharmacokinetics of indacrinone. Indacrinone displays both natriuretic and uricosuric activity. The two optically active isomers have been shown to have differing pharmacological properties: while both enantiomers are natriuretic, the (−) isomer is mainly responsible for the natriuretic activity and the (+) isomer is primarily responsible for the uricosuric activity: A. Lant, *Drugs,* 1985, *29,* 57; idem, 162.

Comparison with hydrochlorothiazide.— C. E. Wilhelmsson *et al., Br. J. clin. Pharmac.,* 1979, *8,* 261.

The response to indacrinone, and to indacrinone plus amiloride, in healthy subjects.— P. J. Ravenscroft *et al., Clin. Pharmac. Ther.,* 1980, *28,* 45.

Comparison with frusemide.— J. D. Irvin *et al., Clin. Pharmac. Ther.,* 1980, *28,* 376.

Comparison with ethacrynic acid and hydrochlorothiazide.— B. A. Brooks *et al., Br. J. clin. Pharmac.,* 1984, *17,* 497.

The effects of different enantiomers.— J. D. Irvin *et al., Clin. Pharmac. Ther.,* 1980, *27,* 260; J. A. Tobert *et al., ibid.,* 1981, *29,* 344; P. H. Vlasses *et al., ibid.,* 798; P. H. Vlasses *et al., Pharmacotherapy,* 1984, *4,* 272; A. K. Jain *et al., ibid.,* 278; K. Williams and E. Lee, *Drugs,* 1985, *30,* 333.

Further references: K. F. Tempero *et al., Clin. Pharmac. Ther.,* 1976, *19,* 116; K. F. Tempero *et al., ibid.,* 1977, *21,* 119; *Nephron,* 1979, *23, Suppl.* 1, 1–66; B. A. Brooks *et al., Br. J. clin. Pharmac.,* 1980, *10,* 249.

Proprietary Names and Manufacturers

Merck Sharp & Dohme, USA.

2335-q

Indapamide *(BAN, USAN, rINN).*

SE-1520. 4-Chloro-*N*-(2-methylindolin-1-yl)-3-sulphamoylbenzamide.

$C_{16}H_{16}ClN_3O_3S$=374.8.

CAS — 26807-65-8 (anhydrous).

Adverse Effects, Treatment, and Precautions

As for Chlorothiazide, p.981.

EFFECTS ON THE ELECTROLYTE BALANCE. A report of very severe hypokalaemia in an elderly man given indapamide for hypertension.— O. Rodat and J. -P. Hamelin, *Nouv. Presse méd.,* 1978, *7,* 3054.

Reductions in plasma-potassium concentration were observed in 8 patients with a mean age of 70 years and 7 patients with a mean age of 36 years following treatment with indapamide 2.5 mg daily for 16 weeks.— D. B. Rowlands and W. A. Littler (letter), *Br. med. J.,* 1982, *284,* 1407.

EFFECTS ON THE SKIN. Sixteen cases of skin rash attributed to indapamide had been reported to the Netherlands Centre for Monitoring of Adverse Reactions to Drugs. All patients had taken indapamide 2.5 mg daily for hypertension. The skin rash was accompanied by fever in 5 cases. In all cases the rash subsided within 14 days of indapamide being stopped, and 11 patients subsequently took thiazides, frusemide, or clopamide without recurrence. Among 188 cases of skin rash attributed to indapamide reported to the WHO Collaborating Centre for International Drug Monitoring were 4 cases of erythema multiforme and 2 of epidermal necrolysis.— B. H. C. Stricker and C. Biriell, *Br. med. J.,* 1987, *295,* 1313.

INTERACTIONS. *Disopyramide.* Cardiac arrhythmias in a 64-year-old hypertensive man with suspected latent coronary insufficiency were considered to have been caused by the hypokalaemic action of indapamide together with the effect of concomitant disopyramide administration.— C. Cosma *et al., Nouv. Presse méd.,* 1978, *7,* 3455.

Absorption and Fate

Indapamide is rapidly and completely absorbed from the gastro-intestinal tract. Elimination is biphasic with a terminal half-life of 14 to 18 hours. It is extensively metabolised. About 60 to 70% of the dose has been reported to be excreted in the urine; only about 5% is excreted unchanged. About 16 to 23% of the administered dose is excreted in the faeces. Indapamide is about 71 to 79% bound to plasma proteins and it is preferentially taken up in the red blood cells. Indapamide is not removed by haemodialysis but does not accumulate in patients with impaired renal function.

Reviews of the pharmacokinetics of indapamide: M. Chaffman *et al.*, *Drugs*, 1984, *28*, 189; B. Beermann and M. Grind, *Clin. Pharmacokinet.*, 1987, *13*, 254.

Uses and Administration

Indapamide is a diuretic which has certain structural similarities to the thiazides and has actions and uses similar to those of chlorothiazide (see p.983). Diuresis is initiated within about 1 to 3 hours and has been reported to last for up to 36 hours. It has little inhibitory action on carbonic anhydrase. In the treatment of oedema it has been given in doses of 2.5 mg daily increasing to 5 mg daily if necessary. In the treatment of hypertension the usual dose is 2.5 mg daily, either alone, or in conjunction with other antihypertensive agents; at higher doses the diuretic effect may become apparent without appreciable additional antihypertensive effect.

When treatment is prolonged, or in susceptible patients, loss of potassium may be sufficient to produce hypokalaemia; potassium supplements should then be given as for chlorothiazide.

A review of the pharmacodynamic properties and therapeutic efficacy of indapamide in hypertension. Indapamide is an indoline derivative of chlorsulphonamide which shares many chemical, pharmacodynamic, and therapeutic similarities with other sulphonamide diuretics. In addition to its diuretic activity, indapamide has been shown to decrease vascular smooth muscle reactivity and peripheral resistance in various *in vitro* and *in vivo* models. Whether these peripheral vascular effects make an important contribution to the antihypertensive activity was unclear. In doses of 2.5 mg, indapamide has demonstrated similar efficacy to the thiazide diuretics in lowering mild to moderately elevated blood pressure. Doses of 5 mg and above have also been effective, but have been associated with significantly greater diuretic responses and tendencies towards biochemical aberrations.— M. Chaffman *et al.*, *Drugs*, 1984, *28*, 189.

Further reviews of indapamide: C. S. Conner, *Drug Intell. & clin. Pharm.*, 1983, *17*, 898; *Med. Lett.*, 1984, *26*, 17.

HYPERCALCIURIA. Indapamide 2.5 mg daily produced a mean reduction in urinary concentrations of calcium of 52% in a study of 26 hypercalciuric patients with kidney stones or recurrent renal colic. The decrease in urinary-calcium concentration was not significantly different from that previously observed with hydrochlorothiazide in 10 patients.— G. Lemieux, *Can. med. Ass. J.*, 1986, *135*, 119.

HYPERTENSION. Indapamide 2.5 mg daily produced a fall in blood pressure similar to that produced by bendrofluazide 5 mg daily. Biochemical changes indicated that indapamide and bendrofluazide lower blood pressure by the same mechanism.— R. F. Bing *et al.*, *Br. J. clin. Pharmac.*, 1981, *12*, 883.

A double-blind placebo-controlled study of 40 patients with mild to moderate hypertension given indapamide 2.5, 5.0, 7.5, and 10 mg. It was concluded that indapamide was an effective antihypertensive and natriuretic agent at all doses tested; kaliuresis was evident only with indapamide 5 mg daily or more.— W. J. Mroczek *et al.*, *Clin. Pharmac. Ther.*, 1984, *35*, 261.

A review of the use of indapamide in hypertension. Indapamide had been found to be effective in the treatment of hypertension and was generally well tolerated. Indapamide had been used alone and in combination with beta blockers, methyldopa, and other antihypertensive drugs. At a dose of 2.5 mg daily, indapamide had not been found to induce biochemical abnormalities.— J. R. Thomas, *Hypertension*, 1985, *7*, *Suppl.* II, 152.

Further references to the use of indapamide in hypertension: M. S. Wheeley *et al.*, *Pharmatherapeutica*, 1982, *3*, 143; P. Capone *et al.*, *Clin. Ther.*, 1983, *5*, 305; C.-B. Abbou, *Curr. med. Res. Opinion*, 1985, *9*, 494; K. Watters and B. Campbell, *Br. J. clin. Pract.*, 1986, *40*, 239.

OEDEMA. In a multicentre double-blind study of 219 patients with oedema of various causes, indapamide 2.5, 5, and 10 mg and hydrochlorothiazide were equally effective.— J. Eff *et al.*, *Clin. Ther.*, 1984, *6*, 778.

Proprietary Preparations

Natrilix *(Servier, UK)*. *Tablets*, indapamide 2.5 mg.

Proprietary Names and Manufacturers

Damide *(Benedetti, Ital.)*; Extur *(Normon, Spain)*; Fludex *(Servier, Denm.; Biopharma, Fr.; Neth.; Servier, Switz.)*; Indaflex *(Lampugnani, Ital.)*; Indamol *(Rorer, Ital.)*; Indolin *(Herdel, Ital.)*; Ipamix *(Gentili, Ital.)*; Lozide *(Servier, Canad.)*; Lozol *(USV Pharmaceutical Corp., USA)*; Millibar *(Lisapharma, Ital.)*; Natrilix *(Servier, Austral.; Itherapia, Ger.; Servier, Ital.; Servier, S.Afr.; Servier, UK)*; Pressural *(Polifarma, Ital.)*; Tertensif *(Servier, Spain)*.

2336-p

Isosorbide *(USAN)*.

AT-101. 1,4:3,6-Dianhydro-D-glucitol.

$C_6H_{10}O_4$=146.1.

CAS — 652-67-5.

Pharmacopoeias. U.S. includes Isosorbide Concentrate.

Isosorbide Concentrate is an aqueous solution containing 70.0 to 80.0% w/w of isosorbide. A colourless to slightly yellow liquid. **Soluble** in water and in alcohol. **Store** in airtight containers. Protect from light.

Adverse Effects and Precautions

These may be anticipated to be as for Mannitol, below Isosorbide has been reported to be less irritant than urea; it is, nevertheless, unpalatable, and gastro-intestinal irritation is common.

Adverse effects noted during isosorbide administration for hydrocephalus included persistent vomiting, marked irritability, doughy skin, failure to gain weight, and elevated blood-urea-nitrogen values.— D. B. Shurtleff and P. W. Hayden, *J. clin. Pharmac.*, 1972, *12*, 108.

EFFECTS ON THE KIDNEYS. Surprisingly, creatinine clearance was significantly increased during isosorbide diuresis (possibly as a result of decreased tubular reabsorption).— J. H. Nodine *et al.*, *Clin. Pharmac. Ther.*, 1973, *14*, 196.

Uses and Administration

Isosorbide is an osmotic diuretic which, unlike mannitol, (p.995) is readily absorbed from the gastro-intestinal tract and, unlike urea (p.1005), is not too irritant for administration by mouth.

Isosorbide is used to lower intraocular pressure in acute glaucoma or prior to surgery in doses of 1 to 3 g per kg body-weight by mouth 2 to 4 times daily. The onset of action is usually within 30 minutes and lasts for up to 5 or 6 hours.

GLAUCOMA. Isosorbide 1.5 g per kg body-weight reduced intra-ocular pressure in 40 glaucomatous eyes and 18 normal eyes. The side-effects were minimal.— O. P. Kulshrestha and R. N. Mittal, *Br. J. Ophthal.*, 1972, *56*, 439.

Further references to the use of isosorbide in glaucoma: *Med. Lett.*, 1974, *16*, 83.

HEPATIC DISORDERS. Isosorbide given to 21 patients with liver cirrhosis or fluid retention, was nearly as effective in producing diuresis as mannitol given intravenously. Since isosorbide produced less increase of plasma volume, it might be safer than mannitol for patients with oesophageal varices, raised central venous pressure, or impending congestive heart failure.— O. Gagnon *et al.*, *Am. J. med. Sci.*, 1967, *254*, 284.

Preparations

Isosorbide Oral Solution *(U.S.P.)*. pH 3.2 to 3.8.

Proprietary Names and Manufacturers

Ismotic *(Alcon Laboratories, USA)*.

2337-s

Lithium Benzoate

$C_7H_5LiO_2$=128.1.

CAS — 553-54-8.

Pharmacopoeias. In *Fr.* and *Port.*

Lithium benzoate has been used as a diuretic and urinary disinfectant. Its use cannot be recommended because of the pharmacological effect of the lithium ion (see Lithium Carbonate, p.365).

2338-w

Mannitol *(USAN)*.

Cordycepic Acid; E421; Manita; Manna Sugar; Mannite. D-Mannitol.

$C_6H_{14}O_6$=182.2.

CAS — 69-65-8.

Pharmacopoeias. In *Aust., Belg., Br., Braz., Chin., Cz., Egypt., Eur., Fr., Ind., It., Jpn, Jug., Nord., Port., Roum., Span., Swiss, Turk.,* and *U.S.*

A hexahydric alcohol related to mannose ($C_6H_{12}O_6$ = 180.2). It is isomeric with sorbitol. A white odourless crystalline powder or granules with a sweetish taste.

Soluble 1 in 6 of water; slightly or very slightly soluble in alcohol; slightly soluble in pyridine; practically insoluble in ether; soluble in solutions of alkali carbonates and hydroxides. A 5.07% solution in water is iso-osmotic with serum. The injection has a pH of 4.5 to 7.0. Any crystals which form during storage of the injection should be dissolved by warming before use. Solutions are **sterilised** by autoclaving or by filtration.

INCOMPATIBILITY. Mannitol solutions, 20% or stronger, could be salted out by potassium or sodium chloride.— J. Jacobs, *J. Hosp. Pharm.*, 1969, *27*, 341.

Flocculent precipitation occurred when a 25% solution of mannitol was allowed to contact plastic.— E. Epperson (letter), *Am. J. Hosp. Pharm.*, 1978, *35*, 1337. Plastic surfaces may act as nuclei for crystallisation to occur at a rapid rate, thereby providing atypically small crystals when supersaturated mannitol injections are used. Resolubilisation with the aid of heat is of no benefit since rapid recrystallisation may occur. Where volume intake is not a major concern this problem may be overcome by diluting the supersaturated injection to 18% or less with water before contact with the plastic container or administration device. In all cases, however, a filtration device should be used during the administration of the fluid.— R. L. Nedich, *Travenol* (letter), *ibid.*

Mannitol should never be added to whole blood for transfusion or given through the same set by which blood is being infused. For details of the adverse effects of mannitol on red blood cells, see Effects on the Blood under Adverse Effects.

STABILITY. There was no physical or chemical change in a mannitol injection nor any change in potency after 5 autoclavings. Mannitol injections could therefore be heated or autoclaved repeatedly if crystals appeared as a result of storage.— B. S. R. Murty and J. N. Kapoor, *Am. J. Hosp. Pharm.*, 1975, *32*, 826.

TABLET EXCIPIENT. For the use of mannitol as a tablet excipient, see Kee-Neng Wai *et al.*, *J. pharm. Sci.*, 1962, *51*, 1076; R. G. Daoust and M. J. Lynch, *Drug Cosmet. Ind.*, 1963, *93*, 26; J. L. Kanig, *J. pharm. Sci.*, 1964, *53*, 188; E. J. Mendell, *Mfg Chem.*, 1972, *43*, (May), 43.

Adverse Effects and Treatment

The most common side-effect associated with mannitol therapy is fluid and electrolyte imbalance including circulatory overload and acidosis at high doses; in patients with diminished cardiac reserve expansion of the extracellular fluid volume is a special hazard. Dehydration of the brain, particularly in patients with renal failure, may give rise to CNS symptoms.

When given by mouth, mannitol causes diarrhoea. Intravenous infusion of mannitol has been associated with nausea, vomiting, thirst, headache, dizziness, chills, fever, tachycardia, chest pain, hyponatraemia, dehydration, blurred vision, urticaria, and hypotension or hypertension. Large doses have been associated rarely with convulsions and acute renal failure. Pulmonary oedema has also been reported and hypersensitivity reactions have occurred.

Extravasation of the solution may cause oedema and skin necrosis; thrombophlebitis may occur.

Severe mannitol intoxication was reported in 8 patients with renal failure who had received large, and sometimes enormous, amounts of mannitol intravenously over 1 to 3 days. These patients had CNS involvement out of proportion to uraemia, severe hyponatraemia, a large osmolality gap, and fluid overload. Six patients were treated with haemodialysis and this was considered to be more effective than peritoneal dialysis, which was used in 1 patient.— H. F. Borges *et al.*, *Archs intern. Med.*, 1982, *142*, 63.

The osmolality of 20% mannitol is 1099 mosmol/kg. Mannitol produces an increase in plasma osmolar load and also induces a hypotonic fluid loss. Symptoms of hyperosmolality include thirst, tachycardia, hypotension, and hyperthermia. Cerebral dehydration causes confusion and coma with convulsions. Symptoms begin at plasma osmolality greater than 320 mosmol/kg with death occurring at plasma osmolality of 350 mosmol/kg.— S. M. Willatts, *Br. J. Hosp. Med.*, 1984, *32*, 8.

ALLERGY. Within 3 to 6 minutes of the commencement of an infusion of 20% mannitol solution, a 65-year-old woman, with a history of allergy to penicillin, procaine, and other agents, showed an allergic reaction including sneezing, rhinorrhoea, swollen tongue, dyspnoea, wheals on the chest, cyanosis, and loss of consciousness. Later, skin testing showed a positive reaction to mannitol solution. Her hypersensitivity could have originated from desensitisation injections containing fungous products with a mannitol content, which had been given 40 years earlier.— G. L. Spaeth *et al.*, *Archs Ophthal., N.Y.*, 1967, *78*, 583.

A sudden allergic reaction with dyspnoea, tightness of the chest, and rash in a patient receiving cisplatin, vinblastine, and bleomycin was attributed to mannitol given to enhance diuresis. Some hypersensitivity reactions attributed to cisplatin could be due to mannitol which is included in commercial cisplatin formulations.— S. P. Ackland and B. L. Hillcoat, *Cancer Treat. Rep.*, 1985, *69*, 562.

Mild respiratory distress, cyanosed lips, and hives attributed to hypersensitivity to mannitol occurred in a 60-year-old patient following two infusions of mannitol.— I. Y. McNeill, *Drug Intell. & clin. Pharm.*, 1985, *19*, 552.

EFFECTS ON THE BLOOD. Agglutination and irreversible crenation of erythrocytes occurred when blood was mixed with varying proportions of a 10% mannitol solution. It was suggested that intravenous infusions should be carefully controlled and administered at a slow rate.— B. E. Roberts and P. H. Smith, *Lancet*, 1966, *2*, 421. The significance of the results in relation to adverse effects in sickle-cell disease.— F. I. D. Konotey-Ahulu (letter), *ibid.*, 591; B. E. Roberts and P. H. Smith (letter), *ibid.* A further comment.— J. H. Samson (letter), *ibid.*, 1191.

EFFECTS ON THE ELECTROLYTE BALANCE. *Sodium.* Severe hyponatraemia in a 69-year-old man who required 30 to 40 litres of mannitol 3% for bladder irrigation during transurethral prostatic resection.— M. A. Kirschenbaum, *J. Urol., Baltimore*, 1979, *121*, 687.

EFFECTS ON THE GASTRO-INTESTINAL TRACT. Potentially explosive intracolonic concentrations of hydrogen gas were detected in 6 out of 10 patients given mannitol prior to colonoscopy.— S. J. La Brooy *et al.*, *Lancet*, 1981, *1*, 634. Data indicating that mannitol is a safe preparation for colonoscopy even when diathermy is to be used.— I. Trotman and R. Walt (letter), *ibid.*, 848. Confirmation that larger amounts of hydrogen are present in pure colonic gas after bowel preparation with mannitol than with castor oil. However, the risk of explosion after mannitol bowel preparation was much lower than previously reported. Air insufflation and suction during colonoscopy of patients prepared with mannitol, reduced the concentrations of colonic gases so that none were in the explosive range. The authors therefore suggested that colonoscopic electrosurgery under air insufflation and suction was safe but recommended that if mannitol bowel preparation was used then oxygen should be excluded by insufflating with a gas that would not support combustion.— A. Avgerinos *et al.*, *Gut*, 1984, *25*, 361.

Prescribers should be aware that mannitol used as a bulk sweetening agent in some foods may cause diarrhoea and flatulence if taken in sufficient quantity.— *Lancet*, 1983, *2*, 1321.

EFFECTS ON THE KIDNEYS. Focal osmotic nephrosis occurred in a patient after the administration of mannitol 20% intravenously.— W. E. Goodwin and H. Latta, *J. Urol., Baltimore*, 1970, *103*, 11.

Acute oliguric renal failure was associated with mannitol intoxication in a 21-year-old man.— T. V. Whelan *et al.*, *Archs intern. Med.*, 1984, *144*, 2053.

Reversible oligoanuric acute renal failure in 2 patients was attributed to infusion of large doses of mannitol.— P. Goldwasser and S. Fotino, *Archs intern. Med.*, 1984, *144*, 2214.

Precautions

Mannitol is contra-indicated in patients with pulmonary congestion or pulmonary oedema, intracranial bleeding (except during craniotomy), congestive heart failure (in patients with diminished cardiac reserve expansion of the extracellular fluid may lead to fulminating congestive heart failure), metabolic oedema with abnormal capillary fragility, and in patients with renal failure unless a test dose has produced a diuretic response (if renal flow is inadequate, expansion of the extracellular fluid may lead to acute water intoxication).

Mannitol should not be added to whole blood.

All patients given mannitol should be carefully observed for signs of fluid and electrolyte imbalance and renal function should be monitored.

INTERFERENCE WITH DIAGNOSTIC TESTS. Evidence that mannitol causes false-positive estimations of ethylene glycol.— I. J. Gilmour *et al.* (letter), *New Engl. J. Med.*, 1974, *291*, 51.

Absorption and Fate

Only small amounts of mannitol are absorbed from the gastro-intestinal tract, but any that is absorbed passes thence to the liver to be metabolised ultimately to carbon dioxide. Following intravenous injection mannitol is excreted rapidly by the kidneys before any very significant metabolism can take place in the liver. Mannitol does not cross the blood-brain barrier or penetrate the eye. An elimination half-life of about 100 minutes has been reported.

Mannitol, given to patients undergoing cardiopulmonary bypass, required over 3 hours for distribution in the extracellular fluid. In the next 24 hours, 83% was recovered in the urine. Approximately 20% of mannitol filtered by the glomeruli was reabsorbed by the tubules.— G. A. Porter *et al.*, *J. Surg. Res.*, 1967, *7*, 447.

A study indicating that mannitol is partially absorbed from the gastro-intestinal tract, and that some of the absorbed mannitol is excreted unchanged in the urine and some is metabolised, presumably in the liver, to carbon dioxide. No difference was noted between the metabolism of mannitol in cirrhotic subjects and those with healthy liver function. As the dose increased, inducing diarrhoea, the proportion of mannitol in the faeces increased. Very little metabolism was noted after intravenous administration of 10 g.— S. M. Nasrallah and F. L. Iber, *Am. J. med. Sci.*, 1969, *258*, 80.

Further references to the pharmacokinetics of mannitol: R. Dominguez *et al.*, *J. Lab. clin. Med.*, 1947, *32*, 1192; J. R. Elkinton, *J. clin. Invest.*, 1947, *26*, 1088; J. K. Clark and H. G. Barker, *Proc. Soc. exp. Biol. Med.*, 1948, *69*, 152; A. N. Wick *et al.*, *ibid.*, 1954, *85*, 188; W. Hindle and C. F. Code, *Am. J. Physiol.*, 1962, *203*, 215; J. C. Cloyd *et al.*, *J. Pharmac. exp. Ther.*, 1986, *236*, 301.

Uses and Administration

Mannitol, an isomer of sorbitol, has little significant energy value, since it is largely eliminated from the body before any metabolism can take place. Mannitol is generally administered by intravenous infusion as an osmotic diuretic but it has also been given by mouth to remove fluid by inducing osmotic diarrhoea. Careful monitoring of fluid balance, electrolytes, renal function, and vital signs is necessary during infusion to prevent fluid and electrolyte imbalance, including circulatory overload and tissue dehydration. Solutions containing more than 18% of mannitol are supersaturated; crystals may be redissolved by warming before use; the administration set should include a filter. Mannitol is not suitable for subcutaneous or intramuscular injection.

Mannitol is mainly used to increase urine flow in patients with acute renal failure, although frusemide is generally preferred, and to reduce raised intracranial pressure. It is also used to reduce intra-ocular pressure prior to ophthalmic procedures, to promote the excretion of toxic substances by forced diuresis, as diluent and excipient in pharmaceutical preparations, and as a bulk sweetener. A 2.5 to 5% solution of mannitol has been used for irrigating the bladder during the transurethral resection of the prostate to reduce haemolysis. It has also been used for the determination of the glomerular filtration-rate which is approximately equivalent to mannitol clearance. Reduction of cerebrospinal and intra-ocular fluid pressure occurs within 15 minutes of the start of a mannitol infusion and lasts for 3 to 8 hours after the infusion is discontinued; diuresis occurs after 1 to 3 hours.

Mannitol may be used to treat patients with renal failure (oliguria) or those suspected of inadequate renal function after correction of plasma volume, provided a test dose of about 200 mg per kg body-weight (about 50 mL of a 25% solution or 100 mL of a 15% solution) given by intravenous infusion over 3 to 5 minutes produces a diuresis of at least 30 to 50 mL per hour during the next 2 to 3 hours; a second test dose is permitted if the response to the first is inadequate. The adult dose of mannitol ranges from 50 to 100 g by intravenous infusion of a 5 to 25% solution, to a maximum of 200 g in 24 hours. The rate of administration is usually adjusted to maintain a urine flow of at least 30 to 50 mL per hour. The total dosage, the concentration, and the rate of administration depend on the fluid requirement, the urinary output, and the nature and severity of the condition being treated. Mannitol infusion may also be used to prevent acute renal failure during cardiovascular and other types of surgery, or following trauma.

To reduce raised intracranial pressure or raised intra-ocular pressure in neurosurgery or ophthamlology, mannitol is given by rapid infusion as a 15 to 25% solution in a dose of 1.5 to 2 g per kg body-weight over 30 to 60 minutes. Rebound increases in intracranial or intra-ocular pressure may occur but are less frequent than with urea.

For children, a dose of 1 to 2 g per kg body-weight has been suggested.

A brief review of the mechanisms of action of mannitol.— A. Lant, *Drugs*, 1985, *29*, 162.

An acceptable daily intake of "not specified" was allocated to mannitol— Thirtieth Report of the Joint FAO/WHO Expert Committee on Food Additives, *Tech. Rep. Ser. Wld Hlth Org. No. 751*, 1987.

ADMINISTRATION IN RENAL FAILURE. Administration of hyperosmotic solutions of mannitol could cause considerable expansion of the extracellular fluid even when urine flow exceeded 5 mL per minute. Severe oliguria could follow and the patient might need dialysis for the relief of pulmonary oedema.— A. Polak and A. G. Morgan (letter), *Lancet*, 1968, *1*, 1310.

A study in 40 patients with glomerular filtration rates ranging from 2 to 100 mL per minute indicated that mannitol can be used successfully as an osmotic diuretic even in patients with low glomerular filtration-rates.— P. Metaxas *et al.*, *Am. J. med. Sci.*, 1970, *259*, 175.

Mannitol is ineffective and hazardous in primary acute or chronic renal failure.— J. S. Cheigh, *Am. J. Med.*, 1977, *62*, 555.

See also under Renal Disorders (below).

CARDIAC DISORDERS. *Heart failure.* Nine patients with chronic heart failure, which had not responded to diuretic therapy, benefited from the administration of 1 litre of mannitol 20% solution by mouth over a period of 2 hours. Diarrhoea began 30 minutes after the first glass of mannitol solution and continued for about 6 hours. Three of the patients (all with cardiac oedema) subsequently responded to diuretic therapy that had previously been ineffective. Six patients with oedema associated with renal failure and one with oedema associated with cirrhosis of the liver also benefited.— J. W. James and R. A. Evans, *Br. med. J.*, 1970, *1*, 463.

DRUG OVERDOSAGE. Of 23 patients with aspirin or barbiturate poisoning given mannitol to induce diuresis, haemodialysis was necessary in 1 due to oliguria and pulmonary oedema. Retention of mannitol occurred in all the patients, ranging from 27 to 314 g. Great caution is necessary during this treatment as retention of mannitol can lead to movement of water into the extracellular fluid.— A. G. Morgan *et al.*, *Q. J. Med.*, 1968, *37*, 589.

GASTRO-INTESTINAL DISORDERS. *Bowel preparation.* Mannitol was effective for preparing the bowel for barium enema. One litre of 10% solution was consumed within 30 minutes early on the day of (afternoon) examination. Bowel clearance was better than that achieved with a 3-day low-residue diet, followed by magnesium sulphate, castor oil, and bisacodyl rectally.— K. R.

Palmer and A. N. Khan, *Br. med. J.*, 1979, *2*, 1038. See also G. L. Newstead and B. P. Morgan, *Med. J. Aust.*, 1979, *2*, 582.

Mannitol provides excellent bowel preparation but because of its potential to cause gas explosion should never be used when electrosurgery is contemplated unless carbon dioxide is used for bowel insufflation. Treatment with metronidazole and tetracycline before mannitol is given can reduce gas production to very low levels. Polyethylene glycol may be a suitable alternative to mannitol.— *Gut*, 1983, *24*, 371.

For bowel preparation in children, senna was preferred to mannitol, which often induces vomiting.— I. W. Booth and J. T. Harries, *Gut*, 1984, *25*, 188.

For further references to the production of explosive gases following oral administration of mannitol, see under Adverse Effects, above.

Diagnosis and testing. References to the use of mannitol in the diagnosis of abnormal intestinal permeability: A. D. J. Pearson *et al.*, *Archs Dis. Childh.*, 1983, *58*, 653; B. T. Cooper (letter), *Lancet*, 1983, *1*, 658.

For a description of a differential sugar absorption test using mannitol and lactulose for the investigation of abnormal intestinal permeability in coeliac disease and other intestinal disorders see Lactulose, p.1093.

RAISED INTRACRANIAL PRESSURE. A review of pharmacokinetic considerations in treating increased intracranial pressure. Osmotic diuretics including mannitol reduce intracranial pressure by establishing an osmotic gradient between the brain and the blood, and their action depends on an intact blood-brain barrier. With intact cerebral autoregulation, mannitol does not change cerebral blood flow. Mannitol increases the specific gravity of cerebral white matter and brain water content is reduced from 80 to 75%. As a consequence of diuresis, blood pressure control, cardiac output, and oxygen transport may be improved.— G. Heinemeyer, *Clin. Pharmacokinet.*, 1987, *13*, 1.

A discussion of the management of raised intracranial pressure after severe head injury. Mannitol may reduce intracranial pressure by increasing the osmotic gradient across the blood-brain barrier, by reducing the volume of CSF in the ventricles possibly by reducing the rate of formation of CSF, and possibly also by improving cerebral blood flow. Mannitol appears to be of less value in patients with defective autoregulation, and this may explain the frequently poor response in paediatric head injury. Osmotherapy remains the therapy of choice for reduction of persistently elevated intracranial pressure. The authors' current practice was to administer mannitol 0.5 g per kg body-weight over 15 to 20 minutes if intracranial pressure exceeds the treatment threshold, combined with frusemide 300 to 600 µg per kg intravenously. After the mannitol infusion circulatory normovolaemia was maintained with plasma-protein infusion. This regimen was repeated every 4 to 6 hours if necessary, while monitoring serum-electrolyte concentrations and osmolality.— N. M. Dearden, *Br. J. Hosp. Med.*, 1986, *36*, 94. Reminder that mannitol should not be given to cases of intracranial bleeding after head injury.— B. Williams (letter), *ibid.*, 1987, *37*, 85.

A brief account of the role of mannitol in the control of cerebral oedema. For the best effects, mannitol should be given rapidly and in an adequate dosage to maximise the osmotic gradient. A typical dose is 1 g per kg body-weight given over approximately 10 minutes, unless the intracranial pressure is being monitored in which case smaller doses may be tried. If mannitol is required more often than every 3 to 4 hours the serum osmolality must be followed closely; if this rises above 320 mosmol per litre and the intracranial pressure remains elevated, administration of more mannitol is likely to lead to renal failure, metabolic acidosis, and death.— J. D. Miller, *Br. J. Hosp. Med.*, 1979, *21*, 152.

In 6 infants with raised intracranial pressure associated with severe perinatal birth asphyxia, the intravenous injection of dexamethasone 4 mg significantly reduced the pressure at 2 hours but produced no improvement in cerebral perfusion pressure. In 4 infants given mannitol 1 g per kg body-weight as 20% solution on 9 occasions intracranial pressure fell usually within 20 minutes and cerebral perfusion pressure (calculated in 6 occasions) was improved at 1 hour and sustained for a further 4 hours. The cautious use of mannitol 20% is recommended.— M. I. Levene and D. H. Evans, *Archs Dis. Childh.*, 1985, *60*, 12.

Further references to the use of mannitol in cerebral oedema: J. Canalese *et al.*, *Gut*, 1982, *23*, 625 (cerebral oedema in hepatic failure); B. A. Bell *et al.*, *Lancet*, 1987, *1*, 66 (reduction in brain water content).

For a recommendation that frusemide be used instead of mannitol when diuresis is required in patients with pre-existing raised intracranial pressure, and in those who have pre-existing cardiac and electrolyte abnormalities, see Frusemide, p.991.

Reye's syndrome. Mannitol was considered to be the single most effective drug for rapidly reducing intracranial pressure in children with Reye's syndrome. A dose of 1 g per kg body-weight intravenously produced an effect within 5 minutes and the intracranial pressure remained low for 90 to 150 minutes thereafter.— B. A. Shaywitz *et al.*, *Pediatrics*, 1977, *59*, 595. Reye's syndrome was successfully treated in 18 children using a specific protocol which included the intravenous infusion of mannitol 2 g per kg body-weight every four hours or more frequently if intraventricular pressure was high. Only 2 patients had neurological sequelae 2 weeks after discharge.— S. L. Newman *et al.* (letter), *New Engl. J. Med.*, 1978, *299*, 1079. A warning of the dangers of mannitol in the treatment of Reye's syndrome. An 11-year-old girl with the syndrome, given mannitol 1 g per kg body-weight every 4 hours and additional doses of up to 0.5 g per kg hourly for rises in intracranial pressure, developed severe hyperosmolarity by the third day which may have contributed to her death.— J. Schmidley *et al.* (letter), *ibid.*, 1979, *301*, 106. Further comment.— S. L. Newman (letter), *ibid.*, 945.

RAISED INTRA-OCULAR PRESSURE. Mention of the use of oral glycerol 50% or intravenous mannitol 20% to treat large increases in intra-ocular pressure after laser trabeculoplasty.— J. Frucht *et al.*, *Br. J. Ophthal.*, 1985, *69*, 771.

RENAL DISORDERS. *Prophylaxis.* Twenty-two men, aged 54 to 73 years, undergoing resection of an aneurysm of the abdominal aorta, were given, as a prophylactic against the renal failure thought to accompany the aortic clamping, either standard pre-operative management (intravenous dextrose-saline solution begun an hour before operation and replaced by blood as required) or 500 mL of 5% mannitol during the 90 minutes before induction, and a further 200 mL of 20% mannitol after the operation had started. No patient in either group developed acute renal failure but 3 who received no mannitol became severely oliguric; there were no comparable cases in the group receiving mannitol.— R. J. Luck and W. T. Irvine, *Lancet*, 1965, *2*, 409.

In a small controlled study, the occurrence of postoperative renal failure in jaundiced patients was reduced by mannitol-induced diuresis. Beginning 1 to 2 hours before operation, 500 mL of a 10% solution was infused, and for 48 hours after operation renal flow was maintained at more than 1 mL per minute with infusions of 5% mannitol.— J. L. Dawson, *Ann. R. Coll. Surg.*, 1968, *42*, 163.

Indication that mannitol infusion prevents radiocontrast-induced acute renal failure.— C. W. Old and L. M. Lehrner (letter), *Lancet*, 1980, *1*, 885. Criticism.— J. A. Becker (letter), *ibid.*, 1147.

Forced alkaline diuresis with bicarbonate and mannitol can help to protect the kidneys in patients with major crush injury.— I. P. Stewart, *Br. med. J.*, 1987, *294*, 854.

Preparations

Mannitol and Sodium Chloride Injection *(U.S.P.)*

Mannitol Injection *(U.S.P.)*

Mannitol Intravenous Infusion *(B.P.)*. Mannitol Injection

Proprietary Preparations

Mannitol Intravenous Infusions *(Boots, UK)*. *Intravenous infusion*, mannitol 10 and 20% in polyethylene containers of 500 mL.

Min-I-Jet Mannitol Injection *(IMS, UK)*. *Injection*, mannitol 25%, in single-use prefilled syringes of 50 mL.

Proprietary Names and Manufacturers

Isotol *(Baxter, Ital.)*; Manicol *(Daniel-Brunet, Fr.)*; Mannistol *(Stholl, Ital.)*; Mannit TM *(Jpn)*; Mede-prep *(Medefield, Austral.)*; Osmitrol *(Travenol, Austral.; Travenol, Canad.; Travenol, UK)*; Osmofundin *(Switz.)*; Osmofundina *(Palex, Spain)*; Osmosal *(Spain)*; Osmosol *(Austral.)*; Resectisol *(McGraw, USA)*; Thomaemannit *(Thomae, Ger.)*

2339-e

Mebutizide *(rINN)*.

6-Chloro-3-(1,2-dimethylbutyl)-3,4-dihydro-2*H*-1,2,4-benzothiadiazine-7-sulphonamide 1,1-dioxide.

$C_{13}H_{20}ClN_3O_4S_2$=381.9.

CAS — 3568-00-1.

Mebutizide is a thiazide diuretic with properties similar to those of chlorothiazide (see p.981).

Proprietary Names and Manufacturers

Neoniagar *(Sintesa, Belg.)*.

2340-b

Mefruside *(BAN, USAN, rINN)*.

Bay-1500; FBA-1500. 4-Chloro-N^1-methyl-N^1-(tetrahydro-2-methylfurfuryl)benzene-1,3-disulphonamide.

$C_{13}H_{19}ClN_2O_5S_2$=382.9.

CAS — 7195-27-9.

Mefruside is a diuretic which has certain structural similarities to the thiazides and has properties similar to those of chlorothiazide (see p.981). Diuresis is initiated in about 2 hours and lasts for about 20 to 24 hours. Its inhibitory action on carbonic anhydrase is only weak.

In the treatment of oedema the usual dose is 25 to 50 mg daily, increasing if necessary to 75 to 100 mg. For long-term therapy a dose of 25 to 50 mg every second or third day is preferable.

In the treatment of hypertension the usual dose is 25 mg daily, either alone, or in conjunction with other antihypertensive agents; initial doses of 25 to 50 mg daily have been recommended; alternate-day maintenance dosage may be used.

When treatment is prolonged, or in susceptible patients, loss of potassium may be sufficient to produce hypokalaemia; potassium supplements or a potassium-sparing diuretic should then be given as for chlorothiazide.

Proprietary Preparations

Baycaron *(Bayer, UK)*. *Tablets*, scored, mefruside 25 mg.

Proprietary Names and Manufacturers

Baycaron *(Arg.; Bayer, Austral.; Belg.; Bayer, Denm.; Bayer, Ger.; Jpn; Neth.; Bayer, Norw.; Bayer, Swed.; Bayer, UK)*; Mefrusal *(Bayropharm, Ital.)*.

2341-v

Meralluride *(BAN, rINN)*.

A mixture of 3-[3-(3-carboxypropionyl)ureido]-2-methoxypropylhydroxomercury and theophylline.

$C_9H_{16}HgN_2O_6$ with $C_7H_8N_4O_2$.

CAS — 113-50-8 (meralluride); 129-99-7; 8069-64-5 (both sodium salt).

Meralluride is a mercurial diuretic with actions and uses similar to those of mersalyl acid (see p.997).

Meralluride was administered by intramuscular injection as a solution of the sodium compound.

Proprietary Names and Manufacturers

Mercuhydrin *(Merrell Dow, USA)*.

2342-g

Mercaptomerin Sodium *(BAN, rINNM)*.

Sodium Mercaptomerin. The disodium salt of carboxymethylthio[3-(3-carboxy-2,2,3-trimethylcyclopentanecarboxamido)-2-methoxypropyl]-mercury.

$C_{16}H_{25}HgNNa_2O_6S$=606.0.

CAS — 20223-84-1 (mercaptomerin); 21259-76-7 (mercaptomerin sodium).

Pharmacopoeias. In *Arg.*, *Jpn*, and *Nord.*

Mercaptomerin sodium is a mercurial diuretic with actions and uses similar to those of mersalyl acid (see p.997).

Mercaptomerin sodium was administered intramuscularly or subcutaneously.

Proprietary Names and Manufacturers

Thiomerin *(Wyeth, Canad.; Wyeth, USA)*.

2343-q

Mercurophylline Sodium *(BAN, rINNM).*

CAS — 8012-34-8.

Pharmacopoeias. Hung. includes Mercamphoramidum, (Mercamphamidum) ($C_{14}H_{25}HgNO_5$ = 487.9).

A mixture of the sodium salt of [3-(3-carboxy-2,2,3-trimethylcyclopentanecarboxamido)-2-methoxypropyl]-hydroxymercury ($C_{14}H_{24}HgNNaO_5$ = 509.9) and theophylline in approximately equimolecular proportions.

Mercurophylline sodium is a mercurial diuretic with actions and uses similar to those of mersalyl acid (see below). It was formerly given by mouth, and by intramuscular or intravenous injection.

Proprietary Names and Manufacturers
Novurit *(Llorens, Spain).*

2344-p

Merethoxylline Procaine
A mixture of the procaine salt of anhydro-*o*-{*N*-[3-hydroxymercuri-2-(2-methoxyethoxy)propyl]carbamoyl}phenoxyacetic acid ($C_{28}H_{39}HgN_3O_8$=746.2) and theophylline in the molecular proportion 1:1.4; available as a solution.

CAS — 8063-37-4.

Merethoxylline procaine has actions and uses similar to those of mersalyl acid (see below) but causes less local irritation. Merethoxylline procaine was administered by deep subcutaneous or intramuscular injection.

Proprietary Names and Manufacturers
Dicurin Procaine *(Lilly, USA).*

2345-s

Mersalyl Acid
Acidum Mersalylicum; Mersal. Acid; Mersalylum Acidum. A mixture of {3-[2-(carboxymethoxy)benzamido]-2-methoxypropyl}hydroxymercury and its anhydrides.
$C_{13}H_{17}HgNO_6$=483.9.

CAS — 486-67-9 ($C_{13}H_{17}HgNO_6$).

Pharmacopoeias. In *Int.*; in *Nord.* which describes the anhydride, $C_{13}H_{15}HgNO_5$.

2346-w

Mersalyl Sodium
Mersalyl *(pINN).* The sodium salt of mersalyl acid.
$C_{13}H_{16}HgNNaO_6$=505.9.

CAS — 492-18-2.

Pharmacopoeias. In *Arg., Jug., Mex.,* and *Turk.*

Adverse Effects
The most frequently occurring adverse effects following the administration of mersalyl are stomatitis, gastric disturbance, vertigo, febrile reactions, and skin eruptions and irritation. Diarrhoea and hypersensitivity reactions may occur. Thrombocytopenia, neutropenia, and agranulocytosis have followed the use of mercurial diuretics. Overdosage may cause severe dehydration and uraemia.
Prolonged administration of mersalyl may cause depletion of electrolytes and water in the body and consequent weakness and hypotension. Hypochloraemic alkalosis is a common feature.
Intravenous injection may cause severe hypotension and cardiac arrhythmias and has been followed by sudden death.
For specific details of adverse effects associated with the administration of mercurials, see under the adverse effects of mercury (p.1587).

Absorption and Fate
Mersalyl acid is incompletely and slowly absorbed from the gastro-intestinal tract and is completely and rapidly absorbed from intramuscular injection sites. Most of an injected dose is rapidly excreted in urine in the form of a mersalyl-cysteine complex; excretion is virtually complete within 24 hours.

Uses and Administration
Mersalyl acid, in the form of its salts, is a powerful diuretic which acts on the renal tubules, increasing the excretion of sodium and chloride, in approximately equal amounts, and of water. Organic mercurial diuretics were widely used prior to the introduction of thiazide and other diuretics but have now been almost completely superseded by these orally active drugs which are both potent and less toxic.
Mersalyl acid was usually given as the sodium salt (mersalyl) in conjunction with theophylline in the form of Mersalyl Injection, as this lessens the local irritant reaction and increases stability. It was given by deep intramuscular injection. A small dose was given initially to test for sensitivity.

ADMINISTRATION IN RENAL FAILURE. Mercurials are ineffective and nephrotoxic in patients with advanced renal disease and should be avoided.— W. M. Bennett, *Drugs,* 1979, *17,* 111.

Proprietary Names and Manufacturers
Salyrgan *(Sterling, USA).*

2347-e

Methazolamide *(BAN, USAN, rINN).*

N-(4-Methyl-2-sulphamoyl-Δ^2-1,3,4-thiadiazolin-5-ylidene)acetamide.
$C_5H_8N_4O_3S_2$=236.3.

CAS — 554-57-4.

Pharmacopoeias. In *U.S.*

A white or faintly yellow crystalline powder with a slight odour. Very slightly **soluble** in water and alcohol; slightly soluble in acetone; soluble in dimethylformamide. **Protect** from light.

Adverse Effects and Precautions
As for Acetazolamide, p.975.

EFFECTS ON THE BLOOD. *Aplastic anaemia.* Non-fatal aplastic anaemia in an 83-year-old man was probably associated with methazolamide administration.— J. L. Gangitano *et al., Am. J. Ophthal.,* 1978, *86,* 138.
Reports of aplastic anaemia in 2 patients and agranulocytosis in 1 patient given methazolamide for the treatment of glaucoma.— T. P. Werblin *et al., J. Am. med. Ass.,* 1979, *241,* 2817.

EFFECTS ON THE LIVER. Cholestatic hepatitis with jaundice, rash, and subsequent pure red cell aplasia was associated with methazolamide in 1 patient.— N. Krivoy *et al., Archs intern. Med.,* 1981, *141,* 1229.

Absorption and Fate
Methazolamide is absorbed from the gastro-intestinal tract more slowly than acetazolamide. It has been reported to be 55% bound to plasma protein, and to have a half-life of about 14 hours. About 25% of the dose is excreted unchanged in the urine; the fate of the remainder is unknown.

Uses and Administration
Methazolamide is an inhibitor of carbonic anhydrase with actions and uses similar to those of acetazolamide (see p.976). Its action is less prompt but of longer duration than that of acetazolamide, lasting for 10 to 18 hours. In the treatment of glaucoma, it is given in doses of 25 to 100 mg two or three times daily.
The diuretic activity of methazolamide is less pronounced than that of acetazolamide.

GLAUCOMA. A study in patients with open-angle glaucoma suggesting that a dose of 100 mg of methazolamide twice daily may represent for most patients a reasonable balance between desired and undesired effects. There were indications that methazolamide may enhance its own metabolism, presumably by enzyme induction.— K. Dahlen *et al., Archs Ophthal., N.Y.,* 1978, *96,* 2214.

MOUNTAIN SICKNESS. Methazolamide produced a beneficial response in a study of acute mountain sickness, but adverse effects occurred in over half the subjects, probably as a result of the high doses (200 mg daily) which were necessary to correct alkalosis.— P. Forster (letter), *Lancet,* 1982, *1,* 1254.

Preparations
Methazolamide Tablets *(U.S.P.)*

Proprietary Names and Manufacturers
Neptazane *(Lederle, Austral.; Lederle, Canad.; Théraplix, Fr.; Lederle, USA).*

2348-l

Methyclothiazide *(USAN, rINN).*
6-Chloro-3-chloromethyl-3,4-dihydro-2-methyl-2*H*-1,2,4-benzothiadiazine-7-sulphonamide 1,1-dioxide.
$C_9H_{11}Cl_2N_3O_4S_2$=360.2.

CAS — 135-07-9.

Pharmacopoeias. In *U.S.*

A white or almost white, odourless or almost odourless, crystalline powder.
Very slightly **soluble** in water and chloroform; soluble 1 in about 90 of alcohol; sparingly soluble in methyl alcohol; freely soluble in acetone.

Adverse Effects, Treatment, and Precautions
As for Chlorothiazide, p.981.

Uses and Administration
Methyclothiazide is a thiazide diuretic with actions and uses similar to those of chlorothiazide (see p.983). Diuresis is initiated in about 2 hours, and lasts for 24 hours or more.
In the treatment of oedema the usual initial dose is 2.5 to 5 mg daily, increasing to a maximum dose of 10 mg daily if necessary. In the treatment of hypertension the usual dose is 2.5 to 5 mg daily, either alone, or in conjunction with other antihypertensive agents; in some cases doses of 10 mg may be necessary.
In children, a dose of 50 to 200 µg per kg body-weight daily has been recommended.
When treatment is prolonged, or in susceptible patients, loss of potassium may be sufficient to produce hypokalaemia; potassium supplements or a potassium-sparing diuretic should then be given as for chlorothiazide.

Preparations
Methyclothiazide Tablets *(U.S.P.)*

Proprietary Preparations
Enduron *(Abbott, UK). Tablets,* scored, methyclothiazide 5 mg.

Proprietary Names and Manufacturers
Aquatensen *(Wallace, USA)*; Duretic *(Abbott, Canad.)*; Enduron *(Abbott, Austral.; Belg.; Spain; Abbott, UK; Abbott, USA)*; Endurona *(Abbott, Swed.)*; Enduron-M *(Abbott, Austral.)*; Thiazidil *(Abbott, Fr.)*; Urimor *(Protea, Austral.).*

The following names have been used for multi-ingredient preparations containing methyclothiazide— Diutensen *(Wallace, USA)*; Diutensen-R *(Wallace, USA)*; Dureticyl *(Abbott, Canad.)*; Enduronyl *(Abbott, UK; Abbott, USA)*; Methyclodine *(Rugby, USA).*

12953-m

Meticrane *(rINN).*
SD-17102. 6-Methylthiochroman-7-sulphonamide 1,1-dioxide.
$C_{10}H_{13}NO_4S_2$=275.3.

CAS — 1084-65-7.

Meticrane is a thiazide diuretic. There have been reports of blood dyscrasias associated with its use.

Report of depression in 8 patients taking diuretics including 4 patients taking meticrane.— F. Okada, *Am. J. Psychiat.,* 1985, *142,* 1101.

Proprietary Names and Manufacturers
Arresten *(Nippon Shinyaku, Jpn)*; Fontilix *(Diamant, Fr.)*; Kastarol *(Tanabe, Jpn).*

2349-y

Metolazone *(BAN, USAN, rINN).*

SR-720-22. 7-Chloro-1,2,3,4-tetrahydro-2-methyl-4-oxo-3-*o*-tolylquinazoline-6-sulphonamide.
$C_{16}H_{16}ClN_3O_3S$=365.8.

CAS — 17560-51-9.

Adverse Effects and Treatment
As for Chlorothiazide, p.981. Metolazone has also been reported to cause palpitations, chest pain, and chills.

Biochemical effects tended to be slightly greater with metolazone than with bendrofluazide in a crossover study in 26 patients.— J. F. Winchester *et al., Clin. Pharmac. Ther.,* 1980, *28,* 611.

CONVULSIONS. Two patients experienced acute muscle cramps with impairment of consciousness and epileptiform movements after taking metolazone 5 mg (single dose) or 2.5 mg daily for 3 days.— M. X. Fitzgerald and N. J. Brennan, *Br. med. J.*, 1976, *1*, 1381. Doubt as to the association with metolazone.— G. H. Gunson, *Pennwalt* (letter), *ibid.*, 1976, *2*, 476.

EFFECTS ON THE ELECTROLYTE BALANCE. See under Precautions (below) for electrolyte imbalance due to metolazone given concurrently with frusemide.

EFFECTS ON GLUCOSE METOBOLISM. Hyperosmolar nonketotic diabetes mellitus was associated with metolazone therapy in a 64-year-old woman.— P. A. Rowe and H. G. Mather, *Br. med. J.*, 1985, *291*, 25. Comment that this patient could have developed non-insulin dependent diabetes unrelated to metolazone treatment.— O. Odugbesan and A. H. Barnett (letter), *ibid.*, 488.

EFFECTS ON THE MUSCLES. Muscle cramps associated with metolazone therapy.— J. L. Cangiano *et al.*, *Curr. ther. Res.*, 1974, *16*, 778.

EFFECTS ON THE SKIN. Cutaneous necrotising vasculitis resembling polyarteritis occurred within 7 days of instituting metolazone therapy in a 75-year-old patient. The reaction was considered to be due to hypersensitivity.— L. A. Weinrauch *et al.*, *Cutis*, 1982, *30*, 83.

Precautions

As for Chlorothiazide, p.982. Metolazone is contra-indicated in patients with hepatic coma or pre-coma and in patients with anuria. Severe electrolyte disturbances may occur when metolazone and frusemide are used concurrently.

INTERACTIONS. *Captopril.* Deterioration in renal function occurred in a 65-year-old woman when metolazone 5 mg daily was added to treatment with captopril, frusemide, spironolactone, and digoxin for congestive heart failure. An interaction between captopril and metolazone was suspected and both drugs were discontinued with a subsequent return to normal renal function. It was suggested that natriuresis and fall in blood pressure caused by the diuretic may have compromised an already low renal perfusion pressure when autoregulatory mechanisms were blocked by captopril.— K. J. Hogg and W. S. Hillis (letter), *Lancet*, 1986, *1*, 501.

Cyclosporin. An increase in serum-creatinine concentration in a renal transplant patient was attributed to a toxic drug interaction between metolazone and cyclosporin. Serum-creatinine concentrations returned to pretreatment values when metolazone was discontinued.— P. Christensen and M. Leski (letter), *Br. med. J.*, 1987, *294*, 578.

Loop diuretics. The synergistic action of metolazone and *frusemide* has been used in the management of patients with gross oedema who are resistant to large doses of loop diuretics. This combination can, however, result in massive diuresis with serious electrolyte disturbances and volume depletion. For these reasons, Ghose and Gupta (*Br. med. J.*, 1981, *282*, 1432) recommended a dose of metolazone 2.5 mg, but Brown and MacGregor (*ibid.*, *283*, 1611) commented that the doses of loop diuretics used were not very large. Allen *et al.* (*ibid.*, *282*, 1873) suggested halving the dose of loop diuretic before adding metolazone, but Bamford (*ibid.*, *283*, 618) found that this did not prevent an uncontrolled diuresis. Brown and MacGregor were unable to avoid massive diuresis in a patient taking frusemide 500 mg daily even when the metolazone dose was reduced to 1.25 mg.

Further references to electrolyte disturbances with metolazone and loop diuretics: W. D. Black *et al.*, *Sth. med. J.*, 1978, *71*, 380; R. F. Gunstone *et al.*, *Postgrad. med. J.*, 1971, *47*, 789.

Absorption and Fate

Metolazone is incompletely absorbed from the gastro-intestinal tract. An average of 65% of the administered dose has been reported to be absorbed following an oral dose in healthy subjects, and an average of about 40% in patients with cardiac disease. About 95% of the drug is bound in the circulation; about 50 to 70% to the red blood cells and between 15 and 33% to plasma proteins. The half-life has been reported to be 8 to 10 hours in whole blood, and 4 to 5 hours in plasma, but the diuretic effect persists for up to 24 hours or more. About 70 to 80% of the amount of metolazone absorbed is excreted in the urine, of which 80 to 95% is excreted unchanged. The remainder is excreted in the bile and some enterohepatic circulation has been reported. Metolazone crosses the placental barrier and is excreted in breast milk.

References on the pharmacokinetics of metolazone: K. N. Modi *et al.*, *Fedn Proc.*, 1970, *29*, 276; W. J. Tilstone *et al.*, *Clin. Pharmac. Ther.*, 1974, *16*, 322.

Uses and Administration

Metolazone is a diuretic which has certain structural similarities to the thiazides and has actions and uses similar to those of chlorothiazide (see p.983). It has no effect on carbonic anhydrase. Unlike other thiazide diuretics, metolazone does not reduce the glomerular filtration-rate or renal blood flow and is reported to be effective in patients with a glomerular filtration-rate of less than 20 mL per minute. Diuresis is initiated in about 1 hour and the effect lasts for 12 to 24 hours.

In the treatment of oedema the usual dose is 5 to 10 mg daily; in some cases doses of 20 mg or more may be required. It has been recommended that not more than 80 mg should be given in any 24-hour period. In refractory cases, metolazone has been used in combination with frusemide, but the electrolyte balance should be monitored closely.

In the treatment of hypertension the usual dose is 2.5 to 5 mg daily, or 5 mg on alternate days, either alone, or in conjunction with other antihypertensive agents.

When treatment is prolonged, or in susceptible patients, loss of potassium may be sufficient to produce hypokalaemia; potassium supplements or a potassium-sparing diuretic should then be given as for chlorothiazide.

References on the combined effect of metolazone and loop diuretics: C. Marone *et al.*, *Eur. J. clin. Invest.*, 1985, *15*, 253; D. C. Brater *et al.*, *J. Pharmac. exp. Ther.*, 1985, *233*, 70; A. Greenberg *et al.*, *J. clin. Pharmac.*, 1985, *25*, 369.

ADMINISTRATION IN RENAL FAILURE. Metolazone has some efficacy in far-advanced renal failure but it is ineffective with glomerular filtration-rates less than 10 mL per minute.— W. M. Bennett, *Drugs*, 1979, *17*, 111. Metolazone can be given in usual doses to patients with renal failure. High doses may be useful in end-stage renal disease. No dosage adjustment is necessary for patients undergoing haemodialysis.— W. M. Bennett *et al.*, *Am. J. Kidney Dis.*, 1983, *3*, 155.

See also Renal Disorders, below.

HYPERTENSION. A study in 57 non-oedematous hypertensive patients indicated that metolazone in doses of 1, 2.5, and 5 mg daily appeared to be equally effective in antihypertensive effect, and much the same as chlorthalidone 100 mg daily. There were no differences in the incidences of hypokalaemia.— S. Fotiu *et al.*, *Clin. Pharmac. Ther.*, 1974, *16*, 318.

Further references to the use of metolazone in hypertension: G. Reda *et al.*, *Curr. ther. Res.*, 1983, *34*, 900.

OEDEMA. Oedema resistant to treatment with loop diuretics in 4 patients responded to the addition of metolazone 2.5 or 5 mg daily. However, treatment with metolazone and loop diuretics produces profound diuresis which may lead to hypovolaemia and hypokalaemia. Ideally, patients should be treated with caution in hospital, as dangerous, uncontrolled losses of fluid and electrolytes may occur.— R. R. Ghose and S. K. Gupta, *Br. med. J.*, 1981, *282*, 1432.

The use of metolazone and frusemide in children with resistant oedema.— W. C. Arnold, *Pediatrics*, 1984, *74*, 872.

See also Precautions (Interaction with Loop Diuretics).

RENAL DISORDERS. In a study in 10 patients with chronic renal failure and 10 patients with the nephrotic syndrome previous diuretic therapy was replaced with metolazone 2.5 to 20 mg once daily; treatment with antihypertensives and corticosteroids was continued. Fluid retention, oedema, and blood pressure were controlled in most patients. One patient with oedema resistant to frusemide alone and to metolazone 40 mg daily responded to frusemide 160 mg daily with metolazone 30 mg. Three patients required potassium supplements.— R. R. Paton and R. E. Kane, *J. clin. Pharmac.*, 1977, *17*, 243.

Further references to the use of metolazone in patients with renal failure: H. Groth *et al.*, *Schweiz. med. Wschr.*, 1985, *115*, 41.

Proprietary Preparations

Metenix 5 *(Hoechst, UK)*. *Tablets*, metolazone 5 mg.

Proprietary Names and Manufacturers

Diondel *(Pharmainvesti, Spain)*; Diulo *(Searle, Austral.; Searle, USA)*; Metenix *(Hoechst, UK)*; Zaroxolyn *(Pennwalt, Canad.; Pennwalt, Eire; Searle, Ger.; ISF, Ital.; Sandoz, S.Afr.; Sterling-Winthrop, Swed.; Pennwalt, USA: Farillon, UK)*; Zaroxolyne *(Sandoz, Switz.)*.

2350-g

Muzolimine *(BAN, USAN, rINN)*.

Bay-g-2821. 3-Amino-1-[1-(3,4-dichlorophenyl)ethyl]-2-pyrazolin-5-one.

$C_{11}H_{11}Cl_2N_3O = 272.1$.

CAS — 55294-15-0.

Although chemically unrelated, muzolimine is a diuretic which has been reported to have actions and uses similar to those of frusemide (see p.989); its duration of action is reported to be more prolonged. Various severe neurological symptoms have been associated with the administration of high doses of muzolimine in patients with renal failure; for this reason muzolimine has been withdrawn worldwide.

In a double-blind study in 12 healthy subjects muzolimine 30 mg was shown to have a similar saliuretic effect to frusemide 40 mg.— D. Loew *et al.*, *Eur. J. clin. Pharmac.*, 1977, *12*, 341.

A brief review of the clinical pharmacokinetics of muzolimine.— B. Beermann and M. Grind, *Clin. Pharmacokinet.*, 1987, *13*, 254.

Report of severe irreversible neuropathy in 2 patients associated with muzolimine.— B. Pohlmann-Eden *et al.* (letter), *Dt. med. Wschr.*, 1987, *112*, 1238.

CARDIAC DISORDERS. *Heart failure.* Single doses of muzolimine 40 mg and frusemide 40 mg were given to 12 patients with heart failure and associated oedema in a double-blind crossover study. In terms of total excretion muzolimine was slightly more effective than frusemide but the difference did not reach statistical significance. The duration of action was prolonged compared to frusemide.— P. Fauchald and E. Lind, *Pharmatherapeutica*, 1977, *1*, 409.

Reports of favourable responses to muzolimine in hypertension: L. A. Ferrara *et al.*, *Eur. J. clin. Pharmac.*, 1985, *28*, 241; P. Wicker and J. Clementy, *Clin. Pharmac. Ther.*, 1986, *39*, 537.

RENAL DISORDERS. In a double-blind crossover study involving 11 patients with advanced renal failure both frusemide and muzolimine had an excellent saliuretic effect. Whereas that of frusemide generally wears off after 12 hours, the effect of muzolimine lasted for a much longer period of time. Muzolimine had a more pronounced effect on potassium excretion in all groups and in all time periods.— P. Schmidt *et al.*, *Eur. J. clin. Pharmac.*, 1978, *14*, 399.

Further references: A. D. Canton *et al.*, *Br. med. J.*, 1981, *282*, 595.

Proprietary Names and Manufacturers

Edrul *(Zyma, Ger.; Bayropharm, Ital.)*;
Manufacturers also include—*Miles Pharmaceuticals, USA.*

13130-a

Piretanide *(BAN, USAN, rINN)*.

Hoe-118; S-734118. 4-Phenoxy-3-(pyrrolidin-1-yl)-5-sulphamoylbenzoic acid.

$C_{17}H_{18}N_2O_5S = 362.4$.

CAS — 55837-27-9.

Adverse Effects

As for Frusemide, p.987. Muscle cramps have been reported following high doses of piretanide.

Piretanide was generally well tolerated in short- and medium-term studies, although more experience was needed of long-term use. Comparison of adverse effects with those of bumetanide and frusemide has suggested that some of the more common acute reactions such as pronounced diuresis, nausea, and thirst are more likely to occur with a conventional tablet formulation of piretanide than with either bumetanide or frusemide. A sustained-release formulation has been shown to reduce the incidence of side-effects. However, in comparative studies the incidence of side-effects with piretanide was similar to or less than those with other diuretics employed. Other adverse effects which have been reported include postural hypotension, hypotonic circulatory disturbance, exanthema, muscle cramps, vertigo, allergic eczema, worsening psoriasis, pruritus, joint pains, and auditory disturbances.— S. P. Clissold and R. N. Brogden, *Drugs*, 1985, *29*, 489.

Precautions

As for Chlorothiazide p.982. Patients with impaired micturition or prostatic hypertrophy may develop retention of urine with piretanide. As with other loop diuretics, piretanide may enhance the nephrotoxicity of cephalosporin antibiotics such as cephalothin and of aminoglycoside antibiotics.

Absorption and Fate

Piretanide has been reported to be almost completely absorbed following oral administration. It is extensively bound to plasma proteins, and is reported to have a half-life of about 1 hour.

A review of the clinical pharmacokinetics of piretanide.— B. Beermann and M. Grind, *Clin. Pharmacokinet.*, 1987, *13*, 254.

Good correlation was found between urinary recovery or renal clearance of piretanide and residual renal function in a study of 10 patients with chronic renal failure. The elimination of piretanide by non-renal mechanisms appeared to be increased when renal function was greatly diminished.— C. Marone *et al.*, *Eur. J. clin. Pharmac.*, 1984, *27*, 589.

Uses and Administration

Piretanide is a loop diuretic with actions and uses similar to those of frusemide (p.989). In the treatment of hypertension it is given in a usual dose of 6 to 12 mg daily as a sustained-release formulation or in conventional tablets.

A review of piretanide. Piretanide is a loop diuretic with a potency intermediate between that of frusemide and bumetanide. Comparative studies have shown that piretanide 6 to 12 mg daily has an antihypertensive effect comparable to hydrochlorothiazide 100 mg daily. Piretanide has generally had less effect on potassium concentrations than thiazides in these studies. Early clinical studies with a conventional tablet formulation of piretanide tended to produce a relatively high incidence of acute adverse effects generally related to pronounced diuretic effects. However, the incidence of these acute reactions has been considerably reduced with a sustained-release formulation of piretanide which has a flatter and more prolonged diuretic profile. In patients with congestive heart failure, single doses of piretanide 6 to 12 mg have comparable efficacy to bumetanide 1 mg and frusemide 40 mg. Results from clinical studies over 3 months have shown that piretanide 6 mg daily was of similar efficacy to frusemide 40 mg daily in reducing the symptoms of congestive heart failure. Piretanide up to 24 mg daily was used to treat 15 patients with moderate to severe congestive heart failure for up to 3 years and was generally well tolerated.

Piretanide has only been investigated in a small number of short-term studies in limited numbers of patients with renal insufficiency. Overall, its natriuretic activity is less pronounced but more prolonged in these patients. It has produced diuresis comparable to bumetanide and frusemide in high-dose comparative studies.— S. P. Clissold and R. N. Brogden, *Drugs*, 1985, *29*, 489.

A brief review of piretanide. Piretanide was not considered to have any advantage over existing diuretics for the treatment of hypertension.— *Drug & Ther. Bull.*, 1985, *23*, 43.

A clear dose-response relationship was found for cumulative urinary output, cumulative excretion of sodium and potassium, and urinary sodium/potassium ratio with piretanide 3-, 6-, and 12-mg doses. A signigicant correlation was found between the net urine volume and excretion of piretanide.— B. H. Meyer *et al.*, *Eur. J. clin. Pharmac.*, 1983, *25*, 783.

Piretanide 18 mg twice daily had similar diuretic effects to bumetanide 3 mg twice daily in 8 patients with renal failure. The onset of action was the same for both drugs, but the duration exceeded 6 hours only for piretanide.— K. J. Berg *et al.*, *Br. J. clin. Pharmac.*, 1983, *15*, 347.

HEART DISEASE. Piretanide in doses of up to 24 mg daily for 28 days produced beneficial responses in 20 patients with mild to moderately severe congestive heart failure compared with 18 patients taking placebo.— L. G. Sherman *et al.*, *Clin. Pharmac. Ther.*, 1986, *40*, 587.

HYPERTENSION. The hypotensive effect of piretanide from a standard tablet and from a sustained-release capsule was compared in 40 patients. Both formulations produced a reduction in blood pressure but the sustained-release capsule produced a more gradual response than the tablet. There were no significant changes in serum-potassium or -magnesium concentrations with either formulation. Three patients withdrew from the study: one patient had an excessive antihypertensive response to the tablet, and 2 patients had allergic reactions while taking the sustained-release capsule.— W. Dols *et al.*, *J. int. med. Res.*, 1985, *13*, 31.

Further references to the use of piretanide in hypertension: M. Verho *et al.*, *Eur. J. clin. Pharmac.*, 1984, *27*, 407; C. Buekert *et al.*, *J. int. med. Res.*, 1984, *12*, 81.

Proprietary Preparations

Arelix *(Hoechst, UK). Capsules*, sustained-release, piretanide 6 mg.

Proprietary Names and Manufacturers

Arelix *(Cassella-Riedel, Ger.; Hoechst, Ital.; Hoechst, UK)*; Diumax *(Cusi, Spain)*; Tauliz *(Hoechst, Ital.)*.

2352-p

Polythiazide *(BAN, USAN, rINN)*.

P-2525. 6-Chloro-3,4-dihydro-2-methyl-3-(2,2,2-trifluoroethylthiomethyl)-2*H*-1,2,4-benzothiadiazine-7-sulphonamide 1,1-dioxide.

$C_{11}H_{13}ClF_3N_3O_4S_3$=439.9.

CAS — 346-18-9.

Pharmacopoeias. In *Br.* and *U.S.*

A white or almost white crystalline powder with an alliaceous odour. *B.P.* **solubilities** are: practically insoluble in water and chloroform; soluble 1 in 40 of alcohol. *U.S.P.* solubilities are: soluble in more than 1000 of water and ether, 1 in 175 of chloroform, and in 150 of alcohol; soluble in methyl alcohol and acetone. **Store** in airtight containers. Protect from light.

Adverse Effects, Treatment, and Precautions

As for Chlorothiazide, p.981.

Report of depression in 8 patients taking diuretics, including 2 patients taking polythiazide.— F. Okada, *Am. J. Psychiat.*, 1985, *142*, 1101.

Absorption and Fate

Polythiazide is fairly readily absorbed from the gastro-intestinal tract, and *animal* studies have indicated that it is fairly extensively metabolised.

In 18 healthy subjects given polythiazide 1 mg the mean plasma half-lives for absorption and elimination were 1.2 and 25.7 hours respectively. Within 48 hours a mean of 20.34% of the administered dose had been excreted unchanged in the urine of 13 subjects. It can be concluded that about 25% of the dose is cleared intact by the kidney, the remainder presumably cleared after metabolic changes as well as by elimination in the faeces. Studies *in vitro* indicated that about 83.5% of polythiazide is bound to plasma proteins.— D. C. Hobbs and T. M. Twomey, *Clin. Pharmac. Ther.*, 1978, *23*, 241.

Uses and Administration

Polythiazide is a thiazide diuretic with actions and uses similar to those of chlorothiazide (see p.983). Diuresis is initiated within about 2 hours after administration, and lasts for 24 to 48 hours.

In the treatment of oedema the usual dose is 1 to 4 mg daily. In the treatment of hypertension the usual dose is 2 to 4 mg daily, either alone, or in conjunction with other antihypertensive agents; doses of 0.5 mg to 1.0 mg may be adequate in some patients.

When treatment is prolonged, or in susceptible patients, loss of potassium may be sufficient to produce hypokalaemia; potassium supplements or a potassium-sparing diuretic should then be given as for chlorothiazide.

Preparations

Polythiazide Tablets *(B.P.)*

Polythiazide Tablets *(U.S.P.)*

Proprietary Preparations

Nephril *(Pfizer, UK). Tablets*, scored, polythiazide 1 mg.

Proprietary Names and Manufacturers

Drenusil *(Pfizer, Ger.; S.Afr.)*; Nephril *(Austral.; Pfizer, UK)*; Rénèse *(Pfizer, Switz.)*; Renese *(Belg.; Canad.; Pfizer, Denm.; Pfizer, Fr.; Neth.; Pfizer, Norw.; Spain; Pfizer, Swed.; Pfizer, USA)*.

The following names have been used for multi-ingredient preparations containing polythiazide— Minizide *(Pfizer, USA)*; Renese-R *(Pfizer, USA)*.

2353-s

Prorenoate Potassium *(BAN, USAN, rINN)*.

Potassium Prorenoate; SC-23992. Potassium 6α,7α-dihydro-17β-hydroxy-3-oxo-3′*H*-cyclopropa[6,7]-17α-pregna-4,6-diene-21-carboxylate.

$C_{23}H_{31}KO_4$=410.6.

CAS — 49848-01-3 (prorenoic acid); 49847-97-4 (potassium salt).

Prorenoate potassium has properties similar to those of spironolactone (see p.1001). It has been given in doses of about 40 mg daily.

In a double-blind study involving 6 healthy subjects aged 18 to 35 years, the responses to prorenoate potassium 40 mg were similar to those to spironolactone 100 mg. Spironolactone had a slightly higher activity as regards sodium excretion whereas potassium retention was greater after prorenoate potassium but the differences were not significant. Prorenoate potassium was, however, significantly more active than spironolactone when the amount of potassium spared was expressed per unit of sodium excreted, thus demonstrating a qualitative difference. Both drugs showed significant activity between 2 to 16 hours after administration.— L. E. Ramsay *et al.*, *Br. J. clin. Pharmac.*, 1976, *3*, 475.

Further references to the actions of prorenoate: L. E. Ramsay *et al.*, *Br. J. clin. Pharmac.*, 1975, *2*, 271; L. E. Ramsay *et al.*, *Clin. Pharmac. Ther.*, 1975, *18*, 391; G. T. McInnes *et al.*, *Br. J. clin. Pharmac.*, 1981, *11*, 114P; G. T. McInnes *et al.*, *ibid.*, 1982, *13*, 187; G. T. McInnes *et al.*, *ibid.*, 1984, *18*, 169.

Proprietary Names and Manufacturers

Searle, USA.

13199-c

Quincarbate *(rINN)*.

DU-23187. Ethyl 10-chloro-3-ethoxymethyl-2,3,6,9-tetrahydro-9-oxo-*p*-dioxino[2,3-*g*]quinoline-8-carboxylate.

$C_{17}H_{18}ClNO_6$=367.8.

CAS — 54340-59-9.

Quincarbate is a diuretic with natriuretic properties.

References: J. van Dijk *et al.*, *J. med. Chem.*, 1976, *19*, 982.

Proprietary Names and Manufacturers

Duphar, Neth.

2354-w

Quinethazone *(BAN, USAN, rINN)*.

Chinethazonum. 7-Chloro-2-ethyl-1,2,3,4-tetrahydro-4-oxoquinazoline-6-sulphonamide.

$C_{10}H_{12}ClN_3O_3S$=289.7.

CAS — 73-49-4.

Pharmacopoeias. In *U.S.*

A white to yellowish-white crystalline powder. Very slightly **soluble** in water; slightly soluble in alcohol; sparingly soluble in pyridine; freely soluble in solutions of alkali hydroxides and carbonates. **Store** in airtight containers.

Quinethazone is a diuretic which has certain structural similarities to the thiazides and has properties similar to those of chlorothiazide (see p.981).

Diuresis is initiated within about 2 hours after administration and lasts for 18 to 24 hours.

In the treatment of oedema the usual dose is 50 to 100 mg daily; in some cases doses of 200 mg daily may be necessary.

In the treatment of hypertension the usual dose is 50 to 100 mg daily, either alone, or in conjunction with other antihypertensive agents.

When treatment is prolonged, or in susceptible patients, loss of potassium may be sufficient to produce hypokalaemia; potassium supplements or a potassium-sparing diuretic should then be given as for chlorothiazide.

Preparations

Quinethazone Tablets *(U.S.P.)*

Proprietary Names and Manufacturers

Aquamox *(Lederle, Austral.; Belg.; Lederle, Canad.; Lederle, Denm.; Ger.; Cyanamid, Ital.; Neth.; Norw.; Lederle, Swed.; Switz.; Lederle, UK)*; Hydromox *(Lederle, USA)*.

The following names have been used for multi-ingredient preparations containing quinethazone— Aquamox with Reserpine *(Lederle, Canad.)*; Hydromox R *(Lederle, USA)*.

2355-e

Spironolactone *(BAN, USAN, rINN)*.

Espironolactona; SC 9420; Spirolactone. 7α-Acetylthio-3-oxo-17α-pregn-4-ene-21,17β-carbolactone acid γ-lactone.

$C_{24}H_{32}O_4S$=416.6.

CAS — 52-01-7.

Pharmacopoeias. In *Br., Braz., Chin., Cz., Egypt., Ind., It., Jpn, Jug., Nord., Swiss,* and *U.S.*

A white to light tan powder; it is odourless or has a slight characteristic odour. Practically **insoluble** in water; soluble 1 in 80 of alcohol, 1 in 3 of chloroform, and 1 in 100 of ether; soluble in ethyl acetate; slightly soluble in methyl alcohol and fixed oils. **Protect** from light.

Adverse Effects

Spironolactone may give rise to headache and drowsiness, and gastro-intestinal disturbances, including cramp and diarrhoea. Ataxia, mental confusion, hirsutism, deepening of the voice, menstrual irregularities, impotence, and skin rashes have been reported as side-effects. Gynaecomastia is not uncommon and in rare cases breast enlargement may persist. Transient increases in blood-urea-nitrogen concentrations may occur and mild acidosis has been reported. Spironolactone has been demonstrated to cause tumours in *rats*.

Spironlactone may cause hyponatraemia and hyperkalaemia.

A survey indicated that of 788 patients who received spironolactone 164 developed side-effects. These included hyperkalaemia in 8.6%, dehydration in 3.4%, hyponatraemia in 2.4%, gastro-intestinal disorders in 2.3%, neurological disorders in 2% and rash, gynaecomastia, and unspecified effects.— D. G. Greenblatt and J. Koch-Weser, *J. Am. med. Ass.*, 1973, *225*, 40.

Spironolactone has recently been used in younger patients at high doses for its anti-androgenic effect. In a study of 44 patients (43 female and 1 male) aged 28 to 50 years who had received treatment with spironolactone commencing at 200 mg daily for 1 to 45 months, the most common side-effect was disturbance of menstruation (66%). Other adverse effects included breast enlargement (27%), breast tenderness (30%), nausea (18%), and dry skin (39%). Two patients complained of abnormal facial pigmentation resembling chloasma. Side-effects tended to occur early and persist throughout treatment. Some cases were managed by reducing the spironolactone dosage, and 4 patients withdrew from treatment.— B. R. Hughes and W. J. Cunliffe, *Br. J. Derm.*, 1987, *117, Suppl.* 32, 38.

ALLERGY. Eosinophilia and a rash developed in 2 patients with alcoholic cirrhosis while taking spironolactone.— C. G. Wathen *et al.* (letter), *Lancet*, 1986, *1*, 919.

CARCINOGENICITY. A report of breast cancer in 5 patients who had taken spironolactone with hydrochlorothiazide for prolonged periods.— S. D. Loube and R. A. Quirk (letter), *Lancet*, 1975, *1*, 1428. Evidence against a substantial association between spironolactone and breast cancer.— H. Jick and B. Armstrong (letter), *ibid.*, *2*, 368.

Long-term studies in *rats* have shown that spironolactone can cause tumours.— *FDA Drug Bull.*, 1976, *6*, 33.

EFFECTS ON THE BLOOD. Agranulocytosis occurred on 2 occasions in a 70-year-old woman and was temporally associated with the administration of spironolactone.— B. H. C. Stricker and T. T. Oei, *Br. med. J.*, 1984, *289*, 731.

EFFECTS ON THE ELECTROLYTE BALANCE. *Magnesium.* Reduced clearance of magnesium by spironolactone.— T. Mountokalakis *et al.*, *Klin. Wschr.*, 1975, *53*, 633. Slight increase in magnesium loss in several cirrhotic patients receiving spironolactone.— J. L. Campra and T. B. Reynolds, *Am. J. dig. Dis.*, 1978, *23*, 1025.

Potassium. Hyperkalaemia was identified in 57 of 783 patients receiving spironolactone (7.3%). Hyperkalaemia was considered to be life-threatening in 5 patients, 3 of whom were also taking potassium supplements. There was an association between hyperkalaemia and raised blood-urea concentrations.— D. H. Lawson *et al.*, *Eur. J. clin. Pharmac.*, 1982, *23*, 21.

A report of a 69-year-old man with near-fatal cardiac arrhythmia caused by spironolactone-induced hyperkalaemia. He had a high dietary potassium intake. Survival followed intravenous therapy with sodium bicarbonate.— C. Pongpaew *et al.*, *Chest*, 1973, *63*, 1023.

Life-threatening hyperkalaemia occurred following bladder decompression in a patient with impaired renal function who had taken spironolactone for several months. Hyperkalaemia responded to withdrawal of spironolactone, administration of calcium polystyrene sulphonate, and a single dose of glucose and insulin.— P. H. O'Reilly *et al.* (letter), *Lancet*, 1987, *2*, 859. Comment on the increased risk of hyperkalaemia due to spironolactone in patients with impaired renal function.— M. G. McGeown (letter), *ibid.*, 1207.

Further references to hyperkalaemia in patients taking spironolactone: E. O. Udezue and B. P. Harrold, *Postgrad. med. J.*, 1980, *56*, 254.

EFFECTS ON ENDOCRINE FUNCTION. A discussion on, and details of, investigations into the oestrogenic effects of spironolactone, which include decreased libido, impotence, and gynaecomastia in men, and menstrual irregularity and painful breast enlargement in women. Spironolactone interferes with testosterone biosynthesis but studies imply that this is inadequate to explain the oestrogen-like side-effects of spironolactone therapy; its anti-androgen action at receptor sites may offer a more convincing explanation. On the other hand, the menstrual irregularity may be explained by its reduction of 17-hydroxylase activity.— D. L. Loriaux *et al.*, *Ann. intern. Med.*, 1976, *85*, 630.

Gynaecomastia developed in 3 of 10 healthy subjects taking spironolactone 100 mg daily and in 5 of 8 subjects taking spironolactone 200 mg daily. No significant changes in androgen metabolism were seen suggesting that alterations in testosterone synthesis or clearance were not the cause of spironolactone-induced gynaecomastia.— D. H. Huffman *et al.*, *Clin. Pharmac. Ther.*, 1978, *24*, 465.

Regrowth of scalp hair was reported in a 56-year-old man with male-pattern baldness during treatment with spironolactone for heart failure.— P. S. Thomas (letter), *Br. med. J.*, 1986, *293*, 698.

Further references to effects of spironolactone on endocrine function: J. I. Levitt, *J. Am. med. Ass.*, 1970, *211*, 2014; L. I. Rose *et al.*, *Ann. intern. Med.*, 1977, *87*, 398; G. Bellati and G. Idéo (letter), *Lancet*, 1986, *1*, 626.

EFFECTS ON LIPID METABOLISM. Spironolactone had a more favourable effect on serum-lipid concentrations than thiazide diuretics in a study of 23 patients.— R. P. Ames and P. B. Peacock, *Archs intern. Med.*, 1984, *144*, 710.

EFFECTS ON THE LIVER. Elevated liver enzymes were associated with spironolactone therapy on 2 occasions in a 53-year-old patient. Liver biopsy showed changes consistent with mild non-specific hepatitis.— J. Shuck *et al.*, *Ann. intern. Med.*, 1981, *95*, 708.

EFFECTS ON SEXUAL FUNCTION. Details of gynaecomastia and impotence complications of spironolactone therapy.— D. J. Greenblatt and J. Koch-Weser, *J. Am. med. Ass.*, 1973, *223*, 82.

A brief review of the effect of spironolactone on sexual function.— J. G. Stevenson and G. S. Umstead, *Drug Intell. & clin. Pharm.*, 1984, *18*, 113.

Further references to the effects of spironolactone on sexual function: P. J. Smith and R. L. Talbert, *Clin. Pharm.*, 1986, *5*, 373.

See also under Effects on Endocrine Function (above).

EFFECTS ON THE SKIN. A report of lichen-planus-like skin eruptions which developed in a 62-year-old woman who was taking digoxin, propranolol, diazepam, spironolactone, and iron tablets. Flares of the lichen-planus-like eruption seemed to be associated with administration of spironolactone and there was evidence of resolution when spironolactone was withdrawn.— T. F. Downham (letter), *J. Am. med. Ass.*, 1978, *240*, 1138.

Cutaneous vasculitis was associated with spironolactone treatment on 3 occasions in an 80-year-old man.— G. W. L. Phillips and A. J. Williams, *Br. med. J.*, 1984, *288*, 368.

EFFECTS ON TASTE PERCEPTION. Reversible ageusia in an 82-year-old man given spironolactone.— M. D. Clee and L. Burrow (letter), *New Engl. J. Med.*, 1983, *309*, 1062. Comment on diuretics and diminished taste perception.— S. S. Schiffman (letter), *ibid.*, 1063.

Precautions

Spironolactone should not be given to patients with hyperkalaemia or progressive renal failure, and should not be given with other potassium-sparing diuretics. Potassium supplements should not be given with spironolactone. It should be given with care to patients with impaired hepatic or renal function. Although spironolactone has not been shown to have any effect on carbohydrate metabolism, it should be given with care to patients with diabetes mellitus, who may be predisposed to hyperkalaemia. It should also be given with care to patients likely to develop acidosis. Serum electrolytes and blood-urea-nitrogen should be estimated periodically.

Spironolactone enhances the effects of other antihypertensive agents and may diminish vascular responses to noradrenaline. Spironolactone is not suitable for nursing mothers.

Severe hyperkalaemia in an insulin-dependent diabetic woman with hyporeninaemic hypoaldosteronism given spironolactone.— D. M. Large *et al.*, *Postgrad. med. J.*, 1984, *60*, 370.

INTERACTIONS. *Ammonium chloride.* A 58-year-old woman receiving spironolactone 25 mg four times a day and potassium chloride about 50 mmol (50 mEq) daily developed acidosis about 20 days after starting ammonium chloride 4 g daily; renal function was adequate. Three factors might have contributed; increased acid load due to ammonium chloride, decreased ability of the kidney to excrete hydrogen ions due to the aldosterone-antagonist effect of spironolactone, and increased acid load due to hyperkalaemia.— M. L. Mashford and M. B. Robertson (letter), *Br. med. J.*, 1972, *4*, 298.

Angiotensin-converting-enzyme inhibitors. Hyperkalaemia causing complete heart block was associated with concomitant administration of spironolactone and captopril (T.C.N. Lo and R.J. Cryer, *Br. med. J.*, 1986, *292*, 1672) in a 72-year-old woman. Lakhani (*ibid.*, *293*, 271) reported a similar fatal reaction in a patient taking spironolactone and enalapril. Hyperkalaemia in a 55-year-old patient taking spironolactone and enalapril (A.R. Morton and S.A. Crook, *Lancet*, 1987, *2*, 1525) persisted for over 48 hours despite discontinuation of the drugs and treatment with ion-exchange resin and intravenous glucose and insulin.

Aspirin. The urinary sodium excretion induced by spironolactone was reduced by 30% in 7 volunteers after a single dose of aspirin 600 mg.— M. G. Tweeddale and R. I. Ogilvie, *New Engl. J. Med.*, 1973, *289*, 198. Prolonged administration of aspirin did not appear to alter the effect of spironolactone on blood pressure, serum electrolytes, urea nitrogen, or plasma-renin activity in a double-blind crossover study of 5 patients with low-renin essential hypertension and 2 with hypertension associated with primary aldosteronism.— J. W. Hollifield, *Sth. med. J.*, 1976, *69*, 1034. In a double-blind study in 6 healthy subjects the administration of aspirin 600 mg with spironolactone 50 mg significantly reduced the urinary excretion and the fractional excretion of its active metabolite, canrenone, 4 to 6 hours later.— L. E. Ramsay *et al.*, *Eur. J. clin. Pharmac.*, 1976, *10*, 43.

Digoxin and other cardiac glycosides. For discussions of the effects of concomitant administration of spironolactone on digoxin pharmacokinetics, see Digoxin, p.828.

For the effect of spironolactone on digitoxin, see Digitoxin, p.824.

Fludrocortisone. For reference to a paradoxical increase in urinary-potassium excretion on concomitant administration of spironolactone and fludrocortisone, see Canrenoate Potassium, p.981.

Mitotane. For a report of the inhibition of the action of mitotane by concomitant administration of spironolactone, see Mitotane, p.643.

Opioid analgesics. An allergic pruritic reaction to a preparation of dextropropoxyphene, aspirin, caffeine, and phenacetin was considered to trigger spironolactone-induced gynaecomastia in one patient. The pruritus and breast swelling resolved when both the preparation and spironolactone were withdrawn. The reintroduction of spironolactone produced no ill effect but the effects returned when the dextropropoxyphene preparation was reinstituted.— A. A. Licata and F. C. Bartter (letter), *Lancet*, 1976, *2*, 905.

Warfarin. For references to the interaction between warfarin and spironolactone, see p.346.

INTERFERENCE WITH LABORATORY ESTIMATIONS. Spironolactone can interfere with assays for plasma-digoxin concentrations (J.M. Horn, *Drug Interact. News.*, 1982, *2*, 51; S. Yosselson-Superstine, *Clin. Pharmacokinet.*, 1984, *9*, 67). There have also been reports of interference with measurements of blood-cortisol concentrations, the diagnosis of low plasma-renin activity, and radioassays for deoxycortone, oestrogen, and progesterone (see *Martindale 28th Edn*, p.610).

PORPHYRIA. Spironolactone was considered to be unsafe in patients with acute porphyria because it has been shown to be porphyrinogenic in *animals* or *in vitro* systems.— M.R. Moore and K.E.L. McColl, *Porphyrias, Drug Lists*, Glasgow, Porphyria Research Unit, University of Glasgow, 1987.

PREGNANCY AND THE NEONATE. In a study of a nursing mother taking spironolactone 25 mg four times daily the estimated maximum quantity of canrenone (the principal metabolite) ingested by the infant in the breast milk was 0.2% of the daily dose.— D. L. Phelps and A. Karim, *J. pharm. Sci.*, 1977, *66*, 1203.

Absorption and Fate

Spironolactone is fairly rapidly absorbed from the gastro-intestinal tract, the extent of absorption depending on particle size and formulation. It is rapidly and extensively metabolised and extensively bound to plasma proteins. Canrenone, which is an active metabolite, has a plasma half-life of about 10 to 35 hours. Spironolactone is excreted in the urine and in the faeces, in the form of metabolites. Spironolactone or its metabolites may cross the placental barrier, and canrenone is excreted in breast milk.

A review of the disposition, metabolism, pharmacodynamics, and bioavailability of spironolactone.— A. Karim, *Drug Metab. Rev.*, 1978, *8*, 151.

Further references to the pharmacokinetics of spironolactone: A. Karim *et al.*, *Clin. Pharmac. Ther.*, 1976, *19*, 158; A. Karim *et al.*, *ibid.*, 177; U. Abshagen *et al.*, *Eur. J. clin. Pharmac.*, 1979, *16*, 255; W. Krause *et al.*, *ibid.*, 1983, *25*, 449; P. C. Ho *et al.*, *ibid.*, 1984, *27*, 435; P. C. Ho *et al.*, *ibid.*, 441.

Study indicating that it was unlikely that spironolactone has a pronounced enzyme-inducing effect.— E. E. Ohnhaus and E. Gerber-Taras (letter), *Br. J. clin. Pharmac.*, 1984, *17*, 485.

BIOAVAILABILITY. Studies in healthy subjects indicated that administration of spironolactone with food increased the amount of canrenone which entered the general circulation.— A. Melander *et al.*, *Clin. Pharmac. Ther.*, 1977, *22*, 100. Study in 9 healthy subjects indicating that food promotes the absorption of spironolactone and possibly decreases first-pass metabolism.— H. W. P. M. Overdiek and F. W. H. M. Merkus, *Clin. Pharmac. Ther.*, 1986, *40*, 531.

A single-blind, randomised, crossover study involving 6 healthy subjects showed no differences in bioavailability between 2 commercial preparations of spironolactone. Following administration of spironolactone 100 mg twice daily for 6 days a mean peak serum-canrenone concentration of about 500 ng per mL occurred about 3 hours after a dose.— H. Rameis *et al.*, *Dt. med. Wschr.*, 1979, *104*, 881.

The bioavailability of spironolactone was higher from tablets containing micronised spironolactone than from standard tablets.— G. T. McInnes *et al.*, *J. clin. Pharmac.*, 1982, *22*, 410.

METABOLISM. Study of the pharmacokinetics of spironolactone following single doses in healthy subjects using a specific HPLC assay. The major metabolite was found to be 7α-thiomethylspirolactone. High concentrations of unchanged spironolactone were found in the serum and spironolactone was still detectable 8 hours after dosing. The half-lives of spironolactone and 7α-thiomethylspirolactone were much shorter than that of canrenone and it was considered possible that relatively higher proportions of canrenone could be present at steady-state.— H. W. P. M. Overdiek *et al.*, *Clin. Pharmac. Ther.*, 1985, *38*, 469.

In a patient taking spironolactone 100 mg daily for 15 days, 7α-thiomethylspirolactone was found to be the major metabolite. Canrenone and 7α-thiomethylspirolactone accumulated, canrenone reaching steady state after 14 days of spironolactone therapy and 7α-thiomethylspirolactone after 9 days. No accumulation was found for the parent drug.— J. W. P. M. Overdiek and F. W. H. M. Merkus (letter), *Lancet*, 1986, *1*, 1103.

Comment that the relative contributions of spironolactone and its metabolites to both anti-mineralocorticoid activity and endocrine side-effects requires further evaluation, and that it is no longer appropriate to consider canrenone to be the major active metabolite.— P. Gardiner (letter), *Lancet*, 1985, *2*, 1432.

Further references to the activity of spironolactone and its metabolites: L. E. Ramsay *et al.*, *Br. J. clin. Pharmac.*, 1976, *3*, 607; L. E. Ramsay *et al.*, *Clin. Pharmac. Ther.*, 1976, *20*, 167; G. T. McInnes *et al.*, *Clin. Pharmac. Ther.*, 1980, *27*, 363.

PROTEIN BINDING. Protein binding of spironolactone and canrenone exceeded 89% at plasma concentrations of 550 and 710 ng per mL respectively.— A. Karim *et al.*, *Clin. Pharmac. Ther.*, 1976, *19*, 158.

Further references: A. S. Ng *et al.*, *J. pharm. Sci.*, 1980, *69*, 30.

Uses and Administration

Spironolactone, a steroid with a structure resembling that of the natural adrenocortical hormone, aldosterone, acts on the distal portion of the renal tubule as a competitive inhibitor of aldosterone. It thus increases sodium and water excretion and reduces potassium excretion. It acts both as a potassium-sparing diuretic and as an antihypertensive agent.

Spironolactone is reported to have a relatively slow onset of action, requiring 2 or 3 days for maximum effect, and a similarly slow diminishment of action over 2 or 3 days on discontinuation.

Spironolactone is used in the treatment of refractory oedema associated with congestive heart failure, cirrhosis of the liver, or the nephrotic syndrome. For these purposes it is frequently given with the thiazides, frusemide, and similar diuretics, where it adds to their natriuretic but diminishes their kaliuretic effects, hence conserving potassium. In hepatic disorders, in view of its slower onset of action, it has been recommended that it be given a few days before concomitant therapy with potassium-losing diuretics in order to prevent induction or exacerbation of hypokalaemia with the associated risk of coma. Spironolactone has also been used as an antihypertensive agent, particularly in the diagnosis and treatment of primary hyperaldosteronism. In the *UK* spironolactone is no longer recommended for use in essential hypertension or idiopathic oedema; doubts have been expressed over its safety during long-term administration.

Spironolactone is usually given in an initial dose of 100 mg daily, subsequently increased as necessary; some patients may require doses of up to 400 mg daily. It is given in doses of 400 mg daily for the diagnosis of hyperaldosteronism; in doses of 100 to 400 mg daily for the pre-operative management of hyperaldosteronism; and in the lowest effective dosage for long-term maintenance therapy in the absence of surgery. A suggested initial dose of spironolactone for children is 3 mg per kg body-weight daily, in divided doses. If necessary a suspension can be made by suspending crushed tablets in cherry syrup or methylcellulose solution (Cologel 20%, water to 100%). Such suspensions are chemically stable for one month when refrigerated.

Spironolactone has also been used for hirsutism.

Potassium supplements should not be given with spironolactone.

A detailed review of the chemistry, pharmacokinetics, mechanisms of action, uses, and unwanted effects of spironolactone.— H. R. Ochs *et al.*, *Am. Heart J.*, 1978, *96*, 389.

A study in patients with primary hyperaldosteronism, indicating that the antihypertensive effect of spironolactone is nonspecific and largely dependent on salt and water balance.— E. L. Bravo *et al.*, *Clin. Pharmac. Ther.*, 1974, *15*, 201.

A study suggesting that mineralocorticoid excess is rarely responsible for essential hypertension, and that the beneficial role of spironolactone cannot be fully explained by mineralocorticoid antagonism.— B. I. Hoffbrand *et al.*, *Br. med. J.*, 1976, *1*, 682.

Absence of correlation between the antihypertensive effect of spironolactone and changes in body-weight or plasma-renin activity.— R. I. Ogilvie *et al.*, *Clin. Pharmac. Ther.*, 1977, *21*, 113.

In a study of 14 patients taking bendrofluazide, the response of the plasma-potassium concentration to spironolactone varied sevenfold. It was suggested that variability in response between patients is such that fixed-dose thiazide-spironolactone tablets are unlikely to prevent hypokalaemia reliably.— L. E. Ramsay and J. Hettiarachchi, *Br. J. clin. Pharmac.*, 1981, *11*, 153.

In the treatment of thiazide-induced hypokalaemia, spironolactone 50 mg was equivalent to triamterene 200 mg and amiloride 20 mg.— P. R. Jackson *et al.*, *Br. J. clin. Pharmac.*, 1982, *14*, 257.

A study of the dose-response relationship of spironolactone in healthy subjects. Dose-response relationships for urinary electrolyte variables were linear between spironolactone 25 and 100 mg as single doses. The mean sodium excretion following spironolactone 200 mg was not greater than that following spironolactone 100 mg, but the response following 400 mg was consistently greater than those to lower doses.— G. T. McInnes *et al.*, *Br. J. clin. Pharmac.*, 1982, *13*, 513.

Under steady-state conditions spironolactone did not influence potassium excretion in a dose-dependent manner.— G. T. McInnes *et al.*, *Br. J. clin. Pharmac.*, 1982, *13*, 596P.

ADMINISTRATION. For reference to the enhanced bioavailability of spironolactone when given with food, see under Absorption and Fate.

ADMINISTRATION IN HEPATIC FAILURE. A study suggesting that the metabolism of spironolactone is unaltered in patients with liver disease.— U. Abshagen *et al.*, *Eur. J. clin. Pharmac.*, 1977, *11*, 169.

In 5 patients with chronic liver disease the mean elimination half-life of canrenone, a major metabolite of spironolactone, was about 59 hours, and in 7 patients with congestive heart failure about 37 hours, compared to 20.5 hours in healthy subjects. However, there was no evidence of accumulation of canrenone in plasma.— L. Jackson *et al.*, *Eur. J. clin. Pharmac.*, 1977, *11*, 177.

See also under Hepatic Disorders (below).

ADMINISTRATION IN RENAL FAILURE. Potassium-sparing diuretics are best avoided in patients with impaired renal function because of the risk of hyperkalaemia and because decline in renal function has been observed with spironolactone, triamterene, and amiloride.— R. R. Bailey (letter), *Br. med. J.*, 1978, *1*, 1618.

Spironolactone could be administered to patients with renal failure by adjusting the dosage interval. A dosage interval of 6 to 12 hours is suitable for patients whose glomerular filtration-rates exceed 50 mL per minute; an interval of 12 to 24 hours between doses is advisable for rates of between 10 and 50 mL per minute. Where the rate is less than 10 mL per minute, spironolactone should be avoided.— W. M. Bennett *et al.*, *Am. J. Kidney Dis.*, 1983, *3*, 155.

CARCINOMA. Suppression of plasma androgens by spironolactone in castrated men with carcinoma of the prostate.— P. C. Walsh and P. K. Siiteri, *J. Urol., Baltimore*, 1975, *114*, 254.

Primary aldosteronism due to adrenocortical cancer was reported in 3 patients. Treatment with spironolactone had transient clinical effects.— E. Arteaga *et al.*, *Ann. intern. Med.*, 1984, *101*, 316.

CARDIAC DISORDERS. A favourable response to spironolactone used concurrently with digoxin and chlorothiazide in infants with congestive heart failure.— S. M. Hobbins *et al.*, *Archs Dis. Childh.*, 1981, *56*, 934.

ENDOCRINE DISORDERS. Beneficial responses to spironolactone were seen in 10 of 12 patients with hirsutism, 6 of 7 patients with androgenic alopecia, and 6 of 8 patients with acne which had not responded to erythromycin or benzoyl peroxide gel. Reductions in sebum excretion rate compared favourably with those previously reported with a combination of cyproterone and oestrogen.— B. M. Burke and W. J. Cunliffe, *Br. J. Derm.*, 1985, *112*, 124.

Decrease in virilisation was seen in a study of 34 women with polycystic ovary syndrome following treatment with spironolactone 100 mg daily for 3 months.— A. Milewicz *et al.*, *Obstet. Gynec.*, 1983, *61*, 429.

Acne. In women with acne vulgaris for whom oestrogen

therapy is contra-indicated spironolactone 100 mg twice daily will suppress sebum excretion and can be of value.— W. J. Cunliffe, *Prescribers' J.*, 1987, *27*, (Aug.), 23.

A preliminary study indicating beneficial response of acne to spironolactone cream 5%.— M. Messina *et al.*, *Curr. ther. Res.*, 1983, *34*, 319. In a study involving 31 patients with moderately severe facial acne topical application of spironolactone 3% or 5% or canrenoate potassium 3% produced no reduction in sebum excretion rate over 2 months, suggesting that topical spironolactone was unlikely to be beneficial in the treatment of acne.— S. Walton *et al.* (letter), *Br. J. Derm.*, 1986, *114*, 261.

In a placebo-controlled, double-blind study of 26 patients with severe acne given spironolactone 50, 100, 150, or 200 mg daily, doses of 150 and 200 mg appeared to confer the greatest benefit. Consistent improvement was recorded in 6 of 9 female patients and 5 of 6 male patients who received spironolactone 100 mg or more daily.— A. Goodfellow *et al.*, *Br. J. Derm.*, 1984, *111*, 209.

Further references to spironolactone in the treatment of acne: M. F. Muhlemann *et al.*, *Br. J. Derm.*, 1986, *115*, 227.

Hirsutism. A review and discussion of hirsutism including treatment with spironolactone. Spironolactone has been used in doses of 75 to 200 mg daily: efficacy is not clearly improved with higher dosages, but adverse reactions appear to be dose-related. Its primary action appears to be at the androgen receptor, because changes in unbound testosterone concentrations are not always seen in patients who have a good therapeutic response.— R. S. Rittmaster and D. L. Loriaux, *Ann. intern. Med.*, 1987, *106*, 95.

In view of the large doses of anti-androgens needed to produce a modest effect in the treatment of hirsutism, the use of weaker anti-androgens such as spironolactone is illogical.— S. Shuster, *Prescribers' J.*, 1985, *25*, 12.

Beneficial response to spironolactone with a combined oral contraceptive in an open study of 23 hirsute women.— M. G. Chapman *et al.*, *Br. J. Obstet. Gynaec.*, 1985, *92*, 983.

Spironolactone 100 mg twice daily was effective in the treatment of hirsutism in 42 of 48 patients with either polycystic ovary syndrome (24) or idiopathic hirsutism (24). Polymenorrhoea, menorrhagia, or oligo-amenorrhoea in 9 patients was sufficiently severe to result in the withdrawal of treatment from 4. Menstrual regularity improved in 12 women whose periods were initially irregular. No electrolyte disturbances were noted.— D. J. Evans and C. W. Burke, *J. R. Soc. Med.*, 1986, *79*, 451.

Further studies of the use of spironolactone in hirsutism: G. Shapiro and S. Evron, *J. clin. Endocr. Metab.*, 1980, *51*, 429; D. G. Cummings *et al.*, *J. Am. med. Ass.*, 1982, *247*, 1295; D. E. Pittaway *et al.*, *Fert. Steril.*, 1985, *43*, 878; P. Serafini and R. A. Lobo, *Fert. Steril.*, 1985, *44*, 595; M. G. Chapman *et al.*, *Acta obstet. gynec. scand.*, 1986, *65*, 349; J. A. Board *et al.*, *Sth. med. J.*, 1987, *80*, 483.

For a report of hair regrowth in a bald male patient during treatment with spironolactone, see under Adverse Effects, above.

HEPATIC DISORDERS. A review of the management of ascites in patients with liver disease. Spironalctone may be regarded as the drug of choice in the management of ascites due to liver disease. It antagonises hyperaldosteronism and avoids the hypokalaemia which other diuretics may induce. If spironolactone alone does not result in a sufficient diuresis, a thiazide diuretic may be added, or, in resistant cases, a loop diuretic. However, the use of these potent diuretics may produce too rapid a diuresis resulting in hepatorenal syndrome or aggravation of encephalopathy and patients should be carefully monitored.— E. Elias, *Prescribers' J.*, 1985, *25*, 26.

A review of the pathology, diagnosis, and management of cirrhotic ascites. If bed rest and sodium restriction does not produce adequate diuresis, spironolactone therapy may be started. Although traditionally used in doses of 25 to 50 mg four times daily, doses of 300 to 600 mg (and occasionally 800 to 1000 mg) per day have been shown to be safe and effective. The urine sodium/potassium ratio may be useful in deciding the initial dose of spironolactone and perhaps also in titrating future doses. Patients with urine sodium/potassium ratios greater than 1 tend to respond to lower doses of spironolactone (100 to 150 mg daily); those with ratios less than 1 usually respond to spironolactone 200 to 1000 mg daily. There is some evidence that spironolactone is more effective than frusemide in non-uraemic cirrhotic patients with ascites. There have been few studies of the use of combined diuretic preparations in cirrhotic patients, but they are not recommended for routine use because of the considerable rate of complications associated with them.— V. K. Rocco and A. J. Ware, *Ann. intern. Med.*, 1986, *105*, 573.

Comment that spironolactone may not be the diuretic of choice in cirrhotic ascites and that frusemide should also be considered. There is a risk of hyperkalaemia in patients with impaired renal function given spironolactone and the effects of the drug persist after it is withdrawn. However, frusemide-induced hypokalaemia could precipitate hepatic encephalopathy.— A. Spital (letter), *Ann. intern. Med.*, 1987, *106*, 169.

Further reviews of the management of hepatic ascites: *Br. med. J.*, 1978, *1*, 66.

References to the use of spironolactone in ascites due to hepatic disease: R. C. Eggert, *Br. med. J.*, 1970, *4*, 401; N. Papadoyanakis *et al.*, *Br. J. clin. Pract.*, 1972, *26*, 27; T. Feher *et al.* (letter), *Lancet*, 1976, *2*, 51; A. A. Mihas *et al.* (letter), *Lancet*, 1977, *1*, 914; J. L. Campra and T. B. Reynolds, *Am. J. dig. Dis.*, 1978, *23*, 1025; D. M. Danks (letter), *J. Pediat.*, 1976, *88*, 695.

For further reports on the use of spironolactone in the treatment of hepatic cirrhosis and cardiac oedema, see Frusemide, p.990.

HIRSUTISM. For references to the treatment of hirsutism with spironolactone, see under Endocrine Disorders, above.

HYPERTENSION. A review of the drugs used in chronic hypertension. Spironolactone has some antihypertensive activity but causes troublesome adverse effects, particularly tender gynaecomastia in men.— *Med. Lett.*, 1984, *26*, 107.

In a double-blind crossover study of 24 hypertensive patients, 13 of whom had normal and 11 of whom had low renin activity, administration of spironolactone had no advantage over hydrochlorothiazide in either group. Side-effects were significantly higher following spironolactone administration and included skin eruption, lassitude, gastro-intestinal complaints, and breast swelling and tenderness in men.— R. K. Ferguson *et al.*, *Clin. Pharmac. Ther.*, 1977, *21*, 62.

Further references to the use of spironolactone in hypertension: G. M. Bell *et al.* (letter), *Br. J. clin. Pharmac.*, 1981, *12*, 585; J. H. Kreeft *et al.*, *Can. med. Ass. J.*, 1983, *128*, 31; S. Freestone *et al.*, *Br. J. clin. Pharmac.*, 1983, *15*, 622P.

Associated with aldosteronism. In 67 patients with hypertension, raised plasma concentrations of aldosterone, and low plasma concentrations of renin, there was an inverse correlation between aldosterone and renin concentrations. After treatment with spironolactone 50 to 400 mg daily for at least 4 weeks, blood pressure was reduced from a mean of 201/122 to 159/101 mmHg 3 to 5 weeks after starting treatment. The response was comparable in those with or without adrenocortical adenoma and was greater in those with lower initial blood-urea concentrations. In 32 patients subjected to surgery, usually for adrenocortical adenoma, there was good correlation between postoperative hypotensive response and prior response to spironolactone.— J. J. Brown *et al.*, *Br. med. J.*, 1972, *2*, 729.

A detailed account of the surgical and medical management of patients with low-renin (primary) hyperaldosteronism. In patients with a good response to pre-operative spironolactone, surgical removal of the tumour-bearing gland is usually the treatment of choice. Long-term spironolactone therapy is, however, an acceptable alternative, and if it is not tolerated, amiloride may be substituted.— J. B. Ferriss *et al.*, *Am. Heart J.*, 1978, *96*, 97.

MENTAL DISORDERS. Six manic-depressive patients who were well maintained on lithium therapy but who found its side-effects unacceptable were changed to spironolactone 25 mg four times daily. Over a follow-up period of 12 to 18 months 5 of the 6 were maintained satisfactorily. Spironolactone might act by stabilising a presynaptic membrane in the hypothalamus against fluctuations of aldosterone seen in manic disease.— N. H. Hendler, *J. nerv. ment. Dis.*, 1978, *166*, 517.

Beneficial response to lithium and spironolactone in a patient with recurrent manic illness suggesting that this combination may be useful in patients resistant to lithium or in whom low doses of lithium are advisable.— M. A. Gillman and F. J. Lichtigfeld, *Br. med. J.*, 1986, *292*, 661.

MOUNTAIN SICKNESS. Two of 6 unacclimatised climbers taking spironolactone 25 mg three times daily starting 48 hours before reaching 3000 m developed acute mountain sickness compared with 5 of 6 similar climbers taking a placebo. A larger study was needed to confirm the value of spironolactone.— G. V. Brown *et al.* (letter), *Lancet*, 1977, *1*, 855.

Further comments on experience with spironolactone in mountain sickness: T. T. Currie *et al.*, *Med. J. Aust.*, 1976, *2*, 168; A. C. McFarlane (letter), *ibid.*, 923; T. T. Currie (letter), *ibid.*, 1977, *1*, 419; J. A. Snell and E. P. Cordner, *ibid.*, 828; A. C. McFarlane (letter), *ibid.*, *2*, 616; G. Turnbull (letter), *Br. med. J.*, 1980, *280*, 1453; D. H. Meyers (letter), *ibid.*, *281*, 1569; L. D. Rutter (letter), *ibid.*, 618.

See also under Acetazolamide Sodium, p.976.

PREMENSTRUAL SYNDROME. A report of a double-blind crossover study, involving 18 women with premenstrual tension and 10 control women, during 4 menstrual cycles, comparing spironolactone 25 mg four times daily from the 18th to the 26th day of the cycle, with placebo. Spironolactone had a beneficial effect on weight gain and mood in most of those with premenstrual syndrome. There was no evidence to support the hypothesis that aldosterone concentrations were higher in the symptomatic group and it is probable that spironolactone acted purely through its diuretic effect.— P. M. S. O'Brien *et al.*, *Br. J. Obstet. Gynaec.*, 1979, *86*, 142.

Further references to the use of spironolactone in premenstrual syndrome: I. D. Vellacott *et al.*, *Curr. med. Res. Opinion*, 1987, *10*, 450.

Preparations

Spironolactone Tablets *(B.P.)*

Spironolactone Tablets *(U.S.P.)*

Proprietary Preparations

Aldactone *(Searle, UK). Tablets*, spironolactone 25, 50, and 100 mg.

Diatensec *(Gold Cross, UK). Tablets*, spironolactone 50 mg.

Laractone *(Lagap, UK). Tablets*, spironolactone 25, 50, and 100 mg.

Spiretic *(DDSA Pharmaceuticals, UK). Tablets*, spironolactone 25 and 100 mg.

Spiroctan *(MCP Pharmaceuticals, UK). Capsules*, spironolactone 100 mg.
Tablets, spironolactone 25 and 50 mg.

Spirolone *(Berk Pharmaceuticals, UK). Tablets*, spironolactone 25, 50, and 100 mg.

Proprietary Names and Manufacturers

Acelat *(Searle, Ger.)*; Aldace *(Searle, Ger.)*; Aldactone *(Searle, Austral.; Searle, Canad.; Denm.; Searle, Fr.; Boehringer Mannheim, Ger.; Lepetit, Ital.; Neth.; Searle, Norw.; Searle, S.Afr.; Searle, Spain; Searle, Swed.; Searle, Switz.; Searle, UK; Searle, USA)*; Aldactone-A *(Arg.; Jpn; Neth.; Spain)*; Aldopur *(Heumann, Ger.)*; Alexan *(Jpn)*; Almatol *(Jpn)*; Alpamed *(Jpn)*; Altex *(USA)*; Aporasnon *(Jpn)*; Aquareduct *(Azupharma, Ger.)*; Diatensec *(Gold Cross, UK)*; Dira *(Jpn)*; Duraspiron *(Durachemie, Ger.)*; Hexalacton *(Durascan, Denm.)*; Hokuraton *(Jpn)*; Idrolattone *(Zoja, Ital.)*; Lacalmin *(Jpn)*; Lacdene *(Jpn)*; Laractone *(Lagap, UK)*; Nefurofan *(Jpn)*; Noidouble *(Jpn)*; Novospiroton *(Novopharm, Canad.)*; Osiren *(Hoechst, Denm.; Hoechst, Norw.; Hoechst, Switz.)*; Osyrol *(Hoechst, Ger.; Jpn)*; Pirolacton *(Jpn)*; Practon *(Biogalenique, Fr.)*; Rolactone Microfine *(Doms, Fr.)*; Sagisal *(Sagitta, Ger.)*; Sincomen *(Berlex, Canad.; Schering, Ger.; Farmades, Ital.; S.Afr.)*; Spiractin *(Lennon, S.Afr.)*; Spiretic *(DDSA Pharmaceuticals, UK)*; Spiridon *(Orion, Swed.; Orion, Switz.)*; Spirix *(Benzon, Denm.; Benzon, Norw.; Benzon, Swed.)*; Spiro *(Beiersdorf, Ger.)*; Spiroctan *(Médicia, Fr.; Neth.; Boehringer Mannheim, Swed.; Boehringer Mannheim, Switz.; MCP Pharmaceuticals, UK)*; Spirolang *(Smith Kline & French, Ital.)*; Spirolone *(Berk Pharmaceuticals, UK)*; Spiron *(Orion, Denm.)*; Spironone *(Clin Midy, Fr.)*; Spiropal *(Nyco, Norw.)*; Spirotone *(Protea, Austral.)*; Supra-Puren *(Klinge-Nattermann, Ger.)*; Suracton *(Jpn)*; Tensin *(Rolab, S.Afr.)*; Uractone *(SPA, Ital.)*; Urusonin *(Jpn)*; Verospirone *(Hung.)*; Xénalon *(Mepha, Switz.)*.

The following names have been used for multi-ingredient preparations containing spironolactone— Aldactazide *(Searle, Canad.; Searle, USA)*; Aldactide *(Gold Cross, UK)*; Lasilactone *(Hoechst, UK)*; Novospirozine *(Novopharm, Canad.)*; Spironazide *(Schein, USA)*; Spiroprop *(Searle, UK)*.

2356-l

Teclothiazide Potassium *(BANM, rINNM).*
Tetrachlormethiazide. The potassium salt of 6-chloro-3,4-dihydro-3-trichloromethyl-2*H*-1,2,4-benzothiadiazine-7-sulphonamide 1,1-dioxide.
$C_8H_6Cl_4KN_3O_4S_2$=453.2.

CAS — 4267-05-4 (teclothiazide); 5306-80-9 (potassium salt).

Teclothiazide potassium is a thiazide diuretic with properties similar to those of chlorothiazide (see p.981). It has been given in doses of 110 to 165 mg daily.

Proprietary Names and Manufacturers
Deplet *(Marshall's Pharmaceuticals, UK).*

2357-y

Tienilic Acid *(BAN, rINN).*
SKF-62698; Ticrynafen *(USAN).* [2,3-Dichloro-4-(2-thenoyl)phenoxy]acetic acid.
$C_{13}H_8Cl_2O_4S$=331.2.

CAS — 40180-04-9.

Adverse Effects
Severe liver damage has been associated with tienilic acid therapy which has resulted in a number of deaths; for this reason tienilic acid has been withdrawn in many countries.
Like chlorothiazide, administration of tienilic acid may be associated with electrolyte imbalances, notably hypokalaemia; it has also been associated with reduced glucose tolerance and increased plasma-triglyceride concentrations. Unlike chlorothiazide, tienilic acid has a uricosuric action and reduces, rather than raises, plasma concentrations of uric acid; its prolonged administration has not therefore been associated with the development of gout. During initial therapy its uric acid mobilising action has precipitated acute attacks of gout in hyperuricaemic subjects. It can also cause renal failure and the production of urate renal stones.

EFFECTS ON THE ELECTROLYTE BALANCE. During a comparative study both hydrochlorothiazide and tienilic acid significantly reduced serum concentrations of potassium and chloride and increased serum bicarbonate content. Four patients developed hypokalaemia; in 2 it was severe enough to require potassium supplements during tienilic acid therapy.— E. D. Frohlich *et al., Postgrad. med. J.,* 1979, *55, Suppl.* 3, 98.

EFFECTS ON ENDOCRINE FUNCTION. A man had to start shaving twice daily three days after starting tienilic acid therapy; he had not done this for 15 years. A woman with previous thining of hair felt that regrowth of fine hair at the hairline slowed when she started tienilic acid.— H. J. Waal-Manning *et al., Postgrad. med. J.,* 1979, *55, Suppl.* 3, 85.

EFFECTS ON THE HEART. A patient complained of chest pain on several occasions after receiving tienilic acid.— M. Nemati *et al., J. Am. med. Ass.,* 1977, *237,* 652.

EFFECTS ON THE KIDNEYS. A 45-year-old woman developed oliguric renal failure 5 days after starting treatment with tienilic acid; acute uric acid nephropathy was probably the cause.— W. M. Bennett *et al.* (letter), *New Engl. J. Med.,* 1979, *301,* 1179. Acute renal failure occurred in 2 patients within hours of a single dose of tienilic acid.— L. H. Cohen *et al.* (letter), *ibid.,* 1180. An untoward reaction to tienilic acid has been reported in about 0.05% of patients; it has usually been limited to hypertensive patients with raised uric-acid concentrations whose treatment has been changed to tienilic acid without a diuretic-free period or adequate hydration. The reaction is characterised by flank or abdominal pain, noted within hours of the first dose, followed by nausea, vomiting, uraemia, transient oliguria, and rarely, anuria. Treatment of the reaction has included hydration and administration of allopurinol with or without loop diuretics although, in general, disturbances have cleared within 7 to 10 days of discontinuing tienilic acid regardless of the measures used. It appears that the reaction may be avoided if patients are adequately hydrated before starting treatment with tienilic acid and other diuretics discontinued 3 days beforehand.— T. Selby, *Smith Kline & French, USA* (letter), *ibid.*

EFFECTS ON LIPID METABOLISM. Significant increases in plasma triglyceride concentrations during tienilic acid therapy.— E. D. Frohlich *et al., Postgrad. med. J.,* 1979, *55, Suppl.* 3, 98.

EFFECTS ON THE LIVER. Tienilic acid had been withdrawn from the *U.S.* market because of strong suspicion of hepatic damage; 56 cases had been reported. Damage was predominantly hepatocellular, with fever, malaise, and abdominal pain; jaundice occurred in about 60% of cases. Toxicity usually occurred 1 to 3 months after starting treatment, and was generally reversible.— *FDA Drug Bull.,* 1980, *10,* 3.
Discussion of the clinicopathological features of hepatic disease caused by tienilic acid in 37 patients.— J. -P. Lafay *et al., Gastroenterol. clin. biol.,* 1983, *7,* 523.
An analysis of 340 cases of hepatic injury associated with tienilic acid.— H. J. Zimmerman *et al., Hepatology,* 1984, *4,* 315.

GOUT. Changing from a thiazide diuretic to tienilic acid appeared to precipitate acute attacks of gout in 2 patients with hyperuricaemia. By increasing excretion and mobilisation of urate, tienilic acid might precipitate acute attacks of gout in a similar manner to uricosuric agents.— R. S. King and B. A. Wichman (letter), *New Engl. J. Med.,* 1979, *301,* 1065.

Precautions
As for Chlorothiazide, p.982.
Severe liver damage has been associated with tienilic acid therapy which has resulted in a number of deaths; for this reason tienilic acid has been withdrawn in many countries.
Despite its uricosuric properties, tienilic acid is not suitable for the treatment of gout, because it is a diuretic. It has been recommended that tienilic acid therapy should not be initiated in patients being treated with other diuretics or within 3 days of stopping such treatment, and should only be initiated in adequately hydrated patients.
The effect of warfarin may be enhanced by concurrent administration of tienilic acid, and the uricosuric action of tienilic acid may be diminished by concurrent administration of aspirin (the plasma concentrations of which may, in turn, be raised by tienilic acid).

INTERACTIONS. *Diuretics.* Acute renal insufficiency occurred in a woman given tienilic acid in addition to amiloride.— D. Hillion *et al., Nouv. Presse méd.,* 1979, *27,* 2284.

Phenytoin and other anti-epileptics. A woman receiving phenytoin 300 mg daily developed dizziness, slurred speech, confusion, and ataxia on addition of tienilic acid. She gradually recovered on withdrawal of tienilic acid.— K. T. Weber and A. P. Fishman, *Postgrad. med. J.,* 1979, *55, Suppl.* 3, 58.

Warfarin. For enhancement of the effect of warfarin by tienilic acid, see Warfarin Sodium, p.346.

Uses and Administration
Although chemically related to ethacrynic acid, tienilic acid is a diuretic with uses similar to those of chlorothiazide (see p.983). Unlike chlorothiazide it also has a uricosuric action, which, it has been considered, might be of benefit to hypertensive patients who are also hyperuricaemic. Diuresis lasts for up to about 12 hours.
Severe liver damage has been associated with tienilic acid therapy which has resulted in a number of deaths; for this reason tienilic acid has been withdrawn in many countries.
Tienilic acid has been given in doses of 250 to 500 mg daily initially then adjusted according to response. Patients must be adequately hydrated and not receiving other diuretic therapy before starting tienilic acid treatment.
When treatment is prolonged, or in susceptible patients, loss of potassium may be sufficient to produce hypokalaemia; potassium supplements should then be given as for chlorothiazide.

A brief review of the clinical pharmacology and therapeutic use of tienilic acid.— A. Lant, *Drugs,* 1985, *29,* 162.

ADMINISTRATION. To avoid possible renal impairment associated with the uricosuric activity of tienilic acid, therapy should be started with low doses and after neutralisation of the urine.— G. Lohmöller *et al., Postgrad. med. J.,* 1979, *55, Suppl.* 3, 68.

HYPERTENSION. In a double-blind randomised study, 240 men with mild to moderate hypertension took either tienilic acid, 250 or 500 mg, or hydrochlorothiazide, 50 or 100 mg, once daily for 6 weeks. All 4 regimens were associated with significant reductions in systolic and diastolic blood pressure although tienilic acid 250 mg daily appeared to be less effective. Serum concentrations of uric acid were significantly reduced by both doses of tienilic acid but rose in patients taking hydrochlorothiazide. Mean serum-potassium concentrations were reduced in all 4 groups. Mean serum-creatinine concentrations rose significantly more in patients on tienilic acid although the absolute increase was not great. Of these patients 189 continued treatment for a total of 6 months, doses being individually titrated up to a maximum of tienilic acid 1 g daily or hydrochlorothiazide 200 mg daily. At the end of 6 months blood pressure had been similarly reduced by both drugs. Treatment was generally well tolerated although there was more postural dizziness in patients taking tienilic acid.— Veterans Administration Cooperative Study Group on Antihypertensive Agents, *New Engl. J. Med.,* 1979, *301,* 293.

Proprietary Names and Manufacturers
Diflurex *(Anphar-Rolland, Fr.; Max Ritter, Switz.)*; Selcryn *(RIT, Belg.; Smith Kline & French, USA).*

17013-f

Tizolemide *(BAN, rINN).*
Hoe-740 (hydrochloride); S-730740B (hydrochloride). 2-Chloro-5-(4-hydroxy-3-methyl-2-methyliminothiazolidin-4-yl)-benzenesulphonamide.
$C_{11}H_{14}ClN_3O_3S_2$=335.8.

CAS — 56488-58-5.

Tizolemide is a diuretic.

References: W. P. Leary and A. J. Reyes, *S. Afr. med. J.,* 1982, *61,* 398; B. Beermann *et al., Clin. Nephrol.,* 1983, *19,* 124; B. Beermann and C. Edelstam, *Eur. Heart J.,* 1984, *5,* 338.

Proprietary Names and Manufacturers
Hoechst, Ger.

1272-d

Torasemide *(BAN, rINN).*
AC-4464; BM-02.015. 1-Isopropyl-3-(4-*m*-toluidinopyridine-3-sulphonyl)urea.
$C_{16}H_{20}N_4O_3S$=348.4.

CAS — 56211-40-6; 72810-59-4 (torasemide sodium).

Torasemide is a loop diuretic with properties similar to those of frusemide (see p.989). It has been used in doses of 10 to 20 mg daily.

In a study of 13 patients with chronic heart failure, a single dose of torasemide 20 mg was more effective than frusemide 40 mg, which was not significantly different from torasemide 10 mg.— A. J. Scheen *et al., Eur. J. clin. Pharmac.,* 1986, *31, Suppl.,* 35.
A study of the pharmacokinetics and pharmacodynamics of torasemide in healthy subjects. An intravenous dose of between 10 and 20 mg had a natriuretic effect similar to frusemide 40 mg. The pharmacokinetic data indicated that the elimination half-life may be dose-dependent, and it is possible that torasemide may have a prolonged action at high doses. There was also evidence of dose-dependent renal excretion.— D. C. Brater *et al., Clin. Pharmac. Ther.,* 1987, *42,* 187.
Further references to the actions of torasemide: Y. Ambroes *et al., Eur. J. clin. Pharmac.,* 1986, *31, Suppl.,* 1; R. Lambe *et al., ibid.,* 9; R. Cuvelier *et al., ibid.,* 15; L. Dodion *et al., ibid.,* 21; J. Broekhuysen *et al., ibid.,* 29.

Proprietary Names and Manufacturers
MCP Pharmaceuticals, UK.

2358-j

Triamterene *(BAN, USAN, rINN).*
SKF-8542; Triamterenum. 6-Phenylpteridine-2,4,7-triamine.
$C_{12}H_{11}N_7$=253.3.

CAS — 396-01-0.

Pharmacopoeias. In *Belg., Br., Braz., Chin., Cz., Egypt., Eur., Fr., Ind., It., Jpn., Jug., Neth., Swiss., and U.S.*

A yellow odourless crystalline powder.
B.P. **solubilities** are: very slightly soluble in water, alcohol, and chloroform; practically insoluble in ether. *U.S.P.* solubilities are: 1 in 30 of formic acid and 1 in 85 of 2-methoxyethanol; very slightly soluble in acetic acid and dilute mineral acids; practically insoluble in water, chlo-

roform, ether, and dilute solutions of alkali hydroxides. Acidified solutions give a blue fluorescence. **Store** in airtight containers. Protect from light.

Adverse Effects

The adverse effects of triamterene are similar to those reported with amiloride (p.977). Triamterene has also been reported to cause photosensitivity reactions, increases in uric acid concentrations, and blood dyscrasias. Nephrolithiasis may occur in susceptible patients, and megaloblastic anaemia has been reported in patients with depleted folic acid stores such as those with hepatic cirrhosis.

ALLERGY. Fever and rigor were associated with the use of triamterene in a 53-year-old woman.— M. A. Safdi (letter), *New Engl. J. Med.*, 1980, *303*, 701.

EFFECTS ON THE BLOOD. A patient with cirrhosis of the liver developed megaloblastosis after 2 weeks' treatment with triamterene. The dihydrofolate reductase activity of bone marrow was inhibited and it was considered that triamterene should be used with caution in patients, such as pregnant women and alcoholics, with reduced stores of folate.— J. Corcino *et al.*, *Ann. intern. Med.*, 1970, *73*, 419.

Acute pancytopenia associated with triamterene therapy in 2 patients.— G. Castellano *et al.*, *Gastroenterol. Hepatol.*, 1983, *6*, 540.

Report of pancytopenia in 2 patients associated with triamterene therapy. A review of the published literature revealed 10 further reports.— A. Remacha *et al.*, *Biol. clin. Hematol.*, 1983, *5*, 127.

EFFECTS ON THE ELECTROLYTE BALANCE. In a study in 16 healthy subjects, triamterene administration caused significant increases in renal clearances of magnesium and sodium and significant decreases in the clearances of creatinine, potassium, and uric acid. Calcium and phosphate clearance was not significantly altered. It is unlikely that triamterene would produce significant elevation of serum-calcium or uric acid concentrations in non-azotaemic patients although magnesium depletion could complicate long-term therapy.— B. R. Walker *et al.*, *Clin. Pharmac. Ther.*, 1972, *13*, 245.

For a report of metabolic acidosis in patients receiving triamterene and total parenteral nutrition, see Amiloride p.977. For a report of hyponatraemia in elderly patients taking thiazide with potassium-sparing diuretics, see Hydrochlorothiazide p.992.

EFFECTS ON THE KIDNEYS. Acute interstitial nephritis was associated with triamterene therapy in a 52-year-old woman.— R. R. Bailey *et al.* (letter), *Lancet*, 1982, *1*, 226.

A review and discussion of the effects of triamterene on the kidneys. An abnormal urinary sediment was described (K.F. Fairley *et al.*, *Lancet*, 1983, *1*, 421) in patients taking triamterene which was thought to represent precipitated triamterene. These observations were expanded in a crossover study by Spence *et al.* (*ibid.*, 1985, *2*, 73). Abnormal urinary sediment was seen in 14 of 26 patients while taking triamterene but in none while taking amiloride. Triamterene and its metabolites had been identified by Ettinger *et al.* (*J. Am. med. Ass.*, 1980, *244*, 2443) in 181 of 50 000 renal calculi. Triamterene either formed the nucleus of the stone or was deposited with calcium oxalate or uric acid. One-third of the 181 stones were entirely or predominantly composed of triamterene and its metabolites. There had been further reports of nephrolithiasis associated with triamterene although Jick *et al.* (*J. Urol., Baltimore*, 1982, *127*, 224) found no evidence that triamterene use was associated with an increased incidence of renal stones.— *Lancet*, 1986, *1*, 424.

A study of the solubility of triamterene and its metabolite. The urinary excretion pattern and metabolism in 11 patients who had passed kidney stones containing triamterene was the same as in 103 other patients taking triamterene regularly or 6 healthy subjects. The solubility of triamterene in urine was approximately one-half of its solubility in buffer solution, whereas the sulphate ester was nearly twice as soluble in urine as in buffer solution: in the majority of subjects studied the concentration of the sulphate ester approached or exceeded apparent solubility limits in urine. Alteration in the metabolism of triamterene was probably not a factor in triamterene nephrolithiasis. The saturation of urine with triamterene and especially with the sulphate ester may be related to stone formation.— F. Sörgel *et al.*, *J. pharm. Sci.*, 1986, *75*, 129. See also B. Ettinger, *J. clin. Pharmac.*, 1985, *25*, 365.

For a report of renal colic induced by triamterene and hydrochlorothiazide, see Hydrochlorothiazide, p.991.

Precautions

As for Amiloride, p.977. Triamterene should be given with caution to patients with hyperuricaemia or gout, or a history of nephrolithiasis. Patients with depleted folic acid stores such as those with hepatic cirrhosis may be at increased risk of megaloblastic anaemia.

Triamterene may interfere with the fluorescent measurement of quinidine; it may slightly colour the urine blue.

INTERACTIONS. Reports of renal failure in patients taking triamterene with non-steroidal anti-inflammatory drugs: L. Favre *et al.*, *Ann. intern. Med.*, 1982, *96*, 317; M. Häkönen and S. Ekblom-Kullberg (letter), *Br. med. J.*, 1986, *293*, 698.

For references on the antagonism of the action of potassium-sparing diuretics by non-steroidal anti-inflammatory drugs, see p.974.

For reports of the effects of triamterene on digoxin, see p.828, and on amantadine, see p.1008.

Absorption and Fate

Triamterene is variably but fairly rapidly absorbed from the gastro-intestinal tract. The bioavailability has been reported to be about 50%. It has been estimated to have a plasma half-life of about 2 hours and is about 60% bound to plasma proteins. It is extensively metabolised and is mainly excreted in the urine in the form of metabolites with some unchanged triamterene. *Animal* studies have indicated that triamterene crosses the placental barrier and is excreted in milk.

Triamterene clearance was markedly decreased in 7 patients with alcoholic cirrhosis and ascites. The diuretic effect lasted for up to 48 hours in cirrhotic patients compared with 8 hours in healthy controls.— J. P. Villeneuve *et al.*, *Clin. Pharmac. Ther.*, 1984, *35*, 831.

Studies of the pharmacokinetics of triamterene indicating that it is rapidly and extensively metabolised. There was some evidence of first-pass hepatic metabolism and entero-hepatic circulation.— A. W. Pruitt *et al.*, *Clin. Pharmac. Ther.*, 1977, *21*, 610; U. Gundert-Remy *et al.*, *Eur. J. clin. Pharmac.*, 1979, *16*, 39.

References to the bioavailability of triamterene: H. J. Gilfrich *et al.*, *Eur. J. clin. Pharmac.*, 1983, *25*, 237; F. Sörgel *et al.*, *Clin. Pharmac. Ther.*, 1985, *38*, 306; R. L. Williams *et al.*, *ibid.*, 1986, *40*, 226.

Uses and Administration

Triamterene is a mild diuretic which has actions and uses similar to amiloride (p.977). It produces a diuresis in about 2 to 4 hours, with a duration of 7 to 9 hours. The full effect may be delayed until after several days of treatment.

Triamterene adds to the natriuretic but diminishes the kaliuretic effects of other diuretics, and is mainly used as an adjunct to the thiazides, frusemide, and similar diuretics, to conserve potassium, in the treatment of refractory oedema associated with hepatic cirrhosis, congestive heart failure, and the nephrotic syndrome.

When given alone, the suggested range of dosage is 150 to 250 mg daily; 100 mg twice daily, after breakfast and lunch, is considered to be the optimum dose, preferably on alternate days for maintenance therapy. More than 300 mg daily should not be given. Smaller doses are suggested initially when other diuretics are being given.

In children, when given alone, a suggested initial dose is 1 to 2 mg per kg body-weight twice daily. Potassium supplements should not be given.

ADMINISTRATION. *In the elderly*. Use of triamterene in association with hydrochlorothiazide in 549 elderly patients. Of 189 who had normal serum-potassium concentrations before treatment, 5% developed hypokalaemia and 12% developed hyperkalaemia.— A. D. Bender *et al.*, *J. Am. Geriat. Soc.*, 1967, *15*, 166.

ADMINISTRATION IN RENAL FAILURE. Triamterene could be given in usual doses in mild or moderate renal failure. It should be avoided in patients with a glomerular filtration-rate of less than 10 mL per minute.— W. M. Bennett *et al.*, *Am. J. Kidney Dis.*, 1983, *3*, 155.

Urinary excretion of triamterene and its hydroxysulphuric acid ester were significantly reduced in patients with renal failure. The results suggested accumulation of the active metabolite.— H. Knauf *et al.*, *Eur. J. clin. Pharmac.*, 1983, *24*, 453.

ADMINISTRATION WITH POTASSIUM-WASTING DIURETICS. In patients taking bendrofluazide, triamterene 100 to 200 mg and spironolactone 50 to 100 mg daily increased serum-potassium concentrations more than administration of potassium chloride in a dose of potassium 32 to 64 mmol daily. Triamterene 200 mg was considered to be equivalent to spironolactone 50 mg. Potassium chloride was considered to be ineffective in correcting moderate diuretic-induced hypokalaemia even at doses of 64 mmol potassium daily.— P. R. Jackson *et al.*, *Br. J. clin. Pharmac.*, 1982, *14*, 257.

In a crossover study of 16 patients with diuretic-induced hypokalaemia, triamterene 50 to 200 mg daily increased plasma-potassium concentrations to 3.5 mmol per litre or above in 10 patients. Potassium supplements of up to 96 mmol daily increased plasma-potassium concentrations to this value in 8 patients. Some patients who failed to respond to one drug did respond to the other.— V. Papademetriou *et al.*, *Archs intern. Med.*, 1985, *145*, 1986.

Reports of the use of triamterene to reduce thiazide-induced hypokalaemia: E. L. Webb *et al.*, *J. int. med. Res.*, 1984, *12*, 133; E. L. Webb *et al.*, *ibid.*, 140; E. L. Webb *et al.*, *ibid.*, 147.

For further references to the use of potassium-sparing diuretics for the prophylaxis or treatment of diuretic-induced hypokalaemia, see p.973.

HEPATIC DISORDERS. A discussion of the use of the potassium-sparing diuretics, including triamterene, in cirrhosis of the liver.— P. Vesin, *Postgrad. med. J.*, 1975, *51*, 545.

Further references to triamterene in hepatic cirrhosis: E. J. Thompson *et al.*, *Clin. Pharmac. Ther.*, 1977, *21*, 392 (with frusemide).

Preparations

Triamterene Capsules *(B.P.)*. Store at a temperature not exceeding 30°.

Triamterene Capsules *(U.S.P.)*. Store in airtight containers. Protect from light.

Proprietary Preparations

Dytac *(Bridge, UK)*. *Capsules*, triamterene 50 mg.

Proprietary Names and Manufacturers

Diesse *(Biosint, Ital.)*; Diucelpin *(Jpn)*; Dyrenium *(Smith Kline & French, Canad.; Smith Kline & French, Switz.; Smith Kline & French, USA)*; Dytac *(Smith Kline & French, Austral.; Belg.; Neth.; S.Afr.; Bridge, UK)*; Jatropur *(Röhm, Ger.)*; Natrium *(Ravizza, Ital.)*; Tériam *(Roussel, Fr.)*; Triamteril *(Ital.)*; Urocaudal *(Jorba, Spain)*.

The following names have been used for multi-ingredient preparations containing triamterene—Apo-Triazide *(Apotex, Canad.)*; Diucomb *(Melusin, Ger.)*; Dyazide *(Smith Kline & French, Austral.; Smith Kline & French, Canad.; Bridge, UK; Smith Kline & French, USA)*; Dytenzide; Dytide *(Bridge, UK)*; Frusene *(Fisons, UK)*; Kalspare *(Rorer, UK)*; Maxzide *(Lederle, USA)*; Novotriamzide *(Novopharm, Canad.)*; Triamco *(Norton, UK)*.

2359-z

Trichlormethiazide *(USAN, rINN)*.

Trichlormethiazidum. 6-Chloro-3-dichloromethyl-3,4-dihydro-2*H*-1,2,4-benzothiadiazine-7-sulphonamide 1,1-dioxide.

$C_8H_8Cl_3N_3O_4S_2$=380.6.

CAS — 133-67-5.

Pharmacopoeias. In *Jpn* and *U.S.*

A white or almost white, odourless or almost odourless, crystalline powder.

Very slightly **soluble** in water, chloroform, and ether; soluble 1 in 48 of alcohol, 1 in about 9 of dioxan, and 1 in about 4 of dimethylformamide; freely soluble in acetone; soluble in methyl alcohol. The *U.S.P.* tablets should be stored in airtight containers.

Adverse Effects, Treatment, and Precautions

As for Chlorothiazide, p.981.

Report of depression in 8 patients taking diuretics, including 2 patients taking trichlormethiazide.— F. Okada, *Am. J. Psychiat.*, 1985, *142*, 1101.

Uses and Administration

Trichlormethiazide is a thiazide diuretic with actions and uses similar to those of chlorothiazide (see p.983). Diuresis is initiated in about 2 hours, and lasts about 24 hours.

In the treatment of oedema the usual dose is 1 to 4 mg daily or intermittently. In the treatment of hypertension the usual dose is 2 to 4 mg daily, either alone, or in conjunction with other antihypertensive agents.

When treatment is prolonged, or in susceptible patients, loss of potassium may be sufficient to produce hypokalaemia; potassium supplements or a potassium-sparing diuretic should then be given as for chlorothiazide.

ADMINISTRATION IN RENAL FAILURE. The plasma half-life of trichlormethiazide and the area under the plasma concentration-time curve were greater in 5 patients with impaired renal function (mean creatinine clearance 48 mL per minute) compared with 7 patients with creatinine clearance greater than 90 mL per minute. There were no differences in the peak plasma concentrations of trichlormethiazide or the time to maximum concentration between the two groups and the amount of trichlormethiazide recovered in the urine in 48 hours was 62 to 70% of the administered dose in both groups. However, a patient with a creatinine clearance of 5 mL per minute only excreted 24.4% of the drug.— I. S. Sketris *et al.*, *Eur. J. clin. Pharmac.*, 1981, *20*, 453.

Preparations

Trichlormethiazide Tablets *(U.S.P.)*

Proprietary Names and Manufacturers

Achletin *(Jpn)*; Anatran *(Jpn)*; Anistadin *(Jpn)*; Aponorin *(Jpn)*; Carvacron *(Jpn)*; Chlopolidine *(Jpn)*; Cretonin *(Jpn)*; Diu-Fortan *(Lazar, Arg.)*; Esmarin *(E. Merck, Ger.)*; Fluitran *(Schering Corp., Denm.*; *SCA, Ital.*; *Schering, Norw.*; *Schering, NZ)*; Flutra *(Schering, Swed.)*; Hidroalogen *(Spain)*; Intromene *(Jpn)*; Kubacron *(Jpn)*; Metahydrin *(Merrell Dow, USA)*; Naqua *(Schering, USA)*; Sanamiron *(Jpn)*; Schebitran *(Jpn)*; Tachionin *(Jpn)*; Tolcasone *(Jpn)*; Triazide *(Legere, USA)*; Triflumen *(Spain)*.

The following names have been used for multi-ingredient preparations containing trichlormethiazide— Metatensin *(Merrell Dow, USA)*; Naquival *(Schering, USA)*.

1293-v

Tripamide *(USAN, rINN)*.

ADR-033; E-614. 4-Chloro-*N*-(*endo*-hexahydro-4,7-methanoisoindolin-2-yl)-3-sulphamoylbenzamide.

$C_{16}H_{20}ClN_3O_3S$=369.9.

CAS — 73803-48-2.

Tripamide is a diuretic structurally related to indapamide.

References: D. C. Brater and S. Anderson, *Clin. Pharmac. Ther.*, 1983, *34*, 79; T. C. Fagan *et al.*, *ibid.*, 1986, *40*, 352; K. A. Conrad *et al.*, *ibid.*, 476.

Proprietary Names and Manufacturers

Adria, USA.

2360-p

Trometamol *(BAN, rINN)*.

THAM; Trihydroxymethylaminomethane; TRIS; Tris(hydroxymethyl)aminomethane; Tromethamine *(USAN)*. 2-Amino-2-(hydroxymethyl)propane-1,3-diol.

$C_4H_{11}NO_3$=121.1.

CAS -- 77-86-1.

Pharmacopoeias. In *Cz.*, *Nord.*, and *U.S.*

A white crystalline powder with a slight characteristic odour.

Soluble 1 in 1.8 of water and 1 in about 45 of alcohol; practically insoluble in carbon tetrachloride and chloroform. A 5% solution in water has a pH of 10.0 to 11.5. **Store** in airtight containers.

The alkalinity of trometamol solutions precluded their sterilisation by heat in glass because of silicate formation.— G. G. Nahas, *Clin. Pharmac. Ther.*, 1963, *4*, 784. Solutions could be sterilised by autoclaving.— C. Rauch *et al.*, *Pharm. Ztg, Berl.*, 1964, *109*, 693.

Adverse Effects and Precautions

Great care must be taken to avoid extravasation at the injection site as solutions may cause tissue damage. Local irritation may follow administration and venospasm and phlebitis have occurred.

Respiratory depression and hypoglycaemia may occur and the respiration may require assistance. Trometamol is contra-indicated in anuria and uraemia and should be administered cautiously in patients with impaired renal function. Hyperkalaemia has been reported in patients with renal impairment. Trometamol is contra-indicated in chronic respiratory acidosis.

Blood concentrations of carbon dioxide, bicarbonate, glucose, and electrolytes, and blood pH should be monitored during infusion of trometamol.

PREGNANCY AND THE NEONATE. *Necrosis.* Haemorrhagic liver necrosis was found at post mortem in 22 of 67 infants who had received hypertonic trometamol (3 to 90 mL of a 1.2M solution) and bicarbonate—2 to 34 mmol (2 to 34 mEq)—in the treatment of the respiratory distress syndrome. The injections were made into the umbilical vein. Those who had injections via the umbilical artery, or who had received bicarbonate only, were not affected.— V. E. Goldenberg *et al.*, *J. Am. med. Ass.*, 1968, *205*, 81. The 1.2M solution had a pH of 10.2. Concentrated alkaline solutions should not be administered in the central or peripheral veins of infants whose circulation might be impaired.— G. G. Nahas (letter), *ibid.*, *206*, 1793.

Accidental intra-arterial injection of trometamol produced severe haemorrhagic necrosis in 2 newborn girls and was fatal in 1.— H. Rehder and E. Heiming, *Archs Dis. Childh.*, 1974, *49*, 76.

Bladder necrosis developed in an infant given trometamol in a 10% glucose solution by umbilical artery catheter.— M. J. Mihatsch *et al.*, *J. Urol., Baltimore*, 1974, *111*, 835.

Uses and Administration

Trometamol is an organic amine proton acceptor which is used as an alkalinising agent in the treatment of metabolic acidosis. It should not be used in patients with chronic respiratory acidosis. It also acts as a weak osmotic diuretic. Trometamol is mainly used during cardiac bypass surgery and during cardiac arrest. It may also be used to reduce the acidity of citrated blood before transfusion.

The dose used should be the minimum required to increase the pH of the blood to within normal limits and is based on the body weight and the base deficit. Trometamol is administered by slow intravenous infusion as a 0.3M solution over a period of not less than 1 hour. Generally, the dose should not exceed 500 mg per kg body-weight.

In shock, acidosis which had led to diminished vascular and cardiac tone could be corrected by administering sodium bicarbonate or trometamol 0.3M solution. Trometamol conferred no sodium ions but influenced intracellular acidosis by undergoing 30% ionisation. Hazards associated with its use included respiratory depression, hypokalaemia, and hypoglycaemia and frequent monitoring was necessary of arterial and venous pH, venous carbon-dioxide tension, and glucose and electrolyte concentrations in blood. The guiding formula for the dose of trometamol was: mmol trometamol = 0.3 × body-weight (kg) × mmol deficiency of bicarbonate ion.— J. J. Byrne, *New Engl. J. Med.*, 1966, *275*, 659.

Stored blood adjusted to approximately normal pH with trometamol, then recalcified and heparinised, was suitable for priming the pump oxygenator and replacing blood losses during open-heart surgery. Its viscosity was less than that of fresh blood, and the osmotic diuresis due to the trometamol would improve renal function.— L. P. Rosky and T. Rodman, *New Engl. J. Med.*, 1966, *274*, 883 and 886.

For a report of the use of trometamol to dissolve cystine stones, see Acetylcysteine p.904.

Preparations

Tromethamine for Injection *(U.S.P.)*. A sterile lyophilised mixture of trometamol with potassium chloride and sodium chloride.

Proprietary Names and Manufacturers

Addex-THAM *(Pharmacia, Swed.)*; Alcaphor *(Bellon, Fr.)*; Basionic *(RIT, Belg.)*; Tham *(Abbott, USA)*; Tham-acetat *(Bellon, Fr.)*; Tham-E *(Abbott, UK*; *Abbott, USA)*; Thamesol *(Baxter, Ital.)*; Trisaminol *(Bellon, Fr.)*.

2361-s

Urea *(BAN, USAN)*.

Carbamide; Ureum.

$NH_2.CO.NH_2$=60.06.

CAS — 57-13-6.

Pharmacopoeias. In *Aust.*, *Br.*, *Cz.*, *Hung.*, *Ind.*, *Jpn*, *Jug.*, *Mex.*, *Neth.*, *Nord.*, *Pol.*, *Port.*, *Swiss*, *Turk.*, and *U.S.*

Colourless, transparent, slightly hygroscopic, odourless or almost odourless, prismatic crystals, or white crystalline powder or pellets. May gradually develop a slight odour of ammonia on prolonged standing.

Soluble 1 in 1 to 1.5 of water, 1 in 10 to 12 of alcohol, and 1 in 1 to 1.5 of boiling alcohol; practically insoluble in chloroform and ether.

Solutions in water are neutral to litmus. Solutions are **sterilised** by filtration. **Incompatible** with nitric acid, nitrites, alkalis, and formaldehyde. Solutions in water hydrolyse during storage, liberating ammonia and carbon dioxide. **Store** in well-closed containers.

An aqueous solution of urea iso-osmotic with serum (1.63%) caused 100% haemolysis of erythrocytes cultured in it for 45 minutes.— E. R. Hammarlund and K. Pedersen-Bjergaard, *J. pharm. Sci.*, 1961, *50*, 24.

Urea should never be added to whole blood for transfusion or given through the same set by which blood is being infused. For details of the adverse effects of urea on red blood cells, see above and see also under Effects on the Blood, under Adverse Effects.

STABILITY. Urea in solution or when moist slowly hydrolysed to carbon dioxide and ammonia, whilst heat, acids, and alkalis increased the rate of hydrolysis. However, little decomposition was evident in solutions stored at either 16° or 4° for 1 month.— R. H. Sutaria and F. H. Williams, *Publ. Pharm.*, 1960, *17*, 168, 225, and 281.

The degree of degradation of 2M, 4M, 6M and 8M solutions of urea at 25°, 35°, and 45° was extremely small.— H. L. Welles *et al.*, *J. pharm. Sci.*, 1971, *60*, 1212.

STERILISATION. Dry sterile urea suitable for intravenous use could be prepared by first sterilising a concentrated solution by filtration and subsequently drying under vacuum at temperatures not exceeding 100°. Irradiation with ultraviolet light and washing with ether were unreliable methods.— R. H. Sutaria and F. H. Williams, *Publ. Pharm.*, 1960, *17*, 168, 225, and 281.

Adverse Effects

Urea may cause gastric irritation with nausea and vomiting when given by mouth. Intravenous administration may cause headache, nausea, vomiting, confusion, and a fall in blood pressure. Continued administration of urea may lead to disturbances of fluid and electrolyte balance.

The intravenous administration of urea may cause venous thrombosis or phlebitis at the site of injection and only large veins should be used for infusion. Rapid intravenous injection of solutions of urea can cause haemolysis; the risk is reduced by using glucose or invert sugar solution as diluent. Extravasation may cause sloughing or necrosis. Thrombosis may occur independently of extravasation.

Topical applications may be irritant to sensitive skin.

EFFECTS ON THE BLOOD AND VASCULAR SYSTEM. Fatal intracranial haemorrhage was provoked in a 54-year-old hypertensive man, suffering from cerebrovascular disease, who was given 90 g of urea in 1 litre of normal saline by slow intravenous infusion as a test of kidney function.— S. Marshall and F. Hinman, *J. Am. med. Ass.*, 1962, *182*, 813.

In healthy subjects the infusion of a 6M solution of urea in 10% invert sugar solution caused intravascular haemolysis similar to that in patients with sickle-cell anaemia.— T. A. Bensinger *et al.*, *Blood*, 1973, *41*, 461.

PREGNANCY AND THE NEONATE. Disseminated intravascular coagulation, attributed to urea, occurred in a 24-year-old woman given urea and oxytocin for termination of pregnancy.— M. F. B. Grundy and E. R. Craven, *Br. med. J.*, 1976, *2*, 677.

A report of haemorrhage due to coagulopathy in 2 women undergoing mid-trimester termination of pregnancy using hyperosmotic urea solution.— R. T. Burkman *et al.*, *Am. J. Obstet. Gynec.*, 1977, *127*, 533.

Raised blood-urea concentrations occurred in 2 infants during topical application of a cream containing urea.— D. W. Beverley and D. Wheeler, *Archs Dis. Childh.*, 1986, *61*, 696. Comment.— B. Z. Garty, *ibid.*, 1245. Condemnation of the topical use of any systemically active agents in neonates.— D. J. Atherton and J. I. Harper (letter), *ibid.*, *62*, 212.

Precautions

As for Mannitol, p.995.

Extreme care is essential to prevent accidental extravasation of urea infusions; to avoid phlebitis and thrombosis urea should not be infused in the veins of the lower limbs of elderly subjects.

Infusions of urea must be given slowly.

Absorption and Fate

Urea is fairly rapidly absorbed from the gastro-intestinal tract but causes gastro-intestinal irritation. Urea is distributed into extracellular and intracellular fluids including lymph, bile, CSF, and blood. It is reported to cross the placenta, and penetrate the eye. It is excreted unchanged in the urine.

Uses and Administration

Urea is an osmotic diuretic. It has been used intravenously in the treatment of acute increases in intracranial pressure due to cerebral oedema, to maintain the output of urine during surgical procedures, and to decrease intra-ocular pressure in acute glaucoma. Urea has been largely superseded by mannitol. Rebound increases in intracranial and intra-ocular pressure may occur after about 12 hours.

Urea is generally administered as an intravenous infusion of a 30% solution in glucose 5 to 10% or invert sugar 10%, at a rate not exceeding 4 mL per minute, in a dose of 1 to 1.5 g per kg body-weight to a maximum of 120 g daily. For children under 2 years a dose of 0.1 g per kg has been suggested and 0.5 to 1.5 g per kg for those over 2 years. Urea has also been given by mouth.

Solutions of urea 40 to 50% have also been given by intra-amniotic injection for the termination of pregnancy. Oxytocin, by intravenous injection, or dinoprost, by intra-amniotic infusion, is often given concomitantly.

Urea is used as a 10% cream for the treatment of ichthyosis and hyperkeratotic skin disorders.

HEPATIC DISORDERS. Beneficial response to urea in the treatment of water retention in hyponatraemic cirrhosis with ascites resistant to diuretics.— G. Decaux *et al.*, *Br. med. J.*, 1985, *290*, 1782.

INAPPROPRIATE SECRETION OF ANTIDIURETIC HORMONE. Although urea has been shown to be effective in acute and chronic treatment of the syndrome of inappropriate secretion of antidiuretic hormone, the use of urea has been limited in clinical practice. Urea acts immediately and may be given by mouth or intravenously. Oral administration of urea 10 to 30 g daily has been shown to increase serum-sodium concentrations, to decrease urinary sodium excretion, and to produce a persistent osmotic diuresis allowing a normal daily intake of water. However, gastro-intestinal complaints are common with urea, and patients are at risk of developing a hypernatraemic dehydration if they do not have an intact thirst mechanism.— C. I. Miyagawa, *Drug Intell. & clin. Pharm.*, 1986, *20*, 527.

Further references to the use of urea for inappropriate secretion of antidiuretic hormone: G. Decaux *et al.*, *J. Am. med. Ass.*, 1980, *244*, 589; G. Decaux *et al.*, *Am. J. Med.*, 1980, *69*, 99; G. Decaux and F. Genette, *Br. med. J.*, 1981, *283*, 1081.

NEOPLASMS. Over a period of 3 years 112 patients with basal or squamous cell skin carcinoma were treated with urea injected around the lesions and later by debridement and the topical application of urea powder. Complete remission occurred in 65 and considerable improvement in 27 of the patients.— E. D. Danopoulos and I. E. Danopoulou, *Lancet*, 1974, *1*, 115. Beneficial results were also obtained in patients with tumours of the liver given 2 to 2.5 g four to six times daily.— *idem* (letter), 132.

Tumours in 8 patients with epibulbar malignancies of the eyes were successfully treated with urea as a sterilised powder applied to the surface of the eye, a 10% subconjunctival injection, and a 10% instillation.— E. D. Danopoulos *et al.*, *Br. J. Ophthal.*, 1975, *59*, 282.

OTITIS MEDIA. Despite early encouraging results following the instillation of urea solution into the ear by paracentesis for the treatment of otitis media with effusion, this treatment has not been widely adopted, perhaps because of the pain of paracentesis and the lack of demonstrated long-term benefit.— D. T. Brown *et al.*, *Ann. Otol. Rhinol. Lar.*, 1985, *94*, 3.

PREGNANCY AND THE NEONATE. *Termination of pregnancy.* Mid-trimester abortion occurred within a mean of 22.3 hours in 257 of 295 patients after the intra-amniotic injection of 200 mL of freshly prepared 45% urea solution, followed by infusion of oxytocin. In 38 in whom abortion had not occurred within 50 hours the foetus was macerated allowing easy evacuation by suction curettage.— W. G. Smith *et al.*, *Am. J. Obstet. Gynec.*, 1977, *126*, 228.

Further references to the use of urea for termination of pregnancy: M. E. Kafrissen *et al.*, *J. Am. med. Ass.*, 1984, *251*, 916; R. V. Haning and B. M. Peckham, *Am. J. Obstet. Gynec.*, 1985, *151*, 92.

For a review from the *USA* of current methods of pregnancy termination including the use of urea, see Dinoprost p.1369.

RAISED INTRACRANIAL PRESSURE. Urea was considered to be of no value in the treatment of cerebral oedema associated with stroke.— *Drug & Ther. Bull.*, 1983, *21*, 21.

SICKLE-CELL DISEASE. Comment on the use of urea in the treatment of sickle-cell anaemia. Although the results of the cooperative studies dampened almost all enthusiasm in the United States for any form of urea therapy, work continues in Africa on the possible effectiveness of long-term oral administration for the prevention of crises.— J. Dean and A. N. Schechter, *New Engl. J. Med.*, 1978, *299*, 804.

Further reviews and comments: *Lancet*, 1974, *2*, 762.

SKIN DISORDERS. Reviews and discussions on the use of urea cream.— *Drug & Ther. Bull.*, 1971, *9*, 29; H. Ashton *et al.*, *Br. J. Derm.*, 1971, *84*, 194; *Med. Lett.*, 1973, *15*, 104.

Epidermal thinning, associated with a decreased number of DNA-synthesising cells, provoked by application of a 10% solution of urea for 8 weeks, suggested that additional or preliminary treatment with urea may enhance the effectiveness of topical drugs.— W. Wohlrab, *Dermatologica*, 1977, *155*, 97.

Eczema. In a double-blind comparison in 50 patients a cream containing urea 10% and hydrocortisone 1% (Calmurid HC) was as effective as betamethasone valerate cream 0.1% in the treatment of atopic eczema. Six patients who had excoriated skin reported initial smarting when urea and hydrocortisone cream was applied.— J. Almeyda and L. Fry, *Br. J. Derm.*, 1973, *88*, 493.

Further references: T. C. Hindson, *Archs Derm.*, 1971, *104*, 284; S. A. Khan, *Practitioner*, 1978, *221*, 265; R. S. Chapman, *ibid.*, 1979, *223*, 713.

Ichthyosis and hyperkeratosis. Excellent results were achieved in all of 17 patients with ichthyosis treated with 10% urea cream and in 10 of 11 patients with hyperkeratosis of the hands and feet. Fewer patients with atopic dermatitis, disseminated neurodermatitis, and hand dermatitis responded, and there was no response in those with psoriasis, solar keratitis, or perioral dermatitis.— M. Rosten, *Aust. J. Derm.*, 1970, *11*, 142.

In a double-blind trial in 55 patients, a cream containing 10% urea (Calmurid) was no more effective than aqueous cream in the treatment of hyperkeratoses.—Report No. 179 of the General Practitioner Research Group, *Practitioner*, 1973, *210*, 294.

In 14 patients with ichthyosis, treatment for 3 weeks with 10% urea cream caused an increase of about 100% in the ability of skin scales to retain water. The effect of urea in ichthyosis was probably due to its hygroscopic effect.— K. Grice *et al.*, *Acta derm.-vener., Stockh.*, 1973, *53*, 114.

Further references: F. M. Pope *et al.*, *Br. J. Derm.*, 1972, *86*, 291 (ichthyosis); C. Blair, *Br. J. Derm.*, 1976, *94*, 145 (ichthyosis).

Preparations

Sterile Urea *(U.S.P.)*. Urea suitable for parenteral use.

Urea Cream *(B.P.)*. Store at 2 to 8°.

Proprietary Preparations

Alphaderm *(Norwich-Eaton, UK)*. *Cream*, urea 10%, hydrocortisone 1%.

Aquadrate *(Norwich-Eaton, UK)*. *Cream*, urea 10%.

Calmurid *(Pharmacia, UK)*. *Cream*, urea 10%, lactic acid 5%.
Topical solution, urea 20%, lactic acid 5%.

Calmurid HC *(Pharmacia, UK)*. *Cream*, urea 10%, hydrocortisone 1%, lactic acid 5%.

Nutraplus *(Alcon, UK)*. *Cream*, urea 10%.

Sential *(Pharmacia, UK)*. *Cream*, urea 4%, hydrocortisone 0.5%.

Proprietary Names and Manufacturers

Aquacare *(Allergan, Austral.; Herbert, USA)*; Aquadrate *(Norwich-Eaton, Austral.; Norwich-Eaton, UK)*; Basodexan *(Röhm, Ger.)*; Calmurid *(Arg.; Pharmacia, Austral.; Belg.; Pharmacia, Canad.; Pharmacia, UK)*; Calmuril *(Pharmacia, Norw.; Pharmacia, Swed.)*; Carbaderm *(Denm.)*; Carmol *(Canad.; Syntex, USA)*; Dermaflex *(Neolab, Canad.)*; Elaqua XX *(Elder, USA)*; Gormel *(USA)*; Hyanit *(Burnus, Ger.)*; Keratinamin *(Jpn)*; Nutraplus *(Alcon, Austral.; Alcon, Canad.; Alcon, Switz.; Alcon, UK; Owen, USA)*; Onychomal *(Hermal, Ger.)*; Pastaron *(Jpn)*; Ultra Mide *(Baker/Cummins, USA)*; Ureacin *(Pedinol, USA)*; Ureaphil *(Abbott, UK; Abbott, USA)*; Urederm *(Hamilton, Austral.)*; Uremol *(Trans Canaderm, Canad.)*; Urepearl *(Jpn)*; Urevert *(Travenol, UK)*; Urisec *(Odan, Canad.)*; Uroderm *(Wilson, Pakistan)*; Velvelan *(Merck Sharp & Dohme, Canad.)*.

The following names have been used for multi-ingredient preparations containing urea—Alphaderm *(Norwich-Eaton, UK; Vivan, USA)*; Amino-Cerv *(Milex, USA)*; Calmurid HC *(Pharmacia, Canad.; Pharmacia, UK)*; Esoban *(Southon-Horton, UK)*; Panafil *(Rystan, USA)*; Psoradrate *(Norwich-Eaton, Austral.; Norwich-Eaton, UK)*; Sential *(Pharmacia, UK)*; Trysul *(Savage, USA)*; Uremol-HC *(Trans Canaderm, Canad.)*.

2362-w

Xipamide *(BAN, USAN, rINN)*.

BE-1293; MJF-10938. 4-Chloro-5-sulphamoylsalicylo-2′,6′-xylidide; 4-Chloro-2-hydroxy-2′,6′-dimethyl-5-sulphamoylbenzanilide.

$C_{15}H_{15}ClN_2O_4S$=354.8.

CAS — 14293-44-8.

Adverse Effects, Treatment, and Precautions

As for Chlorothiazide, p.981.

EFFECTS ON THE ELECTROLYTE BALANCE. Ventricular fibrillation due to hypokalaemia in a patient taking xipamide 20 mg daily.— P. Altmann and J. J. Hamblin, *Br. med. J.*, 1982, *284*, 494.

Further reports of hypokalaemia induced by xipamide: E. B. Raftery (letter), *Br. med. J.*, 1982, *284*, 975; P. Weissberg and M. J. Kendall (letter), *ibid.*; J. Bentley (letter), *ibid.*; A. J. M. Boulton and C. A. Hardisty (letter), *ibid.*

For references on biochemical disturbances produced by xipamide compared with those produced by thiazide diuretics, see under Uses, below.

Absorption and Fate

Unlike chlorothiazide, xipamide has been reported to be well absorbed from the gastro-intestinal tract. Absorption is fairly rapid with peak plasma concentrations occurring within 1 or 2 hours of oral administration. It is 99% bound to plasma proteins, and is excreted in the urine, partly unchanged and partly in the form of the glucuronide metabolite. It is reported to have a plasma half-life of about 5 to 8 hours, its biological half-life being much longer. In patients with renal failure excretion in the bile becomes more prominent, and a plasma half-life of 9 hours has been reported in patients with end-stage renal failure.

The clinical pharmacokinetics of xipamide.— F. W. Hempelmann and P. Dieker, *Arzneimittel-Forsch.*, 1977, *27*, 2143.

An analysis of the pharmacokinetics of xipamide in 19 healthy subjects and 10 patients with chronic renal failure. Following single oral and intravenous doses of xipamide 20 mg the drug appeared to be completely absorbed from the gastro-intestinal tract. The mean elimination half-life in healthy subjects was 7 hours and two-thirds of the clearance was by extrarenal routes. Although there was some accumulation in patients with chronic renal failure, with a calculated elimination half-life of 9 hours in end-stage renal disease this was not thought to be clinically relevant.— H. Knauf and E. Mutschler, *Eur. J. clin. Pharmac.*, 1984, *26*, 513.

Reviews of the pharmacokinetics of xipamide: B. N. C. Prichard and R. N. Brogden, *Drugs*, 1985, *30*, 313; B. Beerman and M. Grind, *Clin. Pharmacokinet.*, 1987, *13*, 254.

Uses and Administration

Xipamide is a diuretic which has certain structural similarities to the thiazides and has uses similar to those of chlorothiazide (see p.983). Diuresis is initiated in about 1 or 2 hours and lasts for about 12 hours.

In the treatment of oedema the usual initial dose is 40 mg daily, subsequently reduced to 20 mg daily, according to the patient's response; in resistant cases doses of 80 mg daily may be required. In the treatment of hypertension the usual dose is 20 mg daily, as a single morning dose, either alone, or in conjunction with other antihypertensive agents; this may be increased to 40 mg daily, as a single morning dose, if necessary.

When treatment is prolonged, or in susceptible patients, loss of potassium may be sufficient to produce hypokalaemia; potassium supplements or a potassium-sparing diuretic should then be given as for chlorothiazide.

A detailed review of xipamide, a non-thiazide salicylic acid derivative resembling chlorthalidone structurally. The diuresis produced by xipamide over 24 hours is equivalent to that of frusemide, but the time course of the diuretic, natriuretic, and kaliuretic effects is similar to that of hydrochlorothiazide. There is evidence that xipamide, like the thiazides, acts on the distal tubule, but it also resembles frusemide by being an effective diuretic in patients with renal failure.— B. N. C. Prichard and R. N. Brogden, *Drugs*, 1985, *30*, 313.

HYPERTENSION. Xipamide 10 to 20 mg had similar effects on supine blood pressure to cyclopenthiazide 0.5 mg in a crossover study of 14 patients with mild to moderate hypertension, but produced greater biochemical disturbances. At the end of 6 weeks 13 out of 14 patients taking xipamide were hypokalaemic compared with only 6 patients on cyclopenthiazide. Increases in plasma uric acid and plasma renin activity were both greater with xipamide.— G. A. MacGregor *et al.*, *Br. J. clin. Pharmac.*, 1982, *13*, 859.

In a study of 20 hypertensive patients taking bendrofluazide 5 mg daily neither the addition of xipamide 20 mg nor doubling the dose of bendrofluazide produced a clinically important additional reduction in blood pressure. However, xipamide produced more pronounced biochemical disturbances including increases in blood urea and serum uric acid concentrations and decreases in serum potassium than bendrofluazide.— S. Freestone and L. E. Ramsay, *Br. J. clin. Pharmac.*, 1984, *18*, 616.

Further references on the use of xipamide in hypertension: R. Pasquel *et al.*, *J. clin. Pharmac.*, 1981, *21*, 316; A. Brochez *et al.*, *Int. J. clin. Pharmac. Ther. Toxic.*, 1983, *21*, 394; S. Dean *et al.*, *Eur. J. clin. Pharmac.*, 1984, *28*, 29.

Proprietary Preparations

Diurexan *(Degussa, UK)*. *Tablets*, scored, xipamide 20 mg.

Proprietary Names and Manufacturers

Aquafor *(Selvi, Ital.)*; Aquaphor *(Beiersdorf, Ger.)*; Demiax *(Igoda, Spain)*; Diurex *(Lacer, Spain)*; Diurexan *(Degussa, UK)*.

Dopaminergic Antiparkinsonian Agents

4540-v

Dopamine is a key neurotransmitter in the central nervous system; in particular, striatal dopamine depletion is associated with the clinical condition of parkinsonism. Dopamine also inhibits prolactin release from the pituitary and is believed to be the prolactin-release inhibiting factor (PRIF or PIF); its deficiency here is associated with conditions characterised by hyperprolactinaemia, for example, the galactorrhoea-amenorrhoea syndrome.

Accordingly, agents which replenish central dopamine or which themselves can act as stimulants of dopamine receptors (dopamine agonists), may alleviate the symptoms of parkinsonism, hyperprolactinaemia, and related disorders.

Dopaminergic agents described in this section include:

1. levodopa, which is converted into dopamine in the body, and which, unlike dopamine itself, can penetrate the blood-brain barrier hence supplying a source of dopamine to the brain;
2. the peripheral decarboxylase inhibitors, benserazide and carbidopa which have no anti-parkinsonian action of their own but enhance the action of levodopa;
3. the aporphine, apomorphine which is structurally related to dopamine and acts as a dopamine agonist;
4. the adamantanamine, amantadine which may augment dopaminergic activity (amantadine is also an antiviral agent);
5. the ergolines, including bromocriptine, lysuride, and pergolide, which are ergot derivatives acting as dopamine agonists;
6. the specific monoamine oxidase type B inhibitor, selegiline which enhances the action of levodopa.

The non-ergot dopamine agonist, piribedil has also been tried in parkinsonism as has the dopamine-β-hydroxylase inhibitor, fusaric acid which prevents the conversion of dopamine into noradrenaline. Other drugs used include antimuscarinic agents (p.522).

For an overview of parkinsonism and its treatment, see Levodopa, p.1019.

For reviews on hyperprolactinaemia and related disorders, see Bromocriptine Mesylate, p.1013.

4542-q

Amantadine Hydrochloride *(BANM, USAN, pINNM).*

1-Adamantanamine Hydrochloride; EXP-105-1; NSC-83653. Tricyclo[3.3.1.$1^{3,7}$]dec-1-ylamine hydrochloride.

$C_{10}H_{17}N,HCl = 187.7$.

CAS — 768-94-5 (amantadine); 665-66-7 (hydrochloride).

Pharmacopoeias. In *Chin., Ind., Swiss.,* and *U.S.*

A white or almost white crystalline powder with a bitter taste.

Soluble 1 in 2.5 of water, 1 in about 5 of alcohol, 1 in 18 of chloroform, and 1 in 70 of macrogol 400. A 20% solution in water has a pH of 3.0 to 5.5.

Adverse Effects

Most side-effects associated with amantadine therapy are dose-related and relatively mild; some resemble those of antimuscarinic drugs. They may be reversed by withdrawing therapy but many resolve despite continuation.

Livedo reticularis, sometimes associated with ankle oedema, is common in parkinsonian patients given amantadine. Mild central nervous system effects such as nervousness, inability to concentrate, dizziness, insomnia, and changes in mood may occur. Psychotic reactions including hallucinations and confusion have been reported, especially in patients with impaired renal function and those also receiving antimuscarinic drugs.

Other side-effects reported have included orthostatic hypotension, urinary retention, slurred speech, ataxia, lethargy, nausea, anorexia, vomiting, dry mouth, constipation, skin rash, and blurred vision. There have been isolated reports of congestive heart failure, arrhythmias, leucopenia, and convulsions.

About 10% of healthy volunteers have mild reactions to an initial single dose of 100 mg of amantadine and 10 to 15% to a single dose of 200 mg. Although the incidence of reactions in healthy volunteers decreased with continuous doses at the same level, side-effects occurred on average in 3 to 7% of healthy adults.— F. Assaad *et al., Bull. Wld Hlth Org.,* 1978, *56,* 229.

Although amantadine primarily has dopamine agonist function and negligible atropine-like effects in *animal* tissue, side-effects such as dry mouth, blurred vision, mydriasis, and urinary retention suggest antimuscarinic activity. Delirium and myoclonus in a patient receiving amantadine for haloperidol-induced extrapyramidal symptoms were reversed by physostigmine.— D. E. Casey (letter), *New Engl. J. Med.,* 1978, *298,* 516.

For studies of the relative toxicities of rimantadine and amantadine, see Rimantadine Hydrochloride, p.699.

EFFECTS ON THE CARDIOVASCULAR SYSTEM. Congestive heart failure associated with amantadine occurred in a patient who had been receiving combined treatment with amantadine, levodopa, and orphenadrine for 4 years.— J. A. Vale and K. S. Maclean (letter), *Lancet,* 1977, *1,* 548. Although amantadine sometimes causes ankle oedema, an association between amantadine and heart failure is not proven. Livedo reticularis, a mottled blue discoloration of the skin due to prominence of the normal pattern of venous drainage, occurs in about 50% of all elderly patients given amantadine 100 to 300 mg daily for 2 to 6 weeks and is associated with oedema in 5 to 10%. Both livedo and oedema are usually confined to the legs and may result from the catecholamine-releasing action of amantadine in certain vascular beds; the oedema is unlikely to be due to heart failure. Angina, dyspnoea, pulmonary congestion, or distension of neck veins developed in 4 of 89 parkinsonian patients on amantadine; only 2 had had ankle oedema before heart failure developed. No patient has been observed in whom heart failure seemed due directly to amantadine.— J. D. Parkes *et al.* (letter), *ibid.,* 904.

See also under Overdosage (below).

EFFECTS ON THE EYES. Sudden loss of vision occurred in a 67-year-old man who had been taking amantadine 200 mg daily for several weeks. Improvement of visual acuity occurred gradually after discontinuation of amantadine.— J. T. Pearlman *et al.* (letter), *J. Am. med. Ass.,* 1977, *237,* 1200. See also *idem, Archs Neurol., Chicago,* 1977, *34,* 199.

EFFECTS ON THE SKIN. A report of photosensitisation by amantadine in a patient who developed a dermatitis on sun-exposed areas of his body.— W. H. H. W. van den Berg and W. G. van Ketel, *Contact Dermatitis,* 1983, *9,* 165.

OVERDOSAGE. A patient with postencephalitic parkinsonism who had taken an estimated 2.8 g of amantadine in a suicide attempt suffered an acute toxic psychosis with disorientation, visual hallucinations, and aggressive behaviour. Convulsions did not occur, possibly because he had been receiving phenytoin which was continued. The patient was treated with hydration and chlorpromazine and recovered in 4 days.— S. Fahn *et al., Archs Neurol., Chicago,* 1971, *25,* 45.

A 2-year-old child who had ingested 600 mg of amantadine hydrochloride developed symptoms of acute toxicity, including agitation and dystonic posturing, despite emesis with 'syrup of ipecac'. She responded immediately to a trial of physostigmine 500 µg intravenously, followed after 10 minutes by a second dose of 500 µg intravenously. Her pupils remained moderately dilated until about 20 hours after the ingestion.— C. D. Berkowitz, *J. Pediat.,* 1979, *95,* 144.

Cardiac arrest developed 6 hours after a 37-year-old woman ingested 2.5 g of amantadine hydrochloride and was treated successfully. However, ventricular arrhythmias, including torsade de pointe, continued over the ensuing 48 hours and may have been exacerbated by administration of isoprenaline and dopamine. The patient was subsequently stabilised on lignocaine by intravenous infusion, but died of respiratory failure 10 days after admission.— M. Sartori *et al., Am. J. Med.,* 1984, *77,* 388.

Precautions

Amantadine should be avoided in severe renal disease and in patients with a history of epilepsy or gastric ulceration. It should be used with caution in patients with cardiovascular or liver disease, impaired renal function, recurrent eczema, or psychosis. Care should be taken in all elderly patients.

The use of amantadine should be avoided in nursing mothers.

Amantadine may enhance the adverse effects of antimuscarinic agents and the dose of these drugs should be reduced when amantadine is given concomitantly; side-effects of levodopa may also be exacerbated. Treatment with amantadine should not be stopped abruptly in parkinsonian patients.

ADMINISTRATION IN RENAL FAILURE. Evidence of extremely poor total body clearance of amantadine in patients with renal failure; only a small fraction of the total body store was removed by haemodialysis.— L. -S. Soung *et al., Ann. intern. Med.,* 1980, *93,* 46.

Reports of psychotic reactions in patients with impaired renal function given amantadine.— T. S. Ing *et al.* (letter), *New Engl. J. Med.,* 1974, *291,* 1257; R. L. Borison, *Am. J. Psychiat.,* 1979, *136,* 111; T. S. Ing *et al., Can. med. Ass. J.,* 1979, *120,* 695.

See also under Absorption and Fate and Administration in Renal Failure in Uses (below).

INTERACTIONS. *Antimuscarinic agents.* Amantadine given with benzhexol or orphenadrine might cause hallucinations and doses of these drugs might need to be reduced during amantadine therapy.— V. Dallos *et al., Br. med. J.,* 1970, *4,* 24.

Diuretics. A 61-year-old man with Parkinson's disease, previously stabilised on amantadine hydrochloride 300 mg daily, developed symptoms of amantadine toxicity, including ataxia, myoclonus, and confusion, 7 days after starting treatment with triamterene in association with hydrochlorothiazide (Dyazide). It was postulated that the effect was due to reduction of the tubular secretion of amantadine.— T. W. Wilson and A. H. Rajput, *Can. med. Ass. J.,* 1983, *129,* 974.

Monoamine oxidase inhibitors. Hypertension occurred about 48 hours after starting treatment with phenelzine sulphate in a patient already receiving amantadine.— R. A. Jack and D. G. Daniel (letter), *Archs gen. Psychiat.,* 1984, *41,* 726.

PREGNANCY AND THE NEONATE. A complex cardiovascular lesion occurred in an infant whose mother had taken amantadine hydrochloride 100 mg daily for the first 3 months of pregnancy. Amantadine has been reported to be embryotoxic and teratogenic in *rats* given high doses, but the manufacturers have received no previous reports of teratogenic effects in humans.— J. J. Nora *et al.* (letter), *Lancet,* 1975, *2,* 607. A recommendation that since amantadine is potentially teratogenic it should not be used in pregnancy.— *Med. Lett.,* 1985, *27,* 93.

WITHDRAWAL. Neuroleptic malignant syndrome occurred in a patient being treated for heat stroke when all his medication, including neuroleptics and amantadine, was withdrawn. It is suggested that dopamine agonists should not be discontinued in patients with hyperpyrexia at risk from this syndrome.— D. M. Simpson and G. C. Davis, *Am. J. Psychiat.,* 1984, *141,* 796.

Absorption and Fate

Amantadine hydrochloride is readily absorbed from the gastro-intestinal tract; peak concentrations in the blood appear after about 4 hours. It is mainly excreted unchanged in the urine. Amantadine is also excreted in breast milk.

Detection of amantadine in the cerebrospinal fluid of patients given the drug by mouth for the treatment of subacute sclerosing panencephalitis.— R. H. A. Haslam *et al., Neurology,* 1969, *19,* 1080.

Following administration of amantadine 100 mg twice daily to physically healthy schizophrenic subjects, plasma concentrations after 7 days ranged from 0.12 to

1.12 μg per mL.— D. J. Greenblatt *et al.*, *J. clin. Pharmac.*, 1977, *17*, 704.

Plasma elimination half-lives ranged from 10.2 to 31.4 hours in 13 healthy young adults who received amantadine 25, 100, or 150 mg every 12 hours for 15 days. Observations on renal clearance suggested that amantadine is actively secreted into urine as well as being eliminated in part by glomerular filtration.— F. Y. Aoki *et al.*, *Clin. Pharmac. Ther.*, 1979, *26*, 729. Following a single 300-mg dose of amantadine hydrochloride by mouth elimination half-lives ranged from 9.7 to 14.5 hours in 6 healthy subjects, from 18.5 hours to 33.8 days in 8 patients with renal insufficiency, and from 7.0 to 10.3 days in 4 patients on chronic haemodialysis.— V. W. Horadam *et al.*, *Ann. intern. Med.*, 1981, *94*, 454.

Uses and Administration

Amantadine may augment dopaminergic activity and is used in the treatment of parkinsonism, usually in conjunction with other therapy. It may improve akinesia and rigidity but usually has less effect on tremor.

Amantadine is also an antiviral agent which inhibits replication of influenza type A virus. Variable activity has been reported *in vitro* against other viruses. It is used prophylactically against infection with influenza type A virus and to ameliorate symptoms when administered during the early stages of infection.

Amantadine has been used in the management of postherpetic neuralgia.

The usual dose of amantadine hydrochloride is 100 mg twice daily by mouth. Dosage should be reduced in patients with renal impairment.

In parkinsonism, treatment is usually started with 100 mg daily and is increased to 100 mg twice daily after a week. Doses up to 400 mg daily have occasionally been used.

In influenza 100 mg is given twice daily for 5 to 7 days. For the prophylaxis of influenza the same dose is given for as long as protection from infection is required; this is usually 7 to 10 days, but prophylaxis for up to 90 days has been recommended. In herpes zoster, treatment may be given for 14 days and for a further 14 days if postherpetic pain continues.

Amantadine sulphate has also been used.

ADMINISTRATION IN RENAL FAILURE. After a loading dose of 200 mg of amantadine on the first day, the following maintenance regimens are suggested for patients with varying degrees of renal impairment in order to achieve steady state blood concentrations of 0.7 to 1.0 μg per mL. Patients with a creatinine clearance of 80 to 100 mL per minute per 1.73 m^2 body-surface, a dose of 200 mg daily; 60 mL per minute per 1.73 m^2, 200 mg/100 mg daily on alternate days; 40 to 50 mL per minute per 1.73 m^2, 100 mg daily; 30 mL per minute per 1.73 m^2, 200 mg twice weekly; 20 mL per minute per 1.73 m^2, 100 mg three times a week; 10 mL per minute per 1.73 m^2 or patients on chronic haemodialysis three times a week, 200 mg/100 mg weekly on alternate weeks.— V. W. Horadam *et al.*, *Ann. intern. Med.*, 1981, *94*, 454.

CHRONIC GRANULOMATOUS DISEASE. Beneficial results with amantadine 25 mg twice daily by mouth in a child of 4 years 9 months with chronic granulomatous disease.— J. O. Warner (letter), *Lancet*, 1985, *2*, 447.

INFLUENZA. Reviews of amantadine and other antiviral agents in the prophylaxis and treatment of influenza.— K. G. Nicholson, *Lancet*, 1984, *2*, 617; A. W. Galbraith, *Br. med. Bull.*, 1985, *41*, 381.

Amantadine inhibits replication of all known human influenza A strains. Occasional drug-resistant viruses have been isolated from the community but have not been reported from persons undergoing prophylaxis or treatment with amantadine or rimantadine. Rimantadine has a similar antiviral spectrum to that of amantadine. Antiviral efficacy of amantadine and rimantadine is comparable at a dosage of 200 mg daily although amantadine appears to cause more side-effects; 100 mg daily may be adequate. There is now considerable evidence that amantadine and rimantadine are effective in the prevention of influenza A infection and illness caused by all known human serotypes of human influenza A virus in all age groups. Reported efficacy is comparable to that of influenza vaccines and appears to be additive to any vaccine-induced effect, however, unlike vaccine, neither drug is effective against influenza B virus. Prophylactic use of amantadine or rimantadine in at-risk individuals can be considered for a period of up to 6 weeks after the onset of an outbreak of influenza A in the community. Both drugs have small but demonstrable therapeutic effects in uncomplicated influenza A infections; they shorten the duration of fever and other symptoms and also reduce virus shedding. Treatment should be started on the first day of symptoms and continued for 3 to 5 days.— *Bull. Wld Hlth Org.*, 1985, *63*, 51.

Recommendations of the Immunization Practices Advisory Committee, of the Centers for Disease Control, for the prevention and control of influenza. The two measures presently available are immunoprophylaxis with vaccines and chemoprophylaxis or therapy with amantadine hydrochloride. Vaccination of high-risk persons each year before the influenza season is the single most important control measure. Amantadine appears to interfere with the uncoating step in the virus replication cycle and also reduces virus shedding. It is 70 to 90% effective in preventing illnesses caused by circulating strains of type A influenza viruses but is not effective against type B influenza and therefore should not be used in lieu of vaccination. Amantadine prophylaxis is particularly recommended to control presumed influenza A outbreaks and should be given as early as possible in an effort to reduce the spread of infection. Amantadine does not interfere with antibody response to influenza vaccine and, since the development of a response following vaccination takes about 2 weeks, it is recommended that amantadine be given during this period as an adjunct to late immunisation of high-risk individuals. It may also be given to supplement vaccination in immunodeficient patients and to persons hypersensitive to influenza vaccine. Early treatment with amantadine should be effective in reducing the severity and duration of illness for high-risk individuals in whom influenza vaccine has not been used or has not prevented infection. For prophylaxis, amantadine must be taken each day for the duration of influenza A activity in the community, generally 6 to 12 weeks. For therapy, amantadine should be started as soon as possible after onset of symptoms and should be continued for 24 to 48 hours after their disappearance, generally 5 to 7 days. The usual adult dosage of amantadine is 200 mg daily; when given in divided doses, as 100 mg twice daily, the incidence of side-effects may be reduced. A dose of 100 mg daily is recommended for persons of 65 years or more. Children aged 1 to 9 years may be given 4.4 to 8.8 mg per kg body-weight daily; the total daily dosage should not exceed 150 mg daily. Doses should be reduced in patients with renal disease.— *Ann. intern. Med.*, 1986, *105*, 399. Criticism of the Centers for Disease Control recommendations for influenza control.— P. J. Imperato, *Lancet*, 1986, *1*, 728. Updated recommendations for 1987–1988. Although not a substitute for vaccination, amantadine was still recommended for the prevention of influenza A infection under specific circumstances and should be considered for therapy in high-risk patients.— *Ann. intern. Med.*, 1987, *107*, 521.

Treatment for 5 days with aspirin 3.25 g daily was compared with amantadine 100 or 200 mg daily in a double-blind study in 47 young adults with naturally acquired influenza A infections who had onset of signs and symptoms of less than 48 hours duration. The aspirin-treated group defervesced most rapidly, but by the second day amantadine recipients had greater symptomatic improvement although the difference was only significant in those receiving 100 mg daily. More subjects discontinued aspirin than amantadine because of side-effects.— S. W. Younkin *et al.*, *Antimicrob. Ag. Chemother.*, 1983, *23*, 577.

During an influenza A outbreak in a boarding school for boys where routine influenza vaccination was carried out, 267 boys were given amantadine 100 mg daily for 14 days, and 269 received no specific treatment. Only 3 boys receiving amantadine developed laboratory-proven influenza A whereas 29 boys in the control group did so. Amantadine was well tolerated, the only side-effect being urticaria in one boy which necessitated withdrawal of treatment.— D. K. Payler and P. A. Purdham, *Lancet*, 1984, *1*, 502.

For a comparison of the activities *in vitro* of amantadine and rimantadine against influenza A viruses, see Rimantadine Hydrochloride, p.700.

For comparisons between rimantadine and amantadine in the treatment and prophylaxis of influenza, see p.700.

Administration. Studies on amantadine administered by aerosol for the treatment of influenza A virus infections.— V. Knight *et al.*, *Antimicrob. Ag. Chemother.*, 1979, *16*, 572; F. G. Hayden *et al.*, *ibid.*, 644; F. G. Hayden *et al.*, *J. infect. Dis.*, 1980, *141*, 535.

MENTAL DISORDERS. For reference to beneficial results with amantadine in pathological laughing and crying, see Levodopa, p.1019.

NEUROLEPTIC MALIGNANT SYNDROME. Reports of beneficial results with amantadine in the treatment of the neuroleptic malignant syndrome.— M. M. McCarron *et al.*, *J. clin. Psychiat.*, 1982, *43*, 381; S. Amdurski *et al.*, *Curr. ther. Res.*, 1983, *33*, 225; J. Woo *et al.* (letter), *Postgrad. med. J.*, 1986, *62*, 809.

PAIN. Amantadine 100 mg twice daily given to elderly patients with herpes zoster of recent onset reduced the duration of postherpetic neuralgia when compared with placebo.— A. W. Galbraith, *Br. J. clin. Pract.*, 1983, *37*, 304. See also *idem*, *Br. med. J.*, 1973, *4*, 693.

PANENCEPHALITIS. A review of 38 patients with subacute sclerosing panencephalitis, 8 of whom were treated with amantadine, suggested that amantadine may produce periods of mild improvement and retard the relentless progression of the disease.— W. C. Robertson *et al.*, *Ann. Neurol.*, 1980, *8*, 422.

PARKINSONISM AND OTHER EXTRAPYRAMIDAL DISORDERS. Amantadine probably acts as an antiparkinsonian agent by augmenting the presynaptic synthesis and release of dopamine, but it also diminishes dopamine re-uptake and may have antimuscarinic properties. It produces similar or slightly more improvement than antimuscarinic agents and benefits about two-thirds of patients with Parkinson's disease. Tolerance to the beneficial effects of amantadine may develop in a small proportion of patients after 6 to 12 weeks. It is less effective than levodopa, but most studies have shown a synergistic action with levodopa. Treatment of Parkinson's disease is currently started with an antimuscarinic drug and/or amantadine, levodopa preparations being added or substituted only when functional disability begins to interfere with the patient's life.— N. P. Quinn, *Drugs*, 1984, *28*, 236.

A brief report of the successful use of amantadine sulphate by intravenous infusion in the management of akinetic crisis in patients with Parkinson's disease.— N. Gadoth *et al.* (letter), *Clin. Pharm.*, 1985, *4*, 146.

For an overview of parkinsonism and its treatment, see Levodopa, p.1019.

Drug-induced extrapyramidal disorders. Antiparkinsonian agents have been used in the management of neuroleptic-induced parkinsonism since, like idiopathic Parkinson's disease, it is due to functional loss of cerebral dopaminergic activity. However, apart from antimuscarinic drugs, only amantadine has undergone any serious clinical examination and results have been conflicting.— P. Jenner and C. D. Marsden, Antiparkinsonian and Antidyskinetic Drugs, in *Drugs in Psychiatric Practice*, P.J. Tyrer(Ed.), London, Butterworths, 1982, p.82.

URINARY INCONTINENCE. Amantadine hydrochloride 50 to 200 mg daily reduced wetting frequency in a preliminary study in 6 children aged 7 to 11 years with nocturnal enuresis.— P. J. Ambrosini and J. Fried, *J. clin. Psychopharmacol.*, 1984, *4*, 223.

Preparations

Amantadine Hydrochloride Capsules *(U.S.P.)*. Store in airtight containers.

Amantadine Hydrochloride Syrup *(U.S.P.)*. Store in airtight containers.

Proprietary Preparations

Mantadine *(Du Pont Pharmaceuticals, UK)*. *Capsules*, amantadine hydrochloride 100 mg.

Symmetrel *(Geigy, UK)*. *Capsules*, amantadine hydrochloride 100 mg. *Syrup*, 50 mg/5 mL.

Proprietary Names and Manufacturers

Amantadin *(Ferrosan, Denm.)*; Amantan *(Belg.)*; Amazolon *(Jpn)*; Antadine *(Du Pont, Austral.; NZ; Boots, S.Afr.)*; Contenton *(Smith Kline Dauelsberg, Ger.; Switz.)*; Mantadan *(De Angeli, Ital.)*; Mantadine *(Du Pont Pharmaceuticals, UK)*; Mantadix *(Belg.; Du Pont de Nemours, Fr.)*; PK-Merz *(Merz, Ger.; Merz, Switz.)*; Protexin *(Landerlan, Spain)*; Solu-Contenton *(Ger.)*; Symmetrel *(Geigy, Austral.; Du Pont, Canad.; Denm.; Geigy, Ger.; Neth.; Geigy, Norw.; Geigy, S.Afr.; Geigy, Swed.; Geigy, Switz.; Geigy, UK; Du Pont, USA)*; Trivaline *(Fr.)*; Virofral *(Ferrosan, Swed.)*; Virosol *(Arg.)*.

4543-p

Apomorphine Hydrochloride *(BANM, USAN)*.

Apomorphini Hydrochloridum. 6aβ-Aporphine-10,11-diol hydrochloride hemihydrate; (*R*)-10,11-Dihydroxy-6a-apomorphinium chloride hemihydrate; (6a*R*)-5,6,6a,7-Tetrahydro-6-methyl-4*H*-dibenzo[*de,g*]quinoline-10,11-diol

hydrochloride hemihydrate.
$C_{17}H_{17}NO_2,HCl,\frac{1}{2}H_2O$=312.8.

CAS — 58-00-4 (apomorphine); 314-19-2 (hydrochloride, anhydrous); 41372-20-7 (hydrochloride, hemihydrate).

Pharmacopoeias. In *Arg., Aust., Belg., Br., Chin., Cz., Eur., Egypt., Fr., Ger., Hung., Int., It., Jug., Mex., Neth., Nord., Pol., Port., Rus., Span., Swiss, Turk.,* and *U.S. Port.* specifies anhydrous; *Rus.* specifies $\frac{3}{4}H_2O$. Also in *B.P. Vet.*

White or faintly yellow to green-tinged greyish crystals or crystalline powder, the green tint becoming more pronounced on exposure to air and light. **Soluble** 1 in 50 of water and 1 in 20 of water at 80°; soluble 1 in 50 of alcohol; very slightly soluble in ether; practically insoluble in chloroform. A 1% solution in water has a pH of 4.0 to 5.0. Aqueous solutions decompose on storage and should not be used if they turn green or brown or contain a precipitate. Solutions for injection should be free from dissolved air and contain 0.1% of sodium metabisulphite; they are **sterilised** by distributing in ampoules, replacing the air with nitrogen or other suitable gas, sealing immediately and autoclaving. **Protect** from light. The *U.S.P.* recommends storage in small airtight containers.

Results indicating that solutions of apomorphine hydrochloride should be sterilised by aseptic filtration rather than by autoclaving. Solutions of 1 mg per mL, also containing sodium metabisulphite 0.1%, were green in colour after autoclaving whereas similar solutions prepared by aseptic filtration remained colourless for at least a year when stored in a refrigerator and protected from light.— T. J. Maloney (letter), *Aust. J. Hosp. Pharm.*, 1985, *15*, 34.

Adverse Effects

Administration of apomorphine may cause both stimulation and depression of the central nervous system. Persistent vomiting, respiratory depression, acute circulatory failure, coma, and death may occur. An opioid antagonist such as naloxone has been given to treat excessive vomiting and CNS and respiratory depression. Although drowsiness is more usual, euphoria, restlessness, and tremors have also been reported. Uraemia has been associated with the high doses required for parkinsonism.

ALLERGY. Allergic reactions developed in 2 persons in contact with apomorphine powder.— I. Dahlquist, *Contact Dermatitis*, 1977, *3*, 349.

Precautions

Apomorphine should be used with extreme caution in children, debilitated or elderly patients, or those with cardiac decompensation, and in persons prone to nausea and vomiting. If vomiting does not result from the first dose of apomorphine being used as an emetic, then a second dose should *not* be given. It should not be used in patients with respiratory or central nervous system depression, or in patients suffering from the effects of corrosive poisons.

The effectiveness of apomorphine as an emetic is diminished by drugs that depress the vomiting centre and they in turn may enhance its central depressant effects.

Uses and Administration

Apomorphine is a morphine derivative with structural similarities to dopamine. It is a dopamine agonist and was used to control the symptoms of parkinsonism.

Apomorphine stimulates the chemoreceptor trigger zone in the brain to produce emesis within a few minutes of administration, but when administered by mouth its emetic action is not dependable. Apomorphine hydrochloride has been given subcutaneously as a single dose of 5 or 6 mg for adults and 70 μg per kg body-weight for children, for the induction of emesis in acute non-corrosive poisoning (a glass of water being given before the injection). This practice is considered dangerous owing to the risk of inducing protracted vomiting and shock and is not recommended by authorities in the *UK*.

Soluble tablets of apomorphine hydrochloride for the preparation of injections are available in the *USA*.

Apomorphine is reported to stimulate postsynaptic dopamine receptors independently of presynaptic dopamine synthesis or stores.— N. P. Quinn, *Drugs*, 1984, *28*, 236.

Apomorphine and its derivatives have no known interaction with the serotonin system.— R. Horowski (letter), *Lancet*, 1986, *2*, 510.

EMESIS IN ACUTE POISONING. Apomorphine has no valid place as an emetic, because of the dangers of toxicity.— *Br. med. J.*, 1977, *2*, 977. Beneficial results with apomorphine hydrochloride 70 μg per kg body-weight given subcutaneously to 20 children who had ingested toxic substances.— F. J. deCastro *et al.*, *Clin. Toxicol.*, 1978, *12*, 65.

EMESIS BEFORE SURGERY. A review of methods available for gastric emptying prior to general anaesthesia. Some have advocated induction of emesis with apomorphine whereas others have considered this method to be hazardous.— M. Morgan, *Br. J. Anaesth.*, 1984, *56*, 47. Apomorphine does not guarantee an empty stomach and has lost popularity.— W. S. Nimmo, *Br. J. Hosp. Med.*, 1985, *34*, 176.

Apomorphine, given to empty the stomach before induction of general anaesthesia in 43 patients in labour, was found to be more pleasant and just as effective as the use of a stomach tube in 37 similar patients. Neither method guaranteed an empty stomach and nor did the absence of vomiting with apomorphine guarantee an empty stomach; no deleterious effects were noted on the infants. The apomorphine was used as follows: 3 mg of apomorphine was diluted in 10 mL of 0.9% sodium chloride injection or Water for Injections, and the solution was injected intravenously at the rate of 1 mL (300 μg) every 15 seconds with the patient sitting up holding a vomit bowl; when the patient retched or vomited the injection was stopped. After a short time atropine 600 μg or hyoscine 600 μg was injected intravenously, and 20 mL of Magnesium Trisilicate Mixture *B.P.C. 1973* given by mouth.— J. D. Holdsworth, *J. int. med. Res.*, 1978, *6*, *Suppl.* 1, 26. Discussion, including comments on the hazards of intravenous atropine, and emphasis that the danger of the acid aspiration cannot be guaranteed to be removed.— *ibid.*, 30–32. Further comment.— J. S. Crawford (letter), *Lancet*, 1979, *2*, 353.

MENTAL DISORDERS. There have been reports of beneficial results with apomorphine in schizophrenia, but in a placebo-controlled study no specific clinical changes were seen following the administration of apomorphine 750 μg by subcutaneous injection apart from a reduction in anxiety in acute schizophrenics.— I. N. Ferrier *et al.*, *Br. J. Psychiat.*, 1984, *144*, 341.

PARKINSONISM AND OTHER EXTRAPYRAMIDAL DISORDERS. Apomorphine in doses of 0.5 to 2 mg by subcutaneous injection has been beneficial in patients with parkinsonism, some of whom also received levodopa; the response was rapid in onset and lasted for 1 to 2 hours (J. Braham *et al.*, *Br. med. J.*, 1970, *3*, 768; S.E. Düby *et al.*, *Archs Neurol.*, *Chicago*, 1972, *27*, 474). The high doses necessary when apomorphine hydrochloride was given by mouth (up to 1.4 g daily) were associated with uraemia, thus precluding further study; symptomatic improvement, without uraemia, was achieved with the apomorphine derivative *N*-propylnoraporphine [$C_{19}H_{21}NO_2$=295.4] in much lower oral doses, but was sustained for only about 3 weeks (G.C. Cotzias *et al.*, *New Engl. J. Med.*, 1976, *294*, 567). In a preliminary study apomorphine-induced side-effects, including nausea, sedation, and hypotension, were prevented by the injection of domperidone prior to the intramuscular administration of apomorphine (G.U. Corsini *et al.*, *Lancet*, 1979, *1*, 954). Nevertheless, adverse effects and the need for administration by injection have meant that apomorphine has no place in routine antiparkinsonian treatment (N.P. Quinn, *Drugs*, 1984, *28*, 236). More recently, sustained improvement has been achieved in parkinsonian patients with severe 'on-off' fluctuations given apomorphine subcutaneously by continuous infusion or repeated injections (C.M.H. Stibe *et al.*, *Lancet*, 1988, *1*, 403).

Unexpectedly there have been reports of improvement with apomorphine in other movement disorders including: haloperidol-induced dyskinetic-dystonic reactions (R. Gessa *et al.*, *Lancet*, 1972, *2*, 981); Huntington's chorea (G.U. Corsini *et al.*, *Archs Neurol.*, *Chicago*, 1978, *35*, 27); and tardive dyskinesia and spasmodic torticollis (E.S. Tolosa, *ibid.*, 459). It has been suggested that the antiparkinsonian effect of apomorphine results from the direct stimulation of postsynaptic dopamine receptors while the antidyskinetic effect results from stimulation of presynaptic dopamine receptors (dopamine autoreceptors) with a consequent reduction in dopamine synthesis and release, but there is insufficient evidence for this at present (J.D. Parkes, in *Research Progress in Parkinson's Disease*, F.C. Rose and R. Capildeo (Ed.), London, Pitman Medical, 1981, p.254).

WITHDRAWAL SYNDROMES. For reference to the use of apomorphine in the treatment of alcohol-withdrawal symptoms, see Bromocriptine Mesylate, p.1014.

Preparations

Apomorphine Hydrochloride Injection *(B.P. Vet.)*. Apomorphine Injection

Apomorphine Hydrochloride Tablets *(U.S.P.)*

Proprietary Names and Manufacturers

Aguettant, Fr.; Chabre, Fr.; Lilly, USA.

4544-s

Benserazide Hydrochloride *(BANM, rINNM).*

Ro-4-4602 (benserazide); Serazide Hydrochloride. DL-Serine 2-(2,3,4-trihydroxybenzyl)hydrazide hydrochloride; DL-2-Amino-3-hydroxy-2′-(2,3,4-trihydroxybenzyl)propionohydrazide hydrochloride.
$C_{10}H_{15}N_3O_5,HCl$=293.7.

CAS — 322-35-0 (benserazide); 14919-77-8 (hydrochloride); 14046-64-1 (hydrochloride).

NOTE. Benserazide is USAN.

Benserazide hydrochloride 28.5 mg is approximately equivalent to 25 mg of benserazide.

SOLUBILITY. Benserazide is highly soluble in water; it is unstable in a neutral, alkaline, or strongly acidic medium.— D. E. Schwartz and R. Brandt, *Arzneimittel-Forsch.*, 1978, *28*, 302.

Benserazide hydrochloride is a peripheral decarboxylase inhibitor with actions similar to those of carbidopa (p.1014) and is used similarly as an adjunct to levodopa in the treatment of parkinsonism. For details of administration and dosage, see Levodopa, p.1018.

ABSORPTION AND FATE. Pharmacokinetic and metabolic studies of benserazide in *animals* and man. Following oral administration to parkinsonian patients benserazide was rapidly absorbed to the extent of about 58%, simultaneous administration of levodopa tending to increase slightly this absorption. It was rapidly excreted in the urine in the form of metabolites, 70 to 77% being excreted within 6 hours, and up to 90% within 12 hours. Benserazide is predominantly metabolised in the gut and appears to protect levodopa against decarboxylation primarily in the gut, but also in the rest of the organism, mainly by way of its metabolite trihydroxybenzylhydrazine. Benserazide did not cross the blood-brain barrier in *rats*.— D. E. Schwartz *et al.*, *Eur. J. clin. Pharmac.*, 1974, *7*, 39. See also D. E. Schwartz and R. Brandt, *Arzneimittel-Forsch.*, 1978, *28*, 302.

PRECAUTIONS. Developmental abnormalities of the *rat* skeleton have been reported with benserazide (E. Theiss and K. Schärer, in *Monoamines Noyaux Gris Centraux et Syndrome de Parkinson*, J. de Ajuriaguerra and G. Gauthier (Eds), Geneva, Georg, 1971, p.497), but Ziegler *et al.* (*ibid.*, p.505) found no evidence of any disorder involving bone metabolism in man. Nevertheless the manufacturers have recommended that benserazide should not be given to patients under 25 years of age or to pregnant women.

Proprietary Preparations

See Levodopa, p.1020.

Proprietary Names and Manufacturers

The following names have been used for multi-ingredient preparations containing benserazide hydrochloride— Madopar *(Roche, Austral.; Roche, UK)*; Madopark *(Roche, Swed.)*; Prolopa *(Roche, Canad.)*.

4546-e

Bromocriptine Mesylate *(BANM, USAN, rINNM).*

2-Bromo-α-ergocryptine Mesylate; 2-Bromoergocryptine Monomethanesulfonate; Bromocriptine Methanesulphonate; Bromocryptine Mesylate; CB-154 (bromocriptine). (5′*S*)-2-Bromo-12′-hydroxy-2′-(1-methylethyl)-5′-(2-methylpropyl)-ergotaman-3′,6′,18-trione methanesulphonate. $C_{32}H_{40}BrN_5O_5,CH_4O_3S=750.7$.

CAS — 25614-03-3 (bromocriptine); 22260-51-1 (mesylate).

Pharmacopoeias. In *Br.* and *U.S.*

A white or greyish-white to pale yellow crystalline powder; odourless or almost odourless. Bromocriptine mesylate 2.87 mg is approximately equivalent to 2.5 mg of bromocriptine. Practically **insoluble** in water; sparingly soluble in dehydrated alcohol; soluble in alcohol; very slightly soluble in chloroform; freely soluble in methyl alcohol. A 1% solution is methyl alcohol has a pH of 3.0 to 4.0. **Store** in airtight containers at a temperature not exceeding -18°. Protect from light. Capsules and tables of bromocriptine mesylate should be stored in airtight containers and protected from light.

Adverse Effects

Nausea is the most common side-effect at the beginning of treatment with bromocriptine, but vomiting, dizziness, and orthostatic hypotension may also occur. Syncope has followed initial doses of bromocriptine.

Side-effects are generally dose-related and may therefore be more frequent with the higher doses that have been used in the treatment of Parkinson's disease and acromegaly. Reduction of the dosage of bromocriptine, followed in a few days by a more gradual increase, causes the reversal of many side-effects. Nausea may be diminished by taking bromocriptine with food.

Bromocriptine is a vasoconstrictor; digital vasospasm induced by cold and leg cramps have been reported, especially with high doses. Other cardiovascular effects have included erythromelalgia, prolonged severe hypotension, arrhythmias, and exacerbation of angina.

Other side-effects reported include headache, nasal congestion, drowsiness, dryness of the mouth, constipation, diarrhoea, and altered liver-function tests. Dyskinesias have occurred in patients suffering from parkinsonism. Gastro-intestinal bleeding has been reported in acromegalic patients. Psychosis, with hallucinations, delusions, and confusion, occurs particularly when high doses are used to treat parkinsonism, but has also been reported with low doses.

In 27 published studies of bromocriptine in the treatment of Parkinson's disease, 217 of the 790 patients given bromocriptine had adverse effects. Mental changes were noted in 90 patients, dyskinesia in 20, orthostatic hypotension in 40, and gastro-intestinal effects in 40. The fewest adverse effects (9%) occurred with low-dose bromocriptine, more occurred with high-dose bromocriptine (27%) or with low-dose bromocriptine with levodopa (26%), and the most occurred with high-dose bromocriptine and levodopa (32%). However, those on high doses had more advanced disease and might be more susceptible to mental changes and dyskinesias.— A. N. Lieberman and M. Goldstein, *Pharmac. Rev.*, 1985, *37*, 217.

An analysis by the manufacturer of published reports on patients treated with bromocriptine for 1 to 10 years. In general, side-effects noted were no different from those associated with short-term treatment. The significance of 2 reports of urinary incontinence and 2 of ergotism was not known and a definite relationship between pleuropulmonary changes in some male parkinsonian patients and bromocriptine could not be established. There was no indication that long-term treatment has harmful effects on hepatic, renal, haematological, or cardiac functions nor that endocrinological complications result from the long-term suppression of prolactin secretion in parkinsonian patients. There was no evident increased risk of uterine neoplasia and teratogenicity was not seen when the use of bromocriptine in pregnancy was analysed.— C. Weil, *Curr. med. Res. Opinion*, 1986, *10*, 25.

CARCINOGENICITY. Despite a report from the manufacturers of an increased incidence of uterine tumours in *rats* given bromocriptine for 2 years (R.W. Griffith, *Br. med. J.*, 1977, *2*, 1605), no evidence of endometrial neoplasia, metaplasia, or hyperplasia, or of cervical abnormalities, was found in 88 women who had taken bromocriptine for up to 6 years (G.M. Besser *et al.*, *ibid.*, 868). Nevertheless an annual gynaecological assessment was recommended.

EFFECTS ON THE BLOOD. Severe leucopenia and mild thrombocytopenia developed in a 23-year-old woman after treatment with bromocriptine 7.5 to 10 mg daily for about 3 months.— O. Giampietro *et al.*, *Am. J. med. Sci.*, 1981, *281*, 169.

EFFECTS ON THE CARDIOVASCULAR SYSTEM. Asymptomatic hypotension occurs in many subjects given bromocriptine. However faintness and dizziness, sometimes accompanied by nausea and vomiting, are common at the start of treatment with bromocriptine and these symptoms rather than an anaphylactic type of reaction are likely to account for the collapse that occurs in a few sensitive patients. Two of 53 patients with Parkinson's disease fainted after an initial dose of 1.25 or 2.5 mg, but the exact incidence of shock-like syndromes is difficult to assess; the manufacturers have stated that 22 of over 10 000 subjects given bromocriptine have had hypotension and collapse, mainly at the start of treatment. It is essential to warn all patients starting treatment of the possibility of fainting. The initial dose should not exceed 1.25 to 2.5 mg and should be taken with food and in bed. If fainting does occur recovery is usually rapid and spontaneous. Tolerance to side-effects such as hypotension and nausea may develop rapidly.— D. Parkes (letter), *New Engl. J. Med.*, 1980, *302*, 749.

Reversible collagenosis-like symptoms and signs, including arthralgia and intermittent claudication, were associated with high-dose long-term bromocriptine therapy in a patient with Parkinson's disease. They were thought to be caused by a large vessel vasculitis rather than arterial spasms.— E. Dupont *et al.* (letter), *Lancet*, 1982, *1*, 850.

The FDA has received 17 reports of postpartum hypertension, seizures, and cerebrovascular accidents associated with the use of bromocriptine to suppress lactation. Mean onset was about 9 days post partum. One patient who suffered a cerebrovascular accident died.— *FDA Drug Bull.*, 1984, *14*, 3.

EFFECTS ON THE EARS. Audiometric evidence of bilateral sensorineural hearing loss in 3 patients receiving bromocriptine 15 or 20 mg daily for chronic hepatic encephalopathy. Hearing improved when the dose was reduced to 10 mg daily.— P. L. Lanthier *et al.*, *J. Lar. Otol.*, 1984, *98*, 399.

EFFECTS ON THE EYES. References to effects on the eyes associated with bromocriptine: D. B. Calne *et al.*, *Lancet*, 1978, *1*, 735 (blurred vision and diplopia); R. S. Manor *et al.* (letter), *ibid.*, 1981, *1*, 102 (myopia); R. J. M. Lane and P. A. Routledge, *Drugs*, 1983, *26*, 124 (visual cortical disturbances).

EFFECTS ON THE GASTRO-INTESTINAL TRACT. Of 96 patients receiving bromocriptine for acromegaly in doses of 10 to 60 mg daily, 6 developed peptic ulcers; 3 had severe gastro-intestinal bleeding.— J. A. H. Wass *et al.* (letter), *Lancet*, 1976, *2*, 851.

For reference to the use of domperidone in the management of nausea and vomiting associated with bromocriptine in patients with Parkinson's disease, see under Precautions and Uses in Domperidone, p.1090.

EFFECTS ON KIDNEY FUNCTION. A report of profound hyponatraemia associated with the use of bromocriptine in a patient with cirrhosis and portosystemic encephalopathy. It was suggested that bromocriptine should be used with extreme caution in patients with cirrhosis and ascites.— A. W. Marshall *et al.*, *Br. med. J.*, 1982, *285*, 1534.

EFFECTS ON MENTAL STATE. Psychotic reactions to high doses of bromocriptine are well known in patients with Parkinson's disease (D.B. Calne *et al.*, *Lancet*, 1978, *1*, 735). However, mania has been associated with the use of bromocriptine post partum (D.N. Vlissides *et al.*, *Br. med. J.*, 1978, *1*, 510; N.M. Brook and I.B. Cookson, *ibid.*, 790) and Pearce and Pearce (*ibid.*, 1402) state that psychological symptoms may occur with doses of only 2.5 to 5 mg daily. They also note that, instead of the relatively mild and transient symptoms associated with levodopa, bromocriptine produces a severe psychosis in which the patient is violent and aggressive, suffering from intense delusions which are often hostile and violent; complete withdrawal of bromocriptine may still leave a residue of severe psychotic illness persisting for 1 to 3 weeks. Psychosis associated with low doses of bromocriptine has often occurred in patients with a history of psychotic illness or considerable changes in behaviour and mood prior to treatment (K.C. Pearson, *New Engl. J. Med.*, 1981, *305*, 173; C.M. Le Feuvre *et al.*, *Br. med. J.*, 1982, *285*, 1315; A.W. Procter *et al.*, *ibid.*, 1983, *286*, 50 and 311; I.F. Pye and R. Abbott, *ibid.*, 50). Drug-related psychotic reactions have also been reported in patients with no psychiatric history given bromocriptine or lysuride for the treatment of acromegaly or prolactinoma (T.H. Turner *et al.*, *Br. med. J.*, 1984, *289*, 1101); 8 of 600 patients developed symptoms including anxiety, depression, auditory hallucinations, delusions, hyperactivity, disinhibition, euphoria, and insomnia and 4 had received doses only previously associated with psychosis in susceptible patients.

EFFECTS ON THE NERVOUS SYSTEM. A report of cerebrospinal-fluid rhinorrhoea associated with the use of bromocriptine to treat prolactinoma.— D. S. Baskin and C. B. Wilson (letter), *New Engl. J. Med.*, 1982, *306*, 178.

EFFECTS ON THE RESPIRATORY TRACT. Reports of pleuropulmonary changes, namely pleurisy, accompanied by effusion, pleural thickening, and pulmonary infiltration, associated with long-term high-dose bromocriptine therapy in patients with Parkinson's disease.— U. K. Rinne (letter), *Lancet*, 1981, *1*, 44; P. A. LeWitt and D. B. Calne (letter), *ibid.*

EFFECTS ON SEXUAL FUNCTION. Severe hypersexuality occurred in a middle-aged man receiving bromocriptine and levodopa for Parkinson's disease. About 3 years after the onset of hypersexuality he developed paranoid-hallucinatory psychoses which subsided on the reduction of dosage. It was apparent that addictive abuse of dopaminergic drugs had occurred.— H. P. Vogel and R. Schiffter, *Pharmacopsychiatry*, 1983, *16*, 107.

A report of sexual dissatisfaction and decreased libido in 3 women receiving bromocriptine for hyperprolactinaemia.— A. K. Saleh and M. A. A. Moussa, *Br. med. J.*, 1984, *289*, 228.

EFFECTS ON THE SKIN AND HAIR. Increased loss of hair was noted by women receiving bromocriptine. It did not progress to alopecia, even after treatment for 3 years.— I. Blum and S. Leiba (letter), *New Engl. J. Med.*, 1980, *303*, 1418.

EFFECTS ON THE URINARY TRACT. Constant dribbling of urine throughout the day and during sleep in a 57-year-old woman receiving bromocriptine.— R. Sandyk and M. A. Gillman (letter), *Lancet*, 1983, *2*, 1260. Bromocriptine has 2 synergistic pharmacological mechanisms, one acting on the detrusor and one on the bladder outflow tract, that could predispose to urinary incontinence.— M. Caine (letter), *ibid.*, 1984, *1*, 228.

FIBROSIS. A report of retroperitoneal fibrosis associated with bromocriptine.— J. V. Bowler *et al.* (letter), *Lancet*, 1986, *2*, 466.

OVERDOSAGE. The most striking symptom in two children aged 2 and 2½ years who accidentally ingested an estimated 25 and 7.5 mg of bromocriptine, respectively, was lethargy with altered mental status. The child who was thought to have ingested 25 mg of bromocriptine vomited and became sleepy. On admission he was markedly lethargic, but combative when disturbed, and also had hypotension, shallow breathing, dilated pupils, and hyperreflexic lower extremities. Nasogastric lavage was promptly performed and actived charcoal and then magnesium citrate administered. Blood pressure and ECG were monitored and glucose and sodium chloride solution infused. The other child vomited, became lethargic, and had dilated pupils. Ipecacuanha was administered and activated charcoal followed by magnesium citrate given by nasogastric tube. Both children recovered completely.— S. H. Vermund *et al.*, *J. Pediat.*, 1984, *105*, 838.

Precautions

Patients with hyperprolactinaemia should be investigated for the possibility of a pituitary tumour before treatment with bromocriptine. Treatment of women with hyperprolactinaemic amenorrhoea results in ovulation; such patients should be advised to use contraceptive measures other than an oral contraceptive. Visual fields should be checked in patients who become pregnant, since there have been reports of the rapid expansion of pre-existing pituitary tumours during pregnancy. Acromegalic patients should be checked for symptoms of peptic ulcer before therapy and should immediately report symptoms of gastro-intestinal discomfort during therapy.

Bromocriptine should be given with caution to patients with cardiovascular disease, liver disease, or a history of psychotic disorders. Liver-function checks have been recommended for patients on long-term therapy; annual gynaecological examinations, or every 6 months for postmenopausal women, are also recommended. Patients who drive or operate machinery should be warned of the possibility of dizziness and fainting during the first few days of treatment.

Dopamine antagonists such as the phenothiazines, butyrophenones, thioxanthenes, and metoclopramide might be expected to reduce the prolactin-lowering effect and, as with levodopa, the antiparkinsonian effect of bromocriptine.

INTERACTIONS. *Alcohol.* Mention of alcohol intolerance in 5 of 73 patients receiving bromocriptine 10 to 60 mg daily for the treatment of acromegaly.— J. A. H. Wass *et al., Br. med. J.*, 1977, *1*, 875.

Gastro-intestinal side-effects with low doses of bromocriptine were markedly reduced in 2 women when they abstained from alcohol.— J. Ayres and M. N. Maisey (letter), *New Engl. J. Med.*, 1980, *302*, 806.

Antibiotics. Drowsiness, dystonia, choreoathetoid dyskinesias, and visual hallucinations occurred when josamycin was given to a patient receiving bromocriptine.— J. L. Montastruc and A. Rascol, *Presse méd.*, 1984, *13*, 2267.

Antifungal agents. The response to bromocriptine was blocked in a patient who was also receiving griseofulvin.— G. Schwinn *et al., Eur. J. clin. Invest.*, 1977, *7*, 101.

Tranquillisers. Serum concentrations of prolactin rose and visual fields deteriorated following administration of thioridazine to a 40-year-old man receiving bromocriptine therapy for a large prolactinoma.— R. J. Robbins *et al., Am. J. Med.*, 1984, *76*, 921.

PREGNANCY AND THE NEONATE. In 19 children born to mothers in whom ovulation had been induced by bromocriptine no numerical or structural chromosomal anomalies which might be ascribed to the maternal use of bromocriptine could be demonstrated.— L. A. Schellekens *et al., Arzneimittel-Forsch.*, 1977, *27*, 2151.

An increased incidence of foetal abnormalities, especially cleft palate, seen in *rabbits* given bromocriptine was not confirmed by subsequent *animal* work and experience has shown bromocriptine to present no teratological potential in pregnant women.— C. Weil, *Curr. med. Res. Opinion*, 1986, *10*, 25.

A surveillance report, from the manufacturer, of all pregnancies reported between 1973 and 1980 in women who had taken bromocriptine after conception. Information was obtained on 1410 pregnancies in 1335 women, the majority of whom had been treated for hyperprolactinaemic conditions, while in 256 pregnancies pituitary tumours and acromegaly were the primary diagnosis. Bromocriptine was generally taken at some time in the first 8 weeks after conception, the mean duration of treatment being 21 days. In 4 patients bromocriptine was not prescribed until late in pregnancy and in 9 with acromegaly and pituitary microadenoma it was taken continuously throughout gestation. There were 157 (11.1%) spontaneous abortions, 12 (0.9%) extrauterine pregnancies, 2 patients with 3 hydatidiform moles, and an incidence of twin pregnancies of 1.8%. Major congenital abnormalities were detected in 12 (1%) infants at birth and minor abnormalities in 31 (2.5%). All of these incidence rates were comparable with those quoted for normal populations and the data indicate that the use of bromocriptine in the treatment of women with infertility is not associated with an increased risk of abortion, multiple pregnancy, or congenital abnormalities. Nevertheless, since the risk of abortion is not increased by interruption of treatment, it is still recommended that bromocriptine therapy be stopped as soon as pregnancy is confirmed unless there is a definite indication for its continuation.— I. Turkalj *et al., J. Am. med. Ass.*, 1982, *247*, 1589. See also C. Weil, *Curr. med. Res. Opinion*, 1986, *10*, 172.

See also under Hyperprolactinaemia and Prolactinomas: Female Infertility in Uses (below).

WITHDRAWAL. Transient galactorrhoea and hyperprolactinaemia occurred in a young woman after withdrawal of bromocriptine therapy for Parkinson's disease. It was suggested the effects were due to a rebound phenomenon.— B. Pentland and J. S. A. Sawers, *Br. med. J.*, 1980, *281*, 716.

A report of hyperthermia following withdrawal of treatment with levodopa/carbidopa and bromocriptine.— L. Figà-Talamanca *et al., Neurology*, 1985, *35*, 258.

Absorption and Fate

Bromocriptine is incompletely absorbed from the gastro-intestinal tract, metabolised in the liver, and mainly excreted in the bile. It has been reported to be 90 to 96% bound to serum albumin *in vitro*.

In a study involving 10 patients with Parkinson's disease, single doses of bromocriptine 12.5, 25, 50, and 100 mg resulted in very variable peak plasma concentrations ranging from 1.3 to 5.3, 1.4 to 3.5, 2.6 to 19.7, and 6.5 to 24.6 ng per mL respectively, 30 to 210 minutes (mean 102 minutes) after dosage. After 4 hours plasma concentrations were about 75% of the peak values. Clinical improvement was evident within 30 to 90 minutes of a dose with peak effect at about 130 minutes and in most patients improvement persisted throughout the 4-hour study period. Peak clinical response, peak fall in blood pressure, and peak rise in plasma concentrations of growth hormone occurred about 30, 60, and 70 minutes respectively after peak plasma-bromocriptine concentrations but there was no significant relationship between them. There was however a significant relationship between plasma concentrations and concurrent changes in clinical response compared with pretreatment scores. Dyskinesias occurred within 90 to 180 minutes of dosage in 5 of 10 patients. Metoclopramide 60 mg given 30 minutes before bromocriptine had no consistent effect on plasma-bromocriptine concentrations.— P. Price *et al., Br. J. clin. Pharmac.*, 1978, *6*, 303.

Further references: S. Flechter *et al., Curr. ther. Res.*, 1979, *25*, 540; M. L. Friis *et al., Eur. J. clin. Pharmac.*, 1979, *15*, 275.

Uses and Administration

Bromocriptine, an ergot derivative or ergoline (see p.1051), is a dopamine agonist acting at receptors in the central nervous system, cardiovascular system, pituitary-hypothalamic axis, and gastro-intestinal tract. It inhibits the secretion of prolactin (see p.1145) from the anterior pituitary and is used to suppress physiological lactation and in endocrinological disorders associated with hyperprolactinaemia, including amenorrhoea in women and impotence in men. Growth-hormone secretion may be suppressed by bromocriptine in some patients with acromegaly. Because of its dopaminergic activity bromocriptine is also used in the management of Parkinson's disease.

It is administered by mouth as bromocriptine mesylate; doses are expressed in terms of the base. It should be taken with food.

For the prevention of puerperal lactation bromocriptine 2.5 mg is given on the day of delivery followed by 2.5 mg twice daily for 14 days. The risk of hypotension and, more rarely, hypertension must be borne in mind and it has been recommended that bromocriptine should not be given until at least 4 hours after delivery. For the suppression of established lactation it is given in a dose of 2.5 mg daily for 2 to 3 days subsequently increased to 2.5 mg twice daily for 14 days.

For the treatment of other conditions the dose of bromocriptine is usually increased gradually as follows: an initial dose of 1 to 1.25 mg at night, increased to 2 to 2.5 mg at night after 2 to 3 days, and subsequently increased by 1 to 2.5 mg at intervals of 2 to 3 days to a dose of 2.5 mg twice daily. Any further increments should be made in a similar manner.

In the treatment of hypogonadism and galactorrhoea syndromes and infertility in both men and women bromocriptine is introduced gradually as described above. Most patients respond to 7.5 mg daily but up to 30 mg daily may be required. Similar doses are given to patients known to have prolactinomas. Infertile patients without raised serum concentrations of prolactin are usually given 2.5 mg twice daily.

In cyclical benign breast and menstrual disorders bromocriptine is introduced gradually up to a usual dosage of 2.5 mg twice daily.

Bromocriptine is used as an adjunct to surgery and radiotherapy to reduce growth-hormone concentrations in plasma in acromegalic patients. It is introduced gradually up to a dose of 2.5 mg twice daily and may then be increased further every 2 to 3 days to a dose of 20 mg daily.

In Parkinson's disease bromocriptine is usually given as an adjunct to levodopa treatment. It should be introduced gradually and in general levodopa dosage should be decreased, also gradually, until an optimal response is achieved. A suggested initial dose is 1 to 1.25 mg of bromocriptine at night during week 1, increased to 2 to 2.5 mg at night for week 2, 2.5 mg twice daily for week 3, and thereafter 2.5 mg three times daily, increased by 2.5 mg every 3 to 14 days depending on response. Most patients require doses within the range of 10 to 40 mg daily.

Studies in *rats* supported the conclusion that bromocriptine acted by stimulating dopamine receptors in the CNS but unlike apomorphine its action depended upon intact catecholamine stores.— A. M. Johnson *et al., Br. J. Pharmac.*, 1976, *56*, 59.

Ergot-derivative dopaminergic drugs such as bromocriptine, lysuride, and pergolide can be considered to be serotonin partial agonists whereas apomorphine and its derivatives have no known interaction with the serotonin system.— R. Horowski (letter), *Lancet*, 1986, *2*, 510.

A review of the actions and uses of drugs which suppress prolactin secretion, including direct-acting dopamine agonists.— E. E. Müller *et al., Drugs*, 1983, *25*, 399.

Reviews of bromocriptine: *Bromocriptine: A Clinical and Pharmacological Review*, M.O. Thorner *et al.* (Ed.), New York, Raven, 1980; M. L. Vance *et al., Ann. intern. Med.*, 1984, *100*, 78.

ACROMEGALY. A review of the treatment of acromegaly. The choice of treatment lies between surgery and irradiation. Bromocriptine is best regarded as an adjuvant and is used to complement radiotherapy, taking advantage of its rapid action, and for patients in whom surgery has either failed or is refused; it is probably the treatment of choice for mild acromegaly. Bromocriptine given alone restores the growth-hormone value to normal in relatively few patients.— J. P. Thomas, *Br. med. J.*, 1983, *286*, 330.

Of 73 patients with acromegaly 71 experienced improvement after treatment for 3 to 25 months with bromocriptine 10 to 20 mg daily, increased if necessary to 60 mg daily. Improvement included reduced sweating, decreased hand, foot, and finger size, relief of headache, and increased libido. Mean growth-hormone concentrations and growth-hormone concentrations during a glucose-tolerance test generally fell and glucose tolerance was improved in 20 of 23 diabetic patients. Serum-prolactin concentrations fell.— J. A. H. Wass *et al., Br. med. J.*, 1977, *1*, 875. Evidence that bromocriptine can reduce the size of growth-hormone-secreting pituitary tumours in some patients with acromegaly.— J. A. H. Wass *et al., Lancet*, 1979, *2*, 66.

A double-blind placebo-controlled crossover study in 18 patients given bromocriptine 20 mg daily for 6 weeks did not confirm earlier reports of a beneficial effect in acromegaly.— J. Lindholm *et al., New Engl. J. Med.*, 1981, *304*, 1450. Criticism of the study. Many authorities consider bromocriptine 20 mg daily to be an inadequate dose in some patients.— M. O. Thorner *et al.* (letter), *ibid.*, *305*, 1092. Reply.— J. Lindholm *et al.*, *ibid.* Further criticism. All authorities who use bromocriptine in acromegaly first test individual responses to the drug and only treat the responding patients who have at least a 50% decrease in growth hormone; nonresponders make up about a third of all patients.— J. Köbberling *et al.* (letter), *ibid.*, 1982, *306*, 748. Reply.— J. Lindholm *et al.* (letter), *ibid.*, 749.

ADMINISTRATION IN RENAL FAILURE. Bromocriptine can be given in usual doses to patients with renal failure.— W. M. Bennett *et al., Am. J. Kidney Dis.*, 1983, *3*, 155.

ANOREXIA NERVOSA AND OBESITY. Elevated growth-hormone concentrations during a glucose-tolerance test were reduced in 8 patients with anorexia nervosa during treatment with bromocriptine 10 mg daily; there was no significant change in body-weight. There were no significant changes in growth-hormone concentrations or body-weight in 9 patients with refractory obesity.— A. D. B. Harrower *et al., Br. med. J.*, 1977, *2*, 156. See also A. D. B. Harrower, *Br. J. Hosp. Med.*, 1978, *20*, 672.

CARDIOVASCULAR DISORDERS. A discussion on the hypotensive actions of bromocriptine. Although it has been used in the treatment of essential hypertension, bromocriptine offers no apparent advantage over other antihypertensive agents.— M. J. Lewis, *Br. J. Hosp. Med.*, 1978, *20*, 661.

Studies on the hypotensive action of bromocriptine: P. Benito *et al.* (letter), *Drug Intell. & clin. Pharm.*, 1984,

18, 80 (independent of the renin-aldosterone system); G. Mercuro *et al.*, *Eur. J. clin. Pharmac.*, 1985, *27*, 671 (inhibition of noradrenaline release).

Symptoms related to congestive heart failure were alleviated in a patient already receiving digoxin, diuretics, and isosorbide dinitrate when she was given bromocriptine, 2.5 mg three times daily for acromegaly.— W. Luqman (letter), *Ann. intern. Med.*, 1985, *103*, 958.

CUSHING'S DISEASE. Remission of ACTH-dependent Cushing's syndrome was maintained for 6 years by bromocriptine 2.5 mg twice daily in a patient who had initially received pituitary irradiation.— A. B. Atkinson *et al.*, *Postgrad. med. J.*, 1985, *61*, 239.

EXTRAPYRAMIDAL DISORDERS. As with levodopa (see p.1019) there have been variable results with bromocriptine in the management of dystonias. Anecdotal reports have included 2 musicians with horn players' palsy who benefited from treatment with bromocriptine (I. James and P. Cook, *Lancet*, 1983, *1*, 1450). In a double-blind crossover study 15 patients with various dystonias were given bromocriptine in doses ranging from 18 to 150 mg daily (R.P. Newman *et al.*, *Clin. Neuropharmacol.*, 1985, *8*, 328). Two dropped out because of nausea and abdominal pain, 7 improved when compared with placebo, 2 worsened, and in 4 there was no change. Improvement was not dose-related and clinical features of patients likely to respond could not be identified. Bromocriptine does not appear to have been studied in drug-induced parkinsonism and results in tardive dyskinesia have been conflicting.

See also Parkinsonism (below).

GLAUCOMA. Bromocriptine reduced intra-ocular pressure in healthy subjects following a single dose of 1.25 mg by mouth (Q.A. Mekki *et al.*, *Lancet*, 1983, *1*, 1250) or topical application of 0.025% and 0.05% eye-drops (Q.A. Mekki *et al.*, *ibid.*, 1984, *1*, 287). It is thought to act by stimulation of D_2 dopamine receptors (Q.A. Mekki and P. Turner, *Br. J. Ophthal.*, 1985, *69*, 909).

HEPATIC ENCEPHALOPATHY. Variable results have been achieved with bromocriptine in the treatment of chronic hepatic encephalopathy. No significant improvement was seen with bromocriptine 5 mg three times daily in 7 cirrhotic patients with severe chronic portosystemic encephalopathy who had previously responded to therapy with neomycin and milk of magnesia (M. Uribe *et al.*, *Gastroenterology*, 1979, *76*, 1347), whereas overall improvement in all of 6 patients who had failed to sustain improvement on standard therapy was reported in another study (M.Y. Morgan, *et al.*, *ibid.*, 1980, *78*, 663). It has been suggested (I.R. Crossley and R. Williams, *Gut*, 1984, *25*, 85) that a trial of bromocriptine 15 mg daily is worthwhile in chronic hepatic encephalopathy when symptoms are not relieved by standard therapy including dietary protein restriction and the administration of neomycin, lactulose, and branched-chain amino acids.

HYPERPROLACTINAEMIA AND PROLACTINOMAS. Prolactinomas are pituitary tumours that secrete prolactin. The main clinical problems due to these tumours are generally secondary to hyperprolactinaemia which causes menstrual disturbances, such as amenorrhoea, oligomenorrhoea, or cycles with a deficient luteal phase, and sometimes galactorrhoea; about one fifth of women with amenorrhoea and the other types of menstrual disorder have hyperprolactinaemia. Prolactinomas in women are almost all less than 1 cm in diameter and are called microadenomas. Using computed tomography techniques small tumours have been found in most patients with hyperprolactinaemia and normal skull radiographs. Prolactinomas in men are less common but usually large; the hyperprolactinaemia causes decreased libido and impotence. Hyperprolactinaemia may be corrected by treatment with bromocriptine or newer ergot derivatives such as pergolide, resulting in the rapid restoration of normal gonadal function in either sex. Without treatment most prolactinomas seem to remain static, some progress, and a few apparently disappear, often after pregnancy. Large tumours often recur even after surgery unless radiotherapy is given. Bromocriptine and related drugs can shrink most prolactinomas as well as reducing serum concentrations of prolactin.— A. Grossman and G. M. Besser, *Br. med. J.*, 1985, *290*, 182.

There has been controversy over the optimal management of macroprolactinomas. Surgery has been recommended (A.G. Robinson and P.B. Nelson, *Ann. intern. Med.*, 1983, *99*, 115) but the recurrence rate is reported to be high and bromocriptine has been used effectively as initial therapy although withdrawal has usually resulted in the return of hyperprolactinaemia and tumour re-expansion (M.L. Vance *et al.*, *ibid.*, 1984, *100*, 78). Tumour expansion, following initial reduction, has also been reported in one patient during treatment with bromocriptine (H.D. Breidahl *et al.*, *Br. med. J.*, 1983, *287*, 451). However, in a study in 15 patients, rapid tumour regrowth was uncommon following withdrawal of long-term therapy with bromocriptine or pergolide, although symptoms and hyperprolactinaemia recurred (D.G. Johnston *et al.*, *Lancet*, 1984, *2*, 187). In another study of long-term treatment (A Liuzzi *et al.*, *New Engl. J. Med.*, 1985, *313*, 656) the authors concluded that although prolonged treatment is rarely curative an attempt should be made to reduce the daily dose progressively once a positive effect has been obtained. Results in 27 patients with large prolactin-secreting macroadenomas given bromocriptine daily for one year (M.E. Molitch *et al.*, *J. clin. Endocr. Metab.*, 1985, *60*, 698) also suggested that bromocriptine should be considered as primary therapy.

Although bromocriptine or lysuride are generally accepted as first-line treatment for microprolactinomas, Landolt *et al.* (*Lancet*, 1982, *2*, 657) reported that pretreatment with bromocriptine might render later surgery less effective. Faglia *et al.* (*ibid.*, 1983, *1*, 133) disagreed and reported no significant effect on surgical outcome. In the light of a retrospective review of 75 women who underwent surgery for microprolactinomas, and pending more extensive studies, it is recommended that dopamine agonists should be discontinued weeks or months before surgery and should not be given at all if microprolactinomas associated with prolactin concentrations higher than 200 ng per mL (usually larger than 7 mm diameter) are to be operated on.— R. Fahlbusch *et al.* (letter), *Lancet*, 1984, *2*, 520.

Pituitary function was improved by treatment with bromocriptine in a study of 6 men with prolactin-secreting pituitary macroadenomas and deficiencies of pituitary hormones other than gonadotrophins. In addition to decreasing serum-prolactin concentrations in all 6 and decreasing adenoma size in 4, bromocriptine restored normal function by the sixth month of treatment in 2 patients who had initially been hypothyroid, 1 who had been hypoadrenal, and 2 of 6 who had had subnormal growth-hormone secretion.— A. Warfield *et al.*, *Ann. intern. Med.*, 1984, *101*, 783.

Acute oestrogen-induced swelling of a large invasive pituitary adenoma in a 45-year-old woman was treated successfully by intramuscular injection of bromocriptine 50 mg in a sustained-release formulation.— A. M. Landolt *et al.* (letter), *Lancet*, 1984, *2*, 111.

Female infertility. A discussion on pregnancy and the hyperprolactinaemic woman. Bromocriptine restores ovulation and fertility and is the treatment of choice for women with idiopathic hyperprolactinaemia. It is also preferred to surgery and to surgery or radiotherapy followed by bromocriptine in patients with a microadenoma; the risk of tumour enlargement is low with bromocriptine alone but patients should be monitored carefully throughout gestation. Bromocriptine is also favoured as primary therapy for women with small intrasellar · or inferiorly extending macroadenomas. In those with larger macroadenomas that may have suprasellar extension there is a 15 to 35% risk of clinically serious tumour enlargement during pregnancy when bromocriptine alone is used; because of this high risk the author's preference is surgery before pregnancy, although in general the larger the tumour the lower the chance of success; late recurrence of hyperprolactinaemia has been reported in 20 to 80% of women following surgery. After surgery bromocriptine is required to restore normal prolactin levels and allow ovulation. Radiotherapy before pregnancy, followed by bromocriptine, reduces the risk of tumour enlargement but is rarely curative and may also result in long-term hypopituitarism. The continuous administration of bromocriptine throughout pregnancy has also been advocated in women with macroadenomas, but the effects on the developing foetus are not yet known and such therapy cannot be recommended. However, existing information is reassuring and discovery of pregnancy at an advanced stage in a woman taking bromocriptine does not justify therapeutic abortion. If symptomatic tumour enlargement occurs during pregnancy reinstitution of bromocriptine is probably less harmful to the mother and child than surgery.— M. E. Molitch, *New Engl. J. Med.*, 1985, *312*, 1364.

A review of the safety of bromocriptine when used to facilitate pregnancy.— C. Weil, *Curr. med. Res. Opinion*, 1986, *10*, 172.

Of 20 hyperprolactinaemic women followed up for 4 years, 3 were unable to tolerate bromocriptine, 5 are still receiving bromocriptine, and one discontinued treatment after 2 successful pregnancies. The remaining 11 patients showed evidence of tumour regression and bromocriptine treatment was stopped. Of these 11 patients, 7 achieved at least one viable pregnancy. One patient with pituitary gonadotrophin failure required exogenous gonadotrophins to become pregnant and remained amenorrhoeic after delivery. Except for one woman in whom recurrence of symptoms necessitated resumption of bromocriptine after 3 months, the remainder continued to ovulate regularly and no re-expansion of prolactinomas was detected. Pregnancy might exercise a synergistic effect with bromocriptine to induce regression of prolactinomas.— K. W. Hancock *et al.*, *Br. med. J.*, 1985, *290*, 117.

There have been reports of beneficial results with bromocriptine in women with normal serum concentrations of prolactin, including restoration of menstruation in patients with secondary amenorrhoea (M. Seppälä *et al.*, *Lancet*, 1976, *1*, 1154), restoration of ovulation in women with anovulation following oral contraceptive withdrawal (H.J. van der Steeg and H.J.T.C. Bennink, *ibid.*, 1977, *1*, 502), relief of galactorrhoea (J.G. Mathur, *Med. J. Aust.*, 1984, *140*, 564), and relief of galactorrhoea and ovulatory dysfunction (S.L. Padilla *et al.*, *Fert. Steril.*, 1985, *44*, 695). However, bromocriptine and placebo were equally effective and restored menstrual function in about half the patients in a study involving 33 amenorrhoeic women with normoprolactinaemia (P.G. Crosignani *et al.*, *Br. J. Obstet. Gynaec.*, 1978, *85*, 773).

Polycystic ovary syndrome probably reflects a primary hypothalamic defect resulting in altered patterns of gonadotrophin and prolactin secretion. Up to one third of women with the syndrome have mild basal hyperprolactinaemia without evidence of a pituitary tumour. Bromocriptine 5 mg daily for up to 2 years was given to 34 women with polycystic ovary syndrome and either normal or increased prolactin levels; none had monthly menses. Improved menstrual patterns were achieved in 28 women and 24 developed monthly menses. Gonadotrophin, prolactin, and dehydroepiandrosterone sulphate levels before treatment were not significantly different in responders and nonresponders. Prolactin levels were uniformly depressed in both groups.— J. J. Pehrson *et al.*, *Ann. intern. Med.*, 1986, *105*, 129.

Male infertility. Bromocriptine had a favourable effect in some men with oligospermia and slight hyperprolactinaemia.— K. Saidi *et al.* (letter), *Lancet*, 1977, *1*, 250.

In a double-blind study bromocriptine was no more effective than placebo in the treatment of oligospermic infertile men, none of whom had marked hyperprolactinaemia.— O. Hovatta *et al.*, *Clin. Endocr.*, 1979, *11*, 377.

Prolactin-secreting pituitary tumours in men produce hypogonadism, impotence, and infertility. They are often large at presentation and there may be symptoms such as visual-field defects or cranial nerve palsies. Bromocriptine 20 mg daily was given as sole therapy for 3 to 11 months to 8 hyperprolactinaemic men, 7 of whom presented with impotence and one with gynaecomastia and galactorrhoea. Serum prolactin fell to within normal limits in 7 subjects and potency was restored in 5 and improved in one. There was evidence of tumour regression in the 6 patients examined.— R. W. G. Prescott *et al.*, *Lancet*, 1982, *1*, 245.

INHIBITION OF LACTATION. A reminder that puerperal lactation is a physiological state and advice that such a powerful drug as bromocriptine be used for its inhibition only when more conservative measures are inadequate.— *Br. med. J.*, 1977, *1*, 189. A review of the suppression of lactation and the view that when suppression is desirable bromocriptine, given after delivery or when full lactation is established, is the most effective method available.— R. J. Pepperell, *Med. J. Aust.*, 1986, *144*, 37.

Breast engorgement and secretion were completely absent in 272 of 370 postpartum women following bromocriptine 2.5 mg twice daily for 14 days. Rebound engorgement and secretion occurred in 26 women; the symptoms disappeared spontaneously in 17 and were completely inhibited in the remainder by treatment with bromocriptine for an additional 7 days.— C. Duchesne and R. Leke, *Obstet. Gynec.*, 1981, *57*, 464.

MALIGNANT NEOPLASMS. Remissions of from 3 to 7 years have been achieved so far in 5 of 18 patients with advanced carcinoma of the cervix treated with bromocriptine 2.5 mg twice daily; a further 3 achieved tumour stasis. Remissions were very slow in onset. One patient with advanced ovarian carcinoma also achieved tumour stasis.— D. Guthrie, *Br. J. Obstet. Gynaec.*, 1982, *89*, 853. Beneficial results with bromocriptine in the treatment of cervical dysplasia.— E. M. Donath and A. E. Schindler (letter), *Lancet*, 1984, *2*, 157.

MASTALGIA. Mastodynia or breast pain is accepted as a normal premenstrual symptom by many women, but some with severe and protracted pain seek medical advice. The value of bromocriptine in severe cyclical mastodynia is now established; in patients with mild symptoms the side-effects of bromocriptine often outweigh the benefits. Non-cyclical mastodynia does not respond to bromocriptine. Controlled studies in patients with premenstrual tension and fibrocystic disease of the breast suggest a selective improvement with bromocriptine.— *Lancet*, 1982, *2*, 590.

A suggestion that the term fibrocystic disease of the breast has lost its specificity and should be abandoned. It has been defined as a condition in which there are palpable lumps in the breast, usually associated with pain and tenderness, that fluctuate with the menstrual cycle, but this description of cystic mastalgia applies to the majority of women of reproductive age.— S. M. Love *et al.*, *New Engl. J. Med.*, 1982, *307*, 1010.

A review of the overall performance of drug treatment in 291 patients with severe mastalgia and recommendations for its management. A good or useful response was obtained in 165 of 215 patients (77%) with cyclical mastalgia and overall 44% had a lasting response. Danazol achieved the highest response rate, but bromocriptine and evening primrose oil were also effective. The recommended dose for bromocriptine is 1.25 mg at night for one week, increasing to 2.5 mg nightly. The response rate in non-cyclical mastalgia was only 44% and individual drugs were no better than placebo overall, but danazol, bromocriptine, and evening primrose oil each appeared to help a different group of patients. Progestagens were ineffective in both types of mastalgia.— J. K. Pye *et al.*, *Lancet*, 1985, *2*, 373.

MENTAL DISORDERS. *Depression and mania.* Treatment with bromocriptine 5 mg three times daily was effective in 48 hours, and without side-effects, for the treatment of severe mania in 2 patients with long-standing manic-depressive psychosis for whom phenothiazines and lithium carbonate were contra-indicated.— C. Dorr and K. Sathananthan (letter), *Br. med. J.*, 1976, *1*, 1342. A double-blind study completed by 20 women with manic-depressive psychosis failed to show any benefit from bromocriptine in mania.— A. H. W. Smith *et al.*, *ibid.*, 1980, *280*, 86.

Bipolar, but not unipolar depression was improved by bromocriptine. Two of the 5 patients with bipolar depression became manic, supporting the view that bipolar depression is associated with a reduction in central dopaminergic neurotransmission and mania with an increase.— T. Silverstone (letter), *Lancet*, 1984, *1*, 903.

NEUROLEPTIC MALIGNANT SYNDROME. Reports of beneficial results with bromocriptine in the treatment of the neuroleptic malignant syndrome.— P. S. Mueller *et al.*, *J. Am. med. Ass.*, 1983, *249*, 386; S. Dhib-Jalbut *et al.* (letter), *ibid.*, *250*, 484.

PARKINSONISM. With the emergence of the late complications associated with levodopa in the treatment of Parkinson's disease attention turned to the dopamine agonists which theoretically might be expected to be preferable to levodopa. Bromocriptine is a potent agonist with relatively selective activity at dopamine D_2 receptors and has a longer duration of action than levodopa. However, despite a decade of clinical experience its use in Parkinson's disease remains controversial. Bromocriptine in adequate doses undoubtedly has antiparkinsonian properties, but is associated with a higher incidence of adverse reactions than levodopa; nausea, vomiting, dizziness, postural hypotension, and psychiatric disturbances are common side-effects and failure to tolerate bromocriptine has accounted for a 30 to 50% withdrawal-rate in most reported studies. The majority of studies have been with bromocriptine as an adjuvant to conventional levodopa therapy in poorly controlled patients. A smoother response has been achieved in some patients with fluctuations in motor performance and single doses of bromocriptine at bedtime have reduced early-morning akinesia and dystonia. Replacement of levodopa by bromocriptine because of intolerance or loss of response has rarely been beneficial. Experience with bromocriptine alone in Parkinson's disease is limited. In a series of 50 previously untreated patients given bromocriptine for more than 5 years (A.J. Lees and G.M. Stern, *J. Neurol. Neurosurg. Psychiat.*, 1981, *44*, 1020) the high failure-rate after one year was attributed to unacceptable adverse reactions at subtherapeutic doses, but in the remaining 28 patients drug-induced dyskinesia occurred in only one and fluctuations were not seen. There was however a tendency towards deterioration after 2 years of treatment and patients then responded poorly to levodopa; only 5 patients showed sustained benefit from bromocriptine after 5 years. Significant benefit with bromocriptine in small daily doses, introduced very slowly, has been claimed in both levodopa-treated and previously untreated patients (P.F. Teychenne *et al.*, *Neurology*, 1982, *32*, 577) and there have been further reports of comparable benefit. However these results are at variance with those of other workers and the outcome of a multicentre long-term study is awaited. At present levodopa remains the treatment of first choice in Parkinson's disease, despite the hazards of late complications, and is well tolerated, effective, and relatively cheap. Bromocriptine, although almost as effective in high doses, does not share the other advantages of levodopa and is more difficult to use in the elderly. Currently the value of bromocriptine appears to be limited to the management of fluctuations developing during long-term levodopa therapy, especially in patients with prominent early-morning disability. Reducing the dose of levodopa and adding a small dose of bromocriptine has been claimed to reduce drug-induced dyskinesia but remains controversial. The benefits of bromocriptine alone in low doses augmented slowly are not yet proved.— R. J. Hardie *et al.*, *Clin. Neuropharmacol.*, 1985, *8*, 150. For a further review of bromocriptine in Parkinson's disease, including reference to its mode of action, see A. N. Lieberman and M. Goldstein, *Pharmac. Rev.*, 1985, *37*, 217.

For an overview of parkinsonism and its treatment, see Levodopa, p.1019.

PREMENSTRUAL SYNDROME. Premenstrual syndrome is commonly characterised by mental symptoms such as depression and irritability, headache, mastodynia, peripheral oedema, and abdominal distension. Conventional therapy has been the administration of diuretics during the latter half of the menstrual cycle. Bromocriptine has also been tried with variable success. Idiopathic oedema is an ill-defined disorder affecting women during the reproductive years and involving fluid retention in the absence of cardiac, hepatic, renal, gastro-intestinal, or allergic disease. Treatment has included salt restriction, wearing of elastic stockings, intermittent diuretic administration, levodopa, carbidopa, and bromocriptine. No treatment is entirely satisfactory although bromocriptine appears to be beneficial in a subgroup of patients who may have either peripheral dopamine deficiency or altered sensitivity to the action of dopamine.— M. L. Vance *et al.*, *Ann. intern. Med.*, 1984, *100*, 78.

A survey of 14 controlled studies did not support the opinion that bromocriptine is effective in the premenstrual syndrome as such, although it appeared to be the treatment of choice for premenstrual mastodynia.— B. Andersch, *Obstetl gynec. Surv.*, 1983, *38*, 643. See also S. F. Pariser *et al.*, *Am. J. Obstet. Gynec.*, 1985, *153*, 599.

See also Mastalgia (above).

RESTLESS LEG SYNDROME. For reference to beneficial results with bromocriptine in the restless leg syndrome, see Levodopa, p.1020.

URINARY INCONTINENCE. A discussion on the treatment of urge incontinence. Dopamine agonists such as bromocriptine have proved disappointing.— *Lancet*, 1983, *1*, 1086.

See also Effects on the Urinary Tract in Adverse Effects (above).

WITHDRAWAL SYNDROMES. Bromocriptine 2.5 mg three times daily reduced the severity of alcohol-withdrawal symptoms in a preliminary study and tended to be more effective than apomorphine 10 mg three times daily.— V. Borg and T. Weinholdt, *Curr. ther. Res.*, 1980, *27*, 170.

Further references to the use of bromocriptine in the treatment of alcoholism: V. Borg, *Acta psychiat. scand.*, 1983, *68*, 100; R. Manopulo *et al.*, *Clin. Ther.*, 1986, *116*, 297.

Preliminary data suggesting that bromocriptine may be effective in the management of cocaine abuse by reducing the craving for cocaine associated with withdrawal.— C. A. Dackis and M. S. Gold (letter), *Lancet*, 1985, *1*, 1151.

Preparations

Bromocriptine Capsules *(B.P.)*. Bromocriptine Mesylate Capsules

Bromocriptine Tablets *(B.P.)*. Bromocriptine Mesylate Tablets

Bromocriptine Mesylate Tablets *(U.S.P.)*

Proprietary Preparations

Parlodel *(Sandoz, UK)*. *Capsules*, bromocriptine 5 and 10 mg (as mesylate).

Tablets, scored, bromocriptine 1 and 2.5 mg (as mesylate). Also available as a Parkinson's Disease Starter Pack.

Proprietary Names and Manufacturers

Bagren *(Serono, Ital.)*; Lactismine *(Serono, Spain)*; Parlodel *(Arg.; Sandoz, Austral.; Belg.; Anca, Canad.; Sandoz, Denm.; Sandoz, Fr.; Sandoz, Ital.; Jpn; Neth.; Sandoz, Norw.; Sandoz, S.Afr.; Sandoz, Spain; Sandoz, Switz.; Sandoz, UK; Sandoz, USA)*; Pravidel *(Sandoz, Ger.; Sandoz, Swed.)*.

4547-l

Carbidopa *(BAN, USAN, rINN)*.

(−)-L-α-Methyldopa Hydrazine; MK-486.
(−)-L-2-(3,4-Dihydroxybenzyl)-2-hydrazinopropionic acid monohydrate.
$C_{10}H_{14}N_2O_4,H_2O = 244.2$.

CAS — 28860-95-9 (anhydrous); 38821-49-7 (monohydrate).

NOTE. The synonym MK-485 has been used for the racemic mixture.

Pharmacopoeias. In *Br.* and *U.S.*

A white or creamy-white, odourless or almost odourless powder. Slightly **soluble** in water and methyl alcohol; very slightly soluble in alcohol; freely soluble in 3M hydrochloric acid; practically insoluble in acetone, chloroform, and ether. A 1% suspension in water has a pH of 4.0 to 6.0. **Protect** from light.

Absorption and Fate

Carbidopa is rapidly but incompletely absorbed from the gastro-intestinal tract. It is rapidly excreted in the urine both unchanged and in the form of metabolites. It does not cross the blood-brain barrier. In *rats*, carbidopa has been reported to cross the placenta and to be excreted in milk.

Pharmacokinetic and metabolic studies of carbidopa in *animals* and man.— S. Vickers *et al.*, *Fedn Proc.*, 1971, *30*, 336; *idem*, *Drug Metab. & Disposit.*, 1974, *2*, 9; *idem*, *J. med. Chem.*, 1975, *18*, 134.

For the effect of decarboxylase inhibitors on the pharmacokinetics and metabolism of levodopa, see Levodopa, p.1017.

Uses and Administration

Carbidopa is a peripheral decarboxylase inhibitor with little or no pharmacological activity when given alone in usual doses. It inhibits the peripheral decarboxylation of levodopa to dopamine and as, unlike levodopa, it does not cross the blood-brain barrier, effective brain concentrations of dopamine are produced with lower doses of levodopa. At the same time reduced peripheral formation of dopamine reduces peripheral side-effects notably, nausea and vomiting, and cardiac arrhythmias, although the dyskinesias and mental effects associated with levodopa therapy tend to develop earlier. Contrary to its effect in patients on levodopa alone, pyridoxine does not inhibit the response to levodopa in patients also receiving a peripheral decarboxylase inhibitor.

It is given with levodopa in the treatment of parkinsonism to enable a lower dosage of the latter to be used and a more rapid response to be obtained, and to decrease side-effects. For details of administration and dosage, see Levodopa, p.1018.

Carbidopa also inhibits the peripheral decarboxylation of the serotonin precursor oxitriptan (see p.376).

A discussion on the influence of the decarboxylase inhibitors carbidopa and benserazide on the pharmacokinetic, pharmacodynamic, and clinical effects of levodopa in parkinsonism.— R. M. Pinder *et al.*, *Drugs*, 1976, *11*, 329. See also B. Boshes, *Ann. intern. Med.*, 1981, *94*, 364 (carbidopa).

There is no difference in efficacy between levodopa with carbidopa or levodopa with benserazide in the treatment of parkinsonism.— G. Stern, *Prescribers' J.*, 1982, *22*, 1.

See also under Parkinsonism in Levodopa, p.1019.

PITUITARY AND HYPOTHALAMIC DISORDERS. Increased serum concentrations of prolactin have been reported following administration of carbidopa or benserazide.— E. E. Müller *et al.*, *Drugs*, 1983, *25*, 399.

PREGNANCY AND THE NEONATE. For a report of normal offspring following the use of levodopa alone or levodopa with carbidopa during pregnancy, see Levodopa, p.1017.

Preparations and Proprietary Preparations

See Levodopa, p.1020.

Proprietary Names and Manufacturers
The following names have been used for multi-ingredient preparations containing carbidopa— Sinemet *(Merck Sharp & Dohme, Austral.; Merck Sharp & Dohme, Canad.; Merck Sharp & Dohme, UK; Merck Sharp & Dohme, USA)*; Sinemet-Plus *(Merck Sharp & Dohme, UK)*.

4548-y

Fusaric Acid
5-Butylpicolinic Acid. 5-Butylpyridine-2-carboxylic acid.
$C_{10}H_{13}NO_2$=179.2.

CAS — 536-69-6.

Fusaric acid is an inhibitor of dopamine-β-hydroxylase, the enzyme responsible for conversion of dopamine into noradrenaline, and was formerly tried in the management of Parkinson's disease.

4549-j

Lergotrile Mesylate *(USAN, rINNM).*
Lilly-79907 (lergotrile); Lilly-83636. (2-Chloro-6-methylergolin-8β-yl)acetonitrile methanesulphonate.
$C_{17}H_{18}ClN_3,CH_4O_3S$=395.9.

CAS — 36945-03-6 (lergotrile); 51473-23-5 (mesylate).

Lergotrile mesylate, an ergot derivative or ergoline, is a dopamine agonist similar to bromocriptine. It was tried in the management of Parkinson's disease and in disorders associated with hyperprolactinaemia, but was found to be hepatotoxic.

Proprietary Names and Manufacturers
Lilly, USA.

4541-g

Levodopa *(BAN, USAN, rINN).*

Dihydroxyphenylalanine; Dopa; Laevo-dopa; Levodopum; L-Dopa. (−)-3-(3,4-Dihydroxyphenyl)-L-alanine.
$C_9H_{11}NO_4$=197.2.

CAS — 59-92-7.

Pharmacopoeias. In *Belg., Br., Braz., Chin., Cz., Egypt., Eur., Fr., Ind., Int., It., Jpn, Jug., Neth., Nord., Swiss,* and *U.S.*

A white or slightly cream-coloured, odourless, crystalline powder. In the presence of moisture it is rapidly oxidised by atmospheric oxygen and darkens.

Slightly **soluble** in water; freely soluble in 1M hydrochloric acid but sparingly soluble in 0.1M hydrochloric acid; practically insoluble in alcohol, chloroform, and ether. A 1% suspension in water has a pH of 4.5 to 7.0. **Protect** from light. The *U.S.P.* recommends **storage** at a temperature not exceeding 40° in airtight containers.

STABILITY. A warning that extemporaneously prepared oral liquid dosage forms may be unstable and manufacturers' formulations should be used where possible. An extemporary formula is available for levodopa syrup.— T. J. Walls *et al., Br. med. J.,* 1985, *290,* 444.

Adverse Effects

Gastro-intestinal effects, notably nausea, vomiting, and anorexia are common early in treatment with levodopa, particularly if the dosage is increased too rapidly. Gastro-intestinal bleeding has been reported in patients with a history of peptic ulcer.

The commonest cardiovascular effect is orthostatic hypotension, which is usually asymptomatic, but may be associated with faintness and dizziness. Cardiac arrhythmias have been reported and hypertension has occasionally occurred.

Psychiatric symptoms occur in a high proportion of patients, especially the elderly, and include agitation, anxiety, euphoria, and insomnia, or sometimes drowsiness and depression. More serious effects, usually requiring a reduction in dosage or withdrawal of levodopa, include aggression, paranoid delusions, hallucinations, delirium, severe depression, with or without suicidal behaviour, and unmasking of dementia. Psychotic reactions are more likely in patients with postencephalitic parkinsonism or a history of mental disorders.

Abnormal involuntary movements or dyskinesias are the most serious dose-limiting adverse effects of levodopa and are very common at the optimum dose required to control Parkinson's disease; their frequency increases with duration of treatment. Involuntary movements of the face, tongue, lips, and jaws often appear first and those of the trunk and extremities later. Severe generalised choreoathetoid and dystonic movements may occur after prolonged administration. Muscle twitching and blepharospasm may be early signs of excessive dosage. Exaggerated respiratory movements and exacerbated oculogyric crises have been reported in patients with postencephalitic parkinsonism. Re-emergence of akinesia, in the form of 'end-of-dose' deterioration and the 'on-off' phenomenon, in patients with Parkinson's disease is a complication of long-term treatment, but is probably due to progression of the disease rather than to levodopa (see also under Parkinsonism in Uses).

A positive response to the direct Coomb's test may occur, usually without evidence of haemolysis although auto-immune haemolytic anaemia has occasionally been reported. Transient leucopenia has occurred rarely. The effects of levodopa on liver and kidney function are generally slight. Levodopa may cause discoloration of the urine and other body fluids.

Some of the adverse effects reported may not be attributable directly to levodopa, but rather to the use of antimuscarinic agents, to increased mobility, or to unmasking of underlying conditions as parkinsonism improves. Concomitant administration of a peripheral decarboxylase inhibitor may reduce the severity of peripheral symptoms such as gastro-intestinal and cardiovascular effects, but central effects such as dyskinesias and mental disturbances may occur earlier in treatment.

Monitoring of clinical laboratory values in a multicentre study of 974 parkinsonian patients receiving levodopa revealed few, if any, abnormalities clearly related to treatment. Blood-urea-nitrogen was abnormal in 34% of 5877 determinations; elevated concentrations generally fell rapidly with increased fluid intake, but a possible relationship with levodopa could not be eliminated. Serum aspartate aminotransferase (SGOT) was abnormal in 9% of 5427 determinations; abnormalities were generally minor transient elevations, but monitoring of liver function in patients on levodopa was considered necessary. Blood concentrations of uric acid were abnormal in 31% of 625 determinations and were generally attributed to the colorimetric technique used, however, a few values were slightly raised even when the uricase method of determination was used. Abnormal fasting blood sugars and protein-bound iodine could not be related to levodopa therapy.— F. McDowell, *Clin. Pharmac. Ther.,* 1971, *12,* 335 (See also under Gout (below)).

The major adverse effects of levodopa are dyskinesia in 75% of patients and psychiatric disturbances in 25%. Nausea and vomiting in 40 to 50% are gradually tolerated and hypotension in 25 to 30% is generally asymptomatic. Other adverse effects include cardiac arrhythmias, particularly atrial and ventricular ectopic beats and less commonly atrial flutter and fibrillation; palpitations and flushing often accompanied by excessive sweating; hypertension; polyuria, incontinence, and urinary retention, although antimuscarinic drugs often contribute to problems with micturition; and dark coloration of the urine and saliva. Rare adverse effects include abdominal pain, constipation, and diarrhoea; mydriasis, blurred vision, diplopia, and precipitation of glaucoma; headache; stridor; tachypnoea; and parasthesias.— D. B. Calne and J. L. Reid, *Drugs,* 1972, *4,* 49.

ABNORMAL COLORATION. Intense black pigmentation confined to the costal cartilages was noted at necropsy in a 70-year-old woman who had taken tablets containing levodopa 250 mg and carbidopa 25 mg to a maximal dose of 8 tablets daily for 13 years. It was suggested that failure to metabolise high plasma concentrations of levodopa in the presence of a dopa-decarboxylase inhibitor had resulted in the deposition of dihydroxyphenylalanine (DOPA) in the cartilage. It is known that DOPA will readily auto-oxidise *in vitro* in the presence of oxygen to a black pigment and this can also happen *in vivo* since black urine is a well known side-effect of levodopa therapy. Dark sweat and pigmentation of the skin and teeth are also side-effects known to the manufacturers of levodopa.— C. E. Connolly *et al.* (letter), *Lancet,* 1986, *1,* 690.

See also Effects on Skin and Hair (below).

DYSGEUSIA. A change in taste sensation was reported by 23 of 514 patients treated with levodopa in association with a decarboxylase inhibitor; 2 of the 23 had total loss of taste initially. The altered taste was often described as insipid, metallic, or plastic, was first observed 3 to 32 weeks after beginning treatment, and lasted for 2 to 40 weeks. In an earlier report (A. Barbeau, *Ariz. Med.,* 1970 *27,* 1) 22 of 100 patients receiving levodopa alone had experienced changes in taste.— J. Siegfried and H. Zumstein, *Z. Neurol.,* 1971, *200,* 345.

EFFECTS ON THE BLOOD. A report of acute non-haemolytic anaemia and a skin rash occurring in 1 patient during treatment with levodopa.— I. Alkalay and T. Zipoli, *Ann. Allergy,* 1977, *39,* 191.

Haemolytic anaemia. Of 365 patients on a mean daily dosage of 4.04 g of levodopa over a period of 10 to 902 days, 32 developed a positive direct Coombs' test but there were no cases of haemolytic anaemia.— C. Joseph, *New Engl. J. Med.,* 1972, *286,* 1401.

References to patients developing auto-immune haemolytic anaemia following administration of levodopa: M. C. Territo *et al., J. Am. med. Ass.,* 1973, *226,* 1347; F. D. Lindström *et al., Ann. intern. Med.,* 1977, *86,* 298; R. M. Bernstein, *Br. med. J.,* 1979, *1,* 1461.

Levodopa did not cause haemolysis in Chinese patients with glucose 6-phosphate dehydrogenase deficiency. These observations do not support the hypothesis that favism, which is found in Mediterranean and Chinese people, is due to the levodopa content of fava beans.— T. K. Chan *et al., Br. med. J.,* 1976, *2,* 1227.

Leucopenia. Transient minor decreases in total leucocyte counts occurred in 3 of 80 parkinsonian patients treated with levodopa.— A. Barbeau, *Can. med. Ass. J.,* 1969, *101,* 791.

Thrombocytopenia. A 63-year-old man developed thrombocytopenia after long-term levodopa and procyclidine therapy. Thrombocytopenia was attributed to levodopa and was amenable to prednisone therapy.— W. M. Wanamaker *et al., J. Am. med. Ass.,* 1976, *235,* 2217.

EFFECTS ON THE CARDIOVASCULAR SYSTEM. There have been conflicting reports on the effects of peripheral decarboxylase inhibitors on orthostatic hypotension attributed to levodopa therapy. Calne *et al.* (*Br. J. Pharmac.,* 1972, *44,* 162) found supine and erect systolic blood pressure to be significantly higher in parkinsonian patients given levodopa in association with carbidopa than in those receiving levodopa alone and suggested that the peripheral actions of dopamine contribute to levodopa-induced hypotension. However, Leibowitz and Lieberman (*Neurology,* 1975, *25,* 917) found no change in the incidence and degree of orthostatic hypotension after levodopa in association with carbidopa and, similary, no difference in the frequency of ventricular arrhythmias.

See also Effects on Kidney Function (below).

EFFECTS ON THE ENDOCRINE SYSTEM. A study of the effects of levodopa therapy on insulin and carbohydrate metabolism indicated that untreated parkinsonian patients have abnormally low rates of glucose utilisation, associated with deficient insulin secretion following intravenous glucose loading, and that oral levodopa therapy does not produce any further impairment of these metabolic parameters.— M. H. Van Woert and P. S. Mueller, *Clin. Pharmac. Ther.,* 1971, *12,* 360. In a similar study, levodopa stimulated the release of growth hormone and after 1 year of levodopa therapy all 19 patients had some impairment of glucose utilisation, associated with a delayed hypersecretion of insulin.— C. R. Sirtori *et al., New Engl. J. Med.,* 1972, *287,* 729. Plasma concentrations of glucose, insulin, growth hormone, and glucagon were increased in healthy subjects following a single dose of levodopa 500 mg by mouth.— E. J. Rayfield *et al., ibid.,* 1975, *293,* 589.

A 66-year-old woman with parkinsonism became febrile and had a very low plasma-cortisol concentration after taking levodopa 250 mg four times a day gradually increased to 2.5 g daily. Her temperature and plasma cortisol returned to normal 4 days after withdrawing levodopa but on challenging with a dose of 250 mg three times daily the symptoms recurred.— S. R. Greenberg (letter), *New Engl. J. Med.*, 1972, *286*, 375.

Postmenopausal bleeding occurred in varying degrees in 12 of 47 women treated with levodopa.— J. Wajsbort (letter), *New Engl. J. Med.*, 1972, *286*, 784.

For an association between levodopa, abnormal cortisol rhythm, and mental disturbances, see Effects on Mental State (below).

For the effects of levodopa on pituitary function, see under Uses (below).

EFFECTS ON THE EYES. In 10 of 11 patients with Parkinson's disease who were receiving levodopa 1 to 6.8 g daily, the pupillary diameter was significantly decreased 4 hours after a dose. The miotic effect might reflect decreased peripheral sympathetic activity following partial noradrenaline depletion at sympathetic nerve endings, or be a central sympatholytic action.— A. S. D. Spiers *et al.*, *Br. med. J.*, 1970, *2*, 639.

Varying degrees of bilateral pupillary dilatation were noted in many of 28 patients with Parkinson's disease on chronic levodopa therapy. One patient was found to have latent Horner's syndrome when anisocoria with dilatation of only the left pupil was noted.— M. I. Weintraub *et al.*, *New Engl. J. Med.*, 1970, *283*, 120.

For a report of the exacerbation of oculogyric crises by levodopa, see Extrapyramidal effects (below).

EFFECTS ON THE GASTRO-INTESTINAL TRACT. Acute melaena and non-specific gastritis were associated with levodopa therapy in a 56-year-old man. Five other cases of gastro-intestinal haemorrhage had been reported.— D. Riddoch (letter), *Br. med. J.*, 1972, *1*, 53.

See also Dysgeusia (above).

EFFECTS ON THE IMMUNE SYSTEM. A hypersensitivity vasculitis characterised by neuromyopathy, periarteriolitis, eosinophilia, and raised concentrations of creatine phosphokinase, antinuclear antibody, and antibodies against gammaglobulin occurred in a man given levodopa therapy for 4 years.— S. Wolf *et al.*, *Archs intern. Med.*, 1976, *136*, 1055.

A lupus-like auto-immune syndrome occurred in a 62-year-old man treated for 2 months with levodopa and benserazide.— G. Massarotti *et al.* (letter), *Br. med. J.*, 1979, *2*, 553.

For references to auto-immune haemolytic anaemia associated with levodopa, see Effects on the Blood, above.

EFFECTS ON KIDNEY FUNCTION. Administration of levodopa 1 to 2 g to 7 patients with idiopathic or postencephalitic Parkinson's disease produced significant increments in renal plasma flow, glomerular filtration-rate, and sodium and potassium excretion. The natriuretic effects could contribute to the orthostatic hypotension commonly noted in patients receiving levodopa.— G. D. Finlay *et al.*, *New Engl. J. Med.*, 1971, *284*, 865.

Confirmation that levodopa has a kaliuretic effect, resulting in hypokalaemia, in some parkinsonian patients. The effect could be prevented by concomitant administration of a peripheral dopa decarboxylase inhibitor.— A. K. Granerus *et al.*, *Acta med. scand.*, 1977, *201*, 291.

EFFECTS ON MENTAL STATE. Psychiatric complications were the single commonest reason for stopping levodopa treatment in a 6-year follow-up study of 178 patients with idiopathic Parkinson's disease. Within 2 years levodopa was withdrawn because of toxic confusional states (21 patients), paranoid psychosis (6), unipolar depression (2), and mania (1). The incidence of visual hallucinations increased as treatment continued but, as with toxic confusional states, patients generally improved when levodopa was withdrawn. Before treatment 40 patients had suffered severe depression and levodopa produced sustained improvement in only 2. After 6 years, 20 of the 81 patients remaining were moderately or severely depressed and were rarely improved by withdrawal or reduction in dosage of levodopa. Increasing dementia affected 26 of the 81 patients after 6 years; withdrawal of levodopa in 5 failed to improve cognitive disabilities, but increased parkinsonism.— K. M. Shaw *et al.*, *Q. J. Med.*, 1980, *49*, 283.

Mental disorders occurred in 141 of 400 patients being treated for Parkinson's disease. Certain acute states, particularly anxiety, on-off hallucinations, and fits of delirium were linked to treatment with levodopa, whereas dementia and depression were not.— P. Rondot *et al.*, *Adv. Neurol.*, 1984, *40*, 259.

Sleep-related complaints were reported by 74 of 100 patients with Parkinson's disease. All 74 were on levodopa and the prevalence of symptoms increased with the duration of treatment. Symptoms included insomnia, excessive daytime somnolence, altered dream phenomena, nocturnal vocalisation, involuntary myoclonic movements, and, rarely, sleep walking. Sleep fragmentation, which includes insomnia and somnolence, was the most common symptom overall. Progression was noted within each symptom category, for example vivid dreaming preceded nightmares and nocturnal terrors and sleep-restricted myoclonus preceded waking myoclonic activity. In an evaluation of cortisol rhythm in parkinsonian patients on chronic levodopa therapy, a strong association between abnormal rhythm and major sleep disruption as well as between abnormal rhythm and hallucinations or psychotic behaviour was found.— P. A. Nausieda *et al.*, *Adv. Neurol.*, 1984, *40*, 271.

See also Effects on Sexual Function (below).

EFFECTS ON RESPIRATION. Respiratory crises, including attacks of gasping, panting, sniffing, puffing, and breath-holding, occurred in 12 of 25 patients with postencephalitic parkinsonism during treatment with levodopa. A further 8 developed respiratory and phonatory tics, including sudden deep breaths, yawns, coughs, giggles, sighing, grunting, and moaning. All 20 patients also suffered tachypnoea, bradypnoea, and asymmetrical movement of both sides of the chest, paradoxical diaphragmatic movements, and reversal of inspiratory and expiratory phases. The induction of respiratory crises may be prompt or greatly delayed; 3 patients only developed crises after more than 9 months of treatment with levodopa. Crises were readily precipitated by psychophysiological arousals such as rage and exertion. Most of the patients who developed marked respiratory disorders had shown slight irregularities of respiratory rhythm, rate, and force before receiving levodopa.— O. W. Sacks *et al.* (letter), *Lancet*, 1970, *1*, 1006.

A distressing dose-related irregularity in the rate and depth of breathing occurred when a patient with Parkinson's disease was given levodopa with benserazide. The respiratory abnormality was completely suppressed by concomitant administration of tiapride, with no reduction in the beneficial effect of levodopa.— J. De Keyser and W. Vincken, *Neurology*, 1985, *35*, 235.

EFFECTS ON SEXUAL FUNCTION. Reports of hypersexuality associated with levodopa: J. J. Korten *et al.* (letter), *J. Am. med. Ass.*, 1973, *226*, 355 (strong hypersexual behaviour and hypergenitalism in a prepubertal boy); H. P. Vogel and R. Schiffter, *Pharmacopsychiatry*, 1983, *16*, 107 (severe hypersexuality in a parkinsonian man on levodopa and bromocriptine; there was evidence of addictive abuse of these drugs).

EFFECTS ON THE SKIN AND HAIR. Two women who were given levodopa, up to 3 g daily, developed diffuse alopecia in addition to nausea, mental agitation, and involuntary choreiform movements.— A. Marshall and M. J. Williams (letter), *Br. med. J.*, 1971, *2*, 47.

Repigmentation of hair occurred in a white-bearded man after being treated with levodopa 1.5 g daily for 8 months.— K. M. Grainger (letter), *Lancet*, 1973, *1*, 97.

See also Melanoma, under Precautions.

EXTRAPYRAMIDAL EFFECTS. A review of problems associated with levodopa in the treatment of Parkinson's disease. With long-term treatment the general tendency is for patients only to tolerate progressively smaller doses at shorter intervals. After 3 to 5 years of therapy 40 to 80% of patients may experience dyskinesias, including chorea, ballism, dystonia, or myoclonus and/or oscillations in motor performance (akinetic 'off-periods'). The periodic re-emergence of akinesia may take various forms, including 'end-of-dose' akinesia ('wearing-off' effect), random 'on-off' oscillations in motor performance, and akinesia paradoxica ('freezing' or 'start hesitation').— M. W. I. M. Horstink, *Clin. Neurol. Neurosurg.*, 1984, *86*, 196.

Choreiform movements were the major dose-limiting complication of long-term treatment with levodopa in a follow-up study of 178 patients with idiopathic Parkinson's disease, 81 of whom were still taking levodopa after 6 years. Dyskinesias usually appeared in the first year and became more severe and generalised with time. Certain distinctive patterns of involuntary movements occurred as follows: peak-dose movements affected 65 of the 81 patients and were dose-related. Movements were usually choreic, affecting the face and limbs, but dystonic and ballistic movements were also seen; characteristically they began 20 to 90 minutes after an oral dose and lasted from 10 minutes to 4 hours with a tendency to be more severe mid-way through the inter-dose period; biphasic movements presenting as 2 distinct episodes of chorea or dystonia within each interdose period occurred in only 3 patients; early morning and 'end-of-dose' dystonia was present in 15 patients after 6 years of treatment with levodopa, but rarely developed during the first 3 years; nocturnal myoclonus occurred in 12 patients. The frequency, intensity, and complexity of spontaneous fluctuations in performance were greatly enhanced by long-term levodopa therapy. Two clinically distinct types of fluctuation, 'end-of-dose' deterioration and the 'on-off' phenomenon, were related to treatment. 'End-of-dose' deterioration or the 'wearing-off' effect affected 52 patients after 6 years of treatment and was characterised by progressive reduction in the duration of benefit from each dose together with a gradual return of nocturnal and early morning disability in some patients. The 'on-off' phenomenon affected 14 patients who experienced completely unpredictable swings from relative mobility, usually accompanied by involuntary movements, to periods of profound bradykinesia and hypotonia. In addition, 'freezing episodes' and abrupt falls became increasingly common and affected 50 patients after 6 years compared to 33 before therapy.— K. M. Shaw *et al.*, *Q. J. Med.*, 1980, *49*, 283.

Oculogyric crisis. After initial remission, oculogyric crises in 5 of 25 patients with postencephalitic parkinsonism recurred and were subsequently severely exacerbated during treatment with levodopa. One patient, who previously had not had oculogyric crises, developed severe crises in the fourth month of therapy with levodopa. During these crises forced gaze deviation was always accompanied by severe neurological and mental symptoms, some of which were scarcely tolerable.— O. W. Sacks and M. Kohl (letter), *Lancet*, 1970, *2*, 215.

GOUT. Three patients treated for parkinsonism with levodopa developed elevated serum concentrations of uric acid, with gout occurring in 2. On cessation of levodopa therapy the serum concentrations returned to normal and did not increase when levodopa 4 g daily was again administered.— H. Honda and R. W. Gindin, *J. Am. med. Ass.*, 1972, *219*, 55. See also D. B. Calne and J. Fermaglich, *Postgrad. med. J.*, 1976, *52*, 232.

OVERDOSAGE. Adverse effects following ingestion of 80 to 100 g of levodopa over a 12-hour period by a parkinsonian patient included hypertension initially, followed by hypotension of a few hours' duration, sinus tachycardia, and symptomatic postural hypotension for more than a week. Marked confusion, agitation, insomnia, and restlessness were the most prominent clinical symptoms and did not disappear completely for over a week; severe anorexia and insomnia persisted for 2 to 3 weeks. After the overdose he had virtually no signs of parkinsonism and received no levodopa or antimuscarinic medication for 6 days; rigidity and akinesia began to recur on the fourth day.— M. M. Hoehn and C. O. Rutledge, *Neurology*, 1975, *25*, 792.

Treatment of Adverse Effects

Reduction in dosage reverses most of the side-effects of levodopa. Nausea and vomiting may be diminished by increasing the dose of levodopa gradually, by taking after meals, and by taking an anti-emetic such as cyclizine hydrochloride or domperidone. Orthostatic hypotension may respond to the use of elastic stockings.

If acute overdosage occurs the stomach should be emptied by aspiration and lavage and supportive measures instituted. If arrhythmias develop anti-arrhythmic therapy may be necessary. Pyridoxine has been given to reverse some effects of levodopa overdosage; it does not reverse the effects of levodopa given in association with a peripheral decarboxylase inhibitor.

EXTRAPYRAMIDAL EFFECTS. Administration of tiapride with levodopa has been reported to reduce levodopa-induced dyskinesias (P. Price *et al.*, *Lancet*, 1978, *2*, 1106), but Lees *et al.* (*ibid.*, 1205) warned of the hazards of irreversibly aggravating parkinsonism and inducing tardive dyskinesias.

See also Effects on Respiration in Adverse Effects (above).

NAUSEA AND VOMITING. For reference to the use of domperidone in the management of nausea and vomiting associated with levodopa in patients with Parkinson's disease, see under Precautions and Uses in Domperidone p.1089 and p.1090.

Precautions

Levodopa is contra-indicated in patients with closed-angle glaucoma. It should be used with caution in patients with cardiovascular disease, diabetes mellitus, psychiatric disturbances, open-angle glaucoma, or a history of gastric or duodenal ulceration. Periodic evaluations of hepatic, haematological, renal, and cardiovascular functions have been advised.

There are recommendations that levodopa should not be given to patients with a history of malignant melanoma nor to patients with the disease

or with skin disorders suggestive of it. However, the association between the use of levodopa and activation of malignant melanoma is only suspected.
Parkinsonian patients who benefit from levodopa therapy should be warned to resume normal activities gradually to avoid the risk of injury. Treatment with levodopa should not be stopped abruptly.
Levodopa inhibits prolactin secretion and may therefore interfere with lactation.
Interactions. The therapeutic or adverse effects of levodopa may be affected by interactions with a variety of drugs. Mechanisms may include effects on catecholamine metabolising enzymes, neurotransmitters, or receptor sites, effects on the endocrine system, and effects on gastro-intestinal absorption (J.R. Bianchine and L. Sunyapridakul, *Drugs*, 1973, *6*, 364). Food interferes with the absorption of levodopa, though it is usually given with or immediately after meals to reduce nausea and vomiting. In addition, drugs which modify gastric emptying may affect the absorption of levodopa.
For beneficial enhancement of the effect of levodopa by the peripheral decarboxylase inhibitors *benserazide* or *carbidopa*, see Uses (below).
Amino acids. Daniel *et al.* (*Lancet*, 1976, *1*, 95) reported that transport of levodopa into the brain is subject to competition from chemically related L-amino acids, especially the other aromatic amino acids *phenylalanine*, *tyrosine*, *tryptophan*, and *histidine*. Later, Nutt *et al.* (*New Engl. J. Med.*, 1984, *310*, 483) demonstrated that a high-protein diet or the large neutral amino acids phenylalanine, *leucine*, or *isoleucine* reduced the therapeutic effect of levodopa given by intravenous infusion to parkinsonian patients and concluded that alterations in the absorption and transport of levodopa may contribute to the fluctuating responses seen in Parkinson's disease, the so-called 'on-off' phenomenon (see also under Absorption and Fate and under Parkinsonism in Uses, below). Other reported interactions with amino acids include: *methionine*-antagonism of the therapeutic effect of levodopa in parkinsonism (L.A. Pearce and L.D. Waterbury, *Neurology*, 1974, *24*, 640); *tryptophan*-reduced blood concentrations of levodopa (W.-U. Weitbrecht and K. Wiegel, *Dt. med. Wschr.*, 1976, *101*, 20).
Antacids. Administration of an antacid reduced the prolonged gastric emptying time of a parkinsonian patient and enhanced the absorption of levodopa (L. Rivera-Calimlim *et al.*, *Br. med. J.*, 1970, *4*, 93) whereas no such effect was found in patients with presumably normal gastric motility (A.S. Leon and H.E. Spiegel, *J. clin. Pharmac.*, 1972, *12*, 263).
Anti-emetics. *Metoclopramide* accelerates gastric emptying and has been reported to increase the rate of levodopa absorption (J.G.L. Morris *et al.*, *Br. J. clin. Pharmac.*, 1976, *3*, 983). Berkowitz and McCallum (*Clin. Pharmac. Ther.*, 1980, *27*, 414) noted the importance of timing since levodopa delayed gastric emptying and metoclopramide antagonised this effect. *Domperidone* has been reported to slightly increase the bioavailability of levodopa (J.S. Shindler *et al.*, *Br. J. clin. Pharmac.*, 1984, *18*, 959).
Antihypertensive agents. Concurrent administration of levodopa with *guanethidine* and other antihypertensive agents may cause increased hypotension. In addition, *clonidine* has been reported to inhibit the therapeutic effect of levodopa, possibly by stimulating central alpha adrenoceptors (I. Shoulson and T.N. Chase, *Neuropharmacology*, 1976, *15*, 25). *Methyldopa* and levodopa may enhance each other's therapeutic or adverse effects, although there has been mention of the inhibitory effect of methyldopa on the therapeutic response to levodopa (G.C. Cotzias *et al.*, *New Engl. J. Med.*, 1969, *281*, 272; O. Kofman, *Can. med. Ass. J.*, 1971, *104*, 483). Methyldopa inhibits the decarboxylation of dopa to dopamine and has been used, similarly to carbidopa, in the treatment of parkinsonism (R.D. Sweet *et al.*, *Clin. Pharmac. Ther.*, 1972, *13*, 23; J. Fermaglich and T.N. Chase, *Lancet*, 1973, *1*, 1261).
Antimuscarinic agents. Antimuscarinic antiparkinsonian agents may enhance the therapeutic effects of levodopa, but by delaying gastric emptying they may reduce its absorption.
Central stimulants. Amphetamine may enhance the effects of levodopa.
Isoniazid. A hypertensive reaction and severe tremor occurred when isoniazid was given to a patient receiving levodopa (J.P. Morgan, *Ann. intern. Med.*, 1980, *92*, 434); it was not certain whether isoniazid was acting as a monoamine oxidase inhibitor.
Monoamine oxidase inhibitors. Administration of levodopa with non-specific monoamine oxidase inhibitors may cause dangerous hypertension; it is suggested that levodopa should not be given within at least 14 days of stopping a monoamine oxidase inhibitor. Teychenne *et al.* (*Clin. Pharmac. Ther.*, 1975, *18*, 273) found that hypertensive reactions to levodopa in association with the monoamine oxidase inhibitor *tranylcypromine* were inhibited by carbidopa, but the manufacturers of preparations containing levodopa with carbidopa or benserazide still contra-indicate the concomitant use of monoamine oxidase inhibitors. For beneficial enhancement of the antiparkinsonian effect of levodopa by a specific monoamine oxidase type B inhibitor, see Selegiline Hydrochloride, p.1022.
Pyridoxine. The enzyme responsible for the decarboxylation of levodopa, L-amino acid decarboxylase is dependent on pyridoxine and pyridoxine supplements have been reported to enhance the peripheral metabolism of levodopa to dopamine leaving less available to cross the blood-brain barrier for central conversion to dopamine; pyridoxine therefore inhibits the action of levodopa but this can be stopped by concurrent administration of a peripheral decarboxylase inhibitor.
Sympathomimetics and general anaesthetics. Sympathomimetic agents such as *adrenaline* or *isoprenaline* may enhance the cardiac side-effects of levodopa. The general anaesthetics *cyclopropane* and *halothane* lower the threshold for ventricular arrhythmias to sympathomimetic amines, including dopamine, and should probably not be used within 6 hours of the administration of levodopa (L.I. Goldberg and T.L. Whitsett, *Clin. Pharmac. Ther.*, 1971, *12*, 376). However, it has been suggested that levodopa can safely be taken before surgery when given with a decarboxylase inhibitor (*Drug & Ther. Bull.*, 1984, *22*, 73).
Tranquillisers. The therapeutic effects of levodopa may be diminished by drugs acting as dopamine inhibitors in the CNS including phenothiazine derivatives such as *chlorpromazine*, butyrophenones such as *haloperidol*, thioxanthenes such as *flupenthixol*, and by *reserpine* or *tetrabenazine*.

Tricyclic antidepressants. Although tricyclic antidepressants have been used safely with levodopa (K.R. Hunter *et al.*, *Lancet*, 1970 *2*, 1283), hypertensive crises have occurred in patients receiving *amitriptyline* or *imipramine* and levodopa with carbidopa (D.S. Rampton, *Br. med. J.*, 1977, *2*, 607— the patient was also on metoclopramide; M. Edwards, *Practitioner*, 1982, *226*, 1447). Imipramine has been reported to impair the rate of levodopa absorption (J.P. Morgan *et al.*, *Neurology*, 1975, *25*, 1029).
Miscellaneous. Other drugs reported to diminish the therapeutic effect of levodopa include: the benzodiazepines, *chlordiazepoxide* (S. Yosselson-Superstine and A.G. Lipman, *Ann. intern. Med.*, 1982, *96*, 259) and *diazepam* (K.R. Hunter *et al.*, *Lancet*, 1970, *2*, 1283; J. Wodak *et al.*, *Med. J. Aust.*, 1972, *2*, 1277); *papaverine* (R.C. Duvoisin, *J. Am. med. Ass.*, 1975, *231*, 845; D.M. Posner, *ibid.*, *233*, 768); *phenylbutazone* (J. Wodak *et al.*, *Med. J. Aust.*, 1972, *2*, 1277); and *phenytoin* (J.S. Mendez *et al.*, *Archs Neurol., Chicago*, 1975, *32*, 44).
Other drugs reported to enhance the effects of levodopa include: *melanostatin* (A. Barbeau, *Lancet*, 1975, *2*, 683).
Interference with diagnostic tests. Depending on the methods used, levodopa may interfere chemically with several diagnostic laboratory tests including those for glucose, ketone bodies, or catecholamines in urine and for glucose or uric acid in blood. Levodopa therapy has been reported to inhibit the response to protirelin in tests of thyroid function.

ADMINISTRATION IN CARDIOVASCULAR DISORDERS. A high incidence of cardiovascular side-effects was reported in early studies of levodopa. However, Jenkins *et al.* (*Br. med. J.*, 1972, *3*, 512) noted that both Parkinson's disease and heart disease are common in the elderly and that adverse cardiac effects of levodopa are less prevalent than was first thought. From a study in 40 patients they concluded that, apart from those with severe postural hypotension or unstable coronary disease, levodopa may be used safely in parkinsonian patients with heart disease. They recommended in-patient monitoring at the start of therapy and the use of anti-arrhythmic agents when necessary. Parkes *et al.* (*Lancet*, 1977, *1*, 904) also considered that levodopa therapy should not be witheld from parkinsonian patients who also have heart disease. They noted that levodopa and bromocriptine cause cardiac arrhythmias in less than 1% of all patients, the incidence for levodopa in association with a decarboxylase inhibitor being lower still, and that increased mobility in treated parkinsonian patients may have been indirectly responsible for signs of ischaemic heart disease.

MELANOMA. There has been concern over the effects of levodopa on melanoma in view of the ability of malignant melanoma cells to convert levodopa to melanin and reports of patients with a history of melanoma experiencing exacerbation of their disease after starting levodopa therapy. However, in a survey of 1099 patients with primary cutaneous malignant melanoma only one had taken levodopa. It was concluded that levodopa therapy is not an important factor in the induction of malignant melanoma.— A. J. Sober and M. M. Wick, *J. Am. med. Ass.*, 1978, *240*, 554.

PREGNANCY AND THE NEONATE. Information from the manufacturers suggests that levodopa alone and with carbidopa has been associated with foetal abnormalities in *animals* given high doses, whereas no teratogenic effect has been noted with carbidopa alone. However, 2 women with parkinsonism who received levodopa with carbidopa or levodopa alone throughout their pregnancies gave birth to normal infants.— D. G. Cook and H. L. Klawans, *Clin. Neuropharmacol.*, 1985, *8*, 93.

WITHDRAWAL. A syndrome similar to the neuroleptic malignant syndrome and characterised by fever, muscle rigidity, profuse diaphoresis, tachycardia, tachypnoea, and muscle enzyme level elevations occurred in 3 patients with Parkinson's disease on withdrawal of levodopa therapy. None of the patients had been exposed to neuroleptics.— J. H. Friedman *et al.*, *J. Am. med. Ass.*, 1985, *254*, 2792. Similar reports: G. Sechi *et al.*, *Neurology*, 1984, *34*, 249; L. Figà-Talamanca *et al.*, *ibid.*, 1985, *35*, 258; W. R. G. Gibb and D. N. W. Griffith, *Postgrad. med. J.*, 1986, *62*, 59.

Absorption and Fate
Levodopa is absorbed from the gastro-intestinal tract, principally from the small intestine, and only a small amount is excreted unchanged in the faeces. It is rapidly decarboxylated to dopamine and about 80% is excreted in the urine within 24 hours of an oral dose, mainly as the dopamine metabolites dihydroxyphenylacetic acid (DOPAC) and homovanillic acid (HVA). Some levodopa is also metabolised to 3-*O*-methyldopa and noradrenaline. Levodopa is actively transported across the blood-brain barrier, but because of extensive peripheral decarboxylation very little is available to enter the central nervous system unless it is given in association with a peripheral decarboxylase inhibitor (see Uses, below).

The pharmacokinetics of levodopa are of special importance since the drug has several unique features: it has a very short plasma half-life because of its rapid metabolism, it is transported across membranes by a saturable carrier system rather than by simple diffusion, and the clinical status of many parkinsonian patients appears to become critically dependent on brain concentrations of levodopa.

Decarboxylation, *O*-methylation, transamination, and oxidation are the major pathways for levodopa metabolism. Decarboxylation to dopamine by aromatic amino acid decarboxylase [peripheral dopa decarboxylase] in the gut, liver, and kidney is the principal metabolic pathway and 69% of urinary levodopa metabolites appear as dopamine and its metabolites. The major end-products are homovanillic acid (HVA) and dihydroxyphenylacetic acid (DOPAC); 5% or less of the dopamine is hydroxylated to noradrenaline and then metabolised to vanillinemandelic acid (VMA). Methoxylation to 3-*O*-methyldopa by catechol-*O*-methyltransferase in liver and other tissues also occurs and since 3-*O*-methyldopa has a 15-hour plasma half-life it will accumulate during chronic treatment. Urinary end-products of transamination by tyrosine aminotransferase are vanillpyruvate, vanillactate, and trihydroxyphenylacetic acid. There is no direct evidence for oxidation of levodopa in humans, but the appearance of cysteinyldopa in the urine of parkinsonian patients suggests that oxidation, with a dopa quinone intermediate, does occur. Several of these metabolic pathways have the potential for producing toxic metabolites, but the relevance of this to the long-term complications associated with levodopa therapy is not known.

Levodopa is almost completely absorbed from the gut, only 2% appearing in the faeces. Absorption, as judged by peak plasma concentrations following oral levodopa, shows marked interpatient, and to a lesser extent intrapatient, variability some of which may be related to timing and content of meals and the administration of antacids or antimuscarinic agents. The non-linear relationship between dose and plasma concentrations means that minor changes in levodopa dosage can have a profound effect on therapeutic response. The stomach has a very limited capacity to absorb levodopa, although it can decarboxylate the drug, and most absorption appears to take place in the proximal small bowel. Excessive gastric acidity, meals, antimuscarinics, and dopaminergics can delay gastric emptying and may reduce levodopa absorption, whereas the dopamine antagonist metoclopramide enhances gastric emptying and has been reported to increase bioavailability [See also Interactions in Precautions, above]. However, Evans *et al.* (*Neurology*, 1981, *31*, 1288) found that although elderly controls and elderly parkinsonian patients had much slower gastric emptying than young controls, the absorption of levodopa was not significantly slowed.

Intact levodopa crosses biological membranes by the saturable transport system for aromatic and branched-chain amino acids and is therefore in competition with them. Levodopa has not been detected in plasma following rectal administration, presumably because the rectal mucosa has no amino-acid transport system. The abundant aromatic amino acid decarboxylase activity in the gastric and intestinal walls is a significant barrier to levodopa absorption. Although the liver has high decarboxylase concentrations and rapidly metabolises levodopa it appears to be a less important site than the gut; metabolism in the intestine is important even after the drug reaches the general circulation. Without concomitant carbidopa only about 30% of a dose of levodopa reaches the circulation intact whereas this is doubled or trebled in the presence of a decarboxylase inhibitor. It has been suggested that altered absorption or peripheral metabolism of levodopa underlies the difference between fluctuating and stable responders to levodopa. Decarboxylase inhibitors have not reduced the incidence or severity of fluctuations, but stabilisation of plasma concentrations by constant intravenous infusion of levodopa has produced a stable clinical response (J.G. Nutt *et al.*, *New Engl. J. Med.*, 1984, *310*, 483).

Evans *et al.* (*Eur. J. clin. Pharmac.*, 1980, *17*, 215; *Neurology*, 1981, *31*, 1288) reported increased absorption of levodopa in elderly healthy subjects or parkinsonian patients when compared with young healthy subjects. This could be explained on the basis of reduced intestinal decarboxylase activity in the elderly, but has not been proved. Evidence for more rapid and complete absorption of levodopa after chronic treatment is conflicting.

Levodopa is transported across the blood-brain barrier in competition with other amino acids; as plasma concentrations fall there is a net flux from brain to blood. It is not bound to plasma proteins to any extent. Plasma concentrations of levodopa are a poor predictor of brain concentrations and complete correlation of plasma concentrations with clinical response has not been found. The levodopa metabolite 3-*O*-methyldopa has a greater affinity for the transport system than does levodopa and the plasma concentrations of 3-*O*-methyldopa achieved during chronic therapy could interfere with transport at the blood-brain barrier.

Levodopa is cleared quickly from plasma. Reported half-lives following oral administration range from 0.77 to 1.08 hours and 70 to 80% of a dose appears in the urine within 24 hours, largely as dopamine metabolites. Concomitant administration of decarboxylase inhibitors has reduced the dose required for a therapeutic response by 60 to 80%, but plasma half-life is only modestly prolonged or unchanged and a reduction in the frequency of levodopa administration is not possible. The metabolic profile of levodopa is altered by these inhibitors: less of an administered dose is metabolised to homovanillic acid and dihydroxyphenylacetic acid and there is an absolute increase in the amount of vanillactic acid and a relative increase in the amount of 3-*O*-methyldopa.

Thus, the pharmacokinetics of levodopa are intricate and their ramifications may be critical to a patient's clinical response to levodopa. It remains to be seen whether some of the adverse effects, especially the fluctuating response ('on-off' phenomenon) can be attributed to the pharmacokinetic behaviour of the drug.— J. G. Nutt and J. H. Fellman, *Clin. Neuropharmacol.*, 1984, *7*, 35.

A review of the clinical pharmacokinetics of antiparkinsonian agents.— J. M. Cedarbaum, *Clin. Pharmacokinet.*, 1987, *13*, 141.

Uses and Administration

Levodopa, a naturally occurring amino acid, is the immediate precursor of the neurotransmitter dopamine. The actions of levodopa are mainly those of dopamine (p.1460).

Unlike dopamine, levodopa readily enters the central nervous system and is used in the treatment of conditions, such as Parkinson's disease, which are associated with depletion of dopamine in the brain. However, high doses are necessary since levodopa is so rapidly decarboxylated that very little unchanged drug is available to cross the blood-brain barrier for central conversion into dopamine. Consequently levodopa is usually given together with a peripheral decarboxylase inhibitor such as benserazide (p.1010) or carbidopa (p.1014) thus permitting a considerably higher proportion of levodopa to enter the brain. This enables the dosage of levodopa to be reduced and may diminish peripheral side-effects, such as nausea and vomiting and cardiac arrhythmias, by blocking the peripheral production of dopamine. It may also provide a more rapid response at the start of therapy.

The majority of patients with Parkinson's disease are benefited by levodopa, but after 2 or more years improvement in disability is gradually lost as the disease progresses and fluctuations in mobility emerge. Postencephalitic parkinsonism responds to levodopa, but a higher incidence of side-effects has been reported than in the idiopathic form and smaller doses are generally used. Levodopa has also been used to control the neurological symptoms of chronic manganese poisoning, which resemble those of parkinsonism. It is not generally considered beneficial in drug-induced parkinsonism.

Levodopa has an effect on pituitary function as a result of its conversion to dopamine. It may enhance growth-hormone secretion and is used diagnostically as a provocative test for growth-hormone deficiency. Levodopa also inhibits prolactin secretion and has been used in disorders associated with hyperprolactinaemia, although dopamine agonists such as bromocriptine are generally preferred.

Response to levodopa varies considerably between patients. Treatment of parkinsonism should commence with small doses increased gradually, ideally to a dose which improves mobility without incurring side-effects. Levodopa should be taken after meals. When given without a peripheral decarboxylase inhibitor a suggested initial dose is 125 mg twice daily by mouth increased gradually every few days, according to response, to a dose within the range of 1 to 8 g daily in divided doses; maximum improvement may take up to 6 months or longer to occur. The intervals between doses should be adjusted to meet individual needs; many patients find 4 or 5 divided doses daily to be satisfactory although some may require smaller more frequent doses in order to control fluctuations in mobility.

When given *with a peripheral decarboxylase inhibitor* lower doses of levodopa are employed. Both beneficial and adverse effects tend to occur more rapidly than with levodopa alone and patients should be monitored carefully. In those already receiving levodopa the drug should be discontinued and benserazide or carbidopa with levodopa started on the following day. *Benserazide hydrochloride* is usually given with levodopa in the ratio of 1 part of benserazide base to 4 parts of levodopa. The suggested initial dose is benserazide 25 mg with levodopa 100 mg twice daily by mouth increased gradually, according to response, to a maintenance dose usually within the range of benserazide 100 to 200 mg with levodopa 400 to 800 mg daily in divided doses. It is rarely necessary to exceed benserazide 250 mg and levodopa 1 g daily. The initial dose of levodopa given with benserazide should be about 15% of the dose previously being taken, thus benserazide 150 mg with levodopa 600 mg would be appropriate for a patient previously taking levodopa 4 g daily.

Full inhibition of peripheral dopa decarboxylase is reported to be achieved by 70 to 100 mg of *carbidopa* daily and a dose of at least 75 mg daily has been recommended. Tablets of carbidopa with levodopa are available in the ratio of 1 to 4 and 1 to 10 which allows dosage adjustments of either drug for individual patients. Doses of carbidopa are expressed in terms of the anhydrous base. A suggested initial dose is carbidopa 25 mg with levodopa 100 mg three times daily by mouth, increased gradually as necessary. The usual maintenance dosage range is carbidopa 75 to 150 mg with levodopa 0.75 to 1.5 g daily in divided doses. Carbidopa doses greater than 200 mg daily are not generally exceeded. The initial dose of levodopa given with carbidopa should be about 20% of the dose previously being taken, thus carbidopa 75 mg with levodopa 750 mg would be appropriate for a patient previously taking levodopa 4 g daily.

ADMINISTRATION IN RENAL FAILURE. Levodopa or levodopa with carbidopa can be given in usual doses to patients with renal failure.— W. M. Bennett *et al.*, *Am. J. Kidney Dis.*, 1983, *3*, 155.

CARDIOVASCULAR DISORDERS. Levodopa is converted *in vivo* to the positive inotropic agent dopamine. Haemodynamic effects resembling those following the intravenous administration of dopamine were seen following the administration of single oral doses of levodopa 1.5 or 2 g to 10 patients with severe chronic congestive heart failure. A sustained improvement in cardiac function was achieved when 5 of these patients were given levodopa 1.5 or 2 g every 6 hours by mouth together with pyridoxine hydrochloride 50 mg daily for 3 to 12 months in addition to their prestudy dosages of digoxin, diuretics, and anti-arrhythmic agents. There was no evidence of serious adverse effects.— S. I. Rajfer *et al.*, *New Engl. J. Med.*, 1984, *310*, 1357. Comment that, since dopamine generated from the peripheral decarboxylation of levodopa is probably responsible for the beneficial haemodynamic responses observed, levodopa would not be expected to improve cardiac performance when given with carbidopa. The investigational nature of levodopa in the treatment of heart failure was also emphasised.— S. I. Rajfer (letter), *ibid.*, *311*, 672.

See also Administration in Cardiovascular Disorders in Precautions (above).

CHOREA. In a discussion on basal ganglia disease, Marsden (*Lancet*, 1982, *2*, 1141) noted that, unlike Parkinson's disease, the striatal concentration of dopamine is increased in Huntington's disease and there is probably a net overactivity of stimulation of the residual dopamine receptors; in a minority of patients with the akinetic-rigid variant striatal dopamine content tends to be lower than normal. Thus, levodopa usually exacerbates Huntington's disease. However, improvement in choreic movements and psychiatric symptoms has followed levodopa therapy in patients with reduced concentrations of homovanillic acid in the cerebrospinal fluid suggestive of reduced dopamine metabolism (C. Loeb *et al.*, *J. Neurol. Neurosurg. Psychiat.*, 1976, *39*, 958) and symptomatic relief with levodopa has also been reported in the juvenile form of Huntington's disease (the Westphal variant) (D. Krishnappa, *Med. J. Aust.*, 1984, *140*, 32). This variant is characterised by rigidity, akinesia, and dysarthria rather than by choreoathetosis.

Presymptomatic diagnosis. Levodopa has been administered as a presymptomatic provocative test to identify those at risk of developing Huntington's disease (H.L. Klawans *et al.*, *New Engl. J. Med.*, 1980, *302*, 1090). However, false-negative results have been reported (R.H. Myers *et al.*, *ibid.*, 1982, *307*, 561) and it was concluded that the levodopa challenge is not valid as a predictor of the carriers of the gene for Huntington's disease and should be abandoned.

EXTRAPYRAMIDAL DISORDERS. Dystonia implies an abnormal position or posture, but is usually taken to mean an abnormal movement or dyskinesia in a group with tremor, chorea, myoclonus, and tic. Dystonias are rare, the commonest cause perhaps being drug therapy and including an acute dystonic reaction to phenothiazines, butyrophenones, or metoclopramide; dystonia associated with levodopa therapy of Parkinson's disease; and chronic tardive dystonia or dyskinesia associated with neuroleptic therapy. Primary dystonias are either generalised, also called dystonia musculorum deformans and usually beginning in childhood, or focal, usually beginning in adult life and including spasmodic torticollis, writer's cramp, oromandibular dystonia, and blepharospasm. Treatment is generally disappointing. Many drugs, including levodopa and lysuride maleate, have been tried in the primary dystonias and although there may be benefit in a small proportion of patients the results are unpredictable.— *Lancet*, 1985, *1*, 321.

Beneficial results with levodopa in the treatment of the extrapyramidal manifestations of various diseases: *phenylketonuria*: K. Bartholomé and D. J. Byrd (letter), *Lancet*, 1975, *2*, 1042; M. D. Macleod *et al.*, *Archs Dis. Childh.*, 1983, *58*, 457. *subacute sclerosing panencephalitis*: B. Halikowiski and M. Piotropawlowska-Weinert (letter), *Lancet*, 1977, *2*, 1033.

See also Chorea, Manganese Poisoning, and Parkinsonism.

Drug-induced extrapyramidal disorders. Neuroleptic drugs can produce a range of extrapyramidal side-effects including drug-induced parkinsonism and the dyskinesias akathisia, acute dystonic reactions, and chronic tardive dyskinesias. Parkinsonism induced by neuroleptics resembles idiopathic Parkinson's disease and similarly is due to dopamine deficiency in the brain. Reserpine and tetrabenazine act presynaptically by preventing dopamine storage whereas the phenothiazine, thioxanthene, butyrophenone, and substituted benzamide classes of neuroleptic drugs act postsynaptically by blocking dopamine receptors in the brain. It is generally reversible on withdrawal of the offending drugs and may sometimes gradually disappear despite continued drug therapy. Although the use of dopamine agonists, especially levodopa, to overcome neuroleptic-induced blockade of dopamine receptors might appear rational, levodopa has generally been reported to be ineffective or to increase psychiatric symptoms and the mainstay of drug treatment has been antimuscarinic agents. There have however been reports suggesting that relatively low doses of levodopa can reverse neuroleptic-induced parkinsonism without serious psychiatric complications. Experience with other dopamine agonists is limited. The drug treatment of akathisia, acute dystonic reactions, and chronic tardive dyskinesias is difficult and the underlying pathophysiology obscure. Tardive dyskinesias are the most serious of these neuroleptic-induced disorders and therapy has been based on the hypothesis that they are due to overactivity of dopaminergic transmission within the brain. Nevertheless treatment with low doses of dopamine agonists has been tried, the theory being that they may act preferentially at presynaptic dopamine receptors and thereby prevent synthesis and release of endogenous dopamine. Apomorphine has been reported to be of limited benefit. Worsening of tardive dyskinesia has been reported with levodopa although improvement has been claimed with low doses. Levodopa has also been tried in high doses in an attempt to decrease the sensitivity of supposedly overactive postsynaptic dopamine receptors and improvement has been reported although initially the tardive dyskinesia is exacerbated. Results with bromocriptine have also been conflicting.— P. Jenner and C. D. Marsden, Antiparkinsonian and Antidyskinetic Drugs in *Drugs in Psychiatric Practice*, P.J. Tyrer (Ed.), London, Butterworths, 1982, p.82.

For a review of the role of antimuscarinic agents in the treatment of drug-induced extrapyramidal disorders, see p.522.

HEPATIC ENCEPHALOPATHY. Temporary arousal from acute hepatic coma has been reported in patients given levodopa (J.D. Parkes *et al.*, *Lancet*, 1970, *2*, 1341; J.E. Fischer and R.J. Baldessarini, *ibid.*, 1971, *2*, 75) and has been attributed to a central effect of its derivative dopamine. Fischer and Baldessarini postulated that accumulation of false neurotransmitters might contribute to the aetiology of hepatic coma. However, from work in *rats* Zieve *et al.* (*Gut*, 1979, *20*, 28) concluded that the beneficial effect of levodopa could be accounted for by a peripheral effect of dopamine on renal function, the excretion of ammonia being increased. There have been differing results from controlled studies of levodopa in chronic hepatic encephalopathy. Lunzer *et al.* (*Gut*, 1974, *15*, 555) reported improvement in 3 of 6 patients resistant to conventional therapy when they were given levodopa in a mean dose of 2.1 g daily, whereas Michel *et al.* (*Gastroenterology*, 1980, *79*, 207) found levodopa, with or without a decarboxylase inhibitor, to be no better than placebo in a study involving 75 patients. Measurement of urinary metabolites indicated that levodopa had not been absorbed by a patient with hepatic coma who failed to respond to the drug (G.M. Tyce *et al.*, *Clin. Pharmac. Ther.*, 1983, *34*, 390).

MANGANESE POISONING. Neurological signs and symptoms of chronic manganese poisoning were relieved or abolished in 7 of 8 patients by levodopa, given initially in a dose of 100 mg six times daily, slowly increased to an optimal dose of up to 8 g daily. Rigidity, hypotonia, and postural reflex disturbances were mainly affected. In 1 patient weakness, hypotonia, tremor, and hypokinesia were aggravated. This patient responded to treatment with DL-5-hydroxytryptophan, up to 3 g daily.— I. Mena *et al.*, *New Engl. J. Med.*, 1970, *282*, 5.

MENTAL DISORDERS. Pathological laughing and/or crying was controlled completely by levodopa 0.6 to 1.5 g daily in 10 of 25 patients with cerebrovascular disease or brain trauma. Amantadine hydrochloride 100 mg daily was also beneficial.— F. Udaka *et al.*, *Archs Neurol., Chicago*, 1984, *41*, 1095.

Dementia. Lewis *et al.* (*Br. med. J.*, 1978, *1*, 550) reported improvement in intellectual function, but not in other areas of behaviour, in patients with senile dementia given levodopa 875 mg daily. At follow-up (K. Johnson *et al.*, *ibid.*, 1625) the small gains made in intellectual performance appeared to be maintained but were of questionable clinical relevance and Hollister (*Drugs*, 1985, *29*, 483) in a review of Alzheimer's disease noted that clinical trials with levodopa in senile brain disease have not been encouraging. Dementia is said to be present in at least a third of patients with Parkinson's disease and the mental state of some of these patients may be indistinguishable from that seen in Alzheimer's disease (A.E. Lang and R.D.G. Blair, *Can. med. Ass. J.*, 1984, *131*, 1031). There is no evidence that levodopa improves symptoms of dementia in patients with Parkinson's disease.

See also Effects on Mental State in Adverse Effects (above).

Depression. Earlier reports of some benefit with levodopa in the treatment of depression were not confirmed by a double-blind controlled study in depressed patients given levodopa in doses of up to 8 g daily.— J. Mendels *et al.*, *Archs gen. Psychiat.*, 1975, *32*, 22.

Depression is common in Parkinson's disease and although it is lifted in some patients when they start levodopa therapy, this is not the case in most patients.— N. P. Quinn, *Drugs*, 1984, *28*, 236.

See also Effects on Mental State in Adverse Effects (above).

NEUROLEPTIC MALIGNANT SYNDROME. A report of the successful use of levodopa in the treatment of the neuroleptic malignant syndrome.— W. Knezevic *et al.*, *Med. J. Aust.*, 1984, *140*, 28.

PAIN. Levodopa 100 mg with benserazide 25 mg given three times daily for 10 days relieved herpes zoster pain when compared with placebo in a double-blind study in 47 patients. Treatment was started within 5 days of the onset of eruptions.— S. Kernbaum and J. Hauchecorne, *J. Am. med. Ass.*, 1981, *246*, 132.

Brief reports of beneficial results with levodopa together with a peripheral decarboxylase inhibitor in the treatment of the thalamic pain syndrome.— R. J. Plasencia *et al.*, *Neurology*, 1984, *34*, *Suppl.* 1, 137; R. Grant and P. O. Behan, *Br. med. J.*, 1984, *289*, 1272.

Contrary to earlier reports of pain relief with levodopa in patients with bone metastases of various malignant diseases (R.P. Dickey and J.P. Minton, *New Engl. J. Med.*, 1972, *286*, 843; J.P. Minton, *Cancer*, 1974, *33*, 358; D.W. Nixon, *New Engl. J. Med.*, 1975, *292*, 1196; M.D. Altschule and Z.L. Hegedus, *ibid.*, 1196), an analgesic effect could not be confirmed in a pilot study involving 14 patients given levodopa 100 mg with carbidopa 25 mg every 4 hours.— S. U. Sjølin and H. Trykker (letter), *New Engl. J. Med.*, 1985, *312*, 650.

PARKINSONISM. The syndrome of parkinsonism is characterised by tremor, rigidity, akinesia, and loss of postural reflexes. It may be classified into primary or idiopathic parkinsonism, usually referred to as Parkinson's disease (formerly paralysis agitans); secondary parkinsonism, including postencephalitic parkinsonism, drug-induced parkinsonism, and symptoms associated with manganese poisoning; and 'parkinsonism-plus' syndromes where parkinsonism is a feature of other degenerative diseases of the central nervous system, such as progressive supranuclear palsy and the Shy-Drager syndrome. 'Arteriosclerotic parkinsonism' has been used to describe parkinsonism associated with cerebrovascular disease although this may be confusing since vascular brain damage is not a cause of Parkinson's disease. The term parkinsonism is often used for the idiopathic form, that is, Parkinson's disease.

In parkinsonism there is reduced dopamine activity in the brain. Parkinson's disease and postencephalitic parkinsonism have been attributed primarily to depletion of striatal dopamine in the basal ganglia as a result of the loss of neurones in the substantia nigra. Striatal dopamine deficiency results in loss of the normal functional balance between dopaminergic and cholinergic activity and treatment aims to increase the former or decrease the latter. Dopaminergic activity may be enhanced by the dopamine precursor levodopa or direct-acting dopamine agonists such as bromocriptine which appear to act by stimulating dopamine D_2 receptors. Cholinergic activity may be reduced by antimuscarinic drugs (formerly termed anticholinergic drugs). There is evidence for the involvement of other neurotransmitters such as noradrenaline. Levodopa is also the precursor of noradrenaline and both dopamine and noradrenaline may contribute to its therapeutic effect.

The cause of Parkinson's disease is not established although environmental and genetic factors superimposed on a background of neuronal loss related to normal ageing has been postulated (D.B. Calne and J.W. Langston, *Lancet*, 1983, *2*, 1457; A. Barbeau *et al.*, *ibid.*, 1985, *2*, 1213). Great interest was aroused by the discovery that ingestion of MPTP (1-methyl-4-phenyl-1,2,5,6-tetrahydropyridine), a contaminant of an illicitly produced pethidine analogue MPPP (1-methyl-4-phenyl-4-propionoxypiperidine), caused irreversible parkinsonism with pathology similar to that of Parkinson's disease and responding to treatment with levodopa (J.W. Langston *et al.*, *Science*, 1983, *219*, 979).

In drug-induced parkinsonism neuroleptic drugs such as the phenothiazines and butyrophenones block postsynaptic dopamine receptors in the striatum and treatment with levodopa is not generally considered effective (but see also under Drug-induced Extrapyramidal Disorders). Levodopa or dopamine agonists are not usually effective in 'parkinsonism-plus' syndromes.

There have been numerous reviews and discussions on Parkinson's disease and its treatment (C.D. Marsden, *Lancet*, 1982, *2*, 1141; N.P. Quinn, *Drugs*, 1984, *28*, 236; D.B. Calne, *New Engl. J. Med.*, 1984, *310*, 523; A.E. Lang and R.D.G. Blair, *Can. med. Ass. J.*, 1984, *131*, 1031; *Drug & Ther. Bull.*, 1984, *22*, 37; J.M.S. Pearce, *Br. med. J.*, 1984, *288*, 1777; *Lancet*, 1984, *1*, 829; R. Hardie, *Br. J. Hosp. Med.*, 1985, *33*, 45; M.J. Eadie, *Med. J. Aust.*, 1985, *142*, 113; J.G.L. Morris, *ibid.*, *143*, 347; *Med. Lett.*, 1986, *28*, 62). The majority of patients respond initially to levodopa and its use has improved the quality and duration of life. However, long-term studies with relatively high doses showed that after 2 or 3 years benefit was reduced as the disease progressed and late complications emerged (C.D. Marsden and J.D. Parkes, *Lancet*, 1977, *1*, 345; K.M. Shaw *et al.*, *Q. J. Med.*, 1980, *49*, 283). Apart from dyskinesias and psychiatric effects (see Adverse Effects, above) a major problem with long-term levodopa treatment is the appearance of fluctuations in mobility, the two predominant forms being 'end-of-dose' deterioration ('wearing-off' effect) and the 'on-off' phenomenon. Thus, although it is generally agreed that levodopa, given with a peripheral decarboxylase inhibitor such as carbidopa or benserazide, is currently the most effective treatment for Parkinson's disease, views differ as to the best time to start treatment and the dosage to employ in order to limit the long-term complications. Those who consider that these long-term effects reflect severity of the disease favour the early use of levodopa, whereas those implicating cumulative exposure to levodopa advocate later use. In practice, treatment is generally started with antimuscarinic agents and/or amantadine while symptoms are relatively mild and levodopa substituted or added as soon as functional disability becomes a problem, usually within 2 or 3 years. Antimuscarinic agents should generally be avoided in elderly patients and levodopa used from the start. In the early days of therapy with levodopa, the dose was usually increased progressively to the maximum tolerated dose and many patients received what might now be considered excessive amounts. The usual practice nowadays is to start with small doses of levodopa, together with a peripheral decarboxylase inhibitor, and increase slowly to a dose which reduces disability to an acceptable level. Variations in response and diminishing effectiveness over the years necessitate careful monitoring of dosage; small relatively frequent doses are preferable to occasional large ones.

Fluctuations in mobility have been reported in more than half of patients on levodopa after 5 years of therapy. They generally proceed through predictable 'end-of-dose' deterioration, necessitating administration of the daily dose in smaller more frequent doses, to the 'on-off' phenomenon with marked very sudden swings from mobility to immobility. The cause of the fluctuations is not known, but multiple factors including desensitisation of dopamine receptors, interference with the response to dopamine by other levodopa metabolites such as 3-*O*-methyldopa, and fluctuating plasma concentrations have been suggested (See also Absorption and Fate, above). Various attempts have been made to overcome the 'on-off' phenomenon. Those speculating that long-term treatment results in altered dopamine receptor sensitivity have advocated controlled withdrawal of levodopa for periods of 7 to 10 days. However, these 'drug holidays' should not be undertaken lightly since deterioration may be dramatic when levodopa is stopped. Any benefit is often transitory and readjustment of dosage rather than complete withdrawal may be more helpful. Dopamine agonists should be effective despite altered receptor responsiveness and some patients do appear to benefit from the concomitant use of bromocriptine (see p.1011) or pergolide (see p.1021). Others have linked the 'on-off' phenomenon to variable plasma concentrations although, since transfer of levodopa into the brain involves active transport mechanisms, concentrations in plasma may not necessarily reflect those in the brain. Slow-release preparations of levodopa have been of no benefit so far, but continuous intravenous infusion of levodopa has been shown to reduce fluctuations in mobility (J.G. Nutt *et al., New Engl. J. Med.*, 1984, *310*, 483) which suggests that dopamine receptors are still sensitive. Intravenous or subcutaneous infusions of the dopamine agonist lysuride below have also been given as has subcutaneous apomorphine (p.1009). Concomitant administration of selegiline (p.1021), a monoamine oxidase type B inhibitor, prolongs the action of levodopa by inhibiting dopamine metabolism and some patients may benefit, especially those with 'end-of-dose' deterioration.

According to Quinn *et al.* (*Lancet*, 1986, *1*, 1366) the severe pain and dystonia suffered by some patients with Parkinson's disease may occur within a certain threshold of dopaminergic stimulation and in all cases is due to the disease or its therapy. They consider that, despite suggestions that these pains could be caused by levodopa or its metabolites, measures to increase 'on' periods will reduce or eliminate pain in most patients. Such measures usually entail increasing the frequency and sometimes the dose of levodopa, often with addition of, or replacement by, longer-acting ergot drugs. Quinn and Marsden (*ibid.*, 1377) have also reported beneficial results with lithium carbonate in patients with painful dystonia; they suggested it might be helpful in those with 'off' period dystonias unresponsive to other treatment.

PITUITARY AND HYPOTHALAMIC DISORDERS. *Diagnosis and testing.* Diminished growth-hormone reserve is one of the earliest functional abnormalities in anterior pituitary failure and, since dopamine is believed to stimulate growth-hormone secretion, the administration of levodopa is used as a provocative test for the diagnosis of growth-hormone deficiency. Levodopa 500 mg is given by mouth after an overnight fast and serum concentrations of growth hormone measured hourly at 0 to 3 hours; children may be given 10 mg per kg body-weight to a maximum of 500 mg. Transient nausea, vomiting, vertigo, and hypotension may occur and the patient should be kept recumbent during the test. A normal response is an increase in serum concentration of growth hormone of more than 5 ng per mL or to a level of more than 10 ng per mL, although 10 to 15% of normal subjects may not respond. Other provocative tests include insulin-induced hypoglycaemia, propranolol-glucagon, arginine infusion, sleep, and exercise.— C. F. Abboud, *Mayo Clin. Proc.*, 1986, *61*, 35.

Sexual function. Four of 7 male parkinsonian patients reported increased libido during administration of levodopa. Hormonal factors appeared to be involved.— E. Brown *et al., Am. J. Psychiat.*, 1978, *135*, 1552.

See also Effects on Sexual Function in Adverse Effects (above).

RESTLESS LEG SYNDROME. Complete symptomatic relief was achieved in 5 patients with restless legs syndrome, 4 of whom received levodopa 200 mg with benserazide 50 mg about an hour before going to sleep; the fifth patient had a daily dosage of 500 to 750 mg. Bromocriptine mesylate was also effective in 3 patients.— S. Akpinar (letter), *Archs Neurol., Chicago*, 1982, *39*, 739. See also C. von Scheele, *Lancet*, 1986, *2*, 426.

Preparations

Carbidopa and Levodopa Tablets *(U.S.P.)*

Levodopa and Carbidopa Tablets *(B.P.)*

Levodopa Capsules *(B.P.)*

Levodopa Capsules *(U.S.P.)*

Levodopa Tablets *(B.P.)*

Levodopa Tablets *(U.S.P.)*

Proprietary Preparations

Brocadopa *(Brocades, UK). Capsules*, levodopa 125, 250, and 500 mg.

Larodopa *(Roche, UK). Tablets*, scored, levodopa 500 mg.

Madopar *(Roche, UK). Capsules* (Madopar 62.5), levodopa 50 mg, benserazide 12.5 mg (as hydrochloride). *Capsules* (Madopar 125), levodopa 100 mg, benserazide 25 mg (as hydrochloride). *Capsules* (Madopar 250), levodopa 200 mg, benserazide 50 mg (as hydrochloride). *Tablets* (Madopar 62.5 dispersible), scored, levodopa 50 mg, benserazide 12.5 mg (as hydrochloride). *Tablets* (Madopar 125 dispersible), scored, levodopa 100 mg, benserazide 25 mg (as hydrochloride).

Sinemet *(Merck Sharp & Dohme, UK). Tablets* (Sinemet-110), scored, levodopa 100 mg, carbidopa 10 mg (as monohydrate). *Tablets* (Sinemet-275), scored, levodopa 250 mg, carbidopa 25 mg (as monohydrate).

Sinemet-Plus *(Merck Sharp & Dohme, UK). Tablets*, scored, levodopa 100 mg, carbidopa 25 mg (as monohydrate).

Proprietary Names and Manufacturers

Bendopa *(ICN, USA)*; Berkdopa *(Berk Pharmaceuticals, UK)*; Brocadopa *(Fr.; Merckle, Ger.; Brocades, UK)*; Cidandopa *(Cidan, Spain)*; Dopaidan *(Ital.)*; Dopaken *(Kairon, Spain)*; Dopalfher *(Spain)*; Dopar *(Norwich Eaton, USA)*; Doparkine *(Arg.)*; Doparl *(Jpn)*; Dopasol *(Jpn)*; Dopaston *(Jpn)*; Dopastral *(Swed.)*; Eldopal *(Belg.; Neth.)*; Eldopar *(Weiders, Norw.)*; Eldopatec *(Switz.)*; Larodopa *(Arg.; Roche, Austral.; Belg.; Roche, Canad.; Roche, Denm.; Roche, Fr.; Roche, Ger.; Roche, Ital.; Neth.; Norw.; Roche, S.Afr.; Roche, Swed.; Roche, Switz.; Roche, UK; Roche, USA)*; Levopa *(Austral.; Canad.; Neth.; Switz.)*; Maipedopa *(Spain)*; Novedopa *(Torlan, Spain)*; Rigakin *(Neth.)*; Syndopa *(Faulding, Austral.)*; Veldopa *(Smith & Nephew Pharmaceuticals, UK)*.

The following names have been used for multi-ingredient preparations containing levodopa— Madopar *(Roche, Austral.; Roche, UK)*; Madopark *(Roche, Swed.)*; Prolopa *(Roche, Canad.)*; Sinemet *(Merck Sharp & Dohme, Austral.; Merck Sharp & Dohme, Canad.; Merck Sharp & Dohme, UK; Merck Sharp & Dohme, USA)*; Sinemet-Plus *(Merck Sharp & Dohme, UK)*.

1510-r

Lysuride Maleate *(BANM)*.

Lisuride Maleate *(rINNM)*; Methylergol Carbamide Maleate. 3-(9,10-Didehydro-6-methylergolin-8α-yl)-1,1-diethylurea hydrogen maleate; 8-Decarboxamido-8-(3,3-diethylureido)-D-lysergamide.

$C_{20}H_{26}N_4O,C_4H_4O_4$=454.5.

CAS — 18016-80-3 (lysuride); 19875-60-6 (maleate).

Pharmacopoeias. In *Cz.*

Lysuride maleate, an ergot derivative or ergoline, is a dopamine agonist with actions and uses similar to those of bromocriptine (p.1011). It has been used similarly in the management of Parkinson's disease, in disorders associated with hyperprolactinaemia, and to inhibit lactation.

Lysuride maleate is given for the prophylaxis of migraine in some countries.

Plasma concentrations varied widely following a single oral dose of lysuride maleate 300 μg in 11 patients with Parkinson's disease. Absorption was rapid and the mean plasma elimination half-life was 2.2 hours. Only a mean of 0.05% of the dose was excreted unchanged in the urine in 24 hours.— R. S. Burns *et al., Clin. Pharmac. Ther.*, 1984, *35*, 548.

EXTRAPYRAMIDAL DISORDERS. Beneficial results with lysuride 2 or 3 mg daily by mouth in divided doses in 3 patients with spasmodic torticollis and 3 of 4 with generalised dystonia.— S. Bassi *et al.* (letter), *Lancet*, 1982, *1*, 514.

See also Parkinsonism (below).

HYPERPROLACTINAEMIA AND PROLACTINOMAS. Plasma-prolactin concentrations were reduced to normal in 4 female patients with macroprolactinomas given lysuride 400 to 800 μg daily for 2 years. Subsequent dosage reduction in 3 was followed by a rise in prolactin values. In the fourth patient prolactin remained in the normal range when the dose was progressively reduced from 400 to 50 μg daily, although complete withdrawal was followed by an increase in prolactin concentration within 3 months.— A. Liuzzi *et al., New Engl. J. Med.*, 1985, *313*, 656.

INHIBITION OF LACTATION. Lactation was prevented in 53 women by lysuride 100 or 200 μg three times daily by mouth started within 24 hours of delivery and continued for 7 days. Rebound lactation occurred in half of the 26 patients given 300 μg daily and a third of the 27 given 600 μg daily and, apart from one woman in the 300- μg group, was controlled by administration of lysuride 600 μg daily for a further week.— L. De Cecco *et al., Br. J. Obstet. Gynaec.*, 1979, *86*, 905.

MIGRAINE. Lysuride maleate 25 μg three times daily was significantly superior to placebo for the prophylaxis of migraine in a 3-month double-blind study involving 132 patients. Side-effects caused 12 and 5 patients receiving lysuride and placebo respectively to withdraw from the study.— B. W. Somerville and W. M. Herrmann, *Headache*, 1978, *18*, 75.

PARKINSONISM. Lysuride maleate is a water-soluble semisynthetic ergot alkaloid with dopaminergic and seratonergic actions. Like apomorphine and pergolide, but unlike bromocriptine its stimulant effect at postsynaptic dopamine receptors is independent of presynaptic dopamine synthesis or stores. Beneficial results have been achieved when doses of up to 5 mg daily have been added to levodopa treatment, with improvement in 'on-off' fluctuations. Side-effects are similar to those of bromocriptine; a higher incidence of somnolence is probably due to serotonergic effects. Despite a prolonged suppressant effect on prolactin secretion, the duration of motor benefit in Parkinson's disease has been reported to be only 2 to 3 hours after a single intravenous dose.— N. P. Quinn, *Drugs*, 1984, *28*, 236.

Lysuride given in a dose of 0.2 to 6 mg daily in three divided doses to 12 parkinsonian patients with levodopa-induced oscillations improved oscillations in only one; 4 patients reported an improvement in mobility during 'on' periods. Adverse effects were frequent and dose-limiting. In 12 similar patients pergolide 1.5 to 8 mg daily in three divided doses was more effective, probably because of its longer duration of action (4 to 8 hours compared with 1 to 3 hours for lysuride).— A. J. Lees and G. M. Stern (letter), *Lancet*, 1981, *2*, 577.

Lysuride by continuous intravenous infusion reduced fluctuations in motor response in 10 patients with Parkinson's disease on oral levodopa therapy. Normal daily treatment with levodopa had to be continued during the infusions.— J. A. Obeso *et al., Ann. Neurol.*, 1986, *19*, 31.

Continuous subcutaneous administration of lysuride by infusion pump considerably improved mobility in 3 patients with Parkinson's disease and severe 'on-off' fluctuations unresponsive to conventional treatment. Two were maintained for several months on a constant infusion of lysuride 2.5 mg in 3.2 mL of solution over 24 hours; the third patient required an increased infusion rate at night. Oral levodopa therapy was continued although in 2 the total daily dose was greatly reduced. Domperidone was given by mouth to prevent nausea and vomiting. All 3 patients had previously received lysuride by intravenous infusion, but only 2 had benefited; these 2 had also gained moderate benefit from lysuride 3 mg daily by mouth in addition to their levodopa therapy.— J. A. Obeso *et al., Lancet*, 1986, *1*, 467. Reports of serious psychiatric side-effects complicating treatment with lysuride by continuous subcutaneous infusion.— A. Castro-Caldas *et al.* (letter), *ibid.*, 1150; D. Chin (letter), *ibid.*, 1151 (intravenous infusion); C. J. Todes (letter), *ibid.*, *2*, 36; S. Ruggieri *et al.* (letter), *ibid.*, 348; S. Bittkau and H. Przuntek (letter), *ibid.*, 349. Motor fluctuations were strikingly improved or abolished by lysuride infusion in 12 parkinsonian patients with severe 'on-off' fluctuations on levodopa therapy, but lysuride had to be withdrawn in 10 patients, solely because of psychosis in 8 and because of psychosis and significantly increased involuntary movements in 2. Mental effects were difficult to manage and decreasing the lysuride dose by 25% in 4 patients had no effect.— P. Critchley *et al.* (letter), *ibid.*, 349. Comment on the psychiatric side-effects of lysuride infusion therapy and the view that they are virtually identical to those seen with all forms of high-dose dopaminergic therapy.— R. Horowski (letter), *ibid.*, 510.

PORPHYRIA. Lysuride maleate was considered to be unsafe in patients with acute porphyria because it has been shown to be porphyrinogenic in *animals* or *in vitro* systems.— M.R. Moore and K.E.L. McColl, *Porphyrias, Drug Lists*, Glasgow, Porphyria Research Unit, University of Glasgow, 1987.

Proprietary Names and Manufacturers
Cuvalit *(Schering, Ger.; Schering, Ital.)*; Dopergin *(Schering, Ger.; Schering, Ital.; Schering, Switz.)*; Lysenyl *(Cz.)*.

4550-q

Memantine *(rINN)*.

3,5-Dimethyl-1-adamantanamine; D-145. 3,5-Dimethyltricyclo[3.3.1.1^{3,7}]dec-1-ylamine.
$C_{12}H_{21}N$=179.3.

CAS — 19982-08-2.

Memantine is a derivative of amantadine used in the treatment of parkinsonism. The hydrochloride is available as 10-mg tablets. It has also been given by injection.

The pharmacology of memantine.— B. Costall and R. J. Naylor, *Psychopharmacologia*, 1975, *43*, 53.

PARKINSONISM. Rigor, tremor, and motor drive in 12 patients with parkinsonism improved after receiving memantine 40 mg by intravenous infusion.— P. -A. Fischer *et al.*, *Arzneimittel-Forsch.*, 1977, *27*, 1487.

Proprietary Names and Manufacturers
Akatinol *(Merz, Ger.)*.

16889-x

Mesulergine *(rINN)*.

CQ-32085; CU-204079; CU-29717; CU-32085. *N′*-(1,6-Dimethylergolin-8α-yl)-*N,N*-dimethylsulfamide.
$C_{18}H_{26}N_4O_2S$=362.4.

CAS — 64795-35-3.

Mesulergine, an ergot derivative or ergoline, is a dopamine agonist similar to bromocriptine. It has been tried in the management of Parkinson's disease and in disorders associated with hyperprolactinaemia, but clinical studies were suspended because of toxicity in *animals*.

Proprietary Names and Manufacturers
Sandoz, Switz.

1511-f

Metergoline *(BAN, rINN)*.

FI-6337; MCE; Methergoline. Benzyl (8*S*,10*S*)-(1,6-dimethylergolin-8-ylmethyl)carbamate.
$C_{25}H_{29}N_3O_2$=403.5.

CAS — 17692-51-2.

Metergoline, an ergot derivative or ergoline, is a dopamine agonist with actions and uses similar to those of bromocriptine (p.1011). It is also a serotonin antagonist. Metergoline has been used similarly to bromocriptine in disorders associated with hyperprolactinaemia and to inhibit lactation. It has also been used in the prophylaxis of migraine.

ACROMEGALY. Plasma concentrations of growth hormone and prolactin were suppressed in 3 patients with acromegaly given metergoline 2 mg four times daily for 6 days.— G. Delitala *et al.*, *J. clin. Endocr. Metab.*, 1976, *43*, 1382.

HYPERPROLACTINAEMIA AND PROLACTINOMAS. Metergoline lowered plasma-prolactin concentrations, although not to normal, in 3 men and 8 women with hyperprolactinaemia who were intolerant of bromocriptine. Galactorrhoea was abolished and/or a regular menstrual cycle established in 5 of the women. Prolactin concentrations and symptoms were unchanged in 3 further women with normoprolactinaemic galactorrhoea. Initial doses of 2 mg daily were increased over 2 weeks to 4 mg three times daily and at monthly re-assessment the dose was increased up to 24 mg daily in divided doses, according to response.— I. F. Casson *et al.*, *Br. med. J.*, 1985, *290*, 1783.

INHIBITION OF LACTATION. Metergoline reduced the elevated plasma-prolactin concentrations in 78 lactating women. Lactation was suppressed within 5 days in 59 of 69 women given 4 mg twice daily for 5 days when started within 24 hours of delivery. In 9 women given metergoline from the 4th day congestion and discomfort were rapidly relieved.— G. Delitala *et al.*, *Br. med. J.*, 1977, *1*, 744.

Metergoline 4 mg three times daily for 5 days inhibited lactation in 20 women when administered within 24 hours of delivery and suppressed lactation in a further 10 when administered within 48 to 72 hours of delivery. After stopping therapy only 3 women showed a mild rebound of lactation, breast engorgement, or pain, which was relieved by a few additional days of treatment. Plasma-prolactin concentrations were significantly reduced.— P. G. Crosignani *et al.*, *Obstet. Gynec.*, 1978, *51*, 113.

Proprietary Names and Manufacturers
Liserdol *(Farmitalia, Ital.)*.

13095-p

Pergolide Mesylate *(BANM, USAN, rINNM)*.

LY-127809. 8β-Methylthiomethyl-6-propylergoline methanesulphonate; Methyl (8*R*,10*R*)-6-propylergolin-8-ylmethyl sulphide.
$C_{19}H_{26}N_2S,CH_4O_3S$=410.6.

CAS — 66104-22-1 (pergolide); 66104-23-2 (mesylate).

Pergolide mesylate, an ergot derivative or ergoline, is a dopamine agonist with actions and uses similar to those of bromocriptine (p.1011). It has been used similarly in the management of Parkinson's disease and in disorders associated with hyperprolactinaemia.

The physiological disposition of pergolide.— A. Rubin *et al.*, *Clin. Pharmac. Ther.*, 1981, *30*, 258.

ACROMEGALY. Serum concentrations of growth hormone were reduced in 7 patients with acromegaly given pergolide in single daily doses ranging from 100 to 350 µg daily by mouth; normal concentrations were achieved in only 2.— D. L. Kleinberg *et al.*, *New Engl. J. Med.*, 1983, *309*, 704.

HYPERPROLACTINAEMIA AND PROLACTINOMAS. A single dose of pergolide mesylate 50 µg by mouth reduced serum-prolactin concentrations for more than 24 hours in patients with hyperprolactinaemia.— S. Franks *et al.*, *Lancet*, 1981, *2*, 659. Confirmation of the efficacy of pergolide in suppressing serum-prolactin concentrations in a long-term study involving 17 women and 8 men with hyperprolactinaemia. Concentrations were reduced in all of the 24 in whom they were measured, to normal in 16. Initial doses of pergolide 25 µg daily were increased at intervals of 2 weeks according to response; in most patients the effective dose was between 50 and 150 µg daily as a single dose. Of the 14 amenorrhoeic women who took pergolide for at least 6 months, menstruation resumed in 12 and ovulation in 11 of these. Clinical response was more difficult to judge in the men, 5 of whom presented with hypogonadism, but a reduction in the size of prolactinoma was noted in 2; effective suppression of prolactin concentrations had no effect on sperm density or fertility in 2 men with oligospermia. Side-effects were similar to those seen with bromocriptine, the most common being nausea (12 patients), nasal congestion (8), and postural dizziness (8); 4 of 8 patients who had previously been unable to tolerate bromocriptine were maintained successfully on pergolide. Conversely, 6 patients had to stop taking pergolide because of nausea and postural dizziness in 3 and, after 6 to 9 months of treatment, persistent nausea and drowsiness in 2 and depression in 1; 2 of the 6 subsequently tolerated bromocriptine.— idem, *Br. med. J.*, 1983, *286*, 1177. See also D. L. Kleinberg *et al.*, *New Engl. J. Med.*, 1983, *309*, 704.

Further references: O. A. Kletzky *et al.*, *Am. J. Obstet. Gynec.*, 1986, *154*, 431 (comparison with bromocriptine).

PARKINSONISM. Pergolide mesylate is a synthetic ergoline with postsynaptic dopamine agonist properties which, like apomorphine and lysuride but unlike bromocriptine, are independent of presynaptic dopamine synthesis or stores. Pergolide has been used, similarly to bromocriptine in the management of parkinsonian patients with the 'wearing-off' effect and 'on-off' fluctuations. When added to existing levodopa therapy pergolide has been given in doses of 2 to 4 mg daily although some patients seem to need higher doses especially if monotherapy is attempted in severely fluctuating patients. Side-effects are similar to those with bromocriptine; earlier concern over the potential of pergolide to cause cardiac arrhythmias has not been substantiated.— N. P. Quinn, *Drugs*, 1984, *28*, 236.

Pergolide 1.5 to 8 mg daily in 3 divided doses was more effective than treatment with lysuride 0.2 to 6 mg daily in separate preliminary studies in parkinsonism patients with levodopa-induced oscillations, probably because of its longer duration of action (4 to 8 hours compared with 1 to 3 hours for lysuride).— A. J. Lees and G. M. Stern (letter), *Lancet*, 1981, *2*, 577.

Significant improvement was seen with both pergolide and placebo in a 6-month double-blind study in 20 patients with Parkinson's disease who had been taking levodopa and carbidopa with a less than optimal response. In those receiving pergolide, mean levodopa/carbidopa dosage had been reduced from 941 to 677 mg daily by the end of the study, but remained essentially unchanged in those on placebo.— S. G. Diamond *et al.*, *Neurology*, 1985, *35*, 291.

A long-term study in 18 patients with Parkinson's disease who received up to 4 mg of pergolide daily by mouth for more than 2 years; 16 were also on levodopa therapy. Pergolide improved motor function in most patients with on-off fluctuations although improvement was less evident after 2 years than after 10 weeks; levodopa dosage was reduced by about 33%. However, sudden freezing episodes and start hesitation did not improve and became more frequent and intense in all but 2 patients. Most patients experienced some adverse reactions including orthostatic lightheadedness, nausea, hallucinations, nervousness, depression, confusion, ankle swelling, insomnia, and nasal stuffiness.— J. Jankovic, *Neurology*, 1985, *35*, 296.

Pergolide was substituted for bromocriptine in 10 patients with Parkinson's disease when the beneficial effects of bromocriptine, which had been maximal at 12 months, waned after a mean of 29 months. Clinical function improved again, with maximal improvement at 12 months, and was maintained after a mean of 29 months of treatment with pergolide. All patients took levodopa throughout the study.— C. G. Goetz *et al.*, *Neurology*, 1985, *35*, 749.

Proprietary Names and Manufacturers
Lilly, USA.

4551-p

Piribedil *(rINN)*.

ET-495; EU-4200. 2-(4-Piperonylpiperazin-1-yl)pyrimidine.
$C_{16}H_{18}N_4O_2$=298.3.

CAS — 3605-01-4.

Piribedil is a non-ergot dopamine agonist and has been tried in the treatment of parkinsonism and in depression. In some countries it is used in the treatment of circulatory disorders and is available as tablets of 20 mg and as an injection containing 3 mg of piribedil mesylate in 1 mL.

Adverse effects reported include nausea and vomiting, dizziness, confusion, drowsiness, hypothermia, dyskinesias, and occasional changes in liver function.

PARKINSONISM. Piribedil may be more effective in reducing tremor than in improving other aspects of Parkinson's disease, but its antiparkinsonian efficacy is considerably less than that of levodopa or bromocriptine. In some countries it has found a role in early treatment.— N. P. Quinn, *Drugs*, 1984, *28*, 236.

Proprietary Names and Manufacturers
Circularina *(Searle, Spain)*; Trivastal *(Eutherapie, Fr.; Itherapia, Ger.; Servier, Spain; Servier, Switz.)*; Trivastan *(Stroder, Ital.)*.

13228-v

Selegiline Hydrochloride *(BANM, rINNM)*.

Deprenyl. (−)-(*R*)-*N*,α-Dimethyl-*N*-(prop-2-ynyl)phenethylamine hydrochloride; (*R*)-Methyl(α-methylphenethyl)-prop-2-ynylamine hydrochloride.
$C_{13}H_{17}N,HCl$=223.7.

CAS — 14611-51-9 (selegiline); 14611-52-0 (hydrochloride).

STABILITY. A warning that extemporaneously prepared oral liquid dosage forms of selegiline may be unstable and manufacturers' formulations should be used where possible. An extemporary formula is available for selegiline syrup.— T. J. Walls *et al.*, *Br. med. J.*, 1985, *290*, 444.

Adverse Effects and Precautions

Selegiline is usually given as an adjunct to levodopa therapy and most of the adverse effects reported can be attributed to enhanced levodopa activity; dosage of levodopa may have to be reduced. Adverse effects have included hypotension, nausea, confusion, agitation, hallucinations, and increased dyskinesias.

Unlike non-selective monoamine oxidase inhibitors such as phenelzine, selegiline is reported not to interact with tyramine in food.

Absorption and Fate

Selegiline is rapidly absorbed from the gastro-intestinal tract and crosses the blood-brain barrier. It is metabolised to methylamphetamine and amphetamine which are excreted in the urine.

Selegiline hydrochloride given by mouth to 6 healthy subjects appeared to be completely metabolised. Within 24 hours of a 5- or 10-mg dose a mean of 63.3% was excreted in the urine as methylamphetamine and 15.1% as amphetamine. It seemed likely that the metabolites would be (−)-isomers.— G. P. Reynolds *et al.* (letter), *Br. J. clin. Pharmac.*, 1978, *6*, 542.

Uses and Administration

Selegiline hydrochloride is a selective inhibitor of monoamine oxidase type B, an enzyme involved in the metabolic degradation of dopamine in the brain. It enhances the effects of levodopa and is used in Parkinson's disease as an adjunct to levodopa therapy, usually when fluctuations in mobility have become a problem. The initial dose is 5 mg of selegiline hydrochloride by mouth each morning, increased to 10 mg daily if necessary. Levodopa dosage may need to be reduced by up to 50%.

Selegiline has also been tried in the treatment of depression.

MENTAL DISORDERS. *Depression.* Clinical improvement in depressed patients given selegiline 5 mg three times daily for 40 days when compared with placebo.— J. Mendlewicz and M. B. H. Youdim, *Br. J. Psychiat.*, 1983, *142*, 508.

Beneficial results with selegiline 5 to 10 mg daily together with phenylalanine 250 mg daily in patients with unipolar depression.— W. Birkmayer *et al.*, *J. neural Transmission*, 1984, *59*, 81.

PARKINSONISM. Early attempts to prolong the effects of levodopa in Parkinson's disease by the concomitant administration of monoamine oxidase inhibitors were unsuccessful because of intolerable side-effects and the hazard of potentially catastrophic hypertension. Following the realisation that monoamine oxidase (MAO) exists in at least 2 forms, A and B, and that dopamine in the human brain is metabolised predominantly by MAO-B, selegiline, a specific MAO-B inhibitor, was found to delay oxidative deamination of dopamine without provoking a 'cheese reaction'. When selegiline is given together with levodopa and a peripheral decarboxylase inhibitor there should be a smoother therapeutic response in about half of patients experiencing 'end-of-dose' akinesia (*Lancet*, 1982, *2*, 695). However, improvement is often short-lived and the place of selegiline in the management of Parkinson's disease is mostly restricted to the early stages of the 'wearing-off' effect ['end-of-dose' deterioration]; it is ineffective in advanced disease with severe levodopa 'on-off' swings (N.P. Quinn, *Drugs*, 1984, *28*, 236). Selegiline has been claimed to slow the progression of Parkinson's disease when added to conventional levodopa therapy (W. Birkmayer *et al.*, *Mod. Problems Pharmacopsychiat.*, 1983, *19*, 170; W. Birkmayer, *et al.*, *J. neural Transmission*, 1985, *64*, 113) although this has been questioned (R. Lewin, *Science*, 1985, *230*, 527).

Results indicating that the clinical effects of selegiline in Parkinson's disease are not dependent on its amphetamine metabolites.— G. M. Stern *et al.*, *Acta neurol. scand.*, 1983, *95*, *Suppl.*, 113.

For an overview of parkinsonism and its treatment, see Levodopa, p.1019.

Proprietary Preparations

Eldepryl *(Britannia Pharmaceuticals, UK)*. *Tablets*, scored, selegiline hydrochloride 5 mg.

Proprietary Names and Manufacturers

Eldepryl *(Britannia Pharmaceuticals, UK)*; Jumex *(Chinoin, Hung.; Chiesi, Ital.)*; Jumexal *(Labatec-Pharma, Switz.)*; Movergan *(Asta Pharma, Ger.)*.

Electrolytes

1150-y

Electrolyte solutions are used to correct disturbances in fluid and electrolyte balance. The principal factors involved in fluid and electrolyte homoeostasis are maintenance of blood volume and osmotic equilibrium, acid-base balance, and the effects of specific ions. The osmotic effects of solutions may be expressed in terms of osmolality which is defined as the 'molal' concentration in moles (or osmoles) per kg of solvent, or in terms of osmolarity which is the 'molar' concentration in moles (or osmoles) per litre of solution. In clinical practice, solute concentrations are measured per litre of solution and are expressed as millimoles (mmol) per litre.

For electrical neutrality to exist in the extracellular fluid, the sum of the concentrations of cations must equal the sum of the concentrations of anions. Measurements of extracellular (plasma or serum) concentration are usually limited to sodium (or sodium and potassium), chloride, and bicarbonate. Assuming measurement only of sodium, bicarbonate, and chloride, the sum of the concentrations of sodium plus unmeasured cations (calcium, magnesium, potassium) equals the sum of the concentrations of bicarbonate and chloride plus unmeasured anions (phosphate, protein, sulphate, derivatives of organic acids). The difference between the concentrations of unmeasured anions and unmeasured cations is known as the *anion gap*; variations in the anion gap are useful diagnostic indications to disorders of acid-base balance.

A discussion on the uses and limitations of measuring serum osmolality.— F. J. Gennari, *New Engl. J. Med.*, 1984, *310*, 102. Comments.— L. H. Hilborne *et al.* (letter), *ibid.*, 1608; R. H. Sterns and A. Spital (letter), *ibid;* M. J. DiNubile (letter), *ibid.*, 1609; V. Batuman and J. K. Maesaka (letter), *ibid.* Reply.— F. J. Gennari (letter), *ibid.*, 1610.

A review of the regulation of water balance in the body.— S. M. Willatts, *Br. J. Hosp. Med.*, 1984, *32*, 8.

A review of the relative merits of colloids and crystalloids for the maintenance of plasma volume.— A. D. Ross and D. M. Angaran, *Drug Intell. & clin. Pharm.*, 1984, *18*, 202. See also K. M. Hillman, *Br. J. Hosp. Med.*, 1986, *35*, 217.

Salt Intake and Hypertension

The relationship between sodium intake and prevalence of hypertension is complicated, and may be confused by other factors such as other cations (potassium, calcium, magnesium), fat intake, alcohol consumption, obesity, and genetic predisposition.

The effect of individual salt intake on individual blood pressure is difficult to study, owing, in part, to problems of variability in measurement. Some data suggest that weight reduction and reduced sodium intake each make an independent contribution to the lowering of the blood pressure and enhance the effect of drug treatment of high blood pressure. The ultimate potential for prevention of high blood pressure in populations is illustrated by its virtually total absence in a few traditional, isolated, subsistence economies. The people are generally physically active, obesity is rare, and the sense of community is strong. Habitual salt intake is usually under 3 g daily. The population data also indicate that with a reduction of 5 g in the average daily salt intake of the population, average diastolic pressure can be lowered by 4 mm Hg and it is recommended that populations should be encouraged to reduce the consumption of salt in the direction of 5 g daily or less.— Report of a WHO Expert Committee on Prevention of Coronary Heart Disease, *Tech. Rep. Ser. Wld Hlth Org. No.678*, 1982.

A discussion on the 'non-drug' treatment of mild hypertension with reference to the roles of sodium restriction, and calcium, magnesium, and potassium supplementation.— N. M. Kaplan, *Ann. intern. Med.*, 1985, *102*, 359.

References to the effects of sodium restriction on blood pressure: G. A. MacGregor, *Hypertension*, 1985, *7*, 628; N. A. Boon and J. K. Aronson, *Br. med. J.*, 1985, *290*, 949; D. E. Grobbee and A. Hofman, *ibid.*, 1986, *293*, 27.

References to the effects of calcium supplementation on blood pressure: L. M. Resnick, *Ann. intern. Med.*, 1985, *103*, 944; H. Heath and C. W. Callaway, *ibid.*, 944 and 946; *Lancet*, 1986, *1*, 359; D. E. Grobbee and A. Hofman, *ibid.*, *2*, 703; N. M. Kaplan and R. B. Meese, *Ann. intern. Med.*, 1986, *105*, 947; R. P. Wedeen (letter), *ibid.*, 1987, *106*, 472; R. M. Lyle *et al.*, *J. Am. med. Ass.*, 1987, *257*, 1772.

References to the effects of potassium supplementation on blood pressure: S. J. Smith *et al.*, *Br. med. J.*, 1985, *290*, 110; *Lancet*, 1985, *1*, 1308; K. -T. Khaw and E. Barrett-Connor, *New Engl. J. Med.*, 1987, *316*, 235; A. Siani *et al.*, *Br. med. J.*, 1987, *294*, 1453.

Multiple Electrolyte Preparations

Elliott's B Solution. Artificial Spinal Fluid. Sodium chloride 730 mg, potassium chloride 30 mg, calcium chloride dihydrate 20 mg, magnesium sulphate 30 mg, sodium phosphate heptahydrate 20 mg, glucose 80 mg, sodium bicarbonate 190 mg, phenol red 10 µg, Water for Injections to 100 mL.—M.J. Duttera *et al.* (letter), *Lancet*, 1972, *1*, 540.

Ringer's Injection *(U.S.P.)*. A sterile solution containing sodium chloride 860 mg, potassium chloride 30 mg, calcium chloride dihydrate 33 mg, and Water for Injections to 100 mL. It contains no antimicrobial agents. pH 5.0 to 7.5. Each litre contains approximately 147.5 mmol of sodium, 156 mmol of chloride, 4 mmol of potassium, and 2.25 mmol of calcium.

Ringer's Irrigation *(U.S.P.)*. A sterile solution containing sodium chloride 860 mg, potassium chloride 30 mg, calcium chloride dihydrate 33 mg, and Water for Injections to 100 mL. It contains no antimicrobial agents. pH 5.0 to 7.5. It should not be used for injection or for irrigations that might result in absorption into the blood.

Proprietary Preparations

Balanced Salt Solution *(Alcon, UK). Solution*, sterile, iso-osmotic, sodium chloride 0.64%, potassium chloride 0.075%, calcium chloride 0.048%, magnesium chloride 0.03%, sodium acetate 0.39%, sodium citrate 0.17% in Water for Injections in single-use disposable containers of 15 and 30 mL. May be used for intraocular and topical irrigation of the eye.

Balanced Salt Solution *(CooperVision, UK). Solution*, sterile, iso-osmotic, sodium chloride 0.64%, potassium chloride 0.075%, calcium chloride 0.048%, magnesium chloride 0.03%, sodium acetate 0.39%, sodium citrate 0.17% in Water for Injections in single-use disposable containers of 15 mL. May be used for intraocular and topical irrigation of the eye.

Plasma-Lyte 50/30 *(Travenol, UK). Intravenous infusion*, hypertonic, anhydrous glucose 50 g, potassium chloride 2.24 g, sodium acetate 1.63 g, sodium chloride 1.52 g, sodium lactate 1.35 g, magnesium chloride 508 mg, calcium chloride 441 mg/litre providing (approximately) sodium 50 mmol, potassium 30 mmol, calcium 3 mmol, magnesium 2.5 mmol, chloride 67 mmol, acetate 12 mmol, lactate 12 mmol.

Plasma-Lyte 148 in Water *(Travenol, UK). Intravenous infusion*, isotonic, sodium chloride 5.26 g, sodium gluconate 5.02 g, sodium acetate 3.68 g, potassium chloride 370 mg, magnesium chloride 300 mg/litre providing (approximately) sodium 140 mmol, potassium 5 mmol, magnesium 1.5 mmol, chloride 98 mmol, acetate 27 mmol, gluconate 23 mmol.

Plasma-Lyte 148 with 5% Dextrose *(Travenol, UK). Intravenous infusion*, hypertonic, anhydrous glucose 50 g, sodium chloride 5.26 g, sodium gluconate 5.02 g, sodium acetate 3.68 g, potassium chloride 370 mg, magnesium chloride 300 mg/litre providing (approximately) sodium 140 mmol, potassium 5 mmol, magnesium 1.5 mmol, chloride 98 mmol, acetate 27 mmol, gluconate 23 mmol.

Plasma-Lyte M with 5% Dextrose *(Travenol, UK). Intravenous infusion*, hypertonic, anhydrous glucose 50 g, sodium acetate 1.61 g, sodium lactate 1.38 g, potassium chloride 1.19 g, sodium chloride 940 mg, calcium chloride 370 mg, magnesium chloride 300 mg/litre providing (approximately) sodium 40 mmol, potassium 16 mmol, calcium 2.5 mmol, magnesium 1.5 mmol, chloride 40 mmol, acetate 12 mmol, lactate 12 mmol.

Plegisol *(Abbott, UK). Solution*, sterile, sodium 110 mmol, potassium 16 mmol, magnesium 16 mmol, calcium 1.2 mmol, chloride 160 mmol in single-use disposable containers of 1 litre. 10 mL of Sodium Bicarbonate Injection 8.4% must be added to each litre immediately before use. For cardioplegia.

Proprietary Names and Manufacturers of Multiple Electrolytes

The following names have been used for multi-ingredient preparations containing multiple electrolytes—Balanced Salt Solution *(Alcon, UK; CooperVision, UK)*; BSS *(Alcon, Canad.)*; BSS Plus *(Alcon, Canad.)*; Cellular Repair Solution (Nabarro's Solution) *(Boots, UK)*; Eye-Stream *(Alcon, Austral.; Alcon, Canad.)*; Paediatric Electrolyte Solution *(Boots, UK)*; Plasma-Lyte *(Travenol, Austral.; Travenol, UK)*; Plegisol *(Abbott, UK)*.

For other electrolyte preparations, see under Dialysis Solutions, Oral Rehydration Therapy, and individual monographs. See also under Infusion Fluids for Parenteral Nutrition, p.1290.

Single and mixed electrolyte preparations may be obtained in the *UK* from Boots, IMS, and Travenol.

3276-x

Dialysis Solutions

Dialysis solutions are solutions of electrolytes formulated in concentrations similar to those of extracellular fluid. Glucose may be added as an osmotic agent. Dialysis solutions are used in the management of renal failure and poisoning; they allow the selective removal of toxic substances, electrolytes, and excessive body fluid from the blood. In haemodialysis, the exchange of ions between the solution and the patient's blood is made across a synthetic semi-permeable membrane. In peritoneal dialysis, the exchange is made across the membranes of the peritoneal cavity.

In dialysis, bicarbonate is best given as acetate or lactate in order to avoid the release of carbon dioxide into solution.

A discussion on haemodialysis and its side-effects.— G. Eknoyan, *New Engl. J. Med.*, 1984, *311*, 915.

A discussion on the respective roles of acetate and bicarbonate in haemodialysis.— M. A. Mansell and A. J. Wing, *Br. med. J.*, 1983, *287*, 308. See also R. Duarte (letter), *New Engl. J. Med.*, 1985, *312*, 513; R. M. Hakim *et al.* (letter), *ibid.*, 515; G. Eknoyan (letter), *ibid.*

A review of continuous ambulatory peritoneal dialysis.— G. Wu *et al.*, *Can. med. Ass. J.*, 1984, *130*, 699.

Preparations

Haemodialysis Solutions *(B.P., Eur. P.)*. These are usually prepared by diluting a concentrated solution with water. Advice on the freshly distilled, purified, or potable water that can be used is provided in an annex to the *B.P.* monograph. The concentrations of salts in **Concentrated Haemodialysis Solutions** are such that, after dilution to the stated volume, the final concentrations of the ions are normally within the following ranges: sodium 130 to 140 mmol per litre; potassium 0 to 3 mmol per litre; calcium 1 to 2 mmol per litre; magnesium 0.25 to 1.0 mmol per litre; acetate or lactate (expressed as bicarbonate) 32 to 40 mmol per litre; chloride 95 to 110 mmol per litre. Store at a sufficiently elevated temperature to prevent formation of crystals.

Proprietary Preparations

Dialaflex 61 *(Boots, UK). Solution*, sterile, sodium chloride 0.56%, sodium lactate 0.5%, calcium chloride dihydrate 0.026%, magnesium chloride 0.015%, anhydrous glucose 1.36%, sodium metabisulphite less than 0.005%. For peritoneal dialysis.

Dialaflex 62 *(Boots, UK). Solution*, sterile, sodium chloride 0.56%, sodium lactate 0.5%, calcium chloride dihydrate 0.026%, magnesium chloride 0.015%, anhydrous glucose 6.36%, sodium metabisulphite less than 0.012%. For peritoneal dialysis.

Dialaflex 63 *(Boots, UK). Solution*, sterile, sodium chloride 0.5%, sodium lactate 0.5%, calcium chloride dihydrate 0.026%, magnesium chloride 0.015%, anhydrous glucose 1.36%, sodium metabisulphite less than 0.005%. For peritoneal dialysis.

Diambulate 61 *(Boots, UK). Solution*, sterile, sodium chloride 0.56%, sodium lactate 0.5%, calcium chloride dihydrate 0.026%, magnesium chloride 0.015%, anhydrous glucose 1.36%, sodium metabisulphite less than

0.005%. For continuous ambulatory peritoneal dialysis or intermittent peritoneal dialysis.

Diambulate 63 *(Boots, UK). Solution*, sterile, sodium chloride 0.5%, sodium lactate 0.5%, calcium chloride dihydrate 0.026%, magnesium chloride 0.015%, anhydrous glucose 1.36%, sodium metabisulphite less than 0.005%. For continuous ambulatory peritoneal dialysis or intermittent peritoneal dialysis.

Diambulate 64 *(Boots, UK). Solution*, sterile, sodium chloride 0.56%, sodium lactate 0.5%, calcium chloride dihydrate 0.026%, magnesium chloride 0.015%, anhydrous glucose 4.25%, sodium metabisulphite less than 0.012%. For continuous ambulatory peritoneal dialysis or intermittent peritoneal dialysis.

Diambulate 65 *(Boots, UK). Solution*, sterile, sodium chloride 0.56%, sodium lactate 0.5%, calcium chloride dihydrate 0.026%, magnesium chloride 0.015%, anhydrous glucose 3.86%, sodium metabisulphite less than 0.012%. For continuous ambulatory peritoneal dialysis or intermittent peritoneal dialysis.

Diambulate 66 *(Boots, UK). Solution*, sterile, sodium chloride 0.5%, sodium lactate 0.5%, calcium chloride dihydrate 0.026%, magnesium chloride 0.015%, anhydrous glucose 3.86%, sodium metabisulphite less than 0.012%. For continuous ambulatory peritoneal dialysis or intermittent peritoneal dialysis.

Difusor P *(Boots, UK). Solution*, sterile, sodium chloride 0.56%, sodium lactate 0.5%, calcium chloride dihydrate 0.026%, magnesium chloride 0.015%, anhydrous glucose 1.36%. For peritoneal dialysis.

Difusor E *(Boots, UK). Solution*, sterile, sodium chloride 0.56%, sodium lactate 0.5%, calcium chloride dihydrate 0.026%, magnesium chloride 0.015%, anhydrous glucose 6.36%. For peritoneal dialysis.

Difusor Y *(Boots, UK). Solution*, sterile, sodium chloride 0.5%, sodium lactate 0.5%, calcium chloride dihydrate 0.026%, magnesium chloride 0.015%, anhydrous glucose 1.36%. For peritoneal dialysis.

Difusor PC *(Boots, UK). Solution*, sterile, sodium chloride 0.53%, sodium acetate 0.61%, calcium chloride dihydrate 0.026%, magnesium chloride 0.015%, anhydrous glucose 1.36%. For peritoneal dialysis.

Difusor PD *(Boots, UK). Solution*, sterile, sodium chloride 0.53%, sodium acetate 0.61% calcium chloride dihydrate 0.026%, magnesium chloride 0.015%, anhydrous glucose 6.36%. For peritoneal dialysis.

Difusor PA *(Boots, UK). Solution*, sterile, sodium chloride 0.53%, sodium acetate 0.54%, calcium chloride dihydrate 0.026%, magnesium chloride 0.015%, anhydrous glucose 1.36%. For peritoneal dialysis.

Dianeal *(Travenol, UK). Solution*, sterile, sodium chloride 0.56%, sodium lactate 0.5%, calcium chloride dihydrate 0.026%, magnesium chloride 0.015%, anhydrous glucose 1.36% or 3.86%. For peritoneal dialysis.

Dianeal 130 *(Travenol, UK). Solution*, sterile, sodium chloride 0.5%, sodium lactate 0.5%, calcium chloride dihydrate 0.026%, magnesium chloride 0.015%, anhydrous glucose 1.36%. For peritoneal dialysis.

Dianeal 130 with Potassium *(Travenol, UK). Solution*, sterile, sodium chloride 0.526%, sodium acetate 0.544%, calcium chloride dihydrate 0.026%, potassium chloride 0.0186%, magnesium chloride 0.015%, anhydrous glucose 1.36%. For peritoneal dialysis.

Dianeal 137 *(Travenol, UK). Solution*, sterile, sodium chloride 0.57%, sodium lactate 0.39%, calcium chloride dihydrate 0.0257%, magnesium chloride 0.0152%, anhydrous glucose 1.36%, 2.27%, or 3.86%. For peritoneal dialysis.

Dianeal PD2 *(Travenol, UK). Solution*, sterile, sodium chloride 0.54%, sodium lactate 0.45%, calcium chloride dihydrate 0.0257%, magnesium chloride 0.0051%, anhydrous glucose 1.36% or 3.86%. For peritoneal dialysis.

Dianeal PD3 *(Travenol, UK). Solution*, sterile, sodium chloride 0.57%, sodium lactate 0.45%, calcium chloride dihydrate 0.0257%, magnesium chloride 0.0051%, anhydrous glucose 1.36% or 3.86%. For peritoneal dialysis.

3277-r

Oral Rehydration Therapy

Administration of fluid and electrolytes by mouth to prevent or treat dehydration due to acute diarrhoeal diseases is known as oral rehydration therapy. There are two basic treatment phases; the rehydration phase, which involves the replacement of fluid and electrolytes lost through diarrhoea and vomiting, and the maintenance phase, which is the replacement of losses due to continuing diarrhoea and vomiting, and of normal losses due to respiration, sweating, and urination which are especially high in infants.

Acute diarrhoea leads to loss of essential water and salts and unless these are adequately replaced dehydration will develop. Prevention of dehydration is therefore the first appropriate response to diarrhoea. It is now firmly established that, regardless of the causative agent of diarrhoea or the age of the patient, an oral rehydration solution containing glucose and essential salts is adequately absorbed and replaces both previous and continuing fluid and salt losses. It does not stop the diarrhoea, but the diarrhoea usually continues for only a limited time. Glucose accelerates the absorption of sodium and water from the small intestine and this process is not impaired during acute diarrhoea. A rational response to diarrhoea involves prevention of dehydration using solutions prepared from ingredients commonly found in the home ("home remedies") and correction of dehydration using a balanced, more complete, glucose-salt solution— Oral Rehydration Salts is the universal solution of this type recommended by WHO and UNICEF [see under Preparations, below]. Home remedies which have been used include coconut water, rice water, various soups, weak tea, and solutions consisting of different salts and sugars. Further studies are required in order to clarify the benefits of such preparations. Severe dehydration, usually defined as loss of 10% or more of body-weight, should be corrected by intravenous therapy; this method should be used in patients who are unconscious or unable to drink *Joint WHO/UNICEF Statement on the Management of Diarrhoea and Use of Oral Rehydration Therapy*, 2nd Edn, Geneva, World Health Organization, 1985. See also *Treatment and Prevention of Dehydration in Diarrhoeal Diseases*, Geneva, World Health Organization, 1976; M. H. Merson, *Chronicle Wld Hlth Org.*, 1986, *40*, 116; B. F. Stanton *et al.*, *Lancet*, 1987, *1*, 33; *Med. Lett.*, 1987, *29*, 63.

Half Darrow's-glucose, made by mixing equal volumes of Darrow's solution (see p.1028) with 5% glucose, has been widely used in developing countries for fluid and electrolyte replacement including the treatment of dehydration due to gastroenteritis in children. It has been observed however, that the "half-strength Darrow's" solution supplied to The Gambia contains no glucose, and is therefore hypo-osmolar. Hypotonic glucose-free solutions appear to have been manufactured and supplied to developing countries inadvertently through a failure to appreciate that "half-Darrow's" is not synonymous with "half-Darrow's in 2.5% glucose", and it is only the latter solution which should be used in hospitals in developing countries.— M. Levin *et al.* (letter), *Lancet*, 1987, *1*, 1204.

Preparations

Oral Rehydration Salts *(B.P.)*. Oral Rehydration Salts-Formula A also known as Compound Sodium Chloride and Dextrose Oral Powder or Compound Sodium Chloride and Glucose Oral Powder contain:

sodium chloride 1 g, potassium chloride 1.5 g, sodium bicarbonate 1.5 g, anhydrous glucose 36.4 g or glucose 40 g; may contain suitable flavouring agents. For solution in 1 litre of water.

Oral Rehydration Salts-Bicarbonate (Formula B) and Oral Rehydration Salts-Citrate (Formula C) correspond to the formulas recommended by WHO/UNICEF (see below).

Oral Rehydration Salts should be protected from moisture. They should be kept in sachets, preferably made of aluminium foil, containing sufficient for a single dose or for a single day's treatment.

Oral Rehydration Salts *(WHO; UNICEF)*. Sodium chloride 3.5 g, potassium chloride 1.5 g, sodium bicarbonate 2.5 g or sodium citrate dihydrate 2.9 g, anhydrous glucose 20 g. For solution in 1 litre of water.

Proprietary Preparations

Dextrolyte *(Cow & Gate, UK). Oral solution*, sodium chloride, sodium lactate, potassium chloride, glucose, providing (approximately) sodium 3.5 mmol, potassium 1.34 mmol, chloride 3.05 mmol, lactate 1.77 mmol, glucose 20 mmol/100 mL. Rehydration solution.

Dioralyte *(Armour, UK). Oral powder*, sodium chloride 200 mg, potassium chloride 300 mg, sodium bicarbonate 300 mg, glucose 8 g/sachet providing (approximately) sodium 7 mmol, potassium 4 mmol, chloride 7.4 mmol, bicarbonate 3.6 mmol, glucose 40 mmol.

To be dissolved in 200 mL. water before administration.

Tablets, one tablet provides the equivalent of half a sachet.

Electrolade *(Nicholas, UK). Oral powder*, sodium chloride 236 mg, potassium chloride 300 mg, sodium bicarbonate 500 mg, glucose 4 g/sachet providing (approximately) sodium 10 mmol, potassium 4 mmol, chloride 8 mmol, bicarbonate 6 mmol, glucose 22 mmol. To be dissolved in 200 mL water before administration.

Electrosol *(Martindale Pharmaceuticals, UK). Oral powder*, sodium chloride 200 mg, potassium chloride 300 mg, sodium bicarbonate 300 mg, glucose 8 g/sachet providing (approximately) sodium 7 mmol, potassium 4 mmol, chloride 7.4 mmol, bicarbonate 3.6 mmol, glucose 40 mmol. To be dissolved in 200 mL water before administration.

NOTE. The name Electrosol is also applied to a veterinary preparation of different composition.

Glucolyte *(Cupal, UK). Oral powder*, sodium chloride 200 mg, potassium chloride 300 mg, sodium bicarbonate 300 mg, glucose 8 g/sachet providing (approximately) sodium 7 mmol, potassium 4 mmol, chloride 7.4 mmol, bicarbonate 3.6 mmol, glucose 40 mmol. To be dissolved in 200 mL water before administration.

Paedialyte MS *(Abbott, UK). Oral solution*, sodium chloride 513 mg, sodium citrate dihydrate 245 mg, potassium citrate 540 mg, glucose 6.9 g/250 mL bottle providing (approximately) sodium 11.3 mmol, potassium 5 mmol, chloride 8.8 mmol, citrate 2.5 mmol, glucose 34.8 mmol. Maintenance solution.

Paedialyte RS *(Abbott, UK). Oral solution*, sodium chloride 950 mg, sodium citrate dihydrate 245 mg, potassium citrate 540 mg, glucose 6.9 g/250 mL bottle providing (approximately) sodium 18.8 mmol, potassium 5 mmol, chloride 16.3 mmol, citrate 2.5 mmol, glucose 34.8 mmol. Rehydration solution.

Rehidrat *(Searle, UK). Oral powder*, sodium chloride 440 mg, potassium chloride 380 mg, sodium bicarbonate 420 mg, citric acid 440 mg, glucose 4.09 g, sucrose 8.07 g, fructose 70 mg/sachet providing (approximately) sodium 12.5 mmol, potassium 5 mmol, chloride 12.5 mmol, bicarbonate 5 mmol, citrate 2.25 mmol, glucose 22.8 mmol, sucrose 23.5 mmol, fructose 0.5 mmol. To be dissolved in 250 mL water before administration.

Proprietary Names and Manufacturers

Dextrolyte *(Cow & Gate, UK)*; Diolyte *(McGloin, Austral.)*; Dioralyte *(Armour, UK)*; Electrolade *(Nicholas, Austral.; Nicholas, UK)*; Electrosol *(Martindale Pharmaceuticals, UK)*; Gastrolyte *(USV, Austral.; Rorer, Canad.; USV Pharmaceutical Corp., USA)*; Glucolyte *(Cupal, UK)*; Infalyte *(Pennwalt, USA)*; Lytren *(Mead Johnson, Canad.)*; Paedialyte *(Abbott, UK)*; Pedialyte *(Ross, Canad.; Ross, USA)*; Rehidrat *(Searle, UK)*; Repalyte *(Drug Houses Austral., Austral.)*; Resol *(Wyeth, USA)*; Staminade *(Nicholas, Austral.)*.

3269-r

Bicarbonate

The normal concentration range of bicarbonate in plasma is 22 to 32 mmol per litre. The average intake of bicarbonate in the diet is negligible and very little is excreted in the urine under normal conditions; bicarbonate ions formed in the body are excreted in biliary, intestinal, pancreatic, and salivary fluids. If bicarbonate is administered therapeutically thus increasing the plasma-bicarbonate concentration above the normal range, then compensatory renal mechanisms come into play and bicarbonate is excreted in the urine. Bicarbonate may be administered as sodium bicarbonate or as acetate, citrate, or lactate salts; allowance should be made for the presence of the cation.

Acid-Base Balance

The pH of plasma is normally maintained at around 7.4 and the partial pressure of carbon dioxide (pCO_2) at 40 mm Hg by means of respiratory, renal, and buffering mechanisms. The most important buffer system is the Bicarbonate-Carbonic Acid System which operates on a compensatory basis in the regulation of the acid-base balance. The system is thrown out of balance in acute, severe metabolic disturbances.

Carbonic acid, the principal acidic end-product of metabolism, exists in a dynamic equilibrium with carbon dioxide and water in body fluids which in turn are in equilibrium with bicarbonate and hydrogen ions as shown in the following equation:

$$H_2CO_3 \rightleftharpoons H_2O + CO_2 \rightleftharpoons H^+ + HCO_3^-$$

There are 4 major acid-base disturbances of clinical importance:

Respiratory alkalosis, resulting from an excessive loss of carbon dioxide from the body;
Respiratory acidosis, caused by retention of excess carbon dioxide in the body;
Metabolic alkalosis, caused by retention of excess bicarbonate in the body;
Metabolic acidosis, resulting from an excessive loss of bicarbonate from the body.

3275-t

Calcium Citrate *(USAN)*.

Tricalcium Citrate. Tricalcium 2-hydroxypropane-1,2,3-tricarboxylate tetrahydrate.
$C_{12}H_{10}Ca_3O_{14},4H_2O$=570.5.

CAS — 5785-44-4.

Pharmacopoeias. In *U.S.*

A white, odourless, crystalline powder. Each g represents approximately 5.3 mmol of calcium and 3.5 mmol of citrate.
Slightly **soluble** in water; insoluble in alcohol. **Store** in well-closed containers.

Calcium citrate is an alkalinising agent with phosphate-binding properties. It is given by mouth in doses of 1.9 to 3.8 g daily (citrate 6.7 to 13.3 mmol; calcium 10 to 20 mmol). Excessive doses may lead to calcium overloading and hypercalcaemia; for symptoms see under Calcium, p.1028.

In a preliminary study involving 26 patients with marked renal impairment, administration of calcium citrate for 6 months resulted in increased serum-calcium and decreased serum-phosphate concentrations. Hypercalcaemia, which developed in a number of patients, was controlled with drug dosage reduction, but was considered to be a potentially major complication.— H. M. Cushner *et al.*, *Curr. ther. Res.*, 1986, *40*, 998.

Proprietary Names and Manufacturers
Citracal *(Mission Pharmacal, USA)*.

The following names have been used for multi-ingredient electrolyte preparations containing calcium citrate—Calcigard *(Advanced Medical Nutrition, USA)*.

1180-t

Potassium Citrate *(BAN, USAN)*.

E332; Kalii Citras; Tripotassium Citrate. Tripotassium 2-hydroxypropane-1,2,3-tricarboxylate monohydrate.
$C_6H_5K_3O_7,H_2O$=306.4 (anhydrous); 324.4 (monohydrate).

CAS — 866-84-2 (anhydrous); 6100-05-6 (monohydrate).

Pharmacopoeias. In *Aust.*, *Br.*, *Chin.*, *Egypt.*, *Eur.*, *Fr.*, *Ger.*, *Hung.*, *Ind.*, *Neth.*, *Nord.*, *Port.*, *Swiss*, and *U.S.* which specifies the anhydrous form.

Transparent, odourless, hygroscopic crystals or a white granular powder. Each g of potassium citrate (anhydrous) represents approximately 9.79 mmol of potassium and 3.26 mmol of citrate.
Each g of potassium citrate (monohydrate) represents approximately 9.25 mmol of potassium and 3.08 mmol of citrate.
Soluble 1 in 1 of water and 1 in 2.5 of glycerol; practically insoluble in alcohol. Aqueous solutions, owing to their slight alkalinity, may be **incompatible** with acidifying agents. **Store** in airtight containers.

Potassium citrate, after absorption, is metabolised to bicarbonate; it then has similar actions to those of sodium bicarbonate (p.1026). It is administered by mouth to alkalinise the urine. A mild diuresis usually occurs after its use. Potassium citrate is used to relieve painful irritation caused by cystitis in divided doses of up to 10 g daily of the monohydrate (citrate 31 mmol; potassium 93 mmol. It may also be used in the treatment of calcium renal calculi associated with hypocitraturia. Like other potassium salts, potassium citrate preparations should be taken after meals with plenty of water, and should be administered with caution to patients with impaired renal function. Excessive doses may lead to potassium overloading and hyperkalaemia; for symptoms see under Potassium, p.1036.

Studies of citrate excretion in healthy subjects and in patients with uric acid or calcium nephrolithiasis, following single-dose and repeated administration of potassium citrate in solution and as sustained-release tablets.— C. Y. C. Pak *et al.*, *J. clin. Pharmac.*, 1984, *24*, 19.

RENAL CALCULI. Citrate forms soluble complexes with calcium, thereby reducing urinary saturation of stone-forming calcium salts. Potassium citrate has a hypocalciuric effect when given by mouth, probably due to enhanced renal calcium absorption. Urinary calcium excretion is unaffected by sodium citrate, since the alkali-mediated hypocalciuric effect is offset by a sodium-linked calciuresis.— *Lancet*, 1986, *1*, 955.

In an uncontrolled long-term study of 37 patients with recurrent calcium-oxalate nephrolithiasis, 17 of whom had hypocitraturia as the sole abnormality, 25 patients received treatment with potassium citrate alone and 12 patients received potassium citrate together with thiazide, allopurinol, or both. Potassium citrate therapy was associated with a sustained rise in urinary pH and citrate and potassium concentrations. The mean urinary pH rose by 0.7 to 1.0 and was maintained at 6.5 to 7.0. There was also a sustained reduction in the urinary saturation of calcium oxalate and a reduction in the stone formation rate of 89.2%.— C. Y. C. Pak and C. Fuller, *Ann. intern. Med.*, 1986, *104*, 33. Criticism.— G. D. Park and R. Spector (letter), *ibid.*, 723. Reply.— C. Y. C. Pak (letter), *ibid.*, 724.

Further references: K. D. Lake and D. C. Brown, *Drug Intell. & clin. Pharm.*, 1985, *19*, 530.

Preparations

Potassium Citrate Mixture *(B.P.)*. Potassium Citrate Oral Solution. Commonly known as Mist. Pot. Cit. Potassium citrate 3 g, citric acid monohydrate 0.5 g, syrup 2.5 mL, quillaia tincture 0.1 mL, lemon spirit 0.05 mL, double-strength chloroform water 3 mL, water to 10 mL. The mixture should be recently prepared and well diluted with water before use. Each 10 mL contains about 28 mmol of potassium.

For a report of incompatibility when Potassium Citrate Mixture was prepared with or diluted with syrup preserved with hydroxybenzoates, see under Sucrose, p.1276.

In a study of various non-sterile pharmaceutical preparations, Potassium Citrate Mixture *B.P.* was found to be inadequately preserved against microbial spoilage as determined by *B.P.* challenge tests.— T. R. R. Kurup and L. S. C. Wan, *Pharm. J.*, 1986, *2*, 761 (The formula for Potassium Citrate Mixture (*B.P. 1980*) is the same as that in *B.P. 1988*).

Potassium Citrate Mixture *(A.P.F.)*. Mist. Pot. Cit. Potassium citrate 2 g, citric acid monohydrate 0.4 g, lemon syrup 1 mL, concentrated chloroform water 0.2 mL or methyl hydroxybenzoate solution 0.1 mL, water to 10 mL. The mixture should be well diluted with water before use. Each 10 mL contains about 18.5 mmol of potassium.

Potassium Citrate Mixture CF *(A.P.F.)*. Potassium Citrate Mixture for Children. Potassium citrate 1 g, citric acid monohydrate 0.2 g, lemon syrup 1 mL, concentrated chloroform water 0.1 mL or methyl hydroxybenzoate solution 0.05 mL, water to 5 mL. The mixture should be well diluted with water before use. Each 5 mL contains about 9 mmol of potassium.

Potassium Citrate and Hyoscyamus Mixture *(B.P.C. 1973)*. Mist. Pot. Cit. et Hyoscy. Potassium citrate 3 g, citric acid monohydrate 0.5 g, hyoscyamus tincture 2 mL, syrup 2.5 mL, quillaia tincture 0.1 mL, lemon spirit 0.05 mL, double-strength chloroform water 2 mL, water to 10 mL. The mixture should be recently prepared and well diluted with water before use. Each 10 mL contains about 28 mmol of potassium.

Potassium Citrate and Sodium Bicarbonate Mixture *(A.P.F.)*. Potassium citrate 1 g, sodium bicarbonate 0.75 g, orange syrup 1 mL, concentrated chloroform water 0.2 mL or methyl hydroxybenzoate solution 0.1 mL, water to 10 mL. The mixture should be well diluted with water before use. Each 10 mL contains about 9 mmol of potassium and of sodium.

Potassium Citrate and Citric Acid Oral Solution *(U.S.P.)*. Contains, in each 100 mL, potassium citrate 20.9 to 23.1 g and citric acid monohydrate 6.34 to 7.02 g in a suitable aqueous vehicle, providing approximately 2 mmol of potassium per mL. pH 4.9 to 5.4.

Tricitrates Oral Solution *(U.S.P.)*. Contains, in each 100 mL, potassium citrate 10.45 to 11.55 g, sodium citrate dihydrate 9.5 to 10.5 g, and citric acid monohydrate 6.34 to 7.02 g in a suitable aqueous vehicle, providing approximately 1 mmol of potassium and 1 mmol of sodium per mL. pH 4.9 to 5.4.

Proprietary Preparations

Effercitrate *(Typharm, UK)*. *Tablets*, effervescent, potassium citrate (equivalent to 1.5 g), citric acid (equivalent to 0.25 g) providing 13.9 mmol of potassium.

Proprietary Names and Manufacturers
Effercitrate *(Typharm, UK)*; Efferkal *(Grossmann, Switz.)*; Kacitrin *(Switz.)*; Kajos *(Hässle, Norw.*; *Hässle, Swed.)*; Kation *(Schiapparelli, Ital.)*; Urocit-K *(Mission Pharmacal, USA)*.

The following names have been used for multi-ingredient electrolyte preparations containing potassium citrate—Bi-K *(USV Pharmaceutical Corp., USA)*; Effervescent Saline Tablets *(Southon-Horton, UK)*; K-Lyte *(Bristol, USA)*; Polycitra *(Willen, USA)*; Polycitra-K *(Willen, USA)*; Quik-Prep *(Jayco, USA)*; Twin-K *(Boots, USA)*; Twin-K-Cl *(Boots, USA)*.

See also under pp.1023-4.

1189-v

Sodium Acetate *(BAN, USAN)*.

E262; Natrii Acetas; Natrium Aceticum.
$CH_3.CO_2Na,3H_2O$=136.1.

CAS — 127-09-3 (anhydrous); 6131-90-4 (trihydrate).

Pharmacopoeias. In *Aust.*, *Br.*, *Braz.*, *Cz.*, *Eur.*, *Fr.*, *Ger.*, *Hung.*, *Ind.*, *It.*, *Jpn*, *Neth.*, *Nord.*, *Pol.*, *Swiss*, and *U.S.* which also allows the anhydrous form.
NOTE. The material described in *B.P.* and *Eur. P.* is not necessarily suitable for preparation of haemodialysis solutions.

Colourless transparent crystals or a white granular crystalline powder or white flakes, odourless or with a slight odour of acetic acid. It effloresces in warm dry air. Each g represents approximately 7.3 mmol of sodium and of acetate.
Soluble 1 in 0.8 of water and 1 in 19 of alcohol. A 5% solution in water has a pH of 7.5 to 9.2. **Store** in airtight containers.

Sodium acetate is used as a source of sodium and acetate ions in solutions for haemodialysis (see also under Dialysis Solutions, p.1023). The usual concentration range of sodium in dialysis fluid is about 130 to 140 mmol per litre. Sodium acetate may be added to total parenteral nutrition solutions as a bicarbonate precursor. It is also used as a food preservative.

Studies *in vitro* on human blood monocytes showed the production of intracellular interleukin-1 and its extracellular release to be higher in the presence of sodium acetate than it was in either sodium chloride or medium alone. The experiments had been carried out following reports of loss of ultrafiltration capacity and of progressive peritoneal fibrosis associated with the use of sodium acetate as a buffer in the exchange fluid of peritoneal dialysis, and it was considered that the widespread use of sodium acetate in haemodialysis solutions may also be contra-indicated.— M. Bingel *et al.*, *Lancet*, 1987, *1*, 14.

Preparations

Sodium Acetate Injection *(U.S.P.)*. pH 6 to 7. To be diluted before use.

Sodium Acetate Solution *(U.S.P.)*

See also under pp.1023-4.

1190-r

Sodium Bicarbonate *(BAN, USAN)*.

500; Baking Soda; Monosodium Carbonate; Natrii Bicarbonas; Natrii Hydrogenocarbonas; Sal de Vichy; Sodium Acid Carbonate; Sodium Hydrogen Carbonate.
$NaHCO_3$=84.01.

CAS — 144-55-8.

Pharmacopoeias. In *Arg., Aust., Belg., Br., Braz., Chin., Cz., Egypt., Eur., Fr., Ger., Hung., Ind., Int., It., Jpn, Jug., Mex., Neth., Nord., Pol., Port., Roum., Rus., Span., Swiss, Turk.*, and *U.S.* Also in *B.P. Vet.*

A white odourless crystalline powder Each g represents approximately 11.9 mmol of sodium and of bicarbonate. When heated or in moist air it decomposes, and is converted progressively into sodium carbonate.

Soluble 1 in 11 to 12 of water; practically insoluble in alcohol. A solution in water is alkaline to litmus; alkalinity increases on standing, agitation, or heating. A 1.39% solution in water is iso-osmotic with serum, and thus in most cases isotonic with blood serum and lachrymal secretions.

Sodium bicarbonate is **incompatible** with acids, acidic salts, and many alkaloidal salts. Sodium bicarbonate solutions should not be mixed with calcium or magnesium salts, cisplatin, dobutamine hydrochloride, labetalol hydrochloride, or oxytetracycline hydrochloride as this may result in the formation of insoluble precipitates. The following drugs have been reported to be susceptible to inactivation on mixing with sodium bicarbonate solution: adrenaline hydrochloride, benzylpenicillin potassium, carmustine, glycopyrronium bromide, isoprenaline hydrochloride, and suxamethonium chloride. **Store** in well-closed containers.

Adverse Effects and Treatment

Administration of sodium bicarbonate by mouth can cause stomach cramps and flatulence. Extravasation of irritant hypertonic sodium bicarbonate solutions resulting in tissue necrosis at injection site has been reported following intravenous administration.

Excessive administration of sodium bicarbonate may lead to metabolic alkalosis, especially in patients with impaired renal function. Symptoms may include shortness of breath, muscle weakness (associated with potassium depletion), and mental disturbances such as restlessness, convulsions, and coma. Muscle hypertonicity, twitching, and tetany may develop especially in hypocalcaemic patients due to increased protein binding and renal reabsorption of calcium. Excessive doses may also lead to sodium overloading and hyperosmolality; for symptoms see under sodium chloride, (p.1039).

Treatment of metabolic alkalosis and hypernatraemia associated with sodium bicarbonate overdose consists mainly of apppropriate correction of fluid and electrolyte balance. Replacement of calcium, chloride, and potassium ions may be of particular importance.

EFFECTS ON THE GASTRO-INTESTINAL TRACT. Spontaneous rupture of the stomach occurred in a 31-year-old man following ingestion of a not excessive dose of sodium bicarbonate which had been taken to relieve abdominal discomfort after a large meal.— M. R. Mastrangelo and E. W. Moore, *Ann. intern. Med.*, 1984, *101*, 649.

A survey of adverse reactions to drugs in children; of 7 children who had been given an effervescent preparation containing citric acid and sodium bicarbonate, there was one report of vomiting.— C. G. Woods *et al.*, *Br. med. J.*, 1987, *294*, 869.

OVERDOSAGE. Hypernatraemia developed in a 3-year-old girl who had been given excessive amounts of sodium bicarbonate for 10 days as a home remedy for abdominal pain. An increased serum-chloride concentration was also noted, the cause of which was not known. The patient survived after fluid therapy.— M. S. Puczynski *et al.*, *Can. med. Ass. J.*, 1983, *128*, 821. A view that this was a case of child abuse.— A. B. MacMillan *et al.* (letter), *ibid.*, *129*, 684. Comment.— M. S. Puczynski *et al.* (letter), *ibid;* B. S. Chang (letter), *ibid.*, 685.

Precautions

Sodium bicarbonate should be administered extremely cautiously to patients with congestive heart failure, renal impairment, cirrhosis of the liver, or hypertension, and to patients receiving corticosteroids. It is generally recommended that sodium bicarbonate should not be administered to patients with metabolic or respiratory alkalosis, hypocalcaemia, or hypochlorhydria.

Alkalinisation of the urine by sodium bicarbonate leads to increased renal clearance of acidic drugs. If this feature is being used to eliminate drugs such as salicylates or barbiturates then it is essential to maintain a high urine output.

See also under Cardiac Resuscitation below, under Uses.

For a report of the development of calcification in the superficial scalp veins of a neonate caused by simultaneous administration of sodium bicarbonate and calcium chloride through the same needle, see p.1029.

Absorption and Fate

Administration of sodium bicarbonate by mouth causes neutralisation of gastric acid with the production of carbon dioxide. Sodium bicarbonate not involved in that reaction is absorbed and in the absence of a deficit of bicarbonate in the plasma, bicarbonate ions are excreted in the urine along with sodium ions; the urine is rendered alkaline and there is an accompanying diuresis.

Uses and Administration

Sodium bicarbonate is an alkalinising agent used in the treatment of metabolic acidosis that can arise from a variety of disorders including diabetic coma, diarrhoea, kidney disturbances and shock; it may also be used to treat severe respiratory acidosis. The dose of sodium bicarbonate required must be calculated on an individual basis, and is dependent on the acid-base balance and electrolyte status of the patient. Sodium bicarbonate 8.4 g provides approximately 100 mmol of bicarbonate and of sodium.

In the treatment of moderate acidosis sodium bicarbonate is given by mouth and doses providing 100 to 200 mmol have been given daily. In acute metabolic acidosis, sodium bicarbonate may be given intravenously; doses providing up to 300 mmol may be necessary. Solutions of sodium bicarbonate available for parenteral use are often hypertonic and it may be necessary to carry out a suitable dilution before administration. Various regimens for administering parenteral sodium bicarbonate have been suggested including the slow intravenous infusion of a 1.26% solution. In the treatment of acidosis associated with cardiac arrest an undiluted hypertonic 8.4% solution may be given by intravenous injection. The subcutaneous route may be used in situations where administration by the intravenous route is not possible.

Overtreatment with bicarbonate should be avoided. It is recommended that the calculated bicarbonate deficit should not be replaced within the first 24 hours of treatment. Frequent monitoring of serum-electrolyte concentrations and acid-base status is essential.

Sodium bicarbonate causes alkalinisation of the urine and is used for example in renal tubular acidosis and cystinuria. It was also used as an adjunct to sulphonamide therapy (to increase solubility). Sodium bicarbonate is also used with a diuretic in the treatment of acute poisoning from weakly acidic drugs such as phenobarbitone and salicylates to enhance their excretion; this process is known as 'forced alkaline diuresis'.

When administered by mouth sodium bicarbonate neutralises acid secretions in the gastro-intestinal tract. It is therefore used as an antacid to relieve dyspepsia in doses of about 1 to 5 g that provide up to 60 mmol. It may also be given in the treatment of severe diarrhoea where there has been significant loss of bicarbonate.

Solutions of sodium bicarbonate are used as eye lotions, to aid the removal of crusts in blepharitis, as ear-drops, to soften and remove ear wax, and as lubricating fluids for contact lenses.

Sodium bicarbonate is also used in various preparations for double-contrast radiography where production of gas (carbon dioxide) in the gastro-intestinal tract is necessary.

A brief discussion on metabolic acidosis and its treatment, including the use of sodium bicarbonate.— D. J. Bihari, *Br. J. Hosp. Med.*, 1986, *35*, 89.

AQUAGENIC PRURITUS. Complete abolition of aquagenic pruritus symptoms was obtained by the addition to bath water of sodium bicarbonate 25 g in the case of one patient, and of 200 g in another. Itching occurred in both patients if the respective amount of sodium bicarbonate was not added.— A. -H. M. Bayoumi and A. S. Highet (letter), *Lancet*, 1986, *2*, 464.

ARRHYTHMIAS. After ingestion of imipramine hydrochloride 5.35 g a 23-year-old woman developed ventricular tachycardia which persisted despite hyperventilation with 100% oxygen. Despite the presence of respiratory alkalosis superimposed on metabolic acidosis administration of sodium bicarbonate 50 mmol immediately restored sinus rhythm. Although the patient had a blood pH greater than 7.35 sodium bicarbonate was successfully used on 2 further occasions to control arrhythmias that recurred despite continued hyperventilation and the administration of physostigmine. The use of sodium bicarbonate in the presence of combined metabolic and respiratory alkalosis is not without risk and should be reserved for life-threatening arrhythmias unresponsive to conventional therapy.— D. W. Molloy *et al.*, *Can. med. Ass. J.*, 1984, *130*, 1457. Comment questioning the proposed pharmacokinetic mode of action of sodium bicarbonate.— B. G. Pollock and J. M. Perel (letter), *ibid.*, *131*, 717. Reply.— K. W. Hall and J. Rabson (letter), *ibid.*

ASTHMA. Although sodium bicarbonate was given almost routinely to patients with severe asthma and respiratory acidosis this treatment was still unproved. Its use could sometimes be deleterious and could delay institution of other important measures. Apart from emergency situations when severe metabolic acidosis accompanies respiratory acidosis, such as may occur in respiratory arrest, respiratory acidosis should be corrected by improving alveolar ventilation.— R. P. McCombs *et al.*, *J. Am. med. Ass.*, 1979, *242*, 1521.

Administration of bicarbonate to 3 patients with severe status asthmaticus led to control of physiological pH despite persistent hypercapnia and allowed mechanical ventilation to be reduced.— S. M. Menitore and R. M. Goldring, *Am. J. Med.*, 1983, *74*, 898.

CARDIAC RESUSCITATION. Bicarbonate should be administered only if there is a measured acidosis. External chest compression produces poor cerebral blood flow and even less peripheral circulation. There is little effective venous return so lactic acid builds up but is not immediately returned to the circulation, this being delayed until the heart has restarted. Serious acid-base problems may occur in the period just after arrest, and it is essential that blood gases are monitored continuously every 15 minutes, possibly for several hours. Sodium bicarbonate provides a large hyperosmolar sodium load to an extremely compromised circulation and can produce sudden reduction in serum-potassium concentrations. It neutralises acid by the release of carbon dioxide, and a rise in the partial pressure of carbon dioxide leads to increased cerebral oedema. Movement of carbon dioxide into the cerebrospinal fluid makes central monitoring of pH by the brain difficult following restoration of cardiac output. If ventilation and restoration of renal function fail to control blood gas and acid-base abnormalities, small doses of bicarbonate can be given provided blood gases are constantly monitored. Hypokalaemia may precipitate cardiac arrest, especially in elderly patients taking digoxin and diuretics, and administration of bicarbonate can cause further reduction in serum-potassium concentrations.— A. D. Redmond, *Br. med. J.*, 1986, *292*, 1444.

Standards and guidelines for cardiopulmonary resuscitation and emergency cardiac care, including recommendations on the use of sodium bicarbonate. Adequate alveolar ventilation is the mainstay of the control of acid-base balance in cardiac arrest, and administration of sodium bicarbonate in the absence of adequate ventilation and intubation to correct acidosis will not lead to improvement in blood pH. Bicarbonate should be used, if at all, only after more proved interventions such as defibrillation, cardiac compression, support of ventilation including intubation, and pharmacologic therapies such as adrenaline and antiarrhythmics have been applied. Patients with pre-existing acidosis with or without hyperkalaemia may benefit from treatment with bicarbonate, but its use must be based on a clearly defined diagnosis. Administration in the postresuscitation phase should be guided by measurements of arterial pH and partial pressure of carbon dioxide in arterial blood. An initial dose of 1 mmol per kg body-weight (1 mL per kg of 8.4% solution) should be given intravenously, and then not more than half of this dose every 10 minutes thereafter.

In *children,* sodium bicarbonate may be used in the patient with prolonged cardiac arrest or in an unstable haemodynamic state with documented metabolic acidosis. An initial dose of bicarbonate 1 mmol per kg body-weight should be given intravenously, including the intra-osseous route. A dilute solution of 0.5 mmol per mL should be used in infants. Further doses of bicarbonate should be based on measured base deficits, but if such measurements are unavailable, subsequent doses of bicarbonate may be considered every 10 minutes of continued arrest.— *J. Am. med. Ass.*, 1986, *255*, 2905. See also R. J. Bray, *Br. J. Hosp. Med.*, 1985, *34*, 72.

CYSTIC FIBROSIS. In young cystic fibrosis patients with gastric acidity a supplement of sodium bicarbonate at meal times of up to 15 g per day may adjust the duodenal pH towards normal.— M. B. Mearns, *Archs Dis. Childh.*, 1985, *60*, 272.

DIABETIC KETOACIDOSIS. There is continuing controversy over the specific role of bicarbonate in the treatment of diabetic ketoacidosis. Untreated severe acidosis can lead to hypotension, peripheral vasodilation, and respiratory depression, while, on the other hand, administration of sodium bicarbonate to patients with diabetic ketoacidosis can lead to hypokalaemia, rebound metabolic alkalosis, and possibly cerebral oedema.

A discussion on diabetic ketoacidosis and its management including the use of bicarbonate.— D. N. W. Griffith and J. S. Yudkin, *Br. J. Hosp. Med.*, 1986, *35*, 82.

Results from a study in 32 patients with diabetic ketoacidosis indicated that administration of sodium bicarbonate did not affect the fall in blood-glucose concentration, but delayed the improvement in concentrations of lactate and total ketone bodies and in the lactate-pyruvate ratio observed during treatment with saline and insulin. The authors concluded that there was no metabolic indication for the use of intravenous bicarbonate in the treatment of diabetic ketoacidosis.— P. J. Hale *et al.*, *Br. med. J.*, 1984, *289*, 1035. Correspondence.— *ibid.*, 1985, *290*, 68. See also J. M. Leigh (letter), *ibid.*, 1984, *289*, 1384.

Neither a beneficial nor a deleterious effect was demonstrated in terms of clinical recovery or biochemical variables following administration of bicarbonate to patients with diabetic ketoacidosis.— L. R. Morris *et al.*, *Ann. intern. Med.*, 1986, *105*, 836. Correspondence. Further studies are needed.— *ibid.*, 1987, *106*, 635.

LACTIC ACIDOSIS. The value of intravenous sodium bicarbonate administration in the treatment of lactic acidosis has been questioned. Stacpoole (*Ann. intern. Med.*, 1986, *105*, 276) put forward the case against its use in an editorial which outlined results from studies carried out in humans and *dogs*. These results indicated that administration of bicarbonate may lack efficacy and could even be potentially deleterious. In a detailed reply to this editorial, Narins and Cohen (*ibid.*, 1987, *106*, 615) presented the case for its continued use. They argued that experiments in *animals* had limited clinical relevance to the treatment of life-threatening lactic acidosis in humans, and believed that the benefits of raising blood pH with bicarbonate in order to alleviate the hazardous cardiovascular effects produced by acidaemia far outweighed any possible risks associated with its administration. Both parties agreed however that further research into the role of bicarbonate therapy in lactic acidosis was required.

OESOPHAGEAL OBSTRUCTION. Administration of effervescent granules containing sodium bicarbonate, activated dimethicone, and anhydrous citric acid to 2 patients with absolute dysphagia due to impaction of a meat bolus in the oesophagus resulted in immediate passage of the bolus into the stomach (N. Campbell and P. Sykes, *Lancet*, 1986, *2*, 1405). However, Durham *et al.* (*ibid.*, 1987,*1*, 108) had found such an approach unsuccessful and suggested that the addition of glucagon to such a regime might be an alternative. Favourable results have been obtained with the use of various carbonated drinks in the non-endoscopic relief of oesophageal obstruction (D.G. John *et al.*, *ibid.*, 107; S.H. Mohammed and V. Hegedüs, *ibid.*, 393). Mohammed and Hegedüs reported an 80% success rate with carbonated drinks, which they considered to be the first line of treatment for impacted oesophageal foreign bodies due to their wide availability and their patient acceptability.

ORAL REHYDRATION. Oral rehydration solution containing bicarbonate or an identical solution containing chloride in place of bicarbonate was administered to 40 children with acute gastroenteritis aged 5 years old or less. Both solutions were found to be equally effective for rehydration and correction of acidosis and it was suggested that replacement of bicarbonate by chloride in such solutions would simplify production, increase stability, and reduce costs.— E. J. Elliott *et al.*, *Gut*, 1986, *27*, A1274.

Preparations

Sodium Bicarbonate Ear Drops *(B.P.).* Sodium bicarbonate 5 g, glycerol 30 mL, freshly boiled and cooled water to 100 mL. The ear-drops should be recently prepared.

Sodium Bicarbonate Ear Drops *(A.P.F.).* Aurist. Sod. Bicarb. Sodium bicarbonate 5 g, glycerol 30 mL, freshly boiled and cooled water to 100 mL. The ear-drops should be recently prepared.

Sodium Bicarbonate Eye Lotion *(A.P.F.).* Collyr. Sod. Bicarb.; Alkaline Eye Lotion. Sodium bicarbonate 3.5% in Water for Injections.

Sodium Bicarbonate Injection *(U.S.P.).* A sterile solution in Water for Injections, the pH of which may be adjusted by the addition of carbon dioxide. pH 7.0 to 8.5.

Sodium Bicarbonate Intravenous Infusion *(B.P.).* Sodium Bicarbonate Injection. A sterile solution in Water for Injections; sterilised by autoclaving.

Paediatric Sodium Bicarbonate Mixture *(B.P.C. 1973).* Mistura Carminativa pro Infantibus. Sodium bicarbonate 50 mg, ginger syrup 0.2 mL, concentrated dill water 0.1 mL, syrup 1.85 mL, double-strength chloroform water 2.5 mL, water to 5 mL. It should be recently prepared.

Sodium Bicarbonate Oral Powder *(U.S.P.)*

Sodium Bicarbonate Tablets *(U.S.P.)*

Compound Sodium Bicarbonate Tablets *(B.P.).* Soda Mint Tablets. Each contains sodium bicarbonate 300 mg. They have a peppermint flavour and should be allowed to dissolve slowly in the mouth. Store at a temperature not exceeding 25°.

Proprietary Preparations

Baritop *(Concept Pharmaceuticals, UK). Tablets,* effervescent, sodium bicarbonate 35 mg, tartaric acid 35 mg, calcium carbonate 5 mg, and dimethicone 3 mg. For production of gas in double-contrast radiography of the gastro-intestinal tract.

Carbex *(Ferring, UK). Oral granules,* sodium bicarbonate 1.26 g, activated dimethicone 42 mg, supplied with solution containing anhydrous citric acid 10%. For production of gas in double-contrast radiography of the gastro-intestinal tract.

Concept Effervescent Granules *(Concept Pharmaceuticals, UK). Oral granules,* effervescent, sodium bicarbonate 1.05 g, tartaric acid 1.05 g, dimethicones 0.15 g. For production of gas in double-contrast radiography of the stomach.

Min-I-Jet Sodium Bicarbonate *(IMS, UK). Injection,* sodium bicarbonate 42 mg/mL (4.2%) and 84 mg/mL (8.4%) in single-use prefilled syringes of 10 and 50 mL.

Nicholas CO_2 Granules *(Nicholas, UK). Granules,* sodium bicarbonate, carbon dioxide generating system for use in double contrast work.

Proprietary Names and Manufacturers

Alkaject *(Remedia, S.Afr.)*; Min-I-Jet Sodium Bicarbonate *(IMS, UK)*; Natriumbikarbonat *(DAK, Denm.)*; Nephrotrans *(Nefro-Pharma, Ger.; Salmon, Switz.)*; Neut *(Abbott, USA)*; Nicholas CO_2 Granules *(Nicholas, UK)*; Normogastryl *(Sabex, Canad.)*; Segmentan *(Hameln, Ger.)*; Sodibic *(Protea, Austral.)*.

The following names have been used for multi-ingredient preparations containing sodium bicarbonate—Actonorm Powder *(Wallace Mfg Chem., UK)*; Alka-Seltzer *(Bayer, UK)*; Alka-Seltzer (Antacid) *(Miles Laboratories, USA)*; Alka-Seltzer (Pain Reliever & Antacid) *(Miles, Canad.; Miles Laboratories, USA)*; Baritop *(Concept Pharmaceuticals, UK)*; Baros *(Mallinckrodt, Canad.)*; Carbalax *(Pharmax, UK)*; Carbex *(Ferring, UK)*; Caved-S *(Muir & Neil, Austral.; Tillotts, UK)*; Ceo-Two *(Beutlich, USA)*; Citrocarbonate *(Upjohn, Canad.)*; Colyte *(Reed & Carnrick, Canad.; Reed & Carnrick, USA)*; Concept *(Concept Pharmaceuticals, UK)*; Cystemme *(Abbott, UK)*; Dexsal *(Reckitt & Colman, Austral.)*; E-Z-Gas *(E-Z-EM, Canad.)*; Gastrocote *(MCP Pharmaceuticals, UK)*; Gastron *(Winthrop, UK)*; Gavigrans *(Reckitt & Colman, Austral.)*; Gaviscon Tablets, Infant Preparations, and Liquid *(Reckitt & Colman, Austral.; Reckitt & Colman Pharmaceuticals, UK)*; Gaviscon Granules *(Reckitt & Colman, Austral.)*; GoLytely *(Braintree, USA)*; Meracote *(Merrell Dow, Austral.)*; Pepsillide *(Cambridge Laboratories, Austral.)*; Pep-Uls-Ade *(Cambridge Laboratories, Austral.)*; Phosphate-Sandoz *(Sandoz, Canad.; Sandoz, UK)*; Prefagyl *(Sabex, Canad.)*; Pyrogastrone Tablets *(Winthrop, UK)*; Quik-Prep *(Jayco, USA)*; Roter *(Four Macs, Austral.; Anglo-French Laboratories, Canad.; Roterpharma, UK)*; Royvac *(Roy, Canad.)*; Unik-Zoru *(Therapex, Canad.)*; Ural *(Abbott, Austral.)*; Uro-Tainer Suby G *(Vifor, Switz.: CliniMed, UK)*.

See also under pp.1023-4.

1192-d

Sodium Acid Citrate *(BAN).*

Disodium Hydrogen Citrate; E331; Natrium Citricum Acidum.

$C_6H_6Na_2O_7,1\frac{1}{2}H_2O=263.1$.

CAS — 144-33-2.

Pharmacopoeias. In *Br.*, *Hung.*, and *Rus.*

A white odourless or almost odourless powder. Each g represents approximately 7.6 mmol of sodium and 3.8 mmol of citrate.

Soluble 1 in less than 2 of water; practically insoluble in alcohol. A 3% solution in water has a pH of 4.9 to 5.2.

1193-n

Sodium Citrate *(BAN, USAN).*

E331; Natrii Citras; Trisodium Citrate. Trisodium 2-hydroxypropane-1,2,3-tricarboxylate.

$C_6H_5Na_3O_7,2H_2O=294.1$.

CAS — 68-04-2 (anhydrous); 6132-04-3 (dihydrate).

Pharmacopoeias. In *Arg., Aust., Belg., Br., Chin., Cz., Egypt., Eur., Fr., Ger., Hung., Ind., Int., It., Jpn, Jug., Mex., Neth., Nord., Pol., Port., Roum., Swiss,* and *Turk. Rus.* and *Span.* specify $5\frac{1}{2}H_2O$. *Braz.* and *U.S.* specify anhydrous or dihydrate. Also in *B.P. Vet.*

White odourless granular crystals or crystalline powder; slightly deliquescent in moist air. Each g of sodium citrate (anhydrous) represents approximately 11.6 mmol of sodium and 3.9 mmol of citrate.

Each g of sodium citrate (dihydrate) represents approximately 10.2 mmol of sodium and 3.4 mmol of citrate.

B.P. **solubilities** are: soluble 1 in less than 2 of water; practically insoluble in alcohol. *U.S.P.* solubilities for the hydrous form are: soluble 1 in 1.5 of water and 1 in 0.6 of boiling water; practically insoluble in alcohol. Aqueous solutions, owing to their alkalinity, may be **incompatible** with acidifying agents. Solutions when stored may cause separation of particles from glass containers and solutions containing such particles must not be used. **Store** in airtight containers.

Sodium citrate, after absorption, is metabolised to bicarbonate; it then has similar actions to those of sodium bicarbonate. Sodium citrate is administered as an oral solution to relieve painful irritation caused by cystitis; up to about 15 g of the dihydrate (citrate 51 mmol; sodium 153 mmol) may be given daily in divided doses. Oral solutions should be taken well-diluted with water and preferably after meals. Sodium citrate has also been given by mouth prior to the induction of anaesthesia in order to prevent acid aspiration pneumonitis.

Solutions of sodium citrate are administered in doses of 450 mg of the dihydrate (citrate 1.5 mmol; sodium 4.6 mmol) as rectal enemas in the treatment of constipation, and solutions may also be used for bladder irrigation.

Sodium citrate has anti-clotting properties and is employed in mixtures as the acid citrate in the anticoagulation and preservation of blood for transfusion purposes.

Sodium citrate has also been used in dentifrices as a desensitising agent and has been added to milk for infant feeding to prevent the formation in the stomach of large curds.

ANTICOAGULATION. A report of the successful use of regional citrate anticoagulation for haemodialysis in 4 patients with acute renal failure complicated by active bleeding. Comparative studies in 4 stable patients with chronic renal failure, who were being maintained on long-term haemodialysis, indicated that citrate anticoagulation was equal to heparinisation in maintaining haemodialyser efficiency.— R. V. Pinnick *et al.*, *New Engl. J. Med.*, 1983, *308*, 258.

The mistaken use of sodium citrate instead of sodium heparin as an anticoagulant in an arterial blood sample led to a set of laboratory results which indicated severe non-respiratory acidosis when in fact the patient had mild respiratory alkalosis.— P. E. Stein and D. W. Goodier (letter), *J. clin. Path.*, 1986, *39*, 1046.

METABOLIC ACIDOSIS. Severe metabolic acidosis and secretory diarrhoea developed in an infant due to a previously undescribed congenital defect in sodium absorption. Citrate supplementation corrected and maintained fluid and electrolyte balance and at the age of nine the patient was reported to be developing normally despite continuing diarrhoea.— C. Holmberg and J. Perheentupa, *J. Pediat.*, 1985, *106*, 56.

Haemodialysis. In a double-blind crossover study 12 patients on chronic haemodialysis received an oral solution containing sodium citrate for 8 weeks and a placebo for 8 weeks. Sodium citrate corrected predialysis metabolic acidosis and was associated with an improvement in the predialysis plasma pH from 7.35 to 7.41 with values for serum bicarbonate and pH remaining within normal limits after dialysis. Similar results were found in patients on acetate dialysis and in those on bicarbonate dialysis. Patients gained 0.4 kg more body-weight between dialysis treatments while taking sodium citrate.— J. C. Van Stone, *Ann. intern. Med.*, 1984, *101*, 199.

Preparations

Acid Citrate Dextrose Solution (ACD) *(B.P.)*. This is included under Anticoagulant and Preservative Solutions for Blood. A sterile solution of sodium citrate and citric acid monohydrate with glucose or anhydrous glucose in Water for Injections. pH 4.5 to 5.0. Protect from light.

Anticoagulant Citrate Dextrose Solution *(U.S.P.)*. A sterile solution of citric acid, sodium citrate, and glucose in Water for Injections.

Anticoagulant Citrate Phosphate Dextrose Solution *(U.S.P.)*. A sterile solution of citric acid, sodium citrate, monobasic sodium phosphate, and glucose in Water for Injections.

Anticoagulant Citrate Phosphate Dextrose Adenine Solution *(U.S.P.)*. A sterile solution of citric acid, sodium citrate, monobasic sodium phosphate, glucose, and adenine in Water for Injections.

Anticoagulant Sodium Citrate Solution *(U.S.P.)*. A sterile solution in Water for Injections containing 3.8 to 4.2% of sodium citrate dihydrate or an equivalent amount of anhydrous sodium citrate. pH 6.4 to 7.5. It contains no antimicrobial agents.

Citrate Phosphate Dextrose Solution (CPD) *(B.P.)*. This is included under Anticoagulant and Preservative Solutions for Blood. A sterile solution of sodium citrate, citric acid monohydrate, and sodium acid phosphate with glucose or anhydrous glucose in Water for Injections. pH5 to 6. Protect from light.

Sterile Sodium Citrate Solution for Bladder Irrigation *(B.P.C. 1973)*. Sodium citrate 3 g, dilute hydrochloric acid 0.2 mL, freshly boiled and cooled water to 100 mL. Sterilised by autoclaving or by filtration. Not suitable for injection.

Sodium Citrate Irrigation *(A.P.F.)*. A sterile solution of sodium citrate 4% in Water for Injections. Sterilised by autoclaving. For use as a bladder irrigation.

Sodium Citrate Mixture *(B.P.C. 1973)*. Sodium citrate 3 g, citric acid monohydrate 500 mg, syrup 2.5 mL, lemon spirit 0.05 mL, quillaia tincture 0.1 mL, double-strength chloroform water 3 mL, water to 10 mL. The mixture should be recently prepared and well-diluted with water before administration. When a dose of less than 5 mL is prescribed, the mixture may be suitably diluted with syrup.

For a report of incompatibility when Sodium Citrate Mixture was prepared with or diluted with syrup preserved with hydroxybenzoates, see under Sucrose, p.1276.

Sodium Citrate Mixture *(A.P.F.)*. Mist. Sod. Cit. Sodium citrate 2 g, citric acid monohydrate 400 mg, lemon syrup 1 mL, concentrated chloroform water 0.2 mL or methyl hydroxybenzoate solution 0.1 mL, water to 10 mL. The mixture should be well-diluted with water before use.

Sodium Citrate Mixture CF *(A.P.F.)*. Sodium Citrate Mixture for Children. Sodium citrate 1 g, citric acid monohydrate 200 mg, lemon syrup 1 mL, concentrated chloroform water 0.1 mL or methyl hydroxybenzoate solution 0.05 mL, water to 5 mL. The mixture should be well-diluted with water before use.

Sodium Citrate Tablets *(B.P.)*. For use in infant feeding; they should be dissolved in water and the solution added to the feed.

Sodium Citrate and Citric Acid Oral Solution *(U.S.P.)*. A solution of sodium citrate dihydrate 9.5 to 10.5% and citric acid monohydrate 6.34 to 7.02% in a suitable aqueous vehicle. pH 4.0 to 4.4. Store in airtight containers.

Proprietary Preparations

Cymalon *(Sterling Health, UK)*. *Oral granules*, sodium citrate dihydrate 4 g in single-dose sachets providing approximately 41 mmol of sodium and 14 mmol of citrate. To be dissolved in water. For relief of symptoms of cystitis in women.

Cystemme *(Abbott, UK)*. *Oral powder*, effervescent, sodium citrate, sodium bicarbonate, in single-dose sachets with a combined alkalinity equivalent to sodium citrate 4 g. To be dissolved in water. For relief of symptoms of cystitis in women.

Micolette *(Ayerst, UK)*. *Rectal solution*, sodium citrate 450 mg, sodium lauryl sulphoacetate 45 mg, glycerol 625 mg, potassium sorbate, sorbitol, citric acid, in single-dose disposable containers of 5 mL.

Micralax *(Smith Kline & French, UK)*. *Rectal solution*, sodium citrate 450 mg, sodium alkylsulphoacetate 45 mg, sorbic acid 5 mg, glycerol, sorbitol, in single-dose disposable containers of 5 mL.

Relaxit *(Pharmacia, UK)*. *Rectal solution*, sodium citrate dihydrate 450 mg, sodium lauryl sulphate 75 mg, sorbic acid 5 mg, glycerol, sorbitol, in single-dose disposable containers of 5 mL.

Urisal *(Winthrop, UK)*. *Oral granules*, effervescent, sodium citrate dihydrate 4 g in single-dose sachets providing approximately 41 mmol of sodium and 14 mmol of citrate. To be dissolved in water. For relief of symptoms of cystitis in women.

Proprietary Names and Manufacturers of Sodium Acid Citrate and Sodium Citrate

Blood Pack-Sodium Citrate *(Fenwal, Denm.)*; Citralka *(Parke, Davis, Austral.*; *Belg.*; *Parke, Davis, Canad.)*; Citravescent *(Protea, Austral.)*; Citrosodina *(Roussel Maestretti, Ital.)*; Citrosodine Longuet *(Belg.)*; Cymalon *(Sterling Health, UK)*; Hi-Alkocit *(High Noon, Pakistan)*; Sodiocitrina *(Biologici Italia, Ital.)*; Urade *(Austral.)*; Urisal *(Winthrop, UK)*;

Manufacturers also include—*Travenol, UK*.

The following names have been used for multi-ingredient electrolyte preparations containing sodium acid citrate and sodium citrate—Bicitra *(Willen, USA)*; Citrocarbonate *(Upjohn, Canad.)*; Cystemme *(Abbott, UK)*; Dexsal *(Reckitt & Colman, Austral.)*; Diarrest *(Galen, UK)*; Micolette *(Ayerst, UK)*; Micralax *(Smith Kline & French, UK)*; Microlax *(Pharmacia, Austral.*; *Pharmacia, Canad.)*; Polycitra *(Willen, USA)*; Quik-Prep *(Jayco, USA)*; Relaxit *(Pharmacia, UK)*; Ural *(Abbott, Austral.)*.

See also under pp.1023-4.

1194-h

Sodium Lactate

E325. Sodium 2-hydroxypropionate.
$C_3H_5NaO_3$=112.1.

CAS — 72-17-3.

Pharmacopoeias. In *Chin.*, *Ger.*, *Nord.*, and *Roum.* with differing percentages of $C_3H_5NaO_3$.

1 g of $C_3H_5NaO_3$ represents approximately 8.9 mmol of sodium and of lactate.

Incompatibility has been reported with oxytetracycline hydrochloride and sodium bicarbonate.

NOTE. Solutions of sodium lactate, on keeping, may cause separation of small solid particles from glass containers; solutions containing such particles must not be used.

Sodium lactate, after absorption, is metabolised in 1 to 2 hours to bicarbonate; it then has similar actions to those of sodium bicarbonate (see p.1026). It has been given as an alternative to sodium bicarbonate in the treatment of metabolic acidosis and to alkalinise urine, usually as a solution containing bicarbonate (as lactate) 167 mmol and by intravenous infusion at a rate not exceeding 300 mL per hour. Compound lactate solutions have been given by mouth or by intravenous infusion in the treatment of metabolic acidosis associated with dehydration (e.g. Ringer-Lactate), or associated with potassium deficiency (e.g. Darrow's). Sodium lactate should not be administered to patients with severely impaired liver function or other seriously ill patients as they are at particularly high risk of developing lactic acidosis.

Sodium lactate also has humectant properties.

Lactate infusions have been reported to induce feelings of anxiety, especially in patients with anxiety states, and have been used as a pharmacological model in the evaluation of mechanisms involved in clinical anxiety.— M. Lader and M. Bruce, *Br. J. clin. Pharmac.*, 1986, *22*, 251.

Preparations

Compound Sodium Lactate Intravenous Infusion *(B.P.)*. Compound Sodium Lactate Injection; Hartmann's Solution for Injection; Ringer-Lactate Solution for Injection. A sterile solution containing sodium lactate 0.25% (prepared from lactic acid), sodium chloride 0.6%, potassium chloride 0.04%, and calcium chloride 0.027% in Water for Injections. It provides, per litre, sodium 131 mmol, potassium 5 mmol, calcium 2 mmol, bicarbonate (as lactate) 29 mmol, and chloride 111 mmol. Sterilised by autoclaving. pH 5 to 7. Store at a temperature not exceeding 25°.

Darrow's Solution. A solution containing sodium chloride 4 g, potassium chloride 2.7 g, and molar solution of sodium lactate 53.3 mL in one litre providing sodium 121 mmol, potassium 35 mmol, chloride 103 mmol, and bicarbonate (as lactate) 53 mmol.

Lactated Ringer's Injection *(U.S.P.)*. A sterile solution of calcium chloride, potassium chloride, sodium chloride, and sodium lactate in Water for Injections providing in each litre sodium approximately 130 mmol, potassium 4 mmol, calcium 2.7 mmol, chloride 104 to 115 mmol, and lactate 26 to 29 mmol. It contains no antimicrobial agents. pH 6.0 to 7.5.

Sodium Lactate Intravenous Infusion *(B.P.)*. Sodium Lactate Injection. A sterile 1.85% solution of sodium lactate in Water for Injections prepared from lactic acid. It provides, per litre, sodium 167 mmol and bicarbonate (as lactate) 167 mmol. The injection is approximately one-sixth molar. Sterilised by autoclaving. pH 5 to 7. Store at a temperature not exceeding 25°.

Sodium Lactate Injection *(U.S.P.)*. Sterile Sodium Lactate Solution *(U.S.P.)* in Water for Injections, or a sterile solution of lactic acid in Water for Injections prepared with the aid of sodium hydroxide. pH 6.0 to 7.3.

Sodium Lactate Solution *(U.S.P.)*. An aqueous solution containing not less than 50% w/w of sodium lactate. pH 5 to 9. Store in airtight containers.

See also under pp.1023-4.

1151-j

Calcium

Ca=40.08.

Calcium is the most abundant mineral in the body and is an essential body electrolyte. Homoeostasis is mainly regulated by the parathyroid hormone, by calcitonin, and by vitamin D. The body contains about 350 to 500 mmol of calcium per kg body-weight, approximately 99% of which is found in the skeleton. The normal concentration of calcium in plasma is between 2.2 to 2.6 mmol per litre. There is an inverse relationship between the concentration of calcium and that of phosphate. The intracellular (cytosol) calcium concentration ranges from 0.1 to 1 μmol per litre.

About 10 to 20 mmol of calcium is ingested daily in the typical diet. The amount absorbed varies depending on the requirements of the body, but is normally only 20 to 30 per cent. Excretion of calcium is mainly in the urine with some faecal loss; a small amount is also lost in sweat.

The amount of calcium required by an adult is about 600 mg (15 mmol) per day. Calcium supplements are seldom necessary except for growing children and pregnant women, whose requirements are greater, and those on parenteral nutrition. The calcium salts discussed below are generally used as a source of calcium.

NOTE. Each g of calcium represents approximately 25 mmol.

Hypercalcaemia

Hypercalcaemia, an increase in plasma-calcium concentration above the normal range, may be due to increased absorption from the gastro-intestinal tract or increased mobilisation from bone. The most common causes of hypercalcaemia are neoplastic disease and primary hyperparathyroidism. Other causes are excessive intake of vitamin D, hyperthyroidism, sarcoidosis, and thiazide diuretics.

Symptoms of hypercalcaemia may include anorexia, nausea, vomiting, constipation, abdominal pain, muscle weakness, mental disturbances, polydipsia, polyuria, bone pain, nephrocalcinosis, renal calculi, and, in severe cases, cardiac arrhythmias and coma.

Hypocalcaemia

Hypocalcaemia, a decrease in plasma-calcium concentration below the normal range, may be due to impaired or reduced absorption from the gastro-intestinal tract, increased deposition in bone, or to excessive losses, for instance during lactation. Hypocalcaemia may also be caused by hypoalbuminaemia which may in turn be the result of cirrhosis or the nephrotic syndrome. Other causes of hypocalcaemia include decreased parathyroid hormone activity, vitamin D deficiency, and hypomagnesaemia. Hyperphosphataemia which leads to hypocalcaemia is described on p.1034.

Symptoms may include paraesthesia, carpopedal spasm, extrapyramidal signs, muscle cramps, increased muscle excitability leading to tetany, convulsions, mental changes, dermatitis, and ECG changes.

1152-z

Calcium Acetate *(BAN).*

Dried Calcium Acetate; E263.

$C_4H_6CaO_4$=158.2.

CAS — 62-54-4.

Pharmacopoeias. In *Br.*

A white, odourless or almost odourless, hygroscopic powder. It may contain up to 7% of water. Each g (anhydrous) represents approximately 6.3 mmol of calcium and the equivalent of bicarbonate. Calcium acetate 3.95 g is approximately equivalent to 1 g of calcium.

Soluble 1 in 3 of water; slightly soluble in alcohol. A 5% solution in water has a pH of 7.2 to 8.2. **Store** in well-closed containers.

INCOMPATIBILITY. As for Calcium Gluconate.

Calcium acetate is used as a source of calcium and as an acetate supply of bicarbonate in haemodialysis and peritoneal dialysis solutions (see also under Dialysis Solutions, p.1023). The concentration of calcium in dialysis fluid ranges between 1 to 2 mmol per litre. However, a narrower range of 1.63 to 1.75 mmol per litre is considered to provide the optimum concentration.

Calcium acetate is also used as a food preservative.

Development of hypercalcaemia in a 35-year-old anuric woman with consumption coagulopathy was associated with the use of resorbable haemostatic compresses containing 4.6 to 6.8% w/w of calcium acetate.— D. Texier *et al.* (letter), *Lancet*, 1982, *1*, 688.

1154-k

Calcium Chloride *(BAN, USAN).*

509; Calcii Chloridum; Calcium Chloratum; Calcium Chloride Dihydrate; Cloreto de Cálcio; Cloruro de Calcio.

$CaCl_2,2H_2O$=147.0.

CAS — 10035-04-8; 10043-52-4 (anhydrous); 7774-34-7 (hexahydrate).

Pharmacopoeias. In *Arg., Aust., Belg., Br., Braz., Chin., Egypt., Eur., Fr., Ger., Ind., It., Jpn, Mex., Neth., Nord., Swiss,* and *U.S. Braz.* and *Nord.* also specify the hexahydrate. *Arg.* also specifies the anhydrous salt. *Cz., Hung., Int., Jug., Pol., Port., Roum., Rus., Span.,* and *Turk.* only specify the hexahydrate.

White, hygroscopic, odourless, crystalline powder or granules. Each g represents approximately 6.8 mmol of calcium and 13.6 mmol of chloride. Calcium chloride (dihydrate) 3.67 g is approximately equivalent to 1 g of calcium.

Soluble 1 in 0.7 to 1.2 of water, 1 in 0.2 of boiling water, 1 in 4 of alcohol, and 1 in 2 of boiling alcohol. A 5% solution in water has a pH of 4.5 to 9.2. **Store** in airtight containers.

INCOMPATIBILITY. As for Calcium Gluconate.

Adverse Effects, Treatment, and Precautions

As for Calcium Gluconate, p.1030.

Solutions of calcium chloride are extremely irritant and should not be injected intramuscularly or subcutaneously. Calcium chloride is irritant to the gastro-intestinal tract and must not be given to infants. Calcium chloride, because of its acidifying nature, is unsuitable for the treatment of hypocalcaemia caused by renal insufficiency.

Calcification of the superficial scalp veins developed in a neonate following the simultaneous administration of calcium chloride and sodium bicarbonate through a pre-existing scalp vein needle during resuscitation for cardiac arrest.— M. E. Speer and A. J. Rudolph, *Cutis*, 1983, *32*, 65.

For a report of vasospastic angina which occurred during general anaesthesia following the intravenous administration of calcium chloride, see under Calcium Gluconate, p.1030.

Uses and Adminstration

Calcium chloride has similar actions and uses to calcium gluconate (see p.1030) and is administered by slow intravenous or intracardiac injection usually as a 10% solution of the dihydrate. As calcium chloride is highly irritant, less irritating calcium salts such as calcium gluconate are often used in preference.

An opinion that calcium chloride rather than calcium gluconate should be the calcium salt of choice for parenteral indications: first, the body's retention of calcium chloride is greater and more predictable than its retention of calcium gluconate; second, the increase in extracellular ionised calcium concentration is unpredictable for the gluconate; finally, the positive inotropic effect of calcium chloride is greater than that of calcium gluconate.— L. I. G. Worthley and P. J. Phillips (letter), *Lancet*, 1980, *2*, 149.

CARDIAC RESUSCITATION. In a randomised double-blind study in a prehospital setting calcium chloride was administered intravenously to 18 patients with cardiac arrest refractory to adrenaline, bicarbonate, and atropine. Only one patient was successfully resuscitated, and it was concluded that the use of calcium chloride is of no value in resuscitation of refractory asystole in the prehospital setting.— H. A. Stueven *et al.*, *Ann. emerg. Med.*, 1984, *13*, 820.

Standards and guidelines for cardiopulmonary resuscitation and emergency cardiac care, including recommendations on the use of calcium. Calcium chloride as a 10% solution of the dihydrate is recommended in a dose of 0.2 mL per kg body-weight which will deliver 5.4 mg per kg of elemental calcium. The dose should be infused slowly and repeated in 10 minutes if required; further doses should be based on measured deficits of calcium.— National Conference on Cardiopulmonary Resuscitation and Emergency Cardiac Care, *J. Am. med. Ass.*, 1986, *255*, 2905.

See also under Calcium Gluconate, p.1030.

Preparations

Calcium Chloride Injection *(U.S.P.).* A sterile solution of calcium chloride in Water for Injections. pH 5.5 to 7.5.

Proprietary Preparations

Min-I-Jet Calcium Chloride *(IMS, UK). Injection,* calcium chloride 100 mg/mL, in single-use prefilled syringes of 10 mL.

Proprietary Names and Manufacturers

Chloro-Calcion *(Fr.)*; Min-I-Jet Calcium Chloride *(IMS, UK).*

The following names have been used for multi-ingredient electrolyte preparations containing calcium chloride—Artisial *(Jouveinal, Canad.)*; Calciforte *(Bio-Chemical Laboratory, Canad.)*; Chibret Iodo-chloride Collyrium *(Merck Sharp & Dohme-Chibret, Fr.)*; Miol (Formula M.I.) Cream *(BritCair, UK)*; Miol (Formula M.I.) Lotion *(BritCair, UK).*

See also under pp.1023-4.

1156-t

Calcium Glubionate *(USAN, rINN).*

Calcium Gluconate Lactobionate Monohydrate; Calcium Gluconogalactogluconate Monohydrate. Calcium D-gluconate lactobionate monohydrate.

$(C_{12}H_{21}O_{12},C_6H_{11}O_7)Ca,H_2O$=610.5.

CAS — 31959-85-0 (anhydrous); 12569-38-9 (monohydrate).

Each g represents approximately 1.6 mmol of calcium. Calcium glubionate monohydrate 15.2 g is approximately equivalent to 1 g of calcium.

INCOMPATIBILITY. As for Calcium Gluconate.

Calcium glubionate has similar actions and uses to calcium gluconate (below) and is administered as an injection or by mouth as a syrup. It may be administered intravenously or intramuscularly, however the intramuscular route is not recommended for children.

Preparations

Calcium Glubionate Syrup *(U.S.P.)*

Proprietary Preparations

Calcium-Sandoz *(Sandoz, UK). Injection,* calcium glubionate 1.375 g/10 mL (equivalent to calcium gluconate 10%) providing calcium 2.32 mmol.

Syrup, calcuim glubionate 3.26g, calcium lactobionate 2.17g/15 mL providing calcium 8.1 mmol in 15 mL.

Proprietary Names and Manufacturers

Calcium-Sandoz *(Sandoz, Austral.; Canad.; Sandoz, Denm.; Sandoz, Fr.; Sandoz, Norw.; Sandoz, Swed.; Sandoz, Switz.; Sandoz, UK)*; Dorcol Calcium Supplement *(Dorsey Laboratories, USA)*; Neo-Calglucon *(Sandoz, USA).*

1157-x

Calcium Gluceptate *(USAN).*

Calcium Glucoheptonate *(pINN).*

$C_{14}H_{26}CaO_{16}$=490.4.

CAS — 17140-60-2; 29039-00-7 (both anhydrous).

Pharmacopoeias. In *U.S.* which allows anhydrous or with varying amounts of water of hydration.

A white to faintly yellow amorphous powder. It is stable in air, but the hydrous forms may lose part of their water of hydration on standing. Each g represents approximately 2 mmol of calcium. Calcium gluceptate (anhydrous) 12.2 g is approximately equivalent to 1 g of calcium.

Freely **soluble** in water; insoluble in alcohol and many other organic solvents. A 10% solution in water has a pH of 6 to 8.

INCOMPATIBILITY. As for Calcium Gluconate.

Calcium gluceptate has similar actions and uses to calcium gluconate (below). It is given by slow intravenous injection as a 22% solution. Calcium gluceptate may be administered by intramuscular injection when administration by the intravenous route is not possible.

Preparations

Calcium Gluceptate Injection *(U.S.P.).* pH 5.6 to 7.0.

Proprietary Names and Manufacturers

The following names have been used for multi-ingredient electrolyte preparations containing calcium gluceptate—Calciforte *(Bio-Chemical Laboratory, Canad.).*

1158-r

Calcium Gluconate *(BAN, USAN).*

578; Calcii Gluconas; Calcium Glyconate. Calcium D-gluconate monohydrate.

$C_{12}H_{22}CaO_{14},H_2O$=448.4.

CAS — 18016-24-5 (monohydrate); 299-28-5 (anhydrous).

Pharmacopoeias. In *Arg., Aust., Belg., Br., Braz., Chin., Cz., Egypt., Eur., Fr., Ger., Hung., Ind., Int., It., Jpn, Jug., Mex., Neth., Nord., Pol., Port., Roum., Rus., Span., Swiss,* and *Turk.* Also in *U.S.* as the anhydrous or the monohydrate form.

Calcium borogluconate is included in *Aust.* and as an injection in *B.P. Vet.*

A white, odourless, crystalline or granular powder. Each g represents approximately 2.2 mmol of calcium. Calcium gluconate 11.2 g is approximately equivalent to 1 g of calcium.

Soluble 1 in 30 of water and 1 in 5 of boiling water. Calcium salts can form complexes with many drugs; this may result in the formation of a precipitate. Calcium salts are **incompatible** with oxidising agents, citrates, soluble carbonates, bicarbonates, phosphates, tartrates, and sulphates. Physical incompatibility has also been reported with amphotericin, cephalothin sodium, cephazolin sodium, cephamandole nafate, novobiocin sodium, dobutamine hydrochloride, prochlorperazine, and tetracyclines.

Adverse Effects

Administration of some calcium salts by mouth can cause gastro-intestinal irritation and constipation. Soft-tissue calcification due to extravasation of calcium solutions has also been reported. Injection of calcium salts intramuscularly or subcutaneously can cause local reactions including sloughing or necrosis of the skin.

Excessive administration of calcium salts leads to hypercalcaemia; for symptoms, see Hypercalcaemia, under Calcium. Too rapid injection of calcium salts may also lead to many of the symptoms of hypercalcaemia as well as a chalky taste, hot flushes, and peripheral vasodilation.

Brain calcification was found at autopsy in 13 of 17 stressed neonates who had survived for at least 5 days; calcium gluconate had been administered parenterally to all infants. It was suggested that a pathophysiologic state exists in such infants which may be exaggerated by parenteral administration of calcium.— D. G. Changaris *et al.*, *J. Pediat.*, 1984, *104*, 941.

A report of 2 cases of vasospastic angina occurring during general anaesthesia following administration of calcium chloride 1 g intravenously. It was suggested that a rapid increase in extracellular calcium concentration could possibly trigger coronary spasm in susceptible individuals.— M. Boulanger *et al.*, *Anesth. Analg.*, 1984, *63*, 1124.

Treatment of Adverse Effects

Severe hypercalcaemia should be treated with administration of sodium chloride by intravenous infusion to expand the extracellur fluid. This may be given with or followed by frusemide or other loop diuretics to increase calcium excretion. Other drugs which may be used if this treatment proves unsuccessful include calcitonin (see p.1338), the biphosphonates (p.1340), plicamycin (p.647), and corticosteroids. Disodium edetate (p.841) has been used. Phosphates (p.1034) may be useful, but should be given by mouth and only to patients with low serum-phosphate concentrations and normal renal function. Haemodialysis may be considered as a last resort. Careful monitoring of serum-electrolyte concentrations is essential throughout therapy.

Precautions

Solutions of calcium salts, particularly calcium chloride, are irritant, and care should be taken to prevent extravasation during intravenous injection. Calcium salts should be given cautiously to patients with impaired renal function, cardiac disease, or sarcoidosis.

Calcium enhances the effects of digitalis on the heart and may precipitate digitalis intoxication; parenteral calcium therapy is contra-indicated in patients receiving cardiac glycosides. Calcium salts reduce the absorption of tetracyclines.

Absorption and Fate

Calcium is absorbed from the small intestine; about one-third of ingested calcium is absorbed although this can vary depending upon dietary factors and the state of the small intestine. Absorbed calcium is excreted mainly in the urine with some faecal loss. Calcium is also excreted in saliva, sweat, breast milk, bile, and pancreatic juice.

Uses and Administration

Calcium salts are used mainly in the treatment of calcium deficiency. In simple deficiency states calcium salts may be given by mouth in doses to provide up to 50 mmol of calcium daily. Vitamin D analogues may be given concomitantly with calcium especially when hypocalcaemia is caused by vitamin D deficiency.

In acute hypocalcaemia and hypocalcaemic tetany parenteral administration is necessary. A typical dose is 2.25 to 4.5 mmol of calcium given by slow intravenous injection and repeated as required. Calcium may also be administered intravenously in this dose as an adjunct in the treatment of severe hyperkalaemia, repeated as required under ECG control. Intravenous injections of calcium have also been used in the treatment of acute colic.

Calcium salts may be given for their inotropic effect in cardiac resuscitation in doses of 2.25 mmol of calcium intravenously, or very occasionally by intracardiac injection. Calcium salts may also be used for the prevention of hypocalcaemia in exchange transfusions, and in long-term electrolyte replacement therapy.

Calcium gluconate is more acceptable for administration by mouth than other calcium salts as it is non-irritant to the stomach. It is usually administered by mouth as tablets; calcium gluconate 11 g provides approximately 25 mmol of calcium. For a more rapid effect calcium gluconate may be given intravenously or intracardially as a 10% solution. It may also be given intramuscularly if intravenous administration is not possible, however intramuscular injections are not recommended for children.

Calcium lactate gluconate, a related salt, is used in some preparations. 3.08 g of calcium lactate gluconate is equivalent to 4.5 g of calcium gluconate.

Calcium gluconate, applied as a gel or injected as a solution, is also used in the treatment of burns from hydrofluoric acid.

For a view that calcium chloride rather than calcium gluconate is the calcium salt of choice for parenteral preparations, see Calcium Chloride, p.1029.

CARDIAC RESUSCITATION. Movement of calcium ions is implicated in vasospasm; administration of calcium during cardiac arrest must therefore be questioned and can be endorsed only for electromechanical dissociation.—A. D. Redmond, *Br. med. J.*, 1986, *292*, 1444.

Standards and guidelines for cardiopulmonary resuscitation and emergency cardiac care, including recommendations on the use of calcium. Experimental evidence for the efficacy of calcium in the treatment of electromechanical dissociation and asystole is lacking. Calcium is indicated only when hypocalcaemia has been documented, and it may be considered in the treatment of hyperkalaemia, hypermagnesaemia, and calcium-channel blocker overdose.— National Conference on Cardiopulmonary Resuscitation and Emergency Cardiac Care, *J. Am. med. Ass.*, 1986, *255*, 2905. See also A. Stempien *et al.*, *Ann. intern. Med.*, 1986, *105*, 603; M. C. Finn (letter), *ibid.*, 1987, *106*, 630; A. M. Katz *et al.* (letter), *ibid.*, 631.

Differences in the calcium concentration of calcium-containing solutions can lead to considerable confusion about the dose administered. Suggestions put forward by the author to decrease the potential risk of underdosage or overdosage included the labelling of all calcium solutions in mmol per mL, and the standardisation of all calcium-containing preparations.— P. Nightingale (letter), *Lancet*, 1987, *1*, 1213.

HYPERTENSION. For references to the effects of calcium supplementation on blood pressure, see p.1023.

OSTEOPOROSIS. Calcium reduces bone loss in some postmenopausal women, but there are no guidelines as to which postmenopausal women may benefit. It also probably prevents further bone loss in established osteoporosis, and should be used where the disease is causing symptoms such as back pain, or a fractured proximal femur. The benefits however are likely to be marginal.— *Drugs for the Elderly*, Copenhagen, World Health Organisation, 1985, p.46.

Drugs that have been used in the treatment of established osteoporosis include calcium, oestrogens, calcitonin, sodium fluoride, and phosphates. The role of calcium supplements in the prevention and treatment of established osteoporosis is controversial and there is doubt about its efficacy. References:; B. L. Riggs and L. J. Melton, *New Engl. J. Med.*, 1986, *314*, 1676; B. Riis *et al.*, *ibid.*, 1987, *316*, 173; R. Smith, *Br. med. J.*, 1987, *294*, 329; *Lancet*, 1987, *1*, 370; P. L. Selby and R. M. Francis (letter), *ibid.*, 747; D. Y. Gillespie (letter), *ibid.*

RICKETS OF PREMATURITY. Results from a study in very low-birthweight infants who were given prophylactic treatment with either vitamin D alone, with phosphate, or with phosphate and calcium, indicated that supplementation with calcium and phosphate did not reduce the incidence of rickets of prematurity.— N. McIntosh *et al.* (letter), *Lancet*, 1986, *2*, 981. Dietary insufficiency of calcium and/or phosphate has been implicated in the pathogenesis of rickets of prematurity, but in any one infant the cause of disease is likely to be multifactorial. In the treatment of established disease one approach is to give extra calcium and phosphate along with an active vitamin D metabolite such as alfacalcidol, titrating the dose against alkaline phosphatase activity and radiographic evidence of healing. The goal is to promote maximum mineral absorption, retention, and utilisation, and to allow for the baby who has enzyme immaturity.— *ibid.*, 1987, *1*, 200. See also A. M. Sutton and F. Cockburn (letter), *ibid.*, 559.

Preparations

Calcium Gluconate Injection *(B.P.)*. A sterile solution of calcium gluconate in Water for Injections; not more than 5% of the calcium gluconate may be replaced with calcium D-saccharate, or other suitable calcium salt, as a stabiliser. Solutions are supersaturated and must be completely free from solid particles.

Calcium Gluconate Injection *(U.S.P.)*. A sterile solution of calcium gluconate, anhydrous or the monohydrate, in Water for Injections. It may contain small amounts of calcium saccharate or other suitable calcium salts as stabilisers; sodium hydroxide may be added to adjust the pH to 6.0 to 8.2.

Calcium Gluconate Tablets *(B.P.)*. If they are intended to be chewed before being swallowed they are prepared in a chocolate-flavoured basis.

Calcium Gluconate Tablets *(U.S.P.)*. Tablets containing calcium gluconate, anhydrous or the monohydrate.

Effervescent Calcium Gluconate Tablets *(B.P.)*. They should be dissolved in water immediately before use. Store at a temperature not exceeding 25° in well-closed containers.

Proprietary Preparations

Chocovite *(Medo, UK)*. *Tablets*, calcium gluconate 500 mg, ergocalciferol 15 μg (600 units), in a chocolate-flavoured basis.

Sandocal *(Sandoz, UK)*. *Tablets*, effervescent, calcium lactate gluconate 3.08 g (equivalent to calcium gluconate 4.5 g) providing calcium 10 mmol, sodium 6 mmol, potassium 4.5 mmol, and bicarbonate 10.5 mmol.

Proprietary Names and Manufacturers of Calcium Gluconate and Related Salts

Calcitrans *(Fresenius, Ger.)*; Dobo *(Wolfer, Ger.)*; Dreisacal *(Gry, Ger.)*; Glucal *(Lennon, S.Afr.)*; Sandocal *(Sandoz, UK)*; Vical *(Ital.)*; Vitaplex Supa-C *(Vitaplex, Austral.)*; Weifa-Kalk *(Weiders, Norw.)*;

The following names have been used for multi-ingredient electrolyte preparations containing calcium gluconate and related salts—Calciforte *(Bio-Chemical Laboratory, Canad.)*; Glucaloids *(Ingram & Bell, Canad.)*; Gramcal *(Anca, Canad.)*; Sandocal 1000 *(Sandoz, Austral.)*; Supac *(Mission Pharmacal, USA)*; Tonic Dellipsoids D 2 *(Pilsworth, UK)*.

1931-t

Calcium Glycerophosphate

Calcium Glycerinophosphate.

$C_3H_7CaO_6P(+xH_2O)=210.1$.

CAS — 27214-00-2 (anhydrous).

Pharmacopoeias. In *Arg.*, *Aust.*, *Belg.*, *Braz.*, *Fr.*, *It.*, *Mex.*, *Port.*, *Roum.*, *Span.*, and *Swiss.*

Calcium glycerophosphate may be administered by mouth as a source of calcium.

Proprietary Names and Manufacturers
The following names have been used for multi-ingredient electrolyte preparations containing calcium glycerophosphate—Calphosan *(Glenwood, USA)*.

See also under glycerophosphoric acid p.1576.

1160-z

Calcium Lactate *(BAN, USAN)*.

Calcii Lactas; E327. Calcium 2-hydroxypropionate.
$C_6H_{10}CaO_6,xH_2O$=218.2 (anhydrous); 308.3 (pentahydrate); 272.3 (trihydrate).

CAS — 814-80-2 (anhydrous); 41372-22-9 (hydrate); 5743-47-5; 63690-56-2 (both pentahydrate).

Pharmacopoeias. In *Arg., Aust., Belg., Br., Braz., Chin., Egypt., Eur., Fr., Ger., Hung., Ind., Int., It., Jpn, Mex., Neth., Nord., Pol., Port., Roum., Rus., Span., Swiss, Turk.,* and *U.S. Br.* has separate monographs for the pentahydrate and the trihydrate. *U.S.* allows anhydrous or hydrous forms. Also in *B.P. Vet.*

A white or almost white crystalline or granular powder. Each g (pentahydrate) represents approximately 3.2 mmol of calcium. Each g (trihydrate) represents approximately 3.7 mmol of calcium. Calcium lactate (pentahydrate) 7.7 g and calcium lactate (trihydrate) 6.8 g are approximately equivalent to 1 g of calcium.
Soluble 1 in 20 of water. The *B.P.* specifies freely soluble in boiling water; soluble 1 in 1500 of alcohol. The *U.S.P.* specifies that the pentahydrate is practically insoluble in alcohol. The pentahydrate effloresces on exposure to air and becomes anhydrous when heated at 120°. **Store** in airtight containers.

INCOMPATIBILITY. As for Calcium Gluconate.

Calcium lactate has similar actions and uses to calcium gluconate (p.1029). It is administered by mouth as tablets or in solution.

Preparations
Calcium Lactate Tablets *(B.P.)*
Calcium Lactate Tablets *(U.S.P.)*. The content of calcium lactate is expressed in terms of the pentahydrate.

Proprietary Names and Manufacturers
Spuman *(Luitpold, Ger.)*; Taxofit *(Anasco, Ger.)*;
Manufacturers also include—*Upjohn, USA.*

The following names have been used for multi-ingredient electrolyte preparations containing calcium lactate—Calciforte *(Bio-Chemical Laboratory, Canad.)*; Calphosan *(Glenwood, USA)*; Citrocarbonate *(Upjohn, Canad.)*.

1161-c

Calcium Laevulinate

Calcii Levulinas; Calcium Laevulate; Calcium Levulinate *(USAN)*; Lévulinate Calcique. Calcium 4-oxovalerate dihydrate.
$C_{10}H_{14}CaO_6,2H_2O$=306.3.

CAS — 591-64-0 (anhydrous); 5743-49-7 (dihydrate).

Pharmacopoeias. In *Aust., Belg., Braz., Egypt., Ind., Nord., Span., Swiss,* and *U.S.*

A white crystalline or amorphous powder with an odour suggestive of burnt sugar. Each g represents approximately 3.3 mmol of calcium. Calcium laevulinate 7.64 g is approximately equivalent to 1 g of calcium.
Freely **soluble** in water; slightly soluble in alcohol; insoluble in chloroform and ether. A 10% solution in water has a pH of 7.0 to 8.5.

INCOMPATIBILITY. As for Calcium Gluconate.

Calcium laevulinate has similar actions and uses to calcium gluconate (p.1029).It has been given by mouth and by intravenous and intramuscular injection.

Preparations
Calcium Levulinate Injection *(U.S.P.)*

Proprietary Names and Manufacturers
Levucal *(Canad.)*.

1159-f

Calcium Hydrogen Phosphate *(BAN)*.

Calcii et Hydrogenii Phosphas; Calcii Hydrogenophosphas; Calcium Hydrophosphoricum; Calcium Monohydrogen Phosphate; Dibasic Calcium Phosphate *(USAN)*; Dicalcium Orthophosphate; Dicalcium Phosphate; E341. Calcium hydrogen orthophosphate dihydrate.
$CaHPO_4,2H_2O$=172.1.

CAS — 7757-93-9 (anhydrous); 7789-77-7 (dihydrate).

Pharmacopoeias. In *Arg., Aust., Belg., Br., Eur., Fr., Ger., Hung., Ind., It., Jpn, Jug., Mex., Neth., Nord., Pol., Port., Rus., Span.,* and *Swiss.* Also in *U.S.* which also permits anhydrous calcium hydrogen phosphate.

A white, odourless, crystalline powder. Each g represents approximately 5.8 mmol of calcium and of phosphate. Calcium hydrogen phosphate 4.3 g is approximately equivalent to 1 g of calcium.
The *B.P.* specifies: practically **insoluble** in cold water and alcohol; soluble in dilute acids. The *U.S.P.* specifies: practically insoluble in water; soluble in 3*N* hydrochloric acid and in 2*N* nitric acid; insoluble in alcohol.
Store in well-closed containers.

1162-k

Calcium Phosphate *(BAN)*.

Calcium Orthophosphate; E341 *(tricalcium diorthophosphate)*; Fosfato Tricalcico; Phosphate Tertiaire de Calcium; Precipitated Calcium Phosphate; Tribasic Calcium Phosphate *(USAN)*; Tricalcium Phosphate.

CAS — 7758-87-4 [$Ca_3(PO_4)_2$].

Pharmacopoeias. In *Arg., Br., Fr., Hung., Ind., Mex., Port., Roum., Span., Swiss,* and *U.S.N.F.*

A white, odourless or almost odourless, amorphous powder. The *B.P.* specifies that it consists mainly of tricalcium diorthophosphate $Ca_3(PO_4)_2$ (310.2), together with calcium phosphates of more acidic or basic character. The *U.S.N.F.* specifies that it consists of a variable mixture of calcium phosphates having the approximate composition $10CaO,3P_2O_5.H_2O$. Each g $Ca_3(PO_4)_2$ represents approximately 9.7 mmol of calcium and 6.4 mmol of phosphate. Calcium phosphate ($Ca_3(PO_4)_2$) 2.6 g is approximately equivalent to 1 g of calcium.
Practically **insoluble** in water and alcohol.

INCOMPATIBILITY. As for Calcium Gluconate.

Calcium phosphate has similar actions and uses to calcium gluconate (p.1029) and is administered by mouth usually as calcium hydrogen phosphate when it may be of use in patients requiring both calcium and phosphorus supplementation.
Calcium phosphate is a useful non-hygroscopic diluent for powders and vegetable extracts but it should not be used as a diluent in ergocalciferol preparations because it may considerably modify the absorption of high doses of the vitamin. It is used as a tablet excipient particularly in compression-coated tablets, and in fine powder as an abrasive in toothpastes.
Calcium phosphate (Calcarea Phosphorica; Calc. Phos.) is used in homoeopathic medicine.

Preparations
Dibasic Calcium Phosphate Tablets *(U.S.P.)*. Tablets containing calcium hydrogen phosphate. Potency is expressed in terms of the dihydrate.

Proprietary Names and Manufacturers
Calcevidol *(Ital.)*; DCP 340 *(Parke, Davis, Austral.; Canad.)*; Emcompress *(Mendell, USA: Forum Chemicals, UK)*; Kafoma *(Ferring, Swed.)*; Kalk *(NAF, Norw.)*; Ostram *(Merck-Clévenot, Fr.)*; Posture *(Ayerst, USA)*; Trikalkol *(Laves, Ger.)*.

12511-d

Calcium Pidolate

Calcium Pyroglutamate. Calcium 5-oxopyrrolidine-2-carboxylate.
$Ca(C_5H_6NO_3)_2$=296.3.

Each g represents approximately 3.4 mmol of calcium. Calcium pidolate 7.4 g is approximately equivalent to 1 g of calcium.

INCOMPATIBILITY. As for Calcium Gluconate.

Calcium pidolate has actions and uses similar to calcium gluconate (p.1029). It is administered by mouth in doses of 2 to 4 g daily (calcium 6.8 to 13.5 mmol).

Proprietary Names and Manufacturers
Efical *(Millot-Solac, Fr.)*; Ibercal *(Boi, Spain)*.

1164-t

Calcium Sodium Lactate *(BAN)*.

$2C_3H_5NaO_3,(C_3H_5O_3)_2Ca,4H_2O$=514.4.

Pharmacopoeias. In *Br.* Also in *B.P. Vet.*

A white deliquescent powder or granules with a slight characteristic odour. Each g represents approximately 1.9 mmol of calcium and 3.9 mmol of sodium. Calcium sodium lactate 12.8 g is approximately equivalent to 1 g of calcium.
Soluble 1 in 14 of water and 1 in 25 of boiling alcohol; practically insoluble in ether. **Store** in well-closed containers.

Calcium sodium lactate has similar actions and uses to calcium gluconate (see p.1029) and is administered by mouth.

Preparations
Calcium Sodium Lactate Tablets *(B.P.C. 1973)*. Store in airtight containers.
Calcium with Vitamin D Tablets *(B.P.C. 1973)*. Each contains calcium sodium lactate 450 mg, calcium phosphate 150 mg, and ergocalciferol 12.5 µg (500 units). The tablets should be crushed before administration. Store in a cool place in airtight containers.

BEE STINGS. A view that Calcium with Vitamin D Tablets were effective in controlling the swelling that follows bee stings. A dose of 2 tablets three times a day had been used.— D. A. Long (letter), *Prescribers' J.*, 1980, *20*, 52.

1168-d

Hydroxyapatite *(BAN)*.

542 *(edible bone phosphate)*. Decacalcium dihydroxide hexakis (orthophosphate).
$3Ca_3(PO_4)_2,Ca(OH)_2$=1004.6.

CAS — 1306-06-5.

A natural mineral with composition similar to that of the mineral in bone.

Hydroxyapatite for therapeutic purposes is prepared from bovine bone and contains, in addition to calcium and phosphate, trace elements, fluoride and other ions, proteins, and glycosaminoglycans. It is administered by mouth to patients requiring both calcium and phosphorus supplementation.

Hydroxyapatite has been used in the management of bone-wasting conditions with some response: K. H. Nilsen *et al.*, *Br. med. J.*, 1978, *2*, 1124 (for prophylaxis of osteoporosis in corticosteroid-treated rheumatoid arthritis); C. E. Dent and I. J. T. Davies, *J. R. Soc. Med.*, 1980, *73*, 780 (with dihydrotachysterol in the treatment of osteoporosis); O. Epstein *et al.*, *Am. J. clin. Nutr.*, 1982, *36*, 426 (in the treatment of cortical bone thinning due to primary biliary cirrhosis); A. Pines *et al.*, *Curr. med. Res. Opinion*, 1984, *8*, 734 (in the prevention of osteoporosis due to corticosteroid therapy); A. Stellon *et al.*, *Postgrad. med. J.*, 1985, *61*, 791 (in the prevention of bone loss in corticosteroid patients with chronic active hepatitis).
Satisfactory results were obtained in 60 patients with ossicular chain defects of the middle ear following reconstruction with hydroxyapatite implants.— J. J. Grote, *Ann. Otol. Rhinol. Lar.*, 1986, *95*, *Suppl.* 123, 10.

Proprietary Preparations
Ossopan *(Labaz Sanofi, UK)*. *Powder*, microcrystalline

hydroxyapatite 820 mg providing calcium 176 mg and phosphorus 82 mg. One level 5 mL spoonful contains approximately 4 g. *Dose.* One or two level 5-mL spoonfuls daily in divided doses, with or before food.

Ossopan 800 *(Labaz Sanofi, UK). Tablets,* microcrystalline hydroxyapatite 830 mg providing calcium 178 mg and phosphorus 83 mg. *Dose.* Four to eight tablets daily in divided doses, before meals.

Proprietary Names and Manufacturers
Ossopan *(Fr.; Berna, Spain; Labaz Sanofi, UK).*

1170-k

Magnesium

Mg=24.305.

Magnesium is the second most abundant cation in intracellular fluid and is an essential body electrolyte. It is a cofactor in numerous enzyme systems and is involved in phosphate transfer, muscle contractility, and neuronal transmission. The body contains about 14 mmol of magnesium per kg body-weight, approximately 50 per cent of which is found in the skeleton. The normal concentration of magnesium in intracellular fluid and plasma is about 15 and 0.75 to 1.1 mmol per litre respectively.

About 10 to 20 mmol of magnesium is ingested daily in the typical diet and 30 to 40 per cent is absorbed, mainly in the small intestine. Excretion of absorbed magnesium is mainly in the urine with some faecal loss; small amounts may also be excreted in breast milk and saliva.

The amount of magnesium required by an adult is 250 to 360 mg (10 to 15 mmol) per day; children require more than this.

NOTE. Each g of magnesium represents approximately 41.1 mmol.

Hypermagnesaemia

Hypermagnesaemia, an increase in plasma-magnesium concentration above the normal range, occurs rarely but has occurred after the excessive use of magnesium-containing antacids and laxatives, and especially in renal insufficiency. Symptoms of hypermagnesaemia may include flushing of the skin, thirst, hypotension due to peripheral vasodilatation, drowsiness, confusion, loss of tendon reflexes due to neuromuscular blockade, muscle weakness, respiratory depression, cardiac arrhythmias, coma, and cardiac arrest.

Hypomagnesaemia

Hypomagnesaemia, a decrease in plasma-magnesium concentration below the normal range, is often associated with deficiency of calcium and potassium. Deficiency may occur due to reduced intake, malabsorption, and excessive loss due to vomiting, diarrhoea, and drainage from fistulas; it is commonly associated with alcoholism, pancreatitis, aldosteronism, and may occur in renal tubular necrosis, after the use of diuretics, after the infusion of magnesium-free fluids, especially in diabetic acidosis.

Symptoms may include nausea, vomiting, abdominal pain, muscle tremor and weakness, lethargy, tetany due to increased muscle excitability, ataxia, mental disturbances, convulsions, cardiac arrhythmias, tachycardia, and cardiac arrest.

1171-a

Magnesium Acetate *(BAN).*

$C_4H_6MgO_4,4H_2O$=214.5.

CAS — 142-72-3 (anhydrous); 16674-78-5 (tetrahydrate).

Pharmacopoeias. In *Br.*

Odourless or almost odourless colourless crystals or a white crystalline powder. Each g represents approximately 4.7 mmol of magnesium and the equivalent of bicarbonate. Magnesium acetate (tetrahydrate) 8.8 g is approximately equivalent to 1 g of magnesium.

Soluble 1 in 1.5 of water and 1 in 4 of alcohol. A 5% solution in water has a pH of 7.5 to 8.5. **Store** in well-closed containers.

Magnesium acetate is used as a source of magnesium and as an acetate supply of bicarbonate in haemodialysis and peritoneal dialysis solutions (see also under Dialysis Solutions, p.1023).

12907-x

Magnesium Ascorbate

$(C_6H_7O_6)_2Mg$=374.5.

CAS — 15431-40-0.

Each g represents approximately 2.7 mmol of magnesium. Magnesium ascorbate 15.4 g is approximately equivalent to 1 g of magnesium.

Magnesium ascorbate may be used similarly to magnesium sulphate (p.1033) in the treatment of hypomagnesaemia.

Proprietary Names and Manufacturers
Magnorbin *(E. Merck, Ger.; Bracco, Ital.).*

600-z

Magnesium Aspartate

Magnesium aminosuccinate tetrahydrate.
$C_8H_{12}MgN_2O_8,4H_2O$=360.6.

CAS — 7018-07-7 (tetrahydrate).

Pharmacopoeias. In *It.*

Magnesium aspartate may be used similarly to magnesium sulphate (p.1033) in the treatment of hypomagnesaemia. Magnesium aspartate hydrochloride is also used.

For reference to the effect of magnesium, administered as magnesium aspartate hydrochloride, on blood pressure, see under Magnesium Sulphate, p.1033.

Proprietary Names and Manufacturers
Magmin *(Vitaplex, Austral.)*; Magnesiocard *(Verla, Ger.; Verla-Pharm, Switz.)*; Magnetrans *(Fresenius, Ger.)*; Mg 5-Granoral *(Artesan, Ger.; Artesan, Switz.)*; Mg 5-Longoral *(Artesan, Ger.; Artesan, Switz.)*; Manufacturers also include—*Sas, UK.*

The following names have been used for multi-ingredient electrolyte preparations containing magnesium aspartate—Aspara *(Jpn)*; K-Mag *(Vitaplex, Austral.)*; Panangin *(Gedeon Richter, Hung.)*; Trommcardin *(Trommsdorff, Ger.)*; Trophicard *(Köhler, Ger.).*

1172-t

Magnesium Chloride *(BAN, USAN).*

Chlorure de Magnésium Cristallisé; Cloreto de Magnésio; Magnesii Chloridum; Magnesium Chloratum.
$MgCl_2,6H_2O$=203.3.

CAS — 7786-30-3 (anhydrous); 7791-18-6 (hexahydrate).

Pharmacopoeias. In *Arg., Aust., Br., Cz., Eur., Fr., Ger., Ind., It., Jug., Neth., Nord., Port., Swiss,* and *U.S.* Also in *B.P. Vet.* Magnesium Chloride specified in the *B.P.* is not necessarily suitable for dialysis.

Colourless odourless hygroscopic crystals or flakes. Each g represents approximately 4.9 mmol of magnesium and 9.8 mmol of chloride. Magnesium chloride (hexahydrate) 8.4 g is approximately equivalent to 1 g of magnesium.

Soluble 1 in 1 of water and 1 in 2 of alcohol. A 5% solution in water has a pH of 4.5 to 7.0. **Store** in airtight containers.

Magnesium chloride is used as a source of magnesium and chloride in haemodialysis and peritoneal dialysis solutions. It may be used similarly to magnesium suphate (p.1033) in the treatment of hypomagnesaemia.

Uraemic pruritus, unresponsive to conventional treatments, in a patient undergoing chronic haemodialysis was promptly relieved when the magnesium concentration of the dialysate was lowered to produce a predialysis serum-magnesium concentration of 0.57 mmol per litre.— H. Graf *et al., Br. med. J.,* 1979, *2,* 1478.

Proprietary Preparations

Miol (Formula M.I.) *(BritCair, UK). Cream,* magnesium chloride 1.5%, sodium chloride 2.1%, calcium chloride 0.2%, alcloxa 1%, chlorphenesin 0.1%, camphor 4%. *Lotion,* magnesium chloride 1.42%, sodium chloride 1.98%, calcium chloride 0.17%, alcloxa 1%, camphor 1%. For pruritic, inflammatory, and ulcerative conditions of the skin and mucosa.

Encouraging results were obtained in 120 patients suffering from stasis ulcers (44), varicose eczema (36), varicose eczema with superimposed contact eczema (20), severe intertrigo (13), cutaneous angiitis (4), Darier's disease (1), widespread capillary haemangioma with ulceration (1), and benign familial chronic pemphigus (1), and treated with a hypertonic cream or lotion containing magnesium chloride, sodium chloride, camphor, and other ingredients (Miol). All lesions were initially infected and 96 patients obtained substantial clinical improvement which was maintained for at least a month.— P. W. M. Copeman and S. Selwyn, *Br. med. J.,* 1975, *4,* 264. Criticism.— K. Haeger (letter), *ibid.,* 1976, *1,* 155. Reply.— S. Selwyn and P. Copeman (letter), *ibid.,* 399.

Proprietary Names and Manufacturers
Slow-Mag *(Glenfair, S.Afr.).*

The following names have been used for multi-ingredient electrolyte preparations containing magnesium chloride—Artisial *(Jouveinal, Canad.)*; Miol (Formula M.I.) Cream *(BritCair, UK)*; Miol (Formula M.I.) Lotion *(BritCair, UK)*; Prefagyl *(Sabex, Canad.).*

See also under pp.1023-4.

12909-f

Magnesium Gluceptate

Magnesium Glucoheptonate.
$C_{14}H_{26}MgO_{16}$=474.7.

Each g represents approximately 2.1 mmol of magnesium. Magnesium gluceptate 19.5 g is approximately equivalent to 1 g of magnesium.

Magnesium gluceptate may be used similarly to magnesium sulphate (p.1033) in the treatment of hypomagnesaemia.

Proprietary Names and Manufacturers
Magnesium-Rougier *(Rougier, Canad.)*; Magneston *(Berenguer-Beneyto, Spain).*

1203-w

Magnesium Gluconate *(USAN).*

Magnesium D-gluconate.
$C_{12}H_{22}MgO_{14}$=414.6.

CAS — 3632-91-5 (anhydrous); 59625-89-7 (dihydrate).

Pharmacopoeias. In *U.S.* which allows either anhydrous or the dihydrate.

Colourless odourless crystals or a white powder or granules. Each g represents approximately 2.4 mmol of magnesium. Magnesium gluconate (anhydrous) 17 g is approximately equivalent to 1 g of magnesium. Freely **soluble** in water; very slightly soluble in alcohol; practically insoluble in ether. A 5% solution in water has a pH of 6.0 to 7.8.

Magnesium gluconate may be used similarly to magnesium sulphate (p.1033) in the treatment of hypomagnesaemia.

Preparations

Magnesium Gluconate Tablets *(U.S.P.).* Potency is

expressed in terms of the equivalent amount of anhydrous magnesium gluconate.

Proprietary Names and Manufacturers
Erimag *(ICN, Canad.)*; GYN *(Amfre-Grant, USA)*; Maglucate *(Pharmascience, Canad.)*; Ultra Mg *(Sopar, Belg.)*.

1938-m

Magnesium Glycerophosphate
Magnesium Glycerinophosphate.
$C_3H_7MgO_6P(+xH_2O)=194.4$.

CAS — 927-20-8 (anhydrous).

Magnesium glycerophosphate may be administered by mouth as a source of magnesium.

12911-c

Magnesium Lactate
Magnesium 2-hydroxypropionate.
$C_6H_{10}MgO_6=202.4$.

CAS — 18917-93-6.

Each g represents approximately 4.9 mmol of magnesium. Magnesium lactate 8.3 g is approximately equivalent to 1 g of magnesium.

Magnesium lactate may be used similarly to magnesium sulphate (below) in the treatment of hypomagnesaemia.

Proprietary Names and Manufacturers
Ionimag *(Valpan, Fr.)*; Magnesioboi *(Boi, Spain)*; Magnespasmyl *(CCP, Belg.; Gerbiol, Fr.; Clin-Midy, Switz.)*.

12912-k

Magnesium Pidolate
Magnesium Pyroglutamate. Magnesium 5-oxopyrrolidine-2-carboxylate.
$(C_5H_6NO_3)_2Mg=280.5$.

CAS — 62003-27-4.

Each g represents approximately 3.6 mmol of magnesium. Magnesium pidolate 11.5 g is approximately equivalent to 1 g of magnesium.

Magnesium pidolate may be used similarly to magnesium sulphate (below) in the treatment of hypomagnesaemia.

Proprietary Names and Manufacturers
Actimag *(Faes, Spain)*; Mag 2 *(Mêram, Fr.; Lirca, Ital.; Casen Fisons, Spain; Sapos, Switz.)*; Solumag *(Biothérax, Fr.)*.

1174-r

Magnesium Sulphate *(BAN)*.

518; Epsom Salts; Magnesii Sulfas; Magnesium Sulfate *(USAN)*; Magnesium Sulfuricum Heptahydricum; Sal Amarum; Sel Anglais; Sel de Sedlitz.
$MgSO_4,7H_2O=246.5$.

CAS — 10034-99-8.

Pharmacopoeias. In *Arg., Aust., Belg., Br., Braz., Chin., Cz., Egypt., Eur., Fr., Ger., Hung., Ind., It., Jpn, Jug., Mex., Neth., Nord., Pol., Port., Roum., Rus., Span., Swiss, Turk.*, and *U.S.* which allows the anhydrous, monohydrate, or heptahydrate form. Also in *B.P. Vet.*

Odourless, brilliant, colourless crystals or a white crystalline powder. It effloresces in warm dry air. Each g represents approximately 4.1 mmol of magnesium and of sulphate. Magnesium sulphate (heptahydrate) 10.1 g is approximately equivalent to 1 g of magnesium.

The *B.P.* specifies: **soluble** 1 in 1.5 of water and very soluble in boiling water; practically insoluble in alcohol. The *U.S.P.* specifies: soluble 1 in 0.8 of water and 1 in 0.5 of boiling water; freely but slowly soluble 1 in 1 of glycerol; sparingly soluble in alcohol. A 5% solution in water has a pH of 5.0 to 9.2.

Magnesium sulphate has been reported to be **incompatible** with polymyxin B sulphate, streptomycin sulphate, tobramycin sulphate, fat emulsion, calcium gluceptate, calcium gluconate, dobutamine hydrochloride, procaine hydrochloride, tetracyclines, soluble phosphates, and with alkali carbonates and bicarbonates. Incompatibility has also been reported with benzylpenicillin and nafcillin due to a pH-dependent effect of magnesium sulphate. **Store** in a cool place in well-closed containers.

Adverse Effects

Magnesium salts are poorly absorbed following oral administration, but in patients with impaired renal function there may be sufficient accumulation to produce toxic effects.

Excessive administration of magnesium leads to the development of hypermagnesaemia; for symptoms, see Hypermagnesaemia above, under Magnesium.

Acute ingestion of magnesium sulphate may also cause gastro-intestinal irritation and watery diarrhoea.

Hypermagnesaemia and hypophosphataemia, without cardiovascular or respiratory symptoms, after the presumed ingestion of an overdose of magnesium sulphate.— P. Garcia-Webb *et al., Br. med. J.*, 1984, *288*, 759.

PREGNANCY AND THE NEONATE. *Effects on the mother.* A report of acute pulmonary oedema in 2 patients given magnesium sulphate and betamethasone to prevent premature labour.— J. P. Elliott *et al., Am. J. Obstet. Gynec.*, 1979, *134*, 717.

Development of paralytic ileus in a 29-year-old patient during the continuous intravenous infusion of magnesium sulphate for premature labour.— W. C. Hill *et al., Am. J. Perinatol.*, 1985, *2*, 47.

Effects on the neonate. Magnesium sulphate 4 g intravenously over 20 minutes followed by 1 g per hour by continuous infusion administered to 16 women with nonasphyxiated term pregnancies complicated by pregnancy-induced hypertension produced elevated neonatal umbilical cord magnesium concentrations. No correlation was found between the neurological performance of the neonate and either cord-magnesium concentrations or the total dose of magnesium administered.— K. W. Green *et al., Am. J. Obstet. Gynec.*, 1983, *146*, 29.

Treatment of Adverse Effects

Calcium gluconate injection 10% should be administered intravenously in a dose of 10 to 20 mL to counteract respiratory depression or heart block. If renal function is normal, adequate fluids should be given to assist removal of magnesium from the body. Dialysis may be necessary in patients with renal impairment or severe hypermagnesaemia.

Precautions

Magnesium sulphate should be administered with caution to patients with impaired renal function or those receiving digitalis glycosides. Parenteral administration of magnesium sulphate may enhance the effects of neuromuscular blocking agents.

A recommendation that patients with heart block or myocardial damage should not receive parenteral magnesium sulphate in the treatment of preterm labour. In addition, it should not be administered concomitantly with high doses of barbiturates, opioids, or hypnotics because of the risk of respiratory depression.—S. N. Caritis, *Drugs*, 1983, *26*, 243.

Hypomagnesaemia was diagnosed in a 69-year-old woman with Crohn's disease whose daily medication included vitamin D and calcium; her serum-calcium concentration was normal. After treatment with magnesium sulphate 10 g intravenously over 48 hours the patient had a generalised seizure and became confused, she was found to be hypercalcaemic. It was likely that the hypercalcaemia in this patient was prevented by concomitant hypomagnesaemia and was precipitated when magnesium was administered.— A. A. Nanji, *Postgrad. med. J.*, 1985, *61*, 47. Recommendations on how hypercalcaemia and tissue calcinosis may be avoided in patients receiving treatment with both vitamin D and magnesium salts. Concomitant calcium (and phosphorus) should not be prescribed, an initially physiological daily dose of vitamin D should not be exceeded, and plasma-calcium concentrations and 24-hour calciuria should be systematically checked for at least one month.— J. Durlach (letter), *ibid.*, 1986, *67*, 239.

Severe hypermagnesaemia and hypercalcaemia developed in 2 patients with hepatic encephalopathy following the administration of magnesium sulphate enemas; both patients died, one during and one after asystole. It was recommended that patients with liver disease who might develop renal impairment or in whom renal failure is established should not be prescribed enemas containing magnesium for treatment of hepatic encephalopathy as serious magnesium toxicity can occur, which may contribute to death.— P. O. Collinson and A. K. Burroughs, *Br. med. J.*, 1986, *293*, 1013.

Absorption and Fate

Approximately one third of magnesium is absorbed from the small intestine following oral administration and even soluble magnesium salts are generally very slowly absorbed. Absorption of magnesium is enhanced by the presence of the vitamin D compound calcitriol. Magnesium salts are excreted mainly in the urine with small amounts being excreted in breast milk and saliva.

Uses and Administration

Magnesium salts are used in the treatment of magnesium deficiency. In simple deficiency states magnesium salts may be given by mouth in doses to provide up to 50 mmol of magnesium daily.

In acute hypomagnesaemia parenteral administration is necessary and doses of up to 16 mmol daily may be given by slow intravenous injection, intravenous infusion, or intramuscular injection. Magnesium salts may also be added to solutions for total parenteral nutrition. Careful monitoring of plasma-magnesium and other electrolyte concentrations is essential.

Magnesium sulphate for parenteral use is usually administered as a 50% solution; magnesium sulphate (heptahydrate) 10 g provides approximately 40 mmol of magnesium.

Magnesium sulphate acts as a saline laxative and is administered by mouth for this purpose in usual daily doses of 15 g in 250 mL of water. Children over 6 years of age may be given up to 10 g in 120 mL of water and children aged 2 to 5 years may be given up to 5 g daily.

A 50% solution of magnesium sulphate in water may be given rectally as an enema and is used in doses of 130 mL as an adjunct in neurosurgery to lower cerebrospinal fluid pressure.

Magnesium sulphate has anticonvulsant properties when administered parenterally and may be used to prevent or control seizures associated with acute uraemia, hypothyroidism, and eclampsia. It may be given intramuscularly in doses of up to 5 g, by slow intravenous injection in doses of up to 4 g, or by intravenous infusion in glucose or saline in doses of up to 4 g per hour. The total daily dose should not exceed approximately 30 g in patients with normal renal function; appropriate reductions in dosage should be made for patients with renal impairment.

Dried magnesium sulphate is described below.

BRONCHIAL ASTHMA. Rapid and marked bronchodilatation following administration of magnesium sulphate by intravenous infusion to 13 asthmatic patients.— H. Okayama *et al., J. Am. med. Ass.*, 1987, *257*, 1076.

CARDIOVASCULAR DISORDERS. *Cardiac arrhythmia.* Successful use of intravenous magnesium sulphate in the treatment of 3 patients with torsades de pointes.— D. Tzivoni *et al., Am. J. Cardiol.*, 1984, *53*, 528.

Hypertension. Hypertension and tachycardia persisted during pre-induction and surgery for removal of a phaeochromocytoma in a 16-year-old girl despite the use of alpha- and beta-adrenergic blockers. Adequate cardiovascular control was achieved with intravenous infusions of magnesium sulphate, administered on the basis that magnesium inhibits the release of catecholamines and exerts a direct effect on adrenergic receptors and blood vessels.— M. F. M. James, *Anesthesiology*, 1985, *62*, 188.

Dyckner and Wester (*Br. med. J.*, 1983, *286*, 1847) reported a decrease in the blood pressure of patients, already receiving long-term diuretic treatment, who were given magnesium supplementation in the form of magnesium aspartate hydrochloride. Their study was criticised in view of the absence of an effect by the magnesium on plasma and urinary electrolyte concentrations, and it was suggested that the decrease in blood pressure may have been mediated by a placebo effect (H.-G. Güllner, *ibid.*, *287*, 363). Two later controlled studies in hypertensive patients reported that magnesium supplementation did not exert an effect on blood pressure either in untreated patients (F.P. Cappuccio, *et al.*, *ibid.*, 1985, *291*, 235) or in patients receiving long-term diuretic treatment (D.G. Henderson *et al.*, *ibid.*, 1986, *239*, 664).

Myocardial infarction. In a double-blind placebo-controlled study involving 130 patients with acute myocardial infarction 56 patients received magnesium (as magnesium chloride) by intravenous infusion and 74 patients received placebo. Results showed that mortality during the first 4 weeks after treatment was 7% in the magnesium group compared with 19% in the placebo group; the incidence of arrhythmias requiring treatment was 21% and 47% respectively.— H. S. Rasmussen *et al.*, *Lancet*, 1986, *1*, 234. Correspondence.—*ibid.*, 551.

PREGNANCY AND THE NEONATE. *Cervical ripening.* Effective use of a synthetic polymer sponge, impregnated with magnesium sulphate 450 mg, in producing cervical ripening prior to induction of labour.— I. R. Johnson *et al.*, *Am. J. Obstet. Gynec.*, 1985, *151*, 604.

Eclampsia. A detailed report on the management of 245 cases of eclampsia, including the use of magnesium sulphate to control convulsions.— J. A. Pritchard *et al.*, *Am. J. Obstet. Gynec.*, 1984, *148*, 951.

Disadvantages of the use of magnesium sulphate in the management of hypertensive crises in pregnancy relate to the risk of cardiovascular and respiratory depression in both the mother and foetus. Elevated serum-magnesium concentrations significantly complicate anaesthetic management since the duration of action of muscle relaxants is increased. Magnesium may also exaggerate the hypotensive effect of anaesthesia. Although magnesium sulphate is used in many centres its use should be restricted to the severely hypertensive patient with imminent or recent eclampsia.— W. F. Lubbe, *Drugs*, 1984, *28*, 170.

Foetal distress. Administration of magnesium sulphate 4 g by rapid intravenous infusion to a 22-year-old woman in early labour with acute intrapartum foetal distress (persistent bradycardia) led to a reduction in uterine activity and recovery of foetal heart-rate within 2 minutes.— E. A. Reece *et al.*, *Am. J. Obstet. Gynec.*, 1984, *148*, 104.

Premature labour. Magnesium sulphate, administered intravenously was considered to be a good substitute in conditions of preterm labour where beta-adrenoceptor agonists, such as ritodrine, are contra-indicated or poorly tolerated. It was considered to be particularly useful in women with diabetes mellitus or hypertension where beta-adrenergic stimulation is not desirable. Magnesium suppresses the release of acetylcholine, inhibits uterine contractions, and blocks transmission at the neuromuscular junction. Magnesium sulphate crosses the placenta causing a loss of beat-to-beat variability in the foetal heart-rate. The concentration in cord blood is similar to that of the mother, but does not indicate the likelihood of neonatal depression. Labour-inhibiting doses of magnesium do not usually compromise the neonate, however there have been occasional reports of neonatal depression.— S. N. Caritis, *Drugs*, 1983, *26*, 243.

In a study carried out by Ferguson *et al.* (*Am. J. Obstet. Gynec.*, 1984, *148*, 166) ritodrine alone or with adjunctive magnesium sulphate was administered to 17 and 24 patients with premature labour respectively. Labour was delayed with a slightly lower dose of ritodrine when used with magnesium sulphate, but the combination was associated with significantly more adverse cardiovascular effects than ritodrine alone. However, Hatjis *et al.* (*ibid.*, *150*, 142) reported beneficial effects when magnesium sulphate was administered to 30 patients with advanced premature labour who had failed to respond to ritodrine.

Preparations

Magnesium Sulfate Injection *(U.S.P.)*. A sterile solution of magnesium sulphate (heptahydrate) in Water for Injections. pH of a 5% solution 5.5 to 7.0.

Magnesium Sulphate Mixture *(B.P.)*. Magnesium Sulphate Oral Suspension. Magnesium sulphate 4 g, light magnesium carbonate 500 mg, concentrated peppermint emulsion 0.25 mL, double-strength chloroform water 3 mL, water to 10 mL. It should be recently prepared. This mixture was known as Mistura Alba.

In a study of various non-sterile pharmaceutical preparations, Magnesium Sulphate Mixture *B.P.* was found to be inadquately preserved against microbial spoilage as determined by *B.P.* challenge tests.— T. R. R. Kurup and L. S. C. Wan, *Pharm. J.*, 1986, *2*, 761 (The *B.P. 1980* formula is identical to that in *B.P. 1988*).

Proprietary Preparations

Fletchers' Magnesium Sulphate Retention Enema *(Pharmax, UK)*. *Solution*, magnesium sulphate 50%, in single-use disposable containers of 130 mL.

Kest *(Rorer, UK)*. *Tablets*, magnesium sulphate 300 mg, phenolphthalein 49 mg.

Proprietary Names and Manufacturers of Magnesium Sulphate and some other Magnesium Compounds

Addex-Magnesium *(Pharmacia, Swed.)*; Fletchers' Magnesium Sulphate Retention Enema *(Pharmax, UK)*; Mg 5-Sulfat *(Artesan, Switz.)*; Mg-Plus *(USA)*; Sulmetin *(Semar, Spain)*.

The following names have been used for multi-ingredient electrolyte preparations containing magnesium sulphate and some other magnesium compounds—Citrocarbonate *(Upjohn, Canad.)*; Kest *(Rorer, UK)*; Osmopak-Plus *(Charton, Canad.)*.

1175-f

Dried Magnesium Sulphate *(BAN)*.

Dried Epsom Salts; Exsiccated Magnesium Sulphate.

CAS — 7487-88-9.

Pharmacopoeias. In *Arg.*, *Aust.*, *Belg.*, *Br.*, *Cz.*, *Hung.*, *Jug.*, *Nord.*, *Pol.*, and *Rus.*

A white odourless or almost odourless powder, prepared by drying magnesium sulphate (heptahydrate) at 100° until it has lost about 25% of its weight; it contains 62 to 70% of $MgSO_4$.

Soluble 1 in 2 of water; more rapidly soluble in hot water. A 7.5% solution in water is neutral to phenol red. **Store** in well-closed containers.

Dried magnesium sulphate is employed when the use of the hydrated salt would be disadvantageous. As Magnesium Sulphate Paste it is used as an application to inflammatory skin conditions such as boils and carbuncles but prolonged or repeated use may damage the surrounding skin.

Magnesium sulphate paste probably prevents bacterial growth through an osmotic action which has been described as "sucking" bacteria dry. It seems to be very effective for cleaning heavily infected ulcers and wounds but must be frequently renewed to prevent overdilution by the exudate. Once a healthy granulating wound base has formed, strong osmotic agents such as magnesium sulphate are best discontinued to avoid overgranulation and excessive scarring. A paste made from sodium sulphate may serve as a possible alternative if magnesium needs to be avoided.— P. Lowthian and S. Barnett (letter), *Lancet*, 1985, *2*, 1186.

Preparations

Magnesium Sulphate Paste *(B.P.)*. Morison's Paste. Dried magnesium sulphate, after drying at 150° or 130°, 45 g, glycerol, heated at 120° for 1 hour and cooled, 55 g, and phenol 500 mg.

Proprietary Names and Manufacturers

The following names have been used for multi-ingredient electrolyte preparations containing dried magnesium sulphate—Agobyl *(Desbergers, Canad.)*; Magnoplasm *(Faulding, Austral.)*.

2898-t

Phosphate

Phosphate is the principal anion of intracellular fluid. It exists in the body mainly as divalent HPO_4 ions (about 80%) and monovalent H_2PO_4 ions (about 20%). Phosphate is involved in many physiological processes including the metabolism of carbohydrates and lipids, the storage and transfer of energy, the formation of buffer systems which influence acid-base balance, and in the renal excretion of hydrogen ions. The body contains about 330 mmol of phosphate per kg body-weight, approximately 80 per cent of which is found in the skeleton and 15 per cent in soft tissue. The normal concentration range of phosphate in plasma is 0.8 to 1.5 mmol per litre. There is an inverse relationship between the concentration of phosphate and that of calcium.

Most foods contain adequate amounts of phosphate hence deficiency is virtually unknown except in patients receiving total parenteral nutrition. About 20 to 40 mmol (0.62 to 1.24 g) of phosphorus is ingested daily in the typical diet. Approximately 70 to 80 per cent of phosphate is absorbed from the small intestine; it is excreted mainly in the urine with some faecal loss.

NOTE. Each g of phosphorus represents approximately 32.3 mmol.

Hyperphosphataemia

Hyperphosphataemia, an increase in plasma-phosphate concentration above the normal range, rarely occurs from excessive intake of phosphate unless there is renal failure. Hyperphosphataemia may also occur in the presence of acidosis, acromegaly, haemolysis, hypoparathyroidism, tissue destruction, or vitamin D toxicity. Hyperphosphataemia leads in turn to hypocalcaemia (see also p.1029), which may be severe, and ectopic calcification. Secondary hyperparathyroidism may develop in the presence of renal failure.

Hypophosphataemia

Hypophosphataemia, a decrease in plasma-phosphate concentration below the normal range, may occur in the presence of chronic alcoholism, extracellular fluid expansion, or renal tubular defects, during the recovery phase of diabetic ketoacidosis, or following the use of phosphate-binding antacids or hyperalimentation. Symptoms of hypophosphataemia may include haemolysis, leucopenia, thrombocytopenia, muscle weakness, paraesthesia, osteomalacia, rickets, rhabdomyolysis, depression of myocardial function, seizures and coma.

1184-d

Dibasic Potassium Phosphate *(USAN)*.

Dipotassium Hydrogen Phosphate; Dipotassium Phosphate; E340; Potassium Phosphate. Dipotassium hydrogen orthophosphate.

K_2HPO_4=174.2.

CAS — 7758-11-4.

Pharmacopoeias. In *U.S.*

Each g represents approximately 11.5 mmol of potassium and 5.7 mmol of phosphate. A 5% solution in water has a pH of 8.5 to 9.6.

1183-f

Monobasic Potassium Phosphate *(USAN)*.

E340; Monopotassium Phosphate; Potassium Acid Phosphate; Potassium Biphosphate. Potassium dihydrogen orthophosphate.

KH_2PO_4=136.1.

CAS — 7778-77-0.

Pharmacopoeias. In *U.S.N.F.*

Colourless crystals or a white odourless granular or crystalline powder. Each g represents approximately 7.3 mmol of potassium and of phosphate. Freely **soluble** in water; practically insoluble in alcohol. A 1% solution in water has a pH of about 4.5. **Store** in airtight containers.

INCOMPATIBILITY. As for Sodium Phosphate.

Dibasic and monobasic potassium phosphates are used as sources of phosphate, and have the actions and uses described under Sodium Phosphate, below.

For a report of the development of hypocalcaemia and hypomagnesaemia following administration of potassium phosphates to a child with diabetic ketoacidosis, see under Sodium Phosphate, p.1035.

Preparations

Potassium Phosphates Injection *(U.S.P.)*. A sterile solution of monobasic potassium phosphate and dibasic potassium phosphate in Water for Injections. It contains no bacteriostatic agent or other preservative. To be diluted before use.

Proprietary Preparations

Addiphos *(KabiVitrum, UK). Solution,* monobasic potassium phosphate 170.1 mg, sodium acid phosphate dihydrate 133.5 mg, potassium hydroxide 14 mg, sorbitol 1 mg, in vials of 20 mL providing phosphate 40 mmol, potassium 30 mmol, and sodium 30 mmol. pH 6.3 to 6.4. For addition to infusion fluids to provide phosphate during total parenteral nutrition.

Proprietary Names and Manufacturers of Dibasic and Monobasic Potassium Phosphate

K-Phos Original *(Beach, USA).*

The following names have been used for multi-ingredient electrolyte preparations containing dibasic and monobasic potassium phosphate—Artisial *(Jouveinal, Canad.)*; K-Phos *(Beach, USA)*; Neutra-Phos *(Willen, USA)*; Neutra-Phos-K *(Willen, USA)*; Phosphates Solution *(Boots, UK)*; Thiacide *(Beach, USA).*

1195-m

Sodium Acid Phosphate *(BAN).*

E339; Monobasic Sodium Phosphate *(USAN)*; Natrii Dihydrogenophosphas; Natrium Phosphoricum Monobasicum; Sodium Dihydrogen Phosphate. Sodium dihydrogen orthophosphate.

NaH_2PO_4,xH_2O.

CAS — 7558-80-7 (anhydrous); 10049-21-5 (monohydrate); 13472-35-0; 10028-24-7 (both dihydrate).

Pharmacopoeias. In *Arg., Aust., Belg., Br., Eur., Fr., Ger., Hung., Ind., Int., Jug., Neth., Nord.,* and *Swiss* (all with $2H_2O$); in *Braz., Chin., Mex.,* and *Pol.* (all with $1H_2O$). The *U.S.P.* specifies that it contains one or two molecules of water of hydration, or is anhydrous. Also in *B.P. Vet.*

Odourless colourless crystals or white crystalline powder; slightly deliquescent.

Each g of sodium acid phosphate (anhydrous) represents approximately 8.3 mmol of sodium and of phosphate.

Each g of sodium acid phosphate (monohydrate) represents approximately 7.2 mmol of sodium and of phosphate.

Each g of sodium acid phosphate (dihydrate) represents approximately 6.4 mmol of sodium and of phosphate.

Soluble 1 in 1 of water; very slightly soluble or practically insoluble in alcohol. A 5% solution in water has a pH of 4.1 to 4.5 and effervesces with sodium carbonate.

Store in well-closed containers.

1196-b

Sodium Phosphate *(BAN).*

Dibasic Sodium Phosphate *(USAN)*; Dinatrii Phosphas; Disodium Hydrogen Phosphate; Disodium Phosphate; E339; Natrii Phosphas. Disodium hydrogen orthophosphate.

Na_2HPO_4,xH_2O.

CAS — 7558-79-4 (anhydrous); 7782-85-6 (heptahydrate); 10039-32-4 (dodecahydrate).

Pharmacopoeias. Aust., Br., Cz., Egypt., Eur., Ger., Hung., Ind., It., Jpn, Neth., Pol., Port., and *Roum.* specify $12H_2O$. *Arg., Fr., Span.,* and *Swiss* specify either anhydrous or $12H_2O$. *Mex.* specifies $7H_2O$. *U.S.* specifies either dried or $7H_2O$. *Belg., Jug.,* and *Nord.* specify $2H_2O$.

The *B.P.* specifies: colourless transparent, strongly efflorescent crystals. The *U.S.P.* specifies for the dried substance: a white powder that readily absorbs moisture, and for the heptahydrate: a colourless or white granular salt.

Each g of sodium phosphate (anhydrous) represents approximately 14.1 mmol of sodium and 7.0 mmol of phosphate.

Each g of sodium phosphate (heptahydrate) represents approximately 7.5 mmol of sodium and 3.7 mmol of phosphate.

Each g of sodium phosphate (dodecahydrate) represents approximately 5.6 mmol of sodium and 2.8 mmol of phosphate.

B.P. solubilities are: very soluble in water; practically insoluble in alcohol. *U.S.P.* solubilities are for the dried substance: soluble 1 in 8 of water; insoluble in alcohol, and for the heptahydrate: freely soluble in water; very slightly soluble in alcohol.

Phosphates are **incompatible** with calcium salts; the mixing of calcium and phosphate salts in parenteral nutrition solutions can lead to the formation of insoluble calcium-phosphate precipitates. Incompatibility has also been reported with magnesium salts.

Store in airtight containers.

INCOMPATIBILITY. Several factors including drug concentration, temperature, salt form, pH, amino acid composition, presence of other additives, and order of mixing have been shown to influence the potential interaction of calcium and phosphate in parenteral nutrition solutions. References: L. D. Eggert *et al., Am. J. Hosp. Pharm.,* 1982, *39,* 49; L. A. Robinson and B. T. Wright, *ibid.,* 120; P. W. Niemiec and T. W. Vanderveen, *ibid.,* 1984, *41,* 893.

Adverse Effects and Treatment

Excessive administration of phosphate, particularly by the intravenous route, may cause hyperphosphataemia (see also Hyperphosphataemia above, under Phosphate). This in turn leads to the development of hypocalcaemia, and ectopic calcification may occur due to precipitation of calcium phosphate.

Adverse effects which may occur after intravenous injection also include hypocalcaemic tetany, hypotension, tachycardia, fever, oedema, and acute renal failure. Adverse effects occur less frequently after oral administration due to poor absorption from the gastro-intestinal tract, but nausea, vomiting, diarrhoea, and abdominal pain have been reported.

Treatment of adverse effects involves withdrawal of phosphate, general supportive measures, and correction of serum-electrolyte concentrations, especially calcium.

EFFECTS ON FLUID AND ELECTROLYTE HOMOEOSTASIS. Development of hypocalcaemia and hypomagnesaemia in a 9-year-old boy with diabetic ketoacidosis following the administration of potassium 225 mmol and phosphate 153 mmol as a mixture of the dibasic and monobasic potassium phosphate salts.— R. J. Winter *et al., Am. J. Med.,* 1979, *67,* 897.

A report of fatal poisoning which occured in an 11-month-old infant following administration of an overdose of hypertonic sodium phosphate enema solution. The enema was retained and the infant developed hypernatraemia, metabolic acidosis, hyperphosphataemia, hypocalcaemia, and cardiac arrest.— R. R. Martin *et al., J. Am. med. Ass.,* 1987, *257,* 2190.

Similar reports.— M. Biberstein and B. A. Parker, *Am. J. Med.,* 1985, *79,* 645 (life-threatening hyperphosphataemia and hypocalcaemia); L. P. Haskell (letter), *Lancet,* 1985, *2,* 1433 (hypocalcaemic tetany).

EFFECTS ON THE RECTUM. Rectal gangrene, which developed in 3 compromised patients with haemorrhoids, all of whom were given phosphate enemas, was attributed to a direct necrotising effect of phosphate on the rectum.— J. L. Sweeney *et al., Med. J. Aust.,* 1986, *144,* 374.

Precautions

Phosphates should not be administered to patients with severely impaired renal function or hyperphosphataemia. They should not be administered concomitantly with aluminium, calcium, or magnesium salts, as they bind phosphate thus impairing its absorption from the gastro-intestinal tract.

Absorption and Fate

Approximately two-thirds of ingested phosphate is absorbed from the gastro-intestinal tract; most of the absorbed phosphate is then filtered by the glomeruli and subsequently undergoes reabsorption. Parathyroid hormone and vitamin D stimulate absorption of phosphate from the small intestine and its reabsorption from the proximal tubule. Virtually all absorbed phosphate is eventually excreted in the urine, the remainder being excreted in the faeces.

Pharmacokinetic data obtained from a case of acute poisoning which had followed ingestion of a phosphate laxative by a 4-month-old infant were analysed in conjunction with data from 4 previous reports of similar poisonings. It was found that in infants with normal renal function after rehydration there is rapid clearance of phosphorus with a plasma half-life of 5 to 11 hours. A nomogram was constructed to predict the peak concentration, the response to treatment, and the expected time for recovery of plasma phosphate and calcium.— J.E. Larson *et al., Hum. Toxicol.,* 1986, *5,* 45.

Uses and Administration

Phosphates may be used in the treatment of hypophosphataemic and hypercalcaemic states. They should be administered by mouth when possible, and the dose and rate of administration should be individualised for each patient. In mild to moderate hypophosphataemic/hypercalcaemic states including rickets and osteomalacia, and for prophylaxis of renal calculi, phosphates may be given by mouth in doses to provide up to 65 mmol or more of phosphate daily. The intravenous route is seldom justified, but up to 100 mmol of phosphate daily may be given by slow intravenous infusion in severe acute hypophosphataemia, severe hypercalcaemia, or when administration by the oral route is not possible. Plasma-electrolyte concentrations, especially phosphate and calcium, and renal function should be carefully monitored. Smaller doses may be necessary in patients with impaired renal function.

Phosphates act as mild saline laxatives when administered by mouth as dilute solutions, or by the rectal route as enemas or suppositories. Doses of up to 111 mmol of phosphate daily have been given for this purpose.

Sodium phosphates lower the pH of urine, and have been given as adjuncts to certain urinary antimicrobial agents which are dependent on an acid urine for their activity against urinary-tract infections.

Solutions of various phosphate salts in proportions to give an approximately neutral pH have been used in the treatment of various disorders of calcium and phosphate metabolism.

Rickets. Treatment with calcitriol 0.25 µg and phosphate 19.4 mmol daily by mouth was commenced in a 2-month-old girl following a diagnosis of familial hypophosphataemic rickets. Doses were increased until alkaline phosphatase concentrations were reduced to normal; this was obtained at doses of 1.25 µg and 71.1 mmol respectively. Treatment at these doses was continued and at age 2½ years bone radiographs remained normal, and the patient had not developed any bone lesions.— M. Roza *et al., Archs Dis. Childh.,* 1983, *58,* 1020.

Treatment with neutral phosphate 32.3 to 80.7 mmol daily in divided doses by mouth was given to 6 patients with a rare syndrome of hereditary hypophosphataemic rickets and hypercalciuria. Long-term treatment resulted in disappearance of bone pain within several weeks and a substantial improvement in muscular strength. Radiological signs of rickets disappeared completely after 4 to 9 months of treatment.— M. Tieder *et al., New Engl. J. Med.,* 1985, *312,* 611.

A discussion on metabolic bone disease in preterm infants (also known as 'rickets of prematurity') based on proceedings sponsored by the British Paediatric Association's Nutrition Group. The main cause of the disease was thought probably to be deficiency of substrates such as calcium and phosphate. Studies have shown that when sufficient phosphate is given to meet soft-tissue needs, hydroxyapatite can again be formed in bone, and calcium absorbed from the diet is avidly retained with consequent reduction in its urinary excretion. Infants weighing less than 1000 g at birth were considered to be most at risk, and it was suggested that such babies, fed on breast milk alone, should receive phosphate supplementation. Infants weighing up to 1200 g at birth may also require supplementation, and although the value of routine supplements for larger, more mature babies had not been established, it was suggested that phosphate supplementation should be continued until the infant reaches a weight of 2000 g.— O. G. Brooke and A. Lucas, *Archs Dis. Childh.*, 1985, *60*, 682.

For a report of a study in which supplementation with calcium and phosphate did not reduce the incidence of rickets of prematurity, see p.1030.

HYPERCALCAEMIA. Hypercalcaemia associated with hypophosphataemia in immature infants of low birth weight failed to respond to reduction of calcium intake but responded to administration of phosphate. It was suggested that the high incidence of rickets of prematurity in such infants may be due to the active mobilisation of calcium and phosphate from bone caused by extreme hypophosphataemia.— A. J. Lyon *et al.*, *Archs Dis. Childh.*, 1984, *59*, 1141. A further report.— A. J. Lyon and N. McIntosh, *ibid.*, 1145.

See also under Rickets, above.

Phosphate was considered to be one of the most effective agents in the treatment of hypercalcaemia of malignancy.— G. R. Munday *et al.*, *Am. J. Med.*, 1983, *74*, 421. See also N. J. Scolding (letter), *Lancet*, 1985, *2*, 1299.

Hyperparathyroidism. A report of a detailed study in 10 patients with primary hyperparathyroidism before and after treatment with oral phosphate for 1 year. Plasma-1,25-dihydroxyvitamin D concentrations were reduced as was calcium excretion, but subjective improvement was reported by only 2 patients.— A. E. Broadus *et al.*, *J. clin. Endocr. Metab.*, 1983, *56*, 953.

Oral phosphate therapy may be an alternative for treating hyperparathyroidism in pregnancy when parathyroidectomy is contra-indicated.— D. T. Wilson *et al.*, *Can. med. Ass. J.*, 1983, *129*, 986.

HYPOPHOSPHATAEMIA. *Acute respiratory failure.* In a study by Aubier *et al.* (*New Engl. J. Med.*, 1985, *313*, 420), administration of phosphate 10 mmol, as monobasic potassium phosphate, by continuous intravenous infusion over 4 hours to 8 patients with acute respiratory failure and hypophosphataemic-related diaphragm weakness resulted in improved contractile properties of the diaphragm. This effect was thought to be of potential clinical importance in the achievement of successful weaning from ventilators. However, Rie (*ibid.*, 1986, *314*, 519) considered, although they had not conducted any formal studies, that when most patients who are undergoing mechanical ventilation have their serum phosphate replenished, no grossly detectable changes occur in their ability to be weaned from the ventilator.

Diabetic ketoacidosis. A discussion on the clinical status of hypophosphataemia including reference to whether the treatment of diabetic ketoacidosis should include administration of phosphate salts. The majority of patients with diabetic ketoacidosis become hypophosphaturic and hypophosphataemic during treatment with fluids and insulin despite normal or elevated serum-phosphate concentrations before treatment. Most of these patients do not have any recognisable hypophosphataemic complications and serum-phosphate concentrations return to normal spontaneously. Occasionally however, hypophosphataemia does occur in the presence of ketoacidosis, and severe hypophosphataemia may develop with treatment; such patients should probably receive phosphate supplementation.— J. P. Knochel, *New Engl. J. Med.*, 1985, *313*, 447.

Preparations

Effervescent Sodium Phosphate *(U.S.P.)*. Oral granules from dried sodium phosphate 20% with sodium bicarbonate, tartaric acid, and citric acid monohydrate. Store in airtight containers.

Phosphates Enema *(B.P.)*. Sodium Phosphates Enema. *Formula A.* Sodium acid phosphate 16 g, sodium phosphate 6 g, freshly boiled and cooled water to 100 mL. *Formula B.* Sodium acid phosphate 10 g, sodium phosphate 8 g, freshly boiled and cooled water to 100 mL. Both formulas may include a suitable preservative.

Sodium Phosphates Enema *(U.S.P.)*. A solution of sodium acid phosphate (monohydrate) 15.2 to 16.8% and sodium phosphate (heptahydrate) 5.7 to 6.3% in water. pH 5.0 to 5.8.

Sodium Phosphates Injection *(U.S.P.)*. A sterile solution of sodium acid phosphate (monohydrate) and sodium phosphate (heptahydrate) in Water for Injections. It contains no bacteriostatic agent or other preservative. To be diluted before use.

Sodium Phosphates Oral Solution *(U.S.P.)*. A solution of sodium acid phosphate (monohydrate) 45.6 to 50.4% and sodium phosphate (heptahydrate) 17.1 to 18.9% in water. pH 4.4 to 5.2. Store in airtight containers.

Proprietary Preparations

Carbalax (formerly known as Beogex) *(Pharmax, UK)*. *Suppositories*, anhydrous sodium acid phosphate 1.32 g (equivalent to sodium acid phosphate dihydrate 1.72 g), sodium bicarbonate 1.08 g in an inert polyethylene glycol base.

Fletchers' Phosphate Enema *(Pharmax, UK)*. *Rectal solution*, sodium acid phosphate dihydrate 12.8 g, sodium phosphate dodecahydrate 10.24 g in single-dose disposable containers of 128 mL.

Phosphate-Sandoz *(Sandoz, UK)*. *Tablets*, effervescent, anhydrous sodium acid phosphate 1.936 g, sodium bicarbonate 350 mg, potassium bicarbonate 315 mg, anhydrous citric acid 800 mg, providing phosphate 16.1 mmol, sodium 20.4 mmol, potassium 3.1 mmol, citrate 4.17 mmol, and bicarbonate 7.3 mmol.

Proprietary Names and Manufacturers of Sodium Acid Phosphate and Sodium Phosphate

The following names have been used for multi-ingredient electrolyte preparations containing sodium acid phosphate and sodium phosphate—Carbalax *(Pharmax, UK)*; Citrocarbonate *(Upjohn, Canad.)*; Effervescent Saline Tablets *(Southon-Horton, UK)*; Fleet Enema *(Frosst, Canad.*; *Fleet, USA)*; Fletchers' Phosphate Enema *(Pharmax, UK)*; K-Phos *(Beach, USA)*; Neutra-Phos *(Willen, USA)*; pHos-pHaid *(Guardian, Canad.*; *Guardian, USA)*; Phosphates Solution *(Boots, UK)*; Phosphate-Sandoz *(Austral.*; *Sandoz, Canad.*; *Sandoz, UK)*; Phospho-Soda *(Fleet, USA)*; Travad *(Travenol, Austral.)*; Uro-Phosphate *(Poythress, USA)*; Uroqid-Acid *(Beach, USA)*.

1176-d

Potassium

K=39.098.

Potassium is an essential body electrolyte. It is the principal cation of intracellular fluid and is involved in numerous enzymatic reactions and physiological processes including nerve conduction, muscle contraction, and carbohydrate metabolism. The body contains about 50 mmol of potassium per kg bodyweight, approximately 75 per cent of which is found in skeletal muscle. The normal concentration of potassium in intracellular fluid and plasma is about 150 and 3.5 to 5 mmol respectively per litre. The concentration of potassium in plasma is often not a reliable indication of total body stores.

About 50 to 100 mmol of potassium is ingested daily in the typical diet and most of this is absorbed from the gastro-intestinal tract. Potassium is excreted mainly in the urine with some faecal loss. Unlike sodium, the renal capacity to conserve potassium is poor, even when there is severe depletion.

The amount of potassium required by an adult is about 1 to 1.5 g per day.

NOTE. Each g of potassium represents approximately 25.6 mmol.

Hyperkalaemia

Hyperkalaemia may occur after excessive intake of potassium (including the excessive transfusion of stored blood), after the improper use of potassium-sparing diuretics, in adrenal cortical insufficiency, renal failure, and acidosis, and after tissue trauma. Symptoms include paraesthesia of the extremities, muscle weakness, paralysis, hypotension, cardiac arrhythmias, heart block, and cardiac arrest.

Hypokalaemia

Hypokalaemia may occur due to inadequate intake of potassium or due to increased gastro-intestinal loss (vomiting, diarrhoea, fistulae). It is often accompanied by hypochloraemia and commonly occurs in acid base disturbances characterised by alkalosis, aldosterone excess, Cushing's syndrome, and renal tubular acidosis. Losses are increased during the use of thiazide diuretics. Symptoms may include abdominal distension, paralytic ileus, muscle weakness, reduced or absent reflexes, paralysis, respiratory failure, polydipsia, polyuria due to renal tubular damage, and cardiac arrhythmias. Hypokalaemia increases the potential toxicity of digitalis glycosides.

1177-n

Potassium Acetate *(BAN, USAN)*.

E261; Kalii Acetas.

$CH_3.CO_2K$=98.14.

CAS — 127-08-2.

Pharmacopoeias. In *Br., Braz., Fr., Pol., Port., Rus., Span.*, and *U.S.*

A solution of potassium acetate (about 33%) is included in *Aust.* and *Pol. Jpn* has 38%.

Colourless crystals or a white crystalline powder; odourless or with a faint acetous odour. It is deliquescent in moist air. Each g represents approximately 10.2 mmol of potassium. Potassium acetate 2.5 g is approximately equivalent to 1 g of potassium. *B.P.* **solubilities** are: soluble 1 in 0.5 of water and 1 in 2 of alcohol. *U.S.P* solubilities are: soluble in 0.5 of water, 1 in 0.2 of boiling water, and 1 in 3 of alcohol. A 5% solution in water has a pH of 7.5 to 9.5. **Store** in airtight containers.

INCOMPATIBILITY. As for Potassium Chloride.

Potassium acetate may be used similarly to potassium chloride for the prevention and treatment of potassium deficiency. It may be administered by mouth or by slow intravenous infusion.

Potassium acetate is used as a source of potassium and acetate in solutions for haemodialysis and peritoneal dialysis (see also under Dialysis Solutions, p.1023). A potassium concentration in dialysis fluid of 1 mmol per litre maintains plasma-potassium concentrations within the normal range when dietary intake is 60 to 80 mmol per day.

Potassium acetate is also used as a food preservative.

Preparations

Potassium Acetate Injection *(U.S.P.)*. A sterile solution of potassium acetate in Water for Injections. pH (of a 1% solution) 5.5 to 8.0. To be diluted before use.

Trikates Oral Solution *(U.S.P.)*. A solution of potassium acetate, potassium bicarbonate, and potassium citrate in water. Store in airtight containers. Protect from light.

1178-h

Potassium Bicarbonate *(USAN)*.

501; Kalii Hydrogenocarbonas; Monopotassium Carbonate; Potassium Hydrogen Carbonate.

$KHCO_3$=100.1.

CAS — 298-14-6.

Pharmacopoeias. In *Arg., Braz., Ger., Mex., Nord., Pol., Port., Span., Swiss*, and *U.S.*

Colourless, odourless, transparent prisms or white granular powder. Each g represents approximately 10 mmol of potassium and of bicarbonate. Potassium bicarbonate 2.6 g is approximately equivalent to 1 g of potassium.

Freely **soluble** in water; practically insoluble in alcohol. **Store** in well-closed containers.

Potassium bicarbonate may be used similarly to potassium chloride for the prevention and treatment of potassium deficiency. It is administered by mouth. As potassium bicarbonate is an alkalinising agent it is useful in the treatment of hypokalaemia occurring with metabolic acidosis.

Preparations

Potassium Bicarbonate Effervescent Tablets for Oral Solution *(U.S.P.)*. Store in airtight containers.

Potassium Bicarbonate and Potassium Chloride for Effervescent Oral Solution *(U.S.P.)*. Store in airtight containers.

Potassium Bicarbonate and Potassium Chloride Effervescent Tablets for Oral Solution *(U.S.P.)*. Store in airtight containers.

Potassium and Sodium Bicarbonates and Citric Acid Effervescent Tablets for Oral Solution *(U.S.P.)*. Store in airtight containers.

Proprietary Names and Manufacturers
Klor-Con-EF *(Upsher-Smith, USA)*.

The following names have been used for multi-ingredient electrolyte preparations containing potassium bicarbonate—Algicon *(Rorer, UK)*; Alka-Seltzer (Antacid) *(Miles Laboratories, USA)*; Brinaldix K *(Sandoz, UK)*; Kloref *(Cox, UK)*; Kloref-S *(Cox, UK)*; Klorvess Effervescent *(Sandoz, USA)*; K-Lyte *(Bristol, Canad.; Bristol, USA)*; K-Lyte/Cl *(Bristol, USA)*; Neo-K *(Neolab, Canad.)*; Phosphate-Sandoz *(Sandoz, Canad.; Sandoz, UK)*; Potavescent *(Protea, Austral.)*.

1179-m

Potassium Chloride *(BAN, USAN)*.

508; Cloreto de Potássio; Kalii Chloridum; Kalium Chloratum.
KCl=74.55.

CAS — 7447-40-7.

Pharmacopoeias. In *Arg., Aust., Belg., Br., Braz., Chin., Cz., Egypt., Eur., Fr., Ger., Hung., Ind., Int., It., Jpn, Jug., Mex., Neth., Nord., Pol., Port., Roum., Rus., Span., Swiss, Turk.*, and *U.S.*

Odourless, colourless, cubical, elongated, or prismatic crystals or white crystalline powder. Each g represents approximately 13.4 mmol of potassium. Potassium chloride 1.9 g is approximately equivalent to 1 g of potassium.

Soluble 1 in 2.8 to 3 of water; practically insoluble in alcohol. The *U.S.P.* also has soluble 1 in 2 of boiling water. A solution in water is neutral to litmus.

Potassium chloride is **incompatible** with amphotericin. Incompatibilities have also been reported with amikacin sulphate, dobutamine hydrochloride, and fixed oil emulsions. **Store** in well-closed containers.

Adverse Effects

Excessive administration of potassium leads to development of hyperkalaemia; for symptoms, see Hyperkalaemia above, under Potassium. Pain or phlebitis may occur during intravenous administration of solutions containing about 30 mmol or more potassium per litre.

Nausea, vomiting, diarrhoea, and abdominal cramps may occur following oral administration of potassium salts. There have been numerous reports of gastro-intestinal ulceration, sometimes with haemorrhage and perforation or with the late formation of strictures, after the use of enteric-coated tablets of potassium chloride. Ulceration has also occurred after the use of sustained-release tablets.

EFFECTS ON THE GASTRO-INTESTINAL TRACT. Results from 2 studies involving endoscopic examination of healthy subjects indicated that wax-matrix potassium chloride tablets were associated with a higher incidence of gastro-intestinal mucosal lesions than had previously been thought, and significantly less mucosal lesions were seen in subjects given microencapsulated potassium chloride (F.G. McMahon *et al.*, *Lancet*, 1982, *2*, 1059; J.S. Barkin, *et al.*, *Ann intern. Med.*, 1983, *98*, 261). The antimuscarinic drug glycopyrronium bromide had been given to most subjects in order to delay gastric emptying. A further study by McLoughlin (*Lancet*, 1985, *1*, 581) comparing wax-matrix, microencapsulated, and controlled-release potassium chloride formulations found considerable differences in the erosive action of different preparations on the upper gastro-intestinal tract; the greatest number of erosions was seen with the wax matrix. However, Aselton and Jick (*ibid.*, 1983, *1*, 184) had examined data from the Boston Collaborative Drug Surveillance Program and their findings had argued against a positive association between the use of wax-matrix potassium chloride and upper gastro-intestinal tract bleeding over a short period of time, although an association with asymptomatic lesions could not be ruled out. Endoscopic findings by Patterson *et al.* (*ibid.*, *2*, 1077) indicated that any solid potassium chloride formulation could cause erosive gastro-intestinal lesions when administered at high doses with an antimuscarinic agent. Two more recent studies (W.R. Alsop, *et al.*, *J. clin. Pharmac.*, 1984, *24*, 235; C. Kendall *et al.*, *Clin. Pharmac. Ther.*, 1985, *38*, 28) found no significant differences between various different potassium chloride formulations with respect to gastro-intestinal lesions. In both studies all subjects, including those in the placebo groups, received glycopyrronium bromide and in view of the high incidence of lesions found in the glycopyrronium bromide—placebo groups it was suggested that the antimuscarinic alone might cause gastro-intestinal mucosal lesions.

Ulceration and perforation of a Meckel's diverticulum in a 65-year-old woman was associated with the administration of a preparation containing slow-release potassium chloride 573 mg and bumetanide 500 mg over a period of 6 months.— G. T. Layer *et al.*, *Postgrad. med. J.*, 1987, *63*, 211.

EFFECTS ON THE SKIN. Skin necrosis in a patient following the accidental subcutaneous infiltration of molar potassium chloride solution; the potassium chloride was administered by an intravenous infusion pump into a peripheral vein but the cannula became dislodged and the solution extravasated.— H. P. E. Williams, *Br. med. J.*, 1984, *289*, 1742.

Analysis, by the Boston Collaborative Drug Surveillance Program, of data on 15 438 patients hospitalised between 1975 and 1982 detected 1 allergic skin reaction attributed to potassium chloride among 3460 recipients of the drug.— M. Bigby *et al.*, *J. Am. med. Ass.*, 1986, *256*, 3358.

Treatment of Adverse Effects

Potassium-containing foods and medications must be discontinued and potassium-retaining diuretics withdrawn. Severe cardiac toxicity may be treated by intravenous administration of calcium gluconate, with ECG monitoring. Serum concentrations of potassium may be reduced by infusions of glucose with or without insulin, or by the infusion of sodium bicarbonate solution. Care should be taken with digitalised patients, as rapid lowering of potassium concentration may precipitate cardiac toxicity.

Mild hyperkalaemia may be treated with sodium polystyrene sulphonate, administered by mouth or as an enema. In severe hyperkalaemia, treatment with haemodialysis or peritoneal dialysis may become necessary.

Hyperkalaemia associated with hyponatraemia may respond to treatment with infusions of sodium salts.

Precautions

Potassium salts should be administered with considerable care to patients with renal or adrenal insufficiency, cardiac disease, acute dehydration, heat cramps, extensive tissue destruction as occurs with severe burns, or to patients receiving potassium-sparing diuretics.

Solid oral dosage forms of potassium salts should not be administered to patients with gastro-intestinal ulceration or obstruction. They should be given with caution to patients in whom passage through the gastro-intestinal tract may be delayed as in pregnant patients or in those receiving antimuscarinic agents. Treatment should be discontinued if severe nausea, vomiting, or abdominal distress develops.

Excessive use of potassium-containing salt substitutes or concurrent administration with potassium supplements may lead to accumulation of potassium especially in patients with renal insufficiency. Attention should be paid to the concurrent use of other drugs that either contain potassium or have the potential for hyperkalaemia.

ADMINISTRATION. Considerable concern has been expressed by several clinicians regarding the procedure for the intravenous administration of potassium chloride (L. Rendell-Baker and J.A. Meyer, *Lancet*, 1985, *2*, 329; M. Lakhani and W.K. Stewart, *ibid.*, 453; C. Hawkins, *ibid.*, 552). Deaths have resulted from the addition of incorrect amounts of concentrated potassium chloride solution to infusions and also from injection of concentrated solutions of potassium chloride, ampoules of which have been mistaken for sodium chloride.—.

BLOOD DISORDERS. Although a 25-year-old woman with sickle-cell haemoglobinopathy had a normal response to acute potassium loading she developed life-threatening hyperkalaemia after receiving only modest amounts of potassium chloride over 3 days. It was recommended that potassium should be administered with caution to patients with sickle-cell haemoglobinopathy.— P. Mitnick *et al.* (letter), *Ann. intern. Med.*, 1979, *91*, 319.

LABORATORY ESTIMATIONS. Elevated serum-potassium concentrations in association with low serum glucose in a patient with a myeloproliferative disease were due to the rapid consumption of glucose and the leakage of potassium during clot formation and serum separation. Glucose and potassium values were normal when measured in plasma separated immediately after collection of blood. Routine analyses on serum samples by large automated laboratories could lead, especially in patients with blood diseases, to overestimation of potassium values and dangerously low potassium concentrations might be overlooked.— N. Ricci and P. M. Toma (letter), *Lancet*, 1985, *1*, 521. See also D. Hyman and N. M. Kaplan (letter), *New Engl. J. Med.*, 1985, *313*, 642.

POTASSIUM-CONTAINING SALT SUBSTITUTES. A report of a 63-year-old man with cardiomyopathy, taking frusemide and spironolactone, who developed hyperkalaemia on using a potassium-containing salt substitute.— D. McCaughan (letter), *Lancet*, 1984, *1*, 513.

A 70-year-old woman with angina pectoris which was controlled with diltiazem, metoprolol, and isosorbide dinitrate developed near-fatal hyperkalaemia following repeated ingestion of soup seasoned with a potassium-containing salt substitute. It was thought that the patients's hyperkalaemia could have been exacerbated by diltiazem.— R. E. Hoyt (letter), *J. Am. med. Ass.*, 1986, *256*, 1726.

Absorption and Fate

Potassium salts other than the phosphate, sulphate, and tartrate are generally readily absorbed from the gastro-intestinal tract. Potassium is excreted mainly by the kidneys; it is secreted in the distal tubules which are also the site of sodium—potassium exchange. The capacity of the kidneys to conserve potassium is poor and urinary excretion of potassium continues even when there is severe depletion. Tubular secretion of potassium is influenced by several factors, including chloride ion concentration, hydrogen ion exchange, acid-base equilibrium, and adrenal hormones. Some potassium is excreted in the faeces and small amounts may also be excreted in saliva, sweat, bile, and pancreatic juice.

Results from pharmacokinetic studies in 5 healthy subjects indicated that the average plasma-potassium concentration 3 hours after administration of potassium chloride 64 mmol by mouth was higher with a syrup preparation than with wax-based tablets. Total 36-hour urinary excretion and overall bioavailability were found to be similar for both formulations.— J. M. Toner and L. E. Ramsay, *Br. J. clin. Pharmac.*, 1985, *19*, 489.

In a study involving 28 healthy subjects no statistical difference was found between wax-matrix and microencapsulated potassium chloride formulations in terms of total amount of potassium excreted in the urine over a 24-hour period or in the rate of potassium excretion.— V. A. Skoutakis *et al.*, *J. clin. Pharmac.*, 1985, *25*, 619.

Uses and Administration

Potassium salts in this section are used in the treatment of potassium deficiency confirmed by plasma-potassium estimations; dosage should be individualised for each patient. In simple deficiency states potassium salts should be given by mouth in doses that provide up to 100 mmol or more of potassium daily. Potassium salts by mouth are more irritating than the corresponding sodium salts and should be taken with or after meals with plenty of fluid; liquid preparations should be well-diluted before administration. Prophylaxis with potassium salts is controversial, but is employed in certain patients, such as those on long-term or intensive therapy with diuretics (see p.983) or corticosteroids, and in patients receiving digitalis glycosides.

Potassium salts have a low renal threshold and excretion promotes diuresis. Potassium citrate (p.1025) is given by mouth as an alkalinising agent. The phosphate, sulphate, and tartrate salts of potassium are poorly absorbed and have been given by mouth to reduce the normal absorption of water from the intestine and, by promoting peristalsis, to cause evacuation of the intestine.

Some potassium salts are used as sodium-free condiments when sodium intake must be restricted.

In acute hypokalaemia, parenteral administration of potassium is necessary and doses of up to 100 mmol or more may be given by slow intravenous infusion under ECG control at a rate not exceeding 20 mmol per hour; the concentration of potassium should not exceed 40 mmol per litre. Adequate urine flow must be ensured and careful monitoring of plasma-potassium and other electrolyte concentrations is essential.

Potassium chloride is usually the potassium salt of choice as hypochloraemic alkalosis, which is often associated with hypokalaemia, can be corrected by the chloride ions. Various oral formulations of potassium chloride are available including syrups, effervescent tablets, and sustained-release tablets and capsules. Potassium chloride 1.9 g provides approximately 26 mmol of potassium.

Potassium chloride may be administered with sodium chloride and/or glucose by slow intravenous infusion to correct severe hypokalaemia occurring in association with sodium and fluid depletion.

There should be careful and thorough mixing when adding concentrated potassium chloride solutions to infusion fluids.

ADMINISTRATION. A comment on the possible hazards of nausea, retching, and vomiting brought on by the unpleasant taste of potassium chloride in solution. Three patients suffered life-threatening cardiovascular complications immediately after or during ingestion of potassium chloride solution; 2 subsequently died. Nausea with eructation or vomiting preceded the complications. When fluctuations in cardiac output and arterial pressure are undesirable, potassium replacement should be given intravenously, especially if the patient complains of nausea.— F. H. Messerli and N. D. Pappas (letter), *Lancet*, 1980, *2*, 919.

A recommendation that acute transient hypokalaemia, which may occur in association with postoperative or accidental hypothermia, should be corrected by administration of potassium by the intravenous route.— H. A. Bruining and R. U. Boelhouwer (letter), *Lancet*, 1982, *2*, 1283.

Potassium chloride was given by hypodermoclysis on 350 occasions to 67 patients. The solutions contained 34 mmol of potassium chloride per litre, was rendered iso-osmotic with glucose or sodium chloride, and contained hyaluronidase 1500 units per litre; one litre was given over 3 or 4 hours. The serum-potassium concentration rose by up to 1 mmol per litre; the procedure was considered to have advantages over intravenous administration in mild hypokalaemia.— R. J. Schen and S. Arieli, *Br. med. J.*, 1982, *285*, 1167.

Forty-six courses of intravenous potassium chloride administration were evaluated in 10 postoperative cardiac patients of mean age 13.7 months. Results indicated that intravenous supplementation of potassium chloride in a dose of 0.7 mmol per kg body-weight administered over 2 hours was safe and effective for paediatric postoperative cardiac patients.— D. E. Schaber *et al.*, *Drug Intell. & clin. Pharm.*, 1983, *17*, 439.

ASTHMA. Low serum-potassium is the most common electrolyte disturbance occurring in acute asthma. Serum-potassium concentrations should be monitored and supplements given as necessary.— J. Rees, *Br. med. J.*, 1984, *288*, 1747.

DIABETIC KETOACIDOSIS. Diabetic ketoacidosis is marked by normal or even increased serum-potassium concentrations despite a reduction in total body potassium. Patients with ketoacidosis require potassium supplementation and this may be necessary even in the presence of oliguria.— G. Kandel and A. Aberman, *Can. med. Ass. J.*, 1983, *128*, 392.

ECTOPIC PREGNANCY. Injection of 0.5 mL potassium chloride solution 20% w/v into the gestation sac under ultrasound control led to resolution of ectopic pregnancy in 3 patients. In 2 patients however, trophoblastic tissue was not completely destroyed and in both cases a necrotic villous tissue mass was subsequently removed by surgery.— D. E. Robertson *et al* (letter), *Lancet*, 1987, *1*, 974.

HYPERTENSION. For references to the effects of potassium supplementation on blood pressure, see p.1023.

LOCAL ANAESTHESIA. Addition of potassium chloride 0.2 mmol to 40 mL of bupivacaine solution 0.25% resulted in more rapid onset of sensory loss than bupivacaine alone in a double-blind study of 20 patients undergoing brachial plexus blockade. No difference in speed of onset of sensory loss was found when potassium chloride was added to prilocaine.— M. R. Parris and W. A. Chambers, *Br. J. Anaesth.*, 1986, *58*, 297.

MYOCARDIAL INFARCTION. Patients who had experienced an acute myocardial infarction within 12 hours received either conventional treatment or 48-hour infusions with glucose 300 g, insulin 500 units, and potassium chloride 80 mmol per litre. Significant decreases in mean blood pressure and pulmonary arterial end-diastolic pressure with improvement in cardiac index were observed in the glucose-insulin-potassium group compared with the control group.— J. A. Mantle *et al.*, *Am. Heart J.*, 1981, *102*, 313. See also *J. Am. med. Ass.*, 1977, *237*, 1070.

Preparations

Potassium Chloride Elixir *(U.S.P.)*. An elixir containing potassium chloride and alcohol about 18%. pH 5.7 to 6.7. Store in airtight containers.

Potassium Chloride Mixture *(A.P.F.)*. Potassium chloride 1 g, lemon syrup 2 mL, concentrated chloroform water 0.25 mL or methyl hydroxybenzoate solution 0.1 mL, water to 10 mL.

Each 10 mL contains 13.4 mmol of potassium and of chloride.

Potassium Chloride Injection *(U.S.P.)*. A sterile solution in Water for Injections. pH 4 to 8. To be diluted before use.

Potassium Chloride in Dextrose Injection *(U.S.P.)*. A sterile solution of potassium chloride and glucose in Water for Injections. Contains no antimicrobial agents. pH 3.5 to 6.5.

Potassium Chloride and Glucose Intravenous Infusion *(B.P.)*. Potassium Chloride and Dextrose Injection; Potassium Chloride and Dextrose Intravenous Infusion; Potassium Chloride and Glucose Injection. A sterile solution of potassium chloride and anhydrous glucose or glucose in Water for Injections. It is sterilised, immediately after preparation, by autoclaving. pH 3.5 to 6.5. Store at a temperature not exceeding 25°.

Potassium Chloride and Sodium Chloride Intravenous Infusion *(B.P.)*. Potassium Chloride and Sodium Chloride Injection. A sterile solution of potassium chloride and sodium chloride in Water for Injections. Sterilised by autoclaving.

Potassium Chloride, Sodium Chloride and Glucose Intravenous Infusion *(B.P.)*. Potassium Chloride, Sodium Chloride and Dextrose Injection; Potassium Chloride, Sodium Chloride and Dextrose Intravenous Infusion; Potassium Chloride, Sodium Chloride and Glucose Injection. A sterile solution of potassium chloride, sodium chloride 0.17 to 0.19%, and anhydrous glucose 3.8 to 4.2% (or the equivalent of glucose) in Water for Injections. Sterilise immediately by autoclaving. pH 3.5 to 6.5. Store at a temperature not exceeding 25°. It may cause the separation of solid particles from glass containers; solutions containing such particles must not be used.

Potassium Chloride for Oral Solution *(U.S.P.)*. A dry mixture of potassium chloride and one or more suitable diluents, colouring, and flavouring agents. Store in airtight containers.

Potassium Chloride Oral Solution *(U.S.P.)*. A solution containing potassium chloride. It may contain up to 7.5% of alcohol. Store in airtight containers.

Effervescent Potassium Chloride Tablets *(B.P.)*. Tablets containing potassium chloride in an effervescent basis. The proportion of chloride ions should be not less than 66 per cent of that of potassium ions. The tablets should be dissolved before administration. Store at a temperature not exceeding 25°.

Potassium Chloride Extended-release Capsules *(U.S.P.)*. Store in airtight containers at a temperature not exceeding 30°.

Potassium Chloride Extended-release Tablets *(U.S.P.)*. Store in airtight containers at a temperature not exceeding 30°.

Potassium Chloride, Potassium Bicarbonate, and Potassium Citrate Effervescent Tablets for Oral Solution *(U.S.P.)*. Store in airtight containers.

Proprietary Preparations

Kay-Cee-L *(Geistlich, UK)*. *Syrup*, sugar-free, potassium chloride 5 mmol/5 mL.

Kloref *(Cox, UK)*. *Tablets*, effervescent, betaine hydrochloride, potassium bicarbonate, potassium chloride, potassium benzoate providing 6.7 mmol of potassium and of chloride (equivalent to 500 mg of potassium chloride) when dissolved in water.

Kloref-S *(Cox, UK)*. *Oral granules*, effervescent, betaine hydrochloride, potassium bicarbonate, potassium chloride, in sachets providing 20 mmol of potassium and of chloride (equivalent to 1.5 g of potassium chloride) when dissolved in water.

Leo K *(Leo, UK)*. *Tablets*, sustained-release, potassium chloride, 600 mg (8 mmol of potassium and of chloride).

MicroK *(E. Merck, UK)*. *Capsules*, controlled-release, potassium chloride 600 mg (8 mmol of potassium and of chloride).

A review of the use of MicroK in the treatment of potassium depletion.— *Med. Lett.*, 1982, *24*, 71.

Nu-K *(Consolidated Chemicals, UK)*. *Capsules*, sustained-release, potassium chloride, 600 mg (8 mmol of potassium and of chloride).

Sando-K *(Sandoz, UK)*. *Tablets*, effervescent, potassium chloride 600 mg, potassium bicarbonate 400 mg, providing potassium 12 mmol and chloride 8 mmol, with anhydrous citric acid 800 mg when dissolved in water.

Slow-K *(Ciba, UK)*. *Tablets*, sustained-release, potassium chloride 600 mg (8 mmol of potassium and of chloride).

Proprietary Names and Manufacturers

Apo-K *(Apotex, Canad.)*; Celeka *(Arg.)*; Chloropotassuril *(Belg.)*; Chlorvescent *(Protea, Austral.)*; Diffu-k *(Delagrange, Fr.)*; Durules-K *(Arg.)*; K-10 Solution *(Beecham, Canad.)*; Kadalex *(Ital.)*; Kaleorid *(Leo, Denm.; Leo, Fr.; Leo, Norw.; Lövens, Swed.)*; Kalienor *(Biosédra, Fr.)*; Kaliglutol *(Switz.)*; Kalilente *(Ciba, Norw.; Ciba, Swed.)*; Kalinor *(Nordmark, Ger.)*; Kalinorm *(Benzon, Denm.; Benzon, Norw.)*; Kalipor *(Sanbolagen, Swed.)*; Kali-Retard *(Collett, Norw.)*; Kalitabs *(Ferrosan, Swed.)*; Kalitrans *(Fresenius, Ger.)*; Kalium Duretter *(Hässle, Norw.; Hässle, Swed.)*; Kalium Durettes *(Belg.; Neth.)*; Kalium Durules *(Astra, Canad.; Astra, UK)*; Kalium-Duriles *(Ger.)*; Kaochlor *(Adria, Canad.; Adria, USA)*; Kaon-Cl *(Adria, USA)*; Kato *(ICN, Canad.; ICN, USA)*; Kay Ciel *(Schering, Austral.; Berlex, Canad.; Forest Pharmaceuticals, USA)*; Kay-Cee-L *(Geistlich, UK)*; KCl-retard *(Zyma, Ital.; Inquinasa, Spain; Hausmann, Switz.; Zyma, Switz.)*; K-Contin Continus *(Napp, UK)*; K-Dur *(Key, USA)*; K-Long *(Adria, Canad.)*; K-Lor *(Abbott, Canad.; Abbott, USA)*; Klor *(Upsher-Smith, USA)*; Klor-Con *(Upsher-Smith, USA)*; Klorfen *(USA)*; Klorvess 10% Liquid *(Sandoz, USA)*; Klotrix *(Mead Johnson Pharmaceutical, USA)*; K-Lyte/Cl *(Bristol, Canad.)*; K-Norm *(Pennwalt, USA)*; K-San *(Prosana, Austral.)*; K-Tab *(Abbott, USA)*; Lento-K *(Propan, S.Afr.)*; Lento-Kalium *(Boehringer Biochemia, Ital.)*; Leo K *(Leo, S.Afr.; Leo, UK)*; MicroK *(Ciba, Austral.; Robins, Canad.; E. Merck, UK; Robins, USA)*; Miopotasio *(Bama, Spain)*; Novolente-K *(Novopharm, Canad.)*; Nu-K *(Consolidated Chemicals, UK)*; Nutek-K *(Script Intal, S.Afr.)*; Pan-Kloride *(Panray, USA)*; Peter-Kal *(S.Afr.)*; PfiKlor *(Pfipharmecs, USA)*; Plenish-K *(Lennon, S.Afr.)*; Potage *(Lemmon, USA)*; Potasion *(Delagrange, Spain)*; Potassion *(Fr.)*; Potassium Hausmann *(Hausmann, Switz.)*; Rekawan *(Giulini, Ger.)*; Roychlor *(Roy, Canad.)*; Rum-K *(Fleming, USA)*; Slo-Pot *(ICN, Canad.)*; Slow-K *(Ciba, Austral.; Ciba, Canad.; Jpn.; Ciba, S.Afr.; Ciba, UK; Ciba, USA)*; Span-K *(Protea, Austral.)*; Steropotassium *(Belg.)*; Swiss-Kal SR *(Hausmann, S.Afr.)*; Ten-K *(Geigy, USA)*; Ultra-K-Chlor *(Belg.)*.

The following names have been used for multi-ingredient electrolyte preparations containing potassium chloride—Artisial *(Jouveinal, Canad.)*; Brinaldix K *(Sandoz, UK)*; Burinex K *(Leo, UK)*; Centyl K *(Leo, UK)*; Colyte *(Reed & Carnrick, Canad.; Reed & Carnrick, USA)*; Diarrest *(Galen, UK)*; Diumide-K *(Degussa, UK)*; Esidrex-K *(Ciba, UK)*; GoLytely *(Braintree, USA)*; HydroSaluric-K *(Merck Sharp & Dohme, UK)*; Hygroton-K *(Geigy, UK)*; Hypertane Forte *(Medo, UK)*; Kloref *(Cox, UK)*; Kloref-S *(Cox, UK)*; Klorvess Effervescent *(Sandoz, USA)*; K-Lyte/Cl *(Bristol, USA)*; Lasikal *(Hoechst, UK)*; Lasix + K *(Hoechst, UK)*; Naturetin-K *(Squibb, Canad.)*; Navidrex-K *(Ciba, UK)*; Neo-K *(Neolab, Canad.)*; Neo-NaClex-K *(Duncan, Flockhart, UK)*; Rautractyl *(Squibb, Canad.)*; Rautrax *(Squibb, UK; Squibb, USA)*; Rautrax-N *(Squibb, USA)*; Salupres *(Merck Sharp & Dohme, UK)*; Sando-K *(Sandoz, UK)*; Serpasil-Esidrex-K *(Ciba, UK)*.

See also under pp.1023-4.

1181-x

Potassium Gluconate *(USAN)*.
577. Potassium D-gluconate.
$CH_2OH.[CH(OH)]_4.CO_2K$=234.2.

CAS — 299-27-4 (anhydrous); 35398-15-3 (monohydrate).

Pharmacopoeias. In *U.S.* which permits anhydrous or the monohydrate. Also in *B.P.C. 1973*.

A white or yellowish-white, odourless, crystalline powder or granules. Each g represents approximately 4.3 mmol of potassium. Potassium gluconate 6 g is approximately equivalent to 1 g of potassium.
Soluble 1 in 3 of water; practically insoluble in dehydrated alcohol, chloroform, and ether. A solution in water is slightly alkaline. **Store** in airtight containers.

Potassium gluconate may be used similarly to potassium chloride for the prevention and treatment of potassium deficiency. It is administered by mouth. As potassium gluconate is an alkalinising agent it may be useful in the treatment of hypokalaemia occurring with metabolic acidosis.

Preparations

Potassium Gluconate Elixir *(U.S.P.)*. Contains potassium gluconate and alcohol 4.5 to 5.5%. Potency is expressed in terms of anhydrous potassium gluconate.

Potassium Gluconate and Potassium Chloride Oral Solution *(U.S.P.)*

Potassium Gluconate and Potassium Chloride for Oral Solution *(U.S.P.)*

Potassium Gluconate and Potassium Citrate Oral Solution *(U.S.P.)*

Potassium Gluconate, Potassium Citrate, and Ammonium Chloride Oral Solution *(U.S.P.)*

Potassium Gluconate Tablets *(U.S.P.)*. Potency is expressed in terms of anhydrous potassium gluconate.

Proprietary Names and Manufacturers of Potassium Gluconate and other Related Salts

Gluconsan *(Jpn)*; Kalium Beta *(Beta, Arg.)*; Kalium-Hausmann *(Asta, Ger.)*; Kaon *(Montpellier, Arg.; Adria, Canad.; Adria, USA)*; Kaoplus *(Fulton, Ital.)*; Katorin *(Boots, UK)*; Potasion *(Delagrange, Spain)*; Potasoral *(Galepharma, Spain)*; Potassion *(Delagrange, Fr.)*; Potassium Égic *(Egic, Fr.)*; Potassium-Rougier *(Rougier, Canad.)*; Potassuril *(Sopar, Belg.)*; Royonate *(Roy, Canad.)*; Sirokal *(Belg.)*; Ultra K *(Sopar, Belg.)*.

The following names have been used for multi-ingredient electrolyte preparations containing potassium gluconate and other related salts—Bi-K *(USV Pharmaceutical Corp., USA)*; Twin-K *(Boots, USA)*; Twin-K-Cl *(Boots, USA)*.

1188-b

Sodium

Na=22.99.

The body contains about 40 to 60 mmol of sodium per kg body-weight, approximately 40 per cent of which is found in the skeleton. Sodium is the principal cation in the extracellular fluid (normal concentration range 135 to 145 mmol per litre) and is the main osmotic component in the control of blood volume. The intracellular sodium concentration is about 5 to 10 mmol per litre.

About 100 to 200 mmol of sodium is ingested daily in the typical diet and a similar amount is excreted, chiefly in the urine. The body can adapt to a wide range of intakes by adjustment of renal excretion through physical and hormonal factors. The amount of sodium lost in the faeces is only about 5 to 10 mmol per day. Loss through the skin is only significant if excessive sweating occurs.

In a temperate climate, the amount of sodium (as sodium chloride) required by an adult is less than 3 g per day (about 130 mmol) and such an intake can be gained from salt already present in food. However, most people are reported to add about 5 to 20 g per day (up to 870 mmol).

Sodium chloride is included in this section as it is used as a source of sodium in the treatment of electrolyte disturbances related to sodium depletion. Other sodium salts, some of which are described in other sections of this chapter, may also contribute to the sodium load. Sodium phosphate (p.1035) and the alkalinising agents sodium acetate, bicarbonate, citrate, and lactate (see under Bicarbonate, p.1024) are included in this chapter.

NOTE. Each g of sodium represents approximately 43.5 mmol.

Sodium Excess

Sodium excess may be caused by inadequate fluids, excessive fluid losses, excessive administration of sodium, impaired renal function, and aldosteronism. Sodium excess may take two forms. The first form, known as *hypernatraemia*, is a rise in extracellular concentration which may be the consequence of too little available water or over-provision of sodium against a low excretion-rate. The second form is too much sodium and water in the body without change in extracellular concentration. Retention of sodium leads to the accumulation of extracellular fluid (oedema) which may affect the cerebral, pulmonary, or peripheral circulations.

Sodium Depletion

Sodium deficit may take two forms. The first form, known as *hyponatraemia*, is associated with an inappropriate ratio of sodium to water in the extracellular space, and is usually the result of an excessive amount of water in the body. The second form of sodium deficit is when sodium and water are both lost. Symptoms of hyponatraemia include headache, anorexia, nausea, vomiting, muscle weakness, apathy, lethargy, confusion, delirium, and, in severe cases, coma and convulsions. Features of iso-osmotic fluid loss include thirst, dizziness, postural hypotension, low urine output, and ultimately shock because of fall in the plasma volume.

1191-f

Sodium Chloride *(BAN, USAN)*.

Chlorure de Sodium; Cloreto de Sódio; Natrii Chloridum; Salt.
NaCl=58.44.

CAS — 7647-14-5.

Pharmacopoeias. In *Arg., Aust., Belg., Br., Braz., Chin., Cz., Egypt., Eur., Fr., Ger., Hung., Ind., Int., It., Jpn, Jug., Mex., Neth., Nord., Pol., Port., Roum., Rus., Span., Swiss, Turk.,* and *U.S.* Also in *B.P. Vet.*

Odourless colourless crystals or white crystalline powder. Each g represents approximately 17.1 mmol of sodium and of chloride. Sodium chloride 2.54 g is approximately equivalent to 1 g of sodium.
Soluble 1 in 3 of water, 1 in 10 of glycerol; slightly soluble in alcohol and dehydrated alcohol. A 0.9% solution in water is iso-osmotic, and thus in most cases isotonic with serum and lachrymal secretions.
Solutions are **sterilised** by autoclaving or by filtration. Solutions, when stored, may cause separation of solid particles from glass containers and solutions containing such particles must not be used.
Store in well-closed containers.

Adverse Effects

Poisoning from sodium chloride has resulted from unsuccessful induction of emesis, gastric lavage with hypertonic saline, and errors in the formulation of infant feeds. Excessive administration of sodium chloride causes hypernatraemia, the most serious effect of which is dehydration of internal organs, especially the brain, which may lead to thrombosis and haemorrhage.

General adverse effects of excess sodium chloride in the body include nausea, vomiting, diarrhoea, abdominal cramps, thirst, reduced salivation and lachrymation, sweating, fever, hypotension, tachycardia, renal failure, peripheral and pulmonary oedema, respiratory arrest, headache, dizziness, restlessness, irritability, weakness, muscular twitching and rigidity, convulsions, coma, and death. Excess chloride in the body may cause a loss of bicarbonate with an acidifying effect.

Infants may appear not to be severely dehydrated, but coma and convulsions may persist due to vascular injury. They may show respiratory distress with tachypnoea and flaring nostrils.

Intra-amniotic injection of hypertonic solutions of sodium chloride can lead to serious adverse effects including disseminated intravascular coagulation, renal necrosis, cervical and uterine lesions, haemorrhage, pulmonary embolism, pneumonia, and death.—

EFFECTS ON BLOOD PRESSURE. For references to the effects of sodium restriction on blood pressure, see p.1023.

EFFECTS ON THE GASTRO-INTESTINAL TRACT. A report of massive necrosis of the gastric, duodenal, and jejunal mucosa in a 27-year-old female after receiving sodium chloride, about 1 kg in 600 mL of water, as an emetic. The patient required 31 weeks of continuous hospital care and 3 laparotomies over a period of 16 months. The hazards of salt emesis were emphasised.— J. Calam *et al., Dig. Dis. Scis,* 1982, *27,* 936.

Treatment of Adverse Effects

In the event of recent acute ingestion of sodium chloride, induction of emesis or gastric lavage should be carried out along with general symptomatic and supportive treatment. Convulsions should be treated with intravenous diazepam.

Normal serum-sodium concentrations should be carefully restored at a rate not exceeding 10 to 15 mmol per day by administration of hypotonic saline solutions intravenously. Dialysis may be necessary if there is significant renal impairment, the patient is moribund, or if the serum-sodium concentration is greater than 200 mmol per litre.

Precautions

Sodium chloride should be administered with caution to patients with congestive heart failure, peripheral or pulmonary oedema, impaired renal function, or pre-eclampsia. Care should also be taken when administering sodium chloride intravenously to very young or elderly patients. Excessive administration should be avoided as this may result in hypokalaemia.

Pseudohyponatraemia, a condition where spuriously low concentrations of sodium are found, occurs when a high concentration of solid matter (such as lipids and protein) is present in the plasma. This has been reported in patients with diabetes mellitus. False readings for plasma concentrations may be obtained as sodium is present only in the aqueous phase of plasma. Correct values are obtained by referring the concentration to plasma water, thus avoiding unnecessary, and possibly dangerous, treatment with sodium chloride.

Uses and Administration

Sodium chloride is used in the treatment of extracellular volume depletion, dehydration, and sodium depletion which may occur for instance following excessive diuresis, gastroenteritis, or salt restriction. A suggested oral replacement dose of sodium chloride is about 1 to 2 g three times daily either with food or as a solution. Sodium chloride 2.54 g provides approximately 43.5 mmol of sodium. Glucose facilitates the absorption of sodium from the gastro-intestinal tract and solutions containing sodium chloride and glucose often with additional electrolytes, are used for oral rehydration in acute diarrhoea and cholera (see p.1024).

The concentration and dosage of sodium chloride solutions for intravenous use is determined by several factors including the age, weight, and clinical condition of the patient. Serum-electrolyte concentrations should be carefully monitored. Isotonic (0.9% w/v) sodium chloride injection is used when sodium and water are depleted in isotonic proportions, for instance in the management of metabolic alkalosis and during and after surgery. It may also be used as a priming fluid for haemodialysis procedures. Intravenous administration of hypotonic sodium chloride, usually 0.45%, is used in solution with glucose in the management of hyperosmolar diabetes mellitus and in the maintenance and replacement of fluid, electrolyte, and carbohydrate in patients who are unable to take fluids and nutrients by mouth. It may also be used to assess renal function. Hypertonic solutions of sodium chloride, 3 or 5%, have been used in emergency situations of extreme sodium depletion (but see below under Hyponatraemia).

Intra-amniotic injection of sodium chloride solution 20 or 30% has been used to induce abortion, but serious side-effects such as haemorrhage have been reported which have led to maternal death (see also under Adverse Effects).

Sodium chloride 0.9% injections are often used as diluents for the infusion of drug additives, and 0.9% solutions of sodium chloride are widely used for sterile irrigation and dilution purposes.

Sodium chloride solutions should not be used to induce emesis; this practice is dangerous and deaths from resulting hypernatraemia have been reported.

Solutions of sodium chloride 0.9% may be used as eye-drops (as an irrigating agent), as nasal drops (to relieve nasal congestion), and as a mouthwash (to remove debris). Sodium chloride has also been included in dermatological preparations as a hydrating agent.

Sodium chloride (Natrium muriaticum; Nat. Mur.) is used in homoeopathic medicine.

CORNEAL EROSION. Recurrent corneal erosion in 60 patients was treated initially with chloramphenicol ointment or eye-drops, with debridement if necessary. Prophylaxis with 5% sodium chloride ointment at night kept 32 patients symptom-free, with improvement in a further 16. Deterioration was common when treatment was stopped. It was not clear whether the lubricant or desiccant effect of the ointment was the more important.— N. Brown and A. Bron, *Br. J. Ophthal.*, 1976, *60*, 84.

CYSTIC FIBROSIS. Inhalation with an aerosol of isotonic or hypertonic saline (7%) used for 10 minutes prior to physiotherapy sometimes aids the clearing of secretions in patients with cystic fibrosis.— M. B. Mearns, *Archs Dis. Childh.*, 1985, *60*, 272.

Cystic fibrosis patients have increased salt loss in sweat, and should be advised to take liberal dietary salt and plenty of fluid especially in hot weather, febrile illness, and vigorous exercise.— C. Smalley, *Prescribers' J.*, 1986, *26*, 122.

Sweat test. The diagnosis of cystic fibrosis is based on the determination of elevated concentrations of chloride ions in sweat; chloride concentrations in stimulated sweat from healthy children are less than 50 mmol per litre whereas concentrations above 60 mmol per litre are seen in children with cystic fibrosis. The sweat test recognises more than 98 per cent of children with cystic fibrosis.— *Bull. Wld Hlth Org.*, 1985, *63*, 1.

DIAGNOSIS AND TESTING. *Asthma diagnosis.* Inhalation of different concentrations of ultrasonically nebulised saline to detect non-immunologically mediated bronchial hyperreactivity.— R. E. Schoeffel *et al.*, *Br. med. J.*, 1981, *283*, 1285.

Blood group serology. Indirect anti-human-globulin tests washed in saline manufactured for irrigation purposes showed variable and at times a profound inhibition of antigen-antibody reactions involving antibodies of known clinical significance.— R. Mitchell *et al.* (letter), *Lancet*, 1983, *1*, 998.

Cystic fibrosis. See under Sweat Test, above.

Primary aldosteronism. Measurement of urinary aldosterone excretion after administration of sodium chloride injection 0.9% intravenously to 35 patients with hypertension and hypokalaemia proved to be a useful test in the identification of primary aldosteronism due to aldosterone-producing adenoma.— G. S. Stokes *et al.*, *Aust. N.Z. J. Med.*, 1984, *14*, 201.

DIET SUPPLEMENTATION. Twenty-two infants of gestational age 27 to 34 weeks given sodium chloride supplementation by mouth to maintain sodium homoeostasis showed improved growth and biochemical status compared with 24 infants given no diet supplementation. It was recommended that babies born before 34 weeks' gestation should either be given salt supplementation or be fed on their own mothers' milk; supplementation was considered to be unnecessary after the second postnatal week.— J. Al-Dahhan *et al.*, *Archs Dis. Childh.*, 1984, *59*, 945.

HYDATID CYST. An account of the management of hydatid disease and mention of preference for hypertonic saline 10% as a scolicidal agent after aspiration of the cyst.— D. L. Morris, *Br. J. Hosp. Med.*, 1981, *25*, 586.

The following recommendations were made for the use of hypertonic saline in the surgical management of hydatid cysts: close postoperative monitoring of electrolyte concentrations, protection of the peritoneal cavity from both the cyst contents and the saline, and careful, accurate injection of cysts.— T. P. Gage and G. Vivian (letter), *Ann. intern. Med.*, 1984, *101*, 405.

HYPONATRAEMIA. The treatment of severe hyponatraemia is controversial and it is still unclear whether resulting neurologic disorders, which can be fatal, are caused by the severity of the hyponatraemia itself or the speed with which it is corrected with intravenous sodium chloride. Arieff (*New. Engl. J. Med.*, 1986, *314*, 1529) reviewed the treatment of 15 women, none of whom had had relevant pre-existing medical conditions, who had developed severe hyponatraemia following elective surgery. The causes of the abrupt fall in serum-sodium concentration were thought to be multiple, with the most important factor being excessive postoperative administration of hypotonic fluid. There was an average delay of 16 hours before therapy for hyponatraemia was initiated, the mean rate of correction being less than 0.7 mmol per litre per hour. In another retrospective study Sterns *et al.* (*ibid.*, 1535) described 8 patients with serious neurological complications believed to have been caused by overly rapid correction of hyponatraemia. They believed, on the grounds of existing data, that worsening of neurological function appeared to be associated with the correction of serum-sodium concentration at a rate of more than 12 mmol per litre per day. There have been 2 critical reviews of these and other reports. Narins (*ibid.*, 1573) concluded that, in the light of previous clinical experience, although very rapid correction of severe hyponatraemia might be dangerous, most experts believed that an increase in the serum-sodium concentration of 2 mmol per litre per hour to a concentration of 120 to 130 mmol per litre was not excessive in symptomatic patients with hyponatraemia. However, Swales (*Br. med. J.*, 1987, *294*, 261) considered that the rate for correcting hyponatraemia suggested by Sterns *et al.* (12 mmol per litre per day) seemed reasonable. Various authors have also expressed views on the therapy of hyponatraemia in correspondence (*New Engl. J. Med.*, 1986, *315*, 1351-5; *Br. med. J.*, 1987, *294*, 837).

Five patients with severe hyponatraemia and seizures thought to be caused by water intoxication from excess fluids were given 50 mL of sodium chloride solution 29.2% over 10 minutes by intravenous infusion in an attempt rapidly to reduce cerebral oedema, control seizures, and reduce the incidence of irreversible neuronal damage. Seizures were controlled in all patients by the sodium chloride, and further saline and frusemide was administered over an average of 10 hours. The total amount of sodium administered was 790 mmol which increased the serum-sodium concentration to an average of 133 mmol per litre. All patients survived, but one patient was left with a permanent neurological defect which may have been due to a prolonged episode of status epilepticus and hypotension, but treatment with 29.2% saline could not be excluded as a cause.— L. I. G. Worthley and P. D. Thomas, *Br. med. J.*, 1986, *292*, 168. Criticism.— G. Gill (letter), *ibid.*, 625.

LAVAGE. Since the absorption of some drugs could be enhanced by the presence of water in the gastro-intestinal tract it was suggested that in the emergency treatment of overdoses of lipid-insoluble drugs, gastric lavage with isotonic saline would be preferable to lavage with water.— G. Williams and J. L. Maddocks (letter), *Br. J. clin. Pharmac.*, 1975, *2*, 543.

Rigid bronchoscopy and cold saline lavage was carried out in 12 patients with massive haemoptysis. All patients stopped bleeding during the procedure, and bleeding in 2 patients who had a second haemorrhage was also controlled by bronchoscopy and lavage with saline.— A. A. Conlan and S. S. Hurwitz, *Thorax*, 1980, *35*, 901.

PAIN. Local infiltration of lignocaine 1.5% or saline 0.9% into pericranial tender spots were both found to have a beneficial effect on attacks of common migraine.— P. Tfelt-Hansen *et al.* (letter), *Lancet*, 1980, *1*, 1140.

In a double-blind study of 28 patients with myofascial pain, local injections of physiological saline tended to achieve better pain relief than mepivacaine 0.5%.— F. A. Frost *et al.*, *Lancet*, 1980, *1*, 499.

RENAL OBSTRUCTION. Sodium chloride depletion following relief of urinary obstruction may be difficult to detect clinically without measurement of central venous pressure, especially in patients who have already experienced a prolonged diuresis due to partial obstruction. Sodium chloride solution 0.9% should be administered intravenously to replace saline losses, and not 5% glucose solution which can lead to severe hyponatraemia.— *Lancet*, 1985, *1*, 1429.

SCLEROTHERAPY. Use of hypertonic sodium chloride solution 23.4% as a sclerosing agent for varicose veins.— E. L. Bodian, *J. dermatol. Surg. Oncol.*, 1985, *11*, 696.

A report on the successful use of hypertonic sodium chloride solution 20% as a sclerosing agent during endoscopic sclerotherapy in 10 children with variceal bleeding.— V. N. Perisic (letter), *Gut*, 1986, *27*, 350.

TATTOO REMOVAL. The use of sodium chloride in the abrasive removal of tattoos.— A. M. M. Strong and I. T. Jackson, *Br. J. Derm.*, 1979, *101*, 693; *Lancet*, 1980, *1*, 577; M. D. Catterall (letter), *ibid.*, 981.

TRANSTRACHEAL INJECTION. Transtracheal injection of isotonic saline proved to be a safe and effective method of obtaining lower respiratory tract secretions from 42 patients with pneumonia who could not produce sputum spontaneously.— J. T. Macfarlane and M. J. Ward, *Br. med. J.*, 1984, *288*, 974. Comment that a guard may be used to prevent over-insertion of the needle thus preventing possible damage to the vocal cords. In addition, patients should be instructed to apply pressure over the puncture site following the procedure in order to prevent subcutaneous emphysema or haematoma developing on coughing.— A. T. Irvine (letter), *ibid.*, 1311.

WOUND HEALING. Results from a study in 12 patients with 18 leg ulcers indicating that continuous irrigation with isotonic saline solution via a special dressing may be a clinically useful method of wound treatment. The temperature, pH, content, and osmotic activity of the fluid used may be changed and substances such as proteolytic enzymes and anti-inflammatory and local anaesthetic substances and, where necessary, antibiotics may be added.— P. Svedman, *Lancet*, 1983, *2*, 532.

Preparations

Sodium Chloride Eye Lotion *(B.P.)*. Sodium chloride 900 mg, water to 100 mL. The solution is filtered, transferred to the final containers, which are then closed to exclude micro-organisms, and sterilised by autoclaving.

NOTE. The *B.P.* permits the title SALINE for single-dose eye-drops containing sodium chloride 0.9%.

Sodium Chloride Ophthalmic Ointment *(U.S.P.)*

Sodium Chloride Ophthalmic Solution *(U.S.P.)*. A sterile solution of sodium chloride; it contains a buffer and may contain suitable antimicrobial and stabilising agents. pH 6 to 8. Store in airtight containers.

Sodium Chloride Inhalation Solution *(U.S.P.)*. A sterile solution of sodium chloride in water containing no antimicrobial agents or other added substances. pH 4.5 to 7.0.

Bacteriostatic Sodium Chloride Injection *(U.S.P.)*. A sterile isotonic solution of sodium chloride in Water for Injections, containing one or more suitable antimicrobial agents.

Sodium Chloride Intravenous Infusion *(B.P.)*. Sodium Chloride Injection. A sterile solution of sodium chloride in Water for Injections. Sterilised by autoclaving. Store at a temperature not exceeding 25°.

NOTE. When Normal Saline Solution for Injection is prescribed, a 0.9% injection is supplied.

Sodium Chloride Injection *(U.S.P.)*. A sterile solution of sodium chloride in Water for Injections containing no antimicrobial agents. pH 4.5 to 7.0. Injections containing more than 0.9% of sodium chloride should be diluted with Water for Injections to give a concentration of 0.9% of sodium chloride.

Dextrose and Sodium Chloride Injection *(U.S.P.)*. A sterile solution of glucose and sodium chloride in Water for Injections containing no antimicrobial agents. pH 3.5 to 6.5.

Sodium Chloride and Glucose Intravenous Infusion *(B.P.).* Sodium Chloride and Dextrose Injection; Sodium Chloride and Dextrose Intravenous Infusion; Sodium Chloride and Glucose Injection. A sterile solution of sodium chloride and anhydrous glucose or glucose in Water for Injections. The solution is sterilised immediately after preparation by autoclaving. pH 3.5 to 6.5. Store at a temperature not exceeding 25°.

Sodium Chloride Irrigation *(U.S.P.)*

Compound Sodium Chloride Mouthwash *(B.P.).* Sodium chloride 1.5 g, sodium bicarbonate 1 g, concentrated peppermint emulsion 2.5 mL, double-strength chloroform water 50 mL, water to 100 mL. To be diluted with an equal volume of warm water before use.

Sodium Chloride Solution *(B.P.).* Sodium chloride 0.9% in freshly boiled and cooled water. The solution is clarified by filtration. It should not be used for injection.
NOTE. When Normal Saline is prescribed, Sodium Chloride Solution is supplied.

Sodium Chloride Tablets for Solution *(U.S.P.).* Tablets containing sodium chloride with no added substance.

Sodium Chloride Tablets *(B.P.).* To be dissolved in water before administration.

Sodium Chloride Tablets *(U.S.P.)*

Sodium Chloride and Dextrose Tablets *(U.S.P.).* Tablets containing sodium chloride and glucose.

Proprietary Preparations

Alcon Opulets Sodium Chloride *(Alcon, UK). Eye-drops,* sodium chloride 0.9%, in single-use disposable applicators.

Minims Sodium Chloride *(Smith & Nephew Pharmaceuticals, UK). Eye-drops,* sodium chloride 0.9%, in single-use disposable applicators.

Normasol *(Seton, UK). Solution,* sterile, sodium chloride 0.9%, in single-use disposable sachets of 25 and 100 mL.

Normasol Undine *(Seton, UK). Solution,* sterile, sodium chloride 0.9%, in single-use disposable dual-opening polypropylene containers of 20 mL.

Topiclens *(Smith & Nephew Pharmaceuticals, UK). Solution,* sterile, sodium chloride 0.9%, in single-use disposable sachets of 25 and 100 mL.

Uro-Tainer Sodium Chloride 0.9% *(Vifor, Switz.: CliniMed, UK). Solution,* sterile, sodium chloride 0.9%, in single-use disposable sachets of 100 mL. For maintenance of indwelling urinary catheters.

Uro-Tainer M Sodium Chloride 0.9% *(Vifor, Switz.: CliniMed, UK). Solution,* sterile, sodium chloride 0.9%, in single-use disposable sachets of 50 and 100 mL. For instillation and retrieval of cytotoxic agents, antibiotics, and antiseptics via indwelling urinary catheters.

Proprietary Names and Manufacturers

Addex-Natriumklorid *(Pharmacia, Swed.)*; Adsorbonac *(Alcon, Canad.; Alcon, Ger.)*; Alcon Opulets Sodium Chloride *(Alcon, UK)*; Coca's Extracting Fluid *(Commonwealth Serum Laboratories, Austral.)*; Fyskosal *(Norw.; Swed.)*; Humist *(Scherer, USA)*; Hypersal *(American Optical, USA)*; Isosol *(Allergan, Austral.)*; Koksalt *(Swed.)*; Minims Sodium Chloride *(Smith & Nephew, Austral.; Smith & Nephew Pharmaceuticals, UK)*; Muro-128 *(Charton, Canad.)*; NaSal *(Winthrop-Breon, USA)*; Natrilentin *(Leo, Norw.; Swed.)*; Normasol *(Seton, UK)*; Ocean Mist *(Fleming, USA)*; Salinex *(Charton, Canad.; Muro, USA)*; Saltvann *(Nyco, Norw.)*; Scanlens Rinse *(Alcon, Austral.)*; Øyebadevann *(Norw.)*; Slow Sodium *(Ciba, S.Afr.; Ciba, UK)*; Topiclens *(Smith & Nephew Pharmaceuticals, UK)*; Uro-Pract *(Schiwa, Ger.)*; Uro-Tainer Sodium Chloride *(Vifor, Switz. : CliniMed, UK)*; Vésirig *(Fr)*;

Manufacturers also include—*Boots, UK.*

The following names have been used for multi-ingredient electrolyte preparations containing sodium chloride—Artisial *(Jouveinal, Canad.)*; Citrocarbonate *(Upjohn, Canad.)*; Colyte *(Reed & Carnrick, Canad.; Reed & Carnrick, USA)*; Diarrest *(Galen, UK)*; Effervescent Saline Tablets *(Southon-Horton, UK)*; GoLytely *(Braintree, USA)*; Iodised Sodium Chloride Tablets *(Southon-Horton, UK)*; Miol (Formula M.I.) Cream *(BritCair, UK)*; Miol (Formula M.I.) Lotion *(BritCair, UK)*; Normol *(Alcon, Austral.)*; Quik-Prep *(Jayco, USA)*; Sclerodex *(Ondee, Canad.)*.

See also under pp.1023-4.

Enzymes

3700-x

This section describes some enzymes of various origins which are used therapeutically.

16956-z

Alteplase

G-11021 (2-chain form); G-11035; G-11044; rt-PA; Tissue Plasminogen Activator; Tissue-type Plasminogen Activator; t-PA.

Units

850 units of tissue plasminogen activator are contained in one ampoule of the second International Standard Preparation (1987).

Adverse Effects, Treatment, and Precautions

As for streptokinase (p.1048). Allergic reactions should be less of a problem with alteplase.

Uses and Administration

Alteplase is a predominantly single-chain form of tissue plasminogen activator produced by recombinant DNA technology. It acts on plasminogen to yield plasmin (p.1047) and has a selective action on fibrin plasminogen.

Alteplase is used as a thrombolytic principally to clear occlusions in coronary vessels in patients with myocardial infarction. It is given by intravenous infusion in a dose of 100 mg over a period of 3 hours. Treatment with anticoagulants then follows.

The role of thrombolytics in thrombo-embolic disorders is discussed under streptokinase (p.1048) and included there are details on alteplase.

Reviews of the actions and uses of alteplase: S. J. Crabbe and C. C. Cloninger, *Clin. Pharm.*, 1987, *6*, 373; *Tissue Plasminogen Activator in Thrombolytic Therapy*, B.E. Sobel, D. Collen, E.B. Grossbard (Eds), New York and Basel, Marcel Dekker, 1987.

Proprietary Names and Manufacturers

Actilyse *(Boehringer Ingelheim, UK)*; Activase *(Genentech, USA)*.

3702-f

Amylase

Diastase. An enzyme catalysing the hydrolysis of α-1,4-glucosidic linkages of polysaccharides such as starch, glycogen, or their degradation products.

CAS — 9000-92-4.

Pharmacopoeias. In *Fr.*and *Ind.*

Amylases may be classified according to the manner in which the glucosidic bond is attacked. Endoamylases attack the α-1,4-glucosidic linkage at random.Alpha-amylases are the only types of endoamylases known and yield dextrins, oligosaccharides, and monosaccharides. The more common alpha-amylases include those isolated from human saliva, mammalian pancreas, *Bacillus subtilis, Aspergillus oryzae*, and barley malt. Exoamylases attack the α-1,4-glucosidic linkage only from the non-reducing outer polysaccharide chain ends. They include beta-amylases and glucoamylases (amyloglucosidases or gamma-amylases) and are of vegetable or microbial origin. Beta-amylases yield beta-limit dextrins and maltose and glucoamylases yield glucose.

Adverse Effects

Hypersensitivity reactions have been reported.

A report of allergic responses in workers exposed to fungal α-amylase derived from *Aspergillus oryzae.* These responses were not obtained with α-amylase derived from *Bacillus subtilis.* These findings have implications for workers in the flour milling and bakery industries.— M. L. H. Flindt (letter), *Lancet*, 1979, *1*, 1407.

Uses.

Amylase is used in the production of predigested starchy foods and for the conversion of starch to fermentable sugars in the brewing and fermentation industries.

Amylase from various sources has also been used as a digestant.

Proprietary Names and Manufacturers

Bilezyme *(Geriatric Pharm. Corp., USA)*; Buccalase *(Winthrop, Austral.)*; Landrase *(Landerlan, Spain)*; Maxilase *(Millot-Solac, Fr.*; *Lesvi, Spain*; *Solac, Switz.)*; Oramyl *(Sandoz, Fr.)*; Taka-Diastasa *(Parke, Davis, Spain)*; Taka-Diastase *(Parke, Davis, UK)*.

The following names have been used for multi-ingredient preparations containing amylase—Preven-zyme *(Legere, USA)*.

16996-d

Anistreplase *(BAN, pINN)*.

Anisoylated Plasminogen Streptokinase Activator Complex; APSAC; BRL-26921. *p*-Anisoylated (human) lys-plasminogen streptokinase activator complex (1:1).

CAS — 81669-57-0.

Units

One unit of anistreplase is approximately equivalent to 1 mg.

Adverse Effects, Treatment, and Precautions

As for streptokinase (p.1048). Hypotension should be less of a problem with anistreplase although it does occur if the injection is given rapidly over a period of less than 3 minutes.

Absorption and Fate

Anistreplase is reported to have a plasma half-life of 90 to 112 minutes. It is metabolised to the plasminogen-streptokinase complex at a steady rate.

Uses and Administration

Anistreplase consists of a complex of the lys-form of plasminogen and streptokinase with the addition of a *p*-anisoyl group that prevents the complex activating plasminogen to plasmin. Following intravenous injection the anisoyl group undergoes deacylation at a steady rate to release the active complex which has a selective action on fibrin plasminogen to produce plasmin (see p.1047).

Anistreplase is used as a thrombolytic principally to clear occlusions in coronary vessels in patients with myocardial infarction. It is given as a single intravenous injection in a dose of 30 units over 4 to 5 minutes within 6 hours of the onset of symptoms of infarction. Treatment with anticoagulants then follows.

A symposium on anistreplase.— J. L. Anderson *et al.* (Ed.), *Drugs*, 1987, *33*, *Suppl.* 3, 1-316.

A review of the actions and uses of anistreplase.— J. P. Monk and R. C. Heel, *Drugs*, 1987, *34*, 25.

For an overview of thrombolytic therapy in thrombo-embolic disorders including a discussion of anistreplase see streptokinase (p.1048).

Proprietary Preparations

Eminase *(Beecham Research, UK)*. *Injection*, powder for reconstitution, anistreplase 30 units per vial.

Proprietary Names and Manufacturers

Eminase *(Beecham-Wülfing, Ger.*; *Beecham Research, UK)*.

3704-n

Brinolase

Astra-1652; Brinase *(rINN)*; CA-7; Protease I. A fibrinolytic enzyme from *Aspergillus oryzae.*

CAS — 9000-99-1.

Brinolase has fibrinolytic and proteolytic activity and lowers the plasmin-inhibitory activity of the serum.

It has been used for clearing blocked haemodialysis cannulas.

Allergic symptoms arising from industrial handling of brinolase.— M. Forsbeck and L. Ekenvall (letter), *Lancet*, 1978, *2*, 524.

Intravenous treatment with brinolase resulted in clinical improvement in 13 of 17 patients suffering from chronic peripheral arterial disease. The condition of 2 patients remained unchanged, and in 2 patients amputation could not be avoided.— F. Lund *et al.*, *Angiology*, 1975, *26*, 534.

Brinolase has a direct effect not only on fibrin but also on other substrates such as fibrinogen, prothrombin, and factors V and VII. It has been claimed to be effective in lysing intravascular fibrin without undue bleeding.— V. V. Kakkar and M. F. Scully, *Br. med. Bull.*, 1978, *34*, 191.

Proprietary Names and Manufacturers

Brinastrase *(Astra, Norw.*; *Astra, Swed.)*.

3705-h

Bromelains *(BAN, USAN, rINN)*.

Bromelins; Plant Protease Concentrate.

CAS — 9001-00-7.

A concentrate of proteolytic enzymes derived from the pineapple plant, *Ananas comosus* (=*A. sativus*) (Bromeliaceae).

The properties and assay methods of bromelains.— Bromelain, in *Pharmaceutical Enzymes*, R. Ruyssen and A. Lauwers (Ed.), Gent, E. Story-Scientia, 1978, p.107.

Units

One Rorer unit of protease activity has been defined as that amount of enzyme which hydrolyses a standardised casein substrate at pH 7 and 25° so as to cause an increase in absorbance of 0.00001 per minute at 280 nm.

One FIP unit of bromelain activity is reported to be contained in that amount of a standard preparation, which hydrolyses a suitable preparation of casein (FIP controlled) under the standard conditions at an initial rate such that there is liberated per minute an amount of peptides, not precipitated by a specified protein precipitation reagent which gives the same absorbance as 1 μmol of tyrosine at 275 nm.

Activity has also been described in terms of milk-clotting units.

Adverse Effects

Bromelains may cause nausea, vomiting, and diarrhoea. Metrorrhagia and menorrhagia have occasionally occurred. Hypersensitivity reactions have been reported and have included skin reactions and asthma.

A report of bronchial asthma experienced by 2 patients after exposure to bromelains.— F. Galleguillos and J. C. Rodriguez, *Clin. Allergy*, 1978, *8*, 21.

Of 6 workers sensitised to papain 5 showed positive skin tests to bromelains and 2 of them also showed immediate asthmatic reactions after bronchial challenge with bromelains.— X. Baur and G. Fruhmann, *Clin. Allergy*, 1979, *9*, 443.

Precautions

Bromelains should be given with care to patients with coagulation disorders or with severely impaired hepatic or renal function.

Uses and Administration

Bromelains is used as an adjunct in the treatment of soft tissue inflammation and oedema associated with trauma and surgery.

The suggested dose by mouth, is 100 000 Rorer units 4 times daily. Bromelains has also been given as an aid to digestion.

Proprietary Preparations

Ananase Forte *(Fisons, UK)*. *Tablets*, enteric-coated, bromelains 100 000 Rorer units.

Proprietary Names and Manufacturers

Ananase *(Austral.*; *Rottapharm, Ital.*; *Lagamed, S.Afr.*; *USA)*; Ananase Forte *(Lagamed, S.Afr.*; *Fisons, UK)*; Dayto Anase *(Dayton, USA)*; Extranase *(Belg.*; *Rorer, Fr.)*; Proteolis *(Benvegna, Ital.)*; Resolvit *(Switz.)*; Rogorin *(Saba, Ital.)*; Traumanase *(Rorer, Ger.*; *Rorer, Switz.)*.

The following names have been used for multi-ingredient preparations containing bromelains— Nutrizym *(E. Merck, UK)*.

3044-b

Catalase

Caperase; Equilase; Optidase.

Catalase is an enzyme obtained from a wide variety of biological sources including animal liver (hepatocatalase) and certain bacteria and fungi. It has been applied to wounds and skin ulcers and has also been used in the treatment of eczema.

Combinations of catalase with superoxide dismutase (see Orgotein, p.1045) have also been investigated.

Proprietary Names and Manufacturers

Biocatalase *(Bilbo, Spain)*.

3708-v

Chymopapain *(BAN, USAN, rINN)*.

Bax-1526; NSC-107079. A proteolytic enzyme isolated from the latex of papaya (*Carica papaya*), differing from papain in electrophoretic mobility, solubility, and substrate specificity. Molecular weight approximately 27 000.

CAS — 9001-09-6.

Units

One nanokatal (nKat) is defined as the amount of chymopapain which produces 1 nanomole of *p*-nitroaniline per second from DL-benzoylarginine-*p*-nitroanilide substrate at pH 6.4 and 37°.

Adverse Effects

The most important adverse effect of chymopapain is anaphylaxis which can occur in up to about 1% of patients. It has resulted in fatalities and restricts its use to only one treatment session per patient. Typical symptoms include angioedema, laryngeal oedema and bronchospasm, shock and cardiac arrest. Allergic skin reactions may also occur. Severe muscle spasm and an increase in back pain are common reactions. Paraplegia, acute transverse myelitis, arachnoiditis, subarachnoid haemorrhage, and pulmonary embolism have occurred. Other reported reactions include headache, nausea and vomiting, paralytic ileus, urinary retention, thrombophlebitis, paraesthesias, foot-drop, and discitis.

In a postmarketing surveillance study on a chymopapain preparation for intradiscal injection (Chymodiactin) data was received on 29 075 patients by January 1984 (representing about 50% of the total number of vials sold to that date). Anaphylactic reactions were confirmed in 194 patients (0.67%), 2 of whom died. The incidence was higher in women than in men. In 52 cases the reaction occurred after the test dose.

Neurological reactions of a serious nature were reported in 22 patients. Six patients had cerebral haemorrhage and 3 died; autopsy revealed that they had underlying cerebrovascular abnormalities. Eleven patients were reported to have developed paraplegia; in 5 of these cases this may have been due to incorrect needle placement. Two patients suddenly developed transverse myelitis with paraplegia after 2 and 3 weeks, with subsequent recovery. Two patients had seizures after the injection of chymopapain, and in another patient this reaction occurred several days after the procedure. Hypersensitivity to the contrast medium and underlying epilepsy may have played a role in 2 of these cases.

Twenty-two patients had discitis with severe back pain and spasm. In 9 cases bacteria could be cultured.

There were 11 deaths. In addition to the 5 deaths mentioned above 1 patient developed a fatal *Staphylococcus aureus* meningitis following discitis at the site of injection. Three patients apparently died of an underlying disease and in 2 other cases the relationship to the administration of chymopapain was not clear.

It was concluded that careful attention to proper patient selection and correct techniques of intradiscal needle placement are the most important factors in avoiding adverse effects with chymopapain.— K. Agre *et al.*, *Spine*, 1984, *9*, 479. See also C. Watts, *Neurosurgery*, 1977, *1*, 2.

A discussion of the various regimens that have been recommended to pretreat patients prior to chymopapain injection to prevent anaphylaxis.— J. Iwatsubo and L. J. Miwa, *Drug Intell. & clin. Pharm.*, 1985, *19*, 26.

Neurotoxicity may arise not only from inadvertent injection into the CSF but following diffusion from the disk, see under Disk Disorders in Uses, below.

Precautions

Chymopapain should not be used in those patients with a known sensitivity to papaya proteins or in patients with paralysis, tumours of the spinal cord, or lesions of the cauda equina. Severe spondylolisthesis is also a contra-indication.

Care is required in administering chymopapain to ensure that the injection is into the disk and not intrathecal. Contrast media used to assist placement of the needle can inactivate chymopapain, so as little as possible should be used.

Various measures are or have been used in an attempt to reduce the risk of allergic reactions including tests to identify those most at risk and the administration of antihistamines and corticosteroids. None of these measures should be considered as an alternative to the necessity of drugs and equipment for the emergency management of anaphylactic reactions always being to hand when giving patients chymopapain. The risk of allergic reactions associated with chymopapain is so high that no patient should ever receive it more than once.

Uses and Administration

Chymopapain is used as an injection into the intervertebral disk in the treatment of sciatic pain secondary to herniation of intervertebral disks of the lumbar spine (chemonucleolysis).

Chymopapain injection should be administered under local anaesthesia rather than under general anaesthesia. A recommended dose for a single intervertebral disk is 3 or 5 nanokatals, with a maximum dose per patient of 10 nanokatals.

DISK DISORDERS. Chymopapain was first tried in the treatment of deranged disks in the early 1960s (chemonucleolysis) and since then hundreds of thousands of patients have been given the enzyme. While it is accepted that chymopapain causes proteoglycan breakdown, what effect that has on the mechanics of the disk is not clear. It is assumed that reduction in nuclear size leads to a reduction in size of the prolapse and a consequent diminution of nerve root pain, but some observations are at odds with such an explanation and the immediate relief of pain is more likely to be due to the initial hydraulic effect of the injection.

It would appear that chymopapain can be expected to give a successful result in about 70% of cases, although a critical review of results could give a lower figure of 50%. Problems with studies to assess the effectiveness of chymopapain have involved the lack of controls or the inappropriate activity of the placebo. Even sodium chloride injection 0.9% as a placebo, which has been shown to be inferior to chymopapain, can be questioned as it can cause a disk to swell. Comparisons of surgery with chymopapain have either shown no difference between the 2 treatments or surgery to be the superior form of treatment. What is not known is how chymopapain compares with no treatment.— *Lancet*, 1986, *2*, 843. A point not made in the above review was that the disastrous complications of paraplegia, quadriplegia, and subarachnoid haemorrhage may not only be a result of inadvertent injection of chymopapain into the CSF but may be due to its passage out of the disk into the vertebral body veins and the internal vertebral venous plexus. This toxicity and its consequences may account for the sharp decline in use of chymopapain in the USA.— H. V. Crock (letter), *ibid.*, 1159.

Reviews and discussions on the use of chymopapain in chemonucleolysis: *Med. Lett.*, 1983, *25*, 41; T. R. Einarson *et al.*, *Drug Intell. & clin. Pharm.*, 1984, *18*, 560; R. D. Fraser, *Med. J. Aust.*, 1985, *142*, 431; C. E. Graham, *ibid.*, 461; T. K. F. Taylor and P. Ghosh, *ibid.*, 462; R. C. Mulholland, *Practitioner*, 1986, *230*, 883.

A report of experience with 2000 patients using chymopapain chemonucleolyis. Results are provided for 225 patients with the clinical criteria for disk herniation; treatment was considered to be successful in 158. Patients with nonorganic spinal pain, spinal stenosis, and poor response to previous surgery are unlikely to respond well to chemonucleolysis.— J. A. McCulloch, *Clin. Orthop.*, 1980, *146*, 128.

There were 15 failures among 55 patients with herniated lumbar disks treated with chymopapain compared with 31 of 53 patients given a placebo injection. Patients who did not respond to placebo were subsequently considered for chymopapain treatment; of 32 so treated 29 responded.— M. J. Javid *et al.*, *J. Am. med. Ass.*, 1983, *249*, 2489.

A significantly higher failure rate with chymopapain than surgery in patients with confirmed intervertebral disk herniation that had failed to respond to conservative measures.— C. Crawshaw *et al.*, *Spine*, 1984, *9*, 195. No difference between surgery and chymopapain.— J. Weinstein *et al.*, *J. Bone Jt Surg.*, 1986, *68A*, 43.

Proprietary Preparations

Discase *(Boots, UK)*. *Injection*, powder for reconstitution, chymopapain 7.5 and 12.5 nanokatals.

Proprietary Names and Manufacturers

Chymodiactin *(Ayerst, Canad.*; *Spain*; *Smith, USA)*; Chymodiactine *(Rorer, Fr.)*; Discase *(Travenol, Canad.*; *Kanoldt, Ger.*; *Boots, UK)*.

3709-g

Chymotrypsin *(BAN, USAN, rINN)*.

α-Chymotrypsin; Chymotrypsinum.

CAS — 9004-07-3.

Pharmacopoeias. In *Aust.*, *Br.*, *Cz.*, *Eur.*, *Fr.*, *Ger.*, *It.*, *Neth.*, *Swiss*, and *U.S.*

A proteolytic enzyme obtained by the activation of chymotrypsinogen extracted from ox pancreas. Chymotrypsin (*B.P.*, *Eur. P.*) contains not less than 5 microkatals in each mg. Chymotrypsin (*U.S.P.*) contains not less than 1000 *U.S.P.* units in each mg, calculated on the dry basis.

A white to yellowish-white odourless crystalline or amorphous powder; the amorphous form is hygroscopic. Sparingly **soluble** in water. A 1% solution has a pH of 3.0 to 5.0. Solutions have a maximum stability at pH 3 and a maximum activity at about pH 8. **Store** at 2° to 8° in airtight containers. Protect from light.

The properties and assay methods of chymotrypsin.— Chymotrypsin, in *Pharmaceutical Enzymes*, R. Ruyssen and A. Lauwers (Ed.), Gent, E. Story-Scientia, 1978, p. 41.

Units

Chymotrypsin (*B.P.*, *Eur. P.*) is assayed for potency, by comparison with a reference standard, in terms of its ability to digest *N*-acetyl-L-tyrosine ethyl ester at 25° and the hydrolysis is followed potentiometrically. The activity is expressed in terms of microkatals and Chymotrypsin (*B.P.*, *Eur. P.*) contains not less than 5.0 microkatals per mg.

Chymotrypsin (*U.S.P.*) is assayed for potency, by comparison with a reference standard, in terms of its ability to digest *N*-acetyl-L-tyrosine ethyl ester at 25°. The hydrolysis is followed spectrophotometrically by measurement of the light absorption at 237 nm and the potency is determined by the average change in absorption per minute. The activity is expressed in terms of *U.S.P.* units and Chymotrypsin (*U.S.P.*) contains not less than 1000 units per mg.

Other units that may be encountered are FIP units, 60 of which have been taken to be equivalent to about one microkatal, Armour units and Denver (or Wallace or Wampole) units. One Armour unit and 2½ Denver (or Wallace or Wampole) units are considered to be equivalent to 1 *U.S.P.* unit.

Adverse Effects

Chymotrypsin is antigenic and severe allergic reactions have occasionally followed its intramuscular injection; where allergy is suspected, a sensitivity test should be made before injection. Increased intra-ocular pressure, corneal oedema, striation, and moderate uveitis have occurred following its use in ophthalmology.

Precautions

It is inadvisable to use chymotrypsin in ocular surgery for patients under 20 years of age or for patients with congenital cataracts with high vitreous pressure and a gaping incisional wound.

Uses and Administration

Chymotrypsin is used in ophthalmology for the dissection of the zonule of the lens, thus facilitating intracapsular cataract extraction and reducing trauma to the eye. For this purpose a 1 in 5000 or 1 in 10 000 solution of chymotrypsin in a sterile diluent such as sodium chloride injection (0.9%) is usually employed.

Chymotrypsin is also given with the intention of reducing soft tissue inflammation and oedema from abscesses and ulcers, or associated with traumatic injuries, and to promote liquefaction of secretions of the upper respiratory tract in patients suffering from asthma, bronchitis, pulmonary diseases, and sinusitis.

Chymotrypsin may be administered by intramuscular injection in doses of of 5000 *U.S.P.* units once to three times daily. Chymotrypsin is administered by mouth in conjunction with trypsin in a combined dose of 100 000 units (*U.S.P.* or Armour) four times a day.

A combination of chymotrypsin and trypsin (Chymoral) given by mouth and the use of polyglycolic acid sutures rather than catgut sutures reduced the level of pain after episiotomy.— A. D. G. Roberts and D. McKay Hart, *Br. J. Obstet. Gynaec.*, 1983, *90*, 650.

Preparations

Chymotrypsin for Ophthalmic Solution *(U.S.P.)*. Sterile chymotrypsin suitable for ophthalmic use. pH 4.3 to 8.7 after reconstitution.

Proprietary Preparations

Chymar *(Rorer, UK)*. *Injection*, powder for reconstitution, chymotrypsin 5000 *U.S.P.* units.
Injection, chymotrypsin 5000 *U.S.P.* units/mL, in vials of 5 mL.

Zonulysin *(Henleys, UK)*. *Injection*, powder for reconstitution, chymotrypsin 300 *U.S.P.* units.

Proprietary Names and Manufacturers

Alfa-Chimo *(Ital.)*; Alfapsin *(Ind.)*; Alpha Chymar *(Barnes-Hind, USA)*; Alpha Chymolean *(Organon, Canad.)*; Alphachymotrypsine *(Choay, Fr.*; *Leurquin, Fr.)*; Alphacutanée *(Leurquin, Fr.)*; Aphlozyme *(Fumouze, Fr.)*; Avazyme *(Wallace, USA)*; Catarase *(Alcon, Austral.*; *Coopervision, Canad.*; *Ger.*; *Coopervision, USA)*; Chymar *(Austral.*; *S.Afr.*; *Semar, Spain*; *Switz.*; *Rorer, UK)*; Chymar-Zon *(USV, Austral.*; *Armour, UK)*; Chymoser *(Switz.)*; Deanase DC *(Consolidated Chemicals, UK)*; Kimopsin *(Difrex, Austral.*; *Jpn)*; Quimotrase *(Canad.*; *Cusi, Spain*; *Switz.)*; Seroquin *(Farma-Lepori, Spain)*; Zolyse *(Alcon, Austral.*; *Canad.*; *Alcon, Switz.)*; Zonulasi *(Arg.*; *ISF, Ital.)*; Zonulyn *(Canad.)*; Zonulysin *(Covan, S.Afr.*; *Henleys, UK)*.

The following names have been used for multi-ingredient preparations containing chymotrypsin— Chymacort Ointment *(Armour, UK)*; Chymocyclar *(Armour, UK)*; Chymoral *(USV, Austral.*; *Armour, UK)*; Orenzyme *(Merrell Dow, USA)*.

12606-q

Collagenase

Clostridiopeptidase A.

CAS — 9001-12-1.

An enzyme derived from the fermentation of *Clostridium histolyticum*.

Preparations containing collagenase are used for the debridement of dermal ulcers and burns, and possibly other necrotic lesions, to facilitate granulation and epithelialisation. Infections may require additional treatment.

Collagenase has also been given by injection into the intervertebral disk in the treatment of herniation of intervertebral disks of the lumbar spine.

Hypersensitivity reactions may occur.

Collagenase potency is expressed in units based on the amount of enzyme required to degrade a standard preparation of undenatured collagen.

One unit of collagenase is measured as nanomole leucine equivalents released per minute from collagen substrate in 1 mL of diluent.— M. D. Brown and J. S. Tompkins, *Spine*, 1986, *11*, 123.

Therapeutic uses and potential of bacterial collagenase.— I. Mandl, *Arzneimittel-Forsch.*, 1982, *32*, 1381.

DISK DISORDERS. There have been a number of reports of collagenase being used for chemonucleolysis in the treatment of herniated disks (B.J. Sussman *et al.*, *J. Am. med. Ass.*, 1981, *245*, 730; J.W. Bromley *et al.*, *Spine*, 1984, *9*, 486; M.D. Brown and J.S. Tompkins, *ibid*, 1986, *11*, 123; R.G. Fisher *et al.*, *J. Neurosurg.*, 1986, *64*, 613). These reports, which include a placebo-controlled study of collagenase versus saline, have involved the same group of workers. Another group provided details of 3 patients who suffered complications arising from enzymatic damage outside the disk (M. Brock *et al.*, *Sur. Neurol.*, 1984, *22*, 124; J. Artigas *et al.*, *J. Neurosurg.*, 1984, *61*, 679), although these effects were not considered by the first group to be attributable to collagenase. An initial increase in the size of the hernia was observed in a series of patients given collagenase and followed up with the aid of computed tomography (E. Wintermantel *et al.*, *Acta neurochir.*, 1985, *78*, 98). See also under chymopapain (p.1043) for a discussion of chemonucleolysis.

PEYRONIE'S DISEASE. Beneficial effects of intralesional collagenase in men with Peyronie's disease.— M. K. Gelbard *et al.*, *J. Urol., Baltimore*, 1985, *134*, 280.

PRESSURE SORES. Collagenase had been suggested for the treatment of pressure sores.— *Drug & Ther. Bull.*, 1977, *15*, 69.

Proprietary Names and Manufacturers

Biozyme-C *(Armour, USA)*; Collagin *(Ikapharm, Israel)*; Santyl *(Pentagone, Canad.*; *Knoll, USA)*.

3717-g

Deoxyribonuclease

Desoxyribonuclease; Pancreatic Dornase.

CAS — 9003-98-9.

An enzyme obtained from beef pancreas.

Units

The unit of activity is based on the rate of decrease in viscosity of a solution of thymus deoxyribonucleic acid when digested by deoxyribonuclease. One dornase viscosity unit of activity has been defined as that amount of enzyme which causes a drop of 1 viscosity unit in the viscosity of thymus deoxyribonucleic acid in 10 minutes at 30°, where the flow-time of water is taken as 1 viscosity unit.

Deoxyribonuclease acts directly upon deoxyribonucleoprotein and deoxyribonucleic acid, causing rapid depolymerisation with a resulting decrease in viscosity of purulent material. Deoxyribonuclease is used topically, often with plasmin, as a debriding agent in a variety of inflammatory and infected lesions. It has also been given by injection. An aerosol inhalation spray has been used to reduce the viscosity of pulmonary secretions.

Proprietary Names and Manufacturers

Deanase *(Liberman, Spain*; *Consolidated Chemicals, UK)*; Dinase *(Ital.)*.

The following names have been used for multi-ingredient preparations containing deoxyribonuclease—Elase *(Parke, Davis, Austral.*; *Parke, Davis, Canad.*; *Parke, Davis, USA)*; Elase-Chloromycetin *(Parke, Davis, Canad.*; *Parke, Davis, USA)*.

3718-q

Dextranase

CAS — 9025-70-1.

An enzyme reported to break down the dextran-binding dental plaque.

For a review of dextranase and dental caries, see S. A. Leach, *Br. dent. J.*, 1969, *127*, 325.

For a discussion of the use of dextranase and proteolytic enzymes in the removal of dental plaque, and some formulas, see P. Alexander, *Mfg Chem.*, 1972, *43* (June), 45.

18650-y

Hyalosidase *(BAN, rINN)*.

GL Enzyme; Hyaluronoglucosaminidase.

Hyalosidase which is a highly purified form of hyaluronidase has been studied in the treatment of myocardial infarction. It is proposed that it may offer benefit in limiting the size of the infarction by increasing the diffusion of nutrients and metabolites.

Hyalosidase given intravenously to patients shortly after the onset of symptoms of myocardial infarction has been reported to decrease the size of the infarction (S. Saltissi *et al.*, *Lancet*, 1982, *1*, 867) and to reduce the mortality rate (E.J. Flint *et al.*, *ibid.*, 1982, *1*, 871). However, while Henderson *et al.* (*ibid.*, 1982, *1*, 874) found signs of decreased infarct size, they found no significant change in mortality. Cairns *et al.* (*Circulation*, 1982, *65*, 764) found no change in infarct size in a study aimed at detecting a 50% reduction. Also the Multicentre Investigation of the Limitation of Infarct Size (MILIS) (*Am. J. Cardiol.*, 1986, *57*, 1236) found no difference between placebo and hyaluronidase given more than 9 hours after the onset of the infarction.

Proprietary Names and Manufacturers

Biorex, UK.

3724-v

Hyaluronidase *(BAN, USAN, rINN)*.

CAS — 9001-54-1.

Pharmacopoeias. In *Arg.*, *Braz.*, *Chin.*, *Cz.*, *Fr.*, and *Ind. Br.*and *U.S.* include Hyaluronidase Injection. *U.S.* also includes Hyaluronidase for Injection.

An enzyme which depolymerises the mucopolysaccharide hyaluronic acid. It is prepared from the testes and semen of mammals and purified so as to remove most of the inert material, the resulting solution is sterilised by filtration and freeze-dried; suitable stabilising agent or agents may be added to the purified preparation.

A sterile, white or yellowish-white, powder, containing not less than 300 International units per mg. *U.S.P.* specifies not more than 0.25 µg of tyrosine for each unit of hyaluronidase, i.e. not less than 4000 units of hyaluronidase for each mg of tyrosine.

Very **soluble** in water; practically insoluble in alcohol, acetone, and ether. A 0.3% solution in water has a pH of 4.5 to 7.5. A 1% solution in water is clear and not more than faintly yellow.

The properties and assay methods of hyaluronidase.— Hyaluronidase, in *Pharmaceutical Enzymes*, R. Ruyssen and A. Lauwers (Ed.), Gent, E. Story-Scientia, 1978, p. 217.

Units

Approximately 2000 units of hyaluronidase, bovine are contained in one ampoule of the first International Standard Preparation (1955). One ampoule contains 10 tablets, each containing approximately 20 mg of dried material.

The International and *U.S.P.* units are equivalent.

One International unit of hyaluronidase was approximately equivalent to 1 Turbidity Reducing unit and to 3.3 Viscosity Reducing Units.— International Commission for the Standardisation of Pharmaceutical Enzymes, *J. mond. Pharm.*, 1965, *8*, 5.

Adverse Effects and Precautions

Sensitivity to hyaluronidase occasionally occurs. Hyaluronidase should be administered with caution to patients with infections; because of the danger of spreading infection, the enzyme generally should not be injected into or around an infected area. It has been suggested that the presence of malignancy may similarly be a contra-indication to the use of hyaluronidase. It should not be administered by intravenous injection.

Uses and Administration

Hyaluronidase is an enzyme which has a specific action on the mucopolysaccharide, hyaluronic acid, a component of the mucoprotein ground substance or tissue cement of the tissue spaces, thereby reducing its viscosity and rendering the tissues more readily permeable to injected fluids. Therapeutically, hyaluronidase is employed to increase the speed of absorption and to diminish discomfort due to subcutaneous or intramuscular injection of fluids, to promote resorption of excess fluids and extravasated blood in the tissues, and to increase the effectiveness of local anaesthesia.

In hypodermoclysis, hyaluronidase is used to aid the subcutaneous administration of relatively large volumes of fluids, especially in infants and young children, where intravenous injection is difficult. Hyaluronidase may be added to the injection fluid or may be injected into the site before the fluid is administered; 1000 mL or more of fluids can be administered subcutaneously with the aid of 1500 International units. Care should be taken in the treatment of children to control the speed and total volume administered and to avoid over-hydration.

Hyaluronidase also allows for the effective intramuscular or subcutaneous administration of other drugs so providing an alternative to the intravenous route. Diodone may be given subcutaneously with the aid of hyaluronidase to provide an alternative to the more common intravenous technique in pyelography.

The diffusion of local anaesthetics is accelerated by the addition of 1500 units of hyaluronidase to 20 mL to 40 mL of the anaesthetic solution. This is of value in the reduction of fractures and in pudendal block in midwifery. It has also been used in ophthalmology as an aid to local anaesthesia.

Hyalosidase (see above) is a highly purified form of hyaluronidase.

CATARACT SURGERY. Results of a pilot study involving 10 cataract patients demonstrated that hyaluronidase could aid the removal from the anterior chamber of the eye of sodium hyaluronate being used as an aid to intra-ocular lens implantation and could counteract the increase in intra-ocular pressure that occurs with sodium hyaluronate.— I. G. Calder and V. H. Smith, *Br. J. Ophthal.*, 1986, *70*, 418.

MYOCARDIAL INFARCTION. For a discussion of hyaluronidase, given mainly as hyalosidase, in myocardial infarction, see above under hyalosidase.

Preparations

Hyaluronidase for Injection *(U.S.P.)*. Sterile hyaluronidase suitable for parenteral use. Store at 15° to 30°.

Hyaluronidase Injection *(B.P.)*. A sterile solution of hyaluronidase. The sealed container should be stored in a cool place. The injection decomposes on storage and should be used immediately after preparation. Not for intravenous injection.

Hyaluronidase Injection *(U.S.P.)*. A sterile solution in Water for Injections. pH 6.4 to 7.4. It may contain suitable stabilisers. Store at 2° to 8°.

Proprietary Preparations

Hyalase *(CP Pharmaceuticals, UK)*. *Injection*, powder for reconstitution, hyaluronidase 1500 units.

Lasonil *(Bayer, UK)*. *Ointment*, hyaluronidase 15 000 units/100 g, heparinoid equivalent to 5000 units of heparin.

A report of oleogranuloma in a 57-year-old man following the rectal administration of Lasonil.— M. G. Greaney and P. R. Jackson, *Br. med. J.*, 1977, *2*, 997.

Proprietary Names and Manufacturers

Hyalas *(Swed.)*; Hyalase *(Austral.; Ondee, Canad.; Bengers, S.Afr.; CP Pharmaceuticals, UK)*; Hyason *(Belg.; Neth.; Switz.)*; Jalovis *(Coli, Ital.)*; Jaluran *(Bioindustria, Ital.)*; Kinaden *(Spain)*; Kinetin *(Schering, Ger.)*; Penetrase *(Leo, Denm.; Leo, Norw.)*; Permease *(Aust.; Switz.)*; Wydase *(Wyeth, Canad.; Wyeth, USA)*.

The following names have been used for multi-ingredient preparations containing hyaluronidase— Lasonil *(Bayer, Austral.; Bayer, UK)*; Xylodase *(Astra, UK)*.

3728-s

Muramidase

Globulin G_1; *N*-acetylmuramide glycanohydrolase; Lysozyme.

CAS — 9001-63-2.

A crystalline polypeptide mucolytic enzyme, widely distributed in nature.

The properties and assay methods of muramidase.— Lysosyme, in *Pharmaceutical Enzymes*, R. Ruyssen and A. Lauwers (Ed.), Gent, E. Story-Scientia, 1978, p. 167.

Muramidase is a mucopolysaccharidase which is active against Gram-positive bacteria, possibly by transforming the insoluble polysaccharides of the cell wall to soluble mucopeptides. It is also active against some viruses and some Gram-negative bacteria. Muramidase has been claimed to enhance the activity of some antimicrobial preparations when given concomitantly. Sensitivity reactions have been reported.

Proprietary Names and Manufacturers of Muramidase and its Salts

Aibel D *(Jpn)*; Antalzyme *(Vifor, Switz.)*; Buco-Lysozima *(Poen, Arg.)*; Debizima *(Miba, Ital.)*; Eggtose *(Jpn)*; Eyebel *(Galenica, Switz.)*; Fisiozima *(Neopharmed, Ital.)*; Leftose *(Jpn)*; Lisobase Lacrimale *(Allergan, Ital.)*; Lisozima *(Wasserman, Spain)*; Lisozimina *(Volpino, Arg.)*; Lysorzym *(Jpn)*; Lysozym *(Prospa, Switz.)*; Neuzym *(Jpn)*; Toyolyzom-DS *(Jpn)*.

13043-t

Orgotein *(BAN, USAN, rINN)*.

Bovine Superoxide Dismutase; Ormetein. A group of water-soluble protein congeners isolated from liver, red blood cells, and other tissues; mol. wt about 33 000 with a compact conformation maintained by about 4 gram-atoms of chelated divalent metal. It is produced from beef liver as Cu-Zn mixed chelate having superoxide dismutase activity.

A human clone version of *N*-acetylsuperoxide dismutase is known as sudismase.

CAS — 9016-01-7 (orgotein); 110294-55-8 (sudismase).

Orgotein has anti-inflammatory properties. It has been given by intra-articular injection in degenerative joint disease, and for bladder disorders and the amelioration of side-effects of radiotherapy.

Human superoxide dismutase is under investigation. The endogenous enzyme scavenges oxygen free radicals which may have a role in tissue damage and ageing.

A review of orgotein.— W. Huber and K. B. Menander-Huber, *Clins rheum. Dis.*, 1980, *6*, 465.

For a series of reports on the actions and uses of orgotein, see *Eur. J. Rheumatol. Inflamm.*, 1981, *4*, 151–270.

JOINT DISORDERS. Favourable comparisons with intra-articular injections of aspirin: K. -M. Goebel *et al.*, *Lancet*, 1981, *1*, 1015. With placebo: K. Lund-Olesen and K. B. Menander-Huber, *Arzneimittel-Forsch.*, 1983, *33*, 1199. With methylprednisolone: W. Gammer and L.-G. Brobäck, *Scand. J. Rheumatol.*, 1984, *13*, 108.

PREGNANCY AND THE NEONATE. *Respiratory distress syndrome.* A preliminary double-blind placebo-controlled study in 45 neonates with severe respiratory distress syndrome showed that orgotein 0.25 mg per kg body-weight every 12 hours by subcutaneous injection was helpful in reducing the severity of bronchopulmonary dysplasia.— W. Rosenfeld *et al.*, *J. Pediat.*, 1984, *105*, 781.

RADIOTHERAPY. A double-blind study in 38 patients given orgotein 4 mg or placebo intramuscularly for 8 weeks after each session of irradiation for bladder tumours indicated that orgotein had a significant effect in ameliorating the side-effects of irradiation.— F. Edsmyr *et al.*, *Curr. ther. Res.*, 1976, *19*, 198.

Further references: H. Marberger *et al.*, *Curr. ther. Res.*, 1975, *18*, 466.

Proprietary Names and Manufacturers

Artrolasi *(Ausonia, Ital.)*; Interceptor *(Isnardi, Ital.)*; Ontosein *(Zambeletti, Spain)*; Orgoten *(Serono, Ital.)*; Oxinorm *(Zambeletti, Ital.)*; Peroxinorm *(Grünenthal, Ger.; Andromaco, Spain; Grünenthal, Switz.)*.

13044-x

Ornicarbase

Ornithine Carbamoyltransferase.

CAS — 9001-69-8.

Ornicarbase has been used in hepatic disorders.

Proprietary Names and Manufacturers

Ociter *(Bracco, Ital.)*; Préortan *(Leurquin, Fr.)*; Protenzima *(Jorba, Spain)*; Regepat *(Llorens, Spain)*.

3731-b

Pancreatin *(BAN, USAN)*.

Pancreatinum.

CAS — 8049-47-6.

Pharmacopoeias. In *Aust.*, *Br.*, *Chin.*, *Egypt.*, *Eur.*, *Fr.*, *Ind.*, *It.*, *Jug.*, *Swiss*, and *U.S.* as pancreatin or another pancreatic extract. *B.P.* includes both. Also in *B.P. Vet.*

A preparation of mammalian pancreas containing enzymes having protease, lipase, and amylase activity.

The *B.P.* describes pancreatin as a white or buff-coloured amorphous powder free from unpleasant odour. Each g of pancreatin contains not less than 1400 units of free protease activity, not less than 20 000 units of lipase activity, and not less than 24 000 units of amylase activity. It may contain sodium chloride. **Soluble** or partly soluble in water forming a slightly turbid solution; practically insoluble in alcohol and ether. **Store** at a temperature not exceeding 15° in well-closed containers.

The *U.S.P.* includes Pancreatin, a cream-coloured amorphous powder with a faint characteristic not offensive odour, containing in each g not less than 25 000 *U.S.P.* units of protease activity, not less than 2000 *U.S.P.* units of lipase activity, and not less than 25 000 *U.S.P.* units of amylase activity. It may be labelled as a whole-number multiple of the 3 minimum activities, or may be diluted with lactose, sucrose containing up to 3.25% of starch, or pancreatin of lower digestive power. Store at a temperature not exceeding 30° in airtight containers.

A comparative assessment *in vitro* of pancreatic extract preparations.— A. M. Howell *et al.*, *J. Hosp. Pharm.*, 1975, *33*, 143.

Assay *in vitro* of 16 different commercial pancreatic preparations for lipase, trypsin, chymotrypsin, proteolytic activity, and amylase demonstrated wide variation between preparations, in particular the lipase content varied from 10 to 3600 units per product unit. *In vivo* studies demonstrated correlation with the *in vitro* results and indicated that, despite theoretical advantages, enteric coating could reduce the clinical effectiveness of pancreatic extracts. Most commercial preparations contained inadequate amounts of lipase and required a lipase supplement.— D. Y. Graham, *New Engl. J. Med.*, 1977, *296*, 1314. Comments.— J. H. Meyer, *ibid.*, 1347; T. L. Yeh and M. L. Rubin (letter), *ibid.*, *297*, 615; R. Kirshen (letter), *ibid.*, 616. From an *in vitro* study simulating the conditions in which orally administered pancreatin is exposed in the human stomach it was concluded that administration of uncoated pancreatin in powder form may result in substantial loss of enzymic activity.— D. T. Graham *et al.*, *Med. J. Aust.*, 1979, *1*, 45. Criticisms of the extrapolation of *in vitro* results to *in vivo* situations.— G. L. Barnes and P. D. Phelan (letter), *ibid.*, 282; B. Allen and G. Giles (letter), *ibid.*

The properties and assay methods of pancreatin.— Pancreatin, in *Pharmaceutical Enzymes*, R. Ruyssen and A. Lauwers (Ed.), Gent, E. Story-Scientia, 1978, p. 57.

Units

The *B.P.* and *U.S.P.* units of protease activity depend upon the rate of hydrolysis of casein, those of lipase activity depend upon the rate of hydrolysis of olive oil, and those of amylase activity depend upon the rate of hydrolysis of starch. The *B.P.* and *U.S.P.* units are not interchangeable and the following equivalent figures should only be used as a guide. One *B.P.* unit of protease activity is approximately equivalent to

62.50 *U.S.P.* units, 1 *B.P.* unit of lipase activity is approximately equivalent to 1 *U.S.P.* unit, and 1 *B.P.* unit of amylase activity is approximately equivalent to 4.15 *U.S.P.* units. *U.S.P.* units are equivalent to the former *U.S.N.F.* units.
FIP and *Eur. P.* units of protease, lipase, and amylase activity are equivalent to *B.P.* units.

Adverse Effects

Pancreatin may cause buccal and perianal soreness, particularly in infants. Hypersensitivity reactions have been reported; these may be sneezing, lachrymation, or skin rashes. Hyperuricaemia or hyperuricosuria have occurred with high doses.

In 3 children taking preparations of pancreatic extracts (Pancrex V powder, Pancrex V Forte), severe mouth ulceration and angular stomatitis, causing dysphagia, loss of weight, and pyrexia, were attributed to digestion of the mucous membrane due to retention of the preparations in the mouth before swallowing.— C. W. Darby (letter), *Br. med. J.*, 1970, *2*, 299.

ALLERGY. Hypersensitivity to pancreatic extracts in parents of patients with cystic fibrosis.— F. J. Twarog *et al.*, *J. Allergy & clin. Immunol.*, 1977, *59*, 35.

Allergy to pancreatin in 6 of 11 nurses caring for children with cystic fibrosis.— G. W. Lipkin and D. W. Vickers (letter), *Lancet*, 1987, *1*, 392.

CONTAMINATION. Reports of *Salmonella* contamination of pancreatin preparations: E. J. G. Glencross, *Br. med. J.*, 1972, *2*, 376; B. Lüssi-Schlatter and P. Speiser, *Pharm. Acta Helv.*, 1974, *49*, 41; A. Lipson (letter), *Lancet*, 1976, *1*, 969; A. Lipson and A. Meikle, *Archs Dis. Childh.*, 1977, *52*, 569.

EFFECT ON FOLIC ACID. Pancreatic extract significantly inhibited folate absorption in healthy subjects and in pancreatic insufficient patients. Testing *in vitro* showed that pancreatic extract formed insoluble complexes with folate. Patients being treated for pancreatic insufficiency should be monitored for folate status or given folic acid supplementation, particularly if pancreatic enzymes and bicarbonate (or cimetidine) were being used together in the treatment regimen.— R. M. Russell *et al.*, *Dig. Dis. Scis*, 1980, *25*, 369.

Uses and Administration

Pancreatin hydrolyses fats to glycerol and fatty acids, changes protein into proteoses and derived substances, and converts starch into dextrins and sugars. It is given by mouth in conditions of pancreatic deficiency such as pancreatitis and cystic fibrosis. Pancreatin may also be given as an aid to digestion following gastrectomy. It is available in the form of powder, capsules which are intended to be opened before use and the contents sprinkled on the food, tablets which are enteric-coated, or granules which may contain suitable enteroprotective substances. If pancreatin is mixed with liquids or feeds the resulting mixture should not be allowed to stand for more than 1 hour prior to use. Antacids and histamine H_2-receptor antagonists, such as cimetidine, have been given in conjunction with pancreatin in an attempt to lessen destruction of pancreatin by the gastric acids.

The dose of pancreatin is adjusted according to the needs of the individual patient. There is a wide range of preparations and dose forms and in the *UK* doses of up to 3360 units of protease activity, 60 000 units of amylase activity, and 60 000 units of lipase activity have been given with each meal. In the *US* doses providing up to 36 000 *U.S.P.* units of lipase activity have been given with each meal.

CYSTIC FIBROSIS. A review of the management of cystic fibrosis with reference to the use of pancreatin for malabsorption.— C. Smalley, *Prescribers' J.*, 1986, *26*, 122.

Long-term cimetidine treatment in children with steatorrhoea associated with cystic fibrosis produced some improvements in intestinal absorption when given with pancreatic enzyme therapy. The improved absorptive function was not reflected in the nutritional state of the patient.— D. M. Chalmers *et al.*, *Gut*, 1983, *24*, A978.

PANCREATIC INSUFFICIENCY. A review of the management of maldigestion associated with pancreatic insufficiency. Pancreatic insufficiency is usually managed by replacement therapy with pancreatic enzymes. Problems with gastric inactivation of the enzymes have prompted the development of enteric-coated tablets and enteric-coated encapsulated microspheres (ECEM). Several studies have shown that some enteric-coated preparations do not deliver enough enzyme to the duodenum for a clinical response. Clinical evaluation of the efficacy of ECEM versus conventional formulations has shown conflicting results.
Histamine H_2-receptor antagonists have been shown to have beneficial effects when used as adjuncts to enzyme therapy, as a result of an increase in both gastric and duodenal pH and a corresponding decrease in the inactivation of administered pancreatic enzymes. Histamine H_2-receptor antagonists may be less effective in patients with cystic fibrosis who secrete large amounts of gastric acid.
Antacids have also been used as adjuncts to enzyme therapy. To be effective, antacids must raise the gastric pH above 4, the level that inactivates enzymes. It has been shown that antacids must be given before or during meals to produce a beneficial effect. In the studies in which antacids were given after meals there was no benefit.— R. S. Perry and J. Gallagher, *Clin. Pharm.*, 1985, *4*, 161. A similar review covering pancreatin and pancrelipase.— Y. W. Cho and D. M. Aviado, *J. clin. Pharmac.*, 1981, *21*, 224.

In a double-blind crossover study in 13 patients with steatorrhoea due to pancreatic insufficiency faecal fat output was significantly reduced when pancreatin was given as 'positioned-release' capsules compared with when given as standard capsules.— R. H. Taylor *et al.*, *Br. med. J.*, 1982, *285*, 1392.

Pancreatic enzyme replacement was successful in preventing diabetic instability after pancreatectomy.— I. P. Linehan *et al.*, *Gut*, 1986, *27*, A1278.

Preparations

Pancreatic Extract *(B.P.)*. Pancreas Powder (*Eur. P.*). A preparation of fresh or frozen mammalian pancreas containing enzymes having protease, lipase, and amylase activity. Contains in each g not less than 1000 units of total protease activity, not less than 15 000 units of lipase activity, and not less than 12 000 units of amylase activity.

Pancreatin Capsules *(U.S.P.)*

Pancreatin Granules *(B.P.)*. They may contain enteroprotective substances.

Pancreatin Tablets *(B.P.)*

Pancreatin Tablets *(U.S.P.)*

Proprietary Preparations containing Pancreatin and some Pancreatic Enzymes

Cotazym *(Organon, UK)*. *Capsules*, pancreatic enzymes, amylase not less than 9000 *B.P.* units, lipase not less than 13 000 *B.P.* units, protease not less than 450 *B.P.* units.

Creon *(Duphar, UK)*. *Capsules*, enteric-coated granules, pancreatin equivalent to amylase 9000 *B.P.* units, lipase 8000 *B.P.* units, protease 210 *B.P.* units.

Nutrizym GR *(E. Merck, UK)*. *Capsules*, containing enteric-coated pellets, pancreatin 300 mg equivalent to amylase 10 000 *B.P.* units, lipase 10 000 *B.P.* units, protease 650 *B.P.* units.

Pancrease *(Ortho-Cilag, UK)*. *Capsules*, enteric-coated granules, pancreatin equivalent to amylase 2900 *B.P.* units, lipase 5000 *B.P.* units, protease 330 *B.P.* units.

Pancrex *(Paines & Byrne, UK)*. *Capsules* (Pancrex V '125'), pancreatin, providing not less than amylase 3300 *B.P.* units, lipase 2950 *B.P.* units, protease 160 *B.P.* units. *Capsules* (Pancrex V), pancreatin, providing not less than amylase 9000 *B.P.* units, lipase 8000 *B.P.* units, protease 430 *B.P.* units.
Granules, enteric-coated, pancreatin, providing not less than amylase 4000 *B.P.* units/g, lipase 5000 *B.P.* units/g, protease 300 *B.P.* units/g.
Powder (Pancrex V), pancreatin, providing not less than amylase 30 000 *B.P.* units/g, lipase 25 000 *B.P.* units/g, protease 1400 *B.P.* units/g.
Tablets (Pancrex V), enteric-coated, pancreatin, providing not less than amylase 1700 *B.P.* units, lipase 1900 *B.P.* units, protease 110 *B.P.* units. *Tablets* (Pancrex V Forte), enteric-coated, pancreatin, providing not less than amylase 5000 *B.P.* units, lipase 5600 *B.P.* units, protease 330 *B.P.* units.

Proprietary Names and Manufacturers of Pancreatic Enzymes

Alcon Enzymatic Cleaner *(Alcon, Austral.)*; Alipase *(Cilag, Fr.)*; Atezym *(Scharper, Ital.)*; Converzyme *(Ascher, USA)*; Cotazym *(Organon, Austral.; Organon, Canad.; Ital.; Organon, UK; Organon, USA)*; Creon *(Latéma, Fr.; Kali-Chemie, Switz.; Duphar, UK; Reid-Rowell, USA)*; Damagal *(Siegfried, Switz.)*; Depropanex *(Merck Sharp & Dohme, UK)*; Fermentogran *(Keimdiät, Ger. : Thomson & Joseph, UK)*; Ilozyme *(Adria, USA)*; Krebsilasi *(IRBI, Ital.)*; Kreon *(Kali-Chemie, Ger.)*; Nutrizym GR *(E. Merck, UK)*; Panar *(Armour, UK)*; Pancrease *(Cilag, Austral.; McNeil, Canad.; Cilag, Ital.; Ortho-Cilag, UK; McNeil Pharmaceutical, USA)*; Pancreon *(Farmades, Ital.)*; Pancrex *(Stansen, Austral.; Paines & Byrne, UK)*; Pankrease *(Johnson & Johnson, S.Afr.)*; Pankreatan *(Brunnengräber, Ger.)*; Pankreon *(Kali-Chemie, Ger.; Kali-Chemie, Norw.; Kali-Farma, Spain; Kali-Chemie, Swed.)*; Pankrotanon *(Hausmann, Switz.)*; Panpur *(Nordmark, Ger.)*; Panteric *(Canad.)*; Panzytrat *(Nordmark, Ger.)*; Protopan *(Pharmaceutical Mfg, UK)*; Viokase *(Robins, Austral.; Robins, Canad.; Continental Ethicals, S.Afr.; Robins, USA)*; Zypanar *(Armour, UK)*.

The following names have been used for multi-ingredient preparations containing pancreatic enzymes—Combizym Co *(Luitpold, Austral.)*; Combizym Compositum *(Panpharma, UK)*; Digepepsin *(Ram, USA)*; Donnazyme *(Robins, Canad.; Robins, USA)*; Entozyme *(Robins, Canad.; Robins, USA)*; Enzobile *(Mallard, USA)*; Enzypan *(Norgine, UK; Norgine, USA)*; Kanulase *(Dorsey Laboratories, USA)*; Karbokoff *(Arlo, USA)*; Phazyme *(Stafford-Miller, Austral.)*; Zypan *(Standard Process, USA)*.

3732-v

Pancrelipase *(USAN)*.

CAS — 53608-75-6.

Pharmacopoeias. In *U.S.*

A preparation obtained from the pancreas of the hog. It is a cream amorphous powder with a faint characteristic, not offensive odour, containing enzymes, principally lipase, with protease and amylase; it contains in each g not less than 100 000 *U.S.P.* units of protease activity, not less than 24 000 *U.S.P.* units of lipase activity, and not less than 100 000 *U.S.P.* units of amylase activity. Its greatest activity is exhibited in neutral or faintly alkaline media. It is inactivated by more than traces of acids, by large amounts of alkali hydroxides, or by excess of alkali carbonate. **Store** in airtight containers.

Units

See Pancreatin, p.1045.

Uses and Administration

Pancrelipase has the actions and uses of pancreatin (see p.1045). The dose is the equivalent of 8000 to 24 000 *U.S.P.* units of lipase activity before each meal or snack, or according to the patient's needs.

A review of pancreatic enzyme preparations with special reference to enterically-coated microspheres of pancrelipase.— Y. W. Cho and D. M. Aviado, *J. clin. Pharmac.*, 1981, *21*, 224.

Preparations

Pancrelipase Capsules *(U.S.P.)*. Capsules containing not less than 30 000 *U.S.P.* units of protease activity, not less than 8000 *U.S.P.* units of lipase activity, and not less than 30 000 *U.S.P.* units of amylase activity. Store at a temperature not exceeding 25° in airtight containers.

Pancrelipase Tablets *(U.S.P.)*. Tablets containing not less than 30 000 *U.S.P.* units of protease activity, not less than 8000 *U.S.P.* units of lipase activity, and not less than 30 000 *U.S.P.* units of amylase activity. Store at a temperature not exceeding 25° in airtight containers.

Proprietary Names and Manufacturers

Proprietary names of pancrelipase are listed with proprietary names of other pancreatic enzymes under pancreatin, above.

3733-g

Papain *(USAN).*

CAS — 9001-73-4.

Pharmacopoeias. In *Arg., Ind.,* and *U.S.*

A proteolytic enzyme or mixture of enzymes prepared from the juice of the unripe fruit of *Carica papaya* (Caricaceae). The *U.S.P.* specifies not less than 6000 *U.S.P.* units per mg.

An amorphous, white to light brown powder.

Soluble in water, the solution being colourless to light yellow and more or less opalescent; practically insoluble in alcohol, chloroform, and ether. A 2% solution in water has a pH of 4.8 to 6.2. **Store** in a cool place in airtight containers. Protect from light.

The properties and assay methods of papain.— Papain, in *Pharmaceutical Enzymes,* R. Ruyssen and A. Lauwers (Ed.), Gent, E. Story-Scientia, 1978, p. 95.

Units

One *U.S.P.* unit of papain activity is the activity that releases the equivalent of 1 μg of tyrosine from a specified casein substrate under the conditions of the assay, using the enzyme concentration that liberates 40 μg of tyrosine per mL of test solution.

One FIP unit of papain is defined as the enzyme activity which under specified conditions hydrolyses 1 μmol of *N*-benzoyl-L-arginine ethyl ester per minute.

Adverse Effects

Allergic reactions have followed repeated inhalations of papain powder.

Extensive destruction of the oesophageal wall, with perforation, resulted from the use of a papain suspension given to treat an obstruction caused by impacted meat. The patient had been given 1.2 g of papain over a 12-hour period. Ten days after a thoracotomy, the descending thoracic aorta ruptured, and she died from haemorrhage.— J. W. Holsinger *et al., J. Am. med. Ass.,* 1968, *204,* 734.

Papain solution caused pruritus in blister-base tests in all of 20 subjects.— J. Kirby *et al., Br. med. J.,* 1974, *4,* 693.

Of 6 workers sensitised to papain 5 showed positive skin tests to bromelains and 2 of them also showed immediate asthmatic reactions after bronchial challenge with bromelains. It was considered that this provided evidence for immunological cross-reaction between bromelains and papain.— X. Baur and G. Fruhmann, *Clin. Allergy,* 1979, *9,* 443.

A case report of ocular and periorbital angioedema within 4 hours of use of a contact lens cleansing solution containing papain.— D. I. Bernstein *et al., J. Allergy & clin. Immunol.,* 1984, *74,* 258.

Uses and Administration

Papain consists chiefly of a mixture of papain and chymopapain, proteolytic enzymes which hydrolyse polypeptides, amides, and esters, especially at bonds involving basic amino acids, or leucine or glycine, yielding peptides of lower molecular weight. It is used as a topical debriding agent in conjunction with urea. It is also used for the removal of protein deposits from the surface of soft contact lenses.

Papain is widely used as a meat tenderiser and in the clarification of beverages.

Papain given as enteric-coated tablets in a dose of 1.98 g with every meal reversed a malabsorption syndrome incompletely controlled by a gluten-free diet and considered to be due to a transient gluten intolerance.— M. Messer and P. E. Baume (letter), *Lancet,* 1976, *2,* 1022.

Preparations

Papain Tablets for Topical Solution *(U.S.P.).* Tablets containing papain. pH of a solution of one tablet in 10 mL of water 6.9 to 8.0.

Proprietary Names and Manufacturers

Benase *(Ferndale, USA)*; Cacital *(Parke, Davis, Spain)*; Carofem *(Winthrop, Canad.)*; Extenzyme *(Allergan, USA)*; Hydrocare Enzymatic Protein Remover *(Allergan, Austral.)*; Papase *(Parke, Davis, USA)*; Soflens *(Allergan, USA)*; Tromasin *(Parke, Davis, Arg.*; *Warner, Austral.*; *Warner, S.Afr.)*; Vermizym *(Schwab, Ger.)*.

The following names have been used for multi-ingredient preparations containing papain—Panafil *(Rystan, USA)*; Prevenzyme *(Legere, USA)*.

3734-q

Pectinase

Pectin-polygalacturonase; Pectolase; PG.

CAS — 9032-75-1.

Pharmacopoeias. In *Aust.* and *Nord.*

An enzyme found widely in plant tissues.

Pectinase hydrolyses pectin and pectic acids (polygalacturonic acids) and is used in wine making and in the manufacture of fruit juices to reduce their viscosity.

3735-p

Penicillinase *(BAN, rINN).*

An enzyme produced by many strains of bacteria. The commercial product is obtained by fermentation from cultures of a strain of *Bacillus cereus* or *Bacillus subtilis.*

CAS — 9001-74-5.

Units

One Levy unit is defined as that amount which inactivates 59.3 units of benzylpenicillin (sodium or potassium salt) per hour *in vitro* at 25° and pH 7 in the presence of an excess of penicillin.

Penicillinase catalyses the hydrolysis of penicillin to produce penicilloic acid which is biologically inactive and is now used, prior to culture, to inactivate any penicillin in clinical specimens.

Proprietary Names and Manufacturers

Compenase *(Commonwealth Serum Laboratories, Austral.)*; Labpenase *(Commonwealth Serum Laboratories, Austral.)*; Neutrapen *(Riker, UK)*.

3736-s

Pepsin

CAS — 9001-75-6.

Pharmacopoeias. In *Arg., Aust., Cz., Egypt., Fr., Hung., Ind., Jug., Pol., Port., Roum.,* and *Span.* In *Chin.* and *Jpn* as Saccharated Pepsin.

A substance containing a proteolytic enzyme present in the gastric juice of animals and obtained from the mucous membrane of the stomach of certain animals commonly used for food.

A review of the properties and assay methods of pepsin. The activity required for pharmaceutical pepsin should fall between 0.5 and 0.7 FIP units per mg.— Pepsin, in *Pharmaceutical Enzymes,* R. Ruyssen and A. Lauwers (Ed.), Gent, E. Story-Scientia, 1978, p. 85.

Units

One FIP unit of pepsin activity is contained in that amount of the standard preparation, which upon incubation at 25° for 1 minute with a suitable preparation of pure haemoglobin will cause the decomposition of the haemoglobin to such an extent that the amount of hydroxyaryl substances liberated will, upon reaction with Folin-Ciocalteu reagent, result in the formation of a coloured solution of equal intensity to that resulting from the reaction of 1 μmol of tyrosine with the reagent.

Uses and Administration

Pepsin is a proteolytic enzyme which is secreted by the stomach and controls the degradation of proteins into proteoses and peptones. It hydrolyses polypeptides including those with bonds adjacent to aromatic or dicarboxylic L-amino-acid residues.

Pepsin was formerly used with dilute hydrochloric acid to increase the digestive power of the gastric juice when there was considered to be a deficiency of pepsin secretion.

Proprietary Preparations

Muripsin *(Norgine, UK). Tablets,* pepsin 35 mg, glutamic acid hydrochloride 500 mg.

Proprietary Names and Manufacturers

The following names have been used for multi-ingredient preparations containing pepsin— Acidol Pepsin *(Winthrop, Austral.*; *Sterling Research, UK)*; Digepepsin *(Ram, USA)*; Donnazyme *(Robins, Canad.*; *Robins, USA)*; Entozyme *(Robins, Canad.*; *Robins, USA)*; Enzobile *(Mallard, USA)*; Enzypan *(Norgine, UK*; *Norgine, USA)*; Kanulase *(Dorsey Laboratories, USA)*; Muripsin *(Norgine, Austral.*; *Norgine, UK*; *Norgine, USA)*; Zypan *(Standard Process, USA)*.

3739-l

Plasmin *(BAN).*

Fibrinolysin (Human) *(pINN)*; Plasmin (Human). A proteolytic enzyme derived from the activation of human plasminogen which converts fibrin into soluble products.

CAS — 9004-09-5 (human).

The properties and assay methods of plasmin.— Plasmin, in *Pharmaceutical Enzymes,* R. Ruyssen and A. Lauwers (Ed.), Gent, E. Story-Scientia, 1978, p. 123.

Units

10 units of human plasmin are contained in 1 mL of a solution of partially purified plasmin in glycerol 50% in one ampoule of the second International Reference Preparation (1982).

One FIP unit of plasmin is defined as the enzyme activity which under the specified standard conditions in the course of 1 minute gives rise to the formation of peptides soluble in perchloric acid with an absorbance at 275 nm equal to that of 1 μmol of tyrosine.

Uses and Administration

Plasmin has fibrinolytic properties and is used in conjunction with deoxyribonuclease for the debridement of wounds. It has also been used for the treatment of thrombotic disorders.

Plasmin has been used in conjunction with streptokinase in the thrombolytic treatment of deep vein thrombosis (G.A. Marbet *et al., Thromb. Haemostasis,* 1982, *48,* 190) although the incidence of adverse effects is high with almost half the patients having to stop treatment (*idem,* 196).

Proprietary Names and Manufacturers

The following names have been used for multi-ingredient preparations containing plasmin—Elase *(Parke, Davis, Austral.*; *Parke, Davis, Canad.*; *Parke, Davis, USA)*; Elase-Chloromycetin *(Parke, Davis, Canad.*; *Parke, Davis, USA)*.

13211-t

Ribonuclease

RNAase.

CAS — 9001-99-4.

An enzyme present in most mammalian tissue.

Ribonuclease is involved in the catalytic cleavage of ribonucleic acid. It has been used in ointments in the treatment of traumatic and articular pain.

Proprietary Names and Manufacturers

Ribalgilasi *(Italfarmaco, Ital.)*.

248-z

Saruplase *(pINN).*

Pro-urokinase; Recombinant Human Single-Chain Urokinase-type Plasminogen Activator; scuPA.

CAS — 99149-95-8.

Saruplase is a urokinase-type plasminogen activator with a single chain structure prepared via recombinant techniques and under investigation in thrombo-embolic disorders. It is reported to have greater selectivity for fibrin-bound plasminogen than for plasma plasminogen.

For an overview of thrombolytic therapy, see under streptokinase (p.1048).

Proprietary Names and Manufacturers

Grünenthal, Ger.

13233-h

Serrapeptase *(rINN).*

A proteolytic enzyme derived from *Serratia* spp.

Serrapeptase has been used in the treatment of inflammatory disorders.

Following surgery for chronic empyema, buccal inflammation was significantly less in patients receiving serrapeptase 30 mg per day by mouth than in patients receiving placebo in a multicentre trial using 174 patients.— M. Tachibana *et al.*, *Pharmatherapeutica*, 1984, *3*, 526.

Proprietary Names and Manufacturers
Aniflazym *(Madaus, Ger.)*; Danzen *(Cyanamid, Ital.)*; Dazen *(Takeda, Fr.)*.

3745-w

Streptodornase *(BAN, rINN).*
Streptococcal Deoxyribonuclease. An enzyme obtained from cultures of various strains of *Streptococcus haemolyticus.*

CAS — 37340-82-2.

Units
2400 units of streptodornase are contained in approximately 1 mg of extract which also contains streptokinase, with lactose 5 mg, in one ampoule of the first International Standard Preparation (1964).

Uses and Administration
Streptodornase catalyses the depolymerisation of polymerised deoxyribonucleoproteins. It liquefies the viscous nucleoprotein of dead cells; it has no effect on living cells. It is used only in conjunction with streptokinase in the topical treatment of lesions, wounds and other conditions that require the removal of clots or purulent matter.

Proprietary Names and Manufacturers
The following names have been used for multi-ingredient preparations containing streptodornase—Varidase *(Lederle, Austral.*; *Lederle, Canad.*; *Cyanamid-Lederle, Ger.*; *Lederle, Swed.*; *Lederle, Switz.*; *Lederle, UK)*.

3746-e

Streptokinase *(BAN, rINN).*

A protein obtained from culture filtrates of certain strains of *Streptococcus haemolyticus* group C, which has the property of combining with human plasminogen to form plasminogen activator, and has been purified to contain not less than 600 International units of streptokinase activity per microgram of nitrogen. After purification it is usually mixed with a buffer and may be stabilised by the addition of suitable substances such as Albumin Solution.

CAS — 9002-01-1.

Pharmacopoeias. In *Br., Eur., Fr., It., Neth.,* and *Swiss.*

A hygroscopic white powder or friable solid. Freely **soluble** in water. A solution in water containing 5000 units per mL has a pH of 6.8 to 7.5. **Store** in sealed containers and protect from light; under these conditions the powder may be expected to retain its potency for 3 years.

The incorporation of albumin in commercial preparations of streptokinase has reduced the incidence of flocculation with streptokinase solutions. However, flocculation has occurred with small volumes prepared with sodium chloride injection (0.9%) in sterilised glass containers apparently because of residual acid buffers that remain in empty evacuated containers following sterilisation.— L. Thibault (letter), *Am. J. Hosp. Pharm.*, 1985, *42*, 278.

Units
3100 units of streptokinase are contained in approximately 1 mg of extract which also contains streptodornase, with lactose 5 mg, in one ampoule of the first International Standard Preparation (1964). The Christensen unit is the quantity of streptokinase that will lyse a standard blood clot completely in 10 minutes. The Christensen unit is equivalent to the International unit.

Adverse Effects
Streptokinase may cause fever and haemorrhage. Cerebral, peripheral, and pulmonary embolisms have occurred. Streptokinase is antigenic and allergic reactions may occur. Liver enzyme abnormalities may occur. Hypotension can occur directly or as a result of reperfusion; arrhythmias may also occur as a result of reperfusion.

A review of adverse reactions to thrombolytic drugs.— J. Nazari *et al.*, *Med. Toxicol.*, 1987, *2*, 274.

Results of a postmarketing surveillance programme on streptokinase (streptase). Reports were received on 306 patients, 50% of whom were reported to have sustained adverse reactions; 149 patients recovered from minor reactions eg. allergy, fever, bleeding; one patient had a neuropathy secondary to femoral haematoma; and three patients with severe bleeding died. It was judged that 70% of patients benefited from treatment.— C. F. Thayer, *Curr. ther. Res.*, 1981, *30*, 129.

EFFECTS ON THE BLOOD. In 5 patients massive blood plasmocytosis occurred 7 to 9 days after beginning therapy with streptokinase. One patient also had clinical signs of serum sickness.— P. W. Straub *et al.*, *Schweiz. med. Wschr.*, 1974, *104*, 1891.

EFFECTS ON THE KIDNEY. A 50-year-old man developed temporary and reversible changes in renal function 10 days after starting therapy with streptokinase.— L. Spangen *et al.*, *Acta med. scand.*, 1976, *199*, 335.

Reports of acute renal failure with streptokinase: F. W. Rieben *et al.*, *Dt. med. Wschr.*, 1979, *104*, 1447; R. A. Pick *et al.*, *West. J. Med.*, 1983, *138*, 878.

EFFECTS ON THE LIVER. Severe intra-abdominal bleeding with spontaneous rupture of the liver and spleen occurred in 3 and 1 patients respectively during treatment with streptokinase for deep vein thrombosis. Liver disease was not found in any of the patients.— B. Eklöf *et al.*, *Vasa*, 1977, *6*, 369. The same study.— L. Norgren *et al.*, *Läkartidningen*, 1978, *75*, 777.

Another report of liver dysfunction associated with streptokinase.— M. K. Sallen *et al.*, *Am. J. Gastroent.*, 1983, *78*, 523.

EFFECTS ON THE NERVOUS SYSTEM. A possible association of the Guillain-Barré syndrome with the intravenous administration of streptokinase by constant infusion for 72 hours.— K. V. Eden (letter), *J. Am. med. Ass.*, 1983, *249*, 2020. A further report.— D. A. Leaf *et al.* (letter), *Ann. intern. Med.*, 1984, *100*, 617. A view that no firm conclusion can be made concerning the association between exposure to streptokinase and subsequent development of Guillain-Barré syndrome. Large increases in the wholesale distribution of streptokinase had not increased the rate of reporting of streptokinase-associated Guillain-Barré syndrome to the FDA.— J. B. Arrowsmith *et al.* (letter), *ibid.*, 1985, *103*, 302.

Subarachnoid haemorrhage, intracerebral haemorrhage, and a thrombo-embolic nonhaemorrhagic stroke were observed respectively in 3 patients who had received streptokinase for vascular occlusion. A retrospective study of 88 further patients similarly treated with streptokinase revealed no additional cerebrovascular complications. It was stated that a number of factors make it difficult to determine the true incidence of cerebrovascular complications from streptokinase use.— M. S. Aldrich *et al.*, *J. Am. med. Ass.*, 1985, *253*, 1777.

EFFECTS ON THE RESPIRATORY SYSTEM. Fatal adult respiratory distress syndrome in one patient given streptokinase. It was suggested that streptokinase may have caused the pulmonary injury by altering vascular permeability due to generation of fibrinolytic products or via reperfusion oedema.— T. R. Martin *et al.*, *Chest*, 1983, *83*, 151.

Treatment of Adverse Effects
Allergic reactions may require treatment with corticosteroids; they have sometimes been given with streptokinase to reduce the risk of such reactions. Haemorrhage may be treated by the administration of fresh blood, tranexamic acid, or plasma volume expanders.

Precautions
Streptokinase should not be given to patients with severe hypertension, coagulation defects, cerebral metastases, visceral carcinoma, or with haemorrhagic diathesis such as peptic ulcer, ulcerative colitis, or to patients following recent surgery, parturition, or trauma. It should not be given for occlusion of the carotid or vertebral arteries. Its use should also be avoided during the first 16 to 18 weeks of pregnancy because of the risk of placental separation. It is also contra-indicated in patients with streptococcal infections or sub-acute bacterial endocarditis and in patients with liver or kidney disease. Streptokinase is not recommended in patients with cerebrovascular accidents, but see the discussion on thrombolytics in stroke under Thrombolytic Therapy for Thromboembolic Disorders in Uses. It has been suggested that streptokinase should not be used during menstruation. It should be used with care in the elderly and in patients with atrial fibrillation. Drugs, such as aspirin or dipyridamole, that affect platelet function as well as heparin and oral anticoagulants can increase the risk of haemorrhage if used during treatment with streptokinase. It has been recommended that during streptokinase therapy invasive procedures, including intramuscular injections, should be avoided.

Overinfusion of streptokinase may occur if a drop-counting infusion pump is employed. This arises as a result of flocculation of the streptokinase solution producing translucent fibres that affect the drop-forming mechanism so increasing the drop size.— R. F. Schad and R. H. Jennings (letter), *Am. J. Hosp. Pharm.*, 1982, *39*, 1850.

Absorption and Fate
Streptokinase is rapidly cleared from the circulation following intravenous administration. Clearance is biphasic with the initial phase being due to specific antibodies.

A study of the pharmacokinetics of streptokinase, based on its amidolytic activity.— D. S. Grierson and T. D. Bjornsson, *Clin. Pharmac. Ther.*, 1987, *41*, 304.

Uses and Administration
Streptokinase rapidly activates plasminogen, indirectly by means of a streptokinase-plasminogen complex, to plasmin (see p.1047), a proteolytic enzyme which has fibrinolytic effects and can be used to dissolve intravascular blood clots. Streptokinase is given by intravenous or intra-arterial infusion in the treatment of thrombo-embolic disorders such as pulmonary embolism and arterial and venous occlusions. It is also used in myocardial infarction when it may be infused intravenously or into the coronary artery. Treatment is most likely to be effective if given as soon as possible after the onset of symptoms.

The usual intravenous dose consists of a loading dose of 250 000 to 600 000 units infused over a period of 30 minutes to 1 hour followed by a maintenance dose of 100 000 units per hour for up to 72 hours; on occasions the maintenance dose has been extended for a further 72 hours. Sodium chloride injection (0.9%) or glucose injection (5%) may be used as vehicles. Treatment should be controlled through measurements of the thrombin clotting time.

Coronary catheterisation with the aid of angiography is required for appropriate intracoronary infusion in myocardial infarction. An initial dose of 10 000 to 25 000 units is given as a bolus injection followed by an infusion of 2000 to 4000 units per minute for up to 60 to 75 minutes. Because thrombolytic activity rapidly fades when treatment ceases, anticoagulant therapy with heparin by intravenous infusion and then with oral anticoagulants must follow. Streptokinase is also used to clear cannulas and shunts of occluding thrombi. It is used topically in conjunction with streptodornase to clear clots and purulent matter.

THROMBOLYTIC THERAPY FOR THROMBO-EMBOLIC DISORDERS. The agents used for the thrombolysis of undesirable clots act as plasminogen activators to produce plasmin which has fibrinolytic properties as well as fibrinogenolytic properties. However, these agents possess different relative activities on fibrin-bound plasminogen and on plasma plasminogen. The newer activators such as the tissue-type plasminogen activator alteplase and the single chain urokinase-type activator saruplase or pro-urokinase demonstrate greater selectivity for fibrin-bound plasminogen than anistreplase (anisoylated plasminogen streptokinase activator) which in turn shows greater selectivity than either streptokinase or urokinase. Activation of plasma plasminogen yields plasmin in a quantity that exceeds the neutralising capacity of the plasma inhibitory proteins and leads to a fibrinolytic state with debatable haemorrhagic consequences

(V.J. Marder and C.W. Francis, *Drugs*, 1987, *33*, *Suppl.* 3, 13). In addition, these thrombolytic agents demonstrate different features with regard to duration and method of administration, the time to obtain a response, and the level of antigenicity.

This review discusses briefly the role of thrombolytic agents in various thrombo-embolic disorders. Streptokinase and to a lesser extent urokinase have shown the value of this type of therapy in deep vein thrombosis, pulmonary embolism, and coronary occlusion in myocardial infarction and it is on this latter condition that many of the investigations have concentrated, especially with the newer agents. There are studies that show reperfusion and improved patency of coronary vessels and some that show improvement in cardiac function and in mortality. While some studies indicate advantages for one thrombolytic over another, the selection of an appropriate agent is not yet straightforward.

Myocardial Infarction.

Streptokinase has been shown to dissolve the thrombi in coronary vessels if given by intravenous infusion or if administered directly into the affected coronary vessel following cardiac catheterisation. Some commentators consider intracoronary administration to provide better clearance than infusion by the intravenous route (*Lancet*, 1987, *2*, 138), while others consider that there is little to choose between the two routes (S. Yusuf *et al.*, *Eur. Heart J.*, 1986, *6*, 556). Associated with the clearance of the coronary occlusion is a reduction in mortality if streptokinase is given within 4 to 6 hours of the onset of pain (M.L. Simoons *et al.*, *Lancet*, 1985, *2*, 578; GISI, *ibid.*, 1986, *1*, 397; *idem*, 1987, *2*, 871; ISIS Steering Committee, *Lancet*, 1987, *1*, 502). The large-scale ISIS-2 study (*Lancet*, 1988, *2*, 349) showed that one dose of streptokinase 1.5 million units given over one hour intravenously even within 24 hours of pain onset significantly reduced mortality; the addition of aspirin 160 mg daily for one month provided added benefit. Others, although finding a reduction in infarct size, have failed to find a significant improvement in mortality (ISAM Study Group, *J. Am. Coll. Cardiol.*, 1987, *9*, 197).

Urokinase causes fewer antigenic problems than streptokinase, but experience in its use in myocardial infarction is less than with streptokinase. The intravenous route has produced improvement in terms of patency (D.G. Mathey *et al.*, *Am. J. Cardiol.*, 1985, *55*, 878). The intracoronary route has also been used, although the benefit was less clear cut (H. Kambara *et al.*, *Cath. Cardiovasc. Diagnosis*, 1985, *11*, 349). Also an earlier collaborative study failed to show an improvement in mortality over 1 year (*Lancet*, 1975, *2*, 624). A single-chain urokinase-type plasminogen activator known as saruplase or pro-urokinase has been produced through recombinant DNA techniques; its effect is awaited with interest.

The human plasminogen-streptokinase complex is the basis for anistreplase which is anisoylated plasminogen streptokinase activator complex (APSAC). Because of its structure, this complex has a more prolonged half-life than streptokinase and can be given as a simple rapid intravenous injection rather than as a prolonged infusion. It also has greater clot selectivity and remains longer in the clot than does streptokinase (*Lancet*, 1988, *1*, 565). Reperfusion occurs with anistreplase as frequently as with intracoronary streptokinase (J.P. Monk and R.C. Heel, *Drugs*, 1987, *34*, 25) and several studies have demonstrated benefit in myocardial infarction (S. Ikram *et al.*, *Br. med. J.*, 1986, *293*, 786; M. Been *et al.*, *Int. J. Cardiol.*, 1986, *11*, 53; J.L. Anderson *et al.*, (Ed.), *Drugs*, 1987, *33*, *Suppl.* 3, 1-316). More recently the APSAC intervention mortality study was halted in view of the large difference in survival in favour of the treatment group (AIMS Trial Study Group, *Lancet*, 1988, *1*, 545). Of 502 patients in the placebo group 61 died in the first 30 days compared with 32 of 502 in the group given anistreplase within 6 hours of the onset of major symptoms of myocardial infarction.

Alteplase or tissue plasminogen activator offers another thrombolytic approach. It has a preferential effect on fibrin-associated plasminogen and plasmin is considered to bind more strongly to fibrin when alteplase is present (*Lancet*, 1988, *1*, 565). When given by intravenous infusion, usually over several hours, it has been shown to be more effective than placebo or intravenous streptokinase in inducing coronary reperfusion (TIMI Study Group, *New Engl. J. Med.*, 1985, *312*, 932; M. Verstraete *et al.*, *Lancet*, 1985, *1*, 842; *idem*, *2*, 965; F.H. Sheehan *et al.*, *Circulation*, 1987, *75*, 817; J.H. Cheseboro *et al.*, *ibid.*, *76*, 142; P.L. Thompson *et al.*, *Lancet*, 1988, *1*, 203). The large-scale ASSET study (R.G. Wilcox *et al.*, *Lancet*, 1988, *2*, 525) showed a reduction in mortality with alteplase when given within 5 hours of the onset of major symptoms of myocardial infarction. This reduction of 26% in the first month was considered to be similar to that observed in other major studies with other thrombolytics. Some studies were carried out using a double-stranded molecule of tissue plasminogen activator. The form made available commercially consists predominantly of a single chain; this form produced by recombinant DNA technology has been shown to be effective in rendering infarct-related arteries patent (E.J. Topol *et al.*, *J. Am. Coll. Cardiol.*, 1987, *9*, 1205), although it has been reported to be less potent but more clot-selective than the 2 chain form (S.Z. Goldhaber *et al.*, *Lancet*, 1986, *2*, 886) and to require more rapid infusion (H.D. Garabedian *et al.*, *J. Am. Coll. Cardiol.*, 1987, *9*, 599). It is this single-chain form that is known by the name alteplase.

A higher rate of re-occlusion has been reported with tissue plasminogen activator than with streptokinase given by the intravenous or intracoronary routes (D.O. Williams *et al.*, *Circulation*, 1986, *73*, 338). Immediate or deferred coronary angioplasty has been considered to be a valuable adjunct to tissue plasminogen activator (E.J. Topol *et al.*, *Circulation*, 1987, *75*, 420; A.D. Guerci *et al.*, *New Engl. J. Med.*, 1987, *317*, 1613). Others have found immediate coronary angioplasty to be of no additional benefit to tissue plasminogen activator (M.L. Simoons *et al.*, *Lancet*, 1988, *1*, 197).

It is common practice to use heparin in conjunction with thrombolytic therapy. The role of anticoagulants in myocardial infarction is discussed on p.338. Antiplatelet agents are also used, see p.6 as are beta blockers, see p.781 and intravenous vasodilators, see p.501 and p.1501.

Deep Vein Thrombosis and Peripheral Arterial Occlusion.

Thrombolysis can be achieved in deep vein thrombosis with streptokinase or urokinase (S.Z. Goldhaber *et al.*, *Am. J. Med.*, 1984, *76*, 393; G. Trübestein *et al.*, *Vasc. Med.*, 1985, *3*, 72). Peripheral arterial occlusions can also be cleared and techniques have been developed for local low-dose thrombolytic therapy aimed directly at the occlusion (H. Hess *et al.*, *New Engl. J. Med.*, 1982, *307*, 1627; T.O. McNamara, *Am. J. Med.*, 1987, *83*, *Suppl.* 2A, 6). Anistreplase has been tried, but Earnshaw *et al.* reported poor results with intravenous or intra-arterial doses for acute peripheral arterial occlusions (J.J. Earnshaw *et al.*, *Thromb. Haemostasis*, 1986, *55*, 259).

Pulmonary Embolisms.

Pulmonary embolisms have also responded to streptokinase or urokinase (*J. Am. med. Ass.*, 1974, *229*, 1606; G.V.R.K. Sharma *et al.*, *New Engl. J. Med.*, 1980, *303*, 842; S. Sherry, *Drug Ther.*, 1983, *13*, 144; UKEP Study Research Group, *Eur. Heart J.*, 1987, *8*, 2). Anistreplase has also been tried (J.H.N. Bett *et al.*, *Aust. N.Z. J. Med.*, 1987, *17*, 77) as has alteplase (H. Bounamcaux *et al.*, *Ann. intern. Med.*, 1985, *103*, 64; S. Z. Goldhaber *et al.*, *Lancet*, 1988, *2*, 293).

Stroke.

As with anticoagulants, the use of thrombolytics in stroke has to be treated with caution because of the risks of haemorrhage. There have, however, been some reports of thrombolytics being used and they have been reviewed by Del Zoppo and his colleagues (G.J. Del Zoppo *et al.*, *Stroke*, 1986, *17*, 595) who argue for the theoretical advantages of thrombus dissolution by local infusion; alteplase and saruplase may also provide effective intravenous therapy.

Pregnancy.

Streptokinase and urokinase have been used for thrombolysis in pregnant patients (R.J.C. Hall *et al.*, *Br. med. J.*, 1972, *4*, 647; H. Ludwig, *Postgrad. med. J.*, 1973, *49*, (Aug.), *Suppl.* 5, 65; G.L. Declos and F. Davila, *Am. J. Obstet. Gynec.*, 1986, *155*, 375) without adverse effect in the foetus.

Preparations

Streptokinase Injection *(B.P.)*

Proprietary Preparations

Kabikinase *(KabiVitrum, UK). Injection*, powder for reconstitution, streptokinase 100 000, 250 000, and 600 000 units per vial.

Streptase *(Hoechst, UK). Injection*, powder for reconstitution, streptokinase 100 000, 250 000, and 750 000 units per vial.

Varidase *(Lederle, UK). Topical powder*, for reconstitution, streptokinase 100 000 units, streptodornase 25 000 units.

Proprietary Names and Manufacturers

Kabikinas *(KabiVitrum, Denm.; KabiVitrum, Norw.; Kabi, Swed.)*; Kabikinase *(Pharmacia, Austral.; Belg.; Kabivitrum, Fr.; Kabi, Ger.; Pierrel, Ital.; Neth.; Kabi, S.Afr.; Fides, Spain; KabiVitrum, Switz.; KabiVitrum, UK; Kabivitrum, USA)*; Streptase *(Hoechst, Austral.; Belg.; Hoechst, Canad.; Behringwerke, Denm.; Hoechst, Fr.; Behringwerke, Ger.; Istituto Behring, Ital.; Neth.; Behring, Norw.; S.Afr.; Behring, Spain; Behring, Switz.; Hoechst, UK; Hoechst, USA)*.

The following names have been used for multi-ingredient preparations containing streptokinase— Varidase *(Lederle, Austral.; Lederle, Canad.; Ger.; Lederle, Swed.; Lederle, Switz.; Lederle, UK)*.

3748-y

Sutilains *(BAN, USAN, rINN).*

BAX-1515.

CAS — 12211-28-8.

Pharmacopoeias. In *U.S.*

A cream-coloured powder containing proteolytic enzymes derived from *Bacillus subtilis*. It contains not less than 2 500 000 *U.S.P.* Casein units of proteolytic activity per g. A 1% solution has a pH of 6.1 to 7.1. **Store** at 2° to 8° in airtight containers.

Units

One *U.S.P.* Casein unit of proteolytic activity is contained in the amount of sutilains which when incubated at 37° with 35 mg of denatured casein, produces in 1 minute a hydrolysate whose absorbance at 275 nm is equal to that of a tyrosine solution containing 1.5 μg of *U.S.P.* Tyrosine Reference Standard per mL.

Adverse Effects

Pain, paraesthesia, bleeding, and dermatitis may occur.

Precautions

Contact with the eyes should be avoided. It should not be used in major body cavities, wounds containing exposed nerves or nervous tissues, or in fungating neoplastic lesions.

Uses and Administration

Sutilains is a proteolytic agent used for wound debridement in moist conditions. The wound should be irrigated with water or sodium chloride solution, and cleansed of antiseptics which may reduce activity.

Preparations

Sutilains Ointment *(U.S.P.)*

Proprietary Names and Manufacturers

Travase *(Flint, Canad.; Flint, USA)*.

3903-p

Thiomucase

C-84-04; Chondroitinsulphatase.

Thiomucase is a mucopolysaccharidase with general properties similar to those of hyaluronidase, p.1044, but which also depolymerises chondroitin sulphate. It has been given to assist the diffusion of local anaesthetic injections.

Proprietary Names and Manufacturers

Funk, Spain.

12779-v

Tilactase *(rINN).*

β-Galactosidase; Lactase.

CAS — 9031-11-2.

Tilactase is the enzyme involved in the hydrolysis of lactose. Deficiency of the enzyme may result in alactasia or lactose intolerance.

A discussion of lactose intolerance.— *Med. Lett.*, 1981, *23*, 67.

Results of a study involving 80 subjects showed that tilactase deficiency is an uncommon cause of intestinal symptoms in subjects with irritable bowel syndrome.— A. D. Newcomer and D. B. McGill, *Mayo Clin. Proc.*, 1983, *58*, 339.

Diagnosis and management of tilactase deficiency.— G. P. Davidson, *Med. J. Aust.*, 1984, *141*, 442.

Proprietary Names and Manufacturers

Galantase *(Noristan, S.Afr.)*; Imulact *(Kali-Farma, Spain)*; LactAid *(Jan, Canad.; Lactaid, USA)*; Lactozyma *(Ital.)*; Lactrase *(Kremers-Urban, USA)*; Lactyme *(Jpn)*; Lamitase *(Jpn)*; Lysolac *(Tosi, Ital.)*; Organase *(Jpn)*.

3751-p

Trypsin

Crystalline Trypsin; Crystallized Trypsin *(USAN)*.

CAS — 9002-07-7.

Pharmacopoeias. In *Chin., Cz., Fr., Roum., Rus.,* and *U.S.*

A proteolytic enzyme (protease) obtained from mammalian pancreas. The *U.S.P.* specifies bovine pancreas and not less than 2500 *U.S.P.* units in each mg.

A white to yellowish-white, odourless, crystalline or amorphous powder. **Store** in a cool place in airtight containers.

The properties and assay methods of trypsin.— Trypsin, in *Pharmaceutical Enzymes,* R. Ruyssen and A. Lauwers (Ed.), Gent, E. Story-Scientia, 1978, p. 33.

Units

Trypsin is assayed for potency on the basis of its proteolytic activity and the potency of commercial products has been expressed in various units based on different methods of assay.

There are 2 principal methods of assay. One is based on the use of a denatured haemoglobin substrate; the other is based on the hydrolysis of *N*-benzoyl-L-arginine ethyl ester by trypsin at the ester linkage. Crystallized Trypsin *U.S.P.* is assayed for potency, by comparison with a reference standard, in terms of its ability to digest *N*-benzoyl-L-arginine ethyl ester hydrochloride at 25°. The hydrolysis is followed spectrophotometrically by measurement of the light absorption at 253 nm and the unit is determined by the average change in absorption per minute. One *U.S.P.* Trypsin unit is the activity causing a change in absorption of 0.003 per minute under the conditions specified in the assay.

One FIP unit of trypsin activity is contained in that amount of the standard preparation which, under specified conditions, hydrolyses 1 μmol of *N*-benzoyl-L-arginine ethyl ester as the hydrochloride per minute. The hydrolysis is followed potentiometrically.

Uses and Administration

Trypsin is a proteolytic enzyme that has been used for the removal of coagulated blood, exudate, and necrotic tissue. It has been applied as a dressing, irrigation, or instillation, or given as an intramuscular injection. It has been used intrapleurally for the liquefaction of viscous sputum. It is also used in conjunction with chymotrypsin when it has been given by mouth or applied topically for its proteolytic effect.

Allergic reactions may occur.

References to studies comparing trypsin with a combination of streptokinase and streptodornase in ulcers showing a similar or better response with the combination.— L. Hellgren, *Eur. J. clin. Pharmac.,* 1983, *24,* 623; O. Suomalainen, *Annls Chir. Gynaec.,* 1983, *72,* 62.

Preparations

Crystallized Trypsin for Inhalation Aerosol *(U.S.P.).* Trypsin Crystallized for Aerosol

Proprietary Preparations

Chymoral *(Rorer, UK). Tablets,* enteric-coated, trypsin and chymotrypsin, total enzyme activity 50 000 Armour units.

Tablets (Chymoral Forte), enteric-coated, trypsin and chymotrypsin, total enzyme activity 100 000 Armour units.

Proprietary Names and Manufacturers

Tryptar *(Austral.; Armour, UK)*; Trypure Novo *(Denm.; Ger.; Ital.; Neth.; Norw.; Novo, Swed.; Switz.; Novo, UK).*

The following names have been used for multi-ingredient preparations containing trypsin— Chymacort Ointment *(Armour, UK)*; Chymocyclar *(Rorer, UK)*; Chymoral *(USV, Austral.; Rorer, UK)*; Granulex *(Hickam, USA)*; Orenzyme *(Merrell Dow, USA)*; Ototrips *(Consolidated Chemicals, UK)*; Stimuzyme Plus *(National Dermaceutical, USA).*

3752-s

Urokinase *(BAN, USAN, rINN).*

An enzyme isolated from human urine, or from tissue cultures of human kidney cells.

CAS — 9039-53-6.

Pharmacopoeias. In *It.*

Several forms with different molecular weights have been described. A single-chain urokinase-type plasminogen activator has also been prepared, see saruplase, p.1047.

The properties and assay methods of urokinase. It was generally admitted that preparations of urokinase obtained from the extraction of human urine must be able to activate plasminogen to plasmin for an activity of 24 FIP units per mg of protein.— Urokinase, in *Pharmaceutical Enzymes,* R. Ruyssen and A. Lauwers (Ed.), Gent, E. Story-Scientia, 1978, p. 133.

The stability of a heparin urokinase mixture suitable for use in maintaining vascular access devices free of thrombi.— G. J. Morgan *et al., Intensive Therapy clin. Monit.,* 1987, *8,* 89.

Units

4800 units of urokinase are contained in approximately 1.8 mg of urokinase, with lactose 5 mg, in one ampoule of the first International Reference Preparation (1968).

In Great Britain potency is also expressed in arbitrary units known as Ploug units. One Ploug unit is approximately equivalent to 1.5 International units.

In the USA, potency has been expressed in CTA Units (National Heart Institute Committee on Thrombolytic Agents). One CTA unit is approximately equivalent to 1 International unit.

One FIP unit of urokinase hydrolyses 1 μmol of *N*-α-acetyl-glycyl-L-lysine methyl ester acetate per minute. One FIP unit is equivalent to 546 Ploug units and approximately to 780 CTA units.

Adverse Effects, Treatment, and Precautions

As for Streptokinase, p.1048. Serious allergic reactions may be less likely to occur with urokinase than with streptokinase.

The conversion of plasminogen to plasmin by urokinase can be inhibited by aminocaproic acid and tranexamic acid but this conversion is not inhibited by aprotinin.— Urokinase, in *Pharmaceutical Enzymes,* R. Ruyssen and A. Lauwers (Ed.), Gent, E. Story-Scientia, 1978, p. 133.

Uses and Administration

Urokinase directly converts plasminogen to plasmin (see p.1047) a proteolytic enzyme which has fibrinolytic effects.

It is used similarly to streptokinase in thromboembolic disorders including pulmonary embolisms and coronary occlusions in myocardial infarction. It also has a specific use in clearing both clots and haemorrhage in the eye.

Like streptokinase it is used to clear cannulas and shunts of occluding thrombi.

For hyphaemia, doses of 5000 International units dissolved in 2 mL of sodium chloride injection (0.9%) are used to irrigate the anterior chamber. Higher doses may be used. For vitreous haemorrhage, solutions of 25 000 International units dissolved in 0.3 mL of Water for Injections may be used. Higher doses may also be used in this condition. The doses of urokinase in hyphaemia and in vitreous haemorrhage are confused by preparations being expressed in either International units or in Ploug units. Despite these units not being equivalent (1.5 International unit is approximately equivalent to 1 Ploug unit), similar numerical dose ranges are quoted for the preparations. The lower dose ranges, i.e. those given in International units are cited here. In the treatment of pulmonary embolism urokinase is given by intravenous infusion in initial doses of 4400 International units per kg body-weight over 10 minutes, followed by 4400 units per kg per hour for 12 hours. Treatment may be monitored through coagulation tests. Doses of 6000 International units have been infused every minute for up to 2 hours into coronary vessels under angiographic control.

For an overview of thrombolytic therapy including urokinase, see under streptokinase (p.1048).

In addition, urokinase has been used locally to clear clots as well as haemorrhage in the eye. Some references to its use in vitreous haemorrhage:; *Br. J. Ophthal.,* 1977, *61,* 499; J. S. Chapman-Smith and G. W. Crock, *ibid.,* 500; *Br. med. J.,* 1978, *1,* 940.

PERITONITIS. A report of successful treatment in 3 consecutive patients with recurrent peritonitis in continuous ambulatory peritoneal dialysis (CAPD) by using urokinase without Tenckhoff catheter removal. Oral and intraperitoneal antibiotics were continued throughout the procedure and for a total of 7 days.— S. J. Pickering *et al.* (letter), *Lancet,* 1987, *1,* 1258.

Proprietary Preparations

Ukidan *(Serono, UK). Injection,* powder for reconstitution, urokinase 5000 or 25 000 International units per vial.

Urokinase *(Leo, UK). Injection,* powder for reconstitution, urokinase 5000 or 25 000 Ploug units per vial.

Proprietary Names and Manufacturers

Abbokinase *(Abbott, Ger.; Dainippon, Jpn; Abbott, Spain; Abbott, Swed.; Abbott, UK; Abbott, USA)*; Actosolv *(Hoechst, Fr.; Behringwerke, Ger.)*; Alphakinase *(Alpha, Ger.)*; Breokinase *(Winthrop-Breon, USA)*; Cultokinase *(Kyorin, Jpn)*; Natel *(Merrell Dow, Spain)*; Persolv *(Lepetit, Ital.)*; Purochin *(Sclavo, Ital.)*; Rheotromb *(Schwarz, Ger.)*; Ukidan *(Serono, Ger.; Serono, Ital.; Serono, Switz.; Serono, UK)*; Uroquidan *(Farma-Lepori, Spain)*; Wakamoto 6000 *(Jpn).*

3755-l

Proprietary Preparations of Other Mixed Enzymes

Vasolastine *(Enzypharm, UK: Phoenix, UK). Injection,* enzymes of lipid metabolism 4000 Enzypharm units/mL, amine oxidase 2000 Enzypharm units/mL, tyrosinase 2000 Enzypharm units/mL in ampoules of 2 mL. For atherosclerosis and associated symptoms.

Local sensitivity may occur at the injection site of Vasolastine. There appeared to be no acceptable evidence that Vasolastine was of help in peripheral vascular disease.— *Drug & Ther. Bull.,* 1981, *19,* 27.

Ergot Alkaloids and Derivatives

1500-t

Ergot is the sclerotium of the fungus *Claviceps purpurea* which grows on rye and other grains. Seven isomeric pairs of alkaloids have been isolated from ergot, all derivatives of the tetracyclic compound 6-methylergoline: ergocristine and ergocristinine, ergotamine and ergotaminine, ergocryptine and ergocryptinine, ergocornine and ergocorninine, ergosine and ergosinine, ergostine and ergostinine, ergometrine (also called ergonovine, ergobasine, ergostetrine, ergotocine) and ergometrinine. Ergocryptine is now known to comprise α-ergocryptine and β-ergocryptine, likewise ergocryptinine comprises α-ergocryptinine and β-ergocryptinine. Ergotoxine, the first active substance to be isolated from ergot was later found to be a mixture of ergocristine, ergocornine, α-ergocryptine, and β-ergocryptine. Similarly ergotonine is a mixture of ergocristinine, ergocorninine, α-ergocryptinine, and β-ergocryptinine.

The first 12 of these alkaloids are derivatives of lysergic or isolysergic acid combined with polypeptide groups and have been called amino-acid alkaloids, peptide alkaloids, or ergopeptines. In ergometrine and ergometrinine the polypeptide group is replaced by propanolamine; they have been called amine alkaloids. The first named of each of the isomeric pairs is laevorotatory, derived from lysergic acid, and physiologically active while the second is dextrorotatory, derived from isolysergic acid, and has little physiological activity. The nature and quantity of the alkaloids present in ergot vary with the geographical source.

Semisynthetic derivatives of ergot alkaloids have been prepared. Hydrogenation of one of the double bonds of lysergic acid produces stable dihydrogenated alkaloids such as dihydroergotamine. Different amides of lysergic acid have been produced, including methylergometrine, the hydroxybutylamide; methylation of the indole nitrogen of methylergometrine has yielded methysergide. The diethylamide, lysergide, is described on p.1584. Ergot alkaloids and derivatives with the same basic tetracyclic structure may all be called ergolines, but in practice the term has often been restricted to compounds used for their dopaminergic activity. The ergolines lergotrile, lysuride, metergoline, and pergolide, together with bromocriptine, a derivative of α-ergocryptine, are described in the section on Dopaminergic Antiparkinsonian Agents (p.1008).

The ergot alkaloids were the first alpha-adrenoceptor blocking agents discovered. Different alkaloids and their derivatives have varying degrees of blocking activity; dihydrogenated alkaloids are potent blocking agents while compounds such as ergometrine and methylergometrine, which lack a polypeptide side-chain in their structure, possess little or none of this activity. However, it is now generally accepted that the varied and complex pharmacological properties of these alkaloids and their derivatives result from their actions as partial agonists or antagonists at dopamine and serotonin receptors as well as alpha-adrenoceptors. The most important effects are due to actions on the central nervous system and direct stimulation of smooth muscle of the uterus and blood vessels. Differences between individual compounds may be due to varying activity at different receptors and the range of effects exhibited can also depend on dosage and the pathophysiological state of the patient. All the natural ergot alkaloids have a qualitatively similar stimulant effect on the uterus, but ergometrine is the most active. The amino-acid alkaloids, especially ergotamine, constrict both arteries and veins. Hydrogenation reduces this effect but dihydroergotamine is still an effective vasoconstrictor; co-dergocrine has considerably less vasoconstrictor activity. The amine alkaloids, such as ergometrine, may raise blood pressure and decrease peripheral blood flow at therapeutic doses.

The ergot alkaloids and their derivatives have varied clinical applications. Ergometrine and methylergometrine are used in the management of postpartum haemorrhage, while ergotamine, dihydroergotamine, and methysergide are used mainly for the relief of migraine. Dihydroergotamine is also given with heparin in the prophylaxis of postoperative deep-vein thrombosis. Co-dergocrine is used in the management of senile dementia and nicergoline has been used similarly.

References: A. Stoll, *Pharm. J.*, 1965, *1*, 605 (chemistry and pharmacology); A. Hofmann, *Pharmacology*, 1978, *16, Suppl.* 1, 1 (historical view); J. R. Boissier, *ibid.*, 12 (pharmacology); *Ergot Alkaloids and Related Compounds*, B. Berde and H.O. Schild (Ed.), *Handbook of Experimental Pharmacology*, Vol. 49, Berlin, Springer-Verlag, 1978.

1503-f

Co-dergocrine Mesylate *(BAN)*.

Co-dergocrine Methanesulphonate; Dihydroergotoxine Mesylate; Dihydroergotoxine Methanesulphonate; Dihydrogenated Ergot Alkaloids; Ergoloid Mesylates *(USAN)*; Hydrogenated Ergot Alkaloids. A mixture in equal proportions of dihydroergocornine mesylate ($C_{31}H_{41}N_5O_5,CH_4O_3S = 659.8$), dihydroergocristine mesylate ($C_{35}H_{41}N_5O_5,CH_4O_3S = 707.8$), and α- and β-dihydroergocryptine mesylates ($C_{32}H_{43}N_5O_5,CH_4O_3S = 673.8$) in the ratio 1.5 to 2.5:1.

CAS — 11032-41-0 (co-dergocrine); 8067-24-1 (mesylate).

Pharmacopoeias. In *Br., Cz., Fr., Swiss,* and *U.S. Jug.* allows mesylate or esylate.

White to yellowish-white odourless or almost odourless powder. *B.P.* **solubilities** are: soluble 1 in 50 of water, 1 in 30 of alcohol, 1 in 10 of acetone, and 1 in 100 of chloroform; practically insoluble in ether. *U.S.P.* solubilities are: slightly soluble in water; soluble in alcohol and methyl alcohol; sparingly soluble in acetone. A 0.5% solution in water has a pH of 4.2 to 5.2.

Protect from light. The *B.P.* recommends **storage** in well-closed containers at a temperature not exceeding 25°. The *U.S.P.* recommends storage in airtight containers; the Oral Solution should be stored at a temperature not exceeding 30°.

SOLUBILITY. Caffeine and several other xanthines increased the aqueous solubility of co-dergocrine mesylate in 0.1 N hydrochloric acid and pH 6.65 phosphate buffer.— M. A. Zoglio and H. V. Maulding, *J. pharm. Sci.*, 1970, *59*, 215.

Adverse Effects

Side-effects occasionally reported with co-dergocrine mesylate include nausea, vomiting, headache, blurred vision, skin rashes, nasal stuffiness, flushing of the skin, dizziness, and orthostatic hypotension.

Local irritation has been reported following sublingual administration.

EFFECTS ON THE CARDIOVASCULAR SYSTEM. Of 8 patients given co-dergocrine mesylate 1.5 mg three times daily for the treatment of dementia, 3 developed severe sinus bradycardia associated with general deterioration in their condition, necessitating withdrawal of the treatment.— A. C. D. Cayley *et al.*, *Br. med. J.*, 1975, *4*, 384. No sinus bradycardia had been observed in 40 elderly patients in whom the dose was built up to 1.5 mg three times daily over 3 weeks.— C. Cohen (letter), *ibid.*, 581.

Absorption and Fate

The absorption and fate of co-dergocrine mesylate is similar to that of ergotamine tartrate, p.1056.

The pharmacokinetics of co-dergocrine mesylate were studied in 8 healthy subjects using a specific and sensitive radio-immunoassay. Following 4.5 mg by mouth, as a solution, co-dergocrine was rapidly absorbed, but oral bioavailability was low and ranged from 5.25 to 12.4% (mean 8.85%). The mean peak plasma concentration was 576 pg per mL at about one hour.— B. G. Woodcock *et al.*, *Clin. Pharmac. Ther.*, 1982, *32*, 622.

Further references: P. Loddo *et al.*, *Boll. chim.-farm.*, 1976, *115*, 570; W. H. Aellig and E. Nüesch, *Int. J. clin. Pharmac. Biopharm.*, 1977, *15*, 106.

Uses and Administration

Unlike the natural ergot alkaloids, co-dergocrine mesylate has only limited vasoconstrictor effects.

It is used with the intention of treating symptoms of mild to moderate impairment of mental function in the elderly in doses of 3 or 4.5 mg daily by mouth, preferably before meals. Higher doses have also been used. It is also given sublingually in doses of 3 mg daily. Doses of 300 μg have been given intramuscularly, subcutaneously, or by intravenous infusion.

Co-dergocrine mesylate has also been used in the treatment of hypertension, particularly in the elderly.

Co-dergocrine esylate has been used similarly to the mesylate.

CEREBROVASCULAR DISORDERS. See Senile dementia.

EXTRAPYRAMIDAL DISORDERS. Co-dergocrine mesylate 4.5 mg once daily for 6 weeks was compared with placebo in a double-blind study in 19 patients with tardive dyskinesia secondary to treatment with neuroleptic drugs. Improvement occurred in both groups, especially towards the end of the 6 weeks, but on follow-up for a further 6 weeks without treatment, only patients who had received co-dergocrine maintained their improvement.— J. Hajioff and M. Wallace, *Psychopharmacology*, 1983, *79*, 1.

Further references: J. Hajioff (letter), *Br. med. J.*, 1978, *2*, 834.

HYPERTENSION. Co-dergocrine mesylate had antihypertensive activity similar to that of nifedipine in a preliminary study in 42 elderly hypertensive patients. An initial dose of 4.5 mg daily by mouth was increased to 4.5 mg twice daily in 11 of the 21 patients taking co-dergocrine mesylate. There were fewer side-effects with co-dergocrine mesylate and there were no symptoms of hypotension with either treatment.— M. Bellani *et al.*, *Curr. ther. Res.*, 1983, *34*, 1014.

SENILE DEMENTIA. There is still much uncertainty about the use of co-dergocrine mesylate in the treatment of senile dementia. It was originally thought to act as a peripheral and cerebral vasodilator and vasodilatation was considered an effective treatment for senile dementia due to cerebral ischaemia. However, cerebral ischaemia is no longer believed to be central to the problem. Co-dergocrine mesylate is now classified as a metabolic enhancer. Optimal dosage has not been established; standard oral doses are 3 mg daily in the US and 4.5 mg daily in Europe and Japan, but in some countries as much as 12 mg daily is used without reports of serious side-effects. J.A. Yesavage *et al.* (*J. Am. Geriat. Soc.*, 1979, *27*, 80) found little difference between doses of 3 and 6 mg daily in patients with senile dementia, whereas M. Yoshikawa *et al.* (*J. Am. Geriat. Soc.*, 1983, *31*, 1) concluded that 6 mg daily was superior in a study of patients with multi-infarct dementias or mental disturbances after stroke. The overall trend seems to be to use larger doses, orally rather than sublingually, for longer periods. J.A. Yesavage *et al.* (*Archs gen. Psychiat.*, 1979, *36*, 220) reviewed 22 controlled studies of co-dergocrine mesylate in senile dementia, but although each study showed significant improvement on some behavioural or psychological measure, conclusions as to the therapeutic usefulness of co-dergocrine mesylate were guarded. Improvements ranging from 11 to 21% were calculated for mood depression, confusion, mental alertness, orientation, recent memory, emotional lability, and self-care from 4 studies submitted to the FDA, but specific clinical effects reported have varied widely. Patients selected for evaluation of co-dergocrine mesylate should be limited to those with senile dementia of the Alzheimer or multi-infarct type and the 2 groups should be considered separately. Patients with advanced disease are unlikely to benefit. Although many clinicians continue to regard co-dergocrine mesylate as a placebo it is one of the few potentially effective treatments available for senile dementia of the Alzheimer type. It is suggested that doses of at least 6 mg daily should be given for 6 months and treatment continued, possibly at a lower dose, if improvement or stabilisation of decline is seen; if treatment has not been successful it should be abandoned.— L. E. Hollister and J. Yesavage, *Ann. intern. Med.*, 1984, *100*, 894.

Further reviews and comments on co-dergocrine mesylate in the treatment of senile dementia: P. Cook and I. James, *New Engl. J. Med.*, 1981, *305*, 1508 and 1560; D. M. Loew and C. Weil, *Gerontology*, 1982, *28*, 54; A. Spagnoli and G. Tognoni, *Drugs*, 1983, *26*, 44; *Drug & Ther. Bull.*, 1984, *22*, 98; *Lancet*, 1984, *2*, 1313; L. E. Hollister, *Drugs*, 1985, *29*, 483.

Reports on the use of co-dergocrine mesylate in elderly patients with impaired mental function: D. B. Rao and J. R. Norris, *Johns Hopkins med. J.*, 1972, *130*, 317 (cerebrovascular insufficiency associated with cerebral arteriosclerosis); A. Arrigo *et al.*, *Curr. ther. Res.*, 1973, *15*, 417 (cerebrovascular insufficiency); C. M. Gaitz *et al.*, *Archs gen. Psychiat.*, 1977, *34*, 839 (organic brain syndrome); J. Kugler *et al.*, *Dt. med. Wschr.*, 1978, *103*, 456 (cerebrovascular insufficiency); R. Spiegel *et al.*, *J. Am. Geriat. Soc.*, 1983, *31*, 549 (ageing process in healthy subjects); S. Köberle and R. Spiegel, *Gerontology*, 1984, *30 Suppl.* 1, 3 (ageing process in healthy subjects); C. M. S. van Loveren-Huyben *et al.*, *J. Am. Geriat. Soc.*, 1984, *32*, 584 (senile mental deterioration).

Preparations

Co-dergocrine Tablets *(B.P.)*. Co-dergocrine Mesylate Tablets

Ergoloid Mesylates Oral Solution *(U.S.P.)*. A solution containing co-dergocrine mesylate.

Ergoloid Mesylates Tablets *(U.S.P.)*. Tablets containing co-dergocrine mesylate.

Proprietary Preparations

Hydergine *(Sandoz, UK)*. *Tablets*, scored, co-dergocrine mesylate 1.5 mg.
Tablets, co-dergocrine mesylate 4.5 mg.

Proprietary Names and Manufacturers

Circanol *(Ger.; Riker, USA)*; Coristin *(San Carlo, Ital.)*; Dacoren *(Ger.)*; DCCK *(Ger.)*; Deapril-ST *(Mead Johnson Pharmaceutical, USA)*; DH-Ergotoxin-forte *(Ger.)*; Dulcion *(Dulcis, Mon.)*; Ergodilat *(Liberman, Spain)*; Ergoplus *(Ger.)*; Hydergin *(Sandoz, Denm.; Ger.; Sandoz, Swed.)*; Hydergina *(Arg.; Sandoz, Ital.; Sandoz, Spain)*; Hydergine *(Sandoz, Austral.; Belg.; Anca, Canad.; Fr.; Sandoz, S.Afr.; Sandoz, Switz.; Sandoz, UK; Sandoz, USA)*; Hydro-ergoloid *(Schein, USA)*; Ischelium *(Polifarma, Ital.)*; Niloric *(Ascher, USA)*; Optamine *(Théraplix, Fr.)*; Perenan *(Millot-Solac, Fr.)*; Progeril *(Midy, Ital.; Clin-Midy, Switz.)*; Redergam *(Hung.)*; Ségolan *(Wyeth-Byla, Fr.)*; Secatoxin *(Cz.)*.

12007-q

Dihydroergocristine Mesylate

Dihydroergocristine Methanesulphonate.
$C_{35}H_{41}N_5O_5,CH_4O_3S=707.8$.

CAS — 17479-19-5 (dihydroergocristine); 24730-10-7 (mesylate).

Pharmacopoeias. In *Cz.*

SOLUBILITY. Caffeine, proxyphylline, or theophylline increased the aqueous solubility of dihydroergocristine mesylate in 0.1 N hydrochloric acid and pH 6.65 phosphate buffer.— H. V. Maulding and M. A. Zoglio, *J. pharm. Sci.*, 1970, *59*, 384.

Dihydroergocristine mesylate is a component of co-dergocrine mesylate (p.1051) and has similar actions. In some countries it has been given in doses of 3 to 6 mg daily by mouth in the symptomatic treatment of mental impairment associated with cerebrovascular disorders and in peripheral vascular disease. Doses of 300 to 600 µg have been given intramuscularly or intravenously.

Findings of a beneficial effect and a low incidence of side-effects from surveillance of 9702 patients with chronic cerebrovascular disease who were given dihydroergocristine 6 mg daily by mouth for 40 days.— F. G. Mailland *et al.*, *Curr. ther. Res.*, 1983, *33*, 997.

HYPERPROLACTINAEMIA. Preliminary findings that dihydroergocristine 1.5 mg by intramuscular injection reduced serum concentrations of prolactin in normoprolactinaemic and hyperprolactinaemic patients appeared to confirm the hypothesis of a potential dopaminergic effect.— M. Poli *et al.*, *Curr. ther. Res.*, 1984, *35*, 169.

Proprietary Names and Manufacturers

Decme *(Zyma, Ger.)*; Decril *(Schwarz, Ital.)*; Diertina *(Poli, Ital.; Switz.)*; Diertine *(Morrith, Spain)*; Enirant *(Desitin, Ger.)*; Ergodavur *(Davur, Spain)*; Insibrin *(Arg.)*; Nehydrin *(TAD, Ger.)*.

12008-p

Dihydroergocryptine Mesylate

Dihydroergocryptine Methanesulphonate; Dihydroergokryptine Mesylate.
$C_{32}H_{43}N_5O_5,CH_4O_3S=673.8$.

CAS — 25447-66-9 (dihydroergocryptine); 19467-62-0 (dihydroergocryptine, β-isomer); 68974-27-6 (hydrochloride); 14271-05-7 (mesylate, α-isomer); 65914-79-6 (mesylate, β-isomer).

Dihydroergocryptine mesylate is a component of co-dergocrine mesylate (p.1051) and has similar actions. In some countries it has been given by mouth in doses of 2 mg twice daily in the symptomatic treatment of mental impairment associated with cerebrovascular disease and in peripheral vascular disease.

References: I. M. James and W. Burgoyne (letter), *Br. J. clin. Pharmac.*, 1983, *15*, 123 (effect on muscle blood flow); C. Ferrari *et al.*, *Eur. J. clin. Pharmac.*, 1985, *27*, 707 (dopaminergic effects on the pituitary).

Proprietary Names and Manufacturers

The following names have been used for multi-ingredient preparations containing dihydroergocryptine mesylate—Vasobral *(Logeais, Fr.)*.

1504-d

Dihydroergotamine Mesylate *(BAN, USAN)*.

Dihydroergotamine Mesilate *(rINNM)*; Dihydroergotamine Methanesulphonate. (5′*S*)-9,10-Dihydro-12′-hydroxy-2′-methyl-5′-benzyl-ergotaman-3′,6′,18-trione methanesulphonate.
$C_{33}H_{37}N_5O_5,CH_4O_3S=679.8$.

CAS — 511-12-6 (dihydroergotamine); 6190-39-2 (mesylate).

Pharmacopoeias. In *Br., Cz., Eur., Jug., Swiss,* and *U.S.*

Colourless crystals or a white or almost white or faintly red crystalline powder; odourless or with a slight odour. *B.P.* **solubilities** are: slightly soluble in water and alcohol; sparingly soluble in chloroform and methyl alcohol. *U.S.P.* solubilities are: soluble 1 in 125 of water, 1 in 90 of alcohol, 1 in 175 of chloroform, and 1 in 2600 of ether. A 0.1% solution in water has a pH of 4.4 to 5.4. Solutions are **sterilised** by filtration.

Store in well-closed containers and protect from light. *B.P.* preparations should be stored at a temperature not exceeding 25°.

Adverse Effects and Treatment

As for Ergotamine Tartrate, p.1055. When given by mouth, adverse effects with dihydroergotamine mesylate are claimed to be less frequent than with ergotamine tartrate.

EFFECTS ON THE CARDIOVASCULAR SYSTEM. A report of severe ischaemia in 2 patients, associated with heparin-dihydroergotamine prophylaxis; one patient died. Despite claims that vasospasm due to dihydroergotamine is very rare and limited to the lower extremities it was considered that ergotism is a serious side-effect which can cause potentially fatal complications in any vascular system.— E. van den Berg *et al.* (letter), *Lancet*, 1982, *1*, 955. Critical comment from the manufacturers. Vasospastic reactions were not seen in 2 studies of heparin-dihydroergotamine therapy involving more than 6600 patients.— P. Krupp and M. Majer (letter), *ibid.*, 1302. Further criticism. In a study of heparin with dihydroergotamine mesylate in 500 patients, many of them elderly, none had symptoms suggestive of vasospasm. — V. V. Kakkar (letter), *ibid.*, *2*, 96. Reply and a report of 3 further patients with arterial vascular spasm during heparin-dihydroergotamine prophylaxis.— E. van den Berg *et al.* (letter), *ibid.*, 268.

Skin and muscle necrosis occurred in 3 elderly patients given heparin and dihydroergotamine prophylactically, but could not be attributed with certainty to drug therapy.— M. Monreal *et al.* (letter), *Lancet*, 1984, *2*, 820.

FIBROSIS. Mention of retroperitoneal fibrosis developing in one patient during treatment with dihydroergotamine.— J. R. Graham *et al.*, *New Engl. J. Med.*, 1966, *274*, 359.

OVERDOSAGE. A 42-year-old woman who had taken dihydroergotamine 10 mg daily for 2 weeks and then 20 mg in a day had symptoms suggestive of chronic renal failure, later considered to be acute renal failure in diuretic phase.— C. D. Pusey and D. J. Rainford, *Br. med. J.*, 1977, *2*, 935.

Precautions

As for Ergotamine Tartrate, p.1056. There may be less risk attached to the use of dihydroergotamine mesylate by mouth than by injection.

INTERACTIONS. A report of ergotism following treatment with dihydroergotamine mesylate and triacetyloleandomycin.— A. Franco *et al.* (letter), *Nouv. Presse méd.*, 1978, *7*, 205.

For reference to glyceryl trinitrate increasing the oral bioavailability of dihydroergotamine, see under Absorption and Fate.

Absorption and Fate

The absorption and fate of dihydroergotamine is similar to that of ergotamine (p.1056).

Dihydroergotamine was rapidly absorbed following intramuscular injection of 1 mg of the mesylate in 10 patients about to undergo spinal anaesthesia. Peak plasma concentrations, measured by radio-immunoassay, of about 7 picomol per mL were achieved at 30 minutes.— H. Hilke *et al.*, *Int. J. clin. Pharmac. Biopharm.*, 1978, *16*, 277.

The low oral bioavailability of dihydroergotamine (range less than 0.1% to 1.5%) in a study of 6 patients with orthostatic hypotension was considered to be determined primarily by extensive first-pass extraction by the liver. When 4 of the patients were given glyceryl trinitrate 1.2 mg by mouth in addition to dihydroergotamine 200 to 300 µg per kg body-weight, also by mouth, plasma concentrations of dihydroergotamine, measured by radio-immunoassay, increased although oral absorption, measured by urinary excretion of tritium, was not affected. Mean increases in blood pressure were greater with glyceryl trinitrate and dihydroergotamine than with dihydroergotamine alone or placebo. It was suggested that glyceryl trinitrate increased the oral bioavailability of dihydroergotamine by reducing first-pass extraction by the liver, presumably by increasing splanchnic blood flow.— A. Bobik *et al.*, *Clin. Pharmac. Ther.*, 1981, *30*, 673.

Following administration of radioactively-labelled dihydroergotamine mesylate 3 mg by mouth to 6 healthy subjects it was rapidly absorbed, the peak plasma concentration of radioactivity occurring at 3.2 hours. The drug was extensively metabolised, and exhibited a biphasic disposition half-life of 2.1 and 32.3 hours. Very little of the drug was excreted in urine. The primary metabolite appeared to be 8′-hydroxydihydroergotamine which was pharmacologically active and should be taken into account in bioavailability studies.— G. Maurer and W. Frick, *Eur. J. clin. Pharmac.*, 1984, *26*, 463.

A study *in vitro* and in *animals* indicating that the dihydroergotamine metabolites 8′-hydroxydihydroergotamine, 8′,10′-dihydroxydihydroergotamine, and dihydrolysergic acid amide all possess considerable venoconstrictor activity and may contribute to the selective therapeutic action of dihydroergotamine.— E. Müller-Schweinitzer, *Eur. J. clin. Pharmac.*, 1984, *26*, 699.

Further references: W. H. Aellig and E. Nüesch, *Int. J. clin. Pharmac. Biopharm.*, 1977, *15*, 106 (comparison with other ergot alkaloids); P. J. Little *et al.*, *Br. J. clin. Pharmac.*, 1982, *13*, 785 (oral bioavailability); B. Lindblad *et al.*, *Eur. J. clin. Pharmac.*, 1983, *24*, 813 (pharmacokinetics of dihydroergotamine by subcutaneous injection given alone and with dextran 70 by infusion).

Uses and Administration

Dihydroergotamine mesylate has diminished oxytocic and vasoconstrictor effects compared with ergotamine. It is used similarly to ergotamine tartrate (p.1056) in the treatment of acute attacks of migraine and is given by subcutaneous or intramuscular injection in doses of 1 mg repeated, if necessary, in 30 to 60 minutes. Administration of up to 2 mg by intravenous injection has been recommended if a more rapid effect is desired. The maximum daily dose is 3 mg and no more than 6 mg should be injected in one week.

In mild attacks, 2 to 3 mg of dihydroergotamine mesylate may be given by mouth and repeated every half hour if necessary to a total daily dose of 10 mg. A dose of 1 or 2 mg has been given three times daily by mouth to reduce the frequency and severity of attacks.

Dihydroergotamine mesylate is also used in conjunction with a low-dose heparin regimen in the prophylaxis of postoperative deep-vein thrombosis. A suggested dose is 500 µg subcutaneously with heparin 5000 units, also subcutaneously, every 8 to 12 hours, starting 1 to 2 hours before surgery and continued not less than 6 hours postoperatively for at least 7 to 10 days.

HYPOTENSION. In 6 patients with autonomic insufficiency and orthostatic hypotension blood pressure was increased after dihydroergotamine given intravenously. Of 4 patients given the drug by mouth one was controlled on 10 mg daily and 3 on 30 mg daily.— G. Jennings *et al.*, *Br. med. J.*, 1979, *2*, 307. The apparent failure of 2 patients with postural hypotension to respond to dihydroergotamine by mouth was attributed to low bioavailability of the drug as both patients greatly improved following dihydroergotamine intravenously.— I. N. Olver *et al.*, *ibid.*, 1980, *281*, 275.

Dihydroergotamine mesylate 1 mg daily intramuscularly relieved severe incapacitating orthostatic hypotension, refractory to usual medical management, in a patient who had ingested a nitrophenylurea rodenticide (Vacor).— N. L. Benowitz *et al.*, *Ann. intern. Med.*, 1980, *92*, 387.

Further references: F. M. Fouad *et al.*, *Clin. Pharmac. Ther.*, 1981, *30*, 782 (short-term intramuscular and long-term oral therapy); G. R. Bellamy and S. N. Hunyor, *Aust. N.Z. J. Med.*, 1984, *14*, 157 (effect on venous distensibility and blood pressure in idiopathic orthostatic hypotension).

THROMBO-EMBOLISM PROPHYLAXIS. In a study of heparin with or without dihydroergotamine in the prevention of postoperative thrombo-embolic complications, 181 patients undergoing major abdominal surgery received either dihydroergotamine mesylate 500 µg with heparin sodium 5000 units, both subcutaneously 1 hour pre-operatively and then twice daily for 7 days, or heparin alone. A fibrinogen-uptake test was performed pre-operatively, immediately postoperatively, and on days 1, 3, 5, and 7 postoperatively. Ascending phlebography was performed when results of the test were abnormal or when clinical signs of thrombo-embolism were present. No significant difference was found between the incidence of thrombo-embolism in the 2 groups, but abnormal results [evidence of thrombo-embolism] of the fibrinogen-uptake test were more frequent in the heparin group. It was concluded that dihydroergotamine with heparin had little if any advantage over heparin alone in the prevention of postoperative thrombo-embolic complications. The results also indicated that dihydroergotamine might have influenced the outcome of the fibrinogen-uptake test which, if true, would invalidate the test as a criterion for deep-vein thrombosis.— P. Wille-Jørgensen *et al.*, *Archs Surg.*, 1983, *118*, 926.

Dihydroergotamine mesylate and heparin, given alone and together, were compared with placebo in a double-blind multicentre study of the prophylaxis of postoperative deep-vein thrombosis in 744 evaluable patients undergoing general surgery. All patients were over 40 years of age. Doses were administered subcutaneously, starting about 2 hours before surgery and continuing postoperatively every 12 hours for 5 to 7 days. The presence or absence of deep-vein thrombosis in the lower extremities, determined postoperatively by a radiofibrinogen-uptake test, was the primary criterion for efficacy of treatment. Incidence-rates of deep-vein thrombosis for each of the 5 treatment groups were: placebo, 24.4%; dihydroergotamine mesylate 500 µg, 19.4%; heparin sodium 5000 units, 16.8%; dihydroergotamine mesylate 500 µg with heparin sodium 2500 units, 16.8%; and dihydroergotamine mesylate 500 µg with heparin sodium 5000 units, 9.4%. Dihydroergotamine mesylate 500 µg with heparin sodium 5000 units was significantly superior to placebo and the other treatment regimens and was considered to have effectively reduced the risk of deep-vein thrombosis of the lower extremities. Adverse effects, including bleeding complications, did not differ significantly between the groups.— A. A. Sasahara *et al.*, *J. Am. med. Ass.*, 1984, *251*, 2960. Comment on the multicentre study.— J. Hirsh, *ibid.*, 2985.

Further references: K. Koppenhagen *et al.*, *Dt. med. Wschr.*, 1977, *102*, 1374; V. V. Kakkar *et al.*, *J. Am. med. Ass.*, 1979, *241*, 39.

Preparations

Dihydroergotamine Injection *(B.P.).* Dihydroergotamine Mesylate Injection

Dihydroergotamine Mesylate Injection *(U.S.P.)*

Dihydroergotamine Oral Solution *(B.P.).* Dihydroergotamine Mesylate Solution; Dihydroergotamine Solution

Dihydroergotamine Tablets *(B.P.).* Dihydroergotamine Mesylate Tablets

Proprietary Preparations

Dihydergot *(Sandoz, UK). Injection*, dihydroergotamine mesylate 1 mg/mL, in ampoules of 1 mL.

Proprietary Names and Manufacturers

Agit *(Midy, Ger.)*; Angionorm *(Schwabe-Farmasan, Ger.)*; Dergolyoc *(Abbott, Fr.)*; Dergotamine *(Abbott, Fr.)*; DET MS *(Rentschler, Ger.)*; D.H.E. 45 *(Sandoz, USA)*; DH-Ergotamin-retard *(Ger.)*; DHE-Tablinen *(Beiersdorf, Ger.)*; Diergo-spray *(Sandoz, Fr.)*; Dihydergot *(Arg.; Sandoz, Austral.; Belg.; Sandoz, Denm.; Sandoz, Ger.; Jpn; Neth.; Sandoz, Norw.; Wander, S.Afr.; Sandoz, Spain; Sandoz, Switz.; Sandoz, UK)*; Diidergot *(Sandoz, Ital.)*; Endophleban *(Rentschler, Ger.)*; Ergomimet *(Klinge, Ger.)*; Ergont *(Desitin, Ger.)*; Ergotonine *(Streuli, Switz.)*; Hydro-Tamin *(Ratiopharm, Ger.)*; Ikaran *(Sinbio, Fr.; Formenti, Ital.; Uhlmann-Eyraud, Switz.)*; Morena *(Kettelhack Riker, Ger.)*; Orstanorm *(Sandoz, Swed.)*; Séglor *(Roland-Marie, Fr.)*; Seglor *(Lirca, Ital.)*; Tamik *(Marcofina, Fr.)*; Tenuatina *(Gamir, Spain)*; Tonopres *(Boehringer Ingelheim, Ger.)*.

The following names have been used for multi-ingredient preparations containing dihydroergotamine mesylate—Embolex *(Sandoz, USA)*; Plexonal *(Sandoz, Canad.)*; Tonolift *(Drug Houses Austral.)*.

1505-n

Dihydroergotamine Tartrate *(BAN, rINNM).*

$(C_{33}H_{37}N_5O_5)_2,C_4H_6O_6=1317.5$.

CAS — 5989-77-5.

Pharmacopoeias. In *Br.*

Odourless or almost odourless colourless crystals or a white or almost white crystalline powder. Very slightly **soluble** in water; sparingly soluble in alcohol; soluble in pyridine. A 0.25% suspension in water has a pH of 4.0 to 5.5. **Store** in well-closed containers and protect from light.

There is little evidence of use of dihydroergotamine tartrate.

1506-h

Ergometrine Maleate *(BAN, rINNM).*

Ergobasine Maleate; Ergometrinhydrogenmaleat; Ergometrini Maleas; Ergometrinii Maleas; Ergonovine Bimaleate; Ergonovine Maleate *(USAN)*; Maleato de Ergonovina. *N*-[(*S*)-2-Hydroxy-1-methylethyl]-D-lysergamide hydrogen maleate; 9,10-Didehydro-*N*-[(*S*)-2-hydroxy-1-methylethyl]-6-methylergoline-8β-carboxamide hydrogen maleate.

$C_{19}H_{23}N_3O_2,C_4H_4O_4=441.5$.

CAS — 60-79-7 (ergometrine); 129-51-1 (maleate).

Pharmacopoeias. In *Arg., Aust., Belg., Br., Braz., Chin., Cz., Egypt., Eur., Fr., Ger., Hung., Ind., Int., It., Jpn, Jug., Mex., Neth., Nord., Pol., Roum., Span., Swiss, Turk.,* and *U.S.*

A white or yellowish, odourless, crystalline powder. It darkens with age and on exposure to light. **Soluble** 1 in 40 of water and 1 in 100 of alcohol; practically insoluble in chloroform and ether. The *B.P.* injection has a pH of 2.7 to 3.5. Solutions for injection are **sterilised** by autoclaving.

Store in airtight glass containers at a temperature of 2° to 8 ° and protect from light.

Adverse Effects

Adverse effects reported with ergometrine maleate, especially following intravenous administration, include headache, dizziness, tinnitus, abdominal pain, nausea, vomiting, hypertension, chest pain, palpitation, dyspnoea, and bradycardia. Ergometrine shows less tendency to produce gangrene than ergotamine (p.1055), but ergotism has been reported and symptoms of acute poisoning are similar.

EFFECTS ON THE CARDIOVASCULAR SYSTEM. Gangrene of the feet developed in a 20-year-old woman given ergometrine maleate 200 µg three times a day by mouth to a total of 3.6 mg.— W. Bross *et al.*, *Lancet*, 1963, *1*, 85.

Hypertension. A 17-year-old girl in labour was given 500 µg of ergometrine maleate intramuscularly as the head crowned and after 12 minutes her blood pressure rose sharply. It fell again 30 minutes after papaveretum 20 mg had been given, and then 25 minutes later she developed severe frontal headache, a further increase in blood pressure, and typical generalised eclamptic convulsions. In reports by H.G. Hamilton (*Am. J. Obstet. Gynec.*, 1953, *65*, 503) and I.R. McFadyen (*Lancet*, 1960, *2*, 1009), ergometrine was also considered the causative factor in cases of postpartum eclampsia in previously normotensive patients.— A. M. Hassim (letter), *Br. med. J.*, 1964, *2*, 1327.

Postpartum administration of ergometrine in 4 patients resulted in hypertension in 3 (with eclampsia in 1) and cardiac arrest in the fourth. Blood pressure rose to 180/130 mmHg, 190/165 mmHg, and 180/120 mmHg respectively and responded to hydralazine in 2 patients and spontaneously in the third. Cardiac arrest responded to cardiac massage. It was suggested that ergometrine should not be used routinely in obstetrics.— D. J. Browning, *Med. J. Aust.*, 1974, *1*, 957.

MUTAGENICITY. Chromosomal aberrations in cultured leucocytes were noted after 4 hours' exposure to a dilute solution of ergometrine maleate.— L. F. Jarvik and T. Kato (letter), *Lancet*, 1968, *1*, 250.

OVERDOSAGE. Convulsions, ventilatory failure, and water intoxication in a neonate following the accidental administration of ergometrine 500 µg with synthetic oxytocin 5 units (Syntometrine) intramuscularly. Following therapy with anticonvulsants and assisted respiration the infant made an uneventful recovery.— M. F. Whitfield and S. A. W. Salfield, *Archs Dis. Childh.*, 1980, *55*, 68.

A newborn infant was accidentally given ergometrine 500 µg by intramuscular injection immediately after birth instead of vitamin K. One hour later she had a brief cyanotic episode and later developed respiratory failure, generalised convulsions, acute renal failure, and temporary lactose interolance. She recovered after intensive treatment including assisted ventilation, anticonvulsants, and peritoneal dialysis.— S. K. Pandey and C. I. Haines, *Br. med. J.*, 1982, *285*, 693. A similar report of convulsions, respiratory failure, and intense peripheral vasoconstriction in a neonate accidentally given ergometrine maleate 200 µg intramuscularly. She was given frusemide because of decreased urine output and was weaned from the ventilator about 24 hours after receiving ergometrine.— A. A. Mitchell *et al.* (letter), *J. Am. med. Ass.*, 1983, *250*, 730.

PREGNANCY AND THE NEONATE. A report of a congenital defect, the Poland anomaly, in the offspring of a woman who had attempted abortion with an unknown dose of ergometrine maleate by mouth.— T. J. David, *New Engl. J. Med.*, 1972, *287*, 487. Comment.— B. MacMahon, *ibid.*, 514.

Treatment of Adverse Effects

As for Ergotamine Tartrate, p.1055.

See Overdosage in Adverse Effects (above).

Precautions

As for Ergotamine Tartrate, p.1056. Ergometrine maleate should not be used for the induction of labour or during the first stage of labour. If used at the end of the second stage of labour, prior to delivery of the placenta, there must be expert obstetric supervision. Its use should be avoided in patients with eclampsia.

The effects of ergometrine on the parturient uterus are diminished by halothane.

Vasoconstrictive effects made the use of ergometrine undesirable for obstetric patients who had cardiovascular, respiratory, or renal diseases, chronic anaemia, or toxaemia of pregnancy; oxytocin was preferable in such cases, its hypotensive effect being less if it was given to patients in the lithotomy position.— M. Johnstone, *Br. J. Anaesth.*, 1972, *44*, 826.

INTERACTIONS. A report of symmetrical gangrene of the extremities associated with the use of dopamine subsequent to ergometrine administration.— N. Buchanan *et al.*, *Intensive Care Med.*, 1977, *3*, 55.

Absorption and Fate

Ergometrine is reported to be rapidly and almost completely absorbed after administration by mouth and by intramuscular injection.

Uses and Administration

Ergometrine has a much more powerful action on the uterus than most of the other alkaloids of ergot, especially on the puerperal uterus. Its main action is the production of sustained contractions, in contrast to the more physiological rhythmic uterine contractions induced by oxytocin; its action is more prolonged than that of oxytocin, but less rapid in onset. Uterine stimulation is said to occur within about 10 minutes of administration by mouth, within 7 minutes of intramuscular injection, and almost immediately after intravenous administration. Following intramuscular injection of ergometrine with oxytocin contractions are reported to occur within 2 or 3 minutes.

Ergometrine maleate is used in the prevention and treatment of postpartum haemorrhage. It is given in doses of 500 µg, generally with oxytocin, in the UK, whereas in the US ergometrine maleate is used alone in doses of 200 µg.

In the UK ergometrine maleate is given with oxytocin under full obstetric supervision in the active management of the third stage of labour of normal confinements. A dose of ergometrine maleate 500 µg and oxytocin 5 units is injected intramuscularly after delivery of the anterior shoulder of the infant. Delivery of the placenta is actively assisted while the uterus is firmly contracted. A similar dose of ergometrine maleate, with or without oxytocin, may be given following delivery of the placenta to prevent or treat postpartum haemorrhage; intravenous doses of 250 or 500 µg of ergometrine maleate have been given in emergencies. In mild secondary postpartum haemorrhage ergometrine maleate has been given by mouth in a dose of 500 µg three times daily.

In the US ergometrine maleate is not generally recommended before delivery of the placenta, although it has been given similarly to ergometrine and oxytocin (above) after delivery of the anterior shoulder. More usually it is given after the third stage of labour in a dose of 200 µg intramuscularly, repeated if necessary in 2 to 4 hours. In emergencies 200 µg may be given intravenously. In late postpartum bleeding 200 to 400 µg may be given twice to four times daily by mouth; it may be taken sublingually.

Ergometrine maleate is not used in the treatment of migraine; it has been reported to be effective, but less so than ergotamine.

CONTRACEPTION. Ergometrine maleate is a powerful stimulant of fallopian tube motility and studies suggested that ergometrine administered immediately after coitus significantly reduced the conception-rate.— E. M. Coutinho *et al.*, *Am. J. Obstet. Gynec.*, 1976, *126*, 48.

ERGOMETRINE PROVOCATION TEST. *Diagnosis of ischaemic heart disease.* Although provocation of coronary spasm with ergometrine appeared reasonably safe when carried out in research centres on carefully selected patients, its diagnostic value in everyday practice was limited.— *Lancet*, 1982, *2*, 805. Comment by the American College of Physicians on ergometrine testing to provoke coronary artery spasm during the evaluation of possible variant angina, and the potential risks and benefits involved.— *Ann. intern. Med.*, 1984, *100*, 151.

Ergometrine testing for variant angina was carried out in a coronary care unit in a study of 100 patients with established or suspected variant angina who had previously undergone coronary arteriography. Incremental bolus intravenous injections of ergometrine were given at 5-minute intervals as follows: 12.5, 25, 50, 100, 200, 300, and 400 µg. A bolus intravenous injection of glyceryl trinitrate 300 µg was given as soon as a positive response (an S-T segment elevation of more than 1 mm) was detected or at the end of a negative test if diastolic pressure exceeded 100 mmHg. The test was positive in all of 17 patients with previously established variant angina, in 18 of 45 with symptoms strongly suggestive of variant angina, and in 1 of 38 with atypical symptoms. Serious complications in 4 of the 36 patients with positive tests included severe hypotension (2 patients), recurrent episodes of angina with S-T elevation (1), and subendocardial infarction (1). The test was considered useful in patients with symptoms highly suggestive of variant angina, but without documented S-T elevation. It was recommended that tests be performed either in a coronary care unit in patients with known coronary anatomy or during coronary arteriography, that patients with multiple severe fixed obstructions should be excluded, that the initial dose of ergometrine should be limited to 12.5 or 25 µg with dosage intervals of not less than 5 minutes, and that angina with S-T elevation be treated immediately with intravenous or intracoronary glyceryl trinitrate.— D. D. Waters *et al.*, *Am. J. Cardiol.*, 1980, *46*, 922.

In a comparative study of 3 provocative tests for variant angina in 34 patients with active disease, angina with ST-elevation was provoked in 32 patients (94%) by ergometrine, in 10 (29%) by exercise testing, and in 3 (9%) by the cold pressor test.— D. D. Waters *et al.*, *Circulation*, 1983, *67*, 310.

Further references: R. C. Curry *et al.*, *Circulation*, 1977, *56*, 803; J. S. Schroeder *et al.*, *Am. J. Cardiol.*, 1977, *40*, 487; F. A. Heupler *et al.*, *ibid.*, 1978, *41*, 631; J. L. Gerry *et al.*, *J. Am. med. Ass.*, 1979, *242*, 2858; M. E. Bertrand *et al.*, *Circulation*, 1982, *65*, 1299 (methylergometrine).

Diagnosis of oesophageal spasm. A study indicating that provocation with ergometrine 500 µg by slow intravenous injection during oesophageal manometry is useful in the diagnosis of oesophageal spasm in patients with severe angina-like pain but no evidence of cardiac abnormality. It was stressed that the ECG should be monitored during the test, that resuscitation facilities should be available, and that the response to 50 µg of ergometrine should be assessed first, followed after 5 minutes by incremental doses.— H. A. Davies *et al.*, *Gut*, 1982, *23*, 89. and *idem* (letter), 1983, *24*, 683. Comment that it was generally considered unsafe to use ergometrine because of its cardiac effects and that the edrophonium oesophageal stress test was the best currently available.— J. N. Blackwell *et al.*, *Br. J. Hosp. Med.*, 1984, *32*, 267.

POSTPARTUM HAEMORRHAGE. A short discussion on the traditional uses of ergot compounds in obstetrics.— A. C. Turnbull, *Postgrad. med. J.*, 1976, *52*, *Suppl.* 1, 15.

In a double-blind study, 250 µg was as effective as 500 µg of ergometrine maleate given intravenously after completion of the second stage of labour for achieving haemostasis in the third stage of labour and in preventing primary postpartum haemorrhage. Postpartum haemorrhage was related to genital tract trauma rather than to the dose of ergometrine administered.— J. D. Paull and G. J. Ratten, *Med. J. Aust.*, 1977, *1*, 178.

For comparisons between oxytocin and ergometrine in the management of postpartum haemorrhage, see Oxytocin, p.1147.

Ergometrine with oxytocin. In a clinical study, the intramuscular injection of ergometrine with oxytocin (Syntometrine), given with the birth of the anterior shoulder in the active management of the third stage of labour and the prophylaxis of postpartum haemorrhage, resulted in a significant reduction in the incidence of postpartum haemorrhage compared with the intramuscular injection of ergometrine; in both primigravidas and multigravidas the frequency of postpartum haemorrhage was approximately halved. There was no increase in the incidence of retention of the placenta.— M. P. Embrey *et al.*, *Br. med. J.*, 1963, *1*, 1387.

A retrospective study of 1392 deliveries indicated that the incidence of postpartum haemorrhage and heavy loss was reduced when ergometrine maleate 500 µg and oxytocin 5 units (Syntometrine 1 mL) was given intramuscularly after delivery of the anterior shoulder, compared to ergometrine 500 µg only.— O. Djahanbakhch *et al.*, *Br. J. clin. Pract.*, 1978, *32*, 137.

Further references: J. McGrath and A. D. H. Browne, *Br. med. J.*, 1962, *2*, 524; W. O. Chukudebelu *et al.*, *ibid.*, 1963, *1*, 1390; J. Kemp, *ibid.*, 1391; S. K. Basu and H. G. I. Shanks, *Practitioner*, 1964, *192*, 784; R. J. Beard *et al.*, *Br. J. clin. Pract.*, 1973, *27*, 13.

Preparations

Ergometrine and Oxytocin Injection *(B.P.).* Contains ergometrine maleate and synthetic oxytocin; pH 2.9 to 3.5. Sterilise by filtration. Store at a temperature not exceeding 25° and protect from light. Under these conditions it may be expected to retain its potency for not less than 2 years.

Ergometrine Injection *(B.P.).* A sterile solution of ergometrine maleate in Water for Injections.

Ergonovine Maleate Injection *(U.S.P.).* A sterile solution of ergometrine maleate in Water for Injections.

Ergometrine Tablets *(B.P.).* Ergonovine Maleate Tablets. Tablets containing ergometrine maleate.

Ergonovine Maleate Tablets *(U.S.P.).* Tablets containing ergometrine maleate.

Proprietary Preparations

Syntometrine *(Sandoz, UK). Injection,* ergometrine maleate 500 µg, oxytocin 5 units/mL, in ampoules of 1 mL.

Proprietary Names and Manufacturers

Ergometron *(Vernleigh, S.Afr.)*; Ergomine *(Austral.)*; Ergotrate *(Arg.; Lilly, Austral.; Lilly, Canad.; Lilly, S.Afr.; Lilly, USA)*; Ermalate *(Austral.)*; Ermetrine *(Belg.; Neth.)*.

The following names have been used for multi-ingredient preparations containing ergometrine maleate— Syntometrine *(Sandoz, Austral.; Sandoz, UK)*.

1507-m

Ergometrine Tartrate *(rINNM)*.

Ergometrini Tartras; Ergonovinum Tartaricum.
$(C_{19}H_{23}N_3O_2)_2,C_4H_6O_6$=800.9.

CAS — 129-50-0.

Ergometrine tartrate has similar actions to the maleate and was formerly used in the management of postpartum haemorrhage.

Proprietary Names and Manufacturers

The following names have been used for multi-ingredient preparations containing ergometrine tartrate— Neo-Femergin *(Sandoz, UK)*.

1501-x

Ergot

Cornezuelo de Centeno; Cravagem de Centeio; Ergot de Seigle; Esporão de Centeio; Grano Speronato; Mutterkorn; Rye Ergot; Secale Cornutum.

Pharmacopoeias. In *Arg., Aust., Fr., Int., Port., Roum., Rus., Span.,* and *Turk.*

The sclerotium of the fungus *Claviceps purpurea* (Hypocreaceae) developed in the ovary of the rye, *Secale cereale* (Gramineae), containing not less than 0.15% of total alkaloids, calculated as ergotoxine, and not less than 0.01% of water-soluble alkaloids, calculated as ergometrine. Some authorities have expressed alkaloidal content in terms of ergotamine and ergometrine.

1502-r

Prepared Ergot

Ergota Praeparata; Prep. Ergot; Secalis Cornuti Pulvis Standardisatus.

Pharmacopoeias. In *Arg., Aust., Int.,* and *Turk.* which all specify about 0.2% of total alkaloids.

Powdered and defatted ergot. A purplish-brown powder with an unpleasant odour and taste.

A comparison of alkaloid contents of Argentine and European ergot.— G. E. Ferraro *et al.* (letter), *J. Pharm. Pharmac.*, 1976, *28*, 729.

Adverse Effects and Treatment

As for Ergotamine Tartrate, p.1055.

Epidemic ergot poisoning, arising from the ingestion of ergotised rye bread, is now seldom seen. Two forms of epidemic toxicity, which rarely occur together, have been described, a gangrenous form characterised by agonising pain of the extremities of the body followed by dry gangrene of the peripheral parts, and a rarer nervous type giving rise to paroxysmal epileptiform convulsions.

A report of an outbreak of ergotism, attributed to the ingestion of infected wild oats (*Avena abyssinica*), in Wollo, Ethiopia.— B. King (letter), *Lancet*, 1979, *1*, 1411.

Uses and Administration

Ergot has the vasoconstricting and oxytocic actions of its constituent alkaloids (see p.1051), especially ergotamine and ergometrine. A liquid extract or tablets of prepared ergot were formerly used as an oxytocic.

1508-b

Ergotamine Tartrate *(BAN, USAN, rINNM).*

Ergotamini Tartras; Ergotaminii Tartras. (5′*S*)-12′-Hydroxy-2′-methyl-3′,6′,18-trioxo-5-benzylergotaman (+)-tartrate.

$(C_{33}H_{35}N_5O_5)_2,C_4H_6O_6$=1313.4.

CAS — 113-15-5 (ergotamine); 379-79-3 (tartrate).

Pharmacopoeias. In *Aust., Belg., Br., Braz., Cz., Egypt., Eur., Fr., Ger., Hung., Ind., Int., It., Jpn, Jug., Mex., Neth., Nord., Pol., Port., Roum., Swiss, Turk.,* and *U.S.*

It may contain 2 molecules of methanol of crystallisation. Slightly hygroscopic colourless odourless crystals or a white or yellowish-white crystalline powder. *B.P.* **solubilities** are: dissolves in water; slightly soluble in alcohol and in chloroform and practically insoluble in ether. *U.S.P.* solubilities are: soluble 1 in about 3200 of water, but soluble 1 in about 500 of water in the presence of a slight excess of tartaric acid; soluble 1 in 500 of alcohol. A 0.25% suspension in water has a pH of 4.0 to 5.5. Solutions for injection are **sterilised** by filtration.

Store in airtight glass containers at a temperature of 2° to 8° and protect from light.

SOLUBILITY. Caffeine increased the solubility of ergotamine tartrate at gastric and intestinal pH *in vitro* so that ergotamine was not precipitated.— M. A. Zoglio *et al., J. pharm. Sci.*, 1969, *58*, 222.

STABILITY IN SOLUTION. The stability and degradation of ergotamine tartrate in aqueous solution.— B. Kreilgård and J. Kisbye, *Arch. Pharm. Chemi, scient. Edn*, 1974, *2*, 1 and 38.

Adverse Effects

Common side-effects with therapeutic doses of ergotamine include nausea and vomiting, weakness in the legs, muscle pains in the extremities, and numbness and tingling of the fingers and toes. Anginal-type pain and transient tachycardia or bradycardia have also been reported. Headache may occur and is also a major withdrawal symptom following the abuse of ergotamine. There may occasionally be localised oedema and itching in hypersensitive patients. The majority of these side-effects do not generally necessitate withdrawal of ergotamine, but treatment should be stopped if symptoms of vasoconstriction such as paraesthesias of the extremities persist.

Susceptible patients, especially those with severe infections, liver disease, kidney disease, or occlusive peripheral vascular disease, may show signs of acute or chronic poisoning with normal doses of ergotamine.

Syptoms of acute poisoning include nausea, vomiting, diarrhoea, extreme thirst, coldness, tingling, and itching of the skin, a rapid and weak pulse, confusion, convulsions, and unconsciousness; fatalities have been reported.

In chronic poisoning or ergotism, resulting from therapeutic overdosage or the use of ergotamine in susceptible patients, severe circulatory disturbances develop as a result of vasoconstriction and thrombi formation. The extremities, especially the feet and legs, become numb, cold, tingling, and pale or cyanotic with muscle pain; there may be no pulse in the affected limb. Eventually gangrene develops in the toes and sometimes the fingers. Anginal pain, tachycardia or bradycardia, and hypertension or hypotension may also occur. Other common symptoms of chronic ergotism include headache, nausea, vomiting, diarrhoea, and dizziness; there may also be weakness. Confusion and drowsiness, and sometimes convulsions, hemiplegia, and a fixed miosis may occur.

A number of patients seen in 2 migraine clinics appeared to be suffering from ergotamine tartrate overdosage. It was considered that ergotamine-induced headache could occur with doses as low as 1 mg daily by mouth or 250 µg daily intramuscularly.— F. C. Rose and M. Wilkinson, *Br. med. J.*, 1976, *1*, 525.

Ergotamine overdosage was encountered in about 3% of patients attending a migraine clinic for the first time. All of 25 patients who had taken 7 to 60 mg of ergotamine tartrate weekly for 1.5 to 30 years were suffering daily headaches and 23 showed overt signs of intoxication. Ergotamine was stopped and although many patients reported withdrawal headaches in the first 3 to 5 days, side-effects had disappeared within 2 weeks in the majority. Ergotamine was subsequently reintroduced in a carefully controlled manner in some patients. Unlike D.A. Orton and R.J. Richardson (*Postgrad. med. J.*, 1982, *58*, 6) who found that adverse reactions occurred more frequently in subjects with concentrations exceeding 1.8 ng per mL, adverse effects could not be correlated with serum concentrations of ergotamine; radio-immunoassay was used in both studies.— A. N. Graham *et al., Hum. Toxicol.*, 1984, *3*, 193.

EFFECTS ON THE CARDIOVASCULAR SYSTEM. Subclinical ergotism was detected in a group of 29 patients who had been taking ergotamine regularly in therapeutic doses for at least one year. They had reduced footsystolic blood pressure indicating a risk of arterial insufficiency. There was a significant rise in blood pressure in all 13 patients who succeeded in stopping ergotamine treatment.— H. Dige-Petersen *et al., Lancet*, 1977, *2*, 65.

Individual reports of adverse cardiovascular effects associated with ergotamine: U. Mintz *et al., Postgrad. med. J.*, 1974, *50*, 244 (venous thrombosis of the leg); G. C. Merhoff and J. M. Porter, *Ann. Surg.*, 1974, *180*, 773 (ischaemia and bilateral foot-drop or transient monocular blindness); N. J. C. Snell *et al., Postgrad. med. J.*, 1978, *54*, 37 (acute myocardial ischaemia); M. Zicot *et al., Angiology*, 1978, *29*, 495 (arterial haemodynamic disturbances); C. R. Benedict and D. Robertson, *Am. J. Med.*, 1979, *67*, 177 (angina pectoris and sudden death); P. Carr, *Postgrad. med. J.*, 1981, *57*, 654 (myocardial infarction following massive overdosage); M. Pajewski *et al.* (letter), *Lancet*, 1981, *2*, 934 (arterial aneurysm); D. A. Joyce and S. S. Gubbay, *Br. med. J.*, 1982, *285*, 260 (arterial occlusion with methysergide in association with high dosage of parenteral ergotamine); L. S. Klein *et al., Chest*, 1982, *82*, 375 (myocardial infarction); R. Corrocher *et al.* (letter), *New Engl. J. Med.*, 1984, *310*, 261 (multiple arterial stenoses).

EFFECTS ON THE LIVER. A report of fatal acute hepatic necrosis, presumably of viral origin, in a patient with ergotism.— M. J. Whelton *et al., Gut*, 1968, *9*, 287.

EFFECTS ON THE NERVOUS SYSTEM. Autonomic dysaesthesia developed in a woman who regularly took up to 24 mg of ergotamine tartrate a week; it was initially mistaken for progression of chronic back pain.— P. J. D. Evans *et al., Br. med. J.*, 1980, *281*, 1621.

FIBROSIS. Fibrotic pleurisy and fibrotic constrictive pericarditis were associated with long-term therapy with ergotamine in a 44-year-old woman. She had taken methysergide for 3 months about 10 years earlier, but had used suppositories containing ergotamine tartrate 2 mg two or three times daily for 19 years.— M. Robert *et al.* (letter), *New Engl. J. Med.*, 1984, *311*, 601. Comment from the manufacturers that the patient took 3 to 4 times the recommended dosage for 19 years and that uncertainty remains about whether fibrotic disorders may result from ergotamine alone.— W. F. Westlin (letter), *ibid.*, 602.

Further reports of fibrosis associated with ergotamine: J. R. Graham *et al., New Engl. J. Med.*, 1966, *274*, 359 (retroperitoneal fibrosis); D. Lepage-Savary and A. Vallières, *Clin. Pharm.*, 1982, *1*, 179 (retroperitoneal fibrosis).

PREGNANCY AND THE NEONATE. A report of jejunal atresia in an infant born prematurely to a woman who had taken ergotamine tartrate 6 to 8 mg daily, as Cafergot tablets, throughout her pregnancy.— J. M. Graham *et al., Clin. Pediat.*, 1983, *22*, 226.

Treatment of Adverse Effects

Treatment of acute poisoning with ergotamine is symptomatic. Following recent ingestion the stomach should be emptied by aspiration and lavage.

In chronic poisoning, withdrawal of ergotamine may be all that is required in some patients. However, in both acute and chronic poisoning, attempts must be made to maintain an adequate circulation to the affected parts in order to prevent the onset of gangrene. In severe arterial vasospasm vasodilators such as sodium nitroprusside by intravenous infusion have been given; heparin and dextran 40 have also been advocated to minimise the risk of thrombosis. Analgesics may be required for severe ischaemic pain.

Convulsions may be controlled with diazepam and nausea and vomiting by intramuscular injection of chlorpromazine or a related phenothiazine.

A woman who had used 18 rectal suppositories containing ergotamine tartrate 2 mg and caffeine 100 mg in 18 hours developed lower extremity cyanosis which was not relieved by hydralazine hydrochloride. An intravenous infusion of sodium nitroprusside was started at a rate of 50 µg per minute. The infusion was stopped after 20 hours but restarted 3 hours later at a rate of 123 µg per minute because of coldness of the feet and continued for 15 hours. The patient recovered fully.— N. H. Carliner *et al., J. Am. med. Ass.*, 1974, *227*, 308. Intra-arterial infusion of sodium nitroprusside 16 µg per minute slowly increased to 300 µg per minute over the next 45 minutes alleviated signs of severe peripheral vasoconstriction of the legs attributed to ergotamine tartrate in a 33-year-old patient. The infusion was continued for 9 hours and gradually decreased to 32 µg per minute and then given at this rate intravenously for a further 96 hours.— C. W. O'Dell *et al., Radiology*, 1977, *124*, 73. A report of the successful treatment of severe ergotamine-induced ischaemia of the lower extremities in 2 women by means of intravenous infusion of sodium nitroprusside 25 µg per minute increased by 25 µg per minute at intervals of 5 to 15 minutes to maximum infusion-rates of 100 and 150 µg per minute. Total doses of 80 and 100 mg were given over about 32 and 16 hours respectively. Epidural block with bupivacaine had been unsuccessful.— P. K. Andersen *et al., New Engl. J. Med.*, 1977, *296*, 1271.

Further references to the use of sodium nitroprusside in ergotamine-induced ischaemia: B. Eurin *et al.* (letter), *New Engl. J. Med.*, 1978, *298*, 632 (intravenous infusion); T. L. Whitsett *et al.* (letter), *Am. Heart J.*, 1978, *96*, 700 (intra-arterial infusion); G. A. Skowronski *et al., Med. J. Aust.*, 1979, *2*, 8 (intravenous infusion); P. Carr, *Postgrad. med. J.*, 1981, *57*, 654 (intravenous infusion).

Ergotamine-induced severe peripheral vascular ischaemia, involving upper and lower extremities, in a 30-year-old woman was successfully treated with intravenous phentolamine 10 mg every 8 hours and intravenous heparin 3000 units every 4 hours for 4 days. Pethidine hydrochloride was used to relieve pain.— C. A. Attah, *N.Y. St. J. Med.*, 1977, *77*, 2257.

Streptokinase was used effectively for the treatment of arterial insufficiency and impending gangrene of the foot, with the risk of thrombosis, in a woman who had for 3 years been using suppositories containing ergotamine tartrate.— B. Brismar *et al., Acta chir. scand.*, 1977, *143*, 319.

Infusion of glyceryl trinitrate successfully alleviated the symptoms of ergotism in a 41-year-old woman admitted with a 12-hour history of pain, coldness, discoloration, and numbness in her right foot. She had been using half a suppository of Gynergen Comp (each suppository containing ergotamine tartrate 2 mg and caffeine 100 mg) up to 5 times weekly for the preceding 10 years and daily for the preceding 5 months; 5 weeks before admission she had also started treatment with propranolol 120 mg daily. She was treated with a continuous intravenous infusion from a glass bottle containing glyceryl trinitrate 50 mg (10 mL of glyceryl trinitrate 0.5% in alcohol) in 500 mL of glucose solution 5.5%. The infusion was discontinued after 11 hours, and the maximum infusion-rate was 3.2 µg per kg body-weight per minute. During the infusion the patient had a brief headache of her usual migraine type; no other untoward effects were noted.— B. Husum *et al.* (letter), *Lancet*, 1979, *2*, 794.

Ergotamine-induced peripheral ischaemia in a patient was successfully treated with prazosin hydrochloride 1 mg three times daily by mouth.— D. S. Cobaugh, *J. Am. med. Ass.*, 1980, *244*, 1360.

In 2 patients with imminent gangrene of the extremities caused by ergotamine-induced arteriospasm arterial dilatation by a balloon-tipped catheter produced an immediate and sustained reversal of the arteriospasm, together with a dramatic relief of symptoms and signs. The patients had not responded to standard therapy.— E. Shifrin *et al.*, *Lancet*, 1980, *2*, 1278.

Peripheral ischaemia due to ergotamine in a 43-year-old man responded rapidly to captopril 50 mg three times daily by mouth for 4 days; all peripheral pulses were palpable within 6 hours of starting treatment.— A. Zimran *et al.*, *Br. med. J.*, 1984, *288* 364.

Further references: S. T. Yao *et al.*, *Br. med. J.*, 1970, *3*, 86 (dextran 40, heparin, and analgesics); C. W. Imrie, *Br. J. clin. Pract.*, 1973, *27*, 457 (lumbar blocks with phenol for ischaemic pain); J. Webb (letter), *Br. med. J.*, 1977, *2*, 1355 (anticoagulants, tolazoline, nerve blocks, phentolamine, sodium nitroprusside, methylprednisolone, and dextran 40 injection).

DIALYSIS. A 13-month-old girl swallowed about 15 mg of ergotamine tartrate and 1 g of phenobarbitone in Bellergal tablets and was unconscious 5 hours later. The stomach was washed out immediately but the respiration-rate continued to fall and peritoneal dialysis was started. The intravenous injection of 2 doses, each of 20 mL of 10% mannitol solution, provided forced diuresis. Nine hours later the child was fully conscious and continued to recover.— E. M. Jones and B. Williams, *Br. med. J.*, 1966, *1*, 466.

Precautions

Ergotamine tartrate is contra-indicated in patients with severe hypertension, severe or persistent sepsis, peripheral vascular disease, ischaemic heart disease, or impaired hepatic or renal function. It is also contra-indicated in pregnancy and should be avoided in nursing mothers.

Symptoms of overdosage may mimic those of migraine and patients should be warned to keep within the recommended dosage. Numbness or tingling of the extremities generally indicates that ergotamine should be discontinued. Ergotamine should not be administered prophylactically, as prolonged use may give rise to gangrene.

The vasoconstrictor effects of ergotamine are enhanced by sympathomimetic agents such as adrenaline.

A 68-year-old woman with headache developed cyanosis of the tongue 3 hours after the administration of ergotamine tartrate 500 µg intramuscularly and again 6 days later after two 1-mg tablets given with an interval of 6 hours. Partial necrosis of the tongue resulted. Temporal arteritis was later diagnosed and it was suggested that ergotamine should be used with caution in elderly patients with headache until temporal arteritis was ruled out.— J. R. Wolpaw *et al.*, *J. Am. med. Ass.*, 1973, *225*, 514.

INTERACTIONS. *Beta blockers.* A 61-year-old man who was regularly using Cafergot suppositories twice daily for migraine was given propranolol 30 mg daily as additional prophylaxis; the patient's feet became progressively more purple and painful.— J. F. Baumrucker (letter), *New Engl. J. Med.*, 1973, *288*, 916. There were no adverse reactions in 50 patients with migraine who received simultaneous doses of ergotamine and propranolol. It was noted that the above patient received 4 mg of ergotamine tartrate daily, which was much higher than the accepted limit and it was suggested that the patient had ergotism rather than an interaction with propranolol.— S. Diamond (letter), *ibid.*, *289*, 159.

Severe bilateral narrowing of the superficial femoral arteries in a 21-year-old man who had taken propranolol 120 mg and methysergide 3 mg both daily for 2 weeks; the condition progressed to gangrene of the feet necessitating bilateral amputation. A second patient had severe spasm of the femoral, brachial, and radial arteries after taking oxprenolol with ergotamine; the condition responded to heparin and glyceryl trinitrate intra-arterially.— C. P. Venter *et al.*, *Br. med. J.*, 1984, *289*, 288.

Caffeine. For a report of caffeine enhancing and accelerating the absorption of ergotamine from the gastro-intestinal tract, see Absorption and Fate, below.

Macrolide antibiotics. A report of minor ergotism in a 34-year-old woman when she took erythromycin ethylsuccinate in addition to ergotamine tartrate.— G. Lagier *et al.*, *Thérapie*, 1979, *34*, 515.

Acute ergotism in 2 patients receiving ergotamine tartrate and triacetyloleandomycin.— N. T. Matthews and J. H. Havill, *N.Z. med. J.*, 1979, *89*, 476.

PORPHYRIA. Ergot preparations should not be used in patients with acute porphyrias since they might precipitate attacks.— M.R. Moore and K.E.L. McColl, *Porphyrias, Drug Lists*, Glasgow, Porphyria Research Unit, University of Glasgow, 1987.

PREGNANCY AND THE NEONATE. Ergot alkaloids in the milk of nursing mothers gave infants symptoms of ergotism, such as vomiting, diarrhoea, weak pulse and unstable blood pressure. Care should be taken when giving nursing mothers preparations containing ergot alkaloids for the treatment of migraine.— J. A. Knowles, *J. Pediat.*, 1965, *66*, 1068.

Ergot alkaloids impaired lactation by inhibition of maternal pituitary prolactin secretion.— *J. Am. med. Ass.*, 1974, *227*, 676.

Absorption and Fate

Ergotamine is incompletely absorbed from the gastro-intestinal tract. There is reported to be considerable individual variation in bioavailability, regardless of the route of administration. It appears to be metabolised extensively in the liver, the majority of metabolites being excreted in the bile. Ergotamine or its metabolites are reported to be secreted in breast milk.

A review of the pharmacokinetics of ergotamine with reference to the problems of interpreting studies in relation to the type of assay used. Overall, published work suggests that ergotamine has a relatively rapid elimination, a high clearance by metabolism, and a very incomplete bioavailability due to a first-pass effect if administered by a route which allows passage through the liver before reaching the general circulation. Biological effects appear to last much longer than its short elimination half-life would suggest. It may be that ergotamine is biologically active at concentrations below those detectable by current assays or its activity may be partly due to one or more metabolites.— M. J. Eadie, *Cephalalgia*, 1983, *3*, 135.

A review of the clinical pharmacokinetics of ergotamine in migraine and cluster headache.— V. L. Perrin, *Clin. Pharmacokinet.*, 1985, *10*, 334.

Studies on the bioavailability and pharmacokinetics of ergotamine have been hampered by the low concentrations found in plasma and the lack of a sufficiently sensitive and specific assay method. W.H. Aellig and E. Nüesch (*Int. J. clin. Pharmac. Biopharm.*, 1977, *15*, 106) used tritium-labelled ergot alkaloids, including dihydroergotamine, co-dergocrine, and ergotamine, in a comparative study. Mean peak plasma concentrations of 1.52 ng per mL occurred 2.1 hours after ergotamine tartrate 1 mg by mouth in 6 subjects, with elimination half-lives from plasma of 2.7 hours for the α-phase and 21 hours for the β-phase. The other drugs tested had qualitatively similar pharmacokinetics. V. Ala-Hurula *et al.* (*Eur. J. clin. Pharmac.*, 1979, *15*, 51) used a radio-immunoassay to assess systemic availability of ergotamine tartrate following oral, rectal, and intramuscular administration in healthy subjects. They found great individual variation in plasma concentrations with mean peak concentrations of 0.36 ng per mL 2 hours after 2 mg by mouth, 0.42 ng per mL 1 hour after 2 mg rectally (as a suppository also containing caffeine 100 mg), and 1.94 ng per mL half an hour after 500 µg intramuscularly. Most subjects showed a second increase in plasma concentrations at 24 to 48 hours which was considered might point to accumulation or to the appearance of immunoreactive metabolites. In a further study, also using radio-immunoassay, V. Ala-Hurula *et al.* (*Eur. J. clin. Pharmac.*, 1979, *16*, 355) found evidence for the accumulation of ergotamine or its metabolites in healthy subjects given doses on 3 consecutive days. They also found a mean concentration of 0.40 ng per mL in the cerebrospinal fluid of 4 patients 1 to 2 hours after ergotamine tartrate 2 mg with caffeine 200 mg by mouth. No ergotamine was detected in the plasma of 7 of 17 migraine patients 1 hour after their usual daily oral or rectal dose, indicating considerable variation in bioavailability. H. Hovdal *et al.* (*Cephalalgia*, 1982, *2*, 145), using the same radio-immunoassay method as V. Ala-Hurula *et al.*, were unable to detect ergotamine in the cerebrospinal fluid of 18 patients given ergotamine 500 µg intramuscularly or rectally as suppositories containing 2 or 4 mg. J.J. Ibraheem *et al.* (*Eur. J. clin. Pharmac.*, 1982, *23.*, 235) used a sensitive and specific high performance liquid chromatography (HPLC) assay (P.O. Edlund, *J. Chromat.*, 1981, *226*, 107) to determine plasma concentrations of unchanged ergotamine following single doses of the tartrate by intravenous and intramuscular injection. The mean terminal half-life was 1.86 hours following 500 µg intravenously in 10 migraine patients. Following 500 µg intramuscularly in 5 patients, ergotamine was rapidly absorbed but bioavailability was low and variable; a mean peak plasma concentration of 0.8 ng per mL was found at the first measurement at 10 minutes. They found no evidence of a second peak. Using the same assay method, J.J. Ibraheem *et al.* (*Br. J. clin. Pharmac.*, 1983, *16*, 695) reported low bioavailability of ergotamine tartrate after oral and rectal administration in migraine patients. Following a 2-mg oral dose in 7 fasting patients ergotamine could not be detected in plasma from 10 minutes up to 54 hours. Low and very variable concentrations were achieved in 9 patients given a 2-mg suppository; bioavailability was increased marginally when a rectal solution was given to 12 patients. Commenting on their results J.J. Ibraheem *et al.* speculated that the very low bioavailability of oral ergotamine must be due to either poor absorption, or high first-pass elimination, or both and that the pharmacodynamic effectiveness of ergotamine might be attributed to active metabolites or an extremely high potency. They also suggested that earlier workers had mostly measured metabolites. P. Tfelt-Hansen and L. Paalzow (*Clin. Pharmac. Ther.*, 1985, *37*, 29), using the HPLC assay, were unable to correlate the pharmacological effect of ergotamine on arteries with plasma concentrations. Following intramuscular injection ergotamine was quickly absorbed, but the effect on arteries developed slowly and was well sustained for up to 29 hours, at which time no ergotamine was measurable in plasma. They considered that ergotamine was probably firmly bound to the arteries.

Results in 6 healthy subjects given tritium-labelled ergotamine tartrate by mouth, with or without caffeine, indicating that the gastro-intestinal absorption of ergotamine is enhanced and accelerated by caffeine.— R. Schmidt and A. Fanchamps, *Eur. J. clin. Pharmac.*, 1974, *7*, 213.

Buccal absorption of ergotamine was estimated in 7 healthy subjects by measuring the loss of ergotamine from buffered solutions circulated around the mouth for up to 5 minutes. The results indicated that therapeutically useful amounts of ergotamine are unlikely to be absorbed across the buccal mucosa and that concurrent administration of caffeine was unlikely to enhance absorption.— J. M. Sutherland *et al.*, *J. Neurol. Neurosurg. Psychiat.*, 1974, *37*, 1116. In a study in 12 subjects, single doses of ergotamine tartrate 2 mg sublingually or 250 µg intramuscularly had similar peripheral vasoconstrictor effects as judged by plethysmographic measurements determined for 90 minutes following administration. It was suggested that at these doses the 2 routes should be therapeutically equivalent.— T. Winsor, *Clin. Pharmac. Ther.*, 1981, *29*, 94. Using a high performance liquid chromatography assay, ergotamine was not detected in the blood of 4 healthy subjects following ergotamine tartrate 2 mg sublingually, whereas mean plasma concentrations of 0.96, 0.80, and 0.57 ng per mL were found in 4 migraine patients 30, 60, and 120 minutes after ergotamine tartrate 500 µg per 70-kg body-weight intramuscularly. It was considered unlikely that ergotamine tartrate 2 mg sublingually and 250 µg intramuscularly have the same bioavailability.— P. Tfelt-Hansen *et al.* (letter), *Br. J. clin. Pharmac.*, 1982, *13*, 239.

Further references to pharmacokinetic studies on ergotamine: V. Ala-Hurula, *Headache*, 1982, *22*, 167 (effervescent ergotamine tablets); D. A. Orton and R. J. Richardson, *Postgrad. med. J.*, 1982, *58*, 6 (adverse effects and plasma concentrations following parenteral, oral, and rectal administration).

Uses and Administration

Ergotamine tartrate has marked vasoconstrictor effects and a powerful action on the uterus, comparable to that of ergometrine but less rapid in onset. It is used in the treatment of acute attacks of migraine and should be given at the first warning of an attack since the earlier it is given the smaller the dose needed and the more effective the treatment. In subsequent attacks the total dose found effective previously may be given immediately symptoms occur.

The usual dose is 1 to 2 mg of ergotamine tartrate by mouth, repeated, if necessary, half an hour later. Usually not more than 6 mg should be administered in 24 hours and not more than 10 mg in a week; some manufacturers suggest a maximum daily dose of 8 mg and a maximum weekly dose of 12 mg. Similar doses may also be administered sublingually. Absorption from oral doses is variable and administration in association with caffeine has been reported to enhance the effect of ergotamine.

Ergotamine tartrate may also be administered

rectally as suppositories, especially if the oral route is not effective or not practicable; suppositories usually also contain caffeine. The rectal dose of ergotamine tartrate is 2 mg repeated, if necessary, once or twice at hourly intervals. Not more than 6 mg should be administered in 24 hours and not more than 10 mg in a week; in the USA the maximum recommended daily dose, given in the form of suppositories, is 4 mg.

A more rapid onset of action may be achieved by oral inhalation. One dose containing 360 μg of ergotamine tartrate may be inhaled at the onset of the attack and repeated, if necessary, after 5 minutes. Not more than 6 inhalation doses should be taken in 24 hours and not more than 15 in a week. Ergotamine tartrate was formerly given by subcutaneous or intramuscular injection in reported doses of 250 to 500 μg, repeated if necessary, but not more than a total dose of 1 mg in a week. Official injections of ergotamine tartrate allow a mixture of alkaloids, thus these doses may represent ergotamine tartrate or a mixture of ergotamine tartrate and other related alkaloids. However, dihydroergotamine mesylate (p.1052) is generally used if parenteral administration is necessary.

Ergotamine tartrate should not be used for the prophylaxis of migraine, but doses of 1 to 2 mg by mouth at bedtime for 10 to 14 days have been given to patients with cluster headache.

MIGRAINE. An account of migraine and its treatment. In acute attacks simple analgesics such as aspirin and paracetamol are often effective. Ergotamine preparations are no longer used as readily now that prophylactic medication for migraine has become more popular. Nevertheless ergotamine remains valuable for patients with infrequent severe attacks. For prophylaxis the drugs of first choice are propranolol and pizotifen; methysergide is effective but has become the drug of third choice because of its more serious side-effects. Cluster headaches are best managed prophylactically. The traditional treatment is ergotamine since the self-limiting nature of the cluster in most patients should not require long-term continuous therapy; most of the other drugs used in migraine have not been effective. Beneficial results have been reported with corticosteroids and with lithium carbonate in the prophylaxis of cluster headaches.— R. Peatfield, *Drugs*, 1983, *26*, 364. and *idem, Br. J. Hosp. Med.*, 1984, *31*, 142.

Further reviews and discussions on migraine and its management: D. Thrush, *Br. med. J.*, 1978, *2*, 1004; W. E. Waters (letter), *ibid.*, 1228; *Lancet*, 1982, *1*, 1338; *Med. Lett.*, 1984, *26*, 95; R. Atkinson and O. Appenzeller, *Postgrad. med. J.*, 1984, *60*, 841; J. N. Blau, *Lancet*, 1984, *1*, 444; R. Joseph (letter), *ibid.*, 742; W. E. Waters (letter), *ibid;* B. J. Repschlaeger and M. A. McPherson, *Clin. Pharm.*, 1984, *3*, 139.

A study indicating that most children with severe frequent migraine recover on an appropriate diet, and that so many foods can provoke attacks that any food or association of foods may be the cause.— J. Egger *et al.*, *Lancet*, 1983, *2*, 865. Comments and criticisms.— G. Hearn and R. Finn (letter), *ibid.*, 1081; R. C. Peatfield (letter), *ibid.*, 1082; M. Wilkinson and J. N. Blau (letter), *ibid;* G. E. Cook and R. Joseph (letter), *ibid.*, 1256; J. B. P. Stephenson (letter), *ibid.*, 1257; J. W. Gerrard (letter), *ibid.*

Preparations

Ergotamine Aerosol Inhalation *(B.P.C. 1973)*. Contains ergotamine tartrate.

Ergotamine Tartrate Inhalation Aerosol *(U.S.P.)*

Ergotamine Injection *(B.P.)*. Of the total alkaloidal content not less than 50% and not more than 70% is present as ergotamine tartrate.

Ergotamine Tartrate Injection *(U.S.P.)*. The content of ergotamine tartrate is 52 to 74% of the total alkaloidal content, and the content of ergotaminine tartrate is not more than 45% of the total alkaloidal content.

Ergotamine Tartrate and Caffeine Suppositories *(U.S.P.)*

Ergotamine Tablets *(B.P.)*. Tablets containing ergotamine tartrate.

Ergotamine Tartrate and Caffeine Tablets *(U.S.P.)*

Ergotamine Tartrate Tablets *(U.S.P.)*

Proprietary Preparations

Cafergot *(Sandoz, UK)*. *Tablets*, ergotamine tartrate 1 mg, caffeine 100 mg. *Dose.* 1 to 2 tablets at the onset of symptoms, repeated if necessary up to a maximum of 4 tablets in 24 hours or 10 in any 1 week. Not to be repeated at intervals of less than 4 days.

Suppositories, ergotamine tartrate 2 mg, caffeine 100 mg. *Dose.* 1 to be administered at the onset of symptoms, repeated if necessary up to a maximum of 2 suppositories in 24 hours or 5 in any 1 week. Not to be repeated at intervals of less than 4 days.

Lingraine *(Winthrop, UK)*. *Tablets*, sublingual, ergotamine tartrate 2 mg. *Dose.* 1 tablet at the onset of symptoms, repeated if necessary after half an hour. Maximum of 3 tablets in 24 hours or 6 in any 1 week.

Medihaler Ergotamine *(Riker, UK)*. *Aerosol inhalation* (oral), ergotamine tartrate 360 μg/metered inhalation. *Dose.* 1 inhalation at the onset of symptoms, repeated if necessary after 5 minutes. Maximum of 6 inhalations in 24 hours or 15 in any 1 week.

Migril *(Wellcome, UK)*. *Tablets*, scored, ergotamine tartrate 2 mg, caffeine hydrate 100 mg, cyclizine hydrochloride 50 mg. *Dose.* 1 or 2 tablets at the onset of symptoms, followed if necessary by ½ to 1 tablet after half an hour. Maximum of 4 tablets for any single attack, or 6 in any 1 week.

Proprietary Names and Manufacturers

Ergate *(Vernleigh, S.Afr.)*; Ergomar *(Fisons, Canad.; Fisons, USA)*; Ergostat *(Parke, Davis, USA)*; Ergotamin Medihaler *(Ger.)*; Ergotamin-medihaler *(Riker, Denm.)*; Ergotan *(Salf, Ital.)*; Exmigra *(Neth.)*; Exmigrex *(Fin.)*; Femergin *(Wander, UK)*; Gravergol *(Horner, Canad.)*; Gynergen *(Neth.)*; Gynergen *(Austral.; Sandoz, Canad.; Denm.; Sandoz, Ger.; Sandoz, Ital.; Switz.; Sandoz, USA)*; Gynergene *(Belg.; Fr.)*; Gynergeno *(Arg.; Sandoz, Spain)*; Lingraine *(Winthrop, Austral.; Winthrop, UK)*; Lingran *(Sterling-Winthrop, Swed.)*; Lingrene *(Norw.)*; Medihaler Ergotamine *(Riker, Austral.; Riker, Canad.; Riker, UK; Riker, USA)*; Megral *(Wellcome, Canad.)*; Migretamine *(Jpn)*; Wigrettes *(Organon, USA)*.

The following names have been used for multi-ingredient preparations containing ergotamine tartrate—Bellergal *(Sandoz, Austral.; Sandoz, Canad.; Sandoz, UK; Sandoz, USA)*; Cafergot *(Sandoz, Austral.; Sandoz, Canad.; Sandoz, UK; Sandoz, USA)*; Cafergot P-B *(Sandoz, USA)*; Cafergot-PB *(Sandoz, Austral.; Sandoz, Canad.)*; Cafetrate-PB *(Schein, USA)*; Effergot *(Wander, UK)*; Ergodryl *(Parke, Davis, Austral.; Parke, Davis, Canad.; Parke, Davis, UK)*; Migral *(Wellcome, Austral.)*; Migril *(Wellcome, UK)*; Orgraine *(Organon, UK)*; Wigraine *(Organon, Canad.; Organon, USA)*; Wigraine-PB *(Organon, USA)*.

1509-v

Ergotoxine

A mixture in equal proportions of ergocornine ($C_{31}H_{39}N_5O_5$ = 561.7), ergocristine ($C_{35}H_{39}N_5O_5$ = 609.7), and ergocryptine, as the α- and β-isomers ($C_{32}H_{41}N_5O_5$ = 575.7).

CAS — 8006-25-5 (ergotoxine); 8047-28-7 (ergotoxine esylate); 564-36-3 (ergocornine); 511-08-0 (ergocristine); 511-09-1 (ergocryptine).

Ergotoxine is a mixture of naturally occurring ergot alkaloids. The esylate was formerly used as an oxytocic and in the treatment of migraine.

1512-d

Methylergometrine Maleate *(BANM, rINNM)*.

Methylergobasine Maleate; Methylergonovine Maleate *(USAN)*. *N*-[(*S*)-1-(Hydroxymethyl)propyl]-D-lysergamide hydrogen maleate; 9,10-Didehydro-*N*-[(*S*)-1-(hydroxymethyl)propyl]-6-methylergoline-8β-carboxamide hydrogen maleate.
$C_{20}H_{25}N_3O_2,C_4H_4O_4$=455.5.

CAS — 113-42-8 (methylergometrine); 57432-61-8 (maleate).

Pharmacopoeias. In *Braz., Ind., Jpn, Jug., Nord., Turk.*, and *U.S.*

A white to pinkish-tan, odourless, microcrystalline powder

Soluble 1 in 100 of water, 1 in 175 of alcohol, 1 in 1900 of chloroform and 1 in 8400 of ether. A 0.02% solution in water has a pH of 4.4 to 5.2. **Store** in airtight containers at a temperature not exceeding 8°. Protect from light.

Adverse Effects, Treatment, and Precautions

As for Ergometrine Maleate, p.1053.

PREGNANCY AND THE NEONATE. See Absorption and Fate for the excretion of methylergometrine in breast milk.

Absorption and Fate

As for Ergometrine Maleate, p.1054.

References: R. Mäntylä *et al.*, *Int. J. clin. Pharmac. Biopharm.*, 1978, *16*, 254 (oral administration); H. Allonen *et al.*, *ibid.*, 340 (oral administration).

PREGNANCY AND THE NEONATE. In a study of 8 women who had been treated with methylergometrine 125 μg three times daily by mouth for 5 days, concentrations in plasma and milk were measured by radio-immunoassay (lower limit 0.50 ng per mL) 1 and 8 hours after a dose of 250 μg by mouth. Concentrations in plasma ranged from 0.6 to 4.4 ng per mL at 1 hour and from 0 to 0.6 ng per mL at 8 hours; those in breast milk ranged from less than 0.5 to 1.3 ng per mL at 1 hour and from 0 to 1.2 ng per mL at 8 hours. It was considered that the amount of methylergometrine excreted in breast milk was unlikely to affect the suckling infant.— R. Erkkola *et al.*, *Int. J. clin. Pharmac. Biopharm.*, 1978, *16*, 579.

Uses and Administration

Methylergometrine maleate has an action on the uterus similar to that of ergometrine maleate (see p.1054) and is used similarly in the prevention and treatment of postpartum haemorrhage in doses of 200 μg. It is given on completion of the third stage of labour in a dose of 200 μg intramuscularly, repeated if necessary at intervals of 2 to 4 hours. In emergencies 200 μg may be given by slow intravenous injection over at least 60 seconds. Although its use before delivery of the placenta is not generally recommended in the US, methylergometrine has been given similarly to ergometrine and oxytocin (see p.1054) after delivery of the anterior shoulder. During the puerperium 200 μg may be given by mouth 3 or 4 times daily for up to 7 days.

Preparations

Methylergonovine Maleate Injection *(U.S.P.)*. A sterile solution of methylergometrine maleate in Water for Injections.

Methylergonovine Maleate Tablets *(U.S.P.)*. Tablets containing methylergometrine maleate.

Proprietary Names and Manufacturers

Basofortina *(Sandoz, Arg.)*; Levospan *(Jpn)*; Methergin *(Sandoz, Austral.; Sandoz-Wander, Belg.; Sandoz, Denm.; Sandoz, Fr.; Sandoz, Ger.; Sandoz, Ital.; Sandoz, Neth.; Sandoz, Norw.; Sandoz, S.Afr.; Sandoz, Spain; Sandoz, Swed.; Sandoz, Switz.)*; Methergine *(Sandoz, USA)*.

1513-n

Methysergide Maleate *(BANM, USAN, rINNM)*.

1-Methyl-D-lysergic Acid Butanolamide Maleate. *N*-[1-(Hydroxymethyl)propyl]-1-methyl-D-lysergamide hydrogen maleate; 9,10-Didehydro-*N*-[1-(hydroxymethyl)propyl]-1,6-dimethylergoline-8β-carboxamide hydrogen maleate.
$C_{21}H_{27}N_3O_2,C_4H_4O_4$=469.5.

CAS — 361-37-5 (methysergide); 129-49-7 (maleate).

Pharmacopoeias. In *Br., Swiss,* and *U.S.*

A white to yellowish-white or reddish-white, odourless or almost odourless, crystalline powder. Methysergide 1 mg is approximately equivalent to 1.33 mg of methysergide maleate.

B.P. **solubilities** are: slightly soluble in water and

in methyl alcohol; practically insoluble in chloroform and in ether. *U.S.P.* solubilities are: soluble 1 in 200 of water, 1 in 165 of alcohol, and 1 in 3400 of chloroform; practically insoluble in ether. A 0.2% solution in water has a pH of 3.7 to 4.7. **Store** in well-closed containers at a temperature of 2° to 8° and protect from light.

SOLUBILITY. The addition of caffeine increased the aqueous solubility of methysergide maleate independently of pH.— M. A. Zoglio and H. V. Maulding, *J. pharm. Sci.*, 1970, *59*, 1836.

Adverse Effects

Gastro-intestinal effects such as nausea, vomiting, diarrhoea, and abdominal pain are common with methysergide maleate, as are dizziness and drowsiness. Other central nervous system effects reported include ataxia, insomnia, weakness, confusion, restlessness, lightheadedness, euphoria, and hallucinations. Peripheral or localised oedema, leg cramps, and weight gain have occurred and there have been occasional reports of skin rashes, loss of hair, joint and muscle pain, neutropenia, and eosinophilia. Orthostatic hypotension and tachycardia have been observed. Arterial spasm has occurred in some patients with manifestations such as paraesthesia of the extremities and anginal pain, similar to those reported with ergotamine (p.1055); if such symptoms occur methysergide should be withdrawn, although rebound headaches may be experienced if it is withdrawn suddenly. Vascular insufficiency of the lower limbs may represent arterial spasm or fibrotic changes. Retroperitoneal fibrosis, with obstruction of abdominal blood vessels and ureters, pleuropulmonary fibrosis, and fibrotic changes in heart valves have occurred in patients on long-term treatment. Methysergide must be withdrawn if fibrosis occurs. Retroperitoneal fibrosis is usually reversible, but other fibrotic changes are less readily reversed.

In 850 patients with migraine, methysergide 1 to 8 mg daily benefited 45% without side-effects; 12% were not benefited. Side-effects in the remaining 43% included weight gain (30%), severe oedema (4%), severe depression (2%), pain in the calves (26%), disturbed vision (1%), and loss of hair (1%); 3% were completely intolerant of the drug.— N. Leyton (letter), *Lancet*, 1964, *1*, 830.

EFFECTS ON THE BLOOD. A report of reversible haemolytic anaemia in a middle-aged woman who took methysergide daily for about 5 years.— P. H. Slugg and R. S. Kunkel, *J. Am. med. Ass.*, 1970, *213*, 297.

EFFECTS ON THE CARDIOVASCULAR SYSTEM. Reports of adverse cardiovascular effects associated with methysergide: G. M. Fenichel and S. Battiata, *J. Pediat.*, 1966, *68*, 632 (thrombophlebitis); R. E. Buenger and J. A. Hunter, *J. Am. med. Ass.*, 1966, *198*, 558 (intestinal ischaemia); J. Katz and R. M. Vogel, *J. Am. med. Ass.*, 1967, *199*, 124 (intestinal ischaemia); P. Hudgson *et al.* (letter), *Lancet*, 1967, *1*, 444 (myocardial infarction); K. Raw and H. Gaylis, *S. Afr. med. J.*, 1976, *50*, 1999 (acute arterial spasm of the lower extremities after methysergide 1 mg daily for 5 days); F. M. Ameli *et al.*, *Can. J. Surg.*, 1977, *20*, 158 (occlusion of brachial artery).

FIBROSIS. Methysergide daily, taken for headaches for periods of 9 to 54 months, was considered to be responsible for the development of retroperitoneal fibrosis in 27 patients; cardiac murmurs developed in 6 of them. Fibrotic changes, affecting the aorta, heart valves, and pulmonary tissues, also occurred in a few of the patients.— J. R. Graham *et al.*, *New Engl. J. Med.*, 1966, *274*, 359.

Endocardial fibrosis indicated by cardiac murmurs developed in 48 patients receiving methysergide. The murmurs gradually regressed in 27 of the patients when methysergide was discontinued. Retroperitoneal fibrosis was present in 9 patients and pleuropulmonary fibrosis in 2.— D. S. Bana *et al.*, *Am. Heart J.*, 1974, *88*, 640.

Further reports of fibrosis associated with methysergide: F. D. Schwartz and G. Dunea, *Lancet*, 1966, *1*, 955 (retroperitoneal fibrosis); H. B. Miles and W. M. Tappan (letter), *J. Am. med. Ass.*, 1968, *203*, 431 (retroperitoneal fibrosis with vasculitis of iliac vessels); W. Hindle *et al.*, *Br. med. J.*, 1970, *1*, 605 (pleural fibrosis); K. A. Misch, *Br. med. J.*, 1974, *2*, 365 (cardiac fibrosis); J. W. Mason *et al.*, *Circulation*, 1977, *56*, 889 (cardiac fibrosis); R. C. Orlando *et al.*, *Ann. intern. Med.*, 1978, *88*, 213 (pleural fibrosis and pericarditis).

LUPUS ERYTHEMATOSUS. Methysergide had been suspected of inducing a syndrome resembling systemic lupus erythematosus.— J. P. Harpey, *Adverse Drug React. Bull.*, 1973, Dec., 140.

Treatment of Adverse Effects

As for Ergotamine Tartrate, p.1055.

A report of the succesful treatment of methysergide-induced retroperitoneal fibrosis by means of corticosteroid therapy.— J. Paccalin *et al.*, *Thérapie* 1976, *31*, 231.

Precautions

As for Ergotamine Tartrate, p.1056. Methysergide maleate is also contra-indicated in valvular heart disease, pulmonary and collagen diseases, and debilitated states. It should be used with caution in patients with peptic ulcer. Patients should be closely supervised and methysergide withdrawn if symptoms of fibrosis or arterial spasm develop.

INTERACTIONS. Arterial occlusion occurred in 2 patients taking methysergide and a high parenteral dosage of ergotamine concomitantly for cluster headache; the combination should be avoided.— D. A. Joyce and S. S. Gubbay, *Br. med. J.*, 1982, *285*, 260.

For a report of gangrene in a patient taking propranolol and methysergide, see Ergotamine Tartrate, p.1056.

Absorption and Fate

Total radioactivity, an indicator of unchanged drug and metabolites, was measured in the plasma and urine of 3 groups of 6 subjects following administration by mouth of single radioactively-labelled doses of methysergide solution, ergotamine capsules, or dihydroergotamine solution. Calculated elimination half-lives were 10.0, 34.3, and 30.3 hours for methysergide, ergotamine, and dihydroergotamine, respectively, and calculated amounts of a dose excreted in the urine were 56.4, 4.23, and 3.06%, respectively. With a dosage regimen of 2 mg of methysergide 3 times daily, a simulated mean steady-state concentration of 40 ng per mL was estimated; similarly, simulated peak and trough plasma concentrations were 60 and 17 ng per mL, respectively. The results indicate that methysergide is eliminated more rapidly than ergotamine or dihydroergotamine, has a smaller volume of distribution, and that metabolism plays a less dominant role in its pharmacokinetics.— J. Meier and E. Schreier, *Headache*, 1976, *16*, 96.

Uses and Administration

Methysergide maleate is a potent serotonin antagonist and, compared with ergotamine, has only feeble vasoconstrictor and oxytocic effects. It is used as a prophylactic agent in the management of severe recurrent migraine, but its mode of action is not established. It is ineffective in the treatment of acute attacks of migraine.

Methysergide maleate is given by mouth in a dosage equivalent to 2 to 6 mg of methysergide base daily in divided doses with meals. It is suggested that treatment should be started with 1 mg at bedtime and doses increased gradually over about 2 weeks; the minimum effective dose should be used. In the US and some other countries doses are expressed in terms of the maleate and 4 to 8 mg daily of methysergide maleate is given; some authorities recommend a maximum dose of 6 mg daily of the maleate. Careful and regular observation of the patient is essential because of the high incidence of side-effects. Treatment should not be continued for more than 6 months, after which it should be gradually reduced over 2 or 3 weeks and then discontinued for at least a month for reassessment. Some authorities consider that treatment courses should not exceed 3 months without a break. In patients receiving methysergide maleate, the dose of ergotamine required to control acute attacks of migraine may need to be reduced.

Methysergide has also been used to control the diarrhoea associated with carcinoid disease.

MIGRAINE. An account of the management of migraine and the view that, although methysergide is effective for the prophylaxis of migraine, propranolol or pizotifen are preferred because of the more serious side-effects of methysergide.— R. Peatfield, *Br. J. Hosp. Med.*, 1984, *31*, 142.

For further reviews on the management of migraine, see Ergotamine Tartrate, p.1057.

Preparations

Methysergide Maleate Tablets *(U.S.P.)*

Methysergide Tablets *(B.P.)*. Tablets containing methysergide maleate.

Proprietary Preparations

Deseril *(Sandoz, UK)*. *Tablets*, methysergide 1 mg (as maleate).

Proprietary Names and Manufacturers

Deseril *(Sandoz, Austral.; Belg.; Sandoz, Denm.; Sandoz, Ger.; Neth.; Sandoz, Norw.; Wander, S.Afr.; Sandoz, Spain; Sandoz, Switz.; Sandoz, UK)*; Désernil *(Sandoz, Fr.)*; Deserril *(Sandoz, Ital.)*; Sansert *(Sandoz, Canad.; Sandoz, Swed.; Sandoz, USA)*.

1514-h

Nicergoline *(BAN, USAN, rINN)*.

FI-6714. 10α-Methoxy-1,6-dimethylergolin-8β-ylmethyl 5-bromonicotinate.

$C_{24}H_{26}BrN_3O_3$=484.4.

CAS — 27848-84-6.

Adverse Effects and Precautions

Gastro-intestinal side-effects, flushing of the skin, drowsiness, dizziness, and insomnia may occur. Hypotension, particularly following parenteral administration of nicergoline, has been reported and the effects of antihypertensive agents may be enhanced.

Of 359 patients with cerebrovascular insufficiency treated with nicergoline for 1 month side-effects occurred in 25, necessitating withdrawal of therapy in 11. The reactions included hot flushes (6), general malaise (8), agitation (2), hyperacidity (3), nausea (1), diarrhoea (3), and dizziness and somnolence (2).— J. Dauverchain, *Arzneimittel-Forsch.*, 1979, *29*, 1308.

INTERACTIONS. A study in healthy subjects indicating that nicergoline enhances the cardiac depressant action of propranolol.— F. Boismare *et al.*, *Methods Find. exp. clin. Pharmacol.*, 1983, *5*, 83.

Uses and Administration

Nicergoline is an ergot derivative. It has been used similarly to co-dergocrine mesylate to treat symptoms of mental deterioration associated with cerebrovascular insufficiency and has also been used in peripheral vascular disease. Nicergoline has been given in doses of 5 to 10 mg three times daily by mouth and by intramuscular injection in doses of 2 to 4 mg once or twice daily; 2 to 8 mg has been given by slow intravenous infusion.

A study on the metabolism of nicergoline.— F. Arcamone *et al.*, *Biochem. Pharmac.*, 1972, *21*, 2205.

BENIGN PROSTATIC HYPERTROPHY. Nicergoline 4 mg twice daily by intramuscular injection for 3 days improved the symptoms of benign prostatic hypertrophy when compared with placebo in a double-blind crossover study in 16 patients.— F. Ronchi *et al.*, *Urol. Res.*, 1982, *10*, 131.

CEREBROVASCULAR DISORDERS. See Senile dementia.

DEAFNESS. A favourable report on the effect of nicergoline 30 mg daily by mouth for 30 days on the reduced hearing of old age in 30 patients.— G. Aliprandi and V. Tantalo, *Arzneimittel-Forsch.*, 1979, *29*, 1287.

DIAGNOSIS. The use of nicergoline in fluorescence retinographic studies in ophthalmology.— M. Borgioli *et al.*, *Arzneimittel-Forsch.*, 1979, *29*, 1311.

PERIPHERAL VASCULAR DISEASE. References: F. Boismare *et al.*, *Thérapie*, 1974, *29*, 925; J. C. Schrub *et al.*, *Thérapie*, 1975, *30*, 407.

SENILE DEMENTIA. Brief comment on nicergoline as a 'cerebroactive' drug. Actions claimed for nicergoline have included vasodilatation, metabolic activation, and platelet aggregation.— A. Spagnoli and G. Tognoni, *Drugs*, 1983, *26*, 44.

Nicergoline 4 mg twice daily by intramuscular injection for 2 weeks followed by 20 mg three times daily by mouth for 12 weeks improved symptoms of mild to moderate senile dementia when compared with placebo in a double-blind crossover study.— A. Arrigo *et al.*, *Int. J. clin. Pharmacol. Res.*, 1982, *2*, *Suppl.* 1, 33.

Further references: F. P. Bernini *et al.*, *Farmaco, Edn*

prat., 1977, *32*, 32 (chronic cerebral insufficiency); L. D. Iliff *et al.*, *J. Neurol. Neurosurg. Psychiat.*, 1977, *40*, 746 (effect on cerebral blood flow); J. Dauverchain, *Arzneimittel-Forsch.*, 1979, *29*, 1308.

Proprietary Names and Manufacturers

Circo-Maren *(Krewel, Ger.)*; Duracebrol *(Durachemie, Ger.)*; Ergobel *(Hormosan, Ger.)*; Fisifax *(Valles Mestre, Spain)*; Memoq *(Gödecke, Ger.)*; Nicergolyn *(ICT-Lodi, Ital.)*; Sermion *(Montedison, Arg.; Specia, Fr.; Farmitalia, Ger.; Farmitalia, Ital.; Farmitalia, Spain; Farmitalia Carlo Erba, Switz.)*; Varson *(Almirall, Spain)*.

Essential Oils

4600-n

Essential oils are volatile odorous mixtures of esters, aldehydes, alcohols, ketones, and terpenes. In many pharmacopoeias volatile oils are described as ethereal oils (aetherolea). Other names used include atherische öle, esencias, essences, essências, essentiae, and olea aetherea.

Taken internally, the volatile oils exert a mild irritant action on the mucous membranes of the mouth and the digestive tract, which induces a feeling of warmth and increases salivation, hence their use as carminatives. They have also been inhaled for the relief of congestive respiratory disorders.

When applied to the intact skin essential oils have an irritant and rubefacient action, causing first a sensation of warmth and smarting, which is followed by a mild local anaesthesia. For this reason they are used as counter-irritants.

Several oils have been reported to possess antimicrobial activity.

Essential oils are used as flavours and are widely used in folk medicine.

STANDARD FOR ESSENTIAL OILS. In addition to those standards noted under the oils included in *Martindale*, the British Standards Institution publishes British Standard Specifications for various other essential oils under BS 2999.

Adverse Effects

Excessive doses of essential oils are irritant to the gastro-intestinal tract and may cause nausea, vomiting, and diarrhoea. There may be irritation of the urinary tract and aggravation of pre-existing inflammatory conditions. The CNS may be depressed leading to stupor and respiratory failure, or stimulated leading to excitement and convulsions.

Essential oils or their extracts may be irritant to the skin and may cause contact dermatitis.

4601-h

Achillea

Milfoil; Millefeuille; Millefolii Herba; Schafgarbe; Yarrow.

Pharmacopoeias. In *Aust.*, *Cz.*, *Hung.*, *Pol.*, and *Swiss. Roum.* includes the oil (Aetheroleum Millefolii).

The dried flowering tops of yarrow, *Achillea millefolium* (Compositae). It contains a volatile oil, alkaloids, flavonoids, and various other compounds including tannins.

Achillea has been used mainly in folk medicine for a great variety of purposes. It has been stated to have diaphoretic, anti-inflammatory, and other miscellaneous properties.

References: J. D. Phillipson and L. A. Anderson, *Pharm. J.*, 1984, *2*, 111.

4606-q

Anethole *(USAN).*

Anethol; Anetol; *p*-Propenylanisole. (*E*)-1-Methoxy-4-(prop-1-enyl)benzene.

$C_{10}H_{12}O$=148.2.

CAS — 104-46-1; 4180-23-8 (E).

NOTE. Distinguish from Anethole Trithione p.1543.

Pharmacopoeias. In *Braz.* Also in *U.S.N.F.*

At or above 23° anethole is a colourless or faintly yellow liquid with a sweet taste and the characteristic odour of aniseed. It is obtained from anise oil or other sources or prepared synthetically.

Very slightly **soluble** in water; soluble 1 in 2 of alcohol; readily miscible with chloroform and with ether. **Store** in airtight containers. Protect from light.

Anethole is used for the same purposes as anise oil.

Temporary estimated acceptable daily intake of *trans*-anethole: up to 2.5 mg per kg body-weight. Adequate long-term feeding studies had still to be completed.— Twenty-eighth Report of the Joint FAO/WHO Expert Committee on Food Additives, *Tech. Rep. Ser. Wld Hlth Org.* No. 710, 1984.

Proprietary Names and Manufacturers

Monasirup *(Rorer, Ger.).*

4607-p

Aniseed *(BAN).*

Anice; Anis Verde; Anis Vert; Anise; Anise Fruit; Anisi Fructus; Fructus Anisi Vulgaris.

Pharmacopoeias. In *Arg.*, *Aust.*, *Belg.*, *Br.*, *Cz.*, *Egypt.*, *Eur.*, *Fr.*, *Ger.*, *Hung.*, *It.*, *Neth.*, *Pol.*, *Port.*, *Roum.*, *Rus.*, *Span.*, and *Swiss.*

The dried ripe fruit of *Pimpinella anisum* (Umbelliferae), containing not less than 2% v/w of volatile oil. **Powdered Aniseed** is greenish yellow or brownish green. **Store** in a dry place. Protect from light.

4608-s

Star Anise

Anís Estrellado; Anis Étoilé; Anisum Badium; Anisum Stellatum; Badiana; Badiane de Chine; Star Anise Fruit; Sternanis.

Pharmacopoeias. In *Arg.*, *Aust.*, *Braz.*, *Chin.*, *Fr.*, and *Port.*

The dried ripe fruit of *Illicium verum* (Magnoliaceae).

4609-w

Anise Oil *(BAN, USAN).*

Aniseed Oil; Esencia de Anís; Essence d'Anis; Oleum Anisi.

CAS — 8007-70-3.

Pharmacopoeias. In *Arg.*, *Aust.*, *Belg.*, *Br.*, *Chin.*, *Cz.*, *Egypt.*, *Fr.*, *Ger.*, *Hung.*, *Jug.*, *Mex.*, *Neth.*, *Nord.*, *Pol.*, *Port.*, *Roum.*, *Span.*, *Swiss*, and *Turk.* Also in *U.S.N.F.*

A colourless or pale yellow oil obtained by distillation from aniseed or star anise. It has a characteristic odour and a sweet aromatic taste.

Soluble 1 in 3 of alcohol (90%), sometimes with a slight opalescence. If the oil has crystallised it should be melted completely and mixed before use. **Store** at a temperature not exceeding 25° in well-filled airtight containers. Protect from light.

The Pharmaceutical Society's Department of Pharmaceutical Sciences found that PVC bottles softened and distorted fairly rapidly in the presence of anise oil, which should not be stored or dispensed in such bottles.— *Pharm. J.*, 1973, *1*, 100.

The solubility of anise oil in macrogol esters.— K. Thoma and G. Pfaff, *J. Soc. cosmet. Chem.*, 1976, *27*, 221.

Aniseed or anise is carminative and mildly expectorant; it is used mainly as anise oil or as preparations of the oil which is a common ingredient of cough preparations. The oil is also a flavouring agent.

A brief review of aniseed.— R. F. Chandler and D. Hawkes, *Can. pharm. J.*, 1984, *117*, 28.

Preparations

Concentrated Anise Water *(B.P.).* Anise Water Concentrated *(A.P.F.).* Anise oil 2 mL, alcohol (90%) 70 mL, water to 100 mL; shaken with 5 g of sterilised talc and filtered.

4611-b

Bay Oil

Myrcia Oil; Oleum Myrciae.

CAS — 8006-78-8.

NOTE. Laurel Leaf Oil (Bay Leaf Oil) is obtained from the leaves of *Laurus nobilis* (Lauraceae).

A yellow oil, darkening rapidly on exposure to air, with a pleasant odour and spicy taste, obtained by distillation from the leaves of *Pimenta acris* (=*P. racemosa*) (Myrtaceae) and probably other allied species.

STANDARD FOR BAY OIL. A British Standard Specification for Bay Oil (BS 2999/16: 1972) is published by the British Standards Institution.

The principal use of bay oil is in the preparation of bay rum, which is used as a hair lotion and as an astringent application.

4612-v

Benzaldehyde *(BAN, USAN).*

C_6H_5.CHO=106.1.

CAS — 100-52-7.

Pharmacopoeias. In *Belg.*, *Br.*, *Braz.*, *Hung.*, *Mex.*, and *Port.* Also in *U.S.N.F.*

A clear colourless strongly refractive liquid with a characteristic odour of bitter almonds and a burning aromatic taste.

Soluble 1 in 350 of water; miscible with alcohol, ether, and fixed and volatile oils. It becomes yellowish on keeping and oxidises in air to benzoic acid. **Store** at a temperature not exceeding 15° in well-filled airtight containers. Protect from light.

Benzaldehyde is used as a flavouring agent in the place of volatile bitter almond oil. It has been postulated that benzaldehyde is derived enzymatically from amygdalin (see p.1582).

Estimated acceptable daily intake: up to 5 mg per kg body-weight as total benzoic acid from all food additive sources.— Eleventh Report of the Joint FAO/WHO Expert Committee on Food Additives, *Tech. Rep. Ser. Wld Hlth Org. No. 383*, 1968.

Preparations

Benzaldehyde Spirit *(B.P.).* Benzaldehyde 1 mL, alcohol (90%) 80 mL, water to 100 mL.

Compound Benzaldehyde Elixir *(U.S.N.F.).* Benzaldehyde 0.05 mL, vanillin 100 mg, orange-flower water 15 mL, alcohol 5 mL, syrup 40 mL, water to 100 mL.

4613-g

Bergamot Oil

Bergamot Essence; Oleum Bergamottae.

CAS — 8007-75-8.

Pharmacopoeias. In *Arg.*, *Fr.*, *Port.*, and *Span.*

A greenish or brownish-yellow oil with a characteristic fragrant odour and a bitter aromatic taste, obtained by expression from the fresh peel of fruit of *Citrus bergamia* (Rutaceae). Constituents include linalyl acetate and 5-methoxypsoralen.

STANDARD FOR BERGAMOT OIL. A British Standard Specification for Bergamot Oil (BS 2999/32: 1971) is published by the British Standards Institution.

Bergamot oil is employed in perfumery and in suntanning preparations. It contains 5-methoxypsoralen whose actions are described on p.928.

An estimated acceptable daily intake of up to 500 µg per kg body-weight was established for citral, geranyl acetate, citronellol, linalol, and linalyl acetate, expressed as citral.— Twenty-third Report of Joint FAO/WHO Expert Committee on Food Additives, *Tech. Rep. Ser. Wld Hlth Org. No. 648*, 1980.

4616-s

Cajuput Oil

Cajuput Essence; Oleum Cajuputi.

CAS — 8008-98-8.

Pharmacopoeias. In *Arg.*, *Port.*, and *Span.* Also in *B.P.C. 1973.*

A colourless, yellow, or green oil with an agreeable

camphoraceous odour and a bitter, aromatic, camphoraceous taste, obtained by distillation from the fresh leaves and twigs of certain species of *Melaleuca* such as *M. cajuputi* and *M. leucadendron* (Myrtaceae). It contains cineole. **Store** in a cool place in well-filled airtight containers. Protect from light.

Cajuput oil obtained from the leaves of *Melaleuca cajuputi* contained about 10% of a crystalline phenolic compound 3,5-dimethyl-4,6-di-*O*-methylphloroacetophenone. This would explain its reputed antiseptic properties and the green colour due to chelation of copper distillation vessels.— J. B. Lowry (letter), *Nature*, 1973, *241*, 61.

Cajuput oil has been applied externally as a stimulant and mild rubefacient in rheumatism. It has been given internally as a carminative.

4617-w

Capsicum

Capsic.; Capsici Fructus; Chillies; Piment Rouge; Pimentão; Spanischer Pfeffer.

CAS — 404-86-4 (capsaicin).

NOTES. Ground cayenne pepper of commerce is normally a blend of varieties. Paprika is from *Capsicum annuum* var. *longum*; it is milder than capsicum.

Pharmacopoeias. In *Aust., Belg., Egypt., Ger., Hung., It., Jpn, Pol., Port., Span.,* and *Swiss.* Also in *B.P.C. 1973. Belg.* and *B.P.C. 1973* also include capsicum oleoresin.

The dried ripe fruits of *Capsicum annuum* var. *minimum* and small-fruited varieties of *C. frutescens* (Solanaceae). Some pharmacopoeias allow different varieties. It contains not less than 0.5% of the pungent principle capsaicin ((*E*)-8-methyl-*N*-vanillylnon-6-enamide, $C_{18}H_{27}NO_3$ = 305.4). **Store** in a cool dry place. Protect from light.

Capsicum has a carminative action but it is mainly used externally as a counter-irritant. Preparations can be very irritant.

The oleoresin is very irritant. The active ingredient capsaicin has local anaesthetic properties and is used as a neuropharmacological tool.

EFFECTS ON THE GASTRO-INTESTINAL TRACT. In a study in 50 patients with endoscopically-proved duodenal ulcer receiving antacids there was no difference in clinical progress, nor in endoscopy 4 weeks later, between those taking a normal hospital diet and those taking also red chilli powder 3 g daily.— N. Kumar *et al.*, *Br. med. J.*, 1984, *288*, 1803.

Proprietary Names and Manufacturers

Zostrix *(Genderm, USA).*

4619-l

Caraway *(BAN, USAN).*

Alcaravia; Caraway Fruit; Caraway Seed; Carum; Cumin des Prés; Fructus Carvi; Kümmel.

Pharmacopoeias. In *Aust., Br., Egypt., Fr., Ger., Hung., Jug., Pol., Port., Roum.,* and *Swiss.* Also in *U.S.N.F.*

The dried ripe fruits of *Carum carvi* (Umbelliferae). The *B.P.* specifies not less than 3.5% v/w of volatile oil. **Powdered Caraway** *(B.P.)* contains not less than 2.5% v/w of volatile oil. **Store** at a temperature not exceeding 25°; the powdered drug should be kept in well-closed containers.

4620-v

Caraway Oil *(BAN, USAN).*

Kümmelöl; Oleum Cari; Oleum Carui; Oleum Carvi.

CAS — 8000-42-8.

Pharmacopoeias. In *Aust., Br., Cz., Egypt., Ger., Hung., Jug.,* and *Roum.* Also in *U.S.N.F.*

A colourless or pale yellow oil with a characteristic odour and taste, obtained by distillation from caraway. The *B.P.* specifies that it contains 53 to 63% w/w of ketones calculated as carvone, $C_{10}H_{14}O$; the *U.S.N.F.* specifies not less than 50% v/v of *d*-carvone. **Soluble** 1 in 7 of alcohol (80%). **Store** at a temperature not exceeding 25° in well-filled airtight containers. Protect from light.

Caraway is an aromatic carminative and is employed as caraway water for the flatulent colic of infants.

Temporary estimated acceptable daily intake of (+)-carvone and (−)-carvone: up to 1 mg per kg body-weight. Further biochemical and metabolic studies are required.— Twenty-seventh Report of Joint FAO/WHO Expert Committee on Food Additives, *Tech. Rep. Ser. Wld Hlth Org. No. 696*, 1983.

Preparations

Concentrated Caraway Water *(B.P.C. 1973).* Aq. Cari Conc. Caraway oil 2 mL, alcohol (90%) 60 mL, water to 100 mL; shaken with 5 g of sterilised talc and filtered.

4621-g

Cardamom Fruit *(BAN).*

Cardam. Fruit; Cardamom Seed *(USAN)*; Cardamomi Fructus.

Pharmacopoeias. In *Br., Jpn,* and *Port.*

Arg., Egypt., and *U.S.N.F.* specify Cardamom Seed recently removed from the fruit.

The dried, nearly ripe fruit of *Elettaria cardamomum* var. *minuscula* (Zingiberaceae). Only the seeds are used in making preparations of cardamom; they are removed from the fruit when required for use; they have a strongly aromatic odour and an aromatic slightly bitter taste and contain not less than 4% v/w of volatile oil. The seeds should not be **stored** after removal from the fruit.

4622-q

Cardamom Oil *(BAN, USAN).*

Ol. Cardamom.

CAS — 8000-66-6.

Pharmacopoeias. In *Br.* Cardamom Oil (*U.S.N.F.*) is distilled from the seeds.

A colourless or pale yellow oil with an aromatic pungent odour and taste, distilled from crushed cardamom fruit (*B.P.*) or seeds (*U.S.N.F.*). **Soluble** 1 in 6 of alcohol (70%) (*B.P.*) or 1 in 5 (*U.S.N.F.*). **Store** at a temperature not exceeding 25° in well-filled airtight containers. Protect from light.

Preparations of cardamom fruit and oil are used as carminatives and as flavouring agents.

Preparations

Aromatic Cardamom Tincture *(B.P.).* Arom. Cardam. Tinct. Cardamom oil 0.3 mL, caraway oil 1 mL, cinnamon oil 1 mL, clove oil 1 mL, strong ginger tincture 6 mL, alcohol (90%) to 100 mL.

Compound Cardamom Tincture *(B.P.).* Co. Cardam. Tinct. Cardamom oil 0.045 mL, caraway oil 0.04 mL, cinnamon oil 0.0225 mL, glycerol 5 mL, with cochineal, in alcohol (60%) to 100 mL.

Compound Cardamom Tincture *(U.S.N.F.).* Prepared by macerating cardamom seed 2 g, cinnamon 2.5 g, and caraway 1.2 g with glycerol 5 mL and diluted alcohol to 100 mL. The tincture may be coloured. Store at a temperature not exceeding 40° in airtight containers. Protect from light.

4624-s

Cassia Oil

Chinese Cinnamon Oil; Cinnamon Oil *(USAN)*; Oleum Cassiae; Oleum Cinnamomi; Oleum Cinnamomi Cassiae.

CAS — 8007-80-5.

Pharmacopoeias. In *Chin., Egypt., Hung.,* and *Jpn.* Also in *U.S.N.F. Chin., Hung., Jpn,* and *Roum.* also include cassia bark.

A mobile yellowish or brownish oil with a fragrant pungent odour and a sweetish, spicy, burning taste, obtained by steam distillation from the leaves and twigs of *Cinnamomum cassia*, and rectified by distillation. It darkens with age or exposure to light, and becomes more viscous. The *U.S.N.F.* specifies not less than 80% v/v of aldehydes.

Soluble 1 in 2 of alcohol (70%) and 1 in 1 of glacial acetic acid. **Store** at a temperature not exceeding 40° in well-filled airtight containers.

STANDARD FOR CASSIA OIL. A British Standard Specification for Cassia Oil (BS 2999/17: 1972) is published by the British Standards Institution.

Cassia Oil has properties resembling those of cinnamon oil and is used similarly as a carminative and flavour.

Temporary estimated acceptable daily intake of cinnamaldehyde: up to 700 µg per kg body-weight. Further studies are required.— Twenty-eighth Report of Joint FAO/WHO Expert Committee on Food Additives, *Tech. Rep. Ser. Wld Hlth Org. No. 710*, 1984.

4628-y

Chamomile Flowers *(BAN).*

Anthemidis Flores; Anthemidis Flos; Anthemis; Camomille Romaine; Chamomile; Flos Chamomillae Romanae; Manzanilla Romana; Roman Chamomile; Roman Chamomile Flowers.

NOTE. German chamomile is known as Matricaria Flowers.

Pharmacopoeias. In *Arg., Aust., Belg., Br., Eur., Fr., Ger., It., Neth., Span.,* and *Swiss.*

The dried flowerheads of the cultivated double variety of *Anthemis nobilis* (Compositae), containing not less than 0.7% v/w of volatile oil. **Store** in well-closed containers. Protect from light.

An infusion of chamomile flowers, 'chamomile tea' is a domestic remedy for indigestion. A poultice of the flowers has sometimes been applied externally in the early stages of inflammation.

There have been rare reports of contact sensitivity and anaphylaxis.

Proprietary Preparations

Kamillosan *(Norgine, UK). Ointment*, extract of chamomile 10%, volatile oil of chamomile 0.5%. For cracked nipples and nappy rash.

4629-j

Cineole

Cajuputol; Eucalyptol. 1,8-Epoxy-*p*-menthane; 1,3,3-Trimethyl-2-oxabicyclo[2.2.2]octane.

$C_{10}H_{18}O$=154.3.

CAS — 470-82-6.

Pharmacopoeias. In *Arg., Egypt., Mex., Port., Span.,* and *Swiss.* Also in *B.P.C. 1973.*

A colourless liquid with an aromatic camphoraceous odour obtained from eucalyptus oil, cajuput oil, and other oils.

Soluble 1 in 2 of alcohol (70%). **Store** in a cool place in airtight containers. Protect from light.

Cineole has the actions and uses of eucalyptus oil. It has been used in counter-irritant ointments and in dentifrices. It has also been used in nasal preparations, but oily solutions inhibit ciliary movement and may cause lipoid pneumonia.

4630-q

Cinnamon *(BAN, USAN).*

Canela; Canela do Ceilão; Cannelle Dite de Ceylan; Ceylon Cinnamon; Ceylonzimt; Cinnam.; Cinnamomi Cortex; Cinnamon Bark; Zimt.

Pharmacopoeias. In *Aust., Belg., Br., Braz., Egypt., Eur., Fr., Mex., Neth., Port., Roum., Span.,* and *Swiss.* Also in *U.S.N.F.*

The *B.P.* specifies the dried bark of the shoots of coppiced trees of *Cinnamomum zeylanicum* Blume [Lauraceae] containing not less than 1.2% v/w of volatile oil. The *U.S.N.F.* specifies the dried bark of *Cinnamomum loureirii* Nees containing not less than 2.5% v/w of volatile oil. **Powdered Cinnamon** (*B.P.*) contains not less than 1% v/w of volatile oil. **Store** in well-closed containers. Protect from light.

4631-p

Cinnamon Oil *(BAN).*

Aetheroleum Cinnamomi Zeylanici; Ceylon Cinnamon Bark Oil; Cinnam. Oil; Esencia de Canela; Essence de Cannelle de Ceylan; Oleum Cinnamomi; Zimtöl.

CAS — 8007-80-5.

Pharmacopoeias. In *Arg., Aust., Belg., Br., Cz., Egypt., Fr., Mex., Roum., Span.,* and *Swiss.*
Cinnamon Oil in *Chin. P., Jpn P.,* and *U.S.N.F.* is Cassia Oil.

A yellow oil with characteristic odour obtained by distillation from cinnamon. It becomes reddish-brown with age. It contains 60 to 80% w/w of aldehydes, calculated as cinnamaldehyde (C_9H_8O).
Store in well-filled well-closed containers, at a temperature not exceeding 25°. Protect from light.

Cinnamon and cinnamon oil are carminative and are largely used as flavouring agents. There have been a number of reports of sensitivity to cinnamon.

Temporary estimated acceptable daily intake of cinnamaldehyde: up to 700 µg per kg body-weight. Further studies are required.— Twenty-eighth Report of Joint FAO/WHO Expert Committee on Food Additives, *Tech. Rep. Ser. Wld Hlth Org. No. 710*, 1984.

For the estimated acceptable daily intake of eugenol, see p.1063.

Preparations

Concentrated Cinnamon Water *(B.P.).* Cinnamon oil 2 mL, alcohol (90%) 60 mL, water to 100 mL; shaken with 5 g of sterilised talc and filtered.

4633-w

Citronella Oil

Oleum Citronellae.

CAS — 8000-29-1.

Pharmacopoeias. In *Aust., Belg., Cz., Roum.,* and *Swiss.* Also in *B.P.C. 1973. Aust.* and *Roum.* give Oleum Melissae Indicum as a synonym for citronella oil.

A pale to deep yellow oil with a pleasant characteristic odour, obtained by distillation from *Cymbopogon nardus* or *C. winterianus* (Gramineae) or varietal or hybrid forms of these species. The chief constituents are geraniol ($C_{10}H_{18}O$) and citronellal ($C_{10}H_{18}O$). **Soluble** 1 in 4 of alcohol (80%) forming a clear or slightly opalescent solution. **Store** in a cool place in well-filled airtight containers. Protect from light.

STANDARD FOR CITRONELLA OILS. British Standard Specifications for Ceylon Citronella Oil (BS 2999/18: 1972) and Java Citronella Oil (BS 2999/19: 1972) are published by the British Standards Institution.

Citronella oil is used as a perfume and insect repellent. Hypersensitivity has been reported.

4634-e

Clove *(BAN).*

Caryoph.; Caryophylli Flos; Caryophyllum; Clou de Girofle; Cloves; Cravinho; Cravo-da-India; Gewürznelke; Giroflier.

Pharmacopoeias. In *Aust., Br., Chin., Egypt., Eur., Fr., Hung., Jpn, Neth., Port.,* and *Swiss.*

The dried flower-buds of *Syzgium aromaticum* (= *Eugenia caryophyllus*) (Myrtacaea), containing not less than 15% v/w of volatile oil. **Powdered Clove** (*B.P.*) contains not less than 12% v/w of volatile oil. Clove has a strong, characteristic, aromatic, spicy odour and an aromatic pungent taste. **Store** in a well-closed container. Protect from light.

4635-l

Clove Oil *(BAN, USAN).*

Esencia de Clavo; Essence de Girofle; Nelkenöl; Ol. Caryoph.; Oleum Caryophylli.

CAS — 8000-34-8.

Pharmacopoeias. In *Arg., Aust., Br., Cz., Egypt., Fr., Ger., Hung., Ind., It., Jpn, Jug., Mex., Neth., Port., Roum., Span.,* and *Swiss.* Also in *U.S.N.F.*

A colourless or pale yellow oil with the characteristic odour and taste of clove, obtained by distillation from clove. It darkens and thickens with age and on exposure to air. The *U.S.N.F.* specifies not less than 85% v/v of total phenolic substances, chiefly eugenol **Soluble** 1 in 2 of alcohol (70%). **Store** at a temperature not exceeding 25° in well-filled airtight containers. Protect from light.

The Pharmaceutical Society's Department of Pharmaceutical Sciences found that PVC bottles softened and distorted fairly rapidly in the presence of clove oil, which should not be stored or dispensed in such bottles.— *Pharm. J.*, 1973, *1*, 100.

The solubility of clove oil in macrogol esters.— K. Thoma and G. Pfaff, *J. Soc. cosmet. Chem.*, 1976, *27*, 221.

STANDARD FOR CLOVE OILS. British Standard Specifications for oils of clove bud, leaf, and stem (BS 2999/20/21/22: 1972) and Indonesian Clove Leaf Oil (BS 2999/54: 1975) are published by the British Standards Institution.

Clove oil is a carminative that is sometimes used in the treatment of flatulent colic. It is also used as a flavouring agent.
Applied externally clove oil is irritant but can produce local anaesthesia. It is used as a domestic remedy for toothache, a plug of cotton wool soaked in the oil being inserted in the cavity of the carious tooth; repeated application may damage the gingival tissues. Mixed with zinc oxide, it is used as a temporary anodyne dental filling, though eugenol (see p.1063) is often preferred.

For the estimated acceptable daily intake of eugenol, see p.1063.

4637-j

Coriander *(BAN).*

Coentro; Coriand.; Coriander Fruit; Coriander Seed; Fruto de Cilantro.

Pharmacopoeias. In *Aust., Belg., Br., Egypt., Fr., Hung., Pol., Port.,* and *Span.*

The dried ripe fruits of *Coriandrum sativum* (Umbelliferae), containing not less than 0.3% v/w of volatile oil.
Powdered Coriander (*B.P.*) contains not less than 0.2% v/w of volatile oil. **Store** at a temperature not exceeding 25° in a dry place; the powdered drug should also be kept in well-closed containers.

4638-z

Coriander Oil *(BAN, USAN).*

Ol. Coriand; Oleum Coriandri.

CAS — 8008-52-4.

Pharmacopoeias. In *Arg., Br.,* and *Cz.* Also in *U.S.N.F.*

A colourless or pale yellow oil with the characteristic odour and taste of coriander, obtained by distillation from coriander.
Soluble 1 in 3 of alcohol (70%). **Store** at a temperature not exceeding 25° in well-filled airtight containers. Protect from light.

STANDARD FOR CORIANDER OIL. A British Standard Specification for Coriander Oil (BS 2999/33: 1971) is published by the British Standards Institution.

Coriander oil is aromatic and carminative.

An estimated acceptable daily intake of up to 500 µg per kg body-weight was established for citral, geranyl acetate, citronellol, linalol, and linalyl acetate, expressed as citral.— Twenty-third Report of the Joint FAO/WHO Expert Committee on Food Additives, *Tech. Rep. Ser. Wld Hlth Org. No. 648*, 1980.

3268-x

Dementholised Mint Oil *(BAN).*

Pharmacopoeias. In *Br.*
Mint oil or Mentha oil is in *Ger.* and *Jpn. Belg.* specifies oil from *Mentha arvensis* var. *piperascens* or *M. piperita. Ind.* allows oil from various species of *Mentha.*

A colourless to pale yellow oil with a characteristic odour obtained by steam distillation followed by partial dementholisation and processing from the flowering tops of *Mentha arvensis* var. *piperascens* (Labiatae). The *B.P.* describes Brazilian Oil which contains between 3 and 10% w/w of esters calculated as menthyl acetate, $C_{12}H_{22}O_2$ and between 35 and 55% of free alcohols calculated as menthol. The *B.P.* also describes Chinese Oil which contains between 3 and 8% of esters calculated as menthyl acetate and between 41 and 58% of free alcohols calculated as menthol.
Soluble 1 in 4 of alcohol (70%); there may be some opalescence on further dilution. **Store** at a temperature not exceeding 25° in well-filled well-closed containers. Protect from light.

STANDARD FOR DEMENTHOLISED MINT OIL. A British Standard Specification for Dementholised Mentha Arvensis Oil (BS 2999/56: 1975) is published by the British Standards Institution.

Dementholised mint oil is used as a flavour.

4642-e

Dill Oil *(BAN).*

European Dill Seed Oil; Oleum Anethi.

CAS — 8016-06-6.

Pharmacopoeias. In *Br.*

A colourless or pale yellow oil obtained by distillation from the dried ripe fruits of dill, *Anethum graveolens* (Umbelliferae). It darkens with age and has a characteristic odour. It contains 43 to 63% of carvone ($C_{10}H_{14}O$).
Soluble 1 in 1 of alcohol (90%) and 1 in 10 of alcohol (80%). **Store** at a temperature not exceeding 25° in well-filled well-closed containers. Protect from light.

Dill oil, usually in the form of dill water, is used as an aromatic carminative.

Temporary estimated acceptable daily intake of (+)-carvone and (−)-carvone: up to 1 mg per kg body-weight. Further biochemical and metabolic studies are required.— Twenty-fifth Report of Joint FAO/WHO Expert Committee on Food Additives, *Tech. Rep. Ser. Wld Hlth Org. No. 669*, 1981.

Preparations

Concentrated Dill Water *(B.P.C. 1973).* Aqua Anethi Concentrata. Dill oil 2 mL, alcohol (90%) 60 mL, water to 100 mL; shaken with 5 g of sterilised talc and filtered.

18370-v

Ethyl Cinnamate *(BAN).*

Ethyl (*E*)-3-phenylprop-2-enoate.
$C_{11}H_{12}O_2$=176.2.

CAS — 103-36-6.

Pharmacopoeias. In *Br.*

A clear colourless or almost colourless liquid with a fruity balsamic odour. Practically **insoluble** in water; miscible with most organic solvents.

Ethyl cinnamate is used as a flavour and perfume.

4644-y

Eucalyptus Oil *(BAN, USAN).*
Esencia de Eucalipto; Essence d'Eucalyptus Rectifiée; Eucalypti Aetheroleum; Oleum Eucalypti.

CAS — 8000-48-4.

Pharmacopoeias. In *Arg., Aust., Belg., Br., Chin., Cz., Egypt., Eur., Fr., Ger., Hung., Ind., It., Jpn, Neth., Pol., Port., Roum., Rus., Span.,* and *Swiss.* Also in *U.S.N.F.*

A colourless or pale yellow oil with a characteristic aromatic camphoraceous odour and a pungent camphoraceous cooling taste, obtained by rectifying the oil distilled from the fresh leaves and terminal branches of various species of *Eucalyptus* (Myrtaceae) (*E. globulus, E. fruticetorum* = *E. polybractea,* and *E. smithii* are used). It contains not less than 70% w/w of cineole (eucalyptol). **Soluble** 1 in 5 of alcohol (70%). **Store** at a temperature not exceeding 25° in well-filled airtight containers. Protect from light.

STANDARD FOR EUCALYPTUS OILS. British Standard Specifications for Eucalyptus Oil obtained from *E. citriodora* (BS 2999/23: 1972) and Eucalyptus Oil from *E. globulus* (BS 2999/53: 1975) are published by the British Standards Institution.

Adverse Effects and Treatment
The symptoms of poisoning with eucalyptus oil include epigastric burning, nausea and vomiting, dizziness and muscular weakness, miosis, and a feeling of suffocation. Cyanosis, delirium and convulsions may occur. Deaths have been recorded from doses as low as 3.5 mL.

A report of severe poisoning in a 3-year-old child who had taken about 10 mL of eucalyptus oil.— S. Patel and J. Wiggins, *Archs Dis. Childh.,* 1980, *55,* 405.

Uses and Administration
Eucalyptus oil has been taken by mouth for catarrh. It has been used as an inhalation often in combination with other volatile substances. Eucalyptus oil has also been applied as a rubefacient.

4645-j

Eugenol *(BAN, USAN).*
4-Allylguaiacol; Eugen.; Eugenic Acid. 4-Allyl-2-methoxyphenol.
$C_{10}H_{12}O_2$=164.2.

CAS — 97-53-0.

Pharmacopoeias. In *Belg., Egypt., Jug., Nord., Pol., Swiss,* and *U.S.*

A colourless or pale yellow liquid with an odour of clove and a spicy pungent taste; it may be obtained from clove oil.
Slightly **soluble** in water; soluble 1 in 2 of alcohol (70%); miscible with alcohol, chloroform, ether, and fixed oils. Eugenol darkens in colour with age or on exposure to air. **Store** at a temperature not exceeding 25° in well-filled airtight containers. Protect from light.

Eugenol is an irritant and sensitiser and can produce local anaesthesia. It is reported to inhibit prostaglandin synthesis.
It is employed in dentistry often mixed with zinc oxide, as a temporary anodyne dental filling.

Estimated acceptable daily intake of eugenol: up to 2.5 mg per kg body-weight. Eugenol was not considered to have carcinogenic potential.— Twenty-sixth Report of the Joint FAO/WHO Expert Committee on Food Additives, *Tech. Rep. Ser. Wld Hlth Org. No. 683,* 1982.

4646-z

Fennel
Fenchel; Fennel Fruit; Fennel Seed; Fenouil; Fenouil Doux; Foeniculum; Fruto de Hinojo; Funcho.

Pharmacopoeias. In *Aust., Belg., Chin., Cz., Egypt., Fr., Ger., Hung., Jpn, Neth., Pol., Port., Roum., Rus., Span.,* and *Swiss.* Also in *B.P.C. 1973.*

The dried fruits of cultivated plants of *Foeniculum vulgare* var. *vulgare* (Umbelliferae), containing not less than 1.2% v/w of volatile oil. **Powdered Fennel** (*B.P.C. 1973*) contains not less than 1% v/w of volatile oil. **Store** in a cool dry place; the powdered drug should be stored in airtight containers. Protect from light.

4647-c

Fennel Oil *(USAN).*
Aetheroleum Foeniculi; Esencia de Hinojo; Essência de Funcho; Oleum Foeniculi.

CAS — 8006-84-6.

Pharmacopoeias. In *Arg., Aust., Cz., Egypt., Ger., Hung., Jpn, Jug., Neth., Nord., Pol., Roum.,* and *Swiss.* Also in *U.S.N.F.*

A colourless or pale yellow oil with the characteristic aromatic odour and taste of fennel, obtained by distillation from fennel. **Soluble** 1 in 1 of alcohol (90%). If solid matter separates it should be melted and mixed before use. **Store** in airtight containers.

Fennel oil is used as an aromatic carminative.

4652-y

Geranium Oil
Aetheroleum Pelargonii; Oleum Geranii; Pelargonium Oil; Rose Geranium Oil.

CAS — 8000-46-2.

Pharmacopoeias. In *Cz.* and *Nord.*

An oil obtained by distillation from the aerial parts of various species and hybrid forms of *Pelargonium* (Geraniaceae).

STANDARD FOR GERANIUM OILS. British Standard Specifications for Kenya, North Africa, and Réunion geranium oils (BS 2999/24/25/26: 1972) are published by the British Standards Institution.

Geranium oil is used to perfume various preparations.

An estimated acceptable daily intake of up to 500 µg per kg body-weight was established for citral, geranyl acetate, citronellol, linalol, and linalyl acetate, expressed as citral.— Twenty-third Report of Joint FAO/WHO Expert Committee on Food Additives, *Tech. Rep. Ser. Wld Hlth Org. No. 648,* 1980.

4653-j

Ginger *(BAN).*
Gengibre; Gingembre; Ingwer; Zingib.; Zingiber.

Pharmacopoeias. In *Aust., Belg., Br., Chin., Egypt., Jpn, Mex., Port.,* and *Swiss.*

The scraped or unscraped rhizome of *Zingiber officinale* (Zingiberaceae), known in commerce as unbleached ginger. It contains not less than 4.5% of alcohol (90%)-soluble extractive and not less than 10% of water-soluble extractive. **Powdered Ginger** (*B.P.*) is light yellow or yellowish-brown. **Store** in a dry place, in well-closed containers. Protect from light.

Ginger has carminative properties. It is also used as a flavouring agent and has been tried in motion sickness.

The reduction of motion sickness by ginger.— D. B. Mowrey and D. E. Clayson, *Lancet,* 1982, *1,* 655.

Preparations

Ginger Syrup *(B.P.C. 1973, A.P.F.).* Syrupus Zingiberis. Strong ginger tincture 5 mL, syrup to 100 mL.

Strong Ginger Tincture *(B.P.).* Strong Ginger Tinct.; Ginger Essence. Prepared by percolating ginger 50 g with alcohol (90%) to 100 mL.

Weak Ginger Tincture *(B.P.).* Weak Ginger Tinct. Strong ginger tincture 20 mL, alcohol (90%) to 100 mL.

Proprietary Names and Manufacturers
Travellers *(Phillips Yeast, UK)*; Zintona *(GPL, Switz.).*

4654-z

Juniper
Baccae Juniperi; Genièvre; Juniper Berry; Juniper Fruit; Juniperi Fructus; Wacholderbeeren; Zimbro.

Pharmacopoeias. In *Aust., Belg., Cz., Ger., Hung., Jug., Port., Roum., Rus.,* and *Swiss.*

The dried ripe fruits of *Juniperus communis* (Cupressaceae).

4655-c

Juniper Oil
Essence de Genièvre; Juniper Berry Oil; Oleum Juniperi; Wacholderöl.

CAS — 8012-91-7.

Pharmacopoeias. In *Aust., Fr., Hung., Jug., Roum.,* and *Swiss.*

The oil distilled from the dried ripe fruits of *J. communis.* **Store** in a cool place in airtight containers. Protect from light.

Juniper oil has been used as a carminative.

4659-x

Lavender Oil *(BAN, USAN).*
Esencia de Alhucema; Esencia de Espliego; Essência de Alfazema; Lavender Flower Oil; Oleum Lavandulae.

CAS — 8000-28-0.

Pharmacopoeias. The title of lavender oil is used in many pharmacopoeias usually to describe oil obtained from *Lavandula officinalis* (=*L. spica* L. =*L. vera*), although the *B.P.* specifies *L. intermedia* or *L. angustifolia.*

A colourless or pale yellow or yellowish-green oil with a characteristic fragrant odour reminiscent of the flowers, obtained by distillation from the fresh flowering tops. Lavender Oil *U.S.N.F.* may also be produced synthetically.
Soluble 1 in 4 of alcohol (70%). Solutions in alcohol may be slightly opalescent. The oils become less soluble with age. *U.S.N.F.* specifies that it contains not less than 35% of total esters calculated as linalyl acetate ($C_{12}H_{20}O_2$). **Store** in airtight containers.

STANDARD FOR LAVENDER OIL. A British Standard Specification for French Lavender Oil (BS 2999/34: 1971) is published by the British Standards Institution.

The solubility of lavender oil in macrogol esters.— K. Thoma and G. Pfaff, *J. Soc. cosmet. Chem.,* 1976, *27,* 221.

Lavender oil has been used as a carminative and as a colouring and flavouring agent. It is sometimes applied externally as an insect repellent. Its chief use is in perfumery and it is occasionally used in ointments and other pharmaceutical preparations to cover disagreeable odours.

An estimated acceptable daily intake of up to 500 µg per kg body-weight was established for citral, geranyl acetate, citronellol, linalol, and linalyl acetate, expressed as citral.— Twenty-third Report of Joint FAO/WHO Expert Committee on Food Additives, *Tech. Rep. Ser. Wld Hlth Org. No. 648,* 1980.

4660-y

Spike Lavender Oil
Ol. Lavand. Spic.; Oleum Lavandulae Spicatae; Spike Oil.

CAS — 8016-78-2.

The oil from *Lavandula latifolia* (= *L. spica* DC.) (Labiatae).

STANDARD FOR SPIKE LAVENDER OIL. A British Standard Specification for Spike Lavender Oil (BS 2999/42: 1971) is published by the British Standards Institution.

Spike lavender oil resembles lavender oil in its properties and is mainly used in perfumery.

An estimated acceptable daily intake of up to 500 µg per kg body-weight was established for citral, geranyl acetate, citronellol, linalol, and linalyl acetate, expressed as citral.— Twenty-third Report of Joint FAO/WHO Expert Committee on Food Additives, *Tech. Rep. Ser. Wld Hlth Org. No. 648,* 1980.

4661-j

Lemon Grass Oil
Essência de Capim-Limão; Indian Melissa Oil; Indian Verbena Oil; Lemongrass Oil; Oleum Graminis Citrati.

CAS — 8007-02-1.

The oil is obtained by distillation from *Cymbopogon flexuosus* or *C. citratus* (Gramineae).

STANDARD FOR LEMON GRASS OILS. British Standard Specifications for East Indian and West Indian Lemon Grass Oils (BS 2999/35/36: 1971) are published by the British Standards Institution.

Lemon grass oil was formerly given as a carminative. It has been used in perfumery and as a flavouring agent.

An estimated acceptable daily intake of up to 500 µg per kg body-weight was established for citral, geranyl acetate, citronellol, linalol, and linalyl acetate, expressed as citral.— Twenty-third Report of Joint FAO/WHO Expert Committee on Food Additives, *Tech. Rep. Ser. Wld Hlth Org. No. 648*, 1980.

4662-z

Lemon Oil *(BAN, USAN).*
Aetheroleum Citri; Citronenöl; Esencia de Cidra; Essência de Limão; Essence de Citron; Ol. Limon.; Oleum Citri; Oleum Limonis.

CAS — 8008-56-8.

Pharmacopoeias. In *Arg., Aust., Belg., Br., Cz., Egypt., Fr., Ger., Hung., It., Jug., Mex., Pol., Port., Roum., Span.,* and *Swiss.* Also in *U.S.N.F.*
The *B.P.* also includes a monograph on dried lemon peel; *Egypt.* includes fresh or dried lemon peel; *Fr.* and *Port.* include fresh lemon peel.

A pale yellow or greenish-yellow oil with a characteristic odour and taste, obtained by expression from the fresh peel of the ripe or nearly ripe fruit of *Citrus limon* (Rutaceae). The *B.P.* specifies not less than 3.5% w/w of aldehydes calculated as citral ($C_{10}H_{16}O$). The *U.S.N.F.* specifies 2.2 to 3.8% of aldehydes, calculated as citral, for California-type Lemon Oil and 3.0 to 5.5% for Italian-type Lemon Oil.
B.P. **solubilities** are: soluble 1 in 12 of alcohol (90%), the solution having a slight opalescence; miscible with dehydrated alcohol. *U.S.N.F.* solubilities are: soluble 1 in 3 of alcohol. **Store** at a temperature not exceeding 25° in well-filled airtight containers. Protect from light.

Lemon oil is chiefly used as a flavouring agent.

An estimated acceptable daily intake of up to 500 µg per kg body-weight was established for citral, geranyl acetate, citronellol, linalol, and linalyl acetate, expressed as citral.— Twenty-third Report of Joint FAO/WHO Expert Committee on Food Additives, *Tech. Rep. Ser. Wld Hlth Org. No. 648*, 1980.
The use of a preparation of *d*-limonene for dissolving gallstones.— H. Igimi *et al., Am. J. dig. Dis.*, 1976, *21*, 926.

4663-c

Terpeneless Lemon Oil *(BAN).*
Oleum Limonis Deterpenatum.

Pharmacopoeias. In *Br.*

A colourless or pale yellow oil with the characteristic odour and taste of lemon, prepared by concentrating lemon oil *in vacuo* until most of the terpenes have been removed, or by solvent partition. It contains not less than 40% w/w of aldehydes calculated as citral.
Soluble 1 in 1 of alcohol (80%). **Store** at a temperature not exceeding 25° in well-filled well-closed containers. Protect from light.

Terpeneless lemon oil is used as a flavouring agent. It has the advantages of being stronger in flavour and odour and more readily soluble than the natural oil and is the oil used in the preparation of lemon spirit and lemon syrup.

An estimated acceptable daily intake of up to 500 µg per kg body-weight was established for citral, geranyl acetate, citronellol, linalol, and linalyl acetate, expressed as citral.— Twenty-third Report of Joint FAO/WHO Expert Committee on Food Additives, *Tech. Rep. Ser. Wld Hlth Org. No. 648*, 1980.

Preparations
Lemon Spirit *(B.P., A.P.F.).* Sp. Limon. Terpeneless lemon oil 10% v/v in alcohol (96%).
Lemon Syrup *(B.P.).* Lemon spirit 0.5 mL, citric acid monohydrate 2.5 g, invert syrup 10 mL, syrup to 100 mL.
A.P.F. has a similar preparation without invert syrup.
Lemon Syrup (*B.P.*) was not considered to be adequately preserved since it failed to pass microbial spoilage tests with 4 different organisms.— T. R. Kurup and L. S. C. Wan, *Pharm. J.*, 1986, *2*, 761.
Lemon Syrup Neutral *(A.P.F.).* Lemon spirit 0.5 mL, syrup to 100 mL.

4667-x

Mace Oil

CAS — 8007-12-3.

NOTE. Mace has also been used as a name for a tear gas.

A volatile oil obtained by distillation from mace, the arillus of the seed of *Myristica fragrans* (Myristicaceae).

Mace is used as a flavour similarly to nutmeg. As with nutmeg, large doses of mace may cause epileptiform convulsions.

4668-r

Matricaria Flowers *(BAN).*
Camomille Allemande; Camomilla; Chamomilla; Flos Chamomillae; Flos Chamomillae Vulgaris; German Chamomile; Kamillenblüten; Manzanilla Ordinaria; Matricaria; Matricariae Flos.

CAS — 8002-66-2 (Matricaria oil).

Pharmacopoeias. In *Arg., Aust., Br., Cz., Egypt., Eur., Fr., Ger., Hung., It., Jug., Neth., Pol., Port., Roum., Rus., Span.,* and *Swiss. Aust.* and *Hung.* also include Matricaria Oil.

The dried flowerheads of *Matricaria recutita* (= *Chamomilla recutita*) (Compositae), containing not less than 0.4% v/w of volatile oil. **Store** in well-closed containers. Protect from light.

Matricaria is used for the same purposes as chamomile (see p.1061).

Ventricular catheterisation studies in 12 patients with heart disease showed that chamomile tea prepared from matricaria had no significant cardiac effects. A marked hypnotic effect was observed; approximately 10 minutes after drinking the tea, 10 patients fell into a deep sleep lasting about 90 minutes.— L. Gould *et al., J. clin. Pharmac.*, 1973, *13*, 475. See also N. R. Farnsworth and B. M. Morgan (letter), *J. Am. med. Ass.*, 1972, *221*, 410.

4670-z

Melissa
Balm; Melissenblatt.

Pharmacopoeias. In *Aust., Belg., Cz., Fr., Ger., Jug., Roum., Span.,* and *Swiss.*

The leaves or leaves and tops of *Melissa officinalis* (Labiatae).

Melissa has been used as a carminative.

An estimated acceptable daily intake of up to 500 µg per kg body-weight was established for citral, geranyl acetate, citronellol, linalol, and linalyl acetate, expressed as citral.— Twenty-third Report of Joint FAO/WHO Expert Committee on Food Additives, *Tech. Rep. Ser. Wld Hlth Org. No. 648*, 1980.

4672-k

Black Mustard
Graine de Moutarde Noire; Mostarda Preta; Moutarde Jonciforme; Schwarzer Senfsame; Semilla de Mostaza; Sinapis Nigra.

Pharmacopoeias. In *Aust., Belg., Egypt., Fr., Jug., Mex., Port., Roum., Span.,* and *Swiss. Fr.* specifies the seeds of *B. juncea. Swiss* allows *B. nigra, B. juncea,* and other species. *Chin.* includes Semen Sinapis.

The dried ripe seeds of *Brassica nigra* (= *B. sinapioides*) (Cruciferae).

4673-a

White Mustard
Sinapis Alba.

Pharmacopoeias. In *Fr.*

The dried ripe seeds of *Brassica alba* (Cruciferae).

4675-x

Volatile Mustard Oil
Allyl Isothiocyanate; Allylsenföl; Essence of Mustard; Oleum Sinapis Volatile.

CAS — 57-06-7.

Pharmacopoeias. In *Aust., Belg., Cz., Hung., Jug., Pol., Port.,* and *Roum. Fr.* includes allyl isothiocyanate.

It may be prepared synthetically or distilled from black mustard seeds after expression of the fixed oil and contains not less than 92% w/w of allyl isothiocyanate, (C_3H_5CNS = 99.15).

CAUTION. *Volatile Mustard Oil is a powerful vesicant and irritant and should not be inhaled or tasted undiluted.*

Black mustard and white mustard are used as condiments. They have been used as emetics and counter-irritants.
Volatile mustard oil is an extremely powerful irritant that has been used as a counter-irritant and rubefacient. Expressed mustard oil contains a smaller proportion of volatile oil and was used as a less powerful counter-irritant.

4676-r

Neroli Oil
Esencia de Azahar; Essência de Flor de Laranjeira; Oleum Neroli; Orange Flower Oil *(USAN)*; Orange-flower Oil.

CAS — 8016-38-4.

Pharmacopoeias. In *Arg., Aust., Belg., Egypt., Mex., Port.,* and *Swiss.* Also in *U.S.N.F. Aust.* also includes a monograph on the dried flowers.

A pale yellow, slightly fluorescent oil, becoming reddish-brown on exposure to air and light, with a characteristic odour and a sweet aromatic taste with a bitter after-taste, obtained by distillation from the flowers of the bitter-orange tree, *Citrus aurantium* (Rutaceae). It may become turbid or solid at low temperatures. It is neutral to litmus.
Soluble 1 in 2 of alcohol (80%), the solution becoming turbid on the addition of more of the alcohol. **Store** in airtight containers. Protect from light.

STANDARD FOR NEROLI OIL. A British Standard Specification for Neroli Oil (BS 2999/8: 1965) is published by the British Standards Institution.

Neroli oil is used as a flavouring agent and in perfumery. *Citrus aurantium* is used in folk medicine.

Estimated acceptable daily intake of methyl anthranilate: up to 1.5 mg per kg body-weight and of methyl *N*-methylanthranilate: up to 200 µg per kg.— Twenty-third Report of Joint FAO/WHO Expert Committee on Food Additives, *Tech. Rep. Ser. Wld Hlth Org. No. 648*, 1980.

Preparations
Orange Flower Water *(U.S.N.F.).* A saturated solution prepared by distilling the fresh flowers of *C. aurantium* with water and removing the excess volatile oil from the clear aqueous portion of the distillate.

4677-f

Niaouli Oil

Essence de Niaouli.

CAS — 8014-68-4.

Pharmacopoeias. In *Arg., Belg., Fr., Neth., Port., Roum.,* and *Span.*

An oil, obtained by distillation from the fresh leaves of *Melaleuca viridiflora* or *Melaleuca quinquenervia* (Myrtaceae).

Niaouli oil contains cineole and has similar actions to eucalyptus oil (p.1063).

4679-n

Nutmeg

Muscade; Myristica; Noz Moscada; Nuez Moscada; Nux Moschata.

Pharmacopoeias. In *Egypt., Port., Span.,* and *Swiss* . In *B.P.C. 1973* which also includes Powdered Nutmeg.

The dried kernels of the seeds of *Myristica fragrans* (Myristicaceae).

4678-d

Nutmeg Oil *(BAN, USAN).*

Ätherisches Muskatöl; Esencia de Nuez Moscada; Essência de Moscada; Essence de Muscade; Myristica Oil; Oleum Myristicae.

CAS — 8008-45-5.

Pharmacopoeias. In *Arg., Aust.,* and *Br.* Also in *U.S.N.F.*

A volatile oil obtained by distillation from nutmeg. It is a colourless, pale yellow or pale green liquid with an odour and taste of nutmeg. It is available as East Indian Nutmeg Oil and West Indian Nutmeg Oil.
East Indian oil is **soluble** 1 in 3 of alcohol (90%), West Indian 1 in 4. **Store** at a temperature not exceeding 25° in well-filled airtight containers. Protect from light.

STANDARD FOR NUTMEG OILS. British Standard Specifications for East Indian and West Indian Nutmeg Oil (BS 2999/37/38: 1971) are published by the British Standards Institution.

Adverse Effects

Nutmeg, taken in large doses may cause nausea and vomiting, flushing, dry mouth, tachycardia, stimulation of the central nervous system possibly with epileptiform convulsions, miosis, mydriasis, euphoria, and hallucinations.

Within 4 hours of taking 28 g of nutmeg in water and orange juice, a 19-year-old woman felt cold and shivery. This was followed after 6 to 8 hours by severe vomiting accompanied by hallucinations. For a week she had poor concentration and was disorientated. The hallucinogen in nutmeg was believed to be myristicin.— D. J. Panayotopoulos and D. D. Chisholm (letter), *Br. med. J.,* 1970, *1,* 754. A similar report.— R. A. Faguet and K. F. Rowland, *Am. J. Psychiat.,* 1978, *135,* 860.

Within 3 days of receiving ground nutmeg 9 teaspoonfuls daily to control the diarrhoea associated with medullary carcinoma of the thyroid, a patient complained of dry eyes and mouth, blurred vision, dizziness, tingling, and feelings of depersonalisation and remoteness. The symptoms gradually subsided as the dose was reduced.— G. S. Venables *et al.* (letter), *Br. med. J.,* 1976, *1,* 96.

Ingestion of freshly ground nutmeg 1.5 to 4 g three to four times daily for 2 days by 2 subjects produced constipation, but no aspirin-like effect on biphasic platelet aggregation was noted. Both subjects also felt lightheaded, slightly disorientated, occasionally nauseated, flushed, and had nasal congestion and very dry mouths; pupil size was unaffected.— W. H. Dietz and M. J. Stuart (letter), *New Engl. J. Med.,* 1976, *294,* 503.

Uses and Administration

Nutmeg and nutmeg oil are aromatic and carminative and are used as flavouring agents. Nutmeg oil and expressed nutmeg oil, a solid fat, are rubefacient. Nutmeg is reported to inhibit prostaglandin synthesis.

Reports of diarrhoea associated with increased plasma-prostaglandin concentrations responding to treatment with nutmeg: J. A. Barrowman *et al., Br. med. J.,* 1975, *3,* 11; *idem* (letter), 160; I. Shafran *et al.* (letter), *New Engl. J. Med.,* 1977, *296,* 694.

4680-k

Orange Oil *(BAN, USAN).*

Arancia Dolce Essenza; Essência de Laranja; Essence of Orange; Essence of Portugal; Sweet Orange Oil.

CAS — 8008-57-9.

NOTE. The oil from the flowers of *Citrus aurantium* is known as neroli oil or orange flower oil (p.1064).

Pharmacopoeias. In *Br., Fr., It.,* and *Jpn.* Also in *U.S.N.F.* Bitter orange oil is included in *Belg., Port.,* and *Span.*

Orange oil is obtained by mechanical means from the fresh peel of the sweet orange *Citrus sinensis* (Rutaceae). The *B.P.* specifies not less than 1% w/w of aldehydes calculated as decanal ($C_{10}H_{20}O$). The *U.S.N.F.* describes California-type Orange Oil and Florida-type Orange Oil and specifies 1.2 to 2.5% of aldehydes calculated as decanal.
A yellow, orange, or yellowish-brown liquid with an odour and taste characteristic of orange.
Soluble 1 in 7 of alcohol (90%) but rarely with the formation of bright solutions on account of the presence of waxy non-volatile substances; soluble 1 in 1 of glacial acetic acid.**Store** at a temperature not exceeding 25° in well-filled airtight containers. Protect from light.

STANDARD FOR ORANGE OIL. A British Standard Specification for Sweet Orange Oil (BS 2999/43: 1971) is published by the British Standards Institution.

Orange oil is used as a flavouring agent and in perfumery.

Preparations

Aromatic Elixir *(U.S.N.F.).* Orange oil *U.S.N.F.* 0.24 mL, lemon oil *U.S.N.F.* 0.06 mL, coriander oil 0.024 mL, anise oil 0.006 mL, syrup 37.5 mL, alcohol about 25 mL, and water to 100 mL; shaken with talc (3 g) and filtered.

Compound Orange Spirit *(U.S.N.F.).* Orange oil *U.S.N.F.* 20 mL, lemon oil *U.S.N.F.* 5 mL, coriander oil 2 mL, anise oil 0.5 mL, alcohol to 100 mL. Store at a temperature not exceeding 8° in airtight containers. Protect from light.

4681-a

Terpeneless Orange Oil *(BAN).*

Oleum Aurantii Deterpenatum.

Pharmacopoeias. In *Br.*

A yellow or orange-yellow oil with the characteristic odour of orange, prepared by concentrating orange oil *in vacuo* until most of the terpenes have been removed, or by solvent partition. It contains not less than 18% w/w of aldehydes calculated as decanal, $C_{10}H_{20}O$.
Soluble 1 in 1 of alcohol (90%). **Store** at a temperature not exceeding 25° in well-filled well-closed containers. Protect from light.

Terpeneless orange oil is used as a flavouring agent.

An estimated acceptable daily intake of up to 500 µg per kg body-weight was established for citral, geranyl acetate, citronellol, linalol, and linalyl acetate, expressed as citral.— Twenty-third Report of Joint FAO/WHO Expert Committee on Food Additives, *Tech. Rep. Ser. Wld Hlth Org. No. 648,* 1980.

Preparations

Compound Orange Spirit *(B.P.).* Terpeneless orange oil 0.25 mL, terpeneless lemon oil 0.13 mL, coriander oil 0.625 mL, anise oil 0.425 mL, alcohol (90%) to 100 mL.

4682-t

Dried Bitter-Orange Peel *(BAN).*

Aurantii Amari Cortex; Aurantii Cortex Siccatus; Corteza de Naranja Amarga; Flavedo Aurantii Amara; Pericarpium Aurantii; Pomeranzenschale.

Pharmacopoeias. Most pharmacopoeias include the dried or fresh peel from either bitter orange or sweet orange (*C. sinensis*).

The dried outer part of the pericarp of the ripe or nearly ripe fruit of the bitter orange, *Citrus aurantium* (Rutaceae).

Dried bitter-orange peel is used as a flavouring agent and for its bitter and carminative properties.

A survey of the use of herbal remedies by some patients in Puerto Rico identified *Citrus aurantium* as the most frequently used plant. Conditions for which it was used included: sleep disorders, gastro-intestinal disorders, respiratory ailments, and raised blood pressure.— L. Hernández *et al., Am. J. Hosp. Pharm.,* 1984, *41,* 2060.

Preparations

Aromatic Syrup *(A.P.F.).* Orange tincture 5 mL, lemon spirit 0.5 mL, syrup to 100 mL.

Concentrated Orange Peel Infusion *(B.P.).* Conc. Orange Peel Inf. Dried bitter-orange peel (1 in 2.7), prepared by maceration in alcohol (25%).
Orange Peel Infusion is prepared by diluting 1 vol. of this concentrated infusion to 10 vol. with water.

Orange Syrup *(B.P.).* Orange tincture 6 mL, syrup to 100 mL.
A.P.F. has a similar formula.

Orange Syrup *(U.S.N.F.).* Sweet orange peel tincture 5 mL, anhydrous citric acid 500 mg, and talc 1.5 g, mixed with water 40 mL, and filtered until clear with enough water to make a filtrate of 45 mL. Dissolve sucrose 82 g in the filtrate without the use of heat, and dilute to 100 mL with water. Store at a temperature not exceeding 8° in airtight containers.

Orange Tincture *(B.P.).* Orange Tinct. Dried bitter-orange peel 11 in 100; prepared by percolation with alcohol (70%).

Sweet Orange Peel Tincture *(U.S.N.F.).* Prepared by macerating fresh sweet-orange peel 1 in 2 of alcohol. Store at a temperature not exceeding 40° in airtight containers. Protect from light.

4690-t

Peppermint Leaf *(BAN).*

Hoja de Menta; Hortelã-Pimenta; Menth. Pip.; Mentha Piperita; Menthae Piperitae Folium; Menthe Poivrée; Peppermint *(USAN)*; Pfefferminzblätter.

Pharmacopoeias. In *Arg., Aust., Belg., Br., Cz., Egypt., Eur., Fr., Ger., Hung., It., Jug., Neth., Pol., Port., Roum., Rus., Span.,* and *Swiss.* Also in *U.S.N.F.*
Chin. P. specifies *M. haplocalyx. Jpn. P.* specifies *M. arvensis* var. *piperascens.*

The dried leaves of *Mentha* × *piperita* (Labiatae), containing not less than 1.2% v/w of volatile oil. Peppermint in the *U.S.N.F.* consists of the dried leaves and flowering tops of *M. piperita.* **Store** in well-closed containers. Protect from light.

4691-x

Peppermint Oil *(BAN, USAN).*

Essência de Hortelã-Pimenta; Essence de Menthe Poivrée; Menthae Piperitae Aetheroleum; Ol. Menth. Pip.; Oleum Menthae Piperitae; Pfefferminzöl.

CAS — 8006-90-4.

Pharmacopoeias. In *Arg., Aust., Br., Cz., Egypt., Eur., Ger., Hung., It., Jug., Mex., Neth., Nord., Pol., Port., Roum., Rus., Span.,* and *Swiss.* Also in *U.S.N.F.* and *B.P. Vet* .
Mentha Oil (*Ind. P.*) is from various species of *Mentha. Belg.* specifies *M. piperita* or *M. arvensis* var. *piperascens.* Oleum Menthae (*Chin. P.*) is from *M. haplocalyx.*

The oil obtained by distillation from the fresh flowering tops of *Mentha* × *piperita* (Labiatae) and rectified if necessary.
It is a colourless, pale yellow, or greenish-yellow liquid with the characteristic odour of peppermint and a pungent aromatic cooling taste. It contains menthol, menthone, and menthyl acetate. The *B.P.* specifies 4.5 to 10% w/w of esters, calculated as menthyl acetate, $C_{12}H_{22}O_2$, not less than 44% w/w of free alcohols calculated as menthol, and 15 to 32% of ketones calculated as menthone, $C_{10}H_{18}O$. The *U.S.N.F.* specifies not less than 5% of esters calculated as menthyl acetate and not less than 50% of total menthol, free and as esters.

Soluble 1 in 4 (*B.P.*) or 1 in 3 (*U.S.N.F.*) of alcohol (70%) with slight opalescence. **Store** at a temperature not exceeding 25° in well-filled airtight containers. Protect from light.

The Pharmaceutical Society's Department of Pharmaceutical Sciences found that PVC bottles softened and distorted fairly rapidly in the presence of peppermint oil, which should not be stored or dispensed in such bottles.— *Pharm. J.*, 1973, *1*, 100.

The solubility of peppermint oil in macrogol esters.— K. Thoma and G. Pfaff, *J. Soc. cosmet. Chem.*, 1976, *27*, 221.

STANDARD FOR PEPPERMINT OIL. A British Standard Specification for Peppermint Oil (BS 2999/39: 1971) is published by the British Standards Institution.

Adverse Effects

Peppermint oil can be irritant and may cause allergic reactions. Heartburn has been reported.

Idiopathic auricular fibrillation in 2 patients addicted to 'peppermints'. Normal rhythm was restored when peppermint-sucking ceased.— J. G. Thomas (letter), *Lancet*, 1962, *1*, 222.

Uses and Administration

Peppermint oil is an aromatic carminative and relieves flatulence. Enteric-coated capsules containing peppermint oil are used for the relief of symptoms of the irritable bowel syndrome. Usual doses are 0.2 or 0.4 mL three times daily by mouth before food.

Peppermint oil is also used as a flavour.

EFFECTS ON THE COLON. Pharmacological studies indicate that peppermint oil exerts its muscle relaxant activity through menthol probably by calcium antagonsim (B.A. Taylor *et al.*, *Gut*, 1983, *24*, A992; *idem*, 1984, *25*, A1168). Administration in enteric-coated capsules can deliver the unmetabolised oil to the colon (K.W. Somerville *et al.*, *Br. J. clin. Pharmac.*, 1984, *18*, 638). When administered in this form pepppermint oil has been reported to improve the symptoms of the irritable bowel syndrome (W.D.W. Rees *et al.*, *Br. med. J.*, 1979, *2*, 835; M.J. Dew *et al.*, *Br. J. clin. Pract.*, 1984, *38*, 394); it has also been reported to be no better than placebo (P. Nash *et al.*, *Br. J. clin. Pract.*, 1986, *40*, 292). The relaxant effect of peppermint oil has been used to reduce colonic spasm during endoscopy by injecting the oil or a diluted suspension of the oil along the biopsy channel of the colonoscope (R.J. Leicester and R.H. Hunt, *Lancet*, 1982, *2*, 989).

Preparations

Concentrated Peppermint Emulsion *(B.P.)*. Peppermint oil 2 mL, polysorbate '20' 0.1 mL, double-strength chloroform water 50 mL, freshly boiled and cooled water to 100 mL. When diluted to 40 times its volume with freshly boiled and cooled water it yields a preparation equivalent in strength to Peppermint Water.

Concentrated Peppermint Emulsion (*B.P.*) was not considered to be adequately preserved since it failed to pass microbial spoilage tests with *Pseudomonas aeruginosa*.— T. R. R. Kurup and L. S. C. Wan, *Pharm. J.*, 1986, *2*, 761.

Concentrated Peppermint Water *(B.P. 1973)*. Conc. Peppermint Water; Peppermint Water Concentrated *(A.P.F.)*; Aq. Menth. Pip. Conc. Peppermint oil 2 mL, alcohol (90%) 60 mL, water to 100 mL; shaken with talc and filtered. It is 40 times as strong as peppermint water.

Peppermint Spirit *(B.P., A.P.F.)*. Peppermint Essence. Peppermint oil 10 mL, alcohol (90%) to 100 mL. Clarify if necessary by shaking with sterilised talc and filtering.

Peppermint Spirit *(U.S.P.)*. Peppermint oil 10% v/v in alcohol in which 1% w/v of coarsely powdered peppermint leaves (previously macerated in water for 1 hour and then expressed) has been macerated for 6 hours. Store in airtight containers. Protect from light.

Peppermint Water *(B.P. 1973)*. Aq. Menth. Pip. Concentrated peppermint water 2.5 mL, freshly boiled and cooled water to 100 mL.

Peppermint Water *(U.S.N.F.)*. A saturated solution of peppermint oil in water. Store in airtight containers.

Proprietary Preparations

Colpermin *(Tillotts, UK). Capsules*, enteric-coated, peppermint oil 0.2 mL.

Mintec *(Bridge, UK). Capsules*, enteric-coated, peppermint oil 0.2 mL.

4696-h

Pulegium Oil

Pennyroyal Oil.

CAS — 8007-44-1.

An oil distilled from pennyroyal herb, *Mentha pulegium* (Labiatae), containing pulegone ($C_{10}H_{16}O$).

STANDARD FOR PULEGIUM OIL. A British Standard Specification for Pennyroyal Oil (BS 2999/50: 1972) is published by the British Standards Institution.

Pulegium oil was formerly used as an emmenagogue. Severe toxic effects have followed its use as an abortifacient with convulsions, hepatotoxicity, and death. It is reported to have insect repellent activity.

4697-m

Pumilio Pine Oil *(BAN)*.

Dwarf Pine Needle Oil; Essence de Pin de Montagne; Latschenöl; Oleum Pini Pumilionis; Pine Needle Oil *(USAN)*.

CAS — 8000-26-8.

Pharmacopoeias. In *Aust.*, *Cz.*, *Hung.*, *It.*, *Roum.*, and *Swiss.* Also in *U.S.N.F.*

A colourless or faintly yellow oil with a pleasant aromatic odour and a bitter pungent taste, obtained by distillation from the fresh leaves of *Pinus mugo* var. *pumilio* (Pinaceae). The *U.S.N.F.* specifies 3 to 10% of esters.

Soluble 1 in 4.5 to 10 of alcohol 90%, with turbidity. **Store** in well-filled airtight containers.

Pumilio pine oil has been inhaled with steam to relieve cough and nasal congestion and has been applied externally as a rubefacient. It has also been used as a perfume.

4699-v

Rose Oil *(USAN)*.

Otto or Attar of Rose; Esencia de Rosa; Oleum Rosae.

CAS — 8007-01-0.

Pharmacopoeias. In *Arg.*, *Port.*, and *Span.* Also in *U.S.N.F.*

Arg. allows the use of *R. damascena*, *R. centifolia*, and other species; *Egypt.*, *Span.*, and *U.S.N.F.* allow the oil of *R. gallica*, *R. damascena*, *R. alba*, *R. centifolia*, and varieties of these species.

An oil obtained by distillation from the fresh flowers of *Rosa damascena* (Rosaceae) and other species. It is a colourless or yellow liquid with the characteristic odour and taste of rose which on cooling becomes a translucent crystalline solid. **Store** in well-filled airtight containers.

Rose oil is largely employed in perfumery and toilet preparations and has been used as a flavouring agent.

An estimated acceptable daily intake of up to 500 µg per kg body-weight was established for citral, geranyl acetate, citronellol, linalol, and linalyl acetate, expressed as citral.— Twenty-third Report of Joint FAO/WHO Expert Committee on Food Additives, *Tech. Rep. Ser. Wld Hlth Org. No. 648*, 1980.

Preparations

Rose Water Ointment *(U.S.P.)*. Cetyl esters wax 12.5 g, white beeswax 12 g, almond oil 56 g, borax 500 mg, stronger rose water 2.5 mL, water 16.5 mL, and rose oil 0.02 mL (to make about 100 g). It must be free from rancidity. Store in airtight containers. Protect from light.

Stronger Rose Water *(U.S.N.F.)*. A saturated solution of the odoriferous principles of the flowers of *R. centifolia*, prepared by distilling the fresh flowers with water and separating the excess volatile oil from the clear aqueous portion of the distillate. It should be stored in containers which allow a limited access of fresh air.

The *U.S.N.F.* states that Stronger Rose Water diluted with an equal volume of water may be supplied when Rose Water is required.

4700-v

Rosemary Oil

Esencia de Romero; Essência de Alecrim; Essence de Romarin; Oleum Roris Marini; Oleum Rosmarini; Rosmarinöl.

CAS — 8000-25-7.

Pharmacopoeias. In *Arg.*, *Aust.*, *Belg.*, *Cz.*, *Fr.*, *Ger.*, *Mex.*, *Port.*, *Span.*, and *Swiss.* Also in *B.P.C. 1973.*

An oil obtained by distillation from the flowering tops or leafy twigs of rosemary, *Rosmarinus officinalis* (Labiatae). It contains 2 to 5% of esters, notably bornyl acetate ($C_{12}H_{20}O_2$) and 10 to 18% of free alcohols including borneol ($C_{10}H_{18}O$) and linalol ($C_{10}H_{18}O$). It is a colourless or pale yellow oil with a characteristic odour and a warm bitter camphoraceous taste.

Soluble 1 in 10 of alcohol (80%), with slight turbidity, and 1 in 1 of alcohol (90%) with not more than slight opalescence. **Store** in a cool place in well-filled airtight containers. Protect from light.

STANDARD FOR ROSEMARY OIL. A British Standard Specification for Rosemary Oil (BS 2999/40: 1971) is published by the British Standards Institution.

Rosemary oil is carminative and mildly irritant and has been used in hair lotions and liniments.

An estimated acceptable daily intake of up to 500 µg per kg body-weight was established for citral, geranyl acetate, citronellol, linalol, and linalyl acetate, expressed as citral.— Twenty-third Report of Joint FAO/WHO Expert Committee on Food Additives, *Tech. Rep. Ser. Wld Hlth Org. No. 648*, 1980.

4702-q

Rue Oil

Oleum Rutae.

CAS — 8014-29-7.

An oil obtained from rue, *Ruta graveolens* (Rutaceae).

Rue oil and infusions of rue were formerly used as antispasmodics and emmenagogues. Rue is a photosensitiser and the oil is a powerful local irritant.

Rue (Ruta grav.) is used in homoeopathic medicine.

4704-s

Sage

Feuilles de Sauge; Salbeiblätter; Salvia.

CAS — 8022-56-8 (sage oil).

Pharmacopoeias. In *Aust.*, *Fr.*, *Ger.*, *Hung.*, *Jug.*, *Pol.*, *Port.*, *Roum.*, *Rus.*, and *Swiss. Cz.* includes sage herb. *Ger.* also specifies *Salvia triloba*. *Jug.* also specifies sage oil.

The dried leaves of *Salvia officinalis* (Labiatae).

STANDARD FOR OIL OF SPANISH SAGE. A British Standard Specification (BS 2999/13: 1965) for Oil of Spanish Sage, from *S. lavandulae*, is published by the British Standards Institution.

Sage has carminative properties and is used as a flavouring agent. It has been used in folk medicine.

4708-y

Sassafras Oil
Oleum Sassafras.

CAS — 8006-80-2.

Pharmacopoeias. In *Port.* and *Span.*

An oil distilled from the root or root bark of *Sassafras albidum* (Lauraceae), or from the wood of certain species of *Ocotea* (Lauraceae). It contains safrole.

STANDARD FOR SASSAFRAS OIL. A British Standard Specification for Brazilian Sassafras Oil (BS 2999/41: 1971) is published by the British Standards Institution.

Neither sassafras nor the oil should be taken internally; the use of herb teas of sassafras may lead to a large dose of safrole. The use of safrole in foods has been banned because of carcinogenic and hepatotoxic risks. The use of safrole in toilet preparations is also controlled.
Sassafras oil has rubefacient properties and was formerly used as a pediculocide.

4712-s

Spearmint *(USAN).*
Mentha Viridis; Mint.

Pharmacopoeias. In *Hung.* which specifies varieties of *M. spicata* and *M. aquatica.* Also in *U.S.N.F.* which specifies *Mentha spicata* (Common Spearmint) or *M. cardiaca* (Scotch Spearmint).

The dried leaves and flowering tops of spearmint, *Mentha spicata* (= *M. viridis*) or of *M. cardiaca* (Labiatae).

4713-w

Spearmint Oil *(BAN, USAN).*
Oleum Menthae Crispae; Oleum Menthae Viridis.

CAS — 8008-79-5.

Pharmacopoeias. In *Br.* Also in *U.S.N.F.*

A colourless, pale yellow or greenish-yellow oil with the characteristic odour of spearmint and a warm and slightly bitter taste, obtained by distillation from fresh flowering spearmint, *Mentha spicata*, or Scotch Spearmint, *Mentha cardiaca* or *Mentha* × *cardiaca* (Labiatae). It becomes darker and viscous on keeping. It contains not less than 55% w/w of carvone ($C_{10}H_{14}O$).
Soluble 1 in 1 of alcohol (80%); the solution may become cloudy when diluted. **Store** at a temperature not exceeding 25° in well-filled airtight containers. Protect from light.

STANDARD FOR SPEARMINT OIL. A British Standard Specification for Spearmint Oil (BS 2999/14: 1965) is published by the British Standards Institution.

Spearmint oil has similar properties to peppermint oil and is used as a carminative and as a flavouring agent.

Temporary estimated acceptable daily intake of (+)-carvone and (−)-carvone: up to 1 mg (as the sum of the isomers) per kg body-weight. Further biochemical and metabolic studies are required.— Twenty-seventh Report of Joint FAO/WHO Expert Committee on Food Additives, *Tech. Rep. Ser. Wld Hlth Org. No. 696,* 1983.

4715-l

Terpineol *(BAN).*

$C_{10}H_{18}O$=154.3.

CAS — 8000-41-7; 98-55-5 (α); 2438-12-2 [(±)-α].

Pharmacopoeias. In *Arg.* and *Br.*

A mixture of isomers in which α-terpineol [*p*-menth-1-en-8-ol] largely predominates.
It is a colourless, slightly viscous liquid which may deposit crystals; it has a pleasant lilac-like odour.
Very slightly **soluble** in water; soluble 1 in 2 of alcohol (70%); soluble in ether.

Terpineol has disinfectant and solvent properties.

4716-y

Thyme
Common Thyme; Garden Thyme; Rubbed Thyme; Thymi Herba; Timo.

Pharmacopoeias. In *Arg., Aust., Cz., Fr., Ger., Hung., Neth., Nord., Pol.,* and *Roum., Jug.* includes the leaves only. *Ger.* also specifies *Thymus zygis. Swiss* includes the leaves, flowers, and stalk-tips of *T. vulgaris* and/or *T. zygis* and specifies a minimum of 1.5% of oil, and 0.5% of phenols.

The dried leaves and flowering tops of the 'garden thyme', *Thymus vulgaris* (Labiatae).

4717-j

Thyme Oil
Esencia de Tomillo; Essência de Tomilho; Ol. Thym.; Oleum Thymi.

CAS — 8007-46-3.

Pharmacopoeias. In *Arg., Aust., Fr., Mex., Pol., Roum., Span.,* and *Swiss* (all from *T. vulgaris* only).

An oil obtained from the leaves and flowering tops of *Thymus vulgaris* and other species of *Thymus* and of species of *Origanum* (Labiatae).

Thyme and its oil have carminative properties and are used as flavouring agents.

4720-s

Turpentine Oil *(BAN).*
Aetheroleum Terebinthinae; Esencia de Trementina; Essence de Térébenthine; Oleum Terebinthinae; Oleum Terebinthinae Depuratum; Rectified Turpentine Oil; Spirits of Turpentine.

CAS — 8006-64-2.

Pharmacopoeias. In *Arg., Aust., Belg., Br., Chin., Cz., Egypt., Fr., Hung., Jpn, Mex., Nord., Pol., Port., Roum., Rus., Span.,* and *Swiss.* Also in *B.P. Vet.*

The oil obtained by distillation and rectification from turpentine, an oleoresin obtained from various species of *Pinus* (Pinaceae).
It is a clear bright colourless liquid with a characteristic odour. **Soluble** 1 in 7 of alcohol (90%) and 1 in 3 of alcohol (96%). **Store** at a temperature not exceeding 25° in well-filled well-closed containers. Protect from light.

Adverse Effects
In poisoning with turpentine oil there may be local burning and gastro-intestinal upset, coughing and choking, pulmonary oedema, excitement, coma, fever, tachycardia, liver damage, haematuria, and albuminuria.
The application to the skin of liniments containing turpentine oil may cause irritation and absorption of large amounts may cause some of the effects listed above. Sensitivity reactions have been reported.
In Great Britain the recommended exposure limits of turpentine oil are 100 ppm (long-term); 150 ppm (short-term).

Uses and Administration
Turpentine oil is widely used as a solvent. It is applied topically as a rubefacient. It was formerly used as an expectorant.

Myiasis in 14 patients caused by maggots in the ear was treated by turpentine oil, given as ear-drops, and douching. The parasite was removed in 6 patients; pain and severe inflammation occurred in 3 patients. Ether ear-drops were effective in the remaining 8 patients and caused no pain.— R. Sharan and D. K. Isser, *J. Lar. Otol.,* 1978, *92,* 705.

Preparations

Turpentine Liniment *(B.P.).* Turpentine oil 65 mL, camphor 5 g, soft soap 7.5 g, and freshly boiled and cooled water 22.5 mL.

An improved method of preparation of Turpentine Liniment (*B.P.*).— L. S. C. Wan (letter), *Pharm. J.,* 1976, *1,* 206.

White Liniment *(B.P.).* White Embrocation. Turpentine oil 25 mL, oleic acid 8.5 mL, dilute ammonia solution 4.5 mL, ammonium chloride 1.25 g, and water 62.5 mL.

White Liniment (*B.P.*) was not stable when the ammonia content was less than 6.5%. Because of problems with the stability of ammonia solutions in the tropics, it is recommended that freshly prepared dilute ammonia solution be used or that the content of ammonia in solution be determined and adjustments made if the ammonia content is slightly less than about 10% w/w.— L. S. C. Wan (letter), *Pharm. J.,* 1984, *1,* 693.

Proprietary Preparations
Cerumol (*Laboratories for Applied Biology, UK*). *Ear drops,* turpentine oil 10%, chlorbutol 5%, paradichlorobenzene 2%.
The name Cerumenol has also been used for this preparation.

Gases

5200-c

This section includes monographs on oxygen, carbon dioxide, carbon monoxide, helium, hydrogen sulphide, and nitrogen. Some compressed and liquefied gases are used as refrigerants and aerosol propellents and some of these are included.

18361-b

Butane

n-Butane.

C_4H_{10}=58.12.

CAS — 106-97-8.

Pharmacopoeias. In *U.S.N.F.*, which also includes Isobutane.

A colourless, odourless, inflammable, explosive gas. It is supplied compressed in metal cylinders. **Store** the cylinders in a cool place free from materials of an inflammable nature.

Butane is used as an aerosol propellent (see p.1072). It is widely used as a fuel.

5202-a

Carbon Dioxide

Carbon Diox.; Carbonei Dioxidum; Carbonei Dioxydum; Carbonic Acid Gas; Carbonic Anhydride; E290.

CO_2=44.01.

CAS — 124-38-9.

Pharmacopoeias. In *Arg., Aust., Br., Braz., Chin., Cz., Egypt., Eur., Fr., Ger., Hung., Int., It., Jpn, Jug., Neth., Pol., Swiss, Turk.*, and *U.S.* Also in *B.P. Vet.*

A colourless odourless gas which does not support combustion. It is supplied liquefied under pressure in metal cylinders. It is about 1½ times as heavy as air. A solution in water has weakly acid properties. Carbon dioxide can be liquefied by pressure at 31° or lower; at 31° a pressure of 72 atmospheres is required.

Soluble 1 in about 1 of water by volume at normal temperature and pressure. **Store** the cylinders in a cool place free from materials of an inflammable nature.

In the *UK* cylinders of carbon dioxide are painted grey. The name of the gas or the chemical symbol 'CO_2' should be stencilled in paint on the shoulder of the cylinder and clearly and indelibly stamped on the cylinder valve.

Liquid carbon dioxide and solid carbon dioxide are described below.

In the *US* and some European countries, cylinders of carbon dioxide are also coded grey. For the colours of cylinders containing a mixture of oxygen and carbon dioxide, see under oxygen, (p.1070).

Adverse Effects

Above a concentration of 6%, carbon dioxide gives rise to headache, dizziness, mental confusion, palpitations, hypertension, dyspnoea, increased depth and rate of respiration, and depression of the central nervous system. Concentrations of about 30% may produce convulsions. Higher concentrations are depressant; inhalation of 50% carbon dioxide is reported to produce central effects similar to anaesthetics. The inhalation of high concentrations may produce respiratory acidosis.

Abrupt withdrawal of carbon dioxide after prolonged inhalation commonly produces pallor, hypotension, dizziness, severe headache, and nausea or vomiting.

In Great Britain the recommended exposure limits of carbon dioxide are 5000 ppm (long-term); 15 000 ppm (short-term). In the *US* the permissible and recommended exposure limits are 9000 mg per m^3 and 18 000 mg per m^3 respectively.

Uses and Administration

Carbon dioxide is added to the oxygen in certain types of pump oxygenators to maintain the carbon dioxide content of the blood.

Although carbon dioxide stimulates respiration, it is seldom used for this purpose. Treatment of carbon monoxide poisoning with carbon dioxide/oxygen mixtures is discouraged due to the risk of respiratory acidosis.

Inhalation of carbon dioxide has been tried for relief of intractable hiccups. Carbonated vehicles are useful for masking the unpleasant taste of saline aperients.

Carbon dioxide gas is sometimes used as an inert gas to replace air in containers holding oxidisable substances when the pH is suitable.

Solid carbon dioxide, or 'dry ice' has a temperature of −80° and is used to treat warts and naevi by cryotherapy.

INVESTIGATIVE PROCEDURES. Carbon dioxide insufflation during colonoscopy should be considered to avoid overdistension in patients with irritable bowel, diverticular disease, or stricture, as well as to avoid the risk of explosion with electrocoagulation if mannitol had been used for bowel preparation.— F. A. Macrae *et al.*, *Gut*, 1983, *24*, 376.

In a study of 151 patients undergoing double contrast barium enema, patients experienced significantly less abdominal pain following the use of carbon dioxide for gas contrast than after the use of air. The authors recommended the routine use of carbon dioxide.— R. A. Frost *et al.*, *Gut*, 1985, *26*, A582. See also *ibid.*, 1983, *24*, 371.

LEISHMANIASIS. A report of 30 patients with cutaneous leishmaniasis treated by the application of solid carbon dioxide. All were cured without noticeable scarring within 4 to 5 weeks, with no relapses.— A. Bassiouny *et al.*, *Br. J. Derm.*, 1982, *107*, 467.

NEURALGIA. Cryocautery using a stick of solid carbon dioxide applied for 1 minute to hyperaesthetic areas has been reported to produce relief of postherpetic neuralgia. Repeated applications were necessary.— P. N. Robinson and N. Fletcher, *J. R. Coll. gen. Pract.*, 1986, *36*, 24.

SUDDEN DEAFNESS. In a study of 29 patients, the inhalation of carbogen (5% carbon dioxide, 95% oxygen) was found to be an effective, non-invasive means of assisting the spontaneous recovery of sudden loss of hearing.— U. Fisch, *Otolaryngol. Head Neck Surg.*, 1983, *91*, 3.

12525-g

Carbon Monoxide

CO=28.01.

CAS — 630-08-0.

A colourless, odourless, tasteless, highly inflammable gas.

Adverse Effects

Sources of carbon monoxide include the incomplete combustion of natural gas and other fuels, coal gas, the exhaust fumes of internal combustion engines, and tobacco smoking. Carbon monoxide is highly toxic when inhaled; infants, small children, and elderly people are particularly susceptible. When inhaled, carbon monoxide combines with haemoglobin in the blood to form carboxyhaemoglobin which is unable to transport oxygen; the symptoms of carbon monoxide poisoning are largely due to anoxia.

Unconsciousness may occur suddenly or may be preceded by dizziness, weakness, nausea, vomiting, headache, skin lesions, excessive sweating, pyrexia, increased respiration, and mental dullness and confusion; there may be involuntary defaecation and urination. Death results from respiratory failure, pulmonary oedema, myocardial infarction, or cerebral damage. Neurological and psychiatric sequelae may develop in the survivors of severe poisoning. The lethal concentration of carboxyhaemoglobin in the blood is about 50% or more. Concentrations over 1000 ppm of carbon monoxide in inspired air may be fatal in 1 hour. Smoking during pregnancy may be hazardous to the foetus due to high maternal blood concentration of carboxyhaemoglobin.

In Great Britain the recommended exposure limits of carbon monoxide are 50 ppm (long-term); 400 ppm (short-term). In the *US* the permissible and recommended exposure limits are 55 mg per m^3 and 40 mg per m^3 respectively.

Carbon Monoxide, *Environmental Health Criteria 13*, Geneva, Wld Hlth Org., 1979.

While there has been a reduction in the incidence of carbon monoxide poisoning in the *UK* (*Lancet*, 1981, *2*, 75), there are still some cases, including some arising from faulty natural gas appliances, and warnings have been given of the continued need for vigilance, especially in the detection of such poisoning (A.R. Buckley, *Lancet*, 1984, *1*, 165; *Drug & Ther. Bull.*, 1984, *22*, 81; M.C. Dolan, *Can. med. Ass. J.*, 1985, *133*, 392 and *134*, 992).

EFFECTS ON THE BLOOD. An association between the raised blood-carboxyhaemoglobin concentrations associated with cigarette smoking, and polycythaemia.— J. R. Smith and S. A. Landaw, *New Engl. J. Med.*, 1978, *298*, 6.

EFFECTS ON THE GASTRO-INTESTINAL TRACT. A report of carbon monoxide poisoning mimicking gastroenteritis.— J. M. Hopkinson *et al.*, *Br. med. J.*, 1980, *281*, 214.

EFFECTS ON THE LIVER. A report of anoxic hepatic and intestinal injury from carbon monoxide poisoning.— A. Watson and R. Williams, *Br. med. J.*, 1984, *289*, 1113.

EFFECTS ON THE MUSCLES. Myonecrosis may develop as a complication of carbon monoxide poisoning.— *J. Am. med. Ass.*, 1976, *236*, 2589.

EFFECTS ON THE NERVOUS SYSTEM. Of 74 patients who had suffered acute carbon monoxide poisoning and who were followed up for an average of 3 years after exposure, 8 had gross neuropsychiatric damage attributable to carbon monoxide, 29 had personality changes, and 27 had memory defects. Many had received treatment only in a casualty department and many had not been followed up. The importance of adequate oxygenation, reduction of cerebral oedema, and follow-up was emphasised.— J. S. Smith and S. Brandon, *Br. med. J.* 1973, *1*, 318.

A report of sensorineural hearing loss from acute carbon monoxide poisoning.— S. R. Baker and D. J. Lilly, *Ann. Otol. Rhinol. Lar.*, 1977, *86*, 323.

Retrobulbar neuritis with neuroretinal oedema as a delayed effect of carbon monoxide poisoning.— N. C. Reynolds and I. Shapiro, *Milit. Med.*, 1979, *144*, 472.

Reports of encephalopathy as a delayed effect of carbon monoxide poisoning: S. Quilliam (letter), *Lancet*, 1984, *2*, 408; D. G. Swain (letter), *ibid.*, 637.

Focal epileptiform seizures in a 55-year-old woman following carbon monoxide poisoning.— C. Durnin (letter), *Lancet*, 1987, *1*, 1319.

EFFECTS ON VENTILATION. A report of carbon monoxide poisoning presenting as hyperventilation syndrome (respiratory alkalosis).— M. S. Skorodin *et al.* (letter), *Ann. intern. Med.*, 1986, *105*, 632.

PREGNANCY AND THE NEONATE. A review of the biological effects of carbon monoxide on the pregnant woman, the foetus, and the newborn infant.— L. D. Longo, *Am. J. Obstet. Gynec.*, 1977, *129*, 69.

A report of fatal foetal carbon monoxide poisoning resulting from accidental nonlethal maternal carbon monoxide intoxication.— C. R. Cramer, *J. Toxicol. clin. Toxicol.*, 1982, *19*, 297.

The view that acute carbon monoxide poisoning is not associated with sudden infant death syndrome (cot deaths).— J. L. Emery (letter), *Lancet*, 1984, *2*, 1101.

Chronic, not acute, carbon monoxide poisoning might be involved in the sudden infant death syndrome.— J. Cleary (letter), *ibid.*, 1403. Criticisms of the proposal that carbon monoxide poisoning is a cause of sudden infant death syndrome: A. Kahn *et al.* (letter), *ibid.*, 1985, *1*, 168; W. Q. Sturner (letter), *ibid.*, 457.

Treatment of Adverse Effects

Remove the patient from the contaminated atmosphere; if necessary, apply suction to remove obstruction (vomitus) from the airway and assist the respiration; give 100% oxygen by mask until blood carboxyhaemogloblin concentration has fallen below dangerous levels (usually 10%). Hyperbaric oxygen is recommended by most authorities, especially in severe poisoning. After a long period of unconsciousness, maintain the circulation with infusions of plasma or suitable electrolyte solutions. Acidosis should be corrected if this does not respond to oxygen treatment. If cerebral oedema is suspected 20% mannitol solution should be given intravenously usually in conjunction with corticosteroids.

Absolute rest should be maintained for 3 days while possible cardiac damage is assessed; in severe poisoning, bed rest for 2 to 4 weeks may minimise neurological sequelae.

It was exceptional for the skin to be pink in the living patient poisoned by carbon monoxide; such patients were commonly cyanosed and pale. The breathing was not usually depressed unless the patient was moribund; it was usually more than adequate although the arterial pCO_2 was usually low and hypoxia had induced such a fall in standard bicarbonate that the arterial pH was below normal. The addition of carbon dioxide in any concentration to the oxygen being administered was clearly irrational as it would tend to reduce arterial pH even further. Similarly blood transfusion in a condition characterised by myocardial damage could be extremely dangerous.— H. Matthew, *Br. med. J.*, 1971, *1*, 519.

A 26-year-old man who was comatose for 5 days after carbon monoxide poisoning with no clinical or electroencephalographic improvement was treated with acetylcysteine by intravenous infusion and allopurinol by mouth. The patient made a steady recovery over the next 3 weeks and neurological and mental examinations were normal at 6 weeks follow-up. The use of allopurinol and acetylcysteine to reduce secondary oxidative damage and so limit neuropsychiatric damage was suggested in cases of carbon monoxide poisoning where hyperbaric oxygen was not available or when treatment had been delayed.— R. J. M. W. Howard *et al.* (letter), *Lancet*, 1987, *2*, 628.

HYPERBARIC OXYGEN. A reminder that carbon monoxide is a leading cause of fire-associated deaths and the view that hyperbaric oxygen therapy is mandatory in confirmed cases of carbon monoxide exposure with evidence of CNS dysfunction.— R. M. Roberts (letter), *Lancet*, 1981, *2*, 816.

Three large studies have confirmed hyperbaric oxygen as the treatment of choice for carbon monoxide poisoning. It reduces the morbidity rate to under 5% and apparently prevents late-onset neurological sequelae. This compares with the 43% morbidity reported from studies not using hyperbaric oxygen. Hyperbaric oxygen is effective even after considerable delays. All victims with a history of unconsciousness or who have symptoms or signs other than headache and nausea should be referred for hyperbaric oxygen regardless of carboxyhaemoglobin level. A carboxyhaemoglobin level of over 40% is also an indication for referral. Victims with carboxyhaemoglobin levels under 40% who are normal on thorough physical examination (including assessment of higher mental function) should be treated with 100% oxygen by tight-fitting mask until the carboxyhaemoglobin level remains below 5%.— J. R. Broome and R. R. Pearson (letter), *Lancet*, 1987, *2*, 225.

For further reports of the use of hyperbaric oxygen in carbon monoxide poisoning, see Hyperbaric Oxygen Therapy under Oxygen, p.1071.

Uses and Administration

Carbon monoxide has been used in low concentrations as a tracer gas in measurements of lung function.

5206-f

Dichlorodifluoromethane *(BAN, USAN).*
Difluorodichloromethane; Propellent 12; Refrigerant 12.
CCl_2F_2=120.9.

CAS — 75-71-8.

Pharmacopoeias. In *Br.* Also in *U.S.N.F.*

A colourless non-inflammable gas with a faint ethereal odour which, when liquefied by compression, forms a clear colourless liquid. It is supplied under compression in metal cylinders. B.p. about −29.8°. In the liquid state it is practically **immiscible** with water but miscible with dehydrated alcohol. **Store** the cyclinders at a temperature of 8 to 15° and away from materials of an inflammable nature.

Dichlorodifluoromethane is a halogenated hydrocarbon which is used as a refrigerant and as an aerosol propellent (see p.1072). A spray is used as a local anaesthetic, the intense cold produced by the rapid evaporation of the spray making the tissues insensitive.

In Great Britain the recommended exposure limits of dichlorodifluoromethane are 1000 ppm (long-term); 1250 ppm (short-term).

Estimated acceptable daily intake up to 1.5 mg per kg body-weight.— Nineteenth Report of the Joint FAO/WHO Expert Committee on Food Additives, *Tech. Rep. Ser. Wld Hlth Org. No. 576,* 1975.

USE IN FOOD. The use of dichlorodifluoromethane is permitted in frozen food under The Miscellaneous Additives in Food Regulations 1980 (SI 1980: No. 1834) for England and Wales and The Miscellaneous Additives in Food (Scotland) Regulations 1980 [SI 1980: No. 1889 (S.176)].

5207-d

Dichlorotetrafluoroethane *(BAN, USAN).*
Cryofluorane *(rINN)*; Propellent 114; Refrigerant 114; Tetrafluorodichloroethane. 1,2-Dichloro-1,1,2,2-tetrafluoroethane.
$CClF_2.CClF_2$=170.9.

CAS — 76-14-2.

Pharmacopoeias. In *Br.* Also in *U.S.N.F.*

A colourless non-inflammable gas with a faint ethereal odour which, when liquefied by compression, forms a clear colourless liquid. It is supplied under compression in metal cylinders. B.p. about 3.5°. In the liquid state it is practically **immiscible** with water, but miscible with dehydrated alcohol. **Store** the cylinders at a temperature of 8 to 15° and away from material of an inflammable nature.

Dichlorotetrafluoroethane is a halogenated hydrocarbon which is used as a refrigerant and aerosol propellent, (see p.1072).

In Great Britain the recommended exposure limits of dichlorotetrafluoroethane are 1000 ppm (long-term); 1250 ppm (short-term).

5203-t

Helium

He=4.0026.

CAS — 7440-59-7.

Pharmacopoeias. In *Br.* and *U.S.*

A colourless odourless tasteless gas which is not combustible and does not support combustion; it has a relative density not greater than 0.16. **Soluble** 1 in 72.5 of water by volume at normal temperature and pressure. **Store** under compression in metal cylinders.

In the *UK* cylinders of helium are painted brown. The name or chemical symbol of the gas or gases should be stencilled in paint on the shoulder of the cylinder and clearly and indelibly stamped on the cylinder valve.

In the *US* and some European countries, cylinders of helium are also coded brown. For the colours of cylinders containing a mixture of oxygen and helium, see under Oxygen, below.

As helium is less dense than nitrogen, breathing a mixture of 80% helium and 20% oxygen requires less effort than breathing air. Such mixtures have been used in patients with acute obstructions of the upper respiratory tract. Due to the low solubility of helium, mixtures of helium and oxygen are used by divers or others working under high pressure to prevent the development of decompression sickness (caisson disease); they are preferred to compressed air since they do not cause nitrogen narcosis. Helium is useful in pulmonary function testing.

Breathing helium increases vocal pitch and causes voice distortion.

Helium and oxygen mixtures in decompression sickness.— C. H. Brookings and N. K. I. McIver (letter), *Lancet*, 1978, *2*, 468; P. B. James *et al.* (letter), *ibid.*, 469.

Decreased respiratory work was noted in 9 of 10 patients with an upper airway obstruction after breathing a helium-oxygen mixture. While aiming for the easing of respiratory work with a high helium concentration, a balance would have to be established that took into account the need for a greater fractional oxygen intake to deal with hypoxaemia.— G. J. Skrinskas *et al.*, *Can. med. Ass. J.*, 1983, *128*, 555.

Helium-oxygen mixtures may reduce the work of breathing in infants with bronchopulmonary dysplasia and subglottic stenosis, but at the expense of a brisk drop in oxygenation.— W. W. Butt *et al.*, *J. Pediat.*, 1985, *106*, 474.

12832-k

Hydrogen Sulphide
Sulphuretted Hydrogen.
H_2S=34.08.

CAS — 7783-06-4.

A colourless inflammable gas with a characteristic odour.

Adverse Effects

Hydrogen sulphide poisoning is a common industrial hazard and is encountered in such places as chemical works, mines, sewage works, and stores of decomposing protein; concentrations of 0.1 to 0.2% in the atmosphere may be fatal in a few minutes. At concentrations of about 0.005% and above hydrogen sulphide causes anosmia and its unpleasant odour is no longer detectable. Pulmonary irritation, oedema, and respiratory failure usually occur after acute poisoning; prolonged exposure to low concentrations may give rise to severe conjunctivitis with photophobia and corneal opacity, irritation of the respiratory tract, cough, nausea, vomiting and diarrhoea, pharyngitis, headache, dizziness, and lassitude. There are some similarities to poisoning with cyanides.

In Great Britain the recommended exposure limits of hydrogen sulphide are 10 ppm (long-term); 15 ppm (short-term). In the *US* the permissible and recommended exposure limits are 20 ppm and 10 ppm respectively.

Hydrogen Sulfide, *Environmental Health Criteria 19*, Geneva, Wld Hlth Org., 1981.

A discussion of poisoning by hydrogen sulphide.— *Lancet*, 1978, *1*, 28. Comments.— A. Downie (letter), *ibid.*, 219; C. H. B. Binns (letter), *ibid.*, 501; A. Downie (letter), *ibid.*

Long-term exposure to hydrogen sulphide produced an illness resembling subacute necrotising encephalopathy in a 20-month-old child.— U. B. Gaitonde *et al.*, *Br. med. J.*, 1987, *294*, 614.

Acute hydrogen sulphide intoxication in a factory worker resulted in a subendocardial infarction and probably induced a change in emotional behaviour.— A. S. Vathenen (letter), *Lancet*, 1988, *1*, 305.

Further references to hydrogen sulphide poisoning: W. W. Burnett *et al.*, *Can. med. Ass. J.*, 1977, *117*, 1277; R. P. Smith (letter), *ibid.*, 1978, *118*, 775; W. W. Burnett and E. G. King (letter), *ibid.*, 776; *J. Am. med. Ass.*, 1978, *239*, 1374; L. N. Osbern and R. O. Crapo, *Ann. intern. Med.*, 1981, *95*, 312.

Treatment of Adverse Effects

After exposure to hydrogen sulphide place the patient in

fresh air, give inhalations of oxygen and, if necessary, assist the respiration. The conjunctival sacs should be carefully washed out if eye irritation is severe.

The successful treatment of a 47-year-old man with severe hydrogen sulphide poisoning using oxygen, amyl nitrite inhalations for 30 seconds out of each minute for 5 minutes, and then sodium nitrite 300 mg intravenously for 3 minutes. Treatment was aimed at producing met-haemoglobinaemia to inactivate the sulphide. In addition he received sodium thiosulphate 12.5 g by intravenous injection.— R. J. Stine *et al.*, *Ann. intern. Med.*, 1976, *85*, 756. See also J. W. Peters, *J. Am. med. Ass.*, 1981, *246*, 1588.

Uses.
Hydrogen sulphide is widely employed in many industrial processes.

5204-x

Nitrogen

Azote; Nitrogenium.
N_2=28.0134.

CAS — 7727-37-9.

Pharmacopoeias. In *Aust.*, *Cz.*, *Fr.*, *Hung.*, *Jpn*, *Jug.*, *Nord.*, and *Swiss.* Also in *U.S.N.F.*

A colourless odourless tasteless gas which is non-inflammable and does not support combustion.

Soluble 1 in 65 of water by volume and 1 in 9 of alcohol by volume, at normal temperature and pressure. **Store** under compression in metal cylinders.

In the *UK* cylinders of nitrogen are painted grey with black neck and shoulder. The name of the gas or the chemical symbol 'N_2' should be stencilled in paint on the shoulder of the cylinder and clearly and indelibly stamped on the cylinder valve. In the *US* and some European countries, cylinders of nitrogen are coded black.

Adverse Effects

Nitrogen narcosis has been reported from nitrogen breathed at high pressure as in deep-water diving. Under high pressure, nitrogen dissolves in blood and lipid. If decompression is too rapid, nitrogen effervesces from body stores producing gas emboli and leading to the syndrome of decompression sickness.

A tingling sensation persisting for 2 days in the last 2 fingers of the hand followed the application of liquid nitrogen to a wart on the elbow of a 21-year-old man; numbness of the hand followed and ulnar neuropathy was apparent 6 months later.— P. F. Finelli, *Archs Derm.*, 1975, *111*, 1340.

Uses and Administration

Nitrogen is used as a diluent for pure oxygen or other active gases and as an inert gas to replace air in containers holding oxidisable substances. Liquid nitrogen is used as a cryotherapeutic agent for the removal of warts and malignant growths, the treatment of cysts in acne vulgaris, and for preservation of tissues and organisms.

DECOMPRESSION THERAPY. Three divers with refractory decompression sickness requiring exposure to compressed air for durations leading to pulmonary oxygen toxicity were satisfactorily treated with nitrogen-oxygen. The use of nitrogen-oxygen mixtures with an inspired pO_2 of 0.5 atmospheres absolute or less allows a potentially indefinite duration of recompression at raised environmental pressure.— J. N. Miller *et al.*, *Lancet*, 1978, *2*, 169. Criticisms.— C. H. Brookings and N. K. I. McIver (letter), *ibid.*, 468; P. B. James *et al.* (letter), *ibid.*, 469. Reply.— T. G. Shields and D. H. Elliott (letter), *ibid.*, 782. Further comment.— J. N. Miller and L. Fagraeus (letter), *ibid.*

TRIGEMINAL NEURALGIA. Liquid nitrogen applied directly to the nerve provided relief of pain in trigeminal neuralgia.— F. F. Nally and J. M. Zakrzewska (letter), *Lancet*, 1984, *1*, 1021.

WARTS. The application of liquid nitrogen was considered to be the treatment of choice for ano-genital warts in pregnant women.— *Med. Lett.*, 1982, *24*, 29.

Although podophyllin remained the most widely used therapy for condyloma acuminata, or veneral warts, application of liquid nitrogen was an alternative and possibly more effective treatment.— *Med. Lett.*, 1986, *28*, 23.

5201-k

Oxygen

Ossigeno; Oxygenium; Sauerstoff.
O_2=31.9988.

CAS — 7782-44-7.

Pharmacopoeias. In *Arg.*, *Aust.*, *Belg.*, *Br.*, *Braz.*, *Chin.*, *Cz.*, *Egypt.*, *Eur.*, *Fr.*, *Ger.*, *Hung.*, *Ind.*, *Int.*, *It.*, *Jpn*, *Jug.*, *Mex.*, *Neth.*, *Nord.*, *Pol.*, *Port.*, *Roum.*, *Span.*, *Swiss*, *Turk.*, and *U.S.* Also in *B.P. Vet.* *U.S.* also includes Oxygen 93 Percent and Compressed Air.

A colourless odourless tasteless gas. It contains not less than 99% v/v of O_2, the residue consisting either of argon with a trace of nitrogen or of hydrogen. Oxygen intended for aviation or mountain rescue must have a sufficiently low moisture content to avoid blocking of valves by freezing.

Soluble 1 in 32 of water by volume and 1 in 7 of alcohol by volume at normal temperature and pressure. **Store** under compression in metal cylinders.

In the *UK* cylinders of oxygen are painted black with a white shoulder. Cylinders of oxygen mixed with carbon dioxide are painted black with grey and white quarterings on neck and shoulder. Cylinders of oxygen mixed with helium are painted black with brown and white quarterings on neck and shoulder. The name or chemical symbol of the gas or gases should be stencilled in paint on the shoulder of the cylinder and clearly and indelibly stamped on the cylinder valve.

In the *US* cylinders of oxygen are coded green, oxygen mixed with carbon dioxide, green and grey, and oxygen mixed with helium, brown and yellow. In some European countries, cylinders of oxygen are coded white, oxygen mixed with carbon dioxide, white and grey, and oxygen mixed with helium, white and brown.

Adverse Effects

Oxygen toxicity depends upon both the inspired pressure (a function of concentration and barometric pressure) and the duration of exposure, the safe duration decreasing as the pressure increases. At lower pressures, of up to 2 atmospheres absolute, pulmonary toxicity occurs before CNS toxicity; at higher pressures, the reverse applies. Symptoms of pulmonary toxicity include a decrease in vital capacity, cough, substernal distress, and later, atelectasis. Symptoms of CNS toxicity include nausea, mood changes, vertigo, twitching, convulsions, and loss of consciousness. Retinopathy of prematurity (retrolental fibroplasia) has occurred in premature infants whose arterial partial pressure of oxygen has been maintained above 70 mmHg. Hyperbaric oxygen can cause retinal damage in adults.

A review of oxygen toxicity.— L. Frank and D. Massaro, *Am. J. Med.*, 1980, *69*, 117.

EFFECTS ON THE BLOOD. Reticulocytopenia and reduced packed cell volume in a patient with sickle-cell anaemia, attributable to hyperoxygenation.— D. L. Solanki, *Br. med. J.*, 1983, *287*, 725.

EFFECTS ON THE EYES. A healthy 44-year-old man exposed for 1 hour to hyperbaric oxygen at 2 atmospheres absolute pressure on 2 occasions sustained a field defect in his left eye.— K. Herbstein and J. B. Murchland, *Med. J. Aust.*, 1984, *140*, 728.

Refraction changed in the direction of myopia in 25 patients during prolonged hyperbaric oxygen therapy for peripheral ischaemic ulcers. The induced myopia was reversible in most patients. Of the 15 patients with clear lens nuclei before treatment, 7 developed nuclear cataracts with visual impairment.— B. -M. Palmquist *et al.*, *Br. J. Ophthal.*, 1984, *68*, 113.

For references questioning the role of oxygen in retinopathy of prematurity (retrolental fibroplasia) in neonates, see under Pregnancy and the Neonate, below.

EFFECTS ON THE LUNGS. Normobaric oxygen toxicity of the lung.— S. M. Deneke and B. L. Fanburg, *New Engl. J. Med.*, 1980, *303*, 76.

For a reference to the role of oxygen in bronchopulmonary dysplasia in preterm infants, see under Pregnancy and the Neonate, below.

PREGNANCY AND THE NEONATE. Comment on the role of oxygen and other factors in the incidence of bronchopulmonary dysplasia in preterm infants.— *Lancet*, 1980, *1*, 690.

The occurrence of retrolental fibroplasia (retinopathy of prematurity) in 14 infants was unrelated to an increase in requirement for, or duration of oxygen therapy, arterial oxygen tensions, or the availability of transcutaneous oxygen monitoring.— V. Y. H. Yu *et al.*, *Archs Dis. Childh.*, 1982, *57*, 247.

Discussions questioning the role of oxygen in retinopathy of prematurity: W. A. Silverman, *Archs Dis. Childh.*, 1982, *57*, 731; B. P. Cats and K. E. W. P. Tan, *Br. J. Ophthal.*, 1985, *69*, 500.

Precautions

Any fire or spark is highly dangerous in the presence of increased oxygen concentrations especially when oxygen is used under pressure.

Metal cylinders containing oxygen should be fitted with a reducing valve by which the rate of flow can be controlled. It is important that the reducing valve should be free from all traces of oil or grease, as otherwise a violent explosion may occur. Combustible material soaked in liquid oxygen is potentially explosive and the low temperature of liquid oxygen may cause unsuitable equipment to become brittle and crack. Liquid oxygen should not be allowed to come into contact with the skin as it produces severe 'cold burns'.

High concentrations of oxygen should be avoided in patients whose respiration is dependent upon hypoxic drive, otherwise carbon dioxide retention and respiratory depression may ensue.

NEBULISER THERAPY. It was felt that although it was safe to use oxygen as the driving gas for nebulisers in patients with obstructive airways disease with normal pCO_2, caution should be exercised in those who already have carbon dioxide retention.— K. A. Gunawardena *et al.*, *Br. med. J.*, 1984, *288*, 272. The view that in chest units oxygen should not be used for nebulisation purposes.— S. J. Austin and C. Chan (letter), *ibid.*, 488. Further comments on the risks of oxygen as a carrier gas for nebulisers: S. Coltart and B. D. W. Harrison (letter), *ibid.*, 646; J. W. Hadfield *et al.* (letter), *ibid.*, 795. In patients with severe chronic lung disease, the danger of aggravating hypoxaemia may outweigh the risks associated with the rise in pCO_2 when nebulisers are driven with air.— H. Cass *et al.* (letter), *ibid.*, 1009. A reply. For most patients with chronic bronchitis, there is little danger from hypoxaemia. If the patients happen to be very hypoxic, it is perhaps wise to use oxygen to drive the nebuliser but then only for the shortest possible period and the patients should be watched carefully if they also have carbon dioxide retention.— K. A. Gunawardena *et al.* (letter), *ibid.*, 1237.

Oxygen is to be preferred for the delivery of nebulised drugs in acute asthma.— B. G. Loftus and J. F. Price (letter), *Lancet*, 1985, *1*, 393.

Uses and Administration

Oxygen is given by inhalation to correct hypoxia in conditions causing under-ventilation of the lungs, such as exacerbations of chronic bronchitis, pneumonia, or pulmonary oedema, where bronchospasm causes hypoxia, as in asthma, in extensive fibrosing alveolitis, after general anaesthesia, and in conditions where the oxygen content of the air breathed is inadequate as at high altitudes; it is also used in circulatory failure associated with conditions such as myocardial infarction or after cardiac arrest or hypothermia. Oxygen is of value in the treatment of carbon monoxide poisoning and in providing enhanced oxygenation in inhalation injury, severe anaemia, or in the treatment of respiratory depression or respiratory failure until more specific treatments are started. It may be useful in the management of abdominal distension, pneumatosis cystoides intestinalis (intestinal gas-filled cysts), and in removing accumulated nitrogen from other cavities. Oxygen is also given by inhalation to subjects working in pressurised spaces and to divers to reduce the concentration of nitrogen inhaled. It is used as a diluent of volatile and gaseous anaesthetics.

The addition of 5 or 7% of carbon dioxide to inhaled oxygen (such mixtures have been given the name carbogen), stimulates the respiratory centre and causes deeper breathing, except in patients who have stopped breathing; this effect may be diminished by depressants.

In chronic obstructive airways disease, in conditions such as bronchitis and emphysema, oxygen is usually administered to give an inspired concentration of about 30%. High concentrations are to be avoided as they may enhance carbon-dioxide retention and narcosis.

In conditions not usually associated with retention of carbon dioxide, such as asthma, pneumonia, pulmonary oedema, fibrosing alveolitis, or circulatory failure, oxygen may be administered in concentrations of up to 100%. The concentration should be reduced as soon as possible. In crush injuries of the chest or in respiratory depression due to poisoning, oxygen may be administered in conjunction with assisted respiration. High concentrations of oxygen may be administered in carbon monoxide poisoning, until treatment with hyperbaric oxygen can be started.

Oxygen is employed in asphyxia in the newborn and in conditions associated with respiratory distress in infants, when arterial blood gas concentrations should be measured.

Oxygen may be administered by means of a nasal catheter, face mask, endotracheal tube, or oxygen tent. Face masks are commonly employed for domiciliary oxygen therapy when flow-rates are 2 or 4 litres per minute. Oxygen concentrators produce oxygen-enriched air and are useful for domiciliary therapy, especially in patients using large quantities of oxygen.

Oxygen may also be supplied at low temperature in insulated containers as liquid oxygen.

Oxygen at a pressure greater than 1 atmosphere absolute, i.e. hyperbaric oxygen, is administered by enclosing the patient in a special high-pressure chamber. It is used to correct hypoxia in conditions such as arterial disease, asphyxia in the newborn, congenital heart disease, severe anaemia, and poisoning by carbon monoxide and cyanide. It is also used to enhance the effectiveness of irradiation in the treatment of malignant disease, as an adjunct in the treatment of severe anaerobic infections, especially gas gangrene, and for the treatment of decompression sickness and gas emboli.

A discussion on acute oxygen therapy.— *Lancet*, 1981, *1*, 980.

ADMINISTRATION. *Long-term domiciliary therapy.* Reviews and discussions on long-term oxygen therapy (LTOT) for outpatients: *Drug & Ther. Bull.*, 1982, *20*, 65; N. R. Anthonisen, *Ann. intern. Med.*, 1983, *99*, 519; *Lancet*, 1985, *2*, 365; A. B. X. Breslin, *Med. J. Aust.*, 1985, *142*, 508; M. S. Skorodin, *J. Am. med. Ass.*, 1986, *255*, 3283; P. Howard, *Prescribers' J.*, 1986, *26*, 115.

The oxygen concentrator appeared to be the most economical means of providing oxygen treatment at home and was much preferred by patients who had previously used oxygen cylinders.— T. W. Evans *et al.*, *Br. med. J.*, 1983, *287*, 459. The benefit of these costly devices remained to be proved.— I. W. B. Grant (letter), *ibid.*, 685.

The mechanics of oxygen concentrators: A. J. Crockett, *Med. J. Aust.*, 1985, *142*, 512; G. Rose, *Pharm. J.*, 1987, *2*, 776.

Percutaneous administration. In 13 preterm infants with severe respiratory distress, the replacement of their surrounding air with 95% oxygen resulted in a substantial increase in arterial oxygen tension due to percutaneous oxygen absorption.— P. H. T. Cartlidge and N. Rutter, *Lancet*, 1988, *1*, 315.

Transtracheal administration. The administration of oxygen through a catheter implanted in the trachea is a practical method of treatment which may have an important role in rehabilitating patients with chronic lung disease.— N. R. Banner and J. R. Govan, *Br. med. J.*, 1986, *293*, 111. Refractory hypoxaemia in 8 patients was successfully treated with transtracheal oxygen therapy, and all experienced improved quality of life.— K. L. Christopher *et al.*, *J. Am. med. Ass.*, 1986, *256*, 494.

CARDIOVASCULAR DISORDERS. Administration of oxygen before or during the slow injection of an intravenous anaesthetic was considered to be highly desirable for patients with severe heart disease.— S. M. Lyons and R. S. J. Clark, *Br. J. Anaesth.*, 1972, *44*, 575.

Pulmonary hypertension. There was little evidence that oxygen therapy produced haemodynamic or clinical benefits in patients with primary pulmonary hypertension.— M. Packer, *Ann. intern. Med.*, 1985, *103*, 258.

See also under Chronic Obstructive Airways Disease, below.

Sickle-cell anaemia. In a study of 3 patients with sickle-cell anaemia, it was concluded that when oxygen therapy is administered to such patients, it should be given intermittently rather than continuously.— S. H. Embury *et al.*, *New Engl. J. Med.*, 1984, *311*, 291. Criticism. There was no evidence that supplemental oxygen had any effect in the treatment of acute painful crises. The only role of oxygen therapy was to improve arterial hypoxaemia, without regard to peripheral blood sickling. In this situation, oxygen therapy must be continuous and not intermittent.— L. L. Schulman (letter), *ibid.*, 1319. Reply. The decision whether to employ oxygen inhalation in the therapy of acute painful episodes required consideration of more than just the generally recognised rheological deficits that result from cellular sickling.— S. H. Embury *et al.* (letter), *ibid.*, 1320.

Life-threatening sickle chest syndrome in one patient was successfully treated with extracorporeal membrane oxygenation when conventional treatment had failed.— D. S. Gillett *et al.*, *Br. med. J.*, 1987, *294*, 81.

DECOMPRESSION SICKNESS. For a report on nitrogen-oxygen mixtures in the treatment of divers with decompression sickness, see Nitrogen, p.1070.

HEADACHE. The author achieved relief of cluster headaches by inhaling oxygen.— J. F. Janks (letter), *J. Am. med. Ass.*, 1978, *239*, 191.

Further reports of the relief of cluster headache through oxygen inhalation: L. Fogan, *Archs Neurol., Chicago*, 1985, *42*, 362; S. Diamond *et al.*, *Headache*, 1986, *26*, 42.

HYPERBARIC OXYGEN THERAPY. A review of the actions and uses of hyperbaric oxygen therapy.— *Hyperbaric Oxygen Therapy: A Committee Report*, R.A.M. Myers, (chairman), Undersea Medical Society, Bethesda, 1986.

Carbon monoxide poisoning. Carbon monoxide poisoning must be treated with hyperbaric oxygen. Normobaric oxygen is not adequate.— P. B. James (letter), *Lancet*, 1984, *2*, 810. Although hyperbaric oxygen should be started as soon as possible after acute carbon monoxide poisoning, it was emphasised that anyone who had been exposed should be treated regardless of the delay between exposure and presentation, to reduce the incidence of late neurological sequelae. Six cases are presented, where treatment commenced 8 to 16 hours after exposure; 5 patients made full mental and physical recoveries.— A. Ziser *et al.*, *Br. med. J.*, 1984, *289*, 960. Criticism. There was no evidence that late neuropsychiatric sequelae are prevented by hyperbaric oxygen.— S. Kumar (letter), *ibid.*, 1315.

Further references to the value of hyperbaric oxygen in the treatment of carbon monoxide poisoning: D. M. Norkool and J. N. Kirkpatrick, *Ann. emerg. Med.*, 1985, *14*, 1168; D. Mathieu *et al*, *Clin. Toxicol.*, 1985, *23*, 315.

Cystitis. The successful use of hyperbaric oxygen in the treatment of radiation-induced cystitis in 3 patients.— J. P. Weiss *et al.*, *J. Urol., Baltimore*, 1985, *134*, 352.

Gas gangrene. A review of 73 cases of gas gangrene managed with hyperbaric oxygen.— I. P. Unsworth and P. A. Sharp, *Med. J. Aust.*, 1984, *140*, 256.

Ischaemic lesions. Hyperbaric oxygenation was beneficial in the treatment of 3 infants with peripheral ischaemic lesions secondary to disseminated intravascular clotting.— E. Rosenthal *et al.*, *Archs Dis. Childh.*, 1985, *60*, 372.

Following hyperbaric oxygen, healing of foot lesions was achieved in 12 of 14 diabetic adults.— T. Porro and E. Faglia, *Br. med. J.*, 1985, *290*, 208.

See also: M. C. Y. Heng, *Br. J. Derm.*, 1983, *109*, 232 (leg ulcers); *idem*, *Aust. N.Z. J. Med.*, 1984, *14*, 618 (pyoderma gangrenosum).

Malignant neoplasms. Results of radiotherapy treatment under hyperbaric oxygen were assessed in 1669 cancer patients registered for study between 1963 and 1976. Hyperbaric oxygen was found significantly to improve the results of radiotherapy, both in terms of survival and local tumour control, for tumours in the head and neck, and in the uterine cervix. Although some improvement in survival appeared to occur in carcinoma of the bronchus the results were not statistically significant; no improvement was noted in carcinoma of the bladder. Side-effects included occasional oxygen convulsions and refusal of therapy owing to claustrophobia.—Report of a Medical Research Council Working Party, *Lancet*, 1978, *2*, 881.

Multiple Sclerosis. Preliminary observations suggested subjective and objective improvement in multiple sclerosis after 10 to 20 treatments of hyperbaric oxygen at pressures of up to 2 atmospheres absolute for 60 to 90 minutes in an uncontrolled study in 250 patients (R.A. Neubauer, *J. Fla med. Assoc.*, 1980, *67*, 498) and in a placebo-controlled double-blind trial in 40 patients (B.H. Fischer *et al.*, *New Engl. J. Med.*, 1983, *308*, 181). However 3 further placebo-controlled double-blind trials involving 120, 41, and 84 patients (M.P. Barnes *et al.*, *Lancet*, 1985, *1*, 297; J. Wood *et al.*, *Med. J. Aust.*, 1985, *143*, 238; C.M. Wiles *et al.*, *Br. med. J.*, 1986, *292*, 367) and 2 uncontrolled studies involving 32 and 12 patients (B.H. Bass, *Br. med. J.*, 1984, *288*, 1230; J.A. Rosen, *Ann. Neurol.*, 1985, *17*, 615), all using 20 sessions of hyperbaric oxygen at up to 2 atmospheres absolute for 1 to 3 hours, failed to show any significant overall improvement. Criticisms of these later trials have included too prolonged an exposure (R.A. Neubauer, *Br. med. J.*, 1984, *288*, 1831), too high a pressure (P.B. James, *Lancet*, 1985, *1*, 572; D.J.D. Perrins *ibid.*; R.A. Neubauer, *ibid*, 810; J. Bolt *et al.*, *Br. med. J.*, 1986, *292*, 691; P.B. James, *ibid.*, 692), faulty methodology and incorrect evaluation of results (P.B. James, *Lancet*, 1985, *1*, 572; R.A. Neubauer, *ibid*, 810).

INVESTIGATIVE PROCEDURES. Oxygen given via nasal cannulae largely prevented hypoxaemia during upper gastro-intestinal endoscopy. The use of supplementary oxygen was strongly suggested in elderly patients, particularly those with a history of cardiovascular disease.— G. D. Bell *et al.*, *Lancet*, 1987, *1*, 1022.

PREGNANCY AND THE NEONATE. Preliminary results from the successful management of 5 cases suggest that maternal oxygen administration could increase the pO_2 of the hypoxic, growth-retarded foetus to normal, which may prevent intra-uterine death and, in some cases, allow delivery to be delayed until the foetus reaches the stage of viability.— K. H. Nicolaides *et al.*, *Lancet*, 1987, *1*, 942.

Respiratory distress syndrome. For the use of oxygen in the management of respiratory distress syndrome, see below.

RESPIRATORY DISORDERS. *Adult respiratory distress syndrome.* Some reviews of the aetiology and management of the adult respiratory distress syndrome including the use of oxygen and mechanical ventilation: C. R. M. Boggis and R. Greene, *Br. J. Hosp. Med.*, 1983, *29*, 167; D. C. Flenley, *Br. med. J.*, 1983, *286*, 871; J. H. Stevens and T. A. Raffin, *Postgrad. med. J.*, 1984, *60*, 505 and 573; B. A. Boucher and T. S. Foster, *Drug Intell. & clin. Pharm.*, 1984, *18*, 862.

Asthma. In severely ill asthmatics, oxygen should be administered in concentrations of 40 to 60%. There was little risk of promoting hypercapnia because respiratory drive was well maintained.— M. A. Branthwaite, *Br. J. Hosp. Med.*, 1985, *34*, 331.

Breathlessness. Breathlessness and exercise tolerance were improved in 'pink and puffing' patients with fixed airways obstruction when they breathed oxygen.— A. A. Woodcock *et al.*, *Lancet*, 1981, *1*, 907.

Chronic obstructive airways disease. In a long-term comparative study of patients with hypoxaemic chronic obstructive lung disease continuous oxygen therapy, provided by oxygen concentrators in some cases, was associated with a lower mortality than 12-hour nocturnal oxygen therapy.— Nocturnal Oxygen Therapy Trial Group, *Ann. intern. Med.*, 1980, *93*, 391. Comment.— S. D. Roberts, *ibid.*, 499. A multicentre controlled study in patients with chronic bronchitis and emphysema complicated by hypoxic cor pulmonale indicated that long-term oxygen therapy for at least 15 hours daily (most using a concentrator) could reduce mortality over 3 years in both men and women but the effect only became evident in men after 500 days had elapsed. —Report of the Medical Research Council Working Party, *Lancet*, 1981, *1*, 681. Comments on long-term oxygen therapy at home in patients with advanced chronic bronchitis and other chronic obstructive lung diseases.— *ibid.*, 701.

Nocturnal hypoxia. Nocturnal oxygen therapy reduced nocturnal hypoxaemia and ameliorated some electrocardiographic signs of cardiac arrhythmia in patients with the 'blue and bloated' form of chronic airways disease.— V. G. Tirlapur and M. A. Mir, *New Engl. J. Med.*, 1982, *306*, 125. Nocturnal oxygen desaturation should be treated if causing the patient ill effects, but prophylactic therapy for preventing such ill effects had not been studied and could not be recommended.— A. J. Block, *ibid.*, 166. In a study of patients with alveolar hypoventilation, including several who resembled 'blue bloaters', nocturnal low-flow oxygen therapy (1 to 3 litres per minute) increased the mean duration of apnoeic events, the length of episodes of low-tidal-volume respiration and end-tidal carbon dioxide values. Intermittent severe hypercapnia occurred. Accurate titration of the appropriate oxygen flow and nocturnal polysomnography was necessary before patients received long-term nocturnal oxygen therapy.— M. J. Thorpy *et al.* (letter), *ibid.*, *307*, 123. Replies suggesting that the risk to the patient of untreated hypoxaemia was greater than the possible risk of hypercapnia and acidosis in an occasional patient and that routine polysomnography was not justified: V. G. Tirlapur and Mir M.A. (letter), *ibid;* A. J. Block (letter), *ibid.*

In a study of 15 hypercapnoeic and hypoxaemic patients with severe but stable chronic obstructive lung disease, supplemental nocturnal oxygen, given to prevent the falls in arterial oxygen saturation that occur during sleep, was associated with only a small and clinically unimportant increase in pCO_2. Low-flow nocturnal oxygen was considered relatively safe, but when obstructive sleep apnoea is present in addition to chronic obstructive lung disease, the effects should be monitored carefully since pCO_2 may be markedly elevated.— R. S. Goldstein *et al.*, *New Engl. J. Med.*, 1984, *310*, 425.

See also under Sleep Apnoea, below.

Respiratory distress syndrome. The management of hyaline membrane disease in infants, with special reference to the use of oxygen.— E. O. R. Reynolds, *Br. med. Bull.*, 1975, *31*, 18.

The domiciliary treatment of neonatal respiratory disease with low-flow oxygen therapy.— A. N. Campbell *et al.*, *Archs Dis. Childh.*, 1983, *58*, 795.

Sleep apnoea. Some studies have suggested that central apnoeas may be prolonged if oxygen is given, but most have indicated that the severity of desaturation and incidence of bradyarrhythmias is decreased.— M. C. P. Apps, *Br. J. Hosp. Med.*, 1983, *30*, 339.

For the use of nocturnal oxygen therapy for obstructive sleep apnoea, see under Nocturnal Hypoxia, above.

Viral respiratory disease. Oxygen administration has been shown repeatedly to be a major life-saving measure in young children with severe acute viral respiratory disease.— A. Pio *et al.*, *Bull. int. Un. Tuberc.*, 1983, *58*, 199.

Whooping-cough. Although seldom required, oxygen and suction should be immediately available for all infants with whooping-cough since they may stop breathing after a paroxysm.— *Lancet*, 1984, *1*, 1162.

Proprietary Names and Manufacturers

The following names have been used for multi-ingredient preparations containing oxygen— Entonox *(BOC, UK).*

16196-j

Propane

Dimethylmethane; Propyl Hydride.
C_3H_8=44.10.

CAS — 74-98-6.

Pharmacopoeias. In *U.S.N.F.*

A colourless, odourless, inflammable gas. It is supplied under compression in metal cylinders. **Store** the cylinders in a cool place free from materials of an inflammable nature.

Propane is used as a refrigerant and as an aerosol propellent (see below). It is also used as fuel.

5205-r

Refrigerants and Aerosol Propellents

A number of compressed and liquefied gases are used as refrigerants and as aerosol propellents; these include nitrogen, nitrous oxide, carbon dioxide, propane, and the butanes. Halogenated hydrocarbons, sometimes called fluorocarbons, were widely used but because of environmental hazards their use has been severely restricted; they are still used in pharmacy.

Adverse Effects

The deliberate inhalation of high concentrations of halogenated hydrocarbons for their euphoriant effect may result in CNS depression, cardiac arrhythmias, respiratory depression, and death. Propane and butane can act as simple asphyxiants. Heat can cause the decomposition of halogenated hydrocarbons into irritant and toxic gases such as hydrogen chloride and phosgene.

ABUSE. Deaths following abuse of aerosols: M. Bass, *J. Am. med. Ass.*, 1970, *212*, 2075; *Pharm. J.*, 1973, *2*, 146.

Further reports of abuse of aerosols: P. J. Thompson *et al.*, *Br. med. J.*, 1983, *287*, 1515; P. O. Brennan (letter), *ibid.*, 1877; H. Wickramasinghe and H. J. Liebeschuetz (letter), *ibid.*

EFFECTS ON THE HEART. Ventricular tachycardia associated with non-Freon aerosol propellents.— S. Wason *et al.*, *J. Am. med. Ass.*, 1986, *256*, 78. Criticisms: H. B. McCain and A. R. Ebrahim (letter), *ibid.*, 1987, *257*, 26; R. D. Stewart *et al.* (letter), *ibid.*

EFFECTS ON THE SKIN. Skin sensitivity to trichlorofluoromethane, as shown by patch tests, in 3 patients, one of whom was also sensitive to dichlorodifluoromethane.— W. G. van Ketel, *Contact Dermatitis*, 1976, *2*, 115.

Absorption and Fate

There appears to be little absorption following inhalation of aerosol propellents or refrigerants.

Proprietary Names and Manufacturers of Refrigerants and Aerosol Propellents

Arcton Propellents *(ICI Mond, UK)*; Arklone *(ICI Mond, UK)*; Calor Aerosol Propellants *(Calor, UK)*; Dermamist *(Austral.)*; Flugene *(Fr.)*; Forane *(Austral.; Fr.; Spain)*; Freeze-O-Derm *(Canad.)*; Freon *(USA)*; Frigen *(Ger.)*; Genetron *(USA)*; Isceon Propellents *(ISC Chemicals, UK)*; Isotron *(USA)*; Kaltron *(Ger.)*; Provotest *(Hoechst, Ger.; Hoechst, Switz.)*; Sterethox *(ICI Mond, UK)*; Ucon *(USA)*.

The following names have been used for multi-ingredient preparations containing refrigerants and aerosol propellents— Coolspray *(Bengué, UK)*; Deep Freeze *(Mentholatum, UK)*; Derm-Freeze *(Eagle, Austral.)*; Frezan *(Drug Houses Austral., Austral.)*; PR Spray *(Crookes Healthcare, UK)*; Skefron *(Smith Kline & French, Austral.; Smith Kline & French, UK)*.

5208-n

Trichlorofluoromethane *(BAN).*

Fluorotrichloromethane; Propellent 11; Refrigerant 11; Trichloromonofluoromethane *(USAN).*
CCl_3F=137.4.

CAS — 75-69-4.

Pharmacopoeias. In *Br.* Also in *U.S.N.F.*

A clear, colourless, non-inflammable, volatile liquid with a faint ethereal odour. B.p. about 23.7°. In the liquid state it is practically **immiscible** with water but miscible with dehydrated alcohol. **Store** under compression in metal cylinders.

Trichlorofluoromethane is a halogenated hydrocarbon which is used as a refrigerant and as an aerosol propellent (see above).

In Great Britain the recommended exposure limits of trichlorofluoromethane are 1000 ppm (long-term); 1250 ppm (short-term).

Gastro-intestinal Agents

670-g

The main groups of drugs included in this section are the antacids, antidiarrhoeal agents, anti-emetics, anti-ulcer agents, and laxatives, and these are discussed in more detail below.

Miscellaneous agents included are mesalazine and its derivatives which are used in the management of patients with ulcerative colitis and mebeverine which is used as a gastro-intestinal antispasmodic.

Many other compounds which may be used in a variety of disease states as well as gastro-intestinal disorders may be found in other sections of *Martindale*.

Antacids

Antacids are used to anticipate and relieve pain in the symptomatic management of gastric and duodenal ulcers and reflux oesophagitis by neutralising hydrochloric acid in the gastric secretion. They are normally given between meals and at bedtime when symptoms will usually occur. Antacids are also used as domestic remedies in conditions affecting the stomach which may not necessarily be related to hyperacidity.

Antacids do not reduce the volume of hydrochloric acid secreted and may increase it, but by increasing the gastric pH they diminish the activity of pepsin in the gastric secretion.

Care is necessary when giving drugs to patients receiving antacids. Gastro-intestinal absorption can be reduced by adsorption on insoluble antacids or changes in gastric emptying time and the effects of a drug may be diminished or enhanced by alterations in the intestinal pH or by the formation of complexes.

In addition to the drugs described in this section, sodium bicarbonate (see p.1025) is a commonly used antacid; though highly effective it can cause systemic alkalosis.

A review of the use of antacids in duodenal ulcers.— R. C. Heading, *Gut*, 1984, *25*, 1195.

A short discussion on the treatment of heartburn and dyspepsia in pregnancy summarising that non-systemic antacids are probably the best drugs in conjunction with reassurance and advice on meals and smoking.— C. W. Howden, *Br. med. J.*, 1986, *293*, 1549.

Antidiarrhoeal Agents

In acute diarrhoeas it should always be remembered that fluid and electrolyte depletion may occur and that rehydration therapy may be necessary, especially in infants and young children. For further details concerning rehydration therapy see p.1024.

Antidiarrhoeal agents may be used, where necessary, as adjuncts in the symptomatic treatment of diarrhoea. The main groupings are the adsorbents such as attapulgite, chalk, and kaolin, and the drugs which reduce intestinal motility such as codeine (see p.1297), diphenoxylate, and loperamide. Bulk laxatives (see below) may also be used in the symptomatic treatment of diarrhoea.

Anti-emetics

Included in this section are some miscellaneous compounds used to treat or prevent nausea and vomiting. Other drugs used as anti-emetics include Antimuscarinic Agents, p.522, Antihistamines, p.443, and Neuroleptics, p.706.

Vomiting follows stimulation of the vomiting centre in the medulla, and closely associated with this is the chemoreceptor trigger zone (CTZ) which is sensitive to many drugs and to certain metabolic disturbances. Stimulation of the vomiting centre also occurs following actions on other areas such as the vestibular apparatus of the ear in motion sickness, the cerebral cortex in psychogenic vomiting, and also multiple peripheral receptors. In adults vomiting is almost invariably preceded by a sensation of nausea. As a protective reflex, vomiting is frequently a symptom of disease and should not be treated until the cause has been found.

If vomiting is prolonged, dehydration, hypokalaemia, and alkalosis may occur and replacement of fluid and electrolytes may be necessary.

Cancer chemotherapy can produce severe nausea and vomiting which still proves difficult to treat, especially in children. Repeated exposure to such emetic agents as well as the anxiety associated with hospital attendance can lead to conditioned vomiting. Many of the drugs used in the control of cytotoxic drug-induced nausea and vomiting exert some effect on the CTZ: high-dose metoclopramide has been used in cisplatin-induced emesis, and domperidone and the phenothiazines such as prochlorperazine, perphenazine, and thiethylperazine have been used against moderately emetic agents. However, chemotherapy-induced emesis may be mediated through multiple sites and therefore other drugs may be of benefit including the cannabinoids dronabinol and nabilone, dexamethasone (see p.887), and, particularly during repeated treatments, tranquillisers such as lorazepam. Combinations of different anti-emetics have been tried. Other cannabinoids that have been developed as potential anti-emetics are levonantradol hydrochloride, naboctate hydrochloride, nonabine, and synhexyl but further investigation of these compounds appears now to have ceased.

Radiation-induced emesis is mediated through the CTZ and anti-emetics are used to control the vomiting.

Postoperative emesis may be caused by anaesthetic agents or opioid analgesics. Antimuscarinic agents such as atropine or hyoscine hydrobromide given as part of pre-operative medication reduce the emetic action of opioid analgesics, but they have a shorter duration of action than morphine. Antihistamines such as cyclizine, butyrophenones such as droperidol, or phenothiazines such as perphenazine have also been used, but again the action of some of these drugs may not last as long as that of morphine. Variable results have been obtained with domperidone and metoclopramide.

Motion sickness and other *labyrinthine disorders* such as vertigo or nausea and vomiting associated with Ménière's disease have been treated with antimuscarinic agents such as hyoscine hydrobromide and antihistamines such as cinnarizine, cyclizine, or dimenhydrinate. For the prevention of motion sickness during short journeys hyoscine hydrobromide is considered adequate, but for longer journeys an antihistamine may be more appropriate. Metoclopramide and domperidone are generally ineffective in motion sickness.

Nausea and vomiting associated with *pregnancy* has been controlled with antihistamines such as promethazine or phenothiazines. They should only be administered, however, if vomiting is severe.

Reviews of nausea and vomiting and its treatment: R. S. J. Clarke, *Br. J. Anaesth.*, 1984, *56*, 19; J. Stonham and S. Ross, *Br. J. Hosp. Med.*, 1984, *31*, 354.

Reviews on the control of nausea and vomiting associated with cancer chemotherapy: *Drugs*, 1983, *25*, *Suppl.* 1, 1-83; C. L. Fortner *et al.*, *Drug Intell. & clin. Pharm.*, 1985, *19*, 21; P. L. Triozzi and J. Laszlo, *Drugs*, 1987, *34*, 136.

Anti-ulcer Agents

Peptic ulceration is a common condition and healing can often be accelerated by simple measures such as bed-rest and stopping smoking; antacids have traditionally been used in the symptomatic management of peptic ulcers.

Several specific anti-ulcer agents with a variety of mechanisms of action are now available and although most have been shown to produce rapid short-term healing of ulcers in the majority of patients, none has convincingly been shown to significantly alter the natural history of the disease whereby relapse occurs in a substantial number of patients once therapy is discontinued. Investigations are being directed at whether intermittent therapy with such agents when relapse occurs or alternatively low-dose maintenance therapy is the best form of management.

Recent reports of the discovery of the bacterium *Campylobacter pylori* (*C. pyloridis*) in the gastric secretions of patients with gastritis or peptic ulceration have focussed attention on the aetiology of the disease. These reports suggest that effective therapies for peptic ulceration may have to include not only agents with mucosal protective properties or an ability to reduce secretion of gastric acid, but also agents with antimicrobial activity. Studies with tri-potassium di-citrato bismuthate, an agent with both mucosal protectant properties and an activity against *C. pylori*, have indeed demonstrated that like many other agents it is effective for short-term healing and have also suggested that a lower relapse-rate may occur although relapse is still a fairly frequent occurrence.

Some of the more widely-used anti-ulcer agents are carbenoxolone, pirenzepine, and sucralfate, as well as the histamine H_2-receptor antagonists, cimetidine, famotidine, nizatidine, ranitidine, and roxatidine; another H_2-antagonist under investigation is sufotidine (AH-25352). Several other H_2-antagonists including burimamide, etintidine (BL-5641A), lamtidine (AH-22216), loxtidine (AH-23844), lupitidine (SKF-93479), metiamide (SKF-92058), oxmetidine (SKF-92994), tiotidine (ICI-125211), and tiquinamide (Wy-24081) have been produced but further investigation and development on many of these compounds appears to have ceased usually following reports of undue toxicity in *animals*.

Another class of agents being investigated in peptic ulceration and allied disorders are the so-called proton-pump inhibitors which also reduce secretion of gastric acid; omeprazole is the most widely studied member of this group.

A brief review of some forms of management of peptic ulceration, concluding that agents relying upon actions other than suppression of gastric acid are unlikely to replace the H_2-antagonists for routine or maintenance therapy but that they do offer useful alternatives.— D. G. Colin-Jones, *Gut*, 1986, *27*, 475.

A review concerning the proposed role of *Campylobacter pylori* (*C. pyloridis*) in causing peptic ulceration.— R. B. Hornick, *New Engl. J. Med.*, 1987, *316*, 1598.

Laxatives

Laxatives (purgatives or cathartics) induce defaecation. They are widely used as self medications to satisfy the patient's desire for an altered or more regular bowel habit. Constipation can often be resolved without recourse to laxatives. An adjustment in diet to increase vegetable fibre and fluid intake may be all that is required. However, the use of a laxative may be necessary in certain conditions, for example to reduce excessive straining in cardiovascular disease or in patients with haemorrhoids, following surgery, or when constipation is due to neurological defects, hormonal changes as in pregnancy, or treatment with certain drugs such as opioid analgesics.

Abuse of laxatives is a well-known phenomenon that may occasionally lead to severe toxicity although the presenting features are not always clear. Most patients are reported to be women and commonly have associated psychiatric disorders such as depression, anorexia nervosa, or a personality problem.

Laxatives may be classified according to their action. There is a certain amount of overlap between the various groups and although the mechanisms of action are not fully understood most laxatives are now considered to act, at least in part, by increasing retention of fluid in the colon.

Bulk-forming laxatives such as psyllium, sterculia, methylcellulose (see p.1436), or bran cause retention of fluid and an increase in faecal mass resulting in stimulation of peristalsis. They usually have an effect within 12 to 24 hours, reaching a maximum after several days. They are used for the treatment of constipation and, due to their hydrophilic nature, they may also be used to control acute diarrhoea and to regulate the effluent in colostomy patients. Bulk-forming laxatives need to be taken with an adequate fluid intake to avoid compaction in the gastro-intestinal tract.

Stimulant laxatives (contact laxatives) include anthraquinone-containing laxatives such as senna or cascara, diphenylmethane derivatives such as bisacodyl, phenolphthalein, or sodium picosulphate, and other miscellaneous agents such as castor oil (see p.1554). They appear to stimulate accumulation of water and electrolytes in the colon and to increase intestinal motility. They usually have an effect within 6 to 12 hours. Stimulant laxatives should only be used in functional constipation that has not responded to dietary measures and they should be withdrawn as soon as possible. They are also used for bowel clearance before radiological examination, endoscopy, surgery, or childbirth.

Osmotic laxatives include saline laxatives such as magnesium sulphate (see p.1033) or magnesium citrate which cause retention of fluid in the bowel. Full cathartic doses cause a semi-fluid evacuation within about 3 hours, but lower doses may take 6 to 12 hours for an effect. They are used for bowel evacuation before radiological, endoscopic, and surgical procedures, and also to expel parasites and toxic materials. Adequate fluid intake is necessary to avoid dehydration. Lactulose may also be classified as an osmotic laxative because its breakdown products increase intra-colonic osmotic pressure. It may take one to three days to have an effect. Also included in this group are hyperosmotic laxatives such as sorbitol (see p.1273) and glycerol (see p.1128).

Other laxatives include faecal softeners (emollient laxatives) such as docusates which soften the faeces by decreasing surface tension and increasing the penetration of intestinal fluids into the faecal mass, and the lubricant laxative liquid paraffin (see p.1322). These may be of value in treating painful anorectal disorders, such as haemorrhoids and anal fissures, or to prevent straining at stool.

Parasympathomimetic agents such as neostigmine (see p.1332) are occasionally used to treat constipation when there is an underlying disorder such as paralytic ileus.

A review of constipation including a suggested approach to management. Mild constipation can often be managed solely by manipulation of diet (increasing the content of vegetables, fruit, whole grain cereal and bread, and ensuring an adequate intake of fluid). Supplements of unprocessed bran have often been used but many patients find bran unpalatable, and if so, other bulking agents, such as ispaghula and sterculia, are available. If the altered diet and an added bulking agent do not produce an acceptable bowel habit further agents such as lactulose or docusate sodium can be added. The stimulant or irritant laxatives such as senna, cascara, danthron, phenolphthalein, and bisacodyl may lead to immediate or long-term side-effects. Lubricants, such as liquid paraffin, as long-term oral medications, are probably best avoided and enemas and suppositories should be reserved primarily for the short-term management of severe constipation or faecal impaction.— R. Smallwood, *Med. J. Aust.*, 1984, *141*, 447.

Further reviews of the use of laxatives and the treatment of constipation: W. G. Thompson, *Drugs*, 1980, *19*, 49; E. W. Godding, *Pharm. J.*, 1984, *1*, 75, 110, 138, 168, 198, and 239; B. Rados and H. Hopkins, *FDA Consumer*, 1985, *19*, (May), 12; A. Li Wan Po, *Chemist Drugg.*, 1985, *224*, 567.

12307-t

Aceglutamide Aluminum *(USAN)*.

Aceglutamide Aluminium *(rINNM)*; KW-110. Pentakis (N^2-acetyl-L-glutaminato)tetrahydroxytrialuminium.
$C_{35}H_{59}Al_3N_{10}O_{24}$=1084.9.

CAS — 12607-92-0.

Aceglutamide aluminum is used in the treatment of peptic ulcer in doses of up to 3 g daily.

Proprietary Names and Manufacturers
Glumal *(Kyowa, Jpn; Liade, Spain)*.

712-d

Alexitol Sodium *(BAN, rINN)*.

Sodium poly(hydroxyaluminium) carbonate-hexitol complex.

CAS — 66813-51-2.

Alexitol sodium is an antacid that is given in doses of 360 to 720 mg.

Proprietary Preparations
Actal *(Winthrop, UK)*. *Tablets*, alexitol sodium 360 mg. *Suspension*, alexitol sodium 360 mg/5 mL.
Droxalin *(Sterling Health, UK)*. *Tablets*, chewable, alexitol sodium 200 mg, magnesium trisilicate 162 mg. *Dose.* 1 or 2 tablets as required.

Proprietary Names and Manufacturers
Actal *(Winthrop, Austral.; Maggioni-Winthrop, Ital.; Winthrop, S.Afr.; Winthrop, UK)*; Actonalt; Talakt *(Winthrop, Denm.)*.

18803-j

Alizapride *(rINN)*.

N-(1-Allyl-2-pyrrolidinylmethyl)-6-methoxy-1*H*-benzotriazole-5-carboxamide.
$C_{16}H_{21}N_5O_2$=315.4.

CAS — 59338-93-1.

16020-y

Alizapride Hydrochloride *(rINNM)*.

$C_{16}H_{21}N_5O_2$,HCl=351.8.

Adverse Effects
Alizapride has been reported to cause muscle spasms, drowsiness, galactorrhoea, amenorrhoea, and cardiovascular disturbances.

Episodes of hypertension were associated with alizapride 14 mg per kg body-weight or prochlorperazine 0.56 mg per kg each administered in 5 divided doses by intravenous infusion to control cisplatin-induced emesis. Nine of 32 patients experienced hypertension in 14 courses: 6 episodes following alizapride and 8 episodes following prochlorperazine.— H. Roche *et al.* (letter), *New Engl. J. Med.*, 1985, *312*, 1125.

For reference to further adverse effects, see below under Uses and Administration.

Absorption and Fate
Alizapride is mainly excreted unchanged in the urine.

Pharamcokinetic studies of alizapride administered by various routes to healthy subjects: G. Houin *et al.*, *J. pharm. Sci.*, 1983, *72*, 71; G. Houin *et al.*, *ibid.*, 1984, *73*, 1450.

Uses and Administration
Alizapride is a substituted benzamide which has been used as the hydrochloride to control nausea and vomiting associated with a variety of disorders. Alizapride hydrochloride has been given in usual doses equivalent to 100 to 200 mg of alizapride daily by mouth; children have been given 5 mg per kg body-weight daily. For patients receiving cancer chemotherapy daily doses equivalent to 100 to 200 mg of alizapride have been administered intravenously or intramuscularly in 2 divided doses, one immediately before and one about 4 hours after cytotoxic drug administration; children have received 2 to 4 mg per kg in 2 divided doses.

NAUSEA AND VOMITING. A dose-finding study of alizapride given to 24 patients receiving strongly emetic cytotoxic therapy. Doses of 4 mg, 6 mg, or 8 mg per kg body-weight were administered as 15-minute infusions 0.5 hour before and 1.5, 3.5, 5.5, and 8.5 hours after chemotherapy; 4 mg per kg appeared to be the optimum dose. All 4 patients given high doses of 8 mg per kg experienced profuse sweating and malaise and in 3 of these patients the treatment had to be interrupted due to adverse effects. Other adverse effects reported during the study included dizziness, hypotension, trembling, dyspnoea, and diarrhoea; in one patient a short-lived extrapyramidal syndrome was observed.— R. A. Joss *et al.*, *Eur. J. clin. Pharmac.*, 1985, *27*, 721.

In a double-blind crossover study of 44 cancer patients, alizapride in doses of 4 mg per kg body-weight was significantly more effective than domperidone 600 µg per kg in reducing nausea and vomiting associated with cisplatin therapy, especially in severe cases; both drugs were administered by intravenous infusion over 15 minutes at 2-hourly intervals for 5 doses. Alizapride and domperidone were well tolerated although sedation, diarrhoea, and hypotension were reported with both drugs; extrapyramidal symptoms were seen in 2 patients on each drug.— J. Huys *et al.*, *Curr. med. Res. Opinion*, 1985, *9*, 400. Another comparative study in similar patients receiving cisplatin or other highly emetic cancer chemotherapy. Alizapride 4 mg per kg was less effective than metoclopramide 2 mg per kg and also demonstrated more side-effects. Of particular concern was a patient who experienced 4 convulsive episodes with apnoea, and another in whom atrial fibrillation and right bundle branch block occurred. Despite its initial promise alizapride could not, in the authors' view, be recommended for further use.— R. A. Joss *et al.*, *Clin. Pharmac. Ther.*, 1986, *39*, 619.

Proprietary Names and Manufacturers of Alizapride and its Salts
Limican *(Vita, Ital.)*; Litican *(Delagrange, Belg.)*; Liticum *(Delagrange, Spain)*; Nausilen *(Inverni della Beffa, Ital.)*; Pesalin *(Prodes, Spain)*; Plitican *(Delagrange, Fr.)*; Vergentan *(Schürholz, Ger.)*.

19021-z

Almagate *(rINN)*.

A hydrated aluminium-magnesium hydroxycarbonate.
$Al_2Mg_6(OH)_{14}(CO_3)_2.4H_2O$=630.0.

CAS — 66827-12-1; 72526-11-5 (anhydrous).

Almagate is an antacid that is given in doses of about 1 g.

A series of papers on almagate.— *Arzneimittel-Forsch.*, 1984, *34*, 1343-83.

Proprietary Names and Manufacturers
Almax *(Almirall, Spain)*.

15333-f

Almasilate *(BAN, rINN)*.

Aluminium Magnesium Silicate Hydrate; Magnesium Aluminosilicate Hydrate; Magnesium Aluminum Silicate Hydrate. An artificial form of aluminium magnesium silicate hydrate.
$Al_2O_3.MgO.2SiO_2,xH_2O$=262.4 (anhydrous).

CAS — 71205-22-6.

Almasilate is an antacid that is given in doses of 1 g. Hydrated native aluminium magnesium silicate (p.1433) is used as a suspending, thickening, and stabilising agent in pharmaceutical preparations.

Proprietary Preparations
Malinal *(Robins, UK)*. *Tablets*, chewable, scored, almasilate 500 mg.
Suspension, almasilate 500 mg/5 mL.

7501-f

Aloes *(BAN)*.

Acibar; Aloe *(USAN)*.

CAS — 8001-97-6; 67479-27-0 (aloe gum).

Pharmacopoeias. In *Arg., Aust., Belg., Br., Braz., Egypt., Eur., Fr., Ger., Hung., It., Jpn, Neth., Nord., Pol., Port., Roum., Span., Swiss, Turk.,* and *U.S. Br.*

also includes Powdered Aloes.
Braz. and *Egypt.* also allow Socotrine aloes.

The residue obtained by evaporating the juice of the leaves of various species of *Aloe* (Liliaceae).
The *B.P.* and *Eur. P.* describe Barbados Aloes (Curaçao aloes) obtained from *Aloe barbadensis* (=*A.vera*) containing not less than 28% of hydroxyanthracene derivatives, calculated as anhydrous barbaloin and Cape Aloes (*Aloe capensis*) obtained mainly from *Aloe ferox* and its hybrids containing not less than 18% of hydroxyanthracene derivatives, calculated as anhydrous barbaloin.
Aloe (*U.S.P.*) is Cape Aloe or Curaçao Aloe, yielding not less than 50% of water-soluble extractive.
Barbados and Cape aloes are partly soluble in boiling water, soluble in hot alcohol, and practically insoluble in chloroform and ether. Powdered Barbados or Cape aloes are almost entirely soluble in alcohol 60%.

Adverse Effects and Precautions
As for Senna, p.1106, although aloes has a more drastic and irritant action.

Uses and Administration
Aloes is an anthraquinone laxative that has been superseded by less toxic agents.

Although *Aloe vera* has for many years been used as an ingredient in cosmetics such as face and hand creams, lotions, and skin moisturisers the FDA has recently become concerned about the widespread distribution of *Aloe vera* products promoted for self-treatment of human complaints. Exaggerated and unsubstantiated claims are being made that these products can cure or alleviate a variety of unrelated conditions including colitis, asthma, glaucoma, haemorrhoids, arthritis, acne, anaemia, tuberculosis, cancer, diabetes, depression, multiple sclerosis, and even blindness. Such products are often sold as food supplements or cosmetics in health stores but the manufacturers are careful to make no health claims on the product labels and in order to remove them from the market the FDA would have to prove them to be adulterated or misbranded. Serious harm may follow when proper medical treatment of serious illness is neglected or abandoned in favour of such products with no proven value.— A. Hecht, *FDA Consumer*, 1981, *15*, Jul.-Aug., 26.

Preparations
Standardised Aloes Dry Extract (*B.P., Eur. P.*). Contains 19.0 to 21.0% of hydroxyanthracene derivatives, calculated as anhydrous barbaloin. Store in well-closed containers. Protect from light and moisture.

Proprietary Names and Manufacturers
The following names have been used for multi-ingredient preparations containing aloes— Nature's Remedy (*Norcliff Thayer, USA*); Opobyl (*Bengué, UK*).

12343-d

Aloglutamol
2-Amino-2-hydroxymethylpropane-1,3-diol gluconate dihydroxyaluminate.
$C_{10}H_{24}AlNO_{12}$=377.3.

Aloglutamol is an antacid that is given in doses of 0.5 to 1 g.

Proprietary Names and Manufacturers
Altris (*Isnardi, Ital.*); Pyreses (*Berenguer-Beneyto, Spain*); Tasto (*Scharper, Ital.*).

7502-d

Aloin (*BAN*).
CAS — 5133-19-7; 8015-61-0; 1415-73-2 (barbaloin).

Pharmacopoeias. In *Arg., Br., Braz.,* and *Span.*

A yellow crystalline substance extracted from aloes and containing not less than 70% of anhydrous barbaloin.

Almost completely **soluble** 1 in 130 of water; soluble in alcohol and in acetone; very slightly soluble in chloroform and in ether. A 1% suspension in water has a pH of 4.0 to 6.5.

Aloin like aloes is very irritant and has been superseded by less toxic laxatives.

Proprietary Names and Manufacturers
The following names have been used for multi-ingredient preparations containing aloin—Alophen (*Parke, Davis, Canad.*; *Warner-Lambert, UK*); Aperient Dellipsoids D9 (*Pilsworth, UK*); Purgoids (*Evans Medical, UK*).

671-q

Aluminium Glycinate (*BAN*).
Dihydroxyaluminum Aminoacetate (*USAN*). (Glycinato-*N,O*)dihydroxyaluminium hydrate.
$C_2H_6AlNO_4(+xH_2O)$=135.1.

CAS — 13682-92-3 (anhydrous); 41354-48-7 (hydrate).

Pharmacopoeias. In *Br.* and *U.S.*

A white or almost white, odourless or almost odourless, powder. The *B.P.* specifies 34.5 to 38.5% of Al_2O_3 calculated on the dried substance, and not more than 12% loss of weight on drying. The *U.S.P.* specifies not more than 14.5% loss on drying.
Practically **insoluble** in water and organic solvents; soluble in dilute mineral acids and solutions of alkali hydroxides. A 4% suspension in water has a pH of 6.5 to 7.5. **Store** in well-closed containers.

Aluminium glycinate is an antacid that is given in doses of about 1 g.

Preparations
Dihydroxyaluminum Aminoacetate Capsules (*U.S.P.*)
Dihydroxyaluminum Aminoacetate Magma (*U.S.P.*). A white viscous suspension of aluminium glycinate. Store in airtight containers. Protect from freezing.
Dihydroxyaluminum Aminoacetate Tablets (*U.S.P.*)

Proprietary Names and Manufacturers
Alcap (*Ital.*); Apercide (*Cinfa, Spain*); Rinveral (*Monik, Spain*); Robalate (*Robins, Canad.*; *Robins, UK*; *USA*).

The following names have been used for multi-ingredient preparations containing aluminium glycinate—Glycinal (*Medo, UK*); Prodexin (*Bencard, UK*).

673-s

Aluminium Hydroxide (*BAN*).
Aluminum Hydroxide (*USAN*).

CAS — 21645-51-2 [Al(OH)₃].

Pharmacopoeias. In *Arg., Aust., Belg., Br., Chin., Cz., Egypt., Eur., Fr., Hung., Ind., It., Jpn., Jug., Mex., Neth., Pol., Port., Rus., Swiss, Turk.,* and *U.S.*

Dried Aluminium Hydroxide (*B.P.*) [Dried Aluminium Hydroxide Gel; Hydrated Aluminium Oxide (*Eur. P.*)] contains the equivalent of 47 to 60% Al_2O_3. It is a white odourless amorphous powder. Practically **insoluble** in water; soluble in dilute mineral acids and in solutions of alkali hydroxides. **Store** in airtight containers at a temperature not exceeding 30°.
Dried Aluminum Hydroxide Gel (*U.S.P.*) is an amorphous form of aluminium hydroxide in which there is a partial substitution of carbonate for hydroxide. It contains the equivalent of not less than 76.5% of $Al(OH)_3$ and may contain varying quantities of basic aluminium carbonate and bicarbonate. In the labelling requirements the *U.S.P.* states that 1 g of dried aluminum hydroxide gel is equivalent to 765 mg of $Al(OH)_3$. It is a white, odourless, tasteless, amorphous powder. Practically **insoluble** in water and alcohol; soluble in dilute mineral acids and in solutions of alkali hydroxides. A 4% aqueous dispersion has a pH of not more than 10.0. **Store** in airtight containers.

Algeldrate (*USAN, pINN*) is defined as a hydrated aluminium hydroxide with the general formula of $Al(OH)_3,xH_2O$.

Adverse Effects and Precautions
Aluminium hydroxide in common with other aluminium compounds is astringent and may cause nausea, vomiting, and constipation; large doses can cause intestinal obstruction.
Excessive doses, or even normal doses in patients with low-phosphate diets, may lead to phosphate depletion accompanied by increased resorption and urinary excretion of calcium with the risk of osteomalacia.
Osteomalacia, and also encephalopathy and dementia, have occurred in patients with chronic renal failure who received relatively high doses of aluminium hydroxide as a phosphate-binding agent. For further details concerning this use as a phosphate-binder, see under Uses. Similar adverse effects are associated with the aluminium content of the dialysis fluids, see under aluminium, (p.1541).
Aluminium hydroxide may alter the absorption of other drugs from the gastro-intestinal tract if administered concomitantly.

References to aluminium toxicity in dialysis patients are included under aluminium (p.1541).

Reports of aluminium intoxication attributed to the use of aluminium-containing phosphate-binders in patients with renal failure but not undergoing dialysis: S. Pedersen and E. Nathan (letter), *Lancet*, 1982, *2*, 1107 (dementia in a child receiving aluminium hydroxide); W. R. Griswold *et al., Pediatrics*, 1983, *71*, 56 (osteomalacia, encephalopathy, and seizures in a child receiving aluminium hydroxide); M. E. Randall (letter), *ibid.*, 1327 (encephalopathy and seizures in a nondialysed infant receiving aluminium carbonate); S. P. Andreoli *et al., New Engl. J. Med.*, 1984, *310*, 1079 (osteomalacia in 3 nondialysed infants receiving aluminium hydroxide); A. B. Sedman *et al., J. Pediat.*, 1984, *105*, 836 (encephalopathy in a child receiving aluminium hydroxide).

Absorption and Fate
The insoluble aluminium compounds that constitute aluminium hydroxide mixture are slowly but perhaps incompletely converted to aluminium chloride in the stomach. Some absorption of soluble aluminium salts occurs from the gastro-intestinal tract with some excretion in the urine. Some unabsorbed aluminium hydroxide combines with phosphates present in the gut to form insoluble aluminium phosphates and some forms carbonates and salts of fatty acids; all these salts are excreted in the faeces.

Studies of the absorption of aluminium hydroxide, aluminium carbonate, aluminium glycinate, and aluminium phosphate by healthy subjects demonstrated that although the gastro-intestinal tract was a formidable barrier to entry of aluminium it was not impervious. Following ingestion of the first 3 compounds plasma-aluminium concentrations rose significantly and urinary excretion rose markedly. Absorption of aluminium phosphate (virtually insoluble at acid pH but slightly more soluble than aluminium hydroxide in alkaline pH) was insignificant which correlated with the hypothesis that aluminium absorption occurred largely in the acid milieu of the proximal duodenum or stomach and very little if at all in the rest of the gastro-intestinal tract.— W. D. Kaehny *et al., New Engl. J. Med.*, 1977, *296*, 1389.

Uses and Administration
Aluminium hydroxide is an antacid that is given in doses of up to about 1 g. In order to reduce the constipating effects, it is often given in association with a magnesium-containing antacid, such as magnesium carbonate, magnesium hydroxide, or magnesium trisilicate. See also almasilate (p.1074).
Aluminium hydroxide may also be used as a phosphate-binder in patients with chronic renal failure. Daily doses of up to 10 g have been given. Because of adverse effects other agents are now preferred, see below.
Aluminium hydroxide is also used as an adjuvant in the manufacture of adsorbed vaccines.

PHOSPHATE BINDING. Secondary hyperparathyroidism is common in patients with chronic renal failure and may lead to the development of associated bone disorders such as osteitis fibrosa and metastatic calcification. Phosphate retention with hyperphosphataemia has been implicated in the development of this hyperparathyroid state and thus aluminium hydroxide, which binds dietary phosphate in the gastro-intestinal tract, has been used in order to reduce the body-phosphate load. However, the relatively large doses of aluminium hydroxide needed in some of these patients with compromised renal function has led to cases of aluminium toxicity (see under Adverse Effects) and alternative phosphate-binders have been sought.

Sucralfate, another aluminium-containing compound not apparently associated with aluminium toxicity, has been found, in doses of 3 to 9 g daily, to produce satisfactory phosphate control in patients on dialysis, (A.C.T. Leung *et al.*, *Br. med. J.*, 1983, *286*, 1379; B. Vucelić *et al.*, *Int. J. clin. Pharmac. Ther. Toxic.*, 1986, *24*, 93) as has magnesium carbonate 0.5 to 1.5 g daily in association with low-magnesium dialysis fluids (R. O'Donovan *et al.*, *Lancet*, 1986, *1*, 880).

Calcium carbonate had been proposed many years ago as a phosphate binder but until recently does not appear to have been widely used. In a crossover study involving children with preterminal chronic renal failure (R.H.K. Mak *et al.*, *Br. med. J.*, 1985, *291*, 623) it was found that at the end of 6 months' treatment calcium carbonate had been as effective as aluminium hydroxide in suppressing secondary hyperparathyroidism; final mean doses were calcium carbonate 3.4 g daily and aluminium hydroxide 5.8 g daily. It was recommended that high dose calcium carbonate should be used as the phosphate-binder after the initial reduction of plasma-phosphate concentrations had been achieved with a low-phosphate diet and aluminium hydroxide. Another study (E. Slatopolsky *et al.*, *New Engl. J. Med.*, 1986, *315*, 157) confirmed that calcium carbonate, in the majority of patients, may be a satisfactory substitute for traditional aluminium-containing phosphate-binders but it was noted that 6 of the 20 patients investigated who were receiving calcium carbonate at a mean dosage of 8.5 g daily needed aluminium hydroxide additionally for satisfactory control of hyperphosphataemia. Further support for the use of calcium carbonate was provided by a study in dialysis patients (J.F. Addison and C.J. Foulks, *Curr. ther. Res.*, 1985, *38*, 241) although some controversy has arisen because of the risk of hypercalcaemia developing (H.D. Stein *et al.*, *New Engl. J. Med.*, 1987, *316*, 109; A.E.G. Raine and D.O. Oliver, *Lancet*, 1987, *1*, 633). Responding to the problem of hypercalcaemia Slatopolsky and colleagues (*New Engl. J. Med.*, 1987, *316*, 110) have emphasized that the dosage of calcium carbonate used should be titrated against the intake of dietary phosphate and that dialysis fluids with lower calcium contents should be employed.

Preparations

Dried Aluminum Hydroxide Gel Capsules *(U.S.P.)*. Capsules containing aluminium hydroxide $[Al(OH)_3]$.

Alumina and Magnesia Oral Suspension *(U.S.P.)*. A mixture containing aluminium hydroxide $[Al(OH)_3]$ and magnesium hydroxide with aluminium hydroxide predominating. pH 7.3 to 7.9. Store in airtight containers. Avoid freezing.

See also Magnesia and Alumina Oral Suspension under Magnesium Hydroxide.

Alumina, Magnesia, and Calcium Carbonate Oral Suspension *(U.S.P.)*. A suspension containing aluminium hydroxide $[Al(OH)_3]$, magnesium hydroxide, and calcium carbonate. Store in airtight containers. Avoid freezing.

Alumina, Magnesia, and Simethicone Oral Suspension *(U.S.P.)*. A suspension containing aluminium hydroxide $[Al(OH)_3]$, magnesium hydroxide, and dimethicones. Store in airtight containers. Avoid freezing.

Alumina and Magnesium Carbonate Oral Suspension *(U.S.P.)*. A suspension containing aluminium hydroxide $[Al(OH)_3]$ and magnesium carbonate. Store in airtight containers. Avoid freezing.

Alumina and Magnesium Trisilicate Oral Suspension *(U.S.P.)*. A suspension containing aluminium hydroxide $[Al(OH)_3]$ and magnesium trisilicate. Store in airtight containers.

Aluminium Hydroxide Oral Suspension *(B.P.)*. Aluminium Hydroxide Gel; Aluminium Hydroxide Mixture. An aqueous suspension of hydrated aluminium oxide together with varying quantities of basic aluminium carbonate containing 3.5 to 4.4% w/w of Al_2O_3. Store at a temperature not exceeding 30°. Avoid freezing.

Aluminium Hydroxide and Belladonna Mixture *(B.P.C. 1973)*. Belladonna tincture 0.5 mL, chloroform spirit 0.25 mL, aluminium hydroxide mixture to 5 mL. *Dose*. 5 mL, suitably diluted.

Aluminium Hydroxide and Kaolin Mixture *(A.P.F.)*. Aluminium Hydroxide Gel with Kaolin. Light kaolin or light kaolin (natural) 2 g, sodium citrate 10 mg, concentrated chloroform water 0.2 mL or compound hydroxybenzoate solution 0.1 mL, aluminium hydroxide mixture to 10 mL. *Dose*. Initial, 15 mL; repeated, 5 to 10 mL.

Aluminum Hydroxide Gel *(U.S.P.)*. A suspension containing 5.5 to 6.7% w/w of aluminium hydroxide $[Al(OH)_3]$, in the form of amorphous aluminium hydroxide in which there is a partial substitution of carbonate for hydroxide. pH 5.5 to 8.0. Store in airtight containers. Avoid freezing.

Alumina and Magnesia Tablets *(U.S.P.)*. Tablets containing aluminium hydroxide $[Al(OH)_3]$ and magnesium hydroxide.

See also Magnesia and Alumina Tablets under Magnesium Hydroxide.

Alumina, Magnesia, and Calcium Carbonate Tablets *(U.S.P.)*. Chewable tablets containing aluminium hydroxide $[Al(OH)_3]$, magnesium hydroxide, and calcium carbonate.

Alumina, Magnesia, and Simethicone Tablets *(U.S.P.)*. Tablets containing aluminium hydroxide $[Al(OH)_3]$, magnesium hydroxide, and dimethicones. Store in well-closed containers.

Alumina, Magnesium Carbonate, and Magnesium Oxide Tablets *(U.S.P.)*. Tablets containing aluminium hydroxide $[Al(OH)_3]$, magnesium carbonate, and magnesium oxide. Store in airtight containers.

Alumina and Magnesium Trisilicate Tablets *(U.S.P.)*. Tablets containing aluminium hydroxide $[Al(OH)_3]$ and magnesium trisilicate.

Aluminium Hydroxide Tablets *(B.P.)*. Chewable tablets with a peppermint flavour containing 500 mg of dried aluminium hydroxide. Store at a temperature not exceeding 25°.

Dried Aluminum Hydroxide Gel Tablets *(U.S.P.)*. Tablets containing aluminium hydroxide $[Al(OH)_3]$.

Proprietary Preparations

Actonorm Gel *(Wallace Mfg Chem., UK)*. *Gel*, dried aluminium hydroxide 220 mg, magnesium hydroxide 200 mg, activated dimethicone 25 mg/5mL. *Dose*. 5 to 20 mL when required.

For Actonorm Powder see under Magnesium Carbonate.

Alu-Cap *(Riker, UK)*. *Capsules*, dried aluminium hydroxide 475 mg.

Aludrox *(Wyeth, UK)*. *Mixture*, Aluminium Hydroxide Mixture (*B.P.*).

For Aludrox Tablets see under Aluminium Hydroxide-Magnesium Carbonate Co-dried Gel.

Aludrox SA *(Wyeth, UK)*. *Suspension*, aluminium hydroxide mixture 4.75 mL, magnesium hydroxide 100 mg, ambutonium bromide 2.5 mg/5mL. *Dose*. 5 to 10 mL between meals and at bedtime.

Aluhyde *(Sinclair, UK)*. *Tablets*, chewable, scored, dried aluminium hydroxide 245 mg, magnesium trisilicate 245 mg, belladonna liquid extract 7.8 mg. *Dose*. 2 tablets three times daily.

Andursil Suspension (*Geigy, UK*). *Suspension*, aluminium hydroxide mixture equivalent to Al_2O_3 200 mg, magnesium hydroxide 200 mg, aluminium hydroxide-magnesium carbonate co-dried gel 200 mg, activated dimethicone 150 mg/5mL. *Dose*. 5 to 10 mL 3 or 4 times daily and at bedtime.

For Andursil Tablets see under Aluminium Hydroxide-Magnesium Carbonate Co-dried Gel.

Asilone (*Rorer, UK*). *Tablets*, chewable, dried aluminium hydroxide 500 mg, activated dimethicone 270 mg.

Gel, dried aluminium hydroxide 420 mg, light magnesium oxide 70 mg, activated dimethicone 135 mg/5 mL.

Suspension, dried aluminium hydroxide 420 mg, light magnesium oxide 70 mg, activated dimethicone 135 mg/5 mL. *Dose*. 1 or 2 tablets, or 5 to 10 mL of gel or suspension before meals and at bedtime.

Asilone for Infants (*Rorer, UK*). *Suspension*, dried aluminium hydroxide 84 mg, light magnesium oxide 14 mg, activated dimethicone 27 mg/5 mL. *Dose*. Infants 1 to 3 months, 2.5 mL three or four times daily before or during feeds; older children, 5 mL three or four times daily before or during feeds.

Dijex Liquid *(Crookes Healthcare, UK)*. *Oral liquid*, aluminium hydroxide mixture 98%, magnesium hydroxide 1.7%.

For Dijex Tablets see under Aluminium Hydroxide-Magnesium Carbonate Co-dried Gel.

Diovol Suspension *(Pharmax, UK)*. *Suspension*, aluminium hydroxide 200 mg, magnesium hydroxide 200 mg, dimethicone 25 mg/5 mL. *Dose*. 10 to 20 mL when required.

Gastrocote *(MCP Pharmaceuticals, UK)*. *Tablets*, chewable, dried aluminium hydroxide 80 mg, magnesium trisilicate 40 mg, sodium bicarbonate 70 mg, alginic acid 200 mg.

Liquid, dried aluminium hydroxide 80 mg, magnesium trisilicate 40 mg, sodium bicarbonate 70 mg, sodium alginate 220 mg. *Dose*. 1 to 2 tablets or 5 to 15 mL of liquid after meals and at bedtime.

Gastron *(Winthrop, UK)*. *Tablets*, chewable, dried aluminium hydroxide 240 mg, sodium bicarbonate 210 mg, magnesium trisilicate 60 mg, alginic acid 600 mg. *Dose*. 1 or 2 tablets after meals and 2 at bedtime.

Gaviscon *(Reckitt & Colman Pharmaceuticals, UK)*. *Tablets*, chewable, dried aluminium hydroxide 100 mg, magnesium trisilicate 25 mg, alginic acid 500 mg, sodium bicarbonate 170 mg. *Dose*. 1 or 2 tablets after meals and at bedtime.

For Liquid Gaviscon see under Calcium Carbonate.

Infant Gaviscon *(Reckitt & Colman Pharmaceuticals, UK)*. *Oral powder*, dried aluminium hydroxide 200 mg, magnesium trisilicate 50 mg, alginic acid 924 mg, sodium bicarbonate 340 mg/sachet. *Dose*. The contents of ½ to 1 sachet mixed with each milk feed or mixed with water and taken after each meal.

NOTE. In view of its high sodium content this preparation should not be used in premature infants or in situations where excess water-loss is likely, such as fever or high room-temperature; some sources have recommended that it should be avoided altogether in children less than 6 months of age.

Gelusil *(Warner-Lambert, UK)*. *Tablets*, chewable, dried aluminium hydroxide 250 mg, magnesium trisilicate 500 mg. *Dose*. 1 or 2 tablets after meals, or when necessary.

Kolanticon *(Merrell, UK)*. *Gel*, dried aluminium hydroxide 200 mg, dicyclomine hydrochloride 2.5 mg, light magnesium oxide 100 mg, activated dimethicone 20 mg/5mL. *Dose*. 10 to 20 mL every 4 hours.

Kolantyl *(Merrell, UK)*. *Gel*, dried aluminium hydroxide 200 mg, dicyclomine hydrochloride 2.5 mg, light magnesium oxide 100 mg/5 mL. *Dose*. 10 to 20 mL every 4 hours.

LoAsid *(Calmic, UK)*. *Tablets*, chewable, dried aluminium hydroxide 230 mg, magnesium hydroxide 230 mg, activated dimethicone 12 mg. *Dose*. 1 or 2 tablets after or between meals and at bedtime.

Maalox *(Rorer, UK)*. *Tablets*, chewable, dried aluminium hydroxide 400 mg, magnesium hydroxide 400 mg.

Suspension, dried aluminium hydroxide 220 mg, magnesium hydroxide 195 mg/5 mL. *Dose*. 1 or 2 tablets, or 10 to 20 mL of suspension after meals and at bedtime.

Maalox Plus *(Rorer, UK)*. *Tablets*, chewable, dried aluminium hydroxide 200 mg, magnesium hydroxide 200 mg, activated dimethicone 25 mg.

Suspension, dried aluminium hydroxide 220 mg, magnesium hydroxide 195 mg, activated dimethicone 25 mg/5 mL. *Dose*. 2 to 4 tablets, or 10 to 20 mL of suspension after meals and at bedtime.

Maalox TC (previously known as Maalox Concentrate) *(Rorer, UK)*. *Tablets*, dried aluminium hydroxide 600 mg, magnesium hydroxide 300 mg.

Suspension, dried aluminium hydroxide 600 mg, magnesium hydroxide 300 mg/5 mL. *Dose*. 15 mL of suspension or 3 tablets in the morning after food and again at bedtime.

Mucaine *(Wyeth, UK)*. *Suspension*, aluminium hydroxide mixture 4.75 mL, oxethazaine 10 mg, magnesium hydroxide 100 mg/5 mL. *Dose*. 5 to 10 mL before meals and at bedtime; to be taken without a drink.

Mucogel *(Pharmax, UK)*. *Tablets*, chewable, dried aluminium hydroxide 400 mg, magnesium hydroxide 400 mg.

Suspension, dried aluminium hydroxide 220 mg, magnesium hydroxide 195 mg/5 mL. *Dose*. 1 or 2 tablets, or 10 to 20 mL of suspension after meals and at bedtime.

Polyalk Revised Formula *(Galen, UK)*. *Suspension*, dried aluminium hydroxide 440 mg, light magnesium oxide 70 mg/5 mL. *Dose*. 10 to 20 mL when required.

Polycrol Gel *(Nicholas, UK)*. *Suspension*, aluminium hydroxide mixture 4.75mL, magnesium hydroxide 100 mg, activated dimethicone 25 mg/5 mL. *Dose*. 5 to 10 mL between meals and at bedtime.

For Polycrol Tablets see under Aluminium Hydroxide-Magnesium Carbonate Co-dried Gel.

Polycrol Forte Gel *(Nicholas, UK)*. *Gel*, aluminium hydroxide mixture 4.75 mL, magnesium hydroxide 100 mg, activated dimethicone 125 mg/5 mL. *Dose*. 5 to 10 mL between meals and at bedtime.

For Polycrol Forte Tablets, see under Aluminium Hydroxide-Magnesium Carbonate Co-dried Gel.

Siloxyl *(Martindale Pharmaceuticals, UK)*. *Tablets*, chewable, dried aluminium hydroxide 500 mg, activated dimethicone 250 mg.

Suspension, dried aluminium hydroxide 420 mg, light

magnesium oxide 70 mg, activated dimethicone 125 mg/5 mL. *Dose.*1 or 2 tablets, or 5 to 10 mL of suspension when required.

Simeco Suspension *(Wyeth, UK). Suspension*, aluminium hydroxide 215 mg, magnesium hydroxide 80 mg, activated dimethicone 25 mg/5 mL. *Dose.* 10 mL after or between meals and at bedtime.

For Simeco Tablets see under Aluminium Hydroxide-Magnesium Carbonate Co-dried Gel.

Topal *(ICI Pharmaceuticals, UK). Tablets*, chewable, dried aluminium hydroxide 30 mg, light magnesium carbonate 40 mg, alginic acid 200 mg. *Dose.* 1 to 3 tablets after meals and at bedtime.

Unigest *(Unigreg, UK). Tablets*, chewable, dried aluminium hydroxide 450 mg, dimethicone 400 mg. *Dose.* 1 or 2 tablets when required.

Some other proprietary preparations containing aluminium hydroxide are described under Magnesium Carbonate and Magnesium Trisilicate.

Proprietary Names and Manufacturers

Adagel *(Nelson, Austral.)*; Aldrox *(Arg.; Belg.)*; Allulose *(Weiders, Norw.)*; Alternagel *(Stuart Pharmaceuticals, USA)*; Alu-Cap *(Kettelhack Riker, Ger.; Riker, UK; Riker, USA)*; Alucol *(Sandoz, Ital.)*; Aludrox *(Wyeth, UK)*; Alugelibys *(IBYS, Spain)*; Alukon *(Remedia, S.Afr.)*; Alumag *(S.Afr.)*; Aluminox *(Neth.)*; Alusorb *(Drug Houses Austral., Austral.)*; Alu-Tab *(Riker, Austral.; Riker, Canad.; Riker, USA)*; Amphojel *(Wyeth, Austral.; Wyeth, Canad.; Wyeth, S.Afr.; Wyeth, USA)*; Amphotabs *(Wyeth, Austral.)*; Anti-Phosphat *(Gry, Ger.)*; Basaljel *(Austral.; Wyeth, Canad.; Wyeth, USA)*; Dialume *(Spain; Armour, USA)*; Gamma-gel *(Ital.)*; Gastracol *(Switz.)*; Gelox *(Prosana, Austral.)*; Lithiagel *(Daniel-Brunet, Fr.)*; Minajel *(Austral.)*; Nephrox *(Fleming, USA)*; Palliacol *(Ger.)*; Pepsamar *(Winthrop, Arg.; Sterwin, Spain)*; Rocgel *(Roques, Fr.)*; Uldecan *(Spain)*.

The following names have been used for multi-ingredient preparations containing aluminium hydroxide—Abacid Plus *(Ticen, Eire)*; Actonorm *(Wallace Mfg Chem., UK)*; Alka Butazolidin *(Geigy, Canad.)*; Alkabutazone *(ICN, Canad.)*; Alka-Donna *(Carlton Laboratories, UK)*; Alkaphenylbutazone *(Pro Doc, Canad.)*; Alk-Donna P *(Carlton Laboratories, UK)*; Alma-Mag No. 4 *(Rugby, USA)*; Alubarb *(Norton, UK)*; Alucone *(Drug Houses Austral., Austral.)*; Aludrox *(Wyeth, Austral.; Wyeth, USA)*; Aludrox SA *(Wyeth, UK)*; Aluhyde *(Sinclair, UK)*; Alumag *(Trianon, Canad.)*; Amphojel 500 *(Wyeth, Canad.)*; Amphojel Plus *(Wyeth, Canad.)*; Ancatropine Gel *(Anca, Canad.)*; Ancatropine Gel Plain *(Anca, Canad.)*; Andursil Suspension *(Geigy, UK)*; Antacid Plus *(Clark, Canad.)*; Antasil *(Stuart, UK)*; Antidiar *(Armour, UK)*; APP Stomach Preparations *(Consolidated Chemicals, UK)*; Ascon *(Cox, UK)*; Asilone *(USV, Austral.; Rorer, UK)*; Caved-S *(Muir & Neil, Austral.; Tillotts, UK)*; Dia-Chek *(Searle, Austral.)*; Diaguard Tablets *(Nelson, Austral.)*; Diareze Tablets *(Key, Austral.)*; Dijene Liquid *(Boots, Austral.)*; Dijex Liquid *(Crookes Healthcare, UK)*; Diovol Ex *(Horner, Canad.)*; Diovol Suspension *(Horner, Canad.; Pharmax, UK)*; Diovol Tablets *(Horner, Canad.; Pharmax, UK)*; Duoquel *(Wellcome, Austral.)*; Gastreze *(Key, Austral.)*; Gastrocote *(MCP Pharmaceuticals, UK)*; Gastrogel *(Fawns & McAllan, Austral.)*; Gastron *(Winthrop, UK)*; Gavigrans *(Reckitt & Colman, Austral.)*; Gaviscon Granules *(Reckitt & Colman, Austral.)*; Gavison Liquid *(Winthrop, Canad.; Marion Laboratories, USA)*; Gaviscon Tablets and Infant Preparations *(Reckitt & Colman, Austral.; Winthrop, Canad.; Reckitt & Colman Pharmaceuticals, UK; Marion Laboratories, USA)*; Gelusil *(Warner, Austral.; Parke, Davis, Canad.; Warner-Lambert, UK; Parke, Davis, USA)*; Glucomagma *(Drug Houses Austral., Austral.)*; Kaogel *(Faulding, Austral.)*; Kaomagma *(Wyeth, Austral.)*; Kolanticon *(Merrell, UK)*; Kolantyl *(Merrell, UK; Merrell Dow, USA)*; LoAsid *(Calmic, UK)*; Maalox *(Rorer, Canad.; Rorer, UK; Rorer, USA)*; Maalox Plus *(Rorer, Canad.; Rorer, UK)*; Meracote *(Merrell Dow, Austral.)*; Merasyn *(Merrell Dow, Austral.)*; Mucaine *(Wyeth, Austral.; Wyeth, Canad.; Wyeth, UK)*; Mucogel *(Pharmax, UK)*; Mucoxin; Mutesa; Muthesa; Mygel *(Geneva, USA)*; Mylanta *(Parke, Davis, Austral.; Parke, Davis, Canad.; Parke, Davis, UK; Stuart Pharmaceuticals, USA)*; Neo-Tropine Alkaline *(Neolab, Canad.)*; Neutralca-S *(Desbergers, Canad.)*; Neutrolactis *(Sandoz, UK)*; Oxaine; Phenylone Plus *(Medic, Canad.)*; Polyalk *(Galen, UK)*; Polyalk Revised Formula *(Galen, UK)*; Polycrol Gel *(Nicholas, UK)*; Pyrogastrone *(Winthrop, UK)*; Regacid *(Riva, Canad.)*; Silocalm *(Concept Pharmaceuticals, UK)*; Siloxyl *(Martindale Pharmaceuticals, UK)*; Simeco Suspension *(Wyeth, Austral.; Wyeth, UK; Wyeth, USA)*; Sodexol *(Schering, Austral.)*; Streptomagma Suspension *(Wyeth, Austral.)*; Sylopal *(Norton, UK)*; Tepilta; Theodrox *(Riker, UK)*; Topal *(ICI Pharmaceuticals, UK)*; Unigest *(Unigreg, UK)*.

674-w

Aluminium Hydroxide-Magnesium Carbonate Co-dried Gel

F-MA 11. A co-precipitate of aluminium hydroxide and magnesium carbonate carefully dried to contain a critical proportion of water for antacid activity.

Aluminium hydroxide-magnesium carbonate co-dried gel is an antacid that is given in doses of up to 1 g.

Proprietary Preparations

Algicon *(Rorer, UK). Tablets*, chewable, aluminium hydroxide-magnesium carbonate co-dried gel 360 mg, magnesium alginate 500 mg, magnesium carbonate 320 mg, potassium bicarbonate 100 mg.
Suspension, aluminium hydroxide-magnesium carbonate co-dried gel 140 mg, magnesium alginate 250 mg, magnesium carbonate 175 mg, potassium bicarbonate 50 mg/5 mL. *Dose.* 1 or 2 tablets or 10 to 20 mL of suspension after meals and at bedtime.

Aludrox Tablets *(Wyeth, UK). Tablets*, chewable, aluminium hydroxide-magnesium carbonate co-dried gel 282 mg, magnesium hydroxide 85 mg. *Dose.* 1 or 2 tablets between meals and at bedtime.

For Aludrox see under Aluminium Hydroxide.

Andursil Tablets *(Geigy, UK). Tablets*, aluminium hydroxide - magnesium carbonate co-dried gel 750 mg, activated dimethicone 250 mg. *Dose.* 1 or 2 tablets three or four times daily and at bedtime.

For Andursil Suspension see under Aluminium Hydroxide.

Dijex Tablets *(Crookes Healthcare, UK). Tablets*, chewable, aluminium hydroxide-magnesium carbonate co-dried gel 400 mg.

For Dijex Liquid see under Aluminium Hydroxide.

Gastrils *(Ernest Jackson, UK). Pastilles*, aluminium hydroxide-magnesium carbonate co-dried gel 500 mg.

Polycrol Tablets *(Nicholas, UK). Tablets*, chewable, aluminium hydroxide-magnesium carbonate co-dried gel, 275 mg, magnesium hydroxide 100 mg, activated dimethicone 25 mg. *Dose.* 1 or 2 tablets between meals and at bedtime.

For Polycrol Gel see under Aluminium Hydroxide.

Polycrol Forte Tablets *(Nicholas, UK). Tablets*, chewable, aluminium hydroxide-magnesium carbonate co-dried gel 275 mg, magnesium hydroxide 100 mg, activated dimethicone 250 mg. *Dose.* 1 or 2 tablets between meals and at bedtime.

For Polycrol Forte Gel see under Aluminium Hydroxide.

Simeco Tablets *(Wyeth, UK). Tablets*, aluminium hydroxide-magnesium carbonate co-dried gel 282 mg, magnesium hydroxide 85 mg, activated dimethicone 25 mg. *Dose.* 2 tablets after or between meals and at bedtime.

For Simeco Suspension see under Aluminium Hydroxide.

Proprietary Names and Manufacturers

Acinorm *(Benzon, Denm.)*; Allulose *(Norw.)*; Almacarb *(Glaxo, Austral.; Duncan, Flockhart, UK)*; Dijene Tablets *(Boots, Austral.)*; Dijex Tablets *(Crookes Healthcare, UK)*; Gastalar *(Armour, UK)*; Gastrils *(Ernest Jackson, UK)*; Link *(A.L., Denm.; Apothekernes Laboratorium, Norw.; A.L., Swed.)*.

The following names have been used for multi-ingredient preparations containing aluminium hydroxide-magnesium carbonate co-dried gel—Algicon *(Rorer, Canad.; Rorer, UK; Rorer, USA)*; Aludrox Tablets *(Wyeth, UK)*; Amphojel Plus *(Wyeth, Canad.)*; Andursil *(Geigy, UK)*; Diloran *(Lipha, UK)*; Diovol *(Horner, Canad.; Pharmax, UK)*; Polycrol Tablets *(Nicholas, UK)*; Simeco Tablets *(Wyeth, Austral.; Wyeth, UK)*; Univol *(Horner, Canad.)*.

676-l

Aluminium Phosphate *(BAN)*.

Aluminum Phosphate *(USAN)*.

CAS — 7784-30-7 ($AlPO_4$).

Pharmacopoeias. Br. includes Dried Aluminium Phosphate.

Dried Aluminium Phosphate (*B.P.*) (Dried Aluminium Phosphate Gel) consists largely of hydrated aluminium orthophosphate and contains not less than 80% of $AlPO_4$. It is a white powder containing some friable aggregates. Practically **insoluble** in water, alcohol, and solutions of alkali hydroxides; soluble in dilute mineral acids. A 4% suspension in water has a pH of 5.5 to 6.5. **Store** in well-closed containers at a temperature not exceeding 30°.

Aluminium phosphate is an antacid that is given in doses of up to about 800 mg.

Aluminium phosphate is also used as an adjuvant in the manufacture of adsorbed vaccines.

Preparations

Aluminium Phosphate Oral Suspension *(B.P.)*. Aluminium Phosphate Gel; Aluminium Phosphate Mixture. A peppermint-flavoured aqueous suspension of aluminium orthophosphate containing 7.0 to 8.0% w/w of $AlPO_4$. Store at a temperature not exceeding 30°. Avoid freezing.

Aluminum Phosphate Gel *(U.S.P.)*. An aqueous suspension containing 4 to 5% w/w of $AlPO_4$. Store in airtight containers.

Aluminium Phosphate Tablets *(B.P.)*. Chewable tablets with a peppermint flavour containing dried aluminium phosphate equivalent to 360 to 440 mg of $AlPO_4$. Store at a temperature not exceeding 30°.

Proprietary Names and Manufacturers

Aluphos Gel *(Fisons, UK)*; Fosfalugel *(Biothérax, Denm.; Biotherax, Norw.; Biotherax, Swed.)*; Fosfalumina *(Essex, Spain)*; Fosfidral *(Angelini, Ital.)*; Fosfoalugel *(IBYS, Spain)*; Phosphaljel *(USA)*; Phosphalugel *(Belg.; Biothérax, Fr.; Biotherax, Ger.; Boehringer Ingelheim, Switz.)*; Phosphalutab *(Ger.)*; Synergel *(Biothérax, Fr.: Servier, UK)*.

677-y

Aluminium Sodium Silicate

554; Sodium Aluminium Silicate; Sodium Aluminosilicate; Sodium Silicoaluminate.

CAS — 1344-00-9.

Aluminium sodium silicate is an antacid that is given in doses of about 1 to 2 g. It is also used as a food additive.

Proprietary Names and Manufacturers

Neutralon *(Schering, Austral.; Schering, Ital.; Spain)*.

The following names have been used for multi-ingredient preparations containing aluminium sodium silicate—Belladonna-Neutralon *(Schering, Austral.)*; Neutradonna *(Nicholas, UK)*; Neutradonna Sed *(Nicholas, UK)*.

679-z

Attapulgite *(BAN)*.

CAS — 1337-76-4.

Pharmacopoeias. In *Br.* Activated Attapulgite is also included in *Br., It.*, and in *B.P. Vet.*

Attapulgite is a purified native hydrated magnesium aluminium silicate essentially consisting of the clay mineral palygorskite. Activated attapulgite is attapulgite which has been carefully heated to increase its adsorptive capacity. Both are light, cream or buff, very fine powders, free or almost free from gritty particles. A 5% suspension of either substance in water has a pH of 7.0 to 9.5.

Attapulgite is highly adsorbent and is mainly used as a pharmaceutical aid.

Activated attapulgite is used as an adsorbent in the treatment of diarrhoea and has been given in doses of up to 12 g daily.

It should be noted that a consequence of diarrhoea may be fluid and electrolyte depletion, and that rehydration therapy may be necessary, especially in infants and young children. For further details concerning rehydration therapy, see p.1024.

Proprietary Names and Manufacturers

Actapulgite *(Belg.; Beaufour, Fr.)*; Atasorb *(Lilly, UK)*; Atasorb N *(Lilly, UK)*; Attasorb *(Lawrence Industries, UK)*; Diasorb *(Key, USA)*; Masigel *(Fher, Spain)*; Pharmasorb *(Lawrence Industries, UK)*; Rheaban *(USA)*.

The following names have been used for multi-ingredient preparations containing attapulgite—Diaguard Tablets *(Nelson, Austral.)*; Diarcalm *(McGloin, Austral.)*; Diareze *(Key, Austral.)*; Diban *(Robins, Canad.)*; Polymagma *(Wyeth, USA)*; Streptomagma Tablets *(Wyeth, Austral.)*; Sulphamagna *(Wyeth, UK)*.

16525-z

Balsalazide *(BAN, rINN).*
BX-661A *(sodium salt)*. 5-[4-(2-Carboxyethylcarbamoyl)phenylazo]salicylic acid.
$C_{17}H_{15}N_3O_6$=357.3.

CAS — 80573-04-2.

NOTE. Balsalazide Sodium is *BANM.*

Balsalazide, which consists of mesalazine (see p.1097) linked to 4-aminobenzylalanine, is a pro-drug of mesalazine and is being investigated for use in ulcerative colitis.

Three men suffered infertility while taking sulphasalazine 2 to 3 g daily; sperm count and motility returned to normal in 2 after taking balsalazide 2 g daily instead of sulphasalazine, and presumably in the third whose wife became pregnant. There was no relapse of their ulcerative colitis.— P. B. McIntyre and J. E. Lennard-Jones, *Br. med. J.*, 1984, *288*, 1652.

Proprietary Names and Manufacturers
Biorex, UK.

6542-d

Benzquinamide Hydrochloride *(BANM, rINNM).*
P-2647 *(benzquinamide)*. 3-Diethylcarbamoyl-1,3,4,6,7,11b-hexahydro-9,10-dimethoxy-2*H*-benzo[*a*]-quinolizin-2-yl acetate hydrochloride.
$C_{22}H_{32}N_2O_5$,HCl=441.0.

CAS — 63-12-7 (benzquinamide); 113-69-9 (hydrochloride).

NOTE. Benzquinamide is USAN.

Incompatibilites have been reported with chlordiazepoxide hydrochloride, diazepam, pentobarbitone sodium, phenobarbitone sodium, quinalbarbitone sodium, and thiopentone sodium.

Adverse Effects
The most common side-effect associated with benzquinamide hydrochloride is drowsiness. Other side-effects reported include antimuscarinic, cardiovascular, and extrapyramidal effects; allergic reactions such as skin rashes have also occurred.

Single cases of acute dystonic reactions following benzquinamide administration: T. E. Rose and S. D. Averbuch (letter), *Ann. intern. Med.*, 1975, *83*, 231; W. R. Grove *et al.*, *Drug Intell. & clin. Pharm.*, 1976, *10*, 638.

A report of delirium following benzquinamide administration.— J. W. Chapin and D. W. Wingard, *Anesthesiology*, 1977, *46*, 364.

Precautions
Since benzquinamide has been associated with adverse cardiovascular effects when given intravenously, this route should not be used in patients with cardiovascular disease or in those receiving premedication or cardiovascular drugs. Because of its mild antimuscarinic activity the precautions described under Diphenidol, p.1087 should be considered.

Absorption and Fate
Following injection benzquinamide is metabolised in the liver and excreted in the urine and bile. Some unchanged benzquinamide is excreted in the urine. About 58% is bound to plasma protein.

References: D. C. Hobbs and A. G. Connolly, *J. Pharmacokinet. Biopharm.*, 1978, *6*, 477.

Uses and Administration
Benzquinamide hydrochloride has been reported to have anti-emetic, antihistaminic, weak antimuscarinic, and sedative properties and is used to control nausea and vomiting usually associated with anaesthesia and surgery. Benzquinamide hydrochloride is administered by deep intramuscular injection in a dose equivalent to 50 mg of benzquinamide. It acts within about 15 minutes of injection and a second dose of 50 mg may be given 1 hour later if necessary; subsequent doses of 50 mg may be repeated every 3 to 4 hours as necessary. It may also be given by slow intravenous injection in a dose of 25 mg administered over a period of 0.5 to 1.0 minute in selected patients; subsequent doses should be given intramuscularly.

NAUSEA AND VOMITING. The use of benzquinamide in the control of cytotoxic drug-induced vomiting.— P. Nietsch, *Arzneimittel-Forsch.*, 1983, *33*, 1694.

Proprietary Names and Manufacturers
Emete-con *(Roerig, USA)*; Promecon *(Searle, Ger.)*.

7503-n

Bisacodyl *(BAN, USAN, rINN).*
4,4′-(2-Pyridylmethylene)di(phenyl acetate).
$C_{22}H_{19}NO_4$=361.4.

CAS — 603-50-9; 1336-29-4 (bisacodyl tannex).

Pharmacopoeias. In *Br., Braz., Cz., Fr., Ind., Jug.,* and *U.S.*

A white or almost white, odourless or almost odourless, crystalline powder.
Practically **insoluble** in water; slightly soluble in alcohol and ether; freely soluble in chloroform; sparingly soluble in methyl alcohol. **Store** in well-closed containers. Protect from light.

CAUTION. Avoid inhalation of the powder and contact with eyes, skin, and mucous membranes.

Adverse Effects
Bisacodyl may cause abdominal discomfort such as colic or cramps. When administered rectally it sometimes causes irritation and repeated use may cause proctitis or sloughing of the epithelium. To avoid gastric irritation bisacodyl tablets are enteric-coated. Prolonged use or overdosage can result in diarrhoea with excessive loss of water and electrolytes particularly potassium; there is also the possibility of developing an atonic non-functioning colon.

Precautions
Bisacodyl should not be given to patients with intestinal obstruction or with undiagnosed abdominal symptoms; care should also be taken in patients with inflammatory bowel disease. The suppositories should be used with caution in patients with rectal fissures or ulcerated haemorrhoids. Prolonged use should be avoided.

Absorption and Fate
Absorption of bisacodyl is variable following administration by mouth; part of a dose is excreted in the urine as the glucuronide. Bisacodyl is mainly excreted in the faeces.

Bisacodyl was hydrolysed to bis(*p*-hydroxyphenyl)pyridyl-2-methane which was responsible for the laxative action.— R. Jauch *et al.*, *Arzneimittel-Forsch.*, 1975, *25*, 1796.

Uses and Administration
Bisacodyl is a diphenylmethane stimulant laxative used for the treatment of constipation and for bowel evacuation before investigational procedures or surgery. Its action is mainly in the large intestine and it is usually effective within 6 to 12 hours following administration by mouth and within 15 to 60 minutes following rectal administration.
It is given in a usual dose of 10 mg daily as enteric-coated tablets administered at night or as a suppository administered in the morning; doses of up to 30 mg have been given by mouth for complete bowel evacuation. A rectal solution is also used in a dose of 5 to 10 mg usually as an adjunct to bowel preparation; it may also be administered together with a barium enema at a dose of bisacodyl 5.5 to 13.7 mg in 1 to 3 litres of enema solution.
Children under 10 years may be given bisacodyl 5 mg daily.
A complex of bisacodyl with tannic acid (bisacodyl tannex) is also used.

A thrice-weekly regimen of a faecal softener followed in 24 hours by rectal administration of a solution of bisacodyl in propylene glycol to evacuate the bowel was used successfully in the management of bowel incontinence in patients with spinal cord injuries.— R. F. Jones and G. J. L. Hall, *Med. J. Aust.*, 1979, *1*, 309.

Bisacodyl suppositories may cause a profound inflammatory reaction in the rectum and so if used prior to sigmoidoscopy the mucosal appearances are difficult to interpret.— D. G. Colin-Jones, *Prescribers' J.*, 1981, *21*, 209.

Preparations
Bisacodyl Suppositories *(B.P.)*
Bisacodyl Suppositories *(U.S.P.)*
Bisacodyl Tablets *(B.P.)*. Enteric-coated.
Bisacodyl Tablets *(U.S.P.)* Enteric-coated.

Proprietary Preparations
Dulcolax *(Boehringer Ingelheim, UK). Tablets*, enteric-coated, bisacodyl 5 mg.
Suppositories, bisacodyl 10 mg.
Paediatric suppositories, bisacodyl 5 mg.

Proprietary Names and Manufacturers
Alaxa *(Angelini, Ital.)*; Anan *(Jpn)*; Babynormo *(Medea, Spain)*; Bisacolax *(ICN, Canad.)*; Bisalax *(Protea, Austral.)*; Bisco-Lax *(Raway, USA)*; Bisco-Zitron *(Biscova, Ger.)*; Capolax *(Vernleigh, S.Afr.)*; Carters pilletjes *(Neth.)*; Contalax *(Riker, Fr.)*; Contlax *(Fr.)*; Darmoletten *(Ger.)*; Deficol *(Vangard, USA)*; Delco-Lax *(USA)*; Dulcolax *(Belg.; Boehringer Ingelheim, Canad.; Pharmacia, Denm.; Boehringer Ingelheim, Fr.; Thomae, Ger.; Boehringer Ingelheim, Ital.; Neth.; Boehringer Ingelheim, Norw.; Boehringer Ingelheim, S.Afr.; Boehringer Ingelheim, Swed.; Boehringer Ingelheim, Switz.; Boehringer Ingelheim, UK; Boehringer Ingelheim, USA)*; Dulco-laxo *(Boehringer Ingelheim, Spain)*; Durolax *(Boehringer Ingelheim, Austral.)*; Ercolax *(Ercopharm, Switz.)*; Eulaxan *(Ger.)*; Evac-Q-Kwik Suppository *(Adria, Canad.; Adria, USA)*; Forrest X-Ray Prep Kit *(Forrest, Austral.: Schering, UK)*; Godalax *(Ger.)*; Laco *(Canad.)*; Laxagetten *(Ger.)*; Laxanin *(Schwarzhaupt, Ger.)*; Laxatets *(Pharmadrug, Ger.)*; Laxbene *(Merckle, Ger.; Switz.)*; Laxit *(ICN, Canad.)*; Med-Laxan *(Ger.)*; Multilax *(Hameln, Ger.)*; Nedalax *(Neda, Ger.)*; Neodrast *(Ger.)*; Normalene *(Montefarmaco, Ital.)*; Nourilax N *(Neth.)*; Obstilax forte *(Ger.)*; Perilax *(ND & K, Denm.; Norw.; Lennon, S.Afr.)*; Prontolax *(Streuli, Switz.)*; Raykit *(Boots, Austral.)*; Rytmil *(Switz.)*; Sanvacual *(Spain)*; Satolax-10 *(Jpn)*; Serax *(Ger.)*; SK-Bisacodyl *(USA)*; Spirolax *(Switz.)*; Stadalax *(Stada, Ger.)*; Theralax *(Beecham Laboratories, USA)*; Toilax *(Erco, Denm.; Neth.; Erco, Norw.; Erco, Swed.)*; Toilex *(Austral.)*; Vinco *(OTW, Ger.)*.

The following names have been used for multi-ingredient preparations containing bisacodyl— Coloxyl Suppositories *(Fawns & McAllan, Austral.)*; Dulcodos *(Boehringer Ingelheim, Canad.; Boehringer Ingelheim, UK)*; Royvac *(Roy, Canad.)*.

5275-l

Bismuth Salicylate
Basic Bismuth Salicylate; Bismuth Oxysalicylate; Bismuth Subsalicylate.

CAS — 14882-18-9.

Pharmacopoeias. In *Arg., Belg., Fr., Hung., Int., It., Mex., Neth., Nord., Port., Roum., Span.,* and *Turk.*

A basic salt of varying composition, corresponding approximately to $C_6H_4(OH).CO_2(BiO)$ and containing about 58% of Bi.

Adverse Effects, Treatment, and Precautions
Absorption of salicylate occurs following the administration of bismuth salicylate by mouth and therefore the adverse effects, treatment of adverse effects, and precautions of aspirin (see p.3) should be considered.
Although it has been stated that no bismuth has been detected in the plasma or urine of patients following recommended doses of bismuth salicylate, excessive dosage or overdosage may result in the adverse effects described under bismuth (see p.1547).
When taken by mouth bismuth salicylate may be converted in the gastro-intestinal tract to bismuth sulphide causing a darkening or blackening of the faeces.
It has been reported that bismuth salicylate reduces the bioavailability of concomitantly-administered tetracycline.

Studies demonstrating absorption of salicylate from a bismuth salicylate preparation: L. K. Pickering *et al.*, *J. Pediat.*, 1981, *99*, 654; S. Feldman *et al.*, *Clin. Pharmac. Ther.*, 1981, *29*, 788.

Bismuth encephalopathy in a patient after prolonged and excessive use of bismuth salicylate.— G. J. Hasking and J. M. Duggan (letter), *Med. J. Aust.*, 1982, *2*, 167.

Uses and Administration
Bismuth salicylate is used in the management of diarrhoea. The usual dose by mouth is about 500 mg repeated as necessary to a maximum of 4 g over a 24-hour period.
It should be noted that a consequence of diarrhoea may be fluid and electrolyte depletion, and that rehydration therapy may be necessary, especially in infants and

young children. For further details concerning rehydration therapy, see p.1024.

Studies confirming the efficacy of a tablet preparation of bismuth salicylate for the prevention of travellers' diarrhoea: R. Steffen *et al.*, *Antimicrob. Ag. Chemother.*, 1986, *29*, 625; H. L. DuPont *et al.*, *J. Am. med. Ass.*, 1987, *257*, 1347.

For further comments regarding the use of bismuth salicylate in travellers' diarrhoea, see under loperamide, p.1094.

For reference to the use of bismuth salicylate in gastritis in which *Campylobacter pylori* was implicated, see under tripotassium dicitratobismuthate, p.1111.

Proprietary Preparations

Pepto-Bismol *(Richardson-Vicks, UK)*. *Oral liquid*, bismuth salicylate 87.6 mg/5 mL.

Proprietary Names and Manufacturers

Pepto-Bismol *(Richardson-Vicks, UK; Procter & Gamble, USA)*; Spiromak *(Valeas, Ital.)*; Vismut *(DAK, Denm.)*.

12446-q

Bisoxatin Acetate *(BANM, USAN, rINNM)*.

Bisoxatin Diacetate; Wy-8138. 2,2-Bis(4-hydroxyphenyl)-1,4-benzoxazin-3(2*H*,4*H*)-one diacetate.

$C_{24}H_{19}NO_6$=417.4.

CAS — 17692-24-9 (bisoxatin); 14008-48-1 (acetate).

Bisoxatin acetate is used as a laxative.

Proprietary Names and Manufacturers

Kritel *(Gramon, Arg.)*; Laxonalin *(Fher, Spain)*; Maratan *(Ravizza, Ital.)*; Wylaxine *(Wyeth, Belg.; Wyeth, Neth.)*.

681-s

Bran

The fibrous outer layers of cereal grains, usually wheat, consisting of the pericarp, testa, and aleurone layer. It contains celluloses, polysaccharides or hemicelluloses, protein, fat, minerals, and moisture and may contain part of the germ or embryo.

It comprises about 12% of the weight of the grain and is a byproduct of flour milling. It is available in various grades.

A review of the importance of fibre. Nutritionalists restricted the term fibre to filamentous material in plant food. The term 'dietary fibre' had been introduced to provide a practical term to cover all structures of the plant cell-wall that were not digested by human alimentary enzymes. Dietary fibre was composed of the unavailable carbohydrates, i.e. cellulose and other plant cell-wall polysaccharides (hemicelluloses), and also lignins H. C. Trowell, *Chemist Drugg.*, 1975, *204*, 692.

Dietary fibre might be defined as the plant polysaccharides and lignin resistant to hydrolysis by the digestive enzymes of man.— H. Trowell *et al.* (letter), *Lancet*, 1976, *1*, 967. In order to avoid the limitation imposed by defining dietary fibre as plant material it could be called edible fibre and defined as polysaccharides, related polymers, and lignin resistant to hydrolysis by the digestive enzymes of man. This would include animal aminopolysaccharides in the diet of Eskimos.— E. W. Godding (letter), *Lancet*, 1976, *1*, 1129.

The term 'plantix' has been coined and used to describe non-fibrous plant polymers such as cellulose, hemicelluloses, and pectins which are resistant to human digestion and are frequently included as dietary fibre.— G. A. Spiller (letter), *Lancet*, 1977, *1*, 198.

Adverse Effects

Large quantities of bran may temporarily increase flatulence and distension, and intestinal obstruction may occur rarely. Interference with iron, zinc, and calcium absorption has been reported; calcium phosphate may be added to bran to neutralise phytic acid present which is considered to be the component responsible for the interference.

Intestinal obstruction occurred in a 53-year-old woman after the prolonged ingestion of excessive amounts of unprocessed bran.— J. Y. Kang and W. F. Doe, *Br. med. J.*, 1979, *1*, 1249. See also.— T. Allen-Mersh and L. R. De Jode (letter), *ibid.*, 1982, *284*, 740.

Bran was unlikely to cause a mineral deficiency provided that a sensible dose was taken and a sensible mixed diet eaten.— K. W. Heaton, *Br. med. J.*, 1983, *286*, 1124. People who increase their fibre intake up to 50 g daily (double the amount usually present in British diets) run no risk of serious adverse effects on their health but enthusiasts who pour large quantities of bran onto their food gain no benefit from the excess and expose themselves unnecessarily to known, and perhaps unknown, hazards.— M. A. Eastwood and R. Passmore, *Lancet*, 1983, *2*, 202.

Precautions

Bran is contra-indicated in patients with intestinal obstruction. Bran should not be eaten dry because of the possibility of oesophageal obstruction. By lowering the transit time through the gut the absorption of other drugs could also be affected.

Uses and Administration

Bran's main use is as a source of dietary fibre in the management of disorders of the gastro-intestinal tract such as constipation, diverticular disease, and the irritable bowel syndrome.

It is used as the basis for some breakfast cereals.

DIETARY FIBRE. Proposals for Nutritional Guidelines for Health Education in Britain: extracts from a discussion paper prepared for the National Advisory Committee on Nutrition Education. Intakes of dietary fibre should be increased to an average of about 30 g daily for adults and the suggestion that this dietary fibre might best be derived from foods, and not from either dietary fibre preparations or from foods to which bran and other fibres have been added.— *Lancet*, 1983, *2*, 835.

Dietary fibre is derived from complex carbohydrates synthesised by plants and the composition of the fibre (the relative amounts of cellulose, lignins, hemicelluloses, mucilages, gums, and pectins) will differ depending on the plant source. In consequence the important properties of dietary fibre may vary considerably between types and this diversity of behaviour appears to have been given insufficient attention when high-fibre diets have been advocated. Dietary fibre is not digested or absorbed in the small intestine. The principal thrust behind increasing the fibre content of Western diets has come from a comparison of the prevalence of certain diseases such as diverticulitis, colonic cancer, coronary artery disease, and diabetes which are much less common in Africans whose dietary fibre intake is higher than in Europeans and North Americans whose fibre intake is generally much lower. Although lines of evidence suggest that a high-fibre diet may be beneficial to health in the long-term, the role in preventive medicine must still be regarded as speculative, particularly since most of the diseases that have been linked with fibre-depleted diets are likely to be multifactorial in origin. It may, however, be considered to be of therapeutic importance, rather than of general prophylactic benefit, to increase dietary fibre in conditions such as diverticular disease and the irritable bowel syndrome.— R. Smallwood, *Med. J. Aust.*, 1984, *141*, 447. See also.— R. H. Taylor, *Br. med. J.*, 1984, *289*, 69.

A review of constipation and the use of dietary fibre in its management including the mechanisms of action of dietary fibre.— J. H. Cummings, *Postgrad. med. J.*, 1984, *60*, 811.

A discussion of the use of bran in the irritable bowel syndrome.— *Lancet*, 1987, *1*, 782.

A series of articles concerning dietary fibre in health and disease: L. A. Simons, *Aust. J. Pharm.*, 1984, *65*, 664; M. L. Wahlqvist, *ibid.*, 892; W. F. Doe, *ibid.*, 956; A. J. McMichael, *ibid.*, 1985, *66*, 53; A. S. Truswell, *ibid.*, 204.

Further reviews and discussions on dietary fibre: M. A. Eastwood and R. Passmore, *Lancet*, 1983, *2*, 202; T. Moore (letter), *ibid.*, 1986, *1*, 1040; M. A. Eastwood, *ibid.*, 1487.

For the use of guar gum, which may be considered to be a type of dietary fibre, as an adjunct in the management of diabetes mellitus, see Guar Gum, p.391.

Proprietary Preparations

Fybranta *(Norgine, UK)*. *Tablets*, chewable, bran 2 g with calcium phosphate.

Lejfibre *(Britannia Pharmaceuticals, UK)*. *Biscuits*, oat bran meal 4.04 g.

Proctofibe *(Roussel, UK)*. *Tablets*, fibrous grain extract 375 mg, fibrous citrus extract 94 mg.

Proprietary Names and Manufacturers of Bran and Fibre Supplements

Fibermed *(Purdue Frederick, USA)*; Fibre Trim *(Schering, USA)*; Fibyrax *(Roussel, Austral.; Roussel, Canad.)*; Fybranta *(Norgine, Austral.; Norgine, UK)*; HC5 *(HR Health Care, UK)*; Infibran *(Jouveinal, Canad.)*; Lejfibre *(Britannia Pharmaceuticals, UK)*; Proctofibe *(Roussel, UK)*; Trifyba *(Labaz Sanofi, UK)*.

The following names have been used for multi-ingredient preparations containing bran and fibre supplements— Anorex-CCK *(Robertson/Taylor, USA)*.

12454-q

Bromopride *(rINN)*.

CM-8252; VAL-13081. 4-Amino-5-bromo-*N*-(2-diethylaminoethyl)-*o*-anisamide.

$C_{14}H_{22}BrN_3O_2$=344.3.

CAS — 4093-35-0.

Bromopride is a substituted benzamide which has been used in a variety of gastro-intestinal disorders, including the relief of nausea and vomiting and motility disturbances. Bromopride hydrochloride has also been used.

Proprietary Names and Manufacturers of Bromopride or Bromopride Hydrochloride

Cascapride *(E. Merck, Ger.)*; Emoril *(Roemmers, Arg.)*; Lemetic *(Novag, Spain)*; Opridan *(Locatelli, Ital.)*; Plesium *(Chiesi, Ital.)*; Praiden *(Ital.)*; Valopride *(Vita, Ital.; Delagrange, Spain)*; Viaben *(Schürholz, Ger.)*; Viadil *(Pharmainvesti, Spain)*.

7504-h

Buckthorn

Bacca Spinae Cervinae; Espino Cerval; Nerprun; Rhamnus.

Pharmacopoeias. In *Arg.*, *Rus.*, and *Span.*

The dried ripe fruit of buckthorn, *Rhamnus cathartica* (Rhamnaceae).

Buckthorn has been used as a laxative.

682-w

Calcium Carbonate *(BAN)*.

Calcii Carbonas; Creta Preparada; E170; Precipitated Calcium Carbonate *(USAN)*; Precipitated Chalk.

$CaCO_3$=100.1.

CAS — 471-34-1.

Pharmacopoeias. In *Arg.*, *Aust.*, *Belg.*, *Br.*, *Braz.*, *Cz.*, *Egypt.*, *Eur.*, *Fr.*, *Ger.*, *Hung.*, *Ind.*, *It.*, *Jpn.*, *Jug.*, *Mex.*, *Neth.*, *Nord.*, *Pol.*, *Port.*, *Roum.*, *Span.*, *Swiss.*, *Turk.*, and *U.S.*

A white, odourless, powder.

Practically **insoluble** in water; its solubility in water is increased by the presence of carbon dioxide or ammonium salts; practically insoluble in alcohol; soluble with effervescence in acetic acid, hydrochloric acid, and nitric acid.

Adverse Effects

Calcium carbonate, like other calcium salts, may cause constipation. Flatulence from released carbon dioxide is not usually a serious problem though eructation may occur in some patients. Hypercalcaemia (see p.1028) can occur as can alkalosis following the regular use of calcium carbonate; the milk-alkali syndrome, which includes both features together with renal dysfunction, has occasionally occurred, usually in patients taking large doses.

A review of the milk-alkali syndrome. Clinical characteristics are variable, but classically the syndrome consists of hypercalcaemia, alkalosis, and renal impairment. It was first described following the use of a regimen consisting of milk or cream with alkaline powders but was later associated with the use of milk with calcium carbonate or calcium carbonate alone. The essential ingredients needed to produce the syndrome are calcium and absorbable alkali; the amounts necessary to produce the syndrome are ill-defined, it having occurred with calcium carbonate in doses ranging from 4 to 60 g daily.— E. S. Orwoll, *Ann. intern. Med.*, 1982, *97*, 242.

Treatment of Adverse Effects

Hypercalcaemia and alkalosis respond to reduction in dosage of calcium carbonate. In the milk-alkali syndrome, fluid and electrolyte losses should also be replaced. See also under calcium gluconate, p.1030.

Precautions

When calcium carbonate is used in large doses, serum-calcium concentrations and kidney function should be determined weekly or at the first sign of hypercalcaemia. Calcium salts may enhance the cardiac effects of digitalis glycosides. Calcium carbonate may interfere with the absorption of other drugs given concomitantly.

Absorption and Fate

Calcium carbonate is converted to calcium chloride by gastric acid. Some of the calcium is absorbed from the intestines but about 80% is reconverted to insoluble calcium salts such as the carbonate and stearate, and excreted.

Uses and Administration

Calcium carbonate is used as an antacid, usually in doses of up to about 1 g. In order to reduce the constipating effects, it is often given in association with a magnesium-containing antacid.

It may also be used as a calcium supplement in deficiency states.

A preparation of a native calcium carbonate (Calcarea Carbonica; Calc. Carb.) is used in homoeopathic medicine.

Calcium carbonate is used as a food additive.

PHOSPHATE BINDING. For the use of calcium carbonate as a phosphate binder in patients with chronic renal failure, see under aluminium hydroxide (p.1076).

Preparations

Calcium Carbonate Mixture Compound *(A.P.F.)*. Calcium carbonate 1 g, magnesium hydroxide mixture 3 mL, syrup 1 mL, concentrated chloroform water 0.25 mL or compound hydroxybenzoate solution 0.1 mL, water to 10 mL. *Dose.* 10 mL.

Paediatric Compound Calcium Carbonate Mixture *(B.P.C. 1973)*. Calcium carbonate 50 mg, light magnesium carbonate 50 mg, sodium bicarbonate 50 mg, aromatic cardamom tincture 0.05 mL, syrup 0.5 mL, double-strength chloroform water 2.5 mL, water to 5 mL. It should be recently prepared. *Dose.* Children, up to 1 year, 5 mL; 1 to 5 years, 10 mL.

Compound Calcium Carbonate Powder *(B.P.C. 1973)*. Calcium carbonate 37.5 g, sodium bicarbonate 37.5 g, light kaolin or light kaolin (natural) 12.5 g, heavy magnesium carbonate 12.5 g. *Dose.* 1 to 5 g.

Calcium Carbonate Tablets *(U.S.P.)*

Calcium and Magnesium Carbonates Tablets *(U.S.P.)*. Tablets containing calcium carbonate and magnesium carbonate.

Calcium Carbonate and Magnesia Tablets *(U.S.P.)*. Chewable tablets containing calcium carbonate and magnesium hydroxide.

Proprietary Preparations

Calcichew *(Shire, UK)*. *Tablets*, chewable, calcium carbonate 1.26g (equivalent to calcium 500 mg).

Liquid Gaviscon *(Reckitt & Colman Pharmaceuticals, UK)*. *Suspension*, calcium carbonate 160 mg, sodium bicarbonate 267 mg, sodium alginate 500 mg/10 mL. *Dose.* 10 to 20 mL after meals and at bedtime.

For Gaviscon tablets, see under Aluminium Hydroxide.

Titralac *(Riker, UK)*. *Tablets*, chewable, calcium carbonate 420 mg, glycine 180 mg.

Tums *(Beecham Proprietaries, UK)*. *Tablets*, chewable, calcium carbonate 500 mg.

Some other proprietary preparations containing calcium carbonate are described under Magnesium Carbonate and Magnesium Trisilicate.

Proprietary Names and Manufacturers

Alka-2 *(Miles Pharmaceuticals, USA)*; Apo-Cal *(Apotex, Canad.)*; Biocal *(Miles, Canad.; Miles Laboratories, USA)*; Calcichew *(Shire, UK)*; Calcidia *(Lefrancq, Fr.)*; Calcilève *(Fr.)*; Calcite *(Riva, Canad.)*; Calsan *(Anca, Canad.)*; Caltab *(Austral.)*; Caltrate *(Lederle, Canad.; Lederle, USA)*; Carbonate De Chaux Adrian *(Fr.)*; Equilet *(Mission Pharmacal, USA)*; Frubiase *(Biotherax, Ger.)*; Mega-Cal *(Jamieson, Canad.)*; Os-Cal *(Ayerst, Canad.; Marion Laboratories, USA)*; Spar-Cal *(Austral.)*; Suplical *(Warner-Lambert, USA)*; Titralac *(Nyco, Norw.)*; Tums *(Beecham Proprietaries, UK; Norcliff Thayer, USA)*.

The following names have been used for multi-ingredient preparations containing calcium carbonate—Actonorm *(Wallace Mfg Chem., UK)*; APP Stomach Preparations *(Consolidated Chemicals, UK)*; Baritop *(Concept Pharmaceuticals, UK)*; Cal-Bid *(Geriatric Pharm. Corp., USA)*; Calcite D-500 *(Riva, Canad.)*; Dical-D *(Abbott, Canad.)*; Gastrobrom *(Fawns & McAllan, Austral.)*; Gaviscon Liquid *(Reckitt & Colman, Austral.; Reckitt & Colman Pharmaceuticals, UK)*; Gramcal *(Anca, Canad.)*; Neutrolactis *(Sandoz, UK)*; Nulacin *(Bencard, UK)*; Os-Cal-Gesic *(Marion Laboratories, USA)*; Rabro *(Sinclair, UK)*; Sandocal 1000 *(Sandoz, Austral.)*; Titralac *(Riker, Austral.; Riker, UK)*; Ulsade *(Cambridge Laboratories, Austral.)*.

683-e

Calcium Silicate *(USAN)*.

552. A naturally occurring mineral, the most common forms being calcium metasilicate ($CaSiO_3$ = 116.2), calcium diorthosilicate (Ca_2SiO_4 = 172.2), and calcium trisilicate (Ca_3SiO_5 = 228.3). It is usually found in hydrated forms containing various amounts of water of crystallisation. Commercial calcium silicate is prepared synthetically.

CAS — 1344-95-2; 10101-39-0 ($CaSiO_3$); 10034-77-2 (Ca_2SiO_4); 12168-85-3 (Ca_3SiO_5).

Pharmacopoeias. In *U.S.N.F.*

Calcium silicate (*U.S.N.F.*) is a compound of calcium oxide and silicon dioxide containing not less than 25% of CaO and not less than 45% of SiO_2. A white to off-white free-flowing powder. Practically **insoluble** in water; with mineral acids it forms a gel. A 5% aqueous suspension has a pH of 8.4 to 10.2.

Calcium silicate is used as an antacid. It is also used as an anticaking agent in the preparation of pharmaceuticals and as a food additive.

Proprietary Names and Manufacturers

Sil-Ca *(Centrallab., Denm.; Felo, Denm.)*.

685-y

Carbenoxolone Sodium *(BANM, USAN, rINNM)*.

Disodium Enoxolone Succinate. The disodium salt of 3β-(3-carboxypropionyloxy)-11-oxo-olean-12-en-30-oic acid.

$C_{34}H_{48}Na_2O_7$=614.7.

CAS — 5697-56-3 (carbenoxolone); 7421-40-1 (disodium salt).

Pharmacopoeias. In *Br.* and *Chin.*

A white or pale cream-coloured hygroscopic powder. **Soluble** 1 in 6 of water and 1 in 30 of alcohol; practically insoluble in chloroform and ether. A 10% solution in water has a pH of 8.0 to 9.2. **Store** in well-closed containers.

CAUTION. *Carbenoxolone sodium powder is irritating to nasal membranes.*

Adverse Effects

Carbenoxolone sodium may produce sodium and water retention, leading to oedema, alkalosis, hypertension, hypokalaemia, and muscular weakness and damage. Renal failure has developed in some patients.

A report of fatal polyarteritis in a patient following a 5-week course of treatment with carbenoxolone sodium. It was considered that the induction of hypertension may have precipitated the onset of polyarteritis in a predisposed subject.— J. Sloan and J. A. Weaver, *Ir. J. med. Sci.*, 1968, *1*, (Nov.), 505.

Three to 7 hours after ingestion of a preparation of carbenoxolone sodium (Duogastrone), a loud noise like a pistol shot would regularly occur in a 40-year-old woman C. C. Evans and J. B. Ridyard (letter), *Br. med. J.*, 1969, *1*, 120.

In patients given carbenoxolone sodium as positioned-release capsules in a dose of 200 mg daily serum-carbenoxolone concentrations varied widely and were above 20 μg per mL in the elderly and in those with healed ulcers. The most severe side-effects occurred in 3 patients with serum concentrations of 82, 82, and 55 μg per mL, in whom diuretics and potassium supplements were required.— W. A. Davies and P. I. Reed, *Gut*, 1977, *18*, 78.

Further reports of adverse effects associated with carbenoxolone: T. N. Morgan *et al.* (letter), *Br. med. J.*, 1966, *2*, 48 (muscle weakness); A. Muir *et al.* (letter), *ibid.*, 1969, *2*, 512 (hypokalaemia and muscle weakness); J. H. Baron (letter), *ibid.*, 1969, *3*, 476 (hypokalaemia; muscle weakness, and myopathy); G. J. Davies *et al.*, *ibid.*, 1974, *3*, 400 (hypokalaemia, muscle weakness, headache, hypertension, and cardiac failure); A. Royston and B. J. Prout, *ibid.*, 1976, *2*, 150 (hypokalaemia; muscle weakness, and arreflexia); C. Descamps *et al.*, *ibid.*, 1977, *1*, 272 (hypokalaemia; muscle weakness, muscle necrosis, and acute tubular necrosis); R. J. Dickinson and R. Swaminathan, *Postgrad. med. J.*, 1978, *54*, 836 (hypokalaemia, muscle weakness, and renal tubular dysfunction).

Treatment of Adverse Effects

Symptoms of sodium and water retention may be relieved by a restricted sodium diet or by the concomitant administration of a thiazide diuretic such as chlorothiazide, with potassium supplements.

Precautions

Carbenoxolone sodium should be used with caution in the elderly and in patients with cardiac disease, hypertension, or impaired hepatic or renal function. It should not be given with digitalis glycosides unless serum-electrolyte concentrations are measured at weekly intervals and measures are taken to avoid hypokalaemia.

Although amiloride or spironolactone relieve sodium and water retention, they should not be used with carbenoxolone as they antagonise the healing properties of carbenoxolone.

ADMINISTRATION IN THE ELDERLY. A comparative study of healthy adults and geriatric patients suggested that protein binding of carbenoxolone was reduced in the elderly, and was associated with lower plasma albumin concentrations; the half-life of carbenoxolone was longer in the elderly subjects. These two factors would contribute to the higher incidence of carbenoxolone side-effects in the elderly.— M. J. Hayes *et al.*, *Gut*, 1977, *18*, 1054.

PREGNANCY AND THE NEONATE. Carbenoxolone, because of its side-effects of sodium and water retention, is contra-indicated in pregnancy.— C. W. Howden, *Br. med. J.*, 1986, *293*, 1549.

Absorption and Fate

Carbenoxolone sodium is absorbed from the gastro-intestinal tract, the main site of absorption being the stomach. Maximum plasma concentrations are obtained about 1 hour after administration in a fasting state but may be delayed for several hours if the dose is taken after food; a second peak appears 2 or 3 hours later probably due to enterohepatic cycling of metabolites. It is bound to proteins in the circulation. Carbenoxolone is mainly excreted in the faeces via the bile.

The absorption of carbenoxolone in 15 patients with gastric ulcer (as Biogastrone) and 8 patients with duodenal ulcer (as Duogastrone) was not affected by concurrent antacid administration after the first few days of treatment. There was no significant difference in serum-carbenoxolone concentration when Biogastrone tablets were taken before or after meals. Serum concentrations were higher in older patients and side-effects could be correlated with them although ulcer healing could not. This suggests that the ulcer-healing effect of carbenoxolone is topical whereas the metabolic effects are systemic.— J. H. Baron *et al.*, *Gut*, 1978, *19*, 330.

Uses and Administration

Carbenoxolone sodium has marked anti-inflammatory actions. It appears to act by stimulating the production of protective mucus, the composition of which may be altered. It is used in the treatment of duodenal and gastric ulcers and, in combination with antacids, in gastric reflux and reflux oesophagitis.

The suggested dose in gastric ulcer is 100 mg

three times daily for one week followed by 50 mg three times daily. Doses should be taken after meals. The dose in duodenal ulcer is 50 mg in a capsule for release in the duodenum, swallowed whole with liquid four times daily 15 to 30 minutes before meals; antacids may be given but antimuscarinics should be discontinued.

Potassium salts should generally be given concomitantly with carbenoxolone. If carbenoxolone is to be given to elderly patients reduced doses should generally be employed.

Carbenoxolone sodium is also used as a gel or as a mouthwash in the treatment of ulcers of the mouth.

References to the effective use of carbenoxolone sodium in the treatment of duodenal ulcer: B. O. Amure, *Gut*, 1970, *11*, 171; *Br. J. clin. Pract.*, 1973, *27*, 50; *Gut*, 1977, *18*, 717; G. S. Nagy, *Gastroenterology*, 1978, *74*, 7.

References to carbenoxolone sodium being no more effective than a placebo in the treatment of duodenal ulcer: J. M. Cliff and G. J. Milton-Thompson, *Gut*, 1970, *11*, 167; P. Brown *et al.*, *Gut*, 1972, *13*, 324; *Br. J. clin. Pract.*, 1973, *27*, 140.

Of 54 patients with endoscopically proven gastric ulcer 27 were randomly allocated to receive cimetidine 200 mg four times daily for 6 weeks while the remainder received carbenoxolone sodium 100 mg thrice daily for a week then 50 mg thrice daily for 5 weeks. Pain was reduced within one week in patients taking cimetidine and within 2 weeks in patients taking carbenoxolone. Ulcers healed in 78% and 52% respectively of patients. Side-effects were minimal with cimetidine but 44% of patients taking carbenoxolone experienced hypokalaemia or oedema.— S. J. La Brooy *et al.*, *Br. med. J.*, 1979, *1*, 1308.

Further references to carbenoxolone and gastric ulcer: R. Doll *et al.*, *Gut*, 1968, *9*, 42; R. D. Montgomery *et al.*, *Practitioner*, 1969, *202*, 398; J. B. Cocking and J. N. MacCaig, *Gut*, 1969, *10*, 219; J. A. C. Wilson, *Br. J. clin. Pract.*, 1972, *26*, 563; W. -P. Fung *et al.*, *Lancet*, 1974, *2*, 10.

Preparations

Carbenoxolone Tablets *(B.P.)*. Contain carbenoxolone sodium.

Proprietary Preparations

Biogastrone *(Winthrop, UK)*. *Tablets*, scored, carbenoxolone sodium 50 mg.

Bioplex *(Biorex, UK)*. *Mouthwash granules*, carbenoxolone sodium 1%. *Administration*. One 5-mL spoonful of granules dissolved in water and used as a mouthwash.

Bioral Gel *(Winthrop, UK)*. *Gel*, carbenoxolone sodium 2%. *Administration*. To be applied thickly to the lesions of mouth ulcers after meals and at bedtime.

Duogastrone *(Winthrop, UK)*. *Capsules*, carbenoxolone sodium 50 mg; the capsules are designed to release their contents into the duodenum. For duodenal ulcer.

Pyrogastrone *(Winthrop, UK)*. *Tablets*, chewable, carbenoxolone sodium 20 mg, alginic acid 600 mg, dried aluminium hydroxide 240 mg, magnesium trisilicate 60 mg, sodium bicarbonate 210 mg.

Liquid, as powder for suspension, carbenoxolone sodium 10 mg, dried aluminium hydroxide 150 mg/5 mL when reconstituted with water. For gastric reflux and reflux oesophagitis. *Dose*. One tablet, or 10 mL of liquid, three times daily after meals and 2 tablets or 20 mL of liquid at bedtime.

Proprietary Names and Manufacturers

Biogastrone *(Smith & Nephew, Austral.; Belg.; Canad.; Ger.; Jpn; Neth.; S.Afr.; Switz.; Winthrop, UK)*; Bioplex *(Biorex, UK)*; Bioral *(Smith & Nephew, Austral.; Fisons, S.Afr.; Winthrop, UK)*; Duogastrone *(Smith & Nephew, Austral.; Belg.; Canad.; Fr.; S.Afr.; Switz.; Winthrop, UK)*; Gastrausil *(Searle, Ital.)*; Neogel *(Ger.)*; Sanodin *(Leo, Spain)*; Sustac *(Arg.)*; Terulcon *(Belg.)*; Ulcus-Tablinen *(Beiersdorf, Ger.)*.

7505-m

Casanthranol *(USAN)*.

A purified mixture of the anthranol glycosides derived from cascara; practically devoid of free anthraquinones. Two active fractions have been identified as casanthranol A and casanthranol B.

CAS — 8024-48-4.

Casanthranol is an anthraquinone laxative. It has been given in doses of 30 to 120 mg daily by mouth, together with a faecal softener.

Proprietary Names and Manufacturers

The following names have been used for multi-ingredient preparations containing casanthranol—Acidobyl with Cascara *(Desbergers, Canad.)*; Comfolax-plus *(Searle, USA)*; Dialose Plus *(Stuart Pharmaceuticals, USA)*; D-S-S Plus *(Parke, Davis, USA)*; Peri-Colace *(Bristol, Canad.; Mead Johnson Pharmaceutical, USA)*.

7506-b

Cascara *(BAN)*.

Cascara Sagrada *(USAN)*; Cascararinde; Chittem Bark; Rhamni Purshianae Cortex; Rhamni Purshiani Cortex; Sacred Bark.

CAS — 8047-27-6; 8015-89-2 (cascara sagrada extract).

Pharmacopoeias. In *Arg., Aust., Br., Belg., Braz., Egypt., Eur., Fr., Ger., Int., It., Mex., Neth., Nord., Port., Span., Swiss, Turk.*, and *U.S. Br.* and *Turk.* also describe Powdered Cascara.

The dried bark of *Rhamnus purshianus* (=*Frangula purshiana*) (Rhamnaceae). The *B.P.* and *Eur. P.* specify that it contains not less than 8% of hydroxyanthracene glycosides of which not less than 60% consists of cascarosides, both calculated as cascaroside A; the *U.S.P.* specifies not less than 7% of total hydroxyanthracene derivatives. **Store** in well-closed containers. Protect from light and moisture.

Adverse Effects and Precautions

As for Senna, p.1106.

Absorption and Fate

The absorption and fate of anthraquinones from cascara is similar to that from senna, see p.1106.

Uses and Administration

Cascara is an anthraquinone laxative with a mild action. The active anthraquinones are liberated into the colon from the glycosides by colonic bacteria; a laxative effect usually occurs 6 to 8 hours after administration. It is usually given at night as an elixir or in tablets.

Preparations

Cascara Elixir *(B.P.)*. Cascara Oral Solution. An aqueous extract of cascara (1 in 1) and liquorice (1 in 8) with glycerol 30% v/v and flavouring agents.

Aromatic Cascara Fluidextract *(U.S.P.)*. An aqueous extract of cascara (1 in 1) with liquorice, flavouring agents, and alcohol 20% v/v. Store in airtight containers.

Cascara Dry Extract *(B.P.)*. Contains not less than 13% of hydroxyanthracene derivatives, of which not less than 40% is cascarosides, calculated as cascaroside A.

Cascara Sagrada Extract *(U.S.P.)*. A dry extract of cascara containing 11% of hydroxyanthracene derivatives. Store in airtight containers.

Cascara Sagrada Fluidextract *(U.S.P.)*. An aqueous percolate of cascara equivalent to 1 in 1 and containing 20% v/v of alcohol. Store in airtight containers.

Cascara and Belladonna Mixture *(B.P.C. 1973)*. Compound Cascara Mixture. Cascara elixir 2 mL, belladonna tincture 0.5 mL, double-strength chloroform water 5 mL, water to 10 mL. *Dose*. 10 to 20 mL.

Cascara Tablets *(B.P.)*. Coated tablets, each containing 17 to 23 mg of total hydroxyanthracene derivatives, of which not less than 40% is cascarosides, calculated as cascaroside A.

Cascara Tablets *(U.S.P.)*. Store (if uncoated) in airtight containers.

Proprietary Names and Manufacturers

Brevilax *(Cassella-med, Ital.)*; Cascara Evacuant *(Parke, Davis, UK)*; Cascara-Salax *(Ferring, Switz.)*; Cas-Evac *(Parke, Davis, Canad.)*; Péristaltine *(Ciba, Fr.; Ciba, Switz.)*.

The following names have been used for multi-ingredient preparations containing cascara—Celluka *(Bio-Chemical Laboratory, Canad.)*; Cholibile *(Bio-Chemical Laboratory, Canad.)*; Kondremul with Cascara *(Fisons, USA)*; Nature's Remedy *(Norcliff Thayer, USA)*.

7507-v

Cassia Pulp

The evaporated aqueous extract of crushed ripe cassia fruits (cassia pods), *Cassia fistula* (Leguminosae).

Cassia pulp was formerly used as a laxative owing to its content of hydroxymethylanthraquinones.

15314-t

Cetraxate Hydrochloride *(USAN, rINNM)*.

DV-1006. 4-(2-Carboxyethyl)phenyl tranexamate hydrochloride; 4-(2-Carboxyethyl)phenyl *trans*-4-aminomethylcyclohexanecarboxylate hydrochloride.

$C_{17}H_{23}NO_4,HCl=341.8$.

CAS — 34675-84-8 (cetraxate); 27724-96-5 (hydrochloride).

Cetraxate hydrochloride is used in the treatment of peptic ulcer in doses of up to 800 mg daily.

Proprietary Names and Manufacturers

Neuer *(Daiichi, Jpn)*.

713-n

Chalk *(BAN)*.

Prepared Chalk.

$CaCO_3=100.1$.

CAS — 13397-25-6.

Pharmacopoeias. In *Br.* and *Egypt.* Also in *B.P.Vet.*

A native calcium carbonate purified by elutriation. It consists of the calcareous shells and detritus of various foraminifera and contains when dried not less than 97% of $CaCO_3$.

White or greyish-white, odourless or almost odourless, amorphous, earthy, friable masses, usually conical in form, or powder.

Practically **insoluble** in water; slightly soluble in water containing carbon dioxide.

Chalk is used as an antacid and in the treatment of diarrhoea.

It should be noted that a consequence of diarrhoea may be fluid and electrolyte depletion, and that rehydration therapy may be necessary, especially in infants and young children. For further details concerning rehydration therapy, see p.1024.

Preparations

Aromatic Chalk with Opium Mixture *(B.P.)*. Aromatic Chalk with Opium Oral Suspension. A suspension containing chalk 3.25% and 5% v/v of opium tincture in a vehicle containing aromatic ammonia solution, compound cardamom tincture, and catechu tincture. Extemporaneous preparations should be freshly prepared according to the following formula: chalk 325 mg, sucrose 650 mg, tragacanth 20 mg, opium tincture 0.5 mL, catechu tincture 0.5 mL, aromatic ammonia solution 0.5 mL, compound cardamom tincture 1 mL, double-strength chloroform water 5 mL, water to 10 mL.

Paediatric Chalk Mixture *(B.P.)*. Paediatric Chalk Oral Suspension. A suspension with a cinnamon flavour containing chalk 2%. Extemporaneous preparations should be frshly prepared according to the following formula: chalk 100 mg, tragacanth 10 mg, syrup 0.5 mL, concentrated cinnamon water 0.02 mL, double-strength chloroform water 2.5 mL, water to 5 mL.

Aromatic Chalk Powder *(B.P.C. 1973)*. Pulvis Cretae Aromaticus. Chalk 25 g, cinnamon 10 g, nutmeg 8 g, clove 4 g, cardamom seed 3 g, and sucrose 50 g. Store in airtight containers. *Dose*. 0.5 to 5 g.

Aromatic Chalk with Opium Powder *(B.P.C. 1973).* Pulvis Cretae Aromaticus cum Opio. Powdered opium 2.5% in aromatic chalk powder. It contains about 2.5 mg of anhydrous morphine in 1 g. Store in airtight containers. *Dose.* 0.5 to 5 g.

Proprietary Names and Manufacturers
The following names have been used for multi-ingredient preparations containing chalk— Triscal *(Nicholas, UK).*

688-c

Chlorbenzoxamine Hydrochloride *(rINNM).*
1-[2-(2-Chlorobenzhydryloxy)ethyl]-4-(2-methylbenzyl)piperazine dihydrochloride dihydrate.
$C_{27}H_{31}ClN_2O,2HCl,2H_2O=544.0.$

CAS — 522-18-9 (chlorbenzoxamine); 5576-62-5 (hydrochloride, anhydrous).

Chlorbenzoxamine hydrochloride is used in the treatment of peptic ulcer in doses of up to 180 mg daily.

Proprietary Names and Manufacturers
Antiulcera Master *(Coli, Ital.)*; Gastomax *(Brocchieri, Ital.)*; Libratar *(UCB, Arg.; UCB, Denm.; UCB, Ger.; UCB, Ital.; Vesta, S.Afr.; IBYS, Spain).*

6117-g

Cimetidine *(BAN, USAN, rINN).*

SKF-92334. 2-Cyano-1-methyl-3-[2-(5-methylimidazol-4-ylmethylthio)ethyl]guanidine.
$C_{10}H_{16}N_6S=252.3.$

CAS — 51481-61-9.

Pharmacopoeias. In *Ind.* and *U.S.*

A white to off-white crystalline powder, odourless or with a slight mercaptan odour. Slightly **soluble** in water and chloroform; soluble in alcohol; freely soluble in methyl alcohol; sparingly soluble in isopropyl alcohol; practically insoluble in ether. **Store** in airtight containers. Protect from light.

Adverse Effects

Adverse reactions to cimetidine are generally infrequent and are usually reversible following a reduction of dosage or withdrawal of therapy. The commonest side-effects reported have been diarrhoea, dizziness, tiredness, and rashes.

Reversible confusional states, especially in the elderly or in seriously ill patients such as those with renal failure, have occasionally occurred. Cimetidine has a weak anti-androgenic effect and gynaecomastia and impotence have also occasionally occurred in men receiving relatively high doses for conditions such as the Zollinger-Ellison syndrome.

Other adverse effects which have been reported rarely are allergic reactions, arthralgia and myalgia, blood disorders including agranulocytosis or granulocytopenia and thrombocytopenia, interstitial nephritis, headache, hepatotoxicity, and pancreatitis.

A review of adverse reactions encountered with H_2-receptor antagonists.— J. Penston and K. G. Wormsley, *Med. Toxicol.*, 1986, *1*, 192.

A postmarketing surveillance survey examining mortality amongst 9928 patients taking cimetidine and 9351 controls, all followed up for one year. Despite a substantially higher number of deaths in the cimetidine group no evidence of any fatal adverse effect from cimetidine emerged.— D. G. Colin-Jones *et al.*, *Br. med. J.*, 1983, *286*, 1713. Follow-up of these patients for a further 3 years, of whom 9377 survivors were traced, still found no fatal disorder which could be attributed to cimetidine treatment.— *idem*, 1985, *291*, 1084. The original cohorts were also studied for cimetidine-associated morbidity during the first year. No side-effects were detected which had not previously been reported. Pruritus or skin rash and diarrhoea were the commonest events. Although the occurrence of gynaecomastia was confirmed, no such clear-cut association was found for impotence.— *idem*, *Q. J. Med.*, 1985, *54*, 253.

Recurrent parotitis in a patient when given cimetidine or ranitidine.— P. Caraman *et al.* (letter), *Lancet*, 1986, *2*, 1455.

ALLERGY. Three episodes of facial oedema and laryngospasm occurred in a 35-year-old woman who was taking cimetidine. Each episode began soon after a dose of cimetidine 300 mg by mouth.— L. Delaunois (letter), *New Engl. J. Med.*, 1979, *300*, 1216.

A 46-year-old woman developed a generalised red rash with moderate pruritus after taking cimetidine for about 3 weeks. This disappeared within 48 hours of stopping cimetidine but recurred when she again took cimetidine and developed into widespread giant urticaria.— W. A. Hadfield (letter), *Ann. intern. Med.*, 1979, *91*, 128.

Pruritus, urticaria, and angioneurotic oedema in 1 patient developed after the third successive dose of cimetidine intravenously.— B. S. Sandhu and R. Requena (letter), *Ann. intern. Med.*, 1982, *97*, 138. Comments including mention that the reaction may have been due to pethidine which was also given and that it may have been exaggerated by or only apparent after the administration of cimetidine.— R. B. Leftwich and R. A. Simon (letter), *ibid.*, 620. Similar comment on the possible implication of pethidine.— P. García-Ortega and A. Cadahía (letter), *ibid.*, 930. Another report of allergy and anaphylaxis in a patient receiving cimetidine and pethidine. Skin testing and rechallenge was considered to have proved cimetidine to be the responsible agent.— A. B. Knapp *et al.*, *Ann. intern. Med.*, 1982, *97*, 374.

See also under Effects on the Skin, below.

EFFECTS ON THE BLOOD. Reports of agranulocytosis or granulocytopenia possibly associated with cimetidine: E. R. Craven and J. M. Whittington (letter), *Lancet*, 1977, *2*, 294 (agranulocytosis); F. H. Al-Kawas *et al.* (letter), *Ann. intern. Med.*, 1979, *90*, 992 (agranulocytosis); G. O. Littlejohn and M. B. Urowitz (letter), *Ann. intern. Med.*, 1979, *91*, 317 (agranulocytosis); R. Rate *et al.* (letter), *Ann. intern. Med.*, 1979, *91*, 795 (granulocytopenia, thrombocytopenia, and a haemolytic disorder); H. W. Carloss *et al.*, *Ann. intern. Med.*, 1980, *93*, 57 (granulocytopenia); E. Sazie and J. P. Jaffe (letter), *Ann. intern. Med.*, 1980, *93*, 151 (granulocytopenia); S. Eridani *et al.* (letter), *Ann. intern. Med.*, 1982, *97*, 620 (granulocytopenia); D. S. Lewis and E. R. Beck, *Postgrad. med. J.*, 1982, *58*, 443 (agranulocytosis).

Reports of thrombocytopenia possibly associated with cimetidine: J. Idvall (letter), *Lancet*, 1979, *2*, 159; J. L. McDaniel and J. J. Stein (letter), *New Engl. J. Med.*, 1979, *300*, 864; A. J. Isaacs, *Br. med. J.*, 1980, *280*, 294; V. M. Yates and R. E. I. Kerr (letter), *Br. med. J.*, 1980, *280*, 1453; M. J. Collen, *West. J. Med.*, 1980, *132*, 257. Mention in a Committee on Safety of Medicines Update that the annual review had shown that during 1985 15 reports of thrombocytopenia associated with H_2-antagonists had been received.— *Br. med. J.*, 1986, *293*, 688.

Reports of other adverse haematological effects possibly associated with cimetidine: N. M. Johnson *et al.* (letter), *Lancet*, 1977, *2*, 1226 (leucopenia); S. A. Klotz and B. F. Kay (letter), *Ann. intern. Med.*, 1978, *88*, 579 (marrow suppression); C. L. Corbett *et al.*, *Br. med. J.*, 1978, *1*, 753 (leucopenia); A. López-Luque *et al.* (letter), *Lancet*, 1978, *1*, 444 (leucopenia); C. James and B. J. Prout (letter), *Lancet*, 1978, *1*, 987 (marrow suppression); C. de Galocsy and C. van Ypersele de Strihou (letter), *Ann. intern. Med.*, 1979, *90*, 274 (pancytopenia); H. K. Chang and S. L. Morrison, *Ann. intern. Med.*, 1979, *91*, 580 (marrow suppression); B. Rotoli *et al.* (letter), *Lancet*, 1979, *2*, 583 (haemolytic anaemia).

EFFECTS ON BONES AND JOINTS. A report of 5 patients who developed severe arthritic complaints in association with cimetidine administration.— T. K. Khong and P. J. Rooney (letter), *Lancet*, 1980, *2*, 1380.

A report of arthritic inflammatory reactions, clinically identical to gout, precipitated by both cimetidine and ranitidine in a patient with a history of gouty arthritis.— T. R. Einarson *et al.*, *Drug Intell. & clin. Pharm.*, 1985, *19*, 201.

EFFECTS ON THE ENDOCRINE SYSTEM. Mention of diabetes insipidus developing in 2 patients taking cimetidine.— *Br. med. J.*, 1981, *282*, 56.

A study investigating the effect of cimetidine on gonadal function in males found that although the mean sperm count was lower during therapy than that after drug withdrawal the motility and morphology of the spermatozoa were not affected.— C. Wang *et al.*, *Br. J. clin. Pharmac.*, 1982, *13*, 791.

Results of a study to examine the ability of cimetidine to cause clinically important anti-androgenic side-effects. Of 22 male patients receiving relatively high doses of cimetidine for gastric hypersecretory states 11 reported the recent onset of impotence, breast tenderness, gynaecomastia, or a combination of these effects; 9 patients had impotence which was complete in 5, 9 had breast changes (breast tenderness in 8 and gynaecomastia in 5), and 7 had both impotence and breast changes. The mean dose of cimetidine tended to be higher in those patients with side-effects (5.3 g daily) than in those without (3.0 g daily) but the difference was not significant. Symptoms in all 11 patients disappeared following withdrawal of cimetidine (1), reduction of dose (1), or transfer to ranitidine (9).— R. T. Jensen *et al.*, *New Engl. J. Med.*, 1983, *308*, 883.

EFFECTS ON THE EYE. Ocular pain, blurred vision, and an increase in intra-ocular pressure in a patient with chronic glaucoma during cimetidine treatment. Ocular symptoms associated with an increased pressure also occurred with ranitidine.— G. Dobrilla *et al.* (letter), *Lancet*, 1982, *1*, 1078. Results in healthy subjects and preliminary results in patients with chronic simple glaucoma suggesting that cimetidine was without effect on intra-ocular pressure.— F. Feldman and M. M. Cohen (letter), *ibid.*, 1359.

EFFECTS ON THE GASTRO-INTESTINAL TRACT. *Gastric cancer.* A review and discussion concerning the safety of drugs for the long-term treatment of peptic ulcers. The most serious hypothetical problem concerns the possibility that prolonged inhibition of gastric secretion may result in the development of gastric cancer; although no confirmation of this association has been provided by rigorous surveillance the matter has aroused widespread public concern. Several mechanisms of gastric carcinogenesis have been proposed. Firstly, that a drug or metabolite may be a genotoxic (initiating) carcinogen. While cimetidine and ranitidine are neither mutagenic nor genotoxic, they can be nitrosated *in vitro* to produce genotoxic derivatives, but this is unlikely to be of any clinical significance since the strongly acid conditions and excess of nitrous acid required for the reaction are not encountered in the stomachs of patients receiving such drug treatment. A second proposed mechanism for gastric carcinogenesis is that therapeutic gastric inhibition may produce conditions which promote the development of gastric cancer as the incidence of such cancers is unexpectedly high in patients with impaired gastric secretions, in conditions such as pernicious anaemia and chronic atrophic gastritis, and after gastric resection. It is proposed in this hypothesis that the decreased secretion of acid permits colonisation of the stomach by bacteria which are capable of reducing salivary or dietary nitrate to nitrite which then ultimately forms carcinogenic nitroso compounds. It has, though, been overlooked that this reaction also requires the presence of hydrogen ions so that conditions associated with achlorhydria would be unsatisfactory. However, nitrogen oxides react experimentally with amines in neutral and alkaline conditions but the relevance of this during anti-ulcer therapy cannot be assessed at present. Factual evidence for this achlorhydria-associated hypothesis remains, therefore, uncertain and much more study is needed to confirm the allegedly increased production of possibly carcinogenic nitroso compounds in the stomach. It is important that the problem should be studied properly in patients treated with antisecretory drugs rather than verbally extrapolated as at present. It should also be emphasised that the proposed connection between decreased or absent gastric secretions and gastric cancer is not established either experimentally or clinically and that the association may merely reflect that the decreased gastric secretion is a manifestation of an already-present severe disease of the gastric mucosa. Another explanation for the increased tendency of diseased gastric mucosa to undergo malignant change must be considered in that marked abnormalities of cell proliferation and differentiation are present. It is the author's view that the noxious effects of drugs on this state of the gastric mucosa is the most important criterion of carcinogenic risk and it therefore seems that both cimetidine and ranitidine are without risk as it has been reported that they do not affect the cellular kinetics of the gastric mucosa nor produce the changes of gastritis. In conclusion it is considered that cimetidine and ranitidine can be, and have been, given to patients safely.— K. G. Wormsley, *Gut*, 1984, *25*, 1416. A similar review concerning antisecretory drugs and gastric cancer and commenting that the belief remains that treatment with cimetidine and ranitidine is generally safe although stronger evidence would be desirable.— M. J. S. Langman, *Br. med. J.*, 1985, *290*, 1850.

EFFECTS ON THE HEART. Individual reports of the effects of cimetidine on the heart.— P. Reding *et al.* (letter), *Lancet*, 1977, *2*, 1227 (bradycardia with atrioventricular dissociation); D. B. Jefferys and J. A. Vale (letter), *Lancet*, 1978, *1*, 828 (bradycardia); M. Ligumsky *et al.* (letter), *Ann. intern. Med.*, 1978, *89*, 1008 (bradycardia); T. Tordjman *et al.* (letter), *Archs intern. Med.*, 1984, *144*, 861 (complete atrioventricular block); W. Dickey and M. Symington (letter), *Lancet*, 1987, *1*, 99 (broad-complex tachycardia); M. Ishizaki *et al.* (letter), *ibid.*, 225 (first-degree atrioventricular block).

Studies and ECG recordings in 7 patients receiving cimetidine 1 g daily for one week suggested that it was not associated with clinically or statistically significant bradycardia.— G. Jackson and J. W. Upward (letter), *Lancet*, 1982, *2*, 265.

See also under Overdosage.

EFFECTS ON THE KIDNEY. A comment that up to the end of 1981 the manufacturers of cimetidine (*Smith Kline and French*) were aware of 20 patients who may have had interstitial nephritis out of an estimated total of 20 million cimetidine-treated patients. On the assumption that only 10% of these adverse effects have been reported, which is a figure consistent with that suggested for a voluntary reporting system, the incidence would be around 1 in 100 000 treated patients. The interstitial nephritis related to cimetidine administration has always been reversed on cessation of therapy.— D. Rowley-Jones and A. C. Flind (letter), *Br. med. J.*, 1982, *285*, 1422.

EFFECTS ON THE LIVER. For a review comparing the incidence of hepatotoxicity reported with cimetidine and ranitidine, see Ranitidine, p.1104.

EFFECTS ON THE MUSCLES. A report implicating cimetidine in the development of polymyositis in one patient.— A. J. S. Watson *et al.*, *New Engl. J. Med.*, 1983, *308*, 142. A comment that further follow-up of the patient, during which time he has continued to have progressive polymyositis, despite the discontinuation of cimetidine 15 months earlier, argues against the role of cimetidine in inducing the disorder.— R. A. Hawkins *et al.* (letter), *ibid.*, *309*, 187. Reply that it may be premature to exclude a possible role of cimetidine in the pathogenesis of polymyositis.— A. J. S. Watson *et al.* (letter), *ibid.*, 188.

EFFECTS ON THE NERVOUS SYSTEM. Individual reports of adverse neurological effects possibly associated with cimetidine and mainly in patients who were elderly, seriously ill, or had impaired renal function.— T. A. Grimson (letter), *Lancet*, 1977, *1*, 858 (confusion); J. C. Delaney and M. Ravey (letter), *Lancet*, 1977, *2*, 512 (confusion); W. Grave *et al.* (letter), *Lancet*, 1977, *2*, 719 (twitching and deepening of unconsciousness); T. J. Robinson and T. O. Mulligan (letter), *Lancet*, 1977, *2*, 719 (confusion); N. Menzies-Gow (letter), *Lancet*, 1977, *2*, 928 (confusion); J. B. Spears (letter), *Am. J. Hosp. Pharm.*, 1978, *35*, 1035 (confusion); T. R. Vickery (letter), *Drug Intell. & clin. Pharm.*, 1978, *12*, 242 (confusion); C. A. Wood *et al.* (letter), *J. Am. med. Ass.*, 1978, *239*, 2550 (confusion); S. K. Agarwal (letter), *J. Am. med. Ass.*, 1978, *240*, 214 (hallucinations); M. L. Levine (letter), *J. Am. med. Ass.*, 1978, *240*, 1238 (coma); W. J. K. Cumming and J. B. Foster (letter), *Lancet*, 1978, *1*, 1096 (reversible brain stem syndrome characterised by headache, ataxia, dysarthria, visual impairment, deafness, paraesthesia, and incontinence); M. A. McMillen *et al.* (letter), *New Engl. J. Med.*, 1978, *298*, 284 (confusion); J. W. Jefferson, *Am. J. Psychiat.*, 1979, *136*, 346 (depression); C. C. Barnhart and C. L. Bowden, *Am. J. Psychiat.*, 1979, *136*, 725 (confusion); J. Johnson and S. Bailey, *Br. J. Psychiat.*, 1979, *134*, 315 (depression); H. G. Kinnell and A. Webb (letter), *Br. med. J.*, 1979, *2*, 1438 (paranoia and confusion); S. R. Mogelnicki *et al.*, *J. Am. med. Ass.*, 1979, *241*, 826 (confusion); M. E. Edmonds *et al.*, *J. R. Soc. Med.*, 1979, *72*, 172 (confusion, muscular twitching and convulsions); L. E. Adler *et al.*, *Am. J. Psychiat.*, 1980, *137*, 1112 (paranoia); T. G. Feest and D. J. Read (letter), *Br. med. J.*, 1980, *281*, 1284 (myopathy); T. J. Walls *et al.*, *Br. med. J.*, 1980, *281*, 974 (motor neuropathy); B. J. Kimelblatt *et al.*, *Gastroenterology*, 1980, *78*, 791 (confusion); A. B. Atkinson *et al.* (letter), *Lancet*, 1980, *2*, 36 (neuropathy; with captopril); J. Totte *et al.* (letter), *Lancet*, 1981, *1*, 1047 (neurological dysfunction and metabolite); M. J. Kushner (letter), *Ann. intern. Med.*, 1982, *96*, 126 (chorea); M. Sonnenblick *et al.*, *Postgrad. med. J.*, 1982, *58*, 415 (confusion and coma); A. R. Rushton (letter), *Ann. intern. Med.*, 1983, *98*, 677 (hallucinations); K. A. Papp and R. M. Curtis, *Can. med. Ass. J.*, 1984, *131*, 1081 (hallucinations and bizarre behaviour); Y. Niv *et al.* (letter), *Ann. intern. Med.*, 1986, *105*, 977 (encephalopathy).

For studies indicating that cimetidine by mouth is suitable for those involved in skilled activity, see under Precautions, below.

EFFECTS ON THE RESPIRATORY SYSTEM. A report of 20 patients who developed work-related respiratory symptoms associated with exposure to cimetidine dust; the effects were most common in those most often exposed.— I. I. Coutts *et al.*, *Br. med. J.*, 1984, *288*, 1418.

EFFECTS ON THE SKIN. Wide-spread erythrosis-like lesions in a 36-year-old man were probably induced by cimetidine.— G. Angelini *et al.* (letter), *Br. med. J.*, 1979, *1*, 1147.

A report of a skin eruption clinically consistent with erythema annulare centrifugum developing in a patient after 6 months of treatment with cimetidine; the eruption resolved after withdrawal of cimetidine and reappeared on rechallenge. The condition had not recurred during therapy with ranitidine.— A. C. Merrett *et al.*, *Br. med. J.*, 1981, *283*, 698.

Analysis, by the Boston Collaborative Drug Surveillance Program, of data on 15 438 patients hospitalised between 1975 and 1982 detected 3 allergic skin reactions attributed to cimetidine among 235 recipients of the drug.— M. Bigby *et al.*, *J. Am. med. Ass.*, 1986, *256*, 3358.

Alopecia. A review of 21 cases of alopecia in patients taking cimetidine reported to the Division of Drug Experience in the *USA*; these were the cases where a temporal relationship to cimetidine use could be established with some degree of certainty.— J. H. Khalsa *et al.* (letter), *Int. J. Derm.*, 1983, *22*, 202.

Exfoliative dermatitis. A report of exfoliative dermatitis associated with the use of cimetidine.— P. L. Yantis, *Dig. Dis. Scis*, 1980, *25*, 73.

Lupus. For reports of lupus in association with cimetidine, see below.

Stevens-Johnson syndrome. For reports of the Stevens-Johnson syndrome in association with cimetidine, see below.

Vasculitis. A rash consistent with urticarial vasculitis in a patient was demonstrated by biopsy and re-challenge to be induced by cimetidine.— G. G. Mitchell *et al.*, *Am. J. Med.*, 1983, *75*, 875.

FEVER. Reports of febrile reactions associated with cimetidine: C. Ramboer (letter), *Lancet*, 1978, *1*, 330; J. C. McLoughlin *et al.* (letter), *ibid.*, 499; C. L. Corbett and C. D. Holdsworth, *Br. med. J.*, 1978, *1*, 753; K. Landolfo *et al.*, *Can. med. Ass. J.*, 1984, *130*, 1580.

LUPUS. Exacerbation of cutaneous lupus erythematosus in 1 patient following the introduction of cimetidine therapy.— B. L. Davidson, *Archs intern. Med.*, 1982, *142*, 166.

Brief details of a patient who had a lupus erythematosus-like eruption on light-exposed skin 10 days after starting cimetidine therapy, which settled on withdrawal and recurred again during a further course of cimetidine. Mention was also made that the Committee on the Safety of Medicines had received one report of an association between cimetidine and a cutaneous manifestation of lupus erythematosus.— K. J. S. Macdonald and K. J. A. Kenicer, *Br. med. J.*, 1984, *288*, 1498.

OVERDOSAGE. A patient who took about 12 g of cimetidine had slurred speech, high pulse-rate, and dilated pupils. Five hours after gastric lavage he was confused, agitated, disorientated and making staccato nonsensical conversation. He recovered from these mental symptoms the next day. There were no changes in ECG, blood indexes, liver or kidney.— P. G. Nelson (letter), *Lancet*, 1977, *2*, 928.

A patient took a 2-month course of cimetidine in one week without untoward effect; this produced a daily dose of about 12 g. His dyspepsia was relieved and his duodenal ulcer healed.— G. V. Gill (letter), *Lancet*, 1978, *1*, 99.

Four men took overdoses (5.2 to 19.6 g) of cimetidine; plasma concentrations of up to 57 μg per mL were recorded, compared with reported peak concentrations of 1 μg per mL after a single 200-mg dose. Apart from dry mouth no patient experienced untoward effects.— R. N. Illingworth and D. R. Jarvie, *Br. med. J.*, 1979, *1*, 453.

Respiratory depression associated with cimetidine overdosage.— J. B. Wilson (letter), *Br. med. J.*, 1979, *1*, 955.

Fatal bradycardia in a 38-year-old woman after an overdose of cimetidine and diazepam. Bradycardia was considered to have been precipitated by cimetidine, and death to be due to the combined effects of cimetidine and diazepam. Traces of digoxin were considered unlikely to have caused the clinical picture.— J. Hiss *et al.* (letter), *Lancet*, 1982, *2*, 982.

Treatment. Experience with 14 adults and 4 children, who had taken cimetidine alone or with alcohol and various other drugs, has not demonstrated any significant toxicity of cimetidine in overdosage. Three of 7 adults who remained completely free of symptoms had taken 20 g of cimetidine, and 3½ hours after ingestion one of these had a blood-cimetidine concentration of 45.8 mg per litre. In view of the apparent lack of toxicity of cimetidine in overdosage it is recommended that treatment should consist of gastric lavage or administration of syrup of ipecacuanha, provided that not more than 4 hours have elapsed since ingestion of the drug, followed by supportive measures and symptomatic treatment only. Forced diuresis is not recommended and, moreover, there appears to be no evidence that it enhances the excretion of cimetidine from the body.— T. J. Meredith and G. N. Volans (letter), *Lancet*, 1979, *2*, 1367.

STEVENS-JOHNSON SYNDROME. After taking cimetidine for 25 days a 38-year-old Asian woman with a history of penicillin allergy developed the Stevens-Johnson syndrome. It was not considered ethically justifiable to confirm the association by readministering cimetidine.— A. H. Ahmed *et al.* (letter), *Lancet*, 1978, *2*, 433. A similar report in which cimetidine may have been the precipitating cause of the Stevens-Johnson syndrome in a patient with a history of allergy to sulphonamides.— R. Guan and P. P. B. Yeo (letter), *Aust. N.Z. J. Med.*, 1983, *13*, 182.

Precautions

Before giving cimetidine to patients with gastric ulcers the possibility of malignancy should be excluded since cimetidine may mask symptoms and delay diagnosis. Cimetidine should be given in reduced dosage to patients with impaired renal function.

Cimetidine has been reported to interact with many other drugs but the full clinical significance of some of these interactions has yet to be established since many of the studies have involved healthy subjects given single or subtherapeutic doses. Those interactions which are generally considered to be of clinical importance are with lignocaine, phenytoin, theophylline, and warfarin where the blood concentrations of these drugs may be increased to such a degree that a reduction in their dosage may be necessary. Increased blood concentrations of some anti-arrhythmics, some benzodiazepines, some beta-blockers, and some vasodilators, have also been reported.

Intravenous injections of cimetidine should be given slowly and intravenous infusion is recommended in patients with cardiovascular impairment.

Results of a study in 7 healthy subjects showing no modulation of CNS function or impairment of performance following single doses of cimetidine 200 and 400 mg and ranitidine 150 and 300 mg by mouth and the suggestion that in individuals free of renal or hepatic disease both drugs would be suitable for those involved in skilled activity.— A. N. Nicholson and B. M. Stone, *Eur. J. clin. Pharmac.*, 1984, *26*, 579. A similar study.— N. Theofilopoulos *et al.*, *Br. J. clin. Pharmac.*, 1984, *18*, 135.

INTERACTIONS. Reviews of drug interactions with cimetidine: E. M. Sorkin and D. L. Darvey, *Drug Intell. & clin. Pharm.*, 1983, *17*, 110; J. Penston and K. G. Wormsley, *Med. Toxicol.*, 1986, *1*, 192; A. Somogyi and M. Muirhead, *Clin. Pharmacokinet.*, 1987, *12*, 321.

Severe headache with transient hypertension subsequent to the ingestion of tyramine-rich foods occurred in an elderly patient receiving cimetidine. Rechallenge was not possible, but it was considered that cimetidine may have interfered with the normal hepatic elimination of tyramine.— M. J. J. Griffin and J. S. Morris (letter), *Drug Intell. & clin. Pharm.*, 1987, *21*, 219.

Antacids. A short review of published studies on the interactions between anti-ulcer medications. Although it has been reported that antacids have a dose-related effect on the bioavailability of cimetidine it would appear that with the usual dosage schedules of cimetidine (with meals and at bedtime) and of antacids (one to three hours after meals), no significant interaction will occur; even if antacids were to be administered at the same time as cimetidine or ranitidine, there is no evidence that efficacy would be decreased. Although a potential exists for an interaction between cimetidine or ranitidine and sucralfate, the inhibition of cimetidine absorption by sucralfate appears to be clinically insignificant and there is no evidence that the activity of sucralfate is reduced.— *Drug Interact. News.*, 1985, *5*, 11.

Anti-arrhythmics. For the effect of cimetidine on some anti-arrhythmic agents, see under flecainide acetate (p.79), procainamide hydrochloride (p.83), quinidine sulphate (p.86), and verapamil hydrochloride (p.90). See also under lignocaine hydrochloride (p.1218).

Antimuscarinics. Some reduction in the bioavailability

of cimetidine on concomitant administration of *metoclopramide* and *propantheline*.— J. Kanto *et al.* (letter), *Br. J. clin. Pharmac.*, 1981, *11*, 629.

Antidepressants. For the effect of cimetidine on some tricyclic antidepressants, see under amitriptyline hydrochloride (p.353).

Antiepileptics. For the effect of cimetidine on some antiepileptic agents, see under carbamazepine (p.401), and phenytoin sodium (p.408).

Antiprotozoals. For the effect of cimetidine on metronidazole, see under metronidazole (p.668).

Benzodiazepines. For the effect of cimetidine on benzodiazepines, see under diazepam (p. 729).

Local anaesthetics. For the effect of cimetidine on lignocaine, see under lignocaine hydrochloride (p.1218); for the effect on bupivacaine, see under bupivacaine hydrochloride (p.1209).

Vasodilators. For the effect of cimetidine on some vasodilators, see under diltiazem hydrochloride (p.1496). See also under verapamil hydrochloride (p.90), and nifedipine (p.1510).

PORPHYRIA. Cimetidine was considered to be unsafe in patients with acute porphyria although there is conflicting experimental evidence on porphyrinogenicity.— M.R. Moore and K.E.L. McColl, *Porphyrias, Drug Lists*, Glasgow, Porphyria Research Unit, University of Glasgow, 1987.

PREGNANCY AND THE NEONATE. Cimetidine was detected in the milk of a nursing mother in concentrations higher than in her plasma. It was calculated that the maximum amount of cimetidine that an infant could ingest assuming an intake of about 1 litre of milk daily and fed at the time of peak concentrations would be about 6 mg.— A. Somogyi and R. Gugler (letter), *Br. J. clin. Pharmac.*, 1979, *7*, 627.

Absorption and Fate

Cimetidine is readily absorbed from the gastro-intestinal tract and peak plasma concentrations are obtained about an hour after administration on an empty stomach and about 2 hours after administration with food.

The bioavailability of cimetidine following oral administration is about 60 to 70% compared to an intravenous dose due to first-pass metabolism. The elimination half-life from plasma is around 2 hours and cimetidine is weakly bound, about 20%, to plasma proteins. Cimetidine is partially metabolised in the liver to the sulphoxide and to hydroxymethylcimetidine but most is excreted unchanged in the urine. Cimetidine crosses the placental barrier and is excreted into breast milk where concentrations are reported to be higher than those in plasma. It does not readily cross the blood-brain barrier.

A review of the clinical pharmacokinetics of cimetidine.— A. Somogyi and R. Gugler, *Clin. Pharmacokinet.*, 1983, *8*, 463.

Uses and Administration

Cimetidine is a histamine H_2-receptor antagonist. Accordingly, it inhibits gastric acid secretion and reduces pepsin output; it has also been shown to inhibit other actions of histamine mediated by H_2-receptors. It is used in conditions where inhibition of gastric acid secretion may be beneficial; such conditions include duodenal and gastric ulcers, oesophageal reflux, selected cases of persistent dyspepsia, and pathological hypersecretory states, such as the Zollinger-Ellison syndrome. Its ability to inhibit acid secretion also means that cimetidine may be used for the prophylaxis of gastro-intestinal haemorrhage as a consequence of stress ulceration and in patients at risk of acid aspiration (Mendelson's syndrome) during general anaesthesia. Cimetidine may also be used to reduce malabsorption and fluid loss in patients with the short bowel syndrome and to reduce the degradation of enzyme supplements given to patients with pancreatic insufficiency.

Cimetidine may be given by mouth, by the nasogastric route, or parenterally by the intravenous or intramuscular routes; the total daily dose by any route should not normally exceed 2.4 g. Although some formulations are prepared with the aid of hydrochloric acid, strengths and doses are expressed in terms of the base.

When cimetidine is given by mouth, day-time doses should generally be taken with meals. The usual dose by mouth is 400 mg twice daily (in the morning and at bedtime); other regimens are 200 mg, or if necessary 400 mg, three times daily with 400 mg at bedtime.

The usual dose of cimetidine by intravenous injection is 200 mg which should be given slowly over at least 2 minutes and may be repeated every 4 to 6 hours. If a larger dose is required, or if the patient has cardiovascular impairment, intravenous infusion is recommended. For an intermittent intravenous infusion the recommended dose is 400 mg (in 100 mL of sodium chloride 0.9%) given over 30 minutes to 1 hour and repeated every 4 to 6 hours if necessary. For a continuous intravenous infusion the recommended rate is 50 to 100 mg per hour. The usual intramuscular dose is 200 mg which may be repeated at intervals of 4 to 6 hours.

In the management of duodenal and gastric ulcers a single daily dose of 800 mg by mouth at bedtime is recommended which should be given initially for at least 4 weeks in the case of duodenal and for at least 6 weeks in the case of gastric ulcers. Where appropriate a maintenance dose of 400 mg may then be given once at bedtime, or both in the morning and at bedtime.

In reflux oesophagitis the recommended dose is 400 mg four times daily (with meals and at bedtime) for 4 to 8 weeks, and in pathological hypersecretory conditions, such as the Zollinger-Ellison syndrome, a dose of 400 mg four times daily may also be required, occasionally increased to a total of 2.4 g daily.

Doses of 200 or 400 mg by mouth, by nasogastric administration, or parenterally (200 mg only for direct intravenous injection) every 4 to 6 hours are recommended for the management of patients at risk from stress-related ulceration of the upper gastro-intestinal tract. In patients at risk of developing the acid aspiration syndrome during general anaesthesia, a dose of 400 mg by mouth may be given 90 to 120 minutes before the induction of anaesthesia or at the start of labour, and doses of up to 400 mg (by the parenteral route if appropriate, see above) may be repeated at intervals of 4 hours if required.

To reduce the degradation of pancreatic enzyme supplements, patients with pancreatic insufficiency may be given cimetidine 0.8 to 1.6 g daily by mouth in 4 divided doses before meals.

The dosage of cimetidine should be reduced in patients with impaired renal function; suggested doses according to creatinine clearance are: creatinine clearance of 0 to 15 mL per minute, 200 mg twice daily; creatinine clearance of 15 to 30 mL per minute, 200 mg three times daily; creatinine clearance of 30 to 50 mL per minute, 200 mg four times daily; creatinine clearance of over 50 mL per minute, normal dosage.

A suggested dose of cimetidine for children over one year of age is 25 to 30 mg per kg body-weight daily by mouth or parenterally.

The doses of cimetidine cited above relate to *UK* use. This is because, depending on the country in which it is marketed, cimetidine is supplied in different dose units; most doses in the *UK* are 200 or 400 mg while most doses in the *USA* are 300 mg. In general the recommended oral dose of cimetidine in the *USA* is 300 mg four times daily (with meals and at bedtime), increased to a maximum total daily dose of 2.4 g in pathological secretory conditions such as the Zollinger-Ellison syndrome. The usual parenteral dose of cimetidine in the *USA* is also 300 mg.

ADMINISTRATION. Results of a study suggesting that continuous infusions of cimetidine are superior to bolus injections in the control of gastric pH since the infusion sustains therapeutic blood concentrations more effectively than intermittent injections.— M. J. Ostro *et al.*, *Gastroenterology*, 1985, *89*, 532.

ADMINISTRATION IN CHILDREN. Although the use of cimetidine in adults has been extensive the corresponding use in children, and particularly in neonates, is limited. Studying the pharmacokinetics of cimetidine in one premature and 2 full-term neonates Ziemniak *et al.* (*Develop. Pharmac. Ther.*, 1984, *7*, 30) considered that dosage adjustments should be made based on renal function with a dose of 15 to 20 mg per kg body-weight daily being adequate for full-term neonates but with lower doses necessary for premature infants and those with renal dysfunction. In further pharmacokinetic studies Lloyd *et al.* (*Drug Intell. & clin. Pharm.*, 1985, *19*, 203) found that the half-life of cimetidine was prolonged in a full-term neonate after doses of 10 mg per kg daily compared with doses of 5 mg per kg daily and Stile *et al.* (*Clin. Ther.*, 1985, *7*, 361) after studying 3 neonates given single doses of cimetidine suggested that a dose of 5 to 7 mg per kg would effectively suppress secretion of gastric acid in neonates but also commented that further studies were needed to determine the lowest effective daily dose and the appropriate dosing interval. In a study of older children aged 4 to 13 years Somogyi *et al.* (*Eur. J. Pediat.*, 1985, *144*, 72) considered a dosage regimen of approximately 30 mg per kg daily in 3 or 4 divided doses to be appropriate.

ADMINISTRATION IN THE ELDERLY. A preliminary report of a marked reduction in the plasma clearance of cimetidine with increasing age.— R. Gugler and A. Somogyi (letter), *New Engl. J. Med.*, 1979, *301*, 435. In a study in 20 healthy subjects aged 22 to 84 years, the bioavailability of cimetidine appeared to be increased in the elderly subjects, possibly due to decreased clearance of the drug. It was suggested that the standard dose of cimetidine could be reduced by about 30% to 50% without loss of efficacy.— A. Redolfi *et al.*, *Eur. J. clin. Pharmac.*, 1979, *15*, 257.

Further references: A. Somogyi *et al.*, *Clin. Pharmacokinet.*, 1980, *5*, 84; D. E. Drayer *et al.*, *Clin. Pharmac. Ther.*, 1982, *31*, 45.

ADMINISTRATION IN HEPATIC FAILURE. Results of a pharmacokinetic study in 16 cirrhotic patients suggesting that patients with a history of portal systemic encephalopathy may require up to 40% reduction in the dosage of cimetidine; in cirrhotic patients with no such history, kinetics and metabolism were similar to healthy subjects.— J. A. Ziemniak *et al.*, *Clin. Pharmac. Ther.*, 1983, *34*, 375.

Further pharmacokinetic studies in patients with impaired hepatic function: R. Gugler *et al.*, *Br. J. clin. Pharmac.*, 1982, *14*, 421 (cirrhosis); J. P. Cello and S. Øie, *Eur. J. clin. Pharmac.*, 1983, *25*, 223 (cirrhosis).

ADMINISTRATION IN RENAL FAILURE. The mean total amount of an intravenous dose of cimetidine removed by haemodialysis in 6 patients with severe chronic renal failure was 13.7% and it was therefore concluded that a major adjustment of the dose on days of dialysis was not necessary.— R. Larsson *et al.*, *Eur. J. clin. Pharmac.*, 1982, *21*, 325.

A study in 6 patients undergoing continuous ambulatory peritoneal dialysis showed that only about 2% of an intravenous dose of cimetidine was removed by dialysis. It was concluded that there was no need to adjust the conventional renal failure dosing regimens in such patients.— F. J. Kogan *et al.*, *J. clin. Pharmac.*, 1983, *23*, 252.

Further references: R. Larsson *et al.*, *Br. J. clin. Pharmac.*, 1982, *13*, 163 (pharmacokinetics in patients with varying degrees of impaired renal function).

ASPIRATION SYNDROME. A comment regarding the prevention of acid aspiration during labour. During labour gastric emptying is slowed and often leads to the accumulation of highly acid stomach contents. These present a serious hazard in that during the induction of general anaesthesia they may be vomited or regurgitated into the pharynx and reach the lungs via the paralysed larynx. The severity of the lung reaction is related to the acidity and volume; if the pH is below 2.5 a fatal outcome is likely. Reduction of gastric acidity in all women in labour is now commonly practised, magnesium trisilicate being most commonly employed. An alternative approach is to use H_2-antagonists. Neither cimetidine nor ranitidine act quickly because of the existing acid and the time to reach an effective therapeutic plasma concentration but when properly timed in relation to the induction of anaesthesia either is acceptable for elective surgery. However, for treatment throughout labour ranitidine, because of its longer duration of action, would seem more appropriate. The effects of both are augmented by the administration of a dose of sodium citrate by mouth immediately before operation.— J. Moore *et al.*, *Br. J. clin. Pharmac.*, 1984, *17*, 226P.

A review of the methods available for reducing gastric acidity and volume in patients presenting for general anaesthesia.— M. Morgan, *Br. J. Anaesth.*, 1984, *56*, 47. A review of studies using cimetidine for the prophylaxis of the acid aspiration syndrome.— S. F. Kowalsky, *Drug Intell. & clin. Pharm.*, 1984, *18*, 382.

See also under Magnesium Trisilicate, p.1096.

CARCINOID SYNDROME. Elimination of flushing attacks associated with a metastatic gastric carcinoid tumour was achieved when diphenhydramine hydrochloride 50 mg and cimetidine 300 mg were both taken 6-hourly by a 54-year-old woman who had suffered attacks every day for the previous 22 years. Diphenhydramine alone reduced the frequency of attacks while cimetidine alone reduced their duration. Over a 6-week period on the combined treatment the patient experienced only about 2 very mild flushes weekly.— L. J. Roberts *et al.*, *New Engl. J. Med.*, 1979, *300*, 236. A 58-year-old woman with carcinoid syndrome associated with metastatic ileal carcinoid tumour was treated similarly without success.— T. D. Wingert *et al.* (letter), *ibid.*, 1980, *302*, 234. The frequency, duration, and intensity of flushing were substantially reduced by treatment with diphenhydramine 25 mg and cimetidine 300 mg, both four times daily, in a man with metastatic ileal carcinoid tumour.— J. D. Pyles *et al.* (letter), *ibid.* Comment.— L. J. Roberts *et al.* (letter), *ibid.*, 235.

CYSTIC FIBROSIS. For reports of cimetidine therapy in cystic fibrosis, see under Pancreatic Disorders (below).

DYSPEPSIA. Results from a double-blind controlled study involving 159 patients with non-ulcer dyspepsia showing that neither an antacid nor cimetidine had any therapeutic advantage over a placebo. It was concluded that neutralisation or suppression of gastric acid is of no clinical value in such patients.— O. Nyrén *et al.*, *New Engl. J. Med.*, 1986, *314*, 339.

A discussion on the treatment of non-ulcer dyspepsia noting the curiosity that cimetidine, but not ranitidine, has been approved by the Committee on Safety of Medicines for use in the *UK* in patients with non-ulcer dyspepsia.— *Lancet*, 1986, *1*, 1306. Reply from the manufacturers of cimetidine stating that the CSM has not approved unrestricted use of cimetidine in non-ulcer dyspepsia but rather that the data sheet allows for the symptomatic treatment of persistent dyspeptic symptoms responsive to reduction of gastric acid secretion whether or not an ulcer is present when treatment starts.— D. A. Boyko and A. C. Flind (letter), *ibid.*, *2*, 113.

Further reviews on the use of cimetidine in non-ulcer dyspepsia.— *Drug & Ther. Bull.*, 1986, *24*, 3.

GASTRO-INTESTINAL BLEEDING. Although histamine H_2-antagonists are commonly used in acute upper gastro-intestinal haemorrhage there is no single study giving reliable evidence of an important benefit. Studies so far performed have been individually too small reliably to assess the effect of treatment on important end-points, such as re-bleeding, surgery, and death. Therefore an attempt has been made to review data from all 27 available randomised controlled trials of H_2-antagonists in acute upper gastro-intestinal haemorrhage. The combined analysis of these results, which included over 2500 patients, indicated overall trends in favour of treatment. However, although this implies that treatment is moderately promising, the available data lack the statistical power to allow any moderate but clinically important effects to be demonstrated with confidence even when combined results are analysed.— R. Collins and M. Langman, *New Engl. J. Med.*, 1985, *313*, 660.

For the effect of cimetidine on stress-induced bleeding, see under Stress Ulceration (below).

HYPERPARATHYROIDISM. A review of the medical management of primary hyperparathyroidism. Although initial reports of cimetidine in both primary and secondary hyperparathyroidism appeared very encouraging they were unsatisfactory in various ways and at least two subsequent controlled studies together with numerous case reports have failed to confirm any clear response to cimetidine other than in the occasional patient; in no case did the treatment produce normocalcaemia.— *Lancet*, 1984, *2*, 727. A comment that the evaluation of cimetidine in parathyroid disease has been obscured by failure to distinguish hyperparathyroidism due to adenomatous disease from a broad category of other conditions which cause hypercalcaemia and/or raised parathyroid hormone concentrations. In the authors' experience it has not been possible to detect any effect of cimetidine in any condition other than primary hyperparathyroidism due to adenomatous disease. It is not suggested that cimetidine should be substituted for definitive surgery, but rather that cimetidine seems to have a role in the management and is also an important tool for research on the disease.— J. K. Sherwood *et al.* (letter), *ibid.*, 1219.

IMMUNOLOGICAL DISORDERS. Cimetidine has been reported (M.E. Osband *et al.*, *Lancet*, 1981, *1*, 636; R.R.M. Gifford *et al.*, *Lancet*, 1981, *1*, 638) to be a successful form of immunotherapy of tumours in *mice* and to be associated with decreased production of suppressor T-lymphocytes. The following reports and references may possibly represent a beneficial response to cimetidine being mediated through an immunomodulatory action.

Candidiasis. Encouraging results with cimetidine in 4 patients with chronic mucocutaneous candidiasis.— J. L. Jorizzo *et al.*, *Ann. intern. Med.*, 1980, *92*, 192.

Eosinophilic fasciitis. Response to cimetidine in a patient with eosinophilic fasciitis, a disorder that may be modulated through an altered immune response. It was emphasized that prednisone must still be regarded as the preferred therapy but that in patients who cannot tolerate steroid therapy, or who need doses which result in unacceptable side-effects, cimetidine may represent a valuable adjunct to therapy, or in selected patients, an alternative primary therapy.— G. Solomon *et al.*, *Ann. intern. Med.*, 1982, *97*, 547. Further reports.— E. B. Loftin (letter), *ibid.*, 1983, *98*, 112 (no benefit in one patient); F. J. Laso *et al.* (letter), *ibid.*, 1026 (response in one patient); O. García-Morteo *et al.* (letter), *ibid.*, 1984, *100*, 318 (response in two patients).

Herpesvirus infections. Although there have been numerous isolated and anecdotal reports of a beneficial response to cimetidine in patients with infections due to various herpes viruses, including genital herpes simplex (D. Wakefield, *Ann. intern. Med.*, 1984, *101*, 882), infectious mononucleosis (J.A. Goldstein, *Ann. intern. Med.*, 1983, *99*, 410; *idem*, 1986, *105*, 139), and herpes zoster (S. Van der Spuy *et al.*, *S. Afr. med. J.*, 1980, *58*, 112; S.T. Hayne and J.B. Mercer, *Can. med. Ass. J.*, 1983, *129*, 1284; R. Shandera, *Can. med. Ass. J.*, 1984, *131*, 279; G.M. Mavligit and M. Talpaz, *New Engl. J. Med.*, 1984, *310*, 318; B.S. George, *Med. J. Aust.*, 1984, *141*, 320; R.S. Arnot, *Med. J. Aust.*, 1984, *141*, 903; J. Fitzhenry, *Med. J. Aust.*, 1985, *142*, 78) some of these reports have been criticised (D.L. Tyrrell, *Can. med. Ass. J.*, 1984, *130*, 1109; K.E. Giles, *Med. J. Aust.*, 1985, *142*, 283) mainly on the grounds that the majority of cases of herpes zoster will resolve within 2 to 3 weeks whether any treatment is given or not. Also, a recently published double-blind placebo-controlled study involving 63 patients with herpes zoster (D.W. Levy *et al.*, *J.R. Coll. Physns* , 1985, *19*, 96) found no evidence that cimetidine relieved the pain or accelerated the rate of healing of lesions.

Hypogammaglobulinaemia. The effects of cimetidine on suppressor-cell function in 5 patients with common variable hypogammaglobulinaemia. In 3 patients who exhibited excessive suppressor activity, treatment with cimetidine resulted in a marked reduction of this activity, and in one of these patients intermittent therapy with cimetidine for 18 months resulted in a nearly infection-free state with only one transfusion of normal immunoglobulin being required. In the other 2 patients who had not exhibited suppressor activity cimetidine resulted in no significant change.— W. B. White and M. Ballow, *New Engl. J. Med.*, 1985, *312*, 198. Another report of a beneficial effect in one patient.— A. P. Efremidis *et al.* (letter), *ibid.*, *313*, 265. The effect of cimetidine on cell counts and function in 2 patients positive for HIV infection. Further investigation was needed to clarify whether immunomodulation by cimetidine would have any beneficial effect on the outcome of AIDS.— N. Brockmeyer *et al.* (letter), *ibid.*

Malignant neoplasms. Beneficial results following cimetidine and other drug therapy in some patients with malignant melanoma.— R. D. Thornes *et al.* (letter), *Lancet*, 1982, *2*, 328 (with coumarin); S. Borgström *et al.* (letter), *New Engl. J. Med.*, 1982, *307*, 1080 (with interferon); N. O. Hill *et al.* (letter), *ibid.*, 1983, *308*, 286 (with interferon).

Response in 5 of 7 patients with solid organ malignant neoplasms given cimetidine with histamine.— C. Burtin *et al.* (letter), *New Engl. J. Med.*, 1983, *308*, 591.

Complete clinical remissions in 2 patients with mycosis fungoides (a cutaneous T-cell lymphoma) occurred during treatment with cimetidine; the disease relapsed following withdrawal of cimetidine and improved again following re-introduction.— S. W. Mamus *et al.* (letter), *Lancet*, 1984, *2*, 409. Lack of benefit with cimetidine in 3 patients with mycosis fungoides. The disease progressed in 2 of the patients and did not change remarkably in the third.— W. Sterry *et al.* (letter), *ibid.*, 1985, *1*, 396.

MASTOCYTOSIS. Reports of a beneficial response of symptoms of systemic mastocytosis to cimetidine: D. M. McCarthy, *Gastroenterology*, 1978, *74*, 453 (gastro-intestinal symptoms); B. I. Hirschowitz and J. F. Groarke, *Ann. intern. Med.*, 1979, *90*, 769 (gastro-intestinal symptoms); R. Linde *et al.* (letter), *Ann. intern. Med.*, 1980, *92*, 716 (gastro-intestinal symptoms); R. A. Simon (letter), *New Engl. J. Med.*, 1980, *302*, 231 (urticaria); M. Frieri *et al.*, *Am. J. Med.*, 1985, *78*, 9 (pruritus and urticaria).

MENETRIER'S DISEASE. Beneficial results with cimetidine in a patient with Menetrier's disease (a protein-losing gastropathy) E. Krag *et al.*, *Scand. J. Gastroenterol.*, 1978, *13*, 635.

PANCREATIC DISORDERS. *Cystic fibrosis.* A review of the treatment of pancreatic insufficiency including the use of H_2-antagonists as adjuncts to pancreatic enzyme therapy in patients with cystic fibrosis. H_2-antagonists can increase the response to enzymes but interpatients response is quite variable. The beneficial effects appear to result from an increase in both gastric and duodenal pH with a corresponding decrease in the inactivation of the enzymes. H_2-antagonists may be less effective in patients who secrete large amounts of gastric acid. An improvement in steatorrhoea is most likely if they are administered with high doses of lipase with each meal.— R. S. Perry and J. Gallagher, *Clin. Pharm.*, 1985, *4*, 161.

Some studies on the use of cimetidine in cystic fibrosis: A. S. Ahuja and N. N. Mann (letter), *Archs Dis. Childh.*, 1978, *53*, 766 (reduction of steatorrhoea); K. L. Cox *et al.*, *J. Pediat.*, 1979, *94*, 488 (reduction of steatorrhoea and azotorrhoea); P. L. Zentler-Munro *et al.*, *Gut*, 1985, *26*, 892 (reduction of steatorrhoea).

Pancreatitis. A comment that although much of the secretory function of the pancreas is controlled by secretin, the main stimulus (or possibly only stimulus) of which is hydrochloric acid, and that it would therefore be logical to expect cimetidine to be of value in the treatment of acute pancreatitis; controlled studies have shown that cimetidine is not superior to a placebo.— C. E. Welch and R. A. Malt, *New Engl. J. Med.*, 1983, *308*, 753.

PARACETAMOL TOXICITY. A study to investigate the effect of cimetidine on the metabolic activation of paracetamol in healthy subjects, prompted by the reports of cimetidine in large doses protecting *rodents* against acute paracetamol hepatotoxicity. Cimetidine, by mouth, did not inhibit the conversion of a non-toxic dose of paracetamol to its hepatotoxic metabolite and it was considered that it was most unlikely to do so after an overdose. There was no evidence to support the use of cimetidine for the treatment of paracetamol poisoning in man.— J. A. J. H. Critchley *et al.*, *Lancet*, 1983, *1*, 1375. See also.— *Lancet*, 1985, *2*, 868. Results of a study in healthy subjects showed that ranitidine did not affect the metabolic disposition of paracetamol and would not be expected to affect the toxicity of paracetamol after overdosage.— D. Jack (letter), *ibid.*, 1067.

PEPTIC ULCERS. Many clinical studies have established that the H_2-antagonists cimetidine and ranitidine are both highly effective for the short-term medical management of duodenal ulcer with a large majority (about 80%) of ulcers being healed after a few weeks of therapy. For those patients whose ulcers do not heal initially with cimetidine or ranitidine a change to a different type of anti-ulcer medication is generally suggested rather than increasing the dose or prolonging the duration of treatment with the H_2-antagonist. In accordance, however, with the natural history of the disease, most patients generally relapse after stopping H_2-antagonist therapy and even with maintenance treatment a substantial proportion (about 25%) will also suffer a recurrence; there has also been some suggestion that the relapse-rate may be slightly higher than with other agents, particularly than with colloidal bismuth. A similar overall picture of healing and possible subsequent relapse is seen with gastric ulcers. Cimetidine and ranitidine have accordingly had a considerable impact on the management of peptic ulcers, but the question of whether lifelong maintenance therapy, or possibly a regimen of limited courses of treatment during relapses, is better than surgical management has not yet been totally resolved.
Some references.— J. J. Misiewicz, *Postgrad. med. J.*, 1984, *60*, 751; R. E. Pounder, *Gut*, 1984, *25*, 697; *Lancet*, 1985, *1*, 23; J. P. Miller and E. B. Faragher, *Br. med. J.*, 1986, *293*, 1117.

For the treatment of stress-induced ulceration, see under Stress Ulceration (below).

REFLUX OESOPHAGITIS. A short discussion on the medical therapy for reflux oesophagitis mentioning that large multicentre studies have provided good evidence that both cimetidine and ranitidine will produce significant alleviation of symptoms during 8 weeks of acute therapy but that in some patients even the most intense combination medical therapy will not produce satisfactory improvement.— D. O. Castell, *Ann. intern. Med.*, 1986, *104*, 112.

SKIN DISORDERS. Reports of the use of cimetidine in various skin disorders: C. A. Commens and M. W. Greaves, *Br. J. Derm.*, 1978, *99*, 675 (no benefit in chronic idiopathic urticaria); P. Phanuphak *et al.*, *Clin. Allergy*, 1978, *8*, 429 (some response in chronic idiopathic urticaria); P. Easton and P. R. Galbraith (letter), *New Engl. J. Med.*, 1978, *299*, 1134 (response of pruritus associated with polycythaemia vera); C. E. Hess (letter), *New Engl. J. Med.*, 1979, *300*, 370 (response of pruritus associated with myeloproliferative disorders); A. R. Harrison *et al.* (letter), *New Engl. J. Med.*, 1979, *300*, 433 (no benefit in cholestatic pruritus); G. L. Scott and R. J. Horton (letter), *ibid.*, 434 and 936 (no benefit in pruritus associated with polycythaemia rubra vera); A. R. Zappacosta and D. Hauss (letter), *ibid.*, 1280 (no benefit in pruritus associated with chronic renal failure); D. V. Schapira and J. M. Bennett (letter), *Lancet*, 1979, *1*, 726 (response of pruritus associated with a myelodysplastic disorder); J. P. Aymard *et al.*, *Br. med. J.*, 1980, *280*, 151 (response of pruritus associated with Hodgkin's disease); H. B. Kaiser *et al.* (letter), *Lancet*, 1980, *2*, 206 (some response in chronic urticaria); J. Boyle and R. M. MacKie, *Br. J. Derm.*, 1982, *107*, *Suppl.* 22, 18 (response of chronic urticaria with dermographism); P. H. Deutsch (letter), *Ann. intern. Med.*, 1984, *101*, 569 (response of pruritus with dermographism).

See also under Immunological Disorders (above).

STRESS ULCERATION. A discussion and review of stress ulceration in the critically ill patient. A large proportion of critically ill patients develop acute upper gastro-intestinal lesions of variable severity; although extremely common and deserving of the term stress ulceration, the clinical significance of these lesions, unless complicated by bleeding, remains uncertain. The likelihood of bleeding or perforation from stress ulceration is increased by a number of risk factors which include sepsis, multiple trauma, fulminant hepatic failure or severe hepatic dysfunction, respiratory failure, severe burns, head injury, and renal failure. Current strategies for the prophylaxis of haemorrhagic stress ulceration rely mainly on the administration of either an antacid or an H_2-antagonist or both on the assumption that a reduction of gastric acidity will result in a reduction in the incidence of bleeding. Although there is evidence to support this thesis in selected groups, there is no evidence that the use of antacids or H_2-antagonists improve the overall survival of critically ill patients. Nevertheless, it is the authors' practice to treat patients having 2 or more risk factors with an H_2-antagonist, ranitidine being chosen.— A. Knight *et al.*, *Br. J. Hosp. Med.*, 1985, *33*, 216. Comments and correspondence regarding the choice of ranitidine rather than cimetidine.— D. A. Boyko and D. Rowley-Jones (letter), *ibid.*, *34*, 186; D. Bihari and A. Knight (letter), *ibid.*,; D. A. Boyko and D. Rowley-Jones (letter), *ibid.*, 1986, *35*, 205.

A statistical combined re-evaluation of 16 prospective randomised studies that had investigated the use of cimetidine or antacid for the prophylaxis of stress-ulcer bleeding; 2133 patients had been involved in all. The analysis indicated that cimetidine and antacid were equally effective for the prevention of overt bleeding and that both were superior to placebo. Thus, the choice would depend on such factors as cost, ease of administration, and side-effects.— R. B. Shuman *et al.*, *Ann. intern. Med.*, 1987, *106*, 562.

ZOLLINGER-ELLISON SYNDROME. A review of the management of the Zollinger-Ellison syndrome. Most patients can be started with cimetidine or ranitidine by mouth but a few patients presenting with severe electrolyte or metabolic abnormalities and complications of the ulcer disease will require appropriate fluid and electrolyte replacement, nasogastric suction, and H_2-antagonists by continuous intravenous infusion initially. For long-term treatment either cimetidine or ranitidine by mouth, alone or with an antimuscarinic agent, should be used; antacids, even in large amounts, are ineffective. In sufficient doses, cimetidine or ranitidine will control gastric hypersecretion in almost every patient with the Zollinger-Ellison syndrome. In most patients with a gastrinoma larger doses than those used in the routine treatment of duodenal ulcer will be required and in recent studies the median doses needed were 3 to 5 g daily of cimetidine or 1 to 1.5 g daily of ranitidine. Some patients with gastrinoma have been treated for more than one year with doses of up to 12 g daily of cimetidine or 6 g daily of ranitidine without evidence of dose-related hepatic, renal, or CNS toxicity. The continued efficacy of antisecretory control should be checked every 6 to 12 months in asymptomatic patients or at any time if symptoms develop and persist for more than one week.— R. T. Jensen *et al.*, *Drugs*, 1986, *32*, 188. See also.— R. T. Jensen *et al.*, *Ann. intern. Med.*, 1983, *98*, 59.

Preparations

Cimetidine Tablets *(U.S.P.)*

Proprietary Preparations

Dyspamet *(Smith Kline & French, UK)*. *Tablets*, chewable, cimetidine 200 mg.
Suspension, cimetidine 200 mg/5 mL.

Tagamet *(Smith Kline & French, UK)*. *Tablets*, cimetidine 200, 400, and 800 mg.
Syrup, cimetidine 200 mg/5 mL.
Injection, cimetidine 100 mg/mL, in ampoules of 2 mL.
Intravenous infusion, cimetidine 4 mg/mL in sodium chloride 0.9%, in infusion bags of 100 mL.

Proprietary Names and Manufacturers

Acibilin *(Arg.)*; Aciloc *(Orion, Swed.)*; Acinil *(GEA, Denm.*; *Tricum, Swed.)*; Brumetidina *(Bruschettini, Ital.)*; Cimal *(Apothekernes Laboratorium, Norw.*; *A.L., Swed.)*; Cimetid *(Nyco, Norw.)*; Cimetin *(Ital.)*; Cimetum *(Arg.)*; Cinulcus *(Wasserman, Spain)*; Citimid *(CT, Ital.)*; Citius *(High Noon, Pakistan*; *Berenguer-Beneyto, Spain)*; Dina *(San Carlo, Ital.)*; Duogastril *(Hosbon, Spain)*; Duractin *(Commonwealth Serum Laboratories, Austral.)*; Dyspamet *(Smith Kline & French, UK)*; Edalene *(Pharmuka, Fr.)*; Eureceptor *(Zambon, Ital.)*; Fremet *(Antibioticos, Spain)*; Gastro H2 *(Lesvi, Spain)*; Gastrobitan *(GEA, Norw.)*; Gastromet *(Sigurtà, Ital.)*; Itacem *(Ital.)*; Mansal *(Vita, Spain)*; Notul *(Dox-Al, Ital.)*; Novocimetine *(Novopharm, Canad.)*; Peptol *(Horner, Canad.)*; Tagagel *(Smith Kline Dauelsberg, Ger.)*; Tagamet *(Arg.*; *Smith Kline & French, Austral.*; *Belg.*; *Smith Kline & French, Canad.*; *Smith Kline & French, Denm.*; *Smith Kline & French, Fr.*; *Smith Kline Dauelsberg, Ger.*; *Smith Kline & French, Ital.*; *Neth.*; *Smith Kline & French, Norw.*; *NZ*; *Smith Kline & French, S.Afr.*; *Smith Kline & French, Spain*; *SK & F, Swed.*; *Smith Kline & French, Switz.*; *Smith Kline & French, UK*; *Smith Kline & French, USA)*; Tametin *(Gipharmex, Ital.)*; Temic *(Aandersen, Ital.)*; Ulcedin *(AGIPS, Ital.)*; Ulcerfen *(Arg.)*; Ulcestop *(Gibipharma, Ital.)*; Ulcimet *(Arg.)*; Ulcodina *(Locatelli, Ital.)*; Ulcomedina *(Von Boch, Ital.)*; Ulcomet *(Italfarmaco, Ital.)*; Ulhys *(Lafare, Ital.)*; Vagolisal *(Janus, Ital.)*; Valmagen *(UCM-Difme, Ital.)*.

16581-d

Cisapride *(BAN, USAN, rINN)*.

R-51619. *cis*-4-Amino-5-chloro-*N*-{1-[3-(4-fluorophenoxy)propyl]-3-methoxy-4-piperidyl}-2-methoxybenzamide.
$C_{23}H_{29}ClFN_3O_4$=466.0.

CAS — 81098-60-4.

Cisapride stimulates gastro-intestinal motility and is reported to be devoid of antidopaminergic activity. It is being investigated in a variety of gastro-intestinal disorders.

Reports of a beneficial response to cisapride in varying disorders: G. Reboa *et al.*, *Eur. J. clin. Pharmac.*, 1984, *26*, 745 (chronic constipation); R. Jian *et al.*, *Gut*, 1985, *26*, 352 (chronic dyspepsia); J. E. Prinsen and M. Thomas (letter), *Lancet*, 1985, *1*, 512 (improvement of stool characteristics in patients with cystic fibrosis); J. W. L. Puntis *et al.* (letter), *ibid.*, 1986, *2*, 108 (pseudo-obstruction in neonatal short gut); P. T. Cullen and F. C. Campbell (letter), *ibid.*, 1987, *1*, 47 (severe postoperative gastroparesis); D. J. Rowbotham and W. S. Nimmo, *Br. J. Anaesth.*, 1987, *59*, 536 (possible prevention of aspiration syndrome); S. Cucchiara *et al.*, *Archs Dis. Childh.*, 1987, *62*, 454 (reflux oesophagitis in children).

Proprietary Names and Manufacturers

Janssen, Belg.

16583-h

Clebopride *(rINN)*.

4-Amino-*N*-(1-benzyl-4-piperidyl)-5-chloro-*o*-anisamide.
$C_{20}H_{24}ClN_3O_2$=373.9.

CAS — 55905-53-8.

Clebopride is a substituted benzamide which is used similarly to metoclopramide in the treatment of nausea and vomiting. It has also been used in a wide range of gastro-intestinal disorders. Usual doses consist of 500 μg three times daily. The malate has also been used.

Extensive metabolism of clebopride given by mouth to one healthy subject.— J. Segura *et al.*, *Drug Metab. & Disposit.*, 1980, *8*, 87.

References to the uses of clebopride: E. Murillo Capitan and J. A. Sánchez Romero, *Curr. ther. Res.*, 1982, *31*, *Suppl.* 1S, S61 (nausea and vomiting due to cancer chemotherapy); H. Pardell *et al.*, *ibid.*, S74 (vomiting and abdominal pain in patients with irritable bowel syndrome); E. Rodríguez Sánchez *et al.*, *ibid.*, S80 (radiological exploration); D. F. Duarte *et al.*, *Clin. Ther.*, 1985, *7*, 365 (postoperative nausea and vomiting); L. Bavestrello *et al.*, *ibid.*, 468 (dyspepsia secondary to delayed gastric emptying); C. Alegre *et al.*, *Curr. ther. Res.*, 1985, *37*, 289 (dyspeptic symptoms associated with non-steroidal anti-inflammatory agents).

Proprietary Names and Manufacturers of Clebopride or Clebopride Malate

Clanzol *(Orfi, Spain)*; Cleboril *(Almirall, Spain)*; Clebutec *(Boehringer Ingelheim, Port.)*; Cleprid *(Recordati, Ital.)*; Motilex *(Guidotti, Ital.)*; Vuxolin *(Farmitalia, Spain)*.

12581-j

Clocanfamide *(rINN)*.

4-Chloro-*N*-(2-hydroxyethyl)-*N*-(3-methyl-8,9,10-trinorborn-2-ylmethyl)benzamide.
$C_{18}H_{24}ClNO_2$=321.8.

CAS — 18966-32-0.

Clocanfamide is used in the treatment of peptic ulcer in doses of up to 525 mg daily.

Proprietary Names and Manufacturers

Clamiren *(Zilliken, Ital.)*.

7508-g

Colocynth

Bitter Apple; Colocynth Pulp; Colocynthis; Coloquinte; Coloquintidas; Koloquinthen.

NOTE. The synonym Bitter Apple has also been applied to the fruits of *Solanum incanum*.

Pharmacopoeias. In *Egypt.* and *Port.*

The dried pulp of the fruit of *Citrullus colocynthis* (Cucurbitaceae).

Colocynth has a drastic purgative and irritant action. It has been superseded by less toxic laxatives.

7509-q

Croton Oil

Oleum Crotonis; Oleum Tiglii.

CAS — 8001-28-3.

Pharmacopoeias. In *Arg.*, *Port.*, and *Span.* *Chin.* includes fruits of *Croton tiglium*.

An oil expressed from the seeds of *Croton tiglium* (Euphorbiaceae). It is an amber-yellow, orange, or brown, viscous liquid with a nauseous odour.

Practically **insoluble** in water; soluble 1 in less than 1 of dehydrated alcohol; freely soluble in carbon disulphide, chloroform, ether, light petroleum, and fixed and volatile oils.

Croton oil has such a violent purgative action that it should not now be employed. Externally, it is a powerful counter-irritant and vesicant.

The possible mechanism of action of tumour promoters such as the phorbol diesters found in croton oil is discussed.— I. B. Weinstein and M. Wigler, *Nature*, 1977, *270*, 659.

7510-d

Danthron *(BAN, USAN)*.

Antrapurol; Chrysazin; Dantron *(rINN)*; Dianthon; Dioxyanthrachinonum. 1,8-Dihydroxyanthraquinone.
$C_{14}H_8O_4$=240.2.

CAS — 117-10-2.

NOTE. Compounded preparations of danthron and poloxamer 188 in the mass proportions 1 part to 8 parts have the British Approved Name Co-danthramer and in the mass proportions 3 parts to 40 parts have the British Approved Name Strong Co-danthramer. Compounded preparations of danthron and docusate sodium in the mass proportions 5 parts to 6 parts have the British Approved Name Co-danthrusate.

Pharmacopoeias. In *Aust., Br., Neth., Pol.,* and *U.S.* Also in *B.P. Vet.*

An orange, odourless or almost odourless, crystalline powder.

Practically **insoluble** in water; very slightly soluble in alcohol; soluble in chloroform; slightly soluble in ether; soluble in hot glacial acetic acid; dissolves in solutions of alkali hydroxides.

Adverse Effects and Precautions

As for Senna, p.1106. Danthron may colour the perianal skin pink or red as well as colour the urine. Superficial sloughing of discoloured skin may occur in incontinent patients or children wearing napkins; danthron should not be used in such patients. The mucosa of the large intestine may be discoloured with prolonged use or high dosage.

Some studies have suggested that chronic administration of very high doses of danthron to *rats* and *mice* may be associated with the development of intestinal and liver tumours.

Leucopenia and liver damage with deposits of IgE were reported in a 24-year-old woman taking a preparation containing danthron with docusate calcium for the treatment of chronic constipation. Neither drug alone caused changes in serum concentrations of bilirubin, alkaline phosphatase, or SGOT, but rechallenge with the combination of the 2 drugs produced elevation of alkaline phosphatase and return of leucopenia.— K. G. Tolman *et al., Ann. intern. Med.,* 1976, *84,* 290.

Greyish-blue discoloration of the skin in a 51-year-old nurse appeared to be associated with the danthron content of Dorbanex.— C. S. Darke and R. G. Cooper, *Br. med. J.,* 1978, *1,* 1188.

Orange vaginal secretions in a woman taking large amounts of a laxative containing danthron.— I. A. Greer (letter), *Br. med. J.,* 1984, *289,* 323.

For a report of melanosis coli following abuse of preparations of senna and of danthron with poloxamer 188, see under Senna, p.1106.

Absorption and Fate

Danthron is absorbed from the small intestine to some extent. It is excreted in the faeces and the urine, and also in other secretions including milk.

Uses and Administration

Danthron is an anthraquinone laxative which is effective within 6 to 12 hours. It is used to treat constipation and also for bowel evacuation prior to investigational procedures or surgery. It is often administered as co-danthrusate (danthron and docusate sodium) and was formerly given as co-danthramer (danthron and poloxamer 188). Danthron is given in usual doses of 25 to 150 mg by mouth at bedtime; children aged 6 to 12 years have been given one-half the adult dose.

The view that the addition of surfactants to danthron preparations is both unnecessary and hazardous. Mixtures of danthron with docusate sodium have been reported to be hepatotoxic.— E. W. Godding, *Pharm. J.,* 1984, *1,* 168.

Preparations

Danthron Tablets *(U.S.P.)*

Proprietary Preparations

Normax *(Bencard, UK). Capsules,* co-danthrusate 110 mg (danthron 50 mg, docusate sodium 60 mg). *Dose.* 1 to 3 capsules at bedtime.

Proprietary Names and Manufacturers

Bancon *(Ital.)*; Dorbane *(Riker, Canad.; 3M, USA)*; Duolax *(USA)*; Fructines-Vichy *(Sidel, Fr.)*; Istizin *(Neth.)*; Modane *(Adria, Canad.)*; Roydan *(Roy, Canad.)*.

The following names have been used for multi-ingredient preparations containing danthron—Agarol Capsules *(Parke, Davis, Canad.)*; Coloxyl with Danthron Tablets *(Fawns & McAllan, Austral.)*; Dorbanate Liquid *(Riker, Austral.)*; Dorbanate Tablets *(Riker, Austral.)*; Dorbanex *(Riker, Canad.; Swed.; Riker, UK)*; Dorbantyl *(Riker, Canad.)*; Doss *(Beecham, Canad.)*; Doxidan *(Hoechst, Canad.; Hoechst, USA)*; Normax *(Bencard, UK)*.

6220-v

Difenoxin Hydrochloride *(BANM, rINNM).*

Difenoxylic Acid Hydrochloride; R-15403. 1-(3-Cyano-3,3-diphenylpropyl)-4-phenylpiperidine-4-carboxylic acid hydrochloride.

$C_{28}H_{28}N_2O_2,HCl=461.0.$

CAS — 28782-42-5 (difenoxin); 35607-36-4 (hydrochloride).

NOTE. Difenoxin is *USAN.*

Difenoxin is the principal metabolite of diphenoxylate (see p.1087). Difenoxin hydrochloride, in conjunction with subclinical amounts of atropine sulphate, is used similarly to diphenoxylate, in the symptomatic treatment of diarrhoea. The usual initial dose for acute diarrhoea is 1 mg three times daily, subsequently adjusted as necessary; a total daily dose of 6 mg should not be exceeded.

It should be noted that a consequence of diarrhoea may be fluid and electrolyte depletion, and that rehydration therapy may be necessary, especially in infants and young children. For further details concerning rehydration therapy, see p.1024.

Proprietary Names and Manufacturers

The following names have been used for multi-ingredient preparations containing difenoxin hydrochloride—Lyspafen *(Protea, Austral.; Fisons, S.Afr.; Cilag, Switz.)*; Motofen *(McNeil Pharmaceutical, USA)*.

689-k

Dihydroxyaluminum Sodium Carbonate *(USAN).*

Aluminium Sodium Carbonate Hydroxide; Dihydroxyaluminium Sodium Carbonate. Sodium (carbonato)dihydroxyaluminate(1-).

$CH_2AlNaO_5=144.0.$

CAS — 12011-77-7; 16482-55-6; 539-68-4.

Pharmacopoeias. In *Nord.* and *U.S.*

A fine white odourless powder. It loses not more than 14.5% of its weight on drying. Practically **insoluble** in water and organic solvents; soluble in dilute mineral acids with the evolution of carbon dioxide. A 4% suspension in water has a pH of 9.9 to 10.2. **Store** in airtight containers.

Dihydroxyaluminum sodium carbonate is an antacid that is given in doses of about 300 to 600 mg.

Preparations

Dihydroxyaluminum Sodium Carbonate Tablets *(U.S.P.).* The tablets should be chewed before swallowing.

Proprietary Names and Manufacturers

Kompensan *(Pfizer, Ger.; Pfizer, Switz.)*; Minicid *(Pharmacia, Norw.; Pharmacia, Swed.)*; Noacid *(Pharmacia, Denm.; Pfizer, Spain)*.

6543-n

Diphenidol Hydrochloride *(BANM, USAN).*

Difenidol Hydrochloride *(pINNM)*; SKF-478. 1,1-Diphenyl-4-piperidinobutan-1-ol hydrochloride.

$C_{21}H_{27}NO,HCl=345.9.$

CAS — 972-02-1 (diphenidol); 3254-89-5 (hydrochloride); 26363-46-2 (embonate).

Adverse Effects

Adverse effects of diphenidol hydrochloride include auditory and visual hallucinations, disorientation, and confusion. Drowsiness, restlessness, depression and antimuscarinic effects may occur. Transient hypotension, headache, and skin rashes have occasionally been reported.

Precautions

Due to the risk of confusional states diphenidol should only be given to patients under close supervision. It is contra-indicated in renal failure and because of weak antimuscarinic activity it should be used cautiously in patients with glaucoma, obstructive lesions of the gastro-intestinal or genito-urinary tracts, or sinus tachycardia.

Absorption and Fate

Diphenidol is absorbed from the gastro-intestinal tract and peak blood concentrations are obtained in 1½ to 3 hours. It is excreted primarily in the urine.

Uses and Administration

Diphenidol hydrochloride is an anti-emetic agent which probably acts through the chemoreceptor trigger zone. It is claimed to control vertigo by means of a specific effect on the vestibular apparatus. Diphenidol also has a weak peripheral antimuscarinic action.

It is used for the symptomatic treatment of vertigo, nausea and vomiting due to Ménière's disease and other labyrinthine disturbances, radiation sickness, and postoperative vomiting.

The usual dose is the equivalent of 25 mg of diphenidol by mouth every 4 hours; doses of 50 mg every 4 hours may sometimes be required.

Proprietary Names and Manufacturers

Ansmin *(Jpn)*; Antiul *(Jpn)*; Avomol *(Landerlan, Spain)*; Cephadol *(Jpn)*; Cerrosa *(Jpn)*; Deanosarl *(Jpn)*; Difenidolin *(Jpn)*; Maniol *(Jpn)*; Mecalmin *(Jpn)*; Meniedolin *(Jpn)*; Meranom *(Jpn)*; Midnighton *(Jpn)*; Pineroro *(Jpn)*; Satanolon *(Jpn)*; Solnomin *(Jpn)*; Tenesdol *(Jpn)*; Verterge *(Jpn)*; Vontril *(Smith Kline & French, Austral.)*; Vontrol *(Smith Kline & French, Arg.; Smith Kline & French, Canad.; Smith Kline & French, S.Afr.; Smith Kline & French, USA)*; Wansar *(Jpn)*; Yesdol *(Jpn)*; Yophadol *(Jpn)*.

6223-p

Diphenoxylate Hydrochloride *(BANM, USAN, rINNM).*

R-1132. Ethyl 1-(3-cyano-3,3-diphenylpropyl)-4-phenylpiperidine-4-carboxylate hydrochloride.

$C_{30}H_{32}N_2O_2,HCl=489.1.$

CAS — 915-30-0 (diphenoxylate); 3810-80-8 (hydrochloride).

Pharmacopoeias. In *Br., Braz., Ind.,* and *U.S.*

A white or almost white odourless or almost odourless crystalline powder. Slightly to sparingly **soluble** in water; soluble 1 in 50 of alcohol, 1 in 40 of acetone, and 1 in 2.5 of chloroform; soluble in methyl alcohol; practically insoluble in ether and light petroleum; slightly soluble in isopropyl alcohol. A saturated solution in water has a pH of about 3.3.

Dependence

Short-term administration of diphenoxylate with atropine in the recommended dosage carries a negligible risk of dependence, although prolonged use or use of high doses may produce dependence of the morphine type (see p.1310).

Adverse Effects

Reported side-effects include anorexia, nausea and vomiting, abdominal distention, paralytic ileus, toxic megacolon, headache, drowsiness, insomnia, dizziness, restlessness, euphoria, depression, numbness of the extremities, and allergic reactions including angioedema, urticaria, pruritus, and swelling of the gums.

After overdosage, symptoms are similar to those of morphine poisoning (see p.1311). Young children are particularly susceptible to the effects of overdosage.

The presence of subclinical doses of atropine sulphate in preparations containing diphenoxylate may give rise to the side-effects of atropine in susceptible individuals or in overdosage—see Atropine Sulphate, p.523.

Acute pancreatitis occurred in a patient, on two occasions, 3 hours after taking diphenoxylate with atropine (Lomotil) for attacks of diarrhoea.— P. A. McCormick *et al.* (letter), *Lancet*, 1985, *1*, 752.

Treatment of Adverse Effects

As for Morphine, p.1311.

Patients should be observed for at least 48 hours after overdosage.

Precautions

Diphenoxylate should be used with caution in patients with hepatic dysfunction. It should also be used with caution in young children because of a greater variability of response in such an age group, and is not generally recommended for use in infants. Patients with inflammatory bowel disease receiving diphenoxylate should be carefully observed for signs of toxic megacolon. It has been recommended that diphenoxylate should not be used for the treatment of diarrhoea associated with antibiotic-induced pseudomembranous entero-colitis.

Diphenoxylate may potentiate the effects of other CNS depressants, such as alcohol, barbiturates, and some tranquillisers, and because of its structural relationship to pethidine a theoretical risk of an interaction with monoamine oxidase inhibitors exists.

Absorption and Fate

Diphenoxylate is well absorbed from the gastro-intestinal tract and extensively metabolised in the liver to diphenoxylic acid (difenoxin, see p.1087) and hydroxydiphenoxylic acid. It is excreted mainly as metabolites in the urine and bile; it may also be excreted in breast milk.

Uses and Administration

Diphenoxylate hydrochloride is a derivative of pethidine but has no analgesic activity. It reduces intestinal motility and is used in the symptomatic treatment of acute and chronic diarrhoea. It is also used to reduce the frequency and fluidity of the stools in patients with colostomies or ileostomies.

The usual initial dose for adults is 5 mg four times daily, later reduced when the diarrhoea is controlled. Suggested doses for children have been: 4 to 8 years, 2.5 mg three times daily; 9 to 12 years, 2.5 mg four times daily; over 12 years, 5 mg three times daily. Diphenoxylate is not generally recommended for use in infants under the age of 4 years.

If no improvement in acute diarrhoea has been observed after 48 hours, diphenoxylate should be discontinued. It has been stated that if clinical improvement of chronic diarrhoea is not observed after 10 days' treatment with the maximum daily dose of 20 mg (in adults) further administration is unlikely to result in any benefit.

It should be noted that a consequence of diarrhoea may be fluid and electrolyte depletion, and that rehydration therapy may be necessary, especially in infants and young children. For further details concerning rehydration therapy, see p.1024.

Preparations of diphenoxylate usually contain subclinical amounts of atropine sulphate in an attempt to prevent abuse by deliberate overdosage.

OPIOID DEPENDENCE AND WITHDRAWAL. References to diphenoxylate being used in the management of opioid dependence and withdrawal syndromes: M. M. Glatt, *Br. med. J.*, 1971, *3*, 105 (diamorphine and other opioids); M. H. Kleinman and D. Arnon, *Br. J. Addict.*, 1977, *72*, 167 (methadone); T. J. Ives and C. C. Stults, *Br. J. Psychiat.*, 1983, *143*, 513 (methadone).

Preparations

Diphenoxylate Hydrochloride and Atropine Sulfate Oral Solution *(U.S.P.)*. Store in airtight containers. Protect from light.

Diphenoxylate Hydrochloride and Atropine Sulfate Tablets *(U.S.P.)*. Protect from light.

Proprietary Preparations

Lomotil *(Gold Cross, UK)*. *Tablets*, diphenoxylate hydrochloride 2.5 mg, atropine sulphate 25 µg. *Liquid*, diphenoxylate hydrochloride 2.5 mg, atropine sulphate 25 µg/5mL.

Proprietary Names and Manufacturers

Lomotil *(Searle, Canad.)*.

The following names have been used for multi-ingredient preparations containing diphenoxylate hydrochloride—Diarsed *(Fr.)*; Di-Atro *(Legere, USA)*; Lomotil *(Searle, Austral.; S.Afr.; Gold Cross, UK; Searle, USA)*; Lomotil with Neomycin *(Searle, UK)*; Lonox *(Geneva, USA)*; Reasec *(Janssen, Austral.; Ital.; Switz.; Janssen, UK)*; Retardin *(Denm.; Norw.; Swed.)*; SK-Diphenoxylate *(Smith Kline & French, USA)*.

6018-m

Docusate Calcium *(USAN)*.

Dioctyl Calcium Sulfosuccinate; Dioctyl Calcium Sulphosuccinate. Calcium 1,4-bis(2-ethylhexyl) sulphosuccinate.

$C_{40}H_{74}CaO_{14}S_2$=883.2.

CAS — 128-49-4.

Pharmacopoeias. In *U.S.*

A white amorphous solid with the characteristic odour of octyl alcohol. **Soluble** 1 in 3300 of water and 1 in more than 1 of alcohol, chloroform, and ether; very soluble in macrogol 400 and maize oil.

6019-b

Docusate Potassium *(USAN)*.

Dioctyl Potassium Sulfosuccinate; Dioctyl Potassium Sulphosuccinate. Potassium 1,4-bis(2-ethylhexyl) sulphosuccinate.

$C_{20}H_{37}KO_7S$=460.7.

CAS — 7491-09-0.

Pharmacopoeias. In *U.S.*

A white amorphous solid with a characteristic odour suggestive of octyl alcohol. Sparingly **soluble** in water; soluble in alcohol and glycerol; very soluble in light petroleum.

6020-x

Docusate Sodium *(BAN, USAN, rINN)*.

Dioctyl Sodium Sulfosuccinate; Dioctyl Sodium Sulphosuccinate; DSS; Sodium Dioctyl Sulphosuccinate. Sodium 1,4-bis(2-ethylhexyl) sulphosuccinate.

$C_{20}H_{37}NaO_7S$=444.6.

CAS — 577-11-7.

NOTE. Compounded preparations of docusate sodium and danthron in the mass proportions 6 parts to 5 parts have the British Approved Name Co-danthrusate.

Pharmacopoeias. In *Arg., Br.* , and *U.S.*

White or almost white hygroscopic waxy masses or flakes with a characteristic odour suggestive of octyl alcohol.

Slowly **soluble** 1 in 70 of water, higher concentrations forming a thick gel; soluble 1 in 3 of alcohol, 1 in 1 of chloroform, and 1 in 1 of ether; very soluble in light petroleum; freely soluble in glycerol. **Store** in well-closed containers.

Adverse Effects and Precautions

Like all laxatives, docusate should not be administered when intestinal obstruction, abdominal pain, nausea or vomiting is present.

Docusate may also facilitate gastro-intestinal absorption or hepatic cell uptake of other drugs, thereby enhancing their activity and possibly increasing their toxicity; it should not be used with liquid paraffin.

For a report of leucopenia and liver damage occurring in a patient taking docusate calcium with danthron for chronic constipation, see Danthron, p.1087.

PREGNANCY AND THE NEONATE. A comment that docusate sodium taken by a nursing mother may cause increased bowel activity in the breast-fed infant.— J. M. Forrest, *Med. J. Aust.*, 1976, *2*, 138.

Hypomagnesaemia, manifested by jitteriness, in a neonate was considered to be secondary to maternal hypomagnesaemia caused by the use of docusate sodium by the mother during pregnancy.— A. M. Schindler (letter), *Lancet*, 1984, *2*, 822.

Absorption and Fate

Docusate sodium is absorbed from the gastro-intestinal tract; there is significant biliary excretion.

Uses and Administration

Docusate, in the calcium, potassium, or sodium form is used as a faecal softening agent in the management of constipation. They are anionic surfactants which are considered to act by stimulating intestinal secretions and by increasing the penetration of fluid into the faeces. The effect is usually seen within 1 to 3 days. The usual daily dose by mouth of docusate as one of the above salts is up to 300 mg given in divided doses although docusate sodium has been given in doses of up to 500 mg daily. Suggested doses for children have been up to 150 mg daily. Docusate sodium is also given rectally as an enema in doses of 50 to 100 mg.

Docusate sodium is also used for softening wax in the ear.

Studies on the mechanism of action of docusate sodium in the human jejunum.— K. J. Moriarty *et al.*, *Gut*, 1985, *26*, 1008.

Preparations

Docusate Calcium Capsules *(U.S.P.)*. Store at 15° to 30° in airtight containers.

Docusate Potassium Capsules *(U.S.P.)*. Store at 15° to 30° in airtight containers.

Docusate Sodium Capsules *(U.S.P.)*. Store at 15° to 30° in airtight containers.

Docusate Sodium Solution *(U.S.P.)*. pH 4.5 to 6.9. Store in airtight containers.

Docusate Sodium Syrup *(U.S.P.)*. pH 5.5 to 6.5. Store in airtight containers. Protect from light.

Docusate Tablets *(B.P.)*. Docusate Sodium Tablets; Dioctyl Sodium Sulphosuccinate Tablets

Docusate Sodium Tablets *(U.S.P.)*

Proprietary Preparations

Audinorm *(Carlton Laboratories, UK)*. *Ear-drops*, docusate sodium 5%, glycerol 10%.

Dioctyl *(Medo, UK)*. *Tablets*, docusate sodium 100 mg. *Syrup*, docusate sodium 50 mg/5 mL. *Paediatric Syrup*, docusate sodium 12.5 mg/5 mL.

Dioctyl Ear-drops *(Medo, UK)*. *Ear-drops*, docusate sodium 5%.

Fletchers' Enemette *(Pharmax, UK)*. *Enema*, docusate sodium 90 mg/5 mL in single-dose containers of 5 mL.

Molcer *(Wallace Mfg Chem., UK)*. *Ear-drops*, docusate sodium 5%.

Soliwax *(Martindale Pharmaceuticals, UK)*. *Ear-capsules*, docusate sodium 5%. *Administration:* the contents of a capsule to be expressed into the ear.

Waxsol *(Norgine, UK)*. *Ear-drops*, docusate sodium 0.5%.

Proprietary Names and Manufacturers of Docusates

Adjust *(Jpn)*; Aerosol OT *(Cyanamid, UK)*; Afko-Lube *(USA)*; Audinorm *(Carlton Laboratories, UK)*; Bu-Lax *(USA)*; Colace *(Bristol, Canad.; Mead Johnson Pharmaceutical, USA)*; Coloxyl Enema *(Fawns & McAllan, Austral.)*; Coloxyl Tablets *(Fawns & McAllan, Austral.)*; Comfolax *(Searle, USA)*; Constiban *(Canad.)*; Dialose *(Stuart Pharmaceuticals, USA)*; Dilax *(Mission Pharmacal, USA)*; Doctocal *(Schein, USA)*; Dioctyl *(Medo, UK)*; Dioctyl Forte *(Belg.)*; DioMedicone *(Medicone, USA)*; Disonate *(Lannett, USA)*; Doxinate *(Hoechst, USA)*; D-S-S *(Parke, Davis, USA)*; Ediclone *(Synlab, Fr.)*; Emcol *(Witco, UK)*; Fletchers' Enemette *(Pharmax, UK)*; Kasof *(Stuart Pharmaceuticals, USA)*; Laxagel *(Everest, Canad.)*; Modane Soft *(Adria, USA)*; Molcer *(Wallace Mfg Chem., UK)*; Mollax *(Dumex, Denm.)*; Norgalax *(Norgan, Fr.)*; Rapilax *(Belg.)*; Rectalad Enema *(Carter-Wallace, Austral.; Wallace, USA)*; Regulex *(Ayerst, Canad.)*; Soliwax *(Martindale Phar-*

maceuticals, UK); Surfak (Hoechst, Canad.; Hoechst, USA); Tirolaxo (Ale, Spain); Wasserlax (Wasserman, Spain); Waxsol (Norgine, Austral.; Camden, S.Afr.; Norgine, UK).

The following names have been used for multi-ingredient preparations containing docusates—Acidobyl (Desbergers, Canad.); Agarol Capsules (Parke, Davis, Canad.); Bilax (Drug Industries, USA); Coloxyl Suppositories (Fawns & McAllan, Austral.); Coloxyl with Danthron Tablets (Fawns & McAllan, Austral.); Comfolax-plus (Searle, USA); Dialose Plus (Stuart Pharmaceuticals, USA); Dorbantyl (Riker, Canad.); Doss (Beecham, Canad.); Doxidan (Hoechst, Canad.; Hoechst, USA); D-S-S Plus (Parke, Davis, USA); Dulcodos (Boehringer Ingelheim, Canad.; Boehringer Ingelheim, UK); Klyx (Ferring, UK); Liqui-Doss (Ferndale, USA); Modane Plus (Adria, USA); Neolax (Central Pharmaceuticals, USA); Normax (Bencard, UK); Peri-Colace (Bristol, Canad.; Mead Johnson Pharmaceutical, USA); Phillips' Laxcaps (Glenbrook, USA); Sarolax (Saron, USA); Senokot-S (Purdue Frederick, Canad.; Purdue Frederick, USA); Trilax (Drug Industries, USA).

6544-h

Domperidone (BAN, USAN, rINN).

R-33812. 5-Chloro-1-{1-[3-(2-oxobenzimidazolin-1-yl)propyl]-4-piperidyl}benzimidazolin-2-one.

$C_{22}H_{24}ClN_5O_2$=425.9.

CAS — 57808-66-9.

Adverse Effects

Domperidone is less likely than metoclopramide to produce central effects such as extrapyramidal reactions or drowsiness, but there have been a few reports of dystonic reactions. Plasma-prolactin concentrations may also be increased which may lead to galactorrhoea or gynaecomastia.

Domperidone by injection has been associated with arrhythmias in patients with cardiac disease or hypokalaemia and in those receiving cancer chemotherapy. Fatalities have restricted administration by this route.

EFFECTS ON THE CARDIOVASCULAR SYSTEM. Sudden death has occurred in cancer patients given domperidone intravenously in doses that have been considered to be too high or administered too rapidly (R.A. Joss *et al.*, *Lancet*, 1982, *1*, 1019; G. Giaccone *et al.*, *ibid.*, 1984, *2*, 1336; A. Weaving *et al.*, *Br. med. J.*, 1984, *288*, 1728). Four cancer patients experienced cardiac arrest following high intravenous doses (J.B. Roussak *et al.*, *Br. med. J.*, 1984, *289*, 1579) and 2 of 4 similar patients experienced ventricular arrhythmias (R.J. Osbourne *et al.*, *Lancet*, 1985, *2*, 385). The manufacturers discontinued the injection in the UK but for a time supplied ampoules for use in named patients (*Pharm. J.*, 1985, *1*, 508).

EFFECTS ON THE ENDOCRINE SYSTEM. A report of gynaecomastia and galactorrhoea together with increased serum concentrations of prolactin in a male infant given domperidone 600 µg per kg body-weight three times daily for 5 days. The symptoms disappeared and serum-prolactin concentrations returned to normal within a week of discontinuation of domperidone.— M. Van der Steen *et al.* (letter), *Lancet*, 1982, *2*, 884.

Five of 30 patients experienced mastalgia and galactorrhoea and 2 mastalgia alone while taking domperidone 20 mg four times daily. Serum-prolactin concentrations were abnormally high in 15 of the 18 patients in whom it was measured; 2 of the patients with breast symptoms had normal concentrations.— P. A. Cann *et al.*, *Br. med. J.*, 1983, *286*, 1395.

EXTRAPYRAMIDAL EFFECTS. Reports of extrapyramidal symptoms in individual patients given domperidone: P. Sol *et al.* (letter), *Lancet*, 1980, *2*, 802; O. Debontridder (letter), *ibid.*, 802 and 1259; M. Casteels-Van Daele *et al.* (letter), *ibid.*, 1984, *1*, 57.

Precautions

If given intravenously domperidone should be used with great caution in patients predisposed to cardiac arrhythmias or hypokalaemia and in those receiving cancer chemotherapy.

Due to similarities in the mode of action, the precautions described under metoclopramide, p.1098 should be observed.

PARKINSONISM. Use of domperidone in the management of nausea arising from the treatment of Parkinson's disease should be viewed with caution because of possible adverse central effects (J. Leeser and D.N. Bateman, *Br. med. J.*, 1985, *290*, 241). In response, the manufacturers stated that reports involving 271 treated patients did not support this view (G. Lake-Bakaar and H.A. Cameron, *ibid.*) while other reports and experience with over 100 patients support the value of domperidone in such nausea and vomiting (P. Critchley *et al.*, *ibid.*, 788). In spite of these comments, it was considered that, as domperidone can cross the blood-brain barrier, there is a risk of central effects and that it should only be used in parkinsonian patients when safer anti-emetic measures have failed (D.N. Bateman, *ibid.*, 1079).

Absorption and Fate

Domperidone is absorbed from the gastro-intestinal tract, but its bioavailability following oral administration is low probably due to first-pass hepatic and intestinal metabolism. It is excreted in the faeces and urine mainly as metabolites. Domperidone is not generally considered to cross the blood-brain barrier but there have been some reports of central adverse effects.

The main faecal metabolite of domperidone given by mouth to 3 healthy subjects was hydroxydomperidone. Urinary metabolites included 2,3-dihydro-2-oxo-1*H*-benzimidazole-1-propanoic acid, which together with its conjugates accounted for 23% of the dose, and 5-chloro-4-piperidinyl-1,3-dihydrobenzimidazol-2-one.— W. Meuldermans *et al.*, *Eur. J. Drug Metab. Pharmacokinet.*, 1981, *6*, 49.

A study in 8 healthy subjects of the pharmacokinetics and bioavailability of domperidone. Following rapid intravenous administration of domperidone 10 mg a triphasic course of the plasma concentrations occurred. Following intramuscular or oral administration of domperidone 10 mg, maximum plasma concentrations of 40 and 23 ng per mL, respectively, were reached within 30 minutes. After rectal administration of 60 mg, plasma concentrations reached a plateau of 20 ng per mL at one hour. Following oral administration to fasted subjects the systemic bioavailability was 5 to 6 times lower than after parenteral administration, probably due to first-pass hepatic and intestinal metabolism. Bioavailability following oral administration was significantly increased when domperidone was given 90 minutes after a meal, although the time to maximum plasma concentration was delayed. Oral bioavailability increased linearly over the 10 to 60 mg dose range. The bioavailability following rectal administration was similar to that obtained with an equal oral dose. About 30% of an oral dose was excreted in the urine over 24 hours with only 0.4% as unchanged drug. About 66% of the dose was excreted in the faeces within 4 days of which 10% was unchanged drug.— J. Heykants *et al.*, *Eur. J. Drug Metab. Pharmacokinet.*, 1981, *6*, 61.

PREGNANCY AND THE NEONATE. Two mothers were given domperidone 10 mg by mouth every 8 hours from day 3 to day 6 of the puerperium. Domperidone was detected at mean concentrations of 10.3 ng per mL in serum samples taken 1.75 to 3 hours after a dose, and mean concentrations of 2.6 ng per mL were found in pooled breast milk which was expressed about 4 times daily.— G. J. Hofmeyr and B. van Iddekinge (letter), *Lancet*, 1983, *1*, 647. In a double-blind crossover study of 10 lactating mothers a single dose of domperidone 20 mg by mouth produced a mean serum-prolactin concentration of 255 ng per mL 2 hours after treatment compared with 150 ng per mL after placebo. Breast milk concentrations of domperidone were 0.24 and 1.1 ng per mL after 2 and 4 hours respectively. In 4 women taking domperidone 10 mg every 8 hours for 1 to 3 months domperidone was detected in breast milk at a mean concentration of 2.3 ng per mL 2 hours after the last dose.— G. J. Hofmeyr *et al.*, *Br. J. Obstet. Gynaec.*, 1985, *92*, 141.

Uses and Administration

Domperidone is a dopamine antagonist with properties similar to those of metoclopramide hydrochloride (p.1099). It is used for the symptomatic relief of acute nausea and vomiting and in the treatment of nausea and vomiting caused by levodopa or bromocriptine administration in Parkinson's disease. It has been stated that domperidone should not be used for chronic nausea and vomiting and that in parkinsonian patients it should be used for periods of up to 12 weeks only. For further comments regarding its use in parkinsonian patients, see under Precautions (above). Indications for its use in children are limited mainly to the control of nausea and vomiting associated with cancer therapy.

It is administered in doses of 10 to 20 mg by mouth or 30 to 60 mg rectally every 4 to 8 hours. In children doses of 200 to 400 µg per kg body-weight may be given by mouth every 4 to 8 hours; approximately 4 mg per kg daily may be given rectally.

Domperidone is used as the maleate in tablet preparations, but doses are expressed in terms of the base.

Domperidone is rarely administered parenterally; doses of 10 mg have been injected up to 5 times daily. Patients at risk of cardiac arrhythmias should not receive a bolus injection; if the intravenous route has to be used, domperidone should be infused over 15 to 30 minutes. Larger doses of up to 2 mg per kg body-weight daily have been infused slowly over at least 6 hours.

A review of the action, pharmacokinetics, and uses of domperidone.— R. N. Brogden *et al.*, *Drugs*, 1982, *24*, 360.

GASTRO-INTESTINAL DISORDERS. *Diabetic gastroparesis.* Successful treatment of severe diabetic gastroparesis and massive colonic dilatation in a 48-year-old woman given domperidone. Gastric stasis had completely disappeared 24 hours after starting domperidone 10 mg intravenously every 4 hours and she was changed to oral medication at the same dose.— M. Heer *et al.* (letter), *Lancet*, 1980, *2*, 1145. Similar benefit in several patients. However, not all gastroparetic patients respond well to dopaminergic receptor antagonist therapy.— S. J. Gordon and R. E. Joseph (letter), *ibid.*, 1981, *1*, 390.

Gastro-oesophageal reflux. Conflicting results have been obtained with domperidone in reflux oesophagitis. Weihrauch *et al.* (*Postgrad. med. J.*, 1979, *55*, *Suppl.* 1, 7) showed that it increased lower oesophageal sphincter pressure whereas Schulze-Delrieu *et al.* (*Lancet*, 1981, *1*, 159) did not find that it prevented exacerbations of chronic reflux oesophagitis. However, Grill *et al.* (*J. Pediat.*, 1985, *106*, 311) found that infants given domperidone 600 µg per kg body-weight four times daily showed improvement in symptoms of gastro-oesophageal reflux.

Irritable bowel syndrome. Domperidone 20 mg four times daily by mouth, half an hour before meals and just before sleep, was no better than placebo for the management of the common symptoms in irritable bowel syndrome. Five of the 31 patients involved in the double-blind crossover study experienced galactorrhoea and/or mastalgia and 4 other patients complained of urinary frequency while receiving domperidone.— P. A. Cann *et al.*, *Gut*, 1983, *24*, 1135. In a study of 22 patients domperidone 10 mg three times daily significantly reduced symptoms of irritable bowel syndrome compared with baseline values. Pinaverium bromide 50 mg three times daily was also found to reduce symptoms although to a lesser extent.— A. Martin *et al.*, *ibid.*, 1984, *25*, A584.

MIGRAINE. In a double-blind crossover study 19 patients with classical migraine were given domperidone 30 mg by mouth before 2 migraine attacks immediately they became aware of the warning signals; a placebo was given on 2 similar occasions. No aura or headache was experienced in 25 of 38 attacks (66%) following domperidone administration but in only 2 of 38 attacks (5%) after placebo. Although the warning signals occurred from 7 to 48 hours before the attacks, domperidone prevented migraine attacks even though its duration of action is about 6 hours.— J. Waelkens, *Br. med. J.*, 1982, *284*, 944.

NAUSEA AND VOMITING. In a 2-week double-blind study of 47 infants and children aged between 3 weeks and 8 years domperidone was more effective than metoclopramide and both drugs were superior to placebo in controlling the symptoms of chronic vomiting after food. The dose of both drugs was 0.3 mg per kg body-weight three times daily given before meals as drops of a solution containing 10 mg per mL.— I. De Loore *et al., Postgrad. med. J.*, 1979, *55, Suppl.* 1, 40.

From cancer chemotherapy. For comparative studies involving domperidone in the control of chemotherapy-induced nausea and vomiting see under alizapride, p.1074 and nabilone, p.1101.

Parkinsonism. In a double-blind placebo-controlled study of 17 patients with parkinsonism domperidone 20 mg three times daily 30 minutes before bromocriptine administration reduced the nausea, vomiting, and hiccups caused by bromocriptine; treatment was on average for 9 days. In 8 patients receiving domperidone, a mean daily dose of 148 mg of bromocriptine was achieved before side-effects intervened, and clinical improvement was observed. Four of 9 patients receiving placebo tolerated high doses of bromocriptine, but the other 5 patients experienced severe nausea, vomiting, and hiccups, and could only continue with high doses of bromocriptine if domperidone was also administered.— Y. Agid *et al., Lancet,* 1979, *1,* 570. In a double-blind crossover study of 8 patients with Parkinson's disease the addition of domperidone 40 mg three times daily to their therapy for 4 weeks produced no significant difference in parkinsonian disability scores when compared with placebo. Two patients withdrew from the study while on domperidone due to akathisia with dyskinesia and worsening parkinsonism.— J. Leeser and D. N. Bateman, *Br. J. clin. Pharmac.,* 1985, *20,* 284P (Because of the risk of central effects, these authors have questioned this recommended use of domperidone, see under Precautions).

Postoperative. A double-blind placebo-controlled study of 100 patients who had vomited postoperatively demonstrated that domperidone 10 mg administered by intravenous injection after vomiting occurred was very effective in the control of postoperative vomiting; 74% of patients who received domperidone had no recurrence of vomiting compared with 38% of patients who received placebo.— L. van Leeuwen and J. H. J. H. Helmers, *Anaesthesist,* 1980, *29,* 490. For an absence of effect with domperidone in the treatment of postoperative nausea and vomiting, see under Metoclopramide, p.1100.

PREGNANCY AND THE NEONATE. *Lactation.* As domperidone increases serum-prolactin concentrations and is excreted in nanogram quantities (that are considerably lower than those observed with metoclopramide) in breast milk, its effect in augmenting inadequate lactation requires further investigation.— G. J. Hofmeyr *et al., Br. J. Obstet. Gynaec.,* 1985, *92,* 141.

Proprietary Preparations

Evoxin *(Sterling Research, UK). Tablets,* domperidone 10 mg (as maleate).
Suppositories, domperidone 30 mg.

Motilium *(Janssen, UK). Tablets,* domperidone 10 mg (as maleate).
Suspension, domperidone 5 mg/5 mL.
Suppositories, domperidone 30 mg.

Proprietary Names and Manufacturers of Domperidone or Domperidone Maleate

Evoxin *(Sterling Research, UK)*; Motilium *(Janssen, Austral.; Janssen, Canad.; Janssen, Denm.; Janssen, Fr.; Byk Gulden, Ger.; Janssen, Ital.; Neth.; Janssen, S.Afr.; Esteve, Spain; Janssen, Switz.; Janssen, UK)*; Nauzelin *(Janssen, Spain)*; Peridon *(Italchimici, Ital.)*; Peridys *(Spret-Mauchant, Fr.)*.

3780-y

Dronabinol *(USAN, rINN).*

NSC-134454; Δ^9-Tetrahydrocannabinol; Δ^9-THC. (6a*R*,10a*R*)-6a,7,8,10a-Tetrahydro-6,6,9-trimethyl-3-pentyl-6*H*-dibenzo[*b,d*]pyran-1-ol.
$C_{21}H_{30}O_2$=314.5.

CAS — 1972-08-3.

Adverse Effects

Dronabinol, being a major psychoactive constituent of cannabis, may produce adverse effects similar to those of cannabis itself (see p.1553). See also under Nabilone (p.1101) for adverse effects associated with the use of cannabinoids as therapeutic agents.

The possibility of dependence similar to that of cannabis itself should be borne in mind.

Precautions

As for Nabilone, p.1101.

Uses and Administration

Dronabinol, a major psychoactive constituent of cannabis (see p.1553), has anti-emetic properties and is used for the control of nausea and vomiting associated with cancer chemotherapy.

The usual initial dose of dronabinol by mouth is 5 mg per m^2 body-surface given 1 to 3 hours before the first dose of the antineoplastic agent with subsequent doses being given every 2 to 4 hours after chemotherapy to a maximum of 4 to 6 doses daily. If necessary, the dose may be increased by increments of 2.5 mg per m^2 to a maximum dose of 15 mg per m^2.

A short discussion on the possible uses of cannabis and cannabinoids. Despite initial hopes the therapeutic use of cannabinoids remains limited. Dronabinol and nabilone have been used as anti-emetics for patients taking cytotoxic drugs; they are as effective as phenothiazines, with which they may be combined, but the incidence of adverse effects is high and immunosuppression is a theoretical risk. Oral cannabinoids are probably unsuitable for lowering intra-ocular tension in glaucoma and topical solutions require further development. Cannabidiol is effective in some cases of generalised epilepsy but further human studies are needed. Cannabinoids may eventually be used for anxiety, insomnia, muscle spasticity, and bacterial and fungal infections, but will probably not be used as antihypertensive agents, bronchodilators, or appetite stimulants for those with anorexia nervosa.— C. H. Ashton, *Br. med. J.,* 1987, *294,* 141.

NAUSEA AND VOMITING. A critical review of published studies assessing the antiemetic efficacy of dronabinol in patients receiving cancer chemotherapy; they show considerable inconsistency in results. The equivocal nature of the results can be partly attributed to differences in the study designs, procedures, and assessments that have been used; other factors that may be important are chemotherapy regimens, age of the patients, and pharmacologic variables such as drug tolerance, dose, schedule, toxicity, route of administration, and drug interactions. The authors believe that dronabinol does have anti-emetic efficacy but that the lack of controlled research does not allow precise knowledge of its true efficacy and toxicity.— M. P. Carey *et al., Ann. intern. Med.,* 1983, *99,* 106. A short review of dronabinol for nausea and vomiting due to cancer chemotherapy. The apparent mechanism of action of dronabinol is through binding to receptors in the forebrain and indirect inhibition of the vomiting centre in the medulla. Dronabinol, by mouth, can prevent nausea and vomiting caused by some cancer chemotherapy regimens, especially in younger patients, but older patients often find it difficult to tolerate; it is not likely to be effective in patients receiving cisplatin.— *Med. Lett.,* 1985, *27,* 97.

Proprietary Names and Manufacturers

Marinol *(Roxane, USA)*.

7511-n

Euonymus

Fusain Noir Pourpré; Wahoo Bark.

The dried root-bark of *Euonymus atropurpureus* (Celastraceae).

Euonymus was formerly used as a laxative.

Proprietary Names and Manufacturers
Opobyl *(Bengué, UK)*.

16598-s

Famotidine *(BAN, USAN, rINN).*

L-643341; MK-208; YM-11170. 3-[2-(Diaminomethyleneamino)thiazol-4-ylmethylthio]-*N*-sulphamoylpropionamidine.
$C_8H_{15}N_7O_2S_3$=337.5.

CAS — 76824-35-6.

Adverse Effects and Precautions

As for Cimetidine, p.1082. However, unlike cimetidine, famotidine is reported to have little or no anti-androgenic effect. Also it is generally considered that the potential for interactions with famotidine is less than with cimetidine.

Absorption and Fate

Famotidine is readily absorbed from the gastro-intestinal tract with peak concentrations in plasma occurring about 2 hours after administration by mouth. The bioavailability of famotidine following oral administration is about 40% compared with an intravenous dose. The elimination half-life from plasma is reported to be between 2.5 and 4 hours and famotidine is weakly bound, about 20%, to plasma proteins. A small proportion of famotidine is metabolised in the liver but most is excreted unchanged in the urine.

Uses and Administration

Famotidine is a histamine H_2-receptor antagonist with actions and uses similar to those of cimetidine (p.1084).

Famotidine may be given by mouth or parenterally by the intravenous route.

In the management of duodenal and gastric ulcers the dose is 40 mg daily by mouth at bedtime, for 4 to 8 weeks, and where appropriate a maintenance dose of 20 mg daily, also at bedtime, may be given.

In the Zollinger-Ellison syndrome the initial dose by mouth is 20 mg every 6 hours.

The usual dose of famotidine by the intravenous route is 20 mg and may be given as a slow injection over at least 2 minutes or as an infusion over 30 minutes; the dose may be repeated every 12 hours.

The dosage of famotidine should be reduced in patients with impaired renal function.

A review of the actions and uses of famotidine.— D. M. Campoli-Richards and S. P. Clissold, *Drugs,* 1986, *32,* 197. See also *Med. Lett.,* 1987, *29,* 17.

ADMINISTRATION IN RENAL FAILURE. A study of the pharmacokinetics of famotidine administered intravenously in healthy subjects and in patients with varying degrees of renal impairment. It was suggested that in patients with a creatinine clearance above 60 mL per minute per 1.48 m^2 body-surface the normal daily dose of famotidine could be employed; in those with a clearance of between 30 and 60 mL per minute per 1.48 m^2 the dose should be reduced by 50%; and in those with a clearance below 30 mL per minute per 1.48 m^2 the dose should be reduced by 75%.— T. Takabatake *et al., Eur. J. clin. Pharmac.,* 1985, *28,* 327.

Proprietary Preparations

Pepcid PM *(Morson, UK). Tablets,* famotidine 20 and 40 mg.

Proprietary Names and Manufacturers

Famodil *(Sigmatau, Ital.)*; Fanox *(Lesvi, Spain)*; Gaster *(Yamanouchi, Jpn)*; Gastridin *(Merck Sharp & Dohme, Ital.)*; Gastrion *(Vita, Spain)*; Motiax *(Neopharmed, Ital.)*; Pepcid *(Morson, UK; Merck Sharp & Dohme, USA)*; Pepcidin *(Merck Sharp & Dohme, Denm.)*; Pepcidine *(Merck Sharp & Dohme, Switz.)*; Pepdul *(Frosst, Ger.)*; Tamin *(Merck Sharp & Dohme, Spain)*.

7512-h

Fig *(BAN).*

Carica; Ficus.

Pharmacopoeias. In *Br.* and *Swiss.*

The sun-dried succulent fruit of *Ficus carica* (Moraceae) containing not less than 60% of water-soluble extractive. **Store** in a dry place.

Fig is a mild laxative and demulcent used medicinally as a syrup, usually with other laxatives.

Preparations

Compound Fig Elixir *(B.P.).* Compound Fig Syrup; Aromatic Fig Syrup. Prepared from fig 32 g, compound rhubarb tincture 5 mL, senna liquid extract 10 mL, cascara elixir 5 mL, sucrose 54 g, and water to 100 mL.

15320-k

Flumeridone *(BAN, USAN, rINN).*
R-45486. 5-Chloro-1-{1-[3-(5-fluoro-2-oxobenzimidazolin-1-yl)propyl]-4-piperidyl}benzimidazolin-2-one.
$C_{22}H_{23}ClFN_5O_2$=443.9.

CAS — 75444-64-3.

Flumeridone is reported to have anti-emetic activity.

Proprietary Names and Manufacturers
Janssen, Belg.

7513-m

Frangula Bark *(BAN).*
Alder Buckthorn Bark; Amieiro Negro; Bourdaine; Faulbaumrinde; Frangulae Cortex; Rhamni Frangulae Cortex.

CAS — 8057-57-6 (frangula extract).

Pharmacopoeias. In *Aust., Belg., Br., Cz., Eur., Fr., Ger., Hung., It., Jug., Neth., Nord., Pol., Roum., Rus., Span.,* and *Swiss. Br.* also describes Powdered Frangula Bark.

The dried bark of the stems and branches of *Rhamnus frangula* (=*Frangula alnus*) (Rhamnaceae). It contains not less than 6% of glucofrangulins, calculated as glucofrangulin A. **Protect** from light and moisture.

Frangula bark is an anthraquinone laxative.

Proprietary Names and Manufacturers
Irgalax *(Geigy, Switz.)*; Solco-Lax *(Solco, Ger.)*.

The following names have been used for multi-ingredient preparations containing frangula bark—Caved-S *(Muir & Neil, Austral.)*; Granocol *(Schering, Austral.)*; Movicol *(Norgine, USA)*; Normacol Plus *(Norgine, UK)*; Normacol Standard *(Norgine, Austral.)*; Pepsillide *(Cambridge Laboratories, Austral.)*; Pep-Uls-Ade *(Cambridge Laboratories, Austral.)*; Rabro *(Sinclair, UK)*; Roter *(Four Macs, Austral.; Anglo-French Laboratories, Canad.; Roterpharma, UK)*.

690-w

Gefarnate *(BAN, rINN).*
Geranyl Farnesylacetate. A mixture of stereoisomers of 3,7-dimethylocta-2,6-dienyl 5,9,13-trimethyltetradeca-4,8,12-trienoate.
$C_{27}H_{44}O_2$=400.6.

CAS — 51-77-4.

Gefarnate is used in the treatment of peptic ulcer in doses of 100 to 300 mg daily by mouth or 50 to 100 mg daily intramuscularly.

Proprietary Names and Manufacturers
Alsanate *(Jpn)*; Andoin *(Spain)*; Arsanyl *(Jpn)*; Dixnalate *(Jpn)*; Farnesil *(AGIPS, Ital.)*; Farnisol *(FIRMA, Ital.)*; Gefalon *(Jpn)*; Gefarnil *(Belg.; De Angeli, Ital.; De Angeli, S.Afr.; Almirall, Spain; de Angeli, Switz.; WB Pharmaceuticals, UK)*; Gefarol *(Ital.)*; Gefulcer *(Jpn)*; Matorozin *(Jpn)*; Nolesil *(Ital.)*; Polyl *(Jpn)*; Salanil *(Jpn)*; Terpanil *(Jpn)*; Ulco *(Ital.)*; Ulcofarm *(Ausonia, Ital.)*; Ulcotrofina *(Ripari-Gero, Ital.)*; Vagogernil *(Benvegna, Ital.)*; Zackal *(Jpn)*; Zenowal *(Jpn)*.

691-e

Hydrotalcite *(BAN, rINN).*
Aluminium magnesium carbonate hydroxide hydrate.
$Mg_6Al_2(OH)_{16}CO_3,4H_2O$=604.0.

CAS — 12304-65-3.

Pharmacopoeias. In *Br.*

A white or almost white, free-flowing, granular powder. It contains not less than 14.4% and not more than 19.4% of Al_2O_3 and not less than 34.0% and not more than 46.0% of MgO. The ratio of Al_2O_3 to MgO is not less than 0.40 and not more than 0.45. Practically **insoluble** in water; it dissolves in dilute mineral acids with slight effervescence. A 4% suspension in water has a pH of 8.0 to 10.0.

Hydrotalcite is an antacid that is given in doses of 1 g.

Preparations
Hydrotalcite Tablets *(B.P.)*

Proprietary Preparations
Altacite Plus *(Roussel, UK). Tablets,* chewable, hydrotalcite 500 mg, activated dimethicone 250 mg.
Suspension, hydrotalcite 500 mg, activated dimethicone 125 mg/5 mL. *Dose.* 2 tablets or 10 mL of suspension between meals and at bedtime.

Hydrotalcite (formerly known as Altacite) *(Roussel, UK). Tablets,* chewable, hydrotalcite 500 mg.
Suspension, hydrotalcite 500 mg/5 mL.

Proprietary Names and Manufacturers
Agastrin *(Rottapharm, Ital.)*; Altacet *(Roussel, Swed.)*; Altacite *(Canad.; Roussel, S.Afr.)*; Hi-Ti *(Jpn)*; Hydrotalcite *(Roussel, UK)*; Nacid *(Jpn)*; Talcid *(Bayer, Ger.; Bayer, Spain)*; Ultacit *(Neth.)*.

The following names have been used for multi-ingredient preparations containing hydrotalcite— Altacaps *(Roussel, UK)*.

7514-b

Ipomoea
Ipomoea Root; Mexican Scammony Root; Orizaba Jalap Root; Scammony Root.

Pharmacopoeias. Radix Scammoniae of *Egypt. P.* and *Span. P.* is Levant scammony root, *Convolvulus scammonia.*

The dried root of *Ipomoea orizabensis* (Convolvulaceae), containing not less than 12% of resin.

7515-v

Ipomoea Resin
Mexican Scammony Resin; Scammony Resin.

CAS — 9000-34-4.

Pharmacopoeias. In *Egypt.* and *Mex. Egypt.* also includes Levant Scammony Resin. Resina Scammoniae of *Arg., Belg., Port., Roum.,* and *Span.* is from Levant scammony.

A mixture of glycosidal resins obtained from ipomoea. Practically **insoluble** in water; soluble in alcohol; almost entirely soluble in ether.

Ipomoea resin has a drastic purgative and irritant action. It has been superseded by less toxic laxatives.

5439-c

Ispaghula

Pharmacopoeias. In *U.S.* under the title of Plantago Seed (see below). See also Psyllium, p.1104.

Ispaghula consists of the dried ripe seeds of *Plantago ovata* (Plantaginaceae).

Plantago Seed (*U.S.P.*) is the cleaned, dried, ripe seed of *Plantago ovata*, known in commerce as Blond Psyllium or as Indian Plantago Seed, or of *Plantago psyllium*, or of *Plantago indica* (*Plantago arenaria*), known in commerce as Spanish Psyllium Seed or as French Psyllium Seed.

5440-s

Ispaghula Husk *(BAN).*

Pharmacopoeias. In *Br.* and *Ind.* Also in *U.S.* under the title of Psyllium Husk (see below). See also Psyllium, p.1104.

Ispaghula Husk (*B.P.*) consists of the epidermis and collapsed adjacent layers removed from the dried ripe seeds of *Plantago ovata*. Small, pale buff, brittle flakes; it loses not more than 12% of its weight on drying. Ispaghula husk swells rapidly in water forming a stiff mucilage.

Psyllium Husk (*U.S.P.*) is the cleaned, dried seed coat (epidermis), in whole or in powdered form, separated by winnowing and thrashing from the seeds of *Plantago ovata*, known in commerce as Blond Psyllium, or as Indian Psyllium, or as Ispaghula, or from *Plantago psyllium* or from *Plantago indica* (*Plantago arenaria*), known in commerce as Spanish Psyllium or as French Psyllium.

Adverse Effects and Precautions
Large quantities of ispaghula and other bulk laxatives may temporarily increase flatulence and distension and there is a risk of intestinal obstruction. Oesophageal obstruction may occur if such compounds are swallowed dry.

Bulk laxatives should not be given to patients with intestinal obstruction or conditions likely to lead to intestinal obstruction. They should be taken with sufficient fluid to prevent faecal impaction or oesophageal obstruction.

Bulk laxatives lower the transit time through the gut and could affect the absorption of other drugs.

Reports of allergic reactions associated with ispaghula or psyllium: W. W. Busse and W. F. Schoenwetter, *Ann. intern. Med.*, 1975, *83*, 361 (rhinitis and wheezing in 3 men following industrial exposure); R. Gross (letter), *J. Am. med. Ass.*, 1979, *241*, 1573 (acute bronchospasm following inhalation); R. Suhonen *et al.*, *Allergy*, 1983, *38*, 363 (urticaria and anaphylaxis following ingestion); G. P. Zaloga *et al.*, *J. Allergy & clin. Immunol.*, 1984, *74*, 79 (urticaria and anaphylaxis following ingestion).

Uses and Administration
Ispaghula and ispaghula husk are used as bulk laxatives since by taking up water in the gastro-intestinal tract the volume of faeces is increased and peristalsis promoted; they may be used in the treatment of chronic constipation and when excessive straining at stool must be avoided following ano-rectal surgery or in the management of haemorrhoids. The ability to increase faecal mass also means that they may be used in the management of diarrhoea and for adjusting faecal consistency in patients with colostomies and in patients with diverticular disease or the irritable bowel syndrome.

The effect of bulk-forming laxatives is usually apparent within 24 hours, but 2 to 3 days of medication may be required to achieve the full effect.

Ispaghula has been administered after soaking for several hours or as a powder in doses of up to 10 g. The husk is given in smaller doses of 3 to 5 g.

Preparations
Psyllium Hydrophilic Mucilloid for Oral Suspension *(U.S.P.).* A dry mixture of Psyllium Husk (*U.S.P.*) with suitable additives. Store in airtight containers.

Proprietary Preparations
Colven *(Reckitt & Colman Pharmaceuticals, UK). Granules,* ispaghula husk 3.5 g, mebeverine hydrochloride 135 mg/sachet. For irritable bowel syndrome. *Dose.* The contents of 1 sachet, in water, 2 or 3 times daily before meals.

Fybogel *(Reckitt & Colman Pharmaceuticals, UK). Granules,* ispaghula husk 3.5 g/sachet. For patients requiring extra dietary fibre. *Dose.* The contents of 1 sachet, in water, twice daily.

Isogel *(Allen & Hanburys, UK). Granules,* ispaghula husk. For chronic constipation and colostomy control. *Dose.* Two 5-mL spoonfuls, in water, once or twice daily.

Manevac *(Galen, UK). Granules,* ispaghula 54.2%, senna fruit 12.4%.
A similar product was formerly marketed in Great Britain under the name Agiolax.

Metamucil *(Searle, UK). Oral powder,* ispaghula husk 49% (3.4 g/7-g sachet). For constipation. *Dose.* One 5-mL spoonful or 1 sachet, in water, one to three times daily.

Regulan *(Gold Cross, UK). Oral powder,* ispaghula husk 3.6 g/sachet. For constipation and for patients requiring extra dietary fibre. *Dose.* The contents of 1 sachet, in water, one to three times daily.

Proprietary Names and Manufacturers of Ispaghula and Ispaghula Husk
Agiofibe *(Schering, Austral.)*; Effersyllium *(Stuart Pharmaceuticals, USA)*; Fiberall *(Rydelle, USA)*; Fibrolax *(Gipharmex, Ital.)*; Fybogel *(Reckitt & Col-*

man, Austral.; Reckitt & Colman, S.Afr.; Reckitt & Colman Pharmaceuticals, UK); Hydrocil Instant *(Rowell, USA)*; Isogel *(Allen & Hanburys, UK)*; Ispaghul *(Fr.)*; Karacil *(ICN, Canad.)*; Konsyl *(Lafayette, USA)*; Konsyl-D *(Lafayette, USA)*; LA Formula *(Lafayette, USA)*; Lexogel *(Wilson, Pakistan)*; Lunelax *(Tika, Norw.; Tika, Swed.)*; Manevac *(Galen, UK)*; Metamucil *(Searle, Austral.; Searle, Canad.; Searle, Denm.; Searle, Ger.; Neth.; Searle, S.Afr.; Searle, Spain; Searle, Swed.; Searle, Switz.; Searle, UK; Procter & Gamble, USA)*; Modane Bulk *(Adria, USA)*; Naturacil *(Mead Johnson Nutritional, USA)*; Novomucilax *(Novopharm, Canad.)*; Nuggets *(Jayco, USA)*; Prodiem *(Rorer, Canad.)*; Regulan *(Gold Cross, UK)*; Siblin *(Parke, Davis, Canad.; Parke, Davis, S.Afr.)*; Spagulax *(Fr.)*; Syllact *(Wallace, USA)*; Vi-Siblin *(Parke, Davis, Denm.; Parke, Davis, Norw.; Parke, Davis, Swed.; Parke, Davis, UK)*.

The following names have been used for multi-ingredient preparations containing ispaghula and ispaghula husk—Agiolax *(Schering, Austral.)*; Colven *(Reckitt & Colman Pharmaceuticals, UK)*; Prompt *(Searle, USA)*.

7516-g

Jalap

Jalap Root; Jalap Tuber; Jalapa; Jalapenwurzel; Vera Cruz Jalap.

Pharmacopoeias. In *Arg., Aust., Belg., Egypt., Mex., Port.,* and *Span.*

Port. also includes Brazilian Jalap, the dried sliced root of *Operculina macrocarpa* (=*O. tuberosa; Ipomoea tuberosa; Piptostegia pisonis*) (Convolvulaceae), containing not less than 15% of resin.

The dried tubercles of *Ipomoea purga* (=*Exogonium purga*) (Convolvulaceae), containing not less than 10% of resin.

7517-q

Jalap Resin

Jalapenharz.

CAS — 9000-35-5.

Pharmacopoeias. In *Arg., Aust., Belg., Egypt., Mex., Port., Roum.,* and *Span.*

A mixture of glycosidal resins obtained by extraction of jalap with alcohol; it contains not less than 85% ether-insoluble resin. Practically **insoluble** in water; soluble in alcohol.

Jalap resin has a drastic purgative and irritant action. It has been superseded by less toxic laxatives.

7518-p

Kaladana

Pharbitis Seeds.

Pharmacopoeias. In *Jpn.*

The dried seeds of *Ipomoea hederacea* (sometimes known as morning glory or *Pharbitis nil*) (Convolvulaceae), containing not less than 14% of alcohol (95%)-soluble extractive.

Kaladana has a purgative action similar to jalap.

694-j

Kaolin *(BAN, USAN).*

Pharmacopoeias. In *Arg., Aust., Belg., Br., Chin., Egypt., Eur., Fr., Ger., Hung., Ind., It., Jpn, Jug., Mex., Neth., Nord., Pol., Port., Rus., Span., Swiss.,* and *U.S.* Also in *B.P. Vet.* Some pharmacopoeias do not differentiate between the heavy and light varieties.

Kaolin is a hydrated aluminium silicate.

Heavy Kaolin (*B.P., Eur. P.*) is a purified natural form of variable composition. It is a fine white or greyish-white unctuous powder. Practically **insoluble** in water and in organic solvents. Labels of containers containing Heavy Kaolin should state whether or not the material is intended for internal use.

Light Kaolin (*B.P., B.P. Vet.*) is a native form, freed from most of its impurities by elutriation, and dried. It contains a suitable dispersing agent. It is a light, white, odourless or almost odourless unctuous powder free from gritty particles. Practically **insoluble** in water and in mineral acids.

Light Kaolin (Natural) (*B.P., B.P.Vet.*) is Light Kaolin which does not contain a dispersing agent.

Kaolin (*U.S.P.*) is a native form, powdered and freed from gritty particles by elutriation. It is a soft, white or yellowish-white powder or lumps with an earthy or clay-like taste and when moistened with water assumes a darker colour and develops a marked clay-like odour. Practically **insoluble** in water, in cold dilute acids, and in solutions of alkali hydroxides.

NOTE. The *B.P.* directs that when Kaolin or Light Kaolin is prescribed or demanded, Light Kaolin must be dispensed or supplied unless it is ascertained that Light Kaolin (Natural) is required.

Light kaolin and light kaolin (natural) are adsorbent, and when given by mouth adsorb toxic and other substances from the alimentary tract and increase the bulk of the faeces. They are employed in the symptomatic treatment of diarrhoea and have been given in doses of up to about 20 g.

It should be noted that a consequence of diarrhoea may be fluid and electrolyte depletion, and that rehydration therapy may be necessary, especially in infants and young children. For further details concerning rehydration therapy, see p.1024.

Externally, light kaolin is used as a dusting-powder. Kaolin is liable to be heavily contaminated with bacteria, and when used in dusting-powders, it should be sterilised.

Light kaolin is also used as a food additive.

Heavy kaolin is used in the preparation of kaolin poultice, which is applied with the intention of reducing inflammation and alleviating pain.

Since kaolin is an adsorbent it should be remembered that the absorption of other drugs from the gastro-intestinal tract may be reduced if administered concomitantly.

A discussion on the merits of simple aspiration to treat spontaneous pneumothorax, and the suggestion that perhaps all pneumothoraces that do not respond to treatment by simple aspiration as described by A.A.D. Hamilton and G.J. Archer (*Thorax*, 1983, *38*, 934) should have kaolin pleurodesis.— *Lancet*, 1984, *1*, 434.

Preparations

Kaolin Dusting-powder Compound *(A.P.F.)*. Conspers. Kaolin. Co. Light kaolin 25, zinc oxide 25, and purified talc 50. Sterilise by heating at a temperature not lower than 160° in a closed container for not less than 2 hours.

Kaolin Mixture *(B.P.)*. Kaolin Oral Suspension. A suspension with a peppermint flavour containing light kaolin or light kaolin (natural) 20% and 5% each of light magnesium carbonate and sodium bicarbonate. Extemporaneous preparations should be prepared according to the following formula: light kaolin or light kaolin (natural) 2 g, light magnesium carbonate 500 mg, sodium bicarbonate 500 mg, concentrated peppermint emulsion 0.25 mL, double-strength chloroform water 5 mL, water to 10 mL. It should be recently prepared, unless the kaolin has been sterilised.

Kaolin and Morphine Mixture *(B.P.)*. Kaolin and Morphine Oral Suspension. A suspension containing light kaolin or light kaolin (natural) 20%, sodium bicarbonate 5%, and chloroform and morphine tincture 4% v/v. Extemporaneous preparations should be prepared according to the following formula: light kaolin or light kaolin (natural) 2 g, sodium bicarbonate 500 mg, chloroform and morphine tincture 0.4 mL, water to 10 mL. It contains 550 to 800 μg of anhydrous morphine in 10 mL. It should be recently prepared, unless the kaolin has been sterilised. Store in well-filled, well-closed glass containers.

Kaolin and Opium Mixture *(A.P.F.)*. Mist. Kaolin. et Opii. Light kaolin or light kaolin (natural) 2.5 g, alum 10 mg, opium tincture 0.5 mL, concentrated chloroform water 0.25 mL or compound hydroxybenzoate solution 0.1 mL, water to 10 mL. It contains 5 mg of anhydrous morphine in each 10 mL. *Dose.* 10 to 20 mL.

Kaolin Powder Compound *(A.P.F.)*. Pulv. Kaolin. Co. Light kaolin or light kaolin (natural) 55, heavy magnesium carbonate 30, sodium bicarbonate 15, peppermint oil 0.2. *Dose.* 2 to 5 g.

Kaolin Poultice *(B.P.)*. Heavy kaolin 52.7%, boric acid 4.5%, with glycerol, methyl salicylate, peppermint oil, and thymol. Store in containers which minimise absorption, diffusion, or evaporation.

Proprietary Preparations

Kaolin Poultice K/L Pack *(K/L Pharmaceutical, UK)*. *Poultice,* kaolin poultice in 100-g pouches.

Kaopectate *(Upjohn, UK)*. *Suspension,* kaolin 1.03 g/5 mL.

Maws KLN *(Ashe, UK)*. *Suspension,* light kaolin 1.15 g, pectin 57.5 mg, peppermint oil 1.15 mg, sodium citrate 17.25 mg. *Dose.* 6 to 12 months, 5 mL; 1 to 3 years, 10 mL; 3 to 10 years, 20 mL.

Proprietary Names and Manufacturers

Kaolin Poultice K/L Pack *(K/L Pharmaceutical, UK)*; Kaopectate *(Upjohn, UK)*; Kao-pront *(Upjohn, Ital.)*; Kaylene *(Dendron, UK)*.

The following names have been used for multi-ingredient preparations containing kaolin—Actonorm *(Wallace Mfg Chem., UK)*; ADM *(Wellcome, Austral.)*; Diaguard *(Nelson, Austral.)*; Diaguard Forte *(Nelson, Austral.)*; Donnagel *(Robins, Austral.; Robins, Canad.)*; Donnagel with Neomycin *(Robins, Canad.; Robins, UK)*; Donnagel-MB *(Robins, Canad.)*; Donnagel-PG *(Robins, Canad.; Robins, USA)*; Glucomagma *(Drug Houses Austral., Austral.)*; Guanimycin *(Allen & Hanburys, UK)*; Kao-Con *(Upjohn, Austral.; Upjohn, Canad.)*; Kaodene *(Crookes Healthcare, UK)*; Kaofort *(Boots, Austral.)*; Kaogel *(Faulding, Austral.)*; Kaomagma *(Wyeth, Austral.)*; Kaomycin *(Upjohn, Austral.; Upjohn, Canad.; Upjohn, UK)*; Kaopectate *(Upjohn, Austral.; Upjohn, Canad.)*; Kaylene-Ol *(Dendron, UK)*; Maws KLN *(Ashe, UK)*; Noratex *(Norton, UK)*; Parepectolin *(Rorer, USA)*; Pectokay *(Bowman, USA)*; Penbritin KS *(Beecham Research, UK)*; Pomalin *(Winthrop, Canad.)*; Streptomagma Suspension *(Wyeth, Austral.)*; Thovaline *(Ilon Laboratories, UK)*.

7519-s

Lactulose *(BAN, USAN, rINN).*

4-*O*-β-D-Galactopyranosyl-D-fructose.

$C_{12}H_{22}O_{11}$=342.3.

CAS — 4618-18-2.

Pharmacopoeias. Br. has a monograph for Lactulose Solution. *U.S.* includes Lactulose Concentrate.

A synthetic disaccharide. Lactulose Concentrate *(U.S.P.)* is **miscible** with water; **store** in airtight containers preferably at a temperature between 2° and 30°. Lactulose Solution *(B.P.)* should be stored at a temperature not exceeding 20°.

Adverse Effects

Lactulose may cause abdominal discomfort associated with flatulence or cramps. Nausea and vomiting have occasionally been reported following high doses. Prolonged use or overdosage may result in diarrhoea with excessive loss of water and electrolytes, particularly potassium.

Hypernatraemia in patients with decompensated liver disease appeared to be due to increased insensible water losses, impaired access to free water, cathartic use (usually lactulose), and occasionally the administration of parenteral solutions high in sodium.— S. E. Warren *et al., J. Am. med. Ass.*, 1980, *243*, 1257. In a retrospective study involving 33 patients with portal-systemic encephalopathy, hypernatraemia developed during 20 of 75 courses of lactulose therapy and was associated with a mortality of 41% (9 deaths) compared with 14% (8 deaths) in those who remained normonatraemic.— D. C. Nelson *et al., J. Am. med. Ass.*, 1983, *249*, 1295.

Severe and intractable lactic acidosis developed in a patient being treated with lactulose for hepatic encephalopathy; the patient was unable to pass stool satisfactorily due to adynamic ileus.— N. S. Mann *et al.* (letter), *Ann. intern. Med.*, 1985, *103*, 637.

Precautions

Lactulose should not be given to patients with intestinal obstruction. It should not be used in patients on a galactose-free diet and care should be taken in patients with lactose intolerance or in diabetic patients because of the presence of some free galactose and lactose.

Diarrhoea, simulating lactose intolerance, had been seen in several children when full-strength milk foods had been re-introduced after gastroenteritis; lactulose had been identified in some prepacked liquid milks and might be present in laxative amounts.— R. G. Hendrickse *et al.*, *Br. med. J.*, 1977, *1*, 1194; R. G. Hendrickse (letter), *ibid.*, 1977, *2*, 187. The lactulose concentrations of various liquid prepacked infant milk feeds ranged from 1.6 to 13.7 mmol per litre. Most infant feeds were subjected to terminal sterilisation which appeared to result in the conversion of 5 to 6% of the lactose to lactulose. However, lactulose in infant feeds promoted a microflora rich in lactobacilli similar to that found in breast-fed infants and there was little evidence that the presence of lactulose was harmful.— R. C. Beach and I. S. Menzies (letter), *Lancet*, 1983, *1*, 425.

Absorption and Fate

Following administration by mouth, lactulose is almost completely unabsorbed from the gastro-intestinal tract. It passes essentially unchanged into the large intestine where it is metabolised by saccharolytic bacteria with the formation of simple organic acids such as lactic and acetic acids. Urinary excretion has been reported to be 3% or less.

Uses and Administration

Lactulose is a synthetic disaccharide which is used in the treatment of constipation and in hepatic encephalopathy. Lactulose is broken down by colonic bacteria mainly into acetic and lactic acids which exert a local osmotic effect in the colon resulting in increased faecal bulk and stimulation of peristalsis. It may take up to 48 hours before an effect is obtained. When larger doses are given for hepatic encephalopathy the pH in the colon is reduced significantly by this acid production and the absorption of ammonium ions and other toxic nitrogenous compounds is decreased leading to a fall in blood-ammonia concentration.

Lactulose is usually administered as a solution containing approximately 3.35 g of lactulose per 5 mL together with other sugars. In the treatment of constipation, the usual initial dose is 10 to 20 g (15 to 30 mL) given daily by mouth in a single dose or in 2 divided doses and gradually reduced according to the patient's needs; maintenance doses of 7 to 10 g (10 to 15 mL) have been given daily. Children aged 6 to 12 years may be given initial doses of 20 mL daily; 1 to 5 years, 10 mL daily; under 1 year, 5 mL daily.

In hepatic encephalopathy, 60 to 100 g (90 to 150 mL) is given daily by mouth in 3 divided doses; initially doses of 20 to 30 g (30 to 45 mL) may be given every hour. The dose is subsequently adjusted to produce 2 or 3 soft stools each day. Lactulose solution 300 mL mixed with 700 mL of water or physiological saline has been used as a retention enema; the enema is retained for 30 to 60 minutes, repeated every 4 to 6 hours until the patient is able to take oral medication.

Lactitol (p.1582) is an analogue of lactulose used similarly in hepatic encephalopathy.

DIAGNOSIS AND TESTING. A discussion on techniques used to investigate abnormal intestinal permeability. The recognition that reduced absorption of monosaccharides in coeliac disease is accompanied by a paradoxical increase in permeability to disaccharides prompted the development of the differential sugar absorption test in which 2 sugars are given simultaneously by mouth and urinary recovery of each is determined. In the presence of mucosal disease the urinary recovery of the disaccharide is increased whilst that of the monosaccharide is decreased. The permeability to sugars is also abnormal in Crohn's disease. Thus tests of intestinal permeability have a wide application in the investigation of intestinal disease and are ready for more general use. At present, a differential sugar absorption test, using mannitol or rhamnose as one component and lactulose as the other seems to be the best buy.— *Lancet*, 1985, *1*, 256.

Reduction of the cholesterol saturation of bile by lactulose.— J. R. Thornton and K. W. Heaton, *Br. med. J.*, 1981, *282*, 1018.

ENCEPHALOPATHY. Reviews on the treatment of hepatic encephalopathy including the use of lactulose: I. R. Crossley and R. Williams, *Gut*, 1984, *25*, 85; C. L. Fraser and A. I. Arieff, *New Engl. J. Med.*, 1985, *313*, 865; *Lancet*, 1987, *2*, 81.

Preparations

Lactulose Syrup *(U.S.P.)*

Proprietary Preparations

Duphalac *(Duphar, UK)*. *Syrup*, lactulose 3.35 g, lactose 300 mg, galactose 550 mg/5 mL.

Proprietary Names and Manufacturers

Acilac *(Technilab, Canad.)*; Bifiteral *(Belg.; Duphar, Ger.)*; Cephulac *(Merrell Dow, Canad.; Merrell Dow, USA)*; Chronulac *(Merrell Dow, Canad.; Merrell Dow, USA)*; Dia-Colon *(Piam, Ital.)*; Duphalac *(Cilag, Austral.; Belg.; Ferrosan, Denm.; Duphar, Fr.; ISM, Ital.; Ferrosan, Norw.; Duphar, S.Afr.; Kali-Farma, Spain; Ferrosan, Swed.; Switz.; Duphar, UK)*; Epalfen *(Zambon, Ital.)*; Eugalac *(Topfer, Ger.)*; Gatinar *(Sandoz, Spain; Wander, Switz.; Sandoz, UK)*; Lactofalk *(Falk, Ger.)*; Lactuflor *(Chephasaar, Ger.)*; Lactulax *(Technilab, Canad.)*; Lactulon *(Arg.)*; Laevilac *(Atmos, Ger.)*; Laevolac *(Boehringer Biochemia, Ital.)*; Levolac *(Laevosan, Norw.)*; Loraga *(Generics, Swed.)*; Monilac *(Jpn)*; Normase *(Molteni, Ital.)*; Portalac.

16875-j

Lidamidine Hydrochloride *(USAN)*.

Lidamide Hydrochloride *(rINNM)*; WHR-1142A. *N*-(2,6-Dimethylphenyl)-*N'*-[imino(methylamino)methyl]-urea hydrochloride.

$C_{11}H_{16}N_4O,HCl=256.7$.

CAS — 66871-56-5 (lidamidine); 65009-35-0 (hydrochloride).

Lidamidine hydrochloride is used in the management of diarrhoea.

It should be noted that a consequence of diarrhoea may be fluid and electrolyte depletion, and that rehydration therapy may be necessary, especially in infants and young children. For further details concerning rehydration therapy, see p.1024.

Reports of the use of lidamidine hydrochloride: J. S. Goff (letter), *Ann. intern. Med.*, 1984, *101*, 874 (encouraging results in 3 diabetic patients with diarrhoea); C. Edwards *et al.*, *Gut*, 1986, *27*, 581 (no benefit in a patient with a tumour-associated secretory diarrhoea); G. Gasbarrini *et al.*, *Arzneimittel-Forsch.*, 1986, *36*, 1843 (comparable to loperamide in acute diarrhoea).

Proprietary Names and Manufacturers

Idealid *(AF, Mex.)*; Lidarral *(Yamanouchi, Jpn; Rorer, Mex.; Rorer, USA)*.

2021-l

Liquorice *(BAN)*.

Alcaçuz; Glycyrrhiza *(USAN)*; Licorice; Liquiritiae Radix; Liquorice Root; Orozuz; Raiz de Regaliz; Süssholzwurzel.

Pharmacopoeias. In *Arg., Aust., Belg., Br., Braz., Chin., Cz., Egypt., Eur., Fr., Ger., Hung., Ind., Jpn, Jug., Neth., Nord., Pol., Port., Roum., Rus., Span.*, and *Swiss*. Many allow peeled or unpeeled liquorice. Also in *U.S.N.F. Br.* also describes Powdered Liquorice.

Liquorice (*B.P.*) and Liquorice Root (*Eur. P.*) consist of the dried unpeeled roots and stolons of *Glycyrrhiza glabra* (Leguminosae) containing not less than 4% of glycyrrhizinic acid. **Store** in airtight containers. Protect from light.

Glycyrrhiza *U.S.N.F.* is the dried rhizome and roots of *Glycyrrhiza glabra*, known in commerce as Spanish Licorice, or of *G. glabra* var. *glandulifera*, known in commerce as Russian Licorice, or of other varieties.

Adverse Effects

Liquorice may cause reversible sodium retention and potassium loss leading to hypertension, water retention, and electrolyte imbalance. Deglycyrrhizinised liquorice is not usually associated with such adverse effects.

Reports of adverse effects, often associated with the ingestion of excessive amounts of liquorice in foods or drinks: E. G. Gross *et al.*, *New Engl. J. Med.*, 1966, *274*, 602 (hypokalaemic myopathy with myoglobinuria: confectionery); T. J. Chamberlain (letter), *J. Am. med. Ass.*, 1970, *213*, 1343 (hypertension, hypokalaemic alkalosis, oedema, headache, muscle weakness, and congestive heart failure: confectionery); L. K. Wash and J. D. Bernard, *Am. J. Hosp. Pharm.*, 1975, *32*, 73 (hypokalaemia and hypertension: confectionery); B. Bannister, *Br. med. J.*, 1977, *2*, 738 (hypokalaemic myopathy: confectionery); S. Werner *et al.* (letter), *Lancet*, 1979, *1*, 319 (hypokalaemia, hyperprolactinaemia, and amenorrhoea: confectionery); A. M. M. Cumming *et al.*, *Postgrad. med. J.*, 1980, *56*, 526 (hypokalaemia, complete flaccid paralysis, and myoglobinuria: liquorice-containing laxative); J. D. Blachley and J. P. Knochel, *New Engl. J. Med.*, 1980, *302*, 784 (hypokalaemia, muscle weakness, and hypertension: chewing-tobacco containing liquorice); F. Lai *et al.* (letter), *New Engl. J. Med.*, 1980, *303*, 463 (hypokalaemic myopathy: over-the-counter medicines); S. Nightingale *et al.*, *Postgrad. med. J.*, 1981, *57*, 577 (hypokalaemic myopathy: confectionery); J. M. Cereda *et al.* (letter), *Lancet*, 1983, *1*, 1442 (muscle weakness and hypertension: soft drinks); J. P. Haberer *et al.* (letter), *ibid.*, 1984, *1*, 575 (hypokalaemia leading to fatal cardiac arrest: soft drinks); I. Nielsen and R. S. Pedersen (letter), *ibid.*, 1305 (hypokalaemia and paralysis: confectionery).

Uses and Administration

Liquorice is used as a flavouring and sweetening agent. It has also been used in cough preparations. It has mild anti-inflammatory and mineralocorticoid properties associated with the presence of glycyrrhizin.

Deglycyrrhizinised liquorice has a reduced mineralocorticoid activity and is used in the treatment of peptic ulcer. It appears to act similarly to carbenoxolone by stimulating the production of mucus.

PEPTIC ULCER. A comparative study involving 100 patients with benign gastric ulceration showing that deglycyrrhizinated liquorice plus antacids (as Caved-S) produced a slightly lower (88%), but not significantly different, healing-rate than cimetidine (94%) after treatment for up to 12 weeks. These results confirmed those obtained by the same group of workers in a previous trial (A.G. Morgan *et al.*, *Br. med. J.*, 1978, *2*, 1323) concerning the efficacy of the deglycyrrhizinated liquorice preparation but contrasted with other studies (K.D. Bardhan *et al.*, *Gut*, 1978, *19*, 779) where a different formulation (Ulcedal) was found to be no better than a placebo. It was considered that the difference in formulation produced the conflicting results in published reports and that although the gelatin capsule of the Ulcedal formulation disintegrated within the stomach the liquorice did not break up and disperse, but passed through intact into the small bowel.— A. G. Morgan *et al.*, *Gut*, 1982, *23*, 545. Follow-up demonstrating that maintenance therapy with either deglycyrrhizinated liquorice plus antacids or cimetidine reduced symptomatic ulcer recurrence.— A. G. Morgan *et al.*, *ibid.*, 1985, *26*, 599. Combination therapy with ranitidine and liquorice had no advantage over ranitidine alone in a further study of the treatment of 100 patients.— A. G. Morgan *et al.*, *ibid.*, 1377.

Preparations

Glycyrrhiza Fluidextract *(U.S.N.F.)*. Store at a temperature not exceeding 40° in airtight containers. Protect from light.

Pure Glycyrrhiza Extract *(U.S.N.F.)*

Liquorice Extract *(B.P.C. 1973)*. Extractum Glycyrrhizae. A soft extract prepared by percolation with chloroform water. *Dose*. 0.6 to 2 g.

Liquorice Liquid Extract *(B.P.)*. A water percolate of liquorice, evaporated to a wt per mL of 1.198 g and mixed with a quarter of its volume of alcohol (90%).

Deglycyrrhizinised Liquorice Extract *(B.P.)*. Prepared by extracting powdered liquorice with water, removing glycyrrhizinic acid from the extract, and evaporating to dryness. A 1% solution in water has a pH of 5.0 to 6.5.

Liquorice Lozenges *(B.P.C. 1973)*. Trochisci Glycyrrhizae; Brompton Cough Lozenges. Each lozenge contains liquorice extract 200 mg, anise oil 0.03 mL.

Compound Liquorice Powder *(B.P.C. 1973)*. Pulvis Glycyrrhizae Compositus. Peeled liquorice 16 g, senna leaf 16 g, fennel 8 g, sublimed sulphur 8 g, and sucrose 52 g. *Dose*. 5 to 10 g.

Proprietary Preparations

Caved-S *(Tillotts, UK)*. *Tablets*, chewable, deglycyrrhizinised liquorice 380 mg, aluminium hydroxide 100 mg, magnesium carbonate 200 mg, sodium bicarbonate

100 mg. *Dose.* Gastric ulcer; 2 tablets three times daily; in duodenal ulcer this dose may be increased if necessary to a maximum of 2 tablets 6 times daily.

Rabro *(Sinclair, UK). Tablets,* chewable, deglycyrrhizinised liquorice 400 mg, magnesium oxide 100 mg, calcium carbonate 500 mg, frangula bark 25 mg. *Dose.* 1 or 2 tablets three times daily after meals.

Proprietary Names and Manufacturers

Ammoniated Glycyrrhizin *(MacAndrews & Forbes, UK)*; Glymocone *(Plantier, Fr.)*; Magnasweet *(MacAndrews & Forbes, UK)*; Rucedal *(Neth.)*; Ulcedal *(Boehringer Ingelheim, UK)*.

The following names have been used for multi-ingredient preparations containing liquorice—Caved-S *(Muir & Neil, Austral.; Tillotts, UK)*; Ceduran *(Tillotts, UK)*; Pepsillide *(Cambridge Laboratories, Austral.)*; Rabro *(Sinclair, UK)*.

5235-b

Loperamide Hydrochloride *(BANM, USAN, rINNM).*

R-18553. 4-(4-*p*-Chlorophenyl-4-hydroxypiperidino)-*NN*-dimethyl-2,2-diphenylbutyramide hydrochloride.

$C_{29}H_{33}ClN_2O_2,HCl=513.5$.

CAS — 53179-11-6 (loperamide); 34552-83-5 (hydrochloride).

Pharmacopoeias. In *U.S.*

A white to slightly yellow powder. Slightly **soluble** in water and dilute acids; freely soluble in chloroform, isopropyl alcohol, and methyl alcohol.

Adverse Effects and Treatment

Abdominal pain and other gastro-intestinal disturbances, including toxic megacolon, dry mouth, dizziness, fatigue, and skin rashes have been reported. Depression of the CNS, to which children may be more sensitive, may be seen in overdosage, and naloxone (see p.845) has been recommended in addition to gastric lavage in the management of poisoning.

Toxic megacolon developed in a patient with ulcerative colitis within 3 weeks of beginning treatment with loperamide.— J. W. Brown, *J. Am. med. Ass.*, 1979, *241*, 501.

Opioid toxicity manifested by respiratory depression and coma in a 15-month-old child given a single dose of loperamide 1 mg. Recovery followed resuscitation with oxygen and naloxone intravenously. The child was well hydrated at the time of the incident but did have a low serum-protein concentration and some evidence of liver disturbance; these might have been contributory factors since loperamide is highly protein bound (97%) and is metabolised in the liver.— N. A. Minton and P. G. D. Smith, *Br. med. J.*, 1987, *294*, 1383.

Precautions

Loperamide should be used with caution in patients with hepatic dysfunction because of its considerable first-pass metabolism in the liver. It should also be used with caution in young children because of a greater variability of response in such an age group, and it is not generally recommended for use in infants.

Patients with inflammatory bowel disease receiving loperamide should be carefully observed for signs of toxic megacolon.

Absorption and Fate

Loperamide, following partial absorption in the gastro-intestinal tract, is reported to undergo considerable first-pass metabolism in the liver and to be excreted predominantly in the faeces. The elimination half-life is reported to be about 10 hours.

Uses and Administration

Loperamide inhibits peristalsis and gastro-intestinal secretions and is used in the treatment of some diarrhoeas. It is also used in ileostomy management to control the volume of discharge.

In acute diarrhoea the usual initial dose for adults is 4 mg followed by 2 mg after each loose stool; the usual daily dose is 6 to 8 mg and 16 mg daily should not be exceeded. For children suggested initial doses for the first day of treatment have been: 2 to 5 years (13 to 20 kg body-weight), 3 mg in divided doses; 5 to 8 years (20 to 30 kg), 4 mg in divided doses; and 8 to 12 years (over 30 kg), 6 mg in divided doses. Suggested subsequent doses have been 1 mg per 10 kg body-weight, administered only after a loose stool with the total daily dose not exceeding that given on the first day of treatment. In the *US* loperamide is not recommended for use in children under the age of 2 years; in the *UK* it is not recommended in children under the age of 4 years. If no improvement in acute diarrhoea has been observed after 48 hours, loperamide should be discontinued.

In chronic diarrhoea the usual initial dose for adults is 4 to 8 mg daily in divided doses subsequently adjusted as necessary; the usual daily dose is also 4 to 8 mg and it has been stated that an increase above a total of 16 mg daily is unlikely to produce further benefit.

It should be noted that a consequence of diarrhoea may be fluid and electrolyte depletion, and that rehydration therapy may be necessary, especially in infants and young children. For further details concerning rehydration therapy, see p.1024.

Results of a double-blind, placebo-controlled, multicentre study of loperamide in acute childhood diarrhoea. The study involved 303 patients aged 3 months to 3 years with acute diarrhoea of less than 2 weeks' duration. All children received oral rehydration therapy, 101 received loperamide 400 μg per kg body-weight daily additionally, 102 received loperamide 800 μg per kg daily additionally and 100 received a placebo; drug administration was continued until diarrhoea resolved or for 7 days, whichever was the sooner. The doses of loperamide used, which were approximately two times and four times the usual recommended doses for children, were chosen since lower doses of about 200 μg per kg daily had previously been reported to have no significant advantage over placebo (A.S. Kassem *et al., J. diarrh. Dis. Res.*, 1983, *1*, 10). Comparison of the groups indicated that the recovery of patients treated with the higher dose of loperamide was hastened by about 24 hours over those receiving a placebo and that a larger proportion of children in the 2 loperamide groups had gained weight compared to those in the placebo group. It was noted that the argument against the use of antimotility agents in acute diarrhoea rests on the premise that reduced motility and stasis favour the multiplication of pathogens in the gastro-intestinal tract, which is potentially harmful, but that this study provided no evidence to suggest that such deleterious effects may be associated with the use of loperamide. It was concluded that loperamide is a safe and potentially useful adjunct to oral rehydration in well-nourished children with acute diarrhoea whose response to oral rehydration alone is slow or unsatisfactory. It was emphasised that loperamide cannot be used as a substitute for oral rehydration therapy and that any extrapolation from this study to malnourished populations in developing countries is unwarranted and must be discouraged.— Diarrhoeal Diseases Study Group of the UK, *Br. med. J.*, 1984, *289*, 1263.

A review and discussion on the chemotherapy and chemoprophylaxis of travellers' diarrhoea. It should be remembered that fluids and electrolytes represent the only essential form of therapy for travellers' diarrhoea (as enteric or typhoid fever are rarely encountered) but that several appropriate and effective drugs are available and that therapy with them should be based upon the severity and nature of the illness. Loose bowel movements (1 to 3 unformed stools daily) without important associated symptoms need not be treated with a pharmacologic agent. When illness is more bothersome (3 to 5 unformed stools daily), the associated symptoms are a concern but not disabling to the patient, and there is no fever, toxicity, or dysentery (passage of bloody stools) then loperamide or bismuth salicylate is a reasonable choice. If the diarrhoea is of greater severity, the symptoms are disabling, and fever or dysentery are present, an antimicrobial agent may be necessary.— H. L. DuPont *et al., Ann. intern. Med.*, 1985, *102*, 260. For a favourable report of the use of loperamide or bismuth salicylate in the treatment of acute travellers' diarrhoea, see P. C. Johnson *et al., J. Am. med. Ass.*, 1986, *255*, 757.

Results of a double-blind placebo-controlled study involving 82 patients with acute infectious diarrhoea showed that although a statistically significant reduction in the number of loose stools passed by the loperamide-treated patients occurred, such a difference could hardly be considered a major clinical advantage.— T. Bergström *et al., J. Infect.*, 1986, *12*, 35.

Preparations

Loperamide Hydrochloride Capsules *(U.S.P.)*

Proprietary Preparations

Arret *(Janssen, UK). Capsules,* loperamide hydrochloride 2 mg.
Syrup, loperamide hydrochloride 2 mg/10 mL.

Imodium *(Janssen, UK). Capsules,* loperamide hydrochloride 2 mg.
Syrup, loperamide hydrochloride 2 mg/10 mL.

Proprietary Names and Manufacturers

AMI-29 *(Bonomelli, Ital.)*; Arret *(Janssen, UK)*; Blox *(Biomedica Foscama, Ital.)*; Brek *(IRBI, Ital.)*; Colifilm *(Arg.)*; Dissenten *(SPA, Ital.)*; Elcoman *(Arg.)*; Fortasec *(Esteve, Spain)*; Imodium *(Aust.; Janssen, Austral.; Belg.; Janssen, Canad.; Janssen, Denm.; Janssen, Fr.; Ger.; Janssen, Ital.; Neth.; Janssen, Norw.; Janssen, S.Afr.; Janssen Pharmaceutica, Swed.; Janssen, Switz.; Janssen, UK; Janssen, USA)*; Imosec *(Janssen, Spain)*; Lopemid *(Gentili, Ital.)*; Loperam *(Septa, Spain)*; Loperyl *(Zambeletti, Ital.)*; Orulop *(Morgens, Spain)*; Pricilone *(Cheminova, Spain)*; Regulane *(Arg.)*; Suprasec *(Arg.)*; Taguinol *(Spyfarma, Spain)*; Tebloc *(Dukron, Ital.)*.

695-z

Magaldrate *(BAN, USAN, rINN).*

Aluminum Magnesium Hydroxide Sulfate; AY-5710.

$Al_5Mg_{10}(OH)_{31}(SO_4)_2,xH_2O$.

CAS — 74978-16-8.

Pharmacopoeias. In *Braz.* and *U.S.*

A combination of aluminium and magnesium hydroxides and sulphate. A white odourless crystalline powder. Practically **insoluble** in water and alcohol; soluble in dilute mineral acids.

Magaldrate is an antacid that is given in doses of 0.8 to 1.6 g.

Preparations

Magaldrate Oral Suspension *(U.S.P.)*. Store in airtight containers.

Magaldrate and Simethicone Oral Suspension *(U.S.P.)*. A suspension containing magaldrate and dimethicones. Store in airtight containers. Keep from freezing.

Magaldrate Tablets *(U.S.P.)*. The label states whether they are to be swallowed or chewed.

Magaldrate and Simethicone Tablets *(U.S.P.)*. Tablets containing magaldrate and dimethicones. Store in well-closed containers.

Proprietary Preparations

Dynese *(Galen, UK). Suspension,* magaldrate 800 mg/5 mL.

Proprietary Names and Manufacturers

Dynese *(Galen, UK)*; Riopan *(Ayerst, Canad.; Byk Gulden, Ger.; Ayerst, Ital.; Ayerst, USA)*; Riopone *(Ayerst, S.Afr.)*.

The following names have been used for multi-ingredient preparations containing magaldrate—Antiflux *(Ayerst, Canad.)*; Extra Strength Riopan Plus *(Ayerst, Canad.; Ayerst, USA)*; Riopan Plus *(Ayerst, Canad.; Ayerst, USA)*.

698-a

Magnesium Carbonate *(BAN, USAN).*

504; Magnesii Subcarbonas.

CAS — 546-93-0 (anhydrous); 23389-33-5 (normal, hydrate); 39409-82-0 (basic, hydrate).

Pharmacopoeias. In *Arg., Aust., Belg., Br., Braz., Chin., Cz., Egypt., Eur., Fr., Ger., Hung., Ind., It., Jpn, Jug., Mex., Neth., Nord., Pol., Port., Roum., Rus., Span., Swiss., Turk.,* and *U.S.*. Also in *B.P. Vet.* Some pharmacopoeias include a single monograph which permits both the light and heavy varieties whilst some have 2 separate monographs for the 2 varieties.

Heavy Magnesium Carbonate (*B.P., Eur. P.*) and Light Magnesium Carbonate (*B.P., Eur. P., B.P. Vet.*) are hydrated basic magnesium carbonates containing the equivalent of 40 to 45% of MgO. Both are white odourless powders and are practically **insoluble** in water but dissolve in dilute acids with strong effervescence. For the heavy variety 15 g occupies a volume of about 30 mL and for the light variety 15 g occupies a volume of about 180 mL.

Magnesium Carbonate (*U.S.P.*) is a basic hydrated magnesium carbonate or a normal hydrated magnesium carbonate containing the equivalent of 40.0 to 43.5% of MgO. It is a bulky white powder or light, white, friable masses. Practically **insoluble** in water and alcohol; soluble in dilute acids with effervescence.

Adverse Effects, Treatment, and Precautions

Magnesium carbonate in common with other magnesium salts may cause diarrhoea. The release of carbon dioxide in the stomach may cause discomfort.

If renal function is impaired hypermagnesaemia may result producing the adverse effects described under Magnesium, p.1032; such adverse effects may be treated by the intravenous administration of calcium salts as described on p.1033.

Magnesium carbonate in common with other magnesium salts may interfere with the absorption of other drugs when these are taken concomitantly.

Absorption and Fate

Magnesium carbonate is converted to magnesium chloride and carbon dioxide in the stomach. In the intestine, magnesium salts act as saline laxatives; they are more soluble at intestinal pH than calcium salts. Any absorbed magnesium is usually excreted rapidly in the urine.

Uses and Administration

Magnesium carbonate is an antacid that is given in doses of up to about 1 g.

Magnesium carbonate also possesses laxative properties and is often given in conjunction with aluminium-containing antacids such as aluminium hydroxide in order to reduce their constipating effects. It has also been given as a laxative in doses of up to 5 g.

Magnesium carbonate is also used as a food additive.

PHOSPHATE BINDING. For the use of magnesium carbonate as a phosphate-binder in patients with chronic renal failure, see under aluminium hydroxide (p.1076).

Preparations

Aromatic Magnesium Carbonate Mixture *(B.P.)*. Aromatic Magnesium Carbonate Oral Suspension. A suspension containing light magnesium carbonate 3%, sodium bicarbonate 5%, and aromatic cardamom tincture. Extemporaneous preparations should be recently prepared according to the following formula: light magnesium carbonate 300 mg, sodium bicarbonate 500 mg, aromatic cardamom tincture 0.3 mL, double-strength chloroform water 5 mL, water to 10 mL.

Magnesium Carbonate Mixture *(B.P.C. 1973)*. Light magnesium carbonate 500 mg, sodium bicarbonate 800 mg, concentrated peppermint emulsion 0.25 mL, double-strength chloroform water 5 mL, water to 10 mL. It should be recently prepared. *Dose.* 10 to 20 mL.

Magnesium Carbonate and Sodium Bicarbonate for Oral Suspension *(U.S.P.)*. Store in airtight containers.

Compound Magnesium Carbonate Powder *(B.P.C. 1973)*. Heavy magnesium carbonate 4, calcium carbonate 4, sodium bicarbonate 3, and light kaolin or light kaolin (natural) 1. *Dose.* 1 to 5 g.

Compound Magnesium Carbonate Tablets *(B.P.C. 1973)*. Chewable tablets containing heavy magnesium carbonate 200 mg, calcium carbonate 200 mg, sodium bicarbonate 120 mg, light kaolin or light kaolin (natural) 60 mg, ginger 60 mg, and peppermint oil 0.006 mL. *Dose.* 1 or 2 tablets.

Proprietary Preparations

Actonorm *(Wallace Mfg Chem., UK)*. *Oral powder*, magnesium carbonate 300 mg, dried aluminium hydroxide 56 mg, atropine sulphate 100 µg, calcium carbonate 145 mg, light kaolin 50 mg, magnesium trisilicate 50 mg, sodium bicarbonate 373 mg, thiamine hydrochloride 1 mg/g. *Dose.* One 5-mL spoonful of powder in liquid after meals and at bedtime.

For Actonorm Gel see under Aluminium Hydroxide.

APP Stomach Preparations *(Consolidated Chemicals, UK)*. *Tablets*, magnesium carbonate 195 mg, magnesium trisilicate 92.5 mg, dried aluminium hydroxide 15 mg, bismuth carbonate 12.5 mg, calcium carbonate 180.5 mg, papaverine hydrochloride 3 mg, homatropine methobromide 1.5 mg.

Oral powder, magnesium carbonate 37.5%, magnesium trisilicate 19.48%, dried aluminium hydroxide 3%, bismuth carbonate 2%, calcium carbonate 37.82%, papaverine hydrochloride 0.1%, homatropine methobromide 0.1%. *Dose.* 1 or 2 tablets after meals or one 5-mL spoonful of powder in water or milk three or four times daily.

Some other proprietary preparations containing magnesium carbonate are described under Aluminium Glycinate, Aluminium Hydroxide, Aluminium Hydroxide-Magnesium Carbonate Co-dried Gel, and Magnesium Trisilicate.

Proprietary Names and Manufacturers

Palmicol *(Neda, Ger.)*.

The following names have been used for multi-ingredient preparations containing magnesium carbonate—Actonorm *(Wallace Mfg Chem., UK)*; Algicon *(Rorer, Canad.*; *Rorer, UK*; *Rorer, USA)*; APP Stomach Preparations *(Consolidated Chemicals, UK)*; Bellocarb *(Sinclair, UK)*; Caved-S *(Muir & Neil, Austral.*; *Tillotts, UK)*; Gastrobrom *(Fawns & McAllan, Austral.)*; Gaviscon Liquid *(Marion Laboratories, USA)*; Nulacin *(Bencard, UK)*; Pepsillide *(Cambridge Laboratories, Austral.)*; Pep-Uls-Ade *(Cambridge Laboratories, Austral.)*; Prodexin *(Bencard, UK)*; Roter *(Four Macs, Austral.*; *Anglo-French Laboratories, Canad.*; *Roterpharma, UK)*; Topal *(ICI Pharmaceuticals, UK)*; Triscal *(Nicholas, UK)*; Uro-Tainer Solution R *(Vifor, Switz. : CliniMed, UK)*.

1173-x

Magnesium Citrate

$C_{12}H_{10}Mg_3O_{14}$=451.1.

CAS — 3344-18-1.

Magnesium citrate is used, usually in the form of Magnesium Citrate Oral Solution *U.S.P.* and in a dose of about 280 mL, as a bowel evacuant prior to radiological examination of the colon. A high fluid intake and low residue diet are needed in conjunction with such bowel preparation.

For the general properties of magnesium salts, see p.1032.

Preparations

Magnesium Citrate Oral Solution *(U.S.P.)*. Prepared by dissolving magnesium carbonate 15 g in a solution of anhydrous citric acid 27.4 g (or the equivalent amount of citric acid monohydrate) in water, adding syrup 60 mL, heating to boiling-point, adding lemon oil 0.1 mL previously triturated with talc 5 g, and filtering while hot. The mixture is cooled, diluted to 350 mL, and potassium bicarbonate 2.5 g or if citric acid monohydrate is used sodium bicarbonate 2.1 g added. The container is immediately stoppered and shaken; the solution may be further carbonated by the use of carbon dioxide under pressure. The solution is sterilised or pasteurised. Store at 8° to 30°.

Proprietary Names and Manufacturers

Citro-Mag *(Rougier, Canad.)*; Evac-Q-Kwik Solution *(Adria, Canad.)*; Evac-Q-Mag *(Adria, USA)*; National Laxative *(Therapex, Canad.)*.

The following names have been used for multi-ingredient preparations containing magnesium citrate— Picolax *(Ferring, UK)*; Royvac *(Roy, Canad.)*.

699-t

Magnesium Hydroxide *(BAN, USAN)*.

528; Magnesii Hydroxidum.

$Mg(OH)_2$=58.32.

CAS — 1309-42-8.

Pharmacopoeias. In *Arg., Belg., Br., Eur., Fr., It., Neth., Span., Swiss,* and *U.S.*

A fine, white, amorphous, odourless, powder. Practically **insoluble** in water, alcohol, chloroform, and ether; dissolves in dilute acids. A solution in water is alkaline to phenolphthalein. **Store** in airtight containers.

Adverse Effects, Treatment, and Precautions

As for Magnesium Carbonate (above), but without the side-effects associated with carbon dioxide release.

For reports of metabolic alkalosis associated with the concomitant administration of sodium polystyrene sulphonate and magnesium hydroxide, see Sodium Polystyrene Sulphonate, p.854.

Uses and Administration

Magnesium hydroxide is an antacid that is given in doses of up to about 800 mg.

Magnesium hydroxide also possesses laxative properties and is often given in conjunction with aluminium-containing antacids such as aluminium hydroxide in order to reduce their constipating effects. It is also given as a laxative in doses of 2 to 4 g.

Magnesium hydroxide is also used as a food additive.

Preparations

Magnesia and Alumina Oral Suspension *(U.S.P.)*. A mixture containing aluminium hydroxide [$Al(OH)_3$] and magnesium hydroxide in equal amounts, or with magnesium hydroxide predominating. pH 7.3 to 8.5.

See also Alumina and Magnesia Oral Suspension under Aluminium Hydroxide.

Magnesium Hydroxide Mixture *(B.P.)*. Cream of Magnesia; Magnesium Hydroxide Oral Suspension. An aqueous suspension of hydrated magnesium oxide. Extemporaneous preparations should be prepared according to the following formula: magnesium sulphate 475 mg, sodium hydroxide 150 mg, light magnesium oxide 525 mg, chloroform 0.025 mL, water to 10 mL. It contains the equivalent of about 550 mg of MgO in 10 mL. It should not be stored in a cold place.

Milk of Magnesia *(U.S.P.)*. A suspension containing magnesium hydroxide 7.0 to 8.5% w/w; Double-strength Milk of Magnesia contains 14.0 to 17.0% w/w of magnesium hydroxide and Triple-strength Milk of Magnesia contains 21.0 to 25.5% w/w of magnesium hydroxide. Store at a temperature not exceeding 35° in airtight containers; avoid freezing.

NOTE. In Great Britain the name Milk of Magnesia is a trade-mark.

In some other countries Phillips' Milk of Magnesia is a trade-mark.

Magnesium Hydroxide Paste *(U.S.P.)*

Magnesia and Alumina Tablets *(U.S.P.)*. Tablets containing magnesium hydroxide and aluminium hydroxide [$Al(OH)_3$].

See also Alumina and Magnesia Tablets under Aluminium Hydroxide.

Magnesia Tablets *(U.S.P.)*. Tablets containing magnesium hydroxide.

Proprietary Preparations

Some proprietary preparations containing magnesium hydroxide are described under Aluminium Hydroxide and Aluminium Hydroxide-Magnesium Carbonate Co-dried Gel.

Proprietary Names and Manufacturers

Aquamag *(Chemical & Insulating Co., UK)*; Chlorumagène *(Thepenier, Fr.*; *Switz.)*; Citrato Espresso S. Pellegrino *(Granelli, Ital.)*; Emgesan *(Ferrosan, Swed.)*; Mablet *(Gunnar Kjems, Denm.)*; Magnesia S. Pellegrino *(Granelli, Ital.)*; Magnesia Volta *(Edmond Pharma, Ital.)*; Phillips' Magnesia Tablets *(Sterling, Canad.)*; Phillips' Milk of Magnesia *(Sterling, Canad.*; *Glenbrook, USA)*.

The following names have been used for multi-ingredient preparations containing magnesium hydroxide—Actonorm Gel *(Wallace Mfg Chem., UK)*; Actonorm-Sed *(Wallace Mfg Chem., UK)*; Alma-Mag No. 4 *(Rugby, USA)*; Alucone *(Drug Houses Austral., Austral.)*; Aludrox *(Wyeth, Austral.*; *Wyeth, UK*; *Wyeth, USA)*; Aludrox SA *(Wyeth, UK)*; Alumag *(Trianon, Canad.)*; Amphojel 500 *(Wyeth, Canad.)*; Amphojel Plus *(Wyeth, Canad.)*; Ancatropine Gel *(Anca, Canad.)*; Ancatropine Gel Plain *(Anca, Canad.)*; Andursil Suspension *(Geigy, UK)*; Antacid Plus *(Clark, Canad.)*; Antasil *(Stuart, UK)*; Carbellon *(Torbet Laboratories, UK)*; Celluka *(Bio-Chemical Laboratory, Canad.)*; Dijene Liquid *(Boots, Austral.)*; Dijex *(Crookes Heal-*

thcare, UK); Diovol Ex *(Horner, Canad.)*; Diovol Suspension *(Horner, Canad.; Pharmax, UK)*; Diovol Tablets *(Horner, Canad.; Pharmax, UK)*; Duoquel *(Wellcome, Austral.)*; Gastrobrom *(Fawns & McAllan, Austral.)*; Gastrogel *(Fawns & McAllan, Austral.)*; Gelusil *(Warner, Austral.; Parke, Davis, Canad.; Parke, Davis, USA)*; LoAsid *(Calmic, UK)*; Maalox *(Rorer, Canad.; Rorer, UK; Rorer, USA)*; Maalox Plus *(Rorer, Canad.; Rorer, UK)*; Maalox TC *(Rorer, UK)*; Magnolax *(Wampole, Canad.)*; Merasyn *(Merrell Dow, Austral.)*; Mucaine *(Wyeth, Austral.; Wyeth, Canad.; Wyeth, UK)*; Mucogel *(Pharmax, UK)*; Mucoxin; Mutesa; Muthesa; Mygel *(Geneva, USA)*; Mylanta *(Parke, Davis, Austral.; Parke, Davis, Canad.; Parke, Davis, UK; Stuart Pharmaceuticals, USA)*; Neo-Tropine Alkaline *(Neolab, Canad.)*; Neutralca-S *(Desbergers, Canad.)*; Oxaine; Polycrol Gel *(Nicholas, UK)*; Polycrol Tablets *(Nicholas, UK)*; Regacid *(Riva, Canad.)*; Simeco Suspension *(Wyeth, Austral.; Wyeth, UK; Wyeth, USA)*; Simeco Tablets *(Wyeth, UK)*; Sodexol *(Schering, Austral.)*; Stomachic Dellipsoids D20 *(Pilsworth, UK)*; Tepilta; Univol *(Horner, Canad.)*.

702-r

Magnesium Oxide *(BAN, USAN)*.

530.

MgO=40.30.

CAS — 1309-48-4.

Pharmacopoeias. In *Arg., Aust., Belg., Br., Chin., Cz., Egypt., Eur., Fr., Ger., Hung., Ind., It., Jpn, Jug., Mex., Neth., Nord., Pol., Port., Roum., Rus., Span., Swiss., Turk.,* and *U.S.* Some pharmacopoeias include a single monograph which permits both the light and heavy varieties whilst some have 2 separate monographs for the 2 varieties.

Heavy Magnesium Oxide (*B.P., Eur. P.*) and Light Magnesium Oxide (*B.P., Eur. P.*) (Light Magnesia) are fine white odourless powders and are practically **insoluble** in water but dissolve in dilute acids with at most slight effervescence. For the heavy variety 15 g occupies a volume of about 30 mL and for the light variety 20 g occupies a volume of about 150 mL. They both produce solutions in water which are alkaline to phenolphthalein. **Store** in well-closed containers.

Magnesium Oxide (*U.S.P.*) is either the heavy or light variety. Heavy magnesium oxide is a relatively dense white powder with 5 g occupying a volume of about 10 to 20 mL and light magnesium oxide is a very bulky white powder with 5 g occupying a volume of about 40 to 50 mL. Both varieties are practically **insoluble** in water and alcohol but soluble in dilute acids. **Store** in airtight containers.

Adverse Effects, Treatment, and Precautions

As for Magnesium Carbonate (above), but without the side-effects associated with carbon dioxide release.

In Great Britain the recommended exposure limit of magnesium oxide fume (as Mg) is 10 mg per m^3 (long-term).

Uses and Administration

Magnesium oxide is an antacid that is given in doses of up to about 500 mg.

Magnesium oxide also possesses laxative properties and is often given in conjunction with aluminium-containing antacids such as aluminium hydroxide in order to reduce their constipating effects. It has also been given as a laxative in doses of up to 5 g.

Magnesium oxide is also used as a food additive.

Reports of the use of magnesium salts given by mouth for the treatment of recurrent renal calcium stones: I. Melnick *et al., J. Urol., Baltimore,* 1971, *105,* 119 (magnesium oxide); G. Johansson *et al., ibid.,* 1980, *124,* 770 (magnesium hydroxide).

Preparations

Magnesium Oxide Capsules *(U.S.P.)*

Magnesium Oxide Tablets *(U.S.P.)*

Proprietary Preparations

Some proprietary preparations containing magnesium oxide are described under Aluminium Hydroxide and Magnesium Trisilicate.

Proprietary Names and Manufacturers

Magnesias Pellegrino *(Gamaprod, Austral.)*; Magnetrans *(Fresenius, Ger.)*; Mag-Ox 400 *(Blaine, USA)*; Oxabid *(Pharmacare, USA)*; Salilax *(Erco, Denm.; Erco, Swed.)*; Uro-Mag *(Blaine, USA)*.

The following names have been used for multi-ingredient preparations containing magnesium oxide—Artéchol *(Anglo-French Laboratories, Canad.)*; Asilone Gel *(Rorer, UK)*; Asilone for Infants *(Rorer, UK)*; Asilone Suspension *(USV, Austral.; Rorer, UK)*; Beelith *(Beach, USA)*; Diloran *(Lipha, UK)*; Kolanticon *(Merrell, UK)*; Kolantyl *(Merrell Dow, Austral.; Merrell, UK)*; Nulacin *(Bencard, UK)*; Polyalk Revised Formula *(Galen, UK)*; Rabro *(Sinclair, UK)*; Siloxyl Suspension *(Martindale Pharmaceuticals, UK)*; Sylopal *(Norton, UK)*; Uro-Tainer Suby G *(Vifor, Switz.: CliniMed, UK)*.

703-f

Magnesium Phosphate *(USAN)*.

Tribasic Magnesium Phosphate; Trimagnesium Phosphate.

$Mg_3(PO_4)_2,5H_2O$=352.9.

CAS — 7757-87-1 (anhydrous); 10233-87-1 (pentahydrate).

Pharmacopoeias. In *U.S.*

A white odourless tasteless powder. Practically **insoluble** in water; readily soluble in dilute mineral acids.

Magnesium phosphate is an antacid that has been used in doses of up to 4 g.

704-d

Magnesium Trisilicate *(BAN, USAN)*.

553(a); Magnesii Trisilicas; Magnesium Silicate; Magnesium Trisilicate Oral Powder; Magnesium Trisilicate Powder.

CAS — 14987-04-3 (anhydrous); 39365-87-2 (hydrate).

Pharmacopoeias. In *Arg., Aust., Br., Braz., Chin., Cz., Egypt., Eur., Fr., Ger., Hung., Ind., It., Jpn, Jug., Mex., Neth., Nord., Rus., Span., Swiss, Turk.,* and *U.S.*

A hydrated magnesium silicate corresponding approximately to the formula $2MgO,3SiO_2$, with water of crystallisation. An odourless, white powder free from gritty particles.

Practically **insoluble** in water and alcohol. It is readily decomposed by mineral acids. **Store** in well-closed containers.

Adverse Effects, Treatment, and Precautions

As for Magnesium Carbonate (above), but without the side-effects associated with carbon dioxide release.

A 68-year-old man with a history of renal calculus passed a 300-mg stone which was found to consist chiefly of silicon dioxide. He had been taking the equivalent of 2 g of magnesium trisilicate daily for many years.— A. M. Joekes *et al., Br. med. J.,* 1973, *1,* 146.

Absorption and Fate

Magnesium chloride and hydrated silica gel are formed during neutralisation. About 5% of the magnesium is absorbed and traces of the liberated silica may be absorbed and excreted in the urine.

Uses and Administration

Magnesium trisilicate is an antacid that is given in doses of up to about 2 g. The antacid action is exerted slowly, so that it does not give such rapid symptomatic relief as the alkali carbonates, bicarbonates, and oxides; however, the action is prolonged.

ASPIRATION SYNDROME. Antacids were recommended before surgery especially in obstetrics to raise the pH of any stomach contents. Aspiration would not be prevented but the dangers might be reduced by the aspirate being of reduced acidity and the acid-aspiration syndrome might be prevented. In obstetrics a dose of 15 mL of Magnesium Trisilicate Mixture was recommended by J.S. Crawford (*Practitioner,* 1974, *212,* 677; see also J.D. Holdsworth *et al., Br. J. Anaesth.,* 1977, *49,* 520); this should be given every 2 hours from the time of admission until completion of the third stage of labour. Associated with this is the application of cricoid pressure before induction. There have, however, been several reports of the acid-aspiration syndrome occurring in patients despite the fact that they were given antacids (G. Taylor, *Br. J. Anaesth.,* 1975, *47,* 615; G.A.H. Heaney and H.D. Jones, *ibid.,* 1979, *51,* 266; R.M. Whittington *et al., Lancet,* 1979, *2,* 228). Although some of the patients had not been treated according to the above recommendations there was a plea that the technique should be reappraised (R.M. Whittington *et al., Lancet,* 1979, *2,* 630). Commenting on a report into maternal deaths F. Reynolds (*Anaesthesia,* 1983, *38,* 391) stated a personal opinion that the use of antacids in labour is not associated with a reduction in death-rate and that the aim should be to keep the stomach empty.

Preparations

Magnesium Trisilicate Mixture *(B.P.)*. Compound Magnesium Trisilicate Mixture; Magnesium Trisilicate Oral Suspension. A peppermint-flavoured suspension containing 5% of each of magnesium trisilicate, light magnesium carbonate, and sodium bicarbonate. Extemporaneous preparations should be recently prepared according to the following formula: magnesium trisilicate 500 mg, light magnesium carbonate 500 mg, sodium bicarbonate 500 mg, concentrated peppermint emulsion 0.25 mL, double-strength chloroform water 5 mL, water to 10 mL.

Magnesium Trisilicate Mixture *(A.P.F.)*. Magnesium trisilicate 1 g, calcium carbonate 500 mg, light magnesium carbonate 500 mg, concentrated peppermint water 0.25 mL, concentrated chloroform water 0.25 mL or compound hydroxybenzoate solution 0.1 mL, water to 10 mL. *Dose.* 10 to 20 mL.

Magnesium Trisilicate and Belladonna Mixture *(B.P.C. 1973)*. Belladonna tincture 0.5 mL, magnesium trisilicate mixture to 10 mL. It must be freshly prepared. *Dose.* 10 to 20 mL.

Compound Magnesium Trisilicate Oral Powder *(B.P.)*. Compound Magnesium Trisilicate Powder. Equal parts of magnesium trisilicate, heavy magnesium carbonate, chalk, and sodium bicarbonate.

Compound Magnesium Trisilicate Tablets *(B.P.)*. Aluminium Hydroxide and Magnesium Trisilicate Tablets. Chewable tablets with a peppermint flavour containing magnesium trisilicate 250 mg and dried aluminium hydroxide 120 mg.

Magnesium Trisilicate Tablets *(U.S.P.)*

Proprietary Preparations

Alka-Donna *(Carlton Laboratories, UK)*. *Tablets,* magnesium trisilicate 500 mg, dried aluminium hydroxide 250 mg, belladonna alkaloids (calculated as hyoscyamine) 8 mg.

Suspension, magnesium trisilicate 342.5 mg, aluminium hydroxide mixture 2.15 mL, belladonna alkaloids (calculated as hyoscyamine) 60 µg/5mL. *Dose.* 1 or 2 tablets sucked slowly before meals, or 5 to 10 mL of suspension between meals.

Alka-Donna P *(Carlton Laboratories, UK)*. *Tablets,* magnesium trisilicate 500 mg, dried aluminium hydroxide 250 mg, belladonna dry extract 8 mg, phenobarbitone 8 mg.

Mixture, magnesium trisilicate 342.5 mg, aluminium hydroxide mixture 2.15 mL, belladonna tincture 0.2 mL, phenobarbitone 8 mg/5 mL. *Dose.* 1 or 2 tablets sucked slowly before meals or 5 to 10 mL of mixture three times daily.

Nulacin *(Bencard, UK)*. *Tablets,* chewable, magnesium trisilicate 230 mg, heavy magnesium oxide 130 mg, calcium carbonate 130 mg, magnesium carbonate 30 mg, with dextrins, maltose, and peppermint oil. *Dose.* 1 or more tablets as required.

Some other proprietary preparations containing magnesium trisilicate are described under Alexitol Sodium, Aluminium Hydroxide, and Magnesium Carbonate.

Proprietary Names and Manufacturers
Gastrobin *(Divapharma, Ger.)*; Mabosil *(Mabo, Spain)*; Magnesiumsilikat *(Denm.)*; Magsorbent *(Dendron, UK)*; Rolo *(Ger.)*; Silimag *(Faes, Spain)*; Trisil *(Austral.)*; Trisillac *(Philip Harris, UK)*.

The following names have been used for multi-ingredient preparations containing magnesium trisilicate—Abacid Plus *(Ticen, Eire)*; Actonorm *(Wallace Mfg Chem., UK)*; Alka Butazolidin *(Geigy, Canad.)*; Alkabutazone *(ICN, Canad.)*; Alka-Donna *(Carlton Laboratories, UK)*; Alka-Donna P *(Carlton Laboratories, UK)*; Alka-phenylbutazone *(Pro Doc, Canad.)*; Aluhyde *(Sinclair, UK)*; APP Stomach Preparations *(Consolidated Chemicals, UK)*; Ascon *(Cox, UK)*; Bellocarb *(Sinclair, UK)*; Droxalin *(Sterling Health, UK)*; Gastreze *(Key, Austral.)*; Gastrobrom *(Fawns & McAllan, Austral.)*; Gastrocote *(MCP Pharmaceuticals, UK)*; Gastrogel *(Fawns & McAllan, Austral.)*; Gastron *(Winthrop, UK)*; Gavigrans *(Reckitt & Colman, Austral.)*; Gaviscon Granules *(Reckitt & Colman, Austral.)*; Gaviscon Infant Preparations *(Reckitt & Colman, Austral.; Reckitt & Colman Pharmaceuticals, UK)*; Gaviscon Tablets *(Reckitt & Colman, Austral.; Winthrop, Canad.; Reckitt & Colman Pharmaceuticals, UK; Marion Laboratories, USA)*; Gelusil *(Warner-Lambert, UK)*; Glycinal *(Medo, UK)*; Meracote *(Merrell Dow, Austral.)*; Neutrolactis *(Sandoz, UK)*; Nulacin *(Bencard, UK)*; Phenylone Plus *(Medic, Canad.)*; Pyrogastrone Tablets *(Winthrop, UK)*.

604-t

Manna

Manne en Larmes.

Pharmacopoeias. In *Aust., Fr., Port.,* and *Span. It.* and *Port.* permit other *Fraxinus* species.

The dried exudation from the stems of the European flowering ash, *Fraxinus ornus* (Oleaceae), containing mannitol.

Manna has been used as a laxative.

5236-v

Mebeverine Hydrochloride *(BANM, USAN, pINNM).*

CSAG-144. 4-[Ethyl(4-methoxy-α-methylphenethyl)amino]butyl veratrate hydrochloride.
$C_{25}H_{35}NO_5,HCl=466.0$.

CAS — 3625-06-7 (mebeverine); 2753-45-9 (hydrochloride).

Pharmacopoeias. In *Br.*

A white or almost white crystalline powder. Very **soluble** in water; freely soluble in alcohol; practically insoluble in ether. A 2% solution in water has a pH of 4.5 to 6.5. **Store** in airtight containers at a temperature not exceeding 30°. Protect from light.

Mebeverine hydrochloride is used as a gastro-intestinal antispasmodic in conditions such as the irritable bowel syndrome in doses of 135 mg three times daily before meals. The embonate is also used in a dose equivalent to 150 mg of the hydrochloride.

Preparations

Mebeverine Tablets *(B.P.)*. Coated tablets containing mebeverine hydrochloride.

Proprietary Preparations

Colofac *(Duphar, UK). Tablets,* mebeverine hydrochloride 135 mg.
Oral Liquid, mebeverine hydrochloride 50 mg (as embonate)/5 mL.

Proprietary Names and Manufacturers of Mebeverine Salts
Colofac *(Cilag, Austral.; Duphar, S.Afr.; Duphar, UK)*; Duspatal *(Duphar, Ger.)*; Duspatalin *(Belg.; Ferrosan, Denm.; Duphar, Fr.; S.Afr.; Kali-Farma, Spain; Duphar, Switz.)*.

The following names have been used for multi-ingredient preparations containing mebeverine salts— Colven *(Reckitt & Colman Pharmaceuticals, UK)*.

16887-a

Mesalazine *(BAN, rINN).*

5-Aminosalicylic Acid; 5-ASA; Fisalamine; Mesalamine *(USAN)*. 5-Amino-2-salicylic acid.
$C_7H_7NO_3=153.1$.

CAS — 89-57-6.

NOTE. Distinguish from 4-aminosalicylic acid (Aminosalicylic Acid, p.554) which is used in the treatment of tuberculosis.

Adverse Effects and Precautions

The side-effects experienced by patients taking sulphasalazine are generally not manifested when the patients are transferred to mesalazine therapy although headache or gastro-intestinal disturbances, such as nausea, diarrhoea, and abdominal pain, may occasionally occur. Patients who experience exacerbation of symptoms of colitis with sulphasalazine may also do so with mesalazine. Unlike sulphasalazine, mesalazine has not been associated with reports of adverse haematological effects or with reports of altered sperm counts or function.

It has been recommended that mesalazine should not be given to patients with impaired renal function and should be used with caution in the elderly.

Preparations in which the formulation is designed to release mesalazine in the colon should not be given with lactulose or similar drugs which lower pH thereby preventing the release of mesalazine.

Of 35 patients unable to tolerate therapy with sulphasalazine because of allergy (rashes, haemolytic anaemia, fever, allergic fibrosing alveolitis) or other adverse reactions (headache, nausea and vomiting, feelings of unreality), 32 took mesalazine without side-effects of any kind; the other 3 patients had side-effects identical to those previously encountered with sulphasalazine.— M. J. Dew *et al.* (letter), *Lancet,* 1983, *2,* 801. Similar reports.— C. A. Austin *et al.* (letter), *ibid.,* 1984, *1,* 917; I. P. Donald and S. P. Wilkinson, *Postgrad. med. J.,* 1985, *61,* 1047.

EFFECTS ON THE BLOOD. A report of pure red-cell aplasia in a patient after treatment with sulphasalazine who, after recovery, received mesalazine without incident.— P. M. Anttila *et al.* (letter), *Lancet,* 1985, *2,* 1006.

EFFECTS ON FERTILITY. Pregnancy occurred in the wife of a 33-year-old man within 2 months of his treatment for ulcerative colitis being changed from sulphasalazine to mesalazine; the wife had failed to conceive during the previous 2 years when the patient was receiving sulphasalazine. The patient also noted that his semen and urine had always been stained yellow while he was taking sulphasalazine but cleared within 2 days of his taking mesalazine.— P. A. Cann and C. D. Holdsworth (letter), *Lancet,* 1984, *1,* 1119. A similar report.— J. L. Shaffer *et al.* (letter), *ibid.,* 1240.

EFFECTS ON THE HAIR. Accelerated hair loss from the scalp in 2 patients receiving mesalazine enemas.— P. K. Kutty *et al.* (letter), *Ann. intern. Med.,* 1982, *97,* 785. A comment that patients with severe inflammatory bowel disease are likely to develop a certain type of hair loss which may be unrelated to drug therapy.— W. H. C. Burgdorf and D. A. Weigand (letter), *ibid.,* 1983, *98,* 419.

EFFECTS ON THE KIDNEY. A report of the nephrotic syndrome developing in one patient after 5 months of therapy with mesalazine.— B. H. Novis *et al., Br. med. J.,* 1988, *296,* 1442.

Absorption and Fate

Oral preparations of mesalazine for use in patients with ulcerative colitis are generally formulated so that the mesalazine is released in the terminal ileum and colon, where partial absorption occurs. Since plasma concentrations at steady-state are relatively low, it is considered that only a proportion of mesalazine is absorbed and available to the systemic circulation and that the mode of action of mesalazine is local rather than systemic. Acetylation, which is not subject to genetic control and is not reversible, occurs in the gastro-intestinal wall during absorption and also in the liver. The acetylated metabolite, which has been reported by some, but not all, workers to be active, is predominantly excreted in the urine. Although mesalazine itself is reported to have a short half-life (about 1 hour) and to be slightly bound to plasma proteins (about 40%) the acetylated metabolite is reported to have a much longer half-life (about 5 to 10 hours) and to be more extensively bound (about 80%).

It has been stated that only negligible quantities of mesalazine cross the placenta and that following therapy with sulphasalazine, no mesalazine is excreted in breast milk.

The clinical pharmacokinetics of mesalazine.— U. Klotz, *Clin. Pharmacokinet.,* 1985, *10,* 285.

Uses and Administration

Mesalazine is a component of sulphasalazine, the latter being broken down into 5-aminosalicylic acid (mesalazine) and sulphapyridine by bacteria in the colon. Sulphasalazine has been widely used in ulcerative colitis and Crohn's disease and in rheumatoid arthritis; mesalazine is considered to be the active moiety in ulcerative colitis, but not however in rheumatoid arthritis.

Mesalazine is used for the maintenance of remission of ulcerative colitis in patients unable to tolerate sulphasalazine. The usual dose, by mouth, is 1.2 to 2.4 g daily in divided doses.

A review of the actions and uses of mesalazine.— *Drug & Ther. Bull.,* 1986, *24,* 38.

In a double-blind study in 67 patients in remission with ulcerative colitis mesalazine (minimum dose 1.2 g daily as tablets coated with an acrylic-based resin) was as effective as sulphasalazine (minimum dose 2 g daily), the drug reported to be the most effective agent for maintaining remission but limited in use by its side-effects.— M. J. Dew *et al., Br. med. J.,* 1982, *285,* 1012. In a further study involving some of the previously investigated patients and some new entrants higher doses of mesalazine (mean dose 2.7 g daily; range 2.4 to 4.4 g daily) were as effective, but not more so, than conventional doses of sulphasalazine (mean dose 2.3 g daily; range 2 to 4 g daily). It was considered that the higher doses of mesalazine had no real advantage over the lower doses of 1.2 g previously used but might possibly be of value in the treatment of acute colitis.— M. J. Dew *et al., ibid.,* 1983, *287,* 23.

Encouraging results with enemas of mesalazine in patients with ulcerative colitis.— M. Campieri *et al.* (letter), *Lancet,* 1984, *1,* 403.

Proprietary Preparations

Asacol *(Smith Kline & French, UK). Tablets,* coated with an acrylic-based resin to ensure release in the terminal ileum and colon, mesalazine 400 mg.

Proprietary Names and Manufacturers
Asacol *(Norwich-Eaton, Canad.; Permamed, Switz.; Smith Kline & French, UK)*; Asacolitin *(Röhm, Ger.)*; Claversal *(Smith Kline Dauelsberg, Ger.)*; Pentasa *(Ferring, Denm.)*; Salofalk *(Interfalk, Canad.; Falk, Ger.; Falk, Switz.)*.

6541-f

Metoclopramide Hydrochloride *(BANM, USAN, rINNM).*

AHR-3070-C; DEL-1267; MK-745. 4-Amino-5-chloro-*N*-(2-diethylaminoethyl)-2-methoxybenzamide hydrochloride monohydrate.
$C_{14}H_{22}ClN_3O_2,HCl,H_2O=354.3$.

CAS — 364-62-5 (metoclopramide); 7232-21-5 (hydrochloride, anhydrous); 54143-57-6 (hydrochloride, monohydrate); 2576-84-3 (dihydrochloride, anhydrous).

Pharmacopoeias. In *Br., Fr., It., Swiss,* and *U.S. Chin.* and *Jpn* include anhydrous metoclopramide. *Cz.* and *Roum.* include anhydrous metoclopramide hydrochloride.

A white or almost white, odourless or almost odourless, crystalline powder. Metoclopramide hydrochloride 10.5 mg is approximately equivalent to 10.0 mg of the anhydrous substance which is approximately equivalent to 8.9 mg of the anhydrous base. **Soluble** 1 in 0.7 of water, 1 in 3 of alcohol, and 1 in 55 of chloroform; practically insoluble in ether. A 10% solution in water has a pH of 4.5 to 6.5; the *B.P.* injection of metoclopramide hydrochloride has a pH of 3.0 to 5.0; the *U.S.P.* injection of metoclopramide hydrochloride has a pH of 2.5 to 6.5. Solutions for injection may be **sterilised** by autoclaving. **Store** in airtight containers. Protect from light.

Some proprietary preparations of metoclopramide have been reported to be **incompatible** with cephalothin sodium, chloramphenicol sodium succinate, and sodium bicarbonate. Other drugs which may be incompatible include ampicillin sodium, benzylpenicillin potassium, calcium gluconate, cisplatin, erythromycin lactobionate, methotrexate sodium, and tetracycline hydrochloride.

Adverse Effects

Metoclopramide may cause extrapyramidal symptoms which usually occur as acute dystonic reactions especially in young patients. The risk may be reduced by keeping the daily dose below 500 µg per kg body-weight. Parkinsonism and/or tardive dyskinesia have occasionally occurred, usually during prolonged treatment in elderly patients.

Other adverse effects include restlessness, drowsiness, dizziness, and bowel upsets such as diarrhoea or constipation.

Metoclopramide stimulates prolactin secretion and may cause galactorrhoea or related disorders. Transient increases in plasma aldosterone concentrations have been reported.

Urinary incontinence in one patient associated with metoclopramide.— B. B. Kumar (letter), *J. Am. med. Ass.*, 1984, *251*, 1553.

Bronchospasm in an asthmatic patient following metoclopramide administration.— M. M. Chung *et al.* (letter), *Ann. intern. Med.*, 1985, *103*, 809.

EFFECTS ON THE CARDIOVASCULAR SYSTEM. Reports of hypotension following the injection of metoclopramide in surgical patients: G. R. Park (letter), *Br. J. Anaesth.*, 1978, *50*, 1268; M. S. Pegg (letter), *Anaesthesia*, 1980, *35*, 615. Transient hypertension has occurred in a few patients receiving metoclopramide in association with cancer chemotherapy: C. Sheridan *et al.* (letter), *New Engl. J. Med.*, 1982, *307*, 1346; D. J. Filibeck *et al.*, *Clin. Pharm.*, 1984, *3*, 548.

EFFECTS ON THE ENDOCRINE SYSTEM. A report of hyperprolactinaemia, galactorrhoea, and pituitary adenoma in a 49-year-old woman with reflux oesophagitis who had received metoclopramide for 3 months. Her plasma-prolactin concentrations fell to normal and her symptoms resolved over 4 months following withdrawal of metoclopramide.— B. T. Cooper *et al.*, *Postgrad. med. J.*, 1982, *58*, 314.

An 82-year-old man suffering from mild congestive heart failure developed oedema during a 2-week course of metoclopramide. This might have been a consequence of metoclopramide increasing plasma concentrations of aldosterone.— B. Zumoff (letter), *Ann. intern. Med.*, 1983, *98*, 557.

In 15 patients with ascites due to cirrhosis of the liver and with high plasma concentrations of aldosterone, metoclopramide 10 mg given by bolus injection caused a further significant increase in plasma-aldosterone concentrations.— G. Mazzacca *et al.* (letter), *Ann. intern. Med.*, 1983, *98*, 1024.

EFFECTS ON MENTAL STATE. Altered sleep patterns in 6 of 15 patients receiving metoclopramide.— T. G. Saxe (letter), *Ann. intern. Med.*, 1983, *98*, 674.

Metoclopramide induced severe depression in a 19-year-old woman. She was managed by withdrawal of metoclopramide and its gradual reintroduction at a lower dose when the depression had resolved.— R. K. Bottner and C. J. Tullio (letter), *Ann. intern. Med.*, 1985, *103*, 482. Similar findings in 2 further patients with diabetic gastroparesis.— C. D. Adams (letter), *ibid.*, 960.

EXTRAPYRAMIDAL EFFECTS. The Adverse Reactions Register of the Committee on the Safety of Medicines for the years 1967-82 contained 479 reports of extrapyramidal reactions in which metoclopramide was the suspected drug: 455 were for dystonic-dyskinetic reactions, 20 for parkinsonism, and 4 for tardive dyskinesia. The acute dystonic-dyskinetic reactions were reported predominantly in younger female patients (particularly aged 12 to 19 years). The parkinsonian reactions occurred predominantly in older patients.— D. N. Bateman *et al.*, *Br. med. J.*, 1985, *291*, 930.

Acute dystonia. Fourteen (3.1%) of 452 patients given high doses of metoclopramide intravenously experienced acute dystonic reactions which were controlled by diphenhydramine. There was a marked difference in incidence of these adverse effects according to age: 6 of 22 patients (27.3%) aged 15 to 29 years experienced dystonic reactions compared with 8 of 430 patients (1.8%) aged 30 to 72 years. It had also been observed in paediatric patients that a higher incidence of extrapyramidal reactions occurred on the second consecutive day of metoclopramide administration and that there was a trend towards fewer extrapyramidal reactions when diphenhydramine was given with the first dose. Concomitant use of intravenous diphenhydramine with the initial dose of metoclopramide should be considered in patients with a history of extrapyramidal reactions and in those under the age of 30 years.— M. G. Kris *et al.* (letter), *New Engl. J. Med.*, 1983, *309*, 433.

Results of double-blind studies involving 98 cancer patients suggested that, in adults, important dystonic reactions to metoclopramide are uncommon, are not dose dependent, and are easy to control.— S. G. Allan *et al.* (letter), *Lancet*, 1984, *1*, 283.

A 50-year-old woman experienced a severe tetanus-like dystonic reaction to metoclopramide 1.5 mg per kg body-weight infused intravenously over 15 minutes. The woman had previously been tolerant to repeated use of metoclopramide.— R. Della Valle *et al.*, *Clin. Pharm.*, 1985, *4*, 102.

Further references to acute dystonic reactions with metoclopramide: I. Wandless *et al.* (letter), *Lancet*, 1980, *1*, 1255 (fever associated with dystonic reactions); L. C. K. Low and K. M. Goel, *Archs Dis. Childh.*, 1980, *55*, 310 (overdosage in children); T. R. E. Barnes *et al.* (letter), *Lancet*, 1982, *2*, 48 (acute akathisia); C. F. Pollera *et al.* (letter), *Lancet*, 1984, *2*, 460 (sudden death; administration in association with hexamethylmelamine).

Parkinsonism or tardive dyskinesia. A report of 18 patients (aged 53 to 76 years) with acute or chronic metoclopramide-induced extrapyramidal disorders seen over a 2-year period. Acute dystonic reactions were observed in 4 patients after treatment for one to 10 days, but these adverse effects disappeared promptly when metoclopramide was withdrawn. Parkinsonism developed in 12 patients who had received metoclopramide treatment for 2 weeks to 4 years (average 8.7 months); following withdrawal of the drug the parkinsonism cleared completely in 9 patients within 3 weeks and in one patient within 4 months, but the other 2 patients although improved still showed features of parkinsonism. Tardive dyskinesia developed in 7 patients (including 5 of the 12 with parkinsonism) following withdrawal of metoclopramide that had been given for 14 months to 4 years; in 4 patients the abnormal involuntary movements ceased within 3 weeks of withdrawal, but in the remaining 3 patients dyskinetic facial and tongue movements were still present 15 months later.— J. D. Grimes *et al.*, *Can. med. Ass. J.*, 1982, *126*, 23. Twelve patients with tardive dyskinesia due to metoclopramide were followed up over the past 3 years; 8 patients experienced persisting involuntary movements for periods ranging from 6 to 36 months (average 18 months).— J. D. Grimes *et al.* (letter), *Lancet*, 1982, *2*, 563.

Eleven cases of tardive dyskinesia associated with the use of metoclopramide had been reported to the Swedish Adverse Drug Reactions Advisory Committee from 1977 to 1981. All patients were women and were over 69 years of age. The median duration of treatment before onset of symptoms was 14 months (range 4 to 44); symptoms appeared after withdrawal of metoclopramide in 3 patients and during treatment in 8 patients.— B. -E. Wiholm *et al.*, *Br. med. J.*, 1984, *288*, 545.

A discussion of tardive dyskinesia associated with the use of metoclopramide in the elderly and recommendations that metoclopramide should not be used for trivial symptoms, and that if necessary it may by used for short term anti-emetic treatment in the elderly provided that the dose is limited to 500 µg per kg body-weight daily.— M. L'E. Orme and R. C. Tallis, *Br. med. J.*, 1984, *289*, 397.

Further reports of and references to tardive dyskinesia associated with metoclopramide: W. Breitbart (letter), *New Engl. J. Med.*, 1986, *315*, 518; A. W. Board (letter), *ibid.*

PORPHYRIA. Metoclopramide induced clinical exacerbation of acute intermittent porphyria in a young girl.— M. Doss *et al.* (letter), *Lancet*, 1981, *2*, 91.

Precautions

Metoclopramide should not be used when stimulation of muscular contractions might adversely affect gastro-intestinal conditions as in intestinal obstruction or immediately after surgery. There have been reports of hypertensive crises in patients with phaeochromocytoma given metoclopramide, thus its use is not recommended in such patients.

Children, young patients, and the elderly should be treated with care; there are specific doses recommended for young people up to the age of about 20 years and these are lower than the doses for adults (see under Uses and Administration). Patients on prolonged therapy should be reviewed regularly. Care should also be taken when metoclopramide is administered to patients with significant renal impairment or to those at risk of fluid retention as in hepatic impairment. It is recommended that metoclopramide should not be given to patients with convulsive disorders. Caution should be observed when using metoclopramide in patients taking other drugs that can also cause extrapyramidal reactions, such as the phenothiazines. The effects of CNS depressants may also be enhanced. Antimuscarinic agents and opioid analgesics antagonise the effects of metoclopramide. The absorption of other drugs may be affected by metoclopramide; it may either diminish absorption from the stomach or enhance absorption from the small intestine. Metoclopramide may also increase prolactin blood-concentrations and therefore interfere with drugs which have a hypoprolactinaemic effect and with some diagnostic tests.

Extrapyramidal symptoms had been observed in 6 pneumocystis patients with the acquired immune deficiency syndrome receiving low doses of metoclopramide or chlorpromazine. Until more information is available, these drugs should be used with caution in such patients.— H. Hollander *et al.* (letter), *Lancet*, 1985, *2*, 1186.

ADMINISTRATION IN RENAL FAILURE. For reference to the precautions to be observed in renal failure, see under Uses, Administration in renal failure.

INTERACTIONS. *Carbamazepine.* For a report of neurotoxicity associated with administration of metoclopramide and carbamazepine, see under Carbamazepine, p.401.

Diazepam. The addition of diazepam to a standard metoclopramide regimen for control of cisplatin-induced emesis in 5 patients resulted in significantly more nausea and emesis than that experienced by other patients receiving the standard regimen.— B. R. Meyer *et al.* (letter), *Ann. intern. Med.*, 1984, *101*, 141.

PORPHYRIA. Metoclopramide was considered to be unsafe in patients with acute porphyria although there is conflicting experimental evidence on porphyrinogenicity.— M.R. Moore and K.E.L. McColl, *Porphyrias, Drug Lists*, Glasgow, Porphyria Research Unit, University of Glasgow, 1987. See also Adverse Effects, above.

Absorption and Fate

Metoclopramide is rapidly absorbed from the gastro-intestinal tract and undergoes variable first-pass hepatic metabolism. It is excreted in the urine as free and as conjugated metoclopramide and as metabolites. It is excreted in breast milk.

The elimination half-life following administration of metoclopramide 10 mg by mouth has been reported to be up to about 6 hours; the half-life is prolonged in patients with renal failure.

A review of the clinical pharmacokinetics of metoclopramide. It appears to be rapidly and well absorbed from the gastro-intestinal tract, but the bioavailability is very variable and has been found to correlate with the ratio of free to conjugated metoclopramide in the urine; sulphate conjugation at the first pass through the gut wall or liver has been suggested as the factor governing bioavailability (D.N. Bateman *et al.*, *Br. J. clin. Pharmac.*, 1980, *9*, 371). Maximum plasma-concentrations of metoclopramide have been found to vary approximately 10-fold following oral administration and akathisia has been reported with maximum plasma-concentrations above 120 ng per mL (D.N. Bateman *et al.*, *Br. J. clin. Pharmac.*, 1979, *8*, 179). However, no difference in plasma concentrations of metoclopramide was observed in 3 children who had dystonic reactions compared with those who did not (D.N. Bateman *et al.*, *Br. J. clin. Pharmac.*, 1983, *15*, 557).

Metoclopramide is rapidly distributed following intravenous administration and an α half-life of between 3 and 21 minutes, and a β half-life of between 2.6 and 5.4 hours have been reported. The apparent volume of distribution at steady state has been reported to range

from 2.2 to 3.4 litres per kg body-weight following intravenous administration to healthy subjects; a large volume of distribution would be expected for metoclopramide which is a lipid-soluble basic compound. Protein binding of metoclopramide has not been thoroughly investigated but protein binding interactions are unlikely to be clinically important.
Urinary excretion appears to be the main route of elimination of metoclopramide and its metabolites; approximately 20% of an intravenous dose of metoclopramide hydrochloride 10 mg has been reported to be recovered unchanged in the urine (C. Graffner *et al.*, *Br. J. clin. Pharmac.*, 1979, *8*, 469; D.N. Bateman *et al.*, *ibid.*, 1980, *9*, 371). It appears that the adverse effects of metoclopramide observed in patients with renal failure are probably due to accumulation of the drug as a result of reduced clearance (D.N. Bateman *et al.*, *Eur. J. clin. Pharmac.*, 1981, *19*, 437) but the reasons for the magnitude of this reduction have not been established. Metoclopramide undergoes significant first-pass metabolism to the N-4 sulphate (D.N. Bateman *et al.*, *Br. J. clin. Pharmac.*, 1980, *9*, 371). The only other metabolites of metoclopramide that have been identified in man are the N-4 glucuronide (less than 2% of a dose) and the side-chain product 4-amino-5-chloro-2-methoxybenzamidoacetic acid.
Single-dose studies have suggested that the elimination of metoclopramide is dose-dependent in man after both intravenous and oral administration (C. Graffner *et al.*, *Br. J. clin. Pharmac.*, 1979, *8*, 469; D.N. Bateman *et al.*, *ibid.*, 1980, *9*, 371); however, studies using high-dose metoclopramide have shown a constant plasma-clearance over a 3-fold dose range (D.N. Bateman *et al.*, *Br. J. Pharmac.*, 1983, *80*, 490P). A high-dose regimen involving metoclopramide 10 mg per kg body-weight administered in 5 divided doses over a 9-hour period has been shown, in a small number of patients to lead to accumulation of the drug (W.B. Taylor and D.N. Bateman, *Br. J. clin. Pharmac.*, 1983, *16*, 341), but steady-state plasma concentrations of metoclopramide can be achieved by a regimen consisting of a loading dose followed by a constant-rate infusion (D.N. Bateman *et al.*, *Br. J. Pharmac.*, 1983, *80*, 490P).— D. N. Bateman, *Clin. Pharmacokinet.*, 1983, *8*, 523.

A review of the pharmacokinetics of high-dose metoclopramide in cancer patients concluding that despite considerable pharmacokinetic variability the intravenous administration of high doses of metoclopramide is relatively safe due to the large therapeutic index.— E. M. McGovern *et al.*, *Clin. Pharmacokinet.*, 1986, *11*, 415.

PREGNANCY AND THE NEONATE. In a study involving 17 mothers undergoing caesarean section, metoclopramide 10 mg administered intramuscularly 12 and 2 hours before the operation and intravenously just before the onset of general anaesthesia was found to cross the placenta rapidly and was detected in varying concentrations in the amniotic fluid. At the time of delivery metoclopramide reached concentrations in the foetal plasma which were about 60 to 70% of those in the maternal plasma.— P. Arvela *et al.*, *Eur. J. clin. Pharmac.*, 1983, *24*, 345.

Metoclopramide 10 mg three times daily by mouth was found to be transferred to breast milk and in 4 of 5 mothers the concentrations were higher than those in the maternal plasma. Peak maternal plasma concentrations occurred 2 to 3 hours after administration of the drug and were accompanied by, or were rapidly followed by peak concentrations in milk. Metoclopramide was only detected in the plasma of one neonate whose mother had the highest plasma and milk concentrations. Following administration of metoclopramide to 18 mothers during the late puerperium the concentration of metoclopramide in the milk was found to be slightly less than that observed in the 5 mothers during the early puerperium. The estimated maximum exposure of the infants to metoclopramide varied from 1 to 13 μg per kg and 6 to 24 μg per kg daily during late and early puerperium, respectively.— A. Kauppila *et al.*, *Eur. J. clin. Pharmac.*, 1983, *25*, 819.

Uses and Administration

Metoclopramide hydrochloride is a substituted benzamide which stimulates the motility of the upper gastro-intestinal tract without affecting gastric acid secretion. Metoclopramide increases gastric peristalsis leading to accelerated gastric emptying. Duodenal peristalsis is also increased which decreases intestinal transit time. The resting tone of the gastro-oesophageal sphincter is increased and the pyloric sphincter is relaxed. Metoclopramide possesses parasympathomimetic activity as well as being a dopamine receptor antagonist with a direct effect on the chemoreceptor trigger zone. Metoclopramide also increases prolactin secretion.
Metoclopramide hydrochloride is used in the treatment of some forms of nausea and vomiting such as that associated with cancer therapy or that following surgery; it is of little benefit in the prevention or treatment of motion sickness. Metoclopramide is also used for gastro-oesophageal reflux or gastric stasis.
Metoclopramide hydrochloride may be used to facilitate intubation procedures and to stimulate gastric emptying during radiographic examinations. There may be some benefit in migraine.
It is usually administered by mouth in a dose equivalent to 10 mg of anhydrous metoclopramide hydrochloride three times daily but may also be given by intramuscular or slow intravenous injection in the same dosage; in the *US* potency is expressed in terms of anhydrous metoclopramide and doses of 10 to 15 mg up to four times daily have been given. Single doses should be considered where appropriate and single doses of up to 20 mg expressed as anhydrous base or anhydrous hydrochloride have been used. Doses should be reduced in young adults and in children. In the *UK* suggested doses for those aged 15 to 19 years are 5 mg three times daily for those weighing 30 to 59 kg and 10 mg three times daily for those weighing 60 kg and over; 9 to 14 years, 5 mg three times daily; 5 to 9 years, 2.5 mg three times daily; 3 to 5 years, 2 mg two or three times daily; 1 to 3 years, 1 mg two or three times daily; and under 1 year 1 mg twice daily.
In general the total daily dose should not exceed 500 μg per kg body-weight. However, high doses are employed in the treatment of the nausea and vomiting associated with cancer chemotherapy. The loading dose of metoclopramide given before cancer therapy is 2 to 4 mg per kg body-weight administered as a continuous intravenous infusion over 15 to 30 minutes and is followed by maintenance doses of 3 to 5 mg per kg, again as a continuous intravenous infusion, administered over 8 to 12 hours. Alternatively, initial doses of up to 2 mg per kg by intravenous infusion over at least 15 minutes may be given before cancer therapy and repeated every 2 hours. The total dosage by either continuous or intermittent infusion should not normally exceed 10 mg per kg in 24 hours.

Reviews of the actions and uses of metoclopramide: K. Schulze-Delrieu, *New Engl. J. Med.*, 1981, *305*, 28; *Med. Lett.*, 1982, *24*, 67; R. Albibi and R. W. McCallum, *Ann. intern. Med.*, 1983, *98*, 86; R. A. Harrington *et al.*, *Drugs*, 1983, *25*, 451; A. F. Shaughnessy, *Drug Intell. & clin. Pharm.*, 1985, *19*, 723.

ADMINISTRATION IN RENAL FAILURE. A study of the pharmacokinetics of metoclopramide 10 mg by mouth and intravenously in 6 patients with chronic renal failure, 2 of whom were anephric. In addition to the reduced or non-existent renal clearance, total body clearance was also found to be substantially reduced in comparison with 7 subjects with normal renal function, and the terminal half-life was prolonged to about 14 hours. This suggests that the dose of metoclopramide in patients with severe renal impairment should be reduced by at least 60% of that normally prescribed.— D. N. Bateman and R. Gokal (letter), *Lancet*, 1980, *1*, 982.

Metoclopramide could be administered to patients with renal failure by adjusting the dose. In patients with glomerular filtration-rates greater than 50 mL per minute no reduction was necessary, for rates of between 10 and 50 mL per minute the dose should be reduced to 75% of the normal dose, and for rates of less than 10 mL per minute the dose should be reduced to 50%.— W. M. Bennett *et al.*, *Am. J. Kidney Dis.*, 1983, *3*, 155.

ASPIRATION SYNDROME. Howard and Sharp (*Br. med. J.*, 1973 *1*, 446) found that gastric emptying in parturient women could be improved by administration of metoclopramide 10 mg intramuscularly and therefore the risk of vomiting during emergency general anaesthesia could be reduced. However, Nimmo *et al.* (*Lancet*, 1975, *1*, 890) who studied 56 women during labour and in the postpartum period found that gastric emptying was markedly delayed in women receiving opioid analgesics and furthermore intramuscular administration of metoclopramide 10 mg at the same time as pethidine 150 mg or diamorphine 10 mg did not increase the rate of gastric emptying. In contrast, Murphy *et al.* (*Br. J. Anaesth.*, 1984, *56*, 1113) found that although gastric emptying was significantly delayed when labour was established and that this delay was further prolonged by the administration of pethidine 50 mg intramuscularly, significant improvement in gastric emptying could be achieved with metoclopramide 10 mg given intravenously after pethidine administration.
In a study of 80 women undergoing laparoscopy, metoclopramide 10 mg alone or in association with cimetidine 300 mg administered by mouth about 2 hours before the induction of anaesthesia resulted in a significant reduction in gastric fluid volume. The combination produced significant decrease in gastric acidity, but so did cimetidine on its own. The administration of the 2 drugs may be beneficial for the prevention of regurgitation and aspiration of gastric contents in patients with increased gastric fluid volume or in patients prone to regurgitation.— T. L. K. Rao *et al.*, *Anesth. Analg.*, 1984, *63*, 1014.

AMENORRHOEA. In 7 of 8 women with amenorrhoea associated with normoprolactinaemia metoclopramide 5 mg four times daily for 10 days followed by 2.5 mg 3 times daily for 20 days then the whole sequence repeated twice produced menstrual bleeding and regular menstruation was restored in 5 patients.— C. Hagen *et al.* (letter), *Lancet*, 1983, *1*, 422.

GASTRO-INTESTINAL DISORDERS. *Diabetic gastroparesis.* In a double-blind crossover study of 10 insulin-dependent diabetics with gastroparesis metoclopramide 10 mg 4 times daily by mouth 30 minutes before meals and before going to sleep improved both gastric emptying and symptoms of gastric stasis when compared with placebo; both metoclopramide and placebo were taken for 3 weeks.— W. J. Snape *et al.*, *Ann. intern. Med.*, 1982, *96*, 444.

Gastro-oesophageal reflux. In a double-blind study in 31 patients with gastro-oesophageal reflux, metoclopramide 10 mg administered by mouth 30 minutes before meals and upon retiring produced a significant and sustained improvement in 10 of 15 patients compared with 7 of 16 patients receiving placebo; the difference was not significant.— A. Paull and A. K. Grant, *Med. J. Aust.*, 1974, *2*, 627.
A 4-week double-blind study involving 20 patients with chronic heartburn demonstrated that metoclopramide 10 mg taken by mouth 15 minutes before meals and 30 minutes before retiring was significantly more effective than placebo in decreasing daytime symptoms of heartburn and regurgitation. One patient withdrew from the study after one week because of restlessness and anxiety.— R. W. McCallum *et al.*, *Am. J. Gastroent.*, 1984, *79*, 165.
In 32 infants with gastro-oesophageal reflux metoclopramide 500 μg per kg body-weight daily by mouth in 4 divided doses 10 to 20 minutes before feeding reduced the frequency of regurgitation compared with 9 similar children who received a placebo.— A. K. C. Leung and P. C. W. Lai, *Curr. ther. Res.*, 1984, *36*, 911.
No clinical advantage was observed when cimetidine in association with metoclopramide was used to treat oesophageal acid reflux disease compared with cimetidine alone.— J. G. Temple *et al.*, *Br. med. J.*, 1983, *286*, 1863. Metoclopramide in association with cimetidine was effective in the management of severe reflux oesophagitis refractory to standard treatment with cimetidine, antacids, diet modification, and bed elevation. Nine of 12 patients improved clinically after 8 weeks' treatment with metoclopramide 10 mg before meals and at bedtime added to a standard regimen with cimetidine 300 mg before meals and at bedtime compared with only 3 of 12 similar patients who received cimetidine with placebo; endoscopic improvement was noted in 9 and 4 patients respectively. One patient who received metoclopramide was withdrawn from the study after 4 weeks because of confusion, visual hallucinations, and disorientation.— D. A. Lieberman and E. B. Keeffe, *Ann. intern. Med.*, 1986, *104*, 21.

HICCUP. For details of a protocol for the control of hiccups which involves the use of metoclopramide, see Chlorpromazine Hydrochloride, p.725.

LACTATION INSUFFICIENCY. Metoclopramide in doses of 10 mg or 15 mg three times daily increased serum-prolactin concentrations and the quantity of breast milk whereas a dose of 5 mg three times daily did not. The study involved 37 women with inadequate lactation and was placebo-controlled. Nine of the 27 mothers taking the effective doses were able to stop supplementary infant feeding. One child of a mother taking 45 mg daily had some intestinal discomfort.— A. Kauppila *et al.*, *Lancet*, 1981, *1*, 1175.

MIGRAINE. Metoclopramide is used in migraine because of its anti-emetic action and its effect on accelerating the absorption of some other drugs (M. Wilkinson, *Prescribers' J.*, 1980, *20*, 57). The use of combinations of metoclopramide with analgesics has been criticised since metoclopramide by mouth was considered to be unlikely to have any effect on the absorption of the analgesic (*Drug & Ther. Bull.*, 1980, *18*, 95). However, it has been shown that the absorption of aspirin in migraine patients is improved by metoclopramide given 3 minutes earlier (L.M. Ross-Lee *et al.*, *Eur. J. clin. Pharmac.*, 1983, *24*, 777).

NAUSEA AND VOMITING. *From cancer chemotherapy.* Early studies with metoclopramide in patients suffering from nausea and vomiting induced by cancer chemotherapy failed to demonstrate a significant anti-emetic effect. The doses might have been too low, for Gralla *et al.* (*New Engl. J. Med.*, 1981, *305*, 905) successfully used a high-dose intravenous regimen of metoclopramide to control nausea and vomiting associated with the administration of cisplatin 120 mg per m^2 body-surface. The dose of metoclopramide was 2 mg per kg bodyweight by intravenous infusion over 15 minutes administered 30 minutes before, and 1.5, 3.5, 5.5, and 8.5 hours after cisplatin. Beneficial results were also obtained with metoclopramide 1 mg per kg for 6 doses in patients receiving lower doses of cisplatin (50 to 100 mg per m^2) (H.D. Homesley *et al.*, *New Engl. J. Med.*, 1982, *307*, 250) and anti-emetic protection was maintained with subsequent courses of up to 8 consecutive cycles of chemotherapy (S.B. Strum *et al.*, *J. Am. med. Ass.*, 1982, *247*, 2683). Accumulation of metoclopramide has occurred following repeated intravenous doses and so a weight-related loading dose followed by a continuous intravenous infusion to achieve steady-state plasma concentrations was suggested (W.B. Taylor and D.N. Bateman, *Br. med. J.*, 1983, *287*, 841); such a technique employing a loading dose of 3 mg per kg followed by a continuous infusion of 4 mg per kg has been found to provide a considerable improvement in anti-emetic effect compared with a total dose of 7 mg per kg given as intermittent infusions (P.S. Warrington *et al.*, *Br. med. J.*, 1986, *293*, 1334 and 1540). Plasma concentrations of 850 ng per mL (B.R. Meyer *et al.*, *Ann. intern. Med.*, 1984, *100*, 393), 800 ng per mL (D.J. Kerr *et al.*, *Br. J. clin. Pharmac.*, 1985, *20*, 426), and 1 µg per mL (E.M. McGovern *et al.*, *J. Pharm. Pharmac.*, 1985, *37*, *Suppl.*, 40P) are associated with emesis control.

High-dose oral administration of metoclopramide 2 mg per kg given 1 hour before, and 1, 3, 5, 8, and 11 hours after initiation of chemotherapy has also been found to be of benefit (M.B. Garnick, *Ann. intern. Med.*, 1983, *99*, 127). Taylor and Bateman (*Br. J. clin. Pharmac.*, 1985, *20*, 296P) suggested that high-dose oral metoclopramide showed less interindividual variation in bioavailability than did standard doses.

Although metoclopramide has been shown to be effective against cisplatin-induced vomiting, probably due to its peripheral action on the gastro-intestinal tract, it might not be the anti-emetic of choice for all chemotherapy-induced nausea and vomiting (G.S. Ogawa, *New Engl. J. Med.*, 1982, *307*, 249). However, Strum *et al.* (*Cancer*, 1984, *53*, 1432) found that various dosage schedules of intravenous metoclopramide possessed significant anti-emetic activity in patients receiving potent, non-cisplatin containing chemotherapy. In contrast, Cunningham *et al.* (*Br. med. J.*, 1985, *290*, 604) found that the superiority of high-dose metoclopramide over the phenothiazines in controlling emesis induced by cisplatin was not apparent in patients receiving cytotoxic regimens without cisplatin.

Combined anti-emetic treatment particularly using drugs with different mechanisms of action might be beneficial (L.J. Seigel and D.L. Longo, *Ann. intern. Med.*, 1981, *95*, 352). Joss *et al.* (*Eur. J. clin. Pharmac.*, 1983, *25*, 35) and Allan *et al.* (*Br. med. J.*, 1984, *289*, 878) found that the addition of methylprednisolone or dexamethasone to a metoclopramide regimen enhanced the anti-emetic effect. Kris *et al.* (*Cancer*, 1985, *55*, 527) also found that metoclopramide with dexamethasone produced an enhanced effect. They also reported that the anti-emetic effect could be improved by infusing metoclopramide 3 mg per kg over 15 minutes for 2 doses, 30 minutes before and 1.5 hours after cisplatin administration and by injecting dexamethasone 20 mg and diphenhydramine 50 mg 30 minutes before cisplatin. A 5-drug regimen of metoclopramide, diphenhydramine, dexamethasone, diazepam, and thiethylperazine has also been found to be beneficial in controlling intractable vomiting while on cisplatin-containing chemotherapy (P.M. Plezia *et al.*, *Cancer Treat. Rep.*, 1984, *68*, 1493), but other workers have found that the addition of diazepam to a standard metoclopramide regimen may increase the vomiting (B.R. Meyer *et al.*, *Ann. intern. Med.*, 1984, *101*, 141).

For a suggestion that nabilone may be preferable to metoclopramide or domperidone in patients with breast cancer see under nabilone, p.1101.

In labour. A double-blind study of 477 mothers in labour demonstrated that either metoclopramide 10 mg or promethazine 25 mg administered intramuscularly with the first dose of pethidine 100 to 150 mg prevented the increase in nausea and vomiting associated with pethidine. Promethazine caused significantly more drowsiness 2 to 4 hours after the pethidine injection and the pain relief from pethidine was significantly reduced when promethazine was given compared with metoclopramide. The results suggested that metoclopramide was to be preferred to promethazine for administration with pethidine in labour, because of improved analgesia and less sedation.— L. Vella *et al.*, *Br. med. J.*, 1985, *290*, 1173.

Postoperative. Results of studies of metoclopramide to control postoperative nausea and vomiting have been variable. Clark and Storrs (*Br. J. Anaesth.*, 1969, *41*, 890) demonstrated a significant reduction in vomiting with metoclopramide 20 mg administered intramuscularly immediately after the operation, and Lind and Breivik (*ibid.*, 1970, *42*, 614) found metoclopramide 10 mg administered intramuscularly at the end of the operation was more effective than perphenazine 5 mg intramuscularly in the prevention of postoperative nausea and vomiting. In contrast, Shah and Wilson (*ibid.*, 1972, *44*, 865) found no significant benefit from metoclopramide 10 mg administered intramuscularly with the pre-anaesthetic medication. However, Assaf *et al.* (*ibid.*, 1974, *46*, 514) demonstrated that metoclopramide 10 or 20 mg given with pethidine 100 mg or morphine 10 mg pre-operatively reduced the incidence of postoperative nausea and vomiting, and that additional doses of metoclopramide postoperatively reduced the emetic effects of pethidine but had very much less effect on morphine. Korttila *et al.* (*Anesth. Analg.*, 1979, *58*, 396) compared metoclopramide 10 mg, domperidone 5 or 10 mg, and droperidol 1.25 mg, all administered intravenously 5 minutes before the end of anaesthesia with, if necessary, an additional dose given intramuscularly during the first 24 hours postoperatively, but found that only droperidol significantly reduced the incidence of nausea and vomiting. Other studies have also demonstrated no significant effect against nausea and vomiting with metoclopramide 10 mg or domperidone 10 mg administered intravenously before spinal anaesthesia (K.R. Spelina *et al.*, *Anaesthesia*, 1984, *39*, 132) or at induction of general anaesthesia (C.S. Waldmann *et al.*, *Br. J. clin. Pharmac.*, 1985, *19*, 307).

PREGNANCY AND THE NEONATE. For references to the use of metoclopramide during labour or post partum, see under Aspiration Syndrome, Lactation Insufficiency, and Nausea and Vomiting.

Preparations

Metoclopramide Injection *(B.P.).* Contains metoclopramide hydrochloride.

Metoclopramide Injection *(U.S.P.).* Contains metoclopramide hydrochloride.

Metoclopramide Tablets *(B.P.).* Contain metoclopramide hydrochloride.

Metoclopramide Tablets *(U.S.P.).* Contain metoclopramide hydrochloride.

Proprietary Preparations

Gastrobid Continus *(Napp, UK). Tablets*, sustained-release, metoclopramide hydrochloride 15 mg.

Gastromax *(Farmitalia Carlo Erba, UK). Capsules*, sustained-release, metoclopramide hydrochloride 30 mg.

Maxolon *(Beecham Research, UK). Tablets*, scored, metoclopramide hydrochloride equivalent to anhydrous metoclopramide hydrochloride 10 mg.
Paediatric Liquid, metoclopramide hydrochloride equivalent to anhydrous metoclopramide hydrochloride 1 mg/mL.
Syrup, metoclopramide hydrochloride equivalent to anhydrous metoclopramide hydrochloride 5 mg/5 mL.
Injection, metoclopramide hydrochloride equivalent to anhydrous metoclopramide hydrochloride 5 mg/mL, in ampoules of 2 mL.

Maxolon 'High Dose' *(Beecham Research, UK). Injection*, metoclopramide hydrochloride equivalent to anhydrous metoclopramide hydrochloride 5 mg/mL, in ampoules of 20 mL.

Maxolon SR *(Beecham Research, UK), Capsules*, sustained-release, metoclopramide hydrochloride 15 mg.

Metox *(Steinhard, UK). Tablets*, scored, metoclopramide hydrochloride equivalent to anhydrous metoclopramide hydrochloride 10 mg.

Metramid *(Nicholas, UK). Tablets*, scored, metoclopramide hydrochloride equivalent to anhydrous metoclopramide hydrochloride 10 mg.

Mygdalon *(DDSA Pharmaceuticals, UK). Tablets*, scored, metoclopramide hydrochloride equivalent to anhydrous metoclopramide hydrochloride 10 mg.

Parmid *(Lagap, UK). Tablets*, scored, metoclopramide hydrochloride equivalent to anhydrous metoclopramide hydrochloride 10 mg.
Syrup, metoclopramide hydrochloride equivalent to anhydrous metoclopramide hydrochloride 5 mg/5 mL.
Injection, metoclopramide hydrochloride equivalent to anhydrous metoclopramide hydrochloride 5 mg/mL, in ampoules of 2 mL.

Primperan *(Berk Pharmaceuticals, UK). Tablets*, scored, metoclopramide hydrochloride equivalent to anhydrous metoclopramide hydrochloride 10 mg.
Syrup, metoclopramide hydrochloride equivalent to anhydrous metoclopramide hydrochloride 5 mg/5 mL.
Injection, metoclopramide hydrochloride equivalent to anhydrous metoclopramide hydrochloride 5 mg/mL, in ampoules of 2 mL.

Proprietary Names and Manufacturers

Ananda *(Bonomelli, Ital.)*; Anausin *(Sarget, Fr.)*; Citroplus *(Irbi, Ital.)*; Clodilion *(Rhone-Poulenc, Ital.)*; Clopamon *(Lennon, S.Afr.)*; Clopan *(FIRMA, Ital.)*; Clopra *(Quantum, USA)*; Contromet *(Propan, S.Afr.)*; Desvomin *(Miquel, Spain)*; Digetres *(Ital.)*; Donopon-GP *(Jpn)*; Duraclamid *(Durachemie, Ger.)*; Emex *(Beecham, Canad.)*; Emperal *(Orion, Denm.)*; Enterosil *(Vis, Ital.)*; Gastrobid Continus *(Napp, UK)*; Gastromax *(Farmitalia Carlo Erba, UK)*; Gastronerton *(Dolorgiet, Ger.)*; Gastrosil *(Heumann, Ger.*; *Heumann, Switz.)*; Gastro-Tablinen *(Beiersdorf, Ger.)*; Gastrotem *(Temmler, Ger.)*; Gastro-Timelets *(Temmler, Ger.*; *Temmler, Switz.)*; Hyrin *(Merckle, Ger.)*; Imperan *(Arg.)*; Maxeran *(Nordic, Canad.)*; Maxolon *(Beecham, Austral.*; *Beecham, S.Afr.*; *Beecham Research, UK*; *Beecham Laboratories, USA)*; Meclopran *(Lagap, Switz.)*; Mepramid *(DAK, Denm.)*; Metagliz *(Prodes, Spain)*; Metamide *(Protea, Austral.)*; Metoclol *(Jpn)*; Metocobil *(Vita, Ital.)*; Metopram *(Leiras, Fin.)*; Metox *(Steinhard, UK)*; Metramid *(Nicholas, UK)*; Moriperan *(Jpn)*; Mygdalon *(DDSA Pharmaceuticals, UK)*; Nadir *(Recordati, Ital.)*; Netaf *(Arg.)*; Parmid *(Lagap, UK)*; Paspertin *(Kali-Chemie, Ger.*; *Kali-Chemie, Switz.)*; Peraprin *(Jpn)*; Placitril *(Ital.)*; Plasil *(Arg.*; *Lepetit, Ital.)*; Pramiel *(Jpn)*; Pramin *(Alphapharm, Austral.)*; Primperan *(USV, Austral.*; *Belg.*; *Lundbeck, Denm.*; *Lundbeck, Fin.*; *Delagrange, Fr.*; *Neth.*; *Nyco, Norw.*; *Fisons, S.Afr.*; *Delagrange, Spain*; *Lundbeck, Swed.*; *Delagrange, Switz.*; *Berk Pharmaceuticals, UK)*; Primperil *(Arg.)*; Prostal *(Rolab, S.Afr.)*; Randum *(Scharper, Ital.)*; Reclomide *(Ultra, USA)*; Regastrol *(Sarm, Ital.)*; Reglan *(Robins, Canad.*; *Continental Ethicals, S.Afr.*; *Robins, USA)*; Reliveran *(Arg.)*; Ulcofar *(Spain)*; Viscal *(Zoja, Ital.)*.

The following names have been used for multi-ingredient preparations containing metoclopramide hydrochloride— Migravess *(Bayer, UK)*; Paramax *(Beecham Research, UK)*.

6545-m

Metopimazine *(BAN, USAN, rINN).*
EXP-999; RP-9965. 1-[3-(2-Methylsulphonylphenothiazin-10-yl)propyl]piperidine-4-carboxamide.
$C_{22}H_{27}N_3O_3S_2$=445.6.

CAS — 14008-44-7.

Pharmacopoeias. In *Fr.*

Metopimazine is a phenothiazine which is used as an anti-emetic usually in doses of 5 to 15 mg daily, by mouth or by rectum, in 2 or 3 divided doses; up to 30 mg daily has been given by mouth. It has also been given by intramuscular injection.

A study of the pharmacokinetics of metopimazine and a comparison of different oral dosage forms.— J. Gaillot and A. Bieder, *Farmaco, Edn prat.*, 1980, *35*, 3.

Use as an anti-emetic in cancer patients: C. G. Moertel and R. J. Reitemeier, *J. clin. Pharmac.*, 1973, *13*, 283; L. Israel and C. Rodary, *J. int. med. Res.*, 1978, *6*, 235.

Proprietary Names and Manufacturers

Vogalen *(Rhone, Spain)*; Vogalene *(Rhodia, Arg.*; *Rhone-Poulenc, Belg.*; *Théraplix, Fr.*; *RBS Pharma, Ital.*; *Théraplix, Neth.)*.

843-e

Nabilone *(BAN, USAN, pINN).*

Lilly-109514. (±)-(6a*R*,10a*R*)-3-(1,1-Dimethylheptyl)-6a,7,8,9,10,10a-hexahydro-1-hydroxy-6,6-dimethyl-6*H*-benzo[*c*]chromen-9-one.
$C_{24}H_{36}O_3$=372.5.

CAS — 51022-71-0.

Adverse Effects

Nabilone, being a synthetic cannabinoid, may produce adverse effects similar to those of cannabis (see p.1553). The most common side-effect is reported to be drowsiness; other neurological side-effects that have been observed are confusion, disorientation, dizziness, euphoria, hallucinations, psychosis, mental depression, headache, decreased concentration, blurred vision, decreased co-ordination, and tremors. Adverse cardiovascular reactions that have occurred are postural hypotension and tachycardia. Dry mouth, decreased appetite, and abdominal cramp have also been reported.

For an estimate of the incidence of some of the commoner side-effects seen with nabilone, see below under Uses and Administration.

Precautions

Nabilone, because of its biliary excretion, is not recommended for use in patients with severe liver impairment. It should be administered cautiously to patients with a history of psychosis.

Because of the possibility of CNS depression patients should be warned not to drive, operate machinery, or consume alcoholic drink.

A study showing that nabilone does not affect concentrations of the beta subunit of human chorionic gonadotrophin (hCG) which is an important staging and monitoring marker in the treatment of testicular cancer. Although a rise in hCG in cannabis smokers has been reported, it is suggested that a rise in hCG should be considered as evidence of a relapse until proven otherwise.— P. Hogan *et al.* (letter), *Lancet*, 1983, *2*, 1144.

Absorption and Fate

Nabilone is absorbed from the gastro-intestinal tract, undergoes metabolism, possibily to active metabolites, and is excreted predominantly by the biliary route.

Following intravenous administration of radioactively labelled nabilone 500 µg to 5 healthy subjects the half-life of the total radioactivity ranged from 17 to 25 hours (mean 20.6 hours); nabilone was rapidly distributed into tissues and metabolised so that relatively little was detected in plasma after 6 hours, the estimated half-life of the parent compound being only 1.7 hours or about one-twelfth that of the total radioactivity. Following administration of 2 mg by mouth to 2 subjects the estimated half-life of total radioactivity was about 35 hours whereas that of unchanged nabilone was only about 2 hours; the estimated half-life of the carbinol metabolite was about 5 to 10 hours. Following intravenous administration about 67% was eliminated in the faeces and 22% in the urine; similar values were obtained following administration by mouth indicating that most of the oral dose was absorbed. Nabilone and its isomeric carbinol metabolites were noted in faeces but not in urine; at least 6 other metabolites were noted but not identified in urine. The short half-life of nabilone did not correspond to its longer duration of action which suggested that one or more of its metabolites was active.— A. Rubin *et al.*, *Clin. Pharmac. Ther.*, 1977, *22*, 85.

Uses and Administration

Nabilone, a synthetic cannabinoid with anti-emetic and anxiolytic properties, is used for the control of nausea and vomiting associated with cancer chemotherapy.

The usual dose for adults is 1 or 2 mg twice daily by mouth. The first dose should be given the evening before initiation of chemotherapy with the second dose of nabilone being given 1 to 3 hours before the first dose of the antineoplastic agent. Nabilone may be given throughout each cycle of chemotherapy and for 24 hours after the last dose of chemotherapy, if required. The dose of nabilone should not exceed 6 mg daily.

For comments on the potential therapeutic uses of synthetic cannabinoids, see under Dronabinol, p.1090.

NAUSEA AND VOMITING. A review of the pharmacological properties and therapeutic use of nabilone. The pharmacological profile of nabilone suggests that its anti-emetic action is possibly effected in the forebrain causing an inhibition of the vomiting control mechanism in the medulla oblongata; a secondary mild anxiolytic activity may contribute to the overall efficacy. It should be noted, when assessing clinical studies conducted with nabilone, that there have been a number of shortcomings of trial design and that the subjective use of 'good' relief has been used many times without standardisation. Overall, it is difficult to assess studies comparing the efficacy of nabilone with prochlorperazine in patients undergoing cancer chemotherapy because of the inconsistency of dosage regimens, patient populations, and chemotherapy regimens. However, having made that qualification it would appear that nabilone has a greater anti-emetic effect than prochlorperazine by mouth. Although the incidence of side-effects associated with nabilone is higher than that with prochlorperazine, patients do mainly prefer nabilone therapy. The overall incidences of many of the side-effects with nabilone are difficult to quantify due to the overlap in terminology and to widely differing methods of obtaining data but the ones most commonly reported at usual therapeutic doses are drowsiness (4 to 89%), dizziness (12 to 65%), and dry mouth (6 to 62%). Most side-effects are mild to moderate in severity with the severity usually lessening with continued treatment although occasionally they are severe enough to warrant discontinuation of nabilone. Postural hypotension is potentially one of the most troublesome adverse effects seen with nabilone, and has been observed in over 5% of patients on several occasions.— A. Ward and B. Holmes, *Drugs*, 1985, *30*, 127.

A brief report stating that because nabilone did not raise basal prolactin concentrations it is a suitable alternative anti-emetic during chemotherapy for breast cancer overcoming the considerable theoretical objections to using anti-emetics such as phenothiazines, metoclopramide, or domperidone which may induce unwanted hyperprolactinaemia.— S. Kumar and R. E. Mansel, *Br. med. J.*, 1984, *288*, 760.

A favourable report on the use of nabilone in combination with prochlorperazine in patients receiving cytotoxic regimens (without cisplatin). Complete control of emesis was achieved in a large proportion of patients whether they received nabilone alone or with prochlorperazine but the incidence of CNS adverse effects associated with nabilone therapy alone was significantly reduced when the combination was used. Of 30 patients who received both anti-emetic regimens 15 preferred the combination therapy, 1 preferred nabilone alone, and 14 expressed no preference.— D. Cunningham *et al.*, *Br. med. J.*, 1985, *291*, 864.

Results of a double-blind crossover study comparing nabilone with domperidone in children receiving emetogenic chemotherapy. Doses of nabilone were: children of less than 18 kg body-weight, 0.5 mg twice daily; 18 to 36 kg, 1 mg twice daily; more than 36 kg, 1 mg three times daily. Corresponding doses of domperidone for the same body-weight groups were 5 mg, 10 mg, and 15 mg all given three times daily. In 18 evaluable patients the frequency of vomiting and nausea scores both showed a significant difference in favour of nabilone; two patients were withdrawn by their parents because vomiting was uncontrolled with nabilone. Adverse effects were more frequent in the nabilone treatment period, but apart from a patient who had treatment interrupted because of disturbing hallucinations, they were thought to be acceptable. Twelve patients or parents, or both, expressed a preference for nabilone, one for domperidone, and 5 did not express a preference.— A. M. Dalzell *et al.*, *Archs Dis. Childh.*, 1986, *61*, 502.

Proprietary Preparations

Cesamet *(Lilly, UK). Capsules*, nabilone 1 mg.

Proprietary Names and Manufacturers

Cesamet *(Lilly, Canad.; Lilly, UK).*

12003-m

Nizatidine *(BAN, USAN, rINN).*

LY-139037. 4-[2-(1-Methylamino-2-nitrovinylamino)ethylthiomethyl]thiazol-2-ylmethyl(dimethyl)amine; *N*-[2-(2-Dimethylaminomethylthiazol-4-ylmethylthio)ethyl]-*N'*-methyl-2-nitrovinylidenediamine.
$C_{12}H_{21}N_5O_2S_2$=331.5.

CAS — 76963-41-2.

Adverse Effects

Adverse effects reported with nizatidine include headache, chest pain, myalgia, abnormal dreams, weakness, somnolence, rhinitis, pharyngitis, cough, pruritus, and sweating. Unlike cimetidine, nizatidine has little or no anti-androgenic effect.

Precautions

As for cimetidine, p.1083. It is generally considered that the potential for interactions with nizatidine is less than with cimetidine.

Uses and Administration

Nizatidine is a histamine H_2-receptor antagonist with actions and uses similar to those of cimetidine (p.1084).

In the management of duodenal and gastric ulcers a single daily dose of nizatidine 300 mg by mouth in the evening is recommended, which should be given initially for 4 weeks and may be extended to 8 weeks if necessary; alternatively 150 mg twice daily in the morning and evening may be given. Where appropriate in duodenal ulcer a maintenance dose of 150 mg daily may be given in the evening.

The dosage of nizatidine should be reduced in patients with impaired renal function; suggested doses according to creatinine clearance are: creatinine clearance of less than 20 mL per minute, 150 mg on alternate days for treatment and 150 mg every third day for maintenance therapy; creatinine clearance of 20 to 50 mL per minute, 150 mg daily for treatment and 150 mg on alternate days for maintenance therapy.

Some references to studies on the activity of nizatidine: J. T. Callaghan *et al.*, *Clin. Pharmac. Ther.*, 1985, *37*, 162; H. Levendoglu *et al.*, *Am. J. Gastroent.*, 1986, *81*, 1167.

Proprietary Preparations

Axid *(Lilly, UK). Capsules*, nizatidine 150 and 300 mg.

Proprietary Names and Manufacturers

Axid *(Lilly, UK)*; Calmaxid *(Lilly, Switz.)*; Nizax *(Lilly, Ital.).*

3779-x

Olsalazine *(BAN, rINN).*

5,5'-Azodisalicylic acid.
$C_{14}H_{10}N_2O_6$=302.2.

CAS — 15722-48-2.

16608-a

Olsalazine Sodium *(BANM, rINNM).*

CI Mordant Yellow 5; CI No. 14130. Disodium azodisalicylate.
$C_{14}H_8N_2Na_2O_6$=323.2.

Olsalazine, which consists of two molecules of mesalazine (see p.1097) linked with an azo bond, is being investigated as the sodium salt for use in ulcerative colitis.

A brief review of olsalazine sodium. The compound has provoked interest because, unlike mesalazine, it is not absorbed in the small intestine but can reach the colon where bacteria split the azo bridge and release free mesalazine; thus olsalazine is effectively a pro-drug for mesalazine. Because olsalazine itself is physically difficult to handle, the sodium salt has been used clinically.— R. A. Levinson *et al.*, *Am. J. Gastroent.*, 1985, *80*, 203.

A study reporting encouraging results with olsalazine in the treatment of mildly active ulcerative colitis.— W. S. Selby *et al.*, *Br. med. J.*, 1985, *291*, 1373. A correction to the dosage stated.— *ibid.*, 1986, *292*, 28. Further encouraging results in a preliminary study of olsalazine for the prevention of relapse.— H. Sandberg-Gertzén *et al.*, *Gastroenterology*, 1986, *90*, 1024.

16938-y

Omeprazole *(BAN, USAN, rINN).*
H-168-68. 5-Methoxy-2-(4-methoxy-3,5-dimethyl-2-pyridylmethylsulphinyl)benzimidazole.
$C_{17}H_{19}N_3O_3S$=345.4.

CAS — 73590-58-6.

Adverse Effects

Adverse effects reported with omeprazole in clinical studies have included nausea, diarrhoea, abdominal colic, paraesthesia, dizziness, and headache and have been stated to be generally mild and transient and not requiring a reduction in dosage.

Findings during early toxicological studies of carcinoid-like tumours of the gastric mucosa in *animals* given very high doses of omeprazole over long periods led to a temporary halt on further investigation with the compound. However, studies so far in patients have found no mucosal changes indicative of such an association.

Absorption and Fate

Omeprazole is acid-labile and consequently various formulations have been developed in an attempt to improve bioavailability from the gastro-intestinal tract. The absorption of omeprazole, as well as being formulation-dependent, also appears to be dose-dependent, as increasing the dosage has been reported disproportionately to increase the plasma concentrations. This has led to suggestions that omeprazole may improve its own absorption and relative bioavailability by inhibiting the secretion of gastric acid.

Following absorption, omeprazole is almost completely metabolised and rapidly eliminated, mostly in the urine. Although the elimination half-life from plasma is short, being reported to be 0.5 to 1.5 hours, its duration of action with regard to inhibition of acid secretion is much longer and it is suggested that its distribution to the tissues, and particularly to the gastric parietal cells, accounts for this action. Omeprazole is highly bound (about 95%) to plasma proteins.

Uses and Administration

Omeprazole inhibits secretion of gastric acid and is considered to do so by irreversibly blocking the enzyme system of hydrogen/potassium adenosine triphosphatase, the so-called proton pump of the gastric parietal cell.

Omeprazole is being studied for use in patients with peptic ulceration and for disorders associated with hypersecretion of gastric acid, such as the Zollinger-Ellison syndrome. Usual doses by mouth in peptic ulceration have been 20 to 40 mg daily as a single dose with larger doses of up to 180 mg daily in divided doses being used in patients with the Zollinger-Ellison syndrome.

A detailed preliminary review of omeprazole, a substituted benzimidazole, the first of a new class of anti-ulcer agents. Omeprazole is thought to reduce acid secretion by inhibiting hydrogen/potassium adenosine triphosphatase (believed to be the proton pump of the parietal cell). This is the first time that intragastric acidity can be reduced independently of the primary stimulus as the mechanism of action of omeprazole is at the terminal stage of the acid-secreting process.

A small number of appropriately-controlled comparative studies have demonstrated that omeprazole produced significantly more rapid healing of ulcers after 2 to 4 weeks of treatment than either cimetidine or ranitidine but in studies following patients after the discontinuation of active treatment no significant difference between omeprazole or the H_2-antagonists in relapse-rate or time to relapse was reported. Preliminary studies in a small number of patients have also demonstrated the efficacy of omeprazole in patients with duodenal ulcers refractory to H_2-antagonists. At present there is no available data concerning the use of omeprazole as maintenance therapy for duodenal ulcers.

The efficacy of omeprazole has also been demonstrated in small groups of patients with gastric ulcers or peptic oesophagitis.

Experience with omeprazole in patients with Zollinger-Ellison syndrome is also limited but most studies, using doses of up to 180 mg daily, have found it effective and many authors consider it will become the drug of choice for this disease.

Questions, however, concerning the safety of omeprazole have arisen. Following long-term toxicological studies in various *animal* species, the findings of carcinoid-like tumours and morphological changes of the gastric mucosa gave rise to a great deal of speculation and they remain a contentious issue amongst gastro-enterologists. Current evidence suggests that the hyperplasia is not directly induced by omeprazole and that omeprazole does not represent a carcinogenic risk to patients during treatment although further studies are needed. In the clinical studies reported so far, omeprazole has been very well tolerated both by patients and healthy subjects.

Independent of its clinical future, omeprazole is already an important pharmacological 'tool' for investigating changes that occur in the gastric mucosa and for evaluating the mechanisms of action of inhibitors of gastric acid.— S. P. Clissold and D. M. Campoli-Richards, *Drugs*, 1986, *32*, 15.

Further references: *Scand. J. Gastroenterol.*, 1986, *21, Suppl.* 118, 1—195; *Lancet*, 1987, *2*, 1187.

Proprietary Names and Manufacturers

Yoshitomi, Jpn; Astra, UK.

6546-b

Oxypendyl Hydrochloride *(rINNM).*
D-706; Oxipendyl Dihydrochloride; Oxypendyl Dihydrochloride; Perthipendyl Dihydrochloride. 2-{4-[3-(Pyrido[3,2-*b*][1,4]benzothiazin-10-yl)propyl]piperazin-1-yl}ethanol dihydrochloride.
$C_{20}H_{26}N_4OS,2HCl$=443.4.

CAS — 5585-93-3 (oxypendyl); 17297-82-4 (hydrochloride).

Oxypendyl hydrochloride has been used as an anti-emetic.

Proprietary Names and Manufacturers

Pervetral *(Homburg, Ger.).*

7520-h

Oxyphenisatin *(BAN).*
Dihydroxyphenylisatin; Oxyphenisatine *(rINN).* 3,3-Bis(4-hydroxyphenyl)indolin-2-one.
$C_{20}H_{15}NO_3$=317.3.

CAS — 125-13-3.

7521-m

Oxyphenisatin Acetate *(USAN).*
Acetphenolisatin; Bisatin; Diacetoxydiphenylisatin; Diacetyldiphenolisatin; Diasatin; Diphesatin; Isaphenin; Oxyphenisatin Diacetate *(BANM)*; Oxyphenisatine Acetate *(rINNM)*; Phenlaxine.
$C_{24}H_{19}NO_5$=401.4.

CAS — 115-33-3.

Pharmacopoeias. In *Cz., Hung., Jug.,* and *Nord.*

Adverse Effects

Liver damage has occurred usually following prolonged use of oxyphenisatin acetate. Abdominal discomfort such as cramps, nausea and vomiting, or diarrhoea may occur. Other adverse effects which have been reported include sweating, tachycardia, and occasionally syncope.

Allergic reaction to oxyphenisatin might induce or activate systemic lupus erythematosus.— D. Alarcón-Segovia, *Drugs*, 1976, *12*, 69.

EFFECTS ON THE LIVER. References to liver impairment associated with oxyphenisatin: T. B. Reynolds *et al.*, *New Engl. J. Med.*, 1971, *285*, 813; E. Gjone and R. Stave (letter), *Lancet*, 1973, *1*, 421; P. Kotha *et al.*, *Br. med. J.*, 1980, *281*, 1530; D. Schmitz *et al.*, *J. Méd. Strasbourg*, 1983, *14*, 155.

Precautions

As for Bisacodyl, p.1078. The concomitant administration of docusate sodium may enhance the liver toxicity of oxyphenisatin.

Uses and Administration

Oxyphenisatin acetate is a stimulant laxative with actions similar to those of bisacodyl, but its use is no longer permitted in some countries.

Oxyphenisatin 50 mg is given rectally in 2 litres of water as an enema for cleansing the large intestine and as an adjunct in barium enema examinations.

Proprietary Preparations

Veripaque *(Sterling Research, UK). Enema,* powder for reconstitution, oxyphenisatin 50 mg/3 g.

Proprietary Names and Manufacturers of Oxyphenisatin or Oxyphenisatin Acetate

Cirotyl *(Spain)*; Laxnormal *(Spain)*; Veripaque *(Switz.; Sterling Research, UK).*

13090-m

Pentaerythritol
Tetramethylolmethane. 2,2-Bis(hydroxymethyl)propane-1,3-diol.
$C_5H_{12}O_4$=136.1.

CAS — 115-77-5.

Pentaerythritol is used in the treatment of constipation.

Proprietary Names and Manufacturers

Auxinutril *(Gallier, Fr.).*

13093-g

Pepstatin *(USAN, rINN).*
Pepstatin A. *N*-[Isovaleryl-L-valyl-L-valyl-4-amino-3-hydroxy-6-methylheptanoyl-L-alanyl]-4-amino-3-hydroxy-6-methylheptanoic acid.
$C_{34}H_{63}N_5O_9$=685.9.

CAS — 26305-03-3.

Pepstatin inhibits the effect of pepsin probably by binding to form a pepsin-pepstatin complex.

It has been tried without great success in patients with peptic ulcer. Other pepstatins, with differing radicals substituted at four places in the molecule, have been identified.

Proprietary Names and Manufacturers

Bristol, USA.

7522-b

Phenolphthalein *(BAN, USAN, rINN).*
Dihydroxyphthalophenone; Fenolftaleina. 3,3-Bis(4-hydroxyphenyl)phthalide.
$C_{20}H_{14}O_4$=318.3.

CAS — 77-09-8.

Pharmacopoeias. In *Arg., Aust., Belg., Br., Braz., Chin., Cz., Hung., It., Jug., Mex., Nord., Pol., Port., Rus., Span., Swiss, Turk.,* and *U.S. U.S.* also includes Yellow Phenolphthalein.

A white or yellowish-white, odourless or almost odourless, crystalline or amorphous powder. Practically **insoluble** in water; soluble 1 in 15 of alcohol and 1 in 100 of ether; soluble in dilute solutions of alkali hydroxides, and in hot solutions of alkali carbonates, forming a red solution.

Adverse Effects

Allergic reactions usually as skin rashes or eruptions have occurred with phenolphthalein. Cardiac and respiratory distress, and albuminuria and haematuria have also been reported. Abdominal discomfort such as cramps or colic may occasionally occur.

Prolonged use or overdosage can result in diarrhoea with excessive loss of water and electrolytes, particularly potassium; there is also the possibility of developing an atonic non-functioning colon.

Phenolphthalein may cause pink or red discoloration of the urine or faeces.

ABUSE. Osteomalacia in a 51-year-old woman was attributed to depletion of body calcium as a result of diarrhoea due to long-term phenolphthalein ingestion.— B. Frame *et al.*, *Archs intern. Med.*, 1971, *128*, 794.

EFFECTS ON THE SKIN. References to skin reactions associated with phenolphthalein: J. A. Savin, *Br. J. Derm.*, 1970, *83*, 546 (fixed drug eruptions); E. D. Lowney *et al.*, *Archs Derm.*, 1967, *95*, 359 (toxic epidermal necrolysis); R. L. Baer and H. Harris, *J. Am. med. Ass.*, 1967, *202*, 710 (eruptions resembling erythema multiforme).

OVERDOSAGE. Tablets containing about 1.8 g of phenolphthalein were taken by a 3-year-old child. Despite gastric lavage she developed pulmonary oedema and became comatose. Death occurred after 13 hours and postmortem examination revealed cerebral and pulmonary oedema, and phenol in the gastric juice.— L. Sarcinelli *et al.*, *Proc. Eur. Soc. Stud. Drug*, 1970, *11*, 261.

Peritoneal dialysis for 24 hours and the administration of isoprenaline was successful treatment for the hypotension, severe acidosis, pulmonary oedema, and oliguria which occurred in a 35-year-old man who had taken phenolphthalein 2 g as a chocolate laxative preparation.— N. Buchanan *et al.*, *S. Afr. med. J.*, 1976, *50*, 1060.

A report of acute pancreatitis occurring in a 34-year-old man who had inadvertently ingested phenolphthalein 2 g. The patient had been taking phenolphthalein for 2 years for the treatment of chronic constipation. There was complete recovery and no sequelae from the pancreatitis.— A. L. Lambrianides and R. D. Rosin, *Postgrad. med. J.*, 1984, *60*, 491.

Precautions

As for Bisacodyl, p.1078. Phenolphthalein should not be given to patients who have previously shown sensitivity to the drug.

Phenolphthalein could interfere with the Acetest and Ketostix qualitative urine tests for ketones to produce a pink colour.— *Drug & Ther. Bull.*, 1972, *10*, 69.

Absorption and Fate

Up to 15% of phenolphthalein given by mouth is absorbed. Enterohepatic circulation occurs and the glucuronide is excreted in the bile. Some excretion occurs in the urine.

Uses and Administration

Phenolphthalein is a diphenylmethane stimulant laxative. It usually has an effect within 6 to 8 hours but because of enterohepatic circulation its action may continue for several days.

It is usually administered in pills or tablets, or it may also be given as an emulsion with liquid paraffin. It is usually given in a dose of 30 to 200 mg taken at bedtime; doses of 270 mg daily should not be exceeded.

Yellow phenolphthalein, an impure form, has been claimed to be more active than phenolphthalein.

Preparations

Compound Phenolphthalein Pills *(B.P.C. 1973)*. Pilulae Phenaloini. Each contains phenolphthalein 30 mg, aloin 15 mg, and belladonna dry extract 5 mg. They are coated with a chocolate-coloured coating. *Dose*. 1 or 2 pills.

Phenolphthalein Tablets *(U.S.P.)*. Store in airtight containers.

Proprietary Preparations

Alophen *(Warner-Lambert, UK)*. *Pills*, phenolphthalein 30 mg, aloin 15 mg, prepared ipecacuanha 4 mg, belladonna dry extract 5 mg.

Proprietary Names and Manufacturers

Bom-Bon *(Montefarmaco, Ital.)*; Darmol *(Ger.; Switz.)*; Euchessina *(Antonetto, Ital.; Switz.)*; Evac-Q-Kwik Tablets *(Adria, Canad.)*; Evac-Q-Tabs *(Adria, USA)*; Evac-U-Gen *(Walker, Corp, USA)*; Fructines Vichy *(Switz.)*; Fructine-Vichy *(Lirca, Ital.)*; Laxante Yer *(Yer, Spain)*; Laxatone *(De-Nol, S.Afr.)*; Laxen Busto *(Busto, Spain)*; Lilo *(Ital.)*; Neo-Prunex *(Neolab, Canad.)*; Neopurghes *(IFCI, Ital.)*; Phenolax *(Upjohn, USA)*; Prulet *(Mission Pharmacal, USA)*; Purganol *(Saunier-Daguin, Fr.)*; Purgante *(Falqui, Ital.)*; Purgante el Aleman *(Puerto Galiano, Spain)*; Purgante Orravan *(Orravan, Spain)*; Purgestol *(Zoja, Ital.)*.

The following names have been used for multi-ingredient preparations containing phenolphthalein—Agarol *(Warner, Austral.; Parke, Davis, Canad.; Warner-Lambert, UK)*; Agoral *(Parke, Davis, USA)*; Alophen *(Parke, Davis, Canad.; Warner-Lambert, UK)*; Anodyne Dellipsoids D4 *(Pilsworth, UK)*; Aperient Dellipsoids D9 *(Pilsworth, UK)*; Boldolaxine *(Simes, Austral.)*; D & M Tablets *(Cambridge Laboratories, Austral.)*; Evactil *(Faulding, Austral.)*; Kest *(Rorer, UK)*; Kondremul with Phenolphthalein *(Fisons, USA)*; Modane *(Adria, USA)*; Modane Plus *(Adria, USA)*; Mucinum *(Sabex, Canad.)*; Paradeine *(Scotia, UK)*; Petrolagar Emulsion (Red Label) *(Wyeth, UK)*; Phillips' Laxcaps *(Glenbrook, USA)*; Purgoids *(Evans Medical, UK)*; Sarolax *(Saron, USA)*; Trilax *(Drug Industries, USA)*; Veracolate *(Warner, Austral.; Parke, Davis, UK)*.

13101-y

Phenolphthalol

2-(4,4'-Dihydroxybenzhydryl)benzyl alcohol.

$C_{20}H_{18}O_3$=306.4.

CAS — 81-92-5.

Phenolphthalol is used as a laxative.

Proprietary Names and Manufacturers

Gentiapol *(Pohl, Ger.)*; Normolax *(Biagini, Ital.)*; Regolax *(Corvi, Ital.)*.

13115-t

Pifarnine *(USAN, rINN)*.

U-27. 1-Piperonyl-4-(3,7,11-trimethyldodeca-2,6,10-trienyl)piperazine.

$C_{27}H_{40}N_2O_2$=424.6.

CAS — 56208-01-6.

Pifarnine is used in the treatment of peptic ulcer in doses of up to 150 mg daily.

Proprietary Names and Manufacturers

Pifazin *(Pierrel, Ital.)*.

13129-h

Pirenzepine Hydrochloride *(BANM, rINNM)*.

LS-519 (pirenzepine); LS-519-CL-2 (hydrochloride). 5,11-Dihydro-11-(4-methylpiperazin-1-ylacetyl)pyrido[2,3-*b*][1,4]benzodiazepin-6-one dihydrochloride.

$C_{19}H_{21}N_5O_2$,2HCl=424.3.

CAS — 28797-61-7 (pirenzepine); 29868-97-1 (hydrochloride).

Adverse Effects

Dry mouth and blurred vision may occur with pirenzepine but other side-effects associated with traditional antimuscarinic agents are stated to be less likely to occur since it binds preferentially to receptors in the gastric mucosa and the penetration across the blood-brain barrier is poor. Other adverse effects reported with pirenzepine include diarrhoea or constipation, headache, and mental confusion.

Thrombocytopenia in one patient and agranulocytosis in another probably associated with the administration of pirenzepine.— B. Stricker *et al.*, *Br. med. J.*, 1986, *293*, 1074.

Absorption and Fate

Pirenzepine is absorbed from the gastro-intestinal tract but the bioavailability is reported to be only about 25% being decreased to about 10 to 20% when taken with food. Very little pirenzepine is metabolised with about 90% of an oral dose being excreted in the faeces.

Pirenzepine has an elimination half-life of about 12 hours and is only slightly (about 12%) bound to plasma proteins. Diffusion across the blood-brain barrier is poor and only minimal amounts are stated to be present in the milk of lactating women.

Uses and Administration

Pirenzepine is a selective antimuscarinic agent which displays preferential binding to the receptors of the gastric mucosa thus causing a reduction in the secretion of gastric acid; it also reduces the secretion of pepsin.

Pirenzepine hydrochloride is used in the treatment of duodenal and gastric ulcers. The usual dose is 50 mg twice daily by mouth for 4 to 6 weeks; if necessary the dose may be increased to 50 mg three times daily. If longer-term therapy is required pirenzepine may be administered for a period of up to 3 months. Pirenzepine should be taken on an empty stomach before meals.

PEPTIC ULCER. A detailed and extensive review of the pharmacodynamic and pharmacokinetic properties and therapeutic efficacy of pirenzepine in peptic ulcer disease. The results from numerous double-blind, placebo-controlled studies in patients with endoscopically verified duodenal ulcers have indicated that the ulcer healing with pirenzepine is dose-related, with doses of 100 to 150 mg daily generally improving healing-rates significantly while smaller doses did not. Healing with doses of pirenzepine 100 to 150 mg daily did not usually differ significantly from that achieved with cimetidine 1 g daily. Some small studies comparing pirenzepine as low-dose (30 to 50 mg daily) long-term prophylactic therapy with placebo or cimetidine (400 mg daily) have not consistently demonstrated any significant differences in recurrence-rates. The efficacy of pirenzepine in benign gastric ulcer has been less extensively studied than in duodenal ulcer and the results are less conclusive.— A. A. Carmine and R. N. Brogden, *Drugs*, 1985, *30*, 85.

A short review of pirenzepine concluding that although pirenzepine is certainly effective in peptic ulcer, it relieves symptoms more slowly than the well-tried H_2-antagonists and offers no advantages over them. It should however, prove a useful second-line treatment.— *Drug & Ther. Bull.*, 1985, *23*, 29.

Proprietary Preparations

Gastrozepin *(Boots, UK)*. *Tablets*, scored, pirenzepine hydrochloride equivalent to anhydrous pirenzepine hydrochloride 50 mg.

Proprietary Names and Manufacturers

Acilec *(Lasa, Spain)*; Duogastral *(ISM, Ital.)*; Durapirenz *(Durachemie, Ger.)*; Gasteril *(Ripari-Gero, Ital.)*; Gastricur *(Heumann, Ger.)*; Gastri-P *(Beiersdorf, Ger.)*; Gastrol *(Tiber, Ital.)*; Gastropiren *(AGIPS, Ital.)*; Gastrosed *(Samil, Ital.)*; Gastrozépine *(Boehringer Ingelheim, Fr.; Boehringer Ingelheim, Switz.)*; Gastrozepin *(Bender, Aust.; Boehringer Ingelheim, Canad.; Thomae, Ger.; Boehringer Ingelheim, Ital.; Boehringer Ingelheim, Norw.; Boehringer Ingelheim, S.Afr.; Boehringer Ingelheim, Spain; Boehringer Sohn, Switz.; Boots, UK)*; Indone *(Hosbon, Spain)*; Leblon *(De Angeli, Ital.)*; Lulcus *(Tosi-Novara, Ital.)*; Maghen *(Caber, Ital.)*; Ulcin *(Ibirn, Ital.)*; Ulcopir *(Aesculapius, Ital.)*; Ulcoprotect *(Azuchemie, Ger.)*; Ulcosafe *(Sagitta, Ger.)*; Ulcosan *(Dompé, Ital.)*; Ulcosyntex *(Francia Farm., Ital.)*; Ulcuforton *(Plantorgan, Ger.)*; Ulgescum *(Dolorgiet, Ger.)*; Ulpir *(IBP, Ital.)*.

5448-k

Plantain Seed

The seed of *Plantago major* var. *asiatica* .

Pharmacopoeias. In *Jpn*.

Plantain seed has been suggested as a substitute for ispaghula.

5008-c

Polycarbophil Calcium *(BANM, rINNM)*.

AHR-3260B; Calcium Polycarbophil *(USAN)*; Polycarbophilum Calcii; WI-140.

CAS — 9003-97-8 (polycarbophil).

Pharmacopoeias. In *U.S.*

The calcium salt of polyacrylic acid cross-linked with divinyl glycol. A white to creamy-white powder. Practically **insoluble** in water, common organic solvents, and dilute acids and alkalis. It loses not more than 10% of its weight on drying and contains not less than 18% and not more than 22% of calcium, calculated on the anhydrous basis. **Store** in airtight containers.

Adverse Effects and Precautions

As for ispaghula, p.1091.

Polycarbophil calcium releases calcium ions in the gastro-intestinal tract and should be avoided by patients who must restrict their calcium intake or by those taking tetracyclines by mouth.

Uses and Administration

Polycarbophil calcium has similar properties to ispaghula (see p.1091) and is used similarly as a bulk laxative and for adjusting faecal consistency. Following ingestion calcium ions are replaced by hydrogen ions from gastric acid and the resultant polycarbophil exerts a hydrophilic effect in the intestines. Polycarbophil is not absorbed from the gastro-intestinal tract.

In the treatment of constipation the usual dose by mouth as chewable tablets is the equivalent of 1 g of polycarbophil four times daily up to a total of 6 g daily. Doses should be taken with about 250 mL of water. Suggested children's doses are: 6 to 12 years, the equivalent of 500 mg three times daily up to 3 g daily; 3 to 6 years, the equivalent of 500 mg twice daily up to 1.5 g daily.
In the treatment of severe diarrhoea individual doses may be repeated at half-hour intervals, but the maximum daily dosage should not be exceeded.

A review of the actions and uses of polycarbophil calcium.— I. E. Danhof, *Pharmacotherapy*, 1982, *2*, 18.

Proprietary Names and Manufacturers
Carbopol EX 55 *(Goodrich, UK)*; Carbopol EX 83 *(Goodrich, UK)*; FiberCon *(Lederle, USA)*; Mitrolan *(Robins, Canad.; Robins, USA)*.

1185-n

Potassium Sulphate
515; Kalium Sulfuricum; Potassii Sulphas; Tartarus Vitriolatus.
K_2SO_4=174.3.

CAS — 7778-80-5.

Pharmacopoeias. In *Arg., Aust., Belg., Fr., Hung., Jpn, Nord., Pol., Port., Span.,* and *Swiss.*

Potassium sulphate has been used, in doses of 1 to 3 g, in dilute solution as a laxative.
It is used as a food additive.
For the general properties of potassium salts, see p.1036.

1186-h

Potassium Acid Tartrate
E336; Kalium Hydrotartaricum; Potassium Bitartrate; Potassium Hydrogen Tartrate; Purified Cream of Tartar; Tártarus Depuratus; Weinstein.
$C_4H_5KO_6$=188.2.

CAS — 868-14-4.

Pharmacopoeias. In *Arg., Aust., Belg., Fr., Neth., Pol., Port., Roum.,* and *Span.* Also in *B.P.C. 1973.*

Odourless or almost odourless colourless crystals or white crystalline powder. It absorbs insignificant amounts of moisture at 25° at relative humidities up to about 90%.
Soluble 1 in 190 of water and 1 in 16 of boiling water; practically insoluble in alcohol.

Potassium acid tartrate has been used, in doses of 1 to 4 g, as a laxative.
It is used as a food additive.
For the general properties of potassium salts, see p.1036.

Proprietary Names and Manufacturers
Evac-Q-Sert *(Adria, USA)*.

The following names have been used for multi-ingredient preparations containing potassium acid tartrate— Ceo-Two *(Beutlich, USA)*; Potavescent *(Protea, Austral.)*.

1187-m

Potassium Tartrate
E336.
$(C_4H_4K_2O_6)_2,H_2O$=470.6.

CAS — 921-53-9 (anhydrous).

Pharmacopoeias. In *Port.*

Potassium tartrate has been used, in doses of 2 to 16 g, in dilute solution as a laxative.
It is used as a food additive.
For the general properties of potassium salts. see p.1036.

Proprietary Names and Manufacturers
K-Med *(Riva, Canad.)*; Nati-K *(Sabex, Canad.; Synlab, Fr.; Nativelle, Switz.)*; Wel-K *(Welcker-Lyster, Canad.)*.

705-n

Proglumide *(BAN, USAN, rINN).*
CR-242; W-5219; Xylamide. (±)-4-Benzamido-*NN*-dipropylglutaramic acid.
$C_{18}H_{26}N_2O_4$=334.4.

CAS — 6620-60-6.

Proglumide has an inhibitory effect on gastric secretion and is reported to be a gastrin-receptor antagonist. It is used in the treatment of peptic ulcer in doses of 0.8 to 1.2 g daily before meals; it is also given by intramuscular or by slow intravenous injection.

Proprietary Names and Manufacturers
Gastridine *(Bernabó, Arg.)*; Gastrotopic *(Perga, Spain)*; Milid *(Opfermann, Ger.; Rottapharm, Ital.; Ethimed, S.Afr.; Max Ritter, Switz.)*; Milide *(Beytout, Fr.; Farma-Lepori, Spain)*; Promid *(Jpn)*; Snol *(Inexfa, Spain)*; Triulco *(Santos, Spain)*; Xyla-Ulco *(Spain)*.

7526-p

Prune
Ameixa; Prunus.

The dried ripe fruits of *Prunus domestica* and other species of *Prunus* (Rosaceae). **Store** in a dry place.

Prune has laxative and demulcent properties.

5452-y

Psyllium

Pharmacopoeias. In *Egypt., Int., Nord.,* and *Swiss.* Also in *B.P.C. 1973.* Also in *U.S.* under the title of Plantago seed (see below). See also Ispaghula and Ispaghula Husk, p.1091.

Psyllium (*B.P.C. 1973*) (Flea Seed) consists of the dried ripe seed of *Plantago afra* (*Plantago psyllium*) or of *Plantago indica* (*Plantago arenaria*) (Plantaginaceae).
Plantago Seed (*U.S.P.*) is the cleaned, dried, ripe seed of *Plantago ovata*, known in commerce as Blond Psyllium or as Indian Plantago Seed, or of *Plantago psyllium*, or of *Plantago indica* (*Plantago arenaria*), known in commerce as Spanish Psyllium Seed or as French Psyllium Seed.

Psyllium has properties similar to those of ispaghula husk (see p.1091). It has been given as a bulk laxative in doses of 5 to 15 g.

For reports of allergic reactions associated with psyllium-containing preparations see under Ispaghula Husk, p.1091.

Proprietary Names and Manufacturers
Mucilar *(Spirig, Switz.)*; Osmolax *(Seclo, Fr.)*; Planten *(Serono, Ital.)*.

3777-a

Ranitidine *(BAN, USAN, rINN).*
AH-19065. *NN*-Dimethyl-5-[2-(1-methylamino-2-nitrovinylamino)ethylthiomethyl]furfurylamine.
$C_{13}H_{22}N_4O_3S$=314.4.

CAS — 66357-35-5.

6162-e

Ranitidine Hydrochloride *(BANM, rINNM).*

$C_{13}H_{22}N_4O_3S,HCl$=350.9.

Adverse Effects
As for cimetidine (p.1082). However, unlike cimetidine, ranitidine has little or no anti-androgenic effect and the incidence of gynaecomastia and impotence in patients treated with higher doses of ranitidine has been reported not to differ from that encountered in the general population. Ranitidine, also, does not appear to be associated with reports of interstitial nephritis.

Although there have been isolated case reports of adverse endocrine effects (unilateral painful gynaecomastia: S. Tosi and M. Cagnoli, *Lancet*, 1982, *1*, 160; impotence: L. Viana, *ibid.*, 1983, *2*, 635) and adverse cardiovascular effects (bradycardia: E. Camarri *et al.*, *Lancet*, 1982, *2*, 160 and R.R. Shah, *ibid.*, 1108) associated with ranitidine the manufacturers (*Glaxo*) responded, generally stating the incidence was no higher than in the general population and doubting such an association with ranitidine (*Lancet* 1982, *2*, 264 and 1281; *ibid.*, 1983, *2*, 798). A review (M.A. Souza Lima, *Ann. intern. Med.*, 1986, *105*, 140) concluding that ranitidine may have a significantly higher incidence of hepatotoxicity than cimetidine also resulted in a reply from *Glaxo* (*ibid.*, 803) in which it was regarded that the relative rate was similar for both drugs.

ALLERGY. Respiratory stridor and urticaria in one patient shortly after taking the first dose of ranitidine; the symptoms responded to adrenaline subcutaneously.— C. M. Brayko (letter), *New Engl. J. Med.*, 1984, *310*, 1601.

EFFECTS ON THE BLOOD. Reports of agranulocytosis or granulocytopenia possibly associated with ranitidine: L. I. Shields *et al.* (letter), *Ann. intern. Med.*, 1986, *104*, 128 (agranulocytosis); L. O. Brenner (letter), *ibid.*, 896 (agranulocytosis).
Reports of thrombocytopenia possibly associated with ranitidine: R. T. Spychal and N. W. R. Wickham, *Br. med. J.*, 1985, *291*, 1687; M. W. Pearson (letter), *ibid.*, 1986, *292*, 489; U. Gafter *et al.* (letter), *Ann. intern. Med.*, 1987, *106*, 477.
Reports of other adverse haematological effects possibly associated with ranitidine: P. A. Lebert *et al.*, *Clin. Pharmac. Ther.*, 1981, *30*, 539 (leucopenia); D. C. Harmon and R. Shuman (letter), *New Engl. J. Med.*, 1984, *310*, 1604 (aplastic anaemia); A. Herrera *et al.* (letter), *ibid.*, 1604 (neutropenia); J. B. Zeldis *et al.* (letter), *ibid.*, 1605 (doubt about the case of aplastic anaemia); D. Jack *et al.* (letter), *ibid.*, 1606 (doubt from Glaxo about the case of aplastic anaemia).

EFFECTS ON THE ENDOCRINE SYSTEM. A study investigating the effect of ranitidine on gonadal function in males found no significant changes in sperm concentration, motility, or morphology.— C. Wang *et al.*, *Br. J. clin. Pharmac.*, 1983, *16*, 430.
Reversible amenorrhoea possibly associated with ranitidine.— L. Lombardo (letter), *Lancet*, 1982, *1*, 224. The amenorrhoea and raised prolactin concentrations were associated with a pituitary microadenoma and not ranitidine. Moreover, in a study of 10 young women with duodenal ulcers ranitidine had no effect on serum-prolactin values and none of the patients exhibited menstrual disorders, or other clinical disturbances. On the basis of these findings and published data the view was no longer held that ranitidine can cause hyperprolactinaemia and amenorrhoea.— *idem*, 1983, *2*, 42.

EFFECTS ON THE EYE. For a report of an increase in intraocular pressure associated with ranitidine, see under Cimetidine (p.1082).

EFFECTS ON THE GASTRO-INTESTINAL TRACT. *Gastric cancer.* For reviews concerning the debate about H_2-antagonists and the development of gastric cancer, see cimetidine (p.1082).

EFFECTS ON THE LIVER. A review of computerised reports of hepatotoxicity associated with ranitidine and cimetidine held by the Division of Drug Experience of the Food and Drug Administration; the reports covered a period of about 2 years for ranitidine and 8 years for cimetidine. Although there were 45 reports of hepatic injury for ranitidine a cause-and-effect relationship could not be established for many, but in 18 cases the circumstantial evidence appeared strong despite a lack of re-challenge with the drug. The time from the start of ranitidine treatment to the onset of hepatic injury ranged from a few days to 2 months and all patients recovered or improved on withdrawal of therapy. Using the same guidelines, however, only 3 cases of cimetidine-associated hepatic injury were identified where the evidence was considered strong. Although it was acknowledged that such retrospective analysis carries inherent flaws it was considered that ranitidine has a significantly higher incidence of hepatotoxicity than does cimetidine especially in view of the shorter lifespan and smaller market share of ranitidine.— M. A. Souza Lima (letter), *Ann. intern. Med.*, 1986, *105*, 140. Reply from *Glaxo* stating that hepatitis can be regarded as a rare and idiosyncratic occurrence with both cimetidine and ranitidine and that the relative rate is similar with both drugs.— J. H. Dobbs *et al.* (letter), *ibid.*, 803.

EFFECTS ON THE NERVOUS SYSTEM. Individual reports of adverse neurological effects possibly associated with ranitidine and mainly in patients who were elderly or seriously ill: J. D. Hughes *et al.*, *Med. J. Aust.*, 1983, *2*, 12 (hallucinations); C. M. Epstein (letter), *New Engl. J. Med.*, 1984, *310*, 1602 (headache); P. H. Silverstone (letter), *Lancet*, 1984, *1*, 1071 (confusion); C. M. Epstein (letter), *ibid* (confusion); C. De Giacomo *et al.* (letter), *ibid.*, *2*, 47 (confusion and loss of colour vision); R. B. Mani *et al.* (letter), *ibid.*, 98 (confusion); W. Price *et al.*, *Eur. J. clin. Pharmac.*, 1985, *29*, 375 (hallucinations); S. K. Mandal, *Br. J. clin. Pract.*, 1986, *40*, 260 (confusion); A. J. MacDermott *et al.* (letter), *Br. med. J.*, 1987, *294*, 1616 (confusion).

For studies indicating that ranitidine by mouth is suitable for those involved in skilled activity, see under Precautions for cimetidine (p.1083).

Precautions

As for cimetidine (p.1083). Although there have been isolated reports of drug interactions with ranitidine, it is generally considered that the potential for such interactions is far less in comparison to cimetidine.

For a study on the effect of ranitidine on performance, see under cimetidine (p.1083).

INTERACTIONS. Reviews comparing the drug interactions of ranitidine with those of cimetidine.— *Drug Interact. News.*, 1983, *3*, 31; W. Kirch *et al.*, *Clin. Pharmacokinet.*, 1984, *9*, 493.

Antacids. For comments on the interaction of ranitidine with antacids, see under cimetidine (p.1083).

Anti-arrhythmics. For the effect of ranitidine on procainamide, see under Procainamide Hydrochloride, p.83. See also under Lignocaine Hydrochloride, p.1218.

Antiepileptics. For the effect of ranitidine on some antiepileptic agents, see under Carbamazepine, p.401 and Phenytoin Sodium, p.408.

Local anaesthetics. For the effect of ranitidine on some local anaesthetics, see under Bupivacaine Hydrochloride, p.1209 and Lignocaine Hydrochloride, p.1218.

Vasodilators. For the effect of ranitidine on diltiazem, see under Diltiazem Hydrochloride, p.1496.

PREGNANCY AND THE NEONATE. Pharmacokinetic study in a lactating mother given multiple doses of ranitidine showed higher concentrations in breast milk than in serum; it was not considered feasible to estimate the dose of ranitidine that the infant may consume in milk.— G. L. Kearns *et al.*, *Clin. Pharm.*, 1985, *4*, 322.

Absorption and Fate

Ranitidine is readily absorbed from the gastro-intestinal tract with peak concentrations in plasma occurring about 2 hours after administration by mouth. The bioavailability of ranitidine following oral administration is about 50% compared to an intravenous dose due to first-pass metabolism. The elimination half-life from plasma is around 2 hours and ranitidine is weakly bound, about 15%, to plasma proteins.

A small proportion of ranitidine is metabolised in the liver to the N-oxide, the S-oxide, and desmethylranitidine but most is excreted unchanged in the urine; there may also be some enterohepatic recycling. Ranitidine crosses the placental barrier and is excreted into breast milk where concentrations are reported to be higher than those in plasma. It does not readily cross the blood-brain barrier.

A review of the clinical pharmacokinetics of ranitidine.— C. J. C. Roberts, *Clin. Pharmacokinet.*, 1984, *9*, 211.

Uses and Administration

Ranitidine is a histamine H_2-receptor antagonist with actions and uses similar to those of cimetidine (p.1084).

Ranitidine may be given by mouth or parenterally by the intravenous or intramuscular routes. Although the preparations contain ranitidine hydrochloride, strengths and doses are expressed in terms of the base.

The usual dose of ranitidine by mouth is 150 mg twice daily (in the morning and at bedtime). The usual dose by intramuscular or intravenous injection is 50 mg which may be repeated every 6 to 8 hours; the intravenous injection should be given slowly over not less than 2 minutes and should be diluted to contain 50 mg in 20 mL. For an intermittent intravenous infusion the recommended dose is 25 mg per hour given for 2 hours which may be repeated at intervals of 6 to 8 hours.

In the management of duodenal and gastric ulcers a single daily dose of 300 mg by mouth at bedtime is suggested as an alternative to twice-daily administration and treatment should be given initially for at least 4 weeks. Where appropriate a maintenance dose of 150 mg daily may be given at bedtime.

In reflux oesophagitis the recommended dose is 150 mg twice daily by mouth for up to 8 weeks.

In pathological hypersecretory conditions, such as the Zollinger-Ellison syndrome, the initial oral dose is usually 150 mg twice or three times daily and may be increased if necessary; doses of up to 6 g daily have been employed.

For the management of patients at risk from stress-related ulceration of the upper gastro-intestinal tract doses of 150 mg twice daily by mouth are suggested or parenteral therapy may be employed (see above). In patients at risk of developing the acid aspiration syndrome during general anaesthesia, a dose of 150 mg by mouth may be given 2 hours before the induction of anaesthesia or at the start of labour and may be repeated at intervals of 6 hours if required; alternatively a dose of 50 mg may be given by intramuscular or slow intravenous injection 45 to 60 minutes before the induction of anaesthesia.

The dosage of ranitidine should be reduced in patients with severely impaired renal function; the suggested doses are 150 mg daily by mouth or 25 mg for parenteral administration.

For reviews, reports, and comments on the use of ranitidine in the Aspiration Syndrome, Gastro-intestinal Bleeding, Pancreatic Disorders, Paracetamol Toxicity, Peptic Ulcers, Reflux Oesophagitis, Stress Ulceration, and the Zollinger-Ellison Syndrome, see under cimetidine (p.1084).

ADMINISTRATION. From results obtained in pharmacokinetic studies in 10 healthy young adults, 9 patients with cirrhosis, and 8 healthy elderly people, it was predicted that concentrations of ranitidine would be approximately 55% higher in the cirrhotics and 60% higher in the elderly compared to the young adults but that a dosage reduction would not be mandatory.— C. J. Young *et al.*, *Gut*, 1982, *23*, 819.

Proprietary Preparations

Zantac *(Glaxo, UK)*. *Tablets*, ranitidine 150 and 300 mg (as hydrochloride).

Tablets, dispersible, scored, ranitidine 150 mg (as hydrochloride).

Syrup, ranitidine 75 mg/5 mL (as hydrochloride).

Injection, ranitidine 25 mg (as hydrochloride)/mL, in ampoules of 2 mL.

Proprietary Names and Manufacturers of Ranitidine or Ranitidine Hydrochloride

Azantac *(Glaxo, Fr.)*; Coralen *(Alter, Spain)*; Mauran *(Coli, Ital.)*; Nodol *(Del Saz & Filippini, Ital.)*; Quantor *(Almirall, Spain)*; Ranacid *(Nyco, Norw.)*; Raniben *(FIRMA, Ital.)*; Ranibloc *(Bonomelli, Ital.)*; Ranidil *(Duncan, Ital.)*; Ranidin *(Faes, Spain)*; Ranilonga *(Lafarquim, Spain)*; Raniplex *(Fournier S.A., Fr.)*; Ranix *(Liade, Spain)*; Ranuber *(Hubber, Spain)*; Sostril *(Cascan, Ger.)*; Tanidina *(Robert, Spain)*; Toriol *(Vita, Spain)*; Trigger *(Polifarma, Ital.)*; Ulcex *(Guidotti, Ital.)*; Ulkobrin *(Zoja, Ital.)*; Zantac *(Glaxo, Austral.*; *Glaxo, Canad.*; *Glaxo, Denm.*; *Glaxo, Ital.*; *Glaxo, Norw.*; *Glaxo, S.Afr.*; *Glaxo, Spain*; *Glaxo, Swed.*; *Glaxo, UK*; *Glaxo, USA)*; Zantic *(Glaxo, Ger.*; *Glaxo, Switz.)*.

7527-s

Rhubarb *(BAN)*.

Chinese Rhubarb; Rabarbaro; Rhabarber; Rhei Radix; Rhei Rhizoma; Rheum; Rhubarb Rhizome; Ruibarbo.

Pharmacopoeias. In *Arg.*, *Aust.*, *Belg.*, *Br.*, *Braz.*, *Chin.*, *Cz.*, *Egypt.*, *Eur.*, *Fr.*, *Ger.*, *Hung.*, *It.*, *Jpn*, *Mex.*, *Neth.*, *Pol.*, *Port.*, *Roum.*, *Rus.*, *Span.*, and *Swiss*. *Chin.* also permits *R. tanguticum* and *Jpn* also permits *R. coreanum*. *Br.* and *Jpn* also describe Powdered Rhubarb.

The dried underground parts of *Rheum palmatum* or *R. officinale* (Polygonaceae) or hybrids of these species, or mixtures of these, separated from the stem, rootlets, and most of the bark. The *B.P.* and *Eur. P.* specify not less than 2.5% of hydroxyanthracene derivatives, calculated as rhein ($C_{15}H_8O_6$=284.2). **Store** in well-closed containers. Protect from light and moisture.

Other rhubarbs include Indian rhubarb (Himalayan rhubarb), the dried rhizome and roots of *R. emodi*, *R. webbianum*, or some other species of *Rheum*, and an adulterant of rhubarb known as Rhapontic rhubarb (Chinese rhapontica), obtained from *R. rhaponticum*. English rhubarb is derived from *R. rhaponticum* and other species of *Rheum*; the leaf-stalks of garden rhubarb are used as a food.

Adverse Effects and Precautions

As for Senna, p.1106.

Uses and Administration

Rhubarb is an anthraquinone laxative. It also exerts an astringent action due to the presence of tannins.

Preparations

Ammoniated Rhubarb and Soda Mixture *(B.P.)*. Rhubarb, Ammonia and Soda Mixture; Ammoniated Rhubarb and Soda Oral Suspension. A peppermint-flavoured suspension containing rhubarb 2.5%, sodium bicarbonate 8%, and ammonium bicarbonate 2%. Extemporaneous preparations should be recently prepared according to the following formula: rhubarb 250 mg, ammonium bicarbonate 200 mg, sodium bicarbonate 800 mg, concentrated peppermint emulsion 0.25 mL, double-strength chloroform water 5 mL, water to 10 mL.

Compound Rhubarb Mixture *(B.P.)*. Compound Rhubarb Oral Suspension. A ginger-flavoured suspension containing compound rhubarb tincture 10% v/v and 5% each of light magnesium carbonate and sodium bicarbonate. Extemporaneous preparations should be recently prepared according to the following formula: compound rhubarb tincture 1 mL, light magnesium carbonate 500 mg, sodium bicarbonate 500 mg, strong ginger tincture 0.3 mL, double-strength chloroform water 5 mL, water to 10 mL.

Paediatric Compound Rhubarb Mixture *(B.P.C. 1973)*. Mistura Rhei Composita pro Infantibus; Rhubarb Mixture for Infants. Compound rhubarb tincture 0.3 mL, light magnesium carbonate 75 mg, sodium bicarbonate 75 mg, ginger syrup 0.5 mL, double-strength chloroform water 2.5 mL, water to 5 mL. *Dose.* Children, up to 1 year, 5 mL; 1 to 5 years, 10 mL.

Rhubarb and Soda Mixture *(A.P.F.)*. Rhubarb 250 mg, light magnesium carbonate 500 mg, sodium bicarbonate 500 mg, ginger syrup 1 mL, concentrated chloroform water 0.25 mL or compound hydroxybenzoate solution 0.1 mL, water to 10 mL. *Dose.* 10 to 20 mL.

Compound Rhubarb Tincture *(B.P.)*. Prepared by percolation from rhubarb 10 g, cardamom oil 0.04 mL, coriander oil 0.003 mL, glycerol 10 mL, and alcohol (60%) to 100 mL.

2430-g

Roxatidine *(BAN, rINN)*.

N-{3-[(α-Piperidino-*m*-tolyl)oxy]propyl}glycolamide.
$C_{17}H_{26}N_2O_3$=306.4.

Roxatidine is a histamine H_2-receptor antagonist with actions and uses similar to those of cimetidine (p.1082).

Proprietary Names and Manufacturers

Altat *(Teikoku, Jpn)*.

7530-b

Senna *(USAN)*.

CAS — 8013-11-4 (senna); 81-27-6 (sennoside A); 128-57-4 (sennoside B); 52730-36-6 (sennoside A, calcium salt); 52730-37-7 (sennoside B, calcium salt).

Pharmacopoeias. Senna fruit, from Alexandrian and Tinnevelly senna is included in *Arg.*, *Aust.*, *Belg.*, *Br.*, *Cz.*, *Egypt.*, *Eur.*, *Fr.*, *Ger.*, *Hung.*, *Ind.*, *Int.*, *It.*, *Neth.*, *Nord.*, and *Swiss*; some have only one monograph covering both varieties; *Port.* includes only Tinnevelly senna fruit. Senna leaf, from Alexandrian or Tinnevelly senna or both, is included in *Arg., Aust., Belg., Br., Braz., Chin., Egypt., Eur., Fr., Ger., Hung., Ind., Int., It., Jpn., Jug., Mex., Neth., Nord., Port., Rus., Span., Swiss,* and *U.S. U.S.* also includes Sennosides.

In commerce senna obtained from *Cassia senna* (=*C. acutifolia*) (Leguminosae) is known as Alexandrian senna or Khartoum senna and that from *Cassia angustifolia* (Leguminosae) as Tinnevelly senna.

Alexandrian Senna Fruit (Alexandrian Senna Pods) of the *B.P.* and *Eur. P.* is the dried fruit of *Cassia senna* containing not less than 3.4% of hydroxyanthracene glycosides calculated as sennoside B. **Protect** from light and moisture.

Tinnevelly Senna Fruit (Tinnevelly Senna Pods) of the *B.P.* and *Eur. P.* is the dried fruit of *Cassia angustifolia* containing not less than 2.2% of hydroxyanthracene glycosides calculated as sennoside B. **Protect** from light and moisture.

Senna Leaf (*B.P., Eur. P.*) is the dried leaflets of *Cassia senna*, or of *Cassia angustifolia* or a mixture of both species containing not less than 2.5% of hydroxyanthracene glycosides calculated as sennoside B. **Protect** from light and moisture.

Senna (*U.S.P.*) is the dried leaflets of *Cassia acutifolia* (=*C.senna*) or *Cassia angustifolia*.

Sennosides (*U.S.P.*) is a partially purified natural complex of anthraquinone glucosides found in senna, isolated from *Cassia acutifolia* (=*C. senna*) or *Cassia angustifolia* as calcium salts. It is a brownish powder. **Soluble** 1 in 35 of water, 1 in 2100 of alcohol, 1 in 3700 of chloroform, and 1 in 6100 of ether.

Adverse Effects

Senna may cause mild abdominal discomfort such as colic or cramps. Prolonged use or overdosage can result in diarrhoea with excessive loss of water and electrolytes, particularly potassium; there is also the possibility of developing an atonic non-functioning colon. Discoloration of the urine may occur with anthraquinone derivatives.

ABUSE. Tetany and finger clubbing in the absence of diarrhoea was believed to be associated with ingestion of large amounts of senna in a patient with anorexia nervosa.— J. Prior and I. White (letter), *Lancet*, 1978, *2*, 947.

Melanosis coli in a 4-year-old child following anthracene abuse using preparations of senna and of danthron with poloxamer 188.— B. A. Price *et al., Postgrad. med. J.*, 1980, *56*, 854.

Finger clubbing and intermittent urinary excretion of aspartylglucosamine in a woman who had taken a senna laxative preparation continuously for 10 years.— J. Malmquist *et al., Postgrad. med. J.*, 1980, *56*, 862.

Senna abuse in one patient associated with reversible cachexia, hypogammaglobulinaemia, and finger clubbing.— D. Levine *et al., Lancet*, 1981, *1*, 919.

Hypertrophic osteoarthropathy associated with excessive use of senna.— R. D. Armstrong *et al., Br. med. J.*, 1981, *282*, 1836.

Precautions

Senna should not be given to patients with intestinal obstruction or with undiagnosed abdominal symptoms; care should also be taken in patients with inflammatory bowel disease. Prolonged use should be avoided.

Although anthraquinone derivatives may be excreted in the milk of lactating mothers, following normal dosage the concentration is usually insufficient to affect the nursing infant.

There is the possibility that by discoloring the urine anthraquinone laxatives may interfere with diagnostic tests.

Colonic perforation with faecal peritonitis resulting in death of 2 patients following the use of a senna preparation containing sennosides 142 mg for bowel preparation prior to a barium enema.— D. Galloway *et al., Br. med. J.*, 1982, *284*, 472. A comment that the implication that the senna preparation used causes greater colonic peristalsis than other laxatives has not been found to be so in the author's experience. Patients who are fit enough to undergo a double-contrast barium-enema examination are fit enough for full bowel preparation including the administration of senna; however, the use of any laxative in acutely inflamed diverticular disease is more debatable.— J. R. Lee (letter), *ibid.*, 740. A further report of a non-fatal colonic perforation following bowel preparation with a senna preparation. To reduce the risk of colonic perforation, patients with suspected stricture, inflammatory bowel disease, or impending obstruction should not receive a bowel stimulant.— D. Cave-Bigley (letter), *ibid.*

Absorption and Fate

There is some absorption of the anthraquinones from senna preparations following hydrolysis by colonic bacteria. Excretion occurs in the urine and the faeces and also in other secretions including milk.

Uses and Administration

Senna is an anthraquinone laxative which is used to treat constipation and for bowel evacuation before radiological procedures. The active anthraquinones are liberated into the colon from the glycosides by colonic bacteria and an effect usually occurs 6 to 12 hours after administration.

For the treatment of constipation senna is usually administered as tablets, granules, or syrup. In the UK the usual adult dose is the equivalent of 15 to 30 mg of total sennosides given as a single dose at bedtime. Children over 6 years of age have been given one-half the adult dose.

For bowel evacuation a dose equivalent to 1 mg per kg body-weight of total sennosides (up to 72 mg) may be given as a liquid preparation by mouth on the day before the examination; doses of 142 mg were previously used.

The use of senna for treating constipation in paediatrics, obstetrics, and geriatrics.— E. W. Godding, *Pharm. J.*, 1984, *1*, 198.

Preparations

Senna Fluidextract *(U.S.P.)*. Prepared by percolation from senna leaf (1 in 1) using a mixture of alcohol 1 part and water 2 parts. Store in airtight containers.

Senna Liquid Extract *(B.P.)*. A 1 in 1 aqueous extract of senna fruit (Alexandrian or Tinnevelly) containing 0.6% v/v of coriander oil and 25% v/v of alcohol (90%).

Senna Syrup *(U.S.P.)*. Senna fluidextract 25 mL, coriander oil 0.5 mL, sucrose 63.5 g, water to 100 mL. Store in airtight containers.

Senna Tablets *(B.P.)*. Tablets containing the powdered pericarp of senna fruit (Alexandrian or Tinnevelly). Potency is expressed in terms of total sennosides calculated as sennoside B.

Sennosides Tablets *(U.S.P.)*

Proprietary Preparations

Senade *(Andard-Mount, UK)*. *Tablets*, sennosides 13.5 mg (as calcium salt).
Syrup, sennosides 13.5 mg (as calcium salt)/5 mL.

Senokot *(Reckitt & Colman Pharmaceuticals, UK)*. *Tablets*, standardised senna equivalent to total sennosides 7.5 mg calculated as sennoside B.
Granules, standardised senna equivalent to total sennosides 15 mg/5 mL calculated as sennoside B.
Syrup, standardised senna extract equivalent to total sennosides 7.5 mg/5 mL calculated as sennoside B.

X-Prep *(Napp, UK)*. *Oral liquid*, standardised extract of senna fruit equivalent to total sennosides 72 mg/72 mL. For the preparation of the intestinal tract prior to radiography.

Proprietary Names and Manufacturers of Senna and Sennosides

Bekunis *(Roha, Ger.; Farmades, Ital.; Jpn)*; Bidrolar *(Armour, UK)*; Blysennid *(Dorsey Laboratories, USA)*; Casafru *(Key, USA)*; Celer-X *(Gobbi-Novag, Arg.)*; Colonorm *(Ger.)*; Depuran *(Nattermann, Ital.)*; Florida Syrup of Prunes *(Lagamed, S.Afr.)*; Floripuran *(Scheurich, Ger.)*; Laxatan *(Divapharma, Ger.)*; Liquidepur *(Nattermann, Ger.)*; Mucinum-Herbal *(Sabex, Canad.)*; Nytilax *(USA)*; Palamkotta *(Bucopa, Ger.)*; Primolax *(Napp, UK)*; Puntual *(Lainco, Spain)*; Pursenid *(Sandoz, Spain)*; Pursennid *(Sandoz, Denm.; Sandoz, Ger.; Sandoz, Ital.; Sandoz, Norw.; Sandoz, Swed.; Sandoz, UK)*; Pursennide *(Belg.; Fr.; Neth.; Sandoz, Switz.)*; Regulato Nr. 1 *(Ger.)*; Senade *(Andard-Mount, UK)*; Sennatin *(Madaus, Ger.)*; Sennocol *(Neth.)*; Sennokott *(Swed.)*; Senokot *(Reckitt & Colman, Austral.; Belg.; Purdue Frederick, Canad.; Sarget, Fr.; Nyco, Norw.; Reckitt & Colman, S.Afr.; Landerlan, Spain; Mundipharma, Switz.; Reckitt & Colman Pharmaceuticals, UK; Purdue Frederick, USA)*; Senpurgin *(Ger.)*; Silaxo *(Dolorgiet, Ger.)*; X-Prep *(Purdue Frederick, Canad.; Mundipharma, Ger.; Chinoin, Ital.; Nyco, Norw.; Lainco, Spain; Sarget, Spain; Mundipharma, Switz.; Napp, UK; Gray, USA)*.

The following names have been used for multi-ingredient preparations containing senna and sennosides— Agiolax *(Schering, Austral.; Madaus, Ger.)*; Mucinum *(Sabex, Canad.)*; Pripsen *(Reckitt & Colman Pharmaceuticals, UK)*; Prompt *(Searle, USA)*; Senokot-S *(Purdue Frederick, Canad.; Purdue Frederick, USA)*.

6427-x

Simethicone *(USAN)*.

Activated Dimethicone; Activated Polymethylsiloxane.

CAS — 8050-81-5.

Pharmacopoeias. In *Ind.* and *U.S.*

A mixture of liquid dimethicones containing finely divided silicon dioxide to enhance the defoaming properties of the silicone. It is a grey, translucent, viscous fluid, containing 4 to 7% w/w of silicon dioxide.

Insoluble in water and dehydrated alcohol; soluble 1 in 10 of chloroform and ether leaving a residue of silicon dioxide. **Store** in airtight containers.

Simethicone reduces the surface tension of gas bubbles, causing them to coalesce. It is used in the treatment of flatulence and meteorism, for the elimination of gas, air, or foam from the gastro-intestinal tract prior to radiography, and for the relief of abdominal distension and dyspepsia. Doses of up to 2 g daily have been used, often in conjunction with antacids such as aluminium hydroxide.

A brief review of the use of simethicone for gastro-intestinal symptoms concluding that although it is commonly prescribed in combination with an antacid, there is no good evidence that it provides additional benefit. When used alone it probably helps to relieve minor postoperative and postprandial symptoms and it is a useful aid in upper gastro-intestinal endoscopy.— *Drug & Ther. Bull.*, 1986, *24*, 21.

ACTION. Froth tests showed that the defoaming properties of dimethicone in antacid preparations were due to the presence of free dimethicone. Omission of silica had little effect on the defoaming action. It was suggested that the aluminium hydroxide and talc components were responsible for dispersing the dimethicone, and silica was not necessary for 'activation'.— J. E. Carless *et al., J. Pharm. Pharmac.*, 1973, *25*, 849.

Preparations

Simethicone Emulsion *(U.S.P.)*. Store in airtight containers.

Simethicone Oral Suspension *(U.S.P.)*. pH 4.4 to 4.6. Store in airtight containers. Protect from light.

Simethicone Tablets *(U.S.P.)*

Proprietary Preparations

Infacol *(Pharmax, UK)*. *Liquid*, simethicone 40 mg/mL.

Phazyme *(Stafford-Miller, UK)*. *Tablets*, outer layer, simethicone 20 mg, core, simethicone 40 mg for release in the small intestine.

Windcheaters *(Napp, UK)*. *Capsules*, simethicone 100 mg.

Further proprietary preparations containing simethicone are described under aluminium hydroxide (p.1076) and aluminium hydroxide-magnesium carbonate co-dried gel (p.1077).

Proprietary Names and Manufacturers

Abulen *(Searle, Swed.)*; Aeropax *(Erco, Denm.; Neth.; Ercopharm, Switz.)*; Be-ma *(Danapharm, Denm.)*; Bicolon *(Ger.)*; Carbogasol Liquido *(Arg.)*; Decubal *(Dumex, Denm.)*; Disflatyl *(Neth.; Inibsa, Spain)*; Emophasil *(Amacon, Denm.)*; Endo-Paractol *(Degussa, Ger.)*; Entero-Silicona *(Estedi, Spain)*; Heydogen *(Denm.; Switz.)*; Infacol *(Rosken, Austral.; Pharmax, UK)*; Kestomal Infantil *(Boizot, Spain)*; Kestomatine *(Ital.)*; Kramik *(Duphar, Ger.)*; Lancepol *(Lancet, UK : Kirby-Warrick, UK)*; Lefax *(Asche, Ger.)*; Medefoam-2 *(Medefield, Austral.)*; Meteorex *(Neth.)*; Minifom *(Tika, Norw.; Tika, Swed.)*; Mylicon *(Parke, Davis, Austral.; Parke, Davis, Denm.; Parke, Davis, Ital.; Stuart Pharmaceuticals, USA)*; Pergastric *(Prodes, Spain)*; Phazyme *(Reed & Carnrick, Canad.; Stafford-Miller, UK; Reed & Carnrick, USA)*; Polycrol S

(Nicholas, UK); Sab *(Parke, Davis, Ger.)*; Silain *(Robins, USA)*; Silan *(Denm.)*; Siloxan *(NAF, Norw.)*; Simecon *(Gen, Canad.)*; Windcheaters *(Napp, UK)*.

The following names have been used for multi-ingredient preparations containing simethicone—Abacid Plus *(Ticen, Eire)*; Actonorm Gel *(Wallace Mfg Chem., UK)*; Alma-Mag *(Rugby, USA)*; Altacaps *(Roussel, UK)*; Altacite Plus *(Roussel, UK)*; Alucone *(Drug Houses Austral., Austral.)*; Amphojel Plus *(Wyeth, Canad.)*; Andursil *(Geigy, UK)*; Antacid Plus *(Clark, Canad.)*; Antasil *(Stuart, UK)*; Asilone *(USV, Austral.; Rorer, UK)*; Baritop *(Concept Pharmaceuticals, UK)*; Carbex *(Ferring, UK)*; Diaguard *(Nelson, Austral.)*; Diaguard Forte *(Nelson, Austral.)*; Diareze Suspension *(Key, Austral.)*; Dijene Liquid *(Boots, Austral.)*; Diloran *(Lipha, UK)*; Diovol Suspension *(Horner, Canad.; Pharmax, UK)*; Diovol Tablets *(Horner, Canad.; Pharmax, UK)*; Duoquel *(Wellcome, Austral.)*; Gastreze *(Key, Austral.)*; Gelusil *(Parke, Davis, USA)*; Infacol-C *(Rosken, Austral.)*; Kolanticon *(Merrell, UK)*; LoAsid *(Calmic, UK)*; Maalox Plus *(Rorer, Canad.; Rorer, UK)*; Merasyn *(Merrell Dow, Austral.)*; Mygel *(Geneva, USA)*; Mylanta *(Parke, Davis, Austral.; Parke, Davis, Canad.; Warner-Lambert, UK; Stuart Pharmaceuticals, USA)*; Ovol *(Pharmax, UK)*; Phazyme *(Stafford-Miller, Austral.)*; Phazyme-PB *(Reed & Carnrick, USA)*; Piptalin *(MCP Pharmaceuticals, UK)*; Polyalk *(Galen, UK)*; Polycrol Gel *(Nicholas, UK)*; Polycrol Tablets *(Nicholas, UK)*; Riopan Plus *(Ayerst, Canad.; Ayerst, USA)*; Silgastrin *(Unimed, UK)*; Silocalm *(Concept Pharmaceuticals, UK)*; Siloxyl *(Martindale Pharmaceuticals, UK)*; Simeco Suspension *(Wyeth, Austral.; Wyeth, UK; Wyeth, USA)*; Simeco Tablets *(Wyeth, Austral.; Wyeth, UK)*; Sodexol *(Schering, Austral.)*; Sylopal *(Norton, UK)*; Unigest *(Unigreg, UK)*.

706-h

Sodium Amylosulphate

SN-263; Sodium Amylopectin Sulphate; Sodium Amylosulfate *(USAN)*. The sodium salt of the sulphated form of amylopectin derived from potatoes, *Solanum tuberosum* (Solanaceae).

CAS — 9010-01-9.

Sodium amylosulphate inhibits the activity of pepsin and has been used for the treatment of peptic ulcer.

Proprietary Names and Manufacturers
Depepsen *(Searle, UK)*.

7533-q

Sodium Picosulphate *(BAN)*.

DA-1773; La-391; Picosulphol; Sodium Picosulfate *(rINN)*. Disodium 4,4′-(2-pyridylmethylene)di(phenyl sulphate).
$C_{18}H_{13}NNa_2O_8S_2$=481.4.

CAS — 10040-45-6.

Adverse Effects
Sodium picosulphate may cause abdominal discomfort such as colic. Prolonged use or overdosage can result in diarrhoea with excessive loss of water and electrolytes, particularly potassium; there is also the possibility of developing an atonic non-functioning colon.

Precautions
As for Bisacodyl, p.1078.

Absorption and Fate
Sodium picosulphate is hydrolysed by colonic bacteria to the active compound bis(*p*-hydroxyphenyl)-2-pyridylmethane.

Uses and Administration
Sodium picosulphate is a stimulant laxative related to bisacodyl used for the treatment of constipation and for evacuation of the colon before investigational procedures or surgery. When taken by mouth it stimulates bowel movements following hydrolysis by colonic bacteria. It is usually effective within 10 to 14 hours although when used with magnesium citrate for bowel evacuation an effect may be seen after only 3 hours.

It is given by mouth as a solution in doses of 5 to 15 mg usually at bedtime. Doses of 2.5 mg have been given to children up to 5 years of age and doses of 2.5 to 5 mg to children 5 to 10 years.

For bowel evacuation, a dose of sodium picosulphate 10 mg with magnesium citrate is given in the morning and again in the afternoon of the day before the examination.

Effective outpatient preparation with sodium picosulphate for colonoscopy.— J. J. Brown and D. P. Jewell (letter), *Lancet*, 1981, *2*, 695. See also.— D. G. Karamanolis *et al.*, *Gut*, 1982, *23*, A883.

In a study of bowel preparation in 160 patients Picolax, with dietary restriction, was significantly better than X-Prep, with dietary restriction, and was recommended for routine bowel preparation before double-contrast barium-enema examination. Colonic lavage had no beneficial effect.— J. R. Lee and J. R. Ferrando, *Gut*, 1984, *25*, 69. Similar results.— G. De Lacey *et al.*, *Br. med. J.*, 1982, *284*, 1021.

Proprietary Preparations

Laxoberal *(Windsor, UK)*. *Oral Liquid*, sodium picosulphate 5 mg/5 mL.

Picolax *(Ferring, UK)*. *Oral powder*, sodium picosulphate 10 mg/sachet, with magnesium citrate formed in solution. For bowel preparation.

Proprietary Names and Manufacturers
Contumax *(Casen Fisons, Spain)*; Elimin *(Cantabria, Spain)*; Evacuol *(Almirall, Spain)*; Gocce Antonetto *(Antonetto, Ital.)*; Gocce Lassative Aicardi *(Schiapparelli, Ital.)*; Gutalax *(Fher, Spain)*; Guttalax *(Belg.; De Angeli, Ital.; Switz.)*; Laxante Azoxico *(Spain)*; Laxoberal *(Pharmacia, Denm.; Biotherax, Ger.; Ferring, Swed.; Windsor, UK)*; Laxoberon *(Belg.; Neth.; Boehringer Ingelheim, Switz.)*; Mendilax *(Cinfa, Spain)*; Neopax *(IFCI, Ital.)*; Skilax *(High Noon, Pakistan; Prodes, Spain)*; Totalaxan *(Arg.)*; Trali *(Arg.)*.

The following names have been used for multi-ingredient preparations containing sodium picosulphate— Picolax *(Ferring, UK)*.

1198-g

Sodium Potassium Tartrate

E337; Kalium-natrium Tartaricum; Potassium Sodium Tartrate *(USAN)*; Rochelle Salt; Seignette Salt; Sodii et Potassii Tartras; Tartarus Natronatus.
$C_4H_4KNaO_6,4H_2O$=282.2.

CAS — 304-59-6 (anhydrous); 6381-59-5 (tetrahydrate); 6100-16-9 (tetrahydrate).

Pharmacopoeias. In *Aust., Belg., Cz., Fr., Hung., Mex., Neth., Port., Roum., Span., Swiss,* and *U.S.* Also in *B.P.C 1973.*

Odourless or almost odourless colourless crystals or white crystalline powder, with a cooling saline taste. It effloresces slightly in warm dry air, the crystals often being coated with a white powder.
Soluble 1 in 1 of water; practically insoluble in alcohol. **Store** in airtight containers.

Sodium potassium tartrate has been used, in doses of 8 to 16 g, as a laxative.
It is used as a food additive.
For the general properties of potassium salts, see p.1036, and of sodium salts, see p.1039.

Preparations

Compound Effervescent Powder *(B.P.C. 1973)*. Seidlitz Powder. Sodium potassium tartrate, in powder, 7.5 g, sodium bicarbonate, in powder, 2.5 g, in blue paper. Tartaric acid, in powder, 2.5 g, in white paper. *Dose.* Dissolve the contents of the blue paper in a tumblerful of cold or warm water, then add the contents of the white paper and drink the liquid while it is effervescing.

Double-strength Compound Effervescent Powder *(B.P.C. 1973)*. Double-strength Seidlitz Powder. Formula as for Compound Effervescent Powder (above) but with double the amount (15 g) of sodium potassium tartrate.

1200-q

Anhydrous Sodium Sulphate *(BAN)*.

Dried Sodium Sulphate; Exsiccated Sodium Sulphate; Natrii Sulfas Anhydricus; Natrium Sulfuricum Siccatum.
Na_2SO_4=142.0.

CAS — 7757-82-6.

Pharmacopoeias. In *Arg., Aust., Belg., Br., Chin., Cz., Egypt., Eur., Fr., Ger., Hung., It., Jug., Neth., Nord., Pol., Port., Span.,* and *Swiss.*

A white odourless hygroscopic powder.
Freely **soluble** in water. **Store** in well-closed containers.

1199-q

Sodium Sulphate *(BAN)*.

514; Glauber's Salt; Natrii Sulfas Decahydricus; Natrii Sulphas; Natrium Sulfuricum Crystallisatum; Sodium Sulfate *(USAN)*; Sodium Sulphate Decahydrate.
$Na_2SO_4,10H_2O$=322.2.

CAS — 7727-73-3.

Pharmacopoeias. In *Arg., Aust., Belg., Br., Braz., Chin., Cz., Egypt., Eur., Fr., Ger., Hung., It., Jug., Mex., Neth., Nord., Pol., Port., Roum., Rus., Span., Swiss, Turk.,* and *U.S.* Also in *B.P. Vet.*

Large colourless odourless transparent crystals or white crystalline powder; efflorescent in dry air. It partially dissolves in its own water of crystallisation at about 33°.

Soluble 1 in 2.5 of water; soluble in glycerol; practically insoluble in alcohol. A 3.89% solution is iso-osmotic, and thus in most cases isotonic with blood, serum, and lachrymal secretions. **Store** in airtight containers, preferably at a temperature not exceeding 30°.

Sodium sulphate is poorly absorbed from the gastro-intestinal tract and retains water in the lumen of the intestine. It has been given by mouth in dilute solution as a saline laxative to produce a prompt watery evacuation of the bowel.
It has also been used as a 3.89% solution administered by slow intravenous infusion in the treatment of severe hypercalcaemia.
Sodium sulphate is used as a food additive.
For the general properties of sodium salts, see p.1039.

Preparations

Sodium Sulfate Injection *(U.S.P.)*. A sterile concentrated solution of sodium sulphate in Water for Injections, which upon dilution is suitable for parenteral use. pH 5.0 to 6.5. It should be diluted to 3.89% before use.

Proprietary Names and Manufacturers
Liquisulf *(Cophar, Switz.)*.

The following names have been used for multi-ingredient preparations containing sodium sulphate—Colyte *(Reed & Carnrick, Canad.; Reed & Carnrick, USA)*; Cuproxil *(Gamaprod, Austral.)*; GoLytely *(Braintree, USA)*; Prefagyl *(Sabex, Canad.)*.

1201-p

Sodium Tartrate

E335; E335 (monosodium tartrate).
$C_2H_4O_2(CO_2Na)_2,2H_2O$=230.1.

CAS — 868-18-8 (anhydrous); 6106-24-7 (dihydrate).

Sodium tartrate has been used as a laxative.
It is used as a food additive.
For the general properties of sodium salts, see p.1039.

Proprietary Names and Manufacturers
Limonade Asepta *(Rodeca, Canad.)*.

16989-n

Sofalcone *(pINN)*.

SU-88. [5-[(3-Methyl-2-butenyl)oxy]-2-[*p*-[(3-methyl-2-butenyl)oxy]cinnamoyl]phenoxy]acetic acid.
$C_{27}H_{30}O_6$=450.5.

CAS — 64506-49-6.

Sofalcone is used in the treatment of peptic ulcer in doses of up to 300 mg daily.

Proprietary Names and Manufacturers
Solon *(Taisho, Jpn)*.

5461-j

Sterculia *(BAN)*.

416; Indian Tragacanth; Karaya; Karaya Gum; Sterculia Gum.

CAS — 9000-36-6.

Pharmacopoeias. In *Br.* and *Fr.* Also in *B.P. Vet.*

Sterculia is the gum obtained from *Sterculia urens* and other species of *Sterculia*(Sterculiaceae). Irregular or vermiform pieces, greyish-white with a brown or pink tinge, with an odour resembling that of acetic acid and containing not less than 14% of volatile acid, calculated as acetic acid. Sparingly **soluble** in water, in which it swells to a homogeneous, adhesive, gelatinous mass; practically insoluble in alcohol.

Powdered Sterculia is a white or buff-coloured powder containing not less than 10% of volatile acid, as acetic acid. **Store** at a temperature not exceeding 25° in a dry place.

Uses and Administration

Sterculia has similar properties to ispaghula (see p.1091) and is similarly used as a bulk laxative and for adjusting faecal consistency.

Sterculia has adhesive properties and is used in the fitting of ileostomy and colostomy appliances and in dental fixative powders.

Sterculia is also used as a food additive.

Proprietary Preparations

Normacol (formerly known as Normacol Special) *(Norgine, UK). Granules*, sterculia 62%. For constipation, diverticular disease, and colostomy and ileostomy control. *Dose.* 1 or 2 sachets, with plenty of water, once or twice daily after meals.

Normacol Antispasmodic *(Norgine, UK). Granules*, sterculia 62%, alverine citrate 0.5%. For spastic and hypertonic constipation and irritable bowel syndrome. *Dose.* One to two 5-mL spoonfuls, with plenty of water, once or twice daily after meals.

Normacol Plus (formerly known as Normacol Standard) *(Norgine, UK). Granules*, sterculia 62%, frangula 8%. For constipation. *Dose.* One to two 5-mL spoonfuls, with plenty of water, once or twice daily after meals.

Prefil *(Norgine, UK). Granules*, sterculia 55%. For appetite suppression. *Dose.* Two 5-mL spoonfuls, with plenty of water, half to one hour before meals.

Proprietary Names and Manufacturers

Colosan mite *(Medichemie, Switz.)*; Decorpa *(Belg.; Norgan, Fr.; Norgine, Ger.)*; Hollister Karaya Paste *(Abbott, Austral.)*; Hollister Karaya Powder *(Abbott, Austral.)*; Inolaxine *(Debat, Fr.; Martindale Pharmaceuticals, UK)*; Inolaxol *(Debat, Norw.; Debat, Swed.)*; Karagum *(Austral.)*; Karaya Gum Powder *(Denyer, Austral.)*; Karaya Paste *(Abbott, Austral.)*; Normacol *(Norgan, Fr.; Norgine, UK)*; Normacol Special *(Norgine, Austral.; Norgine, Switz.; Norgine, UK)*; Normalax *(Swed.)*; Prefil *(Norgine, UK)*; Puraya *(Delalande, Ger.)*; Saltair Karaya Gum Powder *(Salt, UK)*; Tex *(Simpla, UK)*.

The following names have been used for multi-ingredient preparations containing sterculia—Movicol *(Norgine, USA)*; Normacol Antispasmodic *(Norgine, Austral.; Norgine, UK)*; Normacol Plus *(Norgine, UK)*; Normacol Standard *(Norgine, Austral.; Norgine, UK)*.

707-m

Sucralfate *(BAN, USAN, rINN).*

Sucrose hydrogen sulphate basic aluminium salt; Sucrose octakis(hydrogen sulphate) aluminium complex; β-D-Fructofuranosyl-α-D-glucopyranoside octakis (hydrogen sulphate) aluminium complex.

$C_{12}H_mAl_{16}O_nS_8$.

CAS — 54182-58-0.

Adverse Effects

Constipation is the most frequently reported adverse effect of sucralfate although other gastro-intestinal effects such as diarrhoea, nausea, or gastric discomfort may occur. Other adverse effects reported have included dry mouth, dizziness, and skin rashes.

A report of a sucralfate bezoar in a patient given sucralfate in crushed form via a nasogastric tube.— G. J. Algozzine *et al.* (letter), *New Engl. J. Med.*, 1983, *309*, 1387. Comments on methods available for suspending sucralfate tablets prior to administration via a nasogastric tube.— J. S. Schneider and S. M. Ouellette (letter), *ibid.*, 1984, *310*, 990.

Precautions

Sucralfate should be administered with caution to patients with renal disorders.

Sucralfate may interfere with the absorption of other drugs and it has been suggested that there should be an interval of 2 hours between the administration of sucralfate and other concurrent non-antacid medication. The recommended interval between sucralfate and other antacids is 30 minutes.

Uses and Administration

Sucralfate is not significantly absorbed from the gastro-intestinal tract and has a local action providing a protective barrier over the gastric mucosa.

Sucralfate is used in the treatment of gastric and duodenal ulcers. The usual dose is 1 g four times daily or 2 g twice daily by mouth for 4 to 6 weeks; if necessary the dose may be increased to a maximum of 8 g daily. If longer-term therapy is required sucralfate may be administered for a period of up to 12 weeks. Sucralfate should be taken on an empty stomach before meals. Antacids may be taken concurrently, but should not be administered for 30 minutes before or after the dose of sucralfate.

DIAGNOSTIC USE. A study suggesting that sucralfate labelled with technetium-99m may be useful for the detection of inflammatory bowel diseases. It was probable that the labelled sucralfate bound to active lesions in the small intestine and colon in a similar way to its binding in peptic ulcer thus providing a positive scan. It was not suggested that technetium-99m sucralfate scanning would replace radiography or colonoscopy but that it would offer a safe and useful complement to those techniques.— D. J. Dawson *et al.*, *Br. med. J.*, 1985, *291*, 1227.

PEPTIC ULCER. A review of the pharmacodynamic properties of sucralfate and its use in peptic ulcer disease. Although the extent of published therapeutic experience with sucralfate is considerably less than that with cimetidine, controlled studies do indicate that it is effective in accelerating the healing of duodenal ulcers; it has been less well studied in gastric ulcer but has generally been found to be more effective than a placebo. In comparative studies in patients with duodenal or gastric ulcer sucralfate has not been found to be significantly different from cimetidine but the small numbers of patients studied precludes a firm conclusion that the 2 drugs are equally effective. Further studies are needed to determine the optimum dosage regimen for the prevention of duodenal ulcer recurrence and preliminary studies in the prevention of gastric ulcer recurrence are inconclusive. It is concluded that sucralfate offers an effective and well-tolerated alternative form of management for peptic ulcer disease.— R. N. Brogden *et al.*, *Drugs*, 1984, *27*, 194.

PHOSPHATE BINDING. For the use of sucralfate as a phosphate-binder in patients with chronic renal failure, see under aluminium hydroxide.

Proprietary Preparations

Antepsin *(Ayerst, UK). Tablets*, scored, sucralfate 1 g.

Proprietary Names and Manufacturers

Andapsin *(Medipolar, Swed.)*; Antepsin *(Arg.; Farmos, Denm.; Baldacci, Ital.; Farmos, Norw.; Ayerst, UK)*; Carafate *(Marion Laboratories, USA)*; Duracralfat *(Durachemie, Ger.)*; Keal *(Sinbio, Fr.)*; Sucralfin *(Inverni della Beffa, Ital.)*; Sucramal *(Malesci, Ital.)*; Sugast *(Istituto Wassermann, Ital.)*; Sulcrate *(Nordic, Canad.)*; Ulcar *(Houdé, Fr.)*; Ulcogant *(Merck, Belg.; E. Merck, Ger.; E. Merck, Switz.)*; Ulsanic *(Du Pont, Austral.; High Noon, Pakistan; Continental Ethicals, S.Afr.)*; U-one S *(Sawai, Jpn)*.

708-b

Sucralox *(BAN, rINN).*

Manalox AS. A polymerised complex of sucrose and aluminium hydroxide.

CAS — 12040-73-2.

Sucralox is an antacid that has been given in doses of 0.5 to 1 g.

Proprietary Names and Manufacturers

The following names have been used for multi-ingredient preparations containing sucralox— Alusac *(Calmic, UK)*.

13282-e

Sulglycotide *(BAN).*

Sulglicotide *(rINN)*. The sulphuric polyester of a glycopeptide isolated from pig duodenum.

CAS — 54182-59-1.

Sulglycotide is used in the treatment of peptic ulcer.

Proprietary Names and Manufacturers

Gliptid *(Merck, Arg.)*; Gliptide *(Crinos, Ital.)*; Ulcodavur *(Davur, Spain)*.

13283-l

Sulisatin Sodium *(pINNM).*

The disodium salt of 3,3-bis(4-hydroxyphenyl)-7-methylindolin-2-one bis(hydrogen sulphate) (ester).

$C_{21}H_{15}NNa_2O_9S_2$=535.5.

CAS — 54935-03-4 (sulisatin); 54935-04-5 (sodium salt).

Sulisatin sodium is used as a laxative.

Proprietary Names and Manufacturers

Laxitex *(Andreu, Spain)*.

4951-n

Sulphasalazine *(BAN).*

Salazosulfapyridine; Salicylazosulphapyridine; Sulfasalazine *(USAN, rINN)*. 4-Hydroxy-4′-(2-pyridylsulphamoyl)azobenzene-3-carboxylic acid.

$C_{18}H_{14}N_4O_5S$=398.4.

CAS — 599-79-1.

Pharmacopoeias. In *Jpn* and *U.S.*

A fine odourless bright yellow to brownish-yellowish powder.

Practically **insoluble** in water, chloroform, and ether; soluble 1 in 2900 of alcohol and 1 in 1500 of methyl alcohol; soluble in aqueous solutions of alkali hydroxides. **Store** in airtight containers. Protect from light.

Adverse Effects, Treatment, and Precautions

Since sulphasalazine is metabolised to sulphapyridine and 5-aminosalicylic acid (mesalazine), its adverse effects, treatment and precautions are similar to those of sulphonamides (see Sulphamethoxazole, p.306) and of salicylates (see Aspirin, p.3). Many adverse effects have been attributed to the sulphapyridine moiety and appear to be more common if serum-sulphapyridine concentrations are greater than 50 μg per mL or if the daily dose of sulphasalazine is 4 g or more.

Oligospermia, reversible on withdrawal of sulphasalazine, has also been reported. Administration of sulphasalazine may result in yellow-orange discoloration of skin, urine, and other body fluids.

Sulphasalazine may interfere with the absorption of digoxin or folic acid from the gastro-intestinal tract.

A review of adverse effects associated with the administration of sulphasalazine and of desensitisation regimens. Such regimens have begun with doses of sulphasalazine between 1 and 500 mg daily.— S. L. Taffet and K. M. Das, *Dig. Dis. Scis*, 1983, *28*, 833. Twelve of 13 patients who had previously experienced allergic skin rashes with or without fever after administration of sulphasalazine, tolerated doses of 2 g daily after a desensitisation regimen. Doses were slowly increased beginning at a dose of 1 mg daily, and temporarily decreased if a reaction occurred; the time required for desensitisation varied from 32 days to 7 months. During therapy, the clinical condition was improved in 11 and unchanged in one of the 12 patients.— B. H. Purdy *et al.*, *Ann. intern. Med.*, 1984, *100*, 512.

Possible cytogenetic effects with sulphasalazine.— F. Mitelman *et al.* (letter), *Lancet*, 1980, *1*, 1249. See also J. M. Mackay *et al.*, *Gut*, 1986, *27*, A1271.

Raynaud's syndrome was associated with treatment with sulphasalazine 2 to 4 g daily, in a man with ulcerative colitis. Withdrawal of the drug and then re-introduction, on 2 occasions, resulted in successive disappearance and then reappearance of the symptoms.— J. Reid *et al.*, *Postgrad. med. J.*, 1980, *56*, 106.

Irreversible staining of an extended-wear soft contact lens associated with administration of sulphasalazine.— S. A. Riley *et al.* (letter), *Lancet*, 1986, *1*, 972.

Toxicity of sulphasalazine was monitored for 1 to 11 years in 774 patients with rheumatoid arthritis from 3 centres; most patients received 1.5 to 3.0 g daily according to need and tolerability. Treatment was stopped permanently in 205 patients (26%) because of a possible adverse event. A total of 383 (50%) stopped treatment within the first year of treatment; 199 because of toxicity, and most of the remainder because of inefficacy of treatment. Most toxic events were trivial, resolving rapidly when treatment was stopped. Nausea, dyspepsia, headache, dizziness, and abdominal pain often occurred together early in treatment, and the need to withdraw sulphasalazine was reduced by routine use of enteric-coated sulphasalazine, dose manipulation, and the short-term use of anti-emetics. Depression, irritability, and mood disturbances were not infrequent, usually occurring within the first 6 months. Mucocutaneous reactions, most commonly pruritic maculopapular generalised eruptions, were the second commonest events after those affecting the central and gastro-intestinal systems. Leucopenia occurred in 11 patients, thrombocytopenia in 1, and megaloblastic anaemia in 6. Other adverse effects reported included abnormal liver function tests, exacerbation of arthritic symptoms, numb hands, urinary retention, and dyspnoea.

It was concluded that, as with other second-line antirheumatoid drugs, toxicity is a limiting factor in the use of sulphasalazine. Most of the adverse reactions are, however, trivial in their implications, and the type and incidence of events seem to differ little in patients with rheumatological and gastro-enterological conditions. As most potentially serious effects, especially leucopenia, take place early, vigilance in the first 3 months of treatment is advisable. The centres involved in this study carry out blood counts every 2 to 4 weeks in the first 3 months of treatment. Beyond this period it is debatable whether formal monitoring is required; 2 of the centres review patients according to clinical need and perform blood counts at the time, usually at intervals of several weeks to several months in the first year of treatment and less frequently thereafter; in the third centre patients are monitored every 6 weeks for the first year, and every three months subsequently.— R. S. Amos *et al.*, *Br. med. J.*, 1986, *293*, 420.

ALLERGY. For reference to the occurrence of hypersensitivity to sulphasalazine in a patient with AIDS, see Ampicillin Trihydrate, p.117.

EFFECTS ON THE BLOOD. Folate deficiency can occur in patients with inflammatory bowel diseases, but may be further enhanced by administration of sulphasalazine; this may be due to interference by sulphasalazine with absorption of folic acid or to increased folate requirements secondary to minor haemolysis. Although folate deficiency is not usually a significant clinical problem, in the presence of additional aggravating factors such as an intercurrent illness or an exacerbation of the bowel disease, macrocytosis, megaloblastic anaemia, or even pancytopenia due to folic acid deficiency has been reported (C.M. Swinson *et al.*, *Gut*, 1981, *22*, 456; E.C.M. Logan *et al.*, *ibid.*, 1986, *27*, 868). Macrocytic anaemia has also been observed in patients given sulphasalazine for the treatment of rheumatoid arthritis (P.J. Prouse *et al.*, *Br. med. J.*, 1986, *293*, 1407).

In an analysis of adverse drug reaction reports received by the Committee on Safety of Medicines during 1985, sulphasalazine was one of the most commonly reported drugs (18 reports) suspected of causing a depressed peripheral white cell count.— *Br. med. J.*, 1986, *293*, 688.

A study of over 100 patients with rheumatoid arthritis suggested that leucopenia associated with administration of gold may predict a similar adverse reaction to sulphasalazine.— H. Bliddal *et al.* (letter), *Lancet*, 1987, *1*, 390.

EFFECTS ON FERTILITY. Sulphasalazine has been observed to have an adverse effect on semen quality, including oligospermia, reduced motility, and a change in sperm morphology; such changes may result in infertility. Birnie *et al.* (*Gut*, 1981, *22*, 452) noted abnormal semen analyses in 18 of 21 men (86%) treated with sulphasalazine for inflammatory bowel diseases; oligospermia occurred in 15 (75%). Semen quality appears to be improved 2 to 3 months after withdrawal of the drug; pregnancies have occurred after withdrawal of sulphasalazine (S. Toovey *et al.*, *ibid.*, 445) or substitution with mesalazine (S.A. Riley *et al.*, *ibid.*, 1987, *28*, 1008). Studies in *rats* suggest that these effects are caused by a direct toxic effect, possibly due to the sulphapyridine moiety, on the immature and developing spermatozoa (C. Ó'Moráin *et al.*, *ibid.*, 1984, *25*, 1078), although an antiprostaglandin effect of the salicylic acid portion has also been proposed (J.F. Buchanan and L.J. Davis, *Drug Intell. & clin. Pharm.*, 1984, *18*, 122).

EFFECTS ON THE GASTRO-INTESTINAL TRACT. Two patients taking sulphasalazine 2 g daily experienced a metallic taste which abated when the dose was reduced to 1 g or less daily.— R. M. Ogburn, *J. Am. med. Ass.*, 1979, *241*, 837.

Reports of exacerbations of ulcerative colitis caused by administration of sulphasalazine: A. G. Schwartz *et al.*, *New Engl. J. Med.*, 1982, *306*, 409; F. A. Ring *et al.*, *Can. med. Ass. J.*, 1984, *131*, 43. Comment that such exacerbations may be due to the salicylate moiety of sulphasalazine.— F. Shanahan and S. Targan (letter), *New Engl. J. Med.*, 1987, *317*, 455.

Angioimmunoblastic lymphadenopathy and intestinal villous atrophy were diagnosed in a 67-year-old woman 9 months after starting sulphasalazine therapy.— M. A. Smith *et al.*, *Postgrad. med. J.*, 1985, *61*, 337.

For a discussion on the use of enteric-coated sulphasalazine tablets in rheumatoid arthritis in an attempt to decrease gastro-intestinal disturbances, see under Rheumatoid Arthritis in Uses, below.

EFFECTS ON THE IMMUNE SYSTEM. Low serum concentrations of IgA were detected in 3 patients with rheumatoid arthritis taking sulphasalazine. One of these had shown a similar reaction to sodium aurothiomalate. A similar effect has been observed with penicillamine.— J. P. Delamere *et al.*, *Br. med. J.*, 1983, *286*, 1547. IgA deficiency in 4 of 47 children treated with sulphasalazine for ulcerative colitis.— E. Savilahti (letter), *ibid.*, *287*, 759.

For further reference to the action of sulphasalazine on the immune system see under Action in Uses, below.

EFFECTS ON THE LIVER. A report of hepatotoxicity associated with administration of sulphasalazine. The patient had received the drug for ulcerative colitis during the past 15 years without ill effect on the liver.— T. W. J. Lennard and J. R. Farndon, *Br. med. J.*, 1983, *287*, 96.

EFFECTS ON THE RESPIRATORY SYSTEM. Inflammatory lung disorders such as eosinophilic pneumonia and irreversible fibrosing alveolitis may be more common in patients with inflammatory bowel diseases, and may not be attributable to sulphasalazine administration.— R. Pannier, *Bull. int. Un. Tuberc.*, 1984, *59*, 210.

EFFECTS ON THE SKIN. Reports of adverse effects on the skin associated with administration of sulphasalazine: P. T. Dawes and M. F. Shadforth, *Br. med. J.*, 1984, *288*, 194 (Oral lichen planus); E. G. Breen and S. Donnelly, *ibid.*, 1986, *292*, 802 (alopecia).

INTERACTIONS. In 5 subjects given a single dose of sulphasalazine peak serum concentrations were reduced by ferrous sulphate and delayed by calcium gluconate.— K. M. Das and M. A. Eastwood, *Scott. med. J.*, 1973, *18*, 45.

Concomitant antibiotic therapy might possibly alter the patient's response to sulphasalazine by decreasing the intestinal flora necessary for the initial breakdown of sulphasalazine.— K. M. Das and R. Dubin, *Clin. Pharmacokinet.*, 1976, *1*, 406.

In a study of 11 patients maintained on sulphasalazine for treatment of Crohn's disease, mean plasma concentrations of sulphapyridine and acetyl sulphapyridine were decreased while they were receiving rifampicin and ethambutol concurrently. This may be due to induction of hepatic microsomal enzymes by rifampicin or to a reduction in the systemic availability of sulphapyridine by the effect of antibiotic treatment on intestinal microflora; the latter mechanism was considered most likely.— J. L. Shaffer and J. B. Houston (letter), *Br. J. clin. Pharmac.*, 1985, *19*, 526.

For a report that concurrent administration of sulphasalazine reduced the absorption of digoxin, see under Sulphonamides in Digoxin, p.828.

For the possible effects of interference by sulphasalazine with absorption of folic acid, see Effects on the Blood, above.

PREGNANCY AND THE NEONATE. Major congenital abnormalities occurred in 3 infants born of 2 mothers who received treatment with sulphasalazine throughout their pregnancy.— N. M. Newman and J. F. Correy, *Med. J. Aust.*, 1983, *1*, 528. Ventricular septal defect plus coarctation of the aorta in an infant, possibly associated with *in utero* exposure to sulphasalazine.— J. J. Hoo *et al.*, *New Engl. J. Med.*, 1988, *318*, 1128. See also Uses, below.

For reference to the ability of sulphasalazine to displace bilirubin, and hence the risk of kernicterus in neonates, see Sulphamethoxazole, p.307.

Absorption and Fate

Sulphasalazine is partly absorbed from the small intestine and may later enter the enterohepatic circulation but the majority of a dose passes on to the colon where it is broken down to sulphapyridine and 5-aminosalicylic acid (mesalazine) by bacteria. Most of the sulphapyridine is absorbed and, together with its metabolites, appears in the blood 3 to 6 hours after a single 2-g dose of sulphasalazine is given to healthy subjects; a mean peak serum concentration for sulphapyridine of 21 µg per mL has been reported at 12 hours. Sulphapyridine is metabolised by acetylation, the rate being genetically determined, by hydroxylation, and by conjugation with glucuronic acid. Up to 10% of a dose of sulphasalazine is excreted unchanged in the urine and about 60% as sulphapyridine and its metabolites. A small proportion of the sulphapyridine appears in the faeces and unchanged sulphasalazine may be excreted in the faeces of patients with ulcerative colitis.

The majority of 5-aminosalicylic acid is eliminated unchanged in the faeces but some appears in the blood; about 20% is excreted in the urine unchanged and in the acetylated form.

Sulphasalazine has been claimed to be concentrated in connective tissue.

Reviews of the absorption and fate of sulphasalazine: K. M. Das and R. Dubin, *Clin. Pharmacokinet.*, 1976, *1*, 406; U. Klotz, *ibid.*, 1985, *10*, 285.

In 10 healthy men given a single dose of 4 g of sulphasalazine mean peak serum concentrations of about 26 µg per mL were reached in 3 to 7 hours. In 9 of the men given daily doses of 4 g serum concentrations at day 5 were 4.7 to 45 µg per mL with 37 to 92 µg per mL of sulphapyridine and its metabolites—glucuronide and acetylated sulphapyridine and glucuronide. The mean half-life of sulphasalazine after single and repeated doses was 5.7 and 7.6 hours respectively. From 1.7 to 10% of sulphasalazine appeared in the urine with about 10% of sulphapyridine and about 10% of the glucuronide and about 30% of each of the acetyl derivatives. Excretion was not greatly affected by urinary pH. There was no unchanged sulphasalazine in the faeces.— H. Schröder and D. E. S. Campbell, *Clin. Pharmac. Ther.*, 1972, *13*, 539.

In 7 healthy subjects the azo-reduction of sulphasalazine and recovery of 5-aminosalicylic acid in the faeces was substantially decreased during accelerated intestinal transit. In 18 patients with severe colitis, serum-sulphapyridine concentrations were related to the diarrhoeal state and did not correlate with disease activity, suggesting that the reduced therapeutic efficacy of sulphasalazine in severe colitis may be related to accelerated intestinal transit time.— P. A. M. van Hees *et al.*, *Gut*, 1979, *20*, 300.

DRUG METABOLISM. A review of *N*-acetylation pharmacogenetics. Acetylator status affects the degree of acetylation in serum and urine of sulphapyridine derived from sulphasalazine, although this appears to be compensated for in the slow acetylator by more extensive formation and rapid excretion of the sulphapyridine-*O*-glucuronide; hence the average serum concentration of total sulphapyridine (sulphapyridine and its metabolites) is approximately the same for both phenotypes after ingestion of a single dose of sulphasalazine.

The assessment of acetylator status according to the percentage of acetylated sulphapyridine in serum provides a clear distinction between rapid and slow acetylators; the percentage of acetylsulphapyridine in saliva, however, is a less precise index of acetylator phenotype.— W. W. Weber and D. W. Hein, *Pharmac. Rev.*, 1985, *37*, 25.

PREGNANCY AND THE NEONATE. An infant was born to a mother who had taken sulphasalazine 2 g daily throughout pregnancy. Maternal serum concentrations of sulphasalazine, sulphapyridine, and the acetyl and glucuronide conjugates, were generally similar to those in umbilical cord blood and amniotic fluid.— P. A. Hensleigh and R. E. Kauffman, *Am. J. Obstet. Gynec.*, 1977, *127*, 443.

In 5 patients taking sulphasalazine 500 mg four times daily during pregnancy and the puerperium, concentrations of sulphasalazine and its metabolites in cord blood were not greatly different from those in maternal serum. No adverse effect had been seen in 10 years. In 3 patients concentrations in breast milk were lower and were not considered likely to cause harmful effects.— A. K. A. Khan and S. C. Truelove, *Br. med. J.*, 1979, *2*,

1553.

Pharmacokinetic studies indicating that concentrations of sulphasalazine and its metabolite sulphapyridine achieved in the breast milk of nursing mothers taking sulphasalazine were unlikely to present a hazard to their infants.— G. Järnerot and M. -B. Into-Malmberg, *Scand. J. Gastroenterol.*, 1979, *14*, 869; C. M. Berlin and S. J. Yaffe, *Develop. Pharmac. Ther.*, 1980, *1*, 31.

Further references: G. Järnerot *et al.*, *Scand. J. Gastroenterol.*, 1981, *16*, 693.

Uses and Administration

Sulphasalazine is used in the management of inflammatory bowel diseases. In ulcerative colitis it is effective in the maintenance of remissions and has been used alone or as an adjunct to corticosteroids in the treatment of the acute phase of the disease. Sulphasalazine is also effective in the active treatment of Crohn's disease but it does not appear to be of value in maintaining remissions. The usual initial adult dose of sulphasalazine is 1 to 2 g by mouth 4 times daily, although lower doses may be given at first to minimise adverse effects; up to 12 g daily in divided doses has been given but is associated with an increased risk of toxicity. The night-time interval between doses should not exceed 8 hours. On remission the dose is gradually reduced to up to 2 g daily and then generally continued indefinitely. For children doses should be proportional to body-weight; initially 40 to 60 mg per kg body-weight may be given daily in divided doses reduced to 20 to 30 mg per kg daily for the maintenance of remission.

Sulphasalazine is also given rectally, as suppositories, in a dose of 1 g night and morning, either alone or as an adjunct to treatment by mouth; it may also be given by enema in a dose of 3 g at bedtime.

Sulphasalazine is also used in the treatment of severe or progressive rheumatoid arthritis not responding to analgesics or anti-inflammatory drugs. Treatment is usually commenced with a dose of 500 mg daily by mouth for the first week; dosage is then increased by 500 mg each week to a maximum of 3 g daily given in 2 to 4 divided doses.

Enteric-coated tablets are claimed to decrease the adverse gastro-intestinal effects which may be associated with administration of sulphasalazine, and are commonly used in the treatment of rheumatoid arthritis.

A review of the action and uses of sulphasalazine.— M. A. Peppercorn, *Ann. intern. Med.*, 1984, *3*, 377. Correction.— J. -P. Raufman (letter), *ibid.*, 1985, *102*, 139.

A study of the possible use of sulphasalazine to measure mouth/caecal transit time.— M. Kennedy *et al.* (letter), *Br. J. clin. Pharmac.*, 1979, *8*, 372.

A study suggesting an enterogenic origin for reactive synovitis and a beneficial role of sulphasalazine in its treatment.— H. Mielants *et al.*, *Int. J. clin. Pharmacol. Res.*, 1984, *4*, 409.

Beneficial results with sulphasalazine given systemically together with dexamethasone or betamethasone used as a mouth-wash in the treatment of 2 patients with pyostomatitis vegetans (a rare oral condition which manifests itself as intramucosal abscess formation).— D. Wray, *Br. dent. J.*, 1984, *157*, 316.

For reference to the use of sulphasalazine in the determination of acetylator status, see Sulphadimidine Sodium, p.304.

ACTION. Studies of the action of sulphasalazine in inflammatory bowel diseases have generally concluded that sulphasalazine acts as a vehicle for delivery of the active moiety, 5-aminosalicylic acid (mesalazine) to the colon. Sulphapyridine is considered to contribute to the adverse effects of the drug. This has led to the development of the following alternatives to sulphasalazine: topical or delayed-release preparations of salicylates such as mesalazine itself (see p.1097), or the more stable 4-aminosalicylic acid (see p.555), the joining of mesalazine to a more inert carrier as in balsalazide (see p.1078) or ipsalazide (see p.1580), or by joining 2 molecules of mesalazine as in olsalazine (see p.1101). Some studies, however, have suggested that sulphasalazine has intrinsic therapeutic activity as well as acting as a pro-drug. Sulphasalazine inhibits prostaglandin synthesis, prostaglandin degradation, and thromboxane synthesis, as well as interfering with neutrophil chemotaxis and scavenging radicals. One hypothesis is that the anti-inflammatory activity of sulphasalazine involves inhibition of synthesis of the chemotactic substance leukotriene B4 which occurs in excess in active ulcerative colitis (*Lancet*, 1987, *1*, 1299). Other actions which may contribute to the therapeutic effects of sulphasalazine include its interference with folic acid metabolism, its preferential binding to connective tissue, and its alteration of the flora of the gastro-intestinal tract. Mesalazine shares some of the actions of sulphasalazine including inhibition of prostaglandin synthesis, and inhibition of lipoxygenase although to a lesser extent than sulphasalazine (D.S. Rampton and C.J. Hawkey, *Gut*, 1984, *25*, 1399; J.R.S. Hoult, *Drugs*, 1986, *32*, *Suppl.* 1, 18). Both mesalazine and sulphapyridine, like the parent drug, suppress the production of reactive oxygen species (Y. Miyachi *et al.*, *Gut*, 1987, *28*, 190; B. Halliwell, *Lancet*, 1987, *2*, 635). In contrast to inflammatory bowel disease, a study comparing sulphapyridine and mesalazine in the treatment of rheumatoid arthritis has suggested that sulphapyridine is the active moiety contributing to the second-line effect of sulphasalazine in this condition; this may therefore suggest a role for bacterial infection in the causation or perpetuation of the rheumatoid disease process (T. Pullar *et al.*, *Br. med. J.*, 1985, *290*, 1535). Situnayake and McConkey (*ibid.*, *291*, 138) commented on this study and suggested that the effects of sulphasalazine on prostaglandin and lipoxygenase pathways and the anti-inflammatory effects of both sulphasalazine and sulphapyridine, including inhibitory effects on leucocyte migration and superoxide production may contribute to the effects of sulphasalazine in rheumatoid arthritis.

ANKYLOSING SPONDYLITIS. Report of a double-blind, placebo-controlled study of sulphasalazine in the treatment of 60 patients with ankylosing spondylitis. Patients receiving active treatment were given enteric-coated tablets of sulphasalazine in a dose of 2 g daily for 6 months in addition to their current dose of non-steroidal anti-inflammatory drugs (NSAIDs). Seven and 6 patients in the sulphasalazine and placebo groups respectively withdrew from the study because of inefficacy or adverse effects. In an overall assessment of all 60 patients, treatment was considered effective by half of the patients taking sulphasalazine, and one-fifth of those taking placebo. Of several parameters measured in the 47 patients who completed the study, sulphasalazine resulted in a significant decrease in the daily dosage of NSAIDs taken and in serum concentrations of immunoglobulins, and a significant increase in the functional index. The efficacy of sulphasalazine was apparent only after 3 months of treatment suggesting that it may be useful as a slow-acting drug and not as symptomatic treatment.— M. Dougados *et al.*, *Br. med. J.*, 1986, *293*, 911.

Further references to the use of sulphasalazine in ankylosing spondylitis: B. Amor *et al.* (letter), *Ann. intern. Med.*, 1984, *101*, 878; N. Feltelius and R. Hällgren, *Ann. rheum. Dis.*, 1986, *45*, 396.

HEPATITIS. A pilot study of 5 patients with chronic active hepatitis associated with hepatitis B virus who were treated with sulphasalazine 1 g, taken four times daily for one week and then three times daily for a further 6 months. Marked clinical and biochemical improvement occurred in 4; the fifth admitted to non-compliance with therapy.— J. F. Fielding *et al.*, *Ir. med. J.*, 1982, *75*, 91.

INFLAMMATORY BOWEL DISEASES. A review of the use of sulphasalazine in inflammatory bowel diseases.— M. A. Peppercorn, *J. clin. Pharmac.*, 1987, *27*, 260.

Reviews of inflammatory bowel disease, including its management: J. B. Kirsner and R. G. Shorter, *New Engl. J. Med.*, 1982, *306*, 775; J. M. Rhodes, *Prescribers' J.*, 1986, *26*, 1.

Inflammatory bowel disease in childhood.— I. W. Booth and J. T. Harries, *Gut*, 1984, *25*, 188.

Mention of sulphasalazine in the treatment of microscopic total colitis.— A. M. Dawson, *Br. med. J.*, 1982, *285*, 1601.

For a review of the action of sulphasalazine in inflammatory bowel diseases, see Action, above.

For the use of sulphasalazine in inflammatory bowel disease during pregnancy, see Pregnancy and the Neonate, below.

Collagenous colitis. Collagenous colitis is a rare condition which presents as persistent watery diarrhoea and is associated with a thickened band of collagen immediately below the surface epithelium of the colonic mucosa. Response to any medication is generally disappointing although improvement with sulphasalazine has been reported (*Lancet*, 1986, *2*, 1136; G.T. Williams and J. Rhodes, *Br. med. J.* 1987, *294*, 855). Rams *et al.* (*Ann. intern. Med.*, 1987, *106*, 108) have suggested a trial of therapy with sulphasalazine 2 to 3 g daily once the diagnosis is established. If improvement occurs therapy should be continued for several months to ensure that remission is sustained; thereafter the dosage may be adjusted as in patients with other forms of sulphasalazine-responsive colitis.

Crohn's disease. In a multicentre comparative study of treatment for Crohn's disease, a chronic destructive inflammatory disease of the bowel, prednisone or sulphasalazine were more effective than placebo in patients with active disease; azathioprine was ineffective. Sulphasalazine may be the drug of choice for previously untreated patients; overall, it was the least toxic of the three drugs. Sulphasalazine, prednisone, or azathioprine were not of value in quiescent disease or following surgery. When sulphasalazine and prednisone were used together in actively symptomatic patients there was probably less improvement than when prednisone was used alone. Patients in remission relapsed more quickly on the combined treatment and suffered more adverse effects than those taking prednisone, suggesting that the use of sulphasalazine and prednisone in association for active Crohn's disease should be discouraged.—The National Cooperative Crohn's Disease Study, J. W. Singleton (Ed.), *Gastroenterology*, 1979, *77*, 825–944.

As in ulcerative colitis, corticosteroids are commonly used to treat active Crohn's disease. Sulphasalazine is probably of some value if there is colonic involvement, but there is at present no good evidence that it reduces the relapse rate when given over long periods. It is, however, of doubtful benefit in small bowel disease but is worth trying in difficult cases.— J. M. Rhodes, *Prescribers' J.*, 1986, *26*, 1.

Further reviews and discussions on the management of Crohn's disease: *Lancet*, 1983, *2*, 831; *Drug & Ther. Bull.*, 1986, *24*, 13.

For reference to a study showing metronidazole to be slightly more active than sulphasalazine in patients with active Crohn's disease, see Metronidazole, p.671.

Proctitis. A report of the use of high-fibre diet, sulphasalazine, and prednisolone sodium phosphate enemas or suppositories in haemorrhagic proctitis in 74 patients.— A. Myers *et al.*, *Postgrad. med. J.*, 1976, *52*, 224.

Further references: C. Möller *et al.*, *Clin. Trials J.*, 1978, *15*, 199.

Ulcerative colitis. Corticosteroids are the mainstay of treatment for acute attacks of ulcerative colitis and sulphasalazine for the maintenance of remission. Treatment should be prompt as circumstantial evidence suggests that the chance of achieving remission diminishes if treatment is delayed. Sulphasalazine administered by mouth does, however, have some effect in acute colitis and can be started while the results of investigations are awaited, but corticosteroids are considerably more effective and should be used in all but the mildest of attacks. The preferred route of administration of corticosteroids depends on the extent of the disease. Maintenance treatment with sulphasalazine 1 g twice daily reduces the relapse rate by about two-thirds; larger doses are more effective but are likely to cause nausea.— J. M. Rhodes, *Prescribers' J.*, 1986, *26*, 1. Discussion of the use of sulphasalazine in the treatment of ulcerative colitis. Although commonly used together, there are no controlled studies of the role of sulphasalazine as an adjunct to steroid therapy in ulcerative colitis.— M. A. Peppercorn, *J. clin. Pharmac.*, 1987, *27*, 260. See also J. E. Lennard-Jones, *Postgrad. med. J.*, 1984, *60*, 797.

A study in 185 patients with ulcerative colitis indicated that when patients are maintained on the same dose of sulphasalazine, the serum concentration of total sulphapyridine during remission does not influence the liability to relapse. When relapse does occur, serum concentrations of sulphapyridine fall and remain depressed until remission occurs; the fall is most pronounced in patients with colitis affecting the entire colon and least marked in patients with distal colitis.— A. K. A. Khan and S. C. Truelove, *Gut*, 1980, *21*, 706.

A study suggesting that 'on demand' sulphasalazine may be as effective as continuous therapy in the maintenance of remission in ulcerative colitis.— R. J. Dickinson *et al.*, *Gut*, 1984, *25*, A553.

PREGNANCY AND THE NEONATE. In 38 women with ulcerative colitis during 50 pregnancies there were no complications due to treatment with sulphasalazine and oral and/or topical corticosteroids.— H. P. McEwan, *Proc. R. Soc. Med.*, 1972, *65*, 279.

Recommendations for administration of sulphasalazine during pregnancy have differed. Donaldson (*New Engl. J. Med.*, 1985, *312*, 1616) considered that the only benefit of maintenance sulphasalazine therapy in the asymptomatic patient was a slight decrease in the recurrence of mild ulcerative colitis; therefore the continued use of sulphasalazine after suppression of active disease is not justified because of the potential risk, although unsubstantiated in clinical practice, of harm to the foetus. Rhodes (*Prescribers' J.*, 1986, *26*, 1) in reviewing the management of inflammatory bowel disease, however, considered that maintenance therapy with sulphasalazine should be continued after control of active disease. Byron (*Br. med. J.*, 1987, *294*, 236) has recommended that since sulphasalazine impairs absorption of folic acid, supplementation should be given if the drug is used during pregnancy.

See also Absorption and Fate and Adverse Effects, Treatment, and Precautions, above.

RHEUMATOID ARTHRITIS. Sulphasalazine is described as a 'disease-modifying', 'slow-acting', 'remission-inducing' or 'second-line' drug in the treatment of rheumatoid arthritis, as opposed to anti-inflammatory agents which are first-line agents. Because of the differences in action, most patients requiring second-line drugs should also be taking a non-steroidal anti-inflammatory drug and, if necessary, an analgesic. Second-line agents are reserved for patients with severe disease characterised by persistent inflammation failing to respond to anti-inflammatory drugs, or progressive disease with X-ray changes. Their role in altering the long-term progress of rheumatoid arthritis is unclear. They are, however, now being used earlier in the disease in an attempt to prevent erosive X-ray changes.— D. G. I. Scott and J. S. Coppock, *Prescribers' J.*, 1987, *27* (1), 13. Sulphasalazine is now established as an effective second-line drug for the treatment of rheumatoid arthritis. Minor adverse effects are common but serious problems are rare; gold and penicillamine are probably more effective but are more dangerous. Although sulphasalazine is a slow-acting drug its effect is quicker than gold or penicillamine. Clinical improvement, accompanied by a fall in erythrocyte sedimentation-rate and serum C-reactive protein can be apparent within 6 weeks. It was concluded that there is now enough evidence to consider sulphasalazine as first-choice amongst second-line agents.— B. McConkey and R. D. Situnayake, *ibid.*, 27.

Further reviews and discussions of the treatment of rheumatoid arthritis.— *Drug & Ther. Bull.*, 1985, *26*, 101; H. A. Bird, *Br. J. Hosp. Med.*, 1986, *35*, 374.

Proceedings of a symposium on the use of sulphasalazine in rheumatoid arthritis.— *Drugs*, 1986, *32*, *Suppl.* 1, 1–80.

Further reviews and discussions on the use of sulphasalazine in rheumatoid arthritis: V. C. Neumann and K. A. Grindulis, *J. R. Soc. Med.*, 1984, *77*, 169; *Pharm. J.*, 1986, *1*, 456.

A brief review of the variables affecting the efficacy and toxicity of sulphasalazine in rheumatoid arthritis. Although no clear relationship has been demonstrated between efficacy and serum concentrations of sulphasalazine or its metabolites, there does appear to be a direct dose-response relationship with an optimum dose in excess of 40 mg per kg body-weight daily. It appears that while acetylator phenotype is unlikely to have a clinically significant effect on the efficacy of sulphasalazine, slow acetylators are more prone to discontinue therapy because of upper gastro-intestinal symptoms.— T. Pullar and H. A. Capell, *Drugs*, 1986, *32*, *Suppl.* 1, 54. The clinical response to sulphasalazine in rheumatoid arthritis is unpredictable; some patients do very well, but others derive little obvious benefit. Drug dosage per unit of body-weight appears to have no predictive value for treatment outcome. A standard regimen of 2 g daily has been used; higher doses frequently cause more toxicity with few extra therapeutic benefits.— R. S. Amos *et al.*, *ibid.*, 58.

Beneficial effect of sulphasalazine, administered for a period of 4 to 14 months, in the treatment of juvenile rheumatoid arthritis.— H. Özdogan *et al.*, *J. Rheumatol.*, 1986, *13*, 124.

A discussion on the use of enteric-coated sulphasalazine tablets in the treatment of rheumatoid arthritis. All clinical studies have used the enteric-coated tablets rather than the plain tablets usually employed in ulcerative colitis. The rationale for their use is that they may reduce the incidence of adverse gastro-intestinal disturbances which appear to limit compliance in this group of patients and which may be compounded by the use of non-steroidal anti-inflammatory drugs. No evidence exists, however, on the comparative frequency or severity of adverse effects with the two preparations in rheumatoid arthritis. The sulphapyridine component has been implicated as causing gastro-intestinal effects, but a study in healthy subjects has demonstrated similar bioavailability of sulphapyridine from the post-1984 formulations of plain and enteric-coated Salazopyrin tablets, although plasma concentrations of sulphasalazine were higher after the plain tablets. It was concluded that, in principle, there appears to be a good argument for trying plain sulphasalazine in rheumatoid arthritis.— *Drug & Ther. Bull.*, 1987, *25*, 53.

Comparative studies of sulphasalazine with other agents in the treatment of rheumatoid arthritis: V. C. Neumann *et al.*, *Br. med. J.*, 1983, *287*, 1099 (penicillamine); T. Pullar *et al.*, *ibid.*, 1102 (sodium aurothiomalate); D. E. Bax and R. S. Amos, *Drugs*, 1986, *32*, *Suppl.* 1, 73 (sodium aurothiomalate).

For a report of a study monitoring the adverse effects of sulphasalazine during the treatment of rheumatoid arthritis, see Adverse Effects, Treatment, and Precautions, above.

For a discussion of the possible actions of sulphasalazine in rheumatoid arthritis, see Action, above.

SCLERODERMA. All of 19 patients with scleroderma of 1.5 to 20 years' duration obtained subjective improvement after treatment with sulphasalazine; objective improvement occurred in several parameters. The dose was 1 to 7 g daily by mouth for 2 or 3 weeks, then 0.25 to 7 g daily. Side-effects were common but not severe.— N. Dover, *Israel J. med. Scis*, 1971, *7*, 1301.

In 13 patients with scleroderma of about 1 to 28 years' duration, treatment with sulphasalazine for up to 13 months produced marked improvement in 2, mild improvement in 1, some subjective improvement in 3, and no improvement in the remaining 7. Treatment was discontinued because of side-effects in 9 patients.— Z. Šťáva and M. Kobíková, *Br. J. Derm.*, 1976, *96*, 541.

Further references: A. J. Barnett *et al.*, *Aust. J. Derm.*, 1975, *16*, 55.

Preparations

Sulfasalazine Tablets *(U.S.P.)*

Proprietary Preparations

Salazopyrin *(Pharmacia, UK)*. *Tablets*, scored, sulphasalazine 500 mg.

Tablets (Salazopyrin EN-Tabs), enteric-coated, sulphasalazine 500 mg.

Suspension, sulphasalazine 250 mg/5 mL.

Enema, sulphasalazine 3 g in single-dose bottles of 100 mL.

Suppositories, sulphasalazine 500 mg.

Proprietary Names and Manufacturers

Azulfidine *(Arg.; Pharmacia Arzneimittel, Ger.; Pharmacia, USA)*; Colo-Pleon *(Henning Berlin, Ger.)*; Salazopyrin *(Pharmacia, Austral.; Pharmacia, Canad.; Pharmacia, Denm.; Pharmacia, Ital.; Pharmacia, Norw.; Pharmacia, S.Afr.; Pharmacia, Swed.; Pharmacia, Switz.; Pharmacia, UK)*; Salazopyrina *(Lasa, Spain)*; Salazopyrine *(Belg.; Pharmacia, Fr.; Neth.)*; Salisulf *(Gipharmex, Ital.)*; SAS *(ICN, Canad.; Rowell, USA)*.

7534-p

Tamarind

West Indian Tamarind.

Pharmacopoeias. In *Port.*

The fruits of *Tamarindus indica* (Leguminosae) freed from the brittle outer part of the pericarp and preserved with sugar. **Store** in a cool place and avoid contact with copper.

Tamarind was formerly used as a laxative.

17004-r

Teprenone *(rINN)*.

E-671. 6,10,14,18-Tetramethyl-5,9,13,17-nonadecatetraen-2-one, mixture of (5*E*,9*E*,13*E*) and (5*Z*,9*E*,13*E*) isomers.

$C_{23}H_{38}O$=330.6.

Teprenone is used in the treatment of peptic ulcers in doses of up to 150 mg daily.

Proprietary Names and Manufacturers

Selbex *(Eisai, Jpn)*.

13350-q

Tiopropamine Hydrochloride *(rINNM)*.

3,3-Diphenyl-3′-(phenylthio)dipropylamine hydrochloride.

$C_{24}H_{27}NS,HCl$=398.0.

CAS — 39516-21-7 (tiopropamine).

Tiopropamine hydrochloride is used in the treatment of peptic ulcer in doses of up to 400 mg daily.

Proprietary Names and Manufacturers

Redden *(Alfa Farmaceutici, Ital.)*.

3778-t

Tripotassium Dicitratobismuthate

Bismuth Subcitrate.

CAS — 57644-54-9.

Adverse Effects and Precautions

Nausea and vomiting have been reported with tripotassium dicitratobismuthate. Darkening of the tongue has also been reported and blackening of the faeces is stated to occur. Although there have been no reports of bismuth encephalopathy following the use of tripotassium dicitratobismuthate in the recommended doses this possibility should be borne in mind following overdosage and long-term therapy is not recommended. Tripotassium dicitratobismuthate should not be given to patients with renal disorders and should not be taken at the same time as antacids or milk. It is reported to inhibit the efficacy of tetracyclines taken by mouth.

A short comment that bismuth encephalopathy was associated with the prolonged use of high doses of insoluble bismuth salts but has never been described with tripotassium dicitratobismuthate in recommended doses. It has been proposed that bismuth preparations should be discontinued if blood concentrations exceed 100 ng per mL, with 50 to 100 ng per mL being considered an "alerting zone". Patients with encephalopathy have generally had concentrations of several hundred or thousand ng per mL while in nearly 500 patients given therapeutic doses of tripotassium dicitratobismuthate the mean concentration was only 7 ng per mL with only 2 values in the alerting zone.— J. P. Miller (letter), *Br. med. J.*, 1986, *293*, 1501.

Uses and Administration

Tripotassium dicitratobismuthate is used for the treatment of gastric and duodenal ulcers; its activity against such ulcers is reviewed below.

The usual dose by mouth is 240 mg twice daily or 120 mg four times daily taken before food for a period of 4 weeks extended to 8 weeks if necessary. Maintenance therapy with tripotassium dicitratobismuthate is not recommended although treatment may be repeated after a drug-free interval of one month.

A review.— A. J. Wagstaff *et al.*, *Drugs*, 1988, *36*, 132.

PEPTIC ULCER. Studies have shown that tripotassium dicitratobismuthate is capable of producing initial healing comparable with the H_2-antagonists cimetidine or ranitidine in patients with duodenal ulcer (D.F. Martin *et al.*, *Lancet*, 1981, *1*, 7; G. Bianchi Porro *et al.*, *Gut*, 1984, *25*, A565; F.I. Lee *et al.*, *Lancet*, 1985, *1*, 1299; I. Hamilton *et al.*, *Gut*, 1986, *27*, 106) or gastric ulcer (F. Cipollini and F. Altilia, *Br. J. clin. Pract.*, 1987, *41*, 707). These studies also demonstrated on follow-up, that after the initial therapy was discontinued the relapse-rate was significantly lower in the bismuthate-treated patients than in those given an H_2-antagonist. In a review (J.P. Miller and E.B. Faragher, *Br. med. J.*, 1986, *293*, 1117) it was calculated that the combined results of published studies in duodenal ulcer showed that 85% of patients treated with H_2-antagonists relapsed within a year compared with 59% of those treated with tripotassium dicitratobismuthate. These findings have led to some workers suggesting that bismuthate should be the initial form of therapy for duodenal ulcer but to others (K.G. Wormsley, *Br. med. J.*, 1986, *293*, 1501; J.P. Miller, *ibid.*) debating the question of maintenance therapy as bismuthate is not recommended for long-term treatment although a study is reported to be in progress to assess its safety and efficacy for this purpose.

Investigation has been focussed on the mechanism of action of tripotassium dicitratobismuthate in peptic ulcer with particular interest being shown in its action against *Campylobacter pylori* (*Campylobacter pyloridis*). This bacterium was first isolated from the stomachs of patients with gastritis and peptic ulceration (B.J. Marshall and J.R. Warren, *Lancet*, 1984, *1*, 1311) and has since been found to be present in the majority of patients with peptic ulcer but to be rare in healthy persons. As well as being a mucosal protectant bismuthate is bactericidal to *C. pylori* and various suggestions have been made concerning the use of systemic antibiotics in an anti-ulcer regime; the use of an antibiotic with tripotassium dicitratobismuthate has been proposed (B.J. Marshall *et al.*, *Med. J. Aust.*, 1985, *142*, 439; C.A.M. McNulty, *J. Antimicrob. Chemother.*, 1987, *19*, 281) as well as an antibiotic with an H_2-antagonist (McNulty, *ibid.*) and trials of such combined therapies are reported to be in progress. In a placebo-controlled study (C.A.M. McNulty *et al.*, *Br. med. J.*, 1986, *293*, 645) another bismuth salt, bismuth salicylate, was found to be more effective than erythromycin ethylsuccinate in clearing *C. pylori* and improving gastritis in patients without peptic ulceration with the comment being made that larger studies are still needed.

Proprietary Preparations

De-Nol *(Brocades, UK). Oral Liquid*, tripotassium dicitratobismuthate 120 mg/5mL.

De-Noltab *(Brocades, UK). Tablets*, tripotassium dicitratobismuthate 120 mg.

Proprietary Names and Manufacturers

De-Nol *(Brocades, UK)*; De-Noltab *(Brocades, UK)*; Duosol *(Cooper, Switz.)*; Ulcerone *(Riker, S.Afr.)*.

13383-c

Tritiozine *(rINN).*

ISF-2001; Trithiozine. 4-(3,4,5-Trimethoxythiobenzoyl)morpholine.
$C_{14}H_{19}NO_4S$=297.4.

CAS — 35619-65-9.

Tritiozine is used in the treatment of peptic ulcer in doses of up to 800 mg daily.

Proprietary Names and Manufacturers

Clositol *(Novag, Spain)*; Tresanil *(ISF, Ital.)*; Trizinoral *(Alcor, Spain)*.

7535-s

Turpeth

Indian Jalap; Tripolium; Turbit; Turbito Vegetal; Turpeth Root.

Pharmacopoeias. In *Arg.*, *Port.*, and *Span.*

The dried root and stem of *Ipomoea turpethum* (Convolvulaceae) containing not less than 5% resin.

Turpeth resembles jalap in its action and has similarly been superseded by less toxic laxatives.

709-v

Urogastrone

CAS — 9010-53-1.

An inhibitory factor of gastric secretion derived from human urine. There are two forms β and γ urogastrone with the β form being distinguishable from the other by an additional terminal arginine residue. The β form is reported to be identical to human epidermal growth factor.

The characterisation of urogastrone and its equivalence to human epidermal growth factor.— H. Gregory (letter), *Nature*, 1975, *257*, 325.

Urogastrone is used in the treatment of peptic ulcer. Epidermal growth factor is the subject of much investigation, and has potential in wound healing.

In 4 patients with the Zollinger-Ellison syndrome the administration of urogastrone 250 ng per kg body-weight over 1 hour reduced gastric acid output by 50 to 82%; the concentration of intrinsic factor and pepsin in gastric juice rose by 60 to 300%, and the peak plasma-gastrin concentration by 127 to 164%. Ulcer pain was relieved 30 to 60 minutes after the start of the infusion.— J. B. Elder *et al.*, *Lancet*, 1975, *2*, 424. Significant reduction of basal acid secretion without significant effect on basal pepsin and intrinsic factor secretion or on serum-gastrin concentration was observed in 7 patients with duodenal ulceration given an intravenous infusion of urogastrone 250 ng per kg body-weight over 1 hour.— C. G. Koffman *et al.*, *Gut*, 1982, *23*, 951.

A comment on the heterogeneous group of polypeptides known as growth factors and their receptors and role in disease and mentioning that topical administration of recombinant epidermal growth factor is likely to be used to accelerate wound healing after ophthalmic and plastic surgery.— *Lancet*, 1985, *2*, 251.

A report of the use of recombinant epidermal growth factor/urogastrone in an infant with microvillous atrophy (a disorder within the intractable diarrhoea syndrome of infancy with a very poor prognosis); a dosage of 100 ng per kg body-weight per hour was given by intravenous infusion for two 6-day periods with a 5-day rest period between the 2 courses. Although crypt cell proliferation and growth was stimulated there was little effect on absorptive capacity and the drug did not represent a complete treatment for microvillous atrophy.— J. A. Walker-Smith *et al.* (letter), *Lancet*, 1985, *2*, 1239.

Proprietary Names and Manufacturers

Homogarol *(Tobishi, Jpn)*; Supergastrone *(Ital.)*; Ugaron *(Nippon Shinyaku, Jpn)*.

710-r

Zolimidine *(pINN).*

2-(4-Methylsulphonylphenyl)imidazo[1,2-*a*]pyridine.
$C_{14}H_{12}N_2O_2S$=272.3.

CAS — 1222-57-7.

Zolimidine is used in the treatment of peptic ulcer in doses of 600 to 800 mg daily.

Proprietary Names and Manufacturers

Gastronilo *(Aristegui, Spain)*; Solimidin *(Selvi, Ital.)*; U.G.D. *(Beta, Arg.)*.

General Anaesthetics

3100-t

General anaesthetics are administered either by inhalation or by intravenous or occasionally intramuscular injection. Those administered by inhalation and described in this section include: chloroform, cyclopropane, enflurane, ether, fluroxene, halothane, isoflurane, nitrous oxide, trichloroethylene.

Anaesthetic agents given parenterally include: alphaxalone, etomidate, ketamine hydrochloride, methohexitone sodium, metomidate hydrochloride, propanidid, propofol, sodium oxybate, thialbarbitone sodium, thiamylal sodium, thiobutabarbital sodium, thiopentone sodium.

Other compounds that are also used for anaesthetic purposes are included in the chapters on Anxiolytic Sedatives Hypnotics and Neuroleptics p.706 and on Opioid Analgesics p.1294.

Adverse Effects of General Anaesthetics

Adverse effects which may occur during general anaesthesia include involuntary muscle movements, hiccup, coughing, bronchospasm, laryngospasm, hypotension, cardiac arrhythmias, respiratory depression, emergence reactions, and postoperative nausea and vomiting.

Malignant hyperpyrexia has occasionally been reported mainly with the halogenated hydrocarbon anaesthetics; suxamethonium has also been given in many of the cases. The condition is familial and is often fatal. It is characterised by a rapid rise in body temperature usually accompanied by muscle rigidity and myoglobinuria. There may be cardiovascular changes, acidosis, and increases in serum-enzyme concentrations.

Concern has been expressed about the possible danger to anaesthetists and other operating theatre personnel from exposure to anaesthetic agents. There have been reports of an increased incidence of hypertension and liver disorders; an increase in infertility, spontaneous abortion (affecting not only female personnel but the partners of male personnel), still-births, low birth-weight, congenital malformations and development disorders. Other possible effects reported include an effect on the immune response and an increased incidence of cardiac arrhythmias, gall-bladder disease, lumbar disk disease, migraine, neoplasms, peptic ulcer, renal disease, and ulcerative colitis. Reports are not unanimous and the mortality rate of British anaesthetists has been shown to be less than that of other medical personnel and of the general population (see below).

A review of anaesthetic risk, morbidity and mortality.— M. C. Derrington and G. Smith, *Br. J. Anaesth.*, 1987, *59*, 815.

A review of the toxicity of intravenous anaesthetics.— J. W. Sear, *Br. J. Anaesth.*, 1987, *59*, 24.

Reviews of allergic drug reactions during anaesthesia: A. G. Bird, *Adverse Drug React. Bull.*, 1985, Feb., 408; J. Watkins, *Br. J. Hosp. Med.*, 1986, *36*, 45 (intravenous anaesthetics).

DENTAL SURGERY. A randomised study in 60 outpatients undergoing 30-minute dental operations. Two groups of 25 patients were given general anaesthetic techniques and a third group of 10 patients received local anaesthesia with prilocaine. An established anaesthetic method which included suxamethonium, endotracheal intubation, and halothane yielded the highest incidence of minor sequelae when compared with other groups receiving either fentanyl, an nasopharyngeal airway with incremental methohexitone or local anaesthesia. The study supported the efficacy of local anaesthesia for day case dental surgery.— T. W. Ogg *et al.*, *Br. dent. J.*, 1983, *155*, 14.

See also under Fatalities, below.

EFFECTS ON BODY TEMPERATURE. Some reviews of malignant hyperpyrexia: G. A. Gronert, *Anesthesiology*, 1980, *53*, 395; T. E. Nelson and E. H. Flewellen, *New Engl. J. Med.*, 1983, *309*, 416; M. A. Denborough, *Clin. Anaesth.*, 1984, *2*, 669.

For the use of dantrolene sodium in the treatment of malignant hyperpyrexia, see Dantrolene Sodium, p.1233.

For the use of procaine in the treatment of malignant hyperpyrexia, see Procaine Hydrochloride, p.1226.

EFFECTS ON THE HEART. A discussion of cardiac arrest related to anaesthesia in infants and children.— M. R. Salem *et al.*, *J. Am. med. Ass.*, 1975, *233*, 238.

In a 15-year study 449 cardiac arrests occurred during 163 240 anaesthetic administrations and 27 of these were considered to be primarily due to the anaesthetic itself or to the anaesthetic management of the patient. Twelve of these 27 arrests were attributed to inadequate ventilation and 15 to drug overdosage. Overdosage with inhalation anaesthetics was absolute in 9 of the 15; the remaining 6 patients were haemodynamically unstable and did not tolerate normal doses of anaesthetic. The incidence of arrest in children below 12 years of age was approximately 3 times that in adults.— R. L. Keenan and C. P. Boyan, *J. Am. med. Ass.*, 1985, *253*, 2373. Comment.— L. D. Vandam, *ibid.*, 2415.

FATALITIES. Analyses of anaesthetic-related mortality in the *UK*: J.N. Lunn and M.W. Mushin, *Mortality Associated with Anaesthesia*, London, Nuffield Provincial Hospitals Trust, 1982; J. N. Lunn *et al.*, *Anaesthesia*, 1983, *38*, 1090.

A 25-year survey of anaesthesia-attributable mortality in New South Wales, Australia.— R. Holland, *Br. J. Anaesth.*, 1987, *59*, 834. Anaesthetic-related maternal mortality in England and Wales, covering a 30-year period.— M. Morgan, *ibid.*, 842.

There were 120 deaths associated with dentistry in England and Wales during the 10 years 1970 to 1979. Out of these, 100 deaths were associated with general anaesthesia and 6 with local anaesthesia. Of the 100 deaths associated with general anaesthesia, 36 were in hospital inpatients, 8 were in hospital outpatients, 49 were in general dental practice, and 6 in community dental practice. Two distinct types of collapse could be identified in 52 of the deaths in dental practice: a sudden cardiovascular collapse (22), usually during recovery, and collapse associated with respiratory obstruction (30). There was no evidence to show greater risk in patients anaesthetised in the sitting position compared with those in the supine position, although it was felt that it would still be wise to place a patient flat on his side as soon as possible after completion of treatment, irrespective of the posture in which it was undertaken. Data from Dinsdale and Dixon's paper (R.C.W. Dinsdale and R.A. Dixon, *Br. dent. J.*, 1978, *144*, 271) was also considered in this study and indicated that the unsupplemented nitrous oxide and oxygen, which was still being used in dentistry, was associated with the lowest mortality rate. This data also showed a greater risk with conservative than with emergency procedures.— M. P. Coplans and I. Curson, *Br. dent. J.*, 1982, *153*, 357. A view that deaths associated with anaesthetics in the dental chair are commonly caused by the patient being in the upright or semi-upright position.— J. G. Bourne (letter), *Br. dent. J.*, 1983, *155*, 111.

HAZARD TO USER. Some references to surveys and reviews of the hazards of anaesthesia for the operator: M. P. Vessey and J. F. Nunn, *Br. med. J.*, 1980, *281*, 696; E. N. Cohen *et al.*, *J. Am. dent. Ass.*, 1980, *101*, 21; S. D. Schrag and R. L. Dixon, *Annu. Rev. Pharmacol. Toxicol.*, 1985, *25*, 567. In reviewing the major studies Tannenbaum and Goldberg considered that there was no conclusive evidence of occupational anaesthetic exposure increasing the rate of abortion or congenital abnormalities (*J. occup. Med.*, 1985, *27*, 659). Also in a survey carried out by Neil *et al.* (*Br. med. J.*, 1987, *295*, 360) of 3769 male anaesthetists in the *UK* over a total of 51 431 person-years between 1957 and 1983, the mortality rate for the anaesthetists was less than for the general population or for British doctors as a whole. There was no evidence of an increased risk of cancer mortality, including cancer of the pancreas. While there was an increase in suicide rate in the anaesthetists compared with the general population, the suicide rate did not differ from that in other doctors.

Precautions for General Anaesthetics

Patients with impaired function of the adrenal cortex, such as those who are being treated or have recently been treated with corticosteroids, may experience hypotension with the stress of anaesthesia. Treatment with corticosteroids, pre-operatively and postoperatively, may be necessary—see Corticosteroids, p.874.

Diabetics, particularly those with a severe unstable condition, may require adjustment to their diet or therapy prior to anaesthesia.

In patients being treated for hypertension, change in therapy may be necessary to provide better control during anaesthesia. Patients being treated for cardiac arrhythmias should be anaesthetised with special care. For a discussion of beta-adrenoceptor blocking therapy and anaesthesia, see p.781. Sensitisation of the myocardium to beta-adrenergic stimulation occurs with some anaesthetics and ventricular fibrillation may occur if sympathomimetic agents are administered concomitantly, see Sympathomimetics, p.1453.

Serious effects may follow the use of some drugs administered as adjuncts to anaesthesia in patients taking, or having recently taken, some antidepressants, see Amitriptyline Hydrochloride, p.353 and Phenelzine Sulphate, p.378.

A review of drug interactions in anaesthesia.— M. J. Halsey, *Br. J. Anaesth.*, 1987, *59*, 112.

ALCOHOLISM. A discussion of the problems of anaesthesia and the alcoholic patient.— R. Edwards, *Br. med. J.*, 1985, *291*, 423.

AWARENESS. Some discussions of awareness during anaesthesia: J. G. Jones and K. Konieczko, *Br. med. J.*, 1986, *292*, 1291; *Lancet*, 1986, *2*, 553. See also *Lancet*, 1987, *2*, 543.

EFFECT ON DRIVING. A study of recovery from anaesthesia indicating that patients should be advised not to undertake hazardous tasks such as driving a car for at least 48 hours after a general anaesthetic.— M. Herbert *et al.*, *Br. med. J.*, 1983, *286*, 1539.

Uses of General Anaesthetics

General anaesthetics depress the central nervous system and produce loss of consciousness. An ideal anaesthetic agent would produce unconsciousness, analgesia, and muscle relaxation suitable for all surgical procedures and be metabolically inert and rapidly eliminated. No single agent in safe concentrations fulfils all these requirements and it is customary to employ a number of agents to produce the required surgical conditions. A typical anaesthetic sequence is: induction with a short-acting intravenous agent such as thiopentone; intubation after the use of a short-acting muscle relaxant such as suxamethonium chloride, maintenance of unconsciousness with an inhalation anaesthetic, such as halothane vaporised with nitrous oxide and oxygen; supplementary analgesics and muscle relaxants may be given by injection. In simple terms, the activity of any anaesthetic is dependent on its ability to reach the brain. With inhalational anaesthetics there has to be a transfer from the alveolar space to the blood, then to the brain; recovery is a function of the removal of the anaesthetic from the tissues and the blood. With injectable anaesthetics their activity is similarly dependent on their ability to penetrate the blood/brain barrier and recovery in turn is governed by their redistribution and excretion.

The potency of inhalational anaesthetics is often expressed in terms of minimum alveolar concentrations, known as MAC values. The MAC of an anaesthetic is the concentration at 1 atmosphere that will produce immobility in 50% of subjects exposed to a noxious stimulus. The figures provided in the following monographs are based on the anaesthetic being used without nitrous oxide which can affect the MAC as can other factors such as age and body temperature.

Some reviews and discussions of anaesthetic agents: J. W. Dundee and T. J. McMurray, *J. R. Soc. Med.*, 1984, *77*, 669 (total intravenous anaesthesia); F. A. Berry, *Clin. Anaesth.*, 1985, *3*, 515 (inhalation anaesthesia in paediatrics); D. J. Hatch and E. Sumner, *ibid.*, 633 (neonatal anaesthesia); E. Facer, *ibid.*, 697 (anaesthesia for paediatric ENT surgery); *Lancet*, 1986, *2*, 84 (single-breath technique for inhalational induction); J. Kanto, *Clin. Pharmacokinet.*, 1986, *11*, 283 (pharmacokinetics of anaesthetics for obstetric analgesia); *Lancet*, 1987, *1*, 1357 (anaesthesia for tonsillectomy).

3102-r

Alphadolone Acetate *(BANM).*
Alfadolone Acetate *(rINNM)*; GR-2/1574. 3α,21-Dihydroxy-5α-pregnane-11,20-dione 21-acetate.
$C_{23}H_{34}O_5$=390.5.

CAS — 14107-37-0 (alphadolone); 23930-37-2 (acetate).

Pharmacopoeias. In *B.P. Vet.*

Alphadolone acetate has been used to enhance the solubility of alphaxalone. It possesses some anaesthetic properties and is considered to be about half as potent as alphaxalone.

3103-f

Alphaxalone *(BAN).*
Alfaxalone *(rINN)*; GR-2/234. 3α-Hydroxy-5α-pregnane-11,20-dione.
$C_{21}H_{32}O_3$=332.5.

CAS — 23930-19-0.

Pharmacopoeias. In *B.P. Vet.*

Alphaxalone has been widely used in combination with alphadolone acetate (Althesin) as an intravenous anaesthetic for induction and maintenance of anaesthesia. Induction is rapid, as is recovery even after prolonged maintenance.

Commercial preparations of alphaxalone with alphadolone acetate were provided as a liquid in Cremophor EL. Anaphylactoid reactions associated with Cremophor EL have led to the general withdrawal of alphaxalone with alphadolone acetate from use.

Concern over the withdrawal of alphaxalone with alphadolone acetate with regard to its value as an infusion in the management of patients with head injuries or neurological damage.— J. W. Dundee (letter), *Lancet*, 1984, *1*, 909. See also M. Morgan and J. G. Whitwam, *Anaesthesia*, 1985, *40*, 121.

Proprietary Names and Manufacturers of Mixtures of Alphaxalone and Alphadolone Acetate

Alfatésine *(Fr.)*; Alfatesin *(Neth.; Norw.)*; Alfathesin *(Austral.)*; Alphadione *(Jpn)*; Althesin *(Denm.; Ital.; Glaxo, UK).*

3104-d

Chloroform *(BAN, USAN).*

Chloroformium Anesthesicum; Chloroformum; Chloroformum pro Narcosi. Trichloromethane.
$CHCl_3$=119.4.

CAS — 67-66-3.

Pharmacopoeias. In *Arg., Aust., Belg., Br., Chin., Egypt., Fr., Ger., Hung., Ind., Int., Jug., Mex., Nord., Pol., Port., Rus., Span.*, and *Turk.* Also in *U.S.N.F.* and *B.P. Vet.*

Some pharmacopoeias include a grade of chloroform, with less stringent standards, which may be taken by mouth but which must not be used as an anaesthetic.

A colourless mobile volatile liquid with a characteristic odour and a sweet burning taste. It contains 1 to 2% v/v of ethyl alcohol; the *U.S.N.F.* specifies 0.5 to 1% v/v. Not flammable. B.p. about 61°. The addition of the small percentage of alcohol greatly retards the gradual oxidation which occurs when chloroform is exposed to air and light and which results in its becoming contaminated with the very poisonous carbonyl chloride (phosgene) and with chlorine; the alcohol also serves to decompose any carbonyl chloride that may have been formed.

Slightly **soluble** in water; miscible with dehydrated alcohol, ether, fixed and volatile oils, petroleum spirit, and most other organic solvents. **Store** at a temperature not exceeding 30° in airtight containers with glass stoppers or other suitable closures. Protect from light.

STABILITY. There was a loss of about 30% of chloroform from 2-litre samples of Chloroform Water and Double-strength Chloroform Water in bulk containers opened regularly during a study period of 28 days. Once the containers had been opened the contents should be used entirely or discarded within 10 days. Examination of smaller lots likely to be dispensed showed that there would be an acceptable amount of chloroform present for up to 14 days when patients opened their containers thrice daily. If the medicines were to be taken twice or once daily then this period would extend to 3 and 4 weeks respectively.— Pharm. Soc. Lab. Rep. P/75/11, 1975.

There was little loss of chloroform from non-sedimented mixtures stored in filled unopened bulk containers for more than 4 weeks. There could be a 10% reduction in chloroform content after 7 to 9 days if the containers were opened at regular intervals, and a 30 to 40% reduction after 28 days. In freshly prepared mixtures containing sediments the initial concentration of chloroform in the liquid phase was found to be considerably less than the theoretical concentrations, possibly due to sorption of chloroform by the insoluble powders. Further losses could be expected in regularly opened containers. Studies on the antimicrobial effectiveness of chloroform in aqueous mixtures and suspensions were required.— Pharm. Soc. Lab. Rep. P/75/25, 1975.

Chloroform 0.1 to 0.5% was an effective bactericide against small inocula of *Staphylococcus aureus, Escherichia coli,* and *Pseudomonas aeruginosa;* against large inocula chloroform 0.1% was effective against *Ps. aeruginosa,* but higher concentrations were needed against the other organisms. Spores of *Bacillus pumilus* were not killed. From a study of chloroform losses from chloroform water and from 6 typical *B.P.C.* mixtures under various conditions of storage the following shelf-lives were recommended: chloroform solutions and non-sedimented mixtures could be stored in well-closed well-filled containers for 2 months at ambient temperatures; when stored in partially-filled containers periodically opened the shelf-life should not exceed 2 weeks; sedimented mixtures could be stored for 2 months in well-closed well-filled containers, but because loss of chloroform could be expected in containers periodically opened such mixtures should be prepared as required or packed in their final containers; for chloroform-containing mixtures in the home a shelf-life of 2 weeks was suggested.— M. Lynch *et al., Pharm. J.*, 1977, *2*, 507.

Analysis of the chloroform content of dilute and concentrated chloroform solutions by ultraviolet spectrophotometry. On 4 occasions concentrations of chloroform were found to be below 85% of the theoretical concentration. These findings were confirmed by gas chromatography.— M. Silk (letter), *Pharm. J.*, 1986, *1*, 129.

STORAGE. The Pharmaceutical Society's Department of Pharmaceutical Sciences found that PVC bottles softened and distorted rapidly when filled with Chloroform and Morphine Tincture. Free chloroform produced softening, even in low concentrations; this was associated with loss by permeation. Alcoholic solutions of chloroform produced no physical effect. In Chloroform Water stored at room temperature migration of chloroform was slight in 4 weeks, increased after 7 weeks, and after 9 weeks the content of chloroform had fallen to less than 20%. PVC bottles should not be used for storing or dispensing Chloroform and Morphine Tincture, aqueous mixtures containing more than 5% thereof, mixtures or dispersions in which chloroform was present in excess of its aqueous solubility, aqueous mixtures containing chloroform and high concentrations of electrolytes, or Chloroform Water or mixtures containing it if the period of use would exceed 6 weeks.— *Pharm. J.*, 1973, *1*, 100.

Adverse Effects and Precautions

Chloroform is hepatotoxic and nephrotoxic. It depresses respiration and produces hypotension. Cardiac output is reduced and arrhythmias may develop. Poisoning leads to respiratory depression and cardiac arrest; it may take 6 to 24 hours after a dose before appearance of delayed symptoms characterised by abdominal pain, vomiting, and, at a later stage, jaundice.

Liquid chloroform is irritant to the skin and mucous membranes and may cause burns if spilt on them.

In the *UK* medicinal products are limited to a chloroform content of not more than 0.5% (w/w or v/v as appropriate) of chloroform. Exceptions include supply by a doctor or dentist, or in accordance with his prescription, to a particular patient, supply for external use, and supply for anaesthetic purposes.

In the *USA* the FDA have banned the use of chloroform in medicines and cosmetics, because of reported carcinogenicity in *animals*. It has also been withdrawn from systemic use in other countries.

The sale within or import into England and Wales and Scotland of food containing any added chloroform is prohibited.

In Great Britain the recommended exposure limits of chloroform are 10 ppm (long-term); 50 ppm (short-term). In the *US* the permissible and recommended exposure limits are 240 mg per m^3 and 9.78 mg per m^3 respectively.

See also Adverse Effects and Precautions for General Anaesthetics, p.1113.

A review of chloroform, its metabolism, and teratogenic, mutagenic, and carcinogenic potential.— I. W. F. Davidson *et al., Drug chem. Toxicol.*, 1982, *5*, 1.

PORPHYRIA. Chloroform was considered to be unsafe in patients with acute porphyria because it has been shown to be porphyrinogenic in *animals* or *in-vitro* systems.— M.R. Moore and K.E.L. McColl, *Porphyrias, Drug Lists*, Glasgow, Porphyria Research Unit, University of Glasgow, 1987.

Uses and Administration

Chloroform is an anaesthetic administered by inhalation. It possesses good analgesic and muscle relaxant properties. Because of its toxicity chloroform is seldom used as an anaesthetic and other safer agents are preferable.

Chloroform is used as a carminative and as a flavouring agent and preservative. For these purposes it is usually employed as Chloroform Spirit or Chloroform Water but doubts have been cast on the safety of the long-term use of chloroform in mixtures.

Externally, chloroform has a rubefacient action. Chloroform is also used as a solvent.

A historical review of the use of chloroform in clinical anaesthesia.— J. P. Payne, *Br. J. Anaesth.*, 1981, *53*, 11S.

Preparations

Chloroform Spirit *(B.P.).* Chloroform 5% v/v in alcohol (90%).

Chloroform Water *(B.P.).* Chloroform 0.25% v/v in freshly boiled and cooled water.

Double-Strength Chloroform Water *(B.P.).* Chloroform 0.5% v/v in freshly boiled and cooled water.

Chloroform and Morphine Tincture is described on p.1313.

3105-n

Cyclopropane *(BAN, USAN, rINN).*

Trimethylene.
C_3H_6=42.08.

CAS — 75-19-4.

Pharmacopoeias. In *Arg., Aust., Br., Braz., Cz., Egypt., Ind., It., Mex., Nord., Rus., Turk.*, and *U.S.*

A colourless flammable gas with a characteristic odour and pungent taste supplied compressed in metal cylinders.

Very **soluble** in alcohol, chloroform, and ether; soluble in fixed oils; 1 vol. measured at 101.3 kPa and 0° dissolves in 2.85 vol. of water.

Store in metal cylinders in a special room which should be cool and free from flammable materials. The cylinder should be painted orange; the name or chemical symbol of the gas should be stencilled in paint on the shoulder of the cylinder and clearly and indelibly stamped on the cylinder valve.

CAUTION. *Mixtures of cyclopropane with oxygen or air at certain concentrations are explosive. Cyclopropane should not be used in the presence of an open flame or of any electrical apparatus liable to produce a spark. Precautions should be taken against the production of static electrical discharge.*

The incompatibility of cyclopropane with flexible plastic or rubber tubing.— A. Bracken (letter), *Br. J. Anaesth.*, 1976, *48*, 52. See also J. E. MacKenzie (letter), *Pharm. J.*, 1977, *1*, 38.

Adverse Effects

Cyclopropane depresses respiration to a greater extent than many other anaesthetic agents. It may cause bronchospasm under light anaesthesia; laryngospasm may occur. Cardiac arrhythmias, particularly associated with hypercapnia, may occur. Cyclopropane increases the sensitivity of the heart to sympathomimetic amines. Tachycardia gives warning of overdosage.

Postoperative nausea and vomiting are frequent although less severe than with ether. Severe postoperative fall in blood pressure occasionally occurs. Postoperative headache is more common than with other anaesthetics. Cyclopropane has a tendency to increase haemorrhage.

Blood flow to the kidney and liver may be impaired during cyclopropane anaesthesia. Liver necrosis has been reported.

See also Adverse Effects for General Anaesthetics, p.1113.

Over 800 000 anaesthetic administrations were analysed during a 4-year period in the USA in the National Halothane Study. About 147 000 of the procedures involved the use of cyclopropane which was found to be associated with the highest rate of massive hepatic necrosis and the highest crude mortality-rate when compared with halothane, ether, nitrous oxide with barbiturates, and combinations of these anaesthetics.— *J. Am. med. Ass.*, 1966, *197*, 775.

For a report of deaths associated with the abuse of cyclopropane, see p.1118.

MALIGNANT HYPERPYREXIA. One case of malignant hyperpyrexia associated with cyclopropane.— F. J. Lips *et al.*, *Anesthesiology*, 1982, *56*, 144.

Treatment of Adverse Effects

As for Halothane, p.1118.

Precautions

Cyclopropane should be used with caution in patients with bronchial asthma and cardiovascular disorders.

Pre-operation sedation with respiratory depressants should be used with caution. Adrenaline and most other sympathomimetic agents should not be used during cyclopropane anaesthesia. As with halothane (p.1118) routine premedication with atropine may be advisable to reduce vagal tone. The effects of competitive muscle relaxants are enhanced and they should be used in reduced doses.

See also Precautions for General Anaesthetics, p.1113.

Uses and Administration

Cyclopropane is an anaesthetic administered by inhalation. It has a minimum alveolar concentration (MAC) value (see p.1113) of 9.2%. It is non-irritant and induction and recovery are rapid. Because of the risk of explosion, the usual method of administration is by means of a closed circuit.

A review of the actions and uses of the long established anaesthetic agents including cyclopropane.— J. V. Farman, *Br. J. Anaesth.*, 1981, *53*, 3S.

3106-h

Enflurane *(BAN, USAN, rINN)*.

Compound 347; Methylflurether; NSC-115944.

2-Chloro-1,1,2-trifluoroethyl difluoromethyl ether; 2-Chloro-1-(difluoromethoxy)-1,1,2-trifluoroethane.

$C_3H_2ClF_5O$=184.5.

CAS — 13838-16-9.

Pharmacopoeias. In *U.S.*

A clear colourless volatile liquid with a mild sweet odour. Not flammable. B.p. 55.5° to 57.5°. Slightly **soluble** in water; miscible with organic solvents, fats, and oils. **Store** at a temperature not exceeding 40° in airtight containers. Protect from light.

Adverse Effects and Treatment

Enflurane has similar adverse effects to those of halothane (p.1118) except that it has a stimulant effect on the CNS and that the increased sensitivity to beta-adrenergic activity is less. Malignant hyperpyrexia has been reported. There have also been a number of reports of liver damage (see below). Convulsions have occurred. Asthma and bronchospasm have been reported. There have been reports of elevated serum-fluoride concentrations but renal damage appears to be rare. There have been changes in measurements of hepatic enzymes.

See also Adverse Effects for General Anaesthetics, p.1113.

ABUSE. Report of a fatality in a 29-year-old student nurse anaesthetist who had applied enflurane to the herpes simplex lesions of her lower lip. She was found with an empty 250 mL bottle of enflurane.— R. W. Lingenfelter (letter), *Anesthesiology*, 1981, *55*, 603.

ASTHMA. Acute asthma in an anaesthetist on 6 occasions 8 to 12 hours after administering enflurane.— R. S. Schwettmann and C. L. Casterline, *Anesthesiology*, 1976, *44*, 166.

EFFECTS ON THE CARDIOVASCULAR SYSTEM. A study of cardiac arrhythmias during outpatient dental anaesthesia with halothane or enflurane in 75 young female patients. Enflurane induced a much lower frequency of arrhythmia during surgery than halothane, although many arrhythmias occurred before exposure of the patient to anaesthetic agents.— D. G. Willatts *et al.*, *Br. J. Anaesth.*, 1983, *55*, 399. A similar incidence of arrhythmias in patients receiving halothane and nitrous oxide with oxygen or enflurane and nitrous oxide with oxygen in 56 patients undergoing elective laparoscopy.— M. N. E. Harris *et al.*, *ibid.*, 1213. No significant difference in the overall incidence of cardiac arrhythmias was observed between enflurane and halothane in 49 children undergoing dental surgery.— R. M. Haden, *Br. dent. J.*, 1985, *158*, 23.

A study of 11 patients with severe generalised atherosclerotic disease showed that enflurane was a powerful coronary vasodilator and in this respect slightly less potent than isoflurane. Enflurane may produce regional myocardial ischaemia by redistributing coronary blood flow and/or by inducing hypotension.— A. Rydvall *et al.*, *Acta anaesth. scand.*, 1984, *28*, 690.

EFFECTS ON THE KIDNEY. A review of the nephrotoxicity of volatile anaesthetic agents. Although enflurane released inorganic fluoride it appeared to be safe in patients with normal renal function. It had also been given to patients with mild to moderate renal impairment without any further deterioration. There was an increase in serum-fluoride concentrations when enflurane was administered to a group of patients who had been receiving isoniazid, but there was no change in kidney function.— R. I. Mazze, *Clin. Anaesth.*, 1983, *1*, 469.

EFFECTS ON THE LIVER. A review of enflurane hepatotoxicity. Fifty-eight cases of suspected enflurane hepatitis had been traced, 10 published and 48 reported to *US* organisations. Of these 58 patients, 34 were excluded from the review because other factors could have been involved; the review was therefore of 7 previously published and 17 unpublished reports where enflurane was considered to be the likely cause of the liver damage.

Nine of the patients had been previously exposed to enflurane and 7 to halothane. Only 2 patients had developed pyrexia and eosinophilia after their previous exposure (to halothane in both cases). Three patients experienced renal failure in conjunction with their enflurane-induced liver damage. There was biochemical evidence of liver damage in 23 cases. Histology reports were available for 15 patients and all showed some degree of hepatocellular necrosis and degeneration. Five patients died.

While the incidence of liver damage from enflurane seemed to be lower than from halothane, the character of the injury and presumably its mechanism were similar. Because of cross-sensitivity it was recommended that enflurane should not be administered to patients who had developed evidence of hypersensitivity or hepatic injury after previous exposure to any of the haloalkane anaesthetics.— J. H. Lewis *et al.*, *Ann. intern. Med.*, 1983, *98*, 984. Another review of the same cases plus an additional 30 (88 in all) came to different conclusions. Of the 88 patients with suspected enflurane hepatitis, 30 were rejected because of insufficient evidence and 43 were considered to have other factors known to produce liver injury. This left 15 possible cases of enflurane hepatitis compared with the 24 identified by Lewis *et al.* While agreeing that in the rare patient unexplained liver damage follows enflurane anaesthesia, it was considered that the incidence was too small to suggest an association. No consistent histological pattern was identified in this study E. I. Eger *et al.*, *Anesth. Analg.*, 1986, *65*, 21.

EFFECTS ON THE NERVOUS SYSTEM. Seizure activity in 2 patients 6 and 8 days after enflurane anaesthesia. Neither patient had seizures prior to or during anaesthesia.— W. W. Ohm *et al.*, *Anesthesiology*, 1975, *42*, 367.

See also M. Kruczek *et al.*, *Anesthesiology*, 1980, *53*, 175.

Precautions

Enflurane should be used with caution in patients with convulsive disorders. Care is also required if adrenaline and other sympathomimetic agents are given to patients during enflurane anaesthesia. The effects of competitive muscle relaxants are enhanced. High concentrations may cause uterine relaxation.

As with halothane patients who are known or suspected to be susceptible to malignant hyperpyrexia should not be anaesthetised with enflurane.

There have been reports of liver damage with enflurane; their numbers are not as great as with halothane, but the nature of the damage appears to be similar. There are no authoritative warnings as with halothane, although there have been individual calls for caution, see above under Effects on the Liver in Adverse Effects.

See also Precautions for General Anaesthetics, p.1113.

INTERACTIONS. It appeared likely that the enflurane-induced seizure activity observed in 2 patients could have been enhanced by amitriptyline. It may be advisable to avoid the use of enflurane in patients requiring tricyclic antidepressants, especially when the patient has a history of seizures or when hyperventilation or high enflurane concentrations are a desired part of the anaesthetic technique.— D. H. Sprague and S. Wolf, *Anesth. Analg.*, 1982, *61*, 67.

Isoniazid pretreatment enhanced enflurane defluorination in 9 of 20 subjects studied. In some cases this leads to an increased serum-fluoride concentration which may have nephrotoxic potential.— M. J. Halsey, *Br. J. Anaesth.*, 1987, *59*, 112 (See also under Effects on the Kidney in Adverse Effects).

A retrospective study of nalbuphine as a supplement to isoflurane and enflurane in balanced anaesthesia in 108 surgical patients. Nalbuphine appeared to reduce halogenated anaesthetic requirements by approximately 50%.— E. M. Hew *et al.*, *Curr. med. Res. Opinion*, 1987, *10*, 531.

For reports of enflurane enhancing or prolonging the activity of muscle relaxants, see p.1120.

PORPHYRIA. Enflurane was considered to be unsafe in patients with acute porphyria because it has been shown to be porphyrinogenic in *animals* or *in vitro* systems.— M.R. Moore and K.E.L. McColl, *Porphyrias, Drug Lists*, Glasgow, Porphyria Research Unit, University of Glasgow, 1987.

Absorption and Fate

Enflurane is absorbed on inhalation. The blood/gas coefficient is low. It is mostly excreted unchanged through the lungs. That which is metabolised produces inorganic fluoride.

A review of the pharmacokinetics of inhalational anaesthetics including enflurane.— O. Dale and B. R. Brown, *Clin. Pharmacokinet.*, 1987, *12*, 145.

Uses and Administration

Enflurane is a volatile anaesthetic administered by inhalation. It has anaesthetic actions similar to those of halothane (see p.1119). Enflurane has a minimum alveolar concentration (MAC) value (see p.1113) of about 1.7%. Available figures for variations with age show children having a value of 2.4 to 2.5% and young adults a value of 1.9%. MAC values also increase as body temperature increases.

It is administered using a vaporiser to achieve control of the concentration of inhaled vapour. To avoid excitement a short-acting barbiturate or other intravenous induction agent is recommended before the inhalation of enflurane; anaesthesia is induced starting at an enflurane concentration of 0.4% v/v and increasing by increments of 0.5% v/v every few breaths. Anaesthesia may be maintained with a concentration of 0.5 to 3.5% v/v of enflurane given with nitrous oxide; a concentration of 3.0% v/v should not be exceeded during spontaneous respiration. Although enflurane is reported to possess muscle relaxant properties, muscle relaxants may be required. Postoperative analgesia may be necessary.

A review of the actions and uses of enflurane in clinical practice.— A. P. Adams, *Br. J. Anaesth.*, 1981, *53*, 27S.

A comparative review of enflurane, halothane, and isoflurane.— R. M. Jones, *Br. J. Anaesth.*, 1984, *56*, 57S.

Halothane and enflurane each in combination with nitrous oxide and oxygen were compared in 103 adults undergoing tonsillectomy. Anaesthesia was induced with thiopentone, and intubation was facilitated with suxamethonium. Both inhalation anaesthetics were found to be suitable for tonsillectomy but significantly more ECG changes were noted during halothane anaesthesia.— L. Saarnivaara, *Acta anaesth. scand.*, 1984, *28*, 319.

Some further references: W. A. Allen, *Br. dent. J.*, 1981, *151*, 51 (dental surgery); S. Firn, *J. R. Soc. Med.*, 1982, *75*, *Suppl.* 1, 36 (analgesia for burn dressing) *idem, Postgrad. med. J.*, 1983, *59*, 608 (controlled hypotension).

OPHTHALMIC SURGERY. It was concluded from a study in 20 patients that enflurane 1% decreased intra-ocular pressure significantly and could be used in ophthalmic anaesthesia instead of halothane which, in this study, failed to alter mean intra-ocular pressure significantly and produced varying effects in individual patients.— J. C. Runciman *et al.*, *Br. J. Anaesth.*, 1978, *50*, 371.

See also G. Zindel *et al.*, *Br. J. Anaesth.*, 1987, *59*, 440.

PHAEOCHROMOCYTOMA. Enflurane has been used successfully to anaesthetise patients with phaeochromocy-toma.—C. J. Hull, *Br. J. Anaesth*, 1986, *58*, 1453.

PREGNANCY AND THE NEONATE. Amnesia, absence of foetal depression, and absence of excessive bleeding in 50 women given enflurane for caesarean section.— A. J. Coleman and J. W. Downing, *Anesthesiology*, 1975, *43*, 354.

Proprietary Preparations

Enflurane *(Abbott, UK)*. *Anaesthetic inhalation*, enflurane.

Proprietary Names and Manufacturers

Alyrane *(Anaquest, UK)*; Efrane *(Abbott, Denm.*; *Abbott, Norw.*; *Abbott, Swed.)*; Ethrane *(Abbott, Austral.*; *Belg.*; *Anaquest, Canad.*; *Abbott, Ger.*; *Abbott, Ital.*; *Neth.*; *Abbott, S.Afr.*; *Abbott, Spain*; *Switz.*; *Abbott, UK)*; Inhelthran *(Arg.)*.

3107-m

Anaesthetic Ether *(BAN, USAN)*.

Aether ad Narcosin; Aether Anaestheticus; Ȧether pro Narcosi; Aether Purissimus; Diethyl Ether; Êter Puríssimo; Ether; Ether Anesthesicus.

$(C_2H_5)_2O$=74.12.

CAS — 60-29-7.

Pharmacopoeias. In *Arg.*, *Aust.*, *Belg.*, *Br.*, *Braz.*, *Chin.*, *Cz.*, *Egypt.*, *Eur.*, *Fr.*, *Ger.*, *Hung.*, *Ind.*, *Int.*, *It.*, *Jpn*, *Jug.*, *Mex.*, *Neth.*, *Nord.*, *Pol.*, *Port.*, *Roum.*, *Rus.*, *Span.*, *Swiss*, *Turk.*, and *U.S.* Also in *B.P. Vet.*

Diethyl ether to which an appropriate quantity of a non-volatile antioxidant may have been added. It contains not more than 0.2% of water. Ether *U.S.P.* contains 96 to 98% of $(C_2H_5)_2O$, the remainder consisting of alcohol and water. It is slowly oxidised by the action of air and light, with the formation of peroxides. A clear, colourless, volatile, highly flammable, and very mobile liquid with a characteristic odour. B.p. 34° to 35°.

Soluble 1 in 12 to 15 of water; miscible with alcohol, chloroform, petroleum spirit, and fixed and volatile oils. **Store** at a temperature not exceeding 15° in dry airtight containers. Protect from light. Ether remaining in a partly used container may deteriorate rapidly.

CAUTION. *Ether is very volatile and flammable and mixtures of its vapour with oxygen, nitrous oxide, or air at certain concentrations are explosive. It should not be used in the presence of an open flame or any electrical apparatus liable to produce a spark. Precautions should be taken against the production of static electrical discharge.*

The Pharmaceutical Society's Department of Pharmaceutical Sciences found that free ether, even in low concentrations, caused softening of PVC bottles and was associated with loss by permeation.— *Pharm. J.*, 1973, *1*, 100.

Adverse Effects

Ether has an irritant action on the mucous membrane of the respiratory tract; it stimulates salivation and increases bronchial secretion. Laryngeal spasm may occur. Ether causes vasodilatation which may lead to a severe fall in blood pressure and it reduces blood flow to the kidneys; it also increases capillary bleeding. The bleeding time is unchanged but the prothrombin time may be prolonged. Ether may cause malignant hyperpyrexia in certain individuals. Alterations in kidney and liver function have been reported.

Convulsions occasionally occur in children or young adults under deep ether anaesthesia.

Recovery is slow from prolonged ether anaesthesia and postoperative vomiting commonly occurs. Acute overdosage of ether is characterised by respiratory failure and cardiac arrest.

Dependence on ether or ether vapour has been reported. Prolonged contact with ether spilt on any tissue produces necrosis.

In Great Britain the recommended exposure limits of ether are 400 ppm (long-term); 500 ppm (short-term).

See also Adverse Effects for General Anaesthetics, p.1113.

Precautions

Ether anaesthesia is contra-indicated in patients with diabetes mellitus, impaired kidney function, and severe liver disease. Its use is not advisable in hot and humid conditions for patients with fever as convulsions are liable to occur, particularly in children and in patients who have been given atropine.

Ether enhances the action of competitive muscle relaxants to a greater degree than most other anaesthetics. See also Precautions for General Anaesthetics, p.1113.

Uses and Administration

Ether is an anaesthetic administered by inhalation. Ether has a minimum alveolar concentration (MAC) value (see p.1113) of 1.92% and was one of the first successful anaesthetic agents, but has generally been replaced by the halogenated anaesthetic agents. It possesses a respiratory stimulant effect in all but the deepest planes of anaesthesia. Ether also possesses analgesic and muscle relaxant properties.

Premedication with atropine is usually required to inhibit troublesome bronchial and salivary secretions.

Solvent ether is described on p.1427.

A review of the actions and uses of the long established anaesthetic agents, including ether.— J. V. Farman, *Br. J. Anaesth.*, 1981, *53*, 3S.

ASTHMA. In 2 patients with acute severe asthma, administration of ether by inhalation resulted in prompt bronchodilatation with improvement in arterial blood gases and clinical condition. They had failed to respond to conventional treatment, mechanical ventilation, and halothane. No adverse cardiac effects were observed.— C. E. Robertson *et al.*, *Lancet*, 1985, *1*, 187. A change of strategy for the treatment of severe asthma. The strategy had included deep anaesthesia with ether or halothane when conventional ventilator therapy had failed. High-level positive end-expiratory pressure is now chosen when inhalation anaesthesia and intravenous bronchodilator therapy fail.— J. Qvist *et al.* (letter), *New Engl. J. Med.*, 1982, *307*, 1347.

SOLVENT FOR GALL-STONES. A report that ether injections have proved effective in the treatment of 41 of 42 patients with gall-stones. Ether was injected into the gall-bladder via a fine catheter for 5 to 10 minutes and then aspirated. The process was repeated over a period ranging from 3 hours to a few days. The patient who failed to respond to treatment had gall-stones containing an unusually high proportion of calcium, which is insoluble in ether. Because delayed side-effects may occur, this treatment was reserved for patients over 60 with heart disease who were not able to receive general anaesthesia.— *Practitioner*, 1987, *231*, 933. Earlier reports had involved the additional use of papaverine.— C. L. N. Robinson, *Can. med. Ass. J.*, 1966, *95*, 1205. and *idem*, 1967, *96*, 163.

3110-r

Etomidate *(BAN, USAN, rINN)*.

R-16659; R-26490 *(sulphate)*. *R*-(+)-Ethyl 1-(α-methylbenzyl)imidazole-5-carboxylate.

$C_{14}H_{16}N_2O_2$=244.3.

CAS — 33125-97-2.

Adverse Effects and Precautions

Coughing, hiccup, excitement, and convulsions may occur in patients who have not received premedication. Apnoea has been reported. Laryngospasm is rare; skin rash has occasionally occurred. Nausea and vomiting may occur postoperatively.

Involuntary myoclonic muscle movements, sometimes severe, are common, but may be reduced by the prior administration of an opioid analgesic. Pain on injection may be reduced by giving the injection into a large vein in the arm, rather than into the hand.

Etomidate suppresses adrenocortical function (see below) and should not be used in patients with adrenocortical function already reduced or at risk of being reduced.

See also Adverse Effects and Precautions for General Anaesthetics, p.1113.

A review of the toxicity of intravenous anaesthetics including etomidate.— J. W. Sear, *Br. J. Anaesth.*, 1987, *59*, 24.

A randomised comparison in 120 patients of the effects of etomidate 300 µg per kg body-weight and thiopentone 3.5 mg per kg. Pain on injection occurred in 43.3 and 1.7% of patients respectively, with 5 and 3 patients experiencing thrombophlebitis. [The solvent for etomidate was not specified.] Myoclonic movements occurred in 28% of those given etomidate and were severe in about a third; in several they resembled generalised convulsive seizures but no epileptiform discharges were seen in the EEGs of 10 patients studied. There were no myoclonic movements after thiopentone. Seven patients developed tonic movements after etomidate and one after thiopentone. Apnoea occurred in 8 given etomidate and 25 given thiopentone. There was a slight initial reduction in respiration-rate after etomidate, followed by an increase, compared with a greater initial reduction after thiopentone. There were no significant differences between etomidate and thiopentone in respect of slight increases in pulse-rate and slight reductions in blood pressure. No arrhythmias were seen.— M. M. Ghoneim and T. Yamada, *Anesth. Analg. curr. Res.*, 1977, *56*, 479.

A study of etomidate versus thiopentone for induction of anaesthesia. Induction with 0.4 mg per kg body-weight etomidate was found to be associated with a lesser incidence of apnoea, and a greater incidence of myoclonus and pain on injection.— J. L. Giese *et al.*, *Ancsth. Analg.*, 1985, *64*, 871.

ALLERGY. From the introduction of etomidate in 1978 until 1982, after about 3 000 000 induction doses, there were no convincing reports of anaphylactoid reactions to etomidate. Five possible reactions involving immediate widespread cutaneous flushing or urticaria, followed in 2 cases by extensive peri-operative vomiting were investigated. No plasma-protein involvement was detected. This clinical pattern may be typical of etomidate reactions. Two further cases involving anaphylactoid response with hypotension were studied. Etomidate had been used with suxamethonium and/or alcuronium; these were suggestive of neuromuscular blocking drug involvement rather than etomidate.— J. Watkins, *Anaesthesia*, 1983, *38*, *Suppl.*, 34.

A life-threatening anaphylactoid reaction following induction of anaesthesia with etomidate; the patient recovered following dechallenge and intensive treatment. Skin tests confirmed that etomidate was the agent responsible for the adverse reaction.— M. Sold and A. Rothhammer, *Anaesthesist*, 1985, *34*, 208. A similar report.— W. Krumholz *et al.*, *ibid.*, 1984, *33*, 161.

EFFECTS ON BLOOD AND THE CARDIOVASCULAR SYSTEM. In 14 patients given etomidate 200 µg per kg body-weight intravenously, anaesthesia was induced in 10 seconds and lasted for 6 to 8 minutes. There was a slight reduction (8.5%) in mean arterial pressure, a negligible increase (2.8%) in heart-rate, and no significant effect on the mean pulmonary artery pressure. Cardiac output and stroke volume were lowered by 7.6 and 10% respectively and peripheral vascular resistance was lowered by 3.8%.— K. Rifat *et al.*, *Can. Anaesth. Soc. J.*, 1976, *23*, 492.

In a study in 500 patients the frequency of phlebitis, thrombosis, and thrombophlebitis following intravenous administration of etomidate was governed by injection formulation and dose used and was not related to pain on injection. The frequency was greatest (23.1%) with the propylene glycol formulation compared with 10.8% for the aqueous formulation and 7.7% for the macrogol formulation.— M. Zacharias *et al.*, *Br. J. Anaesth.*, 1979, *51*, 779.

Myocardial infarction and asystole reported in a 42-year-old male and 55-year-old female respectively, following induction and maintenance with intravenous etomidate-fentanyl-oxygen anaesthesia. It was suggested that the adverse effects may be due to the propylene glycol diluent.— A. W. van den Hurk and H. J. Teijen, *Anaesthesia*, 1983, *38*, 1183.

Thrombophlebitis developed in 8 of 33 patients (24%) after the intravenous administration of etomidate injection (containing propylene glycol 35%) compared with only 1 of 28 patients (4%) given thiopentone. Pain on injection was experienced by 8 patients given etomidate but none of those given thiopentone.— A. S. Olesen *et al.*, *Br. J. Anaesth.*, 1984, *56*, 171.

EFFECTS ON THE ENDOCRINE SYSTEM. Ledingham and Watt published a warning (*Lancet*, 1983, *1*, 1270) that etomidate used for sedation in an intensive care unit was implicated in an increase in mortality. The *UK* Committee on Safety of Medicines agreed that etomidate could cause a significant fall in circulating plasma-cortisol concentrations, unresponsive to corticotrophin stimulation (*Lancet*, 1983, *2*, 60). The action of etomidate on cortisol production is complex (J.W. Sear, *Br. J. Anaesth.*, 1987, *59*, 24), with different activities following bolus injection and prolonged infusions. As a result of this effect use of etomidate is restricted to induction of anaesthesia and the manufacturers advise that the postoperative rise in serum-cortisol concentration which has been observed after thiopentone induction is delayed for about 3 to 6 hours with etomidate.

EFFECTS ON THE NERVOUS SYSTEM. Epileptiform movements in four patients after variable periods of etomidate infusion. It was virtually impossible to avoid troublesome involuntary movements during etomidate administration without the simultaneous use of substantial doses of opioid or other sedative drugs.— I. S. Grant and G. Hutchison (letter), *Lancet*, 1983, *2*, 511.

A report of prolonged myoclonus in a 75-year-old man following induction of anaesthesia with etomidate and fentanyl and maintenance with etomidate and nitrous oxide with oxygen.— T. P. Laughlin and L. A. Newberg, *Anesth. Analg.*, 1985, *64*, 80.

Generalised epileptiform EEG activity was recorded in approximately 20% of more than 30 patients following etomidate induction.— W. Krieger *et al.* (letter), *Anesth. Analg.*, 1985, *64*, 1226.

EFFECTS ON THE RESPIRATORY SYSTEM. In 30 patients premedicated with diazepam and atropine apnoea lasting for about 30 seconds occurred in 12 after receiving etomidate (as sulphate) 300 µg per kg body-weight; 8 of 30 given papaveretum and hyoscine as premedication became apnoeic. The respiratory-rate was significantly increased in the diazepam group but not in the papaveretum group; there was a transient depression of minute volume in the papaveretum group.— M. Morgan *et al.*, *Br. J. Anaesth.*, 1977, *49*, 233.

PORPHYRIA. Etomidate was considered to be unsafe in patients with acute porphyria because it has been shown to be porphyrinogenic in *animals* or *in vitro* systems.— M.R. Moore and K.E.L. McColl, *Porphyrias, Drug Lists*, Glasgow, Porphyria Research Unit, University of Glasgow, 1987.

Absorption and Fate

After injection, etomidate is rapidly redistributed to other body tissues, and undergoes rapid metabolism. Plasma decay is complex and has been described by a 2- and a 3-compartment model. Etomidate is extensively (about 76%) bound to plasma protein. It is mainly excreted in the urine, but some is excreted in the bile.

A review of the pharmacokinetics and pharmacodynamics of intravenous anaesthetic agents including etomidate.— B. N. Swerdlow and F. O. Holley, *Clin. Pharmacokinet.*, 1987, *12*, 79. See also P. J. Davis and D. R. Cook, *ibid.*, 1986, *11*, 18.

Uses and Administration

Etomidate is administered intravenously as the base or the hydrochloride for the induction of anaesthesia; it is not now used for maintenance. The sulphate has been employed in some studies. Etomidate has no analgesic activity. Anaesthesia is rapidly induced and may last for 6 to 10 minutes with a single usual dose.

The usual dose is 300 µg of etomidate per kg body-weight given slowly, preferably into a large vein in the arm. Opioid analgesics as premedication reduce myoclonic movements. A muscle relaxant is necessary if intubation is required.

Reviews of the actions and uses of etomidate: *Lancet*, 1983, *2*, 24; J. L. Giese and T. H. Stanley, *Pharmacotherapy*, 1983, *3*, 251.

Results of a study in 10 patients with intracranial lesions requiring craniotomy indicated that etomidate could be used for the induction of anaesthesia in patients with intracranial space-occupying lesions without increasing intracranial pressure or seriously reducing cerebral perfusion pressure.— E. Moss *et al.*, *Br. J. Anaesth.*, 1979, *51*, 347. Etomidate was shown to be effective in the treatment of increased intracranial pressure following severe head injury in a double-blind study in 5 patients. Etomidate was given at an initial infusion rate of 50 µg per kg body-weight per minute for 10 minutes, followed by 20 to 40 µg per kg per minute.— N. M. Dearden and D. G. McDowall, *Br. J. Anaesth.*, 1985, *57*, 361.

Rectal administration of etomidate 1.25% in sterile water to 40 children produced a rapid, predictable onset of hypnosis within 4 minutes and allowed rapid recovery. The doses given ranged from 3 mg per kg body-weight to 6.5 mg per kg. This method of administration was considered suitable for outpatient anaesthesia in unpremedicated children who are unsuitable for inhalational or intravenous induction.—D. M. Linton and R. E. Thornington, *S. Afr. med. J.*, 1983, *64*, 309.

The use of etomidate to activate the seizure focus in patients undergoing temporal lobectomy for the treatment of medically refractory complex partial seizures.— W. Krieger *et al.* (letter), *Anesth. Analg.*, 1985, *64*, 1226.

Beneficial effect of etomidate on hypercortisolism in a 53-year-old man. Continuous infusion of etomidate (125 mg/mL alcoholic solution) 15 to 30 mg per hour reduced cortisol and ACTH levels, although the levels of the latter were not reduced to normal values.— R. Gärtner *et al.* (letter), *Lancet*, 1986, *1*, 275.

In 50 patients in whom anaesthesia was induced by either etomidate 0.3 mg per kg body-weight or thiopentone 4 to 5 mg per kg, intra-ocular pressure was reduced by a significantly greater degree by etomidate compared with thiopentone.— S. Calla *et al.*, *Br. J. Anaesth.*, 1987, *59*, 437. See also C. E. Famewo and C. O. Odugbesan, *Can. Anaesth. Soc. J.*, 1978, *25*, 130.

GYNAECOLOGICAL PROCEDURES. A comparison between etomidate, alphaxalone with alphadolone, and methohexitone as induction agents in 100 unpremedicated patients undergoing short gynaecological procedures. Satisfactory operating conditions were not obtained using etomidate alone (0.3 mg per kg body-weight). Administration of methohexitone (1.5 mg per kg) resulted in a more rapid initial awakening than alphaxalone with alphadolone; the addition of fentanyl (100 µg) did not significantly prolong recovery from either anaesthetic. Etomidate with fentanyl was associated with the greatest frequency of complications.— J. Craig *et al.*, *Br. J. Anaesth.*, 1982, *54*, 447.

Forty-four patients undergoing evacuation of retained products of conception were anaesthetized with either etomidate with alfentanil, or thiopentone with fentanyl, along with 70% nitrous oxide in oxygen. Alfentanil 10 µg per kg body-weight was immediately followed by an induction dose of etomidate 20 mg mixed with 1 mL of 2% lignocaine to minimize pain on injection. Fentanyl 1 µg per kg was followed after 2 minutes by induction with thiopentone. There was no difference between the two techniques in indices of immediate recovery, but the rate of return of higher mental functions was significantly better using the etomidate-alfentanil technique. This regime was associated with significantly more pain on injection and a higher frequency of postoperative vomiting.— I. G. Kestin and P. Dorje, *Br. J. Anaesth.*, 1987, *59*, 364.

PREGNANCY AND THE NEONATE. In a study in 60 women undergoing caesarean section etomidate 300 µg per kg body-weight or thiopentone 3.5 mg per kg body-weight was used for induction of anaesthesia. The clinical status of the newborn was considered superior with etomidate.— J. W. Downing *et al.*, *Br. J. Anaesth.*, 1979, *51*, 135. A similar report.— P. J. C. Houlton *et al.*, *S. Afr. med. J.*, 1978, *54*, 773.

Proprietary Preparations

Hypnomidate *(Janssen, UK). Injection*, etomidate 2 mg/mL, in a vehicle containing propylene glycol 35%, in ampoules of 10 mL.
Concentrate for intravenous infusion, etomidate 125 mg (as hydrochloride)/mL, in ampoules of 1 mL. Dilute with at least 50 mL infusion fluid before use.

Proprietary Names and Manufacturers

Amidate *(Abbott, USA)*; Hypnomidat *(Janssen, Denm.)*; Hypnomidate *(Aust.; Belg.; Janssen, Ger.; Neth.; Janssen, S.Afr.; Janssen, Switz.; Janssen, UK)*; Sibul *(Esteve, Spain)*.

3111-f

Fluroxene *(USAN, pINN)*.

(2,2,2-Trifluoroethoxy)ethylene; 2,2,2-Trifluoroethyl vinyl ether.
$C_4H_5F_3O$=126.1.

CAS — 406-90-6.

CAUTION. *Fluroxene is very volatile and flammable and mixtures of its vapour with oxygen or air at certain concentrations are explosive. It should not be used in the presence of an open flame or any electrical apparatus liable to produce a spark. Precautions should be taken against the production of static electrical discharge.*

Adverse Effects and Precautions

Fluroxene depresses the myocardium but the effect may be masked by concomitant sympathetic stimulation; it does not appear to sensitise the myocardium to the effects of catecholamines. As the depth of anaesthesia is increased there is respiratory depression and a fall in arterial pressure. Postoperative nausea and vomiting are common following prolonged deep anaesthesia. *Animal* studies indicate a high level of toxicity. There have been several reports of hepatotoxicity in patients receiving fluroxene.

See also Adverse Effects for General Anaesthetics, p.1113.

PORPHYRIA. Fluroxene was considered to be unsafe in patients with acute porphyria because it has been shown to be porphyrinogenic in *animals* or *in vitro* systems.— M.R. Moore and K.E.L. McColl, *Porphyrias, Drug Lists*, Glasgow, Porphyria Research Unit, University of Glasgow, 1987.

Uses and Administration

Fluroxene has been used as an inhalational anaesthetic; it has been superseded by other agents. It possesses good analgesic but poor muscle relaxant properties and is less flammable than ether.

3101-x

Halothane *(BAN, USAN, rINN)*.

Alotano; Halothanum; Phthorothanum. (*RS*)-2-Bromo-2-chloro-1,1,1-trifluoroethane.
$CHBrCl.CF_3$=197.4.

CAS — 151-67-7.

Pharmacopoeias. In *Aust., Br., Braz., Chin., Cz., Egypt., Eur., Fr., Ger., Int., It., Jpn, Jug., Neth., Nord., Rus., Swiss,* and *U.S.*

A clear, colourless, mobile, dense, non-flammable liquid with a characteristic chloroform-like odour. It contains 0.01% w/w of thymol as a preservative. Distillation range 49° to 51°.

Slightly **soluble** 1 in 400 of water; miscible with dehydrated alcohol, chloroform, ether, trichloroethylene, and fixed oils. Halothane is soluble in rubber. In the presence of moisture it reacts with many metals. **Store** at a temperature of 8° to 15° in airtight containers. Protect from light.

An isolated report of explosion during halothane anaesthesia. Providing the necessary static discharge was produced it appeared that an explosion with halothane could occur.— T. W. May, *Br. med. J.*, 1976, *1*, 692.

The diffusion of halothane through rubber and plastic tubes.— D. H. Enderby *et al.*, *Br. J. Anaesth.*, 1977, *49*, 561.

The adsorption of halothane by 4 different grades of charcoal.— D. H. Enderby *et al.*, *Br. J. Anaesth.*, 1977, *49*, 567.

Adverse Effects

Halothane has a depressant action on the cardiovascular system and reduces blood pressure; signs of overdosage are bradycardia and profound hypotension. It can produce nausea, vomiting and shivering. Cardiac arrhythmias and respiratory depression may occur. Halothane increases the sensitivity of the heart to beta-adrenergic activity.

Hepatic dysfunction, hepatitis, and necrosis have been reported following the use of halothane and have been reported to be more frequent following repeated use (see below). Malignant hyperpyrexia has been reported.

See also Adverse Effects for General Anaesthetics, p.1113.

ABUSE. A review of 16 reported cases of abuse of modern volatile anaesthetics. Halothane was ingested or injected intravenously for suicidal purposes, and sniffed for mood elevation. Of the 15 cases using halothane 11 died.— M. Yamashita *et al.*, *Can. Anaesth. Soc. J.*, 1984, *31*, 76.

Three young hospital workers died after inhaling halothane illicitly. Postmortem examinations showed pulmonary oedema in all 3 and blood levels of 0.36%, 0.15%, and 0.5%. Death was probably due to cardiac arrhythmias.— J. D. Spencer *et al.*, *J. Am. med. Ass.*, 1976, *235*, 1034.

Hepatitis developed in 3 hospital workers following illicit inhalation of halothane. The effects appeared to be slowly reversible in 2 workers, although the third worker who had been sniffing halothane for over a year and who had consumed about 1.25 litres in the previous month died following cardiac arrhythmia.— H. G. Kaplan *et al.*, *Ann. intern. Med.*, 1979, *90*, 797.

A report following-on from a nationwide survey in the *US* of four deaths from abuse of volatile anaesthetics in operating rooms. Two of the deaths were attributed to halothane abuse the other two to cyclopropane.— M. Bass (letter), *J. Am. med. Ass.*, 1984, *251*, 604.

ALLERGY. A report of halothane allergy manifesting as acneiform eruptions in a nurse anaesthetist.— H. Guldager (letter), *Lancet*, 1987, *1*, 1211.

See also below under Effects on the Liver.

EFFECTS ON BODY TEMPERATURE. Some reference to malignant hyperpyrexia, sometimes fatal, in patients who had received halothane as part of their anaesthetic regimen: M. A. Denborough *et al.*, *Lancet*, 1970, *1*, 1137; D. R. Engelman and C. H. Lockhart, *Anesth. Analg. curr. Res.*, 1972, *51*, 98; R. K. Parikh and W. H. S. Thomson, *Br. J. Anaesth.*, 1972, *44*, 742; B. Peltz and J. Carstens, *Anaesthesia*, 1975, *30*, 346.

For references to reviews on malignant hyperpyrexia, see p.1113.

A halothane-associated increase in intracellular ionised calcium in patients with malignant hyperpyrexia might constitute the basis for a non-invasive screening test for this condition.— A. Klip *et al.*, *Lancet*, 1987, *1*, 463.

EFFECTS ON THE CARDIOVASCULAR SYSTEM. For studies showing enflurane and isoflurane producing a similar or lower incidence of cardiac arrhythmias than halothane, see p.1115 and p.1119.

For a study on the comparative effects of halothane, isoflurane, fentanyl, and ketamine on blood-pressure in preterm neonates, see p.1120.

EFFECTS ON THE KIDNEY. Urinary oxalate crystals were detected in 6 of 14 patients given halothane.— R. E. Tobey and R. J. Clubb, *J. Am. med. Ass.*, 1973, *223*, 649.

Postoperative renal failure with increased blood urea and creatinine concentrations, which started 11 days after she was given halothane, oxygen, and nitrous oxide anaesthesia for an aortofemoral bypass operation, was reported in a 65-year-old woman; she required weekly dialysis for the following 10 months. The clinical and pathological findings resembled those of methoxyflurane nephrotoxicity.— J. R. Cotton *et al.*, *Archs Path.*, 1976, *100*, 628.

Two case reports of combined fatal renal and hepatic failure following repeated exposure to halothane.— M. L. Gelman and N. S. Lichtenstein, *Urology*, 1981, *17*, 323.

EFFECTS ON THE LIVER. Liver damage has been recognised as an adverse effect of halothane for many years. Estimates of its incidence vary; recent reviews have cited incidences of 1 in 6000 to 1 in 20 000 (J.G.L. Stock and L. Strunin, *Anesthesiology*, 1985, *63*, 424) or 1 in 7000 to 1 in 30 000 (*Lancet*, 1986, *1*, 1251).

Two types of hepatotoxicity are recognised; the first is where there is an increase in liver enzyme values (type I). As measured by serum aminotransferase activity, this type might occur in up to 20% of patients given halothane (J. Neuberger and R. Williams, *Br. med. J.*, 1984, *289*, 1136). A higher percentage of patients may be affected if activity is measured by glutathione S-transferase (L.G. Allan *et al.*, *Lancet*, 1987, *1*, 771). The second type of hepatotoxicity is massive liver cell necrosis (type II) which is rare according to the incidences given above.

It is still not clear what causes the liver toxicity, nor can one predict who will develop the severe form with its high mortality rate. Obese women may be at special risk (Neuberger and Williams, 1984). Children have been considered to be a low-risk group (Stock and Strunin, 1985), but halothane hepatitis has been reported (J.G. Kenna *et al.*, *Br. med. J.*, 1987, *294*, 1209). Repeated exposure to halothane is a risk factor. This would appear to indicate some involvement with the immune system and certainly halothane antibodies have been detected in patients with hepatitis (Neuberger and Williams, 1984; J.G. Kenna *et al.*, *Br. J. Anaesth.*, 1987, *59*, 1286), but the role of the antibody is not clear (A.A. Spence, *Br. J. Anaesth.*, 1987, *59*, 1202). Biotransformation may play an alternative or additional role as toxic metabolites may act as haptens (Stock and Strunin, 1985). Whatever the cause, the CSM, after receiving 84 further reports of hepatotoxicity in the *UK* between 1978 and 1985, issued the following guidelines on precautions to be taken before using halothane:

1. A careful anaesthetic history should be taken to determine previous exposure and previous reactions to halothane.

2. Repeated exposure to halothane within a period of at least 3 months should be avoided unless there are overriding clinical circumstances.

3. A history of unexplained jaundice or pyrexia in a patient following exposure to halothane is an absolute contra-indication to its future use in that patient (*Current Problems*, 1986, *Sept.* No. 18; A. Goldberg and A.W. Asscher, *Br. med. J.*, 1987, *294*, 1100).

In response to these guidelines a letter from Adams and 12 other professors of anaesthetics in the *UK* (A.P. Adams *et al.*, *Br. med. J.*, 1986, *293*, 1023) emphasised that there was still a need for halothane and that an anaesthetist, who departed from the CSM guidelines having carefully considered the options and the patient's condition, and who recorded the reasons for the choice of halothane would not be acting negligently.

While there have been other arguments expressing concern at the CSM guidelines limiting the choice of anaesthetic (for example A.A. Spence, *Br. J. Anaesth.*, 1987, *59*, 529; A.W.A. Crossley and P.J. McQuillan, *Lancet*, 1987, *2*, 908), there have been others that have supported the move away from halothane towards other anaesthetics as has happened in the *USA* (C.E. Blogg, *Br. med. J.*, 1986, *292*, 1691). The debate continues.

POISONING. A 48-year-old woman who ingested halothane 250 mL with suicidal intent recovered after intensive therapy including artificial ventilation. No hepatitis occurred and hepatic function was normal over a period of 4 months. A second patient who ingested a similar amount also recovered.— I. Curelaru *et al.*, *Br. J. Anaesth.*, 1968, *40*, 283. A similar case.— J. Wig *et al.*, *Anaesthesia*, 1983, *38*, 552.

For a report of suicide by ingestion of halothane, see J. A. E. Spencer and N. M. Green, *J. Am. med. Ass.*, 1968, *205*, 702.

A 16-year-old girl who mistakenly received halothane, 2.5 mL intravenously, had severe pulmonary oedema and right-heart failure. She recovered with oxygen administered by positive-pressure ventilation.— J. Sutton *et al.* (letter), *Lancet*, 1971, *1*, 345. A fatality following the self-injection of 9 mL of liquid halothane.— P. Berman and M. Tattersall (letter), *ibid.*, 1982, *1*, 340.

See also above under Abuse.

Treatment of Adverse Effects

Bradycardia and hypotension may be controlled by the intravenous injection of 200 to 300 µg of atropine. It is common practice to give atropine as a premedicant to prevent or limit bradycardia and hypotension. Methoxamine has been given in severe hypotension.

Malignant hyperpyrexia responds to treatment with dantrolene sodium (p.1233).

For the use of procaine in the treatment of malignant hyperpyrexia, see Procaine Hydrochloride, p.1226.

Precautions

The risk of halothane hepatitis has led to the following guidelines. A careful history should be taken to determine previous exposure and previous reactions to halothane. Repeated exposure within a period of at least 3 months should be avoided unless there are overriding clinical circumstances. Also a history of unexplained jaundice or pyrexia following exposure to halothane is an absolute contra-indication to its future use in that patient. These guidelines are discussed further under Effects on the Liver, in Adverse Effects, above. It is recommended that patients be informed of any reactions and that this be done in addition to the updating of the patients' medical records.

Halothane reduces muscle tone in the pregnant uterus and generally its use is not recommended in obstetrics because of the increased risk of postpartum haemorrhage; the effects of ergometrine on the parturient uterus are diminished.

Routine premedication with atropine 300 to 600 µg by subcutaneous or intramuscular injection has been recommended to reduce vagal tone and to prevent bradycardia and severe hypotension. Assisted ventilation may be advisable to reduce the risk of respiratory depression, but care must then be taken to avoid forcing high concentrations of halothane into the lungs.

Allowance may need to be made for any increase in CSF pressure or in cerebral blood flow.

Adrenaline and most other sympathomimetic agents, except possibly in very dilute solution for the control of local haemorrhage, should be avoided during halothane anaesthesia since they can produce cardiac arrhythmias—see Sympathomimetics, p.1453. The effects of competitive muscle relaxants such as gallamine and tubocurarine, and of ganglion blocking agents such as pentolinium, pempidine, and trimetaphan are enhanced by halothane and if required they should be given in reduced dosage. Morphine increases the depressant effects of halothane on respiration. Chlorpromazine also enhances the depressant effect of halothane.

Patients who are known or are suspected to be susceptible to malignant hyperpyrexia should not be anaesthetised with halothane or any of the other halogenated inhalational anaesthetics.

In the *US*, the recommended exposure limit of halogenated anaesthetic agents (as waste gases) is 2 ppm.

See also Precautions for General Anaesthetics, p.1113.

INTERACTIONS. *Adrenaline.* A report of a fatality associated with ventricular fibrillation and the combined use of halothane and gingival retraction cord impregnated with 8% adrenaline.— M. D. Hilley *et al.*, *Anesthesiology*, 1984, *60*, 587.

Calcium-channel blockers. A report of cardiac arrest in a 56-year-old man associated with halothane anaesthesia preceded by intravenous verapamil. Caution was recommended in the simultaneous use of these two drugs.— I. W. Møller (letter), *Br. J. Anaesth.*, 1987, *59*, 522.

Fenfluramine. For a possible interaction between fenfluramine and halothane anaesthesia, see p.1443.

Phenytoin. For a case of phenytoin intoxication associated with halothane anaesthesia, see p.408.

Skeletal muscle relaxants. A review of drug interactions in anaesthesia, including details of the interactions between halothane and neuromuscular blocking drugs.— M. J. Halsey, *Br. J. Anaesth.*, 1987, *59*, 112.

A report of potentiation of suxamethonium-induced muscle damage by prior anaesthetic induction using halothane.— A. S. Laurence and P. Henderson, *Br. J. Anaesth.*, 1986, *58*, 126P.

See also under Isoflurane, p.1120.

Sodium bicarbonate. Sodium bicarbonate, given to induce metabolic alkalosis, decreased total peripheral resistance during halothane anaesthesia and might lead to severe hypotension.— J. A. Kaplan *et al.*, *Anesthesiology*, 1975, *42*, 550.

Trichlorethane. A report of 2 patients showing evidence of chronic cardiac toxicity following repeated exposure to trichloroethane. In both cases there was circumstantial evidence of a deterioration after routine anaesthetic use of halothane.— A. A. McLeod *et al.*, *Br. med. J.*, 1987, *294*, 727.

PORPHYRIA. Halothane was considered to be unsafe in patients with acute porphyria as it has been associated with acute attacks.— M.R. Moore and K.E.L. McColl, *Porphyrias, Drug Lists*, Glasgow, Porphyria Research Unit, University of Glasgow, 1987.

Absorption and Fate

Halothane is absorbed on inhalation. It has a relatively low solubility in blood and the arterial tension only slowly reaches the alveolar tension. Halothane reaches the highly vascular tissues in concentrations approaching those in arterial blood; it is more soluble in the neutral fats of adipose tissue than in the phospholipids of brain cells. The blood/gas partition coefficient is low.

Up to 80% of administered halothane is excreted unchanged through the lungs. Up to 20% is metabolised by the liver. Urinary metabolites include trifluoroacetic acid and bromide and chloride salts. It diffuses across the placenta.

A review of the pharmacokinetics of inhalational anaesthetics including halothane.— O. Dale and B. R. Brown, *Clin. Pharmacokinet.*, 1987, *12*, 145.

Some references to the pharmacokinetics of halothane: M. M. Atallah and I. C. Geddes, *Br. J. Anaesth.*, 1973, *45*, 464; S. R. Young *et al.*, *Anesthesiology*, 1975, *42*, 451; R. A. Saraiva *et al.*, *Anaesthesia*, 1977, *32*, 240; E. N. Cohen *et al.*, *Anesthesiology*, 1975, *43*, 392; T. Sakai and M. Takaori, *Br. J. Anaesth.*, 1978, *50*, 785; G. K. Gourlay *et al.*, *Br. J. Anaesth.*, 1980, *52*, 331.

Uses and Administration

Halothane is a volatile anaesthetic administered by inhalation. It has a minimum alveolar concentration (MAC) value (see p.1113) of 0.75%. It is non-flammable and is not explosive when mixed with oxygen at normal atmospheric pressure, although see above for a rare report of an explosion. It is not irritant to the skin and mucous membranes and does not produce necrosis when spilt on tissues. It suppresses salivary, mucous, bronchial, and gastric secretions and dilates the bronchioles.

Halothane is given using a vaporiser to provide close control over the concentration of inhaled vapour.

Anaesthesia may be induced with 2 to 4% v/v of halothane in oxygen or mixtures of nitrous oxide and oxygen. It takes up to about 5 minutes to attain surgical anaesthesia and there is little or no excitement in the induction period. The more usual practice is to induce anaesthesia with an intravenous agent followed by a muscle relaxant if intubation is to be carried out, before administering halothane with oxygen. Anaesthesia is maintained with concentrations of 0.5 to 2.0% v/v and recovery, which is dependent on the concentration used and the duration of anaesthesia, is usually rapid. Shivering may occur during recovery; restlessness during this period is an indication for postoperative analgesia.

Adequate muscle relaxation is only achieved with deep anaesthesia so a muscle relaxant is given to increase muscular relaxation if necessary.

A comparative review of halothane, enflurane, and isoflurane.— R. M. Jones, *Br. J. Anaesth.*, 1984, *56*, 57S.

ASTHMA. Two case reports of patients with severe acute asthma who did not improve with conventional treatment and remained severely bronchospastic when mechanically ventilated. Administration of halothane elicited a prompt bronchodilator response.— S. H. Schwartz, *J. Am. med. Ass.*, 1984, *251*, 2688. Another report.— C. D. Bayliff *et al.*, *Drug Intell. & clin. Pharm.*, 1985, *19*, 307. Reference to the use of high level PEEP (Positive End-Expiratory Pressure) in severe asthma when bronchodilators and then inhalational anaesthetics have failed.— J. Qvist *et al.*, *New Engl. J. Med.*, 1982, *307*, 1347.

Proprietary Preparations

Fluothane *(ICI Pharmaceuticals, UK). Anaesthetic inhalation*, halothane, in bottles of 250 mL.

Halothane *(May & Baker, UK). Anaesthetic inhalation*, halothane, in bottles of 250 mL.

Proprietary Names and Manufacturers

Fluopan *(S.Afr.)*; Fluothane *(ICI, Austral.; Ayerst, Canad.; ICI, Denm.; ICI, Ger.; ICI-Pharma, Ital.; Neth.; ICI, Norw.; ICI, S.Afr.; ICI, Spain; ICI, Swed.; ICI, Switz.; ICI Pharmaceuticals, UK; Ayerst, USA)*; Halovis *(Ital.)*; Rhodialothan *(Ger.)*; Somnothane *(Hoechst, Canad.)*.

3112-d

Hydroxydione Sodium Succinate *(BAN, rINN)*.

Sodium 3,20-dioxo-5α-pregnan-21-yl succinate.

$C_{25}H_{35}NaO_6$=454.5.

CAS — 303-01-5 (hydroxydione); 53-10-1 (sodium succinate).

Hydroxydione sodium succinate is a steroid formerly given intravenously for the induction of anaesthesia.

Proprietary Names and Manufacturers

Viadril G *(Pfizer, Fr.)*.

3113-n

Isoflurane *(BAN, USAN, rINN)*.

Compound 469. 1-Chloro-2,2,2-trifluoroethyl difluoromethyl ether; 2-Chloro-2-(difluoromethoxy)-1,1,1-trifluoroethane.

$C_3H_2ClF_5O$=184.5.

CAS — 26675-46-7.

Pharmacopoeias. In *U.S.*

A clear, colourless, volatile liquid with a pungent odour. B.p. about 49°.

Insoluble in water; miscible with common organic solvents and with fats and oils. **Store** in airtight containers. Protect from light.

Adverse Effects

Isoflurane differs from halothane in that it produces less cardiac depression and does not appear to sensitise the myocardium to the effect of catecholamines. Liver damage does not appear to be a problem with isoflurane.

Induction with isoflurane is not as smooth as with halothane and may be connected with its pungency.

See also Adverse Effects for General Anaesthetics, p.1113.

An extensive multicentre study of isoflurane anaesthesia in 6798 patients. Of 1735 reports of adverse effects only 231 were classed as major, with only 13 deaths, none of which appeared to be related to the use of isoflurane. Respiratory and cardiovascular complications were most frequent during induction (46.6% and 47.9% of 531 events, respectively) and during maintenance (15.9% and 76.1% of 623 events, respectively). No deaths were recorded during induction, and only 4 during maintenance in elderly patients with multisystem disease. In the postoperative period 14.6% of complications were considered to be major. Nine patients died. Adverse effects occurred among the various body systems in the following incidences: cardiovascular (23.7%), respiratory (29.0%), gastro-intestinal (15.3%) and CNS (17.4%). Renal problems were rare with only 6 reports in total. Arrhythmias, hypotension, and hypertension accounted for most of the circulatory disorders, about half of which were considered to be related to isoflurane. Of the respiratory events, laryngospasm (23.6%) and bronchospasm (11.0%) were relatively frequent, and more prevalent in younger patients. These complications were often due to the anaesthetic procedure. Prolonged postoperative nausea and vomiting occurred in 36 and 22 patients respectively.

The haemodynamic and reflex behaviour of the patients confirmed the decrease in arterial pressure and increase in heart-rate during isoflurane anaesthesia. Intra-operative arrhythmias and hypertension were most often associated with a prior history of these conditions. Airway reflexes were the predominant form of reflex activity, with coughing being the most frequently observed response.— J. B. Forrest *et al.*, *Can. Anaesth. Soc. J.*, 1982, *29*, *Suppl.*, S1. Further references to this study: K. Rehder, *ibid.*, 544; W. J. Levy, *Br. J. Anaesth.*, 1984, *56*, 1015.

Cattermole *et al.* (*Br. J. Anaesth.*, 1986, *58*, 385) in comparing isoflurane and halothane for outpatient dental anaesthesia in children considered that isoflurane would produce fewer arrhythmias than halothane, but that the ease of induction and the quality of anaesthesia was inferior to that with halothane. McAteer (*Br. J. Anaesth.*, 1986, *58*, 390) also found a higher incidence of coughing, salivation, and laryngospasm with isoflurane than halothane, but felt that it could be used as an alternative.

Comparable respiratory depressant effects with halothane and isoflurane.— K. Alagesan *et al.*, *Br. J. Anaesth.*, 1987, *59*, 1070.

EFFECTS ON BODY TEMPERATURE. Reports of malignant hyperpyrexia with isoflurane: M. M. Joseph *et al.* (letter), *Anesth. Analg.*, 1982, *61*, 711; J. Boheler *et al.*, *ibid.*, 712; D. W. Thomas *et al.*, *Br. J. Anaesth.*, 1987, *59*, 1196.

EFFECTS ON THE CARDIOVASCULAR SYSTEM. In 7 elderly patients given isoflurane 0.75 increased to 1.5% in 70% nitrous oxide and oxygen, blood pressure, peripheral resistance, end-systolic volume, the rate of left-ventricular pressure development, tension time index, and myocardial oxygen consumption fell; there were no changes in other haemodynamic parameters. The main disadvantage of isoflurane was hypotension.— J. Tarnow *et al.*, *Br. J. Anaesth.*, 1976, *48*, 669.

The haemodynamic and plasma-catecholamine responses during isoflurane anaesthesia in 10 patients undergoing coronary artery bypass surgery. The increase in plasma adrenaline paralleled the increase in heart-rate and cardiac output, and the decrease in plasma noradrenaline paralleled the decrease in systemic vascular resistance.— K. Balasaraswathi *et al.*, *Can. Anaesth. Soc. J.*, 1982, *29*, 533.

In a study of 60 healthy infants aged 5 to 26 weeks isoflurane induction (up to 3.5%) depressed heart-rate and blood pressure. Premedication with atropine (20 µg per kg body-weight) minimised the depression of heart-rate, but did not affect the change in blood pressure.— R. H. Friesen and J. L. Lichtor, *Anesth. Analg.*, 1983, *62*, 411.

The incidence of arrhythmia during surgery under anaesthesia with isoflurane was significantly less than with halothane in 76 Chinese patients. Sinus tachycardia was a significant feature under anaesthesia with isoflurane, and ventricular ectopics occurred most frequently with halothane.—M. R. C. Rodrigo *et al.*, *Br. J. Anaesth.*, 1986, *58*, 394.

A study of the haemodynamic effects of halothane, enflurane, and isoflurane in 15 healthy children. Isoflurane was found to cause less myocardial depression than halothane or enflurane.— T. M. Gallagher *et al.*, *Br. J. Anaesth.*, 1986, *58*, 1116. See also R. W. Cattermole *et al.*, *ibid.*, 385.

Isoflurane dilates small coronary vessels and may be dangerous for some patients with coronary artery disease.— L. C. Becker, *Anesthesiology*, 1987, *66*, 259; *idem*, *67*, 287.

EFFECTS ON THE LIVER. An analysis of 45 cases of isoflurane-associated hepatotoxicity reported to the FDA between 1981 and 1984. It could be considered that in 29 of the cases there was some other cause for the liver damage. While isoflurane might have been one of the causes of the damage in the other 16 cases, it was considered that there was not a reasonable likelihood of an association between isoflurane and postoperative liver impairment (R.K. Stoelting *et al.*, *Anesth. Analg.*, 1987, *66*, 147). Halothane hepatitis is considered to be of 2 types (see p.1118) a mild type (type I) and a severe type (type II). Allan *et al.* (*Lancet*, 1987, *1*, 771) found that plasma concentrations of glutathione S-transferase were a more sensitive measure of acute hepatic damage than aminotransferase measurements and indicated that a higher percentage of halothane patients might be affected by type I toxicity than had previously been thought to be the case. None of their patients who had been given isoflurane showed increased glutathione S-transferase concentrations.

EFFECTS ON THE NERVOUS SYSTEM. A report of seizure associated with induction of anaesthesia with isoflurane and nitrous oxide.— T. J. Poulton and R. J. Ellingson, *Anesthesiology*, 1984, *61*, 471. A further report.— J. A. Hymes, *Anesth. Analg.*, 1985, *64*, 367.

Precautions

As with halothane patients who are known or suspected to be susceptible to malignant hyperpyrexia should not be anaesthetised with isoflurane. It has been reported to increase the cerebrospinal pressure and its use in the presence of space-occupying lesions is best avoided. The effects of competitive muscle relaxants such as tubocurarine are enhanced by isoflurane.

See also Precautions for General Anaesthetics, p.1113.

INTERACTIONS. A study of 36 children. Compared with halothane, enflurane was found to cause a significant increase in action of atracurium and vecuronium. Isoflurane caused a significant increase compared with both halothane and enflurane.— M. Leuwer and R. Dudziak, *Br. J. Anaesth.*, 1986, *58*, 82S.

A retrospective study of the intra-operative use of nalbuphine as a supplement to isoflurane and enflurane in balanced anaesthesia in 108 surgical patients. Nalbuphine appeared to reduce halogenated anaesthetic requirements by approximately 50%.— E. M. Hew *et al.*, *Curr. med. Res. Opinion*, 1987, *10*, 531.

In a comparison of the effects of halothane, isoflurane and enflurane on alcuronium, isoflurane showed the greatest potentiation, then halothane; enflurane did not demonstrate any significant effect on the ED50 of alcuronium. The duration of action of alcuronium was not affected by halothane but was prolonged by enflurane and to a greater extent by isoflurane. In discussing these conflicting results it was considered that the fundamental finding of the study was the marked prolongation of alcuronium activity by enflurane and by isoflurane.—S.J. Keens *et al.*, *Br. J. Anaesth.*, 1987, *59*, 1011.

Absorption and Fate

Isoflurane is absorbed on inhalation. The blood/gas coefficient is lower than that of enflurane. About 0.2% of administered isoflurane is metabolised mainly to inorganic fluoride.

A review of the pharmacokinetics of inhalational anaesthetics including isoflurane.— O. Dale and B. R. Brown, *Clin. Pharmacokinet.*, 1987, *12*, 145.

Uses and Administration

Isoflurane is a volatile anaesthetic administered by inhalation. It is an isomer of enflurane and has anaesthetic actions similar to those of halothane (p.1119). Isoflurane has a minimum alveolar concentration (MAC) value (see p.1113) of about 1.15%. Available figures for variation with age show a value of 1.28% for patients in their mid-twenties to 1.05% for patients in their mid-sixties.

Isoflurane is usually administered after an intravenous induction agent starting with a concentration of 0.5%. If used for induction 1.5 to 3.0% generally produces surgical anaesthesia within 10 minutes. Anaesthesia may be maintained with a concentration of 1.0 to 2.5% with oxygen and nitrous oxide; 1.5 to 3.5% may be required if used only with oxygen. Isoflurane is reported to possess analgesic properties.

Reviews of isoflurane: E. I. Eger, *Anesthesiology*, 1981, *55*, 559; J. G. Wade and W. C. Stevens, *Anesth. Analg.*, 1981, *60*, 666; H. W. Linde and M. H. M. Dykes, *J. Am. med. Ass.*, 1981, *245*, 2335; C. Prys-Roberts, *Br. J. Anaesth.*, 1981, *53*, 1243; *Lancet*, 1985, *2*, 537.

A comparative review of halothane, enflurane, and isoflurane.— R. M. Jones, *Br. J. Anaesth.*, 1984, *56*, 57S.

A multicentre study comparing the clinical differences between an intravenous technique using fentanyl/droperidol and an inhalation technique employing isoflurane, in ambulatory surgery patients undergoing procedures of 30 minutes or less duration. It was concluded that fentanyl/droperidol offered clinically useful advantages over isoflurane.— J. Pollard, *Curr. ther. Res.*, 1984, *36*, 617.

Use of isoflurane and vecuronium anaesthesia in a 30-year-old man with Wolff-Parkinson-White syndrome.— C. M. Kumar (letter), *Br. J. Anaesth.*, 1986, *58*, 574.

The use of isoflurane to control intraoperative hypertension in 10 patients undergoing hypothermic cardiopulmonary bypass surgery.—C. W. Loomis *et al.*, *Clin. Pharmac. Ther.*, 1986, *40*, 304. Isoflurane dilates small coronary vessels and may be dangerous for some patients with coronary artery disease.— L. C. Becker, *Anesthesiology*, 1987, *66*, 259; *idem*, *67*, 287.

A study of isoflurane anaesthesia comparing a single-breath induction technique and a conventional regime using nitrous oxide and oxygen in 72 patients. Single-breath induction was associated with fewer problems on induction, but required more patient co-operation.— J. M. Lamberty and I. H. Wilson, *Br. J. Anaesth.*, 1987, *59*, 1214.

DENTAL SURGERY. Isoflurane was compared with halothane as a supplement to anaesthesia with nitrous oxide and oxygen for outpatient dental extractions in 80 children. Induction and maintenance of anaesthesia were satisfactory with both agents, although there was a higher incidence of coughing, salivation, and laryngospasm with isoflurane. Immediate recovery was significantly slower in patients who had received isoflurane, and was complicated by coughing in a significant number of patients.— P. M. McAteer *et al.*, *Br. J. Anaesth.*, 1986, *58*, 390. A similar study. Isoflurane produced significantly fewer arrhythmias than halothane but the induction of anaesthesia took longer and proved more difficult.— R. W. Cattermole *et al.*, *ibid.*, 385.

PREGNANCY AND THE NEONATE. A randomised study comparing the maternal and neonatal effects of 0.5% halothane or 0.75% isoflurane as supplements to 50% nitrous oxide in oxygen for caesarean section in 20 women. Uterine relaxation was similar in the 2 groups and no patient required blood transfusion. Recovery time was significantly shorter in the isoflurane group. No patient had intraoperative recall.— R. G. Ghaly *et al.*, *Br. J. Anaesth.*, 1987, *59*, 136P.

Proprietary Preparations

Forane *(Abbott, UK). Anaesthetic inhalation,* isoflurane.

Proprietary Names and Manufacturers

Ærrane *(Anaquest, UK)*; Forane *(Anaquest, Canad.; Abbott, Ital.; Abbott, S.Afr.; Abbott, Spain; Abbott, UK; Anaquest, USA)*; Forene *(Abbott, Denm.; Abbott, Ger.; Abbott, Norw.; Abbott, Swed.)*.

3114-h

Ketamine Hydrochloride *(BANM, USAN, pINNM)*.

CI-581; CL-369; CN-52,372-2. (±)-2-(2-Chlorophenyl)-2-methylaminocyclohexanone hydrochloride.

$C_{13}H_{16}ClNO,HCl = 274.2$.

CAS — 6740-88-1 (ketamine); 1867-66-9 (hydrochloride).

Pharmacopoeias. In *Chin.*, *Cz.*, *Jpn*, and *U.S.*

A white crystalline powder with a slight characteristic odour. Ketamine hydrochloride 1.15 mg is approximately equivalent to 1 mg of ketamine base. **Soluble** 1 in 4 of water, 1 in 14 of alcohol, 1 in 60 of dehydrated alcohol and chloroform, and 1 in 6 of methyl alcohol; practically insoluble in ether. A 10% solution has a pH of 3.5 to 4.1; the *U.S.P.* injection has a pH of 3.5 to 5.5. **Incompatible** with soluble barbiturates. **Store** in well-closed containers.

Adverse Effects

Emergence reactions are common during recovery from ketamine anaesthesia and include vivid often unpleasant dreams, confusion, hallucinations, and irrational behaviour that respond if necessary to an intravenous benzodiazepine or similar agent. Patients may also experience increased muscle tone, sometimes resembling seizures. Children and elderly patients appear to be slightly less sensitive than other adult patients. Blood pressure and heart-rate may be temporarily increased by ketamine but hypotension, arrhythmias, and bradycardia have occurred rarely. Ketamine may increase intracranial pressure.

The respiration may be depressed, especially during too rapid intravenous injection or with high doses. Apnoea and laryngospasm have occurred. Diplopia and nystagmus may occur. Nausea and vomiting, dizziness, headache, lachrymation, hypersalivation, raised intraocular and cerebrospinal fluid pressure, have also been reported. Transient skin rashes and pain at the site of injection may occur.

See also Adverse Effects for General Anaesthetics, p.1113.

ABUSE. An alert to physicians and health care professionals to the abuse of ketamine hydrochloride in adolescents and young adults in the *US*. Hallucinations may recur and there is a possibility of psychoses resulting from repeated use of ketamine.— *FDA Drug Bull.*, 1979, *9*, 24.

A report of an acute dystonic reaction in a 20-year-old man following self-administration of ketamine intravenously.— J. M. Felser and D. J. Orban, *Ann. emerg. Med.*, 1982, *11*, 673.

EFFECTS ON BODY TEMPERATURE. Ketamine has been associated loosely with malignant hyperpyrexia.— G. A. Gronert, *Anesthesiology*, 1980, *53*, 395.

EFFECTS ON THE CARDIOVASCULAR SYSTEM. While ketamine often has a positive effect on the cardiovascular system there have been reports of reduced activity or of arrhythmias. Some references: K. Waxman *et al.*, *Anesth. Analg.*, 1980, *59*, 355 (decreased cardiac performance and peripheral oxygen transport); E. B. Cabbabe and P. M. Behbahani, *Ann. Plast. Surg.*, 1985, *15*, 50 (arrythmias in 2 patients); R. H. Friesen and D. B. Henry, *Anesthesiology*, 1986, *64*, 238 (smaller reduction of blood pressure in neonates with ketamine than with fentanyl, halothane, or isoflurane).

For inhibition of ketamine's chronotropic and inotropic activity by halothane see under Precautions, below.

EFFECTS ON THE LIVER. Changes in serum-enzyme levels following infusion of large doses of ketamine.— J. W. Dundee *et al.*, *Anaesthesia*, 1980, *35*, 12.

EFFECTS ON MENTAL STATE. Mental disturbances following ketamine anaesthesia may vary in incidence from less than 5% to greater than 30% (P.F.White *et al.*, *Anesthesiology*, 1982, *56*, 119). Grant *et al.* claimed that the frequency of psychic sequelae after ketamine is dose-related and is markedly reduced with the use of the drug in subanaesthetic doses (*Br. J. Anaesth.*, 1981, *53*, 805). However, Ghoneim *et al.* and Sechzer *et al.* reported a high incidence of such effects even at low doses of 0.25 to 1.0 mg per kg body-weight (*J. clin. Psychopharmacol.*, 1985, *5*, 70; *Curr. ther. Res.*, 1984, *35*, 396).

EFFECTS ON RESPIRATION. Depression of the laryngeal-closure reflex occurred in 7 patients anaesthetised with ketamine. It was suggested that endotracheal intubation should be used to prevent the risk of silent aspiration.— P. A. Taylor and R. M. Towey, *Br. med. J.*, 1971, *2*, 688.

A report of aspiration pneumonitis in a child anaesthetised with ketamine.— B. H. Penrose, *Anesth. Analg. curr. Res.*, 1972, *51*, 41.

Aspiration with subsequent respiratory problems occurred in 3 patients anaesthetised with ketamine for surgery in the nasal or oral cavity. Ketamine was contra-indicated as an anaesthetic for such procedures.— W. M. Bryant, *Plastic reconstr. Surg.*, 1973, *51*, 562.

A report of apnoea of 2 hours duration in a 4-month-old girl who had received a premedication of pentobarbitone 25 mg rectally followed by an intramuscular injection of ketamine 60 mg (10 mg per kg body-weight) then ketamine 10 mg was administered slowly by intravenous injection. Recovery was uneventful.— M. van Wijhe *et al.* (letter), *Br. J. Anaesth.*, 1986, *58*, 573.

PREGNANCY AND THE NEONATE. Harlequin-like colour change in a 9-month-old boy during anaesthesia with ketamine 15 mg.— D. L. Wagner and A. D. Sewell, *Anesthesiology*, 1985, *62*, 695.

Precautions

Ketamine hydrochloride is contra-indicated in patients with cardiovascular disease including severe hypertension. Cardiac function should be monitored in patients with mild hypertension or cardiac decompensation. It is best avoided in patients with eclampsia or pre-eclampsia and should be used with caution in patients with a history of convulsive disorders or psychiatric disease.

Ketamine should not be given to patients with increased intra-ocular or CSF pressure or intracranial space-occupying lesions. Alternative anaesthetics should be considered for patients with penetrating wounds of the eye. Verbal, tactile, and visual stimuli should be kept to a minimum during recovery in an attempt to reduce the risk of emergence reactions.

See also Precautions for General Anaesthetics, p.1113.

It has been recommended that ketamine should not be used in combination with ergometrine.

INTERACTIONS. Ketamine enhances the depressant effects of barbiturates and opioid analgesics. Anaesthetising abusers of such drugs might produce potentially fatal

5 mg per kg (N. Mackenzie and I.S. Grant, *Br. J. Anaesth.*, 1985, *57*, 725). When comparing propofol 1.5 or 2.0 mg per kg with thiopentone 4.0 mg per kg, Rolly and Versichelen found apnoea to be similar in both patient groups (*Anaesthesia*, 1985, *40*, 945).

Absorption and Fate

Propofol is rapidly distributed and metabolised following injection. Most of the dose (88%) is excreted in the urine as conjugated metabolites. A 2-compartment and a 3-compartment model have been used to describe the pharmacokinetics of propofol.

Reviews of the pharmacokinetics of propofol: I. D. Cockshott, *Postgrad. med. J.*, 1985, *61*, *Suppl.* 3, 45; P. J. Davis and D. R. Cook, *ibid.*, 1986, *11*, 18; B. N. Swerdlow and F. O. Holley, *Clin. Pharmacokinet.*, 1987, *12*, 79.

Some studies of the pharmacokinetics of propofol: E. Gepts *et al.*, *Postgrad. med. J.*, 1985, *61*, *Suppl.* 3, 51 (continuous intravenous infusion); N. H. Kay *et al.*, *ibid.*, 55 (single induction dose); L. P. Briggs *et al.*, *ibid.*, 58 (single induction dose); I. D. Cockshott *et al.*, *Br. J. Anaesth.*, 1987, *59*, 941P (intravenous infusion); I. D. Cockshott *et al.*, *ibid.*, 1103 (single bolus injections).

Uses and Administration

Propofol is given by intravenous injection for the induction of anaesthesia. It is also used for the maintenance of anaesthesia for short surgical procedures lasting not more than one hour. Induction is rapid, as is recovery. Supplementary analgesics are normally required.

Induction is generally carried out by administering 40 mg every 10 seconds; 20 mg may be used in high-risk patients. Most adults will be anaesthetised by a dose of 2.0 to 2.5 mg per kg body-weight; elderly patients will be anaesthetised usually by a dose that is 20% less. When used for maintenance propofol is infused at a rate of between 100 to 200 µg per kg per minute, alternatively intermittent bolus injections of 25 to 50 mg may be given.

Reviews of the actions and uses of propofol: R. M. Grounds *et al.*, *Postgrad. med. J.*, 1985, *61*, *Suppl.* 3, 90; *Lancet*, 1987, *1*, 1469. See also C. S. Reilly and W. S. Nimmo, *Drugs*, 1987, *34*, 98.

Many of the studies carried out on propofol have involved comparisons with methohexitone when propofol has generally been found to produce faster recovery, but at the expense of a greater incidence of prolonged apnoea and of reduced blood pressure. Some of the studies also show a smoother induction with propofol.

Some references: J. Noble and T. W. Ogg, *Postgrad. med. J.*, 1985, *61*, *Suppl.* 3, 103; B. Kay and T. E. J. Healy, *ibid.*, 108; J. M. Cundy and K. Arunasalam, *ibid.*, 129; I. S. Grant and N. MacKenzie, *ibid.*, 133; N. Mackenzie and I. S. Grant, *Br. J. Anaesth.*, 1985, *57*, 725; *idem*, 1167; E. Jessop *et al.*, *ibid.*, 1173; D. P. O'Toole *et al.*, *ibid.*, 1986, *58*, 1329P; V. A. Doze, *Anesth. Analg.*, 1986, *65*, 1189; M. R. Logan *et al.*, *Br. J. Anaesth.*, 1987, *59*, 179.

Some studies on propofol: G. Rolly *et al.*, *Br. J. Anaesth.*, 1985, *57*, 743 (rate of administration); B. J. McLeod *et al.*, *ibid.*, 822P (induction agent for cardiac procedures); N. W. Lees *et al.*, *Postgrad. med. J.*, 1985, *61*, *Suppl.* 3, 88 (selective enhancement of muscle relaxant activity); J. S. C. McCollum *et al.*, *Br. J. Anaesth.*, 1986, *58*, 1330P (induction dose reduced by papaveretum with hyoscine); K. R. Spelina *et al.*, *ibid.*, 1080 (premedicated with morphine); M. J. Turtle *et al.*, *ibid.*, 1987, *59*, 283 (premedicated with lorazepam); R. K. Mirakhur *et al.*, *ibid.*, 431 (reduction in intra-ocular pressure); J. S. C. McCollum *et al.*, *ibid.*, 654P (possible anti-emetic activity).

SEDATION. Propofol has been used to provide sedation. Grounds *et al.* (*Br. med. J.*, 1987, *294*, 397) found that an infusion of propofol 1% at a rate of 13.13 µg per kg body-weight per minute (0.798 mg per kg per hour) provided a satisfactory level of sedation after cardiac surgery with rapid recovery when compared with midazolam. The slow infusion rate was probably a result of the residual effect of the fentanyl used during induction. For other intensive care patients a higher infusion rate is recommended by Mackenzie and Grant (*Br. med. J.*, 1987, *294*, 774); 3 mg per kg per hour (50 µg per kg per minute) provided good sedation in ventilated patients after noncardiac surgery (they also observed an analgesic effect). However, a mean infusion rate of 32 µg per kg per minute (1.92 mg per kg per hour) employed by Newman *et al.* (*Br. med. J.*, 1987, *294*, 970) was associated with a significant fall in blood pressure and they called for caution in critically ill patients. Also Brown and Edwards (*ibid.*) warned of the risks to the lungs and plasma of infusions of soya oil used in the vehicle for propofol.

Proprietary Preparations

Diprivan *(ICI Pharmaceuticals, UK)*. *Injection*, propofol 10 mg/mL, in a vehicle containing soya oil and purified egg phosphatide, in ampoules of 20 mL.

Proprietary Names and Manufacturers

Diprivan *(Stuart, S.Afr.; ICI Pharmaceuticals, UK)*.

13234-m

Sevoflurane *(USAN, rINN)*.

BAX-3084. Fluoromethyl 2,2,2-trifluoro-1-(trifluoromethyl)ethyl ether; 1,1,1,3,3,3-Hexafluoro-2-(fluoromethoxy)-propane.

$C_4H_3F_7O$=200.1.

CAS — 28523-86-6.

Sevoflurane is a non flammable inhalation anaesthetic.

References: D. A. Holaday and F. R. Smith, *Anesthesiology*, 1981, *54*, 100.

Proprietary Names and Manufacturers

Travenol, USA.

3121-n

Sodium Oxybate *(USAN)*.

NSC-84223; Sodium Gamma-hydroxybutyrate; Wy-3478. Sodium 4-hydroxybutyrate.

$C_4H_7NaO_3$=126.1.

CAS — 502-85-2.

Pharmacopoeias. In *Chin.*

Adverse Effects

Side-effects with sodium oxybate include abnormal muscle movements during the induction period and nausea and vomiting. Occasional emergence delirium has been reported. Bradycardia frequently occurs. Respiration may be slowed and hypokalaemia has been reported.

See also Adverse Effects for General Anaesthetics, p.1113.

A report of severe metabolic disorders occurring during therapy with sodium oxybate and tetracosactrin in 4 patients with severe head injuries. The disorders consisted of hypernatraemia, hypokalaemia, and metabolic acidosis.— J. L. Béal *et al.*, *Thérapie*, 1983, *38*, 569.

Precautions

Sodium oxybate should be administered with caution in patients with severe hypertension, bradycardia, conditions associated with defects of cardiac conduction, epilepsy, and alcoholic delirium. Sodium oxybate enhances the effects of opioid analgesics and skeletal muscle relaxants. See also Precautions for General Anaesthetics, p.1113.

Sodium oxybate was considered to be unsafe in patients with acute porphyria because it has been shown to be porphyrinogenic in *animals* or *in vitro* systems.— M.R. Moore and K.E.L. McColl, *Porphyrias, Drugs Lists*, Glasgow, Porphyria Research Unit, University of Glasgow, 1987.

Uses and Administration

Sodium oxybate has anaesthetic properties and when injected intravenously produces unconsciousness, but little analgesia. It may be used to produce complete anaesthesia, but is generally employed to produce basal anaesthesia and may be used with nitrous oxide and oxygen or with an opioid analgesic such as pethidine. Skeletal muscle relaxants may be necessary.

A solution of sodium oxybate equivalent to 20% of the acid is administered slowly by intravenous injection, usually in a dose of 60 mg per kg body-weight; further smaller doses may be required in long procedures. In children up to 100 mg per kg may be necessary.

Obese subjects undergoing low-protein dietary restriction or therapeutic starvation were given sodium 3-hydroxybutyrate by mouth or intravenously. The compound reduced loss of body protein and appeared to alter the ratio of fat to lean tissue loss G. L. S. Pawan and S. J. G. Semple, *Lancet*, 1983, *1*, 15.

CEREBROVASCULAR DISORDERS. Reduction of raised intracranial pressure by sodium oxybate following severe head injury.— A. J. Strong *et al.*, *Br. J. Surg.*, 1983, *70*, 303. See also.— E. Escuret *et al.*, *Acta neurol. scand.*, 1979, *60*, 38.

NARCOLEPSY. Use of sodium oxybate in the treatment of narcolepsy: R. Broughton and M. Mamelak, *Can. J. neurol. Sci.*, 1979, *6*, 1; M. Mamelak and P. Webster, *Sleep*, 1981, *4*, 105; M. B. Scharf *et al.*, *J. clin. Psychiat.*, 1985, *46*, 222.

Proprietary Names and Manufacturers

Gamma-OH *(Cernep Synthelabo, Fr.; Neth.)*; Somsanit *(Köhler, Ger.)*.

3123-m

Thialbarbitone Sodium *(BANM)*.

Natrium Cyclohexenylallylthiobarbituricum; Thialbarbital Sodium *(rINNM)*; Thiohexallymalnatrium. Sodium 5-allyl-5-(cyclohex-2-enyl)-2-thiobarbiturate.

$C_{13}H_{15}N_2NaO_2S$=286.3.

CAS — 467-36-7 (thialbarbitone); 3546-29-0 (thialbarbitone sodium).

Pharmacopoeias. In *Aust.* and *Jug.*

Thialbarbitone sodium is a barbiturate formerly administered intravenously for the production of complete anaesthesia of short duration or for the induction of general anaesthesia.

3122-h

Thiamylal Sodium *(USAN)*.

Sodium 5-allyl-5-(1-methylbutyl)-2-thiobarbiturate.

$C_{12}H_{17}N_2NaO_2S$=276.3.

CAS — 77-27-0 (thiamylal); 337-47-3 (thiamylal sodium).

Pharmacopoeias. In *Jpn.* *U.S.* includes Thiamylal Sodium for Injection.

Thiamylal sodium is a barbiturate which is administered intravenously for the production of complete anaesthesia of short duration or for the induction of general anaesthesia. It is possibly slightly more potent than thiopentone sodium and has similar actions and uses.

It is given as a 2.5% solution, an initial injection of 3 to 6 mL being sufficient to produce short periods of anaesthesia. During induction the rate of injection should be 1 mL every 5 seconds. A continuous intravenous infusion of a 0.3% solution has been used for maintenance. It has been administered rectally.

Preparations

Thiamylal Sodium for Injection *(U.S.P.)*

Proprietary Names and Manufacturers

Surital *(Parke, Davis, Canad.; Parke, Davis, USA)*.

13323-b

Thiobutabarbital Sodium

Sodium 5-*sec*-butyl-5-ethyl-2-thiobarbiturate.

$C_{10}H_{15}N_2NaO_2S$=250.3.

CAS — 2095-57-0 (thiobutabarbital); 947-08-0 (sodium salt).

Thiobutabarbital sodium has been used for the induction of anaesthesia.

Proprietary Names and Manufacturers

Inactin *(Byk Gulden, Ger.)*.

3124-b

Thiopentone Sodium *(BANM)*.

Natrium Isopentylaethylthiobarbituricum (cum Natrio Carbonico); Penthiobarbital Sodique; Soluble Thiopentone; Thiomebumalnatrium cum Natrii Carbonate; Thiopent. Sod.; Thiopental Sodium *(USAN, rINN)*; Thiopental Sodium and Sodium Carbonate; Thiopentalum Natricum; Thiopentalum Natricum cum Natrii Carbonate; Thiopentalum Natricum et Natrii Carbonas; Thiopentobarbitalum Solubile. Sodium 5-ethyl-

5-(1-methylbutyl)-2-thiobarbiturate.
$C_{11}H_{17}N_2NaO_2S$=264.3.

CAS — 76-75-5 (thiopentone); 71-73-8 (thiopentone sodium).

NOTE. The name thiopental sodium has been applied to thiopentone sodium with or without sodium carbonate; the name thiobarbital has been applied to thiopentone and has also been used to describe a barbiturate of different composition.

Pharmacopoeias. In *Aust., Belg., Br., Cz., Egypt., Eur., Fr., Ger., Ind., Int., Jug., Neth., Nord., Pol., Rus., Swiss,* and *Turk.* (all with anhydrous sodium carbonate). Also in *B.P. Vet.*

In *Arg., Braz., Jpn,* and *U.S.* without admixture with anhydrous sodium carbonate.

In *Arg., Chin., Ind., It., Jpn, Nord., Swiss,* and *U.S.* as a sterile mixture for injection (Thiopental Sodium for Injection; Thiopentone Injection).

A white to yellowish-white crystalline powder, or pale greenish hygroscopic powder with a characteristic alliaceous odour.

Soluble 1 in 1.5 of water; partly soluble in alcohol; practically insoluble in ether and petroleum spirit. An 8% solution for injection has a pH of 10.2 to 11.2. Solutions of thiopentone sodium are **incompatible** with acidic and oxidising substances so that, amongst other drugs, a number of antibiotics, tranquillisers, muscle relaxants, and analgesics should not be mixed with it. Compounds commonly listed as incompatible include amikacin sulphate, benzylpenicillin salts, cefapirin sodium, codeine phosphate, ephedrine sulphate, morphine sulphate, prochlorperazine edisylate, suxamethonium salts, and tubocurarine chloride. Solutions decompose on standing and precipitation occurs on boiling. **Store** in airtight containers. Protect from light.

Thiopentone sodium has been shown to interact with polyvinyl chloride infusion bags; when stored as an aqueous solution in the dark at room temperature there was a substantial loss of thiopentone sodium after one week.— E. A. Kowaluk *et al., Am. J. Hosp. Pharm.*, 1981, *38*, 1308. Loss of thiopentone in plastic intravenous delivery systems.— E. A. Kowaluk *et al., ibid.*, 1982, *39*, 460.

Adverse Effects and Treatment

As for Phenobarbitone, p.405.

Coughing, sneezing, laryngeal spasm, or bronchospasm may occur, particularly during induction with thiopentone sodium. The intravenous injection of concentrated solutions such as 5% may result in thrombophlebitis. Extravasation may cause tissue necrosis. Intra-arterial injection causes burning pain and may cause prolonged blanching of the forearm and hand and gangrene of digits. Hypersensitivity reactions have been reported. Thiopentone can cause respiratory depression. It depresses cardiac output and often causes an initial fall in blood pressure, and overdosage may result in circulatory failure. Postoperative vomiting is infrequent but there may be persistent drowsiness, confusion, and amnesia. Headache has been reported with the barbiturate anaesthetics.

Adverse effects are treated symptomatically.

See also under Adverse Effects for General Anaesthetics, p.1113.

ALLERGY. A case report of an anaphylactic reaction to thiopentone in a 32-year-old female who had previously had at least six uneventful anaesthetics.— P. Westacott *et al., Can. Anaesth. Soc. J.*, 1984, *31*, 434.

A report of haemolytic anaemia and renal failure in association with the development of an anti-thiopentone antibody in a patient who had undergone general anaesthesia induced by thiopentone.— B. Habibi *et al., New Engl. J. Med.*, 1985, *312*, 353 and 1136.

For further references to allergic reactions to thiopentone sodium, see *Martindale 28th Edn*, p.759.

EFFECTS ON THE CARDIOVASCULAR SYSTEM. The cardiovascular effects of bolus or incremental administration of thiopentone.— J. L. Seltzer *et al., Br. J. Anaesth.*, 1980, *52*, 527.

Precautions

Thiopentone sodium is contra-indicated in respiratory obstruction, severe acute asthma, severe shock, dystrophia myotonica, and porphyria.

Thiopentone sodium alone should not be used for peroral endoscopy since laryngeal spasm may cause grave anoxia. It may also precipitate acute circulatory failure in patients with constrictive pericarditis or with gross dyspnoea due to diseases of the heart or lungs. Doses of thiopentone sodium should be greatly reduced in shock and dehydration, severe anaemia, hyperkalaemia, toxaemia, myxoedema and other metabolic disorders, or in severe hepatic or renal disease. Reduced doses are also required in the elderly. Thiopentone sodium should be used with caution in patients with cardiovascular disease, adrenocortical insufficiency, or with increased intracranial pressure.

Difficulty may be experienced in producing anaesthesia with the usual doses in patients accustomed to taking alcohol or some drugs; additional anaesthetic agents may be necessary. Care is required when anaesthetising patients being treated with phenothiazine neuroleptics since there may be increased hypotension. Reduced doses may be required in patients receiving sulphafurazole.

See also Precautions for General Anaesthetics, p.1113.

Barbiturates used intravenously as anaesthetics decreased cerebrospinal fluid pressure.— T. Takahashi *et al., Br. J. Anaesth.*, 1973, *45*, 179.

Significantly less thiopentone was needed to induce anaesthesia following premedication with hyoscine and morphine, than after atropine, diazepam, and pethidine. Furthermore 37 patients taking digoxin and a diuretic required significantly less thiopentone than 37 patients who did not receive this treatment. It was noted that 21 patients who underwent operation for valvular heart disease required only 60% of the thiopentone dose required by patients undergoing operations on limbs.— F. Andreasen and J. H. Christensen, *Br. J. clin. Pharmac.*, 1977, *4*, 640P.

Absorption and Fate

When administered intravenously thiopentone sodium may reach effective concentrations in the brain within 30 seconds. Redistribution to other tissues, particularly fat, occurs and concentrations in the brain and plasma are reduced. Up to 80% of thiopentone may be bound to plasma proteins, although reports show a wide range of figures. Thiopentone is metabolised in the body, chiefly in the liver, at a very slow rate. It readily diffuses across the placenta.

Reviews of the pharmacokinetics of thiopentone: B. N. Swerdlow and F. O. Holley, *Clin. Pharmacokinet.*, 1987, *12*, 79; G. Heinemeyer, *ibid.*, *13*, 1.

A pharmacokinetic evaluation of infusion regimens for thiopentone as a primary anaesthetic agent.— D. P. Crankshaw *et al., Eur. J. clin. Pharmac.*, 1985, *28*, 543.

PREGNANCY AND THE NEONATE. Pregnancy does not significantly affect thiopentone plasma-binding.— D. J. Morgan *et al., Br. J. clin. Pharmac.*, 1983, *15*, 121.

Elimination kinetics of thiopentone in mothers and their newborn infants.— F. Gaspari *et al., Eur. J. clin. Pharmac.*, 1985, *28*, 321.

PROTEIN BINDING. The amount of unbound thiopentone was 28% in 10 healthy subjects, 53% in 10 patients with hepatic disease, and about 55% in patients with renal disease.— M. M. Ghoneim and H. Pandya, *Anesthesiology*, 1975, *42*, 545.

The amount of free (unbound) thiopentone in normal serum was about 52 to 57%; in serum from patients with kwashiorkor, with a reduced albumin concentration, the amount of free thiopentone was about 65 to 68%. In kwashiorkor serum more thiopentone was bound to other protein fractions; the significance of this secondary binding was not clear.— N. Buchanan and L. A. van der Walt, *Br. J. Anaesth.*, 1977, *49*, 247.

Uses and Administration

Thiopentone sodium is a barbiturate which is administered intravenously for the induction of general anaesthesia or for the production of complete anaesthesia of short duration. It is also used for hypnosis. It has poor analgesic and muscle relaxant properties. Small doses have been shown to be anti-analgesic and lower the pain threshold.

Thiopentone sodium is administered intravenously as a 2.5% or occasionally as a 5% solution, the usual dose for inducing anaesthesia being 100 to 150 mg injected over 10 to 15 seconds; if unconsciousness has not occurred within 30 seconds to 1 minute a further 100 to 150 mg may be given. Childrens doses range from 2 to 8 mg per kg body-weight.

Recovery is usually rapid after moderate doses, but the patient may remain sleepy or confused for several hours. Large doses or repeated smaller doses may markedly delay recovery. Rapid injection gives a more pronounced effect and is followed by a more rapid recovery than slow injection. There is no stage of excitement with thiopentone anaesthesia. Its use should be preceded by atropine or similar agent to depress vagal reflexes and mucous secretions. Morphine or pethidine may be given to enhance the poor analgesic effects of thiopentone.

Thiopentone sodium may be given rectally as a solution, suspension, or suppositories for basal anaesthesia in a dose of about 44 mg per kg body-weight; its effects are usually observed in 10 to 12 minutes.

Thiopentone sodium has also been used for the control of convulsions, including drug-induced convulsions.

Prolongation of thiopentone anaesthesia by probenecid.— S. Kaukinen *et al., Br. J. Anaesth.*, 1980, *52*, 603.

Rectal administration of thiopentone (25 to 45 mg per kg body-weight) was found to be an effective alternative to an intramuscular cocktail of pethidine, chlorpromazine, and promethazine for sedating children before computerised tomography.— G. J. Burckart *et al., Am. J. Hosp. Pharm.*, 1980, *37*, 222.

CEREBROVASCULAR DISORDERS. Thiopentone has been used as an anaesthetic in patients with raised intracranial pressure. Also it has been given to reduce such pressure (C.M. Quandt and R.A. de los Reyes, *Drug Intell. & clin. Pharm.*, 1984, *18*, 105) and this use has included children with Reye's syndrome (J.F.T. Glasgow *et al., Br. J. Hosp. Med.*, 1985, *34*, 42). It has been studied in the prevention and treatment of brain ischaemia, but while Nussmeier *et al.* (*Anesthesiology*, 1986, *64*, 165) showed that thiopentone could protect patients against the neuropsychiatric complications of cardiopulmonary bypass, the Brain Resuscitation Clinical Trial I Study Group (*New Engl. J. Med.*, 1986, *314*, 397) found no cerebral benefit from thiopentone in comatose survivors of cardiac arrest. Nor did Eyre and Wilkinson (*Archs Dis. Childh.*, 1986, *61*, 1084) observe any benefit from thiopentone-induced coma in infants with severe birth asphyxia.

STATUS EPILEPTICUS. Details of 5 cases of status epilepticus successfully treated with thiopentone and pentobarbitone after conventional anticonvulsants failed.— *Can. J. neurol. Sci.*, 1980, *7*, 291.

Further references: M. Partinen *et al., Br. med. J.*, 1981, *282*, 520.

Preparations

Thiopental Sodium for Injection *(U.S.P.)*

Thiopentone Injection *(B.P.)*. Contains thiopentone sodium.

Proprietary Preparations

Intraval Sodium *(May & Baker, UK). Injection*, powder for reconstitution, thiopentone sodium, 0.5 and 1 g ampoules, 2.5 and 5 g vials.

IMS Thiopentone Sodium *(IMS, UK). Injection*, thiopentone sodium 25 mg/mL, available in the Min-I-Mix system. *Injection*, powder for reconstitution, thiopentone sodium, 2.5 or 5 g supplied with solvent (Add-A-Med kit).

Proprietary Names and Manufacturers

Farmotal *(Farmitalia, Ital.)*; Hypnostan *(Fin.)*; Intraval Sodium *(May & Baker, Austral.; May & Baker, S.Afr.; May & Baker, UK)*; Leopental *(Leo, Denm.)*; Nesdonal *(Belg.; Neth.)*; Pentothal or Pentothal Sodium *(Arg.; Abbott, Austral.; Belg.; Abbott, Canad.; Abbott, Denm.; Ital.; Abbott, Norw.; Abbott, Spain; Abbott, Swed.; Switz.; Abbott, UK; Abbott, USA)*; Sandothal *(Sandoz, S.Afr.)*;

Thio-Barbityral *(Switz.)*; Tiobarbital *(Spain)*; Trapanal *(Byk Gulden, Ger.)*.

3125-v

Tribromoethyl Alcohol
Tribromoethanol; Tribromoethanolum. 2,2,2-Tribromoethanol.
$C_2H_3Br_3O$=282.8.

CAS — 75-80-9.

Pharmacopoeias. In *Int.*, *Nord.*, and *Turk.*

Tribromoethyl alcohol was formerly given rectally as a basal anaesthetic and to control convulsions in a solution in amylene hydrate known as bromethol. It could cause hypotension, respiratory depression and paralysis, cardiac depression, and liver impairment. Solutions of bromethol readily decomposed and were highly irritant.

Proprietary Names and Manufacturers
Avertin *(Winthrop, UK)*.

3126-g

Trichloroethylene *(BAN, rINN)*.
Trichlorethylene; Trichlorethylenum; Trichloroethene; Trichloroethylenum.
$CHCl:CCl_2$=131.4.

CAS — 79-01-6.

Pharmacopoeias. In *Aust.*, *Cz.*, *Egypt.*, *Fr.*, *Hung.*, *Ind.*, *Int.*, *Jug.*, *Neth.*, *Nord.*, *Swiss*, and *Turk.*

A clear, colourless or pale blue, mobile liquid with a chloroform-like odour. It contains thymol 0.01% w/w as a preservative and may contain not more than 0.001% w/w of a suitable blue colouring matter to distinguish it from chloroform. B.p. 85° to 88°.

Adverse Effects
Trichloroethylene increases the rate and decreases the depth of respiration and may be followed by apnoea. The sensitivity of the heart to beta-adrenergic activity may increase, possibly with ventricular arrhythmias. Nausea, vomiting and lightheadedness may occur during recovery.
Acute exposure to trichloroethylene outside the anaesthetic environment may be followed by dizziness, lightheadedness, lethargy, nausea, and vomiting; hepatic and renal dysfunction may follow. Fatalities have occurred, although temporary unconsciousness is a more common manifestation.
Chronic poisoning may result in visual disturbances, intolerance to alcohol as manifested by transient redness of the face and neck ('trichloroethylene flush'), impairment of performance, hearing defects, and mild liver dysfunction. Prolonged contact with trichloroethylene can cause dermatitis, eczema, burns, and conjunctivitis.
Dependence has been reported in medical personnel and factory workers who regularly inhale trichloroethylene vapour.
In Great Britain the control exposure limits of trichloroethylene are 100 ppm (long-term); 150 ppm (short-term); suitable precautions should be taken to prevent absorption through the skin. In the *US* the permissible and recommended exposure limits are 100 ppm and 25ppm respectively.
See also Adverse Effects for General Anaesthetics, p.1113.

A review of the toxicity of trichloroethylene.— R. J. Fielder *et al.*, Trichloroethylene, *Health and Safety Executive, Toxicity Review* 6, London, HM Stationery Office, 1982. See also *Trichloroethylene: Health and Safety Precautions*, London, HM Stationery Office, 1985.

ABUSE. Acute liver damage developed in 3 teenagers who inhaled a commercial cleaning fluid containing trichloroethylene and was associated with renal tubular necrosis in 2 of them.— R. D. Baerg and D. V. Kimberg, *Ann. intern. Med.*, 1970, *73*, 713.

A report of hemiparesis and cerebral infarction associated with the sniffing of glue containing trichloroethylene.— M. J. Parker *et al.*, *Archs Dis. Childh.*, 1984, *59*, 675.

A report of 2 cases of sudden death in adolescents associated with inhalation of typewriter correction fluids containing trichloroethylene.— G. S. King *et al.*, *J. Am. med. Ass.*, 1985, *253*, 1604.

EFFECTS ON THE LIVER. Although trichloroethylene is carcinogenic in *mice* an analysis of primary liver cancers during 1951–77 in people living around a manufacturing plant yielded no cases where the sufferer had been employed at the plant, though one former employee had died of oesophageal cancer with secondary liver tumour.— G. M. Paddle, *Br. med. J.*, 1983, *286*, 846.

Precautions
Trichloroethylene is contra-indicated in disease of the heart and is best avoided in patients with liver disease.
Trichloroethylene should not be used in a closed-circuit apparatus because the heat produced by the action of carbon dioxide and water vapour on the soda lime causes the trichloroethylene to react with the soda lime to form dichloroacetylene, which may cause cranial nerve paralysis and possibly death.
Adrenaline and most other sympathomimetic agents, except possibly in very dilute solution for the control of haemorrhage, should not be used during trichloroethylene anaesthesia (see Adrenaline, p.1454).
See also Precautions for General Anaesthetics, p.1113.

Absorption and Fate
Trichloroethylene is rapidly absorbed on inhalation. Some of the inhaled trichloroethylene is slowly eliminated through the lungs; most is metabolised to trichloroethanol and trichloroacetic acid which are excreted in the urine. The latter may be used as an indicator of industrial exposure. It diffuses across the placenta.

Uses and Administration
Trichloroethylene is a weak volatile anaesthetic administered by inhalation. It is a potent analgesic but a poor muscle relaxant. It is not flammable.
Trichloroethylene is used mainly in short surgical procedures where light anaesthesia with good analgesia is required, and is usually given in conjunction with nitrous oxide and oxygen.
A concentration of about 0.5 to 2% of the vapour is required to produce light anaesthesia. To produce analgesia a concentration of 0.35 to 0.5% of trichloroethylene in air is recommended.
Trichloroethylene is used in industry in a less pure form as a solvent for oils and fats, for degreasing metals, and for dry cleaning.

A review of the actions and uses of the long established anaesthetic agents including trichloroethylene.— J.V. Farman, *Br. J. Anaesth.*, 1981, *53*, 3S.

Proprietary Preparations
Trilene *(ICI Pharmaceuticals, UK)*. *Anaesthetic inhalation*, trichloroethylene. Available in bottles of 500 mL.

Proprietary Names and Manufacturers
Triklone *(ICI Mond, UK)*; Trilene *(Austral.; Neth.; S.Afr.; ICI Pharmaceuticals, UK)*.

3127-q

Vinyl Ether *(BAN, USAN)*.
Aether Vinylicus; Divinyl Ether; Divinyl Oxide; Éter Vinílico; Ether Vinylicus. 1,1′-Oxybis-ethene.
$(CH_2:CH)_2O$=70.09.

CAS — 109-93-3.

Pharmacopoeias. In *Br.*, *Braz.*, *Int.*, *Nord.*, and *U.S.*

Divinyl ether, to which has been added about 4% v/v of dehydrated alcohol and not more than 0.01% of *N*-phenyl-1-naphthylamine or other suitable stabiliser. *U.S.P.* specifies not more than 0.025% of a suitable stabiliser.
It is a clear, colourless, flammable liquid with a characteristic odour, and often with a purplish fluorescence derived from the stabiliser. Wt per mL 0.770 to 0.778 g. B.p. 28° to 31°.
Soluble 1 in 100 of water; miscible with alcohol, acetone, chloroform, and ether. When shaken with water the aqueous layer is neutral to litmus. On exposure to air and light it decomposes into formaldehyde and formic acid, ultimately polymerising to a jelly; the rate of decomposition is retarded by the presence of a stabiliser. **Store** at a temperature of 8° to 15° in airtight containers of not more than 200-mL capacity. Protect from light. It should not be used if the container has been opened longer than 48 hours.

CAUTION. *Vinyl ether is very volatile and inflammable and mixtures of its vapour with oxygen, nitrous oxide, or air at certain concentrations are explosive. It should not be used in the presence of an open flame or any electrical apparatus liable to produce a spark. Precautions should be taken against the production of static electrical discharge.*

Vinyl ether is a volatile anaesthetic which has been administered by inhalation. It has about 4 times the potency of ether and has comparable effects although it is less irritating to the respiratory tract.

Proprietary Names and Manufacturers
Vinêther *(Robert et Carrière, Fr.)*; Vinesthene *(May & Baker, UK)*; Vinydan *(Lundbeck, Denm.*; *Byk Gulden, Ger.)*.

Glycerol Glycols and Macrogols

1901-y

Glycerol *(BAN, rINN).*

E422; Glicerol; Glycerin *(USAN)*; Glycerolum.
Propane-1,2,3-triol.
$C_3H_8O_3$=92.09.

CAS — 56-81-5.

Pharmacopoeias. In *Arg., Aust., Belg., Br., Braz., Chin., Cz., Egypt., Eur., Fr., Ger., Hung., Ind., Int., It., Jpn, Mex., Neth., Nord., Pol., Port., Roum., Span., Swiss, Turk.,* and *U.S. Br., Eur., It., Jug.,* and *Swiss* also include Glycerol (85 per cent). *B.P. Vet.* includes Glycerol and Glycerol (85 per cent).

A clear, colourless, hygroscopic, syrupy liquid, odourless or with a slight odour and with a sweet taste.

Miscible with water and alcohol; slightly soluble in acetone; practically insoluble in chloroform, ether, and fixed and essential oils. Solutions in water are neutral to litmus. **Store** in airtight containers.

Adverse Effects

Glycerol's adverse effects are mainly due to its dehydrating effects. When taken by mouth it can produce headache, thirst, nausea, and hyperglycaemia. Glycerol may also produce cardiac arrhythmias and hyperosmolar nonketotic coma. Hyperglycaemia may occur. In addition the injection of large doses may induce haemolysis, haemoglobinuria, and renal failure.

In Great Britain the recommended exposure limits of total glycerol mist are 10 mg per m^3 (long-term) and 20 mg per m^3 (short-term); the limit for respirable glycerol mist is 5 mg per m^3 (long-term).

A report of temporary hearing loss after a glycerol test.— D. E. Mattox and R. L. Goode, *Archs Otolar.*, 1978, *104*, 359.

HAEMOLYSIS. Infusion of glycerol 20% in sodium chloride injection given in doses of 70 g in 30 minutes and 80 g in 60 minutes reduced the intracranial pressure in 2 patients but was associated with severe haemolysis and haemoglobinuria. In one of these patients there was prolonged oliguria. A third patient given 60 g in 15 minutes had slight evidence of haemolysis.— K. Hägnevik *et al.*, *Lancet*, 1974, *1*, 75.

In a review of 500 patients given glycerol by intravenous infusion no side-effects were seen when 50 g in 500 mL of sodium chloride injection was administered over 6 hours daily for 7 to 10 days. Haemolysis was observed in 4 of 70 patients when the rate of infusion was increased.— K. M. A. Welch *et al.* (letter), *Lancet*, 1974, *1*, 416.

Precautions

Glycerol should be administered with caution to diabetic patients and to those at risk of dehydration.

Glycerol, administered by mouth to a patient with glaucoma who had previously undergone partial gastrectomy, gave rise to severe headache, prostration, and diarrhoea; it was suggested that a reduced dosage be given to post-gastrectomy patients.— A. W. Sollom, *Br. J. Ophthal.*, 1972, *56*, 506.

Nonketotic hyperosmolar hyperglycaemia developed in a 29-year-old diabetic man with chronic renal failure following the repeated use of glycerol by mouth for acute glaucoma. He recovered after treatment with hypotonic sodium chloride, albumin, packed red blood cells, insulin, and bicarbonate. Glycerol should be avoided, where possible, in patients likely to develop nonketotic hyperosmolar hyperglycaemia such as maturity-onset elderly diabetics with severe intercurrent disease that may predispose to fluid deprivation. In those patients in whom glycerol therapy is necessary adequate fluid intake should be maintained.— D. E. Oakley and P. P. Ellis, *Am. J. Ophthal.*, 1976, *81*, 469. A similar report in 2 patients, a 66-year-old nondiabetic man and a 63-year-old woman with insulin-dependent maturity-onset diabetes mellitus; both developed fatal nonketotic hyperosmolar hyperglycaemia following administration of glycerol by nasogastric tube for cerebral oedema.— E. S. Sears, *Neurology, Minneap.*, 1976, *26*, 89.

Absorption and Fate

Glycerol is readily absorbed from the intestine and is metabolised to carbon dioxide and glycogen or is used in the synthesis of body fats.

Uses and Administration

When taken by mouth, glycerol is demulcent and mildly laxative. It has an energy value of 18.1 kJ (4.32 kcal) per g. Glycerol is employed as a sweetening agent in mixtures and as an ingredient of some linctuses and pastilles.

Glycerol, by mouth, in doses of about 1 to 1.5 g per kg body-weight, usually as a 50% solution, has been used for reducing intra-ocular pressure in glaucoma and before cataract surgery. It is applied topically to reduce corneal oedema.

Glycerol is given intravenously to reduce intracranial pressure in various conditions. It is usually administered by infusion as a 10% solution in sodium chloride injection 0.9% in a dose of 1.2 g per kg body-weight daily for up to 6 days. Oral administration has also been tried.

When glycerol is given by rectal injection or in suppositories it promotes peristalsis and evacuation of the lower bowel by virtue of its irritant action.

Externally, glycerol is used as a humectant and for its emollient properties in dermatological preparations, toilet creams, and jellies. It is employed, in the form of Kaolin Poultice or Magnesium Sulphate Paste, for its hygroscopic action in the treatment of boils, carbuncles, and other inflammatory conditions. Glycerol is used as the solvent vehicle for some ear-drops. It has a weak antimicrobial action.

Sterile glycerol or glycerol-based jellies are used as lubricants for endoscopic instruments.

A brief discussion of cryopreservation with reference to glycerol.— *Lancet*, 1985, *1*, 678.

CEREBROVASCULAR DISORDERS AND RAISED INTRACRANIAL PRESSURE. A brief discussion of glycerol in the management of increased intracranial pressure.— G. Heinemeyer, *Clin. Pharmacokinet.*, 1987, *13*, 1.

Glycerol 1.2 g per kg body-weight was given every 24 hours by intravenous injection as a 10% solution in glucose injection or sodium chloride injection or 1.5 g per kg by mouth in 6 divided doses daily to 36 patients with cerebral infarction. Four patients in coma died and of the remaining 32 patients, 30 improved during and after the glycerol. The mean CSF pressure decreased after 4 days' treatment. Six patients with brain tumours and CNS oedema improved when given glycerol. Another 6 with CNS oedema due to anoxic encephalopathy showed no improvement.— J. S. Meyer *et al.*, *Lancet*, 1971, *2*, 993. See also M. Buckell and L. Walsh, *Lancet*, 1964, *2*, 1151.

In a study of 54 patients with acute cerebral infarction, the 29 who were given daily infusions of glycerol 50 g in 500 mL of glucose 5% in 25% physiological saline improved more rapidly and to a significantly greater extent than did the 25 who received the solution without glycerol: 75% of those given glycerol improved clinically compared with 56% of those given placebo. Treatment for 6 days appeared to be more effective than for 4 days. No benefit was seen in 2 of 5 patients who were given glycerol and survived spontaneous intracerebral haemorrhage.— N. T. Mathew *et al.*, *Lancet*, 1972, *2*, 1327.

A dose of 500 mL of glycerol 10% in sodium chloride injection was infused over 24 hours together with sodium chloride injection or glucose injection and repeated for 6 days in 30 patients with cerebral infarction. This was compared with dexamethasone 4 mg intramuscularly every 6 hours for 6 days together with the infusions of sodium chloride or glucose injection in 31 similar patients. Glycerol produced greater neurological and clinical improvement; 67% of those given glycerol improved clinically compared with 33% of those given dexamethasone. There was 1 death in the glycerol group and 6 deaths in the dexamethasone group. Glycerol was considerably superior to dexamethasone although there was still a risk of haemolysis with the 10% solution.— V. Gilsanz *et al.*, *Lancet*, 1975, *1*, 1049. See also R. Guisado and A. I. Arieff (letter), *ibid.*, *2*, 183.

In a double-blind study in 27 patients with stroke less than 6 hours before treatment there was no difference in mortality or improvement in neurological score between 12 treated intravenously with 500 mL of 10% glycerol in glucose solution over 6 hours on 6 days and 15 treated with glucose as a placebo.— O. Larsson *et al.*, *Lancet*, 1976, *1*, 832.

Clinical experience indicated that treatment with glycerol 1 g per kg body-weight given by mouth every 6 hours produced symptomatic improvement in patients with raised intracranial pressure despite the reduction in pressure not being sustained throughout all the dose interval. A 4-hourly schedule was evaluated in one patient and found paradoxically to increase further the intracranial pressure.— D. A. Rottenberg *et al.*, *Neurology, Minneap.*, 1977, *27*, 600.

Follow-up 4 months after a placebo-controlled double-blind study involving 51 elderly patients treated 48 hours after the onset of an ischaemic cerebral infarction with glycerol 25 g in 250 mL of a sodium chloride and glucose solution by intravenous infusion twice daily for 6 days indicated that improvement occurred in patients with a moderate neurological deficit but no improvement occurred in those with a severe disability.— R. Fawer *et al.*, *Stroke*, 1978, *9*, 484.

A double-blind study in which 85 stroke patients received glycerol and 88 a placebo demonstrated a reduction in deaths within the first week in the glycerol group. Subsequent mortality up to 12 months was similar in the 2 groups. The dose of glycerol was 500 mL of a 10% solution in sodium chloride injection (0.9%) given intravenously over 4 hours daily for 6 consecutive days.— A. J. Bayer *et al.*, *Lancet*, 1987, *1*, 405.

An overview analysis of the published randomised controlled trials of glycerol in acute stroke, including the study by Bayer *et al.*, showed that this treatment reduced the odds of death within 6 weeks by about 36%, but that there was a nonsignificant reduction of 21% within 4 months to 1 year of the stroke.— P. Sandercock, *Br. med. J.*, 1987, *295*, 1224.

DIAGNOSIS OF MÉNIÈRE'S DISEASE. A single dose of glycerol 1.5 g per kg body-weight by mouth caused a transient reduction of the hearing loss in patients with the early stages of Ménière's disease. No effect occurred in patients with other types of cochlear deafness. Clinically this effect could be used to indicate the reversibility of Ménière's disease and that treatment with diuretic drugs may be of value.— I. Klockhoff and U. Lindblom, *Acta oto-lar.*, 1967, *Suppl.* 224, 449. See also J. M. Snyder, *Archs Otolar.*, 1971, *93*, 155. A theory as to how the test works.— L. Naftalin and K. J. H. Mallett (letter), *Lancet*, 1978, *2*, 103.

Glycerol was capable of improving cochlear function in patients suffering from fluctuating sensorineural hearing loss other than that caused by Ménière's disease and therefore the glycerol test could not be considered to be specific for the diagnosis of Ménière's disease.— D. Celestino and A. Orofino, *J. Lar. Otol.*, 1978, *92*, 467.

A comment that side-effects are not uncommon with this test and these have precluded its acceptance in many centres.— G. B. Brookes, *Drugs*, 1983, *25*, 77 (for a reference to hearing loss associated with a glycerol test see under Adverse Effects).

INTRA-OCULAR PRESSURE. In a controlled study involving 176 extractions of senile cataract, one-half the patients were given glycerol, about 180 mL of a 50% solution in flavoured physiological saline, and the other half water as a control. In the latter group vitreous loss during surgery was 5 times more frequent than in the glycerol-treated subjects in whom reduced ocular tension was associated with correspondingly reduced risk of vitreous loss.— P. Awasthi *et al.*, *Br. J. Ophthal.*, 1967, *51*, 130. See also T. Jerndal and V. Kriisa, *ibid.*, 1974, *58*, 927.

LIVER DISORDERS. Experience in 5 patients with fulminant hepatic failure showed that glycerol 50 g per 24 hours intravenously as a 10% solution produced no improvement in the encephalopathy. Higher doses might cause intravascular haemolysis.— C. O. Record *et al.*, *Br. med. J.*, 1975, *2*, 540.

TRIGEMINAL NEURALGIA. Although some neurosurgeons have produced pain relief from trigeminal neuralgia by instilling glycerol among the trigeminal rootlets (retrogasserian glycerol) Sweet (*New Engl. J. Med.*, 1986, *315*, 174) commented that others had not achieved such success. The viscosity and osmolality appear to be crucial factors in the success of this treatment according to Waltz and Copeland (*ibid.*, *316*, 693) who had observed a greatly increased failure rate when the supply of glycerol was changed to a preparation with reduced viscosity and osmolality.

USE IN THE EAR. Glycerol was often effective in preventing the development of scales on the skin of the meatal canal. Glycerol was as effective as any other preparation for the softening of ear wax.— *Br. med. J.*, 1972, *4*, 623.

Preparations

Glycerin Ophthalmic Solution *(U.S.P.)*

Glycerin Oral Solution *(U.S.P.)*

Glycerin Suppositories *(U.S.P.)*. Contain glycerol solidified with sodium stearate.

Glycerin and Rose Water. Glycerol 2 and rose water 3. An agreeable emollient for the skin.

Glycerol Cream Oily *(A.P.F.)*. Crem. Glycer. Oleos; Oily Glycerin Cream. Glycerol 20 g, calcium hydroxide solution 32 mL, arachis oil 22 g, wool fat 26 g.

Glycerol Suppositories *(B.P.)*. Glycerin Suppositories. Prepared from gelatin, glycerol, and water. They contain about 70% w/w of glycerol and 14% w/w of gelatin. In tropical and subtropical countries up to 18% w/w of gelatin may be included. *A.P.F.* has 18% w/w gelatin.

Glyco-gelatin Gel *(A.P.F.)*. Glyco-gelatin Base; Glycogelatin Suppository Base; Glycogelatin Pessary Base. Gelatin 25 g, glycerol 40 g, water to 100 g.

Proprietary Preparations

Polyfusor Glycerol and Saline Intravenous Infusion *(Boots, UK)*. *Intravenous infusion*, glycerol 10 parts (by weight), sodium chloride 0.9% 100 parts (by volume) in containers of 500 mL. Contains 143 mmol per litre of sodium and of chloride.

Massé Breast Cream *(Ortho-Cilag, UK)*. *Cream*, glycerol and hydrous wool fat in an emollient basis.

Proprietary Names and Manufacturers

Babylax *(Dentinox, Ger.)*; Bulboid *(Switz.)*; Cristal *(Switz.)*; Epiwash *(S.Afr.)*; Fleet Babylax *(Fleet, USA)*; Glax *(Llano, Spain)*; Glycerotone *(Belg.; Faure, Fr.)*; Glycilax *(Engelhard, Ger.)*; Glykoderm *(DAK, Denm.)*; Glyrol *(Coopervision, USA)*; Glysolax *(Switz.)*; Luxoral *(Allergan, Ital.)*; Ophthalgan *(Ayerst, USA)*; Osmoglyn *(Alcon Laboratories, USA)*; Practomil *(Vifor, Switz.)*; Pricerine *(Unichema, UK)*; Sopol Soap Substitute *(Austral.)*; Supo-Gliz *(FFF, Spain)*; Vitrosups *(Llorens, Spain)*; Wibi *(Alcon, Austral.; Alcon, Canad.)*.

The following names have been used for multi-ingredient preparations containing glycerol—Egozite *(Ego, Austral.)*; HEB 'A' (Anerythene) *(Waterhouse, UK)*; Hydraderm *(Sigma, Austral.)*; Magnoplasm *(Faulding, Austral.)*; Massé Breast Cream *(Ortho-Cilag, UK)*; Micolette *(Ayerst, UK)*; Micralax *(Smith Kline & French, UK)*; Murine *(Abbott, Austral.; Ross, USA)*; Murine Ear Drops *(Ross, USA)*; Otipyrin *(Kramer, USA)*; Relaxit *(Pharmacia, UK)*.

1902-j

Glycols

Glycols are dihydric alcohols in which the 2 hydroxyl groups are attached to different carbon atoms in a hydrocarbon chain. They occur as almost colourless and odourless liquids with a low vapour pressure. The lower glycols are distinctly hygroscopic, are soluble in water, and are excellent solvents for essential oils, dyes, and a number of gums and resins. Their hygroscopic properties and low evaporation-rate make them valuable as moistening and softening agents. Some of the glycols, particularly ethylene glycol, are used in antifreeze solutions. Some wines have been sweetened illicitly with glycols.

The toxic effects of the glycols following ingestion are similar to those of alcohol, with depression of the CNS, nausea, vomiting, and degenerative changes in the liver and kidney.

The relative toxicity of glycols is reported to increase in the following ascending order: propylene glycol, triethylene glycol, diethylene glycol, ethylene glycol; glycerol is less toxic than propylene glycol. The glycol ethers are reported to be more toxic than their corresponding parent glycols.

With the exception of propylene glycol, the toxicity of the glycols renders them unsuitable for use in pharmaceutical preparations for internal administration, though they are used to some extent in weak concentrations in the cosmetics industry; they should not be used in preparations to be applied extensively. They are metabolised to carboxylic acids in the body.

Some references to the toxicity of glycols and to its treatment: J. A. Vale *et al.*, *Br. med. J.*, 1982, *284*, 557; *Lancet*, 1985, *2*, 254; B. M. Buckley and J. A. Vale, *Prescribers' J.*, 1986, *26*, 110.

1908-x

Propylene Glycol *(BAN, USAN)*.

Glicol Propilênico; Propilenoglicol; Propyleneglycolum. (±)-Propane-1,2-diol.
$CH_3.CHOH.CH_2OH=76.10$.

CAS — 57-55-6; 4254-15-3 (+); 4254-14-2 (−); 4254-16-4 (±).

Pharmacopoeias. In *Aust., Belg., Br., Braz., Cz., Egypt., Eur., Fr., Ger., Hung., Ind., Int., It., Jpn, Jug., Neth., Nord., Port., Swiss, Turk.*, and *U.S.* Also in *B.P. Vet.*

A clear, colourless, odourless or almost odourless, viscous, hygroscopic liquid with a slightly sweet taste, resembling that of glycerol.

Miscible with water, acetone, alcohol, and chloroform; soluble in ether; immiscible with fixed oils but it will dissolve some essential oils. **Store** in airtight containers.

Adverse Effects

Probably owing to its rapid breakdown and excretion, propylene glycol is much less toxic than the other glycols. It produces some local irritation on application to mucous membranes and on subcutaneous or intramuscular injections. There have been reports of hypersensitivity reactions, CNS depression, lactic acidosis, hyperosmolality, and renal failure.

Chloramphenicol sodium succinate 5% in Ringer's solution and propylene glycol 10% both caused irreversible deafness when instilled into the middle-ear cavity in *guinea pigs*. It was recommended that propylene glycol should not be used as a solvent for chloramphenicol ear-drops.— T. Morizono and B. M. Johnstone, *Med. J. Aust.*, 1975, *2*, 634.

A report of severe hyperosmolality, lactic acidosis, central nervous system depression, and haemolysis in a 72-year-old woman with impaired renal function who received large amounts of propylene glycol intravenously as a solvent for infusions of glyceryl trinitrate. She was treated with haemodialysis, and hypertonic saline was administered to prevent a sudden drop in osmolality. It was considered that the haemolysis probably occurred because red blood cells and propylene glycol 50% solution were administered through the same intravenous line.— H. Demey *et al.* (letter), *Lancet*, 1984, *1*, 1360.

Hyperosmolality was identified following cardiorespiratory arrest in an 8-month-old infant being treated over more than 70% of his body surface with a silver sulphadiazine preparation containing propylene glycol (Silvadene). A high concentration of propylene glycol was detected in the patient's serum and subsequent investigation demonstrated that propylene glycol increases serum osmolality.— C. L. Fligner *et al.*, *J. Am. med. Ass.*, 1985, *253*, 1606.

Some references to hypersensitivity reactions to propylene glycol: A. A. Fisher *et al.*, *Archs Derm.*, 1971, *104*, 286; I. Pevny and M. Uhlich, *Hautarzt*, 1975, *26*, 252; M. Hannuksela and L. Förström, *Contact Dermatitis*, 1978, *4*, 41.

Further references: G. Martin and L. Finberg, *J. Pediat.*, 1970, *77*, 877 (CNS toxicity in children following ingestion of propylene glycol); K. Arulanantham and M. Genel, *ibid.*, 1978, *93*, 515 (CNS toxicity in children); A. W. Van den Hurk and H.J. Teijen, *Anaesthesia*, 1983, *38*, 1183 (cardiac toxicity); J. L. Black *et al.*, *Br. J. clin. Pharmac.*, 1984, *18*, 349 (interaction with prazosin); D. W. Denning and D. B. Webster, *J. Pharm. Pharmac.*, 1987, *39*, 236 (immunosuppressive effect).

Absorption and Fate

Propylene glycol is absorbed from the gastro-intestinal tract and is converted in the liver to lactate and single carbon compounds. A large proportion is excreted unchanged or as a glucuronide conjugate in the urine.

Uses and Administration

Propylene glycol is widely used as a solvent and as a preservative in pharmaceutical preparations. Preparations made with propylene glycol are less viscous than those made with glycerol. In certain instances it is a better solvent than glycerol, and its power of inhibiting mould growth and fermentation is equal to that of alcohol.

Propylene glycol may be included in spray solutions to stabilise the droplet size. It is used similarly to glycerol as a humectant.

Estimated acceptable daily intake: up to 25 mg per kg body-weight.— Seventeenth Report of the FAO/WHO Expert Committee on Food Additives, *Tech. Rep. Ser. Wld Hlth Org. No. 539*, 1974.

The addition of 10 or 20% propylene glycol to an oil-water system preserved with chlorocresol increased the partitioning of the chlorocresol into the aqueous phase.— Pharm. Soc. Lab. Rep. P/75/24, 1975.

SKIN DISORDERS. A 40 to 60% aqueous solution of propylene glycol with occlusion rapidly cleared scaling skin in ichthyosis. Treatment every 3 to 5 days kept skin free of scales. No toxic reactions occurred.— L. A. Goldsmith and H. P. Baden, *J. Am. med. Ass.*, 1972, *220*, 579.

Twenty patients with tinea versicolor were successfully treated with propylene glycol 50% in water applied twice daily for 2 weeks. Two patients complained of a slight burning sensation of the skin after application.— J. Faergemann and T. Fredriksson, *Acta derm.-vener., Stockh.*, 1980, *60*, 92.

Preparations

Propylene Glycol Cream. Propylene glycol 15 g, cetomacrogol emulsifying wax 15 g, white soft paraffin 10 g, liquid paraffin 10 g, chlorocresol 100 mg, water to 100 g.

1922-a

Macrogols *(BAN, USAN, rINN)*.

PEGs; Polietilenglicoli; Polyäthylenglykole; Polyaethylenglycola; Polyethylene Glycols; Polyoxaetheni; Polyoxyethylene Glycols.
$CH_2(OH).[CH_2.O.CH_2]_m.CH_2OH$.

CAS — 25322-68-3.

Pharmacopoeias. Macrogols of various molecular weights are included in many pharmacopoeias.

B.P. specifies macrogol 300, macrogol 1540, and macrogol 4000. *U.S.N.F.* describes Polyethylene Glycol; requires that it be labelled with the average molecular weight; requires that the molecular weight varies from the labelled value by not more than 5%, 10%, and 12.5% respectively for material of nominal molecular weight below 1000, between 1000 and 7000, and above 7000; and gives a viscosity range at about 99° for 44 grades.

NOTE. Some authorities use the general formula $H.(CH_2.O.CH_2)_n.OH$ to describe macrogols. In using this formula the number assigned to n for a specified macrogol is 1 more than that of m in the general formula $CH_2(OH).[CH_2.O.CH_2]_m.CH_2OH$ which is used to describe the macrogols in this section.

The macrogols are mixtures of condensation polymers of ethylene oxide and water. Those with an average molecular weight of 200 to 700 are liquid and hygroscopic; those with an average molecular weight of more than 1000 vary in consistence from soft unctuous to hard wax-like solids and hygroscopicity diminishes with increasing molecular weight. The average molecular weight is indicated by a number in the name; thus macrogol 400 has an average molecular weight of about 400.

They are **soluble** in water and alcohol. The macrogols are **incompatible** with phenols and may reduce the antimicrobial action of other preservatives. Penicillin and bacitracin are rapidly inactivated by macrogols. Macrogols are also incompatible with sorbitol, tannic acid, and salicylic acid. Some plastics are attacked by macrogols.

Adverse Effects and Precautions

Contact dermatitis in patients receiving topical therapy has occasionally been attributed to the presence of macrogols in the preparations.

When macrogols are taken with electrolytes for bowel cleansing, patients may experience initial gastro-intestinal discomfort with nausea, vomiting, abdominal cramps, and anal irritation.

Patients with renal impairment are at risk of developing metabolic acidosis, hyperosmolality, and renal failure following the absorption of macrogols applied topically. The application of generous amounts to raw surfaces is also a risk.

The FDA cautioned practitioners about the use of topical preparations of macrogols in burn patients with known or suspected renal impairment. Progressive renal impairment would develop as a result of the compromised kidney not being able to excrete the macrogol normally. Animals and humans had demonstrated similar symptoms to those with ethylene glycol with increased serum-calcium concentrations and serum osmolality, metabolic acidosis with a large anion gap and renal failure.— *FDA Drug Bull.*, 1982, *12*, 25.

Absorption and Fate

Higher molecular weight macrogols are not significantly absorbed from the gastro-intestinal tract. The liquid macrogols of lower molecular weight are absorbed and a large proportion is excreted unchanged in the urine. After injection, higher molecular weight macrogols are quickly excreted unchanged in the urine; the liquid macrogols are excreted more slowly and may be partly metabolised. There is evidence of absorption of macrogols following topical application.

Uses and Administration

The macrogols are strongly hydrophilic compounds and are therefore only poor oil-in-water emulsifying agents but they are useful as stabilisers of emulsions. Since they are stable, relatively non-irritant to the skin, and emollient, they are useful as water-miscible bases for ointments. Mixtures of macrogols are used as bases for pessaries and suppositories. Other pharmaceutical uses include aiding the dispersion of insoluble drugs and use as binders, plasticisers and lubricants.

Mixtures of macrogol 3350 with electrolytes are used to empty the bowel before surgery. The formulation is intended to promote evacuation through the osmotic activity of the macrogol but to prevent any fluid and electrolyte imbalance by the added electrolytes in the solution. The dose is 4 litres of an aqueous solution containing 236 g of macrogol 3350 taken in drinks of 200 to 300 mL every 10 minutes. The first bowel movement usually begins within an hour of the first drink. Patients may find it easier to drink the solution if it is chilled. Alternatively, it may be given by nasogastric tube.

Macrogols have been recommended for the neutralisation of phenol if spilt on the skin.

Estimated acceptable daily intake of macrogols: up to 10 mg per kg body-weight.— Twenty-third Report of Joint FAO/WHO Expert Committee on Food Additives, *Tech. Rep. Ser. Wld Hlth Org. No. 648*, 1980.

Some references to the macrogols with electrolytes in bowel irrigation: G. R. Davis *et al.*, *Gastroenterology*, 1980, *78*, 991; D. Lubowski *et al.* (letter), *Med. J. Aust.*, 1985, *142*, 256; J. T. DiPiro *et al.*, *Clin. Pharm.*, 1986, *5*, 153; R. Nelson *et al.* (letter), *Lancet*, 1986, *1*, 1503; P. R. Durie *et al.*, *ibid.*

Preparations

Macrogol Ointment *(B.P.)*. Macrogol '300' 65 g, macrogol '4000' 35 g. Store at a temperature not exceeding 25°. *A.P.F.* has equal parts by wt.

Polyethylene Glycol Ointment *(U.S.N.F.)*. Macrogol '400' 60 g, macrogol '3350' 40 g. If a firmer ointment is required up to 10 g of macrogol 400 may be replaced with macrogol 3350. If it is intended to incorporate 6 to 25% of an aqueous solution, replace 5 g of macrogol 3350 with stearyl alcohol.

The name Polyethylene Glycol Ointment is also applied to Macrogol Ointment (*A.P.F.*).

Proprietary Names and Manufacturers

Blink-N-Clean *(Allergan, USA)*; Breox Polyethylene Glycols *(BP Chemicals, UK)*; Carbowax *(BP Chemicals, UK)*; Lutrol E *(Blagden, UK)*.

Macrogols form one of the ingredients of GoLytely *(Braintree, USA)*.

Haemostatics

1710-g

This section includes compounds that are used for the treatment or prophylaxis of haemorrhage by inhibiting the breakdown of the fibrin clot. It also includes compounds that form a barrier to bleeding or perhaps act on the capillary wall.

Other agents used in the control of bleeding but not covered in this section include various blood and related products, gelatin and collagen, adrenaline and noradrenaline, and astringents such as alum or iron salts.

12315-t

Acexamic Acid *(rINN)*.
Acidum Acexamicum; CY-153; Epsilon Acetamidocaproic Acid. 6-Acetamidohexanoic acid.
$C_8H_{15}NO_3$=173.2.

CAS — 57-08-9.

Acexamic acid is related structurally to the antifibrinolytic agent aminocaproic acid and is used as the sodium or calcium salt. It has been administered topically and by mouth to promote the healing of ulcers and various other lesions. The zinc salt has also been tried.

Proprietary Names and Manufacturers of Acexamic Acid Salts
Copinal *(Vinas, Spain)*; Plastenan *(Armstrong, Arg.; de Bournonville, Belg.; Choay, Fr.; Italfarmaco, Ital.; Boizot, Spain)*.

1711-q

Adrenalone Hydrochloride *(pINNM)*.
Adrenalonium Chloratum; Adrenoni Hydrochloridum. 3′,4′-Dihydroxy-2-methylaminoacetophenone hydrochloride.
$C_9H_{11}NO_3HCl(+xH_2O)$=217.7.

CAS — 99-45-6 (adrenalone); 62-13-5 (hydrochloride, anhydrous).

NOTE. Adrenalone is *USAN*.

Adrenalone hydrochloride has been used as a local haemostatic and vasoconstrictor.

Proprietary Names and Manufacturers
Stryphnon *(Hauser, Denm.)*; Stryphnonasal *(Ger.)*.

12357-g

Aminaphtone
Aminaftone; Aminaphthone. 2-Hydroxy-3-methylnaphtho-1,4-hydroquinone 2-(4-aminobenzoate); 3-Methylnaphthalene-1,2,4-triol 2-(4-aminobenzoate).
$C_{18}H_{15}NO_4$=309.3.

CAS — 14748-94-8.

Aminaphtone has been given by mouth as a haemostatic agent.

Proprietary Names and Manufacturers
Capillarema *(Baldacci, Ital.)*.

1712-p

Aminocaproic Acid *(BAN, USAN, rINN)*.

CY-116; EACA; Epsilon Aminocaproic Acid; JD-177. 6-Aminohexanoic acid.
$C_6H_{13}NO_2$=131.2.

CAS — 60-32-2.

Pharmacopoeias. In *Br., Ind., Nord., Roum.,* and *U.S.*

Odourless or almost odourless, colourless crystals or white crystalline powder. The *B.P.* states that it is **soluble** 1 in 1.5 of water. *U.S.P.* solubilities are: 1 in 3 of water; slightly soluble in alcohol; 1 in 450 of methyl alcohol; practically insoluble in chloroform and ether; freely soluble in acids and alkalis. A 20% solution in water has a pH of 7.5 to 8.0. The *U.S.P.* injection has a pH of 6.0 to 7.6. **Incompatible** with fructose infusion. **Store** in airtight containers.

Adverse Effects

Aminocaproic acid may cause diarrhoea, headache, hypotension, dizziness, tinnitus, skin rash, nausea, abdominal pain, conjunctival suffusion, and nasal stuffiness.

Painful myopathy, with weakness or fatigue and sometimes myoglobinuria, has occurred in patients generally receiving high doses or therapy lasting more than 4 weeks. Recovery usually follows withdrawal of treatment though it may be slow; occasionally the condition may progress to renal failure.

Aminocaproic acid may inhibit the lysis of existing clots; ureteric clots may result in intrarenal obstruction.

Rapid intravenous injection may cause hypotension, bradycardia, or arrhythmia.

EFFECTS ON THE BLOOD. Some reports of thrombosis associated with aminocaproic acid: D. T. Purtilo *et al.* (letter), *Lancet,* 1975, *1,* 755; E. P. Hoffman and A. H. Koo, *Radiology,* 1979, *131,* 687; M. D. Hayhurst (letter), *S. Afr. med. J.,* 1983, *63,* 797.

EFFECTS ON MENTAL FUNCTION. An acute delirious state in one patient was associated with aminocaproic acid given intravenously as a bolus.— A. J. Wysenbeek *et al.* (letter), *Lancet,* 1978, *1,* 221.

EFFECTS ON THE MUSCLES. There have been a number of cases of reversible myopathy reported with aminocaproic acid. In presenting their case, Brown *et al.* (*J. Neurosurg.,* 1982, *57,* 130) reviewed the other 18 cases that had been reported. Daily doses ranged from 10 to 49 g and treatment lasted for 22 to 90 days. Five of the 19 were reported to have had myoglobinuria and 3 of the 19 acute reversible tubular necrosis. Vanneste and van Wijngaarden (*Eur. Neurol.,* 1982, *21,* 242) also reviewed 9 of the reported cases when they reported their patient who had experienced myopathy and myoglobinuria after 6 weeks' treatment with aminocaproic acid 26 to 36 g daily. They considered that the myopathy was most probably due to a direct dose-critical toxic effect on the muscle fibre.

EFFECTS ON THE NERVOUS SYSTEM. A report of dizziness, weakness, and a grand mal seizure associated with administration of a 6-g infusion of aminocaproic acid in a man with mild haemophilia.— S. E. Feffer *et al., J. Am. med. Ass.,* 1978, *240,* 2468.

EFFECTS ON SEXUAL FUNCTION. Six reports of inhibited ejaculation in haemophiliac patients associated with ingestion of aminocaproic acid. The effect had so far been completely reversible.— B. E. Evans and L. M. Aledort (letter), *New Engl. J. Med.,* 1978, *298,* 166.

Precautions

Aminocaproic acid is contra-indicated in patients with active intravenous clotting and caution is necessary in any condition which may predispose to thrombosis. Use in disseminated intravascular coagulation is potentially dangerous and may result in serious thrombosis. If aminocaproic acid has to be used in this condition, it should be accompanied by heparin.

Aminocaproic acid should be withdrawn if patients develop muscle pain or weakness.

Aminocaproic acid should be used with care in upper urinary-tract bleeding because there is a risk of intrarenal obstruction, particularly in haemophiliacs. Doses should be reduced in renal impairment. Caution is also advised in patients with hepatic or cardiac disorders. Rapid intravenous injection should be avoided.

The risk of clotting may be increased in patients also taking oestrogen-containing oral contraceptives but clinical reports of this are lacking.

Absorption and Fate

Aminocaproic acid is readily absorbed from the gastro-intestinal tract and peak plasma concentrations are reached within 2 hours. It is widely distributed and is rapidly excreted in the urine mainly unchanged, the greater part of a single dose being eliminated within 12 hours.

Uses and Administration

Aminocaproic acid is an antifibrinolytic agent. It acts principally by inhibiting plasminogen activators and to a lesser degree by inhibiting plasmin. It is used only in haemorrhage associated with excessive fibrinolysis. Conditions in which it may be used include haemorrhage occurring in some forms of surgery or as a result of obstetric complications, in selected cases of menorrhagia or haematuria, in neoplasms such as metastatic carcinoma of the prostate and leukaemia, and in liver disorders. It has also been used in the prophylaxis of hereditary angioedema. It may be used before and after dental extraction in patients with congenital bleeding disorders.

Aminocaproic acid may be given by mouth or, after dilution, by slow intravenous infusion. An initial dose of 5 g is followed by 1 to 1.25 g every hour to maintain a plasma concentration of about 130 µg per mL. Alternatively 3 to 6 g has been given 4 to 6 times daily, although in the *USA* it is recommended that the maximum dose over 24 hours should not exceed 30 g. Dosage should be reduced in renal impairment.

A review of aminocaproic acid.— M. Verstraete, *Drugs,* 1985, *29,* 236.

ANGIOEDEMA. A discussion of hereditary angioedema and its management. Although it is not certain how aminocaproic acid works in this disorder, it has been proposed that local trauma may lead to plasmin activation which in turn may lead to activation of complement component C1 which may precipitate attacks. Antifibrinolytic agents may prevent attacks by inhibiting plasmin activation. For long-term prophylaxis of attacks almost all patients would respond to aminocaproic acid 8 to 10 g daily; in general, adults do not respond to less than 7 g daily. Short-term preventative therapy has been used succesfully in several patients, starting 2 to 3 days before surgery.— M. M. Frank *et al., Ann. intern. Med.,* 1976, *84,* 580.

HAEMORRHAGIC DISORDERS. Aminocaproic acid and cryoprecipitate produced improvement in the severe coagulopathy of the Kasabach-Merritt syndrome in one patient; the syndrome is characterised by thrombocytopenia with haemangiomas.— R. P. Warrell and S. J. Kempin, *New Engl. J. Med.,* 1985, *313,* 309.

Cerebral haemorrhage. See under Tranexamic Acid, p.1134.

Hyphaemia. Beneficial results from treatment with aminocaproic acid in traumatic hyphaemia: E. R. Crouch and M. Frenkel, *Am. J. Ophthal.,* 1976, *81,* 355; J. J. McGetrick *et al., Archs Ophthal., N.Y.,* 1983, *101,* 1031.

Preparations

Aminocaproic Acid Effervescent Oral Powder *(B.P.)*

Aminocaproic Acid Injection *(U.S.P.)*

Aminocaproic Acid Oral Solution *(B.P.)*. Aminocaproic Acid Mixture

Aminocaproic Acid Syrup *(U.S.P.)*

Aminocaproic Acid Tablets *(U.S.P.)*

Proprietary Names and Manufacturers

Amicar *(Lederle, Austral.; Lederle, Canad.; Lederle, S.Afr.; Lederle, USA)*; Capracid *(Bonomelli, Ital.)*; Capralense *(Fr.)*; Capramol *(Belg.; Choay, Fr.; Ital.; Switz.)*; Caproamin *(Fides, Spain)*; Caprolisin *(Malesci, Ital.)*; Ekaprol *(Difrex, Austral.)*; Epsamon *(Switz.)*; Epsikapron *(S.Afr.; Kabi, Swed.; Switz.; KabiVitrum, UK)*; Hemocaprol *(Delagrange, Fr.; Delagrange, Spain; Switz.)*; Ipsilon *(Arg.)*.

1713-s

Aminomethylbenzoic Acid

PAMBA. 4-Aminomethylbenzoic acid.
$C_8H_9NO_2=151.2$.

CAS — 56-91-7.

Pharmacopoeias. In *Chin.* which specifies the monohydrate.

Aminomethylbenzoic acid has similar actions and uses to aminocaproic acid (see above). Up to 2 g by mouth or 600 mg by intramuscular or slow intravenous injection has been given daily in divided doses; it has also been given by intravenous infusion in a dosage of 100 mg per hour.

Proprietary Names and Manufacturers
Gumbix *(Kali-Chemie, Ger.)*.

1714-w

Aprotinin *(BAN, USAN, rINN).*

Bayer A-128; Riker 52G; RP-9921. A single-chain polypeptide derived from bovine tissues consisting of 58 amino-acid residues and having a molecular weight of about 6500. It is extracted under conditions designed to minimise microbial contamination and then purified by a suitable process such as gel filtration.

CAS — 9087-70-1.

Pharmacopoeias. In *Br.*

A clear colourless liquid or an almost white hygroscopic powder. The *B.P.* Injection has a pH of 5.0 to 7.0 and is sterilised by filtration. Aprotinin has been reported to be **incompatible** with corticosteroids and nutrient solutions containing amino acids or fat emulsions.

Store in airtight tamper-evident containers.

Units

Potency is expressed in terms of kallikrein (kallidinogenase) inactivator units. One unit inactivates about 500 ng of trypsin, and is contained in 140 ng of the pure substance. Potency is also expressed in terms of trypsin inactivation.

Adverse Effects

Aprotinin is usually well tolerated but nausea and vomiting, diarrhoea, muscle pains, and blood-pressure changes have occurred. Allergic reactions such as erythema, urticaria, and bronchospasm have occasionally been reported. Anaphylaxis has also occurred.

After one year's successful treatment of a diabetic patient with aprotinin and insulin given subcutaneously, loss of effect from the aprotinin was accompanied by development of lipohypertrophy; this was not seen during prior or subsequent use of insulin alone. On continuing treatment glomerulonephritis was detected. It was suggested that development of antibodies against aprotinin might explain these effects.— F. Boag *et al.* (letter), *New Engl. J. Med.*, 1985, *312*, 245.

ALLERGY. Two of 136 courses of aprotinin led to acute allergic reactions; one patient experienced acute anaphylaxis the other an acute urticarial reaction. Such patients might be detected by challenging their reactivity using aprotinin eye-drops.— J. G. Freeman *et al.*, *Curr. med. Res. Opinion*, 1983, *8*, 559. A severe anaphylactic reaction occurred in one patient after the intravenous administration of aprotinin despite negative ocular sensitivity tests.— G. A. LaFerla and W. R. Murray, *Br. med. J.*, 1984, *289*, 1176.

EFFECTS ON THE BLOOD. Consumptive coagulopathy occurred in 2 patients with pancreatitis treated with aprotinin.— M. L. Lewis (letter), *Br. med. J.*, 1974, *3*, 741.

PANCREATITIS. In a study of aprotinin therapy as prophylaxis against postoperative pancreatitis 11 of 49 patients who received aprotinin developed pancreatitis compared with 5 of 50 who received placebo.— D. B. Skinner *et al.*, *J. Am. med. Ass.*, 1968, *204*, 945.

Absorption and Fate

Aprotinin is not absorbed from the gastro-intestinal tract. After intravenous injection or infusion of aprotinin there is an initial rapid clearance. It is excreted in the urine in an inactive form.

Uses and Administration

Aprotinin inhibits proteolytic enzymes including kallidinogenase and trypsin. It also inhibits plasmin and some plasminogen activators.

It has been used in the treatment of haemorrhage due to hyperfibrinolysis and in some types of shock.

In haemorrhage due to hyperfibrinolysis up to 500 000 kallikrein inactivator units may be given immediately by slow intravenous injection followed by 200 000 units every hour by continuous intravenous infusion until haemorrhage is controlled. Similar doses are used in the management of shock. In disseminated intravascular coagulation with secondary hyperfibrinolysis, doses up to 1 000 000 units or more may be necessary. For prophylaxis before upper abdominal surgery in patients with hyperfibrinolysis, 200 000 units may be given pre-operatively by slow intravenous injection and 200 000 units should be given every 4 hours by continuous intravenous infusion or slow intravenous injection on the day of the operation and for the next 2 days. Because it inhibits proteolytic enzymes aprotinin has also been used in acute pancreatitis, although it is doubtful if it produces any benefit.

Aprotinin given by infusion before surgery and continued throughout the operation reduced blood loss in 11 patients undergoing repeat open heart surgery when compared with controls. Also 7 of the 11 patients in the aprotinin group did not require any additional donor blood. The dose of aprotinin was 280 mg as a loading dose given over 20 minutes before opening the previous wound then a continuous infusion of 70 mg per hour until skin closure at the end of the operation. An additional 280 mg was added to the prime volume of the oxygenator.— D. Royston *et al.*, *Lancet*, 1987, *2*, 1289.

A review of aprotinin.— M. Verstraete, *Drugs*, 1985, *29*, 236.

For the use of aprotinin in patients resistant to high doses of insulin, see under Resistance to Insulin, p.394.

PANCREATITIS. Aprotinin has been tried in the treatment of acute pancreatitis with the intention of inhibiting proteolytic activity. Although Trapnell *et al.* (*Br. J. Surg.*, 1974, *61*, 177) reported that aprotinin reduced the mortality in acute pancreatitis other studies have not shown that aprotinin offers any benefit (MRC Multicentre Trial, *Lancet*, 1977, *2*, 632 and *Gut*, 1980, *21*, 334; C.W. Imrie *et al.*, *Gut*, 1977, *18*, A957; C.W. Imrie *et al*, *Gut*, 1980, *21*, A457).

Preparations

Aprotinin Injection *(B.P.)*. Store at a temperature not exceeding 25° and protect from light.

Proprietary Preparations

Trasylol *(Bayer, UK)*. *Injection*, aprotinin 20 000 kallidinogenase inactivator units/mL, in ampoules of 5 and 10 mL.

Proprietary Names and Manufacturers

Antagosan *(Hoechst, Fr.; Behringwerke, Ger.; Istituto Behring, Ital.; Jpn)*; Antikrein *(Jpn)*; Gordox *(Hung.)*; Inhibin *(Thiemann, Ger.)*; Inibil *(Sclavo, Ital.)*; Iniprol *(Choay, Fr.; Italfarmaco, Ital.)*; Kir *(Lepetit, Ital.)*; Midran *(Manetti Roberts, Ital.; S.Afr.)*; Onquinin *(Jpn)*; Repulson *(Jpn)*; Trasylol *(Arg.; Bayer, Austral.; Belg.; Miles, Canad.; Bayer, Denm.; Bayer, Ger.; Bayer, Ital.; Neth.; Bayer, Norw.; Bayer, S.Afr.; Bayer, Spain; Bayer, Swed.; Bayer, Switz.; Bayer, UK)*; Trazinin *(Jpn)*; Tzalol *(Bayropharm, Ital.)*; Zymofren *(Specia, Fr.)*.

12419-b

Batroxobin *(rINN).*

An enzyme obtained from the venom of the viper *Bothrops atrox.*

CAS — 9039-61-6 (batroxobin); 9001-13-2 (haemocoagulase).

NOTE. Batroxobin has also been obtained from *Bothrops moojeni*; a similar preparation is derived from *Bothrops jararaca.* The name haemocoagulase (hemocoagulase) is used for a preparation of batroxobin with a factor-X activator.

Batroxobin is reported to act on fibrinogen to produce a fibrin monomer that can be converted by thrombin to a fibrin clot. It has been used both as a haemostatic and, in larger doses, to induce a hypofibrinogen state. When used as a haemostatic it is usually given with a factor-X activator as haemocoagulase.

Proprietary Names and Manufacturers of Batroxobin or Haemocoagulase
Botropase *(Ravizza, Belg.; Ravizza, Ital.; Rovi, Spain; Ravizza, Switz.)*; Defibrase *(Serono, Ger.; Pentapharm, Switz.)*; Defibrol *(Swed.)*; D-Fibrol *(UK)*; Hemostase *(USA)*; Reptilase *(Merck-Clévenot, Fr.; Knoll, Ger.; Lepetit, Ital.; Llorente, Spain; Kramer-Synthelabo, Switz.; Pentapharm, Switz.)*.

1715-e

Calcium Alginate

E404.

CAS — 9005-35-0.

Pharmacopoeias. In *Fr.* Also in *B.P.C. 1973.*

The calcium salt of alginic acid, a polyuronic acid composed of residues of D-mannuronic and L-guluronic acids. It may be obtained from seaweeds including species of *Laminaria.* It is an odourless or almost odourless, white to pale yellowish-brown powder or fibres.

Practically **insoluble** in water and organic solvents; soluble in dilute solutions of sodium citrate. **Store** in airtight containers.

Uses and Administration

Calcium alginate is an absorbable haemostatic. When applied to bleeding surfaces its fibres act as a matrix for coagulation and swell to a viscous absorbent gel.

Calcium alginate is used in the management of bleeding wounds, as well as leg ulcers, pressure sores, and other exuding wounds.

It is also used in the food industry.

Estimated acceptable daily intake of calcium alginate: up to 25 mg, as alginic acid, per kg body-weight.— Seventeenth Report of the FAO/WHO Expert Committee on Food Additives, *Tech. Rep. Ser. Wld Hlth Org. No. 539*, 1974.

A discussion with case reports on the use of a calcium alginate dressing.— S. Thomas, *Pharm. J.*, 1985, *2*, 188.

Proprietary Preparations

Kaltocarb *(BritCair, UK)*. *Dressing*, calcium alginate fibres and an absorbent layer of activated charcoal cloth.

Kaltostat *(BritCair, UK)*. *Dressing*, calcium alginate fibres.
Wound packing, calcium alginate fibres.

Sorbsan *(Steriseal, UK)*. *Dressing*, calcium alginate fibres.
Wound packing, calcium alginate fibres.

Proprietary Names and Manufacturers

Coalgan-Ouate *(Brothier, Fr.)*; Haemostatiques Pharmadose *(Gilbert, Fr.)*; Kaltocarb *(BritCair, UK)*; Kaltostat *(BritCair, UK)*; Ouate Hemostatique *(Pharmastra, Fr.)*; Sorbsan *(Steriseal, UK)*; Stop Hemo *(Brothier, Fr.)*; Trophiderm *(Brothier, Fr.)*.

1716-l

Carbazochrome *(rINN).*

Adrenochrome Monosemicarbazone. 5,6-Dihydro-3-hydroxy-1-methylindoline-5,6-dione 5-semicarbazone.
$C_{10}H_{12}N_4O_3=236.2$.

CAS — 69-81-8 (carbazochrome); 13051-01-9 (salicylate); 51460-26-5 (sodium sulphonate).

An oxidation product of adrenaline.

Carbazochrome has been given by mouth and by injection as a haemostatic. It has also been used as the salicylate and the sodium sulphonate.

Proprietary Names and Manufacturers of Carbazochrome and its Derivatives
Adcal *(Jpn)*; Adedolon *(Jpn)*; Adenaron *(Jpn)*; Adnamin *(Jpn)*; Adona *(SIT, Ital.; Jpn; Tanabe, Switz.)*; Adorzon *(Jpn)*; Adozon *(Jpn)*; Adrechros *(Jpn)*; Adrenocron *(Arg.)*; Adrenosem Salicylate *(Beecham Laboratories, USA)*; Adrenoxyl *(Labaz, Belg.; Labaz, Fr.; Labaz, Ger.; Labaz, Neth.)*; Adrezon *(Jpn)*; Auzei *(Jpn)*; Blockel *(Jpn)*; Carbazon *(Jpn)*; Chichina *(Jpn)*; Cromadren Zambeletti *(Craveri, Arg.)*; Cromosil *(Zambeletti, Ital.)*; Cromoxin *(R. Rius, Spain)*; Donaseven *(Jpn)*; Emex *(Ital.; Switz.)*; Hubercrom *(Hubber, Spain)*; Olinate *(Jpn)*; Ranobi-V *(Jpn)*; Shiketsumin *(Jpn)*; Tazin *(Jpn)*.

1719-z

Oxidised Cellulose *(BAN)*.

Cellulosic Acid; Oxidized Cellulose *(USAN)*.

CAS — 9032-53-5.

Pharmacopoeias. In *Br., It., Jug.*, and *U.S. U.S.P.* also includes Oxidized Regenerated Cellulose.

A sterile polyanhydroglucuronic acid, prepared by the oxidation of a suitable form of cellulose. It occurs as white or creamy-white gauze, lint, or knitted material, with a faint odour. The *B.P.* specifies not less than 16% and not more than 22% of carboxyl, calculated with reference to the dried substance. *U.S.P.* specifies 16 to 24% of carboxyl.

Soluble in aqueous solutions of alkali hydroxides; practically insoluble in acids and water. **Store** in a cool place in containers sealed to exclude micro-organisms. Protect from light.

Adverse Effects

Foreign body reactions have occurred. Headache, burning, stinging, and sneezing have been reported after use of oxidised cellulose in epistaxis and other rhinological procedures and stinging has been reported after application to surface wounds. Inappropriate use may lead to obstruction or stenosis.

Precautions

Oxidised cellulose should not be used as a surface dressing, except for immediate control of bleeding, as it inhibits epithelialisation; it should not be used for packing or implantation in bone surgery. Its use should be avoided in infected wounds. Silver nitrate or other escharotic chemicals should not be applied prior to use as cauterisation might inhibit absorption of oxidised cellulose. Thrombin is inactivated by oxidised cellulose; it is recommended that oxidised cellulose should not be impregnated with other haemostatics or antibiotics.

Uses and Administration

Oxidised cellulose is an absorbable haemostatic. When applied to a bleeding surface, it swells to form a gelatinous mass that is gradually absorbed by the tissues, usually within 2 to 7 days. Complete absorption of large amounts of such material may take 6 weeks or more. Despite this absorption, removal of oxidised cellulose should be considered once haemostasis is achieved and it should always be removed if it is used in orthopaedic procedures or around the optic nerve.

Oxidised cellulose is employed in surgery as an adjunct in the control of moderate bleeding where suturing or ligation is impracticable or ineffective; it should not be used to control haemorrhage from large arteries.

Oxidised cellulose should be used as the dry material as its haemostatic effect is reduced by moistening.

Proprietary Preparations

Oxycel *(Associated Hospital Supply, UK). Haemostatic gauze*, sterile oxidised cellulose.

Surgicel *(Johnson & Johnson, UK). Haemostatic gauze*, sterile oxidised cellulose.

Proprietary Names and Manufacturers

Oxycel *(Parke, Davis, Austral.; Belg.; Neth.; Norw.; S.Afr.; Associated Hospital Supply, UK)*; Surgicel *(Fr.; Ital.; Johnson & Johnson, UK; Johnson & Johnson, USA)*.

12611-b

Cotarnine Chloride

Cotarnine Hydrochloride; Cotarninium Chloratum.
7,8-Dihydro-4-methoxy-6-methyl-1,3-dioxolo[4,5-*g*]isoquinolinium chloride dihydrate.
$C_{12}H_{14}ClNO_3,2H_2O=291.7$.

CAS — 82-54-2 (cotarnine); 10018-19-6 (chloride).

Pharmacopoeias. In *Aust., Rus.,* and *Span.*

The chloride of cotarnine, an alkaloid obtained by oxidising noscapine with nitric acid.

Cotarnine chloride was formerly used locally and systemically to arrest bleeding.

1720-p

Ethamsylate *(BAN, USAN)*.

Cyclonamine; E-141; Etamsylate *(rINN)*; MD-141. Diethylammonium 2,5-dihydroxybenzenesulphonate.
$C_{10}H_{17}NO_5S=263.3$.

CAS — 2624-44-4.

Pharmacopoeias. In *Chin.*

Adverse Effects

Nausea, headache, and skin rash have occurred. Transient hypotension has been reported following intravenous injection.

EFFECTS ON THE BLOOD. Vere *et al.* (*Br. med. J.*, 1979, *2*, 528) reported that ethamsylate was associated with an increased incidence of deep-vein thromboses in patients undergoing vaginal surgery. Subsequent studies have failed to confirm this finding (R.F. Harrison *et al.*, letter, *Br. med. J.*, 1982, *284*, 901; G.J. Lewis, *ibid.*, 1984, *288*, 899).

PORPHYRIA. Ethamsylate was considered to be unsafe in patients with acute porphyria because it has been shown to be porphyrinogenic in *animals* or *in-vitro* systems.— M.R. Moore and K.E.L. McColl, *Porphyrias, Drug Lists*, Glasgow, Porphyria Research Unit, University of Glasgow, 1987.

Absorption and Fate

Ethamsylate is absorbed from the gastro-intestinal tract. It is excreted unchanged mainly in the urine.

Ethamsylate 500 mg by mouth failed to produce adequate foetal or maternal plasma concentrations in 5 patients in labour. The same dose given intramuscularly to 7 mothers produced concentrations in cord blood that were considered to be within the therapeutic range.— R. F. Harrison and T. Matthews (letter), *Lancet*, 1984, *2*, 296.

Uses and Administration

Ethamsylate is a haemostatic agent that is considered to act on the capillary wall. It is given for the prophylaxis and control of haemorrhages from small blood vessels.

It is administered by intramuscular or intravenous injection in an initial dose of 1 g followed by 500 mg every 4 to 6 hours. The dose by mouth is 500 mg four times a day. Children have been given 250 to 750 mg by injection as the initial dose followed by 250 mg by mouth or injection every 4 to 6 hours. Neonates have been given 12.5 mg per kg body-weight every 6 hours by intramuscular or intravenous injection.

Prevention of periventricular haemorrhage with ethamsylate in very low birthweight infants. The initial dose was 12.5 mg per kg body-weight intravenously or intramuscularly within 1 hour of delivery. This was followed by the same dose every 6 hours intravenously for 4 days to a total dose of 200 mg per kg. There was also a reduction in patent ductus arteriosus in the treated infants.— J. W. T. Benson *et al.*, *Lancet*, 1986, *2*, 1297. See also M. E. I. Morgan, *ibid.*, 1981, *2*, 830; R. W. I. Cooke and M. E. I. Morgan, *Archs Dis. Childh.*, 1984, *59*, 82.

Proprietary Preparations

Dicynene *(Delandale, UK). Tablets*, ethamsylate 250 and 500 mg.

Injection, ethamsylate 125 mg/mL, in ampoules of 2 mL.

Injection (Dicynene 1000), ethamsylate 500 mg/mL, in ampoules of 2 mL.

Proprietary Names and Manufacturers

Aglumin *(Jpn)*; Altodor *(Delalande, Ger.)*; Antihemorragico Fortuny *(Spain)*; Dicinone *(Pensa, Spain)*; Dicynene *(Delandale, UK)*; Dicynone *(Delalande, Fr.; Delalande, Ital.; Om, Switz.)*; Eselin *(Ravizza, Ital.)*; Hemo 141 *(Esteve, Spain)*; Impedil *(Arg.)*.

1723-e

Metacresolsulphonic Acid-Formaldehyde

Dicresulene polymer; *m*-Cresolsulphonic acid-formaldehyde condensation product; Polycresolsulfonate. Dihydroxydimethyldiphenylmethanedisulphonic acid polymer; Methylenebis(hydroxytoluenesulphonic acid) polymer.
$(C_{15}H_{16}O_8S_2)_n$.

Solutions of metacresolsulphonic acid-formaldehyde are highly acidic and are used as local haemostatics and antiseptics. There are a number of vaginal preparations.

Proprietary Names and Manufacturers
Albocresil *(Byk Liprandi, Arg.)*; Albothyl *(Byk Gulden, Ger.)*; Dermido *(Tosse, Ger.)*; Lotagen *(Byk, Neth.)*; Negaderm *(Byk Gulden, Ital.)*; Negatan *(Savage, USA)*; Negatol *(Valpan, Fr.; Byk Gulden, Ital.; Unibios, Spain; Byk Gulden, Switz.)*; Nelex *(Byk Gulden, Denm.; Byk Gulden, Norw.; Byk Gulden, S.Afr.; Byk Gulden, Swed.)*.

1724-l

Naftazone *(BAN, rINN)*.

1,2-Naphthoquinone 2-semicarbazone.
$C_{11}H_9N_3O_2=215.2$.

CAS — 15687-37-3.

Naftazone is a haemostatic agent which appears to increase capillary resistance. It has been suggested for use in the prophylaxis and treatment of various conditions of venous insufficiency and capillary haemorrhage. It has been given in doses of 2.5 to 5 mg three times daily by mouth. It has also been given by injection.

Some references to the use of naftazone: O. Charles and B. Coolsaet, *Annls Urol.*, 1972, *6*, 209 (reduction in bleeding after prostatectomy); I. Berson, *Praxis*, 1977, *66*, 180 (some improvement in varicose conditions).

Proprietary Names and Manufacturers
Haemostop Injection *(Consolidated Chemicals, UK)*; Karbinone *(Biothera-Asperal, Belg.)*; Mediaven *(Syntex, Switz.)*; Metorene *(Pharmainvesti, Spain)*.

1725-y

Russell's Viper Venom

Pharmacopoeias. In *Ind.*

The dried sterile venom obtained from the poison glands of *Vipera russelli* (Viperidae). *Ind. P.* allows also venom from other species of *Viperae*.

Russell's viper venom is a local haemostatic which rapidly activates prothrombin. It was formerly applied as a 1 in 10 000 solution in the treatment of haemorrhage.

13281-w

Sulfonaphtine Glucoside
Naphthionine Glucoside. 4-(β-D-Glucopyranosylamino)naphthalene-1-sulphonic acid.
$C_{16}H_{19}NO_8S$=385.4.

CAS — 1328-93-4 (glucoside, sodium salt).

Sulfonaphtine glucoside was formerly used, as the sodium salt, as a haemostatic agent.

Proprietary Names and Manufacturers
Emostane *(Ital.).*

1726-j

Tranexamic Acid *(BAN, USAN, rINN).*
Acidum Tranexamicum; AMCA; CL-65336; *trans*AMCHA. *trans*-4-(Aminomethyl)cyclohexanecarboxylic acid.
$C_8H_{15}NO_2$=157.2.

CAS — 1197-18-8.

Pharmacopoeias. In *Br., Chin., Jpn,* and *Nord.*

A white, odourless or almost odourless, crystalline powder. Freely **soluble** in water and glacial acetic acid; practically insoluble in alcohol and ether. A 5% solution in water has a pH of 6.5 to 7.5. Solutions for injection are **sterilised** by autoclaving; they are reported to be **incompatible** with benzylpenicillin.

Adverse Effects
Tranexamic acid is considered to be better tolerated than aminocaproic acid. Patients may experience nausea, vomiting, or diarrhoea. There may be a hypotensive reaction to rapid intravenous administration. Like aminocaproic acid, there is a risk of the lysis of existing clots being inhibited, unlike it myopathy does not appear to be a problem.

Precautions
As for Aminocaproic Acid, p.1131.

Absorption and Fate
Tranexamic acid is rapidly absorbed from the gastro-intestinal tract. Up to about 39% of a dose by mouth and at least 90% of a dose by intravenous injection is reported to be excreted in the urine within 24 hours. It diffuses across the placenta.

The pharmacokinetics and bioavailability of tranexamic acid. Absorption did not appear to be affected by food.— Å. Pilbrant *et al., Eur. J. clin. Pharmac.,* 1981, *20,* 65.

PREGNANCY AND THE NEONATE. Serum concentrations of tranexamic acid in 12 healthy pregnant women who received an infusion of 10 mg per kg body-weight 5 to 25 minutes before undergoing caesarean section ranged from 10 to 53 μg per mL at delivery; serum concentrations in the infant's cord ranged from less than 4 μg per mL to 31 μg per mL.— S. Kullander and I. M. Nilsson, *Acta obstet. gynec. scand.,* 1970, *49,* 241.

Uses and Administration
Tranexamic acid is an antifibrinolytic agent. It acts principally by inhibiting plasminogen activators and is used in the treatment of haemorrhage, or threatened haemorrhage, associated with excessive fibrinolysis. It is many times more potent than aminocaproic acid.

Tranexamic acid is used to treat fibrinolytic states that occur in menorrhagia, epistaxis, traumatic hyphaemia, certain neoplasms, obstetric complications, and after various surgical procedures including bladder surgery, prostatectomy, or cervical conisation. It is also used in the management of haemophiliacs undergoing dental extractions and in the prophylaxis of hereditary angioedema. Doses consist of 0.5 to 1 g given 2 to 3 times daily by slow intravenous injection over a period of 5 to 10 minutes or 1 to 1.5 g given by mouth 2 to 3 times daily. These doses should be reduced in patients with renal impairment.

In epistaxis the injection solution may also be applied topically. After prostatectomy or bladder surgery a solution containing 1 g per litre may be used as a daily bladder irrigation for 2 to 5 days.

A review of tranexamic acid.— M. Verstraete, *Drugs,* 1985, *29,* 236.

ADMINISTRATION IN RENAL FAILURE. Following a study of 28 patients with chronic renal disease this dosage scheme was recommended for tranexamic acid: 10 mg per kg body-weight given intravenously, twice daily to patients with a serum-creatinine concentration of 120 to 250 nmol per mL, every 24 hours to patients with a concentration of 250 to 500 nmol per mL, and every 48 hours to patients with a concentration of 500 nmol or more per mL.— L. Andersson *et al., Urol. Res.,* 1978, *6,* 83.

ANGIOEDEMA. Tranexamic acid 1 g given every 6 hours by mouth for 48 hours before surgery and for 48 hours postoperatively enabled 14 patients with hereditary angioedema to undergo dental or surgical procedures. Eight of the patients had experienced 1 or more attacks of angioedema after previous dental extractions without prophylactic therapy.— A. L. Sheffer *et al., J. Allergy & clin. Immunol.,* 1977, *60,* 38.

A report on experience of treating 21 patients with hereditary angioedema over 3½ years. Continuous administration of tranexamic acid 1.5 to 2 g daily has abolished all but the most trivial symptoms. Danazol 300 mg daily is equally successful in abolishing attacks.— P. Naish and J. Barratt (letter), *Lancet,* 1979, *1,* 611.

See also under Urticaria, below.

HAEMORRHAGIC DISORDERS. Tranexamic acid produced improvement in bleeding in 2 patients with α_2-antiplasmin deficiency.— K. Koie *et al., Lancet,* 1978, *2,* 1334; P. Kettle and E. E. Mayne, *J. clin. Path.,* 1985, *38,* 428.

Results of a study in 100 patients undergoing transurethral prostatectomy or endoscopic bladder tumour resection, demonstrating that tranexamic acid reduced the incidence of secondary haemorrhage.— R. A. Miller *et al., Br. J. Urol.,* 1980, *52,* 26.

Cerebral haemorrhage. There have been several studies as well as reviews on antifibrinolytics being used with the intention of reducing rebleeding in subarachnoid haemorrhage. It is difficult to conclude from the reports that these compounds offer any significant benefit. Some references: J. van Rossum *et al., Ann. Neurol.,* 1977, *2,* 242; R. S. Maurice-Williams, *Br. med. J.,* 1978, *1,* 945; H. P. Adams *et al., Archs Neurol., Chicago,* 1981, *38,* 25; M. Ramirez-Lassepas, *Neurology,* 1981, *31,* 316; E. R. Hitchcock, *Br. med. J.,* 1983, *286,* 1299; M. Vermeulen *et al., New Engl. J. Med.,* 1984, *311,* 432.

Gastro-intestinal haemorrhage. Tranexamic acid was no more effective in 76 patients with gastro-intestinal haemorrhage when compared to the 74 who received placebo. When patients with bleeding due to hiatus hernia or oesophageal varices were excluded, treatment failed in 7 of 62 patients given tranexamic acid compared to 17 of 63 given placebo.— F. Cormack *et al., Lancet,* 1973, *1,* 1207. Seven of 103 patients with upper gastro-intestinal haemorrhage given tranexamic acid required surgery, compared with 21 of the 97 controls.— J. C. Biggs *et al., Gut,* 1976, *17,* 729. Another study showing a small beneficial effect.— A. Engqvist *et al., Scand. J. Gastroenterol.,* 1979, *14,* 839.

Tranexamic acid reduced the mortality but not the frequency or severity of recurrent haemorrhage or the operation frequency in a study involving 775 patients admitted with haematemesis or melaena as a medical emergency. Cimetidine treatment was associated with a smaller but still significant reduction in mortality.— D. Barer *et al., New Engl. J. Med.,* 1983, *308,* 1571.

Reduced blood transfusion requirements in gastric and duodenal bleeding in patients given tranexamic acid.— C. C. S. Staël von Holstein *et al., Br. med. J.,* 1987, *294,* 7.

Hyphaemia. Tranexamic acid reduced the incidence of secondary haemorrhage in patients with traumatic hyphaemia.— L. Varnek *et al., Acta Ophthalmol.,* 1980, *58,* 787; R. J. Uusitalo *et al., ibid.,* 1981, *59,* 539.

Pregnancy and the neonate. There were only 6 perinatal deaths and no maternal deaths among 67 women whose deliveries were complicated by abruptio placentae and who were given tranexamic acid 1 g intravenously just before caesarean section. A further 6 women in earlier stages of pregnancy who had less pronounced symptoms were given 1 g four times daily by mouth until delivery and each had a viable foetus delivered with a high Apgar score.— L. Svanberg *et al., Acta obstet. gynec. scand.,* 1980, *59,* 127. The successful management of placental bleeding by tranexamic acid.— M. Walzman and J. Bonnar, *Arch. Tox.,* 1982, *Suppl.* 5, 214.

In a double-blind study in 100 preterm infants tranexamic acid 25 mg per kg body-weight intravenously 6-hourly for 5 days was no more effective than placebo in preventing the development of periventricular haemorrhage although reduced concentrations of fibrin degradation products were found in the blood of treated infants. The results suggested that increased fibrinolysis is not an important mechanism in the pathogenesis of this disorder.— O. J. Hensey *et al., Archs Dis. Childh.,* 1984, *59,* 719.

URTICARIA. Tranexamic acid was no more effective than a placebo in a double-blind crossover study in 17 patients with chronic urticaria.— G. Laurberg, *Acta derm.-vener., Stockh.,* 1977, *57,* 369. Tranexamic acid 1 g given 4 times daily reduced the frequency and severity of attacks in 2 patients with intractable chronic urticaria. The effect was maintained when the dose was reduced to 500 mg twice daily.— D. Tant (letter), *Br. med. J.,* 1979, *1,* 266. See also under Angioedema.

Preparations
Tranexamic Acid Injection *(B.P.)*
Tranexamic Acid Tablets *(B.P.)*

Proprietary Preparations
Cyklokapron *(KabiVitrum, UK). Tablets,* scored, tranexamic acid 500 mg.
Syrup, tranexamic acid 500 mg/5 mL.
Injection, tranexamic acid 100 mg/mL, in ampoules of 5 mL.

Proprietary Names and Manufacturers
Amcacid *(Bonomelli, Ital.)*; Amchafibrin *(Fides, Spain)*; Amstat *(Spain)*; Anvitoff *(Knoll, Ger.; Knoll, Switz.)*; Carxamin *(Jpn)*; Cyclokapron *(Arg.; Belg.)*; Cyklokapron *(Pharmacia, Canad.; KabiVitrum, Denm.; Kabi, Ger.; Neth.; KabiVitrum, Norw.; Kabi, S.Afr.; Kabi, Swed.; KabiVitrum, Switz.; KabiVitrum, UK; Kabivitrum, USA)*; Emorhalt *(Sigurtà, Ital.)*; Exacyl *(Fumouze, Fr.)*; Frénolyse *(Specia, Fr.)*; Hexapromin *(Jpn)*; Hexatron *(Jpn)*; Tranex *(Malesci, Ital.)*; Tranexan *(Jpn)*; Transamin *(Jpn)*; Trasmalon *(Jpn)*; Trasmalon-G *(Jpn)*; Ugurol *(Bayer, Ger.; Bayer, Ital.)*.

Hypothalamic and Pituitary Hormones

5920-h

The pituitary gland or hypophysis is composed of 2 main parts, namely the adenohypophysis and neurohypophysis. The adenohypophysis consists of the anterior lobe and the neurohypophysis of the posterior lobe and the neural stalk, above which lies the hypothalamus. The anterior lobe is linked to the hypothalamus by a portal vascular system but there is no vascular link between the posterior lobe and the hypothalamus.

The following hormones are secreted by the anterior lobe of the pituitary: adrenocorticotrophic hormone or corticotrophin, p.1139; the gonadotrophic hormones, follicle-stimulating hormone and luteinising hormone, p.1144; growth hormone or somatropin, p.1148; lactogenic hormone or prolactin, p.1145; thyroid-stimulating hormone or thyrotrophin, p.1153; and melanocyte-stimulating hormone, p.1145.

Oxytocin and vasopressin are synthesised in the hypothalamus. They become associated with carrier proteins, neurophysins, and are then transported down nerve fibres to the posterior pituitary where they are stored until required. The release of oxytocin and vasopressin appears to be controlled mainly by nervous reflex responses.

The secretion of anterior pituitary hormones, in which the hypothalamus plays a major part, is regulated by a complex interaction between stimulatory and inhibitory neural and hormonal influences. Transmitter substances are secreted within neurones of the hypothalamus, stored in the median eminence, and released into the hypophyseal portal system to reach the anterior pituitary. Extracts of the hypothalamus which contain these substances have been shown to inhibit or stimulate the release of specific anterior pituitary hormones. Conventionally these transmitters are referred to as 'factors' and when their structure is known and they are well established as physiological regulators of anterior pituitary hormone secretion, they are called hormones.

The system regulating growth hormone, or somatropin, for example is relatively well characterised; secretion of somatropin from cells of the anterior pituitary called somatotrophs is stimulated by somatorelin (p.1150) and inhibited by somatostatin (p.1151), both of which are secreted by hypothalamic neurones called neuroendocrine transducers. Secretion of these hypothalamic regulatory hormones in turn appears to be subject to a complex system of regulation, but this is less well understood. The synthesis and release of hypothalamic hormones may be controlled by feedback mechanisms involving target organ hormones, pituitary hormones, and possibly the hypothalamic hormones themselves, as well as by excitatory or inhibitory impulses from different parts of the brain. These impulses may be mediated by dopamine, acetylcholine, gamma-aminobutyric acid, or other neurotransmitters; the hypothalamic hormones and other peptides such as substance P, enkephalins, and endorphins may act as transmitters or modulators in the hypothalamus.

Prolactin and melanocyte-stimulating hormone are thought to be under similar dual systems of hypothalamic regulation although the regulatory factors involved are not yet completely characterised, but it is uncertain whether corticotrophin, thyrotophin, and the gonadotrophic hormones are subject only to stimulatory control by hypothalamic mechanisms. Hypothalamic hormones and factors described below include, in addition to somatorelin and somatostatin: corticotrophin-releasing hormone, p.1140; gonadotrophin-releasing hormone or gonadorelin, p.1142; melanocyte-stimulating-hormone-release-inhibiting factor or melanostatin, p.1146; thyrotrophin-releasing hormone or protirelin, p.1152.

Reviews and studies of the diagnosis of anterior pituitary dysfunction: C. F. Abboud, *Mayo Clin. Proc.*, 1986, *61*, 35; L. M. Sandler *et al.*, *Br. med. J.*, 1986, *292*, 511; A. Grossman *et al.* (letter), *ibid.*, 1272; *Lancet*, 1986, *1*, 839.

Reviews of the management of patients with pituitary disorders during pregnancy: Z. M. van der Spuy, *Postgrad. med. J.*, 1984, *60*, 312; W. M. Hague, *Br. med. J.*, 1987, *294*, 297.

3884-r

Antidiuretic Hormones

The following section includes the natural antidiuretic hormone, Vasopressin; its synthetic forms Argipressin and Lypressin; and some analogues such as Desmopressin, Felypressin, Ornipressin, and Terlipressin. A preparation of the posterior pituitary, Powdered Pituitary (Posterior Lobe), is also included, which possesses both antidiuretic and oxytocic properties.

5922-b

Desmopressin *(BAN, rINN)*.

[1-(3-Mercaptopropionic acid)-8-D-arginine]-vasopressin; [1-Deamino,8-D-arginine]vasopressin.

$C_{46}H_{64}N_{14}O_{12}S_2$=1069.2.

CAS — 16679-58-6.

Pharmacopoeias. In *Br.* and *Cz.*

A white, fluffy powder containing not less than 900 units of desmopressin per mg. **Soluble** in water, alcohol, glacial acetic acid, and methyl alcohol; slightly soluble in chloroform and in ethyl acetate.

Store in well-closed containers at a temperature not exceeding 25°. Protect from light. Under these conditions it may be expected to retain its potency for not less than 3 years.

The *B.P.* requires that preparations should be stored at a temperature of 2° to 8°. The *B.P.* injection has a pH of 3.5 to 5.0 and is sterilised by filtration; the intranasal solution also has a pH of 3.5 to 5.0.

5923-v

Desmopressin Acetate *(BANM, USAN, rINNM)*.

The monoacetate trihydrate of desmopressin.

$C_{46}H_{64}N_{14}O_{12}S_2,C_2H_4O_2,3H_2O$=1183.3.

CAS — 62288-83-9 (anhydrous); 62357-86-2 (trihydrate).

Units

27 units of desmopressin are contained in approximately 27 µg of desmopressin (with 5 mg of human albumin and citric acid) in one ampoule of the first International Standard Preparation (1980).

Adverse Effects and Precautions

As for Vasopressin, p.1138.

The pressor activity of desmopressin is about 2000 times less than that of argipressin and it is generally well tolerated.

Paranoid psychosis after desmopressin therapy for Alzheimer's dementia.— G. B. Collins *et al.* (letter), *Lancet*, 1981, *2*, 808.

Evidence that desmopressin produces thrombocytopenia and platelet aggregation in type IIB von Willebrand's disease and the recommendation that it should not be used in patients with this type of von Willebrand's disease.— L. Holmberg *et al.*, *New Engl. J. Med.*, 1983, *309*, 816. Comment and a report of similar effects in 2 patients with platelet-type (pseudo) von Willebrand's disease, apparently via a different mechanism.— H. Takahashi *et al.* (letter), *ibid.*, 1984, *310*, 722.

Comment on the hypotensive effects of desmopressin given by intravenous infusion. Facial flushing and warmth reflect a vasodilator action. A drop in diastolic blood pressure of about 14 mmHg and an increase in heart-rate of 20 beats per minute are the rule during intravenous infusion of desmopressin in doses of 400 ng per kg body-weight or more.— E. J. P. Brommer *et al.* (letter), *Ann. intern. Med.*, 1985, *103*, 962. See also R. M. Pigache (letter), *Br. J. clin. Pharmac.*, 1984, *17*, 369 (facial flushing).

TOLERANCE. In 3 uraemic patients desmopressin infusion produced an initial shortening of the bleeding time but following repeated infusions this response was reduced and there was even some increase in baseline bleeding times. Two infusions of desmopressin 300 ng per kg body-weight in one day appear to induce a near maximum response; different treatment is required subsequently.— C. Canavese *et al.* (letter), *Lancet*, 1985, *1*, 867.

Absorption and Fate

Desmopressin is absorbed from the nasal mucosa. Following oral administration it is destroyed in the gastro-intestinal tract, although some may be absorbed following very high doses (see under Administration, below).

Confirmation that desmopressin acetate given intranasally induces antidiuresis, in patients with diabetes insipidus, over approximately 12 hours.— P. R. Blackett *et al.*, *Clin. Pharmac. Ther.*, 1981, *29*, 793.

Uses and Administration

Desmopressin as the acetate is used similarly to vasopressin (p.1138) in the diagnosis and treatment of cranial diabetes insipidus. It has greater antidiuretic activity, a more prolonged action, and slight pressor activity compared with vasopressin or lypressin. It is given as a solution intranasally and by injection; the intranasal dose is approximately ten times that required intravenously.

In the control of diabetes insipidus, desmopressin acetate is used intranasally in usual doses of 10 to 40 µg daily as a single dose or in divided doses; children may be given 5 to 30 µg daily. It may also be administered subcutaneously, intramuscularly, or intravenously in a dose of 1 to 4 µg daily; a dose of 0.4 µg may be used in children. Single intranasal or intramuscular doses have been given in the diagnosis of diabetes insipidus and to test renal function.

Desmopressin acetate is also given intranasally in the management of primary nocturnal enuresis, in usual doses of 20 to 40 µg at night.

Desmopressin acetate, by intravenous infusion, is given to boost concentrations of factor VIII prior to surgical procedures in patients with mild to moderate haemophilia or von Willebrand's disease. The usual dose is 0.3 to 0.4 µg (300 to 400 ng) per kg body-weight by slow intravenous infusion a half to 1½ hours before surgery.

A review of desmopressin.— D. W. Richardson and A. G. Robinson, *Ann. intern. Med.*, 1985, *103*, 228.

ADMINISTRATION. A report of 2 new modes (a metered-dose nasal spray and a gelatin-based sublingual lozenge) of administration of desmopressin. A study in 12 patients with confirmed cranial diabetes insipidus indicated that the methods produced a similar antidiuresis and duration of action to that produced by administration by 'rhinyle'. The patients in general preferred the nasal spray method.— A. Grossman *et al.*, *Br. med. J.*, 1980, *280*, 1215.

Evidence of enhanced absorption and bioavailability of desmopressin from a nasal spray compared with nasal drops.— A. S. Harris *et al.*, *J. pharm. Sci.*, 1986, *75*, 1085.

In a neonate with cranial diabetes insipidus and severely deformed oral and nasal cavities, in whom intranasal desmopressin proved unsuitable, oral administration of the nasal solution in a dose of 5 µg twice daily (about 10 times the appropriate nasal dose) proved effective.—

S. M. Stick and P. R. Betts, *Archs Dis. Childh.*, 1987, *62*, 1177. See also D. Cunnah *et al.*, *Clin. Endocr.*, 1986, *24*, 253; U. Westgren *et al.*, *Archs Dis. Childh.*, 1986, *61*, 247; A. Fjellestad-Paulsen *et al.*, *ibid.*, 1987, *62*, 674.

COAGULATION DISORDERS. A discussion of the use of desmopressin in patients with haemophilia and von Willebrand's disease. Desmopressin can be used to treat patients with mild haemophilia, carriers of haemophilia with low factor VIII concentrations, and patients with von Willebrand's disease. It should be given by slow intravenous injection in a dose of 300 ng per kg body-weight and immediately followed by tranexamic acid 10 mg per kg to inhibit the enhanced fibrinolytic activity. The result is a 3- to 5-fold increase in all factor VIII activities and provided the basal concentration of the most deficient factor VIII activity is 7% or more this rise, which reaches a maximum in 60 to 120 minutes, should be sufficient to stop external haemorrhage or to allow minor surgery. More major surgery such as cholecystectomy or thoracotomy may be possible if the basal factor VIII concentrations are higher, particularly in von Willebrand's disease where haemostasis tends to be easier to control. Desmopressin can also be given intranasally to raise factor VIII concentrations but the response is less predictable than with injection; however, it might be given by this route to blood donors in order to improve the supply of factor VIII.— *Lancet*, 1983, *2*, 774.

Further references to the use of desmopressin in haemophilia or von Willebrand's disease: *Med. Lett.*, 1984, *26*, 82; C. R. Rizza, *Prescribers' J.*, 1984, *24*, 71; N. L. Kobrinsky *et al.*, *Lancet*, 1984, *1*, 1145; B. de la Fuente *et al.*, *Ann. intern. Med.*, 1985, *103*, 6; V. Vicente *et al.* (letter), *ibid.*, 807; S. Prince, *Br. dent. J.*, 1987, *162*, 256. Reference to the use of desmopressin in patients with acquired antibodies to factor VIII.— S. M. Naorose-Abidi *et al.* (letter), *Lancet*, 1988, *1*, 366.

Intravenous infusion of desmopressin markedly shortened the prolonged bleeding time in studies in patients with uraemia, and prevented bleeding complications in uraemic patients undergoing surgical procedures.— P. M. Mannucci *et al.*, *New Engl. J. Med.*, 1983, *308*, 8. See also C. Jacquot *et al.* (letter), *Lancet*, 1988, *1*, 420 (with recombinant human erythropoietin).

For a report of tolerance to the effects of repeated doses of desmopressin in uraemic patients see under Adverse Effects and Precautions, above.

Desmopressin acetate 300 ng per kg body-weight by intravenous infusion significantly shortened median bleeding time in 9 patients with liver disease (8 with cirrhosis and one with a hepatic abscess). Five patients had had prolonged bleeding times before the infusion; in 3 of these bleeding time was reduced to normal values of less than 10 minutes while the bleeding times of the other 2 improved from 25.5 and 26 minutes to 18 and 17.5 minutes respectively. The bleeding time in the 4 patients with normal values shortened in 3 and remained unchanged in one. The concentrations of factor VIII, von Willebrand factor, and ristocetin cofactor were all increased after desmopressin infusion and there was an increase in the proportion of von Willebrand factor represented by high-molecular-weight multimeric forms. Similar results were seen in a second study comparing 6 cirrhotic patients given desmopressin acetate infusion with 6 similar patients given placebo; desmopressin significantly shortened bleeding time and increased factor VIII (in particular), von Willebrand factor, and ristocetin cofactor values. Desmopressin may prove a useful addition to the management of liver disease as the first agent shown to shorten bleeding time in cirrhotic patients without major side-effects.— A. K. Burroughs *et al.*, *Br. med. J.*, 1985, *291*, 1377. Comment on the possible mechanism of desmopressin's haemostatic action.— K. Rak *et al.* (letter), *ibid.*, 1986, *292*, 138.

In a study in patients undergoing heart operations involving cardiopulmonary bypass 35 received intravenous desmopressin acetate 300 ng per kg body-weight over 15 minutes once cardiopulmonary bypass was concluded while a further 35 received placebo. Total mean blood loss at operation and in the following 24 hours was only 1317 mL in patients given desmopressin, whereas in those given placebo it was significantly greater at 2210 mL. The ability of desmopressin to offset the haemostatic defect caused by extracorporeal circulation was probably related to its observed effect in elevating von Willebrand factor. If the reduction in blood loss seen in these patients could be extended to other cardiac operations it would represent a substantial saving in banked blood as well as the benefit to the patient of reduced transfusion requirements and a reduced rate of haemorrhagic complications.— E. W. Salzman *et al.*, *New Engl. J. Med.*, 1986, *314*, 1402.

Desmopressin 10 µg per m^2 body-surface intravenously (to a maximum of 20 µg) reduced overall blood loss by 32.5% among 17 patients undergoing spinal fusion for scoliosis compared with 18 similar patients given placebo. Desmopressin also decreased the duration of treatment with analgesic agents postoperatively, presumably by decreasing bleeding into the wound. Patients with scoliosis secondary to neuromuscular disorders showed the greatest benefit. In view of the beneficial results in these haemostatically normal patients the use of desmopressin in other surgical procedures associated with significant blood loss is recommended.— N. L. Kobrinsky *et al.*, *Ann. intern. Med.*, 1987, *107*, 446.

Desmopressin may be useful in non-cardiac surgery associated with significant blood loss but further investigations are required before it can be recommended for general use.— *Lancet*, 1988, *1*, 155.

ENURESIS. There was a significant reduction in the incidence of bed-wetting among 15 children treated with intranasal desmopressin 10 µg at night from a mean of 18.7 out of 30 nights before treatment to occurrences on only 6.5 of 30 nights during desmopressin treatment. Response was prompt and could be seen as early as 1 to 3 days after administration began; results were considered to be excellent in 6 children, satisfactory in 6 and unsatisfactory in 3. In contrast, treatment with placebo in 17 similar children had no significant effect on the overall frequency of nocturnal enuresis; only one child had an excellent, and one a satisfactory response. Among the children treated with desmopressin results were significantly better in older children. Beneficial effects lasted only during the treatment period and following discontinuation of the drug the incidence of bed-wetting rose to its former frequency; nonetheless, desmopressin appears to be a safe and useful tool in the treatment of nocturnal enuresis, particularly in older children.— M. Aladjem *et al.*, *Archs Dis. Childh.*, 1982, *57*, 137. Criticism of the use of drugs to treat nocturnal enuresis.— S. R. Meadow, *ibid.*, 139.

A crossover study in 17 children with intractable enuresis given desmopressin 20 µg intranasally at night showed significant clinical improvement, particularly in older children; osmolality of overnight urine samples was increased in all but 5 of the children and the best results were achieved if overnight urine osmolality after desmopressin was increased beyond 1000 mmol per kg. Patients responding to desmopressin relapsed when treatment was stopped and it was therefore best reserved for situations such as school trips and holidays; it had subsequently been used for this purpose in 12 further children, with success in 7. There were no side-effects and no clinical evidence of overhydration in any of the children. These results demonstrate the safety and efficacy of desmopressin in intractable nocturnal enuresis; the effects are probably mainly due to its antidiuretic effect although other mechanisms such as improved memory and learning may occasionally be involved.— S. B. Dimson, *Archs Dis. Childh.*, 1986, *61*, 1104.

A comparison of intranasal desmopressin with conditioning using an enuresis alarm in a study completed by 46 children with primary nocturnal enuresis. Desmopressin gave better results in the first 3 weeks due to its immediate effects but in the long-term results with the alarm were better. Most of the children responding to desmopressin relapsed when treatment stopped but in this study the frequency of wet nights was still lower than before treatment. No serious adverse effects were registered with desmopressin although some cases of nasal discomfort and dysgeusia occurred and one child developed occasional nose bleeds. The enuresis alarm appears to be the first choice in the treatment of nocturnal enuresis but where it fails or is impractical desmopressin offers a safe, practical alternative.— S. Wille, *Archs Dis. Childh.*, 1986, *61*, 30.

LUMBAR-PUNCTURE HEADACHE. Results of a double-blind crossover study completed by 9 healthy subjects suggested that intramuscular injection of desmopressin 6 µg might reduce the frequency and-or intensity of headaches following lumbar puncture. However, the difference between desmopressin and placebo saline injections was not statistically significant.— E. Widerlöv and L. Lindström (letter), *Lancet*, 1979, *1*, 548. A technique involving tilting the patient prevents the development of such headaches.— J. D. Easton (letter), *ibid.*, 974. See also W. F. Durward and H. Harrington (letter), *Lancet*, 1976, *2*, 1403; A. Sakula (letter), *ibid.*, 1977, *1*, 146.

In a double-blind study involving 79 patients, prophylactic intranasal administration of desmopressin had no significant effect on the incidence of headache or on the consumption of analgesics following lumbar puncture or pneumoencephalography compared with a placebo.— P. E. Hansen and J. H. Hansen, *Acta neurol. scand.*, 1979, *60*, 183.

In a double-blind study in 50 patients undergoing lumbar puncture, desmopressin 4 µg intramuscularly 4 hours before puncture then 12-hourly for a total of 3 doses did not decrease the incidence of headache but significantly reduced the severity. Desmopressin might also be of value for established headache.— J. M. A. Cowan *et al.*, *Br. med. J.*, 1980, *280*, 224.

MEMORY. Desmopressin failed to have any beneficial effect on the impairment of memory arising from severe head injuries in 6 men, aged 24 to 36 years, injured in road traffic accidents 3 to 8 years previously, none of whom had diabetes insipidus. A subsequent course of lypressin also failed to have any beneficial effect.— J. S. Jenkins *et al.* (letter), *Lancet*, 1979, *2*, 1245.

Vasopressin and analogues such as desmopressin, given intranasally, have been found in some studies to enhance memory and learning in both healthy subjects and patients with senile dementia; however, there is little experience of how best to use such compounds and potential side-effects are a disadvantage.— *Drug & Ther. Bull.*, 1984, *22*, 98.

ORTHOSTATIC HYPOTENSION. In 5 patients with autonomic failure desmopressin 2 to 4 µg intramuscularly at night markedly reduced nocturnal polyuria and diminished overnight weight-loss; supine blood pressure was increased, particularly in the morning, and the postural fall reduced. The patients felt considerably better whilst receiving desmopressin due to the reduction or abolition of nocturia and the reduction in postural symptoms, particularly in the morning when they were often at their worst. There were no untoward side-effects in these patients; however, a further patient who had been enrolled in the study was withdrawn due to the development of water intoxication and severe hyponatraemia. Desmopressin may well have a role in the treatment of automonic failure, probably in combination with a mineralocorticoid and salt supplementation, but patients must be carefully monitored for hyponatraemia.— C. J. Mathias *et al.*, *Br. med. J.*, 1986, *293*, 353.

RENAL-FUNCTION TEST. Desmopressin is effective for the assessment of urine-concentrating ability. There was no significant difference between the effect of 2 µg intramuscularly and 40 µg intranasally given overnight; the intranasal dose has also been given at 9 a.m., the bladder being emptied at that time and a second urine specimen being obtained 5 to 9 hours later.— J. P. Monson and P. Richards, *Br. med. J.*, 1978, *1*, 24. Urine-concentrating ability was reduced with advancing age.— J. P. Monson and P. Richards (letter), *Br. med. J.*, 1978, *1*, 1054.

Experience in 32 adults suggests that desmopressin is as effective as vasopressin tannate for assessing urinary concentration; a dose of 40 µg intranasally was suggested at 8 a.m. after 12 hours' water deprivation.— K. Delin *et al.*, *Br. med. J.*, 1978, *1*, 757. Intranasal administration of desmopressin is used routinely and the result checked using the intramuscular route if technical difficulties arise. Maximum concentration of the urine was not achieved when desmopressin 4 µg was given intravenously.— K. Delin *et al.* (letter), *Br. med. J.*, 1979, *1*, 888.

The intramuscular injection of desmopressin 4 µg is suitable for assessing renal concentrating ability in sedentary subjects or hospital inpatients.— J. R. Curtis and B. A. Donovan, *Br. med. J.*, 1979, *1*, 304.

A study indicating that a test of urinary osmolality using desmopressin before and after 14 hours of total restriction of fluid intake is a safe, convenient, and reliable means of estimating renal concentrating capacity in patients treated with lithium.— K. Asplund *et al.* (letter), *Lancet*, 1979, *1*, 491. See also P. Vestergaard and H. E. Hansen, *Acta psychiat. scand.*, 1980, *61*, 152.

SICKLE-CELL DISEASE. Preliminary but encouraging results with desmopressin in 3 patients with severe sickle-cell anaemia. Desmopressin administered intranasally was used to induce hyponatraemia, which resulted in a reduction in mean corpuscular haemoglobin concentration, a decreased degree of sickling, and an increase in oxygen affinity. Sustained treatment appears to reduce the frequency of crises and acute induction of hyponatraemia appears to shorten their duration.— R. M. Rosa *et al.*, *New Engl. J. Med.*, 1980, *303*, 1138. Although results in 4 patients confirmed that hyponatraemia could be induced in hospital and that the use of desmopressin acetate rather than vasopressin was essential, the number of hospital admissions for sickle-cell crisis was not altered nor was the length of hospital stay during crises. There were also neurological complications. Anorexia and listlessness occurred in 3 of the 4 patients, hallucinations in 2, and a grand mal seizure in 1.— M. Leary and N. Abramson (letter), *ibid.*, 1981, *304*, 844. Reply.— F. H. Epstein *et al.* (letter), *ibid.*

Proprietary Preparations

DDAVP *(Ferring, UK). Injection*, desmopressin acetate

4 μg/mL, in ampoules of 1 mL.
Nasal solution, desmopressin acetate 100 μg/mL.

Desmospray *(Ferring, UK)*. *Nasal spray*, desmopressin acetate 10 μg/metered dose.

Proprietary Names and Manufacturers

Adiuretin-SD *(Cz.)*; Dav Ritter *(Switz.)*; DDAVP *(Richmond, Canad.; Ayerst, S.Afr.; Ferring, UK; USV Pharmaceutical Corp., USA)*; Desmospray *(Ferring, UK)*; Minirin *(Protea, Austral.; Ferring, Fr.; Ferring, Ger.; Ferring, Norw.; Ferring, Swed.; Ferring, Switz.)*; Minirin/DDAVP *(Valeas, Ital.)*; Minurin *(Ferring, Denm.; Landerlan, Spain)*; Stimate *(Armour, USA)*.

5924-g

Felypressin *(BAN, USAN, rINN)*.

Phelypressine; PLV2. [2-Phenylalanine,8-lysine]vasopressin.
$C_{46}H_{65}N_{13}O_{11}S_2$=1040.2.
CAS — 56-59-7.

Felypressin is a vasopressor agent with actions similar to those of vasopressin (p.1138). Its antidiuretic effects are less than those of vasopressin. It is used as a vasoconstrictor in local anaesthetic injections for dental use when sympathomimetic agents should be avoided.

For a review of the use of felypressin in local anaesthetic injections, see *Drug & Ther. Bull.*, 1970, *8*, 38.

Proprietary Names and Manufacturers
Octapressin *(Astra, UK)*.

The following names have been used for multi-ingredient preparations containing felypressin— Citanest with Octapressin *(Astra, Austral.; Astra, UK)*.

5938-l

Ornipressin *(rINN)*.

[8-Ornithine]-vasopressin.
$C_{45}H_{63}N_{13}O_{12}S_2$=1042.2.
CAS — 3397-23-7.

Ornipressin is a synthetic derivative of vasopressin with similar actions (see p.1138). It is reported to be a strong vasoconstrictor with only weak antidiuretic properties and has been used to reduce bleeding during surgery. A solution containing up to 5 units in 20 to 60 mL of sodium chloride injection (0.9%) or local anaesthetic solution has been infiltrated into the area involved.

In 12 subjects undergoing anaesthesia with nitrous oxide or nitrous oxide and halothane, ornipressin 5 units intravenously increased peripheral vascular resistance and mean arterial blood pressure and reduced heart-rate and cardiac output. There was no dysrhythmia.— A. J. Coleman and L. W. Baker, *Br. J. Anaesth.*, 1973, *45*, 511.

Infusion of ornipressin 18 units over 4 hours produced temporary improvement in renal function in a patient with cirrhosis of the liver associated with the hepatorenal syndrome, which results in resistant renal failure usually ending in death. After stopping the infusion renal function reverted to its previous low level. The patient was subsequently maintained with a continuous infusion of ornipressin 1.5 units per hour until a liver transplant could be successfully performed.— K. Lenz *et al.*, *Gut*, 1985, *26*, 1385.

Proprietary Names and Manufacturers
Por 8 *(Sandoz, Austral.; Sandoz, Ger.; Sandoz, S.Afr.; Sandoz, Switz.)*.

5943-s

Powdered Pituitary (Posterior Lobe)

Hypophysis Cerebri Pars Posterior; Hypophysis Sicca; Ipofisi Posteriore; Pituitarium Posterius Pulveratum; Pituitary; Posterior Pituitary.

Pharmacopoeias. In *Arg.*, *Aust.*, and *Turk.* (which specify not less than 1 unit of oxytocic activity per mg), and *Jug.* (no strength specified). Also in *B.P.C. 1973. U.S.* includes Posterior Pituitary Injection.

A preparation from the posterior lobes of mammalian pituitary bodies.

Adverse Effects, Treatment, and Precautions
Similar to those for oxytocin (p.1146) and for vasopressin (p.1138). Allergic symptoms, including anaphylaxis, have occasionally been reported. The major protein contained in the preparation is neurophysin and nearly all patients treated have antineurophysin antibodies.

Uses and Administration
Powdered pituitary (posterior lobe) has oxytocic, pressor, antidiuretic, and hyperglycaemic actions and has generally been replaced by compounds or preparations with more specific actions such as Oxytocin Injection (p.1147), Vasopressin (p.1138), and Desmopressin (p.1135).

Preparations
Posterior Pituitary Injection *(U.S.P.)*. A sterile solution, in a suitable diluent, of material containing the polypeptide hormones derived from the posterior lobes of mammalian pituitary bodies. It is standardised in respect of oxytocic and pressor activity. pH 2.5 to 4.5. Avoid freezing.

Proprietary Names and Manufacturers
Acetuber *(Hubber, Spain)*; Di-Sipidin *(Austral.; Samil, Ital.; Switz.; Paines & Byrne, UK)*; Endopituitrina *(Ital.)*; Piton *(Ravasini, Ital.)*; Pituidrol *(Ital.)*; Pituitrin *(USA)*; Thymophysin *(Ger.)*.

12796-g

Terlipressin *(BAN, rINN)*.

Triglycyl-lysine-vasopressin. *N*-[*N*-(*N*-Glycylglycyl)glycyl]lypressin; Gly-Gly-Gly-Cys-Tyr-Phe-Gln-Asn-Cys-Pro-Lys-Gly-NH_2 cyclic (4→9) disulphide.
$C_{52}H_{74}N_{16}O_{15}S_2$=1227.4.
CAS — 14636-12-5.

Adverse Effects, Treatment, and Precautions

As for Vasopressin, p.1138.
Its pressor and antidiuretic effects are reported to be less marked than those of vasopressin.

Uses and Administration

Terlipressin is an inactive pro-drug which is slowly converted in the body to lypressin, and has the general physiological actions of vasopressin (p.1138).
It is used in the control of bleeding oesophageal varices, in doses of 2 mg by intravenous injection, repeated every 4 to 6 hours if necessary, until bleeding is controlled, for up to 72 hours.
The acetate has been used similarly.

The conversion of terlipressin to lypressin following intravenous or intranasal administration in 5 healthy subjects. Following intravenous administration, in a dose of 7.5 μg per kg body-weight plasma concentrations of terlipressin fell rapidly, with a mean half-life of 24.2 minutes, and terlipressin was virtually absent from the plasma by 120 minutes. There was a transient initial peak of biological activity, presumably due to some activity of terlipressin itself, followed by a second peak (due to lypressin) between 60 and 120 minutes which lasted for at least 180 minutes. Injection was associated with skin pallor and increased diastolic blood pressure; the former was greatest after 30 to 45 minutes and lasted about 4 hours. When terlipressin was given by intranasal instillation in doses of 5 mg it was detected in plasma within 5 minutes, reaching a peak after 15; following this plasma concentrations fell more slowly than after injection. The concentrations of lypressin achieved in plasma were much lower than with the intravenous route.— M. L. Forsling *et al.*, *J. Endocr.*, 1980, *85*, 237.

A comparison of terlipressin and vasopressin in the early management of bleeding oesophageal varices. The study involved 21 bleeding episodes in 19 patients. Terlipressin 2 mg every 6 hours as an intravenous bolus, followed by 1 mg every 6 hours for a further 18 hours once active bleeding ceased was given in 10 episodes, while vasopressin was given by intravenous infusion at 0.4 units per minute until bleeding stopped, and then at half this rate for a further 18 hours, in the remaining 11 episodes. Terlipressin was effective in stopping bleeding in 70% of cases while vasopressin was effective only in 9% of cases. There was no significant difference in mortality between the groups but only 1 of the patients given terlipressin died of continued bleeding whereas 3 of those given vasopressin died from this cause. No serious complications of vasoconstrictor therapy occurred in either group. Because of its efficacy, lack of side-effects, and ease of administration terlipressin seems to be useful in the managemnt of bleeding varices.— J. G. Freeman *et al.*, *Lancet*, 1982, *2*, 66.

Proprietary Preparations

Glypressin *(Ferring, UK)*. *Injection*, powder for reconstitution, terlipressin 1 mg, supplied with diluent.

Proprietary Names and Manufacturers

Glipressina *(Valeas, Ital.)*; Glycylpressin *(Ferring, Ger.)*; Glypressin *(Ferring, UK)*; Glypressine *(Ferring, Switz.)*.

5948-j

Vasopressin

ADH; Antidiuretic Hormone; Beta-Hypophamine.

The pressor principle of the posterior lobe of the pituitary gland. It may be prepared by extraction or by synthesis.

5949-z

Argipressin *(BAN, rINN)*.

[8-Arginine]vasopressin; AVP. Cys-Tyr-Phe-Gln-Asn-Cys-Pro-Arg-Gly-NH_2 cyclic (1→6) disulphide.
$C_{46}H_{65}N_{15}O_{12}S_2$=1084.2.
CAS — 113-79-1.

NOTE. Argipressin Tannate is *USAN*.

Vasopressin from most mammals including man but excluding pig. Lypressin (below) is vasopressin from pig.

Units

8.2 units of arginine-vasopressin for bioassay are contained in approximately 20 μg of synthetic peptide (with human albumin 5 mg and citric acid) in one ampoule of the first International Standard Preparation (1978).

5934-p

Lypressin *(BAN, USAN, rINN)*.

L-8; LVP. [8-Lysine]vasopressin; Cys-Tyr-Phe-Gln-Asn-Cys-Pro-Lys-Gly-NH_2 cyclic (1→6) disulphide.
$C_{46}H_{65}N_{13}O_{12}S_2$=1056.2.
CAS — 50-57-7.

A form of vasopressin which is usually prepared synthetically, or may be extracted from the posterior pituitary of pigs.

Units

7.7 units of lysine-vasopressin are contained in approximately 23.4 μg of synthetic peptide (with albumin 5 mg and citric acid) in one ampoule of the first International Standard Preparation (1978).

5935-s

Lypressin Injection *(BAN)*.

Lypressini Solutio Iniectabilis.

Pharmacopoeias. In *Br.*, *Eur.*, *Fr.*, *Ger.*, *It.*, *Neth.*, and *Swiss.*

A clear colourless sterile aqueous solution of lypressin. **Sterilised** by filtration. pH 3.7 to 4.3. **Store** at 2° to 15° and avoid freezing.

5951-s

Vasopressin Injection *(USAN, rINN)*.

Vasopressin; Vasopressini Injectio.

Pharmacopoeias. In *Arg.* and *Nord.* (which specify 10 units per mL); in *Cz.* (which specifies 5 or 10 units per mL); in *Jpn*, *Jug.*, and *U.S.* (no strength specified); and in *Egypt.*, *Ind.*, *Int.*, and *Turk.* (which specify 20 units per mL).

A sterile solution with a faint characteristic odour containing the pressor and antidiuretic principle of the posterior lobe of the pituitary

gland, prepared from the glands of oxen or other mammals, including pigs. *U.S.P.* allows synthetic vasopressin. It contains not more than 1.2 units of oxytocic activity for each 20 units of pressor activity. The solution has a pH of between 2.5 and 4.5.
It should be **stored** so as to avoid freezing.

5950-p

Vasopressin Tannate

The water-insoluble tannate of the pressor principle of the posterior lobe of the pituitary.

Adverse Effects

Large parenteral doses of vasopressin may give rise to marked pallor, nausea, eructation, cramp, and a desire to defaecate. In women it may cause uterine cramps of a menstrual character. Hyponatraemia with water retention and signs of water intoxication can occur and may be more likely with the longer acting tannate.
Hypersensitivity reactions have occurred and include urticaria, fever, angioedema and bronchial constriction, and rashes. Anaphylactic shock and cardiac arrest have been reported.
Vasopressin may constrict coronary arteries. Chest pain, myocardial ischaemia, and infarction have occurred following injection, and fatalities have been reported. Other cardiovascular effects include occasional reports of arrhythmias and bradycardia, as well as hypertension. Peripheral vasoconstriction has resulted in gangrene, and thrombosis as well as local irritation at the injection site may occur.
Following intranasal use (usually as lypressin) nasal congestion, irritation, and ulceration have been reported occasionally; systemic effects at usual intranasal doses are mostly reported to be mild.

EFFECTS ON THE HEART. Ventricular tachycardia and fibrillation developed in a patient with no history of cardiac disorder after she had received vasopressin 20 units intravenously over 15 minutes.— K. J. Kelly *et al.*, *Ann. intern. Med.*, 1980, *92*, 205. Ventricular arrhythmia was induced in a patient who developed bradycardia following vasopressin infusion.— E. Eden *et al.*, *Mt Sinai J. Med.*, 1983, *50*, 49. See also J. D. Fitz (letter), *Archs intern. Med.*, 1982, *142*, 644 (ventricular ectopy and asystole).

ISCHAEMIA. Gangrene occurred in 2 patients after the extravasation of vasopressin given by intravenous infusion. Amputation was necessary in one patient and the other developed clostridial sepsis and died.— R. A. Greenwald *et al.*, *Gastroenterology*, 1978, *74*, 744. Cyanosis and ischaemia of both upper and lower extremities developed in a patient receiving vasopressin at an initial rate of 0.4 units per minute by intra-arterial infusion for gastro-intestinal bleeding. Ischaemia improved when the rate of vasopressin infusion was reduced but gastro-intestinal bleeding recurred. Following surgical treatment and discontinuation of vasopressin, ischaemic changes in the lower extremities and the left hand resolved within 2 hours but remained in the fingers of the right hand which subsequently became gangrenous and required amputation.— P. Colombani, *Dig. Dis. Scis*, 1982, *27*, 367. Acute haemorrhagic necrosis of the bowel wall consistent with ischaemic colitis was seen in a patient who had received an infusion of vasopressin for treatment of variceal haemorrhage. Bloody diarrhoea and necrotic changes subsequently resolved without treatment.— M. Lambert *et al.*, *J. Am. med. Ass.*, 1982, *247*, 666. A report of cutaneous gangrene in 5 patients following peripheral intravenous infusion of vasopressin; there was evidence of extravasation only in one case.— J. R. Anderson and G. W. Johnston, *Br. med. J.*, 1983, *287*, 1657. Two cases (one in a man, one in a woman) of bilateral nipple necrosis following intravenous vasopressin.— K. R. Reddy *et al.*, *Archs intern. Med.*, 1984, *144*, 835.

Treatment of Adverse Effects

The antidiuretic effects on water retention and sodium imbalance may be treated by water restriction and a temporary withdrawal of vasopressin.

A report of the localised intravenous and intra-arterial administration of guanethidine in the treatment of a patient with extravasation of vasopressin. The intra-arterial administration of guanethidine was considered to have helped to avoid necrotic changes.— M. C. Crocker (letter), *New Engl. J. Med.*, 1981, *304*, 1430.

Precautions

Vasopressin should not be used in patients with chronic nephritis with nitrogen retention, and should be avoided or given only with extreme care, and in small doses, to patients with vascular disease, especially of the coronary arteries.
It should be given with care to patients with asthma, epilepsy, migraine, heart failure, or other conditions which might be aggravated by water retention. Fluid intake should be adjusted to avoid hyponatraemia and water intoxication.
Care should be taken to avoid extravasation of parenteral vasopressin. Repeated injections of the tannate may give rise to inflammation and sterile abscess and care should be taken to vary the site of such injections. Nasal absorption of vasopressin may be impaired in patients with rhinitis.
The antidiuretic effects of vasopressins have been reported to be enhanced in some patients receiving chlorpropamide, clofibrate, carbamazepine, or tricyclic antidepressants; lithium, heparin, and alcohol may decrease the antidiuretic effect. Ganglion-blocking agents such as hexamethonium and pentolinium may increase sensitivity to the pressor effects of vasopressins.

The appearance of a raised white line over a peripheral vein used for infusion of vasopressin may be an indicator of incipient skin necrosis.— P. G. Wiles *et al.*, *Br. med. J.*, 1986, *292*, 396.

INTERACTIONS. A report of severe bradycardia and heart block leading to asystole in a patient given combined vasopressin and *cimetidine* therapy.— G. Nikolic and J. B. Singh, *Med. J. Aust.*, 1982, *2*, 435.

RESISTANCE. After 20 years of treatment with vasopressin injection a patient with hypothalamic diabetes insipidus developed resistance associated with a high titre of antibodies.— N. G. Soler *et al.*, *Archs intern. Med.*, 1979, *139*, 677.

Uses and Administration

Vasopressin has a direct antidiuretic action on the kidney. It also constricts peripheral vessels and causes contraction of the smooth muscle of the intestine, gall-bladder, and urinary bladder. It has practically no oxytocic activity.
Vasopressin (argipressin) is used in the treatment and diagnosis of diabetes insipidus due to a deficiency in antidiuretic hormone. It is ineffective in nephrogenic diabetes insipidus. It should not be used to raise the blood pressure. It has also been used in the treatment of abdominal distension, and is sometimes given to remove gas in abdominal visualisation procedures. Vasopressin has been used in the treatment of bleeding oesophageal varices, but with variable results.
In the treatment of diabetes insipidus to control polyuria, Vasopressin Injection or argipressin is usually administered subcutaneously or intramuscularly in doses of 5 to 20 units given at least twice daily. It has also been given intranasally, but desmopressin (p.1135) is usually preferred. Because its actions last only a few hours its main use is in the diagnosis of diabetes insipidus. For a more prolonged effect, suitable for the treatment of diabetes insipidus, vasopressin tannate may be given intramuscularly as an oily suspension, in doses of 1.5 to 5 units at usual intervals of 1 to 3 days. It should not be given intravenously and it is important that the preparation should be warmed and thoroughly shaken before use to ensure even suspension.
Alternatively, if parenteral administration is unsuitable, lypressin may be given as a nasal spray, the usual dose for diabetes insipidus being 2 to 5 units 3 or 4 times daily or more, as required in one or both nostrils.
In the management of variceal bleeding Vasopressin Injection or argipressin may be given by intravenous or occasionally direct intra-arterial infusion. For intravenous use an initial dose of 20 units in 100 mL of glucose (5%) injection, infused over 15 minutes has been suggested for initial control of bleeding.

HAEMORRHAGE. A 3-year retrospective study of the treatment of 70 episodes of gastro-intestinal bleeding in 65 patients. Vasopressin was given by constant arterial infusion in a dose of 0.2 unit per minute, increased to 0.4 unit per minute if bleeding did not stop. Haemorrhage was completely controlled in 43% of variceal bleeds, 67% of episodes of haemorrhagic gastritis, 45% of bleeding ulcers, and 62% of patients with bleeding colons. The infusion was usually tapered off over 24 to 48 hours; the overall incidence of relapse after initial control was 16%. Major complications occurred in 22 patients and especially those with cirrhosis.— L. M. Sherman *et al.*, *Ann. Surg.*, 1979, *189*, 298.

Vasopressin is the most widely known of the current agents for arresting active variceal haemorrhage. It can be injected directly into the mesenteric artery but this is no more effective than the more common intravenous route and carries more risks. A reduction in portal pressure for about 1 hour is produced by 20 units of vasopressin in 100 mL of glucose 5% infused over 10 minutes but a continuous infusion of 0.2 to 0.4 units per minute is probably more effective than bolus administration. Gradual reduction of the concentration of vasopressin in the infusion may lessen the risk of rebound haemorrhage. Absence of side-effects such as abdominal pain, facial pallor, and bowel evacuation indicates an inadequate therapeutic effect. Because of the physiological actions of the drug hyponatraemia and oliguria may be encountered. Other disadvantages of vasopressin include its short duration of action and an adverse influence on systemic haemodynamics which leads to myocardial ischaemia in some patients. The addition of sublingual glyceryl trinitrate has been reported to minimise such reactions and to reduce portal pressure further. Terlipressin has a longer duration of action than vasopressin and may prove more effective.— P. Hayes and I. A. D. Bouchier, *Br. J. Hosp. Med.*, 1984, *32*, 39. While vasopressin or its analogues may have a place in the management of acute variceal bleeding its role is at best subsidiary; sclerotherapy, which prevents rebleeding, may be of greater value in most cases.— R. J. Dickinson *et al.* (letter), *Lancet*, 1982, *2*, 393. The success-rate in controlling variceal haemorrhage with either intravenous or intra-arterial vasopressin is only 50% and even if bleeding is effectively controlled survival is not increased. If bleeding is not controlled quickly by doses up to 0.9 units per minute other methods of stopping bleeding should be instituted without delay.— D. E. Larson and M. B. Farnell, *Mayo Clin. Proc.*, 1983, *58*, 371.

For a comparison of vasopressin and terlipressin in the control of variceal bleeding, see Terlipressin, p.1137. For comparison of argipressin and somatostatin in the control of variceal bleeding see Somatostatin, p.1151.

References to the use of vasopressin to control other forms of haemorrhage: R. E. Pyeritz *et al.*, *J. Urol., Baltimore*, 1978, *120*, 253 (cyclophosphamide-induced haemorrhagic cystitis); J. A. Mellor *et al.*, *Gut*, 1982, *23*, 872 (intra-arterial infusion for massive haemorrhage in Crohn's disease); K. F. Schulz *et al.*, *Lancet*, 1985, *2*, 353 (paracervical injection to reduce blood loss in abortion); T. W. Noseworthy and B. J. Anderson, *Can. med. Ass. J.*, 1986, *135*, 1097 (in haemoptysis).

MEMORY. Results in *animals* have shown that vasopressin appears to improve memory and that different portions of the vasopressin molecule mediate the facilitation of memory and the classical physiological actions. As a result of these findings there have been a number of attempts to give vasopressin analogues to patients with dementia or other memory disorders. Many studies have reported negative results and where benefit has been reported there have usually been indications that this might be due to improvements in mood and attention rather than to a direct effect on cognition. However there is some evidence for improved memory in patients with diabetes insipidus and for facilitation of conditioned responses; lypressin has been given to help smokers acquire an avoidance response to smoking.— M. D. Kopelman and W. A. Lishman, *Br. med. Bull.*, 1986, *42*, 101.

Preparations

Lypressin Nasal Solution *(U.S.P.)*. A solution containing synthetic lypressin in a suitable diluent and supplied in packages which permit nasal administration in controlled dosage. pH 3.0 to 4.3.

Proprietary Preparations

Pitressin *(Parke, Davis, UK). Injection,* argipressin 20 units/mL, in ampoules of 1 mL.

NOTE. Pitressin formerly consisted of Vasopressin Injection.

Syntopressin *(Sandoz, UK). Nasal spray,* lypressin 50 units/mL, supplying 2.5 units/dose.

Proprietary Names and Manufacturers of Vasopressin or its analogues

Diapid *(Sandoz, Fr.; Sandoz, USA)*; Landuren *(Landerlan, Spain)*; Pitressin *(Parke, Davis, Austral.; Parke, Davis, Canad.; Parke, Davis, Ger.; Parke, Davis, UK; Parke, Davis, USA)*; Pitressin Tanato *(Parke, Davis, Spain)*; Pitressin Tannaat *(Substantia, Neth.)*; Pitressin Tannat *(Parke, Davis, Ger.; Parke, Davis, Norw.)*; Pitressin Tannate *(Parke, Davis, Austral.; Belg.; Parke, Davis, Canad.; Parke, Davis, S.Afr.; Parke, Davis, Swed.; Parke, Davis, Switz.; Parke, Davis, USA)*; Pos-Hipon *(Arg.)*; Postacton *(Ferring, Ger.; Ferring, Swed.)*; Syntopressin *(Sandoz, UK)*; Vasopresina-Sandoz *(Sandoz, Spain)*; Vasopressine *(Sandoz, Switz.)*; Vasopressin-Sandoz *(Sandoz, Austral.; Sandoz, Swed.)*.

3885-f

Corticotrophic Hormones

The following section includes the adrenocorticotrophic hormone, Corticotrophin, its hypothalamic releasing hormone, and some synthetic corticotrophin analogues such as Octacosactrin and Tetracosactrin.

In line with the negative feedback principles involved in many homoeostatic processes the hormones of the adrenal cortex are also involved in the hormonal regulation of the adrenal cortex; for the adrenocortical hormones and their analogues see Corticosteroids, p.872.

1461-v

Corticotrophin *(BAN, rINN).*

ACTH; Adrenocorticotrophic Hormone; Adrenocorticotropin; Corticotropin *(USAN)*; Corticotropinum.

CAS — 9002-60-2 (corticotrophin); 9050-75-3 (corticotrophin zinc).

Pharmacopoeias. In *Arg., Aust., Br., Braz., Egypt., Eur., Fr., Ger., Ind., It., Jug., Neth., Swiss,* and *U.S.* Certain pharmacopoeias include only as a preparation in the form of an injection.

Corticotrophin is a substance obtained from the anterior lobe of the pituitary gland of mammals used by man for food and contains the polypeptide corticotrophic principle that increases the rate at which corticoid hormones are secreted by the adrenal gland. It contains not less than 55 units per mg.

Units

5 units of porcine corticotrophin for bioassay are contained in approximately 50 µg (with lactose 5 mg) in one ampoule of the third International Standard Preparation (1962).

Adverse Effects

Corticotrophin stimulates the adrenals to produce cortisol (hydrocortisone) and mineralocorticoids; it therefore has the adverse glucocorticoid and the adverse mineralocorticoid properties of corticosteroids (see p.872).

In particular, its mineralocorticoid properties may produce marked sodium and water retention; considerable potassium loss may also occur.

Although corticotrophin has a marked diabetogenic effect, some other adverse effects, such as gastro-intestinal side-effects and osteoporosis, attributable to its glucocorticoid properties are believed to be less common than with the corticosteroids.

Corticotrophin also stimulates the adrenals to produce androgens with the result that acne and hirsutism occur more frequently than with corticosteroids.

Corticotrophin sometimes induces skin pigmentation. It can induce sensitisation and severe allergic reactions may occur.

Whereas corticosteroids replace endogenous cortisol (hydrocortisone) and thereby induce adrenal atrophy, corticotrophin's stimulant effect induces hypertrophy. Withdrawal of corticotrophin may therefore be easier than withdrawal of corticosteroids; nevertheless, the ability of the hypothalamic-pituitary-adrenal axis to respond to stress is still reduced, and abrupt withdrawal of corticotrophin may result in symptoms of hypopituitarism (see Withdrawal, below).

Reports of the adverse effects observed in children given corticotrophin for infantile spasms: R. Riikonen and M. Donner, *Archs Dis. Childh.*, 1980, *55*, 664; F. Hanefeld *et al.* (letter), *Lancet*, 1984, *1*, 901; R. Riikonen *et al.*, *Archs Dis. Childh.*, 1986, *61*, 671; J. Perheentupa *et al.*, *ibid.*, 750.

ALLERGY. Allergic reactions occurred in 13 patients receiving prednisolone therapy and injections of corticotrophin at 10-day intervals. The reactions usually occurred about half an hour after the sixth injection.— O. Forssman *et al.*, *Acta allerg.*, 1963, *18*, 462.

Thirteen of 19 children, who had been treated with a long-acting preparation of porcine corticotrophin (Acthar Gel) for 5 to 200 weeks, developed circulating antibodies directed mainly against the species-specific part of the molecule. There was no clinical or biochemical evidence that the antibodies impaired the effects of exogenous hormone or blocked endogenous human corticotrophin.— J. Landon *et al.*, *Lancet*, 1967, *1*, 652. For a similar report, see N. Fleischer *et al.*, *J. clin. Invest.*, 1967, *46*, 196.

Corticotrophin is a straight-chain polypeptide consisting of 39 amino acids, only the first 24 of which are biologically active and common to man and cattle, pigs, and sheep. The last 15 amino acids differ between species. The differences could account for the development of antibodies and allergic reactions when animal corticotrophin is injected in man. Amino acids 4 to 11 are identical with the sequence in melanocyte-stimulating hormone and produce the pigmentation of the skin seen in Addison's disease.— *Br. med. J.*, 1969, *2*, 809.

EFFECTS ON BONES AND JOINTS. Aseptic necrosis of the femur occurred in a 23-year-old man 9 months after receiving 1070 units of corticotrophin over 16 days for retrobulbar neuritis due to multiple sclerosis.— A. E. Good, *J. Am. med. Ass.*, 1974, *228*, 497.

EFFECTS ON THE ELECTROLYTE BALANCE. Severe hyponatraemia occurred in 3 patients following intravenous infusion of corticotrophin in glucose injection 5% to diagnose adrenocortical insufficiency. It was recommended that sodium chloride injection should be used as the infusing solution.— L. R. Sheeler and O. P. Schumacher, *Ann. intern. Med.*, 1979, *90*, 798. A previous study had shown that natural corticotrophin preparations were contaminated with sufficient amounts of vasopressin to produce water retention even in normal subjects. However the problem of water intoxication could be entirely avoided by using a synthetic corticotrophin preparation which had not been found to contain vasopressin and did not produce water retention or hyponatraemia even when infused in salt-free solutions.— G. Baumann (letter), *ibid.*, *91*, 499. Further speculation on the reason for the hyponatraemia.— M. Geheb *et al.* (letter), *ibid.*, 792. Reply and emphasis that infusion of 5% glucose seems to cause more problems than infusion of saline.— L. R. Sheeler and O. P. Schumacher (letter), *ibid.*

EFFECTS ON THE EYES. A 50-year-old woman with chronic rheumatoid arthritis who had been treated with corticotrophin, about 20 units intramuscularly daily for 2.5 years, developed posterior subcapsular cataracts and macular lesions in both eyes.— J. Williamson and T. G. Dalakos, *Br. J. Ophthal.*, 1967, *51*, 839.

EFFECTS ON THE SKIN. Exudative erythema multiforme developed after one administration of corticotrophin.— E. N. Soloshenko and A. I. Brailovskiĭ, *Klin. Med., Mosk.*, 1975, *53*, 136.

Treatment of Adverse Effects

Adverse effects should be treated symptomatically and the dosage reduced or the drug withdrawn.

Withdrawal

Corticotrophin administration may depress the natural secretion of the hormone sufficiently to cause pituitary hypoplasia. Abrupt withdrawal of corticotrophin may therefore produce symptoms of hypopituitarism and therapy should be stopped gradually. See also Withdrawal under corticosteroids, p.873.

Precautions

As for corticosteroids, p.873.

Absorption and Fate

Corticotrophin is ineffective when given by mouth. It produces rapid effects when administered intravenously but its biological half-life in plasma is only about 15 minutes. The long-acting depot preparations formulated with gelatin or zinc have, however, much longer durations of action of about 24 hours when administered subcutaneously or intramuscularly.

A review of studies on the distribution and fate of corticotrophin.— H. P. J. Bennett and C. McMartin, *Pharmac. Rev.*, 1978, *30*, 247.

Uses and Administration

Corticotrophin is a naturally occurring hormone of the anterior lobe of the pituitary gland which induces hyperplasia and increase in weight of the adrenal gland. The secretion of adrenocortical hormones, especially cortisol (hydrocortisone), some mineralocorticoids, such as corticosterone, and, to a lesser extent, of androgens is increased. It has little effect on aldosterone secretion which proceeds independently.

Secretion of corticotrophin by the functioning pituitary gland is controlled by the release of corticotrophin-releasing hormone (corticotrophin-releasing factor) in the hypothalamus and is stimulated by a reduction in the concentration of circulating cortisol by an increase in circulating adrenaline, and by conditions of stress. High blood concentrations of cortisol prevent release of corticotrophin and this results in hypofunction of the adrenal gland.

As corticotrophin stimulates the activity of the adrenal cortex and produces a high level of circulating cortisol it has been used therapeutically in most of the conditions (with the exception of the adrenal deficiency states and adrenocortical overactivity) for which systemic corticosteroid therapy is indicated. Its use for such purposes is now, however, fairly limited with corticosteroids themselves being preferred although certain neurological disorders such as Bell's palsy and multiple sclerosis are sometimes treated with corticotrophin. Corticotrophin may also be used diagnostically to investigate adrenocortical insufficiency.

Corticotrophin may be available for injection in two forms. One form is a plain injection that may be administered by the subcutaneous, intramuscular, or intravenous routes. The other form includes the long-acting depot preparations in which the viscosity is increased by the addition of gelatin or in which corticotrophin is combined with zinc hydroxide or carmellose sodium. These long-acting preparations are administered subcutaneously or intramuscularly and should not be given intravenously.

For therapeutic purposes both the plain and the long-acting depot preparations have been used subcutaneously and intramuscularly. Typical initial doses for the plain type of injection have been up to 20 units four times daily and for the depot preparations about 40 to 80 units every 24 to 72 hours. As soon as possible the dosage should be reduced gradually to the minimum necessary to control symptoms.

For diagnostic purposes corticotrophin may be used intramuscularly as a depot preparation or intravenously as the plain preparation. The test is based on the measurement of plasma-cortisol concentrations before and after the injection. The depot preparation has been given in doses of 40 units by intramuscular injection and the plain preparation in doses of 10 to 25 units in 500 mL of glucose 5% infused intravenously over 8 hours (but see Effects on the Electrolyte Balance under Adverse Effects, above, for suggestions that sodium chloride rather than glucose should be used as the infusion fluid).

Studies and comments on the physiology and pharmacology of corticotrophin: K. H. Falchuk, *New Engl. J. Med.*, 1977, *296*, 1129; J. F. Desforges *et al.*, *ibid.*, 1165; J. Volavka *et al.* (letter), *New Engl. J. Med.*, 1979, *300*, 1056.

EPILEPSY. For a review and discussion on the management of infantile spasms, including the use of corticotrophin, see under Corticosteroids (p.877).

MULTIPLE SCLEROSIS. A review of the current concepts in the management of multiple sclerosis. Studies have shown that corticotrophin is useful for treating acute exacerbations of multiple sclerosis and it is now widely used for this purpose but there is no basis for recommending corticotrophin as a long-term treatment. Dosages used for acute treatment vary, but one schedule is 80 units intramuscularly for 5 days followed by 40 units intramuscularly for another 5 days. With regard to retrobulbar neuritis which occurs in about 55% of patients, corticotrophin may be useful in hastening recovery or reducing the degree of residual visual deficit although there is no unequivocal evidence to prove this.— B. Giesser, *Drugs*, 1985, *29*, 88.

Preparations

Corticotrophin for Injection *(U.S.P.)*. A sterile dry mixture which contains corticotrophin and may contain a suitable antimicrobial agent, diluents, and buffers. pH of the reconstituted solution 2.5 to 6.0.

Corticotropin Injection *(U.S.P.)*. A sterile solution in a suitable diluent. It may contain a suitable antimicrobial. pH 3 to 7. Store at a temperature not exceeding 8°.

Corticotrophin for Injection *(Eur. P.)*. Corticotropinum ad Iniectabile. A dry sterile preparation of corticotrophin. It may contain a suitable buffer, stabiliser, and antimicrobial preservative. pH of the reconstituted solution 3 to 5. Store at a temperature not exceeding 25°. Protect from light.

Corticotrophin Gelatin Injection *(B.P.)*. ACTH Gelatin Injection. A sterile aqueous solution of corticotrophin containing suitably hydrolysed gelatin. Sterilised by filtration. pH 4.5 to 7.0. Store at 2° to 8°. Protect from light. Under these conditions it may be expected to retain its potency for 18 months. If necessary, the contents should be warmed before use. For subcutaneous or intramuscular use only.

Corticotrophin Zinc Injection *(B.P.)*. Corticotrophin Zinc Hydroxide Injection *(Eur. P.)*; ACTH Zinc Injection; Corticotropini Zinci Hydroxidi Suspensio Iniectabilis. A sterile aqueous suspension, prepared aseptically, of corticotrophin with zinc hydroxide made iso-osmotic with blood by the addition of sodium chloride. pH 7.5 to 8.5. Store at 2° to 8°. Under these conditions it may be expected to retain its potency for 2 years. The container should be gently shaken before a dose is withdrawn. It is for subcutaneous or intramuscular use only.

Repository Corticotropin Injection *(U.S.P.)*. A sterile solution of corticotrophin in partially hydrolysed gelatin. It may contain a suitable antimicrobial agent. pH 3 to 7.

Sterile Corticotropin Zinc Hydroxide Suspension *(U.S.P.)*. A sterile suspension of corticotrophin adsorbed on zinc hydroxide; it contains sodium phosphate. pH 7.5 to 8.5. Store at 15° to 30°.

Proprietary Preparations

Acthar Gel *(Armour, UK)*. *Injection*, Corticotrophin Gelatin Injection *(B.P.)* 20 units/mL in vials of 5 mL, 40 units/mL in vials of 2 and 5 mL, 80 units/mL in vials of 5 mL.

Proprietary Names and Manufacturers

Acethropan *(Hoechst, Ger.)*; Acortan *(Ferring, Ger.)*; Acthar *(Austral.; Rorer, Canad.; Rorer, Ital.; Armour, S.Afr.; Fisons, S.Afr.; Armour, UK; Armour, USA)*; ACTH/CMC *(Ferring, UK)*; Acthelea *(Elea, Arg.)*; Acton *(Ferring, Swed.)*; Actonar *(Arg.)*; Cortico-Gel *(Crookes Laboratories, UK)*; Cortigel *(Savage, USA)*; Cortrophin ZN *(Austral.; Organon, UK)*; Cortrophine-Z *(Switz.)*; Cortrophin-Zinc *(Organon, USA)*; Crookes acth/cmc *(Crookes Laboratories, UK)*; Depot-Acethropan *(Hoechst, Ger.)*; Durackin *(Canad.)*; H.P. Acthar Gel *(Armour, USA)*; Reacthin *(Swed.)*.

16592-m

Corticotrophin-releasing Hormone

Corticoliberin; Corticotropin-releasing Factor; CRF; CRH.

A 41-amino acid polypeptide isolated from the hypothalamus that stimulates the release of corticotrophin (p.1139) from the anterior pituitary.

Characterisation of the structure of ovine corticotrophin-releasing hormone.— W. Vale *et al.*, *Science*, 1981, *213*, 1394. The human peptide, as determined by gene sequencing, differs by 7 amino acid residues from the ovine molecule; the human hormone is identical to that of *rats*.— G. P. Chrousos *et al.*, *Ann. intern. Med.*, 1985, *102*, 344.

Adverse Effects

Flushing of the face and mild dyspnoea may follow injection of corticotrophin-releasing hormone; hypotension has been reported, especially following large doses.

A warning that hypotensive episodes have followed the use of corticotrophin-releasing hormone in *monkeys*.— N. H. Kalin *et al.* (letter), *Lancet*, 1982, *2*, 1042.

Loss of consciousness, lasting for 10 seconds to 5 minutes, occurred in 3 patients, two of whom had Cushing's disease and one who had secondary adrenal insufficiency, following intravenous injection of corticotrophin-releasing hormone 200 µg. The 2 patients with Cushing's disease had a slight accompanying fall in blood pressure. In a fourth patient, receiving corticosteroid and thyroid hormone replacement therapy, injection of corticotrophin-releasing hormone was associated with a sharp fall in systolic blood pressure and subsequent asystole.— A. Hermus *et al.* (letter), *Lancet*, 1983, *1*, 776. Criticism. No serious adverse effects had been seen among 70 patients with disorders of the hypothalamic-pituitary-adrenal axis, nor among 30 psychiatric patients or 40 healthy subjects all of whom had received intravenous corticotrophin-releasing hormone in doses of 1 µg per kg body-weight. The reactions reported by Hermus *et al.* might have been due to impurities in the synthetic preparation used, or be due to the higher dose (approximately 3 µg per kg).— H. M. Schulte *et al.* (letter), *ibid.*, 1222. Further comment, and the suggestion that human corticotrophin-releasing hormone (hCRH) might be less likely to produce severe adverse effects than the ovine preparation (oCRH).— D. Oppermann (letter), *ibid.*, 1986, *2*, 1031. Reply. No serious side-effects had been seen since the dose had been lowered to 100 µg given over 1 minute. Ovine hormone is prefered to human in everyday practice because of its longer duration of action and lesser hypotensive effects.— A. R. M. M. Hermus *et al.* (letter), *ibid.*, 1032.

Uses and Administration

Corticotrophin-releasing hormone has been investigated in the differential diagnosis of Cushing's syndrome and other adrenal disorders. Doses of 100 µg, or of 1 µg per kg body-weight, have been given by intravenous injection; higher doses have been given but may be associated with an increased risk of adverse effects (see above).

A report of a conference on the clinical applications of corticotrophin-releasing hormone. The hormone has been investigated as a diagnostic agent in the 3 forms of Cushing's syndrome: pituitary Cushing's syndrome (Cushing's disease); ectopic ACTH syndrome; and adrenal syndrome, for example due to adenoma or cancer of the adrenal glands. Testing with corticotrophin-releasing hormone reliably differentiates the ACTH-dependent from the ACTH-independent forms of Cushing's syndrome and provides useful information in the differential diagnosis of pituitary from ectopic ACTH secretion. It has also been investigated, with little success, in Nelson's syndrome, and has been tried in the differential diagnosis of primary and secondary adrenocortical insufficiency; preliminary results suggest that it has the potential to differentiate pituitary from hypothalamic causes of secondary adrenocortical insufficiency. Corticotrophin-releasing hormone has also been used in the investigation of psychiatric states, such as depression, associated with hypercortisolism and it has been suggested that the endogenous hormone may be implicated in the pathophysiology of depressive symptoms.— G. P. Chrousos *et al.*, *Ann. intern. Med.*, 1985, *102*, 344.

A study of the effects of ovine corticotrophin-releasing hormone as a bolus intravenous injection of 1 µg per kg body-weight in 13 patients with Cushing's disease and 9 with other forms of Cushing's syndrome. All of the former group responded to the injection with increases in plasma corticotrophin (ACTH) and cortisol concentration, regardless of whether they were receiving treatment (and hence regardless of basal corticotrophin concentrations). In contrast, patients with ectopic ACTH syndrome showed no response to corticotrophin-releasing hormone, nor did a patient with micronodular adrenal disease or one with untreated metastatic adrenal carcinoma. Control of adrenal carcinoma with mitotane or mitotane and aminoglutethimide resulted in the restoration of some responsiveness to the injection. Similarly one patient with the ectopic ACTH syndrome was treated with metyrapone and subsequently had a response to corticotrophin-releasing hormone, while the response of patients with Cushing's disease successfully treated with surgery was similar to that in healthy subjects. The use of corticotrophin-releasing hormone may prove valuable in differentiating pituitary from ectopic causes of Cushing's syndrome.— G. P. Chrousos *et al.*, *New Engl. J. Med.*, 1984, *310*, 622.

Comparison of the accuracy of the corticotrophin-releasing hormone (CRH) test with that of the high-dose dexamethasone suppression test in the differential diagnosis of Cushing's syndrome. A false-negative response occurred in 2 of 22 patients with (pituitary dependent) Cushing's disease given the CRH test; this compared with 2 of 18 of these patients who gave false negatives in the dexamethasone suppression test. A false-positive response also occurred with the dexamethasone suppression test in 1 patient with ectopic corticotrophin secretion whereas CRH revealed the cause of Cushing's syndrome to be non-pituitary-dependent in this patient and in 3 with adrenal adenoma. It is recommended that routine CRH testing should be used in addition to high-dose dexamethasone testing to discriminate with the highest precision between the various forms of Cushing's syndrome.— A. R. Hermus *et al.*, *Lancet*, 1986, *2*, 540. Criticism of the value and accuracy of corticotrophin-releasing hormone tests in differentiating Cushing's disease from primary adrenal disease; computerised tomographic scanning of the adrenal glands is the most reliable means of demonstrating an adrenal tumour.— P. Kendall-Taylor and P. H. Baylis (letter), *ibid.*, 750. See also T. A. Howlett *et al.* (letter), *ibid.*, 871.

A further comparison of the corticotrophin-releasing hormone test and the dexamethasone suppression test in the differential diagnosis of Cushing's syndrome. The combined use of both tests would appear to yield improved diagnostic accuracy compared with either test alone.— L. K. Nieman *et al.*, *Ann. intern. Med.*, 1986, *105*, 862.

DEPRESSION. References to altered responses to corticotrophin-releasing factor in patients with depression: F. Holsboer (letter), *New Engl. J. Med.*, 1984, *311*, 1127; M. T. Lowy *et al.* (letter), *ibid.*, 1985, *312*, 791; P. W. Gold *et al.*, *ibid.*, 1986, *314*, 1329.

For a discussion of depression and Cushing's syndrome, and the possible uses of corticotrophin-releasing hormone in the investigation of both conditions, see *Lancet*, 1986, *2*, 550.

1463-q

Octacosactrin *(BAN)*.

α^{1-28}-Corticotrophin (human); Tosactide *(rINN)*. [25-Aspartic acid,26-alanine,-27-glycine]corticotrophin-(1–28)-octacosapeptide; Ser-Tyr-Ser-Met-Glu-His-Phe-Arg-Trp-Gly-Lys-Pro-Val-Gly-Lys-Lys-Arg-Arg-Pro-Val-Lys-Val-Tyr-Pro-Asp-Ala-Gly-Glu.

$C_{150}H_{230}N_{44}O_{38}S$=3289.8.

CAS — 47931-80-6.

Octacosactrin is a synthetic polypeptide representing the first 28 amino-acid residues of human corticotrophin.

Octacosactrin was formerly given for diagnostic purposes by intravenous injection.

Proprietary Names and Manufacturers

Actid 1–28 *(Ferring, Ger.)*; Homactid *(Ferring, Swed.)*.

1465-s

Tetracosactrin *(BAN)*.

Cosyntropin *(USAN)*; Tetracosactide *(rINN)*.

$C_{136}H_{210}N_{40}O_{31}S$=2933.5.

CAS — 16960-16-0.

Pharmacopoeias. In *Br.*

Tetracosactrin is a tetracosapeptide that increases the rate at which corticoid hormones are secreted by the adrenal gland. Its amino acid sequence is the same as that of the first 24 residues of human corticotrophin. It contains not less than 800 units per mg. It is available in the acetate form.

Tetracosactrin acetate is a white to yellow amorphous powder. **Soluble** 1 in 70 of water. **Store** at 2° to 8° under an atmosphere of nitrogen. Protect from light.

Units

490 units of tetracosactrin for bioassay are contained in approximately 490 µg of synthetic tetracosactrin with mannitol 20 mg in one ampoule of the first International Reference Preparation (1981).

Adverse Effects and Treatment

As for corticotrophin, p.1139.

ALLERGY. Experience had shown that the hope that tetracosactrin would cause fewer reactions than natural corticotrophin might not be realised. There had been 2 deaths in patients whose treatment had continued after a mild reaction had occurred with an earlier dose, and serious, even fatal, reactions had occurred at various times during courses of therapy with no mild premonitory symptoms. Although reactions had occurred after the patient had left the doctor's surgery none had occurred more than an hour after injection. The manufacturers had agreed to recommend that patients should remain at the hospital or surgery for a recovery period following an injection, and that self-injection should not normally be recommended.— Committee on Safety of Medicines, *Current Problems Series No. 1*, Sept., 1975.

Individual reports of allergic reactions following injection of tetracosactrin: N. E. Jensen and I. Sneddon (letter), *Br. med. J.*, 1969, *2*, 383; G. Fagg, *Br. J. clin. Pract.*, 1970, *24*, 155; G. Patriarca (letter), *Lancet*, 1971, *1*, 138; P. J. Brombacher *et al.* (letter), *ibid.*, 1975, *1*, 456; P. D. Mohr (letter), *Br. med. J.*, 1975, *4*, 162; J. Porter and H. Jick, *Lancet*, 1977, *1*, 587.

Withdrawal

As for corticotrophin, p.1139.

Precautions

As for corticosteroids, p.873.

Since reactions may not occur for up to 1 hour after injection sufficient time should be allowed for recovery after administration at the hospital or surgery. Self-administration is not recommended.

Absorption and Fate

Tetracosactrin is inactivated when administered by mouth. Intravenous administration results in a prompt rise in plasma cortisol (hydrocortisone). After intramuscular injection, blood-cortisol (hydrocortisone) concentrations reach a peak within an hour and decline to the basal concentration after about 4 hours.

The long-acting depot preparations of tetracosactrin are given by intramuscular injection and produce peak blood-cortisol concentrations in about 8 hours, with raised values for more than 24 hours.

Uses and Administration

Tetracosactrin is a synthetic polypeptide with general properties similar to those of corticotrophin (see p.1139).

Although tetracosactrin, like corticotrophin, has been used therapeutically for most of the conditions in which systemic corticosteroid therapy is indicated, its use is now generally limited to only a few of these indications such as Crohn's disease or ulcerative colitis and rheumatoid arthritis. Tetracosactrin may also be used diagnostically to investigate adrenocortical insufficiency.

Tetracosactrin is employed in the form of the acetate although doses are expressed in terms of tetracosactrin itself.

For therapeutic purposes it is given by intramuscular injection in the form of a long-acting depot preparation. The usual initial adult dose is 1 mg daily, reduced after the acute symptoms have been controlled to 1 mg every 2 or 3 days; maintenance doses may be 500 µg every 2 or 3 days or 1 mg weekly. For children suggested initial daily doses and suggested maintenance doses every 2 to 8 days have been 250 µg for those aged 1 month to 2 years, 250 to 500 µg for those aged 2 to 5 years, and 250 µg to 1 mg for those aged 5 to 12 years.

For diagnostic purposes tetracosactrin is used intramuscularly or intravenously but the preparation used is not formulated as a long-acting depot injection. The test is based on the measurement of plasma-cortisol concentrations immediately before and exactly 30 minutes after an intramuscular or intravenous injection of 250 µg; adrenocortical function may be regarded as normal if there is a rise in the cortisol concentration of at least 200 nmol per litre (70 µg per litre). A suggested intravenous dose in children has been 250 µg per 1.73 m^2 body-surface. If the results of this test are equivocal the long-acting depot preparation may be used. In adults a dose of 1 mg is given intramuscularly with adrenocortical function being regarded as normal if plasma-cortisol concentrations have steadily increased to 1000 to 1800 nmol per litre 5 hours after the injection.

Preparations

Tetracosactrin Injection *(B.P.)*. A sterile aqueous solution of Tetracosactrin (*B.P.*) sterilised by heating.

Tetracosactrin Zinc Injection *(B.P.)*. A sterile aqueous suspension of Tetracosactrin (*B.P.*) with zinc hydroxide prepared aseptically. It is for intramuscular injection only.

Proprietary Preparations

Synacthen *(Ciba, UK)*. *Injection*, tetracosactrin 250 µg (as acetate)/mL in ampoules of 1 mL.

Injection (Synacthen Depot), suspension, tetracosactrin 1 mg (as acetate)/mL absorbed onto zinc phospate, in ampoules of 1 mL and vials of 2 mL.

Proprietary Names and Manufacturers

Cortrosinta Depot *(Spain)*; Cortrosyn *(Austral.; Belg.; Organon, Canad.; Ravasini, Ital.; Neth.; Norw.; S.Afr.; Swed.; Organon, Switz.; Organon, USA)*; Cortrosyn Depot *(Organon, UK)*; Nuvacthen *(Ciba, Spain)*; Synacthène *(Ciba, Fr.)*; Synacthen *(Arg.; Ciba, Austral.; Belg.; Ciba, Canad.; Ciba, Denm.; Ciba, Ger.; Ciba, Ital.; Neth.; Ciba, Norw.; Ciba, S.Afr.; Ciba, Swed.; Ciba, Switz.; Ciba, UK)*.

3886-d

Gonad-regulating Hormones

The following section includes substances such as Chorionic Gonadotrophin, Menotrophin, and Urofollitrophin, which have the actions of the gonadotrophic hormones, follicle-stimulating hormone and luteinising hormone. It also includes the hypothalamic releasing hormone of the gonadotrophic hormones, namely Gonadorelin, and a number of its analogues including Buserelin Acetate, Goserelin Acetate, Leuprorelin Acetate, Nafarelin Acetate, and Triptorelin.

The sex hormones are also involved in the hormonal regulation of the gonads—see Sex Hormones, p.1383.

14039-p

Buserelin Acetate *(BANM, USAN, rINNM)*.

D-Ser $(Bu^t)^6$ Pro^9 NEt LHRH acetate; HOE-766; S74-6766 *(buserelin)*. (6-*O*-*tert*-Butyl-D-serine)-des-10-glycinamidegonadorelin ethylamide acetate.

$C_{60}H_{86}N_{16}O_{13},C_2H_4O_2$=1299.5.

CAS — 57982-77-1 (buserelin); 68630-75-1 (acetate).

1.05 g of buserelin acetate is approximately equivalent to 1 g of buserelin.

Adverse Effects and Precautions

As for Gonadorelin (p.1142).

Buserelin or triptorelin was used in the treatment of 46 men with symptomatic locally advanced or metastic prostatic cancer. Various doses were used and produced objective improvement in 26 of 35 given buserelin and 8 of 11 given triptorelin. However 17 of 32 patients who had bone pain at the start of treatment had an increase in bone pain which resolved after the first week; one patient who had no initial bone pain developed such pain on receiving the gonadorelin analogue. Additional symptoms to increased bone pain included lymphoedema in 4, increased serum-creatinine concentration in 1, and one patient who developed signs of compression of the spinal cord with complete sphincter dysfunction and weakness in the legs.— J. Waxman *et al.*, *Br. med. J.*, 1985, *291*, 1387. Patients are routinely pretreated with cyproterone acetate for 3 days before and one week after the initiation of gonadorelin analogue treatment.— J. Waxman (letter), *ibid.*, 1986, *292*, 58.

Reduced bone density and mineral content in pre-menopausal women given buserelin for endometriosis.— W. H. Matta *et al.*, *Br. med. J.*, 1987, *294*, 1523. See also J. -P. Devogelaer *et al.* (letter), *Lancet*, 1987, *1*, 1498.

EFFECTS ON THE CARDIOVASCULAR SYSTEM. Hypertension in one patient associated with buserelin acetate.— J. F. R. Barrett and M. E. Dalton, *Br. med. J.*, 1987, *294*, 1101.

Uses and Administration

Buserelin acetate is an analogue of gonadorelin (see p.1142). It is mainly used for the suppression of testosterone in the treatment of malignant neoplasm of the prostate. Treatment is started with the equivalent of 500 µg of buserelin being injected subcutaneously every 8 hours for 7 days. On the eighth day treatment is changed to the nasal route with 100 µg of buserelin being sprayed into each nostril on 6 occasions throughout the day. A full response should be achieved within 4 to 6 weeks.

ACNE. Resolution of life-long acne conglabata in a patient being treated with buserelin for advanced prostatic cancer.— J. Waxman *et al.*, *Br. J. Derm.*, 1983, *109*, 679.

CONTRACEPTION. Buserelin given intranasally in doses up to 600 µg daily has provided effective contraception in women (C. Berquist *et al.*, *Lancet*, 1979, *2*, 215; *idem*, *Contraception*, 1985, *31*, 111). It could also be used as a postcoital contraceptive (A. Lemay *et al.*, *Fert. Steril.*, 1983, *39*, 661).

ENDOMETRIOSIS. Buserelin or nafarelin have been studied in daily doses of 0.3 to 1 mg intranasally for up to 6 months in patients with endometriosis. Therapy was started in the early follicular phase of the menstrual cycle and up to 9-fold unwanted increases in oestradiol concentrations occurred in the first few weeks. LHRH agonist treatment should start in the luteal phase. Further experience has been gained in 400 patients given up to 1.2 mg of buserelin daily for 6 months. Improvement in endometriosis was noted in 79 of 101 evaluable patients. Plasma-oestradiol concentrations fell as treatment continued, although episodic oestrogen secretion persisted in 10% of women throughout treatment. All treated patients experienced hot flushes once postmenopausal concentrations of oestradiol were achieved; a combination with a progestogen might alleviate this.— *Lancet*, 1986, *2*, 1016.

Further references to buserelin in endometriosis: R. W. Shaw *et al.*, *Br. med. J.*, 1983, *287*, 1667; A. Lemay *et al.*, *Fert. Steril.*, 1984, *41*, 863.

FIBROIDS. Shrinkage of a uterine fibroid after subcutaneous infusion of buserelin.— D. L. Healy *et al.*, *Br. med. J.*, 1984, *289*, 1267.

INFERTILITY, FEMALE. Reports of buserelin followed by gonadotrophic stimulation for the induction of ovulation: R. Fleming *et al.* (letter), *Lancet*, 1984, *1*, 399; R. N. Porter *et al.* (letter), *ibid.*, *2*, 1284; R. W. Shaw *et al.* (letter), *ibid.*, 1985, *2*, 506; M. Armitage *et al.*, *Br. med. J.*, 1987, *295*, 96.

MALIGNANT NEOPLASMS. Twelve patients with advanced prostatic cancer, previously untreated, were treated for up to 9 months with buserelin 200 µg three to five times daily by nasal inhalation. Serum concentrations of testosterone, gonadotrophins, and oestradiol fell, and 9 patients achieved objective and subjective signs of disease regression. Although initially promoting increased secretion of gonadotrophins, long-term use resulted in a decrease of synthesis and secretion. Facial flushing occurred in all patients and lessened in intensity and frequency as treatment continued. No patient was able to attain an erection.— J. H. Waxman *et al.*, *Br. med. J.*, 1983, *286*, 1309.

The manufacturers reported that 77 buserelin-treated cases of advanced prostatic cancer had been recorded and 40 of them had been published. Most patients had been given buserelin by subcutaneous injection for 1 week followed by administration by intranasal spray. Peak serum-testosterone concentrations were obtained after 3 to 6 days; after 2 weeks reductions of 60 to 90% in serum-testosterone concentrations were achieved. A clinical response was noted in 37 of the treated patients.— D. R. Chadha and A. Matroos (letter), *Lancet*, 1983, *2*, 916.

A group of 8 men were selected from 58 with metastatic prostatic carcinoma being treated with buserelin 500 µg by subcutaneous injection every 8 hours for one week than 3 daily intranasal applications of 400 µg. Treatment periods had ranged from 6 to 22 months (mean 13). The 8 patients who were in remission demonstrated castration levels of testosterone, indicating that repeated administration of buserelin over a mean period of 13 months can maintain testosterone suppression. Out of the 8 patients one subsequently relapsed, the other 7 were still responding to buserelin at 13 to 26 months.— M. T. W. T. Lock *et al.* (letter), *Lancet*, 1985, *2*, 1236.

Further references to buserelin in prostatic carcinoma: M. C. Volmer *et al.* (letter), *Lancet*, 1985, *1*, 1507 (clearance of lung metastases); J. G. M. Klign *et al.* (letter), *ibid.*, *2*, 493 (combination with cyproterone acetate); F. Labrie *et al.* (letter), *ibid.*, 1986, 1, 48 (combination with flutamide).

Use of buserelin in metastatic breast cancer.— J. G. M. Klijn and F. H. de Jong, *Lancet*, 1982, *1*, 1213.

PUBERTY, PRECOCIOUS. References to the use of buserelin in precocious puberty: R. Stanhope *et al.*, *Archs Dis. Childh.*, 1985, *60*, 116; P. S. Ward *et al.*, *ibid.*, 872; R. Stanhope *et al.*, *Clin. Endocr.*, 1985, *22*, 795.

Proprietary Preparations

Suprefact *(Hoechst, UK). Injection*, buserelin acetate 1.05 mg equivalent to buserelin 1 mg in ampoules of 1 mL.

Nasal spray, buserelin acetate 10.5 mg equivalent to buserelin 10.0 mg in multidose containers of about 100 doses.

Proprietary Names and Manufacturers

Suprefact *(Hoechst, Belg.; Hoechst, Denm.; Hoechst, Fr.; Hoechst, Ger.; Hoechst, Ital.; Behring, Spain; Hoechst, UK).*

5925-q

Gonadorelin *(BAN, rINN).*

GnRH; Gonadoliberin; Gonadotrophin-releasing Hormone; Hoe471; LH/FSH-RF; LH/FSH-RH; LH-RF; LH-RH; Luliberin. 5-Oxo-L-prolyl-L-histidyl-L-tryptophyl-L-seryl-L-tyrosylglycyl-L-leucyl-L-arginyl-L-prolylglycinamide.

$C_{55}H_{75}N_{17}O_{13}$=1182.3.

CAS — 33515-09-2; 34973-08-5 (diacetate, anhydrous); 52699-48-6 (diacetate, tetrahydrate); 51952-41-1 (xHCl).

NOTE. Gonadorelin Acetate and Gonadorelin Hydrochloride are *USAN*.

Pharmacopoeias. In *Br.*

A decapeptide obtained by synthesis. A white or faintly yellowish-white powder. **Soluble** 1 in 25 of water, 1 in 50 of methyl alcohol, and 1 in 25 of 1% v/v acetic acid.

The *B.P.* injection has a pH of 4.5 to 8.0 and the solution should be stored at a temperature not exceeding 15° and protected from light; the unreconstituted injection can be stored at a temperature not exceeding 25°.

Gonadorelin acetate and hydrochloride have been described.

STABILITY. Gonadorelin stored at 4° in nonsterile solutions of 0.9% sodium chloride or 1% glycine was inactive at 23 or 27 weeks respectively. Similar solutions stored at −20° retained their activity for about a year.— W. C. Dermondy and J. R. Reel (letter), *New Engl. J. Med.*, 1976, *295*, 173. This loss of activity was probably due to bacterial contamination of the solutions. Gonadorelin in lyophilised form and as a sterile solution retained its activity when stored at 4° and 40° for 18 months.— J. Sandow *et al.* (letter), *New Engl. J. Med.*, 1977, *296*, 885. Aqueous solutions of gonadorelin were stable for at least 10 weeks when stored at 37° according to an *in vitro* bioassay and to chromatography. There was no deterioration after 2 years of storage at 4°.— Y. -F. Shi *et al.*, *J. pharm. Sci.*, 1984, *73*, 819.

Units

31 units of gonadorelin for bioassay are contained in approximately 50 µg of gonadorelin acetate with lactose 2.5 mg and human plasma albumin 0.5 mg in one ampoule of the first International Reference Preparation (1980).

Adverse Effects

Gonadorelin and its analogues may cause gastro-intestinal adverse effects, usually nausea and abdominal pain or discomfort. There may be headache or lightheadedness and an increase in menstrual bleeding. Reactions or pain may occur at the site of injection with rash, swelling, or pruritus. Bronchospasm has been reported.

Other effects may be a consequence of the particular use of gonadorelin or its analogues. Tumour flare, for instance, has been reported in the initial stages of treatment for cancer of the prostate. This may occur as an increase in bone pain; occasionally there has been a worsening of urinary-tract symptoms with haematuria and urinary obstruction; some patients have experienced weakness and paraesthesia of the lower limbs. It is common practice to give an antiandrogen such as cyproterone acetate in the first few weeks of treatment with gonadorelin or its analogues when used in prostatic cancer; this will cover the initial surge in testosterone concentrations.

For disease flare in patients with prostatic cancer being treated with gonadorelin analogues, see buserelin acetate (p.1141).

See also buserelin acetate (p.1141) for a report of diminished bone density in pre-menopausal women receiving that analogue for endometriosis.

For a report of a gonadorelin analogue having no effect on antithrombin III, see goserelin acetate (p.1143).

Precautions

Gonadorelin should not be used in women with polycystic disease of the ovary. It is also recommended that patients with weight-related amenorrhoea should not recieve gonadorelin until their weight is corrected. Gonadorelin should be discontinued if the the patient becomes pregnant. Contraceptive measures should be taken to protect against unwanted ovulation. Concomitant drug therapy may alter the response to gonadorelin, especially when being used as a test of pituitary function. Other hormonal therapy can obviously affect the response. Spironolactone and levodopa can stimulate gonadotrophins while phenothiazines, dopamine antagonists, digoxin, and sex hormones can inhibit gonadotrophin secretion.

Absorption and Fate

Gonadorelin has a plasma half-life of only a few minutes after intravenous injection. It is hydrolysed in the plasma and excreted in the urine.

Gonadorelin analogues are also absorbed following oral, intranasal, or rectal administration.

Gonadotrophin-releasing hormone has been detected in milk in concentrations of 0.1 to 3.0 nanograms per mL. Thyrotrophin-releasing hormone appears in smaller concentrations.— T. Baram *et al.*, *Science*, 1977, *198*, 300.

Uses and Administration

Gonadorelin is a hypothalamic releasing hormone, sometimes used as the hydrochloride, which stimulates the synthesis of follicle-stimulating hormone and luteinising hormone in the anterior lobe of the pituitary as well as their release. Gonadorelin secretion which is pulsatile is controlled by several factors including circulating sex hormones.

Gonadorelin is used in the diagnosis of hypothalamic-pituitary-gonadal dysfunction. Assessment is usually based on the response to a dose of gonadorelin 100 µg by intravenous or subcutaneous injection.

Gonadorelin is also used in the treatment of amenorrhoea and infertility associated with hypogonadotrophic hypogonadism and multifollicular ovaries. Weight-related amenorrhoea should have been corrected by diet. Treatment in such conditions is based on an intermittent pulse pump providing 10 to 20 µg over one minute every 90 minutes for up to 6 months or until conception.

Gonadorelin or more usually its analogues (which are more potent and have a longer duration of action) are used in contraception, cryptorchidism, malignant neoplasms (especially of the prostate), and in precocious puberty.

The therapeutic applications of gonadorelin and its analogues.— G. B. Cutler *et al.*, *Ann. intern. Med.*, 1985, *102*, 643; M. Filicori and C. Flamigni, *Drugs*, 1988, *35*, 63.

ACNE. For a report of a gonadorelin analogue producing improvement in acne, see buserelin acetate (p.1141).

CONTRACEPTION. A discussion on gonadorelin analogues, mainly agonists, in contraception. A simple measure involves the daily administration of the agonist and this has been shown to be effective but can produce a high incidence of amenorrhoea; it can also cause oestrogen deficiency with symptoms of hot flushes and vaginal dryness although that may vary with the agonist being used. There is, too, the possibility of loss of bone mineral. The combination of an agonist with a progestogen in a cyclic regimen allows for some oestrogen production and regular bleeds, but at the expense of possible breakthrough bleeding and other adverse effects associated with steroid oral contraceptives.

LHRH agonist contraceptives could be useful in women at risk from combined steroid contraceptives, such as those aged over 35 and particularly those who smoke. They may be useful in women with heavy periods and in lactating women since milk production should not be affected and the small amount excreted in milk would have no effect on the infant since it would be broken down in its gastro-intestinal tract.

LHRH agonists suppress spermatogenesis. However, they also affect libido and cause impotence so that androgen replacement would be required and this in turn could diminish the contraceptive effect.

LHRH antagonists could be used for both male and female contraception, but they have a complex structure which makes them difficult to produce.— *Lancet*, 1987, *1*, 1179.

Further references to gonadorelin analogues being used for contraception are provided under buserelin acetate (p.1141) and nafarelin acetate (p.1143).

CRYPTORCHIDISM. There are several studies of gonadorelin being used to correct cryptorchidism; some showing a useful response (R. Illig *et al.*, *Lancet*, 1977, *2*, 518; A.M. Klidjian *et al.*, *Archs Dis. Childh.*, 1985, *60*, 568), others showing no benefit (J. Rajfer *et al.*, *New Engl. J. Med.*, 1986, *314*, 466; S.M.P.F. De Muinck Keizer-Schrama *et al.*, *Lancet*, 1986, *1*, 876). The opinion has been expressed (*Lancet*, 1986, *1*, 1133) that gonadorelin appears to be ineffective in boys of any age with impalpable testes. In boys under the age of 2 years with palpable testes gonadorelin could be worth trying for this is an age group in whom surgery may be difficult and a small percentage will respond to gonadorelin.

DIAGNOSIS OF HYPOTHALAMIC AND PITUITARY DYSFUNCTION. Some references to gonadorelin in the diagnosis of hypothalamic-pituitary-gonadal dysfunction including one (Adulwahid *et al.*, 1985) suggesting its abandonment: C. H. Mortimer *et al.*, *Br. med. J.*, 1973, *4*, 73; Y. Yoshimoto *et al.*, *New Engl. J. Med.*, 1975, *292*, 242; J. Sagel *et al.*, *Postgrad. med. J.*, 1975, *51*, 611; J. Ginsburg *et al.*, *Br. med. J.*, 1975, *3*, 130; N. A. Adulwahid *et al.*, *ibid.*, 1985, *291*, 1471.

ENDOMETRIOSIS. Improvement in endometriosis consequent on medical oophorectomy by the gonadotrophin releasing hormone D-Trp^6-Pro^9-NEt-LHRH ($LHRH_A$) in 5 women.— D. R. Meldrum *et al.*, *J. clin. Endocr. Metab.*, 1982, *54*, 1081.

See also under buserelin acetate (p.1141) for a reference to buserelin and nafarelin producing improvement in endometriosis.

FIBROIDS. A discussion of gonadotrophin releasing hormone or its analogues in the treatment of uterine fibroids.— *Lancet*, 1986, *2*, 1197.

Further references to gonadorelin analogues being used in the treatment of fibroids are provided under buserelin acetate (p.1141), goserelin acetate (p.1143) and triptorelin (below).

INFERTILITY, FEMALE. A discussion of the practical aspects of pulsatile gonadorelin for the treatment of infertility in women. Patients with hypogonadotrophic hypogonadism and those with weight-related amenorrhoea who remain anovulatory despite adequate weight gain do best with this treatment. Patients with multicystic ovaries also benefit. Those with polycystic ovaries do less well and although they may respond to the addition of clomiphene citrate, the rate of abortion is higher in this group. Multiple folliculogenesis occasionally occurs, particularly during the first cycle and when it dose happen the pulsatile administration of gonadorelin should be discontinued. In patients with hypogonadotrophic hypogonadism this hyperstimulation does not occur as long as gonadorelin is withdrawn before the follicles are mature enough to ovulate, since there is no midcycle surge in LH. A few patients develop a normal follicular growth pattern yet fail to ovulate; an injection of chorionic gonadotrophin may overcome this.
An alternative method of treatment is to give gonadorelin in a similar pulsatile manner, but only until ovulation is induced and then to give 3 injections of chorionic gonadotrophin 2000 units at 3-day intervals to support the luteal phase.— N. A. Armar *et al.*, *Br. J. Hosp. Med.*, 1987, *37*, 429.

References to the induction of ovulation and subsequent pregnancy in women given pulsatile gonadorelin: G. Leyendecker *et al.*, *J. clin. Endocr. Metab.*, 1980, *51*, 1214; D. Bogchelman *et al.* (letter), *Lancet*, 1982, *2*, 45; D. S. Miller *et al.*, *J. Am. med. Ass.*, 1983, *250*, 2937; P. Mason, *Br. med. J.*, 1984, *288*, 181; D. M. Hurley *et al.*, *New Engl. J. Med.*, 1984, *310*, 1069; J. Adams *et al.*, *Lancet*, 1985, *2*, 1375.

Further references to gonadorelin analogues being used in protocols for the induction of ovulation in the management of female infertility are provided under buserelin acetate (p.1141) and triptorelin (below).

INFERTILITY, MALE. Low-dose pulsatile treatment with gonadorelin has induced puberty in men with hypogonadotrophic hypogonadism (A.R. Hoffman and W.F. Crowley, *New Engl. J. Med.*, 1982, *307*, 1237 and 1655) and such treatment has been maintained for up to 36 months (D.I. Spratt *et al.*, *Ann. intern. Med.*, 1986, *105*, 848). Spermatogenesis has been initiated as a result of such treatment and this has been used to treat infertility in selected patients (A.A. Shargil, *Fert. Steril.*, 1987, *47*, 492).

MALIGNANT NEOPLASMS. Gonadorelin analogues are used sometimes with antiandrogens in the treatment of prostatic cancer. They have also been tried in neoplasms of the breast, ovary, and pancreas.
Analogues used include buserelin acetate (p.1141), goserelin acetate, leuprorelin acetate, nafarelin acetate, and triptorelin (all below).
D-Trp[6]-Pro[9]-NEt-LHRH ($LHRH_A$) has also been used (F. Labrie *et al.*, *Br. med. J.*, 1985, *291*, 369).

PREMENSTRUAL SYNDROME. Gonadorelin as the analogue D-Trp[6]-Pro[9]-NEt-LHRH ($LHRH_A$) might confer benefit in the premenstrual syndrome.— K. N. Muse *et al.*, *New Engl. J. Med.*, 1984, *311*, 1345.

PUBERTY, DELAYED. See above under Infertility, Male.

PUBERTY, PRECOCIOUS. The most important long-term consequence of precocious puberty is short stature, since rapid skeletal maturation leads to early epiphyseal fusion. Gonadorelin or its analogues have proved an efficient treatment. They initially produce a transient increase in gonadotrophin secretion but pituitary reserves fall and pulsatile natural gonadotrophin secretion ceases and leads to reversal of gonadal maturation and decreased secretion of gonadal steroids. Larger doses may be required for girls than for boys. Therapy is usually continued until the average age of puberty and/or menarche. When treatment is stopped there is gradual reversion to pulsatile gonadotrophin secretion and a pubertal luteinising hormone response to native gonadotrophin releasing hormone.— *Lancet*, 1986, *2*, 80.
References to the gonadorelin analogue D-Trp[6]-Pro[9]-NEt-LHRH ($LHRH_A$) in a daily dose of 4μg per kg bodyweight for the treatment of precocious puberty.— O. H. Pescovitz *et al.*, *J. Pediat.*, 1986, *108*, 47; F. Comite *et al.*, *J. Am. med. Ass.*, 1986, *255*, 2613.

For further references to gonadorelin analogues being used in the treatment of precocious puberty, see buserelin acetate (p.1142) and triptorelin (p.1144).

Preparations

Gonadorelin Injection *(B.P.)*

Proprietary Preparations

Fertiral *(Hoechst, UK)*. *Injection*, gonadorelin 500 μg/mL, in ampoules of 2 mL. For infusion by intermittent pulsatile pump.

HRF Ayerst *(Ayerst, UK)*. *Injection*, powder for reconstitution, gonadorelin 100 and 500 μg, supplied with diluent.

Relefact LH-RH *(Hoechst, UK)*. *Injection*, gonadorelin 100 μg/mL, in ampoules of 1 mL.

Relefact LH-RH/TRH *(Hoechst, UK)*. *Injection*, gonadorelin 100 μg and protirelin 200 μg/mL, in ampoules of 1 mL.

Proprietary Names and Manufacturers

Factrel *(Ayerst, Canad.; Ayerst, USA)*; Fertiral *(Hoechst, UK)*; HRF *(Ayerst, Austral.; Belg.; Ayerst, Ital.; S.Afr.; Ayerst, UK)*; Kryptocur *(Hoechst, Ger.; Hoechst, Switz.)*; LRH *(Roche, Austral.)*; Luforan *(Serono, Spain)*; Lutamin *(Jpn)*; Lutrelef *(Ferring, Fr.; Ferring, Ger.)*; Relefact LH-RH *(Hoechst, Austral.; Hoechst, Ger.; Hoechst, UK)*; Relisorm L *(Serono, Ital.; Serono, Switz.)*; Stimu-LH *(Roussel, Fr.)*.

16845-p

Goserelin Acetate *(BANM, pINNM)*.

D-Ser (Bu[t])[6] Azgly[10]-LHRH Acetate; ICI-118630. 3-[5-Oxo-L-prolyl-L-histidyl-L-tryptophyl-L-seryl-L-tyrosyl-(3-*O*-*tert*-butyl)-D-seryl-L-leucyl-L-arginyl-L-prolyl]carbazamide acetate.
$C_{59}H_{84}N_{18}O_{14}, C_2H_4O_2$=1329.5.

CAS — 65807-02-5 (goserelin).

NOTE. Goserelin is *USAN*.

1.05 g of goserelin acetate is approximately equivalent to 1 g of goserelin.

Adverse Effects and Precautions

As for gonadorelin (p.1142).

In order to estimate the risk of thrombo-embolic events in men given goserelin for prostatic carcinoma, antithrombin III concentrations were measured in 30 men. No significant change occurred.— E. Varenhorst *et al.*, *Br. med. J.*, 1986, *292*, 935.

Uses and Administration

Goserelin acetate is an analogue of gonadorelin (p.1142). It is used for the suppression of testosterone in the treatment of malignant neoplasms of the prostate. Goserelin acetate is available as a depot preparation such that a dose equivalent to 3.6 mg of goserelin given subcutaneously provides effective suppression of testosterone for 28 days. A full response should be achieved by the end of this period.

A single dose of goserelin 3.6 mg as the acetate suppressed the secretion of luteinising hormone for about 5 weeks in women.— E. J. Thomas *et al.*, *Br. med. J.*, 1986, *293*, 1407.

FIBROIDS. Follow-up of 12 women given goserelin for uterine fibroids showed that return of ovulatory menstruation was accompanied by rapid fibroid regrowth. Agonists such as goserelin may be useful in controlling symptoms before surgery and may facilitate hysterectomy.— M. A. Lumsden *et al.* (letter), *Lancet*, 1987, *1*, 36.

MALIGNANT NEOPLASMS. Use of a depot formulation of goserelin allowing subcutaneous administration once every 28 days in the treatment of prostatic carcinoma: G. Williams *et al.*, *Br. med. J.*, 1984, *289*, 1580; S. R. Ahmed *et al.*, *ibid.*, 1985, *290*, 185.

Further references to goserelin in the treatment of prostatic carcinoma: J. M. Allen *et al.*, *Br. med. J.*, 1983, *286*, 1607; K. J. Walker *et al.*, *Lancet*, 1983, *2*, 413; S. R. Ahmed *et al.*, *ibid.*, 415.

Proprietary Preparations

Zoladex *(ICI Pharmaceuticals, UK)*. *Implant*, goserelin, 3.6 mg (as acetate) in syringe applicator.

12895-s

Leuprorelin Acetate *(BANM, rINNM)*.

Abbott-43818; Leuprolide Acetate *(USAN)*; TAP-144. 5-OxoPro-His-Trp-Ser-Tyr-D-Leu-Leu-Arg-*N*-ethyl-L-prolinamide acetate.
$C_{59}H_{84}N_{16}O_{12}, C_2H_4O_2$=1269.5.

CAS — 74381-53-6.

Adverse Effects and Precautions

As for gonadorelin (p.1142).

Uses and Administration

Leuprorelin acetate is an analogue of gonadorelin. It is used for the suppression of testosterone in the treatment of malignant neoplasms of the prostate. Leuprorelin acetate is given by subcutaneous injection in a usual daily dose of 1 mg.

Single-dose pharmacokinetics of leuprorelin following subcutaneous and intravenous injection.— L. T. Sennello *et al.*, *J. pharm. Sci.*, 1986, *75*, 158.

MALIGNANT NEOPLASMS. Reviews and discussions of leuprorelin in the treatment of malignant neoplasm of the prostate: R. J. Santen, *Ann. intern. Med.*, 1985, *102*, 648; N. J. Wojciechowski *et al.*, *Drug Intell. & clin. Pharm.*, 1986, *20*, 746.

Leuprorelin 1 mg by subcutaneous injection daily was as effective as stilboestrol 3 mg daily by mouth in a multicentre study involving 199 men with metastatic prostatic cancer who had not received previous therapy. The incidence of adverse effects was significantly less with leuprorelin.—The Leuprolide Study Group, *New Engl. J. Med.*, 1984, *311*, 1281.

Proprietary Names and Manufacturers

Carcinil *(Abbott, Ger.)*; Lucrin *(Abbott, Fr.)*; Lupron *(Abbott, Canad.; TAP, USA)*; Procrin *(Abbott, Spain)*.

16907-g

Nafarelin Acetate *(BANM, USAN, pINNM)*.

D-Nal(2)[6]-LHRH acetate hydrate; RS-94991298. 5-Oxo-L-prolyl-L-histidyl-L-tryptophyl-L-seryl-L-tyrosyl-3-(2-naphthyl)-D-alanyl-L-leucyl-L-arginyl-L-prolylglycinamide acetate hydrate.
$C_{66}H_{83}N_{17}O_{13}, xC_2H_4O_2, yH_2O$.

CAS — 86220-42-0; 76932-56-4 (nafarelin).

Nafarelin acetate is a gonadorelin analogue under investigation for the treatment of prostate cancer, endometriosis, and for contraception.

References to nafarelin acetate: J. A. Gudmundsson *et al.*, *Contraception*, 1984, *30*, 107 (contraception); C. A. Peters and P. C. Walsh, *New Engl. J. Med.*, 1987, *317*, 599 (benign prostatic hypertrophy).

16834-v

Triptorelin *(USAN, pINN)*.

AY-25650; D-Trp[6]-LHRH; Triptoreline. 5-Oxo-L-prolyl-L-histidyl-L-tryptophyl-L-seryl-L-tyrosyl-D-tryptophyl-L-leucyl-L-arginyl-L-prolyl glycinamide.
$C_{64}H_{82}N_{18}O_{13}$=1311.5.

CAS — 57773-63-4.

Adverse Effects and Precautions

As for gonadorelin (p.1142).

For a report of disease flare in patients given triptorelin for prostatic cancer, see buserelin acetate, p.1141.

Uses and Administration

Triptorelin is an analogue of gonadorelin used for the suppression of testosterone in the treatment of malignant neoplasms of the prostate. It has been given as a depot preparation.

FIBROIDS. Six patients with uterine leiomyomas were given one injection of triptorelin 4 mg monthly; this depot injection released 100 μg daily. After 2 months, the uterus was reduced to 68% of its former size and after a further 2 months of treatment uterine volume was more than halved.— H. A. I. M. van Leusden (letter), *Lancet*, 1986, *2*, 1213.

INFERTILITY, FEMALE. A carefully timed programme of ovarian stimulation enabled follicular aspiration for *in vitro* fertilisation to be carried out usually on a weekday and avoided the need for clinical and laboratory staff to be on duty 7 days a week. Triptorelin 1.8 mg intramuscularly was added to a schedule of norethisterone and human menopausal gonadotrophin to prevent spontaneous surges of luteinising hormone.— J. R. Zorn (letter), *Lancet*, 1987, *1*, 385.

MALIGNANT NEOPLASMS. Clearance of lung and bone metastases in a patient with prostatic carcinoma given triptorelin daily by subcutaneous injection. The initial dose was 500 µg daily for the first 7 days after which it was reduced to 100 µg daily.— A. M. Gomaru-Schally *et al.* (letter), *Lancet*, 1984, *2*, 281.

In a multicentre study orchidectomy and triptorelin usually as a slow-release preparation given once a month after 3 injections in the first month produced similar responses in the initial treatment of advanced prostatic carcinoma.— H. Parmar *et al.*, *Lancet*, 1985, *2*, 1201. Similar findings in another multicentre study.— F. Boccardo *et al.* (letter), *ibid.*, 1986, *1*, 621.

Some improvement in 5 patients with advanced adenocarcinoma of the pancreas when given triptorelin 1 mg subcutaneously daily for 7 days reduced to 100 µg daily.— D. Gonzalez-Barcena *et al.* (letter), *Lancet*, 1986, *2*, 154.

PUBERTY, PRECOCIOUS. The use of triptorelin in precocious puberty.— M. Roger *et al.*, *J. clin. Endocr. Metab.*, 1986, *62*, 670.

Proprietary Names and Manufacturers

Decapeptyl *(IPSEN, Fr.; Ferring, Ger.)*.

5926-p

Gonadotrophic Hormones

The gonadotrophins secreted by the anterior lobe of the pituitary gland stimulate the normal functioning of the gonads and the secretion of sex hormones in both men and women. The two glycoprotein gonadotrophins that are produced are *follicle-stimulating hormone*(FSH) and *luteinising hormone* or *interstitial-cell-stimulating hormone* (LH; ICSH). The pituitary secretion of FSH and LH is regulated by a complex interaction between the hypothalamic gonadotrophin releasing hormone (see Gonadorelin p.1142), and both positive and negative feedback effects of circulating sex hormones on the pituitary and hypothalamus. This control system can also be influenced by the pituitary hormone prolactin (p.1145).

A gonadotrophin with predominantly luteinising properties is produced by the placenta and obtained from the urine of pregnant women (chorionic gonadotrophin); others with follicle-stimulating properties (urofollitrophin) or with predominantly follicle-stimulating properties (menotrophin) are obtained from the urine of postmenopausal women. A gonadotrophin with predominantly follicle-stimulating properties has also been obtained from the serum of pregnant mares (serum gonadotrophin), but is little used nowadays.

The functional relationship of the gonadotrophic hormones is complicated.

In a normal menstrual cycle follicle-stimulating hormone stimulates the development and maturation of the follicles and ova. As the follicle develops it produces oestrogen in increasing amounts which at mid-cycle stimulate the release of luteinising hormone. This causes rupture of the follicle with ovulation and converts the follicle into the corpus luteum which secretes progesterone.

In men, follicle-stimulating hormone has a role in spermatogenesis while luteinising hormone stimulates the interstitial cells of the testis to secrete testosterone, which in turn has a direct effect on the seminiferous tubules. Spermatogenesis has been reported to promote the secretion of a selective pituitary FSH suppressor, inhibin.

5927-s

Chorionic Gonadotrophin *(BAN, rINN)*.

CG; Choriogonadotrophin; Chorion. Gonadotr.; Chorionic Gonadotropin *(USAN)*; Gonadotrophinum Chorionicum; HCG; Human Chorionic Gonadotrophin; Pregnancy-urine Hormone; PU.

CAS — 9002-61-3.

Pharmacopoeias. In *Aust., Br., Braz., Chin., Egypt., Eur., Hung., Ind., It., Jpn, Jug., Nord., Swiss, Turk.,* and *U.S.* Also in *B.P. Vet.*

A preparation of a glycoprotein substance secreted by the placenta and obtained from the urine of pregnant women. It is a white or almost white amorphous powder. The *B.P.* specifies a sterile preparation containing not less than 2500 units per mg.

Soluble in water. The *B.P.* and *U.S.P.* specify that a 1% solution of the injection has a pH of 6.0 to 8.0. **Store** at a temperature not exceeding 20° in airtight containers sealed to exclude micro-organisms and protected from light; under these conditions it may be expected to retain its potency for not less than 3 years. The *U.S.P.* specifies a potency of not less than 1500 *U.S.P.* units per mg and storage in airtight containers at 2° to 8°.

Units

5300 units of human chorionic gonadotrophin for bioassay are contained in approximately 2 mg (with lactose 5 mg) in one ampoule of the second International Standard Preparation (1963).

650 units of human chorionic gonadotrophin for immunoassay are contained in approximately 70 µg (with human albumin 5 mg) in one ampoule of the first International Reference Preparation for Immunoassay (1975).

70 units of the alpha subunit of human chorionic gonadotrophin for immunoassay are contained in approximately 70 µg (with human albumin 5 mg) in one ampoule of the first International Reference Preparation for Immunoassay (1975).

70 units of the beta subunit of human chorionic gonadotrophin for immunoassay are contained in approximately 70 µg (with human albumin 5 mg) in one ampoule of the first International Reference Preparation for Immunoassay (1975).

Adverse Effects and Precautions

Side-effects that have been reported include headache, tiredness, changes in mood, oedema, and pain on injection. Treatment for cryptorchidism may produce precocious puberty. Gynaecomastia has been reported. Ovarian hyperstimulation may occur.

Chorionic gonadotrophin should be given with care to patients in whom fluid retention might be a hazard as in asthma, epilepsy, migraine, or cardiac or renal disorders. Allergic reactions may occur and it is recommended that patients suspected to be susceptible should be given skin tests before treatment. It should not be given to patients with disorders that might be exacerbated by androgen release such as carcinoma of the prostate.

Uses and Administration

Chorionic gonadotrophin is produced in the placenta and is found in the blood and urine of pregnant women; its action is predominantly that of the pituitary luteinising hormone. In the male, it stimulates the interstitial cells of the testes and consequently the secretion of androgens; it also has an effect on the Sertoli cells.

In women it is given to induce ovulation after follicular development has been stimulated with follicle-stimulating hormone or menotrophin in the treatment of infertility due to absent or low concentrations of gonadotrophins. Duration of therapy varies but the total dose is in the region of 10 000 units, by intramuscular injection.

In males it has been used in the treatment of cryptorchidism in doses of 500 to 4000 units three times weekly by intramuscular injection. It has also been given for hypogonadotrophic hypogonadism due to pituitary deficiency, in the treatment of delayed puberty, and of oligospermia.

Chorionic gonadotrophin has been used in the treatment of obesity but there is no evidence to support its value.

CRYPTORCHIDISM. Poor results with chorionic gonadotrophin in cryptorchidism: J. M. Garagorri *et al.*, *J. Pediat.*, 1982, *101*, 923; J. Rajfer *et al.*, *New Engl. J. Med.*, 1986, *314*, 466. See also under gonadorelin (p.1142).

INFERTILITY, FEMALE. Some references to chorionic gonadotrophin usually in conjunction with other agents in the management of female infertility: L. D. Nash, *Infertility*, 1982, *5*, 87; E. Rosenberg and J. Cortes-Prieto, *Fert. Steril.*, 1983, *40*, 790; R. Zimmermann *et al.*, *ibid.*, 1984, *41*, 714; B. H. Yuen *et al.*, *Am. J. Obstet. Gynec.*, 1985, *151*, 172. See also under gonadorelin (p.1143).

INFERTILITY, MALE. The efficacy of chorionic gonadotrophin alone and in association with human menopausal gonadotrophin in stimulating spermatogenesis in men with hypogonadotrophic hypogonadism.— D. M. Finkel *et al.*, *New Engl. J. Med.*, 1985, *313*, 651.

Preparations

Chorionic Gonadotrophin Injection *(B.P.)*

Chorionic Gonadotropin for Injection *(U.S.P.)*

Proprietary Preparations

Gonadotraphon LH *(Paines & Byrne, UK)*. *Injection*, powder for reconstitution, chorionic gonadotrophin in ampoules of 500, 1000, and 5000 units, with solvent.

Profasi *(Serono, UK)*. *Injection*, powder for reconstitution, chorionic gonadotrophin in ampoules of 500, 1000, 2000, or 5000 units, with solvent.

Proprietary Names and Manufacturers

Antuitrin S *(Austral.; Canad.)*; APL *(Ayerst, Austral.; Ayerst, Canad.; Ital.; Ayerst, S.Afr.; Inibsa, Spain; Ayerst, USA)*; BayHCG *(Bay, USA)*; Choragon *(Ferring, Ger.)*; Choriomon *(Switz.)*; Coriantin *(Ital.)*; Endocorion *(Arg.)*; Follutein *(Squibb, USA)*; Glukor *(Hyrex, USA)*; Gonadex *(Swed.; Switz.; USA)*; Gonadotrafon LH *(Samil, Ital.)*; Gonadotraphon LH *(Paines & Byrne, UK)*; Harvatropin *(USA)*; Neogonadil *(Bruco, Ital.)*; Physex *(Leo, Denm.; Leo, Norw.)*; Predalon *(Organon, Ger.)*; Pregnesin *(Serono, Ger.)*; Pregnyl *(Organon, Austral.; Organon, Denm.; Ravasini, Ital.; Neth.; Organon, Norw.; Organon, S.Afr.; Organon, Spain; Organon, Swed.; Organon, Switz.; Organon, UK; Organon, USA)*; Primogonyl *(Schering, Austral.; Schering, Ger.; S.Afr.; Schering, Switz.)*; Profasi *(Commonwealth Serum Laboratories, Austral.; Pharmascience, Canad.; Serono, Denm.; Serono, Ital.; Neth.; Serono, S.Afr.; Serono, Spain; Serono, Swed.; Serono, Switz.; Serono, UK; Serono, USA)*.

5930-b

Menotrophin *(BAN)*.

Menotropins *(USAN)*.

CAS — 9002-68-0.

Pharmacopoeias. In *Br., Eur., It., Swiss,* and *U.S.*

An extract of the urine of postmenopausal women, containing follicle-stimulating hormone with luteinising hormone.

It is an off-white or slightly yellow powder containing not less than 40 units of follicle-stimulating hormone activity per mg and about 1 unit of luteinising hormone activity per unit of follicle-stimulating hormone activity.

Soluble in water. The injection has a pH of 6.0

to 8.0. **Store** in airtight containers. Protect from light. The *B.P.* recommends storage at a temperature not exceeding 25°; the U.S.P. recommends storage at 2° to 8°.

Units
54 units of human urinary follicle-stimulating hormone and 46 units of human urinary luteinising hormone are contained in approximately 1 mg (with lactose 5 mg) in one ampoule of the first International Standard Preparation for Bioassay (1974).

Adverse Effects
Menotrophin may cause dose-related ovarian hyperstimulation varying from mild ovarian enlargement and abdominal discomfort to severe hyperstimulation with ovarian rupture and intraperitoneal haemorrhage. There may be ascites, pleural effusion, oliguria, hypotension, and arterial thrombo-embolism. Fatalities have been reported.
There is a risk of multiple births. Sensitivity reactions may occur.

Precautions
Menotrophin should not be given to pregnant patients. Use should be avoided in patients with abnormal genital bleeding, intracranial lesions, adrenal or thyroid disorders, or ovarian cysts or enlargement not caused by the polycystic ovary syndrome. Patients who experience ovarian enlargement are at risk of rupture; diagnostic procedures should be carried out with care and the recommendation has been made that sexual intercourse should be avoided while there is such a risk.

Uses and Administration
Menotrophin followed by chorionic gonadotrophin is used in the treatment of anovulatory infertility due to insufficient gonadotrophins. Menotrophin is administered to induce follicular maturation and endometrial proliferation, and is followed by treatment with chorionic gonadotrophin to stimulate ovulation and corpus luteum formation. Clomiphene (p.1394) can also be used to induce ovulation; amenorrhoeic women with hyperprolactinaemia may be treated with bromocriptine (p.1012).
The dosage and schedule of treatment must be determined according to the needs of each patient; it is usual to monitor response by studying the patient's urinary oestrogen excretion. Menotrophin may be given daily by intramuscular injection to provide a dose of 75 units of follicle-stimulating hormone with 75 units of luteinising hormone, until an adequate response, judged on the basis of daily oestrogen determinations, is achieved, followed after 1 or 2 days by chorionic gonadotrophin (see p.1144). A course of menotrophin should not exceed 12 days. Alternatively, three doses may be given on alternate days followed by chorionic gonadotrophin one week after the first dose.
Menotrophin is also used in conjunction with chorionic gonadotrophin to stimulate spermatogenesis in men with hypogonadotrophic hypogonadism in doses of 75 or 150 units of follicle-stimulating hormone with 75 or 150 units of luteinising hormone three times weekly.

INFERTILITY, FEMALE. Some references to the use of menotrophin in conjunction with other agents in the management of infertility: E. Kemmann and J. R. Jones, *Fert. Steril.*, 1983, *39*, 772; R. Zimmermann *et al.*, *ibid.*, 1984, *41*, 714; A. M. M. Afnan *et al.* (letter), *Lancet*, 1984, *1*, 1239; B. H. Yuen *et al.*, *Am. J. Obstet. Gynec.*, 1985, *151*, 172; J. R. Zorn *et al.* (letter), *Lancet*, 1987, *1*, 385.
See also under chorionic gonadotrophin (p.1144).

Preparations
Menotrophin Injection *(B.P.)*
Menotropins for Injection *(U.S.P.)*

Proprietary Preparations
Pergonal *(Serono, UK)*. *Injection*, powder for reconstitution, menotrophin (as follicle-stimulating hormone 75 units and luteinising hormone 75 units) with lactose 10 mg, supplied with solvent.

Proprietary Names and Manufacturers
Fertinorm *(Serono, Ger.; Serono, Spain)*; Human Pituitary Gonadotrophin *(Commonwealth Serum Laboratories, Austral.)*; Humegon *(Organon, Austral.; Belg.; Organon, Denm.; Organon, Fr.; Organon, Ger.; Neth.; Organon, S.Afr.; Organon, Swed.; Organon, Switz.)*; Inductor *(Searle, Fr.)*; Néo-Pergonal *(Fr.)*; Pergonal *(Commonwealth Serum Laboratories, Austral.; Pharmascience, Canad.; Serono, Denm.; Serono, Ger.; Serono, Ital.; Neth.; Serono, S.Afr.; Serono, Swed.; Serono, UK; Serono, USA)*.

12013-v

Urofollitrophin *(BAN)*.
Urofollitropin *(USAN, pINN)*.
CAS — 97048-13-0.

An extract of the urine of postmenopausal women containing follicle-stimulating hormone.

Urofollitrophin is used similarly to menotrophin in the treatment of infertility with the exception that being without luteinising hormone it is used in patients where any increase in luteinising hormone activity is not required as in polycystic ovarian disease. It is given intramuscularly usually in a dose of 150 units (of follicle-stimulating hormone) daily or 375 units on alternate days for up to 3 weeks. When a response is achieved, as determined by oestrogen monitoring, chorionic gonadotrophin is administered.

Proprietary Preparations
Metrodin *(Serono, UK)*. *Injection*, powder for reconstitution, follicle-stimulating hormone 75 units (as urofollitrophin) with solvent.

Proprietary Names and Manufacturers
Metrodin *(Serono, Ital.; Serono, UK; Serono, USA)*.

NOTE. The name Metrodin has also been used to denote a preparation of treoxytocin.

3887-n

Lactotrophic Hormones

The following section includes the natural lactotrophic hormone, Prolactin.
Oxytocin is involved in the ejection but not the secretion of milk—see Oxytocin, p.1147.

5944-w

Prolactin

Galactin; Lactogen; Lactotropin; LMTH; LTH; Luteomammotropic Hormone; Luteotrophic Hormone; Luteotropin; Mammotropin.

CAS — 9002-62-4; 12585-34-1 (sheep); 56832-36-1 (ox); 9046-05-3 (pig).

A water-soluble protein from the anterior pituitary. Sheep prolactin has a molecular weight of about 25 000 and an isoelectric point at pH 5.7. Its activity is readily destroyed by proteolytic enzymes and by cysteine.
The entire amino-acid sequence of linear human prolactin has been reported by B. Shome and A.F. Parlow (*J. clin. Endocr. Metab.*, 1977, *45*, 1112); it consists of 198 amino-acid residues, only 16% of the sequence corresponding with that of human growth hormone and only 13% with that of human placental lactogen.

Units
One unit of ovine prolactin for bioassay is contained in 0.04545 mg of the second International Standard Preparation (1962) which contains 22 units per mg.
0.65 unit of human prolactin for immunoassay is contained in approximately 20 µg (with human albumin 1 mg and lactose 5 mg) in one ampoule of the first International Reference Preparation for Immunoassay (1978).

Uses and Administration
In *animals*, prolactin has a wide variety of actions and is involved in reproduction, parental care, feeding of the young, electrolyte balance, and growth and development. In humans it has a definite role with other hormones in lactation; oxytocin (p.1147) stimulates milk ejection. Relatively high concentrations of prolactin have been found in amniotic fluid. Placental lactogen has been shown to have prolactin-like activity.
Hyperprolactinaemia, sometimes accompanied by galactorrhoea, occurs in many patients with gonadal disorders and may be associated with amenorrhoea in women and impotence in men. More than 70% of patients with pituitary adenomas have been reported to secrete excessive amounts of prolactin.
The hypothalamus can both stimulate and inhibit prolactin secretion by the anterior pituitary; the inhibitory influence is predominant and is thought to be mediated through a dopaminergic system. The hypothalamic inhibitory factor (PIF or PRIF; also known as prolactin release-inhibiting hormone, PRIH) is probably dopamine. Noradrenaline and gamma-aminobutyric acid are also inhibitory as are dopaminergic agents such as bromocriptine. Although protirelin (p.1152) has prolactin-releasing activity, there is evidence for the existence of a separate hypothalamic releasing factor (PRF). Prolactin secretion may also be stimulated by methyldopa, reserpine, opioid analgesics, and neuroleptics of the phenothiazine or butyrophenone type.

EFFECT OF PROLACTIN GIVEN INTRAMUSCULARLY. Sheep prolactin administered by intramuscular injection to 5 healthy subjects in a dose of 8 mg and compared with a placebo reduced the water and sodium excretion significantly and raised plasma-sodium concentration. Individual urinary pH variations were observed and there was an insignificant reduction in potassium excretion. All 5 experienced muscle aches and malaise, 4 noted thirst, and 3 had a craving for salt.— D. F. Horrobin *et al.*, *Lancet*, 1971, *2*, 352.
Controlled studies in 3 subjects given sheep prolactin 8 mg intramuscularly demonstrated the presence of antidiuretic hormone in their urine which could account for the renal retention effect of prolactin.— M. S. Manku *et al.* (letter), *Lancet*, 1972, *1*, 1243.
Daily intramuscular injections of prolactin, 600 to 900 µg per kg body-weight daily for 3 to 6 weeks, provoked an erythropoietic response in 2 patients with chronic bone-marrow failure, but not in 2 patients with acute failure.— J. H. Jepson and E. E. McGarry, *J. clin. Pharmac.*, 1974, *14*, 296.

Proprietary Names and Manufacturers
Ferolactan *(Bioindustria, Ital.)*; Prolatte *(Ital.)*.

3888-h

Melanocyte-regulating Hormones

The following section includes Melanocyte-stimulating Hormone, and its hypothalamic release-inhibiting hormone, Melanostatin.

5936-w

Melanocyte-stimulating Hormone
B Hormone; Chromatophore Hormone; Intermedin; Melanotropin; MSH; Pigment Hormone.
CAS — 9002-79-3.

A polypeptide isolated from the pars intermedia of the pituitary of fish and amphibia.
Melanocyte-stimulating hormone has been isolated in

two chemically distinct forms. Alpha-melanocyte-stimulating hormone (α-MSH) is probably derived from the degradation of adrenocorticotrophic hormone. Beta-melanocyte-stimulating hormone (β-MSH) comprises 18 amino acids in most species but 22 in man; it is considered to be formed by the degradation of the much larger molecule, beta-lipotrophin (β-LPH), which has 91 amino acids and the same peptide core as adrenocorticotrophic hormone. Beta-lipotrophin has been identified in the pituitary in man; it is probably synthesised by the same cells as adrenocorticotrophic hormone and the two hormones may be secreted together.

Melanocyte-stimulating hormone causes dispersal of melanin granules in the skin of fish and amphibia and allows adaptation to the environment. Its function in mammals is uncertain.

Its release is inhibited by melanostatin; there is also evidence for a hypothalamic releasing factor (MRF).

5937-e

Melanostatin

Intermedin-inhibiting Factor; Melanocyte-stimulating-hormone-release-inhibiting Factor; Melanotropin Release-inhibiting Factor; MIF. Pro-Leu-Gly-NH_2.

CAS — 9083-38-9.

A tripeptide obtained from the hypothalamus. It has been suggested that it is derived from oxytocin (below).

Melanostatin is the active principle of the hypothalamus which inhibits the release of melanocyte-stimulating hormone (see above) in animals. However, there is little evidence of its activity in man. It has been tried in the treatment of depression and parkinsonism but with little benefit.

Proprietary Names and Manufacturers
Abbott, USA.

3889-m

Oxytocic Hormones

The following section includes the natural pituitary oxytocic hormone, Oxytocin, and some synthetic analogues such as Demoxytocin and Treoxytocin.

A preparation of the posterior pituitary, Powdered Pituitary (Posterior Lobe), which possesses oxytocic activity, is included under the section on Antidiuretic Hormones, above.

12630-q

Demoxytocin *(rINN).*

Desamino-oxytocin; ODA-914. 1-(3-Mercaptopropionic acid)-oxytocin.
$C_{43}H_{65}N_{11}O_{12}S_2$=992.2.

CAS — 113-78-0.

Demoxytocin is a synthetic derivative of oxytocin below and has similar properties. Its oxytocic action is reported to be more powerful than that of oxytocin and more prolonged. It is given as buccal tablets, for the induction of labour, in doses of 50 units every half-hour until a normal contraction rhythm is established, up to a maximum of 500 units per day. For the stimulation of labour, 25 units every half-hour has been recommended. Twenty-five or 50 units may be given 5 minutes before nursing to stimulate milk ejection.

Proprietary Names and Manufacturers
Sandopart *(Sandoz-Wander, Belg.; Sandoz, Denm.; Sandoz, Ital.; Sandoz, S.Afr.; Sandoz, Switz.).*

5940-g

Oxytocin *(BAN, USAN, rINN).*

Alpha-Hypophamine. Cys-Tyr-Ile-Gln-Asn-Cys-Pro-Leu-Gly-NH_2 cyclic (1→6) disulphide; [2-Leucine, 7-isoleucine]-vasopressin.
$C_{43}H_{66}N_{12}O_{12}S_2$=1007.2.

CAS — 50-56-6.

A cyclic polypeptide comprised of 9 amino acids. The oxytocic principle of the posterior lobe of the pituitary body. It may be prepared by a process of fractionation from the glands of oxen or other mammals or by synthesis.

5941-q

Oxytocin Citrate

$C_{43}H_{66}N_{12}O_{12}S_2,C_6H_8O_7$=1199.3.

5942-p

Oxytocin Injection *(BAN, USAN).*

Oxytocin; Oxytocini Injectio; Oxytocini Solutio Iniectabilis.

Pharmacopoeias. In *Br., Chin., Eur., Fr., Ger., Hung., Ind., It., Jpn, Jug., Neth., Pol., Swiss,* and *U.S.* (no strength specified); in *Arg., Cz., Int., Nord.,* and *Turk.* (which specify 10 units per mL); in *Egypt.*

A clear, colourless, sterile, aqueous solution containing the oxytocic principle of the posterior lobe of the pituitary body, which may be prepared from the glands of oxen or other mammals or by synthesis. The *B.P.* specifies that it contains not more than 0.5 units of vasopressor activity per 20 units of oxytocic activity. The *U.S.P.* specifies not more than 0.01 units of vasopressor activity per unit of oxytocic activity. The *B.P.* injection has a pH of 3.5 to 4.5; the *U.S.P.* preparation has a pH between 2.5 and 4.5.

The *B.P.* states that the solution is **sterilised** by filtration. **Store** at 2° to 15° and avoid freezing. The *B.P.* requires that the label states the animal source of the oxytocin, or that it is synthetic.

INCOMPATIBILITY. Oxytocin 0.5 *U.S.P.* unit was 'physically incompatible' with plasmin 200 mg, or warfarin sodium 10 mg in 100 mL of glucose injection.— R. D. Dunworth and F. R. Kenna, *Am. J. Hosp. Pharm.,* 1965, *22,* 190.

Oxytocin was incompatible with sodium bisulphite and solutions lost 80% of their activity over 6 hours.— C. H. Chang *et al., Can. J. Hosp. Pharm.,* 1972, *25,* 152.

Units

12.5 units of oxytocin for bioassay are contained in approximately 21.4 µg of synthetic peptide (with human albumin 5 mg) in one ampoule of the fourth International Standard Preparation (1978).

Adverse Effects

Excess oxytocin may cause violent uterine contractions leading to uterine rupture and extensive laceration of the soft tissues, foetal bradycardia and arrhythmias, and perhaps foetal or maternal death.

Maternal deaths from severe hypertension and subarachnoid haemorrhage have occurred. Postpartum haemorrhage and fatal hypofibrinogenaemia have been reported but may be due to obstetric complications. Water retention and intoxication with convulsions, coma, and even death may follow oxytocin especially when given intravenously in large doses or over prolonged periods. Vasopressin-like activity (see p.1138) is more likely with oxytocin of natural origin but may occur even with the synthetic peptide.

Anaphylactic and other allergic reactions, pelvic haematomas, and nausea and vomiting may occur.

There are reports of neonatal jaundice and retinal haemorrhage associated with the use of oxytocin in the management of labour.

Comment on the misuse of oxytocin in labour. Statements on the management of labour are often misinterpreted as meaning that all labouring women who fail to make adequate progress in terms of cervical dilatation should be given oxytocin. This is only true if poor progress is due to poor uterine action, and is dangerous where there is disproportion. The decision to use oxytocin requires careful assessment by an experienced obstetrician; in the past 2 years the authors have seen one case of fractured pelvis, 2 of ruptured uterus, and 7 cases of cerebral palsy from foetal hypoxia, all of which were the subject of litigation and were thought to be due to the ill-advised use of oxytocin to augment labour.— R. W. Taylor and M. Taylor (letter), *Lancet,* 1988, *1,* 352.

A report of a possible relation between the use of oxytocin to induce labour and the sudden infant death syndrome.— C. Einspieler and T. Kenner (letter), *New Engl. J. Med.,* 1985, *313,* 1660. Criticism. Other studies have failed to show a relation.— J. Golding (letter), *ibid., 315,* 192; L. J. Resseguie *et al.* (letter), *ibid.,* 193. Reply. Other factors are obviously involved but this does not obviate the need for further attention to the possible relationship.— T. Kenner and C. Einspieler (letter), *ibid.*

JAUNDICE. Analysis of neonatal jaundice in 12 461 single births confirmed a higher incidence in those given oxytocin, independent of gestational age at birth, sex, race, epidural analgesia, method of delivery, and birth weight, each of which was also associated with jaundice.— L. Friedman *et al., Br. med. J.,* 1978, *1,* 1235.

In 40 infants delivered after oxytocin-induced labour the packed cell volume of cord blood, the erythrocyte deformability index (a determinant of erythrocyte life span), the plasma-haptoglobin concentration, and the plasma osmolality were significantly reduced while the plasma-bilirubin concentration and the plasma lactate dehydrogenase activity were significantly increased, compared with 40 infants delivered after spontaneous labour and 15 delivered by caesarean section. Oxytocin *in vitro* had a time-related and dose-related effect on erythrocyte deformability.— P. C. Buchan, *Br. med. J.,* 1979, *2,* 1255.

In 50 infants born to mothers in whom labour had been induced with oxytocin, hyponatraemia, hypo-osmolality, and enhanced osmotic fragility of erythrocytes was observed at birth, and serum-bilirubin concentrations were significantly higher 72 hours after birth than in 50 control infants. Glucose injection, used as the vehicle for oxytocin infusion, may further aggravate these changes. Infants with cord serum-sodium concentrations of less than 125 mmol per litre and/or osmolality of less than 260 mmol per kg body-weight were at risk of developing jaundice and should be considered for prophylactic administration of phenobarbitone.— S. Singhi and M. Singh, *Archs Dis. Childh.,* 1979, *54,* 400.

For a study indicating that neonatal jaundice after induction of labour with dinoprostone or oxytocin is primarily associated with foetal maturity rather than the use of drugs see Dinoprost, p.1368.

WATER INTOXICATION. Oxytocin-induced water intoxication is an unusual but not rare occurrence. It is most likely to arise as a result of prolonged attempts to empty the uterus in missed abortion or mid-trimester termination of pregnancy, but it has also been described after oxytocin infusion in other conditions including induction of labour. Irrespective of the oxytocin concentration, patients in virtually all the reported cases have received more than 3.5 litres of infused fluid. In the only reported exception the patient also received very large quantities of buccal oxytocin. Another factor contributing to hyponatraemia is the antidiuretic effect of the pethidine and morphine commonly used for analgesia with oxytocin infusions. Water intoxication usually presents with fits and loss of consciousness but in some cases there may be preceding signs such as raised venous pressure, bounding pulse, and tachycardia. Diagnosis is confirmed by profound hyponatraemia; the mechanisms appears to be more complex than simply haemodilution by the infused water. Treatment consists of controlling convulsions and maintaining an airway; oxytocin infusion must be stopped and isotonic, or even hypertonic, saline may be infused. Diuresis may then be assisted with frusemide. The prime objective, however, should be prevention; no patient should receive more than 3 litres of fluid containing oxytocin, and a careful fluid balance record is essential.— J. G. Feeney, *Br. med. J.,* 1982, *285,* 243.

Precautions

Oxytocin should not be given to women with severe toxaemia, hypertonic uterine dysfunction, or a predisposition to uterine rupture as in patients of high parity or with uterine scar from previous caesarean section. It should not be given for induction before the head is engaged. Placenta praevia, major cephalopelvic disproportion, malposition of the foetus, or obvious foetal distress are also contra-indications.

Care is necessary in the use of oxytocin in patients being treated with pressor agents as

severe hypertension has been stated to occur. For the induction of labour oxytocin should be infused slowly since bolus injections may cause severe hypotension. The infusion volume should be low in patients with cardiovascular disorders.
It is inadvisable to employ 2 routes of administration simultaneously.
Oestrogens intensify and progesterone may diminish the effect of oxytocin on the uterus. Great care is necessary in combined regimens with other oxytocic agents to avoid excessive uterine stimulation.

A 29-year-old pregnant woman with congenital aortic stenosis who was given oxytocin parenterally during therapeutic abortion developed heart failure and died. Autopsy revealed an extensive myocardial infarction. Extreme care should be taken when more than 2 units per minute of oxytocin are given intravenously to pregnant women with heart disease.— M. Robinson *et al.*, *J. Am. med. Ass.*, 1967, *200*, 378.

Water intoxication occurred in 2 patients given intra-amniotic injections of sodium chloride and oxytocin infusion. It was considered that patients receiving this combination must have fluid intake restricted at the beginning of the oxytocin infusion.— D. R. Gupta and N. H. Cohen, *J. Am. med. Ass.*, 1972, *220*, 681.

Absorption and Fate

Oxytocin is rapidly absorbed from the mucous membranes when administered buccally or intranasally. It is metabolised by the liver and kidneys.

Reference: J. Seitchik *et al.*, *Am. J. Obstet. Gynec.*, 1984, *150*, 225.

Uses and Administration

Oxytocin causes contraction of the uterus, the effect depending on whether or not the uterus is pregnant and on the stage of pregnancy. The response is greatest in the later stages of pregnancy. Small doses increase the tone and amplitude of the uterine contractions; large or repeated doses result in tetany lasting for 5 to 10 minutes. Oxytocin also stimulates the smooth muscle associated with the secretory epithelium of the lactating breast causing the ejection of milk but having no direct effect on milk secretion. It has relatively little pressor or antidiuretic action.
Oxytocin is used for the induction and maintenance of labour, to control postpartum bleeding and uterine hypotonicity in the third stage of labour, and to promote lactation in cases of faulty milk ejection. It is also used in missed abortions, but a prostaglandin may be preferred.
For the induction or stimulation of labour, oxytocin 1 to 10 units in one litre of glucose (5%) injection, or other suitable diluent, may be given by slow intravenous infusion at an initial rate of 1 to 2 milliunits per minute and then gradually increased until a contraction pattern similar to that of normal labour is achieved. Foetal heart-rate and uterine contractions should be monitored continuously.
In the management of postpartum haemorrhage infusion of a solution containing 10 units of oxytocin in 500 mL of glucose (5%) injection or other suitable diluent, at a rate of 20 to 40 milliunits per minute, has been suggested; oxytocin has also been given in doses of 2 to 10 units intramuscularly. However, in general an ergot alkaloid is the drug of first choice in the management of postpartum bleeding (see Ergometrine Maleate, p.1054). Preparations containing oxytocin in association with ergometrine have been given by intramuscular or intravenous injection.
In missed abortion 10 to 20 units in 500 mL of glucose (5%) injection may be infused at the rate of 10 to 30 drops per minute initially, the concentration being increased by 10 to 20 units per 500 mL every hour to a maximum of 100 units per 500 mL.
Oxytocin has also been given, as the citrate, in the form of a buccal tablet to induce labour; however, absorption is irregular following buccal administration and this route has been superseded by intravenous infusion.
Oxytocin spray is used to facilitate lactation; the usual dose is 2 to 4 units intranasally several minutes before suckling.
An oxytocin challenge test has been used in pregnant patients at high-risk; oxytocin is infused until a contraction-rate of 3 per 10 minutes is achieved and the occurrence of late or variable decelerations of foetal heart-rate monitored. A negative response is considered to be indicative of foetal well-being although false-negative tests have been reported.

GASTRIC ATONY. Use of oxytocin in 3 patients with gastric atony. An intravenous infusion of 5 to 20 units of oxytocin in 500 mL of sodium chloride (0.9%) solution was given every 4 hours for 3 days. The patients, who had lacked peristaltic function for 2 to 4 months following vagotomy, developed gastric contractions within 20 to 30 minutes of beginning treatment, although one required a further 3 days treatment before effective peristalsis of the stomach was achieved. Normal gastric emptying was subsequently maintained without further treatment.— M. Hashmonai *et al.*, *Br. J. Surg.*, 1979, *66*, 550.

LABOUR INDUCTION. A study of the effectiveness in nulliparous women of a specific oxytocin dosage regimen. Oxytocin was given at 1 milliunit per minute by intravenous infusion, increased if necessary by 1 milliunit per minute at intervals of at least 30 minutes until either a pre-defined level of myometrial activity was reached, or the oxytocin dose reached 4 milliunits per minute. The dose was then held at that level for 2 hours. In 45 women given oxytocin according to this regimen, significantly smaller doses were required to accomplish a change in cervical dilatation, and significantly smaller mean maximum doses were given compared with 84 controls given oxytocin according to the judgement of the attending physician. The most significant factor determining these results was the rate of incrementation of the oxytocin dose.— J. Seitchik and M. Castillo, *Am. J. Obstet. Gynec.*, 1982, *144*, 899. Similar results using the same regimen in multiparous women.— *idem*, 1983, *145*, 777. An alternative induction regimen for oxytocin. Oxytocin 5 milliunits per minute was given by intravenous infusion in nulliparous patients until a satisfactory myometrial response was demonstrated or 40 minutes elapsed without a response. If the uterus responded within 40 minutes, a maintenance dose was selected according to the time from initiation of oxytocin to the first contraction of the myometrial response: first to ninth minute, 1 milliunit per minute; tenth to seventeenth minute, 2 milliunits per minute; eighteenth to twenty-fifth minute, 3 milliunits per minute; twenty-sixth to thirty-third minute, 4 milliunits per minute; thirty-fourth to fortieth minute, 4 milliunits per minute. If the uterus did not respond in 40 minutes, the dose was increased to 10 milliunits per minute and the maintenance dose selected by the time of response: forty-first to forty-eighth minute, 6 milliunits per minute; forty-ninth to fifty-sixth minute, 7 milliunits per minute. This method effectively identified the proper maintenance dose on the first or second attempt in 58 of 59 patients.— J. Seitchik *et al.*, *ibid.*, 1985, *151*, 757.

For the view that vaginally-administered prostaglandins are replacing oxytocin as the method of choice for induction of labour see under Dinoprost, p.1369.

LABOUR STIMULATION. Discussion of the active management of dystocia. Recent studies have cast doubt upon the necessity for high-dose (as opposed to low-dose) oxytocin infusion, and a conservative approach remains a valid clinical option. At present low-dose oxytocin infusion with careful assessment of uterine activity is the best policy in most cases.— *Lancet*, 1988, *1*, 160. Criticism. The conclusion that low-dose oxytocin is best appears to be based on a single study by Bidgood and Steer (*Br. J. Obstet. Gynaec.*, 1987, 94, 518) and is at variance with experience with many thousands of patients at the National Maternity Hospital, Dublin. It is worth emphasising that within the context of active management of labour high-dose oxytocin is strictly confined to nulliparous women with a cephalic presentation, singleton pregnancy, and no evidence of foetal distress. Restriction of high-dose oxytocin augmentation to such patients continues to be associated with low caesarean section rates without any evidence of harm to the foetus.— P. Boylan *et al.* (letter), *ibid.*, 767.

LACTATION. The use of oxytocin nasal spray to enhance lactation in women who had given birth prematurely.— H. Ruis *et al.*, *Br. med. J.*, 1981, *283*, 340.

OXYTOCIN CHALLENGE TEST. Haemorrhage occurred after two oxytocin challenge tests; the patient was found to have a major placenta praevia.— K. H. Ng and W. P. Wong (letter), *Br. med. J.*, 1976, *2*, 698.

Neonatal hyperbilirubinaemia was associated with an oxytocin challenge test in the mother before labour. This test should be used with caution in women whose babies might be at risk from hyperbilirubinaemia.— D. Peleg and J. A. Goldman (letter), *Lancet*, 1976, *2*, 1026.

The oxytocin challenge test (OCT) was performed on 399 occasions in 305 women with pregnancies at risk and a gestational age of 36 weeks or more. Oxytocin 1 milliunit per minute was given by infusion pump and increased every 5 to 10 minutes until a contraction-rate of 3 per 10 minutes was achieved. Less than 10% of late or variable decelerations of foetal heart-rate (FHR) was judged negative; 10 to 29% was judged equivocal; and 30% or more was judged positive. The finding of a positive or equivocal response to the OCT was considered a prediction of decelerations of the FHR during parturition, though the type of risk might vary. The OCT merited continued usage and refinement.— H. Schulman *et al.*, *Am. J. Obstet. Gynec.*, 1977, *129*, 239.

A report on 100 oxytocin challenge tests performed in 90 pregnant women considered at risk. It was concluded that a negative result is a reliable test of foetal wellbeing encouraging the obstetrician to await spontaneous onset of labour in preference to induction.— S. Sellappah and H. Wagman, *Br. J. clin. Pract.*, 1984, *38*, 255.

Reports of foetal death despite negative oxytocin challenge tests.— R. G. Marcum (letter), *Am. J. Obstet. Gynec.*, 1977, *127*, 894; R. P. Lorenz and J. S. Pagano, *Am. J. Obstet. Gynec.*, 1978, *130*, 232; R. Dittman and J. Belcher (letter), *New Engl. J. Med.*, 1978, *298*, 56.

POSTPARTUM HAEMORRHAGE. In a study in 148 patients who had received oxytocin infusions during the first and second stages of labour and who had received epidural analgesia, blood loss at delivery was similar in those given ergometrine 500 μg intravenously or oxytocin 5 units intravenously; the incidence of nausea, retching, and vomiting was 46% in those receiving ergometrine and nil in those receiving oxytocin. Oxytocin was preferable to ergometrine particularly in patients with heart disease, pre-eclampsia, hypertension, phaeochromocytoma, thyrotoxicosis, and coronary insufficiency.— J. E. Moodie and D. D. Moir, *Br. J. Anaesth.*, 1976, *48*, 571.

In a study in 88 primigravidas who had spontaneous delivery, oxytocin 10 units intravenously was as effective as ergometrine 500 μg intravenously in preventing third stage uterine haemorrhage at delivery. Vomiting or retching occurred in 13% of the mothers who received ergometrine.— D. D. Moir and A. B. Amoa, *Br. J. Anaesth.*, 1979, *51*, 113.

A comparison of relatively high doses of oxytocin with ergometrine in the active management of the third stage of labour. Oxytocin 10 units intravenously was given to 506 women whilst 543 received ergometrine 200 μg intravenously; the drugs were given as soon as possible after delivery of the anterior shoulder. Both these groups were compared with 1513 controls from the previous year who had received 200 μg of ergometrine only after delivery of the placenta. There was no significant difference in the mean duration of the third stage between groups but the blood loss in both oxytocic groups was reduced by about one-third compared with controls. However, partial retention or trapping of the placenta was significantly more frequent among women in the early ergometrine group than in the oxytocin or control groups, whilst total retention occurred more frequently in the latter 2 groups. The rhythmic physiological uterine contraction induced by oxytocin, which affects mainly the upper uterine segment, may have advantages over the prolonged uterine spasm induced by ergometrine, which affects the whole uterus and which increases the likelihood of partial placental separation with bleeding and trapping of the placenta.— B. Sorbe, *Obstet. Gynec.*, 1978, *52*, 694.

Comment on the active management of third-stage labour and the benefit of routine oxytocic agents in preventing postpartum haemorrhage.— *Lancet*, 1986, *2*, 22.

For the use of oxytocin in association with ergometrine in the management of postpartum haemorrhage, see Ergometrine Maleate, p.1054.

Preparations

Oxytocin Nasal Solution *(U.S.P.)*. Contains synthetic oxytocin in a suitable diluent. pH 3.7 to 4.3.

Proprietary Preparations

Syntocinon *(Sandoz, UK). Injection,* oxytocin 1 unit/mL, in ampoules of 2 mL; 5 units/mL, in ampoules of 1 mL; 10 units/mL in ampoules of 1 and 5 mL.

Proprietary Names and Manufacturers of Oxytocin or Oxytocin Citrate

Orasthin *(Hoechst, Ger.)*; Partocon *(Ferring, Ger.; Ferring, Swed.)*; Pitocin *(Austral.; Belg.; Canad.; Denm.; Parke, Davis, Ger.; Parke, Davis, Norw.; S.Afr.; Parke, Davis, Spain; Parke, Davis, UK; Parke, Davis, USA)*; Piton-S *(Neth.)*; Syntocinon *(Arg.; Sandoz, Austral.; Belg.; Sandoz, Canad.; Sandoz, Denm.; Sandoz, Fr.; Sandoz, Ger.; Sandoz, Ital.; Neth.; Sandoz, Norw.; Sandoz, S.Afr.; Sandoz, Spain; Sandoz, Swed.; Sandoz, Switz.; Sandoz, UK; Sandoz, USA)*;
Manufacturers also include—*Wyeth, USA.*

The following names have been used for multi-ingredient preparations containing oxytocin or oxytocin citrate—Syntometrine *(Sandoz, Austral.; Sandoz, UK)*.

13368-k

Treoxytocin

[4-L-Threonine]-oxytocin.
$C_{42}H_{65}N_{11}O_{12}S_2$=980.2.

CAS — 26995-91-5.

A synthetic analogue of oxytocin (p.1146) with similar properties.

Proprietary Names and Manufacturers

Metrodin *(Serono, Ital.)*; Treoxin *(Serono, Ital.)*.

NOTE. The name Metrodin was re-allocated by the manufacturer in 1982; it is now used to denote a preparation of follicle-stimulating hormone.

3890-t

Somatotrophic Hormones

The following section includes the growth hormones Somatropin (natural human growth hormone), and Somatrem, its synthetic methionyl analogue; further included are the hypothalamic releasing and release-inhibiting hormones, Somatorelin and Somatostatin; and an analogue of the latter, Octreotide.

Also included, although not of pituitary origin, are the Somatomedins, via which some of the actions of somatropin are mediated.

NOTE. No universally agreed terminology exists for these substances; in this section the term somatropin has been used to describe human growth hormone, whether endogenous or exogenous (either pituitary-derived or synthesised by means of recombinant DNA technology) in origin.

3882-t

Growth Hormone

GH; Phyone; Somatotrophin; STH.

CAS — 9002-72-6.

An anabolic protein produced by the anterior pituitary which promotes the growth of tissues and has a regulatory effect on various aspects of metabolism. It varies in size and amino acid composition between species; somatropin (below) is human growth hormone.

12012-b

Somatrem *(BAN, USAN, pINN).*

Met-HGH; Methionyl Human Growth Hormone.
$C_{995}H_{1537}N_{263}O_{301}S_8$=22 256.

CAS — 82030-87-3.

An analogue of somatropin containing an additional (methionyl) amino-acid residue. Sometribove (*BAN*) is methionyl bovine growth hormone and sometripor (*BAN*) is methionyl porcine growth hormone.

5933-q

Somatropin *(BAN, USAN, pINN).*

CB-311; HGH; Human Growth Hormone.
$C_{990}H_{1529}N_{263}O_{299}S_7$=22 124.

CAS — 12629-01-5 (human).

Pharmacopoeias. In *Eur.* and *It.*

The active ('little') form of human growth hormone, consisting of a single polypeptide chain of 191 amino acids with disulphide linkages between positions 53 and 165 and between 182 and 189.

The synthesis of human growth hormone fragments with growth-promoting activity.— F. Chillemi *et al., Nature New Biol.*, 1972, *238*, 243.

Two immunoreactive components were identified in plasma or pituitary extracts of human growth hormone (somatropin) and named 'big' HGH and 'little' HGH. Little HGH was eluted as a globular protein of molecular weight 22 000 from Sephadex gel following filtration. Big HGH was less retarded by the gel and was considered to have twice the molecular weight. Big HGH made up 24 to 37% of the total circulating material in healthy subjects and 8 to 14% in acromegalic patients. Big HGH had much less activity in a radioreceptor assay than in the radioimmunoassay in both subjects and patients whereas there was no difference with little HGH.— P. Gorden *et al., Science*, 1973, *182*, 829.

The synthesis of somatropin in bacterial cells using synthetic DNA fragments and human pituitary material.— *J. Am. med. Ass.*, 1979, *242*, 701.

The amino-acid sequence of somatropin.— C. H. Li, *Can. med. Ass. J.*, 1979, *120*, 575.

Spectroscopic comparison of somatrem and somatropin.— H. Larhammar *et al., Int. J. Pharmaceut.*, 1985, *23*, 13.

Units

0.35 units of growth hormone for immunoassay are contained in 175 µg of freeze-dried purified human growth hormone, with sucrose 5 mg and buffer salts, in one ampoule of the first International Reference Preparation (1968).

4.4 units of human growth hormone for bioassay are contained in 1.75 mg of freeze-dried purified human growth hormone, with 20 mg of glycine, 2 mg of mannitol, 2 mg of lactose, and 2 mg of sodium bicarbonate, in one ampoule of the first International Standard Preparation (1982).

Adverse Effects and Precautions

Antibodies have been formed in some patients. Because of the diabetogenic effect of growth hormone it should not be given to patients with diabetes mellitus. Hypothyroidism may develop during treatment, and may result in suboptimal response.

Treatment with glucocorticoids may inhibit the effects of growth hormone.

Reports in 1985 of a small number of deaths from Creutzfeldt-Jakob disease in patients under 40 years of age who had received somatropin extracted from human pituitary glands resulted in the suspension of the distribution of pituitary-derived somatropin by the licensing authorities in a number of countries, including Australia, Canada, the Netherlands, the UK, and the USA. References: P. Brown *et al., New Engl. J. Med.*, 1985, *313*, 728 and 967; J. Powell-Jackson *et al., Lancet*, 1985, *2*, 244; *FDA Drug Bull.*, 1985, *15*, 17; L. Lazarus, *Med. J. Aust.*, 1985, *143*, 57; B. A. Bannister and A. McCormick, *J. Infect.*, 1987, *14*, 7.

Studies and comments on the preparation of somatropin free from contamination with slow viruses such as the Creutzfeldt-Jakob agent: D. M. Taylor *et al., Lancet*, 1985, *2*, 260; P. Brown (letter), *ibid.*, 729; D. M. Taylor and A. G. Dickinson (letter), *ibid.*, 837; J. Tateishi *et al.* (letter), *ibid.*, 1299; D. M. Taylor (letter), *ibid.*, 1986, *1*, 559.

CARCINOGENICITY. Despite fears to the contrary there was no evidence from a study involving 31 patients who had received radiotherapy for brain tumours or CNS leukaemia that therapy with growth hormone increased the relapse-rate.— P. E. Clayton *et al., Lancet*, 1987, *1*, 711.

A report of 5 cases of acute leukaemia among patients in Japan treated with growth hormones; this was calculated to represent a 9.4-fold increase over the expected incidence and strongly suggested a relationship between long-term administration of growth hormones in hypopituitary patients and the development of acute leukaemia.— S. Watanabe *et al.* (letter), *Lancet*, 1988, *1*, 1159. A further report.— H. A. Delemarre-Van de Waal *et al.* (letter), *ibid* (acute lymphocytic leukaemia in a child with isolated growth hormone deficiency). In view of the concern raised by these reports an international workshop was convened in 1988 to review known leukaemia cases in patients treated with growth hormones in Europe, North America, Japan, and Australia since 1959. The observed incidence of leukaemia in growth-hormone-treated patients represents a 2-fold increase over the expected rate. After a careful review of the data it was concluded that there may be a small increase in leukaemia incidence associated with growth hormone treatment of growth hormone-deficient patients, but it is not yet clear that this is actually attributable to growth hormone. If there is any risk it is relatively small, and in view of the essential nature of growth hormone therapy in these children it would be inappropriate and unwise to withold it.— D. A. Fisher *et al.* (letter), *ibid.*

Absorption and Fate

After intravenous injection growth hormone has a half-life of about 30 minutes.

References: M. L. Parker *et al., J. clin. Invest.*, 1962, *41*, 262; B. J. Boucher (letter), *Nature*, 1966, *210*, 1288.

Uses and Administration

Somatropin (growth hormone) is secreted by the anterior lobe of the pituitary. It promotes growth of skeletal, muscular, and other tissues, stimulates protein anabolism, and affects fat and mineral metabolism. The hormone has a diabetogenic action on carbohydrate metabolism.

Secretion is dependent on neural and hormonal influences including a hypothalamic release-inhibiting hormone (Somatostatin, p.1151), and a hypothalamic releasing hormone (Somatorelin, p.1150). Sleep, hypoglycaemia, and physical or emotional stress result in increased secretion of growth hormone. The effects of growth hormone on skeletal growth are mediated by the somatomedins (see p.1150).

Growth hormone is species specific, only somatropin or close analogues such as somatrem being effective in man.

In man, deficient secretion of somatropin during the years of active body growth results in pituitary dwarfism. Overproduction of growth hormone before growth is complete results in gigantism. If it occurs after cessation of growth when the epiphyses have closed, it causes acromegaly, in which the features become coarse and the hands and feet become enlarged.

Somatropin or somatrem is given to children with open epiphyses for the treatment of pituitary dwarfism, following assessment of pituitary function. Doses of 0.5 unit per kg body-weight have been given weekly by intramuscular injection in 2 or 3 divided doses or by subcutaneous injection in 6 or 7 divided doses.

A report of a conference on the uses and possible abuses of biosynthetic growth hormones. The ready availability of hormone from recombinant DNA technology will inevitably lead, in a society that values tallness, to pressure to prescribe the drug far more widely than has been possible before. Diagnosis is usually straightforward in children with severe unequivocal growth hormone deficiency, but patients with growth hormone deficiency appear, on the basis of provocative tests, to represent a continuum with no distinct boundaries between partial and normal response, and indeed no consensus as to what constitutes normal response. Further problems arise in clarifying the use of diagnoses such as bioinactive growth hormone. Patients with familial short stature, or delayed growth (which may represent a small growth hormone deficiency) may benefit from the wider availability of the hormone but it is not clear how best to identify the sub-group who will respond, nor whether any long-term benefit in growth occurs. It is anticipated that demand for the use of growth hormone may come from parents of children who while not truly short are not fulfilling parental expectations in sporting or other achievements. In this context the potential complications of therapy including hypothyroidism, antibody formation and possible glucose intolerance, hyperlipidaemia, hypertension, and other symptoms seen in acromegaly should be borne in mind. It should also be remembered that patients and families often have unrealistic expectations of growth hormone therapy and failure to meet these expectations may lead to depression. Nonetheless the wide availability of biosynthetic growth hormones also offers a wide potential spectrum of new uses: in dwarfing conditions such as Turner's syndrome and intrauterine growth retardation; in burns and other catabolic conditions; in osteoporosis, peptic ulcer disease, and ageing. The most effective way to avoid abuse is through education of both physicians and the public.— L. E. Underwood, *New Engl. J. Med.*, 1984, *311*, 606.

Further discussions of whom to treat with biosynthetic growth hormones: R. D. G. Milner, *Lancet*, 1986, *1*, 483; M. A. Preece, *Br. med. J.*, 1986, *293*, 1185.

ADMINISTRATION. A study suggesting that daily subcutaneous administration of somatropin produced improved growth in growth-hormone deficient children when compared with administration of the same total weekly dose as two or three intramuscular injections.— K. Albertsson-Wikland *et al.*, *Acta paediat. scand.*, 1986, *75*, 89.

In a small study in 4 children with growth hormone deficiency administration of pituitary-derived somatropin in the standard regimen of 4 units intramuscularly 3 times a week was compared with subcutaneous administration of either a bolus dose of 2 units nightly or 3 nightly doses of 0.6 units (given by infusion pump), the subcutaneous dosage regimens being given for 6 nights a week. No difference in growth response could be demonstrated for any of the regimens.— P. J. Smith *et al.*, *Archs Dis. Childh.*, 1987, *62*, 849.

A study of the contribution of dose and frequency of administration to the therapeutic effect of growth hormone. Of 42 prepubertal children with untreated growth hormone deficiency treated with subcutaneous somatrem, 13 received 4 units on three days a week; 21 received 2 units six days a week; and 8 received 1 unit twice daily for six days a week. All children responded with a significant change in height velocity standard deviation score (SDS); mean height velocity SDS for the 3 groups after 1 year were +3.8, +5.3, and +5.9 respectively. Although the differences were not significant there was a trend towards the greatest improvement with the higher frequency regimens but the magnitude of response appeared to be chiefly determined by the pretreatment height velocity SDS and the magnitude of the dose per m^2 body-surface administered weekly. As a result of this study prompt recognition and early treatment of growth hormone insufficiency is advocated: the dose should be maintained at not less than 15 units per m^2 per week throughout childhood, administered as equally divided daily subcutaneous injections.— P. J. Smith *et al.*, *Archs Dis. Childh.*, 1988, *63*, 491.

DOWN'S SYNDROME. Five growth-retarded children with Down's syndrome but with normal growth hormone responses to provocative testing were given pituitary-derived somatropin 0.5 units weekly in 3 divided doses for 6 months. All patients responded with an increase in growth velocity of between about 50 and 200%, the mean growth velocity being 2.5, 4.5, and 2.6 cm per six months before, during, and after treatment respectively. The serum concentration of somatomedin C (IGF-1), which is usually below the normal range in patients with Down's syndrome, was increased during growth hormone treatment to a normal value for this age group; another somatomedin, IGF-2, also increased its serum concentration. There was no accompanying improvement in delayed skeletal maturation. Although growth velocity was increased during treatment in these patients it is not certain that short- or long-term treatment with somatropin will increase final height in Down's syndrome children.— G. Annerén *et al.*, *Archs Dis. Childh.*, 1986, *61*, 48.

GROWTH DISORDERS. A report by an MRC Working Party on clinical experience with pituitary-derived somatropin in children with growth hormone deficiency in the UK. A dosage regimen of 5 units three times weekly was found to give superior stature velocity than regimens of 5 units twice weekly or 10 units twice weekly; all injections being given intramuscularly.— R. D. G. Milner *et al.*, *Clin. Endocr.*, 1979, *11*, 15.

For studies suggesting that a more frequent dosage regimen, given subcutaneously, yields greater improvement in growth hormone deficient children see under Administration, above.

A report of pituitary dwarfism in a 14-year-old patient with normal serum concentrations of growth hormone but an apparently abnormal structure of the growth hormone molecule, resulting in reduced biological activity. Treatment with exogenous somatropin for a year resulted in rapid linear growth for a total of 16 cm; growth was retarded on withdrawal of therapy but resumed immediately after re-institution before arresting due to bone maturation.— L. J. Valenta *et al.*, *New Engl. J. Med.*, 1985, *312*, 214.

Comparison of somatrem with pituitary-derived somatropin in growth-hormone deficient children. The mean rate of linear growth increased approximately 3-fold during the first year among 36 children treated with intramuscular somatrem, from 3.2 cm per year to 10.3 cm per year; this was not significantly different from the results in 10 similar children given somatropin in whom mean linear growth-rate increased from 3.8 to 10.1 cm per year. The metabolic actions of somatrem and somatropin were also equivalent. There was a higher incidence of antibody formation to somatrem, particularly in the initial formulation used in the first 22 patients; changes in the purification process gave a preparation that caused a lower incidence of antibody formation (but still higher than with somatropin). However antibody formation did not appear to be associated with adverse reactions, nor to reach levels, except in one patient, that attenuated the action of growth hormone.— S. L. Kaplan *et al.*, *Lancet*, 1986, *1*, 697. See also R. L. Hintz *et al.*, *ibid.*, 1982, *1*, 1276.

A brief review of somatropin derived from recombinant DNA technology. Recommended maximum doses for growth hormone deficiency are less than those for somatrem, apparently because of the design of the clinical trials, but in fact the two are thought to be equipotent, and optimal dosage is unknown.— *Med. Lett.*, 1987, *29*, 73.

Retesting after completion of growth hormone therapy in 15 patients diagnosed as having radiation-induced growth hormone deficiency and in 19 originally diagnosed as suffering from idiopathic deficiency confirmed the existence of the defect in all of the former group; however, 5 of the latter had normal growth hormone responses to provocative testing suggesting that the original diagnosis was misleading.— P. E. Clayton *et al.*, *Archs Dis. Childh.*, 1987, *62*, 222. Comment on the use of growth hormones in children given radiotherapy. Biochemical growth hormone deficiency is prevalent among patients receiving 24 Gy of irradiation but therapy is not appropriate in all cases.— A. D. Leiper *et al.* (letter), *Lancet*, 1988, *1*, 943.

Short stature. Preliminary findings that some normal children of short stature respond to somatropin therapy with an improvement in growth-rate. Pituitary-derived somatropin 0.1 unit per kg body-weight was given intramuscularly three times a week for 6 months to 15 children aged 4.3 to 15.5 years who were of short stature and slow growth-rate but otherwise normal and to 14 children aged 3.9 to 20.3 years with hypopituitarism and growth hormone deficiency. All of the children with hypopituitarism had an increase in height velocity of at least 2 cm per year; 6 of the 14 short normal children who remained prepubertal also increased their height velocity by more than 2 cm per year during somatropin treatment. The short normal children who responded to therapy were younger and had a greater delay in bone age and a slower pretreatment growth-rate than the nonresponders.— G. Van Vliet *et al.*, *New Engl. J. Med.*, 1983, *309*, 1016.

Sixteen prepubertal children of short stature but without growth hormone deficiency were treated for one year with somatrem as a subcutaneous injection in doses of 2 units on 6 nights a week; 10 similar untreated children acted as controls. The standard deviation scores for both height and height velocity, related to chronological and bone age, were significantly increased in the group given somatrem, whereas there was no significant change in growth variables in the control group. Seven of the treated children developed antibodies to somatrem but binding capacity of these antibodies was low and no growth retardation was observed. It was concluded that giving growth hormones to children growing along or parallel to the third height centile leads to an increase in growth velocity without an untoward advance in bone age, so actual height is improved. The extent to which stature will be improved in the long-term remains to be seen.— P. C. Hindmarsh and C. G. D. Brook, *Br. med. J.*, 1987, *295*, 573.

Further reference to a beneficial effect in short children without growth hormone deficiency.— C. R. Buchanan *et al.*, *Archs Dis. Childh.*, 1987, *62*, 912.

HAND-SCHÜLLER-CHRISTIAN DISEASE. Five patients with Hand-Schüller-Christian disease were given growth hormone 2 units thrice weekly by intramuscular injection for 15 months to 2 years. All responded with a significant increase in growth-rate, which was greater in the 1st year than in the 2nd.— G. D. Braunstein *et al.*, *New Engl. J. Med.*, 1975, *292*, 332.

OBESITY. A brief review of the use of growth hormone as therapy for obesity.— R. S. Rivlin, *New Engl. J. Med.*, 1975, *292*, 26.

For the use of growth hormone to conserve lean body-mass during dietary restriction in obese subjects see D. R. Clemmons *et al.*, *J. clin. Endocr. Metab.*, 1987, *64*, 878.

TURNER'S SYNDROME. A 14-year-old girl with Turner's syndrome and with normal concentrations of growth hormone grew 0.23 cm per month during about a year of observation. In the following year, during which she received somatropin 10 mg weekly, the rate of growth was 0.5 cm per month; and in the third year, during which she received conjugated oestrogens 625 µg daily, the rate of growth was 0.3 cm a month.— M. Tzagournis, *J. Am. med. Ass.*, 1969, *210*, 2373.

A 9-year-old girl with Turner's syndrome and growth hormone deficiency grew only 2.3 cm during a year of observation. The next year she received somatropin 5 units three times weekly and grew 6.4 cm with bone age advancing proportionately.— C. G. D. Brook (letter), *New Engl. J. Med.*, 1978, *298*, 1203.

Further references: N. Stahnke (letter), *New Engl. J. Med.*, 1984, *310*, 925 (benefit in only 2 of 8 patients); C. R. Buchanan *et al.*, *Archs Dis. Childh.*, 1987, *62*, 912 (increased growth in 8 of 9 patients given somatropin).

ULCERS. Improvement in severe necrotic ulceration following topical treatment with somatropin in one patient.— H. Waagø (letter), *Lancet*, 1987, *1*, 1485.

VETERINARY AND AGRICULTURAL USE. Bovine growth hormone or somatrophin (BST) can increase milk yield. Some references to the debate on the safety of this practice: *Lancet*, 1988, *2*, 376; C. Davis (letter), *ibid.*, 629; E. Brunner (letter), *ibid.*

Proprietary Preparations

Somatonorm *(KabiVitrum, UK)*. *Injection*, powder for reconstitution, somatrem equivalent to somatropin 4 units, supplied with solvent.

Proprietary Names and Manufacturers of Growth Hormones

Asellacrin *(Serono, USA)*; Crescormon *(Denm.; Norw.; S.Afr.; Swed.; Switz.; KabiVitrum, UK; Pharmacia, USA)*; Grorm *(Serono, Ger.; Serono, Ital.; Serono, Spain; Serono, Switz.)*; Human Growth Hormone *(Commonwealth Serum Laboratories, Austral.)*; Humatrope *(Lilly, USA)*; Nanormon *(Nordisk Gentofte, Denm.; Hormonchemie, Ger.; Nordisk, Norw.; Nordisk, Spain; Nordisk-UK, UK)*; Protropin *(Genentech, Canad.; Genentech, USA)*; Somacton *(Ger.)*; Somatonorm *(Fides, Spain; KabiVitrum, Switz.; KabiVitrum, UK)*; Somatotrope Choay *(Fr.)*.

16932-q

Octreotide *(BAN, USAN, rINN)*.

SMS-201-995. 2-(D-Phenylalanyl-L-cystyl-L-phenylalanyl-D-tryptophyl-L-lysyl-L-threonyl-L-cystyl)-(2*R*,3*R*)-butane-1,3-diol; D-Phenylalanyl-L-cysteinyl-L-phenylalanyl-D-tryptophyl-L-lysyl-L-threonyl-*N*-[(1*R*,2*R*)-2-hydroxy-1-(hydroxymethyl)propyl]-L-cysteinamide cyclic (2→7) disulphide.

$C_{49}H_{66}N_{10}O_{10}S_2$=1019.3.

CAS — 83150-76-9.

Octreotide is an octapeptide analogue of somatostatin (p.1151) which is reported to have similar properties but a longer duration of action.

It has been tried in the management of islet-cell tumours and other neoplasms of the gastro-intestinal tract associated with ectopic peptide production. Doses of 50 to 100 µg by subcutaneous injection have been given two or three times daily.

Octreotide has also been investigated in the treatment of acromegaly and of diabetes mellitus.

ACROMEGALY. Subcutaneous injection of octreotide 50 µg reduced mean serum-somatropin concentrations from 30 to 1.4 ng per mL over a period of 3 hours from the time of injection in 6 acromegalic patients. Basal concentrations of somatropin were not achieved until 9 hours after the injection. In a further patient, in whom basal serum-somatropin concentrations were extremely high, at about 250 ng per mL, injection of octreotide resulted in only about a 20% reduction. Octreotide was well tolerated and may prove of value in the treatment of acromegaly.— G. Plewe *et al.*, *Lancet*, 1984, *2*, 782.

Further references to the use of octreotide in acromegaly: L. J. C. Ch'ng *et al.*, *Br. med. J.*, 1985, *290*, 284 (long-term maintenance in 2 patients); S. W. J. Lamberts *et al.*, *New Engl. J. Med.*, 1985, *313*, 1576 (100 to 300 µg daily subcutaneously for 8 to 24 weeks in 4 acromegalic patients); L. B. Barnard *et al.*, *Ann. intern. Med.*, 1986, *105*, 856 (benefit with 50 to 100 µg subcutaneously every 12 hours in resistant acromegaly); P. Chanson *et al.* (letter), *Lancet*, 1986, *1*, 1270 (improvement in sleep apnoea of acromegaly); G. Williams *et al.*, *ibid.*, *2*, 774 (good results with 4 to 8 mg three times daily by mouth).

CARCINOID SYNDROME. Carcinoid crisis following induction of anaesthesia in a patient with carcinoid syndrome responded to intravenous injection of octreotide 50 µg, repeated after 15 seconds. The dramatic resolution of life-threatening hypotension in this case suggests that octreotide should be available for emergency use in patients with carcinoid syndrome who are undergoing surgery.— L. K. Kvols *et al.* (letter), *New Engl. J. Med.*, 1985, *313*, 1229.

Initial experience with octreotide in the management of patients with carcinoid syndrome. Octreotide was self-administered by subcutaneous injection in doses of 150 µg three times daily by 25 patients and treatment was continued for up to 18 months. Of the 24 patients who had been experiencing flushing, 7 had complete relief and 12 had at least a 50% reduction in frequency and intensity of the flushes. Similarly, diarrhoea was abolished in 4 patients and reduced by at least 50% in 15; 6 had minor or no response. There was also evidence of biochemical response in the majority of patients. Tolerance to octreotide was excellent; only 2 patients developed mild hyperglycaemia, and this was transient. Octreotide appears to be a useful addition to the available treatments for carcinoid syndrome.— L. K. Kvols *et al.*, *New Engl. J. Med.*, 1986, *315*, 663.

CARDIOVASCULAR DISORDERS. A report of benefit from octreotide in patients with postprandial hypotension and orthostatic hypotension associated with autonomic neuropathy.— R. D. Hoeldtke *et al.*, *Lancet*, 1986, *2*, 602.

EFFECTS ON CARBOHYDRATE METABOLISM. A crossover study in 6 insulin-dependent diabetics given octreotide 50 µg, or placebo, three times daily before meals demonstrated that octreotide significantly lowered post-prandial blood-glucose concentrations, and hence reduced insulin requirements. Octreotide may prove to be a useful adjunct to insulin therapy especially in patients experiencing metabolic instability.— M. S. Rios *et al.*, *J. clin. Endocr. Metab.*, 1986, *63*, 1071.

Octreotide 50 µg per hour by intravenous infusion abolished quinine-induced hyperinsulinaemia and resultant hypoglycaemia in a study in 9 healthy subjects, and in a patient receiving quinine for falciparum malaria.— R. E. Phillips *et al.*, *Lancet*, 1986, *1*, 713.

The short-term management of nesidioblastosis, a condition of inappropriate insulin secretion, in a neonate; doses of 1.5 µg subcutaneously at intervals of 3 to 4 hours prevented hypoglycaemia and normalised the glucose requirement.— P. Hindmarsh and C. G. D. Brook (letter), *New Engl. J. Med.*, 1987, *316*, 221. See also H. A. Delemarre-van de Waal *et al.* (letter), *ibid.*, 222.

For the use of octreotide in diabetic diarrhoea see under Gastro-intestinal Disorders, below.

GASTRO-INTESTINAL DISORDERS. Profuse diarrhoea in a diabetic patient, which had lasted for 15 months and was unresponsive to treatment, responded within 10 days of beginning therapy with octreotide; a dose of 50 µg by subcutaneous injection twice daily was given, subsequently increased to 75 µg twice daily. Improvement continued over the next 4 months. The medication, which was given at the same time as the patient's insulin injection, was well tolerated and diabetic control remained stable.— S. -T. Tsai *et al.* (letter), *Ann. intern. Med.*, 1986, *104*, 894.

In a crossover study in 14 patients with postoperative small-bowel fistula octreotide 225 to 300 µg daily for 2 days in divided doses by subcutaneous injection, resulted in a substantial reduction in fistula output. Spontaneous closure occurred in 11 patients (78%) at a mean of 4.5 days after treatment, whereas up to 30 or 40 days may be needed with conventional treatment.— P. Nubiola-Calonge *et al.*, *Lancet*, 1987, *2*, 672.

A report of a dramatic effect on secretory diarrhoea in a patient with AIDS colonised by cryptosporidia. The patient who had been losing stool volumes of up to 3.2 litres daily, with a stool frequency of 10 to 22 times daily, for 10 months was given octreotide 100 µg by subcutaneous injection three times daily initially. Therapy resulted in a reduction in bowel movements to 2 to 6 times daily and volume was reduced to 0.4 to 1.1 litres daily. The patient has subsequently been maintained for 8 months on octreotide 300 µg three times daily subcutaneously without further diarrhoea and with a weight gain of 10 kg.— D. J. Cook *et al.*, *Ann. intern. Med.*, 1988, *108*, 708.

PANCREATIC DISORDERS. *Endocrine tumours.* Reports of the use of octreotide in the management of pancreatic endocrine tumours: W. C. Santangelo *et al.*, *Ann. intern. Med.*, 1985, *103*, 363 (pancreatic cholera syndrome due to islet-cell tumour); K. Osei and T. M. O'Dorisio, *ibid.*, 223 (insulinoma); D. Clements and E. Elias (letter), *Lancet*, 1985, *1*, 874 (metastatic vipoma); S. Bonfils *et al.* (letter), *ibid.*, 1986, *1*, 554 (Zollinger-Ellison syndrome); J. J. Shepherd and G. B. Senator (letter), *ibid.*, *2*, 574 (malignant gastrinoma); G. Boden *et al.*, *New Engl. J. Med.*, 1986, *314*, 1686 (glucagonoma); L. K. Kvols *et al.*, *Ann. intern. Med.*, 1987, *107*, 162 (gastrinoma, glucagonoma, insulinoma, or other ectopic endocrine tumours); L. D. Juby *et al.*, *Postgrad. med. J.*, 1987, *63*, 287 (vipoma).

PITUITARY ADENOMA. References to the effects of octreotide in patients with pituitary adenoma: G. Williams *et al.* (letter), *New Engl. J. Med.*, 1986, *315*, 1166 (relief of headache); R. J. Comi *et al.*, *ibid.*, 1987, *317*, 12 (control of thyrotrophin secretion and associated hyperthyroidism); P. J. Guillausseau *et al.* (letter), *ibid.*, 53 (visual improvement and decrease in secreted thyrotrophin); G. Williams *et al.*, *Br. med. J.*, 1987, *295*, 247 (relief of headache).

Proprietary Names and Manufacturers
Sandoz, Switz.; Sandoz, USA.

16990-k

Somatomedins

Insulin-like Growth Factors; Sulphation Factors. A group of polypeptide hormones related to insulin with molecular weights of about 7000 to 8000. They are synthesised in the liver, kidney, and other tissues and include somatomedin-C (IGF-I; mecatide) and somatomedin-A.

The somatomedins are a group of polypeptide hormones at least some of which are involved in mediating the effects of somatropin in the body. Somatomedin-C is believed to be responsible for many of the anabolic effects of somatropin; serum concentrations of somatomedin-C have been used diagnostically, and are found to be raised in acromegaly and decreased in pituitary dwarfs and in pygmies. Somatomedin-C derived from recombinant DNA technology is under investigation as an alternative to growth hormone in the treatment of dwarfism and short stature, and has been suggested as a possible therapeutic agent in the management of some bone disorders.

Somatomedin-A is reported to be the foetal analogue of somatomedin-C; it stimulates DNA synthesis in cartilage and enhances incorporation of sulphate into chondroitin. Its function in adults remains to be fully elucidated.

Somatomedin-B differs from the other somatomedins in its structure and is less closely related to insulin. It is reported to enhance DNA synthesis in a number of tissues.

3765-j

Somatorelin *(pINN)*.

GHRF; GHRH; GRF; Growth Hormone-releasing Hormone; Somatoliberin.

CAS — 83930-13-6.

Characterisation of the structure of somatorelin: R. P. Guillemin *et al.*, *Science*, 1982, *218*, 585; J. Rivier *et al.*, *Nature*, 1982, *300*, 276; J. Spiess *et al.*, *Biochemistry, N.Y.*, 1982, *24*, 6037.

Somatorelin is a peptide secreted by the hypothalamus which promotes the release of somatropin (growth hormone) from the anterior pituitary. It was originally characterised from pancreatic neoplastic tissue and found to exist as both 44- and 40-amino acid peptides; the larger form may possibly be converted to the smaller but both are reported to be active, the activity residing in the first 29 amino-acid residues.

Synthetic somatorelin (both 40- and 44-amino acid forms) has been investigated in the diagnosis and treatment of growth hormone deficiency. A 29-amino acid analogue has also been tried.

Response to synthetic human pancreatic somatorelin (hpGRF-40), a 40-residue linear peptide, in 6 healthy subjects given 1 µg per kg body-weight as an intravenous bolus. Serum somatropin concentrations were selectively raised within 5 minutes of administration and reached a peak between 30 and 60 minutes.— M. O. Thorner *et al.*, *Lancet*, 1983, *1*, 24 and 256.

Studies of the effects of synthetic 44-amino-acid somatorelin [GRF(1-44)] on somatropin release. Following intravenous injection of 100 µg of the peptide in 11 healthy subjects there was a measurable rise in somatropin concentration within 5 minutes reaching a peak after a mean of about 30 minutes. No further enhancement of response occurred in any subject given 200 µg. Administration of 100 µg of somatorelin to 6 subjects with acromegaly produced responses similar to those in healthy subjects in 3, but the remaining 3, who had more active disease, had greatly exaggerated and prolonged somatropin responses. Similar doses were given to 8 patients with impaired pituitary function: 2 evinced no response and the remainder had much smaller responses than in normal subjects, comparable to those induced by insulin hypoglycaemia but of more rapid onset. The only side-effect reported was facial warmth and flushing in one patient. Somatorelin as a bolus dose of 100 µg may prove of considerable use in assessing growth hormone deficiency and acromegaly.— S. M. Wood *et al.*, *Br. med. J.*, 1983, *286*, 1687.

Synthetic human pancreatic tumour somatorelin (hpGRF-40) in a dose of 10 µg per kg body-weight intravenously increased serum somatropin concentrations in 3 of 7 patients with isolated growth hormone deficiency and in one with Hand-Schüller-Christian disease, although less than in 6 healthy subjects. None of 4 patients with multiple anterior pituitary hormone deficiencies responded with increased somatropin concentrations although 3 had an elevation in serum somatomedin-C concentrations as did 6 of those with isolated growth hormone deficiency. Somatorelin may be useful in distinguishing pituitary from hypothalamic disease and some growth hormone deficient children may be able to benefit from therapy with somatorelin.— J. L. C. Borges *et al.*, *Lancet*, 1983, *2*, 119. Correction.— *ibid.*, 412. Intravenous administration of 200 µg of synthetic somatorelin (hpGRF-40) was followed by a clear rise in circulating somatropin in all of 4 patients with hypothalamic tumours or idiopathic growth hormone deficiency.— A. Grossman *et al.*, *ibid.*, 137.

The effects of therapy with synthetic (40-amino acid) somatorelin in 2 children with growth hormone deficiency. Somatorelin 1 µg per kg body-weight was given subcutaneously over one minute every 3 hours, via a pump, to the 2 children for a period of 2 months; the dose was then increased to 3 µg per kg for a further 4 months. Both children had accelerated growth velocity over the period of therapy, growth-rate increasing from 4.6 to 7.1 cm per year in one and from 2.1 to 13.7 cm per year in the other. Cessation of growth after 15 weeks in the former coincided with glucocorticoid replacement therapy for cortisol deficiency. Although these data are preliminary they suggest that somatorelin can restore somatropin secretion with consequent acceleration of linear growth-rate in children with growth hormone deficiency. However, more experience is required and it will be necessary to evaluate different doses and frequencies of administration.— M. O. Thorner *et al.*, *New Engl. J. Med.*, 1985, *312*, 4. Subsequent assay of serum samples using immunoelectrophoresis revealed the presence of antibodies to somatorelin in the patient with the less marked response to treatment. The presence of antibodies should not detract from further investigations of somatorelin, but in such studies the titres of any such antibodies should be measured by the most sensitive technique available.— *idem*, 994.

The effects of a 29-amino acid somatorelin analogue ([Nle^{27}]GH-RH(1-29)-NH_2) on somatropin secretion following intravenous, subcutaneous, and intranasal administration in studies involving 19 healthy subjects. The peptide produced a comparable degree of stimulation of somatropin when given intravenously to that which followed the same intravenous dose of synthetic (40-amino acid) somatorelin. A ten-fold higher dose is required subcutaneously to produce results comparable with the intravenous route, while a thirty-fold higher intranasal dose is necessary to stimulate approximately one-fifth of the amount of somatropin release.— M. L. Vance *et al.*, *Clin. Pharmac. Ther.*, 1986, *40*, 627.

The use of a 29-amino acid analogue of somatorelin (GHRH(1-29)NH_2) in the treatment of 18 prepubertal growth-hormone deficient children. The peptide was given by subcutaneous injection twice daily in doses of 250 μg to 8 children weighing less than 20 kg and in doses of 500 μg to 10 children weighing over 20 kg. After 3 to 6 months of therapy 12 of the 18 children showed an increase in height velocity, and in 8 the increase was more than 2 cm per year, which was judged satisfactory. The increase in height velocity was maintained in these 8 patients on continued treatment for between 6 and 18 months. Fourteen of 17 patients tested developed antibodies to the peptide but this did not appear to affect response; no side-effects other than a slight stinging at the site of the injection were noted. Somatorelin analogues offer advantages in the treatment of growth hormone deficiency and are likely to be an important new therapy; other means of administration also need to be assessed.— R. J. M. Ross *et al.*, *Lancet*, 1987, *1*, 5.

Proprietary Names and Manufacturers
Kabi, Swed.

5946-l

Somatostatin *(BAN, rINN)*.

GHRIF; GHRIH; Growth-hormone-release-inhibiting Hormone; Somatotrophin-release-inhibiting Factor. Ala-Gly-Cys-Lys-Asn-Phe-Phe-Trp-Lys-Thr-Phe-Thr-Ser-Cys cyclic (3→14) disulphide.

$C_{76}H_{104}N_{18}O_{19}S_2$=1637.9.

CAS — 51110-01-1; 38916-34-6 (sheep, cyclic); 40958-31-4 (sheep, linear).

A polypeptide obtained from the hypothalamus or by synthesis. The naturally occurring form has a cyclic structure; a non-native linear form is also used.

The isolation and structure of somatostatin from sheep.— P. Brazeau *et al.*, *Science*, 1973, *179*, 77.

Somatostatin is a hypothalamic release-inhibiting hormone which inhibits the release of somatropin (p.1148) from the anterior pituitary. It also inhibits the release of thyrotrophin (p.1153) and corticotrophin (p.1139) from the pituitary, glucagon and insulin from the pancreas, and appears to have a role in the regulation of duodenal and gastric secretions.

It has been tried in a variety of disorders including upper gastro-intestinal haemorrhage, insulin resistance, and the management of hormone-secreting tumours, but it has a very short duration of action and several analogues of somatostatin have been produced in an attempt to prolong its activity as well as making its inhibitory effects more specific: octreotide (p.1149) is such an analogue.

Although somatostatin derived from the hypothalamus was found to be a 14-amino-acid peptide, a longer, 28-amino-acid form also exists in some tissues.

Reviews of the actions and potential uses of somatostatin: S. Reichlin, *New Engl. J. Med.*, 1983, *309*, 1495 and 1556; *Lancet*, 1985, *2*, 77; S. R. Bloom and J. M. Polak, *Br. med. J.*, 1987, *295*, 288.

ACTION ON THE KIDNEYS. Life-threatening water retention and hyponatraemia developed in a patient given a somatostatin infusion; a second, ascitic, patient also developed some signs of water retention. Although the mechanism of this water retention is unknown the effects of somatostatin on the kidney are clearly of clinical importance.— C. Halma *et al.*, *Ann. intern. Med.*, 1987, *107*, 518.

Studies of the antidiuretic effect of somatostatin on the kidney: B. J. Walker *et al.* (letter), *Lancet*, 1983, *1*, 1101; W. Pruszczynski and R. Ardaillou (letter), *ibid.*, *2*, 628; E. René *et al.* (letter), *ibid.*, 689; J. P. Vora *et al.*, *Br. med. J.*, 1986, *292*, 1701.

CARCINOID SYNDROME. The symptoms of a patient with a carcinoid tumour were controlled with methyldopa and somatostatin before surgery. During surgical manipulation of the tumour 3 hypotensive episodes were quickly corrected with bolus intravenous injections of somatostatin. Somatostatin was twice given postoperatively to control hypotensive crises.— L. Thulin *et al.* (letter), *Lancet*, 1978, *2*, 43.

Somatostatin had a beneficial effect on bronchial constriction in a patient with carcinoid syndrome. Bronchial resistance was reduced for more than 90 minutes after the intravenous injection of somatostatin 250 μg.— R. Klapdor (letter), *New Engl. J. Med.*, 1980, *303*, 464.

Further references: R. G. Long *et al.*, *Gut*, 1981, *22*, 549; J. A. Oates *et al.* (letter), *New Engl. J. Med.*, 1984, *310*, 1264.

CARDIOVASCULAR DISORDERS. Sinus rhythm was restored in 5 of 6 patients with paroxysmal supraventricular or junctional tachycardia by the intravenous injection, every 2 minutes, of somatostatin 25 μg to a total of 175 to 200 μg.— A. V. Greco *et al.*, *Br. med. J.*, 1984, *288*, 28.

Somatostatin infused at the rate of 500 μg per hour abolished severe postprandial hypotension in an elderly patient.— R. D. Hoeldtke *et al.*, *Ann. intern. Med.*, 1985, *103*, 889.

EFFECTS ON CARBOHYDRATE METABOLISM. A review of somatostatin and its possible role in carbohydrate homoeostasis and the treatment of diabetes mellitus.— J. E. Gerich, *Archs intern. Med.*, 1977, *137*, 659.

An intravenous infusion of cyclic somatostatin in 10 patients with insulin-dependent diabetes decreased plasma concentrations of glucose and glucagon by about 25% and 50% respectively. Linear somatostatin given subcutaneously had a transient effect. Somatostatin with insulin abolished post-meal hyperglycaemia in 4 diabetic patients and the combination was more effective than insulin alone.— J. E. Gerich *et al.*, *New Engl. J. Med.*, 1974, *291*, 544. See also *idem*, 1975, *292*, 985.

Results following 5-hour infusion of linear somatostatin at a rate of 500 to 720 μg per hour into 8 subjects with maturity-onset diabetes controlled by dietary regimen alone suggested that glucagon was not essential for the development and maintenance of fasting hyperglycaemia. Somatostatin accentuated hyperglycaemia, hyperketonaemia, and hyperaminoacidaemia which argued against its use in maturity-onset diabetics with residual insulin secretion.— W. V. Tamborlane *et al.*, *New Engl. J. Med.*, 1977, *297*, 181.

A study in an infant born to an insulin-dependent diabetic mother suggested that somatostatin may have a role in suppressing hyperinsulinism in such infants.— E. Mallet *et al.* (letter), *Lancet*, 1980, *1*, 776.

EFFECTS ON COAGULATION. Intravenous infusions of cyclic somatostatin in doses of 3.4 to 6 μg per minute for 5.25 to 6 hours in 4 healthy subjects impaired platelet aggregation in all 4. Subjective side-effects including abdominal pain, dizziness, and diarrhoea occurred in the 3 subjects who received doses higher than 3.4 μg per minute. It appeared that somatostatin might be involved in a specific intravascular coagulation process.— G. M. Besser *et al.*, *Lancet*, 1975, *1*, 1166. See also E. Carmina *et al.* (letter), *New Engl. J. Med.*, 1976, *294*, 226.

The infusion of linear or cyclic somatostatin in 8 patients, 7 with diabetes, had no apparent effect on coagulation or platelet function.— C. H. Mielke *et al.*, *New Engl. J. Med.*, 1975, *293*, 480.

GASTRO-INTESTINAL DISORDERS. A 24-hour infusion of cyclic somatostatin dramatically reduced faecal losses in a patient with Verner-Morrison syndrome with the full watery diarrhoea, hypokalaemia, and achlorhydria sequence, high serum concentrations of vasoactive intestinal polypeptide, and a pancreatic tumour. On withdrawal of the somatostatin, however, a marked rebound effect occurred.— S. Bonfils *et al.* (letter), *Lancet*, 1979, *2*, 476.

Intravenous infusion of somatostatin 110 ng per kg per minute suppressed or reduced the symptoms of dumping syndrome in 5 of 6 patients given an oral glucose load. Somatostatin, or perhaps its analogues, offer an attractive new approach in the management of early dumping.— R. G. Long *et al.*, *Br. med. J.*, 1985, *290*, 886. See also P. G. Reasbeck and A. M. Van Rij (letter), *ibid.*, 1147.

Somatostatin infusion was effective in controlling diarrhoea in a patient with colonic pseudo-obstruction when given at a dose of 500 μg per hour, but not in a dose of only 250 μg per hour.— S. Mulvihill *et al.* (letter), *New Engl. J. Med.*, 1984, *310*, 467. Comment.— E. René and S. Bonfils (letter), *ibid.*, *311*, 598 (lower doses are frequently effective in diarrhoea).

A report of complete relief of longstanding symptoms of irritable bowel syndrome in a patient given subcutaneous somatostatin for acromegaly.— N. J. Talley *et al.* (letter), *Lancet*, 1987, *2*, 1144. Comment. A pharmacological effect of the administered somatostatin, namely inhibition of colonic activity and other gastro-intestinal functions, was probably seen but this does not necessarily have any physiological implications.— J. Binimelis *et al.* (letter), *ibid.*, 1533.

See also under Haemorrhage, below.

HAEMORRHAGE. Results of a randomised controlled study of sequential design, comparing cimetidine and somatostatin for the treatment of severe and persistent gastro-intestinal bleeding due to peptic ulcer in patients unsuitable for emergency surgery. Bleeding was stopped by somatostatin in 8 out of 10 patients, whereas cimetidine stopped bleeding in only 1 out of 10 patients. Thus cimetidine failed to control peptic ulcer bleeding, whereas somatostatin is suitable for conservative treatment in patients who are unsuitable for surgery, and when stabilisation of the circulation and patient's general condition will decrease the risk of later surgery. Cyclic somatostatin was given as an intravenous bolus injection of 250 μg followed by infusion of 250 μg per hour for 48 to 120 hours.— L. Kayasseh *et al.*, *Lancet*, 1980, *1*, 844. Doubt as to whether it can be concluded from the data presented, that somatostatin may be suitable for the control of peptic ulcer bleeding.— R. J. S. Thomas and J. F. Forbes (letter), *ibid.*, *2*, 200. Reply.— L. Kayasseh *et al.* (letter), *ibid.*, 861.

Bleeding ceased in 19 of 20 patients with various haemorrhagic gastro-intestinal disorders within 8 to 12 hours after treatment with somatostatin, compared with cessation after 20 to 60 hours in 13 of 20 treated with ranitidine and in 9 of 20 treated with placebo. The dose of somatostatin was 250 μg by intravenous injection initially, followed by 250 μg per hour until bleeding ceased; the dose of ranitidine was 50 mg intravenously every 4 hours.— F. Coraggio *et al.*, *Br. med. J.*, 1984, *289*, 224. Criticism. A rebleeding and operation rate of 11% for peptic ulcers treated with somatostatin is undoubtedly better than would be expected with conventional treatment but a larger study with a better defined protocol will be needed to prove the value of somatostatin in treating bleeding peptic ulcers.— S. Brearley (letter), *ibid.*, 1229. Reply. It should be noted in particular that somatostatin led to a reduction of the bleeding time without any rebleeding after the drug was stopped.— F. Coraggio (letter), *ibid.*

In a double-blind study, 46 patients with massive upper-gastro-intestinal bleeding but no oesophageal varices were given somatostatin 250 μg by bolus injection followed by 250 μg per hour for 72 hours by cyclic infusion; 49 similar patients received placebo. Rebleeding occurred in 6 treated patients and 5 controls but surgery, indicated by the magnitude of blood loss or extent of rebleeding, was necessary in only 5 of the patients given somatostatin compared to 14 of those receiving placebo which was a significant difference. The need for blood transfusions and the mortality rate did not differ significantly between the two groups, but 4 patients treated with somatostatin and one patient given placebo died. No adverse effects during somatostatin treatment were observed.— I. Magnusson *et al.*, *Gut*, 1985, *26*, 221.

In a prospective randomised controlled study acute variceal haemorrhage was successfully controlled in all of 10 patients with portal hypertension given somatostatin compared with 4 of 12 patients given argipressin. Somatostatin was given as an intravenous bolus injection of 250 μg followed by a constant intravenous infusion of 250 μg per hour for 24 hours, argipressin was given as an intravenous infusion at a rate of 0.4 units per minute for 6 hours, and if bleeding stopped, decreased to 0.2 units per minute for the following 6 hours, decreased again to 0.1 units per minute for a further 6 hours, and finally discontinued if no further bleeding occurred. Of the 10 patients given somatostatin 7 were subsequently treated with injection sclerotherapy without any further episodes of bleeding; in the other 3 patients, however, 7 episodes of rebleeding occurred before definitive treatment could be undertaken but were controlled by further infusions of somatostatin. No complications were observed in any of the 10 patients during infusion of somatostatin but administration of argipressin had to be stopped in 2 patients because of undesirable side-effects (pulmonary oedema in one and a chest pain and abdominal colic in the other). It therefore appears that somatostatin is an effective stopgap measure, giving time for the patient's condition to improve and diagnostic measures to be undertaken, before definitive treatment is carried out.— S. A. Jenkins *et al.*, *Br. med. J.*, 1985, *290*, 275.

In a study involving 630 patients with upper gastro-intestinal haemorrhage somatostatin treatment (an initial intravenous bolus of 250 μg followed by infusion of 250 μg per hour for 72 hours) in 315 did not significantly reduce rebleeding episodes, necessity for surgery, or death-rate when compared with placebo in the remaining 315. Analysed on an intention-to-treat basis there were 70 cases of rebleeding, 35 operations and 31 deaths in the somatostatin group compared with 89, 34, and 25 respectively in the placebo group. Exclusion from consideration of 96 patients withdrawn from the study did not significantly affect the results. Treatment was well tolerated and no adverse effects were reported. The results do not confirm those of earlier studies and suggest that somatostatin treatment is unlikely to have any substantial effect on outcome in most patients with acute upper gastro-intestinal bleeding.— K. W. Somerville *et al.*, *Lancet*, 1985, *1*, 130. Criticism of the study design and the conclusions. Somatostatin has been found to be of benefit in selected patients.— K. Gyr *et al.* (letter), *ibid.*, *2*, 155. Reply, and a defence of the conclusions of the study.— M. J. S. Langman and K. W. Somerville (letter), *ibid.*, 394. Further comments.— I. Magnusson and T. Ihre (letter), *ibid.*, *1*, 337; J. N. Baxter *et al.* (letter), *ibid.*

PAIN. A report of a potent analgesic effect of somatostatin following intraventricular, intrathecal, or epidural administration in 9 patients with pain due to terminal cancer or to surgery. Somatostatin was as effective as morphine in relieving pain but appeared to act via a different mechanism since analgesia was not reversed by naloxone.— J. Chrubasik *et al.* (letter), *Lancet*, 1984, *2*, 1208.

PANCREATIC DISORDERS. *Endocrine tumours.* Somatostatin inhibited insulin secretion from non-malignant insulinomas in 2 patients.— S. E. Christensen *et al.* (letter), *Lancet*, 1975, *1*, 1426.

The activity of somatostatin in suppressing the insulin response to tolbutamide in patients with hyperinsulinism due to pancreatic hyperplasia but not to insulinoma could be used as a diagnostic test. Suppression would also occur in healthy subjects.— J. L. Del Arbol *et al.* (letter), *Lancet*, 1978, *1*, 281. The test might not be able to differentiate uniformly between the normal function of pancreatic beta-cells and insulinoma or between hyperplasia and neoplasia of the islet-cells.— F. Van Kersen (letter), *Lancet*, 1978, *1*, 557. See also F. Escobar-Jimenez *et al.* (letter), *ibid.*, 1150.

A report of dramatic improvement of skin lesions in 2 patients with glucagonomas following infusion of cyclic somatostatin.— J. Sohier *et al.* (letter), *Lancet*, 1980, *1*, 40.

Pancreatitis. Preliminary findings which suggest that somatostatin may be beneficial in the treatment of acute pancreatitis.— B. Limberg and B. Kommerell (letter), *New Engl. J. Med.*, 1980, *303*, 284. See also K. -H. Usadel *et al.* (letter), *ibid.*, 999.

Proprietary Names and Manufacturers

Aminopan *(UCB, Ger.)*; Modustatina *(Midy, Ital.)*; Somatofalk *(Falk, Ger.)*; Somiaton *(Serono, Spain)*; Stilamin *(Serono, Ger.*; *Serono, Ital.*; *Serono, Switz.)*; Manufacturers also include—*Ayerst, USA; Wyeth, USA.*

3891-x

Thyrotrophic Hormones

The following section includes the pituitary thyrotrophic hormone, Thyrotrophin, and its hypothalamic releasing hormone, Protirelin.

In line with the negative feedback principles involved in many homoeostatic processes the hormones of the thyroid gland are also involved in its hormonal regulation—see Thyroid Agents, p.1487.

5945-e

Protirelin *(BAN, USAN, rINN).*

Abbott-38579; Lopremone; Thyroliberin; Thyrotrophin-releasing Hormone; TRF; TRH. L-Pyroglutamyl-L-histidyl-L-prolinamide; 1-[*N*-(5-Oxo-L-prolyl)-L-histidyl]-L-prolinamide; Glu-His-Pro-NH_2.

$C_{16}H_{22}N_6O_4$=362.4.

CAS — 24305-27-9.

Pharmacopoeias. In *Jpn* which also includes the tartrate.

A tripeptide obtained from the hypothalamus or by synthesis.

Adverse Effects

Protirelin given by intravenous injection may cause nausea, a desire to micturate, flushing, dizziness, and a strange taste. These effects have been attributed to contraction of smooth muscles by the bolus injection. Hypertension or hypotension have occasionally been reported.

Epileptic seizures induced by protirelin in a patient with a history of convulsions.— K. Maeda and K. Tanimoto (letter), *Lancet*, 1981, *1*, 1058.

Transient amaurosis and headache after protirelin injection.— P. L. Drury *et al.* (letter), *Lancet*, 1982, *1*, 218.

A report of adverse effects including unconsciousness, hypotension, and convulsions in 4 patients following injection of high doses (400 µg) of protirelin.— L. Ø. Dolva *et al.*, *Br. med. J.*, 1983, *287*, 532.

EFFECT ON THE CARDIOVASCULAR SYSTEM. A significant increase in arterial blood pressure and heart-rate occurred about 1 minute after rapid intravenous injection of protirelin 200 µg. The effect lasted less than 5 minutes. Other haemodynamic parameters were unchanged. A direct stimulant effect on the smooth muscle of arteries was suggested.— H. A. Abplanalp, *Arzneimittel-Forsch.*, 1976, *26*, 271.

EFFECT ON THE CENTRAL NERVOUS SYSTEM. Mild euphoria, relaxation, and a sense of increased energy unrelated to thyrotrophin response or somatic effects occurred in a controlled study in 10 healthy women given protirelin.— I. C. Wilson *et al.*, *Archs gen. Psychiat.*, 1973, *29*, 15, per *J. Am. med. Ass.*, 1973, *225*, 325.

Intravenous infusions of protirelin 600 µg had no significant cortical activity in 8 healthy subjects.— H. Ashton *et al.*, *Br. J. clin. Pharmac.*, 1976, *3*, 523.

EFFECTS ON THE RESPIRATORY SYSTEM. Bronchospasm in an asthmatic boy given protirelin intravenously.— R. G. McFadden *et al.* (letter), *Lancet*, 1981, *2*, 758.

See also under Precautions, below.

EFFECT ON SEXUAL FUNCTION. On questioning, 7 of 16 women reported a sensation of mild vaginal sexual arousal occurring 1 to 3 minutes after intravenous injection of protirelin. Four women also experienced urinary sensations, and 3 described an urge to urinate with no sexual component.— M. Blum and M. Pulini (letter), *Lancet*, 1980, *2*, 43. A report of a penile-urethral sensation associated with thyroid-releasing hormone [sic].— P. J. Green (letter), *ibid.*, 199.

HYPERCHOLESTEROLAEMIA. Five of 8 patients had elevated serum-cholesterol concentrations after treatment for 2 to 15 months with protirelin 10 to 40 mg daily.— M. J. E. van der Vis-Melsen and J. D. Wiener (letter), *Br. med. J.*, 1973, *4*, 419.

Precautions

Protirelin should be given with care to patients with cardiac insufficiency, obstructive airways disease, or severe hypopituitarism. Administration of protirelin while the patient is lying down may reduce the incidence of hypotension.

In 2 patients with adrenal medullary phaeochromocytomas, following a standard protirelin test using 200 µg the thyrotrophin response was impaired, which could have led to a misdiagnosis of thyrotoxicosis.— D. C. Linch and E. J. Ross (letter), *Lancet*, 1979, *1*, 210. A report of a similar patient with a normal response. An impaired thyrotrophin response to protirelin is not an invariable finding in patients with phaeochromocytoma.— W. J. Kalk and E. Rogaly (letter), *ibid.*, 1079. See also R. Reid *et al.* (letter), *ibid.*

Preliminary results suggest that in some patients with amyotrophic lateral sclerosis intravenous injection of protirelin may result in acute bronchospasm. Five of 25 patients experienced falls in FEV_1 of more than 20%; in 2, a 15% decrease in arterial oxygen pressure occurred. Patients with sclerosis and weakened respiratory muscles should be warned of this potential side-effect.— S. R. Braun *et al.* (letter), *Lancet*, 1984, *2*, 529.

A report of pituitary apoplexy following combined testing of anterior pituitary function in a patient with a pituitary tumour. Of the drugs given protirelin was thought most likely to have an aetiological role.— A. J. Chapman *et al.*, *Br. med. J.*, 1985, *291*, 26. Comment on the risks of protirelin in patients with pituitary adenomas.— D. P. Mikhailidis *et al.* (letter), *ibid.*, 488.

INTERACTIONS. A brief review of drugs influencing the response to protirelin. The secretion of thyrotrophin appears to be modulated by dopaminergic and noradrenergic pathways at both the hypothalamic and pituitary level. Dopamine and bromocriptine have depressed the response to protirelin; levodopa is a powerful depressant. Partial depression has been reported after the administration of chlorpromazine, thioridazine, and phentolamine, all of which have alpha-receptor blocking properties. Beta-receptors do not appear to be involved in the thyrotrophin response to protirelin whereas the antiserotonin agent, cyproheptadine, has an inhibitory effect. Aspirin and corticosteroids with predominantly glucocorticoid activity have also depressed the response. An enhanced response to protirelin has been seen after the administration of theophylline. Oestrogens may also increase the response in men but not usually in women; when combined with a progestogen a slightly depressed response has been reported.— B. -A. Lamberg and A. Gordin, *Ann. clin. Res.*, 1978, *10*, 171.

Lithium diminished the thyroid response to protirelin.— U. B. Lauridsen *et al.*, *J. clin. Endocr. Metab.*, 1974, *39*, 383.

Ranitidine reduced the response of thyrotrophin to protirelin in a study in 7 healthy subjects.— E. Tarditi *et al.*, *Experientia*, 1983, *39*, 109.

Absorption and Fate

Protirelin is absorbed from the buccal and nasal mucosa and from the upper part of the gastro-intestinal tract. It is rapidly metabolised and excreted in the urine.

Protirelin disappeared rapidly from the plasma of 8 male subjects who were given 400 µg intravenously; over 90% was removed within 20 minutes, with a half-life of about 5.3 minutes. Protirelin was rapidly metabolised in plasma and possibly the tissues. About 5.5% of the dose was excreted in the urine, mostly within 30 minutes.— R. M. Bassiri and R. D. Utiger, *J. clin. Invest.*, 1973, *52*, 1616.

Uses and Administration

Protirelin is a hypothalamic releasing hormone which stimulates the release of thyrotrophin (p.1153) from the anterior lobe of the pituitary. It also has prolactin-releasing activity (see p.1145).

Protirelin is used in the assessment of the hypothalamic-pituitary-thyroid axis in the diagnosis of mild hyperthyroidism, primary hypothyroidism, and ophthalmic Graves' disease. A normal thyrotrophin response excludes thyrotoxicosis and primary hypothyroidism. The response to protirelin may be used for differentiating between primary and secondary hypothyroidism but care is required in interpreting the results of the test and it should not be used alone in establishing the diagnosis. Protirelin is given with gonadorelin (p.1142) in the assessment of anterior pituitary function.

Protirelin is given intravenously usually in doses of 200 to 500 µg. It has also been given in larger doses by mouth.

Analogues of protirelin such as DN-1417, MK-771, and RX-77368 are also under investigation.

A review of thyrotropin-releasing hormone.— I. M. D. Jackson, *New Engl. J. Med.*, 1982, *306*, 145.

Discussion of the extrathyroidal actions of thyrotrophin releasing hormone. Distribution of the hormone in the nervous system suggests that it functions as a neurotransmitter; it releases prolactin, and in some circumstances can release vasopressin, growth hormone, corticotrophin, and somatostatin. It can lower blood calcium and inhibit pancreatic enzyme secretion. Given centrally it increases colonic activity and gastric secretion, affects body temperature regulation, and has analeptic and anti-depressant effects. Although it does not act directly on opioid receptors it functions as a partial physiological opioid antagonist. Of particular importance, however, in view of the increasing clinical use of protirelin, is the potential pressor effect, which although generally moderate may be severe in individual patients.— *Lancet*, 1984, *2*, 560.

DEPRESSION. There have been individual reports and small studies suggesting a beneficial response to injection of protirelin in depressed patients (A.J. Kastin *et al.*, *Lancet*, 1972, *2*, 740; A.J. Prange, *ibid.*, 999; P.T. Loosen *et al.*, *Arzneimittel-Forsch.*, 1976, *26*, 1164) but other studies suggest that it is ineffective as an anti-depressant (C.Q. Mountjoy *et al.*, *Lancet*, 1974, *1*, 958; A. Coppen *et al.*, *ibid.*, *2*, 433; A.A. Sugerman *et al.*, *Curr. ther. Res.*, 1976, *19*, 94).

DIAGNOSIS OF DEPRESSION. Data from 10 patients suggesting that the magnitude of the protirelin-induced thyrotrophin response may be useful in the differentiation of bipolar and unipolar depressed patients.— M. S. Gold *et al.* (letter), *Lancet*, 1979, *2*, 411. These findings could not be confirmed.— N. Bjørum and C. Kirkegaard (letter), *Lancet*, 1979, *2*, 694; J. D. Amsterdam *et al.* (letter), *ibid.*, 904.

Findings of a controlled study in 58 female depressive patients matched with 42 healthy female controls indicated that the deficient thyrotrophin response to protirelin, when present, is useful in the differentiation of bipolar and unipolar disorder in females.— J. Mendlewicz *et al.* (letter), *Lancet*, 1979, *2*, 1079. Criticism.— C. Kirkegaard and N. Bjørum (letter), *ibid.*, 1980, *1*, 152.

Thyrotrophin responses to protirelin were significantly less in 13 patients with primary unipolar depression than those in 5 patients with secondary depression, even after clinical recovery.— G. M. Asnis *et al.* (letter), *Lancet*, 1980, *1*, 424.

A further study. A blunted thyrotrophin response to protirelin was found in 19 of 44 depressed outpatients referred for testing while 6 had augmented responses suggesting some degree of hypothyroidism. The results were considered to confirm the value of the thyrotrophin response to protirelin in the diagnosis of major depression.— H. A. Sternbach *et al.*, *J. Am. med. Ass.*, 1983, *249*, 1618.

DIAGNOSIS OF HYPOTHALAMIC AND PITUITARY DYSFUNCTION. In a study of 76 patients with pituitary-hypothalamic disease given protirelin 200 µg intravenously, 7 of 35 patients with acromegaly, 12 of 26 with other pituitary lesions, and 7 of 15 patients with hypothalamic lesions responded normally. However, 13 of the 15 patients with hypothalamic lesions had a delayed response and this could be used in diagnosis.— R. Hall *et al.*, *Lancet*, 1972, *1*, 759.

The use of protirelin in 100 patients enabled the detection of, and differentiation between, hormonal abnormalities due to hypothalamic and pituitary disease, by assessment of thyrotrophic hormone and lactogenic hormone secretory reserves.— P. J. Synder *et al.*, *Ann. intern. Med.*, 1974, *81*, 751.

In a study of male subjects with isolated gonadotrophin deficiency, boys with delayed puberty, and normal adult men the prolactin response to protirelin was impaired in 9 of the 10 subjects with isolated gonadotrophin deficiency but normal in the other 2 groups. The impaired prolactin response to challenge with protirelin might be used to facilitate the diagnosis of isolated gonadotrophin deficiency and differentiate it from delayed puberty.— I. M. Spitz *et al.*, *New Engl. J. Med.*, 1983, *308*, 575.

DIAGNOSIS OF PITUITARY ADENOMAS. Testing with chlorpromazine and protirelin could be of diagnostic value in distinguishing between those patients with galactorrhoea and amenorrhoea produced by pituitary tumours, idiopathic disease or other causes. Testing with protirelin alone was of no diagnostic value.— A. E. Boyd *et al.*, *Ann. intern. Med.*, 1977, *87*, 165.

In 14 infertile women with hyperprolactinaemia the impaired prolactin responses to stimulation with protirelin 200 µg intravenously or metoclopramide 10 mg intravenously were reliable and clinically useful aids to diagnosis. Suppression tests using levodopa or bromocriptine were less reliable.— E. A. Cowden *et al.*, *Lancet*, 1979, *1*, 1155. The protirelin test is an unreliable discriminant for prolactinoma.— D. Handelsman *et al.* (letter), *Lancet*, 1979, *2*, 581. A similar view.— J. G. M. Klijn *et al.* (letter), *ibid.*

DIAGNOSIS OF THYROID DISORDERS. In a study with 14 healthy subjects, intravenous injection of protirelin acetate (TRH) 50 µg or more caused a variable but significant rise in serum concentrations of thyrotrophin (TSH), the peak effect occurring after about 20 minutes. Side-effects included nausea, a flushing sensation, a desire to micturate, a peculiar taste, and tightness in the chest. After administration of 1 mg or more of TRH by mouth, peak TSH concentrations occurred after 2 hours, but a consistent rise in TSH occurred only after administration of 20 mg or more. Rises in serum protein-bound iodine followed increases in TSH.— B. J. Ormston *et al.*, *Br. med. J.*, 1971, *2*, 199.

Protirelin acetate 200 µg in 2 mL of saline given to 45 healthy subjects produced a rise in serum thyrotrophin. In 24 patients with hypothyroidism, the increase in thyrotrophin following the same dose of protirelin was greater than in the controls; this was not the case in 2 patients with preclinical hypothyroidism. Thyrotrophin concentrations following protirelin 200 µg given to 33 patients with hyperthyroidism did not reach those seen in the control subjects.— B. J. Ormston *et al.*, *Lancet*, 1971, *2*, 10.

Two patients had no response to protirelin 200 µg in spite of being euthyroid. The decision to treat patients who had not responded to protirelin as thyrotoxic should not be based on that test alone.— N. F. Lawton *et al.*, *Lancet*, 1971, *2*, 14. A study in 11 euthyroid patients not responding to intravenous protirelin indicated that oral administration of protirelin, to provide depot stimulation, is a useful diagnostic test for euthyroid patients with impaired thyrotrophin reserve but euthyroid function.— J. J. Stuab *et al.* (letter), *Lancet*, 1979, *1*, 209. Comment.— C. Kirkegaard *et al.* (letter), *ibid.*, 556.

The responses of 11 euthyroid patients with Graves' disease to protirelin were compared with the results of the tri-iodothyronine (T_3) suppression test. Of 5 patients whose thyroid uptake of radio-iodine could not be suppressed, 2 had large increases in serum thyrotrophin in response to protirelin 31 µg or 500 µg and 3 had poor responses. In 6 patients whose radio-iodine uptake was suppressible by tri-iodothyronine there were responses to protirelin. Patients with Hashimoto's thyroiditis or normal glands had exaggerated responses to protirelin. No correlation was found between the responses and the course of the exophthalmos.— P. S. Franco *et al.*, *Metabolism*, 1973, *22*, 1357.

Subclinical hypothyroidism or premyxoedema could be diagnosed by an exaggerated response to protirelin; 88 of 100 patients suspected of having premyxoedema had an exaggerated response compared with none of 20 controls.— J. Alaghband-Zadeh *et al.*, *Lancet*, 1977, *2*, 998.

Evidence that a protirelin dose of 1 µg per kg bodyweight intravenously is the ideal dose for the protirelin test in children. Higher doses do not give any more clinical information.— S. Zabransky (letter), *Lancet*, 1980, *2*, 864.

A study involving 75 elderly patients with atrial fibrillation and 73 with sinus rhythm demonstrated that reduced or absent thyrotrophin responses to protirelin were common in sick, elderly patients. An absent response to protirelin alone is not justification for treatment for hyperthyroidism in elderly patients presenting with atrial fibrillation.— A. B. Davies *et al.*, *Br. med. J.*, 1985, *291*, 773. Comment and a reminder of the usefulness of protirelin testing in general.— A. D. Toft *et al.* (letter), *ibid.*, 1276.

Results suggesting that in evaluating equivocally hyperthyroid patients protirelin testing may be redundant if the thyrotrophin value, as measured by high-sensitivity immunoradiometric assay, is 0.08 milliunits per litre or less.— D. J. Kerr and W. D. Alexander (letter), *Lancet*, 1984, *2*, 1161 and 1290.

A strategy for thyroid function testing, including the use of a high-sensitivity thyrotrophin assay as a first-line test, thus avoiding the need for protirelin testing in some patients.— G. Caldwell *et al.*, *Lancet*, 1985, *1*, 1117. Comments on the use of high-sensitivity immunoradiometric assays as a replacement for, or in combination with, protirelin testing of thyroid function: R. J. Mardell and T. R. Gamlen (letter), *ibid.*, 1455; C. Kirkegaard *et al.* (letter), *ibid;* R. Hoermann *et al.* (letter), *ibid;* P. Beck-Peccoz *et al.* (letter), *ibid.*, 1456.

Discussion of the value of sensitive thyrotrophin assays, and their correct use.— A. D. Toft and J. Seth, *Br. med. J.*, 1987, *295*, 1503.

NEUROLOGICAL DISEASES. Protirelin given to 5 patients with parkinsonism produced improvement in well-being for several hours after an injection in 2 of the 3 who were also taking levodopa.— J. A. McCaul *et al.* (letter), *Lancet*, 1974, *1*, 735.

There were impaired prolactin responses to chlorpromazine and protirelin in patients with Huntington's chorea when compared with controls. This might be of value in early detection of the disorder and suggested that there was a dopaminergic influence.— M. R. Hayden *et al.*, *Lancet*, 1977, *2*, 423. Experience with bromocriptine (a dopaminergic agonist) in patients with Huntington's chorea did not show any evidence of dopaminergic hypersensitivity.— R. J. Chalmers *et al.* (letter), *ibid.*, 824.

Results of a study indicating that protirelin is effective against ataxia of spinocerebellar degeneration.— I. Sobue *et al.* (letter), *Lancet*, 1980, *1*, 418. A study in 13 patients failed to show any beneficial effect from protirelin in mild to severe disability from a variety of progressive degenerative cerebellar disorders; patients received protirelin intravenously in doses of 1 to 6.5 mg.— P. A. LeWitt and J. R. L. Ehrenkranz (letter), *ibid.*, 1982, *2*, 981.

Beneficial effect of protirelin on spinal trauma in *cats*, indicating therapeutic potential in man.— A. I. Faden *et al.*, *New Engl. J. Med.*, 1981, *305*, 1063.

Intravenous infusion of very high doses of protirelin at rates of 2 to 19 mg per minute produced moderate to excellent improvement in neurological deficits in studies involving 17 patients with amyotrophic lateral sclerosis and slight to moderate benefit in a further patient with chronic juvenile proximal spinal muscular atrophy. Benefit was evident within 30 seconds of the start of infusion but was sustained for only half to one hour afterwards. Side-effects consisted mainly of effects on temperature regulation (hyperthermia, sweating, shivering), respiration (tachypnoea), and autonomic sensation in the bladder, rectum, and vagina; some patients had transient increases in blood pressure of 5 to 15%. Side-effects and benefits were both less in female patients. The results suggest that there may be a deficiency of the endogenous hormone in amyotrophic lateral sclerosis, which can be replaced by exogenous protirelin. However the wider application of this treatment will depend on the demonstration of sustained benefit from prolonged administration, and the development of more convenient methods for continuous administration, or of longer-acting analogues of protirelin.— W. K. Engel *et al.*, *Lancet*, 1983, *2*, 73.

For a brief discussion of the role of protirelin in the treatment of CNS injury see A. I. Faden, *J. Am. med. Ass.*, 1984, *252*, 1452.

SHOCK. Discussion of the role of protirelin in the treatment of shock, and its relationship to its opioid antagonist properties.— A. I. Faden, *J. Am. med. Ass.*, 1984, *252*, 1177.

THYROID DISORDERS. A study in 7 patients with central hypothyroidism of hypothalamic origin demonstrated that all had blood concentrations of thyrotrophin which were within the normal range or slightly elevated, but that this thyrotrophin had subnormal biological activity; this was shown in 4 to be associated with reduced ability to interact with plasma membrane receptors. Treatment with protirelin 40 mg daily by mouth in 6, or 500 µg daily by subcutaneous injection in one, for between 20 and 30 days, produced an increase in serum-thyrotrophin concentrations and a clear increase in biological activity and receptor binding activity. A thyroid response to increased thyrotrophin concentrations was evident in all subjects; in 4 patients the concentration of serum total thyroxine returned to normal, but in 2 patients a decline in thyrotrophin response to oral protirelin during the last 10 days of treatment was accompanied by a decline in thyroxine and triiodothyronine concentrations towards pretreatment values. It is clear that endogenous thyrotrophin-releasing hormone regulates not only the release of thyrotrophin but also structural features of the hormone that are essential for appropriate receptor binding and stimulation of adenylate cyclase; long-term protirelin administration resulted in sustained increase in thyrotrophin, followed by a return to normal thyroid hormone concentrations but future studies will need to define optimal doses, route, and schedules of protirelin therapy to avoid the apparent desensitisation observed in some patients in the present study.— P. Beck-Peccoz *et al.*, *New Engl. J. Med.*, 1985, *312*, 1085.

For the use of protirelin in the diagnosis of thyroid disorders see above.

Proprietary Preparations

TRH-Roche *(Roche, UK)*. *Injection*, protirelin 100 µg/mL, in ampoules of 2 mL.

Proprietary Names and Manufacturers

Antepan *(Henning Berlin, Ger.)*; Inithyran *(Denm.)*; Relefact TRH *(Hoechst, Canad.; Hoechst, Ger.; Hoechst, USA)*; Stimu-TSH *(Roussel, Fr.)*; Thypinone *(Abbott, USA)*; Thyrefact *(Hoechst, Denm.; Hoechst, Swed.)*; Tiregan *(Spain)*; TRH Prem *(Frumtost, Spain)*; Trhelea *(Arg.)*; TRH-Roche *(Roche, Austral.; Roche, Norw.; Roche, S.Afr.; Roche, Swed.; Roche, UK)*.

5947-y

Thyrotrophin *(BAN, rINN)*.

Thyroid-stimulating Hormone; Thyrotrophic Hormone; Thyrotropin; TSH.

CAS — 9002-71-5.

A glycoprotein from the anterior pituitary with a mol. wt in man of about 28 000.

Studies on the structure of bovine thyrotrophin. The linear amino-acid sequence of the α and β chains has been determined except for the assignment of some amides.— B. Shome *et al.*, *J. biol. Chem.*, 1971, *246*, 833; T. -H. Liao and J. G. Pierce, *ibid.*, 850.

Units

0.037 units of human thyrotrophin for immunoassay and bioassay are contained in approximately 7.5 µg of thyrotrophin, with albumin and lactose, in one ampoule of the second International Reference Preparation (1983).

Adverse Effects

Infrequent side-effects include nausea, vomiting, headache, urticaria, transitory hypotension, and cardiac arrhythmias. Swelling of the thyroid has followed high doses. Allergic reactions have occurred. There may be menstrual irregularities.

Precautions
Thyrotrophin is contra-indicated in patients with coronary thrombosis or adrenal insufficiency and should be given cautiously to patients with angina pectoris, heart failure, or hypopituitarism, and to those receiving corticosteroids.

Uses and Administration
Thyrotrophin is a glycoprotein secreted by the anterior lobe of the pituitary and with an alpha subunit essentially the same as that of the gonadotrophins (p.1144). Its main actions are to increase the iodine uptake by the thyroid and the formation and secretion of the thyroid hormones. It may produce hyperplasia of thyroid tissue. Thyrotrophin secretion is controlled by a hypothalamic releasing hormone (Protirelin, p.1152) and by circulating thyroid hormones; somatostatin (p.1151) may inhibit the release of thyrotrophin.
Thyrotrophin was formerly used in the diagnosis of hypothyroidism and to differentiate between primary and secondary hypothyroidism but direct radio-immunoassay of circulating endogenous thyrotrophin is now generally preferred. Thyrotrophin increases the uptake of radio-iodine by the thyroid and has been used as an adjunct in the treatment of certain types of thyroid cancer.
The usual dose is 10 units daily by intramuscular or subcutaneous injection.

For reference to the role of high-sensitivity radioimmunoassays for thyrotrophin in the diagnosis of thyroid disorders see under Protirelin, p.1153.

Proprietary Names and Manufacturers
Actyron *(Norw.; Ferring, Swed.)*; Ambinon *(Belg.; Neth.; Organon, Switz.)*; Thyratrop *(Ger.)*; Thyréostimuline *(Organon, Fr.)*; Thyreostimulin *(Ger.)*; Thytropar *(USV, Austral.; Rorer, Canad.; S.Afr.; Switz.; Armour, UK; Armour, USA)*.

Immunological Agents

3892-r

Described in this section are immunological agents used for both active immunisation and passive immunisation.

Active immunisation is a process of increasing resistance to infection whereby micro-organisms or products of their activity act as antigens and stimulate certain body cells to produce antibodies with a specific protective capacity. It may be a natural process following recovery from an infection, or an artificial process following the administration of *vaccines*. It is inevitably a slow process dependent upon the rate at which the antibody formation can be developed. Although the terms vaccination and immunisation are often used synonymously and interchangeably, vaccination is strictly only the administration of a vaccine whereas immunisation results in the demonstrable presence of protective levels of antibodies confirmed usually by serological testing.

Passive immunisation, which results in immediate protection of short duration, may be achieved by the administration of the antibodies themselves in the form of *antisera* (of animal origin) or *immunoglobulins* (of human origin).

Some other immunological products are used only for diagnostic purposes and these are described in the section on Diagnostic Agents, p.938.

7931-r

Antisera

Antisera (immunosera) are sterile preparations containing the specific immunoglobulins obtained from the serum of animals by purification. Antisera have the specific power of combining with venins or bacterial toxins, or with the bacterium, virus, or other antigen used for their preparation.

Antisera are obtained from healthy animals immunised by injections of the appropriate toxins or toxoids, venins, or suspensions of micro-organisms or other antigens. The specific immunoglobulins may be obtained from the immune serum by fractional precipitation and enzyme treatment or by other chemical or physical means. A suitable antimicrobial preservative may be added, and is invariably added if the product is issued in multidose containers. The *B.P.* and *Eur. P.* direct that when antisera contain phenol, the concentration is not more than 0.25%. The antiserum is distributed aseptically into sterile containers which are sealed so as to exclude micro-organisms. Alternatively they may be supplied as freeze-dried preparations for reconstitution immediately before use.

Immunoglobulins obtained from human blood are described below.

Adverse Effects and Precautions

Reactions are liable to occur after the injection of any serum of animal origin. Anaphylaxis may occur, with hypotension, dyspnoea, urticaria, and shock. For detailed recommendations concerning the management of anaphylaxis, see adrenaline p.1455.

Serum sickness may occur frequently 7 to 10 days after the injection of serum of animal origin; symptoms include fever, vomiting, diarrhoea, bronchospasm, and urticaria; there may be nephritis, myocarditis, polyarthritis, neuritis, and uveitis.

Before injecting serum, information should be obtained whenever possible as to whether previous injections of serum have been received and whether the patient is subject to allergic diseases. Sensitivity testing should be performed before the administration of antisera. The patient must be kept under observation after the administration of full doses of antisera and adrenaline injection kept in readiness for emergency use.

Uses and Administration

Antisera are used for passive immunisation. After injection intravenously, they immediately provide immunity which persists for perhaps 2 or 3 weeks until the antiserum is excreted; other routes of injection have a delayed onset of action. Because of the risk of adverse reactions (see above) immunoglobulins (see below), which are of human rather than of animal origin, are preferred as passive immunising agents.

It is generally important to follow the conferment of passive immunity, which is largely an emergency procedure, by the injection of suitable antigens to produce active immunity.

NOTE. Some antisera are not generally available commercially in Great Britain but supplies are kept at designated hospitals and other centres. Changes in distribution arrangements are notified to hospitals from time to time by the Department of Health.

3893-f

Immunoglobulins

Immunoglobulins are preparations containing antibodies against infectious micro-organisms and are prepared from human material, often plasma. Normal immunoglobulin, being prepared from material from blood donors contains several antibodies against infectious diseases circulating in the general population whereas specific immunoglobulins contain minimum specified levels of one antibody and are prepared from material collected from persons either recovering from the infection in question or from persons recently actively immunised (vaccinated) against the disease.

Anti-D immunoglobulins are described in the section on Blood Products (see p.811).

Adverse Effects

Local reactions with pain and tenderness at the site of intramuscular injection may follow the administration of immunoglobulins. Allergic reactions, including rarely anaphylactic reactions, have also been reported; such reactions, though, are far less frequent than following the use of antisera of animal origin.

Precautions

Although immunoglobulins are derived from human material strenuous efforts are made to screen the donor material and the transmission of hepatitis B and HIV (or AIDS), previously associated with the use of certain blood products, does not appear to be a problem with the immunoglobulins currently in use.

TRANSMISSION OF HEPATITIS. Transmission of non-A non-B hepatitis following the use of immunoglobulins has occasionally been reported (R. S. Lane, *Lancet*, 1983, *2*, 974; A.M.L. Lever *et al.*, *ibid.*, 1984, *2*, 1062; H.D. Ochs *et al.*, *ibid.*, 1985, *1*, 404; A.D.B. Webster and A.M.L. Lever, *ibid.*, 1986, *1*, 322; H.D. Ochs *et al.*, *ibid.*; O. Weiland *et al.*, *ibid.*, 976), but other studies (C.L.S. Leen *et al.*, *Lancet*, 1985, *1*, 586; H. Atrah *et al.*, *J. clin. Path.*, 1985, *38*, 1192) have indicated that neither non-A non-B hepatitis nor hepatitis B is transmitted by such products. Much of the discussion focussed on different methods of production and inactivation of possible infectious micro-organisms.

TRANSMISSION OF HIV. Although antibodies to the human immunodeficiency virus (HIV) have occasionally been found in samples of immunoglobulins there appears to be general agreement that currently available preparations do not result in the transmission of infection or in the subsequent development of AIDS in recipients (R.S. Tedder *et al.*, *Lancet*, 1985, *1*, 815; D.J. Gocke *et al.*, *ibid.*, 1986, *1*, 37; C. Bremard-Oury *et al.*, *ibid.*, 1090; R.E. Benveniste *et al.*, *ibid.*, 1091; Y. Ikeda *et al.*, *ibid.*, 1092; R. Hein *et al.*, *ibid.*, 1217; J.-J. Morgenthaler, *ibid.*, 1218; D. Piszkiewicz *et al.*, *ibid.*, 1327; *ibid*, *2*, 644; C.C. Wood *et al.*, *Ann. intern. Med.*, 1986, *105*, 536; A.M. Prince *et al.*, *New Engl. J. Med.*, 1986, *314*, 386; T.F. Zuck *et al.*, *ibid.*, 1454).

Uses and Administration

Immunoglobulins are used for passive immunisation, thus conferring immediate protection against some infectious diseases. They are preferred to antisera of animal origin as the incidence of adverse reactions is less.

7930-x

Vaccines

Vaccines are preparations of antigenic materials which are administered with the object of inducing in the recipient a specific active immunity to specific bacteria or viruses. They may contain living or killed micro-organisms, bacterial toxins or toxoids, or antigenic material from particular parts of the bacterium or virus. Vaccines may be single-component vaccines or mixed combined vaccines.

FORMULATION. The characterisation of aluminium hydroxide for use as an adjuvant in vaccines.— S. L. Hem and J. L. White, *J. parent. Sci. Technol.*, 1984, *38*, 2.

PRESERVATION. The antimicrobial effectiveness of some preservatives in inactivated vaccines.— F. E. N. Hekkens *et al.*, *J. biol. Stand.*, 1981, *9*, 277.

STORAGE. Advice of manufacturers in the *USA* concerning the effects of temperature on vaccines.— L. G. Miller and J. H. Loomis, *Am. J. Hosp. Pharm.*, 1985, *42*, 843.

Stability at room temperature of vaccines normally recommended by the manufacturers in the *UK* for cold storage.— P. W. Longland and P. C. Rowbotham, *Pharm. J.*, 1987, *1*, 147. See also: J. Westaway (letter), *ibid.*, 220.

Adverse Effects

Administration of a vaccine by injection may be followed by a local reaction, possibly with inflammation and lymphangitis. At the site of injected vaccine an induration or sterile abscess may develop. The administration of a vaccine may be followed by fever, headache, and malaise starting a few hours after injection and lasting for 1 or 2 days. Allergic reactions may occur and anaphylaxis has been reported rarely.

Further details, if appropriate, of adverse effects of vaccines may be found in the respective individual monographs.

Transverse myelitis occurred in a 7-month-old girl 6 or 7 days after receiving a diphtheria and tetanus vaccine and an oral poliomyelitis vaccine.— E. Whittle and N. R. C. Roberton, *Br. med. J.*, 1977, *1*, 1450.

A 16-year-old girl developed severe vertigo and tinnitus and deafness in the right ear 2 days after revaccination with an adsorbed diphtheria and tetanus vaccine and an oral poliomyelitis vaccine. Vertigo and tinnitus gradually improved, but the hearing loss persisted.— I. W. S. Mair and H. H. Elverland, *J. Lar. Otol.*, 1977, *91*, 323.

A report of the development of dermatomyositis in children following vaccination against diphtheria and scarlet fever, diphtheria alone, and diphtheria, pertussis, and tetanus. There were also reports in the literature of dermatomyositis after vaccination against diphtheria, pertussis, tetanus, and polio, against smallpox, after administration of a cold vaccine, and after a second inactivated poliomyelitis vaccine. The close temporal relationship between onset of symptoms and vaccinations suggested a causal relationship.— W. Ehrengut (letter), *Lancet*, 1978, *1*, 1040. See also J. A. Cotterill and H. Shapiro (letter), *Lancet*, 1978, *2*, 1158.

Adverse reactions to some vaccines reported in the *USA* during 1979-82.— *Drug Intell. & clin. Pharm.*, 1985, *19*, 330.

Some references to postvaccinal neuropathies, such as the Guillain-Barré syndrome: F. C. Westall and R. Root-Bernstein, *Lancet*, 1986, *2*, 251.

A brief comment on reactions to vaccines attributed to the thiomersal used as a preservative.— N. H. Cox *et al.* (letter), *Br. med. J.*, 1987, *294*, 250.

Precautions

Vaccination should be postponed in patients suffering from any acute illness although minor infections without fever or systemic upset are not regarded as contra-indications.

Enquiry regarding previous hypersensitivity should precede the administration of a vaccine and measures to treat allergic reactions should be immediately available; for detailed recommendations concerning the management of anaphylaxis, see adrenaline, p.1455. Some vaccines contain small amounts of antibiotics and should not be given to patients hypersensitive to them. Additionally some vaccines are prepared using hens eggs and hypersensitivity to the ingestion of eggs is a contra-indication to the use of such vaccines. Asthma, eczema, hay fever, or a history of allergy, should not be regarded as contra-indications to vaccination.

Before injection of a vaccine any alcohol or disinfectant used for cleansing the skin should be allowed to evaporate otherwise inactivation of live vaccines may occur.

It is recommended that immunisation of infants should not be postponed because of prematurity and that the normal schedules and timings be adhered to.

Certain precautions and contra-indications apply specifically to vaccines containing live attenuated micro-organisms.

Live vaccines should not be given to patients receiving high-dose systemic corticosteroid therapy (equivalent to prednisolone 2 mg per kg body-weight daily for more than 1 week); to patients receiving immunosuppressive therapy including general irradiation; to patients suffering from certain malignant conditions such as lymphoma, leukaemia, Hodgkin's disease, or other tumours of the reticuloendothelial system; or to patients with other types of impaired immunological responses, such as hypogammaglobulinaemia. In children, vaccination should also be postponed for at least 6 months after the cessation of antineoplastic chemotherapy and for at least 3 months after high-dose systemic corticosteroid therapy.

Because of a theoretical risk to the foetus, live vaccines should not be administered during pregnancy unless it is considered there is a significant risk of exposure to infection.

Live vaccines should either be administered simultaneously (but at different sites) or an interval of at least 3 weeks allowed between administration. Also, an interval of 3 months should be allowed between the use of live vaccines and the prior administration of immunoglobulins.

HIV-positive individuals may receive, where appropriate, vaccination against cholera, diphtheria, hepatitis B, measles, mumps, pertussis, poliomyelitis, rubella, tetanus, and typhoid; it has been recommended that BCG vaccination should not be given to these persons and that yellow fever vaccines should not be given to symptomatic individuals.

Advice concerning the treatment of people who have accidentally injected themselves with oil-based veterinary vaccines. Because intense vascular pressure (that could lead to the loss of a finger) may develop, prompt surgical treatment, including early incision and irrigation of injected area should be given.— *Br. med. J.*, 1987, *294*, 652.

HIV-POSITIVE PATIENTS. Recommendations of the Advisory Committee on Immunization Practices in the *USA* concerning the immunisation of children infected with the human immunodeficiency virus.— *Ann. intern. Med.*, 1987, *106*, 75.

Reviews and discussions concerning the use of vaccines in HIV-positive persons: N. A. Halsey and D. A. Henderson, *New Engl. J. Med.*, 1987, *316*, 683; C. F. von Reyn *et al.*, *Lancet*, 1987, *2*, 669; I. M. Onorato *et al.* (letter), *ibid.*, 1988, *1*, 354.

INTERACTIONS. Reviews of possible interactions between vaccines and other drugs: P. F. D'Arcy, *Drug Intell. & clin. Pharm.*, 1984, *18*, 697; *Drug Interact. News.*, 1984, *4*, 21.

PREMATURE INFANTS. Some discussions on the immunisation of preterm infants: *Br. med. J.*, 1986, *292*, 1183.

SKIN DISORDERS. Children with eczema should be immunised in the same way as other children. The vaccinations are best done when the skin disease is not active.— S. Lingham and R. S. Wells (letter), *Br. med. J.*, 1978, *2*, 355.

SURGERY. A short comment that immunisation and elective surgery should not generally be carried out close together, although there is little evidence, if any, that either would normally interfere with the other.— N. R. Grist, *Br. med. J.*, 1984, *289*, 428.

Uses and Administration

Vaccines are used for active immunisation as a prophylactic measure against some infectious diseases. They provide partial or complete protection for months or years. For inactivated vaccines the first dose generally produces only a slight and rather slow antibody response but, when a second dose is given after a suitable interval, a prompt antibody response follows and high concentrations occur in the blood. Though the antibody concentration may later fall, a further dose of vaccine promptly restores it. For most live vaccines only one dose is required although 3 doses of live (oral) poliomyelitis vaccines are needed to achieve complete immunisation.

Protection against several infectious diseases may be provided in early life by active immunisation. In the *UK* the following schedule of vaccination and immunisation is recommended. During the first year of life, vaccination with an adsorbed diphtheria, tetanus, and pertussis vaccine (see p.1161) together with a live (oral) poliomyelitis vaccine (see p.1173). The first doses should preferably be given at the age of 3 months, the second after an interval of 6 to 8 weeks, and the third 4 to 6 months later. If pertussis vaccine is contra-indicated an adsorbed diphtheria and tetanus vaccine (see p.1160) should be given. During the second year of life, vaccination with measles, mumps, and rubella vaccine (see p.1168). At school (or nursery school) entry, reinforcing doses of an adsorbed diphtheria and tetanus vaccine and a live (oral) poliomyelitis vaccine are recommended. Between 10 and 14 years of age BCG vaccine may be given to tuberculin-negative children. Girls aged 10 to 14 years should receive a live rubella vaccine (see p.1177). On leaving school or before entering employment or further education, reinforcing doses of an adsorbed tetanus vaccine (see p.1180) and a poliomyelitis vaccine, either oral or inactivated, are recommended.

Other countries may often have a slightly different schedule to that outlined above.

A discussion on the prospects of eradication of disease by vaccination. Eradication is defined as the extinction of the pathogen that causes the infectious disease in question whereas in elimination the disease disappears but the causative agent remains. Of the 6 target diseases of the World Health Organisation's Expanded Programme on Immunization; many of the factors necessary for elimination are present for each of the diseases, but some are not. *Measles* is so highly communicable a disease, that a vaccine efficacy-rate of about 95% is probably not high enough even to eliminate, much less eradicate the disease. *Pertussis* is also highly infectious and the vaccine is almost certainly not effective enough. *Tetanus* is not eradicable as the causative organism is ubiquitous. For *poliomyelitis* countries that are efficient at giving vaccines have proved remarkably successful not only in practically eliminating the disease but also in virtually eradicating the organism. *Tuberculosis* is clearly not eradicable at present and *diphtheria* has many features that suggest it cannot be easily eradicated. Prospects for eradicating *congenital rubella syndrome* are more encouraging and the prospects for elimination or eradication of *mumps* are probably similar to those of rubella.— N. D. Noah and N. T. Begg, *Br. med. J.*, 1987, *295*, 1013.

A recommended schedule for the active immunisation of normal infants and children in the *USA*.— *J. Am. med. Ass.*, 1986, *256*, 2311.

Some schedules for the routine immunisation of adults in the *USA*: *Med. Lett.*, 1985, *27*, 98; F. M. LaForce, *J. Am. med. Ass.*, 1987, *257*, 2464.

EXPANDED PROGRAMME ON IMMUNIZATION. In 1974 the World Health Assembly adopted a resolution creating the Expanded Programme on Immunization, the aim of which was to provide immunisation against six target diseases (diphtheria, measles, pertussis, poliomyelitis, tetanus, and tuberculosis) for all children throughout the world by 1990. Although the attention of the World Health Organization had been focussed primarily on the developing countries, it was emphasised that the programme was not created exclusively for these countries. Besides the WHO, many other organisations, including UNICEF, were involved.

By 1987 it was considered that 50% of the world's children were being vaccinated compared to less than 5% a decade earlier. It was estimated that the programme was resulting in the prevention of more than one million deaths annually from measles, neonatal tetanus, and pertussis, and also in the prevention of over 175 000 cases of poliomyelitis annually. It was emphasised that the vaccine coverage, especially for measles and neonatal tetanus, was still low and that the programme would need to be accelerated over the ensuing 3 years, if the goal of universal childhood immunisation by 1990 was to be attained. It was considered particularly important to immunise children as early in life as possible and not to withhold vaccines from those suffering from minor illness or malnutrition.

A schedule designed to provide protection at the earliest possible age consisted of: trivalent oral poliomyelitis vaccine together with BCG vaccine at birth; trivalent oral poliomyelitis vaccine together with diphtheria, tetanus, and pertussis vaccine at 6, 10, and 14 weeks of age; and measles vaccine at 9 months of age.

Some references to the Expanded Programme on Immunization: A. M. Galazka *et al.*, *Bull. Wld Hlth Org.*, 1984, *62*, 357; *Chronicle Wld Hlth Org.*, 1985, *39*, 92; *Lancet*, 1985, *1*, 438; *ibid.*, 1987, *1*, 578; *Wld Hlth Forum*, 1987, *8*, 551.

IMMUNISATION FOR TRAVELLERS. A booklet entitled *Vaccination Certificate Requirements and Health Advice for International Travel* is published annually by the World Health Organization. In the 1988 edition the following information regarding certification of vaccination was given.

In 1981 the International Health Regulations were amended to include *smallpox* among the diseases for which a vaccination certificate should no longer be required because its global eradication had been confirmed; such vaccination may even be dangerous in some cases.

A *yellow fever* vaccination certificate is now the only one that should be required in international travel, and then only for a limited number of travellers. Travellers who enter areas where the yellow fever virus is endemic should be vaccinated, but it is considered an excessive precaution for health administrations to require a certificate from all travellers from endemic zones when they have only been in large towns where the disease is not occurring. Some countries do, however, require that such an individual does have a valid certificate; although there is no epidemiological justification for this requirement, and it is clearly in excess of the International Health Regulations, travellers may find that it is strictly enforced, particularly for persons going to Asia from Africa or South America. The validity period of international certificates of vaccination against yellow fever is 10 years, beginning 10 days after vaccination.

Although a few countries still require a certificate of *cholera* immunisation, this is in excess of the International Health Regulations as the introduction of cholera into any country cannot be prevented by cholera vaccination. A certificate, if issued, is valid for 6 months.

In addition, the following advice was provided:

Travellers would be well advised to have had *diphtheria* and *tetanus* immunisation within the past 10 years and to be immunised against *poliomyelitis*, *typhoid*, and *measles* if there is any doubt as to their immune status. Medical advice should be sought concerning the need for BCG immunisation of children who are likely to be in intimate contact with persons among whom the prevalence of active *tuberculosis* is high.

Polyvalent immunoglobulin can provide some measure of protection against viral *hepatitis A* but it is only recommended for travellers to high-risk areas outside ordinary tourist routes.

Although a variety of other vaccines are available, they

are only indicated for individuals expected to be at a high risk of exposure.

Further information for international travellers is also often provided by national authorities. In the *UK* a leaflet entitled *Protect your health abroad* is issued by the Department of Health and Social Security and in the *USA* a document entitled *Health Information for International Travel* is published by the Centers for Disease Control.

Further references: *Med. Lett.*, 1987, *29*, 53.

VACCINE DEVELOPMENT. Some references concerning advances and development in vaccine manufacture: *Bull. Wld Hlth Org.*, 1985, *63*, 471; *ibid.*, 479; F. Brown, *Br. med. Bull.*, 1985, *41*, 56; D. C. A. Candy, *Trans. R. Soc. trop. Med. Hyg.*, 1985, *79*, 577; M. R. Hilleman, *Med. J. Aust.*, 1986, *144*, 360; J. W. G. Smith, *Archs Dis. Childh.*, 1986, *61*, 531; *Lancet*, 1987, *2*, 666.

18734-k

AIDS Vaccines

HIV Vaccines.

Many prototype vaccines against the acquired immunodeficiency syndrome have been or are being developed but few, as yet, have been tested in humans in clinical studies.

Reference to the use of an AIDS vaccine in HIV-seronegative human volunteers.— D. Zagury *et al.* (letter), *Nature*, 1987, *326*, 249.

Passive immunoneutralisation of HIV in patients with advanced AIDS.— G. G. Jackson *et al.*, *Lancet*, 1988, *2*, 647.

7933-d

Anthrax Vaccines

Adverse Effects and Precautions

As for vaccines in general, p.1155.

Uses and Administration

In the *UK* an anthrax vaccine which is an alum precipitate of the antigen found in the sterile filtrate of suitable cultures of the Stern strain of *Bacillus anthracis* is available for human use. It is used for active immunisation against anthrax and is recommended for persons exposed to a high risk of infection, such as laboratory workers, veterinary practitioners, and workers handling animal hairs, hides, wool, and bone meal. It is given in 4 doses, each of 0.5 mL, administered by intramuscular injection. The first 3 doses are separated by intervals of 3 weeks and the fourth dose follows after an interval of 6 months. Reinforcing doses are required each year.

Some references to anthrax and anthrax vaccines: P. Hambleton *et al.*, *Vaccine*, 1984, *2*, 125; P. C. B. Turnbull, *Abstr. Hyg.*, 1986, *61*, R1.

Proprietary Preparations

An anthrax vaccine is available from designated holding centres: the Regional Public Health Laboratories in Bridge of Earn, Cardiff, Leeds, and Liverpool and the Central Public Health Laboratory in London.

7936-m

BCG Vaccines

Bacillus Calmette-Guérin Vaccines.

Bacillus Calmette-Guérin Vaccine (*B.P.*) (BCG Vaccine) is a preparation containing live bacteria obtained from a strain derived from the bacillus of Calmette and Guérin and known to protect man against tuberculosis; the strain is maintained so as to preserve its stability, its power of sensitising man and guinea-pigs to tuberculin, its ability to protect animals against tuberculosis, and its relative non-pathogenicity to man and laboratory animals. It is supplied as a dried product (Dried Tub/Vac/BCG; Freeze-dried BCG Vaccine (*Eur.P.*); Vaccinum Tuberculosis (BCG) Cryodesiccatum), which is reconstituted immediately before use by the addition of a suitable sterile liquid. The dried vaccine should be stored at 2° to 8°, not be allowed to freeze, and be protected from light. Under these conditions it may be expected to retain its potency for at least 2 years.

BCG Vaccine (*U.S.P.*) is a dried living culture of the bacillus Calmette-Guérin strain of *Mycobacterium tuberculosis* var. *bovis*; it is grown from a strain that has been maintained to preserve its capacity for conferring immunity. It contains an amount of viable bacteria such that inoculation, in the recommended dose, of tuberculin-negative persons results in an acceptable tuberculin conversion rate. It contains a suitable stabiliser and no antimicrobial agent. The dried vaccine should be stored at 2° to 8° in hermetically-sealed containers. The reconstituted vaccine should be used immediately after preparation and any portion not used within 2 hours should be discarded.

Percutaneous Bacillus Calmette-Guérin Vaccine (*B.P.*) (Percut. BCG Vaccine) is a suspension of living cells of an authentic strain of the bacillus of Calmette and Guérin with a higher viable bacterial count than Bacillus Calmette-Guérin Vaccine. It is supplied as a dried vaccine (Tub/Vac/BCG/(Perc)) and is reconstituted immediately before use by the addition of a suitable sterile liquid. The dried vaccine should be stored at 2° to 8°, not be allowed to freeze, and be protected from light. Under these conditions it may be expected to retain its potency for at least 2 years.

Units

The first International Reference Preparation (1965) of BCG vaccine consists of ampoules containing 5.72 mg of dried material derived from 2.5 mg (semi-dry weight) of bacillary mass of BCG and 5 mg of sodium glutamate.

Adverse Effects

As for vaccines in general, p.1155.

Side-effects occur rarely with BCG vaccines. They include ulceration of the inoculation site, lymphadenitis, osteitis, and keloid formation. Very rarely, lupus vulgaris has occurred. Generalised reactions, possibly allergic, with a few fatalities have been reported. Disseminated BCG infection may occur.

ALLERGY. Reports of anaphylactic reactions to BCG vaccination in infants and children: J. R. Harper (letter), *Lancet*, 1982, *1*, 403; R. T. Tshabalala (letter), *ibid.*, 1983, *1*, 653; A. H. W. van Assendelft and A. Jukkara (letter), *Tubercle*, 1986, *67*, 233.

EFFECTS ON THE BONES. Reports of osteomyelitis or osteitis associated with BCG vaccination: S. Bergdahl *et al.*, *J. Bone Jt Surg.*, 1976, *58-B*, 212; M. Pauker *et al.*, *Archs Dis. Childh.*, 1977, *52*, 330; O. Wasz-Hockert *et al.*, *Bull. int. Un. Tuberc.*, 1979, *54*, 325; G. Boman *et al.*, *ibid.*, 1984, *59*, 198; H. Peltola *et al.*, *Archs Dis. Childh.*, 1984, *59*, 157; K. M. Al-Arabi *et al.*, *Tubercle*, 1984, *65*, 305.

DISSEMINATED INFECTION. A report of fatal disseminated BCG infection in an 18-year-old boy 6 years after BCG vaccination.— A. Mackay *et al.*, *Lancet*, 1980, *2*, 1332.

Tuberculous meningitis in 2 children inoculated with BCG vaccine, 5 and 6 months earlier respectively.— M. Tardieu *et al.* (letter), *Lancet*, 1988, *1*, 440. See also: W. L. Morrison *et al.* (letter), *ibid.*, 654.

EFFECTS ON THE NERVOUS SYSTEM. Guillain-Barré syndrome after the use of BCG vaccine.— J. A. M. J. Wils and G. J. M. M. van Gool (letter), *Lancet*, 1975, *1*, 109.

EFFECTS ON THE SKIN. A report of 2 boys who developed dermatomyositis subsequent to BCG vaccination.— E. Kåss *et al.* (letter), *Lancet*, 1978, *1*, 772.

Erythema multiforme following BCG vaccination.— M. Dogliotti, *S. Afr. med. J.*, 1980, *57*, 332.

A report of lupus vulgaris at the site of BCG vaccination progressing over a 30-year period.— A. K. Izumi and J. Matsunaga, *Archs Derm.*, 1982, *118*, 171.

A discussion of scarring following BCG vaccination. The incidence of scarring in Britain is unknown but elsewhere in the world the incidence of hypertrophic scars has been estimated to be 28 to 33% and that of keloid scars to be 2 to 4%. Measures available for the treatment of such scarring include the application of pressure, surgery, radiotherapy, or corticosteroids. Obtrusive scarring can be overcome or minimised by the choice of alternative sites for inoculation.— R. Sanders and M. G. Dickson, *Br. med. J.*, 1982, *285*, 1679.

A discussion of the local complications of BCG vaccination and their treatment. The incidence of serious complications such as systemic disseminated infection is very small but local complications occur quite frequently. In a small proportion of subjects the reaction to vaccination is excessive and results in an ulcer, a subcutaneous abscess, or suppurative lymphadenitis; these complications are reported to occur more frequently if the vaccine is wrongly administered subcutaneously or if the recipient has a positive tuberculin test. Suppurative lymphadenitis may respond slowly to isoniazid but surgical drainage may be necessary in some cases. For persistent ulcers or abscesses at the injection site a short course of isoniazid is often given although no controlled studies have been reported. Erythromycin has also been recently advocated for the treatment of ulcers and abscesses and it would seem reasonable to use short courses of either erythromycin or isoniazid for such purposes.— K. P. Goldman, *Tubercle*, 1985, *66*, 158. For reference to the use of erythromycin to treat local reactions after BCG vaccination, see p.226.

Precautions

As for vaccines in general, p.1156.

It has been suggested that BCG vaccines may be given concomitantly with oral poliomyelitis vaccines, but that for other live vaccines it is preferable to allow an interval of 3 weeks between administration although the period may be reduced to 10 days if absolutely necessary. No further vaccination should be given in the arm used for BCG vaccination for at least 3 months because of the risk of lymphadenitis. It has been recommended that, because of the possible risk of disseminated infections, BCG vaccines should not be given to persons infected with the human immunodeficiency virus (HIV; AIDS virus).

PREGNANCY AND THE NEONATE. An opinion that, provided general immunological deficiency is absent, BCG vaccination (which uses a live but attenuated strain of *Mycobacterium bovis*) does not constitute a danger to the foetus if given during pregnancy. When the vaccine was newly introduced it was reported that there was no sign of congenital tuberculosis in newborn offspring of pregnant *animals* given massive doses of BCG.— P. Hart, *Br. med. J.*, 1986, *293*, 1292.

Uses and Administration

BCG vaccines are used for active immunisation against tuberculosis, principally for the vaccination of selected groups of the population and of persons likely to be exposed to infection. In some countries it is administered only to persons who give a negative tuberculin reaction, but in countries with a high prevalence of tuberculosis, routine vaccination in infancy is recommended.

In the *UK* vaccination is recommended in the following groups of persons, if found to be tuberculin-negative (see under tuberculins, p.947): contacts of persons suffering from active respiratory tuberculosis, including the children of immigrants in whose communities there is known to be a high incidence of tuberculosis; school children aged 10 to 13 years; health service staff. If vaccination of infants is performed very shortly after birth sensitivity testing to tuberculin need not be performed. The BCG vaccine is given intradermally (intracutaneously) at the insertion of the deltoid muscle in a dose of 0.1 mL or 0.05 mL for infants under 3 months of age. If BCG vaccination is to be offered to a person who is a contact of a tuberculosis patient and is already receiving prophylactic treatment with isoniazid, the use of an isoniazid-resistant form of vaccine should be considered.

Immunisation against tuberculosis forms part of the World Health Organization's Expanded Programme on Immunization (see p.1156).

A short review and discussion on BCG vaccination including requirements for dried BCG vaccine. Various daughter strains, all derived from the bacillus of Calmette and Guérin, are being used by manufacturing establishments in the preparation of BCG vaccine. Whilst these strains differ from one another to minor degrees when investigated in the laboratory, there is no evidence to suggest that they differ significantly in their power to protect man. There is no strain that can be said to be preferable to others or that is known to be definitely superior to the others. A major controlled trial of some of the most frequently used strains of BCG would be of value with the aim of re-establishing the properties of seed lots that are suitable for the preparation of a satisfactory freeze-dried BCG vaccine.— Thirty-sixth Report of the WHO Expert Committee on Biological Standardization, *Tech. Rep. Ser. Wld Hlth Org. No. 745*, 1987,, p.60.

Further references to vaccines produced from differing BCG strains: M. Böttiger *et al.*, *J. biol. Stand.*, 1983, *11*, 1; T. W. Osborn, *Tubercle*, 1983, *64*, 1; J. M. Grange *et al.*, *ibid.*, 129; A. Lind, *ibid.*, 233.

LEPROSY. Although it has been shown that BCG vaccination is capable of inducing a positive reaction to lepromin in persons previously displaying a negative reaction, trials and studies using BCG vaccines for the prophylaxis of leprosy have yielded inconsistent results. Protection against leprosy, in different countries, has been reported to be approximately 20% in Burma (L.M. Bechelli *et al.*, *Bull. Wld Hlth Org.*, 1974, *51*, 93), 80% in Uganda (S.J. Stanley *et al.*, *J. Hyg.*, 1981, *87*, 233), 30% in southern India (S.P. Tripathy, *Ann. Natl. Med. Sci. India*, 1983, *19*, 11) and 50% in northern Malawi (P.E.M. Fine *et al.*, *Lancet*, 1986, *2*, 499). Specific vaccines against leprosy (see p.1167) are now, however, being investigated for use either as single agents or in conjunction with BCG vaccines.

MALIGNANT NEOPLASMS. Immunotherapy with BCG vaccines has been tried in various malignant disorders but in general has proved either disappointing or ineffective. In a recent article the question of the safety and efficacy of such immunotherapy was addressed by an invited panel of experts (*J. Am. med. Ass.*, 1987, *257*, 1238). It was stated that although BCG will stimulate the reticuloendothelial system and will inhibit tumour growth in both man and *animals*, certain criteria are necessary for immunotherapy to succeed. These criteria include : a small localised neoplasm; the host must be able to develop an immune response to the mycobacterial antigens; there must be a close contact of BCG and tumour cells; an adequate number of viable BCG organisms must be given. The human neoplasms that were considered to best fit the above criteria were cutaneous melanomas and transitional cell carcinoma of the bladder.

A warning concerning the incorrect dosage of BCG vaccines cited in some reports and reviews in the medical literature for the treatment of bladder cancer. A dose of 6×10^9 organisms has been stated to have been used but this is actually 10 times the dose of viable organisms given to the patients; a dose of 6×10^9 *viable* organisms could result in severe adverse reactions and possibly even death.— *FDA Drug Bull.*, 1983, *13*, 18.

Bladder. Intravesical administration of BCG vaccine has been used in patients with superficial bladder cancer. Two studies (J. H. Mydlo *et al.*, *Urology*, 1986, *28*, 173; W. J. Catalona *et al.*, *J. Urol., Baltimore.*, 1987, *137*, 220), each involving 100 patients, reported favourable results with BCG vaccines.

Skin. Overall, results of studies investigating the use of adjuvant BCG vaccines in patients with malignant melanoma have proved disappointing with no significant effect being observed in survival-rates (U. Veronesi *et al.*, *New Engl. J. Med.*, 1982, *307*, 913; I.C. Quirt *et al.*, *Can. med. Ass. J.*, 1983, *128*, 929; H.K.B. Silver *et al.*, *ibid.*, 1291; A.H.G. Paterson *et al.*, *ibid.*, 1984, *131*, 744).

TUBERCULOSIS. Some general reviews and discussions on the prevention of tuberculosis and the use of BCG vaccines: G. Dahlstrom, *Bull. int. Un. Tuberc.*, 1983, *58*, 43; J. M. Grange, *Tubercle*, 1986, *67*, 1.

Although contradictory results of clinical studies assessing the value of BCG vaccination have been reported in the past it was usually believed that vaccination was of value. Concern was therefore expressed after publication of a report (*Bull. Wld Hlth Org.*, 1979, *57*, 819) giving preliminary results of the Tuberculosis Prevention Trial in South India which indicated that vaccination had provided no protection during the first 7.5 years of follow-up. Two groups sponsored by the World Health Organization discussed the trial and the findings (*Tech. Rep. Ser. Wld Hlth Org. Nos 651 and 652*, 1980) and considered that the absence of protective effect should not be regarded as automatically applying to other parts of the world and that vaccination programmes should continue and should be appropriate to the epidemiological situation in each country.

Further results of the South India trial covering a total follow-up period of 12.5 years (S.P. Tripathy, *Ann. Natl. Med. Sci., India*, 1983, *19*, 11) showed that although a similar number of cases of tuberculosis had been observed in the vaccinated groups and in the placebo groups, a detailed analysis indicated that vaccination probably did provide some protection. It was suggested that infection in India with *Mycobacterium tuberculosis* results in tuberculin conversion and immunisation, but that only rarely does this progress to clinical disease. Therefore, subjects who are naturally infected with the tubercle bacilli and those vaccinated with BCG both have a similar and low incidence of tuberculosis due to superinfection, whereas tuberculosis due to endogenous re-activation of a primary focus can occur in the group naturally infected but not in those vaccinated. This did not appear to be the case as during the first 5 years there was no evidence of protection afforded by vaccination whereas in the next 7.5 years there was a protection of 48%, a figure in keeping with the predicted protection against tuberculosis due to endogenous re-activation. It was concluded that vaccination could make a significant contribution to the control programmes for the prevention of disease.

Some clinical studies in differing countries on the value of BCG vaccination: V. Romanus, *Tubercle*, 1983, *64*, 101 (Sweden: general vaccination of neonates unnecessary); H. M. Curtis *et al.*, *Lancet*, 1984, *1*, 145 (UK: support for neonatal vaccination); S. Padungchan *et al.*, *Bull. Wld Hlth Org.*, 1986, *64*, 247 (Thailand: support for neonatal vaccination); O. Tidjani *et al.*, *Tubercle*, 1986, *67*, 269 (Togo: support for neonatal vaccination); J. L. Stanford *et al.*, *ibid.*, 1987, *68*, 39 (India: protective effect of vaccination in schoolchildren); I. Sutherland and V. H. Springett, *ibid.*, 81 (UK: protective effect of vaccination at about 13 years of age); J. L. Stanford *et al.*, *ibid.*, 169 (India: protective effect of vaccination in children).

Proprietary Preparations

Bacillus Calmette-Guérin Vaccine (*B.P.*) and Percutaneous Bacillus Calmette-Guérin Vaccine (*B.P.*) are available from *Evans Medical, UK.*

7939-g

Botulism Antitoxins

Botulinum Antitoxin (*B.P.*, *Eur. P.*) (Bot/Ser; Immunoserum Botulinicum) is a sterile preparation containing the specific antitoxic globulins that have the power of neutralising the toxins formed by type A, type B, type E, or any mixture of types A, B, and E, of *Clostridium botulinum*. It contains not less than 500 units of each of type A and type B and not less than 50 units of type E per mL. It should be stored at 2° to 8°, not be allowed to freeze, and be protected from light. The *B.P.* states that when Mixed Botulinum Antitoxin or Botulinum Antitoxin is prescribed or demanded and the types to be present are not stated, Botulinum Antitoxin prepared from types A, B, and E shall be dispensed or supplied. It should be noted, however, that some antitoxins available in the *UK* have not conformed to the requirements of the *B.P.* and *Eur. P.* (having a higher phenol content than the pharmacopoeias allow), and thus have been referred to as botulism rather than botulinum antitoxin.

Botulism Antitoxin (*U.S.P.*) is a sterile solution of the refined and concentrated antitoxic antibodies, chiefly globulins, obtained from the blood of healthy horses that have been immunised against the toxins produced by type A and type B and/or E strains of *Clostridium botulinum*. It should be stored at 2° to 8° and preserved in single-use containers only.

Units

500 units of *Clostridium botulinum* Type A antitoxin (equine) are contained in 68.0 mg of dried hyperimmune horse serum in one ampoule of the first International Standard Preparation (1963).

31 units of Type B antitoxin (equine) are contained in 3.6 mg of dried pepsin-treated and fractionated hyperimmune horse serum in one ampoule of the second International Standard Preparation (1985).

1000 units of Type E antitoxin (equine) are contained in 69.1 mg of dried hyperimmune horse serum in one ampoule of the first International Standard Preparation (1963).

Adverse Effects and Precautions

As for antisera in general, p.1155.

Uses and Administration

Botulism antitoxins are used in the treatment of botulism, caused by the ingestion of infected food. Treatment should be given as early as possible in the course of the disease.

Since the type of botulism toxin is seldom known the polyvalent antitoxin is usually given. Sensitivity testing should always be performed before administration of the antitoxin.

In the *UK* a trivalent antitoxin containing 500 units per mL of each of antitoxins types A, B, and E is employed. For the treatment of botulsim, 20 mL of this antitoxin should be diluted to 100 mL with sodium chloride 0.9% and given by slow intravenous infusion over at least 30 minutes; another 10 mL may be given 2 to 4 hours later if necessary, and further doses at 12- to 24-hour intervals if indicated. Persons who have consumed suspected food and in whom symptoms have not developed should be given 20 mL intramuscularly as a prophylactic measure.

In some countries the mixed antitoxin contains differing amounts of type A, B, and E antitoxin.

Proprietary Preparations

A botulism antitoxin is available from designated holding centres (see p.1155).

Proprietary Names and Manufacturers

Connaught, Canad.; Behringwerke, Ger.; ISM, Ital.

7941-d

Cholera Vaccines

Cholera Vaccine (*B.P.*, *Eur. P.*) (Cho/Vac; Vaccinum Cholerae) is a sterile homogeneous suspension of a suitable killed strain or strains of *Vibrio cholerae*. It consists of a mixture of equal parts of vaccines prepared from smooth strains of 2 main serological types, Inaba and Ogawa of the classical biotype with or without the El-Tor biotype. A single strain or several strains of each type may be included. All strains must contain, in addition to their type O antigens, the heat-stable O antigen common to the Inaba and Ogawa types. If more than one strain each of Inaba and Ogawa are used they may be selected to contain other O antigens. It contains not less than 8000 million *V. cholerae* per dose, which does not exceed 1 mL. It contains not more than 0.5% of phenol. It may also be supplied as a dried vaccine (Dried Cho/Vac) which is reconstituted immediately before use by the addition of a suitable sterile liquid. Phenol may not be used in the preparation of the dried vaccine. *Eur P.* includes the dried vaccine as Freeze-Dried Cholera Vaccine (Vaccinum Cholerae Cryodesiccatum). Both the liquid and the dried vaccine should be stored at 2° to 8°, not be allowed to freeze, and be protected from light. Under these conditions the liquid vaccine may be expected to retain its potency for at least 18 months and the dried vaccine for at least 5 years.

Cholera Vaccine (*U.S.P.*) is a sterile suspension, in sodium chloride injection or other suitable diluent, of killed *Vibrio cholerae* selected for high antigenic efficiency. It is prepared from equal parts of suspensions of cholera vibrios of the Inaba and Ogawa strains. It has a labelled potency of not less than 8 units per serotype per mL. It contains a suitable antimicrobial agent. It should be stored at 2° to 8° and not be allowed to freeze.

Units

The second International Reference Preparations (1971) of cholera vaccine (Inaba) and cholera vaccine (Ogawa) each consist of ampoules of freeze-dried material from monovalent vaccine (4×10^{10} organisms per ampoule).

Adverse Effects and Precautions

As for vaccines in general, p.1155.

Slight swelling, erythema, and tenderness occasionally occur at the injection site. Fever and malaise have been reported and general reactions, including anaphylaxis and hypersensitivity reactions, have occurred. Neurological and psychiatric reactions have occasionally occurred.

A report of a syndrome similar to immune complex disease, characterised by fever, myalgia, arthralgia, abdominal pain, vomiting, serositis, hepatitis, suspected myocarditis, anaemia, and thrombocytopenia, in a patient after cholera re-vaccination.— T. Mall and K. Gyr, *Trans. R. Soc. trop. Med. Hyg.*, 1984, *78*, 106.

For reference to the effect of cholera vaccination on the response to yellow fever vaccines, see under yellow fever vaccines, (p.1182).

Uses and Administration

Cholera vaccines are used for active immunisation against cholera but are not considered to be very effective and the immunity conferred is short-lived.

In the *UK* a vaccine containing 8000 million *V. cholerae* per mL is used and a primary prophylactic course of 2 injections at an interval of at least a week and preferably 4 weeks is given. Further doses should be given at intervals of 6 months. The first dose, given by intramuscular or subcutaneous injection, is: 0.5 mL for adults and children over 10 years of age; 0.3 mL for children aged 5 to 10 years; and 0.1 mL for children aged 1 to 5 years. Subsequent doses (the second dose and the 6-monthly booster doses) may also be given by intramuscular or subcutaneous injection, but intradermal (intracutaneous) injection may also be employed, especially if the initial injection produced side-effects. These subsequent doses are: 1.0 mL intramuscularly or subcutaneously or 0.2 mL intradermally for adults and children over 10 years; 0.5 mL intramuscularly or subcutaneously or 0.1 mL intradermally for children aged 5 to 10 years; and 0.3 mL intramuscularly or subcutaneously or 0.1 mL intradermally for children aged 1 to 5 years.

Some other countries have a slightly different dosage schedule to the one outlined above.

ORAL CHOLERA VACCINES. Memorandum from a WHO Meeting concerning recent advances in cholera research and including discussions on new candidate cholera vaccines. The common feature of these candidate vaccines is that they are administered by the oral route and they consist of either non-living antigens or live attenuated strains. Non-living antigenic types of vaccines have included those consisting of: a combination of the B subunit with killed vibrios; a combination of a pro-choleragenoid with killed vibrios; or a crude fraction of the *V. cholerae* O1 cell wall. Live attenuated oral vaccines have included those developed using recombinant DNA technology to attenuate virulent *V. cholerae* O1.— *Bull. Wld Hlth Org.*, 1985, *63*, 841.

Results of a randomised double-blind field trial of 2 oral cholera vaccines in an area of rural Bangladesh where cholera was endemic. Attention had been turned towards oral vaccines as stimulation of intestinal immunity had been reported to be more efficient than that with parenteral vaccines and because parenteral vaccines had yielded only modest and short-term protection. The 2 oral vaccines consisted of either 1 mg of the B subunit component of cholera toxin together with 1×10^{11} killed whole-cell *V. cholerae* per dose or of just the killed whole cells; three doses of each vaccine were given. The participants in the trial were male and female children aged 2 to 15 years and women aged over 15 years. The combined subunit/whole-cell vaccine was given to 21 141 persons, the whole-cell only vaccine to 21 137, and a placebo to 21 220. The combined vaccine conferred a high degree of protection with only 4 cases of confirmed cholera occurring; the whole-cell only vaccine afforded a statistically significant, though less impressive, protection with 11 cases of confirmed cholera occurring; 26 cases of confirmed cholera occurred in the placebo group. The similar degree of protection afforded to both children and adults was of considerable interest, since in endemic areas children are at the highest risk and single doses of conventional vaccines have conferred disappointing levels of protection in children. It was stressed that this study represented only a short-term evaluation of the biological efficacy of the new oral vaccines and that efficacy must be monitored over longer periods and consideration given to testing of formulations and dosage schedules that might realistically be incorporated into vaccination programmes for developing countries.— J. D. Clemens *et al.*, *Lancet*, 1986, *2*, 124. Comment and further review and discussion on oral cholera vaccines.— *ibid.*, 722. See also J. D. Clemens *et al.*, *ibid.*, 1988, *1*, 1375.

Proprietary Preparations

Cholera Vaccine (*B.P.*) is available from *Wellcome, UK.*

Proprietary Names and Manufacturers

Vibriomune *(Duncan, Flockhart, UK).*

7944-m

Cold Vaccines

Cold vaccines containing mixtures of various bacteria have been given both orally and by injection although there is little evidence that they have prophylactic value.

Proprietary Preparations

A catarrh vaccine is available from *HSL Vaccine Laboratory, UK.*

Proprietary Names and Manufacturers

Esobactulin *(Southon-Horton, UK)*; Lantigen B *(Ashe, UK).*

3865-a

Contraceptive Vaccines

A synthetic contraceptive vaccine which stimulates the production of an antibody against human chorionic gonadotrophin thus preventing implantation of the fertilised ovum is being investigated in clinical trials.

Report of a phase 1 clinical study of a WHO birth control vaccine.— W. R. Jones *et al.*, *Lancet*, 1988, *1*, 1295.

3896-h

Cytomegalovirus Immunoglobulins

Cytomegalovirus immunoglobulins containing high levels of specific antibody against cytomegalovirus have been prepared from human plasma.

Adverse Effects and Precautions

As for immunoglobulins in general, p.1155.

Uses and Administration

Cytomegalovirus immunoglobulins are used for passive immunisation against cytomegalovirus infection and disease. They may be used prophylactically, especially in patients undergoing certain transplant procedures such as bone-marrow or renal transplants or therapeutically for the treatment of established cytomegalovirus disease. Preparations are available for either intramuscular or intravenous administration.

PROPHYLACTIC USE. A report of the successful use of an immunoglobulin with high antibody levels against cytomegalovirus for the prevention of cytomegalovirus infection in seronegative leukaemic patients undergoing marrow transplants; the immunoglobulin was given before transplantation and also for 11 weeks after.— J. D. Meyers *et al.*, *Ann. intern. Med.*, 1983, *98*, 442. Failure of a study to show that a cytomegalovirus immunoglobulin can prevent cytomegalovirus infection or ameliorate cytomegalovirus disease in patients undergoing marrow transplantation.— R. A. Bowden *et al.*, *New Engl. J. Med.*, 1986, *314*, 1006.

A prospective randomised study indicating that the use of cytomegalovirus immunoglobulin provided effective prophylaxis in renal-transplant recipients at risk of primary cytomegalovirus disease.— D. R. Snydman *et al.*, *New Engl. J. Med.*, 1987, *317*, 1049.

THERAPEUTIC USE. Reports of beneficial responses to cytomegalovirus immunoglobulin in patients with cytomegalovirus disease: A. J. Nicholls *et al.* (letter), *Lancet*, 1983, *1*, 532 (renal-transplant recipients); M. J. Smith *et al.* (letter), *Lancet*, 1984, *1*, 447 (3-month-old infant); H. A. Blacklock *et al.* (letter), *Lancet*, 1985, *2*, 152 (bone-marrow transplant recipients).

1883-b

Dental Caries Vaccines

A dental caries vaccine consisting of purified protein from the surface of *Streptococcus mutans* has been developed and is awaiting clinical trial.

A review and discussion concerning the prospects for vaccination against dental caries. Successful experimental vaccines have used intact *Streptococcus mutans* or *Streptococcus sobrinus* as immunogens but current efforts are directed towards defining individual molecular components of the bacteria which may have been responsible for inducing the protection. Although there is an extremely active field of research into oral immunisation, the results available indicate that there is no immediate prospect of a feasible orally administered caries vaccine. Passive immunisation, using topically applied mono- or poly-clonal antibodies previously raised against *Str. mutans*, has been reported but this approach again requires considerable research. An injected, suitably-chosen, non-reactogenic, caries vaccine, however, should be no less acceptable than other vaccines in current use. The authors concluded that although potentially highly effective vaccines were being proposed for efficacy studies no clinical trials in children, to their knowledge, had yet been approved by any national authority.— R. R. B. Russell and N. W. Johnson, *Br. dent. J.*, 1987, *162*, 29.

Proprietary Names and Manufacturers

Wellcome, UK.

7951-h

Diphtheria Antitoxins

Diphtheria Antitoxin (*B.P., Eur. P.*) (Dip/Ser; Immunoserum Diphthericum) is a sterile preparation containing the specific antitoxic globulins that have the power of neutralising the toxin formed by *Corynebacterium diphtheriae*. It has a potency of not less that 1000 units per mL when obtained from horse serum and not less than 500 units per mL when obtained from other species. It should be stored at 2° to 8°, not be allowed to freeze, and be protected from light.

Diphtheria Antitoxin (*U.S.P.*) is a sterile solution of the refined and concentrated proteins, chiefly globulins, containing antitoxic antibodies obtained from the serum or plasma of healthy horses that have been immunised against diphtheria toxin or toxoid. It contains not less than 500 units per mL. It should be stored at 2° to 8°.

Units

One unit of diphtheria antitoxin (equine) is contained in 0.0628 mg of the first International Standard Preparation (1934).

Adverse Effects and Precautions

As for antisera in general, p.1155.

Uses and Administration
Diphtheria antitoxins neutralise the toxin produced by *Corynebacterium diphtheriae* locally at the site of infection and in the circulation but do not affect the pathological changes already induced by the toxin.
Diphtheria is usually treated by the concomitant administration of an antibiotic such as erythromycin or benzylpenicillin.
When the attack is mild or of moderate severity doses of 10 000 to 30 000 units of diphtheria antitoxin may be given intramuscularly, after a test dose to eliminate hypersensitivity; doses of 40 000 to 100 000 units may be given in the severe cases. Doses of more than 40 000 units should be given intravenously about 0.5 to 2 hours after the initial portion of the dose has been given intramuscularly.

Proprietary Preparations
A diphtheria antitoxin is available from *Regent Laboratories, UK*.

3894-d

Diphtheria Immunoglobulins
A diphtheria immunoglobulin containing high levels of specific antibody to the toxin of *Corynebacterium diphtheriae* has been prepared from human plasma.

Adverse Effects and Precautions
As for immunoglobulins in general, p.1155.

Uses and Administration
A diphtheria immunoglobulin, in a dose of 250 units by intramuscular injection, has been suggested for the passive immunisation of asymptomatic, unimmunised contacts of patients with diphtheria in whom active immunisation with a diphtheria vaccine and appropriate antibiotic therapy and observation is not possible.

7961-b

Diphtheria Vaccines
Diphtheria Toxoids.

Diphtheria Vaccine (*B.P.*) (Dip/Vac/FT; Diphtheria Prophylactic) is prepared from diphtheria toxin produced by the growth of *Corynebacterium diphtheriae*. The toxin is converted to diphtheria formol toxoid by treatment with formaldehyde solution. It contains not less than 25 Lf (see under Units, below) in the dose stated on the label. It should be stored at 2° to 8°, not be allowed to freeze, and be protected from light.

Adsorbed Diphtheria Vaccine (*B.P.*) (Adsorbed Diphtheria Prophylactic; Dip/Vac/Ads; Diphtheria Vaccine (Adsorbed) (*Eur. P.*); Vaccinum Diphtheriae Adsorbatum) is prepared from diphtheria formol toxoid containing not less than 1500 Lf per mg of protein nitrogen and a mineral carrier which may be hydrated aluminium hydroxide, aluminium phosphate, or calcium phosphate in a saline solution or other suitable solution isotonic with blood. The antigenic properties are adversely affected by certain antimicrobial preservatives, particularly those of the phenolic type. It contains not less than 30 units per dose. It should be stored at 2° to 8°, not be allowed to freeze, and be protected from light.
Diphtheria Toxoid (*U.S.P.*) is a sterile solution of the formaldehyde-treated products of growth of *Corynebacterium diphtheriae*. It contains a non-phenolic preservative. It should be stored at 2° to 8° and not be allowed to freeze.

Diphtheria Toxoid Adsorbed (*U.S.P.*) is a sterile preparation of plain diphtheria toxoid that has been precipitated or adsorbed by alum, aluminium hydroxide, or aluminium phosphate adjuvants. It should be stored at 2° to 8° and not be allowed to freeze.

Units
200 units of diphtheria toxoid, plain, are contained in 21 mg of formalin-treated diphtheria toxoid, freeze-dried, in one ampoule of the second International Standard Preparation (1975).
132 units of diphtheria toxoid, adsorbed, are contained in 75 mg of diphtheria toxoid adsorbed on aluminium hydroxide (1 mg of aluminium with polygeline 26 mg) in one ampoule of the second International Standard Preparation (1978).
The Limes flocculationis (Lf) of diphtheria toxin, diphtheria toxoid, or diphtheria vaccine is determined by incubation with a standard preparation of diphtheria antitoxin for flocculation test; when the concentration of antitoxin is varied in mixtures of constant volume, the mixture flocculating first is that which contains the most nearly equivalent quantities of toxin, or toxoid, and antitoxin.
There is no simple correlation between international units and Lf equivalents.

Adverse Effects and Precautions
As for vaccines in general, p.1155.
Local reactions occur occasionally but are generally not severe; the frequency of reactions is reported to be less in children under 2 years of age than in older children.
If diphtheria vaccines or vaccines containing a diphtheria component need to be given to children over the age of about 10 years or to adults specially prepared vaccines intended for adult use in which the amount of diphtheria toxoid is already reduced should be used. For further details see under Uses and Administration, below.

Uses and Administration
Diphtheria vaccines are used for active immunisation against diphtheria. The non-adsorbed vaccine has weak immunological properties and its effects are enhanced by administration as an adsorbed preparation.
Active immunisation against diphtheria should preferably be started when the infant is 3 months old. For primary immunisation combined diphtheria, tetanus, and pertussis vaccines (see below) or combined diphtheria and tetanus vaccines (see below) if it is decided not to immunise against pertussis, are usually used; immunisation against poliomyelitis is also generally performed at the same time using a live (oral) poliomyelitis vaccine (see p.1173). If neither immunisation against pertussis nor against tetanus is required a single-component diphtheria vaccine may be used.
In the *UK* a single-component adsorbed vaccine is available and is given by deep subcutaneous or by intramuscular injection in usual doses of 0.5 mL (not less than 30 units). The first dose is followed 6 to 8 weeks later by the second dose and the third dose follows after a further interval of 4 to 6 months. A reinforcing dose should be given at the age of 5 or at school entry.
If it is necessary to provide primary immunisation in children above the age of 10 or in adults a specially diluted adsorbed vaccine should be used without prior Schick testing. Three doses, each of 0.5 mL (1.5 Lf), are given by deep subcutaneous or intramuscular injection at one-month intervals. This diluted vaccine may also be used in single doses of 0.5 mL to provide re-inforcement of immunity in patients over 10 years of age. Such a vaccine does not conform to the requirements of the diphtheria vaccines as described in the *B.P.* which have a higher content of diphtheria toxoid.
In some other countries the strength of the vaccines and dosage schedules differ slightly from that outlined above.
Immunisation against diphtheria forms part of the World Health Organization's Expanded Programme on Immunization (see p.1156).

Recommendation of the Immunization Practices Advisory Committee for the prophylaxis of diphtheria, tetanus, and pertussis in the *USA* (*Ann. intern. Med.*, 1985, *103*, 896; *J. Am. med. Ass.*, 1985, *254*, 895 and 1009).
Vaccines against diphtheria, tetanus, and pertussis are available as single antigens or various combinations and with the exception of the single-component tetanus vaccine, all are only available as adsorbed preparations. Multiple-antigen preparations should be used unless there is a contra-indication to one or more antigens in a preparation. The standard single-dose volume for all the vaccines is 0.5 mL, the route being intramuscular for all adsorbed preparations.

References to the use of low-dose (1.5 Lf) diphtheria re-vaccination in adults: J. Mortimer *et al.*, *Lancet*, 1986, *2*, 1182; E. Walker, *Br. med. J.*, 1986, *292*, 507.

For further references relating to the need for revaccination against diphtheria in adults, see under diphtheria and tetanus vaccines (below).

Proprietary Preparations
Adsorbed Diphtheria Vaccine (*B.P.*) is available from *Wellcome, UK*.
A diluted adsorbed diphtheria vaccine is available from *Regent Laboratories, UK*.

7949-p

Diphtheria and Tetanus Vaccines
Diphtheria and Tetanus Toxoids.

Diphtheria and Tetanus Vaccine (*B.P.*) (Diphtheria-Tetanus Prophylactic; DT/Vac/FT) is a sterile mixture of diphtheria formol toxoid and tetanus formol toxoid. It contains not less than 25 Lf of diphtheria toxoid per dose. It should be stored at 2° to 8°, not be allowed to freeze, and be protected from light.
Adsorbed Diphtheria and Tetanus Vaccine (*B.P.*) (Adsorbed Diphtheria-Tetanus Prophylactic; Diphtheria and Tetanus Vaccine (Adsorbed) (*Eur. P.*); DT/Vac/Ads; Vaccinum Diphtheriae et Tetani Adsorbatum) is prepared from diphtheria formol toxoid containing not less than 1500 Limes flocculationis (Lf) per mg of protein nitrogen, tetanus formol toxoid containing not less than 1000 Lf per mg of protein nitrogen, and a mineral carrier, which may be hydrated aluminium hydroxide, aluminium phosphate, or calcium phosphate in a saline solution or other suitable solution isotonic with blood. The antigenic properties are adversely affected by certain antimicrobial preservatives particularly those of the phenolic type. It contains not less than 30 units of diphtheria toxoid and not less than 40 units of tetanus toxoid per dose. It should be stored at 2° to 8°, not be allowed to freeze, and be protected from light. Under these conditions it may be expected to retain its potency for not less than 5 years from the date on which the potency test was begun.
Diphtheria and Tetanus Toxoids (*U.S.P.*) is a sterile solution prepared by mixing suitable quantities of fluid diphtheria toxoid and fluid tetanus toxoid. The antigenicity or potency and the proportions of the toxoids are such as to provide an immunising dose of each toxoid in the labelled dose. It should be stored at 2° to 8 ° and not be allowed to freeze.
Diphtheria and Tetanus Toxoids Adsorbed

(*U.S.P.*) is a sterile suspension prepared by mixing suitable quantities of plain or adsorbed diphtheria toxoid and plain or adsorbed tetanus toxoid and, if plain toxoids are used, an aluminium adsorbing agent. The antigenicity or potency and the proportions of the toxoids are such as to provide an immunising dose of each toxoid in the labelled dose. It should be stored at 2° to 8° and not be allowed to freeze.

Tetanus and Diphtheria Toxoids Adsorbed for Adult Use (*U.S.P.*) is a sterile suspension prepared by mixing suitable quantities of adsorbed diphtheria toxoid and adsorbed tetanus toxoid using the same precipitating or adsorbing agent for both toxoids. The antigenicity or potency and the proportions of the toxoids are such as to provide, in the labelled dose, an immunising dose of adsorbed tetanus toxoid and one-tenth of the immunising dose of adsorbed diphtheria toxoid specified for children and not more than 2 Lf of diphtheria toxoid. It should be stored at 2° to 8° and not be allowed to freeze.

Units

See under diphtheria vaccines, above, and tetanus vaccines, p.1180.

Adverse Effects and Precautions

As for vaccines in general, p.1155. See also under diphtheria vaccines, above, and tetanus vaccines, p.1180.

Side-effects in adults.— J. P. Middaugh, *Am. J. publ. Hlth*, 1979, *69*, 246.

Polyradiculoneuritis in a patient following the use of a diphtheria-tetanus vaccine; it was considered that the tetanus component was the more likely cause of the reaction but this could not be verified.— P. L. Holliday and R. B. Bauer, *Archs Neurol., Chicago*, 1983, *40*, 56.

A report of several cases of encephalopathy occurring in a small region in Italy in children following immunisation against diphtheria and tetanus. The results did not, however, make it possible to infer a causal relationship.— D. Greco, *Bull. Wld Hlth Org.*, 1985, *63*, 919.

Uses and Administration

Combined adsorbed diphtheria and tetanus vaccines are used for active immunisation of children against diphtheria and tetanus in cases where it is decided not to immunise against pertussis also; immunisation against poliomyelitis is also generally performed at the same time using a live (oral) poliomyelitis vaccine (see p.1173).

In the *UK* a combined adsorbed diphtheria and tetanus vaccine is given for primary immunisation in usual doses of 0.5 mL (not less than 30 units of diphtheria toxoid and not less than 40 units of tetanus toxoid) by deep subcutaneous or intramuscular injection, the first dose being given preferably at the age of 3 months, followed after 6 to 8 weeks by the second dose, and after a further 4 to 6 months by the third dose. A reinforcing dose at the age of 5 or at school entry should be given to children who have previously been immunised against diphtheria and tetanus, or against diphtheria, tetanus, and pertussis and in whom the pertussis component is no longer needed.

The non-adsorbed combined diphtheria and tetanus vaccines should be used only for reinforcing doses; the suggested dose by deep subcutaneous or intramuscular injection is 0.5 mL (not less than 25 Lf of diphtheria toxoid and not less than 3.5 Lf of tetanus toxoid) for children under 10 years of age.

In some other countries the strength of the vaccines and dosage schedules differ slightly from that outlined above.

Immunisation against both diphtheria and tetanus forms part of the World Health Organization's Expanded Programme on Immunization (see p.1156).

Recommendation of the Immunization Practices Advisory Committee for the prophylaxis of diphtheria, tetanus, and pertussis in the *USA* (*Ann. intern. Med.*, 1985, *103*, 896; *J. Am. med. Ass.*, 1985, *254*, 895 and 1009).

Vaccines against diphtheria, tetanus, and pertussis are available as single antigens or various combinations and with the exception of the single-component tetanus vaccine, all are only available as adsorbed preparations. Multiple-antigen preparations should be used unless there is a contra-indication to one or more antigens in a preparation. The standard single-dose volume for all the vaccines is 0.5 mL, the route being intramuscular for all adsorbed preparations.

Although routine primary immunisation of children under the age of 7 years is generally performed with a combined diphtheria, tetanus, and pertussis vaccine (DTP vaccine), in children in whom a contra-indication to immunisation against pertussis either already exists, or develops during a course of DTP, a combined diphtheria and tetanus vaccine should be used. In those in whom a combined diphtheria and tetanus vaccine is used from the outset 4 doses intramuscularly should be given if the child is under one year of age when receiving the first dose and 3 doses if the child is already one year of age or older; the doses should be given at 4- to 8-week intervals with the exception of the last dose which should be given 6 to 12 months after the preceding one. In children still in their first year of life who have already received DTP vaccine but in whom a contra-indication to its further use has arisen a combined diphtheria and tetanus vaccine should be substituted for each of the remaining scheduled DTP doses [see under diphtheria, tetanus, and pertussis vaccines, below]; children of one year of age or older who have received DTP, and for whom further pertussis vaccine is contra-indicated, should receive a total of 3 doses of a preparation containing diphtheria and tetanus components with the last dose administered 6 to 12 months after the second dose. Children who complete a primary immunising course against diphtheria and tetanus before their fourth birthday should receive a single booster dose before entering school.

Persons 7 years of age and older requiring primary immunisation should receive a specially prepared diphtheria and tetanus vaccine in which the concentration of the diphtheria toxoid is reduced in order to lessen the incidence of side-effects. Three doses should be given with the second dose 4 to 8 weeks after the first, and the third 6 to 12 months after the second. This vaccine should also be given as a booster immunisation every 10 years to persons 7 years of age or older.

There is no evidence that diphtheria and tetanus vaccines are teratogenic. Therefore, a previously unimmunised pregnant woman who may deliver a child under unhygienic circumstances or surroundings should receive before delivery, and preferably during the last two trimesters, 2 properly-spaced doses of a diphtheria and tetanus vaccine suitable for adult use. Incompletely immunised pregnant women should complete their course of vaccines. A booster dose should be given to those immunised more than 10 years previously.

With regard to tetanus prophylaxis in wound management the need for tetanus vaccines depends on both the condition of the wound and the patient's immunisation history. In adults and children 7 years of age or older a suitable combined diphtheria and tetanus vaccine is preferred to a single-component tetanus vaccine and in younger children either a combined diphtheria, tetanus, and pertussis vaccine or a combined diphtheria and tetanus vaccine is again preferred to a single-component tetanus vaccine. For all wounds a booster dose should be given if the history is unknown, or less than 3 doses of a vaccine containing a tetanus component have previously been received. If 3 or more doses of an adsorbed vaccine have been given previously a booster is not necessary unless an interval of more than 10 years has elapsed since the last dose in the case of clean, minor wounds, and an interval of more then 5 years has elapsed since the last dose in the case of all other wounds. If only 3 doses of a non-adsorbed tetanus vaccine have previously been received a fourth dose, preferably of an adsorbed vaccine, should be given in all cases. A dose of 250 units of tetanus immunoglobulin by intramuscular injection is recommended for wounds of average severity when the history of tetanus vaccination is unknown or less than 3 doses of a vaccine have previously been received.

As, in some countries, booster doses of combined diphtheria and tetanus vaccines are recommended every 10 years, studies have been conducted to assess whether this is necessary.

A study performed in Denmark (K. Kjeldsen *et al.*, *Lancet*, 1985, *1*, 900) found a sufficiently high proportion of subjects investigated to be unprotected against both diphtheria and tetanus such that it was considered advisable to recommend routine revaccination with a combined vaccine. In contrast, following an analysis of data on the number of cases of, and deaths from, diphtheria and tetanus in Canada over the period 1950 to 1982 (R.G. Mathias and M.T. Schechter, *Lancet*, 1985, *1*, 1089), the view was held that routine boosters of the combined vaccine every 10 years were not necessary.

In a comment on these two reports (*Lancet*, 1985, *1*, 1081) it was pointed out that in countries such as Canada, Denmark, and also the UK, where many adults, on the basis of diphtheria antitoxin titres, appear to be susceptible to diphtheria, the disease is still adequately controlled. It was considered that there is no evidence that the UK is on the verge of a diphtheria epidemic, and that the current policy of immunisation against diphtheria in infancy and at school entry is sufficient.

However, following a report (R. Rappuoli *et al.*, *New Engl. J. Med.*, 1988, *318*, 12) of an outbreak of clinical diphtheria in Sweden after a period of many years when no indigenous cases of diphtheria had occurred and the disease was regarded as being eliminated from the country the question of immunity in adults and the need for revaccination again arose. Addressing the question with regard to the situation in the USA (D.T. Karzon and K.M. Edwards, *New Engl. J. Med.*, 1988, *318*, 41) it was considered that re-immunisation every 10 years with a combined diphtheria and tetanus vaccine was mandatory and that this combined vaccine should be used whenever, as in treating emergency wounds, a tetanus vaccine was indicated.

Proprietary Preparations

Diphtheria and Tetanus Vaccine (*B.P.*) is available from *Wellcome, UK* and Adsorbed Diphtheria and Tetanus Vaccine (*B.P.*) is available from *Evans Medical, UK* and *Wellcome, UK*.

7955-g

Diphtheria, Tetanus, and Pertussis Vaccines

Diphtheria, Tetanus and Pertussis Vaccine (*B.P.*) (Diphtheria-Tetanus-Whooping-cough Prophylactic; DTPer/Vac) is a sterile mixture of diphtheria formol toxoid, tetanus formol toxoid, and a suspension of killed *Bordetella pertussis*. It contains not less than 25 Lf of diphtheria toxoid and not less than 4 units of the pertussis component per dose. It should be stored at 2° to 8°, not be allowed to freeze, and be protected from light.

Adsorbed Diphtheria, Tetanus and Pertussis Vaccine (*B.P.*) (Adsorbed Diphtheria-Tetanus-Whooping-cough Prophylactic; Diphtheria, Tetanus and Pertussis Vaccine (Adsorbed) (*Eur. P.*); DTPer/Vac/Ads; Vaccinum Diphtheriae, Tetani et Pertussis Adsorbatum) is prepared from diphtheria formol toxoid containing not less than 1500 Lf per mg of protein nitrogen, tetanus formol toxoid containing not less than 1000 Lf per mg of protein nitrogen, a suspension of killed *Bordetella pertussis*, and a mineral carrier, which may be hydrated aluminium hydroxide, aluminium phosphate, or calcium phosphate in a saline solution or other suitable solution isotonic with blood. It contains not less than 30 units of diphtheria toxoid, not less than 40 units, or 60 units if the test if performed in *mice*, of tetanus toxoid, and not less than 4 units of the pertussis component per dose. The antigenic properties are adversely affected by certain antimicrobial preservatives particularly those of the phenolic type and some of the quaternary-ammonium type and these should not be added to the vaccine. It should be stored at 2° to 8°, not be allowed to freeze, and be protected from light. Under these conditions it may be expected to retain its potency for not less than 2 years from the date on which the potency test for the pertussis component was begun.

Diphtheria and Tetanus Toxoids and Pertussis Vaccine (*U.S.P.*) is a sterile suspension prepared by mixing suitable quantities of pertussis vaccine component of killed *Bordetella pertussis*, or a fraction of this organism, fluid diphtheria toxoid, and fluid tetanus toxoid. The antigenicity or potency and the proportions of the components are such that the labelled dose provides an immunising dose of each component. It should be stored at 2° to 8° and not be allowed to freeze.

Diphtheria and Tetanus Toxoids and Pertussis Vaccine Adsorbed (*U.S.P.*) is a sterile suspension prepared by mixing suitable quantities of plain or adsorbed diphtheria toxoid, plain or adsorbed tetanus toxoid, plain or adsorbed pertussis vaccine, and, if plain antigen components are used, an aluminium adsorbing agent. The antigenicity or potency and the proportions of the components are such that the labelled dose provides an immunising dose of each component. It should be stored at 2° to 8° and not be allowed to freeze.

Units

See under diphtheria vaccines, above, pertussis vaccines, p.1172, and tetanus vaccines, p.1180.

Adverse Effects and Precautions

As for vaccines in general, p.1155. See also under pertussis vaccines, p.1172, and tetanus vaccines, p.1180.

ALLERGY. Anaphylaxis, presenting with a swollen face and tongue, in a 2-month-old infant about 3 hours after the administration of an adsorbed diphtheria, tetanus, and pertussis vaccine.— A. K. C. Leung (letter), *J. R. Soc. Med.*, 1985, *78*, 175.

EFFECTS ON THE CARDIOVASCULAR SYSTEM. Paroxysmal supraventricular tachycardia in a two-month-old child after the use of a diphtheria, tetanus, and pertussis vaccine and an oral polio vaccine.— J. M. Park *et al.*, *J. Pediat.*, 1983, *102*, 883.

Myocarditis in a child developing several hours after diphtheria, tetanus, and pertussis vaccination.— S. G. Amsel *et al.*, *Archs Dis. Childh.*, 1986, *61*, 403.

EFFECTS ON THE NERVOUS SYSTEM. For reports and discussions concerning adverse central nervous system effects, attributed to the pertussis component of combined diphtheria, tetanus, and pertussis vaccines, see under pertussis vaccines, p.1172.

EFFECTS ON THE SKIN. A report of postvaccination granuloma in 2 patients after immunisation with an adsorbed diphtheria, tetanus, and pertussis vaccine. The tumours were considered to be due to the aluminium hydroxide component of the vaccine.— M. Erdohazi and R. L. Newman, *Br. med. J.*, 1971, *3*, 621. See also: D. N. Slater *et al.*, *Br. J. Derm.*, 1982, *107*, 103.

A report of 2 children who developed erythema multiforme after diphtheria, tetanus, and pertussis vaccines.— A. K. C. Leung (letter), *J. R. Soc. Med.*, 1984, *77*, 1066.

Uses and Administration

Combined diphtheria, tetanus, and pertussis vaccines are used for active immunisation of children against diphtheria, tetanus, and pertussis (whooping cough); immunisation against poliomyelitis is also generally performed at the same time using a live (oral) poliomyelitis vaccine (see p.1173). If it is decided not to immunise against pertussis combined diphtheria and tetanus only vaccines are used (see above). Both the non-adsorbed or adsorbed combined diphtheria, tetanus, and pertussis vaccines may be used although the adsorbed type is usually preferred.

In the *UK* a combined adsorbed vaccine is given by deep subcutaneous or intramuscular injection in usual doses of 0.5 mL (not less than 30 units of purified diphtheria toxoid, not less than 60 units of purified tetanus toxoid, and not more than 20 000 million *Bordetella pertussis*); the first dose is given preferably at the age of 3 months, followed after 6 to 8 weeks by the second dose, and after a further 4 to 6 months by the third dose. Alternatively, in the event of a pertussis epidemic, 3 doses may be given at monthly intervals starting at 3 months of age; in these cases where the primary immunisation against diphtheria and tetanus is completed during the first 6 to 8 months of life, a reinforcing dose of a combined diphtheria and tetanus vaccine (see above) should be given after about a year. The non-adsorbed type of combined diphtheria, tetanus, and pertussis vaccine may also be given in the same doses (0.5 mL) and same dosage schedule as that outlined above for the adsorbed vaccine but it should be noted that the strength of the vaccine is expressed differently; each 0.5 mL dose contains 25 Lf of purified diphtheria toxoid, 3.5 Lf of purified tetanus toxoid, and not more than 20 000 million *B. pertussis*. In all children a booster dose of a combined diphtheria and tetanus vaccine (see above) should be given at school entry.

In some other countries the strength of the vaccines and dosage schedules differ slightly from that outlined above.

Immunisation against diphtheria, pertussis, and tetanus forms part of the World Health Organization's Expanded Programme on Immunization (see p.1156).

Recommendation of the Immunization Practices Advisory Committee for the prophylaxis of diphtheria, tetanus, and pertussis in the *USA* (*Ann. intern. Med.*, 1985, *103*, 896; *J. Am. med. Ass.*, 1985, *254*, 895 and 1009).

Vaccines against diphtheria, tetanus, and pertussis are available as single antigens or various combinations and with the exception of the single-component tetanus vaccine, all are only available as adsorbed preparations. Multiple-antigen preparations should be used unless there is a contra-indication to one or more antigens in a preparation. The standard single-dose volume for all the vaccines is 0.5 mL the route being intramuscular for all adsorbed preparations.

Routine primary immunisation of children under the age of 7 years usually consists of 4 doses of a combined diphtheria, tetanus, and pertussis vaccine (DTP vaccine). The first dose is given at 6 weeks of age or later, with the second and third doses at 4- to 8-week intervals; customarily the first dose is given at 8 weeks of age with the second and third doses at 8-week intervals; the fourth dose is given 6 to 12 months after the third dose. Children who have received all 4 doses of the primary immunising course before their fourth birthday should receive a single booster dose before entering school.

Routine immunisation against pertussis is not recommended for persons 7 years of age or older and in these persons, as in any child in whom a contra-indication to the use of a pertussis-containing vaccine exists, an appropriate combined diphtheria and tetanus vaccine should be used [for these recommendations see under diphtheria and tetanus vaccines, above].

Several suggestions have been made (R.M. Barkin *et al.*, *J. Pediat.*, 1984, *105*, 189; A. Leung, *Can. med. Ass. J.*, 1984, *131*, 844; C.A. Hankins, *ibid.*, 1985, *132*, 96; R.M. Barkin and J.S. Samuelson, *J. Am. med. Ass.*, 1986, *255*, 2026) that the severity and incidence of reactions to combined diphtheria, tetanus, and pertussis vaccines may be reduced by the administration of smaller or fractional doses. Most authorities and official advisory bodies, however, continue to recommend against the use of fractional doses on the grounds that such reduced doses have not been proved to confer adequate immunity (J.R. Waters, *Can. med. Ass. J.*, 1985, *132*, 1254; J. Cameron, *ibid.*, 1986, *134*, 18; S.G.F. Wassilak *et al.*, *J. Am. med. Ass.*, 1986, *255*, 2026).

A review of the epidemiology and control of pertussis. Pertussis is a common, highly infectious, respiratory disease, predominantly affecting children, and for which there is no effective treatment. The World Health Organization has estimated that 60 million cases of pertussis occur annually and that the disease is responsible for half a million to one million deaths each year. The highest incidence of pertussis is observed in developing countries where immunisation is low.

A combined adsorbed diphtheria, tetanus, and pertussis vaccine is now used in most countries but both the strengths of the pertussis component and production methods vary, leading to vaccines of different potencies.

In recent years public concern and conflicting views within the medical profession have raised the question in some developed countries as to whether the benefits of pertussis immunisation outweigh the risks. The occurrence of fever and mild local reactions related to the pertussis component of the combined vaccines is common; the estimated risk of severe neurological illness is 1 in 170 000 administered doses, while that for permanent neurological sequelae is 1 in 470 000 doses. It is thus considered that the benefits do outweigh the risks when the post-vaccination sequelae are compared with the morbidity and mortality caused by the natural disease and that the argument in favour of routine pertussis immunisation is even more cogent in developing nations.

Depending upon the country, the age at which a child is given the first dose of the combined vaccine varies from 5 weeks to 6 months. In countries with a high incidence of pertussis the WHO recommends that immunisation should start at 6 weeks of age and that the schedule involve three doses at monthly intervals. A booster dose should be given one year after the end of the primary series of 3 injections and in some countries a second booster at entry to school is given. Several reports have described the use of a two-dose widely-spaced primary immunisation schedule and this would indeed simplify procedures in developing countries; however, the limitation of such a schedule is the long period of risk between doses without adequate protection and unless the interval can be shortened to 4 weeks, the wide use of such a schedule is not advisable in endemic areas. Although the immune reactions of malnourished children are impaired there is no evidence that the response to the combined diphtheria, tetanus, and pertussis vaccines is inadequate; in general malnutrition is considered an indication, rather than a contra-indication, for immunisation.— A. S. Muller *et al.*, *Bull. Wld Hlth Org.*, 1986, *64*, 321.

Proprietary Preparations

Trivax *(Wellcome, UK)*. Diphtheria, Tetanus and Pertussis Vaccine (*B.P.*).

Trivax-AD *(Wellcome, UK)*. Adsorbed Diphtheria, Tetanus and Pertussis Vaccine (*B.P.*).

Adsorbed Diphtheria, Tetanus and Pertussis Vaccine (*B.P.*) is also available from *Evans Medical, UK*.

Proprietary Names and Manufacturers

Anatoxal Di Te Per *(Berna, Switz.)*; Anatoxal DiTePer *(Berna, Ital.)*; Dif-Per-Tet-All *(Sclavo, Ital.)*; Tri-Immunol *(Lederle, USA)*; Triple Antigen *(Commonwealth Serum Laboratories, Austral.)*; Trivax *(Wellcome, UK)*; Trivax-AD *(Wellcome, UK)*;

Manufacturers also include—*Parke, Davis, Austral.; Armand-Frappier, Canad.; Connaught, Canad.; Behringwerke, Ger.; ISI, Ital.; Istituto Behring, Ital.; Max Ritter, Switz.; Evans Medical, UK; Connaught, USA.*

7956-q

Diphtheria, Tetanus, and Poliomyelitis Vaccines

Diphtheria, Tetanus and Poliomyelitis Vaccine (*B.P.*) (DTPol/Vac) is a sterile mixture of diphtheria formol toxoid, tetanus formol toxoid, and poliomyelitis vaccine (inactivated). It contains not less than 25 Lf of diphtheria toxoid per dose. It should be stored at 2° to 8°, not be allowed to freeze, and be protected from light. Under these conditions it may be expected to retain its potency for at least one year.

Adverse Effects and Precautions

As for vaccines in general, p.1155. See also under diphtheria vaccines, above, poliomyelitis vaccines, p.1173, and tetanus vaccines, p.1180.

Uses and Administration

An adsorbed diphtheria, tetanus, and poliomyelitis vaccine with a reduced amount of diphtheria toxoid (2 Lf per dose) may be used, in older children and adults, for both primary immunisation against diphtheria, tetanus, and poliomyelitis and to reinforce the immunity of those who have previously been immunised. Such a vaccine does not conform to the requirements of Diphtheria, Tetanus and Poliomyelitis Vaccine as described in the *B.P.* which has a higher content of diphtheria toxoid.

Primary immunisation of young children is usually performed with a suitable combined diphtheria and tetanus vaccine (see above) together with a live (oral) poliomyelitis vaccine (see p.1173).

Proprietary Preparations

A diphtheria, tetanus, and poliomyelitis vaccine is available on a named-patient basis from *Connaught, Canad.* and *Merieux, UK*.

7957-p

Diphtheria, Tetanus, Pertussis, and Poliomyelitis Vaccines

The *B.P.* 1973 vaccine consisted of a mixture of diphtheria toxoid, tetanus toxoid, a suspension of killed *Bordetella pertussis*, and inactivated poliomyelitis vaccine.

Adverse Effects and Precautions
As for vaccines in general, p.1155. See also under diphtheria vaccines, above, pertussis vaccines, p.1172, poliomyelitis vaccines, p.1173, and tetanus vaccines, p.1180.

Uses and Administration
Diphtheria, tetanus, pertussis, and poliomyelitis vaccines may be used for active immunisation of infants against diphtheria, tetanus, pertussis, and poliomyelitis. Immunisation is, however, usually performed with a combined diphtheria, tetanus, and pertussis vaccine (see above) together with a live (oral) poliomyelitis vaccine (see p.1173).

Proprietary Preparations

A diphtheria, tetanus, pertussis, and poliomyelitis vaccine is available on a named-patient basis from *Connaught, Canad.* and *Merieux, UK.*

16619-r

Japanese Encephalitis Vaccines

Two types of inactivated Japanese encephalitis vaccine are being used, one derived from mouse brain and the other from primary hamster kidney cells. The vaccines are widely used in Japan and other parts of Asia.

A short review of Japanese encephalitis and the vaccines available.— T. Umenai *et al.*, *Bull. Wld Hlth Org.*, 1985, *63*, 625.

Comments and discussion concerning the vaccination of travellers against Japanese encephalitis: D. W. Denning and Y. Kaneko, *Lancet*, 1987, *1*, 853; R. Steffen (letter), *ibid.*, *2*, 511; T. P. Monath, *New Engl. J. Med.*, 1988, *319*, 641.

Further references: C. H. Hoke *et al.*, *New Engl. J. Med.*, 1988, *319*, 608.

Proprietary Names and Manufacturers
Defence Medical Equipment Depot, UK.

3869-f

Tick-borne Encephalitis Vaccines

A vaccine against tick-borne encephalitis is available consisting of inactivated virus particles.

A report of the use of a tick-borne encephalitis vaccine consisting of 350 ng of tick-borne encephalitis virus antigen (formalin-inactivated virus particles) per dose. Intradermal administration resulted in quicker seroconversion and higher antibody levels than did intramuscular administration.— G. Zoulek *et al.* (letter), *Lancet*, 1984, *2*, 584.

Proprietary Preparations

A tick-borne encephalitis vaccine may be available on a named-patient basis from *Immuno, UK.*

8039-n

Gas-gangrene Antitoxins

Gas-gangrene Antitoxin (Novyi) (*B.P., Eur. P.*) (Gas-gangrene Antitoxin (Oedematiens); Immunoserum Gangraenicum (Clostridium Novyi); Nov/Ser) is a sterile preparation containing the specific antitoxic globulins that have the power of neutralising the alpha toxin formed by *Clostridium novyi*. Potency not less than 3750 units per mL.

Gas-gangrene Antitoxin (Perfringens) (*B.P., Eur. P.*) (Immunoserum Gangraenicum (Clostridium Perfringens); Perf/Ser) is a sterile preparation containing the specific antitoxic globulins that have the power of neutralising the alpha toxin formed by *Clostridium perfringens*. It has a potency of not less than 1500 units per mL.

Gas-gangrene Antitoxin (Septicum) (*B.P, Eur. P.*) (Immunoserum Gangraenicum (Clostridium Septicum); Sep/Ser) is a sterile preparation containing the specific antitoxic globulins that have the power of neutralising the alpha toxin formed by *Clostridium septicum*. It has a potency of not less than 1500 units per mL.

Mixed Gas-gangrene Antitoxin (*B.P., Eur. P.*) (Immunoserum Gangraenicum Mixtum; Gas/Ser) is prepared by mixing Gas-gangrene Antitoxin (Novyi), Gas-gangrene Antitoxin (Perfringens), and Gas-gangrene Antitoxin (Septicum) in appropriate quantities. It has a potency of not less than 1000 units of Gas-gangrene Antitoxin (Novyi), not less than 1000 units of Gas-gangrene Antitoxin (Perfringens), and not less than 500 units of Gas-gangrene Antitoxin (Septicum) per mL.

The above antitoxins should be stored at 2° to 8°, not be allowed to freeze, and be protected from light.

Units

1100 units of gas-gangrene antitoxin (*Clostridium novyi*) (equine) are contained in 91 mg of dried hyperimmune horse serum in one ampoule of the third International Standard Preparation (1966).

270 units of gas-gangrene antitoxin (*Clostridium perfringens*, alpha antitoxin) (equine) are contained in 90.35 mg of dried hyperimmune horse serum in one ampoule of the fifth International Standard Preparation (1963).

500 units of gas-gangrene antitoxin (*Clostridium septicum*) (equine) are contained in 59 mg of a dried 1:3 dilution of hyperimmune horse serum in phosphate-buffered saline in one ampoule of the third International Standard Preparation (1957).

Adverse Effects and Precautions

As for antisera in general, p.1155.

Uses and Administration

Monovalent gas-gangrene antitoxins are little used in practice owing to the difficulty of rapidly identifying the infecting organism and are used mainly in the form of a mixed antitoxin. Suggested doses for a mixed gas-gangrene antitoxin have been 25 000 units intravenously or intramuscularly for prophylaxis and 75 000 units intravenously for treatment; these doses may be repeated if necessary. The antitoxin contains in each mL not less than 1000 units of both the novyi and perfringens components and not less than 500 units of the septicum component.

Proprietary Preparations

A mixed gas-gangrene antitoxin is available from *Servier, UK.*

19267-j

Gonococcal Vaccines

Gonorrhoea Vaccines.

Several experimental gonococcal vaccines produced usually from the surface antigens of *Neisseria gonorrhaeae* have been developed but clinical trials have not yet shown convincing benefit.

Some references to gonococcal vaccines: *Bull. Wld Hlth Org.*, 1983, *61*, 415; E. C. Gotschlich, *ibid.*, 1984, *62*, 671; B. E. Britigan *et al.*, *New Engl. J. Med.*, 1985, *312*, 1683.

16828-q

Haemophilus Influenzae Vaccines

Haemophilus influenzae vaccines are prepared from the purified capsular polysaccharide (polyribosylribitol phosphate; PRP) of *Haemophilus influenzae* type b; strains of *H. influenzae* type b used have been the Eagan strain and the CK (ATCC 31441) strain.

A conjugate vaccine containing in each 0.5-mLdose 25 μg of the polysaccharide (Eagan strain) linked to 18 μg of diphtheria toxoid protein is available in some countries.

Non-conjugate vaccines, containing 25 μg of the polysaccharide (Eagan or CK strain) per 0.5-mLdose, have also been used.

Adverse Effects and Precautions

As for vaccines in general, p.1155.

Uses and Administration

Haemophilus influenzae vaccines are used for active immunisation against *Haemophilus influenzae* type b infections, one of the major causes of meningitis and other severe systemic illnesses in young children. Vaccines have been prepared from the capsular polysaccharide of *H. influenzae* type b and immunogenicity, especially in young children, has been shown to be improved by linking the polysaccharide to an agent such as diphtheria toxoid to form a conjugate vaccine.

In the *USA* a conjugate vaccine is recommended for immunisation of all children at 18 months of age. The dose is 0.5 mL (containing 25 μg of polysaccharide linked to 18 μg of diphtheria toxoid protein) given by intramuscular injection. Non-conjugate vaccines, also containing 25 μg of polysaccharide per 0.5-mL dose, have been given, by intramuscular or subcutaneous injection, to older children of 24 months of age or more. For further details concerning the recommendations in the *USA*, see below.

General reviews on vaccination against *Haemophilus influenzae* type b.— *Lancet*, 1986, *1*, 1074.

Recommendations of the Advisory Committee on Immunization Practices for the use of haemophilus influenzae vaccines in the *USA* (*J. Am. med. Ass.*, 1988, *259*, 798). As studies in children receiving the conjugate vaccine (consisting of the capsular polysaccharide of *Haemophilus influenzae* type b covalently linked to diphtheria toxoid) or the non-conjugate vaccine have revealed that the conjugate vaccine is likely to be more effective in producing antibodies, the use of this conjugate vaccine is recommended for children vaccinated against Haemophilus type b disease. It should be noted that although increases in serum diphtheria antitoxin concentrations can follow administration of the conjugate vaccine, the vaccine should not be considered to be an immunising agent against diphtheria and no changes in the schedule for vaccination against diphtheria should be made.

All children should receive a single dose of the conjugate vaccine at 18 months of age. In children of more than 24 months of age who have not yet received any type of haemophilus vaccine the need for vaccination should be based on an assessment of risk of disease; those with a high risk for Haemophilus b disease, such as those with anatomic or functional asplenia (splenectomy or sickle-cell disease) and those with malignancies associated with immunosuppression, should receive the vaccine. Many children may have received a non-conjugate vaccine between 18 and 23 months of age and they should be revaccinated with a single dose of the conjugate vaccine, allowing at least an interval of 2 months before revaccination; routine revaccination of children who received a non-conjugate vaccine at 24 months of age or more is unnecessary.

Vaccination with either a conjugate or a non-conjugate vaccine probably does not inhibit asymptomatic carriage of *Haemophilus influenzae* type b.

The conjugate haemophilus vaccine and combined diphtheria, tetanus, and pertussis vaccines may be given simultaneously at different sites. Although data are lacking regarding concomitant administration with combined measles, mumps, and rubella vaccines or with oral polio vaccines, simultaneous administration of all vaccines appropriate to the recipient's age and vaccination status is recommended if the patient is unlikely to return for further vaccination.

Some reports of beneficial antibody responses to a conjugate haemophilus influenzae vaccine (capsular polysaccharide of *Haemophilus influenzae* type b linked to diphtheria toxoid): R. A. Insel and P. W. Anderson, *New Engl. J. Med.*, 1986, *315*, 499 (children with IgG_2 deficiency); M. Lepow *et al.*, *J. Pediat.*, 1986, *108*, 882 (healthy children); C. D. Berkowitz *et al.*, *ibid.*, 1987, *110*, 509 (healthy children); J. Eskola *et al.*, *New Engl. J. Med.*, 1987, *317*, 717 (healthy children).

Proprietary Preparations

An haemophilus influenzae vaccine is available on a named-patient basis from *Mead Johnson Pharmaceutical, USA*.

1235-a

Hepatitis B Immunoglobulins

Hepatitis B Immunoglobulin (*B.P.*) is a liquid or freeze-dried preparation containing immunoglobulins, mainly immunoglobulin G (IgG). It is obtained from plasma or serum containing specific antibodies against the hepatitis B surface antigen. Normal Immunoglobulin may be added. Hepatitis B Immunoglobulin is prepared in the same manner as Normal Immunoglobulin (see p.1170) except that the pooled material may be from fewer than 1000 donors. It contains not less than 100 units per mL. The liquid preparation should be stored, protected from light, in a sealed, colourless, glass container at a temperature of 2° to 8°. Under these conditions it may be expected to retain its potency for 3 years. The freeze-dried preparation should be stored, protected from light, under vacuum or under an inert gas at a temperature of 2° to 8°. Under these conditions it may be expected to retain its potency for 5 years.

Hepatitis B Immune Globulin (*U.S.P.*) is a sterile solution consisting of globulins derived from the plasma of human donors who have high titres of antibodies against hepatitis B surface antigen. It contains 10 to 18% of protein, of which not less than 80% is monomeric immunoglobulin G. It contains glycine as a stabilising agent, and a suitable preservative. It should be stored at 2° to 8°.

Units

50 units of antihepatitis B immunoglobulin (fractionated plasma, freeze-dried) are contained in one ampoule of the first International Reference Preparation (1977).

Adverse Effects and Precautions

As for immunoglobulins in general, p.1155.

Uses and Administration

Hepatitis B immunoglobulins are used for passive immunisation of persons exposed to hepatitis B virus. They are not appropriate as a treatment for any type of hepatitis B infection.

In the *UK* a hepatitis B immunoglobulin containing 100 units per mL is available for use in persons who have been exposed to hepatitis B virus. The recommended dose in adults is 500 units by intramuscular injection given preferably within 48 hours of exposure and not more than 10 days after exposure. A second dose should be given after 4 weeks unless the patient's blood sample demonstrates prior hepatitis B infection or unless a course of hepatitis B vaccination is started at the same time as the first dose of immunoglobulin. Hepatitis B immunoglobulin should also be given to newborn infants at risk whose mothers are persistent carriers of hepatitis B surface antigen or who are HBsAg-positive as a result of recent infection. The recommended dose is 200 units by intramuscular injection as soon as possible after birth, and certainly within 48 hours of birth. A second dose of 100 units should be given after 4 weeks unless a course of hepatitis B vaccination is started at the same time as the first dose of immunoglobulin.

For further details concerning the use of hepatitis B vaccines for active immunisation in conjunction with hepatitis B immunoglobulins for passive immunisation, see under hepatitis B vaccines, below.

For the Recommendations of the Advisory Committee on Immunization Practices for protection against viral hepatitis in the *USA*, including the use of hepatitis B immunoglobulins, see under hepatitis B vaccines, below.

Proprietary Preparations

A hepatitis immunoglobulin is available from *Blood Products Laboratory, UK*.

12818-t

Hepatitis B Vaccines

Hepatitis B Virus Vaccine Inactivated (*U.S.P.*) is a sterile preparation consisting of a suspension of particles of hepatitis B surface antigen (HBsAg) isolated from the plasma of HBsAg carriers; it is treated so as to inactivate any hepatitis B virus and other viruses. It is adsorbed onto aluminium hydroxide. It should be stored at 2° to 8° and not be allowed to freeze.

Units

100 units of hepatitis B surface antigen *ad* subtype are contained in the lyophilised residue of 1 mL of a 1 in 300 dilution in PBS, BSA, and Na azide of HBsAg-positive serum in one ampoule of the first International Standard Preparation (1985).

Adverse Effects

As for vaccines in general, p.1155.

A report of severe cephalgia, fever, malaise, myalgia, profound asthenia, polyneuropathic and cholestatic symptoms, pyrosis, and constipation in a 59-year-old physician beginning 2 weeks after his first dose of hepatitis B vaccine.— G. B. Snider and S. A. Gogate (letter), *J. Am. med. Ass.*, 1985, *253*, 1260.

ALLERGY. Hypersensitivity, manifested by pruritus and urticaria, in a patient following the administration of a hepatitis B vaccine intradermally.— P. N. Goldwater (letter), *Lancet*, 1984, *2*, 1156. A further report of an urticarial reaction in a patient given the second dose of a hepatitis B vaccine.— L. De Silva and M. Rogers (letter), *Med. J. Aust.*, 1985, *143*, 323.

Acute exacerbation of eczema in a patient on the day after vaccination against hepatitis B; the pruritus experienced and the exacerbation of the eczema was probably due to the formaldehyde contained in the vaccine.— J. Ring (letter), *Lancet*, 1986, *2*, 522.

EFFECTS ON THE EYE. Acute posterior uveitis occurred in a patient after the booster doses of hepatitis B vaccines.— M. Fried *et al.* (letter), *Lancet*, 1987, *2*, 631.

EFFECTS ON THE LIVER. Abnormal liver function values in one person after hepatitis B vaccination.— V. Rajendran and A. P. Brooks, *Br. med. J.*, 1985, *290*, 1476.

EFFECTS ON THE NERVOUS SYSTEM. Polyneuropathy, marked by paraesthesias of all four extremities, in a patient after the second dose of a hepatitis B vaccine.— E. F. Ribera and A. J. Dutka (letter), *New Engl. J. Med.*, 1983, *309*, 614.

EFFECTS ON THE SKIN. A report of erythema multiforme associated with the administration of a hepatitis B vaccine.— S. D. Feldshon and R. E. Sampliner (letter), *Ann. intern. Med.*, 1984, *100*, 156.

Erythema nodosum provoked in one person by the use of a hepatitis B vaccine.— C. A. Di Giusto and J. D. Bernhard (letter), *Lancet*, 1986, *2*, 1042.

Precautions

As for vaccines in general, p.1156.

ALCOHOLISM. Evidence of a defective response to hepatitis B vaccine in alcoholic patients with histologically proven cirrhosis.— F. Degos *et al.* (letter), *Lancet*, 1983, *2*, 1498.

HIV-POSITIVE PERSONS. A study indicating impaired responsiveness of homosexual men with HIV antibodies to plasma-derived hepatitis B vaccine. Of 17 HIV-seropositive patients, 8 failed to develop detectable hepatitis B surface antibody within 3 months of the third dose of hepatitis B vaccine compared with only one of 18 seronegative patients. The results showed that the efficacy of hepatitis B vaccine, and other vaccines, needs to be studied in HIV-infected patients.— C. A. Carne *et al.*, *Br. med. J.*, 1987, *294*, 866. See also: S. C. Hadler *et al.*, *New Engl. J. Med.*, 1986, *315*, 209.

HIV TRANSMISSION. Data demonstrating that hepatitis B vaccines, especially those of the type derived from plasma, do not transmit the human immunodeficiency virus (HIV): C. E. Stevens *et al.* (letter), *New Engl. J. Med.*, 1985, *312*, 375; J. L. Dienstag (letter), *ibid.*, 376; G. Papaevangelou *et al.* (letter), *ibid.*; S. Kato *et al.* (letter), *J. Am. med. Ass.*, 1985, *254*, 53; J. L. Dienstag *et al.*, *ibid.*, 1064; H. Kessler *et al.* (letter), *Lancet*, 1985, *1*, 1506; L. Muylle *et al.* (letter), *New Engl. J. Med.*, 1986, *314*, 581; J. Desmyter *et al.*, *Br. med. J.*, 1986, *293*, 537; D. P. Francis *et al.*, *J. Am. med. Ass.*, 1986, *256*, 869.

OBESITY. A retrospective analysis of 194 persons who had received hepatitis B vaccine intramuscularly into the buttock indicated that obesity may be a predictor of a poor antibody response to vaccination.— D. J. Weber *et al.*, *J. Am. med. Ass.*, 1985, *254*, 3187. Further data suggesting that obesity may be a key predictor of a poor antibody response to the vaccine, irrespective of the injection site.— D. J. Weber *et al.*, *New Engl. J. Med.*, 1986, *314*, 1393.

Uses and Administration

Hepatitis B vaccines are used for active immunisation against hepatitis B infections. Two types of vaccine are available each containing hepatitis B surface antigen (HBsAg) adsorbed onto aluminium hydroxide. In one type of vaccine the surface antigen is obtained from plasma after purification and inactivation processes and in the second type the surface antigen is produced in yeast cells using recombinant DNA techniques.

Immunisation should be considered in persons at high risk of contracting hepatitis B. High-risk groups include: health care personnel, laboratory workers, or any other personnel who have direct contact with patients or their body fluids; patients requiring haemodialysis; contacts or consorts of carriers of hepatitis B; individuals who frequently change sexual partners; parenteral drug abusers; and some travellers to areas where hepatitis B is endemic. Immunisation should also be performed in infants born to women who are persistent carriers of hepatitis B surface antigen or infants born to women who are HBsAg-positive as a result of recent infection.

The basic immunisation schedule consists of 3 doses of a hepatitis B vaccine, with the second and third doses 1 and 6 months, respectively, after the first. Doses should be given intramuscularly, with the deltoid region being the preferred site in adults and the anterolateral thigh the preferred site in infants; the gluteal region (buttock) should not be used as efficacy may be reduced. In both the *UK* and *USA* each recommended dose of the plasma-derived vaccine, expressed in terms of content of the hepatitis B surface antigen, has been 10 ⟨mu⟩g for all those under 10 years of age and 20 ⟨mu⟩g for older children and adults; doses of 40 ⟨mu⟩g (given into different sites), have been recommended for use in immunocompromised and dialysis patients. For the recombinant vaccine recommended doses in the *UK*

have been 20 μg for all persons irrespective of age whereas in the *USA* a dose of 5 μg has been recommended for those under 10 years of age and a dose of 10 μg for older children and adults.
The recombinant vaccine has also been used where more rapid immunisation, for instance with travellers, is required. This schedule has involved the administration of the third dose 2 months after the initial dose with a further booster at 1 year.
For newborn infants at risk combined active and passive immunisation against hepatitis B is recommended. The first dose of vaccine should preferably be given within 12 hours of birth and at this time a single dose of hepatitis B immunoglobulin (200 units) should be administered into a different site. Additionally, in any patient in whom immediate protection is required, combined active and passive immunisation may be considered with a single dose of 500 units of hepatitis B immunoglobulin being the suggested dose for adults.
Hepatitis B vaccines have also been given in reduced doses of about 2 μg by the intradermal route.

Because hepatitis B virus still eludes reliable propagation *in vitro*, the preparation of a vaccine from virus grown in cell cultures is not possible. Current scientific information, however, indicates that the only hepatitis B antigen eliciting a protective immunity against infection with hepatitis B is the surface antigen (the 'Australia antigen') and inactivated vaccines using this hepatitis B surface antigen (HBsAg), purified from the plasma obtained from antigenaemic carriers of hepatitis B, have been prepared. It is essential in the manufacturing process of this type of vaccine to ensure, as far as possible, that inactivation of a wide range of infectious agents (including the human immunodeficiency virus) occurs and it is now recognised that safe and effective hepatitis B vaccines are being prepared using plasma as a starting material. Alternative methods for the production of hepatitis B surface antigen include recombinant DNA technology and chemical synthesis.— Thirty-fifth Report of a WHO Expert Committee on Biological Standardization, *Tech. Rep. Ser. Wld Hlth Org. No. 725*, 1985.. Details of hepatitis B vaccines made by recombinant DNA techniques in yeast.— Thirty-seventh Report of a WHO Expert Committee on Biological Standardization, *Tech. Rep. Ser. Wld Hlth Org. No. 760*, 1987.

Some reviews and discussions on hepatitis B and hepatitis B vaccines: M. A. Kane *et al.*, *Ann. intern. Med.*, 1985, *103*, 791; R. P. Perrillo, *ibid.*, 793; A. J. Zuckerman, *Br. med. J.*, 1985, *290*, 492; *Drug & Ther. Bull.*, 1985, *23*, 49; T. H. Flewett, *Br. med. J.*, 1986, *293*, 404; *Med. Lett.*, 1986, *28*, 118; E. A. Fagan and R. Williams, *Br. J. clin. Pract.*, 1987, *41*, 569; R. G. Finch, *Br. med. J.*, 1987, *294*, 197; *WHO Drug Inf.*, 1987, *1*, 119; *Lancet*, 1988, *1*, 875.

A study showing no significant difference in the quantity, quality, or specificity of the antibody response induced by a recombinant hepatitis B vaccine and a plasma-derived hepatitis B vaccine.— S. E. Brown *et al.*, *Br. med. J.*, 1986, *292*, 159.

Recommendations of the Advisory Committee on Immunization Practices for protection against viral hepatitis in the *USA* using plasma-derived hepatitis B vaccines (*Ann. intern. Med.*, 1985, *103*, 391; *J. Am. med. Ass.*, 1985, *254*, 29 and 197).
Persons at substantial risk of acquiring hepatitis B virus infection who are demonstrated or judged likely to be susceptible should undergo pre-exposure vaccination. Such groups of persons include: health-care workers; clients and staff of institutions for the mentally retarded; haemodialysis patients; homosexually active men; abusers of injectable drugs; recipients of certain blood products; and household and sexual contacts of hepatitis B virus carriers. Vaccination should also be considered in other groups such as heterosexually active persons with multiple partners and travellers to areas with high levels of endemic disease. Primary vaccination consists of three intramuscular doses, with the second and third doses given 1 and 6 months, respectively, after the first; children under 10 years should receive 10 μg per dose, adults and older children 20 μg per dose, and immunosuppressed patients and patients undergoing haemodialysis 40 μg per dose. The vaccine should only be given into the deltoid muscle in adults and children, or into the anterolateral thigh muscle in infants and neonates.
Prophylactic treatment to prevent hepatitis B infection after exposure to hepatitis B virus should be considered in the following: infants born to HBsAg-positive mothers; and sexual contacts of HBsAg-positive persons. For perinatal exposure 0.5 mL of hepatitis immunoglobulin should be administered intramuscularly within 12 hours of birth and the first dose of 0.5 mL (10 μg) of hepatitis B vaccine should be given concurrently but at a different site; the second and third doses of vaccine should be given 1 and 6 months, respectively, after the first dose. For sexual contacts of persons positive for HBsAg, a single dose of hepatitis immunoglobulin (0.06 mL per kg body-weight) is recommended if it can be given within 14 days of the last sexual contact. Prophylactic treatment, involving the use of immunoglobulin and/or vaccine, is also recommended after the accidental percutaneous or permucosal exposure to blood, the schedules varying according to the source of exposure and vaccination status of the exposed person.
Further recommendations were made by the Committee concerning the recombinant hepatitis B vaccine (*Ann. intern. Med.*, 1987, *107*, 353). The indications for this type of vaccine are the same as those for the plasma-derived product except that until a specially formulated product is available for haemodialysis patients the plasma-derived vaccine should be used. The doses of the recombinant vaccine recommended also differ to those for the plasma-derived product being 5 μg per dose for children under 10 years of age and 10 μg per dose for older children and adults.

ADMINISTRATION. *Intradermal.* An appraisal of hepatitis B vaccines administered intradermally. In most of the studies reported so far, the vaccine was administered intradermally to young healthy subjects in whom the antibody response is known to be good and was also administered by experienced staff under ideal conditions. Careful evaluation and review of the intradermal route (and of low-dose schedules) is essential and data are needed on the longer-term duration of induced antibody and on antibody specificity and affinity.— A. J. Zuckerman, *Lancet*, 1987, *1*, 435.

Favourable reports of the use of hepatitis B vaccines administered intradermally in reduced doses: K. D. Miller *et al.*, *Lancet*, 1983, *2*, 1454; G. Zoulek *et al.* (letter), *ibid.*, 1984, *1*, 568; P. N. Goldwater and D. G. Woodfield, *N.Z. med. J.*, 1984, *97*, 905; R. R. Redfield *et al.*, *J. Am. med. Ass.*, 1985, *254*, 3203; I. H. Frazer *et al.*, *Med. J. Aust.*, 1987, *146*, 242; W. L. Irving *et al.* (letter), *Lancet*, 1987, *2*, 561; S. Nagafuchi and S. Kashiwagi (letter), *ibid.*, 1522.

Intramuscular. A report of low immune responses among 130 healthy subjects given the recommended 3-dose course of hepatitis B vaccine by intramuscular injection into the gluteal region. Serum was generally collected during the second and third months after the last dose; antibody titres were suboptimal in 28 subjects and a further 34 were regarded as vaccine failures. It was suggested that the site of administration may have been responsible for the poor response and that the arm rather than the gluteal region should be used.— P. J. Pead *et al.* (letter), *Lancet*, 1985, *1*, 1152. Similar findings.— T. Ukena *et al.* (letter), *New Engl. J. Med.*, 1985, *313*, 579.

ADMINISTRATION TO DIALYSIS PATIENTS. Beneficial results with hepatitis B vaccines in the prevention of hepatitis B in patients undergoing haemodialysis: J. Desmyter *et al.*, *Lancet*, 1983, *2*, 1323; M. J. Alter *et al.*, *J. Am. med. Ass.*, 1985, *254*, 3200; E. Benhamou *et al.* (letter), *New Engl. J. Med.*, 1986, *314*, 1710.

PREGNANCY AND THE NEONATE. Some reviews and discussions concerning the use of hepatitis B immunoglobulins and hepatitis B vaccines for the prevention of perinatally transmitted hepatitis B infection: *Lancet*, 1984, *1*, 939; D. R. Snydman, *New Engl. J. Med.*, 1985, *313*, 1398.

Reports of clinical studies of differing schedules utilising hepatitis B immunoglobulins and hepatitis B vaccines for the prevention of hepatitis B infections in infants born to women positive for the hepatitis B surface antigen: R. P. Beasley *et al.*, *Lancet*, 1983, *2*, 1099; J. A. Mazel *et al.*, *Br. med. J.*, 1984, *288*, 513; V. C. W. Wong *et al.*, *Lancet*, 1984, *1*, 921; M. Piazzi *et al.*, *ibid.*, 1985, *1*, 949; C. E. Stevens *et al.*, *J. Am. med. Ass.*, 1987, *257*, 2612; H. M. H. Ip *et al.* (letter), *Lancet*, 1987, *2*, 1218.

Proprietary Preparations

Engerix B *(Smith Kline & French, UK)*. A hepatitis B vaccine containing hepatitis B surface antigen 20 μg/mL adsorbed onto aluminium hydroxide, and prepared by recombinant DNA technology.

H-B-Vax *(Merck Sharp & Dohme, UK)*. A hepatitis B vaccine containing hepatitis B surface antigen 20 μg/mL adsorbed on to alum.

16841-b

Herpes Simplex Vaccines

Several types of vaccines against herpes simplex virus types 1 and 2 have been developed and tried in small numbers of patients with both oral and genital herpes infections.

Reports of the use of herpes vaccines: A. Buchan *et al.*, *Vaccine*, 1985, *3*, 49 (type 1 viral vaccine; genital herpes); R. Cappel *et al.*, *J. med. Virol.*, 1985, *16*, 137 (type 2 viral vaccine; genital and oral herpes).

Proprietary Names and Manufacturers
Porton, UK.

7967-w

Influenza Vaccines

Inactivated Influenza Vaccine (*B.P.*) (Flu/Vac; Influenza Vaccine (Inactivated) (*Eur. P.*); Vaccinum Influenzae Inactivatum) is a sterile aqueous suspension of a suitable strain or strains of influenza virus types A and B, either individually or mixed, grown in the allantoic cavity of fertile incubated chick embryos, inactivated so that they are non-infective but retain their antigenic properties. Suitable strains of influenza virus are those recommended by the World Health Organization. It may also be supplied as an adsorbed vaccine (Flu/Vac/Ads). The vaccines should be stored at 2° to 8°, not be allowed to freeze, and be protected from light. The date after which they should no longer be used is subject to the strain of virus included. The *B.P.* directs that when Inactivated Influenza Vaccine is prescribed or demanded and the form is not stated, either the plain or adsorbed vaccine may be dispensed or supplied.

Inactivated Influenza Vaccine (Split Virion) (*B.P.*) (Flu/Vac/Split; Influenza Vaccine (Split Virion) (*Eur. P.*); Vaccinum Influenzae ex Virorum Fragmentis Praeparatum) is a sterile aqueous suspension of a suitable strain or strains of influenza virus types A and B, either individually or mixed, in which the integrity of the virus particles has been disrupted; the viruses are grown in the allantoic cavity of the fertile incubated chick embryos and inactivated so that they are non-infective but retain their antigenic properties. Suitable strains of influenza virus are those recommended by the World Health Organization. It may also be supplied as an adsorbed vaccine (Flu/Vac/Split/Ads). The vaccines should be stored at 2° to 8°, not be allowed to freeze, and be protected from light. The date after which they should no longer be used is subject to the strain of virus included. The *B.P.* directs that when Inactivated Influenza Vaccine (Split Virion) is prescribed or demanded and the form is not stated, either the plain or adsorbed vaccine may be dispensed or supplied.

Inactivated Influenza Vaccine (Surface Antigen) (*B.P.*) (Flu/Vac/SA) is a sterile aqueous suspension of the immunologically active haemagglutinin and neuraminidase surface antigens, of a suitable strain or strains of influenza virus types A and B either individually or mixed; the viruses are grown in the allantoic cavity of fertile incubated chick embryos and inactivated so that they are non-infective but retain their antigenic properties. Suitable strains of influenza virus are those recommended by the World Health Organization. It may also be supplied as an adsorbed vaccine (Flu/Vac/SA/Ads). The vaccines should be stored at 2° to 8°, not be allowed to freeze, and be protected from light. Under these conditions they may be expected to retain their potency for not less than one year from the date of the last determination of antigen content. The *B.P.* directs that when Inactivated Influenza Vaccine (Surface Antigen) is prescribed or demanded and the form is not stated, either the plain or the adsorbed vaccine may be dispensed or supplied.

Influenza Virus Vaccine (*U.S.P.*) is a sterile aqueous suspension of suitably inactivated influenza virus types A and B, either individually or combined, or virus sub-units prepared from the extra-embryonic fluid of virus-infected chick embryos. It should be stored at 2° to 8° and not be allowed to freeze.

The antigenic composition of the influenza virus.— G. C. Schild, *Postgrad. med. J.*, 1979, *55*, 87.

NOMENCLATURE OF STRAINS. Influenza virus strains were formerly classified into types A, B, and C on the basis of their ribonucleoprotein antigens. It was now established that the surface of the virus contained an additional virus-coded antigen, the neuraminidase, which was morphologically and immunologically distinct from the haemagglutinin and which underwent independent antigenic variation. A revised system of nomenclature, designed to be used from the beginning of 1972, was therefore proposed.— *Bull. Wld Hlth Org.*, 1971, *45*, 119. A revised system of nomenclature, based on double immunodiffusion reactions, should be used from the date of publication. The strain designation for influenza virus types A, B, and C contains: a description of the antigenic specificity of the nucleoprotein antigen (types A, B, or C) (an internal antigen, the matrix antigen, has also been described); the host of origin (if not man, including, if appropriate, the inanimate source); the geographical origin; the strain number; and the year of isolation; e.g. A/lake water/Wisconsin/1/79. For type A viruses the antigenic description follows (in parenthesis) including the antigenic character of the haemagglutinin (H1 up to H12) and the antigenic character of the neuraminidase (N1 up to N9). There is no provision for describing subtypes of B and C viruses. Recombination between viruses within a type is readily accomplished; the letter R should be added after the strain description to indicate the recombinant nature of the virus, e.g. A/Hong Kong/1/68(H3N2)R. In addition the strain of origin of the H and N antigens of antigenic hybrid recombinant A and B viruses should be given, e.g. A/BEL/42(H1)—Singapore/1/57(N2)R.— *Bull. Wld Hlth Org.*, 1980, *58*, 585.

Units

One unit of influenza virus haemagglutinin (type A) was contained in 0.093661 mg of the first International Reference Preparation (1967) (now discontinued).

Haemagglutinin activity, as measured by haemagglutination or chick-cell agglutination techniques, does not provide a reliable measure of the haemagglutinin content of influenza vaccines. The International Reference Preparation (1967) was discontinued and should not be used. A reference material would be made available annually containing the haemagglutinin and neuraminidase components of viruses causing prevalent infections and would be known as WHO Influenza Virus Reference Haemagglutinin, with the year of production in brackets. Potency should be expressed as the quantity of haemagglutinin expressed in mg per dose.— Twenty-ninth Report of a WHO Expert Committee on Biological Standardization, *Tech. Rep. Ser. Wld Hlth Org. No. 626*, 1978.

Adverse Effects

As for vaccines in general, p.1155.

Local and general reactions may occur but are usually mild. Fever and malaise sometimes occur and severe febrile reactions have been reported.

A 23-year-old nurse developed thrombotic thrombocytopenic purpura 2 to 3 weeks after receiving influenza vaccine (Flenzavax).— R. C. Brown *et al.* (letter), *Br. med. J.*, 1973, *2*, 303.

ALLERGY. Reports of allergic reactions.— U. N. Kumbar and B. Varkey (letter), *Can. med. Ass. J.*, 1977, *116*, 724; D. A. Moneret-Vautrin and J. P. Grilliat (letter), *Lancet*, 1977, *2*, 666; K. E. L. McColl *et al.* (letter), *Lancet*, 1978, *2*, 434.

EFFECTS ON THE CARDIOVASCULAR SYSTEM. A report of pericarditis following influenza vaccination.— J. J. Streifler *et al.*, *Br. med. J.*, 1981, *283*, 526.

EFFECTS ON THE MUSCLES. Acute polyarteritis leading to generalised muscle wasting and ultimate death was attributed to influenza vaccine.— C. F. P. Wharton and R. Pietroni (letter), *Br. med. J.*, 1974, *2*, 331.

EFFECTS ON THE NERVOUS SYSTEM. Brief details of 9 patients who developed neuropathy after administration of influenza vaccine; symptoms included encephalopathy (3), polyneuropathy, transverse myelopathy, radiculopathy, paraparesis, blurred vision due to occlusion of the central retinal vein, and paraesthesia and pain.— C. E. C. Wells, *Br. med. J.*, 1971, *3*, 755.

One patient developed paraesthesia of the arm and another vague annoying sensations in the arm following influenza vaccination.— T. W. Furlow (letter), *Lancet*, 1977, *1*, 253. Bilateral hand and forearm pain with paraesthesia developed in a patient 3 weeks after vaccination. Investigations led to a diagnosis of carpal-tunnel syndrome.— P. Hasselbacher (letter), *ibid.*, 551.

Four cases of meningo-encephalitis occurring after inoculation with influenza vaccine.— R. D. Gens and H. J. Beecham (letter), *New Engl. J. Med.*, 1978, *299*, 721. These 4 cases had been included in 38 reports of CNS inflammation received as a result of national surveillance following the vaccination of over 45 million people in the USA between October and December 1976.— I. C. Guerrero *et al.* (letter), *ibid.*, 1979, *300*, 565.

Bilateral optic neuritis associated with influenza vaccine.— H. D. Perry *et al.*, *Ann. Ophthal.*, 1979, *11*, 545.

Severe progressive polyneuropathy after trivalent influenza vaccination.— H. Fowler *et al.* (letter), *Lancet*, 1979, *2*, 1193.

Acute necrotic myelopathy, a disorder characterised by irreversible paraplegia or quadriplegia, sensory loss, and sphincter dysfunction, in a previously healthy 45-year-old man developed after influenza vaccination.— F. Graus *et al.*, *Lancet*, 1987, *1*, 1311.

Guillain-Barré syndrome. Comment on the Guillain-Barré syndrome associated with influenza vaccination. In 1976 a limited outbreak of influenza in the *USA* caused by a virus closely resembling the swine influenza virus led to the use of a killed swine influenza virus vaccine. After about 45 million doses of the vaccine had been administered the vaccination programme ceased because there was some evidence of a temporal association between vaccination and the onset of a paralytic polyneuropathy of the Guillain-Barré type. An epidemiologic and clinical evaluation of these cases indicates that there was a definite link between vaccination and the onset of the syndrome with extensive paralysis but no association with the onset of limited motor lesions. Influenza virus vaccines which lack a swine influenza virus component seem not to raise the risk of paralysis above background levels.— *Lancet*, 1984, *2*, 850.

Some case reports of the Guillain-Barré syndrome in patients after administration of vaccines without a swine influenza virus component: R. S. G. Knight *et al.* (letter), *Lancet*, 1984, *1*, 394 (2 patients); J. B. Winer *et al.* (letter), *ibid.*, 1182 (2 patients).

Further references to the Guillain-Barré syndrome and influenza immunisation using vaccines with a swine influenza virus component: *Br. med. J.*, 1977, *1*, 1373; P. M. Boffey, *Science*, 1977, *195*, 155; L. B. Schonberger *et al.*, *Am. J. Epidem.*, 1979, *110*, 105.

Multiple sclerosis. Analysis indicating there was no association between the use in the *USA* during 1976 of influenza vaccines containing a swine virus component and the development of multiple sclerosis.— L. T. Kurland *et al.*, *J. Am. med. Ass.*, 1984, *251*, 2672.

Precautions

As for vaccines in general, p.1156.

A patient who had recovered from a single attack of retrobulbar neuritis received an injection of influenza vaccine 7 years later and soon afterwards became blind and quadriplegic. It was suggested that patients who had had a demyelinating disease should not receive vaccines.— J. Rabin (letter), *J. Am. med. Ass.*, 1973, *225*, 63.

Progression of renal disease in Henoch-Schönlein purpura after influenza vaccination.— I. Damjanov and J. A. Amato (letter), *J. Am. med. Ass.*, 1979, *242*, 2555.

ASTHMA. A study in 28 subjects revealed no evidence for the asthmagenicity of influenza vaccination.— B. G. Campbell and R. L. Edwards, *Med. J. Aust.*, 1984, *140*, 773. A similar study showing influenza vaccination was well tolerated by a group of patients with moderately severe asthma.— M. K. Albazzaz *et al.*, *Br. med. J.*, 1987, *294*, 1196.

INTERACTIONS. For the effect of influenza vaccination on some other drugs see under phenytoin sodium (p.409), theophylline hydrate (p.1530), and warfarin sodium (p.347).

SYSTEMIC LUPUS ERYTHEMATOSUS. A number of studies demonstrated that influenza vaccination did not cause undue exacerbations of systemic lupus erythematosus, although patients with the severe form were not studied. G.W. Williams *et al.* (*Ann. intern. Med.*, 1978, *88*, 729) recorded low antibody titres after immunisation and suggested that protection might be poor but double immunisation carried out by R. Brodman *et al.* (*Ann. intern. Med.*, 1978, *88*, 735) produced similar antibody responses in 37 patients as in 42 controls. Other studies found no overall difference in antibody response in vaccinated patients and controls (S.C. Ristow *et al.*, *Ann. intern. Med.*, 1978, *88*, 786; J.S. Louie *et al.*, *ibid.*, 790). Immunosuppressant therapy did not appear to affect the response.— E. V. Hess and B. Hahn, *Ann. intern. Med.*, 1978, *88*, 833. Criticism.— L. F. Ayvazian (letter), *ibid.*, 1979, *90*, 127.

Uses and Administration

Influenza vaccines are used for active immunisation against influenza.

Three types of the influenza virus occur, types A, B, and C, although type C is considered to be relatively unimportant. Epidemic influenza is usually caused by the type A influenza virus. Outbreaks of influenza due to the type A virus occur in most years whilst those due to the type B virus tend to occur at intervals of several years. Influenza A viruses are antigenically labile with the principal surface antigens, the haemagglutinin and neuraminidase, undergoing antigenic changes. Major changes (antigenic shifts) in these surface antigens of the influenza A virus occur periodically and are responsible for the emergence of the sub-types of virus which may cause pandemic influenza; more minor changes (antigenic drift) occur more frequently and are responsible for the interpandemic outbreaks of influenza.

The formulation and composition of influenza vaccines is therefore constantly reviewed with changes made to accomodate the antigenic shifts and drifts of the influenza virus. Recommendations concerning the antigenic nature of influenza vaccines are made annually by the World Health Organization. Currently, influenza vaccines are of the inactivated type and may be available in three forms, as a whole-virus vaccine, as a split-virus vaccine, or as a surface-antigen vaccine.

Influenza vaccination is recommended for persons considered to be at special risk, such as patients with chronic cardiac disease, chronic pulmonary disease, chronic renal disease, or diabetes, patients receiving immunosuppressive therapy, and residents in closed institutions. Influenza vaccines are administered by deep subcutaneous injection or intramuscular injection. In the *UK* they are generally given in the autumn as a single dose, but a second dose after 4 to 6 weeks is suggested for children aged 4 to 13 years, who will not have been exposed naturally to prevalent strains; influenza vaccines are not recommended in the *UK* for children under 4 years of age.

A discussion of the development and use of influenza vaccines.— D. A. J. Tyrrell *et al.*, *Bull. Wld Hlth Org.*, 1981, *59*, 165.

Some general reviews on influenza and influenza vaccination: *Lancet*, 1986, *2*, 372; G. L. Ada, *Med. J. Aust.*, 1987, *146*, 509; *Drug & Ther. Bull.*, 1987, *25*, 75.

Recommendations of the Advisory Committee on Immunization Practices concerning the prevention and control of influenza in the *USA* (*Ann. intern Med.*, 1987, *107*, 521; *J. Am. med. Ass.*, 1987, *258*, 593). Influenza vaccination is recommended for high-risk persons 6 months of age or older and for their medical-care providers or household contacts and also for children and teenagers receiving long-term aspirin therapy (because of the risk of Reye's syndrome following influenza infection). High-risk groups include adults and children with chronic disorders of the cardiovascular or pulmonary systems and residents of nursing homes.

Proprietary Preparations

Fluvirin *(Servier, UK)*. Inactivated Influenza Vaccine (Surface Antigen) (*B.P.*).

Influvac Sub-Unit *(Duphar, UK)*. Inactivated Influenza Vaccine (Surface Antigen) (*B.P.*).

MFV-Ject *(Merieux, UK)*. Inactivated Influenza Vaccine (Split Virion) (*B.P.*).

16872-e

Leishmaniasis Vaccines

Field trials have been performed using vaccines containing *Leishmania* spp. in an attempt to prevent cutaneous leishmaniasis.

Some reports of field trials of leishmaniasis vaccines: W. Mayrink *et al.* (letter), *Trans. R. Soc. trop. Med. Hyg.*, 1978, *72*, 676; M. S. Green *et al.*, *ibid.*, 1983, *77*, 152; W. Mayrink *et al.* (letter), *ibid.*, 1986, *80*, 1001; L. Monjour *et al.* (letter), *Lancet*, 1986, *1*, 1490.

16874-y

Leprosy Vaccines

Vaccines against leprosy have included those using *Mycobacterium leprae* as well as other mycobacteria and three vaccine field trials are reported to be in progress.

Reviews of the development of leprosy vaccines: S. K. Noordeen and H. Sansarricq, *Bull. Wld Hlth Org.*, 1984, *62*, 1; S. K. Noordeen, *Lepr. Rev.*, 1985, *56*, 1; *Lancet*, 1987, *1*, 1183.

7969-l

Leptospira Antisera

Leptospira Antiserum (*B.P.C. 1973*) (Leptospira Icterohaemorrhagiae Antiserum; Lep/Ser) is a native serum, or a preparation from native serum, containing the antibodies that give a specific protection against strains of *Leptospira icterohaemorrhagiae*. It should be stored at 2° to 10°, not be allowed to freeze, and be protected from light.

Adverse Effects and Precautions

As for antisera in general, p.1155.

Uses and Administration

Leptospira antiserum was formerly used in the treatment of spirochaetal jaundice (Weil's disease), mainly as an adjuvant to chemotherapy. Intravenous administration was used in severe cases with intramuscular administration being employed in patients less severely affected.

16882-y

Malaria Vaccines

Prototype malarial vaccines against the sporozoite and merozoite stage of *Plasmodium falciparum* have been developed and field trials are reported to be under consideration.

Reviews and discussions concerning the prospects for malaria vaccines: *Bull. Wld Hlth Org.*, 1984, *62*, 715; *ibid.*, 1986, *64*, 185; L. H. Miller, *New Engl. J. Med.*, 1986, *315*, 640; L. -J. Bruce-Chwatt, *Lancet*, 1987, *1*, 371; K. Marsh, *Archs Dis. Childh.*, 1988, *63*, 468.

Reports and comments concerning the use of malaria vaccines in human volunteers: S. L. Hoffman *et al.*, *New Engl. J. Med.*, 1986, *315*, 601; W. R. Ballou *et al.*, *Lancet*, 1987, *1*, 1277; D. I. Grove (letter), *ibid.*, *2*, 220; D. A. Herrington *et al.* (letter), *Nature*, 1987, *328*, 257.

1236-t

Measles Immunoglobulins

Measles Immunoglobulin (*B.P.*) (Antimeasles Immunoglobulin Injection; Human Measles Immunoglobulin (*Eur. P.*); Immunoglobulinum Humanum Morbillicum) is a liquid or freeze-dried preparation containing immunoglobulins, mainly immunoglobulin G (IgG). It is obtained from plasma or serum containing specific antibodies against the measles virus. Normal Immunoglobulin may be added. Measles Immunoglobulin is prepared in the same manner as Normal Immunoglobulin (see p.1170) except that pooled material may be from fewer than 1000 donors. It contains not less than 50 units per mL. The liquid preparation should be stored, protected from light, in a sealed, colourless, glass container at a temperature of 2° to 8°. Under these conditions it may be expected to retain its potency for 3 years. The freeze-dried preparation should be stored, protected from light, under vacuum or under an inert gas; the *B.P.* specifies storage at a temperature of 2° to 8° whereas the *Eur. P.* specifies a temperature not exceeding 25°. Under these conditions it may be expected to retain its potency for 5 years.

Units

10 units of anti-measles serum, human are contained in 93.8 mg of dried human serum in one ampoule of the first International Reference Preparation (1964).

Adverse Effects and Precautions

As for immunoglobulins in general, p.1155.

Uses and Administration

Measles immunoglobulins may be used for passive immunisation against measles. They have been used to prevent or modify measles in susceptible persons who have been exposed to infection.

7976-e

Measles Vaccines

Measles Vaccine, Live (*B.P.*) (Meas/Vac (Live); Measles Vaccine (Live) (*Eur. P.*); Vaccinum Morbillorum Vivum) is a preparation of a suitable live modified (attenuated) strain of measles virus grown in cultures of chick-embryo cells or other approved cell cultures. It is prepared immediately before use by reconstitution from the dried vaccine. It does not contain any added antimicrobial preservative. The dried vaccine should be stored at 2° to 8°, not be allowed to freeze, and be protected from light. Under these conditions it may be expected to retain its potency for not less than 12 months from the date of the last determination of the virus titre.

Measles Virus Vaccine Live (*U.S.P.*) is a bacterially sterile freeze-dried preparation of a suitable live strain of measles virus grown in cultures of chick-embryo cells. It contains not less than the equivalent of 1000 TCID50 in each immunising dose, and may contain suitable antimicrobial agents. It should be stored at 2° to 8° and be protected from light.

Adverse Effects

As for vaccines in general, p.1155.

Fever and skin rashes occur frequently following the administration of measles vaccines. The fever generally starts 5 to 10 days after the injection and lasts for about 1 or 2 days. Conjunctivitis, coryza, pharyngitis, and cough may also occur. More serious effects reported after the use of the vaccine include convulsions, encephalitis, and thrombocytopenic purpura.

General reactions occurred in 32%, and were severe in 6%, of 50 children vaccinated with live measles vaccine, but there were no serious complications.— J. E. Miller and B. Harding-Cox, *Practitioner*, 1969, *203*, 352.

Some brief comments on side-effects and adverse reactions to measles vaccines made by the Advisory Committee on Immunization in the *USA* (*J. Am. med. Ass.*, 1987, *258*, 890). An excellent safety record of measles vaccines has been indicated by the experience gained through the use of more than 160 million doses up to 1986. Fever (temperature of 39.4° or more) may develop in 5 to 15% of vaccinees beginning about the fifth day after vaccination and usually lasts several days. Transient rashes have been reported in about 5% of vaccinees. Central nervous system disorders, including encephalitis and encephalopathy, have been reported with a frequency of less than one case per million doses administered. The incidence of encephalitis or encephalopathy following vaccination is lower than the incidence-rate of encephalitis of unknown origin suggesting that such events following vaccination may be only temporally related to, rather than due to, vaccination.

ATYPICAL MEASLES. A brief comment on the atypical-measles syndrome, a syndrome which has occurred in persons vaccinated against measles, but particularly in those in whom a killed measles vaccine was used, when later exposed to the natural infection. Reports that it has been described as arising in people who have had the live vaccine, if confirmed, are disturbing. Atypical measles seems unlikely to arise very often after the attenuated vaccine but as the years pass and immunity begins to wane the possibility must be kept in mind.— *Lancet*, 1979, *1*, 962.

Reports of atypical measles in persons who had previously received live measles vaccines: M. Chatterji and V. Mankad, *J. Am. med. Ass.*, 1977, *238*, 2635; E. M. Nichols, *Am. J. publ. Hlth*, 1979, *69*, 160; V. A. Fulginiti and R. E. Helfer, *J. Am. med. Ass.*, 1980, *244*, 804; J. A. M. Henderson and D. I. Hammond, *Can. med. Ass. J.*, 1985, *133*, 211.

EFFECTS ON THE NERVOUS SYSTEM. A 19-month-old girl developed Guillain-Barré syndrome 5 days after being given live measles and rubella vaccine; after 4 days of progressive weakness motor function returned to normal over the following 8 weeks; a second 10-month-old child became similarly ill after receiving live measles vaccine as well as vaccination against polio, diphtheria, pertussis and tetanus, and she too recovered.— C. Grose and I. Spigland, *Am. J. Med.*, 1976, *60*, 441.

A review of 375 cases of subacute sclerosing panencephalitis occurring in the *USA* suggested that live measles vaccine might be implicated in this condition. However, the risk from vaccination appeared less than the risk from measles and since the introduction of measles vaccination there had been a decline in the incidence of subacute sclerosing panencephalitis.— J. F. Modlin *et al.*, *Pediatrics*, 1977, *59*, 505.

Mention that two studies in the *UK* (Measles Vaccine Committee of the Medical Research Council, *Br. med. J.*, 1966, *1*, 441; C.L. Miller, *Practitioner*, 1982, *226*, 535) found an incidence of about 1 in 1000 for febrile convulsions occurring between the fifth and eleventh days after measles vaccination in children aged one to two years.— C. L. Miller (letter), *Lancet*, 1983, *2*, 215.

A review of suspected neurological reactions to measles vaccine in Canada over the period 1965-76 revealed that the overall rate of encephalitis reported was 1.79 cases per million doses distributed and of convulsions 8.46 per million.— F. White (letter), *Lancet*, 1983, *2*, 683.

Precautions

As for vaccines in general, p.1156.

Although it has been stated that care is necessary in administering measles vaccine to persons with allergic disorders, allergy to hens' eggs is no longer considered to be a contra-indication except in individuals with a history of anaphylactoid reactions to egg ingestion.

In the *UK* it was formerly recommended that children with a personal history of convulsions or those whose parents or siblings have a history of idiopathic epilepsy should receive measles vaccine but simultaneously with a specially diluted human normal immunoglobulin; it is now, however, recommended that such children be vaccinated in the same manner as normal healthy children but that suitable prophylactic treatment

against febrile convulsions be undertaken.
Measles vaccination may temporarily reduce the reaction to tuberculin and other skin tests.

Uses and Administration

Measles vaccines may be used for active immunisation against measles. Vaccination against measles in the *UK* and *USA* is normally performed in infants aged 12 months or more using a combined measles, mumps, and rubella vaccine (see below) but a single-antigen measles vaccine may be employed when vaccination against mumps or rubella is not indicated.

In the *UK* single-antigen measles vaccines prepared either from the Schwarz strain or the Moraten strain (more attenuated line derived from Enders' attenuated Edmonston strain) of the measles virus have been employed. Both have been given to children during the second year of life in a dose of 0.5 mL (not less than 1000 TCID50) by subcutaneous or intramuscular injection.

Measles vaccines are not generally recommended for children below the age of 1 year in whom maternal antibodies might prevent a response; however, in many developing countries the risk of measles is considered to pose such a threat to the health of infants that vaccination at about 9 months of age is recommended. Immunisation against measles forms part of the World Health Organization's Expanded Programme on Immunization (see p.1156).

Single-antigen measles vaccines may also be used for prophylaxis after exposure to measles provided they are given within 72 hours of contact.

Some general reviews and discussions on immunisation policies against measles: N. D. Noah, *Br. med. J.*, 1984, *289*, 1476; *Lancet*, 1986, *2*, 671; T. Smith, *Br. med. J.*, 1987, *294*, 989; *Lancet*, 1987, *2*, 78.

Recommendations of the Advisory Committee on Immunization Practices concerning the prevention of measles in the *USA* (*J. Am. med. Ass.*, 1987, *258*, 890). All vaccines containing measles virus are recommended for use at 15 months of age under routine conditions and a combined measles, mumps, and rubella vaccine is the vaccine of choice for routine vaccination programmes. A single dose of either a monovalent or combination product should be given subcutaneously in the volume specified by the manufacturer. If a measles vaccine is given on or after the first birthday there is no need for a further booster dose but those who received the vaccine before their first birthday should be revaccinated. Persons who, in the past, received an inactivated measles vaccine should also be revaccinated with the current live vaccine. It is considered that the benefits of measles immunisation in children with a personal or family history of convulsions greatly outweigh the risks and that such children should be vaccinated in the same way that children without such histories are vaccinated.

Results of a 21-year follow-up of persons vaccinated with a Schwarz strain of live measles vaccine indicated a high level of protection against measles had been provided throughout the period of study.— C. Miller, *Br. med. J.*, 1987, *295*, 22.

Some clinical studies assessing the response to measles vaccination in infants of differing ages: S. Wu *et al.*, *J. biol. Stand.*, 1982, *10*, 197 (China: 4 months and over); P. W. de Haas *et al.*, *Trans. R. Soc. trop. Med. Hyg.*, 1983, *77*, 267 (Tanzania: 7 months and over); D. L. Heymann *et al.*, *Lancet*, 1983, *2*, 1470 (Cameroon: 6 months and over); F. L. Black *et al.*, *Bull. Wld Hlth Org.*, 1984, *62*, 315 (Brazil: 9 months and over); N. A. Halsey *et al.*, *New Engl. J. Med.*, 1985, *313*, 544 (Haiti: 6 months and over).

VACCINE DEVELOPMENT. Some references to newer measles vaccines in development and/or new methods of administration: A. B. Sabin *et al.* (letter), *Lancet*, 1982, *2*, 604 (inhalation: Edmonston-Zagreb or Schwarz strains); A. B. Sabin *et al.*, *J. Am. med. Ass.*, 1983, *249*, 2651 (inhalation: Edmonston-Zagreb or Schwarz strains); A. B. Sabin *et al.*, *ibid.*, 1984, *251*, 2363 (inhalation: Edmonston-Zagreb or Schwarz strains); H. C. Whittle *et al.*, *Lancet*, 1984, *2*, 834 and 1290 (intradermal, subcutaneous, or inhalation: Edmonston-Zagreb strain); R. Vlatkovic *et al.* (letter), *ibid.*, 1985, *1*, 520 (intranasal: Edmonston-Zagreb strain); J. F. de Castro *et al.*, *J. Am. med. Ass.*, 1986, *256*, 714 (subcutaneous or inhalation: Edmonston-Zagreb or Schwarz strains); S. Khanum *et al.*, *Lancet*, 1987, *1*, 150 (subcutaneous or inhalation: Edmonston-Zagreb or Schwarz strains); H. C. Whittle *et al.*, *ibid.*, 1988, *1*, 963 (subcutaneous: Edmonston-Zagreb or Schwarz strains).

Reports of the use of an Edmonston-Zagreb measles vaccine subcutaneously in young infants of 4 months of age or more.— P. Aaby *et al.*, *Lancet*, 1988, *2*, 809; H. Whittle *et al.*, *ibid.*, 811.

Proprietary Preparations

Attenuvax *(Morson, UK)*. A live measles vaccine derived from the Enders' attenuated Edmonston strain.

Mevilin-L *(Evans Medical, UK)*. Measles Vaccine, Live (*B.P.*) derived from the Schwarz strain.

Rimevax *(Smith Kline & French, UK)*. Measles Vaccine, Live (*B.P.*) derived from the Schwarz strain.

7971-g

Measles and Mumps Vaccines

Measles and Mumps Virus Vaccine Live (*U.S.P.*) is a bacterially sterile preparation of a suitable live strain of measles virus and a suitable live strain of mumps virus. It may contain suitable antimicrobial agents. Each labelled dose provides an immunising dose of each component. It should be stored at 2° to 8° and be protected from light.

Adverse Effects and Precautions

As for vaccines in general, p.1155.
See also under measles vaccines, above, and mumps vaccines, below.

Uses and Administration

Measles and mumps vaccines may be used for active immunisation against measles and mumps. Vaccination against measles and mumps is normally performed in infants aged 12 months or more using a combined measles, mumps, and rubella vaccine (see below) but the bivalent measles and mumps vaccine may be employed when vaccination against rubella is not indicated.

Two types of vaccine have been used. One is prepared from the Moraten strain of measles virus (a more attenuated line of measles virus derived from Enders' attenuated Edmonston strain) grown in chick embryo cells and the Jeryl Lynn (B level) strain of mumps virus also grown in chick embryo cells; it contains not less than 1000 and 5000 TCID50 for each component respectively in each dose. It may be given in a single dose by subcutaneous injection to infants of 15 months of age or more or to other susceptible children or adults considered to be at risk; it has been suggested that if children were vaccinated when under 12 months of age they should receive a second dose after reaching 15 months of age. The second type of vaccine is prepared from the attenuated Schwarz strain of measles virus and the attenuated Urabe Am 9 strain of mumps virus, both grown in chick embryo cells; it contains not less than 1000 and 20 000 TCID50 for each component respectively in each 0.5-mL dose. It may be given in a single dose of 0.5 mL by subcutaneous injection to infants of 12 months of age or more or to other susceptible children or adults considered to be at risk; again it has been suggested that if children were vaccinated when under 12 months of age they should receive a second dose after reaching 12 months of age.

Proprietary Preparations

A measles and mumps vaccine is available on a named-patient basis from *Smith Kline & French, UK*.

7972-q

Measles and Rubella Vaccines

Measles and Rubella Virus Vaccine Live (*U.S.P.*) is a bacterially sterile preparation of suitable live strains of measles virus and live rubella virus. It may contain suitable antimicrobial agents. Each labelled dose provides an immunising dose of each component. It should be stored at 2° to 8° and be protected from light.

Adverse Effects and Precautions

As for vaccines in general, p.1155.
See also under measles vaccines, above, and rubella vaccines, p.1177.

Uses and Administration

Measles and rubella vaccines may be used for active immunisation against measles and rubella. Vaccination against measles and rubella is normally performed in infants aged 12 months or more using a combined measles, mumps, and rubella vaccine (see below) but the bivalent measles and rubella vaccine may be employed when vaccination against mumps is not indicated.

A vaccine used in the *USA* is prepared from the Moraten strain of measles virus (a more attenuated line of measles virus derived from Enders' attenuated Edmonston strain) grown in chick embryo cells and the Wistar RA 27/3 strain of live attenuated rubella virus grown in human diploid cells; it contains not less than 1000 TCID50 of each component in each 0.5-mL dose. It may be given in a single dose of 0.5 mL by subcutaneous injection to infants of 15 months of age or more or to other susceptible children or adults considered to be at risk; it has been suggested that if children were vaccinated when under 12 months of age they should receive a second dose after reaching 15 months of age.

Proprietary Preparations

A live measles and rubella vaccine is available on a named-patient basis from *Merck Sharp & Dohme, USA*.

7973-p

Measles, Mumps, and Rubella Vaccines

Measles, Mumps, and Rubella Virus Vaccine Live (*U.S.P.*) is a bacterially sterile preparation of suitable live strains of measles virus, mumps virus, and rubella virus. It may contain suitable antimicrobial agents. Each labelled dose provides an immunising dose of each component. It should be stored at 2° to 8° and be protected from light.

Adverse Effects and Precautions

As for vaccines in general, p.1155.
See also under measles vaccines, above, mumps vaccines, below, and rubella vaccines, p.1177.

A double-blind placebo-controlled crossover study in 581 pairs of twins showing the vast majority of adverse reactions after administration of a measles, mumps, and rubella vaccine to be only temporally, and not causally, related to vaccination. The true frequency of side-effects was estimated to be between 0.5 and 4.0%, indicating that adverse reactions are much less common than was previously thought.— H. Peltola and O. P. Heinonen, *Lancet*, 1986, *1*, 939.

Uses and Administration

Measles, mumps, and rubella vaccines are used for active immunisation against measles, mumps, and rubella.

In the *UK* a combined vaccine prepared from the Schwarz strain of measles virus, the Urabe Am 9 strain of mumps virus, and the Wistar RA 27/3 strain of rubella virus is available. It is now recommended that all children receive a single dose of 0.5 mL of this vaccine by subcutaneous or intramuscular injection during the second year of life. It is also recommended that older children of 4 to 5 years of age, unless they have previously received this combined vaccine or have laboratory evidence of immunity to measles, mumps, and rubella, receive a single dose before school entry. The combined vaccine may also be used for prophylaxis after exposure to measles provided it is given within 72 hours of contact; it is not, however, considered to be effective for post-exposure prophylaxis against either mumps or rubella. Single-antigen rubella vaccines (see p.1177) continue to be recommended for use in unvaccinated girls of 10 to 14 years of age and non-immune women.

In the *USA* a combined vaccine prepared from the Moraten strain of measles virus (a more attenuated line of measles virus derived from Enders' attenuated Edmonston strain), the Jeryl Lynn (B level) strain of mumps virus, and the Wistar RA 27/3 strain of rubella virus is used. A single dose of 0.5 mL by subcutaneous injection is recommended for children at 15 months of age.

Schedules involving the administration of two doses of the combined vaccine, the first at about 15 to 18 months of age and the second at 6 to 12 years of age, have been introduced in some countries.

Some references to immunisation policies including combined measles, mumps, and rubella vaccines: B. Christenson *et al.*, *Br. med. J.*, 1983, *287*, 389 (two-dose schedule: study); P. A. Brunell *et al.*, *J. Am. med. Ass.*, 1983, *250*, 1409 (single-dose schedule: study); H. Peltola *et al.*, *Lancet*, 1986, *1*, 137 (two-dose schedule: study); *ibid.*, *2*, 671 (single- or two-dose schedule: discussion); N. D. Noah, *Br. med. J.*, 1987, *294*, 1270 (single- and two-dose schedule: discussion).

Proprietary Preparations

A measles (Schwarz strain), mumps (Urabe Am 9 strain), and rubella (RA 27/3 strain) vaccine is available from *Merieux, UK* and *Smith Kline & French, UK* (Pluserix).

7979-j

Meningococcal Vaccines

Meningococcal Polysaccharide Vaccine (*B.P.*, *Eur. P.*) (Neimen/Vac; Vaccinum Meningitidis Cerebrospinalis) consists of one or more purified polysaccharides obtained from suitable strains of *Neisseria meningitidis* group A, group C, group Y, and group W135; it may contain a single type of polysaccharide or any mixture of the types. It is prepared immediately before use by reconstitution from the stabilised dried vaccine with a suitable sterile liquid. The dried vaccine should be stored at 2° to 8°, not be allowed to freeze, and be protected from light. Under these conditions it may be expected to retain its potency for not less than 2 years.

Meningococcal Polysaccharide Vaccine Group A (*U.S.P.*) is a sterile preparation of the group-specific polysaccharide antigen from *Neisseria meningitidis* group A.

Meningococcal Polysaccharide Vaccine Group C (*U.S.P.*) is a sterile preparation of the group-specific polysaccharide antigen from *Neisseria meningitidis* group C.

Meningococcal Polysaccharide Vaccine Groups A and C Combined (*U.S.P.*) is a sterile preparation of meningococcal polysaccharide group A and C specific antigens (see above). All three *U.S.P.* vaccines are supplied as dried vaccines which are reconstituted before use with bacteriostatic sodium chloride injection containing thiomersal. The dried vaccines should be stored at 2° to 8° and the reconstituted vaccines should be used immediately after preparation, or within 8 hours if stored at 2° to 8°.

Adverse Effects and Precautions

As for vaccines in general, p.1155.

PREGNANCY AND THE NEONATE. A mixed meningococcal vaccine (A and C) was evaluated in pregnant women and infants during an epidemic of meningitis in Brazil. Antibodies were detected in the women and there was some placental transfer of antibody although this was irregular. Vaccination of children in the first 6 months of life was unsuccessful.— A. de A. Carvalho *et al.*, *Lancet*, 1977, *2*, 809.

Uses and Administration

Meningococcal vaccines are preparations of purified polysaccharide antigens from *Neisseria meningitidis* and may be monovalent containing the antigen of only one serotype of *N. meningitidis* or polyvalent containing antigens of two or more serotypes. Commonly available vaccines appear to be a bivalent vaccine from groups A and C and a tetravalent vaccine from groups A, C, Y, and W135. Their use is indicated in persons of 2 years of age or older at risk, in epidemic or endemic areas, of meningococcal disease caused by the specific serotypes contained in the vaccine. Vaccination may also be considered for persons travelling to countries where the disease is endemic, and as an adjunct to antibiotic prophylaxis for household contacts of persons with the disease.

The bivalent (groups A and C) and tetravalent (groups A, C, Y, and W135) vaccines contain in each 0.5-mL dose, 50 µg of each of the polysaccharide antigens. The recommended dose is a single injection of 0.5 mL given subcutaneously.

Some general reviews on meningococcal disease and its control with meningococcal polysaccharide vaccines: A. Galazka, *Bull. Wld Hlth Org.*, 1982, *60*, 1; M. L. Lepow and R. Gold, *New Engl. J. Med.*, 1983, *308*, 1158.

A comment that the meningococcus is the only bacterial cause of large-scale epidemics of meningitis and these are usually due to *Neisseria meningitidis* of groups A or C. These types of disease can be controlled by vaccination with material containing their group-specific capsular polysaccharide and a vaccine containing these groups along with those of groups Y and W135 is available. However, in interepidemic periods group B is the predominant serogroup causing disease and unfortunately the polysaccharide of this group is poorly immunogenic. Although there has been some progress with semisynthetic carbohydrate antigens as vaccines against group B meningococci the quest for a good vaccine continues.— *Lancet*, 1985, *2*, 929. Further references to group B meningococcal disease and its possible control with vaccines: W. D. Zollinger *et al.* (letter), *Lancet*, 1984, *2*, 166; M. R. Lifely and C. Moreno (letter), *ibid.*, 1986, *1*, 214; *ibid.*, *2*, 551.

Recommendations of the Immunization Practices Advisory Committee in the *USA* concerning the use of meningococcal vaccines (*Drug Intell. & clin. Pharm.*, 1985, *19*, 615). Routine vaccination of civilians with meningococcal polysaccharide vaccines is not recommended because the risk of infection in the *USA* is low, a vaccine against serotype B, the major cause of meningococcal disease in the *USA*, is not yet available, and a high proportion of meningococcal disease occurs in children too young to benefit from a vaccine. However, during an outbreak immunisation of children above the age of 5 years and of young adults with a vaccine representing the serogroups causing the disease may be warranted. Use of the bivalent vaccine (groups A and C) may also benefit some travellers to countries recognised as having hyperendemic or endemic disease. Routine immunisation with the tetravalent vaccine (groups A, C, Y, and W135), the formulation currently available in the *USA*, is recommended for particular high-risk groups, including individuals with terminal complement component deficiencies and those with anatomic or functional asplenia.

Studies showing a beneficial effect of various meningococcal vaccines in the prevention of meningitis: H. Peltola *et al.*, *New Engl. J. Med.*, 1977, *297*, 686 (group A vaccine); M. H. Wahden *et al.*, *Bull. Wld Hlth Org.*, 1977, *55*, 645 (group A vaccine); G. Jamba *et al.*, *ibid.*, 1979, *57*, 943 (group A vaccine); B. M. Greenwood and S. S. Wali, *Lancet*, 1980, *1*, 729 (groups A and C vaccine); I. Mohammed and K. Zaruba, *ibid.*, 1981, *2*, 80 (groups A and C vaccine); N. Binkin and J. Band, *ibid.*, 1982, *2*, 315 and 454.

Proprietary Preparations

Meningococcal polysaccharide vaccines are available on a named-patient basis from *Connaught, Canad.* (Group A, C, A and C, and A, C, Y, and W135), *Merieux, UK* (Group A and A and C), and *Smith Kline & French, UK* (Group A, A and C, and A, C, Y, and W135).

7982-s

Mumps Vaccines

Mumps Vaccine, Live (*B.P.*) (Mump/Vac (Live); Mumps Vaccine (Live) (*Eur. P.*); Vaccinum Parotitidis Vivum) is a preparation containing a suitable live modified strain of mumps virus (*Paramyxovirus parotitidis*) grown in cultures of chick-embryo cells or other suitable cells. It is prepared immediately before use by reconstitution from the dried vaccine. It does not contain any added antimicrobial preservative. The dried vaccine should be stored at 2° to 8°, not be allowed to freeze, and be protected from light. Under these conditions it may be expected to retain its potency for not less than 2 years.

Mumps Virus Vaccine Live (*U.S.P.*) is a bacterially sterile preparation of a suitable strain of mumps virus grown in cultures of chick-embryo cells. It contains not less than 5000 TCID50 in each immunising dose. It may contain suitable antimicrobial agents. It should be stored at 2° to 8° and be protected from light.

Adverse Effects and Precautions

As for vaccines in general, p.1155.

Unilateral nerve deafness and encephalitis have occured rarely.

Uses and Administration

Mumps vaccines may be used for active immunisation against mumps. Vaccination against mumps is normally performed in infants aged 12 months or more using a combined measles, mumps, and rubella vaccine (see above) but a monovalent mumps vaccine may be employed when vaccination against measles or rubella is not indicated. Mumps vaccines are not generally recommended for children below the age of 1 year in whom maternal antibodies might prevent a response.

In the *UK* and *USA* a vaccine prepared from the Jeryl Lynn (B level) strain of mumps virus and containing not less than 5000 TCID50 per 0.5-mL dose is used. It may be given in a single dose of 0.5 mL by subcutaneous injection to infants of 12 months of age or more or to other susceptible children or adults considered to be at risk; it has been suggested that if children were vaccinated when under 12 months of age they should receive a second dose after reaching 12 months of age.

Several strains of attenuated mumps virus have been developed for use in vaccines. The first to be developed, and that most often used, is the Jeryl Lynn strain, which is grown in chick-embryo cell cultures. By 1985, vaccines based on this strain had been given to nearly 50 million children and adults throughout the world. Seroconversion in at least 97% of children and 93% of adults has occurred irrespective of whether the mumps vaccine was given singly or in combination with measles and rubella vaccines. Vaccines based on the Leningrad-3 strain of attenuated mumps virus are produced in cell cultures of either Japanese quail embryo or chicken embryo and about 20 million doses have so far been used. The Urabe strain of attenuated live mumps vaccine is produced either in the amnion of embryonated hens' eggs or in chick-embryo cell cultures. By 1985 about 5 million persons had been immunised with the Urabe strain and its immunogenic properties are similar to those of the Jeryl Lynn strain. Two additional strains of attenuated mumps virus are the Hoshino and Torii strains, both grown in chick-embryo cell culture, but they have been less extensively used than the Jeryl Lynn, Leningrad-3, and Urabe strains.— Thirty-seventh Report of a WHO Expert Committee on Biological Standardization, *Tech. Rep. Ser. Wld Hlth Org. No. 760*, 1987, p.139.

Recommendations of the Advisory Committee on Immunization Practices concerning the use of mumps vaccine in the *USA* (*Ann. intern. Med.*, 1983, *98*, 192). Mumps vaccine is available both in monovalent form and in combinations such as rubella and mumps vaccine and as measles, mumps, and rubella vaccine. The combined measles, mumps, and rubella vaccine is the vaccine of choice and this should be used in all situations where mumps vaccine is to be used if the recipients are likely to be susceptible to measles or rubella also. Vaccination against mumps is recommended for all children at any age after 12 months. It is of particular value for children approaching puberty and adolescence who have not had mumps. It may also be valuable for adults, especially males, who have not had mumps although most adults are likely to have been infected naturally and generally may be considered to be immune. In infants younger than 12 months of age persisting maternal antibody may interfere with seroconversion and those vaccinated before their first birthday might benefit from revaccination after reaching 1 year of age.

Proprietary Preparations

Mumpsvax *(Morson, UK)*. A mumps vaccine prepared from the Jeryl Lynn (B level) strain of mumps virus which, when reconstituted, contains in each dose not less than 5000 TCID50.

1232-z

Normal Immunoglobulins

Normal Immunoglobulin (*B.P.*) (Normal Immunoglobulin Injection; Human Normal Immunoglobulin (*Eur.P.*); Immunoglobulinum Humanum Normale) is a liquid or freeze-dried preparation containing immunoglobulins, mainly immunoglobulin G (IgG); other proteins may be present. It is obtained from plasma or serum or from normal placentas frozen immediately after collection. The donors must be healthy, and as far as can be ascertained be free from detectable agents of infection transmissible by transfusion of blood or blood derivatives. It is prepared from pooled material from at least 1000 donors by a suitable technique known to yield a product that does not transmit infection and that, at a protein concentration of 16%, contains antibodies for at least two of which (one viral and one bacterial) an International Standard or Reference Preparation is available, the concentration of such antibodies being at least 10 times that of the original pooled material. It is prepared as a stabilised solution and sterilised by filtration. An antimicrobial preservative may be added, except when the preparation is to be freeze-dried. The liquid preparation should be stored, protected from light, in a sealed, colourless, glass container at a temperature of 2° to 8°. Under these conditions it may be expected to maintain its potency for 3 years. The freeze-dried preparation should be stored, protected from light, under vacuum or under an inert gas; the *B.P.* specifies storage at a temperature of 2° to 8° whereas the *Eur. P.* specifies a temperature not exceeding 25°. Under these conditions it may be expected to retain its potency for 5 years.

Immune Globulin (*U.S.P.*) is a sterile solution of globulins that contains many antibodies normally present in human adult blood. It is prepared from pooled material (approximately equal quantities of blood, plasma, serum, or placentas) from not fewer than 1000 donors. It contains 15 to 18% of protein, of which not less than 90% is gamma globulin. It contains glycine as a stabiliser, and a suitable preservative. It contains antibodies against diphtheria, measles, and poliomyelitis. It should be stored at 2° to 8°.

Adverse Effects and Precautions

As for immunoglobulins in general, p.1155.

ALLERGY. Repeated systemic allergic reactions in an 18-month-old infant to normal immunoglobulin given intramuscularly were eliminated when the preparation was given by intravenous infusion.— A. G. Peerless and E. R. Stiehm (letter), *Lancet*, 1983, *2*, 461.

Speculation that the IgE content of normal immunoglobulins may be responsible for allergic reactions.— P.-A. Tovo *et al.* (letter), *Lancet*, 1984, *1*, 458. Disagreement that IgE in commercial preparations may be responsible for the rare immediate or anaphylactoid reactions to unmodified IgG preparations.— A. C. Newland *et al.* (letter), *ibid.*, 1406.

A report of two patients experiencing several episodes of anaphylaxis after intravenous infusion of normal immunoglobulin. It was considered that the IgA content of the immunoglobulin may have caused the development of IgE anti-IgA antibodies and that these antibodies may be implicated in the pathogenesis of the anaphylactic reactions.— A. W. Burks *et al.*, *New Engl. J. Med.*, 1986, *314*, 560. Comments and correspondence generally disagreeing with the proposed mechanism of action involved in allergic reactions.— L. Hammarström and C. I. E. Smith (letter), *ibid.*, *315*, 519; R. Bookman (letter), *ibid;* I. Quinti *et al.* (letter), *ibid.* Reply.— A. W. Burks *et al.* (letter), *ibid.*, 520.

EFFECTS ON THE BLOOD. A report of a temporary reduction in platelet adhesiveness in an 8-year-old boy with acute idiopathic thrombocytopenic purpura given high doses of gammaglobulin intravenously. Despite treatment restoring the platelet count to normal, multiple subcutaneous haematomas occurred when the platelet adhesiveness was only 6% (normal 17-35%).— R. Ljung and I. M. Nilsson (letter), *Lancet*, 1985, *1*, 467.

Thrombotic events occurred in 4 elderly subjects with severe atherosclerotic disease receiving intravenous normal immunoglobulin for auto-immune thrombocytopenia; the events proved fatal in 3 of the patients. It was considered that a rising platelet count during therapy may represent a risk situation in patients with severe atherosclerotic disease.— R. K. Woodruff *et al.* (letter), *Lancet*, 1986, *2*, 217. A review of patients treated with normal immunoglobulin in Scotland indicated that there was no association with an excessive number of thrombotic events.— W. D. Frame and R. J. Crawford (letter), *ibid.*, 468.

A report of the use of normal immunoglobulin given intravenously to a pregnant woman causing ABO alloimmunisation resulting in ABO haemolytic disease of her newborn infant who required exchange transfusion. Analysis of the immunoglobulin used revealed the presence of IgG anti-A and anti-B antibodies and tests also suggested the presence of blood group A and B antigen.— M. Potter *et al.* (letter), *Lancet*, 1988, *1*, 932.

EFFECTS ON THE SKIN. A report of 3 women experiencing diffuse alopecia within 1 to 4 weeks of treatment with intravenous normal immunoglobulin.— D. Chan-Lam *et al.* (letter), *Lancet*, 1987, *1*, 1436.

Severe extensive eczema in an elderly woman after the administration of normal immunoglobulin intravenously.— C. Barucha and J. C. McMillan (letter), *Br. med. J.*, 1987, *295*, 1141.

Uses and Administration

Normal immunoglobulin is available as two distinct preparations and formulations. One type of injection containing about 15 or 16% of protein is used for passive immunisation, and sometimes also for hypogammaglobulinaemia, and should only be given intramuscularly; Normal Immunoglobulin (*B.P.*) and Immune Globulin (*U.S.P.*) are intended for intramuscular use only. The second type of preparation is formulated for intravenous administration and is used in disorders such as hypogammaglobulinaemia and idiopathic thrombocytopenic purpura; solutions generally contain about 3 to 6% of protein. Doses of normal immunoglobulin often appear confusing being expressed variously in terms of weight (protein content) or in terms of volume to be administered; the two do not always appear to correspond.

Normal immunoglobulin, being derived from the pooled plasma of blood donors, contains antibodies to viruses currently prevalent in the general population; in the *UK*, and also in some other countries, typical antibodies present include those against hepatitis A, measles, mumps, rubella, and varicella. Normal immunoglobulin, therefore, may be used to provide passive immunisation against such diseases.

For the pre-exposure prophylaxis against hepatitis A in travellers going to endemic areas doses recommended in the *UK* for intramuscular injection are: for short-term exposure of up to 2 months, 125 mg for children under 10 years of age and 250 mg for older children and adults; for longer-term exposure, 250 mg for children under 10 years of age and 500 mg for older children and adults. Alternative doses, expressed in terms of volume administered, have been 0.02 to 0.04 mL per kg body-weight for short-term exposure in both adults and children and 0.06 to 0.12 mL per kg for longer-term exposure. Normal immunoglobulin may also be used to control outbreaks of hepatitis A, the recommended dose for close contacts being 250 mg in those under 10 years of age and 500 mg in older children and adults.

It may also be used to prevent or possibly modify an attack of measles in children at special risk (such as those who are immunocompromised) but should be given as soon as possible after contact with measles. In the *UK* recommended doses, administered intramuscularly, for the prevention of an attack are 250 mg for those under 1 year of age, 500 mg for those aged 1 to 2 years, and 750 mg for those aged 3 years and over; to modify an attack, recommended doses are 100 mg for those under 1 year of age and 250 mg for older children. Alternatively, doses (expressed in terms of volume) of 0.2 to 0.25 mL per kg have been suggested to prevent an attack and 0.04 mL per kg to modify an attack.

For post-exposure protection against mumps, normal immunoglobulin may be used but its value is considered to be uncertain. Recommended doses in the *UK*, administered intramuscularly, are 250 mg for children up to 5 years of age, 500 mg for those 6 to 10 years of age, 750 mg for those 11 to 14 years of age, and 1 g for all older persons.

Normal immunoglobulin may reduce the likelihood of a clinical attack of rubella in pregnant women exposed to rubella but should be given as soon as possible after exposure. The recommended dose is 750 mg by intramuscular injection. A dose of 20 mL has also been suggested.

Normal immunoglobulin may also be used in the management of patients with agammaglobulinaemia or hypogammaglobulinaemia; the immunoglobulin is given to provide protection against infectious diseases that such patients may suffer. For the intramuscular type of preparation the usual initial dose, expressed in terms of volume, is 1.3 to 1.8 mL per kg body-weight in divided doses over 48 hours; the maximum recommended total initial dose is 60 mL. For maintenance, doses of 0.6 to 0.65 mL per kg may be given every 3 to 4 weeks. For intravenous infusion, the dose, expressed in terms of weight (protein content), is usually 100 to 300 mg per kg every 2 to 4 weeks. The initial infusion should always be given very carefully and slowly with gradual increases in the rate of administration.

Intravenous infusion of normal immunoglobulin is also employed to raise the platelet count in patients with idiopathic thrombocytopenic purpura. Doses of 400 mg per kg are given daily for 5 consecutive days with further doses of 400 mg per kg as required.

Mention that although immune plasma obtained from persons who have survived the infection has been used in the management of patients with viral haemorrhagic fevers such as Lassa fever, Ebola fever, Marburg disease, and Crimean-Congo fever, the efficacy of such treatment has not been established.— *Ann. intern. Med.*, 1984, *101*, 73.

A discussion of intravenous immunoglobulins as therapeutic agents.— E. R. Stiehm *et al.*, *Ann. intern. Med.*, 1987, *107*, 367.

AGRANULOCYTOSIS. A temporary return to normal of the granulocyte count was observed in a neonate with allo-immune agranulocytosis during therapy with high-dose intravenous normal immunoglobulin given because of the risk of serious infection developing. It was not, however, considered that this form of therapy should be employed in other types of non-immune neutropenias.— A. Fasth, *Archs Dis. Childh.*, 1986, *61*, 86.

APLASTIC ANAEMIA. Beneficial response in one patient with aplastic anaemia after the administration of normal immunoglobulin intravenously.— H. I. Atrah *et al.* (letter), *Lancet*, 1985, *2*, 339.

EPILEPSY. A report of the use of high-dose normal immunoglobulin administered intravenously in 16 patients with intractable childhood epilepsy. Response was poor in 8, a moderate improvement in electrical seizures without any clinical improvement occurred in 2, a marked improvement occurred in a further 2, and complete clinical and EEG remission was seen in the remaining 4 patients.— M. Ariizumi *et al.* (letter), *Lancet*, 1983, *2*, 162. A similar report of benefit with intravenous normal immunoglobulin in children with post-encephalitic seizures. Of the 8 children treated, 6 displayed signs of intrathecal immunoglobulin synthesis before treatment and it was only in these patients that improvement was noted.— P. Sandstedt *et al.* (letter), *Lancet*, 1984, *2*, 1154.

HAEMOLYTIC ANAEMIA. Case reports of beneficial responses to normal immunoglobulin in patients with auto-immune haemolytic anaemias: H. Oda *et al.*, *J. Pediat.*, 1985, *107*, 744; M. Pococco *et al.* (letter), *J. Pediat.*, 1986, *109*, 726.

HAEMOLYTIC DISEASE OF THE NEWBORN. A report of the use of high-dose intravenous normal immunoglobulin in an attempt to improve the foetal outcome in a woman with severe rhesus immunisation; long-term plasma exchange had been complicated by inadequate venous access. The immunoglobulin was given during the twenty-fifth week of the pregnancy and appeared to reduce anti-D concentrations in maternal blood for about 6 to 8 weeks. Despite maternal treatment the infant needed two exchange transfusions following birth by caesarean section at 35 weeks.— G. Berlin *et al.* (letter), *Lancet*, 1985, *1*, 1153. Comment that high-dose intravenous immunoglobulins had been used with encouraging results in the management of pregnant women with severe rhesus immunisation until plasma exchange became an available technique.— E. Rewald (letter), *ibid.*, *2*, 208.

For the use of anti-D immunoglobulins to prevent haemolytic disease of the newborn, see p.812.

HEPATITIS A. Recommendations of the Advisory Committee on Immunization Practices of the *USA* concerning protection against viral hepatitis (*Ann. intern. Med.*, 1985, *103*, 391).

Pre-exposure prophylaxis against hepatitis A is recommended for international travellers to developing countries if they will be eating in settings of poor or uncertain sanitation. A single dose of normal immunoglobulin of 0.02 mL per kg body-weight should be given intramuscularly if travel is for less than 2 months and 0.06 mL per kg should be given every 5 months if travel is prolonged.

For postexposure prophylaxis against hepatitis A a single dose of 0.02 mL per kg of normal immunoglobulin intramuscularly is recommended.

Discussion of the need of travellers to receive normal immunoglobulin as prophylaxis against hepatitis A and concluding that because many people already possess antibodies a screening policy should be implemented in order to reduce unnecessary immunisation.— J. H. Cossar and D. Reid, *Br. med. J.*, 1987, *294*, 1503. Agreement with a policy of selective screening.— G. Kudesia and E. A. C. Follett (letter), *ibid.*, *295*, 118.

HYPOGAMMAGLOBULINAEMIA. *Intravenous administration.* A comparison of normal immunoglobulin given intramuscularly and intravenously to 5 patients with hypogammaglobulinaemia and chronic bronchitis; doses were 25 mg per kg body-weight once weekly intramuscularly and 200 mg per kg every 18 days intravenously. Sputum volume and infection scores were significantly better during intravenous therapy and it was concluded that intravenous therapy should be considered for hypogammaglobulinaemic patients with severe chest disease and for those who cannot tolerate intramuscular injections.— A. So *et al.*, *Br. med. J.*, 1984, *289*, 1177.

A study indicating that home administration of normal immunoglobulin intravenously is both feasible and safe for patients with primary immunodeficiency diseases including hypogammaglobulinaemia.— H. D. Ochs *et al.* (letter), *Lancet*, 1986, *1*, 610.

A crossover study in 12 patients with hypogammaglobulinaemia and chronic lung disease indicating that doses higher than the conventional dose of 200 mg per kg body-weight intravenously of normal immunoglobulin provide better protection; a dose chosen should provide a serum-IgG concentration of 500 mg per 100 mL.— C. M. Roifman *et al.*, *Lancet*, 1987, *1*, 1075. Comment that these patients had severe lung disease and rather than using higher doses of immunoglobulin a more aggressive but conventional approach (drainage, physiotherapy, and antibiotics) to avoid infection is suggested.— P. E. Williams *et al.* (letter), *ibid.*, 1435.

Intraventricular administration. A report of a hypogammaglobulinaemic child with echovirus encephalitis unresponsive to intravenous immunoglobulin who was successfully treated with immunoglobulin via the intraventricular route.— K. Erlendsson *et al.*, *New Engl. J. Med.*, 1985, *312*, 351. Failure of intraventricular administration of normal immunoglobulin to eradicate echovirus encephalitis in a child with hypogammaglobulinaemia.— P. R. Johnson *et al.*, *ibid.*, *313*, 1546.

Subcutaneous administration. Some references to the use of normal immunoglobulin by subcutaneous infusion in patients with hypogammaglobulinaemia.— A. G. Ugazio *et al.* (letter), *Lancet*, 1982, *1*, 226; M. F. Leahy (letter), *ibid.*, 1986, *2*, 48.

INFECTION PROPHYLAXIS. A report of the use of normal immunoglobulin administered intramuscularly to neonates to prevent infection during an outbreak in a special-care baby unit caused by echovirus 11.— J. Nagington *et al.*, *Lancet*, 1983, *2*, 443. A similar report of the use of normal immunoglobulin to prevent the spread of echovirus 6 in a baby unit.— D. J. Carolane *et al.*, *Archs Dis. Childh.*, 1985, *60*, 674.

An open study involving 120 premature babies of 32 weeks' gestation or less and investigating whether treatment with intramuscular normal immunoglobulin could decrease the morbidity and/or mortality associated with infection found a substantial difference in the number of infective episodes between the group treated with immunoglobulin (22) and the control group (40) although the evidence did not suggest that treatment had decreased the susceptibility of the baby to infection.— S. P. Conway *et al.*, *Archs Dis. Childh.*, 1987, *62*, 1252.

KAWASAKI DISEASE. A study of the effect of high-dose intravenous immunoglobulin in children with Kawasaki disease (since the vasculitis is believed to be due to an over-exuberant immunological response) suggested that treatment provided an anti-inflammatory effect and prevented coronary aneurysm formation.— K. Furusho *et al.* (letter), *Lancet*, 1983, *2*, 1359. See also: K. Furusho *et al.*, *ibid.*, 1984, *2*, 1055.

Evidence after the use in one adult that intravenous immunoglobulin may speed recovery in Kawasaki disease.— P. Chavanet *et al.* (letter), *Lancet*, 1985, *2*, 1184.

Comparison of the efficacy of intravenous immunoglobulin plus aspirin with that of aspirin alone in reducing the frequency of coronary-artery abnormalities in children with acute Kawasaki syndrome. Immunoglobulin was given in a dose of 400 mg per kg body-weight daily for 4 consecutive days and all children received aspirin in high dosage for the first 14 days, thereafter the dose being reduced. After 2 weeks, coronary-artery abnormalities were present in 8% in the immunoglobulin group and in 23% in the aspirin-only group and after 7 weeks the respective figures were 4% and 18%. It was concluded that high-dose intravenous immunoglobulin is safe and effective in reducing the prevalence of coronary-artery abnormalities when given early in the course of Kawasaki syndrome.— J. W. Newburger *et al.*, *New Engl. J. Med.*, 1986, *315*, 341.

MEASLES. Data indicating the efficacy of normal immunoglobulin administered intramuscularly for the prophylaxis of measles in children being treated for acute lymphoblastic leukaemia who had been in contact with persons suffering from measles.— H. E. M. Kay and A. Rankin (letter), *Lancet*, 1984, *1*, 901.

In 17 children being treated for malignant disease who contracted measles, treatment including the use of immunoglobulin could not be shown to be effective in modifying or ameliorating the attack of measles.— J. Kernahan *et al.*, *Br. med. J.*, 1987, *295*, 15.

MYASTHENIA GRAVIS. Reports of beneficial responses to high-dose intravenous immunoglobulin in patients with myasthenia gravis: P. Gajdos *et al.* (letter), *Lancet*, 1984, *1*, 406; A. Fateh-Moghadam *et al.* (letter), *ibid.*, 848; G. Devathasan *et al.* (letter), *ibid.*, *2*, 809; G. Ippoliti *et al.* (letter), *ibid.*

PEMPHIGOID. Of 11 patients with bullous pemphigoid, a severe auto-immune disease, transient improvement occurred in 7 and longer-term improvement in 1 after the administration of intravenous normal immunoglobulin; no improvement was observed in 3 patients. It was considered that this form of therapy might be tried in association with other treatments.— W. Godard *et al.* (letter), *Ann. intern. Med.*, 1985, *103*, 965.

POLYMYOSITIS. Reversal of chronic polymyositis in one patient following the administration of intravenous normal immunoglobulin.— C. M. Roifman *et al.*, *J. Am. med. Ass.*, 1987, *258*, 513.

THROMBOCYTOPENIA. References to the use of high-dose intravenous normal immunoglobulin in idiopathic (auto-immune) thrombocytopenic purpura in adults and children: P. Imbach *et al.*, *Lancet*, 1981, *1*, 1228; B. Schmidt and J. Forster (letter), *ibid.*, 1982, *2*, 39; J. Fehr *et al.*, *New Engl. J. Med.*, 1982, *306*, 1254; P. Bierling *et al.* (letter), *ibid.*, *307*, 1150; D. Lehoczky and E. Kelemen (letter), *ibid;* A. C. Newland *et al.*, *Lancet*, 1983, *1*, 84; B. Rowbotham and R. L. Brearley (letter), *ibid.*, 410; P. G. Mori *et al.*, *Archs Dis. Childh.*, 1983, *58*, 851; R. R. Carroll *et al.*, *J. Am. med. Ass.*, 1983, *249*, 1748; R. A. Seeler (letter), *Lancet*, 1984, *1*, 961; P. Imbach *et al.*, *ibid.*, 1985, *2*, 464; R. W. Walker and W. Walker (letter), *ibid.*, 1011; H. Ekert (letter), *ibid.*, 1310; M. A. Baumann *et al.*, *Ann. intern. Med.*, 1986, *104*, 808; R. Mansberg and W. W. Coupland, *Med. J. Aust.*, 1987, *146*, 217; J. R. Leclerc *et al.*, *Can. med. Ass. J.*, 1987, *136*, 961.

A report of a response in one patient with thrombotic thrombocytopenic purpura to intravenous normal immunoglobulin.— P. Wong *et al.* (letter), New Engl. J. *Med.*, 1986, *314*, 385.

AIDS-associated. Reports of benefit after intravenous immunoglobulin in patients with immune thrombocytopenia associated with AIDS: J. F. Delfraissy *et al.* (letter), *Ann. intern. Med.*, 1985, *103*, 478; J. Ordi *et al.* (letter), *ibid.*, 1986, *104*, 282; Y. Laurian *et al.* (letter), *ibid.*, *105*, 146; M. Ellis *et al.* (letter), *J. Infect.*, 1986, *13*, 312.

Pregnancy and the neonate. As well as being used for idiopathic thrombocytopenic purpura in adults and children normal immunoglobulin has also been used for the management of auto-immune thrombocytopenia associated with pregnancy. Antenatal administration intravenously to the mother has in some cases been reported to be successful with regard to the newborn infant having either a normal platelet count or only mild transient thrombocytopenia that required no further treatment (G.R. Morgenstern *et al.*, *Br. med. J.*, 1983, *287*, 584; A.C. Newland *et al.*, *New Engl. J. Med.*, 1984, *310*, 261; V.L. Rose and L.I. Gordon, *J. Am. med. Ass.*, 1985, *254*, 2626; C.Pappas, *Lancet*, 1986, *1*, 389) whereas in some other cases (C. Pappas, *Lancet*, 1986, *1*, 389; S.V. Davies *et al.*, *ibid.*, 1098) antenatal therapy was less successful as the neonate also required immunoglobulin or other therapy after birth.

Proprietary Preparations

Gamimune N *(Cutter, UK)*. Normal immunoglobulin 5%, in vials of 10, 50, and 100 mL. For intravenous use.

Gammabulin *(Immuno, UK)*. Normal Immunoglobulin (*B.P.*) in vials of 2, 5, and 10 mL or as powder for reconstitution in vials containing 320 mg supplied with solvent. For intramuscular use.

Intraglobin *(Biotest, UK)*. Normal immunoglobulin, powder for reconstitution, in bottles of 250, 500 mg, and 2.5 g supplied with solvent. For intravenous use.

Kabiglobulin *(KabiVitrum, UK)*. Normal immunoglobulin 16% in ampoules of 2 and 5 mL. For intramuscular use.

Sandoglobulin *(Sandoz, UK)*. Normal immunoglobulin, powder for reconstitution, in packs containing 1, 3, and 6 g of protein supplied with solvent. For intravenous use.

A normal immunoglobulin is also available from *Blood Products Laboratory, UK*.

1237-x

Pertussis Immunoglobulins

Pertussis Immune Globulin (*U.S.P.*) is a sterile solution of globulins derived from the plasma of adult human donors who have been immunised with pertussis vaccine. It contains glycine as a stabilising agent, and a suitable preservative. It should be stored at 2° to 8°.

Adverse Effects and Precautions
As for immunoglobulin in general, p.1155.

Uses and Administration
Pertussis immunoglobulins may be used for passive immunisation against pertussis (whooping cough). They have been used to prevent or modify pertussis in susceptible persons who have been exposed to infection.

A brief comment that although the use of hyperimmune globulin or antibody in pertussis prophylaxis has wide acceptance there is no evidence of efficacy in well-controlled trials.— C. R. Manclark, *Bull. Wld Hlth Org.*, 1981, *59*, 9.

7985-l

Pertussis Vaccines

Pertussis Vaccine (*B.P., Eur. P.*) (Per/Vac; Whooping-cough Vaccine; Vaccinum Pertussis) is a sterile suspension, in a saline or other suitable solution isotonic with blood, of a suitable killed strain or strains of *Bordetella pertussis*. The estimated potency is not less than 4 units per dose which does not exceed 1 mL. It contains a suitable antimicrobial preservative.. It may also be supplied as an adsorbed vaccine (Per/Vac/Ads) adsorbed on aluminium hydroxide, aluminium phosphate, or calcium phosphate. *Eur. P.* includes the adsorbed vaccine as Pertussis Vaccine (Adsorbed); Vaccinum Pertussis Adsorbatum. It should be stored at 2° to 8°, not be allowed to freeze, and be protected from light. Under these conditions it may be expected to retain its potency for at least 2 years from the date of the last test for potency. The *B.P.* directs that when Pertussis Vaccine is prescribed or demanded and the form is not stated, either the plain or the adsorbed vaccine may be dispensed or supplied.

Pertussis Vaccine (*U.S.P.*) is a sterile bacterial fraction or suspension of killed *Bordetella pertussis* of a strain or strains selected for high antigenicity. It contains a preservative. It contains 12 protective units per immunising dose. It should be stored at 2° to 8° and not be allowed to freeze.

Pertussis Vaccine Adsorbed (*U.S.P.*) is a sterile bacterial fraction or suspension of killed *Bordetella pertussis* of a strain or strains selected for high antigenicity, precipitated or adsorbed by the addition of aluminium hydroxide or aluminium phosphate. It contains a preservative. It contains not less than 12 protective units per immunising dose. It should be stored at 2° to 8° and not be allowed to freeze.

Discussion of the varying US and WHO standards for pertussis vaccines.— J. Cameron (letter), *New Engl. J. Med.*, 1980, *303*, 157.

Units

46 units are contained in 25 mg of freeze-dried vaccine in one ampoule of the second International Standard Preparation (1980).

Adverse Effects

As for vaccines in general, p.1155.

Local reactions may occur at the site of injection of pertussis vaccines or pertussis-containing vaccines and administration may be followed by mild fever and irritability.

Severe reactions which have been reported include persistent screaming and generalised collapse but these effects were generally associated with an earlier type of vaccine and the reactions are stated to be rarely observed with the currently available vaccines.

Rare neurological adverse reactions have included convulsions and encephalopathy. It has been reported that the best estimate of risk to an apparently normal infant of suffering a severe neurological reaction after pertussis vaccination is about 1 in 100 000 injections and of suffering permanent brain damage about 1 in 300 000 injections. It should be remembered that neurological complications as a consequence of pertussis infection are more frequent than adverse reactions associated with vaccination.

Anxiety, debate, and controversy has surrounded the possible neurotoxicity of pertussis vaccines or vaccines containing a pertussis component and very widely differing estimates of the risk of neurological complications have sometimes been reported.

In the *UK*, the National Childhood Encephalopathy Study has investigated any possible association between neurological disorders and pertussis vaccination. Of the first 1000 cases of acute neurological illness (including encephalitis or encephalopathy, prolonged convulsions, infantile spasms, and Reye's syndrome) notified to the study (D.L. Miller *et al., Br. med. J.*, 1981, *282*, 1595) only 35 were found to have received pertussis antigen (as combined diphtheria, tetanus, and pertussis vaccines) within 7 days before the onset of illness. Of these 35 children, 32 had no previous neurological abnormality, and a year later 2 had died, 9 had developmental retardation, and 21 were normal. The estimated attributable risk of serious neurological disorders occurring within 7 days after immunisation with combined diphtheria, tetanus, and pertussis vaccines in previously normal children irrespective of outcome was 1 in 110 000 injections (95% confidence limits, 1 in 360 000 to 1 in 44 000); the corresponding rate for previously normal children with neurological sequelae persistent one year later was 1 in 310 000 injections (95% confidence limits, 1 in 5 310 000 to 1 in 54 000). The report also noted that no significant association was found between serious neurological illness and immunisation with combined diphtheria and tetanus vaccines. After a subsequent analysis of 269 cases of infantile spasms notified to the study (M.H. Bellman *et al., Lancet*, 1983, *1*, 1031) it was concluded that pertussis immunisation was not a direct causal factor for infantile spasms in children with structurally normal brains, but that it may precipitate the onset of spasms in those children in whom the disorder is already destined to develop.

In a 7-year survey in the *UK* (T.M. Pollock and J. Morris, *Lancet*, 1983, *1*, 753) disorders attributed to vaccination were investigated in approximately 134 700 children who completed courses of diphtheria, tetanus, and pertussis immunisation and approximately 133 500 children who completed courses of only diphtheria and tetanus immunisation. Of a total of 1172 reports of adverse reactions received, 114 covered anaphylaxis or collapse, convulsions, neurological disorders, and deaths. Although neurological complications were reported more frequently in children vaccinated with combined diphtheria, tetanus, and pertussis vaccines than with combined diphtheria and tetanus vaccines it was suggested that this higher incidence may have been due to the adverse publicity accorded to pertussis vaccines since the difference was not observed when immunisation histories of children admitted to hospital for such conditions was investigated. It was also considered that the voluntary neurological reports were too widely divergent to suggest that a common aetiological agent was responsible and the view was held that the study had provided no convincing evidence that combined diphtheria, tetanus, and pertussis vaccines caused major neurological damage. In a similar, but shorter and smaller, study in a different region of the *UK* (T.M. Pollock *et al., Lancet*, 1984, *2*, 146) again no evidence of symptoms specific to the pertussis component of vaccines was found.

Despite these generally reassuring results concerning the safety of pertussis vaccines and despite the advice of many national authorities and international bodies, such as the World Health Organization, that the benefits of pertussis immunisation for previously healthy children outweigh the risks, some individuals still oppose the inclusion of pertussis vaccines in routine mass immunisation programmes.

Precautions

As for vaccines in general, p.1156. Because of the controversy concerning the potential adverse effects, especially neurotoxicity, of pertussis vaccines (see under Adverse Effects, above) the precautions to be observed and the contra-indications to the use of these vaccines has not always been clear and opinion has been divided.

There does appear to be general agreement that if any severe local or general reaction, such as high fever, angioedema, anaphylaxis, generalised collapse, prolonged altered states of consciousness, prolonged screaming, or convulsions, occurs within 48 to 72 hours of administration of a dose of a pertussis vaccine or a pertussis-containing vaccine, further administration is contra-indicated and that the use of combined diphtheria and tetanus only vaccines should be considered to complete the primary immunisation course in children.

Whether children with a personal or family history of convulsions or epilepsy should receive pertussis vaccines appears to have been the most difficult question to resolve. Some authorities have considered that the balance of risk and benefit of vaccination should be assessed in each individual case and others have considered that children with well-controlled seizures may be vaccinated.

A personal or family history of allergy is not generally considered to be a contra-indication to the use of pertussis vaccines, nor are stable neurologic conditions such as cerebral palsy or spina bifida.

Recommendation of the Advisory Committee on Immunization Practices in the *USA* concerning contra-indications to the use of pertussis vaccines (*J. Am. med. Ass.*, 1984, *251*, 2070). A family history of convulsions is not considered to be a contra-indication to receipt of pertussis vaccines. However, a personal history of a prior convulsion should be evaluated before initiating or continuing immunisation with pertussis-containing vaccines. For those with a history of seizures or those who develop seizures before an immunisation course is completed, administration of pertussis vaccines should be deferred until it can be ascertained that there is not an evolving neurologic disorder present. If such disorders are found, combined diphtheria and tetanus vaccines should be used instead of combined diphtheria, tetanus, and pertussis. For infants and children with stable neurologic conditions, including well-controlled seizures, the benefits of pertussis immunisation outweigh the risk. Hypersensitivity to vaccine components, presence of an evolving neurologic disorder, or a history of serious reaction to a previous dose (collapse or shock, persistent screaming episodes, temperature 40.5° or greater, convulsions with or without fever, severe alterations of consciousness, neurologic signs, or systemic allergic reactions) remain definitive contra-indications to the receipt of pertussis vaccines. Haemolytic anaemia and thrombocytopenic purpura are no longer considered to be contra-indications.

Uses and Administration

Pertussis vaccines are used for active immunisation of infants against pertussis (whooping cough).

Pertussis is most dangerous in early life, and immunisation should be started when the infant is 3 months old. For primary immunisation combined diphtheria, tetanus, and pertussis vaccines (see p.1161) are usually used. If neither immunisation against diphtheria nor against tetanus is required a single-component pertussis vaccine may be used.

In the *UK* a monovalent pertussis vaccine may be given in 3 doses at one-month intervals by deep subcutaneous or intramuscular injection.

Immunisation against pertussis forms part of the World Health Organization's Expanded Programme on Immunization (see p.1156).

Memorandum from a WHO Meeting regarding developments in pertussis vaccines. Although it is generally accepted that the whole-cell pertussis vaccine has been useful in controlling pertussis throughout the world. there is also general agreement that a less reactogenic and more effective vaccine is needed and that the development of such a vaccine is now an achievable goal.

Interest in improved vaccines to replace the current whole-cell vaccine centres, in part, on the acellular vaccine used in Japan. This acellular vaccine, which contains mainly toxoided LPF (lymphocytosis-promoting factor) and FHA (filamentous haemagglutinin), has been used, mixed with diphtheria and tetanus toxoids, in the mass immunisation of mainly 24-month-old children in Japan since 1981; it should, however, be noted that its efficacy is still under study. Comparison of this vaccine with whole-cell vaccine has shown that it is indeed less reactogenic, inducing fewer febrile reactions and less erythema and induration. It should also be noted that there are differences not only in the acellular vaccines produced by different manufacturers but also variations in lot to lot from the same manufacturer.— *Bull. Wld Hlth Org.*, 1985, *63*, 241.

Further discussions concerning the acellular pertussis vaccines used in Japan: E. Miller, *Br. med. J.*, 1986, *292*, 1348; G. R. Noble *et al.*, *J. Am. med. Ass.*, 1987, *257*, 1351; J. D. Cherry and E. A. Mortimer, *ibid.*, 1375.

A placebo-controlled study to determine the protective efficacy of and adverse events associated with the administration of two acellular pertussis vaccines in Sweden. The study involved 3801 children aged 5 to 11 months and fewer adverse reactions were found than had been reported for vaccines containing a whole-cell pertussis component. Overall estimates of vaccine efficacy were lower than expected and it was considered that only experience would show whether mass vaccination with these types of acellular pertussis vaccine would induce sufficient population immunity to reduce the attack-rate of pertussis to a low level.— Ad Hoc Group for the Study of Pertussis Vaccines, *Lancet*, 1988, *1*, 955.

Proprietary Preparations

Pertussis Vaccine (*B.P.*) is available from *Wellcome, UK.*

16951-w

Pigbel Vaccines

A vaccine against pigbel (necrotising enteritis), a disease occurring predominantly in children especially in the highlands of Papua New Guinea, has been developed and tested in clinical trials. The vaccine consists of an adsorbed *Clostridium welchii* type C toxoid.

Some reports of the use of a pigbel vaccine in children in Papua New Guinea: G. Lawrence *et al.*, *Lancet*, 1979, *1*, 227; M. Davis *et al.* (letter), *ibid.*, 1982, *2*, 389.

Proprietary Names and Manufacturers

Wellcome, Austral.

7987-j

Plague Vaccines

Plague Vaccine (*U.S.P.*) is a sterile suspension of formaldehyde-killed *Yersinia pestis* (strain 195/P). Potency is assessed by comparison with a reference substance. It should be stored at 2° to 8° and not be allowed to freeze.

Adverse Effects and Precautions

As for vaccines in general, p.1155.

Local and general reactions of moderate severity sometimes occur, but usually subside after 1 or 2 days.

Uses and Administration

Plague vaccines are used for active immunisation against plague in those occupationally exposed to the organism and in workers in infected areas when normal precautionary measures are not possible.

A plague vaccine containing 2000 million inactivated *Yersinia pestis* (strain 195/P) per mL is administered by intramuscular injection. The initial dose for adults and children over 10 years of age is usually 1 mL, and is followed by two further doses, each of 0.2 mL; these two doses may be given either 4 weeks and 6 months respectively after the first dose or after intervals of 1 to 3 months and 3 to 6 months respectively. Three doses, each of 0.5 mL, at weekly intervals afford some protection. Three booster doses, each of 0.1 to 0.2 mL, may be given at 6-monthly intervals, with further doses every 1 to 2 years. Suggested first, second, third, and booster doses for children are: under one year of age, 0.2, 0.04, 0.04, and 0.02 to 0.04 mL respectively; aged 1 to 4 years, 0.4, 0.08, 0.08, and 0.04 to 0.08 mL respectively; 5 to 10 years, 0.6, 0.12, 0.12, and 0.06 to 0.12 mL respectively.

Proprietary Preparations

A plague vaccine is available on a named-patient basis from *Cutter, UK.*

7988-z

Pneumococcal Vaccines

Pneumococcal vaccines are mixtures of purified polysaccharide capsular antigens from differing serotypes of *Streptococcus pneumoniae*. Vaccines have been prepared from various numbers of the serotypes but a vaccine commonly used is prepared from 23 types. Each 0.5-mL dose of this vaccine contains 25 μg pf each of the 23 polysaccharide types.

Adverse Effects and Precautions

As for vaccines in general, p.1155.

Erythema, soreness, and possibly induration may occur at the injection site. Fever and, rarely, allergic reactions have occurred.

Care should be exercised if pneumococcal vaccines are given to patients with severe cardiac or pulmonary impairment where systemic adverse reactions may pose a risk.

Persons previously immunised with a pneumococcal vaccine should not receive a second dose because of the increased incidence and severity of adverse reactions.

In patients with Hodgkin's disease the use of pneumococcal vaccines is not recommended in those who have received extensive chemotherapy or nodal irradiation and in patients with Hodgkin's disease receiving immunosuppressive therapy pneumococcal vaccines should be given at least 10 days before starting such therapy.

A satisfactory response to pneumococcal vaccines is not obtained in children less than 2 years of age and therefore immunisation of this age group is not recommended.

A report of transient decreases in serum-immunoglobulin and serum-complement concentrations in healthy subjects after administration of a pneumococcal polysaccharide vaccine contaminated with blood-group-A-like substances. It was believed that this was the first report of immunosuppression as an adverse reaction to any vaccine.— T. Nurmi and P. Koskela (letter), *Lancet*, 1988, *1*, 771.

Uses and Administration

Of the many serotypes of *Streptococcus pneumoniae* the 23 from which antigens are obtained for the most commonly available pneumococcal vaccine are considered to cause about 90% of pneumococcal disease.

The use of pneumococcal vaccines may be considered in those at increased risk from infection with the types of *Streptococcus pneumoniae* contained in the vaccine. Such persons include those who have undergone splenectomy and those with splenic dysfunction due to sickle-cell anaemia or other causes. Vaccination may also be considered in the elderly or in persons with cardiac, pulmonary, hepatic, or renal impairment or diabetes. Vaccination may also be considered in patients with Hodgkin's disease (but see under Precautions, above).

An antibody response develops by the third week, and probably lasts some years.

A single dose of 0.5 mL of the 23-type vaccine, containing 25 μg of each of the 23 polysaccharide types, is given by subcutaneous or intramuscular injection. Re-vaccination is not recommended and use in children under the age of 2 years is also not recommended.

Reviews of pneumococcal vaccines: *Med. Lett.*, 1983, *25*, 91; R. Austrian, *New Engl. J. Med.*, 1984, *310*, 651; F. M. LaForce and T. C. Eickhoff, *Ann. intern. Med.*, 1986, *104*, 110; *idem*, 1988, *108*, 757.

After immunisation with pneumococcal vaccine there are 2 phases of the immune response—the appearance of B cells secreting antigen-specific antibodies, and the presence of cells that secrete antigen-specific antibodies only after polyclonal stimulation. The latter depends on a functioning spleen.— F. D. Padova *et al.*, *Br. med. J.*, 1983, *287*, 1829.

Recommendations of the Immunization Practices Advisory Committee of the Centers for Disease Control concerning the use of the 23-valent pneumococcal polysaccharide vaccine in the *USA* (*Ann. intern. Med.*, 1984, *101*, 348; *J. Am. med. Ass.*, 1984, *251*, 3071). Vaccination was particularly recommended for the following persons: adults with cardiovascular and chronic pulmonary disease who sustain increased morbidity with respiratory infections; adults with chronic illnesses such as splenic dysfunction or anatomic asplenia, Hodgkin's disease, multiple myeloma, cirrhosis, alcoholism, renal failure, cerebrospinal fluid leaks, and conditions associated with immunosuppression, which are conditions specifically associated with an increased risk for pneumococcal disease or its complications; older adults, especially those over the age of 65 years who are otherwise healthy; children aged 2 years and older with chronic illnesses, such as anatomic or functional asplenia (splenectomy or sickle-cell disease), nephrotic syndrome, cerebrospinal fluid leaks, and conditions associated with immunosuppression, which again are conditions specifically associated with an increased risk of pneumococcal disease or its complications. Recurrent upper-respiratory-tract diseases, including otitis media and sinusitis, were not considered indications for use in children.

Similar recommendations have also been made by the Health and Public Policy Committee of the American College of Physicians (*Ann. intern. Med.*, 1986, *104*, 118).

Proprietary Preparations

Pneumovax *(Morson, UK)*. A pneumococcal vaccine containing polysaccharide from each of 23 capsular types of pneumococcus.

7992-e

Poliomyelitis Vaccines

Polio Vaccines; Poliovirus Vaccines.

NOTE. Inactivated poliomyelitis vaccines are sometimes termed Salk Vaccine and live (oral) poliomyelitis vaccines are sometimes termed Sabin Vaccine.

Inactivated Poliomyelitis Vaccine (*B.P.*) (Pol/Vac(Inact); Poliomyelitis Vaccine (Inactivated) (*Eur. P.*); Vaccinum Poliomyelitidis Inactivatum) is a sterile aqueous suspension of suitable strains of poliomyelitis virus, types 1, 2, and 3, grown in suitable cell cultures and inactivated by a suitable method. It may contain minimal amounts of permitted antibiotics and preservatives. It should be stored at 2° to 8°, not be allowed to freeze, and be protected from light. Under these conditions it may be expected to retain its potency for at least 18 months from the date on which the test for potency was carried out.

Poliovirus Vaccine Inactivated (*U.S.P.*) is a sterile aqueous suspension of poliomyelitis virus, types 1, 2, and 3, grown in cultures of monkey kidney tissue and inactivated. It may contain suitable antimicrobial agents. It should be stored at 2° to 8 °.

Poliomyelitis Vaccine, Live (Oral) (*B.P.*) (OPV; Pol/Vac (Oral); Poliomyelitis Vaccine (Oral) (*Eur. P.*); Vaccinum Poliomyelitidis Perorale) is an aqueous suspension of suitable live attenuated strains of poliomyelitis virus, types 1, 2, or 3, grown in suitable, approved cell cultures; it may contain any one of the 3 virus types or combinations of them. It is standardised for virus titre which is not less than 5.5 $\log_{10}$ CCID50 for types 1 and 3 and not less than 5.0 $\log_{10}$ CCID50 for type 2 per dose. It should be stored at the temperature indicated on the label. When thawed and stored at 2° to 8°, it should be used within 6 months; when exposed to higher temperatures it should be used within a few hours.

Poliovirus Vaccine Live Oral (*U.S.P.*) is a preparation of a combination of the 3 types of suitable live attenuated polioviruses, grown in cultures of monkey kidney tissue. It contains not less than $10^{5.4}$ to $10^{6.4}$ virus titre for type 1, not less than $10^{4.5}$ to $10^{5.5}$ for type 2, and not less than $10^{5.2}$ to $10^{6.2}$ for type 3. It should be stored at 2° to 8° or in the frozen state. The vaccine should not be thawed and refrozen more than 10 times.

Adverse Effects

As for vaccines in general, p.1155.

Vaccine-associated poliomyelitis has been reported in a small number of recipients of oral poliomyelitis vaccines and in contacts of recipients.

Results of a ten-year study on the relationship between acute persisting spinal paralysis and poliomyelitis vaccines. Of 13 participating countries, 2 employing live poliomyelitis oral vaccine (Sabin) exclusively and 1 employing only inactivated vaccine did not report a single occurrence during the 10-year period. In 6 countries, all employing oral vaccines and each reporting, in most years, a small number of cases in relation to the size of their population, the similarity of the data enabled them to be grouped together for the purpose of analysis. In these 6 countries (total population 403 million) 281 reports of acute persisting spinal paralysis were received over the 10 years and of these 52 were in persons immunised 7 to 30 days earlier, 70 were in persons with a history of contact with vaccinees, and 159 were in persons with no history of contact with vaccines or with vaccinees. In patients with acute persisting spinal paralysis where infection with a single virus type was diagnosed, most of the cases in vaccinees and vaccinee-contacts were associated with poliovirus type 3, but in contacts the proportion of type 2 was higher. In distinct contrast, most cases in persons with no history of contact with vaccine or vaccinees were associated with type 1 and all the strains from those examined had 'wild strain' characteristics. Although it was very difficult to be certain that acute persisting spinal paralysis in any individual was caused by the vaccine virus, the grouping of cases due to poliovirus types 2 and 3 within a short interval after immunisation, the evidence of the relationship between the viruses isolated from the patients and the strains in the vaccine, and the isolation of vaccine-like strains from the CNS in patients who died, warrants the conclusion that most, if not all, of the cases in vaccinees and vaccinee-contacts were vaccine-related. However, the relationship between immunisation schedules and the incidence of vaccine-associated cases was apparently of very minor importance. The risk of developing acute persisting spinal paralysis was expressed in 3 ways: the calculated incidence in relation to total population, if all the cases in vaccinees and contacts were causally related to the vaccine, would be 1 in 100 million per year for vaccinees and 1 in 50 million per year for contacts; the incidence in relation to the child population at risk was calculated as less than 1 per million children receiving the vaccine; and the incidence in relation to doses of vaccine distributed was calculated as 1 vaccinee case per 6.7 million doses distributed and 1 vaccinee-contact case for about 5 million doses distributed. All 3 methods of assessment demonstrate that the risk of paralysis attributable to live poliomyelitis vaccines is very remote. Of patients classified as vaccinee-contacts many were young (and presumably non-immune) parents of children undergoing primary immunisation, indicating that parents without definite evidence of previous effective immunisation should be given vaccine at the same time as their children. In the remaining 4 countries included in the study the incidence of acute persisting spinal paralysis differed not only from the combined incidence of the previous 6 countries but also from each other. In one country only 1 report occurred and poliovirus type 1 isolated from the stools of the patient was considered 'non vaccine-like'. In another country, 5 cases occurred in patients with no history of immunisation and no evidence of contact with persons who had received live vaccines as well as an outbreak of 82 cases in communities with religious objections to immunisation. The 2 other countries reported 164 and 165 cases which accounted for 24 and 25% respectively of the total from all countries in the study. In the first of these 2 the rate began to fall during the second half of the study following the change from monovalent to trivalent oral poliomyelitis vaccines and from a strategy of mass campaigns to one of 'throughout the year' immunisation but in the second a continuing high incidence of vaccine-associated cases cannot be explained despite all the investigations made over the period of study.— WHO Consultative Group, *Bull. Wld Hlth Org.*, 1982, *60*, 231.

During the period 1973-84 there had been 138 cases of paralytic poliomyelitis reported in the *USA* and of these 105 (76%) were vaccine-associated. Of the vaccine-associated cases, 35 occurred in recipients of oral vaccines, 50 in contacts of oral vaccine recipients, 14 in immune deficient individuals, and 6 in individuals who had not received vaccine or had no contact with vaccine recipients. The overall frequency of vaccine-associated poliomyelitis was one case per 2.6 million doses distributed. However, the relative frequency associated with the first dose was higher than with subsequent doses, being one case per 520 000 and one case per 12.3 million doses respectively.— B. M. Nkowane *et al.*, *J. Am. med. Ass.*, 1987, *257*, 1335.

Precautions

As for vaccines in general, p.1156.

Oral poliomyelitis vaccines should not be given to patients with diarrhoea or vomiting.

Because the vaccine virus of oral poliomyelitis vaccines is excreted in the faeces, the contacts of recently vaccinated babies and infants should be advised of the need for strict personal hygiene, particularly hand washing after napkin changing, in order to reduce the possibility of infection in unimmunised contacts.

Oral poliomyelitis vaccines should not be given to contacts of immunosuppressed patients and in these persons an inactivated vaccine should be used (see under Uses and Administration, below).

PREGNANCY AND THE NEONATE. A pregnant woman travelling to a developing area should be immunised against poliomyelitis; the risk of the disease was far greater than any risk to the foetus.— M. M. Levine *et al.*, *Lancet*, 1974, *2*, 34. A similar opinion that there is no reason to withhold either inactivated or oral poliomyelitis vaccines from susceptible women where otherwise justified.— M. Bader (letter), *J. Am. med. Ass.*, 1983, *249*, 2018. A reply stating that there is data suggesting that vaccination of pregnant women with inactivated poliomyelitis vaccines which were formerly available may lead to adverse effects in the offspring. Heinonen *et al.* (*Int. J. Epidemiol.*, 1973, *2*, 229) in a study of 50 897 pregnancies reported that the children of mothers who received inactivated poliomyelitis vaccine while pregnant had a significantly higher rate of malignancy (7.6 per 10 000) compared with unexposed children (3.1 per 10 000). Although there are no convincing data regarding currently available inactivated vaccines the recommendation that they should not be given during pregnancy should be continued. There are, however, no data to indicate that oral poliomyelitis vaccines can harm the developing foetus.— R. A. Goodman *et al.* (letter), *ibid.* Further comment that the data of Heinonen *et al.* is not consistent with other studies. The inactivated poliomyelitis vaccine formerly available in the late 1950's was contaminated by simian virus 40, a tumour-producing agent. As the inactivated vaccines now produced do not contain this virus the contra-indication during pregnancy is excessive.— M. Bader (letter), *ibid.*, 1984, *251*, 728. Agreement that the data of Heinonen *et al.* is not consistent with other studies but defence of the statement that inactivated vaccines should not be used during pregnancy.— W. A. Orenstein *et al.*, *ibid.*

Uses and Administration

Poliomyelitis vaccines are used for active immunisation against poliomyelitis. Both live (oral) poliomyelitis vaccines and inactivated poliomyelitis vaccines are available. The oral vaccine stimulates the formation of antibodies in the blood and also produces a local resistance in the intestinal tissues.

In the *UK* an oral poliomyelitis vaccine, containing the three types of poliovirus, is recommended for the primary immunisation of infants and children. The first dose may be given at the age of 3 months, the second dose 6 to 8 weeks later, and the third dose after an interval of 4 to 6 months; these doses are given at the same time that the combined diphtheria, tetanus, and pertussis vaccine is administered. The dose of the oral poliomyelitis vaccine is 3 drops, being dropped directly into the mouth of an infant or being given on a sugar lump to older children. Reinforcing doses of the oral vaccine are recommended at school entry and at 15 to 19 years of age. Further reinforcing doses are necessary only in adults exposed to infection with a single dose being given every 10 years, if necessary.

For the primary immunisation of susceptible adults a course of 3 doses of the oral poliomyelitis vaccine at intervals of 4 weeks is recommended.

On the occurrence of a single case of paralytic poliomyelitis, a single dose of the oral vaccine is recommended for all persons in the neighbourhood, regardless of whether they have previously been immunised.

Inactivated poliomyelitis vaccine is recommended in the *UK* for the immunisation of persons in whom the use of the live oral vaccine is contra-indicated; inactivated vaccine, rather than the live oral vaccine, is also recommended for contacts of immunosuppressed persons. The inactivated vaccine is given by deep subcutaneous or intramuscular injection but the volume and number of doses may differ according to the formulation employed.

Immunisation against poliomyelitis forms part of the World Health Organization's Expanded Programme on Immunization (see p.1156).

A statement by the Advisory Committee on Immunization Practices concerning the use of the enhanced-potency inactivated poliomyelitis vaccine in the *USA* (*J. Am. med. Ass.*, 1988, *259*, 345). Immunisation against poliomyelitis should still rely primarily on the use of the oral vaccine. A method of producing a more potent inactivated poliomyelitis vaccine with a greater antigenic content has been developed and results of studies from several countries have indicated that a reduced number of doses of this vaccine can be used.

The enhanced-potency inactivated vaccine should be used in the immunocompromised and their contacts. The primary series consists of three 0.5-mL doses administered subcutaneously; the interval between the first two doses should be at least 4 weeks, but preferably 8 weeks; the third dose should follow in at least 6 months, but preferably nearer to 12 months. The primary series may be started as early as 6 weeks of age, but 2 months of age is preferable. If possible, young children should receive the third dose at 15 months of age along with diphtheria, tetanus, and pertussis vaccine and measles, mumps, and rubella vaccine. A booster dose should be given before school entry, unless the final dose of the primary series was administered on or after the fourth birthday.

Discussions on various immunisation policies against poliomyelitis: A. M. McBean and J. F. Modlin, *Pediatr. infect. Dis. J.*, 1987, *6*, 881 (in *USA*); A. B. Sabin, *ibid.*, 887 (in *USA*); J. Salk, *ibid.*, 889 (in *USA*); R. Chamberlain, *Br. med. J.*, 1987, *295*, 158 (in *UK*).

Some clinical studies using newer types of poliomyelitis vaccines: P. A. Patriarca *et al.*, *Lancet*, 1988, *1*, 429 (an enhanced-potency oral vaccine); S. E. Robertson *et al.*, *ibid.*, 897 (an enhanced-potency inactivated vaccine).

Proprietary Preparations

Poliomyelitis Vaccine, Live (Oral) (*B.P.*) is available from *Merieux, UK, Smith Kline & French, UK,* and *Wellcome, UK.*

7993-l

Pseudomonas Vaccines

Pseudomonas vaccines have been prepared from differing serotypes of *Pseudomonas aeruginosa*.

A 16-component vaccine (PEV-01) prepared from 16 serotypes of *Pseudomonas aeruginosa* has been investigated for the prevention of pseudomonal infections in a variety of disease states.

The preparation and characterisation of a 16-component *Pseudomonas* vaccine.— J. M. Miler *et al., J. med. Microbiol.*, 1977, *10*, 19.

Some references to clinical studies using pseudomonas vaccines: L. S. Young, *Ann. intern. Med.*, 1973, *79*, 518 (beneficial effect in reducing infections in cancer patients); R. J. Jones *et al., Lancet*, 1979, *2*, 977 (beneficial effect in reducing infections in burns patients); R. J. Jones *et al., ibid.*, 1980, *2*, 1263 (some beneficial effect in reducing infections in burns patients); D. T. Langford and J. Hiller, *Archs Dis. Childh.*, 1984, *59*, 1131 (no benefit in reducing infections in cystic fibrosis).

Proprietary Preparations

A pseudomonas vaccine is available on a named-patient basis from *Wellcome, UK*.

16972-z

Q Fever Vaccines

Several experimental vaccines against Q fever have been developed and some have been tried in persons professionally exposed to the disease.

Reports of the use of a Q fever vaccine in persons exposed to the disease: J. Kazár *et al., Bull. Wld Hlth Org.*, 1982, *60*, 389; B. P. Marmion *et al., Lancet*, 1984, *2*, 1411.

7995-j

Rabies Antisera

Antirabies Serum (*U.S.P.*) is a sterile solution containing antiviral substances obtained from the serum or plasma of a healthy animal, usually the horse, that has been immunised by vaccine against rabies. It should be stored at 2° to 8°.

Units

86.6 units of rabies antiserum (equine) are contained in approximately 86.6 mg of dried hyperimmune horse serum in one ampoule of the first International Standard Preparation (1955).

Adverse Effects and Precautions

As for antisera in general, p.1155.

Uses and Administration

Rabies antisera may be used to provide passive immunisation to rabies but the use of rabies immunoglobulins (see below) is preferred. For the prevention of rabies in patients who have received bites from rabid animals or animals suspected of being rabid the usual dose of rabies antiserum is 40 units per kg body-weight given at the same time, but at different sites, as the first dose of a rabies vaccine (see below). It has been recommended that up to 50% of the dose should be administered by local infiltration at the site of the wound and the remainder given by intramuscular injection unless the wound involves mucous membranes when the entire dose should be given intramuscularly.

Proprietary Preparations

A rabies antiserum is available from *Swiss Serum and Vaccine Institute, Switz.* (*Inst. Serother. & Vaccinal, Switz.*) and may be obtainable on a named-patient basis through an importer.

1239-f

Rabies Immunoglobulins

Rabies Immunoglobulin (*B.P.*) (Antirabies Immunoglobulin Injection) is a liquid or freeze-dried preparation containing immunoglobulins, mainly immunoglobulin G (IgG). It is obtained from plasma or serum containing specific antibodies against the rabies virus. Normal Immunoglobulin may be added. Rabies Immunoglobulin is prepared in the same manner as Normal Immunoglobulin (see p.1170) except that the pooled material may be from fewer than 1000 donors. It contains not less than 150 units per mL. The liquid preparation should be stored, protected from light, in a sealed, colourless, glass container at a temperature of 2° to 8°. Under these conditions it may be expected to retain its potency for 3 years. The freeze-dried preparation should be stored, protected from light, under vacuum or under an inert gas at a temperature of 2° to 8°. Under these conditions it may be expected to retain its potency for 5 years.

Rabies Immune Globulin (*U.S.P.*) is a sterile solution of globulins derived from plasma or serum from selected adult human donors who have been immunised with rabies vaccine and have developed high titres of rabies antibody. It contains 10 to 18% of protein of which not less than 80% is monomeric immunoglobulin G. It contains glycine as a stabilising agent, and a suitable preservative. It contains not less than 110 units per mL. It should be stored at 2° to 8°.

Units

59 units of anti-rabies immunoglobulin, human are contained in the lyophilised residue of 0.5 mL of an 11% solution of immunoglobulin in glycine buffer in one ampoule of the first International Standard Preparation (1984).

Adverse Effects and Precautions

As for immunoglobulins in general, p.1155.

Uses and Administration

Rabies immunoglobulins are used for passive immunisation against rabies. They are used in conjunction with active immunisation employing rabies vaccines as part of the postexposure treatment for the prevention of rabies in persons who have been bitten by rabid animals or animals suspected of being rabid. For further details concerning the recommended schedules in the *UK*, see under rabies vaccines, below.

For the recommendations of the World Health Organization and the Advisory Committee on Immunization Practices in the *USA* concerning the management of persons bitten by rabid animals, and including the use of rabies immunoglobulins, see under rabies vaccines, below.

Proprietary Preparations

A rabies immunoglobulin is available from *Blood Products Laboratory, UK*.

7997-c

Rabies Vaccines

Rabies Vaccine (*B.P.*) (Rab/Vac; Rabies Vaccine for Human Use Prepared in Cell Cultures (*Eur. P.*); Vaccinum Rabiei ex Cellulis ad Usum Humanum) is a sterile aqueous suspension of inactivated rabies virus; a suitable strain is grown in an approved cell culture. The vaccine is prepared immediately before use, by the addition of a suitable sterile liquid. The estimated potency is not less than 2.5 units per dose. The dried vaccine should be stored at 2° to 8°, not be allowed to freeze, and be protected from light. Under these conditions it may be expected to retain its potency for at least 2 years.

Rabies Vaccine (*U.S.P.*) is a sterile preparation, in dried or liquid form, of inactivated rabies virus obtained from inoculated diploid cell cultures. It has a potency of not less than 2.5 units per dose. It should be stored at 2° to 8°.

Units

7.8 units are contained in approximately 49.45 mg of freeze-dried rabies vaccine prepared in human diploid cells and inactivated with propiolactone in one ampoule of the first International Standard Preparation (1983).

Adverse Effects and Precautions

As for vaccines in general, p.1155.

Patients may experience pain, erythema, and induration at the injection site after the use of any type of rabies vaccine; pruritus, nausea, headache, fever, malaise, or myalgia may also occur.

Anaphylactic reactions and lymphadenopathy have been commonly associated with the use of duck-embryo vaccines and neuroparalytic reactions (transverse myelitis, neuropathy, or encephalopathy) with the use of adult animal brain-tissue vaccines. Side-effects after human diploid-cell vaccine are considerably less common and neuroparalytic reactions do not appear to be a problem.

In an estimated 424 000 patients receiving duck-embryo rabies vaccine in the USA from 1958 to 1971 there were 22 reports of anaphylaxis, 137 of minor transient neurological reactions, and 4 of transverse myelitis, 5 of neuropathy, and 4 of encephalopathy (2 fatal). In a prospective study in 116 patients receiving the vaccine after exposure local reactions were a constant feature; other reactions included regional adenopathy (18%), generalised adenopathy (3%), malaise, myalgia, fever, chills, and anaphylaxis (0.9%).— R. H. Rubin *et al., Ann. intern. Med.*, 1973, *78*, 643.

The incidence of neuroparalytic accidents following a course of nerve-tissue vaccines is known to vary from country to country and it is presently impossible to determine the reasons for the apparent differences but factors such as population type, physiological state of patient, and the type of vaccine used (including amount of myelin present, species of animal used for vaccine production, method of inactivation of the virus, and dosage schedule) must be taken into consideration for any analysis. Paralytic accidents have occurred much less frequently with vaccines produced from brain tissue of mice younger than 9 days of age compared to older animals.

Local reactions, including lymphadenopathy, occur commonly when duck-embryo vaccine is used, and neuroparalytic or other severe generalised reactions may also occur, but less frequently than with nerve-tissue vaccine. Properly prepared human diploid cell vaccines have not been associated with serious adverse effects, although a few persons may experience local redness, pain, headache, and fever.— Seventh Report of a WHO Expert Committee on Rabies, *Tech. Rep. Ser. Wld Hlth Org. No. 709*, 1984. Mention that the generally accepted risk of CNS damage associated with the use of rabies vaccines prepared in the brains of adult animals is about 1 in 2000 doses administered.— Thirty-seventh Report of a WHO Expert Committee on Biological Standardization, *Tech. Rep. Ser. Wld Hlth Org. No. 760*, 1987, p.167.

ALLERGY. An analysis of cases of systemic allergic reactions following immunisation with human-diploid cell rabies vaccine reported to the Centers for Disease Control in the *USA* over the period June 1980 to March

1984. Of the 108 reports received classification, on the basis of clinical observation, revealed 9 cases of presumed type I immediate hypersensitivity (incidence of 1 in 10 000 vaccinees), 87 cases of presumed type III hypersensitivity (9 in 10 000 vaccinees), and 12 cases of indeterminate type. All the reactions presumed to be type I occurred during either primary pre- or postexposure immunisation whereas 93% of the presumed type III reactions were observed following booster immunisations. Presenting features of the type III reaction included generalised or pruritic rash or urticaria, angioedema, arthralgias, fever, nausea, vomiting, and malaise.— *J. Am. med. Ass.*, 1984, *251*, 2194. See also: C. Marwick, *ibid.*, 1985, *254*, 13.

EFFECTS ON THE NERVOUS SYSTEM. A review and discussion on neuroparalytic accidents including the association with certain types of rabies vaccines.— B. G. W. Arnason, *New Engl. J. Med.*, 1987, *316*, 406.

Vaccinations against rabies using a vaccine containing animal nervous tisssue provoked the onset of multiple sclerosis in a patient.— H. Miller *et al.*, *Br. med. J.*, 1967, *2*, 210.

Guillain-Barré syndrome after rabies vaccine produced on suckling mouse brain.— I. Vergara *et al.* (letter), *Archs Neurol., Chicago*, 1979, *36*, 254. After human diploid-cell vaccine.— E. Bøe and H. Nyland, *Scand. J. infect. Dis.*, 1980, *12*, 231.

Peripheral neuropathy in a patient followed the use of a foetal bovine-cell rabies vaccine although it could not be certain that the vaccine was responsible. Frequencies of neurological complications of rabies vaccine were stated to be 1 in 1600 for vaccine prepared from adult animal neural tissue, 1 in 8000 for mouse-embryo vaccine, 1 in 32 000 for duck-embryo vaccine, and 1 in 150 000 for human diploid-cell vaccine.— A. Courrier *et al.* (letter), *Lancet*, 1986, *1*, 1273.

INTERACTIONS. Studies suggesting that continuous antimalarial chemoprophylaxis with chloroquine during primary immunisation with human diploid-cell rabies vaccine administered intradermally for pre-exposure prophylaxis is associated with a poor and inadequate antibody response.— D. N. Taylor *et al.* (letter), *Lancet*, 1984, *1*, 1405; M. Pappaioanou *et al.*, *New Engl. J. Med.*, 1986, *314*, 280.

Uses and Administration

Rabies vaccines are used for active immunisation against rabies. They are used as part of postexposure treatment, for the prevention of rabies in patients who have been bitten by rabid animals or animals suspected of being rabid. Infection does not take place through unbroken skin but it is possible through uninjured mucous membranes and has been reported after the inhalation of virus in the laboratory. Rabies vaccines are also used for pre-exposure prophylaxis against rabies in persons exposed to a high risk of being bitten by rabid or potentially rabid animals.

In the *UK* a rabies vaccine cultured on human diploid cells and containing not less than 2.5 units per mL is used.

For *postexposure therapy*, thorough cleansing of the wound with soap and water is imperative. The recommended schedule in the *UK* for the human diploid-cell vaccine is 6 doses, each of 1 mL, by deep subcutaneous or intramuscular injection on days 0, 3, 7, 14, 30, and 90. Rabies immunoglobulin should also be given at the same time as the first dose of vaccine; the recommended dose is 20 units per kg body-weight, half of which should be infiltrated around the wound with the remainder being given intramuscularly but at a different site to that at which the vaccine was administered. A modified course of vaccine administration should be employed in previously immunised persons or those shown to have developed antibodies.

For *pre-exposure prophylaxis* against rabies the recommended schedule in the *UK* for the human diploid-cell vaccine is 2 doses given 4 weeks apart with a third dose after 12 months; either 1 mL may be given by deep subcutaneous or intramuscular injection or 0.1 mL intradermally. Booster doses should be given every 1 to 3 years depending upon the risk of exposure. It has been suggested that rapid immunisation of personnel engaged in the care of a patient with rabies may be achieved by the intradermal administration of 0.1 mL into each limb (total of 0.4 mL) on the first day of exposure to the patient.

The schedules for administration of rabies vaccines vary according to the type of vaccine employed. For differing recommendations concerning the use of human diploid-cell vaccine and recommendations concerning the use of other types of vaccines, see below.

Some general reviews on rabies and its control: G. W. Beran and A. J. Crowley, *Chronicle Wld Hlth Org.*, 1983, *37*, 192; G. S. Turner, *Abstr. Hyg.*, 1984, *59*, R1; L. J. Anderson *et al.*, *Ann. intern. Med.*, 1984, *100*, 728.

Many different rabies vaccines are available for human use. The three types are: those derived from nerve tissue of adult (sheep, goats, or rabbits) or newborn (rabbits, rats, or mice) animals; those derived from avian tissues (duck embryos); and those prepared in cell cultures (human diploid cell strains or animal cell cultures). Originally the only source of rabies virus available for vaccine production was infected brain tissue from adult animals and although this material is still widely used the production of such vaccines in recent years has been discontinued in a number of European countries. These vaccines contain neuroparalytic factors such as myelin and the Committee supports the trend to limit, or abandon completely, their production. To reduce the hazard from these neuroparalytic and encephalitogenic substances, vaccines are also prepared from the brains of suckling animals since the content of such substances is less. A vaccine prepared from virus grown in duck embryos has been developed but the indications are that, although the neuroparalytic hazards have been reduced, allergenic risks still exist. Vaccines prepared in cell-culture are now available and appear to combine safety with high antigenic content. In a number of countries a vaccine developed from an adapted Pasteur strain of virus grown in a human diploid cell strain is used for both pre- and postexposure immunisation. In France, vaccine is also produced from a Pasteur strain of virus grown in foetal bovine kidney cells, and in the Netherlands from a similar strain grown in dog kidney cells. In Japan, the high egg passage (HEP) Flury strain grown in chick-embryo cell cultures is used. In the USSR, Eastern Europe, and Asia, the Vnukovo-32 strain of virus grown in primary hamster-kidney cell cultures has been widely used. Preliminary clincal studies have also been carried out in some countries with purified chick-embryo cell (PCEC) and Vero-cell rabies vaccines.

For *postexposure treatment* against rabies it is emphasised that the most valuable procedure is prompt local treatment of all bite wounds by thorough flushing and washing of the wound with water, or soap and water, or detergent followed by the application of alcohol (400 to 700 mL per litre), tincture or aqueous solution of iodine, or quaternary ammonium compounds (1 mL per litre). Any vaccination schedule recommended in a given situation depends upon the type and potency of the rabies vaccine used. For brain-tissue vaccine, 14 daily doses, with two booster doses 15 and 65 days after the end of the primary series, should be given; smaller doses are recommended by some of the manufacturers for infants. For suckling mouse brain vaccine, 14 daily doses, with two booster doses 10 and 20 days after the end of the primary series, should be given; in France and in several Latin American countries, reduced schedules, generally consisting of 7 daily doses and boosters given 10, 20, and 90 days after the primary series, are used, but the Committee recommends that if reduced schedules are employed the vaccine should have a potency of 1.3 units and that if rabies antisera have been used a complete schedule of vaccine should be employed. For duck-embryo vaccine, 14 daily doses, with 2 booster doses 10 and 60 days after the end of the primary series, should be given. For tissue-culture vaccine, which should have a minimum potency of 2.5 units, 5 doses on days 0, 3, 7, 14, and 30, with an optional booster on day 90, should be given. Additionally, rabies antisera and rabies immunoglobulins are of proven efficacy as an adjunct to vaccine treatment. The dose of antiserum is 40 units per kg body-weight and that of immunoglobulin, the potency of which should be 150 units per mL, is 20 units per kg.

For *pre-exposure prophylaxis* against rabies the most suitable vaccines for use are those of cell-culture origin but suckling mouse brain vaccine may also be employed. Persons regularly at high risk of exposure, such as certain laboratory workers, veterinarians, animal handlers, and wildlife officers, should be protected by pre-exposure immunisation. The immunisation schedule should preferably consist of 3 injections of a rabies vaccine of potency at least 2.5 units given on days 0, 7, and 28 or on days 0, 28, and 56, but a few days' variation is unimportant. If titres of virus-neutralising antibodies, one month after the third injection, are not 0.5 units or more per mL, booster doses should be administered. Further boosters should be given every 1 to 3 years for as long as the person is exposed to risk. The intradermal administration of the human diploid cell vaccine in doses of 0.1 mL on days 0, 7, and 28 has also been shown to induce seroconversion.— Seventh Report of a WHO Expert Committee on Rabies, *Tech. Rep. Ser. Wld Hlth Org. No. 709*, 1984..

Recommendations of the Advisory Committee on Immunization Practices concerning the prevention of rabies in the *USA* (*J. Am. med. Ass.*, 1984, *252*, 883).

For *postexposure treatment*, immediate and thorough washing of all bite wounds and scratches with soap and water is perhaps the most effective measure for preventing rabies. Human diploid-cell vaccine is the only type of vaccine currently available in the *USA* and postexposure treatment should always include the administration of vaccine, together with rabies immunoglobulin (or rabies antiserum if the immunoglobulin is unavailable); the only exception to this is that persons who have been previously immunised with the recommended regimens of the human diploid-cell vaccine or those who have received other vaccines and have a history of documented adequate rabies antibody titres should receive only the vaccine. The recommended schedule for the vaccine is 5 doses, each of 1 mL, given intramuscularly on days 0, 3, 7, 14, and 28. Other routes of administration, such as the intradermal route, have not been adequately evaluated for postexposure use and should not be used. Rabies immunoglobulin in a single dose of 20 units per kg body-weight, should be given preferably at the commencement of vaccine administration but may be given up to the eighth day after the first dose of vaccine was given; if feasible, up to half the dose of immunoglobulin should be thoroughly infiltrated around the wound and the remainder administered intramuscularly. Alternatively, if immunoglobulin is unavailable, rabies antiserum in a dose of 40 units per kg may be used. Previously immunised persons or those with adequate antibody titres should receive only 2 doses of vaccine, each of 1 mL, given intramuscularly on days 0 and 3 and immunoglobulin or antiserum should not be used.

Pre-exposure prophylaxis may be offered to persons in high-risk groups. Three doses of vaccine on days 0, 7, and 28 should be given; either 1 mL given intramuscularly or 0.1 mL given intradermally may be used. Serum-antibody titres should be determined every 6 months to 2 years, depending upon the level of exposure, and booster doses given as necessary.

A discussion on the reported failures of rabies vaccination. No case of rabies has been reported in anyone given the human diploid-cell rabies vaccine correctly, with hyperimmune serum, on the day of contact with a rabid animal. Patients have, however, died of rabies after vaccination because of a delay in treatment, suboptimum methods of administration, or omission of passive immunisation. The need for an intramuscular injection to be given into the deltoid muscle, rather than intragluteally, was also stressed.— *Lancet*, 1988, *1*, 917.

Data indicating that the safest and most economical method of rapidly stimulating neutralising antibody after exposure to rabies virus is by giving human diploid-cell strain vaccine 0.1 mL intradermally at 8 sites on day 0 and at 4 sites on day 7, with a booster dose on days 28 and 91; defects of technique would not be serious as long as 4 or more doses were accurately delivered on day 0. If passive immunisation is given, endogenous antibody production is less urgent and the subcutaneous route of vaccination gives results comparable to the intradermal route. Nevertheless, multiple-site intradermal inoculation is the optimum method of producing antibody within a week.— M. J. Warrell *et al.*, *Lancet*, 1984, *1*, 874. See also: M. J. Warrell *et al.*, *ibid.*, 1985, *1*, 1059. Further references to schedules of human diploid-cell rabies vaccine given intradermally for postexposure treatment: P. Rees *et al.* (letter), *Lancet*, 1984, *1*, 1469; G. Harverson and C. Wasi, *ibid.*, *2*, 313.

Some references to newer types of rabies vaccines being developed for human use: B. S. Berlin *et al.*, *J. Am. med. Ass.*, 1983, *249*, 2663 (rhesus diploid-cell vaccine); R. Barth *et al.* (letter), *Lancet*, 1983, *1*, 700 (purified chicken-embryo vaccine); R. Glück *et al.* (letter), *ibid.*, 1984, *1*, 844 (purified duck-embryo vaccine); C. Wasi *et al.* (letter), *ibid.*, 1986, *1*, 40 (purified chicken-embryo vaccine); B. Dureux *et al.* (letter), *ibid.*, *2*, 98 (Vero-cell vaccine); P. Suntharasamai *et al.*, *ibid.*, 129 (Vero-cell vaccine).

Proprietary Preparations

Merieux Inactivated Rabies Vaccine *(Servier, UK)*. An inactivated rabies vaccine prepared from the Wistar PM/WI 38 1503-3M virus strain propagated in human diploid cells.

7998-k

Rocky Mountain Spotted Fever Vaccines

Although several different vaccines against rocky mountain spotted fever have been produced in the past none has been considered to be very effective, and research is still continuing in order to produce a safe and effective vaccine.

Some references to rocky mountain spotted fever vaccines and their development: T. H. Maugh, *Science*, 1978, *201*, 604; G. A. McDonald *et al.*, *ibid.*, 1987, *235*, 83.

16981-c

Rotavirus Vaccines

Several rotavirus vaccines for use in the prevention of childhood diarrhoea have been developed and two live oral attenuated vaccines, one developed from a bovine rotavirus (RIT 4237) and one developed from a rhesus monkey rotavirus (MMU-18006) have been tested in clinical trials.

A review of the achievements and prospects of rotavirus vaccines.— T. H. Flewett, *Archs Dis. Childh.*, 1986, *61*, 211.

Reports of the use of the live oral bovine rotavirus vaccine (RIT 4237): T. Vesikari *et al.*, *Lancet*, 1983, *2*, 807; T. Vesikari *et al.*, *ibid.*, 1984, *1*, 977; T. Vesikari *et al.* (letter), *ibid.*, *2*, 700; P. De Mol *et al.* (letter), *ibid.*, 1986, *2*, 108; P. Hanlon *et al.*, *ibid.*, 1987, *1*, 1342; B. Biryahwaho (letter), *ibid.*, *2*, 344; Y. D. Senturia *et al.* (letter), *ibid.*, 1091.

A report of the use of the live oral monkey rotavirus vaccine (MMU-18006): J. Flores *et al.*, *Lancet*, 1987, *1*, 882.

8001-w

Rubella Vaccines

Rubella Vaccine, Live (*B.P.*) (Rub/Vac (Live); Rubella Vaccine (Live) (*Eur. P.*); Vaccinum Rubellae Vivum) is an aqueous suspension of a suitable live attenuated strain of rubella virus grown in suitable cell cultures. It is supplied as a freeze-dried vaccine, which is reconstituted, immediately before use, by the addition of a suitable sterile liquid. Antimicrobial preservatives must not be added; it contains a suitable stabiliser. The dried vaccine should be stored at 2° to 8°, not be allowed to freeze, and be protected from light. Under these conditions it may be expected to retain its potency for at least 2 years.

Rubella Virus Vaccine Live (*U.S.P.*) is a bacterially sterile freeze-dried preparation of a suitable live strain of rubella virus grown in cultures of duck-embryo tissue or human tissue. It contains the equivalent of not less than 1000 TCID50 in each immunising dose. It should be stored at 2° to 8° and be protected from light.

Adverse Effects

As for vaccines in general, p.1155.

Generally, side-effects have not been severe. Those occurring most commonly are skin rashes, pharyngitis, fever, and lymphadenopathy; arthralgia and arthritis may also occur and such joint symptoms are reported to be more common in women than young girls. Neurological symptoms including neuropathy and paraesthesia have also been reported.

After immunisation with RA 27/3 rubella vaccine a 24-year-old woman developed chronic recurrent arthritis, hypogammaglobulinaemia, and persistent rubella viraemia, and failed to seroconvert.— A. J. Tingle *et al.* (letter), *Lancet*, 1984, *1*, 1475.

EFFECTS ON THE NERVOUS SYSTEM. Two patients developed diffuse myelitis, with persistent motor impairment of the legs, after receiving rubella vaccine.— S. Holt *et al.*, *Br. med. J.*, 1976, *2*, 1037.

A 27-year-old woman had paraesthesia of both legs and mild paraparesis 8 days after receiving rubella vaccine; a similar attack occurred 14 months later after exposure to rubella.— P. O. Behan (letter), *Br. med. J.*, 1977, *1*, 166.

Facial paraesthesia in a 35-year-old woman after vaccination with an RA 27/3 rubella vaccine.— L. Morton-Kute (letter), *Ann. intern. Med.*, 1985, *102*, 563.

Precautions

As for vaccines in general, p.1156.

Rubella vaccines should not be given during pregnancy and in the *UK* it is recommended that patients should be advised not to become pregnant within one month of vaccination. However, no case of congenital rubella syndrome has been reported following the inadvertent administration of rubella vaccines shortly before or during pregnancy and it is thus considered that there is no evidence that the vaccines are teratogenic. Inadvertent administration of rubella vaccines during pregnancy should not therefore result in a routine recommendation to terminate the pregnancy. There is no risk to a pregnant woman from contact with recently vaccinated persons as the vaccine virus is not transmitted.

Failure of rubella vaccination evidently due to antibodies in a recent blood transfusion.— R. W. Watt and R. B. McGucken, *Br. med. J.*, 1980, *281*, 977.

PREGNANCY AND THE NEONATE. A follow-up study was conducted in 1964 women who were given rubella vaccine. The vaccine was given within 3 months of conception in 27 instances and pregnancy was terminated in 10 women. In 17 pregnancies continued to term all infants appeared normal at birth and at subsequent follow-up.— J. P. Fox *et al.*, *J. Am. med. Ass.*, 1976, *236*, 837.

A preliminary report on 54 women who conceived within 3 months of vaccination against rubella or who received the vaccine during pregnancy. Of the 51 live births there was no evidence of the congenital rubella syndrome in any infant.— S. Sheppard *et al.*, *Br. med. J.*, 1986, *292*, 727.

A report from the Centers for Disease Control in the *USA* concerning rubella vaccination during pregnancy. Reports had been received of 1176 women who had received rubella vaccine either 3 months before or 3 months after their presumed date of conception during the period 1971-86. Of 560 women who received the RA 27/3 vaccine and for whom the outcome of pregnancy was known, all of the 522 living infants were free of defects indicative of the congenital rubella syndrome. It was noted that the Advisory Committee on Immunization Practices continues to consider pregnancy a contra-indication to rubella vaccination but that inadvertent vaccination of a pregnant woman should not ordinarily be a reason to consider interruption of the pregnancy.— *J. Am. med. Ass.*, 1987, *258*, 753.

Uses and Administration

Rubella vaccines are used for active immunisation against rubella (German measles).

In the *UK* and the *USA* routine vaccination against rubella of all children during the second year of life using a combined measles, mumps, and rubella vaccine is recommended (see p.1168). In the *UK* it is also recommended that until a high uptake of this combined vaccine in young children has been achieved and the elimination of rubella demonstrated, a single-antigen rubella vaccine should be administered to girls aged 10 to 14 years. Vaccine should also be given to women of childbearing age if they are seronegative; women who are found to be seronegative during pregnancy should be vaccinated in the early postpartum period. Effective precautions against pregnancy must be observed for at least one month following vaccination. The rubella vaccine available in the *UK* is prepared from the RA 27/3 strain and is given by subcutaneous injection in a single dose of 0.5 mL.

Recommendations of the Advisory Committee on Immunization Practices for the prevention of rubella in the *USA* (*Ann. intern. Med.*, 1984, *101*, 505; *J. Am. med. Ass.*, 1984, *252*, 192). Rubella vaccination should be given to all children 12 months of age or older; because persisting maternal antibodies may interfere with seroconversion it should not be given to younger infants. A monovalent vaccine may be used but preferably a combination product such as measles, mumps, and rubella should be employed and given at 15 months of age or older to maximise measles seroconversion. Increased emphasis should also continue to be placed on vaccinating susceptible adolescent and adult women of childbearing age.

Proprietary Preparations

Almevax *(Wellcome, UK)*. Rubella Vaccine, Live (*B.P.*) prepared from the Wistar RA 27/3 virus strain propagated in human diploid cells, and containing in each 0.5 mL not less than 1000 TCID50.

Ervevax *(Smith Kline & French, UK)*. Rubella Vaccine, Live (*B.P.*) prepared from the Wistar RA 27/3 virus strain propagated in human diploid cells, and containing in each 0.5 mL not less than 1000 TCID50.

Meruvax II *(Morson, UK)*. A live rubella vaccine prepared from the Wistar RA 27/3 virus strain propagated in human diploid cells, and containing in each dose not less than 1000 TCID50.

7999-a

Rubella and Mumps Vaccines

Rubella and Mumps Virus Vaccine Live (*U.S.P.*) is a bacterially sterile preparation of a suitable live strain of rubella virus and a suitable live strain of mumps virus. It may contain suitable antimicrobial agents. The dried vaccine should be stored at 2° to 8° and be protected from light. The reconstituted vaccine should be used within 8 hours of preparation.

Adverse Effects and Precautions

As for vaccines in general, p.1155.

See also under mumps vaccines, p.1169, and rubella vaccines, above.

Uses and Administration

Rubella and mumps vaccines may be used for active immunisation against mumps and rubella. Vaccination against mumps and rubella is normally performed in infants aged 12 months or more using a combined measles, mumps, and rubella vaccine (see p.1168) but the bivalent rubella and mumps vaccine may be employed when vaccination against measles is not indicated.

A vaccine used in the *USA* is prepared from the Wistar RA 27/3 strain of live attenuated rubella virus grown in human diploid cells and the Jeryl Lynn (B level) strain of mumps virus grown in chick-embryo cells; it contains not less than 1000 and 5000 TCID50 for each component respectively in each 0.5-mL dose. It may be given in a single dose of 0.5 mL by subcutaneous injection to infants of 12 months of age or more or to other children or adults considered to be at risk; it has been suggested that if children were vaccinated when under 12 months of age they should receive a second dose after reaching 12 months of age.

Proprietary Preparations

A live rubella and mumps vaccine is available on a named-patient basis from *Merck Sharp & Dohme, USA*.

8006-z

Scorpion Venom Antisera

Scorpion Venom Antiserum (*B.P.*) is a sterile preparation containing the specific antitoxic globulins that have the power of neutralising the venom of one or more species of scorpion. The species of scorpion against whose venom or venoms the antiserum is intended to be used varies according to the geographical region and for any particular region should include those species prevalent in the region. The potency should be such that the dose stated on the label will completely neutralise the maximum amount of venom likely to be delivered by a single sting. It should be stored at 2° to 8°, not be allowed to freeze, and be protected from light.

Adverse Effects and Precautions

As for antisera in general, p.1155.

Uses and Administration

A scorpion sting is not usually fatal to healthy adults in the African and Middle East areas but the sting of South and Central American scorpions frequently results in death.

The use of a scorpion antiserum suitable for the species of scorpion can prevent symptoms provided it is done with the least possible delay; other general supportive measures may also be needed. The volume stated on the label as the dose should preferably be made directly into the site of the sting but, if this cannot be done, as much as possible should be injected into the site and the remainder intramuscularly into a convenient proximal position.

Proprietary Preparations

A scorpion venom antiserum is available on a named-patient basis from *Merieux, UK*.

8008-k

Smallpox Vaccines

Smallpox Vaccine (*B.P.*) is a suspension of a suitable strain of the living virus of vaccinia prepared from material obtained from the lesions produced by the inoculation of vaccinia virus in the skin of healthy animals; it contains no antibiotics. It contains not less than 1×10^8 pock-forming units per mL, when compared with the first International Reference Preparation (1962). It is supplied as a dried vaccine (Dried Var/Vac) which is reconstituted before use by the addition of a suitable sterile liquid. *Eur. P.* includes the dried vaccine as Freeze-Dried Smallpox Vaccine (Dermal); Vaccinum Variolae Cryodesiccatum Dermicum. The dried vaccine should be stored below 5° when it may be expected to retain its potency for 4 years. The reconstituted vaccine may be expected to retain its potency for 7 days at 2° to 8°.

Smallpox Vaccine (*U.S.P.*) is a suspension or solid containing a suitable strain of the living virus of vaccinia grown in the skin of bovine calves; it may contain a suitable preservative. The liquid vaccine should be stored below 0° and the dried vaccine at 2° to 8°.

Units

The first International Reference Preparation (1962) of smallpox vaccine consists of ampoules containing 14 mg of freeze-dried smallpox vaccine.

Uses and Administration

Smallpox vaccines, when inoculated by multiple pressure or by scarification, stimulate the formation of antibodies, and the resulting immunity persists for a number of years.

Following the global eradication of smallpox, vaccination against smallpox is indicated only for investigators at special risk such as laboratory workers handling certain orthopoxviruses. No country now requires an international certificate of vaccination from travellers.

The World Health Organization has recommended that smallpox vaccination of military personnel be discontinued, that a global reserve stock of smallpox vaccine is no longer required, and that remaining stocks of smallpox (variola) virus be destroyed.

An article on smallpox and its post-eradication surveillance dedicated to the Tenth Anniversary of worldwide freedom from smallpox.— Z. Jezek *et al.*, *Bull. Wld Hlth Org.*, 1987, *65*, 425.

8011-l

Snake Venom Antisera

Snake Antivenins.

European Viper Venom Antiserum (*B.P., Eur.P.*) (Immunoserum Contra Venena Viperarum Europaearum) is a sterile preparation containing the specific antitoxic globulins that have the power of neutralising the venom of one or more species of viper (*Vipera ammodytes*, *V. aspis*, *V. berus*, or *V. ursinii*). The globulins are obtained by fractionation of the serum of animals that have been immunised against the venom or venoms. It should be stored at 2° to 8°, not be allowed to freeze, and be protected from light.

Antivenin (Crotalidae) Polyvalent (*U.S.P.*) is a sterile freeze-dried preparation of specific venom-neutralising globulins obtained from the serum of healthy horses immunised against 4 species of pit vipers, *Crotalus atrox* (Western diamondback), *Crotalus adamanteus*, *Crotalus durissus terrificus* (South American rattlesnake), and *Bothrops atrox* (South American fer de lance). One dose neutralises the venoms in not less than 180 mouse LD50 of *C. atrox*, 1320 of *C. durissus terrificus*, and 780 of *B. atrox*. It may contain a suitable preservative. It should be preserved in single-dose containers and stored at a temperature not exceeding 40°.

Antivenin (Micrurus Fulvius) (*U.S.P.*) is a sterile freeze-dried preparation of specific venom-neutralising globulins obtained from the serum of healthy horses immunised against venom of *Micrurus fulvius* (Eastern Coral snake). One dose neutralises the venom in not less than 250 mouse LD50 of *M. fulvius*. It may contain a suitable preservative. It should be preserved in single-dose containers and stored at a temperature not exceeding 40°.

Units

300 units of *Naja* antivenin, equine, are contained in 807 mg of purified, dried, polyvalent (*Naja* and *Hemachatus* spp.) horse serum in one ampoule of the first International Standard Preparation (1964).

Adverse Effects and Precautions

As for antisera in general, p.1155.

Serum sickness is not uncommon and anaphylactic reactions may occur.

A study on the prediction, prevention, and mechanism of early (anaphylactic) antivenom reactions in victims of snake bites; the study involved 15 patients in Nigeria with systemic envenoming by the saw-scaled or carpet viper (*Echis carinatus*) and a total of 80 patients in Thailand with local or systemic envenoming by green pit vipers (*Trimeresurus albolabris* and *T. macrops*), the monocellate Thai cobra (*Naja kaouthia*), or the Malayan pit viper (*Calloselasma rhodostoma*). Conjunctival or cutaneous (intradermal or subcutaneous) hypersensitivity testing was performed in 35 patients before the administration of the antivenoms but failed to predict reactions to the antivenom. Only 2 patients exhibited a positive reaction to sensitivity testing and neither experienced a reaction to treatment; 12 patients developed anaphylactic reactions to antivenom treatment and none of these had exhibited a positive sensitivity test. In 66 of the Thai patients the incidence and severity of reactions to the antivenom was the same whether it was given by an intravenous injection over 10 minutes or diluted and given by intravenous infusion over 30 minutes. It was considered that conventional hypersensitivity testing has no predictive value for the occurrence of allergic reactions to antivenom and that it is not justifiable to delay treatment for 20 or 30 minutes to read the results of these tests. It was also considered that although the rate of administration of the antivenom can be more easily controlled by intravenous infusion this method has serious practical disadvantages in the rural tropics where most cases of snake bite occur and that an advantage of the intravenous push injection is that the person administering the antivenom must remain with the patient during the period when most severe anaphylactic reactions develop.— P. Malasit *et al.*, *Br. med. J.*, 1986, *292*, 17.

Uses and Administration

Venomous snakes comprise the Viperidae (vipers), Elapidae (cobras, kraits, and mambas), and the Hydrophiidae (sea snakes).

The venom of snakes is a complex mixture chiefly of proteins, many of which have enzymatic activity, and may also provoke local inflammatory reactions. The venom may have profound effects on tissue, blood vessels and other organs, blood cells, coagulation, and myotoxic or neurotoxic effects with sensory, motor, cardiac, and respiratory involvement.

In Great Britain the only poisonous snake is the adder, *Viperus berus*. Zagreb antivenin may sometimes be indicated as part of the overall treatment. The usual dose is two ampoules of the antivenom, diluted with 2 to 3 volumes of sodium chloride 0.9%, and given by intravenous infusion; this may be repeated after about 1 to 2 hours if no clinical improvement has occurred.

In the USA a polyvalent crotaline antivenin against *Bothrops atrox*, *Crotalus adamanteus*, *C. atrox*, and *C. durissus terrificus*, and an antivenin against the Eastern Coral snake, *Micrurus fulvius*, are available. In Australia a polyvalent antivenin against the black snake, brown snake, death adder, taipan, and tiger snake is available as well as individual monovalent antivenins against these snakes. In many other countries a wide variety of antivenins are available.

The use of antivenin is an essential part of the treatment of bites from highly venomous snakes. Antivenin is generally given cautiously by intravenous infusion, after dilution with sodium chloride 0.9%. Resuscitative facilities should be available.

A review of adder bites and their management. It was recommended that Zagreb antivenom should be given if hypotension persisted or recurred unless there was a history of allergy. Antivenom might also be indicated if there was leucocytosis, evidence of acidosis, ECG changes or raised serum creatine phosphokinase concentrations. Extensive swelling seen within 2 hours of a bite was also a possible indication in adults to minimise morbidity. Serum sensitivity tests were not recommended as they had been found to be misleading and adrenaline was always effective when given promptly to treat reactions. The contents of 2 ampoules of Zagreb antivenom was a suitable dose for all ages; this was diluted in 100 mL of sodium chloride injection and infused at an initial rate of 15 drops a minute increased to complete the dose within an hour. Further antivenom might be considered if there was no improvement. Should a reaction occur the drip should be stopped temporarily and 0.5 mL of a 1 in 1000 solution of adrenaline given intramuscularly. Once the reaction was controlled the infusion of antivenom could be restarted.— H. A. Reid, *Br. med. J.*, 1976, *2*, 153.

A review and discussion on the epidemiology, pathophysiology, and treatment of snake bite. Most snake species are non-venomous and belong to the colubrid family although a few colubrids are technically venomous. The three families of venomous front-fanged snakes are the elapids, vipers, and sea snakes. Elapids include cobras, mambas, kraits, coral snakes, and the Australasian venomous land snakes. Vipers are subdivided into crotalids (pit vipers) and viperids. Viper bites are much more common than elapid bites, except in Australasia, where vipers do not occur naturally. Sea snake bites occur among fishermen of the Asian and Western Pacific coastal areas. Only a few snakes are known to be of medical importance. The foremost important vipers are *Bothrops atrox* (Central and South America), *Bitis arietans* (Africa), *Echis carinatus* (Africa and Asia), *Vipera russelli* (Asia), and *Agkistrodon rhodostoma* (south-east Asia). In a few restricted areas of Africa and Asia, cobra bites are common; bites by mambas (Africa) and kraits (Asia) are rare. The carpet or saw-scaled viper, *Echis carinatus*, can justifiably be labelled the most dangerous snake in the world and it causes more deaths and serious poisoning than any other snake. Although there are some notable exceptions, an arbitrary classification of snake bites may be made such that vipers cause vasculotoxicity, elapids cause neurotoxicity, and sea snakes cause myotoxicity.

Management of snake bite involves general supportive

care and monitoring of vital functions but in a systemic snake-bite poisoning, specific antivenom is the most effective therapeutic agent available. If used correctly, it can reverse systemic poisoning when given hours or even days after the bite. It is highly desirable to wait for clear clinical evidence of systemic poisoning before giving an antivenom and therefore antivenom should not be given routinely in all cases of snake bite. Monospecific antivenoms are more effective, and less likely to cause reactions, than polyvalent antivenoms. Depending upon the potency of the antivenom, between 20 and 50 mL should be diluted in 3 volumes of isotonic saline although in severe poisoning, especially neurotoxic envenoming, 100 to 150 mL of antivenom would be a suitable initial dose. The rate of infusion should be progressively increased so that it is completed within 1 to 2 hours. Further antivenom may be considered if there has been little significant improvement.— H. A. Reid and R. D. G. Theakston, *Bull. Wld Hlth Org.*, 1983; *61*, 885.

Further reviews and discussions of the treatment of snake bite: F. E. Russell *et al.*, *J. Am. med. Ass.*, 1975, *233*, 341; S. K. Sutherland (letter), *Med. J. Aust.*, 1977, *2*, 841; *Med. J. Aust.*, 1978, *1*, 137; D. A. Warrell, *Prescribers' J.*, 1979, *19*, 190; *ibid.*, *20* (Apr.); *Med. Lett.*, 1982, *24*, 87.

Accounts of the treatment, including the use of snake venom antisera, of various snake bites: D. A. Warrell *et al.*, *Br. med. J.*, 1975, *4*, 697 (puff-adder: *Bitis arietans*); R. N. H. Pugh *et al.*, *Lancet*, 1979, *2*, 625 (carpet or saw-scaled viper: *Echis carinatus*); D. A. Warrell *et al.*, *Br. med. J.*, 1980, *280*, 607 (carpet viper: *Echis carinatus*); D. A. Warrell *et al.*, *ibid.*, 1983, *286*, 678 (Malayan krait: *Bungarus candidus*); G. W. O. Fulde and F. Smith, *Med. J. Aust.*, 1984, *141*, 44 (unidentified sea snake); P. J. Mirtschin *et al.*, *ibid.*, 850 (inland taipan: *Oxyuranus microlepidotus*); K. O. Lwin *et al.*, *Trans. R. Soc. trop. Med. Hyg.*, 1984, *78*, 165 (Russell's viper: *Vipera russelli*); B. R. Patten *et al.*, *Med. J. Aust.*, 1985, *142*, 467 (rough-scaled snake: *Tropidechis carinatus*); Myint-Lwin *et al.*, *Lancet*, 1985, *2*, 1259 (Russell's viper: *Vipera russelli*); I. Tiwari and W. J. Johnston, *ibid.*, 1986, *1*, 613 (sand viper: *Vipera ammodytes*); G. J. Dobb, *Med. J. Aust.*, 1986, *144*, 112 (unidentified sea snake); D. K. Pawar and H. Singh, *Br. J. Anaesth.*, 1987, *59*, 385 (kraits and cobras).

Proprietary Preparations

Snake venom antiserum (Zagreb antivenom) is available from *Regent Laboratories, UK.*

Emergency stocks of some snake venom antisera, including those for certain foreign and exotic snakes, are also held by The National Poisons Information Centre, London and by Walton Hospital Pharmacy, Liverpool.

8035-x

Spider Antivenoms

Spider Antivenins.

Antivenin (Latrodectus mactans) (*U.S.P.*) is a sterile freeze-dried preparation of specific venom-neutralising globulins obtained from the serum of healthy horses immunised against venom of black widow spiders (*Latrodectus mactans*). One dose neutralises the venom in not less than 6000 mouse LD50 of *L. mactans*. It contains thiomersal 0.01%. It should be preserved in single-dose containers and stored at a temperature not exceeding 40°.

Adverse Effects and Precautions

As for antisera in general, p.1155.

Uses and Administration

The use of a spider antivenom suitable for the species of spider can prevent symptoms provided it is done with the least possible delay; other general supportive measures may also be needed.

An antivenom against the black widow spider (*Latrodectus mactans*) is available and the contents of a vial containing at least 6000 antivenin units are given to severe cases and children under 12 years of age by intravenous infusion in sodium chloride 0.9% over 15 minutes; alternatively, in less severe cases, it may be given by intramuscular injection.

An account of the use of an antivenom to the funnel-web spider (*Atrax robustus*) in the treatment of 9 patients in Australia.— L. J. Hartman and S. K. Sutherland, *Med. J. Aust.*, 1984, *141*, 796.

Proprietary Preparations

A black widow spider antivenom is available on a named-patient basis from *Merck Sharp & Dohme, USA.*

Proprietary Names and Manufacturers

Commonwealth Serum Laboratories, Austral.; Merck Sharp & Dohme, Canad.; Wyeth, Canad.; Merck Sharp & Dohme, USA.

8013-j

Staphylococcal Vaccines

Staphylococcal vaccines, prepared from inactivated *Staphylococcus* spp. have been used orally, topically, and by subcutaneous injection.

Proprietary Preparations

A staphylococcal vaccine is available from *HSL Vaccine Laboratory, UK.*

8016-k

Tetanus Antitoxins

Tetanus Antitoxin (*B.P.*) (Tetanus Antitoxin for Human Use (*Eur. P.*); Immunoserum Tetanicum ad Usum Humanum; Tet/Ser) is a sterile preparation containing the specific antitoxic globulins that have the power of neutralising the toxin formed by *Clostridium tetani*. For prophylactic use, it has a potency of not less than 1000 units per mL, and for therapeutic use not less than 3000 units per mL. It should be stored at 2° to 8°, not be allowed to freeze, and be protected from light.

Tetanus Antitoxin (U.S.P.) is a sterile solution of the refined and concentrated proteins, chiefly globulins, containing antitoxic antibodies obtained from the serum or plasma of healthy horses that have been immunised against tetanus toxin or toxoid. It contains not less than 400 units per mL. It should be stored at 2° to 8°.

Units

1400 units (1000 Lf-equivalents for flocculation) of tetanus antitoxin (equine) are contained in 47 mg of freeze-dried hyperimmune horse serum in one ampoule of the second International Standard Preparation (1969).

Adverse Effects and Precautions

As for antisera in general, p.1155.

Uses and Administration

Tetanus antitoxins neutralise the toxin produced by *Clostridium tetani*; the toxin has a high affinity for nerve cells and antitoxin is unlikely to have an effect on toxin that is no longer circulating.

Tetanus antitoxins have been used to provide temporary passive immunity against tetanus but tetanus immunoglobulins (see below) are preferred.

For prophylaxis after injury non-immune or partially immune persons may be given 3000 to 5000 units of a tetanus antitoxin subcutaneously or intramuscularly; the dose for children of less than 30 kg body-weight is usually 1500 units.

Doses of 50 000 to 100 000 units have been given as part of the regimen of treatment of established tetanus; part of this dose is administered by intravenous injection with the remainder being given intramuscularly.

Whenever a non-immune patient is seen because of injury opportunity should be taken to institute a course of active immunisation.

1241-c

Tetanus Immunoglobulins

Tetanus Immunoglobulin (*B.P.*) (Antitetanus Immunoglobulin Injection; Human Tetanus Immunoglobulin (*Eur.P.*); Immunoglobulinum Humanum Tetanicum) is a liquid or freeze-dried preparation containing immunoglobulins, mainly immunoglobulin G (IgG). It is obtained from plasma or serum containing specific antibodies against the toxin of *Clostridium tetani*. Normal Immunoglobulin may be added. Tetanus Immunoglobulin is prepared in the same manner as Normal Immunoglobulin (see p.1170) except that pooled material may be from fewer than 1000 donors. It contains not less than 50 units per mL. The liquid preparation should be stored, protected from light, in a sealed, colourless, glass container at a temperature of 2° to 8°. Under these conditions it may be expected to retain its potency for 3 years. The freeze-dried preparation should be stored, protected from light, under vacuum or under an inert gas; the *B.P.* specifies storage at 2° to 8° whereas the *Eur.P.* specifies storage at below 25°. Under these conditions it may be expected to retain its potency for 5 years.

Tetanus Immune Globulin (*U.S.P.*) is a sterile solution of globulins derived from the plasma of adult human donors who have been immunised with tetanus vaccine. It contains not less than 50 units of tetanus antitoxin per mL. It contains 10 to 18% of protein of which not less than 90% is gamma globulin. It contains glycine as a stabilising agent, and a suitable preservative. It should be stored at 2° to 8°.

Units

The unit for tetanus immunoglobulin is based on the unit for tetanus antitoxin, see above.

Adverse Effects and Precautions

As for immunoglobulins in general, p.1155.

Tetanus immunoglobulins should not be injected into the same site or in the same syringe as a tetanus vaccine.

Uses and Administration

Tetanus immunoglobulins are used for passive immunisation against tetanus.

The use of tetanus immunoglobulins is recommended in the *UK* as part of the management of tetanus-prone wounds in persons unimmunised or incompletely immunised against tetanus (one dose only of tetanus vaccine received), in persons whose immunisation history is unknown, and in persons who received the last dose of tetanus vaccine more than 10 years previously. Active immunisation with a tetanus vaccine (see below) should also be started simultaneously. The usual dose of tetanus immunoglobulin is 250 units by intramuscular injection but if more than 24 hours have elapsed since the wound was sustained or if there is a risk of heavy contamination 500 units should be given irrespective of the immunisation history.

Tetanus immunoglobulin is also used in the treatment of tetanus, the recommended dose being 30 to 300 units per kg body-weight given intramuscularly into different sites.

For the recommendations of the Immunization Practices Advisory Committee in the *USA* concerning the prophylaxis of tetanus, including the use of tetanus immunoglobulins, see under diphtheria and tetanus vaccines (p.1161).

Proprietary Preparations

Humotet *(Wellcome, UK).* Tetanus Immunoglobulin (*B.P.*) containing tetanus antitoxin 250 units in each mL.

A tetanus immunoglobulin is also available from *Blood Products Laboratory, UK.*

8020-y

Tetanus Vaccines

Tetanus Toxoids.

Tetanus Vaccine (*B.P.*) (Tet/Vac/FT) is prepared from tetanus toxin produced by the growth of *Clostridium tetani*. The toxin is converted to tetanus formol toxoid by treatment with formaldehyde solution. It should be stored at 2° to 8°, not be allowed to freeze, and be protected from light. The *B.P.* directs that when Tetanus Vaccine is prescribed or demanded and the form is not stated, Adsorbed Tetanus Vaccine may be dispensed or supplied.

Adsorbed Tetanus Vaccine (*B.P.*) (Tet/Vac/Ads; Tetanus Vaccine (Adsorbed) (*Eur. P.*); Vaccinum Tetani Adsorbatum) is prepared from tetanus formol toxoid containing not less than 1000 Lf per mg of protein nitrogen and a mineral carrier which may be hydrated aluminium hydroxide, aluminium phosphate, or calcium phosphate in a saline solution or other suitable solution isotonic with blood. The antigenic properties are adversely affected by certain antimicrobial preservatives particularly those of the phenolic type and these should not be added to the vaccine. It contains not less than 40 units per dose. It should be stored at 2° to 8°, not be allowed to freeze, and be protected from light. Under these conditions it may be expected to retain its potency for not less than 5 years from the date on which the potency test was begun.

Tetanus Toxoid (*U.S.P.*) is a sterile solution of the formaldehyde-treated products of growth of *Clostridium tetani*. It contains a non-phenolic preservative. It should be stored at 2° to 8° and not be allowed to freeze.

Tetanus Toxoid Adsorbed (*U.S.P.*) is a sterile preparation of plain tetanus toxoid precipitated or adsorbed by alum, aluminium hydroxide, or aluminium phosphate adjuvants. It should be stored at 2° to 8° and not be allowed to freeze.

Units

833 units of tetanus toxoid, plain, are contained in 25 mg of alcohol-purified tetanus toxoid, plain, with glycine, in one ampoule of the first International Standard Preparation (1951).

340 units of tetanus toxoid, adsorbed, are contained in 27.5 mg of a dried mixture of tetanus toxoid (90 Lf per ampoule) adsorbed to aluminium hydroxide (1 mg Al^{3+} per ampoule) and 22.5 mg of haemacel, in one ampoule of the second International Standard Preparation (1981).

Potency has also been expressed in terms of Limes flocculationis (Lf); there is no simple correlation between international units and Lf equivalents.

A short comment on the problems of standardisation of adsorbed tetanus vaccines. A collaborative study revealed that the potency of the second International Standard Preparation (1981) was higher when assayed in guinea-pigs than when assayed in mice and moreover there were considerable interlaboratory differences in the latter assays. It was therefore decided to establish the potency on the basis of assays in guinea-pigs only even though it was known that most laboratories use the mouse assay.— Thirty-third Report of the WHO Expert Committee on Biological Standardization, *Tech. Rep. Ser. Wld Hlth Org. No. 687*, 1983..

Adverse Effects and Precautions

As for vaccines in general, p.1155.

Local reactions occur occasionally, usually following the use of adsorbed vaccines. The incidence of reactions increases with the second and third injections but the reactions are generally not severe. Reactions are more common in adults than in children and an incidence in adults of 1 to 2% has been reported. Hypersensitivity reactions, possibly associated with skin rashes, have been reported.

A discussion of toxic reactions, particularly local reactions, to tetanus vaccine.— *Br. med. J.*, 1974, *1*, 48.

Reduced incidence of pain, tenderness, swelling, and erythema in children aged 15 to 16 given reinforcing doses of a non-adsorbed tetanus vaccine, compared with those given an adsorbed tetanus vaccine.— L. H. Collier *et al.*, *Lancet*, 1979, *1*, 1364. From extensive experience with plain and adsorbed vaccines in thousands of employees at a motor car factory the wisdom of perpetuating the use of plain vaccine is doubted. The only advantage it appears to have over the adsorbed vaccine is its suitability for intradermal administration in the occasional patient who has had a severe reaction to previous inoculations of adsorbed vaccine, aluminium-containing preparations being unsuitable for intradermal inoculation.— W. G. White (letter), *ibid.*, 1980, *1*, 42.

Granuloma, in 3 patients, at the injection site of adsorbed tetanus vaccines. Biopsy and microscopy proved the granuloma to be due to aluminium used as the adsorbant in the vaccines.— H. A. Fawcett and N. P. Smith, *Archs Derm.*, 1984, *120*, 1318.

In a double-blind comparative study involving 205 healthy subjects there was no difference in side-effects in those given a standard (commercial) tetanus vaccine and those given an antibody-affinity-purified vaccine. The results confirmed that side-effects to tetanus vaccines are not eliminated by purification.— C. L. S. Leen *et al.*, *J. Infect.*, 1987, *14*, 119.

For references implicating the tetanus component of mixed vaccines as the cause of adverse reactions, see under diphtheria and tetanus vaccines (p.1161) and Schick test (p.945).

ALLERGY. A 24-year-old woman developed anaphylactic shock and died 30 minutes after an injection of tetanus vaccine. Previous injections with the vaccine had been well tolerated.— M. Staak and E. Wirth, *Dt. med. Wschr.*, 1973, *98*, 110.

A report of anaphylaxis to an adsorbed tetanus vaccine, the first case described in the *UK*.— D. A. Ratliff and C. J. Burns-Cox, *Br. med. J.*, 1984, *288*, 114.

Further reports of allergic reactions associated with the use of tetanus vaccines: G. P. Zaloga and B. Chernow, *Ann. Allergy*, 1982, *49*, 107 (anaphylactoid reaction).

EFFECTS ON THE NERVOUS SYSTEM. Peripheral neuropathy with paralysis of the right radial nerve developed in a medical student a few hours after he had been given tetanus vaccine.— G. I. Blumstein and H. Kreithen, *J. Am. med. Ass.*, 1966, *198*, 1030.

Uses and Administration

Tetanus vaccines are used for active immunisation against tetanus.

Active immunisation should be started in infants aged 3 months and in the *UK* the vaccine is generally given as a combined diphtheria, tetanus, and pertussis vaccine (see p.1161) or as a combined diphtheria and tetanus vaccine (see p.1160) if it is decided not to immunise against pertussis also; immunisation against poliomyelitis is also generally performed at the same time using a live (oral) poliomyelitis vaccine (see p.1173). For a reinforcing dose at the age of 5 years or at school entry, when immunisation against pertussis is no longer necessary, a combined diphtheria and tetanus vaccine should be given. A further reinforcing dose of a single-component tetanus vaccine is recommended at the age of 15 to 19 years.

If neither immunisation against diphtheria nor against pertussis is required, a situation which is more likely to occur in adults than in children, a single-component tetanus vaccine may be used. The non-adsorbed type of tetanus vaccine is less potent as an antigen than the adsorbed type. In the *UK*, therefore, where both types are available it is recommended that the adsorbed type should always be used for the first dose of an immunisation course; subsequent doses may be of either type, although the adsorbed vaccine is generally preferred. The course consists of 3 doses, each of 0.5 mL (not less than 40 units for adsorbed vaccine, not less than 14 Lf for non-adsorbed vaccine), administered by deep subcutaneous or intramuscular injection; the first dose is followed 6 to 8 weeks later by the second dose, and the third dose follows after an interval of 4 to 6 months. A reinforcing dose is desirable 5 years later with a further dose after a further 5 to 15 years.

In the event of injury in a previously immunised person and where it is considered that a risk of tetanus exists an additional reinforcing dose may be given provided such a dose has not been given in the preceding 12 months. In the event of injury in non-immunised persons opportunity is usually taken to initiate a course of primary immunisation. This provides no immediate protection and prophylactic treatment with tetanus immunoglobulin (see above), possibly with antibiotics, may be needed. The first dose of the vaccine may be given concomitantly, but not into the same limb.

In some other countries the strength of the vaccines and dosage schedules differ slightly from that outlined above.

Immunisation against tetanus forms part of the World Health Organization's Expanded Programme on Immunization (see p.1156).

For the Recommendations of the Immunization Practices Advisory Committee for the prophylaxis of diphtheria, tetanus, and pertussis in the *USA*, see under diphtheria and tetanus vaccines (p.1161) and diphtheria, tetanus, and pertussis vaccines (p.1162).

An account of clinical tetanus in a patient following injury despite the fact he had a reliable history of previous immunisation and a neutralising antibody concentration of 0.16 antitoxin units per mL, sixteen times the concentration considered to afford protection. It was considered that there may be no absolute or universal protective concentration of antibody and that protection may simply result when there is sufficient toxin-neutralising antibody in relation to the toxin load.— E. L. Passen and B. R. Andersen, *J. Am. med. Ass.*, 1986, *255*, 1171.

NEONATAL TETANUS. A review and discussion concerning neonatal tetanus. In many countries all forms of tetanus remain substantially under-reported but it has been estimated that over 500 000 newborn children die each year in developing countries due to neonatal tetanus. Control and elimination of neonatal tetanus may be achieved by ensuring adequate hygiene of both mother and baby during the delivery and neonatal period and by ensuring protective immunity of the mother in late pregnancy. The latter is a shortcut to the elimination of tetanus, but not to other causes of neonatal mortality, and should ultimately become unnecessary as the risk of infection is eliminated. Enough is known about the efficacy of tetanus vaccines to give clear guidelines about the optimum schedules. In those countries where there is a continuing neonatal mortality from tetanus, two doses of the vaccine, at least a month apart, should be given in the course of a pregnancy and should be started as soon as possible. If the woman has received two doses within the previous 5 years, only one further dose during pregnancy is required. Thereafter, protection during subsequent pregnancies will probably be obtained with two further booster doses at 5-yearly intervals. In highly endemic areas it may be of benefit to give a primary two-dose course followed by two boosters to all women of child-bearing age.— J. P. Stanfield and A. Galazka, *Bull. Wld Hlth Org.*, 1984, *62*, 647.

Results of a study to determine the relationship between

the timing of maternal immunisation with adsorbed tetanus vaccines and the presence of protective antitoxin in cord blood indicated that the first injection of a two-dose schedule should be given at least 60 days, and preferably 90 days or more, before delivery, with the second injection 20 days or more before delivery.— S. T. Chen *et al., Bull. Wld Hlth Org.*, 1983, *61*, 159.

Proprietary Preparations

Merieux Tetavax *(Merieux, UK)*. Adsorbed Tetanus Vaccine (*B.P.*).

Tetanus Vaccine (*B.P.*) is available from *Wellcome, UK* and Adsorbed Tetanus Vaccine (*B.P.*) is available from *Servier, UK* and *Wellcome, UK*.

3870-z

Trichomonal Vaccines

A trichomonal vaccine containing inactivated *Lactobacillus acidophilus* is available for the prophylaxis of recurrent trichomoniasis in women. The vaccine is reported to stimulate production of antibodies against the aberrant coccoid forms of the lactobacilli associated with trichomoniasis and also by a cross-reaction against the trichomonads as well. Each 0.5-mL dose of the vaccine contains 7000 million inactivated *L. acidophilus* and three doses are given by intramuscular injection at intervals of 2 weeks.

Proprietary Preparations

Gynatren *(Cabot, UK)*. A trichomonal vaccine containing 7000 million *Lactobacillus acidophilus* per 0.5 mL.

8027-x

Typhoid Vaccines

Typhoid Vaccine (*B.P., Eur.P.*) (Typhoid/Vac; Vaccinum Febris Typhoidi) is a sterile suspension of killed *Salmonella typhi* containing not less than 500 million and not more than 1000 million bacteria per dose which does not exceed 1 mL. It is prepared from a suitable strain of *S. typhi* such as Ty 2. The bacteria are killed by heat or by treatment with acetone, formaldehyde, or phenol or by phenol and heat. It may also be supplied as a dried vaccine (Dried Typhoid/Vac) which is reconstituted immediately before use by the addition of suitable sterile liquid. Phenol may not be used in the preparation of the dried vaccine. *Eur.P.* includes the dried vaccine as Freeze-Dried Typhoid Vaccine (Vaccinum Febris Typhoidi Cryodesiccatum). Both the liquid vaccine and the dried vaccine should be stored at 2° to 8°, not be allowed to freeze, and be protected from light. Under these conditions the liquid vaccine may be expected to retain its potency for at least 2 years and the dried vaccine for at least 5 years.

Typhoid Vaccine (*U.S.P.*) is a sterile suspension or solid containing killed typhoid bacilli (*Salmonella typhosa*) of the Ty 2 strain. It has a labelled potency of 8 units per mL. Dried vaccine contains no preservative; aqueous vaccine and reconstituting fluid contain a preservative. It should be stored at 2° to 8° and not be allowed to freeze.

Units

The first International Reference Preparation (1962) of acetone-inactivated typhoid vaccine consists of ampoules containing 11 mg of dried vaccine (*S. typhi*).

The first International Reference Preparation (1962) of heat-phenol-inactivated typhoid vaccine consists of ampoules containing 34 mg of freeze-dried vaccine (*S. typhi*).

Adverse Effects and Precautions

As for vaccines in general, p.1155.

Uses and Administration

Typhoid vaccines are used for active immunisation against typhoid fever. In the *UK* a vaccine containing 1000 million killed *Salmonella typhi* per mL is used and a primary course of 2 injections at an interval of 4 to 6 weeks is given. The doses, given by deep subcutaneous or intramuscular injection, are 0.5 mL for adults and children over 10 years of age and 0.25 mL for children aged 1 to 10 years. Reinforcing doses are generally given every 3 years. Immunisation of children under the age of 1 year is not generally advised because of the risk of side-effects and the relatively low incidence and mild course of the disease in this age group.

CAPSULAR POLYSACCHARIDE TYPHOID VACCINES. A preliminary report of the use of the capsular polysaccharide of *Salmonella typhi* (Vi) as a vaccine to prevent typhoid fever in villagers in Nepal. The vaccine consisted of 25 µg of the capsular polysaccharide in a single-dose of 0.5 mL administered intramuscularly. The overall efficacy in 3457 recipients was 75% 17 months after immunisation. It was considered that this vaccine had advantages over the oral vaccine using the live attenuated Ty 21a strain and that immunogenity of the capsular polysaccharide could be improved by covalent binding to proteins.— I. L. Acharya *et al., New Engl. J. Med.*, 1987, *317*, 1101. A similar study and results.— K. P. Klugman *et al., Lancet*, 1987, *2*, 1165.

ORAL TYPHOID VACCINES. Some comments and discussion on typhoid vaccines. The typhoid vaccines presently available are not wholly satisfactory. Some killed vaccines given by the parenteral route do confer good and long-lasting protection but they also tend to cause undesired local and systemic reactions. Oral killed vaccines are well-tolerated but their efficacy has never been demonstrated and they cannot be recommended.

An attenuated form of *Salmonella typhi* (strain Ty 21a) has been developed and prepared as a candidate for an oral live typhoid vaccine. Both the safety and protective efficacy of this vaccine have been proved in volunteer challenge studies and large field trials. The only difficulty encountered has been the problem of protecting the vaccine bacteria from inactivation by gastric juice and tests have involved either giving the vaccine as capsules together with sodium bicarbonate or as enteric-coated capsules.— Thirty-fourth Report of a WHO Expert Committee on Biological Standardization, *Tech. Rep. Ser. Wld Hlth Org. No. 700*, 1984,, p.48. See also: R. G. A. Sutton and M. H. Merson, *Lancet*, 1983, *1*, 523.

Report of a large-scale field trial of a live oral typhoid vaccine involving 109 000 schoolchildren in Santiago, Chile, an area with a high endemicity of typhoid fever. The vaccine was prepared from an attenuated strain of *Salmonella typhi* (Ty 21a) and contained 1000 to 3000 million viable organisms per dose. Administration of 3 doses given within a week as an enteric-coated formulation provided 67% efficacy for at least 3 years and no enhanced protection was observed when the interval between the doses was extended to 21 days. Significantly less protection followed administration of the vaccine in plain gelatin capsules together with sodium bicarbonate. It was considered that this live oral vaccine in enteric-coated capsules, with its lack of discernible adverse reactions, and ease of administration to children in mass vaccinations, is presently the vaccine of choice for any country intending to embark upon a systematic typhoid fever control programme.— M. M. Levine *et al., Lancet*, 1987, *1*, 1049.

Proprietary Preparations

Typhoid Vaccine (*B.P.*) is available from *Wellcome, UK*.

8025-a

Typhoid and Tetanus Vaccines

Typhoid and Tetanus Vaccine (*B.P.*) (Typhoid/Tet/Vac) is a sterile mixture of a suspension of killed *Salmonella typhi* and tetanus formol toxoid, containing 1000 or 2000 million typhoid bacteria per mL. The suspension is prepared from a strain or strains of *S. typhi* that are smooth and have a full complement of H, O, and Vi antigens. The bacteria are killed by heat or by treatment with formaldehyde or phenol. It should be stored at 2° to 8 °, not be allowed to freeze, and be protected from light.

A combined typhoid and tetanus vaccine has been used by subcutaneous injection for primary immunisation against typhoid fever and tetanus and by intramuscular injection to reinforce immunity.

8034-t

Typhus Vaccines

Typhus Vaccine (*B.P.*) (Typhus/Vac) is a sterile suspension of killed epidemic typhus rickettsiae [*Rickettsia prowazeki*] prepared in the yolk sacs of fertile eggs, rodent lungs, or the peritoneal cavity of gerbils. It should be stored at 2° to 8°, not be allowed to freeze, and be protected from light. Under these conditions it may be expected to retain its potency for at least 1 year.

Adverse Effects and Precautions

As for vaccines in general, p.1155.

Local reactions are usually mild, but reactions of moderate severity may occur.

Uses and Administration

A killed typhus vaccine may be used for active immunisation against louse-borne typhus. Its use may be considered for those living in or visiting the few endemic areas, for medical workers, and laboratory workers. It does not provide complete protection, but lessens the severity of the disease and the incidence of serious complications. It does not provide protection against scrub typhus.

The primary course for adults and children over 10 years of age is 2 doses (1 mL each) given subcutaneously at an interval of 4 weeks. Suggested schedules for younger children have been 3 doses, again at 4-weekly intervals, but in smaller doses; suggested doses have been 0.12 mL for those under 3 years of age, 0.25 mL for those aged 3 to 6 years, and 0.5 mL for those aged 7 to 10 years. Reinforcing doses should be given annually.

Some comments and discussions on louse-borne typhus vaccines for human use. Killed vaccines give limited protection but may modify the disease and further studies are needed for the development of killed vaccines. A vaccine used in the *USSR* contains both live rickettsiae (E strain) and soluble antigen but is awaiting trial under field conditions. A live attenuated vaccine made from the E strain has been tested under field conditions and a much lower rate of late reactions than previously described has been reported.— Thirty-third Report of the WHO Expert Committee on Biological Standardization, *Tech. Rep. Ser. Wld Hlth Org. No. 687*, 1983,, p.61.

Proprietary Preparations

Typhus Vaccine (*B.P.*) is available on a named-patient basis from *Commonwealth Serum Laboratories, Austral.*

1243-a

Vaccinia Immunoglobulins

Human Vaccinia Immunoglobulin (*Eur.P.*) (Immunoglobulinum Humanum Vaccinum) is a liquid or freeze-dried preparation containing immunoglobulins, mainly immunoglobulin G (IgG). It is obtained from plasma or serum containing specific antibodies against the vaccinia virus. Normal Immunoglobulin may be added. It is prepared in the same manner as Normal Immunoglobulin (see p.1170) except that pooled material may be from fewer than 1000 donors. It contains not less than 500 units of neutralising antibody against the vaccinia virus per mL. The liquid preparation should be stored, protected from light, in a sealed, colourless, glass container at a temperature of 2° to 8°. Under these conditions it may be expected to retain its potency for 3 years. The freeze-dried preparation should be stored, protected from light, under vacuum or under an inert gas at a temperature not exceeding 25°. Under these conditions it may be expected to retain its potency for 5 years.

Vaccinia Immune Globulin (*U.S.P.*) is a sterile solution of globulins derived from the plasma of adult human donors who have been immunised with vaccinia virus (smallpox vaccine). It contains 15 to 18% of protein, of which not less than 90% is gamma globulin. It contains glycine as a stabilising agent, and a suitable antimicrobial agent. It should be stored at 2° to 8°.

Units

The unit for vaccinia immunoglobulin is based on the first International Standard Preparation (1965) of anti-smallpox serum, human; 1000 units are contained in 84.3 mg of freeze-dried pooled human serum in one ampoule.

Adverse Effects and Precautions

As for immunoglobulins in general, p.1155.

Uses and Administration

Vaccinia immunoglobulins have been used in the treatment of patients with generalised vaccinia and also those with accidental vaccinia infection endangering the eye.

17024-h

Varicella-Zoster Immunoglobulins

Varicella-Zoster Immune Globulin (*U.S.P.*) is a sterile solution of globulins derived from the plasma of adult donors selected for high titres of varicella-zoster antibodies. It contains 15 to 18% of globulins, of which not less than 99% is immunoglobulin G with traces of immunoglobulin A. It contains glycine as a stabilising agent and thiomersal as a preservative. It should be stored at 2° to 8°.

Adverse Effects and Precautions

As for immunoglobulins in general, p.1155.

Uses and Administration

Varicella-zoster immunoglobulins are used for passive immunisation against varicella (chickenpox) in susceptible persons considered to be at high risk of developing varicella-associated complications after exposure to varicella or herpes zoster (shingles). Such groups of persons include immunocompromised patients and patients with leukaemia, and certain neonates, including those born within about 5 or 6 days of the onset of maternal chickenpox and those whose mothers developed chickenpox shortly after delivery. Varicella-zoster immunoglobulin does not prevent infection when given after exposure but may modify the course of disease.

The recommended doses, given intramuscularly, of the varicella-zoster immunoglobulin available in the *UK* are: 250 mg for all those up to 5 years of age; 500 mg for those aged 6 to 10 years; 750 mg for those aged 11 to 14 years; and 1 g for all those 15 years of age or older.

Recommendations of the Advisory Committee on Immunization Practices concerning the use of varicella-zoster immunoglobulin for the prevention of chickenpox in the *USA* (*Ann. intern. Med.*, 1984, *100*, 859; *J. Am. med. Ass.*, 1984, *251*, 1401). The most important use is for passive immunisation of susceptible immunocompromised children after significant exposure to chickenpox or zoster. Use is also indicated in neonates whose mothers developed chickenpox within 5 days before and 48 hours after delivery. Premature infants who have significant postnatal exposure should be evaluated on an individual basis. Immunocompromised adults, after careful evaluation, who are believed to be susceptible and who have had significant exposure should receive the immunoglobulin. The decision to use the immunoglobulin in a normal adult should be evaluated on an individual basis. The recommended dose given intramuscularly of varicella-zoster immunoglobulin in children is 125 units per 10 kg body-weight, up to a maximum of 625 units; the minimum dose is 125 units and fractional doses (doses other than multiples of 125 units) are not recommended. Data do not exist to be able to calculate the appropriate dose in adults although it appears likely that 625 units should be sufficient in normal adults but higher doses may be necessary in immunocompromised adults.

A study indicating that although immunoglobulin does not prevent varicella in neonates it may reduce the severity of the infection and eliminate mortality.— K. A. J. Hanngren *et al.*, *Scand. J. infect. Dis.*, 1985, *17*, 343.

Some further references to the use of varicella-zoster immunoglobulins for the prophylaxis of neonatal chickenpox: B. Bose *et al.* (letter), *Lancet*, 1986, *1*, 449; M. M. Ogilvie *et al.* (letter), *ibid.*, 915; J. Haddad *et al.* (letter), *ibid.*, 1494; P. Holland *et al.* (letter), *ibid.*, *2*, 1156; P. E. Carter *et al.* (letter), *ibid.*, 1459; J. A. Sills *et al.* (letter), *ibid.*, 1987, *1*, 161.

Proprietary Preparations

A varicella-zoster immunoglobulin is available from *Blood Products Laboratory, UK*.

14011-t

Varicella-Zoster Vaccines

A commonly used varicella vaccine is prepared from live attenuated varicella virus (OKA strain) and contains 2000 plaque-forming units per immunising dose.

Adverse Effects and Precautions

As for vaccines in general, p.1155.

Uses and Administration

Varicella-zoster vaccines may be used for active immunisation against varicella (chicken pox) in persons considered to be at high risk of either contracting the infection or to be highly susceptible to any complications it may cause; such patients include those with leukaemia or solid tumours.

The usual dose of a live attenuated vaccine (OKA strain) is 0.5 mL (2000 plaque-forming units per mL) administered by subcutaneous injection.

Varicella virus infections, because of associated complications, are of greater importance than is generally recognised and vaccines have an important potential role in their control. Several vaccine strains of attenuated varicella virus have been developed and compared, and of these the OKA strain has been shown to have the most desirable attributes of low virulence while inducing adequate antibody response and protection against the disease. The target groups which might be considered for immunisation include: immunosuppressed persons, especially those with cancer or those receiving immunosuppressive therapy; non-immune adults; susceptible patients in hospital at risk of exposure; susceptible health care professionals; non-pregnant teenage females; and susceptible children.— Thirty-fifth Report of a WHO Expert Committee on Biological Standardization, *Tech. Rep. Ser. Wld Hlth Org. No. 725*, 1985, p.102.

Proceedings of a symposium on active immunisation against varicella including reports of several clinical studies using the OKA strain varicella vaccine.— *Postgrad. med. J.*, 1985, *61*, *Suppl.* 4.

Studies demonstrating a beneficial protective effect of a live attenuated varicella vaccine (OKA strain) in persons at risk and/or exposed to varicella infections: P. A. Brunell *et al.*, *Lancet*, 1982, *2*, 1069 (children with lymphoreticular malignancies); R. E. Weibel *et al.*, *New Engl. J. Med.*, 1984, *310*, 1409 (healthy children); A. M. Arbeter *et al.*, *Am. J. Dis. Child.*, 1984, *138*, 434 (healthy children); P. M. Ndumbe *et al.*, *Lancet*, 1985, *1*, 1144 (healthy nurses caring for children with varicella); R. B. Heath *et al.*, *Archs Dis. Childh.*, 1987, *62*, 569 (children with solid tumours).

8038-d

Yellow Fever Vaccines

Yellow Fever Vaccine, Live (*B.P.*) (Yellow Fever Vaccine (Live) (*Eur.P.*); Yel/Vac; Vaccinum Febris Flavae Vivum) is an aqueous suspension of the 17D strain of yellow fever virus grown in embryonated chicken eggs. It is supplied as a freeze-dried product which is reconstituted before use. The dried vaccine should be stored at 2° to 8°, not be allowed to freeze, and be protected from light. Under these conditions it may be expected to retain its potency for at least 2 years. When reconstituted the vaccine should be used immediately.

Yellow Fever Vaccine (*U.S.P.*) is a freeze-dried preparation of a selected attenuated strain of live yellow fever virus cultured in chick embryos. It is reconstituted, just prior to use, by the addition of sodium chloride injection containing no antimicrobial agent. It should be stored under nitrogen preferably below 0° but not above 5°.

Adverse Effects and Precautions

As for vaccines in general, p.1155.

Local and general reactions are not common after vaccination for yellow fever. Hypersensitivity reactions have occurred in persons allergic to egg protein and, very rarely, encephalitis has followed vaccination, generally in infants under 9 months of age.

Yellow fever vaccine should be given with care to persons hypersensitive to egg protein and it should not generally be given to infants less than 9 months of age.

The 17D yellow fever vaccine is normally well tolerated but minor reactions may be observed a few days after immunisation. About 6 days after immunisation fewer than 5% of vaccinees may present with a low-grade fever and slight headache and backache but there is no inflammation at the injection site or in the regional lymph nodes. More severe reactions include encephalitis and allergic reactions. No more than 17 cases of encephalitis have been recorded over a period of 40 years and all occurred in children; although it is possible that some cases may have gone unrecorded, the number would be very small in proportion to the tens of millions of immunisations performed without known encephalitic complications. The risk of encephalitis is minimal if due consideration is given to the circumstances in which children less than 9 months old may be immunised and the contra-indications to immunisation are respected. There has been one report of immunisation provoking the onset of multiple sclerosis or exacerbating the disease but this report has not been confirmed and no further cases have been recorded. Allergic reactions including skin rash, erythema multiforme, urticaria, angioedema, and asthma have been described but occur very infrequently (about 1 in 1 000 000) and predominantly in persons with a history of allergy, especially to eggs. Very rarely, severe reactions of the immediate hypersensitivity type sometimes accompanied by anaphylactic shock and circulatory collapse may occur suddenly after immunisation. In rare instances allergic reactions of the Arthus phenomenon type, sometimes fatal, have occurred in the 24 hours following immunisation.

The general contra-indications for yellow fever vaccine are those for other live vaccines. Sensitivity tests should be performed in persons known to be suffering from an allergy. As a precaution against possible encephalitic complications, infants under 9 months of age are not generally immunised but it may be advisable to immunise children at 6 months of age if they live in rural areas with a history of yellow fever epidemics, and even at 4 months in an active epidemic focus; no child less than 4 months old should receive yellow fever vaccine. Although live vaccines should not generally be given during the first trimester of pregnancy, inquiries by the WHO have not revealed evidence of any damage to the foetus, and if the risk of natural yellow fever is considered higher than the theoretical risk in pregnancy, immunisation should be performed.

There have been several studies on the combined use of yellow fever vaccine and other vaccines. The administration of smallpox vaccine (now no longer in use), measles vaccine, and yellow fever vaccine at the same site has resulted in a decrease in the rate of seroconversions to yellow fever but the injection was made intradermally. When given at different sites, and when diphtheria, tetanus, and pertussis vaccine was also added, no interference was shown. Cholera vaccines should not be given together with yellow fever vaccine, or in the preceeding 3 weeks, since the yellow fever neutralising antibody response, is reduced at least temporarily. Pooled human immunoglobulin given before, at the same time as, or after yellow fever vaccine does not impair the rate of serological conversion.— *Prevention and control of yellow fever in Africa*, World Health Organization, Geneva, 1986..

Uses and Administration

Yellow fever vaccine produces an active immunity which is usually established within about 10 days of administration and persists for many years. Only 1 dose is required for immunisation and is given by subcutaneous injection; the dose is the volume containing at least 1000 mouse LD50 units. The immunity produced may probably last for life although officially an International Certificate of Vaccination against yellow fever is valid only for 10 years starting 10 days after the primary immunisation and only if the vaccine used has been approved by WHO and administered at a designated vaccinating centre.

The 17D (Rockefeller) yellow fever vaccine is now the only yellow fever vaccine produced. The quantity at present available in the world is limited and its relatively short half-life does not permit the accumulation of large stocks. The demand for the vaccine is also somewhat irregular, being suddenly high during epidemics and low during inter-epidemic periods.

During the past 40 years in Africa two different strategies for yellow fever immunisation have been followed. Firstly, an emergency immunisation programme takes place once an outbreak has begun, in an attempt to limit the spread of infection by immunising all persons in the focus, regardless of their former immune status. One disadvantage is that immunity does not appear until 7 days after immunisation and deaths may be expected to occur in the interim period. Secondly, a routine mass immunisation programme for yellow fever is aimed at immunising in advance all populations considered to be at risk.— *Prevention and control of yellow fever in Africa*, World Health Organisation, Geneva, 1986.

Further reviews and discussions on yellow fever and its control: Recommendations of the Immunization Practices Advisory Committee *USA*, *Ann. intern. Med.*, 1984, *100*, 540; Report of a WHO Expert Committee on Viral Haemorrhagic Fevers, *Tech. Rep. Ser. Wld Hlth Org. No. 721*, 1985,, p.24; Memorandum from a Pan American Health Organization Meeting, *Bull. Wld Hlth Org.*, 1986, *64*, 511; P. L. J. Brès, *ibid.*, 775; *Lancet*, 1986, *2*, 1315.

A booklet entitled *Vaccination Certificate Requirements and Health Advice for International Travel* is published annually by the World Health Organization. Information is provided concerning the countries in Africa and South America where yellow fever is endemic and also countries requiring a traveller to hold a valid vaccination certificate. For some further details see p.1156.

Proprietary Preparations

Arilvax *(Wellcome, UK)*. Yellow Fever Vaccine, Live (*B.P.*).

Iodine and Iodides

4570-e

Iodine in various forms, is used as a disinfectant and antiseptic.

Iodine and inorganic iodide salts are used in the management of various thyroid disorders.

15334-d

Cadexomer-Iodine *(BAN).*

Cadexomer Iodine *(USAN, rINN).* 2-Hydroxytrimethylene cross-linked (1→4)-α-D-glucan carboxymethyl ether containing iodine.

Adverse Effects

There is a risk of adverse effects from the systemic absorption of iodine. Some patients have experienced stinging and erythema following application of cadexomer-iodine to their ulcers.

Uses and Administration

Cadexomer-iodine is available for topical application as a powder of micro-beads containing iodine 0.9%. It is applied to venous leg ulcers and pressure sores to aid healing. Like dextranomer (see p.918) it absorbs fluid and the gel thus formed releases iodine.

Beneficial results with cadexomer-iodine in patients with chronic infected venous ulcers unresponsive to previous treatments.— E. Skog *et al., Br. J. Derm.*, 1983, *109*, 77; M. C. Ormiston *et al., Br. med. J.*, 1985, *291*, 308. Comment on earlier work and a report that cadexomer-iodine did not improve the healing-rate and was no more effective than dextranomer in a comparative study.— C. Moss *et al.* (letter), *Br. med. J.*, 1985, *291*, 902.

Proprietary Preparations

Iodosorb *(Janssen, UK). Topical powder,* cadexomer-iodine, containing iodine 0.9%.

Proprietary Names and Manufacturers

Iodosorb *(Syntex, Denm.; Robilliart, Fr.; Smith Kline Dauelsberg, Ger.; Perstorp, Swed.; Smith Kline & French, Switz.; Janssen, UK).*

4573-j

Calcium Iodide

CaI_2=293.9.

CAS — 10102-68-8.

Calcium iodide was formerly given by mouth as an expectorant.

Proprietary Names and Manufacturers

The following names have been used for multi-ingredient preparations containing calcium iodide—Asthma Dellipsoids D17 *(Pilsworth, UK)*; Bepro *(Wallace Mfg Chem., UK)*; Calcidrine *(Abbott, USA)*; Norisodrine With Calcium Iodide *(Abbott, USA).*

4575-c

Dilute Hydriodic Acid

Acid. Hydriod. Dil.

CAS — 10034-85-2 (hydrogen iodide).

A liquid containing 10% w/w of hydrogen iodide, HI=127.9, with 0.3% w/w of hypophosphorous acid, H_3PO_2, added to prevent discoloration on keeping.

Dilute hydriodic acid has been given by mouth, usually diluted in the form of a syrup, as an expectorant.

4576-k

Iodinated Glycerol *(BAN, USAN).*

Iodopropylidene Glycerol. An isomeric mixture of iodinated dimers of glycerol.

$C_6H_{11}IO_3$=258.1.

CAS — 5634-39-9.

Adverse Effects, Treatment, and Precautions

As for Iodine, below.

Uses and Administration

Iodinated glycerol is used as an expectorant in doses of 60 mg four times daily with fluids.

Proprietary Preparations

Organidin *(Boehringer Ingelheim, UK). Elixir,* iodinated glycerol 60 mg, alcohol 1.25 mL/5 mL.

Proprietary Names and Manufacturers

Mucorama Rectal Infantil *(Spain)*; Organidin *(Horner, Canad.; Boehringer Ingelheim, UK; Wallace, USA).*

The following names have been used for multi-ingredient preparations containing iodinated glycerol—Iophen-C *(Schein, USA)*; Theo-Organidin *(Horner, Canad.; Wallace, USA)*; Tussi-Organidin *(Horner, Canad.; Wallace, USA)*; Tussi-Organidin DM *(Wallace, USA).*

4571-l

Iodine *(USAN).*

Iod.; Iodum; Jodum; Yodo.

I_2=253.809.

CAS — 7553-56-2.

Pharmacopoeias. In *Arg., Aust., Belg., Br., Braz., Chin., Cz., Egypt., Eur., Fr., Ger., Hung., Ind., Int., It., Jpn, Jug., Mex., Neth., Nord., Pol., Port., Roum., Rus., Span., Swiss, Turk.,* and *U.S.* Also in *B.P. Vet.*

Greyish-violet or greyish-black brittle plates or small crystals, with a metallic sheen and a distinctive penetrating irritant odour. It is slowly volatile at room temperature.

*B.P.***solubilities**: very slightly soluble in water, soluble 1 in 8 of alcohol, 1 in 30 of chloroform; slightly soluble in glycerol and very soluble in concentrated solutions of iodides. *U.S.P.* solubilities: soluble 1 in 3000 of water, 1 in 13 of alcohol, 1 in 80 of glycerol, and 1 in 4 of carbon disulphide. With acetone iodine forms a pungent irritating compound. **Store** in glass-stoppered bottles.

Adverse Effects

Iodine and iodides can produce goitre and hypothyroidism as well as hyperthyroidism (the Iod-Basedow or Jod-Basedow phenomenon). Goitre and hypothyroidism have also occurred in infants born to mothers who had taken iodides during pregnancy.

Iodine and iodides, whether applied topically or administered systemically, can also give rise to allergic reactions which may include urticaria, angioedema, cutaneous haemorrhage or purpuras, fever, arthralgia, lymphadenopathy, and eosinophilia.

Prolonged administration may lead to a range of adverse effects, often called iodism although some of the effects could be considered to be due to hypersensitivity. These include adverse effects on the mouth such as metallic taste, increased salivation, burning or pain, and coryza; there may be swelling and inflammation of the throat. Eyes may be irritated and swollen. Pulmonary oedema may develop. Skin reactions include acneform or severe eruptions (ioderma). Other reported effects include gastro-intestinal upsets and diarrhoea.

Inhalation of iodine vapour is very irritating to mucous membranes.

The symptoms of acute poisoning from ingestion of iodine are mainly due to its corrosive effects on the gastro-intestinal tract; a disagreeable metallic taste, vomiting, abdominal pain, and diarrhoea occur. Anuria may occur 1 to 3 days later; death may be due to circulatory failure, oedema of the glottis resulting in asphyxia, aspiration pneumonia, or pulmonary oedema. Oesophageal stricture may occur if the patient survives the acute stage. The fatal dose is usually about 2 or 3 g.

In Great Britain the recommended exposure limit is 0.1 ppm.

EFFECTS ON THE THYROID. Increased incidences of thyrotoxicosis occurred in Tasmania in 1964-5, 1966-7, and 1971; each time older patients accounted for most of the increase. The increase in 1966-7 was known to be precipitated by an increase in dietary iodine, caused by the addition of iodate to bread. The other 2 occurrences were believed to be associated with the use of iodophore-containing disinfectants in the dairy industry. It was considered that dietary iodine should be monitored regularly.— J. C. Stewart and G. I. Vidor, *Br. med. J.*, 1976, *1*, 372.

Comment that continued high doses of iodide may cause myxoedema whereas continued small doses cause hyperthyroidism in some patients who, for unknown reasons, are predisposed.— H. Herxheimer (letter), *New Engl. J. Med.*, 1977, *297*, 171.

PREGNANCY AND THE NEONATE. Of 50 282 children born to mothers monitored by the Collaborative Perinatal Project 489 were found to have been exposed to iodides, and possibly other drugs, at some time during the first 4 months of pregnancy. Four of 5 children with eye or ear malformations had cataract and this suggestion of possible teratogenicity needed independent confirmation.— O. P. Heinonen *et al., Birth Defects and Drugs in Pregnancy,* Littleton MA, Publishing Sciences Group, 1977, p. 401.

Treatment of Adverse Effects

Symptomatic treatment may be required for allergic reactions and iodism although symptoms usually subside rapidly when administration of iodine or iodides is discontinued.

In acute iodine poisoning copious draughts of milk and starch mucilage should be given. If there is no oesophageal damage the stomach may be emptied by aspiration and lavage with dilute starch mucilage or a 1% solution of sodium thiosulphate. The use of gastric lavage with activated charcoal has also been suggested. Electrolyte and water losses should be replaced and the circulation should be maintained. Pethidine or morphine sulphate may be given for pain. A tracheostomy may become necessary.

Precautions

Caution is necessary if preparations containing iodine or iodides are taken for prolonged periods, and such preparations should not be taken regularly during pregnancy or lactation. Iodine or iodides should not be administered to patients with a history of hypersensitivity to such compounds.

Solutions of iodine applied to the skin should not be covered with occlusive dressings.

As iodine and iodides can affect the thyroid gland the administration of such preparations may interfere with tests of thyroid function.

The Committee of Drugs of the American Academy of Pediatrics reviewed the toxicity of iodides used for the treatment of asthma and other pulmonary disorders and recommended: 1) iodides should be used as expectorants in the lowest possible doses, for the shortest time, and only when a response is obtained and less toxic substances are ineffective; 2) iodides should not be used as expectorants in pregnancy and should be withdrawn or the dose reduced during breast-feeding; 3) they should not be used as expectorants in adolescents because of their acneform and thyroid effects; 4) they should not be used as expectorants in patients with goitre.— *Pediatrics,* 1976, *57*, 272.

Absorption and Fate

Iodine is slightly absorbed when applied to the skin. When taken by mouth iodine preparations (which are converted to iodide) and iodides are trapped by the thyroid gland (see p.1487). Iodides are excreted mainly in the urine, with smaller amounts appearing in the faeces, saliva, and sweat. They cross the placenta and are excreted in breast milk.

Uses and Administration

Iodine and iodides are used in conjunction with antithyroid agents such as carbimazole, methimazole, or propylthiouracil in the pre-operative management of hyperthyroidism. The patient is rendered euthyroid with an antithyroid agent and iodine or iodides are then added to the therapy for about 1 to 2 weeks before subtotal thyroidectomy. Iodine may be given as a solution with potassium iodide (Aqueous Iodine Solution *B.P.* or Strong Iodine Solution *U.S.P.*) which contains in each mL 130 mg of free and combined iodine; a dose of 0.1 to 0.3 mL in milk or water three times daily renders the thyroid firm and avoids the increased vascularity and friability with increased risk of haemorrhage that may result from the use of an antithyroid agent alone.

Iodine has a powerful bactericidal action and is used for disinfecting unbroken skin before operation. Iodine is also active against fungi, viruses, protozoa, cysts, and spores. It is generally employed as a 2% or 2.5% solution of iodine. If industrial methylated spirit is used for the solution, it should be free from acetone, with which iodine forms an irritant and lachrymatory compound. Iodine may also be employed as the weak solution for the first-aid treatment of small wounds and abrasions and iodine may be used to sterilise drinking water. The germicidal activity is reduced in the presence of organic matter although the reduction is reported to be less than that observed with other halogen disinfectants.

When iodine combines chemically it is decolorised and so-called colourless iodine preparations do not have the disinfectant properties of iodine.

Iodine stains the skin a deep reddish-brown; the stain can readily be removed by dilute solutions of alkalis or sodium thiosulphate.

Iodine is an essential trace element in the human diet; it is necessary for the formation of thyroid hormones, see p.1487. It is used for the prophylaxis and treatment of iodide deficiency disorders, such as endemic goitre, in areas where the diet is deficient in iodine. It may be administered as potassium or sodium iodide, as iodised oil injection, or as potassium iodate. Iodine as potassium iodide, sodium iodide, or calcium iodate (anhydrous or hexahydrate) is permitted as an additive for animal feeds within the EEC.

Iodinated organic compounds including iodised oil injection are used as X-ray contrast media, see p.862.

DISINFECTION. For general references to the use of iodine as a disinfectant or antiseptic, see under Povidone-Iodine, p.1187.

Disinfection of viruses. Recommendations for the first-aid treatment of wounds involving possible exposure to rabies were immediate washing and flushing with soap and water, detergent, or water alone followed by application of a disinfectant such as tincture or aqueous solutions of iodine.— Seventh Report of a WHO Expert Committee on Rabies, *Tech. Rep. Ser. Wld Hlth Org. No. 709*, 1984.

HUMAN REQUIREMENTS. In the United Kingdom deficiency of iodine is either rare, or associated with certain medical conditions, or has not been described or confirmed in man. Iodine occurs in sufficient quantity in a large number of foods. Therefore, in the light of present knowledge and in the context of the diet in the United Kingdom, recommended daily intakes for iodine have not been set.— Recommended Daily Amounts of Food Energy and Nutrients for Groups of People in the United Kingdom, Report by the Committee on Medical Aspects of Food Policy, *Report on Health and Social Subjects No. 15*, London, HM Stationery Office, 1979.

The US National Research Council made the following recommendations for daily dietary allowances of iodine: infants up to 6 months, 40 µg; 6 to 12 months, 50 µg; children 1 to 3 years, 70 µg; 4 to 6 years, 90 µg; 7 to 10 years, 120 µg; children over 11 years and adults, 150 µg; in pregnancy 175 µg; in lactation 200 µg.— *Recommended Dietary Allowances*, 9th Edn, Washington, The National Research Council, 1980.

IODINE DEFICIENCY DISORDERS. A discussion on the public health significance and prevention of endemic goitre and cretinism. The iodisation of salt for the prevention of goitre has been widely and successfully used. The recommended levels in salt for supplementation vary widely from country to country. Fortunately, there is a wide latitude between the required and the toxic levels of iodide. A concentration of 1 in 10 000 is probably higher than necessary, whereas a 1 in 100 000 may be insufficient. A reasonable concentration might be a 1 in 25 000 to 1 in 50 000. Several different chemical forms of iodine have been used in salt supplementation. Generally, sodium or potassium iodide is used; the latter is better because it is less hygroscopic. However, the use of sodium or potassium iodates may be an improvement over the use of iodides because they are more stable. A useful means of combating endemic goitre and cretinism in areas where salt iodisation cannot be employed is the intramuscular injection of iodised oil containing 475 mg of iodine per mL (37% w/w) [Iodised Oil Fluid Injection]. A recommended dosage schedule is: 0 to 6 months, 0.2 to 0.4 mL; 6 to 12 months, 0.3 to 0.6 mL; 6 months to 6 years, 0.5 to 1.0 mL; 6 to 45 years, 1 to 2 mL. The dosage should be reduced to 0.2 mL for all persons with nodular goitres or those presenting with single thyroid nodules without goitre. Iodised oil should be administered to all females up to the age of 45 years and all males up to the age of 20 years. It should be necessary to repeat the injection programme only about once every 3 years. Thyrotoxicosis has occasionally occurred following iodine supplementation; in all recently reported cases it has been mild and easily managed. Thyrotoxicosis after an injection of iodised oil is much more likely to occur in persons over 40 years of age, and it has been suggested that such injections should be avoided in those over the age of 45. The method of supplementation chosen should ensure a minimum of 100 µg of iodine daily.— J. B. Stanbury *et al.*, *Chronicle Wld Hlth Org.*, 1974, *28*, 220.

A discussion of iodine-deficiency disorders and their eradication. In India, the number of people in known endemic goitre areas is 120 million, of whom about one-third have a goitre. Moreover, other pockets are constantly being discovered and the total population affected is believed to be nearer 300 million, with goitre in over 60 million. In China, Indonesia, the Middle East, Africa, and South America many additional millions are affected. Iodine deficiency of the foetus is the result of iodine deficiency in the mother. The condition is associated with stillbirth, abortion, and congenital abnormalities, and the incidence of these can be reduced by iodisation. Another major effect is endemic cretinism, which occurs with an iodine intake of below 20 µg daily; cretinism, however, can be prevented by correction of the severe iodine deficiency before pregnancy. Iodine deficiency in childhood and adolescence is characteristically associated with endemic goitre and the condition can be effectively prevented by various iodisation methods. The common effect of iodine deficiency in adults is endemic goitre; the typical patient is not clinically hypothyroid. Iodised salt, iodised bread, and iodised oil, have all proved effective in the prevention of goitre in adults and iodine administration, particularly in the form of iodised oil, may also reduce existing goitre in adults. The main resources for mass correction of iodine deficiency are iodised salt and iodised oil. In China, where iodised walnut oil has been developed, large injection programmes have been mounted. Pilot studies in South America and Burma have indicated that iodised oil can be effective by mouth. It is now clear that iodised oil is suitable for use in a mass programme. However, despite the readily available means of supplementation, iodine deficiency has persisted. One important factor in the failure to apply knowledge is the geographic isolation of the iodine-deficient communities. It is suggested, though, that a special reason for social and political neglect is its designation simply as 'goitre'. Goitre alone hardly constitutes a serious health problem in developing countries when compared with bacterial or parasitic infection, but the health effects of iodine deficiency extend far beyond those of goitre. It is suggested that the term iodine-deficiency disorders should replace 'goitre' to reflect the wide spectrum of conditions. With existing technology, iodine deficiency could readily be eradicated by 1990.— B. S. Hetzel, *Lancet*, 1983, *2*, 1126.

In many developing countries the major thyroid problem in pregnancy is that of iodine deficiency and endemic goitre. It is estimated that throughout the world up to 250 million people suffer from endemic goitre. This could be totally prevented by the prophylactic intramuscular injection of iodised oil every 4 or 5 years.— I. Ramsay, Thyroid Disease, in *Medical Disorders in Obstetric Practice*, M. de Swiet (Ed.), London, Blackwell Scientific Publications, 1984, p.385.

A report of the Subcommittee for the Study of Endemic Goitre and Iodine Deficiency of the European Thyroid Association. The Subcommittee documented, as far as possible, the prevalence of goitre and iodine status in all European countries. Goitre prevalence was: practically none in Denmark, Finland, Iceland, Norway, and Sweden; practically none to less than 10% in Belgium, Ireland, and the United Kingdom; less than 10% in Bulgaria, Czechoslovakia, France, the Netherlands, and Switzerland; 10 to 30% or more in Austria, the German Democratic Republic, the German Federal Republic, Greece, Hungary, Poland, Romania, Turkey, and Yugoslavia; from 10 to 30% or more, to a risk of endemic cretinism, in Italy, Portugal, and Spain; no information was available for Albania and the USSR. Iodine prophylaxis was: mandatory in Austria (potassium iodide 10 mg per kg of salt), Bulgaria (potassium iodide 20 mg per kg of salt), Czechoslovakia, Finland (sodium iodide 25 mg per kg of salt), Hungary, the Netherlands (potassium iodide 46 mg per kg of bread salt, but recommendations had been made to increase the content to 60 mg per kg and also suggestions made that all household salt should contain potassium iodide 26.2 mg per kg), Poland, Switzerland (potassium iodide 20 mg per kg of salt), and Yugoslavia; voluntary in Belgium, France, the German Democratic Republic, the German Federal Republic, Greece, Ireland, Italy, Norway, Portugal, and Spain; not practised in Denmark and the United Kingdom; information was not available for Albania, Iceland, Romania, Turkey, and the USSR. Iodine intake, including that obtained by prophylactic measures where applicable, was considered to be: sufficient in Bulgaria, Czechoslovakia, Finland, Iceland, Ireland, the Netherlands, Norway, Sweden, Switzerland, the United Kingdom; sufficient to borderline sufficient in Denmark; borderline sufficient in Austria, Belgium, France, Hungary, Poland, Romania, and Yugoslavia; insufficient in the German Democratic Republic, the German Federal Republic, Greece, Italy, Portugal, Spain, and Turkey; no information was available to permit conclusions to be made regarding Albania and the USSR. The overall results of the survey give grounds for concern.— *Lancet*, 1985, *1*, 1289. Further information pertinent to Spain.— F. Escobar del Ray (letter), *ibid.*, *2*, 149.

Studies using various iodisation methods for the prophylaxis and treatment of iodine deficiency: I. H. Buttfield and B. S. Hetzel, *Bull. Wld Hlth Org.*, 1967, *36*, 243 (iodised oil fluid injection); F. W. Clements *et al.*, *ibid.*, 1968, *38*, 297 (potassium iodate or potassium iodide); F. W. Clements *et al.*, *Lancet*, 1970, *1*, 489 (potassium iodate); P. O. D. Pharoah *et al.*, *ibid.*, 1971, *1*, 308 (iodised oil fluid injection); K. J. Connolly *et al.*, *ibid.*, 1979, *2*, 1149 (iodised oil fluid injection); S. S. Sooch *et al.*, *Bull. Wld Hlth Org.*, 1973, *49*, 307 (potassium iodate or potassium iodide); G. F. Maberly *et al.*, *Lancet*, 1981, *2*, 1270 (iodine); A. Bautista *et al.*, *Am. J. clin. Nutr.*, 1982, *35*, 127 (iodised oil by mouth); Y. -Y. Wang and S. -H. Yang, *Lancet*, 1985, *2*, 518 (iodised salt).

See also under Effects on the thyroid in Adverse Effects (above).

Preparations

Iodine Insufflation *(A.P.F.)*. Iodine 0.8, potassium iodide 0.4, anaesthetic ether 10, and lactose, in fine powder, 98.8.

Non-staining Iodine Ointment *(B.P.C. 1968)*. Unguentum Iodi Denigrescens; Ung. Iod. Denig. Iodine 5% w/w in arachis oil and yellow soft paraffin.

Non-staining Iodine Ointment with Methyl Salicylate *(B.P.C. 1968)*. Ung. Iod. Denig. c. Methyl. Sal. Methyl salicylate 5% v/w in non-staining iodine ointment.

Aqueous Iodine Oral Solution *(B.P.)*. Aqueous Iodine Solution; Lugol's Solution; Strong Iodine Solution *(U.S.P.)*. Iodine 5 g, potassium iodide 10 g, water to 100 mL. It contains in 1 mL 50 mg of free iodine and about 130 mg of total iodine.

NOTE. Diluted solutions may be known as Schiller's Iodine.

Compound Iodine Paint *(B.P.C. 1968)*. Pig. Iod. Co.; Mandl's Paint. Iodine 1.25 g, potassium iodide 2.5 g, water 2.5 mL, peppermint oil 0.4 mL, alcohol (90%) 4 mL, glycerol to 100 mL. It should be well shaken before use.

A.P.F. (Iodine Paint Compound) has a similar formula.

Decolourised Solution of Iodine *(B.P.C. 1934)*. Liq. Iod. Decol.; Decolourised Tincture of Iodine. Iodine 2.86 g, strong ammonia solution 6.25 mL, alcohol (90%) to

100 mL. The alcohol may be replaced by industrial methylated spirit diluted so as to be of equivalent alcoholic strength.

Iodine Tincture *(U.S.P.)*. Iodine 2 g, sodium iodide 2.4 g, alcohol 50 mL, water to 100 mL.

Iodine Topical Solution *(U.S.P.)*. Iodine 2 g, sodium iodide 2.4 g, water to 100 mL.

Strong Iodine Solution *(B.P. 1958)*. Strong Iod. Soln; Liq. Iod. Fort. Iodine 10 g, potassium iodide 6 g, water 10 mL, alcohol (90%) to 100 mL.

Strong Iodine Tincture *(U.S.P.)*. Iodine 7 g, potassium iodide 5 g, water 5 mL, alcohol to 100 mL.

Weak Iodine Solution *(B.P.)*. Iodine Tincture. Iodine 2.5 g, potassium iodide 2.5 g, water 2.5 mL, alcohol (90%) to 100 mL.

Proprietary Names and Manufacturers

Ethiodol *(Savage, USA)*; Guttajod *(Blucher-Schering, Ger.)*; Iodex *(Smith Kline & French, Austral.*; *Switz.)*; Iodex Plain *(Menley & James, UK)*; Iodosan *(Zambeletti, Ital.)*; Jod *(DAK, Denm.)*; Jodan *(Arnaldi, Ital.)*; Jodopax *(Ferrosan, Norw.)*; Jodosan *(Norw.)*; Leukona *(Atzinger, Ger.)*; Roma-Nol *(Jamol, USA)*; Vasogen-Thrombo *(Pearson, Ger.)*.

The following names have been used for multi-ingredient preparations containing iodine or a related substance— Iodex with Methyl Salicylate *(Smith Kline & French, Austral.)*; Iodex with Wintergreen *(Menley & James, UK)*; Sclerodine *(Ondee, Canad.)*.

4577-a

Iodoform

Formène Tri-iodé. Tri-iodomethane.

CHI_3=393.7.

CAS — 75-47-8.

Pharmacopoeias. In *Arg., Aust., Belg., Fr., It., Jpn, Jug., Pol., Port., Rus.*, and *Span.*

Iodoform slowly releases elemental iodine when applied to the tissues and has a mild disinfectant action. It was formerly used as a wound dressing. Iodoform as a paint or varnish has been used as a protective covering. A paste of iodoform with bismuth subnitrate has been applied to wounds and abscesses, the area to be treated being cleaned and smeared with the paste. Sterile gauze impregnated with the paste has also been used for packing cavities after oral and otorhinological surgery.

In Great Britain the recommended exposure limits of iodoform are 0.6 ppm (long-term); 1.0 ppm (short-term).

Preparations

Bismuth Subnitrate and Iodoform Paste *(B.P.C. 1954)*. Past. Bism. Subnit. et Iodof.; BIPP; Bismuth and Iodoform Paste. Bismuth subnitrate 1, iodoform 2, sterilised liquid paraffin 1, by wt.

ADVERSE EFFECTS. Open leg ulcers in a Malay child aged 13 months were treated with Bismuth Subnitrate and Iodoform Paste. They healed but oedema and pain increased. After 9 weeks, X-ray examination showed dense transverse bands of metallic bismuth deposited in metaphyseal growth areas of long bones.— H. N. Krige, *S. Afr. med. J.*, 1963, *37*, 1005.

Two reactions to dental dressings with Bismuth Subnitrate and Iodoform Paste occurred in which crystals of bismuth subnitrate were considered to be the cause rather than the iodoform.— W. A. Miller and G. S. Taylor, *Br. dent. J.*, 1968, *124*, 420.

Symptoms compatible with iodoform toxicity occurred in 1 patient and raised iodine concentrations in 2 further patients following the packing of cavities with gauze impregnated with Bismuth Subnitrate and Iodoform Paste. In a further patient who received a pack soaked in Compound Iodoform Paint no signs of iodoform toxicity were observed. It was suggested that Bismuth Subnitrate and Iodoform Paste was satisfactory for packing small operative cavities but for large cavities Compound Iodoform Paint pastes were safer.— A. F. F. O'Connor *et al.*, *J. Lar. Otol.*, 1977, *91*, 903.

Compound Iodoform Paint *(B.P.C. 1954)*. Pig. Iodof. Co.; Whitehead's Varnish. Iodoform 10 g, benzoin 10 g, prepared storax 7.5 g, tolu balsam 5 g, and solvent ether to 100 mL.

13154-m

Potassium Iodate

KIO_3=214.0.

CAS — 7758-05-6.

Pharmacopoeias. In *It.*

Potassium iodate is used for the prophylaxis and treatment of iodine deficiency disorders, such as endemic goitre, in districts where the diet is deficient in iodides. It is usually given for this purpose as iodised salt or added to bread during processing.

DIAGNOSTIC USE. A report of the use of computerised axial tomography to detect small carcinomas of the thyroid gland after 2 days of pretreatment of patients with a solution of iodine and potassium iodide by mouth. The thyroid gland was visible after selective uptake and organification of the non-radioactive iodine and small lesions showing a decrease in absorption (organification) were easily detected. It was considered that this was a procedure without risk.— C. J. M. Lips *et al* (letter), *New Engl. J. Med.*, 1982, *306*, 1491. Disagreement that the procedure was without risk. Iodides in the doses given (estimated at 1 g) could cause various adverse effects.— R. R. Cavalieri (letter), *ibid.*, *307*, 1346. Reply that over 100 patients have been investigated without any adverse effects although, for practical reasons, potassium iodate 850 mg (equivalent to 500 mg of iodine) by mouth administered with milk is now given every 24 hours before scanning.— C. J. M. Lips *et al.* (letter), *ibid.*, 1347.

IODINE DEFICIENCY DISORDERS. For the use of potassium iodate in the prophylaxis and treatment of iodine deficiency disorders, including endemic goitre and cretinism, see under Iodine, p.1185. For a report of an increased incidence of thyrotoxicosis in older people when potassium iodate was added to bread, see under Adverse Effects of Iodine, p.1184.

RADIATION PROTECTION. In 1962 it was proposed that in radiation emergencies involving members of the general public, stable iodide should be administered to reduce thyroid irradiation resulting from inhalation or ingestion of radioactive iodine. Following discussions with various official bodies, stocks of stable iodine tablets have been kept in readiness for distribution. It was noted that the shelf-life of potassium iodide was limited and tests carried out (A. Cronquist *et al.*, *Hlth Phys.*, 1971, *21*, 393) demonstrated that potassium iodate was equally effective in blocking uptake of iodine by the thyroid. Tablets of potassium iodate containing 100 mg of iodine are held in readiness by the police in the vicinity of UK nuclear reactor sites for use in emergencies. These would be issued on a once-off basis to all members of the general public who might be affected. It is desirable for the stable iodine to be taken within about 2 to 4 hours of exposure.— J. A. Bonnell (letter), *Br. med. J.*, 1980, *281*, 1278. One dose of 200 mg of iodine as potassium iodate is proposed. Stable iodine given as long as 4 hours after ingestion of radio-iodine will reduce the thyroid dose by 80% J. A. Bonnell and G. C. Dale (letter), *Lancet*, 1981, *2*, 207.

A discussion on the use of iodine supplements in the event of accidents at nuclear reactors. Although the uncertainties concerning the degree of risk from iodine-131 release are not resolved, the best interests of the public would appear to be served by the administration of a single dose of potassium iodide or potassium iodate to the population at risk immediately a release of radio-iodine occurs.— *Lancet*, 1983, *1*, 451.

A Report of the Environmental Hazards Committee of the American Thyroid Association regarding the use of iodine as a thyroidal blocking agent in the event of a nuclear reactor accident. The Association concluded that potassium iodide in an appropriate dosage form (130-mg scored tablets or an oral solution) should be manufactured in sufficient quantities to fill anticipated needs if its use was required and that although distribution was not recommended, advance planning for possible distribution might be advisable.— D. V. Becker *et al.*, *J. Am. med. Ass.*, 1984, *252*, 659.

4579-x

Potassium Iodide *(USAN)*.

Iodeto de Potássio; Kalii Iodetum; Kalii Iodidum; Kalii Jodidum; Kalium Iodatum; Kalium Jodatum; Pot. Iod.; Potassii Iodidum; Potassium (Iodure de).

KI=166.0.

CAS — 7681-11-0.

Pharmacopoeias. In *Arg., Aust., Belg., Br., Braz., Chin., Cz., Egypt., Eur., Fr., Ger., Hung., Ind., Int., It., Jpn, Jug., Mex., Neth., Nord., Pol., Port., Roum., Rus., Span., Swiss, Turk.*, and *U.S.* Also in *B.P. Vet.*

Odourless, colourless, transparent or somewhat opaque crystals or white granular powder. It is slightly hygroscopic. Each g represents 6 mmol of potassium and of iodide.

Soluble 1 in 0.7 of water, 1 in about 23 of alcohol, and 1 in 2 of glycerol; *U.S.P.* also has soluble 1 in 0.5 of boiling water. Solutions in water are neutral or alkaline to litmus. Iodine readily dissolves in an aqueous solution of potassium iodide, forming a dark brown solution containing potassium tri-iodide. **Store** in well-closed containers. Protect from light.

Adverse Effects, Treatment, Precautions, and Absorption and Fate

As for Iodine, p.1184.

Uses and Administration

Potassium iodide is used similarly to solutions containing iodine and potassium iodide in the pre-operative management of hyperthyroidism (see under Iodine, p.1185). Suggested doses have ranged from 15 mg daily up to 250 mg three times daily.

Potassium iodide may be given by mouth in doses of 100 to 150 mg before the administration of iodine radionuclides to saturate the thyroid gland when uptake of radio-iodine by the thyroid is not desired. Potassium iodide is also given for up to about 2 weeks after radio-iodine.

Potassium iodide is also used in the treatment of cutaneous lymphatic sporotrichosis. It is usually given in a gradually increasing dosage up to the limit of tolerance, which may be up to 15 g or more daily in divided doses, and should be continued for at least 1 month after the disappearance or stabilisation of the lesions.

Potassium iodide has been used as an expectorant but there is little evidence to show that it is effective.

Potassium iodide is usually administered in mixtures or in solution, freely diluted, since concentrated solutions have an irritant action on the gastric mucosa.

Potassium iodide is used for the prophylaxis and treatment of iodine deficiency disorders, such as endemic goitre, in districts where the diet is deficient in iodides. It is usually given for this purpose as iodised salt.

In veterinary medicine potassium iodide is used in the treatment of actinobacillosis of *cattle*.

FUNGAL INFECTIONS. The successful use of potassium iodide by mouth in 3 patients (1 adult and 2 children) with subcutaneous phycomycosis caused by *Basidiobolus haptosporus* S. Kelly *et al.*, *Trans. R. Soc. trop. Med. Hyg.*, 1980, *74*, 396.

Invasion of muscle tissue in addition to dermis and subcutaneous tissue by *Basidiobolus haptosporus* in one patient cured by oral therapy with potassium iodide 600 mg daily for 2 weeks followed by 1.5 g daily for 5 months.—A. Kamalam and A. S. Thambiah, *Sabouraudia*, 1984, *22*, 273.

Studies *in vitro* on the susceptibility of human and wild-type isolates of *Basidiobolus* and *Conidiobolus* species. As none of the strains tested were inhibited or killed at maximum concentrations of potassium iodide, it was suggested that the reported favourable treatment with potassium iodide may not be due to its direct effect on the fungi but rather to other, undefined factors.— B. G. Yangco *et al.*, *Antimicrob. Ag. Chemother.*, 1984, *25*, 413.

Sporotrichosis. An iodide is the drug of first choice for the treatment of lymphocutaneous fungal infections due to *Sporothrix schenckii*.— *Med. Lett.*, 1984, *26*, 36. Despite the appearance of a number of new antifungal drugs over the past decade, the treatment of choice in subcutaneous sporotrichosis remains potassium iodide. Potassium iodide has no inhibitory activity *in vitro* against *Sporothrix schenckii* and is believed to act directly by enhancing phagocytosis. It is given as a saturated aqueous solution and to improve the patient's tolerance, the dose is increased dropwise each day. Treatment is continued for one month after clinical resolution.— R. J. Hay, *Br. J. Hosp. Med.*, 1984, *31*, 278.

HYPERTHYROIDISM. *Pre-operative use.* Ten women with Graves' disease took propranolol 80 mg every 8 hours for a mean of 40 days pre-operatively and continued until the end of the fifth postoperative day, particular care being taken to ensure that the last dose before operation was not omitted. Potassium iodide 60 mg thrice daily was taken for 10 days pre-operatively and produced a marked fall in serum concentrations of thyroid hormone in all patients. At operation all patients were clinically euthyroid with a resting pulse-rate of less than 90 per minute; there were no complications. There is a possibility of a secondary rise in thyroid hormone concentrations if potassium iodide is taken for longer than 10 days. If these preliminary results are verified in a larger series, the combination of propranolol and potassium iodide may prove to be the treatment of choice in preparation of patients with Graves' disease for surgery. In the meantime, however, the long-established antithyroid drugs and iodides should remain the standard treatment.— C. M. Feek *et al.*, *New Engl. J. Med.*, 1980, *302*, 883. Comments and criticisms: C. H. Emerson and M. M. S. El-Zaheri (letter), *ibid.*, *303*, 527; J. Feely, *ibid.*, 528.

See also under Propranolol, p.806.

Thyroid storm. Thyroid storm is a medical emergency. Treatment includes antithyroid agents (propylthiouracil 300 mg three times daily) to prevent more formation of thyroid hormones and to reduce conversion of thyroxine to tri-iodothyronine, propranolol, and iodine to prevent release of formed hormones from the thyroid.— I. R. McDougall, *J. clin. Pharmac.*, 1981, *21*, 365.

The treatment of thyroid storm, a life-threatening acceleration of hyperthyroidism, has been revolutionised by the use of the beta blockers, given as propranolol 5 to 10 mg intravenously, slowly at intervals, titrated to relieve the signs. Large doses of carbimazole or propylthiouracil are given orally or via a nasogastric tube and iodine is given orally or intravenously as potassium iodide.— R. Wilkinson, *Prescribers' J.*, 1984, *24*, 97.

IODINE DEFICIENCY DISORDERS. For the use of potassium iodide in the prophylaxis and treatment of iodine deficiency disorders, including endemic goitre and cretinism, see under Iodine p.1185.—.

RADIATION PROTECTION. For the use of potassium iodide to block uptake by the thyroid gland of radio-iodine in the event of accidents at nuclear reactors, see under Potassium Iodate, p.1186.

SKIN DISORDERS. Erythema nodosum responded to potassium iodide 360 to 900 mg daily in 24 of 28 patients and nodular vasculitis in 16 of 17.— E. J. Schulz and D. A. Whiting, *Br. J. Derm.*, 1976, *94*, 75.

Preparations

Ammoniated Potassium Iodide Mixture *(B.P.C. 1973).* Potassium Iodide and Ammonia Mixture. Potassium iodide 150 mg, ammonium bicarbonate 150 mg, liquorice liquid extract 1 mL, double-strength chloroform water 5 mL, water to 10 mL. *Dose.* 10 to 20 mL.

Potassium Iodide and Pseudoephedrine Mixture *(A.P.F.).* Potassium iodide 250 mg, pseudoephedrine hydrochloride 30 mg, ammonium bicarbonate 100 mg, liquorice liquid extract 0.5 mL, concentrated chloroform water 0.25 mL or methyl hydroxybenzoate solution 0.1mL, water to 10 mL. *Dose.* 10 to 20 mL.

Potassium Iodide and Pseudoephedrine Mixture CF *(A.P.F.).* Potassium iodide 100 mg, pseudoephedrine hydrochloride 15 mg, stramonium tincture 0.2 mL, aromatic ammonia solution 0.1 mL, liquorice liquid extract 0.2 mL, concentrated chloroform water 0.1 mL or methyl hydroxybenzoate solution 0.05 mL, water to 5 mL. *Dose.* 5 to 10 mL.

Potassium Iodide and Stramonium Mixture Compound *(A.P.F.).* Mist Lobelia and Stramonium. Potassium iodide 250 mg, stramonium tincture 0.5 mL, lobelia ethereal tincture 0.5 mL, aromatic ammonia solution 0.5 mL, liquorice liquid extract 0.5 mL, concentrated chloroform water 0.25 mL or methyl hydroxybenzoate solution 0.1mL, water to 10 mL. *Dose.* 10 to 20 mL.

Potassium Iodide Oral Solution *(U.S.P.).* If the solution is not to be used within a short time, 500 µg of sodium thiosulphate is added for each 1 g of potassium iodide. Crystals of potassium iodide may form under normal conditions of storage, especially if refrigerated. Store in airtight containers. Protect from light.

Potassium Iodide Tablets *(U.S.P.).* They may be enteric-coated.

Proprietary Names and Manufacturers

Jodetten *(Winzer, Ger.)*; Jodid *(E. Merck, Ger.)*; Kaliumjodid *(ACO, Swed.)*; Marco-Jod *(Marcopharma, Denm.)*; Pherajod *(Kanoldt, Ger.)*; Pima *(Fleming, USA)*; Solvejod *(Draco, Swed.)*; SSKI *(Upsher-Smith, USA)*; Thyro-Block *(Horner, Canad.)*.

The following names have been used for multi-ingredient preparations containing potassium iodide—Chibret Iodochloride Collyrium *(Merck Sharp & Dohme-Chibret, Fr.)*; Elixophyllin-KI *(Schering, Austral.; Berlex, Canad.; Forest Pharmaceuticals, USA)*; Ephedramine *(Drug Houses Austral., Austral.)*; IDM *(Rougier, Canad.)*; IDM-Expectorant *(Rougier, Canad.)*; Iodised Sodium Chloride Tablets *(Southon-Horton, UK)*; Isuprel Compound Elixir *(Winthrop, Canad.; Winthrop-Breon, USA)*; Mudrane *(Poythress, USA)*; Mudrane-2 *(Poythress, USA)*; Pediacof *(Winthrop-Breon, USA)*; Pneumogeine *(Gamaprod, Austral.)*; Quadrinal *(Knoll, USA)*.

4580-y

Povidone-Iodine *(BAN, USAN).*

Polyvidone-Iodine; Polyvinylpyrrolidone-Iodine Complex; PVP-Iodine.

CAS — 25655-41-8.

Pharmacopoeias. In *U.S.*

A complex of iodine with povidone, containing 9 to 12% of available iodine calculated on the dried basis. It occurs as a yellowish-brown amorphous powder with a slight characteristic odour. It loses not more than 8% of its weight on drying.

Soluble in water and alcohol; practically insoluble in acetone, carbon tetrachloride, chloroform, ether, and light petroleum. *U.S.P.* solutions have a ph of 1.5 to 6.5; the *B.P.* solution containing 0.85 to 1.20% of available iodine has a pH of 3.0 to 5.5. **Store** in airtight containers.

Adverse Effects

Povidone-iodine may produce local reactions but it is considered to be less irritant than iodine.

The application of povidone-iodine to severe burns or to large areas otherwise denuded of skin may produce the systemic adverse effects associated with iodine.

Reports of acidosis in patients whose burns were treated topically with povidone-iodine.— J. Pietsch and J. L. Meakins, *Lancet*, 1976, *1*, 280; C. Scoggin *et al.* (letter), *ibid.*, 1977, *1*, 959.

A report of false-positive blood cultures in hospital patients attributed to contamination of a povidone-iodine solution by *Pseudomonas cepacia*.— D. E. Craven *et al.*, *New Engl. J. Med.*, 1981, *305*, 621. Peritonitis in 4 patients undergoing chronic peritoneal dialysis and infection at the catheter site in another patient were traced to the contamination by *Pseudomonas aeruginosa* of an iodophore solution (poloxamer-iodine) used for the disinfection of the dialysis connections.— P. L. Parrott *et al.*, *Lancet*, 1982, *2*, 683.

Precautions

Application of povidone-iodine to large areas of broken skin should be avoided as excessive absorption of iodine may occur.

Absorption of iodine from povidone-iodine may interfere with tests of thyroid function.

A report of iodine absorption resulting from irrigation of the peritoneal cavity with 550 mL of a 10% solution of povidone-iodine. The intraperitoneal use of this preparation should be limited.— C. F. Strife *et al.* (letter), *Lancet*, 1977, *1*, 1265. The dose used would provide 5.5 g of available iodine, over 10 times what was considered to be an effective dose.— O. J. A. Gilmore (letter), *ibid.*, 1977, *2*, 37.

DENTAL USE. There was no significant change in the mean wet-weight of plaque in 16 healthy subjects who had used a 0.5% aqueous solution of povidone-iodine as a mouth-wash four times daily for 14 days. However, there was a significant increase in the total serum iodide, protein bound iodide, total thyroxine and free thyroxine index. It was recommended that the use of povidone-iodine in a mouth-wash be restricted to acute situations and that it should not be used over prolonged periods. Brown staining of the teeth occurred in 5 subjects.— M. M. Ferguson *et al.*, *Br. dent. J.*, 1978, *144*, 14.

INTERACTIONS. Dermatological reactions, described as second- and third-degree burns, were observed in 4 patients in whom wounds were covered with a povidone-iodine soaked bandage secured to the skin by compound benzoin tincture. It was suggested that an interaction had occurred resulting in a more acidic pH.— L. J. Schillaci *et al.*, *Am. J. Hosp Pharm.*, 1983, *40*, 1694.

INTERFERENCE WITH DIAGNOSTIC TESTS. Contamination of several types of test cards and tapes used for the detection of occult blood in faeces or urine with povidone-iodine produced false-positive results. The reaction was attributed to the strongly oxidative properties of iodine. These findings have important implications, particularly in trauma victims, with regard to the cleansing of the peri-urethral and anal regions since contamination of specimens is a possibility.— D. Bar-Or and J. A. Mark (letter), *Lancet*, 1981, *2*, 589.

Further references to contamination by povidone-iodine producing false-positive results for occult blood: R. Said, *J. Am. med. Ass.*, 1979, *242*, 748 (urine); J. L. Orchard and R. Lawson (letter), *New Engl. J. Med.*, 1984, *311*, 199 (faeces).

PREGNANCY AND THE NEONATE. Studies involving 40 neonates indicated that topical application of povidone-iodine to the umbilical cord and the surrounding area of normal intact skin resulted in significantly increased plasma-iodine concentrations. Although no alteration in thyroid function was observed it was suggested that until further information was available caution should be exercised in the prolonged use of povidone-iodine in neonates.— S. P. Pyati *et al.*, *J. Pediat.*, 1977, *91*, 825.

A suggestion that vaginitis in pregnant women should not be treated with povidone-iodine because of the possible development of iodine-induced goitre and hypothyroidism in the foetus and neonate due to vaginal absorption of iodine.— H. Vorherr *et al.*, *J. Am. med. Ass.*, 1980, *244*, 2628.

A report of hypothyroidism in a neonate considered to have been associated with the topical administration of povidone-iodine to a surgical wound. This case confirms previously published recommendations that iodine-containing preparations be used with caution in full-term babies and avoided in pre-term infants. Furthermore, it is important to be sure that povidone-iodine is not in use before programmes for screening of congenital hypothyroidism are implemented.— H. J. Jackson and R. M. Sutherland (letter), *Lancet*, 1981, *2*, 992.

Further individual reports of hypothyroidism in neonates associated with the topical administration of povidone-iodine: A. Wuilloud *et al.*, *Z. Kinderchir.*, 1977, *20*, 181; K. R. Lyen *et al.*, *Am. J. Dis. Child.*, 1982, *136*, 369.

Uses and Administration

Povidone-iodine is an iodophore which is used as a disinfectant and antiseptic mainly for the treatment of contaminated wounds and pre-operative preparation of the skin and mucous membranes.

Iodophores are loose complexes of iodine and carrier polymers. Solutions of povidone-iodine gradually release iodine to exert an effect against bacteria, fungi, viruses, protozoa, cysts, and spores; povidone-iodine is thus less potent than preparations containing free iodine but it is less toxic.

The antiseptic activity of povidone-iodine is reduced by alkalis.

DISINFECTION. A review and discussion concerning the local management of sepsis. Iodine is bactericidal and kills all bacterial species at approximately the same concentration. In addition it is sporicidal, fungicidal, and virucidal. Povidone-iodine is the most widely used iodophore and is the iodine antiseptic of choice because it is non-irritant, does not stain, and is highly effective. Iodophores are often applied to traumatic wounds and povidone-iodine proved particularly effective in the Vietnam conflict. In traumatic injuries prone to clostridial infection the authors advocate the use of a combination of aqueous povidone-iodine and hydrogen peroxide in equal proportions (brown bubbly). This mixture froths on contact with the tissues and thus enters all nooks and crannies. In addition, the hydrogen peroxide potentiates the povidone-iodine by increasing the release of available iodine. In the treatment of burns the use of povidone-iodine is popular in some areas and is gaining in popularity because it is fungicidal and does not induce the occasional hypersensitivity and leucopenia seen with silver sulphadiazine. For the prevention of infection of surgical wounds steps must be taken to reduce the number of bacteria, both on the patient's skin and on the surgeon's hands, before gloving. Sterilisation is impossible but washing with a disinfectant such as povidone-iodine detergent eliminates the majority of resident flora. In gastro-intestinal surgery the site of anastomosis must be isolated from the wound and the rest of the abdominal cavity by judicious use of packs, and packs soaked in povidone-iodine are an advantage. Allied to good surgical technique the use of topical povidone-iodine during surgery reduces postoperative wound infection.— O. J. A. Gilmore and R. J. Sprignall, *Br. J. Hosp. Med.*, 1983, *29*, 440. A report of a mixture of povidone-iodine solution and hydrogen peroxide exploding.— E. Dannenberg and J. Peebles (letter), *Am. J. Hosp. Pharm.*, 1978, *35*, 525.

Iodine and iodophores as skin disinfectants have a wide range of activity against bacteria, fungi, and viruses and some activity against bacterial spores; their action is rapid. Iodine may, however, corrode metals and tincture of iodine and aqueous iodine solutions can cause skin reactions. Iodophores do not stain and are non-irritant. Micro-organisms on the skin can, for practical purposes, be classified as 'resident' or 'transient'. The 'resident' flora grow on the skin and are not readily removed by washing or disinfection. The 'transient' flora are organisms deposited on the skin which do not usually grow there and can usually be removed readily by washing or disinfection. Preparations currently used and widely accepted for surgical disinfection of the hands to remove the 'residents' include a povidone-iodine detergent solution containing 0.75% available iodine. They should be used for all hand washes during operating sessions to achieve a cumulative effect on the reduction of 'resident' bacteria. A wash duration of 2 minutes, without scrubbing, should be adequate. Hand disinfectants, such as povidone-iodine, in hospital kitchens, however, should only be used on advice from the microbiologist. As for surgical scrubs, agents used for pre-operative disinfection of the patient's skin should be active mainly against the 'resident' flora. Alcoholic solutions of povidone-iodine containing 1% available iodine or alcoholic solutions of 1% iodine are frequently used. Where there is ingrained dirt or where spores in skin present a special hazard, washing with detergents or grease-solvent gels, followed by application of an aqueous povidone-iodine compress containing 1% available iodine for at least 30 minutes will reduce the number of spores, but prophylactic penicillin should still be given to patients thought to be at risk from gas gangrene. Applications of aqueous solutions of iodine or povidone-iodine are effective for disinfection of oral mucous membranes. A vaginal douche of 0.5% povidone-iodine containing 0.05% available iodine, followed by use of povidone-iodine vaginal gel, can be used for disinfection of the vaginal mucosa. Although thorough cleaning of baths with a detergent, daily and after use, is usually sufficient, antiseptic solutions containing an iodophore may be added to the bathwater of patients with infected staphylococcal lesions to reduce the contamination of the water and reduce deposition of organisms on the surface of the bath; cleaning is still necessary after an antiseptic bath additive has been used. Nasal and skin staphylococcal carriers should also wash routinely and bath daily, at least for 1 week, with an antiseptic detergent such as povidone-iodine.— G. A. J. Ayliffe *et al.*, *Chemical Disinfection in Hospitals*, London, Public Health Laboratory Service, 1984. Iodophores are moderately inactivated by protein but not by soap. They have no corrosive action.— G. A. J. Ayliffe *et al.*, *Hospital acquired Infection, Principles and Prevention*, Bristol, John Wright and Sons Ltd, 1982.

Results of a study suggesting that in order to reduce post-extraction bacteraemia in patients undergoing tooth extraction and at risk of developing infective endocarditis, prior irrigation of the gingival crevice with an aqueous solution of povidone-iodine 1% v/v should be considered as a supplement to antibiotic prophylaxis.— T. W. Macfarlane *et al.*, *Br. dent. J.*, 1984, *156*, 179.

Further references to iodine compounds as antiseptics and disinfectants.— W. Gottardi, Iodine and Iodine Compounds, in *Disinfection, Sterilization, and Preservation*, S.S. Block (Ed.), 3rd Edn, Philadelphia, Lea & Febiger, 1983, p.183.

Disinfectants in agriculture. For a list of disinfectants, including iodophores, and their rate of dilution approved for use in Great Britain in foot-and-mouth disease, swine vesicular disease, fowl pest, and tuberculosis in animals, see The Diseases of Animals (Approved Disinfectants) Order 1978 (SI 1978: No. 32), as amended (SI 1985: No. 24).

For information regarding the use of disinfectants, including iodophores, in the dairying industry, see *British Standard Code of practice for cleaning and disinfecting of plant and equipment used in the dairying industry*, BS5305:1984, London, British Standards Institution, 1984.

Disinfection of equipment. References to the use of povidone-iodine for the disinfection of medical equipment: H. J. Weinstein *et al.*, *Am. Rev. resp. Dis.*, 1977, *116*, 541 (fibreoptic bronchoscopes); K. E. Nelson *et al.*, *Am. Rev. resp. Dis.*, 1983, *127*, 97 (fibreoptic bronchoscopes); *Gut*, 1983, *24*, 1064 (endoscopes); F. M. Parsons *et al.* (letter), *Lancet*, 1983, *2*, 907 (continuous ambulatory peritoneal dialysis connections); W. K. Stewart and L. W. Fleming (letter), *Lancet*, 1983, *2*, 1367 (continuous ambulatory peritoneal dialysis connections); H. J. O'Connor and A. T. R. Axon (letter), *Lancet*, 1984, *1*, 631 (fibreoptic endoscopes).

Disinfection of viruses. Methods for the terminal disinfection of materials in contact with Lassa virus with mention that an iodophore containing 450 ppm available iodine is a suitable disinfectant.— *Memorandum on Lassa Fever*, Dept of Health and Social Security, London, HM Stationery Office, 1976.

Methods for the sterilisation and disinfection of materials in contact with Creutzfeldt-Jakob virus with recommendations that iodophores should not be used.— *Report of an Advisory Group on the Management of Patients with Spongiform Encephalopathy (Creutzfeldt-Jakob Disease (CJD))*, Dept of Health and Social Security, London, HM Stationery Office, 1981.

Preparations

Povidone-Iodine Cleansing Solution *(U.S.P.)*
Povidone-Iodine Ointment *(U.S.P.)*
Povidone-Iodine Solution *(B.P., B.P. Vet.)*
Povidone-Iodine Topical Aerosol Solution *(U.S.P.)*
Povidone-Iodine Topical Solution *(U.S.P.)*

Proprietary Preparations

Betadine *(Napp, UK)*. *Gargle and mouth-wash*, povidone-iodine 1%.
Ointment, povidone-iodine 10%.
Pessaries, povidone-iodine 200 mg.
Vaginal gel, povidone-iodine 10%.
Alcoholic solution, povidone-iodine 10%.
Antiseptic paint, povidone-iodine 10%.
Antiseptic solution, povidone-iodine 10%.
Antiseptic spray, aerosol, povidone-iodine 5%.
Dry powder spray, aerosol, povidone-iodine 2.5%.
Scalp and skin cleanser, povidone-iodine 7.5%.
Shampoo, povidone-iodine 4% with lanolin.
Skin cleanser, povidone-iodine 4%.
Surgical scrub, povidone-iodine 7.5%.

Betadine VC *(Napp, UK)*. *Concentrate solution*, povidone-iodine 10%, in antiseptic vaginal cleansing kit. Dilute before use.

Disadine DP *(Stuart, UK)*. *Dry powder spray*, aerosol, povidone-iodine 0.5%.

Inadine *(Johnson & Johnson, UK)*. *Dressings*, sterile povidone-iodine 10%.

Polydine *(Fischer, Israel: Clinical Specialities, UK)*. *Antiseptic soap*, povidone-iodine 5%.

Videne *(Riker, UK)*. *Disinfectant solution*, povidone-iodine 10%.
Disinfectant tincture, povidone-iodine 10%.
Surgical scrub, povidone-iodine 7.5%.
Topical powder, povidone-iodine 5%.

Proprietary Preparations of some other Iodophores

Steribath *(Stuart, UK)*. *Disinfectant bath concentrate*, solution, iodine-nonoxinol complex providing 4.5% available iodine, in sachets of 14 mL. Dilute in bath water.

Vanodine *(Evans Vanodine, UK)*. *Disinfectant concentrate*, solution, nonylphenyl hydroxypoly (oxyethylene/oxypropylene) iodine complex providing 1.92% available iodine. Dilute 1 vol. in 100 vol. of water before use. For control of foot infections in swimming baths and changing rooms.

Proprietary Names and Manufacturers of Povidone-iodine and other Iodophores

Amyderm *(Schulke & Mayr, Ger.)*; Batticon *(Trommsdorff, Ger.)*; Betadermyl *(Dagra, Neth.)*; Betadine *(Faulding, Austral.; Purdue Frederick, Canad.; Sarget, Fr.; Chinoin, Ital.; Neth.; Keatings, S.Afr.; Mundipharma, S.Afr.; Rio, S.Afr.; Sarget, Spain; Mundipharma, Switz.; Napp, UK; Purdue Frederick, USA)*; Betaisodona *(Mundipharma, Ger.)*; Betaseptic *(Sarget, Fr.)*; Betiadine *(Arg.)*; Braunol *(Braun Melsungen, Ger.)*; Braunovidon *(Braun Melsungen, Ger.)*; Bridine *(Allen & Hanburys, Canad.)*; Chem-o-dine *(Remedia, S.Afr.)*; Cold Sore Paint *(Drug Houses Austral., Austral.; Nyal, Austral.)*; Destrobac *(Zyma, Switz.)*; Disadine DP *(ICI, S.Afr.; Stuart, UK)*; Efodine *(Fougera, USA)*; Final Step *(Marion Laboratories, USA)*; Frepp *(Marion Laboratories, USA)*; Inadine *(Johnson & Johnson, UK)*; Iodine Tri-Test *(Drug Houses Austral., Austral.)*; Iso-Betadine *(Belg.)*; Isobetadine *(Leiras, Denm.)*; Isodine *(Faulding, Austral.; Blair, USA)*; Jodocur *(Farmacologico Milanese, Ital.)*; Neojodin *(Jpn)*; Nutradine *(S.Afr.)*; Orodine *(Orapharm, Austral.)*; Pervinox *(Arg.)*; Pevidine *(Berk Pharmaceuticals, UK)*; Podine *(Lennon, S.Afr.)*; Polydine *(Fischer, Israel: Clinical Specialities, UK; Century, USA)*; Povidine-K *(USV, Austral.)*; Proviodine *(Rougier, Canad.)*; Savlon Dry *(ICI, Austral.)*; Septo-Dyne *(USA)*; Steribath *(Stuart, UK)*; Stoxine *(Smith Kline & French, Austral.)*; Summer's Eve *(Fleet, USA)*; Topionic *(R. Rius, Spain)*; Traumasept *(Smith Kline Dauelsberg, Ger.)*; Vanodine *(Evans Vanodine, UK)*; Videne *(Riker, UK)*.

4581-j

Sodium Iodide *(USAN)*.

Iodeto de Sódio; Natrii Iodetum; Natrii Iodidum; Natrii Jodidum; Natrium Iodatum; Sod. Iod.; Sodii Iodidum; Sodium (Iodure de).

NaI = 149.9.

CAS — 7681-82-5.

Pharmacopoeias. In *Arg., Aust., Belg., Br., Braz., Chin., Cz., Egypt., Eur., Fr., Ger., Hung., Ind., It., Jpn, Jug., Mex., Neth., Nord., Pol., Port., Roum., Rus., Span., Swiss, Turk.,* and *U.S.* Also in *B.P. Vet.*

Colourless crystals or white odourless crystalline powder. It is deliquescent in moist air and develops a brown tint upon decomposition. Each g represents 6.7 mmol of sodium and of iodide.

B.P. and *U.S.P.* **solubilities**: 1 in 0.6 of water and 1 in 2 of alcohol; the *U.S.P.* also states soluble 1 in 1 of glycerol. Solutions may be **sterilised** by autoclaving. Aqueous solutions gradually become coloured on exposure to light and air due to the liberation of iodine. **Store** in airtight containers. Protect from light.

Adverse Effects, Treatment, Precautions, and Absorption and Fate

As for Iodine, p.1184.

Uses and Administration

Sodium iodide may be used for the prophylaxis and treatment of iodine deficiency disorders, such as endemic goitre, in districts where the diet is deficient in iodides. It is usually given for this purpose as iodised salt.

Sodium iodide has been given by intravenous injection as part of the management of thyrotoxic crisis.

Sodium iodide has been used as an expectorant but there is little evidence to show that it is effective.

Iodine radionuclides are often administered as preparations of sodium iodide.

In veterinary medicine sodium iodide is used in the treatment of actinobacillosis and actinomycosis of *cattle*.

IODINE DEFICIENCY DISORDERS. For the use of sodium iodide in the prophylaxis and treatment of iodine deficiency disorders, including endemic goitre and cretinism, see under Iodine, p.1185.

Preparations

Sodium Iodide Solution *(U.S.P.)*. An aqueous solution containing not less than 50%, by weight, of sodium iodide. It may contain not more than 500 mg of sodium metabisulphite per litre. Store in airtight containers.

Proprietary Names and Manufacturers

Davurresolutivo *(Davur, Spain)*; Strumex *(Robugen, Ger.)*.

The following names have been used for multi-ingredient preparations containing sodium iodide— Iodo-Ephedrine *(Philip Harris, UK)*; Sclerodine *(Ondee, Canad.)*.

Iron and Iron Compounds

5030-j

Iron is an essential constituent of the body, being necessary for haemoglobin formation and for the oxidative processes of living tissues. The body contains about 4 g of iron most of which is present as haemoglobin. The remainder is present in the storage forms, ferritin or haemosiderin, in the reticuloendothelial system or as myoglobin with smaller amounts occurring in haem-containing enzymes or in plasma bound to transferrin.

Iron is absorbed chiefly in the duodenum and jejunum, absorption being aided by the acid secretion of the stomach and being more readily effected when the iron is in the ferrous state or is part of the haem complex. Only about 5 to 15% of the iron ingested in food is normally absorbed but the 15 to 20 mg of iron in the average Western diet each day is usually sufficient to maintain normal adults in iron equilibrium. Absorption is increased in conditions of iron deficiency and is decreased if the body stores are overloaded.

Good dietary sources of iron include meat, fish, legumes, and some leafy vegetables, but some products with a high iron content also contain phosphates or phytates which inhibit absorption by the formation of unabsorbable complexes.

Iron oxides and hydroxides are used as colouring agents.

Adverse Effects

The oral administration of iron preparations sometimes produces gastro-intestinal irritation and abdominal pain with nausea, vomiting, diarrhoea, or constipation. These side-effects are related to the amount of elemental iron taken rather than the type of preparation. Side-effects may be reduced by administration immediately after food or by beginning therapy with a small dose and increasing gradually. Sustained-release or enteric-coated products are claimed to produce fewer side-effects but this may only reflect the lower availability of iron from these preparations. Oral liquid preparations may blacken the teeth and should be drunk through a straw. The faeces of patients taking iron salts may be coloured black.

The adverse effects associated with iron given parenterally are described under iron dextran (p.1193).

Iron overdosage may have corrosive effects on the gastro-intestinal mucosa; necrosis and perforation may occur; stricture formation may subsequently follow. Symptoms, which may not appear for several hours, include epigastric pain, diarrhoea, nausea, vomiting, and haematemesis. Circulatory failure may follow if the diarrhoea and haemorrhage are severe. Hours or days later, after apparent recovery, metabolic acidosis, convulsions, and coma may occur. If the patient survives, symptoms of acute liver necrosis may develop and may lead to death due to hepatic coma.

Iron overload, with increased storage of iron in various tissues (haemosiderosis), may occur as a result of excessive oral and parenteral therapy or multiple blood transfusions. Patients mistakenly given iron therapy when not suffering from iron-deficiency anaemia are also at risk as are those with pre-existing iron storage or absorption diseases.

In Great Britain the recommended exposure limits of iron salts (as Fe) are 1 mg per m^3 (long-term); 2 mg per m^3 (short-term).

IRON OVERLOAD. A discussion of iron metabolism with special reference to iron overload.— M. Barry, *Gut*, 1974, *15*, 324. See also A. Jacobs, *Semin. Hematol.*, 1977, *14*, 89.

The risk of major iron overload in non-transfused patients with sideroblastic anaemia. The degree of anaemia was a poor guide to the degree of iron loading.— T. E. A. Peto *et al.*, *Lancet*, 1983, *1*, 375. See also R. E. Marcus (letter), *ibid.*, 1276.

Treatment of Adverse Effects

In treating iron poisoning, speed is essential to block absorption of iron from the alimentary tract. In acute poisoning the procedure described under desferrioxamine (see p.838) should be followed. If desferrioxamine is not available, empty the stomach immediately by emesis and lavage using a 1 to 5% solution of sodium bicarbonate, and leave up to about 300 mL of the solution in the stomach; sodium bicarbonate forms poorly absorbed ferrous carbonate with any ferrous ions. Other measures include correction of lost fluids.

An extensive review of iron poisoning and its management.— A. T. Proudfoot *et al.*, *Med. Toxicol.*, 1986, *1*, 83.

Precautions

Iron salts should not be given to patients receiving repeated blood transfusions or to patients with anaemias not produced by iron deficiency unless iron deficiency is also present. Oral iron therapy should not be administered concomitantly with parenteral iron. Care should be taken when given to patients with iron-storage or iron-absorption diseases, haemoglobinopathies, or existing gastro-intestinal disease.

The absorption of iron salts and tetracyclines is diminished when they are taken concomitantly by mouth. If treatment with both drugs is required, the iron salt should be administered 2 hours before or 3 hours after the tetracycline. The absorption of iron salts may also be decreased by some antacids. Iron salts reduce the effects of penicillamine. The response to iron may be delayed in patients receiving concomitant chloramphenicol therapy.

Mixtures containing iron salts should be well diluted with water and swallowed through a straw to prevent discoloration of the teeth.

A report of oral ferrous sulphate exacerbating rheumatoid disease.— D. Blake and P. A. Bacon (letter), *Lancet*, 1982, *1*, 623. Comment.— E. D. Harris and H. L. Bonkowsky (letter), *ibid.*, 745.

A study demonstrating that iron supplementation contributes to maternal zinc depletion when dietary zinc is marginal.— N. J. Meadows *et al.*, *Gut*, 1982, *23*, A438.

A report confirming the presence of diminished zinc absorption in patients with renal failure, and suggesting that routine administration of ferrous sulphate to such patients may contribute to their zinc deficiency.— D. K. Abu-Hamdan *et al.*, *Ann. intern. Med.*, 1986, *104*, 50.

INFECTIONS. A discussion on the effect of iron in relation to infection. Iron should not be available to invading micro-organisms. Only lactobacilli can grow in the total absence of iron, and many pathogenic bacteria need a substantial amount. Iron overload increases the susceptibility to infectious disease. Normal iron balance seems to achieve a compromise in which iron is not readily accessible to invading micro-organisms but is in sufficient quantity to allow the host's immune system to function optimally.— J. H. Brock, *Br. med. J.*, 1986, *293*, 518.

Of 31 patients with chronic mucocutaneous candidiasis, 23 had evidence of iron deficiency. Four with a haemoglobin concentration greater than 12 g per 100 mL were treated, in a controlled trial, with iron dextran by total-dose infusion, followed by ferrous fumarate 200 mg three times daily for 2 months; 3 showed definite clinical improvement in their candidiasis. Eight further patients were treated with iron, usually with improvement in their candidiasis, though iron stores were not consistently replenished.— J. M. Higgs and R. S. Wells, *Br. J. Derm.*, 1972, *87*, *Suppl.* 8, 88.

During a 5-year period the mean incidence of neonatal sepsis in Polynesian neonates was 11 per 1000 births compared with 0.6 per 1000 for European neonates. The years of high incidence appeared to be confined to periods when intramuscular injections of iron dextran were given. Administration of iron had been stopped and subsequent analysis indicated that the incidence of neonatal sepsis over the 5-year period was 17 per 1000 in those who had received iron and 2.7 per 1000 in those who had not. The data suggested that injections of iron dextran might impair the immunity of the treated infants, making them more susceptible to sepsis produced by *Escherichia coli*.— D. M. J. Barry and A. W. Reeve, *Pediatrics*, 1977, *60*, 908.

A report of *Yersinia enterocolitica* infection in 2 children after treatment with desferrioxamine 5 g for overdoses of iron. The patients were without apparent immune defects; the iron binding capacity in both children during their illness excluded the possibility of iron overload. It was thought that both patients had been colonised with *Y. enterocolitica* before the iron intake. Iron and desferrioxamine may possibly have a pathogenetic role in such circumstances.— K. Melby *et al.*, *Br. med. J.*, 1982, *285*, 467.

Malaria. Iron dextran injection 3 mL (Inferon) was administered intramuscularly to 236 of a cohort of 486 two-month-old infants in Papua New Guinea. Those children not receiving iron dextran became relatively iron deficient, however, malaria rates were lower at 6- and 12-month follow-up in this particular group. The overall evidence was for a protective role of iron deficiency against malaria, and a lack of justification for the routine use of iron supplementation in areas where malaria is endemic.— S. J. Oppenheimer *et al.*, *Trans. R. Soc. trop. Med. Hyg.*, 1986, *80*, 603. See also A. E. J. Masawe *et al.*, *Lancet*, 1974, *2*, 314.

Absorption and Fate

Iron is irregularly and incompletely absorbed from the gastro-intestinal tract, the main sites of absorption being the duodenum and jejunum. Absorption is usually increased in conditions of iron deficiency or when given in the fasting state. Absorption of iron may be reduced in certain disease states.

A review of the physiology of iron absorption and supplementation.— B. S. N. Rao, *Br. med. Bull.*, 1981, *37*, 25.

A review of iron metabolism, deficiency, and overload.— C. A. Finch and H. Huebers, *New Engl. J. Med.*, 1982, *306*, 1520. See also E. Björn-Rasmussen, *Lancet*, 1983, *1*, 914.

Human Requirements

Apart from haemorrhage, iron is mainly lost from the body in the faeces, urine, skin, and sweat, but the total loss is small. In healthy men and non-menstruating women the loss is replaced by the absorption of about 1 mg of iron daily; about 2 mg needs to be absorbed daily by menstruating women. In childhood and adolescence, the need is proportionately greater because of growth. In pregnancy and lactation 3 mg or more must be absorbed daily. In the *UK* the recommended dietary allowance of iron is 10 mg daily for men and non-menstruating women, up to 12 mg daily for children (depending on age) and menstruating women, and up to 15 mg daily for pregnant or lactating women. In the *US* recommendations are higher than those in the *UK*, with supplements of 30 to 60 mg being suggested for pregnant or lactating women. The *WHO* generally recommend a lower dietary intake than those of the *UK* or *US*. For a discussion of prophylactic iron given during pregnancy, see p.1190.

The daily intake of iron of breast fed infants up to the age of 4 months was considered to be adequate. Recommended daily intake of iron in individuals who obtained more than 25% of calories from foods of animal origin: infants 5 to 12 months, 4 mg; children, 1 to 12 years, 5 mg; boys, 13 to 16 years, 9 mg; girls, 13 to 16 years, 12 mg; men and non-menstruating women, 5 mg; menstruating women, 14 mg. For the prevention of anaemia during pregnancy and lactation in populations with and without body iron stores, daily supplements of 30 to 60 and 120 to 240 mg of iron respectively were required. In addition about 500 µg daily of folic acid was required. Supplementation with both iron and folic acid should start not later than the second trimester of pregnancy and should continue until the end of lactation.—Report of a WHO Group of Experts on Nutritional Anaemias, *Tech. Rep. Ser. Wld Hlth Org. No. 503*, 1972.

Provided that the iron status of the mother during pregnancy is satisfactory, the infant is born with stores of iron in the body which together with the iron present in human milk, can satisfy iron requirements for the first 4 to 6 months. Recommended daily intakes of iron: infants up to 1 year, 6 mg; boys and girls, 1 to 2 years, 7 mg; 3 to 4 years, 8 mg; 5 to 8 years, 10 mg; 9 to 17 years, 12 mg; men over 18 years, 10 mg; women 18 to 55 years, 12 mg; over 55 years, 10 mg; during pregnancy, 13 mg; during lactation, 15 mg. The recommended intake of iron may not be sufficient for about 10% of girls and women with large menstrual losses.— *Reports on Health and Social Subjects No. 15*, London, HM Stationery Office, 1979 (Report by the Committee on Medical Aspects of Food Policy).

The US National Research Council made the following recommendations for daily dietary allowances of iron: infants up to 6 months, 10 mg; children 6 months to 3 years, 15 mg; 4 to 10 years, 10 mg; males 11 to 18 years, 18 mg; over 18 years, 10 mg; females 11 to 50 years, 18 mg; over 50 years, 10 mg; in pregnancy the increased requirement could not be met by the iron content of the diet nor by the existing iron stores of many women and the use of 30 to 60 mg of supplemental iron was recommended; in lactation the iron needs were not substantially different from those of nonpregnant women but it was advisable to continue supplementation of the mother for 2 to 3 months after parturition.— *Recommended Dietary Allowances*, 9th Edn, Washington, The National Research Council, 1980.

FORTIFICATION OF FOOD. For a review of the use and suitability of various iron compounds for the iron fortification of food, see Control of Nutritional Anaemia with Special Reference to Iron Deficiency, Report of an IAEA/USAID/WHO Joint Meeting, *Tech. Rep. Ser. Wld Hlth Org. No. 580*, 1975.

A discussion on the fortification of food with iron and the prevention of iron deficiency.— *Lancet*, 1980, *1*, 1117.

Therapy with Iron and Iron Salts

Iron and iron salts should only be given for the treatment or prophylaxis of iron deficiency anaemias. They should not be given for the treatment of other types of anaemia except where iron deficiency is also present. Iron-deficiency anaemias respond readily to iron therapy but the underlying cause of the anaemia should be determined and treated. Iron therapy should be continued after the haemoglobin concentration has returned to normal, to replenish the body stores of iron. With therapy by mouth, the haemoglobin concentration may take up to 10 weeks to reach normal values and 3 to 6 months' treatment may be necessary to replenish iron stores. Failure to respond to oral iron after 3 weeks of therapy may be indicative of non-compliance, continued blood loss with inadequate replacement of iron, malabsorption, wrong diagnosis, or other complicating factors and the treatment should be reassessed.

Compounds of iron are used in the treatment of microcytic anaemia, including simple achlorhydric anaemia, simple anaemia of pregnancy, the nutritional anaemia of infants, anaemia due to excessive haemorrhage, and anaemia associated with infections and malignant disease.

Preparations of iron are administered by mouth, usually as soluble ferrous salts which are better absorbed than ferric salts. Iron may also be administered by intramuscular or intravenous injection. Large doses of iron are necessary to relieve iron deficiency; the daily oral dosage of the soluble salts should contain 100 to 200 mg of iron.

In the treatment of macrocytic anaemia, preparations of iron given alone are of no value but they may be of value as a supplement to hydroxocobalamin therapy whenever the reserves of iron are depleted and the increase in haemoglobin does not parallel the rise in the number of red blood-cells.

Diagnosis of iron deficiency anaemias may involve measurement of iron or ferritin concentrations in serum. Care is required in interpreting the former because normochromic or hypochromic anaemia may be associated with a low serum-iron concentration in the presence of adequate amounts of storage iron. Care is also required in interpreting measurements of serum-ferritin concentrations because certain conditions, such as hepatic disease, Hodgkin's disease, breast carcinoma, and acute leukaemia show falsely-elevated concentrations of circulating ferritin.

Externally, some iron salts are powerfully astringent and styptic, ferric chloride being most commonly used for these purposes.

Some reviews of iron therapy: R. L. C. Cumming, *Practitioner*, 1978, *221*, 184; A. S. Prasad, *Trace Elements and Iron in Human Metabolism*, Chichester, John Wiley, 1978; *Drug & Ther. Bull.*, 1979, *17*, 33; M. J. Pippard, *Prescribers' J.*, 1982, *22*, 56; C. K. Arthur and J. P. Isbister, *Drugs*, 1987, *33*, 171.

ANAEMIA OF PREGNANCY. Although it is customary to give iron prophylactically during pregnancy, this practice is being questioned (*Br. med. J.*, 1978, *2*, 1317; A. Malhotra and R.S. Sawers, *ibid.*, 1986, *293*, 465). In discussing iron supplementation during pregnancy, Lind (in *Nutrition in Pregnancy: Proceedings of the Tenth Study Group of the Royal College of Obstetricians and Gynaecologists*, D.M. Campbell and M.D.G. Gillmer (Ed.), London, Royal College of Obstetricians and Gynaecologists, 1983) put forward four approaches. 1) Provide iron as soon as pregnancy is diagnosed. 2) Give iron from 28 weeks onwards. 3) Give iron for 3 months post delivery. 4) Only give iron if the pregnant woman displays iron insufficiency. The first approach was to be condemned. The second and third approaches were possible and their adoption depended on the type of population. The author favoured the fourth approach.

HAEMODIALYSIS. A view that administration of parenteral iron in haemodialysis patients should be restricted to patients with verified iron deficiency (shown by low serum ferritin and absent marrow iron), and when oral iron cannot be given because of gastro-intestinal intolerance.— L. E. Human, *J. Am. med. Ass.*, 1980, *244*, 371.

HEPATIC FAILURE. A case of orally-administered iron protecting against hepatic failure in a patient with erythropoietic protoporphyria.— V. R. Gordeuk *et al.*, *Ann. intern. Med.*, 1986, *105*, 27.

IRON-DEFICIENCY ANAEMIA. A brief review of iron deficiency anaemia and child health surveillance.— R. S. Illingworth, *Archs Dis. Childh.*, 1986, *61*, 1151.

Data supporting the hypothesis that iron deficiency adversely affects the learning and problem-solving capacity of school-age children. Those who were originally anaemic and were treated with iron became faster and more accurate in their responses.— E. Pollitt *et al.* (letter), *Lancet*, 1985, *1*, 158.

In a study of 97 children with anaemia aged 17 to 19 months, those who received treatment with ferrous sulphate 24 mg daily for 2 months had an increased rate of weight gain and more of them achieved the expected increase in psychomotor skills than those who received placebo.— M. A. Aukett *et al.*, *Archs Dis. Childh.*, 1986, *61*, 849. See also *Lancet*, 1987, *1*, 141; J. Poulton (letter), *Archs Dis. Childh.*, 1987, *62*, 213.

Attitudes to prescribing iron supplements in general practice.— D. G. Waller and A. G. Smith, *Br. med. J.*, 1987, *294*, 94.

Diagnosis. Use of a small-dose iron tolerance test as an indicator of mild iron deficiency.— W. H. Crosby and M. A. O'Neil-Cutting, *J. Am. med. Ass.*, 1984, *251*, 1986.

Dysphagia. A controlled study in an adult Indian hospital population of 2840 patients of the association of anaemia with dysphagia and cricoid webs (a stricture in the upper end of the oesophagus). Of the 6 patients with webs 4 improved with iron therapy.— S. N. Khosla, *Postgrad. med. J.*, 1984, *60*, 346.

MOTOR DISTURBANCES. As there was an association between low serum-iron concentrations and the restless leg syndrome, a similar association between low iron values and akathisia was investigated and found to exist. Iron therapy might be worth investigating.— K. W. Brown *et al.*, *Lancet*, 1987, *1*, 1234.

5031-z

Iron

Ferrum.
Fe=55.847.

CAS — 7439-89-6.

Pharmacopoeias. In *Arg.*, *Belg.*, *Hung.*, *Pol.*, *Port.*, and *Span.*, most of which specify iron filings or powder. Also in *B.P.C. 1973* which specifies iron wire. *Arg.*, *Aust.*, *Belg.*, *Braz.*, *Hung.*, *It.*, *Pol.*, *Port.*, *Roum.*, and *Rus.* include a monograph for reduced iron.

Insoluble in water and alcohol; almost completely soluble in dilute mineral acids.

Iron has been used in the preparation of some solutions and syrups. Reduced iron has been used for food fortification. Iron carbonyl which is a highly purified preparation of elemental iron is also reported to be used for food fortification.

Proprietary Names and Manufacturers

Colliron *(Duncan, Flockhart, UK)*.

5033-k

Dextriferron *(BAN, rINN)*.

Iron-Dextrin Complex.

CAS — 9004-51-7.

A complex of ferric hydroxide with partially hydrolysed dextrin.

Dextriferron has similar actions and uses to iron dextran (see p.1193).

Dextriferron may be given intravenously; it should not be given intramuscularly.

Proprietary Names and Manufacturers

Astrafer *(Astra, Austral.*; *Astra, UK)*; Ferrigen *(Astra, Swed.)*; Ferrum Hausmann *(Degussa, Ger.*; *Hausmann, Switz.)*.

5034-a

Ferric Ammonium Citrate

381; Ferricum Citricum Ammoniatum; Iron and Ammonium Citrate.

CAS — 1185-57-5.

Pharmacopoeias. In *Arg.*, *Chin.*, *Egypt.*, *Ind.*, *Mex.*, *Port.*, and *Span.* (Fe content varying from 16 to 22.5%).

A complex of ammonium ferric citrate containing about 21.5% of iron.

Ferric ammonium citrate has the actions and uses of iron salts (see p.1189) and has been given in doses of up to 6 g (equivalent to about 1.2 g of iron) daily. Typical iron doses are described under ferrous sulphate (p.1192). Mixtures should be well diluted with water before taking and a straw should be used to prevent discoloration of the teeth.

Green ferric ammonium citrate has also been used.

Preparations

Ferric Ammonium Citrate Mixture *(B.P.C. 1973)*. Mist. Ferr. et Ammon. Cit.; Iron and Ammonium Citrate Mixture. Ferric ammonium citrate 2 g, double-strength chloroform water 5 mL, water to 10 mL. It should be recently prepared. *Dose.* 10 mL.

Ferric ammonium citrate mixture *B.P.C. 1973* was not adequately preserved against microbial spoilage as determined by the *B.P.* challenge test.— T. R. R. Kurup and L. S. C. Wan, *Pharm. J.*, 1986, *2*, 761.

Paediatric Ferric Ammonium Citrate Mixture *(B.P.C. 1973)*. Mist. Ferr. et Ammon. Cit. pro Inf.; Ferric Ammonium Citrate Mixture Paediatric; Paediatric Iron and Ammonium Citrate Mixture. Ferric ammonium citrate 400 mg, compound orange spirit 0.01 mL, syrup 0.5 mL, double-strength chloroform water 2.5 mL, water to 5 mL. It should be recently prepared. *Dose.* Children, up to 1 year, 5 mL; 1 to 5 years, 10 mL. To be taken well diluted with water.

Proprietary Preparations

Lexpec with Iron *(R.P. Drugs, UK)*. *Syrup*, elemental iron 80 mg (as ferric ammonium citrate), folic acid 2.5 mg/5 mL.

Syrup (Lexpec with Iron-M), elemental iron 80 mg (as ferric ammonium citrate), folic acid 0.5 mg/5 mL.

For preparations containing multivitamins and minerals, see p.1291.

5036-x

Ferric Chloride
Ferr. Perchlor.; Ferrum Sesquichloratum; Iron Perchloride; Iron Sesquichloride; Iron Trichloride.
$FeCl_3,6H_2O$=270.3.

CAS — 7705-08-0 (anhydrous); 10025-77-1 (hexahydrate).

Pharmacopoeias. In *Aust., Hung., Port., Span.,* and *Swiss.*

Ferric chloride has the general properties of iron salts (see p.1189) but is exceptionally astringent. It has been used mainly by local application for its styptic and astringent properties. Local application of ferric chloride or other iron salts may cause permanent discoloration of the skin.

Preparations

Ferric Chloride Solution *(B.P.C. 1973).* Liquor Ferri Perchloridi. Strong ferric chloride solution 25 mL, water to 100 mL. It contains about 15% w/v of $FeCl_3$.

Strong Ferric Chloride Solution *(B.P.C. 1973).* Liquor Ferri Perchloridi Fortis; Liq. Ferr. Perchlor. Fort. An aqueous solution containing about 60% w/v of $FeCl_3$.

For preparations containing multivitamins and minerals, see p.1291.

5037-r

Red Ferric Oxide *(USAN).*
E172 *(iron oxides or hydroxides).*
Fe_2O_3=159.7.

CAS — 1309-37-1.

Pharmacopoeias. In *Fr.* and *Port. Fr.* also includes black ferric oxide and brown ferric oxide. Also in *U.S.N.F.*

A moderately reddish-brown powder. *Insoluble* in water and in organic solvents; dissolves in hydrochloric acid upon warming, a small amount of insoluble residue usually remaining.

Red ferric oxide is used mainly for tinting calamine. In Great Britain the recommended exposure limits of iron oxide, fume (as Fe) are 5 mg per m^3 (long-term); 10 mg per m^3 (short-term).

5038-f

Yellow Ferric Oxide *(USAN).*
E172 *(iron oxides or hydroxides).*

CAS — 51274-00-1.

Pharmacopoeias. In *Fr.* and *U.S.N.F.*

A moderately yellowish-orange powder. *Insoluble* in water and in organic solvents; dissolves in hydrochloric acid upon warming, a small amount of insoluble residue usually remaining.

Yellow ferric oxide is used mainly for tinting pharmaceutical preparations. In Great Britain the recommended exposure limits of iron oxide, fume (as Fe) are 5 mg per m^3 (long-term); 10 mg per m^3 (short-term).

Estimated acceptable daily intake of iron oxides and hydrated iron oxides: up to 500 µg per kg body-weight. Ferric oxide is less available as a source of biologically active iron than are other forms of iron.— Twenty-third Report of Joint FAO/WHO Expert Committee on Food Additives, *Tech. Rep. Ser. Wld Hlth Org. No. 648,* 1980.

12749-f

Ferrous Ascorbate

$C_{12}H_{14}FeO_{12}$=406.1.

CAS — 24808-52-4.

Ferrous ascorbate has the actions and uses of iron salts (p.1189).

Proprietary Names and Manufacturers
Ascofer *(Desbergers, Canad.; Roland-Marie, Fr.; Sodip, Switz.)*; Cefer *(Phoenix, Arg.)*; Ferro-semar *(Semar, Spain)*; Nedifer *(Servier, Neth.).*

5044-x

Ferrous Aspartate

$C_8H_{12}FeN_2O_8,4H_2O$=392.1.

Ferrous aspartate has the actions and uses of iron salts (see p.1189), and has been used in doses of 350 mg (equivalent to about 50 mg of iron). Typical iron doses are described under ferrous sulphate (p.1192).

Proprietary Names and Manufacturers
Ferofer *(Sigmatau, Ital.)*; Ferroglobine *(Belg.)*; Spartocina *(UCB, Ital.)*; Spartocine *(UCB, Arg.; UCB, Belg.; UCB, Ger.; Spain).*

5055-d

Ferrous Carbonate
Carbonato de Hierro; Ferri Carbonas. It consists chiefly of ferrous carbonate with variable proportions of ferric hydroxide and ferroso-ferric oxide.
$FeCO_3$=115.9.

CAS — 563-71-3 ($FeCO_3$).

Pharmacopoeias. In *Span.*

Ferrous carbonate has the actions and uses of iron salts (see p.1189). Preparations of saccharated ferrous carbonate were known as Blauds pills and Blauds tablets.

Proprietary Names and Manufacturers
Abofer *(Denm.)*; Collett Jerntabletter *(Collett, Norw.)*; Ingoferron *(Boehringer Ingelheim, Ger.).*

5054-f

Ferrous Fumarate *(BAN, USAN).*

$C_4H_2FeO_4$=169.9.

CAS — 141-01-5.

Pharmacopoeias. In *Br., Chin., Cz., Egypt., Ind., Neth., Nord.,* and *U.S.*

A fine reddish-orange to reddish-brown powder, odourless or with a slight odour; 200 mg contains about 65 mg of iron. Slightly **soluble** in water; very slightly soluble in alcohol. **Store** in well-closed containers.

Ferrous fumarate has the actions and uses of iron salts (see p.1189) and is given by mouth in the treatment of iron-deficiency anaemia. A usual dose is 200 mg (equivalent to about 65 mg of iron) three times daily. Typical iron doses are described more fully under ferrous sulphate (below).

Preparations

Ferrous Fumarate Mixture *(B.P.C. 1973).* A suspension of ferrous fumarate in a suitable coloured flavoured vehicle. When a dose less than 5 mL is prescribed, the mixture should be diluted to 5 mL with syrup. Such dilutions must be freshly prepared and not used more than 2 weeks after issue. Protect from light.

Ferrous Fumarate Tablets *(B.P.)*

Ferrous Fumarate Tablets *(U.S.P.)*

Proprietary Preparations

BC 500 with Iron *(Ayerst, UK). Tablets,* ferrous fumarate 200 mg, ascorbic acid 500 mg (as sodium salt), calcium pantothenate 20 mg, nicotinamide 100 mg, pyridoxine hydrochloride 10 mg, riboflavine 12.5 mg, thiamine mononitrate 25 mg.

Ferrocap *(Consolidated Chemicals, UK). Capsules,* sustained-release, ferrous fumarate 330 mg. *Dose.* 1 capsule daily.

Ferrocap-F 350 *(Consolidated Chemicals, UK). Capsules,* sustained-release, ferrous fumarate 330 mg, folic acid 350 µg. *Dose.* 1 capsule daily.

Fersaday *(Duncan, Flockhart, UK). Tablets,* ferrous iron 100 mg (as ferrous fumarate).

Fersamal *(Duncan, Flockhart, UK). Tablets,* ferrous iron 65 mg (as ferrous fumarate).
Syrup, ferrous iron 45 mg (as ferrous fumarate)/5 mL.

Folex-350 *(Rybar, UK). Tablets,* ferrous fumarate 308 mg, folic acid 350 µg.

Galfer *(Galen, UK). Capsules,* ferrous fumarate 290 mg.

Galfer F.A *(Galen, UK). Capsules,* ferrous fumarate 290 mg, folic acid 350 µg.

Galfer-Vit *(Galen, UK). Capsules,* ferrous fumarate 305 mg, nicotinamide 10 mg, pyridoxine hydrochloride 4 mg, riboflavine 2 mg, sodium ascorbate 56 mg, thiamine mononitrate 2 mg.

Givitol *(Galen, UK). Capsules,* ferrous fumarate 305 mg, folic acid 500 µg, nicotinamide 10 mg, pyridoxine hydrochloride 4 mg, riboflavine 2 mg, sodium ascorbate 56 mg, thiamine mononitrate 2 mg.

Meterfer *(Sinclair, UK). Tablets,* ferrous iron 100 mg (as ferrous fumarate).

Meterfolic *(Sinclair, UK). Tablets,* ferrous iron 100 mg (as ferrous fumarate), folic acid 350 µg.

Pregaday *(Duncan, Flockhart, UK). Tablets,* ferrous iron 100 mg (as ferrous fumarate), folic acid 350 µg.

Proprietary Names and Manufacturers
Anemotron *(Rovi, Spain)*; Bramiron *(Austral.)*; Erco-Fer *(Denm.; Erco, Swed.)*; Ercofer *(Ercopharm, Switz.)*; Femiron *(Beecham Laboratories, USA)*; Feostat *(Forest Pharmaceuticals, USA)*; Feroton *(Canad.)*; Ferrocap *(Consolidated Chemicals, UK)*; Ferrofume *(Canad.)*; Ferrokapsul *(Asche, Ger.)*; Ferrolande *(Delalande, Ger.)*; Ferromikron *(Ital.)*; Ferrone *(Belg.)*; Ferrum Hausmann *(Degussa, Ger.; Hausmann, Switz.)*; Ferrum Klinge *(Klinge, Ger.)*; Fersaday *(Duncan, Flockhart, UK)*; Fersamal *(Arg.; Austral.; Glaxo, Canad.; Glaxo, S.Afr.; Duncan, Flockhart, UK)*; Ferumat *(Belg.; Neth.)*; Fumafer *(Labaz, Fr.; Swed.)*; Fumasorb *(Milance, USA)*; Fumiron *(Austral.)*; Galfer *(Galen, UK)*; Hematon *(Canad.)*; Hemocyte *(US Pharmaceutical, USA)*; Laud-Iron *(USA)*; Meterfer *(Sinclair, UK)*; Neo-Fer *(Neolab, Canad.; Nyco, Norw.)*; Novofumar *(Novopharm, Canad.)*; Palafer *(Beecham, Canad.)*; Plancaps *(Unimed, UK)*; Rulofer *(Lomapharm, Ger.)*; Soparon *(Belg.)*; Span-FF *(USA)*; Toleron *(Wallace, USA).*

The following names have been used for multi-ingredient preparations containing ferrous fumarate—Loestrin Fe *(Parke, Davis, USA)*; Norlestrin Fe *(Parke, Davis, USA).*

For preparations containing multivitamins and minerals, see p.1291.

5058-m

Ferrous Gluconate *(BAN, USAN).*

Eisen(II)-Gluconat; Ferrosi Gluconas. Iron(II) di(D-gluconate).
$C_{12}H_{22}FeO_{14},2H_2O$=482.2.

CAS — 299-29-6 (anhydrous); 12389-15-0 (dihydrate).

Pharmacopoeias. In *Arg., Aust., Br., Braz., Egypt., Eur., Fr., Ger., Ind., Int., It., Jug., Neth., Pol., Swiss, Turk.,* and *U.S.*

Greenish-yellow to grey powder or granules. It may have a slight odour resembling that of burnt sugar. It contains not less than 11.8% and not more than 12.5% of ferrous iron calculated on the dried material; about 70 mg in 600 mg of the dihydrate.
The *B.P.* specifies slowly **soluble** 1 in 10 of water producing a greenish-brown solution, but more readily soluble on warming; practically insoluble in alcohol. The *U.S.P.* specifies soluble 1 in 5 of water, with slight heating; practically insoluble in alcohol. A 10% solution in carbon-dioxide free water has a pH of 4.0 to 5.5 3 to 4 hours after preparation. **Store** in airtight containers. Protect from light.

Ferrous gluconate has the actions and uses of iron salts (see p.1189) and is used for the treatment of iron-deficiency anaemia. The usual therapeutic dose is 1.2 to 1.8 g (equivalent to 140 to 210 mg of iron) daily in divided doses. Typical iron doses are described under ferrous sulphate (below).

Preparations

Ferrous Gluconate Capsules *(U.S.P.)*

Ferrous Gluconate Elixir *(U.S.P.)*. An elixir containing ferrous gluconate, with alcohol 6.3 to 7.7%. pH 3.4 to 3.8. Protect from light.

Ferrous Gluconate Mixture CF *(A.P.F.)*. Ferrous Gluconate Mixture for Children. Ferrous gluconate 200 mg, glucose 500 mg, orange syrup 1 mL, benzoic acid solution 0.1 mL, citric acid monohydrate 25 mg, water to 5 mL. *Dose.* Children weighing 12 to 15 kg, 5 mL three times daily.

Ferrous Gluconate Tablets *(B.P.)*. The tablets are coated.

Ferrous Gluconate Tablets *(U.S.P.)*

Proprietary Preparations

Feravol-F *(Carlton Laboratories, UK). Tablets*, ferrous gluconate 300 mg, folic acid 3 mg.

Feravol-G *(Carlton Laboratories, UK). Tablets*, ferrous gluconate 300 mg, ascorbic acid 9 mg, riboflavine 1 mg, thiamine hydrochloride 0.4 mg, copper.

Syrup, ferrous gluconate 300 mg, thiamine hydrochloride 1 mg/5 mL.

Ferfolic S.V *(Sinclair, UK). Tablets*, ferrous gluconate 250 mg, folic acid 5 mg.

Fergon *(Winthrop, UK). Tablets*, ferrous gluconate 300 mg.

Proprietary Names and Manufacturers

Fergon *(Winthrop, Austral.; Winthrop, Canad.; Winthrop, UK; Winthrop-Breon, USA)*; Ferralet *(Mission Pharmacal, USA)*; Ferrlecit *(Nattermann, Ger.)*; Ferro-G *(Austral.)*; Ferronicum *(Spain)*; Fersin *(Austral.)*; Fertinic *(Desbergers, Canad.)*; Glucoferron *(Switz.)*; Glucohaem *(Austral.)*; Hierro Laquifal *(Spain)*; Losferron *(Beiersdorf, Ger.)*; Novoferrogluc *(Novopharm, Canad.)*; Sidros *(Potter & Clarke, UK)*; Simron *(Merrell Dow, USA)*.

For preparations containing multivitamins and minerals, see p.1291.

5059-b

Ferrous Glycine Sulphate

Ferrous Aminoacetosulphate.

CAS — 14729-84-1.

A chelate of ferrous sulphate and glycine containing about 40 mg of ferrous iron in each 225 mg.

Ferrous glycine sulphate has the actions and uses of iron salts (see p.1189). The usual dose is the equivalent of 25 to 50 mg of iron three times daily. Typical iron doses are described under ferrous sulphate (below).

Proprietary Preparations

Ferrocontin Continus *(Napp, UK). Tablets*, sustained-release, ferrous iron 100 mg (as ferrous glycine sulphate). *Dose.* 1 tablet daily.

Ferrocontin Folic Continus *(Napp, UK). Tablets*, sustained-release, ferrous iron 100 mg (as ferrous glycine sulphate), folic acid 500 µg. *Dose.* 1 tablet daily.

Plesmet *(Napp, UK). Syrup*, ferrous iron 25 mg (as ferrous glycine sulphate)/5 mL.

Proprietary Names and Manufacturers

Fe-cap *(MCP Pharmaceuticals, UK)*; Ferro Sanol *(Sanol, Ger.)*; Ferro-Chel *(Austral.)*; Ferrocontin Continus *(Napp, UK)*; Ferrosanol *(Schwarz, Switz.)*; Glutaferro *(Medix, Spain)*; Glycifer *(Pharmacia, Denm.; Swed.)*; Jectoral *(Astra, UK)*; Kelferon *(MCP Pharmaceuticals, UK)*; Plesmet *(Nelson, Austral.; Napp, UK)*.

For preparations containing multivitamins and minerals, see p.1291.

3944-k

Ferrous Iodide

FeI_2 = 309.7.

Ferrous iodide has been used as a source of iron and has the actions of iron salts (p.1189). It was given as a solution, often diluted with syrup. The solution was prepared from iron, iodide, and dilute hypophosphorous acid.
The actions of the iodides are described on p.1184.

5060-x

Ferrous Lactate

Iron Lactate.

$C_6H_{10}FeO_6,3H_2O$=288.0.

CAS — 5905-52-2 (anhydrous); 6047-24-1 (trihydrate).

Pharmacopoeias. In *Pol.* and *Span.*

Ferrous lactate has the actions and uses of iron salts (see p.1189).

Proprietary Names and Manufacturers

Ferro Drops L *(Parke, Davis, S.Afr.)*.

5061-r

Ferrous Oxalate

Ferrum Oxalicum Oxydulatum; Iron Protoxalate.

$C_2FeO_4,2H_2O$=179.9.

CAS — 516-03-0 (anhydrous); 6047-25-2 (dihydrate).

Pharmacopoeias. In *Arg., Belg., Fr.,* and *Port.*

Ferrous oxalate has the actions and uses of iron salts (see p.1189).

5062-f

Ferrous Succinate *(BAN)*.

$C_4H_4FeO_4$=171.9.

CAS — 10030-90-7.

Pharmacopoeias. In *Br.*

A basic salt; it is a brownish-yellow to brown amorphous powder with a slight odour, containing 34 to 36% of ferrous iron; about 70 mg in 200 mg. Practically **insoluble** in water and alcohol; dissolves in dilute mineral acids. **Store** in well-closed containers. Protect from light.

Ferrous succinate has the actions and uses of iron salts (see p.1189). A usual dose is 100 mg (equivalent to 35 mg of iron) three times daily. Typical iron doses are described under ferrous sulphate (below).

Recovery of 2 women who had ingested ferrous succinate equivalent to 2 and 11 g respectively of Fe, after treatment with desferrioxamine and, in 1 patient, partial exchange transfusion.—F. Eriksson *et al., Acta med. scand.*, 1974, *196*, 231.

After taking ferrous succinate 330 mg with multivitamins the absorption in normal subjects was 5.2 mg Fe, in subjects with latent iron deficiency 9.9 mg Fe, and in subjects with manifest iron deficiency 34 mg Fe. No significant increase in the iron absorption-rate was observed in women taking oral contraceptives and not suffering from iron deficiency.—E. Zillessen *et al., Arzneimittel-Forsch.*, 1977, *27*, 1606.

Preparations

Ferrous Succinate Capsules *(B.P.)*

Ferrous Succinate Tablets *(B.P.)*. Store in a cool place.

Proprietary Names and Manufacturers

Cerevon *(Wellcome, Canad.)*; Ferrlecit *(Nattermann, Ger.)*; Ferromyn *(Austral.; Denm.; Calmic, UK)*; Ferromyn S *(Hässle, Swed.)*; Mediron *(Denm.)*; Succifer *(Ger.)*; Wellcofer *(Wellcome, Fr.)*.

For preparations containing multivitamins and minerals, see p.1291.

5063-d

Ferrous Sulphate *(BAN)*.

Eisen(II)-Sulfat; Ferreux (Sulfate); Ferrosi Sulfas; Ferrous Sulfate *(USAN)*; Ferrum Sulfuricum Oxydulatum; Iron Sulphate; Iron(II) Sulphate Heptahydrate.

$FeSO_4,7H_2O$=278.0.

CAS — 7720-78-7 (anhydrous); 7782-63-0 (heptahydrate).

NOTE. Crude ferrous sulphate is known as Green Vitriol or Green Copperas.

Pharmacopoeias. In *Arg., Aust., Belg., Br., Braz., Chin., Cz., Egypt., Eur., Fr., Ger., Hung., Ind., Int., It., Jpn, Jug., Mex., Neth., Nord., Pol., Port., Span., Swiss, Turk.,* and *U.S.*. Also in *B.P. Vet.*

Odourless bluish-green crystals or granules or a pale green crystalline powder, containing about 60 mg of iron in 300 mg. It is efflorescent in dry air; on exposure to moist air it is oxidised and becomes brown in colour due to the formation of basic ferric sulphate.
Completely or almost completely **soluble** 1 in 1.5 of water, 1 in 0.5 of boiling water; practically insoluble in alcohol. The *B.P.* specifies that a 5% solution in water has a pH of 3.0 to 4.0. The *U.S.P.* specifies that a 10% solution in water has a pH of about 3.7. **Store** in airtight containers.

5064-n

Dried Ferrous Sulphate *(BAN)*.

Dried Ferrous Sulfate *(USAN)*; Exsiccated Ferrous Sulphate; Ferrosi Sulfas Exsiccatus.

CAS — 13463-43-9.

Pharmacopoeias. In *Arg., Aust., Br., Egypt., Ind., Int., Mex., Turk.,* and *U.S.*

Ferrous sulphate deprived of part of its water of crystallisation by drying at 40°. A greyish-white to buff-coloured powder. The *B.P.* specifies 80 to 90% of $FeSO_4$; the *U.S.P.* specifies 86 to 89% of $FeSO_4$. Dried ferrous sulphate contains about 60 mg of iron in 200 mg.
Slowly but almost completely **soluble** in freshly boiled and cooled water; practically insoluble in alcohol. **Store** in well-closed containers.

Ferrous sulphate has the actions and uses of iron salts (see p.1189). The dried form is mainly used for the administration of ferrous sulphate in tablets.
The usual dose for the treatment of iron-deficiency anaemia is 120 to 300 mg of iron daily in divided doses; this is equivalent to 600 mg to 1.5 g of ferrous sulphate or 400 mg to 1.0 g of dried ferrous sulphate. The usual prophylactic dose is 60 mg of iron daily (equivalent to 300 mg of ferrous sulphate or 200 mg of dried ferrous

sulphate). There are various recommendations for children's doses. In the *UK* children under 1 year of age may be given 36 mg of iron, those aged 1 to 5 years 72 mg, and those aged 6 to 12 years 120 mg; these are daily therapeutic doses. In the *US* children may be given 2 mg of iron per kg body-weight three times daily for treatment and 1 mg per kg daily for prophylaxis of iron-deficiency anaemia.

Ferrous sulphate oxidised with nitric and sulphuric acids yields ferric subsulphate solution also known as Monsel's solution which has been used as a haemostatic.

Preparations

Compound Ferrous Sulphate Tablets *(B.P.C. 1973).* Ferrous Sulphate Compound Tablets. Each contains dried ferrous sulphate equivalent to 170 mg of $FeSO_4$, copper sulphate 2.5 mg, and manganese sulphate 2.5 mg. The tablets may be coated and coloured. Store in airtight containers. Protect from light. *Dose.* 1 or 2 tablets.

Ferrous Sulfate Oral Solution *(U.S.P.).* A solution containing ferrous sulphate. pH 1.8 to 3.2. Store in airtight containers. Protect from light.

Ferrous Sulfate Syrup *(U.S.P.).* Ferrous sulphate 400 mg, citric acid monohydrate 21 mg, peppermint spirit 0.02 mL, sucrose 8.25 g, water to 10 mL. Store in airtight containers.

Ferrous Sulfate Tablets *(U.S.P.).* Tablets containing ferrous sulphate or dried ferrous sulphate. Potency is expressed in terms of $FeSO_4,7H_2O$. Store in airtight containers.

Ferrous Sulphate Mixture *(B.P.C. 1973).* Ferrous sulphate 300 mg, ascorbic acid 10 mg, orange syrup 0.5 mL, double-strength chloroform water 5 mL, water to 10 mL. It should be recently prepared. *Dose.* 10 mL. To be taken well diluted with water.

If tap water is used in the preparation of this mixture, discoloration may occur.

A.P.F. has a similar mixture with benzoic acid solution 0.2 mL instead of concentrated chloroform water.

Discoloration occurred in Ferrous Sulphate Mixture (*B.P.C. 1973*) after 7 days' storage at room temperature regardless of whether it was stored in daylight or in darkness. When the ascorbic acid concentration was increased to 0.3% no discoloration occurred in samples stored for 39 days in daylight. Use of ascorbic acid concentrations above 0.3% resulted in yellow-brown discoloration, especially in samples stored in daylight, presumably due to a breakdown product of ascorbic acid.— Pharm. Soc. Lab. Rep., P/75/15, 1975.

For a report of incompatibility when Ferrous Sulphate Mixture *B.P.C. 1973* was prepared with or diluted with syrup preserved with hydroxybenzoates, see under Sucrose, p.1276.

Ferrous Sulphate Tablets *(B.P.).* Coated tablets containing dried ferrous sulphate.

Paediatric Ferrous Sulphate Oral Solution *(B.P.).* Paediatric Ferrous Sulphate Mixture. A solution containing 1.2% of ferrous sulphate and a suitable antioxidant in a suitable vehicle with an orange flavour. Each 5 mL contains about 12 mg of ferrous iron. For extemporaneous preparations the following formula may be used: ferrous sulphate 60 mg, ascorbic acid 10 mg, orange syrup 0.5 mL, double-strength chloroform water 2.5 mL, water to 5 mL. It should be recently prepared. To be taken well diluted with water.

If tap water is used in the preparation of this mixture, discoloration may occur.

Paediatric Ferrous Sulphate Mixture *B.P.* was not adequately preserved against microbial spoilage as determined by the *B.P.* challenge test.— T. R. R. Kurup and L. S. C. Wan, *Pharm. J.*, 1986, *2*, 761.

Proprietary Preparations

Fefol *(Smith Kline & French, UK). Spansules,* sustained-release capsules, dried ferrous sulphate 150 mg, folic acid 500 µg. *Dose.* 1 spansule daily.

Fefol-Vit *(Smith Kline & French, UK). Spansules,* sustained-release capsules, dried ferrous sulphate 150 mg, folic acid 500 µg, ascorbic acid 50 mg, nicotinamide 10 mg, pyridoxine hydrochloride 1 mg, riboflavine 2 mg, thiamine mononitrate 2 mg. *Dose.* 1 spansule daily.

Fefol Z *(Smith Kline & French, UK). Spansules,* sustained-release capsules, dried ferrous sulphate 150 mg, zinc sulphate monohydrate 61.8 mg, folic acid 500 µg. *Dose.* 1 spansule daily.

Feospan *(Smith Kline & French, UK). Spansules,* sustained-release capsules, dried ferrous sulphate 150 mg. *Dose.* 1 spansule daily.

A comparison of the absorption of iron from ferrous sulphate tablets *B.P.* and from capsules of Feospan in 12 healthy subjects.— E. J. Fitzsimons *et al.* (letter), *Br. J. clin. Pharmac.*, 1984, *17*, 111.

Feospan Z *(Smith Kline & French, UK). Spansules,* sustained-release capsules, dried ferrous sulphate 150 mg, zinc sulphate monohydrate 61.8 mg. *Dose.* 1 spansule daily.

Feravol *(Carlton Laboratories, UK). Tablets,* ferrous sulphate 200 mg, ascorbic acid 9 mg, riboflavine 1 mg, thiamine hydrochloride 0.4 mg.

Syrup, ferrous sulphate 200 mg, ascorbic acid 9 mg, riboflavine 1 mg, thiamine hydrochloride 0.4 mg/5 mL.

Ferrograd C *(Abbott, UK). Filmtabs,* film-coated tablets, sustained-release, dried ferrous sulphate 325 mg, ascorbic acid 500 mg (as sodium salt). *Dose.* 1 tablet daily.

A case of accumulation of Ferrograd C tablets in the stomach and oesophagus of a 74-year-old woman, discovered at post mortem.— R. M. Whittington and I. McKim Thompson (letter), *Lancet*, 1983, *1*, 184.

Ferrograd Folic *(Abbott, UK). Filmtabs,* film-coated tablets, sustained-release, dried ferrous sulphate 325 mg, folic acid 350 µg. *Dose.* 1 tablet daily.

A report of a woman with Crohn's disease in whom intestinal obstruction was precipitated by the accumulation of unabsorbed matrices of Ferrograd-folic behind a stenosed terminal ileum.— J. L. Shaffer *et al.* (letter), *Lancet*, 1980, *2*, 487.

Ferrograd *(Abbott, UK). Filmtabs,* film-coated tablets, sustained-release, dried ferrous sulphate 325 mg. *Dose.* 1 tablet daily.

A report of the entrapment of 98 plastic matrices of Ferrograd tablets in a patient with neoplastic colonic stricture.— M. Spigelman and R. W. McNabb, *Br. med. J.*, 1971, *4*, 534.

Jejunal diverticular perforation in a 74-year-old woman appeared to be due to Ferrograd; the remains of a tablet were lodged in the perforation and the neighbouring tissues were heavily stained with iron.— C. J. H. Ingoldby, *Br. med. J.*, 1977, *1*, 949. See also A. B. Alaily, *ibid.*, 1974, *1*, 103.

Fesovit *(Wellcome, UK). Spansules,* sustained-release capsules, dried ferrous sulphate 150 mg, ascorbic acid 50 mg, nicotinamide 10 mg, pyridoxine hydrochloride 1 mg, riboflavine 2 mg, thiamine mononitrate 2 mg. *Dose.* 1 spansule daily.

Fesovit Z *(Smith Kline & French, UK). Spansules,* sustained-release capsules, dried ferrous sulphate 150 mg, zinc sulphate monohydrate 61.8 mg, ascorbic acid 50 mg, nicotinamide 10 mg, pyridoxine hydrochloride 1 mg, riboflavine 2 mg, thiamine mononitrate 2 mg. *Dose.* 1 spansule daily.

Folicin *(Paines & Byrne, UK). Tablets,* dried ferrous sulphate 200 mg, copper sulphate 2.5 mg, folic acid 2.5 mg, manganese sulphate 2.5 mg.

Irofol C *(Abbott, UK). Filmtabs,* film-coated tablets, sustained-release dried ferrous sulphate 325 mg, folic acid 350 µg, ascorbic acid 500 mg (as sodium salt). *Dose.* 1 tablet daily.

Ironorm *(Wallace Mfg Chem., UK). Capsules,* dried ferrous sulphate 195 mg, ascorbic acid 15 mg, cyanocobalamin 5 µg folic acid 1.7 mg, concentrated intrinsic factor 10 mg, nicotinamide 10 mg, riboflavine 2 mg, thiamine hydrochloride 1 mg.

Oral drops, ferrous iron 125 mg (as ferrous sulphate)/5 mL.

Pregnavite Forte F *(Bencard, UK). Tablets,* dried ferrous sulphate 84 mg, folic acid 120 µg, ascorbic acid 13.3 mg, calcium phosphate 160 mg, ergocalciferol 133 units, nicotinamide 5 mg, pyridoxine hydrochloride 0.33 mg, riboflavine 0.5 mg, thiamine hydrochloride 0.5 mg, vitamin A 1333 units.

Slow-Fe *(Ciba, UK). Tablets,* sustained-release, dried ferrous sulphate 160 mg. *Dose.* Prophylactic, 1 tablet daily; therapeutic, 2 tablets daily.

Slow-Fe folic *(Ciba, UK). Tablets,* sustained-release, dried ferrous sulphate 160 mg, folic acid 400 µg. *Dose.* 1 tablet daily.

Proprietary Names and Manufacturers of Dried Ferrous Sulphate or other similar compounds

Ce-Ferro *(Nordmark, Ger.)*; Dreisafer *(Gry, Ger.)*; Duroferon *(Hässle, Norw.; Hässle, Swed.)*; Eryfer *(Cassella-med, Ger.; Hoechst, Ital.)*; Feosol *(Smith Kline & French, USA)*; Feospan *(Smith Kline & French, UK)*; Fer-in-Sol *(Arg.; Belg.; Mead Johnson, Canad.; Mead Johnson Nutritional, USA)*; Feritard *(Protea, Austral.)*; Fero-Grad *(Abbott, Canad.)*; Fero-Gradumet *(Belg.; Neth.; Spain; Abbott, USA)*; Feroretard *(Jpn)*; Ferrlecit *(Nattermann, Ger.)*; Ferro *(Hässle, Denm.)*; Ferro 66 *(Promonta, Ger.; Neth.)*; Ferro 66 DL *(Ger.)*; Ferrofer *(Neth.)*; Ferro-Grad *(Abbott, Ital.)*; Ferrograd *(Abbott, UK)*; Ferro-Gradumet *(Abbott, Austral.; Abbott, Spain; Abbott, Switz.; Abbott, UK)*; Ferrolande *(Delalande, Ger.)*; Ferromax *(Weiders, Norw.)*; Ferro-O_2 *(Ger.)*; Ferrophor *(Ger.)*; Ferro-Retard *(Collett, Denm.; Collett, Norw.)*; Ferrosan *(S.Afr.)*; Fesofor *(Smith Kline & French, Canad.; Smith Kline & French, S.Afr.)*; Fespan *(Smith Kline & French, Austral.)*; Kendural *(Abbott, Ger.)*; Microfer *(Neth.)*; Mol-Iron *(Schering, USA)*; Novoferrosulfa *(Novopharm, Canad.)*; Plexafer *(Neth.)*; Resoferix *(Brunnengräber, Ger.)*; Resoferon *(Neth.)*; Siderblut *(Arg.)*; Slow-Fe *(Ciba, Austral.; Ciba-Geigy, Canad.; Ciba, UK; Ciba, USA)*; Tardyferon *(Belg.; Robapharm, Ger.; Neth.; Robapharm, Switz.)*; Tetucur-S *(Jpn)*; Toniron *(Medo, UK)*.

For preparations containing multivitamins and minerals, see p.1291.

5065-h

Ferrous Tartrate

Ferrosi Tartras.

$C_4H_4FeO_6,2\frac{1}{2}H_2O=249.0$.

CAS — 2944-65-2 (anhydrous).

Pharmacopoeias. In *Nord.*

Ferrous tartrate has the actions and uses of iron salts (see p.1189). Typical iron doses are described under ferrous sulphate (above).

Proprietary Names and Manufacturers

Ferroplex *(DAK, Denm.)*.

5066-m

Iron Dextran *(BAN, USAN).*

Iron-Dextran Complex.

CAS — 9004-66-4.

A complex of ferric hydroxide with dextrans of weight average molecular weight between 5000 and 7500. Injections have a pH of 5.2 to 6.5. The *B.P.* injection is **sterilised** by autoclaving.

The structure of iron-dextran complex. The molecular weight of the complex was about 73 000.—J. S. G. Cox *et al.*, *J. Pharm. Pharmac.*, 1972, *24*, 513.

Adsorption of iron dextran on membrane filters.— B. G. Bishop, *N.Z. Pharm.*, 1981, *1*, 49.

Adverse Effects

Severe anaphylactoid reactions may occur after administration of iron dextran and fatalities have been reported. It is therefore recommended that administration takes place where there are facilities for immediate treatment. Patients may experience delayed reactions such as arthralgia, myalgia, regional lymphadenopathy, and fever. The incidence of these delayed effects may be increased when large intravenous doses are given for total-dose infusion.

Intravenous injection is associated with peripheral vascular flushing and hypotension; thrombophlebitis may also occur at the site of injection, although the incidence may be reduced by administering iron dextran in sodium chloride injection rather than glucose injection. Intramuscular injection is associated with local reactions, pain, and staining at the site of injection.

Other adverse effects may include: transient paraesthesia, tachycardia, syncope, seizures, dizziness, circulatory collapse, and malaise. Headache, nausea, vomiting, fever, dyspnoea, and a metallic taste may also occur.

ALLERGY. The Boston Collaborative Drug Surveillance Program monitored consecutively 32 812 medical in-patients. Drug-induced anaphylaxis occurred in 1 of 169 patients given iron dextran.— J. Porter and H. Jick, *Lancet*, 1977, *1*, 587.

EFFECTS ON THE BLOOD. A 1-year-old girl with Down's syndrome and iron-deficiency anaemia was given three intramuscular injections of iron dextran (30 mg per kg body-weight) over 6 days. Pancytopenia developed subsequently, which reappeared when challenged with iron dextran.— H. Hurvitz *et al.*, *Archs Dis. Childh.*, 1986, *61*, 194.

NEOPLASMS. Eight cases of sarcoma after intramuscular injection of iron dextran or iron sorbitol had been reported. In 1 instance the time interval excluded iron from implication. Histological re-examination excluded sarcoma in 2 further cases. In contrast to experimental iron-induced sarcoma there was no common histological pattern in the 5 valid cases. If iron was responsible an increased incidence of sarcoma would by now be expected; no such increase was evident. The association was therefore considered to be remote.— K. Weinbren *et al.*, *Br. med. J.*, 1978, *1*, 683.

OVERDOSAGE. A 29-year-old woman with low serum ferritin was given 32 mL iron dextran (Imferon) intravenously. Twenty-four hours later she developed muscle cramps, bilateral frontal headaches, with subsequent neck stiffness, and marked opisthotonia with photophobia. The serum-haemoglobin concentration did not rise following the infusion of iron which indicated there was no iron deficiency. This resulted in abnormally high concentrations of free iron which was able to cross into the cerebrospinal fluid, and was responsible for the meningitic symptoms.— D. Shuttleworth *et al.* (letter), *Lancet*, 1983, *2*, 453.

Precautions

Iron dextran is contra-indicated in patients with severe liver damage, acute kidney infection, or a history of hypersensitivity to the preparation. Iron dextran is not recommended during early pregnancy or in patients receiving oral iron therapy or transfusions of blood. It should not be used to treat anaemias other than those associated with iron deficiency.

A test dose should be given before administration of a full therapeutic dose and emergency measures for the treatment of allergic reactions should be available. Patients should be kept under observation for at least 1 hour after administration of a test dose or following intravenous infusion. Iron dextran should be administered with caution to patients with a history of allergy or asthma and the total-dose infusion method is contra-indicated in these patients. Patients with rheumatoid arthritis may experience a worsening of symptoms when given an infusion of iron dextran. Large doses of iron dextran by infusion may lead to serum discoloration; this should not be mistaken as evidence of haemolysis.

Iron dextran formulated with phenol as a preservative is intended for administration by the intramuscular route only.

Compared with healthy subjects, the utilisation of iron from iron dextran for haemoglobin formation at 14 days was impaired in patients with uraemia, rheumatoid arthritis, and malignant diseases in whom stainable iron was present in the bone marrow.— A. G. Davies *et al.*, *Br. med. J.*, 1971, *1*, 146.

INFECTIONS. See under iron salts (p.1189).

RHEUMATOID ARTHRITIS. A case report of a 63-year-old woman with rheumatoid disease and a history of iron deficiency. Exacerbation of rheumatoid synovitis occurred 3 days after a total-dose infusion of 1 g of iron dextran, with pronounced effusion of the right knee, and inflammation of other peripheral joints. These changes provided evidence that iron-catalysed oxidative reactions influence the inflammatory process. It was suggested that pre-loading with vitamin E or other antioxidants may be useful in preventing synovial flares in rheumatoid patients requiring treatment with iron dextran.— P. G. Winyard *et al.*, *Lancet*, 1987, *1*, 69. Comment.— D. Roberts and J. Davies (letter), *ibid.*, 391. See also H. Schipper, *Br. med. J.*, 1984, *288*, 1346.

Absorption and Fate

Iron dextran is absorbed after intramuscular injection primarily through the lymphatic system. About 60% of iron dextran is absorbed after 3 days and up to 90% after 1 to 3 weeks. The reticuloendothelial cells gradually separate iron from the iron dextran complex and ferric iron is then incorporated into haemoglobin or stored as ferritin and haemosiderin.

Uses and Administration

Iron dextran is used in the treatment of iron-deficiency anaemia where oral therapy is ineffective or impracticable.

It is given by deep intramuscular injection into the upper outer quadrant of the buttock; to prevent leakage along the injection track, the subcutaneous tissue is drawn to one side before the needle is inserted. It may also be given intravenously.

Total dosage is calculated according to the haemoglobin concentration, body-weight, and usually the sex of the patient; allowance is also made for additional iron to replenish iron stores. Iron dextran injection is usually supplied with a dose table from which doses can be obtained for patients of different weights and haemoglobin (Hb) status. There may be variations between countries in the doses obtained from such tables. Also these tables should not be used to obtain a dose of iron dextran to be given to patients who have suffered severe blood loss. Doses for iron-deficiency anaemia can also be calculated from various formulae. Typical formulae used in the *UK* for a preparation containing 50 mg of iron dextran per mL are as follows:

Dose in mL for women =
{0.0476 × body-weight (kg) × [14.8 − Hb level (g/100 mL)]} + 6

Dose in mL for men =
{0.0476 × body-weight (kg) × [14.8 − Hb level (g/100 mL)]} + 14

A typical formula used in the *US* for a preparation containing 50 mg of iron dextran per mL is as follows:

Dose in mg =
[100 − (Hb level in g/100 mL × 100/14.8)] × 0.3 × body-weight (lb)

Using these formulae a 70-kg man with a haemoglobin value of 5.9 g per 100 mL would be given a total of 2.2 g of iron dextran (44 mL) in the *UK* and 2.8 g (56 mL) in the *US*.

The total dose requirement may be administered as a series of intramuscular injections daily or once or twice a week in inactive patients. A suggested dosage per intramuscular injection for children is: less than 5 kg body-weight, up to 0.5 mL (25 mg); 5 to 9 kg, up to 1 mL (50 mg). Adults normally receive 2 mL up to a maximum of 5 mL per injection.

Iron dextran is also administered intravenously undiluted or by total-dose infusion (TDI), but this route should be restricted to hospital usage and should only be employed following a test dose. In total-dose infusion, the total dose calculated according to the haemoglobin concentration is given by slow intravenous infusion preferably in sodium chloride injection. Patients given iron dextran intravenously should be observed closely for at least one hour after administration.

It is advisable to stop oral administration of iron probably at least 24 hours before giving iron dextran; other parenteral forms of iron should also be withdrawn probably for at least several days beforehand.

A short review of iron dextran in the treatment of anaemia in patients with rheumatoid arthritis.— A. G. Mowat, *Prescribers' J.*, 1975, *15*, 107.

For a study on the role of iron in rheumatoid disease, see D. R. Blake *et al.*, *Lancet*, 1981, *2*, 1142.

A report of the effectiveness and toxicity of iron dextran injections given intravenously to 481 people over a period of 8 years.— R. D. Hamstra *et al.*, *J. Am. med. Ass.*, 1980, *243*, 1726.

Preparations

Iron Dextran Injection *(B.P.)*
Iron Dextran Injection *(U.S.P.)*

Proprietary Preparations

Direx *(Andard-Mount, UK)*. *Injection*, ferrous iron 50 mg/mL (as iron dextran complex), in ampoules of 2 and 5 mL.

Imferon *(CP Pharmaceuticals, UK)*. *Injection*, ferrous iron 50 mg/mL (as iron dextran), in ampoules of 2, 5, and 20 mL.

Niferex *(Tillotts, UK)*. *Tablets*, ferrous iron 50 mg (as polysaccharide-iron complex).
Capsules (Niferex-150), ferrous iron 150 mg (as polysaccharide-iron complex).
Elixir, ferrous iron 100 mg/5 mL (as polysaccharide-iron complex).

Proprietary Names and Manufacturers of Iron Dextran or other similar compounds

Chromagen-D *(Savage, USA)*; Dextraron *(Legere, USA)*; Direx *(Andard-Mount, UK)*; Hierro Gar *(Carol, Spain)*; Hytinic *(Hyrex, USA)*; Imferdex *(Switz.)*; Imferon *(Fisons, Austral.; Belg.; Fisons, Canad.; Denm.; Neth.; Fisons, S.Afr.; Llorente, Spain; CP Pharmaceuticals, UK; Fisons, USA)*; Iron Hy-Dex *(S.Afr.)*; Irotran *(USA)*; Niferex *(Webber, Canad.; Parke, Davis, Spain; Tillotts, UK; Central Pharmaceuticals, USA)*; Nu-Iron *(Mayrand, USA)*; Proferdex *(Fisons, USA)*.

For preparations containing multivitamins and minerals, see p.1291.

5067-b

Saccharated Iron Oxide

Eisenzucker; Ferrum Oxydatum Saccharatum; Oxyde de Fer Sucré.

CAS — 8047-67-4.

Pharmacopoeias. In *Aust.* and *Swiss.*

Saccharated iron oxide has the actions and uses of iron salts (p.1189) and has been given by mouth in the treatment of iron-deficiency anaemia. It has also been given by intravenous injection. It can be irritant and has been largely replaced by iron dextran.

Proprietary Names and Manufacturers

Anemicid *(Jpn)*; Egmofer *(Ger.)*; Ferraton *(Ferraton, Denm.)*; Ferrophor *(TAD, Ger.)*; Ferrum Hausmann *(Manzoni, Ital.; Spain; Hausmann, Switz.)*; Macofer *(Hausmann, Norw.)*.

5068-v

Iron Phosphate

Ferri Phosphas.

Pharmacopoeias. In *B.P.C. 1973.*

A mixture of hydrated ferrous phosphate and ferric phosphate and some hydrated oxides of iron. It is a slate-blue amorphous powder, darkening on exposure to air owing to oxidation. It contains not less than 16% of ferrous iron, calculated as Fe, equivalent to not less than 47.9% of $Fe_3(PO_4)_2,8H_2O$.

Practically **insoluble** in water; soluble in hydrochloric acid. **Store** in airtight containers.

Iron phosphate has the actions and uses of iron salts (see p.1189) and has been included in 'tonic' preparations such as compound ferrous phosphate syrup (also known as Parrish's food) and ferrous phosphate, quinine, and strychnine syrup and tablets (also known as Easton's syrup and tablets), see *Martindale, 28th Edition*, p.881.

An iron phosphate (Ferrum Phosphoricum; Ferr. Phos.) is used in homoeopathic medicine.

Preparations

For preparations containing multivitamins and minerals, see p.1291.

12864-h

Iron Polymaltose
Ferromaltose; Ferrum Polyisomaltose. A complex of ferric hydroxide and isomaltose.

Iron polymaltose is used as a source of iron, usually for intramuscular injection.

Proprietary Names and Manufacturers
Fer Lucien *(Lucien, Fr.)*; Ferrimed DS *(Swisspharm, S.Afr.)*; Ferrum *(Sigma, Austral.; Hausmann, Denm.)*; Ferrum Hausmann *(Biothera-Asperal, Belg.; Wasserman, Spain; Hausmann, Switz.)*; Intrafer *(Manzoni, Ital.)*.

5070-f

Iron Sorbitol *(BAN)*.
Iron Sorbitex *(USAN)*; Iron-Sorbitol-Citric Acid Complex.

CAS — 1338-16-5.

A complex of ferric iron, sorbitol, and citric acid, stabilised with dextrin and sorbitol. The average molecular weight of the complex is less than 5000. Injections have a pH of 7.2 to 7.9. The *B.P.* injection is **sterilised** by autoclaving. **Store** injections at 15° to 30° and avoid freezing or low temperatures.

Adverse Effects, Treatment, and Precautions
As for iron dextran, p.1193. There may be severe systemic reactions with cardiac complications which may be fatal, such as, complete atrioventricular block, ventricular tachycardia, or ventricular fibrillation.

Three patients with the malabsorption syndrome were treated with intramuscular injections of iron sorbitol. One patient, who received 100 mg of iron as iron sorbitol, developed symptoms including severe chest pain, profuse sweating, and heavy breathing, and died shortly afterwards. Toxic symptoms developed in the second patient after each of 3 injections, and she died 3 hours after the onset of ventricular tachycardia followed by asystole. In the third patient, nausea, chest pain, and dizziness followed the sixth injection of iron sorbitol. A further dose 2 weeks later caused a more severe reaction from which she recovered, but a complete atrioventricular block developed, and 1 year later a second-degree atrioventricular block persisted.— P. Karhunen *et al.*, *Br. med. J.*, 1970, *2*, 521.

A patient developed signs and symptoms of myocardial damage following an intramuscular injection of iron sorbitol.— P. Eliasen and A. Bendtsen, *Ugeskr. Laeg.*, 1976, *138*, 1522.

Absorption and Fate
More than 50% of iron sorbitol is absorbed within 8 hours of intramuscular injection. About 20 to 30% of a dose is excreted in the urine within 24 hours.

Uses and Administration
Iron sorbitol is used in the treatment of iron-deficiency anaemia where oral therapy is ineffective or impracticable.
It is given by deep intramuscular injection into the upper outer quadrant of the buttock; to prevent leakage along the injection track, the subcutaneous tissue is drawn to one side before the needle is inserted.
Total dosage is calculated according to the haemoglobin concentration of the blood. The volume and number of injections required to provide the total dosage is related to the condition of the patient, the recommended adult dose per injection being the equivalent of 1.5 mg of iron per kg body-weight daily. It is not recommended in children under 3 kg in body-weight.
It is advisable to stop oral administration of iron for at least 24 hours before giving iron sorbitol and to stop administration of other injectable iron preparations for a week beforehand. After an injection, the urine may become dark on standing.
Iron sorbitol should not be administered intravenously.

Preparations
Iron Sorbitol Injection *(B.P.)*
Iron Sorbitex Injection *(U.S.P.)*

Proprietary Preparations
Jectofer *(Astra, UK)*. *Injection*, ferrous iron 50 mg/mL, (as iron sorbitol), in ampoules of 2 mL.

Proprietary Names and Manufacturers
Jectofer *(Astra, Austral.; Astra, Canad.; Astra, Denm.; Astra, Fr.; Astra, Ger.; Neth.; Astra, Norw.; Astra, Swed.; Switz.; Astra, UK)*; Yectofer *(Knoll-Made, Spain)*.

5071-d

Sodium Ironedetate *(BAN)*.
Sodium Feredetate *(rINN)*. The monohydrated iron chelate of the monosodium salt of ethylenediamine-*NNN'N'*-tetra-acetic acid.
$C_{10}H_{12}FeN_2NaO_8,H_2O=385.1$.

CAS — 15708-41-5 (anhydrous).

Sodium Ironedetate contains about 27.5 mg of iron in 190 mg.

Sodium ironedetate has similar actions and uses to iron salts, see p.1189. It is given initially in doses of the equivalent of 27.5 mg of iron three times daily, gradually increasing to the equivalent of 55 mg three times daily. Children aged up to 1 year may be given 13.75 mg twice daily, but smaller doses should be given initially; children of 1 to 5 years 13.75 mg three times daily; children of 6 to 12 years 27.5 mg three times daily.

Proprietary Preparations
Sytron *(Parke, Davis, UK)*. *Mixture*, ferrous iron 27.5 mg/5 mL (as sodium ironedetate).

Proprietary Names and Manufacturers
Ferrostrane *(Substantia, Fr.)*; Ferrostrene *(Parke, Davis, Switz.)*; Irostrene *(Parke, Davis, Norw.; Parke, Davis, Swed.)*; Sytron *(Parke, Davis, UK)*.

Lipid Regulating Agents

1340-t

Lipids occur in the blood mainly as cholesterol and triglycerides, with smaller amounts of phospholipids, fatty acids, and fatty acid esters. Cholesterol and triglycerides are complexed with proteins and transported in the form of particles termed lipoproteins. The surface of the lipoprotein particle is composed largely of phospholipid, free cholesterol, and protein, and the core contains mostly triglyceride and cholesterol ester. The density, composition, and electrophoretic mobility of the lipoproteins have been used to divide them into 4 major groups:
chylomicrons, which are large triglyceride-rich particles derived from dietary fat, are produced in the intestine and finally ungergo catabolism whereby triglyceride is removed by lipolysis to form free fatty acid;
very low-density lipoproteins (VLDL, pre-β-lipoproteins), which are composed largely of endogenous triglycerides, are synthesised in the liver and again undergo catabolic processes;
low-density lipoproteins (LDL, β-lipoproteins), which are rich in cholesterol and are mainly the end-products of VLDL catabolism;
high-density lipoproteins (HDL, α-lipoproteins), which contain about 50% of protein, are produced in the liver and intestine and act as acceptors of lipids, especially free cholesterol.
The protein components of the lipoproteins are known as *apolipoproteins*.
Factors affecting the lipid composition of the blood include the composition of the diet, physical activity, age, sex, and genetic and cultural factors.
Hyperlipidaemias (or hyperlipoproteinaemias) may be classified in a variety of ways. They may be primary inherited disorders or secondary to a number of causes such as dietary factors, excessive alcohol intake, disease states including hypothyroidism and diabetes mellitus, or drug treatment with agents such as beta-blockers, corticosteroids, oestrogens and oral contraceptives, and thiazide diuretics.
The classification proposed by WHO (*Bull. Wld Hlth Org.*, 1970, *43*, 891) has 6 types of hyperlipoproteinaemia and is based solely upon the patterns of the particular lipoproteins that are elevated; it does not reflect clinical status, nor genetic or metabolic characteristics, and should not be used as a diagnostic classification. The 6 types of hyperlipoproteinaemia included are:
type I (hyperchylomicronaemia) characterised by the presence of chylomicrons and by normal or only slightly increased concentrations of very low-density lipoproteins;
type IIa (hyper-β-lipoproteinaemia) characterised by an elevation in the concentration of low-density lipoproteins;
type IIb characterised by an elevation in the concentration of low-density lipoproteins and of very low-density lipoproteins;
type III ('floating β' or 'broad β' pattern) characterised by the presence of very low-density lipoproteins having an abnormally high cholesterol content and an abnormal electrophoretic mobility;
type IV (hyperpre-β-lipoproteinaemia) characterised by an elevation in the concentration of very low-density lipoproteins, by no increase in the concentration of low-density lipoproteins, and by the absence of chylomicrons;
type V ('hyperpre-β-lipoproteinaemia and chylomicronaemia') characterised by an elevation in the concentration of very low-density lipoproteins and the presence of chylomicrons.
Primary hyperlipidaemias may be classified according to the genetic and metabolic disorder resulting in the following categories:
familial hypercholesterolaemia, which is usually heterozygous but very rarely may be homozygous, is characterised by a type IIa pattern but occasionally a type IIb pattern may be present;
familial hypertriglyceridaemia is usually associated with a type IV or type V pattern;
familial combined hyperlipidaemia may be characterised by elevated cholesterol only, elevated triglyceride only, or elevated cholesterol and triglyceride, and type IIa, type IV, or type IIb patterns may be found;
familial dysbetalipoproteinaemia (remnant hyperlipoproteinaemia or broad-β disease) shows the type III pattern;
and *lipoprotein lipase deficiency* or *apolipoprotein C-II deficiency* show a type I or type V pattern.
The treatment of hyperlipidaemias depends upon appropriate dietary modification, which should be controlled in all patients, the correction of the underlying disease or avoidance of precipitating factors, and the use of hypolipidaemic drugs that have various effects on specific lipoprotein fractions. Drugs not included in this section that are used as hypolipidaemic agents include Nicotinic Acid (p.1268) and Neomycin (p.268).
Some hyperlipidaemias are associated with an increased risk of atherosclerosis, ischaemic heart disease, and related complications. Several studies have been performed to investigate whether the use of hypolipidaemic agents in patients at risk is beneficial in the prevention of such disorders (see Cholestyramine, p.1198, Clofibrate, p.1199, and Colestipol, p.1200). It should be remembered, however, that many other factors are likely to be involved in the development of cardiovascular disease. Elevated concentrations of high-density lipoproteins are considered by most, but not all, workers to have a protective effect against the development of ischaemic heart disease.

A discussion of the lipoproteins.— B. Lewis, *Br. med. J.*, 1983, *287*, 1161.

A review of the clinical aspects of hyperlipidaemias.— P. N. Durrington and J. P. Miller, *Br. J. Hosp. Med.*, 1984, *32*, 28.

Report of the Consensus Conference of the National Institutes of Health, USA on the treatment of hypertriglyceridaemia.— *J. Am. med. Ass.*, 1984, *251*, 1196.

A review of the pathogenesis and management of lipoprotein disorders.— E. J. Schaefer and R. I. Levy, *New Engl. J. Med.*, 1985, *312*, 1300.

A review and discussion on the management of hyperlipoproteinaemias.— J. M. Hoeg *et al.*, *J. Am. med. Ass.*, 1986, *255*, 512.

An overview of the indications and optimum therapeutic use of lipid lowering drugs.— D. R. Illingworth, *Drugs*, 1987, *33*, 259. A review of the adverse effects of lipid lowering drugs.— L. C. Knodel and R. L. Talbert, *Med. Toxicol.*, 1987, *2*, 10.

ISCHAEMIC HEART DISEASE. Report of the Council on Scientific Affairs of the American Medical Association on dietary and pharmacologic therapy for the lipid risk factors.— *J. Am. med. Ass.*, 1983, *250*, 1873.

Report of the Consensus Conference of the National Institutes of Health, USA on the lowering of blood-cholesterol to prevent heart disease.— *J. Am. med. Ass.*, 1985, *253*, 2080. Criticisms.— E. H. Ahrens, *Lancet*, 1985, *1*, 1085; M. F. Oliver, *ibid.*, 1087. Replies.— I. Jacoby and M. Rose (letter), *ibid.*, *2*, 205; D. Steinberg (letter), *ibid.*

Further references to strategies for the prevention of coronary heart disease: European Atherosclerosis Society, *Eur. Heart J.*, 1987, *8*, 77; British Cardiac Society Working Group on Coronary Heart Disease Prevention, *Lancet*, 1987, *1*, 377; J. Shepherd *et al.*, *Br. med. J.*, 1987, *295*, 1245 (guidelines of the British Hyperlipidaemia Association).

9002-t

Acetiromate *(rINN).*
TBF-43. 4-(4-Acetoxy-3-iodophenoxy)-3,5-di-iodobenzoic acid.
$C_{15}H_9I_3O_5$=649.9.

CAS — 2260-08-4.

Acetiromate has been used as a hypolipidaemic agent.

Proprietary Names and Manufacturers
Adecol *(Jpn).*

12316-x

Acipimox *(BAN, rINN).*
K-9321. 5-Methylpyrazine-2-carboxylic acid 4-oxide.
$C_6H_6N_2O_3$=154.1.

CAS — 51037-30-0.

Acipimox is used as a hypolipidaemic agent in usual doses of 450 to 750 mg daily. Reduced doses are recommended for patients with renal impairment. Reported adverse effects include gastro-intestinal disturbances.

Proprietary Preparations
Olbetam *(Farmitalia Carlo Erba, UK). Capsules,* acipimox 250 mg.

Proprietary Names and Manufacturers
Olbemox *(Farmitalia, Ger.)*; Olbetam *(Farmitalia, Ital.; Farmitalia Carlo Erba, UK).*

1342-r

Aluminium Clofibrate *(BAN, rINN).*
Alufibrate. Bis[2-(4-chlorophenoxy)-2-methylpropionato]hydroxyaluminium.
$C_{20}H_{21}AlCl_2O_7$=471.3.

CAS — 24818-79-9.

Aluminium clofibrate is used as a hypolipidaemic agent.

For a report of the absorption and fate of aluminium clofibrate, see Clofibrate, p.1199.

Proprietary Names and Manufacturers
Alofran *(IBE, Spain)*; Arteriopront *(Spain)*; Aterolip *(Fher, Spain)*; Atherolip *(Belg.; Millot-Solac, Fr.; Vifor, Switz.)*; Atherolipin *(Schwarz, Ger.)*; Colesnormal *(Spain)*; Sepik *(Also, Ital.).*

1343-f

Aluminium Nicotinate
A complex of aluminium hydroxydinicotinate and nicotinic acid. Each 625 mg represents approximately 450 mg of aluminium hydroxydinicotinate and 155 mg of nicotinic acid, together equivalent to 500 mg of nicotinic acid.

CAS — 1976-28-9.

Aluminium nicotinate has been used as a hypolipidaemic agent.

Proprietary Names and Manufacturers
Nicalex *(Merrell Dow, USA)*; Nicalex Alunitine *(Merrell Dow, Austral.).*

12421-r

Beclobrate *(BAN, rINN).*
Sgd-24774. Ethyl (±)-2-(4-*p*-chlorobenzylphenoxy)-2-methylbutyrate.
$C_{20}H_{23}ClO_3$=346.9.

CAS — 55937-99-0.

Beclobrate, a clofibrate analogue, is used as a hypolipidaemic agent.

Proprietary Names and Manufacturers
Siegfried, Ger.

12424-n

Benfluorex Hydrochloride *(pINNM).*
JP-992; SE-780. 2-[α-Methyl-3-(trifluoromethyl)phenethylamino]ethyl benzoate hydrochloride.
$C_{19}H_{20}F_3NO_2,HCl=387.8$.

CAS — 23602-78-0 (benfluorex); 35976-51-3 (benfluorex, ±); 23642-66-2 (hydrochloride).

Benfluorex hydrochloride is used as a hypolipidaemic agent.

Absence of interaction with phenprocoumon.— P. De Witte and H. M. Brems, *Curr. med. Res. Opinion,* 1980, *6,* 478.

Proprietary Names and Manufacturers
Balans *(IBP, Ital.)*; Médiator *(Servier, Fr.)*; Mediaxal *(Servier, Ital.; Servier, Switz.)*; Minolip *(Master Pharma, Ital.)*; Modulator *(Servier, Spain).*

12431-d

Benzalamide
β-Benzalbutyramide; β-Benzylidenebutyramide. 3-Methyl-4-phenylbut-3-enamide.
$C_{11}H_{13}NO=175.2$.

CAS — 7236-47-7.

Benzalamide is used as a hypolipidaemic agent.

Proprietary Names and Manufacturers
Kata-Lipid *(Ibi, Ital.; IBE, Spain).*

12441-h

Bezafibrate *(BAN, USAN, rINN).*

BM-15075; LO-44. 2-[4-(2-*p*-Chlorobenzamidoethyl)phenoxy]-2-methylpropionic acid.
$C_{19}H_{20}ClNO_4=361.8$.

CAS — 41859-67-0.

Adverse Effects and Precautions
As for Clofibrate, p.1198. It has, however, been stated that administration of bezafibrate is not associated so far with an increased frequency of gall-stones.
It has also been suggested that bezafibrate may be given to patients with mild to moderate renal impairment in doses reduced to 200 to 400 mg daily depending upon serum-creatinine concentrations.

INTERACTIONS. Enhancement of the effect of phenprocoumon by bezafibrate.— R. Zimmerman *et al., Dt. med. Wschr.,* 1977, *102,* 509.

In 13 well-controlled diabetic patients no change in antidiabetic medication was necessary during bezafibrate administration.— P. Wahl *et al., Dt. med. Wschr.,* 1978, *103,* 1233.

RENAL FAILURE. The plasma half-life of bezafibrate in 12 patients with impaired renal function ranged from 3.1 to 20.1 hours (mean 8.05 hours) compared with 2.1 hours in healthy subjects.— P. Anderson and H. -E. Norbeck, *Eur. J. clin. Pharmac.,* 1981, *21,* 209.

Experience in 9 patients with advanced chronic renal failure, but without the nephrotic syndrome, given bezafibrate 200 mg daily for 1 month suggested that the accelerated decline in renal function seen in 2 patients must question the use of bezafibrate in advanced uraemia, unless the dosage is significantly reduced below that used in the present study.— A. J. Williams *et al., Br. J. clin. Pharmac.,* 1984, *18,* 361.

Absorption and Fate
Bezafibrate is readily absorbed from the gastro-intestinal tract; peak concentrations in plasma are reported to occur within about 2 hours; the plasma half-life is about 2 hours. Most of a dose is excreted in the urine with little appearing in the faeces. Plasma protein binding of bezafibrate is about 94 to 96%.

Disposition pharmacokinetics of bezafibrate in healthy subjects.— U. Abshagen *et al., Eur. J. clin. Pharmac.,* 1979, *16,* 31. See also U. Abshagen *et al., ibid.,* 1980, *17,* 305.

For a report of the half-life in patients with impaired renal function, see Renal Failure under Precautions (above).

Uses and Administration
Bezafibrate, a clofibrate analogue, is used as a hypolipidaemic agent, in conjunction with dietary modification. It is recommended in the treatment of type IIa, type IIb, type III, type IV, and type V hyperlipoproteinaemia. The usual dose, by mouth, is 600 mg daily taken with or after food; 400 mg daily may be adequate for maintenance.

ADMINISTRATION IN RENAL FAILURE. See Renal Failure under Precautions (above).

Proprietary Preparations
Bezalip *(MCP Pharmaceuticals, UK). Tablets,* bezafibrate 200 mg.
Bezalip-Mono *(MCP Pharmaceuticals, UK). Tablets,* modified-release, bezafibrate 400 mg.

Proprietary Names and Manufacturers
Befizal *(Oberval, Fr.)*; Bezalip *(Boehringer Biochemia, Ital.; Boehringer Mannheim, S.Afr.; MCP Pharmaceuticals, UK)*; Bezalip-Mono *(MCP Pharmaceuticals, UK)*; Cedur *(Boehringer Mannheim, Ger.; Boehringer Mannheim, Switz.)*; Difaterol *(Andreu, Spain)*; Eulitop *(Boehringer Mannheim, Spain)*; Reducterol *(Drag, Spain).*

18698-g

Binifibrate *(rINN).*
2-(4-Chlorophenoxyl)-2-methylpropionic acid ester with 1,3-dinicotinoyloxypropan-2-ol.
$C_{25}H_{23}ClN_2O_7=498.9$.

CAS — 69047-39-8.

Binifibrate, a clofibrate ester combined with a nicotinic acid derivative, is used as a hypolipidaemic agent.

Proprietary Names and Manufacturers
Biniwas *(Wasserman, Spain).*

1344-d

Cholestyramine *(BAN).*

Cholestyramine Resin *(USAN)*; Colestyramine *(rINN)*; MK-135. Cholestyramine is a strongly basic anion-exchange resin containing quaternary ammonium functional groups which are attached to a styrene-divinylbenzene copolymer (about 2% divinylbenzene). It is used in the chloride form.

CAS — 11041-12-6.

Pharmacopoeias. In *U.S.*

A white to buff-coloured, hygroscopic, fine powder, odourless or with a slight amine-like odour. It loses not more than 12% of its weight on drying.
Practically **insoluble** in water, alcohol, chloroform, and ether. A 1% aqueous slurry has a pH of 4 to 6. **Store** in airtight containers.

Adverse Effects
The most common side-effect of cholestyramine is constipation; faecal impaction may develop and haemorrhoids may be aggravated. Other gastro-intestinal side-effects, including abdominal discomfort or pain, heartburn, flatulence, nausea, vomiting, and diarrhoea, may also occur but are usually mild and transient.
Cholestyramine may cause steatorrhoea by interfering with the absorption of fats from the gastro-intestinal tract and therefore decreased absorption of fat-soluble vitamins, such as vitamins A, D, and K, may occur. Chronic administration of cholestyramine may thus result in an increased bleeding tendency due to hypoprothrombinaemia associated with vitamin K deficiency or it may lead to osteoporosis due to impaired calcium and vitamin D absorption.
Due to the fact that cholestyramine is the chloride form of an anion-exchange resin, prolonged use may produce hyperchloraemic acidosis, particularly in children.
Skin rashes and pruritus have occasionally occurred.

Results of the Lipid Research Clinics Coronary Primary Prevention Trial involving 3806 men given cholestyramine or placebo for an average of 7.4 years. Gastro-intestinal side-effects occurred frequently in both groups but especially in the cholestyramine group. In the first year 68% of the cholestyramine group experienced at least one gastro-intestinal side-effect compared with 43% of the placebo group; by the seventh year the incidence had diminished so that approximately equal percentages of patients were affected (29% and 26% respectively). Constipation and heartburn, especially, were more frequent in the cholestyramine group which also reported more abdominal pain, belching or bloating, gas, and nausea. These side-effects were usually not severe and could be dealt with by standard clinical means. Diagnoses and procedures involving the gall-bladder were scrutinised in view of the ability of certain lipid-lowering agents to produce gall-stones and gall-bladder disease. Gall-stones and gall-bladder and biliary-tract diseases were reported in 31 and 28 patients respectively in the cholestyramine group (total of 1906 patients) compared to 30 and 23 patients respectively in the placebo group (total of 1900 patients). The numbers of "incident and fatal" cases of malignant neoplasms were similar in the two groups; 57 and 16 in the cholestyramine group and 57 and 15 in the placebo group. The cholestyramine group had a few more in some categories, such as the buccal cavity and pharynx, and less in others (the respiratory system) but the numbers were small. When the various categories of gastro-intestinal tract cancers (buccal cavity, pharynx, oesophagus, stomach, colon, rectum, and pancreas) were considered together the number of "incident and fatal" cases were 21 and 8 respectively in the cholestyramine group and 11 and 1 in the placebo group. The number of "incident" cancers of the colon was identical in each group.— *J. Am. med. Ass.,* 1984, *251,* 351. Comment that the occurrence of 6 rare cancers of the buccal cavity or pharynx in the cholestyramine group compared with none in the placebo group should not pass unnoticed and that a complete post-trial follow-up is essential.— M. F. Oliver, *Br. med. J.,* 1984, *288,* 423.

Precautions
Because of the risk of vitamin deficiencies, supplements of vitamins A and D and possibly K should be given in a water-miscible form by mouth or administered parenterally during prolonged therapy with cholestyramine. Reduced serum-folate concentrations have also been reported and it has been suggested that supplementation with folic acid should be considered in such circumstances.
Cholestyramine may also delay or reduce the absorption of other drugs, particularly acidic drugs, administered concomitantly. Delayed or reduced absorption of chlorothiazide and hydrochlorothiazide, digoxin, hydrocortisone, loperamide, naproxen, paracetamol, phenylbutazone, propranolol, sulphinpyrazone, thyroid hormones, and warfarin, has either been reported or may be expected. It is therefore recommended that other drugs should be taken at least 1 hour before or 4 to 6 hours after the administration of cholestyramine. The ability of cholestyramine to bind to other drugs has, however, been used in the management of some cases of drug overdosage (see Poisoning, under Uses).

Uses and Administration
Cholestyramine is not absorbed from the gastro-intestinal tract but it adsorbs and combines with the bile acids in the intestine to form an insoluble complex which is excreted in the faeces. The normal reabsorption of bile acids is thus prevented and this leads to an increased oxidation of cholesterol to bile acids to replace those partially removed from the enterohepatic circulation. The overall effect is a reduction of serum-cholesterol and low-density lipoprotein concentrations. Since the uses of cholestyramine are based upon the removal of intestinal bile acids it is unlikely that a response will be achieved in patients with complete biliary obstruction.
Cholestyramine is used as a hypolipidaemic agent, in conjunction with dietary modification, in the treatment of hypercholesterolaemia, parti-

cularly type II hyperlipoproteinaemia. The usual dose by mouth is 12 to 24 g daily, administered either as a single dose or in up to 4 divided doses. Dosage should be adjusted according to the patient's response and may be increased to 36 g daily if necessary.

It is also used in similar doses for the relief of diarrhoea associated with ileal resection, Crohn's disease, vagotomy, and diabetic vagal neuropathy and for the management of radiation-induced diarrhoea.

Cholestyramine is also used to relieve the pruritus associated with the deposition in dermal tissue of excess bile acids in patients with partial biliary obstruction. Doses of 4 to 8 g daily are usually sufficient.

A suggested dose of cholestyramine for children over 6 years of age is 240 mg per kg body-weight daily.

Cholestyramine should be administered as a suspension in water or a flavoured vehicle.

BILIARY DISORDERS. Reports of the use of cholestyramine in the management of congenital nonobstructive nonhaemolytic hyperbilirubinaemia (Crigler-Najjar disease).— W. A. Arrowsmith *et al.*, *Archs Dis. Childh.*, 1975, *50*, 197; M. Odièvre *et al.*, *ibid.*, 1978, *53*, 81.

A beneficial effect of cholestyramine in 1 patient with sclerosing cholangitis.— D. E. Polter *et al.*, *Gastroenterology*, 1980, *79*, 326.

DIARRHOEA. Some references to cholestyramine being used to relieve diarrhoea associated with various conditions: T. V. Taylor *et al.*, *Lancet*, 1978, *1*, 635 (postvagotomy); J. R. Condon *et al.*, *Postgrad. med. J.*, 1978, *54*, 838 (radiation-induced); T. Vesikari and E. Isolauri, *Acta paediat. scand.*, 1985, *74*, 650 (infants); O. Jacobsen *et al.*, *Br. med. J.*, 1985, *290*, 1315 (ileal resection and an enteric-coated cholestyramine tablet).

HYPERLIPIDAEMIAS. For the use of cholestyramine in association with mevastatin or probucol in hypercholesterolaemia, see under Mevastatin, and Probucol.

For the use of cholestyramine, as a hypolipidaemic agent, in the prevention of ischaemic heart disease, see Ischaemic Heart Disease (below).

HYPEROXALURIA. Cholestyramine 4 g four times daily was given to 4 patients who had developed hyperoxaluria and nephrolithiasis after resection of the lower small intestine. Urinary excretion of calcium oxalate returned to normal and no new kidney stones formed whilst the patients were taking cholestyramine.— L. H. Smith *et al.*, *New Engl. J. Med.*, 1972, *286*, 1371.

Cholestyramine 4 g given four times daily reduced the high urinary oxalate excretion in 6 patients with regional enteritis who had undergone ileal resection. The severe diarrhoea which was present in 5 patients also improved.— J. Q. Stauffer *et al.*, *Ann. intern. Med.*, 1973, *79*, 383. See also W. F. Caspary (letter), *New Engl. J. Med.*, 1977, *296*, 1357.

ISCHAEMIC HEART DISEASE. Results of the Lipid Research Clinics Coronary Primary Prevention Trial demonstrating that treatment with cholestyramine reduced the incidence of coronary heart disease in patients at high risk. In this multicentre double-blind study 3806 middle-aged (mean 47.8 years) men with primary hypercholesterolaemia (type II hyperlipoproteinaemia) were given cholestyramine or placebo for an average of 7.4 years. Both groups followed a moderate cholesterol-lowering diet. Average plasma concentrations of total and low-density lipoprotein cholesterol were reduced by 13.4% and 20.3% respectively in the cholestyramine group, reductions 8.5% and 12.6% greater than those in the placebo group. There were 155 definite coronary heart disease deaths and/or definite nonfatal myocardial infarctions in the cholestyramine group compared with 187 such events in the placebo group and the incidence of coronary heart disease was estimated to be 19% lower in the cholestyramine group; there was a 24% reduction in risk of coronary heart disease death and a 19% reduction in risk of nonfatal infarction. Inclusion of suspected coronary heart disease death and nonfatal infarction resulted in an overall reduction in risk of 15%, with a 30% reduction for fatal events and a 15% reduction for nonfatal events. Death from all causes was reduced by only 7%.— *J. Am. med. Ass.*, 1984, *251*, 351. Further analysis of the results indicated that the reduced incidence of coronary heart disease in the cholestyramine group was mediated chiefly by cholesterol lowering.— *ibid.*, 365. Comment on the Lipid Research Clinics Coronary Primary Prevention Trial. Extreme caution should be used in extrapolating the results to portions of the population that were not represented by the sample included in the study. The study provided no evidence that would imply that cholestyramine would be beneficial in hyperlipidaemic women or those who were either younger or older than the participants in the trial. Likewise, there is no basis for extending these results to those people with lower cholesterol concentrations who are at a considerably lower risk of cardiovascular disease.— R. A. Kronmal, *ibid.*, 1985, *253*, 2091. Reply by the Lipid Research Clinics Program Investigators. There is little reason to believe that the findings of a reduced incidence of coronary heart disease associated with the lowering of plasma-cholesterol concentrations would be entirely confined to the types of patient investigated. It may, however, be debatable whether such a reduction in coronary heart disease in a lower-risk population would outweigh the potential risks of drug treatment.— *ibid.*, *254*, 263.

Further discussions and comments concerning the results and implications of the Lipid Research Clinics Trial.— M. F. Oliver, *Br. med. J.*, 1984, *288*, 423 (caution against the extrapolation of the findings); *Lancet*, 1984, *1*, 317 (support for the case of dietary or drug-induced cholesterol reduction in the population as a whole); L. A. Simons, *Med. J. Aust.*, 1984, *140*, 316 (support for the view that the principle of lowering blood-cholesterol concentrations should be extended).

Results of the National Heart, Lung and Blood Institute (NHLBI) Type II Coronary Intervention Study which was designed to examine the hypothesis that the lowering of plasma-cholesterol concentration would reduce the rate of progression of coronary artery disease. 59 patients with type II hyperlipoproteinaemia and coronary artery disease received cholestyramine 24 g daily (adjusted in response to side-effects) and 57 similar patients received placebo; all followed a low-cholesterol, low-fat diet. After 5 years of treatment the cholestyramine-treated group achieved a 26% reduction in low-density lipoprotein cholesterol compared with a 5% reduction in the placebo group; the difference was statistically significant. Similar differences were observed for total plasma-cholesterol concentrations. The progression of coronary artery disease, assessed angiographically after 5 years, in the cholestyramine and placebo groups yielded the following results: definite progression in 25.4% and 35.1% respectively; probable progression in 6.8% and 14.0%; mixed response in 8.5% and 1.8%; no change in 52.5% and 42.1%; probable regression in 3.4% and 5.3%; and definite regression in 3.4 and 1.8%. Analysis performed with adjustment for baseline inequalities of risk factors showed a more pronounced effect of cholestyramine treatment. The authors concluded that although the results could not be considered definitive, the evidence suggested that the lowering of cholesterol by diet and cholestyramine inhibits the rate of progression of coronary obstructive lesions.— J. F. Brensike *et al.*, *Circulation*, 1984, *69*, 313. Description of the response of the various lipid fractions observed during the study.— R. I. Levy *et al.*, *ibid.*, 325.

POISONING. Comment that cholestyramine given by mouth in repeated doses may interrupt the enterohepatic circulation of polar high molecular weight compounds that are excreted into bile, thus preventing their intestinal re-absorption. By this means the elimination of drugs, such as phenobarbitone, digitoxin, and phenprocoumon can be considerably enhanced after overdosage.— L. F. Prescott, *Br. med. J.*, 1983, *287*, 274.

Reports of the use of cholestyramine in the management of poisoning and overdosage: T. Meinertz *et al.*, *Br. med. J.*, 1977, *2*, 439 (phenprocoumon); J. Kuhlmann, *Int. J. clin. Pharmac. Ther. Toxic.*, 1984, *22*, 543 (beta acetyldigoxin, digitoxin, and medigoxin); S. Renowden *et al.*, *Br. med. J.*, 1985, *291*, 513 (warfarin).

PRURITUS. References to the use of cholestyramine for the relief of pruritus in various conditions: I. Chanarin and L. Szur, *Br. J. Haemat.*, 1975, *29*, 669 (polycythaemia rubra vera); J. T. Rodriguez *et al.*, *J. Pediat.*, 1976, *88*, 659 (ointment for ostomies); D. S. Silverberg *et al.*, *Br. med. J.*, 1977, *1*, 752 (uraemia and haemodialysis); R. van Leusen *et al.* (letter), *ibid.*, 1978, *1*, 918 (haemodialysis); J. S. Duncan *et al.*, *Br. med. J.*, 1984, *289*, 22 (liver disease).

Preparations

Cholestyramine for Oral Suspension *(U.S.P.)*

Proprietary Preparations

Questran *(Bristol-Myers Pharmaceuticals, UK)*. *Oral powder*, cholestyramine (anhydrous) 4 g/sachet.

Proprietary Names and Manufacturers

Cuemid *(Austral.; Ger.; Norw.; Swed.; Merck Sharp & Dohme, UK)*; Lismol *(Lesvi, Spain)*; Quantalan *(Aust.; Bristol, Ger.; Port.; Bristol, Switz.)*; Questran *(Astra, Austral.; Bristol, Canad.; Bristol-Myers, Denm.; Allard, Fr.; Bristol Italiana Sud, Ital.; Neth.; Bristol, Norw.; Bristol, S.Afr.; Bristol, Swed.; Bristol-Myers Pharmaceuticals, UK; Mead Johnson Laboratories, USA)*; Resincolestiramina *(Rubio, Spain)*.

15316-r

Ciprofibrate *(BAN, USAN, rINN).*

Win-35833. 2-[4-(2,2-Dichlorocyclopropyl)phenoxy]-2-methylpropionic acid.

$C_{13}H_{14}Cl_2O_3$=289.2.

CAS — 52214-84-3.

Ciprofibrate, a clofibrate analogue, is used as a hypolipidaemic agent.

Proprietary Names and Manufacturers

Lipanor *(Winthrop, Fr.)*.

16584-m

Clinofibrate *(rINN).*

S-8527. 2,2′-[Cyclohexylidenebis(4-phenyleneoxy)]bis-[2-methylbutyric acid].

$C_{28}H_{36}O_6$=468.6.

CAS — 30299-08-2.

Clinofibrate, a clofibrate analogue, is used as a hypolipidaemic agent.

Proprietary Names and Manufacturers

Lipoclin *(Sumitomo, Jpn)*.

1341-x

Clofibrate *(BAN, USAN, rINN).*

AY-61123; Clofibratum; Ethyl Chlorophenoxyisobutyrate; Ethyl Clofibrate; ICI-28257; NSC-79389. Ethyl 2-(4-chlorophenoxy)-2-methylpropionate.

$C_{12}H_{15}ClO_3$=242.7.

CAS — 637-07-0.

Pharmacopoeias. In *Br., Braz., Chin., Cz., Egypt., Fr., Ind., Eur., Jpn, Neth., Nord., Roum., Swiss,* and *U.S.*

A clear colourless to pale yellow liquid with a characteristic faintly acrid odour. *B.P.* **solubilities** are: very slightly soluble in water; miscible with alcohol, chloroform, and ether. *U.S.P.* solubilities are: practically insoluble in water; soluble in acetone, alcohol, and chloroform. **Store** in airtight containers. Protect from light.

Adverse Effects

The commonest side-effects of clofibrate therapy are gastro-intestinal upsets including nausea, vomiting, diarrhoea, dyspepsia, flatulence, and abdominal discomfort. Other adverse effects reported to occur less frequently include weight gain, headache, dizziness, fatigue or drowsiness, skin rashes, pruritus, alopecia, and anaemia or leucopenia. Slight abnormalities of liver function tests and hepatomegaly, apparently not indicative of hepatotoxicity, have occasionally occurred.

A syndrome of muscle pain and weakness has been associated with clofibrate, occurring particularly in patients with the nephrotic syndrome.

Large-scale studies using clofibrate have demonstrated an increased incidence of cholecystitis, gall-stones, and sometimes pancreatitis, and some studies, but not all, have indicated an increased incidence of certain cardiovascular disorders, including cardiac arrhythmias.

EFFECTS ON THE BILIARY TRACT. Analysis of data obtained from the WHO Co-operative Trial showed that there were 33 cholecystectomies among 3536 men with high serum-cholesterol concentrations given clofibrate compared with 12 in each of 2 groups of 3552 and 3325 men with high and low cholesterol values respectively but not treated with clofibrate. The formation of gall-stones was considered to be associated with clofibrate and not the serum-cholesterol concentration.— J.

Cooper *et al.* (letter), *Lancet*, 1975, *1*, 1083.

Analysis of data obtained during the Coronary Drug Project indicated a significant increase in the development of gall-bladder disease among patients treated with clofibrate (42 cases in 1051 patients) compared with those treated with a placebo (69 cases in 2680 patients).— Coronary Drug Project Research Group, *New Engl. J. Med.*, 1977, *296*, 1185.

EFFECTS ON THE HEART. Reports of individual cases of adverse cardiac effects in patients taking clofibrate.— J. F. X. McGarvey (letter), *J. Am. med. Ass.*, 1973, *225*, 638 (premature atrial and ventricular contractions); E. K. Chung, *Drug Ther.*, 1975, *5*, 54 (frequent premature atrial and ventricular contractions and paroxysmal atrial tachycardia).

A report of an increased incidence of angina pectoris, intermittent claudication, pulmonary embolism, and cardiac arrhythmias (other than fibrillation) in patients taking clofibrate.— Coronary Drug Project Research Group, *J. Am. med. Ass.*, 1975, *231*, 360.

EFFECTS ON THE KIDNEY. Acute-on-chronic renal failure in 2 patients was precipitated by clofibrate.— S. Dosa *et al.* (letter), *Lancet*, 1976, *1*, 250. Acute reversible renal failure, due to interstitial nephritis, associated with the use of clofibrate.— A. Cumming, *Br. med. J.*, 1980, *281*, 1529.

EFFECTS ON THE LIVER. A multicentre study of liver biopsies performed on 40 patients before and after 3 months of clofibrate therapy demonstrated no significant histological changes in fatty infiltration in 13 patients on clofibrate 500 mg daily; of 17 patients with distinct fatty degeneration before therapy with 1.5 g daily, 6 improved, 3 deteriorated, and 8 remained unchanged. No other histological differences were noted between the effects of the 2 dosage regimens and no adverse effects were observed.— P. Schwandt *et al.* (letter), *Lancet*, 1978, *2*, 325.

Granulomatous hepatitis occurred in a woman who had taken clofibrate for 3 months. Liver function had returned to normal on examination 4 weeks after withdrawal of the drug.— E. H. Pierce and D. L. Chesler (letter), *New Engl. J. Med.*, 1978, *299*, 314.

EFFECTS ON THE RESPIRATORY SYSTEM. Eosinophilic pneumonia in 1 patient associated with the use of clofibrate.— R. M. Hendrickson and F. Simpson (letter), *J. Am. med. Ass.*, 1982, *247*, 3082.

EFFECTS ON SEXUAL FUNCTION. Three men complained of impotence while taking clofibrate; in 2 it resolved when clofibrate was withdrawn; it recurred in one when he was again given clofibrate.— J. Schneider and H. Kaffarnik, *Atherosclerosis*, 1975, *21*, 455.

Among the most frequent complaints reported by patients in the Coronary Drug Project receiving clofibrate were decreased libido and, to a lesser degree, breast tenderness.— Coronary Drug Project Research Group, *J. Am. med. Ass.*, 1975, *231*, 360.

Of about 5000 patients treated for 4 to 8 years with clofibrate 14 ceased treatment because of impotence; a further 58 reported the side-effect significantly more often than in a control group.—Report from the Committee of Principal Investigators, *Br. Heart J.*, 1978, *40*, 1069.

Precautions

Clofibrate should not be given to patients with impaired liver or kidney function, primary biliary cirrhosis, or gall-stones or gall-bladder disorders. Caution has also been advised in patients with hypoalbuminaemic states such as the nephrotic syndrome.

Clofibrate may enhance the effects of anticoagulant drugs; the dose of anticoagulant should be reduced to about a half when treatment with clofibrate is started, and then adjusted gradually if necessary. The dosage of antidiabetic agents may need adjusting during concomitant clofibrate therapy.

RENAL FAILURE. Although clofibrate is not recommended in patients with renal impairment Bennett *et al.* (*Am. J. Kidney Dis.*, 1983, *3*, 155) consider that the interval between doses of clofibrate could be extended to 6 to 12 hours in patients with a glomerular filtration-rate (GFR) above 50 mL per minute, to 12 to 18 hours in those with a GFR of 10 to 50 mL per minute, and to 24 to 48 hours in those with a GFR of less than 10 mL per minute. Also Goldberg *et al.* (*Clin. Pharmac. Ther.*, 1977, *21*, 317) consider that uraemic patients managed by haemodialysis could receive 1 to 1.5 g weekly; this dose had produced the desired decrease in triglyceride concentrations without causing toxicity in 5 such patients.

The plasma half-life of total chlorophenoxyisobutyric acid (free and conjugated) was 86.1, 93, and 98.6 hours in 3 patients with renal failure undergoing dialysis 3 times a week and 188.3 and 199.2 hours in 2 patients with renal failure undergoing twice-weekly dialysis. The mean plasma half-life in 5 healthy controls was 17.2 hours.— E. M. Faed and E. G. McQueen, *Br. J. clin. Pharmac.*, 1979, *7*, 407.

Absorption and Fate

Clofibrate is readily absorbed from the gastro-intestinal tract and is rapidly hydrolysed in the blood to its active metabolite, chlorophenoxyisobutyric acid (clofibric acid), which is extensively bound to plasma proteins. The plasma half-life is about 17 hours. It is excreted in the urine, predominantly in the form of a glucuronide conjugate.

A review of the clinical pharmacokinetics of hypolipidaemic agents, including clofibrate.— R. Gugler, *Clin. Pharmacokinet.*, 1978, *3*, 425.

In 10 patients given single doses of clofibrate, clofibride, and pyridoxine clofibrate equivalent to clofibric acid 900 mg mean half-lives were 21.5, 23.5, and 15.0 hours respectively with maximum serum concentrations of clofibric acid of about 100 µg per mL. Aluminium clofibrate had a much longer half-life of about 63 hours with a maximum serum concentration of only about 30 µg per mL; this was probably a result of slower release of clofibric acid from its aluminium salt in the intestine. Following twice-daily administration for 12 days clofibrate produced serum concentrations of clofibric acid which were slightly higher than after aluminium clofibrate; the serum concentrations of the latter, however, showed less daily variation. The steady-state serum concentrations indicated that the half-life in practice was considerably lower than anticipated from the single-dose studies, probably owing to an increase in the proportion of clofibric acid not bound to plasma proteins.— A. Cailleux *et al.*, *Thérapie*, 1976, *31*, 637.

Mean blood concentrations of clofibrate in about 5000 patients taking 1.6 g daily were 124 to 171 µg per mL.—Report from the Committee of Principal Investigators, *Br. Heart J.*, 1978, *40*, 1069.

For a report of the half-life in both healthy controls and patients with renal failure, see Renal Failure under Precautions (above).

Uses and Administration

Clofibrate reduces elevated plasma concentrations of triglycerides and, to a somewhat smaller extent, elevated plasma concentrations of cholesterol; the effect is particularly evident in a reduction of elevated concentrations of very low-density lipoproteins. The mechanism of clofibrate's hypolipidaemic action is not clear.

Clofibrate is used as a hypolipidaemic agent, in conjunction with dietary modification, in the treatment of type III hyperlipoproteinaemia; it may also be helpful in some patients with type IIb, type IV, or type V hyperlipoproteinaemia. Xanthomas may regress. The usual dose, by mouth, is 20 to 30 mg per kg body-weight daily in 2 or 3 divided doses.

Clofibrate has been used for the prophylaxis of ischaemic heart disease but is no longer recommended for widespread use for this purpose. For further details see under Ischaemic Heart Disease (below).

ADMINISTRATION IN RENAL FAILURE. See Renal Failure under Precautions (above).

CHYLURIA. In 10 patients with recurrent chyluria the condition regressed within 12 days during treatment with clofibrate 500 mg thrice daily for 2 to 3 weeks; there was no recurrence in 12 to 18 months.— A. K. R. Choudhury, *J. Indian med. Ass.*, 1976, *66*, 175.

DIABETES INSIPIDUS. In 6 patients with vasopressin-responsive diabetes insipidus, clofibrate 2 g daily for 3 to 5 days reduced urine output by a mean of 47%; chlorpropamide 250 mg daily reduced output by a mean of 57%; the mean reductions with clofibrate 2 g plus chlorpropamide 125 mg (5 patients) and clofibrate 2 g plus chlorpropamide 250 mg (4 patients) were 54 and 61% respectively. One patient responded only to combined treatment.— P. Thompson *et al.*, *Metabolism*, 1977, *26*, 749.

HYPERLIPIDAEMIAS. In 72 patients with 5 different types of hyperlipidaemia divided on the basis of lipoprotein analysis, clofibrate 2 g daily was beneficial in patients with elevated serum concentrations of low-density lipoproteins without tendinous xanthoma, in those with elevated concentrations of very low-density lipoproteins and tuberous xanthomas, and in patients in whom the concentrations of both classes of lipoproteins were raised, though in the latter group the effect on low-density lipoprotein concentrations was variable. There was little response in patients with tendon xanthomas in addition to elevated serum concentrations of low-density lipoproteins. In patients with raised concentrations of very low-density lipoproteins and normal concentrations of low-density lipoproteins a marked fall in the former occurred usually with a concomitant rise in the latter. When clofibrate caused an increase above normal in low-density lipoprotein concentrations, its use should be discontinued.— E. H. Strisower *et al.*, *Am. J. Med.*, 1968, *45*, 488.

ISCHAEMIC HEART DISEASE. Several studies involving clofibrate have been carried out to investigate whether reduction of elevated serum-lipids would reduce the incidence of ischaemic heart disease. Two early studies (The Five-year study by a Group of Physicians of the Newcastle upon Tyne Region, *Br. med. J.*, 1971, *4*, 767; Report by a Research Committee of the Scottish Society of Physicians, *Br. med. J.*, 1971, *4*, 775) involved both men and women with angina, a history of myocardial infarction, or both. Both studies found a reduced incidence of cardiac deaths in clofibrate-treated patients who had a history of angina or angina plus myocardial infarction but not in those with a history of infarction alone. The Coronary Drug Project Research Group (*J. Am. med. Ass.*, 1975, *231*, 360) studied the effect of various lipid-regulating agents, including clofibrate and nicotinic acid, in men who had experienced one or more episodes of myocardial infarction. They found that neither clofibrate nor nicotinic acid was more effective than placebo in reducing overall or cause-specific mortality and concluded that there was no evidence on which to recommend the use of clofibrate in the treatment of patients with coronary heart disease.

The WHO Co-operative Trial on Primary Prevention of Ischaemic Heart Disease with Clofibrate was a study involving 3 groups each of about 5000 men initially free of ischaemic heart disease. Group 1 consisted of patients with elevated serum-cholesterol concentrations who received clofibrate; groups 2 and 3 had high and low cholesterol concentrations respectively and received placebo, thus serving as controls; about 3500 patients in each group completed 5 years of treatment. The first report from the Committee of Principal Investigators (*Br. Heart J.*, 1978, *40*, 1069) found that cholesterol concentrations were reduced less than had been expected and that the incidence of fatal ischaemic heart disease was not significantly different between the 2 high-cholesterol groups, although the incidence of non-fatal myocardial infarction was significantly reduced in the clofibrate-treated group. The Committee also reported that the total number of deaths during the trial and within one year of leaving the trial were significantly higher in the clofibrate group. The conclusion of this report was that clofibrate could not be recommended as a lipid-lowering agent for the widespread primary prevention of ischaemic heart disease. Two further reports from the Committee (*Lancet*, 1980, *2*, 379 and 490; *Lancet*, 1984, *2*, 600) which covered a mean total follow-up period of 7.9 years showed that an excess mortality due to a wide variety of causes other than ischaemic heart disease had occurred in the clofibrate group during the treatment period but that this excess mortality had not continued after the end of treatment.

Another study on the primary prevention of cardiovascular diseases in men (T.A. Miettinen *et al.*, *J. Am. med. Ass.*, 1985, *254*, 2097) was multifactorial in design and included some patients treated with clofibrate or probucol. Multilogistic analysis, which the authors admit must be interpreted with caution, indicated that for probucol the coronary incidence was lower than predicted on the basis of the risk factor levels but that an increased incidence was associated with clofibrate.

Preparations

Clofibrate Capsules *(B.P.)*

Clofibrate Capsules *(U.S.P.)*

Proprietary Preparations

Atromid-S *(ICI Pharmaceuticals, UK)*. *Capsules*, clofibrate 500 mg.

Proprietary Names and Manufacturers

Amotril; Apolan *(Switz.)*; Arterioflexin *(Protea, Austral.)*; Artevil *(Nuovo, Ital.)*; Ateriosan *(Arg.)*; Aterosol *(Swed.)*; Atheromide *(Jpn)*; Atheropront *(Ger.; Switz.)*; Atroayerst *(Arg.)*; Atrolen *(FIRMA, Ital.)*; Atromidin *(Belg.; ICI, Denm.; ICI-Pharma, Ital.; Neth.; ICI, Swed.)*; Atromid-S *(Arg.; ICI, Austral.; Ayerst, Canad.; ICI, S.Afr.; ICI Pharmaceuticals, UK; Ayerst,*

USA); Azionyl; Bioscleran *(Pfleger, Ger.)*; Cartagyl *(Belg.)*; Citiflus *(Ital.)*; Claripex *(ICN, Canad.)*; Cloberat *(Ital.)*; Clofibral *(Pharma 2000, Fr.*; *Lifepharma, Ital.)*; Clofi-ICN *(Neth.)*; Clofinit *(Gentili, Ital.)*; Clofirem *(Millot-Solac, Fr.)*; Clopir *(IRBI, Ital.)*; Corafen *(Arg.)*; Dabical *(Fr.)*; Elpi *(Arg.)*; Fibramid *(Ital.)*; Geromid *(Zoja, Ital.)*; Ipolipid *(Isnardi, Ital.)*; Lipavil *(Farmades, Ital.)*; Lipavlon *(I.C.I.-Pharma, Fr.)*; Lipidicon *(Ital.)*; Liporan *(Ital.)*; Liprin *(Belg.)*; Liprinal *(Austral.*; *Bristol-Myers Pharmaceuticals, UK)*; Lostat *(Austral.)*; Neo-Atromid *(ICI, Spain)*; Nibratol *(Lampugnani, Ital.)*; Normet *(Ital.)*; Normolipol *(Fr.)*; Novofibrate *(Novopharm, Canad.)*; Recolip *(Denm.*; *Swed.)*; Regelan *(ICI, Ger.*; *ICI, Switz.)*; Sclerovasal *(Ital.)*; Serolipid *(S.Afr.)*; Serotinex *(Arg.)*; Skleromexe *(Merckle, Ger.*; *Switz.)*; Sklero-Tablinen *(Ger.)*; Ticlobran *(Ger.)*; Xyduril *(Ger.)*; Yoclo *(Jpn)*.

1345-n

Clofibride *(rINN)*.

MG-46. 3-Dimethylcarbamoylpropyl 2-(4-chlorophenoxy)-2-methylpropionate.
$C_{16}H_{22}ClNO_4$=327.8.

CAS — 26717-47-5.

Clofibride, a clofibrate analogue, is used as a hypolipidaemic agent.

For a report of the absorption and fate of clofibride, see Clofibrate, p.1199.

Proprietary Names and Manufacturers
Lipenan *(Belg.*; *Bouchara, Fr.)*.

1346-h

Colestipol Hydrochloride *(BANM, USAN, rINNM)*.

U-26597A. The hydrochloride of a copolymer of diethylenetriamine and epichlorohydrin (1-chloro-2,3-epoxypropane).

CAS — 26658-42-4; 50925-79-6 (both colestipol); 37296-80-3 (hydrochloride).

Adverse Effects and Precautions
As for Cholestyramine, p.1197.
It has, however, been stated that colestipol does not interfere with the absorption of warfarin.

EFFECTS ON THE BILIARY TRACT. A patient developed gall-stones 3 weeks after starting treatment with colestipol.— S. M. Grundy and H. Y. I. Mok, *J. Lab. clin. Med.*, 1977, *89*, 354.

Uses and Administration
Colestipol hydrochloride has actions similar to those of cholestyramine (see p.1197).
It is used as a hypolipidaemic agent, in conjunction with dietary modification, in the treatment of hypercholesterolaemia, particularly type II hyperlipoproteinaemia. The usual dose by mouth is 15 to 30 g daily in 2 to 4 divided doses.
Colestipol should be administered as a suspension in water or a flavoured vehicle.

HYPERLIPIDAEMIAS. Enhanced reduction of low-density-lipoprotein cholesterol in patients with heterozygous familial hypercholesterolaemia by treatment with colestipol with nicotinic acid.— D. R. Illingworth *et al.*, *Lancet*, 1981, *1*, 296. A similar report.— J. P. Kane *et al.*, *New Engl. J. Med.*, 1981, *304*, 251.

For the use of colestipol in asociation with lovastatin or probucol, see under Lovastatin (p.1201) and Probucol (p.1203).

For the use of colestipol, as a hypolipidaemic agent, in the prevention of ischaemic heart disease, see Ischaemic Heart Disease (below).

ISCHAEMIC HEART DISEASE. In a single-blind multicentre study involving 2278 patients with hypercholesterolaemia, of whom some had pre-existing coronary heart disease, colestipol 5 g three times daily reduced cholesterol concentrations to a significantly greater extent than a placebo. Patients were treated for up to 3 years. Deaths from coronary heart disease were significantly fewer in men receiving colestipol than in those receiving a placebo. There was no significant difference in mortality in women.— A. E. Dorr *et al.*, *J. chron. Dis.*, 1978, *31*, 5.

Proprietary Preparations
Colestid *(Upjohn, UK)*. *Granules*, colestipol hydrochloride, colloidal silicon dioxide 0.2%, in sachets of 5 g.

Proprietary Names and Manufacturers
Cholestabyl *(Holphar, Ger.)*; Colestid *(Upjohn, Austral.*; *Belg.*; *Upjohn, Canad.*; *Ger.*; *NZ*; *S.Afr.*; *Upjohn, Spain*; *Upjohn, Switz.*; *Upjohn, UK*; *Upjohn, USA)*; Lestid *(Upjohn, Denm.*; *Upjohn, Norw.)*.

12634-e

Detaxtran Hydrochloride

DEAE-dextran Hydrochloride; Diethylaminoethyl-dextran Hydrochloride. The hydrochloride of an anion-exchange resin.

CAS — 9064-91-9.

Detaxtran hydrochloride is used as a hypolipidaemic agent.

Proprietary Names and Manufacturers
Dexide *(Fargal-Pharmasint, Ital.*; *Gamir, Spain)*; Nolipid *(Samil, Ital.)*; Pulsar *(Medosan, Ital.)*; Rationale *(Manetti Roberts, Ital.)*.

9003-x

Detrothyronine *(rINN)*.

3,5,3′-Tri-iodo-D-thyronine; D-T_3; SKF-D2623; D-Tri-iodothyronine. 4-*O*-(4-Hydroxy-3-iodophenyl)-3,5-di-iodo-D-tyrosine.
$C_{15}H_{12}I_3NO_4$=651.0.

CAS — 5714-08-9.

Detrothyronine, which is the D-isomer of liothyronine, has been used as a hypolipidaemic agent.

9004-r

Dextrothyroxine Sodium *(BANM, USAN, rINN)*.

3,5,3′,5′-Tetraiodo-D-thyronine Sodium; D-Thyroxine Sodium; Sodium Dextrothyroxine. Sodium 4-*O*-(4-hydroxy-3,5-di-iodophenyl)-3,5-di-iodo-D-tyrosinate hydrate.
$C_{15}H_{10}I_4NNaO_4(+xH_2O)$=798.9.

CAS — 51-49-0 (dextrothyroxine); 137-53-1 (sodium salt, anhydrous); 7054-08-2 (sodium salt, hydrate).

Pharmacopoeias. In *U.S.*

A light yellow to buff-coloured, odourless, tasteless powder which may assume a slight pink colour on exposure to light. It loses not more than 11% of its weight on drying.
Soluble 1 in 700 of water and 1 in 300 of alcohol; soluble in solutions of alkali hydroxides and in hot solutions of alkali carbonates; practically insoluble in acetone, chloroform, and ether. A saturated solution in water has a pH of about 8.9. A solution in a mixture of sodium hydroxide and alcohol is dextrorotatory. **Store** in airtight containers.

Adverse Effects
Cardiac changes including angina pectoris, extrasystoles, ectopic beats, supraventricular tachycardia, and ECG evidence of ischaemic heart disease have been observed during therapy with dextrothyroxine.
Other adverse effects which have been reported include headache, insomnia, nervousness, tremor, myalgia, paraesthesia, diuresis, nausea, vomiting, decrease in appetite, loss of weight, diarrhoea, constipation, sweating, flushing, fever, skin rashes, alopecia, and pruritus. The development of gall-stones has also occasionally been reported. The adverse effects of thyroid hormones are described on p.1488.

In 3798 patients with a history of myocardial infarction followed up for an average of 36 months, the number of deaths was 18.4% higher in the group of 1083 patients taking dextrothyroxine 6 mg daily to reduce hyperlipidaemia than in those taking a placebo. The mortality-rate increased progressively with duration of medication. The use of dextrothyroxine in the study was stopped.—The Coronary Drug Project Research Group, *J. Am. med. Ass.*, 1972, *220*, 996.

Precautions
Dextrothyroxine is contra-indicated in patients with hypertension or organic heart disease including angina pectoris, myocardial infarction, cardiac arrhythmias, and congestive heart failure. It is also contra-indicated in patients with advanced liver or kidney disease.
Dextrothyroxine may enhance the effects of anticoagulant drugs. Diabetic patients should be monitored for increased requirements of insulin or oral hypoglycaemic agents if dextrothyroxine is administered concurrently. The precautions to be taken with thyroid hormones in general are described on p.1489.

Absorption and Fate
Dextrothyroxine sodium is incompletely absorbed from the gastro-intestinal tract and is bound to plasma proteins. Its plasma half-life is reported to be about 18 hours and it has been reported to be excreted in urine and faeces.

Uses and Administration
Dextrothyroxine sodium reduces elevated plasma-cholesterol concentrations, particularly the low-density lipoprotein fraction.
It is used as a hypolipidaemic agent, in conjunction with dietary modification, in the treatment of type II hyperlipoproteinaemia but this use is severely limited by cardiotoxicity. The initial dose is 1 to 2 mg daily, increased by 1 to 2 mg at monthly intervals until a satisfactory response is achieved, up to a maximum of 8 mg daily. For children, an initial daily dose of 50 μg per kg body-weight increased by up to 50 μg per kg at monthly intervals to a maximum of 4 mg daily has been suggested.
Dextrothyroxine was formerly used to treat hypothyroidism.

Preparations
Dextrothyroxine Sodium Tablets *(U.S.P.)*

Proprietary Preparations
Choloxin *(Travenol, UK)*. *Tablets*, dextrothyroxine sodium 2 mg.

Proprietary Names and Manufacturers
Biotirmone *(Fr.)*; Choloxin *(Flint, Canad.*; *S.Afr.*; *Travenol, UK*; *Flint, USA)*; Débétrol *(Fr.)*; Dethyrona *(IBYS, Spain*; *Switz.)*; Dethyrone *(Belg.*; *Neth.)*; Dynothel *(Henning Berlin, Ger.)*; Eulipos *(Boehringer Mannheim, Ger.)*; Lisolipin *(Bracco, Ital.)*; Nadrothyron-D *(Ger.)*.

12701-g

Etamiphylline Heparinate

CAS — 59547-58-9.

Etamiphylline heparinate has been used as a hypolipidaemic agent.

Proprietary Names and Manufacturers
Milhéparine *(Millot-Solac, Fr.)*.

1347-m

Ethanolamine Oxiniacate

Ethanolamine Nicotinate Oxide; Ethanolamine Oxyniacate. 2-Aminoethyl pyridine-1-oxide-3-carboxylate.
$C_8H_{10}N_2O_3$=182.2.

CAS — 36296-31-8.

Ethanolamine oxiniacate has been used as a hypolipidaemic agent.

Proprietary Names and Manufacturers
Novacyl *(Astra, Fr.)*.

12715-l

Etiroxate Hydrochloride *(rINNM)*.

CG-635. Ethyl DL-2-amino-3-[4-(4-hydroxy-3,5-di-iodophenoxy)-3,5-di-iodophenyl]-2-methylpropionate hydrochloride.
$C_{18}H_{17}I_4NO_4$,HCl=855.4.

CAS — 17365-01-4 (etiroxate); 55327-22-5 (hydrochloride).

Etiroxate is used as a hypolipidaemic agent.

Proprietary Names and Manufacturers
Skleronorm *(Grünenthal, Ger.*; *Grünenthal, Switz.)*.

12719-c

Etofibrate *(rINN).*
2-Nicotinoyloxyethyl 2-(4-chlorophenoxy)-2-methylpropionate.
$C_{18}H_{18}ClNO_5$=363.8.

CAS — 31637-97-5.

Etofibrate, a derivative of clofibrate and nicotinic acid, is used as a hypolipidaemic agent.

Proprietary Names and Manufacturers
Afloyan *(Alter, Spain)*; Ligesin *(Madaus Cerafarm, Spain)*; Lipo-Merz *(Merz, Ger.*; *Merz, Switz.)*.

12733-j

Fenbutyramide
Fenbutiramide; Phenetamide; TH-4128. 2-Phenylbutyramide.
$C_{10}H_{13}NO$=163.2.

CAS — 90-26-6.

Fenbutyramide is used as a hypolipidaemic agent.

Proprietary Names and Manufacturers
Hyposterol *(Vaillant, Ital.)*; Liosterin *(Medici Domus, Ital.)*; Normosterolo *(Salfa, Ital.)*.

1348-b

Fenofibrate *(BAN, rINN).*
LF-178; Procetofene. Isopropyl 2-[4-(4-chlorobenzoyl)phenoxy]-2-methylpropionate.
$C_{20}H_{21}ClO_4$=360.8.

CAS — 49562-28-9.

Fenofibrate, a clofibrate analogue, is used as a hypolipidaemic agent.

Proprietary Names and Manufacturers
Lipanthyl *(Fournier S.A., Fr.*; *Holphar, Ger.*; *Nativelle, Ital.*; *Thylmer, Switz.)*; Liparison *(Frumtost, Spain)*; Lipidax *(UCB, Ital.)*; Lipil *(Ibirn, Ital.)*; Lipoclar *(Crinos, Ital.)*; Lipofene *(Selvi, Ital.)*; Liponat *(Geymonat, Ital.)*; Liposit *(SIT, Ital.)*; Lipovas *(Farmasimes, Spain)*; Nolipax *(Mendelejeff, Ital.)*; Normalip *(Knoll, Ger.)*; Procetoken *(Bernabò, Arg.)*; Scleril *(AGIPS, Ital.)*; Secalip *(Tilfarma, Spain)*; Sigurtil *(Sigurtà, Ital.)*; Tilene *(Francia Farm., Ital.)*; Volutine *(Geymonat, Ital.)*.

1349-v

Gemfibrozil *(BAN, USAN, rINN).*

CI-719. 2,2-Dimethyl-5-(2,5-xylyloxy)valeric acid.
$C_{15}H_{22}O_3$=250.3.

CAS — 25812-30-0.

Pharmacopoeias. In *U.S.*

A white waxy crystalline solid. Very slightly **soluble** in water; practically insoluble in alcohol, chloroform, and methyl alcohol. **Store** in airtight containers.

Adverse Effects and Precautions

As for Clofibrate, p.1198, but no caution has been suggested in the nephrotic syndrome.

INTERACTIONS. No evidence of an undesirable interaction in 14 diabetic patients receiving insulin or oral hypoglycaemic agents (acetohexamide, chlorpropamide, or gliclazide) when they were also given gemfibrozil.— I. de Salcedo *et al.*, *Proc. R. Soc. Med.*, 1976, *69, Suppl.* 2, 64. Of 20 diabetic patients receiving insulin or oral hypoglycaemic agents a slight increase in antidiabetic medication was required in 9 and a decrease in 1 when they were also given gemfibrozil.— A. Konttinen *et al.*, *Ann. clin. Res.*, 1979, *11*, 240.

RENAL FAILURE. Although gemfibrozil is not recommended in patients with renal impairment, W.M. Bennett *et al.* (*Am. J. Kidney Dis.*, 1983, *3*, 155) consider that the doses of gemfibrozil could be reduced to 50% in patients with a glomerular filtration-rate (GFR) of 10 to 50 mL per minute and to 25% in those with a GFR of less than 10 mL per minute.—.

Absorption and Fate

Gemfibrozil is readily absorbed from the gastro-intestinal tract; peak concentrations in plasma occur within 1 to 2 hours; the half-life is about 1.5 hours. About 70% of a dose is excreted in the urine; little is excreted in the faeces.

Uses and Administration

Gemfibrozil has actions on plasma-lipids similar to those of clofibrate (p.1199).

It is used as a hypolipidaemic agent, in conjunction with dietary modification. It is recommended in the treatment of type IIa, type IIb, type III, type IV, and type V hyperlipoproteinaemia. The usual dose, by mouth, is 1.2 g daily in 2 divided doses given 30 minutes before the morning and evening meals. The dosage range may vary between 0.9 and 1.5 g daily.

A review of gemfibrozil.— P. A. Todd and A. Ward, *Drugs*, 1988, *36*, 314.

In the Helsinki Heart Study 4081 asymptomatic middle-aged men with increased serum concentrations of non-HDL cholesterol were randomly assigned to gemfibrozil 600 mg or placebo twice daily for 5 years; 2859 subjects completed the study. There was a 34% reduction in the incidence of coronary heart disease in the gemfibrozil group compared with the placebo group, although there was no difference between the 2 groups in overall death rate.— M. H. Frick *et al.*, *New Engl. J. Med.*, 1987, *317*, 1237. Comments.— B. M. Rifkind, *ibid.*, 1279; *Lancet*, 1988, *1*, 333.

ADMINISTRATION IN RENAL FAILURE. See Renal Failure under Precautions (above).

Preparations

Gemfibrozil Capsules *(U.S.P.)*

Proprietary Preparations

Lopid *(Parke, Davis, UK). Capsules,* gemfibrozil 300 mg.

Proprietary Names and Manufacturers

Decrelip *(Ferrer, Spain)*; Gevilon *(Parke, Davis, Ger.)*; Lipozid *(Pierrel, Ital.)*; Lipur *(Substantia, Fr.)*; Lopid *(Parke, Davis, Canad.*; *Parke, Davis, Denm.*; *Parke, Davis, Ital.*; *Parke, Davis, NZ*; *Parke, Davis, Spain*; *Parke, Davis, UK*; *Parke, Davis, USA)*; Trialmin *(Menarini, Spain)*.

1350-r

Halofenate *(BAN, USAN, rINN).*
MK-185. 2-Acetamidoethyl 4-chloro-α-(3-trifluoromethylphenoxy)phenylacetate.
$C_{19}H_{17}ClF_3NO_4$=415.8.

CAS — 26718-25-2.

Halofenate has been used as a hypolipidaemic agent.

Proprietary Names and Manufacturers
Merck Sharp & Dohme, USA.

12827-x

Homonicotinic Acid
3-Pyridylacetic acid.
$C_7H_7NO_2$=137.1.

CAS — 501-81-5.

Homonicotinic acid is used as a hypolipidaemic agent.

Proprietary Names and Manufacturers
Minedil *(Formenti, Ital.)*; Piridil *(Ital.)*; Piristerol *(Janus, Ital.)*.

16894-k

Lovastatin *(USAN, rINN).*
MB-530B; Mevinolin; MK-803; Monacolin K; MSD-803. (1*S*,7*S*,8*S*,8a*R*)-1,2,3,7,8,8a-Hexahydro-3,7-dimethyl-8-{2-[(2*R*,4*R*)-tetrahydro-4-hydroxy-6-oxo-2*H*-pyran-2-yl]ethyl}-1-naphthyl (*S*)-2-methylbutyrate.
$C_{24}H_{36}O_5$=404.5.

CAS — 75330-75-5.

Lovastatin, which has been isolated from *Aspergillus terreus*, is a hypolipidaemic agent; it acts as a competitive inhibitor of 3-hydroxy-3-methylglutaryl coenzyme A reductase (HMG CoA reductase), the rate-determining enzyme for cholesterol synthesis.

Lovastatin is used in conjunction with dietary modification in the treatment of hypercholesterolaemia. Doses start at 20 mg daily in the evening with food, increased if necessary to 80 mg in single or divided doses. Its use is associated with altered liver-function values. Patients may experience muscle damage.

Lovastatin undergoes extensive first-pass metabolism in the liver and it is in the liver that the metabolites inhibit HMG CoA reductase, thus inhibiting cholesterol synthesis with a reduction in LDL and an increase or no change in HDL. This effect has been borne out in clinical studies. Additional use of a bile-acid sequestrant such as colestipol can further lower LDL concentrations. Compared with cholestyramine or colestipol, lovastatin is not considered unpleasant to take. Reports of adverse reactions include gastro-intestinal disturbances, headache, rash, and pruritus. Myositis with increased values for creatine phosphokinase can occur. Severe muscle effects have been reported in patients with liver impairment as well as in patients receiving lovastatin with gemfibrozil or cyclosporin, both of which interfere with lovastatin's metabolism. There may be increased serum aminotransferase activity and there is a suspicion that cataracts can develop. Other concerns are a possible interference with DNA replication and reports of animal carcinogenicity and teratogenicity.— *Med. Lett.*, 1987, *29*, 99.

A discussion of 3-hydroxy-3-methylglutaryl-coenzyme A reductase inhibitors including lovastatin.— J. M. Hoeg and H. B. Brewer, *J. Am. med. Ass.*, 1987, *258*, 3532.

References to the use of lovastatin: B. Lewis *et al.*, *Br. med. J.*, 1983, *287*, 21 (cerebrotendinous xanthomatosis); D. R. Illingworth, *Ann. intern. Med.*, 1984, *101*, 598 (additive effect with colestipol in hypercholesterolaemia); S. M. Grundy *et al.*, *ibid.*, 1985, *103*, 339 (additive effect with colestipol); Lovastatin Study Group II, *J. Am. med. Ass.*, 1986, *256*, 2829 (nonfamilial hypercholesterolaemia); G. L. Vega and S. M. Grundy, *ibid.*, 1987, *257*, 33 (with colestipol in hypercholesterolaemia); A. Garg and S. M. Grundy, *New Engl. J. Med.*, 1988, *318*, 81 (hypercholesterolaemia in non-insulin-dependent diabetes mellitus).

ADVERSE EFFECTS. Myolysis and acute renal failure associated with lovastatin in a heart-transplant patient.— D. J. Norman *et al.* (letter), *New Engl. J. Med.*, 1988, *318*, 46.

Proprietary Names and Manufacturers
Mevacor *(Merck Sharp & Dohme, USA)*.

18802-y

Meglutol *(rINN).*
CB-337. 3-Hydroxy-3-methylglutaric acid.
$C_6H_{10}O_5$=162.1.

CAS — 503-49-1.

Meglutol is used as a hypolipidaemic agent.

Proprietary Names and Manufacturers
Lipoglutaren *(Ausonia, Ital.)*; Mevalon *(Guidotti, Ital.)*.

16885-c

Melinamide *(rINN).*
AC-223. *N*-(α-Methylbenzyl)linoleamide.
$C_{26}H_{41}NO$=383.6.

CAS — 14417-88-0.

Melinamide is used as a hypolipidaemic agent.

Proprietary Names and Manufacturers
Artes Oil *(Sumitomo, Jpn)*.

16591-h

Mevastatin *(rINN)*.
Compactin; CS-500; ML-236B. (1*S*,7*S*,8*S*,8a*R*)-1,2,3,7,8,8a-Hexahydro-7-methyl-8-{2-[(2*R*,4*R*)-tetrahydro-4-hydroxy-6-oxo-2*H*-pyran-2-yl]ethyl}-1-naphthyl (*S*)-2-methylbutyrate.
$C_{23}H_{34}O_5$=390.5.

CAS — 73573-88-3.

Mevastatin, which has been isolated from *Penicillium citrinum*, is reported to be a hypolipidaemic agent; it acts as a competitive inhibitor of 3-hydroxy-3-methylglutaryl coenzyme A reductase (HMG CoA reductase), the rate-determining enzyme for cholesterol synthesis.

A discussion of 3-hydroxy-3-methylglutaryl-coenzyme A reductase inhibitors including mevastatin.— J. M. Hoeg and H. B. Brewer, *J. Am. med. Ass.*, 1987, *258*, 3532

The hypolipidaemic effects of mevastatin in 7 patients.— H. Mabuchi *et al.*, *New Engl. J. Med.*, 1981, *305*, 478.

Reports of the additive effect of cholestyramine with mevastatin in hypercholesterolaemia.— H. Mabuchi *et al.*, *New Engl. J. Med.*, 1983, *308*, 609; *ibid.*, 1180 (correction); A. Yamamoto *et al.*, *Int. J. clin. Pharmac. Ther. Toxic.*, 1984, *22*, 493.

Mevastatin has been reported to induce lymphomas in *dogs*.— *Med. Lett.*, 1987, *29*, 99.

1351-f

Nafenopin *(BAN, USAN, rINN)*.
Nafenoic Acid; Su-13437. 2-Methyl-2-[4-(1,2,3,4-tetrahydro-1-naphthyl)phenoxy]propionic acid.
$C_{20}H_{22}O_3$=310.4.

CAS — 3771-19-5.

Study in the USA of nafenopin as a hypolipidaemic agent ceased following a report of liver nodules in *rats*.

1352-d

Nicoclonate *(rINN)*.
Chlorophenylisobutyl Nicotinate; S-486. 1-(4-Chlorophenyl)-2-methylpropyl pyridine-3-carboxylate.
$C_{16}H_{16}ClNO_2$=289.8.

CAS — 10571-59-2.

Nicoclonate is used as a hypolipidaemic agent.

Proprietary Names and Manufacturers
Lipidium *(Sedaph, Fr.*; *Rorer, Ital.*; *Zambeletti, Spain)*.

1353-n

Nicofibrate Hydrochloride *(rINNM)*.
Clofenpyride Hydrochloride. 3-Pyridylmethyl 2-(4-chlorophenoxy)-2-methylpropionate hydrochloride.
$C_{16}H_{16}ClNO_3,HCl$=342.2.

CAS — 31980-29-7 (nicofibrate); 17413-51-3 (hydrochloride).

Nicofibrate hydrochloride, a clofibrate analogue, is used as a hypolipidaemic agent.

Proprietary Names and Manufacturers
Arterium *(Llorens, Spain)*; Arterium V *(Schwarz, Ital.)*.

13011-e

Nicomol *(rINN)*.
(2-Hydroxycyclohexane-1,3-diylidene)tetrakis(methylene nicotinate).
$C_{34}H_{32}N_4O_9$=640.6.

CAS — 27959-26-8.

Nicomol is used as a hypolipidaemic agent.

Proprietary Names and Manufacturers
Cholexamin *(Kyorin, Jpn)*.

3897-m

Omega-3 Triglycerides

16610-l

Docosahexaenoic Acid

DHA. Docosahexa-3,6,9,12,15,18-enoic acid.
$C_{22}H_{32}O_2$=328.5.

12685-f

Eicosapentaenoic Acid

EPA. Eicosa-5,8,11,14,17-pentaenoic acid.
$C_{20}H_{30}O_2$=302.5.

CAS — 25378-27-2.

3899-v

Omega-3 Marine Triglycerides *(BAN)*.

A mixture of the triglycerides of the fatty acids from marine fish containing the equivalent of about 18% w/w of eicosapentaenoic acid and 12% w/w of docosahexaenoic acid.

The omega-3 triglycerides are precursors of eicosanoids in *fish* and when taken by man they compete with the precursor arachidonic acid. Their actions in man include a reduction in plasma-triglycerides, cholesterol and very low density lipoprotein, an anti-inflammatory action, and a fibrinolytic or antiplatelet effect.

Fish oils are a source of omega-3 triglycerides and oils such as cod liver oil have been investigated, but consideration has to be given to the other ingredients such as vitamin A and vitamin D. Preparations such as omega-3 marine triglycerides are thus employed and are recommended in patients with severe hypertriglyceridaemia together with appropriate dietary modifications. The usual dose is 5 g twice a day with food.

There are also vegetable sources of omega-3 triglycerides.

Some reviews and discussions on the actions and uses of omega-3 triglycerides: *Lancet*, 1983, *1*, 1139; J. A. Glomset, *New Engl. J. Med.*, 1985, *312*, 1253; R. Ballard-Barbash and C. W. Callaway, *Mayo Clin. Proc.*, 1987, *62*, 113; *Lancet*, 1988, *1*, 1081.

Some references to studies of the effects of omega-3 triglycerides: J. Dyerberg *et al.*, *Lancet*, 1978, *2*, 117 (thrombosis and atherosclerosis); D. Kromhout *et al.*, *New Engl. J. Med.*, 1985, *312*, 1205 (inverse relationship between fish consumption and 20-year mortality from coronary heart disease); B. E. Phillipson *et al.*, *ibid.*, 1210 (reduction of plasma lipids, lipoproteins, and apoproteins by dietary fish oils in patients with hypertriglyceridaemia); T. H. Lee *et al.*, *ibid.*, 1217 (effects on neutrophils and monocytes); H. R. Knapp *et al.*, *ibid.*, 1986, *314*, 937 (effect on platelets); J. R. Marsden, *Hum. Toxicol.*, 1987, *6*, 219 (reduction in retinoid-induced hyperlipidaemia); J. M. Kremer *et al.*, *Ann. intern. Med.*, 1987, *106*, 497 (subjective benefit in active rheumatoid arthritis); *Lancet*, 1987, *2*, 720 (discussion of limited benefit in rheumatoid arthritis); S. B. Bittiner *et al.*, *Lancet*, 1988, *1*, 378 (improvement in psoriasis).

Adverse metabolic effects from omega-3 triglycerides in patients with type II diabetes.— H. Glauber *et al.*, *Ann. intern. Med.*, 1988, *108*, 663.

Proprietary Preparations

Maxepa *(Duncan, Flockhart, UK)*. *Capsules*, containing omega-3 marine triglycerides 1g. Vitamin A content less than 100 units/g, vitamin D content less than 10 units/g. *Oral liquid*, omega-3 marine triglycerides; 5 mL of liquid is approximately equivalent to 5g. Vitamin A content less than 100 units/g, vitamin D content less than 10 units/g.

Proprietary Names and Manufacturers
Maxepa *(Duncan, Flockhart, UK*; *Advanced Medical Nutrition, USA*; *Solgar, USA)*.

The following names have been used for multi-ingredient preparations containing marine fish oils— Efamol Marine (*Britannia Health, UK*); Epatrol (*Kramer, USA); EPOC* (*Evening Primrose Oil Co., UK*); Immune-aid (*Advanced Medical Nutrition, USA*); Naudicelle Plus (*Bio-Oil Research, UK*); Super Gammaoil Marine (*Quest, UK*).

13075-b

Pantethine

(+)-(*R*)-*NN'*-[Dithiobis(ethyleneiminocarbonylethylene)]bis(2,4-dihydroxy-3,3-dimethylbutyramide).
$C_{22}H_{42}N_4O_8S_2$=554.7.

CAS — 16816-67-4.

Pantethine is a component of coenzyme A. It has been tried in the treatment of hyperlipidaemias.

References: F. Bellani *et al.*, *Curr. ther. Res.*, 1986, *40*, 912; J. M. Gleeson *et al.*, *ibid.*, 1987, *41*, 83; D. Prisco *et al.*, *Angiology*, 1987, *38*, 241.

Proprietary Names and Manufacturers
Lipodel *(Delalande, Ital.)*; Obliterol *(Faes, Spain)*; Pantetina *(Maggioni-Winthrop, Ital.)*.

1354-h

Pentaerythritol Tetra-acetate
Pentaerythrityl Tetra-acetate; Tetra-*O*-acetylpentaerythritol. 2,2-Bis(hydroxymethyl)propane-1,3-diol tetraacetate.
$C_{13}H_{20}O_8$=304.3.

CAS — 597-71-7.

Pentaerythritol tetra-acetate has been used as a hypolipidaemic agent.

13134-f

Pirifibrate *(rINN)*.
EL-466. 6-Hydroxymethyl-2-pyridylmethyl 2-(4-chlorophenoxy)-2-methylpropionate.
$C_{17}H_{18}ClNO_4$=335.8.

CAS — 55285-45-5.

Pirifibrate, a clofibrate analogue, has been used as a hypolipidaemic agent.

Proprietary Names and Manufacturers
Bratenol *(Elmu, Spain)*.

3912-s

Pirozadil *(rINN)*.
722-D. 2,6-Pyridinediyldimethylene-bis(3,4,5-trimethoxybenzoate.
$C_{27}H_{29}NO_{10}$=527.5.

CAS — 54110-25-7.

Pirozadil is reported to have hypolipidaemic and platelet-anti-aggregatory properties. It has been given in the treatment of hyperlipidaemias and to patients who have suffered myocardial infarction. Usual doses of 1.5 to 3 g daily in divided doses by mouth have been given.

Proprietary Names and Manufacturers
Calpatil *(Igoda, Spain)*.

13139-b

Plafibride *(rINN)*.
ITA-104. 1-[2-(4-Chlorophenoxy)-2-methylpropionyl]-3-morpholinomethylurea.
$C_{16}H_{22}ClN_3O_4$=355.8.

CAS — 63394-05-8.

Plafibride, a clofibrate analogue, has been used as a hypolipidaemic agent.

Proprietary Names and Manufacturers
Idonor *(Roger, Spain)*; Perifunal *(Spain)*; Plafibrinol *(Fides, Spain)*.

1355-m

Polidexide *(BAN).*
DEAE-Sephadex; PDX Chloride; Poly[2-(diethylamino)ethyl]polyglycerylene Dextran. Dextran cross-linked with epichlorohydrin (1-chloro-2,3-epoxypropane) and *O*-substituted with 2-diethylamino and 2-[2-(diethylaminoethyl)-*N,N*-diethylammonio]ethyl groups.

CAS — 56227-39-5.

NOTE. Polidexide Sulfate is rINN.

Polidexide is an anion-exchange resin which was formerly used as a hypolipidaemic agent in the treatment of hypercholesterolaemia.

Proprietary Names and Manufacturers
Secholex *(Pharmacia, UK).*

3758-z

Pravastatin *(pINN).*
CS-514; Eptastatin; SQ-31000. (+)-(*βR,δR,1S,2S,6S,8S,8aR*)-1,2,6,7,8,8a-hexahydro-*β,δ*,6,8-tetrahydroxy-methyl-1-naphthaleneheptanoic acid, 8-[(2*S*)-2-methylbutyrate].
$C_{23}H_{36}O_7$=424.5.

CAS — 81093-37-0.

Pravastatin which has been isolated from *Nocardia autotrophica* is a hypolipidaemic agent. Like lovastatin it acts as a competitive inhibitor of 3-hydroxy-3-methylglutaryl coenzyme A reductase (HMG CoA reductase).

A discussion of 3-hydroxy-3-methylglutaryl-coenzyme A reductase inhibitors including pravastatin.—J. M. Hoeg and H. B. Brewer, *J. Am. med. Ass.*, 1987, *258*, 3532.

References to the use of pravastatin in the treatment of hypercholesterolaemia: G. Yoshino *et al.* (letter), *Lancet*, 1986, *2*, 740; N. Nakaya *et al.*, *J. Am. med. Ass.*, 1987, *257*, 3088; H. Mabuchi *et al.*, *Metabolism*, 1987, *36*, 475; K. Saku *et al.*, *Curr. ther. Res.*, 1987, *42*, 491.

Proprietary Names and Manufacturers
Sankyo, Jpn; Squibb, USA.

1356-b

Probucol *(BAN, USAN, rINN).*

DH-581. 4,4′-(Isopropylidenedithio)bis(2,6-di-*tert*-butylphenol).
$C_{31}H_{48}O_2S_2$=516.9.

CAS — 23288-49-5.

Pharmacopoeias. In *U.S.*

A white to off-white crystalline powder. **Insoluble** in water; soluble in alcohol and petroleum spirit; freely soluble in chloroform and propyl alcohol. **Store** in well-closed containers. Protect from light.

Adverse Effects

The commonest side-effects of probucol therapy are gastro-intestinal upsets with diarrhoea occurring in about 10% of patients; flatulence, abdominal pain, nausea, and vomiting may also occur. Many other adverse effects have been recorded but the reports appear to be mainly isolated and anecdotal.

Side-effects reported by 29 patients receiving probucol were diarrhoea (2), nausea and vomiting (2), abdominal pain (1), constipation (1), dizziness (3), headache (3), insomnia (1), and visual disturbance (2).— D. T. Nash, *J. clin. Pharmac.*, 1974, *14*, 470.

Side-effects reported during a 1-year study involving 88 patients given probucol decreased after the first 3 months of therapy. The most common was loose stools or diarrhoea; constipation was reported much less frequently. Other side-effects which occurred were flatulence, vertigo, dizziness, a different odour of the skin, and pruritus. No patient withdrew from the study because of side-effects.— D. McCaughan, *Artery*, 1982, *10*, 56.

EFFECTS ON THE BILIARY TRACT. A short-term study in 12 patients with hypercholesterolaemia showed that treatment with probucol did not influence biliary lipid values and concluded that probucol should not be associated with an increased prevalence of cholesterol gallstones.— M. C. Bateson *et al.* (letter), *Br. J. clin. Pharmac.*, 1981, *11*, 531.

EFFECTS ON THE ENDOCRINE SYSTEM. Menstrual irregularity, consisting of a 20-day period of blood loss, associated with probucol in 1 patient.— G. Isaacs (letter), *Br. med. J.*, 1985, *291*, 450.

EFFECTS ON THE HEART. Evaluation, as recommended by the FDA, of 198 patients who had received probucol for 5 years or more, revealed that changes in the QT interval of the ECG had occurred with increases predominating.— G. Troendle *et al.* (letter), *Lancet*, 1982, *1*, 1179. Further correspondence.— B. L. Martz (letter), *ibid.*, 1365; D. McCaughan (letter), *ibid.*, *2*, 161. A double-blind crossover study in 42 type II hyperlipoproteinaemic patients showed no correlation between plasma-concentration of probucol and the lengthening of the QT interval. Over the 18 months to 2 years of the study, nearly half of the patients on probucol showed a lengthening of QT interval but this was not statistically significant, and there was no clinical or electrocardiographic evidence of arrhythmia in any of the patients studied.— C. A. Dujovne *et al.*, *Eur. J. clin. Pharmac.*, 1984, *26*, 735.

Absorption and Fate

The absorption of probucol from the gastro-intestinal tract is limited and variable, and is stated to be at a maximum if taken with food. Peak concentrations in blood are achieved after 3 or 4 months' treatment. Probucol accumulates in adipose tissue and concentrations fall only slowly, over several months, when treatment is withdrawn. Excretion is considered to be chiefly by the biliary system into the faeces.

Uses and Administration

Probucol is used as a hypolipidaemic agent, in conjunction with dietary modification, in the treatment of hypercholesterolaemia, particularly type II hyperlipoproteinaemia. The usual dose by mouth is 500 mg twice daily, given with the morning and evening meals.

Reference to probucol in benign prostatic hyperplasia.— M. I. Resnick *et al.*, *J. Urol., Baltimore*, 1983, *129*, 206.

HYPERLIPIDAEMIAS. For the use of probucol, as a hypolipidaemic agent, in the prevention of ischaemic heart disease, see Ischaemic Heart Disease, under Uses of Clofibrate (p.1199).

With cholestyramine. Beneficial effects following the addition of probucol 500 mg twice daily to therapy in 7 patients with familial type II hyperlipoproteinaemia who had shown an inadequate response to cholestyramine 16 g daily.— J. I. Mann *et al.* (letter), *Lancet*, 1981, *1*, 450. Similar results following the addition of cholestyramine 8 g daily in 6 patients who had not responded satisfactorily to probucol alone.— R. Pasquali *et al.* (letter), *ibid.*, 1368.

Further reports of beneficial responses with a combination of cholestyramine and probucol: T. W. Boyden and L. Totman, *J. clin. Pharmac.*, 1981, *21*, 48; P. J. Nestel (letter), *Ann. intern. Med.*, 1982, *97*, 622.

With colestipol. Results of a double-blind double-placebo diet-controlled crossover study lasting 18 months in 47 patients with type II hypercholesterolaemia comparing the effects of combined therapy with probucol 500 mg twice daily (with lunch and dinner) and colestipol 10 g twice daily (before breakfast and at bedtime) with those of each agent given alone. Mean reduction in serum low-density lipoprotein cholesterol concentration was 12% with probucol, 23% with colestipol, and 29% with the combination. The gastro-intestinal side-effects of each drug were decreased considerably or disappeared when both drugs were given together. It was considered that co-administration of colestipol and probucol may provide a practical, safe, and effective alternative for patients unresponsive to dietary modification or who have unsatisfactory results or side-effects from resins or other hypolipidaemic drugs.— C. A. Dujovne *et al.*, *Ann. intern. Med.*, 1984, *100*, 477.

Proprietary Preparations

Lurselle *(Merrell, UK). Tablets,* scored, probucol 250 mg.

Proprietary Names and Manufacturers

Bifenabid *(Merrell Dow, Spain)*; Lesterol *(Arg.)*; Lorelco *(Dow, Canad.; Merrell Dow, USA)*; Lurselle *(Merrell Dow, Austral.; Lepetit, Fr.; Merrell, Ger.; Lepetit, Ital.; Mer-National, S.Afr.; Merrell Dow, Switz.; Merrell, UK)*; Panesclerina *(Infale, Spain)*; Superlipid *(Berenguer-Beneyto, Spain).*

1357-v

Pyridoxine Clofibrate
4,5-Bis(hydroxymethyl)-3-hydroxy-2-methylpyridine 2-(4-chlorophenoxy)-2-methylpropionate.
$C_8H_{11}NO_3,C_{10}H_{11}ClO_3$=383.8.

CAS — 29952-87-2.

Pyridoxine clofibrate is used as a hypolipidaemic agent.

For a report of the absorption and fate of pyridoxine clofibrate, see Clofibrate, p.1199.

Proprietary Names and Manufacturers
Claresan *(Latema, Belg.; Sarbach, Fr.).*

1358-g

Simfibrate *(rINN).*
CLY-503. Trimethylene bis[2-(4-chlorophenoxy)-2-methylpropionate].
$C_{23}H_{26}Cl_2O_6$=469.4.

CAS — 14929-11-4.

Simfibrate, a clofibrate analogue, is used as a hypolipidaemic agent.

Proprietary Names and Manufacturers
Cholesolvin *(Sanders-Probel, Belg.; Cyanamid, Ital.; Jpn)*; Liposolvin *(Tosi-Novara, Ital.)*; Sinfibrex *(Isnardi, Ital.).*

2452-l

Simvastatin *(BAN, USAN, pINN).*
MK-733; Synvinolin; Velastatin. 2, 2-Dimethylbutyric acid, 8-ester with (4*R*,6*R*)-6-[2-[(1*S*,2*S*,6*R*,8*S*,8a*R*)-1,2,6,7,8,8a-hexahydro-8-hydroxy-2,6-dimethyl-1-naphthyl]ethyl]tetrahydro-hydroxy-2*H*-pyran-2-one.
$C_{25}H_{38}O_5$=418.6.

CAS — 79902-63-9.

Simvastatin which has been isolated from *Aspergillus terreus* is a hypolipidaemic agent. Like lovastatin it acts as a competitive inhibitor of 3-hyroxy-3-methylglutaryl coenzyme A reductase (HMG CoA reductase).

A discussion of 3-hydroxy-3-methylglutaryl-coenzyme A reductase inhibitors including simvastatin.—J. M. Hoeg and H. B. Brewer, *J. Am. med. Ass.*, 1987, *258*, 3532.

References to the use of simvastatin in the treatment of hypercholesterolaemia: A. G. Olsson *et al.* (letter), *Lancet*, 1986, *2*, 390; M. J. T. M. Mol *et al.*, *ibid.*, 936; P. Wersweiler and P. Schwandt, *ibid.*, 1212; L. A. Simons *et al.*, *Med. J. Aust.*, 1987, *147*, 65; P. Schulzeck *et al.*, *Lancet*, 1988, *1*, 611.

Proprietary Names and Manufacturers
Merck Sharp & Dohme, USA.

13237-g

Sitofibrate *(rINN).*
Stigmast-5-en-3*β*-ol 2-(4-chlorophenoxy)-2-methylpropionate.
$C_{39}H_{59}ClO_3$=611.3.

CAS — 55902-94-8.

Sitofibrate, a derivative of clofibrate and sitosterol, is used as a hypolipidaemic agent.

Proprietary Names and Manufacturers
Longeril *(Ferrer, Spain).*

1359-q

Sitosterol
β-Sitosterin; *β*-Sitosterol. Stigmast-5-en-3*β*-ol.
$C_{29}H_{50}O$=414.7.

CAS — 83-46-5.

Sitosterol is used as a hypolipidaemic agent. It has also been used in various disorders of the prostate gland.

Proprietary Names and Manufacturers
Cytellin *(Lilly, USA)*; Harzol *(Hoyer, Ger.)*; Prostasal *(TAD, Ger.)*; Sito-Lande *(Delalande, Ger.).*

13262-q

Sorbinicate *(rINN).*
D-Glucitol hexanicotinate.
$C_{42}H_{32}N_6O_{12}$=812.7.

CAS — 6184-06-1.

Sorbinicate is used as a hypolipidaemic agent.

Proprietary Names and Manufacturers
Nicosterolo *(Guidotti, Ital.).*

13285-j

Sulodexide *(rINN).*
Glucurono-2-amino-2-deoxyglucoglucan sulphate.

CAS — 57821-29-1.

Sulodexide is used as a hypolipidaemic agent.

Proprietary Names and Manufacturers
Aterol *(Morrith, Spain)*; Gulenor *(Guidotti, Ital.)*; Luzone *(Aristegui, Spain)*; Provenal *(Pulitzer, Ital.)*; Vessel *(Alfa Farmaceutici, Ital.).*

13289-a

Surfomer *(USAN, rINN).*
AOMA. Poly(1,2-dicarboxy-3-hexadecyltetramethylene).
$(C_{22}H_{40}O_4)_n$.

CAS — 71251-04-2.

Surfomer is reported to be a hypolipidaemic agent.

Proprietary Names and Manufacturers
Monsanto, USA.

12720-s

Theofibrate *(USAN).*
Etofylline Clofibrate *(rINN)*; ML-1024. 2-(Theophyllin-7-yl)ethyl 2-(4-chlorophenoxy)-2-methylpropionate.
$C_{19}H_{21}ClN_4O_5$=420.9.

CAS — 54504-70-0.

Theofibrate, a clofibrate analogue, is used as a hypolipidaemic agent.

Proprietary Names and Manufacturers
Duolip *(Merckle, Ger.; Mepha, Switz.).*

1360-d

Tiadenol *(rINN).*
LL-1558. 2,2′-(Decamethylenedithio)bisethanol.
$C_{14}H_{30}O_2S_2$=294.5.

CAS — 6964-20-1.

Tiadenol is used as a hypolipidaemic agent.

Proprietary Names and Manufacturers
Braxan *(Bago, Arg.)*; Delipid *(Coop. Farm., Ital.)*; Endol *(Cruz, Spain)*; Eulip *(Boehringer Biochemia, Ital.)*; Fonlipol *(Lafon, Fr.; Recordati, Ital.)*; Meralycin *(Disprovent, Arg.)*; Millaterol *(Andreu, Spain)*; Norlipol *(Ifesa, Spain)*; Tiabrenolo *(Brocchieri, Ital.)*; Tiaclar *(CT, Ital.)*; Tiaden *(Malesci, Ital.)*; Tiaterol *(Midy, Ital.)*; Tiodenol *(Uquifa, Spain).*

1361-n

Tibric Acid *(BAN, USAN, rINN).*
CP-18524. 2-Chloro-5-(*cis*-3,5-dimethylpiperidinosulphonyl)benzoic acid.
$C_{14}H_{18}ClNO_4S$=331.8.

CAS — 37087-94-8.

Tibric acid has been used as a hypolipidaemic agent.

Proprietary Names and Manufacturers
Pfizer, USA.

3916-y

Tocofibrate *(rINN).*
2,5,7,8-Tetramethyl-2-(4,8,12-trimethyltridecyl)-6-chromanyl 2-(*p*-chlorophenoxy)-2-methylpropionate.
$C_{39}H_{59}ClO_4$=627.3.

CAS — 50465-39-9.

Tocofibrate has been given for its hypolipidaemic properties in the treatment of disorders of lipid metabolism, in usual doses of 800 mg by mouth three times daily.

Proprietary Names and Manufacturers
Transferal *(Ferrer, Spain).*

7899-j

Tocopheryl Nicotinate

Vitamin E Nicotinate. (±)-α-Tocopherol nicotinate.
$C_{35}H_{53}NO_3$=535.8.

CAS — 51898-34-1.

Tocopheryl nicotinate is a vitamin E substance which has been used in the treatment of hyperlipidaemia.

Proprietary Names and Manufacturers
Disclar *(Casen Fisons, Spain)*; Juvela Nicotinate *(Jpn)*; Nicobita-E *(Jpn)*; Nicoferol *(Jpn)*; Renascin *(Mack, Illert., Ger.; IFI, Ital.).*

14021-r

Xenbucin *(USAN, rINN).*
MG-1559. 2-(Biphenyl-4-yl)butyric acid.
$C_{16}H_{16}O_2$=240.3.

CAS — 959-10-4.

Xenbucin has been used as a hypolipidaemic agent.

Proprietary Names and Manufacturers
Liposana *(Ital.).*

Local Anaesthetics

7600-h

The local anaesthetics are compounds which produce reversible loss of sensation by preventing or diminishing the conduction of sensory nerve impulses near to the site of their application or injection. Local anaesthetics could also be described as local analgesics as they are most often used to produce loss of pain without loss of nervous control. Also because their mode of action is to decrease permeability of the nerve cell membrane to sodium ions they are considered to have a membrane stabilising effect.

Clinically useful local anaesthetics have the same general chemical configuration of an amine portion joined to an aromatic residue by an ester or amide link. Local anaesthetics with an ester link are usually esters of *p*-aminobenzoic acid. The type of linkage is important in determining the properties of the drug.

Local anaesthetics of the ester type include: amethocaine, p.1208, benzocaine, p.1208, cocaine, p.1213, procaine, p.1225.

Local anaesthetics of the amide type include: bupivacaine, p.1209, cinchocaine, p.1212, etidocaine, p.1215, lignocaine, p.1217, mepivacaine, p.1223, prilocaine, p.1225.

Other drugs with local anaesthetic actions include aerosol propellents, some antihistamines, some beta-adrenoceptor blocking agents, some antimuscarinic agents, some anti-arrhythmic agents, benzyl alcohol, menthol, and phenol.

Adverse Effects of Local Anaesthetics

Side-effects apparent after local anaesthesia may be due to the anaesthetic or to errors in technique or may be the result of blockade of the sympathetic nervous system. Local anaesthetics may have systemic adverse effects as a result of the raised plasma concentrations which ensue when the rate of absorption into the circulation exceeds the rate of breakdown, for example, after excessive dosage or accidental intravenous injection or by absorption of large amounts through mucous membranes or damaged skin or from highly vascular areas. Adverse effects may also occur due to the addition of vasoconstrictors.

Allergic reactions to local anaesthetics are rare and generally limited to agents of the ester type. There appears to be no cross-sensitivity between ester and amide type local anaesthetics. Idiosyncrasy to local anaesthetics has been reported. Vasovagal attacks may be associated with local anaesthesia. Local anaesthetics are potent sensitisers and allergic reactions may occur as a result of repeated handling or topical use. Allergic reactions to preservatives in local anaesthetics preparations have been reported.

The systemic toxicity of local anaesthetics mainly involves the central nervous system and the cardiovascular system. Excitation of the CNS may be manifested by restlessness, excitement, nervousness, dizziness, tinnitus, blurred vision, nausea and vomiting, muscle twitching and tremors, and convulsions. Numbness of the tongue and perioral region may appear as an early sign of systemic toxicity. Excitation may be transient and followed by depression with drowsiness, respiratory failure, and coma. There may be simultaneous effects on the cardiovascular system with myocardial depression and peripheral vasodilatation resulting in hypotension and bradycardia; arrhythmias and cardiac arrest may occur. Hypotension often accompanies spinal and epidural anaesthesia; inappropriate positioning of the patient may be a contributory factor for women in labour.

Some local anaesthetics cause methaemoglobinaemia.

Foetal intoxication has occurred following the use of local anaesthetics in labour, either as a result of the transplacental diffusion or after accidental injection of the foetus.

Reviews of adverse effects of local anaesthetics: M. H. Alper, *New Engl. J. Med.*, 1976, *295*, 1432; F. Reynolds, *Br. J. Anaesth.*, 1987, *59*, 78.

A report of 3 deaths associated with paracervical anaesthesia for first trimester abortion. In the first 2 patients the deaths were associated with lignocaine overdosage and possible intravascular injection, but the third might have been associated with intolerance to mepivacaine. A further 2 deaths have been reported between 1972 and 1975. Paracervical anaesthesia should only be given when resuscitative drugs and equipment and staff skilled in their use are available.— D. A. Grimes and W. Cates, *New Engl. J. Med.*, 1976, *295*, 1397. Comments. Adverse reactions can occur with local anaesthetics when used in recommended doses. Since the paracervical region is highly vascular, the site of injection is more important than 'dose limits'.— R. H. de Jong (letter), *ibid.*, 1977, *296*, 760. In view of the large number of first trimester abortions performed with lignocaine, the safety record of a 200-mg dose of lignocaine is impressive.— M. L. Schwartz (letter), *ibid.*

ALLERGY AND EFFECTS ON THE SKIN. Allergic reactions to local anaesthetics are uncommon and hypotension during dental anaesthesia is usually a vasovagal response and is associated with bradycardia. The vasovagal response is unrelated to the type of anaesthetic used and may be prevented by premedication with atropine sulphate 600 µg intravenously or with a sedative such as diazepam.— *Br. med. J.*, 1980, *280*, 1360. See also *ibid.*, *281*, 211.

Apart from lignocaine, local anaesthetics should not be applied to the skin because of the real danger of their causing contact dermatitis. Sensitised patients may subsequently develop a widespread eruption when similar drugs are given systemically. The use of strong sensitisers such as benzocaine and amethocaine in lozenges and throat sprays may also sensitise patients.— J. Verbov, *Practitioner*, 1979, *222*, 400.

Prilocaine 0.5% solution given intradermally as a test dose to a patient with suspected lignocaine allergy produced a local flare reaction which faded after 15 minutes. However, when bupivacaine was given to the same patient an urticarial rash developed over the upper limbs and chest and there were visual difficulties and a tightness in the throat. This systemic reaction was diagnosed as an antibody-mediated allergic reaction.— D. T. Brown *et al.*, *Br. J. Anaesth.*, 1981, *53*, 435.

A patient who had shown severe anaphylactoid reactions to both lignocaine and prilocaine underwent intradermal testing with dilutions of local anaesthetic agents. Positive wheal and flare reactions occurred at high dilutions with lignocaine, prilocaine, and amethocaine but there was no reaction to bupivacaine, even at low dilution. The patient subsequently received bupivacaine for an episiotomy with no adverse effects.— M. M. Fisher and J. C. Pennington, *Br. J. Anaesth.*, 1982, *54*, 893.

Intradermal skin tests with lignocaine 2% and prilocaine 1% in 37 patients who had a previous history of suspected allergy to local anaesthetics gave a positive wheal and flare response to prilocaine in only 2 patients and to lignocaine in only 1 patient. Lymphocyte proliferation to prilocaine and lignocaine respectively was also noted ***in vitro*** suggesting a cell-mediated immune response.— A. V. Babajews and L. Ivanyi, *Br. dent. J.*, 1982, *152*, 385.

A severe systemic allergic reaction occurred in a 14-year-old child with suspected lignocaine-allergy after an intradermal test dose of diluted lignocaine injection. Blood pressure and pulse were unrecordable and there was gross cyanosis, but symptoms responded to adrenaline injection. The author warns that topical use of local anaesthetics may sensitise patients and subsequently result in anaphylactic reactions.— P. M. Mulvey (letter), ***Med. J. Aust.***, 1980, *1*, 386.

EFFECTS ON THE BLOOD. A report of methaemoglobinaemia in a patient who received topical application of Cetacaine spray (benzocaine 14%, butyl aminobenzoate 2%, amethocaine 2%) and benzocaine ointment for endotracheal intubation. Methylene blue 1% solution, given intravenously produced marked clinical improvement and disappearance of the cyanosis. Rechallenge with topical application of lignocaine 4% and benzocaine ointment also caused methaemoglobinaemia which responded to methylene blue 1 mg per kg body-weight intravenously. Benzocaine was thought to be the causative agent, although lignocaine could not be excluded.— M. L. Olson and G. K. McEvoy, *Am. J. Hosp. Pharm.*, 1981, *38*, 89.

EFFECTS ON THE CARDIOVASCULAR SYSTEM. A review of the cardiotoxicity of local anaesthetic agents from *animal* studies.— S. Reiz and S. Nath, *Br. J. Anaesth.*, 1986, *58*, 736.

EFFECTS ON THE EAR. Transient hearing loss of low-frequency sound occurred in 8 of 100 patients after spinal anaesthesia. Recovery was spontaneous within 1 or 2 days.— B. Panning *et al.* (letter), *Lancet*, 1983, *2*, 582. Comment. Hearing loss may be explained by a fall in cerebrospinal fluid pressure leading to accumulation of fluid in the inner ear.— A. G. Gordon (letter), *ibid.*, 793.

EFFECTS ON THE EYES. Severe contact keratitis can develop from the prolonged use of topical anaesthetics in the eye. Local anaesthetics are known to inhibit the rate of movement of corneal epithelial cells migrating to cover wounds.— R. P. Burns and I. Gipson (letter), *J. Am. med. Ass.*, 1978, *240*, 347.

EFFECTS ON THE NERVOUS SYSTEM. Adverse effects of local anaesthetic agents on the central nervous system are seen most commonly after accidental intravenous injection. Signs and symptoms of toxicity after intravenous administration may progress from numbness of the tongue and mouth, light-headedness, tinnitus, visual disturbances, and slurring of speech through to unconsciousness, convulsions, coma, and apnoea, unless toxicity is recognised and the infusion stopped. Signs and symptoms can change rapidly and convulsions may be the first sign of toxicity. It is suggested that injections of local anaesthetics are always given slowly, even if a test dose has been negative, and rapport with the patient is maintained so as to elicit early symptoms of toxicity.— D. B. Scott, *Br. J. Anaesth.*, 1986, *58*, 732.

A unilateral Horner's syndrome has occurred many times after epidural and caudal analgesia.— D. V. Thomas (letter), *Br. J. Anaesth.*, 1976, *48*, 611. See also L. E. S. Carrie and J. Mohan (letter), *ibid.*

PREGNANCY AND THE NEONATE. There are conflicting views on whether epidural anaesthesia during labour is associated with neonatal jaundice. Although Gould *et al.* (*Br. med. J.*, 1974, *3*, 228) found that bupivacaine had no significant effect on neonatal serum-bilirubin concentrations and Bromage (*Lancet*, 1979, *1*, 669) has insisted that allegations associating epidural anaesthesia with neonatal jaundice are unfounded, other workers (N. Campbell *et al.*, *Br. med. J.*, 1975, *2*, 548; P.J. Lewis and L.A. Friedman, *Lancet*, 1979, *1*, 669; B. Wood *et al.*, *Archs Dis. Childh.*, 1979, *54*, 111) have reported that epidural anaesthesia is associated with an increased frequency of neonatal jaundice.

Comment on maternal deaths attributable to anaesthesia between 1973 and 1975.— D. D. Moir, *Br. J. Anaesth.*, 1980, *52*, 1.

Treatment of Adverse Effects

Absorption of local anaesthetics from the site of injection may be reduced, if necessary, by applying a tourniquet. When systemic reactions to local anaesthetics occur steps should be taken to maintain the circulation and respiration and to control convulsions. A patent airway must be established and oxygen given, together with assisted ventilation if necessary. The circulation should be maintained with infusions of plasma or intravenous fluids. Vasopressor agents have been suggested in the treatment of marked hypotension although their use is accompanied by a risk of CNS excitation. Vasopressors should not be given to patients receiving oxytocic drugs. Convulsions may be controlled by the intravenous administration of diazepam or thiopentone sodium. It should be remembered that anticonvulsant treatment may also depress respiration and the circulation. A short-acting neuromuscular blocking agent, together with endotracheal intubation and artificial respiration, has been used when convulsions persist.

Methaemoglobinaemia may be treated by the intravenous administration of a 1% solution of methylene blue.

For reference to the treatment of neonates injected accidentally with mepivacaine during labour, see Mepivacaine Hydrochloride, p.1223.

Precautions for Local Anaesthetics

The use of local anaesthetics is contra-indicated in patients with known hypersensitivity. It may be possible to avoid reactions by using a local anaesthetic of the alternative chemical type. Small doses have been given as a test for hypersensitivity but the results are not necessarily reliable. Facilities for resuscitation should be available when local anaesthetics are administered. Local anaesthetics should be given cautiously to patients with epilepsy, impaired cardiac conduction, shock, or with liver damage; patients with myasthenia gravis are particularly susceptible to the effects of local anaesthetics. The ester type of local anaesthetic is contra-indicated in patients with low plasma-cholinesterase concentrations or in those receiving anticholinesterases. Techniques such as epidural or spinal anaesthesia should not be employed in patients with cerebrospinal diseases. Doses should generally be reduced in elderly and debilitated patients and in children.

The risk of adverse effects from the absorption of local anaesthetics may be reduced by the inclusion of adrenaline to produce vasoconstriction but the lowest effective concentration of adrenaline should be used. Solutions containing adrenaline should not, however, be used for producing anaesthesia in appendages such as digits, because the profound ischaemia that follows may lead to gangrene. Prilocaine and mepivacaine do not require the addition of a vasoconstrictor and can be used in these cases. If local anaesthetics containing adrenaline are given for caudal, epidural, or paracervical block during labour the use of an oxytocic drug post partum may lead to severe hypertension. For details of the precautions to be observed when local anaesthetics containing adrenaline or noradrenaline are needed in patients receiving monoamine oxidase inhibitors, some volatile anaesthetics, and some other drugs, see p.1454 and p.1471 respectively.

When used in the mouth or throat, local anaesthetics may impair swallowing and increase the risk of aspiration and patients should be cautioned not to eat for at least 60 minutes after the anaesthetic.

The effect of local anaesthetics may be reduced if the injection is made into an inflamed or infected area with a low tissue pH. The cornea may be damaged by prolonged application of anaesthetic eye-drops and ointment, and the anaesthetised eye should be protected from dust and bacterial contamination.

The application of local anaesthetics to the skin for prolonged periods or to extensive areas should be avoided.

EFFECTS ON DRIVING. Minimum times during which driving is not recommneded after outpatient anaesthesia with the following local anaesthetics: lignocaine 500 mg with adrenaline intramuscularly, no limitations; dental local anaesthesia, 1 hour; lignocaine (plain) 200 mg intramuscularly, 1 to 1.5 hours; bupivacaine (plain) 1.3 mg per kg body-weight intramuscularly, 2 to 4 hours; etidocaine (plain) 2.6 mg per kg intramuscularly, 2 to 4 hours.— K. Korttila, *Mod. Problems Pharmacopsychiat.*, 1976, *11*, 91.

INFLAMMATION. A discussion of the failure of local anaesthetics in acute inflammation.— R. D. Brown, *Br. dent. J.*, 1981, *151*, 47.

MALIGNANT HYPERPYREXIA. An extensive search of the literature revealed no specific reference to malignant hyperpyrexia being caused solely by the use of amide local anaesthetics; it is questionable whether there is any evidence that they are contra-indicated in malignant hyperpyrexia.— M. G. Adragna (letter), *Anesthesiology*, 1985, *62*, 99. A recommendation that amide type local anaesthetics should no longer be avoided in patients susceptible to or suspected of having malignant hyperpyrexia.— A. K. W. Brownell and R. T. Paasuke, *Can. med. Ass. J.*, 1986, *134*, 993.

TACHYPHYLAXIS. When 329 epidural injections of 2% solutions of lignocaine, mepivacaine, or prilocaine, with or without adrenaline 1:200 000, were given to 140 patients, in successive injections, each dose of anaesthetic was 25 to 30% less effective than its predecessor when intervals between injections were greater than 10 minutes. Augmentation of anaesthesia was obtained if successive injections were given after an interval of less than 10 minutes.— P. R. Bromage *et al.*, *J. clin. Pharmac.*, 1969, *9*, 30.

THROMBO-EMBOLIC DISORDERS. Local anaesthetics must not be given by the epidural or spinal routes in patients requiring anticoagulants, since a haematoma in the region of the spinal cord may lead to neurological complications.— *Drug & Ther. Bull.*, 1984, *22*, 73.

Absorption and Fate

Most local anaesthetics are readily absorbed through mucous membranes, and through damaged skin. Local anaesthetics are weak bases and at tissue pH can diffuse through connective tissue and cellular membranes to reach the nerve fibre where ionisation can occur. While some local anaesthetics are active in the cationic form, others are active in the non-ionised form.

Anaesthetics of the ester type are hydrolysed by esterases in the plasma and, to a lesser extent, in the liver. The effect of spinal anaesthetics lasts until the drug is absorbed into the blood since there is little esterase in the spinal fluid.

Amide-type anaesthetics are metabolised in the liver and, in some cases, the kidneys. While there is little protein binding with the ester-type anaesthetics, the amide types are considerably bound.

A detailed review of the pharmacokinetics of local anaesthetics.— G. T. Tucker, *Br. J. Anaesth.*, 1986, *58*, 717.

PREGNANCY AND THE NEONATE. Reviews of the pharmacokinetics of local anaesthetics during labour and childbirth, and in neonates: R. L. Nation, *Clin. Pharmacokinet.*, 1980, *5*, 340; P. L. Morselli *et al.*, *Clin. Pharmacokinet.*, 1980, *5*, 485; H. Nau, *Develop. Pharmac. Ther.*, 1985, *8*, 149; J. Kanto, *Clin. Pharmacokinet.*, 1986, *11*, 283.

Uses of Local Anaesthetics

Local anaesthetics act by preventing generation and transmission of impulses along nerve fibres and at nerve endings; depolarisation and ion-exchange are inhibited. The effects are reversible. The lipid-soluble anaesthetic base must penetrate the lipoprotein nerve sheath before it can act. In general, loss of pain (analgesia) occurs before loss of sensory and autonomic function (anaesthesia) and loss of motor function (paralysis), but this may depend on the drug used and the site of administration. The effectiveness of an anaesthetic depends on the concentration attained at the nerve fibre. There is a latent period before the onset of action which varies according to the agent used, the concentration used, and the method of administration.

Local anaesthetics are generally administered as acidic solutions of the water-soluble hydrochloride salts. Formulations employing the carbonated base rather than the hydrochloride have also been used. When adrenaline is added, a solution of about pH 3 to 5 is necessary to ensure stability.

The smallest effective dose and the lowest effective concentration should be used. Smaller doses are needed in elderly and debilitated patients and in children. Meticulous attention to technique is essential particularly in nerve block and spinal procedures. In spinal anaesthesia sterility of the injection and equipment must be meticulously preserved. Injections for central nerve block, such as epidural or caudal block, and spinal anaesthesia should not contain preservatives.

Local anaesthetics may be administered in many different ways, some compounds being more suitable than others for a particular route of administration. The agents described in this chapter vary in their potency and speed of onset and duration of action. For example, lignocaine, etidocaine, mepivacaine, and prilocaine have a fast onset of action and bupivacaine a slower onset of action. When classified according to their duration of action chloroprocaine and procaine are short-acting; lignocaine, mepivacaine, and prilocaine are intermediate-acting; and amethocaine, bupivacaine, cinchocaine, and etidocaine are long-acting. The effect is sometimes prolonged by the addition of a vasoconstrictor and solutions containing adrenaline 1 in 200 000 are generally advocated. Felypressin and noradrenaline are also used. The total amount of adrenaline injected should not exceed 500 µg although some consider that the maximum dose should be 200 µg.

Surface or **topical anaesthesia** blocks the sensory nerve endings in the skin or mucous membranes, but to reach these structures the drug must have good powers of penetration. Many of the local anaesthetics are effective surface anaesthetics, a notable exception being procaine hydrochloride. There are a number of special uses of topical anaesthesia including anaesthetising the cornea during ophthalmological procedures and the throat and larynx before intubation and bronchoscopy. Great care is necessary when employing local anaesthetics to anaesthetise the urethra; if trauma has occurred, rapid absorption of the drug may occur and give rise to serious adverse effects. Absorption from the respiratory tract is also rapid and care is essential to avoid administering a toxic dose.

The local anaesthetics mainly used for surface anaesthesia are amethocaine, benzocaine, cocaine, lignocaine, and prilocaine. In ophthalmological procedures amethocaine, oxybuprocaine, and proxymetacaine are used.

Infiltration anaesthesia is produced by injection of an anaesthetic agent into and around the field of operation. The drug must not be absorbed too rapidly otherwise the anaesthesia will wear off too quickly for practical use; many of the synthetic local anaesthetics require the addition of a vasoconstrictor, such as a small amount of adrenaline. If adrenaline is added to such drugs a larger total dose may be given. In dentistry, infiltration anaesthesia is extensively used.

Chloroprocaine, etidocaine, lignocaine, mepivacaine, prilocaine, and procaine are the compounds mainly used for infiltration anaesthesia.

Regional nerve block anaesthesia may include field block, peripheral nerve block, and central nerve block. In *field block* anaesthesia sensory nerve paths are blocked by subcutaneous injection of local anaesthetic close to nerves around the area to be anaesthetised. *Peripheral nerve block* anaesthesia involves injection into or around a peripheral nerve or plexus supplying the part to be anaesthetised; motor fibres may be blocked as well as sensory fibres. Examples of this type of block include brachial plexus block, intercostal nerve block, paracervical block, and pudendal block. Adrenaline is often added as a vasoconstrictor but it must not be used when producing a nerve block in an appendage, as gangrene may occur.

Epidural anaesthesia (*extradural* or *peridural anaesthesia*) is a form of *central nerve block*. Continuous epidural anaesthesia is employed in obstetrics, local anaesthetic being introduced by means of a cannula into the extradural space in the lumbar region in order to block the roots of sensory nerves supplying the uterus and lower birth canal; lignocaine or bupivacaine are the agents generally used. In *caudal anaesthesia* an epidural injection is made through the sacral hiatus. A test dose at the intended injection site is recommended before starting epidural anaesthesia.

For regional nerve block the compounds mainly used are bupivacaine, chloroprocaine, etidocaine, lignocaine, mepivacaine, prilocaine, and procaine.

Spinal or **subarachnoid** or **intrathecal anaesthesia** is another special form of regional anaesthesia; it is produced by injecting a solution of a suitable drug within the spinal theca, intrathecally, causing temporary paralysis of the nerves with which it comes into contact. The addition of adrenaline is usually avoided because of the danger of restricting the blood supply to the spinal cord.

The somatic level at which anaesthesia occurs depends on the specific gravity of the anaesthetic solution used and the positioning of the patient. **Hypobaric solutions** are lighter than the cerebrospinal fluid and rise, thus producing anaesthesia of thoracic structures in a suitably positioned patient. **Isobaric solutions** have about the same specific gravity as the cerebrospinal fluid and produce their effect at about the level of the intrathecal injection.

Hyperbaric solutions are heavier than the cerebrospinal fluid and thus exert their effects at levels lower than the site of injection. They are used mainly for operations on the lower limbs and the perineum.

For spinal anaesthesia, amethocaine, bupivacaine, cinchocaine, lignocaine, mepivacaine, and prilocaine have been used.

In **intravenous regional anaesthesia** *(Bier's block)*a dilute solution of local anaesthetic is injected into a suitable limb vein after application of a tourniquet, in order to produce anaesthesia distal to it. Arterial flow must remain occluded and adrenaline should not be used. Prilocaine and bupivacaine have been used for this technique.

In **intravenous analgesia,** local anaesthetics have been injected by continuous infusion to produce a general analgesia but the technique is potentially dangerous and seldom employed.

Reviews on the actions and uses of local anaesthetics: M. Concepcion and B. G. Covino, *Drugs*, 1984, *27*, 256; J. A. W. Wildsmith, *Br. J. Anaesth.*, 1986, *58*, 692; B. G. Covino, *ibid.*, 701.

Further references to the use of local anaesthetics: J. M. Kidd *et al.*, *Aust. J. Hosp. Pharm.*, 1977, *7*, 73 (in children); E. D. Allen and A. R. Elkington, *Br. J. Anaesth.*, 1980, *52*, 689 (in anaesthesia of the eye); D. S. Arthur and L. R. McNicol, *ibid.*, 1986, *58*, 760 (in paediatric surgery); M. E. Dodson, *Br. J. Hosp. Med.*, 1987, *37*, 114 (in the elderly).

CAUDAL BLOCK. Analysis of the spread of analgesia after caudal injection in 3 groups totalling 152 children showed a linear relationship between the spread of analgesia and age. A regression line for predicting dose requirements was developed.— O. Schulte-Steinberg and V. W. Rahlfs, *Br. J. Anaesth.*, 1977, *49*, 1027.

EPIDURAL BLOCK. The effects of concentration of local anaesthetic on epidural block for surgery were assessed in a double-blind study of 60 patients. Increasing the concentration of bupivacaine from 0.5 to 0.75% and of etidocaine from 1 to 1.5% appeared to offer significant clinical advantages since there was a more rapid onset of sensory analgesia and motor blockade, a greater frequency of adequate analgesia, a greater depth of motor block, and a longer duration of effect. There was no significant advantage when the concentration of prilocaine was increased from 2 to 3%.— D. B. Scott *et al.*, *Br. J. Anaesth.*, 1980, *52*, 1033.

In obstetrics. A review of epidural analgesia in obstetrics.— *Drug & Ther. Bull.*, 1983, *21*, 29. The use of local anaesthetics for epidural and spinal analgesia in obstetrics, and the effects on the foetus and neonate.— D. D. Moir, *Br. J. Anaesth.*, 1986, *58*, 747.

A discussion of the continuous epidural infusion of local anaesthetics. This technique is preferable to intermittent 'top-up' injections for epidural analgesia, potentially avoiding the painful interval between top-up injections.— *Lancet*, 1987, *1*, 1300. Continuous epidural infusion of a low concentration of local anaesthetic may minimise the rate of forceps delivery thus reducing maternal and foetal trauma and pain.— M. J. Turner *et al.* (letter), *ibid.*, 1497.

In a study of the effects of anaesthesia on the adrenocortical response to caesarean section, maternal plasma cortisol concentrations were found to increase significantly in patients receiving general anaesthesia whereas concentrations did not change significantly in those receiving epidural anaesthesia. The method of anaesthesia did not influence the cortisol response of the foetus.— Y. Namba *et al.*, *Br. J. Anaesth.*, 1980, *52*, 1027. Further references to the effects of epidural anaesthesia on the response to surgical stress: M. R. Brandt *et al.*, *Br. med. J.*, 1978, *1*, 1106; J. Rem *et al.*, *Lancet*, 1980, *1*, 283; P. Whelan and P. J. Morris (letter), *ibid.*, 828; I. W. Fellows and A. M. J. Woolfson, *Br. med. Bull.*, 1985, *41*, 287; *Lancet*, 1985, *1*, 1018.

A survey of maternal satisfaction involving 1000 women who had a vaginal delivery found epidural analgesia to be more effective at reducing pain in labour than any other analgesic method used. However, women who had an epidural were less satisfied with the experience of childbirth than those who received an alternative method of analgesia. Assisted delivery also reduced satisfaction and the data suggested an association between forceps delivery and epidural analgesia produced an unfortunate combination of good analgesia with a poor experience. However, an epidural did make childbirth more 'pleasurable' than did an alternative method of analgesia or no analgesia. The survey suggests that epidural analgesia does not confer an improved maternal experience and a reappraisal of its role in labour is needed.— B. M. Morgan *et al.*, *Lancet*, 1982, *2*, 808. Comments. The data presented cannot be fully interpreted since pain relief in labour is influenced by a number of factors and cannot be considered in isolation.— J. Stronge and D. MacDonald (letter), *ibid.*, 991. The degree of dissatisfaction in the women receiving epidural anaesthesia was remarkably low considering that half these patients required assisted delivery.— K. D. MacRae and J. T. Wright (letter), *ibid.*, 992. A similar study.— B. Morgan *et al.*, *Br. med. J.*, 1982, *285*, 689.

In a double-blind study in 40 women undergoing major gynaecological surgery bupivacaine 0.75%, bupivacaine 0.75% with adrenaline 1 in 200 000, etidocaine 1.5%, and etidocaine 1.5% with adrenaline in 200 000 all produced suitable epidural blockade. Onset of sensory and motor blockade was more rapid with etidocaine than bupivacaine. The addition of adrenaline increased the speed of onset of sensory blockade and its duration. Motor blockade was greatest in patients given etidocaine with adrenaline and least in those given bupivacaine alone. Pain returned sooner after etidocaine than after bupivacaine; adrenaline prolonged this period of subjective analgesia.— C. J. Sinclair and D. B. Scott, *Br. J. Anaesth.*, 1984, *56*, 147.

A study comparing 171 healthy women who had caesarean sections under epidural anaesthesia with 91 who were given a general anaesthetic found that epidural block was associated with less postoperative morbidity than general anaesthesia. Less patients in the epidural group experienced pain and discomfort immediately following operation and the incidence of gastro-intestinal stasis, coughing, pyrexia, tiredness, and depression was lower in this group in the following postoperative days. Mothers in the epidural group were also able to start mobilisation and breast feeding earlier than those in the general anaesthetic group. The authors conclude that epidural block is better than a general anaesthetic in the healthy mother.— B. M. Morgan *et al.*, *Lancet*, 1984, *1*, 328.

No appreciable change in foetal blood flow was observed after epidural analgesia with etidocaine and bupivacaine for caesarean section.— A. Lindblad *et al.*, *Br. med. J.*, 1984, *288*, 1329.

Epidural anaesthesia may be beneficial in pregnancy with congestive heart failure, but general anaesthesia is to be preferred if pregnancy is complicated by aortic stenosis, hypertrophic cardiomyopathy, or pulmonary hypertension. Caesarean section may be performed with lumbar, epidural, or general anaesthesia in pregnant patients with cardiac disease; spinal anaesthesia is not the technique of choice.— J. M. Sullivan and K. B. Ramanathan, *New Engl. J. Med.*, 1985, *313*, 304.

Epidural block should be avoided in toxaemia of pregnancy since it is associated with sudden and marked falls in blood pressure and on occasion with vascular collapse when used in pre-eclampsia.— M. D. Lindheimer and A. I. Katz, *New Engl. J. Med.*, 1985, *313*, 675. Comment. Epidural anaesthesia is the analgesic method of choice in patients with toxaemia if plasma volume deficit has been corrected, blood coagulation is adequate, and blood pressure is controlled by other means.— D. B. Seifer and G. A. Albright (letter), *ibid.*, 1986, *314*, 582. Reply.— M. D. Lindheimer and A. I. Katz, *ibid.*, 583.

INFILTRATION ANAESTHESIA. Local infiltration of a local anaesthetic compared favourably with intravenous regional anaesthesia for manipulation of Colles' fractures in terms of satisfactory anaesthesia, ease and speed of performance, and lack of complications. However, pain scores were higher in those patients receiving local infiltration.— A. G. Cobb and G. R. Houghton, *Br. med. J.*, 1985, *291*, 1683.

Intraligamental injection of a local anaesthetic in patients undergoing various dental procedures was found to produce effective anaesthesia in 81% of cases but there was a risk of acute complications following the use of this technique in conservative treatment.— R. K. Faulkner, *Br. dent. J.*, 1983, *154*, 103. Administration of local anaesthetics into the periodontal membrane by intraligamental injection has a less predictable success rate than other methods used in dentistry, the duration of anaesthesia may be much shorter, and soft tissues are little affected. However, administration was less painful than with most subperiosteal infiltrations and the technique should not be written off until there is some evidence to condemn it.— D. N. Allan (letter), *ibid.*, 161. Intraligamental injection of local anaesthetics into the periodontal membrane was found to be a less painful procedure in dental patients than nerve block or infiltration. It had been used successfully in all types of operative dental procedures.— A. R. Dhanji (letter), *ibid.* Postoperative discomfort and complications following intraligamental injection of a local anaesthetic are probably related to the rate at which the injection is given.— A. G. Miller (letter), *ibid.*, 195. Intraligamental injections were used without haematological side-effects in patients with bleeding disorders undergoing dental treatment.— C. Bishop (letter), *ibid.* Disadvantages of the intraligamental injection of local anaesthetics into the periodontal membrane are given. The technique is likely to have strictly limited use.— A. Cowan (letter), *ibid.*, 278.

INTRAVENOUS REGIONAL ANAESTHESIA. Details of a procedure for intravenous regional anaesthesia of the arm for manipulation of fractures and minor surgical procedures. Major adverse effects are rare, but convulsions have occurred after the use of bupivacaine.— W. A. Wallace *et al.*, *Br. med. J.*, 1982, *285*, 554. Criticism of the described technique, especially the lack of adequate precautions and an underestimate of the risks involved.— J. I. Alexander *et al.* (letter), *ibid.*, 731 (several other letters of criticism and comment follow immediately after this letter).

Five deaths directly attributable to intravenous regional anaesthesia had been reported to the *UK* Department of Health and Social Security between 1979 and 1982, all of them occurred in casualty departments.— M. L. Heath, *Br. med. J.*, 1982, *285*, 913.

Further references J. E. Goold, *Br. J. Hosp. Med.*, 1985, *33*, 335.

PAIN. A review of the management of pain with regional analgesia including the use of local anaesthetics in the diagnosis, prognosis, prophylaxis, and treatment of conditions such as post-amputation pain syndromes, acute myocardial infarction, biliary and ureteral colic, postherpetic neuralgia, and cancer pain.— J. J. Bonica, *Postgrad. med. J.*, 1984, *60*, 897.

Cancer pain. Local anaesthetics are useful in the treatment of cancer pain, especially that which is well-defined and localised. They may be used for temporary and diagnostic nerve blocks, and have been given by epidural infusion for the temporary management of difficult pain syndromes, with the advantages of having no cross-tolerance with opiate analgesia and not affecting motor or autonomic function. Trigger-point injections and focal injections into a painful muscle joint are commonly used and give dramatic relief.— K. M. Foley, *New engl. J. Med.*, 1985, *313*, 84.

Headache and migraine. Local infiltration of lignocaine 1.5% or physiological saline into pericranial tender spots were both found to have a beneficial effect on attacks of common migraine.— P. Tfelt-Hansen *et al.* (letter), *Lancet*, 1980, *1*, 1140.

Local anaesthetics may be used for the diagnosis and treatment of cervical headache.— N. Bogduk *et al.*, *Med. J. Aust.*, 1985, *143*, 202.

Obstetrics. See under Epidural Block, above.

Postherpetic neuralgia. Local anaesthetics have been used alone and with corticosteroids for nerve blockade in the prevention and treatment of postherpetic neuralgia, although results of treatment are conflicting.— P. N. Robinson and N. Fletcher, *J. R. Coll. gen. Pract.*, 1986, *36*, 24.

Postoperative pain. Local anaesthetics for the prevention of postoperative pain: J. White *et al.*, *Br. med. J.*, 1983, *286*, 1934 (use in children undergoing circumcision); L. C. Barr and M. R. Pittam (letter), *ibid.*, 1983, *287*, 364 (use in adults undergoing circumcision); E. N. Armitage, *Br. J. Anaesth.*, 1986, *58*, 790 (techniques used in the prevention of postoperative pain).

REGIONAL NERVE BLOCK. A review of the use of local anaesthetics for regional analgesia in labour.— A. Hollmen, *Br. J. Anaesth.*, 1979, *51*, *Suppl.* 1, 17S.

A review of regional anaesthesia in orthopaedic surgery, including peripheral and central nerve blocks.— P. J. McKenzie and A. B. Loach, *Br. J. Anaesth.*, 1986, *58*, 779.

Further references to regional nerve block anaesthesia: J. E. Galway *et al.*, *Br. J. Anaesth.*, 1975, *47*, 730 (intercostal block); J. A. W. Wildsmith *et al.*, *ibid.*, 1977, *49*, 461 (brachial plexus block).

For further references to the use of local anaesthetics in regional nerve blocks, see under Epidural Block and

Pain, above. See also under Adverse Effects, above.

SPINAL ANAESTHESIA. A discussion of spinal anaesthesia.— F. J. Spielman and C. B. Watson, *J. Am. med. Ass.*, 1983, *249*, 734. Comment. Spinal anaesthesia may offer no advantages over general anaesthesia in the elderly, cardiac, or pulmonary patient.— S. V. Scalia (letter), *ibid.*, *250*, 1842. A comparison of spinal and epidural anaesthesia. For many patients and procedures spinal anaesthesia is the regional method of choice, but with careful technique epidural anaesthesia can provide all the benefits of spinal blockade for certain surgical procedures and avoid some of its problems.— J. A. W. Wildsmith, *Br. J. Anaesth.*, 1987, *59*, 397.

Spinal anaesthesia without additional sedation was used in preference to general anaesthesia in patients with fractures of the proximal femur because of the advantages it offered. Spinal block does not cause confusion, patients can remain orientated in time and space, some postoperative analgesia is provided, and chest complications can be avoided. Spinal anaesthesia has been reported to result in less postoperative bleeding, better fibrinolytic function, and a lower incidence of thrombo-embolism when used in total hip replacement and less hypoxia when used in femoral fracture.— J. M. Sikorski *et al.*, *Br. med. J.*, 1985, *290*, 439. Criticism. There is now convincing evidence that spinal anaesthesia does not have any major intrinsic superiority over general anaesthesia for the repair of the fractured femur.— P. J. McKenzie and H. Y. Wishart (letter), *ibid.*, 856. Agreement with the view that spinal anaesthesia is to be preferred over general anaesthesia for repair of fractured femur.— P. H. P. Harris, *ibid.*, 1286.

7603-v

Amethocaine *(BAN)*.

Tetracaine *(USAN, rINN)*. 2-Dimethylaminoethyl 4-butylaminobenzoate.

$C_{15}H_{24}N_2O_2$=264.4.

CAS — 94-24-6.

Pharmacopoeias. In *U.S.*

A white or light yellow waxy solid. M.p. 41° to 46°. Very slightly **soluble** in water; soluble 1 in 5 of alcohol and 1 in 2 of chloroform and ether. **Store** in airtight containers. Protect from light.

7604-g

Amethocaine Hydrochloride *(BANM)*.

Dicainum; Tetracaine Hydrochloride *(USAN, rINNM)*; Tetracaini Hydrochloridum; Tetracainii Chloridum.

$C_{15}H_{24}N_2O_2$,HCl=300.8.

CAS — 136-47-0.

Pharmacopoeias. In *Arg., Aust., Belg., Br., Braz., Chin., Cz., Egypt., Eur., Fr., Ger., Hung., Int., It., Jpn, Jug., Mex., Neth., Nord., Pol., Port., Rus., Swiss, Turk.*, and *U.S. Nord.* also includes Amethocaine Nitrate.

A white, odourless, slightly hygroscopic, crystalline powder.

Soluble 1 in 7.5 of water; soluble in alcohol; sparingly soluble in chloroform; practically insoluble in ether. A 1% solution in water has a pH of 4.5 to 5.5. Solutions may be **sterilised** by autoclaving. **Incompatible** with alkalis. **Store** in airtight containers. Protect from light. Aqueous solutions should be discarded if they contain crystals or are discoloured or cloudy.

Adverse Effects and Treatment

As for Local Anaesthetics, p.1205.

A stinging sensation may occur when amethocaine is used in the eye.

Absorption of amethocaine from mucous membranes is rapid and adverse reactions can occur abruptly without the appearance of prodromal signs or convulsions. There are early reports of fatalities.

Precautions

As for Local Anaesthetics, p.1206.

Amethocaine is contra-indicated in patients with a known hypersensitivity to the drug, to local anaesthetics of the ester type, or to para-aminobenzoic acid and its derivatives. Prolonged application of ophthalmic preparations is not recommended as severe keratitis and permanent corneal opacification and scarring may occur. Patients should be warned not to rub or touch the eye whilst anaesthesia persists.

Amethocaine is hydrolysed in the body to para-aminobenzoic acid and may antagonise the action of sulphonamides.

Absorption and Fate

See under Local Anaesthetics, p.1206.

Amethocaine is hydrolysed by plasma esterases to para-aminobenzoic acid and other metabolites and is excreted mainly by the kidneys.

Uses and Administration

As for Local Anaesthetics, p.1206.

Amethocaine is a potent local anaesthetic of the ester type.

Amethocaine is used for surface anaesthesia and spinal anaesthesia. It is not recommended in other local anaesthetic techniques because of its slow onset of action and systemic toxicity.

Amethocaine is generally used as the hydrochloride in solutions and creams, and as the base in ointments.

For anaesthesia of the eye, solutions containing 0.25 to 1.0% amethocaine hydrochloride and ointments containing 0.5% amethocaine are used.

Amethocaine is used for topical anaesthesia as a 1% cream and as a 0.5% ointment. These preparations may be used for painful conditions of the anus or rectum. A topical solution is also used for anaesthesia of the mucous membranes of the nose and throat. A 0.25 or 0.5% solution is used which may be applied directly or inhaled by nebulisation and adrenaline may be added to delay absorption; no more than 20 mg should be used.

Amethocaine is also used for spinal anaesthesia usually as a 0.5% solution. For a low spinal block in obstetrics a dose of 2 to 5 mg is used as a hyperbaric solution in glucose. For perineal anaesthesia a dose of 5 mg is used, and for anaesthesia of the perineum and lower extremities a dose of 10 mg is used. These doses may be given as hyperbaric or isobaric solutions in glucose 10% or cerebrospinal fluid respectively, depending upon the technique used. For spinal anaesthesia up to the costal margin an isobaric solution is used in a dose of 15 to 20 mg. Doses greater than 15 mg are rarely required for spinal anaesthesia.

Amethocaine has also been used as lozenges and as medicated lollipops.

SPINAL ANAESTHESIA. References to spinal anaesthesia with amethocaine.— D. T. Brown *et al.*, *Br. J. Anaesth.*, 1980, *52*, 589 (comparison of hyperbaric, isobaric, and hypobaric solutions).

For a comparison between amethocaine and bupivacaine solutions for spinal anaesthesia, see under Bupivacaine Hydrochloride, p.1211.

SURFACE ANAESTHESIA. A mucosa-adhesive, pliant polymer film containing amethocaine 10 mg and antimicrobials was formulated for use in patients with aphthae and erosions on the oral mucosa and tongue resulting from radiation and antineoplastic drugs. The film relieved pain and appeared to aid healing of lesions in 2 patients.— T. Yotsuyanagi *et al.* (letter), *Lancet*, 1985, *2*, 613.

Preparations Containing Amethocaine and Amethocaine Hydrochloride

Amethocaine Eye Drops *(A.P.F.)*

Amethocaine Eye Drops *(B.P.)*. AME. Contain amethocaine hydrochloride.

Sterile Tetracaine Hydrochloride *(U.S.P.)*. Amethocaine hydrochloride suitable for parenteral use. A 1% solution has a pH of 5 to 6.

Tetracaine Hydrochloride Cream *(U.S.P.)*. Amethocaine hydrochloride in a suitable water-miscible basis. pH 3.2 to 3.8.

Tetracaine Hydrochloride Injection *(U.S.P.)*. A sterile solution of amethocaine hydrochloride in Water for Injections. pH 3.2 to 6.0. Store at 2° to 8°.

Tetracaine Hydrochloride in Dextrose Injection *(U.S.P.)*. Contains amethocaine hydrochloride in glucose.

Tetracaine Hydrochloride Ophthalmic Solution *(U.S.P.)*. A sterile aqueous solution of amethocaine hydrochloride. pH 3.7 to 6.0. Store in airtight containers.

Tetracaine Hydrochloride Topical Solution *(U.S.P.)*. An aqueous solution of amethocaine hydrochloride containing a suitable antimicrobial agent. pH 4.5 to 6.0.

Tetracaine Ointment *(U.S.P.)*. Amethocaine in a suitable ointment basis.

Tetracaine Ophthalmic Ointment *(U.S.P.)*. A sterile eye ointment containing amethocaine.

Tetracaine and Menthol Ointment *(U.S.P.)*. Amethocaine and menthol in a suitable ointment basis.

Proprietary Preparations Containing Amethocaine and Amethocaine Hydrochloride

Anethaine *(Evans Medical, UK)*. *Cream*, amethocaine hydrochloride 1%.

Minims Amethocaine Hydrochloride *(Smith & Nephew Pharmaceuticals, UK)*. *Eye-drops*, amethocaine hydrochloride 0.5% and 1.0%, in single-use disposable applicators.

Proprietary Names and Manufacturers of Amethocaine and Amethocaine Hydrochloride

Anethaine *(Glaxo, S.Afr.; Evans Medical, UK)*; Contralgine *(Belg.)*; Covostet *(Covan, S.Afr.)*; Decicain *(Winthrop, Austral.)*; Gingicain *(Hoechst, Spain)*; Lubricante Urologico *(Organon, Spain)*; Minims Amethocaine Hydrochloride *(Smith & Nephew, Austral.; Smith & Nephew, S.Afr.; Smith & Nephew Pharmaceuticals, UK)*; Pantocain *(Denm.; Hoechst, Ger.)*; Pontocaine *(Winthrop, Canad.; Winthrop-Breon, USA)*; Tetrakain Minims *(Smith & Nephew, Norw.; Smith & Nephew, Swed.)*.

The following names have been used for multi-ingredient preparations containing amethocaine or amethocaine hydrochloride—Biosone GA *(Biorex, UK)*; Cetacaine *(Cetylite, USA)*; Eludril Spray *(Concept Pharmaceuticals, UK)*; Locan *(Duncan, Flockhart, UK)*; Norgotin *(Norgine, UK)*; Noxyflex *(Geistlich, UK)*; Riddofan *(Seaford, UK)*; Throsil *(Cox, UK)*; Xylotox Extra *(Pharmaceutical Mfg, UK)*.

7605-q

Amylocaine Hydrochloride *(BANM)*.

Amyleinii Chloridum; Amylocain. Hydrochlor.; Chlorhydrate d'Amyléine. 1-Dimethylaminomethyl-1-methylpropyl benzoate hydrochloride.

$C_{14}H_{21}NO_2$,HCl=271.8.

CAS — 644-26-8 (amylocaine); 532-59-2 (hydrochloride).

Pharmacopoeias. In *Belg., Fr., Port., Roum.*, and *Span.*

Amylocaine hydrochloride is a local anaesthetic of the ester type.

The general actions of local anaesthetics are described on p.1205.

Proprietary Names and Manufacturers

The following names have been used for multi-ingredient preparations containing amylocaine hydrochloride—Locan *(Duncan, Flockhart, UK)*; Phenolaine *(Phenolaine, UK)*.

7606-p

Aptocaine Hydrochloride *(BANM, rINNM)*.

2-(Pyrrolidin-1-yl)propiono-*o*-toluidide hydrochloride.

$C_{14}H_{20}N_2O$,HCl=268.8.

CAS — 19281-29-9 (aptocaine); 19281-32-4 (hydrochloride).

Aptocaine hydrochloride is a local anaesthetic.

The general actions of local anaesthetics are described on p.1205.

References: F. Reynolds *et al.*, *Br. J. Anaesth.*, 1976, *48*, 347; A. H. Beckett and W. Vutthikongsirigool, *J. Pharm. Pharmac.*, 1976, *28*, 54P.

7608-w

Benzocaine *(BAN, USAN, rINN)*.

Anaesthesinum; Anesthamine; Benzocainum; Éthoforme; Ethoform; Ethyl Aminobenzoate; Ethylis Aminobenzoas. Ethyl 4-aminobenzoate.

$C_9H_{11}NO_2$=165.2.

CAS — 94-09-7.

Pharmacopoeias. In *Arg., Aust., Belg., Br., Braz., Chin., Egypt., Eur., Fr., Ger., Hung., Ind., Int., It., Jpn, Jug., Mex., Neth., Pol., Roum., Rus., Span., Swiss, Turk.,* and *U.S.* Also in *B.P. Vet.*

Colourless crystals or a white odourless crystalline powder. M.p. 88° to 92°.

Soluble 1 in 2500 of water, 1 in 8 of alcohol, 1 in 2 of chloroform, and 1 in 4 of ether; soluble in dilute acids; soluble 1 in 30 to 50 of almond oil or olive oil. **Store** in well-closed containers. Protect from light.

Adverse Effects and Treatment

As for Local Anaesthetics, p.1205.

Methaemoglobinaemia has been reported following the use of benzocaine.

ALLERGY AND EFFECTS ON THE SKIN. Of 887 persons with dermatitis or eczema submitted to patch testing with benzocaine 5% in yellow soft paraffin, 5.9% gave a positive reaction.— E. Rudzki and D. Kleniewska, *Br. J. Derm.*, 1970, *83*, 543. See also H. Bandmann *et al.*, *Archs Derm.*, 1972, *106*, 335.

For a report of methaemoglobinaemia being associated with the use of benzocaine in an adult, see under Local Anaesthetics p.1205.

Precautions

As for Local Anaesthetics, p.1206. In addition, benzocaine is contra-indicated in patients with a known hypersensitivity to para-aminobenzoic acid and its derivatives, and to hydroxybenzoate preservatives.

Benzocaine may antagonise the action of sulphonamides.

Absorption and Fate

See under Local Anaesthetics, p.1206.

Uses and Administration

As for Local Anaesthetics, p.1206.

Benzocaine is a surface anaesthetic of the ester type with low systemic toxicity. It is used, often in combination with other drugs such as analgesics, antiseptics, antibacterial and antifungal agents, and antipruritics, for the temporary local relief of pain associated with dental conditions, sore throats, haemorrhoids, anal pruritus, and ear pain. It has also been used for pain relief in minor cuts, scrapes, burns, and sunburn, and muscular pains, strains, and sprains.

Lozenges containing benzocaine in usual doses of up to 10 mg are dissolved slowly in the mouth for the relief of sore throat. They should not be used as self-medication for longer than 2 days. Lozenges, gels, and sprays containing benzocaine in higher doses have been used for surface anaesthesia of the mouth and throat.

Ear-drops containing benzocaine in concentrations of 1 to 20% are used for temporary relief of ear pain. They should not be used in conditions with ear discharge or perforated tympanic membrane.

Benzocaine is used in creams, ointments, lotions, solutions, gels, and suppositories in concentrations up to 20% for topical analgesia and anaesthesia.

Despite the inclusion of benzocaine in some over-the-counter appetite suppressants there is no good evidence of its value in obesity.— *Med. Lett.*, 1979, *21*, 65.

Preparations

Benzocaine Topical Aerosol *(U.S.P.)*

Benzocaine Cream *(U.S.P.)*

Benzocaine Lozenges *(D.P.F.)*. Contain benzocaine 10 mg.

Compound Benzocaine Lozenges *(B.P.C. 1973)*. Benzocaine Compound Lozenges; Trochisci Benzocainae Compositi; Compound Benzocaine Tablets. Contain benzocaine 100 mg and menthol 3 mg.

Benzocaine Ointment *(U.S.P.)*

Compound Benzocaine Ointment *(B.P.C. 1973)*. Benzocaine Compound Ointment; Unguentum Benzocainae Compositum. Benzocaine 10% in equal parts of hamamelis ointment and zinc ointment.

Benzocaine Otic Solution *(U.S.P.)*

Benzocaine Topical Solution *(U.S.P.)*

Proprietary Preparations

AAA Mouth and Throat Spray *(Armour, UK)*. *Throat spray*, aerosol, benzocaine 1.5 mg, cetalkonium chloride 41.3 μg per metered dose.

Dequacaine *(Evans Medical, UK)*. *Lozenges*, benzocaine 10 mg, dequalinium chloride 250 μg.

Intralgin *(Riker, UK)*. *Gel*, benzocaine 2%, salicylamide 5%, in an alcoholic vehicle.

Medilave Gel *(Martindale Pharmaceuticals, UK)*. *Gel*, benzocaine 1%, cetylpyridinium chloride 0.01%, in a water-immiscible protective basis.

Merocaine *(Merrell, UK)*. *Lozenges*, benzocaine 10 mg, cetylpyridinium chloride 1.4 mg.

Proprietary Names and Manufacturers

Americaine *(American Critical Care, USA)*; Anaesthesin *(Ritsert, Ger.)*; Baby Anbesol *(Whitehall, USA)*; Bensokain *(ACO, Swed.)*; Children's Chloraseptic Lozenges *(Richardson-Vicks, USA)*; Gengivarium *(Ital Suisse, Ital.)*; Hurricaine *(Beutlich, USA)*; Spec-T *(Squibb, Canad.)*; Teething Syrup *(Sabex, Canad.)*; Topicaine *(Orapharm, Austral.)*.

The following names have been used for multi-ingredient preparations containing benzocaine—AAA Spray *(USV, Austral. Fisons, S. Afr.; Armour, UK)*; Anbesol *(Whitehall, USA)*; Applicaine Liquid *(Nyal, Austral.)*; Audicort *(Lederle, UK)*; Aurafair *(Pharmafair, USA)*; Auralgan *(Ayerst, Austral.; Ayerst, Canad.; Ayerst, USA)*; Auralgicin *(Fisons, UK)*; Auraltone *(Rorer, UK)*; Aurisan *(Nadeau, Canad.)*; Balminil Pastilles *(Rougier, Canad.)*; Benzease *(Bolton, Canad.)*; Benzets *(Norton, UK)*; Bionet *(Horner, Canad.)*; Caligesic; Calmasol *(Ethipharm, Canad.)*; Cepacaine *(Merrell Dow, Austral.)*; Cepacol *(Dow, Canad.; Merrell Dow, USA)*; Cepacol Anaesthetic Throat Discs *(Merrell ·Dow, Austral.)*; Cepacol Cough and Sore Throat Lozenges *(Merrell Dow, Austral.)*; Cetacaine *(Cetylite, USA)*; Codral Lozenges *(Wellcome, Austral.)*; Cornkil *(Rosken, Austral.)*; Dalidyne *(Dalin, USA)*; Dequacaine *(Evans Medical, UK)*; Dermogesic *(Merck Sharp & Dohme, UK)*; Dermoplast *(Ayerst, Austral.; Ayerst, Canad.; Torbet Laboratories, UK; Ayerst, USA)*; Dieutrim *(Legere, USA)*; Fungi-Nail *(Kramer, USA)*; Ger-O-Foam *(Geriatric Pharm. Corp., USA)*; Hedal HC *(Arlo, USA)*; Hemorex *(Winthrop, Austral.)*; Hibitane Antiseptic Lozenges *(Care, UK)*; Intralgin *(Riker, UK)*; Medicone Derma-HC *(Medicone, USA)*; Medilave Gel *(Martindale Pharmaceuticals, UK)*; Merocaine *(Merrell, UK)*; Nestosyl *(Bengué, UK)*; Osmopak-Plus *(Charton, Canad.)*; Oticane *(Rosken, Austral.)*; Otipyrin *(Kramer, USA)*; Pazo *(Bristol-Myers Products, USA)*; Rectal Medicone-HC *(Medicone, USA)*; Rectinol *(G.P. Laboratories, Austral.)*; Rectogel *(Riva, Canad.)*; Semets *(Beecham Laboratories, USA)*; Spec-T *(Squibb, Canad.)*; Tigan Suppositories *(Beecham Laboratories, USA)*; Transvasin *(Reckitt & Colman, Austral.; Lloyd-Hamol, Reckitt & Colman Pharm., UK)*; Tympagesic *(Adria, USA)*; Tyrosolven *(Warner, UK)*; Tyrozets *(Merck Sharp & Dohme, UK)*; URA *(Protea, Austral.)*.

7609-e

Bupivacaine Hydrochloride *(BANM, USAN, rINNM)*.

AH-2250; LAC-43; Win-11 318. (±)-(1-Butyl-2-piperidyl)formo-2′,6′-xylidide hydrochloride monohydrate.

$C_{18}H_{28}N_2O,HCl,H_2O = 342.9$.

CAS — 2180-92-9 (bupivacaine); 18010-40-7 (hydrochloride, anhydrous); 14252-80-3 (hydrochloride, monohydrate).

Pharmacopoeias. In *Br., Chin., Eur., Int., It.,* and *U.S.*

A white odourless or almost odourless crystalline powder.

Soluble 1 in 25 of water and 1 in 8 of alcohol; slightly soluble in acetone, chloroform, and ether. A 1% solution in water has a pH of 4.5 to 6.0. Solutions are **sterilised** by autoclaving. **Store** in well-closed containers.

STABILITY OF SOLUTIONS. For reference to the decreased solubility of bupivacaine in phosphate buffer with increasing temperature and its possible precipitation at the site of injection, see Lignocaine Hydrochloride, p.1217.

Adverse Effects and Treatment

As for Local Anaesthetics, p.1205.

For an evaluation of the toxicity of bupivacaine, see under Regional Nerve Block in Uses, below.

EFFECTS ON THE HEART. Cardiac arrest occurring in 6 patients during regional anaesthesia with bupivacaine or etidocaine, probably as a result of inadvertent intravascular injection, was not preceded by hypoxia and it appeared that even prompt oxygenation and blood pressure support might not prevent arrest. Marked cardiovascular depression may occur with bupivacaine or etidocaine at plasma concentrations only slightly above those for CNS toxicity.— G. A. Albright, *Anesthesiology*, 1979, *51*, 285.

A report of convulsions and cardiac arrest in a 67-year-old woman following intravenous regional anaesthesia with 0.25% bupivacaine solution in a dose of 40 mL (100 mg).— A. Henderson and P. Sujitkumar (letter), *Br. J. Anaesth.*, 1986, *58*, 362.

There now seems little doubt that bupivacaine is substantially more cardiotoxic than most other commonly used local anaesthetics. The pharmacokinetics of bupivacaine in myocardial tissue are such that electrophysiological changes occur at much lower concentrations than with other local anaesthetics.— *Lancet*, 1986, *2*, 1192.

EFFECTS ON THE NERVOUS SYSTEM. A report of an epileptiform convulsion following accidental intravascular injection of bupivacaine during epidural anaesthesia.— D. W. Ryan, *Br. J. Anaesth.*, 1973, *45*, 907.

Hyperexcitability in a 15-year-old boy following intravenous regional anaesthesia with bupivacaine 95 mg.— A. M. Henderson, *Br. med. J.*, 1980, *281*, 1043.

Convulsions with cyanosis occurred in 2 women given bupivacaine for epidural analgesia during caesarean section.— J. Thorburn and D. D. Moir, *Br. J. Anaesth.*, 1984, *56*, 551.

See also under Effects on the Heart, above.

PREGNANCY AND THE NEONATE. *Effects on the foetus.* Perinatal death and foetal bradycardia associated with bupivacaine in paracervical block for women in labour.— P. J. Murphy *et al.*, *Br. med. J.*, 1970, *1*, 526; F. C. R. Picton (letter), *ibid.*, *2*, 49.

Precautions

As for Local Anaesthetics, p.1206.

Bupivacaine is not recommended for use in intravenous regional anaesthesia, or paracervical block in obstetrics and the 0.75% solution is not recommended for epidural block in obstetrics.

A report of prolonged block of about 72 hours' duration following the use of 18 mL of bupivacaine 0.5% for epidural analgesia of a patient in labour.— G. V. Pathy and M. Rosen, *Br. J. Anaesth.*, 1975, *47*, 520.

The mean plasma-bupivacaine concentration was higher in 9 women who received ranitidine 150 mg by mouth prior to epidural anaesthesia with bupivacaine than in 7 women who were not given ranitidine.— C. M. Wilson *et al.*, *Br. J. Anaesth.*, 1986, *58*, 1330P.

Cimetidine 400 mg by mouth 13 and 3 hours before an intravenous infusion of bupivacaine 50 mg significantly decreased the clearance of bupivacaine in 4 healthy subjects, probably by an effect on bupivacaine's metabolism. Pretreatment with 2 doses of ranitidine 150 mg by mouth caused a smaller decrease in clearance which was not significant. Neither drug significantly increased the elimination half-life of bupivacaine.— D. W. Noble *et al.*, *Br. J. Anaesth.*, 1987, *59*, 735.

For reference to the effect of bupivacaine on the protein binding of lignocaine and mepivacaine respectively, see under lignocaine hydrochloride (p.1218) and mepivacaine hydrochloride (p.1223).

Absorption and Fate

Bupivacaine is about 95% bound to plasma proteins and has a half-life of 1.5 to 5.5 hours in the adult and about 8 hours in neonates. It is metabolised in the liver and is excreted in the urine principally as metabolites with only 5 to 6% as unchanged drug.

Foetal concentrations are lower than maternal concentrations.

See also Local Anaesthetics, p.1206.

Bupivacaine hydrochloride was administered by epidural injection to 12 patients in a dose of 150 mg with adrenaline 1 in 200 000, to 5 without adrenaline, and in a dose of 225 mg with adrenaline to a further 6. Mean peak plasma concentrations of bupivacaine were 1.14, 1.26, and 2.33 μg per mL respectively and occurred 20 minutes after administration; elimination half-lives were 2.8, 2.4, and 3.6 hours. In 5 of the patients given

150 mg of bupivacaine hydrochloride with adrenaline a peak CSF concentration of 30.6 μg per mL was achieved 30 minutes after administration.— G. R. Wilkinson and P. C. Lund, *Anesthesiology*, 1970, *33*, 482.

The absorption of bupivacaine hydrochloride, bupivacaine hydrochloride with adrenaline, and carbonated bupivacaine given during epidural blockade.— T. N. Appleyard *et al.*, *Br. J. Anaesth.*, 1974, *46*, 530.

Half-lives reported after the intravenous injection of bupivacaine were: α, 0.045 hours; β, 0.46 hours; and γ, 3.5 hours.— G. T. Tucker and L. E. Mather, *Br. J. Anaesth.*, 1975, *47*, 213.

Plasma-bupivacaine concentrations were measured during combined regional and general anaesthesia for resection and reconstruction surgery in head and neck cancer. The mean total dose of bupivacaine given for regional blockade was 3.4 mg per kg body-weight; 5 patients received bupivacaine without adrenaline, 1 patient was given bupivacaine with adrenaline 1 in 200 000, and 2 patients were given bupivacaine with adrenaline 1 in 400 000. The mean peak concentration in patients receiving adrenaline-free solutions was 4.95 μg per mL, significantly higher than the mean peak concentration of 3.56 μg per mL in patients given bupivacaine with adrenaline. Peak concentrations occurred within 10 to 20 minutes in all patients. No evidence of toxicity was seen despite plasma-bupivacaine concentrations greater than 4 μg per mL in 6 of the patients, concentrations considered by some to be associated with toxicity.— R. S. Neill and R. Watson, *Br. J. Anaesth.*, 1984, *56*, 485.

A study of bupivacaine absorption in 34 patients given bupivacaine 150 mg per mL or 200 mg per mL by continuous pressure irrigation into the knee during arthroscopy found that absorption from the synovial membrane was rapid but serum-bupivacaine concentrations did not exceed 350 ng per mL and were not associated with toxicity. Accidental escape of solution into the surrounding soft tissue occurred in 13 patients but no toxic symptoms were observed.— D. Debruyne *et al.*, *Eur. J. clin. Pharmac.*, 1985, *27*, 733.

For reference to the pharmacokinetics of bupivacaine in surgical patients following epidural administration, see A. G. L. Burm *et al.*, *Clin. Pharmacokinet.*, 1987, *13*, 191.

PREGNANCY AND THE NEONATE. Studies *in vitro* indicated that plasma alpha-1-lipoproteins had a high affinity for bupivacaine. As foetal plasma contains little alpha-1-lipoprotein, the binding capacity for bupivacaine would be reduced, which probably contributes to the higher concentration of bupivacaine in maternal plasma at delivery.— L. E. Mather and J. Thomas, *J. Pharm. Pharmac.*, 1978, *30*, 653.

Following pudendal block plasma-bupivacaine concentrations in the newborn at delivery were approximately 25% of the maternal concentration.— P. Belfrage *et al.*, *Br. J. Anaesth.*, 1973, *45*, 1067.

Six women were given bupivacaine 30 to 45 mg during labour. The maternal β-phase half-life was 1.25 hours compared with 25 hours for the neonate.— J. Caldwell *et al.*, *Br. J. clin. Pharmac.*, 1976, *3*, 956P.

Less bupivacaine crosses the placenta than either lignocaine or mepivacaine, and of the bupivacaine which does cross, relatively less is available as the active form because of greater protein binding in the neonate.— C. E. Blogg and B. R. Simpson (letter), *Lancet*, 1974, *1*, 1283.

A study of 12 women given an epidural loading dose of bupivacaine 50 mg followed by a continuous epidural infusion of bupivacaine 12.5 mg per hour for analgesia during labour and delivery. Peak serum concentrations of 0.68 μg per mL occurred 0.58 hours after the loading dose. No maternal or foetal accumulation or toxicity occurred and the ratio of foetal to maternal serum concentration was 0.44.— D. D. Denson *et al.*, *Ther. Drug Monit.*, 1984, *6*, 393.

Further references to the pharmacokinetics of bupivacaine in pregnancy and the neonate.— R. L. Nation, *Clin. Pharmacokinet.*, 1980, *5*, 340.

PROTEIN BINDING. It appears that the two major binding proteins for bupivacaine in serum are α-1-acid glycoprotein, the influence of which is predominant at low concentrations, and albumin, which plays the major role at high concentrations. Reduction in pH from 7.4 to 7.0 decreased the affinity of the α-1-acid glycoprotein for bupivacaine but had no effect on albumin affinity.— D. Denson *et al.*, *Clin. Pharmac. Ther.*, 1984, *35*, 409.

Protein binding studies of bupivacaine *in vitro* showed that the addition of nonesterified fatty acids to isolated binding proteins of bupivacaine increased binding to α-1-acid glycoprotein and decreased binding to serum albumin. An elevated progesterone concentration in whole serum did not alter bupivacaine protein binding. Neither of these factors accounted for the observed decrease in protein binding of bupivacaine during childbirth.— D. E. Coyle *et al.*, *Clin. Pharmac. Ther.*, 1986, *39*, 559.

Uses and Administration

As for Local Anaesthetics, p.1206.

Bupivacaine hydrochloride is a long-acting local anaesthetic of the amide type, with a duration of action of up to 10 hours. Onset of action and depth of anaesthesia depend upon the concentration, dose, route, and whether adrenaline is used. Doses of bupivacaine are expressed in terms of the anhydrous hydrochloride. Slow accumulation occurs with repeated doses. It is used mainly for infiltration and regional nerve blocks, particularly epidural block, but is not recommended for topical anaesthesia, obstetric paracervical block, or intravenous regional anaesthesia.

The concentration of bupivacaine solution used affects the extent of motor blockade achieved. A 0.25% solution generally produces incomplete motor block, a 0.5% solution will usually produce motor block and some muscle relaxation, and complete motor block and muscle relaxation can be achieved with a 0.75% solution.

The dose of bupivacaine should be reduced in the elderly, in children, and in debilitated patients, and in cardiac or hepatic disease.

For infiltration anaesthesia bupivacaine is used as a 0.25% solution alone or with adrenaline in a dose of up to 150 to 175 mg (60 to 70 mL). For peripheral nerve blocks solutions with or without adrenaline may be used. The usual dose is 12.5 mg (5 mL) of a 0.25% solution or 25 mg (5 mL) of a 0.5% solution up to 150 to 175 mg as a single dose or 400 mg per day. For sympathetic nerve block 50 to 125 mg (20 to 50 mL) as a 0.25% solution is recommended. When a longer duration of anaesthesia is required, as in surgery of the maxillary and mandibular area, 0.5% solution with adrenaline 1 in 200 000 may be used in a dose of 9 mg (1.8 mL) per injection site. This dose may be repeated after 2 to 10 minutes if needed, but a total dose of 90 mg (18 mL) should not be exceeded over a single dental sitting. A 0.75% solution has been used for retrobulbar block in ophthalmic surgery in a dose of 15 to 30 mg (2 to 4 mL).

For lumbar epidural block in surgery or obstetrics a 0.25% solution may be used in a dose of 25 to 50 mg (10 to 20 mL) or as a 0.5% solution in a dose of 50 to 100 mg (10 to 20 mL) and these doses may be repeated at intervals no shorter than 3 hours to a maximum of 400 mg daily. Lower doses of 15 to 30 mg (6 to 12 mL) of the 0.25% solution or 30 to 60 mg (6 to 12 mL) of the 0.5% solution have been recommended for analgesia during labour. A 0.75% solution is also used for induction of lumbar epidural block in non-obstetric surgery in a single dose of 75 to 150 mg (10 to 20 mL). For caudal block a 0.25% or 0.5% solution may be used in a usual dose of 25 to 150 mg. It is recommended that a test dose is given before commencing epidural block and that subsequent doses are given in small increments. Single doses should not exceed 150 to 175 mg and no more than 400 mg should be given daily.

Hyperbaric solutions of bupivacaine may be used for spinal anaesthesia. Preparations containing 0.5% are available and are given in doses of 10 to 20 mg (2 to 4 mL). Preparations containing 0.75% bupivacaine are also in use, and for anaesthesia of the lower extremities and perineal procedures a dose of 7.5 mg (1 mL) has been recommended and a dose of 12 mg (1.6 mL) for lower abdominal procedures. For spinal anaesthesia in obstetrics a 0.75% hyperbaric solution has been used in doses of 6 mg (0.8 mL) for vaginal delivery and 7.5 to 10.5 mg (1.0 to 1.4 mL) for caesarean section.

Intra-abdominal instillation of bupivacaine 2 mg per kg body-weight shortened the period of postoperative colonic adynamic ileus compared with instillation of saline in a study involving 22 patients undergoing abdominal surgery. Colonic propulsion returned significantly faster in the bupivacaine group but there was no difference in colonic transit time between the 2 groups.— G. Rimbäck *et al.*, *Gut*, 1986, *27*, 170.

For a study on the vasoactivity of bupivacaine, see Lignocaine Hydrochloride, p.1220.

EPIDURAL BLOCK. Factors affecting the spread of local anaesthetic solutions in the extradural space were studied. Extradural analgesia was performed on 334 occasions using bupivacaine 0.75% solution 10 mL, 15 mL, or 20 mL, injected at a rate of 1 mL per second using a technique in which site of injection, bevel direction of needle, and position of the patient were all standardised. Arteriosclerosis in 18 patients had no effect on the spread of 15 mL of bupivacaine solution when compared with 70 patients without evidence of cardiac or vascular disease. There was a slight correlation between height of the patient and the level of analgesia. With increasing age there was a small increase in the spread of bupivacaine. The number of segments blocked was not directly related to the volume of anaesthetic solution injected.— E. M. Grundy *et al.*, *Br. J. Anaesth.*, 1978, *50*, 805. In a double-blind study of epidural anaesthesia with bupivacaine in 30 patients undergoing varicose vein surgery, the spread of epidural anaesthesia was not affected by the injection volume or the dose of bupivacaine or by the patient's age, weight, height, or body-mass index. The duration of sensory analgesia and degree of motor block were found to be related to dose and not concentration of solution.— J. Duggan *et al.*, *ibid.*, 1987, *59*, 128P.

Epidural anaesthesia with bupivacaine 0.5% solution with adrenaline 5 μg per mL [1 in 200 000] in 14 patients undergoing total hip replacement resulted in significantly better fibrinolytic function and a lower tendency to clotting than in a similar group of 16 patients who all received general anaesthesia.— J. Modig *et al.*, *Br. J. Anaesth.*, 1983, *55*, 625. Epidural anaesthesia with bupivacaine 0.5% was found to inhibit platelet aggregation in 10 patients undergoing elective surgery. General anaesthesia in a group of 10 similar patients had no effect on platelet aggregation. This effect on platelet function during epidural anaesthesia may play a role in reducing the incidence of venous thrombolytic complications.— C. P. Henny *et al.*, *Br. J. Anaesth.*, 1986, *58*, 301.

In a study involving 24 patients undergoing upper abdominal surgery under general anaesthesia, epidural administration of bupivacaine suppressed the increase in plasma catecholamines normally seen immediately after surgery and also attenuated the endocrine response in the later postoperative period.— H. Rutberg *et al.*, *Br. J. Anaesth.*, 1984, *56*, 233.

A double-blind crossover study of postoperative epidural analgesia with bupivacaine 0.5% in doses of 4 to 8 mL or with morphine sulphate 4 to 8 mg found that both drugs gave excellent analgesia. The onset of pain relief was seen by 15 minutes for both drugs and the effect was maximal in an average of 22 minutes for bupivacaine and 32 minutes for morphine. The mean duration of analgesia for bupivacaine was 321 minutes, significantly shorter than the 489 minutes for morphine. Hypotension requiring treatment occured in 3 patients given bupivacaine.— T. A. Torda and D. A. Pybus, *Br. J. Anaesth.*, 1984, *56*, 141.

The level of sensory analgesia slowly regressed in 8 patients receiving bupivacaine 0.5% solution by continuous epidural infusion at a constant rate for postoperative analgesia. Morphine 10 mg intravenously was given when reduced analgesia was noted, resulting in pronounced pain relief and an increase in level of sensory analgesia in each case.— C. Lund *et al.*, *Lancet*, 1985, *2*, 1156.

Further references to epidural block with bupivacaine.— G. B. Drummond and D. G. Littlewood, *Br. J. Anaesth.*, 1977, *49*, 999 (respiratory effects of epidural analgesia); D. T. Brown *et al.*, *ibid.*, 1980, *52*, 419 (a lack of benefit with carbonated bupivacaine when compared with the hydrochloride).

See also Regional Nerve Block (below).

In obstetrics. A review of 923 women who had undergone lumbar epidural block with bupivacaine and adrenaline before or during labour showed that only 6% of them received no benefit. The optimum dose appeared to be 8 mL of bupivacaine 0.5% solution, which was effective for about 2 hours. The persistence of sensory and motor nerve block after delivery was decreased when the concentration of bupivacaine in the final dose, given 1 hour before delivery, was reduced to 0.25%.— J. S. Crawford, *Br. J. Anaesth.*, 1972, *44*, 66.

Plasma-bupivacaine concentrations were significantly reduced by adrenaline in a study of 70 mothers undergoing epidural block during delivery. It was considered that, using bupivacaine 0.5%, doses of up to 320 mg could be given without adrenaline before there was any risk of systemic toxicity.— F. Reynolds *et al.*, *Br. J. Anaesth.*, 1973, *45*, 1049.

Criticism of the *US* Food and Drug Administration's recommendation to prohibit the use of bupivacaine 0.75% solution in obstetric practice. The evidence for this decision is conflicting and experienced anaesthetists consider serious toxicity is not a problem if the drug is given properly.— D. B. Scott, *Br. J. Anaesth.*, 1984, *56*, 435. See also J. M. Davies *et al.* (letter), *Can. med. Ass. J.*, 1984, *130*, 1110.

In a study of 240 women given epidural analgesia for pain relief during the first stage of labour using bupivacaine 0.5%, 0.375%, or 0.25%, at a dose of 500 μg per kg body-weight, regular 'top-up' injections at approximately 90 minute intervals produced superior analgesia to that from conventional 'on-demand' therapy. Bupivacaine 0.375% solution was found to be the most suitable concentration for epidural analgesia in labour given as regular top-up injections, providing adequate spread of analgesia without increasing the number of operative deliveries.— G. Purdy *et al.*, *Br. J. Anaesth.*, 1987, *59*, 319.

A study in 100 primigravid mothers receiving an initial epidural injection of bupivacaine 0.5% solution followed by either a continuous epidural infusion of bupivacaine 0.125% with additional top-up injection as required, or top-up injections alone. Continuous infusion prolonged the interval between top-up doses without any apparent adverse effects to the foetus.— D. G. Bogod *et al.*, *Br. J. Anaesth.*, 1987, *59*, 325.

See also under Adverse Effects and Precautions above and Regional Nerve Block, below.

INFILTRATION ANAESTHESIA. Bilateral local infiltration with bupivacaine 0.25% solution in patients undergoing third molar extraction under general anaesthesia reduced the incidence of wide complex extrasystoles during surgery and the severity of dental pain 6 hours after operation compared with general anaesthesia alone.— I. H. Wilson *et al.*, *Br. J. Anaesth.*, 1986, *58*, 401.

INTRAVENOUS REGIONAL ANAESTHESIA. Studies of intravenous regional anaesthesia with bupivacaine hydrochloride in patients with various pain syndromes indicated that 200 mg, as 40 mL of a 0.5% solution, may be the optimal dose for producing safe and prolonged intravenous regional anaesthesia.— F. Magora *et al.*, *Br. J. Anaesth.*, 1980, *52*, 1123; F. Magora *et al.*, *ibid.*, 1131 (but see below).

In a pilot study of intravenous regional anaesthesia with bupivacaine in 5 patients the drug was detected in the general circulation throughout the procedure and it was considered that 2 patients had in effect received bolus injections of bupivacaine into the general circulation. An active interosseous circulation exists, especially in young patients, which will bypass the tourniquet cuff. The cuff would seem to present little or no protection against serious consequences of intravenous regional anaesthesia.— M. A. Mason (letter), *Lancet*, 1983, *2*, 1085. The explanation for toxic reactions following intravenous regional anaesthesia with bupivacaine is probably explained by high venous pressures during injection rather than to intraosseous flow.— D. W. McKeown *et al.* (letter), *ibid.*, 1503.

Because of reports of adverse reactions the Association of Anaesthetists have recommended that bupivacaine should no longer be used for intravenous regional anaesthesia. The agent of choice now appears to be prilocaine.— S. P. K. Linter (letter), *Lancet*, 1983, *2*, 787.

Further references recommending that bupivacaine be used no longer for intravenous regional anaesthesia because of serious adverse effects and fatalities.— D. S. Arthur *et al.* (letter), *Br. med. J.*, 1982, *285*, 890.

See also under Adverse Effects, above.

PAIN. Nerve blocks were carried out successfully on 27 patients with intractable post-herpetic neuralgia, neoplastic pain, and orthopaedic pain using bupivacaine 0.25% with adrenaline 1 in 400 000. All patients reported immediate relief from pain. After one day 18 still had relief, at 7 days 13 were free from pain, and at 21 days 12 were still pain free.— J. G. Hannington-Kiff, *Lancet*, 1971, *2*, 1392. Bupivacaine with corticosteroids has been studied in the treatment of postherpetic neuralgia but long-term pain relief is poor.— M. Thompson and M. Bones, *Clin. Pharm.*, 1985, *4*, 170.

A study in 120 children undergoing inguinal herniotomy under general anaesthesia showed that more of those given bupivacaine 0.5% at a dose of 0.5 mL per year of age for ilioinguinal nerve block were free of pain postoperatively than those receiving no such block.— B. A. C. Smith and S. E. F. Jones, *Br. med. J.*, 1982, *285*, 1466.

Injection of 1.5 mL bupivacaine 0.5% solution with methylprednisolone acetate 20 mg into lumbar facet joint spaces of 34 patients with low back pain produced immediate relief from pain in 19 patients. Significant relief of pain lasted for 6 months or more in 12 of these patients, for between 1 and 6 months in 3 patients, and for less than 1 month in the remaining 4 patients.— L. S. W. Lau *et al.*, *Med. J. Aust.*, 1985, *143*, 563.

A study involving 50 patients who had subcostal wounds from cholecystectomy or splenectomy. Perfusion of the wound with bupivacaine 0.5% solution reduced pain, and increased forced vital capacity to a greater extent than in patients receiving perfusion with physiological saline.— I. D. Levack *et al.*, *Br. J. Anaesth.*, 1986, *58*, 615.

Bites and stings. Bupivacaine is the local anaesthetic of choice for the treatment of pain arising from the stings of venomous fish. In very severe cases regional nerve block may be required.— S. K. Sutherland (letter), *Med. J. Aust.*, 1984, *140*, 503.

PREGNANCY AND THE NEONATE. For references to the use of bupivacaine hydrochloride in pregnancy, see under Epidural Block in Obstetrics, above.

REGIONAL NERVE BLOCK. An evaluation of the tissue and systemic toxicity of bupivacaine based on a review of its use in 7688 regional nerve block procedures indicated that bupivacaine has a wide margin of safety and that its toxic dosage had not yet been established. It was considered that doses of up to at least 225 mg of bupivacaine with adrenaline 1 in 200 000 for single-dose epidural block and up to at least 400 mg with adrenaline 1 in 320 000 or less for peripheral nerve block may be safely used in adults when necessary for rapid establishment of surgical anaesthesia, for complete motor blockade, and for prolonged duration of anaesthesia.— D. C. Moore *et al.*, *Acta anaesth. scand.*, 1977, *21*, 109.

A detailed review of the use of bupivacaine hydrochloride for regional nerve block (caudal, epidural, and peripheral) with guidelines on dosage. Of 11 080 procedures performed from 1966 through 1976 using 0.25, 0.5, or 0.75% solutions, with and without adrenaline, 6599 were for surgical, 3496 were for obstetrical, and 985 were for diagnostic and therapeutic procedures. Solutions containing adrenaline were used in 9304 procedures and a dose of 250 μg of adrenaline was seldom exceeded. Sensory anaesthesia of the integumentary and musculoskeletal systems occurred with all strengths of bupivacaine hydrochloride but only the 0.75% solution eliminated traction reflexes from the pelvic viscera. In epidural or caudal block, onset of sensory anaesthesia was noted in 4 to 10 minutes with 0.25 and 0.5% solutions and maximum sensory anaesthesia in 15 to 35 minutes; results were similar in peripheral nerve block. In epidural or caudal block using a 0.75% solution onset of sensory anaesthesia occurred in 3 to 5 minutes and was at a maximum in 10 to 30 minutes. The degree of motor blockade varied with technique and concentration and usually occurred 4 to 8 minutes after sensory anaesthesia; following caudal and epidural block maximum motor blockade in the lower extremities might take up to 60 minutes. Using the single-injection epidural or caudal block techniques for intra-abdominal surgery, including caesarean section and back surgery, profound muscle relaxation in the abdomen and back occurred consistently only with the 0.75% solution. Bupivacaine was well tolerated apart from the following adverse effects: total spinal anaesthesia following caudal block in one patient who recovered completely and systemic toxicity resulting from unrecognised intravascular injections in 13 patients and from absorption in 2 patients; there were no untoward sequelae.— D. C. Moore *et al.*, *Anesth. Analg. curr. Res.*, 1978, *57*, 42.

Stellate-ganglion blockade with 4 to 5 mL of bupivacaine 0.75% solution instantly and completely relieved chronic, severe itching of the upper arms in a 54-year-old man. A 'placebo block' performed with sodium chloride 0.9% solution containing benzyl alcohol 0.9% also gave immediate and complete relief of itching.— C. C. Rattenbourg *et al.* (letter), *New Engl. J. Med.*, 1983, *309*, 433.

Addition of potassium chloride 0.2 mmol to 40 mL of bupivacaine 0.25% solution resulted in a more rapid onset of sensory loss than the same dose of plain bupivacaine in patients undergoing brachial plexus block for forearm or hand surgery.— M. R. Parris and W. A. Chambers, *Br. J. Anaesth.*, 1986, *58*, 297.

For reference to the advantages of using bupivacaine in association with lignocaine for regional nerve block in ophthalmic surgery, see under Lignocaine Hydrochloride p.1221.

For reference to the use of stellate ganglion block with equal parts of bupivacaine and lignocaine solutions in the treatment of herpes zoster ophthalmicus, see under Lignocaine Hydrochloride p.1221.

See also Epidural Block and Pain (above).

SPINAL ANAESTHESIA. Spinal anaesthesia with hyperbaric bupivacaine 0.5% solutions containing either glucose 5% or glucose 8% or with glucose-free bupivacaine 0.5% solution was studied in 30 women undergoing major gynaecological surgery under general anaesthesia or deep sedation. Both the hyperbaric solutions spread further than the plain solution, but the duration of blockade was not affected by baricity. Diastolic pressure decreased more with the glucose 8% solution than with the plain solution, with 2 patients requiring treatment for hypotension.— W. A. Chambers *et al.*, *Br. J. Anaesth.*, 1981, *53*, 279.

Spinal anaesthesia with 3 mL of bupivacaine 0.75% in a double-blind study involving 20 patients undergoing urological surgery gave a longer duration of sensory analgesia and motor blockade than spinal block with 3 mL of hyperbaric amethocaine 0.5% in glucose 5% solution. The onset and spread of sensory analgesia and the onset time to complete motor blockade were similar in both groups, but cardiovascular changes appeared to be less for the isobaric bupivacaine group.— T. Marstrand *et al.*, *Br. J. Anaesth.*, 1985, *57*, 971. See also P. Skretting *et al.*, *Br. J. Anaesth.*, 1984, *56*, 155.

Spinal anaesthesia with solutions of plain bupivacaine 0.5% or 0.75% in doses of 15 or 20 mg gave an unpredictable and wide range of spread of anaesthesia and analgesia; supplementary anaesthesia was required in 10% of patients. Injection at the L2/3 interspace may reduce the failure rate at the expense of an increased incidence of hypotension.— M. R. Logan *et al.*, *Br. J. Anaesth.*, 1986, *58*, 292.

The height of blockade in spinal anaesthesia was found to correlate with body-weight in a study of 50 patients given bupivacaine 0.5% for spinal anaesthesia.— W. J. D. McCulloch and D. G. Littlewood, *Br. J. Anaesth.*, 1986, *58*, 610.

Onset of sensory analgesia was found to be more rapid in a group of 20 patients with chronic renal failure given 3 mL bupivacaine 0.75% for spinal anaesthesia prior to lower abdominal surgery than in a group of 20 control patients. Both sensory and motor blockades were of shorter duration in the patients with renal failure than in the control group.— R. Orko *et al.*, *Br. J. Anaesth.*, 1986, *58*, 605.

No clinically relevant differences in the onset, maximum spread or duration of analgesia, or incidence of post-spinal headache were found in a study of 39 women given either isobaric glucose-free bupivacaine 0.5% solution or hyperbaric bupivacaine 0.5% in glucose 8% solution for spinal analgesia during caesarean section. The hyperbaric solution caused greater changes in systolic arterial pressure and heart rate but the difference was not clinically important.— I. F. Russell and E. L. O. Holmqvist, *Br. J. Anaesth.*, 1987, *59*, 347.

Further references to the use of bupivacaine in spinal anaesthesia: I. F. Russell, *Br. J. Anaesth.*, 1983, *55*, 309 (in caesarean section); K. H. Axelsson *et al.*, *ibid.*, 1985, *57*, 960 (a comparison of hyperbaric and glucose-free solutions); N. Valentin *et al.*, *ibid.*, 1986, *58*, 284 (a comparison of spinal and general anaesthesia); J. M. Millar *et al.*, *ibid.*, 862 (a comparison of bupivacaine and hyperbaric lignocaine).

SURFACE ANAESTHESIA. Bupivacaine was found to be a safe and effective topical anaesthetic for bronchoscopy in doses of 8 to 25.5 mg for anaesthesia of the upper respiratory tract and a dose of 25 mg for the lower respiratory tract.— A. McBurney *et al.*, *Br. J. clin. Pharmac.*, 1984, *17*, 61.

Preparations

Bupivacaine and Adrenaline Injection *(B.P.)*. Contains bupivacaine hydrochloride and adrenaline acid tartrate. pH 3.0 to 5.5. Protect from light.

Bupivacaine and Epinephrine Injection *(U.S.P.)*. Contains bupivacaine hydrochloride and adrenaline or adrenaline acid tartrate. (not more than 1 in 100 000 of adrenaline). pH 3.3 to 5.5.

Bupivacaine Injection *(B.P.)*. Bupivacaine Hydrochloride Injection. pH 4.0 to 6.5.

Bupivacaine Hydrochloride Injection *(U.S.P.)*. pH 4.0 to 6.5.

Bupivacaine in Dextrose Injection *(U.S.P.)*

Proprietary Preparations

Marcain *(Astra, UK)*. *Injection*, bupivacaine hydrochloride 0.25%, 0.5%, and 0.75%, in ampoules of 10 mL.

Injection, bupivacaine hydrochloride 0.25% and 0.5%, adrenaline 1 in 200 000, in ampoules of 10 mL.

Injection (Marcain Heavy), bupivacaine hydrochloride

0.5%, in glucose 8%, in ampoules of 4 mL. Specific gravity 1.026 at 20°.

Proprietary Names and Manufacturers
Carbostésine *(Astra, Switz.)*; Carbostesin *(Astra, Ger.)*; Duracaine *(Arg.)*; Marcain *(Astra, Austral.; Astra, Denm.; Astra, Norw.; Astra, Swed.; Astra, UK)*; Marcaina *(Pierrel, Ital.)*; Marcaine *(Belg.; Canad.; Bellon, Fr.; Neth.; Winthrop, S.Afr.; Winthrop-Breon, USA)*; Sensorcaine *(Astra, USA)*.

The following names have been used for multi-ingredient preparations containing bupivacaine hydrochloride—Marcain with Adrenaline *(Astra, UK)*; Marcaine with Adrenaline *(Astra, Austral.; Cook-Waite, USA; Winthrop-Breon, USA)*; Sensorcaine with Adrenaline *(Astra, USA)*.

7610-b

Butacaine Sulphate *(BANM, rINNM)*.

Butacain. Sulph.; Butacaine Sulfate. 3-Dibutylaminopropyl 4-aminobenzoate sulphate.
$(C_{18}H_{30}N_2O_2)_2,H_2SO_4=711.0$.

CAS — 149-16-6 (butacaine); 149-15-5 (sulphate).

Pharmacopoeias. In *Braz.*, and *Turk.*

Butacaine sulphate is a local anaesthetic of the ester type with the general actions described under Local Anaesthetics p.1205. It may also be used as the base.

A 4% ointment has been used for surface anaesthesia in the mouth to relieve pain produced by dentures, and it has also been used in ear and nasal drops.

7611-v

Butanilicaine Phosphate *(BANM, rINNM)*.

2-Butylamino-6′-chloroaceto-*o*-toluidide dihydrogen phosphate.
$C_{13}H_{19}ClN_2O,H_3PO_4=352.8$.

CAS — 3785-21-5 (butanilicaine); 2081-65-4 (phosphate).

Butanilicaine phosphate is a local anaesthetic of the amide type with the general actions described under Local Anaesthetics, p.1205. It has been used as a 1% solution for infiltration or nerve block anaesthesia, and as a 3% solution in dentistry. It is also used as the hydrochloride.

Proprietary Names and Manufacturers
Hostacain *(Hoechst, Ger.; Hoechst, Spain)*.

7613-q

Butyl Aminobenzoate *(BAN)*.

Butamben *(USAN)*; Butoforme. Butyl 4-aminobenzoate.
$C_{11}H_{15}NO_2=193.2$.

CAS — 94-25-7.

Pharmacopoeias. In *Fr.*, and *U.S.* Also in *B.P. Vet.*

A white, odourless, crystalline powder. M.p. 57° to 59°. **Soluble** 1 in 7000 of water, 1 in 3 of alcohol, and 1 in 2 of ether; soluble in chloroform, fixed oils, and dilute acids. It slowly hydrolyses when boiled with water. **Protect** from light.

Butyl aminobenzoate is a local anaesthetic of the ester type (p.1205) and has been used for surface anaesthesia.

Butyl aminobenzoate picrate is applied to the skin as a 1% ointment for the relief of pruritus and pain.

Proprietary Names and Manufacturers
Butesin Picrate *(Abbott, USA)*.

The following names have been used for multi-ingredient preparations containing butyl aminobenzoate— Butesin Picrate Ointment with Metaphen *(Abbott, Austral.)*; Cetacaine *(Cetylite, USA)*; Nestosyl *(Bengué, UK)*.

7614-p

Carticaine Hydrochloride *(BANM)*.

40 045; Articaine Hydrochloride *(rINNM)*; Carticain Hydrochloride; Hoe-045. Methyl 4-methyl-3-(2-propylaminopropionamido)thiophene-2-carboxylate hydrochloride.
$C_{13}H_{20}N_2O_3S,HCl=320.8$.

CAS — 23964-58-1 (carticaine); 23964-57-0 (hydrochloride).

Carticaine hydrochloride is a local anaesthetic of the amide type and has the general actions described under Local Anaesthetics, p.1205. It has been used as a 1 or 2% solution for infiltration and regional anaesthesia. A 5% hyperbaric solution of carticaine hydrochloride with glucose has been used for spinal anaesthesia.

Proprietary Names and Manufacturers
Ultracain *(Hoechst, Ger.)*.

The following names have been used for multi-ingredient preparations containing carticaine hydrochloride—Ultracaine D-S *(Hoechst, Canad.)*.

7615-s

Chloroprocaine Hydrochloride *(USAN, rINNM)*.

2-Diethylaminoethyl 4-amino-2-chlorobenzoate hydrochloride.
$C_{13}H_{19}ClN_2O_2,HCl=307.2$.

CAS — 133-16-4 (chloroprocaine); 3858-89-7 (hydrochloride).

Pharmacopoeias. In *U.S.*

A white odourless crystalline powder with a numbing taste.
Soluble 1 in 20 of water and 1 in 100 of alcohol; very slightly soluble in chloroform; practically insoluble in ether. Solutions in water are acid to litmus. Discoloured solutions should not be used.

Adverse Effects, Treatment, and Precautions
As for Local Anaesthetics, p.1205.

Absorption and Fate
Chloroprocaine is hydrolysed rapidly in the circulation by plasma cholinesterase. It has a half-life of about 23 seconds in adults.
See also under Local Anaesthetics, p.1206.

Uses and Administration
As for Local Anaesthetics, p.1206.
Chloroprocaine hydrochloride is a local anaesthetic of the ester type with properties similar to those of procaine hydrochloride (p.1226). It has a rapid onset and short duration of action.
It is used for infiltration and regional nerve block, including paracervical block and epidural or caudal anaesthesia, as a 0.5 to 3% solution, if necessary with adrenaline 1 in 200 000 to delay absorption and reduce toxicity. It is not an effective surface anaesthetic. It should not be used for spinal anaesthesia.
For mandibular nerve block a 2% solution has been used in a dose of 40 to 60 mg (2 to 3 mL) and for infraorbital nerve block a dose of 10 to 20 mg (0.5 to 1.0 mL) as a 2% solution has been suggested. A 2% solution has also been used for brachial plexus block in a dose of 600 to 800 mg (30 to 40 mL). For digital nerve block a 1 or 2% solution without adrenaline has been used in a dose of 30 to 80 mg (3 to 8 mL, 1%; 1.5 to 4 mL, 2%). In obstetrics a dose of 200 mg (10 mL) per side as a 2% solution has been suggested for pudendal block, and for a paracervical block a 1% solution in a dose of 30 mg (3 mL) at each of 4 sites.
For lumbar epidural block 40 to 50 mg (2.0 to 2.5 mL) as a 2% solution or 60 to 75 mg (2.0 to 2.5 mL) as a 3% solution has been used for each segment to be anaesthetised. The usual total dose being 300 to 750 mg with smaller repeat doses being given at 40- to 50-minute intervals. For caudal block a dose of 300 to 500 mg (15 to 25 mL) of a 2% solution or 450 to 750 mg (15 to 25 mL) of a 3% solution has been suggested.
In adults single doses of chloroprocaine without adrenaline should not exceed 800 mg and single doses with adrenaline 1 in 200 000 should not exceed 1 g.

Chloroprocaine hydrochloride, in a dose of 12 mL of a 1% solution containing adrenaline 1 in 200 000, was used for 261 paracervical blocks in 211 patients during childbirth. Apgar scores were depressed in 11 of 213 infants and no foetal deaths were related to chloroprocaine. In 6 of 104 foetuses monitored abnormal heart-rate patterns were recorded *in utero* but none had a depressed Apgar score at birth. In 172 blocks pain relief was excellent in 83%, partially effective in 5%, and ineffective in 12%.— D. W. Freeman and N. I. Arnold, *J. Am. med. Ass.*, 1975, *231*, 56.

Preparations
Chloroprocaine Hydrochloride Injection *(U.S.P.)*. pH 2.7 to 4.0.

Proprietary Names and Manufacturers
Nesacaine *(Astra, USA)*; Nesacaine-CE *(Astra, Canad.; Astra, USA)*.

7616-w

Cinchocaine *(BAN, rINN)*.

Cincainum; Dibucaine *(USAN)*. 2-Butoxy-*N*-(2-diethylaminoethyl)cinchoninamide; 2-Butoxy-*N*-(2-diethylaminoethyl)quinoline-4-carboxamide.
$C_{20}H_{29}N_3O_2=343.5$.

CAS — 85-79-0.

Pharmacopoeias. In *Nord.* and *U.S.* Also in *B.P.C. 1973.*

A white to off-white powder, with a slight characteristic odour. M.p. 62° to 66°.
Soluble 1 in 4600 of water, 1 in less than 1 of alcohol and of chloroform, and 1 in 1.4 of ether. It darkens on exposure to light. **Store** in airtight containers. Protect from light.

7617-e

Cinchocaine Hydrochloride *(BANM, rINNM)*.

Cincaini Chloridum; Dibucaine Hydrochloride *(USAN)*; Dibucainium Chloride; Percainum; Sovcainum.
$C_{20}H_{29}N_3O_2,HCl=379.9$.

CAS — 61-12-1.

NOTE. This compound was originally marketed under the name Percaine, but accidents occurred owing to the confusion of this name with procaine.

Pharmacopoeias. In *Arg., Aust., Br., Braz., Cz., Fr., It., Jpn, Nord., Port., Rus., Swiss,* and *U.S.*

Fine, white, odourless or almost odourless, hygroscopic crystals or white to off-white crystalline powder. M.p. 96° to 100°.
Soluble 1 in 0.5 of water; freely soluble in alcohol and acetone; soluble in chloroform. A 2% solution in water has a pH of 5 to 6. It darkens on exposure to light. **Store** in airtight containers. Protect from light.

Adverse Effects, Treatment, and Precautions
As for Local Anaesthetics, p.1205.

Absorption and Fate
Like other local anaesthetics of the amide type, cinchocaine is metabolised in the liver.
See also under Local Anaesthetics, p.1206.

Uses and Administration
As for Local Anaesthetics, p.1206.
Cinchocaine is a local anaesthetic of the amide type which is suitable for surface or spinal anaesthesia. It is one of the most potent, most toxic, and longest acting of the local anaesthetics in use.
Cinchocaine has vasodilator properties; the risk of adverse effects may be reduced by the inclusion of adrenaline to delay absorption.
For surface anaesthesia cinchocaine has been

used, as the base or hydrochloride, as a 0.5% cream or 1.0% ointment and as suppositories for the temporary relief of pain and itching associated with skin and rectal conditions.

For spinal anaesthesia a hyperbaric solution of cinchocaine hydrochloride 0.25% in glucose 5% has been used in doses of 2.5 to 5 mg (1 to 2 mL). A hypobaric injection containing 0.067% (1 in 1500) has also been used in doses up to about 13 mg and an isobaric 0.5% solution has been used in doses up to 10 mg (2 mL) diluted 1 in 1000 with cerebrospinal fluid.

A report of the beneficial effects of regional nerve block with cinchocaine 0.15% in the treatment of muscular atrophy.— Y. Terauchi (letter), *Lancet*, 1976, *2*, 477.

For a comparison of cinchocaine and lignocaine sprays in the treatment of perineal trauma following childbirth, see under Lignocaine Hydrochloride p.1222.

Preparations of Cinchocaine or Cinchocaine Hydrochloride

Dibucaine Cream *(U.S.P.)*. Cinchocaine in a suitable cream basis.

Dibucaine Hydrochloride Injection *(U.S.P.)*. A sterile solution of cinchocaine hydrochloride in Water for Injections. pH 4.5 to 7.0.

Dibucaine Ointment *(U.S.P.)*. Cinchocaine in a suitable ointment basis.

Proprietary Names and Manufacturers of Cinchocaine or Cinchocaine Hydrochloride

Cincain *(Ferring, Denm.; Ferring, Swed.)*; Cinkain *(Denm.)*; Dermacaine *(Medo, UK)*; Nupercainal *(Belg.; Ciba-Geigy, Canad.; Ciba, Denm.; Ital.; Ciba, Switz.; Ciba, UK; Ciba, USA)*; Nupercaine *(Astra, Austral.; S.Afr.; Ciba, UK; Ciba, USA)*; Percainal *(Spain)*.

The following names have been used for multi-ingredient preparations containing cinchocaine or cinchocaine hydrochloride—Biosone GA *(Biorex, UK)*; Locan *(Duncan, Flockhart, UK)*; Nupercainal Suppositories *(Ciba-Geigy, Canad.)*; Proctosedyl *(Roussel, Austral.; Roussel, Canad.; Roussel, UK)*; Proctosone *(Technilab, Canad.)*; Scheriproct *(Schering, Austral.; Schering, UK)*; Ultraproct *(Schering, Austral.; Schering, UK)*; Uniroid *(Unigreg, UK)*.

7618-l

Coca

Coca Leaves; Hoja de Coca.

Pharmacopoeias. In *Arg., Fr., Port.,* and *Span.*

The dried leaves of *Erythroxylum coca* (Bolivian or Huanuco leaf) or of *E. truxillense* (Peruvian or Truxillo leaf) (Erythroxylaceae), indigenous to Bolivia and Peru and cultivated in Colombia and Indonesia.

The total alkaloid content varies from 0.7 to 1.5%.

Coca was formerly used for its stimulant action and for the relief of gastric pain, nausea, and vomiting, but it has no place in modern medicine.

7619-y

Cocaine *(BAN, USAN)*.

Cocaina; Methyl Benzoylecgonine.

(1*R*,2*R*,3*s*,5*S*)-2-Methoxycarbonyltropan-3-yl benzoate.

$C_{17}H_{21}NO_4$=303.4.

CAS — 50-36-2.

Pharmacopoeias. In *Br., It., Mex., Port., Span., Turk.,* and *U.S.*

Colourless crystals or white crystalline powder obtained from the leaves of *Erythroxylum coca* and other spp. of *Erythroxylum*, or by synthesis. M.p. 96° to 98°. It is slightly volatile. *B.P. solubilities* are: practically insoluble in water; soluble 1 in 7 of alcohol, 1 in 0.5 of chloroform, 1 in 4 of ether, and 1 in 30 of arachis oil; slightly soluble in liquid paraffin. *U.S.P.* solubilities are: soluble 1 in 600 of water, 1 in 7 of alcohol, 1 in 1 of chloroform, 1 in 3.5 of ether, 1 in 12 of olive oil, 1 in 80 to 100 of liquid paraffin. A saturated solution in water is alkaline to phenolphthalein and litmus.

7620-g

Cocaine Hydrochloride *(BAN, USAN)*.

Chloridrato de Cocaína; Cocaine Hydrochlor.; Cocaini Hydrochloridum; Cocainium Chloride.

$C_{17}H_{21}NO_4$,HCl=339.8.

CAS — 53-21-4.

NOTE. The following names have also been used to describe cocaine hydrochloride or cocaine base: bernice, blow, C, charlie, coke, crack, flake, girl, gold dust, her, lady, leaf, nose candy, rock, she, snow, toot, white girl, white lady.

Pharmacopoeias. In *Arg., Aust., Belg., Br., Braz., Chin., Cz., Egypt., Eur., Fr., Ger., Hung., Int., It., Jpn, Jug., Mex., Neth., Nord., Pol., Port., Roum., Rus., Span., Swiss, Turk.,* and *U.S.*

Odourless hygroscopic colourless crystals or white crystalline powder. M.p. about 197° with decomposition. Cocaine hydrochloride 1.12 g is approximately equivalent to 1 g of cocaine.

Soluble 1 in 0.5 of water, 1 in 3.5 to 4.5 of alcohol, 1 in 15 to 18 of chloroform; soluble in glycerol; practically insoluble in ether and fixed oils. Solutions are **sterilised** by autoclaving, maintaining at 98° to 100° for 30 minutes with a bactericide, or by filtration. **Store** in well-closed containers. Protect from moisture and light.

STABILITY OF SOLUTIONS. Aqueous solutions containing cocaine hydrochloride 5% and phenol 0.5% remained clear and colourless for a year at 0° to 4°, room temperature, and 37°. A fall in pH from 4.6 to 3.9, 2.7, and 2.1 respectively suggested chemical change; such solutions should therefore be stored in a cool place.— Pharm. Soc. Lab. Rep. P/75/14, 1975.

Adverse Effects

As for Local Anaesthetics, p.1205.

Symptoms of central nervous stimulation and sympathetic overactivity are very marked in overdosage with cocaine. A single dose of 1.2 g may be fatal, but some persons have a cocaine idiosyncrasy and death may occur quite suddenly after doses of only 20 mg. Systemic absorption of small doses may slow the heart, but with increasing doses tachycardia, hypertension, and ventricular fibrillation may occur.

Topical application of cocaine to the cornea can cause corneal damage with clouding, pitting, sloughing, and ulceration. Topical application to the nose or mouth has been reported to cause loss of smell and taste respectively.

Excessive concentrations should not be used as, in addition to risks of systemic toxicity following absorption, they may produce lasting local damage.

Abuse. Cocaine is abused for its stimulant effects on the central nervous system, producing mood elevation and euphoria which may cause an overwhelming desire to continue taking the drug and a psychological dependence on the drug. It is considered to be the most reinforcing of all psychoactive drugs. Repeated use may result in acute tolerance to some effects. Abrupt cessation after chronic administration usually results in signs and symptoms characteristic of a withdrawal syndrome, including fatigue, lassitude, irritability, and depression. This is now accepted as evidence for physical dependence although gradual withdrawal of cocaine is not necessary, indeed is not recommended, in the treatment of cocaine dependency.

Cocaine abuse may give rise to psychotic states and hallucinations, nausea, vomiting, loss of appetite, weight loss, formication (so-called "cocaine bugs"), decreased fatigue, rapid pulse, increased temperature, and rapid, shallow respiration. Convulsions, coma and death from respiratory or cardiac arrest may occur.

Cocaine is abused by nasal inhalation, termed snorting, which may cause mucosal damage and perforation of the nasal septum on prolonged use, by intravenous injection of the hydrochloride, termed shooting, and more recently by smoking of free-base cocaine, known as freebasing. It is sometimes injected with an opioid such as diamorphine to control toxic symptoms.

A review of the medical complications resulting from cocaine abuse. Acute myocardial infarction has been related to cocaine use, especially in patients with coronary artery disease, and because of its arrhythmogenic effect, cardiac arrythmias may also occur. Complications of the central nervous system include cerebrovascular accidents, seizures, and fungal cerebritis. Cocaine has been reported to cause placental vasoconstriction, abruptio placentae, and an increased risk of spontaneous abortion. Infants exposed to cocaine through maternal use during pregnancy are at increased risk of congenital malformations, perinatal mortality, and neurobehavioural impairments. Other medical complications of cocaine abuse include bowel ischaemia, loss of the sense of smell, spontaneous pneumopericardium, rupture of the ascending aorta, sexual dysfunction, and death.— L. L. Cregler and H. Mark, *New Engl. J. Med.*, 1986, *315*, 1495.

For a report on the adverse effects, treatment, and prevention of cocaine abuse, see *Adverse Health Consequences of Cocaine Abuse*, A. Arif (Ed.), Geneva, World Health Organisation, 1987..

A review of the 60 cocaine-related overdose deaths reported in Miami between July 1978 and December 1982 and a further 180 where cocaine did not directly contribute to death.— R. E. Mittleman and C. V. Wetli, *J. Am. med. Ass.*, 1984, *252*, 1889.

Two deaths due to cocaine intoxication in professional athletes are reported. One athlete died from cocaine-induced seizures and cardiac arrest and the other died as a result of severe pulmonary congestion and oedema due to cocaine intoxication. Both athletes had lethal blood concentrations of cocaine.— V. Cowart, *J. Am. med. Ass.*, 1986, *256*, 2457.

Sudden death in 7 recreational cocaine abusers was associated with hyperthermia, delirium, and agitation followed by late-onset rigidity. Cocaine can acutely release large amounts of dopamine and the clinical features seen in these subjects are suggestive of the neuroleptic malignant syndrome which may follow withdrawal of a dopamine agonist. Although chlorpromazine is the suggested treatment for cocaine overdose, it worsens neuroleptic malignant syndrome and may thus be contra-indicated. Bromocriptine may be used to reduce temperature and avoid a fatal outcome.— T. R. Kosten and H. D. Kleber, *Lancet*, 1987, *1*, 1198.

Further references to adverse effects following abuse of cocaine: E. H. Sawicka and A. Trosser, *Br. med. J.*, 1983, *286*, 1476 (CSF rhinorrhoea); J. M. Jonas and M. S. Gold (letter), *Lancet*, 1986, *1*, 390 (association between cocaine abuse and eating disorders); S. M. Tames and J. M. Goldenring (letter), *New Engl. J. Med.*, 1986, *314*, 1324 (loss of eyebrows and eyelashes following inhalation of free-base cocaine); D. Roth *et al.*, *New engl. J. Med.*, 1988, *319*, 673 (acute rhabdomyolysis and renal failure).

DEPENDENCE. When injected or inhaled cocaine produced a condition of hyperstimulation, of short duration, characterised by overalertness, euphoria, and feelings of great power. Heavy users had been known to inject cocaine intravenously every 10 minutes. In consistent users depression might occur when cocaine was withdrawn. Heavy use led to weight loss, insomnia, and anxiety. Oversuspiciousness and paranoid thinking with hallucinations were not uncommon. Violent behaviour might occur. Increases in the heart-rate, blood pressure, and respiration were the result of sympathetic stimulation. Overdosage produced tremors, convulsions, and delirium.— S. Cohen, *J. Am. med. Ass.*, 1975, *231*, 74.

Cocaine does not produce a true physical dependence with definite withdrawal symptoms, but after continual exposure there is a psychological dependence with an excessively strong craving, especially after intravenous use. A strong compulsion to obtain the drug can occur, resulting in an addictive syndrome. By 1980, 27.5% of Americans in the 18 to 25-year-age group had used cocaine, compared with 19.1% in 1978.— A. M. Nicholi, *New Engl. J. Med.*, 1983, *308*, 925.

Results from a survey of 306 intranasal cocaine users demonstrated that intranasal use offers no guarantee of safety and can still result in addiction and serious adverse consequences.— A. M. Washton *et al.* (letter), *Lancet*, 1983, *2*, 1374.

An almost pure form of free-base cocaine is now widely available through conversion of cocaine hydrochloride back to alkaloidal cocaine. This material is sometimes called 'rock' because of its appearance, or 'crack' because of the sound made by the crystals popping when it is heated. Whereas cocaine hydrochloride limits its own absorption after inhalation due to vasoconstriction and is unsuitable for smoking because it decomposes, 'crack' can be smoked allowing large quantities to be delivered to blood vessels in the lungs to produce an effect comparable to intravenous injection. Smoking of 'crack' produces an almost immediate intense euphoric experience, often quickly followed by a dysphoric 'crash' leading to frequently repeated doses and rapid addiction in susceptible individuals.— *Med. Lett.*, 1986, *28*, 69.

Further references to the greater addiction potential and increased risk of acute toxic reactions to free-base cocaine compared with cocaine hydrochloride: J. F. Jekel *et al.*, *Lancet*, 1986, *1*, 459; A. M. Washton and M. S. Gold (letter), *J. Am. med. Ass.*, 1986, *256*, 711; *Lancet*, 1987, *2*, 1061.

EFFECTS ON THE CARDIOVASCULAR SYSTEM. Following his first use of cocaine a 24-year-old man with no history of heart disease, experienced squeezing retrosternal pain after intravenous injection of an unknown amount of cocaine. Two hours later he had sinus tachycardia with raised blood pressure and soon after had a cardiac arrest with ventricular fibrillation. Resuscitation was successful but ventricular arrythmias continued, in spite of lignocaine and procainamide treatment, and chest pain was severe. A large anterior infarction was confirmed by ECG and radionuclide scan.— I. M. Rollingher *et al.*, *Can. med. Ass. J.*, 1986, *135*, 45.

Seven cases of fatal or potentially fatal cardiac events following abuse of cocaine. There were 4 cases of myocardial infarction, 1 case of conduction disturbance, and 2 deaths. A further 19 previously reported cases of cocaine-related cardiovascular disorders are reviewed. The authors conclude that cardiac complications of cocaine abuse are not unique to parenteral use, underlying heart disease is not a prerequisite for cardiac complications, seizures may not precede or accompany cardiac events, and cardiac disorders are not limited to massive doses of cocaine.— J. M. Isner *et al.*, *New Engl. J. Med.*, 1986, *315*, 1438.

Further references to cardiovascular toxicity associated with the abuse of cocaine.— A. Benchimol *et al.*, *Ann. intern. Med.*, 1978, *88*, 519 (palpitations and accelerated ventricular rhythm); J. S. Schachne *et al.* (letter), *New Engl. J. Med.*, 1984, *310*, 1665 (coronary artery spasm and myocardial infarction); R. E. Howard *et al.*, *J. Am. med. Ass.*, 1985, *254*, 95 (myocardial infarction).

Five cases of intracranial haemorrhage are reported associated with cocaine abuse.— A. J. Tuchman *et al.* (letter), *J. Am. med. Ass.*, 1987, *257*, 1175.

EFFECTS ON THE EYES. The use of homatropine and cocaine eye-drops for mydriasis precipitated closed-angle glaucoma in 5 patients with shallow anterior chamber depths.— A. M. V. Brooks *et al.*, *Med. J. Aust.*, 1986, *145*, 34.

EFFECTS ON THE LUNGS. Reports of adverse pulmonary effects associated with cocaine abuse: A. Adrouny and P. Magnusson (letter), *New Engl. J. Med.*, 1985, *313*, 48; R. C. Patel *et al.*, *Ann. intern. Med.*, 1987, *107*, 186.

EFFECTS ON THE NERVOUS SYSTEM. A toxic psychosis developed in a 22-year-old man treated with cocaine 10% solution, 3 mL every 4 hours for severe oral stomatitis.— L. M. Lesko *et al.* (letter), *New Engl. J. Med.*, 1982, *307*, 1153.

For the effects of cocaine abuse on mental state, see under Dexamphetamine Sulphate p.1440.

Gilles de la Tourette's syndrome. Gilles de la Tourette's syndrome, which had been well controlled for 10 years by haloperidol, was precipitated in a 27-year-old man following intranasal use of cocaine on one occasion.— M. -M. Mesulam (letter), *New Engl. J. Med.*, 1986, *315*, 398.

PREGNANCY AND THE NEONATE. A controlled study of the effects of cocaine abuse during pregnancy. Neonatal gestational age, birth weight, birth length, head circumference, and Apgar scores were not affected by cocaine use. However, 4 women who conceived whilst using cocaine had abruptio placentae immediately after intravenous self-injection of cocaine. One baby was born with prune-belly syndrome to a woman who had used 4 to 5 g of cocaine in a single day at 5 weeks' gestation. The infants born to women who used cocaine showed poor interactive abilities and an impairment of organisational response to environmental stimuli compared with the control group.— I. J. Chasnoff *et al.*, *New Engl. J. Med.*, 1985, *313*, 666.

Mean birth weight, body length, and head circumference were found to be significantly decreased in neonates born to women who abused cocaine during pregnancy compared with neonates whose mothers had not abused any drugs during pregnancy. No statistical difference was found in spontaneous abortion-rate between the groups, but the stillbirth-rate was significantly higher in the group of women who abused cocaine. All stillbirths were related to abruptio placentae. The congenital-malformation-rate was also higher in the cocaine group.— N. Bingol *et al.*, *J. Pediat.*, 1987, *110*, 93.

SEPTICAEMIA. Staphylococcal septicaemia occurred following nasal inhalation of cocaine in a 38-year-old man known to be a nasal carrier for *Staphylococcus aureus* and to have abused cocaine for 2 years.— H. S. Silverman and A. L. Smith (letter), *New Engl. J. Med.*, 1985, *312*, 1706.

Treatment of Adverse Effects

As for Local Anaesthetics, p.1205.

If an overdose of cocaine has been taken by mouth, empty the stomach by lavage or emesis. Activated charcoal has been suggested to delay absorption, but efforts to remove the drug more than 30 minutes after ingestion are probably of no use.

Intravenous propranolol has been suggested for the treatment of serious cardiac arrhythmias.

Phentolamine has been given intravenously for hypertensive reactions. The use of vasopressors may be hazardous in cocaine poisoning.

A view that propranolol hydrochloride should be used to treat overdose with cocaine and related sympathomimetic agents. A 1-mg dose administered intravenously at one-minute intervals up to a total dose of 8 mg was effective and safe in over 50 cases. There was an almost instantaneous titration toward reversal of cardiopressor effects and hypertension, tachycardia, and tachypnoea were resolved. Constant cardiovascular monitoring is vital and the problem of hyperpyrexia must be dealt with.— R. T. Rappolt *et al.* (letter), *New Engl. J. Med.*, 1976, *295*, 448.

The treatment of 75 subjects suspected of ingesting small packages containing cocaine for the purpose of smuggling, so called "body packers", is discussed. All patients with the confirmed presence of cocaine packages were given laxatives and only one patient required surgical removal of the packages, but serious consideration should be given to surgical intervention if early signs of cocaine toxicity appear.— M. M. McCarron and J. D. Wood, *J. Am. med. Ass.*, 1983, *250*, 1417. See also: D. S. Caruana *et al.*, *Ann. intern. Med.*, 1984, *100*, 73; C. A. Suarez *et al.*, *J. Am. med. Ass.*, 1977, *238*, 1391.

For reference to the use of bromocriptine in the treatment of cocaine withdrawal, see under Bromocriptine Mesylate p.1014.

Chlorpromazine reduces the acute paranoia of cocaine intoxication.— *Med. Lett.*, 1983, *25*, 85.

Nitrendipine was found to increase the survival time and lethal cocaine dose in *rats* and appeared to be a good antagonist to the toxic cardiac effects of cocaine.— G. Nahas *et al.* (letter), *New Engl. J. Med.*, 1985, *313*, 519.

Trazodone 100 mg at night, increased after one week to 200 mg at night, markedly reduced cocaine craving and relieved withdrawal symptoms of depression, hypersomnia, and agitation in a 32-year-old man who had a 3-year history of cocaine abuse allowing him to stop his cocaine habit.— G. W. Small and J. J. Purcell (letter), *Archs gen. Psychiat.*, 1985, *42*, 524.

Precautions

As for Local Anaesthetics, p.1206.

Since some patients have a marked sensitivity to cocaine the administration of a test dose before use on mucous membranes has been suggested. Ophthalmic preparations of cocaine should not be applied to the eyes for prolonged periods as damage to the cornea may occur not only from the local action of cocaine, but also from loss of the protective eyelid reflexes.

Patients receiving cocaine for surface anaesthesia should be monitored for possible cardiovascular effects. Cocaine and adrenaline enhance each other's sympathomimetic effects and should preferably not be used in association. Caution is needed if cocaine is used with other drugs that may also potentiate the action of catecholamines such as monoamine oxidase inhibitors.

Cocaine should be used with great caution in patients with hypertension, cardiovascular disease, or thyrotoxicosis.

In view of the dangerous potential interaction between cocaine and catecholamines the mixture of dry cocaine powder moistened with adrenaline solution ('Cocaine mud') was unsafe.— E. N. Willey (letter), *J. Am. med. Ass.*, 1977, *238*, 1813.

Acute dystonic reactions occurred in 6 out of 7 heavy cocaine users after 1 or 2 injections of haloperidol 8 mg intramuscularly. In 4 of the subjects dystonia occurred about 22 hours after the first dose of haloperidol and in the remaining 2 it occurred within 3 hours of the second dose. Dystonic reactions included torticollis, oculogyric crisis, and buccolingual symptoms and were severe enough to require treatment.— K. Kumor *et al.* (letter), *Lancet*, 1986, *2*, 1341.

Precipitation of acute porphyria following intranasal use of cocaine in a man with known porphyria variegata.— A. D. Dick and M. G. Prentice (letter), *Lancet*, 1987, *2*, 1150.

Absorption and Fate

Cocaine may be slowly absorbed from some sites because of the vasoconstriction it produces, but absorption occurs from all sites of application, including mucous membranes and the gastro-intestinal tract, and may be enhanced when there is inflammation. It is hydrolysed by plasma esterases and some is demethylated in the liver; it is excreted in the urine, approximately 10% as unchanged drug.

See also under Local Anaesthetics, p.1206.

In 13 surgical patients peak plasma concentratons of cocaine were reached in from 15 to 60 minutes after the application as a vasoconstrictor of cocaine hydrochloride solution 10%, in doses of 1.5 mg per kg body-weight, to the nasal mucosa before intubation; cocaine was detectable in the nose 3 hours later, and persisted in the plasma for 6 hours in some patients. Diazepam and morphine sulphate had also been given as premedication to patients in the study.— C. Van Dyke *et al.*, *Science*, 1976, *191*, 859.

Studies in 4 healthy subjects used to the effects of cocaine showed that the mean peak plasma concentrations after oral administration of cocaine hydrochloride 2 mg per kg body-weight were 104 to 424 ng per mL, reached in about 1 to 1½ hours, and decreasing gradually over the following 4 to 5 hours. Following intranasal administration of a similar dose as 10% solution, mean peak plasma concentrations were 61 to 408 ng per mL reached 1 to 2 hours after use and decreasing over the next 2 to 3 hours.— C. Van Dyke *et al.*, *Science*, 1978, *200*, 211.

Studies in 10 subjects with a known history of cocaine dependence showed a positive relationship between the peak plasma concentration, increase in heart-rate and the amount of cocaine hydrochloride given either intravenously or intranasally. The peak plasma concentration was reached in 30 to 60 minutes after intranasal administration and fell gradually over the next hour. In all patients the heart-rate returned to pre-drug values before the elimination of cocaine from plasma was complete.— J. I. Javaid *et al.*, *Science*, 1978, *202*, 227.

The pharmacokinetics of cocaine hydrochloride 32 mg by intravenous infusion over 2 minutes was studied in 5 subjects who had used cocaine at least once a week for the 2 months prior to the study but had abstained from cocaine and other drugs for 24 hours before the test dose. The mean clearance values were as follows: non-renal 2065 mL per minute, renal 31 mL per minute. The mean half-life was 48 minutes.— M. J. Chow *et al.*, *Clin. Pharmac. Ther.*, 1985, *38*, 318.

The absorption of cocaine was compared in 9 patients following the nasal application of a paste providing 500 mg or a solution (Moffett's solution containing cocaine and adrenaline) providing 200 mg. Only 5% of the total dose applied in each method was absorbed and the safety of both methods is dependent on nasal vasoconstriction restricting absorption.— R. E. Quiney, *J. Lar. Otol.*, 1986, *100*, 279.

References to the metabolism of cocaine: T. Inaba *et al.*, *Clin. Pharmac. Ther.*, 1978, *23*, 547; D. J. Stewart *et al.*, *ibid.*, 1979, *25*, 464.

Uses and Administration

Cocaine is a surface anaesthetic (see p.1206) of the ester type but, because of systemic adverse effects and the danger of causing dependence its use is now almost entirely restricted to surgery of the ear, nose, and throat. It has been largely replaced by other agents in ophthalmology because of its corneal toxicity although it may still be useful in removal or debridement of the corneal epithelium. Cocaine also blocks the uptake of catecholamines at adrenergic nerve endings and potentiates the action of catecholamines. Its sympathomimetic actions cause tachycardia, peripheral vasoconstriction, a rise in blood pressure, and mydriasis. The use of cocaine in association with drugs such as adrenaline increases the risk of cardiac arrhythmias and should be avoided.

When applied to mucous membranes, surface anaesthesia develops rapidly and persists for 30 minutes or longer depending on the concentration of cocaine used, the dose, and on the vascularity of the tissue.

Systemically, cocaine stimulates the cerebral cortex and gives rise to a feeling of well-being and exhilaration; fatigue is overcome and capacity for work increased. Repeated use of cocaine may lead to dependence.

Cocaine hydrochloride is used for the administration of cocaine in aqueous solutions. Cocaine may be used topically in solutions of 1 to 20% although concentrations no greater than 4% are recommended to reduce the incidence and severity of systemic adverse effects. Solutions containing up to 4% have been used in ophthalmology and 0.25 to 0.5% solutions have been suggested for corneal anaesthesia.

It has been recommended that no more than 1.0 to 1.5 mg per kg body-weight should be applied as a single application to mucous membranes in adults; others have recommended a maximum dose of 50 mg in adults.

Cocaine has also been used in pastes for topical application.

Cocaine has been used in conjunction with diamorphine or morphine for the relief of severe pain, especially in terminal illness but this use is now discouraged.

Cocaine solutions should never be administered by injection for local, regional, or spinal anaesthesia; other local anaesthetics are equally effective and much safer.

SURFACE ANAESTHESIA. The view that a 25% paste of cocaine hydrochloride suspended in soft paraffin is an effective and safe local anaesthetic for the nasal mucosa when used very sparingly.— R. P. E. Barton and R. F. E. Gray, *J. Lar. Otol.*, 1979, *93*, 1201.

Cocaine hydrochloride did not exert any clinically significant sympathomimetic effect when a 10% solution was applied to the nasal mucosa before intubation in a study of 18 patients undergoing coronary artery surgery, under general anaesthesia with nitrous oxide, halothane, and pancuronium bromide.— P. G. Barash *et al.*, *J. Am. med. Ass.*, 1980, *243*, 1437.

Nose bleeds. In severe nose bleeds a 2.5 to 10% solution of cocaine, sprayed onto the nasal mucosa, helps to stop the bleeding by vasoconstriction. It also anaesthetises the mucosa so that any later manoeuvre that may be necessary can be performed without discomfort.— H. Ludman, *Br. med. J.*, 1981, *282*, 967.

Preparations of Cocaine and Cocaine Hydrochloride

Cocaine Eye-drops *(B.P.C. 1973).* Guttae Cocainae; CCN. This solution is adversely affected by alkali.

Cocaine Eye Drops Strong *(A.P.F.)*

Cocaine and Homatropine Eye-drops *(B.P.C. 1973).* Guttae Cocainae et Homatropinae. This solution is adversely affected by alkali.

Cocaine Hydrochloride Tablets for Topical Solution *(U.S.P.)*

Homatropine and Cocaine Eye Drops *(A.P.F.)*

Cocaine and Adrenaline Paste 10% *(A.P.F.).* Cocaine hydrochloride 10, adrenaline acid tartrate 0.18, chlorbutol 1, liquid paraffin (by weight) 45, white soft paraffin to 100.

Cocaine and Adrenaline Paste 25% *(A.P.F.).* Cocaine hydrochloride 25, adrenaline acid tartrate 0.18, chlorbutol 1, liquid paraffin (by weight) 45, white soft paraffin to 100.

7621-q

Cyclomethycaine Sulphate *(BANM, rINNM).*

Cyclomethycaine Sulfate *(USAN).* 3-(2-Methylpiperidino)propyl 4-cyclohexyloxybenzoate hydrogen sulphate.

$C_{22}H_{33}NO_3,H_2SO_4$=457.6.

CAS — 139-62-8 (cyclomethycaine); 50978-10-4 (sulphate); 537-61-1 (hydrochloride).

Pharmacopoeias. In *Br.* and *U.S.*

A white odourless or almost odourless crystalline powder. **Soluble** 1 in 50 of water, 1 in 50 of alcohol, and 1 in about 250 of chloroform; slightly soluble in dilute mineral acids.

Cyclomethycaine sulphate is a local anaesthetic of the ester type (p.1205). It has been used as a surface anaesthetic as a cream, ointment, gel, and suppositories.

Preparations

Cyclomethycaine Sulfate Cream *(U.S.P.)*

Cyclomethycaine Sulfate Jelly *(U.S.P.)*

Cyclomethycaine Sulfate Ointment *(U.S.P.)*

Cyclomethycaine Sulfate Suppositories *(U.S.P.)*

Proprietary Names and Manufacturers

Surfacaine *(Lilly, USA).*

7622-p

Dimethisoquin Hydrochloride *(BANM).*

Chinisocaine Hydrochloride; Dimethisoquinium Chloride; Quinisocaine Hydrochloride *(rINNM).* 2-(3-Butyl-1-isoquinolyloxy)-*NN*-dimethylethylamine hydrochloride.

$C_{17}H_{24}N_2O,HCl$=308.9.

CAS — 86-80-6 (dimethisoquin); 2773-92-4 (hydrochloride).

Dimethisoquin hydrochloride is a local anaesthetic (p.1205) which has been used in the form of an ointment in a concentration of 0.5% for the relief of pruritus associated with haemorrhoids, sunburn, and insect stings.

Proprietary Names and Manufacturers

Haenal *(Wolfer, Ger.)*; Isochinol *(Chemipharm, Ger.; Chemipharm, Switz.)*; Pruralgan *(Pharmacia, Ger.)*; Pruralgin *(Pharmacia, Norw.; Pharmacia, Switz.: Pharmacia, Swed.)*; Quotane *(Smith Kline & French, Austral.; Bellon, Belg.; Smith Kline & French, Canad.; Bellon, Fr.; Bellon, Neth.; Smith Kline & French, S.Afr.; Smith Kline & French, UK; Smith Kline & French, USA).*

7623-s

Diperodon *(BAN, USAN, rINN).*

Diperocaine. 3-Piperidinopropylene bis(phenylcarbamate) monohydrate.

$C_{22}H_{27}N_3O_4,H_2O$=415.5.

CAS — 101-08-6 (anhydrous); 51552-99-9 (monohydrate).

Pharmacopoeias. In *U.S.*

A white to cream-coloured powder with a characteristic odour. Practically **insoluble** in water; soluble 1 in 3 of alcohol, 1 in 10 of chloroform, 1 in 4 of ether, and 1 in 1 of methyl alcohol.

7624-w

Diperodon Hydrochloride *(BANM, rINNM).*

Diperocaine Hydrochloride.

$C_{22}H_{27}N_3O_4,HCl$=433.9.

CAS — 537-12-2.

Diperodon is a local anaesthetic which has been used as the base or hydrochloride for surface anaesthesia.

The general actions of local anaesthetics are described on p.1205.

Preparations

Diperodon Ointment *(U.S.P.)*

Proprietary Names and Manufacturers

Diothane *(Merrell Dow, USA).*

The following names have been used for multi-ingredient preparations containing diperodon hydrochloride— Allersone *(Mallard, USA).*

7625-e

Dyclonine Hydrochloride *(USAN, rINNM).*

Dyclocaini Chloridum. 4′-Butoxy-3-piperidinopropiophenone hydrochloride.

$C_{18}H_{27}NO_2,HCl$=325.9.

CAS — 586-60-7 (dyclonine); 536-43-6 (hydrochloride).

Pharmacopoeias. In *U.S.*

White crystals or white crystalline powder, with a slight odour. **Soluble** 1 in 60 of water, 1 in 24 of alcohol, and 1 in 2.3 of chloroform; soluble in acetone; practically insoluble in ether and hexane. A 1% solution in water has a pH of 4 to 7. **Store** in airtight containers. Protect from light.

Dyclonine hydrochloride is a local anaesthetic used for topical anaesthesia of the skin and mucous membranes as a 0.5 or 1.0% aqueous solution. Single doses in excess of 200 mg should generally not be used. It may cause irritation at the site of application and should not be given by injection or used in the eyes.

The general actions of local anaesthetics are described on p.1205.

Preparations

Dyclonine Hydrochloride Gel *(U.S.P.).* pH 2 to 4. Do not pack in aluminium or tin tubes.

Dyclonine Hydrochloride Topical Solution *(U.S.P.).* Dyclonine Hydrochloride Solution. pH 3 to 5.

Proprietary Names and Manufacturers

Dyclone *(Astra, USA).*

3108-b

Ethyl Chloride *(BAN, USAN).*

Aethylium Chloratum; Chlorethyl; Cloruro de Etilo; Ethylis Chloridum; Hydrochloric Ether; Monochlorethane. Chloroethane.

C_2H_5Cl=64.51.

CAS — 75-00-3.

Pharmacopoeias. In *Arg., Aust., Belg., Br., Cz., Egypt., Hung., Ind., Int., It., Jug., Mex., Nord., Pol., Port., Roum., Rus., Span., Turk.,* and *U.S.*

At ambient temperatures and pressures ethyl chloride is gaseous but condenses, when slightly compressed, into a colourless, mobile, flammable, very volatile liquid with an ethereal odour. If prepared from Industrial Methylated Spirit it contains a small variable proportion of methyl chloride. B.p. 12° to 13°.

Slightly **soluble** in water; miscible with alcohol and ether. It is neutral to litmus. **Store** in airtight containers preferably hermetically sealed at a temperature not exceeding 15°. Protect from light.

CAUTION. *Ethyl chloride is highly flammable and mixtures of the gas with 5 to 15% of air are explosive.*

Adverse Effects and Precautions

As for Chloroform, p.1114.

It may induce laryngeal spasm.

In Great Britain the recommended exposure limits of ethyl chloride are 1000 ppm (long-term); 1250 ppm (short-term).

Uses and Administration

Ethyl chloride was used as an inhalational anaesthetic but has been superseded by other agents.

On account of its low boiling-point and the intense cold produced by evaporation, ethyl chloride has been used as a local anaesthetic in minor surgery but this procedure is not generally recommended. It has also been used topically for the relief of pain.

Proprietary Names and Manufacturers

The following names have been used for multi-ingredient preparations containing ethyl chloride— Frezan *(Drug Houses Austral., Austral.).*

7626-l

Etidocaine Hydrochloride *(BANM, rINNM).*

W-19053. (±)-2-(*N*-Ethylpropylamino)butyro-2′,6′-xylidide hydrochloride.

$C_{17}H_{28}N_2O,HCl=312.9$.

CAS — 36637-18-0 (etidocaine); 36637-19-1 (hydrochloride).

NOTE. Etidocaine is *USAN*.

Adverse Effects, Treatment, and Precautions

As for Local Anaesthetics, p.1205.

EFFECTS ON THE HEART. For a report of cardiac arrest, not preceded by hypoxia, in patients given etidocaine, see Bupivacaine Hydrochloride, p.1209.

PORPHYRIA. Etidocaine was considered to be unsafe in patients with acute porphyria because it has been shown to be porphyrinogenic in *animals* or *in vitro* systems.— M.R. Moore and K.E.L. McColl, *Porphyrias, Drug Lists*, Glasgow, Porphyria Research Unit, University of Glasgow, 1987.

PREGNANCY AND THE NEONATE. Epidural anaesthesia for Caesarean section with etidocaine 1.5% in combination with adrenaline 5 µg per mL [1 in 200 000] had no effect on blood flow in the foetal aorta or the umbilical vein. Foetal heart rate decreased but remained within normal limits. Maternal arterial pressure was decreased and 7 of the 9 women required intravenous administration of ephedrine for imminent hypotension.— A. Lindblad *et al., Br. J. Anaesth.*, 1987, *59*, 1265.

Absorption and Fate

Etidocaine is rapidly absorbed into the circulation after parenteral injection and is about 95% bound to plasma proteins. It crosses the placenta. Etidocaine is metabolised in the liver and the metabolites are excreted in the urine.

See also under Local Anaesthetics, p.1206.

Half-lives reported after the intravenous injection of etidocaine were: α, 0.036 hour; β, 0.31 hour; and γ, 2.6 hours.— G. T. Tucker and L. E. Mather, *Br. J. Anaesth.*, 1975, *47*, 213.

The concentration of etidocaine in the umbilical vein (UV) was 0.07 to 0.45 µg per mL compared with 0.25 to 1.3 µg per mL in maternal (M) arterial or venous plasma. The UV:M ratio was lower for etidocaine than for bupivacaine, mepivacaine, lignocaine, or prilocaine.— P. J. Poppers, *Br. J. Anaesth.*, 1975, *47*, 322.

In a study on the disposition of etidocaine following epidural administration, there were no significant differences between pregnant and non-pregnant women except during delivery when the fraction of unbound etidocaine in plasma increased. Following administration during labour the placental transfer of etidocaine was rapid and the cord/maternal venous blood concentration ratio was nearly always less than 1 (mean 0.342).— D. J. Morgan *et al., Eur. J. clin. Pharmac.*, 1977, *12*, 359.

The pharmacokinetics and metabolism of etidocaine in the neonates of mothers who had received epidural injections during labour. In 5 neonates the mean elimination half-life of etidocaine was 6.42 hours and half-lives of the metabolites PABX, EABX, and 2-amino-2′-butyroxylidide (ABX) were 8.15, 8.60, and 13.3 hours respectively.— D. Morgan *et al., Eur. J. clin. Pharmac.*, 1978, *13*, 365.

Uses and Administration

As for Local Anaesthetics, p.1206.

Etidocaine hydrochloride is a local anaesthetic of the amide type. It has a rapid onset similar to lignocaine, but has a longer duration of action.

Etidocaine is used for infiltration anaesthesia and regional nerve block, usually with adrenaline 1 in 200 000. The maximum dose should not generally exceed 300 mg, or 400 mg when given with adrenaline.

For infiltration anaesthesia a 0.5% solution may be used in a dose of 5 to 400 mg (1 to 80 mL) and for peripheral nerve block a 0.5% solution may be used in a dose of 25 to 400 mg (5 to 80 mL) or a 1.0% solution in a dose of 50 to 400 mg (5 to 40 mL).

When given by epidural injection etidocaine hydrochloride produces a profound degree of motor blockade and abdominal muscle relaxation. Up to 300 mg may be injected as a 1 or 1.5% solution for lumbar epidural block prior to surgery, including caesarean section. Lower doses of up to 200 mg as a 0.5 or 1% solution are suggested for epidural anaesthesia during labour. For caudal anaesthesia up to 300 mg as a 0.5 or 1% solution may be given.

EPIDURAL BLOCK. The quality of spinal epidural anaesthesia was assessed in 246 patients using etidocaine 1 or 1.5%, bupivacaine 0.5%, and lignocaine 1.5 or 2%. All solutions contained adrenaline 1 in 200 000. Etidocaine 1.5% (40 patients) was the only anaesthetic completely to block the S1 segment in all patients and its use was associated with fewer complaints from patients.— A. Galindo *et al., Br. J. Anaesth.*, 1975, *47*, 41.

A double-blind crossover comparison in 5 healthy men of the effects of epidural block at L2 by etidocaine 1.5% or bupivacaine 0.75%, both with adrenaline.— M. Stanton-Hicks *et al., Br. J. Anaesth.*, 1976, *48*, 575.

There was no evidence of significant plasma accumulation of etidocaine in 5 patients given etidocaine hydrochloride 200 mg epidurally (as 1% solution) before surgery followed by 4 doses of 100 mg at 2-hour intervals for postoperative pain relief. Prolonged block in some patients suggested local accumulation.— G. T. Tucker *et al., Br. J. Anaesth.*, 1977, *49*, 237.

In obstetrics. In a double-blind randomised study 100 patients were given a single varying dose of either bupivacaine or etidocaine by epidural injection during the surgical induction of labour. Etidocaine had a quicker onset of action than bupivacaine but its duration of action was shorter and it produced a greater degree of muscle weakness. It was not the drug of choice for use during labour.— G. Phillips, *Br. J. Anaesth.*, 1975, *47*, 1305.

A favourable report of the use of 25 mL of etidocaine 1% with or without adrenaline for epidural block in caesarean delivery in 81 patients. The ratio of the pooled umbilical arterial plus venous blood concentration to maternal venous blood concentration was low at about 0.38 for plain solution and 0.28 for solution containing adrenaline. A dose of 20 mL of 1% etidocaine with adrenaline was probably adequate; 214 patients had now been treated.— P. C. Lund *et al., Br. J. Anaesth.*, 1977, *49*, 457.

REGIONAL NERVE BLOCK. In a double-blind study of ulnar nerve block in 10 subjects etidocaine 0.25% and lignocaine 1%, both with adrenaline 1 in 200 000, had a similar rapid onset and similar duration of action. Etidocaine 0.5% and lignocaine 1%, both with adrenaline, produced analgesia lasting 583 and 262 minutes and motor block lasting 653 and 294 minutes, respectively. Etidocaine 0.5% and lignocaine 1%, both without adrenaline, produced analgesia lasting 320 and 165 minutes and motor block lasting 358 and 139 minutes, respectively.— P. J. Poppers *et al., Anesthesiology*, 1974, *40*, 13.

Proprietary Names and Manufacturers

Dur-Anest *(Astra, Ger.)*; Duranest *(Astra, Austral.; Astra, Swed.; Astra, USA)*.

The following names have been used for multi-ingredient preparations containing etidocaine hydrochloride— Duranest with Adrenaline *(Astra, Austral.; Astra, USA)*.

7627-y

Euprocin Hydrochloride *(USAN, rINNM)*.

Isoamylhydrocupreine Dihydrochloride; Isopentylhydrocupreine Dihydrochloride; Wl-287. (9*R*)-10,11-Dihydro-6′-(3-methylbutoxy)cinchonan-9-ol dihydrochloride monohydrate.

$C_{24}H_{34}N_2O_2,2HCl,H_2O=473.5$.

CAS — 1301-42-4 (euprocin); 18984-80-0 (hydrochloride, anhydrous).

Euprocin hydrochloride is a local anaesthetic formerly used in ear-drops.

The general actions of local anaesthetics are described on p.1205.

7628-j

Fomocaine *(BAN, rINN)*.

Fomocainum. 4-[3-(α-Phenoxy-*p*-tolyl)propyl]morpholine.

$C_{20}H_{25}NO_2=311.4$.

CAS — 17692-39-6.

Fomocaine is a local anaesthetic which has been used for surface anaesthesia as a 4% cream or ointment.

The general actions of local anaesthetics are described on p.1205.

Proprietary Names and Manufacturers

Erbocain *(Heilit, Ger.)*.

7630-p

Hexylcaine Hydrochloride *(USAN, rINNM)*.

Hexylcainium Chloride. 2-Cyclohexylamino-1-methylethyl benzoate hydrochloride.

$C_{16}H_{23}NO_2,HCl=297.8$.

CAS — 532-77-4 (hexylcaine); 532-76-3 (hydrochloride).

Pharmacopoeias. In *U.S.*

A white powder with a slight aromatic odour. **Soluble** 1 in 17 of water; freely soluble in alcohol and chloroform; practically insoluble in ether. A 5% solution in water has a pH of 4 to 6. **Store** in airtight containers.

Adverse Effects, Treatment, and Precautions

As for Local Anaesthetics, p.1205.

Tissue irritation and necrosis have been reported following topical or inadvertent parenteral administration of hexylcaine hydrochloride.

EFFECTS ON THE NERVOUS SYSTEM. Convulsions occurred on 5 of 200 occasions in which hexylcaine was used for epidural anaesthesia.— P. C. Lund *et al., Br. J. Anaesth.*, 1975, *47, Suppl.*, 313.

Uses and Administration

Hexylcaine hydrochloride is a local anaesthetic of the ester type which is used for surface anaesthesia (see p.1206). A solution containing up to 5% has been used.

Preparations

Hexylcaine Hydrochloride Topical Solution *(U.S.P.)*

Proprietary Names and Manufacturers

Cyclaine *(Merck Sharp & Dohme, USA)*.

7631-s

Isobucaine Hydrochloride *(USAN)*.

2-Isobutylamino-2-methylpropyl benzoate hydrochloride.

$C_{15}H_{23}NO_2,HCl=285.8$.

CAS — 14055-89-1 (isobucaine); 3562-15-0 (hydrochloride).

Pharmacopoeias. In *U.S.*

A white odourless crystalline powder. **Soluble** 1 in 1 of water, 1 in 8 of alcohol, and 1 in 6 of chloroform; sparingly soluble in isopropyl alcohol; very slightly soluble in ether. A 2% solution in water has a pH of about 6.

Isobucaine hydrochloride is a local anaesthetic of the ester type with the general actions described under Local Anaesthetics, p.1205.

Preparations

Isobucaine Hydrochloride and Epinephrine Injection *(U.S.P.)*. A sterile solution of isobucaine hydrochloride and adrenaline in Water for Injections.

12882-b

Ketocaine Hydrochloride *(rINNM)*.

Chetocaina Cloridrata. 2′-(2-Diisopropylaminoethoxy)butyrophenone hydrochloride.

$C_{18}H_{29}NO_2,HCl=327.9$.

CAS — 1092-46-2 (ketocaine); 1092-47-3 (hydrochloride).

Ketocaine hydrochloride has been used as a local anaesthetic.

Proprietary Names and Manufacturers

Vericaina *(Recordati, Ital.)*.

7632-w

Leucinocaine Mesylate

Leucinocaine Mesilate *(rINNM)*. 2-Diethylamino-4-methylpentyl 4-aminobenzoate methanesulphonate.

$C_{18}H_{32}N_2O_5S=388.5$.

CAS — 92-23-9 (leucinocaine); 135-44-4 (mesylate).

Leucinocaine mesylate is a local anaesthetic of the ester type (see p.1205).

7602-b

Lignocaine *(BAN)*.

Lidocaine *(USAN, rINN)*; Lidocainum. 2-Diethylaminoaceto-2′,6′-xylidide.
$C_{14}H_{22}N_2O$=234.3.

CAS — 137-58-6.

Pharmacopoeias. In *Braz., Hung., Int., It., Jpn, Roum.,* and *U.S.*

A white to slightly yellow crystalline powder with a characteristic odour. It is stable in air. M.p. 66° to 69°.

Practically **insoluble** in water; very soluble in alcohol and chloroform; freely soluble in ether; soluble in oils.

Lignocaine forms a mixture with prilocaine that has a melting point lower than that of either ingredient. This eutectic mixture is used in the preparation of topical dosage forms.

7601-m

Lignocaine Hydrochloride *(BANM)*.

Lidocaine Hydrochloride *(USAN, rINNM)*; Lidocaini Hydrochloridum; Lignoc. Hydrochlor.
$C_{14}H_{22}N_2O,HCl,H_2O$=288.8.

CAS — 73-78-9 (anhydrous); 6108-05-0 (monohydrate).

Pharmacopoeias. In *Arg., Aust., Belg., Br., Braz., Chin., Egypt., Eur., Fr., Ger., Hung., Ind., Int., It., Jug., Neth., Nord., Pol., Port., Swiss, Turk.,* and *U.S.* Also in *B.P. Vet.*

U.S. also includes Sterile Lidocaine Hydrochloride.

A white crystalline odourless or almost odourless powder. M.p. 74° to 79°. Lignocaine hydrochloride 1.23 g is approximately equivalent to 1 g of lignocaine.

Soluble 1 in 0.7 of water, 1 in 1.5 of alcohol; soluble in chloroform; practically insoluble in ether. A 0.5% solution in water has a pH of 4.0 to 5.5. Solutions or gels are **sterilised** by autoclaving. **Store** in well-closed containers. Protect from light.

CARBONATED SOLUTIONS. For a report on the preparation of carbonated solutions of prilocaine and lignocaine, see Prilocaine Hydrochloride, p.1225.

EUTECTIC MIXTURES. The ratio of lignocaine to prilocaine in a eutectic composition is close to 1:1 with a mean eutectic temperature of 18°.— A. Brodin *et al., J. pharm. Sci.,* 1984, *73,* 481.

INCOMPATIBILITY. Lignocaine hydrochloride caused precipitation of amphotericin.— D. A. Whiting, *Br. J. Derm.,* 1967, *79,* 345.

An immediate precipitate occurred when lignocaine hydrochloride 2 g per litre was mixed with *methohexitone sodium* 2 g per litre, and a crystalline precipitate occurred with *sulphadiazine sodium* 4 g per litre in glucose injection.— B. B. Riley, *J. Hosp. Pharm.,* 1970, *28,* 228.

For reference to the incompatability between lignocaine hydrochloride and glyceryl trinitrate, see p.1499.

STABILITY OF SOLUTIONS. Lignocaine, bupivacaine, and mepivacaine as bases, exhibited decreased solubility in phosphate buffer with increasing temperature. It was suggested that possible precipitation of the base of these local anaesthetics from the hydrochloride salt may occur at the site of injection due to an increase in pH of the base to the tissue pH or due to a lowering of free base solubility at body temperature relative to ambient temperature.— N. I. Nakano (letter), *J. pharm. Sci.,* 1979, *68,* 667.

A study of the stability of lignocaine hydrochloride in intravenous infusion fluids stored at 25° for 14 days. As determined by visual inspection, lignocaine hydrochloride was compatible with aminophylline, bretylium tosylate, calcium gluconate, digoxin, dopamine hydrochloride, insulin, and procainamide hydrochloride for at least 24 hours, but incompatible with phenytoin sodium.— H. L. Kirschenbaum *et al., Am. J. Hosp. Pharm.,* 1982, *39,* 1013. Lignocaine concentration, in buffered cardioplegic solutions, decreased significantly when stored in polyvinyl chloride containers at ambient temperature, but not when stored at 4°. This loss appeared to result from sorption of lignocaine onto the plastic and did not occur when lignocaine solutions were stored in glass bottles.— T. E. Lackner *et al., ibid.,* 1983, *40,* 97.

For a report on the stability of injections containing lignocaine hydrochloride and adrenaline, see Adrenaline, p.1454.

Adverse Effects and Treatment

As for Local Anaesthetics, p.1205.

A survey by the Boston Collaborative Drug Surveillance Program of the use and toxicity of lignocaine given intravenously to 750 patients with a mean age of 65 years for the treatment of cardiac arrhythmias. Treatment was started within 48 hours of admission in 77% of patients and adverse reactions were reported in 47 patients (6.3%) as follows: CNS disturbances, 31 patients; cardiovascular disturbances, 8; CNS and cardiovascular reactions, 4; phlebitis at the injection site, 3; and rash, 1. Twelve reactions were considered life-threatening. The majority of adverse effects were reported within the first 2 days of therapy and were more frequent in elderly patients, in those who died, and in those with long hospitalisations. Diagnoses of acute myocardial infarction or congestive heart failure, and low body-weight were also associated with a higher frequency of unwanted effects. Patients with serious underlying disease or with diminished hepatic clearance of lignocaine appear to be predisposed to adverse effects.— H. J. Pfeifer *et al., Am. Heart J.,* 1976, *92,* 168. See also K. Buckman *et al., Clin. Pharmac. Ther.,* 1980, *28,* 177.

ALLERGY AND ANAPHYLAXIS. Intradermal and subcutaneous test doses of lignocaine in 8 patients with suspected lignocaine hypersensitivity who had been given chlorpheniramine 10 mg intramuscularly gave positive wheal and flare reactions in only 2 patients. The authors concluded that all 8 patients could safely be given plain lignocaine in future and question whether true anaphylaxis to lignocaine has ever been shown.— M. R. Barer and M. K. McAllen, *Br. med. J.,* 1982, *284,* 1229.

A 57-year-old woman became somnolent and had several generalised tonic-clonic seizures, 5 minutes after starting nebulisation with 5 mL of lignocaine 4% solution prior to bronchoscopy. Respiration became laboured with audible wheezing and cyanosis requiring intubation and assisted ventilation. The patient improved allowing a return to spontaneous respiration but 3 days after the first episode, 0.5 mL of lignocaine 1% solution was inadvertently given subcutaneously for local anaesthesia and 5 minutes later the patient was agitated, cyanotic, tachypnoeic, and hypotensive requiring a return to the ventilator until oxygenation and alveolar infiltrates improved. Anaphylactic reaction with the development of adult respiratory distress syndrome seems the most likely explanation for these two episodes.— J. J. Howard *et al., Chest,* 1982, *81,* 644.

A 19-year-old woman received less than 30 mL of lignocaine 1% solution for topical anaesthesia prior to bronchoscopy. Anaesthesia and bronchoscopy were well tolerated but 20 minutes after the procedure the patient became hypotensive, tachycardic, and obtunded. Sodium chloride infusion and naloxone were given intravenously but there was no improvement and respiratory arrest occurred. Despite artificial respiration and supportive therapy hypotension and refractory bradycardia occurred and the patient died. An anaphylactic reaction to lignocaine with cardiovascular collapse and adult respiratory distress syndrome was thought to be the reason for death.— R. A. Promisloff and D. C. Du Pont (letter), *Chest,* 1983, *83,* 585.

Wheezy dyspnoea and cyanosis occurred in a 67-year-old man 2 minutes after the administration of lignocaine spray 20 mg to one nostril and 60 mg to the posterior pharyngeal wall for premedication prior to bronchoscopy. Cardiorespiratory arrest occurred which was treated with sodium bicarbonate infusion, adrenaline, and calcium chloride, resulting in ventricular fibrillation. Cardioversion and lignocaine injection 100 mg produced asystole from which the patient did not recover despite attempts at resuscitation. Death was attributed to a hypersensitivity reaction to topical lignocaine.— S. P. Ruffles and J. G. Ayres, *Br. med. J.,* 1987, *294,* 1658.

Erythema of the upper lip occurred in a 7-year-old girl after buccal and palatal infiltration of a local anaesthetic solution containing lignocaine. The erythematous lesion became crusted and a pigmented area remained faintly visible 7 months later. Skin testing with the constituents of the local anaesthetic solution gave negative results and subsequent local anaesthesia with a procaine solution caused no adverse reactions. It was postulated that this reaction was a type of fixed drug eruption to lignocaine.— R. K. Curley *et al., Br. dent. J.,* 1987, *162,* 113.

EFFECTS ON THE BLOOD. Reports of methaemoglobinaemia associated with the use of lignocaine: D. Burne and A. Doughty (letter), *Lancet,* 1964, *2,* 971; W. J. O'Donohue *et al., Archs intern. Med.,* 1980, *140,* 1508.

Lignocaine 75 mg given intramuscularly to 8 healthy subjects resulted in small, but significant decreases in plasma viscosity and whole blood viscosity at both high and low shear rates. Haematocrit and red-cell deformability remained unchanged.— J. E. Orr *et al., Br. J. Anaesth.,* 1986, *58,* 306.

EFFECTS ON THE EARS. Lignocaine with adrenaline, used by injection for ear-canal anaesthesia or applied directly into the middle ear, could cause severe vertigo lasting 6 to 9 hours.— F. B. Simmons *et al., Archs Otolar.,* 1973, *98,* 42.

EFFECTS ON THE HEART. Sinus standstill and loss of consciousness occurred in a 65-year-old woman given lignocaine 50 mg intravenously for ventricular arrhythmias following myocardial infarction. A pacemaker was activated and sinus rhythm returned. Ischaemic injury of the sinus node after acute myocardial infarction might enhance the inhibitory effect of lignocaine on sinus node activity.— D. Antonelli and L. Bloch (letter), *J. Am. med. Ass.,* 1982, *248,* 827.

Further reports of adverse effects on the heart with lignocaine in patients with cardiac disease.— C. T. Lippestad and K. Forfang, *Br. med. J.,* 1971, *1,* 537 (cessation of sinus node activity); J. R. Wagner and A. R. Hunter (letter), *Lancet,* 1972, *1,* 967 (Cardiac arrest); T. O. Cheng and K. Wadhwa, *J. Am. med. Ass.,* 1973, *223,* 790 (sinus rhythm replaced by junctional rhythm); S. T. Sinatra and R. M. Jeresaty, *ibid.,* 1977, *237,* 1356 (accelerated atrioventricular conduction); S. M. Mohiuddin *et al., Drug Intell. & clin. Pharm.,* 1984, *18,* 498 (atrioventricular heart block).

EFFECTS ON THE NERVOUS SYSTEM. The adverse effects of lignocaine on the central nervous system may be reduced by giving loading bolus doses over several minutes to avoid high peak blood concentrations, by reducing infusion rates if restlessness occurs, and by reducing loading doses and infusion rates by 50% in vulnerable patients such as those with liver disease or low cardiac output, or the small, frail, and elderly patient.— R. J. C. Hall, *Adverse Drug React. Bull.,* 1982, (Dec.), 356.

Six cases of suspected psychotic reactions associated with the use of lignocaine are reported in patients given intravenous lignocaine for the treatment of cardiac arrhythmias.— W. M. Turner (letter), *Ann. intern. Med.,* 1982, *97,* 149.

Tonic-clonic seizures occurred in an 89-year-old man after accidentally swallowing or aspirating an unknown amount of lignocaine 4% topical solution given for oesophageal anaesthesia. The serum-lignocaine concentration, 30 minutes after the seizures, was 7.8 µg per mL. The patient was also taking cimetidine which could have contributed to the raised serum concentration.— R. C. Parish *et al., Drug Intell. & clin. Pharm.,* 1985, *19,* 199.

OVERDOSAGE. A 54-year-old woman, accidentally given a 1-g bolus injection of lignocaine instead of 50 mg, became asystolic and apnoeic within seconds of the injection. Grand mal seizures were eventually controlled with diazepam. Her blood pressure could not be recorded until dopamine and sodium chloride infusions were begun.— F. Finkelstein and J. Kreeft (letter), *New Engl. J. Med.,* 1979, *301,* 50. For similar reports, see P. P. Mayer (letter), *Br. med. J.,* 1972, *3,* 291; B. Burlington and C. R. Freed (letter), *J. Am. med. Ass.,* 1980, *243,* 1036.

See also under Treatment of Adverse Effects, below.

Oral administration. Two cases of prolonged seizures following the oral use of lignocaine 2% viscous solution in children. Both children received lignocaine in excess of the recommended dose.— P. Rothstein *et al., J. Pediat.,* 1982, *101,* 461.

CNS toxicity in an elderly woman after swallowing 30 mL of a 4% solution of lignocaine for topical use.— R. J. Fruncillo *et al.* (letter), *New Engl. J. Med.,* 1982, *306,* 426.

An 11-month-old child experienced generalised seizures after receiving about 80 mL of lignocaine 2% viscous solution over a period of 1 week. Lignocaine had been applied to the gums for teething problems and the blood-lignocaine concentration on admission to hospital was found to be in the toxic range at 10 µg per mL.— H. C. Mofenson *et al., Clin. Pediat.,* 1983, *22,* 190.

For further reports of lignocaine overdosage in children see: R. I. Sakai and J. E. Lattin, *Am. J. Dis. Child.,* 1980, *134,* 323 (seizures and respiratory arrest); M. J. Giard *et al., Clin. Pharm.,* 1983, *2,* 110 (generalised seizures); Y. Amitai *et al.* (letter), *New Engl. J. Med.,* 1986, *314,* 182 (death).

See also under Effects on the Nervous System, above.

Urethral anaesthesia. Two patients collapsed after using urethral anaesthetic jelly; about 225 mg of lignocaine as a 2% preparation was used in 1 case.— V. W. Dix and G. C. Tresidder (letter), *Lancet*, 1963, *1*, 890. A recommendation that lignocaine jelly should not be used for urethral anaesthesia in quantities of more than 15 mL or strengths greater than 1%.— J. T. Flynn and J. P. Blandy, *Br. med. J.*, 1980, *281*, 928. A view that 50 mL of 2% lignocaine gel can be used provided that the patient has no history of allergy to local anaesthetics.— K. Axelsson *et al.*, *ibid.*, 1981, *282*, 153.

PREGNANCY AND THE NEONATE. *Effects on the foetus.* References to the effects of lignocaine on foetal heart rate following maternal paracervical block with lignocaine: W. A. Liston *et al.*, *Br. J. Anaesth.*, 1973, *45*, 750 (bradycardia); K. S. Amankwah and J. M. Esposito, *Am. J. Obstet. Gynec.*, 1972, *112*, 50 (no change in foetal heart rate); R. H. Petrie *et al.*, *ibid.*, 1974, *120*, 791 (bradycardia).

Effects on the neonate. A report of lignocaine intoxication in a newborn infant following accidental injection of the foetal scalp during maternal episiotomy.— W. Y. Kim *et al.*, *Pediatrics*, 1979, *64*, 643.

TREATMENT OF ADVERSE EFFECTS. A review of the treatment for acute overdosage with cardioactive drugs, including lignocaine.— J. Henry and G. Volans, *Br. med. J.*, 1984, *289*, 1062.

Cardiopulmonary bypass. A 58-year-old man undergoing coronary artery bypass surgery was accidentally given an injection of lignocaine 2 g instead of 200 mg, resulting in complete asystole. This was treated successfully by restarting cardiopulmonary bypass support, to produce a satisfactory cardiac output, followed by atrial pacing with inotropic support.— J. Noble *et al.*, *Br. J. Anaesth.*, 1984, *56*, 1439. See also C. R. Freed and M. R. Freedman (letter), *J. Am. med. Ass.*, 1985, *253*, 3094.

Cardiac bypass support is unlikely to be a useful treatment for patients with gradual severe intoxication with lignocaine caused by inappropriately high maintenance infusion rates.— W. F. Nicholson (letter), *J. Am. med. Ass.*, 1985, *254*, 2889.

Precautions

As for Local Anaesthetics, p.1206.

In general lignocaine should not be given to patients with hypovolaemia, heart block or other conduction disturbances, and shouldbe used with caution in patients with congestive heart failure, bradycardia, or respiratory depression. A reduction in dose may be needed in cardiac disease. Lignocaine is metabolised in the liver and must be given with caution to patients with hepatic insufficiency. The plasma half-life of lignocaine may be prolonged in conditions which reduce hepatic blood flow such as cardiac and circulatory failure. Metabolites of lignocaine may accumulate in patients with renal impairment.

The clearance of lignocaine may be reduced by beta-blocking agents and cimetidine, requiring a reduction in lignocaine dosage. The cardiac depressant effects of lignocaine are additive with those of other antiarrhythmics including intravenous phenytoin.

The intramuscular injection of lignocaine may increase creatine phosphokinase concentrations which can interfere with the diagnosis of acute myocardial infarction.

ADMINISTRATION IN CARDIOVASCULAR DISORDERS. The use of lignocaine for ventricular arrhythmias not associated with myocardial infarction could be hazardous, especially in patients with hypoxia. Lignocaine might depress the cough reflex, thereby increasing pooling of secretions, and possibly lead to more severe hypoxia and arrhythmias.— J. J. Adler (letter), *New Engl. J. Med.*, 1973, *288*, 1303.

A study in 53 patients with atrial flutter or fibrillation indicated that there may be potentially serious clinical effects associated with an increased ventricle-rate if lignocaine is given intravenously to patients with atrial arrhythmias.— D. T. Danahy and W. S. Aronow, *Am. Heart J.*, 1978, *95*, 474.

In a study involving 33 patients with cardiac disease who had been given a lignocaine infusion for at least 24 hours, signs of lignocaine toxicity were observed in 6 patients. Plasma-lignocaine concentrations, however, did not provide a reliable means of predicting toxicity, although patients showing toxicity generally had higher serum-monoethylglycinexylidide (MEGX) concentrations. The mean plasma protein binding of MEGX was 15%, that of glycinexylidide 5%, and that of lignocaine 50%. The mean ratio of MEGX to lignocaine in serum water, corrected for protein binding, was 0.68 and MEGX probably contributes to the pharmacological action of lignocaine in a substantial proportion of patients.— D. E. Drayer *et al.*, *Clin. Pharmac. Ther.*, 1983, *34*, 14.

See also Cardiac Arrhythmias under Uses.

Hypotension. Both liver blood flow and lignocaine clearance were found to decrease in proportion to the degree of hypotension in patients with idiopathic orthostatic hypotension. The maximum plasma-lignocaine concentration was raised during hypotensive periods in these patients, and the volume of distribution at steady state was reduced. The results suggest that in the presence of hypotension, the maintenance dose of lignocaine should be reduced, and the initial loading dose should be given slowly to avoid high peak concentrations that might cause toxicity.— J. Feely *et al.*, *New Engl. J. Med.*, 1982, *307*, 866.

ADMINISTRATION IN RENAL FAILURE. See under Uses, below.

INTERACTIONS. A study to determine the effect of basic drugs on the binding of lignocaine to α-1-acid glycoprotein found that the free fraction of lignocaine in serum taken from healthy non-smokers, increased after the addition of chlorpromazine, propranolol, pethidine, bupivacaine, quinidine, disopyramide, amitriptyline, imipramine, or nortriptyline. Bupivacaine was found to be the most potent displacing agent and pethidine the least potent. The combination of bupivacaine and lignocaine should be used with caution.— D. L. Goolkasian *et al.*, *Eur. J. clin. Pharmac.*, 1983, *25*, 413.

Anti-arrhythmic agents. A prolonged Q-T interval, atrioventricular block, and ventricular fibrillation in a woman who had received lignocaine 8.16 g and *disopyramide* 900 mg in 29 hours.— M. T. Rothman, *Br. med. J.*, 1980, *280*, 922.

Anti-epileptic agents. After an intravenous injection of lignocaine 2 mg per kg body-weight, plasma concentrations of lignocaine were lower in 7 epileptic patients taking various anticonvulsants, including *phenytoin, benzodiazepines,* and *barbiturates,* than in 6 healthy subjects.— J. Heinonen *et al.*, *Acta anaesth. scand.*, 1970, *14*, 89.

Beta-blocking agents. A review of the interaction between lignocaine and beta-blocking agents. Significant impairment of lignocaine clearance is most likely to occur with beta blockers lacking intrinsic sympathomimetic activity and with the more lipid-soluble agents.— G. T. Tucker *et al.*, *Br. J. clin. Pharmac.*, 1984, *17*, 21S.

A study demonstrating that, in healthy subjects, both prolonged infusion of lignocaine and co-administration of *propranolol* reduce the plasma clearance of lignocaine. It may be necessary to reduce the dosage of lignocaine when propranolol is given concomitantly and to reduce the rate of infusion when lignocaine is given for prolonged periods.— H. R. Ochs *et al.*, *New Engl. J. Med.*, 1980, *303*, 373.

Pretreatment for one day with propranolol or metoprolol by mouth in 6 healthy non-smokers resulted in a significant reduction in the clearance of lignocaine given by intravenous injection compared with lignocaine clearance when no pretreatment was given.— K. A. Conrad *et al.*, *Clin. Pharmac. Ther.*, 1983, *33*, 133. Pretreatment with metoprolol or atenolol by mouth for one week in seven healthy subjects was found to have no significant effect on the systemic or apparent oral clearance of lignocaine given by mouth or intravenously.— J. O. Miners *et al.*, *Br. J. clin. Pharmac.*, 1984, *18*, 853. Pretreatment with propranolol 80 mg every 12 hours by mouth for 3 days prior to a dose of lignocaine 200 mg by mouth in 6 healthy non-smokers was found to increase the area under the mean plasma-lignocaine concentration-time curve, to increase the terminal elimination half-life, and to increase the peak plasma concentration of lignocaine. A reduction in the clearance of indocyanine green also occurred after propranolol pretreatment. The results supported theoretical predictions that propranolol lowers systemic clearance of lignocaine mainly by direct inhibition of its metabolism rather than by lowering hepatic blood flow.— N. D. S. Bax *et al.*, *Br. J. clin. Pharmac.*, 1985, *19*, 597.

H_2 receptor antagonists. A rise in serum-lignocaine concentrations was observed when cimetidine was given to patients receiving a lignocaine infusion, resulting in toxic concentrations in some cases (A.B. Knapp, *Ann. intern. Med.*, 1983, *98*, 174); the interaction might be mediated by cimetidine's antagonism at the H_2 receptor causing a reduction in hepatic blood flow. However, these results were criticised, since plasma-lignocaine concentrations might rise during a continuous infusion in the absence of cimetidine (J.R. Powell, *ibid.*, *99*, 279; W.O. Frank *et al.*, *ibid.*, 414). Ranitidine was also found to alter lignocaine kinetics due to a small reduction in hepatic blood flow in healthy subjects (R.A. Robson *et al.*, *Br. J. clin. Pharmac.*, 1985, *20*, 170), but in a separate study in healthy subjects ranitidine had no effect on lignocaine kinetics and the authors concluded that the interaction between lignocaine and cimetidine could not be explained by H_2-receptor antagonism (J. Feely and E. Guy, *ibid.*, 1983, *15*, 378).

Further references on the interaction between lignocaine and H_2 receptor antagonists: A. B. Knapp, *J. clin. Pharmac.*, 1985, *25*, 562 (cimetidine); J. H. Patterson *et al.*, *ibid.*, 607 (cimetidine in myocardial infarction).

Smoking. In smokers the systematic bioavailability of lignocaine was decreased secondary to a marked increase in clearance after oral administration, reflecting an induction of drug-metabolising activity.— P. -M. Huet and J. LeLorier, *Clin. Pharmac. Ther.*, 1980, *28*, 208.

PORPHYRIA. Lignocaine was considered to be unsafe in patients with acute porphyria because it has been shown to be porphyrinogenic in *animals* or *in vitro* systems.— M.R. Moore and K.E.L. McColl, *Porphyrias, Drug Lists*, Glasgow, Porphyria Research Unit, University of Glasgow, 1987.

PREGNANCY AND THE NEONATE. CNS and cardiac toxicity may occur in the foetus and neonate if lignocaine is given in the presence of foetal acidosis; this has been attributed to ion trapping.— H. H. Rotmensch *et al.*, *Ann. intern. Med.*, 1983, *98*, 487.

A warning of dangers in using lignocaine in the presence of foetal hypoxia.— K. R. Lees and P. C. Rubin, *Br. med. J.*, 1987, *294*, 358.

Absorption and Fate

Lignocaine is readily absorbed from the gastro-intestinal tract, from mucous membranes, and through damaged skin. Absorption through intact skin is poor. It is rapidly absorbed from injection sites including muscle.

After an intravenous dose lignocaine is rapidly and widely distributed into highly perfused tissues followed by redistribution into skeletal muscle and adipose tissue. Lignocaine is bound to plasma proteins, including α-1-acid glycoprotein (AAG). The extent of binding is variable, depending in part on the concentrations of both lignocaine and AAG, but is approximately 70%.

Plasma concentrations decline rapidly after an intravenous dose with an initial half-life of less than 30 minutes; the elimination half-life is 1-2 hours but may be prolonged if infusions are given for longer than 24 hours or if hepatic blood flow is reduced.

The therapeutic plasma concentration range is reported to be 1 to 6 µg per mL in the treatment of arrhythmias.

Lignocaine undergoes first-pass metabolism in the liver and bioavailability is about 35% after oral administration. Metabolism in the liver is rapid and approximately 90% of a given dose is dealkylated to form monoethylglycinexylidide (MEGX) and glycinexylidide (GX). Both of these metabolites may contribute to the therapeutic and toxic effects of lignocaine and since their half-lives are longer than that of lignocaine, accumulation, particularly of glycinexylidide, may occur during prolonged infusions. Further metabolism occurs and metabolites are excreted in the urine with less than 10% of unchanged lignocaine.

Lignocaine readily crosses the placenta and blood brain barrier.

See also under Local Anaesthetics, p.1206.

The pharmacokinetics of lignocaine may be altered by disease states, and other factors. During prolonged lignocaine infusions the hepatic extraction of lignocaine decreases and therefore infusion rate should be reduced if infusions are continued for longer than 24 hours. Lignocaine metabolites may have antiarrhythmic effects and also contribute to CNS toxicity; although patients with renal disease may be given regular loading and maintenance doses of lignocaine, glycinexylidide may accumulate in these patients and cause CNS toxicity, and patients with congestive heart failure may accumulate monoethylglycinexylidide which has antiarrhythmic activity. Congestive heart failure also causes a reduction in the volume of distribution of the central compartment of lignocaine and reduced clearance, so both loading doses and infusion rates must be decreased. Lignocaine clearance is also reduced in hepatic disease but does not appear to be altered in the elderly and neither loading doses nor maintenance doses need to be altered for age.— E. S. Waller, *J. clin. Pharmac.*, 1981, *21*, 181.

The mean elimination half-life of lignocaine was 3.22 hours in 12 patients with uncomplicated *myocardial infarction* after they had received an intravenous bolus injection of lignocaine 1 mg per kg body-weight followed by an intravenous infusion of 20 µg per kg per minute for between 25 and 60 hours. It was recommended that even in patients without cardiac or hepatic failure the rate of infusion of lignocaine should be reduced by one half after the first 24 hours to compensate for the decrease in the rate of elimination.— J. LeLorier *et al.*, *Ann. intern. Med.*, 1977, *87*, 700.

For the influence of disease states and other factors on lignocaine pharmacokinetics, see: P. D. Thomson *et al.*, *Ann. intern. Med.*, 1973, *78*, 499 (in heart failure, renal failure, or liver disease); J. A. H. Forrest *et al.*, *Br. med. J.*, 1977, *1*, 1384 (in chronic liver disease); R. L. Williams *et al.*, *Clin. Pharmac. Ther.*, 1976, *20*, 290 (in viral hepatitis); P. -M. Huet and J. LeLorier, *Clin. Pharmac. Ther.*, 1980, *28*, 208 (in chronic hepatitis); R. L. Nation *et al.*, *Br. J. clin. Pharmac.*, 1977, *4*, 439 (in the elderly).

Hepatic blood flow was found to be related to plasma-lignocaine concentrations in 8 cardiac patients and 5 healthy subjects receiving a lignocaine infusion. Early subtherapeutic lignocaine concentrations were found in all the healthy subjects and in 3 of the patients with minimal heart disease; the data suggest that early lignocaine kinetics may be significantly altered by clinical conditions that affect hepatic blood flow.— R. A. Zito and P. R. Reid, *J. clin. Pharmac.*, 1981, *21*, 100.

A high protein meal was found to increase the hepatic clearance of intravenous lignocaine in 9 healthy subjects.— A. T. Elvin *et al.*, *Clin. Pharmac. Ther.*, 1981, *30*, 455.

Lignocaine concentrations may be considerably higher than normal in the first hour after a bolus injection during cardiopulmonary bypass. The free fraction of lignocaine may also be elevated, producing a potentially greater therapeutic effect.— F. O. Holley and D. R. Stanski, *Clin. Pharmac. Ther.*, 1984, *35*, 247.

For reference to the pharmacokinetics of lignocaine in surgical patients following epidural administration, see A. G. L. Burm *et al.*, *Clin. Pharmacokinet.*, 1987, *13*, 91.

ABSORPTION. Lignocaine 400 mg intramuscularly for intercostal block gave a mean plasma concentration of 6.48 µg per mL, compared with 4.91 µg per mL after subcutaneous vaginal injection, 4.27 µg per mL following epidural injection, and 1.95 µg per mL after subcutaneous abdominal injection. The concentration of lignocaine in an injection did not affect the maximum plasma concentration reached but increasing the speed of administration produced a slightly higher plasma concentration.— D. B. Scott *et al.*, *Br. J. Anaesth.*, 1972, *44*, 1040.

The absorption of lignocaine 2 mg per kg body-weight following subcutaneous injection in the lumbar region before lumbar puncture, was studied in 10 patients in whom the blood brain barrier was undamaged. Serum-lignocaine concentrations were measured in all 10 patients and the maximum concentration was seen 25 minutes after injection. The lignocaine metabolite monoethylglycinexylidide (MEGX) was measured in serum, but glycinexylidide (GX) could not be detected. Slow penetration of lignocaine and MEGX into cerebrospinal fluid (CSF) occurred. CSF concentrations of lignocaine and MEGX were measurable in 8 and 5 patients respectively, the peak lignocaine concentration occurring 70 minutes after injection. The ratio of CSF-lignocaine to serum total lignocaine increased steadily throughout the 120-minute study period.— E. Laurikainen *et al.*, *Eur. J. clin. Pharmac.*, 1983, *25*, 639.

Serum-lignocaine concentrations were below detectable limits in 30 patients given subcutaneous injections of lignocaine 1% solution in doses ranging from 10 to 300 mg for the management of lacerations. Absorption characteristics of lignocaine following subcutaneous injection in traumatised tissue appear to differ from those in healthy tissue.— J. A. Barone *et al.*, *Clin. Pharm.*, 1984, *3*, 281.

See also: S. Nattel *et al.*, *New Engl. J. Med.*, 1979, *301*, 418.

Relative bioavailability of lignocaine was found to be higher following administration to the upper respiratory tract than after administration to the lower respiratory tract during fibreoptic bronchoscopy. The time to peak plasma concentration and apparent clearance of lignocaine did not differ between the two routes of administration.— A. McBurney *et al.*, *Br. J. clin. Pharmac.*, 1984, *17*, 61.

A double-blind crossover study of the effect of ultrasound on the percutaneous absorption of lignocaine following application of a 25% cream to the forearm of 10 healthy subjects showed that there was only a marginal trend towards increased lignocaine absorption in the presence of ultrasound.— J. C. McElnay *et al.*, *Br. J. clin. Pharmac.*, 1985, *20*, 421.

For a comparative study of serum concentrations following maxillary buccal infiltrations of mepivacaine hydrochloride or lignocaine hydrochloride, see Mepivacaine Hydrochloride, p.1223.

METABOLISM. The blood concentrations of lignocaine and its active metabolite monoethylglycinexylidide (MEGX) were measured in 31 patients, and higher concentrations of MEGX were found in those with congestive heart failure. In 3 patients who were studied intensively the elimination half-life of MEGX was considered to be similar to that of lignocaine. In 1 patient who experienced CNS toxicity the MEGX concentration probably contributed to the reaction although the contribution of other metabolites of lignocaine could not be discounted.— H. Halkin *et al.*, *Clin. Pharmac. Ther.*, 1975, *17*, 669.

PREGNANCY AND THE NEONATE. Lignocaine has been shown to cross the placenta after epidural and intravenous administration to the mother with a ratio of umbilical to maternal venous lignocaine concentration of 0.5 to 0.6. The foetus appears to be capable of metabolising lignocaine at term and the elimination half-life in the newborn, of drug received *in utero*, is about 3 hours compared with 100 minutes in adults.— H. H. Rotmensch *et al.*, *Ann. intern. Med.*, 1983, *98*, 487.

A review of the use of anti-arrhythmic drugs during pregnancy. Moderate doses of lignocaine over short periods in late pregnancy appear to be safe. Foetal blood concentrations are about half of the maternal values and by term the foetus is capable of metabolising lignocaine K. R. Lees and P. C. Rubin, *Br. med. J.*, 1987, *294*, 358.

See also below under Protein Binding.

Excretion into breast milk. The concentration of lignocaine in the breast milk of a mother given 2 intravenous injections of lignocaine followed by an intravenous infusion was 0.8 µg per mL, 7 hours after starting treatment. The maternal serum-lignocaine concentration at 5 hours was 2 µg per mL. It was concluded that a nursing mother could probably continue to breast feed with safety while on parenteral lignocaine, although there is a remote possibility of an idiosyncratic or allergic reaction in the infant.— J. A. Zeisler *et al.*, *Drug Intell. & clin. Pharm.*, 1986, *20*, 691.

PROTEIN BINDING. A review of the relationship between plasma-lignocaine binding and α-1-acid glycoprotein (AAG). Plasma-lignocaine binding has been shown to be closely related to the plasma concentration of AAG, and this helps to explain the accumulation of lignocaine in the plasma of patients with acute myocardial infarction given a constant infusion of lignocaine, since AAG concentrations are shown to increase with a similar time course following myocardial infarction. The relationship between lignocaine binding and AAG has also been studied with regard to age, sex, renal disease, cirrhosis, and concomitant drug therapy. In situations where AAG concentration is altered the usual therapeutic range for total plasma lignocaine concentrations may not apply, providing a strong rationale for monitoring free-lignocaine concentrations.— D. G. Shand, *Clin. Pharmacokinet.*, 1984, *9*, *Suppl.* 1, 27.

Serum protein binding of lignocaine was found to be increased in the serum of smokers at a final lignocaine concentration of 1.4 µg per mL. This could be due to elevation of serum α-1-acid glycoprotein in smokers.— P. J. McNamara *et al.* (letter), *J. pharm. Sci.*, 1980, *69*, 749. The mean percentage of unbound lignocaine in the plasma of male subjects was 31.8% compared with 37.2% in females taking oral contraceptives and 33.6% in females not taking oral contraceptives. Plasma α-1-acid glycoprotein (AAG) was significantly related to lignocaine plasma binding. AAG concentration in plasma appears to be the major determinant of the sex-related differences in lignocaine binding.— P. A. Routledge *et al.*, *Br. J. clin. Pharmac.*, 1981, *11*, 245.

In a study to evaluate age-related changes in α-1-acid glycoprotein and the influence on plasma drug binding in the newborn, the concentration of α-1-acid glycoprotein was found to be 3 times greater in the maternal plasma than in the plasma of the neonate. The free fraction of lignocaine in neonatal plasma was higher than that in maternal plasma at delivery, indicating reduced protein binding in the newborn, and could be explained, at least in part, by the lower α-1-acid glycoprotein concentration. The free fraction of lignocaine was also greater in pregnant women than in non-pregnant women and greater in women taking the oral contraceptive pill than in an age-matched group of women not taking oral contraceptives.— M. Wood and A. J. J. Wood, *Clin. Pharmac. Ther.*, 1981, *29*, 522.

Total plasma-lignocaine concentrations were found to be raised in the presence of an inflammatory process in patients given lignocaine prior to bronchoscopy. The plasma concentration of α-1-acid glycoprotein was also raised in these patients because of the presence of inflammation, thus allowing increased lignocaine binding. Low plasma concentrations of free lignocaine with high concentrations of total lignocaine may explain in part the absence of adverse effects at potentially toxic lignocaine concentrations in the presence of local inflammation.— B. Bruguerolle *et al.* (letter), *Br. J. clin. Pharmac.*, 1985, *20*, 180.

THERAPEUTIC DRUG MONITORING. *Plasma concentrations.* The optimum therapeutic range for lignocaine has not been well defined although minimum plasma concentrations of 2 µg per mL are usually needed to eliminate ventricular ectopic beats after myocardial infarction and concentrations of 3 to 4 µg per mL are considered relatively safe for prevention of ventricular fibrillation. Toxicity may be expected with lignocaine concentrations greater than 6 µg per mL.— F. Follath *et al.*, *Clin. Pharmacokinet.*, 1983, *8*, 63.

The relationship between dosage and serum-lignocaine concentration appears linear in most patients but is difficult to predict because of large interindividual variability. Several factors can influence the pharmacokinetics of lignocaine and thus serum-drug concentration, including hepatic blood flow, the intrinsic metabolic capacity of the liver, and protein binding. Serum-lignocaine concentration correlates usefully with clinical response and toxicity, supporting the measurement of serum-drug concentrations for individualising lignocaine dosage and several Bayesian methods have been tried for dosing patients to a specified serum-lignocaine concentration to achieve the desired clinical response. The therapeutic range of lignocaine serum concentrations has been accepted as 2 to 5 µg per mL and toxicity appears to be related to serum concentrations greater than 5 µg per mL and accumulation of the lignocaine metabolite, monoethylglycinexylidide.— M. E. Burton *et al.*, *Clin. Pharmacokinet.*, 1985, *10*, 1.

The clinical application of a Bayesian method for predicting individual lignocaine dosage requirements in the treatment of ventricular arrhythmias in patients without liver disease or severe congestive heart failure. Serum-lignocaine concentrations were accurately predicted on the basis of one serum-lignocaine concentration obtained 2 to 4 hours after starting a lignocaine infusion. It was recommended that 2 serum concentrations should routinely be used to reduce the effect of errors.— S. Vozeh *et al.*, *Clin. Pharmacokinet.*, 1984, *9*, 354.

In 16 patients receiving prophylactic lignocaine total plasma-lignocaine concentrations and plasma concentrations of α-1-acid glycoprotein were used to develop a method of predicting the free lignocaine concentration in a further 41 patients receiving lignocaine. There was a close relationship between observed and predicted free-lignocaine concentration.— P. A. Routledge *et al.*, *Br. J. clin. Pharmac.*, 1985, *20*, 695.

A discussion of the rationale and current status of free lignocaine concentration monitoring in clinical practice.— C. K. Svensson *et al.*, *Clin. Pharmacokinet.*, 1986, *11*, 450.

Factors affecting the measurement of free lignocaine serum concentrations: K. V. Ponganis and D. R. Stanski, *Clin. Pharmacokinet.*, 1984, *9*, *Suppl.* 1, 95 (pH); H. R. Ha *et al.*, *ibid.*, 96 (pH, heparin).

Saliva concentrations. In a study involving 6 patients with acute myocardial ischaemia receiving lignocaine by infusion, saliva-lignocaine concentrations were found to be unhelpful in therapeutic drug monitoring because saliva flow was difficult to standardise in these patients. Very high salivary concentrations of lignocaine in these patients may explain the frequent anaesthesia of the tongue and metallic taste which occurred during the infusion.— E. Laurikainen and J. Kanto (letter), *Br. J. clin. Pharmac.*, 1983, *16*, 199. See also J. Kanto *et al.* (letter), *ibid.*, 1982, *13*, 736.

Uses and Administration

As for Local Anaesthetics, p.1206.

Lignocaine is a local anaesthetic of the amide type and is widely used by injection and for local application to mucous membranes. It has a rapid onset of action when injected (about 1 minute following intravenous injection and 15 minutes following intramuscular injection) and rapidly spreads through surrounding tissues. The speed of onset and duration of action of lignocaine are increased by the addition of a vasoconstrictor and absorption into the circulation from the site of injection is reduced. The effect lasts about 10 to 20 minutes and about 60 to 90 minutes following intravenous and intramuscular injections respectively.

Lignocaine is a useful surface anaesthetic. The base is generally used in creams, ointments, and sprays and the hydrochloride in solutions and gels. Lignocaine ointment is used for anaesthesia of mucous membranes with a maximum recommended single dose of 250 mg, calculated as the base. Gels are used for anaesthesia of the urinary tract: in females 60 to 100 mg of lignocaine hydrochloride is inserted into the urethra several minutes before examination; in males 100 to 200 mg is used before catheterisation and 600 mg before sounding or cystoscopy. Not more than 600 mg should be given in the form of a gel in any 12 hour period. Topical solutions are also used for surface anaesthesia of mucous membranes of the mouth, throat, and upper gastro-intestinal tract. For painful conditions of the mouth and throat a 2% solution may be used: 100 mg (5 mL) may be swished around the mouth and swallowed or 300 mg (15 mL) swished and spat out; for pharyngeal pain the solution is gargled and swallowed if necessary. It should not be used more frequently than every 3 hours. A 200 mg (10 mL) dose has been recommended for the treatment of hiccough. A maximum daily dose of 2.4 g has been recommended in the *US* and 600 mg in the *UK*. Doses of 40 to 200 mg (2 to 10 mL) are used prior to bronchoscopy, bronchography, laryngoscopy, endotracheal intubation, and biopsy. Lignocaine has also been used as a spray for application to the oral mucous membranes, with a maximum recommended dose of 30 mg per quadrant over 30 minutes or a total dose of 200 mg. Lignocaine is used rectally as suppositories, ointments, and creams in the treatment of haemorrhoids and other painful perianal conditions.

For percutaneous infiltration anaesthesia 0.5% or 1.0% solutions may be used in doses of 5 to 300 mg (1 to 60 mL of a 0.5% solution, or 0.5 to 30 mL of a 1.0% solution). For local infiltration anaesthesia in children doses up to 4.5 mg per kg body-weight as a 0.25 to 0.5% solution have been recommended.

The dosage of lignocaine in peripheral nerve block depends on the route of administration: for brachial plexus block 225 to 300 mg (15 to 20 mL) as a 1.5% solution may be given; for intercostal nerve block 30 mg (3 mL) is given as a 1% solution; for paracervical block a 1% solution is used in a dose of 100 mg (10 mL) on each side, repeated not more frequently than every 90 minutes; for paravertebral block a 1% solution may be used in doses of 30 to 50 mg (3 to 5 mL); a 1% solution is recommended for pudendal block in doses of 100 mg (10 mL) on each side; for retrobulbar block a 4% solution may be used in doses of 120 to 200 mg (3 to 5 mL).

Lignocaine solutions containing adrenaline 1 in 200 000 or less are used for infiltration anaesthesia and nerve blocks; higher concentrations are seldom necessary, except in dentistry. For dental use a solution of lignocaine 2% with adrenaline 1 in 100 000 to 1 in 50 000 may be used in doses of 20 to 100 mg (1 to 5 mL) for infiltration or nerve block. The maximum recommended dose of lignocaine for dental use is 300 to 500 mg as a single dose or a total dose of 6.6 mg per kg body-weight as a solution containing adrenaline.

Lignocaine is also used for sympathetic nerve block as a 1% solution in doses of 50 mg (5 mL) for cervical block and 50 to 100 mg (5 to 10 mL) for lumbar block.

For epidural anaesthesia 2 to 3 mL of solution is needed for each dermatome to be anaesthetised but usual total doses and recommended concentrations are: lumbar epidural 250 to 300 mg (25 to 30 mL) of a 1% solution for analgesia and 225 to 300 mg (15 to 20 mL) as a 1.5% solution or 200 to 300 mg (10 to 15 mL) as a 2% solution for anaesthesia, and for thoracic epidural a 1% solution may be used at doses of 200 to 300 mg (20 to 30 mL). In obstetric caudal anaesthesia 200 to 300 mg (20 to 30 mL) is used as a 1% solution and in surgical caudal anaesthesia a 1.5% solution may be used in doses of 225 to 300 mg (15 to 20 mL). For continuous epidural anaesthesia, the maximum doses should not be repeated more frequently than every 90 minutes.

A hyperbaric solution of 1.5% or 5% lignocaine hydrochloride in glucose 7.5% solution has been used for spinal anaesthesia. Doses of 50 to 75 mg (1.0 to 1.5 mL) of a 5% solution and 9 to 15 mg (0.6 to 1.0 mL) of a 1.5% solution have been used.

For intravenous regional anaesthesia a 0.5% solution has been used in doses of 50 to 300 mg (10 to 60 mL). A maximum dose of 200 mg is recommended in the *UK* and 4 mg per kg body-weight in the *US*. A maximum dose of 3 mg per kg as a 0.25 or 0.5% solution has been recommended in children.

Lignocaine is a class Ib anti-arrhythmic agent (see p.70). It suppresses spontaneous automaticity in the ventricles and His-Purkinje system; both action potential duration and effective refractory period are decreased but the effect on action potential duration is much greater. It is the drug of choice for ventricular arrhythmias associated with acute myocardial infarction, digitalis toxicity, or cardiac surgery. It is given as the hydrochloride, usually as a loading dose followed by an infusion. It is given in usual doses of 1.0 to 1.5 mg per kg body-weight as a direct intravenous injection at a rate of 25 to 50 mg per minute. If no effect is seen within 5 minutes of this loading dose, it may be repeated to a maximum dose of 200 to 300 mg in 1 hour. A continuous intravenous infusion is usually commenced during loading at a dose of 20 to 50 μg per kg body-weight at 1 to 4 mg per minute up to a maximum of 300 mg in 1 hour. It is rarely necessary to continue this infusion for longer than 24 hours. A suggested paediatric intravenous loading dose is 0.5 to 1.0 mg per kg body-weight repeated if necessary to a maximum of 3 to 5 mg per kg, followed by a continuous infusion of 10 to 50 μg per kg per minute.

Lignocaine has also been given for arrhythmias by intramuscular injection into the deltoid muscle in doses of 4 to 5 mg per kg body-weight repeated if necessary after 60 to 90 minutes to a maximum of 300 mg in 1 hour. However, this route should only be used when ECG monitoring is not available.

Lignocaine has been given by intravenous infusion in the treatment of refractory status epilepticus. It has been used in creams with hyaluronidase for use in dentistry, and with prilocaine for surface anaesthesia prior to venepuncture. It is included in some injections, such as depot corticosteroids, to prevent pain, itching, and other local irritation.

In a double-blind study of the vasoactivity of bupivacaine hydrochloride 0.125, 0.25, and 0.5% and lignocaine hydrochloride 0.5, 1, and 2%, given intradermally to healthy subjects, vasoconstriction was seen more frequently at low concentrations and vasodilation at high concentrations. The duration of action of lignocaine was unaffected by concentration whereas the effect of bupivacaine was more prolonged at a concentration of 0.5%.— C. Aps and F. Reynolds, *Br. J. Anaesth.*, 1976, *48*, 1171.

In a patient presenting with a cockroach in each ear, lignocaine 2% spray in one ear was compared with liquid paraffin in the other ear for effectiveness of cockroach removal. Lignocaine spray caused the insect to exit immediately at a rapid speed but liquid paraffin required subsequent manual removal of the dead insect.— K. O'Toole *et al.* (letter), *New Engl. J. Med.*, 1985, *312*, 1197. A recommendation that liquid paraffin is to be preferred for removing insects from the ear canal after a report of prolonged vertigo following the use of lignocaine 2% spray to remove a cockroach from the ear canal. The patient was found to have a small traumatic perforation of the tympanic membrane allowing lignocaine to enter the middle ear.— H. Cantrell (letter), *ibid.*, 1986, *314*, 720.

ADMINISTRATION. A chart for calculating the maximum safe volume of lignocaine solution, without adrenaline, based on body-weight and the concentration of solution to be used is presented.— D. A. Kelly and A. M. Henderson, *Br. med. J.*, 1983, *286*, 1784. Criticism. The maximum safe dose of lignocaine cannot be consistently related to body-weight; it also depends on the site of injection and type of procedure.— B. Dennison (letter), *ibid.*, *287*, 361.

Intrapleural administration. The discomfort caused by intrapleural instillation of tetracycline in a woman with pleural effusions was drastically reduced by adding 15 mL of a 1% lignocaine hydrochloride solution to the tetracycline solution.— G. N. Fox (letter), *J. Am. med. Ass.*, 1979, *242*, 1362. Following the occurrence of severe chest pain in a patient given a mixture of tetracycline and lignocaine intrapleurally the technique has been amended and 15 to 30 mL of a 1% lignocaine hydrochloride solution, followed by 20 mL of physiological saline, is instilled intrapleurally 30 minutes before the tetracycline. During this 30 minutes the patient is rotated through various positions in order to anaesthetise the pleura fully before instillation of the sclerosing agent.— R. G. Harbecke (letter), *ibid.*, 1980, *244*, 1899.

ADMINISTRATION IN RENAL FAILURE. Data for predicting removal of lignocaine and glycinexylidide by conventional haemodialysis.— T. P. Gibson and H. A. Nelson, *Clin. Pharmacokinet.*, 1977, *2*, 403. See also C. C. Lee and T. C. Marbury, *ibid.*, 1984, *9*, 42.

Normal half-lives for lignocaine of 1.2 to 2.2 hours are reported to be increased to 1.3 to 3 hours in end-stage renal failure. It can be given in usual doses to patients with renal failure. Lignocaine is not removed by haemodialysis.— W. M. Bennett *et al.*, *Am. J. Kidney Dis.*, 1983, *3*, 155. See also K. A. Collinsworth *et al.*, *Clin. Pharmac. Ther.*, 1975, *18*, 59.

CARDIAC ARRHYTHMIAS. Reviews on anti-arrhythmic agents, including lignocaine: J. L. Anderson *et al.*, *Drugs*, 1978, *15*, 271; W. S. Hillis and B. Whiting, *Br. med. J.*, 1983, *286*, 1332; K. A. Muhiddin and P. Turner, *Postgrad. med. J.*, 1985, *61*, 665; *Med. Lett.*, 1986, *28*, 111.

References to the use of lignocaine in the Wolff-Parkinson-White syndrome: M. E. Josephson *et al.*, *Ann. intern. Med.*, 1976, *84*, 44.

The classification of anti-arrhythmic agents, including lignocaine, according to their action on cardiac action potentials.— E. M. Vaughan Williams, *J. clin. Pharmac.*, 1984, *24*, 129. Classification of anti-arrhythmic agents according to the cardiac tissue which each affects.— J. K. Aronson, *Br. med. J.*, 1985, *290*, 487.

For reference to lignocaine in the classification of anti-arrhythmic agents, see Anti-arrhythmic Agents, p.70.

Administration. A pharmacokinetic approach to the clinical use of lignocaine intravenously. Single 50- or 100-mg loading doses of lignocaine hydrochloride may fail to maintain therapeutic plasma concentrations in the first hour of therapy and it is suggested that two bolus doses of 100 mg separated by 20 to 30 minutes or rapid infusion of the total loading dose over 15 to 60 minutes will achieve and maintain adequate concentrations.— D. J. Greenblatt *et al.*, *J. Am. med. Ass.*, 1976, *236*, 273.

A review of the evidence for a concentration-effect relationship for lignocaine in the treatment of cardiac arrhythmias.— F. Follath *et al.*, *Clin. Pharmacokinet.*, 1983, *8*, 63.

A method of maintaining a constant lignocaine plasma concentration using a loading dose followed by an exponentially decreasing infusion is described.— J. G. Riddell *et al.*, *Ann. intern. Med.*, 1984, *100*, 25. See also R. J. Sebaldt *et al.*, *ibid.*, *101*, 632.

Dosing recommendations for lignocaine in the prophylaxis and treatment of cardiac arrhythmias, including those complicted by circulatory failure.— P. Pentel and N. Benowitz, *Clin. Pharmacokinet.*, 1984, *9*, 273.

Endotracheal administration for cardiac resuscitation is discussed below.

Cardiac resuscitation. Standards and guidelines produced at the 1985 National Conference on Cardiopulmonary Resuscitation and Emergency Cardiac Care included recommendations concerning lignocaine. Lignocaine is the drug of choice for the management of ventricular ectopy, including ventricular tachycardia and ventricular fibrillation. Prophylactic administration of lignocaine in patients at high risk of myocardial infarction is recommended since it has been shown to reduce the incidence of primary ventricular fibrillation. Loading doses of lignocaine are necessary: initially 1 mg per kg body-weight as an intravenous bolus followed by additional bolus injections of 0.5 mg per kg every 8 to 10 minutes if necessary to a total of 3 mg per kg. After successful resuscitation, a continuous infusion should be started at 2 to 4 mg per minute, reducing the rate after 24 hours if infusion is continued. Similar doses may be used for prophylaxis against ventricular fibrillation, but additional 0.5 mg per kg bolus doses should be given to a total of only 2 mg per kg unless arrhythmias persist. Lignocaine may be used to treat children with ventricular fibrillation or tachycardia, or symptomatic ventricular ectopy by giving a 1 mg per kg body-weight intravenous bolus dose. It may also be given prior to cardioversion, but if ventricular tachycardia or fibrillation do not respond to cardioversion and bolus lignocaine therapy, a lignocaine infusion should be started at a rate of 20 to 50 µg per kg per minute with an additional bolus of lignocaine 1 mg per kg at the onset of infusion. The dose of lignocaine should be reduced in conditions of decreased cardiac output, in patients over 70 years of age and those with hepatic dysfunction, and in cardiac arrest.—American Heart Association and the National Academy of Sciences-National Research Council, *J. Am. med. Ass.*, 1986, *255*, 2905.

Endotracheal administration of 4% lignocaine hydrochloride solution, 1.5 mg per kg body-weight was assessed as a possible route for cardiopulmonary resuscitation in 6 patients undergoing surgery under general anaesthesia. This route resulted in rapid absorption and may be considered when vascular access cannot be secured. In 4 patients serum-lignocaine concentrations in the usual therapeutic range for the treatment of cardiac arrhythmias (1.5 to 4.0 µg per mL) were observed within 1 to 15 minutes, but were maintained only transiently and supplemental doses are probably necessary to maintain protection against arrhythmias.— M. J. Melby *et al.*, *Clin. Pharm.*, 1986, *5*, 228. See also C. L. Raehl, *ibid.*, 572.

Guidelines from the Resuscitation Council of the United Kingdom recommend administration of lignocaine 100 mg intravenously before the fourth defibrillation shock in prolonged cardiac arrest. Lignocaine may alternatively be given by endotracheal administration at twice the intravenous dose.— D. Chamberlain, *Br. med. J.*, 1986, *292*, 1068. See also B. Steggles, *ibid.*, 1187.

Myocardial infarction. The *prophylactic* use of lignocaine to prevent primary ventricular fibrillation in patients with myocardial infarction has been widely debated. Some studies have indicated a reduction in the incidence of fibrillations but not necessarily in mortality-rate whereas others have been unable to show any beneficial effect. Many cardiologists recommend prophylaxis in patients with suspected infarction (*Med. Lett.*, 1978, *20*, 113), others are less certain (*Lancet*, 1979, *1*, 193). In an evaluation of 15 randomised trials DeSilva *et al.* (*Lancet*, 1981, *2*, 855) considered that lignocaine treatment does provide prophylaxis and that the failure of most trials to demonstrate such an effect is due to small sample sizes and inadequate treatment protocols. An evaluation of published trials was also undertaken by Lown (*J. Am. med. Ass.*, 1981, *246*, 2482) who concluded that although the studies were mostly seriously flawed in design and implementation, the weight of evidence argued persuasively for the effectiveness of lignocaine prophylaxis in acute myocardial infarction. The protective effect of lignocaine in preventing death from ventricular arrhythmias was suggested in a case-control study by Horowitz and Feinstein (*ibid.*, 1981, *246*, 2455) and prophylactic lignocaine for all patients with suspected myocardial infarction was recommended by Harrison and Berte (*ibid.*, 1982, *247*, 2019) to decrease the incidence of ventricular fibrillation, although they acknowledged that many physicians did not recommend prophylactic use because of the potential for adverse effects. A more recent study (R.W. Koster and A.J. Dunning, *New Engl. J. Med.*, 1985, *313*, 1105) suggested that lignocaine might be of value in patients with suspected infarction; that raised some critical comments (B. Lown *ibid.*, 1154; J.S. Edelsberg and W.H. Gullen *ibid.*, 1986, *314*, 1116). On the other hand Carruth and Silverman (*Am. Heart J.*, 1982, *104*, 545) concluded that the frequency of ventricular fibrillation in patients with suspected acute myocardial infarction was so low that they did not recommend the routine use of prophylactic lignocaine if adequate monitoring and prompt treatment of ventricular fibrillation were available. Also Pentecost *et al.* (*Br. Heart J.*, 1981, *45*, 42), after a survey of 3 two-year treatment periods involving 1483 patients, have concluded that myocardial infarction damage, not lignocaine prophylaxis appears to be the main determinant of death or survival.

The ability of neutrophils to release superoxide anion was impaired in patients with coronary disease receiving lignocaine infusion. This could possibly reduce infarct size in patients with acute myocardial infarction.— S. L. Peck *et al.*, *J. Pharmac. exp. Ther.*, 1985, *235*, 418.

DENTAL USE. A study comparing intraligamental injection of lignocaine 2% solution containing adrenaline 1 in 80 000 with a plain lignocaine 2% solution in 98 patients undergoing dental procedures found 70.8% of patients given the solution containing adrenaline had satisfactory analgesia after one injection compared with only 28% in the adrenaline-free group. A repeat injection increased the success rates to 91.6 and 42% respectively.— R. J. M. Gray *et al.*, *Br. dent. J.*, 1987, *162*, 263.

DIALYSIS PRURITUS. In a preliminary study lignocaine 200 mg in 100 mL of physiological saline given during haemodialysis as an infusion through the arterial line of the artificial kidney over a 20-minute period provided some relief of itching to all of 20 patients with persistent severe pruritus during haemodialysis; none responded to physiological saline alone. In a subsequent double-blind study 8 of 10 patients obtained relief of pruritus following lignocaine therapy whereas only 1 of 6 did so after saline placebo.— L. Tapia *et al.*, *New Engl. J. Med.*, 1977, *296*, 261.

DUMPING SYNDROME. Lignocaine hydrochloride 2% viscous solution in doses of 15 mL three times daily an hour before meals prevents the dumping syndrome by dampening the mechanical shock of food ingestion.— A. A. Concon (letter), *Lancet*, 1981, *1*, 1429.

EPILEPSY. Lignocaine 3 mg per kg body-weight as an intravenous bolus injection at a rate not exceeding 25 to 50 mg per minute may be given to control status epilepticus in children when diazepam, phenytoin, and phenobarbitone are ineffective. The bolus dose should be followed by a constant intravenous infusion in a dose of 5 to 10 mg per kg body-weight per hour for 1 to 3 days, gradually reducing the infusion rate.— P. R. Camfield, *Can. med. Ass. J.*, 1983, *128*, 671. Lignocaine may be given to control status epilepticus in adults when diazepam, phenytoin, and phenobarbitone are ineffective. After an intravenous bolus dose of lignocaine 50 to 100 mg, an infusion of 2 to 4 mg per kg body-weight per hour should be given continuing for 1 to 3 days if necessary.— J. Bruni, *ibid.*, 531.

Further references to the use of lignocaine as an anticonvulsant: A. V. Delgado-Escueta *et al.*, *New Engl. J. Med.*, 1982, *306*, 1337.

INTRAOCULAR PRESSURE. Pretreatment with lignocaine 1.5 mg per kg body-weight intravenously failed to prevent the rise in intraocular pressure accompanying tracheal intubation in patients undergoing intraocular surgery given suxamethonium or pancuronium to facilitate intubation (D.F. Murphy *et al.*, *Br. J. Ophthal.*, 1986, *70*, 596). However in 17 children undergoing minor eye surgery with general anaesthesia and no muscle relaxants, lignocaine 2 mg per kg intravenously prior to tracheal intubation resulted in a rise in intraocular pressure of 0.7 mmHg compared with a rise of 5.1 mmHg in 18 patients receiving a saline control (B. Drenger and J. Pe'er *ibid.*, 1987, *71*, 546).

PAIN. Based on experience of more than 1000 patients with craniocervical injuries and symptoms of nerve entrapment, injection of 1 or 2% alcohol in 3 to 5 mL of 2% lignocaine with 2 mL of a depot preparation of methylprednisolone acetate gave rapid relief of pain in all but 10 patients who were considered to have non-organic disease.— R. Cilento (letter), *Br. med. J.*, 1972, *4*, 789.

Pain associated with translumbar aortography can be eliminated by adding 2 mL of 2% lignocaine per 40 mL of contrast medium to be injected intra-arterially.— R. S. Dossetor (letter), *Br. med. J.*, 1978, *2*, 127.

The direct injection of lignocaine into metastatic bone lesions has been used to control intractable bone pain in 9 cancer patients.— J. I. Zweig *et al.*, *J. Am. med. Ass.*, 1980, *244*, 2445.

Mastalgia arising from Tietze's syndrome did not respond to danazol, bromocriptine, or evening-primrose oil in 10 women, but injection of 1 mL of lignocaine 1% with hydrocortisone 50 mg around the affected costochondral junction gave a substantial or excellent reduction in pain in 7 of the 10 patients.— J. K. Pye *et al.*, *Lancet*, 1985, *2*, 373.

The commonest and most satisfactory conservative treatment of tennis elbow is injection of a steroid and local anaesthetic into the tender site. Methylprednisolone 0.5 mL combined with 0.5 mL lignocaine 2% is a useful combination which has also been used with general anaesthesia for manipulation in cases resistant to conservative measures.— T. G. Wadsworth, *Br. med. J.*, 1987, *294*, 621.

At the first request for analgesia following hysterectomy 18 women were given either lignocaine 1.5 mg per kg body-weight by intravenous injection followed by a lignocaine infusion of 2 mg per kg per hour for 2 hours, or saline in the same volumes. Lignocaine had no effect on the intensity of postoperative pain, or on the adrenocortical and hyperglycaemic responses to surgery. Plasma concentrations of lignocaine during the study were between 1.5 and 2.0 µg per mL.— K. Birch *et al.*, *Br. J. Anaesth.*, 1987, *59*, 721.

Diabetic neuropathy. In a double-blind crossover study involving 15 patients with moderate or severe painful diabetic neuropathy, lignocaine 5 mg per kg body-weight by intravenous infusion improved symptoms more effectively than placebo. In the 11 patients who responded to lignocaine, relief of symptoms lasted from 1 to 21 days.— J. Kastrup *et al.*, *Br. med. J.*, 1986, *292*, 173.

Headache. Lignocaine 1 mg per kg body-weight intravenously was found to give rapid relief of acute migraine reducing throbbing, visual disturbances, and peripheral neurological symptoms such as tingling. Tension headaches are only poorly relieved suggesting the effect of lignocaine is one of vascular stabilisation.— P. G. Barker (letter), *Med. J. Aust.*, 1986, *144*, 53.

Herpes infections. Local application of gels containing lignocaine may give considerable pain relief in the symptomatic treatment of genital herpes simplex, but the duration of pain relief is only brief.— J. K. Oates, *Br. J. Hosp. Med.*, 1983, *29*, 13.

Topical anaesthetics are of little value in the treatment of pain from herpes simplex infection, except for mouth ulcers when the application of lignocaine 5% ointment every 5 hours may provide sufficient temporary relief to sustain adequate hydration.— S. E. Straus *et al.*, *Drugs*, 1984, *27*, 364.

Stellate ganglion block was performed in 15 patients with herpes zoster ophthalmicus within 14 days of the onset of the rash using 9.5 mL of equal parts 1% lignocaine and 0.5% bupivacaine, after a test dose of 0.5 mL. The mean pain score assessed on a 100 mm visual analogue scale was 41.9 mm before block and 5.2 mm one hour after block. Mean pain scores remained significantly reduced for at least 8 weeks. In a similar group of patients who did not receive stellate ganglion block there was no significant reduction in pain during the first 8 weeks.— S. P. Harding *et al.*, *Br. med. J.*, 1986, *292*, 1428.

PREGNANCY AND THE NEONATE. The use of lignocaine in the smallest effective doses for the treatment of ventricular arrhythmias was considered to be safe for both mothers and babies.— H. H. Rotmensch *et al.*, *Ann. intern. Med.*, 1983, *98*, 487. See also K. R. Lees and P. C. Rubin, *Br. med. J.*, 1987, *294*, 358.

See also under Absorption and Fate above for use during breast feeding.

REGIONAL NERVE BLOCK. Blocking of the medial and lateral plantar nerves at the ankle by the use of 3 to 6 mL of lignocaine 1% with adrenaline 1 in 200 000 was successful in establishing anaesthesia prior to curetting plantar warts.— W. G. R. M. Laurie (letter), *Br. med. J.*, 1972, *3*, 116. See also E. G. Bradshaw and C. M. Earlam (letter), *ibid.*, 1982, *285*, 977.

Ninety patients undergoing cataract surgery under local anaesthesia received either lignocaine 2% solution or bupivacaine 0.5% solution, or a mixture of equal volumes for retrobulbar block, facial nerve block and eye lid paralysis before surgery. Of the patients receiving bupivacaine alone 37% had eye movements which interfered with surgery, but this was reduced to 17% in patients receiving lignocaine alone and patients who received a mixture of the drugs had almost complete akinesia. Patients receiving bupivacaine alone or the drug combination required little analgesia in the 12 hours following surgery, but all the patients receiving lignocaine alone required analgesia during this time. A mixture of lignocaine and bupivacaine in equal volumes gave the best results for both akinesia and pain relief, minimising the disadvantages of the two drugs used individually.— E. Oji and A. Oji, *Br. J. Ophthal.*, 1987, *71*, 66.

RESPIRATORY DISORDERS. *Cough.* Severe intractable cough was relieved for periods of between 1 and 6 weeks in 4 patients after the inhalation of 400 mg of lignocaine administered by nebuliser as 4 mL of a 10% solution in saline.— P. Howard *et al.*, *Br. J. Dis. Chest*, 1977, *71*, 19. Intractable cough was relieved similarly in 3 cancer patients. The lignocaine was preceded by the inhalation of 2 to 5 mg of salbutamol. Inhalations of lignocaine were needed at intervals of 5 to 7 days.— C. J. Stewart and T. J. Coady (letter), *Br. med. J.*, 1977, *1*, 1660.

Inhalation of lignocaine 400 mg provided dramatic suppression of chronic disabling cough in a 34-year-old man with pulmonary sarcoid. Cough suppression lasted for 7 to 9 weeks.— R. V. Sanders and M. B. Kirkpatrick, *J. Am. med. Ass.*, 1984, *252*, 2456.

SPINAL ANAESTHESIA. Spinal analgesia with hyperbaric 5% lignocaine 1.5 mL was compared with plain 0.5% bupivacaine 3 mL at the L3/4 or L2/3 level in a study involving 102 patients undergoing transurethral prostatectomy. Four patients given lignocaine required general anaesthesia because of inadequate block and 5 required additional analgesia compared to 2 and 3 respectively in the bupivacaine group. The duration of blockade was greater in the bupivacaine treated group, only one patient requiring postoperative analgesia in the first 6 hours compared with 9 patients in the lignocaine group. Time of onset, height of block, degree of hypotension, blood loss, and post-spinal headache were similar in both groups.— J. M. Millar *et al.*, *Br. J. Anaesth.*, 1986, *58*, 862.

STINGS. Successful treatment of the severe pain from a stingray injury with lignocaine nerve block.— F. M. Dormon (letter), *Lancet*, 1985, *2*, 1131.

Limited value of lignocaine application in box-jellyfish sting.— J. A. Williamson *et al.*, *Med. J. Aust.*, 1984, *141*, 851.

Lignocaine 1% cream applied locally had no significant effect on the development of the wheal response induced by the intradermal injection of diluted wasp venom to simulate a wasp sting.— L. J. McLeod *et al.* (letter), *Med. J. Aust.*, 1986, *144*, 220.

SURFACE ANAESTHESIA. Local anaesthesia over the site of minor operations had been induced in over 8000 patients, without adverse effect, by the application under occlusive dressings of 30% lignocaine cream.— H. M. Lubens *et al.*, *Am. J. Dis. Child.*, 1974, *128*, 192.

The use of lignocaine 25% cream for the separation of preputial adhesions in boyhood.— D. M. Griffiths and N. V. Freeman (letter), *Lancet*, 1984, *2*, 344. This procedure is unnecessary since preputial adhesions diminish with age in childhood.— T. Esscher (letter), *ibid.*, 581.

Endoscopy. In 6 patients the mean maximum plasma-lignocaine concentration was 1.03 µg per mL after the endotracheal application of ten 10-mg metered doses of lignocaine; in 5 patients paralysed with suxamethonium the maximum concentration of lignocaine following the application of 100 mg was 1.6 µg per mL. These values were below those at which toxicity was likely to occur.— D. B. Scott *et al.*, *Br. J. Anaesth.*, 1976, *48*, 899.

Serum-lignocaine concentrations were found to be below the sensitivity of the assay method used (0.1 µg/mL) in 14 of 15 patients who gargled and expectorated 15 mL (300 mg) of lignocaine 2% viscous solution.— A. Fazio *et al.* (letter), *Drug Intell. & clin. Pharm.*, 1987, *21*, 752.

Perineal trauma. In a study involving 76 women with moderate to severe postepisiotomy pain an alcoholic lignocaine 5% spray was found to be a more effective analgesic than alcoholic cinchocaine 2% spray and both local anaesthetics gave superior pain relief to distilled water administered as a spray. Pain relief occurred within 30 minutes of administration and was maintained for 3 to 4 hours with both local anaesthetics. Two patients experienced stinging after application of the lignocaine spray.— R. F. Harrison and M. Brennan, *Curr. med. Res. Opinion*, 1987, *10*, 364. An aqueous lignocaine 5% spray provided a superior level of pain relief to an alcoholic lignocaine 5% spray or placebo after a single application in 103 primiparous women with perineal pain associated with episiotomy. Lignocaine 5% aqueous spray provided a similar level of pain relief to mefenamic acid 500 mg by mouth.— *idem*, 375. See also *idem*, 370.

Rectal use. Lignocaine gel alone was found to be as effective as lignocaine gel used with an anal dilator in patients with posterior anal fissure and the use of anal dilators in these patients should be abandoned.— M. J. Gough and A. A. M. Lewis, *Gut*, 1982, *23*, A902.

Urethral anaesthesia. For reference to recommended doses of lignocaine gel in urethral anaesthesia, see under Overdosage in Adverse Effects, above.

Venepuncture. A review of a preparation containing a eutectic mixture of lignocaine and prilocaine for topical anaesthesia of intact skin. Application of a thick layer of the preparation to intact skin under an occlusive dressing for at least 60 minutes allows the local anaesthetics to reach the terminal nerve endings in the skin and produce a reliable anaesthesia, allowing painless needle penetration. The anaesthetics are absorbed and metabolised in the usual way and even after treating large areas or leaving the cream in place for many hours produces only very low plasma concentrations. However care is needed in very small children to avoid excessive absorption of prilocaine which may cause methaemoglobinaemia. After removal of the occlusive dressing and excess cream, the anaesthetised skin will often be much paler than the surrounding skin, but changes in skin circulation do not affect the ease of performing venepuncture and the procedure is made easier for everyone by reducing pain.— D. B. Scott, *Br. J. parent. Ther.*, 1986, *7*, 134.

A double-blind study in 60 children aged 4 to 10 years of a eutectic mixture of lignocaine and prilocaine in a cream basis compared to placebo cream found that the pain of venous cannulation was significantly less after the active cream than after placebo, assessed by both the anaesthetist and the child on a verbal rating scale.— E. -L. Maunuksela and R. Korpela, *Br. J. Anaesth.*, 1986, *58*, 1242.

A study involving 15 children with leukaemia who required repeated venepunctures found that liberal application of a cream containing a eutectic mixture of lignocaine base and prilocaine base under an occlusive dressing for at least 60 minutes significantly reduced the pain of venepuncture measured on a visual analogue scale and a verbal rating scale compared to a placebo cream.— S. Clarke and M. Radford, *Archs Dis. Childh.*, 1986, *61*, 1132.

Reference to the successful use of a cream containing lignocaine and prilocaine for local anaesthesia in adults prior to lumbar puncture.— A. C. Young (letter), *Lancet*, 1987, *2*, 1533.

Further references to the use of a cream containing lignocaine and prilocaine as a eutectic mixture: C. Wahlstedt *et al.* (letter), *Lancet*, 1984, *2*, 106; H. Evers *et al.*, *Br. J. Anaesth.*, 1985, *57*, 997; J. G. Hannington-Kiff (letter), *Lancet*, 1986, *2*, 1031.

TINNITUS. Lignocaine significantly reduced tinnitus when assessed audiometrically and subjectively in a double-blind crossover study in 32 patients. Lignocaine 2% was given intravenously in a dose of 1.5 mg per kg body-weight and was compared with an equal volume of sodium chloride injection.— F. W. Martin and B. H. Colman, *Clin. Otolaryngol.*, 1980, *5*, 3. Intravenous lignocaine can relieve tinnitus in some patients, especially those with damage to the cochlea, but the beneficial effect is transient and some patients do not benefit whilst others have untoward reactions.— S. N. Busis (letter), *J. Am. med. Ass.*, 1985, *253*, 2119. See also E. Perucca and P. Jackson, *J. Lar. Otol.*, 1985, *99*, 657.

VASECTOMY. An injection of 10 mL of 1% lignocaine solution into each vas at the time of vasectomy hastened sterility.— B. B. Errey (letter), *Med. J. Aust.*, 1977, *1*, 642.

Preparations of Lignocaine and Lignocaine Hydrochloride

Lidocaine and Epinephrine Injection *(U.S.P.)*. A sterile solution prepared from lignocaine or lignocaine hydrochloride and adrenaline with the aid of hydrochloric acid in Water for Injections or a sterile solution of lignocaine hydrochloride and adrenaline acid tartrate in Water for Injections. It contains not more than 1 in 50 000 of adrenaline. pH 3.3 to 5.5.

Lidocaine Hydrochloride Injection *(U.S.P.)*. A sterile solution of lignocaine hydrochloride in Water for Injections, or of lignocaine in Water for Injections prepared with the aid of hydrochloric acid. pH 5 to 7.

Lidocaine Hydrochloride and Dextrose Injection *(U.S.P.)*. A sterile solution containing lignocaine hydrochloride and glucose in Water for Injections. pH 3 to 7.

Lidocaine Hydrochloride Jelly *(U.S.P.)*. Lignocaine hydrochloride in a suitable sterile water-soluble viscous basis. pH 6 to 7. Store in airtight containers.

Lidocaine Hydrochloride Topical Solution *(U.S.P.)*. Contains lignocaine hydrochloride. pH 5 to 7. Store in airtight containers.

Lidocaine Hydrochloride Oral Topical Solution *(U.S.P.)*. Contains lignocaine hydrochloride.

Lidocaine Ointment *(U.S.P.)*. Contains lignocaine in a suitable hydrophilic ointment basis. Store in airtight containers.

Lidocaine Oral Topical Solution *(U.S.P.)*. Contains lignocaine with a suitable flavour. Store in airtight containers.

Lidocaine Topical Aerosol *(U.S.P.)*. Lidocaine Aerosol. A solution of lignocaine in a suitable flavoured vehicle.

Lignocaine and Adrenaline Injection *(B.P.)*. A sterile solution containing lignocaine hydrochloride and adrenaline acid tartrate. pH 3.0 to 4.5.

Lignocaine and Adrenaline Ointment *(A.P.F.)*. Contains lignocaine hydrochloride.

Lignocaine and Chlorhexidine Gel *(A.P.F.)*. Contains lignocaine hydrochloride and chlorhexidine gluconate.

Lignocaine and Chlorhexidine Gel *(B.P.)*. Lignocaine Hydrochloride and Chlorhexidine Gluconate Gel. A sterile preparation of lignocaine hydrochloride containing 0.25% v/v of Chlorhexidine Gluconate Solution. Discard after single application. Store in tamper-proof containers at a temperature of 8° to 15°.

Lignocaine Eye Drops *(A.P.F.)*. A sterile solution containing lignocaine hydrochloride and chlorhexidine acetate in Water for Injections.

Lignocaine Gel *(B.P.)*. Lignocaine Hydrochloride Gel. Sterile. Discard after single application. Store in tamper-proof containers at a temperature of 8° to 15°.

Lignocaine Injection *(B.P.)*. Lignocaine Hydrochloride Injection

Proprietary Preparations of Lignocaine and Lignocaine Hydrochloride

Emla *(Astra, UK)*. *Cream*, lignocaine 2.5%, prilocaine 2.5%, in a eutectic mixture.

Hemocane *(Intercare, UK)*. *Cream*, lignocaine hydrochloride 0.65%, zinc oxide 10%, bismuth oxide 2%, benzoic acid 0.4%, cinnamic acid 0.45%.
Suppositories, lignocaine hydrochloride 11 mg, zinc oxide 300 mg, bismuth oxide 25 mg, benzoic acid 8 mg, cinnamic acid 9 mg.

Instillagel *(Farco-Pharma, Ger.: CliniMed, UK)*. *Gel*, sterile, lignocaine hydrochloride 2%, chlorhexidine gluconate solution 0.25%, in single-use disposable syringe.

Laryng-O-Jet *(IMS, UK)*. *Topical solution*, lignocaine hydrochloride 2% in single-dose 3 mL vial and lignocaine hydrochloride 4% in single-dose 4 mL vial, with laryngotracheal cannula and attached vial injector.

Lidocaton *(Pharmaton, Switz.: Claudius Ash, UK)*. *Injection*, lignocaine hydrochloride 2%, adrenaline 1 in 80 000 in cartridges of 1.8 mL.

Lignostab *(Boots, UK)*. *Injection*, lignocaine hydrochloride 2% in cartridges of 2 mL.
Injection (Lignostab-A), lignocaine hydrochloride 2%, adrenaline 1 in 80 000 in cartridges of 2 mL.
Injection (Lignostab-A100), lignocaine hydrochloride 2%, adrenaline 1 in 100 000 in cartridges of 2 mL.
Injection (Lignostab-N), lignocaine hydrochloride 2%, noradrenaline 1 in 80 000 in cartridges of 2 mL.

Min-I-Jet Lignocaine Hydrochloride *(IMS, UK)*. *Injection*, lignocaine hydrochloride 1% in single-use syringes of 10 mL, 2% in single-use syringes of 5 mL.

Min-I-Jet Lignocaine Hydrochloride with Adrenaline 1:200 000 *(IMS, UK)*. *Injection*, lignocaine hydrochloride 5 mg (as monohydrate), adrenaline 0.005 mg (as hydrochloride)/mL in single-use prefilled syringes of 5 mL.

Minims Lignocaine and Fluorescein *(Smith & Nephew Pharmaceuticals, UK)*. *Eye-drops*, lignocaine hydrochloride 4%, fluorescein sodium 0.25%, in single-use disposable applicators.

NOTE. The code LIGFLN is permitted in Great Britain for single-dose eye-drops of lignocaine and fluorescein.

Neo-Lidocaton 2% *(Pharmaton, Switz.: Claudius Ash, UK)*. *Injection*, lignocaine hydrochloride 2%, noradrenaline 1 in 50 000, vasopressin 0.25 units per mL, in cartridges of 1.8 mL.

Oral-B Dental Gel *(Oral-B, UK)*. *Gel*, lignocaine 0.6%, cetylpyridinium chloride 0.02%, menthol 0.06%, cineole 0.1%.

Select-A-Jet Lignocaine Hydrochloride *(IMS, UK)*. *Injection*, lignocaine hydrochloride 20%, in single-use syringes of 5 mL, for intravenous infusion after dilution.

Xylocaine *(Astra, UK)*. *Injection*, lignocaine hydrochloride, anhydrous, 0.5% in ampoules of 10 mL and vials of 20 mL and 50 mL, 1.0% in ampoules of 2 mL and 10 mL and vials of 20 mL and 50 mL, 1.5% in ampoules of 25 mL, 2.0% in ampoules of 5 mL and vials of 20 mL and 50 mL.

Xylocaine with Adrenaline *(Astra, UK)*. *Injection*, lignocaine hydrochloride, anhydrous, 0.5%, adrenaline 1 in 200 000 in multi-dose vials of 50 mL; lignocaine hydrochloride, anhydrous, 1.0%, adrenaline 1 in 200 000, in ampoules of 10 mL and multi-dose vials of 20 and 50 mL; lignocaine hydrochloride, anhydrous, 2%, adrenaline 1 in 200 000, in multi-dose vials of 20 and 50 mL; lignocaine hydrochloride, anhydrous, 2%, adrenaline 1 in 80 000, in standard and self-aspirating cartridges of 2.2 mL.

Xylocaine *(Astra, UK)*. *Gel*, lignocaine hydrochloride, anhydrous, 2%.

Gel, lignocaine hydrochloride, anhydrous, 2%, chlorhexidine gluconate solution 0.25% v/v.
Ointment, lignocaine 5%.
Topical spray, lignocaine 0.1%, cetylpyridinium chloride 0.0001% (lignocaine 10 mg per metered dose).
Topical solution, lignocaine hydrochloride, anhydrous, 4%.
Topical solution, viscous, lignocaine hydrochloride, anhydrous, 2%.
Xylocaine Accordion *(Astra, UK)*. *Gel*, lignocaine hydrochloride, anhydrous, 2%, in single-use bellows-syringe.
Gel, lignocaine hydrochloride, anhydrous, 2%, chlorhexidine gluconate solution 0.25% v/v, in single-use bellows-syringe.
Xylocard *(Astra, UK)*. *Injection*, lignocaine hydrochloride, anhydrous, 20 mg/mL, in disposable syringe of 5 mL.
Injection, lignocaine hydrochloride, anhydrous, 200 mg/mL for intravenous infusion, in disposable syringes of 5 and 10 mL.
Xylodase *(Astra, UK)*. *Cream*, lignocaine 5%, hyaluronidase 0.015%.
Xyloproct *(Astra, UK)*. *Ointment*, lignocaine 5%, hydrocortisone acetate 0.275%, zinc oxide 18%, aluminium acetate 3.5%.
Suppositories, lignocaine 60 mg, hydrocortisone acetate 5 mg, zinc oxide 400 mg, aluminium acetate 50 mg.
Xylotox *(Pharmaceutical Mfg, UK)*. *Injection*, lignocaine hydrochloride 2%, adrenaline 1 in 80 000, in cartridges of 1.8 and 2.2 mL.

Proprietary Names and Manufacturers of Lignocaine and Lignocaine Hydrochloride

Abbott Dental Ointment *(Abbott, Austral.)*; Anestacon *(Webcon, USA)*; BayCaine *(Bay, USA)*; Cito-Optadren *(Switz.)*; Dalcaine *(Forest Pharmaceuticals, USA)*; Democaine *(Canad.)*; Heweneural *(Hevert, Ger.)*; Laryng-O-Jet *(Commonwealth Serum Laboratories, Austral.; IMS, UK)*; Leostesin *(Austral.; Leo, Denm.; Leo, Norw.; S.Afr.)*; Lida-Mantle *(Miles Pharmaceuticals, USA)*; Lidocarb *(NAF, Norw.)*; LidoPen *(Survival Technology, USA)*; Lidothesin *(Pharmaceutical Mfg, UK)*; Lignostab *(Boots, UK)*; Luan *(Molteni, Ital.)*; Neo-Novutox *(Braun Melsungen, Ger.)*; Odontalg *(Giovanardi, Ital.)*; Ortodermina *(Tiber, Ital.)*; Peterkaien *(S.Afr.)*; Rapidocaine *(Switz.)*; Remicaine *(Remedia, S.Afr.)*; Remicard *(Remedia, S.Afr.)*; Sarnacaine *(Austral.)*; Ultracaine *(Ulmer, USA)*; Uro-Jet *(IMS, UK)*; Xylesine *(Amino, Switz.)*; Xylocain *(Astra, Denm.; Astra, Ger.; Astra, Norw.; Astra, Swed.)*; Xylocaina *(Arg.; Byk Gulden, Ital.)*; Xylocaine *(Astra, Austral.; Belg.; Astra, Canad.; Bellon, Fr.; Jpn; Neth.; Astra, S.Afr.; Astra, Switz.; Astra, UK; Astra, USA)*; Xylocard *(Astra, Austral.; Belg.; Astra, Canad.; Bellon, Fr.; Neth.; Hässle, Norw.; Astra, S.Afr.; Hässle, Swed.; Astra, Switz.; Astra, UK)*; Xyloneural *(Stroschein, Ger.)*; Xylotox *(Austral.; Neth.; Astra, S.Afr.; Switz.; Pharmaceutical Mfg, UK)*.

The following names have been used for multi-ingredient preparations containing lignocaine or lignocaine hydrochloride—Anucaine *(Searle, Canad.)*; Anucaine-HC *(Searle, Canad.)*; Bactine *(Miles, Canad.)*; BayCaine-E *(Bay, USA)*; Betnovate Compound Suppositories *(Glaxo, UK)*; Betnovate Rectal Ointment *(Glaxo, UK)*; Bismodyne *(Loveridge, UK)*; Bradosol Plus *(Ciba Consumer, UK)*; Caladryl *(Parke, Davis, Austral.)*; Calistaflex *(Glaxo, Austral.)*; Dequadin Mouth Ulcer Paint *(Glaxo, Austral.)*; Dermocaine *(Ego, Austral.)*; Emla *(Astra, UK)*; Gynaflex *(Geistlich, UK)*;
Hemocane *(Key, Austral.; Intercare, UK)*; Instillagel *(Farco-Pharma, Ger. : CliniMed, UK)*; Lidocaton with Adrenaline *(Pharmaton, Switz.; Claudius Ash, UK)*; Lidosporin *(Wellcome, Canad.)*; Lidothesin Antiseptic Gel *(Pharmaceutical Mfg, UK)*; Lidothesin with Adrenaline *(Pharmaceutical Mfg, UK)*; Lidothesin with Noradrenaline *(Pharmaceutical Mfg, UK)*; Lignostab-A *(Boots, UK)*; Lignostab-N *(Boots, UK)*; Lip-Sed Cold Sore Lotion *(Rosken, Austral.)*; Medi Creme *(Rosken, Austral.)*; Medijel *(Key, Austral.; DDD, UK)*; Minims Fluorescein Sodium and Lignocaine *(Smith & Nephew, Austral.)*; Minims Lignocaine and Fluorescein *(Smith & Nephew Pharmaceuticals, UK)*; Neo-Lidocaton *(Claudius Ash, UK)*; Nurocain *(Astra, Austral.)*; Octocaine with Epinephrine *(Canad.)*; Oral-B Dental Gel *(Oral-B, UK)*; Ora-Sed Lotion *(Rosken, Austral.)*; Otizol-HC *(Nadeau, Canad.)*; Paxyl *(Faulding, Austral.)*; Seda-Gel Lotion *(Nelson, Austral.)*; SM-33 *(Nicholas, Austral.)*; Tuscodin *(Schering, Austral.)*; Tusselix Cough Silencers *(Key, Austral.)*; Xylocaine Gel *(Astra, UK)*; Xylocaine with Adrenaline *(Astra, Austral.; Astra, UK; Astra, USA)*; Xylocaine with Dextrose *(Astra, USA)*; Xylocaine with Hibitane *(Astra, Austral.)*; Xylodase *(Astra, UK)*; Xyloproct *(Astra, Austral.; Astra, UK)*; Xylotox 2% E.80 *(Pharmaceutical Mfg, UK)*; Xylotox 4% *(Pharmaceutical Mfg, UK)*; Xylotox Extra *(Pharmaceutical Mfg, UK)*.

7633-e

Mepivacaine Hydrochloride *(BANM, USAN, rINNM)*.

Mepivacaini Chloridum. (1-Methyl-2-piperidyl)formo-2′,6′-xylidide hydrochloride.
$C_{15}H_{22}N_2O,HCl = 282.8$.

CAS — 96-88-8 (mepivacaine); 1722-62-9 (hydrochloride).

Pharmacopoeias. In *Braz., Jpn, Nord.*, and *U.S.*

A white odourless crystalline powder.
Freely **soluble** in water and methyl alcohol; very slightly soluble in chloroform; practically insoluble in ether. A 2% solution in water has a pH of about 4.5.

STABILITY OF SOLUTIONS. For reference to the decreased solubility of mepivacaine in phosphate buffer with increasing temperature and its possible precipitation at the site of injection, see Lignocaine Hydrochloride, p.1217.

Adverse Effects, Treatment, and Precautions
As for Local Anaesthetics, p.1205.

Studies *in vitro* showed that bupivacaine dramatically reduced the binding of mepivacaine to α-1-acid glycoprotein through competitive inhibition for the same binding site, resulting in a higher than expected free concentration of mepivacaine C. T. Hartrick *et al., Clin. Pharmac. Ther.*, 1984, *36*, 546.

ALLERGY. Death in a patient following administration of mepivacaine for paracervical anaesthesia might have been due to mepivacaine intolerance.— D. A. Grimes and W. Cates, *New Engl. J. Med.*, 1976, *295*, 1397.

PORPHYRIA. Mepivacaine was considered to be unsafe in patients with acute porphyria because it has been shown to be porphyrinogenic in *animals* or *in vitro* systems.— M.R. Moore and K.E.L. McColl, *Porphyrias, Drug Lists*, Glasgow, Porphyria Research Unit, University of Glasgow, 1987.

PREGNANCY AND THE NEONATE. Changes in foetal heart-rate had been observed in 30% of more than 1000 cases where paracervical block had been induced by mepivacaine. After 200 mg of mepivacaine, the mean arterial blood concentration in 13 patients reached 2.3 μg per mL, while foetal scalp blood concentrations averaging 4 μg per mL had accompanied bradycardia. Where no bradycardia had occurred, foetal blood concentrations had averaged 1 μg per mL.— S. M. Shnider *et al.* (letter), *New Engl. J. Med.*, 1968, *279*, 947.

A characteristic syndrome including neonatal depression, seizures, often associated with apnoea and beginning before 6 hours of age, and other neurological findings was seen at birth in 7 infants who had been injected accidentally with mepivacaine during paracervical and/or pudendal block. Promotion of urinary excretion appeared to be the treatment of choice; only small amounts of mepivacaine were recovered by exchange transfusion or by gastric lavage or drainage. Although the infants were critically ill on the first day of life their outcome was generally good and the 6 survivors were subsequently free of seizures and neurologically and developmentally normal.— L. S. Hillman *et al., J. Pediat.*, 1979, *95*, 472.

Absorption and Fate
Mepivacaine is highly bound to plasma proteins. It is rapidly metabolised in the liver and less than 10% of a dose is reported to be excreted unchanged in the urine. Several metabolites are also excreted via the kidneys and include glucuronide conjugates of hydroxy compounds and an *N*-demethylated compound, 2′,6′-pipecoloxylidide (PPX). Small amounts are excreted in the faeces.

See also under Local Anaesthetics, p.1206.

Half-lives reported after the intravenous injection of mepivacaine were: α, 0.012 hour; β, 0.12 hour; and γ, 1.9 hours.— G. T. Tucker and L. E. Mather, *Br. J. Anaesth.*, 1975, *47*, 213.

A comparative study in 5 healthy subjects of serum concentrations obtained following maxillary buccal infiltrations of 36 mg of mepivacaine hydrochloride or lignocaine hydrochloride, administered as 2% solutions. A mean peak serum concentration of 400 ng per mL was achieved 30 minutes after injection of mepivacaine and of 310 ng per mL 15 minutes after injection of lignocaine; there was considerable intersubject variation. Although mepivacaine has been considered to have inherent vasoconstrictor activity it was not apparent in this study.— W. M. Goebel *et al., Br. dent. J.*, 1980, *148*, 261. The finding that mean serum-mepivacaine concentrations were slightly higher than those of lignocaine and the suggestion that mepivacaine does not have vasoconstrictor activity should not deter people from using it.— J. P. Rood (letter), *ibid.*,.

For a comparison of the pharmacokinetics of mepivacaine and prilocaine, see Prilocaine Hydrochloride, p.1225.

PREGNANCY AND THE NEONATE. References to the pharmacokinetics of mepivacaine in pregnancy and the neonate: A. O. Lurie and J. B. Weiss, *Am. J. Obstet. Gynec.*, 1970, *106*, 850; P. Meffin *et al., Clin. Pharmac. Ther.*, 1973, *14*, 218; R. L. Nation, *Clin. Pharmacokinet.*, 1980, *5*, 340 (in childbirth).

Uses and Administration
As for Local Anaesthetics, p.1206.
Mepivacaine hydrochloride is a local anaesthetic of the amide type used for infiltration, peripheral nerve block, and epidural anaesthesia. It has a rapid onset of action and an intermediate duration of action. Vasoconstrictors have been added to delay absorption and prolong duration, and to promote local haemostasis.
An adult dose of mepivacaine hydrochloride should not generally exceed 400 mg and the total dose in 24 hours should not exceed 1 g.
For infiltration anaesthesia up to 400 mg of a 1% (40 mL) or 0.5% (80 mL) solution is used. For dental infiltration a 2% solution with a vasoconstrictor or a 3% plain solution is used. For anaesthesia at a single site in the jaw a dose of 36 mg (1.8 mL) of the 2% solution or 54 mg (1.8 mL) of the 3% solution is used. For anaesthesia of the entire oral cavity 180 mg (9 mL) of the 2% solution or 270 mg (9 mL) of the 3% solution is used.
For cervical, brachial plexus, intercostal and pudendal blocks 1 or 2% solutions may be used in doses of 50 to 400 mg (5 to 40 mL) as a 1% solution, or 100 to 400 mg (5 to 20 mL) as a 2% solution. For paracervical block a dose of 100 mg (10 mL) of a 1% solution on each side has been suggested which may be repeated at an interval of not less than 90 minutes, and for a combined paracervical and pudendal block up to 150 mg (15 mL) of a 1% solution is injected on each side. For therapeutic nerve block in the management of pain 10 to 50 mg (1 to 5 mL) of a 1% solution or 20 to 100 mg (1 to 5 mL) of a 2% solution may be given.
For epidural or caudal anaesthesia usual doses are: 150 to 300 mg (15 to 30 mL) of a 1% solution, 150 to 375 mg (10 to 25 mL) of a 1.5% solution, or 200 to 400 mg (10 to 20 mL) of a 2% solution.
A suggested maximum dose for children is 5 to 6 mg per kg body-weight. Concentrations of less than 2% should be used for children less than 3 years of age.
Mepivacaine has also been used as a surface anaesthetic but other local anaesthetics such as lignocaine are more effective.

Local vasoconstriction occurred after intradermal injection of mepivacaine 0.1, 0.33, and 1.0% solutions in 10 healthy subjects compared with a saline control. Vasocontrictor activity appeared to decline with increasing concentration of mepivacaine. The duration of analgesia increased with concentration.— D. G. Willatts and F. Reynolds, *Br. J. Anaesth.*, 1985, *57*, 1006.

Preparations

Mepivacaine Hydrochloride and Levonordefrin Injection *(U.S.P.)*

Mepivacaine Hydrochloride Injection *(U.S.P.)*

Proprietary Names and Manufacturers

Carbocain *(Astra, Denm.; Astra, Norw.; Astra, Swed.)*; Carbocaina *(Pierrel, Ital.)*; Carbocaine *(Astra, Austral.; Winthrop, Canad.; Winthrop, S.Afr.; Cook-Waite, USA; Winthrop-Breon, USA)*; Chlorocain *(Pharmaceutical Mfg, UK)*; Isocaine *(Bolton, Canad.)*; Meaverin *(Rorer, Ger.)*; Mepicaton *(Pharmaton, Switz.)*; Mepivastesin *(Espe, Ger.)*; Polocaine *(Astra, USA)*; Scandicaïne *(Astra, Switz.)*; Scandicain *(Astra, Ger.; Spain; Switz.)*; Scandicaine *(Belg.; Neth.)*; Scandinibsa *(Inibsa, Spain)*.

The following names have been used for multi-ingredient preparations containing mepivacaine hydrochloride— Carbocaine with Neo-Cobefrin *(Cook-Waite, USA)*.

7634-l

Meprylcaine Hydrochloride *(USAN, rINNM)*.

Meprylcaini Chloridum. 2-Methyl-2-propylaminopropyl benzoate hydrochloride.
$C_{14}H_{21}NO_2,HCl=271.8$.

CAS — 495-70-5 (meprylcaine); 956-03-6 (hydrochloride).

Pharmacopoeias. In *U.S.*

A white odourless crystalline powder. **Soluble** 1 in 6 of water, 1 in 5 of alcohol, 1 in 3 of chloroform, and 1 in 12 of ether; slightly soluble in acetone. A 2% solution in water has a pH of about 5.7.

Meprylcaine hydrochloride is a local anaesthetic of the ester type (see p.1205) which has been used in dentistry.

Preparations

Meprylcaine Hydrochloride and Epinephrine Injection *(U.S.P.)*. A sterile solution of meprylcaine hydrochloride and adrenaline in Water for Injections. Protect from light.

12986-l

Myrtecaine *(rINN)*.

Nopoxamine. 2-[2-(10-Norpin-2-en-2-yl)ethoxy]triethylamine.
$C_{17}H_{31}NO=265.4$.

CAS — 7712-50-7.

Myrtecaine is a local anaesthetic which has been used topically. Myrtecaine lauryl sulphate has also been used. The general actions of local anaesthetics are described on p.1205.

13036-x

Octacaine Hydrochloride *(pINNM)*.

3-Diethylaminobutyranilide hydrochloride.
$C_{14}H_{22}N_2O,HCl=270.8$.

CAS — 13912-77-1 (octacaine); 59727-70-7 (hydrochloride).

Octacaine hydrochloride has been used as a local anaesthetic.

The general actions of local anaesthetics are described on p.1205.

Proprietary Names and Manufacturers

Amplicain *(Geistlich, Switz.)*.

7638-c

Oxethazaine *(BAN, USAN)*.

Oxetacaine *(rINN)*; Wy-806. 2,2′-(2-Hydroxyethylimino)bis[*N*-(αα-dimethylphenethyl)-*N*-methylacetamide].
$C_{28}H_{41}N_3O_3=467.7$.

CAS — 126-27-2.

Pharmacopoeias. In *Jpn.*

Oxethazaine is a surface anaesthetic of the amide type which is stated to have a prolonged action. It is administered by mouth in conjunction with antacids for the symptomatic relief of oesophagitis. It is an ingredient of Mucaine, p.1076. It has also been used as the hydrochloride.

The general actions of local anaesthetics are described on p.1205.

Proprietary Names and Manufacturers

Emoren *(IFI, Ital.)*.

The following names have been used for multi-ingredient preparations containing oxethazaine— Mucaine *(Wyeth, Austral.; Wyeth, Canad.; Wyeth, UK)*; Mucoxin; Mutesa; Muthesa; Oxaine; Tepilta.

7639-k

Oxybuprocaine Hydrochloride *(BANM, rINNM)*.

Benoxinate Hydrochloride *(USAN)*. 2-Diethylaminoethyl 4-amino-3-butoxybenzoate hydrochloride.
$C_{17}H_{28}N_2O_3,HCl=344.9$.

CAS — 99-43-4 (oxybuprocaine); 5987-82-6 (hydrochloride).

Pharmacopoeias. In *Jpn* and *U.S.*

White or off-white crystals or crystalline powder, odourless or with a slight characteristic odour. **Soluble** 1 in 0.8 of water, 1 in 2.6 of alcohol, and 1 in 2.5 of chloroform; practically insoluble in ether. Solutions in water are neutral to litmus.

Adverse Effects, Treatment, and Precautions

As for Local Anaesthetics, p.1205.

EFFECTS ON THE EYES. Repeated topical application of oxybuprocaine resulted in keratitis and serious corneal lesions of the eye in 3 patients. One patient also developed allergic eczema of the eyelids and fingers.— H. E. Henkes and T. N. Waubke, *Br. J. Ophthal.*, 1978, *62*, 62.

Uses and Administration

Oxybuprocaine hydrochloride is a surface anaesthetic (see p.1206) of the ester type, less irritant than amethocaine hydrochloride (p.1208) when applied to the conjunctiva in similar concentrations.

It is an effective surface anaesthetic when used as a 0.4% solution in short ophthalmological procedures. One drop instilled into the conjunctival sac anaesthetises the surface sufficiently to allow tonometry after 60 seconds and a further drop after 90 seconds provides adequate anaesthesia for the fitting of contact lenses. Three drops at 90-second intervals produces sufficient anaesthesia after 5 minutes for a foreign body to be removed from the corneal epithelium, or for incision of a Meibomian cyst through the conjunctiva. The sensitivity of the cornea is normal again after about 1 hour. The solution has no effect on the pupil.

Preparations

Benoxinate Hydrochloride Ophthalmic Solution *(U.S.P.)*. A sterile solution of oxybuprocaine hydrochloride in water. pH 3 to 6. Store in airtight containers.

Proprietary Preparations

Alcon Opulets Benoxinate *(Alcon, UK)*. *Eye-drops*, oxybuprocaine hydrochloride 0.4%, in single-use disposable applicators.

NOTE. The *B.P.* permits the title BNX for single-dose eye-drops containing oxybuprocaine.

Minims Benoxinate Hydrochloride *(Smith & Nephew Pharmaceuticals, UK)*. *Eye-drops*, oxybuprocaine hydrochloride 0.4%, in single-use disposable applicators.

NOTE. The *B.P.* permits the title BNX for single-dose eye-drops containing oxybuprocaine.

Proprietary Names and Manufacturers

Alcon Opulets Benoxinate *(Alcon, UK)*; Cébésine *(Chauvin-Blache, Fr.)*; Conjuncain *(Mann, Ger.)*; Minims Benoxinate Hydrochloride *(Smith & Nephew, S.Afr.; Smith & Nephew Pharmaceuticals, UK)*; Minims Oxybuprocaine Hydrochloride *(Smith & Nephew, Austral.)*; Novesin *(Dispersa, Switz.)*; Novesina *(Sandoz, Ital.)*; Novesine *(Austral.; Belg.; Merck Sharp & Dohme-Chibret, Fr.; Wander, Ger.; Neth.; Wander, Switz.)*; Oftalmocaina *(Arg.)*; Oxibuprokain Minims *(Smith & Nephew, Norw.; Smith & Nephew, Swed.)*; Poen Caina *(Arg.)*; Prescaina *(Llorens, Spain)*.

The following names have been used for multi-ingredient preparations containing oxybuprocaine hydrochloride— Fluress *(Barnes-Hind, Austral.; Barnes-Hind, Canad.; Barnes-Hind, USA)*.

13082-m

Parethoxycaine Hydrochloride *(rINNM)*.

2-Diethylaminoethyl 4-ethoxybenzoate hydrochloride.
$C_{15}H_{23}NO_3,HCl=301.8$.

CAS — 94-23-5 (parethoxycaine); 136-46-9 (hydrochloride).

Parethoxycaine hydrochloride is a local anaesthetic of the ester type. It is used as pastilles for topical anaesthesia of the mouth and throat.

The general actions of local anaesthetics are described on p.1205.

Proprietary Names and Manufacturers

Maxicaïne *(Delagrange, Fr.)*.

7640-w

Phenacaine Hydrochloride *(USAN, pINNM)*.

Phenacainium Chloride; Phenetidylphenacetin Hydrochloride. *NN′*-Bis(4-ethoxyphenyl)acetamidine hydrochloride monohydrate.
$C_{18}H_{22}N_2O_2,HCl,H_2O=352.9$.

CAS — 101-93-9 (phenacaine); 620-99-5 (hydrochloride, anhydrous); 6153-19-1 (hydrochloride, monohydrate).

Pharmacopoeias. In *U.S.*

White odourless crystals. **Soluble** 1 in 50 of water; freely soluble in alcohol and chloroform; practically insoluble in ether.

Phenacaine hydrochloride is a local anaesthetic with the general actions described under Local Anaesthetics, p.1205. It has been used as a surface anaesthetic for the eye.

Proprietary Names and Manufacturers

Holocaine *(City Chemical Corp., USA)*.

7641-e

Piperocaine Hydrochloride *(BANM, rINNM)*.

Piperocaini Hydrochloridum; Piperocainium Chloride. 3-(2-Methylpiperidino)propyl benzoate hydrochloride.
$C_{16}H_{23}NO_2,HCl=297.8$.

CAS — 136-82-3 (piperocaine); 24561-10-2 (hydrochloride).

Pharmacopoeias. In *Int.*

Piperocaine hydrochloride is a local anaesthetic of the ester type and has the general actions described under Local Anaesthetics, p.1205. It has been used for surface anaesthesia, infiltration anaesthesia, and regional nerve block.

Proprietary Names and Manufacturers

Metycaine Hydrochloride *(Lilly, USA)*.

7642-l

Pramoxine Hydrochloride *(BANM, USAN)*.

Pramocaine Hydrochloride *(rINNM)*; Pramoxinium Chloride. 4-[3-(4-Butoxyphenoxy)propyl]morpholine hydrochloride.
$C_{17}H_{27}NO_3,HCl=329.9$.

CAS — 140-65-8 (pramoxine); 637-58-1 (hydrochloride).

Pharmacopoeias. In *U.S.*

A white or almost white crystalline powder; it may have a faint aromatic odour.

Freely **soluble** in water and alcohol; soluble 1 in 35 of chloroform; very slightly soluble in ether. A 1% solution in water has a pH of about 4.5. **Store** in airtight containers.

Pramoxine hydrochloride is a surface anaesthetic without the usual ester or amide linkage. It is used on the skin and less delicate mucous membranes. It is irritant and initial burning or stinging may occur. It should not be used for the nose or eyes or by injection, and should not be used for bronchoscopy or gastroscopy since it does not abolish the gag reflex.

Pramoxine hydrochloride is used as a 1% cream, ointment, gel, lotion, or suppositories to relieve pain and pruritus associated with dermatoses, and for minor cuts and abrasions, haemorrhoids and other anorectal disorders. It has also been used topically with hydrocortisone.

The general actions of local anaesthetics are described on p.1205.

A review of an aerosol foam containing pramoxine 1% with hydrocortisone 1% (Epifoam) for the relief of perineal pain and discomfort following childbirth, concluded that it did not offer any advantages over the more traditional remedies and its routine use could not be recommended on the evidence available.— *Drug & Ther. Bull.*, 1987, *25*, 37.

Preparations

Pramoxine Hydrochloride Cream *(U.S.P.)*

Pramoxine Hydrochloride Jelly *(U.S.P.)*

Proprietary Names and Manufacturers of Pramoxine or Pramoxine Hydrochloride

Fleet Relief *(Fleet, USA)*; Prax *(Ferndale, USA)*; Proctofoam *(Reed & Carnrick, USA)*; Tronolane *(Ross, USA)*; Tronotene *(Abbott, Ital.)*; Tronothane *(Abbott, Canad.; Abbott, Fr.; Abbott, Switz.; Abbott, USA)*.

The following names have been used for multi-ingredient preparations containing pramoxine or pramoxine hydrochloride—Analpram-HC *(Ferndale, USA)*; Anugesic-HC *(Parke, Davis, Canad.)*; Anugesic-HC Cream *(Parke, Davis, UK)*; Anugesic-HC Suppositories *(Parke, Davis, UK)*; Anusol Plus *(Parke, Davis, Canad.)*; Derma-Sone *(Hill, USA)*; Epifoam *(Stafford-Miller, UK; Reed & Carnrick, USA)*; F-E-P Creme *(Boots, USA)*; Otic-HC *(Hauck, USA)*; Oticol *(Arlo, USA)*; PrameGel *(Genderm, USA)*; Pramosone *(Ferndale, USA)*; Pricort Lotion *(Arlo, USA)*; Proctofoam HC *(Reed & Carnrick, Canad.; Stafford-Miller, UK; Reed & Carnrick, USA)*; Zone-A *(UAD, USA)*.

7643-y

Prilocaine Hydrochloride *(BANM, USAN, rINNM).*

Astra-1512; L67; Propitocaine Hydrochloride.
2-Propylaminopropiono-*o*-toluidide hydrochloride.
$C_{13}H_{20}N_2O,HCl=256.8$.

CAS — 721-50-6 (prilocaine); 1786-81-8 (hydrochloride).

Pharmacopoeias. In *Br.* and *U.S.*

A white odourless or almost odourless crystalline powder. M.p. 166° to 169°.

B.P. **solubilities** are: soluble 1 in 5 of water, 1 in 6 of alcohol; practically insoluble in ether. *U.S.P.* solubilities are: 1 in 3.5 of water, 1 in 4.2 of alcohol, 1 in 175 of chloroform; very slightly soluble in acetone; practically insoluble in ether. **Store** in well-closed containers.

Prilocaine forms a mixture with lignocaine that has a melting point lower than that of either ingredient. This eutectic mixture is used in the preparation of topical dosage forms.

CARBONATED SOLUTIONS. Carbonate salts of prilocaine and lignocaine were prepared to give 1.72% and 1.74% solutions respectively of the bases and were sealed in ampoules at a pressure of 600 to 700 mmHg of carbon dioxide. Opened ampoules lost carbon dioxide relatively slowly and its partial pressure fell from 700 to 500 mmHg in 40 minutes. In use, the ampoules were opened and the contents aspirated immediately through a wide-bore needle.— P. R. Bromage, *Can. med. Ass. J.*, 1967, *97*, 1377.

The ratio of lignocaine to prilocaine in a eutectic composition is close to 1:1 with a eutectic temperature of 18°.— A. Brodin *et al.*, *J. pharm. Sci.*, 1984, *73*, 481.

Adverse Effects, Treatment, and Precautions

As for Local Anaesthetics, p.1205.

Methaemoglobinaemia and cyanosis, attributed to the metabolite *o*-toluidine, may occur particularly when doses of prilocaine hydrochloride exceed 600 mg. Methaemoglobinaemia has been observed in neonates whose mothers received prilocaine shortly before delivery.

Prilocaine should be avoided in patients with anaemia, congenital or acquired methaemoglobinaemia, cardiac or ventilatory failure, or hypoxia.

ALLERGY. Three reports of prilocaine allergy are described and an additional case is reported in which the allergy was confirmed by a nasal mucosal test and intradermal skin tests.— C. M. Yeoman, *Br. dent. J.*, 1982, *153*, 69.

See also p.1205.

EFFECTS ON THE BLOOD. Methaemoglobinaemia occurred in a 12-week-old boy after application of about 5 g of a cream containing prilocaine 2.5% and lignocaine 2.5% as a eutectic mixture (EMLA) to the back of the hands and to the forearms prior to venepuncture. Because the operation was delayed, the cream remained on the skin for 5 hours after which time the boy was noted to be pale with "brownish" cyanotic lips; treatment with methylene blue 1 mg per kg body-weight was given intravenously with complete recovery within 30 minutes. The child had also been receiving co-trimoxazole by mouth for 2 months and it was thought that methaemoglobinaemia was probably a result of an additive interaction between prilocaine and the sulphamethoxazole portion of co-trimoxazole.— B. Jakobson and A. Nilsson, *Acta anaesth. scand.*, 1985, *29*, 453.

An increase in the concentration of methaemoglobin is a recognised reaction to prilocaine due to the hydrolysis product *o*-toluidine. A dose of 8 mg per kg body-weight is usually needed to produce symptoms, but the very young are considerably more susceptible. Patients with haemoglobinopathies and glucose-6-phosphate dehydrogenase deficiency and those taking oxidising drugs, such as sulphonamides and antimalarials, may also be predisposed to methaemoglobinaemia.— F. Reynolds, *Br. J. Anaesth.*, 1987, *59*, 78.

Absorption and Fate

Prilocaine hydrochloride is rapidly metabolised mainly in the liver and also in the kidneys. It is excreted in the urine mainly as metabolites. The principal metabolite excreted in the urine is *o*-toluidine, which is believed to cause the methaemoglobinaemia observed after large doses. Prilocaine crosses the placenta and during prolonged epidural anaesthesia may produce methaemoglobinaemia in the foetus.

See also under Local Anaesthetics, p.1206.

After the intravenous injection of 250 mg of prilocaine hydrochloride or mepivacaine hydrochloride in 5 healthy male subjects, plasma concentrations of prilocaine were substantially less than those of mepivacaine and mean elimination half-lives were 93 and 125 minutes respectively, although there was considerable intersubject variation. Total body clearance of prilocaine was consistently greater than that for mepivacaine.— G. R. Arthur *et al.*, *Br. J. Anaesth.*, 1979, *51*, 481.

Plasma prilocaine concentrations were measured after infiltration injections of prilocaine 60 mg, with and without felypressin 0.03 units per mL, in the upper premolar region in 2 subjects. The addition of felypressin did not limit plasma concentrations of prilocaine.— H. Cannell and R. Whelpton, *Br. dent. J.*, 1986, *160*, 47.

Uses and Administration

As for Local Anaesthetics, p.1206.

Prilocaine hydrochloride is a local anaesthetic of the amide type which is used for infiltration, intravenous regional anaesthesia, and nerve block. It has a rapid onset of action, but slower than that of lignocaine, and has less vasodilator activity than lignocaine with a slightly longer duration of action.

The suggested maximum adult dosage of prilocaine hydrochloride is 400 to 600 mg over 2 hours.

For infiltration anaesthesia and nerve blocks in dental procedures it is used in a dose of 30 to 60 mg (1 to 2 mL) as a 3% solution with felypressin 0.03 units per mL, or 40 to 80 mg (1 to 2 mL) as a 4% solution with or without adrenaline 1 in 200 000.

For peripheral nerve block up to 600 mg (30 mL) has been used as a 2% solution or 450 to 600 mg (15 to 20 mL) as a 3% solution and for epidural or caudal anaesthesia 1 to 3% solutions have been used in doses of 150 to 600 mg.

Prilocaine 0.1, 0.33, and 1.0% solutions were each given by intradermal injection to 10 healthy subjects; only the 1.0% solution produced significantly more vasoconstriction than a saline control. Analgesic activity and duration of action increased with concentration.— D. G. Willatts and F. Reynolds, *Br. J. Anaesth.*, 1985, *57*, 1006.

Irrigation of the knee with prilocaine 1 g per litre in isotonic saline at an applied pressure of 100 mm Hg was used in 200 arthroscopies without any toxic effects on the central nervous system or cardiovascular system and without methaemoglobinaemia occurring.— D. Debruyne *et al.*, *Clin. Pharmac. Ther.*, 1985, *38*, 549.

INTRAVENOUS REGIONAL ANAESTHESIA. The agent of choice for intravenous regional anaesthesia appears to be prilocaine in a dose of 2 mg per kg body-weight, or less, at which dose methaemoglobinaemia is not significant and overall toxicity is low.— S. P. K. Linter (letter), *Lancet*, 1983, *2*, 787. Prilocaine 0.5% had been used by the authors in intravenous regional anaesthesia for over 15 years without ever seeing methaemoglobinaemia as a complication. Cyanosis due to methaemoglobinaemia is unlikely in adults at prilocaine doses less than 600 mg and the likely maximum dose in intravenous regional anaesthesia is 250 mg.— D. W. McKeown *et al.* (letter), *ibid.*, 1503.

SURFACE ANAESTHESIA. *Venepuncture.* For references to the use of prilocaine and lignocaine as a eutectic mixture for topical anaesthesia of intact skin prior to venepuncture, see under Lignocaine Hydrochloride, p.1222.

Preparations

Prilocaine Hydrochloride Injection *(U.S.P.)*. pH 6 to 7.

Prilocaine and Epinephrine Injection *(U.S.P.)*. A sterile solution prepared from prilocaine hydrochloride and adrenaline with the aid of hydrochloric acid in Water for Injections or a sterile solution of prilocaine hydrochloride and adrenaline acid tartrate in Water for Injections. It contains not more than 1 in 50 000 of adrenaline. pH 3.3 to 5.5. Protect from light.

Proprietary Preparations

Citanest *(Astra, UK)*. *Injection*, prilocaine hydrochloride 0.5% in single-dose vials of 50 mL; prilocaine hydrochloride 0.5% and 1.0%, methylhydroxybenzoate 0.1% in multi-dose vials of 20 mL and 50 mL.

Injection (Citanest with octapressin), prilocaine hydrochloride 3%, felypressin 0.03 unit/mL in standard and self-aspirating cartridges of 2.2 mL.

Injection, prilocaine hydrochloride 4% in cartridges of 2.2 mL.

Proprietary Names and Manufacturers of Prilocaine or Prilocaine Hydrochloride

Citanest *(Ciba, Austral.; Belg.; Astra, Canad.; Denm.; Bellon, Fr.; Astra, Norw.; Astra, Swed.; Astra, UK; Astra, USA)*; Xylonest *(Astra, Ger.; Astra, Switz.)*.

The following names have been used for multi-ingredient preparations containing prilocaine or prilocaine hydrochloride—Citanest Forte *(Astra, Canad.)*; Citanest with Adrenaline *(Astra, Austral.; Astra, UK)*; Citanest with Octapressin *(Astra, Austral.; Astra, UK)*; Emla *(Astra, UK)*.

7644-j

Procaine Hydrochloride *(BANM, USAN, rINNM).*

Allocaine; Ethocaine Hydrochloride; Novocainum; Procaini Hydrochloridum; Procainii Chloridum; Procainium Chloride; Syncaine. 2-Diethylaminoethyl 4-aminobenzoate hydrochloride.
$C_{13}H_{20}N_2O_2,HCl=272.8$.

CAS — 59-46-1 (procaine); 51-05-8 (hydrochloride).

Pharmacopoeias. In *Arg., Aust., Belg., Br., Braz., Chin., Cz., Egypt., Eur., Fr., Ger., Hung., Ind., Int., It., Jpn, Jug., Mex., Neth., Nord., Pol., Port., Roum., Rus., Span., Swiss, Turk.,* and *U.S. U.S.* also includes Sterile Procaine Hydrochloride. *Port. P.* applies the title Procaine to the hydrochloride.

Colourless odourless crystals or a white crystalline powder.

Soluble 1 in 1 of water; slightly soluble in chloroform; practically insoluble in ether. The *B.P.* specifies soluble 1 in 25 of alcohol and the *U.S.P.* specifies soluble 1 in 15 of alcohol. A 2% solution in water has a pH of 5.0 to 6.5. **Incompatibility** has been reported with aminophylline, barbiturates, magnesium sulphate, phenytoin sodium, sodium bicarbonate, and amphotericin. **Protect** from light.

STABILITY OF SOLUTIONS. Degradation of procaine in a cardioplegic solution containing magnesium, sodium, potassium, and calcium salts was found to be temperature dependent. At a storage temperature of 6° the shelf-life of the solution was 5 weeks and this was increased to 9 weeks when the storage temperature was −10°. Using carbon dioxide instead of nitrogen in the head space did not affect stability of procaine.— R. Synave *et al.*, *J. clin. Hosp. Pharm.*, 1985, *10*, 385.

Adverse Effects and Treatment

As for Local Anaesthetics, p.1205.

ALLERGY AND EFFECTS ON THE SKIN. Of 600 persons with dermatitis or eczema submitted to patch testing with 2% aqueous solution of procaine hydrochloride, 4.8% gave a positive reaction.— E. Rudzki and D. Kleniewska, *Br. J. Derm.*, 1970, *83*, 543.

Severe hypotension leading to death developed in 1 patient following the infusion of 600 mg of procaine for malignant hyperthermia.— D. MacLachlan and A. L. Forrest (letter), *Lancet*, 1974, *1*, 355.

Precautions

As for Local Anaesthetics, p.1206.

Procaine is hydrolysed in the body to *p*-aminobenzoic acid and may antagonise the action of sulphonamides. There is cross-sensitivity between procaine, *p*-aminobenzoic acid and hydroxybenzoate preservatives.

Views on the use of procaine for local anaesthesia in patients who have had procainamide-induced systemic lupus erythematosus. E.L. Dubois considered that, in view of the lack of specific information, it might be safer to use a general anaesthetic whereas D. Alarcón-Segovia thought that the short-term use of procaine derivatives were permissible in such patients. S.L. Lee also felt that procaine could be used but suggested a single test dose 48 hours before the contemplated surgery.— *J. Am. med. Ass.*, 1977, *238*, 2201.

ADMINISTRATION IN RENAL IMPAIRMENT. For reference to the rate of procaine hydrolysis being reduced in patients with renal failure, see under Absorption and Fate, below.

INTERACTIONS. *Anticholinesterases.* Since procaine is hydrolysed by plasma cholinesterase it should not be used in the presence of anticholinesterase drugs.— M. de Swiet, *Prescribers' J.*, 1979, *19*, 59.

Diuretics. Evidence that concomitant administration of *acetazolamide* extends the plasma half-life of procaine.— R. Calvo *et al.*, *Clin. Pharmac. Ther.*, 1980, *27*, 179.

Absorption and Fate

Procaine is readily absorbed following parenteral administration and rapidly hydrolysed by plasma cholinesterase to *p*-aminobenzoic acid and diethylaminoethanol; some may also be metabolised in the liver. About 80% of the *p*-aminobenzoic acid is excreted unchanged or conjugated in the urine. About 30% of the diethylaminoethanol is excreted in the urine, the remainder being metabolised in the liver.

See also under Local Anaesthetics, p.1206.

The serum half-life of procaine was prolonged in newborn infants, patients with liver disease, and in some uraemic patients.— M. M. Reidenberg *et al.*, *Clin. Pharmac. Ther.*, 1972, *13*, 279.

Maximal procaine hydrolysis was found to be 40% less in plasma from patients with renal failure than in a control group, due to a low concentration of plasma esterases R. Calvo *et al.*, *Eur. J. clin. Pharmac.*, 1983, *24*, 533.

Uses and Administration

As for Local Anaesthetics, p.1206.

Procaine is a local anaesthetic of the ester type. Because of its poor penetration of intact mucous membranes, it is ineffective for surface application and has been chiefly used by injection although in general it has been replaced by lignocaine and other local anaesthetics of the amide type. It has an onset of action of around 2 to 5 minutes with a short duration of about 1 hour. It has vasodilator activity and therefore a vasoconstrictor may be added to delay absorption and increase the duration of action.

For infiltration anaesthesia 0.25 to 1.0% solutions of procaine hydrochloride may be used in doses of 250 to 600 mg.

For peripheral nerve block a usual dose of 500 mg is given as a 0.5% (100 mL), 1.0% (50 mL), or 2.0% (25 mL) solution. Doses up to 1 g have been used. For infiltration and peripheral nerve block adrenaline may be added to solutions in general to give a final concentration of 1 in 200 000.

For spinal anaesthesia procaine hydrochloride is given as a 10% solution diluted with sodium chloride injection (0.9%), Water for Injections, cerebrospinal fluid, or for a hyperbaric solution, with glucose. For anaesthesia of the perineum a 50 mg dose is given as 0.5 mL of a 10% solution mixed with an equal volume of the chosen diluent; for anaesthesia of the perineum and lower extremities 100 mg (1 mL) is diluted with an equal volume of diluent; and for anaesthesia up to the costal margin 200 mg (2 mL) is given mixed with 1 mL of diluent.

Procaine hydrochloride has been used with propoxycaine in dentistry (see below).

Procaine forms poorly soluble salts or conjugates with some drugs, for example penicillin, and is used to prolong their action after injection. It may also reduce the pain of injection.

Procaine was reported to be a strong prostaglandin antagonist and weak agonist.— M. S. Manku and D. F. Horrobin, *Lancet*, 1976, *2*, 1115.

Intradermal injection of procaine 0.3 and 1.0% solutions produced significantly more vasodilatation than a saline control in 10 healthy subjects. A 0.1% solution did not show greater vasodilator activity than saline.— D. G. Willatts and F. Reynolds, *Br. J. Anaesth.*, 1985, *57*, 1006.

MALIGNANT HYPERPYREXIA. References to the use of procaine in the treatment of malignant hyperpyrexia: J. E. S. Relton *et al.*, *Can. Anaesth. Soc. J.*, 1972, *19*, 200; G. M. Hall and D. Lister (letter), *Lancet*, 1974, *1*, 208; B. Höivik and J. Stovner (letter), *ibid.*, 1975, *2*, 185; I. M. C. Clarke and F. R. Ellis, *Br. J. Anaesth.*, 1975, *47*, 17.

PAIN. Procaine hydrochloride has been given by intravenous injection for the relief of pain in acute pancreatitis. It may in addition inhibit the enzyme phospholipase A which causes the parenchymal necrosis and possibly shock lung, both of which occur in acute pancreatitis.— P. G. Lankisch, *Drugs*, 1984, *28*, 554.

'H3' (Aslan's Treatment of Old Age). Professor Anna Aslan and her colleagues at the Parhon Institute of Geriatrics, Bucharest, in a series of papers (1956 et seq.), claimed remarkable beneficial results in a wide range of disorders, including the rejuvenation of senile patients, from the intramuscular injection of a 2% solution of procaine, buffered at pH 4.3. This solution, which Aslan called 'H3', was injected in 5-mL doses three times weekly in a series of 12 injections with a 10-day interval between each course, the treatment being continued more or less indefinitely. The remarkable claims for this treatment were not supported by any scientifically valid evidence or by subsequent trials carried out by other workers (see *Martindale, 28th Edn*, p.922).

Gerovital H3 (GH3), an injection consisting of a 2% procaine hydrochloride solution with small amounts of benzoic acid, potassium metabisulphite, and sodium phosphate has been claimed to retard the ageing process but although many uncontrolled studies have described great benefits from the use of GH3, controlled studies have failed to demonstrate any improvement in the physical or mental status of elderly patients with cerebral arteriosclerosis or chronic degenerative disorders, including senile dementia. It has been suggested that procaine acts as a monoamine oxidase inhibitor and Zung *et al.* (*Psychosomatics*, 1974, *15*, 127) found GH3 to be a superior antidepressant to placebo. However in further studies reported by Zwerling *et al.* (*J. Am. Geriat. Soc.*, 1975, *23*, 355) and Olsen *et al.* (*J. Geront.*, 1978, *33*, 514), GH3 did not relieve depression.— *Med. Lett.*, 1979, *21*, 4.

An oral form of procaine bound to haemotoporphyrin, KH_3, has been studied for its use in improving mental function in elderly people. Side-effects of KH_3 included migrainous headache and a systemic lupus erythematosus syndrome.— P. H. Millard, *Br. med. J.*, 1984, *289*, 1094. See also M. R. Hall *et al.*, *Age & Ageing*, 1983, *12*, 302.

Preparations

Procaine and Phenylephrine Hydrochlorides Injection *(U.S.P.).* pH 3.0 to 5.5.

Procaine and Tetracaine Hydrochlorides and Levonordefrin Injection *(U.S.P.).* A sterile solution of procaine hydrochloride, amethocaine hydrochloride, and levonordefrin in Water for Injections. pH 3.5 to 5.0.

Procaine Hydrochloride and Epinephrine Injection *(U.S.P.).* A sterile solution of procaine hydrochloride and adrenaline hydrochloride in Water for Injections. It contains not more than 1 in 50 000 of adrenaline. pH 3.0 to 5.5.

Procaine Hydrochloride Injection *(U.S.P.).* pH 3.0 to 5.5.

Sterile Procaine Hydrochloride *(U.S.P.)*

Proprietary Names and Manufacturers

Anuject *(Hauck, USA)*; Casticaina *(Spain)*; Gero *(U.R.P.A.C., Fr.)*; Gero H3 Aslan *(Phoenix, Arg.; Chefaro, Ger.)*; Lenident *(Zeta, Ital.)*; Novocain *(Vandos, Austral.; Winthrop, Canad.; Hoechst, Ger.; Winthrop-Breon, USA)*; Novutox *(Willows Francis, UK: Pharmaceutical Mfg, UK)*; Recorcaina *(Recordati, Ital.)*; Syntocaine *(Sintetica, Switz.)*; Venocaina *(Andalucia, Spain)*.

7645-z

Propanocaine Hydrochloride *(rINNM).*
467D_3. 3-Diethylamino-1-phenylpropyl benzoate hydrochloride.
$C_{20}H_{25}NO_2,HCl=347.9$.

CAS — 493-76-5 (propanocaine); 1679-79-4 (hydrochloride).

Propanocaine hydrochloride is a local anaesthetic of the ester type which has been used topically.

The general actions of local anaesthetics are described on p.1205.

7646-c

Propoxycaine Hydrochloride *(USAN, rINNM).*
Propoxycainium Chloride. 2-Diethylaminoethyl 4-amino-2-propoxybenzoate hydrochloride.
$C_{16}H_{26}N_2O_3,HCl=330.9$.

CAS — 86-43-1 (propoxycaine); 550-83-4 (hydrochloride).

Pharmacopoeias. In *U.S.*

A white odourless crystalline powder. It discolours on prolonged exposure to light and air.

Soluble 1 in 2 of water, 1 in 10 of alcohol, and 1 in 80 of ether; practically insoluble in acetone and chloroform. A 2% solution in water has a pH of about 5.4. **Protect** from light.

Propoxycaine hydrochloride is a local anaesthetic of the ester type with a longer duration of action than procaine hydrochloride. It has been used in a concentration of 0.4% in combination with procaine 2% solution with a vasoconstrictor for infiltration anaesthesia and nerve block in dental procedures. Usual doses are 7.2 mg of propoxycaine hydrochloride for anaesthesia at a single site and 36 mg for anaesthesia of the entire oral cavity.

The general actions of local anaesthetics are described on p.1205.

Preparations

Propoxycaine and Procaine Hydrochlorides and Norepinephrine Bitartrate Injection *(U.S.P.)*. A sterile solution of propoxycaine hydrochloride, procaine hydrochloride, and noradrenaline acid tartrate in Water for Injections. pH 3.5 to 5.0.

Propoxycaine and Procaine Hydrochlorides and Levonordefrin Injection *(U.S.P.)*. pH 3.5 to 5.0.

7647-k

Proxymetacaine Hydrochloride *(BANM, rINNM)*.

Proparacaine Hydrochloride *(USAN)*. 2-Diethylaminoethyl 3-amino-4-propoxybenzoate hydrochloride.

$C_{16}H_{26}N_2O_3,HCl=330.9$.

CAS — 499-67-2 (proxymetacaine); 5875-06-9 (hydrochloride).

Pharmacopoeias. In *Br.* and *U.S.*

A white or faintly buff-coloured, odourless or almost odourless, crystalline powder. **Soluble** in water, alcohol, chloroform, and methyl alcohol; very soluble in dehydated alcohol; practically insoluble in ether. A 1% solution in water has a pH of 5.7 to 6.4. **Store** in well-closed containers. Protect from light.

Adverse Effects, Treatment, and Precautions

As for Local Anaesthetics, p.1205.

A severe immediate-type corneal reaction may rarely occur. Allergic contact dermatitis has also been reported.

A skin reaction occurred in a woman with the Stevens-Johnson syndrome after ophthalmic anaesthesia with proxymetacaine hydrochloride.— B. Ward *et al.*, *Am. J. Ophthal.*, 1978, *86*, 133.

Absorption and Fate

See under Local Anaesthetics, p.1206.

Uses and Administration

Proxymetacaine hydrochloride is a surface anaesthetic (see p.1206) of the ester type and is used in ophthalmology. It is of similar potency to amethocaine in equal concentrations. Instillation of 1 or 2 drops of a 0.5% solution permits tonometry in 20 to 30 seconds; anaesthesia lasts about 15 minutes. For removal of foreign bodies or sutures from the cornea 1 or 2 drops are instilled every 5 to 10 minutes for 1 to 5 doses or 1 or 2 drops are instilled 2 to 3 minutes before the procedure, and for deeper anaesthesia as needed. For cataract extraction 1 drop is instilled every 5 to 10 minutes to a total of 5 to 7 applications.

Preparations

Proparacaine Hydrochloride Ophthalmic Solution *(U.S.P.)*. A sterile aqueous solution of proxymetacaine hydrochloride. pH 3.5 to 6.0.

Proxymetacaine Eye Drops *(B.P.)*. PROX; Proxymetacaine Hydrochloride Eye Drops. Store at 2° to 8° and avoid freezing.

Proprietary Preparations

Ophthaine *(Squibb, UK)*. *Eye-drops*, proxymetacaine hydrochloride 0.5%, chlorbutol 0.2%, benzalkonium chloride 0.01%, in bottles of 15 mL. Store in a refrigerator.

Proprietary Names and Manufacturers

Ak-taine *(Akorn, Canad.; Akorn, USA)*; Alcaine *(Alcon, Austral.; Alcon, Canad.; Alcon, Norw.; Alcon, Switz.; Alcon Laboratories, USA)*; Kainair *(Pharmafair, USA)*; Kéracaine *(Fr.)*; Kerakain *(Chibret, Ger.)*; Ocu-caine *(Ocumed, USA)*; Ophthaine *(Squibb, Austral.; Squibb, Canad.; Squibb, UK; USA)*; Ophthetic *(Allergan, Austral.; Allergan, Canad.; Allergan, Ger.; Allergan, S.Afr.; Allergan, USA)*; Piloptic *(Ger.)*.

The following names have been used for multi-ingredient preparations containing proxymetacaine hydrochloride— Fluorocaine *(Akorn, USA)*.

7648-a

Pyrrocaine Hydrochloride *(BANM, rINNM)*.

EN-1010; NSC-52644. Pyrrolidin-1-ylaceto-2′,6′-xylidide hydrochloride.

$C_{14}H_{20}N_2O,HCl=268.8$.

CAS — 2210-77-7 (pyrrocaine); 2210-64-2 (hydrochloride).

NOTE. Pyrrocaine is *USAN*.

Pyrrocaine hydrochloride is a local anaesthetic of the amide type which was formerly used in dentistry.

The general actions of local anaesthetics are described on p.1205.

7649-t

Tolycaine Hydrochloride *(BANM, rINNM)*.

Methyl 2-(2-diethylaminoacetamido)-*m*-toluate hydrochloride.

$C_{15}H_{22}N_2O_3,HCl=314.8$.

CAS — 3686-58-6 (tolycaine); 7210-92-6 (hydrochloride).

Tolycaine hydrochloride was formerly used as a local anaesthetic.

The general actions of local anaesthetics are described on p.1205.

Muscle Relaxants

5700-y

The skeletal muscle relaxants included in this section are of 2 main types: those generally with a selective action on the central nervous system, principally used for relieving painful muscle spasms or spasticity occurring in musculoskeletal and neuromuscular disorders; and those affecting neuromuscular transmission which are used as adjuncts in anaesthesia, particularly to enable adequate muscle relaxation to be achieved with light anaesthesia.

The drugs used as adjuncts to anaesthesia are of 2 types—competitive or non-depolarising agents, and depolarising agents.

The competitive agents interrupt neuromuscular transmission by competing with acetylcholine for receptor sites on the motor end-plate, thus reducing the response of the end-plate to acetylcholine released following the nerve impulse; if sufficient blocking drug is present, the end-plate potential will fail to reach the threshold needed to trigger muscular contraction, and neuromuscular block occurs. The action of these drugs can be opposed by increasing the local concentration of acetylcholine, e.g. by giving an anticholinesterase such as neostigmine.

The depolarising agents block neuromuscular transmission by producing a sustained partial depolarisation of the motor end-plate which renders the tissues incapable of responding to the transmitter. Their action is not reversed by anticholinesterases.

Generally, the competitive agents, with a prolonged action, are used in major operations, while the depolarising agents, with a much shorter effect, are used for minor operations or manipulations.

It is common practice to use a short-acting depolarising drug, such as suxamethonium, for intubation, followed by a longer-acting competitive drug, such as pancuronium to maintain muscle relaxation throughout an operation. Sometimes a depolarising drug may be given to facilitate closure of the muscular tissue. In such instances neostigmine should not be given to reverse the action of the competitive agent until the effects of the depolarising drug have ceased; the procedure is accordingly not recommended for routine practice.

Phase I and **Phase II Block**. Repeated doses of depolarising agents may cause a change in response of the motor end-plate so that a competitive block (phase II block) follows the primary depolarising block (phase I block).

Prolonged apnoea or respiratory depression may follow the use of competitive or of depolarising agents. After a competitive blocker, prolonged apnoea, unresponsive to neostigmine, may develop due to metabolic acidosis. Metabolic acidosis is generally considered to have been a major factor in cases formerly described as *neostigmine-resistant curarisation*. After the continuous infusion of a depolarising blocker the resulting dual block may give prolonged respiratory depression related to the prolonged muscular relaxation, but apnoea rarely develops. Prolonged respiratory depression may also occur in patients with low serum-pseudocholinesterase concentrations or with atypical pseudocholinesterase who are given suxamethonium.

For antimuscarinic agents used to relax visceral smooth muscle, see p.522. There are also a number of miscellaneous compounds used as antispasmodics, mainly in gastro-intestinal and genito-urinary spasm; these are described in the section on Gastro-intestinal Agents, p.1073 and in Part 2.

Concern at the use of neuromuscular blockers in intensive therapy units, although they are not sedative or analgesic agents, and a reminder of the horrors of being awake and intubated. Muscle relaxants should only be used for controlled ventilation in intensive therapy units if sedation proves inadequate or if a sleeping patient is not synchronising with a ventilator. The only limitation to the dose of opioid (or other sedative) given, is an untoward reaction or an unsatisfactory haemodynamic state. Worries about addiction are unnecessary.— C. M. H. M. Jones (letter), *Lancet*, 1980, *1*, 312. Agreement. Moreover anaesthetists commonly administer a neuro-muscular blocker, rather than an opioid or other analgesic, when patients make spontaneous coordinated limb movements during general anaesthesia. Although it is not known whether such movements indicate inadequate depression of conscious level, it is known that awareness during general anaesthesia is common.— A. Gilston (letter), *ibid*., 480. A view that muscle relaxants are useful adjuncts to intensive care.— D. Green (letter), *ibid*., 715.

A detailed discussion of competitive neuromuscular blockade as practised in the *USA*. In general neuromuscular blockers are used conservatively: new agents are introduced later; the dosage schedule is more restrained; nerve stimulators are probably used more often; and hypotension following tubocurarine is met with more concern than in the *UK*.

Pancuronium has been the most-used competitive relaxant because its effects tended to offset bradycardia and hypotension due to other agents. Large doses may be used for intubation where suxamethonium is undesirable, with acceptance of the prolonged block that follows. When suxamethonium is used for intubation the initial paralysing dose of pancuronium is reduced, especially where the relaxant is intended only as a supplement in a patient already somewhat relaxed by inhalation anaesthetics.

Tubocurarine is being used less and less in the *USA* and is particularly unpopular in large bolus doses, but it is occasionally chosen intentionally for its hypotensive effects: under such circumstances it may be mixed with pancuronium.

The newer competitive agents atracurium and vecuronium have met with widespread acceptance in the *USA* although their final place remains to be determined.

Maintenance doses of competitive blocking agents are of the order of one-fifth of the intubation dose, and are commonly given when spontaneous recovery has reached 25% of full muscle strength. Monitoring of neuromuscular blockade using peripheral nerve stimulators is relatively common.

Small doses of competitive agents may be used for the relief of laryngospasm, although suxamethonium is preferred because of its more rapid onset of action. To reduce or prevent fasciculation associated with suxamethonium, pancuronium may be given usually in a dose of about 1 mg: subsequent doses of suxamethonium are usually increased by 50%. The use of small doses of a competitive agent as 'priming doses' to potentiate a subsequent dose of the same or another competitive relaxant is currently still considered innovative and is not in common practice.

When pancuronium, tubocurarine, or metocurine are used, anaesthesiologists in the *USA* almost always reverse the block afterwards with an anticholinesterase, always accompanied by atropine or glycopyrronium bromide. Edrophonium has been recommended as the drug of choice for reversal of the short-acting agents atracurium and vecuronium.— C. Lee and R. L. Katz, *Clin. Anaesth*., 1985, *3*, 387.

A discussion of competitive blockade as practised in the *UK*. Alcuronium has increased in popularity, especially among younger anaesthetists, but tubocurarine and pancuronium appear to remain equal first choice. Suxamethonium is used to facilitate endotracheal intubation in most short operations unless there is a specific contra-indication, but if an alternative with non-depolarising characteristics and an equally rapid onset of action were available there is little doubt that it would be preferred. The virtual abandonment of suxamethonium infusions but the persistence of intermittent suxamethonium injections for operations such as endoscopies and appendectomies reflects the reluctance of *UK* anaesthetists to use continuous infusions.

Vecuronium, and to a lesser extent atracurium are finding increasing favour as the most suitable muscle relaxant in frail, debilitated, and elderly patients, although overall pancuronium is still the most-used drug in this group of patients. It is to be anticipated that vecuronium and atracurium will eventually replace other competitive relaxants as agents of choice in patients with renal failure, and that atracurium will become the competitive agent of choice in patients with liver disease.

Although there are marked differences in practice within the *UK*, the use of atropine or hyoscine as an antisialogogue vagolytic agent with the premedication is usual except in patients presenting for cardiac surgery. Intravenous induction of anaesthesia is virtually universal and is followed immediately by a relaxant for endotracheal intubation, usually suxamethonium.

Once intubation is achieved, maintenance of relaxation for abdominal surgery is achieved using a dose of neuromuscular blocker at least 2 times, and in longer cases 4 times, the ED_{95} dose. If a volatile anaesthetic is used for maintenance, then a 10 to 15% reduction in the dose of relaxant is common. With these initial doses relaxation can be maintained for 40 to 80 minutes, sufficient for most general surgical procedures, and the need for a further dose is infrequent.

In spite of papers on the advantages of adequate doses of edrophonium, nearly all patients receiving a competitive relaxant, other than those ventilated postoperatively, receive atropine with neostigmine for reversal of residual blockade.

In recent years differences in anaesthetic practice between the *UK* and the *USA* have been reduced, and it seems likely that existing differences will continue to diminish.— S. A. Feldman, *Clin. Anaesth*., 1985, *3*, 397.

A review of the adverse effects of neuromuscular blocking drugs.— J. M. Hunter, *Br. J. Anaesth*., 1987, *59*, 46.

PREGNANCY AND THE NEONATE. The effect of muscle relaxants in the newborn.— D. R. Cook, *Drugs*, 1976, *12*, 212.

The use of muscle relaxants in neonatal surgery.— E. Vivori and G. H. Bush, *Br. J. Anaesth*., 1977, *49*, 51.

SPASTICITY. For a brief review of the treatment of spasticity, see *Drug & Ther. Bull*., 1983, *21*, 1.

Muscle spasm. A review of oral muscle relaxants used in the management of musculoskeletal disorders. Based on symptomatic response, muscle relaxants appear to be better than placebo in treating the acute painful muscle spasm of musculoskeletal disorders, but superiority of any one agent has not been established. Combination products containing in addition an analgesic appear to provide better symptom relief than the individual agents, indicating that none of the available muscle relaxants is ideal. Additional clinical evaluation of skeletal muscle relaxants is needed the better to identify their role relative to each other, to sedatives and analgesics, and to physical therapy.— J. K. Elenbaas, *Am. J. Hosp. Pharm*., 1980, *37*, 1313.

12331-t

Afloqualone *(rINN)*.

HQ-495. 6-Amino-2-fluoromethyl-3-*o*-tolylquinazolin-4(3*H*)-one.

$C_{16}H_{14}FN_3O$=283.3.

CAS — 56287-74-2.

Afloqualone is reported to be a muscle relaxant used in the management of muscle spasm.

5701-j

Alcuronium Chloride *(BAN, USAN, rINN)*.

Allnortoxiferin Chloride; Diallylnortoxiferine Dichloride; Diallyltoxiferine Chloride; Ro-4-3816. *NN'*-Diallylbisnortoxiferinium dichloride pentahydrate.

$C_{44}H_{50}Cl_2N_4O_2,5H_2O$=827.9.

CAS — 23214-96-2 (alcuronium); 15180-03-7 (chloride).

The manufacturer reports that alcuronium is incompatible with solutions of thiopentone sodium and should not be administered in the same syringe.

Adverse Effects, Treatment, and Precautions

As for Tubocurarine Chloride, p.1241.

Alcuronium chloride has a smaller histamine-releasing effect than tubocurarine chloride.

ALLERGY. Discussions of anaphylactoid reactions to alcuronium: M. Fisher and B. Baldo, *Med. J. Aust*., 1983, *1*, 630; M. M. Fisher and I. Munro, *Anesth. Analg*.,

1983, *62,* 559.

See also under suxamethonium chloride (p.1238).

PORPHYRIA. Alcuronium was considered to be unsafe in patients with acute porphyria because it has been shown to be porphyrinogenic in *animals* or *in vitro* systems.— M.R. Moore and K.E.L. McColl, *Porphyrias, Drug Lists*, Glasgow, Porphyria Research Unit, University of Glasgow, 1987.

Absorption and Fate

When given intravenously, alcuronium is widely distributed throughout the body tissues. It is excreted unchanged, mainly by the kidneys. Small amounts are also present in bile.

Up to 2 hours after an intravenous injection of alcuronium in man the plasma concentration fell rapidly due to redistribution of the drug from the central to the peripheral compartment. The plasma concentration then fell more slowly, the half-life being about 3.3 hours. Alcuronium was not metabolised and about 80 to 85% was eliminated by the kidneys. About 10 to 15% was secreted into the bile and eliminated in the faeces. The half-life of the drug in an anuric patient was 16 hours.— J. Raaflaub and P. Frey, *Arzneimittel-Forsch.*, 1972, *22,* 73.

The elimination half-life of alcuronium was markedly prolonged, and clearance reduced, in 10 patients undergoing surgery involving cardiopulmonary bypass compared with non-cardiac patients in previous studies. Plasma concentrations of alcuronium rose from a mean of 0.55 µg per mL immediately before the start of extracorporeal circulation to one of 1.02 µg per mL in the apparent steady-state achieved after cardiopulmonary bypass was begun. Closer monitoring of neuromuscular function may be necessary in cardiac patients undergoing cardiopulmonary bypass.—J. S. Walker and K. F. Brown, *Br. J. clin. Pharmac.*, 1983, *15,* 237.

Further references: J. Walker *et al.*, *Eur. J. clin. Pharmac.*, 1980, *17,* 449; J. S. Walker *et al.*, *Clin. Pharmac. Ther.*, 1983, *33,* 510.

PREGNANCY AND THE NEONATE. Alcuronium, in a dose of 10 to 15 mg, was administered intravenously to 19 patients undergoing caesarean section. In 12 patients the alcuronium was administered over a few seconds; alcuronium 200 to 400 ng per mL was detected in the cord plasma of 11 of 13 neonates. In 7 patients in whom the administration time ranged from 2 to 6 minutes, the same amounts were detected in the cord plasma of 2 of 7 neonates. Neonatal plasma concentrations of alcuronium appeared to be independent of the maternal plasma concentrations at delivery, but related to the rate of injection. No evidence of neuromuscular block was seen in the neonates.— J. Thomas *et al.*, *Br. J. Anaesth.*, 1969, *41,* 297.

Uses and Administration

Alcuronium chloride is a competitive (non-depolarising) muscle relaxant with effects similar to those of tubocurarine chloride (see p.1241).

Alcuronium is used mainly as an adjuvant to anaesthesia to obtain greater muscle relaxation in surgical operations. An initial dose of 200 to 250 µg per kg body-weight intravenously is usually adequate to achieve 95% neuromuscular blockade. Muscle relaxation is obtained within about 2 minutes and the effect lasts for about 20 to 30 minutes. An initial dose of 300 µg per kg intravenously is reported to provide muscle relaxation for about 40 minutes. Supplementary doses of one-sixth to one-quarter the initial dose are reported to provide relaxation for additional periods of similar duration to the first. Somewhat smaller doses are required in patients anaesthetised with halothane or other potent inhalational anaesthetics that may potentiate neuromuscular blockade produced by alcuronium. Children may be given an initial dose of 125 to 200 µg per kg body-weight.

ADMINISTRATION IN RENAL FAILURE. Alcuronium 160 µg per kg body-weight intravenously gave adequate muscle relaxation in 10 anuric patients with chronic renal failure undergoing nitrous oxide-halothane anaesthesia for renal transplantation. Further doses of 1 to 2 mg were given as required. All patients had complete reversal with neostigmine.— S. Kaushik *et al.*, *Br. J. Anaesth.*, 1984, *56,* 1229.

OCULAR SURGERY. A study in 20 healthy subjects indicated that alcuronium may be a reasonable alternative to pancuronium for routine surgery of the open eye, particularly in elderly patients with limited cardiac reserve.— R. George *et al.*, *Br. J. Anaesth.*, 1979, *51,* 789.

TETANUS. Alcuronium was effective in controlling the spasms of tetanus; the problem of residual curarisation did not arise.— M. A. K. Omar (letter), *Br. med. J.*, 1979, *2,* 274.

Proprietary Preparations

Alloferin *(Roche, UK). Injection,* alcuronium chloride 5 mg/mL, in ampoules of 2 mL.

Proprietary Names and Manufacturers

Alloférine *(Roche, Fr.; Roche, Switz.)*; Alloferin *(Arg.; Roche, Austral.; Roche, Denm.; Roche, Ger.; Neth.; Roche, Norw.; Roche, S.Afr.; Roche, Swed.; Roche, UK)*; Aloferin *(Roche, Spain).*

12405-r

Atracurium Besylate *(BAN, USAN).*

33A74; Atracurium Besilate *(rINN)*; BW-33A.
2,2′-(3,11-Dioxo-4,10-dioxatridecamethylene)bis(1,2,3,4-tetrahydro-6,7-dimethoxy-2-methyl-1-veratrylisoquinolinium) di(benzenesulphonate).
$C_{53}H_{72}N_2O_{12},2C_6H_5O_3S = 1243.5.$

CAS — 64228-81-5.

Store in a cool place at 2 to 8°. Protect from light.

INCOMPATIBILITY. Atracurium besylate is incompatible with alkalis.

Adverse Effects, Treatment, and Precautions

As for Tubocurarine Chloride, p.1241. Atracurium besylate should not be administered by the intramuscular route, which may result in tissue irritation.

Unlike tubocurarine, reduction in body temperature may necessitate a reduction in the dose of atracurium besylate since cooling reduces the rate of its inactivation; however, it can be given in usual doses to patients with impaired renal function.

ALLERGY. Either bronchospasm or a full anaphylactoid reaction had been reported in 27 patients given atracurium, of whom 4 had suffered cardiac arrest but recovered. It may be unwise to use atracurium in people with atopy or asthma.— *Drug & Ther. Bull.*, 1985, *23,* 51.

Atracurium and metocurine were highly cross-reactive with serum IgE antibodies from 6 patients who had experienced life-threatening anaphylactoid reactions to other neuromuscular blocking drugs. Fazadinium was also weakly cross-reactive while vecuronium was intermediate in potency. Results suggest that exposure of sensitive patients to these drugs may result in an adverse reaction.— D. G. Harle *et al.*, *Br. J. Anaesth.*, 1985, *57,* 1073. See also: D. G. Harle and B. A. Baldo (letter), *Med. J. Aust.*, 1986, *144,* 220.

EFFECTS ON THE HEART. A report of 4 cases of profound bradycardia in patients given atracurium during surgical anaesthesia; all 4 responded to atropine.— M. L. Carter, *Br. med. J.*, 1983, *287,* 247. Severe criticism. The surgical operations all involved some degree of vagal traction which could result in a possible fall in heart-rate whatever the anaesthetic technique. Furthermore, one patient received halothane, and all received opioids, which are known to reduce heart-rate. In addition, it should be noted that the bradycardias did not develop immediately on administration of atracurium but during the course of the operation.— J. M. Hunter (letter), *ibid.*, 759. Two of the four cases mentioned had been given doses above the range suggested by the manufacturers but this was unlikely to have had an appreciable effect on heart-rate; nor was it likely that the observed bradycardias were due to a metabolite. If the vagus nerve is not blocked, bradycardia will occur when it is stimulated. Atracurium unlike most other competitive neuromuscular blocking agents has no appreciable vagal blocking effect in clinical doses, and no patient received an effective dose of an antimuscarinic agent before bradycardia developed.— A. P. Madden (letter), *ibid.*, 760. In a series of 626 anaesthetics in which atracurium was used bradycardia occurred on 19 occasions, accompanied by a fall in systolic blood pressure in 5 cases. All responded promptly to the intravenous administration of 600 µg of atropine. Provided a close watch is kept on heart-rate and prompt action taken should it fall and remain below 50 beats per minute there is no need to administer atropine as part of the premedication or induction sequence when using atracurium.— D. E. Rowlands (letter), *ibid.* In 68 elderly patients given atracurium as part of anaesthesia there were 9 cases of bradycardia : 5 were probably due to halothane and 4 were probably related to abdominal traction or vigorous orthopaedic manipulations. It is unlikely that atracurium or its main metabolite laudanosine played any part in producing bradycardia in these patients.— H. Didier (letter), *ibid.*, 984.

MUSCULAR DYSTROPHIES. Atracurium produced neuromuscular blockade uneventfully in a patient with dystrophia myotonica. The case suggests that such patients retain normal sensitivity to atracurium and in view of its rapid elimination, which obviates the need for an anticholinesterase, it is felt that atracurium should be considered when neuromuscular blockade is required for such patients.— P. Nightingale *et al.*, *Br. J. Anaesth.*, 1985, *57,* 1131.

Absorption and Fate

Following intravenous injection atracurium besylate undergoes spontaneous degradation via Hofmann elimination, a non-enzymatic breakdown process occurring at physiological pH and temperature, to produce laudanosine and other metabolites. There is also some ester hydrolysis by non-specific plasma esterases.

It is excreted in urine and bile, mostly as metabolites. The elimination half-life has been reported to be approximately 20 minutes.

It was estimated from *in vitro* work that at 40 minutes, two-thirds of atracurium in plasma was degraded by ester hydrolysis and only one third by the Hofmann reaction. Although ester hydrolysis is clearly the major pathway for the degradation of atracurium, contrary to the suggestion that Hofmann elimination contributes substantially to the total elimination, the latter reaction is a "safety net" in patients with severely impaired liver or renal function.— R. L. Stiller *et al.*, *Br. J. Anaesth.*, 1985, *57,* 1085.

Mean plasma laudanosine concentrations were significantly higher from 90 to 240 minutes after an intravenous bolus injection of atracurium 500 µg per kg body-weight in 8 patients with renal failure undergoing transplantation than in 8 surgical patients with normal kidney function. In view of the CNS-stimulant effects of laudanosine in a variety of species, further studies should be undertaken.— M. R. Fahey *et al.*, *Br. J. Anaesth.*, 1985, *57,* 1049.

See also under Administration, below.

Uses and Administration

Atracurium besylate is a competitive (non-depolarising) muscle relaxant with effects similar to those of tubocurarine chloride (see p.1241), but having a shorter duration of action. Following an intravenous dose muscle relaxation begins in about 2 minutes and lasts for 15 to 35 minutes depending on the dose.

Atracurium besylate is used to provide muscle relaxation in general anaesthesia for surgical procedures and to aid controlled ventilation. It is given by intravenous injection in usual initial doses of 300 to 600 µg per kg body-weight, depending on the duration of block required. Subsequent doses of 100 to 200 µg per kg may be given as necessary.

Atracurium may also be given by continuous intravenous infusion at a rate of 5 to 10 µg per kg per minute to maintain neuromuscular block during prolonged procedures.

Sources in the *USA* advocate a reduction in usual doses of atracurium besylate of up to one-third when it is administered to patients anaesthetised with potent inhalation anaesthetics. Doses may also need to be reduced in the hypothermic patient. However, it may be given in usual doses to patients with impaired renal function, in whom it may be the neuromuscular blocker of choice.

A review of atracurium. The course of action of atracurium is intermediate between that of suxamethonium and the established competitive blocking drugs. Although the duration of full block is dose-related, once recovery of muscle activity has begun the rate of recovery appears to be independent of dose. The rapid rate of recovery may lead to undesirable fluctuations in levels of neuromuscular blockade unless increments are given promptly at regular intervals and the patient monitored: administration by continuous intravenous infusion may have advantages. Atracurium may offer advantages in day-stay surgery, in the management of pregnant patients undergoing caesarean section, in patients with impaired renal function, the elderly, and the severely ill patient.— R. Hughes, *Clin. Anaesth.*, 1985, *3*, 331.

Further reviews: *Lancet*, 1983, *1*, 394; C. J. Hull, *Br. J. Hosp. Med.*, 1983, *30*, 273; C. S. Conner, *Drug Intell. & clin. Pharm.*, 1984, *18*, 714; R. D. Miller *et al.*, *Anesthesiology*, 1984, *61*, 444; *Med. Lett.*, 1984, *26*, 53; *Drug & Ther. Bull.*, 1985, *23*, 51; C. S. Reilly and W. S. Nimmo, *Drugs*, 1987, *34*, 98.

ADMINISTRATION. *In old people.* The mean steady-state dose of atracurium required to maintain constant neuromuscular blockade in 8 patients with a mean age of 76 years was not significantly different at 15 mg per m^2 per hour from that of 13.6 and 14.7 mg per m^2 per hour in 2 similar groups with mean ages of 53 and 26 years respectively. All groups had received an initial bolus dose of atracurium of 300 µg per kg. Atracurium's rate of inactivation, twitch height recovery time and dose requirements appear to be independent of age.— A. A. D'Hollander *et al.*, *Anesthesiology*, 1983, *59*, 237.

In renal failure. A preliminary report of the use of atracurium in 20 anephric patients. Atracurium was given in an initial dose of 500 µg per kg body-weight intravenously, with additional doses of 200 µg per kg as required to maintain adequate blockade. Block was rapidly reversed at the end of surgery by neostigmine in association with atropine and there was no evidence of residual curarisation suggesting that atracurium is the muscle relaxant of choice in patients with renal failure.— J. M. Hunter *et al.*, *J. R. Soc. Med.*, 1982, *75*, 336.

OCULAR SURGERY. Although atracurium lowered intra-ocular pressure to a greater degree than pancuronium, a desirable thing in intra-ocular surgery, the difference was unlikely to be significant in clinical practice, and neither agent prevented the rise in intra-ocular pressure associated with intubation.— D. F. Murphy *et al.*, *Br. J. Ophthal.*, 1985, *69*, 673.

Proprietary Preparations

Tracrium *(Calmic, UK). Injection*, atracurium besylate 10 mg/mL, in ampoules of 2.5, 5, and 25 mL.

Proprietary Names and Manufacturers

Tracrium *(Wellcome, Canad.; Wellcome, Denm.; Wellcome, S.Afr.; Wellcome, Swed.; Wellcome, Switz.; Calmic, UK; Wellcome, USA).*

5702-z

Baclofen *(BAN, USAN, rINN).*

Aminomethyl Chlorohydrocinnamic Acid; Ba-34647. β-Aminomethyl-*p*-chlorohydrocinnamic acid; 4-Amino-3-(4-chlorophenyl)butyric acid.
$C_{10}H_{12}ClNO_2$=213.7.

CAS — 1134-47-0.

Pharmacopoeias. In *Br.* and *U.S.*

A white or creamy-white, odourless or practically odourless, crystalline powder. Slightly **soluble** in water; very slightly soluble in methyl alcohol; practically insoluble in chloroform and organic solvents; soluble in dilute mineral acids and alkali hydroxides. **Store** in airtight containers.

Adverse Effects

The most common side-effect is drowsiness; nausea, vomiting, confusion, fatigue, and hypotonia may also occur. Other side-effects include dizziness, hypotension, euphoria, hallucinations, depression, headache, tinnitus, paraesthesias, slurred speech, diarrhoea or constipation, tremors, insomnia, visual disturbances, allergic skin reactions, pruritus, urinary disturbances, and hepatic impairment.
Baclofen is teratogenic in *animals*.

OVERDOSAGE. Use of atropine in baclofen overdosage.— R. E. Ferner, *Postgrad. med. J.*, 1981, *57*, 580.

Orofacial dyskinesias, including pursing and smacking of the lips, protrusion of the tongue, chewing movements, and frequent blinking, developed in a 60-year-old hypothyroid patient receiving thyroxine, who was given baclofen 40 mg daily for hemifacial spasm; in addition, the patient experienced vivid dreams and unpleasant visual hallucinations while falling asleep and on awakening. Symptoms disappeared on reduction of the dosage to 10 mg twice daily.— R. Sandyk, *Clin. Pharm.*, 1986, *5*, 109.

Deep coma with loss of spontaneous ventilation and reflexes followed increase in dosage of intrathecal baclofen from an infusion rate of 1.2 mg daily to 2 mg daily to treat tetanic muscle spasms in a 25-year-old man. The therapeutic range of intrathecal baclofen in severe tetanus may be very narrow, and this side-effect could prove fatal in the absence of ventilatory support.— J. A. Romijn *et al.* (letter), *Lancet*, 1986, *2*, 696.

WITHDRAWAL. The abrupt withdrawal of baclofen in a patient being treated for parkinsonism resulted in distressing hallucinations. This effect might have been due to altered dopamine metabolism.— A. J. Lees *et al.* (letter), *Lancet*, 1977, *1*, 858. Similar reports: O. B. Skausig and S. Korsgaard (letter), *ibid.*, 1258; R. Stien (letter), *ibid.*, 1977, *2*, 44; S. A. Harrison and C. A. Wood, *Drug Intell. & clin. Pharm.*, 1985, *19*, 747.

Grand mal convulsions, resulting in gastric aspiration and cardiac arrest, occurred in a patient with no history of seizures following abrupt withdrawal of baclofen.— I. Barker and I. S. Grant (letter), *Lancet*, 1982, *2*, 556.

Precautions

Baclofen should be used with caution in patients with a history of gastric and duodenal ulcer, severe psychiatric disorders, or in those with a history of epilepsy or convulsive disorders. Care is also required in the elderly, in patients with renal impairment, and in those receiving anti-hypertensive therapy. It has been suggested that patients with stroke tolerate baclofen poorly.
Patients taking baclofen should not drive or operate machinery where loss of attention may lead to accidents. The CNS effects of baclofen may be exacerbated by alcohol or other CNS depressants.
It is recommended that baclofen should be used with caution in patients in whom spasticity is used to maintain posture or to increase function.
Withdrawal of baclofen should be gradual.

Results of a study of baclofen-stimulated gastric acid secretion in 10 healthy subjects given 600 µg per kg body-weight intravenously suggested that patients on baclofen might be at risk from baclofen-induced hyperacidity.— S. Pugh *et al.*, *Gut*, 1985, *26*, A545.

Acute bradycardia and hypotension occurred following rib retraction in 3 patients given baclofen 30 mg by mouth 90 minutes before thoracic surgery under general anaesthesia, but not in a further 3 patients given placebo. Administration of atropine and ephedrine relieved bradycardia and hypotension in 2 patients, but a brief cardiac arrest occurred in 1. Administration of baclofen may disturb autonomic control of the circulation during general anaesthesia and surgery.— J. C. Sill *et al.*, *Anesthesiology*, 1986, *64*, 255.

Absorption and Fate

Baclofen is rapidly absorbed from the gastro-intestinal tract following an oral dose. The rate and extent of absorption vary between patients, and reportedly vary inversely with the dose. Baclofen is primarily excreted unchanged in the urine; small amounts are metabolised in the liver.

A crossover study in 5 healthy subjects given baclofen 20 mg by mouth after an overnight fast or a standardised breakfast showed that baclofen was rapidly absorbed in both cases, and the rate and extent of absorption were not significantly altered by the presence of food. There is no need to modify the current practice of giving baclofen with food to minimise gastro-intestinal side-effects.— G. M. Peterson *et al.*, *Med. J. Aust.*, 1985, *142*, 689.

Uses and Administration

Baclofen is an analogue of aminobutyric acid (p.1541). Its mode of action is not fully understood. It inhibits monosynaptic and polysynaptic transmission at the spinal level, and also depresses the CNS.
It is used for the symptomatic relief of muscular spasm due to conditions such as multiple sclerosis, and lesions of the spinal cord.
The initial dose is 5 mg three times daily increased by 15 mg daily every fourth day to 20 mg three times daily or until the desired therapeutic effect has been obtained. Doses of more than 80 to 100 mg daily are not generally recommended although higher doses have been given to carefully supervised patients in hospital.
In the *UK*, initial doses of 5 to 10 mg daily, in 3 or 4 divided doses, gradually increased to a maximum of 40 mg daily, have been suggested for children under 8 years; in children over 8 years of age, 10 mg daily in divided doses initially, increased to a maximum of 60 mg daily, has been recommended.
If no benefit is apparent within 6 weeks of achieving the maximum dosage, therapy should probably be withdrawn.

ADMINISTRATION. A report of a dramatic response to intrathecal administration of baclofen in doses of 5 to 25 µg to 2 patients with severe spasticity associated with midthoracic spinal cord injuries. Depending on the dose, the effects lasted for 5 to 8 hours.— R. D. Penn and J. S. Kroin (letter), *Lancet*, 1984, *1*, 1078. Six patients who had not responded to baclofen given by mouth or who had experienced adverse effects were given baclofen intrathecally by continuous infusion, or in 3 or 4 daily doses from a subcutaneous drug delivery system. Initial doses ranged from 12 to 200 µg daily, increased up to 400 µg daily in some patients over several months. Spasms were controlled in all patients, but only one patient had an improvement in voluntary-muscle control, and this did not provide any important functional gain.— idem., 1985, *2*, 125. A report of the use of intrathecal baclofen 150 µg daily in spasticity caused by diffuse cerebral damage following drowning and resuscitation in a 4-year-old child.— D. Dralle *et al.* (letter), *ibid.*, 1003.

ILEUS. Recurrent vomiting due to duodenal ileus in an adolescent with Duchenne muscular dystrophy, and unresponsive to metoclopramide, was markedly reduced in frequency when baclofen 10 mg was taken 3 times daily. The symptoms were felt to be due to a combination of severe weight loss, lordosis, and muscle spasm causing the superior mesenteric vessels to compress the duodenum; baclofen was given to improve the muscle spasm.— J. A. S. Dickson and G. Hosking (letter), *Lancet*, 1983, *2*, 227.

PAIN. Baclofen 20 mg by mouth was not significantly better than placebo in relieving pain after dental surgery in a study involving 33 patients.— C. F. Terrence *et al.*, *Clin. Neuropharmacol.*, 1983, *6*, 241.

A study suggesting that baclofen can potentiate fentanyl-induced opioid analgesia in surgical patients.— A. E. Panerai *et al.*, *Br. J. Anaesth.*, 1985, *57*, 954.

See also under Trigeminal neuralgia, below.

SCHIZOPHRENIA. Beneficial results were achieved in 13 chronic schizophrenic patients treated with baclofen.— P. K. Frederiksen (letter), *Lancet*, 1975, *1*, 702. Unfavourable reports: G. M. Simpson *et al.* (letter), *ibid.*, 1976, *1*, 966; K. L. Davis *et al.* (letter), *ibid.*, 1245; R. Kuhn, *Arzneimittel-Forsch.*, 1976, *26*, 1187; J. Wålinder *et al.* (letter), *New Engl. J. Med.*, 1977, *296*, 452.

SPASTICITY. A review on the treatment of spasticity including the use of baclofen. Baclofen is particularly effective in reducing the frequency and severity of painful or disturbing flexor or extensor muscle spasms, and its principal use is in paraplegic or quadriplegic patients with lesions of the spinal cord, the most common of which are multiple sclerosis or traumatic lesions. Baclofen is undoubtedly the most effective agent for the treatment of spasticity of this kind. It may also improve bladder and bowel control in patients with spinal lesions, but benefit is less dramatic than the effect on spasms. Despite sporadic reports that baclofen is useful in patients with hemiplegic spasticity, parkinsonism, or Huntington's chorea this has not been the general impression, and patients with cerebral lesions of these sorts are much more prone to side-effects.— R. R. Young and P. J. Delwaide, *New Engl. J. Med.*, 1981, *304*, 28 and 96.

In view of the range of adverse effects of baclofen and of their possible severity the Australian Drug Evaluation Committee recommended that its use be restricted to suppression of voluntary muscle spasm in multiple sclerosis and in spinal lesions causing skeletal hypertonus and bladder dysfunction.— *Med. J. Aust.*, 1976, *1*, 322.

Baclofen was used in the long-term management of spasticity and muscle spasm in 113 patients for up to 6 years, in doses ranging from 30 to 200 mg daily. Of 9 patients with spasticity of cerebral origin only 3 experienced any relief of symptoms. Of 79 patients with spasticity due to spinal lesions improvement was slight in 28 and good in 41. In 87 patients with spasms, 51 showed marked improvement and 25 some improvement.

Only 5 of 16 patients with urinary retention showed improvement. Side-effects occurred in 23 patients.— R. F. Jones and J. W. Lance, *Med. J. Aust.*, 1976, *1*, 654.

Since relief of spasticity alone was unlikely to produce significant functional improvement, baclofen was probably best used in the management of non-ambulant patients not requiring their spasticity for support. Its role in ambulant patients was questionable.— *Lancet*, 1977, *2*, 594.

Cerebral palsy. In a double-blind crossover study in 20 children with cerebral palsy, baclofen was significantly more effective than placebo in relieving spasticity. A suggested dose for children aged 2 to 7 years was 5 to 10 mg daily in divided doses gradually increased to a maximum of 30 to 40 mg daily; older children could tolerate 60 mg daily.— P. J. Milla and A. D. M. Jackson, *J. int. med. Res.*, 1977, *5*, 398.

Multiple sclerosis. A review of the management of multiple sclerosis. Spasticity is often best left untreated in the mobile patient with a mild paraparesis as reducing it can accentuate weakness and make walking more difficult. In more severe cases baclofen, in initial doses of 5 mg three times daily, increased gradually to a maximum of about 20 mg three times daily, is the preferred drug. Dantrolene may be substituted or added if baclofen alone is ineffective, usually in an initial dose of 25 mg daily increased if necessary to a maximum of 75 mg three times daily.— *Drug & Ther. Bull.*, 1986, *24*, 41. See also: B. Giesser, *Drugs*, 1985, *29*, 88.

Stroke. Spasticity following stroke can sometimes be distressing but although antispastic drugs such as baclofen or dantrolene do benefit a few patients symptomatically, they have not been shown convincingly to improve functional ability or motor control.— R. Langton-Hewer and D. T. Wade, *Prescribers' J.*, 1984, *24*, 66.

A further reference: *Drug & Ther. Bull.*, 1985, *23*, 9.

TARDIVE DYSKINESIA. In a 6-week study involving 31 patients with neuroleptic-induced tardive dyskinesias addition of baclofen in doses of 10 to 30 mg three times daily to neuroleptic medication in 16 did not significantly reduce the frequency of abnormal movements compared with placebo in the remaining 15 patients. The efficacy of baclofen for tardive dyskinesia is at best controversial.— W. M. Glazer *et al.*, *Psychopharmacology*, 1985, *87*, 480.

For a study indicating an initial benefit with baclofen in patients with tardive dyskinesia, followed by a loss of efficacy with long-term therapy, see R. M. Stewart *et al.*, *Clin. Neuropharmacol.*, 1982, *5*, 365.

TETANUS. A report of the use of baclofen by continuous intrathecal infusion in the management of 2 patients with tetanus. Local spinal application of baclofen might prove to be an advance in the treatment of tetanus, as long-term sedation and respirator therapy can be avoided, and in these patients the disease appeared to run a shorter course.— H. Müller *et al.* (letter), *Lancet*, 1986, *1*, 317.

See also under Adverse Effects.

TRIGEMINAL NEURALGIA. Baclofen significantly decreased the number of painful episodes in 7 of 10 patients with trigeminal neuralgia given doses up to 60 mg daily in a double-blind crossover study. In an open trial in 50 patients with trigeminal neuralgia refractory to carbamazepine or intolerant of it, 12 obtained relief with baclofen alone in doses of 40 to 80 mg and a further 25 became free of pain when baclofen was added to previously ineffective doses of carbamazepine or phenytoin. Long-term follow-up of 1 to 5 years in both sets of patients indicated that 18 of the 60 remained pain-free while receiving baclofen; 10 went into remission after 3 to 6 months of therapy and 13 became refractory to baclofen after 1 to 18 months.— G. H. Fromm *et al.*, *Ann. Neurol.*, 1984, *15*, 240. Comment.— L. A. Hershey, *Ann. intern. Med.*, 1984, *100*, 905.

URINARY DISORDERS. In 15 paraplegic patients the mean volume of residual urine fell from 115 to 63 mL with an accompanying fall in sphincter resistance, after treatment for 2 days with baclofen 20 mg daily by intravenous injection. The incidence of adverse reactions was low. Treatment was considered useful for active bladder training. Oral medication was not effective.— H. J. Hachen and V. Krucker, *Eur. Urol.*, 1977, *3*, 237.

Preparations

Baclofen Tablets *(B.P.)*

Baclofen Tablets *(U.S.P.)*

Proprietary Preparations

Lioresal *(Ciba, UK). Tablets*, scored, baclofen 10 mg. *Oral liquid*, baclofen 5 mg/5 mL.

Proprietary Names and Manufacturers

Lioresal *(Arg.; Ciba, Austral.; Belg.; Geigy, Canad.; Ciba, Denm.; Ciba, Fr.; Geigy, Ger.; Ciba, Ital.; Neth.; Ciba, Norw.; Ciba, S.Afr.; Ciba, Spain; Ciba, Swed.; Geigy, Switz.; Ciba, UK; Geigy, USA)*.

5703-c

Carbolonium Bromide *(BAN)*.

Choline Bromide Hexamethylenedicarbamate; Hexacarbacholine Bromide; Hexcarbacholine Bromide *(rINN)*; Hexcarbocholine Bromide. *NN'*-Hexamethylenebis[(2-carbamoyloxyethyl)trimethylammonium] dibromide.

$C_{18}H_{40}Br_2N_4O_4$=536.3.

CAS — 13309-41-6 (carbolonium); 306-41-2 (bromide).

Carbolonium bromide is a muscle relaxant which produces an initial depolarising neuromuscular block that is rapidly converted to a phase II (non-depolarising type) blockade. Its actions are more prolonged than those of other depolarising muscle relaxants such as suxamethonium (see p.1239).

Proprietary Names and Manufacturers

Imbretil *(Chemie-Linz, Aust.; Hormonchemie, Ger.; Österreichische Stickstoffwerke, Switz.)*.

5704-k

Carisoprodol *(BAN, USAN, rINN)*.

Isopropylmeprobamate. 2-Methyl-2-propyltrimethylene carbamate isopropylcarbamate.

$C_{12}H_{24}N_2O_4$=260.3.

CAS — 78-44-4.

Pharmacopoeias. In *U.S.*

A white crystalline powder with a slight characteristic odour. M.p. 91° to 94°.

Soluble 1 in 2083 of water, 1 in 2.5 of alcohol and of acetone, and 1 in 2.3 of chloroform. **Store** in airtight containers.

Adverse Effects, Treatment, and Precautions

As for Meprobamate, p.750.

Overdosage may result in stupor, coma, shock, respiratory depression and death.

PORPHYRIA. Carisoprodol was considered to be unsafe in patients with acute porphyria as it has been associated with acute attacks.— M.R. Moore and K.E.L. McColl, *Porphyrias, Drug Lists*, Glasgow, Porphyria Research Unit, University of Glasgow, 1987.

Absorption and Fate

Carisoprodol is absorbed from the gastro-intestinal tract. It is metabolised in the liver and excreted in urine as metabolites, including meprobamate. It crosses the placenta and is distributed in substantial amounts into breast milk.

Uses and Administration

Carisoprodol is a centrally-acting muscle relaxant whose mechanism of action is not completely understood. It also has sedative actions. Following administration by mouth its effects begin within about 30 minutes and last for 4 to 6 hours. It is used as an adjunct for the symptomatic treatment of musculoskeletal conditions associated with painful muscle spasm, in usual doses of 350 mg four times daily by mouth.

Carisoprodol had not been found of value in the treatment of painful musculoskeletal conditions; it had sedative effects, but did not relax muscles directly.— *Med. Lett.*, 1975, *17*, 42.

For a comparison of the value of carisoprodol with that of cyclobenzaprine in back strain, see under Cyclobenzaprine Hydrochloride, p.1232.

Preparations

Carisoprodol Tablets *(U.S.P.)*

Carisoprodol and Aspirin Tablets *(U.S.P.)*

Carisoprodol, Aspirin, and Codeine Phosphate Tablets *(U.S.P.)*

Proprietary Preparations

Carisoma *(Pharmax, UK). Tablets*, carisoprodol 125 and 350 mg.

Proprietary Names and Manufacturers

Caprodat *(Ferrosan, Swed.)*; Carisoma *(Pharmax, UK)*; Flexartal *(Clin Midy, Fr.)*; Mioxom *(Ital.)*; Rela *(Schering, USA)*; Relaxo-Powel *(Spain)*; Sanoma *(Heilit, Ger.)*; Soma *(Horner, Canad.; Ital.; Wallace, USA)*; Somadril *(Dumex, Denm.; Dumex, Norw.; Dumex, Swed.)*; Somalgit *(Inibsa, Spain)*; Soprodol *(Schein, USA)*.

The following names have been used for multi-ingredient preparations containing carisoprodol— Carisoma Compound *(Pharmax, UK)*; Soma Compound *(Wallace, USA)*; Soma Compound with Codeine *(Wallace, USA)*.

5705-a

Chlorphenesin Carbamate *(USAN)*.

U-19646. 3-(4-Chlorophenoxy)propane-1,2-diol 1-carbamate.

$C_{10}H_{12}ClNO_4$=245.7.

CAS — 104-29-0 (chlorphenesin); 886-74-8 (carbamate).

Adverse Effects, Treatment, and Precautions

As for Mephenesin, p.1235.

Excitement and nervousness have been reported and allergic reactions have occurred. It should be given with caution to patients with impaired hepatic function. Patients should not drive or operate machinery.

Absorption and Fate

Chlorphenesin carbamate is readily absorbed from the gastro-intestinal tract and metabolised by the liver. About 85% is excreted in the urine as the glucuronide within 24 hours.

Uses and Administration

Chlorphenesin carbamate is a centrally-acting muscle relaxant related to mephenesin. It is used as an adjunct in the symptomatic treatment of musculoskeletal conditions associated with painful muscular spasm. The usual initial dose is 800 mg three times daily reduced to 400 mg four times daily or less once a response is achieved.

Chlorphenesin itself is used as an antifungal agent. It has been recommended that chlorphenesin carbamate should not be administered for longer than 8 weeks.

TRIGEMINAL NEURALGIA. Chlorphenesin carbamate gave marked relief of pain in 4 patients with trigeminal neuralgia and to 2 further patients whose symptoms were only partially controlled with carbamazepine or phenytoin. The initial dosage of 400 mg morning and midday and 800 mg at bedtime was gradually reduced, after pain was controlled, to the lowest effective dose.— D. J. Dalessio, *J. Am. med. Ass.*, 1973, *225*, 1659.

Proprietary Names and Manufacturers

Maolate *(Upjohn, USA)*; Rinlaxer *(Jpn)*.

5706-t

Chlorzoxazone *(BAN, USAN, rINN)*.

Chlorobenzoxazolinone. 5-Chlorobenzoxazol-2(3*H*)-one.

$C_7H_4ClNO_2$=169.6.

CAS — 95-25-0.

Pharmacopoeias. In *Nord.* and *U.S.*

A white or almost white, practically odourless crystalline powder.

Slightly **soluble** in water; sparingly soluble in alcohol, isopropyl alcohol, and in methyl alcohol; soluble in solutions of alkali hydroxides and ammonia. **Store** in airtight containers.

Adverse Effects and Treatment

The most common side-effects of chlorzoxazone are drowsiness and dizziness or lightheadedness. There may also be gastro-intestinal irritation with nausea, vomiting, heartburn, abdominal discomfort, constipation or diarrhoea; gastro-intestinal bleeding has been reported. Other effects that have occurred are headache, excitement, restlessness, irritability, and sensitivity reactions including skin rashes, petechiae, echymoses, urticaria and pruritus; very rarely, angioedema or anaphylactoid reactions may occur. Anaemia and granu-

locytopenia have been reported. Some patients taking chlorzoxazone have developed jaundice and liver damage suspected to be due to the drug.
Following overdosage there may be malaise or sluggishness followed by marked loss of muscle tone, hypotension, and respiratory depression. Treatment consists of emptying the stomach by gastric lavage or emesis, and supportive therapy. The administration of activated charcoal to adsorb any remaining drug after emptying the stomach has been suggested.

A report of a patient with a spasmodic toricollis-like syndrome, consisting of tonic deviation of the head to the right, clenching of the teeth and dysarthria, which developed repeatedly within 2 hours of ingesting chlorzoxazone for low back pain. Intravenous injection of benztropine mesylate 1 mg gave rapid relief of symptoms.— M. A. Rosin (letter), *J. Am. med. Ass.*, 1981, *246*, 2575.

Precautions
Chlorzoxazone should not be given to patients with impaired liver function and should be discontinued if skin rash, pruritus, or signs of liver damage appear. As chlorzoxazone may cause drowsiness and impaired concentration patients should not drive or operate machinery. The adverse CNS effects of chlorzoxazone may be enhanced by other CNS-depressants such as alcohol.
The urine of patients taking chlorzoxazone may be coloured orange or reddish-purple by a metabolite.

PORPHYRIA. Chlorzoxazone was considered to be unsafe in patients with acute porphyria because it has been shown to be porphyrinogenic in *animals* or *in vitro* systems.— M.R. Moore and K.E.L. McColl, *Porphyrias, Drug Lists*, Glasgow, Porphyria Research Unit, University of Glasgow, 1987.

Absorption and Fate
After oral administration chlorzoxazone is rapidly and completely absorbed. It is metabolised in the liver to 6-hydroxychlorzoxazone and excreted in the urine as the glucuronide.

In a study in 23 healthy subjects given chlorzoxazone 750 mg with paracetamol 900 mg as an oral suspension, mean elimination half-life of chlorzoxazone was 1 hour. The apparent volume of distribution of approximately 14 litres suggested that chlorzoxazone was not widely distributed and was confined to the circulatory system and perhaps extracellular fluid.— R. K. Desiraju *et al.*, *J. pharm. Sci.*, 1983, *72*, 991.

Uses and Administration
Chlorzoxazone is a centrally-acting muscle relaxant that has been claimed to exert an effect primarily at the level of the spinal cord and subcortical areas of the brain to inhibit reflex arcs responsible for muscle spasm. Following oral administration its effects begin within an hour and last for 3 to 4 hours.
It is used as an adjunct in the symptomatic treatment of musculoskeletal conditions associated with painful muscle spasm. The usual initial dose is 500 mg three or four times daily by mouth, alone or in association with paracetamol; the dose can often be subsequently reduced to 250 mg, although doses of up to 750 mg three or four times daily may be given if necessary. Doses of 125 to 500 mg three or four times a day, depending on age and weight, have been recommended in children.

Preparations
Chlorzoxazone Tablets *(U.S.P.)*
Chlorzoxazone and Acetaminophen Capsules *(U.S.P.)*. Contain chlorzoxazone and paracetamol.
Chlorzoxazone and Acetaminophen Tablets *(U.S.P.)*. Contain chlorzoxazone and paracetamol.

Proprietary Names and Manufacturers
Biomioran *(Bioindustria, Ital.)*; Escoflex *(Streuli, Switz.)*; Paraflex *(Cilag-Chemie, Belg.; Astra, Denm.; Cilag, Ger.; Cilag, Ital.; Cilag-Chemie, Neth.; Astra, Norw.; Johnson & Johnson, S.Afr.; Astra, Swed.; Cilag, Switz.; McNeil Pharmaceutical, USA)*; Parafon Forte DSC *(McNeil Pharmaceutical, USA)*; Solaxin *(Jpn)*.
The following names have been used for multi-ingredient preparations containing chlorzoxazone—Algisin *(Ram, USA)*; Blanex *(Edwards, USA)*; Chlorzone *(Schein, USA)*; Parafon Forte *(McNeil, Canad.; McNeil Pharmaceutical, USA)*; Parafon Forte C8 *(McNeil, Canad.)*; Saroflex *(Saron, USA)*.

5708-r

Cyclobenzaprine Hydrochloride *(USAN, rINNM)*.

MK-130 *(cyclobenzaprine)*; Proheptatriene Hydrochloride; Ro-4-1557 *(cyclobenzaprine)*; RP-9715 *(cyclobenzaprine)*. 3-(5*H*-Dibenzo[*a,d*]-cyclohepten-5-ylidene)-*NN*-dimethylpropylamine hydrochloride.
$C_{20}H_{21}N,HCl=311.9$.

CAS — 303-53-7 (cyclobenzaprine); 6202-23-9 (hydrochloride).

Pharmacopoeias. In *U.S.*

A white or off-white odourless crystalline powder. Freely **soluble** in water, alcohol, and methyl alcohol; sparingly soluble in isopropyl alcohol; slightly soluble in chloroform and methylene chloride; practically insoluble in hydrocarbons.

Adverse Effects and Treatment
Cyclobenzapine is structurally related to the tricyclic antidepressants, and shares many of their antimuscarinic and other adverse effects. The commonest side-effects are drowsiness, dizziness, and dry mouth; fatigue and weakness, nausea, vomiting, dyspepsia, constipation, gastro-intestinal pain, dysgeusia, tachycardia and arrhythmias may also occur. Other effects may include headache, nervousness or anxiety, confusion, disorientation, depression, agitation, hallucinations, paraesthesias, tremor, blurred vision, and tinnitus. Liver disorders, urinary frequency, urinary retention, rashes, urticaria, and oedema of face and tongue have also been reported.
Overdosage should be treated symptomatically. Dialysis is not considered to be of value because of the low plasma concentrations of cyclobenzaprine.

OVERDOSAGE. A report of acute poisoning, with paradoxical sweating, agitation and confusion, following ingestion of an unknown quantity of cyclobenzaprine. Diaphoresis, as well as the expected antimuscarinic anhidrosis should be considered as part of the spectrum of cyclobenzaprine poisoning.— P. S. Heckerling and T. J. Bartow (letter), *Ann. intern. Med.*, 1984, *101*, 881.

Precautions
As for Amitriptyline Hydrochloride, p.352.

Absorption and Fate
Cyclobenzaprine hydrochloride is readily absorbed from the gastro-intestinal tract although plasma concentrations vary considerably in different individuals given the same dose. It is extensively bound to plasma proteins and has a reported half-life of 1 to 3 days. It is extensively metabolised, and excreted via the kidneys. Some unchanged drug appears in the bile.

Results suggesting that cyclobenzaprine may be metabolised in the intestinal tract or undergo a 'first-pass' effect in the liver.— H. B. Hucher *et al.*, *J. clin. Pharmac.*, 1977, *17*, 719.

Uses and Administration
Cyclobenzaprine hydrochloride is a centrally-acting muscle relaxant, related to the tricyclic antidepressants. It appears to act primarily at brain stem, rather than at spinal cord, levels. Following oral administration its effects begin within 1 hour; the effects of a single dose have been reported to last as long as 12 to 24 hours.
It is used as an adjunct in the symptomatic treatment of musculoskeletal conditions associated with painful muscle spasm. The usual dose is 10 mg three times daily; the daily dose should not exceed 60 mg. Treatment for more than 2 or 3 weeks is not recommended.

The effectiveness of cyclobenzaprine hydrochloride in the treatment of muscle spasm was assessed by means of a postmarketing surveillance programme. In 4657 patients assessed, an excellent or good response was reported in 70%. Side-effects reported in the 4749 patients treated were drowsiness in 14.9%, dry mouth in 6.9%, dizziness in 2.8%, nervousness in 1.1%, fatigue in 1.5%, confusion in 1.5%, and nausea in 1.3%. Other side-effects reported included taste disturbance, tachycardia, disorientation, and hallucinations (all less than 1%). Cyclobenzaprine was discontinued in 101 patients because of adverse reactions.— D. W. Nibbelink and S. C. Strickland, *Curr. ther. Res.*, 1979, *25*, 564.

Little difference in improvement obtained with cyclobenzaprine or placebo in a double-blind study of 54 patients with muscle spasm associated with osteoarthritis of the neck or back.— N. A. Bercel, *Curr. ther. Res.*, 1977, *22*, 462.

A controlled double-blind study lasting 2 weeks in 49 patients with long-term intractable pain of cervical and lumbar origin indicated comparable effectiveness of cyclobenzaprine hydrochloride 10 mg and diazepam 5 mg, both three times daily. Dry mouth and drowsiness occurred more often with cyclobenzaprine than with diazepam.— B. R. Brown and J. Womble, *J. Am. med. Ass.*, 1978, *240*, 1151.

In a study involving 58 patients with thoracolumbar strain or sprain, 30 of whom received cyclobenzaprine and 28 carisoprodol, there was no significant difference in efficacy between cyclobenzaprine hydrochloride 10 mg and carisoprodol 350 mg, both taken 4 times daily and reduced to 3 times a day if indicated. Treatment was for 7 days. Both treatments gave effective relief of pain and muscle spasm and there was no significant difference in the overall incidence of adverse effects, although more patients taking cyclobenzaprine had dry mouth.— H. E. Rollings *et al.*, *Curr. ther. Res.*, 1983, *34*, 917.

Preparations
Cyclobenzaprine Hydrochloride Tablets *(U.S.P.)*

Proprietary Names and Manufacturers
Flexeril *(Merck Sharp & Dohme, Canad.; Merck Sharp & Dohme, USA)*; Flexiban *(Merck Sharp & Dohme, Ital.)*; Yurelax *(Organon, Spain)*.

5709-f

Dantrolene Sodium *(BANM, USAN, rINNM)*.

F-368 *(dantrolene)*; F-440. The hemiheptahydrate of the sodium salt of 1-[5-(4-nitrophenyl)furfurylideneamino]imidazolidine-2,4-dione.
$C_{14}H_9N_4NaO_5,3\frac{1}{2}H_2O=399.3$.

CAS — 7261-97-4 (dantrolene); 14663-23-1 (sodium salt, anhydrous); 24868-20-0 (sodium salt, hemiheptahydrate).

Adverse Effects
The most common side-effects of dantrolene sodium are drowsiness, dizziness, weakness, general malaise, fatigue, and diarrhoea. Other side-effects reported include nausea and vomiting, constipation, gastro-intestinal bleeding, abdominal cramps, tachycardia, phlebitis, pleural effusion, and pericarditis. Haematuria, crystalluria, urinary frequency, retention and incontinence, rashes, myalgia, backache, convulsions, headache, visual disturbances, confusion, and depression have also been reported.
Hepatotoxicity may occur: changes in liver-function tests, jaundice, and hepatitis, sometimes fatal, have been reported.
Dantrolene sodium in high doses is carcinogenic in some *animals*.

Abdominal distension and intestinal obstruction developed in 3 patients who were taking 50 mg or more of dantrolene four times a day.— S. A. Shaivitz (letter), *J. Am. med. Ass.*, 1974, *229*, 1282.

A report of the development of lymphocytic lymphoma in a patient associated with prolonged dantrolene therapy for progressive spastic paraplegia.— H. H. Wan and J. S. Tucker, *Postgrad. med. J.*, 1980, *56*, 261.

EFFECTS ON THE LIVER. An analysis of cases of liver

injury associated with dantrolene reported to the manufacturer or to the FDA. Fifty cases had been reported, with jaundice in 22; there were 14 fatalities. All the fatalities occurred in patients over 30 years of age who had taken dantrolene for at least 2 months. Eleven of the fatalities were in females. No liver damage occurred in patients under the age of 10 or treated for less than 1 month. Most of the cases and fatalities were in patients who had taken 300 mg or more daily. Damage was mainly hepatocellular with no evidence of hypersensitivity. It was estimated that the incidence of hepatic adverse reactions, reflected by elevated serum transaminase, was about 1.8%, and that of overt hepatitis about 0.6%.— R. Utili *et al.*, *Gastroenterology*, 1977, *72*, 610.

Precautions

It is recommended that dantrolene sodium should not be used where spasticity is used to maintain posture or function and in patients with active liver disease. Liver-function tests should be performed in all patients before and during treatment; if values rise treatment should generally be discontinued. It should be used with caution in patients with cardiac or pulmonary disorders.

Patients should not drive or operate machinery where loss of attention could cause accidents.

The CNS effects of dantrolene sodium may be enhanced by tranquillisers or other CNS-depressants such as alcohol. Concomitant administration with oestrogens may possibly increase the risk of liver damage.

INTERACTIONS. A significant reduction in the binding of dantrolene to human serum albumin occurred in the presence of the tightly bound drugs, warfarin and clofibrate, but tolbutamide, which would similarly have been expected to displace dantrolene, increased the binding.— J. J. Vallner *et al.*, *J. pharm. Sci.*, 1976, *65*, 873.

A study of the effects of dantrolene sodium on *guinea-pig* isolated skeletal, smooth, and cardiac muscle. Reflex sympathetic activity might be an important factor in maintaining cardiac output in patients chronically treated with dantrolene. Serious interaction might occur following concurrent administration of drugs that impaired the activity of the sympathetic nervous system, such as adrenergic neurone blocking agents and beta-adrenoceptor blocking agents, or agents that interfered with calcium ion flux across cardiac cell membranes, such as verapamil or nifedipine. Experimental studies were needed.— W. C. Bowman and H. H. Khan, *J. Pharm. Pharmac.*, 1977, *29*, 628.

A report of marked elevation of serum potassium with hypotension, decreasing cardiac output, atrioventricular block, and cardiac arrest following concomitant administration of dantrolene sodium and verapamil to *pigs*.— L. S. Saltzman *et al.*, *Anesth. Analg.*, 1984, *63*, 473.

Absorption and Fate

Dantrolene sodium is incompletely absorbed from the gastro-intestinal tract. It is metabolised in the liver and excreted in the urine mainly as the hydroxylated and acetamide metabolites with a small amount of unchanged dantrolene; some appears in the bile. Dantrolene is bound to plasma proteins.

In adults and children peak blood concentrations of dantrolene were obtained 4 to 6 hours after a single dose by mouth. The mean half-life was 8.7 hours.— M. H. M. Dykes, *J. Am. med. Ass.*, 1975, *231*, 862.

Plasma concentrations of dantrolene were assayed in 6 patients receiving chronic dantrolene therapy. In 4 patients dantrolene concentrations were fairly stable and remained between about 30 and 90 ng per mL, while concentrations fluctuated between 30 and 212 ng per mL in the other 2 patients. Plasma concentrations of 5-hydroxydantrolene ranged from about 100 to 300 ng per mL.— J. J. Vallner *et al.*, *Curr. ther. Res.*, 1979, *25*, 79.

Uses and Administration

Dantrolene sodium is a muscle relaxant with a direct action on skeletal muscle. It uncouples muscular contraction from excitation, probably by interfering with the release of calcium from the sarcoplasmic reticulum.

It is used for the symptomatic relief of spasticity due to conditions such as stroke, multiple sclerosis, spinal cord injury, and cerebral palsy.

The initial dose is 25 mg daily increased gradually over about 7 weeks to 100 mg four times daily or until the desired therapeutic effect has been obtained; dosage in excess of 400 mg daily is not recommended. If no response is achieved in 45 days treatment should be discontinued.

Dantrolene sodium is also used intravenously together with supportive measures, in the treatment of malignant hyperpyrexia. The initial dose is 1 mg per kg body-weight intravenously given rapidly, repeated, if necessary, to a total dose of 10 mg per kg. In the *US*, doses of 1 to 2 mg per kg by mouth 4 times daily have been recommended for up to 3 days after the crisis to prevent recurrence, and similar doses have been given for 1 to 2 days before surgery in individuals thought to be at risk of developing the syndrome.

A detailed review of the actions and uses of dantrolene sodium.— A. Ward *et al.*, *Drugs*, 1986, *32*, 130. A further review.— B. A. Britt, *Can. Anaesth. Soc. J.*, 1984, *31*, 61.

HEAT STROKE. A beneficial response to dantrolene in heat stroke.— J. S. Lydiatt and G. E. Hill (letter), *J. Am. med. Ass.*, 1981, *246*, 41.

See also: R. T. Paasuke (letter), *Can. med. Ass. J.*, 1984, *130*, 341.

HYPERPYREXIA. Rapid diagnosis and intravenous administration of dantrolene 1 mg per kg body-weight, repeated to a maximum of 10 mg per kg, will bring about successful resolution of symptoms in almost every case of malignant hyperpyrexia or neuroleptic malignant syndrome. Before the introduction of dantrolene these disorders, although rare, were associated with a high risk of mortality. To ensure the best outcome, treatment should be started within a few minutes of onset of symptoms, and should be combined with immediate cessation of triggering agents, cooling techniques for raised temperature and correction of blood gas levels and metabolic acidosis with oxygen, and sodium bicarbonate injection. Other supportive measures should be given as appropriate.

Although there is also a strong case for avoidance of triggering agents, dantrolene may be given prophylactically to individuals susceptible to malignant hyperpyrexia, usually in doses totalling 4 to 8 mg per kg daily by mouth for 1 or 2 days before surgery: however, there is a trend towards limiting prophylactic therapy to intravenous administration of 2.5 mg per kg before surgers.— A. Ward *et al.*, *Drugs*, 1986, *32*, 130.

Further references to the use of dantrolene in malignant hyperpyrexia: T. E. Nelson and E. H. Flewellen, *New Engl. J. Med.*, 1983, *309*, 416.

Neuroleptic malignant syndrome. The use of dantrolene sodium 80 mg intravenously, together with cooling and diuretics, to treat a patient with neuroleptic malignant syndrome. Within 2 hours of initiating treatment his temperature, which had been fluctuating between 38.6 and 39.1° fell to 37.4°; there was a much slower fall in creatine phosphokinase values. Muscle rigidity also responded only slowly, returning to its previous intensity after 4 days.— J. G. Goekoop and P. A. T. Carbaat (letter), *Lancet*, 1982, *2*, 49.

Further reports and discussions of the use of dantrolene sodium in the treatment of neuroleptic malignant syndrome: P. Daoudal and J. L. Delacour (letter), *Lancet*, 1982, *2*, 217; D. C. May *et al.* (letter), *Ann. intern. Med.*, 1983, *98*, 183; C. S. Conner, *Drug Intell. & clin. Pharm.*, 1983, *17*, 639; L. J. Birkhimer and C. L. DeVane, *ibid.*, 1984, *18*, 462; F. Konikoff *et al.* (letter), *Br. med. J.*, 1984, *289*, 1228; B. H. Guzé and L. R. Baxter, *New Engl. J. Med.*, 1985, *313*, 163.

PAIN. The use of dantrolene sodium to relieve exercise-induced muscle pain in a patient with muscle phosphorylase deficiency and in a child with Duchenne muscular dystrophy. There was no provocation of muscle weakness in either patient.— T. Bertorini *et al.* (letter), *Lancet*, 1982, *1*, 616.

SPASTICITY. A review of the treatment of spasticity including the use of dantrolene. Dantrolene is particularly useful for the treatment of spasticity in patients whose nursing care is made difficult by severe, prolonged muscle contractions and who will not be troubled by any concomitant decrease in voluntary power. Theoretically it makes little difference what type of spasticity is being treated with dantrolene or where the lesion is located. Dantrolene is said to have been of approximately equal efficacy to diazepam in published studies; it may be more useful in patients in whom the sedative side-effects of diazepam are more of a problem, such as the elderly and persons with CNS lesions, whereas diazepam may be more useful in patients whose strength is already barely sufficient for everyday activities R. R. Young and P. J. Delwaide, *New Engl. J. Med.*, 1981, *304*, 28 and 96.

Dantrolene sodium 25 mg daily controlled muscle spasms and resulting pain in a 65-year-old man with advanced adenocarcinoma of the rectum and pelvic area.— A. Myers (letter), *J. Am. med. Ass.*, 1977, *237*, 2378.

For a discussion of the management of spasticity in multiple sclerosis, see under Baclofen, p.1231.

Proprietary Preparations

Dantrium *(Norwich-Eaton, UK)*. *Capsules*, dantrolene sodium 25 and 100 mg.

Injection, powder for reconstitution, dantrolene sodium 20 mg.

Proprietary Names and Manufacturers

Danlene *(SIT, Ital.)*; Dantamacrin *(Röhm, Ger.; Boehringer Mannheim, Switz.)*; Dantralen *(Lafarquim, Spain)*; Dantrium *(Norwich-Eaton, Austral.; Belg.; Norwich-Eaton, Canad.; Norwich Eaton, Denm.; Oberval, Fr.; Formenti, Ital.; Neth.; NZ; Eaton, S.Afr.; Norwich-Eaton, UK; Norwich Eaton, USA)*.

5710-z

Decamethonium Bromide *(rINN)*.

NN'-Decamethylenebis(trimethylammonium) dibromide.

$C_{16}H_{38}Br_2N_2$=418.3.

CAS — 156-74-1 (decamethonium); 541-22-0 (bromide).

5711-c

Decamethonium Iodide *(BAN)*.

C-10; Decameth. Iod.; Decamethonium Biiodatum; Decametonium Iodidum. *NN'*-Decamethylenebis(trimethylammonium) di-iodide.

$C_{16}H_{38}I_2N_2$=512.3.

CAS — 1420-40-2.

Pharmacopoeias. In *Cz.*, *It.*, and *Pol.*

Adverse Effects, Treatment, and Precautions

As for Suxamethonium Chloride, p.1238.

Decamethonium iodide may produce allergic reactions in patients sensitive to iodine.

Uses and Administration

Decamethonium is a depolarising muscle relaxant with actions similar to suxamethonium (see p.1239), which has been used to obtain muscular relaxation during surgical operations and electroconvulsive therapy. The effect of a single intravenous injection lasts for 15 to 20 minutes, but onset of action is slower than with suxamethonium. Doses of the bromide have ranged from 2.0 to 2.5 mg and of the iodide from 3 to 5 mg.

Proprietary Names and Manufacturers of Decamethonium Bromide

Syncurine *(Wellcome, Austral.; Wellcome, Canad.; Wellcome, USA)*.

5714-t

Fazadinium Bromide *(BAN, rINN)*.

AH-8165D. 1,1'-Azobis(3-methyl-2-phenyl-1*H*-imidazo-[1,2-*a*]pyridinium) dibromide.

$C_{28}H_{24}Br_2N_6$=604.3.

CAS — 36653-54-0 (fazadinium); 49564-56-9 (bromide).

Fazadinium bromide 1.36 mg is approximately equivalent to 1 mg of fazadinium.

INCOMPATIBILITY. Fazadinium bromide was incompatible with alkaline solutions and should not be administered mixed in the same syringe with thiopentone.

Adverse Effects, Treatment, and Precautions

As for Tubocurarine Chloride, p.1241.

Tachycardia may occur after the use of fazadinium bromide, even after low doses, and may be persistent. Hypotension and hypertension have been reported. Local irritation at the site of injection has occurred. Allergic reactions such as bronchospasm or urticaria have occasionally occurred, but histamine release does not appear to be a problem.

For results suggesting that administration of fazadinium to patients sensitive to other neuromuscular blocking drugs might result in an adverse reaction, see Adverse Effects under Atracurium Besylate, p.1229.

Absorption and Fate
Following intravenous injection fazadinium is mainly excreted unchanged in the urine. Small amounts of unchanged drug and metabolites are excreted in bile. Fazadinium crosses the placenta in insignificant amounts.

A study of the pharmacokinetics of fazadinium in 10 anaesthetised patients given a single intravenous dose of 1.5 mg per kg body-weight. The serum half-life of the elimination phase was about 76 minutes and the mean plasma clearance, 132 mL per minute. About 50% of the dose was excreted, essentially unchanged, in the urine within 24 hours. Trace amounts of metabolites accounted for no more than 3% of the injected dose.— P. Duvaldestin *et al.*, *Br. J. Anaesth.*, 1978, *50*, 773.

A new model of the pharmacodynamics and pharmacokinetics of fazadinium.— A. A. d'Hollander *et al.*, *Eur. J. clin. Pharmac.*, 1983, *24*, 407.

Uses and Administration
Fazadinium bromide is a competitive (non-depolarising) muscle relaxant, with a dose-dependent rapid onset and prolonged duration of action. Relaxation is evident in half to one minute; the effect lasts for up to 60 minutes after doses equivalent to 1 mg of fazadinium per kg body-weight. Fazadinium has ganglion-blocking properties. It does not appear to increase intra-ocular pressure. Fazadinium bromide has been used to facilitate endotracheal intubation and to provide muscular relaxation during surgery. The usual initial dose is the equivalent of 0.75 to 1 mg of fazadinium per kg, given intravenously; a subsequent dose one-quarter of the initial dose may be expected to prolong the effect for a further 10 to 20 minutes. Neuromuscular blockade may be reversed by neostigmine methylsulphate.

Proprietary Names and Manufacturers
Fazadon *(Glaxo, Ital.; Glaxo, Spain; Duncan, Flockhart, UK).*

5720-k

Gallamine Triethiodide *(BANM, USAN, rINN).*

Bencurine Iodide; Gallamini Triethiodidum; Gallamone Triethiodide. 2,2′,2″-(Benzene-1,2,3-triyltrioxy)tris(tetraethylammonium) tri-iodide.
$C_{30}H_{60}I_3N_3O_3$=891.5.

CAS — 153-76-4 (gallamine); 65-29-2 (triethiodide).

Pharmacopoeias. In *Arg., Br., Braz., Cz., Egypt., Eur., Fr., Ger., Ind., Int., It., Jug., Neth., Nord., Swiss, Turk.*, and *U.S.*

A white, or almost white, hygroscopic odourless powder.
Soluble 1 in 0.6 of water; slightly soluble in alcohol; very slightly soluble in chloroform; practically insoluble in ether. A 2% solution in water has a pH of 5.3 to 7.0. The *B.P.* injection has a pH of 5.5 to 7.5 and the *U.S.P.* injection a pH of 6.5 to 7.5. Solutions for injection are **sterilised** by autoclaving. **Store** in airtight containers. Protect from light.

INCOMPATIBILITY. Solutions of gallamine triethiodide were compatible with thiopentone when the gallamine triethiodide solution was added to the thiopentone but not *vice versa*; they were incompatible with pethidine hydrochloride solutions.

Adverse Effects and Treatment
As for Tubocurarine Chloride, p.1241. Tachycardia often develops and may be persistent. Blood pressure may be raised. It has a smaller histamine-releasing effect than tubocurarine chloride but occasional anaphylactoid reactions have been reported.

Accidental subarachnoid injection of gallamine in a 48-year-old man, who subsequently underwent general anaesthesia and surgery, was followed 2 hours later by violent muscle spasms, pyrexia, profuse sweating, and increasing arterial pressure and heart-rate. About 4 hours later 15 mL of cerebrospinal fluid was withdrawn and was found still to contain gallamine. Treatment included intravenous injection of diazepam, hydrocortisone, dexamethasone, and infusion fluids. The patient survived.— T. W. Goonewardene *et al.*, *Br. J. Anaesth.*, 1975, *47*, 889.

ALLERGY. For reviews and discussions of allergy and anaphylactoid reactions to neuromuscular blocking agents, including gallamine, see under Suxamethonium Chloride, p.1238.

Precautions
As for Tubocurarine Chloride, p.1241.

INTERACTIONS. *Diazepam.* The intensity and duration of the neuromuscular block induced by gallamine was profoundly enhanced when diazepam, 150 to 200 µg per kg body-weight, was administered intravenously S. A. Feldman and B. E. Crawley (preliminary communication), *Br. med. J.*, 1970, *2*, 336. Diazepam did not enhance the neuromuscular blockade produced by tubocurarine or gallamine; in *rat* phrenic-nerve diaphragm it caused an increased contraction by a direct action on the muscle.— G. Moudgil and B. J. Pleuvry (letter), *ibid.*, 734. There was no evidence in *cats* of diazepam altering the depth or duration of neuromuscular blockade induced by tubocurarine or gallamine.— S. N. Webb and E. G. Bradshaw (letter), *ibid.*, 1971, *3*, 640. Investigations in *dogs* showed that diazepam significantly reversed the neuromuscular blockade induced by non-depolarising agents such as gallamine but augmented that of depolarising agents such as suxamethonium.— K. K. Sharma and U. C. Sharma, *J. Pharm. Pharmac.*, 1978, *30*, 64.

Absorption and Fate
Following intravenous administration gallamine triethiodide is distributed throughout body tissues. It is not metabolised, and is excreted in the urine as unchanged drug. It crosses the placenta.

The clinical pharmacokinetics of gallamine triethiodide.— L. B. Wingard and D. R. Cook, *Clin. Pharmacokinet.*, 1977, *2*, 330.

A preliminary investigation of the renal and hepatic excretion of gallamine in 15 patients undergoing surgery showed that it was primarily excreted unchanged in the urine with negligible amounts in the bile. Observations in 3 patients indicated that poor urinary excretion of gallamine did not invariably result in persistent high serum concentrations or prolonged duration of neuromuscular effects.— S. Agoston *et al.*, *Br. J. Anaesth.*, 1978, *50*, 345.

The relationship between gallamine-plasma concentration and neuromuscular paralysis in 10 surgical patients.— I. M. Ramzan *et al.*, *J. clin. Pharmac.*, 1983, *23*, 243.

The pharmacokinetics of gallamine in patients undergoing surgery involving cardiopulmonary bypass did not differ significantly from those in control patients.— C. A. Shanks *et al.*, *Clin. Pharmac. Ther.*, 1983, *33*, 792.

IN RENAL FAILURE. In a study involving 8 patients with chronic renal failure, mean elimination half-life was 752.40 minutes compared with 130.96 minutes in 17 healthy controls when both groups were given intravenous gallamine in initial doses of 2 mg per kg body-weight. Clearance was markedly reduced in patients with renal failure and despite limited data there appeared to be a tendency to a delayed recovery from neuromuscular blockade, even at the modest doses of gallamine that were used. Use of gallamine in patients with renal failure cannot be advocated.— M. I. Ramzan *et al.*, *Br. J. clin. Pharmac.*, 1981, *12*, 141.

Uses and Administration
Gallamine triethiodide is a competitive (non-depolarising) muscle relaxant with effects similar to those of tubocurarine chloride (p.1241). Muscle relaxation commences within about 1 to 2 minutes of administration and lasts for about 20 to 30 minutes.
Gallamine triethiodide is used mainly as an adjuvant to anaesthesia to obtain greater muscular relaxation in surgical operations. In the *UK*, initial doses of 80 to 120 mg by intravenous injection have been recommended, with further doses of 20 to 40 mg as required. Some sources advocate that an initial dose of 20 mg should be given to the patient before anaesthesia to determine undue susceptibility. In children, a dose of 1.5 mg per kg body-weight has been recommended.
In the *USA* lower doses have generally been employed; an initial dose of 1 mg per kg intravenously, up to a maximum of 100 mg, with additional doses of 0.5 to 1 mg per kg after about 40 minutes if required.
Where intravenous administration is not feasible, gallamine triethiodide may be given intramuscularly, with or without hyaluronidase.
The standard doses of gallamine may need to be reduced in the presence of certain potent inhalation anaesthetics which potentiate competitive neuromuscular blockade.
Small doses of gallamine triethiodide have been employed similarly to tubocurarine in the diagnosis of myasthenia gravis, but such a procedure is extremely hazardous.

In 40 patients gallamine, 300 µg per kg body-weight given 3 minutes before induction of anaesthesia, was more effective than atropine, 6 µg per kg in 40 patients, in preventing slowing of the heart-rate after a second injection of suxamethonium—the incidence was 1 in 39 compared with 14 of 40. Both gallamine and atropine prevented junctional rhythm. Visible muscle fasciculations after the first dose of suxamethonium occurred in 1 of 40 patients after gallamine and in 33 of 40 after atropine.— R. K. Stoelting, *Anesth. Analg. curr. Res.*, 1977, *56*, 493.

ADMINISTRATION IN RENAL FAILURE. Gallamine could be given in normal doses to patients with glomerular filtration-rates above 50 mL per minute but its use should be avoided in patients with glomerular filtration-rate below this figure. Recurarisation could occur up to 24 hours after dosage: dialysis might be useful if blockade was unresponsive to neostigmine.— W. M. Bennett *et al.*, *Am. J. Kidney Dis.*, 1983, *3*, 155.

Preparations
Gallamine Injection *(B.P.).* A sterile solution of gallamine triethiodide in Water for Injections.

Gallamine Triethiodide Injection *(U.S.P.)*

Proprietary Preparations
Flaxedil *(May & Baker, UK). Injection,* gallamine triethiodide 40 mg/mL, in ampoules of 2 mL.

Proprietary Names and Manufacturers
Flaxedil *(Arg.; May & Baker, Austral.; Belg.; Rhône-Poulenc, Canad.; Ger.; Neth.; May & Baker, S.Afr.; Spain; May & Baker, UK)*; Miowas G *(Wasserman, Spain)*; Relaxan *(GEA, Denm.).*

5721-a

Hexafluorenium Bromide *(USAN).*

Hexafluronium Bromide *(rINN)*; NSC-19477. *NN′*-Hexamethylenebis(fluoren-9-yldimethylammonium) dibromide.
$C_{36}H_{42}Br_2N_2$=662.5.

CAS — 4844-10-4 (hexafluorenium); 317-52-2 (bromide).

Pharmacopoeias. In *U.S.*

A white crystalline powder. Sparingly **soluble** in water; soluble in alcohol; practically insoluble in chloroform and ether. **Protect** from light.

Hexafluorenium bromide has been used to prolong the relaxant effects of suxamethonium chloride (see p.1239) by inhibiting plasma cholinesterase and so delaying the enzymatic hydrolysis of the latter; it is also reported to possess some competitive (non-depolarising) neuromuscular blocking actions. It has been claimed to reduce suxamethonium-induced muscle fasciculations and prevent increases in intra-ocular pressure.
It has been given in doses of 100 to 400 µg per kg body-weight intravenously 2 or 3 minutes before injection of suxamethonium; subsequent doses are 100 to 200 µg per kg as required.

Preparations
Hexafluorenium Bromide Injection *(U.S.P.).* A sterile solution in an aqueous solution of macrogols. When diluted with 4 volumes of water, the injection has a pH of 4 to 7.

Proprietary Names and Manufacturers
Mylaxen *(Wallace, USA).*

12842-t

Idrocilamide *(rINN).*
LCB-29. *N*-(2-Hydroxyethyl)cinnamamide.
$C_{11}H_{13}NO_2$=191.2.

CAS — 6961-46-2.

Adverse Effects
Idrocilamide is reported to produce abdominal pain, nausea, and drowsiness. Excitement, euphoria and hallucinations, and mental depression may occur.

Precautions
Idrocilamide is contra-indicated in patients with a history of peptic ulcer. It may cause drowsiness: patients so affected should not drive or operate machinery.
Idrocilamide is stated to inhibit the metabolism of caffeine.

Uses and Administration
Idrocilamide is a central muscle relaxant that is used in the symptomatic treatment of musculoskeletal conditions associated with painful muscle spasm. It has been given in initial doses of 200 mg three times daily after meals, gradually increased, according to response, to a maximum of 1.2 to 1.6 g daily in divided doses. It has also been given by intramuscular injection.

Proprietary Names and Manufacturers
Brolitène *(Médicia, Fr.)*; Srilane *(Médicia, Fr.)*; Talval *(Lipha, Switz.).*

12923-x

Meladrazine *(BAN, rINN).*
Ba-13155 *(tartrate)*; Hydramitrazine. NNN′N′-Tetraethyl-6-hydrazinotriazin-2,4-diyldiamine.
$C_{11}H_{23}N_7$=253.4.

CAS — 13957-36-3; 20423-87-4 (tartrate).

Meladrazine is a central muscle relaxant that was formerly given as the tartrate.

Proprietary Names and Manufacturers
Lisidonil *(Ciba, Denm.; Ciba, Norw.).*

5722-t

Mephenesin *(BAN, rINN).*
Cresoxydiol; Glykresin. 3-(*o*-Tolyloxy)propane-1,2-diol.
$C_{10}H_{14}O_3$=182.2.

CAS — 59-47-2.

Pharmacopoeias. In *Braz., Ind.,* and *It.* Also in *B.P.C. 1973*

White, odourless or almost odourless, crystals or crystalline aggregates. M.p. 70° to 73°.
Soluble 1 in 100 of water, 1 in 8 of alcohol, 1 in 12 of chloroform, and 1 in 7 of propylene glycol. Solutions are **sterilised** by autoclaving or by filtration.

Adverse Effects
Given by mouth, mephenesin may produce lassitude, anorexia, nausea, and vomiting. Allergic reactions may occur. Overdosage may produce nystagmus, blurred vision, and motor incoordination; in gross overdosage there may be hypotonia, a fall in blood pressure and respiratory paralysis.
Intravenous administration of alcoholic solutions of mephenesin may be associated with intravascular haemolysis, haemoglobinuria, and anuria. Local thrombosis may also occur at the site of injection.

In 4 women and 2 men, the colour of the hair changed from brunette to blonde during the first 3 to 4 months of treatment with mephenesin up to 10 to 12 g daily. Normal hair colour was restored about 3 months after withdrawal of the drug.— J. D. Spillane, *Br. med. J.,* 1963, *1,* 997.

Precautions
Mephenesin may enhance the effects of barbiturates and opioids. It may cause drowsiness: patients so affected should not drive or operate machinery.

PORPHYRIA. Mephenesin was considered to be unsafe in patients with acute porphyria because it has been shown to be porphyrinogenic in *animals* or *in vitro* systems.— M.R. Moore and K.E.L. McColl, *Porphyrias, Drug Lists,* Glasgow, Porphyria Research Unit, University of Glasgow, 1987.

Absorption and Fate
Mephenesin is readily absorbed from the gastro-intestinal tract and distributed throughout most tissues of the body. It is mainly metabolised in the liver and excreted in urine as metabolites and a small amount of unchanged drug.

Uses and Administration
Mephenesin is a centrally acting muscle relaxant believed to act primarily at spinal cord level although supraspinal effects may contribute to its action.
Mephenesin is used for the symptomatic treatment of musculoskeletal conditions associated with painful muscle spasm; however, its clinical usefulness is considered to be limited by its brief duration of action. It has been given by mouth in doses of 0.5 to 1 g one to six times daily, preferably after food.
Mephenesin was formerly also given by the intramuscular or intravenous routes.
The carbamate has been used similarly, and has been stated to have a longer duration of action than the parent compound.

Proprietary Names and Manufacturers
Decontractyl *(Synthelabo, Belg.; Robert et Carrière, Fr.; Robert et Carrière, Switz.)*; Myanesin *(Duncan, Flockhart, UK)*; Relaxar *(Bouty, Ital.)*; Rhex *(Hobein, Ger.).*

The following names have been used for multi-ingredient preparations containing mephenesin—Decontractyl-Baume *(Anglo-French Laboratories, Canad.)*; Menopax Forte *(Nicholas, UK)*; Neo-Zoline-M *(Neolab, Canad.)*; Salimed Compound *(Medo, UK).*

5724-r

Metaxalone *(BAN, USAN, rINN).*
AHR-438. 5-(3,5-Xylyloxymethyl)oxazolidin-2-one.
$C_{12}H_{15}NO_3$=221.3.

CAS — 1665-48-1.

Adverse Effects, Treatment, and Precautions
As for Chlorzoxazone, p.1231.
Patients taking metaxalone excrete in the urine a metabolite which gives a false positive reaction to copper sulphate-based tests for glycosuria.

Uses and Administration
Metaxalone is used for the symptomatic treatment of musculoskeletal conditions associated with painful muscle spasm; its mode of action is not fully understood. The usual dose is 800 mg three or four times daily.

Proprietary Names and Manufacturers
Skelaxin *(Robins, Canad.; Carnrick, USA).*

5725-f

Methocarbamol *(BAN, USAN, rINN).*

Guaiphenesin Carbamate. 2-Hydroxy-3-(2-methoxyphenoxy)propyl carbamate.
$C_{11}H_{15}NO_5$=241.2.

CAS — 532-03-6.

Pharmacopoeias. In *Port.* and *U.S.*

A white powder, odourless or with a slight characteristic odour. M.p. about 94° or, if previously ground to a fine powder, about 90°. **Soluble** 1 in 40 of water; sparingly soluble in chloroform; soluble in alcohol only with heating; practically insoluble in *n*-hexane. The *U.S.P.* injection has a pH of 3.5 to 6.0. **Store** in airtight containers.

Adverse Effects
Side-effects reported with methocarbamol include nausea, lightheadedness, dizziness, drowsiness, blurred vision, fever, headache, and allergic reactions including rashes.
After injection patients may experience flushing, and a metallic taste; incoordination, vertigo, syncope, hypotension, bradycardia, and anaphylaxis have been reported. There may be sloughing and thrombophlebitis due to extravasation at the site of injection.
Convulsions have occurred rarely.

Precautions
Methocarbamol is contra-indicated in hypersensitive patients, in coma or pre-coma states, brain damage, myasthenia gravis, or in patients with a history of epilepsy. It may impair concentration: patients so affected should not drive or operate machinery. The CNS effects of methocarbamol may be potentiated by concomitant administration of other CNS depressants such as alcohol. Methocarbamol has also been stated to potentiate the effects of anorectics, antimuscarinics, and some psychotropic agents.
Preparations for injection may contain, as a solvent, a macrogol which could increase existing acidosis and urea retention in patients with renal impairment; such preparations should not be used in patients with known or suspected renal disease.

Methocarbamol could cause discoloration of the urine, which became brown to black or green on standing.— R. B. Baran and B. Rowles, *J. Am. pharm. Ass.,* 1973, *NS13,* 139.

Methocarbomol could produce false-positive results in tests for raised urinary 5-hydroxyindoleacetic acid (5-HIAA) concentrations, intended to diagnose carcinoid syndrome:— B. Clarke and H. J. F. Hodgson, *Br. J. Hosp. Med.,* 1986, *35,* 146.

Absorption and Fate
Methocarbamol is rapidly absorbed from the gastro-intestinal tract following oral administration. It is metabolised, probably in the liver, and excreted in urine primarily as the glucuronide and sulphate conjugates of its metabolites. A small amount is excreted in faeces.

Uses and Administration
Methocarbamol is a muscle relaxant whose mode of action is not established; it may be due to general depressant effects on the CNS. Its effects occur within about half an hour of a dose by mouth.
Methocarbamol is used in the symptomatic treatment of musculoskeletal conditions associated with painful muscle spasm. The usual initial dose is 1.5 g four times daily later reduced to a maintenance dose of about 4 g daily. If necessary it may be given by injection in doses of 1 g; up to 5 mL of a 10% solution (500 mg) may be given intramuscularly into each gluteal region. It may also be given intravenously at a rate of not more than 3 mL per minute, or by infusion in sodium chloride or glucose injection. The parenteral dose should not exceed 3 g daily for 3 days. The patient should remain lying down during, and for 10 minutes after, intravenous administration. Extravasation should be avoided.
As an adjunct in the management of tetanus, methocarbamol has been given in doses of 1 to 2 g by direct intravenous injection, supplemented by intravenous infusion up to a total dose of 3 g; doses may be repeated every 6 hours until oral therapy becomes possible. Doses of 15 mg per kg body-weight have been given in the management of tetanus in children.

SPIDER BITE (ARACHNIDISM). Methocarbamol was used in latrodectism to produce muscle relaxation and to relieve pain, nausea, and respiratory distress.— W. P. Horen, *Clin. Med.,* 1966, *73* (Aug.), 41.

Preparations
Methocarbamol Injection *(U.S.P.).* A sterile solution of methocarbamol in an aqueous solution of macrogol 300.
Methocarbamol Tablets *(U.S.P.)*

Proprietary Preparations
Robaxin *(Robins, UK). Tablets* (Robaxin-750), scored, methocarbamol 750 mg.
Injection, methocarbamol 100 mg/mL, in a vehicle containing 50% aqueous macrogol 300, in ampoules of 10 mL.
Robaxisal Forte *(Robins, UK). Tablets,* methocarbamol 400 mg, aspirin 325 mg.

Proprietary Names and Manufacturers
Delaxin *(Ferndale, USA)*; Lumirelax *(Gallier, Fr.)*; Methocabal *(Jpn)*; Miowas *(IFI, Ital.; Wasserman, Spain)*; Relax Llano *(Llano, Spain)*; Robamol *(USA)*; Robaxin *(Arg.; Robins, Austral.; Robins, Canad.; Denm.; Neth.; Norw.; Continental Ethicals, S.Afr.; Lasa, Spain; Robins, Swed.; Robins, Switz.; Robins, UK; Robins,*

USA); Traumacut *(Brenner, Ger.)*; Tresortil *(GEA, Denm.)*.

The following names have been used for multi-ingredient preparations containing methocarbamol— Robaxacet *(Robins, Canad.)*; Robaxisal *(Robins, Canad.*; *Robins, USA)*; Robaxisal-C *(Robins, Canad.)*; Robaxisal-Forte *(Robins, UK)*.

5726-d

Metocurine Iodide *(USAN)*.

Dimethyl Tubocurarine Iodide; Dimethyltubocurarine Iodide; (+)-*O,O'*-Dimethylchondrocurarine Di-iodide. (+)-6,6',7',12'-Tetramethoxy-2,2,2',2'-tetramethyltubocuraranium di-iodide.

$C_{40}H_{48}I_2N_2O_6$=906.6.

CAS — 5152-30-7 (metocurine); 7601-55-0 (iodide).

NOTE. The name dimethyltubocurarine iodide was based on the old empirical formula for tubocurarine (see p.1240).

Pharmacopoeias. In *U.S.*

A white to pale yellow crystalline powder. **Soluble** 1 in 400 of water and 1 in 10 000 of alcohol, chloroform, and of ether; slightly soluble in dilute acids and alkalis. **Store** in airtight containers.

INCOMPATIBILITY. Metocurine iodide is unstable in alkaline solutions and when combined with barbiturate solutions precipitation may occur. Solutions of barbiturates, pethidine, or morphine sulphate should not be administered in the same syringe with metocurine.

Adverse Effects, Treatment, and Precautions

As for Tubocurarine Chloride, p.1241.

Metocurine iodide has been reported to have a smaller histamine-releasing effect than tubocurarine chloride but may produce allergic reactions in patients sensitive to iodine.

ALLERGY. For results suggesting that administration of metocurine to patients sensitive to other neuromuscular blocking drugs might result in an adverse reaction, see Adverse Effects under Atracurium Besylate, p.1229.

Absorption and fate

Following intravenous administration metocurine is rapidly distributed, and largely excreted unchanged in urine; a small amount is excreted in bile. It crosses the placenta.

PREGNANCY AND THE NEONATE. In 18 women undergoing caesarean section the concentration of metocurine in the umbilical vein compared with that in the maternal vein was 4, 7, 12, and 12% when metocurine was given, 2, 4, 6, and 10 minutes before delivery. It might be wise to avoid metocurine if the foetus was at risk.— I. Kivalo and S. Saarikoski, *Br. J. Anaesth.*, 1976, *48*, 239.

Uses and Administration

Metocurine iodide is a competitive (non-depolarising) muscle relaxant with actions and uses similar to those of tubocurarine chloride (see p.1241) but is about twice as potent. Following a single dose muscle relaxation is maintained for 25 to 90 minutes.

The initial dose of metocurine iodide is usually 100 to 300 µg per kg body-weight by intravenous injection over 1 minute, and further doses of 0.5 to 1 mg may be given as required. For muscle relaxation during electroconvulsive therapy average doses totalling 2 to 3 mg have been employed.

The standard doses of metocurine may need to be reduced when given with potent inhalation anaesthetics which can potentiate its competitive neuromuscular blocking action.

ADMINISTRATION. In 15 patients undergoing surgery a dose of metocurine 300 µg per kg body-weight was necessary for consistent and adequate surgical relaxation. The effect was prolonged, more than 3 hours being needed for 50% recovery. Heart-rate and blood pressure were unchanged.— R. Hughes *et al.*, *Br. J. Anaesth.*, 1976, *48*, 969.

In renal failure. A study involving 5 patients with renal failure undergoing transplantation showed that the mean elimination half-life of metocurine was 11.4 hours, compared to 6.0 hours in 5 normal subjects and plasma clearance was significantly reduced. However, the serum concentration required to produce 90% blockade was significantly elevated in patients with renal failure. There was considerable variation in the duration of neuromuscular blockade in patients with renal failure, one remaining well relaxed for 6 hours while one was well relaxed for only 10 minutes. If patients with renal failure are given metocurine, monitoring is imperative to ensure adequate relaxation without overdosage.— W. P. Brotherton and R. S. Matteo, *Anesthesiology*, 1981, *55*, 273.

Preparations

Metocurine Iodide Injection *(U.S.P.)*. A sterile solution in isotonic sodium chloride solution.

Proprietary Names and Manufacturers

Metubine *(Lilly, Canad.*; *Lilly, USA)*.

5727-n

Pancuronium Bromide *(BAN, USAN, rINN)*.

NA-97; Org-NA-97. 1,1'-(3α,17β-Diacetoxy-5α-androstan-2β,16β-ylene)bis(1-methylpiperidinium) dibromide.

$C_{35}H_{60}Br_2N_2O_4$=732.7.

CAS — 15500-66-0.

Pharmacopoeias. In *Br.*

White or almost white, odourless, hygroscopic crystals or crystalline powder. **Soluble** 1 in 1 of water, 1 in 5 of alcohol and chloroform, 1 in 4 of dichloromethane, and 1 in 1 of methyl alcohol; practically insoluble in ether. The *B.P.* injection is **sterilised** by filtration and has a pH of 3.8 to 4.2. **Store** at 2° to 8° in well-closed containers.

Pancuronium bromide injection did not produce a visible precipitate when mixed in a syringe with thiopentone, methohexitone, propanidid, suxamethonium, pethidine, papaveretum, neostigmine, gallamine, tubocurarine, alcuronium, hydrocortisone, or promethazine.— D. Komesaroff and J. E. Field, *Med. J. Aust.*, 1969, *1*, 908.

Commercially formulated pancuronium bromide injection was reportedly stable for 6 months at room temperature (15° to 30°).— F. R. Vogenberg and P. F. Souney, *Am. J. Hosp. Pharm.*, 1983, *40*, 101.

Adverse Effects and Treatment

As for Tubocurarine Chloride, p.1241.

Tachycardia, and a slight elevation of blood pressure, may occur with pancuronium. It has a smaller histamine-releasing effect than tubocurarine chloride. Local reactions at the site of injection have been reported.

Following administration of pancuronium bromide 100 or 150 µg per kg body-weight intravenously to 100 infants, side-effects included excessive oral, pharyngeal, and tracheal secretions within 2 minutes of administration, and severe sweating in some patients.— E. J. Bennett *et al.*, *Anesth. Analg. curr. Res.*, 1971, *50*, 798.

ALLERGY. Bronchospasm, pulmonary oedema, hypotension, bradycardia, cyanosis, and hypoxaemia occurred in a 57-year-old man given thiopentone and pancuronium bromide and recurred after a second injection of pancuronium several hours later. He had received pancuronium 6 weeks previously and a skin test was positive.— F. S. Brauer and C. R. Ananthanarayan, *Anesthesiology*, 1978, *49*, 434. See also: R. W. Buckland and A. F. Avery, *Br. J. Anaesth.*, 1973, *45*, 518; D. G. Tweedie and P. M. Ordish (letter), *ibid.*, 1974, *46*, 244; S. Mishima and T. Yamamura, *Anesth. Analg.*, 1984, *63*, 865; C. Conil *et al.*, *Annls fr. Anesth. Réanim.*, 1985, *4*, 241.

EFFECTS ON BODY TEMPERATURE. A report of malignant hyperpyrexia occurring in conjunction with the use of pancuronium.— P. M. Waterman *et al.*, *Anesth. Analg.*, 1980, *59*, 220.

EFFECTS ON THE HEART AND BLOOD PRESSURE. Pancuronium 20 to 80 µg per kg body-weight induced tachycardia in patients receiving balanced anaesthesia. Tachycardia was more pronounced when droperidol was also given.— P. Parmentier and P. Dagnelie, *Br. J. Anaesth.*, 1979, *51*, 157.

Hypotension. A report of significant falls in blood pressure in a premature neonate given pancuronium in doses of 50 µg to aid assisted ventilation. If an infant has only a marginally adequate circulating volume the abolition of muscular activity will cause a fall in venous return and cardiac output with a fall in blood pressure.— N. McIntosh (letter), *Lancet*, 1985, *2*, 279.

EFFECTS ON THE JOINTS. Severe joint contractures developed in 3 of 13 newborn infants after neuromuscular blockade with pancuronium bromide in intermittent doses of 100 µg per kg body-weight as needed. A full range of movements had not returned by the age of 2 to 3 months. One infant was born prematurely with joint contractures that became more extensive. The 2 mature infants were both given gentamicin and phenobarbitone which may have potentiated the effect of pancuronium.— S. K. Sinha and M. I. Levene, *Archs Dis. Childh.*, 1984, *59*, 73. Comment. Over the past 3 years none of 85 infants paralysed during ventilation had developed contractures despite the use of the same dosage regimen and, in many cases, simultaneous administration of gentamicin.— A. Greenough (letter), *ibid.*, 390.

Precautions

As for Tubocurarine Chloride, p.1241. Pancuronium should be used with care in patients with raised catecholamine concentrations, including those receiving tricyclic antidepressants, in whom it may result in cardiovascular side-effects, particularly when given in association with halothane.

INTERACTIONS. *Corticosteroids.* Partial recovery from pancuronium neuromuscular blockade after corticosteroids.— E. F. Meyers, *Anesthesiology*, 1977, *46*, 148; M. J. Laflin, *Anesthesiology*, 1977, *47*, 471.

Lithium. Prolonged neuromuscular blockade had been reported in a patient given pancuronium bromide while taking lithium carbonate, and had been confirmed in *dogs*.— J. W. Jefferson (letter), *Ann. intern. Med.*, 1978, *88*, 577.

Neuromuscular blockers. While tubocurarine antagonised the onset and duration of suxamethonium block, pancuronium antagonised its onset but prolonged its duration.— A. D. Ivankovich *et al.*, *Can. Anaesth. Soc. J.*, 1977, *24*, 228.

In a study of the interactions between pancuronium bromide and vecuronium it was shown that after an initial dose of pancuronium the maintenance dose requirements for either pancuronium itself or vecuronium were less than those required when the initial dose was of vecuronium, and the duration of blockade was longer. Conversely, when vecuronium was given initially, maintenance dose requirements were increased and duration of blockade decreased. Anaesthetists should be aware that interactions between competitive muscle relaxants depend not only on the specific drugs but the sequence in which they are given.— O. M. Rashkovsky *et al.*, *Br. J. Anaesth.*, 1985, *57*, 1063.

Parasympathomimetics. In 54 healthy patients undergoing minor surgery the frequency of bradycardia during antagonism of neuromuscular blockade with neostigmine was greater in patients given pancuronium than in those who had received alcuronium. There was no significant difference in patients given tubocurarine or pancuronium.— J. Heinonen and O. Takkunen, *Br. J. Anaesth.*, 1977, *49*, 1109.

Tricyclic antidepressants. Ventricular tachycardia occurred in 2 patients given pancuronium bromide while taking tricyclic antidepressants. The effect was reproduced experimentally in 4 of 10 *dogs*.— M. F. Roizen and T. W. Feeley, *Ann. intern. Med.*, 1978, *88*, 64.

PREGNANCY AND THE NEONATE. Following administration of pancuronium 40 µg per kg body-weight to induce paralysis, 4 infants developed an alarming fall in transcutaneous oxygen tension, although ventilatory support had been adequate beforehand. Patients undergoing paralysis to improve oxygenation might experience significant and potentially injurious hypoxaemia.— J. B. Philips *et al.* (letter), *Lancet*, 1979, *1*, 877.

Radiography in a neonate paralysed with pancuronium for assisted ventilation suggested an almost completely gas-free abdomen; a previous radiograph had been normal. Although babies paralysed with pancuronium cannot swallow, the relative absence of autonomic blocking activity allows peristalsis to continue and evacuate much of the gas present at the onset of drug therapy. The benign nature of this finding needs to be appreciated with the increasing use of pancuronium in neonatal ventilation.— S. Thomas *et al.* (letter), *Lancet*,

1984, *2*, 870.

For a warning of the possibility of hypotension in infants paralysed for ventilatory management see under Adverse Effects.

Absorption and Fate

Following intravenous injection pancuronium is rapidly redistributed into body tissues. It is partially metabolised in the liver and is excreted in urine as unchanged drug and metabolites. Some is also excreted in bile. Small amounts of pancuronium cross the placenta.

The clinical pharmacokinetics of pancuronium bromide.— L. B. Wingard and D. R. Cook, *Clin. Pharmacokinet.*, 1977, *2*, 330.

A pharmacodynamic model for pancuronium.— C. J. Hull *et al.*, *Br. J. Anaesth.*, 1978, *50*, 1113.

For a study of the pharmacokinetics and pharmacodynamics of pancuronium and vecuronium in anaesthetised patients, see under Vecuronium Bromide, p.1242.

PREGNANCY AND THE NEONATE. In 15 patients undergoing caesarean section given pancuronium bromide 100 µg per kg body-weight intravenously with other agents, mean maternal arterial and umbilical venous serum concentrations of pancuronium bromide and metabolites were 520 and 120 ng per mL respectively at delivery (mean of 13 minutes after injection).— L. B. Wingard, *J. pharm. Sci.*, 1979, *68*, 914.

See also: A. J. Cummings, *Clin. Pharmacokinet.*, 1983, *8*, 344.

Uses and Administration

Pancuronium bromide is a competitive (nondepolarising) muscle relaxant with effects similar to those of tubocurarine chloride (p.1241). Muscle relaxation commences within about 1 to 3 minutes of intravenous administration and lasts for about 45 minutes.

Pancuronium bromide is used mainly as an adjuvant to anaesthesia to obtain greater muscular relaxation in surgical operations and in the management of patients on assisted ventilation. The initial dose is usually 40 to 100 µg per kg body-weight by intravenous injection, with supplementary doses of 10 to 20 µg per kg. Children may be given similar doses. Doses of 30 to 40 µg per kg initially have been suggested in neonates, with supplementary doses of up to 20 µg per kg; in the *USA*, dosage based on an initial test dose of 20 µg per kg has been advocated. Patients under intensive care including those with intractable status asthmaticus or tetanus may be given 60 µg per kg intravenously every 1 to 1½ hours or 30 to 60 µg per kg intramuscularly every 1 to 2 hours.

The standard doses of pancuronium bromide may need to be reduced when given with potent inhalation anaesthetics which can potentiate its neuromuscular blocking action. A reduction in dosage is also recommended when pancuronium is given following administration of suxamethonium: initial doses of 20 to 60 µg per kg have been suggested.

A study *in vitro* of serum from 14 subjects, aged 4 to 60 years, with normal reactions to suxamethonium demonstrated that pancuronium caused a powerful and highly selective inhibition of serum cholinesterase. The inhibition was reversible and competitive. Serum-cholinesterase activity decreased by about 60% three minutes after injection of pancuronium 100 µg per kg body-weight in 4 subjects. There was still a 40% depression 45 minutes after injection.— J. Stovner *et al.*, *Br. J. Anaesth.*, 1975, *47*, 949.

ADMINISTRATION. An intravenous bolus injection and concomitant infusion of pancuronium was proposed for use in prolonged anaesthesia. Doses were calculated using pharmacokinetic principles to achieve a plasma concentration of 200 ng per mL which it was considered would provide adequate relaxation. Pancuronium, at an initial intravenous bolus dose of about 62.5 µg per kg body-weight was given to 16 surgical patients with constant infusion at about 350 ng per kg per minute as a solution containing 5 mg in 100 mL of sodium chloride injection. The regimen generally produced and maintained a predictable plasma concentration of pancuronium but monitoring of neuromuscular transmission was necessary to detect the excessive or inadequate dosage which might occur in some patients.— A. A. Somogyi *et al.*, *Br. J. Anaesth.*, 1978, *50*, 575.

In old people. Results of a study of the effects of ageing on the pharmacokinetics of pancuronium suggested that as patients aged the rate of decline of the plasma concentration of pancuronium following a single intravenous dose decreased, so that an increase in recovery time would be expected. However, the study did not support the concept that elderly patients have reduced distribution volumes and therefore require smaller doses of drug to achieve the desired effect.— K. McLeod *et al.*, *Br. J. Anaesth.*, 1979, *51*, 435.

In liver disease. A study in 32 patients with chronic liver disease who underwent surgery concluded that pancuronium bromide could be substituted safely for tubocurarine. All patients exhibited pancuronium 'resistance' and required a mean total dose of 14.9 mg. Reversal effect was difficult in 2 patients with severe obstructive jaundice.— M. E. Ward *et al.*, *Br. J. Anaesth.*, 1975, *47*, 1199.

A study of the pharmacokinetics of pancuronium in 14 cirrhotic patients and 12 controls indicated that a prolonged duration of action of pancuronium could be expected in patients with cirrhosis of the liver. However, the increased distribution volume in these patients might necessitate a higher initial dose although the rate of disappearance of pancuronium from plasma would be slower than in patients without liver disease.— P. Duvaldestin *et al.*, *Br. J. Anaesth.*, 1978, *50*, 1131.

In renal failure. Pancuronium could be given in usual doses to patients with a glomerular filtration-rate (GFR) above 10 mL per minute; its use should be avoided in those with a GFR of less than 10 mL per minute; recurarisation might occur up to 24 hours after administration.— W. M. Bennett *et al.*, *Am. J. Kidney Dis.*, 1983, *3*, 155.

ASTHMA. Pancuronium bromide was a useful neuromuscular blocking agent in the treatment of medically irreversible status asthmaticus.— N. Levin and J. B. Dillon, *J. Am. med. Ass.*, 1972, *222*, 1265.

HYPERPYREXIA. Halothane-induced contracture of muscle strips from patients susceptible to malignant hyperpyrexia was inhibited by methylprednisolone and pancuronium in concentrations equivalent to doses of 495 and 990 mg and 6 and 12 mg respectively. It was considered that pancuronium could be used cautiously in susceptible patients.— P. A. Cain and F. R. Ellis, *Br. J. Anaesth.*, 1977, *49*, 941. But see under Adverse Effects.

PREGNANCY AND THE NEONATE. Pancuronium bromide was a safe and well-tolerated muscle relaxant for anaesthesia in 25 neonates. It was 9 times as potent as tubocurarine at birth and 6 times as potent at 1 month old. Recommended intravenous doses of pancuronium were 30 µg per kg body-weight up to 1 week old, 60 µg per kg at 1 to 2 weeks, and 90 µg per kg at 2 to 4 weeks. Doses were reduced in prematurity, acidosis, hypothermia, and during antibiotic therapy, especially with kanamycin and gentamicin, when increased sensitivity was observed. Neuromuscular block was reversed with atropine 18 µg per kg body-weight and neostigmine 80 µg per kg intravenously.— E. J. Bennett *et al.*, *Br. J. Anaesth.*, 1975, *47*, 75.

Respiratory distress syndrome. There was no significant difference in the incidence of pneumothorax and interstitial emphysema in 24 neonates with hyaline membrane disease who were given pancuronium, in doses of 30 µg per kg body-weight intravenously as required, and 26 similar controls, during mechanical ventilation. However, there was a marked difference in the length of time that added oxygen was required: at 30 days of age all the surviving treated infants were breathing air, but 7 control infants were still oxygen-dependent.— M. J. Pollitzer *et al.*, *Lancet*, 1981, *1*, 346. Pneumothorax developed in only 1 of 11 preterm infants with respiratory distress syndrome who were paralysed with pancuronium 100 µg per kg body-weight every 2 hours, preventing them from actively expiring against ventilator inflation; all of 11 unparalysed controls who similarly expired against artificial ventilation developed pneumothoraces. In 34 infants not entered into the study because they were not breathing against the ventilator no pneumothoraces developed.— A. Greenough *et al.*, *Lancet*, 1984, *1*, 1. Pancuronium paralysis had had no significant effect on frequency of pneumothorax, survival, or intraventricular haemorrhage in ventilated infants below 26 weeks of gestation considered to be at risk. In those of 27 to 32 weeks' gestation the frequency of pneumothorax fell significantly, but there was no change in the incidence of intraventricular haemorrhage, and the reduction in mortality was not significant.— R. W. I. Cooke and J. M. Rennie (letter), *ibid.*, 286.

Muscle paralysis with pancuronium bromide 100 µg per kg body-weight intravenously in 14 of 24 preterm infants requiring ventilation for respiratory distress syndrome resulted in conversion of cerebral blood-flow velocity to a stable pattern from fluctuations that had been previously shown (J. M. Perlman *et al.*,*New Engl. J. Med.*, 1983, *309*, 204) to be associated with the development of intraventricular haemorrhage; paralysis was maintained until the infants were 72 hours old and only one suffered intraventricular haemorrhage during this time. All of the 10 infants with fluctuating cerebral blood-flow velocity who did not receive pancuronium developed intraventricular haemorrhage. Following cessation of paralysis 4 of the infants who had received pancuronium developed intraventricular haemorrhage but in 2 cases this was associated with other disorders; severity of haemorrhage was less in these 4 than in the 10 controls and outcome not so poor.— J. M. Perlman *et al.*, *New Engl. J. Med.*, 1985, *312*, 1353. Comment.— L. R. Ment, *ibid.*, 1385. A similar trial involving infants with gestational ages as low as 26 weeks had had to be abandoned because of serious derangements of fluid balance, oedema and fatal renal failure in 2 very immature infants given pancuronium. Pancuronium might be hazardous in the least mature infants and this strategy could conceivably increase the risk of hypoxic-ischaemic damage to the brain.— E. O. R. Reynolds *et al.* (letter), *ibid.*, *313*, 955. Reply. The procedure requires caution and should only be used in carefully selected high-risk patients, but there is only anecdotal evidence of an increased risk of hypoxic-ischaemic damage to the brain with pancuronium.— J. M. Perlman and J. J. Volpe (letter), *ibid.*, 956.

Discussion of mechanical ventilation of the newborn. Pancuronium should be used with caution, and only when sufficient staff and equipment are availabe for close monitoring of clinical state, respiratory pattern, and blood pressure.— W. Tarnow-Mordi and A. Wilkinson, *Br. med. J.*, 1986, *292*, 575. See also: *Lancet*, 1984, *1*, 831.

SNAKE BITE. The use of pancuronium, in association with diazepam and antivenom, in the management of painful muscular spasms with opisthotonus following sea-snake envenomation.— G. J. Dobb (letter), *Med. J. Aust.*, 1986, *144*, 112.

Preparations

Pancuronium Injection *(B.P.)*. Contains pancuronium bromide in sodium chloride injection. Store at 2° to 8°.

Proprietary Preparations

Pavulon *(Organon Teknika, UK)*. *Injection*, pancuronium bromide 2 mg/mL in ampoules of 2 mL.

Proprietary Names and Manufacturers

Pavulon *(Arg.; Organon, Austral.; Organon, Canad.; Organon, Denm.; Organon, Fr.; Ravasini, Ital.; Neth.; Organon, Norw.; Organon, S.Afr.; Organon, Spain; Organon, Swed.; Organon Teknika, Switz.; Organon Teknika, UK; Organon, USA)*.

5729-m

Pridinol Mesylate

C-238 *(pridinol)*; Pridinol Mesilate *(rINNM)*. 1,1-Diphenyl-3-piperidinopropan-1-ol methanesulphonate.

$C_{20}H_{25}NO,CH_3SO_3H$=391.5.

CAS — 511-45-5 (pridinol); 968-58-1 (hydrochloride); 6856-31-1 (mesylate).

Pridinol mesylate has been used in the symptomatic treatment of muscle spasm.

The hydrochloride has been used in the management of parkinsonism.

Proprietary Names and Manufacturers

Hikicenon *(Jpn)*; Loxeen *(Jpn)*; Lyseen *(Exa, Arg.; CCP, Belg.; Hommel, Ger.; Zyma, Ital.; Zyma, Switz.)*; Mitanoline *(Jpn)*; Nonpressin *(Jpn)*; Parks *(Hommel, Ger.; Hommel, Switz.)*; Tirashizin *(Jpn)*; Trilax *(Jpn)*.

5730-t

Styramate *(BAN, rINN)*.

β-Hydroxyphenethyl carbamate.

$C_9H_{11}NO_3$=181.2.

CAS — 94-35-9.

Styramate is a centrally acting muscle relaxant that has been used in the symptomatic treatment of musculoskeletal conditions associated with painful muscle spasm, in usual doses of 400 mg four times daily.

Proprietary Names and Manufacturers
Sinaxar *(Fawns & McAllan, Austral.; Christiaens, Belg.; Armour, Denm.; Armour, S.Afr.; Armour, UK).*

5731-x

Suxamethonium Bromide *(BAN).*

Choline Bromide Succinate; Succinylcholine Bromide; Suxameth. Brom. 2,2′-Succinyldioxybis(ethyltrimethylammonium) dibromide dihydrate.
$C_{14}H_{30}Br_2N_2O_4,2H_2O$=486.2.

CAS — 306-40-1 (suxamethonium); 55-94-7 (bromide).

Pharmacopoeias. In *Br.*

A white or creamy-white hygroscopic, odourless or almost odourless powder. Suxamethonium 1 mg (1 mg cation) is equivalent to 1.67 mg of suxamethonium bromide dihydrate and to 1.55 mg of anhydrous suxamethonium bromide.
Soluble 1 in 0.3 of water and 1 in 5 of alcohol; practically insoluble in chloroform and ether. Solutions deteriorate on storage and should be used immediately after preparation. It is rapidly hydrolysed by alkalis and therefore should not be mixed with alkaline injections such as thiopentone sodium. **Protect** from light.

5732-r

Suxamethonium Chloride *(BAN, pINN).*

Choline Chloride Succinate; Succicurarium Chloride; Succinylcholine Chloride *(USAN)*; Suxameth. Chlor.; Suxamethonii Chloridum; Suxametonklorid. 2,2′-Succinyldioxybis(ethyltrimethylammonium) dichloride dihydrate.
$C_{14}H_{30}Cl_2N_2O_4,2H_2O$=397.3.

CAS — 71-27-2 (anhydrous); 6101-15-1 (dihydrate); 541-19-5 (suxamethonium iodide).

Pharmacopoeias. In *Aust., Br., Braz., Chin., Egypt., Eur., Fr., Ger., Ind., Int., It., Jpn, Jug., Neth., Nord., Pol., Roum., Swiss, Turk.,* and *U.S. Braz.* has the dihydrate or anhydrous salt; *Arg.* has the anhydrous salt. *Cz., Pol.,* and *Rus.* include the iodide.

A white or almost white, odourless or almost odourless, hygroscopic, crystalline powder. Suxamethonium 1 mg (1 mg cation) is equivalent to 1.37 mg of suxamethonium chloride dihydrate and to 1.24 mg of anhydrous suxamethonium chloride.
Soluble 1 in 1 of water and 1 in 350 of alcohol; practically insoluble in chloroform and ether. The *B.P.* injection has a pH of 3.0 to 5.0 and is **sterilised** by autoclaving. The *U.S.P.* injection has a pH of 3.0 to 4.5. It is rapidly destroyed by alkalis and therefore should not be mixed with alkaline injections such as thiopentone sodium. **Store** in well-closed containers. Protect from light.

STABILITY. A study of the loss of potency of suxamethonium chloride 20 mg per mL in water indicated that decomposition occurred at a considerably higher rate at 40° than at 25° and that the pH range of maximum stability was 3.75 to 4.50 for unbuffered solutions. Assuming the usual conditions of manufacturing, transit, and storage the total loss of potency was estimated to be 7% and 9% respectively for injections kept at room temperature for 4 and 6 weeks. If unbuffered suxamethonium chloride injection complying with *U.S.P.* pH limits (3.0 to 4.5) must be stored at room temperature, it should not be kept for longer than 4 weeks.— J. J. Boehm *et al., Am. J. Hosp. Pharm.,* 1984, *41,* 300. See also: B. E. Kirschenbaum and C. J. Latiolais, *ibid.,* 1976, *33,* 767.

Adverse Effects

Prolonged apnoea may occur in patients with low serum concentrations of pseudocholinesterase and in those with an atypical pseudocholinesterase. It has also been reported after high or repeated doses when a dual block (see p.1228) has occurred. Tachyphylaxis may occur with repeated doses.
Administration of suxamethonium results in transient muscle fasciculations before relaxation, which may be associated with hyperkalaemia, rhabdomyolysis, and myoglobinuria and which may produce a transient rise in intra-ocular and intra-gastric pressure. There may also be postoperative muscle pain which is sometimes severe but is not directly related to the degree of fasciculation or the dose of suxamethonium.
Administration of suxamethonium may be followed by bradycardia and hypotension, often associated with cardiac arrhythmias, and may be exacerbated by the raised plasma-potassium concentrations; cardiac arrest may occur. Tachycardia and an increase in blood pressure have also been reported.
Suxamethonium has some muscarinic actions and may cause increase in bowel movements and in salivary, bronchial, and gastric secretion. Salivary gland enlargement has occurred.
There have been hypersensitivity reactions, including rarely, bronchospasm or shock; a higher incidence of anaphylactoid reactions may be associated with the use of the iodide.
Suxamethonium administration may be implicated in the development of malignant hyperpyrexia in those patients with a genetic predisposition to the syndrome.

ALLERGY. In a study involving 158 patients who had had a systemic reaction during general anaesthesia, skin tests showed that 28 of 85 had a strong reaction to suxamethonium; 11 of 37 were sensitive to alcuronium, 15 of 54 to gallamine and 21 of 43 to tubocurarine. Sensitivity appeared more common in women than in men. Subsequent testing in 15 of the patients giving a positive skin test to suxamethonium showed that 13 were still positive after up to 4 years; 10 close relatives, and a further 60 controls who had undergone uneventful anaesthesia gave negative skin tests. Of the 13 suxamethonium-sensitive patients 10 also reacted to gallamine, 10 to tubocurarine, and 5 to alcuronium. All patients who have systemic reactions during anaesthesia should be tested for sensitivity to muscle relaxant drugs: many sensitive cases may be being missed and the reasons for their collapse under anaesthesia not appreciated.— P. R. Youngman *et al., Lancet,* 1983, *2,* 597. Comment. These results confirm previous studies on the value of skin tests, cross-sensitivity between muscle relaxants, and the release of histamine *in vitro* in some instances. The mechanism of reaction is probably IgE-mediated.— D. Vervloet (letter), *ibid.,* 1197. Detection of IgE antibodies to suxamethonium after anaphylactoid reactions during anaesthesia.— D. G. Harle, *ibid.,* 1984, *1,* 930.

A detailed review of life-threatening anaphylactoid reactions during general anaesthesia. Anaphylactoid reactions are defined as clinical manifestations mimicking anaphylactic shock, where massive histamine liberation is the primary cause of the pathophysiological events. Muscle relaxants and hypnotics are the substances most frequently responsible: suxamethonium and alcuronium appear to be the muscle relaxants most often incriminated. More and more reactions are occurring at first exposure to a muscle relaxant because of cross reaction and it is difficult to foresee and prevent such a reaction.— M. C. Laxenaire *et al., Annls fr. Anesth. Réanim.,* 1985, *4,* 30.

EFFECTS ON MUSCLE. In a study in 36 adult males undergoing elective surgery, suxamethonium was administered intravenously at 6 rates, from 0.25 mg per second to 20 mg per second. The time to the first muscle fasciculation and the total fasciculation score were related to the rate of infusion, with the slowest rate having the lowest fasciculation score and the longest latency time. Infusion rates below 2 mg per second appear to offer a clinical method of reducing fasciculations and might diminish some of the deleterious sequelae of the administration of suxamethonium.— A. Feingold and J. L. Velazquez, *Br. J. Anaesth.,* 1979, *51,* 241.

Evidence to suggest that administration of suxamethonium in divided doses reduces muscle fasciculation but does not reduce postoperative muscle pain.— D. B. Wilson and J. W. Dundee, *Anesthesiology,* 1980, *52,* 273.

Postoperative muscle pain. Suxamethonium-induced muscle pain generally, but not always appears on the first day after operation and persists 2 or 3 days, although it occasionally lasts as long as 6 days. The reported incidence of pains ranges from near zero to near 100%. It is generally accepted that early, especially immediate, ambulation after operation increases the likelihood of development of pain and its severity, and that women are more prone than men, and adults than children under the age of 10. Apart from the prior use of competitive relaxants in small doses no drug or combination of drugs has been found that consistently reduces the incidence of pain.— J. E. Riding, *Br. J. Anaesth.,* 1975, *47,* 91.

EFFECTS ON PLASMA-POTASSIUM CONCENTRATION. In 6 patients, 2 of whom died, intravenous injection of suxamethonium was followed by circulatory arrest and-or severe hyperkalaemia. Increases in serum-potassium concentrations of up to 3.6 mmol per litre occurred within a few minutes of injection. Three of the patients had severe tetanus and 2 had uraemia. It was suggested that uraemia, with increased serum-potassium concentrations, and tetanus were contra-indications for the use of suxamethonium.— F. Roth and H. Wüthrich, *Br. J. Anaesth.,* 1969, *41,* 311.

The effect of different anaesthetics on suxamethonium-induced hyperkalaemia was studied in 101 patients. Maximum increases in serum-potassium concentrations were: trichloroethylene 21.4%, chloroform 17.2%, halothane 15.1%, thiopentone 19.7%, and nitrous oxide controls 4.4%. Ten patients given tubocurarine 3 mg before induction with thiopentone and suxamethonium had a reduced maximum increase in serum potassium of 10.6%. It was concluded that hyperkalaemia was a combined effect of suxamethonium and the anaesthetic used.— V. J. Dhanaraj *et al., Br. J. Anaesth.,* 1975, *47,* 516.

Fifty-four patients undergoing surgery and 21 patients with chronic renal disease were given suxamethonium or suxethonium. Plasma-potassium concentrations rose in those given suxamethonium but not in those given suxethonium.— S. Day, *Br. J. Anaesth.,* 1976, *48,* 1011.

Treatment of Adverse Effects

Prolonged apnoea should be treated by assisted respiration with nitrous oxide and oxygen until spontaneous respiration is fully restored. Transfusion of fresh whole blood, frozen plasma, or other source of pseudocholinesterase will help the destruction of the suxamethonium. Neostigmine should not be used.
Sometimes, though not always, when the action of suxamethonium is prolonged, the neuromuscular block ceases to be depolarising in type and acquires some features of the paralysis produced by tubocurarine, (see p.1228). In these cases, assisted respiration should be continued until spontaneous respiration begins to return. A short-acting anticholinesterase such as edrophonium 10 mg may then be given intravenously. If an obvious improvement is maintained for several minutes, neostigmine, 1 to 2 mg, may be given with atropine.
A small dose of a competitive blocker such as tubocurarine 5 mg intravenously may be given before suxamethonium in order to reduce muscle fasciculations and subsequent pain; however, increased doses of suxamethonium are then required for neuromuscular blockade (see also under Precautions, below).
If malignant hyperpyrexia develops immediate cooling should be instituted, and any metabolic acidosis corrected. Respiration should be supported and dantrolene sodium may be given by rapid intravenous injection (see p.1233).

POSTOPERATIVE MUSCLE PAIN. Results in a study involving 240 patients given suxamethonium as a muscle-relaxant during thiopentone-induced anaesthesia suggested that ascorbic acid given by mouth before and after anaesthesia reduced the incidence and severity of suxamethonium-induced pain.— S. R. Gupte and N. S. Savant, *Anaesthesia,* 1971, *26,* 436. In a double-blind study in 53 patients undergoing bronchoscopy ascorbic acid 2 g daily for 2.5 days before and after examination had no effect on suxamethonium-induced pain.— J. B. Wood *et al., Anaesthesia,* 1977, *32,* 21.

Diazepam 10 mg intravenously, given 5 minutes before suxamethonium, reduced the incidence, severity and duration of suxamethonium-induced muscle pain, compared with control, in a study in 50 patients.— R. S. Verma *et al., Anesth. Analg. curr. Res.,* 1978, *57,* 295. A study indicating that pretreatment with diazepam prevented suxamethonium-induced muscle fasciculations, hyperkalaemia, increased CPK concentrations, increased heart-rate and arterial pressure, and postoperative myalgia.— N. R. Fahmy *et al.*, *Clin. Pharmac. Ther.*, 1979, *26*, 395. Diazepam 10 mg by mouth 90 minutes preoperatively was associated with a 15% incidence of suxamethonium-induced myalgia in 20 patients, compared with 50% incidence in 20 similar patients given placebo.— A. O. Davies, *Can. Anaesth. Soc. J.*, 1983, *30*, 603. For a study indicating that tubocurarine is superior to diazepam or midazolam in the prevention of suxamethonium-induced muscle pain, see p.1241.

A view that efforts to reduce the frequency of suxamethonium-induced muscle pains in patients having major abdominal operations are not justified.— J. B. Brodsky and J. Ehrenwerth, *Br. J. Anaesth.*, 1980, *52*, 215.

'Self-taming' by administration of a dose of suxamethonium 10 mg immediately after induction of anaesthesia and prior to a neuromuscular blocking dose of 1 mg per kg body-weight (as used by A. Baraka, *Anesthesiology*, 1977, *46*, 292) was employed in 25 surgical patients. This resulted in a significant decrease in plasma-potassium concentrations compared with a slight increase in 25 similar patients not given the initial dose. Despite these results, self-taming of fasciculations has been shown in other studies not to prevent postoperative muscle pain or protect against arrhythmias and the technique appears to have limited clinical applicability.— D. A. Magee and E. G. Gallagher, *Br. J. Anaesth.*, 1984, *56*, 977. Comment. Similar studies in children had shown an increase in plasma-potassium concentrations in those given 'self-taming' doses compared with controls. The difference might be age-related, or due to differences in anaesthetic used (halothane, nitrous oxide, oxygen rather than thiopentone). The multitude of proposed preventive measures and contradictory clinical studies suggest that side-effects of suxamethonium on the skeletal muscles cannot be solved by a single comprehensive method.— J. Plötz and W. Schreiber (letter), *ibid.*, 1985, *57*, 1044.

RAISED INTRA-OCULAR PRESSURE. Failure of tubocurarine or gallamine to prevent suxamethonium-induced increase in intra-ocular pressure.— E. F. Meyers *et al.*, *Anesthesiology*, 1978, *48*, 149.

Pretreatment with lignocaine 1.5 mg per kg body-weight intravenously was not found to have any effect on the rise in intra-ocular pressure following suxamethonium in patients undergoing cataract surgery but results suggested that the rise in intra-ocular pressure associated with intubation was of such magnitude as to render the suxamethonium effect unimportant; further studies should rather be aimed at preventing this intubation-associated response.— D. F. Murphy *et al.*, *Br. J. Ophthal.*, 1986, *70*, 596.

Precautions

Suxamethonium chloride is contra-indicated in patients who are burnt, severly hyperkalaemic, or known to have atypical pseudocholinesterase. Suxamethonium chloride is also contra-indicated in patients with penetrating wounds of the eye or while the globe is open, in patients with a personal or family history of malignant hyperpyrexia, in massively traumatised patients or those with extensive muscle degeneration, such as in recent paraplegia. Its use is inadvisable in patients with low serum-pseudocholinesterase concentrations such as may occur in liver disease, malnutrition, severe anaemia, and in persons exposed to organophosphorus insecticides or weedkillers. Serum-pseudocholinesterase concentrations are reduced in pregnancy and pregnant patients may show increased sensitivity. Its use is also inadvisable in patients with advanced myasthenia gravis, neurological defects, or myopathies.

It is not generally recommended in uraemic patients especially those with high serum-potassium concentrations. It should be used with caution in patients with cardiac disease. An antimuscarinic may be given before administration of suxamethonium chloride to prevent excessive bradycardia, bronchial secretion, or other muscarinic effects.

Administration of suxamethonium before or after the use of a competitive (non-depolarising) relaxant such as tubocurarine may cause a mixed block, but small doses of tubocurarine are sometimes given prior to suxamethonium to reduce muscle fasciculations and hyperkalaemia.

The effects of suxamethonium may be enhanced by some aminoglycoside or polypeptide antibiotics, some antineoplastics, beta blockers, opioid analgesics, oral contraceptives, propanidid, quinidine, and by a decreased body temperature. The depolarising effects of suxamethonium may also be enhanced by neostigmine and other anticholinesterases; it has been recommended that eye-drops containing a long-acting anticholinesterase such as ecothiopate should be discontinued several weeks before the administration of suxamethonium. Bradycardia due to suxamethonium may be enhanced by halothane or cyclopropane. The effects of cardiac glycosides may be enhanced by suxamethonium, leading to cardiac arrhythmias.

Serum-cholinesterase concentrations were similar in 52 patients with chronic renal failure, 39 similar patients undergoing peritoneal dialysis, and 64 undergoing haemodialysis. Suxamethonium 50 to 100 mg was used in 81 of 90 patients undergoing renal transplantation. Although 26 had reduced cholinesterase values no problems were encountered except in 1 patient who experienced prolonged apnoea and who was found to have atypical cholinesterase inheritance.— D. W. Ryan, *Br. J. Anaesth.*, 1977, *49*, 945.

Plasma-cholinesterase concentrations were significantly reduced in 9 patients who underwent plasmaphaeresis. Suxamethonium should be used with caution in such patients.— G. J. Wood and G. M. Hall, *Br. J. Anaesth.*, 1978, *50*, 945. See also J. Lumley, *ibid.*, 1980, *52*, 1149.

Approximately 0.04% of the population were homozygous and 4.5% heterozygous for atypical cholinesterase; such individuals might develop apnoea following administration of suxamethonium.— F. M. Williams, *Clin. Pharmacokinet.*, 1985, *10*, 392.

GASTRO-INTESTINAL DISORDERS. A study in 15 patients undergoing surgery for duodenal ulcer and 14 patients with a normal gastro-intestinal tract concluded that there was no increased tendency to regurgitate during fasciculations induced by suxamethonium. This conclusion was not valid when there was an abnormality such as hiatus hernia in the gastro-oesophageal region.— G. Smith *et al.*, *Br. J. Anaesth.*, 1978, *50*, 1137.

A 56-year-old woman with Crohn's disease had prolonged apnoea following suxamethonium administration. Pseudocholinesterase values in this patient and in 2 others with Crohn's disease were subsequently found to be low. The low concentration of pseudocholinesterase found in Crohn's disease may be due to the disease itself, malnutrition, low serum albumin, or liver involvement. The frequency is not known, but anaesthetists should consider asking for measurement of pseudocholinesterase activity in Crohn's disease patients for whom surgery is planned.— S. N. Khalil *et al.* (letter), *Lancet*, 1980, *2*, 267.

INFECTIONS. Nine patients with severe intra-abdominal infection underwent repeat surgery with the use of suxamethonium; in 4, whose infection was of at least 14 days' duration, hyperkalaemia occurred with a rise of up to 2.95 mmol per litre; no significant rise occurred in the 5 with infection of not more than 9 days' duration. Those with severe intra-abdominal or systemic infection lasting longer than 1 week should be added to categories at risk from suxamethonium which should be avoided or, if essential, preceded by a non-depolarising muscle relaxant.— B. Kohlschütter *et al.*, *Br. J. Anaesth.*, 1976, *48*, 557.

INTERACTIONS. *Antineoplastics.* Report of respiratory insufficiency and prolonged apnoea in a patient given tubocurarine and suxamethonium during anaesthesia who was also receiving cyclophosphamide; when suxamethonium was omitted, anaesthesia was uneventful. Serum pseudocholinesterase concentrations were subsequently found to be significantly depressed in this patient, and in 7 of 8 others taking cyclophosphamide.— I. R. Walker *et al.*, *Aust. N.Z. J. Med.*, 1972, *3*, 247.

Studies *in vitro* of the effects of cytotoxic agents on serum pseudocholinisterase. Of those studied, only the alkylating agents possessed significant anticholinesterase effects; tretamine was the most potent, followed by cyclophosphamide, mustine, and thiotepa. The dose of suxamethonium should be reduced in patients treated with these drugs.— E. K. Zsigmond and G. Robins, *Can. Anaesth. Soc. J.*, 1972, *19*, 75.

Aprotinin. A report of 3 cases of prolonged or recurring apnoea following intravenous administration of aprotinin during or immediately after surgery in patients given suxamethonium or suxamethonium and tubocurarine for neuromuscular blockade. Aprotinin may potentiate the effect of muscle relaxants and the anaesthetist should be aware of the possibility of apnoea.— G. Chasapakis and C. Dimas, *Br. J. Anaesth.*, 1966, *38*, 838.

Halothane. A study involving 39 children indicated that use of halothane to induce anaesthesia greatly potentiated suxamethonium-induced muscle damage, as measured by serum myoglobin concentrations; however, children in this study did not appear to be more sensitive than adults in previous studies following intravenous induction with thiopentone. Pretreatment with alcuronium produced a large degree of protection.— A. S. Laurence and P. Henderson, *Br. J. Anaesth.*, 1986, *58*, 126P.

Lithium. Prolongation of suxamethonium-induced neuromuscular blockade in a woman taking lithium carbonate. This interaction was confirmed in *dogs*.— G. E. Hill *et al.*, *Anesthesiology*, 1976, *44*, 439.

Trimetaphan. Prolonged apnoea and depolarising neuromuscular blockade in a patient given trimetaphan, tubocurarine, and suxamethonium. The case might be due to cholinesterase inhibition by trimetaphan.— T. J. Poulton *et al.*, *Anesthesiology*, 1979, *50*, 54.

MUSCULAR DYSTROPHIES. Suxamethonium should be avoided in patients known to have Duchenne's progressive muscular dystrophy.— C. L. Smith and G. H. Bush, *Br. J. Anaesth.*, 1985, *57*, 1113.

A 3-year-old child who developed sudden ventricular fibrillation under general anaesthesia, which included the use of suxamethonium and halothane, was subsequently found to have Duchenne type muscular dystrophy.— A. M. Oudesluys-Murphy *et al.* (letter), *Lancet*, 1985, *1*, 696.

Absorption and Fate

After injection, suxamethonium is hydrolysed by pseudocholinesterases in plasma and body tissues. One molecule of choline is split off rapidly to form succinylmonocholine which is then slowly hydrolysed to succinic acid and choline. Only a small proportion of suxamethonium is excreted unchanged in the urine. Succinylmonocholine has weak muscle-relaxant properties mainly of a competitive (non-depolarising) nature.

The gene responsible for the expression of pseudocholinesterase may have 1 of 4 allelomorphic forms, known as usual, atypical, fluoride-resistant, and silent; of the 10 possible phenotypes that may be formed, the atypical and silent homozygotes, and the atypical-silent heterozygote, will produce variant forms of the enzyme that hydrolyse suxamethonium more slowly, thus prolonging its effects.

Suxamethonium does not readily cross the placenta following usual doses.

The pharmacokinetics of suxamethonium.— D. R. Cook *et al.*, *Clin. Pharmac. Ther.*, 1976, *20*, 493; L. B. Wingard and D. R. Cook, *Clin. Pharmacokinet.*, 1977, *2*, 330.

Uses and Administration

Suxamethonium is a depolarising muscle relaxant. It acts in about 30 seconds following intravenous injection and has a duration of action averaging 4 to 6 minutes. It is used in surgical, anaesthetic, and other procedures in which a brief period of muscle relaxation is called for, as in intubation, endoscopies, orthopaedic manipulations, and electroconvulsive therapy.

As the onset of relaxation is often preceded by a short period of painful muscle fasciculation, an intravenous anaesthetic, such as thiopentone sodium, should be given before suxamethonium is injected. Premedication with an antimuscarinic agent may be of value in reducing excessive salivation and bradycardia. Assisted respiration is necessary.

The usual single dose of suxamethonium chloride for an adult is 20 to 80 mg intravenously, but response varies considerably. An initial test dose of 10 mg may be given intravenously to determine the patient's response. Doses may be repeated if necessary. A suggested dose for children is 1 to 2 mg per kg intravenously.

When a suitable vein is inaccessible suxamethonium may occasionally be given intramuscularly. A suggested intramuscular dose for adults and children is up to 2.5 mg per kg body-weight to a maximum total of 150 mg; the effect may be prolonged after intramuscular injection.

For prolonged procedures, as an alternative to repeated intravenous injections, sustained relaxation may be obtained by continuous intravenous infusion of a 0.1 to 0.2% solution, the rate of flow being adjusted as necessary. It has been suggested that continuous infusion is unsafe in children and neonates because of the risk of inducing malignant hyperpyrexia.

The duration of effect of suxamethonium has been increased by concomitantly administering hexafluorenium (see p.1234). High or repeated doses of suxamethonium may lead to development of phase II block and prolonged apnoea.

The iodide has also been used.

A review of suxamethonium. The primary clinical indication for the use of suxamethonium is for a rapid onset and short duration of neuromuscular block. It is particularly suited for rapid induction techniques. However, once intubation has been accomplished maintenance of muscle relaxation is usually achieved with a competitive neuromuscular blocking agent. There is little indication for the use of a continuous infusion of suxamethonium. Suxamethonium has also been used with success for the control of muscle activity during electroconvulsive therapy.— N. N. Durant and R. L. Katz, *Br. J. Anaesth.*, 1982, *54*, 195.

ADMINISTRATION IN RENAL FAILURE. Suxamethonium could be given in usual doses to patients with renal failure, but in end-stage renal disease acute hyperkalaemia could occur.— W. M. Bennett *et al.*, *Am. J. Kidney Dis.*, 1983, *3*, 155.

SQUINT. The value of suxamethonium in surgery for squint.— J. D. Abrams (letter), *Br. J. Ophthal.*, 1984, *68*, 218.

Preparations

Sterile Succinylcholine Chloride *(U.S.P.)*

Succinylcholine Chloride Injection *(U.S.P.)*. A sterile solution of suxamethonium chloride in Water for Injections. Potency is expressed in terms of anhydrous material. Store at 2° to 8°.

Suxamethonium Bromide Injection *(B.P.)*. Succinylcholine Bromide Injection. Prepared by dissolving, immediately before use, the sterile contents of a sealed container (Suxamethonium Bromide for Injection) in the requisite amount of Water for Injections.

Suxamethonium Chloride Injection *(B.P.)*. Succinylcholine Chloride Injection. Store at as low a temperature as possible above its freezing point and not exceeding 4°. Under these conditions it should meet the requirements of the monograph for not less than 18 months after preparation.

Proprietary Preparations

Anectine *(Calmic, UK)*. *Injection*, suxamethonium chloride 50 mg/mL, in ampoules of 2 mL.

Brevidil M *(May & Baker, UK)*. *Injection*, powder for reconstitution, suxamethonium bromide, 67 mg.

Scoline *(Duncan, Flockhart, UK)*. *Injection*, suxamethonium chloride 50 mg/mL, in ampoules of 2 mL.

Proprietary Names and Manufacturers of Suxamethonium Salts

Anectine *(Wellcome, Austral.; Wellcome, Canad.; Gayoso Wellcome, Spain; Calmic, UK; Wellcome, USA)*; Brevidil M *(May & Baker, Austral.; S.Afr.; May & Baker, UK)*; Célocurine *(Kabivitrum, Fr.)*; Celocurin *(Ital.; ACO, Swed.)*; Celocurin-Chlorid *(Switz.)*; Celocurin-klorid *(ACO, Swed.)*; Curacit *(GEA, Denm.; Nyco, Norw.)*; Curalest *(Neth.)*; Lysthenon *(Hormonchemie, Ger.; Chemie-Linz, Switz.)*; Midarine *(Wellcome, Ital.; Switz.)*; Mioflex *(Andalucia, Spain)*; Muscuryl *(Neth.)*; Myoplegine *(Belg.)*; Myotenlis *(Farmitalia, Ital.)*; Pantolax *(Ger.)*; Paranoval *(Arg.)*; Quelicin *(Abbott, Canad.; Abbott, USA)*; Scoline *(Glaxo, Austral.; Ital.; Glaxo, S.Afr.; Duncan, Flockhart, UK)*; Succinolin *(Amino, Switz.)*; Succinyl *(Neth.)*; Succinyl-Asta *(Asta, Ger.; Degussa, Switz.)*; Sucostrin *(Squibb, USA)*; Sux-Cert *(Travenol, USA)*.

5734-d

Suxethonium Bromide *(BAN)*.
2,2′-Succinyldioxybis(diethyldimethylammonium) dibromide.
$C_{16}H_{34}Br_2N_2O_4$=478.3.

CAS — 111-00-2.

1 mg Suxethonium (1 mg cation) is equivalent to 1.5 mg of suxethonium bromide.

INCOMPATIBILITY. Suxethonium bromide is incompatible with alkalis and should not be mixed with solutions of barbiturates.

Suxethonium bromide is a depolarising muscle relaxant with the same actions and uses as suxamethonium chloride (see p.1238) but it has only about half the potency and a rather shorter duration of action, namely, 2 to 4 minutes. It is administered by intravenous injection, the dose being calculated on the basis of 1 to 1.25 mg cation (1.5 to 1.875 mg salt) per kg bodyweight.

Proprietary Names and Manufacturers
Brevidil E *(Austral.; S.Afr.; May & Baker, UK)*.

13324-v

Thiocolchicoside *(rINN)*.
3,10-Di(demethoxy)-3-glucopyranosyloxy-10-methylthiocolchicine.
$C_{27}H_{33}NO_{10}S$=563.6.

CAS — 602-41-5.

Pharmacopoeias. In *Fr.*

Thiocolchicoside is a muscle relaxant which has been claimed to possess GABA-mimetic and glycinergic actions. It has been used as an adjunct in the management of spasticity, and in the symptomatic treatment of musculoskeletal conditions associated with painful muscle spasm; it has also been given for gynaecological disorders. The usual initial dose is 4 mg four times daily by mouth. It has also been given intramuscularly, in doses of 4 to 8 mg daily, or applied as cream or ointment.

Proprietary Names and Manufacturers
Coltramyl *(Roussel, Belg.; Roussel, Fr.)*; Liviane *(Knoll-Made, Spain)*; Musco-Ril *(Inverni della Beffa, Ital.)*.

13357-j

Tizanidine Hydrochloride *(BANM, rINN)*.
DS-103-282 *(tizanidine)*. 5-Chloro-*N*-(2-imidazolin-2-yl)-2,1,3-benzothiadiazol-4-ylamine hydrochloride.
$C_9H_8ClN_5S,HCl$=290.2.

CAS — 51322-75-9 (tizanidine).

Tizanidine hydrochloride 1.14 mg is approximately equivalent to 1 mg of tizanidine.

Adverse Effects and Precautions
Tizanidine hydrochloride may cause drowsiness; patients so affected should not drive or operate machinery. Other side-effects include dry mouth, fatigue, dizziness, muscle pain and weakness, tremor, gastro-intestinal disturbances, and hypotension: in view of the latter, it should be given with care to patients receiving antihypertensive therapy. Caution is required in patients with renal or hepatic insufficiency.

Uses and Administration
Tizanidine hydrochloride is a muscle relaxant which is used as an adjunct in the management of spasticity, and in the symptomatic treatment of musculoskeletal conditions associated with painful muscle spasm. It is given in a usual initial dose equivalent to 2 mg of the base three times daily, increased as necessary according to the response of the patient, up to a maximum of 36 mg daily.

A crossover study in 26 patients with spasticity showed that tizanidine, in doses up to 16 mg daily was as effective as baclofen, in doses up to 40 mg daily, in producing improvement. Nine patients improved while receiving tizanidine and 8 while taking baclofen but patients who responded to one drug did not always respond to the other. A further 8 patients were withdrawn from the study due to side-effects, 6 while receiving baclofen and 2 whilst on tizanidine. In a subsequent open study completed by 11 of 14 spastic patients, the optimum dose of tizanidine was found to be from 12 to 24 mg daily. Ten of the 11 had previously received another antispastic drug, and 8 of these preferred tizanidine. Tizanidine may be a useful alternative to baclofen in patients with spasticity related to spinal cord disease.— P. M. Newman *et al.*, *Eur. J. clin. Pharmac.*, 1982, *23*, 31. See also: U. K. Rinne, *Curr. ther. Res.*, 1980, *28*, 827; C. Smolenski *et al.*, *Curr. med. Res. Opinion*, 1981, *7*, 374; O. L. Hennies, *J. int. med. Res.*, 1981, *9*, 62 (comparisons with diazepam or baclofen).

Proprietary Names and Manufacturers
Sirdalud *(Sandoz, Denm.; Wander, Ger.; Wander, Switz.)*.

5735-n

Tolperisone Hydrochloride *(BANM, rINNM)*.
N-553. 2,4′-Dimethyl-3-piperidinopropiophenone hydrochloride.
$C_{16}H_{23}NO,HCl$=281.8.

CAS — 728-88-1 (tolperisone); 3644-61-9 (hydrochloride).

Pharmacopoeias. In *Cz.* and *Jpn.*

Tolperisone hydrochloride is a muscle relaxant that has been used for the symptomatic treatment of musculoskeletal conditions associated with painful muscle spasm, in doses of 150 mg three times daily.

Proprietary Names and Manufacturers
Abbsa *(Jpn)*; Arantoick *(Jpn)*; Atmosgen *(Jpn)*; Besnoline *(Jpn)*; Colmaite *(Jpn)*; Isocalm *(Jpn)*; Kineorl *(Jpn)*; Lasmon *(Jpn)*; Magnine *(Jpn)*; Menopatol *(Jpn)*; Metosomin *(Jpn)*; Minacalm *(Jpn)*; Miodom *(Dominguez, Arg.)*; Mio-Relax *(Spain)*; Muscalm *(Jpn)*; Mydocalm *(Richter, Denm.; Choay, Fr.; Gedeon Richter, Hung.; Katwijk, Neth.; Labatec-Pharma, Switz.)*; Naismeritin *(Jpn)*; Nichiperizone *(Jpn)*; Renbert *(Jpn)*; Rencarl *(Jpn)*; Roystajin *(Jpn)*; Sagereal *(Jpn)*; Sinorum *(Jpn)*; Tolisartine *(Jpn)*.

5736-h

Tubocurarine Chloride *(BAN, USAN, rINN)*.

d-Tubocurarine Chloride; Tubocurar. Chlor.; (+)-Tubocurarine Chloride Hydrochloride Pentahydrate; Tubocurarini Chloridum; Tubocurarinii Chloridum. (+)-7′,12′-Dihydroxy-6,6′-dimethoxy-2,2′,2′-trimethyltubocuraranium dichloride pentahydrate.
$C_{37}H_{42}Cl_2N_2O_6,5H_2O$=771.7 (The empirical formula of tubocurarine chloride was formerly considered to be $C_{38}H_{44}Cl_2N_2O_6,5H_2O$).

CAS — 57-95-4 (tubocurarine); 57-94-3 (chloride, anhydrous); 6989-98-6 (chloride, pentahydrate).

Pharmacopoeias. In *Arg., Aust., Br., Braz., Cz., Egypt., Eur., Fr., Ger., Ind., Int., It., Jpn, Jug., Mex., Neth., Span., Swiss, Turk.,* and *U.S.*

The chloride of (+)-tubocurarine. It may be obtained from extracts of the stems of *Chondodendron tomentosum* (Menispermaceae)and is one of the active principles of curare, by which name it is sometimes referred to in anaesthetic literature. It is a white or slightly yellowish-white or greyish-white, crystalline powder.

Soluble 1 in 20 of water; soluble in solutions of alkali hydroxides; practically insoluble in acetone, chloroform and ether.The *B.P.* specifies a solubility of 1 in 30 of alcohol, the *U.S.P.* 1 in 45. The *B.P.*also specifies that a 1% solution in water has a pH of 4.0 to 6.0; the *U.S.P.* injection has a pH of 2.5 to 5.0. The *B.P.* injection is **sterilised** by autoclaving. **Store** in airtight containers.

INCOMPATIBILITY. Tubocurarine hydrochloride solution, 15 mg per mL, could usually be mixed with thiopentone sodium 2.5% solution in the proportion 1:19. If the pH of the resultant solution fell below 9.7, thiopentone was precipitated; above pH 9.7 the shelf-life of the mixture was limited to 48 hours.— C. Riffkin, *Am. J. Hosp. Pharm.*, 1963, *20*, 19.

A haze developed over 3 hours when tubocurarine chloride 60 mg per litre was mixed with trimetaphan camsylate 1 g per litre in glucose injection.— B. B. Riley, *J. Hosp. Pharm.*, 1970, *28*, 228.

A haze developed in 15 minutes when methohexitone sodium 100 mg in 10 mL was mixed with tubocurarine chloride 12 mg in 4 mL.

Adverse Effects

In the doses commonly employed during anaesthesia, tubocurarine produces few side-effects provided efficient respiratory exchange is maintained. A fall in blood pressure usually occurs, probably due in part to ganglionic blockade and the release of histamine; there may be a slight increase in heart-rate but some authorities have also reported a slight fall. Reduction in gastro-intestinal motility and tone may occur; in patients undergoing surgery in the Trendelenburg position, in which the lower body is elevated above the head, the stomach contents may be regurgitated into the pharynx.

Tubocurarine-induced histamine release may lead to wheal-and-flare effects at the site of injection, flushing, and occasionally bronchospasm.

In overdosage there is prolonged apnoea due to paralysis of the intercostal muscles and diaphragm, with cardiovascular collapse and the effects of histamine release.

Postoperative apnoea resistant to reversal with neostigmine has sometimes occurred (but see p.1228).

ALLERGY. In common with many drugs, neuromuscular blocking agents may cause histamine release which on most occasions is of little clinical importance, but anaphylactoid reactions have been encountered and there may be cross-sensitivity between different agents. However, the incidence of life-threatening reactions is low and in most cases patients respond to conventional cardiorespiratory support.— *Lancet*, 1985, *1*, 1195.

For the view that anaphylactoid reactions to neuromuscular blocking agents may be a commonly undiagnosed condition, see under Suxamethonium Chloride, p.1238.

EFFECTS ON BODY TEMPERATURE. Two cases of malignant hyperpyrexia where tubocurarine was probably the triggering drug. Each episode developed in a member of a known malignant hyperpyrexia family and developed despite preventive measures such as prophylactic cooling, and avoidance of potent inhalational anaesthetic agents and depolarising muscle relaxants.— B. A. Britt *et al.*, *Can. Anaesth. Soc. J.*, 1974, *21*, 371.

PREGNANCY AND THE NEONATE. A young woman, about 28 weeks pregnant, with status epilepticus was given 15- to 30-mg doses of tubocurarine as needed, then every 2 hours, to control the fits. The total dose of tubocurarine was 245 mg. Premature labour occurred and after delivery the infant's heart beat was normal but there was no spontaneous activity or effort to breathe. Edrophonium 200 µg was injected through an umbilical catheter and within a few seconds the baby showed vigorous movements and began to breathe normally although it died 5½ hours after birth.— P. O. Older and J. M. Harris, *Br. J. Anaesth.*, 1968, *40*, 459.

Treatment of Adverse Effects

In respiratory paralysis or depression due to tubocurarine respiration should be assisted; in addition, neostigmine methylsulphate 2 to 3 mg should be given in association with atropine sulphate 0.6 to 1.2 mg. Additional neostigmine may be given if required but a dose of 5 mg should not be exceeded.

Severe hypotension may require intravenous fluid replacement and cautious administration of a pressor agent; the patient should be positioned to facilitate venous return from the muscles.

Administration of an antihistamine before induction of neuromuscular blockade may be of value in preventing histamine-induced adverse effects.

In 3 patients with renal failure given tubocurarine, recurring dyspnoea or apnoea after neuromuscular blockade had apparently been reversed by neostigmine probably represented recurarisation. Pyridostigmine, with its longer action, might be preferable in such patients.— R. D. Miller and D. J. Cullen, *Br. J. Anaesth.*, 1976, *48*, 253.

Precautions

Tubocurarine chloride should be used with great care, if at all, in patients with myasthenia gravis, who are extremely sensitive to its effects, in respiratory insufficiency or pulmonary disease, and in the dehydrated or severely ill patient. Care is also required in patients with a history of asthma or allergy, in the presence of renal impairment, or when tubocurarine has to be given to a patient on 2 occasions within 24 hours. Doses should be reduced in neonates, who are particularly sensitive to the effects of competitive neuromuscular blocking agents. Patients with hepatic impairment may be relatively resistant to the effects of tubocurarine.

The effects of tubocurarine are increased by acidosis and hypokalaemia. Competitive neuromuscular blockade may also be enhanced by raised body temperature and reduced in the presence of hypothermia.

The effects of tubocurarine are enhanced to some extent by inhalational anaesthetics; the hypotension produced by halothane anaesthesia is increased by tubocurarine. The effects of tubocurarine may be enhanced by certain aminoglycoside and polypeptide antibiotics; they may also be enhanced by beta-blockers, magnesium salts, potassium-depleting diuretics, opioid analgesics, and quinidine.

Administration of tubocurarine either with or before a depolarising neuromuscular blocker such as suxamethonium may cause a muscle relaxation which is irreversible by neostigmine (see p.1228).

INTERACTIONS. *Aprotinin.* For a report of the interaction of neuromuscular blockers with aprotinin, see under Suxamethonium Chloride, p.1239.

Diazepam. For reports of the effects of diazepam on competitive neuromuscular blocking agents, see Gallamine Triethiodide, p.1234.

Ketamine. The effect of tubocurarine was enhanced by ketamine; pancuronium and suxamethonium were not affected.— R. R. Johnston *et al.*, *Anesth. Analg. curr. Res.*, 1974, *53*, 496.

Absorption and Fate

Tubocurarine chloride is a quaternary ammonium compound and absorption from the gastro-intestinal tract following oral administration is extremely poor. Absorption is slow and irregular when given intramuscularly. Following intravenous injection tubocurarine is widely distributed throughout body tissues. When given in usual doses it does not pass the blood-brain barrier, and does not appear to cross the placenta in significant amounts. Half to two-thirds of a dose is excreted unchanged in the urine over several hours, and a small amount in bile. A small proportion of a dose is metabolised in the liver.

A detailed review of the clinical pharmacokinetics of muscle relaxants, including tubocurarine chloride.— L. B. Wingard and D. R. Cook, *Clin. Pharmacokinet.*, 1977, *2*, 330.

Pharmacokinetics of tubocurarine administered by combined intravenous bolus injection and infusion.— M. I. Ramzan *et al.*, *Br. J. Anaesth.*, 1980, *52*, 893.

Uses and Administration

Tubocurarine is a competitive (non-depolarising) muscle relaxant and when given by injection produces paralysis of voluntary muscle by blocking impulses at the neuromuscular junction. The action is rapid, effects beginning to appear within a minute or so after intravenous injection and lasting for 30 to 40 minutes on average; the maximum effect is attained within 3 to 5 minutes.

In the dosage used clinically, tubocurarine chloride has no central stimulant, depressant, or analgesic action. It has histamine-releasing properties, and it blocks the action of acetylcholine at the autonomic ganglia to some degree.

Tubocurarine is used as an adjuvant to anaesthesia to obtain greater muscular relaxation in surgical operations and in orthopaedic manipulations. Response to tubocurarine is variable: in the *UK*, it has been suggested that dosage should be based on an initial intravenous dose of 10 to 15 mg, although initial doses of up to 30 mg or more are used. Additional doses of 5 mg may be given at intervals of about 25 minutes if required: it has been recommended that the total dose should not exceed 40 mg. Some sources advocate that an initial dose of 5 mg should be given to the patient before anaesthesia to determine undue susceptibility. In the *USA* lower doses have generally been employed: an initial dose of 6 to 9 mg intravenously, followed by 3 to 4.5 mg after 3 to 5 minutes if necessary; additional doses of 3 mg may be given as required for prolonged procedures.

In children, doses in the range 300 to 500 µg per kg body-weight intravenously have been employed in the *UK* and the *USA*, but in premature infants and neonates, who are more sensitive to the effects of tubocurarine, a dose of 200 to 250 µg per kg is suggested.

These standard doses of tubocurarine should be decreased in the presence of certain inhalation anaesthetics which may potentiate competitive neuromuscular blockade.

In most patients who have had large doses of tubocurarine over a long period, there will be some residual effect which will require reversal with neostigmine; the use of an additional dose of 5 to 10 mg of tubocurarine chloride to facilitate closure of the abdominal wall does not materially affect the ease with which this reversal can be accomplished.

Tubocurarine chloride is also used to control the muscle spasms and convulsions of tetanus, by intravenous or intramuscular injection.

The trauma in electroconvulsive therapy may be minimised by the intravenous administration, 5 minutes before induction of the shock, of tubocurarine chloride to the anaesthetised patient.

Tubocurarine chloride has been used as a diagnostic agent for myasthenia gravis by provoking exacerbation of myasthenic symptoms but the procedure is extremely hazardous and should only be used if other tests are indecisive.

Pretreatment with tubocurarine 3 mg abolished the fasciculations produced by suxamethonium without impairment of relaxation of hand, jaw, and respiratory muscles although 70 to 75% more suxamethonium was required for the same degree of block. Conditions for endotracheal intubation were excellent.— A. L. Pauca *et al.*, *Br. J. Anaesth.*, 1975, *47*, 1067. A study in patients undergoing minor surgery, who received suxamethonium 1 mg per kg body-weight, showed that pretreatment with tubocurarine 50 µg per kg 3 minutes previously virtually abolished visible fasciculations, and reduced severity and frequency of postoperative muscle pain, when compared with placebo; pretreatment with diazepam or midazolam failed to reduce fasciculations and protect against muscle pain.— W. N. Chestnutt *et al.*, *Br. J. clin. Pharmac.*, 1984, *17*, 222P.

ADMINISTRATION IN RENAL FAILURE. Tubocurarine could be given in normal doses to patients with renal failure.— W. M. Bennett *et al.*, *Am. J. Kidney Dis.*, 1983, *3*, 155.

OCULAR SURGERY. Reduction of intra-ocular pressure by tubocurarine.— M. H. Al-Abrak and J. R. Samuel, *Br. J. Ophthal.*, 1974, *58*, 806.

PREGNANCY AND THE NEONATE. A report of a technique of curarisation of the foetus to prevent movement during procedures for intra-uterine diagnosis and foetal treatment. Doses of 3 mg per kg body-weight, based on estimated foetal weight, were given by intramuscular injection into the foetal thigh, using a high-resolution ultrasound scanner to view the procedure, and abolished foetal movement within 30 minutes, for a period of some 3 to 5 hours. The procedure had been used on 12 occasions in 5 foetuses; there was no evidence of local soft tissue damage at the injection site or of nerve or muscle damage at birth.— L. C. de Crespigny *et al.* (letter), *Lancet*, 1985, *1*, 1164.

TETANUS. In the treatment of severe tetanus tubocurarine was given intramuscularly in doses sufficient to give freedom from spasm for 2 hours at a time.— J. Macrae, *Br. med. J.*, 1973, *1*, 730. See also G. Clough and J. R. W. Dykes, *Br. J. Anaesth.*, 1973, *45*, 617.

Preparations

Tubocurarine Chloride Injection *(U.S.P.)*

Tubocurarine Injection *(B.P.)*. Tubocurar. Inj. Contains tubocurarine chloride 1% in Water for Injections.

Proprietary Preparations

Jexin *(Duncan, Flockhart, UK). Injection,* tubocurarine chloride 10 mg/mL, in ampoules of 1.5 mL.

Tubarine *(Calmic, UK). Injection,* tubocurarine chloride 10 mg/mL, in ampoules of 1.5 mL.

Proprietary Names and Manufacturers

Curarin *(Ger.; Ital.)*; Curarine *(Neth.)*; Intocostrine-T *(Belg.)*; Intocostrin-T *(Ital.)*; Jexin *(Duncan, Flockhart, UK)*; Tubarine *(Arg.; Wellcome, Austral.; Wellcome, Canad.; Wellcome, Ital.; Wellcome, S.Afr.; Switz.; Calmic, UK)*; Tubocuran *(ND & K, Denm.)*.

14012-x

Vecuronium Bromide *(BAN, USAN, rINN).*

Org-NC-45. 1-(3α,17β-Diacetoxy-2β-piperidino-5α-androstan-16β-yl)-1-methylpiperidinium bromide.

$C_{34}H_{57}BrN_2O_4$=637.7.

CAS — 50700-72-6.

Adverse Effects, Treatment, and Precautions

As for Tubocurarine Chloride, p.1241. It has a smaller histamine-releasing effect then tubocurarine and fewer cardiovascular effects.

Following intravenous injection of vecuronium bromide in a non-atopic surgical patient a flare developed immediately and was followed by urticarial wheals lasting roughly 4 hours but there were no systemic adverse effects.— A. G. Spence and R. S. Barnetson (letter), *Lancet*, 1985, *1*, 979.

For results suggesting that administration of vecuronium to patients sensitive to other neuromuscular blocking drugs might result in an adverse reaction, see under Atracurium Besylate, p.1229.

INTERACTIONS. *Neuromuscular blockers.* For a study of the interaction between vecuronium and pancuronium bromide, see under Precautions in Pancuronium Bromide, p.1236.

Verapamil. Difficulty in reversing vecuronium-induced neuromuscular blockade with usual doses of neostigmine in a patient with renal insufficiency was attributed to the coincidental use of verapamil.— J. F. Van Poorten *et al., Anesth. Analg.*, 1984, *63*, 155.

Absorption and Fate

Following intravenous administration vecuronium is rapidly distributed into extracellular fluid. It is partly metabolised in the liver and is excreted mainly in bile as unchanged drug and metabolites; some is also excreted in urine. Small amounts may cross the placenta.

A comparison of the pharmacokinetics of pancuronium and vecuronium. Vecuronium had a significantly faster clearance rate and a shorter mean elimination half-life of 71 minutes in 5 patients than did similar doses of pancuronium in a further 4 patients, with a mean elimination half-life of 140 minutes. Measurable concentrations of pancuronium were present in serum at 24 hours whereas concentrations of vecuronium could not be detected after 5 to 6 hours.— R. Cronnelly *et al., Anesthesiology*, 1983, *58*, 405.

See also under Administration, below.

Uses and Administration

Vecuronium bromide is a competitive (non-depolarising) neuromuscular blocker with effects similar to those of tubocurarine chloride (see p.1241), but having a shorter duration of action. Following intravenous injection muscle relaxation begins in about 2 to 3 minutes and lasts for 20 to 30 minutes.

It is used as an adjunct to general anaesthesia for muscle relaxation during surgical procedures. The usual initial dose is 80 to 100 µg per kg body-weight by intravenous injection; additional doses of 30 to 50 µg per kg, or in the *US*, 10 to 15 µg per kg, may be given as required during prolonged procedures. It may also be given by intravenous infusion in doses of 50 to 80 µg per kg per hour.

The standard doses of vecuronium bromide may need to be reduced when given with potent inhalation anaesthetics that can potentiate its neuromuscular blocking action.

A review of vecuronium. Because it has little or no cardiovascular effect vecuronium may be an appropriate neuromuscular blocker for cardiac surgery but its short duration of action may not be appropriate for a procedure that requires several hours of paralysis. It does not readily cross the placenta and has been used successfully in caesarean section, and in patients with renal failure.— R. D. Miller, *Pharmacotherapy*, 1984, *4*, 238. Comment. In many institutions vecuronium will replace suxamethonium as the muscle relaxant used to facilitate endotracheal intubation. At other institutions, suxamethonium will continue to be used but vecuronium will probably replace tubocurarine, pancuronium, and metocurine. Although the other 4 muscle relaxants mentioned are effective and have minimal side-effects in the majority of patients, vecuronium is more specific and has fewer side-effects than any, and the author has more or less abandoned the older muscle relaxants and changed to vecuronium, or atracurium, which is similar in terms of action and lack of side-effects. At present, there is no basis for choosing atracurium over vecuronium or vice versa, and both are used, with tubocurarine being employed only when hypotension is desirable and pancuronium when it is wished to increase heart-rate. There seems no reason for using metocurine, decamethonium, or gallamine, and suxamethonium is used by the author only when one must intubate in less than 1 minute, or must provide relaxation almost immediately and for a very brief period of time.— R. L. Katz, *ibid.*, 247.

Further reviews of vecuronium and atracurium C. J. Hull, *Br. J. Hosp. Med.*, 1983, *30*, 273; C. S. Conner, *Drug Intell. & clin. Pharm.*, 1984, *18*, 714; R. D. Miller *et al., Anesthesiology*, 1984, *61*, 444; C. S. Reilly and W. S. Nimmo, *Drugs*, 1987, *34*, 98.

ADMINISTRATION. In a study in surgical patients given either vecuronium 50, 70, or 90 µg per kg body-weight initially, or suxamethonium 1 mg per kg, each in 10 patients, suxamethonium produced 100% block after 90 seconds and provided excellent intubating conditions whereas the 3 doses of vecuronium were associated with 7.5, 18.7, and 30.7% block respectively, and gave acceptable intubation conditions in only 30% of subjects. Although the lack of cumulation and ease of reversibility with vecuronium offer advantages over currently available competitive relaxants, the onset of action of vecuronium is too slow for rapid intubation, such as may be required in an emergency.— A. Williams *et al., Can. Anaesth. Soc. J.*, 1982, *29*, 567.

In a comparative study in surgical patients requiring at least 2 hours of anaesthesia, muscle relaxation was achieved in 29 with vecuronium in initial doses of 100 µg per kg body-weight, with supplemental doses of 25 µg per kg as required, while 22 were given similar doses of pancuronium. Mean duration of effect of the initial dose was 3 times longer with pancuronium than with vecuronium; 5 patients receiving pancuronium required no supplemental dose, and only 1 required more than 3, whereas patients given vecuronium required between 1 and 15 supplemental doses. However, in contrast to pancuronium, there was no evidence of cumulation in those given multiple doses of vecuronium. Vecuronium's lack of cumulation suggests that it could conveniently be given by intravenous infusion.— W. Buzello and G. Nöldge, *Br. J. Anaesth.*, 1982, *54*, 1151. A similar study.— W. J. Kerr and W. L. M. Baird, *ibid.*, 1159.

In renal failure. Results of a study in 5 patients with renal failure given vecuronium 140 µg per kg body-weight and 8 patients with normal kidney function of whom 4 received the same dose and 4, 280 µg per kg, indicated no significant difference in elimination half-life and clearance between normal patients and those with renal failure. Despite the high doses of vecuronium there was no significant difference in duration of neuromuscular blockade in the 2 groups given equivalent doses, nor in the recovery time: mean values were 103.8 and 20.7 minutes in healthy patients, and 104.1 and 28.7 minutes in those with renal failure. Vecuronium bromide may be a suitable competitive muscle relaxant for use in patients with impaired renal function.— M. R. Fahey *et al., Br. J. Anaesth.*, 1981, *53*, 1049.

Proprietary Preparations

Norcuron *(Organon Teknika, UK). Injection,* powder for reconstitution, vecuronium bromide 10 mg, supplied with solvent.

Proprietary Names and Manufacturers

Norcuron *(Organon, Canad.; Organon, Denm.; Organon, Fr.; Organon, Norw.; Organon, Swed.; Organon Teknika, Switz.; Organon Teknika, UK; Organon, USA)*.

Nonionic Surfactants

430-y

A surfactant is a compound that can reduce the interfacial tension between 2 immiscible phases and this is due to the molecule containing 2 localised regions, one being hydrophilic in nature and the other hydrophobic.

The properties of nonionic surfactants are largely dependent on the proportions of these 2 groups in the molecule. Hydrophilic groups include the oxyethylene group ($-O.CH_2.CH_2-$) and the hydroxyl group ($-OH$). By varying the number of these groups in a hydrophobic molecule, such as a fatty acid, substances are obtained which range from strongly hydrophobic and water-insoluble compounds, such as glyceryl monostearate, to strongly hydrophilic and water-soluble compounds, such as the macrogols. These 2 extreme types are not satisfactory as emulsifying agents, though they are useful stabilisers in the presence of efficient emulsifying agents. Between these extremes are the nonionic emulsifying agents in which the proportions of hydrophilic and hydrophobic groups are more evenly balanced; these include some of the macrogol esters and ethers and sorbitan derivatives.

Nonionic surfactants differ from anionic surfactants (see p.1416) by the absence of charge on or ionisation of the molecule; they are generally less irritant than anionic or cationic surfactants.

In addition to their use as emulsifiers some nonionic surfactants may be used in pharmacy as solubilising and wetting agents and nonionic surfactants in general are widely used in various industries. The use of nonionic surfactants as emulsifiers or stabilisers in food is controlled in Great Britain.

Since nonionic surfactants do not ionise to any great extent in solution, they are generally compatible with both anionic and cationic substances, but they reduce the antimicrobial action of many preservatives.

Nonionic surfactants may be classified according to their hydrophilic-lipophilic balance (HLB). This is an arbitrary scale of values denoting the relative affinity of the surfactant for oil and water. Lipophilic surfactants have low HLB values (less than 10) and are generally used as antifoaming agents, water-in-oil emulsifying agents, and as wetting agents; hydrophilic surfactants have higher HLB values (greater than 10) and are generally used as oil-in-water emulsifying agents and solubilising agents.

Glycol and glycerol esters are a group of nonionic surfactants consisting of fatty acid esters of glycols and glycerol. Hydrophobic properties predominate and these compounds are poor emulsifying agents if used alone, though they are useful stabilisers for both oil-in-water and water-in-oil emulsions. If a small amount of soap, sulphated fatty alcohol, or other surfactant is added to the esters, a 'self-emulsifying' product is formed which is capable of producing satisfactory oil-in-water emulsions. **Acetoglycerides** are mixed glyceryl esters in which the glycerol is esterified partly with a fatty acid and partly with acetic acid.

Macrogol esters are polyoxyethylene esters of fatty acids, mainly stearates. The hydrophilic properties of the oxyethylene group are weaker than those of the hydroxyl group but by introducing a sufficient number into a fatty acid molecule, substances are produced in which the hydrophilic and hydrophobic properties are sufficiently well balanced for the esters to act as efficient oil-in-water emulsifying agents. They may also be used as wetting and solubilising agents. Since the ester linkage is prone to hydrolysis, these compounds are less resistant to acids and alkalis than the macrogol ethers.

Macrogol ethers are condensation products prepared by reaction between fatty alcohols or alkylphenols and ethylene oxide. The ether linkage confers good stability to acids and alkalis. Macrogol ethers are widely used in the preparation of oil-in-water emulsions and as wetting and solubilising agents.

NOTE. Two systems of nomenclature are used for macrogol ethers. The number '9' in the name 'Nonoxinol 9' refers to the approximate polymer length in oxyethylene units. The number '1000' in 'Cetomacrogol 1000' refers to the average molecular weight of the polymer chain.

Sorbitan derivatives are derivatives of the cyclic mono- or di-anhydrides of sorbitol. They consist of *sorbitan esters* which are prepared by esterification of one or more of the hydroxyl groups in the anhydrides with a fatty acid such as stearic, palmitic, oleic, or lauric acid, and *polysorbates* which are polyoxyethylene derivatives of the sorbitan esters. Sorbitan esters are oil-soluble, water-dispersible, nonionic surfactants which are effective water-in-oil emulsifiers. Polysorbates are more hydrophilic, water-soluble compounds and are used as oil-in-water emulsifying agents. By varying the number of oxyethylene groups in the molecule (indicated by the number following the word polyoxyethylene), and the type of fatty acid in the sorbitan ester, surfactants with a wide range of properties may be obtained.

In addition to the nonionic surfactants and formulas for emulsion bases given in this section, other nonionic compounds with surface activity such as the higher fatty alcohols and formulas are given in the section on Paraffins and Similar Bases (see p.1322).

445-x

Cetomacrogol 1000 *(BAN, rINN).*

Polyethylene Glycol 1000 Monocetyl Ether.

CAS — 9004-95-9 (m=15).

Pharmacopoeias. In *Br.*

A macrogol ether containing 20 to 24 oxyethylene groups in the polyoxyethylene chain. It is represented by the formula $CH_3.[CH_2]_m.$-$[O.CH_2.CH_2]_n.OH$, where m may be 15 or 17 and n may be 20 to 24.

An almost odourless cream-coloured waxy unctuous mass which melts, when heated, to a clear brownish-yellow liquid. M.p. not lower than 38°. **Soluble** in water, acetone, and alcohol; practically insoluble in petroleum spirit. It has been reported to be **incompatible** with phenols and to reduce the antibacterial activity of quaternary ammonium compounds. Cetomacrogol may separate from solutions in the presence of a high concentration of electrolytes.

Factors affecting autoxidation of aqueous cetomacrogol included temperature, concentration, initial pH, light, metallic impurities, and prior heat treatment or bleaching. Autoxidation could result in an appreciable decrease in solubility.— R. Hamburger *et al.*, *Pharm. Acta Helv.*, 1975, *50*, 10.

INCOMPATIBILITY. Benzocaine hydrochloride solution (0.25M) was incompatible with 3% cetomacrogol; a yellow colour developed on storage and could be retarded by the addition of antoxidants. Other oxidisable substances were likely to be similarly affected in the presence of macrogol groups.— E. Azaz *et al.*, *Pharm. J.*, 1973, *2*, 15.

Uses and Administration

Cetomacrogol 1000 is a macrogol ether which is used with cetostearyl alcohol as an emulsifying agent for making oil-in-water emulsions that are unaffected by moderate concentrations of electrolytes and are stable over a wide pH range.

Cetomacrogol 1000 is also used to disperse volatile oils in water to form transparent sols.

Preparations

Cetomacrogol Cream *(B.P.).* It may be prepared according to the following formulas for use as a diluent where specified: *Formula A,* Cetomacrogol emulsifying ointment 30 g, chlorocresol 100 mg, freshly boiled and cooled water, 69.9 g; *Formula B,* Cetomacrogol emulsifying ointment 30 g, benzyl alcohol 1.5 g, methyl hydroxybenzoate 150 mg, propyl hydroxybenzoate 80 mg, freshly boiled and cooled water 68.27 g. It must be recently prepared. Aluminium tubes should not be used for Formula B creams unless the inner surface of the tubes is coated with a suitable lacquer.

Cetomacrogol Cream Aqueous *(A.P.F.).* Non-ionic Cream; Sorbolene Cream. Cetomacrogol emulsifying wax 15 g, liquid paraffin 10 g, white soft paraffin 10 g, chlorocresol 100 mg, propylene glycol 5 mL, freshly boiled and cooled water to 100 g.

Cetomacrogol Lotion *(A.P.F.).* Cleansing Lotion. Cetomacrogol emulsifying wax 3, liquid paraffin 10, glycerol 10, chlorhexidine gluconate solution 0.1, purified water, freshly boiled and cooled to 100.

Cetomacrogol Emulsifying Ointment *(B.P.).* Cetomacrogol emulsifying wax 30 g, liquid paraffin 20 g, and white soft paraffin 50 g.

Cetomacrogol Emulsifying Wax *(B.P., B.P. Vet.).* Non-ionic Emulsifying Wax. Cetomacrogol '1000' 20 g, cetostearyl alcohol 80 g.

Non-ionic Soap *(A.P.F.).* White soft paraffin 20, cetomacrogol emulsifying wax 80.

Proprietary Names & Manufacturers

Brij *(ICI Speciality Chemicals, UK)*; Collone NI *(ABM Chemicals, UK)*; Crodex N *(Croda, UK)*; Cyclogol 1000 *(Witco, UK)*; Cyclogol NI *(Witco, UK)*; Texofor A1P *(ABM Chemicals, UK)*; Volpo CS20 *(Croda, UK)*.

486-g

Diacetylated Monoglycerides *(USAN).*

Pharmacopoeias. In *U.S.N.F. U.S.N.F.* also includes Mono- and Di-acetylated Monoglycerides.

Consists of glycerol esterified with edible fat-forming fatty acids and acetic acid. A clear liquid. Very **soluble** in alcohol 80%, vegetable oils, and mineral oils; sparingly soluble in alcohol 70%. **Store** in airtight containers. Protect from light.

Diacetylated monoglycerides is an acetoglyceride used as an emulsifying and stabilising agent.

Proprietary Names and Manufacturers of Diacetylated Monoglycerides and Related Compounds

Acetoglycerides *(Bush Boake Allen, UK)*; Myvacet *(Eastman, UK)*.

432-z

Diethylene Glycol Monostearate

Diéthylène Glycol (Stéarate de); Diglycol Stearate.

CAS — 106-11-6 (monostearate); 36381-62-1 (monopalmitate).

Pharmacopoeias. In *Fr.*

A white, odourless, wax-like solid consisting of a mixture of the palmitic and stearic acid esters of diethylene glycol and containing not less than 40% of monoesters and not more than 7.5% of free glycol. M.p. 44° to 46°. Practically **insoluble** in water; soluble in hot alcohol. It is obtainable in the pure, non-dispersible form, or in the self-emulsifying form containing a small proportion of soap or other primary emulsifying agent.

Diethylene glycol monostearate has the properties of and is used for the same purposes as glyceryl monostearate (p.1244) or self-emulsifying glyceryl monostearate (p.1244). Diethylene glycol monolaurate and monooleate are also available commercially.

For the estimated acceptable daily intakes of fatty and other acid esters of glycerol and polyglycerol esters, see Seventeenth Report of FAO/WHO Expert Committee on Food Additives, *Tech. Rep. Ser. Wld Hlth Org. No. 539,* 1974.

Proprietary Names and Manufacturers
Cithrol DGMS *(Croda, UK)*; Emcol CAD *(Witco, UK)*.

433-c

Ethylene Glycol Monostearate
Éthylène Glycol (Stéarate d'); Ethylene Glycol Stearate.

CAS — 111-60-4 (monostearate); 4219-49-2 (monopalmitate).

Pharmacopoeias. In *Fr.*

A white, odourless, wax-like solid consisting of a mixture of the palmitic and stearic acid esters of ethylene glycol and containing not less than 50% of monoesters and not more than 5% of free ethylene glycol. M.p. 54° to 57°. Slightly **soluble** in water; soluble in hot alcohol. It is obtainable in the pure non-dispersible form or in the self-emulsifying form.

Ethylene glycol monostearate has the properties of and is used for the same purposes as glyceryl monostearate (p.1244) or self-emulsifying glyceryl monostearate (p.1244). Ethylene glycol monolaurate and mono-oleate are also available commercially.

Proprietary Names and Manufacturers
Cerasynt M *(Black, UK; Van Dyk, USA)*; Cithrol EGMS *(Croda, UK)*.

3270-j

Glyceryl Behenate *(USAN)*.
Pharmacopoeias. In *U.S.N.F.*

A mixture of glycerides of fatty acids, mainly behenic acid. A fine powder with a faint odour. M.p. about 70°. Practically **insoluble** in water and in alcohol; soluble in chloroform. **Store** in airtight containers at a temperature not exceeding 35°.

Glyceryl behenate is used as a lubricant and binder in tablet-making.

Proprietary Names and Manufacturers
Compritol 888 *(Alfa, UK)*.

434-k

Glyceryl Mono-oleate
Monolein.

CAS — 25496-72-4 (mono-oleate).

Pharmacopoeias. In *Aust.* and *Nord. Aust.* specifies not less than 40% of α-monoglycerides calculated as glyceryl mono-oleate with variable amounts of di- and triglycerides; *Nord.* specifies not less than 90% of chloroform-soluble glycerides.

A mixture of the glycerides of oleic acid and other fatty acids, consisting mainly of the mono-oleate.
A yellow to brownish-yellow oily liquid or unctuous mass with a characteristic odour. Practically **insoluble** in water; miscible with alcohol. **Protect** from light. Glyceryl mono-oleate is obtainable in the non-dispersible form or in the self-emulsifying form.

Glyceryl mono-oleate has similar properties to and is used for the same purposes as glyceryl monostearate (p.1244) or self-emulsifying glyceryl monostearate (p.1244).

Proprietary Names and Manufacturers
Cithrol GMO *(Croda, UK)*.

435-a

Glyceryl Monostearate *(BAN, USAN)*.
Glycérol (Stéarate de); Glyceroli Monostearas; GMS; Monostearin.

CAS — 31566-31-1 (monostearate); 26657-96-5 (monopalmitate).

Pharmacopoeias. In *Aust., Br., Eur., Fr., Ger., Hung., Ind., It., Jpn, Neth., Pol.,* and *Swiss. Br.* and *Eur.* specify 40 to 50% of 1-monoacylglycerols calculated as 2,3-dihydroxypropyl stearate ($C_{21}H_{42}O_4$). Also in *U.S.N.F.* which specifies not less than 90% of monoglycerides.

A mixture of the monoglycerides of stearic and palmitic acids, together with variable quantities of di- and triglycerides.
A white or almost white hard waxy mass, powder, or flakes, greasy to the touch; odourless or with a slight fatty odour. M.p. about 57°. *B.P.* **solubilities** are: practically insoluble in water; soluble in ether and at 60° in alcohol. *U.S.N.F.* **solubilities** are: practically insoluble in water but may be dispersed in hot water with the aid of a small amount of soap or other suitable surfactant; soluble 1 in 10 of chloroform, 1 in 100 of ether and methyl alcohol, 1 in 33 of isopropyl alcohol; soluble in hot organic solvents. The *U.S.N.F.* allows a suitable antoxidant. **Store** in airtight containers. Protect from light.

Uses and Administration
Glyceryl monostearate is a poor water-in-oil emulsifying agent but it is a useful stabiliser of water-in-oil and oil-in-water emulsions in preparations for internal and external use. It has emollient properties. It is usual to add a small amount of soap, sulphated fatty alcohol, or other surfactant, which has the effect of making the product self-emulsifying (see Self-Emulsifying Glyceryl Monostearate) and capable of producing satisfactory oil-in-water emulsions.
Glyceryl monostearate is also used in the food and cosmetic industries.

Propriary Names and Manufacturers
Abracol SLG *(Bush Boake Allen, UK)*; Cerasynt SD *(Van Dyk, USA: Black, UK)*; Cithrol GMS *(Croda, UK)*; Empilan GMS NSE *(Albright & Wilson, Marchon Division, UK)*; Imwitor *(Dynamit Nobel, UK)*; Precirol *(Alfa, UK)*.

436-t

Self-Emulsifying Glyceryl Monostearate *(BAN)*.
Self-Emulsifying Mono- and Di-glycerides of Food Fatty Acids; Monostearin Emulsificans; Self-Emulsifying Monostearin.

Pharmacopoeias. In *Belg.* and *Br.*

A mixture consisting principally of mono-, di- and triglycerides of stearic and palmitic acids, and of minor proportions of other fatty acids; it may also contain free fatty acids, glycerol, and soap. It contains not less than 30% of monoglycerides, not more than 7% of free glycerol, and not more than 6% of soap, calculated as sodium oleate, all calculated with reference to the anhydrous substance.
A white to cream-coloured, hard, waxy solid with a faint fatty odour. Practically **insoluble** in water; dispersible in hot water; soluble in hot dehydrated alcohol and hot liquid paraffin; soluble in hot vegetable oils, but may give turbid solutions at concentrations below 20%. A 5% dispersion in hot water has a pH of 8.0 to 10.0 after cooling.
Because of the presence of soap, it is **incompatible** with acids and high concentrations of ionisable salts, hard water, calcium compounds, zinc oxide, and oxides of heavy metals.

Uses and Administration
Self-emulsifying glyceryl monostearate is used as an emulsifying agent for oils, fats, solvents, and waxes in the preparation of bases of the non-emulsified, emulsified, and vanishing-cream types.
It is not intended for inclusion in preparations for internal use.
Aqueous preparations containing self-emulsifying glyceryl monostearate should contain a preservative to prevent fungal or bacterial growth.

Proprietary Names and Manufacturers
Abracol GMS *(Bush Boake Allen, UK)*; Abracol GSP *(Bush Boake Allen, UK)*; Arlacel 165 *(ICI Speciality Chemicals, UK)*; Cerasynt 945 *(Black, UK; Van Dyk, USA)*; Cerasynt Q *(Black, UK; Van Dyk, USA)*; Cerasynt WM *(Black, UK; Van Dyk, USA)*; Empilan GMS *(Albright & Wilson, Marchon Division, UK)*; Imwitor *(Dynamit Nobel, UK)*.

447-f

Laureth 4 *(USAN)*.
CAS — 9002-92-0.

A mixture of monolauryl ethers of macrogols containing an average of 4 oxyethylene groups in the polyoxyethylene chain.

448-d

Laureth 9 *(USAN)*.
Polidocanol *(rINN)*.

CAS — 9002-92-0; 3055-99-0; 9015-55-8 (lauromacrogol 400).

NOTE. Lauromacrogol 400 has sometimes been described as containing 8 oxyethylene groups, but it is probably identical to laureth 9.

A mixture of monolauryl ethers of macrogols containing an average of 9 oxyethylene groups in the polyoxyethylene chain.

Adverse Effects
Extensive lichenified and excoriated dermatitis of the perianal and vulval skin in a woman following the use of Anacal Rectal Ointment was attributed, following sensitivity testing, to an ingredient of the ointment, laureth 9.— C. D. Calnan, *Contact Dermatitis*, 1978, *4*, 168.

A 63-year-old man developed pulmonary oedema, a dramatic fall in heart-rate, transient left pyramidal syndrome and died following sclerotherapy with laureth 9 to control gastric variceal bleeding; the fatality was attributed to the action of the drug that had passed into the systemic circulation.— A. Paterlini *et al.* (letter), *Lancet*, 1984, *1*, 1241.

Nasal irritation associated with intranasal insulin was dependent on the concentration of the surfactant, laureth 9.— R. Salzman *et al., New Engl. J. Med.*, 1985, *312*, 1078.

Uses and Administration
Lauromacrogols have been used as surfactants and spermicides. Laureth 9 is used as a sclerosing agent in the treatment of oesophageal and gastric varices, and has been used as a local anaesthetic.

ANTIMICROBIAL ACTIVITY. Laureth 9 suppressed the intrinsic resistance to some penicillins in *Staphylococcus aureus in vitro*.— W. Bruns *et al., Antimicrob. Ag. Chemother.*, 1985, *27*, 632.

OESOPHAGEAL VARICES. Laureth 9 is one of several sclerosants used to control variceal bleeding. Injections in some studies have consisted of 30 mg of laureth 9 in 1 mL of water with 0.05 mL of alcohol and 1 mL of this is injected into several sites at each session. These injections may be into the submucosa or directly into the varix. Galambos (*Ann. intern. Med.*, 1983, *98*, 1009) briefly reviewed several studies that showed paravariceal or intravariceal injection controlled the haemorrhage. However, he considered that the role of prophylactic endoscopic sclerotherapy was not yet defined. Terblanche (*Lancet*, 1986, *1*, 961) reviewed more recent work and considered that prophylactic sclerotherapy was unlikely to improve survival if the best available treatment is used for the first acute variceal haemorrhage.

Proprietary Names and Manufacturers of Lauromacrogols
Aethoxysklérol *(Kreussler, Switz.)*; Aethoxysklerol *(Aust.; Belg.; Kreussler, Denm.; Kreussler, Ger.; Neth.; Rus.; Kreussler, Swed.)*; Aetoxisclérol *(Dexo, Fr.)*; Atossisclerol *(Also, Ital.)*; Brij *(ICI Speciality Chemicals, UK)*; Empilan KB *(Albright & Wilson, Marchon Division, UK)*; Etoxisclerol *(Bama, Spain)*; Phlebodestal *(Ger.)*; Sclerovein *(Switz.)*; Sotravarix *(Belg.; Switz.)*.

The following names have been used for multi-ingredient preparations containing lauromacrogols— Alcos-Anal *(Norgine, Austral.)*.

748-l

Menfegol *(rINN).*
Menphegol. α-[p-(p-Menthyl)phenyl]-ω-hydroxypoly(oxyethylene).

CAS — 57821-32-6.

Menthylphenyl ethers of macrogols represented by the formula $C_{16}H_{23}.[O.CH_2.CH_2]_n.OH$.

Menfegol is a nonionic surfactant used as a spermicide.

Proprietary Names and Manufacturers
Neo Sampoon *(Eisai, Indon.)*; Neo-Sampoon *(Eisai, Malaysia; Eisai, Thai.)*.

487-q

Mono- and Di-glycerides *(USAN).*

Pharmacopoeias. In *U.S.N.F.*

A mixture of glyceryl mono- and di-esters, with small amounts of tri-esters, of fatty acids from edible oils. It contains not less than 40% of monoglycerides. It may contain suitable stabilisers. Practically **insoluble** in water; soluble in alcohol, chloroform, and ethyl acetate. **Store** in airtight containers. Protect from light.

Mono- and di-glycerides is an emulsifying and stabilising agent.

Proprietary Names and Manufacturers
Arlacel 186 *(ICI Speciality Chemicals, UK).*

450-k

Nonoxinols *(BAN, rINN).*

Macrogol Nonylphenyl Ethers; Nonoxynols *(USAN).* α-(4-Nonylphenyl)-ω-hydroxypoly(oxyethylene).

CAS — 26027-38-3; 7311-27-5 (nonoxinol 4).

Pharmacopoeias. U.S.P. includes Nonoxynol 9 and *U.S.N.F.* includes Nonoxynol 10.

A series of nonylphenyl ethers of macrogols of differing chain lengths, represented by the formula $C_{15}H_{23}.[O.CH_2.CH_2]_n.OH$. Each nonoxinol name is followed by a number indicating the approximate number of oxyethylene groups in the polyoxyethylene chain. Available nonoxinols include nonoxinol 4, nonoxinol 9, nonoxinol 10, nonoxinol 11, nonoxinol 15, and nonoxinol 30.

Nonoxinol 9 is a colourless to light yellow, clear viscous liquid. **Soluble** in water, alcohol, and maize oil. It has a pH of not greater than 0.2. **Store** in airtight containers.

Nonoxinol 10 is a colourless to light amber viscous liquid with an aromatic odour. **Soluble** in water and in polar organic solvents. **Store** in airtight containers.

Adverse Effects

Nonoxinols used as vaginal spermicides may cause local irritation. There have been a few reports of a toxic shock syndrome occurring in women who have used a contraceptive sponge impregnated with nonoxinol 9.

CYSTITIS. Severe cystitis occurred in a woman who had a contraceptive pessary containing nonoxinol 9 placed inadvertently in her bladder.— J. E. Gottesman (letter), *New Engl. J. Med.*, 1980, *302*, 633.

PREGNANCY AND THE NEONATE. Epidemiological evidence against an association between the use of spermicidal contraceptives and birth defects.— M. B. Bracken, *Am. J. Obstet. Gynec.*, 1985, *151*, 552.

Further references: C. Louik *et al.*, *New Engl. J. Med.*, 1987, *317*, 474; D. Warburton *et al.*, *ibid.*, 478.

TOXIC SHOCK SYNDROME. Thirteen cases of the toxic shock syndrome associated with the use of a vaginal contraceptive sponge impregnated with nonoxinol 9 were reviewed. These had been reported in the *USA* up to November 1984. In 4 of the cases, there were other predisposing conditions; postpartum use, use during menstruation, and prolonged retention.— G. Faich *et al.*, *J. Am. med. Ass.*, 1986, *255*, 216. See also.— A. L. Reingold, *ibid.*, 242.

Uses and Administration

Nonoxinols are used as surfactants. Some nonoxinols, especially nonoxinol 9, are used as spermicides.

ANTIMICROBIAL ACTIVITY. Although reported to be antiviral *in vitro* there was no beneficial effect from nonoxinol 9 cream in a double-blind placebo-controlled study in patients with genital herpes simplex.— L. A. Vontver *et al.*, *Am. J. Obstet. Gynec.*, 1979, *133*, 548.

Reports of *in vitro* activity of nonoxinol 9 against *Chlamydia trachomatis*.— S. Benes and W. M. McCormack, *Antimicrob. Ag. Chemother.*, 1985, *27*, 724; J. P. Kelly *et al.*, *ibid.*, 760.

A report of rapid *in vitro* inactivation of HIV-infected cultures of normal human lymphocytes by nonoxinol 9.— D. R. Hicks *et al.* (letter), *Lancet*, 1985, *2*, 1422. See also.— B. Voeller (letter), *ibid.*, 1986, *1*, 1153.

CONTRACEPTION. Reviews of the use of vaginal spermicides including nonoxinol 9 and octoxinol 9.— R. M. Pearson, *Pharm. J.*, 1985, *1*, 686; D. A. Grimes, *J. Am. med. Ass.*, 1986, *255*, 69; W. Bounds, *Pharm. J.*, 1986, *1*, 521.

Proprietary Preparations

C-Film *(Arun, UK). Vaginal film,* nonoxinol 67 mg/film.

Delfen *(Ortho-Cilag, UK). Vaginal cream,* nonoxinol '9' 5%.
Vaginal foam, aerosol, nonoxinol '9' 12.5%.

Double-Check *(Family Planning Sales, UK). Pessaries,* nonoxinol '9' 6%.

Duracreme *(LRC Products, UK). Vaginal cream,* nonoxinol '11' 2%.

Duragel *(LRC Products, UK). Vaginal gel,* nonoxinol '11' 2%.

Gynol II *(Ortho-Cilag, UK). Vaginal jelly,* nonoxinol '9' 2%.

Ortho-Creme *(Ortho-Cilag, UK). Vaginal cream,* nonoxinol '9' 2%.

Orthoforms *(Ortho-Cilag, UK). Pessaries,* nonoxinol '9' 5%.

Today *(Family Planning Sales, UK). Vaginal sponge,* nonoxinol '9' 1 g/sponge.

Two's Company *(Family Planning Sales, UK). Pessaries,* nonoxinol '9' 5%, supplied with sheaths.

Proprietary Names and Manufacturers

Antarox CO *(GAF, UK)*; Because Contraceptor *(Schering, USA)*; C-Film *(Hommel, Switz.; Arun, UK)*; Conceptrol *(Ortho Pharmaceutical, USA)*; Delfen *(Arg.; Austral.; Belg.; Ortho, Canad.; Cilag, Ger.; Neth.; Johnson & Johnson, S.Afr.; Cilag, Switz.; Ortho-Cilag, UK; Ortho Pharmaceutical, USA)*; Double-Check *(Family Planning Sales, UK)*; Duracreme *(LRC Products, UK)*; Duragel *(LRC Products, UK)*; Emko *(Schering, Canad.; Syntex, UK; Schering, USA)*; Empilan NP *(Albright & Wilson, Marchon Division, UK)*; Encare *(Thompson, USA)*; Genexol *(Rendell, UK)*; Gynol II *(Ortho-Cilag, UK)*; Igepal CO *(USA)*; Koromex *(Youngs, USA)*; Koromex II-A *(Youngs, USA)*; Lubrol N13 *(ICI Organics, UK)*; Ortho-Creme *(Canad.; Cilag, Ger.; Ortho-Cilag, UK; Ortho Pharmaceutical, USA)*; Orthodelfen *(Denm.; Fr.; Norw.)*; Orthoforms *(Ortho-Cilag, UK)*; Patentex *(CCD, Fr.; Patentex, Ger.; Patentex, Switz.)*; Ramses *(Schmid, USA)*; Rendells *(Rendell, UK)*; Semicid *(Bottu, Fr.; Whitehall, USA)*; S'Positive *(USA)*; Staycept Pessaries *(Syntex, UK)*; Synperonic *(ICI Petrochemicals, UK)*; Today *(Family Planning Sales, UK)*; Two's Company *(Family Planning Sales, UK)*; Ultrasure *(Warner, UK)*; Yadalan *(Llorente, Spain)*.

456-d

Octoxinols *(BAN, rINN).*
Macrogol Tetramethylbutylphenyl Ethers; Octoxynols *(USAN)*; Octylphenoxy Polyethoxyethanol. α-[4-(1,1,3,3-Tetramethylbutyl)phenyl]-ω-hydroxypoly(oxyethylene).

CAS — 9002-93-1.

Pharmacopoeias. U.S.N.F. includes Octoxynol 9.

A series of tetramethylbutylphenyl ethers of macrogols of differing chain lengths, represented by the formula $C_{14}H_{21}.[O.CH_2.CH_2]_n.OH$. Each octoxinol name is followed by a number indicating the approximate number of oxyethylene groups in the polyoxyethylene chain.

Octoxinol 9 is a clear, pale yellow, viscous liquid with a faint odour. **Miscible** with water, alcohol, and acetone; soluble in toluene; practically insoluble in petroleum spirit. **Store** in airtight containers.

Octoxinols are used as surfactants and spermicides.

Proprietary Preparations

Ortho-Gynol *(Ortho-Cilag, UK). Vaginal jelly, p*-di-iso-butyl-phenoxypolyethoxyethanol 1%.

Staycept Jelly *(Syntex, UK). Vaginal jelly,* octoxinol 1%.

Proprietary Names and Manufacturers
Antemin *(Napp, UK)*; Cirrasol AEN-XZ *(ICI Speciality Chemicals, UK)*; Koromex II *(Youngs, USA)*; Ortho-Gynol *(Cilag, Austral.; Ortho, Canad.; Fr.; Cilag, Ger.; Ortho-Cilag, UK; Ortho Pharmaceutical, USA)*; Preceptin *(Ortho-Cilag, UK)*; Staycept Jelly *(Syntex, UK)*; Synperonic *(ICI Petrochemicals, UK)*; Triton *(Rohm & Haas, UK)*.

The following names have been used for multi-ingredient preparations containing octoxinols— InterVir-A *(USA).*

463-f

Poloxamers *(BAN, USAN, rINN).*

Polyethylene-polypropylene glycol. α-Hydro-ω-hydroxypoly(oxyethylene)poly(oxypropylene)poly-(oxyethylene) block copolymer.

CAS — 9003-11-6.

Pharmacopoeias. In *U.S.N.F.*

A series of nonionic polyoxyethylene-polyoxypropylene copolymers with the general formula $HO(C_2H_4O)_a(C_3H_6O)_b(C_2H_4O)_aH$, in which a=2 to 130 and b=15 to 67. Each poloxamer name is followed by a number, e.g. poloxamer 188. The first 2 digits, when multiplied by 100, correspond to the approximate average molecular weight of the polyoxypropylene portion of the molecule; the third digit, when multiplied by 10, corresponds to the percentage by weight of the polyoxyethylene portion.

The available grades vary from liquids through pastes to flakes or powders. Their properties range from hydrophobic liquids practically **insoluble** in water to solids which are very soluble in water and have high HLB values; they are freely soluble in alcohol. A 2.5% solution or dispersion in water has a pH of 5.0 to 7.5. Poloxamers have been reported to be **incompatible** with phenols. **Store** in airtight containers.

Poloxalene (SKF-18,667) is a poloxamer in which a in the general formula averages 12 and b averages 34; it has a molecular weight of about 3000.

Poloxamer 188 (poloxalkol) is a poloxamer in which a in the general formula averages 75 and b averages 30; it has a molecular weight of about 8350 and is a waxy solid.

Precautions

Poloxamers may increase the absorption of liquid paraffin and other fat-soluble substances.

Uses and Administration

Poloxamers are used as emulsifying agents for intravenous fat emulsions, as solubilising agents to maintain clarity in elixirs and syrups, and as wetting agents for antibiotics.

Poloxalene is used as a defoaming agent in the treatment of bloat in ruminants.

Poloxamer 188 is used as a wetting agent in the

treatment of constipation. It is usually administered in combination with a laxative such as danthron.

Proprietary Names and Manufacturers of Poloxamers and Related Compounds
Alaxin *(USA)*; Alkènide *(Bottu, Fr.)*; Coloxyl Drops *(Fawns & McAllan, Austral.)*; Falkas *(Arg.)*; Idrocol *(Lafon, Fr.)*; Pliagel *(USA)*; Pluronic *(Pechiney, UK)*; Supronic *(ABM Chemicals, UK)*; Tetronic *(Pechiney, UK)*.

The following names have been used for multi-ingredient preparations containing poloxamers and related compounds— Dorbanex *(Riker, Canad.*; *Swed.*; *Riker, UK)*.

NOTE. Compounded preparations of danthron and poloxamer 188 in the mass proportions of 1 part to 8 parts have the British approved name co-danthramer.

18355-g

Polyoxyl 35 Castor Oil *(USAN)*.

Pharmacopoeias. In *U.S.N.F.*

A mixture of the triricinoleate ester of ethoxylated glycerol with smaller amounts of macrogol ricinoleate and the corresponding free glycols. It is produced by reacting 1 mole of glycerol ricinoleate with about 35 moles of ethylene oxide.

A yellow oily liquid with a faint characteristic odour. Sp. gr. 1.05 to 1.06; viscosity at 25°, 650 to 850 cP. Very **soluble** in water; soluble in alcohol and ethyl acetate; practically insoluble in liquid paraffin. **Store** in airtight containers.

Adverse Effects
Polyethoxylated castor oils (Cremophor EL) used as vehicles in various intravenous injections have been associated with severe anaphylactoid reactions and hyperlipidaemias.

References to the adverse effects, including anaphylaxis and hyperlipidaemias, associated with polyoxyl 35 castor oil.— A. G. Bagnarello *et al.*, *New Engl. J. Med.*, 1977, *296*, 497; A. R. W. Forrest *et al.* (letter), *Br. med. J.*, 1977, *2*, 1357; D. Dye and J. Watkins, *Br. med. J.*, 1980, *280*, 1353; D. L. Howrie *et al.*, *Drug Intell. & clin. Pharm.*, 1985, *19*, 425; B. Chapuis *et al.*, *New Engl. J. Med.*, 1985, *312*, 1259.

Uses and Administration
Polyoxyl 35 castor oil is a macrogol ester which is used as an emulsifying and solubilising agent. It has been used in vehicles for various intravenous injections.

Proprietary Names and Manufacturers of Polyoxyl 35 Castor Oil and Related Compounds
Cremophor EL *(BASF, Ger.*; *Blagden, UK)*; Etocas *(Croda, UK)*.

459-m

Polyoxyl 20 Cetostearyl Ether *(USAN)*.

Pharmacopoeias. In *U.S.N.F.*

A mixture of the monocetostearyl (mixed hexadecyl and octadecyl) ethers of mixed macrogols, the average polymer length being equivalent to 17.2 to 25 oxyethylene units.

A cream-coloured waxy unctuous mass melting, when heated, to a clear brownish-yellow liquid. **Soluble** in water, alcohol, and acetone; practically insoluble in petroleum spirit. A 10% solution in water has a pH of 4.5 to 7.5. **Store** in a cool place in airtight containers.

Polyoxyl 20 cetostearyl ether is a macrogol ether used as a surfactant.

18356-q

Polyoxyl 40 Hydrogenated Castor Oil *(USAN)*.

Pharmacopoeias. In *U.S.N.F.*

A mixture of the trihydroxystearate ester of ethoxylated glycerol, with smaller amounts of macrogol trihydroxystearate and the corresponding free glycols. It is produced by reacting 1 mole of glycerol trihydroxystearate with about 40 to 45 moles of ethylene oxide.

A white to yellowish paste or pasty liquid with a faint odour. Congealing range 20° to 30°. Very **soluble** in water; soluble in alcohol and ethyl acetate; practically insoluble in liquid paraffin. **Store** in airtight containers.

Polyoxyl 40 hydrogenated castor oil is a nonionic surfactant which is used as an emulsifying and solubilising agent.

Proprietary Names and Manufacturers of Polyoxyl 40 Hydrogenated Castor Oil and Related Compounds
Cremophor RH *(BASF, Ger.*; *Blagden, UK)*; Croduret *(Croda, UK)*.

460-t

Polyoxyl 10 Oleyl Ether *(USAN)*.

Polyethylene Glycol Mono-oleyl Ether.

CAS — 9004-98-2.

Pharmacopoeias. In *U.S.N.F.*

A mixture of the mono-oleyl ethers of mixed macrogols, the average polymer length being equivalent to 8.6 to 10.4 oxyethylene units. It may contain suitable stabilisers.

A soft white semisolid or pale yellow liquid with a bland odour. **Soluble** in water and alcohol; dispersible in liquid paraffin and propylene glycol with possible separation on standing. **Store** in a cool place in airtight containers.

Polyoxyl 10 oleyl ether is a macrogol ether used as a surfactant.

ANTIMICROBIAL ACTIVITY. A report of beneficial effects (faster crusting and healing times and rapid complete relief of symptoms) obtained with topical application of an ointment containing polyoxyl 10 oleyl ether and another surfactant in a double-blind study involving 69 patients with recurrent genital, perianal, or orofacial herpes simplex infection.— C. B. Goldberg, *Lancet*, 1986, *1*, 703.

Proprietary Names and Manufacturers of Polyoxyl 10 Oleyl Ether and Related Compounds
Ameroxol OE *(Anstead, UK*; *Amerchol, USA)*; Brij *(ICI Speciality Chemicals, UK)*; Crodafos *(Croda, UK)*; Volpo N *(Croda, UK)*.

The following names have been used for multi-ingredient preparations containing polyoxyl 10 oleyl ether and related compounds— InterVir-A *(USA)*.

440-z

Polyoxyl 8 Stearate *(BAN, USAN)*.

430; Macrogol Ester 400 *(rINN)*; Macrogol Stearate 400; Polyoxyethylene 8 Stearate; Polyoxyethylene Glycol 400 Stearate.

CAS — 9004-99-3.

NOTE. Two systems of nomenclature are used for these compounds, which have the general formula $C_{17}H_{35}COO.[O.CH_2CH_2]_n.H$. The number '8' in the name 'Polyoxyethylene 8 Stearate' refers to the approximate polymer length in oxyethylene units. The number '400' in the name 'Polyoxyethylene Glycol 400 Stearate' refers to the average molecular weight of the polymer chain.

Pharmacopoeias. Substances of similar composition are included in *Aust.*, *Ger.*, and *Swiss. Fr.* includes Stéarate de Polyoxyéthylène-glycol 300, which consists of a mixture of mono- and di-esters of palmitic and stearic acids with macrogol 300. *Fr.* also includes Glycérides Polyoxyéthylénés Glycolysés, which are the products obtained by partial esterification of natural vegetable oils with macrogols of molecular weight between 200 and 400. They consist of glycerides with a certain proportion of macrogol esters.

A mixture of the monostearate and distearate esters of mixed macrogols and the corresponding free glycols, the average polymer length being equivalent to about 8 oxyethylene units.

A cream-coloured, soft, waxy solid. M.p. about 29°. **Dispersible** in warm water. It has been reported to be **incompatible** with strong acids and alkalis, phenols, potassium iodide, tannins, and salts of bismuth, mercury, and silver.

441-c

Polyoxyl 40 Stearate *(BAN, USAN)*.

431; Estearato de Polioxila 40; Macrogol Ester 2000 *(rINN)*; Macrogol Stearate 2000; Polyoxyaethenum Stearinicum; Polyoxyethylene 40 Stearate; Stearethate 40.

CAS — 9004-99-3.

Pharmacopoeias. In *Arg.*, *Braz.*, *Hung.*, *Jpn*, and *Turk.* Also in *U.S.N.F.* Some describe only the monostearate ester.

A mixture of the monostearate and distearate esters of mixed macrogols and the corresponding free glycols, the average polymer length being equivalent to about 40 oxyethylene units.

A waxy solid which is white to light tan in colour and is odourless or has a faint fatty odour. Congealing range 37° to 47°.

Soluble in water, alcohol, acetone, and ether; practically insoluble in liquid paraffin and fixed oils. **Store** in airtight containers.

442-k

Polyoxyl 50 Stearate *(USAN)*.

Polyoxyethylene 50 Stearate.

CAS — 9004-99-3.

Pharmacopoeias. In *U.S.N.F.*

A mixture of the monostearate and distearate esters of mixed macrogols and the corresponding free glycols, the average polymer length being equivalent to about 50 oxyethylene units.

A cream-coloured soft waxy solid with a faint fatty odour. M.p. about 45°. **Soluble** 1 in 0.7 of water, 1 in 13 000 of dehydrated alcohol, 1 in 0.45 of chloroform, and 1 in 14 000 of ether. Soluble in isopropyl alcohol. **Store** in airtight containers.

Uses and Administration
Polyoxyl stearates are macrogol esters which are used as emulsifying and solubilising agents. Polyoxyl 8 monolaurate, and the mono-oleate and di-oleate esters are also available commercially.

Estimated acceptable total daily intake of polyoxyl 8 stearate and polyoxyl 40 stearate used in combination: up to 25 mg per kg body-weight.— Seventeenth Report of FAO/WHO Expert Committee on Food Additives, *Tech. Rep. Ser. Wld Hlth Org. No. 539*, 1974.

Proprietary Names and Manufacturers of Polyoxyl Stearates and Related Compounds
Cerasynt 616 *(Black, UK*; *Van Dyk, USA)*; Cerasynt 660 *(Black, UK*; *Van Dyk, USA)*; Cerasynt 840 *(Black, UK*; *Van Dyk, USA)*; Cithrol *(Croda, UK)*; Cremophor S9 *(BASF, Ger.*; *Blagden, UK)*; Crodet *(Croda, UK)*; Empilan AQ100 *(Albright & Wilson, Marchon Division, UK)*; Empilan BQ100 *(Albright & Wilson, Marchon Division, UK)*; Emulsynt *(Black, UK*; *Van Dyk, USA)*; Myrj *(ICI Speciality Chemicals, UK)*; Nonex *(BP Chemicals, UK)*.

472-d

Polysorbate 20 *(BAN, USAN, rINN)*.

432; Polyoxyethylene 20 Sorbitan Monolaurate; Polysorbatum 20; Sorbimacrogol Laurate 300; Sorboxaethenum Laurinicum.

$C_{58}H_{114}O_{26}$ (approximate).

CAS — 9005-64-5.

Pharmacopoeias. In *Aust.*, *Br.*, *Eur.*, *Fr.*, *Ger.*, *Hung.*, *Ind.*, *It.*, *Neth.*, and *Swiss.* Also in *U.S.N.F.*

A mixture of partial lauric esters of sorbitol and its mono- and di-anhydrides copolymerised with approximately 20 moles of ethylene oxide for each mole of sorbitol and its anhydrides.

The lauric acid used for esterification may contain variable amounts of other fatty acids.

A clear or slightly opalescent yellowish or brownish-yellow oily liquid with a faint characteristic

odour. Relative density about 1.1; viscosity, at 25°, about 400 cP.
Miscible with water, alcohol, dioxan, and ethyl acetate; practically insoluble in liquid paraffin and fixed oils. **Store** in airtight containers. Protect from light.

427-a

Polysorbate 40 *(BAN, USAN, rINN).*

434; Polyoxyethylene 20 Sorbitan Monopalmitate; Sorbimacrogol Palmitate 300.
$C_{62}H_{122}O_{26}$ (approximate).

CAS — 9005-66-7.

Pharmacopoeias. In *U.S.N.F.*

A mixture of partial palmitic esters of sorbitol and its mono-and di-anhydrides copolymerised with approximately 20 moles of ethylene oxide for each mole of sorbitol and its anhydrides. A yellow oily liquid with a faint characteristic odour.
Soluble in water and alcohol; practically insoluble in liquid paraffin and in fixed oils. **Store** in airtight containers.

474-h

Polysorbate 60 *(BAN, USAN, rINN).*

435; Polyoxyethylene 20 Sorbitan Mono-stearate; Polysorbatum 60; Sorbimacrogol Stearate 300; Sorboxaethenum Stearinicum.
$C_{64}H_{126}O_{26}$ (approximate).

CAS — 9005-67-8.

Pharmacopoeias. In *Aust., Br., Cz., Eur., Fr., Ger., Hung., It., Neth.,* and *Swiss.* Also in *U.S.N.F.*

A mixture of partial stearic esters of sorbitol and its mono-and di-anhydrides copolymerised with approximately 20 moles of ethylene oxide for each mole of sorbitol and its anhydrides. The stearic acid used for esterification may contain variable amounts of other fatty acids especially palmitic acid.
An opaque lemon-coloured or yellowish-brown semi-gel which becomes a clear liquid above 25°; it has a faint characteristic odour. Relative density about 1.1.
Miscible with water, alcohol, methyl alcohol, and ethyl acetate; practically insoluble in liquid paraffin and fixed oils. **Store** in airtight containers. Protect from light.

475-m

Polysorbate 65 *(BAN, USAN, rINN).*

436; Polyoxyethylene 20 Sorbitan Tristearate; Sorbimacrogol Tristearate 300.
$C_{100}H_{194}O_{28}$ (approximate).

CAS — 9005-71-4.

A mixture of partial stearic and palmitic esters, mainly tristearate, of sorbitol and its mono- and di-anhydrides copolymerised with approximately 20 moles of ethylene oxide for each mole of sorbitol and its anhydrides.
A tan-coloured waxy solid with a faint characteristic odour.
Dispersible in water; soluble in alcohol, liquid paraffin, and fixed oils. **Store** in airtight containers.

476-b

Polysorbate 80 *(BAN, USAN, rINN).*

433; Olethytan 20; Polyäthylenglykol-Sorbitan-oleat; Polyoxyethylene 20 Sorbitan Mono-oleate; Polysorbatum 80; Polysorbitanum 80 Oleinatum; Sorbimacrogol Oleate 300; Sorboxaethenum Oleinicum; Sorethytan 20 Mono-oleate.
$C_{64}H_{124}O_{26}$ (approximate).

CAS — 9005-65-6.

Pharmacopoeias. In *Arg., Aust., Br., Braz., Chin., Cz., Eur., Fr., Ger., Hung., Ind., It., Jpn, Neth., Nord., Port., Roum.,* and *Swiss.* Also in *U.S.N.F.*

A mixture of partial oleic esters of sorbitol and its mono- and di-anhydrides copolymerised with approximately 20 moles of ethylene oxide for each mole of sorbitol and its anhydrides.
A clear yellowish or brownish-yellow oily liquid with a faint characteristic odour. Relative density about 1.08; viscosity, at 25°, about 400 cP.
Miscible with water, alcohol, ethyl acetate, and methyl alcohol; practically insoluble in liquid paraffin and fixed oils. **Store** in airtight containers. Protect from light.

477-v

Polysorbate 85 *(BAN, USAN, rINN).*

Polyoxyethylene 20 Sorbitan Trioleate; Sorbimacrogol Trioleate 300.
$C_{100}H_{188}O_{28}$ (approximate).

CAS — 9005-70-3.

A mixture of partial oleic esters, mainly trioleate, of sorbitol and its mono- and di-anhydrides copolymerised with approximately 20 moles of ethylene oxide for each mole of sorbitol and its anhydrides.
An amber-coloured oily liquid with a faint characteristic odour.
Dispersible in water; soluble in alcohol.
Polysorbates have been reported to be **incompatible** with alkalis, heavy metal salts, phenols, and tannic acid; they may reduce the activity of many preservatives.

STABILITY IN SOLUTION. Aqueous solutions of polysorbates underwent autoxidation on storage.— M. Donbrow *et al., J. pharm. Sci.,* 1978, *67,* 1676.

Adverse Effects and Precautions

Polysorbates may increase the absorption of fat-soluble substances. Allergic reactions following topical application of preparations containing polysorbates have occasionally been reported.

EFFECTS ON THE LIVER. Eight preterm infants developed progressively deteriorating symptoms, chiefly characterised by liver failure and massive ascites, and 5 of them died after receiving vitamin E supplements intravenously in the total parenteral nutrition solution. The solubilising agents in the vitamin E preparation were polysorbate 80 and polysorbate 20 and it was recommended that caution should be observed in using any injectable product containing large amounts of polysorbate when treating low birth-weight infants.— J. Butler *et al.* (letter), *Am. J. Hosp. Pharm.,* 1984, *41,* 1514.

Uses and Administration

Polysorbates are hydrophilic nonionic surfactants which are used as emulsifying agents for the preparation of stable oil-in-water emulsions in pharmaceutical products, cosmetics, insecticides, and other products; they are frequently used with a sorbitan ester in varying proportions to produce products with a range of texture and consistency. They are also used as emulsifiers in the food industry.
Polysorbates are used as solubilising agents for a variety of substances including essential oils and oil-soluble vitamins such as vitamins A, D, and E; they are also used as wetting agents in the formulation of oral and parenteral suspensions.
Polysorbates have been used to promote increased absorption of dietary fat in conditions in which steatorrhoea is prominent, such as coeliac disease or sprue.

Estimated acceptable daily intake of polysorbates 20, 40, 60, 65, and 80; up to 25 mg per kg body-weight as total polysorbate esters.— Seventeenth Report of FAO/WHO Expert Committee on Food Additives, *Tech. Rep. Ser. Wld Hlth Org. No. 579,* 1974.

DEFICIENCY IN FAT ABSORPTION. A study in 12 patients with steatorrhoea due to bile-salt deficiency suggested that a diet containing polysorbates may result in improved fat absorption.— R. F. G. J. King *et al., Gut,* 1977, *18,* A-426.

Preparations

Emulsifying Wax *(U.S.N.F.).* A waxy solid prepared from cetostearyl alcohol containing a polysorbate. M.p. 48° to 52°. A 3% dispersion in water has a pH of 5.5 to 7.0.

For Emulsifying Wax (*B.P.*), see p.1325.

Proprietary Names and Manufacturers of Polysorbates
Crillet *(Croda, UK)*; Oleosorbate 80 *(Merck Sharp & Dohme-Chibret, Fr.; Chibret, Switz.)*; Oleosorbato 80 *(Spain)*; Sorbanox *(Witco, UK)*; Tween *(ICI Speciality Chemicals, UK).*

468-b

Polyvinyl Alcohol *(USAN).*

CAS — 9002-89-5.

Pharmacopoeias. In *Jug.* and *U.S.*

A synthetic resin represented by the formula $(-CH_2CHOH-)_n$, where the average value of n is 500 to 5000. It is prepared by 87 to 89% hydrolysis of polyvinyl acetate. A range of polyvinyl alcohols of varying viscosity and saponification value are available commercially.
White to cream-coloured odourless granules or powder. Freely **soluble** in water; more rapidly soluble at higher temperatures. A 4% solution in water has a pH of 5.0 to 8.0. **Store** in airtight containers.

Uses and Administration

Polyvinyl alcohol is a nonionic surfactant which is used as a stabilising agent and as a lubricant in various ophthalmic preparations such as artificial tears and contact lens solutions. It has also been used to increase the viscosity of ophthalmic preparations thus prolonging contact of the active ingredient with the eye. Polyvinyl alcohols of various grades are used for a wide variety of industrial applications.
Polyvinyl alcohols have also been used in the preparation of jellies which dry rapidly when applied to the skin to form a soluble plastic film.

Proprietary Preparations

Hypotears *(CooperVision, UK). Eye-drops,* polyvinyl alcohol 1%, macrogol '8000' 2%.

Liquifilm Tears *(Allergan, UK). Eye-drops,* polyvinyl alcohol 1.4%.

Sno Tears *(Smith & Nephew Pharmaceuticals, UK). Eye-drops,* polyvinyl alcohol 1.4%.

Proprietary Names and Manufacturers

Contafilm *(Allergan, Ger.)*; Hypotears *(Coopervision, Canad.; Cooper-Vision, UK)*; Kunstig Tarevaeske PVA *(NAF, Norw.)*; Lacril *(Allergan, Denm.)*; Liquifilm Tears *(Arg.; Allergan, Austral.; Belg.; Allergan, Canad.; Allergan, Ger.; Allergan, UK)*; Neo Tears *(Barnes-Hind, Canad.)*; Polyviol *(Wacker Chemicals, UK)*; Pre-Sert *(Allergan, Austral.)*; Sno Tears *(Smith & Nephew Pharmaceuticals, UK)*; Total *(Allergan, Austral.).*

The following names have been used for multi-ingredient preparations containing polyvinyl alcohol—Tears Plus *(Allergan, Canad.).*

437-x

Propylene Glycol Monostearate *(USAN).*

Propylèneglycol (Stéarate de); Propylene Glycol Stearate; Prostearin.

CAS — 1323-39-3 (monostearate); 29013-28-3 (monopalmitate).

Pharmacopoeias. In *Fr.* Also in *U.S.N.F.*
U.S.N.F. specifies not less than 90% of monoesters and not more than 1% of free glycerol and propylene glycol; *Fr. P.* specifies not less than 50% of monoesters and not more than 8% of free propylene glycol.

A variable mixture of the propylene glycol mono- and di-esters of stearic and palmitic acids, consisting mainly of the monoesters.
White wax-like solid, beads, or flakes, with a slight agreeable fatty odour. F.p. not less than 45°. Practically **insoluble** in water but it may be dispersed in hot water with the aid of a small amount of soap or other suitable surfactant; soluble in alcohol, acetone, ether, and in

fixed and mineral oils. It is obtainable in the pure, non-dispersible form, or in the self-emulsifying form containing a small proportion of soap or other primary emulsifying agent.

Propylene glycol monostearate is used as a stabiliser or emulsifier similarly to glyceryl monostearate (p.1244) or self-emulsifying glyceryl monostearate (p.1244). Propylene glycol monolaurate and mono-oleate are also available commercially.

Estimated acceptable daily intake of propylene glycol esters of fatty acids; up to 25 mg, as propylene glycol, per kg body-weight.— Seventeenth Report of FAO/WHO Expert Committee on Food Additives, *Tech. Rep. Ser. Wld Hlth Org. No. 539*, 1974.

Proprietary Names and Manufacturers
Cerasynt PA *(Van Dyk, USA: Black, UK)*; Cithrol PGMS *(Croda, UK)*.

469-v

Quillaia *(BAN)*.
Panama Wood; Quillaia Bark; Quillaiae Cortex; Seifenrinde; Soap Bark.

CAS — 631-01-6 (quillaic acid).

Pharmacopoeias. In *Arg., Aust., Br., Egypt., Nord., Port.,* and *Swiss. Br.* also includes Powdered Quillaia.

The dried inner part of the bark of *Quillaja saponaria* and other species of *Quillaja* (Rosaceae), containing not less than 22% of alcohol (45%)-soluble extractive. It is odourless but the dust or powder is strongly sternutatory. It contains 2 amorphous saponin glycosides, quillaic acid and quillaiasapotoxin.

Adverse Effects
Quillaia taken by mouth has been reported to produce severe gastro-intestinal irritation. The ingestion of large amounts may result in systemic poisoning with liver damage, respiratory failure, convulsions, and coma.
Quillaia has been reported to cause haemolysis of red blood cells after intravenous administration.

Uses and Administration
Quillaia is used as an emulsifying agent and frothing agent; it is often used in combination with tragacanth mucilage or other thickening agent.

Estimated acceptable daily intake of quillaia extract: up to 5 mg per kg body-weight.— Twenty-ninth Report of FAO/WHO Expert Committee on Food Additives, *Tech. Rep. Ser. Wld Hlth Org. No. 733*, 1986.

Preparations
Quillaia Liquid Extract *(B.P.)*. 1 in 1; prepared by percolation with alcohol (45%).
Quillaia Tincture *(B.P.)*. Quillaia liquid extract 5 mL, alcohol (45%) to 100 mL.

Proprietary Names and Manufacturers
Ceylania *(Deglaude, Fr.)*.

478-g

Sorbitan Monolaurate *(BAN, USAN)*.
493; Sorbitan Laurate *(rINN)*.
$C_{18}H_{34}O_6$ (approximate).

CAS — 1338-39-2.

Pharmacopoeias. In *Br.* Also in *U.S.N.F.*

A mixture of the partial esters of sorbitol and its mono- and di-anhydrides with lauric acid.
An amber-coloured viscous oily liquid with an odour characteristic of fatty acids. Wt per mL about 1.0 g; viscosity, at 25°, about 4500 cP.
Practically **insoluble** but dispersible in water; miscible with alcohol; slightly soluble in cottonseed oil. **Store** in airtight containers.

479-q

Sorbitan Mono-oleate *(BAN)*.
494; Sorbitan Monooleate *(USAN)*; Sorbitan Oleate *(rINN)*.
$C_{24}H_{44}O_6$ (approximate).

CAS — 1338-43-8.

Pharmacopoeias. In *Br.* Also in *U.S.N.F.*

A mixture of the partial esters of sorbitol and its mono- and di-anhydrides with oleic acid.
An amber-coloured viscous oily liquid with an odour characteristic of fatty acids. Wt per mL about 1.0 g; viscosity, at 25°, about 1000 cP.
Practically **insoluble** but dispersible in water; miscible with alcohol. **Store** in airtight containers.

480-d

Sorbitan Monopalmitate *(BAN, USAN)*.
495; Sorbitan Palmitate *(rINN)*.
$C_{22}H_{42}O_6$ (approximate).

CAS — 26266-57-9.

Pharmacopoeias. In *U.S.N.F.*

A mixture of the partial esters of sorbitol and its mono- and di-anhydrides with palmitic acid.
A cream-coloured, waxy solid with a faint fatty odour.
Practically **insoluble** in water; soluble in warm dehydrated alcohol; soluble with haze in warm liquid paraffin. **Store** in airtight containers.

481-n

Sorbitan Monostearate *(BAN, USAN)*.
491; Sorbitan Stearate *(rINN)*.
$C_{24}H_{46}O_6$ (approximate).

CAS — 1338-41-6.

Pharmacopoeias. In *Br.* Also in *U.S.N.F.*

A mixture of the partial esters of sorbitol and its mono- and di-anhydrides with stearic acid.
A pale yellow waxy solid with a faint oily odour. F.p. about 50°.
B.P. **solubilities** are: practically insoluble but dispersible in water; slightly soluble in alcohol. *U.S.N.F.* solubilities are: insoluble in cold water and in acetone; dispersible in warm water; soluble with haze, above 50°, in ethyl acetate and liquid paraffin. **Store** in airtight containers.

482-h

Sorbitan Sesquioleate *(BAN, USAN, rINN)*.

$C_{33}H_{60}O_{6.5}$ (approximate).

CAS — 8007-43-0.

Pharmacopoeias. In *Jpn* and *Swiss.*

A mixture of the partial mono- and di-esters of sorbitol and its mono- and di-anhydrides with oleic acid.

483-m

Sorbitan Trioleate *(BAN, USAN, rINN)*.

$C_{60}H_{108}O_8$ (approximate).

CAS — 26266-58-0.

A mixture of the partial tri-esters of sorbitol and its mono-and di-anhydrides with oleic acid.
Practically **insoluble** in water; soluble in alcohol and liquid paraffin.

484-b

Sorbitan Tristearate *(BAN, USAN, rINN)*.
492.
$C_{60}H_{114}O_8$ (approximate).

CAS — 26658-19-5.

A mixture of the partial tri-esters of sorbitol and its mono-and di-anhydrides with stearic acid.

Adverse Effects
There have been occasional reports of allergic skin reactions following the topical application of creams containing sorbitan esters.

A 59-year-old woman who developed contact dermatitis after application of Alphaderm cream to the legs produced a positive patch test to sorbitan monolaurate 5% which was used as an emulsifier in the preparation.— O. A. Finn and A. Forsyth, *Contact Dermatitis*, 1975, *1*, 318. See also.— J. Boyle and C. T. C. Kennedy, *Contact Dermatitis*, 1984, *10*, 178.

Of 486 patients with eczema, 2 gave positive patch tests to Arlacel '83' 20% and to a combination of Span '60' 5% and Span '80' 5%. In 412 of the patients, one gave a positive patch test to a combination of Tween '40' 5% and Tween '80' 5%.— M. Hannuksela *et al.*, *Contact Dermatitis*, 1976, *2*, 105.

A report of allergic contact dermatitis attributed to sorbitan mono-oleate.— J. Austad, *Contact Dermatitis*, 1982, *8*, 426.

Uses and Administration
Sorbitan esters are lipophilic nonionic surfactants which are used as emulsifying agents in the preparation of emulsions, creams, and ointments for pharmaceutical and cosmetic use. When used alone they produce stable water-in-oil emulsions but they are frequently used in combination with a polysorbate in varying proportions to produce water-in-oil or oil-in-water emulsions or creams with a variety of different textures and consistencies. Sorbitan esters are also used as emulsifiers and stabilisers in food.

Estimated acceptable daily intake of sorbitan monopalmitate, monostearate, and tristearate: up to 25 mg, as total sorbitan esters, per kg body-weight Seventeenth Report of FAO/WHO Expert Committee on Food Additives, *Tech. Rep. Ser. Wld Hlth Org. No. 539*, 1974. The sorbitan monoesters of lauric acid and oleic acids were considered and it was decided to include them in the group estimated acceptable daily intake for other sorbitan esters, namely up to 25 mg per kg.— Twenty-sixth Report of FAO/WHO Expert Committee on Food Additives, *Tech. Rep. Ser. Wld Hlth Org. No. 683*, 1982.

Proprietary Names and Manufacturers of Sorbitan Esters
Arlacel *(ICI Speciality Chemicals, UK)*; Crill *(Croda, UK)*; Nutra-D *(Alcon, Austral.)*; Span *(ICI Speciality Chemicals, UK)*.

NOTE. The name Arlacel has also been used to denote preparations of self-emulsifying glyceryl monostearate and a mixture of mono- and di-glycerides of fatty acids.

485-v

Sucrose Esters
Esterification of 1 or more hydroxyl groups in sucrose with a fatty acid such as stearic or palmitic acid produces nonionic compounds which possess surface-active properties. Commercial sucrose esters are mixtures of the mono-, di-, and tri-esters of palmitic and stearic acids with sucrose; various grades are available.

Uses and Administration
The sucrose esters are used as dispersing and emulsifying agents in food and cosmetic preparations.

Temporary estimated acceptable daily intake of sucrose esters of fatty acids and sucroglycerides: up to 2.5 mg per kg body-weight either individually or as the sum of both. Further metabolic and toxicity studies were required.— Twentieth Report of the Joint FAO/WHO Expert Committee on Food Additives, *Tech. Rep. Ser. Wld Hlth Org. No. 599*, 1976.

Properties of sucrose ester surfactants.— L. Chalmers, *Soap Perfum. Cosm.*, 1977, *50*, 191.

Proprietary Names and Manufacturers
Crodestas *(Croda, UK)*.

461-x

Tyloxapol *(BAN, USAN, rINN)*.
Superinone.

CAS — 25301-02-4.

Pharmacopoeias. In *U.S.*

A polymer of 4-(1,1,3,3-tetramethylbutyl)phenol with ethylene oxide and formaldehyde.
A viscous amber liquid, sometimes slightly turbid, with a slight aromatic odour. Slowly but freely **miscible** with water; soluble in chloroform, glacial acetic acid, carbon

disulphide, carbon tetrachloride, and toluene. A 5% solution in water has a pH of 4.0 to 7.0. Tyloxapol should not be allowed to come into contact with metals. **Store** in airtight containers.

Adverse Effects

Slight inflammation of the eyelids has been reported after prolonged use of aqueous inhalations. It has been reported that occasional febrile reactions may occur.

Uses and Administration

Tyloxapol is a nonionic surfactant of the alkyl aryl polyether alcohol type. Solutions have been used as an aqueous inhalation as a mucolytic agent for tenacious bronchopulmonary secretions. A 0.125% solution is nebulised as a fine dry spray from a suitable device. It is also used as a vehicle for irrigation solutions.

Proprietary Preparations

Alevaire *(Winthrop, UK). Solution,* tyloxapol 0.125%. For nebulisation or irrigation of bone or joint infections.

Proprietary Names and Manufacturers

Alevaire *(Winthrop, Canad.*; *Winthrop, Denm.*; *Swed.*; *Winthrop, Switz.*; *Winthrop, UK)*; Enuclene *(Alcon, Canad.)*; Lacermucin *(Lacer, Spain)*.

The following names have been used for multi-ingredient preparations containing tyloxapol—NTZ Superinone *(Winthrop, Austral.)*.

Nutritional Agents and Vitamins

570-h

The nutritional substances described in this chapter include amino acids, carbohydrates, certain fixed oils and trace elements, sweeteners, vitamins, and some miscellaneous substances with nutritional value. Compounds related to nutritional agents but which are described in other chapters include alcohol p.950, electrolytes p.1023, and iron compounds p.1189.

3839-c

Nutrition in Health

The principal constituents of food are carbohydrates, fats, minerals, proteins, vitamins, indigestible fibre, and water. Energy is provided by the metabolism of carbohydrates, fats, surplus protein, and alcohol.

The three main groups of **carbohydrate** found in food are sugars, starches, and cellulose and related materials; all of these are made up only of carbon, hydrogen, and oxygen.

Fats have the same elemental composition as carbohydrates, but with a lower proportion of oxygen.

Proteins are made up of carbon, hydrogen, oxygen, and nitrogen; most proteins also contain sulphur and some contain phosphorus. They are required for the regulation of body processes such as growth and tissue maintenance, and excess protein can be converted into carbohydrate and used to provide energy.

Proteins consist of chains of **amino acids** of which there are **essential** and **non-essential** types. Essential amino acids cannot be synthesised in sufficient amounts in the body and must therefore be present in food; non-essential amino acids can be synthesised in the body. There are eight essential amino acids: isoleucine, leucine, lysine, methionine, phenylalanine, threonine, tryptophan, and valine. Histidine and arginine are essential also for infant growth, and recent evidence has suggested that histidine may also be essential for adults.

Several inorganic elements, or minerals, are essential dietary constituents; those which are required in relatively small amounts are known as **trace elements**. Their main function is to act as essential cofactors in various enzyme systems.

Vitamins and their role in health are described on p.1253.

ENERGY AND PROTEIN REQUIREMENTS. The energy requirement of an individual is the level of energy intake from food that will balance energy expenditure consistent with long-term good health. The protein requirement of an individual is the lowest level of dietary protein that will balance the losses of nitrogen from the body in persons maintaining energy balance at modest levels of physical activity. In children and pregnant or lactating women the energy and protein requirements include the needs associated with the deposition of tissues or secretion of milk at rates consistent with good health. In the majority of cases the largest component of energy expenditure is the basal metabolic rate (BMR) which is determined principally by body-size, composition, and age; for practical purposes the most useful index of BMR is body-weight. Daily average energy requirements (derived as an estimate of energy expenditure) range from 6700 kJ (1650 kcal) to 17700 kJ (4200 kcal) in men, and from 6000 kJ (1400 kcal) to 14800 kJ (3500 kcal) in women. For adults the protein requirement per kg body-weight is considered to be the same for both sexes at all ages and body-weights within the acceptable range. The value accepted for the safe level of intake is 750 mg per kg per day, in terms of proteins with the digestibility of milk or egg.— Report of a Joint FAO/WHO/UNU Expert Consultation on Energy and Protein Requirements, *Tech. Rep. Ser. Wld Hlth Org. No. 724*, 1985.

See also *Recommended Daily Amounts of Food Energy and Nutrients for Groups of People in the United Kingdom, Report on Health and Social Subjects No. 15*, London, HM Stationery Office, 1979; *Recommended Dietary Allowances*, 9th Edn, Washington, The National Research Council, 1980; *Manual of Nutrition, Ministry of Agriculture, Fisheries, and Food*, London, HM Stationery Office, 1985.

TRACE ELEMENTS. Fourteen trace elements are believed to be essential for animal life. These are iron, iodine, copper, zinc, manganese, cobalt, molybdenum, selenium, chromium, nickel, tin, silicon, fluorine, and vanadium. All the essential elements become toxic at sufficiently high intakes and the margin between levels that are beneficial and those that are harmful may be small. In general however, deficiency in humans is unlikely and dietary intake is well below that required to cause toxic effects. Increased environmental exposure to several of the more toxic elements, notably lead, cadmium, mercury, and arsenic, as a result of increased industrialisation and motorisation of urban communities is also a matter of public health concern. Little is known of the maximum safe levels for man of long-term exposure to these elements in the food and water supply and the air.— *Trace Elements in Human Nutrition*, Report of a WHO Expert Committee, *Tech. Rep. Ser. Wld Hlth Org. No. 532*, 1973.

A review of the potential importance of trace elements in human nutrition with particular reference to zinc and vanadium.— M. H. N. Golden and B. E. Golden, *Br. med. Bull.*, 1981, *37*, 31.

3840-s

Dietary Modification

Diet may have to be modified or supplemented with respect to the requirements of particular groups of people such as infants, children, elderly people, pregnant or lactating women, and in patients with disorders such as Crohn's disease, diabetes mellitus, and hepatic or renal failure. Special diets may also have to be followed in conditions such as coeliac disease and food allergy.

AMINO ACID METABOLIC DISORDERS. A review of the dietary treatment in selected inherited metabolic disorders. In order to counteract the high blood concentrations of phenylalanine found in *phenylketonuria*, natural protein is restricted and replaced with either hydrolysates of natural protein or mixtures of synthetic L-amino acids. Since phenylalanine is an essential amino acid some natural protein must be given, but only enough to allow the blood-phenylalanine concentration to remain normal. The protein substitute cannot be utilised unless adequate energy and phenylalanine are provided at each meal, and regular monitoring of phenylalanine is essential. *Maple-syrup-urine disease*, involves accumulation of the three essential branched-chain amino acids leucine, valine, and isoleucine in the blood. The dietary treatment requires restriction of all three amino acids and is difficult to manage. A mixture of synthetic L-amino acids excluding these three provides a substitute for most of the protein, and regular monitoring of the branched-chain amino acids in the blood is essential. In this condition adequate energy is especially important as a catabolic state leads to severe acidosis. Glucose polymers and fats are useful for this purpose. Low-protein products as used in the treatment of phenylketonuria allow some variety in this difficult diet.— B. E. Clayton, *Prescribers' J.*, 1984, *24*, 26.

CANCER. A 2-part review on the relationship between diet and cancer. Evidence suggests that dietary factors have important causative and protective roles in carcinogenesis, but information about specific dietary factors is generally inconsistent or incomplete.— W. C. Willett and B. MacMahon, *New Engl. J. Med.*, 1984, *310*, 633 and 697.

Comment on food intake and energy expenditure in patients with cancer cachexia.— *Lancet*, 1984, *1*, 833.

CARBOHYDRATE METABOLIC DISORDERS. Results from a study in 6 children of mean age 4.2 years with glycogen storage disease Type I indicated that the minimal nasogastric infusion rate of carbohydrate (glucose and glucose polymer) needed to maintain plasma-glucose concentrations and suppress organic acidaemia was about 8 to 9 mg per kg per minute; this rate was associated with a plasma-glucose concentration of about 900 µg per mL.— W. F. Schwenk and M. W. Haymond, *New Engl. J. Med.*, 1986, *314*, 682.

CARDIOVASCULAR DISEASE. Dietary recommendations for the prevention of cardiovascular disease.—Report by the Committee on Medical Aspects of Food Policy, *Diet and Cardiovascular Disease, Report on Health and Social Subjects No. 28*, London, HM Stationery Office, 1984.

DIABETES MELLITUS. Dietary fat should be limited to approximately 30% of total daily energy intake, and foods containing polyunsaturated vegetable oils should be substituted for those containing saturated fats. Protein should account for approximately 15 to 20% of the daily intake, and carbohydrates rich in natural fibre should constitute the remaining food energy.— Report of a WHO Study Group on Diabetes Mellitus, *Tech. Rep. Ser. Wld Hlth Org. No. 727*, 1985.

Further references: *Lancet*, 1983, *1*, 741; J. I. Mann, *Br. med. J.*, 1984, *288*, 1025; *Lancet*, 1986, *1*, 720; M. E. J. Lean and W. P. T. James, *ibid.*, 723; W. P. Stephens, *Pharm. J.*, 1986, *1*, 670; J. Cantrill, *ibid.*, 1988, *1*, 390.

FOOD ALLERGY. A discussion on the diagnosis and management of food allergy. Food allergy is thought to play a significant role in urticaria, eczema, cows' milk protein enteropathy, infantile colitis, colic, migraine, and hyperactivity, while asthma and inflammatory bowel disease may sometimes be associated with food allergic reactions. However, the proportion of patients in whom it is important is unclear. The mainstay of treatment is total avoidance of offending foods, but keeping to a diet may be difficult and exclusion is often not absolute.— A. Cant, *Archs Dis. Childh.*, 1986, *61*, 730.

Further references: A. M. Denman, *Br. med. J.*, 1983, *286*, 1164; *Lancet*, 1984, *1*, 900; J. W. Gerrard (letter), *ibid.*, *2*, 413; S. Lingam, *Br. J. clin. Pract.*, 1985, *39*, 49; R. Finn, *ibid.*, 375.

GASTRO-INTESTINAL DISORDERS. *Crohn's disease*. In a randomised study of 21 patients with Crohn's disease treatment with an elemental diet was as effective as treatment with prednisolone in inducing remission; 80% of patients in each group were in remission by 4 weeks.— C. O'Moráin *et al.*, *Br. med. J.*, 1984, *288*, 1859.

A study of 70 patients with non-stenosing Crohn's disease who received either a low-residue diet or a normal Italian diet for a mean period of 29 months found no significant difference in outcome between the 2 groups. However, most patients had eliminated one or more foods from their diet because of presumed exacerbation of symptoms. It was concluded that a balanced diet is more appetising and richer in vitamins than one free of fibre.— S. Levenstein *et al.*, *Gut*, 1985, *26*, 989. See also A. J. Levi, *ibid.*, 985.

Cystic fibrosis. Steatorrhoea occurring in patients with cystic fibrosis is seldom controlled by pancreatin alone and reduction of fat in the diet is necessary. Elemental diets have been devised in order to supply all nutritional requirements but they are unpleasant to take and socially inconvenient. They have led to little change in the clinical status of patients studied and there may be an increased risk of deficiency of essential fatty acids and trace elements.— M. B. Mearns, *Archs Dis. Childh.*, 1985, *60*, 272.

Supplementary high-calorie feedings are increasingly used in cystic fibrosis patients with growth failure in an attempt to provide easier control of chest infection, better respiratory function, and extended survival. Feeds may be given by mouth (the preferred route), or by intravenous or enteral routes; nasogastric tubes and gastrostomy or jejunostomy tubes are used for enteral feeding.— *Lancet*, 1986, *1*, 249.

See also under Enteral and Parenteral Nutrition, below.

Short bowel syndrome. No apparent benefit was found from using a chemically-defined low-fat diet, as compared with a simpler whole protein fat-containing feed, in a study in 6 patients with short bowel syndrome. Patients with short bowel syndrome may absorb only a small proportion of calories administered, even though given as a liquid feed by slow infusion.— P. B. McIntyre *et al.*, *Gut*, 1983, *24*, A990.

HEPATIC ENCEPHALOPATHY. Protein restriction has become a cornerstone of treatment of hepatic encephalopathy but failure to provide adequate protein may lead to progressive depletion of body protein, and in turn to a reduced host defence to infection. Attention has therefore been focused on alternative ways of providing adequate protein without precipitating encephalopathy and some beneficial effect has been found with vegetable-protein, as opposed to animal-protein, diets. Vegetable diets may contain less, as yet unidentified, comagenic substances, may change bowel flora or bioavailability of other amino acids or, because of their bulk, alter bowel transit time and smooth out absorption from the bowel lumen. The major disadvantage of vegetable diets is that they are bulky and may not be well-tolerated because of abdominal bloating and gaseous distension.— I. R. Crossley and R. Williams, *Gut*, 1984, *25*, 85. See also *Lancet*, 1983, *1*, 625.

For reference to the use of branched-chain amino acids in the treatment of hepatic encephalopathy, see under Enteral and Parenteral Nutrition, p.1252.

HYPERKINETIC STATES. A discussion on food additives and hyperactivity.— *Lancet*, 1982, *1*, 662. See also D. J. Rapp (letter), *ibid.*, 1128; W. G. Crook (letter), *ibid.*

A discussion on diet and behaviour, with special reference to the Feingold diet.— E. Taylor, *Archs Dis. Childh.*, 1984, *59*, 97.

HYPERLIPOPROTEINAEMIA. Control of inherited Type V hyperlipoproteinaemia in a child by restriction of dietary fat and refined carbohydrates but without restriction of total calories.— G. N. Thompson *et al.*, *Archs Dis. Childh.*, 1987, *62*, 967.

MUSCULAR AND NEUROMUSCULAR DISORDERS. In a study in a patient with McArdle's syndrome (myophosphorylase deficiency) who had muscle weakness and wasting there was no improvement in exercise performance following carbohydrate ingestion but a marked improvement after ingestion of protein, or protein with carbohydrate. Long-term high-protein therapy produced a progressive improvement in muscle function, manifested primarily as improved endurance while muscle strength remained essentially unchanged.— A. E. Slonim and P. J. Goans, *New Engl. J. Med.*, 1985, *312*, 355. Comments.— R. B. Layzer, *ibid.*, 370; P. D. Thompson and M. M. Flynn (letter), *ibid.*, 1518. Reply.— A. E. Slonim and P. J. Goans (letter), *ibid.*, 1519.

NERVOUS SYSTEM DISORDERS. Beneficial neurological results following treatment with branched-chain amino acids in a preliminary study of 22 patients with amyotrophic lateral sclerosis.— A. Plaitakis *et al.*, *Lancet*, 1988, *1*, 1015.

PREGNANCY AND THE NEONATE. *In pregnancy.* Foetal condition is known to be affected by the quality of maternal diet, a better diet being associated with better condition of the offspring. However, investigations of the effects of additional calories or a high-protein diet during pregnancy have given conflicting results. Marginal imbalances in the diet are not fully understood; in developing nations with their immense problems of malnutrition the benefits of supplementation may be dramatic, but in affluent Western society its value is less certain. Little is known of the beneficial role trace elements and minerals play in human pregnancy. The heart of the problem is that, while the limitations of diagnosing deficiency states in daily practice are clearly recognised, routine supplementation with vitamins and other nutrients must be considered with caution.— A. Malhotra and R. S. Sawers, *Br. med. J.*, 1986, *293*, 465.

Further references: *Lancet*, 1983, *1*, 1142; J. V. G. A. Durnin *et al.*, *ibid.*, 1985, *2*, 823.

The neonate and infant feeding. The *preterm* infant's requirements for vitamins and trace elements are not known and supplementation is largely guesswork. Even the desirable intakes of major nutrients such as protein and principal energy sources are uncertain because, although minimum intakes have been defined and a certain amount is known about the protein and energy cost of growth, there is no agreement about the desirable rate and quality of growth. Breast milk is empirically safe in that potentially toxic metabolic disturbances are unlikely, and has the advantage of biological compatibility. However, human milk, especially preterm milk, is highly variable in composition and often deficient in important nutrients and many preterm infants therefore receive formula feeds at some stage. Commercial "premature" formulas have various common features: a higher protein content with a predominance of whey proteins, slightly higher energy, and more sodium, calcium, phosphorus, and other minerals than "full-term" formulas. Absorption of total energy, fat, and protein is comparable with that for breast milk. Detractors of formula feeding in the very immature point out the metabolic stress caused by a higher protein intake and an amino acid composition which differs from that of breast milk, the possibility of causing necrotising enterocolitis and cows' milk protein allergies, and the absence of the many substances which have anti-infective properties in raw human milk. For the moment, most neonatal paediatricians sit on the fence, being happy to feed the premature infants in their care on the babies' own mothers' milk with the addition of supplements or change to a formula when nutrient deficiencies occur.— O. G. Brooke, *Lancet*, 1983, *1*, 514.

At least 95% of mothers are able to breast-feed their infants for 4 to 6 months and can provide sufficient milk over this period to allow their babies to grow to their full potential. Attention is shifting to special "follow-up" formulas for babies over 4 to 6 months of age, the justification of which is to permit adequate protein, calcium, and iron intake. However, this can be naturally and effectively achieved either by continuing some breast-feeding or by giving about 500 mL of cows' milk daily and in both instances supplementing these milks with suitable weaning foods which may be prepared in the kitchen or by food manufacturers.— *Lancet*, 1986, *1*, 17.

Further references: R. G. Whitehead, *Lancet*, 1983, *1*, 167; *ibid.*, 1987, *1*, 843; Present Day Practice in Infant Feeding: Third Report, Report of a Working Party of the Panel on Child Nutrition, Committee on Medical Aspects of Food Policy, *Report on Health and Social Subjects*, *32*, London, HM Stationery Office, 1988.

RENAL FAILURE. A review in the form of questions on the dietary treatment of chronic renal failure (A.M. El Nahas and G.A. Coles, *Lancet*, 1986, *1*, 597) was followed by a review of answers on behalf of the steering committee of the European Study Groups for the Conservative Treatment of Chronic Renal Failure (S. Giovannetti, *ibid.*, *2*, 1140). Reasons for the existence of many low-protein diets include the attempts to adjust the degree of restriction to the severity of the renal failure and to adapt the low-protein diet to local dietary habits. The principles are the same whatever the diet: to reduce protein intake to the minimum required to maintain nitrogen balance, and with severe protein restriction essential amino acid supplements are required to prevent protein malnutrition; to reduce phosphorus intake to obtain normal serum-phosphate concentrations; to satisfy caloric requirements; to give calcium, iron, and multivitamin supplements. El Nahas and Coles favoured less restricted diets (standard 0.6 g of protein per kg body-weight daily) for future studies. The European Study Group disagreed with this preference on the grounds that if protein and phosphorus restrictions are beneficial for chronic uraemic patients, then the degree of such restrictions should be directly proportional, within certain limits, to the severity of the renal insufficiency. Correspondence.— A. M. El Nahas (letter), *Lancet*, 1987, *1*, 325; S. Giovannetti (letter), *ibid.*

WEIGHT-REDUCING DIETS. In general, few of the diets devised specifically for weight-reduction in obesity have been particularly successful. Reduction in sugar and fat intake with maintenance of starch and fibre is logical for preventive health and appropriate in view of the obese person's tendency to gain weight on fat-enriched diets. Weight-reducing regimens should ensure a sufficient intake of essential nutrients including vitamins and minerals. It is generally recommended that the diet should not be reduced below 4060 kJ (1000 kcal) except on medical advice and with close supervision.

Very low calorie diets have many disadvantages including the production of hypotension in susceptible individuals. Schedules consisting of as much protein and fat as is desired, along with an avoidance of sugar and starch, lead to a reduction in total energy intake and an increase in plasma-cholesterol concentrations which in the long-term may be conducive to atherosclerosis and other diseases.

Artificial sweeteners or other non-sucrose sweeteners are often used as part of weight-reducing diets as well as being widely used in the food industry. Intense and bulk sweeteners are included in this chapter, although some such as lactitol (p.1582) and mannitol (p.994) have additional uses and are described in other chapters.

Some other compounds that are used or been investigated as sweetening agents include monellin, stevioside, sucralose, and volemitol.

Reviews, studies, and discussions on very low calorie diets: T. A. Wadden *et al.*, *Ann. intern. Med.*, 1983, *99*, 675; P. Felig, *New Engl. J. Med.*, 1984, *310*, 589; *Lancet*, 1984, *2*, 500; V. Vertes, *Postgrad. med. J.*, 1984, *60*, *Suppl.* 3, 56; G. L. Blackburn, *ibid.*, 59; J. G. Wechsler *et al.*, *ibid.*, 66; A. J. Isaacs and P. S. Parry, *ibid.*, 74; A. J. Moss, *Ann. intern. Med.*, 1985, *102*, 121; J. V. G. A. Durnin, *Br. med. J.*, 1987, *294*, 1565; *Lancet*, 1987, *2*, 491.

Preparations

For Proprietary Preparations for Modified Diets, see p.1289.

3841-w

Enteral and Parenteral Nutrition

The main objective in providing nutritional support is to maintain the complex nitrogen-energy balance which may be altered by nutritional depletion and trauma. This support consists of administering nitrogen in the form of protein or amino acids and energy as carbohydrate or fat. Fluid and electrolyte, trace element, and vitamin requirements should also be met, particularly in long-term treatment. In general, larger doses are required by the enteral route than by the parenteral route because only a fraction of that given enterally is absorbed.

Enteral Nutrition, also known as Enteral Feeding, includes feeding by mouth, by nasoenteric or nasogastric tube, and through a gastrostomy, duodenostomy, or jejunostomy. Nitrogen is usually given as protein, except for elemental diets which contain amino acid mixtures. Carbohydrate and/or fat provide the non-protein energy. Nutritionally incomplete supplements can be used if there is a specific deficiency or if the deficiency is only likely to be short-term. Complications and adverse effects of enteral nutrition include diarrhoea, vomiting, abdominal pain, hyperglycaemia, fluid and electrolyte disturbances, infection, and mechanical problems as a result of tube insertion such as oesophagitis, regurgitation, and aspiration.

Parenteral Nutrition should only be used when it is impossible to meet nutritional requirements by the enteral route. It is more costly and has a higher incidence of adverse effects. It may be given either as a supplement to other forms of nutrition or on its own when it is often referred to as total parenteral nutrition (TPN). In the short-term, parenteral nutrition may be given via a peripheral vein, but for longer periods a central venous line must be used due to the high osmolarity of most TPN solutions. Simultaneous infusion of nitrogen and energy sources is necessary in order to maximise the rate of protein synthesis. Nitrogen is provided in the form of essential and non-essential amino acids, either as protein hydrolysates such as hydrolysates of casein but nowadays more often as mixtures of synthetic L-amino acids. Energy is provided by carbohydrate (glucose is the carbohydrate of choice) and fat in the form of lipid emulsions which have a relatively high energy content, low osmolarity, and also provide essential fatty acids. The fat emulsions have sometimes been administered from containers separate from the other ingredients. However, problems of stability have been overcome with some preparations where all the ingredients of a TPN solution can be administered from the one bag. Trace element and vitamin deficiencies which may occur during long-term TPN can be prevented by appropriate supplementation. Insulin may be required to prevent or correct hyperglycaemia caused by administration of large amounts of glucose. Complications of parenteral nutrition include catheter-related infection, pneumothorax, haemothorax, air embolism, extravasation, and arterial injury. Thrombophlebitis is often a problem when a peripheral vein is used.

The complex nature of solutions for parenteral nutrition renders them susceptible to compatibility problems. Stability is dependent upon several factors including pH and relative concentrations of the components. Amino acids exert a buffering effect on the overall pH of mixed solutions containing amino acids, glucose, and fat emulsion. Solutions containing electrolytes, particularly divalent cations, are not stable, and aggregation will eventually occur. Additives should be added only if there is known compatibility, and any additions performed aseptically before the start of the infusion. In general mixed parenteral nutrition solutions should be used immediately after preparation and administered to the patient within 24 hours.

The commercial source of different infusions and additives can have an important impact on the stability and compatibility of mixed solutions for parenteral nutrition. Small differences in composition of pH of the amino acid infusion can cause the preparation to become unstable. The most significant losses occurring in filled 3-litre bags are vitamins, especially vitamins A, B_1 (thiamine), and C.— M. C. Allwood, *J. clin. Hosp. Pharm.*, 1984, *9*, 181. See also P. W. Niemiec and T. W. Vanderveen, *Am. J. Hosp. Pharm.*, 1984, *41*, 893.

A discussion on the preparation and properties of fat emulsions for parenteral nutrition.— P. K. Hansrani *et al.*, *J. parent. Sci. Technol.*, 1983, *37*, 145.

A discussion on 10 years' experience of the use of disposable 3-litre bags for total parenteral nutrition.— G. Hardy, *Pharm. J.*, 1987, *2*, HS26.

Further references on the characteristics and content of parenteral nutrition mixtures: M. C. Allwood, *Br. J. parent. Ther.*, 1984, *5*, 113; C. R. Pennington *et al.*, *ibid.*, 1985, *6*, 37; V. A. Parry *et al.*, *Am. J. Hosp. Pharm.*, 1986, *43*, 3017.

Reviews, reports, and discussions on nutrition, malnutrition, and nutritional support with enteral and parenteral nutrition: M. Irving, *Br. med. J.*, 1985, *291*, 1404 (enteral and parenteral nutrition); S. M. Willatts, *Br. J. Anaesth.*, 1986, *58*, 201 (enteral and parenteral nutrition); R. L. Koretz, *Gut*, 1986, *27*, *Suppl.* 1, 85 (enteral and parenteral nutrition); S. B. Heymsfield *et al.*, *Ann. intern. Med.*, 1983, *98*, 168 (home nasoenteric feeding for malabsorption and weight loss); D. B. A. Silk, *Postgrad. med. J.*, 1984, *60*, 779 (enteral nutrition); *Drug & Ther. Bull.*, 1986, *24*, 61 (enteral feeds for adults); D. B. A. Silk, *Gut*, 1986, *27*, *Suppl.* 1, 40 (diet formulation and choice of enteral diet); *idem*, 116 (enteral nutrition); G. P. Young *et al.*, *Med. J. Aust.*, 1985, *143*, 597 (parenteral nutrition); American College of Physicians, *Ann. intern. Med.*, 1987, *107*, 252 (perioperative parenteral nutrition); M. A. Jackson, *Br. J. Hosp. Med.*, 1983, *29*, 105 (long-term home parenteral nutrition); M. W. N. Ward *et al.*, *Practitioner*, 1984, *228*, 831 (home parenteral nutrition); M. Mughal *et al.*, *Lancet*, 1986, *2*, 383 (home parenteral nutrition); D. A. Kelly *et al.* (letter), *ibid.*, 746 (home parenteral nutrition for children); M. Turner and L. A. Goldberg, *Intensive Therapy clin. Monit.*, 1987, *8*, 18 (home parenteral nutrition).

ADVERSE EFFECTS AND PRECAUTIONS. *Enteral nutrition.* Many of the problems encountered with enteral feeding can be avoided by using a fine bore tube, administering the feed by continuous infusion, and by careful monitoring of the patient for metabolic abnormalities. Fine bore tubes are easily misplaced or dislodged from the stomach, and it is important to ensure their correct positioning.— M. D. Bastow, *Gut*, 1986, *27*, *Suppl.* 1, 51.

An interaction between nutrients and antacids with formation of solid masses of protein-aluminium complexes and oesophageal obstruction occurred during enteral tube feeding in 3 patients. It was suggested that for enteric feeding, high molecular protein solutions should not be mixed with or followed by antacids, and that if an antacid is required it should be given some time after the nutrients with vigorous flushing of the tube beforehand.— C. Valli *et al.* (letter), *Lancet*, 1986, *1*, 747.

A report of an unusual oesophageal obstruction during nasogastric feeding with a nutritionally-complete feed (Osmolite) in a 74-year-old patient who had undergone a Polya gastrectomy 15 years previously. Rigid oesophagoscopy revealed blockage of the entire lower third of the oesophagus with a solid white substance which had the same macroscopic appearance as solidified Osmolite. Subsequent tests *in vitro* showed that solidification of Osmolite could be prevented by high concentrations of pepsin. Pepsin concentrations are reduced in patients with a partial gastrectomy, and the gastric pH may be low enough to cause this solidification.— A. Myo *et al.*, *Br. med. J.*, 1986, *293*, 596.

Parenteral nutrition. The principal complication of parenteral nutrition is infection of the intravenous feeding catheter which can produce septicaemia. If this happens the catheter must be removed. Thrombosis of the vessel into which the infusion is being delivered can occur. Extravasation of the infused fluid due to misplacement of the catheter tip is preventable by screening at the time of placing the catheter. Metabolic problems such as hyperglycaemia can arise from infusion of the glucose load, although this usually settles as the patient's body adapts to this form of treatment. In the long-term, trace element deficiencies can create problems, but these are preventable by careful monitoring.— M. Irving, *Br. med. J.*, 1985, *291*, 1404.

Cholestatic liver disease may develop during long-term TPN. It is reported to be most common in premature infants, with severity increasing with immaturity of the infant. Much controversy surrounds the cause but contributory factors may include essential fatty acid deficiency, protein hydrolysate toxicity (although liver disease has also occurred in infants receiving amino acids and lipid emulsion), and a build-up of sludge in the gallbladder.

Acute fatal right ventricular infarction which occurred in a 74-year-old patient was believed to have resulted from inadvertent intracardiac infusion of hyperosmotic parenteral nutrition solutions. The catheter had been inserted into the right subclavian vein but at autopsy the tip was found to have extended into the right ventricular cavity and the myocardium was necrotic and inflamed.— T. C. King and J. E. Saffitz, *Am. J. Cardiol.*, 1985, *55*, 1659.

Results from a retrospective study involving 50 medical and 50 surgical neonates indicated that serious complications from parenteral nutrition in the newborn period were relatively uncommon. Sepsis remained an unsolved problem and even when initial microbiological cultures are sterile the possibility of underlying fungal infection should be considered. Lack of enteral feeding was thought to be an important aetiological factor in the pathogenesis of parenteral-nutrition associated cholestasis, and the higher incidence which was found in surgical babies may have reflected the often necessary delay in starting milk when compared with medical neonates. The authors believed that in this respect it was important to reduce the period of absolute enteral starvation to a minimum, even if only a nutritionally insignificant amount of feed may be given by this route. Experience demonstrated that the incidence of major parenteral nutrition-related side-effects was not so high as to inhibit its use in the nutritional support of neonates.— J. W. L. Puntis *et al.*, *Intensive Therapy clin. Monit.*, 1987, *8*, 48.

A microscopic focus of hepatocellular carcinoma found at autopsy in a 6-month-old non-cirrhotic infant was believed to be associated with the prolonged administration of parenteral nutrition.— K. Patterson *et al.*, *J. Pediat.*, 1985, *106*, 797.

CANCER. Enteral and parenteral nutrition has revolutionised the management of the malnourished surgical patient. Wasting may now be corrected, with increase in body-weight, positive nitrogen balance, and restoration of immune response. Unequivocal evidence of clinical benefit is hard to obtain.— *Lancet*, 1983, *1*, 1025. The indications for using TPN in postoperative cancer patients are ill-defined. Data from retrospective studies were therefore used to form the basis of guidelines in order to avoid its overuse and indications were subsequently outlined. Postoperative TPN was not advocated in patients with pre-operative factors such as well-nourished state, age less than 60 years, and benign disease states of the organ systems undergoing resection. TPN was recommended, starting about 48 hours after surgery, in patients with pre-operative factors such as malnourished state, benign gastroduodenal disease, and malignant disease involving certain defined organ systems.— M. M. Meguid *et al.* (letter), *ibid.*, *2*, 231. Further references: M. Shike *et al.*, *Ann. intern. Med.*, 1984, *101*, 303; P. J. Friedman (letter), *ibid.*, 1985, *102*, 556; M. Shike and K. N. Jeejeebhoy (letter), *ibid.*

CYSTIC FIBROSIS. Invasive enteral techniques appear to be of little value in improving chronic respiratory disease in patients with cystic fibrosis. Growth can be stimulated and wellbeing improved in the short-term but for long-term benefit it seems likely that supplemental feeding would have to be continued for long periods, perhaps indefinitely. Nutritional support during periods of acute illness while giving intensive chest therapy appears to be worthwhile. Slackening of weight-gain is an important pointer to underlying deterioration in respiratory function which may not be obvious clinically. There is a role for supplemental feedings when impairment of growth is first noted and chest infection can be improved by intensive therapy. The intravenous route in hospital followed by nasogastric feedings at home, until growth catches up, seems reasonable, but even this should only be used if oral supplementation fails.— *Lancet*, 1986, *1*, 249.

References: R. Shepherd *et al.*, *J. Pediat.*, 1980, *97*, 351 (supplemental parenteral nutrition); A. L. Mansell *et al.*, *ibid.*, 1984, *104*, 700 (parenteral nutrition); R. W. Shepherd *et al.*, *J. pediatr. Gastroenterol. Nutr.*, 1983, *2*, 439 (enteral feeding via nasogastric tube); J. M. Bertrand *et al.*, *J. Pediat.*, 1984, *104*, 41 (enteral feeding via nasogastric tube); L. D. Levy *et al.*, *ibid.*, 1985, *107*, 225 (enteral feeding via gastrostomy tube); M. P. Boland *et al.*, *Lancet*, 1986, *1*, 232 (enteral feeding via jejunostomy tube).

GASTRO-INTESTINAL DISORDERS. *Inflammatory bowel disease.* Enteral and parenteral nutrition play important roles in severely malnourished patients with Crohn's disease. However, its use is limited as a supplement to other standardised regimens including surgery and it is of little value in ulcerative colitis, for which steroids and surgery are still the principal forms of treatment. Elemental diets may be a suitable way of treating acute Crohn's disease, and more importantly, their use may throw some light on the aetiology and pathogenesis of this disease.— M. L. Clark, *Gut*, 1986, *27*, *Suppl.* 1, 72.

Discussions and studies of nutritional support in inflammatory bowel disease: J. Rhodes and J. Rose, *Gut*, 1986, *27*, 471 (parenteral nutrition, elemental diets, and exclusion diets); P. B. McIntyre *et al.*, *ibid.*, 481 (controlled trial of parenteral nutrition and oral diet); M. A. Gassull *et al.*, *ibid.*, *Suppl.* 1, 76 (a study on the role of enteral nutrition); C. Matuchansky, *ibid.*, 81 (parenteral nutrition); I. R. Sanderson *et al.*, *Archs Dis. Childh.*, 1987, *61*, 123 (remission induced by a nasogastric elemental diet in small bowel Crohn's disease).

Short bowel syndrome. Parenteral nutrition should be started following small bowel resection in order to avoid the development of malnutrition while oral feeding is being attempted. The aim should be to progress as the patient adapts from parenteral nutrition with variable oral intake, through oral diet with parenteral fluids and electrolytes, then defined-formula diets on an ambulatory basis, to a normal or modified oral diet, separating solids from liquids. Patients with less than 60 cm of small bowel remaining require home parenteral nutrition on an indefinite basis; the infusion rate and caloric intake are gradually reduced as the patient can maintain his weight on an oral diet. The decision to reduce intravenous feeding is made on the observations that weight gain is occurring beyond desired limits and that reduced infusion does not result in electrolyte and fluid imbalance.— K. N. Jeejeebhoy, *Lancet*, 1983, *1*, 1427.

HEPATIC ENCEPHALOPATHY. In chronic hepatic encephalopathy there is a 2- to 4-fold increase in the plasma concentrations of aromatic amino acids, together with a decrease in those of the branched-chain amino acids, valine, leucine, and isoleucine. In patients with established chronic hepatic encephalopathy mixtures supplemented with branched-chain amino acid seem to induce positive nitrogen balance to about the same degree as an equivalent amount of dietary protein, without inducing encephalopathy as often. Infusions of branched-chain amino acids alone in patients with cirrhosis and acute encephalopathy do not seem to confer any advantage either in terms of encephalopathy or survival. In contrast, there is a suggestion that survival can be improved, at least if the encephalopathy is not precipitated by significant gastro-intestinal haemorrhage, by administering a specially-formulated amino acid solution which was originally devised by Fischer *et al.* (*Surgery*, 1976, *80*, 77). This contains considerably decreased amounts of phenylalanine, tryptophan, methionine, and glycine, increased amounts of the branched-chain amino acids leucine, isoleucine, and valine, as well as arginine, but contains no tyrosine or cysteine. However, in some patients with cirrhosis, lack of tyrosine and cysteine has been shown to prevent achievement of positive nitrogen balance despite provision of adequate essential amino acid precursors. In addition, the rationale for infusing even small amounts of tryptophan, phenylalanine, and methionine in patients with hepatic encephalopathy is questionable.

It is not certain that the beneficial responses attributed to such a mixture are not due to the increase in arginine content, as there is evidence to suggest that arginine (or ornithine, its precursor as well as its metabolic product) may counteract the hyperammonaemia in hepatic encephalopathy by stimulation of ureagenesis. Further long-term studies are needed before any firm conclusions can be made about the true clinical benefits of branched-chain amino acid supplementation in patients with established subclinical or latent encephalopathy.— D. B. A. Silk, *Gut*, 1986, *27*, *Suppl.* 1, 103. The branched-chain amino acids isoleucine, leucine, and valine are preferentially metabolised at extrahepatic sites and thus, where hepatic function is poor, plasma and CNS concentrations do not increase. Branched-chain amino acids may reduce muscle catabolism, which is a characteristic of poor hepatic function and may also be involved in the active transport of potentially neurotoxic amino acids such as phenylalanine and tyrosine from the CNS.— I. Corall and R. Williams, *Br. J. Anaesth.*, 1986, *58*, 234. See also *Med. Lett.*, 1983, *25*, 72.

MUSCULAR AND NEUROMUSCULAR DISORDERS. Long-term high-protein enteral nutrition administered overnight with daytime high-protein feeds by mouth to 7 patients aged 2 months to 26 years with debrancher enzyme deficiency and myopathy led to improvement in physical activity and endurance in all patients, improvement in muscle strength in 5, and the return to normal of EMG and ECG patterns in 2 and 1 respectively. Marked improvement in growth rate was noted in 4 patients who had also had growth failure. The results obtained from this study support the concept that myopathy in debrancher enzyme deficiency may be at least partly due to reversible muscle amino acid depletion.— A. E. Slonim *et al.*, *J. Pediat.*, 1984, *105*, 906.

For reference to the use of long-term high-protein therapy by mouth in a patient with McArdle's syndrome, see under Dietary Modification, p.1251.

PREGNANCY AND THE NEONATE. *In pregnancy.* No complications unique to the pregnant patient were observed in a retrospective study of 10 patients who had received various TPN regimens during pregnancy; 1 in the first, 3 in the second, and 5 in the third trimester. One patient received TPN in both the second and third trimesters. Of the 10 patients, 9 delivered at or beyond 36 weeks. The tenth pregnancy was terminated at 34 weeks for maternal indications. All infants were judged to be normal and were above the tenth percentile in weight for gestational age. The patient given TPN during the first trimester had been seen at 9 weeks' gestation with hyperemesis gravidarum accompanied by a weight loss of 6.4 kg. Her weight was maintained with a lipid-based regimen for 7 days until symptoms resolved. Labour was induced at 36 weeks due to severe pre-eclampsia and she delivered an infant weighing 2265 g with Apgar scores of 4 and 8. Parenteral nutrition appears to be as safe and effective a method of nutritional support during the second and third trimesters of pregnancy as in non-pregnant patients. Experience with TPN in the first trimester is limited.— D. B. Seifer *et al.*, *J. Am. med. Ass.*, 1985, *253*, 2073.

Successful conception and completion of pregnancy in a patient with Crohn's disease who was maintained throughout pregnancy on home parenteral nutrition.— J. C. Tresadern *et al.*, *J. parenter. enteral Nutr.*, 1984, *8*, 199. See also *idem*, *Br. med. J.*, 1983, *286*, 602. Comment.— M. C. Brown (letter), *ibid.*, 1060. A similar report.— K. J. Breen *et al.*, *Med. J. Aust.*, 1987, *146*, 215.

The neonate. Results from a 2-year study of very low birth-weight (less than 1500 g) infants showed the incidence of necrotising enterocolitis to be reduced from 18.2% (8 of 44) in infants born during the first year and fed exclusively on expressed breast milk, to 3.5% (3 of 85) in infants born during the second year who were not fed enterally for the first 2 to 3 weeks of life, but given peripheral total parenteral nutrition.— F. Eyal *et al.*, *Archs Dis. Childh.*, 1982, *57*, 274. Criticism. The well-known tendency for cases of necrotising enterocolitis to occur in clusters makes the 'historical' controls which were used particularly unsuitable.— R. Cooke (letter), *ibid.*, 889. Reply. The simultaneous increase in the incidence of the disease in preterm infants weighing more than 1500 g, in whom no change in feeding policy was made, rules out that explanation.— F. Eyal *et al.*, *ibid.* Further criticism.— M. R. Drayton *et al.*, *ibid.*, 890. Reply.— F. Eyal, *ibid.*, 961.

For reference to complications associated with parenteral nutrition in the neonate, see under Adverse Effects and Precautions, above.

RENAL FAILURE. The infusion of essential amino acid and glucose solutions has been found to be effective in maintaining a positive nitrogen balance in some patients with acute renal failure but not in others. Severely stressed patients with acute renal failure will generally need higher amounts of essential and non-essential amino acids as well as non-protein calories to reduce the hypercatabolism associated with this disorder. Aggressive nutritional therapy can be less effective when complicated by such factors as sepsis, disseminated intravascular coagulation, shock, and other trauma. In addition, repeated dialysis may affect the ability of these patients to respond to therapy, since amino acids can be lost during dialysis. Increased amounts of these amino acids may have to be used in order to avoid excessive loss.— M. Thompson, *Drug Intell. & clin. Pharm.*, 1985, *19*, 106.

Preliminary results obtained during continuous venovenous haemofiltration in a patient with acute renal failure who was receiving parenteral nutrition indicated that amino acid losses were increased at higher rates of haemofiltration; this loss was not reflected in serum concentrations.— A. Davenport and N. B. Roberts (letter), *Lancet*, 1986, *2*, 685.

SICKLE-CELL ANAEMIA. Results from a preliminary study in 5 children with sickle-cell anaemia and associated retarded growth suggested that nutritional supplementation via a nasogastric tube could provide an effective, simple, relatively non-invasive approach to the prophylaxis and management of inadequate growth and other complications in children with sickle-cell disease.— M. B. Heyman *et al.*, *Lancet*, 1985, *1*, 903. Severe criticism.— L. Luzzatto (letter), *ibid.*, *2*, 37.

TRACE ELEMENTS. Inadequate amounts of zinc, copper, iron, and manganese were found in 2, 5, 2, and 7 enteral feeds respectively out of a total of 14 different commercial preparations studied. It was considered that products which are likely to be the main source of nutrition, sometimes for long periods, should contain at least the lower limits for the recommended quantities of trace elements.— V. W. Bunker and B. E. Clayton, *Lancet*, 1983, *2*, 426.

A review of trace elements in adult total parenteral nutrition. Minimal intravenous requirements closely match the amount of recommended oral intake actually absorbed, but most patients receiving TPN will require more than the minimal amount; many of them are already in a deficiency state as a result of malnourishment and others have major losses from fistulas. Trace elements interact with each other at the absorptive and excretory level and should not be considered for TPN on an individual basis.— A. N. Kingsnorth, *Br. J. parent. Ther.*, 1984, *5*, 8.

Further references: A. Shenkin, *Intensive Therapy clin. Monit.*, 1987, *8*, 38.

For reference to the potential toxicity and deficiency of the essential trace elements, see under Trace Elements, in Nutrition in Health, p.1250.

Preparations

Protein Hydrolysate Injection *(U.S.P.)*. A sterile solution of amino acids and short-chain peptides which represent the approximate nutritive equivalent of the casein, lactalbumin, plasma, fibrin, or other suitable protein from which it is derived by acid, enzymatic, or other method of hydrolysis. It may be modified by partial removal and restoration or addition of one or more amino acids. It may contain alcohol, glucose, or other carbohydrate suitable for intravenous infusion. Not less than 50% of the total nitrogen present is in the form of α-amino nitrogen. pH 4 to 7.

For Proprietary Preparations for Enteral and Parenteral Nutrition, see p.1289.

7820-j

Vitamins

Vitamins are organic substances required by the body in small amounts for various metabolic processes. They are not synthesised in the body, or are synthesised in small or insufficient quantities. Vitamin deficiency may result from an inadequate diet, perhaps due to increased requirements such as during pregnancy, or may be induced by disease or drugs.

Vitamins may be used clinically for the prevention and treatment of specific vitamin deficiency states. Large doses of vitamins (megavitamin therapy) have been used, but adequate evidence of their value is lacking. Excessive intakes of most water-soluble vitamins have little effect due to their rapid excretion in urine, but excessive intakes of fat-soluble vitamins accumulate in the body and are potentially dangerous.

Water-soluble vitamins are liable to degrade in solution especially if exposed to light. Addition of vitamin mixtures to infusion solutions for parenteral nutrition should therefore be carried out as soon as possible before infusion. Solutions should be used within 24 hours of preparation and be protected from light.

A view that vitamins and trace elements should not be mixed together in solutions for parenteral nutrition.— V. D. Gupta (letter), *Am. J. Hosp. Pharm.*, 1986, *43*, 2132. Comment and support for this recommendation unless data prove particular mixtures to be reasonably stable. However, the addition of vitamins and trace elements to the TPN solution on alternating days was suggested.— M. C. Allwood (letter), *ibid.*, 2138. Factors that contribute to instability and incompatibility as well as vitamin dosage requirements in total parenteral nutrition therapy have yet to be fully identified.— N. Louie (letter), *ibid.*

Comment on the use and misuse of vitamins, with special reference to megadoses.— D. Rudman and P. J. Williams, *New Engl. J. Med.*, 1983, *309*, 488.

A review of vitamin therapy in non-deficiency states.— L. Ovesen, *Drugs*, 1984, *27*, 148.

Functions, effects, deficiency, excess, and dietary sources of vitamins.— *Manual of Nutrition*, Ministry of Agriculture, Fisheries and Food, London, HM Stationery Office, 1985.

Reviews, reports, and discussions on the use of vitamin supplementation: *Drug & Ther. Bull.*, 1984, *22*, 33; D. A. Bender, *Pharm. J.*, 1984, *2*, 637; *Med. Lett.*, 1985, *27*, 66; A. S. Truswell, *Br. med. J.*, 1985, *291*, 1033 and 1103; M. L. Wahlqvist, *Med. J. Aust.*, 1987, *146*, 30; D. Colquhoun (letter), *ibid.*, 558; M. L. Wahlqvist (letter), *ibid.*, 559; The Council on Scientific Affairs of the American Medical Association, *J. Am. med. Ass.*, 1987, *257*, 1929; C. D. Jensen and G. M. Briggs (letter), *ibid.*, *258*, 908; D. Kesden (letter), *ibid.*, 909; W. R. Hendee (letter), *ibid;* D. Temple, *Pharm. J.*, 1987, *2*, 206.

ADVERSE EFFECTS AND PRECAUTIONS. A review of the toxic effects of vitamin overdosage. Large overdoses of water-soluble vitamins are readily excreted in the urine; fat-soluble vitamins (A, D, E, and K) are stored and therefore are more likely to cause adverse effects when taken in excess. The fat-soluble vitamins A and D are most likely to cause serious toxicity. However, even some water-soluble vitamins can be toxic, especially when large amounts are taken for prolonged periods.— *Med. Lett.*, 1984, *26*, 73.

Clinicians should be aware that patients may take abnormal doses of vitamins as a pathological feature of a psychiatric illness (perhaps typically an eating disorder) or that they may take them with insight in a misguided attempt to treat a psychiatric illness. In either case the toxicity of the vitamin may exacerbate the psychiatric disorder and introduce new features.— C. D. H. Evans and J. H. Lacey, *Br. med. J.*, 1986, *292*, 509.

CYSTIC FIBROSIS. The fat-soluble vitamins A, D, E, and K may be inadequately absorbed in patients with cystic fibrosis. Classic signs of vitamin A deficiency are rare. Rickets is practically unknown but it is common practice to give vitamins A and D in twice the normal daily dosage. Vitamin K deficiency is seen in patients with appreciable liver dysfunction or severe steatorrhoea; a dose of 5 to 10 mg is usually sufficient. Neurological signs associated with low concentrations of vitamin E have been reported in a few patients; the need for routine use of this vitamin is still to be established.— M. B. Mearns, *Archs Dis. Childh.*, 1985, *60*, 272.

MENTAL FUNCTION. Lack of benefit of megavitamin and mineral supplementation on intellectual functioning of children with Down's syndrome.— G. F. Smith *et al.* (letter), *Lancet*, 1983, *2*, 41. Criticism.— B. Rimland (letter), *ibid.*, 744; H. Turkel (letter), *ibid.*, 745. Reply.— G. F. Smith (letter), *ibid.* Further comments.— T. Mork (letter), *ibid.*, 1255; B. Rimland (letter), *ibid.*

Administration of vitamin/mineral supplements to 30 children for an 8-month period resulted in increased scores of non-verbal intelligence; no increase in score was observed in 30 children who had received placebo or in 30 children who received no supplementation.— D. Benton and G. Roberts, *Lancet*, 1988, *1*, 140. Comments and criticism: *ibid.*, 407.

Psychiatric disorders. Deficiencies of specific vitamins produce consistent symptoms of psychiatric disorder. The use of vitamins has been most prominent in psychiatry in the treatment of schizophrenia, where large doses of nicotinic acid were initially given alone and later combined with other vitamins and minerals. While the therapeutic effects of high-dose vitamins are questionable, at best, it is well known that these agents may produce occasional adverse effects of consequence. The theoretical basis of orthomolecular and megavitamin therapies, which were attractive 30 years ago, have not been supported by time. Caution is advised in the assumption that selected schizophrenic patients may benefit from vitamin therapy. Similar claims have been made (unsuccessfully) for insulin coma, psychoanalysis, and other treatments of schizophrenia which have now been largely abandoned. Vitamin therapy of schizophrenia will no doubt continue, but it should be viewed by clinician and patient alike as unproven.— W. M. Petrie and T. A. Ban, *Drugs*, 1985, *30*, 58.

See also under Adverse Effects and Precautions, above.

PERIPHERAL NEUROPATHY. Nutritional polyneuropathy may be due to the development of an immune state caused by the accumulation of antibodies to vitamin receptors, or apoenzymes. Since the latter consist of protein, they are potentially antigenic. The presence of antibodies to apoenzymes would necessarily increase the daily requirements of the vitamin involved, and the patient would be more susceptible to nutritional depletion. Whether or not significant concentrations of antibodies to vitamins can actually be blamed for a polyneuropathy remains to be demonstrated. Clinical investigations of nutritional polyneuropathies are very difficult, for several reasons. The disease process, both onset and recovery, is very slow, being measured in terms of weeks or months. By the time a patient comes to the attention of a physician, the underlying biochemical defect may already have been corrected, yet the disease continues to evolve. It is not unusual for patients to complain of severe weakness, sensory loss, or troublesome dysaesthesiae while electrical studies and pathological changes suggest improvement of the underlying disease. The measurement of vitamin concentrations in the blood or the estimation of vitamin-dependent enzyme activity may be very misleading. The treatment of nutritional polyneuropathies involves improved nutrition, supplemental vitamins, and the removal of noxious substances; however, prevention would seem more effective than treatment.— Report of a WHO Study Group on Peripheral Neuropathies, *Tech. Rep. Ser. Wld Hlth Org. No. 654*, 1980, p.65.

PREGNANCY AND THE NEONATE. *The neonate.* All standard milk formulae are fortified with vitamins. A separate supplement is unnecessary for bottle-fed babies and probably unnecessary for full-term babies breast feeding from healthy mothers. Preterm babies need a supplementary vitamin preparation and babies of very low birth-weight need additional vitamin D. The role of vitamin E supplements in preventing retrolental fibroplasia and intraventricular haemorrhage is still controversial.— D. A. Curnock, *Prescribers' J.*, 1985, *25*, 62. See also J. G. Bissenden (letter), *Br. med. J.*, 1987, *294*, 880.

For reference to the possible prevention of neural-tube defects by periconceptional vitamin supplementation, see under Folic Acid, p.1263.

Preparations

For Multivitamin Preparations, see p.1291.

14035-b

Acesulfame Potassium *(BANM, rINNM).*

Acesulfame K; H73-3293; HOE-095K. The potassium salt of 6-methyl-1,2,3-oxathiazin-4(3*H*)-one 2,2-dioxide.
$C_4H_4KNO_4S$=201.2.

CAS — 33665-90-6 (acesulfame).

White odourless crystalline powder or granules with an intensely sweet taste.

Acesulfame potassium is an intense sweetener permitted in the *UK* and other countries for use in food. It does not appear to be affected by cooking.

Estimated acceptable daily intake of acesulfame potassium: up to 9 mg per kg body-weight.— Twenty-seventh Report of the Joint FAO/WHO Expert Committee on Food Additives, *Tech. Rep. Ser. Wld Hlth Org. No. 696*, 1983.

Proprietary Names and Manufacturers

Diamin *(Vitalia, UK)*; Hermesetas Gold *(Jenks Brokerage, UK)*; Sunett *(Hoechst, UK)*; Sweetex Plus *(Crookes Healthcare, UK)*.

12309-r

Acetiamine Hydrochloride *(rINNM).*

Acethiamine Hydrochloride; Diacethiamine Hydrochloride. *N*-(5-Acetoxy-3-acetylthiopent-2-en-2-yl)-*N*-(4-amino-2-methylpyrimidin-5-ylmethyl)formamide hydrochloride monohydrate.
$C_{16}H_{22}N_4O_4S,HCl,H_2O$=420.9.

CAS — 299-89-8 (acetiamine).

Acetiamine is a vitamin B_1 substance with the general properties of thiamine hydrochloride (see p.1277).

Proprietary Names and Manufacturers

Névriton *(Spret-Mauchant, Fr.)*; Thianeuron *(Badische, Ger.)*.

572-b

Alanine *(USAN, pINN).*

Ala; L-Alanine. L-2-Aminopropionic acid.
$C_3H_7NO_2$=89.09.

CAS — 56-41-7.

Pharmacopoeias. In *U.S.*

A white odourless crystalline powder. Freely **soluble** in water; slightly soluble in 80% alcohol; insoluble in ether. A 5% solution in water has a pH of 5.5 to 7.0.

Alanine is an aliphatic amino acid. It is used as a dietary supplement.

Preparations

For multi-ingredient preparations containing nutritional agents and vitamins, see p.1289.

18365-p

Ammonium Molybdate *(USAN).*

Hexaammonium molybdate tetrahydrate.
$(NH_4)_6Mo_7O_{24},4H_2O$=1235.9.

CAS — 12054-85-2.

Pharmacopoeias. In *U.S.*

Store in airtight containers.

Molybdenum is an essential trace metal, although there have been no reports of deficiency states in man. Molybdenum has been used to treat copper poisoning in *sheep*.

Preparations

Ammonium Molybdate Injection *(U.S.P.)*. To be diluted before use. pH 3 to 6.

573-v

Arginine *(USAN, rINN).*

Arg; L-Arginine. L-2-Amino-5-guanidinovaleric acid.
$C_6H_{14}N_4O_2$=174.2.

CAS — 74-79-3.

Pharmacopoeias. In *Cz.* and *U.S.*

White, almost odourless crystals. Freely **soluble** in water; sparingly soluble in alcohol; insoluble in ether.

574-g

Arginine Glutamate *(BAN, USAN, rINNM).*

L-Arginine L-glutamate.
$C_6H_{14}N_4O_2,C_5H_9NO_4$=321.3.

CAS — 4320-30-3.

575-q

Arginine Hydrochloride *(USAN, rINNM).*

L-Arginine Monohydrochloride.
$C_6H_{14}N_4O_2,HCl$=210.7.

CAS — 1119-34-2.

Pharmacopoeias. In *U.S.*

A white almost odourless crystalline powder. Each g of monograph substance represents approximately 4.7 mmol of chloride. Freely **soluble** in water. The *U.S.P.* injection which is a 10% solution has a pH of 5.0 to 6.5.

Adverse Effects and Precautions

Nausea, vomiting, flushing, headache, numbness, and local venous irritation may occur if arginine solutions are infused too rapidly. Arginine should be administered with caution to patients with renal disease or anuria. Arginine hydrochloride should be administered cautiously to patients with electrolyte disturbances as its high chloride content could lead to the development of hyperchloraemic alkalosis.

A 10-year-old boy experienced an anaphylactic reaction 5 minutes after the start of an infusion of a 5% arginine hydrochloride solution in a test for growth-hormone output.— C. M. Tiwary *et al.* (letter), *New Engl. J. Med.*, 1973, *288*, 218.

Two alcoholic patients with severe liver disease and moderate renal insufficiency developed severe hyperkalaemia following administration of arginine hydrochloride and one died. Both patients had received a total dose of 300 mg of spironolactone some time before arginine hydrochloride administration, but the contribution of spironolactone to the hyperkalaemia was not known.— D. A. Bushinsky and F. J. Gennari, *Ann. intern. Med.*, 1978, *89*, 632.

Uses and Administration

Arginine is an aliphatic amino acid which is essential for infant growth. It is used as a dietary supplement.

Arginine hydrochloride may be used in the treatment of hyperammonaemia refractory to conventional therapy, but the presence of a chloride ion may be detrimental in some conditions. The usual dose of arginine hydrochloride is 10 g by intravenous infusion over 30 minutes.

Arginine stimulates the release of growth hormone by the pituitary gland and the hydrochloride is used as a test of pituitary function in usual doses of 30 g by intravenous infusion of a 10% solution; children should be given 500 mg per kg body-weight.

Arginine oxoglutarate has been used in the treatment of hepatic encephalopathy.

The aspartate, glucose-1-phosphate, thiazolidinecarboxylate, and tidiacicate have also been used.

HYPERAMMONAEMIA. Arginine may be used to treat hyperammonaemia associated with inborn errors of the urea cycle such as carbamoyl phosphate synthetase deficiency, ornithine carbamoyl transferase deficiency, argininosuccinate synthetase deficiency, and argininosuccinate lysase deficiency. Arginine replenishes ornithine and improves the control of plasma-ammonium concentrations.— J. H. Walter and J. V. Leonard, *Br. J. Hosp. Med.*, 1987, *38*, 176.

INFERTILITY. A study in 18 men with infertility, of whom 15 were followed up, did not confirm early reports of the value of arginine. The sperm count rose in only one patient after treatment for 1 to 2 months with arginine 4 g daily.— M. L. Jungling and R. G. Bunge, *Fert. Steril.*, 1976, *27*, 282. See also J. P. Pryor *et al.*, *Br. J. Urol.*, 1978, *50*, 47.

LIVER DISORDERS. Vigorous medical management of acute fulminant hepatitis included the intravenous administration of arginine hydrochloride for rapid correction of alkalosis.— M. O. Auslander and G. L. Gitnick, *Archs intern. Med.*, 1977, *137*, 599.

For reference to the role of arginine in the treatment of hepatic encephalopathy, see under Enteral and Parenteral Nutrition, p.1252.

Preparations

Arginine Hydrochloride Injection *(U.S.P.)*

Proprietary Names and Manufacturers of Arginine and its Salts

Apermargin *(Farber-Ref, Ital.)*; Argamin *(Rio, S.Afr.)*; Arginil *(SPA, Ital.)*; Bioarginina *(Damor, Ital.)*; Biofons *(IBYS, Spain)*; Eucol *(Lefrancq, Fr.)*; Fosfarginil *(Wasserman, Spain)*; Leberam *(Chephasaar, Ger.)*; Potenciator *(Iquinosa, Spain)*; R-Gene *(Kabivitrum, USA)*; Sargenor *(Sarget, Fr.; Sarget, Spain)*; Sorbenor *(Casen Fisons, Spain)*; Spermargin *(Farber-Ref, Ital.)*.

For multi-ingredient preparations containing nutritional agents and vitamins, see p.1289.

12393-w

Arrowroot

Amylum Marantae; Araruta; Maranta.

Pharmacopoeias. In *Belg., Port.,* and *Span.* Also in *B.P.C. 1973.*

The starch granules of the rhizomes of *Maranta arundinacea* (Marantaceae).

Arrowroot has the general properties of starch and has been used as a gruel in the treatment of diarrhoea. It has been used as a suspending agent in the preparation of barium meals and is sometimes used in place of starch in tablet manufacture.

7881-b

Ascorbic Acid *(BAN, USAN, rINN).*

Acidum Ascorbicum; Cevitamic Acid; E300; L-Ascorbic Acid; Vitamin C. The enolic form of 3-oxo-L-gulofuranolactone; 2,3-Didehydro-L-*threo*-hexono-1,4-lactone.
$C_6H_8O_6$=176.1.

CAS — 50-81-7.

Pharmacopoeias. In *Arg., Aust., Belg., Br., Braz., Chin., Cz., Egypt., Eur., Fr., Ger., Hung., Ind., Int., It., Jpn, Jug., Mex., Neth., Nord., Pol., Port., Roum., Rus., Span., Swiss, Turk.,* and *U.S.* Also in *B.P. Vet.*

Odourless or almost odourless, colourless crystals or white or slightly yellow crystalline powder.

B.P. **solubilities** are: soluble 1 in 3.5 of water and 1 in 25 of alcohol; practically insoluble in chloroform, ether, and light petroleum. *U.S.P.* solubilities are: soluble 1 in 3 of water and 1 in 40 of alcohol; insoluble in chloroform and ether. A 5% solution in water has a pH of 2.1 to 2.6. The *U.S.P.* injection has a pH of 5.5 to 7.0. Solutions of ascorbic acid deteriorate rapidly in air. **Store** in airtight non-metallic containers. Protect from light.

7880-m

Sodium Ascorbate *(BANM, USAN, rINN).*

E301; Monosodium L-ascorbate. 3-Oxo-L-gulofuranolactone sodium enolate.

$C_6H_7NaO_6$=198.1.

CAS — 134-03-2.

Pharmacopoeias. In *Ind.* and *U.S.*

White or very faintly yellow, odourless or almost odourless, crystals or crystalline powder. It gradually darkens on exposure to light. Each g of monograph substance represents about 5 mmol of sodium.

Soluble 1 in 1.3 of water; very slightly soluble in alcohol; insoluble in chloroform and ether. A 10% solution in water has a pH of 7 to 8. **Store** in airtight containers. Protect from light.

STABILITY IN SOLUTION. A review of the compatibility and stability of components of total parenteral nutrition solutions when mixed in 1- or 3-litre flexible containers. Ascorbic acid is likely to be one of the least stable additives, although its degradation depends on a number of inter-related factors. It is oxidised in aqueous solutions by reaction with dissolved oxygen. The most important factors with respect to the rate and extent of degradation are dissolved oxygen and the presence of catalysts, especially copper ions. A second stage of ascorbic acid degradation occurs due to the permeation of oxygen through plastic which can lead to the degradation of 2.0 to 2.5 mg ascorbic acid per hour at room temperature. Another factor that influences degradation is the observation that cysteine and cystine inhibit the catalytic effect of copper. Therefore, if the infusion includes these amino acids, degradation rates can be lower. Ascorbic acid losses in TPN mixtures have been estimated from various studies. Following the addition of 500 mg ascorbic acid to the 3-litre bag, approximately 10% loss has been recorded in 24 hours at ambient temperature with exclusion of copper; with addition of trace elements to the 3-litre bag, up to 40% of the vitamin may be degraded within 2 to 3 hours. If less than 200 mg ascorbic acid is added to each bag, the patient may receive negligible amounts. Either a large excess of ascorbic acid must be added to ensure adequate daily requirements are met, or vitamins and trace elements are administered on alternate days. It should also be noted that one degradation product of ascorbic acid is oxalic acid which may be present in clinically significant quantities if considerable amounts of ascorbic acid have degraded.— M. C. Allwood, *J. clin. Hosp. Pharm.*, 1984, *9*, 181. See also *idem*, 75.

A study of the stability of ascorbic acid in total parenteral nutrition solutions indicated that its degradation followed first-order kinetics. Half-lives were 1.1 hours, 2.9 hours, and 8.9 hours when stored at 24° by daylight, 24° protected from light, and 4° protected from light, respectively.— K. Nordfjeld *et al.*, *J. clin. Hosp. Pharm.*, 1984, *9*, 293.

Adverse Effects and Precautions

Ascorbic acid is usually well tolerated. Large doses are reported to cause diarrhoea and other gastro-intestinal disturbances and are associated with the formation of renal calcium oxalate calculi. Ascorbic acid should be given with care to patients with hyperoxaluria. Tolerance may be induced with prolonged use of large doses.

ALLERGY. A report of an allergic response to ascorbic acid in 3 patients, presenting as eczema, urticaria, or asthma.— P. Vassal, *Revue fr. Allerg.*, 1976, *16*, 103.

DEPENDENCE. A 32-year-old man with migraine apparently became dependent on ascorbic acid which he had substituted for methysergide and codeine. Interrupting an intake of ascorbic acid 6 g daily resulted in acute onset of headache.— L. Bali and E. Callaway (letter), *New Engl. J. Med.*, 1978, *299*, 364.

A brief discussion of rebound scurvy in infants born to mothers taking high doses of ascorbic acid.— V. D. Herbert, *J. Am. pharm. Ass.*, 1977, *NS17*, 764.

EFFECTS ON THE BLOOD. A report of the development of intravascular haemolysis and acute renal failure in a 68-year-old patient with glucose-6-phosphate dehydrogenase deficiency following the administration of ascorbic acid 80 g intravenously on each of 2 consecutive days.— G. D. Campbell *et al.* (letter), *Ann. intern. Med.*, 1975, *82*, 810.

EFFECTS ON THE EYE. At usual therapeutic doses rutin improved colour vision whereas rutin in association with ascorbic acid caused a slight deterioration. This confirmed previous findings of an adverse effect of ascorbic acid on colour vision.— J. Laroche and C. Laroche, *Annls pharm. fr.*, 1977, *35*, 173.

EFFECTS ON THE KIDNEY. Reports of renal impairment associated with excessive oxalate excretion following the administration of large doses of ascorbic acid: V. M. Reznik *et al.* (letter), *New Engl. J. Med.*, 1980, *302*, 1418 (abrupt loss of renal function in an infant with congenital nephrotic syndrome); R. D. Swartz *et al.*, *Ann. intern. Med.*, 1984, *100*, 530 (hyperoxaluria and renal insufficiency during total parenteral nutrition); P. Balcke *et al.*, *ibid.*, *101*, 344 (aggravation of secondary hyperoxalaemia by ascorbic acid in patients on chronic haemodialysis); J. M. Lawton *et al.*, *Archs intern. Med.*, 1985, *145*, 950 (a fatal case of acute oxalate nephropathy).

Comment on ascorbic acid administration and urinary oxalate. Studies carried out by the author have indicated that ingestion of large amounts of ascorbic acid by healthy subjects leads to relatively small increases in oxalate excretion.— C. S. Tsao (letter), *Ann. intern. Med.*, 1984, *101*, 405.

See also under Effects on the Blood, above.

EFFECTS ON THE TEETH. A report of dental enamel erosion which was attributed to the daily ingestion of chewable ascorbic acid tablets over a period of 3 years.— J. L. Giunta, *J. Am. dent. Ass.*, 1983, *107*, 253.

INTERACTIONS. For the effect of ascorbic acid on various drugs see under desferrioxamine (p.838), ethinyloestradiol (p.1398), fluphenazine (p.740), and warfarin (p.348).

INTERFERENCE WITH LABORATORY TESTS. Ascorbic acid, a strong reducing agent, interferes with laboratory tests involving oxidation and reduction reactions. Falsely elevated or false-negative measurements may be obtained in plasma, faeces, or urine depending on such factors as the concentration of ascorbic acid, pH, and specific method employed.

Absorption and Fate

Ascorbic acid is readily absorbed from the gastro-intestinal tract and is widely distributed in the body tissues. It is reported to be about 25% bound to plasma proteins. The amount of ascorbic acid in the body in health is about 1.5 g. The concentration is higher in leucocytes and platelets than in erythrocytes and plasma. In deficiency states the concentration in leucocytes declines later and at a slower rate, and has been considered to be a better criterion for the evaluation of deficiency than the concentration in plasma.

Ascorbic acid is reversibly oxidised to dehydroascorbic acid; some is metabolised to ascorbate-2-sulphate, which is inactive, and oxalic acid which are excreted in the urine. Ascorbic acid in excess of the body's needs is also rapidly eliminated in the urine. Ascorbic acid crosses the placenta and is distributed into breast milk. It is removed by haemodialysis.

In 5 healthy subjects, previously saturated with ascorbic acid, the mean half-life of ascorbic acid after a 1-g dose intravenously was 3.37 hours. About 83% of the dose was recovered in the urine, chiefly (84%) as ascorbic acid.— S. Yung *et al.* (letter), *J. pharm. Sci.*, 1978, *67*, 1491.

Human Requirements

A daily dietary intake of about 30 to 60 mg ascorbic acid has been recommended for adults. There is, however, wide variation in individual requirements. Humans are unable to form their own ascorbic acid and so a dietary source is necessary. Most dietary ascorbic acid is obtained from fruit and vegetable sources; only small amounts are present in milk and animal tissues. Relatively rich sources include rose hips (rose fruit), black currant, citrus fruits, leafy vegetables, tomatoes, potatoes, and green peppers. Ascorbic acid is readily destroyed during cooking processes. Considerable losses may also occur during storage.

The recommended daily intake of ascorbic acid was: from birth to 12 years, 20 mg; 13 years and over, 30 mg; in the second and third trimesters of pregnancy and during lactation, 50 mg.— Report of a Joint FAO/WHO Expert Group, *Tech. Rep. Ser. Wld Hlth Org. No. 452,* 1970.

Estimated acceptable daily intake for ascorbic acid and sodium ascorbate as antoxidants in food: up to 15 mg per kg body-weight in addition to that naturally present in food.— Seventeenth Report of FAO/WHO Expert Committee on Food Additives, *Tech. Rep. Ser. Wld Hlth Org. No. 539,* 1974.

Recommended daily intake of ascorbic acid: boys and girls, up to 8 years, 20 mg; 9 to 17 years, 25 to 30 mg; men and women 18 years and over, 30 mg; during pregnancy and lactation, 60 mg.— Recommended Daily Amounts of Food Energy and Nutrients for Groups of People in the United Kingdom, Report by the Committee on Medical Aspects of Food Policy, *Report on Health and Social Subjects, No. 15,* London, HM Stationery Office, 1979.

The recommendation that infant feeds should provide a minimum of 30 µg ascorbic acid per mL reconstituted feed.— Artificial Feeds for the Young Infant: 1980, Report of the Working Party on the Composition of Foods for Infants and Young Children, Committee on Medical Aspects of Food Policy, *Report on Health and Social Subjects, 18,* London, HM Stationery Office, 1980.

The recommended daily dietary allowance of ascorbic acid for adults is 60 mg; for infants in the first week of life 100 mg; for older breast- or bottle-fed infants 35 mg; for children up to 11 years of age 45 mg; for pregnant women 80 mg; for lactating women 100 mg.— *Recommended Dietary Allowances,* 9th Edn, Washington, The National Research Council, 1980, p. 75.

Very high concentrations of ascorbic acid were found in samples of fruit from *Terminalia ferdinandiana*, a wild tropical tree of the Combretaceae family found in the Australian bush. This fruit may be the richest natural source of the vitamin in the world.— J. C. Brand *et al.* (letter), *Lancet*, 1982, *2*, 873.

A discussion of the biology and biochemistry of ascorbic acid in relation to its recommended daily requirements.— J. S. Flier and L. H. Underhill, *New Engl. J. Med.*, 1986, *314*, 892.

Uses and Administration

Ascorbic acid, a water-soluble vitamin, is essential for the synthesis of collagen and intercellular material. Ascorbic acid deficiency develops when the dietary intake is inadequate. It is rare in adults, but may occur in infants, alcoholics, or the elderly. Deficiency leads to the development of a well-defined syndrome known as scurvy. This is characterised by capillary fragility, bleeding (especially from small blood vessels and the gums), anaemias, cartilage and bone lesions, and slow healing of wounds.

Ascorbic acid is used in the treatment and prevention of ascorbic acid deficiency. It completely reverses symptoms of deficiency. It is usually given by mouth, the preferred route, and is often given to infants in the form of a suitable fruit juice such as orange juice. Ascorbic acid may be administered, as sodium ascorbate, by the intramuscular route, and also by the intravenous or subcutaneous routes. Doses of 0.25 to 1 g daily in divided doses have been recommended.

Ascorbic acid has been used to acidify urine and has also been tried in the treatment of idiopathic methaemoglobinaemia and many other disorders but there is little evidence of beneficial effect. Eye-drops containing potassium ascorbate have been used for the treatment of chemical burns.

Ascorbic acid and sodium ascorbate are used as antoxidants in pharmaceutical manufacturing and in the food industry.

The addition of ascorbic acid to raw and unprocessed meat intended for human consumption is prohibited in Great Britain. This prohibition extends to isoascorbic acid, nicotinic acid, nicotinamide, and any derivative of these substances or of ascorbic acid.

A review of vitamin therapy in non-deficiency states. A beneficial effect of 'megadose' ascorbic acid therapy has been claimed for an extraordinary number of conditions, including infective, allergic, and toxic states of almost every kind. These conditions include the common cold, asthma, atherosclerosis, cancer, psychiatric disorders, infections due to abnormal leucocyte function, infertility, and osteogenesis imperfecta; it has also been tried in treatment of wound healing, pain in Paget's disease, and opioid withdrawal. However, there are only few properly controlled studies which substantiate these claims, and confirmation by controlled studies is required.— L. Ovesen, *Drugs*, 1984, *27*, 148.

AMINO ACID METABOLIC DISORDERS. Benefit following administration of ascorbic acid 0.5 to 1 g daily to an infant with hawkinsinuria (a defect of tyrosine metabolism).— B. Wilcken *et al.*, *New Engl. J. Med.*, 1981, *305*, 865.

DEFICIENCY STATES. Scurvy in 1 patient with Crohn's disease and low leucocyte-ascorbic acid concentrations in a further 9 suggested that patients with Crohn's disease should receive regular treatment with ascorbic acid at a dose of 50 to 100 mg daily.— B. D. Linaker, *Postgrad. med. J.*, 1979, *55*, 26.

A report of adult scurvy in 3 patients with special reference to its epidemiology and clinical features.— J. B. Reuler *et al.*, *J. Am. med. Ass.*, 1985, *253*, 805. Comment.— E. Cheraskin (letter), *ibid.*, *254*, 2894.

Further references: M. Hughes *et al.*, *Br. med. J.*, 1986, *293*, 366; D. R. Morgan, *Practitioner*, 1987, *231*, 450; S. K. Mandal and A. K. Ray, *J. int. med. Res.*, 1987, *15*, 96.

MALIGNANT NEOPLASMS. In a double-blind randomised study ascorbic acid 10 g daily by mouth showed no benefit in 51 patients with advanced colorectal cancer when compared with placebo in 49 similar patients. None of the patients had received previous chemotherapy, and only 4 had had prior radiation treatment; body protective mechanisms were presumably as intact as possible in the presence of incurable cancer. Compliance was good in all but 5 patients taking ascorbic acid and 3 taking placebo. The median duration of therapy was 2.5 months in the ascorbic acid group and 3.6 months in the placebo group. No patient had any evidence of tumour regression, nor were disease progression or patient survival improved in the ascorbic acid group; ascorbic acid performed no better than a dummy medication.— C. G. Moertel *et al.*, *New Engl. J. Med.*, 1985, *312*, 137. Comment.— R. E. Wittes, *ibid.*, 178.

Further references: W. C. Willett and B. MacMahon, *New Engl. J. Med.*, 1984, *310*, 633.

Preparations

Ascorbic Acid Injection *(B.P.C. 1973).* Ascorbic acid 10% and sodium bicarbonate 4.8% in Water for Injections. Sterilise by filtration.

Ascorbic Acid Injection *(U.S.P.).* Contains ascorbic acid prepared with the aid of sodium hydroxide, sodium carbonate, or sodium bicarbonate.

Ascorbic Acid Oral Solution *(U.S.P.).* Contains ascorbic acid in a hydroxylic organic solvent or an aqueous mixture thereof.

Ascorbic Acid Tablets *(B.P.).* Vitamin C Tablets. Tablets containing 500 mg or more of ascorbic acid should be chewed then swallowed.

Ascorbic Acid Tablets *(U.S.P.)*

Proprietary Preparations

Redoxon *(Roche, UK). Tablets*, ascorbic acid 25, 50, 200, and 500 mg.
Tablets, effervescent, ascorbic acid 1 g.

Proprietary Names and Manufacturers

Abbo-C *(Belg.)*; Abboce *(Spain)*; Abriscor *(Fr.)*; Acidylina *(Panthox & Burck, Ital.)*; Adenex *(Canad.)*; Agrumina *(Also, Ital.)*; Agruvit *(Arg.; Lepetit, Ital.)*; Alba-Ce *(USA)*; Amplex-C *(Spain)*; Aran C *(Alfa Farmaceutici, Ital.)*; Asco-C *(Lusofarmaco, Ital.)*; Ascomed *(Ripari-Gero, Ital.)*; Ascor *(Ital.)*; Ascorb *(Protea, Austral.)*; Ascorbef *(Cox, UK)*; Ascorbin *(Switz.)*; Ascorbina *(Carlo Erba, Ital.)*; Ascorbivit *(Ital.)*; Ascorgil *(Biomedica Foscama, Ital.)*; Askorbinsyre *(DAK, Denm.)*; Aster C *(Corvi, Ital.)*; Biocatines C *(Garcia Suarez, Spain)*; Bio-Ci *(Ceccarelli, Ital.)*; C Monovit *(Esseti, Ital.)*; Cantil *(Faes, Spain)*; CC-Kaps *(USA)*; Cebion *(Aust.; Belg.; Merck-Clévenot, Fr.; E. Merck, Ger.; Greece; Bracco, Ital.; Neth.; Merck, S.Afr.; Igoda, Spain; E. Merck, Swed.; Switz.)*; Cecon *(Austral.; Abbott, Ital.)*; Cecrisina *(Syntex-Latino, Spain)*; Cedoxon *(Roche, Ger.)*; Ce-Fortin *(Ger.)*; Ceglycon *(Braun Melsungen, Ger.)*; Cegrovit *(Grossmann, Switz.)*; Cemill *(Miller, USA)*; Cenol *(Belg.)*; Cenolate *(Abbott, USA)*; Cetamin *(Austral.)*; Cetane *(Forest Pharmaceuticals, USA)*; Cetasan *(Spain)*; Cetebe *(Wolfer, Ger.)*; Cetin *(Spain)*; Ceuno *(Andromaco, Spain)*; Cevalin *(Lilly, USA)*; Cevi-Bid *(Geriatric Pharm. Corp., USA)*; Cevigen *(Gentili, Ital.)*; Ce-vi-sol *(Mead Johnson, Canad.; Mead Johnson Nutritional, USA)*; Cevit *(Italfarmaco, Ital.)*; Cevitan *(Belg.)*; Cevitasi Fuerte *(Spain)*; Cevitil *(Swed.)*; Cevitine *(Belg.)*; Cevitol 500 *(Belg.)*; Cewin *(Arg.)*; Ci-Agro *(Ravizza, Ital.)*; Cidalma *(Ital.)*; Cith *(Ital.)*; Citran *(Ital.)*; Citrets *(Fawns & McAllan, Austral.)*; Citrion *(Austral.)*; Citrovit *(Abello, Spain)*; Citrovitamina *(Ital.)*; C-Lisa *(Lisapharma, Ital.)*; C-Span *(Edwards, USA)*; C-Tard *(Ital.)*; C-Tron *(Switz.)*; C-Vicotrat-forte *(Ger.)*; C-vimin *(Astra, Swed.)*; C-Vit *(Spain)*; C-Will *(Belg.)*; Dextamina C *(Spain)*; Dif-Vitamin C *(Spain)*; Duo-C *(Geymonat, Ital.)*; Duoscorb *(USA)*; Esurvit *(Ital.)*; Euvit C *(IBIS, Ital.)*; Farmobion C *(Ital.)*; Flavettes *(Parke, Davis, Austral.)*; Frubiose 500 *(Boehringer Ingelheim, Fr.; Wild, Switz.)*; Godabion C *(Igoda, Spain)*; Gradalin C *(Spain)*; Gregovite C *(Unigreg, UK)*; Hermes *(Hermes, Ger.)*; Hicee *(Jpn)*; Hybrin *(Pharmacia, Swed.)*; Ido-C *(Ferrosan, Swed.)*; Idro-C *(Blue Cross, Ital.)*; Invite-C *(Nelson, Austral.)*; Iskia C *(Spain)*; Junce *(Inibsa, Spain)*; Juva-C *(Austral.)*; Kamu Jay *(Jamieson, Canad.)*; Kosmo-C *(Ital.)*; Kronoletas C Lenta *(Spain)*; Lacivit *(Tiber, Ital.)*; Laroscorbine *(Roche, Fr.)*; Ledovit-C *(Bama, Spain)*; Lemonvit *(Ital.)*; Lifaton-C Normal *(Spain)*; Megascorb *(Canad.)*; Megavit C *(Vitaplex, Austral.)*; Mephacevin *(Switz.)*; Multi-C *(Austral.)*; Orange *(Ital.)*; Orantine *(Belg.)*; Pancervo-C *(Spain)*; Pasta Al Cebion *(Bracco, Ital.)*; Pronto-C *(Edmond Pharma, Ital.)*; Redoxon *(Roche, Canad.; Roche, Ital.; Roche, S.Afr.; Roche, Spain; Roche, Swed.; Roche, Switz.; Roche, UK)*; Roscorbic *(Roche, UK)*; Scorbex *(Lennon, S.Afr.)*; Sergovit-C *(Inexfa, Spain)*; Taxofit *(Anasco, Ger.)*; Viascor *(Belg.)*; Vicemex *(Polcopharma, Austral.; Switz.)*; Vici *(Monico, Ital.)*; Vicisin *(Ital.)*; Vicitina *(CT, Ital.)*; Vicomin-C *(Gayoso Wellcome, Spain)*; Vigovit C *(IFCI, Ital.)*; Vio-C *(Belg.)*; Vita-Cé *(Chemedica, Switz.)*; Vitaceland *(Landerlan, Spain)*; Vitadomus C *(Medici Domus, Ital.)*; Vitafardi-C *(Spain)*; Vitascorb *(Austral.)*; Vitascorbal *(Switz.)*; Vitascorbol *(Belg.; Fr.)*; Viterra C *(Spain; USA)*; Vitoran *(Austral.)*; Vymol-C *(Landerlan, Spain)*; Wil-Cee *(Wilson, Pakistan)*; Xitix *(Woelm, Ger.)*; Yoguis-C *(Pedemonte, Spain)*.

Multivitamin and mineral preparations containing ascorbic acid or ascorbates are included in the lists on pp.1289-93. The following names have been used for preparations containing ascorbic acid or ascorbates and not considered to be a multivitamin or mineral preparation—Cal-Bid *(Geriatric Pharm. Corp., USA)*; Duo-CVP *(Rorer, Canad.)*; Peridin-C *(Hamilton, Austral.; Beutlich, USA)*; Varicyl *(Nadeau, Canad.)*.

2374-j

Aspartame *(BAN, USAN, rINN).*

APM; SC-18862. Methyl *N*-L-α-aspartyl-L-phenylalaninate; 3-Amino-*N*-(α-methoxycarbonylphenethyl)succinamic acid.
$C_{14}H_{18}N_2O_5$=294.3.

CAS — 22839-47-0.

Pharmacopoeias. In *It.* and *U.S.N.F.*

An off-white almost odourless crystalline powder with an intensely sweet taste.

Sparingly **soluble** in water at pH 5.2; more soluble in acidic solutions and hot water; slightly soluble in alcohol; very slightly soluble in chloroform; practically insoluble in oils. A 0.8% solution in water has a pH of about 5.3.

In the presence of moisture it hydrolyses to form aspartylphenylalanine and a diketopiperazine derivative, with a resulting loss of sweetness. It is most stable in solution at about pH 4.3. **Store** in airtight containers.

Adverse Effects and Precautions

Excessive use of aspartame should be avoided by patients with phenylketonuria. Its sweetness is lost during prolonged cooking.

Some discussions of various official bodies' acceptance of the safety of aspartame: H. Yellowlees (letter), *Br. med. J.*, 1983, *287*, 912; *Lancet*, 1983, *2*, 921; *FDA Consumer*, 1985, Feb., 22; Council on Scientific Affairs, *J. Am. med. Ass.*, 1985, *254*, 400.

These considerations had taken into account concerns such as those on the risks of neurochemical changes expressed by Wurtman (*New Engl. J. Med.*, 1983, *309*, 429). However, some concern continues to be expressed (W.M. Pardridge, *J. Am. med. Ass.*, 1986, *256*, 2678; *idem*, 1987, *258*, 206). There have been a few reports of individual reactions to aspartame (see below).

Reports of adverse effects associated with aspartame: N. L. Novick, *Ann. intern. Med.*, 1985, *102*, 206 (a case of granulomatous panniculitis that recurred on aspartame challenge); R. J. Wurtman (letter), *Lancet*, 1985, *2*, 1060 (an association between aspartame and seizures in 3 patients); A. Kulczycki, *Ann. intern. Med.*, 1986, *104*, 207 (aspartame-induced urticaria in 2 patients that recurred on challenge); J. E. Blundell and A. J. Hill (letter), *Lancet*, 1986, *1*, 1092 (paradoxical increase in appetite in a study involving 95 subjects); M. E. Drake (letter), *ibid.*, *2*, 631 (panic attacks in one patient associated with excessive aspartame ingestion in soft drinks); D. R. Johns (letter), *New Engl. J. Med.*, 1986, *315*, 456 (migraine in one patient associated with aspartame and recurring on challenge); S. S. Schiffman *et al.*, *ibid.*, 1987, *317*, 1181 (no association with aspartame and headache in a controlled study).

ADMINISTRATION IN PHENYLKETONURIA. Findings that aspartame may imperil dietary control of phenylketonuria. Unexpectedly high serum concentrations of phenylalanine occurred in a child with well-controlled phenylketonuria following the ingestion of aspartame in soft drinks. When three 9-year-old children with classical phenylketonuria were loaded with aspartame 34 mg per kg body-weight serum-phenylalanine concentrations rose significantly, in contrast to findings in adolescents with phenylketonuria (R. Koch *et al.*, *J. Toxic. environ. Hlth*, 1976, *2*, 459). Concentrations remained high for several days.— F. Güttler and H. Lou (letter), *Lancet*, 1985, *1*, 525.

Uses and Administration

Aspartame is an intense sweetening agent about 200 times as sweet as sucrose used in foods and beverages. Each g provides approximately 17 kJ (4 kcal).

Estimated acceptable daily intake for aspartame: up to 40 mg per kg body-weight. The acceptable daily intake of diketopiperazine (an impurity found in aspartame) is up to 7.5 mg per kg.— Twenty-fifth Report of the Joint FAO/WHO Expert Committee on Food Additives, *Tech. Rep. Ser. Wld Hlth Org. No. 669*, 1981.

Proprietary Names and Manufacturers

Canderel *(Searle, Belg.; Searle, Fr.; Searle, UK)*; D sucril *(Pierre Fabre, Fr.)*; Equal *(Searle, USA)*; Flix *(Searle, UK)*; Glucal Aspartam *(Fournier S.A., Fr.)*; Nozucar *(Prodes, Spain)*; Nutrasweet *(Searle, USA)*; Pouss-suc *(Human-Pharm, Fr.)*; Sukami *(Soekami, Fr.)*.

576-p

Aspartic Acid *(USAN, pINN).*

Asp; L-Aspartic acid. L-Aminosuccinic acid.
$C_4H_7NO_4$=133.1.

CAS — 56-84-8.

Aspartic acid is an aliphatic amino acid. It is used as a dietary supplement.

A study of the use of aspartic acid in the management of opioid withdrawal.— A. I. Sener *et al.*, *Arzneimittel-Forsch.*, 1986, *36*, 1684.

Proprietary Names and Manufacturers of Aspartates
Cogitum *(Merrell Dow, Spain)*.

For multi-ingredient preparations containing nutritional agents and vitamins, see p.1289.

7831-k

Benfotiamine *(rINN).*
S-Benzoylthiamine *O*-Monophosphate. *N*-(4-Amino-2-methylpyrimidin-5-ylmethyl)-*N*-(2-benzoylthio-4-dihydroxyphosphinyloxy-1-methylbut-1-enyl)formamide.
$C_{19}H_{23}N_4O_6PS$=466.4.

CAS — 22457-89-2.

Benfotiamine is a vitamin B_1 substance with the general properties of thiamine hydrochloride (see p.1277).

Proprietary Names and Manufacturers
Berdi *(Elea, Arg.)*; Neuroluy Retard *(Spain)*; Neurostop *(Lacer, Spain)*; Tabiomyl *(Roussel, Belg.)*; Vitanévril *(Midy, Fr.)*.

7824-a

Betacarotene *(rINN).*
Beta Carotene *(USAN)*; all-*trans*-β-Carotene; E160(a). β,β-Carotene; (*all-E*)-1,1′-(3,7,12,16-Tetramethyl-1,3,5,7,9,11,13,15,17-octadecanonaene-1,18-diyl)bis-[2,6,6-trimethylcyclohexene].
$C_{40}H_{56}$=536.9.

CAS — 7235-40-7.

Pharmacopoeias. In *U.S.*

Red or reddish brown to violet-brown crystals or crystalline powder. **Insoluble** in water, acid, or alkalis; soluble in chloroform and carbon disulphide; sparingly soluble in ether, solvent hexane, and vegetable oils; practically insoluble in methyl alcohol and alcohol. **Store** in airtight containers. Protect from light.
Carotene exists in 3 isomeric forms, all of which are converted to some extent into vitamin A in the livers of man and animals. Of the 3 isomers of carotene, the *beta* compound is more active than the *alpha*- or *gamma*-isomers. The vitamin A activity of plants is due to the presence of *alpha*-, *beta*-, and *gamma*-carotenes and to kryptoxanthine; that of animal tissues is due to both vitamin A and carotene, while fish-liver oils contain vitamin A but no carotene.

Units
See under Vitamin A, p.1278.

Betacarotene is a precursor of vitamin A (p.1278). It has been given by mouth to reduce the severity of photosensitivity reactions in patients with erythropoietic protoporphyria in doses of 30 to 300 mg daily. Betacarotene and other carotenoids are used as colouring agents for foods.

PHOTOSENSITIVITY. Although some studies have shown beneficial results with the use of betacarotene to improve tolerance to sunlight in patients with erythropoietic protoporphyria (M. M. Mathews-Roth *et al.*, *J. Am. med. Ass.*, 1974, *228*, 1004; S.T. Zaynoun *et al.*, *Br. J. Derm.*, 1977, *97*, 663; G. Goerz and H. Ippen, *Dt. med. Wschr.*, 1977, *102*, 1051) others have found that it had no more effect than placebo (M.F. Corbett *et al.*, *Br. J. Derm.*, 1977, *97*, 655). Betacarotene has been found to afford little photoprotection in patients with actinic reticuloid and idiopathic solar urticaria (A. Kobza *et al.*, *Br. J. Derm.*, 1973, *88*, 157) and in patients with polymorphous light eruption (J.A. Parrish *et al.*, *ibid.*, 1979, *100*, 187; J.J. Nordlund *et al.*, *Archs Derm.*, 1973, *108*, 710). However, Fusaro and Johnson reported some benefit in 5 patients with hereditary polymorphous light eruption (*J. Am. med. Ass.*, 1980, *243*, 231).

Preparations
Beta Carotene Capsules *(U.S.P.)*. Contain betacarotene.
Arocin *(Modern Health Products, UK)*. *Capsules*, betacarotene 2.7 mg (equivalent to vitamin A 4500 units).

Proprietary Names and Manufacturers
Arocin *(Modern Health Products, UK)*; Beta-Carotene Biorganic *(Gisand, Switz.)*; Carotaben *(Hermal, Ger.; Hermal, Switz.)*; Carotin *(Prosana, Austral.)*; Solatene *(Roche, Austral.; Roche, Canad.; Roche, USA)*.

For multi-ingredient preparations containing nutritional agents and vitamins, see p.1289.

7859-g

Biotin *(USAN, pINN).*
Coenzyme R; Vitamin H. *cis*-5-(Hexahydro-2-oxo-1*H*-thieno[3,4-*d*]imidazol-4-yl)valeric acid.
$C_{10}H_{16}N_2O_3S$=244.3.

CAS — 58-85-5.

Pharmacopoeias. In *Swiss* and *U.S.*

A practically white, crystalline powder. Very slightly **soluble** in water and in alcohol; insoluble in other common organic solvents. **Store** in airtight containers.

Biotin is traditionally considered to be a vitamin B substance. It is an essential coenzyme in fat metabolism and in other carboxylation reactions. Deficiency of biotin is very unlikely in man because of its widespread distribution in food. Egg yolk and offal are especially good sources. Biotin deficiency has been reported however during long-term parenteral nutrition and in patients with multiple carboxylase deficiency.
Biotin combines with avidin, a glycoprotein present in raw egg-white, to form an inactive compound. Prolonged ingestion of large quantities of raw egg-white could therefore lead to biotin deficiency.

A review of vitamin therapy in non-deficiency states. Symptoms of biotin deficiency include seborrhoeic dermatitis, anorexia, muscle pain, and alopecia. Spontaneous deficiency has only been observed in subjects consuming raw egg-whites which contain avidin. Ignoring the rare cases of deficiency, no clearly defined therapeutic uses of biotin exist.— L. Ovesen, *Drugs*, 1984, *27*, 148.

Comment on biotin, including mention of its potential role in diagnostic procedures.— B. Dixon, *Br. med. J.*, 1986, *292*, 1677.

AMINO ACID METABOLIC DISORDERS. Treatment with biotin, 10 mg daily by mouth, was begun at age 11 weeks in a presymptomatic child with biotinadase deficiency. Subsequent physical and biochemical monitoring up to 14 months reflected normal development.— S. J. Wallace, *Archs Dis. Childh.*, 1985, *60*, 574. Further references: B. Wolf *et al.*, *New Engl. J. Med.*, 1985, *313*, 16; W. L. Nyhan, *ibid.*, 43.

HUMAN REQUIREMENTS. In the United Kingdom deficiency of biotin is rare. Biotin occurs in sufficient quantity in a large number of foods. Therefore, in the light of present knowledge and in the context of the diet in the UK, recommended daily intakes for biotin have not been set.— Recommended Daily Amounts of Food Energy and Nutrients for Groups of People in the United Kingdom, Report by the Committee on Medical Aspects of Food Policy, *Report on Health and Social Subjects No. 15*, London, HM Stationery Office, 1979.

A recommended dietary allowance could not be established for biotin. Conventional dietary intake of 100 to 300 μg daily appeared satisfactory for adults. Infants and children should be adequately provided for with 50 μg per 4.18 MJ; human milk provides 10 μg per 4.18 MJ, milk formulas provide 15 μg per 4.18 MJ.— *Recommended Dietary Allowances*, 9th Edn, Washington, The National Research Council, 1980, p. 120.

The recommendation that foods for the young infant should contain biotin in amounts not less than 5 ng per mL (based on the lower limit of the range in pooled samples of human milk).— Artificial Feeds for the Young Infant: Report of the Working Party on the Composition of Foods for Infants and Young Children, Committee on Medical Aspects of Food Policy, *Report on Health and Social Subjects, 18*, London, HM Stationery Office, 1980.

Proprietary Names and Manufacturers
Biodermatin *(Lafare, Ital.)*; Doctodermis *(Medea, Spain)*; Medebiotin *(Medea, Spain)*.

For multi-ingredient preparations containing nutritional agents and vitamins, see p.1289.

7832-a

Bisbentiamine *(rINN).*
O-Benzoylthiamine Disulphide. *NN′*-{Dithiobis[2-(2-benzoyloxyethyl)-1-methylvinylene]}bis[*N*-(4-amino-2-methylpyrimidin-5-ylmethyl)formamide].
$C_{38}H_{42}N_8O_6S_2$=770.9.

CAS — 2667-89-2.

Bisbentiamine is a vitamin B_1 substance with the general properties of thiamine hydrochloride (see p.1277).

Proprietary Names and Manufacturers
Beston *(Triosol, Belg.; Jpn)*; Bithiamin *(Jpn)*; Supra B_1 *(Esteve, Spain)*.

7833-t

Bisbutiamine
O-Butyrylthiamine Disulphide. *NN′*-{Dithiobis[2-(2-butyryloxyethyl)-1-methylvinylene]}bis[*N*-(4-amino-2-methylpyrimidin-5-ylmethyl)formamide].
$C_{32}H_{46}N_8O_6S_2$=702.9.

CAS — 18481-23-7.

Bisbutiamine is a vitamin B_1 substance with the general properties of thiamine hydrochloride (see p.1277).

Proprietary Names and Manufacturers
Beston *(Jpn)*.

7882-v

Black Currant
Rib. Nig; Ribes Nigrum.

Pharmacopoeias. In *Br.*

The fresh ripe fruit of *Ribes nigrum* (Grossulariaceae) together with their pedicels and rachides. It has a strong, characteristic odour and a pleasantly acidic taste. The ascorbic acid content of the fruit varies between about 100 to 300 mg per 100 g.

Black currant is rich in ascorbic acid and is used in the form of a syrup as a dietary supplement, particularly for children. The syrup is also used as a flavouring agent.

Preparations
Black Currant Syrup *(B.P.)*. Prepared by dissolving sucrose 70 g in 56 mL of clarified juice from fresh black currants, previously diluted to a weight per mL of 1.045 g, or in 56 mL of a similarly diluted solution of concentrated black currant juice of commerce; benzoic acid (equivalent to not more than 800 ppm), or sodium metabisulphite or other suitable sulphite (equivalent to not more than 350 ppm of SO_2) is added. Permitted food-grade colours may be added. It contains not less than 0.055% w/w of ascorbic acid (about 7.5 mg in 10 mL) but this standard does not apply to syrup used for pharmaceutical purposes as a flavouring agent. Store at a temperature not exceeding 25° in well-filled, well-closed containers. Protect from light.

12528-s

Carnitine *(rINN).*
Vitamin B_T (L-carnitine). (3-Carboxy-2-hydroxypropyl)trimethylammonium hydroxide, inner salt.
$C_7H_{15}NO_3$=161.2.

CAS — 461-06-3; 541-14-0 (D); 541-15-1 (L); 406-76-8 (DL).

Adverse Effects
Gastro-intestinal disturbances such as nausea, vomiting, diarrhoea, and abdominal cramps have been reported following the administration of L-carnitine.

Administration of carnitine to 3 patients on long-term dialysis was associated with development of severe weakness and myasthenia-like symptoms.— G. Bazzato *et al.* (letter), *Lancet*, 1979, *1*, 1041. A myasthenia-like syndrome occurred after DL-but not L-carnitine.— G. Bazzato *et al.* (letter), *ibid.*, 1981, *1*, 1209.

Uses and Administration
L-Carnitine is an amino acid derivative which is an essential cofactor of fatty acid metabolism.
Carnitine is used in the treatment of primary carnitine deficiency and has also been shown to be of some value in carnitine deficiency secondary to a variety of defects of intermediary metabolism or other conditions. Both the L- and the DL-isomers have been used, but it is believed that only L-carnitine is effective and in addition, that DL-carnitine supplementation can lead to carnitine deficiency.
The usual dose by mouth of L-carnitine is 1 g up to three times daily with food. Children may be given 50 to 100 mg per kg body-weight daily in divided doses up to a maximum of 3 g.

A preliminary review of the pharmacokinetics and therapeutic use of L-carnitine. Administration of L-carnitine in doses of up to 4 g daily to patients with primary systemic carnitine deficiency reverses such clinical symptoms as severe muscle weakness, hypoglycaemia, and intellectual retardation seen in the more severely afflicted patients, and in some instances can be life-saving. In patients with the less debilitating myopathic deficiency there has been objective and subjective evidence of improved muscle strength within one week of the commencement of therapy. There is some evidence to indicate that the elevated plasma concentrations of triglycerides and total cholesterol in patients undergoing chronic intermittent haemodialysis can be decreased by L-carnitine supplementation, whether administered orally, intravenously, or to the dialysate. However, results have been variable and further studies are needed to determine the optimum dose in such patients. A few small studies in patients with symptoms of the 'post-dialysis syndrome' have demonstrated symptomatic improvement after 2 or more months' treatment with L-carnitine 0.99 to 2.0 g daily, although objective measurements in one study did not alter significantly. The addition of L-carnitine to total parenteral nutrition regimens in neonates has increased plasma concentrations of total and free carnitine which are lower than in infants fed enterally. Carnitine supplementation may result in better metabolism of intravenously administered fat emulsion, especially in premature infants. L-Carnitine may also be useful in the treatment of carnitine deficiencies secondary to hyperlipidaemias and in the prevention of toxicity induced by anthracyclines and valproate, however such findings should be regarded as preliminary. Administration of L-carnitine to patients with ischaemic heart disease has been shown to produce beneficial effects on myocardial function and metabolism and an improvement of exercise tolerance in patients with angina pectoris.— K. L. Goa and R. N. Brogden, *Drugs*, 1987, *34*, 1.

References: *Med. Lett.*, 1986, *28*, 88 (review of carnitine); C. J. Rebouche and A. G. Engel, *Mayo Clin. Proc.*, 1983, *58*, 533 (carnitine metabolism and deficiency syndromes); *Lancet*, 1987, *2*, 429 (role of carnitine in Reye's syndrome).

METABOLIC DISORDERS. In patients with defects of intermediary metabolism (organic acidurias) such as propionic acidaemia, methylmalonic aciduria, and isovaleric acidaemia, the accumulation of short chain acyl coenzyme A compounds within the mitochondria results in muscle weakness, incoordination, and retarded growth. L-Carnitine has been shown to be of benefit in children with such defects who display impaired motor skills and low plasma-carnitine concentrations.— K. L. Goa and R. N. Brogden, *Drugs*, 1987, *34*, 1. See also C. R. Roe and T. P. Bohan (letter), *Lancet*, 1982, *1*, 1411 (propionic acidaemia); R. J. Allen *et al.* (letter), *ibid.*, *2*, 500 (various disorders of organic acid metabolism); D. W. Seccombe *et al.* (letter), *ibid.*, 1401 (methylmalonic aciduria); C. R. Roe *et al.*, *Archs Dis. Childh.*, 1983, *58*, 916 (methylmalonic aciduria); J. A. Wolff *et al.*, *Lancet*, 1986, *1*, 289 (propionic acidaemia and methylmalonic aciduria).

Proprietary Names and Manufacturers

Bicarnesine *(Labaz, Fr.; Lennon, S.Afr.)*; Biocarn *(Nefro-Pharma, Ger.)*; Biomux *(Chiesi, Ital.)*; Cardiogen *(Mediolanum, Ital.)*; Carn *(Benvegna, Ital.)*; Carnicor *(Sigma Tau, Spain)*; Carnitolo *(Biochimica Zanardi, Ital.)*; Carnitor *(Sigma-Tau, USA)*; Carnosulen *(Inkey, Spain)*; Carnovis *(Duncan, Ital.)*; Carrier *(Chiesi, Ital.)*; Flatistine *(Sauba, Fr.)*; Framil *(Francia Farm., Ital.)*; L-Carn *(Hormonchemie, Ger.)*; Lefcar *(Glaxo, Ital.)*; Levocarvit *(Mitim, Ital.)*; Metina *(ISOM, Ital.)*; Miocardin *(Magis, Ital.)*; Monocamin *(Jpn)*; Nicetile *(Sigmatau, Ital.)*; Secabiol *(Normon, Spain)*; Vitacarn *(McGaw, USA)*; Zibren *(Duncan, Ital.)*.

7835-r

Cetotiamine Hydrochloride *(rINNM)*.

DCET; Dicethiam Hydrochloride; *O,S*-Bis(ethoxycarbonyl)thiamine Hydrochloride. *N*-(4-Amino-2-methylpyrimidin-5-ylmethyl)-*N*-[4-(ethoxycarbonyloxy)-2-(ethoxycarbonylthio)-1-methylbut-1-enyl]formamide hydrochloride.

$C_{18}H_{26}N_4O_6S,HCl$=462.9.

CAS — 137-76-8 (cetotiamine); 616-96-6 (hydrochloride).

Cetotiamine is a vitamin B_1 substance with the general properties of thiamine hydrochloride (see p.1277).

Proprietary Names and Manufacturers

Dicetamin *(Jpn)*.

7875-g

Choline Chloride *(rINN)*.

Cholinii Chloridum. 2-Hydroxyethyltrimethylammonium chloride.

$C_5H_{14}ClNO$=139.6.

CAS — 67-48-1; 62-49-7 (choline).

Pharmacopoeias. In *Aust.*, *Belg.*, *Fr.*, *Ger.*, and *Hung.*

Choline is an acetylcholine precursor. It is involved in lipid metabolism and acts as a methyl donor in various other metabolic processes. Choline has traditionally been considered to be a vitamin B substance although its functions do not justify its classification as a vitamin. A deficiency syndrome has not been identified in man and daily requirements have not been established. Sources of choline, which occurs mostly as lecithin, include egg yolk and vegetable and animal fat.

Choline has been used to treat fatty liver and cirrhosis. It has also been used in the treatment of dementia and in various extrapyramidal disorders. Choline may be used as the bitartrate and dihydrogen citrate salts as well as the chloride.

ALZHEIMER'S DISEASE. Choline and lecithin are naturally occurring dietary constituents that are precursors for the synthesis of acetylcholine. Clinical trials have attempted to improve cognitive function in patients with Alzheimer's disease by administering large doses of choline and lecithin; up to 16 g daily of choline and 25 to 100 g daily of lecithin have been given by mouth. The concentration of the active ingredient in lecithin, phosphatidyl choline, varies depending on the mixture. Lecithin, the principal source of choline in the diet, is often used in clinical studies as a substitute for choline. It does not produce a fishy odour, as does choline, but has been associated with nausea, bloating, diarrhoea, and fatty stools. Results of most studies using choline and lecithin generally show little or no benefit in memory enhancement.— K. L. Rathmann and C. S. Conner, *Drug Intell. & clin. Pharm.*, 1984, *18*, 684. See also E. Hollander *et al.*, *Br. med. Bull.*, 1986, *42*, 97.

Lack of success of choline and lecithin in the treatment of Alzheimer's disease may be explained by the fact that increasing choline availability has not been shown to increase acetylcholine release, probably because acetylcholine synthesis is linked to a high-affinity choline transport system which is close to saturation under normal conditions.— *Lancet*, 1987, *1*, 139. Comment and criticism. Choline has a dual role in cholinergic neurones, serving as the precursor for both acetylcholine and membrane phosphatidyl choline, and since membrane phosphatide is a reservoir of choline to be used for acetylcholine synthesis, it is conceivable that supplemental choline would significantly enhance acetylcholine release in Alzheimer's disease only after prolonged treatment, sufficient to restore the putative depletion of the membrane phosphatidyl choline reservoir. Whether supplemental choline is found to be of value in Alzheimer's disease, when given alone or as a supplement to anticholinesterases and other drugs, its ability to enhance acetylcholine release from normal neurones would appear to be beyond question.— I. H. Ulus and R. J. Wurtman (letter), *ibid.*, 624.

TARDIVE DYSKINESIA. A review of the management of tardive dyskinesia. Although cholinergic drugs such as choline and lecithin increase choline concentrations in blood, it is unclear whether this affects central cholinergic transmission. Initial results from clinical trials have not been promising.— *Drug & Ther. Bull.*, 1986, *24*, 27.

Proprietary Names and Manufacturers of Choline Chloride or other Choline Salts

Becholine D *(Medical Research, Austral.)*; Colyne *(Ital.)*; Neurotropan *(Itting, Ger.)*; Sulfarlem *(Charton, Canad.)*.

Multivitamin and mineral preparations containing choline are included in the lists on pp.1289-93. The following names have been used for preparations containing choline and not considered to be a multivitamin or mineral preparation— Lipotrope *(Rougier, Canad.)*.

16582-n

Citrulline

N^5-(Aminocarbonyl)-L-ornithine; N^δ-Carbamylornithine. α-Amino-δ-ureidovaleric acid.

$C_6H_{13}N_3O_3$=175.2.

CAS — 372-75-8.

Citrulline is an amino acid which is involved in the urea cycle. The malate is available in preparations that have been given in doses by mouth of 6 g daily with meals for asthenia.

The use of citrulline 0.18 g per kg daily as a substitute for arginine in the treatment of the inborn errors of urea synthesis, carbamyl phosphate synthetase and ornithine transcarbamylase deficiency.— M. Msall *et al.*, *New Engl. J. Med.*, 1984, *310*, 1500. A report of a beneficial response to therapy with L-citrulline by mouth with meals in a child with lysinuric protein intolerance presenting as childhood osteoporosis.— T. O. Carpenter *et al.*, *ibid.*, 1985, *312*, 290.

Proprietary Names and Manufacturers

Stimol *(Biocodex, Fr.)*.

7890-v

Cod-liver Oil *(BAN)*.

Aceite de Hígado de Bacalao; Cod Liver Oil *(USAN)*; Huile de Foie de Morue; Lebertran; Óleo de Bacalhau; Ol. Morrh.; Oleum Jecoris Aselli; Oleum Morrhuae; Olio di Fegato di Merluzzo.

CAS — 8001-69-2.

Pharmacopoeias. In *Arg.*, *Aust.*, *Belg.*, *Br.*, *Cz.*, *Egypt.*, *Hung.*, *Int.*, *Jpn*, *Jug.*, *Mex.*, *Nord.*, *Pol.*, *Port.*, *Roum.*, *Rus.*, *Span.*, *Swiss*, *Turk.*, and *U.S.* Also in *B.P. Vet.* Some pharmacopoeias permit oil from other species of the family Gadidae and several specify higher minima than the *B.P.* for vitamin A and vitamin D.

The oil obtained from the fresh liver of the cod, *Gadus callarias* (=*G. morrhua*) and other species of *Gadus* (Gadidae), refined, and clarified by filtration at about 0°. The *B.P.* specifies not less than 600 units of vitamin A activity per g and not less than 85 units of antirachitic activity (vitamin D) per g and may contain up to 100 ppm of dodecyl gallate, octyl gallate, or propyl gallate, or any mixture of these as an antoxidant. The *U.S.P.* specifies not less than 850 units of vitamin A and not less than 85 units of vitamin D per g, and permits up to 1% of a suitable flavour or flavours.

A pale yellow oil with a slightly fishy but not rancid odour.

B.P. **solubilities** are: practically insoluble in alcohol; miscible with chloroform, ether, and light petroleum. *U.S.P.* solubilities are: slightly soluble in alcohol; freely soluble in ether and chloroform. **Store** in well-filled airtight containers. Protect from light.

Cod-liver oil is a rich source of vitamin D and is also a good source of vitamin A. It also contains several unsaturated fatty acids which are essential food factors and do not occur in vitamin A and D concentrates.

Cod-liver oil dressings or ointment have been advocated to accelerate healing in burns, ulcers, pressure sores, and superficial wounds, but controlled observations have failed to substantiate claims of their value.

Proprietary Preparations

Morhulin *(Napp, UK)*. *Ointment*, cod-liver oil 11.4%, zinc oxide 38% in a wool fat and soft paraffin basis. For minor wounds, varicose ulcers, and pressure sores.

Proprietary Names and Manufacturers

Alk-anal *(Med. y Prod. Quím., Spain)*; Dermovitamina *(Difer, Ital.)*; Gelosellan *(Ger.)*; Jecovitol *(Neth.)*; Merluzzina *(Scherer, Ital.)*; M & M Tulle *(Malam, UK)*; Swansolan-Lebertransalbe *(Ger.)*; Ung-Morrhuol-Lohr *(Austral.)*; Unguentolan *(Heyl, Ger.*; *Siegfried, Switz.)*.

The following names have been used for multi-ingredient preparations containing cod-liver oil— Morhulin *(Napp, UK)*; Morrhuol Acridine Cream *(Hamilton, Austral.)*; Noratex *(Norton, UK)*; Thovaline *(Ilon Laboratories, UK)*; Ung. Morrhuae Co *(Philip Harris, UK)*.

5284-y

Copper

Cu=63.546.

CAS — 7440-50-8.

A reddish-coloured metal with a bright lustre; it is malleable and ductile.

Adverse Effects

Adverse effects from copper have tended to arise following absorption of the metal from cooking utensils and during dialysis. Ingestion of copper from cooking utensils is associated mainly with hepatotoxicity. Dialysis procedures may supply copper through the water supply or from parts of the equipment and when this happens patients may suffer haemolysis and other haematological reactions with kidney involvement as well as hepatotoxicity.

Adverse effects attributed to copper have been reported in women with copper-containing intra-uterine devices. There have been isolated case reports of various effects such as allergy and endometrial changes. However, with these devices it is difficult to separate those adverse effects that are due to the device from those due solely to the copper.

The symptoms of Wilson's disease (hepatolenticular degeneration) are due to an accumulation of copper in various parts of the body.

Copper salts if ingested can produce severe gastro-intestinal effects and there may be systemic absorption of copper leading to the effects discussed above. The use of sprays of copper salts in agriculture has been associated with lung changes. Treatment of copper poisoning is symptomatic and may involve the use of a chelating agent to remove any absorbed metal. Dialysis has been tried.

In Great Britain the recommended exposure limit of copper fume is 0.2 mg per m^3 (long-term) and of copper dusts and mists, 1 mg per m^3 (long-term) and 2 mg per m^3 (short-term).

Provisional maximum tolerable daily intake of copper from all sources: up to 500 µg per kg body-weight.— Twenty-sixth Report of the Joint FAO/WHO Expert Committee on Food Additives, *Tech. Rep. Ser. Wld Hlth Org. No. 683*, 1982.

Uses and Administration

Copper has a contraceptive effect when present in the uterus and is added to some intra-uterine contraceptive devices. It is also reported to have an antimicrobial action.

Copper supplements (usually administered in the form of the sulphate) are occasionally required in malnourished infants or in patients receiving total parenteral nutrition.

Copper bracelets are worn as a folk remedy for rheumatic disorders; there is no good evidence to justify such a practice.

Copper (Cuprum Metallicum; Cuprum Met.) is used in homoeopathic medicine.

CONTRACEPTION. There were several early reports of calcification and corrosion of intra-uterine contraceptive devices containing copper and of reduced effectiveness after 2 years *in situ* (J. Newton *et al., Br. med. J.*, 1977, *1*, 197; C. Gosden *et al., ibid.*, 202). Others doubted whether these changes in the devices reduced their contraceptive activity and felt that the devices could be retained for longer than 2 years (M. Cohen, *ibid.*, 1087; J.F. Miller and M. Elstein, *ibid.*, 1289). As of 1987, manufacturers were recommending that copper-containing devices could remain *in situ* for 2 to 5 years. It has also been reported that diabetic women fitted with copper intra-uterine devices are at greater risk of pregnancy than nondiabetic women (C. Gosden *et al., Lancet*, 1982, *1*, 530). However, others have reported no greater risk (S.O. Skouby and L. Mølsted-Pedersen, *ibid.*, 968; M. Thiery *et al., ibid.*, *2*, 883).

There have been reports of the copper-containing devices causing a lower incidence of tubal disease and tubal infertility compared with other devices (J.R. Daling *et al., New Engl. J. Med.*, 1985, *312*, 937; D.W. Cramer *et al., ibid.*, 941). In contrast Snowden and Pearson had already reported that there was no difference in pelvic infection rates between several types of device including one containing copper (*Br. med. J.*, 1984, *288*, 1570).

The mechanism of action, safety, and efficacy of intra-uterine devices.— Report of a WHO Scientific Group, *Tech. Rep. Ser. Wld Hlth Org. No. 753*, 1987.

DEFICIENCY. Acquired copper deficiency is very rare and the small number of cases have usually involved patients on parenteral nutrition or premature infants. The World Health Organisation (WHO) in 1973 (*Tech. Rep. Ser. Wld Hlth Org. No. 532*, 1973) arrived at a suggested minimum requirement of 50 µg (0.79 µmol) per kg body-weight daily for infants and young children, but felt that this did not provide an adequate margin of safety since copper deficiency had occurred in infants and children on diets providing 48 µg (0.76 µmol) per kg daily. As a result, WHO suggested that 80 µg (1.26 µmol) per kg daily might be a more realistic allowance for this group. An intake of 40 µg (0.63 µmol) per kg daily was considered probably adequate for older children and 30 µg (0.47 µmol) per kg daily for adult males. In a survey of copper in food (Survey of Copper and Zinc in Food, *Food Surveillance Paper No. 5, Minist. Agric. Fish. Fd*, London, H.M. Stationery Office, 1981) it was reported that the estimated daily intake of copper from the 1.46 kg of food consumed daily by the average person is under 1.8 mg (28.33 mmol). This is slightly less than the 30 µg per kg considered adequate for adult males by WHO.

Menkes' kinky hair syndrome is a genetic copper deficiency. References: A. M. Sutton *et al., Archs Dis. Childh.*, 1985, *60*, 644 and 1107 (deficiency in preterm infants); S. Salim *et al., ibid.*, 1986, *61*, 1068 (copper intake in artificially fed infants); *Lancet*, 1987, *1*, 900 (review of copper deficiency in the infant); S. M. Oppenheimer *et al., Postgrad. med. J.*, 1987, *63*, 205 (copper deficiency due to hypogammaglobulinaemia).

Proprietary Preparations

Gravigard *(Gold Cross, UK). Intra-uterine contraceptive device*, copper-wound plastic, copper approximately 200 mm^2. Mini-gravigard is a smaller version.

Multiload *(Organon, UK). Intra-uterine contraceptive device* (Cu250 and Cu250 SHORT), copper-wound plastic, copper approximately 250 mm^2.

Intra-uterine contraceptive device (Cu375), copper-wound plastic, copper approximately 375 mm^2.

Novagard *(KabiVitrum, UK). Intra-uterine contraceptive device*, silver-cored copper-wound plastic, copper approximately 200 mm^2.

Nova-T *(Schering, UK). Intra-uterine contraceptive device*, silver-cored copper-wound plastic, copper approximately 200 mm^2.

Ortho Gyne-T *(Ortho-Cilag, UK). Intra-uterine contraceptive device*, copper-wound plastic, copper approximately 200 mm^2.

Intra-uterine contraceptive device (380 Slimline), copper-wound plastic, copper approximately 380 mm^2.

Proprietary Names and Manufacturers

Copper-T 200 *(Neth.)*; Cu-7 *(Searle, USA)*; D.I.U. ML Cu 250 *(Fr.)*; Gravigard *(Searle, Austral.; Searle, Denm.; Searle, Ger.; Neth.; Searle, Switz.; Gold Cross, UK)*; Gravigarde *(Fr.)*; Gyne-T *(Cilag, Austral.; Fr.; Cilag, Ger.; Neth.)*; Mini-Gravigard *(Searle, Austral.; Searle, Ger.; Searle, Switz.; Gold Cross, UK)*; Multiload *(Organon, Austral.; Nourypharma, Ger.; Neth.; Multilan, Switz.; Organon, UK)*; Novagard *(KabiVitrum, UK)*; Nova-T *(Schering, Ger.; Schering, Switz.; Schering, UK)*; Ortho Gyne-T *(Ortho-Cilag, UK)*; Stérilet T Au Cuivre 200 *(Fr.)*; Sterlys *(Fr.)*; Tatum-T *(Searle, USA)*.

12505-h

Calcium Copperedetate *(BAN).*

Calcium [ethylenediaminetetra-acetato{4—}-*N,N′,O,O′*]-copper (II) dihydrate.

$C_{10}H_{12}CaCuN_2O_8,2H_2O$=427.9.

CAS — 66317-91-7 (anhydrous).

Pharmacopoeias. In *B.P. Vet.*

A blue, almost odourless, crystalline powder. It contains 9.1 to 9.7% of Ca and 14.4 to 15.3% of Cu. **Soluble** 1 in 7 of water, the solution gradually precipitating the insoluble tetrahydrate; practically insoluble in alcohol.

Calcium copperedetate is used by subcutaneous injection in the prevention and treatment of copper deficiency in cattle and sheep.

Proprietary Veterinary Names and Manufacturers

Coprin *(Glaxovet, UK)*.

5288-k

Copper Chloride

Cupric Chloride *(USAN)*.

$CuCl_2,2H_2O$=170.5.

CAS — 7447-39-4 (anhydrous); 10125-13-0 (dihydrate).

Pharmacopoeias. In *U.S.*

Bluish-green deliquescent crystals. Freely **soluble** in water; soluble in alcohol; slightly soluble in ether. **Store** in airtight containers.

Copper chloride is used as a source of copper.

Preparations

Cupric Chloride Injection *(U.S.P.)*. Copper Chloride Injection

Proprietary Names and Manufacturers

Coppertrace *(Armour, USA)*.

For multi-ingredient preparations containing nutritional agents and vitamins, see p.1289.

18507-g

Copper Gluconate *(USAN).*

Copper D-gluconate (1:2); Bis (D-gluconato-O^1,O^2) copper.

$C_{12}H_{22}CuO_{14}$=453.8.

Pharmacopoeias. In *U.S.*

Store in well-closed containers.

Copper gluconate is used as a source of copper.

Preparations

For multi-ingredient preparations containing nutritional agents and vitamins, see p.1289.

5285-j

Copper Sulphate

Copper Sulph.; Cuivre (Sulfate de); Cupr. Sulph.; Cupri Sulphas; Cupric Sulfate *(USAN)*; Kupfersulfat; Sulfato de Cobre. Copper (II) sulphate pentahydrate.

$CuSO_4,5H_2O$=249.7.

CAS — 7758-98-7 (anhydrous); 7758-99-8 (pentahydrate).

NOTE. Crude copper sulphate is sometimes known as 'blue copperas', 'blue stone', and 'blue vitriol'.

Pharmacopoeias. In *Arg., Aust., Belg., Fr., Hung., Jug., Mex., Nord., Pol., Port., Rus., Span., Swiss,* and *U.S.* Also in *B.P. Vet.* and *B.P.C. 1973.*

Blue crystals or crystalline odourless or almost odourless powder. It slowly effloresces in air. The exsiccated salt is nearly white.

Soluble 1 in 3 of water, 1 in 0.5 of boiling water, and 1 in 500 of alcohol; soluble 1 in 3 of glycerol. The *B.P. Vet.* specifies that a 5% solution in water has a pH of not less than 3.8; the *U.S.P.* injection has a pH of 2.0 to 3.5. **Store** in airtight containers.

Copper sulphate and other soluble salts of copper have an astringent action on mucous surfaces and in strong solutions they are corrosive. Their adverse effects are described under copper (above).

Copper sulphate is used as a source of copper in the management of deficiency states when it is usually given with parenteral feeds. The dose should be governed by the serum-copper concentration which in healthy adults ranges between 0.7 and 1.6 µg per mL (0.01 to 0.025 µmol per mL). Doses that have been employed range from 0.5 to 1.5 mg (7.9 to 23.6 µmol) per kg body-weight; infants have received 20 µg (0.3 µmol) per kg.

A 0.1% aqueous solution of copper sulphate has sometimes been used, with care, for gastric lavage and emesis in phosphorus poisoning; a 1% solution has also been used to wash phosphorus burns.

Copper sulphate has been used to prevent the growth of algae in reservoirs, ponds, and swimming pools and as a molluscicide in the control of fresh-water snails that act as intermediate hosts in the life-cycle of the parasites causing schistosomiasis and fascioliasis.

Reagents containing copper sulphate are used in tests for reducing sugars.

Preparations

Cupric Sulfate Injection *(U.S.P.)*. Copper Sulphate Injection

Proprietary Names and Manufacturers

Métacuprol *(Lemoine, Fr.)*.

For multi-ingredient preparations containing nutritional agents and vitamins, see p.1289.

15331-x

Cuproxoline *(BAN, USAN, rINN).*
Copper(II) bis(5,7-disulpho-8-quinolyl oxide)—diethylamine (1:4).
$C_{34}H_{56}CuN_6O_{14}S_4$=964.6.
CAS — 13007-93-7.

Cuproxoline is used in veterinary medicine by subcutaneous injection for the prevention and treatment of copper deficiency in cattle and sheep.

Proprietary Veterinary Names and Manufacturers
Cujec *(Coopers Animal Health, UK).*

7853-d

Cyanocobalamin *(BAN, USAN, rINN).*

Cobamin; Cyanocobalaminum; Cycobemin.
Coα-[α-(5,6-Dimethylbenzimidazolyl)]-*Coβ*-cyanocobamide.
$C_{63}H_{88}CoN_{14}O_{14}P$=1355.4.
CAS — 68-19-9.

NOTE. Vitamin B_{12} is the name generally used for a group of related cobalt-containing compounds, also known as cobalamins, of which cyanocobalamin and hydroxocobalamin are the principal forms in clinical use.

Pharmacopoeias. In *Arg., Aust., Belg., Br., Braz., Chin., Cz., Egypt., Eur., Fr., Hung., Ind., Int., It., Jpn, Jug., Mex., Neth., Nord., Pol., Port., Roum., Rus., Swiss, Turk.*, and *U.S.* Also in *B.P. Vet.*

Dark red crystals or crystalline or amorphous powder. In the anhydrous form it is very hygroscopic and when exposed to air it may absorb about 12% of water.
Soluble 1 in 80 of water; sparingly soluble in alcohol; practically insoluble in acetone, chloroform, and ether. The *B.P.* injection has a pH of 3.8 to 5.5. The *U.S.P.* injection has a pH of 4.5 to 7.0. Solutions are **sterilised** by autoclaving. **Store** in airtight containers. Protect from light.

7854-n

Hydroxocobalamin *(BAN, USAN, rINN).*

Hydroxocobalaminum; Idrossocobalamina. *Coα*-[α-(5,6-Dimethylbenzimidazolyl)]-*Coβ*-hydroxocobamide.
$C_{62}H_{89}CoN_{13}O_{15}P$=1346.4.
CAS — 13422-51-0.

Pharmacopoeias. In *Br., Fr., Ind., It.*, and *U.S.*
Fr. also includes Hydroxocobalamin Acetate and Chloride. *Jpn* has Hydroxocobalamin Acetate. Also in *B.P. Vet.*

Hydroxocobalamin occurs either as aquocobalamin chloride (*Coα*-[α-(5,6-dimethylbenzimidazolyl)]*Coβ*-aquocobamide chloride), which when dried contains 96 to 102% of $C_{62}H_{90}ClCoN_{13}O_{15}P$, or as aquocobalamin sulphate, which when dried contains 96 to 102% of $C_{124}H_{180}Co_2N_{26}O_{34}P_2S$. Dark red, odourless or almost odourless crystals or crystalline powder. Some decomposition may occur on drying. The anhydrous form is very hygroscopic.
Soluble 1 in 50 of water, 1 in 100 of alcohol, and 1 in 10 000 of chloroform and ether; sparingly soluble in methyl alcohol; practically insoluble in acetone. A 2% solution in water has a pH of 8 to 10. The *B.P.* injection has a pH of 3.8 to 5.5. The *U.S.P.* injection has a pH of 3.5 to 5.0. Solutions are **sterilised** by filtration. **Store** at a temperature not exceeding 15° in well-closed containers. Protect from light.

Adverse Effects and Precautions

Allergic hypersensitivity reactions have occurred rarely following the administration of the vitamin B_{12} compounds cyanocobalamin and hydroxocobalamin.
Cyanocobalamin or hydroxocobalamin should, if possible, not be given to patients without first confirming the diagnosis, and should not be used to treat megaloblastic anaemia of pregnancy. Administration of doses greater than 10 μg daily may produce a haematological response in patients with folate deficiency; indiscriminate use may mask the precise diagnosis.
Absorption of vitamin B_{12} from the gastro-intestinal tract may be reduced by aminoglycosides, aminosalicylic acid, anticonvulsants, biguanides, chloramphenicol, cholestyramine, cimetidine, colchicine, potassium salts, and methyldopa. Serum concentrations may be decreased by concurrent administration of oral contraceptives.

Analysis, by the Boston Collaborative Drug Surveillance Program, of data on 15 438 patients hospitalised between 1975 and 1982 detected 3 allergic skin reactions attributed to cyanocobalamin among 168 recipients of the drug. For the purposes of the study, reactions were defined as being generalised morbilliform exanthems, urticaria, or generalised pruritus only.— M. Bigby *et al., J. Am. med. Ass.*, 1986, *256*, 3358.

Malabsorption of protein-bound vitamin B_{12}, which cannot be detected by the Schilling test, may lead to vitamin B_{12} deficiency of clinical importance.— D. W. Dawson *et al., Br. med. J.*, 1984, *288*, 675. See also J. Laustsen and J. Fallingborg (letter), *Lancet*, 1983, *2*, 518.

Absorption and Fate

Vitamin B_{12} substances bind to intrinsic factor and are then actively absorbed from the gastro-intestinal tract. Absorption is impaired in patients with an absence of intrinsic factor, with a malabsorption syndrome or with disease or abnormality of the gut, or after gastrectomy. Vitamin B_{12} is extensively bound to specific plasma proteins called transcobalamins; transcobalamin II appears to be involved in the rapid transport of the cobalamins to tissues. It is stored in the liver, excreted in the bile, and undergoes enterohepatic recycling; part of a dose is excreted in the urine, most of it in the first 8 hours. Vitamin B_{12} diffuses across the placenta and also appears in breast milk.

After injection of cyanocobalamin a large proportion is excreted in the urine within 24 hours; the body retains only 55% of a 100-μg dose and 15% of a 1000-μg dose. Body stores of vitamin B_{12} amount to 2000 to 3000 μg which is believed to be enough for 3 to 4 years. If 1000 μg is injected monthly, the 150 μg retained lasts for about 1 month. Hydroxocobalamin is better retained than cyanocobalamin; 90% of a 100-μg dose and 30% of a 1000-μg dose is retained which is believed to be enough for 2 to 10 months.— *Drug & Ther. Bull.*, 1984, *22*, 43.

Human Requirements

For adults, the daily requirement of vitamin B_{12} is probably about 2 to 3 μg and this amount is present in most normal diets. Vitamin B_{12} occurs only in animal products, it does not occur in vegetables, therefore strict vegetarian diets that exclude dairy products may provide an inadequate amount. Meats, especially liver and kidney, milk, eggs, and other dairy products, and fish are good sources of vitamin B_{12}.

The following daily intakes of vitamin B_{12} were recommended: up to 1 year of age, 0.3 μg; 1 to 3 years, 0.9 μg; 4 to 9 years, 1.5 μg; 10 years and over, 2 μg; in pregnancy, 3 μg; during lactation, 2.5 μg.— Report of a Joint FAO/WHO Expert Group, *Tech. Rep. Ser. Wld Hlth Org. No. 452*, 1970.

In the United Kingdom deficiency of vitamin B_{12} is rare. Vitamin B_{12} occurs in sufficient quantity in a large number of foods. Therefore, in the light of present knowledge and in the context of the diet in the *UK*, recommended daily intakes for vitamin B_{12} have not been set.— Recommended Daily Amounts of Food Energy and Nutrients for Groups of People in the United Kingdom, Report by the Committee on Medical Aspects of Food Policy, *Report on Health and Social Subjects No. 15*, London, HM Stationery Office, 1979.

The recommended daily dietary allowance of vitamin B_{12} for adults is 3 μg; for breast-fed infants, 0.5 μg daily; for infants fed on milk formulas and for children up to adolescence, 0.15 μg per 418 kJ; for pregnant or lactating women, 4 μg.— *Recommended Dietary Allowances*, 9th Edn, Washington, The National Research Council, 1980, p. 117.

The recommendation that foods for the young infant should contain vitamin B_{12} in amounts not less than 0.1 ng per mL (based on the lower limit of the range in pooled samples of human milk).— Artificial Feeds for the Young Infant: Report of the Working Party on the Composition of Foods for Infants and Young Children, Committee on Medical Aspects of Food Policy, *Report on Health and Social Subjects, 18*, London, HM Stationery Office, 1980.

Uses and Administration

Vitamin B_{12}, water-soluble vitamin, occurs in the body mainly as methylcobalamin (mecobalamin) and as adenosylcobalamin (cobamamide) and hydroxocobalamin. Mecobalamin and cobamamide act as coenzymes in nucleic acid synthesis. Mecobalamin is also closely involved with folic acid in several important metabolic pathways.
Vitamin B_{12} deficiency may occur in strict vegetarians with an inadequate dietary intake, in patients with malabsorption syndromes or metabolic disorders, nitrous oxide-induced megaloblastosis, or following gastrectomy. Deficiency leads to the development of megaloblastic anaemias and neurological damage. A specific anaemia known as pernicious anaemia develops in patients with an absence of intrinsic factor.
Vitamin B_{12} preparations are used in the treatment and prevention of vitamin B_{12} deficiency. It is desirable to identify the exact cause of deficiency before commencing therapy. In the *UK*, hydroxocobalamin is the drug of choice as it binds more firmly to plasma proteins and is retained in the body longer. In the *US* however, cyanocobalamin is preferred due to the fact that administration of hydroxocobalamin has resulted in the formation of antibodies to the transcobalamin II-vitamin B_{12} complex in some patients. Cyanocobalamin and hydroxocobalamin are generally administered by the intramuscular route, although cyanocobalamin has been given by mouth in nutritional deficiency where the gastro-intestinal absorption is normal.
In the absence of neurological involvement, cyanocobalamin and hydroxocobalamin may be administered in doses of 250 to 1000 μg intramuscularly on alternate days for 1 to 2 weeks, then 250 μg weekly until the blood count returns to normal. Maintenance doses of 1000 μg are administered monthly (for cyanocobalamin) or every 2 to 3 months (for hydroxocobalamin). Hydroxocobalamin may also be given in these doses in the treatment of tobacco amblyopia and Leber's optic atrophy. If there is neurological involvement, cyanocobalamin or hydroxocobalamin may be given in doses of 1000 μg on alternate days and continued for as long as improvement occurs. Cyanocobalamin has been given by mouth in doses of 35 to 150 μg daily. Lower doses for the administration of both cyanocobalamin and hydroxocobalamin are recommended in the *US*.
Treatment usually results in rapid haematological improvement and a striking clinical response. However, neurological symptoms respond more slowly and in some cases remission may not be complete.

Vitamin B_{12} is necessary for the synthesis of thymidylate, which is the characteristic base of DNA. The vitamin plays a biochemical role in the maintenance of myelin in the nervous system. Deficiency results in megaloblastic anaemia and demyelination involving the posterior and lateral columns of the spinal cord (subacute combined degeneration of the spinal cord). 'Megadose' therapy with vitamin B_{12} has been used for a wide variety of conditions, including neurological and psychiatric disorders, cutaneous sarcoid, and as a roborant for patients complaining of tiredness. However, there is no scientific evidence for a beneficial effect in any of these conditions.— L. Ovesen, *Drugs*, 1984, *27*, 148.

The only available oral preparation of vitamin B_{12} is cyanocobalamin which is manufactured from non-animal sources. Only about 2 μg can be absorbed through the ileum from a conventional oral dose, although about 1% of a large dose can be absorbed passively. Oral treatment cannot provide enough to replenish body stores, so initial treatment should be by injection.— *Drug & Ther. Bull.*, 1984, *22*, 43. See also *ibid.*, 33.

AMINO ACID METABOLIC DISORDERS. References to the use of hydroxocobalamin in the treatment of inborn errors of vitamin B_{12} metabolism: S. Schuh *et al.*, *New Engl. J. Med.*, 1984, *310*, 686 (homocystinuria and megaloblastic anaemia without methylmalonic aciduria); A. V. Hoffbrand *et al.*, *ibid.*, 789 (functionally inactive transcobalamin II); S. Shinnar and H. S. Singer, *ibid.*, *311*, 451 (cobalamin C mutation with methylmalonic aciduria and homocystinuria); D. S. Rosenblatt *et al.*, *Lancet*, 1985, *1*, 1127 (mecobalamin deficiency (cobalamin E disease)); H. R. Bhatt *et al.* (letter), *ibid.*, 1986, *2*, 465 (treatment of hydroxocobalamin-resistant methylmalonic acidaemia with cobamamide).

DIAGNOSIS AND TESTING. Macrocytosis may be found in about one in every 25 routine blood counts, commonly without anaemia, and of these perhaps one in 20 is related to vitamin B_{12} deficiency. The only practical way of assessing the cobalamin state of patients in a general hospital is by measuring the serum concentration which used to be determined by microbiological assay. Most laboratories now use the radioisotope dilution assay. The radioisotope dilution assay confirms the deficiency and will usually differentiate it from folate deficiency. Both a dietary history and an absorption test are required in patients of all races with one exception–those with antibody to intrinsic factor with a low serum concentration of cobalamin which confirms a diagnosis of pernicious anaemia. In general, the Schilling test with plasma uptake is a practical combination of absorption tests. A spot faeces test, based on the excretion of isotope in a single sample, may be as accurate.— D. W. Dawson, *Br. med. J.*, 1984, *289*, 938.

It is unclear whether hydroxocobalamin is as effective as cyanocobalamin as the flushing injection in the Schilling test of vitamin B_{12} malabsorption. Only cyanocobalamin is available with a radioactive label for use in the Schilling test and in laboratory radioassays.— *Drug & Ther. Bull.*, 1984, *22*, 43.

Further references: V. F. Fairbanks and L. R. Elveback, *Mayo Clin. Proc.*, 1983, *58*, 135; V. F. Fairbanks *et al.*, *ibid.*, 541; I. L. Salom (letter), *ibid.*, 839; V. F. Fairbanks (letter), *ibid;* R. Colebunders and E. Van Royen, *ibid.*, 1984, *59*, 53; R. Carmel and D. S. Karnaze, *J. Am. med. Ass.*, 1985, *253*, 1284.

MULTIPLE SCLEROSIS. Persistence of macrocytosis despite vitamin B_{12} therapy in 2 of 3 patients with multiple sclerosis and vitamin B_{12} deficiency, one of whom had juvenile pernicious anaemia. The relationship between vitamin B_{12} deficiency and multiple sclerosis is not clear; multiple sclerosis is not a recognised complication of vitamin B_{12} deficiency. None of these patients had any of the usually recognised neurological or psychiatric complications and all had normal peripheral nerve studies. Further studies of the possible role of vitamin B_{12} in multiple sclerosis are needed.— E. H. Reynolds and J. C. Linnell, *Lancet*, 1987, *2*, 920.

Preparations

Cobalamin Concentrate *(U.S.P.)*. Vitamin B_{12} Activity Concentrate. The dried partially purified product resulting from the growth of selected *Streptomyces* cultures or other cobalamin-producing micro-organisms. It contains not less than 500 µg of cobalamin (measured as cyanocobalamin) per g, and it may contain harmless diluents and stabilising agents. A 0.5% solution in water has a pH of 4 to 8.

A less purified form of vitamin B_{12} suitable for use in oral preparations.

Cyanocobalamin Injection *(B.P.)*. Contains sufficient acetic acid or hydrochloric acid to adjust the pH to about 4. Potency is expressed in terms of the equivalent amount of anhydrous cyanocobalamin.

Cyanocobalamin Injection *(U.S.P.)*. A sterile solution of cyanocobalamin in Water for Injections, or in Water for Injections rendered iso-osmotic by the addition of sodium chloride. Potency is expressed in terms of the equivalent amount of anhydrous cyanocobalamin.

Hydroxocobalamin Injection *(B.P.)*. Contains sufficient acetic acid or hydrochloric acid to adjust the pH to about 4. Potency is expressed in terms of the equivalent amount of anhydrous hydroxocobalamin.

Hydroxocobalamin Injection *(U.S.P.)*. Potency is expressed in terms of the equivalent amount of anhydrous hydroxocobalamin.

Proprietary Preparations

Cobalin-H *(Paines & Byrne, UK)*. *Injection*, hydroxocobalamin 1000 µg/mL, in ampoules of 1 mL.

Cytacon *(Duncan, Flockhart, UK)*. *Liquid*, cyanocobalamin 35 µg/5 mL.
Tablets, cyanocobalamin 50 µg.

Cytamen *(Duncan, Flockhart, UK)*. *Injection*, cyanocobalamin 1000 µg/mL, in ampoules of 1 mL.

Neo-Cytamen *(Duncan, Flockhart, UK)*. *Injection*, hydroxocobalamin 250 and 1000 µg/mL, in ampoules of 1 mL.

Proprietary Names and Manufacturers of Cyanocobalamin, Hydroxocobalamin, and other Vitamin B_{12} Substances

Acimexan *(Switz.)*; Activanat *(Arg.)*; Acuo-Godabion B12 *(Spain)*; Aima *(Ital.)*; Algobaz *(Labaz, Fr.)*; alphaRedisol *(Merck Sharp & Dohme, USA)*; Alpha-Ruvite *(USA)*; Ambritan *(Farmasimes, Spain)*; Anabasi *(Pierrel Hospital, Ital.)*; Anabolizante Hermes *(Organon, Spain)*; Anabozima *(Santos, Spain)*; Anacobin *(Allen & Hanburys, Canad.)*; Anahaemin *(Duncan, Flockhart, UK)*; Anazym *(Ital.)*; Aquo-Cytobion *(E. Merck, Ger.)*; Aquodavur *(Spain)*; Asimil B12 *(Torlan, Spain)*; Augmentan *(Spain)*; Axlon *(Ger.)*; B12-Framan *(Oftalmiso, Spain)*; Balamin forte *(S.Afr.)*; BayBee-12 *(Bay, USA)*; Bedocefarm *(Kairon, Spain)*; Bedoz *(Nadeau, Canad.)*; Behepan *(KabiVitrum, Denm.*; *Kabi, Swed.)*; Be-Livita *(Spain)*; Benydiol *(Spain)*; Berubi *(Redel, Ger.)*; Berubigen *(Upjohn, USA)*; Berubilong *(Redel, Ger.)*; Betalin 12 *(Lilly, USA)*; Betarin *(Beta, Ital.)*; Betolvex *(Dumex, Denm.*; *Dumex, Neth.*; *Dumex, Norw.*; *Dumex, Swed.*; *Dumex, Switz.)*; Bimil *(Ital.)*; B_{12} Dépôt *(Siegfried, Switz.)*; Bio-12 *(Canad.)*; Biocobal VCA *(Bergamon, Ital.)*; Bradirubra *(Ital.)*;

Calomide-ME *(Jpn)*; Campolon Forte *(Belg.)*; Ciclozim *(Ital.)*; Cincomil Bedoce *(Spain)*; Cobafor *(Arg.)*; Cobaforte *(Roussel Maestretti, Ital.)*; Cobaldocemetil *(Clariana, Spain)*; Cobalidrina 1000 *(Ital.)*; Cobalin *(Ital.*; *Paines & Byrne, UK)*; Cobalin-H *(Paines & Byrne, UK)*; Cobalion *(Fr.)*; Cobalparen *(Saarstickstoff-Fatol, Ger.)*; Cobalparen-Depot *(Saarstickstoff-Fatol, Ger.)*; Cobaltamin-S *(Jpn)*; Cobalvit *(Tosi-Novara, Ital.)*; Cobamain *(Jpn)*; Cobametin 500 *(Jpn)*; Cobamide *(UCB, Ital.)*; Cobamyde *(Jpn)*; Cobanzyme *(Bouchara, Fr.)*; Cobazina *(Terapeutico M.R., Ital.)*; Cobazymase *(Bouchara, Switz.)*; Coben B_{12} *(Coli, Ital.)*; Cobimetil-B12 *(Spain)*; Cobolin-M *(Legere, USA)*; Coezim-B_{12} *(Tosi-Novara, Ital.)*; Conzibi 12 *(Ital.)*; Co-Vitam B12 *(Smaller, Spain)*; Cromazim *(Lafare, Ital.)*; Cyanabin *(Stickley, Canad.)*; Cykobemin *(Swed.)*; Cytacon *(Glaxo, Austral.*; *Glaxo, S.Afr.*; *Duncan, Flockhart, UK)*; Cytaman *(Belg.)*; Cytamen *(Arg.*; *Glaxo, Austral.*; *Glaxo, S.Afr.*; *Duncan, Flockhart, UK)*; Cytobion *(E. Merck, Ger.)*;

Depinar *(Petersen, S.Afr.)*; Depogamma *(Ger.)*; Dibencozan *(Houdé, Fr.)*; Dimazin *(Ital.)*; Dobetin *(Angelini, Ital.)*; Docémine *(Roussel, Fr.)*; Docetasan *(Santos, Spain)*; Docevita *(Spain)*; Docigram 1000 *(Lipha, Ital.)*; Docivit *(Ger.)*; Docivit Depot *(Ger.)*; Dodécavit *(L'Arguenon, Fr.)*; Dodecozim B_{12} *(Ital.)*; Dodevitina *(CT, Ital.)*; Dodex *(USA)*; Dolonevran *(Dausse, Fr.)*; Dosixbe *(Arg.)*; Droxodoce 10 000 *(Arg.)*; Droxofor *(Arg.)*; Dunyl *(Exa, Arg.)*; Emazian *(Ital.)*; Ener-B *(Nature's Bounty, USA)*; Eocill B12 *(Nessa, Spain)*; Eparmone *(Ital.)*; Epatomaster *(Ital.)*; Epatormon *(Ital.)*; Eritrovit B_{12} *(Lisapharma, Ital.)*; Eupakriton *(Ital.)*; Extrabolin *(Ital.)*; Ficarmore *(Fr.)*; Fisiocobal *(Ausonia, Ital.)*; Fiviton B12 *(Carol, Spain)*; Forta-B12 *(Belg.)*; Fortezim *(Crosara, Ital.)*; Fravit B_{12} *(Francia Farm., Ital.)*; Glade *(Also, Ital.)*; Gradalin Co-B_{12} *(Ralay, Spain)*; Hépatophal *(Laphal, Fr.)*; Hepacon *(Consolidated Chemicals, UK)*; Hepanorm Fortissimum *(Wallace Mfg Chem., UK)*; Heraclene *(Belg.*; *Fr.)*; Hidroxuber *(Spain)*; Higadin *(Inibsa, Spain)*; Hitocobamin-M *(Jpn)*; Hormantoxone *(Fr.)*; Hycobal *(Jpn)*; Hydrocobamine *(Neth.)*; Hydroxo *(Anphar-Rolland, Fr.*; *Rolland, Switz.*; *USA)*; Hydroxobase *(Lipha, Ger.)*; Idro Apavit *(Locatelli, Ital.)*; Idrobamina *(Tiber, Ital.)*; Idrocobalamin *(Ital.)*; Idrospes B_{12} *(Ausonia, Ital.)*; Idrozima *(Ital.)*; Indusil *(Diamant, Fr.*; *Recordati, Ital.*; *Roussel, Spain)*; Isopto B12 *(Alcon, Spain)*; Lagavit B_{12} *(Switz.)*; Lifaton B12 *(Sabater, Spain)*; Liodozal *(Switz.)*; Liofhem *(Vir, Spain)*; Lipohepal *(Spain)*; Livron *(Medic, Canad.)*; Longicobal *(Farber-Ref, Ital.)*; Lophakomp *(Ger.)*;

Macrabin H *(Ind.)*; Makara *(Makara, Ger.)*; Marvizim *(Ital.)*; Maximal *(Ecobi, Ital.)*; Medozim *(Medosan, Ital.)*; Mega-B12 *(Belg.)*; Megamil Bedoce *(Andromaco, Spain)*; Mepharubin *(Switz.)*; Methycobal *(Jpn)*; Methylcobaz *(Labaz, Fr.)*; Metil-Vitelix *(Emyfar, Spain)*; Milbedoce *(Spain)*; Milbedoce Depot *(Spain)*; Millevit *(Nordmark, Ger.)*; Natur B_{12} *(Panthox & Burck, Ital.)*; Néoton *(Pentapharm, Switz.)*; Névrizide *(Rorer, Fr.)*; Neo-Betalin 12 *(USA)*; Neocobal *(CT, Ital.)*; Neo-Cytamen *(Arg.*; *Glaxo, Austral.*; *Glaxo, Ital.*; *S.Afr.*; *Duncan, Flockhart, UK)*; Neo-Rubex *(Canad.)*; Neuro Liser B12 *(Spain)*; Neurobaltina *(Ital.)*; Norivite-12 *(Ethimed, S.Afr.)*; Noventabedoce *(Spain)*; Novidroxin *(Saarstickstoff-Fatol, Ger.)*; Novobedouze *(Belg.*; *Bouchara, Fr.*; *Bouchara, Switz.)*; Nubee 12 *(Propan, S.Afr.)*; Nutricon *(Ital.)*; OH B_{12} *(Pierrel Hospital, Ital.)*; Optovite B12 *(Normon, Spain)*;

Paidozim *(Ital.)*; Panalamine *(Austral.)*; Panhor *(Casen Fisons, Spain)*; Parenamps *(Paines & Byrne, UK)*; Paxom *(Synlab, Fr.)*; Pharmatovit B_{12} *(Ger.*; *Switz.)*; Plentasal *(Wasserman, Spain)*; Protemi *(Kairon, Spain)*; Radiozima *(Ital.)*; Red 1000 *(Neopharmed, Ital.)*; Redisol *(Canad.*; *Merck Sharp & Dohme, USA)*; Reedvit *(Arg.)*; Reticulogen *(Lilly, Ital.)*; Retidex B12 *(Spain)*; Ripason *(Ascot, Austral.*; *Berna, Spain*; *Robapharm, Switz.* : *Welbeck, UK)*; Robaden *(Robapharm, Switz.* : *Welbeck, UK)*; Robelvit B_{12} *(Ital.)*; Robuden *(Ascot, Austral.*; *Robapharm, Switz.)*; Rossobivit 1000 *(Ital.)*; Rotamin *(Ital.)*; Rubenzim Forte *(Ital.)*; Rubesol *(Central Pharmaceuticals, USA)*; Rubion *(Desbergers, Canad.)*; Rubitard B_{12} *(Proter, Ital.)*; Rubraluy *(Spain)*; Rubramin *(Squibb, Canad.)*; Rubramin PC *(Squibb, USA)*; Rubrovit 1000 *(Switz.)*; Ruvite *(Savage, USA)*;

Sartoenzim *(Spain)*; Sorbevit B12 *(Casen Fisons, Spain)*; Sorbigen B_{12} *(Ital.)*; Surgevit *(Maipe, Spain)*; Sytobex *(Parke, Davis, USA)*; Thencel *(Spain)*; Trillovit *(Boniscontro & Gazzone, Ital.)*; Trofozim *(Ital.)*; Unifort *(Ital.)*; Vancomin-S *(Jpn)*; Vibeden *(GEA, Denm.)*; Vicapan B_{12} *(Merckle, Ger.)*; Viemin 12 *(Valeas, Ital.)*; Vita-Brachont *(Azuchemie, Ger.)*; Vit-Alboform *(Merckle, Ger.)*; Vitarubin *(Streuli, Switz.)*; Vitosit *(Spain)*; Xobaline *(Ger.*; *Spain)*; Zervital *(Ital.)*; Zidovit *(IBP, Ital.)*; Zimadoce *(Rubio, Spain)*.

For multi-ingredient preparations containing nutritional agents and vitamins, see p.1289.

7837-d

Cycotiamine *(rINN)*.

CCT; Cyclocarbothiamine. *N*-(4-Amino-2-methylpyrimidin-5-ylmethyl)-*N*-[1-(2-oxo-1,3-oxathian-4-ylidene)ethyl]formamide.
$C_{13}H_{16}N_4O_3S$=308.4.

CAS — 6092-18-8.

Cycotiamine is a vitamin B_1 substance with the general properties of thiamine hydrochloride (see p.1277).

Proprietary Names and Manufacturers
Cometamin *(Jpn)*.

579-e

Cysteine Hydrochloride *(USAN, pINNM)*.

920; Cys Hydrochloride; L-Cysteine Hydrochloride. L-2-Amino-3-mercaptopropionic acid hydrochloride monohydrate.
$C_3H_7NO_2S,HCl,H_2O$=175.6.

CAS — 52-90-4 (cysteine); 52-89-1 (hydrochloride, anhydrous); 7048-04-6 (hydrochloride, monohydrate).

Pharmacopoeias. In *Cz.* and *U.S. Fr.* permits anhydrous or monohydrate. *Cz.* also includes DL-Cysteine Hydrochloride.

White crystals or crystalline powder. **Soluble** in water, alcohol, and acetone. The injection has a pH of 1.0 to 2.5.

Cysteine is an aliphatic amino acid. It is used as a dietary supplement. It is also used topically in ophthalmology.

For reference to the role of cysteine in the treatment of hepatic encephalopathy, see under Enteral and Parenteral Nutrition, p.1252.

CORNEAL ULCERATION. Perforations of the cornea occurred in only 1 of 33 eyes severely burnt with alkali which were treated with 0.2M cysteine solution applied as 2 drops 6 times daily after 7 days' routine treatment with antibiotics and cycloplegics; perforations occurred in 5 of 7 eyes not treated with cysteine. Progress of corneal ulcers in 3 badly burnt eyes was arrested immediately after the use of cysteine eye-drops.— S. I. Brown *et al.*, *Am. J. Ophthal.*, 1972, *74*, 316.

LEG ULCERATION. Overall degree of healing and

decrease in pain were significantly better in 11 patients with hypostatic leg ulcers treated topically for 12 weeks with a cream containing cysteine, glycine, and racemic threonine than in 10 similar patients treated with the vehicle only.— S. G. Harvey *et al.*, *Pharmatherapeutica*, 1985, *4*, 227.

Preparations

Cysteine Hydrochloride Injection *(U.S.P.)*

Proprietary Names and Manufacturers

Cystein Gel oculaire *(Medipharm, Switz.)*; Narutin *(Angelopharm, Ger.)*; Phakosklerom *(Thilo, Ger.)*.

Multi-ingredient nutritional preparations containing cysteine are included in the lists on pp.1289-93. The following names have been used for preparations containing cysteine and not considered to be such multi-ingredient preparations—Aminoderm *(Desbergers, Canad.)*; Cantothen *(Cantassium Co., UK)*; Cicatrin *(Wellcome, Austral.*; *Wellcome, Canad.*; *Calmic, UK)*.

580-b

Cystine *(USAN)*.

β,β'-Dithiodialanine; Di(α-aminopropionic)-β-disulphide; L-Cystine. L-3,3'-Dithiobis(2-aminopropionic acid).

$C_6H_{12}N_2O_4S_2$=240.3.

CAS — 56-89-3.

Cystine is an aliphatic amino acid. It is used as a dietary supplement. It has been used in the treatment of congenital homocystinuria.

A diet providing only 10 mg of methionine daily per kg body-weight in conjunction with treatment with cystine 1.5 g daily and choline dihydrogen citrate 10 g daily in divided doses, decreased plasma concentrations of methionine and homocystine in 3 children with homocystinuria. In addition, a 3-year-old child treated with a low-methionine diet and cystine since early infancy had remained mentally and physically normal. Choline might facilitate enzymic remethylation of homocystine to methionine.— T. L. Perry *et al.*, *Lancet*, 1968, *2*, 474.

Three children with homocystinuria responded to treatment with a low-methionine diet and supplements of cystine over an 8-month period.— I. B. Sardharwalla *et al.*, *Can. med. Ass. J.*, 1968, *99*, 731.

Proprietary Names and Manufacturers

Cistidil *(IDI, Ital.)*; Gélucystine *(Pharmeurop, Fr.)*.

Multi-ingredient nutritional preparations containing cystine are included in the lists on pp.1289-93. The following names have been used for preparations containing cystine and not considered to be such multi-ingredient preparations—Amino-Cerv *(Milex, USA)*.

581-v

Dextrin *(BAN, USAN)*.

British Gum; Dextrinum Album; Starch Gum.

CAS — 9004-53-9.

Pharmacopoeias. In *Aust.*, *Br.*, *Chin.*, *Cz.*, *Fr.*, *Ger.*, *Jpn*, *Jug.*, *Pol.*, *Port.*, and *Span.* Also in *U.S.N.F.*

An intermediate product in the ultimate hydrolysis of starch, made by heating starch with or without the aid of suitable acids and buffers.

A white, pale yellow, or brown powder with a slight characteristic odour. *B.P.* **solubilities** are: very soluble in boiling water forming a mucilaginous solution; slowly soluble in cold water; practically insoluble in alcohol and ether. The *U.S.N.F.* states that the solubility of dextrin varies; that it is usually very soluble, but often contains an insoluble portion.

Dextrin, a glucose polymer, is a source of carbohydrate often used in oral dietary supplements and tube feeding. It is used as a tablet and capsule diluent, and as a binding, suspending, and viscosity-increasing agent.

Dextrin has also been used as an adhesive and stiffening agent for surgical dressings.

Fourteen neonates weighing less than 1.5 kg at birth gained weight faster when water-soluble dextrin powder 6 g per kg body weight was added to their milk feeds for 7-day periods than when it was omitted.— A. Raffles *et al.*, *Br. med. J.*, 1983, *286*, 935. Addition of protein-free energy supplements to low-protein milk may result in a very low protein:energy ratio. Energy supplements should be used with caution where the protein content of the basic feed is unknown.— O. G. Brooke (letter), *ibid.*, 1143.

Proprietary Names and Manufacturers

Caloreen *(Austral.*; *Roussel, Canad.*; *Denm.*; *Roussel, UK)*; Crystal Gum S *(Laing-National, UK)*; Poly-Joule *(Sharpe, Austral.)*.

2390-j

Dulcin

Phenetolurea. (4-Ethoxyphenyl)urea.

$C_9H_{12}N_2O_2$=180.2.

CAS — 150-69-6.

Pharmacopoeias. In *Span.*

Lustrous colourless crystals or a white crystalline powder with a very sweet taste. **Soluble** 1 in 800 of water and 1 in 50 of boiling water.

Dulcin is an intense sweetening agent and has been used in some countries as a substitute for sucrose, being about 250 times as sweet.

Dulcin should not be used as a food additive because of its tumorigenic potentialities.— Eleventh Report of the Joint FAO/WHO Expert Committee on Food Additives, *Tech. Rep. Ser. Wld Hlth Org. No. 383*, 1968.

7860-f

Folic Acid *(BAN, USAN, rINN)*.

Acidum Folicum; Folacin; Folinsyre; PGA; Pteroylglutamic Acid; Pteroylmonoglutamic Acid.

N-[4-(2-Amino-4-hydroxypteridin-6-ylmethylamino)benzoyl]-L(+)-glutamic acid.

$C_{19}H_{19}N_7O_6$=441.4.

CAS — 59-30-3; 6484-89-5 (sodium folate).

Pharmacopoeias. In *Arg.*, *Aust.*, *Belg.*, *Br.*, *Braz.*, *Chin.*, *Cz.*, *Egypt.*, *Eur.*, *Fr.*, *Ger.*, *Ind.*, *Int.*, *It.*, *Jpn*, *Jug.*, *Mex.*, *Neth.*, *Nord.*, *Pol.*, *Port.*, *Rus.*, *Swiss*, *Turk.*, and *U.S.*

A yellow to orange brown, odourless or almost odourless crystalline powder.

B.P. **solubilities** are: practically insoluble in water and most organic solvents. *U.S.P.* solubilities are: very slightly soluble in water; insoluble in alcohol, acetone, chloroform, and ether. It dissolves in dilute acid solutions and in solutions of alkali hydroxides and carbonates. The *U.S.P.* injection has a pH of 8 to 11. **Store** in well-closed containers. Protect from light.

STABILITY IN SOLUTION. A review of the compatibility and stability of components of total parenteral nutrition solutions when mixed in 1- or 3-litre flexible containers. Folic acid has been reported to precipitate in some proprietary amino acid solutions and in the presence of high concentrations of calcium ions, but it appears to be stable and remain in solution provided the pH remains above 5. There have also been reports of folic acid being absorbed by the polyvinyl chloride container and administration set, however other studies have not substantiated such observations.— M. C. Allwood, *J. clin. Hosp. Pharm.*, 1984, *9*, 181. See also P. W. Niemiec and T. W. Vanderveen, *Am. J. Hosp. Pharm.*, 1984, *41*, 893.

Adverse Effects

Folic acid is generally well tolerated. Gastro-intestinal disturbances may occur. Allergic reactions have been reported rarely.

Precautions

Folic acid should never be given alone or in conjunction with inadequate amounts of vitamin B_{12} for the treatment of undiagnosed megaloblastic anaemia. Although folic acid may produce a haematopoietic response in patients with a megaloblastic anaemia due to vitamin B_{12} deficiency, it fails to prevent the onset of subacute combined degeneration of the cord. Therefore, the inclusion of folic acid in multivitamin preparations may be dangerous as an improvement in vitamin B_{12}-dependent megaloblastic anaemia may mask the true deficiency state.

Caution is advised in patients who may have folate-dependent tumours.

DIAGNOSIS AND TESTING. Serum-folate concentration does not indicate the severity of folate deficiency since it may be equally low in grossly anaemic patients and in patients without anaemia. A more reliable index of tissue depletion of folate is measurement of folate in red blood cells.— D. G. Lambie and R. H. Johnson, *Drugs*, 1985, *30*, 145. A study emphasising the need for considerable caution in interpretation of data required for the assessment of folate status.— F. J. Stanley *et al.*, *Lancet*, 1982, *2*, 1100.

INTERACTIONS. A review of drugs affecting folate metabolism. Anticonvulsant drugs, oral contraceptives, antituberculous drugs, alcohol, and folic acid antagonists including aminopterin, methotrexate, pyrimethamine, trimethoprim, and sulphonamides are all reported to produce folate deficiency states.— D. G. Lambie and R. H. Johnson, *Drugs*, 1985, *30*, 145.

For a report of folate deficiency due to the induction of microsomal enzymes after 2 to 5 years' treatment with anticonvulsants, phenothiazines or tricyclic antidepressants with a benzodiazepine, see p.709.

For the interaction between folic acid and phenytoin, see Effects on the Blood in Phenytoin, Adverse Effects, p.407. See also under Pregnancy and the Neonate, below.

MENTAL DISORDERS. Two patients showed exacerbation of psychotic behaviour during treatment with folic acid.— R. Prakash and W. M. Petrie, *Am. J. Psychiat.*, 1982, *139*, 1192.

PREGNANCY AND THE NEONATE. In 133 pregnancies in 125 epileptic women all taking folic acid supplements, folic acid concentrations were inversely related to those of phenytoin and phenobarbitone, but not to those of carbamazepine. There was no evidence of folic acid deficiency in the group, no correlation between folic acid concentrations and seizures and no foetal malformations attributable to lowered concentrations of folic acid.— V. K. Hiilesmaa *et al.*, *Br. med. J.*, 1983, *287*, 577.

A study of 46 pregnant epileptic women, all of whom were taking anticonvulsants, and in which a folate supplement was taken in 31 of 49 pregnancies. Decreased maternal serum-folate and red cell-folate concentrations were significantly associated with adverse pregnancy outcome. Of the 49 pregnancies, there were 10 abnormalities: 4 spontaneous abortions (8.2%) and 6 major congenital malformations (12.2%).— L. V. Dansky *et al.*, *Ann. Neurol.*, 1987, *21*, 176.

Absorption and Fate

Folic acid is absorbed mainly from the proximal part of the small intestine. The naturally occurring folate polyglutamates are largely deconjugated and reduced prior to absorption. It is the 5-methyltetrahydrofolate which appears in the portal circulation, where it is extensively bound to plasma proteins.

Folic acid is rapidly absorbed from normal diets and is distributed in body tissues. The principal storage site is the liver. There is an enterohepatic circulation for folate; about 4 to 5 μg is excreted in the urine daily. Administration of larger doses of folic acid leads to proportionately more of the of the vitamin being excreted in the urine. Folate is distributed into breast milk.

In a study of 15 healthy subjects, eight of whom smoked cigarettes, serum-folate concentrations were significantly lower in smokers than in non-smokers. The possibility that the reduction in serum folate may be related to elevated hepatic microsomal enzyme activity in smokers is discussed.— Y. Nakazawa *et al.*, *Drug & Alcohol Depend.*, 1983, *11*, 201.

Human Requirements

Body stores of folate in healthy persons have been reported as being between 5 to 10 mg, but may be much higher. About 400 μg of folate a day is considered a suitable average intake. Folate is present, chiefly combined with several L(+)-glutamic acid moieties, in many foods, particularly liver, kidney, yeast, nuts, and leafy green vegetables. The vitamin is readily oxidised to unavailable forms and is easily destroyed during cooking.

The recommended daily intakes of total folate were: infants up to 6 months, 40 to 50 μg; 7 to 12 months, 120 μg; children 1 to 12 years, 200 μg; persons 13 years and over, 400 μg; pregnant women, 800 μg; lactating women, 600 μg. All pregnant women needed daily supplements of about 500 μg of folic acid.— Report of a WHO Group of Experts on Nutritional Anaemias, *Tech. Rep. Ser. Wld Hlth Org. No. 503*, 1972.

Recommended daily intake of total folate: infants under 1 year, 50 μg; children 1 to 4 years, 100 μg; boys 5 to 11 years 200 μg; girls 5 to 8 years, 200 μg; older persons 300 μg; during pregnancy 500 μg; during lactation, 400 μg.— Recommended Daily Amounts of Food Energy and Nutrients for Groups of People in the United Kingdom, Report by the Committee on Medical Aspects of Food Policy, *Report on Health and Social Subjects No. 15*, London, HM Stationery Office, 1979.

The recommended daily dietary allowance of folate is 400 μg for adults and adolescents; for infants 5 μg per kg body-weight; for children 8 to 10 μg per kg; for pregnant women 800 μg; for lactating women 500 μg.— *Recommended Dietary Allowances*, 9th Edn, Washington, The National Research Council, 1980, p. 109.

The recommendation that foods for the young infant should contain folic acid in amounts not less than 30 ng per mL (based on the lower limit of the range in pooled samples of human milk).— Artificial Feeds for the Young Infant: Report of the Working Party on the Composition of Foods for Infants and Young Children, Committee on Medical Aspects of Food Policy, *Report on Health and Social Subjects, 18*, London, HM Stationery Office, 1980.

For further comments on folate requirements during pregnancy, see under Deficiency States, in Uses.

Uses and Administration

Folic acid is a member of the vitamin B group. Folic acid is reduced in the body to tetrahydrofolate, which is a coenzyme for various metabolic processes including the synthesis of purine and pyrimidine nucleotides, and hence in the synthesis of DNA; it is also involved in some amino-acid conversions, and in the formation and utilisation of formate. Deficiency, which can result in megaloblastic anaemia, develops when the dietary intake is inadequate, as in malnutrition, from malabsorption, from increased utilisation as in pregnancy or conditions such as haemolytic anaemia, and as a result of the administration of folate antagonists and other drugs which interfere with normal folate metabolism (see under Precautions, above).

Folic acid is used in the treatment and prevention of the folate deficiency state. It does not correct folate deficiency due to dihydrofolate reductase inhibitors; calcium folinate (p.1264) is used for this purpose.

For the treatment of megaloblastic anaemia in the *UK* it is recommended that folic acid is given by mouth in an initial dosage of 10 to 20 mg daily for 14 days, or until a haematopoietic response has been obtained; the daily maintenance dose is 2.5 to 10 mg. Children may be given 5 to 15 mg daily according to the severity of the deficiency state. Some authorities have recommended that in folate-deficient megaloblastic anaemia due to causes other than a malabsorption syndrome, folic acid 5 mg daily by mouth for 4 months is sufficient to bring about a haematological remission and replenish body stores. Prophylactic administration of folic acid 5 mg daily or weekly by mouth may be necessary in chronic haemolytic states such as thalassaemia major or sickle-cell anaemia, depending on the diet and rate of haemolysis.

In the *US* much lower doses are recommended. For the treatment of proven folate deficiency, folic acid 0.25 to 1.0 mg daily by mouth may be given until a haematopoietic response has been obtained; the daily maintenance dose is 0.4 mg daily.

In the prophylaxis of megaloblastic anaemia of pregnancy, the usual dose is 200 to 500 μg daily. Folic acid may also be administered by intramuscular, intravenous, or subcutaneous injection as the sodium salt.

ADMINISTRATION IN RENAL FAILURE. For reference to folic acid in renal failure see under Deficiency States (Dialysis), below.

CHROMOSOME DISORDERS. Preliminary findings suggesting that folic acid may be of benefit in improving "psychosis-like" symptoms in patients with the fragile X syndrome.— J. Lejeune (letter), *Lancet*, 1982, *1*, 273. See also H. G. Kinnell, *Br. med. J.*, 1987, *295*, 564.

DEFICIENCY STATES. A detailed review of folic acid and its use in the treatment of conditions associated with folate deficiency.— R. E. Davis, *Clin. Chem.*, 1986, *25*, 233. See also *Drug & Ther. Bull.*, 1984, *22*, 33.

Blood disorders. A report of 2 patients who developed thrombocytopenia and severe haemorrhage associated with folic acid deficiency.— D. J. Easton, *Can. med. Ass. J.*, 1984, *130*, 418.

Dialysis. There appears to be no justification for routine folic acid supplementation in adequately nourished patients receiving either regular haemodialysis (V.L. Sharman *et al.*, *Br. med. J.*, 1982, *285*, 96; C.P. Swainson and R.J. Winney, *Lancet*, 1983, *1*, 239) or continuous ambulatory peritoneal dialysis (Swainson and Winney, 1983; C.R.V. Tomson, *Lancet*, 1988, *1*, 473) despite earlier studies which recommended the administration of folic acid 1 mg after each haemodialysis (V.A. Skoutakis *et al.*, *Clin. Pharmac. Ther.*, 1975, *18*, 200).

In children. In a double-blind controlled study of 62 infants with low birth-weight folic acid 50 μg daily from the age of 2 weeks to 6 months produced no greater benefit than placebo.— A. C. Kendall *et al.*, *Archs Dis. Childh.*, 1974, *49*, 736.

Folic-acid deficiency may be the cause of reduced birth-weight and growth in erythroblastic infants. Folic acid supplementation in 17 such infants improved weight gain although when folic acid was stopped some regressed.— G. Gandy and W. Jacobson, *Archs Dis. Childh.*, 1977, *52*, 1, 7, and 16.

Folic acid treatment of megaloblastosis in preterm infants and warning to avoid excess.— M. K. Strelling *et al.*, *Archs Dis. Childh.*, 1979, *54*, 699; D. Stevens *et al.*, *Pediatrics*, 1979, *64*, 333.

In the elderly. In a study of 200 consecutive patients admitted to a geriatric unit, 46 subjects had low serum concentrations of vitamin B_{12} (15), red-cell folate (26), or both (5). A nutritionally depleted diet may have been responsible for many of the low vitamin values.— E. L. Blundell *et al.*, *J. clin. Path.*, 1985, *38*, 1179.

Infections. In patients infected with *Plasmodium falciparum*, folate requirements may be increased as a consequence of an increased rate of erythropoiesis. The relative folic acid deficiency which may develop in such persons can give rise to megaloblastic marrow changes. Folic acid in doses of 5 mg daily for 2 to 3 weeks will counteract both this effect and any myelotoxic effect resulting from the use of pyrimethamine.— The Clinical Management of Acute Malaria, *WHO Regional Publications, South-East Asia Series No. 9*, 1986.

In a study of 260 patients with viral and mycoplasmal infections, a low serum-folate concentration (less than 3 μg per litre) was reported in 60% of subjects. The authors suggested that lassitude and the need for prolonged convalescence following a viral infection could be associated with acute folate depletion.— W. Jacobson *et al.*, *J. Infect.*, 1987, *14*, 103.

Inflammatory bowel diseases. The causes of folate deficiency in Crohn's disease are multifactorial; anorexia, malabsorption, disease activity, and drug-induced haemolysis from sulphasalazine are all important mechanisms.— R. V. Heatley, *Postgrad. med. J.*, 1983, *59*, 690.

See also *idem*, *Gut*, 1986, *27*, *Suppl.* S1, 61.

Nervous system and psychiatric disorders. It is generally believed that deficiency of folic acid, in contrast to that of vitamin B_{12}, does not produce neuropathy. However, neurological disease, which sometimes has included symptoms indistinguishable from subacute combined degeneration of the spinal cord, has been related to folic acid deficiency.— L. Ovesen, *Drugs*, 1984, *27*, 148.

In a study of 49 depressed patients with low plasma- and cerebrospinal fluid-folate concentrations, the administration of folic acid 10 mg daily by mouth for 7 to 11 months produced a significant improvement in neuropsychological rating scores as evidenced by Wechsler subtests.— M. I. Botez *et al.*, *Psychol. Med.*, 1984, *14*, 431.

A review of folate deficiency in psychiatric patients and the use of folic acid in therapeutic trials. Folate deficiency is a common occurrence in both organic and functional psychiatric disorders. It is a common association of depressive symptoms in a variety of settings including primary endogenous or non-endogenous depression, and in alcoholic, lithium-treated, and anorectic patients.— M. T. Abou-Saleh and A. Coppen, *J. Psychiat. Res.*, 1986, *20*, 91.

Further references: *Lancet*, 1975, *1*, 1283 (folate-responsive schizophrenia); E. H. Reynolds (letter), *ibid.*, 1975, *2*, 189.

See also under Chromosome Disorders, above.

Pregnancy and the neonate. It has been claimed that the risk of foetal neural-tube defect may be reduced by the administration of folic acid and other vitamins in the periconceptional period (R.W. Smithells *et al.*, *Archs Dis. Childh.*, 1981, *56*, 911; K.M. Laurence *et al.*, *Br. med. J.*, 1981, *282*, 1509; R. W. Smithells *et al.*, *Lancet*, 1983, *1*, 1027). The studies by Smithells and co-workers were criticised as the trials were not randomised and the controls may have represented different socioeconomic groups (J.M. Elwood, *Can. med. Ass. J.*, 1983, *129*, 1088; *ibid.*, 1984, *130*, 1116 (correction); G. P. Oakley *et al.*, *Lancet*, 1983, *2*, 798; N.J. Wald and P.E. Polani, *Br. J. Obstet. Gynaec.*, 1984, *91*, 516). The study by Laurence *et al.* (1981) was a double-blind randomised trial, but still attracted criticism because of the small number of subjects and the manner in which the data was analysed (J.M. Elwood (1983); N.J. Wald and P.E. Polani (1984); P. McCullagh, *Med. J. Aust.*, 1985, *142*, 328). However, the possibilities raised by the two studies led to the Medical Research Council (MRC) in the *UK* initiating a multinational, multicentre, controlled clinical trial to study the effects of folate and multivitamin administration in the prevention of neural-tube defects. The MRC study has attracted considerable attention with regard to its necessity, feasibility, and ethics (*Nature*, 1982, *300*, 396; *ibid.*, 565; P. McCullagh (1985); D. Simpson and E. Robertson, *Med. J. Aust.*, 1985, *142*, 706; J.A. Davis, *ibid.*, *143*, 51). However, by August 1987, the MRC trial had recruited only 1046 women 52% of the total needed. It was considered that a further 5 years would elapse before the trial was completed (*Lancet*, 1987, *2*, 376).

See also under Precautions, above.

Mention of the controversy concerning the Committee on Safety of Medicines approval for the use of Pregnavite Forte F [a multivitamin and iron preparation containing folic acid 120 μg] to reduce the risk of spina bifida or anencephaly in babies born to women who have previously given birth to one or more babies (or aborted a foetus) with a neural-tube defect.— *Lancet*, 1987, *2*, 376. Comment.— N. C. Nevin *et al.* (letter), *ibid.*, 516.

DIAGNOSIS AND TESTING. The hydrolytic deconjugation of a triglutamate derivative of folic acid to the monoglutamate form and its subsequent absorption was used as a measure of enterocyte function. The deconjugation step was significantly impaired in 19 patients with progressive systemic sclerosis, relative to a control group of 14 subjects. Absorption of folic acid was similar in both groups.— L. Hendel *et al.*, *Gut*, 1987, *28*, 435.

Preparations

Folic Acid Injection *(U.S.P.)*. A sterile solution of folic acid in Water for Injections prepared with the aid of sodium hydroxide or sodium carbonate.

Folic Acid Tablets *(B.P.)*

Folic Acid Tablets *(U.S.P.)*

Proprietary Preparations

Lexpec *(R.P. Drugs, UK)*. *Syrup*, sucrose-free, folic acid 2.5 mg/5 mL.

Proprietary Names and Manufacturers of Folic Acid and its Salts

Acfol *(Torlan, Spain)*; Folacid *(Neth.)*; Folaemin *(Neth.)*; Folasic *(Nelson, Austral.)*; Foldine *(Fr.)*; Folettes *(Austral.)*; Folicid *(USV, Austral.)*; Folico *(Ecobi, Ital.)*; Folina *(Tosi, Ital.)*; Folsan *(Kali-Chemie, Ger.)*; Folvite *(Lederle, Canad.; Lederle, Switz.; Lederle, USA)*; Lexpec *(R.P. Drugs, UK)*; Nifolin *(Denm.)*; Novofolacid *(Novopharm, Canad.)*; Speciafoldine *(Specia, Fr.)*.

For multi-ingredient preparations containing nutritional agents and vitamins, see p.1289.

7862-n

Folinic Acid

Citrovorum Factor; Formyl Tetrahydropteroylglutamic Acid; Leucovorin. 5-Formyltetrahydropteroylglutamate; *N*-[4-(2-Amino-5-formyl-5,6,7,8-tetrahydro-4-hydroxypteridin-6-ylmethylamino)benzoyl]-L(+)-glutamic acid.

$C_{20}H_{23}N_7O_7$=473.4.

CAS — 58-05-9.

7863-h

Calcium Folinate *(BAN, rINN).*

Calcium Folinate-SF; Calcium Leucovorin; Leucovorin Calcium *(USAN)*; NSC-3590. Calcium 5-formyltetrahydropteroylglutamate; Calcium *N*-[4-(2-amino-5-formyl-5,6,7,8-tetrahydro-4-hydroxypteridin-6-ylmethylamino)benzoyl]-L(+)glutamate.

$C_{20}H_{21}CaN_7O_7$=511.5.

CAS — 1492-18-8 (anhydrous); 41927-89-3; 6035-45-6 (both pentahydrate).

Pharmacopoeias. In *Braz.* and *U.S.*

A yellowish-white or yellow, odourless powder. Very **soluble** in water; practically insoluble in alcohol. The *U.S.P.* injection has a pH of 6.5 to 8.5. **Store** in well-closed containers. Solutions of calcium folinate in glucose injection (5%), sodium chloride injection (0.9%), or compound sodium lactate injection are reported to be stable for 24 hours when stored at 15 to 30°. Protect from light.

Adverse Effects

Occasional allergic reactions have been reported; pyrexia has occurred after injections.

Precautions

Folinic acid should not be administered simultaneously with a folic acid antagonist as this may nullify the effect of the antagonist. See also under Folic Acid, above.

Uses and Administration

Folinic acid is the 5-formyl derivative of tetrahydrofolic acid, the active form of folic acid. Folinic acid is used principally as an antidote to folic acid antagonists, such as methotrexate, which block the conversion of folic acid to tetrahydrofolate by binding the enzyme dihydrofolate reductase.

In cases of inadvertent overdosage of a folic acid antagonist, folinic acid should be administered as soon as possible; if a period of more than 4 hours intervenes, the treatment may not be effective. Where large doses of methotrexate have been given calcium folinate may be given by intravenous infusion in a dose equivalent to 75 mg of folinic acid within 12 hours, followed by 12 mg intramuscularly every 6 hours for 4 doses. Doses equal to or greater than the dose of methotrexate have been recommended. In less severe overdosage 6 to 12 mg of folinic acid intramuscularly every 6 hours for 4 doses may be adequate.

Folinic acid is used in conjunction with methotrexate to reduce the toxicity of the methotrexate ('folinic acid rescue'; 'calcium leucovorin rescue'). Folinic acid is given after an appropriate interval, usually of up to 24 hours, has elapsed for methotrexate to exert its antineoplastic effect. Doses of up to 120 mg have been given over 12 to 24 hours, by intramuscular injection or intravenous injection or infusion, followed by 12 to 15 mg intramuscularly, or 15 mg by mouth, every 6 hours for the next 48 hours. With lower doses of methotrexate folinic acid 15 mg by mouth every 6 hours for 48 to 72 hours may suffice. For further details see under Methotrexate, p.639.

Folinic acid, like folic acid, is effective in the treatment of megaloblastic anaemia. Doses of 15 mg daily by mouth or not greater than 1 mg intramuscularly have been suggested for the treatment of megaloblastic anaemias.

Preparations

Leucovorin Calcium Injection *(U.S.P.)*. Contains calcium folinate. Sodium hydroxide or hydrochloric acid may be added to adjust the pH; it may contain suitable preservatives. Potency is expressed in terms of the equivalent amount of folinic acid.

Proprietary Preparations

Calcium Leucovorin *(Lederle, UK)*. *Injection*, folinic acid (as the calcium salt) 3 mg/mL, in ampoules of 1 mL. *Injection*, powder for reconstitution, folinic acid (as the calcium salt) 15 and 30 mg.
Tablets, folinic acid (as the calcium salt) 5 and 15 mg.

Refolinon *(Farmitalia Carlo Erba, UK)*. *Injection*, folinic acid (as the calcium salt) 3 mg/mL, in ampoules of 2 and 10 mL.
Tablets, scored, folinic acid (as the calcium salt) 15 mg.

Rescufolin *(Nordic, UK)*. *Injection*, powder for reconstitution, folinic acid (as the calcium salt) 15, 50, and 100 mg.
Tablets, folinic acid (as the calcium salt) 15 mg.

Proprietary Names and Manufacturers

Chemifolin *(Bracco, Ital.)*; Citrec *(Laakefarmos, Swed.)*; Disintox *(IRBI, Ital.)*; Lederfolin *(Cyanamid, Ital.; Cyanamid, Spain)*; Lederfoline *(Lederle, Fr.)*; Ledervorin *(Neth.)*; Ledervorin Calcium *(Belg.)*; Refolinon *(Farmitalia Carlo Erba, UK)*; Rescufolin *(Nordic, UK)*; Rescuvolin *(Medac, Ger.; Nyco, Norw.; Nycomed, Swed.)*; Tonofolin *(ABC, Ital.)*; Wellcovorin *(Wellcome, USA)*.

595-e

Fructose *(BAN, USAN).*

Fruit Sugar; Laevulose; Laevulosum (Fructosum); Levulose; D-Fructose. D-(−)-Fructopyranose.

$C_6H_{12}O_6$=180.2.

CAS — 57-48-7.

Pharmacopoeias. In *Aust., Br., Cz., Egypt., Eur., Fr., Ger., It., Jpn, Jug., Neth., Port., Swiss,* and *U.S.*
NOTE. *Nord.* includes Laevulose for Infusion (Fructosum ad Infundibilia).

Odourless colourless crystals or a white crystalline powder with a sweet taste.

B.P. **solubilities** are: 1 in 0.3 of water and 1 in 15 of alcohol. *U.S.P.* solubilities are: freely soluble in water; soluble 1 in 15 of alcohol and 1 in 14 of methyl alcohol. A 5.05% solution in water is iso-osmotic with serum. Solutions are **sterilised** immediately after preparation by autoclaving. **Store** in well-closed containers.

Adverse Effects

Large doses of fructose given by mouth may cause flatulence, abdominal pain and diarrhoea. Lactic acidosis and hyperuricaemia may follow intravenous infusions; fatalities have occurred.

A report of urticaria induced by ingestion of D-psicose, a byproduct of high-fructose syrup.— K. Nishioka *et al.* (letter), *Lancet*, 1983, *2*, 1417.

For reference to the role of sugars, including fructose, in the development of dental caries, see under Sucrose, p.1276.

Precautions

Fructose should not be given to patients with hereditary fructose intolerance.

It should be given with caution to patients with impaired kidney function or severe liver damage.

A report of raised glycosylated haemoglobin values in a 17-year-old diabetic which were incompatible with blood-glucose estimations. The patient regularly ate fructose-containing substances and on elimination of these from the diet her glycosylated haemoglobin values fell to normal.— A. C. Burden (letter), *Lancet*, 1984, *2*, 986. Comment. The patient might have essential fructosuria, an enzyme disorder characterised by a lack of hepatic fructokinase activity.— A. Bär and H. Schneider (letter), *ibid.*, 1985, *1*, 57. Reply.— A. C. Burden (letter), *ibid.*

Absorption and Fate

Fructose is absorbed from the gastro-intestinal tract but more slowly than glucose. It is metabolised more rapidly than glucose, mainly in the liver where it is phosphorylated and a part is converted to glucose. Insulin is considered not to be necessary for its conversion to glycogen.

In 31 children aged 1 month to 16 years, absorption of fructose 2 g per kg body-weight (to a maximum of 50 g) was incomplete in 22 (as judged by the hydrogen concentration in breath); only one of 17 aged less than 9 years absorbed fructose completely. Absorption was complete in 6 of 7 given glucose concomitantly, and in 3 of 3 given galactose concomitantly.— C. M. F. Kneepkens *et al.*, *Archs Dis. Childh.*, 1984, *59*, 735.

Uses and Administration

Fructose is sweeter than sucrose or sorbitol. It has been employed as an alternative to glucose in parenteral nutrition but its use is not recommended because of the risk of lactic acidosis.

Fructose has been given by intravenous infusion in the treatment of severe alcohol poisoning.

Fructose has also been used in the treatment of vomiting of pregnancy.

Because of its slow absorption and rapid metabolism fructose has been used in limited quantities as a source of carbohydrate for the diabetic.

The use of fructose as a carbohydrate source does not appear to help control of diabetes. Its other effects on metabolism need further assessment. It may be useful as a sweetener for diabetics, provided its caloric contribution is appreciated.— *Drug & Ther. Bull.*, 1980, *18*, 67.

Special diabetic products containing fructose and sorbitol are sometimes taken in the mistaken belief that they contain fewer calories. The British Diabetic Association in its dietary recommendations has advised that fructose and sorbitol intake should each be limited to 25 g a day. Diabetic food products containing these substances are expensive, do not have an important role in diabetic diets, and their use is generally not encouraged.— B. F. Clarke (letter), *Br. med. J.*, 1987, *294*, 422.

Preparations

Fructose Injection *(U.S.P.)*. It contains no antimicrobial agents. pH 3 to 6.

Fructose Intravenous Infusion *(B.P.)*. Fructose Injection; Laevulose Intravenous Infusion. pH 3.0 to 5.5. Store at a temperature not exceeding 25°.

Fructose and Sodium Chloride Injection *(U.S.P.)*. It contains no antimicrobial agents. pH 3 to 6.

Proprietary Preparations

Emetrol *(Radiol, UK)*. *Oral solution*, fructose 1.87 g, glucose 1.87 g, phosphoric acid 21.5 mg in each 5 mL.

Proprietary Names and Manufacturers

Esafosfina *(Biomedica Foscama, Ital.)*; Fructal *(Stholl, Ital.)*; Fructo-Fosfan *(SPA, Ital.)*; Fructopiran *(Monico, Ital.)*; Fructosteril *(Fresenius, Ger.)*; Inulon *(Spain)*; Laevoral *(Ger.; Ital.; Switz.)*; Laevosan *(Austral.; Belg.; Ger.; Boehringer Biochemia, Ital.; Switz.)*; Laevuflex 20 *(Geistlich, UK)*; Levo-Husci 20% *(Fidia, Ital.)*; Levugen *(Travenol, UK)*; Levupan *(Ital.)*; Venosio *(Ital.)*.

The following names have been used for multi-ingredient preparations containing fructose—Anvatrol *(Nelson, Austral.)*; Emetrol *(Boots, Austral.; Rorer, Canad.; Radiol, UK; Adria, USA)*; Ethulose *(Geistlich, UK)*.

7838-n

Fursultiamine *(rINN).*

Thiamine Tetrahydrofurfuryl Disulphide; TTFD. *N*-(4-Amino-2-methylpyrimidin-5-ylmethyl)-*N*-[4-hydroxy-1-methyl-2-(tetrahydrofurfuryldithio)but-1-enyl]formamide.

$C_{17}H_{26}N_4O_3S_2$=398.5.

CAS — 804-30-8.

Fursultiamine is a vitamin B_1 substance with the general properties of thiamine hydrochloride (see p.1277).

Proprietary Names and Manufacturers

Alinamin-F *(Jpn)*; Judolor *(Woelm, Ger.; Woelm, Switz.)*.

582-g

Anhydrous Glucose *(BAN).*

Anhydrous Dextrose; Anhydrous Glucose for Parenteral Use; Dextrose *(USAN)*; Dextrosum (Glucosum) Anhydricum; Saccharum Amylaceum; D-Glucose. D-(+)-Glucopyranose.
$C_6H_{12}O_6$=180.2.

CAS — 50-99-7.

Pharmacopoeias. In *Aust., Belg., Br., Cz., Egypt., Eur., Fr., Ger., Hung., Jpn, Neth., Pol., Port., Roum., Span.,* and *Swiss.* Also in *B.P. Vet.*

A white odourless crystalline powder with a sweet taste.

Soluble 1 in 1 of water; sparingly soluble in alcohol. A 5.05% solution in water is iso-osmotic with serum. Solutions are **sterilised,** immediately after preparation, by autoclaving. **Store** in well-closed containers. Glucose solutions for intravenous use should be stored at 2 to 25°, and should not be used unless clear and free from particles.

584-p

Glucose *(BAN).*

Dextrose *(USAN)*; Dextrose Monohydrate for Parenteral Use; Glucose for Parenteral Use; Glycosum; Grape Sugar; D-Glucose Monohydrate. D-(+)-Glucopyranose monohydrate.
$C_6H_{12}O_6,H_2O$=198.2.

CAS — 5996-10-1.

Pharmacopoeias. In *Aust., Br., Chin., Eur., Fr., Ger., Hung., Mex., Neth., Nord., Rus., Swiss,* and *Turk.* Also in *B.P. Vet. Arg., Braz., Ind., Int., It., Jug.,* and *U.S.* permit anhydrous or monohydrate. *U.S.N.F.* includes a monograph for Dextrose Excipient, for non-parenteral use, specified as the monohydrate. *Fr., Egypt.,* and *Hung.* include a monograph for Liquid Glucose (Corn Syrup), which consists chiefly of a mixture of glucose, maltose, dextrins, and water.

A white odourless crystalline or granular powder with a sweet taste. Glucose monohydrate 1.1 g is approximately equivalent to anhydrous glucose 1 g.

B.P. **solubilities** are as for Anhydrous Glucose (above). *U.S.P.* solubilities (for anhydrous or monohydrate) are: soluble 1 in 1 of water and 1 in 100 of alcohol; very soluble in boiling water; soluble in boiling alcohol. A 5.51% solution in water is iso-osmotic with serum.

Sterilisation and **storage** are as for Anhydrous Glucose (above).

DEGRADATION ON HEAT STERILISATION. Furfural had been identified as a decomposition product of glucose solution after prolonged heating.— H. Ogata *et al.* (letter), *J. Pharm. Pharmac.,* 1978, *30,* 668.

Identification of 2 acids, 5-hydroxymethylfuroic acid and furan-2,5-dicarboxylic acid, in addition to the major decomposition product 5-hydroxymethylfurfuraldehyde (5-HMF), in glucose solutions following autoclaving.— D. G. Durham *et al., Int. J. Pharmaceut.,* 1982, *12,* 31.

Adverse Effects

Intravenous administration of hypertonic glucose solutions may cause local pain, vein irritation, and thrombophlebitis. Intravenous infusion of glucose solutions can lead to the development of fluid and electrolyte disturbances including oedema, hypokalaemia, hypomagnesaemia, and hypophosphataemia.

For reference to the role of sugars, including glucose, in the development of dental caries, see under Sucrose, p.1276.

Precautions

The use of hypertonic glucose solutions is contra-indicated in patients with anuria, intracranial or intraspinal haemorrhage, and in delirium tremens where there is dehydration.

Glucose solutions should not be mixed with whole blood as haemolysis and clumping can occur.

PREGNANCY AND THE NEONATE. Results from a study involving 47 fasting women undergoing elective caesarean section indicated that the inclusion of glucose in intravenous infusions of sodium chloride 0.9% did not decrease the incidence of hypotension. Rapid infusions of solutions containing 25 g of glucose or more were associated with foetal acidosis and neonatal hyperinsulinaemia, hypoglycaemia, and jaundice. Until a safe rate of administration is established, it is recommended that glucose infusions immediately before delivery be limited to not more than 6 g per hour.— N. B. Kenepp *et al., Lancet,* 1982, *1,* 1150. Comment and results supporting the suggestion that glucose infusions during labour may be associated with a higher incidence of neonatal jaundice. This effect may not be limited to caesarian-born babies; it has also been observed in infants delivered vaginally.— S. Singhi *et al.* (letter), *ibid., 2,* 335.

Hyponatraemia occurred in 71 of 180 infants (39%) born to mothers who had received an intravenous infusion of glucose solution with or without oxytocin during labour, compared with 6 of 103 (6%) whose mothers received no intravenous hydration. Eleven of the 71 hyponatraemic infants had transient neonatal tachypnoea.— S. C. Singhi and E. Chookang, *Archs Dis. Childh.,* 1984, *59,* 1155.

Absorption and Fate

Glucose is rapidly absorbed from the gastro-intestinal tract. Peak plasma concentrations of glucose occur about 40 minutes after oral administration of glucose to hypoglycaemic patients. It is metabolised to carbon dioxide and water with the release of energy.

Uses and Administration

Glucose, a monosaccharide, is administered by mouth or by intravenous infusion in the treatment of carbohydrate and fluid depletion. It is also used in the treatment of hypoglycaemia-see under Treatment of Insulin-induced Hypoglycaemia, p.393.

Glucose is the preferred source of carbohydrate in parenteral nutrition regimens (see under Enteral and Parenteral Nutrition, p.1251).

For reference to the use of glucose and electrolyte solutions in the prevention and treatment of dehydration due to acute diarrhoeal diseases, see under Oral Rehydration Therapy, p.1024.

Glucose solution 5% is iso-osmotic with blood and may be administered via a peripheral vein. Glucose solutions with a concentration greater than 5% are hypertonic and should be administered by slow intravenous infusion via a central vein. The dose of glucose is variable and is dependent on individual patient requirements; serum-glucose concentrations should be carefully monitored. The maximum rate of glucose utilisation is about 800 mg per kg body-weight per hour. Glucose solution 50% may be administered at a rate of 3 mL per minute; the rate may be doubled for the 25% solution.

Strongly hypertonic glucose solutions (25 to 50%) have been used to reduce cerebrospinal pressure and cerebral oedema caused by delirium tremens or acute alcohol intoxication. Glucose injection 50% has been used as a sclerosing agent in the treatment of varicose veins and as an irritant to produce adhesive pleuritis.

Glucose is also used as a tablet excipient and may be added to injections and dialysis fluids in order to increase their osmotic pressure.

For reference to the use of the oral glucose tolerance test as a diagnostic aid for diabetes mellitus, see under Antidiabetic Agents, p.386.

In a double-blind study, intravenous infusion of 50 mL or less of hypertonic glucose solution (50%) over 5 minutes relieved 17 of 26 episodes of dialysis-induced muscle cramps in 15 chronically uraemic patients. Infusion of 50 mL sodium chloride solution (0.9%) relieved only 5 of 18 similar episodes of muscle cramps.— J. Milutinovich *et al., Ann. intern. Med.,* 1979, *90,* 926.

For a recommendation on the minimal rate of administration of glucose with glucose polymer by nasogastric infusion in patients with glycogen storage disease Type I, see under Dietary Modification, p.1250.

Preparations

Glucose and Glycerol Instillation *(A.P.F.).* Dextrose and Glycerin Nasal Drops. Glucose 20 g, glycerol to 100 mL. Store in well-filled airtight containers.

Glucose Intravenous Infusion *(B.P.).* Dextrose Injection; Glucose Injection; Dextrose Intravenous Infusion. A sterile solution of anhydrous glucose or glucose monohydrate. Potency is expressed in terms of anhydrous glucose. pH of a solution containing not more than 5% of anhydrous glucose, 3.5 to 5.5. Store at a temperature not exceeding 25°. In *Martindale,* glucose injection is 5% unless otherwise specified.

NOTE. The *B.P.* directs that when glucose injection is required as a diluent for official injections, Glucose Intravenous Infusion 5% shall be used.

Dextrose Injection *(U.S.P.).* A sterile solution of anhydrous glucose or glucose monohydrate; it contains no antimicrobial agents. Potency is expressed in terms of glucose monohydrate. pH of a solution containing not more than 5% of glucose, 3.5 to 6.5.

Proprietary Preparations

Glucodin *(Crookes Laboratories, UK). Powder,* glucose monohydrate, with ascorbic acid 50 mg in each 100 g.

Min-I-Jet Dextrose *(IMS, UK). Injection,* glucose 500 mg/mL, in single-use prefilled syringes of 50 mL.

Proprietary Names and Manufacturers

Dextro Med *(Maizena, Ger.)*; Dextromon *(Maizena, Ger.)*; Dextropur *(Denm.)*; Glucodin *(Crookes Laboratories, UK)*; Glucosteril *(Fresenius, Ger.)*; Glutose *(Paddock, USA)*; Min-I-Jet Dextrose *(IMS, UK)*; Nutrosa *(Arg.)*; Manufacturers also include—*Bio-Medical, UK; Boots, UK; Travenol, UK.*

The following names have been used for multi-ingredient preparations containing glucose—Anvatrol *(Nelson, Austral.)*; Dexsal *(Reckitt & Colman, Austral.)*; Emdex *(Mendell, USA : K & K-Greeff, UK)*; Emetrol *(Boots, Austral.; Rorer, Canad.; Radiol, UK; Adria, USA)*; Gastrobrom *(Fawns & McAllan, Austral.)*; Glucomagma *(Drug Houses Austral., Austral.)*; Pal-A-Dex *(Diamed, UK)*; Sclerodex *(Ondee, Canad.)*; Xylocaine with Dextrose *(Astra, USA)*.

For multiple electrolyte solutions, many of which contain glucose, see p.1023. See also preparations for enteral and parenteral nutrition, p.1289.

586-w

Glutamic Acid *(rINN).*

620; Glu; Glutaminic Acid. L-(+)-2-Aminoglutaric acid.
$C_5H_9NO_4$=147.1.

CAS — 56-86-0.

Pharmacopoeias. In *Aust., Belg., Chin., Jug., Pol., Port., Roum., Rus.,* and *Swiss.*

587-e

Glutamic Acid Hydrochloride *(rINNM).*

Aciglumin; Glu Hydrochloride. L-(+)-2-Aminoglutaric acid hydrochloride.
$C_5H_9NO_4,HCl$=183.6.

CAS — 138-15-8.

Pharmacopoeias. In *Nord.* and *Roum.*

Glutamic acid is an aliphatic amino acid which is degraded readily in the body to form levoglutamide (glutamine). It is used as a dietary supplement. It has been given by mouth in the treatment of hyperammonaemia in conditions such as hepatic encephalopathy.

Glutamic acid hydrochloride is used in the symptomatic treatment of gastric hydrochloric acid deficiency in usual doses by mouth of 0.5 to 1 g with meals.

Proprietary Preparations

Muripsin *(Norgine, UK). Tablets,* glutamic acid hydrochloride 500 mg, pepsin 35 mg.

Proprietary Names and Manufacturers of Glutamic Acid and Glutamic Acid Hydrochloride

Acidogene *(Spain)*; Acidulin *(Austral.; Lilly, Canad.; S.Afr.; Lilly, USA)*; Glutacid *(Nyco, Norw.)*; Glutacide *(Treupha, Switz.)*; Glutamin *(Verla, Ger.)*; Glutaminol *(Laroche Navarron, Fr.)*; Hypochylin *(Ferrosan, Swed.)*; Muripsin Plain *(Norgine, UK)*.

For multi-ingredient preparations containing nutritional agents and vitamins, see p.1289.

589-y

Glycine *(USAN).*

Aminoacetic Acid; Gly; Glycocoll; Sucre de Gélatine.
$NH_2.CH_2.CO_2H$=75.07.

CAS — 56-40-6.

Pharmacopoeias. In *Arg., Br., Braz., Cz., Fr., Jpn, Mex., Turk.,* and *U.S.*

A white odourless crystalline powder. **Soluble** 1 in 4 of water; very slightly soluble in alcohol and ether. A 5% solution in water has a pH of 5.9 to 6.3. Irrigation solutions have a pH of 4.5 to 6.5. Solutions may be **sterilised** by autoclaving.

Adverse Effects and Precautions

Systemic absorption of glycine irrigation solutions can lead to disturbances of fluid and electrolyte balance and cardiovascular and pulmonary disorders. Glycine irrigation should be used cautiously in patients with hepatic impairment and should not be used in anuric patients.

For reference to the role of glycine in the treatment of hepatic encephalopathy, see under Enteral and Parenteral Nutrition, p.1252.

Massive hyperglycinaemia and transient loss of vision may occur following the use of glycine as an irrigating fluid during transurethal resection of the prostate.— J. Moelgaard (letter), *Lancet,* 1983, *2,* 793.

Irrigation of the retroperitoneal space with 20 litres of glycine solution 1.5% in a 68-year-old patient undergoing percutaneous ultrasonic lithotripsy for renal stone disease led to an increase in inflation pressure, an increase in intravascular volume with hypertension, hyponatraemia, and hyperkalaemia.— J. F. Sinclair *et al., Br. med. J.,* 1985, *291,* 691. Criticism.— N. M. Goble *et al.* (letter), *ibid.,* 966; R. A. Miller and H. N. Whitfield (letter), *ibid.,* 967.

Uses and Administration

Glycine is the simplest of the amino acids. It is used as a dietary supplement.

Glycine is sometimes used in conjunction with antacids in the treatment of gastric hyperacidity. It is also used as an ingredient of some aspirin tablets with the object of reducing gastric irritation.

Sterile solutions of glycine 1.5% in water which are hypotonic and non-conductive may be used as urogenital irrigation solutions during certain surgical procedures.

For a report of the use of glycine in combination with cysteine and racemic threonine in the topical treatment of leg ulcers, see under Cysteine Hydrochloride, p.1261.

A view that the only indication for the use of glycine irrigation is the use of diathermy, when the irrigation period should be kept to an absolute minimum.— R. A. Miller and H. N. Whitfield (letter), *Br. med. J.,* 1985, *291,* 967.

Preparations

Glycine Irrigation *(U.S.P.)*

Glycine Irrigation Solution *(B.P.)*

Proprietary Names and Manufacturers

Glicoamin *(Ital.)*; Glykokoll *(Swed.)*;

Manufacturers also include—*Boots, UK; Travenol, UK.*

Multi-ingredient nutritional preparations containing glycine are included in the lists on pp.1289-93. The following names have been used for preparations containing glycine and not considered to be such multi-ingredient preparations—Aminoderm *(Desbergers, Canad.)*; Cal.Sup *(Riker, USA)*; Cicatrin *(Wellcome, Austral.; Wellcome, Canad.; Calmic, UK)*; Paynocil *(Beecham Research, UK)*; Titralac *(Riker, Austral.; Riker, UK)*; Ulsade *(Cambridge Laboratories, Austral.)*.

7825-t

Halibut-liver Oil

Aceite de Higado de Hipogloso; Heilbuttleberöl; Ol. Hippogloss.; Oleum Hippoglossi; Oleum Jecoris Hippoglossi.

CAS — 8001-46-5.

Pharmacopoeias. In *Aust., Br., Egypt., Int.,* and *Mex.* Also in *B.P. Vet.*

The fixed oil extracted from the fresh or suitably preserved liver of the halibut species belonging to the genus *Hippoglossus* (Pleuronectidae). It contains not less than 30 000 units of vitamin A activity per g. Halibut-liver oil may contain up to about 3000 units of vitamin D activity per g. Halibut-liver oil containing 30 000 units of vitamin A in 1 g contains approximately 4000 units in 0.15 mL.

A pale to golden-yellow liquid with a fishy but not rancid odour and taste. Practically **insoluble** in alcohol; miscible with chloroform, ether, and light petroleum. **Store** at a temperature not exceeding 20° in well-closed, well-filled containers. Protect from light.

Halibut-liver oil is used as a means of administering vitamins A and D; the proportion of vitamin A to vitamin D is usually greater in halibut-liver oil than in cod-liver oil. It is usually given in capsules.

Preparations

Halibut-liver Oil Capsules *(B.P.).* Contain halibut-liver oil diluted, if necessary, with a suitable fixed oil to a volume of 0.12 to 0.18 mL. Each capsule contains halibut-liver oil equivalent to about 4000 units of vitamin A activity.

591-q

Histidine *(USAN, pINN).*

His; L-Histidine. L-2-Amino-3-(1*H*-imidazol-4-yl)propionic acid.
$C_6H_9N_3O_2$=155.2.

CAS — 71-00-1 (histidine); 645-35-2 (hydrochloride, anhydrous).

Pharmacopoeias. In *U.S. Aust., Fr.,* and *Span.* specify the hydrochloride.

White odourless crystals. **Soluble** in water; very slightly soluble in alcohol; insoluble in ether. A 2% solution in water has a pH of 7.0 to 8.5.

Histidine is an aromatic amino acid which is essential for infant growth. Recent evidence suggests that histidine may be essential for adults. It is used as a dietary supplement.

It has been given by mouth in the investigation of folate deficiency.

Proprietary Names and Manufacturers

Histicaps *(Geistlich, UK)*; Histinorm *(A.S., Ger.)*; Histiplus *(Gry, Ger.)*; Laristine *(Roche, Fr.)*; Larostidine *(Roche, Belg.)*; Plexamine *(Biodica, Fr.)*; Ulcusemol *(Spain)*.

For multi-ingredient preparations containing nutritional agents and vitamins, see p.1289.

592-p

Purified Honey

Clarified Honey; Gereinigter Honig; Mel Depuratum; Mel Despumatum; Miel Blanc; Strained Honey.

CAS — 8028-66-8 (honey).

Pharmacopoeias. In *Arg., Br., Chin., Egypt., Fr., Jpn, Port.,* and *Span.*

Purified honey is obtained by purification of the honey from the comb of the bee, *Apis mellifera* and other species of *Apis* (Apidae). The honey is extracted by centrifugation, pressure, or other suitable procedure, melted at a temperature not exceeding 80° and allowed to stand, skimming off the scum rising to the surface, and adjusting the wt per mL to 1.35 to 1.36 g by adding water.

It is a thick syrupy translucent pale yellow or yellowish-brown liquid with a sweet characteristic taste and a pleasant characteristic odour. It contains 70 to 80% of glucose and fructose, together with water and traces of other nutrients.

Honey is used as a demulcent and sweetening agent, especially in linctuses and cough mixtures.

ANTIMICROBIAL ACTION. Demonstration of broad-spectrum antimicrobial activity in a fraction of honey distillate.— E. E. Obaseiki-Ebor *et al., J. Pharm. Pharmac.,* 1983, *35,* 748. *In vitro* antimycotic activity of a fraction in honey.— E. E. Obaseiki-Ebor and T. C. A. Afonya, *ibid.,* 1984, *36,* 283.

ORAL REHYDRATION THERAPY. The use of honey as a substitute for glucose in oral rehydration therapy for the treatment of infantile gastroenteritis.— I. E. Haffejee and A. Moosa, *Br. med. J.,* 1985, *290,* 1866. Criticism; honey is a risk factor for infant botulism.— A. Clarke (letter), *ibid., 291,* 415.

WOUND HEALING. Honey was preferred to sugar for packing infected wounds because of its lower pH and greater osmotic effect (B. Bose, *Lancet,* 1982, *1,* 963). However, the use of honey to soothe dermal lesions and necrotic malignant breast ulcers has been deprecated (D.A.A. Mossel, *ibid.,* 1980, *2,* 1091).

Preparations

Oxymel *(B.P.C. 1973).* Acetic acid 15 mL, freshly boiled and cooled water 15 mL, purified honey to 100 mL.

10169-s

Hydrogenated Glucose Syrup

A mixture of maltitol, sorbitol, and other polyols, with maltitol being the major ingredient.

Hydrogenated glucose syrup is a bulk sweetener considered to be less cariogenic than sucrose. The ingestion of large quantities may produce flatulence and diarrhoea.

Estimated temporary acceptable daily intake: up to 25 mg per kg body-weight.— Twenty-seventh Report of the Joint FOA/WHO Expert Committee on Food Additives, *Tech. Rep. Ser. Wld Hlth Org. No. 696,* 1983.

Proprietary Names and Manufacturers

Lycasin *(Roquette, UK).*

7877-p

Inositol

i-Inositol; *meso*-Inositol. *myo*-Inositol.
$C_6H_{12}O_6$=180.2.

CAS — 87-89-8.

Pharmacopoeias. In *Aust., Belg.,* and *Fr.*

Inositol, an isomer of glucose, is involved in lipid metabolism. The optically inactive isomer, *myo*-inositol, is the form which has an active role in nutrition. Inositol has traditionally been considered to be a vitamin B substance although it has an uncertain status as a vitamin and a deficiency syndrome has not been identified in man. Sources of inositol include whole-grain cereals, fruits, and plants, in which it occurs as the hexaphosphate, phytic acid. It also occurs in both vegetables and meats in other forms. The usual daily intake of inositol is about 1 g.

Inositol has been tried in the treatment of lipid metabolic disorders and in the management of complications resulting from diabetes mellitus.

Results from a preliminary study indicated that inositol is an important nutrient in immature preterm infants.— M. Hallman *et al., Archs Dis. Childh.,* 1986, *61,* 1076.

A review of the role of inositol in the pathogenesis of diabetic complications. Inositol and its phospholipid metabolites (the phosphoinositides) have emerged as key elements in intracellular regulation. Experiments in *animals* have implicated inositol as a fundamental link between hyperglycaemia and functional impairment in a variety of tissues susceptible to diabetic complications, including peripheral nerves.— D. A. Greene *et al., New Engl. J. Med.,* 1987, *316,* 599.

Proprietary Names and Manufacturers

Multi-ingredient nutritional preparations containing inositol are included in the lists on pp.1289-93. The following names have been used for preparations containing inositol and not considered to be such multi-ingredient preparations—Amino-Cerv *(Milex, USA).*

593-s

Isoleucine *(USAN, pINN).*

Ile; L-Isoleucine. L-2-Amino-3-methylvaleric acid.
$C_6H_{13}NO_2$=131.2.

CAS — 73-32-5.

Pharmacopoeias. In *Cz.*, *Jpn*, and *U.S.*

An almost odourless white crystalline powder. **Soluble** in water; slightly soluble in hot alcohol; insoluble in ether. A 1% solution in water has a pH of 5.5 to 7.0.

Isoleucine is a branched-chain amino acid which is an essential constituent of the diet. It is used as a dietary supplement.

For reference to the role of aromatic and branched-chain amino acids in the treatment of hepatic encephalopathy, see under Enteral and Parenteral Nutrition, p.1252.

Preparations

For multi-ingredient preparations containing nutritional agents and vitamins, see p.1289.

14038-q

Isomalt *(BAN).*
BAY i-3930; Isomaltitol. An approximately equimolar mixture of 6-*O*-(α-D-glucopyranosyl)-D-glucitol ($C_{12}H_{24}O_{11}$ = 344.3) and 1-*O*-(α-D-glucopyranosyl)-D-mannitol ($C_{12}H_{24}O_{11}$,$2H_2O$ = 380.3).

A white, odourless, crystalline, slightly hygroscopic solid with a sweet taste.

Isomalt is used as a bulk sweetener in foods. When ingested it is partly metabolised in the small intestine to glucose, mannitol and sorbitol. Remaining isomalt is metabolised by the flora of the large intestine. The ingestion of large quantities may produce flatulence and have a laxative effect.

Isomalt was assigned an acceptable daily intake of "not specified".— Twenty-ninth Report of the Joint FAO/WHO Expert Committee on Food Additives, *Tech. Rep. Ser. Wld Hlth Org. No. 733*, 1986.

594-w

Lactose *(BAN, USAN).*

Lactosum; Lattosio; Milk Sugar; Saccharum Lactis. 4-*O*-β-D-Galactopyranosyl-α-D-glucopyranose monohydrate.
$C_{12}H_{22}O_{11}$,H_2O=360.3.

CAS — 63-42-3 (anhydrous); 5989-81-1 (monohydrate); 10039-26-6 (monohydrate, cyclic); 64044-51-5 (monohydrate, open form).

Pharmacopoeias. In *Arg., Aust., Belg., Br., Braz., Chin., Cz., Egypt., Eur., Fr., Ger., Hung., Ind., It., Jpn, Jug., Mex., Neth., Nord., Pol., Port., Roum., Rus., Span., Swiss,* and *Turk.*. Also in *U.S.N.F. Braz. P.* and *U.S.N.F.* specify anhydrous or monohydrate. Also in *B.P. Vet.*

A disaccharide obtained from the whey of milk. White or creamy-white odourless crystalline masses or powder with a slightly sweet taste. It readily absorbs odours. Lactose exists in 2 modifications corresponding to the α- and β-isomerides. Lactose used in pharmacy is chiefly α-lactose. β-Lactose is also obtainable; it is anhydrous, more soluble than α-lactose, and passes into the α-form in solution.

B.P. **solubilities** are: soluble 1 in 6 of water; practically insoluble in alcohol. *U.S.N.F.* solubilities are: slowly soluble 1 in 5 of water and soluble 1 in 2.6 of boiling water; very slightly soluble in alcohol; insoluble in chloroform and ether. A 9.75% solution in water is iso-osmotic with serum.

Store in well-closed containers.

Studies *in vitro* indicated that solubility of a drug was the major factor controlling its release from hard gelatin capsules; for soluble drugs, lactose, rather than starch or Primojel, would be the better diluent if required for use in large quantities.— J. M. Newton and F. M. Razzo, *J. Pharm. Pharmac.*, 1977, *29*, 205.

Thermal treatment of α-lactoses involves changes in β-content and in crystal structure.— C. F. Lerk *et al.* (letter), *J. pharm. Sci.*, 1984, *73*, 856. α-Lactose monohydrate loses its water of crystallisation and, like β-lactose, changes into an amorphous state on intensive grinding. Thermal treatment of both amorphous lactose and uncrystallised α-lactose monohydrate results in crystallisation of a crystalline β/α-lactose compound. This is in contrast to uncrystallised β-lactose, which crystallises into β-lactose.— *idem*, 857.

Adverse Effects and Precautions

Lactose intolerance occurs due to a deficiency of the intestinal enzyme lactase. Ingestion of lactose by patients with lactase deficiency leads to a clinical syndrome of abdominal pain, diarrhoea, distension, and flatulence.

Lactose is contra-indicated in patients with galactosaemia, the glucose-galactose malabsorption syndrome, or lactase deficiency.

Absorption and Fate

Lactose is hydrolysed by lactase in the small intestine to glucose and galactose, which are then absorbed. Lactose is excreted unchanged when given intravenously.

Uses and Administration

Lactose, the carbohydrate component of milk, is less sweet than sucrose. It has been used in infant feeding to adjust the carbohydrate content of diluted cows' milk to that of human milk.

Lactose has been tried in the treatment of hepatic encephalopathy.

Lactose is widely used as a diluent to give bulk to powders and as a diluent in compressed tablets.

597-y

Leucine *(USAN, pINN).*
α-Aminoisocaproic Acid; Leu; L-Leucine. L-2-Amino-4-methylvaleric acid.
$C_6H_{13}NO_2$=131.2.

CAS — 61-90-5.

Pharmacopoeias. In *Jpn* and *U.S.*

A white practically odourless crystalline powder. Sparingly **soluble** in water; insoluble in ether. A 1% solution in water has a pH of 5.5 to 7.0.

Leucine is a branched-chain amino acid which is an essential constituent of the diet. It is used as a dietary supplement.

For reference to the role of aromatic and branched-chain amino acids in the treatment of hepatic encephalopathy, see under Enteral and Parenteral Nutrition, p.1252.

598-j

Levoglutamide *(pINN).*
Gln; L-Glutamine. L-Glutamic acid 5-amide; L-(+)-2-Aminoglutaramic acid.
$C_5H_{10}N_2O_3$=146.1.

CAS — 56-85-9.

Levoglutamide is an amino acid which has been used similarly to glutamic acid (see p.1265).

Administration of levoglutamide by mouth to 3 patients with cystinuria induced a reduction in cystine excretion only after an elevation which was associated with a high sodium intake. Despite results from earlier studies to the contrary, levoglutamide is probably not of any practical use in the treatment of cystinuria.— P. Jaeger *et al.*, *New Engl. J. Med.*, 1986, *315*, 1120.

Proprietary Names and Manufacturers
Energlut *(Ital Suisse, Ital.)*; Glutacerebro *(AFOM, Ital.)*; Glutaven *(Ital.)*; Iperphos *(Kalopharma, Ital.)*; Memoril *(Recordati, Ital.)*; Multidin *(Radiumfarma, Ital.)*; Sintoglutam *(Von Boch, Ital.)*.

669-y

Lysine Acetate *(USAN, pINNM).*
Lys Acetate; L-Lysine Monoacetate. L-2,6-Diaminohexanoic acid acetate.
$C_6H_{14}N_2O_2$,$C_2H_4O_2$=206.2.

CAS — 57282-49-2.

Pharmacopoeias. In *U.S.*

White odourless crystals or crystalline powder. Freely **soluble** in water.

599-z

Lysine Hydrochloride *(USAN, pINNM).*
Lys Hydrochloride; L-Lysine Monohydrochloride. L-2,6-Diaminohexanoic acid hydrochloride.
$C_6H_{14}N_2O_2$,HCl=182.6.

CAS — 56-87-1 (lysine); 657-27-2 (hydrochloride).

Pharmacopoeias. In *Cz.* and *U.S.* Also in *Fr.* which specifies the DL form and in *Jpn* which does not state the configuration.

A white odourless powder. Each g of monograph substance represents approximately 5.5 mmol of chloride. Freely **soluble** in water.

Lysine is an aliphatic amino acid which is an essential constituent of the diet. It is used as a dietary supplement. Lysine hydrochloride has been used in the treatment of hypochloraemic alkalosis.

HERPES SIMPLEX. Although some studies have shown a beneficial response following administration of lysine by mouth in the treatment of recurrent herpes simplex virus infections (C. Kagan, *Lancet*, 1974, *1*, 137; R.S. Griffith *et al.*, *Dermatologica*, 1978, *156*, 257; R.S. Griffith *et al.*, *ibid.*, 1987, *175*, 183), others have failed to show a useful effect (N. Milman *et al.*, *Lancet*, 1978, *2*, 942; C.A. Simon *et al.*, *Archs Derm.*, 1985, *121*, 167). Adler and Mindel (*Br. med. Bull.*, 1985, *41*, 361) considered that lysine did not warrant further consideration in the treatment of genital herpes infections.

HYPERARGININAEMIA. Administration of lysine 250 mg per kg body-weight daily and ornithine 100 mg per kg daily for 6 months to an 11-year-old patient with hyperargininaemia resulted in decreased plasma-ammonia and urinary-orotic acid concentrations. However, an increase in plasma- and CSF-arginine concentrations were observed.— S. -S. Kang *et al.*, *J. Pediat.*, 1983, *103*, 763.

Proprietary Names and Manufacturers
Enisyl *(Person & Covey, USA)*.

Multi-ingredient nutritional preparations containing lysine are included in the lists on pp.1289-93. The following names have been used for preparations containing lysine and not considered to be such multi-ingredient preparations— Klorvess Effervescent *(Sandoz, USA)*; K-Lyte/Cl *(Bristol, USA)*.

NOTE. Not all K-Lyte/Cl preparations contain lysine.

601-c

Malt Extract
Extractum Bynes.

CAS — 8002-48-0.

Pharmacopoeias. In *Arg.* and *Ind.* Both incorporate 10% w/w of glycerol. Also in *B.P.C. 1973.*

It contains 50% or more of maltose, together with dextrin, glucose, and small amounts of other carbohydrates. It is prepared from malted grain of barley (*Hordeum distichon* or *H. vulgare*) or a mixture of this with not more than 33% of malted grain of wheat (*Triticum aestivum*).

Malt extract has nutritive properties. It is chiefly used as a vehicle in preparations containing cod-liver oil and halibut-liver oil. It is a useful flavouring agent for masking bitter tastes.

Preparations

Malt Extract with Cod-liver Oil *(B.P.C. 1973).* Extractum Malti cum Oleo Morrhuae. Cod-liver oil 10% w/w (about 4.5 mL in 30 mL) in malt extract. Store in a cool place in well-filled airtight containers. Protect from light.

Malt Extract with Halibut-liver Oil *(B.P.C. 1973).* Extractum Malti cum Oleo Hippoglossi. Malt extract with 2.5% v/w of a mixture of arachis oil and sufficient halibut-liver oil to give not less than 60 units of vitamin-A activity per g (not less than 2500 units in 30 mL). Store in a cool place in well-filled airtight containers. Protect from light.

For multi-ingredient preparations containing nutritional agents and vitamins, see p.1289.

602-k

Maltodextrin

A glucose polymer composed of a mixture of dextrins and maltose and prepared by the limited hydrolysis of starch.

CAS — 9050-36-6.

Maltodextrin is used as a carbohydrate source. It has been used in infant feeding in place of lactose for adjusting the carbohydrate content of diluted cows' milk to that of human milk.

Proprietary Names and Manufacturers

Fortical *(Cow & Gate, UK)*; Maxijul *(Sharpe, Austral.; Scientific Hospital Supplies, UK)*; Polycal *(Cow & Gate, UK)*.

603-a

Maltose

4-*O*-α-D-Glucopyranosyl-β-D-glucopyranose monohydrate.
$C_{12}H_{22}O_{11},H_2O$=360.3.

CAS — 69-79-4 (anhydrous); 6363-53-7 (monohydrate).

It is obtained from starch by hydrolysis with diastase.

Maltose, a disaccharide composed of two glucose molecules, is less sweet than sucrose. It is used as a carbohydrate source and sweetening agent, and has also been used in bacteriological culture media.

5303-d

Manganese

Mn=54.938.

CAS — 7439-96-5.

A greyish- or reddish-white, hard and brittle, metal.

Adverse Effects

Acute poisoning due to ingestion is rare owing to poor absorption of manganese. The main symptoms of chronic poisoning, either from injection or usually inhalation, include extrapyramidal symptoms that can lead to progressive deterioration in the central nervous system similar to the parkinsonian syndrome. Psychotic symptoms may also develop.

In Great Britain the recommended exposure limits of manganese are: manganese or manganese compounds (as Mn) 5 mg per m^3 (long-term); 5 mg per m^3 (short-term); manganese, fume (as Mn) 1 mg per m^3 (long-term); 3 mg per m^3 (short-term).

For a brief review of manganese toxicity see Recommended Health-Based Limits in Occupational Exposure to Heavy Metals, *Tech. Rep. Ser. Wld Hlth Org. No. 647*, 1980, p.80. See also Manganese, *Environmental Health Criteria 17*, Geneva, Wld Hlth Org., 1981.

Uses and Administration

Manganese is a trace element (see p.1250) and small amounts of a salt such as manganese sulphate are sometimes added to solutions for total parenteral nutrition. Manganese salts are occasionally used for their supposed effect in increasing the haematinic action of iron in the treatment of microcytic anaemia.

Manganese compounds or salts that have been used in therapeutics in addition to the sulphate include manganese aspartate complex, manganese amino acid chelate, manganese chloride, manganese dioxide, and manganese gluconate.

A review of the actions of manganese as a trace element covering the effects of deficiency, its pharmacokinetics, and its toxicity.— R. E. Burch *et al.*, *Clin. Chem.*, 1975, *21*, 501.

Preparations

For multi-ingredient preparations containing nutritional agents and vitamins, see p.1289.

5304-n

Manganese Sulphate *(BAN).*

Manganese Sulfate *(USAN)*. Manganese (II) sulphate tetrahydrate.
$MnSO_4,4H_2O$=223.1.

CAS — 7785-87-7 (anhydrous); 10034-96-5 (monohydrate); 10101-68-5 (tetrahydrate).

Pharmacopoeias. In *Br.* and *Fr.* Also in *B.P. Vet. Fr.* and *U.S.* include the monohydrate.

Pale pink odourless or almost odourless crystals or crystalline powder. **Soluble** 1 in 1 of water; practically insoluble in alcohol. **Store** in airtight containers.

Manganese sulphate is an ingredient of Compound Ferrous Sulphate Tablets *B.P.C. 1973*. Doses of 0.5 to 2.5 mg have been given. Manganese sulphate is used to prevent or treat manganese deficiency. It is used similarly in veterinary practice.

Preparations

Manganese Sulfate Injection *(U.S.P.)*. A sterile solution of manganese sulphate in Water for Injections. Dilute before use. pH 2.0 to 3.5.

617-n

Monosodium Glutamate *(USAN).*

621; Chinese Seasoning; MSG; Natrii Glutamas; Sodium Glutamate. Sodium hydrogen L-(+)-2-aminoglutarate monohydrate.
$C_5H_8NNaO_4,H_2O$=187.1.

CAS — 142-47-2 (anhydrous).

Pharmacopoeias. In *Pol.* Also in *U.S.N.F. Chin.* includes the injection.

A white, practically odourless, free-flowing crystalline powder. It may have either a slightly sweet or slightly salty taste. Monosodium glutamate 32 g is approximately equivalent to anhydrous monosodium glutamate 29 g or glutamic acid 25 g. Each g of monograph substance represents 5.3 mmol of sodium. Freely **soluble** in water; sparingly soluble in alcohol. A 5% solution in water has a pH of 6.7 to 7.2. **Store** in airtight containers.

Adverse Effects

Excessive doses of monosodium glutamate may lead to sodium overloading; for symptoms see under sodium chloride (p.1039). Intravenous administration has produced vomiting.

There have been several reports linking the ingestion of monosodium glutamate by susceptible individuals with a syndrome usually consisting of flushing, facial pressure, and chest pain; the association however is doubtful.— M. E. Gore and P. R. Salmon (letter), *Lancet*, 1980, *1*, 251.

References: D. H. Allen and G. J. Baker (letter), *New Engl. J. Med.*, 1981, *305*, 1154 (asthma); A. G. Ebert (letter), *ibid.*, 1982, *306*, 1180 (asthma); S. Garattini (letter), *ibid.*, 1181 (asthma); D. H. Allen and G. J. Baker (letter), *ibid* (asthma); K. W. Heaton (letter), *Br. med. J.*, 1984, *289*, 489 (burning sensation); A. G. Ebert (letter), *ibid.*, 1626 (doubts as to the role of glutamate); J. W. Cochran and A. H. Cochran (letter), *J. Am. med. Ass.*, 1984, *252*, 899 (ataxia and confusion in a 3-year-old child); E. N. Squire (letter), *Lancet*, 1987, *1*, 988 (angioedema of the face and extremities).

Uses and Administration

Monosodium glutamate is widely used as a flavour enhancer and imparts a meaty flavour.

Estimated acceptable daily intake for adults, and children aged over 12 weeks: up to 120 mg, as glutamic acid, additional to glutamic acid from all natural dietary sources, per kg body-weight.— Seventeenth Report of the FAO/WHO Expert Committee on Food Additives, *Tech. Rep. Ser. Wld Hlth Org. No. 539*, 1974.

13003-e

Neohesperidin Dihydrochalcone

3,5-Dihydroxy-4-[3-(3-hydroxy-4-methoxyphenyl)propionyl]phenyl 2-*O*-(6-deoxy-α-L-mannopyranosyl)-β-D-glucopyranoside.
$C_{28}H_{36}O_{15}$=612.6.

CAS — 20702-77-6 (neohesperidin dihydrochalcone); 18916-17-1 (naringin dihydrochalcone); 65520-51-6 (neoeriocitrin dihydrochalcone).

Neohesperidin dihydrochalcone is an intense sweetening agent derived from naringin present in citrus peel. Other dihydrochalcone sweeteners that have been studied include hesperetin dihydrochalcone glucoside ($C_{22}H_{26}O_{11}$ = 466.4), naringin dihydrochalcone ($C_{27}H_{34}O_{14}$ = 582.6), neoeriocitrin dihydrochalcone ($C_{27}H_{34}O_{15}$ = 598.6), and poncirin dihydrochalcone ($C_{28}H_{36}O_{14}$ = 596.6).

7865-b

Nicotinic Acid *(BAN, rINN).*

375; Acidum Nicotinicum; Niacin *(USAN)*; Nikotinsäure. Pyridine-3-carboxylic acid.
$C_6H_5NO_2$=123.1.

CAS — 59-67-6.

Pharmacopoeias. In *Aust., Belg., Br., Braz., Chin., Egypt., Eur., Fr., Ger., Hung., Ind., Int., It., Jpn, Mex., Neth., Nord., Port., Roum., Rus., Span., Swiss, Turk.*, and *U.S.* Also in *B.P. Vet.*

White, odourless or almost odourless, crystals or crystalline powder.

Soluble 1 in 60 of water; soluble in boiling water and boiling alcohol and in dilute aqueous solutions of alkali hydroxides and carbonates; very slightly soluble in chloroform; practically insoluble in ether. The *U.S.P.* injection has a pH of 4 to 6. **Store** in well-closed containers. Protect from light.

7864-m

Nicotinamide *(BAN, rINN).*

Niacinamide *(USAN)*; Nicotinamidum; Nicotinic Acid Amide; Nicotylamide; Vitamin PP. Pyridine-3-carboxamide.
$C_6H_6N_2O$=122.1.

CAS — 98-92-0.

Pharmacopoeias. In *Arg., Aust., Belg., Br., Braz., Chin., Cz., Egypt., Eur., Fr., Ger., Hung., Ind., Int., It., Jpn, Jug., Mex., Neth., Nord., Pol., Port., Roum., Rus., Span., Swiss, Turk.*, and *U.S.* Also in *B.P. Vet.*

A white crystalline powder or colourless crystals, odourless or with a faint characteristic odour.

B.P. **solubilities** are: soluble 1 in 1 of water and 1 in 1.5 of alcohol; slightly soluble in chloroform and ether. *U.S.P.* solubilities are: soluble 1 in 1.5 of water, 1 in 10 of boiling water, and 1 in 5.5 of alcohol; soluble in glycerol. A 5% solution in water has a pH of 6.0 to 7.5. The *U.S.P.* injection has a pH of 5 to 7. **Store** in airtight containers. Protect from light.

Adverse Effects

Nicotinic acid has a vasodilator action and when given by mouth or by injection in therapeutic doses it may cause flushing, a sensation of heat, faintness, and a pounding in the head. These symptoms are transient and may be avoided by substituting nicotinamide which does not have a vasodilator action.

Other adverse effects which have been reported, especially following high doses of nicotinic acid, include dryness of the skin, pruritus, hyperpigmentation, abdominal cramps, diarrhoea, nausea and vomiting, anorexia, activation of peptic ulcer, amblyopia, jaundice and impairment of liver function, decrease in glucose tolerance, hyperglycaemia, and hyperuricaemia. Most of these effects subside on withdrawal of the drug.

Nicotinic acid produces frequent adverse effects, but they are usually not serious, tend to decrease with time, and can be managed easily. Dermal and gastro-intestinal reactions are most common. Truncal and facial flushing are reported in 90 to 100% of treated patients in large clinical trials. Significant elevations of liver enzymes, serum glucose, and serum uric acid are occasionally seen with nicotinic acid therapy. Liver enzyme elevations are

more common in patients given large dosage increases over short periods of time, and in patients treated with sustained-release formulations. Effects on glucose and uric acid appear to be problematic, primarily in patients with pre-existing diabetes mellitus or gout.
Flushing and itching associated with nicotinic acid therapy appear to be prostaglandin-mediated, and can be reduced by aspirin 325 mg given shortly before ingestion of nicotinic acid. Since flushing appears to be more closely related to the continuous rise in plasma-nicotinic acid concentrations rather than the absolute dose, some investigators recommend taking nicotinic acid with meals or slowly tapering the dose upward to minimise these effects.
Patients experiencing marked elevations in liver function enzymes frequently benefit from a temporary reduction in nicotinic acid dosage. Flushing is reported to only occur at plasma concentrations of 0.1 to 0.2 mg per litre, but resolves when constant concentrations are attained. Gastro-intestinal effects appear to be related to formulation, and some patients may benefit from a change from the sustained-release to the conventional tablet.— L. C. Knodel and R. L. Talbert, *Med. Toxicol.*, 1987, *2*, 10.

Precautions

Nicotinic acid should be given cautiously to patients with a history of peptic ulceration, and to patients with diabetes mellitus, gout, or impaired liver function.

Absorption and Fate

Nicotinic acid and nicotinamide are readily absorbed from the gastro-intestinal tract following oral administration and widely distributed in the body tissues. Nicotinic acid appears in breast milk. The main route of metabolism is their conversion to *N*-methylnicotinamide and the 2-pyridone and 4-pyridone derivatives; nicotinuric acid is also formed. Small amounts of nicotinic acid and nicotinamide are excreted unchanged in urine following therapeutic doses, however the amount excreted unchanged is increased with larger doses.

A review of the clinical pharmacokinetics of nicotinic acid.— R. Gugler, *Clin. Pharmacokinet.*, 1978, *3*, 425.

Further references: M. Weiner, *Drug Metab. Rev.*, 1979, *9*, 99.

Human Requirements

The daily human requirement of nicotinic acid, though not definitely known, is probably about 15 to 20 mg. Yeast, meat, fish, potatoes, green vegetables, and wholemeal cereals are good sources of nicotinic acid and nicotinamide. However they may be present in a bound, unabsorbable form in cereals, especially maize. Nicotinic acid can also be obtained from the conversion of tryptophan in the body, so requirements are influenced by dietary protein intake. There is generally little loss of nicotinic acid from foods during cooking.

To allow for the metabolic conversion of tryptophan into nicotinic acid, the recommended intake of the vitamin should be expressed as 'niacin equivalents' per 1000 kcal; 6.6 niacin equivalents were required for every 1000 kcal. One such equivalent was equal to 1 mg of nicotinic acid or 60 mg of tryptophan.— Report of a Joint FAO/WHO Expert Group, *Tech. Rep. Ser. Wld Hlth Org. No. 362*, 1967.

Recommended daily intake of nicotinic acid, calculated on resting metabolism: boys and girls up to 8 years, 5 to 11 mg; 9 to 17 years, 14 to 19 mg; men 18 years and over, 18 mg; women 18 years and over, 15 mg; during pregnancy, 18 mg; during lactation, 21 mg. One mg of available nicotinic acid was considered equivalent to 60 mg of tryptophan.— Recommended Daily Amounts of Food Energy and Nutrients for Groups of People in the United Kingdom, Report by The Committee on Medical Aspects of Food Policy, *Report on Health and Social Subjects No. 15*, London, HM Stationery Office, 1979.

Recommended daily dietary allowances of nicotinic acid: up to 6 months, 6 mg; 6 to 12 months, 8 mg; 1 to 3 years, 9 mg; 4 to 6 years, 11 mg; 7 to 10 years, 16 mg; males 11 to 18 years and 23 to 50 years, 18 mg; males 19 to 22 years, 19 mg; males 51 years and over, 16 mg; females 11 to 14 years, 15 mg; 15 to 22 years, 14 mg; 23 years and over, 13 mg; in pregnancy, an additional 2 mg; in lactation, an additional 5 mg. The allowances are calculated as nicotinic acid equivalents; one nicotinic acid equivalent equals 1 mg of nicotinic acid or 60 mg of dietary tryptophan.— *Recommended Dietary Allowances*, 9th Edn, Washington, The National Research Council, 1980.

The recommendation that foods for the young infant should contain nicotinic acid/nicotinamide in amounts not less than 2.3 µg per mL (based on the lower limit of the range in pooled samples of human milk).— Artificial Feeds for the Young Infant: Report of the Working Party on the Composition of Foods for Infants and Young Children, Committee on Medical Aspects of Food Policy, *Report on Health and Social Subjects, 18*, London, HM Stationery Office, 1980.

Uses and Administration

Nicotinic acid and nicotinamide, the form which occurs naturally in the body, are water-soluble vitamin B substances which are converted to nicotinamide adenine dinucleotide (NAD) and nicotinamide adenine dinucleotide phosphate (NADP). These coenzymes are involved in electron transfer reactions in the respiratory chain.

Nicotinic acid deficiency develops when the dietary intake is inadequate. Deficiency leads to the development of a syndrome known as pellagra, characterised by skin lesions, especially on areas exposed to sunlight, with hyperpigmentation and hyperkeratinisation. Other symptoms include diarrhoea, abdominal pain, glossitis, stomatitis, loss of appetite, headache, lethargy, and mental and neurological disturbances. Nicotinic acid deficiency may occur in association with other vitamin B-complex deficiency states.

Nicotinic acid and nicotinamide are used in the treatment and prevention of nicotinic acid deficiency. Nicotinamide is preferred as it does not cause vasodilatation. They are usually given by mouth, the preferred route, but may also be administered by the intramuscular route or by slow intravenous administration. Doses of up to 500 mg daily (of either compound) in divided doses have been recommended.

Nicotinic acid has been employed for its vasodilator action in the treatment of a variety of disorders; its value is not considered to be established.

Nicotinic acid has been used, often in association with other lipid-regulating agents, in type II, III, IV, and V hyperlipoproteinaemias. Doses of 600 mg daily by mouth in divided doses, gradually increased over 2 to 4 weeks to doses of up to 6 g daily have been given; side-effects may be a limiting factor.

The addition of any of the following substances to raw and unprocessed meat intended for human consumption is prohibited in Great Britain by the Meat (Treatment) Regulations, 1964: ascorbic acid, isoascorbic acid, nicotinic acid, nicotinamide, and any derivative of these substances.

For reference to the lack of effect of nicotinic acid in the treatment of ischaemic heart disease, see Clofibrate, p.1199.

A review of vitamin therapy in non-deficiency states. The effectiveness of massive doses of nicotinic acid, usually 3 to 6 g daily as a hypolipidaemic agent has been demonstrated in several clinical trials. Nicotinamide does not share this effect. Nicotinic acid lowers plasma concentrations of both total cholesterol and triglyceride, probably by reducing the synthesis of very low-density lipoprotein (VLDL) and LDL. Nicotinic acid can enhance the lipid-lowering effect of other drugs, particularly clofibrate and bile acid-binding resins. With combined drug regimens and diet, it is often possible to normalise increased lipid concentrations in patients with primary hyperlipidaemia. However, studies aimed at reducing the recurrence rate of atherosclerotic heart disease by nicotinic acid have been disappointing. In addition, disagreeable side-effects have limited its potential usefulness in reducing cardiovascular morbidity and mortality.
Nicotinic acid was the first vitamin to be used by orthomolecular psychiatrists in the treatment of various mental diseases, particularly schizophrenia. The beneficial results obtained by advocates of 'megadose' nicotinic acid therapy have not been confirmed in controlled studies.— L. Ovesen, *Drugs*, 1984, *27*, 148. See also W. M. Petrie and T. A. Ban, *Drugs*, 1985, *30*, 58.

ADMINISTRATION IN RENAL FAILURE. The dose of nicotinic acid should be reduced to 50% in patients with a glomerular filtration-rate (GFR) of 10 to 50 mL per minute, and to 25% in those with a GFR of less than 10 mL per minute.— W. M. Bennett *et al.*, *Am. J. Kidney Dis.*, 1983, *3*, 155.

DIABETES MELLITUS. Results from a study in 16 patients with newly-diagnosed insulin-dependent diabetes mellitus indicated that nicotinamide slows down the destruction of β-cells and enhances their regeneration, thus extending remission time.— P. Vague *et al.* (letter), *Lancet*, 1987, *1*, 619.

Preparations

Niacin Injection *(U.S.P.)*. Nicotinic Acid Injection. Contains nicotinic acid and sodium nicotinate; prepared with the aid of sodium carbonate or sodium hydroxide.

Niacinamide Injection *(U.S.P.)*. Contains nicotinamide.

Niacin Tablets *(U.S.P.)*. Contain nicotinic acid.

Niacinamide Tablets *(U.S.P.)*. Contain nicotinamide.

Nicotinic Acid Tablets *(B.P.)*

Nicotinamide Tablets *(B.P.)*. Niacinamide Tablets

Proprietary Names and Manufacturers

Akotin 250 *(Glaxo, Arg.)*; Farmobion PP *(Ital.)*; Nicangin *(Astra, Swed.)*; Nico-400 *(Marion Laboratories, USA)*; Nicobid *(USV Pharmaceutical Corp., USA)*; Nicobion *(Astra, Fr.; E. Merck, Ger.; Switz.)*; Nicolar *(USV Pharmaceutical Corp., USA)*; Niconacid *(Wander, Ger.)*; Nicorol *(Paramed, Switz.)*; Nico-Span *(Key, USA)*; Nicotilamida *(Igoda, Spain)*; Nicotinex *(Fleming, USA)*; Nicyl *(Astra, Fr.)*; Nikacid *(USV, Austral.)*; SK-Niacin *(Smith Kline & French, USA)*; Tri-B3 *(Bioglan, Austral.; Anabolic, Canad.)*; Vasotherm *(Nutrition Control Products, USA)*.

Multivitamin and mineral preparations containing nicotinic acid or nicotinamide are included in the lists on pp.1289-93. The following names have been used for preparations containing nicotinic acid or nicotinamide and not considered to be a multivitamin or mineral preparation—Antivert *(Pfizer, Canad.)*; Chilblain Treatment Dellipsoids D27 *(Pilsworth, UK)*; Equivert *(Pfizer, UK)*; Migranol *(Alcon, Austral.)*; Pernivit *(Duncan, Flockhart, UK)*; Tryptoplex *(Tyson, USA)*; Verstat *(Saron, USA)*; Vi-Pernic *(Sigma, Austral.)*; Vitaplex Chilblain Formula *(Vitaplex, Austral.)*.

7839-h

Octotiamine *(rINN)*.

TATD; Thioctothiamine. *N*-[2-(3-Acetylthio-7-methoxycarbonylheptyldithio)-4-hydroxy-1-methylbut-1-enyl]-*N*-(4-amino-2-methylpyrimidin-5-ylmethyl)formamide.

$C_{23}H_{36}N_4O_5S_3$=544.8.

CAS — 137-86-0.

Octotiamine is a vitamin B_1 substance with the general properties of thiamine hydrochloride (see p.1277).

Proprietary Names and Manufacturers

Neuvita *(Jpn)*.

608-d

Ornithine *(pINN)*.

α,δ-Diaminovaleric Acid; Orn; L-Ornithine. L-2,5-Diaminovaleric acid.

$C_5H_{12}N_2O_2$=132.2.

CAS — 70-26-8.

Ornithine is an aliphatic amino acid. It is used as a dietary supplement. The aspartate, hydrochloride, and α-ketoglutarate, have been used in the treatment of hyperammonaemia.

For reference to the role of ornithine in the treatment of hepatic encephalopathy, see under Enteral and Parenteral Nutrition, p.1252.

For a report of the use of ornithine with lysine in the treatment of hyperargininaemia, see under Lysine Hydrochloride, p.1267.

Proprietary Names and Manufacturers

Hepa-Merz *(Merz, Ger.)*; Hepato-Spartan *(Craveri, Arg.)*; Ornicetil *(Logeais, Fr.; Nordmark, Ger.; Geymonat, Ital.; Semar, Spain; Logeais, Switz.)*.

7866-v

Pantothenic Acid *(BAN).*
(+)-(*R*)-3-(2,4-Dihydroxy-3,3-dimethylbutyramido)propionic acid.
$C_9H_{17}NO_5$=219.2.

CAS — 79-83-4.

7867-g

Calcium Pantothenate *(BANM, USAN, pINN).*
Calcii Pantothenas; Dextro Calcium Pantothenate. The calcium salt of (+)-pantothenic acid.
$(C_9H_{16}NO_5)_2Ca$=476.5.

CAS — 137-08-6; 6381-63-1 (calcium (±)-pantothenate); 599-54-2 ((±)-pantothenic acid).

Pharmacopoeias. In *Arg., Aust., Belg., Braz., Chin., Cz., Egypt., Eur., Fr., Ger., Ind., It., Jpn, Jug., Neth., Pol., Port., Swiss,* and *U.S.*, which also has a monograph for Racemic Calcium Pantothenate.

A white, odourless, slightly hygroscopic powder. **Soluble** 1 in 3 of water; soluble in glycerol; practically insoluble in alcohol, chloroform, and ether. The *U.S.P.* specifies that the physiological activity of racemic calcium pantothenate is approximately one-half that of calcium pantothenate. **Store** in airtight containers.

Adverse Effects
Pantothenic acid is reported to be generally nontoxic.

Absorption and Fate
Pantothenic acid is readily absorbed from the gastro-intestinal tract following oral administration. It is widely distributed in the body tissues and appears in breast milk. About 70% of pantothenic acid is excreted unchanged in the urine and about 30% in the faeces.

Human Requirements
Pantothenic acid is widely distributed in foods. Meat, legumes, and whole grain cereals are particularly rich sources; other good sources include eggs, milk, vegetables, and fruits. Recommended daily intakes of pantothenic acid have not been set in the *UK* or in the *US*, but human requirements are adequately met by a daily intake of about 4 to 10 mg.

The recommendation that foods for the young infant should contain pantothenic acid in amounts not less than 2 µg per mL (based on the lower limit of the range in pooled samples of human milk).— Artificial Feeds for the Young Infant: Report of the Working Party on the Composition of Foods for Infants and Young Children, Committee on Medical Aspects of Food Policy, *Report on Health and Social Subjects, 18,* London, HM Stationery Office, 1980.

Uses and Administration
Pantothenic acid is traditionally considered to be a vitamin B substance. It is a component of coenzyme A which is essential in the metabolism of carbohydrate, fat, and protein.
Deficiency of pantothenic acid is unlikely in man because of its widespread distribution in food.
Pantothenic acid has no accepted therapeutic uses in human medicine, though it has been used, with variable results, in a variety of conditions including streptomycin intoxication, postoperative ileus, and rheumatoid conditions. It is administered by mouth as a nutritional supplement, often as the calcium salt and usually in conjunction with other vitamins of the B group.
See also Dexpanthenol, p.1563.

A review of vitamin therapy in non-deficiency states. No spontaneous deficiency of pantothenic acid occurs in man. Experimentally-induced deficiency produces intermittent diarrhoea, insomnia, leg cramps, and paraesthesias. There is no persuasive evidence that pantothenic acid has therapeutic efficacy. In a double-blind trial carried out by the General Practitioner Research Group, patients with various forms of arthritic disease were treated with calcium pantothenate 2 g daily for 8 weeks (*Practitioner*, 1980, *224*, 208). No overall benefit was demonstrated, but analysis of the results revealed highly significant effects in reducing symptoms in patients with rheumatoid arthritis.— L. Ovesen, *Drugs*, 1984, *27*, 148.

Preparations
Calcium Pantothenate Tablets *(U.S.P.).* Potency is expressed in terms of the dextrorotatory isomer.

Proprietary Names and Manufacturers
Cal-Pan *(Canad.)*; Cantopal *(Cantassium Co., UK)*; Cantothen *(Cantassium Co., UK)*; Dexol T.D. *(Legere, USA)*; Galamila *(Ger.)*; Megapantho *(Canad.)*; Modane *(Galepharma, Spain)*; Pantenil *(Quimica Medica, Spain)*; Pantholin *(Lilly, USA)*; Pantogen *(Austral.)*.

Multivitamin and mineral preparations containing pantothenic acid or pantothenate are included in the lists on pp.1289-93. The following names have been used for preparations containing pantothenic acid or pantothenate and not considered to be a multivitamin or mineral preparation—Dorbanate Tablets *(Riker, Austral.)*.

610-k

Phenylalanine *(USAN, pINN).*
α-Aminohydrocinnamic acid; Phe; L-Phenylalanine. L-2-Amino-3-phenylpropionic acid.
$C_9H_{11}NO_2$=165.2.

CAS — 63-91-2.

Pharmacopoeias. In *Cz., Jpn,* and *U.S.*

A white odourless crystalline powder. Sparingly **soluble** in water; very slightly soluble in alcohol, methyl alcohol, and dilute mineral acids. A 1% solution in water has a pH of 5.4 to 6.0.

Phenylalanine is an aromatic amino acid which is an essential constituent of the diet. It is used as a dietary supplement.

For reference to the role of aromatic and branched-chain amino acids in the treatment of hepatic encephalopathy, see under Enteral and Parenteral Nutrition, p.1252.

HYPERPHENYLALANINAEMIA. Some reports have indicated that total parenteral nutrition given to sick, preterm, and newborn infants might be associated with potentially dangerous hyperphenylalaninaemia and solutions for paediatric use with a lower phenylalanine content have been developed. Phenylalanine is metabolised in the liver and reports of raised phenylalanine concentrations could indicate impaired liver function. Monitoring of phenylalanine concentration in conjunction with TPN is important.— O. Björkman and M. Lindholm (letter), *Lancet*, 1987, *1*, 1311. Criticism and the view that reports of raised phenylalanine concentrations have been used to support a commercial drive for the introduction of amino acid solutions specially designed for infants.— P. R. Stutchfield *et al.* (letter), *ibid.*, *2*, 1027.

MENTAL DISORDERS. In a double-blind crossover study involving 13 patients with attention deficit disorder, administration of DL-phenylalanine in an average daily dose of 587 mg for 2 to 4 weeks produced a moderate to marked therapeutic response in 6, as compared to 2 on placebo. However, all patients who had initially responded became tolerant to the therapeutic effect after 2 to 3 months on open trial.— D. R. Wood *et al.*, *Psychiatry Res.*, 1985, *16*, 21. Further references: E. Fischer *et al.*, *Arzneimittel-Forsch.*, 1975, *25*, 132; H. Beckmann and E. Ludolph, *ibid.*, 1978, *28*, 1283.

PARKINSONISM. Tremor and rigidity in 7 of 8 patients with parkinsonism were exacerbated when DL-phenylalanine 1.6 to 12.6 g daily was given by mouth.— G. C. Cotzias *et al.*, *New Engl. J. Med.*, 1967, *276*, 374.
Rigidity, walking disability, speech difficulty, and psychic depression greatly improved in 15 patients with parkinsonism after receiving D-phenylalanine 200 to 500 mg daily for 4 weeks.— B. Heller *et al.*, *Arzneimittel-Forsch.*, 1976, *26*, 577.

VITILIGO. Administration of phenylalanine 100 mg per kg body-weight by mouth in conjunction with UVA/sunlight led to beneficial results in more than 90 per cent of 200 patients with vitiligo. Optimal repigmentation of the vitiliginous macules was noted in early disease, but prolonged treatment still induced repigmentation in long-standing cases. Repigmentation occurred mainly in areas rich in follicles. Phenylalanine loading in increasing doses did not influence the serum-tyrosine concentrations. Such treatment is contra-indicated in phenylketonuria and in pregnancy.— R. H. Cormane *et al.*, *Br. J. Derm.*, 1986, *115*, 587.

Proprietary Names and Manufacturers
Endorphenyl *(Tyson, USA)*; Sabiden *(Beta, Arg.)*.

For multi-ingredient preparations containing nutritional agents and vitamins, see p.1289.

13145-h

Polydextrose *(USAN).*
CP-31081. A randomly bonded glucose polymer, of average molecular weight 1500, with some sorbitol end-groups, and with citric acid residues attached to the polymer by mono- or di-ester bonds.

CAS — 68424-04-4.

Polydextrose has potential as a low-energy replacement for sugar and fats in foods.

Polydextroses are poorly absorbed and are metabolised by gut flora to their normal metabolites, primarily carbon dioxide and volatile fatty acids. Polydextroses, at very high doses, exert a laxative effect, and this should be taken into account when considering appropriate levels for their use either alone or in combination with other substances causing laxative effects by osmotic action.
The report provides an estimated acceptable daily intake for polydextroses (polydextrose A and polydextrose N) of "not specified".— Thirty-first Report of the Joint FAO/WHO Committee on Food Additives, *Wld Hlth Org. Tech. Rep. Ser. No. 759*, 1987, p.31.

Proprietary Names and Manufacturers
Pfizer, USA.

613-x

Proline *(USAN, pINN).*
Pro; L-Proline. L-Pyrrolidine-2-carboxylic acid.
$C_5H_9NO_2$=115.1.

CAS — 147-85-3.

Pharmacopoeias. In *U.S.*

White odourless crystals. Freely **soluble** in water and dehydrated alcohol; insoluble in butyl alcohol, ether, and isopropyl alcohol.

Proline is an amino acid. It is used as a dietary supplement.

Preparations
For multi-ingredient preparations containing nutritional agents and vitamins, see p.1289.

13182-q

Prosultiamine *(rINN).*
DTPT; Thiamine Propyl Disulphide. *N*-(4-Amino-2-methylpyrimidin-5-ylmethyl)-*N*-(4-hydroxy-1-methyl-2-propyldithiobut-1-enyl)formamide.
$C_{15}H_{24}N_4O_2S_2$=356.5.

CAS — 59-58-5.

Prosultiamine is a vitamin B_1 substance with the general properties of thiamine hydrochloride (p.1277).

Proprietary Names and Manufacturers
Binova *(Gentili, Ital.)*; Jubedel Fuerte *(Septa, Spain)*; Taketron *(Neth.)*; Trofotiamin *(IBP, Ital.)*.

7847-h

Pyridoxine Hydrochloride *(BAN, USAN, rINNM).*

Adermine Hydrochloride; Piridossina Cloridrato; Pyridoxini Hydrochloridum; Pyridoxinii Chloridum; Pyridoxinium Chloride; Pyridoxol Hydrochloride; Vitamin B_6. 3-Hydroxy-4,5-bis(hydroxymethyl)-2-picoline hydrochloride.
$C_8H_{11}NO_3,HCl$=205.6.

CAS — 65-23-6 (pyridoxine); 58-56-0 (hydrochloride).

NOTE. Pyridoxine is only one of 3 similar compounds that may be referred to as vitamin B_6; the other two are pyridoxal and pyridoxamine.

Pharmacopoeias. In *Arg., Aust., Belg., Br., Braz., Chin., Cz., Egypt., Eur., Fr., Ger., Hung., Ind., Int., It., Jpn, Jug., Neth., Nord., Port., Roum., Rus., Swiss, Turk.,* and *U.S.* Also in *B.P. Vet.*

A white or almost white odourless or almost odourless crystalline powder, or crystals.

Soluble 1 in 5 of water and 1 in 100 to 115 of alcohol; practically insoluble in chloroform and ether. A 5% solution in water has a pH of 2.4 to 3.0. The *U.S.P.* injection has a pH of 2.0 to 3.8. **Store** at a temperature not exceeding 30° in airtight containers. Protect from light.

STABILITY IN SOLUTION. A review of the compatibility and stability of components of total parenteral nutrition solutions when mixed in 1- or 3-litre flexible containers. Pyridoxine is light sensitive although degradation is far less than is observed with vitamin A or riboflavine. Exposure to direct sunlight has been reported to lead to destruction of more than 80% of the added pyridoxine in 8 hours. Under normal conditions therefore, pyridoxine losses would be small.— M. C. Allwood, *J. clin. Hosp. Pharm.*, 1984, *9*, 181.

Adverse Effects and Precautions

Long-term administration of large doses of pyridoxine is associated with the development of severe peripheral neuropathies. Pyridoxine reduces the effects of levodopa (see p.1017), but this does not occur if a dopa decarboxylase inhibitor is also given.

For reports on the effect of pyridoxine on amiodarone-induced photosensitivity, see under Amiodarone Hydrochloride, p.72.

EFFECTS ON THE NERVOUS SYSTEM. Severe sensory neuropathy occurred in 7 patients who had consumed large daily doses of pyridoxine. Daily consumption of pyridoxine ranged from 2 to 6 g for periods of 2 to 40 months and resulted in gradually progressive sensory ataxia and profound distal limb impairment of position and vibration sense. Neurological disability gradually improved on withdrawal of pyridoxine and 2 patients followed up for a prolonged period had almost completely recovered after 2 and 3 years respectively.— H. Schaumburg *et al.*, *New Engl. J. Med.*, 1983, *309*, 445. Comments.— D. Rudman and P. J. Williams, *ibid.*, 488; L. Pauling (letter), *ibid.*, 1984, *310*, 197; H. Baker and O. Frank (letter), *ibid.*

A report of sensory ataxia in a 34-year-old patient who had been taking pyridoxine 500 mg daily (with an additional 300 mg not more than once weekly) over a period of one year, and 200 mg daily for another 2 years previously.— A. Berger and H. H. Schaumburg (letter), *New Engl. J. Med.*, 1984, *311*, 986. Further references: G. J. Parry and D. E. Bredesen, *Neurology*, 1985, *35*, 1466; J. A. Waterston and B. S. Gilligan, *Med. J. Aust.*, 1987, *146*, 640.

INTERACTIONS. Pyridoxine requirements have been reported to be increased by oral contraceptives, hydralazine, isoniazid, and penicillamine.— *Med. Lett.*, 1985, *27*, 66.

PREGNANCY AND THE NEONATE. A report of phocomelia in an infant whose mother had taken, in addition to the multivitamin preparation prescribed, an assortment of over-the-counter vitamin and nutritional preparations. During the first 7 months of pregnancy she had taken pyridoxine 50 mg daily as well as unknown doses of lecithin and cyanocobalamin.— L. I. Gardner *et al.* (letter), *Lancet*, 1985, *1*, 636.

Absorption and Fate

Pyridoxine, pyridoxal, and pyridoxamine are readily absorbed from the gastro-intestinal tract following oral administration and are converted to the active forms pyridoxal phosphate and pyridoxamine phosphate. They are stored mainly in the liver where there is oxidation to 4-pyridoxic acid which is excreted in the urine. Pyridoxal crosses the placenta and also appears in breast milk.

Human Requirements

For adults, the daily requirement of pyridoxine is probably about 2 mg and this amount is present in most normal diets. Meats, especially liver, cereals, eggs, fish, and certain vegetables and fruits are good sources of pyridoxine.

In the United Kingdom deficiency of pyridoxine is rare. Pyridoxine occurs in sufficient quantity in a large number of foods. Therefore, in the light of present knowledge and in the context of the diet in the *UK*, recommended daily intakes for pyridoxine have not been set.— Recommended Daily Amounts of Food Energy and Nutrients for Groups of People in the the United Kingdom, Report by the Committee on Medical Aspects of Food Policy, *Report on Health and Social Subjects No.15*, London, HM Stationery Office, 1979.

Recommendations for allowances for vitamin B_6 are difficult to make since requirements increase as the protein content of the diet increases. A daily dietary allowance of 2.2 mg should be suitable for men and 2 mg for women; 300 µg daily should be suitable for infants up to 6 months and 600 µg for children from 6 months to 1 year. Older children can be given up to 2 mg daily. Pregnant women should generally take 2.6 mg daily and lactating women 2.5 mg. Supplementation with vitamin B_6 did not appear to be necessary in women taking oral contraceptives.— *Recommended Dietary Allowances*, 9th Edn, Washington, The National Research Council, 1980, p. 96.

The recommendation that foods for the young infant should contain pyridoxine hydrochloride in amounts not less than 50 ng per mL (based on the lower limit of the range in pooled samples of human milk).— Artificial Feeds for the Young Infant: Report of the Working Party on the Composition of Foods for Infants and Young Children, Committee on Medical Aspects of Food Policy, *Report on Health and Social Subjects, 18*, London, HM Stationery Office, 1980.

Uses and Administration

Pyridoxine, a water-soluble vitamin, is involved principally in amino acid metabolism, but is also involved in carbohydrate and fat metabolism. It is also required for the formation of haemoglobin.

Deficiency of pyridoxine is rare in humans due to its widespread distribution in foods. Pyridoxine deficiency may however be drug-induced and can occur, for instance, during isoniazid therapy. Inadequate utilisation of pyridoxine may result from certain inborn errors of metabolism. Pyridoxine deficiency in adults leads to the development of peripheral neuritis; deficiency in children also affects the CNS.

Pyridoxine is used in the treatment and prevention of pyridoxine deficiency states. It is usually given by mouth, the preferred route, but may also be administered by the intramuscular or intravenous routes. Doses of 100 to 400 mg daily have been used in the treatment of sideroblastic anaemias and similar doses have been used to treat certain metabolic disorders. Pyridoxine has also been used to treat seizures due to hereditary syndromes of pyridoxine deficiency or dependency in infants.

Pyridoxine has also been tried in a wide variety of other disorders, including the treatment of depression and other symptoms associated with the premenstrual syndrome and the use of oral contraceptives.

For the use of pyridoxine in the prophylaxis of isoniazid-induced peripheral neuritis and for the treatment of acute isoniazid toxicity, see under Isoniazid, p.565.

A review of vitamin therapy in non-deficiency states. It has been theorised that pyridoxine by its function as a coenzyme in DOPA decarboxylation may increase the hypothalamic content of dopamine with a resultant decrease in prolactin concentrations. Consequently, massive doses of pyridoxine have been proposed in the treatment of hyperprolactinaemic amenorrhoea and galactorrhoea. However, several studies have been unable to demonstrate a dopaminergic effect of acute and chronic pyridoxine administration, and it is presently regarded as an ineffective drug for the management of hyperprolactinaemia.

Pyridoxine has also been thought to have a potential role as an antithrombotic agent by its ability to prolong clotting time and inhibit platelet aggregation. The mechanism seems to be independent of its function as a coenzyme but is probably caused by the binding of pyridoxal phosphate to fibrinogen, and to specific platelet surface amino groups through the formation of a Schiff base.

Idiopathic carpal tunnel syndrome, with swelling of the synovia and compression of the median nerve by the transverse carpal ligament, has been attributed to a deficiency of pyridoxine. The syndrome appears to be reversible upon treatment with pyridoxine 100 to 150 mg daily for 12 or more weeks.

It has also been reported that pyridoxine is effective in treating pregnancy sickness, symptoms of the premenstrual syndrome, muscular weakness, recurrent oxalate urolithiasis, and the hyperkinetic syndrome in children. These possible therapeutic effects need confirmation in properly controlled clinical trials.— L. Ovesen, *Drugs*, 1984, *27*, 148. See also H. Schaumburg *et al.*, *New Engl. J. Med.*, 1983, *309*, 445.

AMINO ACID METABOLIC DISORDERS. Treatment with pharmacologic doses of pyridoxine as a cofactor for cystathionine synthetase might prevent a number of serious clinical sequelae caused by homocystinuria. Six weeks of treatment with pyridoxine led to a substantial reduction in homocysteinaemia which occurred after methionine loading in 10 of 11 heterozygous patients with premature vascular damage; values became normal in 6. The clinical relevance of these observations awaits long-term evaluation.— G. H. J. Boers *et al.*, *New Engl. J. Med.*, 1985, *313*, 709.

Further reports of the beneficial use of pyridoxine in the management of various inborn errors of metabolism: P. Alinei *et al.* (letter), *New Engl. J. Med.*, 1984, *311*, 798 (infantile type I primary hyperoxaluria); E. R. Yendt and M. Cohanim, *New Engl. J. Med.*, 1985, *312*, 953 (type I primary hyperoxaluria); S. Hayasaka *et al.*, *Br. J. Ophthal.*, 1985, *69*, 283 (hyperornithinaemia in association with gyrate atrophy of the choroid and retina); F. de Zegher *et al.* (letter), *Lancet*, 1985, *2*, 392 (infantile type I primary hyperoxaluria complicated by pyrodoxine toxicity).

PSYCHIATRIC DISORDERS. Although oral contraceptives may lead to a functional deficiency of pyridoxine there is no evidence that this deficiency is a cause of depression or that concurrent prescription of pyridoxine lowers the incidence of depression.— P. J. Tyrer, *Prescribers' J.*, 1981, *21*, 237.

In conditions of pyridoxine deficiency, γ-aminobutyric acid (GABA) concentrations are reduced and the resultant convulsive activity may be controlled by administration of GABA. Although psychiatric symptoms have not been classically described in pyridoxine deficiency (except in alcoholics), the changes in serotonin and GABA metabolism are of theoretical interest to psychiatry. Disturbances in serotonin metabolism are accepted as a viable hypothesis in the pathogenesis of affective illness, and GABA has been related to anxiety disorders. Thus, pyridoxine has been administered to depressed patients, both alone and in combination with antidepressant agents. Although anecdotal reports indicate potential efficacy, no conclusive clinical trial has been undertaken. Data are also lacking on the use of pyridoxine in anxiety disorders.— W. M. Petrie and T. A. Ban, *Drugs*, 1985, *30*, 58.

See also under Premenstrual Syndrome, below.

PREMENSTRUAL SYNDROME. Pyridoxine 100 mg daily by mouth is effective for the relief of psychological symptoms attributed to the premenstrual syndrome, although it may act only as a placebo.— H. Massil and P. M. S. O'Brien, *Br. med. J.*, 1986, *293*, 1289.

Pyridoxine is widely prescribed in the management of the premenstrual syndrome. In theory depressive symptoms may be provoked by pyridoxine deficiency because of its role as a coenzyme in the production of certain neurotransmitters. It is difficult to attribute any of the other symptoms of the premenstrual syndrome to pyridoxine deficiency and at a dose of 50 mg daily pyridoxine is no more effective than a placebo.— C. P. West, *Prescribers' J.*, 1987, *27*, 9.

Further references: B. L. True *et al.*, *Drug Intell. & clin. Pharm.*, 1985, *19*, 714; *Aust. J. Pharm.*, 1985, *66*, 853.

Preparations

Pyridoxine Hydrochloride Injection *(U.S.P.)*

Pyridoxine Hydrochloride Tablets *(U.S.P.)*

Pyridoxine Injection *(B.P.C. 1973)*. Pyridoxine Hydrochloride Injection. Contains pyridoxine hydrochloride.

Pyridoxine Tablets *(B.P.)*. Pyridoxine Hydrochloride Tablets; Vitamin B_6 Tablets. Contain pyridoxine hydrochloride.

Proprietary Preparations

Benadon *(Roche, UK)*. *Tablets*, pyridoxine hydrochloride 20 mg.
Tablets, scored, pyridoxine hydrochloride 50 mg.

Comploment Continus *(Napp, UK)*. *Tablets*, sustained-release, pyridoxine hydrochloride 100 mg.

Paxadon *(Steinhard, UK)*. *Tablets*, scored, pyridoxine hydrochloride 50 mg.

Proprietary Names and Manufacturers

Aminoxin *(Tyson, USA)*; Aspardoxine *(Laphal, Fr.)*; Bécilan *(Specia, Fr.)*; Bedoxine *(Belg.)*; Beesix *(Lennon, S.Afr.)*; Benadon *(Arg.; Belg.; Roche, Ger.; Roche, Ital.; Roche, Spain; Roche, Swed.; Roche, Switz.; Roche, UK)*; B_6-Vicotrat *(Ger.)*; Bivit-6 *(Ital.)*; Bonasanit *(Weimer, Ger.)*; Comploment Continus *(Napp, UK)*; Dermo 6 *(Chabre, Fr.)*; Dextamina B6 *(Spain)*; Farmobion B_6 *(Ital.)*; Godabion B6 *(Igoda, Spain)*; Hexa-Betalin *(Lilly, Canad.;*

Lilly, USA); Hexapyral *(Swed.)*; Hexavibex *(Canad.)*; Hexobion *(E. Merck, Ger.; Spain)*; Himitan *(Jpn)*; Hysix *(Jpn)*; Lactosec 200 *(Continental Ethicals, S.Afr.)*; Paxadon *(Steinhard, UK)*; Pidopidon *(Jpn)*; PMT *(Hamilton, Austral.)*; Pydox *(Protea, Austral.)*; Pyricamphre *(Fr.)*; Pyroxin *(USV, Austral.)*; Rodex *(Legere, USA)*; Rodex T.D. *(Legere, USA)*; Sechvitan *(Jpn)*; Seibion *(Ital.)*; Sibevit *(Delagrange, Spain)*; Vitanoxi B6 *(Spain)*; Xanturenasi *(Alfa Farmaceutici, Ital.)*.

Multivitamin and mineral preparations containing pyridoxine are included in the lists on pp.1289-93. The following names have been used for preparations containing pyridoxine and not considered to be a multivitamin or mineral preparation—Ancoloxin *(Duncan, Flockhart, UK)*; Beelith *(Beach, USA)*; Bendectin *(Merrell Dow, USA)*; Debendox *(Merrell, UK)*; Decadol *(Cambridge Laboratories, Austral.)*; Diclectin *(Duchesnay, Canad.)*; Herpecin-L *(Campbell, USA)*; Tryptoplex *(Tyson, USA)*.

7843-r

Riboflavine *(BAN)*.

E101; Lactoflavin; Riboflavin *(USAN, rINN)*; Riboflavinum; Vitamin B_2; Vitamin G. 7,8-Dimethyl-10-(1′-D-ribityl)isoalloxazine; 3,10-Dihydro-7,8-dimethyl-10-(D-*ribo*-2,3,4,5-tetrahydroxypentyl)benzopteridine-2,4-dione.

$C_{17}H_{20}N_4O_6$=376.4.

CAS — 83-88-5.

Pharmacopoeias. In *Arg., Aust., Belg., Br., Braz., Chin., Cz., Egypt., Eur., Fr., Ger., Hung., Ind., Int., It., Jpn, Jug., Mex., Neth., Nord., Pol., Port., Roum., Rus., Span., Swiss, Turk.*, and *U.S.* Also in *B.P. Vet.*

A yellow to orange-yellow crystalline powder with a slight odour.

Very slightly **soluble** in water; more soluble in 0.9% sodium chloride solution than in water; practically insoluble in alcohol, acetone, chloroform, and ether; very soluble in dilute alkali solutions. A saturated solution in water has a pH of about 7.0; the *U.S.P.* injection has a pH of 4.5 to 7.0. **Store** in airtight containers. Protect from light. When dry it is not appreciably affected by light, but in solution, especially in the presence of alkali, it deteriorates rapidly, the decomposition being accelerated by light.

7842-x

Riboflavine Sodium Phosphate *(BANM)*.

Natrii Riboflavinophosphas; Riboflavin 5′-Phosphate Sodium *(USAN)*; Riboflavin Sodium Phosphate *(rINNM)*; Riboflavine 5′-Phosphate Sodium; Riboflavine Phosphate *(Sodium Salt)*; Vitamin B_2 Phosphate. The dihydrate of the sodium salt of riboflavine 5′-phosphate.

$C_{17}H_{20}N_4NaO_9P,2H_2O$=514.4.

CAS — 130-40-5 (anhydrous).

Pharmacopoeias. In *Br., Ind., Jug., Nord.*, and *U.S. Jpn* specifies the anhydrous salt.

A fine yellow to orange-yellow, odourless or almost odourless, crystalline hygroscopic powder. Riboflavine sodium phosphate 1.37 g is approximately equivalent to 1 g of riboflavine. **Soluble** 1 in 20 of water; very slightly soluble in alcohol; practically insoluble in chloroform and ether. The *B.P.* specifies that a 2% solution in water has a pH of 4.0 to 6.3. The *U.S.P.* specifies that a 1% solution in water has a pH of 5.0 to 6.5. **Store** in well-closed containers. Protect from light. When dry, it is not affected by diffused light, but when in solution light induces rapid deterioration.

STABILITY IN SOLUTION. A review of the compatibility and stability of components of total parenteral nutrition solutions when mixed in 1- or 3-litre flexible containers. Unpublished studies have indicated that daylight-induced losses can amount to 40% after 8 hours, and 55% after a typical 24-hour administration period. Losses during passage through the administration set can lead to a further 2% loss. It is important, therefore, to include an adequate overage in a parenteral nutrition regimen to allow for these losses. As with other losses caused by exposure to daylight, commencing infusion in the evening ensures that the patient receives greater amounts of this vitamin.— M. C. Allwood, *J. clin. Hosp. Pharm.*, 1984, *9*, 181.

Adverse Effects and Precautions

No adverse effects have been reported with the use of riboflavine. Large doses of riboflavine result in a bright yellow discoloration of the urine which may interfere with certain laboratory tests.

Absorption and Fate

Riboflavine is readily absorbed from the gastro-intestinal tract. Although riboflavine is widely distributed to body tissues little is stored in the body.

Riboflavine is converted in the body to the coenzyme flavine mononucleotide (FMN; riboflavine 5′-phosphate) and then to another coenzyme flavine adenine dinucleotide (FAD). About 60% of FMN and FAD are bound to plasma proteins. Riboflavine is excreted in urine, mainly as metabolites. As the dose increases, larger amounts are excreted unchanged. Riboflavine crosses the placenta.

Human Requirements

The riboflavine requirement is often related to the energy intake but it appears to be more closely related to resting metabolic requirements. A daily dietary intake of about 1.3 to 1.8 mg of riboflavine is recommended. Liver, kidney, eggs, milk, cheese, yeast, and some green vegetables are the richest sources of riboflavine. In general, little loss of riboflavine occurs during cooking, but considerable losses may occur if foods, especially milk, are exposed to sunlight.

The basic recommended intake of riboflavine was 550 μg per 4200 kJ (1000 kcal) of diet, so that men required 1.8 mg of riboflavine and women required 1.3 mg of riboflavine.— Report of a Joint FAO/WHO Expert Group, *Tech. Rep. Ser. Wld Hlth Org. No. 362*, 1967.

Estimated acceptable daily intake of riboflavine: up to 500 μg per kg body-weight.— Thirteenth Report of FAO/WHO Expert Committee on Food Additives, *Tech. Rep. Ser. Wld Hlth Org. No. 445*, 1971.

In a nutrition survey of elderly subjects aged 65 or over, 57 of 778 had angular stomatitis and cheilosis and a riboflavine intake of 1.2 mg a day compared with 1.3 mg for those without lip lesions; 4 of 23 subjects with a riboflavine intake of less than 700 μg daily for men or less than 550 μg daily for women had lip lesions.— Report by the Panel on Nutrition of the Elderly, *A Nutrition Survey of the Elderly*, London, HM Stationery Office, 1972.

Recommended daily intake of riboflavine calculated on resting metabolism: boys and girls up to 8 years of age, 0.4 to 1 mg; boys and girls 9 to 17 years, 1.2 to 1.7 mg; men over 17 years, 1.6 mg; women over 17 years, 1.3 mg; during pregnancy, 1.6 mg; during lactation 1.8 mg.— Recommended Daily Amounts of Food Energy and Nutrients for Groups of People in the United Kingdom, Report by the Committee on Medical Aspects of Food Policy, *Report on Health and Social Subjects No. 15*, London, HM Stationery Office, 1979.

Recommended daily dietary allowance for riboflavine: up to 6 months, 0.4 mg; 6 to 12 months, 0.6 mg; 1 to 3 years, 0.8 mg; 4 to 6 years, 1 mg; 7 to 10 years, 1.4 mg; males 11 to 14 years and 23 to 50 years, 1.6 mg; males 15 to 22 years, 1.7 mg; males 51 years and over, 1.4 mg; females 11 to 22 years, 1.3 mg; 23 years and over, 1.2 mg; in pregnancy, an additional 0.3 mg; in lactation, an additional 0.5 mg.— *Recommended Dietary Allowances*, 9th Edn, Washington, The National Research Council, 1980.

The recommendation that foods for the young infant should contain riboflavine in amounts not less than 300 ng per mL (based on the lower limit of the range in pooled samples of human milk).— Artificial Feeds for the Young Infant: Report of the Working Party on the Composition of Foods for Infants and Young Children, Committee on Medical Aspects of Food Policy, *Report on Health and Social Subjects, 18*, London, HM Stationery Office, 1980.

Uses and Administration

Riboflavine, a water-soluble vitamin, is essential for the utilisation of energy from food. The active, phosphorylated forms, flavine mononucleotide and flavine adenine dinucleotide, are involved as coenzymes in oxidative/reductive metabolic reactions.

Riboflavine deficiency develops when the dietary intake is inadequate. Deficiency leads to the development of a well-defined syndrome known as ariboflavinosis, characterised by cheilosis, angular stomatitis, glossitis, and seborrhoeic keratosis of the nose and ano-genital region. There may also be ocular symptoms including itching and burning of the eyes, photophobia, and corneal vascularisation. Riboflavine deficiency may occur in association with other vitamin B-complex deficiency states such as pellagra.

Riboflavine is used in the treatment and prevention of riboflavine deficiency. It is usually given by mouth, the preferred route, but may also be administered by the intramuscular or intravenous routes. Doses of up to 30 mg daily in single or divided doses have been recommended.

Riboflavine is a permitted colouring agent for food.

AMINO ACID METABOLIC DISORDERS. Reports of the successful use of riboflavine in the treatment of various organic acid metabolic disorders: J. -P. Harpey and C. Charpentier (letter), *Lancet*, 1983, *1*, 586 (multiple acyl-CoA dehydrogenase deficiency resembling acute fatty liver of pregnancy); W. F. M. Arts *et al.* (letter), *ibid.*, *2*, 581 (NADH-CoQ reductase-deficient myopathy in a 13-year-old patient); B. Francois *et al.* (letter), *ibid.*, 1986, *1*, 380 (metabolic acidosis with organic aciduria in 3 premature infants, suggestive of a multiple acyl-CoA dehydrogenase deficiency syndrome); R. J. Pollitt, *Archs Dis. Childh.*, 1987, *62*, 6 (ethylmalonic-adipic aciduria).

A report of multiple acyl Co-A dehydrogenase deficiency in a neonate which was unresponsive to treatment with riboflavine.— J. -P. Harpey *et al.*, *Lancet*, 1986, *1*, 391.

BLOOD DISORDERS. In view of the possible association between prolonged ascorbic acid administration and hyperoxaluria, a 33-year-old man and a 4-month-old infant with recessive congenital methaemoglobinaemia, were both successfully transferred from ascorbic acid therapy to riboflavine therapy. The maintenance doses of riboflavine of 30 mg daily and 20 mg daily respectively, depressed methaemoglobin concentrations to about 5%.— J. C. Kaplan and M. Chirouze (letter), *Lancet*, 1978, *2*, 1043.

Preparations

Riboflavin Injection *(U.S.P.)*. Contains riboflavine. It may contain nicotinamide or other suitable solubilising agents.

Riboflavin Tablets *(U.S.P.)*. Contain riboflavine.

Riboflavine Tablets *(B.P.C. 1973)*

Proprietary Names and Manufacturers

Adeflavin *(Jpn)*; B2-Elite-10 *(Jpn)*; Beflavin *(Roche, Ger.)*; Beflavina *(Roche, Ital.)*; Beflavine *(Roche, Belg.; Roche, Fr.)*; Beflavit *(Roche, UK)*; Berivine *(Meuse, Belg.)*; Bisulase *(Jpn)*; Fademin *(Jpn)*; Fladd *(Jpn)*; Flamitajin-R *(Jpn)*; Flanin F *(Jpn)*; Flavinin *(Jpn)*; Flavitan *(Jpn)*; Flaziren D *(Jpn)*; Hokurabin *(Jpn)*; Mohaflan *(Jpn)*; Ribofosforil *(Nessa, Spain)*; Wakedenin *(Jpn)*.

For multi-ingredient preparations containing nutritional agents and vitamins, see p.1289.

7844-f

Riboflavine Tetrabutyrate

Riboflavine Butyrate.

$C_{33}H_{44}N_4O_{10}$=656.7.

CAS — 752-56-7.

Riboflavine tetrabutyrate is a vitamin B_2 substance with the general properties of riboflavine. It has also been tried as a hypolipidaemic agent.

Proprietary Names and Manufacturers

Bisanorin *(Jpn)*; Bituvitan *(Jpn)*; Bonabon B_2 *(Jpn)*; Butirid *(Jpn)*; Eyekas *(Jpn)*; Hibon *(Jpn)*; Liperox *(Byk Liprandi, Arg.)*; Multiscleran *(Boehringer Mannheim,*

Spain); Ribobis *(Jpn)*; Ribobutin *(Jpn)*; Riboract *(Jpn)*; Wakaflavin-L *(Jpn)*.

2404-b

Saccharin *(BAN, USAN)*.

Benzosulphimide; Gluside; Sacarina; Saccarina; Zaharina. 1,2-Benzisothiazolin-3-one 1,1-dioxide. $C_7H_5NO_3S$=183.2.

CAS — 81-07-2.

Pharmacopoeias. In *Arg., Br., Egypt., Fr., Hung., Ind., It., Pol., Port., Roum., Span.,* and *Swiss.* Also in *U.S.N.F.*

White odourless or faintly aromatic crystals or crystalline powder with an intensely sweet taste. Slightly **soluble** in water; soluble 1 in 25 of boiling water, 1 in 12 of acetone, and 1 in 30 of alcohol; slightly soluble in chloroform and ether; readily soluble in dilute ammonia solution and in solutions of alkali hydroxides and, with the evolution of carbon dioxide, in solutions of alkali bicarbonates and carbonates. A saturated solution in water is acid to litmus. **Store** in well-closed containers.

2405-v

Saccharin Calcium *(USAN)*.

Calcium Benzosulphimide; Calcium Saccharin. The hydrate of the calcium salt of 1,2-benzisothiazolin-3-one 1,1-dioxide. $C_{14}H_8CaN_2O_6S_2,3\frac{1}{2}H_2O$=467.5.

CAS — 6485-34-3 (anhydrous); 6381-91-5 (hydrate).

Pharmacopoeias. In *U.S.*

White odourless or faintly aromatic crystals or crystalline powder with an intensely sweet taste. Freely **soluble** in water. **Store** in well-closed containers.

2406-g

Saccharin Sodium *(BAN, USAN)*.

Saccharin Sod.; Saccharinnatrium; Saccharoidum Natricum; Sodium Benzosulphimide; Sodium Saccharin; Soluble Gluside; Soluble Saccharin. The dihydrate of the sodium salt of 1,2-benzisothiazolin-3-one 1,1-dioxide. $C_7H_4NNaO_3S$=205.2.

CAS — 128-44-9 (anhydrous); 6155-57-3 (dihydrate).

Pharmacopoeias. In *Arg., Aust., Br., Chin., Egypt., Fr., Ger., Hung., Ind., It., Jpn, Jug., Mex., Neth., Nord., Port., Span., Swiss, Turk.,* and *U.S.* Some pharmacopoeias including *Br.* specify the anhydrous form; others including *U.S.* specify $2H_2O$.

White efflorescent crystals or a white, odourless or faintly aromatic, crystalline powder with an intensely sweet taste. **Soluble** 1 in 1.5 of water and 1 in 50 of alcohol. **Store** in well-closed containers.

Adverse Effects

There have been rare reports of allergic and photosensitivity reactions with saccharin.

Saccharin-associated bladder tumours in *rats* have been the cause of much concern and investigation (see *Martindale 28th Edn*, p.429). However, it is now generally accepted that this is not applicable to saccharin use as a sweetener by man.

Absorption and Fate

Saccharin is readily absorbed from the gastro-intestinal tract. It is almost all excreted unchanged in the urine within 24 to 48 hours.

References: E. W. McChesney and L. Golberg, *Toxic. appl. Pharmac.*, 1973, *25*, 494; W. A. Colburn *et al.*, *Clin. Pharmac. Ther.*, 1981, *30*, 558.

Uses and Administration

Saccharin and its salts are intense sweeteners being several hundred times sweeter than sucrose and are used as food additives. They have no food value. The salts are more often used as they are considered to be the most palatable; salts in use include saccharin potassium as well as the calcium and sodium salts.

An injection of saccharin sodium has been used to measure the arm-to-tongue circulation time.

Estimated temporary acceptable daily intake for saccharin, including its calcium, potassium, and sodium salts: up to 2.5 mg per kg body-weight.— Twenty-eighth Report of the Joint FAO/WHO Expert Committee on Food Additives, *Tech. Rep. Ser. Wld Hlth Org. No. 710*, 1984.

Preparations

Saccharin Sodium Oral Solution *(U.S.P.)*. A solution containing saccharin sodium. pH 3 to 5. Store in airtight containers.

Saccharin Sodium Tablets *(U.S.P.)*

Proprietary Names and Manufacturers

Gaosucryl *(Pharminter, Fr.)*; Oda *(Lafon, Fr.)*; Skun-suc *(Human-Pharm, Fr.)*; Sucline *(Soekami, Fr.)*; Sucredulcor *(Pierre Fabre, Fr.)*; Sucrettes *(Vernin, Fr.)*; Sucromat *(Mayoly-Spindler, Fr.)*; Sun-suc *(Human-Pharm, Fr.)*.

7367-s

Safflower Oil

CAS — 8001-23-8.

Pharmacopoeias. In *U.S. Chin.* and *Jpn* include Safflower, the flower of *Carthamus tinctorius*.

The refined fixed oil obtained from the seeds of the safflower, or false (bastard) saffron, *Carthamus tinctorius*(Compositae). It contains about 75% of linoleic acid as well as various saturated fatty acids.

It has similar characteristics to linseed oil (see p.1584). It thickens and becomes rancid on prolonged exposure to air. **Store** in airtight containers. Protect from light.

Uses and Administration

Safflower oil has similar actions and uses to those of soya oil, p.1274. Emulsions containing a mixture of safflower oil 5% and soya oil 5%, or 10% and 10% respectively, are given as part of total parenteral nutrition regimens.

For reference to the association of lipid emulsion administration, as part of a parenteral nutrition regimen, with the development of sinus bradycardia, see under Soya Oil, p.1274.

Proprietary Names and Manufacturers

Liposyn *(Abbott, Austral.; Ross, Canad.)*; Obesitol *(Carter Bros, UK)*; Safflor *(Wisconsin Pharmacal, USA)*.

The following names have been used for multi-ingredient preparations containing safflower oil—Efamol Plus *(Britannia Health, UK)*.

13231-d

Serendipity Berry

The fruit of *Dioscoreophyllum cumminsii* (Menispermaceae).

Serendipity berries contain a water-soluble proteinaceous sweet principle, many times sweeter than sucrose, but labile to heat.

616-d

Serine *(USAN, pINN)*.

β-Hydroxyalanine; Ser; L-Serine. L-2-Amino-3-hydroxypropionic acid. $C_3H_7NO_3$=105.1.

CAS — 56-45-1.

Pharmacopoeias. In *U.S.*

White odourless crystals. **Soluble** in water; practically insoluble in dehydrated alcohol and ether.

Serine is an aliphatic amino acid. It is used as a dietary supplement.

Preparations

For multi-ingredient preparations containing nutritional agents and vitamins, see p.1289.

2409-s

Sodium Cyclamate *(BAN, rINN)*.

Cyclamate Sodium; Sod. Cyclam.; Sodium Cyclohexanesulphamate. Sodium *N*-cyclohexylsulphamate. $C_6H_{12}NNaO_3S$=201.2.

CAS — 139-05-9.

Pharmacopoeias. In *Fr., Neth., Roum.,* and *Swiss.*

White odourless or almost odourless crystals or crystalline powder with an intensely sweet taste, even in dilute solution.

Soluble 1 in 5 of water.

Sodium cyclamate is an intense sweetening agent. In dilute solutions (up to about 0.17%) sodium cyclamate is about 30 times as sweet as sugar but this factor decreases at higher concentrations. When the concentration approaches 0.5%, a bitter taste becomes noticeable. Cyclamic acid and calcium cyclamate possess similar properties.

Sodium cyclamate has been used as a substitute for sucrose by diabetics and others needing to restrict their intake of carbohydrates but its use as an artificial sweetener in food, soft drinks, and artificial sweetening tablets is no longer permitted in Great Britain and in many other countries because of concern about its metabolite cyclohexylamine. The ban on cyclamates has been reappraised in the *USA* and it appears that early doubts about their carcinogenicity may not have been confirmed.

Temporary estimated acceptable daily intake of sodium or calcium cyclamate: up to 4 mg, as cyclamic acid, per kg body-weight. The following studies were required: 1) determination of the no-effect level for cyclohexylamine (CHA) -induced embryotoxicity in the *mouse* 2) determination of the effect of dose on the degree of cyclamate absorption before conversion to CHA; 3) more precise identification of the no-effect level for CHA effects on *rat* testes; and 4) more precise identification in humans of the amount of cyclamate converted to CHA in the gastro-intestinal tract.— Twenty-first Report of the Joint FAO/WHO Expert Committee on Food Additives, *Tech. Rep. Ser. Wld Hlth Org. No. 617*, 1978.

For early references to the possible hazards and to the pharmacokinetics of the cyclamates, see *Martindale 28th Edn*, p.430.

Proprietary Names and Manufacturers of Cyclamates

Azucrona *(Roger, Spain)*; Sucaryl *(Abbott, Canad.; Abbott, Fr.)*; Sucrum 7 *(Sauba, Fr.)*.

619-m

Sorbitol *(BAN, USAN)*.

E420; D-Sorbitol. D-Glucitol. $C_6H_{14}O_6$=182.2.

CAS — 50-70-4.

Pharmacopoeias. In *Aust., Belg., Br., Cz., Egypt., Eur., Ger., Hung., Ind., It., Jpn, Jug., Neth., Roum.,* and *Swiss.* Also in *U.S.N.F.*

The *B.P.* specifies a white odourless crystalline powder. The *U.S.N.F.* specifies a white hygroscopic powder, granules, or flakes with a sweet taste; it permits small amounts of other polyhydric alcohols.

B.P. **solubilities** are: soluble 1 in 0.5 of water and 1 in 25 of alcohol; practically insoluble in chloroform and ether. *U.S.N.F.* solubilities are: soluble 1 in 0.45 of water; slightly soluble in acetic acid, alcohol, and methyl alcohol. A 5.48% solution of sorbitol hemihydrate is iso-osmotic with serum. Solutions for injection are **sterilised** by autoclaving. **Store** in airtight containers.

Adverse Effects and Precautions

As for fructose, p.1264.

Absorption and Fate

Sorbitol is poorly absorbed from the gastro-intestinal tract following oral or rectal administration. It is metabolised mainly in the liver, to fructose (see p.1264), a reaction catalysed by the enzyme sorbitol dehydrogenase. Some sorbitol may be converted directly to glucose by the enzyme aldose reductase.

Uses and Administration

Sorbitol is a polyhydric alcohol with half the sweetening power of sucrose. It occurs naturally in many fruits and vegetables and is prepared commercially by the reduction of glucose.

It has been employed as a 30% solution as an alternative to glucose in parenteral nutrition but its use is not recommended because of the risk of lactic acidosis.

Sorbitol has been given intravenously as a 50% solution as an osmotic diuretic.

Sorbitol may be administered by mouth or rectally as an osmotic laxative; doses of 20 to 50 g have been suggested.

Sorbitol also acts as a bulk sweetening agent. It is used in limited quantities as a source of carbohydrate in diabetic food products and in sugar-free preparations for the prevention of dental caries.

Sorbitol also has humectant and stabilising properties and is used in various pharmaceutical and cosmetic products including toothpaste.

For reference to the use of diabetic food products containing fructose and sorbitol, see under Fructose, p.1264.

The Food Standards Committee considered that sorbitol was an undesirable ingredient for general use in soft drinks since some individuals had a low gastric tolerance for sorbitol. It was recommended that its use in soft drinks be limited to those intended for consumption by diabetics.— *Review of the Soft Drinks Regulations 1964 (as amended)*, FSC/REP/65, Ministry of Agriculture, Fisheries and Food, London, HM Stationery Office, 1976.

Preparations

Sorbitol Intravenous Infusion *(B.P.)*. Sorbitol Injection. A 30% solution provides 4710 kJ (1125 kcal) per litre and should be administered through a plastic catheter.

Sorbitol Solution *(U.S.P.)*. An aqueous solution containing not less than 64% w/w of sorbitol. A clear, colourless, syrupy liquid with a sweet taste. It is neutral to litmus.

Sorbitol Solution (70 per cent) (Crystallising) *(B.P.)*. A clear colourless, odourless, viscous liquid containing 68 to 72% w/w of hexitols expressed as D-glucitol. Miscible with water, glycerol, and propylene glycol; soluble in alcohol.

Sorbitol Solution (70 per cent) (Non-crystallising) *(B.P.)*. An aqueous solution of hydrogenated, partly hydrolysed starch. A clear colourless, odourless, viscous liquid containing 68 to 72% w/w of solid matter and not less than 62% w/w of polyols expressed as D-glucitol. Miscible with water, glycerol, and propylene glycol.

Proprietary Preparations

Klyx *(Ferring, UK)*. *Enema*, sorbitol 25%, docusate sodium 0.1% in single-dose disposable containers of 120 and 240 mL.

Proprietary Names and Manufacturers

Cinecolex R-X *(Spain)*; Howsorb 1 *(Laporte, UK)*; Howsorb 2 *(Laporte, UK)*; Neosorb *(Roquette, UK)*; Sorbex *(Hefti, Switz. : Steetley Berk, UK)*; Sorbilande *(Austral.; Delalande, Ital.)*; Sorbitur *(Pharmacia, Swed.)*; Sorbostyl *(Delalande, Fr.; Switz.)*; Syn MD *(Belg.; Delalande, Switz.)*.

The following names have been used for multi-ingredient preparations containing sorbitol—Agofell *(Janssen, Ger.; Janssen, S.Afr.)*; Bilagol *(Leo, Swed.)*; Do-Bil *(Dompè, Ital.)*; Galbil *(Janssen, Denm.)*; Klyx *(Ferring, UK)*; Mégabyl *(Janssen, Fr.)*; Medevac *(Medefield, Austral.)*.

For multi-ingredient preparations containing nutritional agents and vitamins, see p.1289.

7369-e

Soya Oil *(BAN)*.

Oleum Sojae; Soja Bean Oil; Soya Bean Oil; Soyabean Oil; Soybean Oil *(USAN)*.

CAS — 8001-22-7.

Pharmacopoeias. In *Br.*, *Chin.*, *Fr.*, *Jpn*, and *U.S.*

The *B.P.* specifies: the refined, deodorised, and clarified oil obtained from the seeds of *Glycine max* (Leguminosae) which may contain a suitable antoxidant; it is odourless or almost odourless. The *U.S.P.* specifies: the refined fixed oil obtained from the seeds of the soya plant *Glycine soja* (Leguminosae); it has a characteristic odour. It is a pale yellow oil. Almost **insoluble** in alcohol; miscible with chloroform, ether, and light petroleum. **Store** in well-filled, well-closed containers at a temperature not exceeding 25°. Protect from light.

For mention of the compatibility and stability of solutions and emulsions for parenteral nutrition see under Enteral and Parenteral Nutrition, p.1251.

Adverse Effects

Fever and chills have been reported following the infusion of soya oil emulsion. Pigmentation of tissues after prolonged therapy with lipid emulsion infusions has also been reported.

The prolonged infusion of soya oil emulsion or its administration to patients with impaired fat metabolism has been associated with the 'overload syndrome' manifested by bone-marrow depression, anaemia, thrombocytopenia, spontaneous bleeding, hepatosplenomegaly, and hyperlipidaemia.

Infected subdural collection of soya oil emulsion in a premature infant during total parenteral nutrition via the common facial vein.— M. J. Stine and H. Harris, *Clin. Pediat.*, 1985, *24*, 40.

A pulmonary fat microembolus was found at necropsy in an infant who had suffered a fatal cardiac arrest 8 hours after the start of infusion with fractionated soya oil emulsion. The patient's serum agglutinated the fat emulsion and contained a high concentration of C-reactive protein at the time of infusion. This finding supported the hypothesis that microemboli are formed by agglutination of fat emulsion in the bloodstream by C-reactive protein. The precise pathogenesis is unclear, nor it is known whether the condition is preventable, but it may be prudent either to ensure that the C-reactive protein concentration is normal (less than 10 mg per litre) or perform a creaming test to determine which babies may embolise the infused fat emulsion.— G. Hulman and M. Levene, *Archs Dis. Childh.*, 1986, *61*, 702. Further reports of pulmonary fat emboli following the administration of soya oil emulsion: A. J. Barson *et al.*, *ibid.*, 1978, *53*, 218; M. I. Levene *et al.*, *Lancet*, 1980, *2*, 815.

EFFECTS ON THE CARDIOVASCULAR SYSTEM. Development of sinus bradycardia in a 16-year-old patient receiving total parenteral nutrition was associated with the administration of a soya oil-based emulsion (A. Sternberg *et al.*, *New Engl. J. Med.*, 1981, *304*, 422). The authors suggested that it might be wise to administer fat emulsion only through a peripheral vein. However, sinus bradycardia has been reported following the administration of a safflower oil-based emulsion via a peripheral vein as part of a TPN regimen (S.L. Traub *et al.*, *J. parenter. enteral Nutr.*, 1985, *9*, 358).

EFFECTS ON IMMUNE RESPONSE. A report of a specific IgE-antibody response to the allergen Kunitz soybean trypsin inhibitor in a patient with anaphylactic reactions after ingestion of soybean products.— L. A. Moroz and W. H. Yang, *New Engl. J. Med.*, 1980, *302*, 1126.

Generalised pruritic urticaria occurred in a 9-year-old boy an hour after the start of infusion with soya oil emulsion. He had previously received this emulsion for 19 days without ill effect. A skin test proved negative but an urticarial reaction developed when a test dose of 1 mL of Intralipid was given intravenously.— K. R. Kamath *et al.* (letter), *New Engl. J. Med.*, 1981, *304*, 360.

EFFECTS ON THE NERVOUS SYSTEM. A report of cerebral disorders in 2 patients during infusion of fractionated soya oil emulsion. Occasional high blood pressures followed by headache, convulsions, coma, retinal and skin haemorrhages, and cortical blindness developed in a 22-year-old woman. The second patient, a 76-year-old man, developed quadriplegia, complete motor aphasia, apraxia, and spasmodic limb weakness.— E. H. Jellinek (letter), *Lancet*, 1976, *2*, 967.

Precautions

Soya oil emulsion should not be given to patients with severe liver disease, acute shock, or hyperlipidaemia, or with other conditions when the ability to absorb or metabolise fat may be impaired. However, if administration is considered in such patients, the fat elimination capacity must be checked daily.

NEONATAL HYPERBILIRUBINAEMIA. The use of intravenous lipid emulsions in hyperbilirubinaemic neonates and the relationship between the resulting increase in plasma free fatty acids and bilirubin remains controversial (P.C. Walker, *Clin. Pharmacokinet.*, 1987, *13*, 26). It has been suggested that because fat particles can bind free bilirubin, intravenous fat may help decrease the risk for kernicterus, but intravenous fat is metabolised to free fatty acids. Long chain fatty acids are tightly bound to albumin and it has been proposed that bilirubin displacement may occur during fat therapy, increasing the infant's risk for bilirubin encephalopathy. However, a study in 20 preterm infants of less than 30 weeks gestation, showed that fat emulsion 1 g per kg body-weight infused over a 15-hour period had minimal risk of significantly decreasing bilirubin binding to albumin since the free fatty acid to albumin ratio remained at approximately 2:1 (M.L. Spear *et al.*, *J. parenter. enteral Nutr.*, 1985, *9*, 144). A later study carried out by Brans *et al.* (*Archs Dis. Childh.*, 1987, *62*, 156) involving 38 neonates of 27 to 34 weeks gestation, demonstrated that varying the administration regimen with different infusion rates and intermittent and constant dosing appeared to have little effect on serum concentrations of total and apparent unbound bilirubin, although there was a trend towards greater variability in apparent unbound concentrations with the intermittent regimen. Serum concentrations of apparent unbound bilirubin as high as 45 nmol per litre were observed without any detectable clinical signs of encephalopathy.

Uses and Administration

Emulsions of fractionated soya oil containing 10 or 20% are given by slow intravenous infusion as part of total parenteral nutrition regimens, either alone or in conjunction with amino acid and carbohydrate solutions (see also under Enteral and Parenteral Nutrition p.1251). Fat emulsions provide a high energy intake in a relatively small volume, and may also be used to prevent or correct essential fatty acid deficiency. The usual daily dose of soya oil emulsion is 500 to 1500 mL of a 10% or 500 to 1000 mL of a 20% emulsion.

The dose on the first day should not usually exceed the equivalent of 1 g of soya oil per kg body-weight, increased on subsequent days to 2, or, if necessary, 3 g per kg over 24 hours. The infusion should be started at the rate of 20 drops per minute and then increased slowly to a maximum of 60 drops per minute of a 10% emulsion or to 40 drops per minute of a 20% emulsion. It is recommended that 500mL of a 10% emulsion should be administered over a period of not less than 3 hours, and 500mL of a 20% emulsion should be administered over not less than 5 hours.

A suggested dose for infants is 0.5 to 4 g per kg over 24 hours.

Preparations made from whole soya beans, utilising soya oil and soya protein are used as the basis of lactose-free vegetable milks for infants and patients with an allergy to cow's milk protein.

Soya oil has emollient properties and is used as a bath additive in the treatment of dry skin conditions.

Soya oil is used as an edible oil and is also used as a lamp oil and in the manufacture of soaps, paints, and varnishes.

FOOD ALLERGY. There is conflicting evidence on whether soya-based infant feeding leads to a lower incidence of allergy in infants predisposed to atopy, but it may benefit some infants with atopic eczema. In genuine gastro-intestinal cows' milk-protein intolerance it is doubtful whether soya is appropriate because of concerns regarding its own allergenicity. The indiscriminate use of soya for vague symptoms and signs not proved to be due to cows' milk intolerance is to be avoided.— L. S. Taitz, *Archs Dis. Childh.*, 1982, *57*, 814. A warning from the FDA against the use of soya-based drinks intended for adults as the sole source of nutrition for infants. Soya drinks can lead to severe protein and calorie malnutrition, multiple vitamin and mineral deficiency, and death in infants who receive no other source of nourishment, and should not be confused with soya-based infant formulas, which are specially formulated to meet the nutritional needs of infants.— *J. Am. med. Ass.*, 1985, *254*, 1428.

See also under Dietary Modification, p.1250.

HYPERCHOLESTEROLAEMIA. A low-lipid low-cholesterol soya protein-based diet produced a reduction of serum-cholesterol concentration in 12 children with familial hypercholesterolaemia who continued the diet for 18 weeks. Serum-cholesterol concentrations stabilised after about 12 weeks with a mean overall reduction of 21.6% against the baseline values. The cholesterol reduction appeared to be limited to changes in low density lipoprotein concentrations and a slight increase in high density lipoprotein concentrations was noted.— A. Gaddi *et al.*, *Archs Dis. Childh.*, 1987, *62*, 274.

Proprietary Preparations

Balneum *(E. Merck, UK). Bath additive*, soya oil 84.75%.

Balneum with Tar *(E. Merck, UK). Bath additive*, soya oil 55%, coal tar distillate 30%.

Proprietary Names and Manufacturers

Balneum *(Hermal, Ger.; Hermal, Switz.; E. Merck, UK)*; Intralipid *(Pharmacia, Austral.; Pharmacia, Canad.; Kabi, Ger.; KabiVitrum, Norw.; Fides, Spain; Kabi, Swed.; KabiVitrum, UK)*; Lipofundin *(Braun Melsungen, Ger.; Braun, Norw.)*; Oelbad Cordes *(Ichthyol, Switz.)*; Tutolipid *(Pfrimmer, Spain)*.

See also under Proprietary Preparations for Enteral and Parenteral Nutrition, p.1289..

1641-s

Starch

Almidón; Amido; Amidon; Amilo; Amylum; Stärke.

CAS — 9005-25-8 (starch); 9005-82-7 (α-amylose); 9004-34-6 (β-amylose); 9037-22-3 (amylopectin).

NOTE. Starches (*B.P.*) may be maize starch, rice starch, potato starch, wheat starch, or tapioca starch (cassava starch). Starch (*U.S.N.F.*) is maize starch, wheat starch, or potato starch.

Pharmacopoeias. Some or all of the starches described are included in *Arg., Aust., Belg., Br., Braz., Chin., Cz., Egypt., Eur., Fr., Ger., Hung., Ind., It., Jpn, Jug., Mex., Neth., Nord., Pol., Port., Roum., Span., Swiss,* and *Turk.* Also in *U.S.N.F.* and *B.P. Vet. U.S.P.* includes Topical Starch.

Polysaccharide granules obtained from the caryopsis of maize, *Zea mays*, rice, *Oryza sativa*, wheat, *Triticum aestivum* (*T. vulgare*), from the tubers of potato, *Solanum tuberosum* or from the rhizomes of cassava, *Manihot esculenta* (=*M.utilissima*). Maize starch is also known as corn starch. Starch contains amylose and amylopectin, both polysaccharides based on α-glucose.

A fine, white, odourless, powder which creaks when pressed between the fingers, or irregular angular masses.

Practically **insoluble** in cold water and alcohol. **Store** in airtight containers.

Adverse Effects

Granulomatous lesions have been reported following the use of starch glove powders. In Great Britain the recommended exposure limits of starch are 10 mg per m^3 (long-term) for total dust, and 5 mg per m^3 (long-term) for respirable dust.

The formation of starch gastroliths in some women who ate large quantities of starch during pregnancy.— E. M. Boyd and S. J. Liu, *Can. med. Ass. J.*, 1968, *98*, 492.

A report of a meningeal reaction to starch glove powder in the CSF after craniectomy.— B. Dunkley and T. T. Lewis, *Br. med. J.*, 1977, *2*, 1391.

A report of granulomatous peritonitis caused by glove starch in a 52-year-old diabetic man.— M. Michowitz *et al.*, *Postgrad. med. J.*, 1983, *59*, 593.

EFFECTS OF CASSAVA ON CARBOHYDRATE METABOLISM. Cassava (or tapioca) is the staple food in many areas where tropical diabetes occurs, and it has been suggested that this, together with malnutrition, is the major cause of the disease. Cassava contains 0.4% protein, 95% starch, and linamarin–a cyanogenic glycoside that, on hydrolysis, releases hydrocyanic acid. Pancreatic diabetes has been found in a patient after prolonged daily consumption of fresh cassava root without associated malnutrition. This patient also acquired a goitre– a better substantiated effect of cassava toxicity. Different methods of preparing and cooking cassava may well result in ingestion of different quantities of cyanide. The cassava/malnutrition hypothesis is attractive but has yet to be proven, and there is strong evidence against it being the only cause of tropical diabetes.— A. Abu-Bakare *et al.*, *Lancet*, 1986, *1*, 1135.

Further references to the association of cassava with malnutrition-related diabetes: T. Teuscher *et al.*, *Lancet*, 1987, *1*, 765; J. C. Brand *et al.* (letter), *ibid.*, 1326; A. G. Alias (letter), *ibid;* M. Rolfe (letter), *ibid;* P. Garcia-Webb (letter), *ibid.*, 1496; T. Teuscher and A. Teuscher (letter), *ibid;* T. van der Werf *et al.* (letter), *ibid.*, *2*, 638.

EFFECTS OF CASSAVA ON THE NERVOUS SYSTEM. Results of a study carried out in Mozambique attributing an epidemic of spastic paraparesis in children to cyanide exposure from cassava in association with a low intake of sulphur amino acids.— J. Cliff *et al.*, *Lancet*, 1985, *2*, 1211. Further references on cassava neurotoxicity: M. J. Hall (letter), *ibid.*, 1986, *1*, 95; A. G. Freeman (letter), *ibid.*, 441; N. W. Pirie (letter), *ibid.*, 561.

Uses and Administration

Starch is absorbent and is widely used in dusting-powders, either alone or mixed with zinc oxide or other similar substances. Starch is used as a surgical glove powder; because starch granulomas have occurred care should be taken to minimise contamination of the wound.

Ointments containing starch may be used as protective applications in skin diseases. Starch Mucilage has been employed as an emollient application to the skin, has formed the basis of some enemas, and has been used in the treatment of iodine poisoning. Starch has been used as a poultice (10%) and is incorporated in many tablets as a disintegrating agent.

Rice-based solutions have been tried in the prevention and treatment of dehydration due to acute diarrhoeal diseases. See also under Oral Rehydration Therapy, p.1024.

An evaluation of sorghum starch, prepared from the seeds of *Sorghum bicolor*, as a tablet disintegrant and binder.— A. V. Deshpande and L. B. Panya, *J. Pharm. Pharmac.*, 1987, *39*, 495.

GLYCOGEN STORAGE DISEASES. A report of the use of uncooked corn starch in the treatment of 12 patients with Type I glycogen storage disease, as an alternative to continuous nocturnal infusion of a glucose-containing solution and frequent day-time feedings. All except one 8-month-old infant responded satisfactorily; failure was considered due to the relatively low pancreatic amylase activity in infancy. The results indicated that uncooked corn starch suspensions prepared with tap water at room temperature and taken every 6 hours in doses of 1.75 to 2.5 g per kg body-weight maintained normoglycaemia and could be used as an alternative therapy for patients with Type I glycogen storage disease.— Y. -T. Chen *et al.*, *New Engl. J. Med.*, 1984, *310*, 171. Comment.— G. L. Wergowske and T. J. Carmody (letter), *ibid.*, *311*, 128. Reply.— Y. -T. Chen and J. B. Sidbury (letter), *ibid.*

PANCREATIC DISORDERS. A report of the use of oral cassava starch and zinc protamine glucagon in the management of postoperative nesidioblastosis.— S. R. Rose *et al.*, *J. Pediat.*, 1986, *108*, 97.

Preparations

Starch Mucilage *(B.P.C. 1973).* Mucilago Amyli. Starch 2.5 g, triturated with water to 20 mL, added to boiling water 80 mL, and again raised to boiling. It should be freshly prepared.

Pregelatinized Starch *(U.S.N.F.).* Starch which has been chemically and/or mechanically processed to rupture all or part of the granules in the presence of water and subsequently dried. Some types are modified to render them compressible and free-flowing. pH of a 10% slurry 4.5 to 7.0. Tablet excipient.

Pregelatinised Maize Starch *(B.P.).* A white to pale cream-coloured, odourless or almost odourless powder, dispersible in cold water; prepared by heating an aqueous slurry of maize starch and removing the water from the resulting paste. It contains no added substances but may be modified to render it compressible and to improve its flow characteristics. A 5% dispersion in water has a pH of 4.5 to 7.0. Tablet excipient.

Sterilisable Maize Starch *(B.P.).* A white, odourless or almost odourless, free-flowing powder, prepared by treating maize starch by chemical and physical means so that it does not gelatinise on exposure to moisture. It contains not more than 2.2% of magnesium oxide. A 10% suspension in water has a pH of 9.5 to 10.8.

The *B.P.* requires that when Absorbable Dusting Powder is demanded, Sterilisable Maize Starch must be supplied. Lubricant for surgical gloves.

Absorbable Dusting Powder *(U.S.P.).* Prepared by processing maize starch. It contains not more than 2% of magnesium oxide. A 10% suspension in water has a pH of 10.0 to 10.8. Lubricant for surgical gloves.

Zinc, Starch, and Talc Dusting-powder *(B.P.C. 1973).* See under Zinc Oxide, p.936.

Proprietary Names and Manufacturers

Bio-Sorb *(Surgikos, UK)*; Capsul *(Laing-National, UK)*; Encapsul *(Laing-National, UK)*; Instant Clearjel *(Laing-National, UK)*; Jalan *(Laing-National, UK)*; National 1551 *(Laing-National, UK)*; Nutregen *(Energen, UK)*; Vulca 90 *(Laing-National, UK)*.

16994-r

Stevioside

Eupatorin; Rebaudin; Stevin; Steviosin.

$C_{38}H_{60}O_{18}$=804.9.

CAS — 57817-89-7.

A glycoside extracted from the leaves of yerba dulce, *Stevia rebaudiana* (Compositae).

Stevioside has about 300 times the sweetness of sucrose and has been used as a sweetening agent in foods. An extract of the leaves of *Stevia rebaudiana* which contains other glycosides including rebaudioside A, has been used similarly.

660-b

Sucrose *(BAN, USAN).*

Azúcar; Cane Sugar; Refined Sugar; Sacarosa; Saccharose; Saccharum; Sucre; Sucrosum; Zucker. β-D-Fructofuranosyl-α-D-glucopyranoside.

$C_{12}H_{22}O_{11}$=342.3.

CAS — 57-50-1.

Pharmacopoeias. In *Arg., Aust., Belg., Br., Chin., Cz., Egypt., Eur., Fr., Ger., Hung., Ind., It., Jpn, Jug., Mex., Neth., Nord., Pol., Port., Roum., Span., Swiss,* and *Turk.* Also in *U.S.N.F. U.S.N.F.* also includes Compressible Sugar, which contains sucrose 95 to 98% and may contain starch, maltodextrin, or invert sugar, and a suitable lubricant; Confectioner's Sugar, which contains sucrose not less than 95% with maize starch, in fine powder; and Sugar Spheres, which contain 62.5 to 91.5% of sucrose, the remainder consisting chiefly of starch.

Colourless or white, odourless, lustrous, dry crystals, crystalline masses, or white crystalline powder, with a sweet taste, obtained from sugar-cane, *Saccharum officinarum* (Gramineae), sugar-beet, *Beta vulgaris* (Chenopodiaceae), and other sources.

B.P. **solubilities** are: soluble 1 in 0.5 of water; slightly soluble in alcohol; freely soluble in alcohol (70%). *U.S.P.* solubilities are: soluble 1 in 0.5 of water, 1 in 0.2 of boiling water, and 1 in 170 of alcohol; insoluble in chloroform and ether. A solution in water is neutral to litmus. A 9.25% solution in water is iso-osmotic with serum. **Store** in well-closed containers.

Adverse Effects

Sucrose consumption increases the incidence of dental caries. Renal tubular damage may be caused by repeated intravenous injections of sucrose. In Great Britain the recommended exposure limits of sucrose are 10 mg per m^3 (long-term) and 20 mg per m^3 (short-term).

A report by the British Nutrition Foundation has found sugars to be relatively harmless apart from their connection with dental caries. A similar report from the FDA's Sugars Task Force also concluded that apart from the contribution to dental caries, there was no conclusive evidence to demonstrate a hazard to the general public with current levels of sugar consumption. This report acknowledged that there may be a link between obesity and overconsumption of sugary foods and that obesity is a risk factor in the development of heart disease, however, any connection between consumption of sugar and heart disease was denied.— *Lancet*, 1987, *1*, 819. Comments and criticisms: A. J. Vlitos (letter), *ibid.*, 918; J. Yudkin (letter), *ibid;* D. M. Conning (letter), *ibid;* M. J. Campbell *et al.* (letter), *ibid.*, 1311; J. C. Waterlow (letter), *ibid.*, *2*, 397; J. Scott (letter), *ibid.*

See also under Effects on the Teeth, below.

EFFECTS ON THE BILIARY TRACT. A study on the effects of dietary sucrose on factors influencing the formation of cholesterol gall-stones. Twelve patients with radiolucent gall-stones were given diets high and low in refined sugar, each for a 6-week period. There was no difference between the effect of the two diets on bile lipid composition or rate of cholesterol secretion but plasma triglyceride concentrations were higher with the sugar-rich diet. Over a 6-week period a high-sugar diet had no adverse effect on bile lipid composition but in the long term the effects on plasma lipids and energy intake might increase the risk of gall-stones.— D. Werner *et al.*, *Gut*, 1984, *25*, 269.

EFFECTS ON THE KIDNEYS. A report of acute renal failure with severe hyponatraemia in a 64-year-old patient following the use of granulated sugar to treat an infected pneumonectomy wound cavity. Mild renal insufficiency before sucrose intoxication may have contributed to the nephrosis.— A. Debure *et al.* (letter), *Lancet*, 1987, *1*, 1034. Comment. The nephrotoxicity may have been caused by gentamicin, a solution of which had been used to irrigate the cavity prior to packing the wound.— H. Archer *et al.* (letter), *ibid.*, 1485.

EFFECTS ON THE TEETH. A review on the role of sugars in the development of dental decay. The main sugars implicated in dental caries, in decreasing order of cariogenicity, are sucrose, glucose, and fructose; there is little evidence that invert sugar is significantly less cariogenic than sucrose. Sucrose causes the most damage because it is the sugar most commonly eaten, and it encourages the colonisation and growth in dental plaque of *Streptococcus mutans*, a cariogenic bacterium. Other sugars have a similar property but to a lesser extent, and they encourage the growth of less cariogenic bacteria. The level of sugar consumption at which most of the population will not get dental caries is 15 kg per person per year. The soundest method of prevention is to reduce the quantity and frequency of consumption of products containing added sugars.— A. Sheiham, *Lancet*, 1983, *1*, 282. Comments and criticism: J. A. C. Hugill (letter), *ibid.*, 598; B. G. Bibby and M. E. J. Curzon (letter), *ibid;* A. R. P. Walker (letter), *ibid.*, 599; D. Howarth (letter), *ibid.*, 827. Reply.— A. Sheiham (letter), *ibid.*, 873.

Precautions

Sucrose should be administered with care to patients with diabetes mellitus. It is contra-indicated in patients with the glucose-galactose malabsorption syndrome, fructose intolerance, or sucrase-isomaltase deficiency.

Absorption and Fate

Sucrose is hydrolysed in the small intestine by the enzyme sucrase to glucose and fructose, which are then absorbed. Sucrose is excreted unchanged in the urine when given intravenously.

Uses and Administration

Sucrose, a disaccharide, is used as a sweetening agent. If the sweetness of sucrose is taken as 100, fructose has a value of about 173, glucose 74, maltose 32, galactose 32, and lactose 16. Syrups prepared from concentrated solutions of sucrose form the basis of many linctuses. It is commonly used as household sugar.

A 30% solution of sucrose has been used as eye-drops as a hypertonic agent in the reduction of corneal oedema.

Sucrose is used as a tablet excipient and lozenge basis, and as a suspending and viscosity-increasing agent.

HICCUPS. Administration of a teaspoon of dry granulated sugar resulted in the immediate cessation of hiccups in 19 of 20 patients who had had hiccups for up to 6 weeks.— E. G. Engleman *et al.* (letter), *New Engl. J. Med.*, 1971, *285*, 1489.

WOUND HEALING. In 19 critically ill patients with open mediastinitis following cardiac surgery, packing the wound with granulated sugar resulted in near-complete debridement and rapid formation of granulation tissue after 5 to 9 days of treatment. The explanation for the success of sugar treatment was, however, still being debated and probably complex. Chirife *et al.* (*Antimicrob. Ag. Chemother.*, 1983, *23*, 766) have proposed, on the basis of *in-vitro* experiments, that sugar creates an environment of low water activity in the wound which inhibits or impairs bacterial growth, since bacteria, like other forms of life, require water for growth.— J. L. Trouillet *et al.*, *Lancet*, 1985, *2*, 180.

Further reports of the successful use of sucrose in wound healing: H. Gordon *et al.* (letter), *Lancet*, 1985, *2*, 663; A. Quatraro *et al.* (letter), *ibid.*, 664; K. R. Middleton and D. Seal, *Pharm. J.*, 1985, *2*, 757.

Sugar is not always sterile; however, since it is a convenient and inexpensive treatment for wounds, an inexpensive method of sterilisation would be most welcome.— M. K. Addison and J. N. Walterspiel (letter), *Lancet*, 1985, *2*, 665. The lack of sterility of sugar is probably attributable to dirt mixed with sugar crystals. When a thick syrup of sugar is cultured the osmotic effect will almost certainly inactive such contaminants.— P. Lowthian and S. Barnett (letter), *ibid.*, 1186.

See also: J. Chirife *et al.* (letter), *Lancet*, 1982, *1*, 560; R. D. Forrest (letter), *ibid.*, 861; J. Chirife and L. Herszage (letter), *ibid.*, *2*, 157.

Preparations

Simple Linctus *(A.P.F.)*. Citric acid monohydrate 125 mg, concentrated anise water 0.05 mL, amaranth solution 0.1 mL, syrup to 5 mL.

Simple Linctus *(B.P.)*. Citric acid monohydrate 125 mg, concentrated anise water 0.05 mL, chloroform spirit 0.3 mL, amaranth solution 0.075 mL, syrup to 5 mL. Store at a temperature not exceeding 25°.

Simple Linctus *B.P.* was not adequately preserved against microbial spoilage as determined by the *B.P.* challenge test.— T. R. R. Kurup and L. S. C. Wan, *Pharm. J.*, 1986, *2*, 761.

Paediatric Simple Linctus *(B.P.)*. Simple linctus 1.25 mL, syrup to 5 mL. Store at a temperature not exceeding 25°.

Syrup *(A.P.F.)*. Sucrose 66.7% w/w in water.

Syrup *(B.P.)*. Simple Syrup. Sucrose 66.7% w/w in water. It may contain one or more suitable antimicrobial preservatives. Syrup should not be exposed to undue fluctuations in temperature.

There was evidence of physical incompatibility (turbidity or precipitation) when the following of the *B.P.C. 1973* preparations were prepared with or diluted with syrup preserved with 0.05% of a combination of hydroxybenzoate esters (Nipastat) or with syrup preserved with methyl hydroxybenzoate 0.03% and propyl hydroxybenzoate 0.015%: Paediatric Belladonna and Ephedrine Mixture, Paediatric Belladonna and Ipecacuanha Mixture, Ferrous Sulphate Mixture, Paediatric Ferrous Sulphate Mixture, Paediatric Ipecacuanha Mixture, Methadone Linctus, Noscapine Linctus, Paediatric Opiate Ipecacuanha Mixture, Paediatric Opiate Squill Linctus, Potassium Citrate Mixture, and Sodium Citrate Mixture. Incompatibility for Cloxacillin Elixir had not been established.— Pharm. Soc. Lab. Rep. P/79/2, 1979. A similar conclusion in respect of Methadone Mixture 1 mg/1 mL (*D.T.F.*). [Now Methadone Mixture (*B.N.F.*) 1 mg/mL].— Pharm. Soc. Lab. Rep. P/80/1, 1980.

Syrup *(U.S.N.F.)*. Sucrose 85% w/v in water. Store, preferably in a cool place, in airtight containers.

661-v

Invert Sugar

CAS — 8013-17-0.

An equimolecular mixture of glucose and fructose which may be prepared by the hydrolysis of sucrose with a suitable mineral acid such as hydrochloric acid.

Adverse Effects and Precautions

As for Fructose, p.1264.

For reference to the role of sugars, including invert sugar, in the development of dental caries, see under Sucrose, above.

Uses and Administration

Invert sugar has similar actions to those of glucose (p.1265) and fructose (p.1264). Like fructose, it has been used as an alternative to glucose in parenteral nutrition. It may be given by intravenous infusion as a 10% solution.

Invert Syrup is used as a stabilising agent.

Preparations

Invert Sugar Injection *(U.S.P.)*. A sterile solution of a mixture of equal amounts of glucose and fructose, or an equivalent sterile solution produced by the hydrolysis of sucrose. It contains no antimicrobial agents. pH 3.0 to 6.5.

Invert Syrup *(B.P.)*. A clear, colourless to pale straw-coloured, odourless or almost odourless, syrupy liquid with a sweet taste containing not less than 67% w/w of invert sugars. It is prepared by hydrolysing a 66.7% solution of sucrose with a suitable mineral acid, and neutralising the solution with, for example, calcium carbonate or sodium carbonate. The degree of inversion is at least 95%. pH 5 to 6. Miscible with water forming a clear solution; it dissolves in alcohol with the formation of an insoluble residue. Store at 35 to 45°.

Proprietary Names and Manufacturers

Inverdex *(Swed.)*; Invertos *(Pharmacia, Swed.)*; Invertose *(DAK, Denm.; NLH, Norw.)*; Invert-Oso *(Ital.)*; Travert *(Travenol, UK)*.

7834-x

Sulbutiamine *(rINN)*.

Bisibutiamine; *O*-Isobutyrylthiamine Disulphide. *NN'*-{Dithiobis[2-(2-isobutyryloxyethyl)-1-methylvinylene]-}bis[*N*-(4-amino-2-methylpyrimidin-5-ylmethyl)formamide].

$C_{32}H_{46}N_8O_6S_2$=702.9.

CAS — 3286-46-2.

Sulbutiamine is a vitamin B_1 substance with the general properties of thiamine hydrochloride (see p.1277).

Proprietary Names and Manufacturers

Arcalion *(Servier, Fr.; Servier, Spain)*; Neodaian *(Jpn)*; Surmenalit *(Faes, Spain)*; Vitaberin *(Jpn)*.

12877-q

Thaumatin *(BAN)*.

Katemfe.

CAS — 53850-34-3.

A mixture in the ratio of 2:1 of two polypeptides thaumatin I and thaumatin II derived from the fruit of *Thaumatococcus daniellii* (Scitamineae).

Thaumatin is a protein whose amino-acid range excludes histidine. It is an intense sweetener considered to be by far the sweetest of such compounds in use. Its anticipated daily intake as a food additive is about 2 mg daily.

Thaumatin was assigned an acceptable daily intake of "not specified".— Twenty-ninth Report of the Joint FAO/WHO Expert Committee on Food Additives, *Tech. Rep. Ser. Wld Hlth Org. No. 733*, 1986.

7829-d

Thiamine Hydrochloride *(BANM, USAN, rINNM).*

Aneurine Hydrochloride; Thiamin Hydrochloride; Thiamine Chloride; Thiamini Hydrochloridum; Thiaminii Chloridum; Vitamin B_1. 3-(4-Amino-2-methylpyrimidin-5-ylmethyl)-5-(2-hydroxyethyl)-4-methylthiazolium chloride hydrochloride. $C_{12}H_{17}ClN_4OS,HCl=337.3$.

CAS — 59-43-8 (thiamine); 67-03-8 (hydrochloride).

Pharmacopoeias. In *Arg., Aust., Belg., Br., Braz., Chin., Cz., Egypt., Eur., Fr., Ger., Hung., Ind., Int., It., Jpn, Jug., Mex., Neth., Nord., Pol., Port., Roum., Rus., Span., Swiss, Turk.*, and *U.S. Rus.* also has the bromide (Thiamini Bromidum), $C_{12}H_{17}BrN_4OS,HBr,\frac{1}{2}H_2O=435.2$. Also in *B.P. Vet.*

Colourless or white crystals or white or almost white crystalline powder with a faint characteristic odour.

Soluble 1 in 1 of water and 1 in 20 of glycerol; practically insoluble in chloroform and ether. The *B.P.* specifies soluble 1 in 100 of alcohol; the *U.S.P.* specifies 1 in 170 of alcohol. The *B.P.* specifies that a 2.5% solution in water has a pH of 2.7 to 3.3; the *B.P.* injection has a pH of 2.8 to 3.4. The *U.S.P.* specifies that a 1% solution in water has a pH of 2.7 to 3.4; the *U.S.P.* injection has a pH of 2.5 to 4.5. Solutions are **sterilised** by filtration. **Store** in airtight nonmetallic containers. Protect from light.

Sterile solutions of pH 4 or less lose activity only very slowly but neutral or alkaline solutions deteriorate rapidly, especially in contact with air. When exposed to air, the anhydrous material rapidly absorbs about 4% of water.

STABILITY IN SOLUTION. A review of the compatibility and stability of components of total parenteral nutrition solutions when mixed in 1- or 3-litre flexible containers. Thiamine is incompatible with reducing agents such as sulphites. The thiamine molecule is cleaved into pyrimidine and thiazole moieties. The rate of hydrolytic cleavage increases with increasing pH, and may be rapid at pH 6. Some studies have shown that thiamine degrades rapidly in amino acid infusion solutions containing thiosulphite, especially above pH 6.5. More recent studies have suggested that the degradation effect of thiosulphite is concentration-dependent. Negligible losses were reported after storage of 3-litre containers in the refrigerator for 7 days, especially in the absence of trace elements. Thiamine has been found to be more stable if the sulphite concentration does not exceed 0.05%. It can be concluded that thiamine losses will be insignificant under normal conditions of the preparation, storage, and administration of 3-litre parenteral nutrition solutions.— M. C. Allwood, *J. clin. Hosp. Pharm.*, 1984, *9*, 181. Further references: B. B. Bowman and P. Nguyen, *J. parenter. enteral Nutr.*, 1983, *7*, 567; P. W. Niemiec and T. W. Vanderveen, *Am. J. Hosp. Pharm.*, 1984, *41*, 893.

Adverse Effects and Precautions

Adverse effects seldom occur following administration of thiamine, but hypersensitivity reactions have occurred, mainly after parenteral administration. These reactions have ranged in severity from very mild to, very rarely, fatal anaphylactic shock.

Absorption and Fate

Thiamine is well absorbed from the gastro-intestinal tract following oral administration, although the absorption of large doses is limited. It is also rapidly absorbed following intramuscular administration. It is widely distributed to most body tissues, and appears in breast milk. Thiamine is not stored to any appreciable extent in the body and amounts in excess of the body's requirements are excreted in the urine as unchanged thiamine or as metabolites.

Thiamine demonstrated nonlinear renal elimination kinetics following oral and intravenous doses of thiamine hydrochloride 50, 100, and 200 mg to 8 men.— W. Weber and H. Kewitz, *Eur. J. clin. Pharmac.*, 1985, *28*, 213.

Human Requirements

Thiamine requirements are directly related to the carbohydrate intake and the metabolic-rate. A daily dietary intake of 1 to 1.3 mg of thiamine is recommended for healthy men and 0.7 to 1 mg for healthy women. Cereals, nuts, peas, beans, and yeast are rich sources of thiamine. Green vegetables, roots, pork and other meats, fruits, milk and other dairy products (except butter), fish, and eggs contain significant amounts. Fats, refined sugar, and alcoholic drinks contain no thiamine. Considerable losses of thiamine may result from cooking processes.

The basic recommended intake of thiamine was 400 µg per 4200 kJ (1000 kcal) of diet, so that men required 1.3 mg of thiamine and women required 900 µg daily.— Report of a Joint FAO/WHO Expert Group, *Tech. Rep. Ser. Wld Hlth Org. No. 362,* 1967.

Recommended daily intake of thiamine: boys and girls up to 8 years of age, 300 to 800 µg; boys 9 to 17 years, 0.9 to 1.2 mg; girls 9 to 17 years, 800 to 900 µg; men 18 to 64 years, 1 to 1.3 mg; over 65 years, 0.9 to 1 mg; women over 18 years, 0.7 to 1 mg; during pregnancy, 1 mg; during lactation, 1.1 mg.— Recommended Daily Amounts of Food Energy and Nutrients for Groups of People in the United Kingdom, Report by the Committee on Medical Aspects of Food Policy, *Report on Health and Social Subjects No. 15*, London, HM Stationery Office, 1979.

Recommended daily dietary allowance of thiamine: up to 6 months, 0.3 mg; 6 to 12 months, 0.5 mg; 1 to 3 years, 0.7 mg; 4 to 6 years, 0.9 mg; 7 to 10 years and males 51 years and over, 1.2 mg; males 11 to 18 years, and 23 to 50 years, 1.4 mg; males 19 to 22 years, 1.5 mg; females 11 to 22 years, 1.1 mg; females 23 years and over, 1 mg; in pregnancy, an additional 0.4 mg; in lactation, an additional 0.5 mg.— *Recommended Dietary Allowances*, 9th Edn, Washington, The National Research Council, 1980.

The recommendation that foods for the young infant should contain thiamine in amounts not less than 130 ng per mL (based on the lower limit of the range in pooled samples of human milk).— Artificial Feeds for the Young Infant: Report of the Working Party on the Composition of Foods for Infants and Young Children, Committee on Medical Aspects of Food Policy, *Report on Health and Social Subjects, 18,* London, HM Stationery Office, 1980.

Results from a study of tissue thiamine status in an age-stratified group of 42 adults indicated that the thiamine fortification concentrations of low-extraction bread and flour in the *UK* should be raised, not withdrawn, as has been proposed. Withdrawal of thiamine fortification of processed cereals could have serious implications for public health.— S. H. Anderson *et al., Lancet,* 1986, *2,* 85.

Uses and Administration

Thiamine, a water-soluble vitamin, is an essential coenzyme for carbohydrate metabolism. Thiamine deficiency develops when the dietary intake is inadequate; severe deficiency leads to the development of a syndrome known as beri-beri. Chronic 'dry' beri-beri is characterised by peripheral neuritis, bradycardia, muscle weakness, and paralysis. Acute 'wet' beri-beri is characterised by cardiac failure and oedema. Wernicke's encephalopathy (demyelination of the central nervous system) may develop in severe cases of thiamine deficiency.

Thiamine is used in the treatment and prevention of thiamine deficiency. It is usually given by mouth, the preferred route, but may also be administered by the intramuscular or intravenous routes. In the treatment of mild chronic thiamine deficiency doses of 5 to 30 mg daily in single or divided doses have been recommended. In severe thiamine deficiency doses of up to 300 mg daily have been given.

A review of vitamin therapy in non-deficiency states. The physiologically active form of thiamine, thiamine pyrophosphate (cocarboxylase), serves as the coenzyme of carboxylase and is involved in the decarboxylation of α-keto acids, such as pyruvic acid and α-ketoglutaric acid. The most important targets for therapy with 'megadoses' of thiamine have been for disorders with a peripheral resemblance to beri-beri, namely peripheral neuritis, neuralgias, and diseases of the cardiovascular and central nervous systems. Recently, high-dose thiamine therapy has been suggested in lead intoxication, fibrocystic breast disease, and recurrent febrile adenopathy. However, there are no scientifically acceptable data to support the usefulness of thiamine in these non-deficiency disorders.— L. Ovesen, *Drugs*, 1984, *27*, 148.

BLOOD DISORDERS. Administration of thiamine to 2 patients with Shwachman-Diamond syndrome led to the correction of defective neutrophil chemotaxis.— P. Szüts *et al.* (letter), *Lancet*, 1984, *1*, 1072.

A report of a beneficial response to high-dose thiamine treatment in a 3-month-old child who presented with a syndrome consisting of severe megaloblastic anaemia, diabetes, deafness, tachycardia, heart failure, and convulsions. Symptoms recurred on 3 occasions when thiamine was discontinued and responded again when therapy was resumed. It was suggested that the child had an autosomal-recessive genetic disorder which caused thiamine insensitivity.— H. Mandel *et al., New Engl. J. Med.*, 1984, *311*, 836. Comment. The syndrome may not be the result of a genetic disorder. It could possibly be caused by acute or subacute arsenic intoxication, which is known to produce similar symptoms.— M. Beaugrand (letter), *ibid.*, 1985, *312*, 447.

WERNICKE'S ENCEPHALOPATHY. Thiamine deficiency, seen commonly in alcoholism, leads to an accumulation of pyruvate in the blood and might cause neuropathy and encephalopathy (Wernicke's syndrome). It has also been hypothesised that thiamine produces a 'diphosphate effect' and increases transketolase activity in thiamine-deficient individuals. The clinical symptoms of Wernicke's encephalopathy (global confusional state, ophthalmoplegia, nystagmus, ataxia) are generally attenuated with immediate thiamine treatment. The symptoms of Korsakoff's psychosis (memory loss, learning deficits, confabulation) are thought to be on the continuum of the same pathological process as Wernicke's encephalopathy. It has been noted that thiamine must be administered early in the course of illness to produce improvement in the psychiatric symptoms of the Wernicke-Korsakoff syndrome. Thiamine has also been used to treat nutritionally-deficient, non-alcoholic patients with apparently neurotic symptoms.— W. M. Petrie and T. A. Ban, *Drugs*, 1985, *30*, 58.

Given the high risk of cardiovascular collapse and sudden death associated with acute disease, Wernicke's encephalopathy must be viewed as a medical emergency, even if other central nervous system processes, which it may mimic, are being considered. Thiamine should be administered parenterally, preferably intravenously, to ensure adequate absorption. Although as little as 2 or 3 mg may be enough to reverse the ocular symptoms, which generally begin to improve in 1 to 6 hours, doses of at least 100 mg should be given initially. The ataxia and acute confusional state may also resolve dramatically although improvement may not be noted for days or months.— J. B. Reuler *et al., New Engl. J. Med.*, 1985, *312*, 1035. Comments.— M. C. Meilgaard (letter), *ibid.*, *313*, 637; J. Ross and C. L. Birmingham (letter), *ibid;* D. A. Frommer and J. Marx (letter), *ibid.*, 638; T. Pearlman (letter), *ibid.* Reply.— J. B. Reuler *et al.* (letter), *ibid.*

A report of successful treatment of Wernicke's encephalopathy with thiamine 250 mg daily intravenously, although Korsakoff's psychosis and ataxia persisted. It was suggested that thiamine should be given to all patients with undiagnosed coma, before glucose, to susceptible patients in coma, and to patients receiving naso-gastric or parenteral feeding or fluid regimens of longer than 2 weeks duration.— W. R. G. Gibb *et al., Postgrad. med. J.*, 1985, *61*, 607. Comment.— R. Iacono and R. Sandyk (letter), *ibid.*, 1986, *62*, 315.

Further references: B. Wood *et al., Med. J. Aust.*, 1986, *144*, 12; P. M. Yellowlees, *ibid.*, *145*, 216; B. Wood (letter), *ibid.*, 1987, *146*, 170.

Preparations

Thiamine Hydrochloride Elixir *(U.S.P.)*

Thiamine Hydrochloride Injection *(U.S.P.)*

Thiamine Injection *(B.P.).* Thiamine Hydrochloride Injection; Vitamin B_1 Injection. Contains thiamine hydrochloride.

Thiamine Hydrochloride Tablets *(U.S.P.)*

Thiamine Tablets *(B.P.).* Thiamine Hydrochloride Tablets; Vitamin B_1 Tablets. Contain thiamine hydrochloride.

Proprietary Preparations

Benerva *(Roche, UK). Tablets*, thiamine hydrochloride 3, 10, 25, 50, 100, and 300 mg.

Proprietary Names and Manufacturers

Aberil *(Ital.)*; Algoneurina *(IBIS, Ital.)*; Aneurin *(A.S., Ger.)*; Aneurol *(Belg.)*; BayBee-1 *(Bay, USA)*; B-Carbossilasi *(Ital.)*; Bévitine *(Specia, Fr.)*; Bemarr Fortisimo

(Spain); Benavit *(Belg.)*; Benerva *(Arg.; Belg.; Roche, Denm.; Roche, Fr.; Roche, Ger.; Roche, Ital.; Roche, Spain; Roche, Swed.; Roche, Switz.; Roche, UK)*; Beneurol 300 *(Belg.)*; Benol *(Belg.)*; Berolase *(Roche, Belg.; Roche, Ger.; Roche, Ital.; Roche, Switz.)*; Bester *(Salvat, Spain)*; Betabion *(E. Merck, Ger.; Bracco, Ital.; Spain)*; Betalin S *(Lilly, USA)*; Betamin *(USV, Austral.)*; Betamine *(Belg.)*; Betar *(Ital.)*; Beta-Sol *(Fawns & McAllan, Austral.)*; Betaxin *(Winthrop, Canad.)*; Bewon *(Austral.; Wyeth, Canad.)*; Bicholase *(Jpn)*; Bioxilasi *(Zyma, Ital.)*; Bisolvit *(Nuovo, Ital.)*; Bivitasi *(ISI, Ital.)*; Co-B_1 *(Bruco, Ital.)*; Cocalose *(Jpn)*; Cocarbasi *(Ital.)*; Cocarbil *(Spain)*; Cocarbose *(Jpn)*; Co-Carbox *(Wasserman, Spain)*; Cocarvit *(CT, Ital.)*; Co-Enzyme B *(Inwood, USA)*; Coneurina *(Ital.)*; Dextamina B_1 *(Spain)*; Extraneurina *(Spain)*; Farmobion B_1 *(Ital.)*; Invite B_1 *(Nelson, Austral.)*; Juvabe '300' *(Austral.)*; Lifaton B_1 *(Spain)*; Magnesiocarbina *(FIRMA, Ital.)*; Megamin *(Canad.)*; Paraboramin *(Jpn)*; Pirofosfasi *(Benvegna, Ital.)*; Proffit *(Jpn)*; Thiminone *(Eagle, Austral.)*; Trifosfaneurina *(Bruschettini, Ital.; Spain)*; Vitaendil Cocarboxilasa 500 *(Boizot, Spain)*; Vitaneurin *(Switz.)*; Vitantial *(Delagrange, Spain)*.

Multivitamin and mineral preparations containing thiamine hydrochloride are included in the lists on pp.1289-93. The following names have been used for preparations containing thiamine hydrochloride and not considered to be a multivitamin or mineral preparation—Aneurone *(Philip Harris, UK)*; Cholibile *(Bio-Chemical Laboratory, Canad.)*.

7830-c

Thiamine Nitrate *(BANM, rINNM)*.

Aneurine Mononitrate; Thiamine Mononitrate *(USAN)*; Vitamin B_1 Mononitrate. 3-(4-Amino-2-methylpyrimidin-5-ylmethyl)-5-(2-hydroxyethyl)-4-methylthiazolium nitrate.
$C_{12}H_{17}N_5O_4S$=327.4.

CAS — 532-43-4.

Pharmacopoeias. In *Br., Braz., Eur., Ger., Ind., Jpn, Swiss,* and *U.S.*

Small white or colourless crystals or a white or almost white crystalline powder with a slight characteristic odour. *B.P.* **solubilities** are: sparingly soluble in water; freely soluble in boiling water; slightly soluble in alcohol and in methyl alcohol. *U.S.P.* solubilities are: soluble 1 in 44 of water; slightly soluble in alcohol and chloroform. A 2% solution in water has a pH of 6.0 to 7.6. **Store** in well-closed, nonmetallic containers. Protect from light.

Thiamine nitrate is a vitamin B_1 substance with the general properties of thiamine hydrochloride.

Preparations

Thiamine Mononitrate Elixir *(U.S.P.)*. Contains thiamine nitrate.

Proprietary Names and Manufacturers

B_1-Vicotrat *(Heyl, Ger.)*; Dagravit B_1 Retard *(Belgana, Belg.; Medinsa, Spain)*; Juvabe '300' *(Cambridge Laboratories, Austral.)*; Neurifosforil *(Nessa, Spain)*.

For multi-ingredient preparations containing nutritional agents and vitamins, see p.1289.

662-g

Threonine *(USAN, pINN)*.

β-Methylserine; L-Threonine; Thr. L-2-Amino-3-hydroxybutyric acid.
$C_4H_9NO_3$=119.1.

CAS — 72-19-5.

Pharmacopoeias. In *Jpn* and *U.S.*

A white odourless crystalline powder. Freely **soluble** in water; insoluble in dehydrated alcohol, chloroform, and ether. A 5% solution in water has a pH of 5.0 to 6.5.

Threonine is an aliphatic amino acid which is an essential constituent of the diet. It is used as a dietary supplement.

For a report of the use of racemic threonine in combination with cysteine and glycine in the topical treatment of leg ulcers, see under Cysteine Hydrochloride, p.1261.

Proprietary Names and Manufacturers

The following names have been used for multi-ingredient preparations containing threonine— Aminoderm *(Desbergers, Canad.)*; Cicatrin *(Wellcome, Austral.; Wellcome, Canad.; Calmic, UK)*.

For multi-ingredient preparations containing nutritional agents and vitamins, see p.1289.

665-s

Tyrosine *(USAN, pINN)*.

L-Tyrosine; Tyr. L-2-Amino-3-(4-hydroxyphenyl)propionic acid.
$C_9H_{11}NO_3$=181.2.

CAS — 60-18-4.

Pharmacopoeias. In *U.S.*

White odourless crystals or crystalline powder. Very slightly **soluble** in water; insoluble in alcohol and ether.

Tyrosine is an aromatic amino acid. It is used as a dietary supplement.

Possible use of tyrosine in depression.— I. K. Goldberg (letter), *Lancet*, 1980, *2*, 364. See also J. A. Hoskins (letter), *ibid.*, 597; A. J. Gelenberg and R. J. Wurtman (letter), *ibid.*, 863.

For reference to the role of aromatic and branched-chain amino acids in the treatment of hepatic encephalopathy, see under Enteral and Parenteral Nutrition, p.1252.

For reference to the use of tyrosine and tryptophan in the treatment of phenylketonuria see under Tryptophan, p.384.

Preparations

For multi-ingredient preparations containing nutritional agents and vitamins, see p.1289.

666-w

Valine *(USAN, pINN)*.

α-Aminoisovaleric Acid; L-Valine; Val. L-2-Amino-3-methylbutyric acid.
$C_5H_{11}NO_2$=117.1.

CAS — 72-18-4.

Pharmacopoeias. In *Jpn* and *U.S.*

A white odourless crystalline powder. **Soluble** in water; practically insoluble in alcohol, acetone, and ether. A 5% solution in water has a pH of 5.5 to 7.0.

Valine is a branched-chain amino acid which is an essential constituent of the diet. It is used as a dietary supplement.

For reference to the role of aromatic and branched-chain amino acids in the treatment of hepatic encephalopathy, see under Enteral and Parenteral Nutrition, p.1252.

Preparations

For multi-ingredient preparations containing nutritional agents and vitamins, see p.1289.

7823-k

Vitamin A

Antixerophthalmic Vitamin; Axerophtholum; Oleovitamin A; Vitaminum A. Consists of 15-apo-β-caroten-15-ol (3,7-dimethyl-9-(2,6,6-trimethylcyclohex-1-enyl)nona-2,4,6,8-*all-trans*-tetraen-1-ol) or its esters.

Pharmacopoeias. In *Arg., Aust., Braz., Egypt., Eur., Fr., Ger., Ind., It., Neth., Pol., Port., Swiss, Turk.,* and *U.S. Chin., Jug., Roum.,* and *Rus.* include a monograph for the acetate. *Cz., Jpn,* and *Pol.* include monographs for the acetate and the palmitate. *Br.* and *B.P. Vet.* include a monograph for Vitamin A Ester Concentrate (Natural). *Br., Eur., Fr.,* and *Neth.* also include monographs for Synthetic Vitamin A Concentrate (Oily Form), Synthetic Vitamin A Concentrate (Powder Form), and Synthetic Vitamin A Concentrate (Water-dispersible Form).

A suitable form of retinol (vitamin A alcohol; $C_{20}H_{30}O$ = 286.5; 68-26-8) which may consist of retinol or its esters formed from edible fatty acids, principally acetic and palmitic acids. It is a light yellow to red oil which may solidify upon refrigeration; practically odourless or with a mild fishy odour but no rancid odour or taste.

In liquid form, it is **insoluble** in water and in glycerol; very soluble in chloroform and in ether; soluble in dehydrated alcohol and in vegetable oils. In solid form, may be dispersible in water. It may be diluted with edible oils or be incorporated in solid edible carriers or excipients, and may contain suitable antoxidants, dispersants, and antimicrobial agents.

Store in airtight containers, preferably under an atmosphere of inert gas. Protect from light.

STABILITY IN SOLUTION. A review of the compatibility and stability of components of total parenteral nutrition solutions when mixed in 1- or 3-litre flexible containers. Retinol is known to be rapidly broken down by exposure to ultraviolet light, and daylight causes rapid degradation. Covering the bag reduces or prevents degradation, depending on the effectiveness of the cover although simple shading on the side of the bag nearest to the daylight can be beneficial. However, up to 50% of the vitamin can be degraded during passage through the administration set. It has been shown that the presence of amino acids offers some protection and the presence of a fat emulsion affords considerable protection.

A number of studies have shown that vitamin A binds to plastics, especially polyvinyl chloride. It is now clear that sorption to bags and administration sets depends on the ester used. While the acetate ester is strongly bound, the palmitate shows little or no tendency to adsorb to polyvinyl chloride. It must be concluded that vitamin A losses will occur during parenteral nutrition, although not during storage in the refrigerator if light-protected.— M. C. Allwood, *J. clin. Hosp. Pharm.*, 1984, *9*, 181. See also P. F. D'Arcy, *Drug Intell. & clin. Pharm.*, 1983, *17*, 726; P. W. Niemiec and T. W. Vanderveen, *Am. J. Hosp. Pharm.*, 1984, *41*, 893.

Further references: W. L. Chiou and P. Moorhatch (letter), *J. Am. med. Ass.*, 1973, *223*, 328; R. L. Nedich (letter), *ibid.*, 1973, *224*, 1531; P. Moorhatch and W. L. Chiou, *Am. J. Hosp. Pharm.*, 1974, *31*, 72.

Units

The International Standards for vitamin A and for provitamin A were discontinued in 1954 and 1956 respectively but the International units for these substances have continued to be widely used. In 1960–1, the WHO Expert Committee on Biological Standardization redefined the International unit for vitamin A as the activity of 0.000344 mg of pure all-*trans* vitamin A acetate and the International unit for provitamin A as the activity of 0.0006 mg of pure all-*trans* β-carotene.

The activity of one International unit is contained in 0.0003 mg of all-*trans* retinol, in 0.00055 mg of all-*trans* retinol palmitate, and in 0.000359 mg of all-*trans* retinol propionate.

Vitamin A Ester Concentrate (Natural) *B.P.* contains not less than 485 000 units of vitamin A in 1 g. Synthetic Vitamin A Concentrate (Oily Form) *B.P.* contains not less than 500 000 units of vitamin A in 1 g. Synthetic Vitamin A Concentrate (Powder Form) *B.P.* contains not less than 250 000 units of vitamin A in 1 g. Synthetic Vitamin A Concentrate (Water-dispersible Form) *B.P.* contains not less than 100 000 units of vitamin A in 1 g.

The *U.S.P.* unit is defined as the specific biologic activity of 0.0003 mg of the all-*trans* isomer of retinol, and is equivalent to the International unit.

Adverse Effects and Precautions

The administration of excessive amounts of vitamin A over long periods can lead to toxicity, known as hypervitaminosis A. This is characterised by fatigue, irritability, anorexia and loss of weight, vomiting and other gastro-intestinal disturbances, low-grade fever, hepatosplenomegaly, skin changes, alopecia, dry hair, cracking and bleeding lips, anaemia, headache, hypercalcaemia, subcutaneous swelling, and pains in bones and joints. Symptoms of chronic toxicity in children may also include raised intracranial pressure and papilloedema mimicking brain tumours, tinnitus, visual disturbances which may be severe, and painful swelling over the long bones. Symptoms usually clear on withdrawal of vitamin A, but in children premature closure of the epiphyses of the long bones may result in arrested bone growth.

Acute vitamin A intoxication may occur with very high doses and is characterised by sedation, dizziness, nausea and vomiting, erythema, pruritus, and desquamation.

Excessive doses of vitamin A should be avoided in pregnancy because of potential teratogenic effects.

Absorption of vitamin A from the gastro-intestinal tract may be reduced by the presence of neomycin, cholestyramine, or liquid paraffin; absorption may also be impaired in cholestatic jaundice and fat-malabsorption conditions.

Usual diets in the *USA* contain about 5000 to 10 000 international units (IU) per day; 25 000 to 50 000 IU per day for 8 months or longer may be toxic. A single dose of 1 500 000 IU has caused poisoning in adults. Acute poisoning causes drowsiness, headache, vomiting, papilloedema and, in infants, a bulging fontanelle. Patients with chronic hypervitaminosis A typically have dry, coarse, scaly skin, hair loss, fissures of the lips, and pruritus. Other signs and symptoms include sore tongue or mouth, clubbing of the fingers, hyperostoses, nystagmus, brittle nails, hypercalcaemia, hepatosplenomegaly, increased intracranial pressure, and low-grade fever. In children, anorexia, pruritus, and failure to gain weight are followed by increasing irritability, tenderness and swelling of bones, and limitation of movement. Large doses of vitamin A are teratogenic.— *Med. Lett.*, 1984, *26*, 73.

Patients with severe hypertriglyceridaemia associated with type V hyperlipoproteinaemia may be at increased risk for hypervitaminosis A.— J. K. Ellis, *Ann. intern. Med.*, 1986, *105*, 877.

EFFECTS ON THE BLOOD. A report of neutropenia associated with hypercarotenaemia in a patient whose diet included a high intake of carrot juice. The neutropenia improved when the patient went on a low carotene diet and recurred when the high carotene diet was resumed.— Y. Shoenfeld *et al.* (letter), *Lancet*, 1982, *1*, 1245. Comments. Administration of pure (crystalline) betacarotene will not cause leucopenia. It was considered likely that the neutropenia was due to other constituents of carrots.— M. M. Mathews-Roth (letter), *ibid.*, *2*, 222; M. J. Stampfer *et al.* (letter), *ibid.*, 615.

Normochromic macrocytic anaemia developed in a patient who had been receiving vitamin A 150 000 IU daily by mouth for several months. The patient's haemoglobin returned to normal when vitamin A was discontinued, and the accompanying symptoms of perioral dermatitis and glossitis also disappeared.— J. M. White (letter), *Lancet*, 1984, *2*, 573.

EFFECTS ON THE LIVER. Excess administration of vitamin A can lead to fibrosis in the Dissë space and obstruction of sinusoidal blood flow, causing non-cirrhotic portal hypertension and hepatocellular dysfunction.— S. Sherlock, *Lancet*, 1986, *2*, 440.

EFFECTS ON THE MUSCULOSKELETAL SYSTEM. Excessive doses of vitamin A can result in osteosclerosis which may be accompanied by ectopic calcification involving tendons, as well as muscle, ligaments, and subcutaneous tissue.— D. M. Davies, *Adverse Drug React. Bull.*, 1985, (Jun.), 416.

EFFECTS ON THE SKIN. Yellow pigmentation of the skin may result from an unusually high consumption of carrots or other source of carotene. Hypercarotenaemia can be distinguished from jaundice by the fact that the sclerae retain their normal white colour. Pigmentation occurs first on the palms and soles and may extend to the nasolabial folds. The condition is harmless as the body converts carotene to retinol only in amounts as required; hypervitaminosis A cannot therefore occur from overconsumption of carotene.— I. M. Sharman, *Br. med. J.*, 1985, *290*, 95. See also D. A. T. Southgate (letter), *ibid.*, 1986, *292*, 1191.

OVERDOSAGE. A report of hypercarotenaemia and vitamin A overdosage in a 10-month-old child associated with a diet which consisted largely of proprietary baby food containing carrot and added vitamin A. Although the serum-vitamin A concentration was raised, serum bilirubin and liver function tests were normal. The vitamin A intake was estimated at about 3000 μg per day, considerably above the recommended limits.— H. F. Stirling *et al.* (letter), *Lancet*, 1986, *1*, 1089.

See also under Effects on the Skin, above.

PREGNANCY AND THE NEONATE. The human teratogenicity of synthetic vitamin A derivatives such as isotretinoin is now well accepted. This has prompted concern about the potential teratogenicity of megadoses of vitamin A. Results from an epidemiological case-controlled study on prenatal exposure to vitamin A alone or in combination with other vitamins, have indicated that a teratogenic effect could exist for exposures to high doses of vitamin A.— M. L. Martínez-Frías and J. Salvador (letter), *Lancet*, 1988, *1*, 236.

See also under Isotretinoin, p.924.

Absorption and Fate

Vitamin A is readily absorbed from the gastro-intestinal tract but absorption may be reduced in the presence of fat malabsorption, low protein intake, or impaired liver or pancreatic function. Vitamin A esters are hydrolysed by pancreatic enzymes to retinol, which is then absorbed. Some retinol is stored in the liver. It is released from the liver bound to a specific α_1-globulin (retinol-binding protein) in the blood. The retinol not stored in the liver undergoes glucuronide conjugation and subsequent oxidation to retinal and retinoic acid; these and other metabolites are excreted in urine and faeces. Vitamin A does not readily diffuse across the placenta but is present in the milk of nursing mothers.

Human Requirements

A daily dietary intake of about 750 μg of vitamin A is recommended for healthy adults. Dietary vitamin A is derived from 2 sources, *preformed retinol* from animal sources such as liver, kidney, dairy produce, and eggs (fish-liver oils is the most concentrated natural source), and *provitamin carotenoids* which can be obtained from many plants; these are converted to retinol in the body but are less effectively utilised. α-, β-, and γ-Carotenes are major sources and of these, β-carotene (betacarotene) has the highest vitamin A activity and is the most plentiful in food. Variable amounts of β-carotenes are found in carrots and dark green or yellow vegetables. Red palm oil is a good source of α- and β-carotenes.

The average daily recommended intake of vitamin A for adults was 750 μg of retinol (vitamin A alcohol). For infants, children, and young people, recommended daily intakes ranged from 300 μg at 6 to 12 months to 725 μg at 13 to 15 years.— Report of a Joint FAO/WHO Expert Group, *Tech. Rep. Ser. Wld Hlth Org. No. 362*, 1967.

Recommended daily intake of vitamin A or its equivalent: boys and girls up to 1 year, 450 μg; 1 to 6 years, 300 μg; 7 to 8 years, 400 μg; boys and girls 9 to 17 years, 575 to 750 μg; men and women 18 years or over, 750 μg; during pregnancy, 750 μg; during lactation, 1.2 mg. One μg of retinol was considered equivalent to 6 μg of β-carotene or 12 μg of other biologically active carotenoids.— *Report on Health and Social Subjects No. 15*, London, HM Stationery Office, 1979.

The recommendation that any infant formula should contain not less than 0.4 μg and not more than 1.5 μg retinol equivalent per mL reconstituted feed.— Artificial Feeds for the Young Infant: 1980, Report of the Working Party on the Composition of Foods for Infants and Young Children, Committee on Medical Aspects of Food Policy, *Report on Health and Social Subjects, 18*, London, HM Stationery Office, 1980.

Recommended daily dietary allowance of vitamin A: up to 6 months, 420 retinol equivalents (RE); 6 months to 3 years, 400 RE; 4 to 6 years, 500 RE; 7 to 10 years, 700 RE; males 11 years and over, 1000 RE; females 11 years and over, 800 RE; in pregnancy, 1000 RE; in lactation, 1200 RE. One retinol equivalent represents 1 μg of retinol, 6 μg of β-carotene, or 12 μg of other provitamin A carotenoids.— *Recommended Dietary Allowances*, 9th Edn, Washington, The National Research Council, 1980.

Uses and Administration

Vitamin A, a fat-soluble vitamin, is essential for growth, for the development and maintenance of epithelial tissue, and for vision, particularly in dim light. Vitamin A deficiency develops when the dietary intake is inadequate. It is rare in developed countries but remains a major problem in many developing countries. Prolonged deficiency leads to xerophthalmia or 'dry eye', the initial symptom of which is night blindness which may progress to severe eye lesions and blindness. Other symptoms include changes in the skin and mucous membranes.

Vitamin A is used in the treatment and prevention of vitamin A deficiency. It may be administered by mouth in an oil- or water-based form, or by intramuscular injection of a water-miscible form. Oil-miscible preparations of vitamin A are poorly absorbed from injection sites following intramuscular injection.

In the treatment of xerophthalmia, vitamin A palmitate 110 mg or vitamin A acetate 66 mg (200 000 units of vitamin A) should be given by mouth immediately on diagnosis. The dose should be repeated the following day with an additional dose administered 1 to 2 weeks later. Children with severe protein-energy deficiency should be given an additional dose every 2 weeks until protein status improves. Water-miscible vitamin A palmitate 55 mg (100 000 units) should be given by intramuscular injection instead of the first oral dose when there is repeated vomiting or severe diarrhoea. These doses should be halved for children under 1 year old. Higher doses have been recommended by the manufacturers.

In the prophylaxis of blinding xerophthalmia, vitamin A palmitate 110 mg or vitamin A acetate 66 mg (200 000 units) may be given by mouth every 4 to 6 months. This dose should be halved for children under 1 year old.

Vitamins A and D have been used together as cream or ointment in the treatment of minor skin disorders including abrasions. Vitamin A has also been used alone to treat various skin disorders including acne and psoriasis.

A review of vitamin A and retinoids. Despite achievements which have been obtained in the treatment of various skin diseases and preneoplastic, benign, and malignant neoplasm lesions, we are still far from the point where we can be satisfied with the practical clinical progress. The toxicity of retinoids remains the main handicap to their practical use. Further chemical manipulations may lead to compounds with more favourable therapeutic margins. It would be desirable to find substances with a more selective action on proliferation, differentiation, malignant transformation, keratinisation, sebum production, inflammation, and immune reactions. These developments would perhaps open new perspectives not only in skin diseases and the prevention and therapy of cancer but also in other branches of medicine.— W. Bollag, *Lancet*, 1983, *1*, 860. See also D. S. Goodman, *New Engl. J. Med.*, 1984, *310*, 1023.

ABETALIPOPROTEINAEMIA. For reference to the use of vitamin A with vitamin E in the treatment of abetalipoproteinaemia, see under vitamin E, p.1285.

ACTION. The effect of vitamin A and its derivatives on collagen production and chemotactic response of fibroblasts.— R. Hein *et al.*, *Br. J. Derm.*, 1984, *111*, 37.

ADMINISTRATION IN RENAL FAILURE. For reference to vitamin A in renal failure see under Dialysis, below.

BILIARY CIRRHOSIS. Vitamin A deficiency continues to cause night blindness in patients with primary biliary cirrhosis. Overt deficiency should be treated initially with oral vitamin A 50 000 units daily. The maintenance dose varies from 5000 to 25 000 units daily depending upon the underlying condition.— *Drug & Ther. Bull.*, 1984, *22*, 33.

Three patients with night blindness associated with primary biliary cirrhosis responded to vitamin A by mouth; 2 had received previous treatment with intramuscular injections of vitamin A.— R. P. Walt *et al.*, *Br. med. J.*, 1984, *288*, 1030.

Results from a study involving 25 patients suggested that patients with primary biliary cirrhosis should not receive regular parenteral or even oral vitamin A supplementation unless dark adaptometry or electro-oculography yields an abnormal result.— A. N. Shepherd *et al.*, *Br. med. J.*, 1984, *289*, 1484.

CROHN'S DISEASE. Of 52 patients with Crohn's disease investigated for evidence of vitamin A deficiency, none of whom were receiving vitamin A supplements, 11 patients had low plasma-retinol concentrations and 3 had impaired dark adaptation, only 2 of whom complained of night blindness. None of the patients had conjunctival or retinal signs of xerophthalmia. Results indicated that vitamin A deficiency was a significant problem in severe Crohn's disease and was associated with extensive small bowel disease, very low plasma-retinol concentrations, and depletion of plasma proteins, especially retinol binding protein and prealbumin. The authors suggested that patients with extensive small bowel Crohn's disease weighing less than 80% of ideal weight should have biochemical tests performed including measurement of plasma retinol and plasma proteins. If dark adaptation testing is not possible, vitamin A supplements should be given. Protein depletion which is likely to be present should also be corrected.— A. N. H. Main *et al.*, *Gut*, 1983, *24*, 1169.

DIAGNOSIS AND TESTING. A simple method for the detection of vitamin A deficiency in underdeveloped areas using impression cytology of the bulbar conjunctival epithelium.— O. Amédée-Manesme *et al.* (letter), *Lancet*, 1987, *1*, 1263.

DIALYSIS. Studies on the raised plasma concentrations of vitamin A in patients on maintenance haemodialysis, and advice that supplements of vitamin A should be avoided: K. Farrington *et al.*, *Br. med. J.*, 1981, *282*, 1999; M. O'Fearghail *et al.* (letter), *ibid.*, *283*, 919; W. K. Stewart and L. W. Fleming (letter), *ibid.*, 1187.

MEASLES. WHO and UNICEF have produced a joint statement outlining the importance of the link between outcome of measles and vitamin A deficiency, and ways in which countries can reduce the impact of measles by giving high doses of vitamin A to young children (*Wkly epidem. Rec.*, 1987, *62*, 133). It has been recommended that high dosage vitamin A supplementation should be provided to all children diagnosed with measles in communities in which vitamin A deficiency is a recognised problem. In countries where the fatality rate of measles is 1% or higher it is considered sensible on the basis of current evidence to provide vitamin A supplements to all children diagnosed with measles.— *Lancet*, 1987, *1*, 1067.

Further references: A. J. G. Barclay *et al.*, *Br. med. J.*, 1987, *294*, 294; M. A. Monnickendam and S. Darougar, *Br. J. Ophthal.*, 1987, *71*, 325.

XEROPHTHALMIA. Vitamin A deficiency and xerophthalmia are among the most widespread and serious nutritional disorders that affect mankind. For many years the problem remained unchecked and continued to exact a devastating, although uncertain, toll in blindness and death among young children. More recently there has been an increasing realisation of the enormity of the problem and concerted efforts have been made in the areas of research, field surveys, action programmes, and educational activities.

It has long been recognised that vitamin A deficiency does not occur as an isolated problem, but is almost invariably accompanied by protein-energy malnutrition and infections. Numerous studies have shown that a variety of infections impair absorption. Malabsorption of vitamin A has been demonstrated in acute gastro-enteritis, ascariasis in adults and children, giardiasis, severe hookworm infestation, and salmonellosis and schistosomiasis. Although vitamin A absorption is also impaired in children with respiratory infections, the mechanism is unclear.

Measles tends to take an especially severe form in the child with protein-energy malnutrition in whom immunocompetence is markedly impaired. Even in mild cases there is viral infection of the cornea, which is unique to measles among the common childhood infections. In the presence of vitamin A deficiency, such infection may facilitate the changes that lead to liquefaction. (See also under Measles, above).— Control of Vitamin A Deficiency and Xerophthalmia, Report of a Joint WHO/UNICEF/USAID/Helen Keller International/International Vitamin A Consultative Group Meeting, *Tech. Rep. Ser. Wld Hlth Org. No 672*, 1982

Uncomplicated, gradual depletion of vitamin A stores results in xerophthalmia or "dry eye" of increasing severity: night blindness, conjunctival xerosis and Bitot's spot, corneal xerosis, and corneal ulceration/keratomalacia. All usually respond rapidly to vitamin A therapy, the milder manifestations usually clearing without significant sequelae. The loss of deep corneal tissue, however, from ulceration/keratomalacia generally results in scarring and residual opacification.

Effective therapy requires prompt recognition of children with, or at high risk of developing, active disease; immediate administration of massive doses of vitamin A with concomitant treatment of underlying systemic illnesses and protein-energy malnutrition, and prevention of any recurrence. Oral administration is just as effective as parenteral administration. As oral dosing does not require sterile needles, syringes, and special water-miscible preparations, it is safe, cheap, and increasingly available.

Oil- or water-miscible vitamin A palmitate 110 mg or vitamin A acetate 66 mg (200 000 units of vitamin A) should be administered by mouth immediately upon diagnosis and the dose repeated the following day. An additional dose should be given 1 to 2 weeks later to boost liver reserves. Because children with severe protein-energy deficiency handle a massive dose poorly, they should receive an additional dose, every 2 weeks, until protein status improves. For children unable to swallow, or suffering from repeated vomiting or profuse diarrhoea, an intramuscular injection of water-miscible vitamin A palmitate 55 mg (100 000 units) should be substituted for the first oral dose. Oil-miscible preparations should never be given by injection as they are poorly absorbed from the injection site. For children aged less than 12 months the dose should be halved.

Only by ensuring that children receive adequate supplies of vitamin A will the underlying cause of deficiency be removed. For the prevention of blinding xerophthalmia in developing countries such supplies must be greater than "recommended daily allowances" established for healthy children. Periodic dosing takes advantage of the fact that large quantities of vitamin A can be stored in the liver for future use. Oral administration of vitamin A palmitate 110 mg or vitamin A acetate 66 mg (200 000 units), and half this dose for children under 12 months, every 4 to 6 months will protect the vast majority of recipients from blinding xerophthalmia. Vitamin A palmitate 27.5 mg (50 000 units) may be administered to newborn infants, and 165 mg (300 000 units) to the mother. Because of the potential risk of teratogenicity from a massive dose, a woman of child-bearing age should receive a massive dose only when it is absolutely certain she is not pregnant (i.e. within one month of giving birth). It is safe and advisable for lactating and pregnant women in high-risk communities to receive frequent low-dose vitamin A supplementation where feasible, for instance vitamin A palmitate 2.75 mg (5000 units) once daily, or 11 mg (20 000 units) once a week.— A. Sommer, Field Guide to the Detection and Control of Xerophthalmia, 2nd Edn, Geneva, *Wld Hlth Org.*, 1982.

Further references: A. S. Truswell, *Br. med. J.*, 1985, *291*, 587; A. Foster and A. Sommer, *Bull. Wld Hlth Org.*, 1986, *64*, 619; A. Sommer *et al.*, *Lancet*, 1986, *1*, 1169; *ibid.*, 1191; A. M. de L. Costello (letter), *ibid.*, *2*, 161; R. H. Gray (letter), *ibid.*; H. Martinez *et al.* (letter), *ibid.*, *2*, 451; A. Sommer and K. P. West (letter), *ibid.*

A report of bilateral keratomalacia and endophthalmitis with a right perforated cornea in a 39-year-old previously undiagnosed chronic schizophrenic. The patient had been observing a strict vegan diet for 7 years resulting in severe nutritional deficiencies. Vitamin A replacement therapy in association with a high-protein high-calorie vegan diet with multivitamin supplementation resulted in rapid improvement of the eyes with clearing of corneal haze over 2 weeks.— J. Olver, *Br. J. Ophthal.*, 1986, *70*, 357.

Preparations

Vitamin A Capsules *(U.S.P.)*

Proprietary Preparations

Morsep *(Napp, UK)*. *Cream*, cetrimide 0.5%, vitamin A 70 units/g, ergocalciferol 10 units/g in a non-greasy basis. For napkin rash.

Ro-A-Vit *(Roche, UK)*. *Injection*, vitamin A as the palmitate 300 000 units (equivalent to retinol 90 mg)/mL, in an oily vehicle, in ampoules of 1 mL.

Tablets, vitamin A as the acetate 50 000 units (equivalent to retinol 15 mg).

Proprietary Names and Manufacturers of Vitamin A and its Esters

A 313 *(Chabre, Fr.)*; Acaren *(Belg.)*; Afaxin *(Canad.)*; AFI-A diagnostikum *(Nyco, Norw.)*; Alfa Monovit *(Ital.)*; Alfatar *(Arnaldi, Ital.)*; Alphalin *(Lilly, USA)*; Amirale *(IDI, Ital.)*; Amplex-A *(Spain)*; A-Mulsin *(Mucos, Ger.)*; Anol Standard *(Belg.)*; A-Om *(Spain)*; Aquasol A *(Arg.; Rorer, Canad.; Armour, USA)*; Ariovit *(Roche, Denm.)*; Arovit *(Belg.; Roche, Fr.; Roche, Ger.; Roche, Ital.; Neth.; S.Afr.; Roche, Spain; Roche, Swed.; Roche, Switz.)*; Atunol *(Arg.)*; Auxina A Masiva *(Gayoso Wellcome, Spain)*; Avibon *(Théraplix, Fr.)*; A-Vicotrat *(Heyl, Ger.)*; Avimin *(Ferrosan, Denm.)*; Avita *(S.Afr.)*; Avitam Masivo *(Spain)*; A-vitamin *(DAK, Denm.)*; Avitina *(CT, Ital.)*; Axérol *(Wander, Switz.)*; Bagoderm A *(Arg.)*; Bagovit-A *(Arg.)*; Biominol A *(Alter, Spain)*; Dagravit A *(Belgana, Belg.; Neth.)*; Davitamon A *(Neth.)*; Dohyfral A *(Neth.)*; Dolce A *(Labaz, Spain)*; Euvit A *(IBIS, Ital.)*; Euvitol *(Zambeletti, Ital.)*; Evitex A *(Alcon, Spain)*; Fabavit *(S.Afr.)*; Farmobion A *(Ital.)*; Fiviton A *(Carol, Spain)*; Ido-A *(Leo, Spain; Swed.)*; Idrurto A *(Ripari-Gero, Ital.)*; Mulsal-A *(Vitapharm, Spain)*; Neo-Dohyfral A *(Belg.)*; Neominas A *(Spain)*; Oculotect *(Dispersa, Ger.; Switz.)*; Ophtosan *(Winzer, Ger.)*; Optovit-A *(Hermes, Ger.)*; Pedi-Vit A *(Pedinol, USA)*; Perlaminas A Masivas *(Spain)*; Primavit *(IBP, Ital.)*; Ro-A-Vit *(Arg.; Roche, Austral.; Roche, UK)*; Vi-Dom A *(USA)*; Vitaendil A *(Spain)*; Vit-A-Plos *(Arg.)*; Vogan *(E. Merck, Ger.)*.

Multivitamin and mineral preparations containing vitamin A are included in the lists on pp.1289-93. The following names have been used for preparations containing vitamin A and not considered to be a multivitamin or mineral preparation—Aquasol A Cream *(Rorer, Canad.)*; Lazer *(Pedinol, USA)*; Morsep *(Napp, UK)*; Paxyl Cream *(Faulding, Austral.)*.

7892-q

Vitamin D

The term vitamin D is used for a range of closely related sterol compounds which possess the property of preventing or curing rickets. These include alfacalcidol, calcifediol, calcitriol, cholecalciferol, dihydrotachysterol, and ergocalciferol.

7885-p

Alfacalcidol *(BAN, pINN)*.

1α-Hydroxycholecalciferol; 1α-Hydroxyvitamin D_3; 1α-OHD_3; EB-644. (5*Z*,7*E*)-9,10-Secocholesta-5,7,10(19)-triene-1α,3β-diol.

$C_{27}H_{44}O_2$=400.6.

CAS — 41294-56-8.

7886-s

Calcifediol *(USAN, rINN)*.

25-Hydroxycholecalciferol; 25-Hydroxyvitamin D_3; 25-$(OH)D_3$; U-32070E. (5*Z*,7*E*)-9,10-Secocholesta-5,7,10(19)-triene-3β,25-diol monohydrate.

$C_{27}H_{44}O_2,H_2O$=418.7.

CAS — 19356-17-3 (anhydrous); 63283-36-3 (monohydrate).

Pharmacopoeias. In *U.S.*

Store in airtight containers. Protect from light.

7887-w

Calcitriol *(BAN, USAN, rINN)*.

1,25-Dihydroxycholecalciferol; 1α,25-Dihydroxycholecalciferol; 1α,25-Dihydroxyvitamin D_3; 1α,25$(OH_2)D_3$; Ro 21-5535. (5*Z*,7*E*)-9,10-Secocholesta-5,7,10(19)-triene-1α,3β,25-triol.

$C_{27}H_{44}O_3$=416.6.

CAS — 32222-06-3.

7888-e

Cholecalciferol *(BAN, USAN)*.

Cholecalciferolum; Colecalciferol *(rINN)*; Activated 7-Dehydrocholesterol; Vitamin D_3. (5*Z*,7*E*)-9,10-Secocholesta-5,7,10(19)-trien-3β-ol.

$C_{27}H_{44}O$=384.6.

CAS — 67-97-0.

Pharmacopoeias. In *Arg., Aust., Belg., Br., Chin., Cz., Eur., Fr., Hung., Ind., Int., It., Jpn, Neth., Pol., Roum., Swiss,* and *U.S.* Also in *B.P. Vet. Br.* and *Eur.* also include monographs for Cholecalciferol Concentrate (Oily Form) and Cholecalciferol Concentrate (Powder Form).

The naturally occurring form of vitamin D. It is produced from 7-dehydrocholesterol, a sterol present in mammalian skin, by ultraviolet irradiation. White or almost white, odourless or almost odourless crystals which are sensitive to air and light. M.p. 82 to 87°.

Practically **insoluble** in water; freely soluble in alcohol, acetone, chloroform, and ether; soluble in fixed oils. Solutions in volatile solvents are unstable and should be used immediately. **Store** at a temperature of 2 to 8° in hermetically sealed containers in which the air has been replaced by an inert gas. The contents of an opened container should be used immediately. Protect from light.

7891-g

Dihydrotachysterol *(BAN, USAN, rINN).*

Dichysterol. (5*E*,7*E*,22*E*)-10α-9,10-Secoergosta-5,7,22-trien-3β-ol.

$C_{28}H_{46}O$=398.7.

CAS — 67-96-9.

Pharmacopoeias. In *Br., Jug.*, and *U.S.*

Odourless or almost odourless colourless crystals or white crystalline powder. M.p. 123.5° to 129°. May also occur in a form melting at about 113°. Practically **insoluble** in water; soluble 1 in 20 of alcohol, 1 in 0.7 of chloroform, 1 in 3 of ether, and 1 in 50 of arachis oil. **Store** at a temperature not exceeding 15° in hermetically sealed glass containers in which the air has been replaced by an inert gas. Protect from light.

7884-q

Ergocalciferol *(BAN, USAN, rINN).*

Calciferol; Irradiated Ergosterol; Ergocalciferolum; Viosterol; Vitamin D_2. (5*Z*,7*E*,22*E*)-9,10-Secoergosta-5,7,10(19),22-tetraen-3β-ol.

$C_{28}H_{44}O$=396.7.

CAS — 50-14-6.

Pharmacopoeias. In *Arg., Aust., Belg., Br., Braz., Chin., Cz., Egypt., Eur., Fr., Ger., Hung., Ind., Int., It., Jpn, Jug., Neth., Nord., Port., Roum., Swiss., Turk.*, and *U.S.* Also in *B.P. Vet.*

An antirachitic substance obtained from ergosterol, a sterol present in fungi and yeasts, by ultraviolet irradiation. Odourless or almost odourless, colourless or slightly yellow crystals or white or slightly yellow crystalline powder. It is sensitive to air, heat, and light.

Practically **insoluble** in water; soluble 1 in 2 of alcohol, 1 in 10 of acetone, 1 in 0.7 of chloroform, 1 in 2 of ether; slightly soluble in fixed oils. **Store** at a temperature of 2 to 8° in hermetically sealed containers in which the air has been replaced by an inert gas. The contents of an opened container should be used immediately. Protect from light.

Expulsion of ergocalciferol injection from plastic syringes was found to be difficult; the use of glass syringes however, allowed satisfactory administration.— K. G. Halsall (letter), *Pharm. J.*, 1985, *2*, 99.

STABILITY IN SOLUTION. A review of the compatibility and stability of components of total parenteral solutions when mixed in 1- or 3-litre flexible containers. Vitamin D may bind strongly to plastic which can lead to significant losses to the bag and administration set. Vitamin D losses from paediatric TPN mixtures have been estimated to be about 30 to 36% over a 24-hour administration period. The quantity of vitamin D delivered depends on infusion rate, type of administration set, composition of mixture, and total volume infused.— M. C. Allwood, *J. clin. Hosp. Pharm.*, 1984, *9*, 181.

Units

The Second International Standard Preparation (1949) of vitamin D consists of bottles containing approximately 6 g of a solution of cholecalciferol in vegetable oil (1000 units per g).

NOTE. One unit of vitamin D is contained in 25 ng of cholecalciferol or ergocalciferol.

In England and Wales, the Labelling of Food Regulations 1970 (SI 1970: No. 400) as amended (SI 1972: 1510) require that in any food labelled as containing vitamins D, D_2 or D_3 the vitamin must be calculated as micrograms of cholecalciferol.

The eventual discontinuation of the International Standard for Vitamin D (and International Unit) was recommended by the WHO Expert Committee on Biological Standardization.— *Chronicle Wld Hlth Org.*, 1973, *27*, 31.

Adverse Effects

Excessive intake of vitamin D leads to the development of hypercalcaemia and its associated symptoms which are described under Calcium, p.1028. Interindividual tolerance to vitamin D varies considerably; infants and children are generally more susceptible to its toxic effects.

A report of the development of deafness after long-term treatment with ergocalciferol 2.5 mg daily.— H. N. Cohen *et al.* (letter), *Lancet*, 1979, *1*, 985.

Vitamin D is the most likely of all vitamins to cause overt toxicity. Doses of 60 000 units (1.25 mg) per day can cause hypercalcaemia, with muscle weakness, apathy, headache, anorexia, nausea and vomiting, bone pain, ectopic calcification, proteinuria, hypertension, and cardiac arrhythmias. Chronic hypercalcaemia can lead to generalised vascular calcification, nephrocalcinosis, and rapid deterioration of renal function.— *Med. Lett.*, 1984, *26*, 73.

A report of prolonged hypercalcaemia in a 32-year-old laboratory technician following industrial exposure to cholecalciferol.— M. Jibani and N. H. Hodges, *Br. med. J.*, 1985, *290*, 748.

A report of a study involving 18 children with chronic renal failure and histological evidence of renal osteodystrophy who were treated with either calcitriol or ergocalciferol. Although both compounds proved to be of equal efficacy, hypercalcaemia occurred more often following treatment with calcitriol (11 episodes) than with ergocalciferol (3 episodes).— E. M. Hodson *et al.*, *Clin. Nephrol.*, 1985, *24*, 192.

Treatment of Adverse Effects

The treatment of hypercalcaemia is described under Calcium Gluconate, p.1030.

Treatment of vitamin D overdose in a 5-month-old infant with phenytoin 5 mg per kg body-weight daily for 17 days and phenobarbitone 5 mg per kg daily for 133 days (but discontinued for 14 days on the 44th day) to induce hepatic microsomal enzymes, as well as initial frusemide therapy, resulted in the return of serum- and urine-calcium concentrations to normal.— J. Łukaszkiewicz *et al.*, *Br. med. J.*, 1987, *295*, 1173. See also S. J. Iqbal and W. H. Taylor, *ibid.*, 1982, *285*, 541 (similar use of glutethimide).

Precautions

Vitamin D should not be administered to patients with hypercalcaemia. It should be administered with caution to infants as they may have increased sensitivity to its effects.

It is advised that, if possible, women receiving vitamin D do not breast feed their infants as this may lead to the development of hypercalcaemia in the infant.

The effects of vitamin D may be reduced in patients taking barbiturates or anticonvulsants.

For recommendations on how hypercalcaemia and tissue calcinosis may be avoided in patients receiving treatment with both vitamin D and magnesium salts, see under Magnesium Sulphate, p.1033.

INTERACTIONS. Three patients receiving dihydrotachysterol and calcium for postoperative hypoparathyroidism, following thyroidectomy, developed hypercalcaemia when their concomitant thyroxine therapy was discontinued before a radio-iodine scan. The dose of dihydrotachysterol should be reduced and serum-calcium concentrations should be monitored when thyroid treatment is interrupted, since elimination of dihydrotachysterol may be delayed in hypothyroidism.— B. -A. Lamberg and M. J. Tikkanen, *Br. med. J.*, 1981, *283*, 461.

Absorption and Fate

Vitamin D substances are well absorbed from the gastro-intestinal tract. The presence of bile is essential for adequate intestinal absorption; absorption may be decreased in patients with decreased fat absorption.

Vitamin D and its metabolites circulate in the blood bound to a specific α-globulin. Vitamin D can be stored in adipose and muscle tissue for long periods of time. Vitamin D compounds generally have a slow onset and a long duration of action; the newer analogues and metabolites, however, have a more rapid action and shorter half-lives.

Cholecalciferol and ergocalciferol are hydroxylated in the liver by the enzyme vitamin D 25-hydroxylase to form 25-hydroxycholecalciferol (calcifediol) and 25-hydroxyergocalciferol respectively. These compounds undergo further hydroxylation in the kidneys by the enzyme vitamin D 1-hydroxylase to form the active metabolites 1,25-dihydroxycholecalciferol (calcitriol) and 1,25-dihydroxyergocalciferol respectively. Further metabolism also occurs in the kidneys, including the formation of the 1,24,25-trihydroxy derivatives.

Vitamin D compounds and their metabolites are excreted mainly in the bile and faeces with only small amounts appearing in urine. Certain vitamin D substances may be excreted into breast milk.

In 4 healthy subjects given calcitriol 4 μg, peak concentrations were achieved at 4 hours and had returned to normal 27 hours after administration. In 3 subjects given 24,25-dihydroxycholecalciferol 250 μg peak concentrations were achieved at 6 hours and were still considerably raised at 48 hours. In 1 subject studied the concentration returned to the normal range in 9 days but not to the pre-treatment value by 21 days.— R. S. Mason *et al.*, *Br. med. J.*, 1980, *280*, 449.

A discussion of the effects of bilateral nephrectomy on the production of vitamin D metabolites.— G. R. D. Catto and N. Muirhead, *Br. med. J.*, 1984, *289*, 146.

Results of an investigation of vitamin D metabolites in bile, in 6 patients with T-tube biliary drainage after cholecystectomy, confirmed that a significant proportion of cholecalciferol given by mouth or intravenously is excreted in bile as biologically inactive polar metabolites; less than 4% of the metabolites were present as 25-hydroxycholecalciferol or its glucuronide conjugate. The concept of S.B. Arnaud *et al.* (*Proc. Soc. exp. biol. Med.*, 1975, *149*, 570) of a large conservative enterohepatic circulation of 25-hydroxycholecalciferol is clearly untenable. Interference with an enterohepatic circulation cannot therefore be the cause of unexplained vitamin D deficiency.— M. R. Clements *et al.*, *Lancet*, 1984, *1*, 1376. Comment. The possibility of a small, but functionally significant, conservative enterohepatic circulation should not be dismissed. The absence of significant amounts of free 25-hydroxycholecalciferol in bile does not exclude a conservative enterohepatic circulation since biliary products may be metabolised in the small intestine, releasing 25-hydroxycholecalciferol which would then be available for reabsorption. A small conservative enterohepatic circulation of 25-hydroxycholecalciferol might well become functionally significant in the presence of two coexisting factors; one is increased faecal metabolite loss due to malabsorption or high fibre intake and the other is low or borderline endogenous vitamin D synthesis. Under these circumstances, increased losses of 25-hydroxycholecalciferol from an enterohepatic circulation might, over a period of time, be an important factor in the development of vitamin D deficiency.— J. Compston and J. E. Ledger (letter), *ibid.*, *2*, 516. See also J. E. Ledger *et al.*, *Gut*, 1985, *26*, 1240.

Further studies of the metabolism of vitamin D: E. B. Mawer *et al.*, *Clin. Sci.*, 1985, *68*, 135 (in patients intoxicated with ergocalciferol); E. B. Mawer *et al.*, *ibid.*, *69*, 561 (in patients with primary biliary cirrhosis and alcoholic liver disease).

Human Requirements

The daily requirements of vitamin D in adults are small and are met mainly by exposure to sunlight and/or obtained from the diet. A daily dietary intake of about 100 to 200 units (2.5 to 5 μg) of vitamin D is generally considered adequate for healthy adults. The requirements are greater in infants and children and during pregnancy and lactation. Requirements may also be higher in people who are not exposed to adequate sunlight such as the elderly or housebound.

Vitamin D is present in few foods. Fish-liver oils, especially cod-liver oil, are good sources of vitamin D. Other sources, which contain much smaller amounts, include butter, eggs, and liver.

The following daily intakes of vitamin D were recommended: from birth to 6 years of age, 400 units (10 μg); 7 years and over, 100 units (2.5 μg); during the second and third trimesters of pregnancy, and during lactation, 400 units (10 μg).— Report of a Joint FAO/WHO Expert Group, *Tech. Rep. Ser. Wld Hlth Org. No. 452*, 1970.

Studies indicated that babies received substantial

amounts of vitamin D during the first 6 to 12 months of life, though there was considerable variation. In some older children the amount of vitamin D received was well below the allowance of 400 units suggested by most countries. It seemed that the use of unfortified cow's milk for young babies should be discouraged. As the main source of vitamin D in older children was margarine, and its consumption was variable, further research was required to indicate whether deficiency of vitamin D necessitated a revision of the scheme for fortifying foods.— *Interim Report on Vitamin D by the Panel on Child Nutrition*, London, HM Stationery Office, 1970.

In a nutrition survey of 879 elderly subjects aged 65 or over the average content of vitamin D in the diet was 104 units and was considered to match recommended intake. However, it was felt that the elderly might be less able to obtain vitamin D from sunlight and that those who were housefast might be at special risk.— Report by the Panel on Nutrition of the Elderly, *A Nutrition Survey of the Elderly*, London, HM Stationery Office, 1972.

The following daily intakes of vitamin D (as cholecalciferol) were recommended: infants under 1 year, 7.5 µg; children 1 to 4 years, 10 µg; in pregnancy and lactation, 10 µg; dietary sources might not be necessary for children and adults sufficiently exposed to sunlight; adults insufficiently exposed to sunlight might need 10 µg daily; children and adolescents should receive that amount during winter.— Daily Amounts of Food and Energy and Nutrients for Groups of People in the United Kingdom, Report by the Committee on Medical Aspect of Food Policy, *Report on Health and Social Subjects No. 15*, London, HM Stationery Office, 1979.

The recommendation that any infant feed should provide about 10 ng vitamin D (0.4 i.u.) per mL reconstituted feed and acceptance of the range 7 to 13 ng vitamin D per mL feed. The recommendation that the vitamin be added as ergocalciferol (vitamin D_2) or cholecalciferol (vitamin D_3).— Artificial Feeds for the Young Infant: 1980, Report of the Working Party on the Composition of Foods for Infants and Young Children, Committee on Medical Aspects of Food Policy, *Report on Health and Social Subjects, 18*, London, HM Stationery Office 1980.

Recommended daily dietary allowance of vitamin D (as cholecalciferol) for infants, children, and adolescents is 10 µg (400 units); for adults aged 19 to 22 years 7.5 µg (300 units); for adults more than 22 years of age 5 µg (200 units); pregnant or lactating women require an additional 5 µg (200 units).— *Recommended Dietary Allowances*, 9th Edn, Washington, The National Research Council, 1980, p. 61.

Uses and Administration

Vitamin D compounds are fat-soluble sterols, sometimes considered to be hormones, which are involved in the regulation of calcium and phosphate homoeostasis and bone mineralisation.

Vitamin D deficiency develops when there is inadequate exposure to sunlight; it may also result from a lack of the vitamin in the diet. Deficiency leads to the development of a syndrome characterised by hypocalcaemia, hypophosphataemia, bone softening and bone pain, and known in adults as osteomalacia. In children, in whom there may be skeletal deformity, especially of the long bones, it is known as rickets.

Vitamin D compounds are used in the treatment and prevention of vitamin D deficiency states including those associated with malabsorption, hypocalcaemia, hypoparathyroidism, and metabolic disorders. Vitamin D is administered as cholecalciferol or ergocalciferol, or as alfacalcidol, calcifediol, calcitriol, or dihydrotachysterol which do not require renal hydroxylation and are therefore useful in patients with renal failure. It has also been given as a cholecalciferol-cholesterin complex. Dosage must be individualised for each patient. Plasma-calcium concentrations should be monitored at regular intervals, initially weekly and then every 2 to 4 weeks, in order to achieve optimum clinical response and to avoid hypercalcaemia.

Cholecalciferol and **ergocalciferol** are usually given by mouth, the preferred route, but may also be administered by intramuscular injection. A dose of 25 µg (1000 units) daily in the treatment of rickets usually results in normal plasma-calcium and plasma-phosphate concentrations in about 10 days. Doses of 75 to 100 µg (3000 to 4000 units) may be given for rapid healing. For vitamin D-dependent rickets, doses of 0.25 to 1.25 mg (10 000 to 50 000 units) or more daily may be required. Doses of 1.25 to 5 mg (50 000 to 200 000 units) or more daily may be used in the treatment of hypocalcaemia due to hypoparathyroidism or in patients with renal osteodystrophy.

Alfacalcidol, an analogue of calcitriol, is given in initial doses of 1 to 3 µg daily by mouth. A starting dose of 0.5 µg is recommended for elderly patients. Doses of 0.25 to 1 µg daily may be given for maintenance.

Calcifediol, the 25-hydroxylated metabolite of cholecalciferol, is given in doses of 50 to 100 µg daily or 300 to 350 µg weekly by mouth.

Calcitriol, the 1,25-dihydroxylated metabolite of cholecalciferol, has the greatest antirachitic activity of the vitamin D metabolites. It is given by mouth or by intravenous injection in initial doses of 0.25 to 2 µg daily, increased if necessary to a maximum of 3 µg daily.

Dihydrotachysterol, although chemically closely-related to calcitriol, has relatively weak antirachitic activity. It is given in initial doses of 0.2 to 2.5 mg daily by mouth. Doses of 0.25 to 1.75 mg weekly may be given for maintenance.

The use of vitamin D_2 and D_3 as additives in animal feeding stuffs is controlled in Great Britain by The Fertilisers and Feeding Stuffs Regulations 1973 (SI 1973: No.1521) as amended (SI 1976: No.840; SI 1977: No.115).

A review of the uses of vitamin D.— D. A. Heath, *Prescribers' J.*, 1981, *21*, 164.

A review of vitamin therapy in non-deficiency states. There are no claims that pharmacological doses of vitamin D are of any benefit in the treatment of disorders other than those caused by vitamin deficiency. However, the new synthetic analogues and vitamin D metabolites are presently the drugs of choice in disorders caused by a defect in vitamin D metabolism, such as uraemic and hepatic osteodystrophy, hypoparathyroidism, and some inborn errors of metabolism. It has been suggested that vitamin D and its metabolites may be of use in postmenopausal and senile osteoporosis, diseases in which there is less clear evidence of a disordered vitamin D metabolism. Balance studies have indicated that the daily administration of 0.5 µg of calcitriol improves calcium balance in osteoporotic females. However, it is unknown whether this improvement in balance will result in an improved bone mass.— L. Ovesen, *Drugs*, 1984, *27*, 148.

ACTION. Over the past 15 years, at least 15 natural metabolites of cholecalciferol have been isolated and identified. Of these, calcitriol (1,25-dihydroxycholecalciferol) appears to carry out all the functions attributed to the vitamin D hormone system. Vitamin D deficiency impairs the mineralisation of bone in children (rickets) and adults (osteomalacia). Treatment with vitamin D restores mineralisation and bone formation; whether this is due to a direct stimulatory effect of a vitamin D metabolite, or an indirect effect due to stimulation of the intestinal absorption of calcium and phospate, remains equivocal.— L. G. Raisz and B. E. Kream, *New Engl. J. Med.*, 1983, *309*, 29. See also L. V. Avioli and J. G. Haddad, *ibid.*, 1984, *311*, 47.

Vitamin D serves as a precursor molecule for the potent calcium-regulating steroid hormone, calcitriol. The paramount function of vitamin D is to permit normal bone mineralisation but, paradoxically, the bulk of experimental evidence indicates that calcitriol is a potent bone-resorbing agent. Even more unexpected is new evidence suggesting that calcitriol has only an indirect effect on osteoblasts, that its principal target bone cells are in fact osteoclasts, and that its bone-resorbing activity is mediated via stimulation of osteoblast-derived factors. There is also a growing body of evidence suggesting that calcitriol has a role in the control of cellular proliferation and differentiation.— *Lancet*, 1987, *1*, 1122. Comment.— S. C. Manolagas (letter), *ibid.*, *2*, 639.

Further references to the action and physiological role of vitamin D: A. M. Pierides, *Drugs*, 1981, *21*, 241; D. R. Fraser, *Br. med. Bull.*, 1981, *37*, 37; S. C. Manolagas and L. J. Deftos, *Ann. intern. Med.*, 1984, *100*, 144; *Lancet*, 1984, *1*, 1105; I. P. Braidman and D. C. Anderson (letter), *ibid.*, 1415; T. J. Chambers and M. A. Horton (letter), *ibid.*, 1298; M. Audran and R. Kumar, *Mayo Clin. Proc.*, 1985, *60*, 851; I. MacIntyre, *Br. med. Bull.*, 1986, *42*, 343.

DEFICIENCY STATES. A discussion of the physiological role of vitamin D in nutrition. The single most important factor determining vitamin D status is the extent of solar irradiation of the skin. However, factors other than a lack of sunlight may play a part in the development of clinical deficiency disease, and further research is needed to assess their significance.— D. R. Fraser, *Lancet*, 1983, *1*, 969.

Calcitriol is effective in promoting calcium absorption and raising the plasma-calcium concentration in patients whose endogenous calcitriol production is impaired. This is the case in renal failure, in hypoparathyroidism (parathyroid hormone is required for the 1-hydroxylation step in vitamin D metabolism), and in a rare inherited disorder, vitamin D-dependent rickets. In these disorders calcitriol is effective in microgram doses compared with the milligram doses needed with cholecalciferol or ergocalciferol.

A useful analogue of calcitriol is *alfacalcidol* (1α-hydroxycholecalciferol); this is hydroxylated at the 25 postion in the liver to give calcitriol. As with calcitriol, microgram doses are effective in patients with renal failure or hypoparathroidism. Both drugs increase the plasma-calcium concentration in a newly-diagnosed patient with hypoparathyroidism in a few days. However, while the speed of action of calcitriol and alfacalcidol is an advantage, it may contribute to the ease with which patients can be poisoned by an unwary physician. The plasma half-life of calcitriol is about 3 hours and appreciable fluctuations in plasma-calcium concentrations are therefore likely to occur in patients taking the drug irregularly. For this reason, preparations with longer half-lives such as alfacalcidol, dihydrotachysterol, cholecalciferol or ergocalciferol are preferable. *Dihydrotachysterol* has long been recognised as an effective alternative to cholecalciferol or ergocalciferol. It has a shorter half-life and requires only a 25-hydroxylation in the liver to produce a metabolite that mimics the action of calcitriol.— C. R. Paterson and J. Feely, *Br. med. J.*, 1983, *286*, 1625.

In the elderly. Low plasma-25-hydroxyvitamin D (25-OHD) concentrations, indicating vitamin D deficiency, are common in elderly people, especially women. Several reports have indicated an increased prevalence of osteomalacia in elderly people, including some with hip fracture, suggesting that osteomalacia might increase the risk of hip fracture in such patients. The finding of low plasma-25-OHD concentrations in a proportion of patients with hip fracture, and the demonstration of a seasonal variation in histological features in such patients similar to the seasonal fluctuation of plasma-25-OHD concentrations, support the suggestion that vitamin D deficiency may increase the risk of hip fracture in the elderly. Because of the high human and financial cost of these fractures, a strong case can be made for vitamin D supplementation in the elderly, at least for high-risk groups. Correction or prevention of vitamin D deficiency in the elderly population can be achieved in various ways. Exposure to ultraviolet irradiation from artificial sources has been shown to increase plasma-25-OHD concentrations in elderly patients on long-stay hospital wards. The use of a single dose of 2.5 mg (100 000 units) by mouth has been reported to maintain normal plasma-25-OHD concentrations for at least 6 months without producing vitamin D toxicity (Y. Weisman *et al.*, *J. Am. Geriat. Soc.*, 1986, *34*, 515). Alternatively, smaller doses, for instance 12.5 µg (500 units) can be given daily. Larger oral doses or parenteral therapy may be required in some patients with malabsorption. Single intramuscular injections of 15 mg (600 000 units) of vitamin D will initiate and sustain a biochemical response in elderly osteomalacic patients, including some who have had a gastrectomy, for up to 6 months; normal plasma-25-OHD concentrations are maintained for up to a year in some subjects. The case for routine vitamin D supplementation in all elderly people remains unproven. Nevertheless, the increased frequency of vitamin D deficiency among certain groups, together with the ease and safety with which normal vitamin D status can be restored, strongly favour supplementation for high-risk patients.— *Lancet*, 1987, *1*, 306.

In renal failure. The availability of vitamin D compounds such as calcitriol and alfacalcidol which do not require activation by the kidney has made clear the importance of vitamin D deficiency in chronic renal failure. These compounds are used most widely in dialysis patients, in whom possible deleterious effects on renal function are of little importance, but they may also be useful before dialysis treatment begins. In early renal failure, before hyperphosphataemia appears, they may prevent the development of renal osteodystrophy and secondary hyperparathyroidism. They are especially useful in children. In moderate or late renal failure, their use in hyperphosphataemic subjects is hazardous. However, if phospate concentrations can be brought under control before these compounds are given, substantial benefit may be achieved.— M. Walser, *Lancet*, 1983, *1*, 340.

Patients with chronic renal failure develop skeletal abnormalities referred to as renal osteodystrophy. Increased parathyroid hormone concentrations and decreased calcitriol concentrations play a primary role in its pathogenesis. Vitamin D therapy in patients with renal osteodystrophy is usually reserved for patients with gross evidence of bone disease, pathologic fractures, and bony symptoms. It may have a place, however, in the therapeutic regimen of uraemic patients earlier on, especially those with high parathyroid hormone concentrations and hypocalcaemia. Long term benefits from early use of vitamin D need to be studied further.— K. F. Landsberg and D. N. Landsberg, *Can. J. Hosp. Pharm.*, 1985, *38*, 10.

Further references to the use of vitamin D analogues in patients with renal failure: F. U. Eke and M. H. Winterborn, *Archs Dis. Childh.*, 1983, *58*, 810 (alfacalcidol); K. Shimamatsu *et al., Curr. ther. Res.*, 1987, *41*, 374 (alfacalcidol).

See also under Deficiency States, above.

Hyperparathyroidism. Disturbances of vitamin D metabolism play an important role in determining the clinical presentation of primary hyperparathyroidism. Circulating concentrations of 1,25-dihydroxyvitamin D are usually raised in primary hyperparathyroidism, because parathyroid hormone, by causing hypophosphataemia, stimulates the renal 1α-hydroxylase enzyme system, thereby enhancing 1,25-dihydroxyvitamin D production. Patients presenting with bone disease and severe hypercalcaemia have decreased circulating concentrations of 25-hydroxyvitamin D. A few patients have overt vitamin D deficiency, with serum-calcium values that may be normal or only slightly increased and these findings are often mistaken for osteomalacia or rickets. In response to vitamin D treatment, the bone lesions heal and frank hypercalcaemia is unmasked, pointing to the correct diagnosis of primary hyperparathyroidism. Recent findings have provided an explanation for the development of vitamin D deficiency in primary hyperparathyroidism. Patients with masked hyperparathyroidism and clinically apparent osteomalacia are likely to be those with a precarious state of vitamin D balance to begin with. In this situation, any increase in metabolic clearance of 25-hydroxyvitamin D induced by hyperparathyroidism would have profound consequences. Moreover, the accelerated catabolism of 25-hydroxyvitamin D induced by hyperparathyroidism is important not only in primary hyperparathyroidism but also in other conditions such as dietary calcium deficiency, malabsorption, intestinal resection, and chronic liver disease. The traditional view was that secondary hyperparathyroidism associated with these conditions was a consequence of vitamin D deficiency. The reverse would now appear to be true. The vitamin D deficiency may, at least in part, be a consequence of hyperparathyroidism.— *Lancet*, 1988, *1*, 451.

See also under Hypoparathyroidism (below).

Hypocalcaemia. See under Hypoparathyroidism, below.

Hypoparathyroidism. The hypocalcaemia of hypoparathyroidism has traditionally been treated with cholecalciferol or ergocalciferol and calcium. Although these drugs are effective they may lead to prolonged hypercalcaemia. With the 1α-hydroxylated derivatives, hypercalcaemia, should it occur, usually subsides rapidly on stopping the drug. However, patients who are well controlled on one of the older drugs should continue with it. Acute hypoparathyroidism presenting after thyroidectomy with stridor and tetany is an emergency which must be treated with intravenous calcium. The fast acting calcitriol will stabilise serum-calcium concentrations within 24 hours, but an adequate oral calcium intake must be maintained. Hypocalcaemia after parathyroidectomy for adenoma appears 2 to 3 days after surgery and is usually less acute, but it is easier to control with the rapid and short-acting derivatives than their precursors.— *Drug & Ther. Bull.*, 1981, *19*, 103.

Hypoparathyroidism in *pregnancy* poses severe risks of foetal hyperparathyroidism with neonatal hypocalcaemic rickets, which may be fatal. Treatment with calcium 1.6 to 2.0 mg daily and either cholecalciferol or ergocalciferol in doses of 1.25 to 2.5 mg daily, or dihydrotachysterol 0.25 to 1.0 mg daily is essential.— W. M. Hague, *Br. med. J.*, 1987, *294*, 297. See also Z. M. van der Spuy and H. S. Jacobs, *Postgrad. med. J.*, 1984, *60*, 245.

See also Hyperparathyroidism, above.

Malignant neoplasms. Preliminary studies in 10 patients indicated that alfacalcidol had considerable antitumour activity and may have a potential role in the management of low-grade non-Hodgkin's lymphoma.— D. Cunningham *et al., Br. med. J.*, 1985, *291*, 1153. See also D. R. Spriggs *et al., Clin. Haematol.*, 1986, *15*, 1081.

Osteomalacia. Subclinical osteomalacia in 41 elderly patients was corrected following treatment for 3 months with either alfacalcidol 0.5 µg daily or ergocalciferol 25 µg daily. There was no evidence of significant hypercalcaemia or renal impairment.— D. J. Hosking *et al., Br. med. J.*, 1984, *289*, 785.

Results of a study in 7 elderly women indicated that a single depot intramuscular injection of ergocalciferol 15 mg was effective in initiating and sustaining healing of osteomalacia for at least 6 months.— J. Burns and C. R. Paterson, *Br. med. J.*, 1985, *290*, 281.

Osteomalacia is a well known but not always recognised complication of gastrectomy. Some authorities have advocated the prophylactic use of low doses of vitamin D in all patients who have had a gastrectomy, though the cost-effectiveness of this strategy is questionable in view of the low prevalence of the disorder and its long latency after operation. For treatment, a low dose of vitamin D is likewise sufficient. The degree of vitamin D malabsorption in these patients is mild and parenteral doses as low as 2.5 µg (100 units) daily are sufficient to bring about healing. Ergocalciferol in a dose of 25 µg (1000 units) by mouth produces clear improvement in histological changes in elderly osteomalacic subjects who have not had a gastrectomy; even with allowance for a degree of malabsorption, therefore, 37.5 to 50 µg (1500 to 2000 units) daily, or the equivalent of 3 to 4 Calcium with Vitamin D Tablets (*B.P.C. 1973*) daily, ought to suffice. Small therapeutic doses of vitamin D appear safe for 3 months, after which the dose can be reduced to a maintenance level of for example 12.5 µg (500 units) daily.— *Lancet*, 1986, *1*, 77.

Osteoporosis. For reference to the use of vitamin D in postmenopausal osteoporosis see under Oestrogens, p.1386.

Pregnancy and the neonate. A study of ergocalciferol supplements in Asian women during pregnancy; such supplements should be given to all pregnant Asian women, for at least the last trimester, in the UK.— O. G. Brooke *et al., Br. med. J.*, 1980, *280*, 751 and 1168.

It is rare for Western breast-fed infants of mothers with adequate dietary vitamin D to get rickets, although there have been reports of decreased bone mineralisation and a few cases of clinical rickets in breast-fed infants without vitamin D supplementation. Concentrations of 25-hydroxyvitamin D in maternal plasma and in the plasma of suckling infants have been shown to be directly related, implying that metabolites of vitamin D can be transferred from mother to child in breast milk. Paediatricians should be aware that the suggestion that large quantities of vitamin D sulphate may be present in breast milk is largely a myth, and that while vitamin D sulphate may be present in small concentrations, unless hydrolysed to vitamin D it probably contributes nothing to the total antirachitic activity. There is no evidence to support the presence of appreciable amounts of water-soluble vitamin D in breast milk and thus the question of whether or not it needs to be supplemented so that breast-fed children receive the recommended 400 units daily still needs to be considered. It is probably fair to say that term infants of mothers with adequate dietary vitamin D can survive on unsupplemented breast milk without considerable deficiency in bone mineralisation. There may, however, be a case for giving vitamin D supplements to children of mothers without adequate dietary vitamin D, preterm infants, infants with pigmented skin, and those from deprived social backgrounds.— H. L. J. Makin *et al., Archs Dis. Childh.*, 1983, *58*, 750.

Further references to the use of vitamin D in newborn infants: R. C. Tsang, *Lancet*, 1983, *1*, 1370; O. G. Brooke, *Archs Dis. Childh.*, 1983, *58*, 573.

See also under Human Requirements, above.

For reference to the use of vitamin D in the treatment of hypoparathyroidism in pregnancy, see under Hypoparathyroidism, above.

Rickets of prematurity. Results from a study in low-birthweight preterm infants indicated that inadequate vitamin D supplementation did not lead to the development of rickets.— N. McIntosh *et al., Archs Dis. Childh.*, 1982, *57*, 848. Comment.— C. McCowen and E. Hey (letter), *ibid.*, 1983, *58*, 476. Reply.— N. McIntosh *et al.* (letter), *ibid.*

Rickets is common in preterm infants of very low birthweight, even with adequate vitamin D supplementation, normal or high serum-25-hydroxyvitamin D concentrations, and apparently normal or high serum-1,25-dihydroxyvitamin D concentrations. Vitamin D supplements are certainly needed by preterm infants. Cholecalciferol or ergocalciferol in doses of at least 25 µg (1000 units), and possibly 50 µg (2000 units), may be required for maximum calcium absorption, and even then rickets may still occur. If the infant is ill as a result of rickets, however, healing may be more rapid if alfacalcidol is given in doses of 0.1 to 0.2 µg per kg daily. There is no evidence that the routine administration of alfacalcidol to preterm infants is necessary or desirable.— O. G. Brooke, *Archs Dis. Childh.*, 1983, *58*, 573. See also O. G. Brooke and A. Lucas, *ibid.*, 1985, *60*, 682.

For further reference to the treatment of rickets of prematurity see under Calcium Gluconate, p.1030.

Rickets, prophylaxis. Prophylactic supplementation with vitamin D may be required by children who are exposed little to sunlight, who are severely handicapped and housebound, or by children taking an anticonvulsant.— *Drug & Ther. Bull.*, 1984, *22*, 33.

Mean plasma concentrations of 25-hydroxyvitamin D were lower in 107 Asian children than in 221 non-Asian controls; lowest values were in Asian girls aged 13 to 15 years. An autumnal dose of ergocalciferol 2.5 mg for Asian adolescent girls is suggested.— A. E. O'Hare *et al., Archs Dis. Childh.*, 1984, *59*, 766.

Reduction in the prevalence of rickets in Asian children given long-term prophylactic low-dose vitamin D supplementation.— M. G. Dunnigan *et al., Br. med. J.*, 1985, *291*, 239.

See also under Rickets of Prematurity, above.

Preparations of Vitamin D Compounds

Calcifediol Capsules *(U.S.P.)*

Calciferol Injection *(B.P.)*. Contains ergocalciferol or cholecalciferol in ethyl oleate, 7.5 mg (300 000 units) in 1 mL. Sterilised by filtration. Store at a temperature not exceeding 25°. For intramuscular use only.

Calciferol Oral Solution *(B.P.)*. Calciferol Oral Drops; Calciferol Solution. Contains ergocalciferol or cholecalciferol in a suitable vegetable oil, such as arachis oil, 75 µg (3000 units) in 1 mL. It may be prepared by warming a 1% w/v suspension to 40°, bubbling carbon dioxide through it to facilitate solution, and adding a sufficient quantity of the oil. It is a pale yellow oily liquid with a slight but not rancid odour. Store at a temperature not exceeding 25° in well-filled, well-closed containers.

Calciferol Tablets *(B.P.)*. Contain ergocalciferol or cholecalciferol. Store at a temperature not exceeding 25°.

When High-strength Calciferol Tablets are prescribed or demanded, tablets containing 250 µg should be dispensed or supplied.

When Strong Calciferol Tablets are prescribed or demanded, it should be confirmed that tablets containing 1.25 mg are intended.

Calcium with Vitamin D Tablets *(B.P.C. 1973)*. See under Calcium Sodium Lactate, p.1031.

Dihydrotachysterol Capsules *(U.S.P.)*. Contain a solution of dihydrotachysterol in a suitable vegetable oil. Store in well-closed containers.

Dihydrotachysterol Oral Solution *(U.S.P.)*. Store in airtight containers.

Dihydrotachysterol Tablets *(U.S.P.)*. Store in well-closed containers.

Ergocalciferol Capsules *(U.S.P.)*. Usually an edible vegetable oil solution of ergocalciferol, encapsulated with gelatin. Store in airtight containers.

Ergocalciferol Oral Solution *(U.S.P.)*. Contains ergocalciferol in an edible vegetable oil, in polysorbate 80, or in propylene glycol. Store in airtight containers.

Ergocalciferol Tablets *(U.S.P.)*. Store in airtight containers.

Proprietary Preparations of Vitamin D Compounds

AT 10 *(Sterling Research, UK)*. *Solution*, oily, dihydrotachysterol 250 µg/mL.

One-Alpha *(Leo, UK)*. *Capsules*, alfacalcidol 0.25 and 1 µg.
Solution, alfacalcidol 0.2 µg/mL.

Rocaltrol *(Roche, UK)*. *Capsules*, calcitriol 0.25 and 0.5 µg.

Tachyrol *(Duphar, UK)*. *Tablets*, scored, dihydrotachysterol 200 µg.

Proprietary Names and Manufacturers of Vitamin D Compounds

Actifral D3 *(Duphar, Spain; Kali-Farma, Spain)*; AFI-d[2] forte *(Nyco, Norw.)*; Aqua-Sterogyl D3 *(Roussel, Belg.)*; AT 10 *(Winthrop, Austral.; Belg.; Bayer, Ger.; Bayer, Ital.; Neth.; Bayer, S.Afr.; Bayer, Switz.; Sterling Research, UK)*; Atecen *(Swed.)*; Calcamine *(Fr.)*; Calderol *(Organon,*

USA); D-cure *(SMB, Belg.)*; Dediol *(Rorer, Ital.)*; Dedrogyl *(Roussel, Fr.; Albert-Roussel, Ger.; Roussel, Switz.)*; Delakmin *(Albert-Roussel, Ger.)*; Deltar *(Arnaldi, Ital.)*; Detin D3 *(Spain)*; DHT *(Roxane, USA)*; Didrogyl *(Roussel Maestretti, Ital.)*; Dihydral *(Belg.; Iraq; Neth.; Spain)*; D_3-Vicotrat *(Heyl, Ger.)*; Diseon *(Smith Kline & French, Ital.)*; D-Mulsin *(Mucos, Ger.)*; Drisdol *(Winthrop, Canad.)*; D-Tracetten *(Albert-Roussel, Ger.)*; D-Vi-Sol *(Mead Johnson, Canad.)*; Dygratyl *(Ferrosan, Denm.; Ferrosan, Swed.)*; EinsAlpha *(Thomae, Ger.)*; Endo D *(Ital.)*; Esterosol *(Spain)*; Etalpha *(Leo, Denm.; Neth.; Leo, Norw.; Alter, Spain; Lövens, Swed.)*; Farmobion D_2 *(Ital.)*; Fiviton D *(Spain)*; Genevis D_2 *(Switz.)*; Hidroferol *(Juventus, Spain)*; Hytakerol *(Winthrop, Canad.; Winthrop-Breon, USA)*; Iper D_3 *(Zambon, Ital.)*; Neo-Dohyfral D_3 *(Philips-Duphar, Belg.; Duphar, Neth.)*; One-Alpha *(Leo, Canad.; Eire; Lennon, S.Afr.; Leo, UK)*; Ostelin *(Glaxo, Austral.; Glaxo, Ital.)*; Radiosterina *(Ital.)*; Radiostol *(Allen & Hanburys, Canad.)*; Raquiferol *(Arg.)*; Rocaltrol *(Aust.; Roche, Austral.; Belg.; Roche, Canad.; Roche, Denm.; Roche, Fr.; Roche, Ger.; Roche, Ital.; Roche, Norw.; Roche, S.Afr.; Roche, Spain; Roche, Swed.; Roche, Switz.; Roche, UK; Roche, USA)*; Sterogyl *(Roussel, Austral.; Belg.; Roussel, Fr.; S.Afr.; Roussel, Spain; Switz.; Roussel, UK)*; Tachyrol *(Duphar, UK)*; Tridelta *(Ceccarelli, Ital.)*; Un-alfa *(Leo, Fr.)*; Vi-De-3 *(Sandoz, S.Afr.; Wander, Switz.)*; Vidue *(Ital.)*; Vigantol *(E. Merck, Ger.; Igoda, Spain)*; Vigantoletten *(E. Merck, Ger.)*; Vigantolo *(Ital.)*; Vigorsan *(Albert-Roussel, Ger.)*; Vitaendil D-3 *(Boizot, Spain)*; Vitanoxi D-2 *(Spain)*; Vitavera D *(Spain)*.

Multivitamin and mineral preparations containing vitamin D are included in the lists on pp.1289-93. The following names have been used for preparations containing vitamin D and not considered to be a multivitamin or mineral preparation—Cal-Bid *(Geriatric Pharm. Corp., USA)*; Calcigard *(Advanced Medical Nutrition, USA)*; Calcite D-500 *(Riva, Canad.)*; Glucaloids *(Ingram & Bell, Canad.)*; Morsep *(Napp, UK)*.

7893-p

Vitamin E

Alpha Tocopherols.

Pharmacopoeias. In *Arg., Aust., Br., Braz., Chin., Cz., Egypt., Eur., Fr., Ger., Hung., Ind., It., Jpn, Jug., Neth., Nord., Pol., Roum., Rus., Swiss,* and *U.S.* Also in *B.P. Vet.* The nomenclature in some pharmacopoeias is confusing.

Alpha Tocopheryl Acetate (*B.P.*) (α-Tocopheryl Acetate; $C_{31}H_{52}O_3$=472.8) is *all-rac-α*-tocopherol acetate. It is a clear, slightly greenish-yellow, viscous oily liquid. It is practically **insoluble** in water, freely soluble in dehydrated alcohol, acetone, chloroform, ether, and fixed oils, and soluble in alcohol.

Vitamin E (*U.S.P.*) includes the following: *d-* or *dl*-alpha tocopherol ($C_{29}H_{50}O_2$); *d-* or *dl*-alpha tocopheryl acetate ($C_{31}H_{52}O_3$); *d-* or *dl*-alpha tocopheryl acid succinate ($C_{33}H_{54}O_5$). It is practically odourless. The alpha tocopherols and alpha tocopheryl acetate occur as clear, yellow, or greenish yellow, viscous oils. *d*-Alpha tocopheryl acetate may solidify in the cold. Alpha tocopheryl acid succinate occurs as a white powder; the *d*-isomer melts at about 75° and the *dl*-form melts at about 70°. The alpha tocopherols are unstable to air and to light, particularly when in alkaline media. The esters are stable to air and to light, but are unstable to alkali; the acid succcinate is also unstable when held molten. Alpha tocopheryl acid succinate is insoluble in water; slightly soluble in alkaline solutions; soluble in alcohol, ether, acetone, and vegetable oils; very soluble in chloroform. The other forms of vitamin E are insoluble in water; soluble in alcohol; miscible with ether, acetone, vegetable oils, and chloroform.

Vitamin E should be **stored** in airtight containers; *d-* or *dl*-alpha tocopherol should be stored in an atmosphere of inert gas. Protect from light.

STABILITY IN SOLUTION. A review of the compatibility and stability of components of total parenteral nutrition solutions when mixed in 1- or 3-litre flexible containers. Vitamin E may bind strongly to plastic which can lead to significant losses to the bag and administration set. Vitamin E losses from paediatric TPN mixtures have been estimated to be about 30 to 36% over a 24-hour administration period. The quantity of vitamin E delivered depends on infusion rate, type of administration set, composition of mixture, and total volume infused.— M. C. Allwood, *J. clin. Hosp. Pharm.*, 1984, *9*, 181.

Units

Though the potency of preparations of vitamin E is still sometimes expressed in units, the International standard for vitamin E was discontinued in 1956. The International unit was the activity contained in 1 mg of a standard preparation of α-tocopheryl acetate.

The *U.S.P.* states that in expressing vitamin E activity of tocopherol products, the following equivalents of 1 mg are employed:
dl-alpha tocopheryl acetate, 1 unit;
dl-alpha tocopheryl acid succinate, 0.89 unit;
dl-alpha tocopherol, 1.1 units;
d-alpha tocopheryl acetate, 1.36 units;
d-alpha tocopherol, 1.49 units;
d-alpha tocopheryl acid succinate, 1.21 units.

Adverse Effects and Precautions

Vitamin E is usually well tolerated. Large doses may cause diarrhoea, abdominal pain, and other gastro-intestinal disturbances, and have also been reported to cause fatigue and weakness. Contact dermatitis has occurred following topical application.

Vitamin E has been reported to antagonise the effects of vitamin K leading to an increase in blood clotting time in predisposed patients such as those taking oral anticoagulants or oestrogens. However, the clinical significance of these effects is not known.

Absorption and Fate

Absorption of vitamin E from the gastro-intestinal tract is dependent on the presence of bile. It enters the bloodstream via the lymph, is widely distributed to all tissues, and stored in adipose tissue. Some vitamin E is metabolised in the liver to glucuronides of tocopheronic acid and its γ-lactone and is excreted in the urine, but most of a dose is slowly excreted in the bile. Vitamin E appears in breast milk but is poorly transferred across the placenta.

A study of the pharmacokinetics of *d*-alpha tocopherol in a water-soluble base in 10 healthy subjects.— N. E. Bateman and D. A. Uccellini, *J. Pharm. Pharmac.*, 1985, *37*, 728.

Human Requirements

The daily requirement of vitamin E has not been clearly defined but is probably about 3 to 15 mg. There appears to be no evidence that supplements are required in subjects on balanced diets. Requirements increase with increased dietary amounts of polyunsaturated fatty acids. Vitamin E is widely distributed in food. The richest sources are vegetable oils especially wheat-germ oil, sunflower oil, and cottonseed oil; cereals and eggs are also good sources. It does not appear to be destroyed by cooking processes.

Estimated acceptable daily intake as an antoxidant: up to 2 mg per kg body-weight of α-tocopherol or mixed tocopherol concentrate (as α-tocopherol).— Seventeenth Report of FAO/WHO Expert Committee on Food Additives, *Tech. Rep. Ser. Wld Hlth Org. No. 539*, 1974.

In the United Kingdom deficiency of vitamin E is rare. Vitamin E occurs in sufficient quantity in a large number of foods. Therefore, in the light of present knowledge and in the context of diet in the *UK*, recommended daily intakes for vitamin E have not been set.— Recommended Daily Amounts of Food Energy and Nutrients for Groups of People in the United Kingdom, Report by the Committee on Medical Aspects of Food Policy, *Report on Health and Social Subjects No.15*, London, HM Stationery Office, 1979.

Human milk contains 2 to 5 units of vitamin E per litre and provides an adequate intake for nursing infants. Milk formulas used for feeding low-birth-weight infants should provide 0.7 units for 0.42 MJ and at least 1 unit per g of linoleic acid. An oral supplement of 5 units of water-soluble vitamin E is also recommended. For children an intake of 5 units daily at 9 kg body-weight increasing to 12 units at 40 kg should be satisfactory in diets providing 4 to 7% of calories as linoleic acid. Most adult diets in the USA provide adequate amounts of vitamin E; balanced diets providing about 10 to 20 units and high-fat diets about 25 units. The increased calorie intake in pregnancy should normally be accompanied by sufficient additional vitamin E.— *Recommended Dietary Allowances*, 9th Edn, Washington, The National Research Council, 1980, p. 63.

The recommendation that the amount of α-tocopherol should be such as to ensure that the ratio of α-tocopherol (mg) to polyunsaturated fatty acids (g) is at least 0.4 : 1.0. The recommendation that an infant feed should contain not less than 3 µg α-tocopherol per mL of reconstituted feed, i.e., the amount found on average in mature human milk.— Artificial Feeds for the Young Infant: 1980, Report of the Working Party on the Composition of Foods for Infants and Young Children, Committee on Medical Aspects of Food Policy, *Report on Health and Social Subjects, 18*, London, HM Stationery Office, 1980.

Uses and Administration

The biochemical role of vitamin E, a fat-soluble vitamin, is not completely understood. It acts as an antoxidant for certain fats and is involved in metabolic reactions.

Vitamin E deficiency develops when the dietary intake is inadequate. Deficiency is rare but may occur in patients with malabsorption syndromes or genetic blood disorders, or in premature infants on unsupplemented artificial feeds. Deficiency in humans has been associated with the development of neurological syndromes similar to those produced by vitamin E deprivation in *animals*.

Vitamin E is used in the treatment and prevention of vitamin E deficiency. It is usually given by mouth, generally the preferred route, but may also be given by intramuscular or intravenous routes. It may be given as *d* or *dl* alpha tocopherol or as the respective acetates or acid succinates. The racemate has also been given as the calcium succinate. Other compounds with vitamin-E activity include other tocopherols and tocotrienols. Vitamin E has been used in the treatment of intermittent claudication and many other disorders but there is little evidence of beneficial effect. Doses used in intermittent claudication have ranged from 300 to 600 mg daily by mouth for periods of 3 months or longer.

A review of vitamin therapy in non-deficiency states. Vitamin E has been tried in the treatment of various disorders including angina pectoris, hypercholesterolaemia, intermittent claudication, fibrocystic breast disease, cancer, nocturnal leg cramps, porphyria cutanea tarda, discoid lupus erythematosus, epidermolysis bullosa, post-herpetic neuralgia, osteoarthritis, contracture formation around silicone breast implants, Raynaud's phenomenon, and polymyositis. Therapeutic doses of vitamin E may also protect genetically defective red blood cells against *in-vivo* oxidative damage in patients with β-thalassaemia major, glutathione synthetase deficiency, and glucose-6-phosphate dehydrogenase deficiency. Vitamin E has also been claimed to enhance athletic performance and to improve sexual arousal and behaviour. The beneficial effects in these conditions have not been confirmed in clinically-controlled studies.— L. Ovesen, *Drugs*, 1984, *27*, 148.

DEFICIENCY STATES. A discussion of the rationale for vitamin E therapy in which the vitamin may have positive clinical effects. It should be recognised at the outset that nutritional inadequacy or frank deficiency of vitamin E is only found in patients with various genetic or acquired diseases, with the exception of premature children, in whom the deficiency may be iatrogenous.— J. G. Bieri *et al.*, *New Engl. J. Med.*, 1983, *308*, 1063.

Vitamin E deficiency is common in patients with steatorrhoea from any cause but seems harmless except perhaps in children with biliary atresia, abetalipoproteinaemia, or cystic fibrosis in whom it may cause spinal cord damage.— *Drug & Ther. Bull.*, 1984, *22*, 33.

Chronic vitamin E deficiency may cause neurological syndromes due to lack of its protective antoxidant action. This may lead to peroxidation of membrane phospholipids rich in polyunsaturated fatty acids. Interaction between vitamin E and other exogenous and endogenous peroxidants and antoxidants (e.g. ascorbic acid, cupric ions, selenium) may influence the protective function of the vitamin. The possibility of vitamin E deficiency should be thought of in any condition associated with lipid malabsorption, and also in spinocerebellar syndromes of unknown cause.— *Lancet*, 1986, *1*, 423. Comment.— A. Burns and T. Holland (letter), *ibid.*, 805.

Further references: D. P. R. Muller *et al.*, *Lancet*, 1983, *1*, 225; H. J. Dworken, *Ann. intern. Med.*, 1983, *98*, 253; D. P. R. Muller, *Postgrad. med. J.*, 1986, *62*, 107; M. G. Traber *et al.*, *New Engl. J. Med.*, 1987, *317*, 262.

Individual reports of the beneficial use of vitamin E in the treatment of neurological symptoms associated with low serum concentrations of vitamin E: J. G. Bieri *et al.*, *Ann. intern. Med.*, 1984, *100*, 238 (abetalipoproteinaemia; administration with vitamin A); R. A. Hegele and A. Angel, *Can. med. Ass. J.*, 1985, *132*, 41 (abetalipoproteinaemia); A. E. Harding *et al.*, *New Engl. J. Med.*, 1985, *313*, 32 (in deficiency where there was no evidence of generalised fat malabsorption); R. J. Sckol *et al.*, *ibid.*, 1580 (chronic cholestasis in children); P. Runge *et al.*, *Br. J. Ophthal.*, 1986, *70*, 166 (abetalipoproteinaemia); R. J. Stead *et al.*, *Gut*, 1986, *27*, 714 (cystic fibrosis); G. Davidai *et al.*, *Archs Dis. Childh.*, 1986, *61*, 901 (exocrine pancreatic failure).

NEONATAL HAEMORRHAGE. In a randomised, controlled study involving 228 premature neonates, administration of vitamin E 20 mg per kg body-weight by intramuscular injection for the first 3 days of life was associated with a rise in plasma-vitamin E concentration and with a reduction in hydrogen peroxide haemolysis *in vitro*. Overall mortality was unaffected by vitamin E supplementation, but among babies who died the frequency of intraventricular or parenchymal haemorrhage was significantly lower in the supplemented group; the precise contribution of haemorrhage to mortality is unclear. Surviving supplemented babies had a lower frequency of intraventricular and parenchymal haemorrhage. The importance of the latter observation cannot be judged until the neurodevelopment of survivors is assessed.— S. Sinha *et al.*, *Lancet*, 1987, *1*, 466. Comment.— R. J. Welch and D. W. A. Milligan (letter), *ibid.*, 1041.

Further references: M. L. Chiswick *et al.*, *Br. med. J.*, 1983, *287*, 81. Correction.— *ibid.*, 383.

RETINOPATHY OF PREMATURITY. The hope that vitamin E would eliminate retinopathy of prematurity has waxed and waned since the late 1940s. The proposition has been subjected to a number of randomised clinical trials in recent years, but unfortunately there is still no convincing answer. There is insufficient information available on the administration of vitamin E to premature infants, and many unresolved questions concerning important side-effects.— W. A. Silverman, *Archs Dis. Childh.*, 1986, *61*, 522.

Some studies indicating that administration of vitamin E in high doses reduces the severity of retinopathy of prematurity in preterm infants requiring oxygen: H. M. Hittner *et al.*, *New Engl. J. Med.*, 1981, *305*, 1365 (oral administration); N. N. Finer *et al.*, *Lancet*, 1982, *1*, 1087 (intramuscular administration).

Preparations

Vitamin E Capsules *(U.S.P.)*. Capsules containing Vitamin E or Vitamin E Preparation.

Vitamin E Preparation *(U.S.P.)*. A combination of a single form of vitamin E with one or more inert substances; it may be in liquid or solid form. Preparations containing the *dl*-form may also contain a small amount of the *d*-form occurring as a minor constituent of an added substance.

Proprietary Preparations

Ephynal *(Roche, UK)*. *Tablets*, tocopheryl acetate 3 and 10 mg.
Tablets, scored, tocopheryl acetate 50 and 200 mg.

Vita-E *(Bioglan, UK)*.
Gels (capsules), *d*-alpha tocopheryl acetate 75, 200, and 400 units.
Gelucaps (tablets), *d*-alpha tocopheryl acetate 75 units.
Tablets, *d*-alpha tocopheryl succinate 50 units.

Proprietary Names and Manufacturers

AFI-E *(Nyco, Norw.)*; Aquasol E *(Rorer, Canad.; Armour, USA)*; Atlagran K 70 *(Keimdiät, Ger.: Thomson & Joseph, UK)*; Atlagran-D *(Keimdiät, Ger. : Thomson & Joseph, UK)*; Auxigran *(Keimdiät, Ger. : Thomson & Joseph, UK)*; Auxina E *(Gayoso Wellcome, Spain)*; Bioglan Micelle E *(Bioglan, Austral.)*; Dal-E *(Dal-Vita, Austral.)*; Daltose *(Canad.)*; Davitamon E *(Neth.)*; Detulin *(Woelm, Ger.)*; Dextamina-E Fuerte *(Spain)*; Dif-Vitamin E *(Andreu, Spain)*; E Perle *(INTES, Ital.)*; E Sir *(Farmades, Ital.)*; E-Caps *(Parke, Davis, Austral.)*; Eferol *(Forest Pharmaceuticals, USA)*; Egermol *(UPB, Belg.)*; E-Grandelan 8470 *(Keimdiät, Ger. : Thomson & Joseph, UK)*; E-Grandelat *(Ger.)*; Embial *(E. Merck, Ger.)*; E-Mulsin *(Mucos, Ger.)*; Ephynal *(Arg.; Austral.; Belg.; Roche, Denm.; Roche, Fr.; Roche, Ger.; Roche, Ital.; Roche, S.Afr.; Roche, Spain; Roche, Swed.; Roche, Switz.; Roche, UK)*; Eplonat *(Nattermann, Ger.)*; Eprolin *(Dista, Switz.)*; Eta-Monovit *(Ital.)*; E-Tap-S *(Jpn)*; Eusovit *(Wolfer, Ger.)*; Everol *(Kin, Spain)*; E-Vicotrat *(Heyl, Ger.)*; E-vimin *(Astra, Swed.)*; Evion *(E. Merck, Ger.; Bracco, Ital.; Igoda, Spain)*; E-Vit *(IBP, Ital.)*; Evit *(Chefaro, Ger.)*; Evitina *(CT, Ital.)*; E-vitum *(Lipha, Ital.)*; Farmobion E *(Ital.)*; Fertilan *(Denm.)*; Fertilvit *(Lafare, Ital.)*; Fravit E *(Francia Farm., Ital.)*; Godabion E *(Igoda, Spain)*; Ido-E *(Ferrosan, Norw.; Ferrosan, Swed.)*; Ilitia *(Biologici Italia, Ital.)*; Invite E *(Nelson, Austral.)*; Juvela *(Jpn)*; Lethopherol *(Nutrition Control Products, USA)*; Multaben *(Priorin, Switz.)*; Na-To-Caps *(SIT, Ital.)*; Optovit *(Hermes, Ger.)*; Pheryl E *(Miller, USA)*; Propan E *(Propan, S.Afr.)*; Redoxogran *(Keimdiät, Ger. : Thomson & Joseph, UK)*; Sanavitan *(Bottger, Ger.)*; Solucap E *(Jamieson-McKames, USA)*; Spondyvit *(Efeka, Ger.)*; Tocerol *(Prosana, Austral.)*; Toco 500 *(Pharma 2000, Fr.)*; Tocoferina E *(Lisapharma, Ital.)*; Tocogen *(Gentili, Ital.)*; Tocomine *(Clin Midy, Fr.)*; Tocopherex *(Ital.)*; Tocovite *(Austral.)*; Tokols *(USA)*; Vita-E *(Bioglan, Austral.; Bioglan, UK)*; Vitagutt *(Schwarzhaupt, Ger.)*; Vitamin E Biorganic *(Gisand, Switz.)*; Viteril *(Panthox & Burck, Ital.)*; ZE Caps *(Everett, USA)*.

The following names have been used for multi-ingredient preparations containing vitamin E—Efamol *(Efamol, Canad.; Britannia Health, UK)*; Efamol Marine *(Britannia Health, UK)*; Efamol Plus *(Britannia Health, UK)*; Epatrol *(Kramer, USA)*; EPOC *(Evening Primrose Oil Co., UK)*; Gammaoil *(Quest, UK)*; Lazer *(Pedinol, USA)*; Naudicelle *(Bio-Oil Research, UK)*; Naudicelle Plus *(Bio-Oil Research, UK)*; Q-Vel *(Rugby, USA)*; Super Gammaoil Marine *(Quest, UK)*.

For multi-ingredient preparations containing nutritional agents and vitamins, see p.1289.

7902-c

Vitamin K

The term vitamin K is used for a range of naphthoquinone compounds which are necessary for the biosynthesis of blood clotting factors. These include acetomenaphthone, menadiol, menadione, menatetrenone, and phytomenadione.

7904-a

Acetomenaphthone *(BAN)*.
Acetomenadione; Acetomenaph.; Menadiol Diacetate. 2-Methylnaphthalene-1,4-diyl diacetate.
$C_{15}H_{14}O_4$=258.3.

CAS — 573-20-6.

Pharmacopoeias. In *Ind.* and *Jug.*

7905-t

Menadiol Sodium Phosphate *(BANM)*.

Menadiol Sodium Diphosphate *(USAN)*; Menadiolum Solubile. 2-Methylnaphthalene-1,4-diyl bis(disodium phosphate) hexahydrate.
$C_{11}H_8Na_4O_8P_2,6H_2O$=530.2.

CAS — 6700-42-1; 131-13-5 (anhydrous); 481-85-6 (menadiol); 84-98-0 (menadiol diphosphate).

Pharmacopoeias. In *Arg.*, *Br.*, *Cz.*, and *U.S.*

A white to pink hygroscopic crystalline powder with a characteristic odour. **Soluble** 1 in less than 1 of water; practically insoluble in alcohol. A solution in water has a pH of about 8. The *U.S.P.* injection has a pH of 7.5 to 8.5. **Store** at a temperature not exceeding 8° in airtight containers. Protect from light.

7906-x

Menadione *(BAN, USAN)*.

Menadionum; Menaph.; Menaphthene; Menaphthone; Methylnaphthochinonum; Vitamin K_3. 2-Methyl-1,4-naphthoquinone.
$C_{11}H_8O_2$=172.2.

CAS — 58-27-5.

Pharmacopoeias. In *Arg.*, *Aust.*, *Belg.*, *Br.*, *Braz.*, *Eur.*, *Fr.*, *Ger.*, *Ind.*, *Int.*, *It.*, *Mex.*, *Neth.*, *Swiss*, *Turk.*, and *U.S.*

A pale yellow or bright yellow practically odourless crystalline powder. It decomposes on exposure to light.

Practically **insoluble** in water. The *B.P.* specifies: sparingly soluble in alcohol and methyl alcohol; soluble in ether; freely soluble in chloroform. The *U.S.P.* specifies: soluble 1 in 60 of alcohol; sparingly soluble in chloroform; soluble in vegetable oils. **Store** in well-closed containers. Protect from light.

CAUTION. *The powder is irritating to the respiratory tract and to the skin. The alcoholic solution has vesicant properties.*

7907-r

Menadione Sodium Bisulphite
Kavitanum; Menadione Sodium Bisulfite *(rINN)*; Menaph. Sod. Bisulphite; Menaphthone Sodium Bisulphite; Methylnaphthochinonumnatrium Bisulfurosum; Vikasolum; Vitamin K_3 Sodium Bisulphite. Sodium 1,2,3,4-tetrahydro-2-methyl-1,4-dioxonaphthalene-2-sulphonate trihydrate.
$C_{11}H_8O_2NaHSO_3,3H_2O$=330.3.

CAS — 130-37-0 (anhydrous); 6147-37-1 (trihydrate).

Pharmacopoeias. In *Arg.*, *Belg.*, *Braz.*, *Hung.*, *Jug.*, *Nord.*, *Pol.*, *Port.*, and *Rus. Braz.* specifies a mixture containing 63 to 75% menadione sodium bisulphite and 30 to 38% sodium bisulphite. *Nord.* specifies $2H_2O$.

7903-k

Phytomenadione *(BAN, rINN)*.

Methylphytylnaphthochinonum; Phylloquinone; Phytomenad.; Phytonadione *(USAN)*; Vitamin K_1. 2-Methyl-3-phytyl-1,4-naphthoquinone.
$C_{31}H_{46}O_2$=450.7.

CAS — 84-80-0.

Pharmacopoeias. In *Arg.*, *Br.*, *Braz.*, *Chin.*, *Cz.*, *Egypt.*, *Fr.*, *Jpn*, *Turk.*, and *U.S.* Also in *B.P. Vet.*

A clear, deep yellow to amber, very viscous, odourless or almost odourless oil which is stable in air but decomposes on exposure to light.

B.P. **solubilities** are: practically insoluble in water; soluble 1 in 70 of alcohol; freely soluble in chloroform, ether, and fixed oils. *U.S.P.* solubilities are: insoluble in water; soluble in dehydrated alcohol, chloroform, ether, and vegetable oils; slightly soluble in alcohol. The *B.P.* injection has a pH of 5.0 to 7.5; the *U.S.P.* injection has a pH of 3.5 to 7.0. Aqueous dispersions for injection may be **sterilised** by filtration. **Store** in airtight containers. Protect from light. Aqueous dispersions of phytomenadione for injection should not be allowed to freeze.

INCOMPATIBILITY. A review of the compatibilities of nutritional agents and drugs in parenteral nutrition solutions. Phytomenadione is reported to be visually compatible for 24 hours in parenteral nutrition solutions containing typical additives. Although concern has been expressed about the instability of phytomenadione to light, only 10 to 15% loss of potency occurs over 24 hours on exposure to sunlight or fluorescent light. Phytomenadione passes through an inline filter with negligible loss.— P. W. Niemiec and T. W. Vanderveen, *Am. J. Hosp. Pharm.*, 1984, *41*, 893.

Adverse Effects and Precautions

Too rapid intravenous administration of phytomenadione has caused severe reactions, including facial flushing, sweating, chest constriction and chest pain, dyspnoea, cyanosis, and cardiovascular collapse; fatalities have been reported. It is not clear if these reactions were caused by phytomenadione itself or by the surfactant included in the formulation. Pain and swelling may occur at the injection site following administration of phytomenadione. Allergic skin reactions have been reported following intramuscular or subcutaneous injection of phytomenadione.

Administration of menadione and its water-soluble derivatives such as menadiol sodium phosphate to neonates, especially premature infants, has been associated with the development of haemolytic anaemia, hyperbilirubinaemia, kernicterus, and haemoglobinaemia. These compounds have also been reported to cause haemolysis in patients with glucose-6-phosphate dehydrogenase deficiency.

Cerebral arterial thrombosis developed in 2 patients with malabsorption syndromes due to coeliac disease during treatment with vitamin K for severe deficiency of vitamin-K-dependent coagulation factors.— J. Florholmen *et al., Br. med. J.*, 1980, *281*, 541.

INTERACTIONS. For reference to the reduction of anticoagulant activity by acetomenaphthone and phytomenadione, see under Warfarin, p.348.

Absorption and Fate

The fat-soluble vitamin K compounds phytomenadione and menadione require the presence of bile for their absorption from the gastro-intestinal tract; the water-soluble derivatives of menadione can be absorbed in the absence of bile. Vitamin K accumulates mainly in the liver but is stored in the body only for short periods of time. Vitamin K does not appear to cross the placenta readily and it is poorly distributed into breast milk. Phytomenadione is rapidly metabolised to more polar metabolites and is excreted in bile and urine as glucuronide and sulphate conjugates.

Human Requirements

The minimum daily requirements of vitamin K are not clearly defined but an intake of about 2 µg per kg body-weight daily appears to be adequate. Vitamin K requirements in normal adults can be met from the average diet and from the synthesis of menaquinones (also known as vitamin K_2) by bacterial action in the intestine. Vitamin K occurs naturally as phytomenadione (vitamin K_1) which is present in many foods, especially leafy green vegetables such as cabbage and spinach, and is also present in beef liver, cows' milk, egg yolk, and some cereals.

In the United Kingdom deficiency of vitamin K is rare. Vitamin K occurs in sufficient quantity in a large number of foods. Therefore, in the light of present knowledge and in the context of diet in the *UK*, recommended daily intakes for vitamin K have not been set.— Recommended Daily Amounts of Food Energy and Nutrients for Groups of People in the United Kingdom, Report by the Committee on Medical Aspects of Food Policy, *Report on Health and Social Subjects No.15*, London, HM Stationery Office, 1979.

No specific recommended dietary allowance could be made for vitamin K. A daily intake of 2 µg per kg body-weight appeared satisfactory. Even if intestinal synthesis contributed little to the intake, most diets could still provide adequate amounts and this included both breast- and bottle-fed infants; current artificial feeds contain 4 µg per 0.42 MJ and breast milk 15 µg per litre.— *Recommended Dietary Allowances*, 9th Edn, Washington, The National Research Council, 1980, p. 69.

The suggestion that an infant feed should contain not less than 15 ng per mL vitamin K.— Artificial Feeds for the Young Infant: 1980, Report of the Working Party on the Composition of Foods for Infants and Young Children, Committee on Medical Aspects of Food Policy, *Report on Health and Social Subjects, 18*, London, HM Stationery Office, 1980.

Uses and Administration

Vitamin K is an essential cofactor in the hepatic synthesis of prothrombin (factor II) and other blood clotting factors (factors VII, IX, and X). Vitamin K deficiency may develop in patients with malabsorption syndromes, obstructive jaundice, or in those receiving treatment with coumarin anticoagulants which interfere with vitamin K metabolism. Deficiency leads to the development of hypoprothrombinaemia, in which the clotting time of the blood is prolonged and spontaneous bleeding can occur. Deficiency may also occur in neonates and can lead to a syndrome known as haemorrhagic disease of the newborn.

Vitamin K compounds are used in the treatment and prevention of haemorrhage associated with vitamin K deficiency. The dose of vitamin K should be carefully controlled by prothrombin-time estimations.

Phytomenadione is a naturally occurring vitamin K substance. It is the only vitamin K compound used to reverse hypoprothrombinaemia and haemorrhage caused by anticoagulant overdose. It is not effective in overdosage with heparin. Phytomenadione may be given by mouth, the preferred route, but may also be administered by subcutaneous, intramuscular, or slow intravenous injection. It may be given by mouth or by intramuscular injection in doses of up to 20 mg, repeated after 8 to 12 hours if necessary. In severe bleeding it may be given intravenously at a rate not greater than 1 mg per minute in doses of 2.5 to 10 mg; up to 20 mg has been given. For further details see p.344. In some countries not all commercial injections are suitable for intravenous use.

In the treatment of haemorrhagic disease of the newborn phytomenadione may be given in a dose of 1 mg intramuscularly and, if necessary, further doses may be given 8-hourly. As a prophylactic measure, a single dose of 0.5 to 1 mg may be given intramuscularly to the newborn infant.

Menadiol sodium phosphate is a water-soluble derivative of menadione; menadione is a synthetic lipid-soluble vitamin K analogue. It may be used for the prevention of vitamin K deficiency in patients with malabsorption syndromes. It is given in usual doses of about 10 mg daily by mouth.

For reference to the use of vitamin K in the reversal of the hypoprothrombinaemia caused by certain cephalosporins, and to the role of cephalosporin-induced vitamin K deficiency in the aetiology of hypoprothrombinaemia, see under Cephamandole Sodium, p.179.

A review of vitamin therapy in non-deficiency states. The only rational use of vitamin K is correction of bleeding tendency due to its deficiency. However, there may be a future for vitamin K in the treatment of non-deficiency disorders, in that it has been shown to inhibit the growth of mammalian tumour cells in culture and to interfere with normal leucocyte function *in vitro*.— L. Ovesen, *Drugs*, 1984, *27*, 148.

ACTION. References to the action of vitamin K and the role of vitamin K-dependent coagulation proteins: P. A. Friedman, *New Engl. J. Med.*, 1984, *310*, 1458; L. H. Clouse and P. C. Comp, *ibid.*, 1986, *314*, 1298 (protein C).

For reference to the antagonistic actions of warfarin with vitamin K and the vitamin K-dependent coagulation proteins, see under Warfarin, p.348.

HAEMORRHAGIC DISEASE OF THE NEWBORN. Although haemorrhagic disease of the newborn is preventable, deaths are increasing because more babies are being breast fed with consequent delay (compared with bottle feeding) in the development of intestinal flora responsible for producing vitamin K. All newborn babies should receive phytomenadione 1 mg, for which there are no contra-indications. Even babies with glucose-6-phosphate dehydrogenase deficiency can be given this dose of phytomenadione without risk of haemolysis. A suitable oral preparation is not yet available but the injectable preparation can be given orally and is well absorbed.— D. A. Curnock, *Prescribers' J.*, 1985, *25*, 62.

A further recommendation that all newborn infants should receive vitamin K prophylaxis. Prophylaxis by the oral route is potentially less certain than that by the intramuscular route as the dose may not be swallowed, absorbed, or metabolised, particularly if the infant has underlying disease yet undiagnosed, for example cystic fibrosis. An oral dose of phytomenadione 1 mg gives peak plasma concentrations of about 300 times the normal adult concentrations (which in turn exceed cord blood concentrations by a factor of 10^{13}) but only 5% of those achieved after intramuscular injection of the same dose. If the intramuscular dose is not considered to be excessive it could be inferred that a larger dose should be used orally for equally effective prophylaxis. It is not certain, however, that peak plasma concentrations after prophylaxis relate to either the total amount of phytomenadione absorbed or retained, and there is good evidence that a 1-mg oral dose gives protection. If considered necessary an increased oral load of phytomenadione could be achieved in several ways, including a larger single dose at birth, repeated oral doses for breast-fed infants, or supplementation of breast feeding mothers to increase the vitamin K content of their milk. The latter methods, requiring repeated doses to either baby or mother, have the attraction that effective prophylaxis may be more reliably extended into the second and third months of life, when there is still risk of late onset haemorrhagic disease and stores from a single prophylactic dose at birth may be exhausted. Compliance with a regimen of repeated doses, however, may be poor and the authors' preference is to give a single prophylactic dose at birth. For reasons of acceptability to parents, safety, convenience, and cost the authors currently use a 1-mg oral dose of phytomenadione for routine prophylaxis and continue to use intramuscular prophylaxis in infants at special risk from haemorrhagic disease of the newborn—that is, those born prematurely or admitted to the special care baby unit for any other reason and those born by traumatic delivery or to mothers taking oral antiepileptics.— J. H. Tripp and A. W. McNinch, *Archs Dis. Childh.*, 1987, *62*, 436. Comment, and the view that intramuscular administration of phytomenadione is more likely to prevent haemorrhagic disease of the newborn than oral administration.— B. L. Priestley (letter), *ibid.*, 979.

The long-term consequences of high blood concentrations of vitamin K immediately after birth are not known; kernicterus was linked with excessive doses of menadiol sodium phosphate but so far as is known that is the only long-term problem reported. It is somewhat of a philosophical decision balancing the possible mistakes made by the routine injection of vitamin K to all newborn babies against the odd case of haemorrhagic disease of the newborn still occurring when adequate blood concentrations have not been achieved by the oral route. The decision must be taken locally depending on the practicalities.— J. G. Bissenden (letter), *Br. med. J.*, 1987, *294*, 430.

Further references: A. W. McNinch *et al., Lancet*, 1983, *1*, 1089; G. C. Bridgman (letter), *ibid.*, 1279; C. M. Verity *et al.* (letter), *ibid.*, 1439; S. Ware and M. Mills (letter), *ibid.*,; P. A. Lane and W. E. Hathaway, *J. Pediat.*, 1985, *106*, 351; A. W. McNinch *et al., Archs Dis. Childh.*, 1985, *60*, 814; I. A. Choonara and B. K. Park (letter), *ibid.*, 1203; A. W. McNinch *et al.* (letter), *ibid.;* R. von Kries *et al.* (letter), *Lancet*, 1985, *1*, 1035; B. A. Behrmann *et al., Can. med. Ass. J.*, 1985, *133*, 884; K. J. Robertson *et al., Intensive Therapy clin. Monit.*, 1987, *8*, 13; A. C. Fenton and P. G. F. Swift (letter), *ibid.*, 108; J. A. Sills (letter), *ibid.*, 110; K. J. Robertson and J. S. Forsyth (letter), *ibid.*

Diagnosis and testing. Significantly raised concentrations of PIVKA (protein induced by vitamin K absence), the circulating prothrombin precursor, in 16 adult epileptic patients on maintenance antiepileptic therapy, when compared with 10 controls, was presumptive evidence for an apparently subclinical coagulation defect similar to that found in vitamin K deficiency. There was no correlation with the particular antiepileptic used. These findings were considered to strengthen the case for antenatal vitamin K supplementation in pregnant epileptics.— V. A. Davies *et al., Lancet*, 1985, *1*, 126.

References to the methods used in the diagnosis of vitamin K deficiency in newborn infants: K. Motohara *et al., Lancet*, 1985, *2*, 242 (measurement of acarboxyprothrombin (PIVKA II) concentrations); R. von Kries *et al.* (letter), *ibid.*, 728 (measurement of PIVKA II); F. Forestier *et al.* (letter), *ibid.*, 729 (measurement of PIVKA II); R. von Kries *et al.* (letter), *ibid.*, 1421 (measurement of PIVKA II); D. Garrow *et al., Archs Dis. Childh.*, 1986, *61*, 349 (measurement of vitamin K-dependent clotting factors); K. Motohara *et al., ibid.*, 1987, *62*, 370 (measurement of PIVKA II); E. Ishii and K. Ueda (letter), *ibid.*, 540 (measurement of vitamin K-dependent clotting factors); R. von Kries *et al., ibid.*, 938 (measurement of PIVKA II and factor II clotting activity).

PRURITUS. In a preliminary study involving 19 patients with pruritus, 10 of whom had intrahepatic cholestasis,

5 extrahepatic cholestasis, and 4 lymphomas, parenteral administration of phytomenadione led to complete remission of pruritus in 12, and a clear improvement in 4. Response was poor or doubtful in 3 patients, all of whom had extrahepatic cholestasis.— F. J. Laso and J. Gonzalez-Macias (letter), *Lancet*, 1982, *2*, 394.

Preparations

Menadiol Sodium Diphosphate Injection *(U.S.P.)*. Contains menadiol sodium phosphate.

Menadione Injection *(U.S.P.)*. A sterile solution of menadione in oil.

Phytomenadione Injection *(B.P.)*. Vitamin K_1 Injection. If oil droplets have appeared or separation has occurred, it should not be used.

Phytonadione Injection *(U.S.P.)*. Contains phytomenadione with suitable solubilising and/or dispersing agents.

Menadiol Phosphate Tablets *(B.P.)*. Contain menadiol sodium phosphate. Potency is expressed in terms of menadiol phosphate.

Menadiol Sodium Diphosphate Tablets *(U.S.P.)*. Contain menadiol sodium phosphate.

Phytomenadione Tablets *(B.P.)*. Vitamin K_1 Tablets. To be chewed before swallowing or allowed to dissolve slowly in the mouth.

Phytonadione Tablets *(U.S.P.)*. Contain phytomenadione.

Proprietary Preparations

Konakion *(Roche, UK)*. *Tablets*, phytomenadione 10 mg. To be chewed or allowed to dissolve slowly in the mouth.

Injection, phytomenadione 1 mg/0.5 mL and 10 mg/mL in ampoules of 0.5 and 1 mL respectively.

Synkavit *(Roche, UK)*. *Tablets*, scored, menadiol sodium phosphate 12.63 mg equivalent to menadiol phosphate 10 mg.

Proprietary Names and Manufacturers of Vitamin K Compounds

Amisyn *(Armour, UK)*; Aquamephyton *(Austral.; Merck Sharp & Dohme, Canad.; Neth.; Merck Sharp & Dohme, UK; Merck Sharp & Dohme, USA)*; Bilkaby *(Bailly, Fr.)*; K Thrombin *(Fawns & McAllan, Austral.)*; Kaergona *(IBYS, Spain)*; Kappadione *(USA)*; Karanum *(Igoda, Spain)*; Katerap *(Sintyal, Arg.)*; Kaytwo *(Jpn)*; Kaywan *(Jpn)*; Kephton-Two *(Jpn)*; Konakion *(Arg.; Roche, Austral.; Belg.; Roche, Canad.; Roche, Denm.; Roche, Ger.; Roche, Ital.; Neth.; Roche, Norw.; Roche, S.Afr.; Roche, Spain; Roche, Swed.; Roche, Switz.; Roche, UK; Roche, USA)*; Menadion *(DAK, Denm.)*; Mephyton *(Canad.; Merck Sharp & Dohme, USA)*; Nuvit *(Propan, S.Afr.)*; Synkavit *(Arg.; Austral.; Belg.; S.Afr.; Switz.; Roche, UK)*; Synkavite *(Roche, Canad.)*; Synkayvite *(Roche, USA)*; Vita-K1 *(Jpn)*; Vita-Noxi K *(Spain)*; Zimema-K *(Spain)*.

The following names have been used for multi-ingredient preparations containing vitamin K compounds— Chilblain Treatment Dellipsoids D 27 *(Pilsworth, UK)*; Pernivit *(Duncan, Flockhart, UK)*; Vi-Pernic *(Sigma, Austral.)*; Vitaplex Chilblain Formula *(Vitaplex, Austral.)*.

7910-c

Vitamin P

The name vitamin P has been applied to a group of flavone derivatives which have also been known as citrus flavonoid compounds, but which are now generally described as bioflavonoids.

Bioflavonoids are claimed to increase the resistance of the capillaries and to reduce their permeability to red blood cells.

Compounds claimed to possess such activity include hesperidin (see p.1577), rutin (see p.1610), and troxerutin (see p.1626).

The source, actions, and uses of compounds with bioflavonoid activity.— *Br. med. J.*, 1969, *1*, 235.

Proprietary Names and Manufacturers

The following names have been used for multi-ingredient preparations containing vitamin P— Duo-CVP *(Rorer, Canad.)*.

For multi-ingredient preparations containing nutritional agents and vitamins, see p.1289.

667-e

Xylitol

Xylit.

$C_5H_{12}O_5$=152.1.

CAS — 87-99-0; 16277-71-7(D).

Pharmacopoeias. In *Cz.* and *Jpn*.

A polyhydric alcohol related to the pentose sugar, xylose (p.948). A white, odourless, hygroscopic, crystalline powder with a sweet taste. **Soluble** in water and alcohol.

Adverse Effects

Large amounts taken by mouth may cause diarrhoea and flatulence. Ingestion of xylitol is not likely to lead to hyperoxaluria which can occur with intravenous infusion. Hyperuricaemia, changes in liver-function tests, and acidosis (including lactic acidosis) have occurred after intravenous infusion.

References to adverse effects following intravenous infusions of xylitol: J. F. Donahoe and R. J. Powers (letter), *New Engl. J. Med.*, 1970, *282*, 690 (hyperuricaemia, hyperuricosuria, and hyperbilirubinaemia); D. W. Thomas *et al.*, *Med. J. Aust.*, 1972, *1*, 1238 (diuresis, renal failure, renal calculi, acidosis, liver function changes, hyperuricaemia, and cerebral disturbances); *idem*, 1246 (diuresis, lactic acidosis); J. F. Donahoe and R. J. Powers, *J. clin. Pharmac.*, 1974, *14*, 255 (hyperuricaemia).

Uses and Administration

Xylitol is used as a bulk sweetener in foods; about 20% of ingested xylitol is absorbed.

Xylitol was formerly considered as a substitute for glucose in intravenous nutrition but such use has generally been abandoned.

Xylitol was assigned an acceptable daily intake of "not specified".— Twenty-seventh Report of the Joint FAO/WHO Expert Committee on Food Additives, *Tech. Rep. Ser. Wld Hlth Org. No. 696*, 1983.

Reduced plaque growth with xylitol chewing gum compared with sucrose chewing gum.— T. H. Grenby *et al.*, *Br. dent. J.*, 1982, *152*, 339.

Proprietary Names and Manufacturers

Eutrit *(Jpn)*; Klinit *(Jpn)*; Kylit *(Jpn)*; Newtol *(Jpn)*; Xyranit *(Jpn)*.

7840-a

Dried Yeast

Cerevisiae Fermentum Siccatum; Faex Siccata; Fermento de Cerveja; Levedura Sêca; Levure de Bière; Saccharomyces Siccum; Trockenhefe.

Pharmacopoeias. In *Aust., Braz., Chin., Cz., Ind., Jpn, Mex., Port.*, and *Span*.

Unicellular fungi belonging to the family Saccharomycetaceae, dried by a process which avoids decomposition of the vitamins present. The chief species are *Saccharomyces cerevisiae*, *S. carlsbergensis*, and *S. monacensis*. Dried yeast contains thiamine, nicotinic acid, riboflavine, pyridoxine, pantothenic acid, biotin, folic acid, cyanocobalamin, aminobenzoic acid, and inositol.

Dried yeast is a rich source of vitamins of the B group. It has been used for the prevention and treatment of vitamin B deficiency in doses of 1 to 8 g daily by mouth.

A report of pseudoporphyria associated with the consumption of brewers' yeast; much of the excess of porphyrins was derived from the ingested tablets.— C. K. Lim *et al.*, *Br. med. J.*, 1984, *288*, 1640.

Addition of yeast to a defined sucrose intake in 8 children with congenital sucrase-isomaltase deficiency led to an improvement of clinical sucrose tolerance with complete elimination of symptoms (diarrhoea, abdominal distension and cramps) in 4.— H. -K. Harms *et al.*, *New Engl. J. Med.*, 1987, *316*, 1306.

Preparations

Yeast Tablets *(B.P.C. 1973)*. Tabellae Cerevisiae Fermenti; Dried Yeast Tablets. Store in airtight containers.

Proprietary Names and Manufacturers

Aquroflora *(S.Afr.)*; DCL Vitamin B_1 Yeast *(Distillers Co., UK)*; Forvite *(Lennon, S.Afr.)*; Grandilase *(Keimdiät, Ger.: Thomson & Joseph, UK)*; Inteflora *(Biocodex, S.Afr.)*; Marmite *(Beecham Bovril, UK)*; Perenterol *(Thiemann, Ger.)*; Proper-Myl *(Consolidated Chemicals, UK)*; Ultra-Levure *(Biocodex, Fr.; Biocodex, Switz.)*.

For multi-ingredient preparations containing nutritional agents and vitamins, see p.1289.

5327-p

Zinc

Zn=65.38.

CAS — 7440-66-6.

A white metal with a bluish tinge; it is not very malleable or ductile.

Adverse Effects

Chronic zinc poisoning in man has not been identified with certainty, although prolonged use may lead to copper deficiency and anaemia which has responded to withdrawal of zinc and symptomatic therapy. Metal fume fever, with nausea, dyspnoea, and chest pain follows inhalation of zinc-containing dust.

Zinc sulphate which is the form of zinc often used for oral administration causes adverse gastro-intestinal effects. It can be converted to the corrosive zinc chloride, and it is this corrosive action that accounts for the acute toxicity of the soluble zinc salts.

A patient who took zinc sulphate 660 mg daily for just over a year for coeliac disease presented with profound hypochromic macrocytic anaemia, associated cardiac failure, and copper deficiency. Treatment consisted of slow transfusion of packed cells, copper sulphate 4 mg daily, and the withdrawal of zinc sulphate. The blood picture was normal 4 weeks later.— K. G. Porter *et al.* (letter), *Lancet*, 1977, *2*, 774.

Impaired immune responses associated with excessive zinc intake (150 mg of zinc as zinc sulphate twice a day by mouth for 6 weeks).— R. K. Chandra, *J. Am. med. Ass.*, 1984, *252*, 1443.

Precautions

Concurrent administration of a zinc salt with penicillamine might diminish the effect of penicillamine. The absorption of zinc, although poor, may be decreased by various compounds including some foods. Chelation may occur with tetracycline.

Iron reduces the bioavailability of zinc (N.J. Meadows *et al.*, *Br. med. J.*, 1983, *287*, 1013; D.K. Abu-Hamdan *et al.*, *Ann. intern. Med.*, 1986, *104*, 50), but there are opposing views (K. Mitchell and W.S. Watson, *Br. med. J.*, 1983, *287*, 1629). Mitchell and Watson also provided a reminder that folic acid may influence the absorption of zinc.

Zinc can reduce the bioavailability of copper (M. Abdulla, *Lancet*, 1979, *1*, 616; W.P. Patterson *et al.*, *Ann. intern. Med.*, 1985, *103*, 385) although Samman and Roberts have reported that zinc supplementation did not affect plasma-copper concentrations in healthy subjects (*Med. J. Aust.*, 1987, *146*, 246). Zinc's effect on copper is put to use in the management of Wilson's disease (see below).

Absorption and Fate

Zinc and its salts are poorly absorbed from the gastro-intestinal tract; only a small proportion of dietary zinc is absorbed. Zinc is distributed widely throughout the body and is excreted in the faeces with only traces appearing in the urine since the kidneys have little or no role in regulating the content of zinc in the body.

Uses and Administration

Zinc is an essential element of nutrition and traces are present in a wide range of foods. It is a constituent of many enzyme systems and is an integral part of insulin. Zinc salts (generally zinc sulphate) are used as supplements to correct zinc deficiency; they have been tried in the treatment of a large number of conditions because of an associated reduced concentration of zinc in the body. Some zinc salts, such as zinc carbonate and zinc oxide, are used topically in a variety of skin conditions mainly for their astringent properties. Zinc hydroxybenzene sulphonate is employed in deodorants and antiperspirants. Zinc gluconate is available in preparations for the relief of the common cold.

References to zinc salts inhibiting dental plaque through antibacterial activity: G. J. Harrap *et al.*, *Arch. oral Biol.*, 1984, *29*, 87; C. A. Saxton *et al.*, *J. clin. Periodontol.*, 1986, *13*, 301.

Zinc potentiation of preservatives.— T. J. McCarthy, *Cosmet. Toilet.*, 1985, *100*, 69.

DEFICIENCY. Recommendations for the daily requirement of zinc range from 5.5 to 22 mg (84.1 to 336.5 µmol) daily. In its 26th report, the Joint FAO/WHO Expert Committee on Food Additives proposed a provisional maximum daily tolerable intake for zinc of 1 mg (15.3 µmol) per kg body-weight and commented that man can tolerate 200 mg of zinc sulphate per day (*Tech. Rep. Ser. Wld Hlth Org. No. 683*, 1982). In the *UK* the average total dietary zinc intake is estimated to be about 10.5 mg (160.6 µmol) daily with meat, cereal products, and milk being the main sources. Vegetarians could have a condsiderably lower zinc intake (Survey of Copper and Zinc in Food, *Food Surveillance Paper No. 5, Minist. Agric. Fish. Fd*, London, H.M. Stationery Office, 1981).

It is difficult to obtain a reliable figure for the amount of zinc in the body.

Zinc's involvement in the senses of sight, smell, and taste.— R. M. Russell *et al.*, *Ann. intern. Med.*, 1983, *99*, 227.

There was a relationship between zinc and serum concentrations of thymic factor.— N. Fabris *et al.*, *Lancet*, 1984, *1*, 983.

Acne. While there have been reports of acne improving with oral zinc therapy (G. Michaëlsson *et al.*, *Archs Derm.*, 1977, *113*, 31; *idem*, *Br. J. Derm.*, 1977, *97*, 561; L. Hillström *et al.*, *ibid.*, 1977, *97*, 681), other studies have failed to show any benefit (K. Weismann *et al.*, *Acta derm.-vener., Stockh.*, 1977, *57*, 357; L. Orris *et al.*, *Archs Derm.*, 1978, *114*, 1018; W.J. Cunliffe *et al.*, *Br. J. Derm.*, 1979, *101*, 321). Topical zinc therapy has also been tried sometimes with erythromycin and has also produced conflicting results (J.H. Exner *et al.*, *Curr. ther. Res.*, 1983, *34*, 762; R.J. Cochran *et al.*, *Int. J. Derm.*, 1985, *24*, 188). In commenting on this conflict, Savin (*Br. med. J.*, 1984, *289*, 1476) makes the point that zinc seems to work better in Scandinavia than elsewhere.

Acrodermatitis enteropathica. Acrodermatitis enteropathica was considered to be a zinc-deficiency disorder. Nine children treated with zinc sulphate were completely free from symptoms. A small daily dose—35 mg of zinc sulphate providing about 8 mg of zinc—might suffice but the optimum daily dose appeared to be 150 mg providing 34 mg of zinc daily.— E. J. Moynahan (letter), *Lancet*, 1974, *2*, 399.

Two successful pregnancies in a woman with acrodermatitis enteropathica treated by zinc supplement.— D. P. Brenton *et al.*, *Lancet*, 1981, *2*, 500.

Alopecia. A double-blind study involving 42 patients showed zinc sulphate to be of no benefit in the treatment of alopecia.— R. D. Ead, *Br. J. Derm.*, 1981, *104*, 483. When zinc metabolism is abnormal and serum-zinc concentrations are reduced, one of the signs is diffuse hair loss. The administration of zinc to individuals with hair loss but no zinc deficiency has no rational basis and is not indicated.— R. P. R. Dawber, *Br. med. J.*, 1987, *294*, 1533.

Anorexia nervosa. Two case reports of zinc administration leading to improvement in anorexia nervosa: D. Bryce-Smith and R. I. D. Simpson (letter), *Lancet*, 1984, *2*, 350; S. Safai-Kutti and J. Kutti (letter), *Ann. intern. Med.*, 1984, *100*, 317. Evidence of a disturbance of zinc metabolism in anorexia nervosa.— W. W. Dinsmore *et al.* (letter), *Lancet*, 1985, *1*, 1041 and 1159.

Aphthous ulcers. Twelve of 17 patients with recurrent aphthous ulcers improved when treated with 50 to 150 mg of zinc daily given as zinc sulphate; ulcers were completely eradicated in 5 patients. Improvement appeared to be associated with zinc treatment in those patients with initial serum-zinc concentrations below 1.1 μg per mL.— H. W. Merchant *et al.*, *Sth. med. J.*, 1977, *70*, 559.

Coeliac disease. Correction of severe zinc deficiency in 6 patients with unresponsive coeliac disease produced immediate and sustained improvement subsequently maintained by a gluten-free diet.— M. Elmes *et al.*, *Q. J. Med.*, 1976, *45*, 696.

Common cold. Zinc gluconate lozenges reduced the average duration of common colds by about 7 days when compared with placebo in a double-blind study of 65 patients.— G. A. Eby *et al.*, *Antimicrob. Ag. Chemother.*, 1984, *25*, 20. Zinc salts including zinc gluconate did not display any *in-vitro* activity against rhinoviruses.— F. C. Geist *et al.*, *ibid.*, 1987, *31*, 622. While some cold symptoms were reduced by zinc gluconate, there was no change in virus titre. Prolonged use was not recommended by Tyrrell (MRC common cold unit).— *Pharm. J.*, 1987, *2*, 210.

A study suggesting that zinc gluconate therapy is not therapeutically useful in the treatment of rhinovirus colds.— B. M. Farr, *Antimicrob. Ag. Chemother.*, 1987, *31*, 1183.

Zinc gluconate lozenges appeared to have a significant effect on the signs and symptoms of rhinovirus colds, although the mechanism of action remained obscure.— W. Al-Nakib *et al.*, *J. antimicrob. Chemother.*, 1987, *20*, 893.

Furunculosis. Reduced serum concentrations of zinc were found in 15 patients with recurrent furunculosis. Treatment with zinc sulphate in 8 of the patients was associated with regression of active lesions and no recurrence. This was superior to treatment by incision and antibiotic therapy in the other 7 patients.— I. Brody (letter), *Lancet*, 1977, *2*, 1358.

Hepatic encephalopathy. Correction of zinc deficiency produced some improvement in hepatic encephalopathy.— P. Reding *et al.*, *Lancet*, 1984, *1*, 493.

Herpes simplex. Conflicting reports of topical zinc sulphate having a beneficial effect in recurrent herpes simplex: I. Brody, *Br. J. Derm.*, 1981, *104*, 191; R. M. Graham *et al.* (letter), *ibid.*, 1985, *112*, 123.

Hyperprolactinaemia. Reduction of serum-prolactin concentrations by zinc supplementation in male haemodialysis patients with hyperprolactinaemia.— S. K. Mahajan *et al.*, *Lancet*, 1985, *2*, 750.

Leprosy. Zinc oxide tape has been reported to be of value in leprosy (p.936). Oral zinc has also been reported to produce some benefit (N.K. Mathur *et al.*, *Int. J. Lepr.*, 1984, *52*, 331). Application of zinc sulphate did not produce any improvement in one study (V.R. Subramanyam, *Lepr. Rev.*, 1986, *57*, 72).

Peptic ulcer. Improved ulcer healing-rate in patients with benign gastric ulcers given zinc sulphate. There was no evidence of zinc deficiency in any of the patients.— D. J. Frommer, *Med. J. Aust.*, 1975, *2*, 793.

Improvement in duodenal ulcers with zinc acexamate.— R. Alcalá-Santaella *et al.* (letter), *Lancet*, 1985, *2*, 157.

Pregnancy and the neonate. Zinc supplementation in pregnancy is a matter of debate, especially as there have been difficulties in measuring zinc values which casts doubt on some of the early figures for serum concentrations. There are a number of reports of reduced zinc concentrations in pregnancy and of reduced foetal growth. However, the view has been expressed that there is no good evidence that zinc supplementation has been of benefit. Another view is that for some women there is as good a case for zinc supplementation as for iron supplementation.

Some references to these arguments: N. J. Meadows *et al.*, *Lancet*, 1981, *2*, 1135; *ibid.*, 1985, *2*, 1046; D. Bryce-Smith and N. I. Ward (letter), *ibid.*, 1297; J. O. Drife, *Br. med. J.*, 1986, *292*, 674; A. Malhotra and R. S. Sawers, *ibid.*, *293*, 465; G. Kynast and E. Saling, *Gynec. Obstet. Invest.*, 1986, *21*, 117.

Rheumatoid arthritis. In a preliminary double-blind study of 24 patients with chronic, active, refractory rheumatoid arthritis, the addition of zinc sulphate 220 mg (equivalent to 50 mg of zinc) thrice daily produced beneficial results when compared with placebo. After 12 weeks all patients were given zinc sulphate for a further 12 weeks; those who had already received zinc continued to improve while those who had been on placebo began to improve.— P. A. Simkin, *Lancet*, 1976, *2*, 539. No long-lasting benefit in a study involving 22 patients with rheumatoid arthritis given zinc sulphate by mouth for up to 2 years.— J. J. Rasker and S. H. Kardaun, *Scand. J. Rheumatol.*, 1982, *11*, 168.

Sexual dysfunction. Reversal of zinc deficiency in 4 men with impotence associated with uraemia improved sexual function although not to the predialysis level. There was no improvement in 4 control patients. Initially zinc replacement was with zinc sulphate given by mouth but as this was inefficient zinc chloride was added to the dialysis bath.— L. D. Antoniou *et al.*, *Lancet*, 1977, *2*, 895. A report of reduced serum-zinc concentrations in 6 of 10 infertile men. Zinc sulphate increased plasma-testosterone concentration in 9 and sperm count in 8 men. One wife became pregnant.— T. R. Hartoma *et al.* (letter), *ibid.*, 1125.

In a double-blind study 7 male patients on regular haemodialysis had zinc solution added to the dialysis fluid to attain a final concentration of 400 μg per litre (6.1 μmol per litre); 7 similar control patients had distilled water added. No beneficial effect was noted on any aspect of sexual function in those given supplementary zinc.— A. C. Brook *et al.*, *Lancet*, 1980, *2*, 618. The poor results may have been due to the associated antihypertensive therapy the men were taking.— L. D. Antoniou and R. J. Shalhoub (letter), *ibid.*, 1034.

Sickle-cell anaemia. Zinc deficiency in sickle-cell disease.— A. S. Prasad *et al.*, *Clin. Chem.*, 1975, *21*, 582. See also: O. F. Ballester and A. S. Prasad, *Ann. intern. Med.*, 1983, *98*, 180; A. S. Prasad and Z. T. Cossack, *ibid.*, 1984, *100*, 367.

Trichomoniasis. Sensitivity of *Trichomonas vaginalis* to zinc.— J. N. Krieger and M. F. Rein, *J. infect. Dis.*, 1982, *146*, 341. A case of recalcitrant trichomoniasis responding to correction of reduced plasma-zinc concentrations.— F. Willmott *et al.* (letter), *Lancet*, 1983, *1*, 1053.

Wound healing. References to zinc being of benefit in wound or ulcer healing: W. J. Pories *et al.*, *Lancet*, 1967, *1*, 121; *idem*, *Ann. Surg.*, 1967, *165*, 432; S. L. Husain, *Lancet*, 1969, *1*, 1069; M. H. N. Golden *et al.* (letter), *ibid.*, 1980, *1*, 1256. No benefit for acute tropical ulcers from zinc supplementation.— M. Watkinson *et al.*, *Am. J. clin. Nutr.*, 1985, *41*, 43.

See also under Leprosy, above.

WILSON'S DISEASE. Zinc increased the rate of excretion of faecal copper in 5 patients with Wilson's disease and could be used as an alternative to penicillamine if patients are intolerant of that chelating agent.— G. J. Brewer *et al.*, *Ann. intern. Med.*, 1983, *99*, 314. Further reports of zinc being effective in Wilson's disease: T. U. Hoogenraad *et al.*, *Br. med. J.*, 1984, *289*, 273; M. Van Caillie-Bertrand *et al.*, *Archs Dis. Childh.*, 1985, *60*, 656. No effect in 3 patients.— J. M. Walshe (letter), *Br. med. J.*, 1984, *289*, 558.

5329-w

Zinc Chloride *(BAN, USAN).*

Zinci Chloridum; Zincum Chloratum.

$ZnCl_2$=136.3.

CAS — 7646-85-7.

Pharmacopoeias. In *Arg.*, *Aust.*, *Belg.*, *Br.*, *Egypt.*, *Eur.*, *Fr.*, *Ger.*, *Hung.*, *Ind.*, *It.*, *Jpn*, *Mex.*, *Neth.*, *Nord.*, *Pol.*, *Port.*, *Roum.*, *Span.*, *Swiss*, and *U.S.*

A white or almost white, odourless, deliquescent, crystalline powder or granules or opaque white masses or sticks.

Soluble 1 in 0.5 of water, 1 in 1.5 of alcohol, and 1 in 2 of glycerol. An approximately 10% solution in water has a pH of 4.6 to 5.5. The *U.S.P.* injection has a pH of 1.5 to 2.5. **Store** in airtight non-metallic containers.

Zinc chloride almost always contains some oxychloride which produces a slightly turbid aqueous solution. Turbid solutions, except when intended for ophthalmic use, may be cleared by adding gradually a small amount of dilute hydrochloric acid. Solutions of zinc chloride should be filtered through asbestos or sintered glass, since they dissolve paper and cotton wool.

Zinc chloride is a powerful caustic and astringent. Its adverse effects arise from its corrosive action following ingestion or application. Weak solutions have been used as astringent preparations and as injections for zinc replacement. It has also been used as an obtundent in dentistry.

In Great Britain the recommended exposure limits of zinc chloride fume are 1 mg per m^3 (long-term) and 2 mg per m^3 (short-term).

Preparations

Zinc Chloride Injection *(U.S.P.)*

Proprietary Names and Manufacturers

Zinctrace *(Armour, USA).*

For multi-ingredient preparations containing nutritional agents and vitamins, see p.1289.

17035-v

Zinc Gluconate *(USAN).*

$C_{12}H_{22}O_{14}Zn$=455.7.

CAS — 4468-02-4.

Pharmacopoeias. In *U.S.*

A 1% solution has a pH of 5.5 to 7.5. **Store** in well-closed containers.

Zinc gluconate is used as a zinc supplement. Doses of up to 230 mg daily by mouth (equivalent to 30 mg zinc) are used to alleviate the common cold (see under Zinc).

Proprietary Preparations

Zincold 23 *(Vitalia, UK). Tablets*, zinc gluconate 23 mg, ascorbic acid 50 mg.

Proprietary Names and Manufacturers

Orazinc *(Mericon, USA)*; Zinc-50 *(Solgar, USA).*

For multi-ingredient preparations containing nutritional agents and vitamins, see p.1289.

5330-m

Zinc Sulphate *(BAN)*.
Zinc Sulfate *(USAN)*; Zinci Sulfas; Zincum Sulfuricum.
$ZnSO_4,7H_2O$=287.5.

CAS — 7733-02-0 (anhydrous); 7446-20-0 (heptahydrate).

NOTE. 'White vitriol' or 'white copperas' is crude zinc sulphate.

Pharmacopoeias. In *Arg., Aust., Belg., Br., Braz., Chin., Cz., Egypt., Eur., Fr., Ger., Hung., Ind., Int., It., Jpn, Jug., Mex., Neth., Nord., Pol., Port., Rus., Span., Swiss,* and *Turk. U.S.* includes the monohydrate and the heptahydrate.

Odourless, colourless, transparent, efflorescent crystals or white crystalline powder. Each g of zinc sulphate represents 3.5 mmol of zinc. Zinc sulphate 220 mg is approximately equivalent to 50 mg of zinc.
Soluble 1 in 0.6 of water; practically insoluble in alcohol. A 5% solution in water has a pH of 4.4 to 5.6. The *U.S.P.* injection has a pH of 2.0 to 4.0.
Store in airtight non-metallic containers.

Adverse Effects
Zinc sulphate may cause nausea and vomiting. In overdosage it has corrosive effects which may be explained by its conversion to zinc chloride.

A 72-year-old woman died 47 days after the inadvertent infusion of zinc sulphate 7.4 g over 60 hours. Initial symptoms included hypotension, pulmonary oedema, diarrhoea and vomiting, jaundice, and oliguria; other features were cardiac arrhythmias, hyperamylasaemia, anaemia, and thrombocytopenia. Treatment included sodium calciumedetate (discontinued because of poor renal function), intravenous fluids, frusemide, and haemodialysis.— A. Brocks *et al., Br. med. J.,* 1977, *1,* 1390.

A 15-year-old girl experienced epigastric discomfort on each occasion after taking zinc sulphate 220 mg as capsules twice daily; after 7 days she developed melaena and anaemia; endoscopy showed a haemorrhagic gastric erosion.— R. Moore, *Br. med. J.,* 1978, *1,* 754.

Precautions
As for Zinc (above).

Absorption and Fate
Zinc sulphate is partially absorbed from the gastro-intestinal tract. For further details, see under Zinc (above).

Uses and Administration
Zinc sulphate has been given internally in doses of up to 220 mg three times daily in the treatment of conditions associated with zinc deficiency such as acrodermatitis enteropathica.
Externally, zinc sulphate is used as an astringent in lotions and eye-drops.

For references to the use of zinc sulphate, see under Zinc (above).

Preparations
Zinc and Adrenaline Eye Drops *(A.P.F.)*. See under Adrenaline, p.1457.

Zinc Sulfate Injection *(U.S.P.)*. A sterile solution of zinc sulphate monohydrate or heptahydrate in Water for Injections.

Zinc Sulfate Ophthalmic Solution *(U.S.P.)*. A sterile aqueous solution of zinc sulphate monohydrate or heptahydrate made isotonic by the addition of suitable salts; pH 5.8 to 6.2 or, if it contains sodium citrate, 7.2 to 7.8. Store in airtight containers.

Zinc Sulphate Eye Drops *(A.P.F.)*. Gutt. Zinc. Sulph.; Zinc and Boric Acid Eye Drops. Zinc sulphate 250 mg, boric acid 1.5 g, chlorbutol 500 mg, glycerol 1 mL, Water for Injections to 100 mL. Sterilised by autoclaving.

Zinc Sulphate Eye Drops *(B.P.)*. ZSU. A sterile solution of zinc sulphate 0.22 to 0.28%, in water.

Zinc Sulphate Lotion *(B.P.)*. Lotio Rubra. Zinc sulphate 1 g, amaranth solution 1 mL, water to 100 mL.

The liability of zinc sulphate lotion to microbial spoilage.— T. R. R. Kurup and L. S. C. Wan, *Pharm. J.,* 1986, *2,* 761.

Proprietary Preparations
Solvazinc *(Thames, UK). Tablets,* effervescent, zinc sulphate 200 mg.

Z Span *(Smith Kline & French, UK). Spansules,* sustained-release capsules, zinc sulphate monohydrate 61.8 mg (equivalent to 22.5 mg of Zn).

Zincomed *(Medo, UK). Capsules,* zinc sulphate 220 mg.

Zincosol *(Bioceuticals, UK). Tablets,* effervescent, zinc sulphate 220 mg.

Proprietary Names and Manufacturers
Anusol *(Parke, Davis, Canad.)*; Solvazinc *(Thames, UK)*; Z Span *(Smith Kline & French, UK)*; Zincomed *(Medo, UK)*; Zincosol *(Bioceuticals, UK)*.
The following names have been used for multi-ingredient preparations containing zinc sulphate—Anucaine *(Searle, Canad.)*; Anucaine-HC *(Searle, Canad.)*; Anugesic-HC *(Parke, Davis, Canad.)*; Anusol Plus *(Parke, Davis, Canad.)*; Anusol-HC *(Parke, Davis, Canad.)*; Hemcort HC *(Technilab, Canad.)*; Ocusol *(Boots, UK)*; Prefrin-Z *(Allergan, Austral.)*; Rectogel *(Riva, Canad.)*; Tri-ac *(Ciba Consumer, UK)*; Vasoclear *(Coopervision, USA)*; Visine A.C. *(Leeming, USA)*; Visine Plus *(G.P. Laboratories, Austral.)*; Welder's Flash Drops *(Industrial Pharmaceutical, UK)*; Zincfrin *(Alcon, Austral.; Alcon, Canad.; Alcon, UK)*; Zincfrin-A *(Alcon, Canad.)*.

For multi-ingredient preparations containing nutritional agents and vitamins, see below.

3866-t

Proprietary Preparations for Modified Diets

Aglutella *(G.F. Dietary Supplies, UK). Pasta* and *Wafers,* low-protein, gluten-free.

Albumaid *(Scientific Hospital Supplies, UK). Powder,* amino acid mixture.

Aminex *(Cow & Gate, UK). Biscuits,* low-protein, low-phenylalanine, lactose- and sucrose-free.

Aminogran *(Allen & Hanburys, UK). Powder,* essential amino acid mixture, phenylalanine-free.

Aproten *(Ultrapharm, UK). Food products,* low-protein, gluten-free.

Bi-Aglut *(Ultrapharm, UK). Food products,* gluten-free.

Caloreen *(Roussel, UK). Powder,* water-soluble dextrins, predominantly polysaccharides containing an average of 5 glucose molecules, with sodium less than 1.8 mmol/100 g and potassium less than 0.3 mmol/100 g.

Carobel *(Cow & Gate, UK). Powder,* carob seed flour.

Casilan *(Crookes Healthcare, UK). Powder,* whole protein, containing all essential amino acids.

Complan *(Crookes Healthcare, UK). Food products,* complete food.

Complete *(Health Care, UK). Food products,* complete food.

Dialamine *(Scientific Hospital Supplies, UK). Powder,* essential amino acids with carbohydrate, ascorbic acid, minerals, and trace elements.

dp *(G.F. Dietary Supplies, UK). Biscuits,* low-protein.

Duocal *(Scientific Hospital Supplies, UK). Liquid* and *powder,* low-electrolyte, gluten-, lactose-, and protein-free.

Ener-G *(General Designs, UK). Food products,* gluten-free.

Enervit *(David Anthony, UK). Food products,* complete food, lactose-free.

Farley's *(Crookes Healthcare, UK). Biscuits,* gluten-free.

Forceval Protein *(Unigreg, UK). Powder,* lactose- and gluten-free.

Formance *(Abbott, UK). Food products,* nutritional supplement.

Formula S *(Cow & Gate, UK). Powder,* soya protein isolate, glucose syrup, vegetable oil, vitamins, minerals.

Fortical *(Cow & Gate, UK). Liquid,* glucose polymer (maltodextrin), low-electrolyte, protein-free.

Galactomin *(Cow & Gate, UK). Powder,* low-lactose content and/or reduced fat.

Glutenex *(Cow & Gate, UK). Biscuits,* gluten-free.

Hycal *(Beecham Bovril, UK). Liquid,* glucose syrup solids, protein-free, low-electrolyte.

Isomil *(Abbott, UK). Powder,* lactose-free.

Juvela *(G.F. Dietary Supplies, UK). Food products,* gluten-free or low-protein.
NOTE. The name Juvela is also applied to a preparation of vitamin E.

Liquigen *(Scientific Hospital Supplies, UK). Emulsion,* medium chain triglycerides.

Locasol New Formula *(Cow & Gate, UK). Powder,* low-calcium.

Lofenalac *(Bristol-Myers Pharmaceuticals, UK). Powder,* gluten-, lactose-, and sucrose-free.

Maxamaid XP *(Scientific Hospital Supplies, UK). Powder,* essential and non-essential amino acids, carbohydrates, vitamins, minerals, trace elements, phenylalanine-free.

Maxamum XP *(Scientific Hospital Supplies, UK). Powder,* essential and non-essential amino acids, carbohydrates, vitamins, minerals, trace elements, phenylalanine-free. Not for children under 8 years old.

Maxijul *(Scientific Hospital Supplies, UK). Liquid* and *soluble powder,* glucose polymer (maltodextrin), gluten-, lactose-, and fructose-free.

Maxipro HBV *(Scientific Hospital Supplies, UK). Powder,* whey protein isolate with added amino acids and minerals.

MCT Oil *(Bristol-Myers Pharmaceuticals, UK).* Medium chain triglycerides.

MCT(1) *(Cow & Gate, UK). Powder,* medium chain triglycerides, protein, carbohydrate, low-lactose, sucrose-free.

Medium Chain Triglyceride (MCT) Oil *(Cow & Gate, UK).* Medium chain triglycerides.

Metabolic Mineral Mixture *(Scientific Hospital Supplies, UK). Powder,* essential mineral salts.

Minafen *(Cow & Gate, UK). Powder,* low-phenylalanine.

Modifast *(Wander, UK). Powder,* nutritionally complete supplement, gluten-free.

MSUD Aid *(Scientific Hospital Supplies, UK). Powder,* amino acids except leucine, isoleucine, and valine, with vitamins, minerals, and trace elements.

Nutramigen *(Bristol-Myers Pharmaceuticals, UK). Powder,* gluten- and lactose-free.

PK Aid I *(Scientific Hospital Supplies, UK). Powder,* essential and non-essential amino acids, phenylalanine-free.

PKU 3 *(Milupa, UK). Granules,* essential and non-essential amino acids, vitamins, minerals, trace elements, phenylalanine-free.

Polial *(Ultrapharm, UK). Biscuits,* gluten- and lactose-free. Also free from egg, milk protein, and wheat starch.

Polycal *(Cow & Gate, UK). Powder,* glucose polymer (maltodextrin).

Polycose *(Abbott, UK). Powder,* glucose polymers, gluten-, lactose-, and sucrose-free.

Pregestimil *(Bristol-Myers Pharmaceuticals, UK). Powder,* gluten-, lactose-, and sucrose-free.

ProMod *(Abbott, UK). Powder,* gluten-free.

Prosobee *(Bristol-Myers Pharmaceuticals, UK). Liquid concentrate* and *powder,* gluten-, lactose-, and sucrose-free.

Protifar *(Cow & Gate, UK). Powder,* low-lactose, gluten- and sucrose-free.

Rite-Diet *(Welfare Foods, UK). Food products,* gluten-free and/or low-protein.

Trufree *(Cantassium Co., UK). Food products,* flours, gluten-free, wheat-free.

Verkade *(G.F. Dietary Supplies, UK). Biscuits,* gluten-free.

Wysoy *(Wyeth, UK). Powder,* lactose-free.

3867-x

Proprietary Preparations for Enteral and Parenteral Nutrition

NOTE. One kcal is equivalent to 4.184 kJ.

Nutritionally Complete Preparations for Oral or Tube Feeding

Amin-Aid *(McGaw, USA: Boots, UK). Liquid,* low-protein with a high calorie-to-nitrogen ratio, energy 2782 kJ (665 kcal)/90-mL package.

Clinifeed *(Roussel, UK). Liquid,* complete feeds, gluten-free, energy 1674 kJ (400 kcal)/375-mL container *(Clinifeed 400),* energy 1575 kJ (376 kcal)/375-mL container *(Clinifeed Favour),* energy 1575 kJ (376 kcal)/375-mL container *(Clinifeed Iso),* energy 2092 kJ (500 kcal)/375-mL container *(Clinifeed Protein Rich).*

Elemental 028 *(Scientific Hospital Supplies, UK). Powder,* complete feed, energy 1673 kJ (400 kcal)/100 g sachet.

Enrich *(Abbott, UK). Liquid,* complete feed, with fibre, lactose- and gluten-free, energy 1090 kJ (260 kcal)/237-mL can.

Ensure *(Abbott, UK). Liquid,* complete feed, lactose- and gluten-free, energy 1050 kJ (253 kcal)/250 mL.
Powder, composition when reconstituted as for the liquid.

Ensure Plus *(Abbott, UK). Liquid,* complete feed, lactose- and gluten-free, energy 1570 kJ (375 kcal)/250 mL.

Flexical *(Bristol-Myers Pharmaceuticals, UK). Powder,* complete feed, lactose- and gluten-free, low-residue, energy 1856 kJ (444 kcal)/100 g.

Fortisip *(Cow & Gate, UK). Liquid,* complete feed, lactose- and gluten-free, energy 1260 kJ (300 kcal)/200 mL (*Energy-plus*), or energy 840 kJ (200 kcal)/200 mL (*Standard*).

Fortison *(Cow & Gate, UK). Liquid,* complete feed, lactose- and gluten-free, energy 3150 kJ (750 kcal)/500 mL (*Energy-plus*), or energy 2100 kJ (500 kcal)/500 mL (*Standard*).
Liquid, complete feed, gluten-free, energy 2100 kJ (500 kcal)/500 mL (*Soya*).

Fresubin *(Fresenius, UK). Liquid,* complete feed, gluten-free, low-lactose, low-cholesterol, energy 840 kJ (200 kcal)/200 mL.

Fresubin Plus F *(Fresenius, UK). Liquid,* complete feed, high-fibre, low sodium, lactose, and cholesterol, energy 2100 kJ (500 kcal)/500 mL; gluten-free preparation also available.

Hepatic-Aid *(McGaw, USA: Boots, UK). Liquid,* high in branched chain amino acids, low in aromatic amino acids and methionine, energy 1674 kJ (400 kcal)/60-mL package.

Isocal *(Bristol-Myers Pharmaceuticals, UK). Liquid,* complete feed, lactose- and gluten-free, energy 1062 kJ (254 kcal)/250 mL.

Liquisorb *(E. Merck, UK). Liquid,* complete feed, gluten-free, low-lactose, energy 2095 kJ (500 kcal)/500 mL.

Liquisorbon, MCT *(E. Merck, UK). Liquid,* complete feed, gluten-, purine-, and fructose-free, low-lactose, low-cholesterol, with the majority of the fat (77%) present in the form of medium chain triglycerides, energy 2095 kJ (500 kcal)/500 mL.

Osmolite *(Abbott, UK). Liquid,* complete feed, gluten- and lactose-free, energy 1050 kJ (250 kcal)/250 mL.

Pepti-2000 LF *(Cow & Gate, UK). Powder,* complete feed, elemental, low-fat, energy 1700 kJ (400 kcal)/100 g. (Formerly called Nutranel).

Peptisorb *(E. Merck, UK). Liquid,* complete feed, fructose- and gluten-free, low-lactose, energy 2100 kJ (500 kcal)/500 mL.

Peptisorbon *(E. Merck, UK). Powder,* complete feed, fructose- and gluten-free, low-lactose, energy 1393 kJ (333 kcal)/83.3-g sachet.

Portagen *(Bristol-Myers Pharmaceuticals, UK). Powder,* lactose- and glucose-free, energy 2040 kJ (488 kcal)/100 g.

Reabilan *(Roussel, UK). Liquid,* complete feed, lactose- and gluten-free, energy 1575 kJ (375 kcal)/375 mL.

Triosorbon *(E. Merck, UK). Powder,* complete feed, gluten-free, energy 1673 kJ (400 kcal)/85-g sachet.

Vivonex *(Norwich-Eaton, UK). Powder,* complete feed, energy 1256 kJ (300 kcal)/80-g sachet.

Infusion Fluids for Parenteral Nutrition

Aminofusin L Forte *(E. Merck, UK).* Contains nitrogen 15.2 g/litre, energy 1700 kJ (406 kcal)/litre, also contains vitamins.

Aminoplasmal *(Braun, UK).* Contains nitrogen 4.82 g/litre, energy 510 kJ (122 kcal)/litre (*Aminoplasmal L3*), nitrogen 8.03 g/litre, energy 850 kJ (203 kcal)/litre (*Aminoplasmal L5*), nitrogen 16.06 g/litre, energy 1700 kJ (406 kcal)/litre (*Aminoplasmal L10*), nitrogen 7.4 g/litre, energy 850 kJ (203 kcal)/litre (*Aminoplasmal Ped*).

Aminoplex *(Geistlich, UK).* Contains nitrogen 5 g/litre, energy 4200 kJ (1004 kcal)/litre, also contains alcohol 5% and sorbitol (*Aminoplex 5*), nitrogen 12.44 g/litre, energy 1300 kJ (311 kcal)/litre (*Aminoplex 12*), nitrogen 13.4 g/litre, energy 1400 kJ (335 kcal)/litre, also contains vitamins (*Aminoplex 14*), nitrogen 24.9 g/litre, energy 2600 kJ (621 kcal)/litre (*Aminoplex 24*).

Aminoven 12 *(MCP Pharmaceuticals, UK).* Contains nitrogen 12.44 g/litre, energy 1300 kJ (311 kcal)/litre.

FreAmine III *(Boots, UK).* Contains nitrogen 13 g/litre, energy 1400 kJ (335 kcal)/litre (*FreAmine III 8.5%*), nitrogen 15.3 g/litre, energy 1650 kJ (394 kcal)/litre (*FreAmine III 10%*).

Glucoplex *(Geistlich, UK).* Contains energy 4200 kJ (1004 kcal)/litre (*Glucoplex 1000*), energy 6700 kJ (1601 kcal)/litre (*Glucoplex 1600*).

Glucoven *(MCP Pharmaceuticals, UK).* Contains energy 4200 kJ (1004 kcal)/litre (*Glucoven 1000*), energy 6720 kJ (1606 kcal)/litre (*Glucoven 1600*).

Intralipid *(KabiVitrum, UK).* Contains fractionated soya oil 100 g, glycerol 22.5 g, energy 4600 kJ (1099 kcal)/litre (*Intralipid 10%*), fractionated soya oil 200 g, glycerol 22.5 g, energy 8400 kJ (2008 kcal)/litre (*Intralipid 20%*).

Laevuflex 20 *(Geistlich, UK).* Contains fructose, energy 3400 kJ (813 kcal)/litre.

Nephramine *(Boots, UK).* Contains essential amino acids only, nitrogen 6.5 g/litre, energy 840 kJ (201 kcal)/litre.

Perifusin *(E. Merck, UK).* Contains nitrogen 5 g/litre, energy 550 kJ (131 kcal)/litre.

Synthamin (known in *USA* as Travasol) *(Travenol, UK).* Contains nitrogen 9.1 g/litre, energy 1000 kJ (239 kcal)/litre (*Synthamin 9*), nitrogen 14 g/litre, energy 1600 kJ (382 kcal)/litre (*Synthamin 14*), nitrogen 14 g/litre, energy 1600 kJ (382 kcal)/litre (*Synthamin 14 without electrolytes*), nitrogen 16.5 g/litre, energy 1900 kJ (454 kcal)/litre (*Synthamin 17*).

Vamin *(KabiVitrum, UK).* Contains nitrogen 9.4 g/litre, energy 1000 kJ (239 kcal)/litre (*Vamin 9*), nitrogen 9.4 g/litre, energy 2700 kJ (645 kcal)/litre (*Vamin 9 Glucose*), nitrogen 13.5 g/litre, energy 1400 kJ (335 kcal)/litre (*Vamin 14*), nitrogen 13.5 g/litre, energy 1400 kJ (335 kcal)/litre (*Vamin 14 Electrolyte-free*), nitrogen 18 g/litre, energy 1900 kJ (454 kcal)/litre (*Vamin 18 Electrolyte-free*), nitrogen 9.3 g/litre, energy 1000 kJ (239 kcal)/litre (*Vamin Infant*).

Supplementary Preparations for Parenteral Nutrition

Addamel *(KabiVitrum, UK). Solution,* electrolytes, trace elements. For addition to the Vamin solutions.

Addiphos *(KabiVitrum, UK).* See under Monobasic Potassium Phosphate, p.1035.

Additrace *(KabiVitrum, UK). Solution,* trace elements. For addition to the Vamin solutions.

Multibionta *(E. Merck, UK). Solution,* fat-soluble and water-soluble vitamins. For addition to infusion solutions.

Ped-El *(KabiVitrum, UK). Solution,* electrolytes, trace elements. For addition to Vamin Infant or Vamin 9 Glucose solutions in the intravenous nutrition of neonates and infants.

Solivito N *(KabiVitrum, UK). Solution,* powder for reconstitution, water-soluble vitamins. For addition to glucose solution or Intralipid.

Vitlipid N *(KabiVitrum, UK). Emulsion,* fat-soluble vitamins. Available as *Vitlipid N Adult* or *Vitlipid N Infant.* For addition to Intralipid.

Proprietary Names and Manufacturers of Preparations for Modified Diets and for Enteral and Parenteral Nutrition

Addamel *(KabiVitrum, UK)*; Addiphos *(KabiVitrum, UK)*; Additrace *(KabiVitrum, UK)*; Advance *(Ross, USA)*; Aglutella *(G.F. Dietary Supplies, UK)*; al 110 *(Nestlé, UK)*; Albumaid *(Sharpe, Austral.; Scientific Hospital Supplies, UK)*; Alfare *(Nestle, Austral.)*; Allergilac *(Cow & Gate, UK)*; Alpha-Plus *(Tyson, USA)*; Alprem *(Nestle, Austral.)*; Amin-Aid *(McGaw, USA; Boots, UK)*; Aminex *(Cow & Gate, UK)*; Aminofusin *(Pfrimmer, Austral.; E. Merck, UK)*; Aminogran *(Glaxo, Austral.; Allen & Hanburys, UK)*; Aminolette *(Tyson, USA)*; Aminomine *(Tyson, USA)*; Aminoplasmal *(Braun, UK)*; Aminoplex *(Tyson, USA; Geistlich, UK)*; Aminosine *(Tyson, USA)*; Aminosol *(KabiVitrum, UK)*; Aminostasis *(Tyson, USA)*; Aminosyn *(Abbott, Austral.; Ross, Canad.)*; Aminotate *(Tyson, USA)*; Aminoven 12 *(MCP Pharmaceuticals, UK)*; Aminutrin *(Geistlich, UK)*; Aproten *(Key, Austral.; Ultrapharm, UK)*; Azeta *(G.F. Dietary Supplies, UK)*; Azonutril 25 *(Bellon, Fr.)*;

BCAA Stresstein *(Sandoz Nutrition, USA)*; Bi Aglute *(Key, Austral.)*; Bi-Aglut *(Ultrapharm, UK)*; C & GV Formula *(Cow & Gate, UK)*; Calonutrin *(Geistlich, UK)*; Caloreen *(Austral.; Roussel, Canad.; Denm.; Roussel, UK)*; Cantabread *(Cantassium Co., UK)*; Carnation *(Carnation Foods, UK)*; Carobel *(Key, Austral.; Cow & Gate, UK)*; Casilan *(Crookes Healthcare, UK)*; Citrotein *(Sandoz Nutrition, USA)*; Clinifeed *(Roussel, UK)*; Complan *(Glaxo, Austral.; Crookes Healthcare, UK)*; Compleat *(Sandoz Nutrition, USA)*; Compleat-B *(Sandoz Nutrition, USA)*; Complete *(Health Care, UK)*; Controlyte *(Doyle, USA: Sandoz Nutrition, USA)*; Criticare H.N. *(Mead Johnson, Austral.)*; Cymogran *(Allen & Hanburys, UK)*; De-Lact *(Sharpe, Austral.)*; Dialamine *(Sharpe, Austral.; Scientific Hospital Supplies, UK)*; Digestelact *(Sharpe, Austral.)*; dp *(G.F. Dietary Supplies, UK)*; Duacal *(Scientific Hospital Supplies, UK)*; Edosol *(Muir & Neil, Austral.; Cow & Gate, UK)*; Eledon *(Nestlé, UK)*; Elemental 028 *(Scientific Hospital Supplies, UK)*; Ener-G *(General Designs, UK)*; Energen *(RHM Foods, UK)*; Enervit *(David Anthony, UK)*; Enfalac *(Mead Johnson, Austral.)*; Enfamil *(Mead Johnson, Austral.)*; Enrich *(Abbott, Austral.; Ross, Canad.; Abbott, UK; Ross, USA)*; Ensure *(Abbott, Austral.; Ross, Canad.; Abbott, UK; Ross, USA)*;

Farley's *(Crookes Healthcare, UK)*; Flexical *(Mead Johnson, Canad.; Bristol-Myers Pharmaceuticals, UK)*; Forceval Protein *(Unigreg, UK)*; Formance *(Abbott, UK)*; Formula S *(Cow & Gate, UK)*; Forta *(Ross, USA)*; Fortical *(Cow & Gate, UK)*; Fortisip *(Cow & Gate, UK)*; Fortison *(Cow & Gate, UK)*; Frailac *(Cow & Gate, UK)*; FreAmine III *(Boots, UK)*; Fresubin *(Fresenius, UK)*; Galactomin *(Key, Austral.; Cow & Gate, UK)*; Glucoplex *(Geistlich, UK)*; Glucoven *(MCP Pharmaceuticals, UK)*; Glutenex *(Cow & Gate, UK)*; Hepatic-Aid *(McGaw, USA: Boots, UK)*; Himaizol *(Cow & Gate, UK)*; Hycal *(Beecham Bovril, UK)*; Immune-aid *(Advanced Medical Nutrition, USA)*; Infasoy *(Wyeth, Austral.)*; Intralipid *(Pharmacia, Austral.; Pharmacia, Canad.; Kabi, Ger.; KabiVitrum, Norw.; Fides, Spain; Kabi, Swed.; KabiVitrum, UK)*; Isocal *(Mead Johnson, Austral.; Mead Johnson, Canad.; Bristol-Myers Pharmaceuticals, UK)*; Isomil *(Abbott, Austral.; Ross, Canad.; Abbott, UK; Ross, USA)*; Isotein HN *(Sandoz Nutrition, USA)*; Juvela *(G.F. Dietary Supplies, UK)*; Ketoperlen *(Pfrimmer, Austral.)*; Kidnamin *(KabiVitrum, UK)*; Komplexogran *(Keimdiät, Ger.: Thomson & Joseph, UK)*; Lactogen *(Nestle, Austral.; Nestlé, UK)*; Laevuflex 20 *(Geistlich, UK)*; Lipex *(Advanced Medical Nutrition, USA)*; Liquigen *(Sharpe, Austral.; Scientific Hospital Supplies, UK)*; Liquisorb *(E. Merck, UK)*; Liquisorbon MCT *(E. Merck, UK)*; Locasol New Formula *(Key, Austral.; Cow & Gate, UK)*; Lofenalac *(Mead Johnson, Canad.; Bristol-Myers Pharmaceuticals, UK)*;

Maxamaid XP *(Sharpe, Austral.; Scientific Hospital Supplies, UK)*; Maxamum XP *(Scientific Hospital Supplies, UK)*; Maxijul *(Sharpe, Austral.; Scientific Hospital Supplies, UK)*; Maxipro HBV *(Scientific Hospital Supplies, UK)*; MBF *(Gerber, USA)*; MCT(1) *(Cow & Gate, UK)*; MCT Oil *(Mead Johnson, Austral.; Mead Johnson, Canad.; Bristol-Myers Pharmaceuticals, UK)*; Medium Chain Triglyceride (MCT) Oil *(Cow & Gate, UK)*; Meritene *(Sandoz Nutrition, USA)*; Metabolic Mineral Mixture *(Scientific Hospital Supplies, UK)*; Milumil *(Milupa, Canad.; Milupa, UK)*; Minafen *(Cow & Gate, UK)*; Modifast *(Wander, Austral.; Wander, UK)*; MSUD Aid *(Sharpe, Austral.; Scientific Hospital Supplies, UK)*; Multibionta *(E. Merck, UK)*; Nan *(Nestle, Austral.)*; Nefranutrin *(Geistlich, UK)*; Nenatal *(Cow & Gate, UK)*; Nephramin *(Pfrimmer, Austral.)*; Nephramine *(Boots, UK)*; Nursoy *(Wyeth, USA)*; Nutramigen *(Mead Johnson, Austral.; Mead Johnson, Canad.; Bristol, Switz.; Bristol-Myers Pharmaceuticals, UK)*; Nutranel *(Roussel, UK)*; Nutrauxil *(KabiVitrum, UK)*; Nutrisource *(Sandoz Nutrition, USA)*; Nutrox *(Tyson, USA)*; Osmolite *(Abbott, Austral.; Ross, Canad.; Abbott, UK; Ross, USA)*; Osterfeed *(Crookes Healthcare, UK)*; Ostermilk Complete Formula *(Crookes Healthcare, UK)*; Ostermilk Two Improved Formula *(Crookes Healthcare, UK)*;

Ped-El *(Pharmacia, Canad.; KabiVitrum, UK)*; Pepti-2000 LF *(Cow & Gate, UK)*; Peptisorb *(Pfrimmer, Austral.; E. Merck, UK)*; Peptisorbon *(E. Merck, UK)*; Perifusin *(E. Merck, UK)*; PK Aid I *(Sharpe, Austral.; Scientific Hospital Supplies, UK)*; PK Aid II *(Sharpe, Austral.)*; PKU 3 *(Milupa, UK)*; Pluritene *(Lipha, UK)*; Plus *(Cow & Gate, UK)*; Polial *(Ultrapharm, UK)*; Polycal *(Cow & Gate, UK)*; Polycose *(Abbott, Austral.; Abbott, UK; Ross, USA)*; Polyjoule *(Sharpe, Austral.)*; Portagen *(Mead Johnson, Austral.; Mead Johnson, Canad.; Bristol-Myers Pharmaceuticals, UK)*; Precision Diet *(Doyle, USA: Sandoz Nutrition, USA)*; Pregestimil *(Mead Johnson, Austral.; Mead Johnson, Canad.; Bristol-Myers Pharmaceuticals, UK)*; Prematalac *(Cow & Gate, UK)*; Premium *(Cow & Gate, UK)*; Progress *(Wyeth, UK)*; ProMod *(Abbott, UK)*; Prosobee *(Mead Johnson, Austral.; Bristol-Myers Pharmaceuticals, UK)*; Prosol *(Cow & Gate, UK)*; Protifar *(Cow & Gate, UK)*; Pulmocare *(Ross, USA)*; RCF *(Ross, USA)*; Reabilan *(Roussel, UK)*; Rite-Diet *(Welfare Foods, UK)*; Ross SLD *(Ross, USA)*;

Similac *(Ross, USA)*; SMA *(Wyeth, Austral.; Wyeth, UK; Wyeth, USA)*; Sobee *(Mead Johnson, UK)*; Solivito N *(KabiVitrum, UK)*; Soypliment *(Vitaplex, Austral.)*; Supro *(Eucomark, UK)*; Survimed *(Tuta, Austral.; Fresenius, Switz.)*; Sustacal *(Mead Johnson, Canad.)*; Sustagen *(Mead Johnson, Austral.; Mead Johnson, Canad.)*; Synthamin *(Travenol, Austral.; Travenol, UK)*; Traumacal *(Mead*

Johnson, Austral.); Travamulsion *(Travenol, UK)*; Travasol *(Travenol, USA)*; Triosorbin *(Pfrimmer, Austral.)*; Triosorbon *(E. Merck, UK)*; Trophysan *(Egic, Fr.: Servier, UK)*; Trufood *(Cow & Gate, UK)*; Trufree *(Cantassium Co., UK)*; Twocal *(Ross, USA)*; Tyrosinaid *(Scientific Hospital Supplies, UK)*; Vamin *(Pharmacia, Austral.; KabiVitrum, UK)*; Velactin *(Wander, UK)*; Verkade *(G.F. Dietary Supplies, UK)*; Vital *(Ross, USA)*; Vitlipid N *(KabiVitrum, UK)*; Vivonex *(Norwich-Eaton, Austral.; Norwich-Eaton, UK; Norwich Eaton, USA)*; Wysoy *(Wyeth, UK)*.

7911-k

Multivitamin Preparations

Decavitamin Capsules *(U.S.P.)*. Contain vitamin A (as retinol), vitamin D (as ergocalciferol or cholecalciferol), ascorbic acid or its equivalent as sodium ascorbate, calcium pantothenate or its equivalent as racemic calcium pantothenate, dexpanthenol, or racemic panthenol, cyanocobalamin, folic acid, nicotinamide, pyridoxine hydrochloride, riboflavine, thiamine hydrochloride or its equivalent as thiamine mononitrate, and a suitable form of alpha tocopherol. Store in airtight containers. Protect from light.

Hexavitamin Capsules *(U.S.P.)*. Contain not less than 5000 units of vitamin A (as retinol), 400 units of vitamin D (as ergocalciferol, cholecalciferol, or from natural sources), 75 mg of ascorbic acid or the equivalent amount of sodium ascorbate, 2 mg of thiamine hydrochloride or an equivalent amount of thiamine mononitrate, 3 mg of riboflavine, and 20 mg of nicotinamide. Store in airtight containers. Protect from light.

Oleovitamin A and D Capsules *(U.S.P.)*. Contain oleovitamin A and D (see below). Store in airtight containers in a dry place. Protect from light.

Vitamins Capsules *(B.P.C. 1973)*. Contain vitamin A 2500 units, thiamine hydrochloride 1 mg, riboflavine 500 µg, nicotinamide 7.5 mg, ascorbic acid 15 mg, and vitamin D 300 units. Store in a cool place. Protect from light.

Vitamins A and D Capsules *(B.P.C. 1973)*. Contain vitamin A 4000 units, vitamin D 400 units. Store in a cool place. Protect from light.

Vitamins B and C Injection *(B.P.C. 1973)*. Contains thiamine hydrochloride, riboflavine or the equivalent amount of riboflavine sodium phosphate, nicotinamide, sodium ascorbate, with either anhydrous glucose (for Strong or Weak Vitamins B and C Injection for intravenous use), or benzyl alcohol (for Strong or Weak Vitamins B and C Injection for intramuscular use). It is prepared, immediately before use, by mixing the contents of a pair of ampoules. Sterilised by autoclaving, by heating with a bactericide, or by filtration. Store in a cool place. Protect from light. The air in ampoules containing ascorbic acid is replaced with nitrogen or other suitable gas.

Compound Vitamin B Tablets *(B.P.C. 1973)*. Compound Thiamine Tablets; Compound Aneurine Tablets. Contain nicotinamide 15 mg, riboflavine 1 mg, thiamine hydrochloride 1 mg. Store in airtight containers and avoid contact with metal. Protect from light.

Strong Compound Vitamin B Tablets *(B.P.C. 1973)*. Strong Compound Thiamine Tablets; Strong Compound Aneurine Tablets. Contain nicotinamide 20 mg, pyridoxine hydrochloride 2 mg, riboflavine 2 mg, thiamine hydrochloride 5 mg. Store in airtight containers and avoid contact with metal. Protect from light.

Decavitamin Tablets *(U.S.P.)*. Contain the same ingredients as Decavitamin Capsules (*U.S.P.*), above. Store in well-closed containers. Protect from light.

Hexavitamin Tablets *(U.S.P.)*. Contain the same ingredients as Hexavitamin Capsules (*U.S.P.*), above. Store in airtight containers.

Concentrated Vitamins A and D Solution *(B.P.C. 1973)*. A fish-liver oil or blend of fish-liver oils, or a solution of sources of vitamins A and D in a vegetable oil such as arachis oil, containing vitamin A 50 000 units and vitamin D 5000 units in 1 g. Store in a cool place in well-filled airtight containers. Protect from light.

Oleovitamin A and D *(U.S.P.)*. A solution of vitamin A and vitamin D in fish-liver oil or in an edible vegetable oil; the vitamin D is present as ergocalciferol or cholecalciferol, or from natural sources. Store in a dry place, preferably under an atmosphere of an inert gas, in airtight containers. Protect from light.

Proprietary Multivitamin and Mineral Preparations

Abidec *(Warner-Lambert, UK)*. *Capsules*, vitamin A 4000 units, thiamine hydrochloride 1 mg, riboflavine 1 mg, pyridoxine hydrochloride 0.5 mg, ascorbic acid 25 mg, ergocalciferol 400 units, nicotinamide 10 mg.
Oral drops, vitamin A 4000 units, thiamine hydrochloride 1 mg, riboflavine 0.4 mg, nicotinamide 5 mg, ascorbic acid 50 mg, ergocalciferol 400 units, pyridoxine hydrochloride 0.5 mg/0.6 mL.

Adexolin *(Seven Seas, UK)*. *Drops*, vitamin A 12 000 units, ergocalciferol 1200 units, ascorbic acid 30 mg/mL.

Allbee with C *(Robins, UK)*. *Capsules*, calcium pantothenate 10 mg, nicotinamide 50 mg, pyridoxine hydrochloride 5 mg, riboflavine 10 mg, thiamine mononitrate 15 mg, ascorbic acid 300 mg.

BC 500 *(Ayerst, UK)*. *Tablets*, calcium pantothenate 20 mg, cyanocobalamin 5 µg, nicotinamide 100 mg, pyridoxine hydrochloride 10 mg, riboflavine 12.5 mg, thiamine mononitrate 25 mg, sodium ascorbate equivalent to ascorbic acid 500 mg.

BC 500 with Iron *(Ayerst, UK)*. *Tablets*, calcium pantothenate 20 mg, nicotinamide 100 mg, pyridoxine hydrochloride 10 mg, riboflavine 12.5 mg, thiamine mononitrate 25 mg, sodium ascorbate equivalent to ascorbic acid 500 mg, ferrous fumarate 200 mg.

Becosym *(Roche, UK)*. *Syrup*, nicotinamide 20 mg, pyridoxine hydrochloride 2 mg, riboflavine 2 mg, thiamine hydrochloride 5 mg/5 mL.
Tablets, nicotinamide 20 mg, pyridoxine hydrochloride 2 mg, riboflavine 2 mg, thiamine hydrochloride 5 mg.
Tablets (*Becosym Forte*), nicotinamide 50 mg, pyridoxine hydrochloride 10 mg, riboflavine 15 mg, thiamine hydrochloride 15 mg.

Benerva Compound *(Roche, UK)*. *Tablets*, nicotinamide 15 mg, riboflavine 1 mg, thiamine hydrochloride 1 mg.

Calcimax *(Wallace Mfg Chem., UK)*. *Syrup*, thiamine hydrochloride 500 µg, riboflavine 125 µg, pyridoxine hydrochloride 125 µg, cyanocobalamin 0.125 µg, ascorbic acid 5 mg, ergocalciferol 400 units, nicotinamide 2 mg, calcium pantothenate 125 µg, calcium glycine hydrochloride 500 mg/5 mL.

Ce-Cobalin *(Paines & Byrne, UK)*. *Syrup*, cyanocobalamin 30 µg, ascorbic acid 10 mg/5 mL.

Celaton CH3 *(Celaton, UK)*. *Tablets*, para-aminobenzoic acid 7.5 mg, biotin 1 µg, vitamin A acetate 0.5 mg, thiamine 0.6 mg, riboflavine 0.6 mg, pyridoxine 0.7 mg, nicotinamide 6 mg, calcium pantothenate 2.5 mg, cyanocobalamin 1 µg, ascorbic acid 25 mg, cholecalciferol 2.5 µg, vitamin E acetate 10.5 mg.

Concavit *(Wallace Mfg Chem., UK)*. *Capsules*, vitamin A 5000 units, thiamine hydrochloride 2.5 mg, riboflavine 2.5 mg, pyridoxine hydrochloride 1 mg, ascorbic acid 40 mg, cyanocobalamin 5 µg, ergocalciferol 500 units, vitamin E 2 units, calcium pantothenate 5 mg, nicotinamide 20 mg.
Drops containing in each 0.5 mL and *syrup* containing in each 5 mL vitamin A 5000 units, thiamine hydrochloride 2 mg, riboflavine 1 mg, pyridoxine hydrochloride 1 mg, ascorbic acid 50 mg, cyanocobalamin 5 µg, ergocalciferol 500 units, dexpanthenol 2 mg, and nicotinamide 12.5 mg.

Dalivit *(Paines & Byrne, UK)*. *Capsules*, vitamin A 7500 units, vitamin D 1000 units, thiamine mononitrate 3 mg, riboflavine 3 mg, pyridoxine hydrochloride 1 mg, ascorbic acid 75 mg, nicotinamide 25 mg, calcium pantothenate 5 mg.
Oral drops, vitamin A 5000 units, vitamin D 400 units, thiamine hydrochloride 1 mg, riboflavine 400 µg, pyridoxine hydrochloride 500 µg, ascorbic acid 50 mg, nicotinamide 5 mg/0.6 mL
Syrup, vitamin A 5000 units, vitamin D 1000 units, thiamine hydrochloride 2.5 mg, riboflavine 1 mg, pyridoxine hydrochloride 1 mg, ascorbic acid 25 mg, nicotinamide 10 mg, calcium pantothenate 5 mg/5 mL.

Dayovite *(Cox, UK)*. *Oral granules*, effervescent, thiamine nitrate 25 mg, riboflavine (as riboflavine sodium phosphate) 12.5 mg, nicotinamide 20 mg, pyridoxine hydrochloride 10 mg, calcium pantothenate 20 mg, cyanocobalamin 5 µg, ascorbic acid (as sodium ascorbate) 500 mg/sachet.

Effico *(Pharmax, UK)*. *Syrup*, tonic, nicotinamide 2.1 mg, thiamine hydrochloride 180 µg, caffeine 20.2 mg, compound gentian infusion 0.31 mL/5 mL.

Forceval *(Unigreg, UK)*. *Capsules*, ferrous fumarate 30.8 mg, vitamin A 5000 units, vitamin D 600 units, vitamin E 10 mg, thiamine mononitrate 10 mg, riboflavine 5 mg, pyridoxine hydrochloride 500 µg, cyanocobalamin 2 µg, ascorbic acid 50 mg, nicotinamide 20 mg, calcium pantothenate 2 mg, calcium 70 mg, lysine hydrochloride 60 mg, inositol 60 mg, choline bitartrate 40 mg, copper 500 µg, phosphorus 55 mg, magnesium 2 mg, potassium 3 mg, zinc 500 µg, iodine 100 µg, and manganese 500 µg.

Gevral *(Lederle, UK)*. *Capsules*, ferrous fumarate 30.8 mg, vitamin A 5000 units, vitamin D 500 units, cyanocobalamin 1 µg, thiamine mononitrate 5 mg, riboflavine 5 mg, nicotinamide 15 mg, pyridoxine hydrochloride 500 µg, calcium pantothenate 5 mg, choline bitartrate 50 mg, inositol 50 mg, ascorbic acid 50 mg, vitamin E (as *d*-alpha tocopheryl acetate) 10 units, lysine hydrochloride 25 mg, iodine (as potassium iodide) 100 µg, calcium (as calcium hydrogen phosphate) 145 mg, phosphorus (as calcium hydrogen phosphate) 110 mg, copper (as oxide) 1 mg, manganese (as dioxide) 1 mg, magnesium (as oxide) 1 mg, potassium (as sulphate) 5 mg, and zinc (as oxide) 500 µg.

Haliborange *(Evans Medical, UK)*. *Tablets*, vitamin A 2500 units, cholecalciferol 200 units, ascorbic acid 25 mg.

Halycitrol *(Laboratories for Applied Biology, UK)*. *Emulsion*, vitamin A 4600 units, vitamin D 380 units/5 mL.

Ironorm *(Wallace Mfg Chem., UK)*. *Capsules*, dried ferrous sulphate 195 mg, folic acid 1.7 mg, thiamine hydrochloride 1 mg, riboflavine 2 mg, nicotinamide 10 mg, cyanocobalamin 5 µg, ascorbic acid 15 mg, intrinsic factor concentrate 10 mg, liver fraction II 130 mg.
Tonic with iron, elixir, proteolysed liver extract equivalent to fresh liver 2 g, ferric ammonium citrate 250 mg, calcium glycerophosphate 10.75 mg, manganese glycerophosphate 1 mg, potassium glycerophosphate 1.75 mg, sodium glycerophosphate 21.25 mg, calcium pantothenate 125 µg, cyanocobalamin 2.5 µg, nicotinamide 3.75 mg, pyridoxine hydrochloride 125 µg, riboflavine 250 µg, thiamine hydrochloride 500 µg/5 mL.

Ironplan *(Menley & James, UK)*. *Capsules*, sustained release, exsiccated ferrous sulphate 150 mg, vitamin B_1 3 mg.

Ketovite *(Paines & Byrne, UK)*. *Tablets*, thiamine hydrochloride 1 mg, riboflavine 1 mg, pyridoxine hydrochloride 330 µg, nicotinamide 3.3 mg, calcium pantothenate 1.16 mg, ascorbic acid 16.6 mg, alpha tocopheryl acetate 5 mg, acetomenaphthone 500 µg, inositol 50 mg, biotin 170 µg, folic acid 250 µg.
Liquid, sugar-free, vitamin A 2500 units, vitamin D 400 units, choline chloride 150 mg, cyanocobalamin 12.5 µg/5 mL.

Labiton *(Laboratories for Applied Biology, UK)*. *Elixir*, thiamine 375 µg, caffeine 3.5 mg, dried extract of kola nuts 3.025 mg, alcohol 1.4 mL/5 mL.

Lipoflavonoid *(Lipomed, UK)*. *Capsules*, dexpanthenol 330 µg, nicotinamide 3.33 mg, pyridoxine hydrochloride 330 µg, riboflavine 330 µg, thiamine hydrochloride 330 µg, hydroxocobalamin 1.66 µg, choline bitartrate 233 mg, inositol 111 mg, methionine 28 mg, ascorbic acid 100 mg, lemon bioflavonoid complex 100 mg.

Lipotriad *(Lipomed, UK)*. *Capsules*, containing in each dose of 3, dexpanthenol 1 mg, nicotinamide 10 mg, pyridoxine hydrochloride 1 mg, riboflavine 1 mg, thiamine hydrochloride 1 mg, cyanocobalamin 5 µg, choline bitartrate 700 mg, inositol 334 mg, racemethionine 84 mg.
Liquid containing the equivalent of 3 capsules in each 5 mL.

Minadex *(Seven Seas, UK)*. *Syrup*, vitamin A 650 units, vitamin D 65 units, iron (as ferric ammonium citrate) 12 mg, calcium glycerophosphate 11.25 mg, potassium glycerophosphate 1.25 mg, manganese sulphate 500 µg, copper sulphate 500 µg/5 mL.

Minamino *(Consolidated Chemicals, UK)*. *Syrup*, cyanocobalamin 5 µg, nicotinamide 20 mg, pyridoxine hydrochloride 1.75 mg, riboflavine 2 mg, thiamine hydrochloride 15 mg, with ferric citrate, manganese sulphate, copper sulphate, amino acids, extracts of liver, spleen, and gastric mucosa/5mL.

Multivite *(Duncan, Flockhart, UK)*. *Pellets*, vitamin A 2500 units, vitamin D 250 units, thiamine 500 µg, ascorbic acid 12.5 mg.

Octovit *(Smith Kline & French, UK)*. *Tablets*, vitamin A acetate 2500 units, thiamine 1 mg (as mononitrate), nicotinamide 20 mg, riboflavine 1.5 mg, pyridoxine 2 mg (as hydrochloride), cyanocobalamin 2 µg, ascorbic acid 30 mg, cholecalciferol 100 units, alpha tocopherol 10 mg (as acetate), calcium 100 mg (as hydrogen phosphate), magnesium 10 mg (as hydroxide), zinc 5 mg (as sulphate), dried ferrous sulphate 32 mg.

Orovite *(Bencard, UK)*. *Syrup*, nicotinamide 80 mg, pyridoxine hydrochloride 2 mg, riboflavine 2 mg, thiamine hydrochloride 20 mg, ascorbic acid 40 mg/5 mL.
Tablets nicotinamide 200 mg, pyridoxine hydrochloride 5 mg, riboflavine 5 mg, thiamine hydrochloride 50 mg, ascorbic acid 100 mg.

Orovite 7 *(Bencard, UK)*. *Granules*, vitamin A palmitate 2500 units, ascorbic acid 60 mg, ergocalciferol 100 units, nicotinamide 18 mg, pyridoxine hydrochloride 2 mg, riboflavine sodium phosphate 1.7 mg, thiamine mononitrate 1.4 mg/sachet.

Pabrinex *(Paines & Byrne, UK)*. *Injection*, Vitamins B and C Injection (*B.P.C. 1973*), Strong, for intravenous use (*High Potency*), in a pair of ampoules each containing 5 mL.

Injection, Vitamins B and C Injection (*B.P.C. 1973*), Strong, for intramuscular use (*High Potency*), in a pair of ampoules containing 5 mL and 2 mL.
Injection, Vitamins B and C Injection (*B.P.C. 1973*), Weak, for intramuscular use (*Maintenance*), in a pair of ampoules each containing 2 mL.

Parentrovite (*Bencard, UK*). *Injection*, Vitamins B and C Injection (*B.P.C. 1973*), Strong, for intravenous use (*IVHP*), in a pair of ampoules each containing 5 mL.
Injection, Vitamins B and C Injection (*B.P.C. 1973*), Strong, for intramuscular use (*IMHP*), in a pair of ampoules containing 5 mL and 2 mL.
Injection, Vitamins B and C Injection (*B.P.C. 1973*), Weak, for intramuscular use (*IMM*), in a pair of ampoules each containing 2 mL.

Pharmaton (*Unichem, UK*). *Capsules*, dimethylaminoethanol bitartrate 26 mg, ginseng complex 40 mg, vitamin A palmitate 4000 units, thiamine mononitrate 2 mg, riboflavine 2 mg, pyridoxine hydrochloride 1 mg, cyanocobalamin 1 µg, ascorbic acid 60 mg, ergocalciferol 400 units, vitamin E 10 mg, nicotinamide 15 mg, calcium pantothenate 10 mg, rutin 20 mg, dried ferrous sulphate 33 mg, dibasic calcium phosphate 307.5 mg, calcium fluoride 0.42 mg, anhydrous copper sulphate 2.8 mg, anhydrous potassium sulphate 18 mg, anhydrous manganese sulphate 71 mg, with choline, inositol, linoleic acid and linolenic acid.

Phyllosan (*Beecham Proprietaries, UK*). *Tablets*, ferrous fumarate 35 mg, nicotinic acid 8.5 mg, thiamine mononitrate 166 µg, riboflavine 333 µg, ascorbic acid 5 mg.

Polyvite (*Medo, UK*). *Capsules*, vitamin A 4500 units, ergocalciferol 11 µg, thiamine hydrochloride 2.5 mg, riboflavine 1.5 mg, pyridoxine hydrochloride 1.5 mg, calcium pantothenate 2 mg, nicotinamide 15 mg, ascorbic acid 30 mg.

Redelan (*Roche, UK*). *Tablets*, effervescent, vitamin A 5500 units, thiamine mononitrate 1.2 mg, riboflavine sodium phosphate 1.8 mg, pyridoxine hydrochloride 1.6 mg, cyanocobalamin 1.4 µg, nicotinamide 15 mg, calcium pantothenate 13 mg, ascorbic acid 75 mg, ergocalciferol 400 units, DL-alpha-tocopheryl acetate 10 mg.

Supradyn (*Roche, UK*). *Tablets*, effervescent, vitamin A 1500 µg, thiamine 15 mg, riboflavine 5 mg, nicotinic acid 50 mg, pyridoxine 10 mg, pantothenic acid 11.6 mg, biotin 250 µg, cyanocabalamin 5 µg, folic acid 300 µg, ascorbic acid 150 mg, vitamin D 10 µg, vitamin E 10 mg, with calcium, iron, magnesium, phosphorus, copper, zinc, molybdenum, manganese.

Surbex T (*Abbott, UK*). *Tablets*, thiamine mononitrate 15 mg, riboflavine 10 mg, nicotinamide 100 mg, pyridoxine hydrochloride 5 mg, ascorbic acid 500 mg.

Tonivitan (*Medo, UK*). *Capsules*, vitamin A 4500 units, thiamine hydrochloride 1 mg, nicotinic acid 15 mg, ascorbic acid 15 mg, ergocalciferol 600 units, dried yeast 50 mg.

Tonivitan B (*Medo, UK*). *Syrup*, nicotinamide 2.5 mg, pyridoxine hydrochloride 16.5 µg, riboflavine 400 µg, thiamine hydrochloride 500 µg, calcium glycerophosphate 20 mg, manganese glycerophosphate 5 mg/5 mL.

Tonivitan A & D (*Medo, UK*). *Syrup*, vitamin A 700 units, ergocalciferol 70 units, ferric ammonium citrate 150 mg, calcium glycerophosphate 25 mg, manganese glycerophosphate 400 µg, copper sulphate 400 µg/5 mL.

Vi-Daylin (*Abbott, UK*). *Syrup*, vitamin A palmitate 3000 units, ergocalciferol 400 units, thiamine hydrochloride 1.5 mg, riboflavine 1.2 mg, ascorbic acid 50 mg, nicotinamide 10 mg, pyridoxine hydrochloride 1 mg/5 mL.

Vigranon B (*Wallace Mfg Chem., UK*). *Syrup*, dexpanthenol 3 mg, nicotinamide 20 mg, pyridoxine 2 mg, riboflavine 2 mg, thiamine 5 mg/5 mL.

Proprietary Names and Manufacturers of Multivitamin and Mineral Preparations

Abdec (*Parke, Davis, Austral.*; *Parke, Davis, Canad.*); Abidec (*Warner-Lambert, UK*); Accomin (*Lederle, Austral.*); ACE + Z (*Legere, USA*); ACN (*Person & Covey, USA*); Added Protection (*Prof. Hlth Prod., USA*); Adeflor (*Upjohn, Canad.*; *Upjohn, USA*); Adexolin (*Seven Seas, UK*); Albafort (*Bart, USA*); Alba-Lybe (*Bart, USA*); Alcovite (*Booker Health, UK*); Alertonic (*Merrell Dow, Austral.*; *Merrell Dow, Canad.*); Allbee (*Robins, Canad.*; *Robins, Austral.*; *Robins, UK*); Altorvite (*Nicholas, Austral.*); Al-Vite (*Drug Industries, USA*); Anabex (*Nordic, Canad.*); Anorvit (*Cox, UK*); Apetil (*Ram, USA*); Apisate (*Wyeth, UK*); Appedrine (*Thompson, USA*); Aquasol A and D (*Rorer, Canad.*); BayBee Complex (*Bay, USA*); BC 500 (*Ayerst, UK*); B Stress (*Stanley, Canad.*); B-Totum (*Desbergers, Canad.*); B-C-Bid (*Geriatric Pharm. Corp., USA*); BCM (*G.P. Laboratories, Austral.*); B-Complex (*Drug Houses Austral., Austral.*); Becosym (*Roche, UK*); Becotin (*Dista, USA*); Beminal (*Ayerst, USA*;*Ayerst, Canad.*); Benerva Compound (*Roche, UK*); Berocca (*Roche, Austral.*; *Roche, Canad.*; *Roche, USA*;); Betalin Compound (*Lilly, USA*); Betaplex (*Winthrop, Austral.*); Bioglan (*Bioglan, Austral.*); Biotin Forte (*Vitaline, USA*); Biovital (*Fisons, UK*); Bravit (*Galen, UK*); Budodouze (*Cambridge Laboratories, Austral.*);

Calavite (*Carlton Laboratories, UK*); Calcet (*Mission Pharmacal, USA*); Calcevitone (*Roche, Austral.*); Calcimax (*Wallace Mfg Chem., UK*); Calcinate (*LRC Products, UK*); Caldecium (*Kerfoot, UK*); Calel-D (*Rorer, USA*); Calsotone (*Southon-Horton, UK*); Caltrate 600 + Vitamin D (*Lederle, Canad.*; *Lederle, USA*); Calvita (*Nicholas, Austral.*); Catovit (*Boehringer Ingelheim, Austral.*); Ce-Cobalin (*Paines & Byrne, UK*); Cefol (*Abbott, USA*); Celathon CH3 (*Celaton, UK*); Centrum (*Lederle, Canad.*); Cevi-Fer (*Geriatric Pharm. Corp., USA*); Chews-eze (*Solgar, USA*); Chocovite (*Medo, UK*); Chromagen (*Savage, USA*); Chromagen OB (*Savage, USA*); Ciron (*Hamilton, Austral.*); Citramins (*3M Health Care, UK*); Clusivol (*Ayerst, USA*); Coba-12 (*Nordic, Canad.*); Co-Ferol (*Cox, UK*); Combex (*Parke, Davis, Austral.*); Compete (*Mission Pharmacal, USA*); Concavit (*Wallace Mfg Chem., UK*); Crysti-Liver (*Hauck, USA*); Dalivit (*Paines & Byrne, UK*); Dayalets (*Abbott, USA*); Dayamin (*Abbott, Austral.*); Dayovite (*Cox, UK*); Dermacaps (*Cambden, Austral.*); Dexatrim Preparations (*Thompson, USA*); Dexkaf (*Nelson, Austral.*); Dical-D (*Abbott, Canad.*; *Abbott, USA*);

ECEE Plus (*Edwards, USA*); Efavite (*Britannia Health, UK*); Effico (*Pharmax, UK*); Eldec (*Parke, Davis, Austral.*; *Parke, Davis, USA*); Eldercaps (*Mayrand, USA*); Eldertonic (*Mayrand, USA*); En-Cebrin (*Lilly, USA*); Enviro-Stress (*Vitaline, USA*); Eso-Tabs (*Southon-Horton, UK*); Esotone (*Southon-Horton, UK*); ET The Extra-Terrestrial (*Squibb, USA*); Extralin (*Lilly, USA*); FEAC (*Robins, UK*); Fe-cap C (*MCP Pharmaceuticals, UK*); Fe-cap Folic (*MCP Pharmaceuticals, UK*); Fefol (*Smith Kline & French, Austral.*; *Smith Kline & French, UK*); Femin-9 (*Seven Seas, UK*); Feosol Plus (*Smith Kline & French, USA*); Feospan Z (*Smith Kline & French, UK*); Ferancee (*Stuart Pharmaceuticals, USA*); Feravol (*Carlton Laboratories, UK*); Ferfolic (*Sinclair, UK*); Fergluvite (*Sinclair, UK*); Fergon B (*Winthrop, Austral.*); Fergon with Liver (*Winthrop, Austral.*); Feritard-Folic (*Protea, Austral.*); Ferlucon (*Duncan, Flockhart, UK*); Ferocal Cor-Tab (*Faulding, Austral.*); Fero-Folic (*Abbott, Canad.*; *Abbott, USA*); Fero-Grad-500 (*Abbott, USA*); Ferraplex B (*Bencard, UK*); Ferritrinsic (*Upjohn, Canad.*); Ferrlecit 100 (*Rorer, UK*); Ferrocap-F 350 (*Consolidated Chemicals, UK*); Ferrocontin Folic Continus (*Napp, UK*); Ferrograd C (*Abbott, UK*); Ferrograd Folic (*Abbott, UK*); Ferromyn (*Calmic, UK*); Ferro-Sequels (*Lederle, USA*); Ferroton B_{12} (*Simes, Austral.*); Fesovit (*Wellcome, UK*); Fetrin (*Lasalle, USA*); FGF (*Abbott, Austral.*); Filibon (*Lederle, USA*); Flar (*Consolidated Chemicals, UK*); Fluorac (*Rorer, Canad.*); Folex-350 (*Rybar, UK*); Folfer (*Faulding, Austral.*); Folicin (*Paines & Byrne, UK*); Folvron (*Lederle, UK*); Forceval (*Unigreg, UK*); Formula-B (*Solgar, USA*); Formula-VM (*Solgar, USA*); Fortamines (*Rougier, Canad.*); Fortior-2B (*Purdue Frederick, Canad.*); Fosfree (*Mission Pharmacal, USA*); Furonatal FA (*Metro Med, USA*);

Galfer F.A. (*Galen, UK*); Galfer-Vit (*Galen, UK*); Gastrovite (*MCP Pharmaceuticals, UK*); Geravite (*Hauck, USA*); Gerimed (*Fielding, USA*); Geriplex (*Parke, Davis, Austral.*; *Parke, Davis, Canad.*); Geriplex-FS (*Parke, Davis, USA*); Geritonic (*Geriatric Pharm. Corp., USA*); Gerobion (*Huffman, USA*); Geroton (*Ram, USA*); Gerovit (*Faulding, Austral.*); Gevrabon, (*Lederle, Canad.*); Gevral (*Lederle, Austral.*; *Lederle, UK*); Givitol (*Galen, UK*); Glutofac (*Kenwood, USA*); Glykola (*Sinclair, UK*); Glykola Infans (*Sinclair, UK*); Glytinic (*Boyle, USA*); Haliborange (*Evans Medical, UK*); Halivol (*Parke, Davis, Austral.*); Halycitrol (*Laboratories for Applied Biology, UK*); Hemocyte Plus (*US Pharmaceutical, USA*); Hemocyte-F (*US Pharmaceutical, USA*); Hemoplex (*Paines & Byrne, UK*); Hemo-Vite (*Drug Industries, USA*); Hepacon-Plex (*Consolidated Chemicals, UK*); Hepanorm (*Wallace Mfg Chem., UK*); Heparos (*Desbergers, Canad.*); Hepasol (*G.P. Laboratories, Austral.*); Hep-Forte (*Marlyn, USA*); Hepicebrin (*Lilly, USA*); Heptuna Plus (*Roerig, USA*);

Hormodausse (*Charton, Canad.*); HY-C (*Solgar, USA*); H_3 Plus (*Eucomark, UK*); Iberet (*Abbott, USA*; *Abbott, Canad.*); Iberol (*Abbott, UK*); ILX B_{12} (*Kenwood, USA*); Incremin (*Lederle, Austral.*; *Lederle, Canad.*); Infantol (*Horner, Canad.*); Intraderm-19 Oral Acne Supplement (*Robertson/Taylor, USA*); Intra-Vite (*Nicholas, Austral.*); Iodo-Niacin (*Forest Pharmaceuticals, USA*); Ircon-FA (*Key, USA*); Irofol C (*Abbott, UK*); Iromin-G (*Mission Pharmacal, USA*); Ironorm (*Wallace Mfg Chem., UK*); Ironplan (*Wellcome, UK*); Irospan (*Fielding, USA*); Irradol-A (*Parke, Davis, Austral.*); Iso-B (*Tyson, USA*); Juvel (*Bencard, UK*); Kelfolate (*MCP Pharmaceuticals, UK*); Ketovite (*Stansen, Austral.*; *Paines & Byrne, UK*);

Labiton (*Laboratories for Applied Biology, UK*); Lance B+C (*Kirby-Warrick, UK*); Larobec (*Roche, USA*); Latan (*Ayerst, Canad.*); Lederplex (*Lederle, UK*); Lextron (*Lilly, USA*); Libidinal (*Everett, USA*); Lipo-B-C (*Legere, USA*); Lipoflavonoid (*Lipomed, UK*); Lipo-Nicin (*Brown, USA*); Lipotriad (*Lipomed, UK*); Litrison (*Roche, Austral.*); Lysin-Vit (*Charton, Canad.*); Lyte-C (*Tyson, USA*); Macro (*Macro Vitamin, Austral.*); Malteval (*Horner, Canad.*); Materna (*Lederle, USA*; *Lederle, Canad.*); Maxi-6 (*Desbergers, Canad.*); Maxi-10 (*Desbergers, Canad.*); Maxovite (*Tyson, USA*); May-Vita (*Mayrand, USA*); Mediatric (*Ayerst, USA*); Mediplex (*US Pharmaceutical, USA*); Medi-Tec 90 (*Robertson/Taylor, USA*); Mega-B (*Arco, USA*); Megadose (*Arco, USA*); Megavit (*Vitaplex, Austral.*); Menopace (*Vitabiotics, UK*); Metaboline (*Desbergers, Canad.*); Metatone (*Parke, Davis, Austral.*; *Warner-Lambert, UK*); Meterfolic (*Sinclair, UK*); Mi-Cebrin (*Dista, USA*); Minadex (*Seven Seas, UK*); Minamino (*Consolidated Chemicals, UK*); Mission (*Mission Pharmacal, USA*); Multi-B (*G.P. Laboratories, Austral.*); Multicebrin (*Lilly, Canad.*; *Lilly, USA*); Multi-Vi-Min (*Sisu, Canad.*); Multivite (*Duncan, Flockhart, UK*); Mulvidren-F (*Stuart Pharmaceuticals, USA*); MVC 9+3 (*Lyphomed, Canad.*); MVI (*Armour, USA*; *Rorer, Canad.*; *USV, Austral.*); MVM (*Tyson, USA*); Myadec (*Parke, Davis, Austral.*; *Parke, Davis, USA*); Mycolactine (*Wilcox, UK*); N.29 (*Norton, UK*); Natabec (*Parke, Davis, Canad.*; *Parke, Davis, USA*); Natafort (*Parke, Davis, USA*); Natalins (*Mead Johnson Laboratories, USA*); Neovita (*Savoy Laboratories, UK*); Nephrocaps (*Fleming, USA*); Nervidox (*Bart, USA*); Nestabs FA (*Fielding, USA*); Neuro B-12 (*Lambda Pharmacal, USA*); Neurogem (*Dal-Vita, Austral.*); Niferex Forte (*Central Pharmaceuticals, USA*); Niferex-PN (*Central Pharmaceuticals, USA*); Noravita (*Wallace Mfg Chem., UK*); Norfer (*Norton, UK*); Norvits (*R.P. Drugs, UK*); Novorenal (*Novopharm, Canad.*); Nutrifer (*Ayerst, Canad.*); Nutril (*Faulding, Austral.*); Nutrilmin (*Faulding, Austral.*);

Octovit (*Smith Kline & French, UK*); Optilets (*Abbott, Canad.*); Orabex-TF (*Lasalle, USA*); Orexin (*Stuart Pharmaceuticals, USA*); Orifer (*Dow, Canad.*); Orovite (*Beecham, Austral.*; *Bencard, UK*); Os-Cal (*Marion Laboratories, USA*); Os-Cal D (*Ayerst, Canad.*); Os-Cal-Gesic (*Marion Laboratories, USA*); Pabrinex (*Paines & Byrne, UK*); Paladac (*Parke, Davis, Austral.*); Pardec (*Parke, Davis, Canad.*); Parentrovite (*Beecham, Austral.*; *Bencard, UK*); Penta-3B (*Berlex, Canad.*); Penta-Vite (*Nicholas, Austral.*); Perihemin (*Lederle, USA*); Peritinic (*Lederle, USA*); Pernexin (*Schering, Austral.*); Pharmaton (*Key, Austral.*; *Unichem, UK*); Pholrexone (*Philip Harris, UK*); Phyllosan (*Beecham Proprietaries, UK*); Plastules (*Wyeth, UK*); Pluravit (*Nyal, Austral.*); Plurivite (*Boots, UK*); Poly-Vi-Flor (*Mead Johnson, Canad.*; *Mead Johnson Nutritional, USA*); Poly-Vi-Sol (*Mead Johnson, Austral.*; *Mead Johnson, Canad.*); Polyvitamins B-ADEC (*Sabex, Canad.*); Polyvite (*Medo, UK*; *Geneva, USA*); Posture-D (*Ayerst, USA*); Potaba+6 (*Glenwood, UK*); Pramet FA (*Ross, USA*); Pramilet FA (*Ross, USA*); Precare FA (*Russ, USA*); Pregaday (*Duncan, Flockhart, UK*); Pregamal (*Glaxo, UK*); Pregfol (*Wyeth, UK*); Pregnacare (*Vitabiotics, UK*); Pregnavite Forte (*Bencard, UK*); Pregnavite Forte F (*Bencard, UK*); Premence-28 (*Vitabiotics, UK*); Prenate 90 (*Bock, USA*); Prenavite (*Allen & Hanburys, Canad.*); Pre-Psorin (*Cambden, Austral.*); Probec-T (*Stuart Pharmaceuticals, USA*); Pronemia (*Lederle, USA*); Reactivan (*E. Merck, UK*); Redelan (*Roche, UK*); Reticulex (*Lilly, USA*); Ri-B-Con (*Riva, Canad.*); Rogenic (*Forest Pharmaceuticals, USA*); Rovigon (*Roche, UK*); Rubiron (*Ascot, Austral.*);

S-26 (*Wyeth, Austral.*); Sanatogen (*Fisons, UK*); Selenium-ACE (*Wassen, UK*); Senilezol (*Edwards, USA*); Sigtab (*Upjohn, USA*); Slow-Fe folic (*Ciba, UK*); Solu-Zyme (*Upjohn, Canad.*); Spartus (*Lederle, Austral.*); Stresscaps

(Lederle, Canad.); Stresstabs *(Lederle, Canad.)*; Stuart Prenatal *(Stuart Pharmaceuticals, USA)*; Stuartinic *(Stuart Pharmaceuticals, USA)*; Stuartnatal *(Stuart Pharmaceuticals, USA)*; Sun Safe-A *(Eagle, Austral.)*; Sunnimax *(Warne, UK)*; Super B Complex *(Sisu, Canad.)*; Super D *(Upjohn, USA)*; Super-B *(Parke, Davis, Austral.)*; Super Plenamins *(Riker, UK)*; Suplevit *(Riva, Canad.)*; Supradyn *(Roche, Austral.; Roche, UK)*; Surbex *(Abbott, Canad.; Abbott, USA)*; Surbex T *(Abbott, UK)*; Tabron *(Parke, Davis, USA)*; Tab-Vita-B *(Nicholas, Austral.)*; Tetracyn SF *(Pfizer, UK)*; The Stuart Formula *(Stuart Pharmaceuticals, USA)*; Therabid *(Mission Pharmacal, USA)*; Theracebrin *(Lilly, USA)*; Thera-Combex H-P *(Parke, Davis, USA)*; Theragran *(Squibb, USA)*; Thiafer *(Medic, Canad.)*; Tia-Doce *(Bart, USA)*; Tifolic *(Ticen, Eire)*; Tolfrinic *(Ascher, USA)*; Tonivitan *(Medo, UK)*; Total Formula *(Vitaline, USA)*; TriHemic *(Lederle, USA)*; Trinsicon *(Glaxo, USA)*; Triplevite *(Geneva, USA)*; Tri-Vi-Flor *(Mead Johnson Nutritional, USA)*; Troph-Iron *(Smith Kline & French, Canad.)*; Trophite *(Smith Kline & French, Canad.)*; Tycopan *(Lilly, USA)*; Unicap-T *(Upjohn, Austral.)*; Valonorm *(Wallace Mfg Chem., UK)*; Verdiviton *(Squibb, UK)*; Vicon *(Glaxo, USA)*; Vi-Daylin *(Abbott, UK; Ross, USA)*; Vigranon B *(Wallace Mfg Chem., UK)*; Vikonon *(Savoy Laboratories, UK)*; Villescon *(Boehringer Ingelheim, UK)*; Vio-Bec Forte *(Rowell, USA)*; Vi-Penta *(Roche, USA)*; Viraxatone *(Faulding, Austral.)*; Virol *(Crookes Healthcare, UK)*; Virvina *(Merck Sharp & Dohme, UK)*; Vita-21 *(Cambridge Laboratories, Austral.)*; Vitaminorum *(Sigma, Austral.)*; Vitanorm *(Wallace Mfg Chem., UK)*; Vita-Numonyl *(Bart, USA)*; Vitaphen *(Faulding, Austral.)*; Vitaplus *(Evans Medical, UK)*; Vita-Six *(Paines & Byrne, UK)*; Vitavel *(Bencard, UK)*; Vita-Zinc *(Vitaplex, Austral.)*; Viten *(Nicholas, Austral.)*; Vitin *(Faulding, Austral.)*; Vitocee *(Boots, UK)*; Vitrite *(Seven Seas, UK)*; Vitron-C *(Fisons, USA)*; Vi-Zac *(Glaxo, USA)*; Vykmin *(Beecham Proprietaries, UK)*; Wallachol *(Wallace Mfg Chem., UK)*; Zenate *(Reid-Rowell, USA)*; Zentinic *(Lilly, USA)*; Zentron *(Lilly, USA)*; Zincvit *(Ram, USA)*; Zinvit *(Vitaplex, Austral.)*.

Opioid Analgesics

6200-n

Opioid analgesics sometimes known as opiate analgesics and formerly as narcotic analgesics are mainly used for the relief of moderate to severe pain. The opioids have been found to interact with several closely related receptors, and possess some of the properties of certain naturally occurring peptides.

These naturally occurring or endogenous peptides include the **enkephalins**, met- and leu-enkephalin; the **endorphins**, particularly beta-endorphin; and the **dynorphins**. The endogenous opioid peptides are widely distributed in the CNS with specific groups of peptides being found in other organs. They appear to function as neurotransmitters, modulators of neurotransmission, or neurohormones.

A number of analogues of opioid peptides are being or have been investigated for their biological activities, these include:

FK-33-824 [DAMME (D-Ala^2, MePhe^4, Met(O)-ol)enkephalin], metkephamid acetate (LY-127623), (Des-Tyr)-γ-endorphin, DADL (D-Ala^7-D-leu^{10}-enkephalin), DADLE (D-Ala^2-D-leu^5-enkephalin), DSIP (delta sleep-inducing peptide), morphiceptin, nifalatide (BW-942C), and ICI-154129.

There are several types of opioid receptors. Four of them have been designated μ (mu), κ (kappa), δ (delta), and σ (sigma). Activities attributed to stimulation of these receptors are considered to be as follows:

μ morphine-like analgesia, euphoria, respiratory depression, physical dependence.

κ pentazocine-like analgesia, sedation, miosis.

σ dysphoria, hallucinations, respiratory and vasomotor stimulation.

δ selective for enkephalins, respiratory depression.

Opioid analgesics may act at one or more of these receptors. Those with agonist and antagonist properties exert an inhibitory action at some and a stimulant action at others. Also there may be a partial agonist activity at one or more receptors. Morphine for example is considered to be an agonist for the μ and κ receptors, pentazocine is an agonist for κ and σ and an antagonist for μ, and buprenorphine a partial agonist for μ. Naloxone, which is used as an antagonist, acts at μ and κ receptors and to a certain extent at σ receptors.

In addition to being used for the relief of moderate to severe pain a number of the opioid analgesics are used in anaesthesia for premedication, induction, or maintenance. They are often used in conjunction with an anaesthetic gas and a muscle relaxant in what is known as balanced anaesthesia. When used with a compound such as droperidol they can produce a state of mild sedation with analgesia called neuroleptanalgesia.

Compounds such as codeine are much less liable to produce dependence and are used for less severe pain as well as for cough suppression.

Discussions of opioid peptides: *Lancet*, 1982, *2*, 305; J. W. Thompson, *Br. med. J.*, 1984, *288*, 259; K. W. Hindmarsh and K. Sankaran, *Can. med. Ass. J.*, 1985, *132*, 331. See also *Br. med. Bull.*, 1983, *39*, 1–106.

Reviews and discussions on the actions and uses of opioid analgesics in severe pain of various sources: *The Management of Terminal Disease*, C.M. Saunders (Ed.), London, Edward Arnold, 1984.; R.G. Twycross and S.A. Lack, *Therapeutics In Terminal Cancer*, London, Pitman Publishing Ltd., 1984; G. K. Gourlay and M. J. Cousins, *Drugs*, 1984, *28*, 79; K. M. Foley, *New Engl. J. Med.*, 1985, *313*, 84; L. E. Mather, *Med. J. Aust.*, 1986, *144*, 424; L. E. Mather and M. J. Cousins, *ibid.*, 475; F. D. Hart, *Drugs*, 1987, *33*, 85; J. G. Bovill, *ibid.*, 520.

ADMINISTRATION, EPIDURAL AND INTRATHECAL. A review of the epidural and intrathecal administration of opioids.— M. J. Cousins and L. E. Mather, *Anesthesiology*, 1984, *61*, 276.

ADMINISTRATION, PATIENT-CONTROLLED. Some reviews and discussions concerning patient-controlled analgesia: D. A. Graves *et al.*, *Ann. intern. Med.*, 1983, *99*, 360; K. A. Lehmann, *Arzneimittel-Forsch.*, 1984, *34*, 1108; M. Rosen, *Br. med. J.*, 1984, *289*, 640; R. E. S. Bullingham, *Drugs*, 1985, *29*, 376.

ADVERSE EFFECTS. A review of the adverse effects of opioid analgesic drugs.— D. J. R. Duthrie and W. S. Nimmo, *Br. J. Anaesth.*, 1987, *59*, 61.

12339-b

Alfentanil Hydrochloride *(BANM, USAN, rINNM).*

R-39209. *N*-{1-[2-(4-Ethyl-5-oxo-2-tetrazolin-1-yl)ethyl]-4-(methoxymethyl)-4-piperidyl}propionanilide hydrochloride monohydrate.

$C_{21}H_{32}N_6O_3,HCl,H_2O$=471.0.

CAS — 71195-58-9 (alfentanil); 69049-06-5 (hydrochloride, anhydrous); 70879-28-6 (hydrochloride, monohydrate).

Dependence

Prolonged use of alfentanil may lead to dependence of the morphine type (see p.1310).

Adverse Effects, Treatment, and Precautions

As for morphine (p.1311). Respiratory depression which occurs especially with high doses responds to naloxone. Atropine has been used for bradycardia induced by alfentanil. Muscle rigidity may occur and require treatment with a muscle relaxant.

Alfentanil or fentanyl, in doses approximating to those used in clinical practice, was added to the priming fluid of an extracorporeal circuit before the institution of cardiopulmonary bypass. The concentration of alfentanil in the priming fluid was unaffected; the concentration of fentanyl decreased at neutral or high pH values.— M. Skacel *et al.*, *Br. J. Anaesth.*, 1986, *58*, 947.

ADMINISTRATION IN LIVER DISORDERS. A study of the pharmacokinetics of alfentanil in 11 patients with alcoholic cirrhosis. Owing to its delayed elimination and increased free fraction, alfentanil will exert a prolonged and pronounced effect in patients with cirrhosis after the administration of a large single or cumulated dose.— C. Ferrier *et al.*, *Anesthesiology*, 1985, *62*, 480.

ADMINISTRATION IN RENAL FAILURE. A brief report of a study of the disposition of alfentanil in uraemic patients. When compared with healthy anaesthetised patients the dose-corrected plasma-alfentanil concentrations were significantly lower at 5 to 180 minutes after injection but not at 5, 10, and 24 hours. Plasma protein binding was 87.2% in the uraemic group and 89.9% in the healthy group. Free drug clearance was similar in both groups; total clearance was greater in the uraemic group.— J. W. Sear *et al.*, *Br. J. Anaesth.*, 1986, *58*, 812P.

EFFECTS ON THE CARDIOVASCULAR SYSTEM. Clinically significant decreases in blood pressure are not seen in healthy patients when anaesthesia is induced with large doses of alfentanil, even with rapid administration. Significant decreases are seen in patients with cardiovascular instability when an induction dose of alfentanil is given very rapidly.— M.R. Murphy, Hypotension during Anaesthetic Induction with Alfentanil, in *Opioids in Anaesthesia*, F.G. Estafanous (Ed.), Boston, Butterworth Publishers, 1984.

A study of 44 patients during major vascular, head and neck, or thoracoabdominal surgery, who received alfentanil 10 µg or 40 µg per kg body-weight or placebo. Alfentanil at both dose levels prevented any increase in heart-rate and arterial pressure after tracheal intubation. Alfentanil 40 µg per kg produced profound hypotension and bradycardia. The use of alfentanil at both doses was associated with a decrease in plasma-adrenaline concentrations after tracheal intubation.— D. C. Crawford *et al.*, *Br. J. Anaesth.*, 1987, *59*, 707.

A report of 2 cases of sinus arrest during intubation following administration of alfentanil 30 µg per kg body-weight.— J. K. Maryniak and V. A. Bishop (letter), *Br. J. Anaesth.*, 1987, *59*, 390.

See also under Anaesthesia: Cardiovascular Surgery in Uses.

EFFECTS ON THE RESPIRATORY SYSTEM. A double-blind study in 40 young subjects of the ventilatory and mental effects of alfentanil and fentanyl. Low and high-dose fentanyl caused significant respiratory depression up to 30 and 80 minutes post-treatment, respectively, while there was no depression with low-dose alfentanil and only at 4 minutes with high-dose alfentanil. The fentanyl to alfentanil potency ratio for respiratory depression was 13:1. High-dose fentanyl caused more intense and prolonged mental effects than other treatments. Neither drug affected learning or recall, although high-dose fentanyl impaired motor activity. Nausea and vomiting rates were similar between high-dose alfentanil and low-dose fentanyl.— F. L. Scamman *et al.*, *Acta anaesth. scand.*, 1984, *28*, 63.

Sudden respiratory arrest, after initial rapid clear recovery from anaesthesia, occurred in 2 patients within 63 and 70 minutes respectively of the end of an alfentanil intravenous infusion. Both patients responded to administration of naloxone.— P. S. Sebel *et al.*, *Br. med. J.*, 1984, *289*, 1581. A comment from the manufacturers supporting the recommendation that respiration should be monitored very closely in the postoperative period following alfentanil infusion. An adequate loading dose of alfentanil should be given at induction, and maintenance infusion rates should be titrated to the patients response and kept below 1 µg per kg body-weight per minute.— H. A. Waldron and R. F. Cookson (letter), *ibid.*, 1985, *290*, 319.

Some studies on the ventilatory effects of alfentanil: C. J. H. Andrews *et al.*, *Br. J. Anaesth.*, 1983, *55*, 211S (continuous infusion: comparison with fentanyl); M. O'Connor *et al.*, *ibid.*, 217S (continuous infusion).

Absorption and Fate

Alfentanil is highly protein bound (about 90%) and has a small volume of distribution. Its pharmacokinetics can be described by a three-compartment model in which the terminal elimination half-life has ranged from about 40 to 137 minutes (longer in patients undergoing cardiac bypass surgery and in the elderly). It is metabolised in the liver to inactive metabolites which are excreted in the urine.

Reviews of the pharmacokinetics of alfentanil: D. R. Stanski and C. C. Hug, *Anesthesiology*, 1982, *57*, 435; C. J. Hull, *Br. J. Anaesth.*, 1983, *55*, 157S; L. E. Mather, *Clin. Pharmacokinet.*, 1983, *8*, 422; P. J. Davis and D. R. Cook, *ibid.*, 1986, *11*, 18.

References to pharmacokinetic studies of alfentanil: S. Bower and C. J. Hull, *Br. J. Anaesth.*, 1982, *54*, 871; F. Camu *et al.*, *Anesth. Analg.*, 1982, *61*, 657; M. Michiels *et al.*, *J. Pharm. Pharmac.*, 1983, *35*, 86; H. Helmers *et al.*, *Clin. Pharm.*, 1984, *36*, 239; K. M. Collins and O. M. Plantevin, *J. R. Soc. Med.*, 1985, *78*, 456; J. A. Reitz *et al.*, *J. clin. Pharmac.*, 1986, *26*, 60.

See also under Administration in Liver Disorders and under Administration in Renal Failure, above.

Uses and Administration

Alfentanil is a short-acting opioid analgesic related to fentanyl (p.1305) and like fentanyl it has actions similar to those of morphine (p.1312) and pethidine (p.1318).

It is administered as the hydrochloride by intravenous injection as an adjunct to anaesthesia or as an induction agent in patients with assisted ventilation. A peak effect may be seen within 1.5 to 2 minutes of an injection and analgesia can be expected to last for up to 10 minutes; dose supplements are therefore required if it is to be used for more prolonged surgical procedures.

An initial dose in patients with spontaneous respiration may be up to 500 µg given slowly over about 30 seconds; supplementary doses of 250 µg may be given. Ventilated patients may be given 30 to 50 µg per kg body-weight over 10 minutes with supplements of 15 µg per kg. When given by infusion to ventilated patients there is an initial loading dose of 50 to 100 µg per kg given over 10 minutes and this is followed by 0.5 to 1.0 µg per kg per minute. Doses are adjusted according to the needs of the patient so that lower or higher doses than those mentioned above, which are the doses recommended in the *UK*, may be required. Recommended dose ranges in the *USA* tend to be higher. Patients with spontaneous respiration may be given 8 to 20 μg per kg initially with supplements of 3 to 5 μg per kg. Ventilated patients may be given doses by injection similar to those recommended in the *UK*, but, when given as an infusion, the initial dose may range from 50 to 245 μg per kg followed by 0.5 to 3.0 μg per kg per minute.

Reviews of alfentanil: R. F. Cookson *et al.*, *Br. J. Anaesth.*, 1983, *55*, 147S; *Drug & Ther. Bull.*, 1986, *24*, 51; *Med. Lett.*, 1987, *29*, 59; G. E. Larijani and M. E. Goldberg, *Clin. Pharm.*, 1987, *6*, 275.

Satisfactory sedation was achieved with an infusion rate of between 0.4 and 0.5 μg of alfentanil per kg body-weight per minute with midazolam supplementation in patients requiring overnight ventilation in an intensive therapy unit. The study involved 30 patients given either pethidine or alfentanil (P.M. Yate *et al.*, *Br. J. Anaesth.*, 1986, *58*, 1091). One patient in the alfentanil group suffered prolonged recovery; this patient was subsequently shown to have a prolonged elimination half-life (P.M. Yate and P.S. Sebel, *ibid.*, 1987, *59*, 808).

A study of the cardiovascular responses to large doses of alfentanil and fentanyl in patients undergoing lower abdominal surgery. Fentanyl produced a more prolonged stable cardiovascular pattern than alfentanil.— M. Rucquoi and F. Camu, *Br. J. Anaesth.*, 1983, *55*, 223S.

A study of the dose effects of alfentanil in human analgesia. Alfentanil was given in subanaesthetic doses to 10 subjects in a laboratory setting.— H. Hill *et al.*, *Clin. Pharmac. Ther.*, 1986, *40*, 178.

ADMINISTRATION, EPIDURAL. A study of 16 primiparous patients requesting pain relief during labour. Alfentanil 30 μg per kg body-weight per hour was administered as a continuous infusion via an epidural catheter. Supplementary bolus doses (30 μg per kg) were administered when considered necessary. Excellent pain relief was rapidly obtained early in labour in all patients. However, analgesia was inadequate in the latter part of stage 1 and during the second stage in 5 of the 16 patients, notwithstanding several additional doses of alfentanil, and bupivacaine. Although all neonatal Apgar scores were between 7 and 10, the Amiel-Tison test clearly indicated the existence of neonatal hypotonia. The continuous epidural administration of alfentanil proved to be unsatisfactory for pain relief in labour.— L. Heytens *et al.*, *Br. J. Anaesth*, 1987, *59*, 331.

ANAESTHESIA. Alfentanil is considered to be associated with a more rapid recovery from anaesthesia when compared with fentanyl (B. Kay and P. Venkataraman, *Br. J. Anaesth.*, 1983, *55*, 169S; J.C. Scott *et al.*, *Anesthesiology*, 1985, *62*, 234). However, Cooper *et al.* (*Br. J. Anaesth.*, 1983, *55*, 179S) could not discriminate between recovery from either opioid. Nor could Brown *et al.* (*Can. Anaesth. Soc. J.*, 1984, *31*, 251) demonstrate a difference in the duration of anaesthesia produced by each opioid with thiopentone. Also Moss *et al.* (*Br. J. Anaesth.*, 1987, *59*, 970) reported that psychomotor function did not return to normal for some hours after use of alfentanil and confirmed the need to warn patients not to drive for at least 24 hours after day-case anaesthesia.

References to alfentanil anaesthesia for a variety of surgical procedures: C. J. Hull and L. Jacobson, *Br. J. Anaesth.*, 1983, *55*, 173S; M. E. Ausems and C. C. Hug, *ibid.*, 191S; K. M. Collins and O. M. Plantevin, *J. R. Soc. Med.*, 1985, *78*, 456; M. Hynynen *et al.*, *Acta anaesth. scand.*, 1985, *29*, 168; J. -P. Dechène, *Can. Anaesth. Soc. J.*, 1985, *32*, 346; J. C. Raeder and A. Hole, *Br. J. Anaesth.*, 1986, *58*, 108S.

Cardiovascular surgery. Continuous infusions of alfentanil in coronary artery bypass patients produced greater cardiovascular stability than the administration of frequent intravenous boluses.— S. De Lange *et al.*, *Anesthesiology*, 1981, *55*, A42.

A study of the use of alfentanil as an anaesthetic induction agent in 20 unsedated patients premedicated with atropine about to undergo general surgical operations with halothane-nitrous oxide anaesthesia (Group I) and in 22 patients premedicated with lorazepam and atropine (Group II), and 13 with coronary artery disease (Group III), about to undergo open-heart surgery with alfentanil-oxygen anaesthesia. Alfentanil resulted in a transient small decrease in systolic arterial blood pressure with loss of consciousness in Groups II and III but with no change in right atrial and mean pulmonary arterial pressure or cardiac output. Patients in Group I had no change in any cardiovascular variable measured. The only significant undesirable side-effect was chest wall rigidity, which occurred in 50% of Group I and 22% and 31% of Groups II and III respectively. No patient remembered any aspect of laryngoscopy, endotracheal intubation, or surgery, and only 1 thought the anaesthetic induction was unpleasant. The authors concluded that rapid infusion with alfentanil results in a rapid, pleasant anaesthetic induction with little change in cardiovascular dynamics and a minimum of side-effects.— J. Nauta *et al.*, *Anesth. Analg.*, 1982, *61*, 267.

A study of the haemodynamic responses to anaesthesia and surgery in 3 groups of 20 patients undergoing heart valve replacement surgery. Anaesthesia was induced with either alfentanil (125 μg per kg body-weight), fentanyl (75 μg per kg), or sufentanil (15 μg per kg). All 3 opioids were found to provide satisfactory anaesthesia for patients having valve replacement surgery.— J. G. Bovill *et al.*, *Anesth. Analg.*, 1984, *63*, 1081.

Suppression of cortisol and arginine vasopressin responses to surgery in patients receiving continuous infusions of alfentanil for coronary artery surgery.— M. Hynynen *et al.*, *Br. J. Anaesth.*, 1986, *58*, 1260.

Successful use of alfentanil 35 μg per kg body-weight in a patient with severe aortic stenosis, in order to minimise the haemodynamic responses to intubation and surgery during Caesarean section. The baby was delivered apnoeic, unresponsive with poor muscle tone, but responded rapidly to naloxone. Free drug concentrations were similar in mother and neonate, but maternal plasma proteins had a higher affinity for alfentanil. Only 67.26% of neonatal plasma alfentanil was bound to plasma protein.— N. Redfern *et al.*, *Br. J. Anaesth.*, 1987, *59*, 1309.

References to alfentanil in cardiovascular surgery: P. S. Sebel *et al.*, *Br. J. Anaesth.*, 1982, *54*, 1185; S. De Lange and N. P. De Bruijn, *ibid.*, 1983, *55*, 183S; M. G. A. Palazzo *et al.*, *Can. Anaesth. Soc. J.*, 1984, *31*, 517; M. Hynynen *et al.*, *Br. J. Anaesth.*, 1986, *58*, 1252.

See also above and under Effects on the Cardiovascular System in Adverse Effects.

Ophthalmic surgery. A double-blind controlled study of 50 consecutive patients undergoing routine ophthalmic surgery. After general anaesthesia patients were given 2.5 μg per kg body-weight of fentanyl or 10 μg per kg of alfentanil. Blood pressure and heart-rate fell to the same extent with both regimens but the fall in intra-ocular pressure in the alfentanil group was significantly greater than in the fentanyl group and the onset of maximum reduction in intra-ocular pressure was quicker with alfentanil than fentanyl; alfentanil is preferred to fentanyl for ophthalmic anaesthesia.— S. M. Mostafa *et al.*, *Anaesthesia*, 1986, *41*, 493.

Phaeochromocytoma. A review of the anaesthetic management of phaeochromocytoma including a brief discussion that as alfentanil does not release histamine it may be used freely. Alfentanil may be the drug of choice, having a very rapid onset of action, good vasodilating properties, and a shorter elimination half-life than other opioids.— C. J. Hull, *Br. J. Anaesth.*, 1986, *58*, 1453.

Pregnancy and the neonate. See above under Cardiovascular Surgery.

Proprietary Preparations

Rapifen *(Janssen, UK)*. *Injection*, alfentanil 500 μg (as hydrochloride)/mL, in ampoules of 2 and 10 mL. *Injection* (Rapifen paediatric), alfentanil 100 μg (as hydrochloride)/mL, in ampoules of 5 mL.

Proprietary Names and Manufacturers

Alfenta *(Janssen, USA)*; Rapifen *(Janssen, Denm.; Janssen, Fr.; Janssen, Ger.; Janssen, S.Afr.; Janssen, Switz.; Janssen, UK)*.

6203-b

Alphaprodine Hydrochloride *(BANM, USAN, rINNM)*.

Nu-1196. (±)-1,3-Dimethyl-4-phenyl-4-piperidyl propionate hydrochloride.

$C_{16}H_{23}NO_2,HCl$=297.8.

CAS — 77-20-3 (alphaprodine); 14405-05-1 (hydrochloride); 561-78-4 (hydrochloride, ±).

Pharmacopoeias. In *U.S.*

A white crystalline powder with a slight odour. **Soluble** 1 in 2 of water, 1 in 7 of alcohol, 1 in 47 of acetone, and 1 in 3 of chloroform; very slightly soluble in ether. The *U.S.P.* injection has a pH of 4 to 6.

Alphaprodine hydrochloride is an analgesic chemically related to and with an action resembling that of pethidine, but more rapid in onset and of shorter duration. It has been used in obstetrics and as pre-operative medication in surgery and for minor surgical procedures in usual doses of 20 to 60 mg subcutaneously every 2 hours to a maximum of 240 mg in 24 hours.

Preparations

Alphaprodine Hydrochloride Injection *(U.S.P.)*

Proprietary Names and Manufacturers

Nisentil *(Roche, Canad.; Roche, USA)*.

6204-v

Anileridine *(BAN, USAN, rINN)*.

Ethyl 1-(4-aminophenethyl)-4-phenylpiperidine-4-carboxylate.

$C_{22}H_{28}N_2O_2$=352.5.

CAS — 144-14-9.

Pharmacopoeias. In *U.S.*

A white to yellowish-white, odourless or almost odourless, crystalline powder. When exposed to light and air it oxidises and darkens in colour. There are 2 crystalline forms, melting at about 80° and about 89° respectively. Very slightly **soluble** in water; soluble 1 in 2 of alcohol and 1 in 1 of chloroform; soluble in ether but solutions may be turbid. **Store** in airtight containers. Protect from light.

6205-g

Anileridine Hydrochloride *(BANM, USAN, rINNM)*.

$C_{22}H_{28}N_2O_2,2HCl$=425.4.

CAS — 126-12-5.

Pharmacopoeias. In *U.S.*

A white or almost white odourless crystalline powder. Anileridine hydrochloride 30 mg is approximately equivalent to 25 mg of anileridine. **Soluble** 1 in 5 of water and 1 in 80 of alcohol; practically insoluble in chloroform and ether. A 5% solution in water has a pH of 2.5 to 3.0. **Store** in airtight containers. Protect from light.

6206-q

Anileridine Phosphate *(BANM, rINNM)*.

$C_{22}H_{28}N_2O_2,H_3PO_4$=450.5.

CAS — 4268-37-5.

Anileridine phosphate 32 mg is approximately equivalent to 25 mg of anileridine.

Dependence

Use of anileridine is liable to produce dependence of the morphine type (see p.1310).

Uses and Administration

Anileridine is an analgesic chemically related to and with an action resembling that of pethidine (see p.1318). The usual dose as the hydrochloride by mouth is 25 to 50 mg every 6 hours.

The usual subcutaneous or intramuscular dose for pain is 25 to 50 mg of anileridine, as the phosphate, every 4 to 6 hours, though for severe pain single doses of 75 to 100 mg may be given. The total daily dosage should not exceed 200 mg.

To support anaesthesia, 50 to 100 mg of anileridine, as the phosphate, is added to 500 mL of glucose injection (5%) and the equivalent of 5 to 10 mg of anileridine is given by slow intravenous infusion followed by slow intravenous infusion of the solution at the rate of about 600 μg of anileridine per minute.

Preparations of Anileridine and its Salts

Anileridine Hydrochloride Tablets *(U.S.P.)*

Anileridine Injection *(U.S.P.)*. A sterile solution of anileridine, prepared with the aid of phosphoric acid, in Water for Injections. pH 4.5 to 5.0.

Proprietary Names and Manufacturers of Anileridine and its Salts

Leritine *(Frosst, Canad.)*.

6208-s

Bezitramide *(BAN, rINN).*
R-4845. 4-[4-(2,3-Dihydro-2-oxo-3-propionyl-1*H*-benzimidazol-1-yl)piperidino]-2,2-diphenylbutyronitrile.
$C_{31}H_{32}N_4O_2$=492.6.

CAS — 15301-48-1.

Bezitramide is an opioid analgesic which has been used in doses of 5 mg in the treatment of severe pain. It has a slow onset of action which lasts for about 8 hours.

Significant reduction in pain was achieved with bezitramide 10 mg although this was less than that achieved with dextromoramide 10 mg in a study covering 47 patients. The study was ended prematurely because of the unacceptable level of side-effects with bezitramide which induced nausea, vomiting, drowsiness, dizziness, and sweating.— B. Kay, *Br. J. Anaesth.*, 1973, *45*, 623.

Further references: Sixteenth Report of the WHO Expert Committee on Drug Dependence, *Tech. Rep. Ser. Wld Hlth Org. No. 407*, 1969.

Proprietary Names and Manufacturers
Burgodin *(Janssen, Belg.; Janssen, Neth.).*

6209-w

Buprenorphine Hydrochloride *(BANM, USAN, rINNM).*

CL-112302; NIH-8805; RX-6029-M (buprenorphine); UM-952. (6*R*,7*R*,14*S*)-17-Cyclopropylmethyl-7,8-dihydro-7-[(1*S*)-1-hydroxy-1,2,2-trimethylpropyl]-6-*O*-methyl-6,14-ethano-17-normorphine hydrochloride; (2*S*)-2-[(−)-(5*R*,6*R*,7*R*,14*S*)-9a-Cyclopropylmethyl-4,5-epoxy-3-hydroxy-6-methoxy-6,14-ethanomorphinan-7-yl]-3,3-dimethylbutan-2-ol hydrochloride.
$C_{29}H_{41}NO_4$,HCl=504.1.

CAS — 52485-79-7 (buprenorphine); 53152-21-9 (hydrochloride).

Dependence
Buprenorphine may have lower potential for producing dependence than morphine. However, it has been subject to abuse.

Discussion and reports of abuse of buprenorphine: A. D. Wodak, *Med. J. Aust.*, 1984, *140*, 389; A. J. Quigley *et al.*, *ibid.*, 425; J. Strang (letter), *Lancet*, 1985, *2*, 725; T. Lebedevs (letter), *Pharm. J.*, 1985, *2*, 641; A. C. W. Curran (letter), *ibid.*, 1986, *1*, 5; N. C. Varey (letter), *ibid.*, 1987, *1*, 425.

Adverse Effects
Buprenorphine appears to have similar adverse effects to morphine, with the possible exception of constipation. The most frequent side-effects of buprenorphine are drowsiness, nausea, vomiting, sweating, and dizziness. Respiratory depression, euphoria, miosis, headache, and dry mouth may also occur.

Over 12 months 8187 patients were monitored for efficacy and untoward effects following administration of buprenorphine. Adverse effects reported were, nausea (8.8%), vomiting (7.4%), drowsiness (4.3%), sleeping (1.9%), dizziness (1.2%), sweating (0.98%), headache (0.55%), confusion (0.53%), lightheadedness (0.38%), blurred vision (0.28%), euphoria (0.27%), dry mouth (0.11%), depression (0.09%), and hallucinations (0.09%). Other adverse effects reported included amnesia, bloating, cough, cramp, diarrhoea, diplopia, and flatulence.— A. W. Harcus *et al.*, *Br. med. J.*, 1979, *2*, 163.

Buprenorphine was given sublingually in doses of 150 to 800 µg to 141 patients with cancer pain. Of 94 patients who discontinued buprenorphine in less than 1 week, 50 did so because of side-effects and 29 because their previous analgesic was preferred. The remaining 47 patients continued taking buprenorphine for an average of 12 weeks. The main side-effects were dizziness, nausea, vomiting, drowsiness, dry mouth, and lightheadedness. Constipation was not reported and dependence and withdrawal did not occur in any patient.— D. S. Robbie, *Br. J. clin. Pharmac.*, 1979, *7, Suppl.* 3, 315S.

Two patients suffered shock 2 hours after the administration of buprenorphine by epidural injection.— F. R. Christensen and L. W. Andersen (letter), *Br. J. Anaesth.*, 1982, *54*, 476.

Temporary self-limiting urinary retention after buprenorphine 1.2 mg sublingually over 18 hours, recurring after a further 400 µg dose.— K. Murray, *Br. med. J.*, 1983, *286*, 763.

A brief report of an 82-year-old woman who developed a painless ulcer on the upper surface of her tongue 4 days after starting buprenorphine which she put on rather than under her tongue.— S. P. Lockhart and J. H. Baron, *Br. med. J.*, 1984, *288*, 1346.

Buprenorphine 30 and 40 µg per kg body-weight when given as the sole intravenous analgesic in balanced anaesthesia caused significant and severe respiratory depression 15 minutes after pre-operative loading in 12 patients undergoing cholecystectomy. In the immediate postoperative period 6 patients were in pain; they were treated with naloxone 80 to 400 µg which produced a long lasting period of pain relief (median 22 hours).— J. F. Schmidt *et al.*, *Anaesthesia*, 1985, *40*, 583. See also.— J. E. Pedersen *et al.* (letter), *Br. J. Anaesth.*, 1985, *57*, 1045; F. Reynolds (letter), *ibid.*, 1986, *58*, 688; J. E. Pedersen *et al.* (letter), *ibid.*

Treatment of Adverse Effects
Treatment is similar to that of morphine (see p.1311), *but* nalorphine and levallorphan are not antagonists. Naloxone (see p.845) and doxapram (see p.1442) may be of benefit.

Three of the first 16 patients entering a study involving buprenorphine showed signs of late-onset respiratory depression after the second dose of buprenorphine sublingually. The depression did not respond to naloxone. The study was abandoned.— S. -E. Thörn *et al.* (letter), *Lancet*, 1988, *1*, 179.

Precautions
As for Morphine, p.1311.
Buprenorphine has opioid antagonist actions and may precipitate withdrawal symptoms if given to patients who have recently used other opioid analgesics.
Buprenorphine should be used with caution in women during labour since the foetus is at risk from the absence of a dependable antagonist.

Absorption and Fate
Following intramuscular injection, buprenorphine rapidly produces peak plasma concentrations. It is metabolised chiefly in the liver and is excreted predominantly in the faeces; there is some urinary excretion. Absorption also takes place through the buccal mucosa following sublingual administration. Buprenorphine is about 96% bound to plasma proteins. Buprenorphine is subject to considerable first-pass metabolism following oral administration.

A review of the clinical pharmacokinetics of opioid agonist-antagonist drugs including buprenorphine.— R. E. S. Bullingham *et al.*, *Clin. Pharmacokinet.*, 1983, *8*, 332.

The pharmacokinetics of buprenorphine given sublingually.— R. E. S. Bullingham *et al.*, *Br. J. clin. Pharmac.*, 1982, *13*, 665.

Uses and Administration
Buprenorphine hydrochloride is an analgesic with actions and uses similar to those of morphine (see p.1312). It is classified as a partial opioid agonist. Following intramuscular injection analgesia is apparent within 30 minutes and lasts up to 6 hours. A slower response is achieved following sublingual administration.
The dose by intramuscular or slow intravenous injection for moderate to severe pain is the equivalent of 300 to 600 µg of buprenorphine repeated every 6 to 8 hours as required. Doses of up to 400 µg are given sublingually every 6 to 8 hours.

A double-blind study in 26 consecutive patients with ureteric colic. Buprenorphine 300 µg or pethidine 100 mg were administered intramuscularly. Buprenorphine was found to be superior to pethidine as an analgesic in ureteric colic.— I. G. Finlay *et al.*, *Br. med. J.*, 1982, *284*, 1830.

A double-blind comparative study of 27 patients with moderate to severe chronic pain of malignant origin . Patients received single-dose buprenorphine 300 µg and morphine 10 mg intramuscularly. There were no significant differences in the peak analgesic effects or in the time to reach these effects. However, buprenorphine had a significantly longer duration of action than morphine. Buprenorphine was associated with a significantly higher incidence, greater severity, earlier onset, and longer duration of dizziness, nausea, and vomiting than morphine.— M. Kjaer *et al.*, *Br. J. clin. Pharmac.*, 1982, *13*, 487.

In a comparative double-blind study using a patient-controlled demand apparatus buprenorphine, meptazinol, morphine, or pethidine was given intramuscularly to 39 patients for 24 hours after cholecystectomy. The set dose-increments were: buprenorphine 150 µg, meptazinol 50 mg, morphine 5 mg, and pethidine 50 mg. Relief of pain was overall adequate. Buprenorphine showed the longest median duration of effect and correspondingly the lowest number of demands (range 4 to 23). Buprenorphine also had the lowest pain score. The average amount of analgesic demanded by each group was more than they would have received with conventional prescribing and administration, though there was no overt evidence of overdosage.— M. Harmer *et al.*, *Br. med. J.*, 1983, *286*, 680.

A study in 32 patients with acute pancreatitis showed that buprenorphine 300 µg and pethidine 100 mg intramuscularly are comparable in terms of pain relief and duration of effect.— S. L. Blamey *et al.*, *Br. med. J.*, 1984, *288*, 1494.

See also D. C. Carter (letter), *ibid.*, 1998.

Two independent crossover studies of 185 cancer patients with moderate to severe pain. Sublingual or intramuscular buprenorphine 0.05 to 1.6 mg was compared with intramuscular morphine 4 to 16 mg. Intramuscular buprenorphine proved above 25 times as potent as intramuscular morphine. The duration of effect was similar for both drugs. Buprenorphine given sublingually was considered to be 15 times as potent as morphine given intramuscularly; pain relief was more delayed with sublingual buprenorphine, but lasted longer.— S. L. Wallenstein *et al.*, *Pharmacotherapy*, 1986, *6*, 228.

Further references to studies comparing buprenorphine with other analgesics mainly in the control of postoperative pain: B. C. Hovell, *Br. J. Anaesth.*, 1977, *49*, 913 (superior to pethidine and to pentazocine; all given intramuscularly); M. M. Kamel and I. C. Geddes, *ibid.*, 1978, *50*, 599 (comparable analgesia with pethidine; intravenous routes); K. Chakravarty *et al.*, *Br. med. J.*, 1979, *2*, 895 (600 times more potent than pethidine; intravenous); M. Freedman, *S. Afr. med. J.*, 1986, *69*, 27 (more potent than pentazocine; intramuscular); M. V. Shah *et al.*, *Br. J. Anaesth.*, 1986, *58*, 508 (sublingual and intramuscular administration of buprenorphine both effective); G. Rolly *et al.*, *J. int. med. Res.*, 1986, *14*, 148 (similar results with buprenorphine and a mixture of buprenorphine and naloxone; intramuscular); G. G. Pugh and G. B. Drummond, *Br. J. Anaesth.*, 1987, *59*, 133P (more effective than nalbuphine; intravenous).

ADMINISTRATION IN THE ELDERLY. A study of 51 patients aged over 65 years with chronic pain to assess the efficacy and tolerance of a low-dose (100 µg) of sublingual buprenorphine administered 3 to 4 times a day over a 14-day period. There was significant improvement in symptoms during the treatment period and the drug was well tolerated, with good compliance. Patients aged over 80 years responded comparatively better than those aged between 65 and 80 years.— M. A. Nasar *et al.*, *Curr. med. Res. Opinion*, 1986, *10*, 251.

ANAESTHESIA. *Premedication.* In a study of 120 adults who received either buprenorphine 300 µg or morphine 10 mg as a premedicant before elective surgery, the frequency of nausea, vomiting, and giddiness was greater in the buprenorphine group.— J. W. Sear *et al.* (letter), *Br. J. Anaesth.*, 1979, *51*, 71.

Further references: B. Kay, *Br. J. Anaesth.*, 1980, *52*, 453 (comparison with fentanyl in analgesic supplemented anaesthesia); H. J. McQuay *et al.*, *ibid.*, 1013 (clinical effects during and after operation); A. Risbo *et al.*, *Acta anaesth. scand.*, 1985, *29*, 180 (comparison with morphine and pethidine as a premedication and postoperative analgesic).

CARDIOVASCULAR DISORDERS. Measurement of the haemodynamic effects of buprenorphine, 5 µg per kg body-weight given intravenously over 30 seconds, in 11 patients after open-heart surgery suggested that it was a suitable analgesic for patients with an unstable circulation.— F. L. Rosenfeldt *et al.*, *Br. med. J.*, 1978, *2*, 1602. See also F. L. Rosenfeldt *et al.*, *Br. J. clin. Pharmac.*, 1978, *5*, 362P. Comments.— D. W. Bethune (letter), *Br. med. J.*, 1979, *1*, 345; D. J. Coltart *et al.* (letter), *ibid;* D. J. Coltart and A. D. Malcolm, *Br. J. clin. Pharmac.*, 1979, *7*, *Suppl.* 3, 309S.

Myocardial infarction. In 10 patients with myocardial infarction buprenorphine 300 µg intravenously caused a fall in systolic blood pressure which was not considered significant. In 43 further patients the effect of buprenorphine 400 μg sublingually was delayed compared with that of 300 μg intravenously. In a double-blind study in 118 patients the effect of buprenorphine 300 μg intravenously was significantly less, at 5 minutes, than that of diamorphine 5 mg intravenously, but at 15 minutes the effects were comparable. Buprenorphine was considered suitable for the relief of pain in myocardial infarction.— M. J. Hayes *et al.*, *Br. med. J.*, 1979, *2*, 300.

DEPRESSION. Significant improvement in depression rating scores occurred in a study involving 13 patients with a major depressive illness given buprenorphine. Central opiate receptors might have a role in the drug treatment of endogenous depression; buprenorphine could be an additional form of treatment.— H. M. Emrich *et al.* (letter), *Lancet*, 1982, *2*, 709.

TREATMENT OF DEPENDENCE. Successful use of buprenorphine in the treatment of diamorphine dependence.— N. K. Mello and J. H. Mendelson, *Science*, 1980, *207*, 657. See also.— S. S. W. Seow *et al.*, *Med. J. Aust.*, 1986, *144*, 407.

Preparations

Temgesic *(Reckitt & Colman Pharmaceuticals, UK)*. *Injection*, buprenorphine 300 μg (as hydrochloride)/mL, in ampoules of 1 and 2 mL.
Sublingual tablets, buprenorphine 200 μg (as hydrochloride).

Proprietary Names and Manufacturers

Buprenex *(Norwich Eaton, USA)*; Buprex *(Esteve, Spain)*; Finibron *(Midy, Ital.)*; Prefin *(Miquel, Spain)*; Temgesic *(Reckitt & Colman, Austral.; Reckitt & Colman, Denm.; Eire; Boehringer Mannheim, Ger.; Boehringer Biochemia, Ital.; Reckitt & Colman, Norw.; Reckitt & Colman, S.Afr.; Reckitt & Colman, Swed.; Reckitt & Colman, Switz.; Reckitt & Colman Pharmaceuticals, UK)*.

6210-m

Butorphanol Tartrate *(BANM, USAN, rINNM)*.

Levo-BC-2627 Tartrate. (−)-17-(Cyclobutylmethyl)morphinan-3,14-diol hydrogen tartrate.
$C_{21}H_{29}NO_2,C_4H_6O_6$=477.6.

CAS — 42408-82-2 (butorphanol); 58786-99-5 (tartrate).

Pharmacopoeias. In *U.S.*

A white powder. Sparingly **soluble** in water; slightly soluble in methyl alcohol; practically insoluble in alcohol, chloroform, ether, ethyl acetate, and hexane; soluble in dilute acids. A solution in water is slightly acidic. The *U.S.P.* injection has a pH of 3.0 to 5.5. **Store** in airtight containers. The *U.S.P.* injection should be protected from light.

Dependence

Prolonged use of butorphanol may lead to dependence of the morphine type (see p.1310).

There have been several case reports of butorphanol abuse and physical dependence (R.P. Austin, *Am. J. Hosp. Pharm.*, 1983, *40*, 1306; W.S. Evans, *et al.*, *J. Am. med. Ass.*, 1985, *253*, 2191; G.R. Brown, *ibid.*, *254*, 910). Abuse of butorphanol by intravenous injection with diphenhydramine has been reported by Smith and Davis (*J. Am. med. Ass.*, 1984, *252*, 1010).

Adverse Effects

As for Morphine, p.1311.

Results suggesting a ceiling effect to the respiratory depression induced by butorphanol.— H. Nagashima *et al.*, *Clin. Pharmac. Ther.*, 1976, *19*, 738; T. Kallos and F. Caruso, *ibid.*, 1977, *21*, 107.

For a study of the respiratory effects of butorphanol or fentanyl following barbiturate induction, see p.1305.

PREGNANCY AND THE NEONATE. Two instances of sinusoidal foetal heart-rate pattern out of 188 consecutive cases of butorphanol administration in active-phase labour.— S. I. Welt (letter), *Am. J. Obstet. Gynec.*, 1985, *152*, 362.

Treatment of Adverse Effects

Treatment is similar to that for Morphine (see p.1311), with the administration of the specific antagonist naloxone.

Precautions

As for Morphine, p.1311.
Butorphanol has opioid antagonist actions and may precipitate withdrawal symptoms if given to patients who have recently used other opioid analgesics.

Absorption and Fate

Butorphanol is absorbed from the gastro-intestinal tract but it undergoes extensive first-pass metabolism. Peak plasma concentrations occur 0.5 to 1 hour after intramuscular and 1 to 1.5 hours after oral administration. It is extensively metabolised through hydroxylation, *N*-dealkylation, and conjugation, less than 5% being excreted unchanged. Butorphanol and its metabolites are excreted mainly in the urine; about 11 to 14% of a parenteral dose is excreted in the bile. It crosses the placenta.

A review of the clinical pharmacokinetics of butorphanol and other opioid agonist-antagonist drugs.— R. E. S. Bullingham *et al.*, *Clin. Pharmacokinet.*, 1983, *8*, 332.

Uses and Administration

Butorphanol tartrate is an analgesic with actions and uses similar to those of morphine (see p.1312). In addition, it has opioid antagonist properties. Analgesia is usually apparent 30 to 60 minutes following intramuscular injection and may last for 3 to 4 hours.
For the relief of moderate to severe pain, butorphanol tartrate is given in doses of 1 to 4 mg every 3 to 4 hours by intramuscular injection. It may also be given in doses of 0.5 to 2 mg by intravenous injection.
Butorphanol tartrate has also been given by mouth.

Reviews of the actions and uses of butorphanol.— R. C. Heel *et al.*, *Drugs*, 1978, *16*, 473; B. Ameer and F. J. Salter, *Am. J. Hosp. Pharm.*, 1979, *36*, 1683; L. D. Vandam, *New Engl. J. Med.*, 1980, *302*, 381; I. J. Pachter and R. P. Evens, *Drug & Alcohol Depend.*, 1985, *14*, 325.

A review of the comparative effects and analgesic efficacy of buprenorphine, butorphanol, pentazocine, and nalbuphine.— E. M. Zola and D. C. McLeod, *Drug Intell. & clin. Pharm.*, 1983, *17*, 411.

ANAESTHESIA. A retrospective study comparing butorphanol with morphine for use in a balanced anaesthetic technique. Patients in the butorphanol group proved to have less postoperative respiratory depression, nausea, and vomiting compared with patients receiving morphine. Neither group had any recall of procedure, hallucination, or dysphoria.— Y. -F. Sung *et al.*, *Sth. med. J.*, 1984, *77*, 180.

A comparative study of 31 women undergoing outpatient gynaecological surgery. Butorphanol tartrate 40 μg per kg body-weight or fentanyl nitrate 2 μg per kg were administered intravenously following methohexitone induction of anaesthesia. Seven of 15 patients who received fentanyl had significant respiratory depression that required assisted ventilation, compared with 1 of the butorphanol patients who experienced a 45-second self-limited respiratory depression. The incidence of adverse effects was greater with fentanyl.— G. E. Dryden, *J. clin. Pharmac.*, 1986, *26*, 203.

Premedication. A double-blind study of butorphanol 2 mg compared with morphine 10 mg intramuscularly as the sole premedication in 40 women undergoing total abdominal hysterectomy. Butorphanol was as effective as morphine with fewer side-effects, although 1 patient complained of hallucinations. There was no clinically significant antagonism between butorphanol and fentanyl which was used in the induction of anaesthesia.— D. A. Laffey and N. H. Kay, *Br. J. Anaesth.*, 1984, *56*, 363.

A study in 96 patients comparing butorphanol and pethidine as premedication in patients undergoing biliary surgery. Butorphanol 2 mg or pethidine 100 mg was administered intramuscularly. There were no significant differences in side-effects between butorphanol and pethidine. Butorphanol did not provoke biliary spasm and produced a comparable level of sedation to pethidine.— R. J. Noveck *et al.*, *Clin. Pharmac. Ther.*, 1984, *35*, 263.

Effective premedication with butorphanol and hydroxyzine.— B. K. Basak, *Curr. ther. Res.*, 1981, *29*, 12.

Preparations

Butorphanol Tartrate Injection *(U.S.P.)*

Proprietary Names and Manufacturers

Stadol *(Canad.; Bristol-Myers Pharmaceuticals, UK; Bristol, USA)*; Stadole *(Bristol Europe, Ital.)*; Verstadol *(Bristol-Myers, Spain)*.

12574-z

Ciramadol *(USAN, rINN)*.

WY-15705. (−)-2-(α-Dimethylamino-3-hydroxybenzyl)cyclohexanol.
$C_{15}H_{23}NO_2$=249.4.

CAS — 63269-31-8.

NOTE. Ciramadol Hydrochloride is *USAN*.

Ciramadol is an opioid analgesic with mixed agonist-antagonist activity.

A dose-response study involving 111 postoperative patients demonstrated that single oral doses of ciramadol 15 mg produced greater pain relief than doses of 30 and 60 mg. Adverse effects included dizziness and vertigo.— L. Lasagna and J. F. Calimlim, *Clin. Pharmac. Ther.*, 1985, *38*, 176.

Clinical studies of ciramadol in the treatment of moderate to severe pain: R. J. Fragen and N. J. Caldwell, *J. clin. Pharmac.*, 1982, *22*, 459 (post-operative; oral administration); W. Oosterlinck and H. Minnaert, *Curr. med. Res. Opinion*, 1982, *8*, 290 (renal colic; intravenous administration); P. Defoort *et al.*, *ibid.*, 1983, *8*, 481 (post-episiotomy; oral administration, comparison with codeine); R. J. Fragen *et al.*, *J. clin. Pharmac.*, 1983, *23*, 219 (postoperative; intramuscular administration); W. Oosterlinck *et al.*, *Curr. med. Res. Opinion*, 1984, *9*, 93 (renal colic; intravenous administration); D. F. Graf *et al.*, *J. clin. Pharmac.*, 1985, *25*, 590 (postoperative; oral administration); H. D. Reines *et al.*, *ibid.*, 1986, *26*, 111 (postoperative; oral administration); D. van Steenberghe *et al.*, *Eur. J. clin. Pharmac.*, 1986, *31*, 355 (postoperative; oral administration); J. E. Stambaugh and J. McAdams, *J. clin. Pharmac.*, 1987, *27*, 162 (cancer; oral administration).

For a comparative study of the haemodynamic and respiratory effects of ciramadol, dezocine, and morphine, see p.1302.

Proprietary Names and Manufacturers

Wyeth, USA.

6211-b

Codeine *(BAN, USAN)*.

Metilmorfina; Morphine Methyl Ether. 7,8-Didehydro-4,5-epoxy-3-methoxy-17-methylmorphinan-6-ol.
$C_{18}H_{21}NO_3,H_2O$=317.4.

CAS — 76-57-3 (anhydrous); 6059-47-8 (monohydrate).

Pharmacopoeias. In *Arg., Belg., Br., Eur., Fr., Ger., Int., It., Mex., Neth., Pol., Port., Roum., Rus., Span., Swiss, Turk.*, and *U.S.*

Codeine is obtained from opium or made by methylating morphine. It occurs as odourless colourless crystals or white crystalline powder. It effloresces slowly in dry air and is affected by light.
Soluble 1 in 120 of water and soluble in boiling water; soluble 1 in 2 of alcohol, 1 in 0.5 of chloroform, and 1 in 50 of ether. A 0.5% solution in water has a pH of more than 9. **Store** in airtight containers. Protect from light.

INCOMPATIBILITY. In the presence of moisture at 60°, aspirin acetylated codeine to 6-acetylcodeine. There was no reaction at room temperature at low moisture levels. The apparent activity and toxicity should not be altered by the acetylation according to the work of W.R. Buckett and others (*J. Pharm. Pharmac.*, 1964, *16*, 174).— A. L. Jacobs *et al.*, *J. pharm. Sci.*, 1966, *55*, 893. See also R. N. Galante *et al.*, *ibid.*, 1979, *68*, 1494.

6212-v

Codeine Hydrochloride *(BANM)*.

$C_{18}H_{21}NO_3,HCl,2H_2O$=371.9.

CAS — 1422-07-7 (anhydrous).

Pharmacopoeias. In *Aust., Br., Hung., Roum.*, and *Swiss.*

Small colourless crystals or a white crystalline

powder. **Soluble** 1 in 20 of water; slightly soluble in alcohol; practically insoluble in chloroform and ether. **Store** in well-closed containers. Protect from light.

6213-g

Codeine Phosphate *(BANM, USAN).*

Codeine Phosphate Hemihydrate; Codeini Phosphas; Codeini Phosphas Hemihydricus; Codeinii Phosphas; Methylmorphine Phosphate.
$C_{18}H_{21}NO_3,H_3PO_4,\frac{1}{2}H_2O=406.4$.

CAS — 52-28-8 (anhydrous); 41444-62-6 (hemihydrate); 5913-76-8 (sesquihydrate).

NOTE. Compounded preparations of codeine phosphate and aspirin in the mass proportions 1 part to 50 parts have the British Approved Name Co-codaprin. Compounded preparations of codeine phosphate and paracetamol in the mass proportions 2 parts to 125 parts have the British Approved Name Co-codamol.

Pharmacopoeias. In *Arg., Aust., Belg., Br., Braz., Chin., Cz., Egypt., Eur., Fr., Ger., Hung., Ind., Int., It., Jpn, Jug., Mex., Neth., Nord., Pol., Port., Roum., Rus., Span., Swiss, Turk.,* and *U.S.* Also in *B.P. Vet.*
It. permits $1\frac{1}{2}H_2O$ or $\frac{1}{2}H_2O$.
Belg., Br., Egypt., Eur., Fr., Int., Neth., and *Swiss* also have a monograph for Codeine Phosphate Sesquihydrate ($C_{18}H_{21}NO_3,H_3PO_4,1\frac{1}{2}H_2O$ = 424.4).

The hemihydrate and the sesquihydrate consist of small odourless colourless crystals or a white crystalline powder.
B.P. **solubilities** are: soluble 1 in 4 of water; slightly soluble in alcohol; practically insoluble in chloroform and in ether. *U.S.P.* solubilities are: soluble 1 in 2.5 of water and 1 in 0.5 of water at 80°; soluble 1 in 325 of alcohol and 1 in 125 of boiling alcohol. A 4% solution in water has a pH of 4 to 5. **Store** in airtight containers. Protect from light.

6214-q

Codeine Sulphate *(BANM).*

Codeine Sulfate *(USAN).*
$(C_{18}H_{21}NO_3)_2,H_2SO_4,3H_2O=750.9$.

CAS — 1420-53-7 (anhydrous); 6854-40-6 (trihydrate).

Pharmacopoeias. In *U.S.*

White crystals, usually needle-like, or white crystalline powder. **Soluble** 1 in 30 of water, 1 in 6.5 of water at 80°, and 1 in 1300 of alcohol. Store in airtight containers. Protect from light.

The effect of pH, buffer, and temperature on the degradation of codeine sulphate in aqueous solution.— M. F. Powell, *J. pharm. Sci.*, 1986, *75,* 901.

Dependence

Prolonged use of high doses of codeine has produced dependence of the morphine type (see p.1310) in a small proportion of users. Codeine is subject to abuse but produces less euphoria and sedation than morphine and is not a completely satisfactory substitute for morphine in morphine addicts.

For an extensive review of the incidence of codeine dependence, tolerance, withdrawal symptoms, and risk of abuse, indicating a low risk to public health from the common use of codeine and its preparations, see N. B. Eddy *et al., Codeine and its Alternates for Pain and Cough Relief,* Geneva, World Health Organization, 1970.

A report on the use of codeine and glutethimide in combination by addicts.— J. N. DiGiacomo and C. L. King, *Int. J. Addict.*, 1970, *5,* 279. See also.— W. R. Lange and R. E. Johnson, *J. clin. Pharmac.*, 1985, *25,* 455.

A report of opioid dependence following the administration of opioids for a considerable period of time in the treatment of chronic pain. The most common opioids of dependence were codeine, dextropropoxyphene, and oxycodone. Detoxification was difficult without opioid maintenance and adjunctive analgesia.— F. S. Tennant and R. A. Rawson, *Archs intern. Med.*, 1982, *142,* 1845.

Comment on the increased incidence of codeine abuse in California.— F. S. Tennant (letter), *New Engl. J. Med.*, 1983, *308,* 288.

Codeine-containing preparations were used by drug abusers in New Zealand to produce demethylated products known as "Homebake" that contained variable amounts of morphine.— J. P. Shaw (letter), *Pharm. J.*, 1987, *1,* 607.

Adverse Effects and Treatment

As for Morphine, p.1311.

In therapeutic doses codeine is much less liable than morphine to produce adverse effects. Following large doses of codeine, excitement and convulsions may occur.

OVERDOSAGE. A report of acute codeine overdosage in 1 patient.— D. H. Huffman and R. L. Ferguson, *Johns Hopkins med. J.*, 1975, *136,* 183.

Blood concentrations of codeine ranged from 1.4 to 5.6 µg per mL in 8 adults whose deaths were attributed primarily to codeine overdosage. Pulmonary oedema was the main drug-related finding at autopsy.— J. A. Wright *et al., Clin. Toxicol.*, 1975, *8,* 457. A report of pulmonary oedema occurring as a result of codeine overdosage.— J. Sklar and R. M. Timms, *Chest,* 1977, *72,* 230.

An evaluation of codeine intoxication in 430 children. Symptoms in decreasing order of frequency included sedation, rash, miosis, vomiting, itching, ataxia, and swelling of the skin. Respiratory failure occurred in 8 children and 2 died. All 8 had taken 5 mg or more per kg body-weight. In spite of this it was considered that a single overdose of 5 to 15 mg per kg would generally be tolerated by small children producing symptoms of overdosage without fatality. Treatment should include attention to respiration, emesis or gastric lavage, naloxone and, in all cases, charcoal and laxatives.— K. E. von Mühlendahl *et al., Lancet,* 1976, *2,* 303.

The serum-concentration of codeine in a 3-month-old infant treated with a cough mixture containing codeine phosphate 10 mg per 5 mL was 12 µg per mL 3 days after the last dose. The infant subsequently died.— H. H. Ivey and J. Kattwinkel, *Pediatrics,* 1976, *57,* 164. A 3-month-old infant who had been born prematurely developed near fatal apnoea after two 5-mL doses of Actifed Compound Linctus [each 5 mL contained 10 mg of codeine phosphate; the linctus has been reformulated and no longer contains codeine]. T. C. R. Wilkes *et al.* (letter), *Lancet,* 1981, *1,* 1166.

Two case reports of opioid toxicity in addition to severe salicylate toxicity after overdoses of aspirin and codeine tablets providing 300 mg of aspirin and 8 mg of codeine. Both patients responded to naloxone.— P. J. Leslie *et al., Br. med. J.*, 1986, *292,* 96.

PREGNANCY AND THE NEONATE. Of 50 282 children born to mothers monitored by the Collaborative Perinatal Project, 1564 were found to have been exposed to opioid analgesics, and possibly other drugs, at some time during the first 4 months of the pregnancy. Although there was little evidence of association between malformations and opioid analgesic exposure in general a possible association between respiratory malformations and codeine (563 exposures) was noted.— O. P. Heinonen *et al., Birth Defects and Drugs in Pregnancy,* Littleton MA, Publishing Sciences Group, 1977, p. 286.

A significant association between congenital heart malformations and maternal use of codeine.— S. Zierler and K. J. Rothman, *New Engl. J. Med.*, 1985, *313,* 347. See also.— M. B. Bracken, *ibid.*, 1986, *314,* 1120.

Precautions

As for Morphine, p.1311.

Codeine phosphate 50 mg alone and in combination with alcohol 0.5 g per kg body-weight had a deleterious effect on driving skills in both normal and emergency situations in a simulated driving test.— M. Linnoila and S. Häkkinen, *Clin. Pharmac. Ther.*, 1974, *15,* 368.

INTERACTIONS. Codeine phosphate was adsorbed by light kaolin *in vitro.*— S. K. S. Yu *et al., Aust. J. Pharm.*, 1976, *57,* 468.

Absorption and Fate

Codeine and its salts are absorbed from the gastro-intestinal tract. Ingestion of codeine phosphate produces peak plasma-codeine concentrations in about one hour. Codeine is metabolised by *O-* and *N*-demethylation in the liver to morphine and norcodeine. Codeine and its metabolites are excreted almost entirely by the kidney, mainly as conjugates with glucuronic acid.

The plasma half-life has been reported to be between 3 and 4 hours after administration by mouth or intramuscular injection.

After the administration of codeine phosphate 10 or 20 mg to 5 volunteers, normorphine was detected in the urine, in addition to other known metabolites. The quantities of each were total codeine 70%, total morphine 10%, total norcodeine 9%, and normorphine less than 4%.— W. O. R. Ebbighausen *et al., J. pharm. Sci.*, 1973, *62,* 146.

The maximal rate of codeine metabolism appeared to be 30 mg per hour.— N. Nomof *et al., Clin. Pharmac. Ther.*, 1974, *15,* 215.

In 6 healthy male subjects given radioactive codeine phosphate 30 mg by mouth peak plasma radioactivity occurred about 1 hour after administration and fell with a half-life of 3.1 hours. Within 4 hours a mean of 55.2% of the administered dose had been excreted in the urine with 95.1% being eliminated after 2 days. Similar results were obtained when the subjects were given 2 doses of 25 mg in solution 4 hours apart.— W. D. Bechtel and K. Sinterhauf, *Arzneimittel-Forsch.*, 1978, *28,* 308.

Following the administration of codeine 30 mg by mouth to 2 healthy subjects hydrocodone, norhydrocodone, 6α-hydrocodol, and 6β-hydrocodol in addition to known metabolites were detected in the urine.— E. J. Cone *et al., J. Pharm. Pharmac.*, 1979, *31,* 314.

PROTEIN BINDING. Codeine was about 25% bound to human serum proteins.— J. Judis, *J. pharm. Sci.*, 1977, *66,* 803.

Uses and Administration

Codeine is an analgesic with uses similar to those of morphine (see p.1312) but it is much less potent as an analgesic and has only mild sedative effects.

It is administered by mouth as the phosphate or sulphate in the form of linctuses for the relief of cough and as tablets for the relief of mild to moderate pain. The hydrochloride has also been given by mouth. The phosphate is also given by injection for the relief of pain.

Codeine and its salts are given in doses of 15 to 60 mg up to 6 times a day for the relief of pain. If these doses fail to relieve pain, larger doses rarely succeed and may give rise to restlessness and excitement. Children may be given 500 µg per kg body-weight 4 to 6 times daily.

Codeine and its salts are used to allay unproductive cough, usually in doses of 10 to 20 mg every 4 to 6 hours, to a maximum total of 120 mg in 24 hours. Children may be given up to 250 µg per kg every 4 to 6 hours. It is less constipating than morphine but it is used as tablets or in mixtures for the relief of diarrhoea.

Codeine, usually as the phosphate, is often administered by mouth with aspirin or paracetamol (sometimes known as co-codaprin and co-codamol, see note above).

Codeine polistirex (a codeine and sulphonated diethenylbenzene-ethenylbenzene copolymer complex) is also used.

A comprehensive review of codeine as an analgesic and antitussive in relation to its dependence-producing potential and adverse effects compared with similar drugs. For mild to moderate pain codeine was effective in relatively non-toxic doses but the side-effects of high doses made it less useful than alternative drugs for severe pain. For cough suppression, alternatives were available with a lower dependence-producing liability and less side-effects but none of them had yet been proved to be therapeutically superior to codeine.— N. B. Eddy *et al., Codeine and its Alternates for Pain and Cough Relief,* Geneva, World Health Organization, 1970; *idem, Bull. Wld Hlth Org.*, 1968, *38,* 673; *idem,* 1969, *40,* 1, 425, 639, and 721.

In a double-blind, crossover study of 16 patients with chronic stable cough, 2 doses of codeine phosphate or dextromethorphan hydrobromide 20 mg by mouth were given at night 4 hours apart. Both suppressed cough frequency and intensity to a greater extent than placebo as measured by a pressure transducer placed over the trachea. Dextromethorphan hydrobromide had a greater effect than codeine phosphate on cough intensity, but their effects on frequency were similar.— H. Matthys *et al.*, *J. int. med. Res.*, 1983, *11*, 92.

ADMINISTRATION. *In infants and children.* On the basis of available data, codeine and other opioid cough suppressants should rarely be administered to children less than 6 to 12 months old. They should not be given in productive cough. When indicated for the treatment of nonproductive cough which interferes with sleep or school attendance, either codeine or dextromethorphan should be recommended in the form of single-ingredient preparations.— S. Segal *et al.*, *Pediatrics*, 1978, *62*, 118.

ANALGESIA.

There have been a number of studies of codeine's effect against pain. Many have involved pain following dental procedures, other surgical operations, or childbirth. Many also have been single-dose studies comparing codeine with analgesics such as ibuprofen or comparing codeine combined with another analgesic such as paracetamol with one of the analgesics alone. The results of such studies could be used to support arguments for and against codeine as a useful analgesic in such painful states.

Some references to studies in dental pain: P. Skjelbred and P. Løkken, *Br. J. clin. Pharmac.*, 1982, *14*, 539; P. J. Desjardins *et al.*, *J. clin. Pharmac.*, 1984, *24*, 35; U. Ahlström *et al.*, *Eur. J. clin. Pharmac.*, 1985, *27*, 693; P. A. Moore *et al.*, *Int. J. clin. Pharmac. Ther. Toxic.*, 1985, *23*, 573; A. D. Giles *et al.*, *J. oral maxillofac. Surg.*, 1986, *15*, 727; S. Sagne *et al.*, *J. int. med. Res.*, 1987, *15*, 83.

Some references to studies of codeine in postoperative pain: H. Quiding and S. -O. Häggquist, *Eur. J. clin. Pharmac.*, 1983, *24*, 475; S. Honig and K. A. Murray, *J. clin. Pharmac.*, 1984, *24*, 96; M. Cater *et al.*, *Clin. Ther.*, 1985, *7*, 442; R. D. Ouellette *et al.*, *Curr. ther. Res.*, 1986, *39*, 839; S. D. Gertzbein *et al.*, *Pharmacotherapy*, 1986, *6*, 104.

Some references to studies of codeine in postpartum pain: C. M. Gruber, *J. Am. med. Ass.*, 1977, *237*, 2734; S. S. Bloomfield *et al.*, *Clin. Pharmac. Ther.*, 1977, *21*, 414; S. S. Bloomfield *et al.*, *ibid.*, 1983, *34*, 488; M. Cater and P. M. S. O'Brien, *Clin. Ther.*, 1985, *7*, 442; S. L. Norman *et al*, *ibid.*, 549; J. Jacobson and S. O. Bertilson, *J. int. med. Res.*, 1987, *15*, 89.

GASTRO-INTESTINAL DISORDERS. In a comparison of the effects of codeine phosphate, diphenoxylate (as Lomotil), and ispaghula (as Isogel), taken before meals, on ileostomy output in 18 patients only codeine produced a significant fall in output. This was achieved by a reduction of water and electrolyte output with consequent thickening of its consistency. With Isogel, ileostomy output was more viscid but water and electrolyte output was increased and there was danger of exacerbating water and electrolyte depletion.— C. R. Newton, *Gut*, 1978, *19*, 377.

In a double-blind study in 11 patients with chronic diarrhoea, loperamide 2 mg, diphenoxylate 5 mg with atropine, and codeine phosphate 30 mg had comparable antidiarrhoeal activity.— C. D. Shee and R. E. Pounder, *Br. med. J.*, 1980, *280*, 524.

Preparations of Codeine and its Salts

For some other preparations containing codeine phosphate, see under Aspirin, p.7, and Paracetamol, p.33.

Codeine Phosphate Injection *(U.S.P.)*. pH 3 to 6. It should not be used if it is more than slightly discoloured or contains a precipitate.

Codeine Linctus *(B.P.)*. Codeine phosphate 15 mg, a suitable flavoured vehicle to 5 mL.

The title Diabetic Codeine Linctus may be used for a preparation formulated with a vehicle appropriate for administration to diabetics.

Codeine Linctus *(A.P.F.)*. Codeine phosphate 25 mg, water 0.5 mL, glycerol 1 mL, concentrated chloroform water 0.15 mL or methyl hydroxybenzoate solution 0.05 mL, syrup to 5 mL.

For reports of cardiac glycoside toxicity and myopathy associated with the abuse of Codeine Linctus (*A.P.F.*), which used to contain squill oxymel, see under the Adverse Effects of Squill, p.914.

Paediatric Codeine Linctus *(B.P.)*. Codeine phosphate 3 mg, a suitable flavoured vehicle to 5 mL.

Codeine Syrup *(A.P.F.)*. Codeine phosphate 50 mg, purified water, freshly boiled and cooled 0.15 mL, syrup to 10 mL.

Codeine Phosphate Syrup *(B.P.C. 1973)*. Syr. Codein. Phos. Codeine phosphate 25 mg, chloroform spirit 0.125 mL, freshly boiled and cooled water 0.075 mL, syrup to 5 mL.

Codeine Phosphate Tablets *(B.P., U.S.P.)*. Compressi Codeini Phosphatis.

Codeine Sulfate Tablets *(U.S.P.)*

Proprietary Preparations of Codeine Salts

For some other proprietary preparations containing codeine phosphate, see under Aspirin, p.7, and Paracetamol, p.33.

Bepro *(Wallace Mfg Chem., UK)*. *Syrup*, codeine phosphate 6.75 mg, papaverine hydrochloride 0.625 mg, calcium iodide 50 mg/5 mL.

Diarrest *(Galen, UK)*. *Liquid*, codeine phosphate 5 mg, dicyclomine hydrochloride 2.5 mg, sodium chloride 50 mg, potassium chloride 40 mg, sodium citrate 50 mg/5 mL.

Galcodine *(Galen, UK)*. *Linctus*, codeine phosphate 15 mg/5 mL.
Paediatric linctus, codeine phosphate 3 mg/5 mL.

Kaodene *(Crookes Healthcare, UK)*. *Suspension*, codeine phosphate 10 mg, light kaolin 3 g/10 mL.

Proprietary Names and Manufacturers of Codeine and its Salts

Actacode *(Sigma, Austral.)*; Codate *(USV, Austral.)*; Codeinfos *(Spain)*; Codeisan *(Abello, Spain)*; Codelix *(Drug Houses Austral., Austral.)*; Codicept *(Sanol, Ger.)*; Codicompren *(Cascan, Ger.)*; Codipertussin *(Fink, Ger.; Fink, Switz.)*; Codlin *(Nelson, Austral.)*; Codyl *(Boehringer Ingelheim, Ger.)*; Galcodine *(Galen, UK)*; Paveral *(Desbergers, Canad.)*; Perduretas Codeina *(Medea, Spain)*; Solcodein *(Inibsa, Spain)*; Tricodein *(Zyma, Ger.; Solco, Switz.)*.

The following names have been used for multi-ingredient preparations containing codeine and its salts—222 Tablets *(Frosst, Canad.)*; 282 Mep *(Frosst, Canad.)*; 282 Tablets *(Frosst, Canad.)*; 292 Tablets *(Frosst, Canad.)*; 293 Tablets *(Frosst, Canad.)*; A.C. & C. *(Pharmascience, Canad.)*; Acetaco *(Legere, USA)*; Actifed with Codeine *(Wellcome, USA)*; Actifed-C *(Wellcome, USA)*; Amaphen with Codeine *(Trimen, USA)*; Ambenyl *(Parke, Davis, Canad.; Forest Pharmaceuticals, USA)*; Anacin with Codeine *(Whitehall, Canad.)*; Ancasal *(Anca, Canad.)*; Anexsia with Codeine *(Beecham Laboratories, USA)*; Anodyne Dellipsoids D4 *(Pilsworth, UK)*; Antoin *(Cox, UK)*; Asco-Tin *(Faulding, Austral.)*; Ascriptin with Codeine *(Rorer, USA)*; Aspalgin *(Fawns & McAllan, Austral.)*; Asprodeine *(Nicholas, Austral.)*; Atasol-15 *(Horner, Canad.)*; Atasol-30 *(Horner, Canad.)*; Atasol-8 *(Horner, Canad.)*;

B-A-C 3 *(Mayrand, USA)*; Bancap with Codeine *(Forest Pharmaceuticals, USA)*; Becolyte *(McGloin, Austral.)*; Benylin with Codeine *(Warner-Lambert, UK)*; Bepro *(Wallace Mfg Chem., UK)*; Bex *(Nicholas, Austral.)*; Bromanyl *(Schein, USA)*; Bromphen DC *(Schein, USA)*; Broncodeine *(Nadeau, Canad.)*; Bufferin with Codeine *(Bristol, USA)*; Calcidrine *(Abbott, UK; Abbott, USA)*; Calmylin with codeine *(Technilab, Canad.)*; Capital with Codeine *(Carnrick, USA)*; Chemhisdex C *(Clark, Canad.)*; Cheracol *(Upjohn, Canad.)*; CoActifed *(Wellcome, Canad.)*; CoActifed Expectorant *(Wellcome, Canad.)*; Codalan *(Lannett, USA)*; Codalgin *(Fawns & McAllan, Austral.)*; Codalin *(Clark, Canad.)*; Coda-Med *(Dep, UK)*; Codamin *(Clark, Canad.)*; Codaminophen *(Clark, Canad.)*; Codimal PH *(Central Pharmaceuticals, USA)*; Codiphen *(G.P. Laboratories, Austral.)*; Codis *(Reckitt & Colman, Austral.; Reckitt & Colman Pharmaceuticals, UK)*; Codispril; Codisprina; Codral Blue Label *(Wellcome, Austral.)*; Codral Flu and Cold *(Wellcome, Austral.)*; Codral Forte *(Wellcome, Austral.)*; Codral Linctus *(Wellcome, Austral.)*; Codral Pain Relief *(Wellcome, Austral.)*; Conex with Codeine *(Forest Pharmaceuticals, USA)*; Copavin *(Lilly, USA)*; Coricidin with Codeine *(Schering, Canad.)*; Coryphen-Codeine *(Rougier, Canad.)*; Coterpin *(Ayrton, Saunders, UK)*;

D & M Tablets *(Cambridge Laboratories, Austral.)*; Decrin *(Nicholas, Austral.)*; Deproist with Codeine *(Geneva, USA)*; Dia-Chek *(Searle, Austral.)*; Diaguard Forte *(Nelson, Austral.)*; Diarcalm *(McGloin, Austral.)*; Diarrest *(Galen, UK)*; Dimetane Expectorant-C *(Robins, Canad.)*; Dimetane-DC *(Robins, USA)*; Dimetapp-C *(Robins, Canad.)*; Dimotane CO *(Robins, UK)*; Dimotane with Codeine *(Robins, UK)*; Dolprn *(Bock, USA)*; Dymadon Co *(Wellcome, Austral.)*; Empirin with Codeine *(Wellcome, USA)*; Empracet *(Wellcome, Canad.; Wellcome, USA)*; Emtec *(Technilab, Canad.)*; Exdol *(Frosst, Canad.)*; Fiorinal *(Sandoz, Austral.)*; Fiorinal with Codeine *(Sandoz, USA)*; Fiorinal-C *(Sandoz, Canad.)*; G-2/G-3 Capsules *(Hauck, USA)*; Glucomagma *(Drug Houses Austral., Austral.)*; Guiatuss A-C *(Schein, USA)*; Hedamol *(Nicholas, UK)*; Histadyl EC *(Lilly, UK)*; Hycodin *(Faulding, Austral.)*; Hypon *(Calmic, UK)*; Iophen-C *(Schein, USA)*; Kaodene *(Crookes Healthcare, UK)*; Kaofort *(Boots, Austral.)*; Lenoltec with Codeine *(Technilab, Canad.)*; Linctifed *(Wellcome, UK)*;

Maxigesic *(Mastar, USA)*; Medocodene *(Medo, UK)*; Mersyndol *(Merrell Dow, Austral.; Merrell Dow, Canad.)*; Migraleve *(International Laboratories, UK)*; Migralift *(International Laboratories, UK)*; Myolgin *(Cox, UK)*; Naldecon-CX *(Bristol, USA)*; Nembudeine *(Abbott, Austral.)*; Neo-Pectol *(Neolab, Canad.)*; Neo-Synephrine Linctus *(Winthrop, Austral.)*; Neurodyne *(Fisons, UK)*; Novahistex C *(Dow, Canad.)*; Novahistine DH *(Lakeside, USA)*; Novahistine Expectorant *(Lakeside, USA)*; Novogesic *(Novopharm, Canad.)*; Nucofed *(Beecham Laboratories, USA)*; Nucofed Expectorant *(Beecham Laboratories, USA)*; Nucosef *(Beecham, Austral.)*; Omni-Tuss *(Pennwalt, Canad.)*; Orthoxicol *(Upjohn, UK)*; Orthoxicol Cold & Flu Caps *(Upjohn, Austral.)*; Orthoxicol Cough Suppressant *(Upjohn, Austral.)*;

Panadeine *(Winthrop, Austral.; Winthrop, UK)*; Panadeine Co. *(Winthrop, UK)*; Panamax Co *(Winthrop, Austral.)*; Paracodol *(Fisons, UK)*; Paradeine *(Scotia, UK)*; Parafon Forte C8 *(McNeil, Canad.)*; Parahypon *(Calmic, UK)*; Parake *(Galen, UK)*; Paralgin *(Norton, UK)*; Pardale *(Martindale Pharmaceuticals, UK)*; Pediacof *(Winthrop-Breon, USA)*; Penntuss *(Pennwalt, Canad.; Pennwalt, USA)*; Pentalgin *(Fawns & McAllan, Austral.)*; Pharmidone *(Farmitalia Carlo Erba, UK)*; Phenaphen with Codeine *(Robins, USA)*; Phenephrin *(Nelson, Austral.)*; Phenergan Expectorant with Codeine *(Rhône-Poulenc, Canad.)*; Phenergan VC Expectorant with Codeine *(Rhône-Poulenc, Canad.)*; Phenergan VC with Codeine *(Wyeth, USA)*; Phenergan with Codeine *(Wyeth, USA)*; Phensedyl *(May & Baker, UK)*; Phrenilin with Codeine *(Carnrick, USA)*; Poly-Histine CS *(Bock, USA)*; Poly-Histine Expectorant with Codeine *(Bock, USA)*; Prodismen *(Prosana, Austral.)*; Propain *(Panpharma, UK)*; Pulmo Bailly *(Bengué, UK)*; Rheumatic Dellipsoids D10 *(Pilsworth, UK)*; Robaxisal-C *(Robins, Canad.)*; Robitussin A-C *(Robins, Canad.; Robins, USA)*; Robitussin AC *(Robins, UK)*; Robitussin-DAC *(Robins, USA)*; Ru-Tuss Expectorant *(Boots, USA)*;

Safapryn-Co *(Pfizer, UK)*; Sedapap 3 *(Mayrand, USA)*; Sigma Relief Cold Tablets *(Sigma, Austral.)*; Sinutab with Codeine *(Warner, Austral.; Parke, Davis, Canad.)*; SK-APAP with Codeine *(Smith Kline & French, USA)*; SK-Terpin Hydrate and Codeine *(Smith Kline & French, USA)*; Solcode *(Reckitt & Colman, Austral.)*; Solpadeine *(Winthrop, Austral.; Sterling Research, UK)*; Soma Compound with Codeine *(Wallace, USA)*; Sonalgin *(May & Baker, Austral.; May & Baker, UK)*; Stopayne *(Springbok, USA)*; Syndol *(Merrell, UK)*; Tecnal C *(Technilab, Canad.)*; Tercoda *(Sinclair, UK)*; Tercolix *(Norton, UK)*; Terpalin *(Norton, UK)*; Terpoin *(Hough, Hoseason, UK)*; Thenfacol *(Winthrop, Austral.)*; Triafed-C *(Schein, USA)*; Triaminic Expectorant with Codeine *(Dorsey Laboratories, USA)*; Tussaminic C *(Ancalab, Canad.)*; Tussar *(USV Pharmaceutical Corp., USA)*; Tussi-Organidin *(Horner, Canad.; Wallace, USA)*; Tussirex *(Scot-Tussin, USA)*; Tylenol No. 1 *(McNeil, Canad.)*; Tylenol with Codeine *(McNeil Pharmaceutical, USA)*; Tylex *(Ortho-Cilag, UK)*; Uniflu *(Unigreg, UK)*; Veganin *(Warner, Austral.; Parke, Davis, Canad.; Warner-Lambert, UK)*.

NOTE. The *UK* preparation Actifed Compound Linctus has been reformulated to exclude codeine.

12603-b

Conorphone Hydrochloride *(USAN)*.

Codorphone Hydrochloride; Conorfone Hydrochloride *(rINNM)*; TR-5109. 17-Cyclopropylmethyl-4,5α-epoxy-8β-ethyl-3-methoxymorphinan-6-one hydrochloride.
$C_{23}H_{29}NO_3,HCl = 403.9$.

CAS — 72060-05-0 (conorphone); 70865-14-4 (hydrochloride).

Conorphone hydrochloride is an opioid analgesic with mixed agonist-antagonist activity.

The analgesic efficacy of 2 doses of conorphone (20 and 40 mg), were compared with 2 doses of codeine for postoperative dental pain. Both doses of conorphone and the 60-mg dose of codeine were superior to 30 mg of codeine for the various indices of analgesic activity. The

40-mg dose of conorphone produced side-effects in 25 of 30 subjects that included drowsiness, dizziness, nausea, and vomiting. The low dose of conorphone resulted in side-effects similar to 60 mg of codeine with the exception of a greater incidence of drowsiness. Conorphone 20 mg may be an alternative to 60 mg of codeine for postoperative pain.— R. A. Dionne *et al.*, *Anesth. Prog.*, 1984, *31*, 77.

A report of two studies evaluating single oral doses of conorphone in 50 women with postepisiotomy pain.— E. D. Nelson *et al.*, *Curr. ther. Res.*, 1987, *41*, 276.

Proprietary Names and Manufacturers
Miles Pharmaceuticals, USA.

6215-p

Dextromoramide *(BAN, rINN).*

Dextrodiphenopyrine; *d*-Moramid; Pyrrolamidol. (+)-1-(3-Methyl-4-morpholino-2,2-diphenylbutyryl)pyrrolidine.
$C_{25}H_{32}N_2O_2$=392.5.

CAS — 357-56-2.

6216-s

Dextromoramide Tartrate *(BANM, rINNM).*

Bitartrate de Dextromoramide; Dextromoramide Acid Tartrate; Dextromoramidi Tartras.
$C_{25}H_{32}N_2O_2,C_4H_6O_6$=542.6.

CAS — 2922-44-3.

Pharmacopoeias. In *Belg., Br., Egypt., Eur., Fr., Neth.*, and *Swiss.*

A white odourless crystalline or amorphous powder. Dextromoramide tartrate 6.9 mg is approximately equivalent to 5 mg of dextromoramide.

Soluble 1 in 25 of water and 1 in 85 of alcohol; slightly soluble in chloroform; very slightly soluble in ether. A 1% solution in water has a pH of 3.0 to 4.0. Solutions may be **sterilised** by autoclaving.

Dependence

The use of dextromoramide may produce dependence of the morphine type (see p.1310). It is subject to abuse.

In a case of marked dependence on dextromoramide a 68-year-old man with severe pain had 4400 tablets over 10½ months. Substitution with dihydrocodeine was unsuccessful but levorphanol 1.5 mg four times daily in conjunction with dihydrocodeine, chlorpromazine, and amitriptyline appeared to control the pain.— J. Cormack (letter), *Br. med. J.*, 1967, *1*, 362. Another similar report.— B. A. Juby (letter), *ibid.*

Gross abuse of dextromoramide in Australia.— D. B. Newgreen, *Aust. J. Pharm.*, 1980, *61*, 641.

Adverse Effects, Treatment, and Precautions

As for Morphine, p.1311. It is reported to be less sedating than morphine.

Uses and Administration

Dextromoramide tartrate is an analgesic related to methadone used in the treatment of severe pain. It is not recommended for use in obstetric analgesia. It is given by mouth, by rectum, or by subcutaneous or intramuscular injection, and similar analgesic effects are claimed for the same dose whether given by mouth or by injection. The analgesic effect begins after about 20 to 30 minutes and its duration of action is about 2 to 3 hours.

The usual dose is the equivalent of dextromoramide 5 mg by mouth or by injection increased if necessary up to 20 mg by mouth or 15 mg by injection.

Dextromoramide is also given rectally as suppositories containing the equivalent of 10 mg.

A dose equivalent to not more than 80 µg per kg body-weight has been suggested for use in children.

Manufacturer's comments mainly on the analgesic effects of dextromoramide.— A. J. Grace (letter), *Br. med. J.*, 1980, *281*, 1285. Criticism. Dextromoramide was considered less suitable as an analgesic than morphine, diamorphine, or phenazocine for the control of pain in terminal illness.— A. T. Judd *et al.* (letter), *ibid.*, 1981, *282*, 75.

Preparations

Dextromoramide Injection *(B.P.).* Dextromoramide Tartrate Injection

Dextromoramide Tablets *(B.P.).* Tablets containing dextromoramide tartrate.

Proprietary Preparations

Palfium *(MCP Pharmaceuticals, UK). Injection,* dextromoramide 5 mg and 10 mg(as tartrate)/mL, in ampoules of 1.1 mL.
Tablets, scored, dextromoramide 5 mg and 10 mg (as tartrate).
Suppositories, dextromoramide 10 mg (as tartrate).

Proprietary Names and Manufacturers of Dextromoramide and Dextromoramide Tartrate

Jetrium *(Hek, Ger.)*; Narcolo *(Lusofarmaco, Ital.)*; Palfium *(Faulding, Austral.; Belg.; Janssen, Denm.; Delalande, Fr.; Ger.; Neth.; S.Afr.; Switz.; MCP Pharmaceuticals, UK).*

6217-w

Dextropropoxyphene Hydrochloride *(BANM, rINNM).*

Propoxyphene Hydrochloride *(USAN).* (+)-(1*S*,2*R*)-1-Benzyl-3-dimethylamino-2-methyl-1-phenylpropyl propionate hydrochloride.
$C_{22}H_{29}NO_2,HCl$=375.9.

CAS — 469-62-5 (dextropropoxyphene); 1639-60-7 (hydrochloride).

NOTE. Compounded preparations of dextropropoxyphene hydrochloride and paracetamol in the mass proportions 1 part to 10 parts have the British Approved Name Co-proxamol.

Pharmacopoeias. In *Br., Braz., Cz., Ind.*, and *U.S.* Also in *B.P. Vet.*

A white or slightly yellow odourless or almost odourless powder.

Soluble 1 in 0.3 of water, 1 in 1.5 of alcohol, and 1 in 0.6 of chloroform; soluble in acetone; practically insoluble in ether. **Store** in airtight containers.

6218-e

Dextropropoxyphene Napsylate *(BANM).*

Dextropropoxyphene Napsilate *(rINNM)*; Propoxyphene Napsylate *(USAN).* Dextropropoxyphene naphthalene-2-sulphonate monohydrate.
$C_{22}H_{29}NO_2,C_{10}H_8O_3S,H_2O$=565.7.

CAS — 17140-78-2 (anhydrous); 26570-10-5 (monohydrate).

Pharmacopoeias. In *Br., Ind.*, and *U.S.*

An odourless or almost odourless white powder. Dextropropoxyphene napsylate 100 mg is approximately equivalent to 66 mg of dextropropoxyphene hydrochloride. Practically **insoluble** in water; soluble 1 in 13 to 15 of alcohol and 1 in 3 to 10 of chloroform; soluble in acetone and methyl alcohol. **Store** in airtight containers.

The napsylate is more stable than the hydrochloride in formulations containing aspirin.

Dependence

Prolonged use of dextropropoxyphene may lead to dependence of the morphine type (see p.1310).

A brief review of the abuse liability of dextropropoxyphene.— M. Lader, *Hum. Toxicol.*, 1984, *3*, 229S.

During an epidemic of dextropropoxyphene abuse among American soldiers 13 died, pulmonary oedema being the primary finding at post mortem. Respiratory arrest, psychotic reactions, and dependence also occurred. In 7 patients who became dependent on the intravenous use of dextropropoxyphene, abscesses, cellulitis, thrombophlebitis, or sclerosis of the veins developed within 6 to 12 weeks despite the use of sterile vehicles and techniques. Withdrawal symptoms were mild.— F. S. Tennant, *Archs intern. Med.*, 1973, *132*, 191.

PREGNANCY AND THE NEONATE. Withdrawal symptoms occurred in an infant born to a woman who had taken dextropropoxyphene during pregnancy, the last dose being taken 11 hours before delivery.— W. W. Quillian and C. A. Dunn, *J. Am. med. Ass.*, 1976, *235*, 2128. See also H. K. Tyson, *J. Pediat.*, 1974, *85*, 684.

TREATMENT OF DEPENDENCE. Treatment of dextropropoxyphene dependence in a 41-year-old woman who had a history of multiple drug abuse consisted of withdrawing dextropropoxyphene and giving methadone on a reducing scale for 10 days.— R. Wall *et al.*, *Br. med. J.*, 1980, *280*, 1213. Comments.— N. Mellor (letter), *ibid.*, *281*, 617. Reply.— R. Wall (letter), *ibid.*

Successful detoxification of a 45-year-old woman with a long history (5 years) of dextropropoxyphene abuse. Administration of clonidine over a 9-day period reduced or eliminated most of the symptoms of dextropropoxyphene withdrawal.— D. A. Johnson and M. E. Bohan, *Am. J. Psychiat.*, 1983, *140*, 1217.

A report of 6 cases of dextropropoxyphene dependence presenting with difficult treatment problems. The patients' subjective discomfort and concomitant craving during gradual withdrawal was more intense and more poorly tolerated than that observed with other opioid analgesic agents.— N. B. D'Abadie and J. D. Lenton, *Sth. med. J.*, 1984, *77*, 299.

Adverse Effects

As for Morphine, p.1311, although in the recommended dosage the adverse effects of dextropropoxyphene are less marked. Gastro-intestinal effects are the most common. Liver impairment has been reported.

There are a disturbing number of fatalities from either accidental or intentional overdosage with dextropropoxyphene. Many reports emphasize the rapidity with which death ensues; death within an hour of overdosage is considered by some not to be uncommon. Overdosage is often complicated by patients also taking alcohol and using mixed preparations such as dextropropoxyphene with paracetamol or aspirin.

Symptoms of overdosage are similar to those of morphine poisoning (see p.1311). In addition patients may experience convulsions and psychotic reactions. There may be pulmonary oedema and cardiac arrhythmias.

Dextropropoxyphene injections are painful and have a very destructive effect on soft tissues and veins.

The proceedings of a symposium on the safety and efficacy of dextropropoxyphene. Many of the participants dealt with the problems of dextropropoxyphene overdosage, often in conjunction with paracetamol and sometimes with alcohol. Profound and even fatal CNS depression can develop rapidly as a result of the dextroproxyphene content and in many cases death has occurred within an hour (A.T. Proudfoot, p.85S). The quantity likely to be fatal is small. Whittington (p.175S) suggested that 15 tablets or less of dextropropoxyphene hydrochloride with paracetamol (co-proxamol) could lead to death and this is close to the figure of 20 tablets suggested by Young and Lawson (*Br. med. J.*, 1980, *280*, 1045). A number of papers reviewed the cases of poisoning in different countries; one of these on poisoning in the *USA* (B.S. Finkle, p.115S) demonstrated that the incidence of dextroproxyphene-associated deaths reached a peak in 1977 and has been falling since then at a rate that is not matched by a decline in prescribing. Also Finkle could not demonstrate a connection between the metabolite norpropoxyphene and the fatalities. One suggestion made during the discussion (E. Anggard, p.181S) and picked up by others (A.T. Proudfoot, p.182S; P. Turner, p.237S) was that changing from the hydrochloride to the more slowly absorbed napsylate might reduce morbidity and mortality.— *Hum. Toxicol.*, 1984, *3*, *Suppl.*, 1S-238S. Some other reviews of poisoning cases: P. S. Madsen *et al.*, *Acta anaesth. scand.*, 1984, *28*, 661; E. Segest, *Hum. Toxicol.*, 1987, *6*, 203. See also R. J. Young, *Drugs*, 1983, *26*, 70.

Neonatal Distalgesic poisoning.— J. O. Beattie *et al.* (letter), *Lancet*, 1981, *2*, 49.

A view that the membrane stabilising activity of dextropropoxyphene is a major factor responsible for its severe cardiac depressant effect and is a major cause of fatal poisoning.— J. A. Henry and S. L. Cassidy, *Lancet*, 1986, *1*, 1414.

EFFECTS ON THE LIVER. Reports of jaundice in patients taking dextropropoxyphene without paracetamol.— G. K. Daikos and J. C. Kosmidis, *J. Am. med. Ass.*, 1975, *232*, 835; T. H. Lee and P. J. Rees, *Br. med. J.*, 1977, *2*, 296; M. J. Ford *et al.*, *ibid.*, 674; *Med. J. Aust.*, 1979, *2*, 494.

Reports of recurrent jaundice, upper abdominal pain, and rigors in 3 patients taking co-proxamol; the effects were attributable to dextropropoxyphene hepatotoxicity.

The diagnosis was established in each patient by rechallenge. Dextropropoxyphene toxicity should be considered in patients with relapsing jaundice mimicking biliary disease, in whom gall stones have been excluded.— M. F. Bassendine *et al.*, *Gut*, 1986, *27*, 444.

Eleven patients on long-term co-proxamol therapy for pain showed no abnormalities of liver or renal function, as assessed by serum-prealbumin concentrations and blood enzyme and electrolyte activities. Although the preparation is hepatotoxic when taken acutely in overdose, in chronic therapeutic dosage it appears to be free from this hazard.— D. R. Hutchinson *et al.*, *J. Pharm. Pharmac.*, 1986, *38*, 242.

Treatment of Adverse Effects

As for Morphine, p.1311.

Rapid treatment of overdosage with naloxone and assisted respiration is essential. Administration of activated charcoal or gastric lavage may be of value but dialysis is of little value.

Convulsions may be controlled with an anticonvulsant. Stimulants should not be used because of the risk of inducing convulsions.

Patients taking overdoses of dextropropoxyphene with paracetamol will also require treatment for paracetamol poisoning, and this is described on p.32.

Mixtures of dextropropoxyphene and aspirin may be involved; the treatment of aspirin poisoning is described on p.5.

A review of the pharmacological considerations and clinical management of dextropropoxyphene overdosage.— R. J. Young, *Drugs*, 1983, *26*, 70.

A review of the clinical features and management of Distalgesic overdose.— A. T. Proudfoot, *Hum. Toxicol.*, 1984, *3*, *Suppl.*, 85S.

A case report of successful treatment of a dextropropoxyphene napsylate and paracetamol overdose with 90 tablets in a 28-year-old patient. The patient recovered following treatment with acetylcysteine and haemodialysis despite a 20-hour delay in therapy.— S. M. Pond *et al.*, *J. Toxicol. clin. Toxicol.*, 1982, *19*, 1.

A case report of successful treatment of dextropropoxyphene overdose by intravenous infusion of naloxone. It was suggested that continuous naloxone infusion is a safe and effective treatment for opiate overdose and that it may be preferable to intermittent boluses as potentially fatal respiratory depression is less likely to occur.— S. G. Parker and D. G. Thomas (letter), *Br. med. J.*, 1983, *287*, 1547.

Precautions

As for Morphine, p.1311.

Central depressants may contribute to the hazards of dextropropoxyphene. The convulsant action of high doses of dextropropoxyphene may be enhanced by central nervous system stimulants.

Dextropropoxyphene interacts with several other drugs through inhibition of liver metabolism. Drugs reported to be affected include benzodiazepines, beta blockers, carbamazepine, phenytoin, and warfarin.

ADMINISTRATION IN RENAL FAILURE. The dose of dextropropoxyphene should be reduced to 25% in patients with a glomerular filtration-rate of less than 10 mL per minute.— W. M. Bennett *et al.*, *Am. J. Kidney Dis.*, 1983, *3*, 155.

PORPHYRIA. Dextropropoxyphene was considered to be unsafe in patients with acute porphyria although there is conflicting experimental evidence on porphyrinogenicity.— M. R. Moore and K. E. L. McColl, *Porphyrias, Drug Lists*, Glasgow, Porphyria Research Unit, University of Glasgow, 1987.

Absorption and Fate

Dextropropoxyphene is readily absorbed from the gastro-intestinal tract, but it is subject to considerable first-pass metabolism. It is rapidly distributed and concentrated in the liver, lungs, brain, and kidneys. Dextropropoxyphene crosses the placenta and has been detected in breast milk. Peak plasma concentrations occur about 1 to 2 hours after ingestion.

Dextropropoxyphene is *N*-demethylated to norpropoxyphene in the liver. It is excreted in the urine mainly as metabolites. It is now recognised that dextropropoxyphene and norpropoxyphene have prolonged elimination half-lives.

A review of the pharmacokinetics of dextropropoxyphene.— R. M. Pearson, *Hum. Toxicol.*, 1984, *3*, *Suppl.*, 37S.

Evidence from a study in 8 healthy subjects that the single-dose kinetics of dextropropoxyphene follow a three-compartment model. Following single oral and intravenous doses of dextropropoxyphene estimated half-life using this model was 18 hours; data analysis according to the two-compartment model yielded much shorter half-lives and a systemic clearance that was on average 30% higher. Prediction of steady-state levels on the basis of a two-compartment analysis would result in an underestimate of the degree of accumulation by an average of 25%.— L. F. Gram *et al.*, *Eur. J. clin. Pharmac.*, 1984, *26*, 749. See also W. A. Colburn and C. E. Inturrisi, *ibid.*, 1985, *28*, 725; L. F. Gram *et al.*, *ibid.*, 726.

Some further references to the pharmacokinetics of dextropropoxyphene: C. E. Inturrisi *et al.*, *Clin. Pharmac. Ther.*, 1982, *31*, 157; P. Crome *et al.*, *Hum. Toxicol.*, 1984, *3*, *Suppl.*, 41S; K. Brøsen *et al.*, *Eur. J. clin. Pharmac.*, 1985, *29*, 79.

Uses and Administration

Dextropropoxyphene is an analgesic related to methadone. It is administered by mouth as the hydrochloride or napsylate to alleviate mild to moderate pain. It has little antitussive activity.

Dextropropoxyphene is mainly used in conjunction with other analgesics with anti-inflammatory and antipyretic effects, such as aspirin and paracetamol. The usual dose is 65 mg of dextropropoxyphene hydrochloride or 100 mg of the napsylate three or four times daily. Compounded preparations of dextropropoxyphene hydrochloride (1 part) and paracetamol (10 parts) have the British Approved Name co-proxamol.

In a detailed review of the analgesic effectiveness of dextropropoxyphene given at a symposium on the analgesics, Beaver (*Hum. Toxicol.*, 1984, *3*, *Suppl.*, 191S) observed that with respect to single oral doses, the weight of evidence points to the recommended doses of dextropropoxyphene being no more and probably less effective than usual doses of paracetamol, aspirin, or other non-steroidal anti-inflammatory agents. However, the comparative effectiveness may vary substantially depending on the cause of the pain. When it comes to comparative studies involving combinations of dextropropoxyphene with other analgesics, findings are even less clear-cut; there are studies showing some benefit from such a combination and there are studies showing no benefit. Sturrock in his review at the same meeting (*ibid.*, 221S) highlighted the problems of carrying out studies on the effectiveness of dextropropoxyphene with paracetamol (co-proxamol). Of the 18 studies on this combination that he reviewed, only 5 were controlled, and of these only 3 included a placebo. There was a need, he considered, for placebo-controlled studies especially in the long-term use of the combination in chronic pain.

In summarising the meeting Turner (*ibid.*, 237S) felt that it was not reasonable to ask for placebo-controlled studies. He also voiced the opinion of various people who used co-proxamol that the combination gives a greater degree of control and effectiveness than is possible with either agent alone. Such a view is a matter of debate and there is the contrary opinion that the benefits of co-proxamol have not been shown to outweigh the risks (*Drug & Ther. Bull.*, 1983, *21*, 17).

For reference to the administration of dextropropoxyphene in renal failure see under Precautions, above.

Preparations of Dextropropoxyphene Salts

Dextropropoxyphene Capsules *(B.P.)*. Capsules containing dextropropoxyphene napsylate.

Propoxyphene Hydrochloride and Acetaminophen Tablets *(U.S.P.)*. Tablets containing dextropropoxyphene hydrochloride and paracetamol.

Propoxyphene Hydrochloride, Aspirin, and Caffeine Capsules *(U.S.P.)*. Capsules containing dextropropoxyphene hydrochloride, aspirin, and caffeine.

Propoxyphene Hydrochloride Capsules *(U.S.P.)*. Capsules containing dextropropoxyphene hydrochloride.

Propoxyphene Napsylate and Acetaminophen Tablets *(U.S.P.)*. Tablets containing dextropropoxyphene napsylate and paracetamol. Store at 15° to 30°.

Propoxyphene Napsylate and Aspirin Tablets *(U.S.P.)*. Tablets containing dextropropoxyphene napsylate and aspirin. Store at 15° to 30°.

Propoxyphene Napsylate Oral Suspension *(U.S.P.)*. A suspension containing dextropropoxyphene napsylate with alcohol 0.5 to 1.5%. Avoid freezing. Protect from light.

Propoxyphene Napsylate Tablets *(U.S.P.)*. Tablets containing dextropropoxyphene napsylate.

Proprietary Preparations

Cosalgesic *(Cox, UK)*. *Tablets*, co-proxamol 357.5mg (dextropropoxyphene hydrochloride 32.5 mg, paracetamol 325 mg).

Distalgesic *(Dista, UK)*. *Tablets*, co-proxamol, 357.5 mg (dextropropoxyphene hydrochloride 32.5 mg, paracetamol 325 mg).

Doloxene *(Lilly, UK)*. *Capsules*, dextropropoxyphene napsylate 100 mg.

Doloxene Compound *(Lilly, UK)*. *Capsules*, dextropropoxyphene napsylate 100 mg, aspirin 375 mg, caffeine 30 mg.

Paxalgesic *(Steinhard, UK)*. *Tablets*, co-proxamol 357.5 mg (dextropropoxyphene hydrochloride 32.5 mg, paracetamol 325 mg).

Proprietary Names and Manufacturers

642 Tablets *(Frosst, Canad.)*; Abalgin *(Denm.)*; Algafan *(Arg.)*; Algaphan *(Austral.; Belg.)*; Algodex *(Canad.)*; Antalvic *(Houdé, Fr.)*; Daraphen *(USA)*; Darvon *(Lilly, Spain; Lilly, USA)*; Darvon-N *(Lilly, Canad.; Lilly, USA)*; Deprancol *(Parke, Davis, Spain)*; Dépronal *(Belg.; Fr.)*; Dépronal retard *(Warner-Lambert, Switz.)*; Depronal *(Neth.)*; Depronal SA *(Canad.; Warner, UK)*; Depronal-SA *(S.Afr.)*; Develin *(Gödecke, Ger.)*; Dolene *(Lederle, USA)*; Dolocap *(USA)*; Dolorphen *(Neth.)*; Dolotard *(Benzon, Swed.)*; Doloxene *(Lilly, Austral.; Lilly, Denm.; Norw.; Lilly, S.Afr.; Lilly, Swed.; Lilly, UK)*; Erantin *(Ger.)*; Lenigesial *(Ital.)*; Liberen *(Lisapharma, Ital.)*; Mardon *(USA)*; Novopropoxyn *(Novopharm, Canad.)*; Pro-65 *(Canad.)*; Proxagesic *(Reid-Provident, USA)*; SK-65 *(Smith Kline & French, UK; Smith Kline & French, USA)*.

The following names have been used for multi-ingredient preparations containing dextropropoxyphene salts—692 Tablets *(Frosst, Canad.)*; Capadex *(Fawns & McAllan, Austral.)*; Cosalgesic *(Cox, UK)*; Darvocet-N *(Lilly, USA)*; Darvon Compound *(Lilly, USA)*; Darvon with A.S.A. *(Lilly, USA)*; Darvon-N Compound *(Lilly, Canad.)*; Darvon-N with A.S.A. *(Lilly, Canad.; Lilly, USA)*; Dextrogesic *(Unimed, UK)*; Di-Gesic *(Dista, Austral.)*; Distalgesic *(Dista, UK)*; Dolasan *(Lilly, UK)*; Dolene AP-65 *(Lederle, USA)*; Dolene Compound-65 *(Lederle, USA)*; Doloxene Compound *(Lilly, UK)*; Doloxene Co *(Lilly, Austral.)*; Lorcet *(UAD, USA)*; Napsalgesic *(Dista, UK)*; Paradex *(Protea, Austral.)*; Paxalgesic *(Steinhard, UK)*; Propacet *(Lemmon, USA)*; SK-65 APAP *(Smith Kline & French, USA)*; Wygesic *(Wyeth, USA)*.

12637-j

Dezocine *(USAN, rINN)*.

Wy-16225. (−)-13β-Amino-5,6,7,8,9,10,11α,12-octahydro-5α-methyl-5,11-methanobenzocyclodecen-3-ol.

$C_{16}H_{23}NO = 245.4$.

CAS — 53648-55-8.

Dezocine is an analgesic with opioid agonist and antagonist properties which has been given by intramuscular, intravenous, and subcutaneous injection for the relief of severe pain.

Reviews of the actions and uses of dezocine: D. J. Petro, *Clin. Anaesth.*, 1983, *1*, 159; M. Weintraub and A. Bakst, *Hosp. Formul.*, 1986, *21*, 667.

After a single intravenous injection of dezocine 20 mg, 21 of 25 patients with severe pain remained free of pain for a mean of 3.5 hours. Doses of 10 or 15 mg were less effective. Pronounced dizziness occurred in 23 of the 25 patients. Other side-effects included nausea, vomiting, aching of the nose (each in 1 patient), and sweating (2 patients).— W. Oosterlinck and A. Verbaeys, *Curr. med. Res. Opinion*, 1980, *6*, 472.

In a double-blind controlled study of 20 cancer patients suffering continuous pain, dezocine 10 mg by intramuscular injection was significantly more effective than placebo in relieving pain. Side-effects reported included nausea, slight perspiration, and sensation of heat.— M. Staquet, *Curr. med. Res. Opinion*, 1980, *6*, 634.

A double-blind study in 160 patients indicated that dezocine was efficient and safe for the relief of moderate pain after lower abdominal obstetric or gynaecological surgery. Dezocine 10 mg was equipotent with morphine 10 mg, both given by intramuscular injection.— J.

W. Downing *et al.*, *Br. J. Anaesth.*, 1981, *53*, 59.

In equivalent analgesic doses (10 mg per 70 kg body-weight intravenously) respiratory depression induced by dezocine was approximately the same as that of morphine, although dezocine was associated with a more rapid onset and a brief higher peak activity. Unlike morphine, a ceiling effect for respiratory depression by dezocine occurred at 30 mg per 70 kg body-weight and an additional 10 mg per 70 kg did not increase respiratory depression. Subjective effects of dezocine were in many ways similar to those of morphine but were considered less pleasant; at high doses symptoms suggestive of psychotomimetic effects occurred more frequently after dezocine.— A. Romagnoli and A. S. Keats, *Clin. Pharmac. Ther.*, 1984, *35*, 367.

A comparative study of the haemodynamic and respiratory effects of dezocine, ciramadol, and morphine in 30 patients undergoing diagnostic cardiac catheterization. Dezocine (0.125 mg per kg body-weight), ciramadol (0.6 mg per kg), or morphine (0.125 mg per kg) was administered as a single intravenous injection. Dezocine, ciramadol, and morphine were found to have no clinically important haemodynamic or respiratory effects.— R. L. Rothbard *et al.*, *Clin. Pharmac. Ther.*, 1985, *38*, 84.

A double-blind study in 198 patients with moderate or severe postoperative pain. The analgesic efficacy of single intravenous injections of dezocine (2.5, 5.0, and 10.0 mg), morphine (5.0 mg), and placebo was assessed at regular intervals for 6 hours after administration. All active treatments provided greater pain relief than placebo. Pain relief with dezocine 5 and 10 mg was significantly greater than with placebo for up to 4 and 5 hours, respectively, and with morphine up to one hour. Pain relief scores were significantly higher with morphine than with placebo at all observations except that of the fifth hour, and higher with dezocine 2.5 mg than with placebo for the first 30 minutes. Dezocine was favoured in a dose-dependent order, with morphine 5 mg rated lower than dezocine 5 mg and higher than dezocine 2.5 mg.— U. A. Pandit *et al.*, *J. clin. Pharmac.*, 1986, *26*, 275.

A double-blind study of 60 hospitalized patients with chronic moderate to severe cancer pain comparing single doses and multiple doses of intramuscular dezocine (10 mg) with butorphanol (2 mg) and placebo. After an initial dose, the peak analgesia of both analgesics was similar, but the duration of analgesia was longer with dezocine. After multiple doses, dezocine was superior to butorphanol in terms of length of treatment; dezocine also produced less incidence of adverse effects compared with butorphanol.— J. E. Stambaugh and J. McAdams, *Clin. Pharmac. Ther.*, 1987, *42*, 210. See also B. T. Finucane *et al.*, *Sth. med. J.*, 1986, *79*, 548.

Further references to comparative studies of dezocine: R. J. Fragen and N. Caldwell, *Anesth. Analg.*, 1978, *57*, 563 (with pethidine); H. P. Wuest and J. W. Bellville, *J. clin. Pharmac.*, 1979, *19*, 205 (with pentazocine); J. S. Gravenstein, *Int. J. clin. Pharmac. Ther. Toxic.*, 1984, *22*, 502 (with morphine and placebo); M. M. Warren *et al.*, *J. Urol., Baltimore*, 1985, *134*, 457 (with morphine).

ABUSE. The abuse potential of dezocine (15, 30, and 60 mg subcutaneously) was studied and compared with that of morphine (15 and 30 mg subcutaneously) and placebo in a double-blind study in 10 adult non-dependent drug abusers. Dezocine appears to have the potential for abuse, although this potential seems to be less than that of morphine.— D. R. Jasinski and K. L. Preston, *Clin. Pharmac. Ther.*, 1985, *38*, 544.

Proprietary Names and Manufacturers

Dalgan *(Wyeth, USA)*.

6219-1

Diamorphine Hydrochloride *(BANM)*.

Diacetylmorphine Hydrochloride; Heroin Hydrochloride. 4,5-Epoxy-17-methylmorphinan-3,6-diyl diacetate hydrochloride monohydrate.

$C_{21}H_{23}NO_5,HCl,H_2O=423.9$.

CAS — 561-27-3 (diamorphine); 1502-95-0 (hydrochloride, anhydrous).

Pharmacopoeias. In *Br.* and *Port.*

An almost white crystalline powder, odourless when freshly prepared but develops an odour of acetic acid on storage.

Soluble 1 in 1.6 of water, 1 in 12 of alcohol, and 1 in 1.6 of chloroform; practically insoluble in ether. Solutions for injection are prepared by dissolving, immediately before use, the sterile contents of a sealed container in Water for Injections.

Incompatible with mineral acids and alkalis. **Store** in well-closed containers. Protect from light. Diamorphine hydrolyses in aqueous solution to 3-*O*- and 6-*O*-acetylmorphine and morphine to a significant extent at room temperature; the rate of decomposition is at a minimum at about pH 4.

Degradation of diamorphine in solution.— E. A. Davey and J. B. Murray, *Pharm. J.*, 1969, *2*, 737. See also.— V. A. Jones *et al.*, *Br. J. clin. Pharmac.*, 1987, *23*, 651P.

Stability of diamorphine in chloroform water.— H. Cooper *et al.*, *Pharm. J.*, 1981, *1*, 682. Comment, including a reminder that the degradation product of diamorphine, monoacetyl morphine, is as potent as morphine, so that the 'efficacy half-life' is far longer than the more strictly interpreted pharmaceutical half-life.— R. G. Twycross (letter), *ibid.*, *2*, 218; I. M. Beaumont (letter), *ibid.*, 41.

Diamorphine was found to be compatible with metoclopramide hydrochloride, haloperidol, hyoscine, prochlorperazine maleate, cyclizine lactate, and methotrimeprazine for at least 24 hours when stored in plastic syringes at ambient temperature away from light.— M. C. Allwood, *Br. J. pharm. Pract.*, 1984, *6*, 88. See also.— M. K. A. Irvine *et al.* (letter), *Pharm. J.*, 1984, *1*, 464.

Solutions of diamorphine hydrochloride and haloperidol in prefilled syringes kept under refrigeration for 7 days showed no loss of haloperidol, and only a loss of 1.5% diamorphine. The solutions kept at room temperature for 24 hours showed no significant loss of diamorphine or haloperidol, either protected or unprotected from light.— A. J. Collins *et al.*, *J. Pharm. Pharmac.*, 1986, *38*, *Suppl.*, 51P.

Dependence

Use of diamorphine is liable to produce dependence of the morphine type (see p.1310).

PREGNANCY AND THE NEONATE. Some references to diamorphine dependence in pregnant women and the effects on the foetus and neonate: M. M. Desmond *et al.*, *J. Pediat.*, 1972, *80*, 190; A. P. Amarose and M. J. Norusis, *Am. J. Obstet. Gynec.*, 1976, *124*, 635; H. S. Fricker and S. Segal, *Am. J. Dis. Child.*, 1978, *132*, 360; E. M. Ostrea and C. J. Chavez, *J. Pediat.*, 1979, *94*, 292; M. H. Lifschitz *et al.*, *ibid.*, 1983, *102*, 686; H. Kalter and J. Warkany, *New Engl. J. Med.*, 1983, *308*, 491; H. M. Klenka, *Br. med. J.*, 1986, *293*, 745.

TOLERANCE. Cross-tolerance between methadone and diamorphine.— J. Volavka *et al.*, *J. nerv. ment. Dis.*, 1978, *166*, 104.

Adverse Effects, Treatment, and Precautions

As for Morphine, p.1311.

Pulmonary oedema after overdosage is a common cause of fatalities among diamorphine addicts. Nausea and vomiting, constipation, and hypotension are claimed to be less common than with morphine.

There are many reports of adverse effects associated with the abuse of diamorphine, usually obtained illicitly in an adulterated form.

Most of the reports of adverse effects with diamorphine involve its abuse. In addition to the central effects, there are effects caused by the administration methods and by the adulterants. Thus in many instances it is difficult to identify the factor causing the toxicity. Most body systems are involved and some representative references are as follows:

Effects on the cardiovascular system.— S. M. Deglin *et al.*, *Drugs*, 1977, *14*, 29; F. L. Glauser *et al.*, *Bull. Narcot.*, 1977, *29*, (Jan.–Mar.), 85.

Effects on the kidneys.— E. E. Cunningham *et al.*, *J. Am. med. Ass.*, 1983, *250*, 2935.

Effects on the liver.— I. V. D. Weller *et al.*, *Gut*, 1984, *25*, 417.

Effects on muscle.— G. Husby, *Ann. intern. Med.*, 1975, *83*, 801.

Effects on the respiratory system.— D. B. Louria, *J. Am. med. Ass.*, 1982, *248*, 2536.

See also Pregnancy and the Neonate under Dependence, above.

Absorption and Fate

Diamorphine hydrochloride is well absorbed from the gastro-intestinal tract and following subcutaneous or intramuscular injection. Following injection it is rapidly converted to 6-*O*-monoacetylmorphine in the blood and then to morphine. Morphine has also been detected in the blood following oral administration of diamorphine. Both diamorphine and monoacetylmorphine readily cross the blood-brain barrier. Morphine and morphine glucuronide are the main excretion products in the urine.

A review of the metabolism of diamorphine and morphine in man.— U. Boerner *et al.*, *Drug Metab. Rev.*, 1975, *4*, 39.

Following administration of diamorphine 10 mg per 70 kg body-weight intravenously to healthy, post-addict subjects the metabolites identified in urine were morphine, 6-acetylmorphine, normorphine, morphine 3-glucuronide, 6-acetylmorphine 3-glucuronide, and normorphine glucuronide. Morphine 3-glucuronide accounted for about 50% and morphine about 7% of the dose of diamorphine.—S. Y. Yeh *et al.*, *J. pharm. Sci.*, 1977, *66*, 201.

The pharmacokinetics of diamorphine hydrochloride 2 mg given intrathecally to 3 patients undergoing cardiopulmonary bypass.— A. Moore *et al.*, *Clin. Pharmac. Ther.*, 1984, *35*, 40.

A study of the pharmacokinetics of diamorphine in 11 patients with chronic pain following intravenous, intramuscular, and oral administration of diamorphine hydrochloride. Parenteral administration provided measurable blood concentrations of diamorphine, and its active metabolites 6-acetylmorphine, and morphine. Maximal blood concentrations of diamorphine and 6-acetylmorphine were reached within minutes and were cleared rapidly. The mean half-life of diamorphine after intravenous injection or infusion was about 3 minutes. Morphine concentrations rose more gradually, and morphine was cleared much more slowly. Oral administration of diamorphine resulted in measurable blood concentrations of morphine but not of diamorphine or 6-acetylmorphine. The amount of circulating morphine provided by an oral dose of diamorphine was only 79% of that available from an equal amount of morphine. It was concluded that diamorphine is a pro-drug that serves to determine the distribution of its active metabolites. Parenteral diamorphine is rapidly converted to 6-acetylmorphine, which contributes to rapid pain relief. Oral diamorphine is converted to morphine and appears to be an efficient means of providing morphine to the systemic circulation.— C. E. Inturrisi *et al.*, *New Engl. J. Med.*, 1984, *310*, 1213.

Uses and Administration

Diamorphine hydrochloride resembles morphine in its action (see p.1312). It is a more potent analgesic than morphine but it has a shorter duration of action, its effect lasting only about 3 hours. However, it is more soluble than the morphine salts so that small volumes can be given by injection when it is used for the relief of severe pain especially in terminal illnesses. Doses by subcutaneous or intramuscular injection are 5 to 10 mg. Similar doses may be used by mouth. Doses of 5 mg have been given intravenously to patients with a myocardial infarction.

Diamorphine was often used in analgesic 'cocktails', such preparations are now seldom used.

Diamorphine has a powerful cough suppressant effect but other suppressants are preferred.

Because of its abuse potential diamorphine is carefully controlled and in many countries it is not available for clinical use since by dose adjustment morphine can provide equivalent analgesia, albeit in a larger injection volume. Some references to the morphine/diamorphine debate: R. G. Twycross, *Pain*, 1977, *3*, 93; *Lancet*, 1984, *1*, 1449; E. N. Brandt, *New Engl. J. Med.*, 1984, *311*, 530; A. M. Mondzac, *ibid.*, 532; M. N. Levine *et al.*, *Archs intern. Med.*, 1986, *146*, 353.

A patient developed acute tolerance to intravenous diamorphine given for chronic cancer pain. Relief of pain was achieved with morphine 100 to 120 mg rectally every four hours.— G. W. Hanks and E. A. Thomas, *Br. med. J.*, 1985, *291*, 1124.

ADMINISTRATION BY CONTINUOUS INFUSION. A discussion of the use of continuous subcutaneous infusions of drugs by syringe driver. This technique may be used successfully in the terminal care of patients when drugs cannot be given orally. Diamorphine, which is more water soluble than morphine, is the opioid of choice, although morphine may be used. Diamorphine 1 g can be dissolved in 1.6 mL of water to give a solution with a

volume of 2.4 mL (415 mg/mL), but the maximum suggested concentration is 250 mg per mL. The equianalgesic dose of subcutaneous diamorphine corresponds to one third of the total daily dose of oral morphine, whether in solution or sustained-release tablets.
If the analgesic requirement is not known the following protocol is recommended:
(1) Start injections every 4 hours of 2.5 or 5 mg diamorphine, or if the patient has already been taking opioids a dose that is equivalent to the last dose.
(2) If this is unsatisfactory increase this dose in 50% increments until the patient reports even a little pain relief.
(3) Calculate the 24-hour requirement by multiplying by six, and start the infusion at this level.
(4) Increase the 24-hour dosage in the pump by 50% increments until the pain is controlled. Note that requirements may vary from less than 20 mg to more than 5 g per 24 hours.
When starting an infusion it is important not to allow any breakthrough pain. This may be achieved either by starting the infusion more than 2 hours before the previous oral dose wears off or by giving a loading dose injection of the 4-hourly requirement.— S. B. Dover, *Br. med. J.*, 1987, *294*, 553. See also H. T. Hutchinson *et al.* (letter), *Lancet*, 1981, *2*, 1279; V. Jones *et al.* (letter), *Pharm. J.*, 1985, *2*, 426.

ADMINISTRATION, EPIDURAL AND INTRATHECAL. A double-blind study comparing diamorphine 5 mg intramuscularly with the same dose epidurally and with phenoperidine 2 mg epidurally for pain following caesarean section. Analgesia was of rapid onset in all groups but its duration was significantly greater with epidural phenoperidine and diamorphine than with intramuscular diamorphine. Itching was reported by 50% of patients undergoing epidural analgesia.— D. J. Macrae *et al.*, *Br. J. Anaesth.*, 1987, *59*, 354.

Further references to intraspinal diamorphine: H. J. McQuay *et al.* (letter), *Lancet*, 1980, *1*, 768; L. Kaufman (letter), *ibid.*, 1981, *2*, 1341.

MYOCARDIAL INFARCTION. A discussion of immediate primary care of a suspected heart attack. The drug of choice for pain relief is diamorphine 5 to 10 mg, preferably by slow intravenous injection. It relieves pain and anxiety and may improve left ventricular function. Intramuscular administration may work too slowly. Acute left ventricular failure should be treated with diamorphine, oxygen, and an intravenous diuretic such as frusemide.— *Drug & Ther. Bull.*, 1986, *24*, 89.

Preparations

Diamorphine and Cocaine Elixir *(B.P.C. 1973)*. Diamorphine hydrochloride 5 mg, cocaine hydrochloride 5 mg, syrup 1.25 mL, alcohol (90%) 0.625 mL, chloroform water to 5 mL. When specified by the prescriber, the proportion of diamorphine may be varied. It should be freshly prepared.

Diamorphine, Cocaine, and Chlorpromazine Elixir *(B.P.C. 1973)*. Diamorphine hydrochloride 5 mg, cocaine hydrochloride 5 mg, chlorpromazine elixir 1.25 mL (containing chlorpromazine hydrochloride 6.25 mg), alcohol (90%) 0.625 mL, chloroform water to 5 mL. When specified by the prescriber, the proportion of diamorphine may be varied. It should be freshly prepared. Protect from light.
NOTE. The administration of cocaine with diamorphine or morphine has been reported to be of no apparent benefit.

Diamorphine Injection *(B.P.)*. Contains diamorphine hydrochloride. Prepared immediately before use by dissolving the sterile contents of a sealed container in the requisite amount of Water for Injections.

Diamorphine Linctus *(B.P.C. 1973)*. Diamorphine hydrochloride 3 mg, oxymel 1.25 mL, glycerol 1.25 mL, compound tartrazine solution 0.06 mL, syrup to 5 mL. It should be recently prepared. When a dose less than, or not a multiple of, 5 mL is prescribed the linctus should be diluted to 5 mL, or a multiple, with syrup. Such dilutions must be freshly prepared and not used more than 2 weeks after issue. *Dose.* 2.5 to 10 mL.

Proprietary Names and Manufacturers

Evans Medical, UK; Roche, UK.

6221-g

Dihydrocodeine Phosphate *(BANM, rINNM)*.
Hydrocodeine Phosphate.
$C_{18}H_{23}NO_3,H_3PO_4$=399.4.

CAS — 24204-13-5.

Pharmacopoeias. In *Jpn.*

6222-q

Dihydrocodeine Tartrate *(BANM, rINNM)*.

Dihydrocodeine Acid Tartrate; Dihydrocodeine Bitartrate; Drocode; Hydrocodeine Bitartrate.
7,8-Dihydro-3-*O*-methylmorphine hydrogen tartrate; 4,5-Epoxy-3-methoxy-17-methylmorphinan-6-ol hydrogen tartrate.
$C_{18}H_{23}NO_3,C_4H_6O_6$=451.5.

CAS — 125-28-0 (dihydrocodeine); 5965-13-9 (tartrate).

NOTE. Compounded preparations of dihydrocodeine tartrate and paracetamol in the mass proportions 1 part to 50 parts have the British Approved Name Co-dydramol.

Pharmacopoeias. In *Aust.*, *Br.*, *Ger.*, and *Hung. Pol.* has the monohydrate.

Odourless, or almost odourless, colourless crystals or white crystalline powder. **Soluble** 1 in 4.5 of water; sparingly soluble in alcohol; practically insoluble in ether. A 10% solution in water has a pH of 3.2 to 4.2. Solutions for injection are **sterilised** by autoclaving. **Protect** from light.

Dependence

Prolonged use of dihydrocodeine may produce dependence of the morphine type (see p.1310).

Withdrawal symptoms occurred in a 6-week-old infant on stopping dihydrocodeine which had been given in a dose of 2.5 mg per kg body-weight daily for 2 weeks.— H. J. Hiller and E. Gladtke, *Dt. med. Wschr.*, 1974, *99*, 1502.

Case reports of 5 patients who had morphine-like side-effects when taking dihydrocodeine or withdrawal symptoms when medication ceased; doses were generally 60 to 90 mg four times daily.— P. Marks *et al.*, *Br. med. J.*, 1978, *1*, 1594.

Adverse Effects, Treatment, and Precautions

As for Morphine, p.1311, though side-effects from dihydrocodeine are less pronounced.

Five of 112 medical or surgical patients taking dihydrocodeine in usual doses had hallucinations and a further 4 had vivid dreams: 2 of 93 controls had hallucinations and 4 of 190 had vivid dreams.— M. Taylor *et al.*, *Br. med. J.*, 1978, *2*, 1198.

Single doses of intravenous dihydrocodeine 25 and 50 mg were assessed in 24 patients who had undergone bilateral third molar surgery. Patients reported significantly more pain after dihydrocodeine than after placebo and the hyperalgesia was greater and of longer duration after 50 mg dihydrocodeine than after 25 mg dihydrocodeine.— R. A. Seymour *et al.*, *Lancet*, 1982, *1*, 1425. A comment that dihydrocodeine might increase dental pain by acting as an antagonist in situations where acute pain is accompanied by high opioid activity.— J. A. Henry (letter), *ibid.*, *2*, 223.

ADMINISTRATION IN RENAL FAILURE. A woman with chronic renal failure, on maintenance haemodialysis, who had received dihydrocodeine 600 mg by mouth over a period of 4 days showed marked signs of CNS depression during the succeeding 24 hours. The condition responded dramatically to naloxone. The plasma-dihydrocodeine concentration 3 days after the last dose was 700 μg per litre. Caution is needed in giving dihydrocodeine to patients with severe renal impairment.— J. N. Barnes and F. J. Goodwin, *Br. med. J.*, 1983, *286*, 438.

See also under Absorption and Fate, below.

OVERDOSAGE. Toxicological investigations in 6 deaths associated with codeine or dihydrocodeine overdosage.— M. A. Peat and A. Sengupta, *Forensic Sci.*, 1977, *9*, 21.

A 29-year-old man who had taken 2.1 g of dihydrocodeine, and who had renal and hepatic impairment, required 46.6 mg of naloxone over 106 hours.— N. Redfern, *Br. med. J.*, 1983, *287*, 751. See also.— S. G. Parker and D. G. Thomas (letter), *ibid.*, 1547.

Absorption and Fate

The pharmacokinetics of dihydrocodeine may be similar to those of codeine.

Studies in 7 healthy subjects indicated that the rate of absorption of dihydrocodeine following oral administration was independent of dose. It was considered likely that the substantially reduced bioavailability observed was due to presystemic metabolism in the gut wall or liver.— F. J. Rowell *et al.*, *Eur. J. clin. Pharmac.*, 1983, *25*, 419.

The pharmacokinetics of dihydrocodeine given by mouth differed between subjects with normal renal function and patients with chronic renal failure treated with haemodialysis. It was suggested that the kidney has an important role in the elimination of opioid analgesics.— J. N. Barnes *et al.*, *Br. med. J.*, 1985, *290*, 740 and 1287.

Uses and Administration

Dihydrocodeine tartrate is used for the relief of moderate to severe pain. The usual dose by mouth is 30 mg after food every 4 to 6 hours. Children over 4 years of age may be given 0.5 to 1 mg per kg body-weight.
Dihydrocodeine tartrate may also be given by deep subcutaneous or intramuscular injection in doses of up to 50 mg.
Dihydrocodeine tartrate may also be given by mouth as a cough suppressant in doses of 10 mg every 4 to 6 hours. A recommended children's dose is 200 μg per kg every 4 to 6 hours.
Dihydrocodeine phosphate has also been used as an analgesic.
Dihydrocodeine tartrate and paracetamol in combination have been used as an analgesic and cough suppressant. Compounded preparations of dihydrocodeine tartrate (1 part) and paracetamol (50 parts) have the British Approved Name Co-dydramol.

For a review of the uses and side-effects of dihydrocodeine as an analgesic and cough suppressant in comparison with codeine, see N. B. Eddy, *Codeine and its Alternates for Pain and Cough Relief*, Geneva, World Health Organization, 1970; *idem*, *Bull. Wld Hlth Org.*, 1969, *40*, 1 and 639.

Eighteen patients with severe airflow obstruction took dihydrocodeine 15 mg or placebo 30 minutes before anticipated exercise during a double-blind crossover study. When the patients assessed their own responses at home their mean daily breathlessness score was significantly improved by the dihydrocodeine but there was only marginal improvement in walking distance, and no significant change in spirometric test values. Hospital assessment showed significant improvement after dihydrocodeine in both treadmill exercise tolerance and breathlessness on walking, but again no significant change in spirometry values. Dihydrocodeine may offer some benefit in normocapnic patients who are severely disabled by breathlessness.— M. A. Johnson, *Br. med. J.*, 1983, *286*, 675. See also.— A. A. Woodcock *et al.*, *New Engl. J. Med.*, 1981, *305*, 1611.

Preparations

Dihydrocodeine Injection *(B.P.)*. Contains dihydrocodeine tartrate.

Dihydrocodeine Tablets *(B.P.)*. Contain dihydrocodeine tartrate.

Proprietary Preparations of Dihydrocodeine Tartrate

DF 118 *(Duncan, Flockhart, UK)*. *Tablets*, dihydrocodeine tartrate 30 mg.
Elixir, dihydrocodeine tartrate 10 mg/5 mL.
Injection, dihydrocodeine tartrate 50 mg/mL, in ampoules of 1 mL.

DHC Continus *(Napp, UK)*. *Tablets*, scored, controlled-release, dihydrocodeine tartrate 60 mg.

Paramol (formerly known as Paramol-118) *(Duncan, Flockhart, UK)*. *Tablets*, co-dydramol 510 mg (dihydrocodeine tartrate 10 mg, paracetamol 500 mg).

Proprietary Names and Manufacturers of Dihydrocodeine Salts

Bicodein *(Spain)*; DF 118 *(Austral.; Allen & Hanburys, S.Afr.; Duncan, Flockhart, UK)*; DHC Continus *(Napp, UK)*; Fortuss *(Austral.)*; Paracodin *(Schering, Austral.; Knoll, Ger.; Knoll, S.Afr.; Knoll, Switz.)*; Paracodina *(Knoll, Ital.; Knoll-Made, Spain)*; Remedacen *(Rorer, Ger.)*; Rikodeine *(Riker, Austral.)*; Tiamon *(Temmler, Ger.)*.

The following names have been used for multi-ingredient preparations containing dihydrocodeine salts— Codox *(Glaxo, Austral.)*; Compal *(Reid-Rowell, USA)*; Onadox-118 *(Duncan, Flockhart, UK)*; Paramol *(Duncan, Flockhart, UK)*; Synalgos-DC *(Wyeth, USA)*; Tuscodin *(Schering, Austral.)*; Tuscodin Cold Capsules *(Schering, Austral.)*.

6224-s

Dipipanone Hydrochloride *(BANM, rINNM)*.

Phenylpiperone Hydrochlorde; Piperidyl Methadone Hydrochloride; Piperidylamidone Hydrochloride. (±)-4,4-Diphenyl-6-piperidinoheptan-3-one hydrochloride monohydrate.
$C_{24}H_{31}NO,HCl,H_2O$=404.0.

CAS — 856-87-1 (hydrochloride); 467-83-4 (dipipanone).

Pharmacopoeias. In *Br.*

An almost odourless, white, crystalline powder. M.p. 124° to 127°.
Soluble 1 in 40 of water, 1 in 1.5 of alcohol, and 1 in 6 of acetone; practically insoluble in ether. A 2.5% solution in water has a pH of 4 to 6. Solutions are **sterilised** by autoclaving.

Dependence
Prolonged use of dipipanone may produce dependence of the morphine type (see p.1310). Preparations of dipipanone hydrochloride with cyclizine hydrochloride are subject to abuse.

References: I. P. James *et al.* (letter), *Br. med. J.*, 1976, *2*, 1448; D. H. Marjot (letter), *ibid.*, 1978, *1*, 1214; *ibid.*, 1980, *281*, 290.

Adverse Effects, Treatment, and Precautions
As for Morphine, p.1311.
Intravenous injection may cause an alarming fall in blood pressure, and is not recommended. Cyclizine hydrochloride is often given with dipipanone hydrochloride to reduce the incidence of nausea and vomiting.

Uses and Administration
Dipipanone hydrochloride is an opioid analgesic related to methadone. It is used in the treatment of moderate or severe pain.
It is usually given by mouth in a dose of 10 mg, with cyclizine hydrochloride, repeated every 6 hours. The dose may be increased if necessary in increments of 5 mg; it is seldom necessary to exceed a dose of 30 mg. Following administration by mouth the effect begins within an hour and lasts about 6 hours. It has also been given by subcutaneous or intramuscular injection.

Preparations
Dipipanone and Cyclizine Tablets *(B.P.)*. Contain dipipanone hydrochloride and cyclizine hydrochloride.

Proprietary Preparations
Diconal *(Calmic, UK)*. *Tablets*, scored, dipipanone hydrochloride 10 mg, cyclizine hydrochloride 30 mg.

Proprietary Names and Manufacturers
The following names have been used for multi-ingredient preparations containing dipipanone hydrochloride— Diconal *(Calmic, UK)*; Wellconal.

12679-n

Doxpicomine Hydrochloride *(USAN, rINNM)*.

Doxpicodin Hydrochloride; LY-108380. (−)-α-1,3-Dioxan-5-yl-*N,N*-dimethyl-3-pyridylmethylamine hydrochloride.
$C_{12}H_{18}N_2O_2,HCl$=258.7.

CAS — 62904-71-6 (doxpicomine); 69494-04-8 (hydrochloride).

Doxpicomine hydrochloride is an analgesic that appears to act through opioid receptors. It has been given by intramuscular injection in doses of up to 400 mg.

References: M. S. Mok *et al.*, *Clin. Pharmac. Ther.*, 1981, *29*, 266 (comparison with pethidine); R. I. H. Wang and N. Robinson, *ibid.*, 771 (comparison with morphine); *idem*, *J. clin. Pharmac.*, 1983, *23*, 44 (comparison with pethidine).

Proprietary Names and Manufacturers
Lilly, USA.

12698-b

Eptazocine *(rINN)*.

ST-2121. (−)-(1*S*,6*S*)-2,3,4,5,6,7-Hexahydro-1,4-dimethyl-1,6-methano-1*H*-4-benzazonin-10-ol.
$C_{15}H_{21}NO$=231.3.

CAS — 72522-13-5.

Eptazocine is reported to be an opioid analgesic.

Proprietary Names and Manufacturers
Sedapain *(Jpn)*.

6225-w

Ethoheptazine Citrate *(BANM, rINNM)*.

Wy-401. Ethyl 1-methyl-4-phenylperhydroazepine-4-carboxylate dihydrogen citrate.
$C_{16}H_{23}NO_2,C_6H_8O_7$=453.5.

CAS — 77-15-6 (ethoheptazine); 6700-56-7 (citrate); 2085-42-9 (citrate, ±).

Adverse Effects
Nausea, vomiting, drowsiness, and dizziness may occur following administration of ethoheptazine citrate. Stimulation of the central nervous system has been reported following administration of large doses.

Uses and Administration
Ethoheptazine citrate is structurally related to pethidine. It is employed as an analgesic in the treatment of mild to moderate pain, usually in conjunction with other compounds such as aspirin and meprobamate. The usual dose is 150 mg three or four times daily.

ANALGESIA. For a review of the clinical efficacy of ethoheptazine, and comparisons of its analgesic effects with codeine, see N. B. Eddy *et al.*, *Codeine and its Alternates for Pain and Cough Relief*, Geneva, World Health Organization, 1970. See also *idem*, *Bull. Wld Hlth Org.*, 1969, *40*, 1.

Proprietary Preparations
Equagesic *(Wyeth, UK)*. *Tablets*, ethoheptazine citrate 75 mg, meprobamate 150 mg, aspirin 250 mg.

Proprietary Names and Manufacturers
Panalgin *(Ital.)*.

The following names have been used for multi-ingredient preparations containing ethoheptazine citrate— Ecuagesico; Equagesic *(Wyeth, Canad.; Wyeth, UK)*; Zactane; Zactipar *(Wyeth, UK)*; Zactirin *(Wyeth, UK)*; Zactrin; Zamintol.

6226-e

Ethylmorphine Hydrochloride *(BANM)*.

Aethylmorphinae Hydrochloridum; Aethylmorphini Hydrochloridum; Chlorhydrate de Codéthyline; Ethylmorphini Hydrochloridum; Ethylmorphinium Chloride. 3-*O*-Ethylmorphine hydrochloride dihydrate; 7,8-Didehydro-4,5-epoxy-3-ethoxy-17-methylmorphinan-6-ol hydrochloride dihydrate.
$C_{19}H_{23}NO_3,HCl,2H_2O$=385.9.

CAS — 76-58-4 (ethylmorphine); 125-30-4 (hydrochloride).

Pharmacopoeias. In *Arg., Aust., Belg., Br., Chin., Cz., Egypt., Eur., Fr., Ger., Hung., Ind., Jpn, Jug., Mex., Neth., Nord., Pol., Port., Roum., Rus., Span.,* and *Swiss.*

A white or almost white crystalline powder. **Soluble** in water and in alcohol; slightly soluble in chloroform; practically insoluble in ether. A 2% solution in water has a pH of 4.3 to 5.7. **Store** in well-closed containers. Protect from light.

Ethylmorphine hydrochloride has been used similarly to codeine as an analgesic and cough suppressant. It was also given in eye-drops as a lymphagogue.

Proprietary Names and Manufacturers
Codéthyline *(Houdé, Fr.)*; Dionina *(Llorens, Spain)*; Diosan Comp. *(Abello, Spain)*; Diptol *(Navarro, Spain)*; Renotin *(Lane & Stedman, UK)*; Trachyl *(Beytout, Fr.)*.

The following names have been used for multi-ingredient preparations containing ethylmorphine hydrochloride— Cosanyl *(Parke, Davis, Austral.)*; Natirose *(Lipomed, UK)*; Terpo-Dionin *(Winthrop, Canad.)*.

6227-l

Etorphine Hydrochloride *(BANM, rINNM)*.

19-Propylorvinol Hydrochloride; M-99. (6*R*, 7*R*, 14*R*)-7,8-Dihydro-7-(1-*R*-1-hydroxy-1-methylbutyl)-6-*O*-methyl-6,14α-ethenomorphine hydrochloride; (2*R*)-2-[(−)-(5*R*, 6*R*, 7*R*, 14*R*)-4,5-Epoxy-3-hydroxy-6-methoxy-9a-methyl-6,14-ethenomorphinan-7-yl]pentan-2-ol hydrochloride.
$C_{25}H_{33}NO_4,HCl$=448.0.

CAS — 14521-96-1 (etorphine); 13764-49-3 (hydrochloride).

Pharmacopoeias. In *B.P. Vet.*

A white or almost white microcrystalline powder. **Soluble** 1 in 40 of water, 1 in 30 of alcohol, very slightly soluble in chloroform; practically insoluble in ether. A 2% solution in water has a pH of 4.0 to 5.5. **Store** in well-closed containers. Protect from light.

Dependence
Etorphine hydrochloride has the potential for abuse and dependence of the morphine type (see p.1310).

References: D. R. Jasinski *et al.*, *Clin. Pharmac. Ther.*, 1975, *17*, 267.

Adverse Effects and Treatment
As for Morphine, p.1311. Spillage on the skin or splashes in the eyes or mouth should be treated immediately by lavage with copious quantities of water. Etorphine hydrochloride is highly potent and rapid acting; minute amounts can exert serious effects leading to coma. It may be absorbed through skin and mucous membranes. It is thus advisable to inject an antagonist immediately following contamination of skin or mucous membranes with preparations containing etorphine hydrochloride and to wash the affected areas copiously. Accidental injection or needle scratch should also be treated immediately by injecting an antagonist. Naloxone is preferred as the antagonist in medical treatment. However, veterinary preparations of etorphine are supplied with a preparation containing diprenorphine hydrochloride and this should be used for immediate first-aid antagonism if naloxone is not available.

The accidental injection of some or all of the contents of a 2-mL syringe containing etorphine 2.45 mg and acepromazine 10 mg per mL (Immobilon, for use in large animals) in a healthy 41-year-old man produced dizziness, nausea, and coma. Two doses of nalorphine 10 mg with supportive measures were required to reverse the coma, and metoclopramide 10 mg was given intravenously to treat the nausea. The patient was out of danger in 6 hours.— S. Firn (letter), *Lancet*, 1973, *2*, 95. It was found later that the syringe contained 1 mL both before and after the accident. The effects were due to solution present on the needle.— *idem*, 1974, *1*, 577.
Further reports of etorphine (Immobilon) poisoning in man.— *Vet. Rec.*, 1976, *98*, 513; P. G. E. Goodrich (letter), *ibid.*, 1977, *100*, 458; C. M. Orr (letter), *ibid.*, 574; H. M. A. Omersa (letter), *ibid.*, 1986, *118*, 466.

Uses and Administration
Etorphine hydrochloride is a highly potent analgesic and narcotic. It is used with acepromazine maleate as a sedative to assist in the control of large animals and with methotrimeprazine for small animals. The duration of action of etorphine is 1 to 2 hours in animals but it may be longer in man, especially if the large animal preparation is involved.

Proprietary Veterinary Names and Manufacturers
Immobilon (also contains acepromazine maleate or methotrimeprazine) *(C-Vet, UK)*.

6228-y

Fentanyl Citrate *(BANM, USAN, rINNM)*.

Phentanyl Citrate; R-4263. *N*-(1-Phenethyl-4-piperidyl)propionanilide dihydrogen citrate.
$C_{22}H_{28}N_2O,C_6H_8O_7$=528.6.

CAS — 437-38-7 (fentanyl); 990-73-8 (citrate).

Pharmacopoeias. In *Br., Braz., Egypt.,* and *U.S.* Also in *B.P. Vet. Cz.* includes Fentanyl.

White granules or a white crystalline powder. **Soluble** 1 in 40 of water, 1 in 140 of alcohol, 1 in 350 of chloroform, 1 in 10 of methyl alcohol; slightly soluble in ether. The *U.S.P.* injection has a pH of 4.0 to 7.5. **Incompatible** with thiopentone and methohexitone. **Store** in well-closed containers. Protect from light.

CAUTION. *Avoid contact with skin and the inhalation of particles of fentanyl citrate.*

INCOMPATIBILITY. Intravenously administered nafcillin sodium shortly followed by a combination of fentanyl citrate and droperidol, resulted in the formation of a thick, white precipitate in the intravenous tubing which completely occluded the lumen.— E. L. Jeglum *et al.*, *Am. J. Hosp. Pharm.*, 1981, *38*, 462.

STABILITY IN SOLUTION. Fentanyl was hydrolysed in acid solution by the cleavage of propionic acid but was unchanged in alkaline solution.— C. A. Janicki *et al.*, *J. pharm. Sci.*, 1968, *57*, 451.

Dependence

Prolonged use of fentanyl may lead to dependence of the morphine type (see p.1310).

Adverse Effects and Treatment

As for Morphine, p.1311. Respiratory depression which occurs especially with high doses responds to naloxone. Atropine may be used to block the vagal effects of fentanyl such as bradycardia. Muscle rigidity may occur and has been reported to be alleviated by muscle relaxants.

A view that the fixed-ratio combination of fentanyl and droperidol is irrational and can cause distressing and potentially lethal adverse effects.— *Med. Lett.*, 1981, *23*, 74.

A study of the haemodynamic changes in 80 preterm neonates receiving fentanyl, isoflurane, halothane, or ketamine.— R. H. Friesen and D. B. Henry, *Anesthesiology*, 1986, *64*, 238.

EFFECTS ON THE NERVOUS SYSTEM. A case report of seizure-like muscle movements in a 73-year-old patient during a fentanyl infusion with simultaneous EEG recording. Cortical seizure activity was found to be absent, the abnormal motor activity was attributed to myoclonus produced by opioid depression or to a pronounced form of opioid-induced rigidity. In all previously reported cases of "seizures" the patients have received less than 50 µg per kg body-weight fentanyl, which suggests that low to moderate doses are responsible.— J. C. Scott and F. H. Sarnquist, *Anesthesiology*, 1985, *62*, 812.

EFFECTS ON RESPIRATORY FUNCTION. A detailed review of the postoperative respiratory complications of opioids, with details of the risk of delayed respiratory depression following fentanyl anaesthesia.— M. R. D. Bennett and A. P. Adams, *Clin. Anesth.*, 1983, *1*, 41.

A double-blind study of the respiratory effects of fentanyl or butorphanol following barbiturate induction in 31 healthy women undergoing outpatient gynaecologic surgery. Seven of the 15 patients receiving fentanyl had significant respiratory depression that required assisted ventilation. One of the butorphanol patients experienced a 45-second self-limited respiratory depression. It was concluded that fentanyl and butorphanol have comparable anaesthetic effects, but butorphanol is safer in terms of respiratory and adverse effects.— G. E. Dryden, *J. clin. Pharmac.*, 1986, *26*, 203.

Precautions

As for Morphine, p.1311.

While using fentanyl citrate and droperidol for hypotensive anaesthesia it was noted in 22 patients that after an initial rapid fall, the systolic blood pressure could not be reduced below 90 to 100 mmHg, even by using concentrations of up to 6% of halothane.— P. J. Thompson (letter), *Br. med. J.*, 1969, *3*, 300.

In 8 patients undergoing neuroleptanalgesia with droperidol, diazepam, and fentanyl prior to carotid angiography, laryngeal reflex closure was repressed permitting aspiration of a test contrast medium. Neuroleptanalgesia should not be used without safeguarding the airway in patients liable to regurgitation and aspiration of gastric contents.— J. G. Brock-Utne *et al.*, *Br. J. Anaesth.*, 1976, *48*, 699. See also C. J. Kopriva *et al.*, *Anesthesiology*, 1974, *40*, 596; V. M. F. Hey and A. H. M. Z. Mollah (letter), *Lancet*, 1979, *1*, 552; L. Strunin and I. M. Corall (letter), *ibid.*, 673.

Unexpectedly high plasma-fentanyl concentrations occurred in a patient following epidural administration.— R. E. S. Bullingham *et al.* (letter), *Lancet*, 1980, *1*, 1361.

ADMINISTRATION DURING CARDIOPULMONARY BYPASS. Several studies have shown that plasma-fentanyl concentrations decrease during cardiopulmonary bypass. Bentley *et al.* demonstrated that fentanyl was sequestered by the lungs (*Clin. Pharmac. Ther.*, 1983, *34*, 703). Whereas, a study *in vitro* showed that the plasma decrease of fentanyl was largely due to its removal by the membrane oxygenator and to a minor extent by the silicone tubing. (G. Koren *et al.*, *Eur. J. clin. Pharmac.*, 1984, *27*, 51). A decrease in concentration of fentanyl in the priming fluid at neutral or high pH values has also suggested adsorption onto the circuit (M. Skacel *et al.*, *Br. J. Anaesth.*, 1986, *58*, 947).

EFFECT ON INTRACRANIAL PRESSURE. Fentanyl and droperidol given by injection reduced the CSF pressure of 8 of 9 patients with space-occupying intracranial lesions and in patients with normal CSF pathways. The CSF pressure was unaffected by phenoperidine and droperidol.— W. Fitch *et al.*, *Br. J. Anaesth.*, 1969, *41*, 800.

In 8 anaesthetised normocapnic patients with space-occupying intracranial lesions droperidol 7.5 to 12.5 mg caused an increase of intracranial pressure (ICP) in 4; a decrease in mean arterial pressure (MAP) (for the 8) from 99.9 to 85 mmHg resulted in a significant decrease from 79.9 to 57.8 mmHg in cerebral perfusion pressure (CPP). When fentanyl 200 to 300 µg was added there were minimal changes in ICP but a further decrease in MAP to 71.1 mmHg resulted in a further reduction in CPP to 47.8 mmHg. Neuroleptanalgesics should be used in patients with intracranial hypertension only if hypocapnia was established and if arterial pressure was near normal.— B. B. Misfeldt *et al.*, *Br. J. Anaesth.*, 1976, *48*, 963.

Fentanyl 200 µg was given intravenously to 10 anaesthetised patients, 9 of whom were hypocapnic, with space-occupying intracranial lesions. Increases or decreases in intracranial pressure occurred but were small and not significant. Mean arterial pressure and cerebral perfusion pressure were significantly reduced by fentanyl, although the changes were small unless the patient was already hypotensive. Fentanyl should not be given to such patients but otherwise it was a valuable adjunct to anaesthesia.— E. Moss *et al.*, *Br. J. Anaesth.*, 1978, *50*, 779.

Absorption and Fate

Fentanyl citrate is absorbed from the gastro-intestinal tract. After parenteral administration it has a rapid onset and short duration of action. It is rapidly metabolised, probably by oxidative *N*-dealkylation, and excreted mainly in the urine. The short duration of action is probably due to redistribution rather than metabolism and excretion. Up to 70% has been reported to be bound to plasma proteins.

A detailed review of the clinical pharmacokinetics of fentanyl.— L. E. Mather, *Clin. Pharmacokinet.*, 1983, *8*, 422.

There were considerable interindividual variations in the pharmacokinetics of fentanyl and plasma concentrations following intravenous bolus injections were shown to be unreliable predictors of both analgesic and respiratory depressant effects in anaesthetic practice. Halothane and enflurane inhibited fentanyl degradation.— K. A. Lehmann, *Fortschr. Med.*, 1985, *103*, 938.

A study in 45 patients of the pharmacokinetics of fentanyl during constant-rate intravenous infusion for the relief of pain following surgery.— D. J. R. Duthrie *et al.*, *Br. J. Anaesth.*, 1986, *58*, 950.

A study of the influence of hypothermia on the disposition of fentanyl in 18 children undergoing cardiac surgery.— G. Koren *et al.*, *Eur. J. clin. Pharmac.*, 1987, *32*, 373.

Fentanyl citrate and base were absorbed transdermally in a study of 10 subjects; the systemic availability of fentanyl by this route was approximately 30% of that found using the intravenous route.— P. S. Sebel *et al.*, *Eur. J. clin. Pharmac.*, 1987, *32*, 529.

For results of a study of transdermal absorption of fentanyl see under Sufentanil Citrate, p.1320.

PREGNANCY AND THE NEONATE. A study of the pharmacokinetics and haemodynamic effects of fentanyl in preterm infants during ligation of patent ductus arteriosus.— C. Collins *et al.*, *Anesth. Analg.*, 1985, *64*, 1078.

A study of the pharmacokinetics of fentanyl in 14 neonates undergoing major surgical procedures.— D. E. Koehntop *et al.*, *Anesth. Analg.*, 1986, *65*, 227.

Uses and Administration

Fentanyl citrate is a potent opioid analgesic, chemically related to pethidine, with actions similar to those of morphine (see p.1312) and pethidine (see p.1318).

Following intravenous injection of 100 µg the effect begins almost immediately, although maximum analgesia and respiratory depression may not occur for several minutes, and the average duration of action is 30 to 60 minutes although analgesia may only last for 10 to 20 minutes. Increasing the dose to 50 µg per kg body-weight can give pain relief for 4 to 6 hours.

Fentanyl is used as an analgesic, an adjunct to general anaesthetics, and as an anaesthetic for induction and maintenance. When used with a neuroleptic such as droperidol it can induce a state of neuroleptanalgesia in which the patient is calm and indifferent to his surroundings and is able to cooperate with the surgeon.

Fentanyl is usually given by intravenous injection, but the intramuscular route is used for premedication and postoperative pain as well as for maintenance of anaesthesia. Dosage recommendations show a wide range depending on the technique. Patients with spontaneous respiration may be given 50 to 200 µg of fentanyl as an initial dose with supplements of 50 µg. In the *USA* it is recommended that doses above 2 µg per kg body-weight should be used in conjunction with assisted ventilation. Patients whose ventilation is assisted may be given 300 to 3500 µg (up to 50 µg per kg) as an initial dose with supplements of 100 to 200 µg or higher depending on the patient's response. These high doses have been reported to moderate or attenuate the response to surgical stress.

Reduced doses are used in children and the elderly. In the *UK* recommended initial doses for children range from 3 to 5 µg per kg for those with spontaneous respiration; supplements of 1 µg per kg may be given. When ventilation is assisted, the initial recommended dose is 15 µg per kg. In the *USA* doses as low as 2 to 3 µg per kg are employed in children between the ages of 2 to 12 years.

A study of the cardiovascular responses to large doses of fentanyl and alfentanil in patients undergoing lower abdominal surgery. Fentanyl produced a more prolonged stable cardiovascular pattern than alfentanil.— M. Rucquoi and F. Camu, *Br. J. Anaesth*, 1983, *55*, 223S.

Administration of high-dose fentanyl was found to have little effect on the established metabolic response to surgery, compared with the marked changes observed when the same dose is given before the onset of surgical stimulation.— J. M. Bent *et al.*, *Anaesthesia*, 1984, *39*, 19.

Haemodynamic responses during induction and intubation in geriatric patients using low-dose fentanyl. Respiratory depression was observed in 3 of 16 patients. There was a significant attenuation of the cardiovascular stress response in those who received fentanyl.— F. Chung and D. Evans, *Can. Anaesth. Soc. J.*, 1985, *32*, 622.

Further references to fentanyl suppressing endocrine or metabolic responses to surgery: M. Hynynen *et al.*, *Br. J. Anaesth.*, 1986, *58*, 1260; C. Klingstedt *et al.*, *ibid.*, 1987, *59*, 184; S. Lacoumenta *et al.*, *ibid.*, 713.

ADMINISTRATION. A case report of unilateral analgesia in an 83-year-old woman who received an injection of fentanyl into the lumbosacral plexus for postoperative pain relief following amputation.— B. Smith *et al.* (letter), *Lancet*, 1987, *1*, 1497.

ADMINISTRATION, EPIDURAL. References to fentanyl being given epidurally for relief of pain of various sources: M. J. Wolfe and A. D. G. Nicholas (letter), *Lancet*, 1979, *2*, 150; H. J. McQuay *et al.* (letter), *ibid.*, 1980, *1*, 768; T. A. Torda and D. A. Pybus, *Br. J. Anaesth.*, 1982, *54*, 291; E. A. Shipton (letter), *S. Afr. med. J.*, 1984, *65*, 193; J. Tisdale, *Can. J. Hosp. Pharm.*, 1986, *39*, 170.

See also under Precautions, above.

ANAESTHESIA. A study comparing fentanyl, morphine, pethidine, and sufentanil as supplements to nitrous oxide anaesthesia in 72 patients undergoing surgery. Following premedication patients received either fentanyl (50 µg per mL), morphine (4 mg per mL), pethidine (33.3 mg per mL), or sufentanil (10 µg per mL) to a total dose of 0.15 mL per kg body-weight, plus 1 mg pancuronium. During the operation, significantly fewer supplementary doses of sufentanil were required to maintain anaesthesia than pethidine or morphine. Among the 64 patients involved in analysis, those who received pethidine exhibited a significant increase in heart-rate on arrival in the recovery room. Fentanyl and sufentanil administration significantly decreased blood pressure and this reduction was maintained until after extubation, thus suppressing the haemodynamic responses to laryngoscopy and intubation. Sufentanil was the only opioid which maintained median noradrenaline levels below the control value until postextubation. Recovery data for 61 patients showed that those who received fentanyl or sufentanil became oriented to their surroundings more rapidly and performed better in a battery of psychological tests than those on pethidine or morphine. Sufentanil and fentanyl were considered to be preferable to pethidine and morphine both in terms of haemodynamic changes to stress and rates of recovery, with no differences apparent between the two opioids.— M. M. Ghoneim *et al.*, *Anesth. Analg.*, 1984, *63*, 405.

A study comparing the anaesthetic requirements, incidences of chest wall rigidity and intraoperative hypertension, and time for recovery from anaesthesia after high-dose fentanyl-oxygen anaesthesia in patients with and without histories of smoking, alcoholic intake, and caffeine consumption who were undergoing coronary artery bypass grafting. Patients without a history of smoking and alcohol or caffeine intake required less fentanyl for induction and maintenance of anaesthesia and experienced less chest wall rigidity and hypertension than similar patients who had been chronically exposed to and/or consumed these agents. Pretreatment with more pancuronium prior to anaesthetic induction and increased fentanyl 'sleep' dose administered after anaesthetic induction but before incision reduced the incidences of chest wall rigidity and intraoperative hypertension in patients with positive histories of exposure to the agents to values similar to patients without histories of exposure.— T. H. Stanley and S. de Lange, *Can. Anaesth. Soc. J.*, 1984, *31*, 368.

A study of female patients admitted for outpatient sterilization by laparoscopy. Thirty patients receiving intravenous alfentanil 50 µg per kg body-weight and atracurium 0.5 mg per kg had significantly less pain during analgesic injection, compared with 32 patients receiving fentanyl 5 µg per kg and pancuronium 0.07 µg per kg. The alfentanil/atracurium group also had less coughing during intubation, and faster and more pronounced neuromuscular blockade during induction of anaesthesia.— J. C. Raeder and A. Hole, *Br. J. Anaesth.*, 1986, *58*, 108S.

For references to fentanyl reducing the responses to the stress of surgery, see above.

For a comparative study of the effects of fentanyl or butorphanol during outpatient gynaecologic surgery, see p.1297.

Cardiovascular surgery. Some references to fentanyl being used usually in high doses in cardiovascular surgery: A. M. Florence (letter), *Br. med. J.*, 1978, *1*, 650; T. H. Stanley and L. R. Webster, *Anesth. Analg.*, 1978, *57*, 411; J. E. Wynands *et al.*, *ibid.*, 1983, *62*, 661; M. Hynynen *et al.*, *Br. J. Anaesth.*, 1986, *58*, 1252; K. M. Vermeyen *et al.*, *ibid.*, 1987, *59*, 1115.

For a comparative study of fentanyl and sufentanil anaesthesia in patients undergoing coronary artery bypass grafting, see p.1320.

Ophthalmic surgery. For a study of the effects of fentanyl and alfentanil on intra-ocular pressure in patients undergoing routine ophthalmic surgery, see p.1295.

Phaeochromocytoma. A review of the anaesthetic management of patients with phaeochromocytoma. A brief mention that as fentanyl does not release histamine it may be used freely.— C. J. Hull, *Br. J. Anaesth.*, 1986, *58*, 1453.

Pregnancy and the neonate. Successful use of fentanyl citrate (30 to 50 µg per kg body-weight) in 10 premature infants, used in conjunction with pancuronium, as the sole anaesthetic for ligation of patent ductus arteriosus.— S. Robinson and G. A. Gregory, *Anesth. Analg.*, 1981, *60*, 331.

A randomised controlled study of preterm babies undergoing ligation of a patent ductus arteriosus who were given nitrous oxide and tubocurarine, with (n=8) or without (n=8) the addition of fentanyl (10 µg per kg body-weight intravenously) to the anaesthetic regimen. Major hormonal responses to surgery were significantly greater in the non-fentanyl than in the fentanyl group. Compared with the fentanyl group, the non-fentanyl group had circulatory and metabolic complications postoperatively. The findings indicated that preterm babies mount a substantial stress response to surgery under anaesthesia with nitrous oxide and curare and that prevention of this response by fentanyl anaesthesia may be associated with an improved postoperative outcome.— K. J. S. Anand *et al.*, *Lancet*, 1987, *1*, 243. Comments: I. S. Gauntlett (letter), *ibid.*, 1090.

Preparations

Fentanyl Citrate Injection *(U.S.P.)*

Proprietary Preparations

Sublimaze *(Janssen, UK)*. *Injection*, fentanyl 50 µg/mL, in ampoules of 2 and 10 mL.

Thalamonal *(Janssen, UK)*. *Injection*, fentanyl 50 µg, droperidol 2.5 mg/mL, in ampoules of 2 mL.

Proprietary Names and Manufacturers

Fentanest *(Carlo Erba, Ital.; Syntex-Latino, Spain)*; Haldid *(Janssen, Denm.)*; Leptanal *(Janssen, Norw.; Janssen Pharmaceutica, Swed.)*; Sublimaze *(Janssen, Austral.; Janssen, Canad.; Janssen, S.Afr.; Janssen, UK; Janssen, USA)*.

The following names have been used for multi-ingredient preparations containing fentanyl citrate— Innovar *(Janssen, Canad.; Janssen, USA)*; Thalamonal *(Janssen, UK)*.

6229-j

Hydrocodone Hydrochloride *(BANM, rINNM)*.

Dihydrocodeinone Hydrochloride.

$C_{18}H_{21}NO_3,HCl,2\frac{1}{2}H_2O=380.9$.

CAS — 25968-91-6 (anhydrous).

6230-q

Hydrocodone Phosphate *(BANM, rINNM)*.

$C_{18}H_{21}NO_3,1\frac{1}{2}H_3PO_4=446.4$.

CAS — 34366-67-1.

Pharmacopoeias. In *Rus.*

6231-p

Hydrocodone Tartrate *(BANM, rINNM)*.

Dihydrocodeinone Acid Tartrate; Hydrocodone Acid Tartrate; Hydrocodone Bitartrate *(USAN)*; Hydrocodoni Bitartras; Hydrocone Bitartrate. 6-Deoxy-3-*O*-methyl-6-oxomorphine hydrogen tartrate hemipentahydrate; (−)-(5*R*)-4,5-Epoxy-3-methoxy-9a-methylmorphinan-6-one hydrogen tartrate hemipentahydrate.

$C_{18}H_{21}NO_3,C_4H_6O_6,2\frac{1}{2}H_2O=494.5$.

CAS — 125-29-1 (hydrocodone); 143-71-5 (tartrate, anhydrous); 34195-34-1 (tartrate, hemipentahydrate).

Pharmacopoeias. In *Aust., Belg., Cz., Ger., Hung., Int., Nord., Port., Swiss,* and *U.S. Turk.* has anhydrous.

Fine, white crystals or crystalline powder.

Soluble in water, slightly soluble in alcohol; insoluble in chloroform and ether. A 2% solution in water has a pH of 3.2 to 3.8. **Store** in airtight containers. Protect from light.

Dependence

Prolonged use of hydrocodone may lead to dependence of the morphine type (see p.1310).

ABUSE. Hydrocodone with phenyltoloxamine as cation exchange resin complexes (Tussionex) was being abused; its psychotropic effects lasted for about 8 hours.— Y. J. Berry (letter), *New Engl. J. Med.*, 1976, *295*, 286.

Adverse Effects, Treatment, and Precautions

As for Morphine, p.1311.

OVERDOSAGE. Three deaths from pulmonary oedema associated with high concentrations of hydrocodone and phenyltoloxamine in body fluids following ingestion of a slow-release liquid preparation.— D. Vivian, *Drug Intell. & clin. Pharm.*, 1979, *13*, 445.

Uses and Administration

Hydrocodone tartrate has actions similar to those of codeine (see p.1298) but is more potent on a weight for weight basis. It is used chiefly for the relief of irritant cough, though it has no particular advantage over codeine. It is also used for the relief of moderate to moderately severe pain. Hydrocodone tartrate is taken by mouth in doses of 5 to 10 mg every 4 to 6 hours.

Hydrocodone is also used as the hydrochloride, the phosphate, and the polistirex (a hydrocodone and sulphonated diethenylbenzene-ethenylbenzene copolymer complex).

Preparations

Hydrocodone Bitartrate Tablets *(U.S.P.)*. Tablets containing hydrocodone tartrate.

Proprietary Names and Manufacturers of Hydrocodone Salts

Biocodone *(Bios, Belg.)*; Broncodid *(Belg.)*; Codinovo *(Nourypharma, Neth.)*; Codone *(Lemmon, USA)*; Corutol DH *(Dow, Canad.)*; Dicodid *(Schering, Austral.; Knoll, Belg.; Knoll, Ger.; Knoll, Switz.; Knoll, USA)*; Hycodan *(Du Pont, Canad.)*; Hycon *(Du Pont, Austral.)*; Hydrokon *(DAK, Denm.; NAF, Norw.)*; Nyodid *(Nyco, Norw.)*; Robidone *(Robins, Canad.)*; Solucodan *(Nadeau, Canad.)*.

The following names have been used for multi-ingredient preparations containing hydrocodone salts—Adatuss *(Mastar, USA)*; Amacodone *(Trimen, USA)*; Anexsia *(Beecham Laboratories, USA)*; Anexsia-D *(Beecham Laboratories, USA)*; Bancap HC *(Forest Pharmaceuticals, USA)*; Biohisdex DHC *(Everest, Canad.)*; Biohisdine DHC *(Everest, Canad.)*; Caldomine-DH *(Technilab, Canad.)*; Calmydone *(Technilab, Canad.)*; Chemhisdex-DHC *(Clark, Canad.)*; Chemhisdex-DHC-Expectorant *(Clark, Canad.)*; Chemhisdine-DHC-Child *(Clark, Canad.)*; Chemhisdine-DHC-Expectorant *(Clark, Canad.)*; Citra Forte Capsules *(Boyle, USA)*; Citra Forte Syrup *(Boyle, USA)*; Codiclear DH *(Central Pharmaceuticals, USA)*; Codimal DH *(Central Pharmaceuticals, USA)*; Co-Gesic *(Central Pharmaceuticals, USA)*; Coristex-DH *(Technilab, Canad.)*; Coristine-DH *(Technilab, Canad.)*; Damacet-P *(Mason, USA)*; Damason-P *(Mason, USA)*; Detussin *(USA)*; Detussin Expectorant *(USA)*; Dia-Gesic *(Central Pharmaceuticals, USA)*; Dimetane Expectorant-DC *(Robins, Canad.)*; Dimotane Expectorant DC *(Robins, UK)*; Dolacet *(Hauck, USA)*; Donatussin DC *(Laser, USA)*; Duradyne DHC *(Forest Pharmaceuticals, USA)*; Entuss *(Hauck, USA)*; Entuss-D *(Hauck, USA)*; Hycodan *(Du Pont, USA)*; Hycodaphen *(Ascher, USA)*; Hycomine *(Du Pont, Austral.; Du Pont, Canad.; Du Pont, USA)*; Hycomine Compound *(Du Pont, USA)*; Hyco-Pap *(Lasalle, USA)*; Hycotuss *(Du Pont, USA)*; Hydrocet *(Carnrick, USA)*; Hydrogesic *(Edwards, USA)*; Hy-Phen *(Ascher, USA)*; Kwelcof *(Ascher, USA)*; Lorcet-HD *(UAD, USA)*; Lortab *(Russ, USA)*; Lortab ASA *(Russ, USA)*; Mercodol with Decapryn *(Dow, Canad.)*; Norcet *(Holloway, USA)*; Novahistex DH *(Dow, Canad.)*; Novahistine DH *(Dow, Canad.)*; Promist HD *(Russ, USA)*; Propain HC *(Springbok, USA)*; Pseudo-Hist Expectorant *(Holloway, USA)*; P-V-Tussin *(Reid-Provident, USA)*; Ru-Tuss with Hydrocodone *(Boots, USA)*; S-T Forte *(Scot-Tussin, USA)*; T-Gesic *(T.E. Williams, USA)*; Triaminic Expectorant DH *(Ancalab, Canad.; Dorsey Laboratories, USA)*; Tussaminic DH *(Ancalab, Canad.)*; Tussend *(Merrell Dow, USA)*; Tussend Expectorant *(Merrell Dow, USA)*; Tussionex *(Pennwalt, Canad.; Pennwalt, USA)*; Vasofrinic DH *(Trianon, Canad.)*; Vicodin *(Knoll, USA)*; Zydone *(Du Pont, USA)*.

6232-s

Hydromorphone *(BAN, rINN)*.

7,8-Dihydromorphinone. 6-Deoxy-7,8-dihydro-6-oxomorphine; (−)-(5*R*)-4,5-Epoxy-3-hydroxy-9a-methylmorphinan-6-one.

$C_{17}H_{19}NO_3=285.3$.

CAS — 466-99-9.

6233-w

Hydromorphone Hydrochloride *(BANM, USAN, rINNM)*.

Dihydromorphinone Hydrochloride.

$C_{17}H_{19}NO_3,HCl=321.8$.

CAS — 71-68-1.

Pharmacopoeias. In *Arg., Aust., Braz., Egypt., Ger., Int., Nord., Roum., Span.,* and *U.S.*

A fine white or almost white odourless crystalline powder. **Soluble** 1 in 3 of water; sparingly soluble in alcohol (90%); practically insoluble in ether. The *U.S.P.* injection has a pH of 3.5 to 5.5. **Store** in airtight containers. Protect from light.

Dependence

The use of hydromorphone may lead to dependence of the morphine type (see p.1310).

Adverse Effects, Treatment, and Precautions
As for Morphine, p.1311.
Pain may occur at the injection site and local tissue irritation and induration may follow subcutaneous injection.

Absorption and Fate
Hydromorphone is absorbed from the gastro-intestinal tract. It is metabolised and excreted in the urine mainly as conjugated hydromorphone.

Following administration of hydromorphone hydrochloride by mouth to 5 healthy former narcotic addicts, conjugated hydromorphone, hydromorphone, dihydroisomorphine, and dihydromorphine were identified in the urine. Conjugated hydromorphone was the major metabolite identified and was present in amounts ranging from 22 to 51% of the administered dose.— E. J. Cone *et al.*, *J. pharm. Sci.*, 1977, *66*, 1709.

Further references: J. J. Vallner *et al.*, *J. clin. Pharmac.*, 1981, *21*, 152.

Uses and Administration
Hydromorphone hydrochloride has a greater analgesic potency than morphine (see p.1312); following injection the analgesic effect usually occurs within 30 minutes and lasts about 5 hours.
It may be used for the relief of moderate and severe pain and is usually administered by subcutaneous or intramuscular injection in doses of 2 mg every 4 to 6 hours as necessary. It may be given by slow intravenous injection or by mouth in similar doses, or rectally in doses of 3 mg. In severe pain up to 4 mg every 4 to 6 hours may be required. Higher doses may be given to opioid-tolerant patients using a highly concentrated solution containing 10 mg per mL.
It has also been given, as a syrup, in doses of 1 mg repeated every 3 to 4 hours for the relief of non-productive cough.

Studies with epidural hydromorphone hydrochloride in healthy subjects, indicated that spinal opiate analgesia confined to the upper thoracic segments may modulate the afferent pathways of the Valsalva sympathetic response.— J. Leslie *et al.* (letter), *Lancet*, 1979, *2*, 151.

A comparative study in 42 patients with acute attacks of biliary stone pain. Subcutaneous injection of hydromorphone 2 mg produced no significant difference in analgesia compared with indomethacin 50 mg injected intravenously.— P. Udén *et al.*, *Curr. ther. Res.*, 1984, *36*, 1228.

TREATMENT OF DEPENDENCE. A study of self-administration of hydromorphone in 6 patients undergoing methadone detoxification. Hydromorphone significantly decreased opioid withdrawal symptoms when compared with a placebo. Neither clonidine nor oxazepam exerted a significant effect.— K. L. Preston *et al.*, *Clin. Pharmac. Ther.*, 1985, *38*, 219.

Preparations
Hydromorphone Hydrochloride Injection *(U.S.P.)*
Hydromorphone Hydrochloride Tablets *(U.S.P.)*

Proprietary Names and Manufacturers
Dilaudid *(Schering, Austral.*; *Knoll, Canad.*; *Knoll, Ger.*; *Knoll, Switz.*; *Knoll, USA)*.

6234-e

Ketobemidone *(BAN, rINN)*.
Cetobemidone. 1-(4-*m*-Hydroxyphenyl-1-methyl-4-piperidyl)propan-1-one.
$C_{15}H_{21}NO_2$=247.3.

CAS — 469-79-4.

Ketobemidone is an opioid analgesic with actions and uses similar to those of morphine (see p.1310). Ketobemidone has been given by mouth, by injection, or rectally, in association with an antispasmodic; the usual dose has been 5 to 10 mg.

Obstetric analgesia with ketobemidone.— C. Carlsson *et al.*, *Br. J. Anaesth.*, 1980, *52*, 827.

A study of the clinical pharmacokinetics and bioavailability of intravenous and rectal ketobemidone in 6 patients following surgery.— P. Anderson *et al.*, *Eur. J. clin. Pharmac.*, 1981, *19*, 217.

Proprietary Names and Manufacturers
Cliradon *(Ciba, Ger.*; *Ciba, Switz.)*.

The following names have been used for multi-ingredient preparations containing ketobemidone— Ketogan *(Lundbeck, Swed.)*.

6235-l

Levomethadyl Acetate *(USAN)*.
l-Acetylmethadol; LAAM; LAM; Levacetylmethadol *(rINN)*. (−)-4-Dimethylamino-1-ethyl-2,2-diphenylpentyl acetate.
$C_{23}H_{31}NO_2$=353.5.

CAS — 1477-40-3 (levomethadyl); 34433-66-4 (acetate).

The laevo isomer of methadyl acetate.

Dependence, Adverse Effects, Treatment, and Precautions
As for Morphine, p.1310.

Absorption and Fate
Levomethadyl acetate is absorbed from the gastro-intestinal tract. It has a slow onset and long duration of action. It is metabolised to compounds which have morphine-like activity and a long half-life. The metabolites *l*-α-noracetylmethadol and *l*-α-dinoracetylmethadol have been identified in plasma while methadol and normethadol have been identified in urine.

A study of the disposition of methadyl acetate in relation to pharmacological action.— R. F. Kaiko and C. E. Inturrisi, *Clin. Pharmac. Ther.*, 1975, *18*, 96.

In a study of acute and chronic administration of levomethadyl acetate to replace oral methadone in 5 subjects and diamorphine in a further 5 subjects, the plasma decay curve was biexponential with an initial half-life of about 6 hours and a further half-life of about 50 hours. During chronic administration plasma concentrations of the metabolites noracetylmethadol acetate and dinoracetylmethadol acetate increased 5 and 13 times respectively and their half-lives were about 30 and more than 100 hours respectively; there appeared, however, to be little accumulation of levomethadyl acetate, no change occurring in the plasma decay curve. The findings suggested that the biological distribution of levomethadyl acetate was complex and its long duration of pharmacological action might be associated with at least 3 factors: *in vivo* generation of active metabolites, drug-tissue binding, and possibly enterohepatic recycling.— G. L. Henderson *et al.*, *Clin. Pharmac. Ther.*, 1977, *21*, 16.

Uses and Administration
Levomethadyl acetate is a long-acting opioid analgesic which has been used in the management of opioid dependence.

TREATMENT OF DEPENDENCE. A comparative study in 193 heroin addicts indicated that levomethadyl acetate was as effective as methadone in the treatment of heroin addiction. Levomethadyl acetate induction was more difficult than methadone induction. Levomethadyl acetate was given on 3 days per week. There was a higher incidence of gastro-intestinal complaints in the levomethadyl acetate group while in the methadone group aching bones and joints, runny nose, and insomnia occurred more often.— E. C. Senay *et al.*, *J. Am. med. Ass.*, 1977, *237*, 138.

A comparative 40-week clinical study in 636 heroin addicts demonstrated that levomethadyl acetate was as effective as methadone for maintenance treatment of addicts. Side-effects were similar for both drugs. Levomethadyl acetate was given according to need in doses not exceeding 100 mg three days a week.— W. Ling *et al.*, *Archs gen. Psychiat.*, 1978, *35*, 345.

Further references: A. Zaks *et al.*, *J. Am. med. Ass.*, 1972, *220*, 811; S. K. Sim, *Can. med. Ass. J.*, 1973, *109*, 615; R. Levine *et al.*, *J. Am. med. Ass.*, 1973, *226*, 316; W. Ling *et al.*, *Archs gen. Psychiat.*, 1976, *33*, 709; J. Panell *et al.*, *Med. J. Aust.*, 1977, *2*, 150; J. H. Mendelson *et al.*, *Clin. Pharmac. Ther.*, 1984, *35*, 545.

6236-y

Levorphanol Tartrate *(BANM, USAN, rINNM)*.
Levorphanol Bitartrate; Methorphinan Tartrate. (−)-9a-Methylmorphinan-3-ol hydrogen tartrate dihydrate.
$C_{17}H_{23}NO,C_4H_6O_6,2H_2O$=443.5.

CAS — 77-07-6 (levorphanol); 125-72-4 (tartrate, anhydrous); 5985-38-6 (tartrate, dihydrate).

Pharmacopoeias. In *Br.*, *It.*, and *U.S.*

A white odourless or almost odourless crystalline powder. M.p. about 116°. *B.P.* **solubilities** are: soluble 1 in 45 of water and 1 in 50 of ether; slightly soluble in alcohol. *U.S.P.* solubilities are: soluble 1 in 50 of water and 1 in 120 of alcohol; insoluble in chloroform and ether. A 0.2% solution in water has a pH of 3.4 to 4.0. The *B.P.* injection has a pH of 5.5; the *U.S.P.* injection has a pH of 4.1 to 4.5. Solutions are **sterilised** by autoclaving. **Store** in well-closed containers.

Levorphanol tartrate is an opioid analgesic with effects similar to those of morphine (see p.1312), differing mainly in that it is almost as effective by mouth as by injection. The analgesic effect usually begins after about 10 to 30 minutes and lasts up to about 8 hours.
For severe pain, a dose of 1.5 to 4.5 mg may be given by mouth once or twice daily; the usual single dose by subcutaneous or intramuscular injection is 2 to 4 mg; it has been given by slow intravenous injection in a dose of 1 to 2 mg. It may also be used for supplementing nitrous oxide and oxygen anaesthesia in a dose of 250 or 500 µg intravenously repeated to a maximum total dose of 1.5 to 2.0 mg.

Preparations
Levorphanol Injection *(B.P.)*. A sterile solution of levorphanol tartrate in Water for Injections. Protect from light.
Levorphanol Tartrate Injection *(U.S.P.)*
Levorphanol Tablets *(B.P.)*. Tablets containing levorphanol tartrate.
Levorphanol Tartrate Tablets *(U.S.P.)*

Proprietary Preparations
Dromoran *(Roche, UK)*. *Tablets*, levorphanol tartrate 1.5 mg.
Injection, levorphanol tartrate 2 mg/mL, in ampoules of 1 mL.

Proprietary Names and Manufacturers
Dromoran *(Austral.*; *Ger.*; *Roche, UK)*; Levo-Dromoran *(Roche, Canad.*; *Roche, USA)*.

12900-y

Lofentanil Oxalate *(BANM, USAN, rINNM)*.
R-34995. (−)-Methyl *t*-3-methyl-1-phenethyl-4-(*N*-phenylpropionamido)piperidine-*r*-4-carboxylate oxalate.
$C_{25}H_{32}N_2O_3,C_2H_2O_4$=498.6.

CAS — 61380-40-3 (lofentanil); 61380-41-4 (oxalate).

Lofentanil oxalate is an opioid analgesic reported to have a long duration of action.

Lofentanil 5 µg in 11 mL of sodium chloride injection given via an epidural catheter provided effective pain relief that was significantly better than after buprenorphine 300 µg in a placebo-controlled study of 60 postoperative orthopaedic patients. Drowsiness occurred in three patients in both treatment groups. Lofentanil was considered to have a rapid onset of action and a prolonged effect.— P. Bilsback *et al.*, *Br. J. Anaesth.*, 1985, *57*, 943.

Proprietary Names and Manufacturers
Janssen, Belg.

12932-r

Meptazinol Hydrochloride *(BANM, USAN, rINNM)*.
IL-22811; Wy-22811. 3-(3-Ethyl-1-methylperhydroazepin-3-yl)phenol hydrochloride.
$C_{15}H_{23}NO,HCl$=269.8.

CAS — 54340-58-8 (meptazinol); 59263-76-2 (hydrochloride); 34154-59-1 (hydrochloride, ±).

Dependence, Adverse Effects, Treatment, and Precautions
As for Morphine, p.1310. As meptazinol possesses antagonist as well as agonist properties, treatment of meptazinol overdose with nalorphine or levallorphan is not recommended. A response may be obtained with naloxone.

A review of the *UK* experience with oral meptazinol. The major side-effects were nausea, vomiting, and dizziness. Other side-effects included stomach ache, indigestion, headache, bad taste, drowsiness, diarrhoea, faintness, and constipation. Euphoria and hallucinations were uncommon and the potential for addiction was reported to be low.— J. A. Henry, *Postgrad. med. J.*, 1985, *61 Suppl.* 2, 29.

ADMINISTRATION IN THE ELDERLY. See below under Absorption and Fate.

ADMINISTRATION IN LIVER DISORDERS. See below under Absorption and Fate.

EFFECTS ON THE RESPIRATORY SYSTEM. Meptazinol 100 mg per 70 kg body-weight intramuscularly caused substantially less respiratory depression than morphine 10 mg per 70 kg or pentazocine 60 mg per 70 kg in 7 healthy subjects. Nausea and vomiting occurred in 5 subjects after meptazinol but euphoria or dysphoria did not.— C. Jordan *et al.*, *Br. J. Anaesth.*, 1979, *51*, 497.

A profound reduction in minute volume was observed after the start of surgery in fit young adults with meptazinol given in doses of 100 mg intravenously. One patient became apnoeic for 10 minutes and required manual ventilation. It was suggested that respiratory function required careful monitoring when meptazinol has been given, especially in patients receiving other depressant drugs.— P. A. J. Hardy (letter), *Lancet*, 1983, *2*, 576.

A case report of respiratory arrest in a 61-year-old woman who was found unconscious approximately 2 hours after taking an overdose of 50 meptazinol tablets and a quarter of a bottle of whisky. She made a full recovery following supportive measures and a total cumulative dose of 10 mg naloxone given intravenously.— A. G. Davison *et al.*, *Hum. Toxicol.*, 1987, *6*, 331.

A study of the ventilatory effects of intravenous meptazinol (20 mg, 30 mg, and 48 mg) in anaesthetised patients compared with those of pethidine 20 mg. Each of 24 female patients received a first dose of drug which was followed after 5 minutes by a second identical dose. After the first injection there was a significant decrease in minute volume with all doses and the ventilatory effects of meptazinol 20 mg were similar to those of pethidine 20 mg. The second injection produced a further decrease only in the pethidine group.— A. Lee and G. B. Drummond, *Br. J. Anaesth.*, 1987, *59*, 1127. See also D. J. Wilkinson *et al.*, *ibid.*, 1985, *57*, 1077.

Absorption and Fate

Following oral administration meptazinol is extensively metabolised in the liver and is excreted mainly in the urine as the glucuronide conjugate.

A review of the pharmacodynamic and pharmacokinetic properties of meptazinol.— B. Holmes and A. Ward, *Drugs*, 1985, *30*, 285.

When 11 healthy fasting subjects were given meptazinol hydrochloride 50, 100, or 200 mg by mouth the drug was rapidly and almost completely absorbed, less than 10% appearing in the faeces. The drug was rapidly excreted and more than 60% appeared in the urine in the first 24 hours. Plasma concentrations of unchanged meptazinol remained below a detectable value of 20 ng per mL following administration by mouth. Intravenous administration of 20 mg to 2 subjects produced peak plasma concentrations of 53 and 60 ng per mL with an elimination half-life of about 2 hours. Meptazinol was considered to undergo extensive first-pass metabolism, its main metabolite being the glucuronide.— R. A. Franklin *et al.*, *Br. J. clin. Pharmac.*, 1976, *3*, 497. Meptazinol hydrochloride 50 or 75 mg was rapidly absorbed and produced peak plasma concentrations of 39 to 190 ng per mL 30 minutes after rectal administration. The elimination half-life was approximately 2 hours. No obvious dose and concentration relationship was evident. Gastric emptying is seriously slowed by meptazinol. It is metabolised in the liver. In a study on 2 subjects given 50 mg by mouth peak plasma concentrations remained below 10 ng per mL.— *idem*, 1977, *4*, 163.

A study of single- and multiple-dose kinetics of meptazinol in elderly patients. Following a single dose of meptazinol 200 mg by mouth, peak plasma concentrations in 10 elderly patients were achieved within 0.5 to 3 hours, and declined with a mean half-life of 3.39 hours, which was not significantly different from 4.97 hours following subsequent dosage with meptazinol 200 mg every 6 hours for 3 days. There was no evidence of accumulation following multiple dosage, and maximum plasma concentrations were similar to those previously reported in younger subjects. There appears no pharmacokinetic reason for recommending a reduction in meptazinol dosage when treating elderly patients.— H. M. Norbury *et al.*, *Eur. J. clin. Pharmac.*, 1984, *27*, 223.

A study suggesting enhanced bioavailability of oral meptazinol in cirrhotic patients.— G. G. Birnie *et al.*, *Gut*, 1987, *28*, 248.

PREGNANCY AND THE NEONATE. In a study of 13 women given an intramuscular injection of 100 to 150 mg during labour, meptazinol was found to cross the placenta readily but was rapidly eliminated from the neonate. This contrasted with pethidine which was known to be excreted very slowly from neonates.— R. A. Franklin *et al.* (letter), *Br. J. clin. Pharmac.*, 1981, *12*, 88. See also P. S. Dowell *et al.* (letter), *ibid.*, 1982, *14*, 748.

Uses and Administration

Meptazinol hydrochloride is a partial opioid agonist used in the treatment of moderate to severe pain. It may be given by intramuscular injection in doses equivalent to 75 to 100 mg of meptazinol every 2 to 4 hours; for obstetric pain a dose of 2 mg per kg body-weight (100 to 150 mg) may be used.

Meptazinol hydrochloride may also be given by slow intravenous injection in doses equivalent to 50 to 100 mg of meptazinol every 2 to 4 hours.

For the short-term treatment of moderate pain meptazinol may be given by mouth in a dose of 200 mg every 3 to 6 hours.

The proceedings of a symposium on the actions and uses of meptazinol.— *Postgrad. med. J.*, 1985, *61*, *Suppl.* 2. See also *ibid.*, 1983, *59*, *Suppl.* 1.

Reviews of the actions and uses of meptazinol: *Lancet*, 1983, *2*, 384; B. Holmes and A. Ward, *Drugs*, 1985, *30*, 285. Comment on the Lancet editorial.— M. Weinstock (letter), *Lancet*, 1983, *2*, 1027.

The analgesic activity of meptazinol in selected doses and routes has been assessed against a range of opioid and nonopioid analgesics. There are studies that report meptazinol to be as effective as or more effective than pentazocine or pethidine, to be as effective as or less effective than morphine, or to be less effective than buprenorphine. Other analgesics involved in these assessments include co-proxamol, diflunisal, and paracetamol, and in such instances meptazinol was reported to produce equivalent analgesia. References:

Buprenorphine.— M. Harmer *et al.*, *Br. med. J.*, 1983, *286*, 680.

Co-proxamol.— R. J. K. Price and A. N. Latham, *Curr. med. Res. Opinion*, 1982, *8*, 54; L. Orö, *ibid.*, 1984, *9*, 240.

Diflunisal.— T. Videman *et al.*, *ibid.*, 246.

Morphine.— D. G. Cohen *et al.*, *Postgrad. med. J.*, 1983, *59*, *Suppl.* 1, 35; R. E. Westcombe and R. K. J. Price, *Curr. ther. Res.*, 1985, *37*, 969.

Paracetamol.— A. G. Wade and P. J. Ward, *Curr. med. Res. Opinion*, 1982, *8*, 191.

Pentazocine.— N. J. Paymaster, *Br. J. Anaesth.*, 1977, *49*, 1139; V. Pearce and P. J. Robson, *Postgrad. med. J.*, 1980, *56*, 474; M. J. Griffiths and T. A. Thomas, *Br. dent. J.*, 1985, *158*, 19.

Pethidine.— N. J. Paymaster, *Br. J. Anaesth.*, 1977, *49*, 1139; A. Hedges *et al.*, *ibid.*, 1980, *52*, 295; P. J. Slatterly *et al.*, *ibid.*, 1981, *53*, 927; P. R. H. Barnes *et al.*, *Postgrad. med. J.*, 1985, *61*, 221; S. A. Ridley *et al.*, *Anaesthesia*, 1986, *41*, 263. See also under Pregnancy and the Neonate, below.

The prolonged use of meptazinol with midazolam for postoperative analgesia and sedation.— A. D. Jardine *et al.* (letter), *Lancet*, 1983, *2*, 395.

ADMINISTRATION, EPIDURAL. Meptazinol 90 mg was administered by the epidural or intramuscular route to 32 postoperative patients. The epidural route was found to be superior with regard to onset, quality, and duration of pain relief. Meptazinol decreased the ventilatory rate equally with both routes, but no incidence of overt respiratory depression was noted. There was a slight decrease in heart-rate with both routes and in blood pressure with the epidural route.— C. Verborgh *et al.*, *Br. J. Anaesth.*, 1987, *59*, 1134.

HERXHEIMER REACTION. A double-blind placebo-controlled study of naloxone and meptazinol in 24 Ethiopian patients with the Jarisch-Herxheimer reaction following treatment of louse-borne relapsing fever. Naloxone 30 to 40 mg intravenously was not effective, but the reaction was diminished by meptazinol, 300 to 500 mg intravenously. Meptazinol was stated to be the first effective treatment of this reaction of louse-borne relapsing fever.— B. Teklu *et al.*, *Lancet*, 1983, *1*, 835. Conjecture on the mechanism of action of meptazinol in this reaction.— D. J. M. Wright, *ibid.*, 1135. A comment that besides a beneficial antipyretic power of meptazinol, there is a cholinergic mechanism which may exert the hypothermic action responsible for an antagonism of the pyretic aspects of the Jarisch-Herxheimer reaction.— M. M. Ben-Sreti *et al.* (letter), *ibid.*, 1389.

PREGNANCY AND THE NEONATE. A double-blind study in 358 healthy pregnant women in the first stage of labour. Meptazinol or pethidine were administered intramuscularly, both in doses of up to 150 mg. Pain relief was consistently better with meptazinol than with pethidine at 60 minutes post-injection, with statistically significant differences at 45 and 60 minutes. After this time pain relief was similar with both drugs. Significantly more infants with Apgar scores of 8 or more at 1 minute were delivered from mothers on meptazinol analgesia than from mothers on pethidine analgesia. Meptazinol seemed to have advantages over pethidine for both mothers and babies.— A. D. G. Nicholas and P. J. Robson, *Br. J. Obstet. Gynaec.*, 1982, *89*, 318.

A double-blind study of 205 pregnant women who received either intramuscular pethidine 100 mg or intramuscular meptazinol 100 mg during the first stage of labour. Every woman receiving one injection of meptazinol complained of moderate to severe pain after 2 hours; and 64 of 65 women receiving pethidine complained of moderate to severe pain after 2 hours. Two further doses of each drug were available for administration if necessary, the interval between each dose being 2 hours and surprisingly only 29 mothers were given a second dose of opioid. There was no difference between the two drugs with regard to pain relief or side-effects both in mother and baby. Meptazinol had no advantage over pethidine in the management of pain relief of labour.— A. Sheikh and M. E. Tunstall, *Br. J. Obstet. Gynaec.*, 1986, *93*, 264.

A comparative double-blind study of meptazinol and pethidine as an analgesic in labour carried out on 1035 women. Women over 70 kg were given 150 mg meptazinol and the remainder 100 mg. Effective analgesia was similar in both drug groups. Significantly more of the meptazinol-treated group (37%) vomited compared with the pethidine-treated group (28%). Meptazinol did not appear to have any clinical advantages over pethidine as a routine analgesic in labour.— C. E. Morrison *et al.*, *Anaesthesia*, 1987, *42*, 7.

Proprietary Preparations

Meptid *(Wyeth, UK). Tablets*, meptazinol 200 mg. *Injection*, meptazinol 100 mg (as hydrochloride)/mL, in ampoules of 1 mL.

6237-j

Methadone Hydrochloride *(BANM, USAN, rINNM).*

Amidine; Amidone Hydrochloride; Phenadone. (±)-6-Dimethylamino-4,4-diphenylheptan-3-one hydrochloride.

$C_{21}H_{27}NO,HCl=345.9$.

CAS — 76-99-3 (methadone); 297-88-1 (methadone, ±); 1095-90-5 (hydrochloride); 125-56-4 (hydrochloride, ±).

Pharmacopoeias. In *Arg., Aust., Belg., Br., Braz., Chin., Cz., Egypt., Eur., Ger., Hung., Ind., Int., It., Jug., Neth., Nord., Port., Rus., Swiss, Turk.,* and *U.S.* Also in *B.P. Vet.*

Odourless colourless crystals or white crystalline powder.

Soluble in water; freely soluble in alcohol and chloroform; practically insoluble in ether and in glycerol. A 1% solution in water has a pH of 4.5 to 6.5. The *U.S.P.* injection has a pH of 3.0 to 6.5 and the oral concentrate a pH of 3.0 to 6.0. Solutions are **sterilised** by autoclaving.

Store in airtight containers. Protect from light.

Dependence

Prolonged use of methadone may lead to dependence of the morphine type (see p.1310). The withdrawal symptoms are less intense but more prolonged than those produced by morphine or diamorphine. They develop more slowly and do not usually appear until 24 to 48 hours after the last dose. Methadone is used for substitution therapy in those dependent on diamorphine and morphine (see under Uses).

Methadone hydrochloride produced subjective changes similar to those produced by diamorphine. It was about as potent as morphine by subcutaneous injection and half as potent by mouth. Chronic administration produced sedation, lethargic apathy, haemodilution, oedema, and reduced sexual interest and activity. Patients receiving and tolerant to methadone 100 mg daily still exhibited drug-seeking behaviour. At a dosage of 100 mg daily physical dependence and an abstinence syndrome developed similar to that produced by morphine except that the onset of the syndrome was slower. As in morphine-dependent subjects the acute syndrome was followed by a protracted syndrome.— W. R. Martin *et al.*, *Archs gen. Psychiat.*, 1973, *28*, 286.

PREGNANCY AND THE NEONATE. In a comparison of 15 infants born to mothers receiving methadone maintenance and 38 born to untreated diamorphine addicts, withdrawal symptoms in the methadone group were more severe and more prolonged (6 to 16 days as against 2 to 8 days). It was considered that this might be due to greater placental passage and delayed renal excretion of methadone. Hypoglycaemia was present in 3 full-term infants in the methadone group.— B. K. Rajegowda *et al.*, *J. Pediat.*, 1972, *81*, 532.

In 105 pregnancies in patients dependent on methadone, mortality, complications of pregnancy, and neonatal growth and development were normal; one-third of the infants were premature, and most showed some signs of withdrawal symptoms.— G. Blinick *et al.*, *J. Am. med. Ass.* 1973, *225*, 477. See also M. H. Lifschitz *et al.*, *J. Pediat.*, 1983, *102*, 686.

Withdrawal symptoms appeared in all except 1 of the infants born to 22 women taking methadone. The severity of withdrawal symptoms was related to the total dose of methadone ingested over the last 12 weeks of pregnancy, to the daily maternal dose at delivery, and to the maternal serum-methadone concentration at parturition. Concentrations in cord blood were lower than those in maternal serum. Concentrations in neonatal urine were 10 to 60 times those in cord blood. Infants were of lower birth weight than controls; a higher incidence of smoking might have been a contributory factor.— R. G. Harper *et al.*, *Am. J. Obstet. Gynec.*, 1977, *129*, 417.

A study of children in the first 18 months of life born to 57 methadone-maintained mothers and to a matched drug-free comparison group of 31 mothers. Findings for the methadone group during the neonatal period were: a moderate-to-severe opioid abstinence syndrome in 75% of infants, reduced head circumferences, and elevated systolic blood pressure. In follow-up, the methadone children had a significantly higher incidence of otitis media, of reduced head circumferences and of abnormal eye findings. They also had lower scores on mental and motor developmental indices.— T. S. Rosen and H. L. Johnson, *J. Pediat.*, 1982, *101*, 192.

Some further references to the behavioural effects of maternal methadone ingestion on their offspring: D. E. Hutchings, *Neurobehav. Toxicol. Teratol.*, 1982, *4*, 429; H. L. Johnson and T. S. Rosen, *Pediat. Pharmacol.*, 1982, *2*, 113.

TOLERANCE. A study of cross-tolerance between methadone and diamorphine in man.— J. Volavka *et al.*, *J. nerv. ment. Dis.*, 1978, *166*, 104.

Adverse Effects and Treatment

As for Morphine, p.1311.

Methadone has a relatively greater respiratory depressant effect than morphine. After gross overdosage symptoms are similar to those of morphine poisoning. Pulmonary oedema after overdosage is a common cause of fatalities among addicts.

Methadone causes pain at injection sites; subcutaneous injection causes local tissue irritation and induration.

A morphine-like sleep arousal by methadone. With long-term administration morphine induces a small but persistent arousal but methadone does not.— W. B. Pickworth *et al.*, *Clin. Ther.*, 1981, *30*, 796.

Findings in 5 methadone-addicted subjects consistent with deficient ACTH production and subsequent secondary hypoadrenalism.— C. A. Dackis *et al.* (letter), *Lancet*, 1982, *2*, 1167. Comment that the blunted cortisol release after ACTH administration may have been due to methadone-induced primary adrenal cortical hypofunction rather than to depletion of the ACTH/beta-endorphin system. More detailed studies, with prolonged ACTH stimulation will be necessary to distinguish these two possibilities with certainty.— P. T. Pullan *et al.* (letter), *ibid.*, 1983, *1*, 714.

For a comparison between isomers of methadone with regard to adverse effects, see under Uses.

EFFECTS ON SEXUAL FUNCTION. In 29 men receiving methadone maintenance therapy sexual function was markedly impaired. The ejaculate volume and seminal vesicular and prostatic secretions were reduced by over 50% in subjects receiving methadone compared with 16 diamorphine addicts and 43 control subjects. Serum-testosterone concentrations were about 43% lower in subjects receiving methadone than in diamorphine users or controls. The sperm count of subjects receiving methadone was over twice that of the controls reflecting a lack of sperm dilution by secondary-sex-organ secretions and the motility was markedly lower than normal.— T. J. Cicero *et al.*, *New Engl. J. Med.*, 1975, *292*, 882.

Further reports on the effect of methadone on sexual function.— F. Azizi *et al.*, *Steroids*, 1973, *22*, 467; J. Mintz *et al.*, *Archs gen. Psychiat.*, 1974, *31*, 700; R. Hanbury *et al.*, *Am. J. Drug Alcohol Abuse*, 1977, *4*, 13; S. Lafisca *et al.*, *Drug & Alcohol Depend.*, 1981, *8*, 229.

PREGNANCY AND THE NEONATE. A review of congenital malformations and aetiological factors. Methadone and diamorphine have not been convincingly associated with congenital malformations, although increased stillbirth-rates, reduced birth weight, and neonatal withdrawal symptoms have consistently been found in studies of methadone and diamorphine.— H. Kalter and J. Warkany, *New Engl. J. Med.*, 1983, *308*, 491.

See also under Dependence, above.

Precautions

As for Morphine, p.1311.

Methadone is not recommended for use in labour because its prolonged duration of action increases the risk of neonatal depression.

An 81-year-old woman with bony metastases from carcinoma of the breast was given methadone 5 mg three times daily for 2 days; she became deeply unconscious but awoke immediately when given naloxone 400 µg intravenously.— P. Symonds (letter), *Br. med. J.*, 1977, *1*, 512. A further report of an enhanced effect of methadone in 3 patients with cancer.— D. S. Ettinger *et al.*, *Cancer Treat. Rep.*, 1979, *63*, 457.

INTERACTIONS. *Cimetidine*. A case report of a potentially serious drug interaction considered to be between methadone and cimetidine. A 76-year-old man was given methadone (5 mg every 8 hours by mouth), and morphine (8 mg subcutaneously as required). After 6 days treatment the patient was commenced on cimetidine (300 mg intravenously every 6 hours). A further 6 days later and 3 hours after a dose of morphine the patient was unresponsive. Naloxone reversed the state but its effect wore off in 6 hours when a second dose was given and was followed by immediate arousal.— E. M. Sorkin and G. S. Ogawa, *Drug Intell. & clin. Pharm.*, 1983, *17*, 60.

Monoamine oxidase inhibitors. A report of the successful use of tranylcypromine in a patient receiving methadone maintenance therapy. No adverse interaction was observed.— G. Mendelson (letter), *Med. J. Aust.*, 1979, *1*, 400.

Phenytoin. A patient's usual dose of methadone failed to prevent withdrawal symptoms when he was also given phenytoin.— P. F. Finelli (letter), *New Engl. J. Med.*, 1976, *294*, 227. See also T. G. Tong *et al.*, *Ann. intern. Med.*, 1981, *94*, 349.

Pregnancy tests. A report of methadone interfering with pregnancy tests.— C. A. Horwitz *et al.*, *J. Reprod. fert.*, 1973, *33*, 489.

Rifampicin. Of 30 patients receiving methadone maintenance, 21 developed withdrawal symptoms following concurrent administration of rifampicin. In a study of 6 whose symptoms were severe, rifampicin was noted to lower plasma-methadone concentrations and to increase urinary excretion of the major metabolite.— M. J. Kreek *et al.*, *New Engl. J. Med.*, 1976, *294*, 1104.

Rifampicin 450 mg daily given as part of an antituberculous regimen involving streptomycin and isoniazid produced symptoms of methadone withdrawal in a patient receiving methadone maintenance at 40 mg daily. Withdrawal effects were abolished by increasing the methadone dose from 40 to 60 mg daily.— M. R. Bending and P. O. Skacel (letter), *Lancet*, 1977, *1*, 1211.

PREGNANCY AND THE NEONATE. The death of a 5-week-old infant might have been the result of methadone ingestion in breast milk from the mother who received maintenance doses of methadone. The methadone-blood concentration of the infant at autopsy was 400 ng per mL.— J. E. Smialek *et al.*, *J. Am. med. Ass.*, 1977, *238*, 2516.

The amount of methadone in breast milk was unlikely to have any pharmacologic effect on the infant.— *Med. Lett.*, 1979, *21*, 52.

See also under Dependence and Adverse Effects, above.

Absorption and Fate

Methadone is readily absorbed from the gastro-intestinal tract. It is widely distributed in the tissues and diffuses across the placenta. It is extensively protein bound. Methadone is metabolised in the liver, mainly by *N*-demethylation and cyclisation, and the metabolites are excreted in the bile and urine. It has a prolonged half-life and is subject to accumulation.

The mean peak plasma-methadone concentration of 74 ng per mL in 5 subjects given 15 mg by mouth occurred at 4 hours. Over the first 24 hours 25% of the dose was excreted in the urine as almost equal parts of methadone and 1 of the 2 metabolites detected and during the next 72 hours an additional 25% of the dose was recovered. The renal clearance was found to be pH-dependent, the lower the pH the greater the clearance.— C. E. Inturrisi and K. Verebely, *Clin. Pharmac. Ther.*, 1972, *13*, 923. The mean apparent plasma half-life of methadone was calculated as 25 hours (range 13 to 47 hours).— *idem*, 633.

Binding of methadone to human plasma proteins *in vitro* ranged from 71.7 to 87.5% over a range of methadone concentrations. The percent bound decreased as methadone concentrations increased.— G. D. Olsen, *Clin. Pharmac. Ther.*, 1973, *14*, 338.

In a study of 17 patients receiving methadone maintenance therapy plasma concentrations fluctuated widely from day to day and week to week in individual patients. There was only rarely any relationship between symptom complaints and plasma-methadone concentrations so that determination of methadone concentrations was unlikely to be of any benefit.— W. H. Horns *et al.*, *Clin. Pharmac. Ther.*, 1975, *17*, 636.

Plasma concentrations and analgesia following deltoid and gluteal injections of methadone and morphine. Administration of methadone into the deltoid muscle produced higher concentrations and greater pain relief than administration into the gluteal muscle.— P. Y. Grabinski *et al.*, *J. clin. Pharmac.*, 1983, *23*, 48.

Further references to the pharmacokinetics of methadone: A. E. Robinson and F. M. Williams, *J. Pharm. Pharmac.*, 1971, *23*, 353; R. C. Baselt and L. J. Casarett, *Clin. Pharmac. Ther.*, 1972, *13*, 64; B. A. Berkowitz, *Clin. Pharmacokinet.*, 1976, *1*, 219; G. D. Bellward *et al.*, *Clin. Pharmac. Ther.*, 1977, *22*, 92; M. -I. Nilsson, *Acta pharm. suec.*, 1982, *19*, 472; M. -I. Nilsson, *Eur. J. clin. Pharmac.*, 1983, *25*, 497; J. Säwe, *Clin. Pharmacokinet.*, 1986, *11*, 87.

PREGNANCY AND THE NEONATE. Methadone pharmacokinetics in methadone-maintained pregnant women. Plasma concentrations of methadone were reduced probably due to enhanced metabolism. It was suggested that the dose of methadone might need to be increased in such patients.— S. M. Pond *et al.*, *J. Pharmac. exp. Ther.*, 1985, *233*, 1.

Uses and Administration

Methadone hydrochloride is a potent analgesic with actions and uses similar to those of morphine (see p.1312) but having a less marked sedative action. The analgesic effect begins about 15 minutes after subcutaneous injection and about 45 minutes after administration by mouth, the effect usually lasting about 4 hours. As accumulation occurs following repeated doses, the effects become more prolonged.

The dose of methadone hydrochloride ranges from 2.5 to 10 mg given at intervals of 3 to 8 hours depending on the pain. A commonly used range is 5 to 10 mg every 6 to 8 hours. It may be given by mouth or by subcutaneous or intramuscular injection; the intravenous route is not recommended and if repeated injections are required the intramuscular route is preferred to the subcutaneous.

Methadone hydrochloride also has a depressant action on the cough centre and is given to control non-productive coughing of intractable disorders, such as lung cancer. For this purpose it is usually given in the form of a linctus in a dose of 1 to 2 mg every 4 to 6 hours, but reduced to twice daily on prolonged use.

Methadone hydrochloride is used as part of the treatment of dependence on opioid drugs (see also under Dependence, p.1308). In the treatment of opioid withdrawal, or detoxification, methadone is given initially in doses sufficient to suppress withdrawal symptoms. A mixture containing 1 mg per mL of methadone hydrochloride is used in the *UK* for drug dependent persons. A dose of 15 to 20 mg by mouth is usually sufficient, although higher doses may be required in some patients. After stabilisation, which can often be achieved with a daily dose of 40 mg, the dose of methadone is gradually decreased until total withdrawal is achieved. Some treatment schedules for opioid dependence involve prolonged maintenance therapy with methadone where the daily dose is adjusted carefully for the individual;

there are reports of some patients receiving 120 mg or more daily. The problems of methadone dependence are discussed under Dependence, see above.

In a study of the clinical effects and pharmacokinetics of racemic methadone compared with its isomers in 30 male subjects the half-life of (±)-methadone in blood was an average of about 22 hours compared with 24 hours for (−)-methadone and 25 hours for (+)-methadone. Further studies on the subjects in groups of 6 indicated that the effects of (+)-methadone 7.5 mg on respiration were not significantly different from a placebo response whereas (−)-methadone 7.5 mg and (±)-methadone 15 mg produced intense respiratory depression with a peak response after an average of about 4 hours and a return to control values at 72 hours for racemic methadone and a peak after an average of about 12 hours and a return to control values after an average of about 75 hours (variation 30 to 118 hours) in the case of (−)-methadone; 2 subjects given (+)-methadone 50 and 100 mg respectively both had small net depressions. The effects of (+)-methadone on pupillary constriction were again not significantly different from placebo but (±)- and (−)-methadone induced marked constriction with a peak effect at 2 hours and a duration lasting an average of 72 hours for racemic methadone and an average of 86 hours for (−)-methadone. Potency ratios for (−)- to (±)-methadone from blood concentration data were 3 for respiratory depression and 2.7 for miosis. The antidiuretic effect of racemic methadone was also more prolonged than the analgesic effect.— G. D. Olsen *et al.*, *Clin. Pharmac. Ther.*, 1977, *21*, 147.

A double-blind comparative study of the efficacy of methadone or diamorphine with cocaine as analgesics in 46 patients with terminal cancer suggested that although methadone was a satisfactory substitute for diamorphine in some patients, diamorphine should be used in very ill patients since it did not accumulate in the body to the same extent as methadone, thereby making dosage adjustment easier. The dangers of accumulation of methadone were stressed particularly in the elderly or debilitated.— R. G. Twycross (letter), *Br. J. clin. Pharmac.*, 1977, *4*, 691.

The use of methadone, on patient demand, for the relief of chronic cancer pain; by the 6th day the dose was 10 to 40 mg daily.— J. Säwe *et al.*, *Br. med. J.*, 1981, *282*, 771.

Methadone was found to produce prolonged postoperative analgesia of about 25 hours when given as a 20-mg intravenous bolus to 19 patients.— G. K. Gourlay *et al.*, *Br. med. J.*, 1982, *284*, 630.

ADMINISTRATION, EPIDURAL AND INTRATHECAL. Analgesia with intraspinal methadone.— T. A. Torda and D. A. Pybus, *Br. J. Anaesth.*, 1982, *54*, 291 (epidural); M. B. Max *et al.*, *Clin. Pharmac. Ther.*, 1985, *38*, 631 (epidural and intrathecal); M. Nyska *et al.*, *Br. med. J.*, 1986, *293*, 1347 (epidural).

TREATMENT OF DEPENDENCE. A review of methadone maintenance treatment of opioid addicts. Research has demonstrated that therapeutic communities are associated with long-lasting improvements in functioning for the few drug abusers who stay in treatment at least 3 months. A principal limitation of this modality is that few patients remain in treatment long enough to acquire the changed values that produce long-lasting effects. Research on methadone maintenance continues to show that this treatment produces immediate decreases in criminality and drug abuse; however, patients who taper off maintenance are prone to relapse. The aspects of treatment that appear to prevent relapse include minimising withdrawal symptoms during tapering and providing support during and after completing maintenance. The strengths of these 2 treatment modalities can be combined to enable opioid addicts to taper off methadone maintenance in a therapeutic community and remain drug-free.— J. L. Sorensen *et al.*, *Am. J. Drug Alcohol Abuse*, 1984, *10*, 347.

A survey supporting the contention that patients receiving prescriptions of methadone continue to abuse illicit drugs and that methadone is itself abused.— M. S. Lipsedge and C. C. H. Cook (letter), *Lancet*, 1987, *2*, 451.

A discussion defining and evaluating the success of methadone treatment for opioid addiction.— R. G. Newman, *New Engl. J. Med.*, 1987, *317*, 447.

Some references to methadone maintenance treatment of opioid addicts: V. P. Dole and M. E. Nyswander, *J. Am. med. Ass.*, 1976, *235*, 2117; N. E. Zinberg, *New Engl. J. Med.*, 1977, *296*, 1000; R. G. Newman and W. B. Whitehill, *Lancet*, 1979, *2*, 485; M. L. Stitzer *et al.*, *Clin. Pharmac. Ther.*, 1983, *34*, 29; J. Cami *et al.*, *Clin. Pharmac. Ther.*, 1985, *38*, 336; G. E. Woody *et al.*, *Archs gen. Psychiat.*, 1981, *38*, 898.

For reference to the control of methadone-withdrawal symptoms by administration of clonidine, see Clonidine, p.475.

For a report on the use of diphenoxylate during withdrawal from methadone maintenance, see Diphenoxylate Hydrochloride, p.1088.

Preparations

Methadone Hydrochloride Injection *(U.S.P.)*

Methadone Injection *(B.P.)*

Methadone Linctus *(B.P.)*. Methadone hydrochloride 2 mg per 5 mL of a suitable vehicle with a tolu flavour.

For a report of incompatibility when Methadone Linctus was prepared with or diluted with syrup preserved with hydroxybenzoates, see under Sucrose, p.1276.

Methadone Mixture 1mg/1ml.. A formula is provided in the *B.N.F.*

NOTE. This preparation is 2.5 times the strength of Methadone Linctus (B.P.) and is intended only for drug-dependent persons.

Methadone Hydrochloride Oral Concentrate *(U.S.P.)*. Contains methadone hydrochloride 9 to 11 mg in each mL. To be diluted.

Methadone Hydrochloride Tablets *(U.S.P.)*

Methadone Tablets *(B.P.)*. Tablets containing methadone hydrochloride.

Proprietary Preparations

Physeptone *(Calmic, UK)*. *Tablets*, scored, methadone hydrochloride 5 mg.
Injection, methadone hydrochloride 10 mg/mL, in ampoules of 1 mL.

Proprietary Names and Manufacturers

Cloro-nona *(Vinsi, Spain)*; Dolophine *(Lilly, USA)*; Eptadone *(Tosi, Ital.)*; Heptanal *(Switz.)*; Ketalgine *(Amino, Switz.)*; Mephenon *(Belg.; Lipha, Ital.)*; Metasedin *(Esteve, Spain)*; Physeptone *(Wellcome, Austral.; Wellcome, Ital.; Wellcome, S.Afr.; Calmic, UK)*; Sedamidone *(Lifepharma, Ital.)*; Sedo Rapide *(Rapide, Spain)*; L-Polamidon *(Hoechst, Ger.)*; Symoron *(Neth.)*; Tussol *(Belg.)*.

6239-c

Morphine *(BAN)*.

7,8-Didehydro-4,5-epoxy-17-methylmorphinan-3,6-diol.

$C_{17}H_{19}NO_3,H_2O$=303.4.

CAS — 57-27-2 (anhydrous); 6009-81-0 (monohydrate).

The principal alkaloid of opium.

6240-s

Morphine Acetate *(BANM)*.

$C_{17}H_{19}NO_3,C_2H_4O_2,3H_2O$=399.4.

CAS — 596-15-6 (anhydrous); 5974-11-8 (trihydrate).

Freeze-dried morphine acetate was stable and because of its solubility could be used to produce intramuscular injections providing up to 200 mg in a suitable volume.— G. K. Poochikian *et al.* (letter), *J. Am. med. Ass.*, 1980, *244*, 1434.

6241-w

Morphine Hydrochloride *(BANM)*.

Morphinii Chloridum; Morphinum Chloratum.

$C_{17}H_{19}NO_3,HCl,3H_2O$=375.8.

CAS — 52-26-6 (anhydrous); 6055-06-7 (trihydrate).

Pharmacopoeias. In *Arg., Aust., Belg., Br., Braz., Chin., Cz., Egypt., Eur., Fr., Ger., Hung., Ind., Int., It., Jpn, Jug., Mex., Neth., Nord., Pol., Port., Roum., Rus., Span., Swiss,* and *Turk.* Also in *B.P. Vet.*

Colourless, silky crystals, cubical masses or a white or almost white, crystalline powder. **Soluble** 1 in 24 of water, 1 in 10 of boiling alcohol (90%); practically insoluble in chloroform and ether. At 15° soluble 1 in 100 of alcohol and at 10° soluble 1 in 50 of alcohol. **Store** in well-closed containers. Protect from light.

6242-e

Morphine Sulphate *(BANM)*.

Morphine Sulfate *(USAN)*; Morphini Sulfas.

$(C_{17}H_{19}NO_3)_2,H_2SO_4,5H_2O$=758.8.

CAS — 64-31-3 (anhydrous); 6211-15-0 (pentahydrate).

Pharmacopoeias. In *Br., Egypt., Ind., Int., Mex., Port., Turk.*, and *U.S.* Also in *B.P. Vet.*

Odourless or almost odourless, white, acicular crystals, cubical masses, or crystalline powder. When exposed to air it gradually loses water of crystallisation. It darkens on prolonged exposure to light.

Soluble 1 in 21 of water and 1 in 1000 of alcohol; practically insoluble in chloroform and ether. The *U.S.P.* injection has a pH of 2.5 to 6.5. Solutions of morphine salts are **sterilised** by autoclaving.

Morphine salts are sensitive to changes in pH and morphine is liable to be precipitated out of solution in an alkaline environment. Compounds reported to be **incompatible** with morphine salts include some barbiturates, pethidine, phenytoin, promethazine, and thiopentone. **Store** in airtight containers. Protect from light.

INCOMPATIBILITY. Morphine sulphate injection containing chlorocresol 0.2% was incompatible with chlorpromazine hydrochloride injection. Morphine injection without chlorocresol should be compatible.— J. B. Crapper, *Br. med. J.*, 1975, *1*, 33.

Morphine sulphate and heparin solutions were incompatible only at morphine concentrations greater than 5 mg per mL. The incompatibility was prevented by using 0.9% sodium chloride solution as the admixture diluent.— D. E. Baker *et al.*, *Am. J. Hosp. Pharm.*, 1985, *42*, 1352.

STABILITY. Stability of morphine in Kaolin and Morphine Mixture *B.P.*— K. Helliwell and P. Game, *Pharm. J.*, 1981, *2*, 128.

The effects of containers on the stability of morphine in Kaolin and Morphine Mixture *(B.P.)*.— K. Helliwell and P. Jennings, *Pharm. J.*, 1984, *1*, 682.

6243-l

Morphine Tartrate *(BANM)*.

$(C_{17}H_{19}NO_3)_2,C_4H_6O_6,3H_2O$=774.8.

CAS — 302-31-8 (anhydrous); 6032-59-3 (trihydrate).

Dependence of the Morphine Type

The opioid analgesics are liable to be subject to abuse.

Drug dependence of the morphine type is a state arising from repeated administration of morphine or a drug with morphine-like effects; it is characterised by an overwhelming need to continue taking the drug or one with similar properties, by a tendency to increase the dose owing to the development of tolerance, and by psychological and physical dependence on the drug.

Abrupt withdrawal of opiates from persons physically dependent on them precipitates a withdrawal syndrome, the severity of which depends on the individual, the drug used, the size and frequency of the dose, and the duration of drug use. *Withdrawal symptoms* usually begin within a few hours, reach a peak within 36 to 72 hours, and then gradually subside. Withdrawal symptoms develop more slowly with methadone. Symptoms include yawning, mydriasis, lachrymation, rhinorrhoea, sneezing, muscle tremor, weakness, sweating, irritability, disturbed sleep or insomnia, restlessness, anorexia, nausea, vomiting, loss of weight, diarrhoea, dehydration, leucocytosis, bone pain, abdominal and muscle cramps, increases in heart-rate, respiratory-rate, and blood pressure, rise in temperature, and gooseflesh and vasomotor disturbances.

Withdrawal symptoms may be terminated by a suitable dose of morphine or related drug.

Some physiological values may not return to normal for several months following the acute withdrawal syndrome.

Withdrawal therapy requires sustained surveillance and the patient should be persuaded to enter hospital or be referred to a treatment centre. Withdrawal may be effected slowly or rapidly. The usual method is to replace the drug of dependence with methadone (see p.1309).

Reviews and discussions on the treatment of opioid dependence: B. Davies, *Pharm. J.*, 1986, *2*, 525; J. E. Peachey, *Med. J. Aust.*, 1986, *145*, 395; R. Batey (letter), *ibid.*, 1987, *146*, 172; J. E. Peachey (letter), *ibid.*

See also under Clonidine Hydrochloride, p.475.

PREGNANCY AND THE NEONATE. An extensive review of neonatal opioid withdrawal and the outcome of children born to women dependent upon opioids.— L. P. Finnegan, *Adv. Alcohol Subst. Abuse*, 1982, *1*, 55.

A brief review of neonatal opiate withdrawal.— R. P. A. Rivers, *Archs Dis. Childh.*, 1986, *61*, 1236. See also P. Caviston, *Br. med. J.*, 1987, *295*, 285.

Treatment of neonatal dependence. Symptoms of diamorphine withdrawal occurred in 259 of 384 infants born to diamorphine-dependent mothers. Of these, 178 required treatment. All signs of withdrawal were effectively relieved by administration of chlorpromazine in a daily dose of 2.2 mg per kg body-weight in divided doses at 6-hourly intervals by mouth or by injection. The dose of chlorpromazine was gradually reduced over 10 to 40 days.— C. Zelson *et al.*, *Pediatrics*, 1971, *48*, 178.

Of 110 infants born to mothers, almost all of whom were taking methadone, diamorphine, or both, sometimes with other agents, 103 showed withdrawal symptoms; 51 needed treatment. There were no significant differences between those treated with methadone 250 µg six-hourly, increased to 500 µg six-hourly, phenobarbitone 5 to 8 mg per kg body-weight daily in 3 divided doses, or diazepam 0.5 to 2 mg eight-hourly. Withdrawal symptoms were less common in those whose mothers were taking less than 20 mg of methadone daily.— J. D. Madden *et al.*, *Am. J. Obstet. Gynec.*, 1977, *127*, 199.

The management of the neonatal opioid withdrawal syndrome includes general supportive therapy as well as specific drug therapy. A quiet darkened environment may help calm the infant while adequate fluid and nutrient intake must be ensured. Camphorated opium tincture (Paregoric *U.S.P.*) has been widely used to treat withdrawal symptoms. An initial dose of 0.2 mL every 3 hours has been used. It is rarely necessary to exceed 0.7 mL per dose. After stabilisation the dose is gradually reduced over 25 to 45 days. The main adverse effects are constipation and lethargy. Diazepam has also been used in doses of 1 to 2 mg intramuscularly every 8 hours. Withdrawal can usually be accomplished within a week. Chlorpromazine has been given in doses of 2 to 3 mg per kg body-weight daily in divided doses by mouth or intramuscularly. Chlorpromazine can usually be withdrawn after 2 to 3 weeks. Phenobarbitone has been given to control symptoms of insomnia and irritability but it does not control gastro-intestinal disorders.— R. G. Harper and G. B. Edwards, in *Drug Abuse in Pregnancy and Neonatal Effects*, J.L. Rementería (Ed.), Saint Louis, C.V. Mosby, 1977, p. 103.

Adverse Effects

In normal doses the commonest side-effects of morphine and other opioid analgesics are nausea, vomiting, constipation, drowsiness, and confusion. Micturition may be difficult and there may be ureteric or biliary spasm; there is also an antidiuretic effect. Dry mouth, sweating, facial flushing, vertigo, bradycardia, palpitations, orthostatic hypotension, hypothermia, restlessness, changes of mood, and miosis also occur. These effects occur more commonly in ambulant patients than in those at rest in bed. Raised intracranial pressure occurs in some patients. The euphoric activity of morphine and similar compounds has led to their abuse. Dependence is discussed above.

Larger doses produce respiratory depression and hypotension, with circulatory failure and deepening coma. Convulsions may occur in infants and children. Death may occur from respiratory failure. Toxic doses vary considerably with the individual and regular users may tolerate large doses.

Due to the histamine-releasing effect, reactions such as urticaria and pruritus, occur in some individuals. Contact dermatitis has been reported and pain and irritation may occur on injection. Anaphylactic reactions following intravenous injection of morphine and codeine have been reported.

Muscle rigidity has been reported following the administration of morphine and some other opioids.

Experience with epidural morphine (chloride) (2 mg in 10 mL physiological saline) for postoperative pain relief in 1200 patients, the first 242 of whom received a commercial preparation containing preservatives, and the remainder of whom were treated with preservative-free filtered solution. Side-effects regarded as related to epidural morphine were: nausea or vomiting (204 patients; 17%), blood pressure drop of 20 mmHg or more (24 patients; 2%), itching in the first 242 patients (36 patients; 15%), itching in the rest (9 patients; 1%), urinary retention (181 patients; 15%), and respiratory depression (1 patient). The 17% incidence of nausea and vomiting was considerably less than in a control group given morphine chloride 2 mg in physiological saline intravenously (57% incidence), as was the fall in blood pressure (2% against 14% in the controls). Itching was not affected by antihistamines and was probably caused by the preservatives; urinary retention might be a local anaesthetic effect; its frequency did not decrease with preservative-free solution. Although the incidence of respiratory depression is low following epidural morphine, it may still occur long after epidural infusion and patients must be closely monitored.— S. Reiz and M. Westberg (letter), *Lancet*, 1980, *2*, 203. Adverse effects of epidural and intrathecal opiates, a report of a nationwide survey in Sweden. Up to May 1981 epidural morphine had been given to approximately 6000 to 9150 patients, and intrathecal morphine to 90 to 150 patients. Ventilatory depression requiring treatment with naloxone was reported in 23 patients treated with epidural morphine (0.25-0.4%) and in 6 given intrathecal morphine (4-7%).— L. L. Gustafsson *et al.*, *Br. J. Anaesth.*, 1982, *54*, 479.

Case reports of 3 patients in whom facial itching was provoked by intrathecal opiate. The itching responded to intravenous naloxone.— P. V. Scott and H. B. J. Fischer, *Br. med. J.*, 1982, *284*, 1015.

A study suggesting that histamine plays an important role in the acute haemodynamic and plasma-adrenaline response to morphine.— N. R. Fahmy *et al.*, *Clin. Pharmac. Ther.*, 1983, *33*, 615.

A study comparing the adverse effects (sedation, nausea, vomiting) following morphine administration either intramuscularly or orally using slow-release tablets. More adverse effects were reported by the patients in the intramuscular group and for similar degrees of analgesia there were fewer side-effects in the oral group.— D. R. Derbyshire *et al.*, *Br. J. Anaesth.*, 1985, *57*, 858.

Increases in prolactin and growth hormone secretion induced by morphine.— T. Duka *et al.*, *Br. J. clin. Pharmac.*, 1986, *21*, 611P.

EFFECTS ON THE LIVER. Serum concentrations of amylase and hydroxybutyric acid dehydrogenase may be raised after administration of opiates due to spasm of the sphincter of Oddi. Serum-aspartate aminotransferase (SGOT) and serum-alanine aminotransferase (SGPT) concentrations can be raised by opioids and they could induce an increase in serum-lactic dehydrogenase concentration of hepatic origin by increasing intrabiliary pressure.— F. Clark, *Adverse Drug React. Bull.*, 1977, Oct., 232.

EFFECTS ON SEXUAL FUNCTION. For the effects of opioid analgesics on sexual function, see under Methadone Hydrochloride, p.1309.

OVERDOSAGE. Morphine overdosage resulting in the death of a 69-year-old woman who had received four 60-mg sustained-release tablets at 8-hourly intervals.— D. Brahams, *Lancet*, 1984, *1*, 1083. Comment.— D. Vere (letter), *ibid.*, 1477.

A report of rhabdomyolysis associated with acute poisoning in 3 patients, following overdosage with opiates. One patient, who had taken dipipanone in association with cyclizine (Diconal), was oliguric and developed renal failure requiring haemodialysis, but renal function subsequently returned to normal— P. G. Blain *et al.*, *Hum. Toxicol*, 1985, *4*, 71.

A case report of prolonged analgesia after inadvertent morphine overdose.— A. P. Fisher *et al.* (letter), *Lancet*, 1987, *1*, 573.

Treatment of Adverse Effects

In acute poisoning by an opioid taken by mouth the stomach should be emptied by aspiration and lavage. A laxative may be given to aid peristalsis.

Intensive supportive therapy may be required to correct respiratory failure and shock. In addition, the specific antagonist naloxone hydrochloride is used to counteract very rapidly the severe respiratory depression and coma produced by excessive doses of opioid analgesics. A dose of 0.4 to 2 mg is given intravenously, repeated at intervals of 2 to 3 minutes if necessary, up to 10 mg. Naloxone may also be given by subcutaneous or intramuscular injection. The effect of naloxone may be of shorter duration than that of the opioid analgesic and additional doses may be required to prevent relapses. For further details concerning the dosage and administration of naloxone in opioid poisoning, see p.845.

Nalorphine hydrobromide (p.844) and levallorphan tartrate (p.842) have also been used to antagonise the adverse effects of opioid analgesics.

The use of opioid antagonists such as naloxone, nalorphine, and levallorphan in persons physically dependent on morphine or related drugs may induce withdrawal symptoms.

A discussion of acute opioid toxicity and its management.— J. Henry and G. Volans, *Br. med. J.*, 1984, *289*, 990.

Precautions

Morphine is not usually given pre-operatively to children under 1 year of age, and it should be given with extreme care to newborn or premature infants for other conditions. The dosage should be reduced in elderly and debilitated patients.

Morphine is generally contra-indicated in respiratory depression, especially in the presence of cyanosis and excessive bronchial secretion. It is also contra-indicated in the presence of acute alcoholism, head injuries, and conditions in which intracranial pressure is raised. It should not be given during an attack of bronchial asthma or in heart failure secondary to chronic lung disease. It should be given with caution or in reduced doses to patients with hypothyroidism, adrenocortical insufficiency, impaired kidney or liver function, prostatic hypertrophy, or shock. It should be used with caution in patients with obstructive bowel disorders. Opioid analgesics should be used with caution in patients with myasthenia gravis.

As serious and sometimes fatal reactions have occurred following administration of pethidine to patients receiving monoamine oxidase inhibitors, pethidine and related drugs are contra-indicated in patients taking monoamine oxidase inhibitors or within 14 days of stopping such treatment; morphine and other opioid analgesics should be given with extreme caution. The depressant effects of morphine are enhanced by depressants of the central nervous system such as alcohol, anaesthetics, hypnotics and sedatives, tricyclic antidepressants, and phenothiazines. The actions of opioids may in turn affect the activities of other compounds. For instance, their gastro-intestinal effects may delay absorption as with mexilitine or may be counteractive as with metoclopramide.

The administration of opioid analgesics during labour may cause respiratory depression in the newborn infant.

ADMINISTRATION IN RENAL FAILURE. Severe and prolonged respiratory depression may occur in patients with renal impairment given morphine; this is attributed to the accumulation of morphine-6-glucuronide.— R. J. Osborne *et al.*, *Br. med. J.*, 1986, *292*, 1548. and *idem*, *293*, 1101.

See also under Absorption and Fate.

INTERACTIONS. Morphine and diamorphine were effective microsomal enzyme depletors.— L. W. Masten *et al.*

(letter), *Nature*, 1975, *253*, 200.

A study demonstrating that cimetidine does not alter morphine disposition in man.— P. Mojaverian *et al.*, *Br. J. clin. Pharmac.*, 1982, *14*, 809.

A study in 24 patients aged 45 to 75 years, who were taking oral morphine solution for the treatment of cancer pain. Plasma concentrations of free morphine were measured after the administration of morphine alone, or after clomipramine or amitriptyline (20 or 50 mg daily) had been administered orally with morphine for 3 days. Both clomipramine and amitriptyline significantly increased the plasma availability of morphine.— V. Ventafridda *et al.* (letter), *Lancet*, 1987, *1*, 1204.

PHAEOCHROMOCYTOMA. Opiates were contra-indicated in patients with a phaeochromocytoma as such drugs could liberate endogenous histamine and stimulate the release of catecholamines.— N. C. Chaturvedi *et al.*, *Br. med. J.*, 1974, *2*, 538.

Absorption and Fate

Morphine salts are absorbed from the gastro-intestinal tract but their effects by this route are not entirely predictable; after subcutaneous or intramuscular injection morphine is readily absorbed into the blood. It undergoes significant first-pass metabolism in the liver. Morphine is distributed throughout the body but mainly in the kidneys, liver, lungs, and spleen, with lower concentrations in the brain and muscles. Morphine diffuses across the placenta and traces also appear in milk and sweat. About 35% is protein bound.

Conjugation to morphine 3- and 6-glucuronides occurs in the liver. About 10% of a dose of morphine is excreted through the bile into the faeces and the remainder is excreted in the urine, mainly as conjugates. About 90% of total morphine is excreted in 24 hours with traces up to 48 hours.

The pharmacokinetics of morphine administered by intraspinal routes: L. L. Gustafsson *et al.* (letter), *Lancet*, 1982, *1*, 796; A. Moore *et al.*, *Clin. Pharmac. Ther.*, 1984, *35*, 40; M. B. Max *et al.*, *ibid.*, 1985, *38*, 631; G. Nordberg *et al.*, *Br. J. Anaesth.*, 1986, *58*, 598.

Some references to the pharmacokinetics of controlled-release forms of morphine: C. A. Pinnock *et al.*, *Br. J. Anaesth.*, 1986, *58*, 868; J. J. Savarese *et al.*, *Clin. Pharmacokinet.*, 1986, *11*, 505.

References to the pharmacokinetics of morphine: J. A. Owen *et al.*, *Clin. Pharmac. Ther.*, 1983, *34*, 364 (age-related pharmacokinetics); J. Säwe *et al.*, *Eur. J. clin. Pharmac.*, 1983, *24*, 537 (steady-state kinetics); P. Y. Grabinski *et al.*, *J. clin. Pharmac.*, 1983, *23*, 48 (equivalent analgesia following deltoid or gluteal injection); T. D. Walsh and B. V. Kadam, *Br. J. clin. Pharmac.*, 1984, *17*, 641P (kinetics during repeated oral administration); A. Moore *et al.*, *Clin. Pharmac. Ther.*, 1984, *35*, 641 (pharmacokinetics during and after renal transplantation); C. S. Waldmann *et al.*, *Anaesthesia*, 1984, *39*, 768 (similar serum concentrations with continuous subcutaneous infusion or intravenous infusion); G. W. Hanks and G. W. Aherne (letter), *Lancet*, 1985, *1*, 221 (liver, kidney, and gastro-intestinal metabolism); G. Nordberg *et al.*, *Eur. J. clin. Pharmac.*, 1985, *27*, 677 (CSF concentrations with intramuscular injection); F. Moolenaar *et al.*, *ibid.*, *29*, 119 (rectal absorption with a solution of pH 7 to 8); J. Säwe, *Clin. Pharmacokinet.*, 1986, *11*, 87 (pharmacokinetics of high oral doses); L. P. Claffey and W. P. Blunnie, *Br. J. Anaesth.*, 1986, *58*, 1324P (CSF and plasma concentrations with oral and intramuscular administration).

ADMINISTRATION IN INFANTS AND CHILDREN. The pharmacokinetics of morphine were studied in 12 neonates given infusions of the sulphate postoperatively. Four received a loading dose of 50 to 100 µg per kg body-weight followed by 6.2 to 40 µg per kg per hour; the other 8 received no loading dose but an infusion of 18.2 to 24 µg per kg per hour. The periods of infusion ranged from 3.5 to 105 hours. After 20 hours the dose correlated with plasma concentrations, but large variability existed. Elimination half-life for 8 infants was 13.9 ± 6.4 hours; in 4 of them the terminal half-life was 24.8 ± 4.6 hours. Two infants with serum-morphine concentrations of 61 and 90 ng per mL suffered generalised seizures and bradycardia; their infusion rates were 32 and 40 µg per kg per hour respectively. It was recommended that the infusion rate should not exceed 15 µg per kg per hour.— G. Koren *et al.*, *J. Pediat.*, 1985, *107*, 963. See also A. M. Lynn and J. T. Slattery, *Anesthesiology*, 1987, *66*, 136.

A study of the pharmacokinetics of morphine in 2 children before and after liver transplantation. Both children metabolised morphine but one who also had renal failure accumulated metabolites.— M. P. Shelly *et al.*, *Br. J. Anaesth.*, 1986, *58*, 1218.

ADMINISTRATION IN RENAL FAILURE. There have been reports of increased plasma concentrations of morphine in patients with renal failure (M. Ball *et al.*, *Lancet*, 1985, *1*, 784; M. Shelly and G.R. Park, *ibid.*, 1100). However. Säwe *et al.* (*Lancet*, 1985, *2*, 211) using high-performance liquid chromatography have observed an increase in morphine glucuronide metabolites and not morphine and have reported that the metabolism of morphine is not impaired in patients with renal failure (J. Säwe and I. Odar-Cederlöf, *Eur. J. clin. Pharmac.*, 1987, *32*, 377). Also, Woolner *et al.* (*Br. J. clin. Pharmac.*, 1986, *22*, 55) have reported that renal failure does not impair the elimination of morphine but does slow the elimination of its glucuronides. An accumulation of morphine-6-glucuronide has been associated with severe respiratory depression in 3 patients with renal failure (R.J. Osborne *et al.*, *Br. med. J.*, 1986, *292*, 1548).

METABOLISM. Discussions on the analgesic role of morphine-6-glucuronide and on extrahepatic metabolism: G. W. Hanks *et al.*, *Lancet*, 1987, *2*, 723; C. W. Hand *et al.* (letter), *ibid.*, 1987, *2*, 1207; H. J. McQuay *et al.* (letter), *ibid.*, 1458; G. W. Hanks *et al.*, *ibid.*, 1988, *1*, 469.

A demonstration of the analgesic activity of morphine-6-glucuronide.— R. Osborne *et al.* (letter), *Lancet*, 1988, *1*, 828.

Further references to the metabolism of morphine: J. Säwe *et al.*, *Br. J. clin. Pharmac.*, 1983, *16*, 85 (no evidence of increased morphine metabolism during long-term treatment with increasing doses); J. Säwe *et al.*, *ibid.*, 1985, *19*, 495 (hepatic glucuronidation).

PREGNANCY AND THE NEONATE. See above under Administration in Infants and Children.

Uses and Administration

Morphine is an opioid analgesic. It acts mainly on the central nervous system and smooth muscle. Although morphine is predominantly a central nervous system depressant it has some central stimulant actions which result in nausea and vomiting and miosis. Morphine generally increases smooth muscle tone, especially the sphincters of the gastro-intestinal tract.

Morphine and related analgesics may produce both physical and psychological dependence and should therefore be used with discrimination (see p.1310). Tolerance may also develop.

Morphine is an analgesic used for the symptomatic relief of moderate to severe pain, especially that associated with neoplastic disease, myocardial infarction, and surgery. When pain is likely to be of short duration, a short-acting analgesic is usually preferred. In addition to relieving pain, morphine also alleviates the anxiety associated with severe pain. It is useful as a hypnotic where sleeplessness is due to pain, and may also relieve the pain of biliary or renal colic, although an antispasmodic may also be required since morphine may increase smooth muscle tone.

Morphine reduces intestinal motility and is used in the symptomatic treatment of diarrhoea. It also relieves the dyspnoea of left ventricular failure and of pulmonary oedema. It is effective for the suppression of cough, but codeine is usually preferred as there is less risk of dependence. Morphine has been used pre-operatively as an adjunct to anaesthesia for pain relief and to allay anxiety. It has also been used in high doses as a general anaesthetic in specialised procedures.

Morphine is usually administered as the sulphate, although the hydrochloride and the tartrate are used in similar doses; the acetate has also been used. Routes of administration include the oral, subcutaneous, intramuscular, intravenous, intraspinal, and rectal routes. Parenteral doses may be intermittent injections or continuous or intermittent infusions adjusted according to individual analgesic requirements.

The usual dose by subcutaneous or intramuscular injection is 5 to 20 mg every 4 hours. Children up to 1 month of age may be given 150 µg per kg body-weight; those aged 1 to 12 months, 200 µg per kg; 1 to 5 years, 2.5 to 5 mg; 6 to 12 years, 5 to 10 mg.

Doses of up to 15 mg have been given by slow intravenous injection, sometimes as a loading dose for continuous or patient-controlled infusion. Continuous administration is discussed further below, however, doses have generally ranged from 0.8 to 80 mg per hour, although some patients have required and been given much higher doses.

Doses by mouth are usually in the range of 5 to 20 mg every 4 hours; with controlled-release preparations the 24-hour dose may be given in 2 divided doses. As with the other routes, high oral doses may be required for effective analgesia, especially in terminal care.

Morphine is sometimes administered rectally generally as suppositories in doses of 10 to 30 mg every 4 hours.

Intraspinal doses are in the region of 5 mg for an initial epidural injection or 2 to 4 mg over 24 hours to start an epidural infusion which may be increased by up to 2 mg daily. Intrathecal doses are smaller being in the range of 0.2 to 1 mg and should only involve the administration of a single dose.

The use of oral morphine in cancer pain.— R.G. Twycross and S.A. Lack, *Oral Morphine In Advanced Cancer*, Beaconsfield, Bucks, England, Beaconsfield Publishers Ltd, 1984; T. D. Walsh, *Pain*, 1984, *18*, 1.

A reminder of the important therapeutic principle that pain is the physiological antagonist of the respiratory depressant effects of opioid analgesics. The practical implication of this for those treating cancer pain patients with oral opioids is that, as long as the patient has pain, it is possible safely to titrate up the dose without fear of significant respiratory depression.— G. W. Hanks and R. G. Twycross (letter), *Lancet*, 1984, *1*, 1477.

For a study comparing the effects of morphine, nalbuphine, and fentanyl on common-bile-duct pressure in patients undergoing cholecystectomy, see p.1314.

ADMINISTRATION, BUCCAL. A double-blind study in 40 patients who experienced pain after orthopaedic operations comparing the effects of buccal and intramuscular morphine. The analgesic effects were equivalent; adverse effects were less with the buccal route.— M. D. D. Bell *et al.*, *Lancet*, 1985, *1*, 71.

ADMINISTRATION BY CONTINUOUS INFUSION. Morphine has been reported to provide effective analgesia when given by continuous intravenous or subcutaneous infusion (C.F. Campbell *et al.*, *Ann. intern. Med.*, 1983, *98*, 51; T.A. Goudie, *Anaesthesia*, 1985, *40*, 1086). Marshall *et al.* (*Br. med. J.*, 1985, *291*, 19) in a study involving intramuscular injections and intravenous infusions of morphine or morphine sulphate suggested that the greater requirement for morphine in the intravenous group might be explained by the development of tolerance. While the methodology of this study was criticised (G.R. Park *et al.*, *Br. med. J.*, 1985, *291*, 345; M.E.H. Barrow *et al.*, *ibid.*; M.H. Ornstein, *ibid.*, 346; N.M. Denny *et al.*, *ibid.*), McQuay and Moore (*Br. med. J.*, 1985, *291*, 346) agree that tolerance can develop on continuous administration and stress the need to titrate the administration to the effect. More recent developments have included patient-controlled analgesia by a series of bolus injections (D.P. Wermeling *et al.*, *Clin. Pharm.*, 1987, *6*, 307).

ADMINISTRATION BY CONTROLLED-RELEASE FORMS. Some comparative studies of the effects of controlled-release forms of morphine sulphate: D. Fell *et al.*, *Br. med. J.*, 1982, *285*, 92 (similar analgesic effects with oral administration of a controlled-release form and intramuscular injection, but more sedation with the tablets); C. A. Pinnock *et al.*, *Anaesthesia*, 1985, *40*, 1082 (equivalent analgesia with controlled-release form and intramuscular form as a premedication but less sedation and more nausea postoperatively with the tablets); S. D. Meed *et al.*, *J. clin. Pharmac.*, 1987, *27*, 155 (equivalent or superior analgesia with a controlled-release form compared with an immediate-release form of morphine sulphate).

ADMINISTRATION IN THE ELDERLY. Studies and discussions concerning the administration of opioids to the elderly. Age should be taken into account in deciding the dose frequency as well as the initial dose.— R. F. Kaiko *et al.*, *Med. Clins N. Am.*, 1982, *66*, 1079.

ADMINISTRATION, EPIDURAL AND INTRATHECAL. In a discussion of the use of spinal opiates it was considered that until a difference in the quality of analgesia between conventional and spinal routes is proved, the balance between morbidity and quality remains tipped in favour of the conventional routes, at least for general use.— *Lancet*, 1986, *1*, 655.

A nationwide follow-up survey of the use of epidural and intrathecal opioids for analgesia in Sweden. During 1984 over 14 000 patients received epidural, and over 1100 patients intrathecal opioids. Morphine was the predominant opioid for epidural administration and was used in 96% of patients. Epidural opioid analgesia constitutes about 25% of all epidural blocks performed in Sweden. Pruritus and urinary retention were considered as minor problems; however, the risk was considerably higher after intrathecal morphine. The incidence of delayed ventilatory depression was about 1:1100 (0.9%) following epidural morphine and 1:275 (0.36%) following intrathecal morphine. Administration of epidural morphine for postoperative pain relief in patients undergoing major surgery is considered a high benefit-low risk technique by most Swedish anaesthetists.— N. Rawal *et al.*, *Br. J. Anaesth.*, 1987, *59*, 791.

A report on the use of a subcutaneous access port for the epidural administration of opioids.— H. B. Andersen *et al.* (letter), *Lancet*, 1985, *1*, 511 (see also under Anginal Pain and Postoperative Pain, below).

For the preparation of a suitable injection of morphine for epidural administration, see under Preparations, below.

Anginal pain. The use of epidural morphine in 7 patients with severe anginal pain. An epidural system of analgesia was implanted subcutaneously, and the morphine was administered by the patients themselves or members of their family.— S. E. Clemensen *et al.*, *Br. med. J.*, 1987, *294*, 475 and 904.

Fractured ribs. Use of intrathecal morphine in the control of pain caused by fractured ribs.— G. R. Dickson and A. J. Sutcliffe (letter), *Br. J. Anaesth.*, 1986, *58*, 1342.

Labour. Disappointing results with epidural morphine in labour.— R. P. Husemeyer *et al.*, *Lancet*, 1979, *2*, 583.

A study of the use of intrathecal morphine sulphate 1.5 mg as the sole analgesic during labour in 12 women. The injection abolished pain during the first stage of labour in all patients and the pain of the second stage was abolished in 4 and reduced in another 3. No loss of the 'pushing reflex' occurred so that full maternal co-operation in the second stage was achieved. Side-effects including itching of the face, mouth, eyes, and nose, and nausea and vomiting occurred but these were generally mild and easily treated.— P. V. Scott *et al.*, *Br. med. J.*, 1980, *281*, 351. This technique was not considered suitable for pain in labour in view of the high incidence of side-effects.— J. A. T. Duncan (letter), *ibid.*, 515; B. W. Perriss and A. F. Malins, *ibid.*

Postoperative pain. Disappointing results were obtained with epidural morphine in doses of 5 mg or 2 mg in a double-blind placebo-controlled study in 30 women on the day after abdominal hysterectomy. Acute pain may be more resistant to the method than chronic pain.— J. H. McClure *et al.*, *ibid.*, 1980, *1*, 975.

Epidural, on-demand, low-dose morphine infusion for effective alleviation of acute postoperative pain. No patient experienced respiratory depression.— J. Chrubasik (letter), *Lancet*, 1984, *1*, 107, 738, and 793. See also E. M. Delhaas *et al.* (letter), *ibid.*, 690.

Comparisons of epidural morphine and bupivacaine: T. A. Torda and D. A. Pybus, *Br. J. Anaesth.*, 1984, *56*, 141; H. Rutberg *et al.*, *ibid.*, 233.

A retrospective clinical study in 125 patients following epidural morphine for postoperative pain.— E. H. Busch and P. M. Stedman, *Anesthesiology*, 1987, *67*, 101.

Further references to morphine given by epidural injection for postoperative pain: J. Kanto *et al.*, *Int. J. clin. Pharmac. Ther. Toxic.*, 1985, *23*, 43 (caesarean section); *Lancet*, 1985, *1*, 1018 (effect on hormonal and metabolic response to surgery).

Postoperative pain in children. Intrathecal morphine provided satisfactory postoperative analgesia for at least 22 hours in 37 of 56 children (aged 1 to 17 years) undergoing open-heart surgery; in 22 children analgesia lasted for over 24 hours. Preservative-free morphine sulphate was injected intrathecally just before the start of surgery. The first 27 patients were given morphine 30 µg per kg body-weight and the following 29 patients were given 20 µg per kg. There was no significant difference in the duration of analgesia between these 2 doses but 6 children given the larger dose developed respiratory depression and required naloxone compared with 3 children in the lower-dose group. This respiratory depression generally occurred about 3.5 to 4.5 hours after administration and it was considered that children receiving intrathecal morphine should be observed closely for at least 8 hours.— S. E. F. Jones *et al.*, *Br. J. Anaesth.*, 1984, *56*, 137.

Morphine 70 to 160 µg per kg body-weight was given epidurally to 9 children aged 4 to 18 years old, to provide pain relief following thoracic or abdominal surgery. The mean duration of analgesia per dose was 10.8 ± 4.0 hours; increasing the dose did not prolong the duration of action but did increase the incidence of side-effects. The postoperative opioid requirements were significantly lower in these children who received epidural morphine compared with 12 similar children who received morphine or pethidine parenterally.— J. A. Glenski *et al.*, *Mayo Clin. Proc.*, 1984, *59*, 530.

ADMINISTRATION IN INFANTS AND CHILDREN. See under Absorption and Fate, above.

ADMINISTRATION IN RENAL FAILURE. See above under Precautions and Absorption and Fate.

MYOCARDIAL INFARCTION. A study on the haemodynamic effects of intravenous morphine in 10 patients with acute myocardial infarction complicated by severe left ventricular failure suggested that the useful action of morphine in relieving distressing cardiac dyspnoea is not adequately explained by systemic venous pooling but rather that the effects of morphine on the central nervous system are more important.— A. D. Timmis *et al.*, *Br. med. J.*, 1980, *280*, 980.

In a study in 6 patients with severe pain, associated with acute myocardial infarction and unresponsive to up to 15 mg of intravenous morphine or other opioids, or both, morphine hydrochloride 1.2 to 2.4 mg by lumbar epidural injection relieved pain in 5 within 30 minutes; the remaining patient needed another 1.2 mg. Four patients required one to three injections of 1.0 to 2.0 mg, at intervals of 4 to 12 hours, but 2 remained free of pain with only the initial dose.— M. Skoeld *et al.* (letter), *New Engl. J. Med.*, 1985, *312*, 650.

PREGNANCY AND THE NEONATE. For reference to the use of morphine in labour see under Administration, Epidural and Intrathecal, above.

TETANUS. Morphine 1 to 2 mg per kg body-weight to a total of 3.1 g over 22 days was used to control autonomic hyperactivity in a patient who had developed generalised tetanus following injury. Dosage was reduced to 60 mg per day on the 23rd day and then discontinued.— M. A. Rie and R. S. Wilson, *Ann. intern. Med.*, 1978, *88*, 653.

Morphine 5 mg intravenously every 6 hours significantly reduced spontaneous sympathetic overactivity but had little effect on spasms induced by handling in 9 adults with tetanus.— N. Buchanan *et al.*, *Intensive Care Med.*, 1979, *5*, 65.

Morphine sulphate starting at a dose of 10 mg intravenously every 6 hours and adjusted according to the response was used to control sympathetic activity in 9 patients with tetanus. Eight patients survived. The mean daily dose of morphine sulphate was 103 mg given for a mean of 10.5 days. The beneficial effects of morphine were due to a reduction in arterial pressure, heart-rate, and systemic vascular resistance.— D. A. Rocke *et al.*, *S. Afr. med. J.*, 1986, *70*, 666.

Preparations of Morphine and its Salts

In addition to the preparations below, further official preparations containing morphine may be found under Ammonium Chloride, Kaolin, and Ipecacuanha.

Morphine and Cocaine Elixir *(B.P.C. 1973).* Morphine hydrochloride 5 mg, cocaine hydrochloride 5 mg, syrup 1.25 mL, alcohol (90%) 0.625 mL, chloroform water to 5 mL. When specified by the prescriber, the proportion of morphine may be varied. It should be recently prepared.

Morphine, Cocaine, and Chlorpromazine Elixir *(B.P.C. 1973).* Morphine hydrochloride 5 mg, cocaine hydrochloride 5 mg, chlorpromazine elixir 1.25 mL, alcohol (90%) 0.625 mL, chloroform water to 5 mL. When specified by the prescriber, the proportion of morphine may be varied. It should be recently prepared.

NOTE. The administration of cocaine with diamorphine or morphine has been reported to be of no apparent benefit.

Morphine and Atropine Injection *(B.P.)* morphine sulphate 1.0% and atropine sulphate 0.06%. Sterilised by filtration.

Morphine Sulfate Injection *(U.S.P.)*

Morphine Sulphate Injection *(B.P.)*

Morphine Sulphate Epidural Injection. An injection of morphine sulphate suitable for epidural administration without preservative or antoxidant could be prepared by packing 10 mL of a solution of morphine sulphate 2 mg in sodium chloride injection (0.9%) into 10 mL ampoules. Filtered oxygen-free nitrogen is bubbled through the solution for 5 seconds immediately before sealing the ampoule which is then autoclaved at 115° for 30 minutes. No breakdown of morphine has been detected in such ampoules after storage at room temperature for 4 months.— R.J. Bunn and R.M. Hobbs (letter), *Pharm. J.*, 1980, *1*, 334. Operating-theatre procedure demanded that the outside of the ampoule be sterile and to this end ampoules were being re-autoclaved in theatre with subsequent breakdown of the morphine. This problem was solved by suitably wrapping the ampoules in the pharmacy before the initial and sole autoclaving.— S. Turner and S. Potter, *ibid.*, *2*, 108.

Stability of an intrathecal morphine injection formulation.— T. Deeks *et al.*, *Pharm. J.*, 1983, *1*, 495. Comment.— J. B. Taylor and M. J. Sherwood (letter), *ibid.*, 543. Reply.— T. Deeks, *ibid.*, 656.

The preparation and dilution of stock solutions of morphine sulphate for epidural infusion.— E. S. Rippe and J. J. Kresel (letter), *Am. J. Hosp. Pharm.*, 1986, *43*, 1420.

Morphine Mixture *(A.P.F.).* Morphine hydrochloride 10 mg, glycerol 1 mL, concentrated chloroform water 0.25 mL or compounded hydroxybenzoate solution 0.1 mL, purified water to 10 mL.

Morphine Mixture Forte *A.P.F.* contains morphine hydrochloride 50 mg/10 mL.

Chloroform and Morphine Tincture *(B.P.).* Chlorodyne. Chloroform 12.5 mL, morphine hydrochloride 229 mg, alcohol (90%) 12.5 mL, liquorice liquid extract 12.5 mL, treacle of commerce 12.5 mL, water 5 mL, anaesthetic ether 3 mL, peppermint oil 0.1 mL, syrup to 100 mL. It contains the equivalent of 0.157 to 0.191% w/v of anhydrous morphine. Store in airtight containers.

For opioid dependence, see under Morphine, p.1310.

Morphine Tablets *(B.P.).* Morphine Sulphate Tablets

Proprietary Preparations of Morphine and its Salts

Cyclimorph *(Calmic, UK). Injection* (Cyclimorph 10), morphine tartrate 10 mg, cyclizine tartrate 50 mg/mL, in ampoules of 1 mL.

Injection (Cyclimorph 15), morphine tartrate 15 mg, cyclizine tartrate 50 mg/mL, in ampoules of 1 mL.

Duromorph *(Laboratories for Applied Biology, UK). Injection*, long-acting microcrystalline form in aqueous suspension, morphine 64 mg/mL, in ampoules of 1 mL.

MST Continus *(Napp, UK). Tablets*, sustained-release, morphine sulphate 10, 30, 60 and 100 mg.

Nepenthe *(Evans Medical, UK). Oral solution*, anhydrous morphine 0.84% (0.05% from opium tincture and 0.79% from morphine alkaloid).

Injection, anhydrous morphine 0.84% (0.05% from papaveretum and 0.79% from morphine hydrochloride), in ampoules of 0.5 mL.

CAUTION. *Nepenthe Oral Solution may become concentrated through evaporation of the solvent. It should be stored in a cool place in airtight containers. If evaporation occurs during storage the solution should not be used because of risk of overdosage.*

Oramorph *(Boehringer Ingelheim, UK). Oral solution*, morphine sulphate 10 mg/5 mL (2 mg/mL).

Concentrated oral solution, morphine sulphate 20 mg/mL.

Proprietary Names and Manufacturers of Morphine and its Salts

Contalgin *(Pharmacia, Denm.)*; Dolcontin *(Pharmacia, Norw.)*; Duramorph *(Elkins-Sinn, USA)*; Duromorph *(Laboratories for Applied Biology, UK)*; Epimorph *(Robins, Canad.)*; Morphitec *(Technilab, Canad.)*; MOS *(ICN, Canad.)*; Moscontin *(Sarget, Fr.)*; MS Contin *(Purdue Frederick, Canad.*; *Purdue Frederick, USA)*; MSIR *(Purdue Frederick, USA)*; MST *(Mundipharma, Ger.)*; MST Continus *(Mundipharma, S.Afr.*; *Mundipharma, Switz.*; *Napp, UK)*; Nepenthe *(Evans Medical, UK)*; Oramorph *(Boehringer Ingelheim, UK)*; RMS *(Upsher-Smith, USA)*; Roxanol *(Organon, Canad.*; *Roxane, USA)*; Statex *(Pharmascience, Canad.)*.

The following names have been used for multi-ingredient preparations containing morphine and its salts—Cyclimorph *(Calmic, UK)*; Linituss *(Ayrton, Saunders, UK)*; Morphalgin *(Fawns & McAllan, Austral.)*; Mortha *(Woods, Austral.)*; Sedol *(Rhône-Poulenc, Canad.)*; Syrup Tussi Hydrobrom *(Philip Harris, UK)*.

6244-y

Nalbuphine Hydrochloride *(BANM, USAN, rINNM).*

EN-2234A. 17-Cyclobutylmethyl-7,8-dihydro-14-hydroxy-17-normorphine hydrochloride; (−)-(5*R*,6*S*,14*S*)-9a-Cyclobutylmethyl-4,5-epoxy-morphinan-3,6,14-triol hydrochloride.

$C_{21}H_{27}NO_4,HCl = 393.9$.

CAS — 20594-83-6 (nalbuphine); 23277-43-2 (hydrochloride).

Intravenously administered nafcillin sodium shortly followed by a combination of nalbuphine hydrochloride and diazepam resulted in the formation of a thick, white precipitate in the intravenous tubing which completely occluded the lumen.— E. L. Jeglum *et al., Am. J. Hosp. Pharm.*, 1981, *38*, 462.

Solutions of diazepam, pentobarbitone, and thiethylperazine were each found to be incompatible with nalbuphine hydrochloride. It was suggested that combinations of nalbuphine with other pre-operative medications should be used as soon after mixture as possible.— W. G. Jump *et al., Am. J. Hosp. Pharm.*, 1982, *39*, 841.

Dependence

Nalbuphine hydrochloride may produce dependence of the morphine type (p.1310). Its abuse potential is generally considered to be equivalent to that of pentazocine, p.1316.

An evaluation of nalbuphine for its abuse potential.— D. R. Jasinski and P. A. Mansky, *Clin. Pharmac. Ther.*, 1972, *13*, 78.

Adverse Effects, Treatment, and Precautions

As for Morphine, p.1311. Because of its opioid agonist and antagonist activity, naloxone is the recommended antagonist for the treatment of overdose.

In a review of the actions and uses of nalbuphine by the manufacturer, data is presented on the adverse reactions observed in 1066 patients treated with injectable nalbuphine. Incidences were: sedation (36%), sweaty/clammy feelings (9%), nausea and vomiting (6%), dizziness and vertigo (5%), dry mouth (4%), and headache (3%). Other adverse reactions had an incidence of 1% or less. Primary dependence studies demonstrated that physical dependence is possible at high dose levels that produce marked side-effects. Six-month studies in patients with chronic pain have confirmed that analgesic tolerance and physical dependence are uncommon. Reports of suspected misuse have been rare.— W. K. Schmidt *et al., Drug & Alcohol Depend.*, 1985, *14*, 339.

For hazards and cautions in using nalbuphine to reverse respiratory depression caused by fentanyl, see below under Uses.

EFFECTS ON THE GASTRO-INTESTINAL TRACT. Premedication with nalbuphine and morphine was found to delay gastric emptying in the period after operation in a study of 40 female patients. Nalbuphine and morphine delayed co-ordinated intestinal motility, although nalbuphine did so for less than half as long as morphine.— M. Shah *et al., Br. J. Anaesth.*, 1984, *56*, 1235.

Studies of the emetic tendency of nalbuphine compared with pethidine or saline being given as premedication or to volunteers. The incidence of nausea and vomiting with nalbuphine was similar to that with pethidine in both groups.— W. N. Chestnutt *et al., Br. J. clin. Pharmac.*, 1985, *19*, 580P.

EFFECTS ON THE RESPIRATORY SYSTEM. Equianalgesic doses of nalbuphine and morphine produced similar respiratory depression. Low doses of nalbuphine produced more respiratory depression than low doses of morphine; with high doses the reverse occurred, with nalbuphine producing less respiratory depression than morphine and with the highest dose less even than with its own lower doses.— I. D. Klepper *et al., Br. J. Anaesth.*, 1986, *58*, 625.

A comparison of the respiratory depressant effects of intramuscular nalbuphine and papaveretum as the sole analgesic agent in patients undergoing gynaecological operations. Nalbuphine was considered to be a practical alternative to papaveretum, but nalbuphine did not appear to produce less respiratory depression, and it was considered that there was no significant advantage in using nalbuphine over papaveretum.— G. G. R. Rutter *et al., Br. J. Anaesth*, 1986, *58*, 121P.

Similar depression of ventilation with 15, 30, or 60 mg per 70 kg body-weight, although naloxone failed to reverse the respiratory depression at the highest nalbuphine dose of 60 mg per 70 kg.— G. C. Pugh *et al., Br. J. Anaesth.*, 1987, *59*, 929P.

PREGNANCY AND THE NEONATE. See under Absorption and Fate, below.

Absorption and Fate

Following intramuscular injection nalbuphine has been reported to produce peak plasma concentrations after 30 minutes. It is metabolised chiefly in the liver and is excreted predominantly in the faeces.

There appears to be considerable first-pass metabolism of nalbuphine following its administration by mouth.

A review of the clinical pharmacokinetics of opioid agonist-antagonist drugs including nalbuphine.— R. E. S. Bullingham *et al., Clin. Pharmacokinet.*, 1983, *8*, 332.

Some references to the pharmacokinetics of nalbuphine: J. W. Sear *et al., Br. J. Anaesth.*, 1987, *59*, 572; B. Kay *et al., ibid.*, 1327P.

PREGNANCY AND THE NEONATE. Studies carried out at delivery in 22 patients receiving pethidine and in 38 patients receiving nalbuphine for analgesia in labour. Nalbuphine produced more maternal sedation than pethidine and produced a greater degree of drowsiness in the infants following its use. Nalbuphine demonstrated a greater placental transfer compared with pethidine. This did not favour the use of nalbuphine in obstetrics.— C. M. Wilson *et al., Br. J. clin. Pharmac.*, 1986, *21*, 571P.

Uses and Administration

Nalbuphine hydrochloride is an analgesic with actions and uses similar to morphine (see p.1312). It is classified as a partial opioid agonist. It is used for the relief of moderate to severe pain and as an adjunct to anaesthesia. It is given subcutaneously, intramuscularly, or intravenously in doses of 10 to 20 mg every 3 to 6 hours. Doses of up to 30 mg have been given intravenously in myocardial infarction and if that failed to produce analgesia a second dose of 20 mg has been given after 30 minutes. Nalbuphine is reported to act within 15 minutes of subcutaneous or intramuscular injection or within 2 to 3 minutes of intravenous injection and generally to produce analgesia for 3 to 6 hours.

Children may be given up to 300 µg per kg body-weight initially, repeated once or twice as necessary. When used in anaesthesia doses of 0.3 to 1.0 mg per kg body-weight are given intravenously over 10 to 15 minutes for induction. Maintenance doses of 250 to 500 µg per kg are given at half-hourly intervals. Premedication has been carried out using doses of 100 to 200 µg per kg.

Some reviews of the actions and uses of nalbuphine hydrochloride: J. K. Errick and R. C. Heel, *Drugs*, 1983, *26*, 191; W. K. Schmidt *et al., Drug & Alcohol Depend.*, 1985, *14*, 339.

For a report of the use of nalbuphine with droperidol, see: D. S. Klein (letter), *Anesthesiology*, 1983, *58*, 397.

Nalbuphine hydrochloride 20 mg reversed diamorphine-induced late-onset respiratory depression in an elderly patient.— J. E. Hammond (letter), *Lancet*, 1984, *2*, 1208. Nalbuphine, when used in small doses of less than 10 mg to reverse respiratory depression due to high-dose fentanyl anaesthesia, was associated with an increase in pain and a number of patients developed tachycardia and/or hypertension. The response to nalbuphine was unpredictable. It was concluded that nalbuphine might be hazardous after a large dose of fentanyl, especially in patients whose myocardial oxygen balance is critical and for whom sympathetic responses are undesirable.— J. G. Ramsay *et al., Can. Anaesth. Soc. J.*, 1985, *32*, 597.

A study in 30 patients undergoing cholecystectomy indicated that whereas doses of morphine or fentanyl produced a significant rise in common-bile-duct pressure an equinanalgesic dose of nalbuphine produced no increase from control values.— E. Vatashsky and Y. Haskel, *Curr. ther. Res.*, 1985, *37*, 95.

A dose-response study with nalbuphine hydrochloride for pain after upper abdominal surgery in 6 subjects. The analgesic effect of nalbuphine appeared to be reversed at high doses and the maximum analgesic effect was considered to be exerted at a plasma concentration between 70 and 115 ng per mL.— G. C. Pugh and G. B. Drummond, *Br. J. Anaesth.*, 1987, *59*, 132P.

Some references to comparative analgesic assessments of nalbuphine:

Buprenorphine.— G. G. Pugh, *Br. J. Anaesth.*, 1987, *59*, 133P (less effective than buprenorphine for analgesia following abdominal surgery).

Morphine.— J. E. Stambaugh, *Curr. ther. Res.*, 1982, *31*, 393 (equivalent analgesia to morphine in chronic pain of malignancy with fewer complications); M. M. Brady *et al., Br. J. Anaesth.*, 1986, *58*, 1332P (inferior to morphine for postoperative pain following hip replacement); S. Christiansen, *Curr. ther. Res.*, 1987, *41*, 933 (equivalent to morphine for patient-controlled analgesia for postoperative pain).

Paracetamol.— A. K. Jain *et al., Clin. Pharmac. Ther.*, 1986, *39*, 295 (more effective analgesia with nalbuphine in combination with paracetamol than with paracetamol alone in postoperative pain).

Pethidine.— J. S. Sprigge and P. E. Otton, *Can. Anaesth. Soc. J.*, 1983, *30*, 517 (equivalent to pethidine in patient-controlled analgesia for postoperative pain); J. G. Brock-Utne *et al., S. Afr. med. J.*, 1985, *68*, 391 (longer duration of analgesia than with pethidine and fewer complications when used for postoperative pain relief after orthopaedic surgery); A. Thornilev *et al., ibid.*, 1986, *69*, 682 (equivalent to pethidine for post-caesarean pain).

See also below under Cardiovascular Disorders and Pregnancy and the Neonate.

ANAESTHESIA. Nalbuphine appeared to reduce isoflurane and enflurane anaesthetic requirements by approximately 50% in a retrospective study of 108 surgical patients.— E. M. Hew *et al., Curr. med. Res. Opinion*, 1987, *10*, 531.

Premedication. Nalbuphine was assessed as being less effective than pethidine as a premedicant in patients undergoing colonoscopy.— J. D. Waye and S. F. Braunfeld, *Gastrointest. endosc.*, 1982, *28*, 86. Nalbuphine was considered a suitable alternative to pethidine as a premedicant for minor gynaecological surgery. Complications of nalbuphine included pain on injection, nausea, and vomiting.— W. N. Chestnutt *et al., Br. J. Anaesth.*, 1987, *59*, 576.

Equivalent sedation to morphine when used as a premedicant for minor gynaecological surgery.— C. A. Pinnock *et al., Anaesthesia*, 1985, *40*, 1078.

CARDIOVASCULAR DISORDERS. A study in 60 patients with ischaemic chest pain randomly treated with intravenous nalbuphine 20 mg or morphine 10 mg. Both treatments significantly decreased pain for the duration of the observation period. Over 60% of the patients had complete pain relief.— E. Hew *et al., Curr. ther. Res.*, 1987, *41*, 394.

Nalbuphine produced comparable analgesia to diamorphine in suspected myocardial infarction with little haemodynamic or respiratory upset.— R. A. Greenbaum *et al., J. R. Soc. Med.*, 1987, *80*, 418.

PREGNANCY AND THE NEONATE. Evidence of efficacy of nalbuphine 15 mg by mouth as a single dose in postpartum pain caused by uterine cramp or episiotomy.— T. G. Kantor and M. Hopper, *Clin. Pharmac. Ther.*, 1984, *35*, 46.

Nalbuphine given intravenously in a patient-controlled device was preferred to pethidine given similarly for labour pain.— E. J. McAteer *et al., Br. J. Anaesth.*, 1986, *58*, 122P.

Intramuscular nalbuphine showed no advantage over pethidine for labour pain.— C. M. Wilson *et al., Anaesthesia*, 1986, *41*, 1207.

Proprietary Preparations

Nubain *(Du Pont Pharmaceuticals, UK). Injection,* nalbuphine hydrochloride 10 mg/mL, in ampoules of 1 or 2 mL.

Proprietary Names and Manufacturers

Nubain *(Du Pont, Canad.; Du Pont de Nemours, Fr.; Boots, S.Afr.; Du Pont de Nemours, Switz.; Du Pont Pharmaceuticals, UK; Du Pont, USA).*

13012-l

Nicomorphine Hydrochloride *(BANM, rINNM).*

3,6-Di-*O*-nicotinoylmorphine hydrochloride; (−)-(5*R*,6*S*)-4,5-Epoxy-9a-methylmorphin-7-en-3,6-diyl dinicotinate hydrochloride.

$C_{29}H_{25}N_3O_5,HCl = 532.0$.

CAS — 639-48-5 (nicomorphine); 12040-41-4 (hydrochloride); 35055-78-8 (xHCl).

Nicomorphine hydrochloride is an opioid analgesic.

Proprietary Names and Manufacturers

Vilan *(Lannacher, Denm.; Nourypharma, Neth.; Synmedic, Switz.).*

13033-k

Normethadone Hydrochloride *(BANM, rINNM).*
Desmethylmethadone Hydrochloride; Hoechst-10582; Phenyldimazone Hydrochloride. 6-Dimethylamino-4,4-diphenylhexan-3-one hydrochloride.
$C_{20}H_{25}NO,HCl=331.9$.

CAS — 467-85-6 (normethadone); 847-84-7 (hydrochloride).

Normethadone is closely related to methadone (p.1308). The hydrochloride has been used as a cough suppressant.

An accidental overdose of 4 mg of normethadone per kg body-weight in a 2-year-old child. Naloxone treatment was effective but for a period had to be given by continuous infusion at a rate of 300 µg per hour. A total dose of 7 mg of naloxone was eventually given.— G. K. Gourlay and K. Coulthard, *Br. J. clin. Pharmac.*, 1983, *15*, 269.

Proprietary Names and Manufacturers
The following names have been used for multi-ingredient preparations containing normethadone hydrochloride— Cophylac *(Hoechst, Canad.)*; Cophylac Expectorant *(Hoechst, Canad.)*; Ticarda *(Hoechst, Austral.)*.

6246-z

Opium *(BAN, USAN).*
Gum Opium; Raw Opium.

Pharmacopoeias. In *Arg., Aust., Belg., Br., Chin., Cz., Egypt., Fr., Ger., Hung., Ind., Int., It., Mex., Neth., Nord., Pol., Port., Roum., Span., Swiss, Turk.,* and *U.S.* The specified minimum content of anhydrous morphine varies slightly but is usually 9.5%.

The dried or partly dried latex obtained by incision from the unripe capsules of *Papaver somniferum* (Papaveraceae). It has a strong characteristic odour and a bitter taste and contains not less than 9.5% of anhydrous morphine. Opium contains a variable mixture of other alkaloids including noscapine, codeine, and papaverine.

The exuded latex is dried, by spontaneous evaporation or by artificial heat, and is manipulated to form cakes of uniform composition, variously shaped according to the country of origin, and known in commerce as Turkish, Indian, or European opium. The *B.P.* specifies Indian opium.

NOTE. The *B.P.* directs that when Opium is prescribed, Prepared Opium shall be dispensed.

6247-c

Prepared Opium *(BAN).*
Opii Pulvis Standardisatus; Opium Pulveratum; Opium Titratum; Pdrd. Opium; Powdered Opium *(USAN)*; Pulvis Opii; Standardised Opium Powder.

Pharmacopoeias. In *Arg., Aust., Belg., Br., Chin., Cz., Ger., Hung., Ind., Int., It., Jpn, Jug., Mex., Neth., Nord., Pol., Port., Roum., Rus., Span., Turk.,* and *U.S. Mex.* and *U.S.* specify 10 to 10.5% of anhydrous morphine. *Jpn* also includes a diluted opium powder containing 1% of anhydrous morphine.

Opium, dried, powdered, and adjusted to contain 9.5 to 10.5% of anhydrous morphine. The *B.P.* specifies that the powdered diluent may be lactose; the *U.S.P.* allows any of its diluents for powdered extracts with the exception of starch. **Store** in well-closed containers.

Dependence
Prolonged use of opium may lead to dependence of the morphine type (see p.1310).

Adverse Effects, Treatment, and Precautions
As for Morphine, p.1311.

Uses and Administration
Opium has analgesic and narcotic actions which are due mainly to its content of morphine (see p.1312).

It acts less rapidly than morphine since opium appears to be more slowly absorbed; the relaxing action of the papaverine and noscapine on intestinal muscle makes it more constipating than morphine.

Camphorated Opium Tincture (Paregoric) is given with expectorants for coughs. For its intestinal action opium is given as Aromatic Chalk with Opium Mixture (see p. 1081).

TREATMENT OF NEONATAL OPIOID DEPENDENCE. A comparative study of paregoric [*U.S.P.*] and phenobarbitone in the treatment of neonatal drug abstinence syndrome. Forty-nine neonates received paregoric by mouth at a dose of 0.2 mL every 3 hours. The dose was increased by 0.05 mL to provide adequate control. The dosage remained at that level for 5 days and was then reduced by 0.05 mL every other day. Phenobarbitone was administered to 62 neonates at a dosage of 5 mg per kg body-weight per day intramuscularly in 3 divided doses, and this was increased by 1 mg per kg per day until the severity score was less than 6. Phenobarbitone was then given by mouth at that dosage for 5 days and subsequently reduced by 1 mg per kg every other day. Seven of the 62 phenobarbitone-treated neonates had abstinence-associated seizures within the first month of life, while none of the 49 paregoric-treated neonates had seizures. Paregoric was considered to be the treatment of choice for the neonatal abstinence syndrome.— S. R. Kandall *et al.*, *Am. J. Dis. Child.*, 1983, *137*, 378.

Preparations

Camphorated Opium Tincture *(B.P.).* Tinct. Opii Camph.; Paregoric; Tinct. Camph. Co. Opium tincture 5 mL, benzoic acid 500 mg, camphor 300 mg, anise oil 0.3 mL, alcohol (60%) to 100 mL. It contains 0.045 to 0.055% w/v of anhydrous morphine; about 5 mg in 10 mL.

Paregoric *(U.S.P.)* is similar and contains 0.035 to 0.045% of anhydrous morphine.

Concentrated Camphorated Opium Tincture *(B.P.).* Tinct. Opii Camph. Conc.; Liquor Opii Camphoratus Concentratus. Opium tincture 40 mL, benzoic acid 4 g, camphor 2.4 g, anise oil 2.4 mL, alcohol 40 mL, water to 100 mL. It is about 8 times as strong as Camphorated Opium Tincture *(B.P.)*.

Compound Camphorated Opium Mixture *(B.P.C. 1973).* Mist. Opii Camph. Co.; Mist. Camph. Co. Camphorated opium tincture 1 mL, ammonium bicarbonate 100 mg, strong ammonium acetate solution 1 mL, water to 10 mL. It should be recently prepared. It contains about 500 µg of anhydrous morphine in 10 mL.

Opiate Squill Linctus *(B.P.).* Linctus Scillae Opiatus; Compound Squill Linctus; Gee's Linctus; Squill Opiate Linctus. Equal volumes of camphorated opium tincture, squill oxymel, and tolu syrup. It contains about 800 µg of anhydrous morphine in 5 mL.

A case report of squill-associated cardiac toxicity resulting from abuse of Opiate Squill Linctus.— W. Smith *et al.*, *Br. med. J.*, 1986, *292*, 868. A similar report.— D. Thurston and K. Taylor (letter), *Pharm. J.*, 1984, *2*, 63.

Paediatric Opiate Squill Linctus *(B.P.).* Linctus Scillae Opiatus pro Infantibus; Squill Opiate Linctus Paediatric; Opiate Linctus for Infants. Camphorated opium tincture 0.3 mL, squill oxymel 0.3 mL, tolu syrup 0.3 mL, glycerol 1 mL, syrup to 5 mL. It contains about 150 µg of anhydrous morphine in 5 mL.

For a report of incompatibility when Paediatric Opiate Squill Linctus was prepared with or diluted with syrup preserved with hydroxybenzoates, see under Sucrose, p.1276.

Opium Tincture *(B.P.).* Laudanum. Prepared by maceration with water (boiling) and with alcohol and adjusted to contain 0.95 to 1.05% w/v of anhydrous morphine; about 20 mg in 2 mL.

The *U.S.P.* includes a tincture containing 1% w/v anhydrous morphine.

Proprietary Names and Manufacturers
The following names have been used for multi-ingredient preparations containing prepared opium— B & O Supprettes *(Webcon, USA)*; Diban *(Robins, Canad.)*; Donnagel-PG *(Robins, Canad.; Robins, USA)*; Linituss *(Ayrton, Saunders, UK)*; Parepectolin *(Rorer, USA)*; Pomalin *(Winthrop, Canad.)*.

6248-k

Oxycodone Hydrochloride *(BANM, USAN, rINNM).*
7,8-Dihydro-14-hydroxycodeinone hydrochloride; Dihydrone Hydrochloride; Oxycone Hydrochloride; Thecodine. 6-Deoxy-7,8-dihydro-14-hydroxy-3-*O*-methyl-6-oxomorphine hydrochloride trihydrate; (−)-(5*R*,6*S*,14*S*)-4,5-Epoxy-14-hydroxy-3-methoxy-9a-methylmorphinan-6-one hydrochloride trihydrate.
$C_{18}H_{21}NO_4,HCl,3H_2O=405.9$.

CAS — 76-42-6 (oxycodone); 124-90-3 (hydrochloride, anhydrous).

Pharmacopoeias. In *Aust., Belg., Cz., Fr., Ger., Int., Jpn, Jug., Nord., Port., Rus., Turk.,* and *U.S.* (mostly as trihydrate).

Store in airtight containers.

Dependence, Adverse Effects, Treatment, and Precautions
As for Morphine, p.1310.

Absorption and Fate
Oxycodone is absorbed from the gastro-intestinal tract. It is metabolised to noroxycodone and both metabolite and unchanged drug are excreted in urine.

Noroxycodone was the major metabolite of oxycodone.— S. H. Weinstein and J. C. Gaylord, *J. pharm. Sci.*, 1979, *68*, 527.

Uses and Administration
Oxycodone is an opioid analgesic used similarly to morphine (see p.1312) for the relief of pain. Oxycodone hydrochloride may be given by mouth in a dose of 5 mg every 6 hours. The pectinate is also given rectally as suppositories. Oxycodone terephthalate is also used by mouth and by injection.

Indomethacin given intravenously was more effective in 148 patients than oxycodone intravenously in 20 patients for relieving pain after surgery for varicose veins or orthopaedic disorders. Doses of 25 mg and 5 mg respectively were given immediately after surgery, followed by 5 mg and 2 mg respectively per hour, with supplementary doses as required. The mean total doses were 123 mg and 38.1 mg respectively. Significantly more patients given indomethacin had no pain and significantly more patients given oxycodone had severe pain.— M. A. K. Mattila *et al.*, *Br. med. J.*, 1983, *287*, 1026.

A study of 61 patients with acute renal colic who received indomethacin 50 mg or a combination of oxycodone 5 mg and papaverine 50 mg as single intravenous doses. There was no significant difference in the mean pain relief provided by the 2 treatments.— P. -E. Jönsson *et al.*, *Br. J. Urol.*, 1987, *59*, 396.

Preparations

Oxycodone and Acetaminophen Capsules *(U.S.P.).* Capsules containing oxycodone hydrochloride and paracetamol, or oxycodone hydrochloride, oxycodone terephthalate, and paracetamol. Store in airtight containers. Protect from light.

Oxycodone and Acetaminophen Tablets *(U.S.P.).* Tablets containing oxycodone hydrochloride and paracetamol. Store in airtight containers. Protect from light.

Proprietary Preparations

Oxycodone Suppositories (formerly known as Proladone) *(Boots, UK)*. Oxycodone pectinate, available as suppositories each containing the equivalent of 30 mg of oxycodone.

Proprietary Names and Manufacturers of Oxycodone Salts
Endone *(Du Pont, Austral.)*; Eubine *(Fr.)*; Eukodal *(E. Merck, Ger.)*; Oxanest *(Leiras, Fin.)*; Pancodone Retard *(Fr.)*; Proladone *(Boots, Austral.)*; Roxicodone *(Roxane, USA)*; Supeudol *(Sabex, Canad.)*.

The following names have been used for multi-ingredient preparations containing oxycodone salts—Oxycocet *(Technilab, Canad.)*; Oxycodan *(Technilab, Canad.)*; Percocet *(Du Pont, Canad.; Du Pont, USA)*; Percodan *(Du Pont, Austral.; Du Pont, Canad.; Du Pont, USA)*; SK-Oxycodone with Acetaminophen *(Smith Kline & French, USA)*; SK-Oxycodone with Aspirin *(Smith Kline & French, USA)*; Tylox *(McNeil Pharmaceutical, USA)*.

6249-a

Oxymorphone Hydrochloride *(BANM, USAN, rINNM).*
7,8-Dihydro-14-hydroxymorphinone hydrochloride; Oximorphone Hydrochloride. 6-Deoxy-7,8-dihydro-14-hydroxy-6-oxomorphine hydrochloride; (−)-(5*R*,6*S*,14*S*)-4,5-Epoxy-3,14-dihydroxy-9a-methylmorphinan-6-one hydrochloride.
$C_{17}H_{19}NO_4,HCl=337.8$.

CAS — 76-41-5 (oxymorphone); 357-07-3 (hydro-

chloride).

Pharmacopoeias. In *U.S.*

A white or slightly off-white odourless powder, darkening on exposure to light. **Soluble** 1 in 4 of water, 1 in 100 of alcohol, and 1 in 25 of methyl alcohol; very slightly soluble in chloroform and ether. The *U.S.P.* injection has a pH of 2.7 to 4.5. **Store** in airtight containers. Protect from light.

Dependence

Prolonged use of oxymorphone may lead to dependence of the morphine type (see p.1310).

Adverse Effects, Treatment, and Precautions

As for Morphine, p.1311.

Uses and Administration

Oxymorphone hydrochloride is an opioid analgesic with actions and uses similar to those of morphine (see p.1312), apart from an absence of cough suppressant activity. It is usually administered by subcutaneous or intramuscular injection in the treatment of moderate and severe pain, including pain in obstetrics, when it is reported to provide analgesia for 3 to 6 hours. It is also used as an adjunct to anaesthesia, generally by intravenous injection. Oxymorphone is given in doses of 1 to 1.5 mg every 4 to 6 hours by intramuscular or subcutaneous injection; 500 µg may be given by intravenous injection.

Oxymorphone is given rectally in a suppository in a dose of 5 mg every 4 to 6 hours. It has also been given by mouth.

In a double-blind crossover study in cancer patients, a single dose of oxymorphone given by mouth was considered to have one-sixth the potency of the same dose given by intramuscular injection. In a further study, oxymorphone had about 9 times the analgesic potency of morphine given by intramuscular injection.— W. T. Beaver *et al., J. clin. Pharmac.*, 1977, *17*, 186. Oxymorphone administered as a suppository was estimated to have one-tenth the analgesic effect of the same dose given by intramuscular injection.— W. T. Beaver and G. A. Feise, *J. clin. Pharmac.*, 1977, *17*, 276.

Preparations

Oxymorphone Hydrochloride Injection *(U.S.P.)*

Oxymorphone Hydrochloride Suppositories *(U.S.P.).* Store at 2° to 8°.

Proprietary Names and Manufacturers

Numorphan *(Du Pont, Canad.; Boots, S.Afr.; Du Pont, USA).*

6250-e

Papaveretum *(BAN).*

Alkaloidorum Opii Hydrochloridum; Extractum Concentratum Opii; Omnoponum; Opialum; Opium Concentratum. The hydrochlorides of alkaloids of opium, containing the equivalent of anhydrous morphine 47.5 to 52.5%, anhydrous codeine 2.5 to 5%, noscapine 16 to 22%, and papaverine 2.5 to 7%.

CAS — 8002-76-4.

Pharmacopoeias. In *B.P.C. 1973.* Similar preparations of mixed opium alkaloids are included in *Jpn, Pol., Roum.,* and *Rus.*

Dependence, Adverse Effects, Treatment, and Precautions

As for Morphine, p.1310.

Uses and Administration

Papaveretum has the analgesic and narcotic properties of morphine (see p.1312) and is used in the treatment of moderate to severe pain and for pre-operative sedation usually in conjunction with hyoscine.

In adults it is generally administered by subcutaneous or intramuscular injection in doses of 10 to 20 mg every 4 hours. Papaveretum may also be given intravenously by slow injection in acute pain when doses may be a quarter to a half of those employed intramuscularly.

Infants aged up to 1 month may be given 150 µg per kg body-weight and infants aged up to 1 year, 200 µg per kg. Children aged 1 to 12 years may be given 200 to 300 µg per kg.

For pre-operative medication papaveretum is given intramuscularly or subcutaneously in a dose of 10 to 20 mg 45 to 60 minutes before anaesthesia often in conjunction with 200 to 400 µg of hyoscine hydrobromide.

Papaveretum may also be given by mouth in doses of 10 to 20 mg.

Preparations

Papaveretum Injection *(B.P.C. 1973).* A sterile solution of papaveretum 2% w/v and glycerol 1.4% w/v in Water for Injections. It may contain a bactericide; phenylmercuric nitrate 0.002% is suitable. It is supplied in single-dose containers. Protect from light.

Papaveretum Tablets *(B.P.C. 1973)*

Proprietary Preparations

Aspav *(Cox, UK). Tablets,* dispersible, papaveretum 10 mg, aspirin 500 mg.

Formerly known as Soluble Aspirin and Papaveretum Tablets.

Omnopon *(Roche, UK). Injection,* papaveretum 20 mg/mL, in ampoules of 1 mL.

Injection (Omnopon Paediatric), papaveretum 10 mg/mL, in ampoules of 1 mL.

Omnopon-Scopolamine *(Roche, UK). Injection,* papaveretum 20 mg, hyoscine hydrobromide 400 µg/mL, in ampoules of 1 mL.

Proprietary Names and Manufacturers

Escopon *(Switz.)*; Omnopon *(Roche, Austral.; Roche, S.Afr.; Roche, UK)*; Pantopon *(Belg.; Roche, Canad.; Ger.; Roche, UK; Roche, USA).*

The following names have been used for multi-ingredient preparations containing papaveretum—Aspav *(Cox, UK)*; Omnopon-Scopolamine *(Roche, Austral.; Roche, UK)*; Soluble Aspirin and Papaveretum Tablets *(Cox, UK).*

6251-l

Pentazocine *(BAN, USAN, rINN).*

NIH-7958; NSC-107430; Win-20,228.

(2*R**,6*R**,11*R**)-1,2,3,4,5,6-Hexahydro-6,11-dimethyl-3-(3-methylbut-2-enyl)-2,6-methano-3-benzazocin-8-ol.

$C_{19}H_{27}NO$=285.4.

CAS — 359-83-1.

Pharmacopoeias. In *Br., It., Jpn, Nord.,* and *U.S.*

A white or creamy-white odourless or almost odourless powder. Pentazocine 100 mg is approximately equivalent to 112.8 mg of pentazocine hydrochloride or 131.6 mg of pentazocine lactate.

B.P. **solubilities** are: practically insoluble in water; soluble 1 in 15 of alcohol, 1 in 2 of chloroform, and 1 in 33 of ether. *U.S.P.* solubilities are: soluble 1 in 1000 of water, 1 in 11 of alcohol, 1 in 2 of chloroform, and 1 in 42 of ether. **Store** in airtight containers. Protect from light.

6252-y

Pentazocine Hydrochloride *(BANM, USAN, rINNM).*

$C_{19}H_{27}NO,HCl$=321.9.

CAS — 2276-52-0; 64024-15-3.

Pharmacopoeias. In *Br., Cz., Ind., It., Nord.,* and *U.S.*

A white or pale cream odourless or almost odourless crystalline powder. *B.P.* **solubilities** are: soluble 1 in 42 of water, 1 in 16 of alcohol, 1 in 8 of chloroform; practically insoluble in ether. *U.S.P.* solubilities are: soluble 1 in 30 of water, 1 in 7 of alcohol, 1 in 4 of chloroform; practically insoluble in ether. A 1% solution in water has a pH of 4 to 6. **Store** in airtight containers. Protect from light.

6253-j

Pentazocine Lactate *(BANM, USAN, rINNM).*

$C_{19}H_{27}NO,C_3H_6O_3$=375.5.

CAS — 17146-95-1.

Pharmacopoeias. In *Nord.*

Solutions for injection are **sterilised** by autoclaving. The *B.P.* and the *U.S.P.* injections have a pH of 4 to 5. **Protect** from light.

INCOMPATIBILITY. Commercial injections of pentazocine lactate are reported to be incompatible with soluble barbiturates and other alkaline substances including sodium bicarbonate. Diazepam and chlordiazepoxide are also reported to be incompatible.

Pentazocine lactate injection (Talwin) was found to be incompatible with glycopyrrolate injection.— T. Ingallinera *et al., Am. J. Hosp. Pharm.*, 1979, *36*, 508.

Intravenously administered nafcillin sodium shortly followed by a combination of pentazocine lactate and atropine sulphate, resulted in the formation of a thick, white precipitate in the intravenous tubing which completely occluded the lumen.— E. L. Jeglum *et al., Am. J. Hosp. Pharm.*, 1981, *38*, 462.

Dependence

Prolonged use of high doses of pentazocine may produce dependence. It is subject to abuse.

A discussion of the intravenous abuse of pentazocine and tripelennamine ('T's and Blues').— A. Poklis and P. L. Whyatt, *J. forens. Sci.*, 1980, *25*, 72.

A case report of a fatal intracranial haemorrhage due to an overdose from drug abuse of pentazocine, phenylpropanolamine, and tripelennamine by a 30-year-old man.— C. Jackson *et al., J. emerg. Med.*, 1985, *3*, 127.

A case report of a 27-year-old woman who developed severe hypertension following her routine intravenous injection of solubilised pentazocine and tripelennamine tablets. To counteract pentazocine's abuse potential, the manufacturers had in 1983 incorporated naloxone into their tablets of pentazocine hydrochloride (Talwin Nx). The naloxone will precipitate withdrawal symptoms in addicts, which is what happened in this case.— S. Reinhart and S. M. Barrett, *Ann. emerg. Med.*, 1985, *14*, 591. The introduction of Talwin Nx tablets, containing 0.5 mg of naloxone, appeared to have greatly decreased the abuse of T's and Blues.— E. C. Senay, *Drug & Alcohol Depend.*, 1985, *14*, 305. Report of two cases of abuse of Talwin Nx and tripelennamine.— D. A. Reed and S. H. Schnoll, *J. Am. med. Ass.*, 1986, *256*, 2562.

A report of intravenous abuse of pentazocine in a 30-year-old theatre sister over a period of 4 years.— R. Hunter and I. M. Ingram (letter), *Lancet*, 1983, *2*, 227.

PREGNANCY AND THE NEONATE. Withdrawal symptoms developed, 10 hours after delivery, in an infant whose mother had taken pentazocine 50 mg three times daily during the last 6 weeks of pregnancy.— O. Preis *et al., Am. J. Obstet. Gynec.*, 1977, *127*, 205.

Adverse Effects

The most frequent side-effects of pentazocine are light-headedness, dizziness, nausea and vomiting, sedation, and sweating. It may also cause headache, dry mouth, constipation, flushing of the skin, respiratory depression, tachycardia, hypotension, raised intracranial pressure, transient hypertension, mood changes, nightmares, paraesthesia, pruritus, and urinary retention. Changed uterine contractions, muscle tremor, convulsions, insomnia, disorientation, hallucinations, disturbances of vision, transient eosinophilia, chills, and allergic reactions have also occurred.

Pentazocine injections may be painful. Local tissue damage may occur at injection sites particularly after subcutaneous injection or multiple doses. There have been reports of muscle fibrosis.

Toxic epidermal necrolysis in a 62-year-old man was attributed to pentazocine; he had taken 50 to 75 mg every 4 hours for 8 days. He was severely dehydrated and had a blood-urea concentration of 4.3 mg per mL, but recovered after fluid replacement and other intensive treatment.— J. A. A. Hunter and A. M. Davison, *Br. J. Derm.*, 1973, *88*, 287.

Six patients who had been given pentazocine intramuscularly for less than 3 months suffered severe induration of soft tissues at pentazocine injection sites. In 1 patient induration was severe and produced ankylosis of the knee joints and limited the range of motion in the hips and shoulders. Four patients had not exceeded the recommended doses.— T. F. Beckner (letter), *J. Am. med. Ass.*, 1974, *227*, 1383.

EFFECTS ON THE BLOOD. Reports of agranulocytosis associated with pentazocine: A. Marks and N. Abramson (letter), *Ann. intern. Med.*, 1980, *92*, 433; H. Haibach *et al., Can. med. Ass. J.*, 1984, *130*, 1165; M. Sheehan *et al., ibid.*, 1985, *132*, 1401.

EFFECTS ON THE MENTAL STATE. Some references to hallucinations with normal doses of pentazocine: A. J. J. Wood *et al., Br. med. J.*, 1974, *1*, 305; J. I. Alexander and A. A. Spence (letter), *ibid.*, *2*, 224; M. Taylor *et al., ibid.*, 1978, *2*, 1198.

Treatment of Adverse Effects

Treatment is similar to that for morphine (see p.1311), *but* nalorphine and levallorphan are not antagonists and may add to the depressant effects of pentazocine. Naloxone should be used as an antagonist.

Precautions

As for Morphine, p.1311.

Pentazocine has weak opioid antagonist actions and may precipitate withdrawal symptoms if given to patients who have recently used other opioid analgesics. Some authorities recommend that pentazocine should be avoided after myocardial infarction as it may increase pulmonary and aortic blood pressure as well as cardiac work. Some also recommend that it should be avoided in arterial or pulmonary hypertension and in heart failure.

When frequent injections are needed, pentazocine should be given intramuscularly and the injection sites should be varied.

Serum creatine kinase values rose significantly in 3 of 15 patients given pentazocine 30 mg intramuscularly; this could cause confusion when these values were used for the assessment of cardiac infarction.— B. B. Scott *et al., Br. med. J.*, 1974, *4*, 691.

ADMINISTRATION IN LIVER DISORDERS. Enhanced bioavailability and decreased clearance of pentazocine in patients with cirrhosis.— E. A. Neal *et al., Gastroenterology*, 1979, *77*, 96.

ANTAGONIST EFFECTS. Not only was pentazocine an antagonist to morphine but to some extent it was also an antagonist to itself. If an initial dose was followed too closely by a second dose some loss of pain relief could occur. Pentazocine should be used only when it was clear that no other analgesic would be needed in the immediate future or had been administered in the immediate past.— A. R. Hunter, *Practitioner*, 1973, *211*, 476.

EFFECT ON THE BILIARY TRACT. The rise in biliary pressure in 31 patients was less with pentazocine than with pethidine or phenazocine and much less than with morphine.— G. Economou and J. N. Ward-McQuaid, *Gut*, 1971, *12*, 218. A study assessing the effects of intravenously administered pentazocine on bile duct sphincter motor activity. Pentazocine adversely affected the bile duct sphincter and was considered not to be the premedication of first choice for endoscopic procedures involving the sphincter of Oddi. It should be avoided in patients with pancreatic and biliary disorders.— M. Staritz *et al., ibid.*, 1986, *27*, 567.

INTERACTIONS. A study in 70 urban subjects indicated that smokers metabolised about 40% more pentazocine than non-smokers, although there was large inter-subject variation. It was suggested that tobacco smoking induces liver enzymes responsible for drug oxidation.— D. P. Vaughan *et al., Br. J. clin. Pharmac.*, 1976, *3*, 279.

PORPHYRIA. Pentazocine was considered to be unsafe in patients with acute porphyria as it has been associated with acute attacks.— M.R. Moore and K.E.L. McColl, *Porphyrias, Drug Lists*, Glasgow, Porphyria Research Unit, University of Glasgow, 1987.

Absorption and Fate

Pentazocine is absorbed from the gastro-intestinal tract; following administration by mouth, peak plasma concentrations are reached in 1 to 3 hours and the half-life is reported to be 2 to 3 hours. After intramuscular injection, peak plasma concentrations are reached in 15 minutes to 1 hour. Pentazocine is metabolised in the liver and only a small proportion of the dose administered appears unchanged in the urine. It diffuses across the placenta.

A review of the clinical pharmacokinetics of opioid agonist-antagonist drugs including pentazocine.— R. E. S. Bullingham *et al., Clin. Pharmacokinet.*, 1983, *8*, 332.

The range of pentazocine binding to plasma protein in the blood from 20 healthy subjects was 56 to 66% whereas in 22 patients the range extended to 48 to 75%. *In vitro* studies on the blood of healthy subjects indicated that 48% of the total amount of pentazocine in whole blood was in the red blood-cells, 33% was bound to the plasma proteins, and 19% was in the plasma water. In subjects with abnormally high or low red blood-cell counts, response to pentazocine might therefore be altered.— M. Ehrnebo *et al., Clin. Pharmac. Ther.*, 1974, *16*, 424.

Measurements of the mean plasma concentration of pentazocine in 5 healthy subjects, made for up to 6 hours after administration indicated that the bioavailability of the dose given by mouth was 18.4% (range 11.1 to 31.6%) of the administered dose. Plasma half-lives of the intravenously and orally administered doses were 203 and 177 minutes respectively.— M. Ehrnebo *et al., Clin. Pharmac. Ther.*, 1977, *22*, 888.

Uses and Administration

Pentazocine is an opioid analgesic with actions and uses similar to those of morphine (see p.1312); it also has antagonist activity . It is used for the relief of moderate to severe pain. Its analgesic effect declines more rapidly than that of morphine.

Pentazocine is administered by mouth as the hydrochloride. The usual dose is the equivalent of 25 to 100 mg of pentazocine every 3 to 4 hours after food. Children aged 6 to 12 may be given 25 mg every 3 to 4 hours.

Pentazocine is also administered by subcutaneous, intramuscular, and intravenous injection as the lactate. The usual dose is the equivalent of pentazocine 30 to 60 mg every 3 to 4 hours; it should not be necessary to exceed 360 mg daily. Intravenous doses of 30 mg are also used. For children, the maximum single dose subcutaneously or intramuscularly should not exceed 1 mg per kg body-weight, or 500 µg per kg intravenously.

Pentazocine is also given rectally as the lactate in suppositories usually in a dose of the equivalent of pentazocine 50 mg up to 4 times daily.

A brief review of pentazocine.— G. Goldstein, *Drug & Alcohol Depend.*, 1985, *14*, 313.

A report of the clinical effects of pentazocine given by mouth in 616 hospitalised medical patients and parenterally in 816.— R. R. Miller, *J. clin. Pharmac.*, 1975, *15*, 198 and 719.

A study in 40 patients of the antagonistic effect of pentazocine on fentanyl-induced respiratory depression. Pentazocine had a weaker antagonist effect than either nalorphine or naloxone and did not improve postoperative analgesia.— L. Kaukinen *et al., Ann. clin. Res.*, 1981, *13*, 396.

A double-blind study with 324 women who received intravenous sedation with pentazocine and diazepam. The results suggested that the optimum dosage of pentazocine to reduce the mean dose of diazepam required to produce sedation was 30 mg, but that 15 mg is often an effective dose. One patient given pentazocine 45 mg and diazepam 5 mg showed severe respiratory depression.— J. I. Murray Lawson and M. K. Milne, *Br. dent. J.*, 1981, *151*, 379.

Some references to comparisons of the analgesic effectiveness of pentazocine and other analgesics: G. Soave *et al., J. int. med. Res.*, 1983, *11*, 354 (inferior to indoprofen); A. Sartani *et al., J. clin. Pharmac.*, 1985, *25*, 596 (inferior to indoprofen); M. J. Griffiths and T. A. Thomas, *Br. dent. J.*, 1985, *158*, 19 (inferior to meptazinol).

ADMINISTRATION, EPIDURAL. A study of the use of epidural pentazocine 300 µg per kg body-weight for the relief of postoperative pain in 20 women who had undergone gynaecological operations. Onset of analgesia was rapid, within 3 minutes in 85% of patients; peak analgesic effect occurred at a mean of 15.3 minutes; duration of analgesia averaged 10.6 hours.— P. K. Kalia *et al., Anesth. Analg.*, 1983, *62*, 949.

ADMINISTRATION, PATIENT-CONTROLLED. Satisfactory management of postoperative pain using patient-controlled analgesia with intravenous pentazocine in 16 patients for the first 48 hours after abdominal surgery.— M. Reedy *et al., Drug Intell. & clin. Pharm.*, 1985, *19*, 457.

EFFECT ON THE COLON. In 5 healthy men, 5 patients with the irritable bowel syndrome, and 5 with diverticular disease, colonic motor activity was significantly reduced after they were given pentazocine 300 µg per kg body-weight intravenously or 500 µg per kg intramuscularly.— C. Stanciu and J. R. Bennett, *Br. med. J.*, 1974, *1*, 312.

Preparations of Pentazocine Salts

Pentazocine Hydrochloride and Aspirin Tablets *(U.S.P.)*. Store in airtight containers. Protect from light.

Pentazocine Hydrochloride Tablets *(U.S.P.)*

Pentazocine Injection *(B.P.)*. Pentazocine Lactate Injection. Potency is expressed in terms of the equivalent amount of pentazocine.

Pentazocine Lactate Injection *(U.S.P.)*. Potency is expressed in terms of the equivalent amount of pentazocine.

Pentazocine and Naloxone Hydrochlorides Tablets *(U.S.P.)*

Pentazocine Tablets *(B.P.)*. Tablets containing pentazocine hydrochloride. They may be film-coated.

Proprietary Preparations of Pentazocine Salts

Fortagesic *(Sterling Research, UK)*. *Tablets*, pentazocine 15 mg (as hydrochloride), paracetamol 500 mg.

Fortral *(Sterling Research, UK)*. *Capsules*, pentazocine hydrochloride 50 mg.
Tablets, pentazocine hydrochloride 25 mg.
Injection, pentazocine 30 mg (as lactate)/mL, in ampoules of 1 or 2 mL.
Suppositories, pentazocine 50 mg (as lactate).

Proprietary Names and Manufacturers of Pentazocine and its Salts

Algopent *(Ital.)*; Fortal *(Sterling Winthrop, Fr.)*; Fortalgesic *(Sterling-Winthrop, Swed.; Winthrop, Switz.)*; Fortral *(Aust.; Winthrop, Austral.; Belg.; Winthrop, Denm.; Winthrop, Ger.; Iceland; Neth.; Sterling Research, UK)*; Fortralin *(Fin.; Winthrop, Norw.)*; Fortwin *(Ind.)*; Liticon *(Lagap, Ital.)*; Pentafen *(Zoja, Ital.)*; Pentalgina *(Pierrel, Ital.)*; Sosegon *(Arg.; Winthrop, S.Afr.; Sterwin, Spain)*; Talwin *(Winthrop, Canad.; Maggioni-Winthrop, Ital.; Winthrop-Breon, USA)*.

The following names have been used for multi-ingredient preparations containing pentazocine and its salts—Fortagesic *(Sterling Research, UK)*; Talacen *(Winthrop-Breon, USA)*; Talwin Compound *(Winthrop, Canad.; Winthrop-Breon, USA)*; Talwin Nx *(Winthrop-Breon, USA)*.

6254-z

Pethidine Hydrochloride *(BANM, rINNM)*.

Meperidine Hydrochloride *(USAN)*; Operidine. Ethyl 1-methyl-4-phenylpiperidine-4-carboxylate hydrochloride.

$C_{15}H_{21}NO_2,HCl=283.8$.

CAS — 57-42-1 (pethidine); 50-13-5 (hydrochloride).

Pharmacopoeias. In *Arg., Aust., Belg., Br., Braz., Chin., Cz., Egypt., Eur., Fr., Ger., Hung., Ind., Int., It., Jpn, Jug., Mex., Neth., Nord., Port., Roum., Swiss, Turk.,* and *U.S.* Also in *B.P. Vet.*

A fine white odourless crystalline powder.

Very **soluble** in water; freely soluble in alcohol and chloroform; practically insoluble in ether. The *U.S.P.* injection has a pH of 3.5 to 6.0; the *U.S.P.* syrup has a pH of 3.5 to 3.9. Solutions are **sterilised** by autoclaving. **Incompatible** with barbiturates. **Store** in airtight containers. Protect from light.

STABILITY. Pethidine hydrochloride was stable for at least 24 hours at room temperature in glucose 5% and 4% and in sodium chloride injection (0.9%) and sodium chloride injection (0.9%) diluted 1 in 5.— L. Rudd and P. Simpson (letter), *Med. J. Aust.*, 1978, *2*, 34.

Dependence

Prolonged use of pethidine may lead to dependence of the morphine type (see p.1310). Doses as large as 3 or 4 g daily may be taken by addicts. As tolerance to the central nervous system stimulant and anticholinergic effects is not complete with these very large doses, muscle twitching, tremor, mental confusion, dilated pupils, and sometimes convulsions may be present.

Withdrawal symptoms appear more rapidly than with morphine and are of shorter duration.

Adverse Effects and Treatment

As for Morphine, p.1311.

Constipation occurs less frequently than with morphine. After overdosage, symptoms are generally similar to those of morphine poisoning, however stimulation of the central nervous system and convulsions may also occur, especially in tolerant individuals or following toxic doses by mouth. Local reactions often follow injection of pethidine; general hypersensitivity reactions occur rarely.

Of 26 294 consecutive patients monitored in the Boston Collaborative Drug Surveillance Program, 366 received pethidine by mouth and adverse reactions were reported in 16, mainly involving the gastro-intestinal tract. A further 3268 patients received pethidine by injection, and adverse effects were reported in 102, involving the central nervous system in 38.— R. R. Miller and H. Jick, *J. clin. Pharmac.*, 1978, *18*, 180.

EFFECTS ON THE NERVOUS SYSTEM. A discussion of Kaiko *et al.*'s study (*Ann. Neurol.*, 1983, *13*, 180) of pethidine-induced central neurotoxicity.— L. A. Hershey, *Ann. intern. Med.*, 1983, *98*, 548.

A report of severe reversible parkinsonism following administration of 4 g of pethidine, over 9 days, to an elderly patient with postoperative pain after removal of an adenocarcinoma of the rectum. Symptoms progressed after withdrawal of pethidine but responded to treatment with carbidopa in association with levodopa.— A. N. Lieberman and M. Goldstein (letter), *New Engl. J. Med.*, 1985, *312*, 509.

Some further reports of pethidine neurotoxicity: V. F. Mauro *et al.*, *Clin. Pharm.*, 1986, *5*, 837; L. Morisy and D. Platt (letter), *J. Am. med. Ass.*, 1986, *255*, 467.

PREGNANCY AND THE NEONATE. In a retrospective study of 34 term infants who had perinatal asphyxia and generalised seizures within 48 hours of birth, and 68 controls, there was no association between the incidence of seizures and epidural anaesthesia or the use of pethidine in labour.— R. J. Derham *et al.*, *Archs Dis. Childh.*, 1985, *60*, 809.

References to the effects of maternal pethidine on the foetal or neonatal heart: H. Epstein *et al.*, *Obstet. Gynec.*, 1982, *59*, *Suppl.*, 22S; M. Ron *et al.*, *Int. J. Gynaecol. Obstet.*, 1982, *20*, 301; J. M. Barrett and F. H. Boehm, *Sth. med. J.*, 1983, *76*, 1480; V. M. Miall-Allen and A. G. L. Whitelaw, *Archs Dis. Childh.*, 1987, *62*, 1179.

Precautions

As for Morphine, p.1311.

It should be given cautiously to patients with supraventricular tachycardia.

Very severe reactions, including coma, severe respiratory depression, cyanosis, and hypotension have occurred in patients receiving monoamine oxidase inhibitors and given pethidine. There are also reports of hyperexcitability, convulsions, tachycardia, hyperpyrexia, and hypertension. Pethidine should not be given to patients receiving monoamine oxidase inhibitors or within 14 days of their discontinuation. Concurrent administration of pethidine and phenothiazines has produced severe hypotensive episodes and may prolong the respiratory depression due to pethidine.

Prolongation of elimination half-life and decreased plasma clearance of pethidine peroperatively compared with postoperatively.— A. Tamsen *et al.*, *Clin. Pharmacokinet*, 1982, *7*, 149.

ADMINISTRATION IN LIVER DISORDERS. Investigations in 8 healthy subjects and 10 patients with cirrhosis of the liver who were given single rapid intravenous injections of pethidine 800 µg per kg body-weight indicated that the elimination of pethidine was prolonged in cirrhosis, probably due to impairment of the drug-metabolising activity in the liver. The terminal pethidine-plasma half-life was an average of about 3 hours in the healthy subjects and 7 hours in the patients.— U. Klotz *et al.*, *Clin. Pharmac. Ther.*, 1974, *16*, 667. See also E. A. Neal *et al.*, *Gastroenterology*, 1979, *77*, 96; S. M. Pond *et al.*, *Clin. Pharmac. Ther.*, 1981, *30*, 183.

ADMINISTRATION IN RENAL FAILURE. Tremors, myoclonus, seizures, and depressed consciousness have been associated with the use of pethidine in patients with renal insufficiency, presumably due to the accumulation of the metabolite norpethidine.— H. H. Szeto *et al.*, *Ann. intern. Med.*, 1977, *86*, 738.

In a study of 10 healthy subjects and 18 patients with renal dysfunction mean plasma protein binding of pethidine ranged from 58.2% in the healthy subjects to 31.8% in 7 anuric patients.— K. Chan *et al.*, *J. Pharm. Pharmac.*, 1983, *35*, *Suppl.* (Dec.), 94P.

A case report of pethidine-related neurologic deterioration in the setting of renal insufficiency due to high-dose parenteral acyclovir treatment.— R. Johnson *et al.* (letter), *Ann. intern. Med.*, 1985, *103*, 962 (see also L. Corey and J. Douglas, *ibid.*, 1986, *104*, 449).

INTERACTIONS. *Acyclovir.* See above under Administration in Renal Failure.

Barbiturates. Stambaugh *et al.* reported a case of prolonged sedation with pethidine in the presence of phenobarbitone therapy (120 mg daily) (*Lancet*, 1977, *1*, 398). They also reported that phenobarbitone pretreatment enhanced the formation of norpethidine, but did not affect the serum concentrations or half-life of pethidine (J.E. Stambaugh *et al.*, *J. clin. Pharmac.*, 1978, *18*, 482). The interaction with barbiturates has another aspect for opioid analgesics have also been shown to enhance the CNS depressant effects of barbiturates (J.W. Bellville *et al.*, *Clin. Pharmac. Ther.*, 1971, *12*, 607).

Histamine H_2 antagonists. A study in 8 healthy male volunteers of the effect of concurrent administration of pethidine and cimetidine. The subjects received pethidine hydrochloride 70 mg intravenously before and during treatment with cimetidine 1200 mg daily by mouth. Pethidine clearance and volume of distribution were reduced and it was suggested that cimetidine induced a reduction in pethidine oxidation to norpethidine.— D. R. P. Guay *et al.*, *Br. J. clin. Pharmac.*, 1984, *18*, 907.

A study in 8 healthy male volunteers of the effect of concurrent administration of pethidine and ranitidine. The subjects received 70-mg intravenous pethidine hydrochloride doses before and during ranitidine treatment (150 mg twice daily by mouth). Ranitidine was found not to interact pharmacokinetically with pethidine.— D. R. P. Guay *et al.*, *Br. J. clin. Pharmac.*, 1985, *20*, 55.

Isoniazid. A case report of hypotension associated with the concurrent use of pethidine and isoniazid in a 54-year-old man.— R. Gannon *et al.* (letter), *Ann. intern. Med.*, 1983, *99*, 415.

Phenothiazines. A study in 6 healthy subjects demonstrated that concurrent administration of prochlorperazine with pethidine prolonged the respiratory depression due to pethidine.— S. N. Steen and M. Yates, *Clin. Pharmac. Ther.*, 1972, *13*, 153.

Chlorpromazine given with pethidine to 10 subjects produced a greater decrease in diastolic and systolic blood pressure than was seen with pethidine and placebo. There was increased lethargy with the combination of chlorpromazine with pethidine. There was also an increase in urinary norpethidine with the combination and it was considered that chlorpromazine enhanced N-demethylation of pethidine.— J. E. Stambaugh and I. W. Wainer, *J. clin. Pharmac.*, 1981, *21*, 140.

Phenytoin. Reduced half-life and bioavailability of pethidine on concomitant administration of phenytoin. Blood concentrations of norpethidine were increased.— S. M. Pond and K. M. Kretschzmar, *Clin. Pharmac. Ther.*, 1981, *30*, 680.

PHAEOCHROMOCYTOMA. Pethidine provoked episodes of hypertension on 5 occasions when given postoperatively to a patient with non-resectable phaeochromocytoma. The effect was suppressed when labetalol was being given.— C. A. Lawrence, *Br. med. J.*, 1978, *1*, 149.

PREGNANCY AND THE NEONATE. Signs of foetal depression were not apparent when delivery occurred within 1 hour of pethidine administration. Depression was present in 6 of 24 infants delivered 1 to 3 hours after injection, and in all of 5 infants delivered 3 to 6 hours after injection.— J. C. Morrison *et al.*, *Am. J. Obstet. Gynec.*, 1973, *115*, 1132.

The pO_2 fell immediately after the administration of pethidine 50 mg in 4 of 9 women in late pregnancy or labour, and in 13 of 19 similar women after the administration of 100 mg with levallorphan 1.25 mg. Abnormal heart-rate patterns were recorded in 8 foetuses.— A. Huch *et al.*, *J. Obstet. Gynaec. Br. Commonw.*, 1974, *81*, 608.

Maternally administered pethidine reduced neonatal serum-bilirubin concentrations, although the magnitude of the effect was small.— J. H. Drew and W. H. Kitchen, *J. Pediat.*, 1976, *89*, 657.

The effects of analgesia during labour were assessed in 920 neonates on the first and second days of life. In infants whose mothers had received pethidine, responses were depressed on both days; the depression was greatest with the highest dose of pethidine (75 to 150 mg within 4 hours of delivery). Depression produced by pethidine and anaesthetic agents was additive. Babies delivered under chloroprocaine epidural anaesthesia suffered least depression.— R. Hodgkinson *et al.*, *Can. Anaesth. Soc. J.*, 1978, *25*, 405.

A study was conducted in 145 women who received either pethidine or epidural bupivacaine or no analgesic during labour. Apgar scores of 7 or less at 1 minute occurred in 10 infants in the pethidine group, in 2 infants in the bupivacaine group and no infants in the control group. There was no significant difference in Apgar scores at 5 minutes. The elimination half-lives of pethidine and bupivacaine in infants were 22.4 hours and 14 hours respectively. There were no significant behavioural differences in infants during the first 6 weeks of life.— B. A. Lieberman *et al.*, *Br. J. Obstet. Gynaec.*, 1979, *86*, 598.

Comment on behavioural studies on the effect on the infant of pethidine analgesia in labour.— *Lancet*, 1981, *2*, 291.

Absorption and Fate

Pethidine hydrochloride is absorbed from the gastro-intestinal tract, but availability is less with the oral than the parenteral routes. It is partly bound to plasma proteins. Pethidine is metabolised in the liver by hydrolysis to pethidinic acid or demethylation to norpethidine and hydrolysis to norpethidinic acid, followed by conjugation with glucuronic acid. At the usual values of urinary pH or if the urine is alkaline, excretion of unchanged pethidine is negligible; urinary excretion of pethidine and norpethidine is enhanced by acidification of the urine. Pethidine crosses the placenta and appears in milk.

Some references to the pharmacokinetics of pethidine.— L. E. Mather *et al.*, *Clin. Pharmac. Ther.*, 1975, *17*, 21; J. E. Stambaugh *et al.*, *J. clin. Pharmac.*, 1976, *16*, 245; L. E. Mather and P. J. Meffin, *Clin. Pharmacokinet.*, 1978, *3*, 352; K. L. Austin *et al.*, *Br. J. clin. Pharmac.*, 1981, *1*, 25; C. La Rosa *et al.*, *ibid.*, 1984, *17*, 405; C. La Rosa *et al.*, *ibid.*, 411; K. Chan *et al.*, *ibid.*, 1985, *20*, 531P; I. Odar-Cederlöf *et al.*, *Eur. J. clin. Pharmac.*, 1985, *28*, 171.

See also under Precautions, above.

PREGNANCY AND THE NEONATE. Twelve women in labour were given one dose of pethidine 150 mg intramuscularly 1 to 4 hours before delivery and most of the infants at birth had plasma concentrations of 500 ng per mL or less. When pethidine was given within 1 hour of delivery, infant plasma concentrations were much higher as they also were when 3 mothers were given 2 doses of pethidine within 8 hours of delivery. The ratio of cord to maternal plasma concentrations for all 19 was 0.74. All babies eliminated pethidine from the blood within 148 hours.— L. V. Cooper *et al.*, *Archs Dis. Childh.*, 1977, *52*, 638.

A study of the excretion of pethidine and norpethidine by 7 neonates, whose mothers had received pethidine intramuscularly or intravenously, showed that the amounts excreted increased significantly with the dose-delivery interval up to 5 hours. Most of the placentally-transferred pethidine should be excreted by the 3rd day.— M. I. J. Hogg *et al.*, *Br. J. Anaesth.*, 1977, *49*, 891.

A further study of the maternal kinetics and transplacental passage of pethidine during labour.— G. Tomson *et al.*, *Br. J. clin. Pharmac.*, 1982, *13*, 653.

Uses and Administration

Pethidine hydrochloride is an analgesic which has the actions and uses of morphine (p.1312) and can be used for the relief of most types of moderate to severe pain including the pain of labour. It is also used as pre-operative medication and as an adjunct to anaesthesia. It has little effect on cough or on diarrhoea.

The analgesic effect of pethidine hydrochloride is shorter than for morphine and usually lasts for 2 to 4 hours.

For the relief of pain, pethidine hydrochloride is given in doses of 50 to 150 mg by mouth every 4 hours. Pethidine may also be given by intramuscular and subcutaneous injection in doses of 25 to 100 mg and by slow intravenous injection in doses of 25 to 50 mg. In children, doses of 0.5 to 2.0 mg per kg body-weight may be given by mouth or by intramuscular injection.

In obstetric analgesia 50 to 100 mg may be given by intramuscular or subcutaneous injection as soon as contractions occur at regular intervals. This dose may be repeated after 1 to 3 hours if necessary.

A study of the minimum effective analgesic blood concentration (MEABC) of pethidine in 16 patients with intractable pain. One patient failed to obtain analgesia with pethidine. In the remaining 15 the minimum effective concentration ranged from 100 to 820 ng per mL (median 250 ng per mL). Additional measures were required where the effective concentration was greater than 400 ng per mL.— L. E. Mather and C. J. Glynn, *Br. J. clin. Pharmac.*, 1982, *14*, 385.

ADMINISTRATION, EPIDURAL AND INTRATHECAL. To obviate the need for repeated subarachnoid injections to obtain analgesia in severe intractable pain, pethidine was injected through an indwelling epidural catheter. In 7 patients with severe postoperative pain, preservative-free pethidine hydrochloride in physiological saline 100 mg in 10 mL, provided onset of pain relief at 5 minutes which corresponded to high CSF-pethidine concentrations of 0.5 to 2 µg per mL. Complete pain relief occurred in all patients in 12 to 20 minutes and corresponded to CSF-pethidine concentrations of 10 to 20 µg per mL. Typical peak blood-pethidine concentrations occurred after approximately 40 minutes with a mean absorption half-life of 25 minutes. Over periods of 2 to 4 days pethidine given as required provided analgesia lasting 4.5 to 20 hours (mean 6 hours). In 6 patients with chronic intractable cancer pain, complete relief was obtained after pethidine hydrochloride 30 mg in 6 mL; blood-pethidine concentrations were less than those previously determined by intravenous infusion to be analgesic in these patients, and analgesia lasted 4.5 to 18 hours (mean 8 hours). Absence of increased analgesia when analgesic concentrations in the blood were eventually reached following the 100-mg injections and reversal only of concomitant transitory mild sedation by intravenous injection of naloxone, strongly suggested that the initial analgesic effect of the high doses of epidural pethidine was due to a spinal action. No changes in sensory, sympathetic, or motor function were detected, indicating that this form of analgesia may have considerable advantages for relief of severe pain.— M. J. Cousins *et al.* (letter), *Lancet*, 1979, *1*, 1141. A note of caution regarding the high dose of pethidine used. A frail 76-year-old woman given pethidine 50 mg in 10 mL epidurally developed virtual apnoea, and a heavy 42-year-old woman given 100 mg developed very slow respiration.— D. B. Scott and J. McClure (letter), *ibid.*, 1410.

Saddle blockade with pethidine hydrochloride in 111 patients undergoing short surgical operations on the perineum, by intrathecal administration. Sensory blockade lasted for 141±26.06 minutes and was followed by postoperative analgesia, the mean duration of which was 301±98.38 minutes. Postoperative neurological complications were recorded in 3 patients. Seven patients complained of itching, 5 patients of nausea and vomiting, and 2 developed urinary retention.— I. Acalovschi *et al.*, *Br. J. Anaesth.*, 1986, *58*, 1012.

Labour. Twelve mothers received 28 doses of pethidine epidurally ranging from 25 to 100 mg. Overall, 14 doses gave good pain relief and 12 gave some relief and the duration of action increased with the dose, being 55 minutes with 25 mg and 150 minutes with 100 mg. There was a feeling that third and subsequent doses of pethidine in any one patient had a diminished effect, although this was not demonstrated if only the 50-mg doses were considered. Five patients were fully satisfied postpartum and 7 were helped.— B. W. Perriss, *Anaesthesia*, 1980, *35*, 380.

A study of pethidine kinetics and analgesia in women in labour following intravenous, intramuscular, and epidural administration. It is suggested that the analgesia produced by the epidural route, which is greater than that produced with the other 2 routes, is due to a mixture of systemic analgesia and a local anaesthetic effect R. P. Husemeyer *et al.*, *Br. J. clin. Pharmac.*, 1982, *13*, 171.

ADMINISTRATION IN LIVER DISORDERS. See under Precautions.

ADMINISTRATION, PATIENT-CONTROLLED. In a small trial in patients who had had upper abdominal surgery the demand for pethidine, from a patient demand apparatus, fell quickly over the first 24 hours. No patient made a demand near the maximum. The average dose was 8.1 mg per kg body-weight in 24 hours with a range of 2.9 to 23 mg per kg.— M. Rosen and M. D. Vickers (letter), *Br. med. J.*, 1979, *1*, 1278.

In a study of 20 patients using patient-controlled intravenous administration of pethidine following surgery, small intravenous doses at short intervals were found to alleviate pain better than large infrequent doses. Almost a constant plasma level of pethidine was maintained by the patient during the first postoperative day and gave a subjectively satisfactory analgesia. It was concluded that postoperative analgesic administration should be individualised according to perceived analgesic effects, and that the rational adult patient is the best judge of therapeutic success.— A. Tamsen *et al.*, *Clin. Pharmacokinet.*, 1982, *7*, 164.

ADMINISTRATION IN RENAL FAILURE. See under Precautions.

Preparations

Meperidine Hydrochloride Injection *(U.S.P.)*. A sterile solution of pethidine hydrochloride in Water for Injections.

Meperidine Hydrochloride Syrup *(U.S.P.)*. A syrup containing pethidine hydrochloride.

Meperidine Hydrochloride Tablets *(U.S.P.)*. Tablets containing pethidine hydrochloride.

Pethidine Injection *(B.P.)*. A sterile solution of pethidine hydrochloride in Water for Injections.

Pethidine Tablets *(B.P.)*. Tablets containing pethidine hydrochloride.

Proprietary Preparations

Pamergan P100 *(Martindale Pharmaceuticals, UK)*. *Injection*, pethidine hydrochloride 50 mg, promethazine hydrochloride 25 mg/mL, in ampoules of 2 mL.

Proprietary Names and Manufacturers

Centralgine *(Amino, Switz.)*; Demer-Idine *(Canad.)*; Demerol *(Arg.; Winthrop, Canad.; Winthrop-Breon, USA)*; Dolanquifa *(Uquifa, Spain)*; Dolantin *(Hoechst, Ger.)*; Dolantina *(Bayer, Spain)*; Dolantine *(Belg.; Hoechst, Switz.)*; Doloneurin *(Neth.)*; Dolosal *(Belg.; Specia, Fr.)* Pethoid *(Austral.)*.

The following names have been used for multi-ingredient preparations containing pethidine hydrochloride— Demerol Apap *(Winthrop-Breon, USA)*; Mepergan *(Wyeth, USA)*; Pamergan *(Rhône-Poulenc, Canad.)*; Pamergan AP100/25 *(Martindale Pharmaceuticals, UK)*; Pamergan P100 *(Martindale Pharmaceuticals, UK)*; Pethilorfan *(Roche, UK)*.

6256-k

Phenazocine Hydrobromide *(BANM, rINNM)*.

1,2,3,4,5,6-Hexahydro-6,11-dimethyl-3-phenethyl-2,6-methano-3-benzazocin-8-ol hydrobromide hemihydrate.

$C_{22}H_{27}NO,HBr,½H_2O=411.4$.

CAS — 127-35-5 (phenazocine); 1239-04-9 (hydrobromide, anhydrous).

Phenazocine hydrobromide is an opioid analgesic with actions and uses similar to those of morphine (see p.1312). It is considered to be less sedating.

Phenazocine acts within 20 minutes after administration by mouth and the analgesic effect may last up to 6 hours. The usual dose by mouth is 5 mg every 4 to 6 hours, though single doses of 20 mg may be given. Phenazocine hydrobromide has been given parenterally and buccally.

EFFECT ON THE BILIARY TRACT. A reference to the suitability of phenazocine for biliary pain.— D. S. Hopton and H. B. Torrance, *Gut*, 1967, *8*, 296.

Proprietary Preparations

Narphen *(Smith & Nephew Pharmaceuticals, UK)*. *Tablets*, scored, phenazocine hydrobromide 5 mg.

6257-a

Phenoperidine Hydrochloride *(BANM, rINNM)*.

R-1406. Ethyl 1-(3-hydroxy-3-phenylpropyl)-4-phenylpiperidine-4-carboxylate hydrochloride.

$C_{23}H_{29}NO_3,HCl=403.9$.

CAS — 562-26-5 (phenoperidine); 3627-49-4 (hydrochloride).

Incompatible with propanidid and solutions of methohexitone sodium and thiopentone sodium.

Dependence, Adverse Effects, Treatment, and Precautions

As for Morphine, p.1310.

Muscular rigidity may require treatment with muscle relaxants. Some cases of jaundice have been reported.

In a study of 7 patients with severe head injury, intravenous bolus doses of phenoperidine alone or in combination with pancuronium resulted in a decrease in cerebral perfusion pressure. It was suggested that phenoperidine should be avoided in traumatic coma.— R. M. Bingham and C. J. Hinds, *Br. J. Anaesth.*, 1987, *59*, 592.

ADMINISTRATION IN LIVER DISORDERS. Liver disease significantly modified the distribution, clearance, excretion, and hepatic extraction ratio of phenoperidine.— C. N. Isherwood *et al.*, *Br. J. clin. Pharmac.*, 1982, *13*, 612P.

INTERACTIONS. Prior beta-blockade with propranolol probably contributed to severe hypotension in a patient with tetanus given phenoperidine; earlier doses of phenoperidine had not caused hypotension.— K. L. Woods (letter), *Br. med. J.*, 1978, *2*, 1164.

Absorption and Fate

Although normally given by injection, there is some absorption of phenoperidine from the gastro-intestinal tract. It is extensively metabolised in the liver to pethidine and norpethidine, which are mainly excreted in the urine.

Five anaesthetised patients were given phenoperidine 2 mg intravenously. The distribution half-life (in 4 patients) ranged from 3.19 to 14.23 minutes while the elimination half-life ranged from 47.31 to 162.30 minutes.— L. Milne *et al.*, *Br. J. Anaesth.*, 1980, *52*, 537.

Further references to the pharmacokinetics of phenoperidine: T. N. Calvey *et al.*, *Br. J. clin. Pharmac.*, 1981, *11*, 124P; *idem*, 1982, *13*, 293P; K. Chan *et al.*, *ibid.*, 1983, *15*, 154P; L. A. Milne *et al.*, *ibid.*, *16*, 101.

See also Administration in Liver Disorders, above.

Uses and Administration

Phenoperidine hydrochloride is an opioid analgesic related to pethidine with similar actions (see p.1318 and morphine p.1312). By injection its effects last for up to 1 hour.

Phenoperidine hydrochloride produces surgical analgesia and when a major tranquilliser or neuroleptic agent such as droperidol is added, the patient can be maintained in a state of neuroleptanalgesia in which he is calm and indifferent to his surroundings and is able to cooperate with the surgeon.

In anaesthesia where spontaneous respiration is maintained, an average initial intravenous dose of phenoperidine hydrochloride is up to 1 mg; supplements of 500 µg may be given approximately every 40 to 60 minutes. In similar conditions children have been given 30 to 50 µg per kg body-weight. In anaesthesia with controlled respiration, the initial dose is 2 to 5 mg with supplementary doses of 1 mg; children have been given 100 to 150 µg per kg.

Intramuscular injections may be given for analgesia.

Phenoperidine has also been used to depress respiration in long-term assisted ventilation.

ADMINISTRATION, EPIDURAL. Effective analgesia with epidural phenoperidine 2 mg for pain following caesarean section. Its duration was less than with diamorphine 5 mg epidurally but greater than after diamorphine 5 mg intramuscularly.— D. J. Macrae *et al.*, *Br. J. Anaesth.*, 1987, *59*, 354.

ANAESTHESIA. In 25 patients whose anaesthesia included phenoperidine 2 mg with supplements of 0.5 to 1 mg, postoperative pain was less at 1 and 2 hours than in 25 patients whose anaesthesia included halothane 0.5%, but the number of doses of opioid analgesics in the first 24 hours was not reduced and the pain scores over the first 3 days were not significantly different. Phenoperidine might have a cumulative effect after opioid premedication or a sedative effect.— J. J. Henderson and G. D.

Parbrook, *Br. J. Anaesth.*, 1976, *48*, 587.

Phaeochromocytoma. Experience of surgery in 102 patients with phaeochromocytoma. Droperidol with phenoperidine had been used for anaesthesia in 38 patients with a decrease in the incidence of arrhythmia and a greater stability of blood pressure. Maintenance of blood pressure after removal of the tumour by maintenance of blood volume was superior to the use of noradrenaline.— J. M. Desmonts *et al.*, *Br. J. Anaesth.*, 1977, *49*, 991.

Proprietary Preparations

Operidine *(Janssen, UK). Injection,* phenoperidine hydrochloride 1 mg/mL, in ampoules of 2 and 10 mL.

Proprietary Names and Manufacturers

Lealgin *(Janssen Pharmaceutica, Swed.)*; Operidine *(Janssen, Austral.; Janssen, UK)*.

6259-x

Piritramide *(BAN, rINN).*

Pirinitramide; R-3365. 1-(3-Cyano-3,3-diphenylpropyl)-4-piperidinopiperidine-4-carboxamide.
$C_{27}H_{34}N_4O$=430.6.

CAS — 302-41-0.

Piritramide is an opioid analgesic with actions similar to those of morphine (see p.1312).

It has a duration of action of about 6 hours after intramuscular injection. It is given in the treatment of postoperative pain in a dose of 15 mg by intramuscular or subcutaneous injection, and may be repeated, if necessary, after half an hour to a maximum daily dosage of 45 mg.

Piritramide may also be administered as the hydrogen tartrate.

In a double-blind study of 240 patients with postoperative pain piritramide 20 mg intramuscularly appeared to be equal in analgesic effect to morphine 15 mg intramuscularly. At this strength the hypnotic effect of piritramide was greater but there was a smaller incidence of other side-effects.— B. Kay, *Br. J. Anaesth.*, 1971, *43*, 1167.

Some further references to piritramide: M. E. Tunstall and T. W. Ogg, *Anaesthesia*, 1974, *29*, 728; E. Knoche *et al.*, *Clin. Ther.*, 1983, *5*, 585.

PORPHYRIA. Piritramide was considered to be unsafe in patients with acute porphyria because it has been shown to be porphyrinogenic in *animals* or *in vitro* systems.— M.R. Moore and K.E.L. McColl, *Porphyrias, Drug Lists*, Glasgow, Porphyria Research Unit, University of Glasgow, 1987.

Proprietary Names and Manufacturers

Dipidolor *(Belg.; Janssen, Ger.; Neth.; Janssen, UK)*; Piridolan *(Janssen, Norw.; Janssen Pharmaceutica, Swed.)*.

6260-y

Poppy Capsule

Dormideiras; Fruit du Pavot; Fruto de Adormidera; Mohnfrucht; Poppy Heads.

Pharmacopoeias. In *Fr., Port.,* and *Span.*

The dried fruits of *Papaver somniferum* (Papaveraceae), collected before dehiscence has occurred, containing about 0.1 to 0.3% of morphine with traces of other opium alkaloids.

Poppy capsule is mildly sedative and has been used as a liquid extract or syrup in cough mixtures.

2695-p

Propiram Fumarate *(BANM, USAN, rINNM).*

Bay-4503; FBA-4503. *N*-(1-Methyl-2-piperidinoethyl)-*N*-(2-pyridyl)propionamide hydrogen fumarate.
$C_{16}H_{25}N_3O,C_4H_4O_4$=391.5.

CAS — 15686-91-6 (propiram); 13717-04-9 (fumarate).

Propiram fumarate is a partial opioid agonist with analgesic properties. It has been given by mouth in doses equivalent to 75 to 150 mg of propiram daily in divided doses. It has also been used as suppositories containing the equivalent of 50 mg of propiram.

Some references to propiram fumarate: W. H. Forrest *et al.*, *J. clin. Pharmac.*, 1972, *12*, 440; *Arzneimittel-Forsch.*, 1974, *24*, 583-722; A. Sunshine *et al.*, *Pharmacotherapy*, 1983, *3*, 299; P. J. Desjardins *et al.*, *J. clin. Pharmac.*, 1984, *24*, 35.

Proprietary Names and Manufacturers

Algeril *(Bayropharm, Ital.)*.

13274-e

Sufentanil Citrate *(BANM, USAN, rINNM).*

R-30730 (sufentanil); R-33800. *N*-{4-(Methoxymethyl)-1-[2-(2-thienyl)ethyl]-4-piperidyl}propionanilide citrate.
$C_{22}H_{30}N_2O_2S,C_6H_8O_7$=578.7.

CAS — 60561-17-3; 56030-54-7 (sufentanil).

Dependence

Prolonged use of sufentanil may lead to dependence of the morphine type (see p.1310).

Adverse Effects, Treatment, and Precautions

As for Morphine, p.1311. Atropine has been used for bradycardia induced by sufentanil. Muscle rigidity may require treatment with muscle relaxants.

High doses produce prolonged respiratory depression and in overdosage an opioid antagonist plus assisted ventilation is recommended.

Elimination of 'opioid bowel syndrome' (adynamic ileus) by changing from sufentanil to fentanyl in balanced anaesthesia.— S. Gelman (letter), *J. Am. med. Ass.*, 1985, *254*, 1721.

A report of muscle rigidity of the chest wall occurring with sufentanil and affecting ventilation.— M. Goldberg *et al.*, *Anesthesiology*, 1985, *63*, 199. See also.— J. Chang and K. J. Fish, *ibid.*, 710.

Absorption and Fate

Following parenteral administration sufentanil citrate is metabolised by *N*-dealkylation and *O*-demethylation to pharmacologically inactive metabolites which are excreted in the urine. The elimination half-life of sufentanil is considerably shorter than that of fentanyl. It is extensively bound to plasma proteins.

Reviews of the pharmacokinetics of sufentanil: L. E. Mather, *Clin. Pharmacokinet.*, 1983, *8*, 422; P. J. Davis and D. R. Cook, *ibid.*, 1986, *11*, 18.

Following the development of new radio-immunoassay methods, plasma concentrations of sufentanil were measured in 2 subjects after an intravenous bolus of sufentanil 5 µg per kg body-weight. The mean terminal elimination half-life was 140 minutes and 6 hours after administration plasma-sufentanil concentrations were 0.26 ng per mL.— M. Michiels *et al.*, *J. Pharm. Pharmac.*, 1983, *35*, 86.

A study of the transdermal absorption of fentanyl (citrate and base) and sufentanil citrate. Sufentanil was found to be absorbed transdermally; the excretion of sufentanil citrate in the first 12-hour period was statistically greater than that of fentanyl citrate.— P. S. Sebel *et al.*, *Eur. J. clin. Pharmac.*, 1987, *32*, 529.

Uses and Administration

Sufentanil citrate is an opioid analgesic used as an adjunct in anaesthesia and as an induction agent. Recovery is considered to be more rapid than with fentanyl.

Doses of up to 8 µg of sufentanil per kg body-weight produce profound analgesia. Doses of 8 µg or more per kg produce a deep level of anaesthesia.

When used in anaesthesia with nitrous oxide and oxygen for surgical procedures lasting up to 8 hours, total dosage requirements should not exceed 1 µg per kg per hour. It is customary to give up to 75% of the dose before intubation and to follow this with increments of 10 to 50 µg as required during surgery. Thus, for an operation lasting 1 to 2 hours the total dose would be 1 to 2 µg per kg with 0.75 to 1.5 µg per kg being given before intubation.

Doses of 8 to 30 µg per kg are employed with 100% oxygen for the induction of anaesthesia which may be maintained with increments of 25 to 50 µg. While useful for cardiovascular surgery and neurosurgery, such high doses are associated with prolonged respiratory depression calling for assisted ventilation in the postoperative stage.

Reviews of the actions and uses of sufentanil.— C. E. Rosow, *Pharmacotherapy*, 1984, *4*, 11; J. P. Monk *et al.*, *Drugs*, 1988, *36*, 286.

ADMINISTRATION, EPIDURAL. An assessment of epidural sufentanil in 10 healthy subjects. A dose of 50 µg produced analgesia for 3 hours. This was intensified and extended to 5 hours by the addition of adrenaline 1 in 200 000 to a second dose given to 8 of the subjects 2 to 3 months later. Respiratory depression was not increased by adrenaline and other side-effects such as drowsiness were decreased.— I. D. Klepper *et al.*, *Br. J. Anaesth.*, 1987, *59*, 1147.

ANAESTHESIA. A double-blind study comparing sufentanil, fentanyl, morphine, and pethidine in balanced anaesthesia. The patients who received sufentanil demonstrated least haemodynamic disturbance and sympathoadrenal activity intra-operatively, and did not require additional inhalational anaesthesia.— J. W. Flacke *et al.*, *Anesth. Analg.*, 1985, *64*, 897.

A comparative study in 40 patients undergoing coronary artery bypass grafting. Muscle relaxation just before induction and intubation was with pancuronium. Patients were induced by the administration of sufentanil 5 µg per kg body-weight or fentanyl 25 µg per kg intravenously. Following intubation supplementary doses of sufentanil 2.5 µg per kg or fentanyl 12.5 µg per kg were administered 1 minute before skin incision, and 1 minute before sternotomy. Sufentanil produced satisfactory induction of anaesthesia and a lower mean arterial pressure compared with fentanyl.— H. M. L. Mathews *et al.*, *Br. J. Anaesth.*, 1987, *59*, 939P.

For a study comparing fentanyl, morphine, pethidine, and sufentanil as supplements to nitrous oxide anaesthesia in patients undergoing surgery, see p.1305.

Proprietary Names and Manufacturers

Sufenta *(Janssen, Canad.; Janssen, USA)*.

6262-z

Tilidate Hydrochloride *(BANM).*

Gö 1261-C; Tilidine Hydrochloride *(USAN, rINNM)*; W-5759A. (±)-Ethyl *trans*-2-dimethylamino-1-phenylcyclohex-3-ene-1-carboxylate hydrochloride hemihydrate.
$C_{17}H_{23}NO_2,HCl,\frac{1}{2}H_2O$=318.8.

CAS — 20380-58-9 (tilidate); 27107-79-5 (hydrochloride, anhydrous); 24357-97-9 (+-trans-hydrochloride).

Dependence, Adverse Effects, Treatment, and Precautions

As for Morphine, p.1310. Tilidate hydrochloride is subject to abuse.

DEPENDENCE. Study of tilidate abuse and dependence.— H. Beil and A. Trojan, *Münch. med. Wschr.*, 1976, *118*, 634.

EFFECTS ON THE RESPIRATORY SYSTEM. A crossover study of the comparative respiratory depression of tilidate and morphine in 6 healthy subjects. The respiratory depression of both drugs was effectively antagonised by naloxone.— A. Romagnoli and A. S. Keats, *Clin. Pharmac. Ther.*, 1975, *17*, 523.

PORPHYRIA. Tilidate was considered to be unsafe in patients with acute porphyria because it has been shown to be porphyrinogenic in *animals* or *in vitro* systems.— M.R. Moore and K.E.L. McColl, *Porphyrias, Drug Lists*, Glasgow, Porphyria Research Unit, University of Glasgow, 1987.

Absorption and Fate

Tilidate is absorbed from the gastro-intestinal tract. It is metabolised and excreted in the urine mainly as metabolites.

Following administration of radioactive tilidate 50 mg by mouth to a healthy subject 93.6% of the radioactivity had been eliminated in the urine within 48 hours with a half-life of 8 hours. Less than 0.2% of the urinary radioactivity corresponded to unchanged tilidate and 2 and 3% respectively to nortilidate and bisnortilidate.— K.-O. Vollmer and A. v. Hodenberg, *Arzneimittel-Forsch.*, 1977, *27*, 1706.

Further references: K. -O. Vollmer and H. Achenbach, *Arzneimittel-Forsch.*, 1974, *24*, 1237; H. Hengy *et al.*, *J. pharm. Sci.*, 1978, *67*, 1765.

Uses and Administration

Tilidate hydrochloride is an opioid analgesic used in the control of moderate to severe pain. Tilidate hydrochloride may be given by intramuscular, intravenous, or subcutaneous injection in doses of up to 400 mg daily; or as a suppository in doses of 75 mg up to four times daily. It may also be given by mouth in doses of 50 mg up to four times daily.

Some references to tilidate: G. Navarro *et al.*, *Clin. Pharmac. Ther.*, 1974, *15*, 215; A. L. Mauro and M. Shapiro, *Curr. ther. Res.*, 1974, *16*, 725; T. Tammisto and I. Tigerstedt, *Acta anaesth. scand.*, 1975, *19*, 296; N. Maranetra and M. C. F. Pain, *Med. J. Aust.*, 1976, *1*, 397.

Proprietary Names and Manufacturers

Analgesic *(ISOM, Ital.)*; Kitadol *(Spain)*; Lak *(Bernabó, Arg.)*; Lucayan *(Corvi, Ital.)*; Tilibac *(Kairon, Spain)*; Tilitrate *(Parke, Davis, Spain)*; Tilsa *(Ferrer, Spain)*; Valoron *(Belg.; Warner, S.Afr.; Warner-Lambert, Switz.)*.

13363-l

Tonazocine Mesylate *(USAN, rINNM).*

Win-42156-2. (±)-1-[(2R^*,6S^*,11S^*)-1,2,3,4,5,6-Hexahydro-8-hydroxy-3,6,11-trimethyl-2,6-methano-3-benzazocin-11-yl]octan-3-one methanesulphonate.

$C_{23}H_{35}NO_2,CH_4O_3S=453.6$.

CAS — 71461-18-2 (tonazocine); 73789-00-1 (mesylate).

Tonazocine mesylate is an opioid analgesic with mixed agonist-antagonist activity.

A study in 150 postoperative patients with moderate to severe pain. Doses of tonazocine mesylate 2, 4, and 8 mg given intramuscularly were compared with morphine sulphate 10 mg and placebo. The results indicated that tonazocine mesylate 3.2 mg produced equivalent analgesia to morphine sulphate 10 mg.— M. Lippmann *et al.*, *Clin. Pharmac. Ther.*, 1984, *35*, 257.

Proprietary Names and Manufacturers

Winthrop-Breon, USA.

6263-c

Tramadol Hydrochloride *(USAN, rINNM).*

CG-315E; U-26225A. (±)-*trans*-2-Dimethylaminomethyl-1-(3-methoxyphenyl)cyclohexanol hydrochloride.

$C_{16}H_{25}NO_2,HCl=299.8$.

CAS — 27203-92-5 (tramadol); 22204-88-2 (hydrochloride).

Dependence

Tramadol may have lower potential for producing dependence than morphine.

Adverse Effects, Treatment, and Precautions

As for Morphine, p.1311.

A double-blind crossover study in 262 patients suffering from moderate to severe pain comparing intramuscular tramadol 50 to 100 mg with pentazocine 30 to 60 mg. Both drugs caused considerable sedation, although tramadol 50 mg appeared to be tolerated best.— I. Arend *et al.*, *Arzneimittel-Forsch.*, 1978, *28*, 199.

A report of severe cerebral depression in a 6-month-old infant who had erroneously been given a suppository of tramadol 100 mg. The child had a dramatic response to an intravenous injection of naloxone, but the effect was only of short duration. After repeating the same dose of naloxone the child wakened and artificial respiration was stopped a few hours later.— F. Riedel and H. -B. von Stockhausen, *Eur. J. clin. Pharmac.*, 1984, *26*, 631.

A comparative study of equianalgesic doses of morphine, pentazocine, pethidine, piritramide, and tramadol All but tramadol depressed respiration.— R. Fechner *et al.*, *Anaeth. Intensivmed.*, 1985, *26*, 126.

A study of the effect of analgesics on the sphincter of Oddi in 23 healthy subjects. The duration of contractions of the sphincter was increased by pentazocine but not by tramadol, buprenorphine, or physiological saline.— M. Staritz *et al.*, *Gut*, 1986, *27*, 567.

Uses and Administration

Tramadol hydrochloride is an opioid analgesic. It is given by mouth, by intramuscular, subcutaneous, or intravenous injection, and by suppository. Usual doses are 50 mg orally, 50 to 100 mg by injection, and 100 mg rectally. Total daily doses should not exceed 400 mg.

Some clinical studies of tramadol in the treatment of various painful conditions: E. G. Schenck and I. Arend, *Arzneimittel-Forsch.*, 1978, *28*, 209 (pain of various origins); G. Rettig and L. Kropp, *Therapiewoche*, 1980, *30*, 5561 (myocardial infarction); A. Fassolt, *Schweiz. Rundsch. Med. Prax.*, 1981, *70*, 435 (comparison with morphine and pentazocine in postoperative pain); P. O. Prasertsawat *et al.*, *Curr. ther. Res.*, 1986, *40*, 1022 (comparison with morphine and pethidine in obstetric analgesia); K. Padmasuta, *ibid.*, 1987, *41*, 899 (as supplement to anaesthesia).

Proprietary Names and Manufacturers

Crispin *(Jpn)*; Tramal *(Grünenthal, Ger.; Grünenthal, Switz.)*.

Paraffins and similar Bases

6400-s

This section includes a number of substances used mainly as bases for the preparation of creams, emulsions, ointments, and suppositories. They are used either as inert carriers for drugs or for their various emulsifying and emollient properties. Some are also used to improve the texture, stability or water repellent properties of the final preparation. Other substances used in the preparation of bases can be found in the sections on Soaps and other Anionic Surfactants (p.1416). Glycerol, Glycols and Macrogols (p.1128), and on Nonionic Surfactants (p.1243).

6401-w

Hard Paraffin *(BAN)*.

905 *(mineral hydrocarbons)*; Hartparaffin; Paraff. Dur.; Paraffin *(USAN)*; Paraffin Wax; Paraffinum Durum; Paraffinum Solidum.

CAS — 8002-74-2.

NOTE. Paraffinum Solidum (*Jug. P.*, *Span. P.*, and *Swiss P.*) is ceresin.

Pharmacopoeias. In *Aust., Belg., Br., Chin., Egypt., Fr., Ger., Hung., Ind., It., Jpn, Neth., Nord., Pol.,* and *Port.* Also in *U.S.N.F.* and *B.P. Vet.*

A mixture of solid hydrocarbons obtained by distillation from petroleum or from the oil produced in the destructive distillation of shale.

It is a colourless or white, odourless or almost odourless, translucent, wax-like solid, frequently showing a crystalline structure, and is slightly greasy to the touch. The *B.P.* specifies a solidifying point of 50° to 57°; the *U.S.N.F.* specifies 47° to 65°.

Practically **insoluble** in water and alcohol; soluble in chloroform, ether, volatile oils, and most warm fixed oils. An alcoholic extract is neutral to litmus. **Store** in well-closed containers at a temperature not exceeding 40°.

Adverse Effects

Injection of paraffins into tissues may cause a granulomatous reaction which may be considerably delayed in onset.

In Great Britain the recommended exposure limits of paraffin wax fumes are 2 mg per m^3 (long-term); 6 mg per m^3 (short-term).

Uses and Administration

Hard paraffin is employed principally as a stiffening ingredient in ointment bases.

A variety of hard paraffin is employed in physiotherapy for the relief of pain in inflamed joints and sprains. For this purpose it is used in the form of paraffin-wax baths or may be applied by means of a brush or spray.

6402-e

Liquid Paraffin *(BAN)*.

905 *(mineral hydrocarbons)*; Dickflüssiges Paraffin; Heavy Liquid Petrolatum; Huile de Vaseline Épaisse; Liquid Petrolatum; Mineral Oil *(USAN)*; Oleum Petrolei; Oleum Vaselini; Paraffinum Liquidum; Paraffinum Subliquidum; Vaselinöl; Vaselinum Liquidum; White Mineral Oil.

CAS — 8012-95-1.

Pharmacopoeias. In *Arg., Aust., Belg., Br., Braz., Chin., Cz., Egypt., Eur., Fr., Ger., Hung., Ind., It., Jpn, Jug., Mex., Neth., Nord., Pol., Port., Roum., Rus., Span., Swiss, Turk.,* and *U.S.*

Liquid paraffin is a mixture of liquid saturated hydrocarbons obtained from petroleum. The *U.S.P.* permits a suitable stabiliser.

It is a transparent, colourless, odourless, or almost odourless, oily liquid, free from fluorescence by daylight.

Practically **insoluble** in water and insoluble or sparingly soluble in alcohol. The *B.P.* also has soluble in chloroform and ether while the *U.S.P.* also has miscible with fixed oils (except castor oil) and soluble in volatile oils. **Store** in airtight containers. Protect from light.

Adverse Effects

Excessive dosage by mouth may result in anal seepage and irritation. Liquid paraffin is absorbed to a slight extent, especially if emulsified, and may give rise to granulomatous reactions. Similar reactions follow the injection of liquid paraffin and may be considerably delayed in onset. Injection may also cause vasospasm and prompt surgical removal may be required to prevent severe damage. Lipoid pneumonia has been reported following the use of liquid paraffin nasal drops or spray solutions or following inhalation of oil taken by mouth.

Prolonged use should be avoided. In Great Britain the recommended exposure limits of mineral oil mist are 5 mg per m^3 (long-term); 10 mg per m^3 (short-term).

GRANULOMA. References to granulomas or similar reactions to injections of liquid paraffin: E. L. Lame *et al., Milit. Med.*, 1974, *139*, 818; J. J. Bloem and I. van der Waal, *Oral Surg.*, 1974, *38*, 675; C. Thiels and K. Dumke, *Fortschr. Geb. RöntgStrahl. NuklMed.*, 1977, *126*, 173; D. D. Albers *et al., J. Urol., Baltimore*, 1984, *132*, 114.

LIPOID PNEUMONIA. References: B. Varkey and A. V. P. Kutty (letter), *Ann. intern. Med.*, 1976, *84*, 176; *New Engl. J. Med.*, 1977, *296*, 1105; B. Beermann *et al., Br. med. J.*, 1984, *289*, 1728; D. L. Becton *et al., J. Pediat.*, 1984, *105*, 421.

Precautions

Prolonged ingestion of liquid paraffin may interfere with normal gastro-intestinal processes and should be avoided. It should not be used when abdominal pain, nausea, or vomiting is present.

Uses and Administration

Taken internally, liquid paraffin acts as a lubricant and, since it keeps the stools soft, it has been employed in chronic constipation, especially in the presence of haemorrhoids or other painful conditions of the anus and rectum. For this purpose, up to 45 mL has been given daily, either in divided doses or at bedtime. It has also been given as an enema.

Externally, liquid paraffin may be used as an ingredient of ointment bases, as an emollient to the skin in irritant conditions, and to remove crusts.

A food grade of liquid paraffin is allowed in certain food processes.

Preparations

Liquid Paraffin Emulsion with Cascara *(B.P.C. 1973)*. Liquid Paraffin and Cascara Mixture. Cascara elixir 0.625 mL, liquid paraffin emulsion to 10 mL. *Dose.* 10 to 30 mL.

Liquid Paraffin and Magnesium Hydroxide Oral Emulsion *(B.P.)*. Emuls. Paraff. Liq. et Mag. Hydrox.; Liquid Paraffin and Magnesium Hydroxide Emulsion; Liquid Paraffin and Magnesium Hydroxide Mixture; Mixture of Magnesium Hydroxide and Liquid Paraffin; Mist. Mag. Hydrox. et Paraff. Liq. Liquid paraffin 2.5 mL, chloroform spirit 0.15 mL, and magnesium hydroxide mixture 7.35 mL. *Dose.* 5 to 20 mL.

Liquid Paraffin Oral Emulsion *(B.P.)*. Liquid Paraffin Emulsion; Liquid Paraffin Mixture; Emulsio Paraffini Liquidi; Emuls. Paraff. Liq. Liquid paraffin 5 mL, methylcellulose '20' 200 mg, chloroform 0.025 mL, benzoic acid solution 0.2 mL, vanillin 5 mg, saccharin sodium 500 µg, water to 10 mL. Mix the methylcellulose with 1.2 mL of boiling water and, when the powder is thoroughly hydrated add sufficient water in the form of ice to produce 3.5 mL, and stir until homogeneous; add the other ingredients (except the liquid paraffin), the saccharin sodium being first dissolved in water, adjust to 5 mL with water, and mix; add the liquid paraffin with constant stirring and pass through a homogeniser. *Dose.* 10 to 30 mL.

The liability of Liquid Paraffin Emulsion (*B.P.* 1980) and Liquid Paraffin and Magnesium Hydroxide Emulsion (*B.P.* 1980) to microbial spoilage.— T. R. R. Kurup and L. S. C. Wan, *Pharm. J.*, 1986, *2*, 761.

Mineral Oil Emulsion *(U.S.P.)*. Liquid paraffin 50 mL, acacia 12.5 g, syrup 10 mL, vanillin 4 mg, alcohol 6 mL, water to 100 mL. The vanillin may be replaced by not more than 1% of other official flavouring substances; sweet orange-peel tincture 6 mL or benzoic acid 200 mg may replace the alcohol as a preservative. Store in airtight containers.

Proprietary Preparations

Agarol *(Warner-Lambert, UK)*. *Emulsion*, liquid paraffin 1.6 mL, phenolphthalein 66 mg, agar 10 mg/5 mL. *Dose.* 5 to 15 mL, according to age, at night, and repeated 2 hours after breakfast if necessary.

Alcoderm *(Alcon, UK)*. *Cream* and *Lotion*, liquid paraffin, water, cetyl alcohol, stearyl alcohol, sodium lauryl sulphate, carbomer, polysorbate 60, triethanolamine, methyl and propyl hydroxybenzoates. For dry skin conditions.

Alpha Keri *(Bristol-Myers Pharmaceuticals, UK)*. *Bath oil*, liquid paraffin 91.7%, liquid lanolin ('lanolin oil') 3%. For dry skin conditions and infant bathing; may be either added to bath water or put on to wet skin.

Keri *(Bristol-Myers Pharmaceuticals, UK)*. *Lotion*, liquid paraffin 16% and liquid lanolin ('lanolin oil').

Locobase *(Brocades, UK)*. *Cream*, liquid paraffin, white soft paraffin, cetostearyl alcohol, cetomacrogol '1000', citric acid, anhydrous sodium citrate, and methyl hydroxybenzoate.

Ointment, liquid paraffin/polythene gel. Used as diluents for Locoid preparations (see p.895).

Oilatum Emollient *(Stiefel, UK)*. *Bath additive*, liquid paraffin 63.4%, acetylated wool alcohols 5%. For ichthyosis and related dry skin conditions.

Petrolagar *(Wyeth, UK)*. *Emulsion*, liquid paraffin 7%, light liquid paraffin 18%.

Proprietary Names and Manufacturers

Agoral Plain *(Parke, Davis, USA)*; Emuliquen Simple *(Lainco, Spain)*; Granugenol *(Knoll, Ger.)*; Granugenolo *(Ital.)*; Hodernal *(Gamir, Spain)*; Kondremul *(Fisons, USA)*; Lansoÿl *(Jouveinal, Canad.*; *Jouveinal, Fr.)*; Laxamalt *(Licardy, Fr.)*; Laxil *(Vis, Ital.)*; Lubath *(Parke, Davis, Canad.)*; Lubentyl *(Vaillant-Defresne, Fr.)*; Neo-Cultol *(Fisons, USA)*; Nujol *(Fumouze, Fr.)*; Nutraderm *(Owen, USA)*; Obstinol *(Thiemann, Ger.)*; Parlax *(Lefrancq, Fr.)*; Sanato-Lax *(Hotz, Ger.)*; Tersa Bath Oil *(Trans Canaderm, Canad.)*; Uni Salve *(United, USA)*; Ventricol *(Spain)*.

The following names have been used for multi-ingredient preparations containing liquid paraffin—Agarol *(Warner, Austral.*; *Parke, Davis, Canad.*; *Warner-Lambert, UK)*; Agoral *(Parke, Davis, USA)*; AKWA Tears Ointment *(Akorn, USA)*; Alcoderm *(Alcon, UK)*; Alpha Keri *(Bristol-Myers Pharmaceuticals, UK)*; Alpha-Keri *(Westwood, Canad.)*; Argobase EU *(Westbrook, UK)*; Diprobase *(Kirby-Warrick, UK)*; Duolube *(Charton, Canad.*; *Muro, USA)*; Duratears *(Alcon, Canad.*; *Alcon Laboratories, USA)*; Emulsiderm *(Dermal Laboratories, UK)*; Evactil *(Faulding, Austral.)*; Hartolite *(Croda, UK)*; HEB Waterproof *(Waterhouse, UK)*; Hydromol *(Quinoderm, UK)*; Kaylene-Ol *(Dendron, UK)*; Keri *(Bristol-Myers Pharmaceuticals, UK)*; Kondremul with Cascara *(Fisons, USA)*; Kondremul with Phenolphthalein *(Fisons, USA)*; Lacri-Lube *(Allergan, Austral.*; *Allergan, Canad.*; *Allergan, UK*; *Allergan, USA)*; Liqui-Doss *(Ferndale, USA)*; Locobase Cream and Ointment *(Brocades, UK)*; Lubentyl *(Uhlmann-Eyraud, Switz.)*; Lubrifair Ointment *(Pharmafair, USA)*; Magnolax *(Wampole, Canad.)*; Oilatum Emollient *(Stiefel, Austral.*; *Stiefel, UK)*; Petrolagar *(Wyeth, UK)*; Polytar Emollient *(Stiefel, Austral.*; *Stiefel, UK)*; Tar Doak *(Trans Canaderm, Canad.)*; Tearfair Ointment *(Pharmafair, USA)*; Translet Skin Cream *(Franklin Medical, UK)*; Ultrabase *(Schering, UK)*; Unguentum Merck *(E. Merck, UK)*.

NOTE. The name Ostomy Plus Three has also been used to denote the preparation now known in the UK as Translet Skin Cream.

6403-l

Light Liquid Paraffin *(BAN)*.
Dünnflüssiges Paraffin; Huile de Vaseline Fluide; Light Liquid Petrolatum; Light Mineral Oil *(USAN)*; Light White Mineral Oil; Paraff. Liq. Lev.; Paraffinum Liquidum Leve; Paraffinum Liquidum Tenue; Paraffinum Perliquidum; Spray Paraffin; Vaselina Liquida.

NOTE. The name Parolein has been applied to light liquid paraffin, particularly when used as eye-drops.

Pharmacopoeias. In *Arg., Br., Eur., Fr., Ger., Ind., It., Jpn, Neth., Port., Span.,* and *Swiss.* Also in *U.S.N.F. U.S.* also includes Topical Light Mineral Oil.

A variety of liquid paraffin of lower kinematic viscosity than the oil for internal administration. **Store** in airtight containers. Protect from light.

Light liquid paraffin is used as an emollient and cleanser in certain skin conditions. It is also used as a lubricant and to facilitate the removal of dermatological preparations.

Proprietary Preparations

Hydromol Emollient *(Quinoderm, UK). Bath additive,* light liquid paraffin 37.8%, isopropyl myristate 13%.

Proprietary Names and Manufacturers

Astrolene *(Astor, UK)*; Salus-öl *(Salushaus, Ger.)*.

The following names have been used for multi-ingredient preparations containing light liquid paraffin— Argobase 125 *(Westbrook, UK)*; Hydromol Emollient *(Quinoderm, UK)*; Hypotears Ointment *(Coopervision, USA)*; Petrolagar *(Wyeth, UK)*.

6404-y

White Soft Paraffin *(BAN)*.

905 *(mineral hydrocarbons)*; Paraff. Moll. Alb.; Paraffinum Molle Album; Vaseline Officinale; White Petrolatum *(USAN)*; White Petroleum Jelly.

Pharmacopoeias. In *Arg., Aust., Belg., Br., Chin., Cz., Egypt., Fr., Ger., Hung., Ind., It., Jpn, Jug., Mex., Neth., Nord., Pol., Port., Roum., Span., Swiss, Turk.,* and *U.S.* Also in *B.P. Vet. U.S.* permits a suitable stabiliser. *Chin. P.* does not differentiate between white and yellow soft paraffin. Many pharmacopoeias use the title Vaselinum Album; in Great Britain the name 'Vaseline' is a trade-mark.

White soft paraffin is bleached yellow soft paraffin.
Protect from light.

6405-j

Yellow Soft Paraffin *(BAN)*.

Paraff. Moll. Flav.; Paraffinum Molle Flavum; Petrolatum *(USAN)*; Petroleum Jelly; Yellow Petrolatum; Yellow Petroleum Jelly.

Pharmacopoeias. In *Aust., Br., Chin., Cz., Egypt., Hung., Ind., Jpn, Jug., Mex., Neth., Nord., Pol., Swiss,* and *U.S.* Also in *B.P. Vet. U.S.* permits a suitable stabiliser. *Chin. P.* does not differentiate between white and yellow soft paraffin. Many pharmacopoeias use the title Vaselinum Flavum; in Great Britain the name 'Vaseline' is a trade-mark.

A purified semi-solid mixture of hydrocarbons obtained from petroleum. It is a pale yellow to light amber-coloured, translucent, soft, unctuous mass, not more than slightly fluorescent by daylight even when melted, and odourless when rubbed on the skin. The *B.P.* specifies m.p. 38° to 56°. The *U.S.P.* specifies 38° to 60°.
Practically **insoluble** in water and in alcohol; soluble in carbon disulphide, chloroform, ether, petroleum spirit, and most fixed and volatile oils, the solutions sometimes showing a slight opalescence. An alcoholic extract is neutral to litmus. **Protect** from light.

Adverse Effects

As for Hard Paraffin, p.1322.

Uses and Administration

Soft paraffin is not readily absorbed by the skin. It is used as an emollient and protective ointment basis for surface action. Sterilised dressings containing yellow soft paraffin or its preparations are often used for wound dressings as they are easily removed.

Preparations

Hydrophilic Ointment *(U.S.P.)*. White soft paraffin 25 g, stearyl alcohol 25 g, propylene glycol 12 g, sodium lauryl sulphate 1 g, methyl hydroxybenzoate 25 mg, propyl hydroxybenzoate 15 mg, and water 37 g. Store in airtight containers.

Hydrophilic Petrolatum *(U.S.P.)*. Cholesterol 3, stearyl alcohol 3, white beeswax 8, white soft paraffin 86.

Paraffin Gauze Dressing *(B.P.)*. Tulle Gras Dressing. A cotton, cotton and viscose, or viscose gauze, impregnated with yellow or white soft paraffin, sealed in suitable containers, and sterilised by a suitable sterilisation process. The degree of loading with paraffins may be 'light' or 'normal'. The soft paraffin may be replaced by a mixture of soft paraffin and hard paraffin when the dressing is required for use in tropical countries.
It is used in the treatment of wounds, such as burns and scalds, and for skin grafts.

Paraffin Ointment *(B.P.)*. Unguentum Paraffini. Hard paraffin 3, white beeswax 2, cetostearyl alcohol 5, and white soft paraffin 90. Store at a temperature not exceeding 25°.

Petrolatum Gauze *(U.S.P.)*. Sterilised absorbent cotton or cotton and viscose gauze saturated with sterilised white soft paraffin; it contains 70 to 80% by weight of soft paraffin.

Simple Eye Ointment *(B.P.)*. Eye Ointment Basis; Eye Ointment Base *(A.P.F.)*; Oculentum Base. Liquid paraffin 10, wool fat 10, yellow soft paraffin 80. Sterilised by maintaining at 150° for 1 hour; *A.P.F.* specifies 150° to 160° for not less than 2 hours.
In *B.P.* and *B.P.C. 1973* eye ointments intended for use in tropical or subtropical climates the proportion of paraffins may be varied or hard paraffin may be included when prevailing high temperatures would otherwise make the ointment too soft.
The *B.P.C. 1973* states that when Non-medicated Eye Ointment is ordered or prescribed, this ointment is supplied.

Simple Ointment *(B.P.)*. Unguentum Simplex; Ung. Simp. Wool fat 5, hard paraffin 5, cetostearyl alcohol 5, and white or yellow soft paraffin 85. Unless otherwise directed, when simple ointment is used in a white ointment it should be prepared with white soft paraffin and when used in a coloured ointment it should be prepared with yellow soft paraffin. Store at a temperature not exceeding 25°.
A.P.F. (Simple Ointment White) has the same formula made only with white soft paraffin.

White Ointment *(U.S.P.)*. White beeswax 5, white soft paraffin 95.

Yellow Ointment *(U.S.P.)*. Yellow beeswax 5 and yellow soft paraffin 95.

Proprietary Preparations

Diprobase *(Kirby-Warrick, UK)*. *Cream,* white soft paraffin 15%, liquid paraffin 6%, cetomacrogol '1000' 2.25%, cetostearyl alcohol 7.2%, chlorocresol 0.1%. *Ointment,* white soft paraffin 95%, liquid paraffin 5%. For dermatoses and for dilution of corticosteroid preparations.

Jelonet *(Smith & Nephew, UK)*. *Impregnated dressing,* Paraffin Gauze Dressing *(B.P.)*.

Lacri-Lube *(Allergan, UK)*. *Ophthalmic ointment,* white soft paraffin, liquid paraffin, lanolin derivatives, chlorbutol 0.5%.

Ultrabase *(Schering, UK)*. *Cream,* white soft paraffin, liquid paraffin, stearyl alcohol, polyoxyl 40 stearate.

Unguentum Merck *(E. Merck, UK)*. *Cream,* white soft paraffin 32%, liquid paraffin 3%, cetostearyl alcohol 9%, polysorbate '40' 8%, glyceryl monostearate 3%, propylene glycol 5%, saturated neutral oil 2%, silicic acid 0.1%, sorbic acid 0.2%. For use as an emollient and as a diluent for dermatological preparations.
Erythematous deterioration of psoriasis lesions in a 31-year-old woman receiving treatment was found to be due to sorbic acid present in Unguentum Merck used as a diluent of the steroid ointment prescribed.— E. M. Saihan and R. R. M. Harman, *Br. J. Derm.*, 1978, *99,* 583.

Proprietary Names and Manufacturers of White and Yellow Soft Paraffin

Dermosa Cusi Lubricante *(Spain)*; Jelonet *(Smith & Nephew, Austral.; Smith & Nephew, S.Afr.; Smith & Nephew, UK)*; Ocu-Lube *(Ocumed, USA)*; Paratulle *(Leo, S.Afr.)*; Peritex *(Southon-Horton, UK)*; Petro-Phylic *(Trans Canaderm, Canad.)*; Unitulle *(Roussel, Austral.)*.

The following names have been used for multi-ingredient preparations containing white and yellow soft paraffin—AKWA Tears Ointment *(Akorn, USA)*; Argobase EU *(Westbrook, UK)*; Diprobase *(Kirby-Warrick, UK)*; Duolube *(Charton, Canad.; Muro, USA)*; Duratears *(Alcon, Canad.; Alcon Laboratories, USA)*; HEB Waterproof *(Waterhouse, UK)*; Hypotears Ointment *(Coopervision, USA)*; Lacri-Lube *(Allergan, Austral.; Allergan, Canad.; Allergan, UK; Allergan, USA)*; Locobase Cream *(Brocades, UK)*; Lubrifair Ointment *(Pharmafair, USA)*; Prevex *(Trans Canaderm, Canad.)*; Tearfair Ointment *(Pharmafair, USA)*; Ultrabase *(Schering, UK)*; Unguentum Merck *(E. Merck, UK)*.

6406-z

Barrier Creams

The term 'barrier creams' is used to describe ointments, creams, or lotions that are applied to prevent damage to the skin. Barrier creams vary widely in composition. They should be non-irritant, easy to apply, easily washed off with soap and water, bacteriostatic, non-hygroscopic, non-transferable, non-sticky, and stable (to avoid the necessity of frequent application), and they must not act as heat insulators. There are many preparations available for use in different industries.

Proprietary Preparations

Kerodex *(Lever Industrial, UK)*. A range of water-resistant and water-soluble barrier creams.

Rozalex *(Sterling Health, UK)*. A range of water-resistant and oil-resistant barrier creams.

See also under Dimethicones, p.1325.

Proprietary Names and Manufacturers

HEB Waterproof *(Waterhouse, UK)*; Kerodex *(Lever Industrial, UK; Ayerst, USA)*; Rozalex *(Sterling Health, UK)*.

6407-c

White Beeswax *(BAN)*.

901 *(beeswax)*; Cêra Branca; Cera Alba; Cera Blanca; Cire Blanche; Gebleichtes Wachs; White Wax *(USAN)*.

CAS — 8012-89-3.

Pharmacopoeias. In *Arg., Aust., Belg., Br., Cz., Egypt., Eur., Fr., Ger., Hung., Ind., It., Jpn, Jug., Mex., Neth., Nord., Pol., Port., Roum., Span.,* and *Swiss.* Also in *U.S.N.F.* and *B.P. Vet.*

Bleached yellow beeswax. A white or yellowish-white solid, translucent in thin layers, with a faint characteristic odour. M.p. 61° to 65°. **Store** in well-closed containers.

6408-k

Yellow Beeswax *(BAN)*.

901 *(beeswax)*; Cêra Amarela; Cera Amarilla; Cera Flava; Cire Jaune; Gelbes Wachs; Yellow Wax *(USAN)*.

CAS — 8012-89-3.

Pharmacopoeias. In *Arg., Aust., Belg., Br., Chin., Egypt., Eur., Fr., Ger., Ind., It., Jpn, Jug., Mex., Neth., Nord., Pol., Port., Roum., Span.,* and *Swiss.* Also in *U.S.N.F.*

The wax obtained by melting with hot water the walls of the honeycomb of the bee, *Apis mellifera* (Apidae), and removing the foreign matter.

It is a yellow or light brown solid with an agreeable honey-like odour, brittle when cold, plastic when warmed in the hand. M.p. 61° to 65°.
B.P. **solubilities** are: practically insoluble in water; partially soluble in alcohol and in chloroform; completely soluble in fixed and volatile oils. *U.S.P.* solubilities are: insoluble in water; sparingly soluble in alcohol; completely soluble in chloroform, in ether, in fixed and volatile oils, and in warm carbon disulphide.
Store in well-closed containers.

Yellow beeswax is used as an ingredient of ointments and enables water to be incorporated to produce water-in-oil emulsions. White beeswax is similarly employed; it is occasionally used to adjust the melting-point of suppositories.
Hypersensitivity to beeswax has been reported.

Preparations

Cold Cream *(A.P.F.)*. Ceratum Hydrosum; Crem. Refrig. Oleos.; Ung. Refrig. White beeswax 17 g, liquid paraffin 45 g, borax 1 g, and freshly boiled and cooled water 37 mL.

Proprietary Preparations

Bonewax *(Ethicon, UK)*. *Surgical wax*, refined white beeswax 90%, isopropyl palmitate 10% in 2.5-g slabs, individually wrapped and sterilised.
This preparation should not be confused with Aseptic Surgical Wax *(B.P.C. 1949)*, also known as Bone Wax or Horsley's Wax, which contained yellow beeswax, olive oil, and phenol in a mercuric chloride solution and has also been used to prevent haemorrhage in cranial surgery.

Proprietary Names and Manufacturers

Gelucire 62/05 *(Alfa, UK)*.

6410-e

Cetostearyl Alcohol *(BAN, USAN)*.

Alcohol Cetylicus et Stearylicus; Cetostearyl Alc.; Cetylstearylalkohol.

CAS — 8005-44-5.

Pharmacopoeias. In *Aust*., *Belg*., *Br*., *Cz*., *Ger*., *Ind*., *Jug*., and *Roum*. Also in *U.S.N.F.* and *B.P. Vet*.

A mixture of solid aliphatic alcohols, mainly stearyl and cetyl alcohols, obtained by the reduction of the appropriate fatty acids, or from sperm oils. *U.S.N.F.* specifies not less than 90% of stearyl and cetyl alcohols and not less than 40% of stearyl alcohol.
A white or cream unctuous mass, or almost white flakes or granules, with a faint characteristic odour. It melts to a clear colourless or pale yellow liquid, free from cloudiness or suspended matter. The *B.P.* specifies a solidifying-point of 45° to 53°; the *U.S.N.F.* specifies a melting-point of 48° to 55°.
Practically **insoluble** in water; soluble in ether; less soluble in alcohol and petroleum spirit.
Store in well-closed containers.

The composition of cetostearyl alcohol.— A. W. Mace, *J. Pharm. Pharmac.*, 1975, *27*, 209.

Cetostearyl alcohol has similar properties to cetyl alcohol. In conjunction with suitable hydrophilic substances, such as sulphated fatty alcohols as in Emulsifying Wax (see p.1325) and cetomacrogol as in Cetomacrogol Emulsifying Wax (see p.1243), it produces oil-in-water emulsions which are stable over a wide pH range. It increases the viscosity of water-in-oil emulsions, thereby improving their stability, and improves the emollient properties of paraffin ointments.
Cetostearyl alcohol can cause hypersensitivity.

Proprietary Names and Manufacturers

Crodacols *(Croda, UK)*; Laurex CS *(Albright & Wilson, Marchon Division, UK)*.

6411-l

Cetyl Alcohol *(BAN, USAN)*.

1-Hexadecanol; Alcool Cetílico; Cetanol; Hexadecyl Alcohol.

CAS — 36653-82-4.

Pharmacopoeias. In *Aust*., *Br*., *Cz*., *Eur*., *Fr*., *Jpn*, *Jug*., *Neth*., *Nord*., *Port*., *Span*., and *Swiss*. Also in *U.S.N.F.*

A mixture of solid aliphatic alcohols consisting chiefly of cetyl alcohol, $C_{16}H_{33}OH$. *U.S.N.F.* specifies not less than 90% of cetyl alcohol, the remainder consisting chiefly of related alcohols.
It occurs as white unctuous flakes, cubes, or granules, with a faint characteristic odour. The *B.P.* specifies a melting-point of 46° to 52°; the *U.S.N.F.* specifies 45° to 50°.
Practically **insoluble** in water; freely to sparingly soluble in alcohol; freely soluble in ether; miscible when melted with animal and vegetable oils, liquid paraffin, and melted wool fat. **Store** in well-closed containers.

Cetyl alcohol is used as a constituent of ointments and creams, especially those in which it is desired to incorporate water or an aqueous solution. It can cause hypersensitivity.

Proprietary Names and Manufacturers

Crodacols *(Croda, UK)*; Laurex 16 *(Albright & Wilson, Marchon Division, UK)*.

6412-y

Cholesterol *(USAN)*.

Cholesterin. Cholest-5-en-3β-ol.
$C_{27}H_{46}O$=386.7.

CAS — 57-88-5.

Pharmacopoeias. In *Aust*., *Braz*., *Cz*., *Fr*., *Jpn*, *Pol*., *Roum*., and *Span*. Also in *U.S.N.F.*

White or faintly yellow, almost odourless, pearly leaflets, needles, powder, or granules. It acquires a yellow to pale tan colour on prolonged exposure to light. Wool Alcohols (see p.1327) contains not less than 30% of cholesterol.
Insoluble in water; slowly soluble 1 in 100 of alcohol and 1 in 50 of dehydrated alcohol; soluble in acetone, chloroform, dioxan, ether, ethyl acetate, light petroleum, and vegetable oils. **Store** in well-closed containers. Protect from light.

Cholesterol imparts water-absorbing power to ointments and is used as an emulsifying agent.
Cholesterol has a physiological role.

Topical cholesterol treatment of recessive x-linked ichthyosis: G. Lykkesfeldt and H. Høyer, *Lancet*, 1983, *2*, 1337; H. H. Ibsen *et al.* (letter), *ibid*., 1984, *2*, 645.

6413-j

Coconut Oil *(BAN)*.

Aceite de Coco; Coconut Butter; Oleum Cocois; Oleum Cocos Raffinatum; Oleum Cocosis.

CAS — 8001-31-8.

Pharmacopoeias. In *Br*. and *Jpn*.

A white or pearl-white unctuous mass, odourless or with an odour of coconut, obtained by expression from the dried solid part of the endosperm of the coconut, the fruit of *Cocos nucifera* (Palmae). M.p. 23° to 26°.
Soluble 1 in 2 of alcohol (at 60°); freely soluble in chloroform and in ether. It readily becomes rancid on exposure to air. **Store** at a temperature not exceeding 25° in well-filled well-closed containers. Protect from light.

NOTE. Fractionated coconut oil is used as a source of medium-chain triglycerides, see p.1560.

Coconut oil forms a readily absorbable ointment basis. Coconut-oil soaps are not easily precipitated by sodium chloride and have been used as sea-water soaps.

A study of 28 patients suggesting that topical application of coconut oil might alter the cutaneous bacterial flora, allowing dominance of *Pityrosporum* spp. and the development of pityriasis versicolor.— V. K. Dave *et al.* (letter), *Lancet*, 1987, *2*, 685.

Proprietary Names and Manufacturers

Cobee *(PVO International, USA*: *Alfa, UK)*.

6428-r

Dimethicones *(BAN)*.

900; Dimethicone *(USAN)*; Dimethyl Silicone Fluid; Dimethylpolysiloxane; Dimethylsiloxane; Dimeticone *(rINN)*; Dimeticonum; Huile de Silicone; Methyl Polysiloxane; Permethylpolysiloxane; Silicone Oil; Siliconum Liquidum.
Poly(dimethylsiloxane).
$CH_3.[Si(CH_3)_2.O]_nSi(CH_3)_3$.

CAS — 9006-65-9.

Pharmacopoeias. In *Br*., *Chin*., *Eur*., *Fr*., *It*., *Neth*., and *Swiss*. Also in *U.S.N.F.* and *B.P. Vet*. *U.S.N.F.* lists requirements for a range of different types of dimethicone.

Dimethicone may be prepared by hydrolysing a mixture of dichlorodimethylsilane, $(CH_3)_2SiCl_2$, and chlorotrimethylsilane, $(CH_3)_3SiCl$. The products of hydrolysis contain active silanol groups (SiOH) through which condensation polymerisation proceeds. By varying the proportion of chlorotrimethylsilane, which acts as a chain terminator, silicones of varying molecular weight may be prepared.
As the molecular weight increases, the products become more viscous, and fluids are available throughout the viscosity range of 0.65 centistokes to 3 million centistokes. The various grades are distinguished by numbers, each number approximately corresponding to the viscosity in centistokes.
Clear colourless, odourless liquids, **immiscible** with water, alcohol, acetone, and methyl alcohol, and miscible with chlorinated hydrocarbons, ether, and xylene; very slightly soluble in absolute alcohol and isopropyl alcohol; also miscible with amyl acetate, cyclohexane, kerosene, toluene, and ethyl acetate. Their viscosities, in centistokes, at 25° are: dimethicone '20'—18 to 22; dimethicone '200'—190 to 220; dimethicone '350'—332.5 to 367.5; dimethicone '500'—475 to 525. **Store** in airtight containers.

Adverse Effects

Injection of silicones, including dimethicones, into tissues may cause a granulomatous reaction.

White plugs which contained fat, dimethicone, and silica were found in the retinal vessels of 2 patients who underwent open-heart surgery. A defoaming agent containing dimethicone fluid and silica gel (Antifoam A, *Dow Corning*) had been used in the perfusion.— I. M. Williams, *Br. J. Ophthal.*, 1975, *59*, 81.

Migration of silicone and granulomatous hepatitis occurred in 2 patients who had received silicone injections to the breasts, malar areas, and trochanters. Another developed rock-hard red breasts with skin changes and an enlarged liver after injections of silicone to the breasts. A fourth patient died shortly after receiving silicone injections to the breasts; death appeared to result from severe bilateral pulmonary oedema.— R. Ellenbogen *et al.*, *J. Am. med. Ass.*, 1975, *234*, 308.

An estimate that at least 12 000 women in the Las Vegas area had received 'bootleg silicone injections' (using a nonmedical-grade silicone) mostly in the breast area for cosmetic purposes, at least 1% of them developed complications each year. Infections which had occurred after the injections usually developed within a short time but had been reported up to 5 years later. Some infections responded to antibiotic therapy while others resulted in necrosis and sloughing of the skin and involved tissue. Migration of the injected material had occasionally occurred. Cyst formation was probably the most frequent complication occurring either shortly after injection or years later. Granuloma formation was less common but was considered to be a more formidable problem and was sometimes accompanied by skin changes including pigment changes, lymphoedema, silicoma of the skin, vesicle formation, and ulceration. Complications occurred irrespective of the site and had developed up to 9 years later. Medical-grade silicone was probably little safer than other types of silicone.— E. H. Kopf *et al.*, *Rocky Mtn med. J.*, 1976, *73*, 77.

Over a period of 10 years 92 patients received injections of medical-grade silicone. Granulomas subsequently developed in 13 injection sites, usually within 1 year but some took a few years to develop and one appeared after 7 years.— T. F. Wilkie, *Plastic reconstr. Surg.*, 1977, *60*, 179.

Malignant lymphoma with intranodal refractile particles after insertion of silicone prostheses.— J. M. Digby and A. L. Wells (letter), *Lancet*, 1981, *2*, 580.

Refractile particles in the livers of haemodialysis patients. Silicone used in the dialysis equipment might have been the cause.— A. S. -Y. Leong *et al.* (letter), *Lancet*, 1981, *1*, 889. Silicone-induced splenomegaly in a dialysis patient. The dialysis equipment contained silicone and histologic examination showed foreign-body inclusions in the spleen.— J. Bommer *et al.*, *New Engl. J. Med.*, 1981, *305*, 1077.

Discussion of the complications of long-term silicone implant arthroplasty, including synovitis and lymphadenopathy: R. M. Nalbandian *et al.*, *J. Am. med. Ass.*, 1983, *250*, 1195. Comment: A. R. Schned *et al.* (letter), *ibid.*, 1985, *253*, 635.

Acute pneumonitis after subcutaneous injections of silicone.— J. Chastre *et al.*, *New Engl. J. Med.*, 1983, *308*, 764. A reminder of an earlier report (B. Celli *et al.*, *Am. J. med. Sci.*, 1978, *275*, 81) in which a patient developed adult respiratory distress syndrome after subcutaneous injection of silicone for mammary augmentation.— B. R. Celli and D. M. Kovnat (letter), *ibid.*, *309*, 856. Comment.— J. Chastre *et al.* (letter), *ibid.*, 857. Comment on silicone pneumonitis.— *Lancet*, 1983, *2*, 833. A report of bilateral pleural effusions in a 40-year-old woman after the implantation of silicone breast prostheses.— J. M. Manresa and F. Manresa (letter), *ibid.*, 1373.

Hypercalcaemia associated with silicone-induced granulomas.— G. A. Kozeny *et al.*, *New Engl. J. Med.*, 1984, *311*, 1103. Comment.— J. Lemann and R. W. Gray, *ibid.*, 1115.

Widespread florid urticaria developed in a 20-year-old patient immediately after the use of Silastic foam dressing as a wound packing, and resolved within 24 hours of its removal.— C. W. Pattison and S. C. Kennedy, *Br. med. J.*, 1985, *290*, 1394. Comment. The authors had not met an example of allergy to Silastic foam in 21 years' experience. Allergy was most likely due not to the foam itself, but to residual catalyst or an organic acid produced during the curing process. These substances could be removed by a thorough initial flushing with water.— L. E. Hughes *et al.* (letter), *ibid.*, *291*, 1052.

Silastic foam dressing had been taken off the market in Germany because of suggestions of carcinogenic effects in *animal* studies.— *Pharm. J.*, 1987, *2*, 157. Inflammatory carcinoma of the breast following silicone injections for cosmetic purposes has been reported (C.M. Lewis, *Plastic reconstr. Surg.*, 1980, *66*, 134). Silastic breast prostheses have been linked with subsequent tumours, but a causal association was unlikely (D.G. Bowers and C.B. Radlauer, *ibid.*, 1969, *4*, 541; M. Johnson and H.E.D. Lloyd, *ibid.*, 1974, *53*, 88; T. de Cholnoky, *ibid.*, 1970, *45*, 573).— G. E. Diggle, *Adverse Drug React. Bull.*, 1987, (Jun.), 464.

Uses and Administration

Dimethicones and silicones are water-repellent and have a low surface tension. They are used in barrier creams for protecting the skin against water-soluble irritants. Creams, lotions, and ointments containing 10 to 30% of a dimethicone are employed for the prevention of bedsores and napkin rash and to protect the skin against trauma due to incontinence or colostomy discharge.

Silicone preparations should not be applied where free drainage is necessary or to inflamed or abraded skin. Silicones are also used topically as wound dressings.

Silicones are used as lubricants for hypodermic syringes. Glassware may be coated with a thin film of silicone, allowing solutions and suspensions to be drained completely.

Silicones have also been tried by intra-articular injection in rheumatic disorders, by intra-ocular injection for retinal detachment, and by subcutaneous injection or implantation in plastic surgery.

Dimethicones and simethicone (activated dimethicone) are used in the treatment of flatulence, see p.1106.

Tentative estimated acceptable daily intake of dimethicones with a relative molecular mass in the range of 200 to 300: up to 1.5 mg per kg body-weight.— Twenty-third Report of the Joint FAO/WHO Expert Committee on Food Additives, *Tech. Rep. Ser. Wld Hlth Org. No. 648*, 1980.

SURGICAL PROCEDURES. References to the use of silicones in plastic surgery: R. C. Webster *et al.*, *Arch. Otolaryngol. Head Neck Surg.*, 1986, *112*, 269 and 290.

WOUND DRESSINGS. The use of silicone foam sponge as a wound dressing.— R. A. B. Wood and L. E. Hughes, *Br. med. J.*, 1975, *4*, 131. See also J. Macfie and J. McMahon, *Br. J. Surg.*, 1980, *67*, 85; R. H. P. Williams *et al.*, *Br. med. J.*, 1981, *282*, 21; T. Gledhill and W. E. Waterfall, *Can. med. Ass. J.*, 1983, *128*, 685.

Preparations

Dimethicone Cream *(B.P.C. 1973)*. Cremor Dimethiconi; Crem. Dimethic.; Dimethicone Cream Aqueous *(A.P.F.)*; Silicone Cream. Dimethicone '350' 10 g, chlorocresol 100 mg, cetrimide 500 mg, cetostearyl alcohol 5 g, liquid paraffin 40 g, and freshly boiled and cooled water 44.4 g. Store in a cool place in well-closed containers.

Proprietary Preparations

Rikospray Silicone *(Riker, UK)*. *Dressing*, aerosol spray, aldioxa 0.5%, cetylpyridinium chloride 0.02%, in a basis of dimethicone '1000'. For bedsores and napkin rash and for colostomy hygiene.

Silastic Foam Dressing *(Dow Corning, UK)*. *Dressing*, silicone polymer foam, supplied as liquid silicone base with stannous octoate as a curing agent. For the management of open granulating wounds.

Siopel *(Care, UK)*. *Cream*, dimethicone 10%, cetrimide 0.3%. For protection of the skin in occupational dermatoses and incontinence, and in colostomy and similar conditions.

Sprilon *(Pharmacia, UK)*. *Dressing*, aerosol spray, dimethicone 1.2 g, zinc oxide 14.4 g, and ointment basis to 60 g. For eczema and leg ulcers, the prevention of bedsores, and protection of the skin in incontinence.

Translet *(Franklin Medical, UK)*. *Cream*, dimethicone 2.5%, stearic acid 18.5%, liquid paraffin 3.2%, glyceryl monostearate 0.5%, propylene glycol alginate 0.5%, glycerol 2.1%. For protection of the skin in colostomy and similar conditions.

Vasogen *(Pharmax, UK)*. *Cream*, dimethicone 20%, zinc oxide 7.5%, calamine 1.5%. For bedsores, napkin rash, and dermatoses.

Proprietary Names and Manufacturers of Dimethicones and other Silicones

Aero-Red *(Rocador, Spain)*; Aerosilane *(Spain)*; Barriere *(Allen & Hanburys, Canad.)*; Ceolat *(Kali-Chemie, Denm.*; *Kali-Chemie, Ger.*; *Neth.*; *Kali-Chemie, Norw.*; *Kali-Chemie, Swed.*; *Switz.)*; Dermafilm *(Parke, Davis, Austral.)*; Dermalase-S *(Hamilton, Austral.)*; Dimethicream *(Hamilton, Austral.)*; Dimetikon *(ACO, Swed.)*; Dipoxane *(Jpn)*; Dow Corning 360 Medical Fluid *(Dow Corning, UK)*; Dow Corning Antifoam M Compound *(Dow Corning, UK)*; Elugan *(Menadier, Ger.)*; Factor A-G Comprimidos *(Arg.)*; Hamilton Skin Repair Cream *(Hamilton, Austral.)*; Instru-Safe *(Eagle, Austral.)*; Nogasilan *(Spain)*; Ovol *(Horner, Canad.)*; Polisilon *(Midy, Ital.)*; Polysilane *(Gamaprod, Austral.*; *Midy, Fr.*; *Clin-Midy, Switz.)*; Polysilon Gel *(Belg.)*; Protecto-Derm *(Ingram & Bell, Canad.)*; Repelcote *(Hopkin & Williams, UK)*; Savlon Hand Care *(ICI, Austral.)*; Silastic 382 Medical Grade Elastomer *(Dow Corning, UK)*; Silastic Foam Dressing *(Dow Corning, UK)*; Silbar *(Sigma, Austral.)*; Silcon *(Faulding, Austral.)*; Silic 15 *(Ego, Austral.)*; Silican *(Lafare, Ital.)*; Silicone Fluids F 111 *(ICI Organics, UK)*; Silicone Skin Spray *(Eagle, Austral.)*; Siligaz *(Fr.)*; Siopel *(ICI, Austral.*; *S.Afr.*; *Care, UK)*; Skin Repair *(Rosken, Austral.)*; Stuart Silicone Protective *(Stuart, UK)*.

The following names have been used for multi-ingredient preparations containing dimethicones and other silicones—Barriere-HC *(Allen & Hanburys, Canad.)*; Complex-15 *(Dormer, Canad.)*; Conotrane *(Boehringer Ingelheim, UK)*; Epicare *(Rosken, Austral.)*; Prevex *(Trans Canaderm, Canad.)*; Rikospray Silicone *(Riker, UK)*; Silicone 555 *(Aerosol Marketing & Chemical Co., UK)*; Silon *(Pharmacia, Canad.)*; Sprilon *(Pharmacia, UK)*; Syl *(Reckitt & Colman Pharmaceuticals, UK)*; Translet Skin Cream *(Franklin Medical, UK)*; Vasogen *(Pharmax, UK)*.

NOTE. The name Ostomy Plus Three has been used to denote the preparation now known in the *UK* as Translet Skin Cream.

6021-r

Emulsifying Wax *(BAN)*.

Anionic Emulsifying Wax; Cera Emulsificans; Cetylanum; Emulsif. Wax.

CAS — 8014-38-8.

Pharmacopoeias. In *Br.*, *Ind.*, *Jug.*, *Nord.*, and *Swiss*. *Belg. P.* has cetostearyl alcohol 9 parts and sodium cetostearyl sulphate 1 part. *Ger. P.* has cetostearyl alcohol about 12.5 parts and sodium cetostearyl sulphate 1 part.

For Emulsifying Wax (*U.S.N.F.*), see under Polysorbates, p.1247.

It is prepared from 9 parts of cetostearyl alcohol and 1 part of sodium lauryl sulphate or sodium salts of similar sulphated higher primary aliphatic alcohols.

It is an almost white or pale yellow waxy solid or flakes, becoming plastic when warm, with a faint characteristic odour. Practically **insoluble** in water, forming an emulsion; partly soluble in alcohol.

Emulsifying wax added to fatty or paraffin bases facilitates the preparation of oil-in-water emulsions which are absorbed, are non-greasy when rubbed into the skin, and protect against dirt and grease. It is a constituent of many hydrophilic ointment bases for so-called 'washable' ointments.

Preparations

Aqueous Cream *(B.P.)*. It may be prepared from emulsifying ointment 30 g, phenoxyethanol 1 g, and freshly boiled and cooled water 69 g. Store at a temperature not exceeding 25° in well-closed containers which minimise evaporation and contamination. *A.P.F.* specifies the addition of glycerol 5% and permits the replacement of phenoxyethanol by chlorocresol 100 mg.

Aqueous cream is sometimes known as hydrous emulsifying ointment or as simple cream.

The liability of aqueous cream (*B.P.* 1980) to microbial spoilage.— T. R. R. Kurup and L. S. C. Wan, *Pharm. J.*, 1986, *2*, 761.

Buffered Cream *(B.P.)*. Buffered Cream Aqueous *(A.P.F.)*. Sodium phosphate 2.5 g, citric acid monohydrate 500 mg, chlorocresol 100 mg, emulsifying ointment 30 g, and freshly boiled and cooled water 66.9 g. pH 5.7 to 6.3. Store at a temperature not exceeding 25° in well-closed containers which minimise evaporation and contamination. Aluminium containers should be internally lacquered.

A reformulation of buffered cream (*B.P.* 1980) suitable for the tropics.— L. S. C. Wan (letter), *Pharm. J.*, 1984, *2*, 508.

Emulsifying Ointment *(B.P., A.P.F.)*. Emulsifying wax 3, white soft paraffin 5, and liquid paraffin 2, all by wt. Store at a temperature not exceeding 25°.

Proprietary Names and Manufacturers

Collone HV *(ABM Chemicals, UK)*; Collone SE *(ABM Chemicals, UK)*; Collone SEC *(ABM Chemicals, UK)*; Crodex A *(Croda, UK)*; Cyclochem *(Witco, UK)*; Cyclonette Wax *(Witco, UK)*; Empiwax SK *(Albright & Wilson, Marchon Division, UK)*; Empiwax SK/BP *(Albright & Wilson, Marchon Division, UK)*; Lanette Wax SX *(Ronsheim & Moore, UK)*.

6415-c

Hard Fat *(BAN)*.

Adeps Neutralis; Adeps Solidus; Glycérides Semi-synthétiques Solides; Hartfett; Massa Estearínica; Neutralfett.

Pharmacopoeias. In *Aust.*, *Belg.*, *Br.*, *Eur.*, *Fr.*, *Ger.*,

Hung., It., Neth., Nord., Port., and *Swiss.* Also in *U.S.N.F.* and *B.P. Vet.*

A mixture of mono-, di-, and triglycerides of the saturated fatty acids $C_9H_{19}COOH$ to $C_{17}H_{35}COOH$.

A white brittle, solid which is greasy to the touch, almost odourless and free from rancid odour. The *B.P.* specifies a melting point of 33° to 36°; the *U.S.N.F.* specifies 27° to 44°. The melted substance is colourless or slightly yellowish and forms a stable white emulsion when shaken with an equal amount of hot water.

Practically **insoluble** in water; slightly soluble in alcohol; freely soluble in ether. **Store** in airtight containers. Protect from light.

The name Hard Fat is applied to a range of bases with varying degrees of hardness and differing melting ranges used for the preparation of suppositories.

Proprietary Names and Manufacturers

Coberine *(Loders & Nucoline, UK)*; Massa Estarinum *(Dynamit Nobel, UK)*; Massuppol *(Loders & Nucoline, UK)*; Suppocire *(Alfa, UK)*; Witepsol Suppository Bases *(Dynamit Nobel, UK)*.

6416-k

Isopropyl Myristate *(BAN, USAN).*

Isopropyl Myrist.

$(CH_3)_2CH.O.CO.(CH_2)_{12}.CH_3=270.5$.

CAS — 110-27-0.

Pharmacopoeias. In *Aust.* and *Br.* Also in *U.S.N.F.* which specifies esters of isopropyl alcohol and saturated high molecular weight fatty acids, principally myristic acid; it contains not less than 90% of $C_{17}H_{34}O_2$. *U.S.N.F.* also includes isopropyl palmitate.

A clear colourless or almost colourless, almost odourless, mobile oily liquid. F.p. about 5°.

Insoluble in water, glycerol, and propylene glycol; soluble 1 in 3 of alcohol; miscible with liquid hydrocarbons, fixed oils, and most organic solvents. **Store** in airtight containers. Protect from light.

Isopropyl myristate is resistant to oxidation and hydrolysis and does not become rancid; it is free from irritant and sensitising properties and is absorbed fairly readily by the skin.

It may be used in external preparations in place of vegetable oils, and in emollient ointments and creams, yielding products which are relatively free from greasiness.

It is a solvent for many substances applied externally and is of value as a vehicle when direct contact and penetration of the medicament are required.

Other isopropyl fatty acid esters, including di-isopropyl adipate, isopropyl laurate, isopropyl linoleate, and isopropyl palmitate have similar properties and are used for similar purposes to those of isopropyl myristate.

Proprietary Preparations

Emulsiderm *(Dermal Laboratories, UK). Emulsion,* isopropyl myristate 25%, liquid paraffin 25%, benzalkonium chloride 0.5%. For skin application or as a bath additive in dry skin conditions.

Proprietary Names and Manufacturers of Isopropyl Fatty Acid Esters

Ceraphyl 230 *(Van Dyk, USA : Black, UK)*; Ceraphyl IPL *(Van Dyk, USA : Black, UK)*; Crodamol DA *(Croda, UK)*; Crodamol IPL *(Croda, UK)*; Crodamol IPM *(Croda, UK)*; Crodamol IPP *(Croda, UK)*; Lexol IPP-NF *(Black, UK)*; Promyr *(Amerchol, USA : Anstead, UK)*; Propal *(Amerchol, USA : Anstead, UK)*.

The following names have been used for multi-ingredient preparations containing isopropyl fatty acid esters—Domol *(Miles, Canad.; Miles Pharmaceuticals, USA)*; Emulsiderm *(Dermal Laboratories, UK)*; Hydromol *(Quinoderm, UK)*; Hydromol Emollient *(Quinoderm, UK)*.

16870-s

Laurocapram *(USAN, rINN).*

N-0252. 1-Dodecylazacycloheptan-2-one; 1-Dodecylhexahydro-2*H*-azepin-2-one.

$C_{18}H_{35}NO=281.5$.

CAS — 59277-89-3.

Laurocapram has been used to enhance the penetration of drugs through the skin.

References: S. L. Spruance *et al., Antimicrob. Ag. Chemother.,* 1984, *26,* 819 (increased penetration of trifluridine through human and *animal* skin); P. K. Wotton *et al., Int. J. Pharmaceut.,* 1985, *24,* 19 (increased penetration of metronidazole through human skin *in vitro*); K. S. Ryatt *et al., J. pharm. Sci.,* 1986, *75,* 374 (increased percutaneous penetration of hexyl nicotinate in healthy subjects); A. Kumar *et al., Curr. ther. Res.,* 1987, *41,* 802 (increased percutaneous penetration of acyclovir in *animals*).

6422-z

Microcrystalline Wax *(USAN).*

907 *(refined microcrystalline wax).*

Pharmacopoeias. In *Fr.* and *Swiss.* Also in *U.S.N.F.*

A mixture of straight-chain, branched-chain, and cyclic hydrocarbons, obtained by solvent fractionation of the still bottom fraction of petroleum by suitable dewaxing or de-oiling means.

A white or cream-coloured odourless waxy solid. Melting range 54° to 102°. **Insoluble** in water; sparingly soluble in dehydrated alcohol; soluble in chloroform, ether, volatile oils, and in most warm fixed oils. **Store** in airtight containers. Ceresin is a mixture of solid hydrocarbons obtained by the purification of ozokerite, a naturally occurring solid paraffin.

Microcrystalline wax is a stiffening agent and tablet-coating agent.

6423-c

Oleyl Alcohol *(USAN).*

CAS — 143-28-2.

Pharmacopoeias. In *U.S.N.F.*

A mixture of unsaturated and saturated high molecular weight fatty alcohols consisting chiefly of oleyl alcohol, $C_{18}H_{36}O = 268.5$.

A clear colourless to light yellow oily liquid with a faint characteristic odour. **Insoluble** in water; soluble in alcohol, ether, isopropyl alcohol, and light liquid paraffin. **Store** at 15° to 30° in well-filled airtight containers.

Oleyl alcohol has been used as an emulsion stabiliser and as a skin emollient.

Oleic acid and oleyl alcohol each enhanced the penetration of acyclovir in propylene glycol across human skin *in vitro.*— E. R. Cooper *et al., J. pharm. Sci.,* 1985, *74,* 688.

Proprietary Names and Manufacturers

Novol *(Croda, UK).*

The following names have been used for multi-ingredient preparations containing oleyl alcohol— Polytar Liquid *(Stiefel, Austral.; Stiefel, UK)*; Polytar Plus *(Stiefel, UK)*.

6425-a

Fractionated Palm Kernel Oil *(BAN).*

Pharmacopoeias. In *Br.* The standards of the *B.P.* monograph encompass several different suppository bases.

A white, solid, odourless or almost odourless, brittle fat, obtained by selective solvent fractionation and hydrogenation of the natural oil from the kernels of *Elaeis guineensis* (Palmae). M.p. 31° to 36°.

Practically **insoluble** in water and alcohol; miscible with chloroform, ether, and petroleum spirit. **Store** at a temperature not exceeding 25°.

Fractionated palm kernel oil is used as a basis for suppositories. It has also been used in chocolate. The unfractionated oil has been used as an ointment basis.

Proprietary Names and Manufacturers

Extracoa *(Loders & Nucoline, UK)*; Supercoa *(Loders & Nucoline, UK)*.

13235-b

Shea Butter

A natural fat obtained from the shea tree *Butyrospermum parkii* (Sapotaceae) indigenous to W. Africa.

Shea butter is used as an ointment and cream basis.

Physico-chemical properties of shea butter.— H. C. Mital and F. R. Dove, *Planta med.,* 1971, *20,* 283.

Pharmaceutical and cosmetic applications of creams and ointments prepared from shea butter.— H. C. Mital, *Drug Cosmet. Ind.,* 1977, *120* (May), 30.

Salicylic acid and benzoic acid were released from an ointment basis prepared from shea butter 75%, arachis oil 25%, and hard paraffin 10% at a faster rate than from white soft paraffin *B.P.* or simple ointment *B.P.*— G. H. Konning and H. C. Mital, *J. pharm. Sci.,* 1978, *67,* 374.

NASAL DECONGESTION. Shea butter was an effective nasal decongestant when applied to the nostrils of 21 subjects suffering from allergic rhinitis. The airways cleared within 0.5 to 1.5 minutes of application and remained clear for 5 to 8.5 hours. Xylometazoline 0.1% cleared the nasal airways within 1 minute of application and the effect lasted for 2 to 4.5 hours in 7 similar patients. Shea butter did not irritate the nasal mucosa or cause rebound congestion.— A. Tella, *Br. J. clin. Pharmac.,* 1979, *7,* 495.

6429-f

Spermaceti

Blanc de Baleine; Cetaceum; Cire de Cachalot; Esperma de Ballena; Espermacete; Walrat.

CAS — 8002-23-1.

Pharmacopoeias. In *Arg., Aust., Belg., Cz., Egypt., Fr., Hung., It., Jug., Nord., Pol., Port., Roum., Span.,* and *Turk.*

A solid wax obtained from the mixed oils from the head, blubber, and carcase of the sperm whale, *Physeter catodon* (=*P. macrocephalus*) (Physeteridae), and the bottle-nosed whale, *Hyperoödon rostratus* (Ziphiidae).

COMPOSITION. An accurate description of the composition of spermaceti, based on thin-layer and gas chromatography, would be a mixture of hexadecyl (cetyl) esters of fatty acids between C_{26} and C_{38} with cetyl laurate, cetyl myristate, cetyl palmitate, and cetyl stearate comprising at least 85% of the total esters.— P. J. Holloway, *J. Pharm. Pharmac.,* 1968, *20,* 775.

6430-z

Cetyl Esters Wax *(USAN).*

Synthetic Spermaceti.

Pharmacopoeias. In *U.S.N.F.*

A mixture consisting primarily of esters of saturated fatty alcohols (C_{14} to C_{18}) and saturated fatty acids (C_{14} to C_{18}). White to off-white translucent flakes with a crystalline structure and a pearly lustre when caked; it has a faint odour. M.p. 43° to 47°.

Insoluble in water; practically insoluble in cold alcohol; soluble in chloroform, ether, fixed and volatile oils, and boiling alcohol. **Store** in well-closed containers in a dry place at a temperature not exceeding 40°.

Spermaceti has been used as an ingredient of some cold creams; a synthetic version is now used.

Preparations

Cold Cream *(U.S.P.).* Cetyl esters wax 12.5 g, white beeswax 12 g, liquid paraffin 56 g, borax 500 mg, water 19 mL.

Proprietary Names and Manufacturers

Crodamol SS *(Croda, UK)*; Cyclol SPS *(Witco, UK)*.

6431-c

Squalane *(USAN).*

Cosbiol; Dodecahydrosqualene; Perhydrosqualène; Spinacane. 2,6,10,15,19,23-Hexamethyltetracosane.

$C_{30}H_{62}=422.8$.

CAS — 111-01-3.

Pharmacopoeias. In *Fr.* Also in *U.S.N.F.*

A saturated hydrocarbon obtained by hydrogenation of squalene, an aliphatic triterpene occurring in some fish oils.

It is a colourless, almost odourless, transparent oil. **Insoluble** in water; very slightly soluble in dehydrated alcohol; miscible with chloroform and with ether; slightly soluble in acetone. **Store** in well-closed containers.

Squalane is miscible with human sebum of which it may possibly be a constituent. It is used as an ingredient of ointment bases to which it imparts increased skin permeability.

Proprietary Preparations

Dermalex *(Labaz Sanofi, UK). Skin lotion,* squalane 3%, hexachlorophane 0.5%, allantoin 0.25%. For prevention of bedsores and for incontinence rash.

Natuderm *(Leo, UK). Cream,* emollient, with a lipid component stated to be similar in composition to human sebum.

Proprietary Names and Manufacturers

Natuderm *(Leo, UK)*; Robane *(Robeco Chemicals, USA: Anstead, UK)*.

6432-k

Stearyl Alcohol *(USAN).*

Alcool Stéarylique; Octadecyl Alcohol.

CAS — 112-92-5.

Pharmacopoeias. In *Fr., It.,* and *Jpn.* Also in *U.S.N.F.*

The *U.S.N.F.* specifies not less than 90% of stearyl alcohol $C_{18}H_{37}OH$, the remainder consisting chiefly of related alcohols.

White unctuous flakes or granules with a faint characteristic odour. M.p. 55° to 60°. **Insoluble** in water; soluble in alcohol and ether. **Store** in well-closed containers.

Stearyl alcohol is used to thicken ointments and creams and to increase their water-holding capacity. It can cause hypersensitivity.

Proprietary Names and Manufacturers

Crodacols *(Croda, UK)*; Laurex 18 *(Albright & Wilson, Marchon Division, UK)*.

6435-x

Theobroma Oil *(BAN).*

Beurre de Cacao; Burro di Cacao; Butyrum Cacao; Cacao Butter; Cocoa Butter *(USAN)*; Kakaobutter; Manteca de Cacao; Manteiga de Cacau; Ol. Theobrom.; Oleum Cacao; Oleum Theobromatis.

CAS — 8002-31-1.

Pharmacopoeias. In *Arg., Aust., Belg., Br., Cz., Egypt., Fr., Ger., Hung., It., Jpn, Jug., Mex., Neth., Nord., Pol., Port., Roum., Rus., Span.,* and *Turk.* Also in *U.S.N.F.* and *B.P. Vet.*

A solid fat expressed from the roasted seeds of *Theobroma cacao* (Sterculiaceae). It is a yellowish-white, somewhat brittle solid with a slight odour of cocoa. M.p. 31° to 34°.

Slightly **soluble** in alcohol; freely soluble in chloroform, ether, and petroleum spirit; soluble in boiling dehydrated alcohol. **Store** in well-closed containers at a temperature not exceeding 25°.

Theobroma oil is employed as a basis for suppositories and similar dosage forms. Theobroma oil exhibits polymorphism and if the basis is heated to more than 36° during preparation the solidification point will be appreciably lowered due to the formation of metastable states, leading to subsequent difficulty in setting. White beeswax is sometimes used to increase the melting-point of theobroma oil.

It is a major ingredient of chocolate.

6436-r

Wool Alcohols *(BAN).*

Alcoholia Lanae; Alcolanum; Lanalcolum; Lanolin Alcohols *(USAN)*; Wollwachsalkohole; Wool Wax Alcohols.

CAS — 8027-33-6.

Pharmacopoeias. In *Aust., Br., Cz., Egypt., Ger., Hung., Jug., Roum.,* and *Swiss.* Also in *U.S.N.F.*

A golden-brown solid, somewhat brittle when cold but plastic when warm, with a faint characteristic odour. The *B.P.* specifies m.p. not below 58°; the *U.S.N.F.* specifies not below 56°. It consists of the alcoholic fraction of the product obtained by saponification of the wool grease of the sheep, and contains not less than 30% of cholesterol. The *B.P.* specifies 500 to 1000 ppm of butylated hydroxytoluene as an antoxidant; the *U.S.N.F.* permits up to 1000 ppm of a suitable antoxidant. It also contains 10 to 13% of isocholesterol with other steroid and triterpene alcohols.

Practically **insoluble** or insoluble in water; slightly soluble in alcohol; completely soluble 1 in 25 of boiling dehydrated alcohol; freely soluble in chloroform, ether, and petroleum spirit. **Store** in well-closed containers at a temperature not exceeding 25°. Protect from light.

Wool alcohols is used in the preparation of water-in-oil creams and ointments.

The addition of 5% of wool alcohols permits a threefold increase in the amount of water which can be incorporated in soft paraffin and such emulsions are not 'cracked' by the addition of weak acids.

Wool alcohols may cause hypersensitivity.

Preparations

Hydrous Ointment *(B.P.).* Oily Cream *(A.P.F.)*; Unguentum Aquosum; Ung. Aquos.; Wool Alcohols Cream. Wool alcohols ointment 50 g, phenoxyethanol 1 g, dried magnesium sulphate 500 mg, water 48.5 g.

Store at a temperature not exceeding 25° in non-absorbent containers. Any aqueous liquid which separates may be reincorporated by stirring. When hydrous ointment is used in a white ointment it should be prepared from wool alcohols ointment made with white soft paraffin and when used in a coloured ointment it should be prepared from wool alcohols ointment made with yellow soft paraffin.

Wool Alcohols Ointment *(B.P.).* Ung. Alcoh. Lan. Wool Alcohols 6%, with hard paraffin, white soft paraffin or yellow soft paraffin, and liquid paraffin. The proportions of the paraffins may be varied to produce an ointment having suitable properties. When wool alcohols ointment is used in a white ointment it should be prepared with white soft paraffin and when used in a coloured ointment it should be prepared with yellow soft paraffin. Store at a temperature not exceeding 25°.

A.P.F. has wool alcohols 6 g, hard paraffin 17 g, white soft paraffin 17 g, liquid paraffin 60 g.

Proprietary Names and Manufacturers of Wool Alcohols or Wool Alcohol Derivatives

Acetulan *(Amerchol, USA: Anstead, UK)*; Aqualose W20 *(Westbrook, UK)*; Argonol ACE 2 *(Westbrook, UK)*; Argonol ACE 5 *(Westbrook, UK)*; Argowax *(Westbrook, UK)*; Crodalan AWS *(Croda, UK)*; Crodalan LA *(Croda, UK)*; Fluicol *(Croda, UK)*; Hartolan *(Croda, UK)*; Liquid Base CB3896 *(Croda, UK)*; Polychols *(Croda, UK)*; Solulans *(Amerchol, USA: Anstead, UK)*; Solulans PB *(Amerchol, USA: Anstead, UK)*; Super Hartolan *(Croda, UK)*.

The following names have been used for multi-ingredient preparations containing wool alcohols or wool alcohols derivatives—Argobase 125 *(Westbrook, UK)*; Argobase EU *(Westbrook, UK)*; Argonol ISO *(Westbrook, UK)*; Hartolite *(Croda, UK)*; Oilatum Emollient *(Stiefel, Austral.; Stiefel, UK)*; Polylan *(Amerchol, USA : Anstead, UK)*.

6437-f

Wool Fat *(BAN).*

Adeps Lanae; Anhydrous Lanolin *(USAN)*; Cera Lanae; Graisse de Suint Purifiée; Lanoléine; Lanolina; Purified Lanolin; Refined Wool Fat; Suarda; Wollfett; Wollwachs.

CAS — 8006-54-0.

Pharmacopoeias. In *Arg., Aust., Belg., Br., Braz., Chin., Cz., Egypt., Eur., Fr., Ger., Hung., Ind., It., Jpn, Jug., Mex., Neth., Nord., Pol., Port., Roum., Rus., Span., Swiss, Turk.,* and *U.S.* Also in *B.P. Vet.*

A pale yellow, tenacious, unctuous substance with a faint characteristic odour. It is the purified anhydrous waxy substance obtained from the wool of the sheep, *Ovis aries* (Bovidae). M.p. 38° to 44°. The *B.P.* permits not more than 200 ppm of butylated hydroxytoluene. 10 g absorbs not less than 20 mL of water.

Practically **insoluble** in water; sparingly soluble in cold alcohol; slightly soluble in boiling alcohol; soluble in chloroform and in ether. **Store** in well-closed containers at a temperature not exceeding 25°.

Wool fat is not readily absorbed, but when mixed with a suitable vegetable oil or with soft paraffin it gives emollient creams which penetrate the skin. It can absorb about 30% of water and is of value in the preparation of water-in-oil emulsions.

Derivatives and modifications of wool fat include liquid lanolin, water-soluble lanolins, and hydrogenated wool fat. Wool fat can cause sensitivity reactions.

Hydrous wool fat (lanolin or hydrous lanolin) is an ointment basis prepared by the addition of water to wool fat. The *B.P.* specifies wool fat 75 g and water 25 mL, but other pharmacopoeias specify various water contents, sometimes with the addition of liquid paraffin.

A review of the preparation and uses of lanolin.— G. Barnett, *Cosmet. Toilet.,* 1986, *101,* 23 and 30.

Preparations

Hydrous Wool Fat Ointment *(B.P.C. 1973).* Unguentum Adipis Lanae Hydrosi. Equal parts of hydrous wool fat and yellow soft paraffin. It should be kept in containers which prevent evaporation.

Proprietary Names and Manufacturers of Wool Fat or Wool Fat Derivatives

Acetadeps *(Westbrook, UK)*; Acylan *(Croda, UK)*; Albalan *(Westbrook, UK)*; Alcolose W2 *(Westbrook, UK)*; Amerchols *(Amerchol, USA : Anstead, UK)*; Amerlate LFA *(Amerchol, USA : Anstead, UK)*; Amerlate P *(Amerchol, USA : Anstead, UK)*; Amerlate W *(Amerchol, USA : Anstead, UK)*; Aqualose *(Westbrook, UK)*; Aqualose L30 *(Westbrook, UK)*; Aqualose L75 *(Westbrook, UK)*; Argonol LIN *(Westbrook, UK)*; Corona *(Croda, UK)*; Coronet *(Croda, UK)*; Crestalan *(Croda, UK)*; Crodalan IPL *(Croda, UK)*; Fluilan *(Croda, UK)*; Fluilanol *(Croda, UK)*; Golden Fleece *(Westbrook, UK)*; Lanesta *(Westbrook, UK)*; Lanex *(Croda, UK)*; Lanexol AWS *(Croda, UK)*; Lanocerin *(Amerchol, USA : Anstead, UK)*; Lanogels *(Amerchol, USA : Anstead, UK)*; Lanogene *(Amerchol, USA : Anstead, UK)*; Lanolin Deodorized AAA Anhydrous *(Amerchol, USA : Anstead, UK)*; Liquid Base CB3929 *(Croda, UK)*; Massé *(Ortho, Canad.)*; Modulan *(Amerchol, USA : Anstead, UK)*; Nutraspa *(Alcon, Austral.)*; OHlan *(Amerchol, USA : Anstead, UK)*; Satulan *(Croda, UK)*; Solan E *(Croda, UK)*; Solulans *(Amerchol, USA : Anstead, UK)*; Super Sterol Ester *(Croda, UK)*; White Swan *(Croda, UK)*; Yeoman *(Croda, UK)*.

The following names have been used for multi-ingredient preparations containing wool fat or wool fat derivatives—AKWA Tears Ointment *(Akorn, USA)*; Alpha Keri *(Bristol-Myers Pharmaceuticals, UK)*; Alpha-Keri *(Westwood, Canad.)*; Argonol ISO *(Westbrook, UK)*; Argonol RIC-2 *(Westbrook, UK)*; Cremba *(Croda, UK)*; Duratears *(Alcon, Canad.; Alcon Laboratories, USA)*; HEB Waterproof *(Waterhouse, UK)*; Iscolan *(Croda, UK)*; Isocreme Absorption Base *(Croda, UK)*; Isopropylan 33 *(Amerchol, USA : Anstead, UK)*; Keri *(Bristol-Myers Pharmaceuticals, UK)*; Lubrifair Ointment *(Pharmafair, USA)*; Massé Breast Cream *(Ortho-Cilag, UK)*; Sebase *(Westbrook, UK)*; Tearfair Ointment *(Pharmafair, USA)*.

Parasympathomimetics

4500-x

Parasympathomimetic agents may be classified into 2 distinct pharmacological groups: cholinergic agonists, such as bethanechol (below), carbachol (p.1329), methacholine (p.1331), and pilocarpine (p.1335); and anticholinesterases.

The former group act directly on effector cells to mimic the effects of acetylcholine (see below) and are sometimes referred to as cholinomimetics or true parasympathomimetics.

The anticholinesterases inhibit the enzymic hydrolysis of acetylcholine by cholinesterases, thereby prolonging and enhancing its actions in the body, and may be further classified by the length of time taken to restore active enzyme following binding of enzyme to drug. The 'reversible' anticholinesterases such as ambenonium (below), neostigmine (p.1331), physostigmine (p.1333), and pyridostigmine (p.1336) generally produce enzyme inhibition for 3 to 4 hours, whereas 'irreversible' anticholinesterases such as dyflos (p.1330), and ecothiopate (p.1330) produce extremely prolonged inhibition, and return of cholinesterase activity depends on synthesis of new enzyme.

4503-d

Aceclidine Hydrochloride *(rINNM)*.

3-Acetoxyquinuclidine hydrochloride; 3-Quinuclidinyl acetate hydrochloride.
$C_9H_{15}NO_2,HCl = 205.7$.

CAS — 827-61-2 (aceclidine); 6109-70-2 (hydrochloride); 6821-59-6 (salicylate).

NOTE. Aceclidine is USAN.

Pharmacopoeias. Rus. includes the salicylate, under the title Aceclidinum.

Adverse Effects, Treatment, and Precautions

As for Neostigmine Methylsulphate, p.1332.

Uses and Administration

Aceclidine hydrochloride is a parasympathomimetic agent with little if any anticholinesterase activity. It is used to lower intra-ocular pressure in patients with open-angle glaucoma. The salicylate has also been used.

Proprietary Names and Manufacturers

Glaucostat *(Merck Sharp & Dohme-Chibret, Belg.; Merck Sharp & Dohme-Chibret, Fr.; Bournonville, Neth.; Merck Sharp & Dohme, Spain; Chibret, Switz.)*; Glaucotat *(Chibret, Ger.)*; Glaunorm *(Farmigea, Ital.)*.

4506-m

Acetylcholine Chloride *(USAN, rINN)*.

Acetylcholini Chloridum. (2-Acetoxyethyl)trimethylammonium chloride.
$C_7H_{16}ClNO_2 = 181.7$.

CAS — 51-84-3 (acetylcholine); 60-31-1 (chloride).

Pharmacopoeias. In *Aust., Belg., Cz., Fr., Jug., Mex., Span., Swiss, Turk.,* and *U.S. Jpn* includes Acetylcholine Chloride for Injection.

A white crystalline powder. Very **soluble** in water; freely soluble in alcohol; practically insoluble in ether. It is decomposed by hot water. **Incompatible** with alkalis. **Store** in airtight containers.

Adverse Effects

Because it is rapidly hydrolysed in the body by cholinesterases the toxicity of acetylcholine is normally relatively low.

Adverse effects of the choline esters include nausea and vomiting, abdominal pain, flushing, sweating, salivation, lachrymation, rhinorrhoea, eructation, involuntary defaecation and urination, bradycardia and peripheral vasodilatation leading to hypotension, transient heart block, bronchoconstriction, and a feeling of constriction under the sternum.

Treatment of Adverse Effects

Atropine sulphate, usually in doses of 600 µg, may be given intravenously, intramuscularly, or subcutaneously to control the muscarinic effects of the choline esters. Supportive treatment may be required.

Precautions

As for Neostigmine Methylsulphate, p.1332.

Acetylcholine is hydrolysed in the body by cholinesterase and its effects are markedly prolonged and enhanced by prior administration of anticholinesterases.

A report of severe bronchospasm with subsequent pulmonary oedema following intra-ocular injection of acetylcholine chloride in a patient also receiving metoprolol.— D. Rasch *et al., Anesthesiology,* 1983, *59,* 583.

Uses and Administration

Acetylcholine is a chemical transmitter with a very wide range of actions in the body; it is a powerful quaternary ammonium parasympathomimetic agent but its action is transient as it is rapidly destroyed by cholinesterase. It is released from post-ganglionic parasympathetic nerves and also from some post-ganglionic sympathetic nerves to produce peripheral actions which correspond to those of muscarine. It is accordingly a vasodilator and cardiac depressant, a stimulant of the vagus and parasympathetic nervous system, and it has a tonic action on smooth muscle. It also increases lachrymal, salivary, and other secretions. All the muscarinic actions of acetylcholine are abolished by atropine.

Acetylcholine also has nicotinic actions and is accordingly a stimulant of skeletal muscle, the autonomic ganglia, and the adrenal medulla. The nicotinic actions of acetylcholine on skeletal muscle are blocked by tubocurarine; they are also inhibited by massive administration or discharge of acetylcholine itself.

Acetylcholine chloride is instilled as a freshly prepared 1% solution as a miotic in cataract surgery to constrict the pupil in seconds; it may also be used in penetrating keratoplasty and in simple iridectomy.

It has also been used in a wide variety of conditions such as Raynaud's disease, intermittent claudication, trophic ulcers, gangrene, postoperative distension and paralytic ileus, paroxysmal tachycardia, and (by subconjunctival injection) in spasm of the retinal arteries and chronic glaucoma, but with variable results, probably owing to its transient action.

A review of the treatment of primary pulmonary hypertension, including mention of the role of acetycholine.— M. Packer, *Ann. intern. Med.,* 1985, *103,* 258. See also C. M. Oakley, *Br. Heart J.,* 1985, *53,* 1.

Preparations

Acetylcholine Chloride for Ophthalmic Solution *(U.S.P.)*

Proprietary Preparations

Miochol *(CooperVision, UK). Intra-ocular irrigation,* powder for reconstitution, acetylcholine chloride 20 mg, supplied in a 2-chambered vial (Univial) with diluent to produce 2 mL of a 1% solution.

Proprietary Names and Manufacturers

Covochol *(S.Afr.)*; Miochol *(Alcon, Austral.; Coopervision, Canad.; CooperVision, Swed.; CooperVision, UK; Coopervision, USA)*.

4507-b

Ambenonium Chloride *(BAN, rINN)*.

Ambestigmini Chloridum; Win-8077. *NN'*-[Oxalylbis(iminoethylene)]bis[(2-chlorobenzyl)diethylammonium] dichloride.
$C_{28}H_{42}Cl_4N_4O_2 = 608.5$.

CAS — 7648-98-8 (ambenonium); 115-79-7 (chloride, anhydrous); 52022-31-8 (chloride, tetrahydrate).

Pharmacopoeias. Rus. P. includes the ethanolate under the title Oxazylum.

An equilibrium mixture of anhydrous material and the tetrahydrate. A white odourless powder. It loses not more than 11.5% of its weight on drying. **Soluble** in water and alcohol; slightly soluble in chloroform; practically insoluble in acetone and ether. **Store** in airtight containers.

Adverse Effects, Treatment, and Precautions

As for Neostigmine Methylsulphate, see p.1332.

It produces fewer muscarinic side-effects than neostigmine. As there is only slight warning of overdosage, routine administration of atropine with ambenonium is contra-indicated because the muscarinic symptoms of overdosage may be suppressed leaving only the more serious nicotinic effects (fasciculation and paralysis of voluntary muscle).

Uses and Administration

Ambenonium is an inhibitor of cholinesterase activity with actions similar to those of neostigmine (see p.1332), but of longer duration. Ambenonium chloride is given by mouth in the treatment of myasthenia gravis and may be of value in patients who cannot tolerate neostigmine or pyridostigmine bromide. It is administered 3 to 4 times daily, usually in doses of 5 to 25 mg.

Proprietary Names and Manufacturers

Mytelase *(Winthrop, Austral.; Belg.; Winthrop, Denm.; Fin.; Winthrop, Fr.; Winthrop, Ger.; Ital.; Neth.; Sterling-Winthrop, Swed.; Winthrop, Switz.; Sterling Research, UK; USA)*.

4509-g

Bethanechol Chloride *(USAN)*.

Carbamylmethylcholine Chloride. (2-Carbamoyloxypropyl)trimethylammonium chloride.
$C_7H_{17}ClN_2O_2 = 196.7$.

CAS — 674-38-4 (bethanechol); 590-63-6 (chloride).

Pharmacopoeias. In *Jpn, Turk.,* and *U.S.*

Colourless or white hygroscopic crystals or white crystalline powder usually having a slight amine-like odour. There are two crystalline forms.

Freely **soluble** in water and alcohol; practically insoluble in chloroform and ether. A 1% solution in water has a pH of 5.5 to 6.5; the *U.S.P.* injection has a pH of 5.5 to 7.5. **Store** in airtight containers.

Adverse Effects and Treatment

As for Acetylcholine Chloride, above. Untoward effects related to the cardiovascular system are less liable to occur.

Precautions

As for Neostigmine Methylsulphate, p.1332. Bethanechol should not be given by the intravenous or intramuscular routes as severe cholinergic adverse effects are liable to occur.

Uses and Administration

Bethanechol chloride is a quaternary ammonium parasympathomimetic agent with the muscarinic actions of acetylcholine (see above). It is not readily inactivated by cholinesterases so that its actions are more prolonged than those of acetylcholine.

Because it has little if any nicotinic actions, bethanechol may be preferred to carbachol for the treatment of gastric atony and retention following vagotomy, in postoperative abdominal distension, and in some forms of urinary retention, including that following surgery. It has also been tried in the treatment of congenital megacolon, and oesophageal reflux.

It is given, usually in doses of 5 mg subcutaneously or 10 to 50 mg by mouth, both up to 4 times daily, but dosage must be adjusted individually. Oral doses should be taken on an empty stomach. The effects usually occur within 5 to 15 minutes of a subcutaneous, or 30 to 90 minutes of an oral dose, and disappear within 2 hours.

ALZHEIMERS DISEASE. A report of the use of bethanechol chloride in doses of 50 to 700 µg daily by continuous intracranial infusion from an implanted pump to treat 4 patients with Alzheimer's disease. Preliminary results were encouraging.— R. E. Harbaugh *et al.*, *Neurosurgery*, 1984, *15*, 514.

GASTRO-OESOPHAGEAL REFLUX. Although some studies indicate that addition of bethanechol to antacid therapy of reflux oesophagitis appears to offer no advantage over the use of antacids alone (L.S. Saco *et al.*, *Gastroenterology*, 1982, *82*, 1369) others show that it is effective in the relief of symptoms of heartburn and oesophageal reflux that are poorly controlled or refractory to antacid therapy (R.L. Farrell *et al.*, *Ann. intern. Med.*, 1974, *80*, 573; K.D. Thanik *et al.*, *ibid.*, 1980, *93*, 805) and is of similar efficacy to cimetidine (K. Thanik *et al.*, *Archs intern. med.*, 1982, *142*, 1479). However, while some workers have found it to be suitable for use in infants and children (A.D. Strickland and J.H.T. Chang, *J. Pediat.*, 1983, *103*, 311) others consider that this role may need reassessing as they found that it could aggravate the condition in some children (S.R. Orenstein *et al.*, *J. pediatr. Gastroenterol. Nutr.*, 1986, *5*, 549).

MALAKOPLAKIA. Administration of bethanechol chloride 40 mg daily corrected the decreased bactericidal activity of mononuclear cells of a patient with malakoplakia and monocyte functional defects. Although the association between malakoplakia and monocyte functional defects was not fully understood it was clear that cholinergic agonists could be helpful in the therapy of malakoplakia.— N. I. Abdou *et al.*, *New Engl. J. Med.*, 1977, *297*, 1413.

REVERSAL OF ANTIMUSCARINIC ACTION. A report of the beneficial use of bethanechol chloride to alleviate side-effects, including salivary gland inhibition, bladder inhibition, and constipation, due to tricyclic antidepressant therapy.— H. C. Everett, *Am. J. Psychiat.*, 1975, *132*, 1202. See also *idem* (letter), *New Engl. J. Med.*, 1984, *310*, 1122.

STUTTERING. A report of bethanechol producing beneficial results in the control of stuttering in 2 patients.— P. Hays (letter), *Lancet*, 1987, *1*, 271.

URINARY INCONTINENCE. A brief discussion of urinary incontinence. It is important to note the type of urinary incontinence before attempting drug therapy; classifications vary but the one that seems most useful comprises: stress incontinence, due to increased intra-abdominal pressure; urge incontinence, where leakage occurs when a patient is unable to delay voiding long enough to reach a toilet; overflow incontinence, due to some anatomical obstruction that prevents emptying of the bladder; and functional incontinence in patients with impaired mobility or mental function. Urge incontinence is the most responsive to drug therapy. Cholinergic drugs such as bethanechol have been used effectively for the treatment of overflow, stress, and urge incontinence but in many older patients bethanechol creates urinary frequency and urgency and therefore exacerbates incontinence.— P. A. L. Haber, *Ann. intern. Med.*, 1986, *104*, 429. In an earlier review it was concluded that although many articles and case reports suggested that bethanechol was sometimes effective in promoting bladder emptying, clinical testing has not shown it to be effective, regardless of dose of bethanechol, route of administration, or disease state, and in fact several studies suggest that it is ineffective.— A. E. Finkbeiner, *J. Urol., Baltimore*, 1985, *134*, 443.

Preparations

Bethanechol Chloride Injection *(U.S.P.)*

Bethanechol Chloride Tablets *(U.S.P.)*

Proprietary Preparations

Myotonine *(Glenwood, UK)*. *Tablets*, scored, bethanechol chloride 10 and 25 mg.

Proprietary Names and Manufacturers

Besacolin *(Jpn)*; Duvoid *(Norwich-Eaton, Canad.; Norwich Eaton, USA)*; Mechothane *(Macarthys, UK)*; Muscaran *(Belg.)*; Myo Hermes *(Organon, Spain)*; Myocholine *(Glenwood, Switz.)*; Myotonachol *(Glenwood, USA)*; Myotonine *(Glenwood, UK)*; Urecholine *(Merck Sharp & Dohme, Austral.; Frosst, Canad.; Merck Sharp & Dohme, Ital.; Merck Sharp & Dohme, S.Afr.; Merck Sharp & Dohme, Switz.; Merck Sharp & Dohme, USA)*; Urocarb *(Hamilton, Austral.)*; Vesicholine *(Star, USA)*.

4511-d

Carbachol *(USAN, rINN)*.

Carbach.; Carbacholine; Carbacholum; Carbacholum Chloratum; Carbamylcholine Chloride; Choline Chloride Carbamate. *O*-Carbamoylcholine chloride; (2-Carbamoyloxyethyl)trimethylammonium chloride.

$C_6H_{15}ClN_2O_2$=182.7.

CAS — 51-83-2.

Pharmacopoeias. In *Arg.*, *Aust.*, *Braz.*, *Int.*, *It.*, *Mex.*, *Nord.*, *Rus.*, *Swiss*, *Turk.*, and *U.S.* Also in *B.P.C. 1973.*

White or faintly yellow hygroscopic crystals or crystalline powder, odourless or with a faint amine-like odour.

Soluble 1 in 1 of water and 1 in 50 of alcohol; practically insoluble in chloroform and in ether. Solutions in water are neutral to litmus. **Store** in airtight containers.

INCOMPATIBILITY. Chlorocresol (0.025 to 0.1%) and chlorbutol (0.5%) were both found to be incompatible with a solution of carbachol (0.8%) and sodium chloride (0.69%), very slight precipitates forming on heating and increasing on standing.— Pharm. Soc. Lab. Rep. No. 911, 1962.

Adverse Effects and Treatment

As for Acetylcholine Chloride, p.1328. Untoward effects related to the cardiovascular system are less liable to occur. Carbachol has substantial nicotinic activity which may be unmasked by the use of atropine to counteract muscarinic effects.

A report of life-threatening attacks of profuse sweating, intestinal cramps, explosive defaecation, hypothermia, hypotension, and bradycardia in a 36-year-old man due to carbachol intoxication. A 10-year-old boy had died following similar attacks associated with repeated carbachol ingestion.— B. Sangster *et al.*, *Neth. J. Med.*, 1979, *22*, 27.

Precautions

As for Neostigmine Methylsulphate, p.1332.

Uses and Administration

Carbachol is a quaternary ammonium parasympathomimetic agent with the muscarinic and nicotinic actions of acetylcholine (see p.1328). It is not readily inactivated by cholinesterases so that its actions are more prolonged than those of acetylcholine.

Carbachol has a miotic action and eye-drops containing 0.75 to 3% have been used to lower intra-ocular pressure in glaucoma, sometimes in conjunction with other miotics such as physostigmine.

Carbachol has also been used by intra-ocular irrigation, 0.4 to 0.5 mL of a 0.01% solution being instilled into the anterior chamber of the eye, to produce miosis in cataract surgery.

Carbachol has been used in the treatment of postoperative intestinal atony and urinary retention, and has been given to stop supraventricular paroxysmal tachycardia.

In the treatment of simple glaucoma, carbachol was considered to be a useful alternative to pilocarpine and to other miotics where resistance or intolerance had developed.— J. J. Kanski, *Br. J. Ophthal.*, 1968, *52*, 936.

Preparations

Carbachol Eye-drops *(B.P.C. 1973)*. CAR. An aqueous solution containing up to 3% of carbachol. Sterilised by autoclaving or by filtration or by maintaining at 98° to 100° for 30 minutes. This solution is adversely affected by alkali.

Carbachol Intraocular Solution *(U.S.P.)*

Carbachol Ophthalmic Solution *(U.S.P.)*

Carbachol Injection *(B.P. 1973)*. A sterile solution in Water for Injections, with the addition of 5% of anhydrous glucose.

Proprietary Preparations

Isopto Carbachol *(Alcon, UK)*. *Eye-drops*, carbachol 3%.

Proprietary Names and Manufacturers

Carbyl *(Ital.)*; Doryl *(E. Merck, Ger.; Neth.; E. Merck, Switz.)*; Isopto Carbachol *(Alcon, Austral.; Alcon, Canad.; Alcon, Ger.; Neth.; Alcon, Norw.; S.Afr.; Switz.; Alcon, UK; Alcon Laboratories, USA)*; Isopto-Karbakolin *(Alcon, Swed.)*; Karbakolin Isopto *(Alcon, Denm.)*; Miostat *(Alcon, Canad.; Norw.; Alcon Laboratories, USA)*; Spersacarbachol *(Dispersa, Switz.)*.

4512-n

Demecarium Bromide *(BAN, USAN, rINN)*.

BC-48. 3,3'-[*NN'*-Decamethylenebis(methylcarbamoyloxy)]bis(*NNN*-trimethylanilinium) dibromide.

$C_{32}H_{52}Br_2N_4O_4$=716.6.

CAS — 56-94-0.

Pharmacopoeias. In *U.S.*

A white or slightly yellow, slightly hygroscopic, crystalline powder. Freely **soluble** in water and alcohol; soluble in ether; sparingly soluble in acetone. A 1% solution in water has a pH of 5 to 7. **Store** in airtight containers. Protect from light.

Adverse Effects

As for Neostigmine Methylsulphate, p.1332 and Ecothiopate Iodide p.1330. The anticholinesterase action of demecarium, and hence its adverse effects, may be prolonged.

Treatment of Adverse Effects

As for Ecothiopate Iodide, p.1330. Pralidoxime has been reported to be more active in counteracting the effects of dyflos and ecothiopate than of demecarium.

Precautions

As for Ecothiopate Iodide, p.1330.

Uses and Administration

Demecarium is an inhibitor of cholinesterase with actions similar to those of ecothiopate. Its miotic action begins within about 15 to 60 minutes of its application and may persist for a week or more. It causes a reduction in intra-ocular pressure which is maximal in 24 hours and may persist for 9 days or more.

Demecarium bromide has been used in the treatment of open-angle glaucoma particularly in aphakic patients, and those in whom other agents have proved inadequate. The dosage varies, 1 to 2 drops of a 0.125% or 0.25% solution being instilled from twice weekly to twice daily, preferably at bedtime.

Demecarium bromide has also been used in the management of accommodative convergent strabismus (esotropia).

Preparations

Demecarium Bromide Ophthalmic Solution *(U.S.P.)*

Proprietary Preparations

Tosmilen *(Sinclair, UK)*. *Eye-drops*, demecarium bromide 0.25%.

Proprietary Names and Manufacturers

Humorsol *(Merck Sharp & Dohme, USA)*; Tonilen *(Spain)*; Tosmilène *(Fr.)*; Tosmilen *(Austral.; Chemie-Linz, Denm.; Ger.; Neth.; Chemie Linz, Swed.; Switz.; Sinclair, UK)*; Visumiotic *(Arg.)*.

4513-h

Distigmine Bromide *(BAN, rINN)*.

BC-51; Bispyridostigmine Bromide; Hexamarium Bromide. 1,1'-Dimethyl-3,3'-[*NN'*-hexamethylenebis(methylcarbamoyloxy)]dipyridinium dibromide.

$C_{22}H_{32}Br_2N_4O_4$=576.3.

CAS — 15876-67-2.

Pharmacopoeias. In *Jpn.*

Adverse Effects, Treatment, and Precautions

As for Neostigmine Methylsulphate, p.1332. The anticholinesterase action of distigmine, and hence its adverse effects, may be prolonged, and if treatment with atropine is required it should be maintained for at least 24 hours.

Absorption and Fate
Distigmine is poorly absorbed from the gastro-intestinal tract.

Uses and Administration
Distigmine is an inhibitor of cholinesterase with actions similar to those of neostigmine (see p.1332) but more prolonged. Maximum inhibition of plasma cholinesterase occurs 9 hours after a single intramuscular dose, and persists for about 24 hours.
It is used in the prevention and treatment of postoperative intestinal atony and urinary retention; 500 µg of distigmine bromide may be injected intramuscularly about 12 hours after surgery and may be repeated every 24 hours until normal function is restored. It may also be given by mouth in a dose of 5 mg daily thirty minutes before breakfast. A similar dose by mouth, given daily or on alternate days, has been employed in the management of neurogenic bladder.
Distigmine bromide in conjunction with short-acting parasympathomimetics has been given for the treatment of myasthenia gravis, but should only be given by mouth. Doses of up to 20 mg daily for adults and 10 mg daily for children have been used.

Proprietary Preparations
Ubretid *(Berk Pharmaceuticals, UK). Tablets,* scored, distigmine bromide 5 mg.
Injection, distigmine bromide 500 µg/mL, in ampoules of 1 mL.

Proprietary Names and Manufacturers
Ubretid *(USV, Austral.*; *Hormonchemie, Ger.*; *Neth.*; *Fisons, S.Afr.*; *Chemie-Linz, Switz.*; *Berk Pharmaceuticals, UK).*

4514-m

Dyflos *(BAN).*

DFP; Di-isopropyl Fluorophosphate; Di-isopropylfluorophosphonate; Fluostigmine; Isoflurophate *(USAN).* Di-isopropyl phosphorofluoridate.
$C_6H_{14}FO_3P$=184.1.

CAS — 55-91-4.

Pharmacopoeias. In *Arg.* and *U.S.*

A clear, colourless, or faintly yellow liquid. Specific gravity about 1.05. Sparingly **soluble** in water; soluble in alcohol and vegetable oils. Solutions in water are unstable and are hydrolysed, with the evolution of hydrogen fluoride. **Store** at 8° to 15° in sealed containers.

CAUTION. *The vapour of dyflos is very toxic. Contaminated material should be immersed in a 2% aqueous solution of sodium hydroxide for several hours. Dyflos can be removed from the skin by washing with soap and water.*

Adverse Effects
As for Neostigmine Methylsulphate, p.1332 and Ecothiopate Iodide, below.
The anticholinesterase action of dyflos, and hence its adverse effects, may be prolonged.
Systemic toxicity also occurs after inhalation of the vapour.

Treatment of Adverse Effects and Precautions
As for Ecothiopate Iodide, below.

Absorption and Fate
Dyflos is readily absorbed from the gastro-intestinal tract, from skin and mucous membranes, and from the lungs. Dyflos interacts with cholinesterases producing stable phosphonylated and phosphorylated derivatives which are then hydrolysed by phosphorylphosphatases. These products of hydrolysis are excreted mainly in the urine.

Uses and Administration
Dyflos is an irreversible inhibitor of cholinesterase with actions similar to those of ecothiopate. Dyflos has a powerful miotic action which begins within 5 to 10 minutes and may persist for up to 4 weeks; it causes a reduction in intra-ocular pressure which is maximal in 24 hours and may persist for a week.
Dyflos is used mainly in the treatment of glaucoma when other agents have proved inadequate, particularly in open-angle glaucoma as well as glaucoma following cataract extraction and in other aphakic patients. It is also employed in the management of accommodative convergent strabismus (esotropia).
It is administered usually as a 0.025% ointment. Since the application causes blurring of vision, advantage should be taken of the fact that dyflos can be applied at night before retiring.

Preparations
Isoflurophate Ophthalmic Ointment *(U.S.P.).* A sterile eye ointment containing dyflos 0.0225 to 0.0275%.

Proprietary Names and Manufacturers
DFP-Oel *(Winzer, Ger.)*; Diflupyl *(Labaz, Fr.*; *Labaz, Neth.)*; Floropryl *(Merck Sharp & Dohme, USA).*

4515-b

Ecothiopate Iodide *(BAN, rINN).*

Echothiophate Iodide *(USAN)*; Ecostigmine Iodide; MI-217. (2-Diethoxyphosphinylthioethyl)trimethylammonium iodide.
$C_9H_{23}INO_3PS$=383.2.

CAS — 6736-03-4 (ecothiopate); 513-10-0 (iodide).

Pharmacopoeias. In *Br.* and *U.S.*

A white crystalline hygroscopic powder with an alliaceous odour. **Soluble** 1 in 1 of water, 1 in 25 of alcohol, and 1 in 3 of methyl alcohol; practically insoluble in other organic solvents. A solution in water has a pH of about 4. The *B.P.* requires **storage** between 2° and 8°; the *U.S.P.* requires storage preferably at a temperature below 0°. Store in airtight containers. Protect from light.

Adverse Effects
As for Neostigmine Methylsulphate, p.1332.
Ecothiopate is an 'irreversible' cholinesterase inhibitor; its action, and hence its adverse effects, may be prolonged.
Plasma and erythrocyte cholinesterases may be diminished by treatment with eye-drops of ecothiopate, or other long-acting anticholinesterases.
Acute iritis, retinal detachment, or precipitation of acute glaucoma may occasionally follow treatment with ecothiopate and iris cysts (especially in children) or lens opacities may develop following prolonged treatment.

Treatment of Adverse Effects
In systemic poisoning, atropine sulphate may be given parenterally, usually in a dose of 2 mg. Pralidoxime chloride may be given concomitantly in a dose of 1 to 2 g by slow intravenous injection over 5 to 10 minutes, or by infusion, in order to reactivate cholinesterase; subconjunctival injection of pralidoxime has been employed to reverse severe ocular adverse effects. Supportive treatment, including assisted ventilation, should be given as necessary.
To prevent or reduce development of iris cysts in patients receiving ecothiopate eye-drops, phenylephrine eye-drops may be given simultaneously.

Precautions
In general ecothiopate, in common with other long-acting anticholinesterases, should be used only where therapy with other agents has proved ineffective.
It should be used with great care if at all in patients with a history of retinal detachment or iodine hypersensitivity.
Treatment with ecothiopate eye-drops should be stopped if persistent diarrhoea, urinary incontinence, sweating, cardiotoxicity, or muscle weakness occurs. Long-acting anticholinesterases should not be used in patients with bronchial asthma, cardiovascular disease, parkinsonism, peptic ulcer, epilepsy, or intestinal or urinary-tract obstruction. They are contra-indicated in the treatment of closed-angle glaucoma prior to surgery or glaucoma associated with iridocyclitis or uveal inflammation. If possible, treatment should be discontinued prior to surgery on the eye as there is an increased risk of hyphaemia.

INTERACTIONS. Prolonged apnoea following suxamethonium administration in an elderly patient undergoing general anaesthesia was probably secondary to a low concentration of serum cholinesterase resulting from long-term use of ecothiopate eye-drops.— L. P. Kramer (letter), *Can. med. Ass. J.*, 1982, *127*, 1078. Comment.— G. R. Laroche (letter), *ibid.*, 1983, *128*, 894; H. W. Bauld (letter), *ibid.*

Uses and Administration
Ecothiopate is an irreversible inhibitor of cholinesterase with actions similar to those of neostigmine, but much more prolonged. Its miotic action begins within 10 to 30 minutes of its application and may persist for 1 to 4 weeks; it causes a reduction in intra-ocular pressure which is maximal after 24 hours and may persist for days or weeks.
Ecothiopate iodide is used mainly in the treatment of open-angle glaucoma particularly in aphakic patients, and when other agents have proved inadequate. It is administered as drops of a 0.03 to 0.25% solution, usually once or twice daily; doses are given at bedtime where possible. Pilocarpine eye-drops should be administered for at least 2 months before starting high strengths of ecothiopate eye-drops.
Ecothiopate iodide has also been used in the management of accommodative convergent strabismus (esotropia).

GLAUCOMA. Satisfactory control occurred with ecothiopate iodide in 14 of 17 eyes with chronic *closed-angle glaucoma* which was previously not controlled with pilocarpine and acetazolamide.— J. D. Sussman, *Am. J. Ophthal.*, 1965, *59*, 308.

Preparations
Echothiophate Iodide for Ophthalmic Solution *(U.S.P.)*

Proprietary Preparations
Phospholine Iodide *(Ayerst, UK). Eye-drops,* powder for reconstitution, ecothiopate iodide 1.5, 3, 6.25, and 12.5 mg, supplied with diluent, to produce a 0.03, 0.06, 0.125, and 0.25% solution.

Proprietary Names and Manufacturers
Echodide *(USA)*; Ecofilina *(Venez.)*; Iodeto de fosfolina *(Braz.)*; Phospholine *(Sodip, Switz.)*; Phospholine Iodide *(Ayerst, Austral.*; *Belg.*; *Ayerst, Canad.*; *Ayerst, Denm.*; *Promedica, Fr.*; *Chinoin, Ital.*; *Ayerst, Norw.*; *S.Afr.*; *Ayerst, UK*; *Ayerst, USA)*; Phospholinjodid *(Winzer, Ger.)*; Yoduro de fosfolina *(Mex.).*

4516-v

Edrophonium Chloride *(BAN, USAN, rINN).*

Edrophonii Chloridum. Ethyl(3-hydroxyphenyl)dimethylammonium chloride.
$C_{10}H_{16}ClNO$=201.7.

CAS — 312-48-1 (edrophonium); 116-38-1 (chloride).

Pharmacopoeias. In *Br.*, *Int.*, and *U.S.*

A white odourless or almost odourless crystalline powder.
Soluble 1 in 0.5 of water and 1 in 5 of alcohol; practically insoluble in chloroform and ether. A 10% solution in water has a pH of 4 to 5; injections have a pH of 5 to 6. The *B.P.* requires solutions for injection to be **sterilised** by autoclaving. **Store** in well-closed containers. Protect from light.

Adverse Effects, Treatment, and Precautions
As for Neostigmine Methylsulphate, p.1332.

Atropine appears to be more suitable than glycopyrronium bromide for the antagonism of the muscarinic effects of edrophonium in patients undergoing reversal of neuromuscular blockade.— R. K. Mirakhur, *Br. J. Anaesth.*, 1985, *57*, 1213.

DIAGNOSIS OF MYASTHENIA GRAVIS. A warning against the use of 10 mg of edrophonium intravenously as a test for myasthenia gravis; it might cause failure of respiratory and bulbar muscles and excessive secretion of saliva and bronchial secretions.— D. L. McLellan (letter), *Br. med. J.*, 1973, *3*, 634.

Uses and Administration

Edrophonium has actions similar to those of neostigmine (see p.1332) but its effect on skeletal muscle is claimed to be particularly prominent. Its action is rapid in onset and of short duration.

Edrophonium chloride is of particular value in the diagnosis of myasthenia gravis. It is given by intravenous injection; the usual procedure is to inject 2 mg and, if no adverse reaction occurs within 30 to 45 seconds, to continue with the injection of a further 8 mg. Children may be given suggested doses usually in the range 100 to 150 µg per kg body-weight, one-fifth of the dose being given initially, followed by the remainder if no adverse effect develops. In patients in whom intravenous injection is difficult, edrophonium may be given by intramuscular injection; the normal dose in adults is 10 mg while children below 34 kg in weight may be given 2 mg and heavier children 5 mg. Atropine should always be available when the test is carried out to treat any severe muscarinic reactions that may occur.

In patients with myasthenia gravis, there is immediate subjective improvement and muscle strength increases. This effect usually lasts only for about 5 to 15 minutes, after which time the typical signs and symptoms return; because of its brief action the drug is not suitable for the routine treatment of myasthenia gravis.

Lower doses of edrophonium chloride are used to distinguish severe symptoms of myasthenia gravis, due to inadequate therapy, from the effects of overdosage with anticholinesterase drugs. If treatment has been inadequate, edrophonium chloride will produce an immediate amelioration of symptoms, whereas in cholinergic crises due to over-treatment the symptoms will be aggravated.

Edrophonium chloride was originally introduced for the reversal of the effects of tubocurarine and other non-depolarising muscle relaxants. A dose of 5 to 10 mg was given by intravenous injection and repeated every 5 to 10 minutes up to 40 mg if necessary. The briefness of its action limits its usefulness and neostigmine is preferred. Where prolonged apnoea occurs in a patient treated with a depolarising muscle relaxant, such as suxamethonium, edrophonium 10 mg may be given intravenously to determine the presence of a dual block.

Suggested doses of 10 to 20 mg have been given intravenously in the treatment of paroxysmal tachycardia.

ABSORPTION AND FATE. A study in 5 surgical patients on the plasma elimination half-lives of edrophonium chloride after intravenous injection indicated that an initial rapid phase of elimination (range 0.54 to 1.92 minutes) was followed by a much slower decline (range 24.23 to 45.00 minutes). It was suggested that the rapid fall in the plasma concentration of edrophonium was not primarily due to metabolism and excretion but to the rapid uptake of the drug by other tissues.— T. N. Calvey *et al.*, *Clin. Pharmac. Ther.*, 1976, *19*, 813.

DIAGNOSIS OF OESOPHAGEAL DISORDERS. Edrophonium may be recommended as a useful provocative test for evaluating non-cardiac chest pain of possible oesophageal origin and may be preferred to ergometrine.— J. E. Richter *et al.*, *Ann. intern. Med.*, 1985, *103*, 14 and 482. Criticism. Whereas edrophonium almost certainly has advantages over ergometrine as a provocative drug for evaluating oesophageal chest pain it is much inferior in the far commoner clinical problem of determining the cause of chest pain not yet known to be cardiac or oesophageal in origin.— D. L. Oshin (letter), *ibid.*, 958. Reply. Ergometrine testing for coronary artery spasm has a very low yield when chest pain is not associated with ST-segment abnormalities or T-wave inversion and cannot be administered for diagnostic purposes to patients receiving long-acting nitrates or calcium channel blockers.— B. T. Hackshaw *et al.* (letter), *ibid.*, 959. See also J. N. Blackwell and D. O. Castell, *Gut*, 1984, *25*, 1; H. A. Davies *et al.* (letter), *ibid.*, 801.

MYASTHENIA GRAVIS. A discussion of controversies in the treatment of myasthenia gravis. The edrophonium test to determine optimal dosage of another cholinergic drug in myasthenia gravis has never been assessed formally. The author has not found it a reliable guide to oral therapy and it does not seem to be used very often. There are still however occasional references to the use of edrophonium to determine whether weakness is 'myasthenic' or 'cholinergic' but again the interpretation was never assessed formally and in the author's institution the distinction becomes inconsequential, since it is standard practice to discontinue all cholinergic drug therapy in patients requiring respiratory support.— L. P. Rowland, *J. Neurol. Neurosurg. Psychiat.*, 1980, *43*, 644.

REVERSAL OF NEUROMUSCULAR BLOCKADE. Although edrophonium has been considered to be less effective than neostigmine in reversing neuromuscular blockade its role has been re-evaluated following the increased use of shorter acting neuromuscular blocking agents such as atracurium and vecuronium (C.S. Reilly and W.S. Nimmo, *Drugs*, 1987, *34*, 98). It was suggested that because of its shorter duration of action and lesser effect on the vagus, edrophonium might be the more suitable agent (C.J. Hull, *Br. J. Hosp. Med.*, 1983, *30*, 273). However, although it has a more rapid onset of action (R.M. Jones *et al.*, *Br. J. Anaesth.*, 1984, *56*, 453; J.E. Caldwell *et al.*, *ibid.*, 1987, *59*, 478) than neostigmine and does not appear to re-induce blockade on repeated administration (B.A. Astley *et al.*, *Br. J. Anaesth.*, 1987, *59*, 983) its antagonism is not adequately and reliably sustained especially following profound block (J.E. Caldwell *et al.*, *Br. J. Anaesth.*, 1986, *58*, 1285; R.K. Mirakhur *et al.*, *ibid.*, 1987, *59*, 473) and some workers consider that neostigmine is still the agent of choice for use with these agents (J.E. Caldwell *et al.*, *Br. J. Anaesth.*, 1987, *59*, 478). It has been suggested that the use of edrophonium may be preferable to neostigmine in patients undergoing colorectal surgery (A.R. Hunter, *Br. J. Anaesth.*, 1986, *58*, 825).

SNAKE BITE. Results of a placebo-controlled crossover study indicated that the use of edrophonium was beneficial in the management of 10 patients bitten by the Philippine cobra (*Naja naja philippinensis*).— G. Watt *et al.*, *New Engl. J. Med.*, 1986, *315*, 1444.

For reference to the use of edrophonium in a patient bitten by a Malayan krait, see under Neostigmine Methylsulphate, p.1333.

TETRODOTOXIN POISONING. In 3 patients with respiratory distress and paresis or reduced muscle power following ingestion of puffer fish (*Sphaeroides maculatus* or *Arothron stellatus*) a significant increase in motor power was observed immediately following edrophonium 10 mg by intravenous injection and was maintained in one without further anticholinesterase treatment. In the other 2 recovery was accelerated following introduction of neostigmine after the initial dose of edrophonium. In a further 13 cases, with mild poisoning uncomplicated by respiratory distress or paralysis, a single dose of neostigmine 0.5 mg intramuscularly produced marked improvement of paraesthesia and numbness.— S. K. Chew *et al.* (letter), *Lancet*, 1984, *2*, 108. See also T. A. Torda *et al.*, *Med. J. Aust.*, 1973, *1*, 599.

Preparations

Edrophonium Chloride Injection *(U.S.P.)*

Edrophonium Injection *(B.P.)*. Contains edrophonium chloride.

Proprietary Preparations

Tensilon *(Roche, UK)*. *Injection*, edrophonium chloride 10 mg/mL, in ampoules of 1 mL.

Proprietary Names and Manufacturers

Anticude *(UCB, Spain)*; Enlon *(Anaquest, USA)*; Tensilon *(Roche, Canad.; Roche, UK; Roche, USA)*.

4517-g

Galantamine Hydrobromide *(rINNM)*.

Galanthamine Hydrobromide; Galanthamini Hydrobromidum.

$C_{17}H_{21}NO_3,HBr = 368.3$.

CAS — 357-70-0 (galantamine); 1953-04-4 (hydrobromide).

Pharmacopoeias. In *Chin.* and *Rus.*

The hydrobromide of galantamine, an alkaloid which has been obtained from the Caucasian snowdrop (Voronov's snowdrop), *Galanthus woronowii* (Amaryllidaceae) and related species.

Galantamine hydrobromide is an inhibitor of cholinesterase activity, with actions similar to those of neostigmine (see Neostigmine Methylsulphate, p.1332). It has been used in the USSR in myasthenia and other neuromuscular disorders, and to curtail the muscle relaxation produced by non-depolarising muscle relaxants such as tubocurarine and gallamine.

A study of the pharmacokinetics of galantamine hydrobromide.— P. Westra *et al.*, *Br. J. Anaesth.*, 1986, *58*, 1303.

Proprietary Names and Manufacturers

Nivalina *(UCB, Ital.)*.

4520-n

Methacholine Chloride *(BAN, USAN, rINN)*.

Acetyl-β-methylcholine Chloride; Amechol Chloride; Methacholinium Chloratum. (2-Acetoxypropyl)trimethylammonium chloride.

$C_8H_{18}ClNO_2 = 195.7$.

CAS — 55-92-5 (methacholine); 62-51-1 (chloride).

Pharmacopoeias. In *Braz.*, *Fr.*, *Ind.*, *It.*, *Mex.*, *Swiss*, and *U.S.* Also in *B.P.C. 1973*. *Nord.* includes the bromide.

Colourless, or white, very hygroscopic crystals, or a white crystalline powder, odourless or with a slight odour. Very **soluble** in water; freely soluble in alcohol and in chloroform. Solutions in water are neutral to litmus. **Store** in airtight containers.

Adverse Effects and Treatment

As for Acetylcholine Chloride, p.1328.

Precautions

As for Neostigmine Methylsulphate, p.1332. Methacholine is hydrolysed by cholinesterase, and its effects are markedly enhanced by prior administration of anticholinesterases.

Uses and Administration

Methacholine is a quaternary ammonium parasympathomimetic agent with the muscarinic actions of acetylcholine (see p.1328). It is hydrolysed at a considerably slower rate than acetylcholine by cholinesterase so that its actions are more prolonged.

Methacholine chloride has been used to terminate attacks of supraventricular paroxysmal tachycardia, the usual dose being 10 to 25 mg subcutaneously. It should not be given by intravenous or intramuscular injection.

Methacholine has been used by mouth and subcutaneously in the treatment of Raynaud's syndrome, and other vasospastic conditions. It has been given as eye-drops for the diagnosis of Adie's pupil, and in the treatment of simple glaucoma.

Inhalation of nebulised solutions is used to provoke bronchoconstriction in studies of airway function.

The bromide has also been used similarly.

Administration of methacholine chloride by inhalation is used as a challenge test in the diagnosis of bronchial airway hypersensitivity in patients who do not have clinically apparent asthma (S.L. Nightingale, *J. Am. med. Ass.*, 1987, *257*, 732). While some clinicians consider that methacholine is too dangerous for routine use in the diagnosis of asthma and that its use should rarely be necessary (*Med. Lett.*, 1987, *29*, 60) others report that it is of use in carefully selected patients and rarely dangerous if used according to the directions (*Med. Lett.*, 1987, *29*, 74).

Proprietary Names and Manufacturers

Provocholine *(Roche, USA)*.

4501-r

Neostigmine Bromide *(BAN, USAN, pINN)*.

Neostig. Brom.; Neostigmini Bromidum; Neostigminii Bromidum; Neostigminum Bromatum; Synstigmine Bromide. 3-(Dimethylcarbamoyloxy)-*NNN*-trimethylanilinium bromide.

$C_{12}H_{19}BrN_2O_2 = 303.2$.

CAS — 59-99-4 (neostigmine); 114-80-7 (bromide).

Pharmacopoeias. In *Aust., Belg., Br., Braz., Chin., Cz., Egypt., Eur., Fr., Ger., Hung., Ind., Int., Jug., Mex., Neth., Nord., Roum., Swiss, Turk.,* and *U.S.*

Hygroscopic, odourless, colourless crystals or a white crystalline powder.

Soluble 1 in 0.5 of water and 1 in 8 of alcohol; freely soluble in chloroform; practically insoluble in ether. A solution in water is neutral to litmus. **Store** in airtight containers. Protect from light.

4502-f

Neostigmine Methylsulphate *(BAN)*.

Neostig. Methylsulph.; Neostigmine Methylsulfate *(USAN)*; Neostigmini Methylsulfas; Proserinum.

$C_{13}H_{22}N_2O_6S$=334.4.

CAS — 51-60-5.

Pharmacopoeias. In *Arg., Aust., Br., Braz., Chin., Cz., Egypt., Fr., Ger., Hung., Ind., Int., It., Jpn, Jug., Mex., Pol., Port., Rus., Turk.,* and *U.S.*

Odourless colourless crystals or a white crystalline powder.

Soluble 1 in 0.5 of water and 1 in 6 of alcohol. A solution in water is neutral to litmus. The *B.P.* requires solutions for injection to be **sterilised** by autoclaving; the *B.P.* injection has a pH of 4.5 to 6.5 and the *U.S.P.* injection a pH of 5 to 6.5. **Store** in airtight containers. Protect from light.

Degradation kinetics of neostigmine bromide in aqueous solutions.— H. Porst and L. Kny, *Pharmazie*, 1985, *40*, 713.

Adverse Effects

The side-effects of neostigmine are chiefly due to excessive cholinergic stimulation and most commonly include increased salivation, nausea and vomiting, abdominal cramps, and diarrhoea. Allergic reactions have been reported.

Overdosage may lead to a 'cholinergic crisis', characterised by both muscarinic and nicotinic effects. These effects may include excessive sweating, lachrymation, increased peristalsis, involuntary defaecation and urination or desire to urinate, miosis, ciliary spasm, nystagmus, headache, bradycardia and other arrhythmias, hypotension, muscle cramps, fasciculations, weakness and paralysis, tight chest, wheezing, and increased bronchial secretion combined with bronchoconstriction. CNS effects include confusion, ataxia, convulsions, coma, slurred speech, restlessness, agitation, and fear. Death may result from respiratory failure, due to a combination of the muscarinic, nicotinic and central effects, or cardiac arrest.

It has been stated that a paradoxical increase in blood pressure and heart-rate may result from nicotinic stimulation of sympathetic ganglia, especially where atropine has been given to reverse the muscarinic effects (see under Treatment of Adverse Effects, below).

In patients with myasthenia gravis, in whom other symptoms of overdosage may be mild or absent, the major symptom of cholinergic crisis is increased muscular weakness, which must be differentiated from the muscular weakness caused by an exacerbation of the disease itself.

Treatment of Adverse Effects

If neostigmine has been taken by mouth the stomach should be emptied by aspiration and lavage. Atropine sulphate, usually in doses of 1 to 2 mg, may be given preferably intravenously, or else intramuscularly or subcutaneously to control the muscarinic effects. This dose may be repeated as necessary. Nicotinic effects, including muscle weakness and paralysis, are not antagonised by atropine; small doses of tubocurarine may be used to control muscle twitching. Supportive treatment should be given as required.

Precautions

Neostigmine is contra-indicated in patients with mechanical intestinal or urinary-tract obstruction, or peritonitis. It should be used with caution in patients with cardiovascular disorders including arrhythmias, bradycardia, and hypotension, as well as in patients with vagotonia, Addison's disease, epilepsy, hyperthyroidism, parkinsonism, bronchial asthma, or peptic ulcer. When neostigmine is given by injection, atropine should always be available to counteract any excessive reactions to neostigmine; atropine may also be given before, or with, neostigmine to prevent or minimise muscarinic side-effects but this may mask the initial symptoms of overdosage and lead to cholinergic crisis.

Neostigmine should not be used in conjunction with depolarising muscle relaxants such as suxamethonium. It should not be used during cyclopropane or halothane anaesthesia, although it may be used after withdrawal of these agents.

Large doses by mouth should be avoided in conditions where there may be increased absorption from the gastro-intestinal tract. Neostigmine should be avoided in patients known to be hypersensitive; the bromide ion from neostigmine bromide may contribute to the allergic reaction.

Postoperative leakage from ileorectal anastomoses occurred in 12 out of 33 patients with chronic ulcerative colitis who received neostigmine during anaesthesia to reverse the muscle relaxant compared with 2 leakages out of 50 similar patients who did not receive neostigmine.— C. M. A. Bell and C. B. Lewis, *Br. med. J.*, 1968, *3*, 587. An intravenous injection of 2 to 2.5 mg of neostigmine with, or preceded by 0.6 to 1.2 mg of atropine, greatly increased bowel activity in unanaesthetised patients and in 38% of patients anaesthetised with anaesthetics other than halothane. In patients anaesthetised with 1 to 2% of halothane, this effect on the bowel was reduced or abolished. It was suggested that recently constructed ileorectal anastomoses were particularly at risk when neostigmine was used to reverse muscle relaxation; atropine did not reduce the risk.— J. L. Wilkins *et al.*, *Br. med. J.*, 1970, *1*, 793. Suture line leakage has been associated with the use of neostigmine in anaesthetic regimens for patients undergoing colorectal surgery. If reversal of muscle relaxation due to non-depolarising muscle relaxants is required in these patients then edrophonium may be preferable.— A. R. Hunter, *Br. J. Anaesth.*, 1986, *58*, 825.

Treatment of residual non-depolarising neuromuscular block by administration of neostigmine in association with atropine to a patient with dystrophia myotonica was only partly effective, and following a second dose of both drugs complete neuromuscular block developed. In a second patient, with a history of progressive muscle dystrophy, the administration of neostigmine to reverse residual non-depolarising blockade gave rise to a tonic response in the indirectly stimulated muscle. The type and degree of the response to neostigmine, and probably other anticholinesterases, cannot be predicted in patients with neuromuscular disease.— W. Buzello *et al.*, *Br. J. Anaesth.*, 1982, *54*, 529.

See also under Reversal of neuromuscular blockade, below.

INTERACTIONS. Decrease in muscle strength occurred in 30 of 42 courses of methylprednisolone given to 9 severely myasthenic patients also receiving either neostigmine methylsulphate intramuscularly or pyridostigmine bromide by mouth; in 24 courses, weakness was very marked, necessitating continual assisted ventilation. During courses accompanied by a decrease in strength, previously effective doses of anticholinesterase either had less effect or produced a decrease in muscle strength with concomitant increase in muscarinic side-effects.— N. G. Brunner *et al.*, *Neurology*, 1972, *22*, 603. See also W. Jubiz and A. W. Meikle, *Drugs*, 1979, *18*, 113.

REVERSAL OF NEUROMUSCULAR BLOCKADE. The neuromuscular block induced by tubocurarine, metocurine, or gallamine, during halothane anaesthesia was antagonised by a single dose of neostigmine preceded by atropine but was potentiated by a second dose given 2 to 3 minutes later. A possible explanation was that the tetanus had fully recovered after the first dose and that the second dose was acting on normal unblocked muscle. It was suggested that neostigmine in doses used clinically may produce an acetylcholine-induced block which could be a potential hazard in clinical anaesthesia.— R. Hughes *et al.*, *Br. J. Anaesth.*, 1979, *51*, 568P; J. P. Payne *et al.*, *ibid.*, 1980, *52*, 69.

Absorption and Fate

Neostigmine is a quaternary ammonium compound and as the bromide is poorly absorbed from the gastro-intestinal tract. Following parenteral administration as the methylsulphate, neostigmine is rapidly eliminated and is excreted in the urine both as unchanged drug and metabolites. It is metabolised partly by hydrolysis of the ester linkage.

Neostigmine was rapidly eliminated from the plasma of 5 patients to whom 5 mg of the methylsulphate had been given to antagonise residual neuromuscular block. The plasma concentration of neostigmine declined to about 8% of its initial value after 5 minutes with a distribution half-life of less than one minute. Elimination half-life ranged from about 15 to 30 minutes. Trace amounts of neostigmine could be detected in the plasma after one hour.— N. E. Williams *et al.*, *Br. J. Anaesth.*, 1978, *50*, 1065.

In 4 non-myasthenic patients given neostigmine 2.5 or 3 mg intravenously to antagonise the neuromuscular block after general surgery the mean plasma half-life of neostigmine was 0.89 hours (range 0.79 to 1.01 hours). In 3 fasting myasthenic patients peak plasma concentrations occurred 1 to 2 hours after a single dose of neostigmine 30 mg by mouth and mean plasma half-life was 0.87 hours. Comparison of these results suggested a bioavailability of 1-2% of the oral dose, although considerable individual differences in absorption were found.— S. -M. Aquilonius *et al.*, *Eur. J. clin. Pharmac.*, 1979, *15*, 367.

In patients with myasthenia gravis given a single dose of neostigmine methylsulphate intramuscularly the mean plasma half-life was 71.9 minutes. Approximately 50% of the dose was eliminated unchanged in the urine within 24 hours with 15% appearing as 3-hydroxyphenyltrimethylammonium and about 15% as other metabolites. It was suggested that metabolism and biliary excretion may play significant roles in the elimination of neostigmine.— S. M. Somani *et al.*, *Clin. Pharmac. Ther.*, 1980, *28*, 64.

The mean elimination half-life of neostigmine was 39 minutes following administration of 100 µg per kg body-weight intravenously to reverse neuromuscular blockade in 5 infants aged 2 to 10 months; in 5 children aged 1 to 6 years, and 5 adults, who received 70 µg per kg, mean elimination half-lives were 48 and 67 minutes respectively. The larger dose in infants was to prolong the time period over which neostigmine was detectable in serum. The results demonstrated that elimination half-life of neostigmine was significantly lower in infants and children than in adults, although this was not related to duration of effect in antagonising neuromuscular blockade.— D. M. Fisher *et al.*, *Anesthesiology*, 1983, *59*, 220.

Uses and Administration

Neostigmine inhibits cholinesterase activity and thus prolongs and intensifies the physiological actions of acetylcholine (see p.1328). It probably also has direct effects on skeletal muscle fibres. The anticholinesterase actions of neostigmine are reversible.

In the treatment of myasthenia gravis neostigmine is given where possible by mouth as the bromide in a total daily dose usually between 75 and 300 mg, divided throughout the day, and if necessary the night, according to individual response; larger portions of the total dose may be given at times of greater fatigue. In some instances, larger total daily doses may be required. In patients in whom oral therapy is impractical neostigmine methylsulphate has been employed in doses of 1 to 2.5 mg by intramuscular or subcutaneous injection at intervals, giving a total daily dose usually in the range 5 to 20 mg. Administration by the intravenous route is hazardous; if used, administration must be by very slow injection and atropine must be held ready to counteract any severe muscarinic reactions. The manufacturers state that 0.5 mg by intravenous injection is approximately equivalent in effect to 1 to 1.5 mg by intramuscular or subcutaneous injection, or 15 mg of the bromide by mouth.

In some patients, improved response has been achieved by concomitant administration of an ephedrine salt with neostigmine bromide.

In the treatment of neonatal myasthenia doses in the range 50 to 250 μg of the methylsulphate by injection, or 1 to 5 mg of the bromide by mouth, have been given every 4 hours; treatment is rarely needed beyond 8 weeks of age.

Neostigmine has also been used in the diagnosis of myasthenia gravis.

Neostigmine methylsulphate is used to curtail the muscular relaxation produced by non-depolarising muscle relaxants such as tubocurarine and gallamine; for adults the usual dose is 2 to 3 mg given concomitantly with 0.6 to 1.2 mg of atropine sulphate by slow intravenous injection over a period of 60 seconds. Additional neostigmine may be given until the muscle power is normal but a total of 5 mg should not be exceeded. The recommended ratio of atropine to neostigmine given varies from 1:2 to 1:3. A suggested dose for children is 50 μg per kg body-weight. Lower doses of neostigmine are used in the USA.

It is also used in the treatment of paralytic ileus and postoperative urinary retention, in doses of 15 to 30 mg of the bromide by mouth, or more usually 0.5 to 1 mg of the methylsulphate by subcutaneous or intramuscular injection.

A 3% solution of the methylsulphate has been instilled to lower intra-ocular pressure in the treatment of glaucoma.

ADMINISTRATION IN RENAL FAILURE. Studies during anaesthesia indicated that the mean serum elimination half-life of neostigmine was 79.8 minutes in 8 patients with normal renal function but was prolonged to a mean of 181.1 minutes in 4 anephric patients.— R. Cronnelly *et al., Anesthesiology*, 1979, *51*, 222.

The interval between doses of neostigmine should be extended from 6 hours to 12 to 18 hours in patients with a glomerular filtration-rate of less than 10 mL per minute.— W. M. Bennett *et al., Am. J. Kidney Dis.*, 1983, *3*, 155.

CONSTIPATION. References to the use of neostigmine in severe constipation: H. J. Dworken, *Ann. intern. Med.*, 1984, *100*, (Apr.), I-7 (following spinal cord injury); L. S. Miller (letter), *ibid.*, *101*, 279; O. A. Thurtle *et al., J. R. Soc. Med.*, 1984, *77*, 327 (with alpha-adrenoceptor blockers in intractable constipation due to malignant phaeochromocytoma).

MYASTHENIA GRAVIS. A review of the pathogenesis of myasthenia gravis, and of current concepts in its management. The disorder is characterised by defective neuromuscular transmission and consequent muscular weakness due to formation of auto-antibodies to acetylcholine receptors. The thymus appears to be involved. There are several varieties: generalised, affecting muscles other than the extra-ocular muscles; ocular, clinically confined to the extra-ocular muscles; neonatal, which may persist for 1 to 6 weeks in the infants of myasthenic mothers due to transplacental passage of receptor antibodies; penicillamine-induced; and congenital, for which no effective treatment is available— anticholinesterase drugs are unhelpful, and 4-aminopyridine is too toxic.

There is still debate about the management of generalised myasthenia gravis. Symptomatic treatment is by anticholinesterases, most commonly oral pyridostigmine, although neostigmine, with a shorter duration of action but quicker onset, may offer an advantage at the beginning of the day. The dose must be adjusted to give the maximum therapeutic response: this may not restore muscle strength to normal and some patients must live with a degree of disability. Edrophonium, which has a short duration of action, may be employed between doses to establish whether the patient is under- or overdosed.

Corticosteroids and azathioprine are the main immunosuppressive drugs used. The place of the former is for patients who are seriously ill prior to thymectomy, for those unsuitable for thymectomy, and those who are insufficiently improved postoperatively. They are also useful in patients with ocular myasthenia, who as a group respond poorly to anticholinesterases and to thymectomy, provided that their disability is severe enough to warrant long-term corticosteroid treatment with its attendant side-effects. Oral prednisolone 1 mg per kg body-weight daily is used; a regimem of 2 mg per kg on alternate days is often employed to decrease side-effects.

Azathioprine 2.5 mg per kg daily is also effective, although response is slower than with corticosteroids. It should be reserved for use in patients with severe disease unresponsive to other treatment, or as a steroid-sparing agent in patients receiving high corticosteroid dosages. It is also useful in association with plasma exchange to prevent rebound hypersecretion of antibodies.

Plasma exchange provides a dramatic but short-lived improvement in muscular strength, and is useful as a short-term measure to improve ill patients while other therapies take effect, but there is no evidence that repeated plasma exchange combined with immunosuppression is superior to immunosuppression alone.

Thymectomy is of increasing importance in the management of myasthenia gravis and is offered to all patients sufficiently fit to undergo surgery unless they have minimal symptoms, purely ocular disease, or are prepubertal (there is evidence suggesting that response to surgery is not as good as in adults, and that symptomatic treatment with anticholinesterases should be continued until adolescence, when the disease often improves spontaneously) or elderly. Complete remission or improvement may be expected in 80% of patients without thymomas, although this may take some years.

Other forms of treatment, such as irradiation or use of antithymocyte immunoglobulin, are mostly nonspecific and have been used only in patients refractory to all other treatment; however, recent work has suggested that specific immunotherapy may become possible in the future.— C. W. H. Havard and G. K. Scadding, *Drugs*, 1983, *26*, 174. For a discussion of controversies in the treatment of myasthenia gravis, including critical reference to the differentiation between cholinergic and myasthenic crisis, see L. P. Rowland, *J. Neurol. Neurosurg. Psychiat.*, 1980, *43*, 644. See also: G. K. Scadding and C. W. H. Havard, *Br. med. J.*, 1981, *283*, 1008; *Lancet*, 1982, *2*, 135.

PAIN. For a report of the relief of chronic pain following administration of anticholinesterases in 3 patients see under Physostigmine Sulphate, p.1335.

PANCREATITIS. Although elevation of blood amylase or lipase concentrations, abdominal pain, or both, following injection of morphine with neostigmine (the 'morphine-Prostigmin test') has been used to diagnose dysfunction of the sphincter of Oddi, a study showed that 6 of 10 healthy controls and 3 of 5 control patients with irritable bowel syndrome had significant rises in serum amylase and lipase concentrations following intramuscular injection of morphine sulphate 10 mg and neostigmine methylsulphate 1 mg; one of the latter 3 had abdominal pain as well, and one of the patients with irritable bowel syndrome had abdominal pain without a rise in enzyme values. Of a further 4 patients with chronic abdominal pain of unknown origin, the results of the test were reproducible on separate days only in 2. Major clinical decisions should not be made on the basis of this test.— W. M. Steinberg *et al., Gastroenterology*, 1980, *78*, 728. See also.— I. C. Roberts-Thomson and J. Toouli, *Gut*, 1985, *26*, 1367.

REVERSAL OF NEUROMUSCULAR BLOCKADE. When reversal of curarisation in 31 patients was undertaken using simultaneous intravenous injections of atropine 20 μg per kg body-weight and neostigmine 50 μg per kg, no serious cardiac hazards were encountered if hyperventilation was maintained throughout the recovery period.— A. Baraka, *Br. J. Anaesth.*, 1968, *40*, 30. See also *idem.*, 27.

Simultaneous injection of atropine with neostigmine intravenously over 60 seconds appeared to be the most suitable method for the reversal of neuromuscular blockade.— V. Rosner *et al., Br. J. Anaesth.*, 1971, *43*, 1066.

In a study involving 12 infants between 3 and 48 weeks of age, and 15 children aged 1 to 8 years, all undergoing nitrous oxide-halothane anaesthesia, neuromuscular blockade by continuous infusion of tubocurarine was antagonised by intravenous injection of neostigmine 6.25, 12.5, or 25 μg per kg body-weight with atropine 5, 10, or 20 μg per kg respectively. The calculated dose required to produce 50% antagonism of neuromuscular blockade was 13.1 μg per kg for infants and 15.5 μg per kg for children, compared with reported values for adults (R.D. Miller *et al., Anesthesiology*, 1974, *41*, 27) indicating a calculated dose of 22.9 μg per kg. Although it is commonly believed that infants and children require larger doses for their weight than adults these results suggest that neostigmine dose requirements are smaller in paediatric patients.— D. M. Fisher *et al., Anesthesiology*, 1983, *59*, 220.

For references to the use of glycopyrronium bromide with neostigmine for reversing neuromuscular block, see Glycopyrronium Bromide, p.533.

See also under Precautions (above).

SNAKE BITE. Neostigmine 500 μg intravenously, repeated on 2 occasions, was successfully used in the treatment of snake bite [probably cobra] in a 10-year-old child; it was considered to have reversed respiratory paralysis caused by the neurotoxin component of the venom.— R. W. Naphade and R. N. Shetti, *Br. J. Anaesth.*, 1977, *49*, 1065. Neostigmine would be of no value in the treatment of bites from snakes of which the venom has neurotoxins which act presynaptically, including the Asian krait, the Australian tiger snake, and the taipan.— T. Brophy and S. K. Sutherland (letter), *Br. J. Anaesth.*, 1979, *51*, 264. Of 2 patients bitten by a Malayan krait (*Bungarus candidus*) one, who responded to polyspecific antivenom, had no objective improvement in muscle power following subcutaneous injection of neostigmine 1 mg, preceded by atropine 0.6 mg; a second patient, who did not respond to *B. fasciatus* antivenom, improved markedly following an initial dose of edrophonium 10 mg intravenously after atropine 0.6 mg. More sustained improvement was provided by continuous infusion of neostigmine 0.5 mg per hour with atropine 0.15 mg per hour. In view of conflicting reports, further critical clinical studies are needed of adjuvant treatment such as anticholinesterases in neurotoxic envenoming.— D. A. Warrell *et al., Br. med. J.*, 1983, *286*, 678.

TETRODOTOXIN POISONING. For reference to the use of neostigmine and edrophonium in the treatment of tetrodotoxin poisoning caused by eating puffer fish, see under Edrophonium Chloride, p.1331.

Preparations

Neostigmine Injection *(B.P.)*. Contains neostigmine methylsulphate.

Neostigmine Methylsulfate Injection *(U.S.P.)*

Neostigmine Bromide Tablets *(U.S.P.)*

Neostigmine Tablets *(B.P.)*. Tablets containing neostigmine bromide.

Proprietary Preparations

Prostigmin *(Roche, UK)*. *Tablets*, scored, neostigmine bromide 15 mg.

Injection, neostigmine methylsulphate 0.5 and 2.5 mg/mL, in ampoules of 1 mL.

Proprietary Names and Manufacturers of Neostigmine Bromide and Neostigmine Methylsulphate

Intrastigmina *(Lusofarmaco, Ital.)*; Juvastigmin *(Austral.; Switz.)*; Prostigmin *(Roche, Austral.; Roche, Canad.; Roche, Denm.; Roche, Ger.; Neth.; Roche, Norw.; Roche, S.Afr.; Swed.; Roche, UK; Roche, USA)*; Prostigmina *(Roche, Ital.)*; Prostigmine *(Belg.; Roche, Fr.; Roche, Spain; Roche, Switz.)*.

4521-h

Physostigmine *(USAN)*.

Eserine. (3a*S*,8a*R*)-1,2,3,3a,8,8a-Hexahydro-1,3a,8-trimethylpyrrolo[2,3-*b*]indol-5-yl methylcarbamate.

$C_{15}H_{21}N_3O_2$=275.4.

CAS — 57-47-6.

Pharmacopoeias. In *U.S.* Also in *B.P.C. 1973.*

An alkaloid obtained from the calabar bean (ordeal bean; chopnut), the seed of *Physostigma venenosum* (Leguminosae). It occurs as a white, odourless, microcrystalline powder which becomes pink on exposure to heat, light, air, or contact with traces of metals. M.p. not lower than 103°. Slightly **soluble** in water; very soluble in chloroform or dichloromethane; freely soluble in alcohol; soluble in fixed oils. Sterile oily solutions are prepared aseptically. **Store** in airtight containers. Protect from light.

4523-b

Physostigmine Salicylate *(BAN, USAN)*.

Eserine Salicylate; Eserinii Salicylas; Physostig. Sal.; Physostigmine Monosalicylate; Physostigmini Salicylas; Physostigminii Salicylas.

$C_{15}H_{21}N_3O_2,C_7H_6O_3$=413.5.

CAS — 57-64-7.

Pharmacopoeias. In *Arg., Aust., Belg., Br., Cz., Eur., Fr., Ger., Hung., Ind., Int., It., Jpn, Jug., Mex., Neth., Nord., Pol., Port., Roum., Rus., Swiss, Turk.*, and *U.S.*

Colourless or white odourless crystals or white powder. The crystals and their aqueous solution become red on exposure to heat, light, air, and contact with traces of metals.

The *B.P.* states that it is **soluble** 1 in 90 of water and 1 in 25 of alcohol. Soluble in chloroform and very slightly soluble in ether. A 0.9% solution in water free of carbon dioxide has a pH of 5.1 to 5.9. The *U.S.P.* solubilities are: 1 in 75 of water, 1 in 16 of alcohol, 1 in 6 of chloroform, and 1 in 250 of ether. The pH of the *U.S.P.* injection is between 3.5 and 5.0. **Store** in airtight containers. Protect from light.

Solutions are unstable and should be freshly prepared or, if kept, stored in hermetically sealed containers. Solutions for injection should not be used if more than slightly discoloured.

4524-v

Physostigmine Sulphate *(BAN)*.

Eserine Sulphate; Physostig. Sulph.; Physostigmine Sulfate *(USAN)*.

$(C_{15}H_{21}N_3O_2)_2,H_2SO_4$=648.8.

CAS — 64-47-1.

Pharmacopoeias. In *Br., Braz., Port., Span., Swiss,* and *U.S.* Also in *B.P. Vet.*

A white or almost white, deliquescent, odourless or almost odourless, microcrystalline powder. The powder and its aqueous solution become red on exposure to heat, light, air, and contact with traces of metals.

B.P. **solubilities** are: 1 in less than 1 of water or alchohol; slightly soluble in ether. *U.S.P.* solubilities are: 1 in 4 of water, 1 in 0.4 of alcohol, and 1 in 1200 of ether. A 1% solution has a pH of 3.5 to 5.5. Solutions for use in eye-drops may be **sterilised** by heating at 98° to 100° for 30 minutes with a bactericide. **Store** in airtight containers. Protect from light. Solutions should be freshly prepared or, if kept, stored in hermetically sealed containers.

The degradation products of physostigmine which might be formed after heat sterilisation of eye-drops were eseroline, rubreserine, eserine blue, and eserine brown. The anticholinesterase activity *in vitro* of eseroline and rubreserine was 1000 to 5000 times less than that of physostigmine. Eserine blue was the most potent degradation product and was 100 to 500 times less active than physostigmine.— B. A. Hemsworth and G. B. West (letter), *J. Pharm. Pharmac.*, 1968, *20,* 406.

Physostigmine eye-drops 0.25, 0.5, or 1%, prepared to the *B.P.C. 1973* formula (pH 3.6 to 3.8) and sterilised by heating or by filtration retained more than 99% of their activity after storage at 25° for 1 year. A faint pink colour occurred after sterilisation by heat, and in all samples after storage for 1 year.— A. R. Rogers and G. Smith, *Pharm. J.*, 1973, *2,* 353.

Preliminary results indicating that, in the opinion of the authors, eye-drop formulations of pilocarpine hydrochloride with physostigmine sulphate could be successfully sterilised by autoclaving at 115° for 30 minutes.— A. E. Mair and J. H. M. Miller, *J. clin. Hosp. Pharm.*, 1984, *9,* 217.

Adverse Effects, Treatment, and Precautions

As for Neostigmine Methylsulphate, p.1332.

Toxic effects are usually more severe than those occurring with neostigmine.

Atropine was not successful in the management of a patient who had taken 1 g of physostigmine salicylate; it was associated with tachycardia and multifocal ventricular ectopic beats.— G. Cumming *et al.*, *Lancet*, 1968, *2,* 147. A slow intravenous injection of 5 mg of propranolol might reduce the heart-rate and avert the danger of ventricular fibrillation in physostigmine poisoning. Propranolol in conjunction with atropine had been found a safe procedure, slowing the heart-rate to its low intrinsic level.— A. Valero (letter), *ibid.*, 459. Results of a study in *mice* suggested that hyoscine might be more appropriate than atropine in the treatment of poisoning caused by very high doses of centrally acting anticholinesterases such as physostigmine.— D. Janowsky *et al.* (letter), *Lancet*, 1984, *2,* 747.

Interactions. A prolonged response to suxamethonium occurred in a 25-year-old woman undergoing caesarean section who had, about 15 minutes earlier, received physostigmine salicylate 2 mg intravenously followed by 2 mg intramuscularly to control the adverse effects of the premedication.— A. F. Kopman *et al.*, *Anesthesiology*, 1978, *49,* 142.

Absorption and Fate

Physostigmine is readily absorbed from the gastro-intestinal tract, subcutaneous tissues, and mucous membranes. It is largely destroyed in the body by hydrolysis of the ester linkage by cholinesterases; a 1-mg dose injected subcutaneously has been claimed to be destroyed in 2 hours. It crosses the blood-brain barrier. Little is excreted in the urine.

A preliminary study of the pharmacokinetics of physostigmine. Following doses of physostigmine salicylate 1 or 2 mg as a solution by mouth in a healthy subject, physostigmine concentrations in the blood were below the detectable level of 50 pg per mL, although low concentrations were measurable in urine. A dose of 4 mg produced measurable blood concentrations with a peak after 45 minutes, and an apparent first-order half-life of 25 to 30 minutes. Measurable blood concentrations were associated with changes in blood pressure and there was a non-linear relationship between the size of the dose and urinary excretion.— M. Gibson *et al.* (letter), *Lancet*, 1985, *1,* 695. Physostigmine was clearly measurable in plasma within 15 minutes of ingestion of a tablet of physostigmine salicylate 2 mg by a healthy subject. A peak concentration of 1.03 ng per mL was achieved at 30 minutes; concentrations then fell and were undetectable by 2 hours after ingestion. These results show that there are marked differences in the absorption and metabolism of physostigmine in individual subjects.— N. S. Sharpless and L. J. Thal (letter), *ibid.*, 1397. Following oral doses of 2 or 3 mg of physostigmine salicylate in water, and intravenous infusion of 0.6 or 1.2 mg, availability of the oral dose in 3 healthy subjects was 11.7, 5.2, and 7.8%. High values of clearance indicated extrahepatic metabolism.— R. Whelpton and P. Hurst (letter), *New Engl. J. Med.*, 1985, *313,* 1293.

A study of the pharmacokinetics of physostigmine following oral administration of physostigmine aminoxide oral drops or granules.— A. Astier and O. Petitjean, *J. Pharmac. clin.*, 1985, *4,* 521.

Uses and Administration

Physostigmine is an inhibitor of cholinesterase activity with actions similar to those of neostigmine (see p.1332).

Physostigmine is used as a miotic. It may be used to counteract the dilatation of the pupil caused by atropine, homatropine, or cocaine; in these circumstances it may, however, produce considerable irritation and pain due to spasm. Physostigmine has also been used, alone or more usually in combination with other miotics such as pilocarpine, to decrease intra-ocular pressure in glaucoma.

Unlike neostigmine, physostigmine crosses the blood-brain barrier and can reverse the central as well as the peripheral effects of antimuscarinic agents such as atropine. Physostigmine, 0.5 to 2 mg subcutaneously, intramuscularly, or by slow intravenous injection, repeated every 1 or 2 hours as necessary, has been advocated for the reversal of antimuscarinic poisoning associated with overdosage of antimuscarinic agents and tricyclic antidepressants. In general, however, such treatment is not recommended (see Antimuscarinic Poisoning, below).

A 0.25% ointment has been employed in the treatment of pediculosis of the eyelashes.

Studies of the effects of physostigmine on memory: *J. Am. med. Ass.*, 1978, *239,* 2419; K. L. Davis *et al.*, *Science*, 1978, *201,* 272; K. L. Davis *et al.* (letter), *New Engl. J. Med.*, 1979, *301,* 946.

ALZHEIMER'S DISEASE. Physostigmine has been administered to small groups of patients with Alzheimer's disease in an effort to improve the cholinergic deficit found in the brains of such patients. Davis and Mohs (*Am. J. Psychiat.*, 1982, *139,* 1421) found a significant improvement in memory processes in 8 of 10 patients with moderately severe disease, following intravenous infusion of previously-determined optimum individual doses of physostigmine. In view of the limitations of parenteral therapy various researchers have given physostigmine by mouth: Jotkowitz (*Ann. Neurol.*, 1983, *14,* 690) reported no clinical improvement in 10 patients with mild to severe disease given 1.25 mg every 3 hours, increased to 2.0 to 2.5 mg, over a period of up to 10 months. However, Davis *et al.* (*New Engl. J. Med.*, 1983, *308,* 721) found that administration of individualised doses of physostigmine in the range 0.25 to 2 mg every 2 hours produced improvements in memory performance or disease assessment score in 10 of 12 patients when compared with placebo but the effect was considered clinically meaningful in only 2. A similar study (L. J. Thal and P.A. Fuld, *ibid.*, 720) reported improved results in a memory test in 8 of 12 patients with early disease who were given physostigmine in association with lecithin, the peak performance being associated with physostigmine doses of 1.0 to 2.5 mg six times daily at 2-hour intervals. Although no benefit has been demonstrated in studies giving lecithin alone, Peters and Levin (*Ann. Neurol.*, 1979, *6,* 219) found physostigmine with lecithin enhanced memory storage and retrieval compared with physostigmine alone, and it has been suggested (R.J. Wurtman, *New Engl. J. Med.*, 1983, *309,* 555) that until more is known about the extent to which cholinergic brain neurones use the choline in their own membrane lecithins for acetylcholine synthesis, generous quantities of lecithin or another choline source should be supplied when patients with Alzheimer's disease are given anticholinesterases.

For a report of the use of bethanechol infusion in patients with Alzheimer's disease, see under Bethanechol Chloride, p.1329.

ANAESTHESIA. Studies on physostigmine for the reversal of postanaesthetic or postanalgesic effects.— J. Brebner and L. Hadley, *Can. Anaesth. Soc. J.*, 1976, *23,* 574; H. G. R. Balmer and S. R. Wyte (letter), *Br. J. Anaesth.*, 1977, *49,* 510 (reversal of ketamine-induced sedation without loss of analgesia); M. Weinstock *et al.*, *ibid.*, 1982, *54,* 429 (reversal of morphine-induced sedation and enhanced or unaffected analgesia).

ANTIMUSCARINIC POISONING. Although physostigmine can reverse effects of antimuscarinic and tricyclic antidepressant poisoning, most reviewers agree that in general such a use is inappropriate and hazardous. Some clinicians consider that its use should be reserved for treatment of life-threatening symptoms such as uncontrollable convulsions, coma with respiratory depression, or severe hypertension (*Med. Lett.*, 1987, *29,* 83). Newton (*J. Am. med. Ass.*, 1975, *231,* 941) concluded from a study of 21 patients suffering from tricyclic overdosage that in the routine management of tricyclic poisoning the hazards of the cholinergic properties of physostigmine, in particular the risk of inducing respiratory difficulty, outweigh any benefits of an early return to consciousness. In order to counteract the peripheral cholinergic actions of physostigmine, yet benefit from its central cholinergic properties, Aquilonius and Hedstrand (*Acta anaesth. scand.*, 1978, *22,* 40) administered propantheline bromide to 10 patients with tricyclic poisoning before giving physostigmine; as anticipated successful reversal of central effects of the tricyclics was achieved without significant peripheral cholinergic toxicity, but the beneficial effect of physostigmine on consciousness lasted less than 1 hour and one patient suffered grand mal seizures. They concluded that the use of physostigmine had not been shown to affect the mortality-rate in tricyclic poisoning and might exacerbate the risk of grand mal seizures. Indeed seizures have been reported by Knudsen and Heath (*Br. med. J.*, 1984, *288,* 601) in 6 of 7 patients treated with physostigmine for maprotiline overdosage.

Nevertheless Pall *et al.* (*Acta pharmac. tox.*, 1977, *41, Suppl.* 2, 171) do consider that seriously poisoned patients may benefit from physostigmine administration and that not only does it have a beneficial effect on the central aspects of antimuscarinic poisoning but that some of the adverse cardiac effects of tricyclics may be also reversed. However, as a serious complication of physostigmine administration, they pointed out that 2 patients, both known chronic alcoholics, developed acute pancreatitis. Physostigmine has a shorter duration of action than most antimuscarinic agents, and a considerably shorter duration of action than most tricyclics, therefore reports of the successful use of physostigmine have highlighted the need for repeated doses over periods of hours or days (see R.H. Brier, *Ann. intern. Med.*, 1978, *89,* 579). Briefly discussing the difficulties in the diagnosis and treatment of antimuscarinic poisoning Caine (*New Engl. J. Med.*, 1979, *300,* 1278) suggested that although physostigmine can be beneficial when absolutely necessary to maintain the patient's safety, its use could lead to severe cardiac and respiratory effects, and that in uncomplicated cases of overdosage, to await the spontaneous remission of toxicity could be the safest treatment of all. Crome (*Drugs*, 1982, *23,* 431) in another brief review felt that while physostigmine may be helpful in comatose patients with complications such as pneumonia there is insufficient evidence to recommend the general use of physostigmine in tricyclic-induced coma.

ATAXIA. A report of the beneficial effect of physostigmine in patients with familial ataxias.— R. A. P. Kark et al., *Neurology*, 1977, *27*, 70.

DELIRIUM TREMENS. A report of the use of intravenous physostigmine in the management of 2 patients with delirium tremens.— J. S. Powers *et al.*, *J. clin. Pharmac.*, 1981, *21*, 57.

GILLES DE LA TOURETTE'S SYNDROME. The reduction of tics after treatment with physostigmine in patients with the Tourette syndrome appears to be due to an increase in central cholinergic activity. Six patients with frequent and relatively constant motor tics given physostigmine 50 µg per kg body-weight infused intravenously over one hour had a significant decrease in tic frequency with the greatest effect 30 minutes after the infusion. Patients were pretreated with propantheline to prevent peripheral cholinergic effects.— S. M. Stahl and P. A. Berger (letter), *New Engl. J. Med.*, 1980, *302*, 1311. See also *idem*, 298.

PAIN. Three of 12 patients with severe chronic pain of neurological origin obtained marked improvement following slow intravenous injection of physostigmine 0.5 to 1 mg. Of the 3 responders 2 had thalamic pain and one of these was subsequently maintained pain-free on pyridostigmine 30 and 60 mg alternately by mouth every 3 hours; the other received no benefit from pyridostigmine, but was much improved following physostigmine 0.5 mg or neostigmine 15 mg by mouth, given every 3 hours. Despite subsequent withdrawal of medication in the latter patient due to side-effects, severe pain did not return. The third patient, with causalgia due to the shoulder-hand syndrome, achieved sustained pain relief by self administration of physostigmine 0.5 mg subcutaneously four times daily.— G. D. Schott and L. Loh, *Pain*, 1984, *20*, 201.

Preparations

Physostigmine and Pilocarpine Eye-drops *(B.P.C. 1973)*. Eserine and Pilocarpine Eye-drops. A sterile solution containing up to 0.5% of physostigmine sulphate and up to 4% of pilocarpine hydrochloride. The solution is adversely affected by alkalis.

Physostigmine Eye Drops *(A.P.F.)*. Eserine Eye-drops. Contain physostigmine sulphate 0.5%.

Physostigmine Eye Drops *(B.P.)*. Eserine Eye Drops; ESR. Contain physostigmine sulphate.

Physostigmine Salicylate Injection *(U.S.P.)*. pH 3.5 to 5.0.

Physostigmine Salicylate Ophthalmic Solution *(U.S.P.)*. pH 2 to 4.

Physostigmine Sulfate Ophthalmic Ointment *(U.S.P.)*. A sterile eye ointment containing physostigmine sulphate.

Proprietary Names and Manufacturers of Physostigmine and its derivatives

Anticholium *(Köhler, Ger.)*; Antilirium *(Forest, Canad.; Forest Pharmaceuticals, USA)*; Fisostin *(Allergan, Ital.)*; Génésérine 3 *(Amido, Fr.)*; Isopto-Eserine *(Alcon Laboratories, USA)*.

4525-g

Pilocarpine *(USAN)*.

(3*S*,4*R*)-3-Ethyldihydro-4-[(1-methyl-1*H*-imidazol-5-yl)methyl]furan-2(3*H*)-one.
$C_{11}H_{16}N_2O_2$=208.3.

CAS — 92-13-7.

Pharmacopoeias. In *U.S. Braz.*, *Fr.*, *Port.*, and *Span.* include monographs for Jaborandi.

An alkaloid obtained from the leaflets of jaborandi, *Pilocarpus microphyllus* (Rutaceae) and other species of *Pilocarpus*. A viscous, hygroscopic, oily liquid or crystals. M.p. about 34°. **Soluble** in water, alcohol, and chloroform; sparingly soluble in ether; practically insoluble in light petroleum. **Store** at a temperature not exceeding 8° in airtight containers. Protect from light.

4526-q

Pilocarpine Hydrochloride *(BAN, USAN)*.

Pilocarp. Hydrochlor.; Pilocarpine Monohydrochloride; Pilocarpini Chloridum; Pilocarpini Hydrochloridum; Pilocarpinium Chloratum.
$C_{11}H_{16}N_2O_2$,HCl=244.7.

CAS — 54-71-7.

Pharmacopoeias. In *Arg.*, *Aust.*, *Br.*, *Braz.*, *Cz.*, *Hung.*, *Int.*, *It.*, *Jpn*, *Jug.*, *Mex.*, *Nord.*, *Pol.*, *Port.*, *Roum.*, *Rus.*, *Span.*, *Swiss*, and *U.S.* Also in *B.P.Vet.*

Odourless or almost odourless hygroscopic colourless crystals or white crystalline powder with a slightly bitter taste.
Soluble 1 in 0.3 of water, 1 in 3 of alcohol, and 1 in 360 of chloroform; practically insoluble in ether. A 0.5% solution in water has a pH of 3.8 to 5.2. **Store** in airtight containers. Protect from light.

4527-p

Pilocarpine Nitrate *(BAN, USAN)*.

Pilocarp. Nit.; Pilocarpine Mononitrate; Pilocarpini Nitras; Pilocarpinii Nitras; Pilocarpinium Nitricum.
$C_{11}H_{16}N_2O_2$,HNO_3=271.3.

CAS — 148-72-1.

Pharmacopoeias. In *Arg.*, *Aust.*, *Belg.*, *Br.*, *Braz.*, *Eur.*, *Fr.*, *Ger.*, *Ind.*, *Int.*, *It.*, *Mex.*, *Neth.*, *Port.*, *Roum.*, *Span.*, *Swiss*, *Turk.*, and *U.S.*

Odourless colourless or white crystals, or white crystalline powder.
B.P. **solubilities** are: soluble 1 in 8 of water; sparingly soluble in alcohol; practically insoluble in chloroform and in ether. *U.S.P.* solubilities are: soluble 1 in 4 of water and 1 in 75 of alcohol; practically insoluble in chloroform and in ether. A 5% solution in water has a pH of 3.5 to 4.5. **Store** in airtight containers. Protect from light.

Pilocarpine hydrochloride solutions packaged in syringes for single-dose delivery were found to be contaminated with the vulcanising agent 2-mercaptobenzothiazole, presumably leached from the rubber closure. Other tests showed this agent to be a common contaminant for a variety of drug solutions in similar packaging.— J. C. Reepmeyer and Y. H. Juhl, *J. pharm. Sci.*, 1983, *72*, 1302.

Adverse Effects, Treatment, and Precautions

As for Neostigmine Methylsulphate, p.1332.
Following ocular administration pilocarpine is usually better tolerated than the anticholinesterases, but in common with other miotics may produce ciliary spasm, ocular pain and irritation, blurred vision, and headache.

The dementia of Alzheimer's disease may be exacerbated by the use of pilocarpine eye-drops and withdrawal of their use may lead to substantial symptomatic improvement.— P. F. Reyes *et al.* (letter), *J. Neurol. Neurosurg. Psychiat.*, 1987, *50*, 113.

EFFECTS ON THE EYES. A review and discussion on the use of miotics and the incidence of retinal detachment.— J. J. Alpar, *Ann. Ophthal.*, 1979, *11*, 395. See also H. Beasley and F. T. Fraunfelder, *Ophthalmology*, 1979, *86*, 95.

A paradoxical increase in intra-ocular pressure occurred in a patient with unilateral angle-recession glaucoma given pilocarpine eye-drops.— B. S. Bleiman and A. L. Schwartz, *Archs Ophthal., N.Y.*, 1979, *97*, 1305.

Superficial punctate keratitis developed over the lower portion of the cornea in 26 of 59 patients who received pilocarpine gel. It occurred primarily in the first weeks of gel use, but usually cleared spontaneously. Of the 53 patients who received pilocarpine gel for more than 2 months, 15 developed a subtle corneal haze, in the majority after 9 to 12 months of therapy; 9 of the 15 had previously experienced the keratitis. The haze has persisted in 13 patients for 2 years after stopping gel therapy and regressed in 2. None of 14 patients receiving pilocarpine eye-drops had the corneal haze. The long-term significance of these corneal changes is uncertain.— D. H. Johnson *et al.*, *Am. J. Ophthal.*, 1986, *101*, 13.

The use of pilocarpine should be avoided if possible at any time after drainage operations for glaucoma because it can increase the occurrence of posterior pupillary synechiae. A topical beta-blocking agent is usually adequate if control of intra-ocular pressure is required.— C. I. Phillips *et al.*, *Br. J. Ophthal.*, 1987, *71*, 428.

Uses and Administration

Pilocarpine is a parasympathomimetic agent with primarily the muscarinic effects of acetylcholine (see p.1328). Following topical application to the eye miosis occurs in about 10 to 30 minutes and lasts 4 to 8 hours while peak reduction in intra-ocular pressure occurs within 75 minutes and the reduction usually persists for 4 to 14 hours.
Pilocarpine is most commonly used to reduce intra-ocular pressure in the treatment of open-angle glaucoma. It is used as the hydrochloride or the nitrate, usually as a 0.5 to 4% solution, the dose being adjusted individually. A sustained-release system inserted into the conjunctival sac and releasing 20 or 40 µg per hour has also been used. Pilocarpine may also be used in the emergency treatment of acute attacks of closed-angle glaucoma prior to surgery.
The miotic action of pilocarpine may also be employed to antagonise the effects of mydriatics on the eye and in surgical procedures on the eye.

Pilocarpine 1% counteracted the mydriatic effects of sympathomimetic agents, such as phenylephrine and hydroxyamphetamine in concentrations usually used in ophthalmology, within 30 minutes. After mydriasis with antimuscarinic agents, such as tropicamide and homatropine, pilocarpine did not cause effective miosis.— L. M. Anastasi *et al.*, *Archs Ophthal., N.Y.*, 1968, *79*, 710.

See also.— M. E. Nelson and H. P. Orton, *ibid.*, 1987, *105*, 486.

ADMINISTRATION. In a study involving 83 glaucomatous patients treatment with 4% pilocarpine hydrochloride gel once daily was as effective as previous therapy with pilocarpine eye-drops.— D. H. Johnson *et al.*, *Am. J. Ophthal.*, 1984, *97*, 723.

For adverse effects associated with the administration of pilocarpine gel, see under Adverse Effects, above.

DIAGNOSIS OF CYSTIC FIBROSIS. Diagnosis of cystic fibrosis relies heavily on a single pointer, the electrolyte content of sweat. The most accurate and widely-used method has been that described by Gibson and Cooke (*Pediatrics*, 1959, *23*, 545) in which sweating is promoted by pilocarpine iontophoresis. Pilocarpine nitrate, as 4 drops of a 0.2% solution on filter paper was delivered to the skin by iontophoresis with a 2 mA current for 5 minutes, and sweat subsequently collected from the area by application of a weighed filter paper disc under a plastic square for 30 minutes. Following tests in 11 patients with cystic fibrosis and 5 related and 39 unrelated controls an average of 76 mg of sweat was obtained in each collection. Polarographic analysis revealed mean chloride concentrations of 94.8, 32.5, and 21.1 µEq per mL respectively. An alternative method, using gauze squares instead of filter paper, and employing 4 mL of a 0.05 or 0.1% pilocarpine nitrate solution delivered over 15 minutes by a 4 mA current was found less convenient but permitted collection of an average of 692 mg of sweat in 14 patients, 12 relatives, and 8 unrelated controls, with mean chloride concentrations of 110.1, 33.9, and 45.4 µEq per mL respectively. The test was considered by Gibson and Cooke to be quite safe and it also avoided the danger of heat stress and the pain of local cholinergic injection. It appeared to be well adapted to testing fairly large numbers of patients consecutively, while giving good diagnostic evidence for or against cystic fibrosis. However, it has been found that the most common reason for incorrect diagnosis of cystic fibrosis is an inaccurately-performed sweat test. It is therefore recommended that testing should only be performed by an experienced person (*Lancet*, 1982, *2*, 1196). Furthermore, as the test not only demands scrupulous techniques but is also time-consuming, standardisation and monitoring of the procedures are important. Although the sweat test has been reported to recognise more than 98% of children with cystic fibrosis it is recommended that a diagnosis should not be based upon a single test; testing should always be repeated with borderline cases being tested at least 3 or 4 times (*Bull. Wld Hlth Org.*, 1985, *63*, 1). Laboratories may vary in the sodium and chloride concentrations considered abnormal but they usually use a minimum weight of sweat of 100 mg. However, it is often difficult to obtain an adequate amount in small infants and children and the use of this test may be impractical during the first 6 weeks of life and in very premature infants (*Bull. Wld Hlth Org.*, 1985, *63*, 1; *Lancet*, 1987, *1*, 24). There is also doubt as to whether fluid loss from premature babies represents true sweat. A technique to improve sweat collection in children has been described by Carter et al (*Archs Dis. Childh.*, 1984, *59*, 919) but is not considered to be applicable to very immature infants (*Lancet*, 1987, *1*, 24). For children, the area of overlap for sweat electrolyte concentrations between those with or without cystic fibrosis is small but with increasing age, concentrations for the healthy population approach those concentrations associated with cystic fibrosis. Administration of fludrocortisone reduces sweat sodium concentrations in healthy individuals to a greater extent than in patients with cystic fibrosis and it has been used in an attempt to reduce the number of false-positive results when testing is required in adults or following borderline results in children (J. M. Littlewood *et al.*, *Archs Dis. Childh.*, 1986, *61*, 1041).

GLAUCOMA. A review of the treatment of open-angle glaucoma. Treatment aims to reduce the intra-ocular pressure enough to prevent further loss of visual field, usually to below 21 mmHg, and involves topical or systemic ocular hypotensive drugs and conventional or laser surgery. Pilocarpine, usually instilled 4 times daily, is still regarded by many as the drug of first choice in patients with glaucoma, particularly for the older patient with a normal lens. Delivery by soft contact lens reservoirs and conjunctival inserts seems to be of limited value. Patients who are not controlled by pilocarpine or by timolol alone, may require a combination of pilocarpine and timolol or pilocarpine and adrenaline, and oral acetazolamide may be required as a short-term measure to reduce intra-ocular pressure. If topical drugs do not control the disease, surgery is indicated.— *Drug & Ther. Bull.*, 1983, *21*, 85. A further review of the treatment of glaucoma.— R. A. Hitchings, *Prescribers' J.*, 1983, *23*, 106.

Medical treatment has traditionally been the first-line therapy for open-angle glaucoma but drugs that need to be instilled every 6 hours, such as pilocarpine, are apt to be instilled irregularly, allowing intermittent pressure spikes with progressive visual damage.— *Lancet*, 1984, *2*, 81.

LEPROSY. The use of pilocarpine nitrate intradermally to assess the therapeutic efficacy of dapsone in patients with maculoanaesthetic leprosy.— P. B. Joshi, *Lepr. India*, 1976, *48*, 55.

REVERSAL OF ANTIMUSCARINIC ACTION. Reference to the use of pilocarpine in patients with blurred vision as a consequence of antipsychotic therapy.— J. G. Carter *et al.* (letter), *Am. J. Psychiat.*, 1977, *134*, 941.

Preparations of Pilocarpine or one of its salts

Pilocarpine Eye Drops *(A.P.F.)*. A solution containing pilocarpine hydrochloride in Water for Injections. Sterilise by autoclaving.

Pilocarpine Eye Drops *(B.P.)*. PIL. Contain pilocarpine hydrochloride.

Pilocarpine Eye Drops Buffered *(A.P.F.)*. A buffered solution containing pilocarpine hydrochloride. pH 6.5. Sterilised by maintaining at 98° to 100° for 30 minutes. They should be recently prepared. Store below 25° and use within 2 months.

Pilocarpine Hydrochloride Ophthalmic Solution *(U.S.P.)*. pH 3.5 to 5.5.

Pilocarpine Nitrate Ophthalmic Solution *(U.S.P.)*. pH 4.0 to 5.5.

Pilocarpine Ocular System *(U.S.P.)*. A sterile device containing pilocarpine intended to permit the gradual release of pilocarpine.

Proprietary Preparations

Alcon Opulets Pilocarpine *(Alcon, UK)*. *Eye-drops*, pilocarpine hydrochloride 1, 2, and 4%, in single-use disposable applicators.

Isopto Carpine *(Alcon, UK)*. *Eye-drops*, pilocarpine hydrochloride 0.5, 1, 2, 3, and 4%.

Minims Pilocarpine Nitrate *(Smith & Nephew Pharmaceuticals, UK)*. *Eye-drops*, pilocarpine nitrate 1, 2, and 4%, in single-use disposable applicators.

Ocusert Pilocarpine *(May & Baker, UK)*. *Ocular inserts* (Pilo-20), sustained-delivery system, pilocarpine 5 mg, releasing approximately 20 µg/hour for 1 week. *Ocular inserts* (Pilo-40), sustained-delivery system, pilocarpine 11 mg, releasing approximately 40 µg/hour for 1 week.

Sno Pilo *(Smith & Nephew Pharmaceuticals, UK)*. *Eye-drops*, pilocarpine hydrochloride 1, 2, and 4%.

Proprietary Names and Manufacturers of Pilocarpine or its Salts

Adsorbocarpine *(Canad.; Alcon Laboratories, USA)*; Akarpine *(Akorn, USA)*; Alcon Opulets Pilocarpine *(Alcon, UK)*; Almocarpine *(Ayerst, USA)*; Chibro-Pilocarpine *(Fr.; Switz.)*; Dropil *(Bruschettini, Ital.)*; Dulcicarpine *(Dulcis, Mon.)*; Faring-S *(Spain)*; Isopto Carpina *(Arg.; Spain)*; Isopto Carpine *(Alcon, Austral.; Alcon, Canad.; Neth.; Switz.; Alcon, UK; Alcon Laboratories, USA)*; Isopto Pilocarpin *(Alcon, Ger.)*; Isopto Pilocarpine *(Alcon, Denm.; Fr.)*; Isopto-Carpine *(Alcon, Norw.; S.Afr.)*; Isopto-Pilokarpin *(Alcon, Swed.)*; Licarpin *(Allergan, Swed.)*; Liocarpina *(SIFI, Ital.)*; Marticarpine *(Fr.)*; Minims Pilocarpina *(Smith & Nephew, Austral.)*; Minims Pilocarpine Nitrate *(Smith & Nephew, S.Afr.; Smith & Nephew Pharmaceuticals, UK)*; Miocarpine *(Coopervision, Canad.)*; Miopos *(Ursapharm, Ger.)*; Mi-Pilo *(USA)*; Neutracarpine *(Austral.)*; Ocu-Carpine *(Ocumed, USA)*; Ocusert P40 *(Recordati, Ital.)*; Ocusert Pilo *(Protea, Austral.; Canad.; May & Baker, UK; Alza, USA)*; Ocusert Pilocarpine *(May & Baker, UK)*; Pilo *(Fr.)*; Pilocar *(Ger.; Holpro, S.Afr.; Coopervision, USA)*; Pilocarpol *(Winzer, Ger.)*; Pilogel *(Alcon, Ger.)*; Pilokair *(Pharmafair, USA)*; Pilokarpin Minims *(Smith & Nephew, Denm.; Smith & Nephew, Norw.)*; Pilomann *(Mann, Ger.)*; Pilopine HS *(Alcon, Canad.; Alcon Laboratories, USA)*; Piloplos *(Arg.)*; Pilopos *(Ursapharm, Ger.)*; Pilopt *(Sigma, Austral.)*; Pilosyst 20/40 Ocusert *(Switz.)*; Pilotonina *(Farmila, Ital.)*; PV Carpine *(Allergan, Austral.; Allergan, Canad.; Allergan, S.Afr.; Allergan, USA)*; Sno Pilo *(Smith & Nephew Pharmaceuticals, UK)*; Spersacarpin *(Dispersa, Ger.)*; Spersacarpine *(Denm.; Dispersa, Swed.; Dispersa, Switz.)*; Spersakarpin *(Dispersa, Norw.)*; Thilo-Carpin *(Thilo, Ger.)*; Veriscarpina *(Spain)*; Vistacarpin *(Allergan, Ger.)*.

The following names have been used for multi-ingredient preparations containing pilocarpine or its salts—E-Carpine *(Alcon, Austral.)*; E-Pilo *(Coopervision, Canad.; Coopervision, USA)*.

4528-s

Pyridostigmine Bromide *(BAN, USAN, rINN)*.

Pyridostig. Brom.; Pyridostigmini Bromidum.
3-Dimethylcarbamoyloxy-1-methylpyridinium bromide.
$C_9H_{13}BrN_2O_2$=261.1.

CAS — 155-97-5 (pyridostigmine); 101-26-8 (bromide).

Pharmacopoeias. In *Br., Egypt., Int., Jpn, Jug., Nord.,* and *U.S.*

A white or almost white deliquescent crystalline powder with an agreeable characteristic odour. **Soluble** 1 in less than 1 of water or of alcohol, and 1 in 1 of chloroform; slightly soluble in light petroleum; practically insoluble in ether. The *B.P.* injection has a pH of 5.7 to 6.3; that of the *U.S.P.* injection is 4.5 to 5.5. Solutions for injection may be **sterilised** by autoclaving. **Store** in airtight containers. Protect from light.

Adverse Effects, Treatment, and Precautions

As for Neostigmine Methylsulphate, p.1332. It has been stated that adverse effects occur less frequently with pyridostigmine treatment than with neostigmine.

ALOPECIA. Toxic alopecia associated with pyridostigmine therapy.— L. M. Field (letter), *Archs Derm.*, 1980, *116*, 1103.

Absorption and Fate

Pyridostigmine is poorly absorbed from the gastro-intestinal tract; it is excreted mainly in the urine as unchanged drug and metabolites. It has been reported to have a plasma half-life of 1.9 hours following intravenous administration.

Pyridostigmine and three metabolites were isolated from the urine of 3 patients with myasthenia gravis given pyridostigmine. One metabolite was found to be 3-hydroxy-*N*-methylpyridinium; the other two were not identified.— S. M. Somani *et al.*, *Clin. Pharmac. Ther.*, 1972, *13*, 393.

In a study of the pharmacokinetics of pyridostigmine the mean plasma elimination half-life following intravenous injection of 2.5 mg in 2 healthy subjects was 1.52 hours, while that following a dose of 120 mg by mouth in 5 fasting subjects was 1.78 hours. The calculated bioavailability was 7.6%, and it did not change significantly when the dose was given with food, although time to peak plasma concentration was delayed from 1.7 to 3.2 hours after ingestion. In 6 patients with myasthenia gravis, in whom steady-state pyridostigmine plasma concentrations were studied, there was a 7-fold variation in concentration between patients, which cannot be explained on the basis of the pharmacokinetic data obtained from healthy subjects.— S. -M. Aquilonius, *Eur. J. clin. Pharmac.*, 1980, *18*, 423.

A study of the kinetics of intravenous pyridostigmine in 10 anaesthetised patients suggested that although it is generally assumed that pyridostigmine is eliminated more slowly than neostigmine, the clearance of pyridostigmine is in fact greater than that previously found for neostigmine, and equal doses of the drugs have a similar half-life.— T. N. Calvey *et al.* (letter), *Br. J. clin. Pharmac.*, 1981, *11*, 406.

Pyridostigmine was present in breast milk from 2 lactating mothers receiving maintenance therapy for myasthenia gravis in a concentration between 36 and 113% of that in maternal plasma, but in both cases the dose ingested per kg body-weight by the nursing infant was 0.1% or less of that ingested by the mother. Maternal medication with pyridostigmine should be no obstacle to breast feeding, at least with doses in the range of 180 to 300 mg daily.— L. -I. Hardell *et al.* (letter), *Br. J. clin. Pharmac.*, 1982, *14*, 565.

Uses and Administration

Pyridostigmine bromide is an inhibitor of cholinesterase activity with actions similar to those of neostigmine (see p.1332), but is slower in onset and of longer duration.

Pyridostigmine bromide is mainly used in the treatment of myasthenia gravis, usually in total daily doses of 0.3 to 1.2 g by mouth although more may be required; the dose should be divided throughout the day and, if necessary, the night according to the response of the patient and larger portions of the total daily dose may be given at times of greater fatigue. A suggested dose for children is 7 mg per kg body-weight daily in 6 divided doses. It has been given as sustained-release tablets, usually at bed time but these offer less flexibility of dosage. It may also be given by subcutaneous or intramuscular injection. In severe cases it can also be given by very slow intravenous injection. The manufacturers state that 2 mg by subcutaneous, intramuscular, or intravenous injection is approximately equivalent in effect to 60 mg by mouth.

In the treatment of neonatal myasthenia doses in the range 0.2 to 0.4 mg by intramuscular injection or 5 to 10 mg by mouth have been given every 4 hours; however, neostigmine has generally been preferred. Treatment is rarely needed beyond 8 weeks of age.

Pyridostigmine bromide has also been employed in the treatment of paralytic ileus and postoperative urinary retention.

Pyridostigmine is generally considered less satisfactory than neostigmine in the reversal of neuromuscular blockade produced by non-depolarising muscle relaxants such as tubocurarine and gallamine. A dose of 2 to 5 mg given intravenously, preceded by atropine 1.2 mg, and repeated to a total of 10 mg of pyridostigmine has been suggested, but doses of 10 to 20 mg have been employed.

ADMINISTRATION IN RENAL FAILURE. In patients receiving pyridostigmine for the reversal of non-depolarising muscular blockade following anaesthesia pyridostigmine kinetics were not significantly different in 5 following renal transplantation from those in 5 with normal renal function but in 4 anephric patients the elimination half-life was significantly increased and the plasma clearance significantly decreased. It appeared that approximately 75% of the plasma clearance of pyridostigmine depended on renal function.— R. Cronnelly *et al.*, *Clin. Pharmac. Ther.*, 1980, *28*, 78.

The normal half-life for pyridostigmine of 1.5 to 2 hours was prolonged in end-stage renal failure. It could be given in usual doses to patients with renal failure.— W. M. Bennett *et al.*, *Am. J. Kidney Dis.*, 1983, *3*, 155.

CONSTIPATION. A report of the use of pyridostigmine, generally in doses of 60 mg up to 3 times daily, to relieve severe constipation in patients with Parkinson's disease. No interaction has been observed with other drugs used for the management of Parkinson's disease.— K. Sadjadpour (letter), *J. Am. med. Ass.*, 1983, *249*, 1148.

REVERSAL OF NEUROMUSCULAR BLOCKADE. Investigations in 100 surgical patients indicated that pyridostigmine bromide 10 to 20 mg effectively antagonised pancuronium and appeared to be a safe alternative to neostigmine for the reversal of neuromuscular blockade due to pancuronium bromide.— M. Lippmann and R. C. Rogoff, *Anesth. Analg. curr. Res.*, 1974, *53*, 20.

Preparations

Pyridostigmine Bromide Injection *(U.S.P.)*

Pyridostigmine Bromide Syrup *(U.S.P.)*. A syrup containing 1.08 to 1.32 g of pyridostigmine bromide in each 100 mL.

Pyridostigmine Bromide Tablets *(U.S.P.)*

Pyridostigmine Injection *(B.P.)*. Contains pyridostigmine bromide.

Pyridostigmine Tablets *(B.P.)*. Tablets containing pyridostigmine bromide.

Proprietary Preparations

Mestinon *(Roche, UK)*. *Tablets*, scored, pyridostigmine bromide 60 mg.

Proprietary Names and Manufacturers

Mestinon *(Roche, Austral.*; *Belg.*; *Roche, Canad.*; *Roche, Denm.*; *Roche, Fr.*; *Roche, Ger.*; *Roche, Ital.*; *Neth.*; *Roche, Norw.*; *Roche, S.Afr.*; *Roche, Spain*; *Roche, Swed.*; *Roche, Switz.*; *Roche, UK*; *Roche, USA)*; Regonol *(Organon, Canad.*; *Organon, USA)*.

1447-q

Tacrine Hydrochloride *(BANM, rINNM)*.

Tetrahydroaminoacrine Hydrochloride. 1,2,3,4-Tetrahydroacridin-9-ylamine hydrochloride.
$C_{13}H_{14}N_2$,HCl=234.7.

CAS — 321-64-2 (tacrine); 1684-40-8 (hydrochloride).

Tacrine hydrochloride is an anticholinesterase with actions similar to those of neostigmine (p.1332). It has been used to prolong the action of suxamethonium and to antagonise competitive (non-depolarising) muscle relaxants. It has also been used as a respiratory stimulant usually in conjunction with opioid analgesics.

Doses have ranged from 10 to 120 mg usually given intravenously.

It has been investigated in Alzheimer's disease.

ALZHEIMER'S DISEASE. Anticholinesterases such as physostigmine (see p.1334) and tacrine hydrochloride have been used in an attempt to correct the cholinergic deficit found in the brains of patients with Alzheimer's disease. Encouraging improvements in some symptoms of senile dementia have been obtained by Summers *et al.* (*New Engl. J. Med.*, 1986, *315*, 1241) using tacrine given by mouth but there have been criticisms that this study lacked the rigour and control to make the results more convincing (F.J. Pirozzolo *et al.*, *New Engl. J. Med.*, 1987, *316*, 1603; N. Herrmann *et al.*, *ibid.*). It has also been pointed out that these patients were also receiving lecithin but opinion varies as to the effect it may have had on the results (G. W. Small *et al.*, *New Eng. J. Med.*, 1987, *316*, 1604; *Lancet*, 1987, *1* 139). Consequently, caution has been urged in using these findings for the prediction of any therapeutic benefit and further studies are being performed in an attempt to replicate the results.

Proprietary Names and Manufacturers

THA *(Woods, Austral.*; *WB Pharmaceuticals, UK)*.

The following names have been used for multi-ingredient preparations containing tacrine hydrochloride— Mortha *(Woods, Austral.)*.

Parathyroid Calcitonin and Biphosphonates

8050-t

The agents covered in this section are the calcium-regulating hormones, parathyroid hormone and calcitonin, and the biphosphonates. Parathyroid hormone and calcitonin are both involved in the regulation of plasma-calcium concentration, parathyroid hormone having a hypercalcaemic, and calcitonin a hypocalcaemic effect. Calcitonin is used in the treatment of hypercalcaemia, but parathyroid hormone is no longer used in the treatment of hypocalcaemia; agents used for hypocalcaemia include calcium salts (p.1028) and vitamin D substances (p.1282).

Calcitonin and the biphosphonates inhibit bone resorption and are used in the treatment of conditions associated with increased bone resorption and re-formation, such as Paget's disease of bone (osteitis deformans). The biphosphonates have been tried in the treatment of hypercalcaemia. Other agents used in the treatment of hypercalcaemia include corticosteroids (p.878), phosphate salts (p.1035), sodium sulphate (p.1107), and sodium cellulose phosphate (p.853). See also sodium fluoride (p.1616). Plicamycin (p.647) is used as an inhibitor of bone resorption.

A review of the hormonal regulation of plasma-calcium concentrations.— I. MacIntyre, *Br. med. Bull.*, 1986, *42*, 343.

Studies and discussions on the possible role of calcium-regulating hormones in the regulation of blood pressure.— A. K. Sangal and D. G. Beevers, *Br. med. J.*, 1983, *286*, 498; A. Goulding (letter), *ibid.*, 1053; T. Christensson, *ibid.*, 1899; D. E. Grobbee and A. Hofman, *Lancet*, 1986, *2*, 703; G. M. A. Palmieri *et al.*, *ibid.*, 1106; L. M. Resnick *et al.*, *Ann. intern. Med.*, 1986, *105*, 649.

A review of the design, biological evaluation, and potential uses of parathyroid hormone antagonists.— M. Rosenblatt, *New Engl. J. Med.*, 1986, *315*, 1004.

8051-x

Parathyroid Hormone

Parathyrin; PTH.

CAS — 9002-64-6.

Parathyroid hormone is a single-chain polypeptide isolated from the parathyroid glands. It contains 84 amino acids and in man the first 34 appear to be responsible for the hormonal activity. The amino-acid sequence varies according to the source.

Solutions of parathyroid hormone for injection may be diluted with glucose 2.5 to 5%. Sodium chloride solutions should not be used as they often cause precipitation. They should be **stored** at a temperature not greater than 8°.

Units

200 units of parathyroid hormone, bovine, for bioassay are contained in approximately 0.6 mg of freeze-dried trichloroacetic acid extract of bovine parathyroid glands, with lactose 5 mg in one ampoule of the first International Reference Preparation (1974).

2 units of parathyroid hormone, bovine, for immunoassay are contained in approximately 1 µg of freeze-dried purified isohormone I from bovine parathyroid, with human albumin 200 µg and lactose 1 mg in one ampoule of the first International Reference Preparation (1974).

0.1 units of human parathyroid hormone for immunoassay are contained in 100 ng of freeze-dried purified hormone with human serum albumin 250 µg and lactose 1.25 mg in one ampoule of the first International Reference Preparation (1981). One *U.S.P.* parathyroid unit represents one-hundredth of the amount of Parathyroid Injection (*U.S.P.*) required to raise the calcium content of 100 mL of the blood serum of normal *dogs* 1 mg within 16 to 18 hours after administration. The first International Standard Preparation (1985) of parathyroid hormone, bovine, for *in vitro* bioassay consists of ampoules containing the lyophilised residue of about 10 µg of parathyroid hormones, bovine, in solution in 0.01 mol per litre acetic acid and 0.1% w/v mannitol buffer.

MRC and *U.S.P.* units are approximately equivalent to international units.

Adverse Effects and Precautions

Overdosage with parathyroid hormone causes hypercalcaemia (see under Calcium, Hypercalcaemia, p.1028). Hypersensitivity reactions may occur, therefore skin tests for sensitisation should be carried out before intravenous administration.

Parathyroid hormone should be used with caution in patients with renal or cardiac disease.

Absorption and Fate

As parathyroid hormone is destroyed by proteolytic enzymes it is given by injection. Cleavage to peptide fragments occurs after administration, probably in the liver and kidney. Less than 1% of the parathyroid hormone is excreted in the urine.

Although the half-life of parathyroid hormone has been reported to be only a few minutes, the onset of action is slow. It has been stated that the response may last up to 36 hours.

Uses and Administration

Parathyroid hormone is involved in the maintenance of plasma-calcium concentrations through its actions on bone, kidney, and the gastro-intestinal tract. It increases bone resorption and stimulates production of 1,25-dihydroxycholecalciferol in the kidney. Renal excretion of inorganic phosphate is increased but overall that of calcium is decreased. It acts on the wall of the gut to increase absorption of calcium and phosphate and this is probably an indirect result of stimulating 1,25-dihydroxycholecalciferol production.

The response to an intravenous injection of parathyroid hormone may be used in the differential diagnosis of hypoparathyroidism and pseudo-hypoparathyroidism.

Parathyroid hormone was formerly used to raise the plasma-calcium concentration in acute hypoparathyroidism with tetany.

Synthetic preparations of the first 34 amino acids of human and bovine parathyroid hormones (PTH 1-34) are also in use, and other peptide fragments have been used investigationally.

Reviews of the actions of parathyroid hormone and its role in the regulation of plasma-calcium concentrations and of bone formation.— L. G. Raisz and B. E. Kream, *New Engl. J. Med.*, 1983, *309*, 29; I. MacIntyre, *Br. med. Bull.*, 1986, *42*, 343.

A review of the management of parathyroid disorders in pregnancy.— Z. M. Van Der Spuy and H. S. Jacobs, *Postgrad. med. J.*, 1984, *60*, 245.

DIAGNOSIS OF PSEUDOHYPOPARATHYROIDISM. The absence of a phosphaturic response to the exogenous administration of parathyroid hormone has been used in the diagnosis of pseudohypoparathyroidism Type II. False positive responses have been described, however, and it was therefore suggested that the effect of parathyroid hormone on 1,25-dihydroxycholecalciferol concentrations should be measured in preference.— J. Thode and S. N. Holmegaard (letter), *New Engl. J. Med.*, 1983, *308*, 104. The response of 1,25-dihydroxycholecalciferol concentrations to parathyroid hormone in this condition has not been sufficiently demonstrated, and several indices of parathyroid hormone-responsiveness, including phosphaturia, calcaemia, and the rise in 1,25-dihydroxycholecalciferol should probably be measured.— A. M. Spiegel *et al.* (letter), *ibid.*

OSTEOPOROSIS. Twenty patients with severe vertebral crush fractures and one patient with a history of fractures of the long bones were given synthetic human parathyroid hormone fragment (PTH 1-34) as once-daily subcutaneous injections for 6 to 24 months. Calcium and phosphate balances improved in some patients but there was no significant improvement overall. There were, however, substantial increases in iliac trabecular bone volume and this new bone was histologically normal. It was suggested that as vertebrae are normally more than 75% composed of trabecular bone this hormone fragment might usefully increase the strength of the vertebrae in patients with axial osteoporosis.— J. Reeve *et al.*, *Br. med. J.*, 1980, *280*, 1340; *ibid.*, *281*, 198. See also J. Reeve *et al.*, *Lancet*, 1976, *1*, 1035.

Further references: J. Reeve *et al.*, *Bone*, 1986, *7*, 160 (PTH 1-34 and oestrogens); D. M. Slovik *et al.*, *J. Bone Mineral Res.*, 1986, *1*, 377 (PTH 1-34 and calcitriol).

Preparations

Parathyroid Injection *(U.S.P.)*. A sterile solution in Water for Injections of the water-soluble hormone from the parathyroid glands of mammals, which has the property of increasing the calcium content of the blood. pH 2.5 to 3.5. It possesses a potency per mL of not less than 100 *U.S.P.* parathyroid units.

Proprietary Names and Manufacturers

Parathorm *(Hormonchemie, Ger.)*; Para-Thor-Mone *(Lilly, Austral.; Lilly, UK)*.

8052-r

Calcitonin *(BAN, USAN, rINN)*.

Thyrocalcitonin.

CAS — 9007-12-9.

A hormone, extracted from the mammalian thyroid parafollicular cells and the ultimobranchial gland in non-mammalian vertebrates, or obtained by synthesis, which has the property of lowering the calcium content of blood. It is a polypeptide containing 32 amino acids. The amino-acid sequence varies greatly from species to species. Forms used include: calcitonin (pork), calcitonin (salmon) or salcatonin, a synthetic human calcitonin, and a synthetic analogue of eel calcitonin (elcatonin).

8053-f

Calcitonin (Pork) *(BANM)*.

CAS — 12321-44-7.

Pharmacopoeias. In *Br.* and *It.*

A polypeptide hormone extractable from pork thyroid. It contains not less than 60 units per mg calculated with reference to the dried material.

A white or almost white powder. **Soluble** in water and in solutions of alkali hydroxides; practically insoluble in acetone, alcohol, chloroform, and ether; sparingly soluble in solutions of mineral acids. The *B.P.* states that it is prepared in conditions designed to minimise microbial contamination.

Store at a temperature not exceeding 25° in a well-closed container. Protect from light. Under these conditions it may be expected to retain its potency for not less than 2 years. Solutions for injection should be used within 24 hours of preparation or, if stored at 2° to 8°, within 7 days.

19126-n

Elcatonin *(rINN)*.

CAS — 60731-46-6.

A synthetic analogue of eel calcitonin.

8054-d

Salcatonin *(BAN)*.

Calcitonin (Salmon); SCT-1.

CAS — 47931-85-1.

Pharmacopoeias. In *Br.* and *Eur. Swiss* includes Human Calcitonin.

A polypeptide having the structure of salmon calcitonin I. It contains not less than 4000 units per mg calculated with reference to the peptide content.

A white or almost white, light powder. Freely **soluble** in water. Solutions are **sterilised** by filtration.

Store at 2° to 8° in a well-closed container. Protect from light. Under these conditions it may be expected to retain its potency for not less than 2 years.

Units

One unit of calcitonin, porcine, for bioassay is contained in approximately 10 µg of freeze-dried purified porcine calcitonin, with mannitol 5 mg in one ampoule of the first International Reference

Preparation (1974).
80 units of calcitonin, salmon, for bioassay are contained in approximately 20 μg of freeze-dried purified synthetic salmon calcitonin, with mannitol 2 mg in one ampoule of the first International Reference Preparation (1974).
One unit of calcitonin, human, for bioassay is contained in approximately 8.5 μg of freeze-dried synthetic human calcitonin peptide with mannitol 10 mg in one ampoule of the first International Reference Preparation (1978).
Potency is estimated by comparing the hypocalcaemic effect, in *rats*, with that of the standard preparation, and is expressed in international or MRC units which are considered to be equivalent. The first International Standard Preparation (1985) of elcatonin consists of ampoules containing approximately 3 μg of elcatonin, 0.25 mg of albumin, and 2 mg of trehalose.

Adverse Effects, Treatment, and Precautions
Calcitonin (pork) or salcatonin may cause nausea and tingling or flushing of the face or hands. Other gastro-intestinal disturbances and urinary frequency occur less often. These side-effects usually settle as treatment progresses. An unpleasant taste, inflammatory reactions at the injection site, and skin rash have also been reported. Circulating antibodies may develop after prolonged treatment but resistance to treatment does not necessarily follow. Synthetic human calcitonin may be effective in overcoming resistance to other calcitonins.
In patients with a history of allergy a skin test with a 1:100 (in the *UK*) or 1:20 (in the *US*) dilution should be performed before administration.
Calcitonin should be used with caution during pregnancy. It is better avoided during lactation.
Troublesome side-effects may be reduced by administration at bed-time or by prior administration of an anti-emetic.

Formation of antibodies to synthetic human calcitonin during treatment of Paget's disease.— F. M. Dietrich *et al.*, *Acta endocr., Copenh.*, 1979, *92*, 468.

Beneficial effect of pizotifen by mouth on the adverse effects of salcatonin in 3 patients.— A. J. Crisp (letter), *Lancet*, 1981, *1*, 775.

From a study in 36 patients receiving synthetic salcatonin or synthetic human calcitonin 100 units intramuscularly daily, or placebo, for 15 days, it was suggested that adverse effects are more common and more severe with the human than the salmon preparation.— C. Gennari *et al.* (letter), *Lancet*, 1983, *1*, 594. A comment that these differences may reflect a difference in biological activity of the preparations at the dosages used. The author had not observed a high frequency of adverse effects in his experience of over 200 patient-years of treatment using a 'non-antigenic' synthetic human calcitonin.— J. C. Stevenson (letter), *ibid.*, 926. Each batch of a synthetic calcitonin preparation may contain small amounts of contaminant peptides each with its own spectrum of pharmacological activity.— D. R. Bangham and J. M. Zanelli, *ibid.*, 926.

EFFECT ON GLUCOSE METABOLISM. Blood-sugar concentrations were increased by a single subcutaneous injection of salcatonin in 9 patients.— A. Gattereau *et al.* (letter), *Lancet*, 1977, *2*, 1076. It was very unlikely that long-term treatment with calcitonin would cause diabetes mellitus.— I. M. A. Evans *et al.* (letter), *ibid.*, 1978, *1*, 280.

Marked deterioration in control occurred during treatment with calcitonin (pork) in a diabetic patient previously well controlled with tolbutamide.— D. W. Thomas *et al.* (letter), *Med. J. Aust.*, 1979, *2*, 699.

INTERACTIONS. For the effect of salcatonin on serum-potassium concentrations in a patient receiving hydrochlorothiazide, see Hydrochlorothiazide p.992.

Absorption and Fate
Calcitonin is rapidly inactivated when given by mouth. After injection it is rapidly degraded mainly in the kidneys. The inactive metabolites, and a small proportion of unchanged drug are excreted in the urine.
Calcitonin is reported not to cross the placenta.

The distribution and clearance of calcitonin in *animals* and man.— H. P. J. Bennett and C. McMartin, *Pharmac. Rev.*, 1978, *30*, 247.

Uses and Administration
Calcitonin has a hypocalcaemic action due to inhibition of bone resorption. Naturally-occurring porcine calcitonin and synthetic salmon calcitonin (salcatonin) are in clinical use and salcatonin is the more potent. Synthetic human calcitonin is also being used. Elcatonin, a synthetic derivative of eel calcitonin, is available in some countries.
Calcitonins are used in the treatment of selected patients with diseases characterised by bone resorption and re-formation, such as Paget's disease of bone (osteitis deformans).
In Paget's disease of bone the usual dose range for calcitonin (pork) by subcutaneous or intramuscular injection is 80 units three times weekly to 160 units daily. For salcatonin given by similar routes the range is 50 units three times weekly to 100 units daily in single or divided doses. The higher dosage is recommended for patients with bone pain or nerve compression. Human calcitonin is given by subcutaneous or intramuscular injection in a dose range of 0.5 mg three times weekly to 0.5 mg daily. Biochemical improvement may be monitored by measurement of serum-alkaline phosphatase and urinary-hydroxyproline excretion values; dosage may be reduced as these values fall.
Calcitonins are used for the treatment of hypercalcaemia from a variety of causes including vitamin D intoxication, neoplastic disease, thyrotoxicosis, and hyperparathyroidism. They have a rapid effect which is greatest in patients with an increased bone turnover. Calcitonin (pork) may be given in a dose of 4 units per kg body-weight daily by intramuscular or subcutaneous injection according to the patient's needs. Larger doses may be required but would be more conveniently administered as salcatonin. Salcatonin may be given by subcutaneous or intramuscular injection in a dosage regimen of 4 units per kg body-weight given every 12 hours, increased if necessary to a maximum of 8 units per kg every 6 hours. Doses greater than 8 units per kg are considered to have no additional benefit. Plasma-calcium concentrations should be monitored during treatment.
Salcatonin has been used in the treatment of postmenopausal osteoporosis in a dose of 100 units daily by subcutaneous or intramuscular injection in association with an equivalent of elemental calcium 600 mg daily and vitamin D 400 units daily both given by mouth.
Salcatonin has also been administered by subcutaneous or intramuscular injection in a dose of 200 units every 6 hours or 400 units every 12 hours for a period of 48 hours, in the treatment of pain due to metastatic bone disease.

Reviews of the actions and uses of calcitonins.— J. C. Stevenson and I. M. A. Evans, *Drugs*, 1981, *21*, 257; L. A. Austin and H. Heath, *New Engl. J. Med.*, 1981, *304*, 269; L. J. Deftos and B. P. First, *Ann. intern. Med.*, 1981, *95*, 192.

Salcatonin had a beneficial influence on the clinical course of 51 patients with acute pancreatitis compared to 52 similar patients used as controls.— F. Paul *et al.*, *Dt. med. Wschr.*, 1979, *104*, 615. Calcitonin concentrations were considered to be above normal in 21 patients with acute pancreatitis. It was therefore suggested that the administration of supplementary calcitonin intended to inhibit pancreatic secretion is unnecessary.— C. W. Imrie *et al.*, *Gut*, 1983, *24*, A597.

A beneficial effect of human calcitonin on the pain of Tietze's syndrome in 5 patients unresponsive to conventional therapy.— G. Ricevuti, *Clin. Ther.*, 1985, *7*, 669.

Report of improvement in 30 patients with migraine after treatment with daily intramuscular injections of salcatonin for 30 days.— F. Patti *et al.*, *Headache*, 1986, *26*, 172.

ACTION. A review of the actions of calcitonin and its role in the regulation of plasma-calcium concentrations. Plasma levels of calcitonin in women are lower than in men, however there is disagreement over the supposed decline of plasma-calcitonin with age. The resolution of these problems depends on the development of improved assays.— I. MacIntyre, *Br. med. Bull.*, 1986, *42*, 343.

Studies of the structure-activity relationship of calcitonin.— E. T. Kaiser and F. J. Kézdy, *Science*, 1984, *223*, 249; J. W. Taylor and E. T. Kaiser, *Pharmac. Rev.*, 1986, *38*, 291.

A study in 8 healthy subjects indicating an absence of diurnal variation in serum-calcitonin concentrations.— S. C. Manolagas and L. J. Deftos (letter), *New Engl. J. Med.*, 1985, *312*, 122.

ADMINISTRATION. A study comparing the effect of intravenous and intranasal human calcitonin on plasma-calcium concentrations in 6 healthy subjects.— A. E. Pontiroli *et al.*, *Br. med. J.*, 1985, *290*, 1390. Criticisms.— J. C. Stevenson (letter), *ibid.*, *291*, 54. Reply.—A. E. Pontiroli *et al.* (letter), *ibid.* The effect of calcitonin on serum-calcium concentrations in healthy subjects is controversial and seems an inappropriate variable for the testing of the effectiveness of intranasal administration. In an investigation of the effect of salcatonin on the hourly urinary excretion of electrolytes, 200 units administered as an intranasal spray induced significant excretion of sodium, chloride, calcium, and potassium. Although this dose was less potent than salcatonin 100 units administered intramuscularly it did not produce any of the unpleasant adverse effects. The authors have also demonstrated decreased bone turnover in Paget's disease of bone and a reconstructive action on the osteolytic lesions after intranasal administration of salcatonin.— C. Nagant de Deuxchaisnes *et al.* (letter), *ibid.*, 544.

BONE PAIN AND METASTASIS. A gradual decrease in analgesic consumption, with improvement in general condition and in mobility, occurred in 5 of 6 patients with bone pain due to osteolytic metastases given salcatonin 100 units daily by subcutaneous injection for 28 days, and in 1 of 6 patients treated with a placebo.— J. Szántó and J. Sándor, *Clin. Trials J.*, 1983, *20*, 266.

Addition of calcitonin to treatment of multiple myeloma with chemotherapy and stanolone was considered to have a beneficial effect on bone pain.— A. Fremiotti *et al.*, *Curr. ther. Res.*, 1984, *36*, 627.

Although calcitonin has been shown experimentally to possess a central analgesic action, the relevance of this action to bone pain relief is not established.— I. MacIntyre, *Br. med. Bull.*, 1986, *42*, 343.

HYPERCALCAEMIA. The hypocalcaemic effect of calcitonin may wear off after about 48 to 72 hours, possibly due to a down-regulation of receptors. However, its action may be prolonged by the simultaneous administration of glucocorticoids. Calcitonin has been administered as an intravenous infusion in the treatment of hypercalcaemia, but the subcutaneous route is preferred to avoid the adverse effect of nausea. If calcitonin is given as an intravenous infusion, protein must be added to the solution to prevent its adsorption on to delivery systems.— J. C. Stevenson, *Br. med. J.*, 1985, *291*, 421.

Further reviews of hypercalcaemia, including its treatment with calcitonin.— G. T. Elliott and M. W. McKenzie, *Drug Intell. & clin. Pharm.*, 1983, *17*, 12; G. R. Mundy *et al.*, *New Engl. J. Med.*, 1984, *310*, 1718; P. C. Selby *et al.*, *Br. J. Hosp. Med.*, 1984, *31*, 186; R. A. Evans, *Drugs*, 1986, *31*, 64.

A study of the renal effects of salcatonin in 18 patients with hypercalcaemia of malignancy. Overall there was considerable variation in response and no close correlation with tumour type or between the dose and response. The renal effects of salcatonin did not decrease with time.— D. J. Hosking and S. R. Heller, *Eur. J. clin. Pharmac.*, 1986, *31*, 27.

A partial or complete response to salcatonin given by rectal suppositories for 5 to 7 days was observed in 9 of 10 patients with mild malignancy-associated hypercalcaemia.— D. Thiébaud *et al.*, *Am. J. Med.*, 1987, *82*, 745.

For reports of the use of salcatonin in association with prednisolone in the treatment of hypercalcaemia of malignancy, see Disodium Aminohydroxypropylidenediphosphonate, p.1340.

MENTAL DISORDERS. Salcatonin controlled 2 episodes of catatonia with hyperthermia in one patient with malignant catatonia. The results suggest a role for calcium in hyperthermic crises.— J. S. Carmen and R. J. Wyatt (letter), *Lancet*, 1977, *2*, 1124.

Salcatonin administered to patients with primary psychotic disorders tended to worsen depression but to reduce agitation during the succeeding 24 hours.— J. S. Carman and R. J. Wyatt, *Archs gen. Psychiat.*, 1979, *36*, 72.

In a preliminary study of 9 patients with various psychopathological syndromes, the intramuscular administration of salcatonin appeared to have a beneficial effect on some of the symptoms. The possible mechanisms of this action are discussed.— M. Mussini *et al.*, *J. int. med. Res.*, 1984, *12*, 23.

OSTEOGENESIS IMPERFECTA. Studies indicating that calcitonin may be of benefit in the treatment of osteogenesis imperfecta.— S. Castells *et al.*, *J. Pediat.*, 1979, *95*, 807; Y. Nishi *et al.*, *Pediatrics*, 1984, *73*, 538.

OSTEOPOROSIS. Reviews of the management of osteoporosis: calcitonin was generally not recommended for the treatment of this condition.— *Drug & Ther. Bull.*, 1984, *22*, 1; A. S. J. Dixon, *Drugs*, 1984, *28*, 565; R. Smith, *Postgrad. med. J.*, 1984, *60*, 383; S. F. Bauwens *et al.*, *Clin. Pharm.*, 1986, *5*, 639; B. L. Riggs and L. J. Melton, *New Engl. J. Med.*, 1986, *314*, 1676; R. Smith, *Br. med. J.*, 1987, *294*, 329.

Report of a multicentre open study investigating the effect of synthetic human calcitonin on bone pain and functional impairment in 530 patients with primary or secondary osteoporosis or Sudeck's disease.— V. Maresca, *J. int. med. Res.*, 1985, *13*, 311.

Postmenopausal osteoporosis. A review of the use of calcitonin in the treatment of postmenopausal osteoporosis.— *Med. Lett.*, 1985, *27*, 53.

Results suggesting that women with postmenopausal osteoporosis may have a calcitonin deficiency as defined by an inadequate calcitonin response to hypercalcaemia. Thus, the administration of exogenous calcitonin may be of benefit in such patients.— H. M. Taggart *et al.*, *Lancet*, 1982, *1*, 475. Contradictory results which appear to establish that calcitonin deficiency is not associated with, and therefore probably does not cause, postmenopausal osteoporosis.— R. D. Tiegs *et al.*, *New Engl. J. Med.*, 1985, *312*, 1097.

In a 2-year study of 45 women with postmenopausal osteoporosis, all patients received ergocalciferol 400 units in association with calcium carbonate 1.2 g, both given by mouth four times daily. Twenty-four women also received injections of salcatonin 100 units daily. Two treated patients and 3 controls failed to complete the study. Although there were no significant differences between mean treated and control total body-calcium values throughout the study period, treated patients tended to show an increase and control patients a decrease in this parameter throughout the first 18 months. During the final 8 months, however, this trend was reversed. Women treated with salcatonin also showed an increase in bone mass, as indicated by the difference in the percent trabecular bone area, as compared with control patients after 26 months. No lowering in fracture-frequency was observed, although it was considered that a large number of patients would need to be studied over a long period to assess fracture-incidence accurately. Salcatonin produced some rapid metabolic changes, such as an increase in urinary-calcium concentrations at 4 months, but these changes were not maintained throughout the treatment period.— H. E. Gruber *et al.*, *Metabolism*, 1984, *33*, 295.

Further references: R. Franceschini *et al.*, *Curr. ther. Res.*, 1983, *34*, 795; L. Zorzin and M. Capone, *ibid.*, 1984, *36*, 473; J. Y. Reginster *et al.*, *Lancet*, 1987, *2*, 1481; I. MacIntyre *et al.*, *ibid.*, 1988, *1*, 900 and 1278.

PAGET'S DISEASE OF BONE. A review of the actions and use of calcitonin in the management of Paget's disease of bone (osteitis deformans). The major indication for treatment of Paget's disease is uncontrolled bone pain and increased bone turnover. Improvement in bone pain generally begins within 4 to 6 weeks of starting therapy with calcitonin. Neurological compression syndromes may respond to treatment with calcitonin, however a beneficial response on hearing loss is only seldom observed. Calcitonin therapy may improve the high-output heart failure which sometimes occurs due to an increase in bone blood flow. There is no clear relationship between the clinical response and the reduction in bone turnover. When treatment is stopped serum-alkaline phosphatase and urinary-hydroxyproline concentrations usually return to pretreatment values within 6 months although many patients stay in clinical remission for at least a year. Primary non-response to calcitonin therapy in Paget's disease is rare. However, in most patients serum-alkaline phosphatase and urinary-hydroxyproline concentrations fall by 40 to 50% within 6 months of treatment but further reductions thereafter are unusual (plateau response). The cellular basis for this response is unclear, but may be reflected *in vitro* by the phenomenon of 'escape' in which the suppressive effect of calcitonin on osteoclastic resorption decreases with time. Down-regulation of calcitonin receptors during treatment has also been suggested. Incidences of resistance to calcitonin treatment due to the development of antibodies ranging between 5 and 40% have been reported, however resistance may have been overestimated in the past. Clinical resistance is related to high antibody titres and is usually a problem of prolonged treatment. The diagnosis of resistance should be based on the antibody titre and on the demonstration that control of bone turnover can be re-established by changing to a species of calcitonin to which antibodies are absent. The effect of calcitonin on the structure of bone may be assessed histologically and radiographically. Radiographic improvements usually occur over 8 to 12 months.— D. J. Hosking, *Drugs*, 1985, *30*, 156. The duration of treatment with calcitonin is controversial. Where pain is the indication for treatment, calcitonin can be given for an initial period of 6 to 8 weeks. If there is no improvement it is stopped; if pain is alleviated and there is satisfactory biochemical response calcitonin can be continued for up to a year and then stopped. Further calcitonin may be given if symptoms recur.— R. Smith, *Prescribers' J.*, 1982, *22*, 25. In patients in whom the indication for treatment is pain, calcitonin is usually ceased after 6 months if the patient is free of symptoms. When the indication for treatment is a high cardiac output, neurological symptoms, or deformity in a young person, treatment should be continued indefinitely three times a week while biochemical remission and clinical improvement are maintained.— R. A. Melick, *Med. J. Aust.*, 1985, *143*, 394. See also *Lancet*, 1986, *1*, 1255; *Med. Lett.*, 1987, *29*, 47.

In a study of 20 patients with Paget's disease of bone the 12 patients who received salcatonin for 3 years did not demonstrate the gradual decrease in bone-mineral content of non-pagetic bone showed by the 8 patients receiving no treatment. Thus calcitonin may protect against the bone loss associated with ageing.— S. H. Toh *et al.*, *J. clin. Endocr. Metab.*, 1983, *56*, 405.

For references to the use of a combination of calcitonin and disodium etidronate and for their sequential use in the treatment of Paget's disease of bone, see Disodium Etidronate p.1343.

A review of calcitonin. Treatment of familial idiopathic hyperphosphatasaemia [a juvenile condition resembling adult Paget's disease of bone] with calcitonin was considered to be highly beneficial, especially if begun before gross deformities have developed. Since treatment may be lifelong use of human calcitonin is specifically indicated.— J. C. Stevenson and I. M. A. Evans, *Drugs*, 1981, *21*, 257.

Preparations

Calcitonin (Pork) Injection *(B.P.)*. pH 3.5 to 5.5.

Salcatonin Injection *(B.P.)*. pH 3.9 to 4.5.

Proprietary Preparations

Calcitare *(Armour, UK). Injection*, powder for reconstitution, calcitonin (pork) 160 units, supplied with gelatin diluent.

Calsynar *(Armour, UK). Injection*, salcatonin 100 units/mL, in ampoules of 1 mL. *Injection*, salcatonin 200 units/mL, in vials of 2 mL.

Proprietary Names and Manufacturers of Calcitonins

Calcimar *(Rorer, Canad.*; *USV Pharmaceutical Corp., USA)*; Calcitar *(Rorer, Fr.*; *Rorer, Ital.*; *Jpn)*; Calcitare *(USV, Austral.*; *Belg.*; *Armour, Denm.*; *Neth.*; *Norw.*; *S.Afr.*; *Armour, UK)*; Calcitonina *(Ital.)*; Calcitonine-Sandoz *(Sandoz, Switz.)*; Calcitonin-Sandoz *(Sandoz, S.Afr.)*; Calsyn *(Rorer, Fr.)*; Calsynar *(USV, Austral.*; *Armour, Denm.*; *Rorer, Ger.*; *Neth.*; *S.Afr.*; *Armour, UK)*; Carbicalcin *(Smith Kline & French, Ital.)*; Cibacalcin *(Ciba, Austral.*; *Ciba, Ital.*; *Neth.*; *NZ*; *Ciba, Swed.*; *Ciba, USA)*; Cibacalcin DC *(Neth.)*; Cibacalcine *(Ciba, Fr.*; *Ciba, Switz.)*; Elcitonin *(Toyo Jozo, Jpn)*; Karil *(Sandoz, Ger.)*; Miacalcic *(Sandoz, Austral.*; *Sandoz, Denm.*; *Sandoz, Fr.*; *Sandoz, Norw.*; *NZ*; *Sandoz, Swed.*; *Sandoz, UK)*; Osteotonina *(Guidotti, Ital.)*; Staporos *(Roussel, Fr.*; *Roussel Maestretti, Ital.)*; Tonocalcin *(Schiapparelli, Ital.)*; Turbocalcin *(ISF, Ital.)*.

12672-k

Disodium Aminohydroxypropylidenediphosphonate

Aminohydroxypropylidenebisphosphonate Disodium; APD; CGP-23339. Disodium 3-amino-1-hydroxypropylidenediphosphonate.
$C_3H_9NNa_2O_7P_2$=279.0.

CAS — 57248-88-1; 40391-99-9 (aminohydroxypropylidenediphosphonic acid).

Disodium aminohydroxypropylidenediphosphonate is a biphosphonate which is being investigated in the treatment of Paget's disease of bone (osteitis deformans) and hypercalcaemia. It is reported to inhibit bone resorption while having less effect on mineralisation than disodium etidronate. It may be administered by mouth or intravenously.

Report of the treatment of serious skeletal lesions due to Gaucher's disease in an 18-year-old man with disodium aminohydroxypropylidenediphosphonate 600 mg by mouth daily. There was rapid biochemical and clinical improvement, and radiographic changes consistent with an arrest or even a reversal of the bone lesion.— H. I. J. Harinck *et al.* (letter), *Lancet*, 1984, *2*, 513.

ADVERSE EFFECTS. In 169 patients treated for a mean of 8.5 months with disodium aminohydroxypropylidenediphosphonate, in a dose of 6 to 8.2 mg per kg body-weight daily by mouth, side-effects were: gastric intolerance interrupting treatment (8 patients), minor gastro-intestinal disturbances (6), skin rash (2), mild leucopenia (11). One patient developed idiopathic thrombocytopenic purpura.— C. A. Mautalen *et al.*, *Br. med. J.*, 1984, *288*, 828.

Disodium aminohydroxypropylidenediphosphonate has been reported to cause a transient lymphopenia. This may be due to an action on the mononuclear phagocyte system.— D. J. Hosking, *Drugs*, 1985, *30*, 156.

Symptomatic hypocalcaemia occurred in a woman who was given an intravenous infusion of disodium aminohydroxypropylidenediphosphonate 30 mg in 500 mL sodium chloride 0.9% over 6 hours for the treatment of hypercalcaemia due to malignancy.— D. I. Jodrell *et al.* (letter), *Lancet*, 1987, *1*, 622.

BONE PAIN AND METASTASIS. Reduced morbidity from skeletal metastases in breast cancer patients during long-term disodium aminohydroxypropylidenediphosphonate treatment.— A. T. van Holten-Verzantvoort *et al.*, *Lancet*, 1987, *2*, 983.

HYPERCALCAEMIA. Beneficial results, including a dramatic fall in serum concentrations of parathyroid hormone, in a 63-year-old woman with metastatic parathyroid carcinoma who was given intravenous disodium aminohydroxypropylidenediphosphonate 15 to 75 mg daily followed by maintenance on 300 mg daily by mouth. She had previously received disodium clodronate without significant effect.— K. Mann (letter), *Lancet*, 1985, *1*, 101.

Results of a prospective study of intravenous disodium aminohydroxypropylidenediphosphonate (APD) in 30 patients with tumour-induced hypercalcaemia, with special emphasis on renal function. In 11 of the patients, detailed metabolic studies were carried out to define the respective effects of volume repletion and APD treatment. Volume repletion (with at least 3 litres of saline; 462 mmol NaCl daily) was only partially effective in lowering serum calcium and raising glomerular filtration-rate and it increased the tendency towards hypomagnesaemia; the raised calcium production persisted, the slight improvement noted being due to a decrease in tubular resorption of calcium. In all but one of the 30 patients, normal serum-calcium values were obtained within 6 days of starting treatment with APD and this was due to reduced production of calcium from bone; in contrast to volume repletion, serum-magnesium concentrations were raised. It was noteworthy that APD improved renal function in all patients and that it was effective at a dosage of less than 1% of the lowest doses of disodium clodronate and disodium etidronate reported by H.M. Bounameaux *et al.* (*Lancet*, 1983, *1*, 471) to be associated with renal failure. The overall efficacy of all doses tested (ranging from 1.75 to 30 mg daily) and the great variability of initial serum-calcium concentrations made it impossible to draw any conclusions about a dose-effect relation; no adverse effects were noted.— H. P. Sleeboom *et al.*, *Lancet*, 1983, *2*, 239.

Report of a study of 39 patients with hypercalcaemia (adjusted serum-calcium concentration above 2.8 mmol per litre) due to malignant diseases. Patients received rehydration with sodium chloride 0.9% followed by treatment with either disodium aminohydroxypropylidenediphosphonate (APD), a combination of salcatonin and prednisolone, or plicamycin (13 patients in each group). APD 15 mg in 250 mL sodium chloride 0.9% was given as an infusion daily until the serum-calcium concentration was normal (2.6 mmol per litre) or until a nadir was reached. Salcatonin 400 units every 8 hours was administered by subcutaneous injection in association with prednisolone 40 mg daily by mouth in divided doses, (or an equivalent intravenous dose in patients unable to swallow) for 9 days. Plicamycin 25 µg per kg body-weight was given as an infusion in 500 mL glucose 5% and repeated after 2 days if the serum-calcium concentration remained above 2.9 mmol per litre. Data were not included in the analysis from 2 patients in the APD group who had surgical resection of the tumour on day 7. Two, one, and one patients from the 3 groups respectively died of complications of the tumour before the end of the study period; 2 patients receiving salcatonin and prednisolone were withdrawn because of clinical deterioration and successfully treated with plicamycin; one patient treated with plicamycin died of hypercalcaemic crisis despite repeated plicamycin and aggressive sodium chloride diuresis. All three regimens produced a significant decrease in serum-calcium concentration from that achieved with rehydration. A median decrease of 0.35 mmol per litre was achieved after 24 hours in the group treated with salcatonin and prednisolone, 48 hours in the plicamycin group, and 72 hours in the APD group. The slow onset of action of APD was compensated for by a progressive and consistent control of hypercalcaemia. Serum-calcium concentrations were lower in patients treated with APD than in those treated with salcatonin and prednisolone at days 6 and 9 of the study, and lower than in patients treated with plicamycin at day 9. Approximately half of the patients treated with plicamycin had begun to relapse by day 9 of the study; repeated daily doses could not be justified in view of the potential toxicity. The mechanisms of the calcium-lowering effect of these treatments were investigated by studies of urinary calcium and hydroxyproline excretion. APD progressively reduced bone resorption with little change in renal tubular handling of calcium. The rapid effect of the combination of salcatonin and prednisolone was mainly due to a reduction in renal tubular calcium reabsorption, and the continued effect to an improvement in the glomerular filtration rate rather than a substantial decrease in bone resorption. The initial effect of plicamycin was due mainly to a decrease in bone resorption, however from day 3 onwards there was also a reduction in renal tubular calcium reabsorption. It was concluded that although APD was most effective in the medium-term control of malignancy-associated hypercalcaemia, it was less suitable for the rapid control of severe hypercalcaemia.— S. H. Ralston *et al.*, *Lancet*, 1985, *2*, 907. In a similar study, 8 patients with hypercalcaemia due to malignancies received, after initial rehydration, APD 15 mg by intravenous infusion daily in association with salcatonin 100 units every 8 hours by subcutaneous injection for 6 days. There was a rapid decrease in serum-calcium concentrations which was maintained for 6 days after treatment was stopped. The initial rapid action was due to a reduction in both bone resorption and renal calcium tubular reabsorption. After treatment was stopped renal tubular calcium reabsorption rose, but decreased bone resorption was maintained; this was attributed to the sustained action of APD. It was therefore concluded that combination therapy would be suitable for the treatment of severe hypercalcaemia where a quick but sustained reduction in the serum-calcium concentration is desired.— S. H. Ralston *et al.*, *Br. med. J.*, 1986, *292*, 1549.

Ten patients with hypercalcaemia due to malignant neoplasms were treated with a single infusion of disodium aminohydroxypropylidenediphosphonate (APD) 30 mg in 500 mL sodium chloride 0.9% over 2 hours. Five patients also received hydration with 3 to 4 litres of sodium chloride 0.9% daily, and 3 also received corticosteroids. Normocalcaemia was achieved in 8 patients, and was maintained for more than 5 weeks in 3. Three patients had mild transient fever within one day of administration. It was suggested that single infusions of APD every 2 to 3 weeks may be adequate to treat mild to moderate cancer-associated hypercalcaemia.— B. Cantwell and A. L. Harris (letter), *Lancet*, 1986, *1*, 165. Similar results in a further 16 patients treated with the same regimen.—*idem*, *Br. med. J.*, 1987, *294*, 467. Comment on the first group of patients emphasising the importance of volume expansion in the management of hypercalcaemia, and doubting that the rapid attainment of normocalcaemia and the sustained remission was related solely to the action of APD.— J. A. Kanis *et al.* (letter), *Lancet*, 1986, *1*, 615.

Further reports and discussions of the use of disodium aminohydroxypropylidenediphosphonate in hypercalcaemia.— H. C. R. Brandenburg and P. Vermeij, *Pharm. Weekbl. Ned.*, 1984, *119*, 1189; P. C. Selby *et al.*, *Br. J. Hosp. Med.*, 1984, *31*, 186; C. J. Gibbs and M. Peacock, *Postgrad. med. J.*, 1986, *62*, 937.

OSTEOPOROSIS. In a study of the effects of disodium aminohydroxypropylidenediphosphonate (APD) on 14 patients with Paget's disease of bone there was a significant increase in the ratio of bone mineral content to bone width in the midshaft radius in both men and women after a mean duration of treatment of 15.3 and 7.7 months respectively; there was also a similar trend in the distal radius. Thus APD could be useful in the treatment of bone loss due to osteoporosis.— C. Nagant de Deuxchaisnes *et al.* (letter), *Br. med. J.*, 1983, *286*, 1648.

Prevention of steroid-induced osteoporosis with disodium aminohydroxypropylidenediphosphonate.— I. R. Reid *et al.*, *Lancet*, 1988, *1*, 143.

PAGET'S DISEASE OF BONE. In a study of the use of disodium aminohydroxypropylidenediphosphonate, by mouth in the treatment of 18 patients with Paget's disease of bone, bone resorption generally became normal within a few days but return to normal bone formation required a few months, this difference creating a positive calcium balance associated with transient secondary hyperparathyroidism.— W. B. Frijlink *et al.*, *Lancet*, 1979, *1*, 799. See also O. L. M. Bijvoet *et al.* (letter), *ibid.*, 1980, *1*, 1416.

A study of the use of disodium aminohydroxypropylidenediphosphonate (APD) by mouth in patients with Paget's disease of bone, of whom 26 had received no previous treatment, and 28 had previously been treated with disodium etidronate alone or in association with calcitonin. APD was administered in a dosage of 300 to 800 mg daily given as enteric-coated tablets half an hour before meals. Of 39 who had bone pain at the beginning of treatment, 34 reported relief of or diminished symptoms. Previously untreated patients received treatment for 4 to 6 months, which was prolonged if biochemical indices were still abnormal after this time. After 2 months' treatment there was a significant decrease in serum-alkaline phosphatase concentrations and urinary-hydroxyproline excretion in these patients, followed by a more gradual decline for up to 4 months, but with no further significant change after prolongation of therapy to 6 months. In terms of urinary-hydroxyproline excretion, 23 and 3 patients were considered to have a complete or partial response respectively; in terms of serum-alkaline phosphatase concentrations the equivalent figures were 22 and 4. The biochemical response was slower in patients who had received previous treatment.

The duration of remission was studied in 43 patients; about half were still in remission 10.6 months after stopping APD therapy. Remissions were longer in those who had achieved a complete biochemical response than in those who had a partial response. Nine of 11 who had a biochemical relapse responded to retreatment. A mild, and rapidly reversible leucopenia was observed in 3 patients.— C. A. Mautalen *et al.*, *Bone*, 1985, *6*, 429.

Beneficial biochemical response in 20 patients with Paget's disease of bone after administration of disodium aminohydroxypropylidenediphosphonate 15 mg by intravenous infusion daily for 5 days or weekly for 12 weeks. Eight patients experienced transient exacerbation of pain after the first injection and 7 developed transient hypophosphataemia.— J. A. Cantrill *et al.*, *Ann. rheum. Dis.*, 1986, *45*, 1012. See also D. C. Anderson *et al.* (letter), *Lancet*, 1986, *1*, 1442; H. I. J. Harinck *et al.*, *Br. med. J.*, 1987, *295*, 1301.

Proprietary Names and Manufacturers
Henkel, Ger.; Ciba-Geigy, UK.

12673-a

Disodium Clodronate

BM-06011; Cl_2MDP; Clodronate Disodium; Clodronate Sodium; Dichloromethane Diphosphonate Disodium; Dichloromethylene Diphosphonate Disodium; Sodium Clodronate *(BANM)*. Disodium (dichloromethylene)diphosphonate.
$CH_2Cl_2Na_2O_6P_2$=288.9.

CAS — 22560-50-5; 10596-23-3 (clodronic acid).

NOTE. Clodronic Acid is *BAN*, *USAN*, and *rINN*.

Disodium clodronate is a biphosphonate which is administered by mouth or intravenously in the treatment of Paget's disease of bone (osteitis deformans) and in hypercalcaemia. It is reported to inhibit bone resorption while having less effect on mineralisation than disodium etidronate. Gastro-intestinal disturbances have been reported after its administration by mouth.

Beneficial effect in one patient of disodium clodronate by mouth in association with intravenous plicamycin on the paraparesis caused by carcinoma of the prostate.— R. C. Percival *et al.*, *Postgrad. med. J.*, 1985, *61*, 551.

ABSORPTION AND FATE. From studies in 9 healthy subjects using C^{13}-labelled disodium clodronate, the bioavailability of the drug from a solution was calculated to be 1 to 2%. Disodium clodronate was primarily excreted in the urine as unchanged drug, and had a half-life of 2 hours.— G. J. Yakatan *et al.*, *Clin. Pharmac. Ther.*, 1982, *31*, 402. See also K. A. Conrad and S. M. Lee, *ibid.*, 1981, *30*, 114.

ADVERSE EFFECTS. In a study of the use of disodium clodronate in the treatment of Paget's disease of bone (P.D. Delmas *et al.*, *J. clin. Endocr. Metab.*, 1982, *54*, 837), an acute myeloblastic leukaemia developed in a 68-year-old man given 400 mg daily by mouth for 6 months. He had, however, been exposed to benzene over many years. Heath (*Br. med. J.*, 1987, *294*, 1048) mentioned in a review of agents used in Paget's disease of bone that disodium clodronate had been linked with several cases of leukaemia but that subsequent studies had questioned the causal relationship of this adverse effect. Several clinical studies of disodium clodronate have monitored haematological indices during treatment and have observed no deleterious effects (I. Elomaa *et al.*, *Lancet*, 1983, *1*, 146; I. Elomaa *et al.*, *ibid.*, 1985, *1*, 1155; A.D. Paterson *et al.*, *Br. J. Haematol.*, 1983, *54*, 121).

BONE PAIN AND METASTASIS. Results of a study of 34 normocalcaemic women with multiple osteolytic bone metastases due to breast cancer treated with disodium clodronate 1.6 to 3.2 g daily by mouth for 3 to 9 months (17 patients) or placebo (17). All patients received the same cancer therapy as they had received for the 3 months before the study. Analgesic consumption decreased in 15 and 3 patients in the 2 groups respectively. Biochemical indices of bone resorption decreased only in the patients receiving active treatment; serum-parathyroid hormone concentrations also increased slightly in patients in this group. Bone scan studies appeared to indicate that disodium clodronate inhibits the extension of bone metastases and retards the formation of new osteolytic foci. The drug also prevented the development of severe hypercalcaemia.— I. Elomaa *et al.*, *Lancet*, 1983, *1*, 146. In a follow-up study, bone metastases developed after withdrawal of disodium clodronate. It was suggested that it may be given continuously in cancer patients.— I. Elomaa *et al.* (letter), *ibid.*, 1985, *1*, 1155.

Twelve normocalcaemic patients with metastatic bone disease were treated with placebo or disodium clodronate 8 mg per kg body-weight daily by intravenous infusion for 14 days followed by 1.2 g twice daily by mouth for one month. In the final month all patients received calcium gluconate 1 g and vitamin D 800 units daily by mouth. Twenty-day calcium balance and kinetic studies performed before and after treatment indicated a favourable effect of disodium clodronate on calcium balance and an increase in calcium absorption compared with placebo. It was concluded that disodium clodronate may be a useful adjuvant in the management of metastatic bone disease.— A. Jung *et al.*, *New Engl. J. Med.*, 1983, *308*, 1499.

Further references: E. S. Siris *et al.*, *Am. J. Med.*, 1983, *74*, 401.

HYPERCALCAEMIA. Disodium clodronate 1 to 3.2 g daily by mouth for up to 32 weeks was given to 9 elderly patients with primary hyperparathyroidism. There was some relief of skeletal pain (2 patients of 3), and complete relief of loin pain from renal calculi (3 of 3). Serum-calcium concentrations fell to normal or near-normal in the 8 patients who were treated for at least 5 weeks and there was a fall in excretion of hydroxyproline, indicating reduced bone resorption. Disodium clodronate is a promising agent for the short-term management of hyperparathyroidism.— D. L. Douglas *et al.*, *Br. med. J.*, 1983 *286*, 587. See also E. Shane *et al.*, *Ann. intern. Med.*, 1981, *95*, 23; *Lancet*, 1984, *2*, 727.

Reports of the use of disodium clodronate to control hypercalcaemia due to various causes.— T. P. Jacobs *et al.*, *Ann. intern. Med.*, 1981, *94*, 312 (hypercalcaemia of malignancy); A. Jung, *Am. J. Med.*, 1982, *72*, 221 (malignancy); A. D. Paterson *et al.*, *Br. J. Haemat.*, 1983, *54*, 121 (multiple myeloma); D. Jüngst (letter), *Lancet*, 1984, *2*, 1043 (parathyroid carcinoma); A. J. P. Yates *et al.*, *Br. med. J.*, 1984, *289*, 1111 (immobilisation).

For a report of the possible renal toxicity of disodium clodronate, and its use in the treatment of hypercalcaemia, see Disodium Etidronate p.1342.

PAGET'S DISEASE OF BONE. Results of a study of 76 patients with Paget's disease of bone treated with disodium clodronate 1.6 g daily by mouth for 6 months (45 patients), or administered as a daily intravenous infusion over 3 hours of 300 mg in 500 mL sodium chloride 0.9% for 5 days (31). In the patients treated orally, urinary excretion of hydroxyproline fell within 1 month followed by a later fall in serum-alkaline phosphatase concentrations. After 6 months of treatment these values were 38% and 34% of initial values respectively. Bone pain was reduced in 90% of the patients. In the 16 patients given intravenous disodium clodronate, and who had not received previous treatment with biphosphonates, the suppression of serum-alkaline phosphatase concentrations was similar to that in those treated by mouth; the decrease in hydroxyproline excretion, however, was not so great. The remaining 15 patients who had previously received treatment with biphosphonates appeared to have an attenuated biochemical response. However, when the results were expressed as a proportion of biochemical values before any treatment had been received, the response to the 5-day intravenous course of disodium clodronate was no different to those who had no previous biphosphonate treatment. Bone pain improved in 20 patients. Examination of bone biopsies taken from 5 patients treated by mouth and 9 treated intravenously indicated no significant impairment of bone mineralisation. A short intravenous course of disodium clodronate appears to produce inhibition of bone resorption followed by an inhibition of bone formation (as judged by urinary hydroxyproline and serum-alkaline phosphatase values) which does not depend on continued administration of the drug.— A. J. P. Yates *et al.*, *Lancet*, 1985, *1*, 1474.

Proprietary Names and Manufacturers
MCP Pharmaceuticals, UK; Procter & Gamble, USA.

12674-t

Disodium Etidronate *(BANM, rINNM).*

EHDP; Etidronate Disodium *(USAN)*. Disodium dihydrogen 1-hydroxyethylidenediphosphonate.
$C_2H_6Na_2O_7P_2$=250.0.
CAS — 7414-83-7; 2809-21-4 (etidronic acid).

NOTE. Other etidronic acid sodium salts are designated as etidronate monosodium, etidronate trisodium, and etidronate tetrasodium. The name sodium etidronate is used only where the salt cannot be identified more precisely.

Pharmacopoeias. In *U.S.*

A 1% solution has a pH of 4.2 to 5.2. **Store** in airtight containers.

Adverse Effects and Precautions

Adverse effects of disodium etidronate include nausea and diarrhoea. Impairment of bone mineralisation, associated with increased bone pain, osteomalacia, and fractures has been reported; these effects appear to be dose-related. Transient loss or alteration of taste has been reported during and after infusion. Disodium etidronate should be discontinued if a fracture occurs. It should be given with great care to patients with impaired renal function. Intravenous treatment with disodium etidronate should be withheld in patients with a serum creatinine concentration greater than 440 µmol per litre.

A report of gastric ulceration associated with the use of disodium etidronate.— R. L. Saunders, *Sth. med. J.*, 1977, *70*, 1327.

EFFECTS ON THE BONES. For reports of the effects of disodium etidronate on bone mineralisation and a possible increase in fracture rates, see under Uses, Paget's Disease of Bone, below.

EFFECTS ON THE KIDNEYS. A report of progressive renal failure in 3 patients associated with the intravenous administration of biphosphonates for the treatment of hypercalcaemia due to malignant neoplasms. Two patients were given disodium etidronate; patient 1 received an infusion of 1 g in 100 mL sodium chloride 0.9% on 2 successive days, and patient 2 received 500 mg daily for 5 days. Patient 3 was given disodium clodronate 200 to 1500 mg daily to a total of 19.9 g intravenously over 30 days. Patients 2 and 3 had increased serum-creatinine concentrations on admission, and hypercalcaemia (patients 2 and 3) or the malignancy itself (patient 3) may have contributed to the renal failure. It was recommended that in the treatment of hypercalcaemia biphosphonates should be infused slowly in doses of no more than 1 g daily with monitoring of renal function.— H. M. Bounameaux (letter), *Lancet*, 1983, *1*, 471. The nephrotoxicity of drugs in patients with progressive renal impairment is difficult to assess, however a causal relationship with intravenous disodium etidronate in patient 1 seems likely. The authors use doses of biphosphonates of up to 300 mg daily by intravenous infusion over 2 to 3 hours for the treatment of hypercalcaemia or for the rapid control of Paget's disease of bone. They consider that the hypocalcaemic effect is unlikely to be increased by higher doses. They have not observed progressive renal impairment in more than 40 patients treated with disodium etidronate or disodium clodronate up to a total dose of 14.5 g. Transient proteinuria was observed in 3 patients with normal renal function immediately after an infusion of disodium clodronate. They have treated 9 patients with impaired renal function with disodium clodronate without deleterious effect. They have not given intravenous disodium etidronate to any patients with significantly impaired renal function.— J. A. Kanis *et al.* (letter), *ibid.*, 1328.

Absorption and Fate

From 1 to 6% of a dose of disodium etidronate is absorbed from the gastro-intestinal tract. It is not metabolised. The majority of absorbed drug disappears from the blood within 6 hours. About 50% is excreted in the urine within 24 hours, the remainder being chemically adsorbed on bone and slowly eliminated. Unabsorbed disodium etidronate is excreted in the faeces.

Uses and Administration

Disodium etidronate is a biphosphonate which inhibits the growth and dissolution of hydroxyapatite crystals in bone and may also directly impair osteoclast activity. It diminishes bone resorption and bone formation.

Disodium etidronate is used in the treatment of Paget's disease of bone (osteitis deformans). Bone pain is generally relieved but has occasionally been exacerbated, especially with high doses. The reduction of accelerated bone turnover may be monitored by measurement of the fall in serum concentrations of alkaline phosphatase and urinary excretion of hydroxyproline. Serum-phosphate concentrations usually rise during therapy and have been used as an indication of adequate absorption of disodium etidronate, and as a guide to possible dosage adjustment.

In the treatment of Paget's disease of bone, disodium etidronate is given by mouth in doses of 5 to 20 mg per kg body-weight daily. The usual dose is 5 mg per kg daily for not more than 6 months. Retreatment should only be given after a drug-free interval of at least 3 months, after evidence of relapse, and should not be continued for more than 6 months. Doses above 10 mg per kg daily should not be given for more than 3 months. Disodium etidronate is usually administered as a single dose 2 hours before a meal and food should be avoided for 2 hours before and after the meal, especially milk and other products with a high calcium content. The response to disodium etidronate may be slow in onset and may continue for several months after cessation of therapy; doses should therefore not be increased prematurely. Generally no further benefit can be obtained by extending the treatment period beyond 6 months.

Disodium etidronate by mouth or intravenously is used in the treatment of hypercalcaemia, especially that due to neoplastic diseases. The recommended dose of disodium etidronate by slow intravenous infusion is 7.5 mg per kg body-weight daily for 3 successive days. This daily dose should be diluted in at least 250 mL of sodium chloride injection (0.9%). All infusions should be given over at least 2 hours and there should be at least a 7-day interval between courses of treatment. Doses may need to be reduced in renal impairment (see under Precautions, above).

Disodium etidronate has also been used for the prevention and treatment of heterotopic ossification associated with specified conditions. For that complicating hip replacement it is given in a dose of 20 mg per kg for one month before and 3 months after the operation. For heterotopic ossification due to spinal cord injury it has been given in a dose of 20 mg per kg for 2 weeks followed by 10 mg per kg for 10 weeks.

Radioactively labelled etidronate has been used as a bone scanning agent.

A review of the actions and uses of biphosphonates.— *Lancet*, 1981, *2*, 1326.

ADMINISTRATION IN RENAL FAILURE. See under Adverse Effects, above.

BONE PAIN AND METASTASIS. In 6 patients with painful bony metastases treated with disodium etidronate 5 to 7 mg per kg body-weight daily, bone pain improved within 3 weeks as demonstrated by a decrease in analgesic requirements.— W. Schnur (letter), *Med. J. Aust.*, 1983, *2*, 15.

ECTOPIC CALCIFICATION. A report of 2 double-blind placebo-controlled studies to assess the effect of disodium etidronate on heterotopic ossification following hip replacement or spinal cord injury. Patients undergoing hip replacement received disodium etidronate 20 mg per kg body-weight daily by mouth for one month before and 3 months after surgery, and those who had sustained spinal cord injuries received 20 mg per kg daily for 2 weeks followed by 10 mg per kg daily for 10 weeks, treatment being commenced between 20 and 121 days after the injury. In both studies, treatment with disodium etidronate decreased the incidence of heterotopic bone formation and of clinically significant lesions. Although heterotopic ossification may occur after cessation of therapy, lesions that subsequently developed were less severe than in patients receiving placebo.— G. A. M. Finerman and S. L. Stover, *Metab. Bone Dis. relat. Res.*, 1981, *4 and 5*, 337.

Mention that results with disodium etidronate in the treatment of post-traumatic myositis ossificans had been disappointing.— *Br. med. J.*, 1986, *293*, 437.

HYPERCALCAEMIA. Control of skeletal bone pain, and a decrease in serum-calcium concentrations and alkaline phosphatase levels in a patient with primary hyperparathyroidism treated with disodium etidronate 5 mg per kg body-weight daily by mouth.— A. A. Licata and E. O'Hanlon, *J. Am. med. Ass.*, 1983, *249*, 2063. In a review of the medical management of primary hyperparathyroidism, it was considered that the use of disodium etidronate had overall been unsatisfactory, and its routine use could not be recommended.— *Lancet*, 1984, *2*, 727.

In a study of 8 patients with severe hypercalcaemia due to malignancies, the administration of disodium etidronate 10 mg per kg body-weight daily by mouth after inital treatment with rehydration and an intravenous injection of plicamycin 25 µg per kg, increased the interval required between subsequent doses of plicamycin.— D. H. Shevrin *et al.*, *Clin. Pharm.*, 1985, *4*, 204. See also A. Jung, *Am. J. Med.*, 1982, *72*, 221 (intravenous use in hypercalcaemia of malignancy).

Further references to the use of disodium etidronate in hypercalcaemia of various causes: E. Hägg *et al.*, *Br. med. J.*, 1984, *288*, 607 (two patients with hypercalcaemia due to immobilisation); R. B. Thomson and J. K. Johnson, *Postgrad. med. J.*, 1986, *62*, 1025 (a family with vitamin D intoxication).

For references to the doses of intravenous disodium etidronate recommended for the treatment of hypercalcaemia, see under Effects on the Kidneys in Adverse Effects, above.

PAGET'S DISEASE OF BONE. Reviews of Paget's disease of bone and its treatment with disodium etidronate.— R. Smith, *Prescribers' J.*, 1982, *22*, 25; *Drug & Ther. Bull.*, 1982, *20*, 25; S. M. Krane, *Ann. intern. Med.*, 1982, *96*, 619; O. L. M. Bijvoet, *Pharm. Weekbl. Ned.*, 1984, *119*, 557; R. A. Melick, *Med. J. Aust.*, 1985, *143*, 394; D. J. Hosking, *Drugs*, 1985, *30*, 156; *Lancet*, 1986, *1*, 1255; D. A. Heath, *Br. med. J.*, 1987, *294*, 1048.

Preston *et al.* (*Br. med. J.*, 1986, *292*, 79), treated 12 patients with Paget's disease of bone with disodium etidronate 20 mg per kg body-weight daily by mouth for one month. Biopsies of the transiliac bone were performed before, and 4 to 12 months after, completing treatment in 5 patients, and 2 weeks after completing treatment in 4. Mean urinary-hydroxyproline excretion fell to 40% of initial values after treatment, and continued to fall to 32% of initial values 5 months later. Mean serum-alkaline phosphatase concentrations remained unchanged during treatment, but fell to 39% and 36% of the initial values 5 and 11 months after ceasing treatment respectively. Bone pain improved considerably in 8 of 11 patients by 5 months after ceasing treatment. None of the patients developed bone pain or sustained a fracture. Examination of the biopsy specimens indicated that mineralisation was halted during treatment but was reversible on stopping of treatment. They considered that the regimen induced suppression of disease activity, comparable to that observed after longer treatment, with only transient impairment of bone mineralisation. Gibbs *et al.* (*ibid.*, 1227) treated 11 patients with the same dosage for either 2 or 4 weeks; Serum-alkaline phosphatase concentrations and urinary-hydroxyproline excretion rates decreased during the course of treatment and remained suppressed for 3 months. In the 6 patients who received treatment for 4 weeks, transiliac crest biopsy specimens indicated pronounced mineralisation defects, osteomalacia being present in 5. The 5 patients treated for only 2 weeks had one biopsy performed either at the end of treatment or 10 to 16 weeks later. The results of these suggested a mineralisation defect which spontaneously resolved on stopping treatment. They, however, doubted that any manipulation of dose or duration of treatment could dissociate the beneficial effect of disodium etidronate on resorption from its adverse effects on mineralisation, and therefore considered that this dosage regimen is not ideal for the long-term management of Paget's disease. The first group (J.A. Kanis *et al.*, *ibid.*, 1667) commented that any risk from fracture is probably due to the prolonged and marked suppression of bone formation and the delayed repair of fatigue damage. Therefore the clinical importance of a transient delay in mineralisation may be negligible; short-term high-dose treatment exploits the sustained biochemical control of disodium etidronate and the relatively rapid rate of offset of any inhibition of mineralisation. From analysis of results from patients who had received 20 mg per kg daily for 1 or 6 months they suggested that extending treatment beyond 1 month confers no advantage for either the degree of biochemical suppression attained or the duration of the response. The second group (M. Peacock and C.J. Gibbs, *ibid.*, *293*, 207) replied that this analysis was inappropriate, and reaffirmed their initial conclusions.

A retrospective study of 737 patients with Paget's disease of bone who had been treated in various studies with one or more courses of disodium etidronate and observed over periods of up to 8 years. Analysis of fracture rates suggested that untreated patients and patients treated with disodium etidronate and observed for less than a year are at about equal risk of fracture, and that this risk is similar to that noted in patients with postmenopausal osteoporosis, although the types of fracture differed. The fracture rate decreased with time after initiation of treatment whether additional courses of therapy were received or not. Pretreatment urinary-hydroxyproline concentrations were more strongly related to fracture risk than either dosage regimen or serum-alkaline phosphatase concentration. While some patients had received prolonged therapy it was considered that doses greater than 10 mg per kg body-weight daily are rarely warranted for continuous periods longer than 6 months.— C. C. Johnston *et al.*, *Clin. Orthop.*, 1983, *172*, 186.

Evaluation of the histological, biochemical, and clinical responses in 13 patients with Paget's disease of bone given disodium etidronate 400 mg once daily for 6 months; the dosage ranged from 5 to 8 mg per kg body-weight daily. Nine of the 13 experienced overall symptomatic improvement during treatment but 2 of these also noted, for the first time, painful fissure fractures; a pre-existing fissure fracture in a third did not improve during treatment. In all of 9 in whom post-therapy biopsy specimens were taken through pagetic bone, there was evidence of focal osteomalacia, and in the remaining 4 in whom specimens were taken through non-pagetic bone a significant mineralisation defect was present.— B. F. Boyce *et al.*, *Lancet*, 1984, *1*, 821.

From a comparison of fracture rates before and after treatment of Paget's disease of bone with disodium etidronate, using figures from various studies, it was concluded that disodium etidronate increased the fracture rate considerably at various dosage regimens.— C. Nagant de Deuxchaisnes *et al.* (letter), *Lancet*, 1985, *2*, 610.

Further comments and discussions on the relationship between disodium etidronate and the development of fractures.— S. M. Krane, *Ann. intern. Med.*, 1982, *96*, 619; R. A. Evans (letter), *Med. J. Aust.*, 1984, *140*, 182; C. J. Mugglestone (letter), *Lancet*, 1985, *1*, 1393.

Intravenous administration. A rapid improvement was observed in a patient with spinal cord dysfunction with progressive impairment of sensory function and paraplegia related to Paget's disease of bone of the sixth thoracic vertebra, when he was treated daily with disodium etidronate 4.3 mg per kg body-weight in sodium chloride 0.9% infused intravenously over 3 hours.— S. Charhon *et al.* (letter), *Lancet*, 1982, *1*, 391.

For a reference to the use of intravenous disodium etidronate for the rapid control of Paget's disease of bone, see under Effects on the Kidneys in Adverse Effects, above.

Use with calcitonin. Reports of the use of disodium etidronate by mouth in association with calcitonin in the treatment of Paget's disease of bone.— D. J. Hosking *et al.*, *Lancet*, 1976, *1*, 615; O. L. M. Bijvoet *et al.* (letter), *Lancet*, 1980, *1*, 1416.

Results of a study involving 37 patients with Paget's disease of bone suggested that patients treated with disodium etidronate followed by salcatonin each given for 6 months, showed a better clinical and biochemical response than patients treated with salcatonin followed by disodium etidronate.— H. M. Perry *et al.*, *Archs intern. Med.*, 1984, *144*, 929.

Preparations

Etidronate Disodium Tablets *(U.S.P.)*

Proprietary Preparations

Didronel *(Norwich-Eaton, UK). Tablets*, disodium etidronate 200 mg.

Concentrate for intravenous infusion, disodium etidronate 50 mg/mL in ampoules of 6 mL. Dilute before use.

Proprietary Names and Manufacturers

Calcimux *(Arg.)*; Didronate *(A.L., Denm.; A.L., Swed.)*; Didronel *(Norwich-Eaton, Austral.; Norwich-Eaton, Canad.; Nativelle, Fr.; Procter & Gamble, Switz.; Norwich-Eaton, UK; Norwich Eaton, USA)*; Difosfen *(Rubio, Spain)*; Diphos *(Boehringer Mannheim, Ger.)*; Etidron *(Gentili, Ital.)*; Osteum *(Vinas, Spain).*

Pesticides and Repellents

3560-n

Most of the compounds in this section are insecticides used to treat insect and mite infestation or infection, such as pediculosis or scabies, or to control insect vectors of disease, such as blackflies, fleas, lice, and mosquitoes. Molluscicides and rodenticides are also used to control disease vectors as with the insecticides and those compounds with no other significant uses are included in this section; for this reason compounds such as crotamiton (p.918), niclosamide (p.60), and warfarin sodium (p.344) appear in other sections.

A number of pesticides are of interest because of their toxicity which explains the inclusion of compounds like paraquat.

Insect repellents are included. Some compounds such as diethyltoluamide and dimethyl phthalate are effective as repellents while others such as benzyl benzoate and some of the pyrethroids are effective both as insecticides and repellents. There are biological methods of control such as larvicidal fish and organisms such as *Bacillus thuringiensis* that are outside the scope of *Martindale*.

This section only includes a small selection of proprietary names of pesticides. Reference books devoted solely to pesticides are better suited to providing such nomenclature. A useful source for *UK* names is: Pesticides 1986, *Reference Book 500, Minist. Agric. Fish. Fd. Hlth & Safety Executive*, London, HM Stationery Office, 1987.

Resistance

Resistance by disease vectors is a problem with the common groups of pesticides and has extended to cover the newer groups, including the pyrethroids, hormone mimics, and other insect development inhibitors. Also most if not all vector groups are now involved.

References: Resistance of Vectors of Disease to Pesticides, Fifth Report of the WHO Expert Committee on Vector Biology and Control, *Tech. Rep. Ser. Wld Hlth Org. No. 655*, 1980; *Chronicle Wld Hlth Org.*, 1981, *35*, 141.

Pesticides in the Body and Diet

Pesticides can be absorbed during application, by consumption of treated products, or by accidental contamination and they may be stored or retained in the tissues. International regulations and controls operate to reduce the risk to both public and user.

Values for acceptable daily intakes of pesticides are provided by the Food and Agriculture Organization of the United Nations and the World Health Organization (WHO) through the WHO Technical Report series of publications or, more recently, through *Pesticides Residues in Food: yearly evaluations*, FAO Plant Production and Protection Papers, Rome.. A review of the dietary intake of chemical contaminants, including pesticides.—H. G. Gorchev and C. F. Jelinek, *Bull. Wld Hlth Org.*, 1985, *63*, 945; P. J. I. Snell and K. J. Nicol, *Pesticide Residues and Food: The Need for Real Control*, London, The London Food Commission, 1986; The Effects of Pesticides on Human Health, *Second Special Report of the House of Commons Agriculture Committee*, London, H.M. Stationery Office, 1987.

3561-h

Carbamate Pesticides

The carbamate pesticides are *N*-substituted esters of carbamic acid and can be classified as insecticides, herbicides, and fungicides. There are a large number of these compounds; those selected for inclusion in *Martindale* are: bendiocarb, carbaryl, and propoxur.

Carbamate Pesticides: A General Introduction, *Environmental Health Criteria 64*, Geneva, Wld Hlth Org., 1986.

Adverse Effects

As for Organophosphorus Pesticides, below.

The carbamates are cholinesterase inhibitors, differing from the organophosphorus insecticides in that the inhibition they produce is generally less intense and more rapidly reversible. Also they do not appear to enter the CNS as readily so that severe central effects are uncommon.

The related dithiocarbamate fungicides are considered to be less toxic. They are also related to disulfiram (p.1565) and thus could produce a similar reaction with alcohol.

Treatment of Adverse Effects

If carbamates have been ingested the stomach should be emptied by aspiration and lavage. Activated charcoal and a saline laxative have also been given. Contaminated clothing should be removed and the skin washed with soap and water. Symptomatic treatment includes atropine generally in doses of 2 mg. Diazepam is sometimes given. Pralidoxime or other oximes should *not* be given.

3562-m

Chlorinated Pesticides

The chlorinated or organochlorine pesticides form a wide group of compounds that were widely used as insecticides. Because of persistence in man their use has been restricted; dicophane (DDT) has been banned by several countries. Those selected for inclusion in *Martindale* are: chlordane, dicophane, dieldrin, endosulfan, endrin, heptachlor, and lindane.

Polychlorinated Biphenyls and Terphenyls, *Environmental Health Criteria 2*, Geneva, Wld Hlth Org., 1976.

Adverse Effects

Chlorinated or organochlorine pesticides form a very wide group and the toxicity of individual members varies widely. Aldrin, dieldrin, and endrin are considered to be the members that commonly cause poisoning. In general these insecticides produce symptoms consistent with central nervous system stimulation. They may be absorbed through the respiratory and gastro-intestinal tracts and through the skin.

Symptoms of acute poisoning include nausea and vomiting, paraesthesia, giddiness, tremors, convulsions, coma, and respiratory failure. Liver, kidney, and myocardial toxicity have been reported. Effects on the blood include agranulocytosis and aplastic anaemia. Symptoms may be complicated by the effects of the solvent.

Chlorinated pesticides have been reported to enhance microsomal hepatic enzyme activity. Skin reactions can follow contact with pesticides.

For further information on the toxic effects of chlorinated insecticides, see under dicophane (p.1347), dieldrin (p.1348), and lindane (p.1350).

Polychlorinated biphenyl (PCB) and terphenyl compounds were formerly used as insecticides in many countries, but because of their toxicity they now have only a few industrial applications. They are stored in body fat and not readily excreted except in breast milk and possibly through the placenta; because of this and because of accidental contamination as happened in Japan, they remain a cause for concern. The related polybrominated biphenyl compounds (PBB) which have no insecticidal uses have also been absorbed by the public following accidental contamination of the food chain. In Great Britain the recommended exposure limits of chlorinated biphenyls (54% chlorine) are 0.5 mg per m^3 (long-term); 1 mg per m^3 (short-term); suitable precautions should be taken to prevent absorption through the skin. In the *US* the permissible and recommended exposure limits are 0.5 mg per m^3 and 0.001 mg per m^3 respectively.

Treatment of Adverse Effects

Ingested material should be removed by aspiration and lavage. Activated charcoal may be given and a saline laxative has also been used. Contaminated clothing should be removed and the skin washed with soap and water. Treatment thereafter is symptomatic.

Milk and oily substances should not be given, nor generally should adrenaline since it may precipitate arrhythmias in a heart sensitised by chlorinated insecticides.

3564-v

Organophosphorus Pesticides

These pesticides which are widely used as insecticides are derivatives of phosphoric or phosphonic acid. Those selected for inclusion in *Martindale* are: chlorphoxim, chlorpyrifos, diazinon, dichlofenthion, dichlorvos, dioxathion, fenitrothion, fenthion, iodofenphos, malathion, parathion, pirimiphos-methyl, pyrimitate, and temefos.

Organophosphorus Insecticides: A General Introduction, *Environmental Health Criteria 63*, Geneva, Wld Hlth Org., 1986.

Adverse Effects

Organophosphorus pesticides are potent cholinesterase inhibitors and can be very toxic. This inhibition results in both muscarinic and nicotinic effects with some central involvement.

Toxic effects may include abdominal cramps, nausea, vomiting, diarrhoea, urinary incontinence, eye changes, weakness, respiratory disturbances, lachrymation, increased salivation and sweating, bradycardia or tachycardia, hypotension or hypertension, cyanosis, muscular twitching, and convulsions. Some organophosphorus compounds cause delayed neuropathy. Central nervous system symptoms include restlessness, anxiety, dizziness, confusion, coma, and depression of the respiratory or cardiovascular system. Patients may experience mental disturbances. Inhalation or external contact can cause local as well as systemic effects.

Repeated exposure may have a cumulative effect though the organophosphorus insecticides are, in contrast to the chlorinated insecticides, rapidly metabolised and excreted and are not appreciably stored in body tissues.

Treatment of Adverse Effects

Rapid treatment is essential. Ingested organophosphorus pesticides should be removed by aspiration and lavage. Activated charcoal and a saline laxative have also been given. Contaminated clothing should be removed and the skin, including any areas contaminated by vomiting or hypersecretion, should receive copious and prolonged washing with soap and water. Contamination of the eye is treated by washing of the conjunctiva. The patient should be treated with atropine and pralidoxime (p.851) and symptomatic treatment should be instituted. Diazepam is sometimes given. The patient should be observed for signs of deterioration due to delayed absorption. Morphine and phenothiazines must *not* be given nor must aminophylline.

3861-j

Pyrethroid Pesticides

The pyrethrins in the form of pyrethrum extract have a long history of use as insecticides. Synthetic analogues known as pyrethroids have now been developed; those included in *Martindale* are: cyfluthrin, cypermethrin, decamethrin, permethrin, phenothrin, and tetramethrin.

The pyrethroids possess potent insecticidal activity with low mammalian toxicity. Exposure may lead to local irritation; poisoning does not appear to be a problem.

Concern has been expressed that resistance might limit the value of these new insecticides.

The Pyrethroid Insecticides, J.P. Leahey (Ed.), London, Taylor & Francis, 1985.

16410-b

Aluminium Phosphide

Aluminum Phosphide.

AlP=57.96.

CAS — 20859-73-8; 7803-51-2 (phosphine); 1314-84-7 (zinc phosphide).

Aluminium phosphide releases phosphine (PH_3) in the presence of moisture and this accounts for its pesticidal activity. It is used for the fumigation of grain and as a rodenticide. Phosphine gas has a garlic-like odour repulsive to man and domestic animals but apparently not to *rats*. Zinc phosphide is used similarly.

A report of 15 cases of poisoning with aluminium phosphide, amounts ingested ranging from 1.5 to 9.0 g. All patients suffered repeated vomiting and hypotension; 13 were in shock and 11 of these patients died despite dopamine treatment. Other symptoms included restlessness, oliguria, anuria, jaundice, respiratory complications, cardiac arrhythmias, and metabolic acidosis.— S. Singh, *Br. med. J.*, 1985, *290*, 1110.

Acute phosphine poisoning aboard a grain freighter.— R. Wilson *et al.*, *J. Am. med. Ass.*, 1980, *244*, 148.

Proprietary Names and Manufacturers

Phostoxin *(Rentokil, UK).*

16411-v

Antu

1-Naphthylthiourea.

$C_{11}H_{10}N_2S$=202.3.

CAS — 86-88-4.

Antu has been used as a rodenticide. The carcinogenic risk from naphthylamine impurities has restricted its use; its use is not recommended by WHO.

A study of deaths from bladder tumours in rodent operators who had handled antu. The material is believed to have contained about 0.2% of the carcinogen β-naphthylamine; judgment is reserved about the safety of material currently used in some countries.— J. M. Davies *et al.*, *Br. med. J.*, 1982, *285*, 927.

18020-g

Bendiocarb

2,3-Isopropylidenedioxyphenyl methylcarbamate.

$C_{11}H_{13}NO_4$=223.2.

CAS — 22781-23-3.

Bendiocarb is a carbamate pesticide (p.1344) effective against a wide range of insects including flies, fleas, and mosquitoes. It is used as a public health insecticide as well as in industry and agriculture.

Bendiocarb has been shown to possess residual activity against mosquitoes at a concentration that does not produce any visible deposit or odour.

Action of bendiocarb against triatomine (Hemiptera: Reduviidae) vectors of Chagas' disease.— I. A. Sherlock *et al.*, *J. med. Entomol.*, 1983, *20*, 440.

Like other *N*-methylcarbamates, bendiocarb is a fast-acting anticholinesterase compound with a relatively high acute mammalian toxicity mitigated by rapid spontaneous reactivation of carbamoylated cholinesterase and relatively flat dose-response curve. Studies in humans have shown that the threshold oral dose for reducing whole-blood cholinesterase activity with typical symptoms such as vertigo, nausea, and sweating lies between 150 to 200 μg per kg body-weight. These symptoms disappear within 30 minutes while cholinesterase activity returns to normal within 4 hours. Ingestion of 100 μg per kg at hourly intervals did not cause symptoms. A spraying experiment identified a dermal exposure for 4.5 hours of spraying of 6.1 to 157 mg with a mean of 31.8 mg. This was achieved when applying bendiocarb at a concentration of 400 mg per m^2 surface area. This concentration provided residual activity against malaria vectors and because of a lack of any visible deposit or odour is acceptable to the householder.— Safe Use of Pesticides, Ninth Report of the WHO Expert Committee on Vector Biology and Control, *Tech. Rep. Ser. Wld Hlth Org. No. 720*, 1985.

Proprietary Names and Manufacturers

Ficam D *(FBC, UK)*; Ficam W *(FBC, UK)*; Garvox *(FBC, UK)*; Seedox *(FBC, UK).*

The following names have been used for multi-ingredient preparations containing bendiocarb— Ficam Plus *(FBC, UK).*

3569-w

Benzyl Benzoate *(BAN, USAN).*

Benzoato de Bencilo; Benzoesäurebenzylester; Benzyl Benz.; Benzylis Benzoas.

$C_6H_5.CO.O.CH_2.C_6H_5$=212.2.

CAS — 120-51-4.

Pharmacopoeias. In *Arg., Aust., Br., Braz., Cz., Egypt., Fr., Hung., Ind., Int., It., Jpn, Jug., Mex., Neth., Nord., Pol., Port., Span., Swiss, Turk.,* and *U.S.* Also in *B.P. Vet.*

Colourless crystals or a clear colourless oily liquid with a faintly aromatic odour. The *B.P.* specifies f.p. not below 17°; the *U.S.P.* specifies not below 18°. Practically **insoluble** in water and glycerol; miscible with alcohol, chloroform, and ether. **Store** at a temperature not exceeding 40° in well-filled airtight containers. Protect from light.

Adverse Effects and Treatment

Benzyl benzoate is irritant to the eyes and mucous membranes and it may be irritant to the skin. Hypersensitivity reactions have been reported. When ingested, benzyl benzoate may cause stimulation of the CNS and convulsions. Treatment of poisoning involves aspiration and lavage and appropriate symptomatic measures.

Uses and Administration

Benzyl benzoate is an acaricide used in the treatment of scabies. It is customary to apply benzyl benzoate as a 25% application to the whole body from the neck down immediately after a bath; a second application may be made within 5 days. Alternatively 3 applications may be made at 12-hourly intervals. Clothing and bedding should be changed to prevent reinfestation. Other acaricides are preferred for infants and children, but if benzyl benzoate is used, then the application should be diluted to minimise the risk of irritation.

Benzyl benzoate has also been used as a pediculicide.

Benzyl benzoate is used as an insect repellent and as a solubilising agent.

SCABIES. Burrows only appear from the neck down in scabies, although there may be exceptions in infants. Because benzyl benzoate stings, the application should be diluted with water to 12.5% for children or to one-third strength (approximately 8%) for infants. Lindane is preferred in long-standing and secondarily infected scabies.— J. Verbov, *Practitioner*, 1987, *231*, 732.

For a study showing a malathion emulsion to be more effective than a benzyl benzoate emulsion in the treatment of scabies, see Malathion, p.1351.

Preparations

Benzyl Benzoate Application *(B.P., A.P.F.).* Benzyl benzoate 25 g, emulsifying wax 2 g, freshly boiled and cooled water to 100 mL.

Benzyl Benzoate Lotion *(U.S.N.F.).* Benzyl benzoate 25 mL, triethanolamine 500 mg, oleic acid 2 g, and water 75 mL. pH 8.5 to 9.2.

Proprietary Preparations

Ascabiol *(May & Baker, UK). Application,* benzyl benzoate 25% as an emulsion.

Proprietary Names and Manufacturers

Antiscabiosum *(Mago, Ger.)*; Ascabiol *(May & Baker, Austral.; May & Baker, S.Afr.; May & Baker, UK)*; Benzemul *(McGloin, Austral.)*; Scabanca *(Anca, Canad.).*

The following names have been used for multi-ingredient preparations containing benzyl benzoate—Anugesic-HC *(Parke, Davis, UK)*; Anusol *(Warner, Austral.; Parke, Davis, USA)*; Anusol HC *(Warner, Austral.)*; Anusol-HC *(Parke, Davis, UK; Parke, Davis, USA).*

16545-t

Brodifacoum

WBA-8119. 3-[3-(4′-Bromobiphenyl-4-yl)-1,2,3,4-tetrahydro-1-naphthyl]-4-hydroxycoumarin.

$C_{31}H_{23}BrO_3$=523.4.

CAS — 56073-10-0.

Brodifacoum is an anticoagulant rodenticide. It is reported to inhibit prothrombin synthesis.

Brodifacoum, a second-generation anticoagulant rodenticide, inhibits prothrombin synthesis to cause bleeding that may be occult. It is absorbed from the gastro-intestinal tract; dermal absorption is possible. Baits containing 100 mg per kg are not hazardous to man; more concentrated forms are particularly hazardous and their availability should be restricted. Baits, which should be prepared only by trained personnel, should contain a suitable marker dye and should not be used in domestic, public, or industrial situations where they can come into contact with food and water. Unnecessary distribution into the environment should be avoided.— Safe Use of Pesticides, Ninth Report of the WHO Expert Committee on Vector Biology and Control, *Tech. Rep. Ser. Wld Hlth Org. No. 720*, 1985.

Proprietary Names and Manufacturers

Klerat *(ICI Plant Protection, UK)*; Mouser *(ICI Plant Protection, UK).*

3862-z

Bromadiolone

3-[3-(4′-Bromobiphenyl-4-yl)-3-hydroxy-1-phenylpropyl]-4-hydroxycoumarin.

$C_{30}H_{23}BrO_4$=527.4.

CAS — 28772-56-7.

Bromadiolone like brodifacoum is an anticoagulant rodenticide reported to inhibit prothrombin synthesis.

Bromadiolone, a second-generation anticoagulant rodenticide, inhibits prothrombin synthesis to cause bleeding that may be occult. It is absorbed from the gastro-intestinal tract; dermal absorption is possible. Baits containing 100 mg per kg are not hazardous to man; more concentrated forms are particularly hazardous and their availability should be restricted. Baits, which should be prepared only by trained personnel, should contain a suitable marker-dye and should not be used in domestic, public, or industrial situations where they can come into contact with food and water. Unnecessary distribution into the environment should be avoided.— Safe Use of Pesticides, Ninth Report of the WHO Expert Committee on Vector Biology and Control, *Tech. Rep. Ser. Wld Hlth Org. No. 720*, 1985.

Prolonged anticoagulation in 2 children due to poisoning with bromadiolone.— M. C. Greeff *et al.* (letter), *Lancet*, 1987, *2*, 1269.

Proprietary Names and Manufacturers

Slaymor *(Ciba-Geigy Agrochemicals, UK).*

2551-z

Butopyronoxyl
Indalone. Butyl 3,4-dihydro-2,2-dimethyl-4-oxo-2*H*-pyran-6-carboxylate.
$C_{12}H_{18}O_4$=226.3.

CAS — 532-34-3.

Butopyronoxyl is an insect repellent which is effective against ticks, but it may be mildly irritating to the skin. It has been used mainly in conjunction with dimethyl phthalate and ethohexadiol.

The effectiveness of butopyronoxyl against sandflies.— F. P. Fossati and M. Maroli, *Trans. R. Soc. trop. Med. Hyg.*, 1986, *80*, 771.

2552-c

Butylethylpropanediol

$C_9H_{20}O_2$=160.3.

Butylethylpropanediol is an insect repellent used for the treatment of clothing. It should not be applied directly to the skin. It is effective against blackflies, mosquitoes, and other biting Diptera.

3570-m

Carbaryl
Carbaril (*pINN*); OMS-29. 1-Naphthyl methylcarbamate.
$C_{12}H_{11}NO_2$=201.2.

CAS — 63-25-2.

The manufacturers report that carbaryl is sensitive to heat and is degraded at temperatures above 30°.

Adverse Effects and Treatment
As for Carbamate Pesticides, p.1344. Carbaryl may be absorbed following ingestion, inhalation, or skin contamination.
In Great Britain the recommended exposure limits of carbaryl are 5 mg per m^3 (long-term); 10 mg per m^3 (short-term). In the *US* the permissible and recommended exposure limits are 5 mg per m^3. The production of carbaryl is not without hazard; the release of lethal vapour at Bhopal in 1984 occurred during the synthesis of carbaryl.

A review of the effects of carbaryl on health.— Recommended Health-based Limits in Occupational Exposure to Pesticides, *Tech. Rep. Ser. Wld Hlth Org. No. 677*, 1982.

Uses and Administration
Carbaryl is a carbamate pesticide. It is widely used as an insecticide in agriculture as well as public health where it is employed to control disease vectors such as lice and fleas. Carbaryl is used clinically as an 0.5 or 1.0% application or shampoo in the treatment of pediculosis capitis. Some authorities recommend that carbaryl should be rotated with malathion in the treatment of pediculosis in an attempt to restrict the development of resistance.

Carbaryl for head lice.— *Drug & Ther. Bull.*, 1982, *20*, 59.

Discussions on 2-hour applications versus 12-hour applications of carbaryl and of malathion preparations for head lice: J. W. Maunder (letter), *Pharm. J.*, 1984, *2*, 708; D. M. Merrington (letter), *ibid.*, 1985, *1*, 33.

Proprietary Preparations
Carylderm *(Napp, UK). Lotion,* carbaryl 0.5% in an alcoholic basis.
Shampoo, carbaryl 1%.
Clinicide *(De Witt, UK). Lotion,* carbaryl 0.5% in an alcoholic basis.
Derbac *(International Laboratories, UK). Shampoo,* carbaryl 0.5%.
Suleo-C *(International Laboratories, UK). Lotion,* carbaryl 0.5% in an alcoholic basis.
Shampoo, carbaryl 0.5%.

Proprietary Names and Manufacturers
Carylderm *(Napp, UK)*; Clinicide *(De Witt, UK)*; Derbac *(International Laboratories, UK)*; Murvin *(Murphy Chemical, UK)*; Sevin *(Union Carbide, UK)*; Suleo-C *(International Laboratories, UK)*; Thinsec *(ICI Plant Protection, UK)*.

18055-k

Chlordane
1,2,4,5,6,7,8,8-Octachloro-2,3,3a,4,7,7a-hexahydro-4,7-methanoindene.
$C_{10}H_6Cl_8$=409.8.

CAS — 57-74-9.

Chlordane is a chlorinated pesticide (p.1344) effective against a range of insects. Its use is limited in some countries to the control of termites.
In Great Britain the recommended exposure limits of chlordane are 0.5 mg per m^3 (long-term); 2 mg per m^3 (short-term); suitable precautions should be taken to prevent absorption through the skin.

Chlordane, *Environmental Health Criteria 34*, Geneva, Wld Hlth Org., 1984.

A report of fatal chlordane poisoning.— F. W. Kutz *et al.*, *J. Toxicol. clin. Toxicol.*, 1983, *20*, 167.

Progressive motor neurone disease in a patient exposed to an insecticide containing chlordane with permethrin.— H. S. Pall *et al.* (letter), *Lancet*, 1987, *2*, 685.

Proprietary Names and Manufacturers
Nippon Ant Destroyer Powder *(Synchemicals, UK)*; Sydane *(Synchemicals, UK)*.

12554-e

Chloropicrin
Nitrochloroform. Trichloronitromethane.
CCl_3NO_2=164.4.

CAS — 76-06-2.

A slightly oily liquid with an intense odour.

Chloropicrin is a lachrymatory agent and is intensely irritating to the skin and mucous membranes. It is an insecticide and is used for fumigating stored grain and soil. Chloropicrin is also added to other fumigants as a warning gas.
In Great Britain the recommended exposure limits of chloropicrin are 0.1 ppm (long-term); 0.3 ppm (short-term).

18110-p

Chlorphoxim
2-(2-Chlorophenyl)-2-(diethoxyphosphinothioyloxyimino)acetonitrile.
$C_{12}H_{14}ClN_2O_3PS$=332.7.

CAS — 14816-20-7.

Chlorphoxim is an organophosphorus pesticide (p.1344) with a residual effect against mosquitoes; resistance has been reported. It is also an effective blackfly larvicide.

18112-w

Chlorpyrifos *(BAN).*
O,O-Diethyl *O*-3,5,6-trichloro-2-pyridyl phosphorothioate.
$C_9H_{11}Cl_3NO_3PS$=350.6.

CAS — 2921-88-2.

Chlorpyrifos is an organophosphorus pesticide (p.1344) effective against a range of insects. It has high residual activity against mosquito larvae although resistance is emerging. The methyl derivative chlorpyrifos-methyl is effective against blackfly larvae.
In Great Britain the recommended exposure limits of chlorpyrifos are 0.2 mg per m^3 (long-term); 0.6 mg per m^3 (short-term); suitable precautions should be taken to prevent absorption through the skin.

Chlorpyrifos: pharmacokinetics in human volunteers.— R. J. Nolan *et al.*, *Toxic. appl. Pharmac.*, 1984, *73*, 8.

Five cases of organophosphorus poisoning arising from use of chlorpyrifos with methylcarbamic acid.— M. J. Hodgson and D. K. Parkinson (letter), *New Engl. J. Med.*, 1985, *313*, 329.

Proprietary Names and Manufacturers
Dursban *(Dow Agriculture, UK)*; EF121 *(May & Baker Agrochemicals, UK)*; Spannit *(Pan Britannica, UK)*.

The following names have been used for multi-ingredient preparations containing chlorpyrifos— Chlorophos *(Pan Britannica, UK)*.

12608-s

Copper Oleate

$Cu(C_{18}H_{33}O_2)_2$=626.5.

CAS — 1120-44-1.

Copper oleate has been used in a concentration of 0.03% for the treatment of pediculosis.

Emerald-green urine associated with copper oleate therapy.— K. D. Grant *et al.* (letter), *Sth. med. J.*, 1985, *78*, 365.

Proprietary Names and Manufacturers
Cuprex *(Merck, Arg.)*.

12620-v

Cycloheximide *(USAN).*
Cicloheximide (*rINN*); U-4527. 3-{(*R*)-2-[(1*S*,3*S*,5*S*)-3,5-Dimethyl-2-oxocyclohexyl]-2-hydroxyethyl}glutarimide.
$C_{15}H_{23}NO_4$=281.4.

CAS — 66-81-9.

An antimicrobial substance produced by strains of *Streptomyces griseus*.

Cycloheximide has antifungal properties and has been used for the treatment and control of certain mycotic plant diseases. It may be added to bacteriological media to facilitate the isolation or counting of bacteria in the presence of yeasts or moulds; similarly, it has been used in the detection and isolation of *Chlamydia trachomatis*. Cycloheximide has demonstrated antiviral activity. It is a potent skin irritant and if spilled on the skin should be washed off immediately with soap and water.

Proprietary Names and Manufacturers
Acti-dione *(Upjohn, USA)*.

3855-c

Cyfluthrin *(BAN).*
Bay-Vl-1704; Cyfluthin. (*RS*)-α-Cyano-4-fluoro-3-phenoxybenzyl (1*RS*,3*RS*;1*RS*,3*SR*)-3-(2,2-dichlorovinyl)-2,2-dimethylcyclopropanecarboxylate.
$C_{22}H_{18}Cl_2FNO_3$=434.3.

CAS — 68359-37-5.

Cyfluthrin is a pyrethroid insecticide (p.1345). It is used in public health to control disease vectors such as tsetse flies.

19015-k

Cypermethrin *(BAN).*
NRDC-149. (*RS*)-α-Cyano-3-phenoxybenzyl (1*RS*,3*RS*)-(1*RS*,3*RS*)-3-(2,2-dichlorovinyl)-2,2-dimethylcyclopropanecarboxylate.
$C_{22}H_{19}Cl_2NO_3$=416.3.

CAS — 52315-07-8.

Cypermethrin is a pyrethroid insecticide (p.1345) widely used in agriculture. It is used in the control of disease vectors such as mosquitoes, where resistance has developed to organophosphorus compounds, and tsetse flies.
Cypermethrin is also used as a reaction mixture of the 2 stereoisomers when the name alphamethrin was sometimes used.

Nausea, prolonged vomiting with colicky pain, tenesmus, diarrhoea, convulsions, coma, respiratory failure, and death occurred in a 45-year-old man after ingesting an unknowm quantity of cypermethrin.— L. Poulos *et al.* (letter), *J. Toxicol. clin. Toxicol.*, 1982, *19*, 519.

Proprietary Names and Manufacturers
Ambush C *(ICI Plant Protection, UK)*; Cymbush *(ICI Plant Protection, UK)*; Ripcord *(Shell Chemicals, UK)*; Toppel *(ICI Plant Protection, UK)*.

16614-c

Decamethrin
Deltamethrin; NRDC-161. (*S*)-α-Cyano-3-phenoxybenzyl (1*R*,3*R*)-3-(2,2-dibromovinyl)-2,2-dimethylcyclopropanecarboxylate.
$C_{22}H_{19}Br_2NO_3$=505.2.

CAS — 52918-63-5.

Decamethrin is a pyrethroid (p.1345) active against a wide range of insects. Its residual insecticidal effect has been demonstrated against mosquitoes and their larvae as well as tsetse flies and blackflies.
A field study of decamethrin for malaria control.— P. Taylor *et al.*, *Trans R. Soc. trop. Med. Hyg.*, 1986, *80*, 537.

Proprietary Names and Manufacturers
Crackdown *(Wellcome, UK)*; Decis *(Hoechst Animal Health, UK)*.

18132-j

Diazinon *(BAN)*.
Dimpylate *(rINN)*. *O,O*-Diethyl *O*-(2-isopropyl-6-methylpyrimidin-4-yl) phosphorothioate.
$C_{12}H_{21}N_2O_3PS$=304.4.

CAS — 333-41-5.

Diazinon is an organophosphorus pesticide (p.1344) used as an insecticide in agriculture, horticulture, and veterinary practice.
In Great Britain the recommended exposure limits of diazinon are 0.1 mg per m^3 (long-term); 0.3 mg per m^3 (short-term); suitable precautions should be taken to prevent absorption through the skin.

Reports of poisoning with diazinon: S. A. Soliman *et al.*, *Archs environ. Hlth*, 1982, *37*, 207; K. S. Hui (letter), *Archs Path. lab. Med.*, 1983, *107*, 154.

Proprietary Names and Manufacturers
Basudin *(Ciba-Geigy Agrochemicals, UK)*; Flytrol *(Rentokil, UK)*; Murphy Root Guard *(Fisons Horticultural Division, UK)*.

The following names have been used for multi-ingredient preparations containing diazinon—Chlorophos *(Pan Britannica, UK)*; Insectrol *(Rentokil, UK)*.

12642-e

Dibromochloropropane
1,2-Dibromo-3-chloropropane.
$C_3H_5Br_2Cl$=236.3.

CAS — 96-12-8.

Dibromochloropropane has been used as a pesticide. Low sperm counts have occurred in workers exposed to dibromochloropropane.
In the US the permissible and recommended exposure limits of dibromochloropropane are 1 ppb and 10 ppb respectively.

References: D. Whorton *et al.*, *Lancet*, 1977, *2*, 1259; *ibid.*, 1978, *2*, 79; R. I. Glass *et al.*, *Am. J. Epidem.*, 1979, *109*, 346; D. Whorton *et al.*, *J. occup. Med.*, 1979, *21*, 161.

2553-k

Dibutyl Phthalate
Butyl Phthalate; DBP. Dibutyl benzene-1,2-dicarboxylate.
$C_{16}H_{22}O_4$=278.3.

CAS — 84-74-2.

Pharmacopoeias. In *Ind.*

Dibutyl phthalate is slightly less effective than dimethyl phthalate as an insect repellent but it is more effective against the mite vector of scrub typhus.
It is less volatile and less easily removed by washing than dimethyl phthalate, and its chief use is for the impregnation of clothing. As with other phthalates contact with plastics should be avoided.
Dibutyl phthalate has occasionally caused hypersensitivity reactions. In Great Britain the recommended exposure limit of diisobutyl phthalate is 5 mg per m^3 (long-term).

12644-y

Dichlofenthion *(BAN)*.
V-C-13. *O*-2,4-Dichlorophenyl *O,O*-diethyl phosphorothioate.
$C_{10}H_{13}Cl_2O_3PS$=315.2.

CAS — 97-17-6.

Pharmacopoeias. In *B.P. Vet.*

A colourless or pale yellow oily liquid. **Immiscible** with water; miscible with alcohol and chloroform.

Dichlofenthion is an organophosphorus compound (p.1344), used as an insecticide in veterinary practice.

3576-s

Dichlorophenoxyacetic Acid
2,4-D. 2,4-Dichlorophenoxyacetic acid.
$C_8H_6Cl_2O_3$=221.0.

CAS — 94-75-7.

Adverse Effects
Most cases of poisoning with dichlorophenoxyacetic acid have involved the ingestion of it with other herbicides; the solvent may also play a part in any toxicity. There is little pattern to the range of adverse effects which may occur following ingestion, inhalation, or topical exposure. Death has followed the ingestion of 6 g, yet in another patient 7 g was not fatal. It is considered that 36 mg per kg body-weight might be a threshold dose above which adverse effects could be expected.
Observed adverse effects have involved the central and peripheral nervous system, muscles, and the cardiovascular system. Gastro-intestinal effects are common with poisoning. Hepatotoxicity, nephrotoxicity, and pulmonary disorders have been observed but it is not clear that dichlorophenoxyacetic acid contributed to the toxicity. The role of phenoxyacetic acids in cancer is discussed under trichlorophenoxyacetic acid (p.1354).
In Great Britain the recommended exposure limits of dichlorophenoxyacetic acid are 10 mg per m^3 (long-term); 20 mg per m^3 (short-term).
2,4-Dichlorophenoxyacetic Acid (2,4-D), *Environmental Health Criteria 29*, Geneva, Wld Hlth Org., 1984.

A fatality following ingestion of not less than 6 g.— K. Neilsen *et al.*, *Acta pharmac. tox.*, 1965, *22*, 244. Recovery after the ingestion of 7 g.— P. Berwick, *J. Am. med. Ass.*, 1970, *214*, 1114.

Three cases of poisoning with dichlorophenoxyacetic acid taken with other herbicides; two of the patients died.— L. J. Onyon *et al.*, *Hum. Toxicol.*, 1986, *5*, 127.

Treatment of Adverse Effects
Ingested material should be removed by aspiration and lavage. Contaminated clothing should be removed and the skin washed with soap and water. Forced diuresis has been reported to be effective in removing dichlorophenoxyacetic acid. Further treatment is symptomatic.

A report of prolonged coma and delayed peripheral neuropathy in a 61-year-old man following ingestion of a weedkiller containing dichlorophenoxyacetic acid and trichlorophenoxyacetic acid in a hydrocarbon solvent. Despite gastric lavage he became drowsy and within 6 hours was responsive only to pain. Within 24 hours he became unresponsive to pain and was unconscious for 4 days. During this time he was treated with continuous oxygen and forced diuresis with intravenous glucose 5%, isotonic saline, and potassium. He regained consciousness on the fifth day and was discharged 2 days later. One month later he presented with progressive difficulty in walking and peripheral neuropathy was confirmed. Three months later he had made a full spontaneous recovery.— J. F. O'Reilly, *Postgrad. med. J.*, 1984, *60*, 76.

Uses.
Dichlorophenoxyacetic acid is a systemic herbicide widely used in cereals and other crops. It is usually used as its salts or esters in combination with other herbicides.

Proprietary Names and Manufacturers
Dicotox Extra *(May & Baker Agrochemicals, UK)*; Fernimine *(ICI Plant Protection, UK)*; For-Ester *(Synchemicals, UK)*; Planotox *(May & Baker Agrochemicals, UK)*; Silvapron D *(BP Chemicals, UK)*; Syford *(Synchemicals, UK)*; Weedon LV4 *(A.H. Marks, UK)*.

The following names have been used for multi-ingredient preparations containing dichlorophenoxyacetic acid—Kilnet *(May & Baker Agrochemicals, UK)*.

3577-w

Dichlorvos *(BAN, USAN, rINN)*.
DDVP; OMS-14; SD-1750. 2,2-Dichlorovinyl dimethyl phosphate.
$C_4H_7Cl_2O_4P$=221.0.

CAS — 62-73-7.

Adverse Effects and Treatment
As for Organophosphorus Pesticides p.1344.
In Great Britain the recommended exposure limits of dichlorvos are 0.1 ppm (long-term); 0.3 ppm (short-term); suitable precautions should be taken to prevent absorption through the skin.

A 54-year-old pest control operator whose clothing became contaminated with dichlorvos developed erythema and bullae on areas of the skin exposed to dichlorvos. He also complained of tiredness and constipation and had blood-cholinesterase concentrations 36% of normal. He recovered with conservative treatment.— J. A. Bisby and G. R. Simpson, *Med. J. Aust.*, 1975, *2*, 394.

Five children with aplastic anaemia and one with acute lymphoblastic leukaemia had been exposed to dichlorvos with propoxur; one of the children had also been exposed to a pyrethrin. A seventh child with aplastic anaemia had been exposed to malathion.— J. D. Reeves *et al.* (letter), *Lancet*, 1981, *2*, 300. Criticism (from the manufacturers) of a causal relationship.— H. G. S. v. Raalte and J. D. Jansen (letter), *ibid.*, 811.

Uses and Administration
Dichlorvos is an organophosphorus pesticide of short persistence, effective against a wide range of insects. It is used in the form of impregnated strips or blocks which slowly release vapour. Impregnated animal collars may contain dichlorvos. It has also been used for the extermination of insects in aircraft (disinsection).
Dichlorvos is used as a veterinary anthelmintic and for the eradication of other intestinal parasites. It has been tried in human helminthiasis.

Proprietary Names and Manufacturers
Insectigas-D *(BOC, UK)*; Mafu Fly Killer *(Bayer Agrochem, UK)*; Mafu Small Space *(Bayer Agrochem, UK)*; Nuvan *(Ciba-Geigy Agrochemicals, UK)*.

The following names have been used for multi-ingredient preparations containing dichlorvos—Blattenex Aerosol *(Bayer Agrochem, UK)*; Defest *(Asche, UK)*; Mafu Fly Spray *(Bayer Agrochem, UK)*; Nuvan Fly Killer *(Ciba-Geigy Agrochemicals, UK)*.

3578-e

Dicophane
Chlorofenotano; Chlorophenothane; Chlorphenothanum; Clofenotane *(rINN)*; DDT; Dichlorodiphenyltrichloroethane; Dichophanum. 1,1,1-Trichloro-2,2-bis(4-chlorophenyl)ethane.
$C_{14}H_9Cl_5$=354.5.

CAS — 50-29-3.

Pharmacopoeias. In *Arg.*, *Aust.*, *Egypt.*, *Ind.*, *It.*, *Nord.*, *Pol.*, *Span.*, and *Turk.* The content of $C_{14}H_9Cl_5$ ranges from not less than 70% to not less than 99%.

Adverse Effects and Treatment
As for Chlorinated Pesticides, p.1344.
In Great Britain the recommended exposure limits of dicophane are 1 mg per m^3 (long-term); 3 mg per m^3 (short-term). In the *US* the permissible and recommended exposure limits are 1 mg per m^3 and 0.5 mg per m^3 respectively; suitable precautions should be taken to prevent absorption through the skin.

DDT and its Derivatives, *Environmental Health Criteria 9*, Geneva, Wld Hlth Org., 1979.

Absorption and Fate
Dicophane may be absorbed after ingestion or

inhalation or through the skin. Dicophane is stored in the body, particularly in body fat, and is very slowly eliminated. It crosses the placenta and appears in breast milk. It is metabolised in the body to the ethylene derivative (DDE); the acetic acid derivative (DDA) also appears in the urine.

Uses.
Dicophane is a chlorinated pesticide used as an insecticide and larvicide. It is a stomach and contact poison and retains its activity for long periods under a variety of conditions. It is effective against disease vectors such as fleas, lice, and mosquitoes.
Because of the extreme persistence of dicophane, concern in respect of its effect in the environment, and the problem of resistance, the widespread use of dicophane is now generally discouraged. It is no longer used in some countries while in others it is limited to those applications for which there is no effective or suitable alternative.

In order to maintain and extend malaria eradication programmes dicophane should remain available. Its withdrawal from public health use could lead to great problems, and expose considerable populations to outbreaks of endemic and epidemic malaria. It was considered that the liver tumours found in *mice* given dicophane did not provide an adequate basis for recommending the withdrawal of dicophane where its use could be life-saving and where any possible risk to man would be outweighed by the benefits arising from its controlled use.— Safe Use of Pesticides, Twentieth Report of the WHO Expert Committee on Insecticides, *Tech. Rep. Ser. Wld Hlth Org. No. 513*, 1973. Liver tumours had not been produced in any other species tested and the limited epidemiological evidence available in man, including intermittent exposure over 30 years, gave no evidence that dicophane might be a human carcinogen.— Pesticide Residues in Food, *Tech. Rep. Ser. Wld Hlth Org. No. 574*, 1975.

Proprietary Names and Manufacturers
Benzochloryl *(Delalande, Fr.)*; Nosa Locion Parasiticida *(Sokatarg, Spain)*.

The following names have been used for multi-ingredient preparations containing dicophane— Esoderm *(Napp, UK)*.

3579-l

Dieldrin *(BAN, pINN)*.

CAS — 60-57-1 (HEOD).

Dieldrin contains about 85% of (1*R*,4*S*,5*S*,8*R*)-1,2,3,4,10,10-hexachloro-6,7-epoxy-1,4,4a,5,6,7,8,8a-octahydro-1,4:5,8-dimethanonaphthalene (HEOD), $C_{12}H_8Cl_6O$ = 380.9. The remaining 15% is mainly chlorinated organic compounds related to HEOD.

Adverse Effects and Treatment
As for Chlorinated Pesticides, p.1344.
Dieldrin is more toxic than dicophane and is readily absorbed through the skin. Fish, birds, dogs, and other animals are susceptible to dieldrin.
In Great Britain the recommended exposure limits of dieldrin are 0.25 mg per m^3 (long-term); 0.75 mg per m^3 (short-term); suitable precautions should be taken to prevent absorption through the skin. Similar limits apply to aldrin.

Uses.
Dieldrin is a chlorinated pesticide formerly used as a sheep dip. Its use is now limited to a few specified purposes such as termite control.

2554-a

Diethyltoluamide *(BAN, USAN)*.

Deet. *NN*-Diethyl-*m*-toluamide.
$C_{12}H_{17}NO$=191.3.

CAS — 134-62-3.

Pharmacopoeias. In *Ind.* and *U.S.*

A colourless or faintly yellow liquid, odourless or with a faint pleasant odour. Practically **insoluble** in water and glycerol; miscible with alcohol, carbon disulphide, chloroform, ether, isopropyl alcohol, and propylene glycol. **Store** in airtight containers.

Adverse Effects and Precautions
Occasional hypersensitivity has been reported. There have been rare reports of encephalopathy in children. Diethyltoluamide should not be applied near the eyes, to mucous membranes, to broken skin, or to areas of skin flexion as irritation or blistering may occur.
A 35-year-old woman developed contact urticaria (considered to be an immediate-type hypersensitivity) after application of diethyltoluamide; this was confirmed by patch testing.— H. I. Maibach and H. L. Johnson, *Archs Derm.*, 1975, *111*, 726. A report of anaphylactic hypersensitivity to diethyltoluamide.— J. D. Miller (letter), *New Engl. J. Med.*, 1982, *307*, 1341.
Reports of toxic encephalopathy in children receiving liberal applications of diethyltoluamide: H. M. C. Heick *et al.*, *J. Pediat.*, 1980, *97*, 471; E. H. Roland *et al.*, *Can. med. Ass. J.*, 1985, *132*, 155.
Severe toxicity in 5 subjects who swallowed large amounts of diethyltoluamide. Symptoms included coma, seizures, and hypotension. Two patients died.— M. Tenenbein, *J. Am. med. Ass.*, 1987, *258*, 1509.

Uses.
Diethyltoluamide is an insect repellent which is effective against blackflies, harvest-bugs or chiggers, midges, mosquitoes, ticks, and fleas. It has also been used as a repellent against leeches. It may be applied to skin and clothing.
A brief discussion of diethyltoluamide.— *Lancet*, 1988, *2*, 610.
The effectiveness of diethyltoluamide against sandflies.— F. P. Fossati and M. Maroli, *Trans. R. Soc. trop. Med. Hyg.*, 1986, *80*, 771.

Preparations
Diethyltoluamide Topical Solution *(U.S.P.)*. A solution containing diethyltoluamide in alcohol or isopropyl alcohol.

Proprietary Names and Manufacturers
Autan *(Bayer, UK)*; Jungle Formula *(Jungle Formula Co., UK)*; Metadelphene *(Hercules, UK)*.

3864-k

Difenacoum

3-(3-Biphenyl-4-yl-1,2,3,4-tetrahydro-1-naphthyl)-4-hydroxycoumarin.
$C_{31}H_{24}O_3$=444.5.

CAS — 56073-07-5.

Difenacoum, like bromadiolone and brodifacoum is an anticoagulant rodenticide reported to inhibit prothrombin synthesis.

Difenacoum, a second-generation anticoagulant rodenticide inhibits prothrombin synthesis to cause bleeding that may be occult. It is absorbed from the gastro-intestinal tract; dermal absorption is possible. Baits containing 100 mg per kg are not hazardous to man; more concentrated forms are particularly hazardous and their availability should be restricted. Baits, which should be prepared only by trained personnel, should contain a suitable marker-dye and should not be used in domestic, public, or industrial situations where they can come into contact with food and water. Unnecessary distribution into the environment should be avoided.— Safe Use of Pesticides, Ninth Report of the WHO Expert Committee on Vector Biology and Control, *Tech. Rep. Ser. Wld Hlth Org. No. 720*, 1985.
A report of a suicidal attempt using difenacoum; phytomenadione was required at intervals for more than 6 weeks.— A. M. Barlow *et al.*, *Br. med. J.*, 1982, *285*, 541.

Proprietary Names and Manufacturers
Fentrex *(Rentokil, UK)*; Fentrol *(Rentokil, UK)*; Neosorexa *(Sorex, UK)*; Ratak *(ICI Plant Protection, UK)*.

18066-x

Diflubenzuron

1-(4-Chlorophenyl)-3-(2,6-difluorobenzoyl)urea.
$C_{14}H_9ClF_2N_2O_2$=310.7.

CAS — 35367-38-5.

Diflubenzuron is an insecticide or larvicide that acts as a growth regulator by interfering with the formation of cuticle. It is used in agriculture.
Diflubenzuron possesses residual activity against mosquito larvae.

Activity of diflubenzuron against murine melanoma cell cultures.— J. O. Norman and S. M. Meola, *Antimicrob. Ag. Chemother.*, 1983, *23*, 313.

Proprietary Names and Manufacturers
Antec Larvakill *(Antec, UK)*; Dimilin *(ICI Plant Protection, UK)*.

2555-t

Dimethyl Phthalate *(BAN)*.

DMP; Methyl Phthalate. Dimethyl benzene-1,2-dicarboxylate.
$C_{10}H_{10}O_4$=194.2.

CAS — 131-11-3.

Pharmacopoeias. In *Br.* and *Nord.*

A colourless or faintly coloured liquid, odourless or almost odourless.
Slightly **soluble** in water; miscible with alcohol, ether, and most organic solvents.

Adverse Effects
Dimethyl phthalate may cause temporary smarting and should not be applied near the eyes or to mucous membranes. Ingestion may cause CNS depression.
In Great Britain the recommended exposure limits of dimethyl phthalate are 5 mg per m^3 (long-term); 10 mg per m^3 (short-term).

Uses
Dimethyl phthalate is an insect repellent which is effective against blackflies, harvest-bugs or chiggers, mosquitoes, midges, mites, ticks, and fleas. It is usually applied to the skin as a cream or lotion containing at least 40% of dimethyl phthalate.
Some synthetic clothing and spectacle frames may be damaged by dimethyl phthalate.

Proprietary Names and Manufacturers
Affel *(Fr.)*; Shoo *(Torbet Laboratories, UK)*; Sketofax *(Wellcome, UK)*.

18085-d

Dinitro-*o*-cresol

DNOC. 4,6-Dinitro-*o*-cresol.
$C_7H_6N_2O_5$=198.1.

CAS — 534-52-1.

Dinitro-*o*-cresol is a dinitrophenol insecticide and herbicide (see below). It has also been used in obesity and fatal poisoning has occurred.
In Great Britain the recommended exposure limits of dinitro-*o*-cresol are 0.2 mg per m^3 (long-term); 0.6 mg per m^3 (short-term); suitable precautions should be taken to prevent absorption through the skin. In the *US* the permissible and recommended exposure limits are 0.2 mg per m^3.

A review of the effects of dinitro-*o*-cresol on health.— Recommended Health-based Limits in Occupational Exposure to Pesticides, *Tech. Rep. Ser. Wld Hlth Org. No. 677*, 1982.

Proprietary Names and Manufacturers
Sandolin *(Sandoz Agrochem, UK)*.

3580-v

Dinitrophenol

2,4-Dinitrophenol.
$C_6H_4N_2O_5$=184.1.

CAS — 51-28-5.

Dinitrophenol and some other nitrophenols are used as pesticides and herbicides, although for some such as dinoseb use is restricted. Since dinitrophenol increases metabolism it was formerly used in the treatment of obesity. Fatal poisoning has occurred.

3581-g

Dioxathion *(BAN).*
Dioxation *(rINN).* It consists mainly of *cis* and *trans* isomers of *S,S'*-1,4-dioxane-2,3-diyl bis(*O,O*-diethyl phosphorodithioate).
$C_{12}H_{26}O_6P_2S_4$=456.5.

CAS — 78-34-2.

CAUTION. *Contact with dioxathion is hazardous, see below under Adverse Effects.*

Adverse Effects and Treatment
As for Organophosphorus Pesticides, p.1344.
Dioxathion is very toxic when inhaled, swallowed, or spilled on the skin. It can be removed from the skin by washing with soap and water. Contaminated material should be immersed in a 2% aqueous solution of sodium hydroxide for several hours.
In Great Britain the recommended exposure limit of dioxathion is 0.2 mg per m^3 (long-term); suitable precautions should be taken to prevent absorption through the skin.

Uses
Dioxathion is an agricultural insecticide and acaricide. It has been used for the control of cattle ticks as well as other parasites.

3583-p

Diquat
9,10-Dihydro-8a,10a-diazoniaphenanthrene ion; 1,1'-Ethylene-2,2'-bipyridyldiylium ion.
$C_{12}H_{12}N_2$=184.2.

CAS — 2764-72-9.

3584-s

Diquat Dibromide

$C_{12}H_{12}Br_2N_2$=344.0.

CAS — 85-00-7.

Diquat is a contact herbicide used usually as the dibromide in agriculture and horticulture. It has similar adverse effects to those of paraquat (p.1352). In Great Britain the recommended exposure limits of diquat dibromide are 0.5 mg per m^3 (long-term); 1 mg per m^3 (short-term).

Paraquat and Diquat, *Environmental Health Criteria 39*, Geneva, Wld Hlth Org., 1984.

Proprietary Names and Manufacturers
Reglone *(ICI Plant Protection, UK).*

The following names have been used for multi-ingredient preparations containing diquat dibromide— Cleansweep *(Shell Chemicals, UK)*; Groundhog *(ICI Plant Protection, UK)*; New Weedol *(ICI Plant Protection, UK)*; Pathclear *(ICI Plant Protection, UK)*; Soltair *(ICI Plant Protection, UK)*; Weedol *(ICI Plant Protection, UK).*

19131-r

Endod
A preparation from the dried fruits of *Phytolacca dodecandra* (phytolaccaceae).
Endod has molluscicidal properties. A related plant, *Phytolacca americana* (=*P. decandra*) known as phytolacca or poke root has emetic, laxative, and mildly sedative properties; in powdered form it is sternutatory.

18067-r

Endosulfan
1,4,5,6,7,7-Hexachloro-8,9,10-trinorborn-5-en-2,3-ylene-bismethylene sulphate.
$C_9H_6Cl_6O_3S$=406.9.

CAS — 115-29-7.

Endosulfan is a chlorinated pesticide (p.1344) active against a range of insects and mites. Susceptible insects include the tsetse fly.
In Great Britain the recommended exposure limits of endosulfan are 0.1 mg per m^3 (long-term); 0.3 mg per m^3 (short-term); suitable precautions should be taken to prevent absorption through the skin.

Endosulfan, *Environmental Health Criteria 40*, Geneva, Wld Hlth Org., 1984.

Tolerance to Endosulfan by tsetse flies.— W. H. Kwan *et al., Bull. entomol. Res.,* 1982, *72,* 391.

18068-f

Endrin
(1*R*,4*S*,4a*S*,5*S*,6*S*,7*R*,8*R*,8a*R*)-1,2,3,4,10,10-Hexachloro-1,4,4a,5,6,7,8,8a-octahydro-6,7-epoxy-1,4:5,8-dimethanonaphthalene.
$C_{12}H_8Cl_6O$=380.9.

CAS — 72-20-8.

Endrin is a chlorinated pesticide (p.1344) used as an insecticide. It has been associated with a number of poisonings.
In Great Britain the recommended exposure limits of endrin are 0.1 mg per m^3 (long-term); 0.3 mg per m^3 (short-term); suitable precautions should be taken to prevent absorption through the skin.

Some references to fatal endrin poisoning: *J. Am. med. Ass.,* 1985, *253,* 334; E. A. Runhaar *et al., Hum. Toxicol.,* 1985, *4,* 241.

2556-x

Ethohexadiol
Ethylhexanediol; Rutgers-612. 2-Ethylhexane-1,3-diol.
$C_8H_{18}O_2$=146.2.

CAS — 94-96-2.

Ethohexadiol is an insect repellent which is effective against blackflies, harvest-bugs or chiggers, and mosquitoes. It may be applied topically to the skin and to clothing. It has been used in conjunction with dimethyl phthalate and butopyronoxyl.

12710-q

Ethylene Dibromide
EDB. 1,2-Dibromoethane.
$C_2H_4Br_2$=187.9.

CAS — 106-93-4.

A heavy colourless non-inflammable liquid.

Ethylene dibromide is an insecticidal fumigant and a lead scavenger used in the petroleum industry. Its use has been restricted in certain areas because of carcinogenicity in experimental *animals* and because of evidence of persistence in fruit and cereals that have undergone fumigation. Ethylene dibromide is more toxic than carbon tetrachloride or ethylene dichloride. It is irritant to the eyes, skin, and mucous membranes. Inhalation leads to drowsiness, CNS depression, and possibly pulmonary oedema. Contact with the skin causes blistering and it is readily absorbed. Kidney and liver damage may occur.
In Great Britain the control exposure limit of ethylene dibromide is 1 ppm (long-term); suitable precautions should be taken to prevent absorption through the skin. In the *US* the permissible and recommended exposure limits are 20 ppm and 0.045 ppm respectively.

A study in *rats* showed an increased incidence of morbidity and mortality in animals exposed to a combination of ethylene dibromide and disulfiram. The clinical significance was not known but the advisability of continued occupational exposure to ethylene dibromide by patients receiving disulfiram was uncertain.— H. B. Plotnick (letter), *J. Am. med. Ass.,* 1978, *239,* 1609. See also R. E. Yodaiken, *ibid.,* 2783.

Two fatalities associated with acute occupational exposure to ethylene dibromide.— G. A. Letz *et al., J. Am. med. Ass.,* 1984, *252,* 2428.

12711-p

Ethylene Dichloride
Brocide; Dutch Liquid. 1,2-Dichloroethane.
$C_2H_4Cl_2$=98.96.

CAS — 107-06-2.

A colourless inflammable liquid with a chloroform-like odour.
Ethylene dichloride is used as an industrial solvent and, usually in conjunction with carbon tetrachloride, as an insecticide by fumigation. Exposure to the vapour may cause lachrymation and corneal clouding, nasal irritation, and vertigo due to the depressant effect on the CNS. Contact with the skin may cause dermatitis. Kidney and liver damage may follow absorption after inhalation, topical application, or ingestion.
In Great Britain the recommended exposure limits of ethylene dichloride are 10 ppm (long-term); 15 ppm (short-term). In the *US* the permissible and recommended exposure limits are 50 ppm and 1 ppm respectively.
Ethylene dichloride has been reported to be carcinogenic in experimental *animals.*

18142-c

Fenitrothion *(BAN).*
O,O-Dimethyl *O*-4-nitro-*m*-tolyl phosphorothioate.
$C_9H_{12}NO_5PS$=277.2.

CAS — 122-14-5.

Fenitrothion is an organophosphorus pesticide (p.1344) effective against a wide range of insects. It is used in the control of disease vectors including mosquitoes and fleas.

Malaria control with residual fenitrothion.— S. Gandahusada *et al., Bull. Wld Hlth Org.,* 1984, *62,* 783.

Fenitrothion in bedbug control.— B. D. Varma and K. K. Gupta, *J. commun. Dis.,* 1983, *15,* 126.

Proprietary Names and Manufacturers
Dicofen *(Pan Britannica, UK)*; Fentro *(Murphy Chemical, UK)*; Folithion *(Bayer Agrochem, UK)*; Insectigas-F *(BOC, UK).*

3586-e

Fenthion *(BAN).*
Bayer 29493; S-752. *O,O*-Dimethyl *O*-4-methylthio-*m*-tolyl phosphorothioate.
$C_{10}H_{15}O_3PS_2$=278.3.

CAS — 55-38-9.

Pharmacopoeias. In *B.P. Vet.*

A yellowish-brown almost odourless oily liquid. Practically **immiscible** with water; miscible with alcohol and chloroform.

An organophosphorus pesticide (see p.1344). In veterinary practice it is used for the control of warble fly and lice. It is also used as a crop insecticide.
Fenthion has been used as a mosquito larvicide but resistance has developed in several countries.

A study of retinal changes in workers regularly exposed to pesticides. None of 18 subjects engaged in spraying dicophane had any macular changes, whereas 15 of 79 exposed to fenthion had macular lesions of varying severity; this compared with only 3 of 100 control subjects who had such changes. Seven of the 15 affected reported visual impairment, and in severely affected patients visual acuity, colour vision, and field of vision were all impaired; the remaining eight were asymptomatic. Workers exposed to fenthion should undergo periodic ophthalmoscopic examination, and there is a need for long-term studies on subjects exposed to different organophosphorus compounds to assess their role in producing macular changes.— U. K. Misra *et al., Hum. Toxicol.,* 1985, *4,* 135.

Further references to fenthion poisoning: P. Mahieu *et al., J. Toxicol. clin. Toxicol.,* 1982, *19,* 425.

7731-y

Fluoroacetamide
Compound 1081.
$FCH_2.CONH_2$=77.06.

CAS — 640-19-7.

Fluoroacetamide is used as a rodenticide and produces adverse effects similar to those of sodium fluoroacetate (p.1354).
In Great Britain, the use of fluoroacetamide is restricted to the destruction of rodents in ships, sewers, and specified dock warehouses. When supplied for use as a rodenticide it must contain a distinctive colouring matter.
Fluoroacetamide and its analogues bromoacetamide and chloracetamide are reported to have high molluscicidal activity.

For recommendations on the use of fluoroacetamide as a rodenticide and precautions to be taken in its use, see under sodium fluoracetate (p.1354).

Proprietary Names and Manufacturers
Fluorakil *(Rentokil, UK).*

18074-x

Heptachlor
1,4,5,6,7,8,8-Heptachloro-3a,4,7,7a-tetrahydro-4,7-methanoindene.
$C_{10}H_5Cl_7$=373.3.

CAS — 76-44-8.

Heptachlor is a chlorinated pesticide (p.1344) effective against a wide range of insects although its use is becoming restricted to termite control.
In Great Britain the recommended exposure limits of heptachlor are 0.5 mg per m^3 (long-term); 2 mg per m^3 (short-term); suitable precautions should be taken to prevent absorption through the skin.

Heptachlor, *Environmental Health Criteria 38*, Geneva, Wld Hlth Org., 1984.

12823-c

Hexachlorobenzene

C_6Cl_6=284.8.

CAS — 118-74-1.

NOTE. Hexachlorobenzene should not be confused with Benzene Hexachloride.

Hexachlorobenzene has been used as an agricultural fungicide. It is not biodegradable to any significant extent and hexachlorobenzene residues in food have arisen as a result of its occurrence in industrial wastes as well as its use as a fungicide.
Hexachlorobenzene is reported to be excreted in breast milk.

Porphyria cutanea tarda in 348 patients was traced to consumption of wheat for planting which had been treated with a fungicide containing 10% of hexachlorobenzene. The patients had probably ingested 50 to 200 mg daily. Acute manifestations disappeared without specific therapy 20 to 30 days after consumption had ceased.— C. Cam and G. Nigogosyan, *J. Am. med. Ass.*, 1963, *183,* 88. Symptoms persisted for up to 30 years after consumption.— D. J. Cripps *et al.*, *Br. J. Derm.*, 1984, *111,* 413. Parkinsonism had been observed in subjects taking seed corn treated with hexachlorobenzene.— L. J. Chapman *et al.* (letter), *Lancet,* 1987, *1,* 332.

7751-k

Hydrocyanic Acid
Prussic Acid.

CAS — 74-90-8.

An aqueous solution containing hydrogen cyanide, HCN = 27.03. A colourless liquid with a characteristic almond odour.

CAUTION. *Hydrocyanic acid and its vapour are intensely poisonous.*

Adverse Effects
Cyanides interfere with the oxygen uptake of cells by inhibition of cytochrome oxidase, an enzyme necessary for cellular oxygen transport.
Poisoning by cyanides may occur from inhalation of the vapour, ingestion, or absorption through the skin. Poisoning may arise from cyanide pesticides, industrial accidental exposure, or the inhalation of fumes from some burning plastics. Poisoning may also occur from cyanide-containing plants or fruits.
When large doses of hydrocyanic acid are taken, unconsciousness occurs within a few seconds and death within a few minutes. With smaller toxic doses the symptoms, which occur within a few minutes, may include constriction of the throat, nausea, vomiting, giddiness, headache, palpitation, hyperpnoea then dyspnoea, bradycardia, (initially there may be tachycardia), unconsciousness, and violent convulsions, followed by death. The characteristic smell of bitter almonds may not be obvious. Cyanosis is not prominent. Similar but usually slower effects occur with cyanide salts.
The fatal dose of hydrocyanic acid (HCN) for man is considered to be about 50 mg and of the cyanides about 250 mg.
In Great Britain the control exposure limit of hydrogen cyanide is 10 ppm (short-term). The recommended exposure limit of cyanides (as CN) is 5 mg per m^3 (long-term). Suitable precautions should be taken to prevent absorption through the skin. In the *US* the permissible and recommended exposure limits of hydrogen cyanide are 11 mg per m^3 and 5 mg per m^3 respectively; for cyanides both limits are 5 mg CN per m^3.

Treatment of Adverse Effects
Treatment must be given rapidly but should not involve the use of antidotes unless it is certain that cyanide has been absorbed. No case should be considered hopeless if the heart is still beating.
Cyanide is absorbed very rapidly on inhalation and the poisoned patient should be removed from the area and given oxygen (hyperbaric oxygen may be used). Steps should be taken to ensure that the airway is adequate. Contaminated clothing should be removed and skin washed. If the patient is conscious, amyl nitrite inhalations should be given for up to 30 seconds every 2 or 3 minutes; up to 6 ampoules have been used. Should the patient be unconscious or nearly so, then in the *UK* and some other countries it is the practice to give dicobalt edetate (p.839) by injection when it forms a stable complex with the cyanide ion. Absence of cyanide puts the patient at risk from the adverse effects of dicobalt edetate. The recommended dose is 300 mg given intravenously over about 1 to 5 minutes depending on the severity of the poisoning and repeated once or twice depending on the response. It is customary to give 50 mL of glucose injection (50%) after each injection, although the value of this has been questioned. An alternative treatment and one used in some countries is to inject as soon as possible 10 mL of sodium nitrite injection (3%) intravenously at the rate of 2.5 to 5 mL per minute; using the same needle and vein continue with an injection of 12.5 g of sodium thiosulphate (50 mL of a 25% solution or 25 mL of a 50% solution) administered over a period of about 10 minutes. Sodium nitrite converts haemoglobin to methaemoglobin, which competes with cytochrome oxidase for cyanide with the formation of cyanmethaemoglobin; sodium thiosulphate aids the conversion or inactivation of cyanide from cyanmethaemoglobin to thiocyanate. If toxic symptoms recur, the injections of nitrite and thiosulphate may be repeated at half the initial doses. Appropriate measures should be instituted to correct hypotension and acidosis.
If cyanide has been ingested, one of the above procedures should be instituted and the stomach then rapidly emptied by aspiration and lavage.

Some recent references to the management of cases of cyanide poisoning: G. L. Mouzas *et al.*, *Br. J. clin. Pract.*, 1983, *37,* 245; J. L. Bonsall, *Hum. Toxicol.*, 1984, *3,* 57; C. Dodds and C. McKnight, *Br. med. J.*, 1985, *291,* 785; N. R. Peden *et al.*, *ibid.*, 1986, *293,* 538.

Uses
Cyanides have various industrial applications. Hydrocyanic acid and cyanide salts produce hydrogen cyanide which is used as a gas for the eradication of rabbits, rodents, and some other pests. Cyanide salts that might be encountered include calcium cyanide, potassium cyanide, potassium ferricyanide, potassium sodium cyanide, and sodium cyanide.

Proprietary Names and Manufacturers
Cyanocil *(Rentokil, UK).*

3863-c

Iodofenphos *(BAN).*
Jodfenphos. *O*-2,5-Dichloro-4-iodophenyl *O,O*-dimethyl phosphorothioate.
$C_8H_8Cl_2IO_3PS$=413.0.

CAS — 18181-70-9.

Iodofenphos is an organophosphorus insecticide and acaricide (p.1344) used in agriculture, industry, and public health. It is an effective mosquito larvicide.

Proprietary Names and Manufacturers
Dermanol *(Harkers, UK)*; Elocril *(Ciba-Geigy Agrochemicals, UK)*; Waspex *(Rentokil, UK).*

The following names have been used for multi-ingredient preparations containing iodofenphos— Defest *(Ashe, UK).*

3587-l

Lindane *(BAN, USAN, rINN).*
666; Benhexachlor; Gamma Benzene Hexachloride; Gamma-BHC; Gamma-HCH; HCH; Hexicide. 1α,2α,3β,4α,5α,6β-Hexachlorocyclohexane.
$C_6H_6Cl_6$=290.8.

CAS — 58-89-9.

Pharmacopoeias. In *Arg., Aust., Br., Braz., Egypt., Fr., Ind., Int., Nord., Pol.,* and *U.S.* Also in *B.P. Vet.*

A white crystalline powder with a slight musty odour. Crystallising-point not less than 112°. Practically **insoluble** in water; soluble 1 in 19 of dehydrated alcohol, 1 in 2 of acetone, and 1 in 5.5 of ether; freely soluble in chloroform; slightly soluble in ethylene glycol. **Store** in well-closed containers. Protect from light.

Adverse Effects and Treatment
As for Chlorinated Pesticides, p.1344.
There has been some concern over the application of higher than normal concentrations of lindane to the skin in the treatment of scabies and pediculosis; children are considered to be particularly at risk.
In Great Britain the recommended exposure limits of lindane are 0.5 mg per m^3 (long-term); 1.5 mg per m^3 (short-term); suitable precautions should be taken to prevent absorption through the skin.

A review of the toxicity of lindane. It should not be applied after a hot soapy bath; application for less than 24 hours might be effective; a concentration of less than 1% might be sufficient, especially for excoriated skin; the 1% preparation should be used with extreme caution, if at all, in pregnancy, in very small infants, in the presence of massive excoriation; retreatment should not take place before 8 days and then only if infection could be demonstrated.— L. M. Solomon *et al.*, *Archs Derm.*, 1977, *113,* 353.

A review of reported cases of adverse drug reactions to lindane. It was concluded that a 1% solution of lindane is an extraordinarily safe preparation when used according to instructions.— M. S. Kramer *et al.*, *Clin. Pharmac. Ther.*, 1980, *27,* 149.

A review of the effects of lindane on health.— Recommended Health-based Limits in Occupational Exposure to Pesticides, *Tech. Rep. Ser. Wld Hlth Org. No. 677,* 1982.

The absorption of lindane by infants and children following the application of a 1% lotion.— C. M. Ginsburg *et al.*, *J. Pediat.*, 1977, *91,* 998. Transcutaneous lindane absorption and toxicity in infants and children.— A. K. Pramanik and R. C. Hansen, *Archs Derm.*, 1979, *115,* 1224.

Some recent reports of poisoning with lindane following ingestion or excessive application: J. E. Davies *et al.*, *Archs Derm.*, 1983, *119,* 142; J. D. Etherington, *Br. med. J.*, 1984, *289,* 228; V. T. Kelly (letter), *ibid.*, 837; U. Jaeger *et al.*, *Vet. hum. Toxicol.*, 1984, *26,* 11; W. Daerr *et al.*, *Dt. med. Wschr.*, 1985, *110,* 1253.

Uses and Administration
Lindane is an insecticide, larvicide, and acaricide. It is used topically in concentrations of 0.1 to 1% for pediculosis and in a concentration of 1% for scabies. However other agents are now preferred.

It is also used for the control of disease vectors including mosquitoes, lice, and fleas but resistance has developed.
Benzene hexachloride has several isomers apart from lindane. Mixtures of these isomers have been used but are more toxic than lindane.

PEDICULOSIS. Removal of crab lice from the eyelashes with neomycin and lindane.— M. H. Kirschner (letter), *J. Am. med. Ass.*, 1982, *248*, 428.

In a comparison of malathion lotion with lindane shampoo in the treatment of 62 children with head lice no difference was detected between treatments.— R. G. Mathias *et al.*, *Can. med. Ass. J.*, 1984, *130*, 407.

Lindane was shown to possess residual activity *in vitro* against human lice; malathion did not demonstrate residual activity.— S. P. Weisbroth and S. Cancellieri (letter), *New Engl. J. Med.*, 1984, *310*, 1668. Criticism. Because no time was allowed for the alcohol present in the preparation to evaporate no malathion was left on the hair being tested. Also using fresh lice each day meant that even if a residue was left, the lice would have had insufficient time to accumulate a lethal dose.— B. C. Fine (letter), *ibid.*, 801.

Preparations

Lindane Application *(B.P.)*. Lindane 100 mg (or a suitable quantity), emulsifying wax 4 g, xylene of commerce 15 mL, lavender oil 1 mL, freshly boiled and cooled water to 100 mL.

Lindane Cream *(B.P.)*. Lindane 1 g (or a suitable quantity), cetomacrogol emulsifying wax 14 g, liquid paraffin 8 g, freshly boiled and cooled water to 100 g.

Lindane Cream *(U.S.P.)*. pH of a 20% dilution 8 to 9. Store in airtight containers.

Lindane Lotion *(U.S.P.)*. pH 6.5 to 8.5. Store in airtight containers.

Lindane Shampoo *(U.S.P.)*. pH 6.2 to 7.0. Store in airtight containers.

Proprietary Preparations

Lorexane *(Care, UK)*. *Cream*, lindane 1%.
Shampoo, lindane 2%.
Quellada *(Stafford-Miller, UK)*. *Lotion*, lindane 1%.
Shampoo(Application PC), lindane 1%.

Proprietary Names and Manufacturers

Aphtiria *(Debat, Fr.)*; Atan *(Switz.)*; Desantin *(Fin.; Port.)*; Élentol *(Aguettant, Fr.)*; Gambex *(Continental Ethicals, S.Afr.)*; Gamene *(USA)*; Gamma-Col *(ICI Plant Protection, UK)*; Gammasan *(ICI Plant Protection, UK)*; GBH *(Rorer, Canad.)*; Hexicid *(Denm.; NAF, Norw.)*; Inexit *(Boehringer Ingelheim, UK)*; Jacutin *(Hermal, Ger.; Neth.; Hermal, Norw.; Hermal, Swed.; Hermal, Switz.)*; Kwell *(Reed & Carnrick, USA)*; Kwellada *(Reed & Carnrick, Canad.; Greece; Stafford-Miller, Switz.)*; Lencid *(Belg.)*; Liceonil *(Wilson, Pakistan)*; Lindacol *(Boehringer Ingelheim, UK; Shell Chemicals, UK)*; Lorexane *(ICI, Austral.; Care, UK)*; New Kotol *(Shell Chemicals, UK)*; Nexa Lotte *(Boehringer Ingelheim, UK)*; Quellada *(Stafford-Miller, Austral.; Stafford-Miller, S.Afr.; Stafford-Miller, UK)*; Scabecid *(Stiefel, Fr.)*; Scabene *(Stiefel, USA)*; Skabex *(S.Afr.)*; Yacutin *(Igoda, Spain)*.

The following names have been used for multi-ingredient preparations containing lindane— Esoderm *(Napp, UK)*; Gammalex *(ICI Plant Protection, UK)*; Mergamma *(ICI Plant Protection, UK)*; Sentry *(Union Carbide, UK)*.

3590-q

Malathion *(BAN, USAN)*.

Carbofos; Compound 4047; OMS-1. Diethyl 2-(dimethoxyphosphinothioylthio)succinate.
$C_{10}H_{19}O_6PS_2$=330.4.

CAS — 121-75-5.

Pharmacopoeias. In *Int.* and *U.S.*

A yellow to deep brown liquid with a characteristic odour. Slightly **soluble** in water; miscible with alcohols, ethers, aromatic and alkylated aromatic hydrocarbons, and vegetable oils. **Store** in airtight containers. Protect from light.

The manufacturers report that malathion is sensitive to heat and is degraded at temperatures above 30°.

Adverse Effects and Treatment

As for Organophosphorus Pesticides, p.1344.
Malathion is one of the safer organophosphorus insecticides.
In Great Britain the recommended exposure limit of malathion is 10 mg per m^3 (long-term); suitable precautions should be taken to prevent absorption through the skin. In the *US* the permissible and recommended exposure limits are 15 mg per m^3.

A review of the effects of malathion on health.— Recommended Health-based Limits in Occupational Exposure to Pesticides, *Tech. Rep. Ser. Wld Hlth Org. No. 677*, 1982.

Chlorine was reported to inactivate malathion; patients should not go swimming for one week after treatment.— M. Tamblyn, *Br. med. J.*, 1977, *2*, 1292.

Among 7500 field workers exposed to malathion during malaria control operations in Pakistan, poisoning occurred in probably more than 2500, of whom 5 died. Poisoning was attributed to the presence of other organophosphorus compounds as impurities in some batches of malathion powder. Isomalathion was implicated as the main cause of increased toxicity.— Chemistry and Specifications of Pesticides, Second Report of the WHO Expert Committee on Vector Biology and Control, *Tech. Rep. Ser. Wld Hlth Org. No. 620*, 1978. See also E. L. Baker *et al.*, *Lancet*, 1978, *1*, 31.

Acute renal failure in one patient associated with excessive exposure to a malathion spray.— R. K. Albright *et al.* (letter), *J. Am. med. Ass.*, 1983, *250*, 2469.

Of 75 patients with malathion poisoning, 47 had raised serum amylase values and 3 also had mild hyperglycaemia. Serum amylase values had returned to normal in all patients by 60 hours after hospital admission without specific treatment for pancreatic involvement, suggesting that in organophosphorus pesticide poisoning pancreatic involvement is mild and transient.— A. J. Dagli and W. A. Shaikh, *Br. J. clin. Pract.*, 1983, *37*, 270.

Uses and Administration

Malathion is an organophosphorus pesticide. It is used as an insecticide and acaricide in the treatment of pediculosis and scabies in concentrations of 0.5% as well as in veterinary care, agriculture, and horticulture. It is widely used for adult and larval mosquito control although resistance occurs.
Some authorities recommend that malathion be rotated with carbaryl in the treatment of pediculosis.

Some reports of resistance to malathion: P. R. J. Herath and G. Davidson, *Bull. Wld Hlth Org.*, 1981, *59*, 383; J. Hemingway, *Trans. R. Soc. trop. Med. Hyg.*, 1983, *77*, 106; *idem*, 477.

PEDICULOSIS. Malathion for head lice: *Med. Lett.*, 1983, *25*, 30; D. Taplin *et al.*, *J. Am. med. Ass.*, 1982, *247*, 3103.
R. G. Mathias *et al.*, *Can. med. Ass. J.*, 1984, *130*, 407.

Discussions on 2-hour applications versus 12-hour applications of malathion and carbaryl preparations for head lice: J. W. Maunder (letter), *Pharm. J.*, 1984, *2*, 708; D. M. Merrington (letter), *ibid.*, 1985, *1*, 33.

SCABIES. Malathion 0.5% in aqueous emulsion showed significantly better results than benzyl benzoate 25% emulsion in the treatment of scabies in a study involving 112 patients 67 of whom could be assessed satisfactorily.— I. Burgess *et al.*, *Br. med. J.*, 1986, *292*, 1172.

Preparations

Malathion Lotion *(U.S.P.)*. Malathion in a suitable isopropyl alcohol vehicle. Store in airtight glass containers.

Proprietary Preparations

Derbac-M *(International Laboratories, UK)*. *Liquid*, malathion 0.5%.
Prioderm Lotion *(Napp, UK)*. *Lotion*, malathion 0.5% in an alcoholic basis.
Shampoo, malathion 1%.
Suleo-M *(International Laboratories, UK)*. *Lotion*, malathion 0.5% in an alcoholic basis.

Proprietary Names and Manufacturers

Ban-Mite *(Johnsons, UK)*; Derbac-M *(International Laboratories, UK)*; Duramitex *(Crown, UK)*; KP 24 *(Nelson, Austral.)*; Noury Hoofdlotion *(Neth.)*; Organoderm *(Mundipharma, Ger.)*; Prioderm *(Pharmacia, Denm.; Plantier, Fr.; Neth.; Pharmacia, Norw.; NZ; Pharmacia, Swed.; Mundipharma, Switz.; Napp, UK; Purdue Frederick, USA)*; Suleo-M *(International Laboratories, UK)*.

3591-p

Metaldehyde

A polymer of acetaldehyde.
$(C_2H_4O)_x$.

CAS — 9002-91-9.

A white crystalline solid, burning readily and subliming at 100°.

Adverse Effects and Treatment

Symptoms of poisoning by metaldehyde may be delayed and include vomiting and diarrhoea, fever, drowsiness, convulsions, and coma. Death from respiratory failure may occur within 48 hours. Kidney and liver damage may occur.
Treatment is symptomatic.

Metaldehyde poisoning from slug bait ingestion.— W. T. Longstreth and D. J. Pierson, *West. J. Med.*, 1982, *137*, 134.

Uses.

Metaldehyde is a molluscicide used in pellets against slugs and snails. It is also reported to be an ingredient of some firelighters.
'Meta' is compressed metaldehyde which has been used as a solid fuel burning with a non-luminous carbon-free flame.

Proprietary Names and Manufacturers

Helarion *(Fisons Horticultural Division, UK)*.

3592-s

Methoprene

ZR-515. Isopropyl 11-methoxy-3,7,11-trimethyldodeca-2(*E*),4(*E*)-dienoate.
$C_{19}H_{34}O_3$=310.5.

CAS — 40596-69-8.

Methoprene is an insect growth regulator which mimics the action of insect juvenile hormones causing death by preventing the transformation of larva to pupa, if applied at the appropriate period of sensitivity. It is used against a variety of insects including fleas and mosquitoes.

Proprietary Names and Manufacturers

Acclaim Flea Control *(Ceva, UK)*; Altocid *(Zoecon, USA)*; Cevrin *(Ceva, UK)*; Pharorid *(Zoecon, UK)*; Precor *(Zoecon, UK)*.

2257-s

Methyl Bromide

Bromomethane; Monobromomethane.
CH_3Br=94.94.

CAS — 74-83-9.

A colourless non-inflammable gas with a burning taste; odourless in low concentrations or with a chloroform-like odour at high concentrations. B.p. 4.5°.

Adverse Effects and Treatment

Methyl bromide is a vesicant. Toxic effects after inhalation or percutaneous absorption include dizziness, headache, anorexia, nausea, vomiting, abdominal pain, blurred vision, weakness, ataxia, confusion, hyperactivity, convulsions, pulmonary oedema, and coma. Renal failure may occur and death may be due to circulatory collapse or respiratory failure. Onset of symptoms may be preceded by a latent period. Concentrations of 1% or more are irritant to the eyes. Treatment is symptomatic.

Rubber absorbs and retains methyl bromide and should not therefore be used in protective clothing.
In Great Britain the recommended exposure limits of methyl bromide are 5 ppm (long-term); 15 ppm (short-term); suitable precautions should be taken to prevent absorption through the skin. In the *US* the permissible exposure limit is 80 mg per m^3.

Methyl bromide optic atrophy.— C. T. Chavez *et al.*, *Am. J. Ophthal.*, 1985, *99*, 715.

Uses.
Methyl bromide is used as an insecticidal fumigant for soil and some foodstuffs.
Methyl bromide has been used as a gaseous disinfectant; it has low antimicrobial activity but good penetrating power.
When supplied for fumigation it may contain not less than 2% w/w of chloropicrin as a lachrymatory warning agent.
Methyl bromide has been used with carbon tetrachloride in some fire extinguishers. It is also used as a refrigerant.

3595-l

Monosulfiram *(BAN)*.

Sulfiram *(rINN)*; Sulfiramum. Tetraethylthiuram monosulphide.
$C_{10}H_{20}N_2S_3$=264.5.

CAS — 95-05-6.

Pharmacopoeias. In *Aust.* and *Br.* Also in *B.P. Vet.*

A yellow or yellowish-brown solid with a sulphurous odour. F.p. 28.5° to 32°. Practically **insoluble** in water, acids, and alkalis; freely soluble in organic solvents. **Store** in a cool place. Protect from light.

Adverse Effects
An erythematous rash has occasionally been reported. Monosulfiram produces effects similar to those of disulfiram (p.1565) if ingested with alcohol. As there may be a risk of absorption following the application of monosulfiram to the whole body, patients are advised to abstain from alcohol for at least 48 hours.

Uses and Administration
Monosulfiram is a pesticide and acaricide used clinically in the treatment of scabies. It has also been used as a veterinary pesticide.
A 25% alcoholic solution is used in the treatment of scabies. This solution is diluted with 2 or 3 parts of water immediately before use. After a hot bath, the diluted preparation is applied over the whole of the body, with the exception of the face and scalp, rubbed well in and allowed to dry. If necessary the treatment may be repeated daily for 2 or 3 days. It is considered suitable for children. A soap containing monosulfiram is used in place of toilet soap for controlling the spread of scabies, especially in closed communities such as schools and hospitals.

Preparations
Monosulfiram Solution *(B.P.)*. A solution of monosulfiram in alcohol (or industrial methylated spirit) containing a suitable dispersing agent. Crystals which may deposit at low temperatures may be redissolved by warming. Flammable: keep away from an open flame.

Proprietary Preparations
Tetmosol *(ICI Pharmaceuticals, UK). Solution*, monosulfiram 25%, in industrial methylated spirit.
Soap, monosulfiram 5%.

Proprietary Names and Manufacturers
Tetmosol *(ICI, Austral.; ICI, S.Afr.; ICI Pharmaceuticals, UK)*.

3596-y

Naphthalene

Naphthalin.
$C_{10}H_8$=128.2.

CAS — 91-20-3.

Pharmacopoeias. In *Port.*

Adverse Effects and Treatment
Ingestion of naphthalene can produce headache, nausea and vomiting, diarrhoea, profuse perspiration, dysuria, haematuria, acute haemolytic anaemia, coma, and convulsions. It is toxic to the eye. Doses as low as 2 g have proved fatal to the small child. Treatment is symptomatic and includes emptying the stomach by aspiration and lavage. Blood transfusions may be required.
In Great Britain the recommended exposure limits of naphthalene are 10 ppm (long-term); 15 ppm (short-term).

For reports of haemolytic anaemia due to naphthalene in patients with a deficiency in glucose-6-phosphate dehydrogenase, see *Chronicle Wld Hlth Org.*, 1974, *28*, 25.

Uses.
Naphthalene is used in lavatory deodorant discs and in old-fashioned mothballs. It was formerly used as an anthelmintic and in the treatment of pediculosis and scabies.

Proprietary Names and Manufacturers
Scent Off *(Synchemicals, UK)*.

3597-j

Norbormide

McN-1025. 5-[α-Hydroxy-α-(2-pyridyl)benzyl]-7-[α-(2-pyridyl)benzylidene]-8,9,10-trinorborn-5-ene-2,3-dicarboximide.
$C_{33}H_{25}N_3O_3$=511.6.

CAS — 991-42-4.

Norbormide is a selective rodenticide effective against most species of rats, in which it produces extreme irreversible peripheral vasoconstriction. It is not very toxic to other rodents. The concentration in baits is usually 0.5 to 1%.

Norbormide was considered to be one of the safest rodenticides and its use was endorsed. It was reported to have low toxicity to other mammals; the LD50 for *rabbits* was around 1 g per kg body-weight and *dogs* had been fed a dietary concentration of 1% without harm.— *Safe Use of Pesticides,* Twentieth Report of the WHO Expert Committee on Insecticides, *Tech. Rep. Ser. Wld Hlth Org. No. 513,* 1973.

Proprietary Names and Manufacturers
Dithoxin *(Gerhardt, UK)*.

3598-z

Orthodichlorobenzene

1,2-Dichlorobenzene.
$C_6H_4Cl_2$=147.0.

CAS — 95-50-1; 106-46-7(paradichlorobenzene).

Orthodichlorobenzene is a pesticide used as a wood and furniture preservative.
It is an irritant volatile liquid; lens opacities have occurred.
In Great Britain the recommended exposure limit of orthodichlorobenzene is 50 ppm (long-term and short-term).
Paradichlorobenzene (1,4-dichlorobenzene) is used similarly but is considered to be less irritant. It is also used in mothballs and in lavatory deodorant blocks.
In Great Britain the recommended exposure limits of paradichlorobenzene are 75 ppm (long-term); 110 ppm (short-term).

Clastogenic chromosomal aberrations in 26 individuals accidentally exposed to orthodichlorobenzene vapour.— C. Zapata-Gayon *et al.*, *Archs environ. Hlth*, 1982, *37*, 231.

3600-c

Paraquat

1,1′-Dimethyl-4,4′-bipyridyldiylium ion.
$C_{12}H_{14}N_2$=186.3.

CAS — 4685-14-7.

3601-k

Paraquat Dichloride

$C_{12}H_{14}Cl_2N_2$=257.2.

CAS — 1910-42-5.

A white crystalline solid. Very **soluble** in water. Hydrolysed by alkalis.

Adverse Effects
Concentrated solutions of paraquat may cause irritation of the skin, inflammation, and possibly blistering; cracking and shedding of the nails; and delayed healing of cuts and wounds. It is not significantly absorbed from undamaged skin. A few fatalities have occurred following skin contact but these appear to have been associated with prolonged contact and concentrated solutions.
Splashes in the eye cause severe inflammation, which may be delayed for 12 to 24 hours, corneal oedema, reduced visual acuity, and extensive superficial stripping of the corneal and conjunctival epithelium, which usually slowly heals.
Inhalation of dust or spray may cause nasal bleeding.
Paraquat weedkillers available for use in domestic gardens (e.g. Weedol; Pathclear) contain 2.5% w/v paraquat sometimes in association with other herbicides such as diquat. While this strength of paraquat can cause nausea and vomiting as well as some respiratory changes when ingested, it is not considered to be a lethal form.
Most of the cases of severe poisoning follow the ingestion or sometimes injection of the concentrated forms of paraquat herbicide (20% w/v), the distribution of which is restricted to agriculturalists and horticulturalists. In many cases this ingestion is intentional. It is considered that patients who ingest 20 to 40 mg per kg body-weight suffer moderate to severe poisoning; most but not all die up to about 2 or 3 weeks after ingestion. Severe acute poisoning occurs with ingestion of higher doses. The irritant effects of paraquat are reflected in oesophageal ulceration and gastro-intestinal effects. There is widespread organ damage, most notably involving the kidneys, liver, lungs and pancreas. In such poisoning death is certain and occurs rapidly.
Several preparations of paraquat now contain an emetic or a laxative and some contain a stench.
In Great Britain the recommended exposure limit of paraquat dichloride, respirable dust is 0.1 mg per m^3 (long-term).

Paraquat and Diquat, *Environmental Health Criteria 39*, Geneva, Wld Hlth Org.,.

A review of the features of paraquat poisoning.— J. A. Vale *et al.*, *Hum. Toxicol.*, 1987, *6*, 41.

Plasma-paraquat concentrations were measured in 79 patients suffering from paraquat poisoning. It was found that patients whose plasma concentrations did not exceed 2.0, 0.6, 0.3, 0.16, and 0.1 mg per litre at 4, 6, 10, 16, and 24 hours after ingestion, survived. Minimally poisoned patients should be protected from unnecessary treatment.— A. T. Proudfoot *et al.*, *Lancet*, 1979, *2*, 330. A report of 2 patients with plasma-paraquat concentrations greatly in excess of the critical values, who survived after charcoal haemoperfusion. They were haemoperfused with acrylic-hydrogel-coated activated charcoal for an average of 8 hours daily for 2 to 3 weeks.— S. Okonek *et al.* (letter), *ibid.*, 1980, *2*, 589. A report of a further patient who survived paraquat poisoning despite blood concentrations well above the limit for an expected fatal result. The implications are that active treatment should be given to all patients.— J. D. R. Rose (letter), *ibid.*, 924. A further reference to the value of using plasma-paraquat concentrations with a probability curve as a guide to the likelihood of survival even in minimally poisoned patients.— T. B. Hart *et al.* (letter), *Lancet*, 1984, *2*, 1222. See also *ibid.*, 1985, *1*, 395.

Methaemoglobinaemia in a woman who had taken paraquat, as Gramonol, was considered to be due to its monolinuron content.— A. T. Proudfoot (letter), *Br. med. J.*, 1982, *285*, 812.

A 44-year-old farmer developed non-fatal renal and respiratory failure, hepatic damage, and a skin lesion after accidental application of paraquat dichloride 20% to intact perineal and scrotal skin.— K. Tungsanga *et al.*, *Postgrad. med. J.*, 1983, *59*, 338.

Treatment of Adverse Effects
Following contact with paraquat, contaminated clothing should be removed and the skin washed with soap and water. The eyes, if splashed, should be irrigated and treated with antibiotics to control infection. After regrowth of corneal and conjunctival epithelium, corticosteroids may be necessary to promote resolution of granulation tissue.
There is no specific treatment for paraquat poisoning and there is some controversy surrounding most routine procedures. The immediate aim in managing the poisoned patient is to remove or inactivate the paraquat. A number of authorities recommend emesis and in the *UK* the manufacturer has incorpor-

ated an emetic PP796 into both the dilute and the concentrated preparation. Emesis should be followed as soon as possible by gastric aspiration and lavage. The patient is then usually given 200 to 250 mL of a suspension of Fuller's Earth 30% together with a laxative such as magnesium sulphate 15 g. Sorbitol is sometimes used. Further doses of Fuller's Earth may be given every 4 hours and additional doses of the laxative may be considered. Alternative adsorbents include bentonite and activated charcoal; sodium polystyrene sulphonate has also been tried. Some authorities have used Fuller's Earth 15%, instead of 30%. Others use 300 mL of 30%, and may repeat it after 2 hours. Patients may require intensive supportive therapy, but oxygen should not be given as it appears to enhance the pulmonary toxicity of paraquat.
Haemodialysis, peritoneal dialysis, and haemoperfusion have been tried without greatly affecting the mortality rate. Forced diuresis has also been employed, although it may put the patients at greater risk. Specific treatments that have been tried include immunosuppressants, irradiation, ascorbic acid, dexpropranolol, and orgotein; these treatments require further study but generally do not appear to be applicable to human poisoning.

For a series of papers on paraquat poisoning and its treatment, see the Proceedings of the Second European Symposium on Paraquat Poisoning, 27th January 1986, Guy's Hospital, London, in *Hum. Toxicol.*, 1987, *6*, 3.
Some references to various techniques tried in the treatment of paraquat poisoning, many of which were discussed at the above symposium:
Cyclophosphamide with a corticosteroid E. Addo and T. Poon-King, *Lancet*, 1986, *1*, 1117; J. A. Vale *et al.* (letter), *ibid.*, 1439; *ibid.*, *2*, 375.
Haemoperfusion B. H. Mascie-Taylor *et al.*, *Lancet*, 1983, *1*, 1376; J. F. Winchester *et al.* (letter), *ibid.*, *2*, 277; R. Garnier *et al.* (letter), *ibid.*
Methylene Blue for methaemoglobinaemia L. L. Ng *et al.*, *Br. med. J.*, 1982, *284*, 1445; A. Yardley-Jones (letter), *ibid.*, *285*, 735.
Radiotherapy D. B. Webb *et al.*, *Br. med. J.*, 1984, *288*, 1259; *idem*, *289*, 12; A. T. Proudfoot *et al.* (letter), *ibid.*, 112; D. B. Webb *et al.* (letter), *ibid.*
Rehydration P. S. Williams *et al.* (letter), *Lancet*, 1984, *1*, 627.
Vitamin E E. Shahar *et al.* (letter), *Archs Dis. Childh.*, 1980, *55*, 830.

Uses.
Paraquat is a contact herbicide widely used as the dichloride in agriculture and horticulture. Liquid concentrates are supplied in the *UK* only to approved users.

Proprietary Names and Manufacturers
Dextrone X *(Chipman, UK; ICI Plant Protection, UK)*; Gramoxone *(FBC, UK; ICI Plant Protection, UK)*; Scythe *(Cyanamid, UK)*; Speedway *(ICI Plant Protection, UK)*.

The following names have been used for multi-ingredient preparations containing paraquat dichloride— Cleansweep *(Shell Chemicals, UK)*; Dexuron *(Chipman, UK)*; Gramazine *(ICI Plant Protection, UK)*; Gramonol *(Hoechst Animal Health, UK; ICI Plant Protection, UK)*; Groundhog *(ICI Plant Protection, UK)*; New Weedol *(ICI Plant Protection, UK)*; Pathclear *(ICI Plant Protection, UK)*; Soltair *(ICI Plant Protection, UK)*; Weedol *(ICI Plant Protection, UK)*.

18168-m

Parathion
O,O-Diethyl *O*-4-nitrophenyl phosphorothioate.
$C_{10}H_{14}NO_5PS=291.3$.

CAS — 56-38-2; 298-00-0 (parathion-methyl).

Parathion is an organophosphorus pesticide (p.1344) with insecticidal and acaricidal properties. It has been associated with a number of poisonings. Its metabolite diethyl nitrophenyl phosphate (pavaoxon) contributes to its toxicity.
The methyl form, parathion-methyl is also used.
In Great Britain the recommended exposure limits of parathion are 0.1 mg per m^3 (long-term); 0.3 mg per m^3 (short-term); suitable precautions should be taken to prevent absorption through the skin. Corresponding figures for parathion-methyl are 0.2 and 0.6 mg per m^3. In the *US* the permissible and recommended exposure limits are 0.1 mg per m^3 and 0.05 mg per m^3 respectively. The recommended exposure limit for parathion-methyl is 0.2 mg per m^3.

Some references to poisoning with parathion: C. J. Anastassiades and M. Ioannides, *Br. med. J.*, 1984, *289*, 290; H. Golsousidis and V. Kokkas (letter), *Hum. Toxicol.*, 1985, *4*, 339.

13097-w

Permethrin *(BAN, USAN, rINN)*.
3-Phenoxybenzyl 3-(2,2-dichlorovinyl)-2,2-dimethylcyclopropanecarboxylate.
$C_{21}H_{20}Cl_2O_3=391.3$.

CAS — 52645-53-1.

Permethrin is a pyrethroid insecticide (p.1345) with wide agricultural and veterinary uses. It is used clinically against lice and is reported to be active against nits. A 1% application is also considered to provide protection for up to 14 days.
Permethrin is active against mosquitoes, and blackflies in the adult and larval stages; it is also effective against tsete flies. It is suitable for aircraft disinsection.

In a study involving 508 patients with pediculosis capitis, a single 10-minute application of permethrin cream rinse 1% was highly effective and therapeutically superior to a single 4-minute application of lindane shampoo 1%.— K. Brandenburg *et al.*, *Am. J. Dis. Child.*, 1986, *140*, 894.
For a report of progressive motorneurone disease associated with exposure to permethrin and chlordane, see under chlordane (p.1346).

Proprietary Names and Manufacturers
Ambush Fog *(ICI Plant Protection, UK)*; Cooper Coopex *(Wellcome, UK)*; Muscatrol *(Rentokil, UK)*; Nix *(Wellcome, USA)*; Permit *(Pan Britannica, UK)*; Picket *(ICI Plant Protection, UK)*; Sybol 2 Aerosol *(ICI Plant Protection, UK)*.

The following names have been used for multi-ingredient preparations containing permethrin— Dragon *(ICI Plant Protection, UK)*; Nippon Ant & Crawling Insect Killer *(Synchemicals, UK)*.

3602-a

Phenothrin *(BAN, rINN)*.
3-Phenoxybenzyl (1*RS*)-*cis,trans*-chrysanthemate.
$C_{23}H_{26}O_3=350.5$.

CAS — 26002-80-2.

Phenothrin is a pyrethroid pesticide (p.1345) active against a variety of insects and mites. It is used in human medicine, in agriculture and for disinsection of public areas.

Proprietary Names and Manufacturers
The following names have been used for multi-ingredient preparations containing phenothrin— R&C Spray *(Reed & Carnrick, USA)*.

3603-t

Piperonyl Butoxide *(BAN)*.
5-[2-(2-Butoxyethoxy)ethoxymethyl]-6-propyl-1,3-benzodioxole.
$C_{19}H_{30}O_5=338.4$.

CAS — 51-03-6.

Pharmacopoeias. In *B.P. Vet.*

A yellow or pale brown oily liquid with a faint characteristic odour.
Very slightly **soluble** in water; miscible with alcohol, chloroform, ether, petroleum oils, and liquefied aerosol propellents such as dichlorodifluoromethane, dichlorotetrafluoroethane, and trichlorofluoromethane.
Piperonyl butoxide is unstable in sunlight.— Resistance of Vectors of Disease to Pesticides, Fifth Report of the WHO Expert Committee on Vector Biology and Control, *Tech. Rep. Ser. Wld Hlth Org. No. 655*, 1980.

Piperonyl butoxide is used as a synergist for pyrethrins and pyrethroids. Mixtures of piperonyl butoxide and pyrethrins are used in the treatment of pediculosis. Piperonyl butoxide possesses activity against mites and some insects.
Piperonyl butoxide is considered to cause a variety of gastro-intestinal effects as well as CNS depression.

Proprietary Names and Manufacturers
The following names have been used for multi-ingredient preparations containing piperonyl butoxide—A-200 Pyrinate *(Norcliff Thayer, USA)*; Ficam Plus *(FBC, UK)*; Lyban Foam *(USV, Austral.)*; Para Spray *(Stiefel, Canad.)*; Pre-vent *(Agropharm, UK)*; Pronto *(Commerce Drug, USA)*; Pyrifoam *(Schering, Austral.)*; Pyrinyl *(Schein, USA)*; RID *(Leeming, USA)*.

18181-d

Pirimiphos-methyl
O-2-Diethylamino-6-methylpyrimidin-4-yl *O,O*-dimethyl phosphorothioate.
$C_{11}H_{20}N_3O_3PS=305.3$.

CAS — 29232-93-7; 23505-41-1 (pirimiphos-ethyl).

Pirimiphos-methyl is an organophosphorus insecticide, larvicide, and acaricide (p.1344). It is used against vectors of disease including mosquitoes, fleas, and blackflies. Pirimiphos-ethyl is also in use.

A large-scale evaluation of pirimiphos-methyl for malaria control.— S. M. Nasir *et al.*, *J. trop. Med. Hyg.*, 1982, *85*, 239.

Proprietary Names and Manufacturers
Actellic *(ICI Plant Protection, UK)*; Blex *(ICI Plant Protection, UK)*; Sybol 2 *(ICI Plant Protection, UK)*.

The following names have been used for multi-ingredient preparations containing pirimiphos-methyl— Kerispray *(ICI Plant Protection, UK)*.

18039-k

Propoxur
2-Isopropoxyphenyl methylcarbamate.
$C_{11}H_{15}NO_3=209.2$.

CAS — 114-26-1.

Propoxur is a carbamate pesticide (p.1344) used against a wide range of insects including mosquitoes and lice.
In Great Britain the recommended exposure limits of propoxur are 0.5 mg per m^3 (long-term); 2 mg per m^3 (short-term).

Proprietary Names and Manufacturers
Blattanex 20 *(Bayer Agrochem, UK)*.

The following names have been used for multi-ingredient preparations containing propoxur— Blattanex Aerosol *(Bayer Agrochem, UK)*.

3604-x

Pyrethrum Flower
Chrysanthème Insecticide; Dalmatian Insect Flowers; Insect Flowers; Insektenblüten; Piretro; Pyrethri Flos.

CAS — 8003-34-7 (pyrethrum); 121-21-1 (pyrethrin I); 121-29-9 (pyrethrin II); 25402-06-6 (cinerin I); 121-20-0 (cinerin II).

Pharmacopoeias. In *Arg.*, *Aust.*, and *Fr.* In *B.P. Vet.* which also includes Pyrethrum Extract.

The dried flowerheads of *Chrysanthemum cinerariaefolium* (Compositae), containing not less than 1% of pyrethrins of which not less than one-half consists of pyrethrin I.

Adverse Effects
Pyrethrum is irritant to the eyes and mucosa. Hypersensitivity reactions have been reported.
In Great Britain the recommended exposure limits of pyrethrins are 5 mg per m^3 (long-term); 10 mg per m^3 (short-term).

Uses.
Pyrethrum flower is mainly used for the preparation of pyrethrum extract that contains about 25% w/w of pyrethrins.
Pyrethrum is rapidly toxic to many insects. It has a much quicker knock-down effect than dicophane or lin-

dane, but it is less persistent and less stable. Its action can be enhanced by certain substances such as piperonyl butoxide (see above) and pyrethrins with piperonyl butoxide are used in the treatment of pediculosis.
Pyrethrum is widely used in domestic and agricultural insecticidal sprays and dusting-powders.

Proprietary Names and Manufacturers of Pyrethrum or a Pyrethrin
Alfadex *(Ciba-Geigy Agrochemicals, UK)*.

The following names have been used for multi-ingredient preparations containing pyrethrum or a pyrethrin—A-200 Pyrinate *(Norcliff Thayer, USA)*; Ficam Plus *(FBC, UK)*; Insectrol *(Rentokil, UK)*; Kerispray *(ICI Plant Protection, UK)*; Lyban Foam *(USV, Austral.)*; Nuvan Fly Killer *(Ciba-Geigy Agrochemicals, UK)*; Prevent *(Agropharm, UK)*; Pyrifoam *(Schering, Austral.)*; Pyrinyl *(Schein, USA)*; RID *(Leeming, USA)*.

3605-r

Pyrimitate *(BAN, rINN)*.

Dimethoate; ICI-29,661; Pyrimithate. *O*-2-Dimethylamino-6-methylpyrimidin-4-yl *O,O*-diethyl phosphorothioate.
$C_{11}H_{20}N_3O_3PS=305.3$.

CAS — 5221-49-8.

CAUTION. *Pyrimitate is very toxic when inhaled, swallowed, or spilled on the skin. It can be removed from the skin by washing with soap and water. Contaminated material should be immersed in a 2% aqueous solution of sodium hydroxide for several hours.*

Pyrimitate is an organophosphorus pesticide (p.1344) used in agriculture for the control of lice and ticks in cattle and sheep as well as for fly control.

2028-t

Red Squill

CAS — 507-60-8 (scilliroside).

A red variety of *Urginea maritima*, which contains, in addition to cardiac glycosides, an active principle, scilliroside.

Red squill is very toxic to rats and is incorporated in rat pastes; it acts on the central nervous system. Its use as a poison is prohibited in theUK.

3606-f

Rotenone

Rotenonum. (−)-1,2,12,12a-Tetrahydro-2-isopropenyl-8,9-dimethoxy-6a*H*-furo[2,3-*h*][1]benzopyrano[3,4-*b*][1]-benzopyran-6-one.
$C_{23}H_{22}O_6=394.4$.

CAS — 83-79-4.

Pharmacopoeias. In *Nord.*

Rotenone is a non-systemic insecticide. It has been used in agriculture for control of lice, fleas, and as a larvicide. It has also been used in horticulture.
Rotenone is the active ingredient of derris (the dried rhizome and roots of *Derris elliptica*; also known as tuba root or aker-tuba) and of lonchocarpus (the dried root of *Lonchocarpus utilis*; also known as cube root, timbo, or barbusco). Powdered forms of derris and of lonchocarpus have been used as insecticides.
In Great Britain the recommended exposure limits of rotenone are 5 mg per m^3 (long-term); 10 mg per m^3 (short-term).

Proprietary Names and Manufacturers
Abol Derris Dust *(ICI Plant Protection, UK)*.

7734-c

Sodium Fluoroacetate

Compound 1080; Sodium Monofluoroacetate.
$FCH_2.CO_2Na=100.0$.

CAS — 62-74-8.

Adverse Effects and Treatment
Sodium fluoroacetate is highly toxic, the lethal dose being about 2 to 10 mg per kg body-weight. Toxic effects may be delayed for several hours after absorption by mouth or inhalation, and include nausea and vomiting, apprehension, muscle twitching, cardiac irregularities, convulsions, respiratory failure, coma, and death.
Treatment is generally supportive and symptomatic. Monoacetin administered parenterally or by mouth has been suggested as an antidote on the basis of *animal* experiments; as an acetate donor it may be a competitive antagonist to fluoroacetate metabolism. Acetamide or alcohol might fulfil the same function but their clinical value is unproven.
In Great Britain the recommended exposure limits of sodium fluoroacetate are 0.05 mg per m^3 (long-term); 0.15 mg per m^3 (short-term); suitable precautions should be taken to prevent absorption through the skin.

Uses.
Sodium fluoroacetate is a highly effective rodenticide but must be used with great caution because of its toxicity to other animals and to man.
In Great Britain, the use of sodium fluoroacetate is restricted to the destruction of rodents in ships, sewers, and specified dock warehouses. When supplied for use as a rodenticide it must contain a distinctive colouring matter.

For the use of fluoroacetamide and sodium fluoroacetate as rodenticides, see *Use of Fluoroacetamide and Sodium Fluoroacetate as Rodenticides; Precautionary Measures*, Ministry of Agriculture, Fisheries and Food, London, HM Stationery Office, 1970.

It was recommended, in view of the extreme hazard to other mammals, that fluoroacetamide and sodium fluoroacetate should only be used by trained pest control operators in areas such as locked warehouses and sewers to which access by unauthorised persons and useful animals could be prevented completely.— Safe Use of Pesticides, Twentieth Report of the WHO Expert Committee on Insecticides, *Tech. Rep. Ser. Wld Hlth Org. No. 513*, 1973.

3609-h

Temefos *(USAN, rINN)*.

Temephos. *O,O'*-(Thiodi-*p*-phenylene) *O,O,O',O'*-tetramethyl bis(phosphorothioate).
$C_{16}H_{20}O_6P_2S_3=466.5$.

CAS — 3383-96-8.

Temefos is an organophosphorus pesticide (p.1344) effective against the larvae of mosquitoes, blackflies, and other insects. It is effective against lice and fleas as well as the guinea worm and is used in the control of dracontiasis; treatment of drinking water is both effective and acceptable. Resistance has emerged in several countries using temefos for larval mosquito control.

The use of temefos for the control of guinea worm.— *Chronicle Wld Hlth Org.*, 1980, *34*, 159; C. K. Rao *et al.*, *J. commun. Dis.*, 1982, *14*, 36; *Wkly epidem. Rec.*, 1983, *58*, 21.

The use of temefos larvicide in solid form for the control of onchocerciasis in Guatemala.— K. Matsuo, *Bull. Pan Am. Hlth Org.*, 1984, *18*, 58.

3610-a

Tetramethrin *(rINN)*.

4,5,6,7-Tetrahydrophthalimidomethyl (1*RS*)-*cis,trans*-chrysanthemate.
$C_{19}H_{25}NO_4=331.4$.

CAS — 7696-12-0.

Tetramethrin is a pyrethroid insecticide (p.1345) usually used in conjunction with a synergist such as piperonyl butoxide (see p.1353).

Proprietary Names and Manufacturers
The following names have been used for multi-ingredient preparations containing tetramethrin—Dragon *(ICI Plant Protection, UK)*; Nippon Ant & Crawling Insect Killer *(Synchemicals, UK)*.

3611-t

Trichlorophenoxyacetic Acid

2,4,5-T. 2,4,5-Trichlorophenoxyacetic acid.
$C_8H_5Cl_3O_3=255.5$.

CAS — 35915-18-5.

Trichlorophenoxyacetic acid is a selective weedkiller with similar actions to dichlorophenoxyacetic acid (see p.1347). It is usually used in ester formulations. It was used as a defoliating agent in the Vietnam conflict in conjunction with dichlorophenoxyacetic acid.
In Great Britain the recommended exposure limits of trichlorophenoxyacetic acid are 10 mg per m^3 (long-term); 20 mg per m^3 (short-term). The content of TCDD (dioxin) which may be formed during production should be less than 1 ppm.

Swedish studies have indicated that there was an increased incidence of soft tissue sarcoma, Hodgkin's disease, and non-Hodgkin's lymphoma with phenoxy herbicides. Other studies have failed to demonstrate such a connection or have only confirmed it for non-Hodgkin's lymphoma. These herbicides were used for defoliation in Vietnam as agent orange, which consisted of a mixture of dichlorophenoxyacetic acid, trichlorophenoxyacetic acid, and the impurity TCDD (dioxin), and concern has been expressed that they may have contributed to an increased incidence of cancer among exposed subjects as well as an adverse effect on the offspring of those subjects. This is a matter of considerable debate, although an Australian judicial review has failed to confirm any association.
References: *Lancet*, 1982, *1*, 105; D. Coggon and E. D. Acheson, *ibid.*, 1057; L. Hardell and O. Axelson (letter), *ibid.*, 1408; S. Milham (letter), *ibid.*, 1464; R. Kilpatrick *et al.*, Advisory Committee on Pesticides, *Minist. Agric. Fish Fd.*, 1982.; F. A. LaVecchio *et al.* (letter), *New Engl. J. Med.*, 1983, *308*, 719; A. Lipson (letter), *ibid.*, *309*, 491; W. R. Gaffey (letter), *ibid.*, 492; F. LaVecchio *et al.* (letter), *ibid.*,; P. H. Casey and W. R. Collie, *J. Pediat.*, 1984, *104*, 313; W. Hall, *Med. J. Aust.*, 1986, *145*, 219; S. K. Hoar *et al.*, *J. Am. med. Ass.*, 1986, *256*, 1141; D. Coggon, *Br. med. J.*, 1987, *294*, 725.

Proprietary Names and Manufacturers
The following names have been used for multi-ingredient preparations containing trichlorophenoxyacetic acid—Kilnet *(May & Baker Agrochemicals, UK)*.

3612-x

Trifenmorph

WL-8008. *N*-Tritylmorpholine.
$C_{23}H_{23}NO=329.4$.

CAS — 1420-06-0.

Trifenmorph has been used as molluscicide for the control of snail vectors of schistosomiasis.

Trifenmorph has been superseded as a molluscicide by niclosamide. It can be supplied but only if large quantities are ordered in advance, as a special production plant must be set up at the factory.— F. S. McCullough *et al.*, *Bull. Wld Hlth Org.*, 1980, *58*, 681.

Preservatives

6630-d

This section includes compounds principally used as antimicrobial preservatives or antoxidants in pharmaceutical preparations, cosmetics, and foods. Many other compounds having antimicrobial and antoxidant properties may be found throughout *Martindale*.

Antimicrobial Preservatives

Antimicrobial preservatives are included in preparations to kill or inhibit the growth of micro-organisms inadvertently introduced during manufacture or use. They are used in sterile preparations such as eye-drops and multidose injections to maintain sterility during use and in cosmetics, foods, and non-sterile pharmaceutical products such as oral liquids and creams to prevent microbial spoilage.

In Great Britain the antimicrobial preservatives which may be added to foods, animal feeding stuffs, and cosmetics are controlled.

Some compounds which are used for both disinfection and preservation, such as benzalkonium chloride, chlorocresol, and thiomersal are described in the section on Disinfectants p.949. Other compounds used as preservatives include alcohol p.950, chloroform p.1114, glycerol p.1128, and sucrose p.1275.

The choice of a suitable preservative for a preparation depends on pH, compatibility with other ingredients, the route, dose and frequency of administration of the preparation, partition coefficients with ingredients and containers or closures, degree and type of contamination, concentration required, and rate of antimicrobial effect.

Antimicrobial preservatives in pharmaceuticals.— J.A. Happel in *Disinfection, Sterilization, and Preservation*, S.S. Block (Ed.), Philadelphia, Lea and Feabiger, 1983, p.918. (review). See also: M. J. Akers, *Pharmaceut. Technol.*, 1984, *8*, 36 (in parenteral products).

Preservation of cosmetics.— F. Sharpell and M. Manowitz in *Disinfection, Sterilization, and Preservation*, S.S. Block (Ed.), Philadelphia, Lea and Feabiger, 1983, p.589..

Antoxidants

Antoxidants may be classified in 3 groups. The first group, sometimes known as *true antoxidants*, or 'anti-oxygens', probably inhibit oxidation by reacting with free radicals. They are effective against autoxidation but not in reversible oxidation (redox) reactions. Examples are the alkyl gallates, butylated hydroxyanisole, butylated hydroxytoluene, nordihydroguaiaretic acid, and the tocopherols.

The second group consists of *reducing agents*; these substances have a lower redox potential than the drug or adjuvants which they are intended to protect and are therefore more readily oxidised than the drug. They are effective against oxidising agents. Reducing agents may act also by reacting with free radicals. Examples are ascorbic acid, the potassium and sodium salts of sulphurous acid, and sodium formaldehyde sulphoxylate.

The third group consists of *antoxidant synergists* which usually have little antoxidant effect themselves but probably enhance the action of antoxidants in the first group by reacting with heavy-metal ions which catalyse oxidation. Examples of synergists are citric acid, edetic acid and its salts, lecithin, and tartaric acid. Mixtures of true antoxidants or true antoxidants and reducing agents may also show synergism.

The choice of a suitable antoxidant for a preparation depends on the route, dose and frequency of administration, the chemical and physical properties of the other ingredients and the container and closure.

ADVERSE EFFECTS. Adverse reactions to pharmaceutical excipients including preservatives and antoxidants.— J. M. Smith and T. R. P. Dodd, *Adverse Drug React. Ac. Pois. Rev.*, 1982, *1*, 93.

Allergy and intolerance. Preservatives and antoxidants have been implicated in food additive intolerance which commonly manifests as urticaria and angioedema (G. Michaëlsson and L. Juhlin, *Br. J. Derm.*, 1973, *88*, 525; A.-M. Ros *et al.*, *ibid.*, 1976, *95*, 19). Results of provocation tests with various food additives in patients with recurrent urticaria revealed that about one-third had one or more positive reactions; in 172 patients tested with benzoates, reactions were positive in 11% and uncertain in 18%; in 156 patients tested with butylated hydroxyanisole or butylated hydroxytoluene, reactions were positive in 15% and uncertain in 12%; and in 115 patients tested with sorbic acid, reactions were positive in 9% and uncertain in 14% (L. Juhlin, *ibid.*, 1981, *104*, 369). Treatment of artificial food additive intolerance includes antihistamines when necessary, oral sodium cromoglycate in some individuals, and avoidance of the causal factors. Supramaniam and Warner (*Lancet*, 1986, *2*, 907) found that about 75% of patients with allergic skin reactions for which a causal agent could not be identified had a good response to a modified diet free of azo-dyes and benzoate preservatives. Of 43 children with urticaria and angioedema who had improved on such a modified diet, 24 reacted when challenged with 1 or more artificial food additives in a double-blind study; 4 of 27 children tested had reactions to sodium benzoate and 1 of 12 reacted to sodium metabisulphite. All but 3 of the 24 children who had a positive reaction were successfully managed on a diet free from just the additives that initiated a positive response and 18 children who had no reactions were able to revert to a normal diet; one child reacted to placebo and was withdrawn from the study.

A relatively high incidence of adverse reactions had been reported in susceptible individuals to certain groups of food additives such as the benzoates and sulphites. It was not clear if these reactions were manifestations of immunological hypersensitivity or of idiosyncratic hyper-reactivity, but both types of reaction could be regarded as forms of intolerance. Since a number of food additives could cause allergic manifestations, the Committee considered that the only feasible means of offering protection to susceptible individuals was appropriate labelling.— Twenty-seventh Report of the Joint FAO/WHO Expert Committee on Food Additives, *Tech. Rep. Ser. Wld Hlth Org. No. 696*, 1983.

A number of preservatives have been associated with contact allergy when applied topically or with generalised allergic reactions such as flushing, rigors, hypotension, and bronchospasm when administered parenterally to susceptible individuals. Sensitivity to excipients in pharmaceutical preparations should therefore be considered whenever patients present with recurrent or unexplained allergies.— J. M. Smith, *Practitioner*, 1987, *231*, 580.

Hyperactivity. Although hyperactivity in some children has been associated with certain colouring agents and preservatives used in foods, evidence from controlled trials has generally been lacking. References: J. Egger *et al.*, *Lancet*, 1985, *1*, 540; T. J. David, *Archs Dis. Childh.*, 1987, *62*, 119.

6633-m

Ascorbyl Palmitate *(USAN).*

E304; Vitamin C Palmitate. L-Ascorbic acid 6-palmitate; 3-Oxo-L-gulofuranolactone 6-palmitate.

$C_{22}H_{38}O_7$=414.5.

CAS — 137-66-6.

Pharmacopoeias. In *U.S.N.F.*

A white to yellowish-white powder with a characteristic odour. M.p. 107° to 117°. Very slightly **soluble** in water, chloroform, ether, and vegetable oils; soluble in alcohol. **Store** in a cool, dry place in airtight containers.

Ascorbyl palmitate is used as an antoxidant in food.

Estimated acceptable daily intake of ascorbyl palmitate: up to 1.25 mg per kg body-weight.— Seventeenth Report of the Joint FAO/WHO Expert Committee on Food Additives, *Tech. Rep. Ser. Wld Hlth Org. No. 539*, 1974.

6634-b

Benzoic Acid *(BAN, USAN).*

Acidum Benzoicum; Benzoesäure; E210.

$C_6H_5.CO_2H$=122.1.

CAS — 65-85-0.

Pharmacopoeias. In *Arg., Aust., Belg., Br., Braz., Chin., Cz., Egypt., Eur., Fr., Ger., Hung., Ind., Int., It., Jpn, Jug., Mex., Neth., Nord., Pol., Port., Roum., Rus., Span., Swiss, Turk.*, and *U.S.*

Colourless or white crystals or white scales, needles, or crystalline powder; odourless or with a slight characteristic odour. Somewhat volatile at moderately warm temperatures; freely volatile in steam.

Soluble 1 in 300 of water, 1 in 3 of alcohol, 1 in 5 of chloroform, and 1 in 3 of ether; soluble in boiling water; freely soluble in fixed oils. **Incompatible** with ferric salts and salts of heavy metals; its activity may be reduced in the presence of nonionic surfactants. **Store** in well-closed containers.

Benzoic acid was adsorbed by light kaolin; adsorption was maximal at about pH 5.— C. D. Clarke and N. A. Armstrong, *Pharm. J.*, 1972, *2*, 44.

Adverse Effects and Precautions

Allergic reactions to benzoic acid have been reported. Large doses by mouth may produce gastric irritation. It can be irritant to the eyes, skin, and mucous membranes.

The antimicrobial activity of benzoic acid may be diminished through incompatibility, interactions, and adsorption (see above) with a resulting reduction in effectiveness.

PREGNANCY AND THE NEONATE. Neonates with fatal toxic syndrome attributable to benzyl alcohol (see p.1356) have been reported to have elevated urinary-concentrations of its metabolites, benzoic acid and hippuric acid; the accumulation of benzoic acid in blood, possibly due to the livers' diminished metabolic capacity in premature infants, might be responsible for the metabolic acidosis observed in this syndrome (J. Gershanik *et al.*, *New Engl. J. Med.*, 1982, *307*, 1384; W.J. Brown *et al.*, *Lancet*, 1982, *1*, 1250). In view of the neonatal morbidity and mortality associated with the syndrome, Edwards and Voegeli (*Am. J. Hosp. Pharm.*, 1984, *41*, 658) suggested that the use of caffeine and sodium benzoate injection in neonates should be reconsidered. In addition, benzoate could also displace bilirubin from albumin binding sites which might induce kernicterus (D. Schiff *et al.*, *Pediatrics*, 1971, *48*, 139).

For the disposition of sodium benzoate in newborn infants, the association of benzoates with increased free bilirubin concentrations in serum, and recommendations on the precautions necessary, especially in jaundiced neonates, see under Absorption and Fate, below.

Absorption and Fate

When taken by mouth, benzoic acid is absorbed from the gastro-intestinal tract. It is conjugated with glycine in the liver to form hippuric acid which is rapidly excreted in the urine; it may also be excreted as benzoylglucuronic acid.

PREGNANCY AND THE NEONATE. The disposition of sodium benzoate was investigated in 4 newborn infants with hyperammonaemia who were receiving treatment which included intravenous sodium benzoate 3.5 mmol per kg body-weight daily, intravenous arginine hydrochloride 2 to 4 mmol per kg daily, peritoneal dialysis, and haemodialysis. The volume of distribution of benzoate ranged from 0.086 to 0.244 litres per kg and the elimination half-life was 0.75 to 7.4 hours. Clearance of benzoate was largely attributable to metabolism with urinary and dialysis clearance accounting for only a small fraction. Hippurate, the major metabolite of benzoate, was predominantly cleared by renal elimination. Steady-state serum-benzoate concentrations of 2.14 to 16.0 mmol per litre found in this study were calculated to be capable of producing a 4- to 25-fold increase in expected free bilirubin concentrations in serum. As there was considerable interpatient variability, monitoring of serum concentrations was warranted to identify patients with impaired formation of hippurate who could accumulate potentially toxic concentrations of benzoate.

Until further data was available, it was also suggested that jaundiced neonates should receive reduced doses of sodium benzoate and that serum concentrations be maintained below 1.6 mmol per litre.— T. P. Green *et al.*, *J. Pediat.*, 1983, *102*, 785.

Uses.

Benzoic acid has antibacterial and antifungal properties. Its antimicrobial activity is due to the undissociated acid; it is therefore effective at an acid pH of 4 or below but relatively inactive above a pH of about 5.

It is used as a preservative in pharmaceutical formulations including oral preparations at concentrations of 0.05% to 0.1% and as a preservative in cosmetics in usual concentrations of 0.1% to 0.5%. Benzoic acid is also used as a preservative in foods, usually at concentrations of 0.03% to 0.1% (as sodium benzoate). Salts of benzoic acid, for example sodium benzoate (p.1362) or potassium benzoate (p.1362), may be preferred for some formulations or products because of their greater solubility in water. However, as benzoate salts have an astringent taste, lower concentrations may be necessary in some oral preparations, though they can often be used in combination with other preservatives. To avoid discoloration and oxidative changes due to benzoates, an antoxidant such as sulphurous acid may be added.

Benzoic acid is applied topically for the treatment of fungal infections of the skin such as ringworm, usually as a compound ointment with salicylic acid. It is also used in desloughing and cleansing preparations for wounds and ulcers.

It was formerly employed as a urinary antiseptic.

Estimated sum acceptable daily intake of benzoic acid, sodium benzoate, and potassium benzoate: up to 5 mg per kg body-weight (expressed as benzoic acid).— Seventeenth Report of the Joint FAO/WHO Expert Committee on Food Additives, *Tech. Rep. Ser. Wld Hlth Org. No. 539*, 1974. Extended to cover calcium benzoate.— Twenty-seventh Report of the Joint FAO/WHO Expert Committee on Food Additives, *Tech. Rep. Ser. Wld Hlth Org. No. 696*, 1983.

ANTIMICROBIAL ACTIVITY. Studies on the mechanism of the antifungal action of benzoate.— H. A. Krebs *et al.*, *Biochem. J.*, 1983, *214*, 657. See also.— *Lancet*, 1983, *2*, 1124.

Preparations

Benzoic and Salicylic Acids Ointment *(U.S.P.)*. Contains benzoic acid and salicylic acid, in the ratio of about 2:1, in a suitable ointment basis. Store at a temperature not exceeding 30°.

Benzoic Acid Solution *(B.P., A.P.F.)*. Benzoic acid 5 g, propylene glycol 75 mL, freshly boiled and cooled water to 100 mL.

Compound Benzoic Acid Ointment *(B.P.)*. Ung. Acid. Benz. Co.; Benzoic Acid Compound Ointment; Benzoic Acid Ointment Compound *(A.P.F.)*; Benzoic and Salicylic Acid Ointment; Whitfield's Ointment. Benzoic acid 6% and salicylic acid 3% in emulsifying ointment.

NOTE. Whitfield's original formula was that of Compound Benzoic Acid Ointment (*B.P.C. 1934*), i.e. benzoic acid 5%, salicylic acid 3%, white soft paraffin 27.6%, and coconut oil 64.4%.

Proprietary Preparations

Aserbine *(Bencard, UK)*. *Cream*, benzoic acid 0.024%, malic acid 0.36%, salicylic acid 0.006%, propylene glycol 1.7%.

Topical solution, benzoic acid 0.15%, malic acid 2.25%, salicylic acid 0.0375%, propylene glycol 40%.

Malatex *(Norton, UK)*. *Cream*, benzoic acid 0.024%, malic acid 0.36%, salicylic acid 0.006%, propylene glycol 1.7%.

Topical solution, benzoic acid 0.15%, malic acid 2.25%, salicylic acid 0.0375%, and propylene glycol 40%.

Proprietary Names and Manufacturers

The following names have been used for multi-ingredient preparations containing benzoic acid—Antinea *(American Dermal, USA)*; Aserbine *(Bencard, UK)*; Egomycol *(Ego, Austral.)*; Malatex *(Norton, UK)*; Mycozol *(Parke, Davis, Austral.)*; Trac Tabs *(Hyrex, USA)*; Urised *(Webcon, USA)*; Uroblue *(Geneva, USA)*.

554-h

Benzyl Alcohol *(BAN, USAN, rINN)*.

Alcohol Benzylicus; Alcool Benzylique; Benzenemethanol; Phenylcarbinol; Phenylmethanol.

$C_6H_5.CH_2OH=108.1$.

CAS — 100-51-6.

Pharmacopoeias. In *Arg., Aust., Belg., Br., Egypt., Eur., Fr., Hung., Ind., Jpn, Neth., Nord., Port.,* and *Swiss.* Also in *U.S.N.F.*

A clear, colourless, oily liquid with a slightly aromatic odour.

Soluble 1 in 25 of water; miscible with alcohol, chloroform, ether, and fixed and volatile oils. It is neutral to litmus. **Store** in completely filled airtight containers and prevent exposure to excessive heat. Protect from light.

Adverse Effects and Precautions

A fatal toxic syndrome occurring in low birth-weight neonates and attributed to benzyl alcohol, present as a bacteriostatic in intravenous formulations, has been described. There have also been reports of hypersensitivity reactions to benzyl alcohol.

ALLERGY AND INTOLERANCE. A 55-year-old man developed fatigue, nausea, and diffuse angioedema following an intramuscular injection of cyanocobalamin. He was later found to be hypersensitive to benzyl alcohol which had been present as a preservative.— J. A. Grant *et al.* (letter), *New Engl. J. Med.*, 1982, *306*, 108.

Allergic contact dermatitis to benzyl alcohol which was present as a preservative in an injectable solution.— E. Shmunes, *Archs Derm.*, 1984, *120*, 1200.

EFFECTS ON THE NERVOUS SYSTEM. Rapid development of flaccid areflexic paraplegia, total anaesthesia below the groin, and radicular abdominal pain in a 64-year-old man following a lumbar intrathecal injection of cytarabine which contained 1.5% benzyl alcohol. Intrathecal injections of cytarabine dissolved in sterile distilled water before and after the episode of paraplegia caused no neurologic symptoms.— A. F. Hahn *et al.*, *Neurology*, 1983, *33*, 1032.

PREGNANCY AND THE NEONATE. The FDA had received reports of 16 deaths attributed to benzyl alcohol in neonates weighing less than 2.5 kg. Bacteriostatic sodium chloride for injection containing 0.9% benzyl alcohol had been used for flushing intravenous catheters; some infants had also received benzyl alcohol from solutions used for diluting or reconstituting medications. A syndrome consisting of metabolic acidosis, central nervous system depression, respiratory distress progressing to gasping respirations, hypotension, renal failure, and sometimes seizures and intracranial haemorrhages was observed and preceded death. It was advised that the use in neonates of such solutions containing benzyl alcohol or other preservatives be discontinued.— *FDA Drug Bull.*, 1982, *12*, 10. Further references: J. Gershanik *et al.*, *New Engl. J. Med.*, 1982, *307*, 1384. The American Academy of Pediatrics, Committees on Fetus/Newborn and on Drugs *Pediatrics*, 1983, *72*, 356; C. W. Anderson *et al.*, *Am. J. Obstet. Gynec.*, 1984, *148*, 344.

Absorption and Fate

Benzyl alcohol is oxidised to benzoic acid which is conjugated with glycine in the liver to form hippuric acid which is then excreted in the urine.

Uses.

Benzyl alcohol is used as an antimicrobial preservative. It also has weak local anaesthetic and antipruritic properties. In the *UK* the use of benzyl alcohol in cosmetics is restricted by law.

Estimated acceptable daily intake of the benzyl/benzoic moiety: up to 5 mg per kg body-weight.— Twenty-third Report of the Joint FAO/WHO Expert Committee on Food Additives, *Tech. Rep. Ser. Wld Hlth Org. No. 648*, 1980.

Proprietary Names and Manufacturers

Topic *(Syntex, USA)*.

6635-v

Benzyl Hydroxybenzoate *(BAN)*.

Benzylparaben. Benzyl 4-hydroxybenzoate.

$C_{14}H_{12}O_3=228.2$.

CAS — 94-18-8.

Pharmacopoeias. In *Br.*

A white to creamy-white, odourless or almost odourless, crystalline powder. Practically **insoluble** in water; soluble 1 in 2.5 of alcohol and 1 in 6 of ether. It dissolves in solutions of alkali hydroxides.

6637-q

Butyl Hydroxybenzoate *(BAN)*.

Butylis Paraoxybenzoas; Butylparaben *(USAN)*. Butyl 4-hydroxybenzoate.

$C_{11}H_{14}O_3=194.2$.

CAS — 94-26-8.

Pharmacopoeias. In *Br.* and *Jpn.* Also in *U.S.N.F.*

Odourless or almost odourless colourless crystals or white crystalline powder. Very slightly **soluble** in water; soluble 1 in 1 of alcohol; freely soluble in acetone, ether, and propylene glycol; slightly soluble in glycerol. It dissolves in solutions of alkali hydroxides. **Store** in well-closed containers.

6648-w

Ethyl Hydroxybenzoate *(BAN)*.

Aethylum Hydroxybenzoicum; E214; Ethylis Paraoxybenzoas; Ethylparaben *(USAN)*. Ethyl 4-hydroxybenzoate.

$C_9H_{10}O_3=166.2$.

CAS — 120-47-8.

Pharmacopoeias. In *Br., Chin., Fr.,* and *Jpn.* Also in *U.S.N.F.*

Odourless or almost odourless colourless crystals or white crystalline powder. Very slightly **soluble** in water; soluble 1 in 2 of alcohol and 1 in 3.5 of ether; freely soluble in acetone and propylene glycol; slightly soluble in glycerol. It dissolves in solutions of alkali hydroxides. **Store** in well-closed containers.

6651-v

Methyl Hydroxybenzoate *(BAN)*.

E218; Metagin; Methyl Parahydroxybenzoate; Methylis Oxybenzoas; Methylis Parahydroxybenzoas; Methylis Paraoxibenzoas; Methylparaben *(USAN)*; Metilparabeno. Methyl 4-hydroxybenzoate.

$C_8H_8O_3=152.1$.

CAS — 99-76-3.

Pharmacopoeias. In *Aust., Belg., Br., Braz., Egypt., Eur., Fr., Ger., Hung., Ind., It., Jpn, Jug., Mex., Neth., Nord., Pol., Port., Roum., Span.,* and *Swiss.* Also in *U.S.N.F.*

Colourless crystals or a white crystalline powder; odourless or with a faint odour. **Soluble** 1 in 400 of water, 1 in 3 of alcohol, and 1 in 10 of ether; freely soluble in methyl alcohol. **Store** in well-closed containers.

6665-e

Propyl Hydroxybenzoate *(BAN)*.

E216; Propagin; Propyl Parahydroxybenzoate; Propylis Oxybenzoas; Propylis Parahydroxybenzoas; Propylis Paraoxibenzoas; Propylparaben *(USAN)*. Propyl 4-hydroxybenzoate.

$C_{10}H_{12}O_3=180.2$.

CAS — 94-13-3.

Pharmacopoeias. In *Aust., Belg., Br., Braz., Cz., Egypt., Eur., Fr., Ger., Hung., Ind., It., Jpn, Jug., Mex., Neth., Nord., Pol., Roum.,* and *Swiss.* Also in *U.S.N.F.*

Colourless crystals or a white crystalline powder.

Soluble 1 in 2500 of water, 1 in 400 of boiling water, 1 in 1.5 of alcohol, and 1 in 3 of ether; freely soluble in methyl alcohol. **Store** in well-closed containers.

6667-y

Sodium Butyl Hydroxybenzoate *(BAN)*.

Sodium Butylparaben. The sodium salt of butyl 4-hydroxybenzoate.

$C_{11}H_{13}NaO_3$=216.2.

CAS — 36457-20-2.

Pharmacopoeias. In *Br.*

A white, odourless or almost odourless, hygroscopic powder. **Soluble** 1 in 1 of water and 1 in 10 of alcohol. A 0.1% solution in water has a pH of 9.5 to 10.5. **Store** in well-closed containers.

6674-l

Sodium Methyl Hydroxybenzoate *(BAN)*.

E219; Methylparaben Sodium *(USAN)*; Sodium Methylparaben; Soluble Methyl Hydroxybenzoate. The sodium salt of methyl 4-hydroxybenzoate.

$C_8H_7NaO_3$=174.1.

CAS — 5026-62-0.

Pharmacopoeias. In *Br.* Also in *U.S.N.F.*

A white, odourless or almost odourless, hygroscopic, crystalline powder. **Soluble** 1 in 2 of water and 1 in 50 of alcohol; practically insoluble in fixed oils. A 0.1% solution has a pH of 9.5 to 10.5. **Store** in airtight containers.

6676-j

Sodium Propyl Hydroxybenzoate *(BAN)*.

E217; Propylparaben Sodium *(USAN)*; Sodium Propylparaben; Soluble Propyl Hydroxybenzoate. The sodium salt of propyl 4-hydroxybenzoate.

$C_{10}H_{11}NaO_3$=202.2.

CAS — 35285-69-9.

Pharmacopoeias. In *Br.* Also in *U.S.N.F.*

A white, odourless or almost odourless, hygroscopic, crystalline powder. **Soluble** 1 in 1 of water, 1 in 50 of alcohol, and 1 in 2 of alcohol (50%); practically insoluble in fixed oils. A 0.1% solution in water has a pH of 9.5 to 10.5. **Store** in airtight containers.

Methyl, ethyl, propyl, and butyl hydroxybenzoates, used as preservatives in oral liquid preparations, were found to partition into flavouring oils. The partitioning effect depended on the concentration of the oils, pH of the aqueous medium, and the nature of other additives. Depletion of the hydroxybenzoates from the aqueous phase could lower their concentration below that required for preservative action.— P. B. Chemburkar and R. S. Joslin, *J. pharm. Sci.*, 1975, *64*, 414.

INCOMPATIBILITY. The antibacterial activity of methyl hydroxybenzoate against *Staphylococcus aureus* was reduced by 75 to 100% in the presence of aluminium magnesium silicate (Veegum), talc, polysorbate 80, or magnesium trisilicate.— R. T. Yousef *et al.*, *Can. J. pharm. Sci.*, 1973, *8*, 54. The adsorption of esters of *p*-hydroxybenzoic acid onto magnesium trisilicate increased with increasing ester chain length but decreased as the pH increased and the ester molecule became ionised. Further microbiological studies were required to elucidate the significance of adsorption on the preservative capacity of the hydroxybenzoates in magnesium trisilicate mixtures. Esters of *p*-hydroxybenzoic acid were reported not to be adsorbed by kaolin.— M. C. Allwood, *Int. J. Pharmaceut.*, 1982, *11*, 101.

For evidence of physical incompatibility when certain *B.P.C. 1973* preparations were prepared with or diluted with syrup preserved with hydroxybenzoates, see under Sucrose, p.1276.

For a report of incompatibility between atropine sulphate and hydroxybenzoate preservatives resulting in decreased concentrations of atropine in an oral mixture, see Atropine Sulphate, p.523.

Nonionic surfactants. The antimicrobial activity of hydroxybenzoate preservatives may be reduced in the presence of nonionic surfactants.

The effect of solubilisation by various nonionic surfactants in aqueous solution on the antimicrobial activity of butyl hydroxybenzoate was studied. The more hydrophobic the surfactant used, the more butyl hydroxybenzoate solubilised, and the greater the reduction of its antimicrobial activity against *Candida albicans*; in this case the antimicrobial activity was possibly due only to the free preservative. In contrast, free and solubilised butyl hydroxybenzoate contributed to the antimicrobial activity against *Pseudomonas aeruginosa*.— M. Yamaguchi *et al.*, *J. Soc. cosmet. Chem.*, 1982, *33*, 297.

SOLUBILITY. Solubilities of hydroxybenzoates over a range of temperatures: K. S. Alexander *et al.*, *J. pharm. Sci.*, 1977, *66*, 42 (in aliphatic alcohols); K. S. Alexander *et al.*, *ibid.*, 1978, *67*, 624 (in water); D. J. W. Grant *et al.*, *Int. J. Pharmaceut.*, 1984, *18*, 25 (in water).

SORPTION. Sorption by nylon 6 (capran polyamide) of methyl and propyl hydroxybenzoates decreased their antimicrobial activity against *Aspergillus niger, Klebsiella aerogenes,* and *Pseudomonas aeruginosa*.— N. K. Patel and N. Nagabhushan, *J. pharm. Sci.*, 1970, *59*, 264.

Studies on the adsorption of hydroxybenzoate preservatives by plastics.— K. Kakemi *et al.*, *Chem. pharm. Bull., Tokyo,* 1971, *19*, 2523.

See also under Incompatibility, above.

STABILITY. Studies of the effect of pH and temperature on the hydrolysis of hydroxybenzoates and relevance to heat sterilisation: N. N. Raval and E. L. Parrott, *J. pharm. Sci.*, 1967, *56*, 274; S. M. Blaug and D. E. Grant, *J. Soc. cosmet. Chem.*, 1974, *25*, 495; V. B. Sunderland and D. W. Watts, *Int. J. Pharmaceut.*, 1984, *19*, 1.

Degradation of hydroxybenzoates was accelerated by transesterification with polyols such as sorbitol.— B. Runesson and K. Gustavii, *Acta pharm. suec.*, 1986, *23*, 151.

Effect of freeze-drying. A report of the loss of hydroxybenzoate preservatives (methyl hydroxybenzoate and propyl hydroxybenzoate) during freeze-drying of aqueous solutions. The loss was dependent on the vacuum of the system, the length of drying cycle, the temperature of the product, and the amount and chemical entity of the materials present. Analysis of hydroxybenzoate-containing freeze-dried products for both active ingredient and preservative appeared warranted.— K. P. Flora *et al.*, *J. Pharm. Pharmac.*, 1980, *32*, 577.

Adverse Effects and Precautions

The hydroxybenzoate preservatives have similar adverse effects to those of Benzoic Acid (p.1355). The antimicrobial activity of hydroxybenzoates may be diminished through incompatibility, interactions, and adsorption (see above) with a resulting reduction in effectiveness.

ALLERGY AND INTOLERANCE. Report of cutaneous allergy induced by systemic administration of pharmaceutical preparations containing hydroxybenzoate preservatives. A review indicated that the incidence of allergic skin reactions following topical application of hydroxybenzoates had ranged from 0.8% (W.F. Schorr, *J. Am. med. Ass.*, 1968, *204*, 859) to 3% (North American Contact Dermatitis Group, *Archs Derm.*, 1973, *108*, 537) in patients with chronic dermatitis but side-effects after systemic administration had been reported less frequently. Cross-sensitivity between hydroxybenzoate esters appeared to be common.— R. M. Chichmanian *et al.*, *Thérapie*, 1985, *40*, 365.

Further reports of hypersensitivity reactions to hydroxybenzoate preservatives: J. E. Nagel *et al.*, *J. Am. med. Ass.*, 1977, *237*, 1594 (pruritus and bronchospasm in an asthmatic provoked by the hydroxybenzoate preservatives present in an intravenous hydrocortisone preparation); Y. Kaminer *et al.*, *Clin. Pharm.*, 1982, *1*, 469 (urticarial maculopapular rash associated with the oral administration of a syrup preserved with methyl hydroxybenzoate).

Evidence of cross-sensitivity between local anaesthetics of the para-aminobenzoate group and methyl hydroxybenzoate.— J. A. Aldrete and D. A. Johnson, *J. Am. med. Ass.*, 1969, *207*, 356.

PREGNANCY AND THE NEONATE. An *in vitro* study on serum from neonates with hyperbilirubinaemia indicated that methyl hydroxybenzoate present in gentamicin injections increased the concentration of free unconjugated bilirubin and interfered with the binding of bilirubin to serum proteins; gentamicin or propyl hydroxybenzoate had no significant effect.— C. J. Loria *et al.*, *J. Pediat.*, 1976, *89*, 479. Urinary excretion of methyl hydroxybenzoate in 6 preterm infants given multiple intramuscular doses of a gentamicin formulation preserved with hydroxybenzoates was variable. Whether there was accumulation of the preservative in some infants and whether the albumin binding capacity for bilirubin was affected remained to be determined.— K. W. Hindmarsh *et al.*, *J. pharm. Sci.*, 1983, *72*, 1039. See also under Benzoic Acid, p.1355.

Uses.

The hydroxybenzoate preservatives (parabens) are alkyl esters of *p*-hydroxybenzoic acid with antibacterial and antifungal properties. They have the advantage that they are active over a broad pH range (4 to 8) though they are generally more active in acidic solutions. Activity increases with increasing alkyl chain length but aqueous solubility decreases.

They are used as preservatives in pharmaceutical preparations including oral liquids, creams, and lotions in concentrations of up to 0.3%. Some authorities consider that the hydroxybenzoates are not satisfactory preservatives for ophthalmic preparations because of their relative lack of efficacy against some Gram-negative bacteria, particularly *Pseudomonas aeruginosa*.

The hydroxybenzoate preservatives are widely used in cosmetics and are also used for food preservation in usual concentrations of up to 0.1%.

Two or more hydroxybenzoate esters are often used together to combine their antimicrobial spectrum and solubilities thus increasing efficacy. The sodium salts of the alkyl esters may sometimes be preferred because of their greater solubility in water.

Estimated sum acceptable daily intake of ethyl, methyl, and propyl hydroxybenzoates: up to 10 mg per kg body-weight.— Seventeenth Report of the Joint FAO/WHO Expert Committee on Food Additives, *Tech. Rep. Ser. Wld Hlth Org. No. 539*, 1974.

ANTIMICROBIAL ACTIVITY. Hugo and Foster (*J. Pharm. Pharmac.*, 1964, *16*, 209) found that a strain of *Pseudomonas aeruginosa*, originally isolated from an infected human eye, would grow readily in a solution containing methyl hydroxybenzoate 0.0229% and propyl hydroxybenzoate 0.0114%. Higher concentrations (0.08% or 0.1% total hydroxybenzoates) were reported to be effective as preservatives in eye-drops (A.K. McIver, *Pharm. J.*, 1964, *1*, 429) but Foster (*ibid.*, 429 and 461) found that a total ester concentration of 0.08% (in the proportion of 2 of methyl to 1 of propyl hydroxybenzoate) was only just bacteriostatic for *Ps. aeruginosa* and a total ester concentration of at least 0.2% was required in order to be bactericidal; eye-drops containing this concentration were considered to be too irritant to use.

In a comparison of the effectiveness of various preservatives in different insulin injections, the most poorly preserved preparations as assessed by the survival of *Pseudomonas aeruginosa* and *Staphylococcus aureus* were soluble insulin injections preserved with 0.1% methyl hydroxybenzoate at neutral pH.— M. C. Allwood, *Pharm. J.*, 1982, *2*, 340. Eleven of 265 used vials of soluble insulin injection were found to be contaminated, representing a contamination rate of approximately 4%. Very heavy contamination in some vials indicated that some organisms were able to survive and multiply in certain insulin injections despite the presence of preservatives. In almost every instance of contamination, the preservative was 0.1% methyl hydroxybenzoate, reinforcing the previous view that this preservative system was unsuitable for soluble insulin injection.— *idem*, 1985, *1*, 320.

Action. The effect of hydroxybenzoate preservatives on the growth and uptake processes of *Escherichia coli, Bacillus subtilis,* and *Pseudomonas aeruginosa.* The results supported the hypothesis of uptake inhibition as the primary mechanism of action.— T. Eklund, *J. appl. Bact.*, 1980, *48*, 423.

Preparations

Compound Hydroxybenzoate Solution *(A.P.F.).* Methyl hydroxybenzoate 8 g, propyl hydroxybenzoate 2 g, propylene glycol to 100 mL.

Hydroxybenzoate Gel *(A.P.F.).* Catheter Lubricant; Surgical Lubricant. See under Tragacanth, p.1438.

Methyl Hydroxybenzoate Solution *(A.P.F.).* Methyl hydroxybenzoate 5 g, propylene glycol to 100 mL.

Proprietary Names and Manufacturers of Hydroxybenzoates

Methyl Chemosept *(USA)*; Nipabenzyl *(Nipa, UK)*; Nipabutyl *(Nipa, UK)*; Nipabutyl Sodium *(Nipa, UK)*; Nipacombin SK *(Nipa, UK)*; Nipagin A *(Nipa, UK)*; Nipagin A Sodium *(Nipa, UK)*; Nipagin M *(Nipa, UK)*; Nipagin M Sodium *(Nipa, UK)*; Nipasept *(Nipa, UK)*; Nipasept Sodium *(Nipa, UK)*; Nipasol M *(Nipa, UK)*; Nipasol M Sodium *(Nipa, UK)*; Nipastat *(Nipa, UK)*.

6636-g

Bronopol *(BAN, rINN)*.
2-Bromo-2-nitropropane-1,3-diol.
$C_3H_6BrNO_4$=200.0.

CAS — 52-51-7.

Pharmacopoeias. In *Br.*

White or almost white crystals or crystalline powder, odourless or almost odourless. **Soluble** 1 in 4 of water and 1 in 2 of alcohol; slightly soluble in glycerol and in liquid paraffin. A 1% solution in water has a pH of 5 to 7.

Store in well-closed containers. Protect from light.

Although bronopol showed little adsorption on to several powders widely used in pharmaceutical and cosmetic preparations, the alkaline pH of the aqueous suspensions of some of these powders adversely affected its antibacterial activity. A similar effect was obtained with some thickening agents.— J. A. Myburgh and T. J. McCarthy, *Cosmet. Toilet.*, 1978, *93*, (Feb.), 47.

Adverse Effects

Bronopol may be irritant to skin and eyes.

Reports of contact dermatitis to bronopol: F. J. Storrs and D. E. Bell, *J. Am. Acad. Derm.*, 1983, *8*, 157; C. E. H. Grattan and R. R. M. Harman, *Br. J. Derm.*, 1985, *113*, *Suppl.* 29, 43.

Uses.

Bronopol is active against a wide range of bacteria, including *Pseudomonas aeruginosa*, but is less active against moulds and yeasts. Its activity does not vary much over the range pH 5 to 8. Concentrations of 0.02 to 0.05% are bacteriostatic. Bronopol is used as a preservative in shampoos, cosmetics, and pharamaceutical preparations.

Proprietary Names and Manufacturers

Boots, UK.

6638-p

Butylated Hydroxyanisole *(BAN, USAN)*.

BHA; Butilidrossianisolo; E320. 2-*tert*-Butyl-4-methoxyphenol.
$C_{11}H_{16}O_2$=180.2.

CAS — 25013-16-5.

Pharmacopoeias. In *Br.*, *Fr.*, *Ind.*, and *It.* Also in *U.S.N.F.*

A white or almost white crystalline powder or a yellowish-white waxy solid with an aromatic odour. It contains a variable proportion of 3-*tert*-butyl-4-methoxyphenol.

B.P. **solubilities** are: practically insoluble in water; soluble in alcohol, propylene glycol, and arachis oil. It dissolves in solutions of alkali hydroxides. *U.S.N.F.* solubilities are: practically insoluble in water; soluble 1 in 4 of alcohol, 1 in 2 of chloroform, and 1 in 1.2 of ether; freely soluble in propylene glycol. **Store** in well-closed containers. Protect from light.

Adverse Effects and Precautions

Butylated hydroxyanisole can be irritant to the eyes, skin, and mucous membranes. Contact sensitivity and allergic skin reactions have been reported.

ALLERGY AND INTOLERANCE. Of 112 patients with eczematous dermatitis patch tested with butylated hydroxyanisole 2%, 3 had positive reactions.— J. Roed-Petersen and N. Hjorth, *Br. J. Derm.*, 1976, *94*, 233.

METHAEMOGLOBINAEMIA. A small outbreak of toxic methaemoglobinaemia in a paediatric ward was thought to be due to the antoxidants (butylated hydroxyanisole, butylated hydroxytoluene, and propyl gallate) used to preserve the oil in a soybean infant feed formula.— M. Nitzan *et al.*, *Clin. Toxicol.*, 1979, *15*, 273.

Absorption and Fate

Butylated hydroxyanisole is absorbed from the gastro-intestinal tract and excreted in the urine as metabolites; less than 1% is excreted in the urine as unchanged drug within 24 hours of ingestion.

A study *in vitro* indicated that following ingestion of usual doses, butylated hydroxyanisole was highly bound to plasma proteins.— R. El-Rashidy and S. Niazi, *J. pharm. Sci.*, 1978, *67*, 967.

Studies in 2 healthy subjects given butylated hydroxyanisole 100 mg by mouth indicated that although it was rapidly absorbed, the bioavailability and rate of absorption could differ greatly between subjects.— R. El-Rashidy and S. Niazi, *J. pharm. Sci.*, 1979, *68*, 103.

Study on the disposition kinetics of butylated hydroxyanisole 100 mg administered by mouth to 2 healthy subjects. Less than 1% of the dose was excreted in the urine unchanged over 24 hours; a mean of 44.2% and 26.0% was excreted as the glucuronide and sulphate respectively. There was significant conversion of butylated hydroxyanisole to its *O*-demethylated metabolite, a tert-butyl hydroquinone, prior to conjugation and the mean recovery of the tert-butyl hydroquinone glucuronide and sulphate in the urine over 24 hours was 21.5% and 22.5% of the dose respectively.— R. El-Rashidy and S. Niazi, *Biopharm. Drug Disposit.*, 1983, *4*, 389.

Uses.

Butylated hydroxyanisole has antoxidant properties; it has also been reported to have antimicrobial activity. It is employed as an antoxidant in cosmetics and foods, particularly to delay or prevent oxidative rancidity of fats and oils in concentrations of up to 0.02%; higher concentrations have been used for essential oils. It is also used to prevent the loss of activity of oil-soluble vitamins.

To improve efficacy, butylated hydroxyanisole is frequently used in combination with other antoxidants such as butylated hydroxytoluene or an alkyl gallate and with sequestrants and synergists such as citric acid.

A review of the uses and efficacy of butylated hydroxyanisole as an antoxidant.— *Fd Add. Ser. Wld Hlth Org. No. 3*, 1972.

A temporary estimated acceptable daily intake for butylated hydroxyanisole of up to 300 µg per kg body-weight was established.— Thirtieth Report of the Joint FAO/WHO Expert Committee on Food Additives, *Tech. Rep. Ser. Wld Hlth Org. No. 751*, 1987.

ANTIMICROBIAL ACTIVITY. An *in vitro* study of the antibacterial activity of butylated hydroxyanisole against *Staphylococcus aureus*, *Bacillus subtilis*, *Bacillus cereus*, *Escherichia coli*, *Pseudomonas aeruginosa*, and *Serratia marcescens*. Gram-positive organisms were generally more susceptible than Gram-negative organisms but the minimum inhibitory concentrations for all the organisms were quite low suggesting appreciable bacteriostatic and bactericidal activity against the organisms studied.— A. Lamikanra and T. A. Ogunbayo, *Cosmet. Toilet.*, 1985, *100*, (Oct.), 69. See also: A. L. Shih and N. D. Harris, *ibid.*, 1980, *95*, (Feb.), 75; J. J. Zeelie and T. J. McCarthy, *ibid.*, 1982, *97*, (Nov.), 61.

Proprietary Names and Manufacturers

Embanox 4 *(May & Baker, UK)*; Embanox 5 *(May & Baker, UK)*; Embanox BHA *(May & Baker, UK)*; Nipantiox 1-F *(Nipa, UK)*; Tenox A *(Eastman, UK)*; Tenox 4A *(Eastman, UK)*; Tenox BHA *(Eastman, UK)*; Tenox R *(Eastman, UK)*.

The following names have been used for multi-ingredient preparations containing butylated hydroxyanisole— Embanox 102 *(May & Baker, UK)*; Embanox 106 *(May & Baker, UK)*; Embanox 2 *(May & Baker, UK)*; Embanox 3 *(May & Baker, UK)*; Embanox 6 *(May & Baker, UK)*; Embanox 7 *(May & Baker, UK)*; Embanox EC30M *(May & Baker, UK)*; Tenox 2 *(Eastman, UK)*; Tenox 22 *(Eastman, UK)*; Tenox 26 *(Eastman, UK)*; Tenox 27 *(Eastman, UK)*; Tenox 4 *(Eastman, UK)*; Tenox 6 *(Eastman, UK)*; Tenox 7 *(Eastman, UK)*.

6639-s

Butylated Hydroxytoluene *(BAN, USAN)*.

BHT; Butylhydroxitoluenum; E321. 2,6-Di-*tert*-butyl-*p*-cresol.
$C_{15}H_{24}O$=220.4.

CAS — 128-37-0.

Pharmacopoeias. In *Br.*, *Fr.*, *Ind.*, and *Nord.* Also in *U.S.N.F.*

Colourless crystals or white crystalline powder, odourless or with a faint odour. *B.P.* **solubilities** are: practically insoluble in water, glycerol, propylene glycol, and solutions of alkali hydroxides; soluble 1 in 4 of alcohol, 1 in 0.5 of ether, 1 in 5 of liquid paraffin, and 1 in 3 of fixed oils. *U.S.N.F.* solubilities are: practically insoluble in water and propylene glycol; soluble 1 in 4 of alcohol, 1 in 1.1 of chloroform, and 1 in 1.1 of ether. **Store** in well-closed containers.

Adverse Effects and Precautions

Butylated hydroxytoluene can be irritant to the eyes, skin, and mucous membranes. Contact sensitivity and allergic skin reactions have been reported.

A 22-year-old woman experienced severe epigastric cramping, nausea and vomiting, and generalised weakness, followed by dizziness, confusion, and a brief loss of consciousness after ingesting 4 g of butylated hydroxytoluene on an empty stomach.— D. M. Shlian and J. Goldstone (letter), *New Engl. J. Med.*, 1986, *314*, 648.

ALLERGY AND INTOLERANCE. Of 112 patients with eczematous dermatitis patch tested with butylated hydroxytoluene 2%, 3 had positive reactions.— J. Roed-Petersen and N. Hjorth, *Br. J. Derm.*, 1976, *94*, 233.

Report of a cutaneous, urticarial, disseminated eruption associated with the regular use of a chewing-gum containing butylated hydroxytoluene. The eruption subsided within a week of stopping the gum but cutaneous signs returned a few hours after an oral challenge with butylated hydroxytoluene.— D. A. Moneret-Vautrin *et al.* (letter), *Lancet*, 1986, *1*, 617.

METHAEMOGLOBINAEMIA. For a report of methaemoglobinaemia associated with the antoxidants (butylated hydroxyanisole, butylated hydroxytoluene, and propyl gallate) used to preserve the oil in a soybean infant feed formula, see under Adverse Effects in Butylated Hydroxyanisole above.

Absorption and Fate

Butylated hydroxytoluene is readily absorbed from the gastro-intestinal tract. It is extensively metabolised and excreted in the urine mainly as metabolites.

The carboxylic acid of butylated hydroxytoluene and its ester glucuronide were the only major metabolites detected in human urine. The aldehyde compound isolated by Daniel *et al.* (*Food & Cosmet. Toxicol.*, 1967, *5*, 475) could not be found.— G. M. Holder *et al.* (letter), *J. Pharm. Pharmac.*, 1970, *22*, 375.

Uses.

Butylated hydroxytoluene has antoxidant properties; it has also been reported to have antimicrobial activity. It is employed as an antoxidant in cosmetics and foods, particularly to delay or prevent oxidative rancidity of fats and oils in concentrations of up to 0.02%. It is also used to prevent the loss of activity of oil-soluble vitamins.

To improve efficacy, butylated hydroxytoluene is frequently used in combination with other antoxidants such as butylated hydroxyanisole and with sequestrants and synergists such as citric acid.

A review of the uses and efficacy of butylated hydroxytoluene as an antoxidant.— *Fd Add. Ser. Wld Hlth Org. No. 3*, 1972.

A temporary estimated acceptable daily intake for butylated hydroxytoluene of up to 125 µg per kg body-weight was established.— Thirtieth Report of the Joint FAO/WHO Expert Committee on Food Additives, *Tech. Rep. Ser. Wld Hlth Org. No. 751*, 1987.

ANTIMICROBIAL ACTIVITY. *In vitro* and *animal* studies on the antiviral activity of butylated hydroxytoluene: W. Snipes *et al.*, *Science*, 1975, *188*, 64; P. Wanda *et al.*, *Antimicrob. Ag. Chemother.*, 1976, *10*, 96; M. Brugh, *Science*, 1977, *197*, 1291; A. D. Keith *et al.*, *Proc. Soc.*

exp. Biol. Med., 1982, *170*, 237; J. T. Richards *et al.*, *Antiviral Res.*, 1985, *5*, 281.

HERPES. In a double-blind study in 30 patients with recurrent herpes labialis, 16 applied butylated hydroxytoluene 15% in mineral oil topically to the lesion 4 times a day for 5 days and 14 applied a placebo. The median time for dry crust formation was slightly shorter in the butylated hydroxytoluene recipients than in controls. Other clinical measures of lesion severity showed a trend in favour of the active treatment, but differences were not significant. Butylated hydroxytoluene had no effect on the duration or degree of pain. Topical butylated hydroxytoluene was well tolerated and there was no evidence of local or systemic toxicity.— D. J. Freeman *et al.*, *Clin. Pharmac. Ther.*, 1985, *38*, 56. See also under Antimicrobial Activity, above.

Proprietary Names and Manufacturers

Anullex BHT *(BTP Cocker Chemicals, UK)*; Embanox BHT *(May & Baker, UK)*; Tenox BHT *(Eastman, UK)*.

The following names have been used for multi-ingredient preparations containing butylated hydroxytoluene—Embanox 2 *(May & Baker, UK)*; Embanox EC30M *(May & Baker, UK)*; Tenox 26 *(Eastman, UK)*; Tenox 4 *(Eastman, UK)*; Tenox 6 *(Eastman, UK)*.

6640-h

Chlorbutol *(BAN)*.

Acetone-Chloroforme; Alcohol Trichlorisobutylicus; Chlorbutanol; Chlorbutanolum; Chlorbutanolum Hydratum; Chloretone; Chlorobutanol *(USAN, rINN)*; Chlorobutanolum; Trichlorbutanolum. 1,1,1-Trichloro-2-methylpropan-2-ol hemihydrate.

$C_4H_7Cl_3O,\frac{1}{2}H_2O$=186.5.

CAS — 57-15-8 (anhydrous); 6001-64-5 (hemihydrate).

Pharmacopoeias. In *Belg.*, *Chin.*, *Cz.*, *Egypt.*, *Hung.*, *Ind.*, *Jug.*, *Nord.*, *Pol.*, and *Span.* (all with ½H_2O). In *Arg.*, *Braz.*, *Int.*, *Mex.*, *Port.*, and *U.S.N.F.* (anhydrous or with ½H_2O).

Aust., *Br.*, *Eur.*, *Fr.*, *Ger.*, *It.*, *Neth.*, and *Swiss* have separate monographs for anhydrous and hemihydrate. *Jpn* permits up to 6% of water. *Turk.* has anhydrous.

Colourless or white crystals or a white crystalline powder with a characteristic, somewhat camphoraceous odour. It sublimes readily. *B.P.* m.p. about 78°; *U.S.N.F.* m.p. about 76°; anhydrous chlorbutol melts at about 95°.

B.P. solubilities are: slightly **soluble** in water; soluble 1 in 0.6 of alcohol; freely soluble in chloroform; very soluble in ether; soluble in glycerol. *U.S.N.F.* solubilities are: soluble 1 in 125 of water, 1 in 1 of alcohol, and 1 in 10 of glycerol; freely soluble in ether, in chloroform, and in volatile oils. A 2% suspension in water is neutral to litmus. **Store** in a cool place in airtight containers. Protect from light.

In the presence of magnesium trisilicate 1%, chlorbutol 0.5% had no antibacterial activity against *Staphylococcus aureus*. Bentonite 1% and carmellose 1% both reduced its activity by between 20 and 30%.— R. T. Yousef *et al.*, *Can. J. pharm. Sci.*, 1973, *8*, 54.

SORPTION. References to the sorption of chlorbutol by polyethylene and polypropylene containers: W. T. Friesen and E. M. Plein, *Am. J. Hosp. Pharm.*, 1971, *28*, 507; N. E. Richardson *et al.*, *J. Pharm. Pharmac.*, 1977, *29*, 717; H. D. Blackburn *et al.* (letter), *ibid.*, 1978, *30*, 666; N. E. Richardson *et al.*, *Pharm. J.*, 1979, *2*, 462; D. G. Holdsworth *et al.*, *J. clin. Hosp. Pharm.*, 1984, *9*, 29.

Chlorbutol was reversibly sorbed from aqueous solution into contact lenses manufactured from polyhydroxyethylmethacrylate.— N. E. Richardson *et al.*, *J. Pharm. Pharmac.*, 1978, *30*, 469.

STABILITY. The half-life at 25° for chlorbutol in a solution buffered at pH 3 was calculated to be 90 years whereas at pH 7.5 it was 0.23 year. Similarly, the decomposition in aqueous solution when heated for 30 minutes at 115° was calculated to be 13% at pH 5 and 58% at pH 6.— A. D. Nair and J. L. Lach, *J. Am. pharm. Ass., scient. Edn*, 1959, *48*, 390.

A 0.5% solution of chlorbutol with a pH of 5 to 6 lost 10% of its potency when stored for six weeks at 25° to 30°. Neutral or alkaline solutions were less stable.— N. V. Patwa and C. L. Huyck, *J. Am. pharm. Ass.*, 1966, *NS6*, 372.

Polysorbate 20 and lauromacrogol [1000] reduced the rate of hydrolysis of chlorbutol at pH 9.2 but macrogol 4000 had no effect.— R. A. Anderson and A. H. Slade, *J. Pharm. Pharmac.*, 1966, *18*, 640.

Adverse Effects

Acute poisoning with chlorbutol may produce central nervous system depression with weakness, loss of consciousness, and depressed respiration. Treatment is symptomatic.

ALLERGY AND INTOLERANCE. A report of a hypersensitivity reaction to chlorbutol used to preserve heparin injection.— S. Dux *et al.* (letter), *Lancet*, 1981, *1*, 149. See also A. Itabashi *et al.* (letter), *ibid.*, 1982, *1*, 108 (hypersensitivity to chlorbutol in desmopressin intra-nasal solution).

EFFECTS ON THE CARDIOVASCULAR SYSTEM. For a report of a sharp fall in blood pressure after the injection of heparin containing chlorbutol, see under Precautions in Heparin, p.340.

EFFECTS ON MENTAL FUNCTION. Symptoms of chlorbutol intoxication developed in a 40-year-old man with a history of alcoholism who had been taking between 6 and 10 sedative capsules daily each containing chlorbutol 150 mg and salicylamide 300 mg. During treatment the elimination half-life of chlorbutol was found to be 13.2 days.— T. Borody *et al.*, *Med. J. Aust.*, 1979, *1*, 288.

It was considered that accumulation of chlorbutol, present as a preservative in the morphine infusion, may have contributed to the somnolence seen in a 19-year-old woman receiving a high-dose morphine infusion.— R. DeChristoforo *et al.*, *Ann. intern. Med.*, 1983, *98*, 335.

Uses and Administration

Chlorbutol has antibacterial and antifungal properties and it is used at a concentration of 0.5% as a preservative in injections and in eye-drops. At this concentration it is close to its saturation point at low temperatures, and crystallisation may occur. It is unstable in alkaline solution, it is more stable in acid solution at room temperature and it decomposes appreciably on autoclaving or steaming.

Chlorbutol has been used as a mild sedative and local analgesic as well as in motion sickness but other compounds are preferred. It has also been used as a dusting powder, in nose drops and as a dental preparation for exposed or infected pulps.

In the *UK* the maximum concentration of chlorbutol in cosmetics, other than foams, is restricted by law to 0.5%, and is not to be used in aerosol dispensers.

Proprietary Names and Manufacturers

Chlorbutone *(Orapharm, Austral.)*.

The following names have been used for multi-ingredient preparations containing chlorbutol—Applicaine Liquid *(Nyal, Austral.)*; Auralgicin *(Fisons, UK)*; Aurisan *(Nadeau, Canad.)*; Cerumol *(Salmond & Spraggon, Austral.; Kingswood, Canad.; Laboratories for Applied Biology, UK)*; Cetanorm *(Norma, UK)*; Eludril Mouthwash *(Concept Pharmaceuticals, UK)*; Monphytol *(Salmond & Spraggon, Austral.; Laboratories for Applied Biology, UK)*; Mycozol *(Parke, Davis, Austral.)*; Pentaid *(Pennwalt, Canad.)*; Sedonan *(Sigma, Austral.; Napp, UK)*.

6641-m

Cinnamic Acid *(BAN)*.

Cinnam. Acid; Cinnamylic Acid. *trans*-3-Phenylpropenoic acid.

$C_6H_5.CH:CH.CO_2H$=148.2.

CAS — 621-82-9.

Pharmacopoeias. In *Br.*

Colourless crystals with a faint balsamic odour. Very slightly **soluble** in water; soluble 1 in 6 of alcohol, 1 in 15 of chloroform, and 1 in 15 of ether.

Cinnamic acid has preservative properties similar to those of benzoic acid (see p.1356). It is used with benzoic acid to simulate the flavour of tolu.

Preparations

Tolu-flavour Solution *(B.P.)*. Prepared by adding a solution of cinnamic acid 500 mg, benzoic acid 250 mg, ethyl cinnamate 30 mg, vanillin 10 mg, and cinnamon oil 0.002 mL in alcohol 10 mL to a solution of sucrose 50 g in water 32 mL and alcohol 25 mL, diluting to 100 mL with water, mixing, and allowing to stand for a few hours before use. Store in well-closed containers.

Tolu Syrup *(B.P.)*. Tolu-flavour solution 10 mL, syrup to 100 mL.

Paediatric Compound Tolu Linctus *(B.P.)*. Paediatric Compound Tolu Oral Solution. A solution containing 0.6% w/v of citric acid monohydrate in a suitable vehicle with a tolu flavour. Store at a temperature not exceeding 25°.

6642-b

Dehydroacetic Acid *(USAN)*.

Methylacetopyronone. 3-Acetyl-6-methyl-2*H*-pyran-2,4(3*H*)-dione (keto form); 3-Acetyl-4-hydroxy-6-methyl-2*H*-pyran-2-one (enol form).

$C_8H_8O_4$=168.1.

CAS — 520-45-6 (keto form); 771-03-9 (enol form).

Pharmacopoeias. In *U.S.N.F.*

A white or nearly white crystalline powder; odourless or practically odourless. Very slightly **soluble** in water; sparingly soluble in alcohol; freely soluble in acetone and benzene; soluble in aqueous solutions of fixed alkalis. **Store** in well-closed containers.

6668-j

Sodium Dehydroacetate *(USAN)*.

The sodium salt of 3-acetyl-6-methyl-2*H*-pyran-2,4(3*H*)-dione.

$C_8H_7NaO_4$=190.1.

CAS — 4418-26-2.

Pharmacopoeias. In *U.S.N.F.*

A white or practically white, odourless powder. Freely **soluble** in water, propylene glycol, and glycerol. **Store** in well-closed containers.

Dehydroacetic acid inhibits the growth of many bacteria, fungi, and yeasts.

Dehydroacetic acid and sodium dehydroacetate have been used in the preservation of cosmetics and shampoos.

6643-v

Diethyl Pyrocarbonate

DEPC; Diethyl Polycarbonate.

$C_6H_{10}O_5$=162.1.

CAS — 1609-47-8.

Diethyl pyrocarbonate is a preservative which is mainly effective against yeast. It was formerly used for the preservation of soft drinks and wine, but it had been reported that there was a risk of the carcinogen diethylurethane being produced with ammonium ions.

6644-g

Diphenyl

E230; Phenylbenzene. Biphenyl.

$C_{12}H_{10}$=154.2.

CAS — 92-52-4.

Diphenyl is fungistatic against a limited number of moulds and has been employed for impregnating the material used for wrapping citrus fruits.

In Great Britain the recommended exposure limits of diphenyl are 0.2 ppm (long-term); 0.6 ppm (short-term).

Though primarily used for treating wrappers for fruit, diphenyl penetrated into the skin of the fruit and might consequently be included in food or drink prepared from the fruit.— Sixth Report of the Joint FAO/WHO Expert Committee on Food Additives, *Tech. Rep. Ser.*

Wld Hlth Org. No. 228, 1962.

Adverse effects, including nausea, vomiting, and irritation of the eyes and nose occurred in workers exposed to diphenyl.— E. Weil *et al., Archs Mal. prof. Med. trav.,* 1965, *26,* 405.

Nine workers exposed to diphenyl developed toxic symptoms which included headache, nausea, diffuse abdominal pain, aching of limbs, and general fatigue. Six had liver damage and 1 of the 6 workers who also had psychic symptoms, somnolence, icterus, ascites, and oedema of the legs died with yellow liver atrophy.— I. Häkkinen *et al., Archs environ. Hlth,* 1973, *26,* 70.

6645-q

Dodecyl Gallate *(BAN).*

E312; Lauryl Gallate; Laurylum Gallicum. Dodecyl 3,4,5-trihydroxybenzoate.
$C_{19}H_{30}O_5$=338.4.

CAS — 1166-52-5.

Pharmacopoeias. In *Aust.* and *Br.*

A white or creamy-white, odourless or almost odourless powder. Practically **insoluble** in water; soluble 1 in 3.5 of alcohol, 1 in 2 of acetone, 1 in 60 of chloroform, 1 in 4 of ether, 1 in 1.5 of methyl alcohol, 1 in 60 of propylene glycol, and 1 in 30 of arachis oil. **Store** in well-closed containers and avoid contact with metals. Protect from light.

6647-s

Ethyl Gallate *(BAN).*

Ethyl 3,4,5-trihydroxybenzoate.
$C_9H_{10}O_5$=198.2.

CAS — 831-61-8.

Pharmacopoeias. In *Br.*

A white to creamy-white, odourless or almost odourless, crystalline powder. Slightly **soluble** in water; soluble 1 in 3 of alcohol and 1 in 3 of ether; practically insoluble in arachis oil. **Store** in well-closed containers and avoid contact with metals. Protect from light.

6654-p

Octyl Gallate *(BAN).*

E311. Octyl 3,4,5-trihydroxybenzoate.
$C_{15}H_{22}O_5$=282.3.

CAS — 1034-01-1.

Pharmacopoeias. In *Br.*

A white or creamy-white, odourless or almost odourless powder. Practically **insoluble** in water; soluble 1 in 2.5 of alcohol, 1 in 1 of acetone, 1 in 30 of chloroform, 1 in 3 of ether, 1 in 0.7 of methyl alcohol, 1 in 7 of propylene glycol, and 1 in 33 of arachis oil. **Store** in well-closed containers and avoid contact with metals. Protect from light.

6664-w

Propyl Gallate *(BAN, USAN).*

E310; Propylis Gallas; Propylum Gallicum. Propyl 3,4,5-trihydroxybenzoate.
$C_{10}H_{12}O_5$=212.2.

CAS — 121-79-9.

Pharmacopoeias. In *Aust., Belg., Br., Cz., Egypt., Ind.,* and *Nord.* Also in *U.S.N.F.*

A white to creamy-white, odourless or almost odourless, crystalline powder. Very slightly **soluble** in water; soluble 1 in 3 of alcohol and 1 in 3 of ether; very slightly soluble in arachis oil. **Store** in airtight containers and avoid contact with metals. Protect from light.

Adverse Effects and Precautions

The alkyl gallates may cause contact sensitivity and skin reactions.

ALLERGY AND INTOLERANCE. Reports of contact sensitivity to alkyl gallates: G. Kahn *et al., Archs Derm.,* 1974, *109,* 506; J. Roed-Petersen and N. Hjorth, *Br. J. Derm.,* 1976, *94,* 233.

METHAEMOGLOBINAEMIA. For a report of methaemoglobinaemia associated with the antoxidants (butylated hydroxyanisole, butylated hydroxytoluene, and propyl gallate) used to preserve the oil in a soybean infant feed formula, see under Adverse Effects in Butylated Hydroxyanisole, p.1358.

Uses.

The alkyl esters of gallic acid (3,4,5-trihydroxybenzoic acid) have antoxidant properties and are employed in cosmetics and foods. They are particularly useful at preventing deterioration and rancidity of fats and oils in usual concentrations of 0.001 to 0.02%.

To improve acceptability and efficacy, the alkyl gallates are frequently used in combination with other antoxidants such as butylated hydroxyanisole or butylated hydroxytoluene and with sequestrants and synergists such as citric acid.

A review of the uses and efficacy of alkyl gallates as antoxidants.— *Fd Add. Ser. Wld Hlth Org. No. 3,* 1972.

Estimated acceptable daily intake of propyl gallate: up to 2.5 mg per kg body-weight. There was insufficient data available to establish an acceptable daily intake for dodecyl gallate and octyl gallate. The Committee noted that octyl gallate could cause reactions in the buccal mucosa of individuals previously sensitised by cutaneous contact with this compound and the use of octyl gallate in beer and other widely consumed beverages was not recommended.— Thirtieth Report of the Joint FAO/WHO Expert Committee on Food Additives, *Tech. Rep. Ser. Wld Hlth Org. No. 751,* 1987.

Proprietary Names and Manufacturers of Alkyl Gallates

Progallin A *(Nipa, UK)*; Progallin BU *(Nipa, UK)*; Progallin LA *(Nipa, UK)*; Progallin O *(Nipa, UK)*; Progallin P *(Nipa, UK)*; Tenox PG *(Eastman, UK)*; Tenox S-1 *(Eastman, UK)*.

The following names have been used for multi-ingredient preparations containing alkyl gallates—Embanox 3 *(May & Baker, UK)*; Embanox 6 *(May & Baker, UK)*; Embanox 7 *(May & Baker, UK)*; Tenox 2 *(Eastman, UK)*; Tenox 6 *(Eastman, UK)*; Tenox 7 *(Eastman, UK)*.

6646-p

Ethoxyquin

6-Ethoxy-1,2-dihydro-2,2,4-trimethylquinoline.
$C_{14}H_{19}NO$=217.3.

CAS — 91-53-2.

Ethoxyquin has been used as an antoxidant for the prevention of common scald of apples and pears during storage. There is debate as to the safety of this practice.

A report of 2 cases of contact dermatitis attributed to ethoxyquin.— D. Burrows, *Br. J. Derm.,* 1975, *92,* 167.

Proprietary Names and Manufacturers

Santoquin *(Monsanto, USA)*.

6652-g

Monothioglycerol *(USAN).*

α-Monothioglycerol; Thioglycerol. 3-Mercaptopropane-1,2-diol.
$C_3H_8O_2S$=108.2.

CAS — 96-27-5.

Pharmacopoeias. In *U.S.N.F.*

A colourless or pale yellow, viscous, hygroscopic liquid with a slight odour of sulphide.

Freely **soluble** in water; miscible with alcohol; practically insoluble in ether. A 10% solution in water has a pH of 3.5 to 7. **Store** in airtight containers.

Monothioglycerol is used as an antoxidant.

References to the antibacterial action of monothioglycerol *in vitro*: K. K. Jensen and G. T. Javor, *Antimicrob. Ag. Chemother.,* 1981, *19,* 556; G. T. Javor, *ibid.,* 1983, *24,* 860 and 868.

2260-b

Myristyl-gamma-picolinium Chloride

4-Methyl-1-tetradecylpyridinium chloride.
$C_{20}H_{36}ClN$=326.0.

CAS — 7631-49-4 (myristyl-gamma-picolinium); 2748-88-1 (chloride).

Myristyl-gamma-picolinium chloride is a cationic surfactant which is used as an antimicrobial preservative in some pharmaceutical products.

6653-q

Nordihydroguaiaretic Acid

Acidum Nordihydroguaiareticum; NDGA. 4,4′-(2,3-Dimethyltetramethylene)bis(benzene-1,2-diol).
$C_{18}H_{22}O_4$=302.4.

CAS — 500-38-9.

Pharmacopoeias. In *Nord.*

Nordihydroguaiaretic acid has been used as an antoxidant for oils and fats. Contact dermatitis has been reported.

The available biological data were inadequate to evaluate its use as an antoxidant in food.— Seventeenth Report of the Joint FAO/WHO Expert Committee on Food Additives, *Tech. Rep. Ser. Wld Hlth Org. No. 539,* 1974.

Evidence that nordihydroguaiaretic acid may have antimicrobial as well as antoxidant activity.— A. L. Shih and N. D. Harris, *Cosmet. Toilet.,* 1980, *95,* 75.

6661-q

Orthophenylphenol

2-Hydroxybiphenyl; E231; E232 (Sodium-*o*-phenylphenol); *o*-Hydroxydiphenyl.
$C_{12}H_{10}O$=170.2.

CAS — 90-43-7.

Orthophenylphenol has antibacterial and antifungal properties and has many industrial uses as a preservative for a wide range of materials, particularly against moulds and rots. Its antimicrobial properties are similar to those of chloroxylenol (see p.959) and it is used in disinfectants. Sodium-*o*-phenylphenol has been used similarly.

Proprietary Names and Manufacturers

Winseptic *(Winthrop, Austral.)*.

6655-s

Pentachlorophenol

PCP; Penta.
C_6HCl_5O=266.3.

CAS — 87-86-5.

NOTE. The name PCP has also been used as a synonym for phencyclidine hydrochloride.

Adverse Effects, Treatment, and Precautions

Pentachlorophenol may be absorbed in toxic amounts through the skin or by inhalation, as well as by ingestion. The fatal dose in man is about 1 g. Pentachlorophenol and its aqueous solutions are irritant to the eyes, mucous membranes, and to the skin and may produce caustic burns. Acute poisoning with pentachlorophenol increases metabolic rate, leading to raised temperature with copious sweating and thirst, restlessness, fatigue, increased rate and depth of respiration, and tachycardia. There may be abdominal pain and nausea, and death has occurred from respiratory failure.

Treatment is symptomatic; it has been suggested that forced alkaline diuresis may be useful.

In Great Britain the recommended exposure limits of pentachlorophenol are 0.5 mg per m^3 (long-term); 1.5 mg per m^3 (short-term); suitable precautions should be taken to prevent absorption through the skin.

Reviews of the toxicity of chlorinated phenols, including pentachlorophenol: *Toxicity Review No. 5: Pentachlorophenol,* Health and Safety Executive, London, HM Stationery Office, 1982; J. H. Exon, *Vet. hum. Toxicol.,* 1984, *26,* 508.

Reports of poisoning by pentachlorophenol: H. Bergner *et al., Can. med. Ass. J.,* 1965, *92,* 448; J. B. Chapman and P. Robson, *Lancet*, 1965, *1*, 1266; M. A. D. Crawford (letter), *ibid.*, 1966, *1*, 875; *Can. med. Ass. J.*, 1968, *98*, 424.

A pharmacokinetic study of poisoning with pentachlorophenol in an elderly patient suggested that forced diuresis was the treatment of preference in adults.— J. F. Young and T. J. Haley, *Clin. Toxicol.*, 1978, *12*, 41.

Aplastic anaemia due to pentachlorophenol.— H. J. Roberts (letter), *New Engl. J. Med.*, 1981, *305*, 1650.

Exposure to pentachlorophenol was considered the likely cause of pancreatitis in a 51-year-old man.— R. G. Cooper and M. B. Macaulay (letter), *Lancet*, 1982, *1*, 517.

A 56-year-old woman developed intravascular haemolysis after handling a pentachlorophenol-containing insecticide.— A. B. Hassan *et al.*, *Br. med. J.*, 1985, *291*, 21.

A report of urticaria in a 39-year-old man from contact with sodium pentachlorophenate.— P. M. Kentor (letter), *J. Am. med. Ass.*, 1986, *256*, 3350.

MALIGNANT NEOPLASMS. Hodgkin's disease and, possibly, nasal cancer among workers in the wood industry might be associated with exposure to chemical preservatives, notably pentachlorophenol.— M. H. Greene *et al.* (letter), *Lancet*, 1978, *2*, 626.

Malignant lymphoma of the histiocytic type in one patient exposed to pentachlorophenol and in 3 exposed to parachlorophenol.— L. Hardell (letter), *Lancet*, 1979, *1*, 55.

Absorption and Fate

Pentachlorophenol may be absorbed after ingestion or inhalation or through the skin. Following ingestion the majority of a dose is eliminated in the urine within 7 days as unchanged pentachlorophenol and its glucuronide with small amounts appearing in the faeces.

The pharmacokinetics and metabolism of pentachlorophenol in 4 healthy male subjects.— W. H. Braun *et al.*, *Toxic. appl. Pharmac.*, 1978, *45*, 278.

An absorption study of pentachlorophenol in persons working with wood preservatives.— R. D. Jones *et al.*, *Hum. Toxicol.*, 1986, *5*, 189.

Uses.

Pentachlorophenol has been used mainly as the sodium salt (C_6Cl_5NaO = 288.3), as a preservative for a wide range of industrial and agricultural products, including woods, textiles, glues and starch. It has also been used for the control of slime and algae, and as a molluscicide.

Proprietary Names and Manufacturers

Santobrite *(Monsanto, UK)*.

6656-w

Phenethyl Alcohol *(BAN)*.

Benzyl Carbinol; Phenethanolum; Phenylethyl Alcohol *(USAN)*. 2-Phenylethanol.

$C_6H_5.CH_2.CH_2OH$=122.2.

CAS — 60-12-8.

Pharmacopoeias. In *Nord.* and *U.S.*

A colourless liquid with a rose-like odour.

Soluble 1 in 60 of water, 1 in less than 1 of alcohol, chloroform, ether, benzyl benzoate, and diethyl phthalate; slightly soluble in liquid paraffin; very soluble in glycerol, propylene glycol, and fixed oils. **Store** in a cool, dry place in airtight containers. Protect from light.

Phenethyl alcohol is more active against Gram-negative than Gram-positive organisms. It is used as a preservative in ophthalmic solutions at a concentration of 0.25 to 0.5%, in conjunction with another bactericide. It is also used in flavouring essences and perfumes.

Solutions of fluorescein sodium 2% inoculated with *Pseudomonas aeruginosa* were sterile within 3 hours in the presence of phenylmercuric nitrate 0.002% and within 1 hour when phenethyl alcohol 0.4% was also present.— R. M. E. Richards *et al.*, *J. Pharm. Pharmac.*, 1969, *21*, 681.

In sterile ophthalmic solutions containing chlorhexidine acetate 0.01% as preservative, the time taken for the solution to become sterile after contamination with *Ps. aeruginosa* was reduced by the addition of phenethyl alcohol 0.4% from 60 to 15 minutes for pilocarpine hydrochloride solution and from 180 to 30 minutes for physostigmine salicylate solution. With phenylmercuric nitrate 0.002% as preservative the resterilisation time was reduced from 240 to 60 minutes for pilocarpine solution, from 24 hours to 90 minutes for atropine solution and from 90 to 45 minutes for physostigmine sulphate or salicylate solution. With benzalkonium chloride 0.01% the resterilisation time was reduced from 60 to 15 minutes for atropine solution but did not improve the times of 15 minutes for pilocarpine and physostigmine sulphate.— R. M. E. Richards and R. J. McBride, *J. Pharm. Pharmac.*, 1972, *24*, 145.

Phenethyl alcohol-resistant strains of *Ps. aeruginosa* were more sensitive to the actions of benzalkonium chloride, chlorhexidine acetate, and phenylmercuric nitrate than phenethyl alcohol-sensitive strains.— R. M. E. Richards and R. J. McBride, *J. pharm. Sci.*, 1972, *61*, 1075.

Proprietary Names and Manufacturers

The following names have been used for multi-ingredient preparations containing phenethyl alcohol—Ceanel Concentrate *(Quinoderm, UK)*.

6657-e

Phenoxyethanol *(BAN)*.

β-Phenoxyethyl Alcohol; Ethyleneglycol Monophenylether; Phenoxyaethanol. 2-Phenoxyethanol.

$C_8H_{10}O_2$=138.2.

CAS — 122-99-6.

Pharmacopoeias. In *Br.*

A colourless slightly viscous liquid with a faint pleasant odour.

Soluble 1 in 43 of water, 1 in 50 of arachis oil and of olive oil; miscible with acetone, alcohol, and glycerol.

Phenoxyethanol absorption by polyvinyl chloride.— M. G. Lee, *J. clin. Hosp. Pharm.*, 1984, *9*, 353.

Phenoxyethanol is effective against strains of *Pseudomonas aeruginosa* but is less effective against other Gram-negative and Gram-positive organisms. It has been used as a preservative at a concentration of 1%. A wider spectrum of antimicrobial activity is obtained with preservative mixtures of phenoxyethanol and hydroxybenzoates.

Phenoxyethanol may be used as a 2.2% solution or a 2% cream for the treatment of superficial wounds, burns, or abscesses infected by *Ps. aeruginosa*. In skin infections, derivatives of phenoxyethanol are used with either salicylic acid or zinc undecenoate.

A solution of phenoxyethanol 2% was more active than Resiguard or chlorhexidine gluconate against 5 different species of Gram-negative bacteria grown in urine. It was considered that chlorhexidine gluconate would not be effective for the prevention of infection and cross-infection in the urinary tract when Gram-negative organisms (especially *Providencia stuarti*) were involved; phenoxyethanol might be a suitable alternative but its lack of activity against Gram-positive organisms might necessitate its being used with another antibacterial agent.— B. Thomas *et al.*, *J. clin. Path.*, 1978, *31*, 929.

PRESERVATIVES FOR VACCINES. A review of different preservative systems compatible with 2 multiple component vaccines with particular reference to the combined use of phenoxyethanol, neomycin and streptomycin.— J. Cameron, *Develop. biol. Stand.*, 1974, *24*, 155.

Proprietary Preparations of Phenoxyethanol and Related Compounds

Phytocil *(Fisons, UK)*. *Cream*, 1-phenoxypropan-2-ol 2%, 2-*p*-chlorophenoxyethanol 1%, salicylic acid 1.5%, menthol 1%.

Powder, 1-phenoxypropan-2-ol 2%, 2-*p*-chlorophenoxyethanol 1%, zinc undecenoate 5.8%. For fungous infections of the skin.

Proprietary Names and Manufacturers of Phenoxyethanol and Related Compounds

Dermasept *(Stickley, Canad.)*; Lanohex *(Rougier, Canad.)*; Para-Chloro-Phenoxetol *(Nipa, UK)*; Phenoxetol *(Nipa, UK)*; Propylene Phenoxetol *(Nipa, UK)*.

6658-l

Phenylmercuric Acetate *(USAN)*.

Phenylhydrargyri Acetas; PMA. (Acetato)phenylmercury.

$C_8H_8HgO_2$=336.7.

CAS — 62-38-4.

Pharmacopoeias. In *Aust.* and *Ind.* Also in *U.S.N.F.*

A white or creamy-white, odourless, crystalline powder or small prisms or leaflets. *U.S.N.F.* **solubilities** are: soluble 1 in 180 of water, 1 in 225 of alcohol, 1 in 6.8 of chloroform, and 1 in 200 of ether; soluble in acetone. **Incompatibilities** as for phenylmercuric nitrate. **Store** in airtight containers. Protect from light.

6659-y

Phenylmercuric Borate *(BAN, rINN)*.

Hydrargyrum Phenyloboricum; Phenomerborum; Phenylhydrargyri Boras.

$C_6H_5HgOH, C_6H_5HgOB(OH)_2$ = 633.2 or $C_6H_5HgOH, C_6H_5HgBO_2$ = 615.2.

CAS — 8017-88-7 ($C_{12}H_{13}BHg_2O_4$); 6273-99-0 ($C_{12}H_{11}BHg_2O_3$); 102-98-7 ($C_6H_7BHgO_3$).

Pharmacopoeias. In *Aust.*, *Belg.*, *Br.*, *Cz.*, *Eur.*, *Fr.*, *Hung.*, *It.*, *Jug.*, *Neth.*, *Swiss*, and *Turk.*

A compound consisting of equimolecular proportions of phenylmercuric orthoborate and phenylmercuric hydroxide ($C_{12}H_{13}BHg_2O_4$) or of the dehydrated form (metaborate, $C_{12}H_{11}BHg_2O_3$) or a mixture of the two compounds.

Colourless shiny crystals or a white or slightly yellowish crystalline powder; odourless or almost odourless. Slightly **soluble** in water and in alcohol. **Incompatibilities** as for phenylmercuric nitrate. **Store** in well-closed containers. Protect from light.

6660-g

Phenylmercuric Nitrate *(BAN, USAN)*.

Basic Phenylmercury Nitrate; Nitrato Fenilmercúrico; Phenylhydrargyri Nitras; PMN. Nitratophenylmercury.

$C_6H_5HgOH,C_6H_5HgNO_3$=634.4.

CAS — 8003-05-2; 55-68-5 ($C_6H_5HgNO_3$).

Pharmacopoeias. In *Br.*, *Braz.*, *Egypt.*, *Fr.*, *Int.*, *Jug.*, *Nord.*, *Port.*, and *Turk.* Also in *U.S.N.F.* and *B.P. Vet.*

A mixture of phenylmercuric nitrate and phenylmercuric hydroxide.

White or yellowish-white, lustrous plates or a white, crystalline powder; odourless or almost odourless. *B.P.* **solubilities** are: very slightly soluble in water and alcohol; dissolves in glycerol and fixed oils. *U.S.N.F.* solubilities are: soluble 1 in 600 of water; slightly soluble in alcohol and glycerol; more soluble in the presence of nitric acid or alkali hydroxide.

Incompatible with halides with which it forms less soluble halogen compounds and with aluminium, iron, and other metals. It combines with amino acids and sulphides to form inactive derivatives; its activity may also be reduced in the presence of certain anionic compounds, edetates, and some thickening and suspending agents. Phenylmercuric nitrate is adsorbed from solution by rubber and polyethylene.

Store in airtight containers. Protect from light.

INCOMPATIBILITY. The antibacterial activity of phenylmercuric nitrate solutions was reduced by the addition of disodium edetate, and also by the addition of sodium thiosulphate.— R. M. E. Richards and J. M. E. Reary, *J. Pharm. Pharmac.*, 1972, *24*, *Suppl.*, 84P.

Study indicating that phenylmercuric acetate might be incompatible with sodium metabisulphite in autoclaved eye-drop preparations.— A. J. Collins *et al.*, *J. Pharm. Pharmac.*, 1985, *37*, *Suppl.*, 123P.

SORPTION. The losses by adsorption of phenylmercuric nitrate from 30 mL of 0.002% aqueous solution filtered through sintered glass, unglazed porcelain candle, asbestos pad, or membrane filter were 7.2, 100, 9, and 13% respectively. In 0.2M acetate buffer (pH 5.9) the respective losses were 2.3, 62, 11, and 3.3%. In aqueous solution with disodium edetate 0.1% the respective losses were 1.9, 77, 39, and 4%.— N. T. Naido *et al.*, *Aust. J. pharm. Sci.*, 1972, *1*, 16.

Bentonite and magnesium trisilicate reduced the antibacterial activity of phenylmercuric nitrate against *Staphylococcus aureus* by more than 60%, while tragacanth, starch, talc, and kaolin reduced it by more than 30%. The antibacterial activity of phenylmercuric nitrate was completely lost in the presence of aluminium magnesium silicate (Veegum).— R. T. Yousef *et al.*, *Can. J.*

pharm. Sci., 1973, *8*, 54. The concentration of a solution of phenylmercuric nitrate 0.002% decreased by over 40% when in contact with powders of colloidal silicon dioxide (Aerosil), light kaolin, magnesium trisilicate, starch, or titanium dioxide, with or without autoclaving.— N. R. Horn *et al.*, *Cosmet. Toilet.*, 1980, *95*, 69.

Low-density polyethylene containers were considered unsuitable for eye-drop formulations containing phenylmercuric acetate as a preservative. In all the formulations studied there was a significant loss of phenylmercuric acetate from solution by sorption through these containers to the atmosphere.— J. A. Aspinall *et al.*, *J. clin. Hosp. Pharm.*, 1980, *5*, 21. The sorption of phenylmercuric acetate by low-density polyethylene eye-drop bottles could be inhibited by the addition of phosphate ions to the solution.— J. E. Aspinall *et al.*, *ibid.*, 1983, *8*, 233.

Adverse Effects, Treatment, and Precautions

As for inorganic mercury p.1587. Phenylmercuric salts are irritant to the skin and may give rise to erythema and blistering. Hypersensitivity reactions have been reported. Topical application to eyes has been associated with mercurialentis and atypical band keratopathy; prolonged use of eye-drops containing phenylmercuric preservatives is not recommended.

The antimicrobial activity of phenylmercuric preservatives may be diminished through incompatibility interactions and adsorption (see above) with a resulting reduction in effectiveness.

EFFECTS ON THE EYE. Review of primary atypical band keratopathy associated with the use of eye-drops containing phenylmercuric nitrate.— R. E. Kennedy *et al.*, *Trans. Am. ophthal. Soc.*, 1974, *72*, 107.

Report on 31 patients who developed pigmentation of the anterior capsule of the lens (mercurialentis) after using eye-drops containing phenylmercuric preservatives for 3 to 15 years. The lens pigmentation did not appear to impair vision and its incidence was probably low; observed pigmentation was estimated to have occurred in approximately 6% of the patients who had used mercury-containing eye-drops for more than 6 years. The pigment appeared to be primarily of melanin derivation but might possibly contain minute amounts of mercury.— L. K. Garron *et al.*, *Trans. Am. ophthal. Soc.*, 1976, *74*, 295.

For a study into the penetration of organic mercurials into the eye, see Thiomersal, p.970.

PORPHYRIA. Mercury compounds were considered to be unsafe in patients with acute porphyria because they have been shown to be porphyrinogenic in *animals* or *in vitro* systems.— M.R. Moore and K.E.L. McColl, *Porphyrias, Drug Lists*, Glasgow, Porphyria Research Unit, University of Glasgow, 1987.

Uses.

Phenylmercuric salts have antibacterial and antifungal properties. They are primarily bacteriostatic compounds although they also have a slow bactericidal action. Their activity has been reported to be pH dependent.

Phenylmercuric compounds are used as preservatives in cosmetic, ophthalmic, or pharmaceutical preparations and as antiseptics. They have also been used as spermicides.

When employed as a preservative in eye-drops, a concentration of 0.002% is usually used; in injection solutions the concentration is 0.001%. For sterilisation by heating with a bactericide a concentration of 0.002% is required. As with all bactericides, they must **not** be used in solutions for intrathecal, intracisternal, peridural, or any other route of injection giving access to the cerebrospinal fluid; for intracardiac or intra-ocular injections; or for injections when a single dose is greater than 15 mL.

In the *UK* the use of phenylmercuric compounds as preservatives in cosmetics and toiletries is restricted by law.

For a reference to the ineffectiveness of phenylmercuric borate in equipment disinfection, see under Uses in Chlorine, p.958.

Preparations

Phenylmercuric Nitrate Gel *(A.P.F.)*. See under Tragacanth, p.1438.

Proprietary Names and Manufacturers of Phenylmercuric Compounds

Aderman *(Schulke & Mayr, Ger.)*; Exomycol *(Geigy, Arg.; Zyma-Galen, Belg.; Zyma, Ger.; Zyma, S.Afr.; Zyma, Switz.)*; Glycero-Merfen *(Zyma, Ger.; Zyma, Switz.)*; Gyne-Merfen *(Zyma, Ger.)*; Hydro-Mercuryl *(Streuli, Switz.)*; Hydro-Merfen *(Zyma, Ger.; Zyma, Switz.)*; Mercuryl-Orange *(Streuli, Switz.)*; Merfène *(Zyma, Fr.)*; Merfen *(Zyma-Galen, Belg.; Zyma, Ger.; Zyma, Switz.)*; Nylmerate *(Austral.; USA)*; Septiféne *(Syntex, Switz.)*; Spersasept *(Dispersa, Switz.)*; Volpar *(Duncan, Flockhart, UK)*.

10287-z

Potassium Benzoate *(USAN)*.

E212.

$C_6H_5.CO_2K$=160.2.

CAS — 582-25-2.

Pharmacopoeias. In *U.S.N.F.*

A white, odourless or practically odourless, granular or crystalline powder. **Soluble** 1 in 2 of water, 1 in 75 of alcohol, and 1 in 50 of alcohol 90%. **Store** in well-closed containers.

Potassium benzoate has the actions and uses of benzoic acid (p.1355). Its antimicrobial ativity is dependent on the concentration of undissociated benzoic acid achieved and it is not very effective above about pH 5.

For the estimated acceptable daily intake of potassium benzoate, see under Benzoic Acid, p.1356.

6663-s

Potassium Sorbate *(BAN, USAN)*.

E202. Potassium hexa-2,4-dienoate.

$C_6H_7KO_2$=150.2.

CAS — 590-00-1; 24634-61-5.

Pharmacopoeias. In *Br.* and *It.* Also in *U.S.N.F.* Some pharmacopoeias specify the *(E,E)*-hexa-2,4-dienoate.

White or creamy-white crystals or powder with a faint characteristic odour. *B.P.* solubilities are: **soluble** 1 in less than 1 of water and 1 in 70 of alcohol; very slightly soluble in acetone. *U.S.N.F.* solubilities are: soluble 1 in 4.5 of water and 1 in 35 of alcohol; very slightly soluble in chloroform and ether. **Store** at a temperature not exceeding 15° in airtight containers. Protect from light.

At acid pH, potassium sorbate has the actions and uses of sorbic acid p.1363. It has also been used for the temporary relief of minor vaginal itching and irritation as a 1% vaginal douche or 3% pessary.

For the estimated acceptable daily intake of potassium sorbate, see under Sorbic Acid, p.1364.

ANTIMICROBIAL ACTIVITY. Sorbate had previously been reported as inhibitory to *Clostridium botulinum* because it delayed or prevented spore germination but results indicated that potassium sorbate also inhibited the growth of vegetative cells of *C. botulinum in vitro* at concentrations proposed for use in cured meats.— J. C. Blocher and F. F. Busta, *J. Fd Sci.*, 1983, *48*, 574.

A study of the effect of dilution and temperature on the bactericidal activity of potassium sorbate against *Escherichia coli* determined that the concentration exponent was approximately 3 and the temperature coefficient (Q_{10}) was 2.3. These results indicated that the preservative capabilities of potassium sorbate could be seriously reduced on dilution but that an increase in temperature of 10° could approximately double its bactericidal activity.— P. Lusher *et al.*, *J. appl. Bact.*, 1984, *57*, 179.

Proprietary Names and Manufacturers

Sorbistat-K *(Pfizer, UK)*; Summer's Eve *(Fleet, USA)*.

6666-l

Sodium Benzoate *(BAN, USAN)*.

E211; Natrii Benzoas; Natrium Benzoicum; Sodii Benzoas.

$C_6H_5.CO_2Na$=144.1.

CAS — 532-32-1.

Pharmacopoeias. In *Arg., Aust., Belg., Br., Braz., Chin., Cz., Egypt., Eur., Fr., Hung., Ind., It., Jpn, Jug., Mex., Neth., Nord., Pol., Port., Roum., Rus., Span., Swiss,* and *Turk.* Also in *U.S.N.F.*

A white, odourless or practically odourless, granular or crystalline powder or flakes; slightly hygroscopic.

B.P. solubilities are: **soluble** 1 in 2 of water and 1 in 90 of alcohol. *U.S.N.F.* solubilities are: soluble 1 in 2 of water, 1 in 75 of alcohol, and 1 in 50 of alcohol 90%. **Incompatible** with ferric salts, calcium salts, and salts of heavy metals; its activity may be reduced in the presence of nonionic surfactants. **Store** in well-closed containers.

Sodium benzoate has the actions and uses of benzoic acid (p.1355). Its antimicrobial activity is dependent on the concentration of undissociated benzoic acid achieved and it is not very effective above about pH 5.

It has also been employed in a test of liver function.

For the estimated acceptable daily intake of sodium benzoate, see under Benzoic Acid, p.1356.

HYPERAMMONAEMIA. Children with inborn errors of urea synthesis such as deficiencies in carbamyl phosphate synthetase, ornithine transcarbamylase, or argininosuccinate synthetase accumulate ammonium and other nitrogenous precursors of urea which can result in fatal neonatal hyperammonaemic coma. Brusilow *et al.* (*Lancet*, 1979, *2*, 452) proposed that alternative endogenous pathways for the excretion of waste nitrogen might be exploited in these children and one possibility was that the administration of sodium benzoate might divert waste nitrogen from the defective urea pathway to hippuric acid synthesis and excretion. In a collaborative study by Batshaw *et al.* (*New Engl. J. Med.*, 1982, *306*, 1387) in 26 neonates with or at risk of developing hyperammonaemic coma due to an inborn error of urea synthesis, 61 of 64 post-neonatal episodes of hyperammonaemia were successfully controlled by intravenous arginine and sodium benzoate therapy and long-term maintenance treatment with arginine, sodium benzoate, and dietary protein modification appeared to prolong life and improve neurological outcome; 22 of the 26 infants were alive at ages ranging from 7 to 62 months. Further studies (M. Msall *et al.*, *New Engl. J. Med.*, 1984, *310* 1500; S.W. Brusilow *et al.*, *ibid.*, 1630) used sodium benzoate as an adjunct in the management of hyperammonaemia in children with inborn errors of urea synthesis and treatment protocols have been suggested (S.W. Brusilow *et al.*, *New Engl. J. Med.*, 1984, *310*, 1630; J.H. Walter and J.V. Leonard, *Br. J. Hosp. Med.*, 1987, *38*, 176). However Brusilow *et al.* (1984) concluded that the role of benzoate in neonatal hyperammonaemic coma or other hyperammonaemic states remained to be determined.

Bohan and Roe (*New Engl. J. Med.*, 1982, *307*, 1212) considered that although the use of benzoate for the treatment of primary hyperammonaemias due to congenital defects in the urea cycle seemed appropriate, sodium benzoate could be contra-indicated in several types of hyperammonaemia secondary to other metabolic disorders such as Reye's syndrome or propionic or methylmalonic acidaemia. However, the preliminary experience of Brusilow *et al.* (1984) suggested that treatment with benzoate was not deleterious in these diseases and might be of value in ameliorating hyperammonaemia though caution was indicated and further studies were required. Prompt initiation of aggressive haemodialysis and intravenous sodium benzoate and sodium phenylacetate infusion have been reported to control transient severe hyperammonaemia in an adult patient receiving therapy for relapse of leukaemia; 2 similar patients treated with haemodialysis alone died (A.J. Watson *et al.*, *Lancet*, 1985, *2*, 1271; Correction, *ibid.*, 1986, *1*, 112).

For the absorption and fate of sodium benzoate in 4 newborn infants with hyperammonaemia and recommendations on precautions, monitoring, and dosage adjustments, see under Benzoic Acid, p.1355.

NONKETOTIC HYPERGLYCINAEMIA. For a report of administration of strychnine as an adjunct to sodium benzoate in the treatment of nonketotic hyperglycinaemia, see Strychnine Sulphate, p.1449.

PREGNANCY AND THE NEONATE. For a comment on the inadvisability of using caffeine and sodium benzoate injection in neonates, see under Benzoic Acid, p.1355.

6669-z

Sodium Diacetate

E262. Sodium hydrogen diacetate.
$CH_3COONa,CH_3COOH(+xH_2O)$.

CAS — 126-96-5 (anhydrous).

Sodium diacetate is used as an inhibitor of moulds and rope-forming micro-organisms in bread.

Estimated acceptable daily intake of sodium diacetate: up to 15 mg per kg body-weight.— Seventeenth Report of the Joint FAO/WHO Expert Committee on Food Additives, *Tech. Rep. Ser. Wld Hlth Org. No. 539*, 1974.

6671-s

Sodium Formaldehyde Sulphoxylate

Sodium Formaldehyde Sulfoxylate *(USAN)*. Sodium hydroxymethanesulphinate dihydrate.
$CH_3NaO_3S,2H_2O$=154.1.

CAS — 149-44-0 (anhydrous); 6035-47-8 (dihydrate).

Pharmacopoeias. In *Fr.* Also in *U.S.N.F.*

White crystals or hard white masses with an alliaceous odour. The *U.S.N.F.* allows a suitable stabiliser, such as sodium carbonate.
Soluble 1 in 3.4 of water, 1 in 510 of alcohol, 1 in 175 of chloroform, and 1 in 180 of ether. A 2% solution in water has a pH of 9.5 to 10.5. **Store** in well-closed containers at 15° to 30°. Protect from light.

Sodium formaldehyde sulphoxylate is used as a preservative and antoxidant. It is used in the treatment of acute mercury poisoning (see p.1588).

6673-e

Sodium Metabisulphite *(BAN)*.

Disodium Pyrosulfite; Disodium Pyrosulphite; E223; E224 *(potassium metabisulphite)*; Natrii Pyrosulfis; Natrium Pyrosulfurosum; Sodium Metabisulfite *(USAN)*; Sodium Pyrosulphite.
$Na_2S_2O_5$=190.1.

CAS — 7681-57-4 (sodium metabisulphite); 7631-90-5 (sodium bisulphite); 16731-55-8 (potassium metabisulphite).

Pharmacopoeias. In *Aust., Belg., Br., Cz., Egypt., Hung., Ind., Int., Jpn, Jug., Neth., Nord.,* and *Turk.* Also in *U.S.N.F.* and *B.P. Vet.*
Jpn also includes Sodium Bisulfite ($NaHSO_3$ = 104.1), described as a mixture of sodium bisulphite and sodium metabisulphite. *Port. P.* and *Span. P.* have monographs for sodium bisulphite (Natrii Bisulfis, Bissulfito de Sódio, Natrii Sulphis Acidus) but this is probably the metabisulphite or a mixture of the bisulphite and the metabisulphite.
U.S.N.F. also includes Potassium Metabisulfite.

Colourless or white prismatic crystals or a white or yellowish crystalline powder. It has a sulphurous odour. On exposure to air and moisture, it is slowly oxidised to sulphate with disintegration of the crystals.
Soluble 1 in 2 of water; slightly soluble in alcohol; freely soluble in glycerol. A solution in water is acid to phenol red. **Store** at a temperature not exceeding 40° in well-filled airtight containers.

INCOMPATIBILITY. For the inactivation of cisplatin by sulphite antoxidants, see under Cisplatin, p.607.
For a study indicating that phenylmercuric acetate might be incompatible with sodium metabisulphite, see under Phenylmercuric Nitrate, p.1361.

Adverse Effects and Precautions

Gastric irritation due to liberation of sulphurous acid follows ingestion of sodium metabisulphite and other sulphites. Large doses of sulphites may cause gastro-intestinal upsets, respiratory or circulatory failure, and central nervous system disturbances. Concentrated solutions of salts of sulphurous acid are irritant to skin and mucous membranes.
Allergic reactions including anaphylaxis have occurred, particularly in patients with asthma, and deaths have been reported. Patients with a known sensitivity to sulphites should avoid sulphite-containing foods and drugs.
Treatment of foods with sulphites reduces their thiamine content.
In Great Britain the recommended exposure limit of sodium metabisulphite is 5 mg per m³ (long-term).

ALLERGY AND INTOLERANCE. Sulphites, including sulphur dioxide, sodium sulphite, potassium bisulphite, sodium bisulphite, potassium metabisulphite, and sodium metabisulphite may cause hypersensitivity reactions in some patients, particularly asthmatics. The most common reaction is bronchospasm but tachypnoea, dyspnoea, wheezing, tachycardia, dizziness, and weakness may occur. Severe flushing, urticaria, angioedema, tingling, pruritus, rhinitis, conjunctivitis, dysphagia, nausea, and diarrhoea have also been reported. Severe reactions have resulted in anaphylactic shock and loss of consciousness. Symptoms appear to be dose-related and generally occur less than 30 minutes after ingestion of sulphite-containing food or less than 5 minutes after inhalation or intravenous injection.— *Med. Lett.*, 1986, *28*, 74. Further reviews: M. F. Dalton-Bunnow, *Am. J. Hosp. Pharm.*, 1985, *42*, 2220; W. H. Yang and E. C. R. Purchase, *Can. med. Ass. J.*, 1985, *133*, 865.
In the *US*, from June 1987, a warning about possible allergic-type reactions, including anaphylaxis, was required in the physician package insert for prescription drugs to which sulphites had been added to the final dosage form.— *FDA Drug Bull.*, 1987, *17*, 2.
Individual reports of hypersensitivity reactions associated with sulphites: B. M. Prenner and J. J. Stevens, *Ann. Allergy*, 1976, *37*, 180 (ingested with foods); G. J. Baker *et al.*, *Med. J. Aust.*, 1981, *2*, 614 (ingested with foods and administered intravenously in a corticosteroid injection); F. J. Twarog and D. Y. M. Leung, *J. Am. med. Ass.*, 1982, *248*, 2030 (inhaled with isoetharine and administered intravenously in an injection of metoclopramide); A. S. Huang and W. M. Fraser (letter), *New Engl. J. Med.*, 1984, *311*, 542 (ingested with foods and administered in a local anaesthetic injection); J. W. Koepke *et al.*, *J. Am. med. Ass.*, 1984, *251*, 2982 (inhaled in a bronchodilator nebuliser solution).

CARCINOGENICITY. Although sulphiting agents may induce mutations in *bacteria*, *in vivo* mutagenicity studies in *mammals* were negative, as were long-term carcinogenicity studies on potassium and sodium metabisulphite in *mice* and *rats*, respectively.— Thirtieth Report of the Joint FAO/WHO Expert Committee on Food Additives, *Tech. Rep. Ser. Wld Hlth Org. No. 751*, 1987.

Absorption and Fate

Sulphites and metabisulphites are oxidised in the body to sulphate and excreted in the urine.

Uses.

Sodium metabisulphite is a strong reducing agent and is used as an antoxidant in pharmaceutical preparations usually in a concentration of 0.1% though concentrations of 0.01% to 1% have been employed. It decomposes in air, especially on heating and injections containing sodium metabisulphite may therefore be filled into containers in which the air has been replaced by an inert gas such as nitrogen before heat sterilisation. Since it may react with the rubber caps used to close multidose containers, the caps should be pretreated with sodium metabisulphite solution.
Sodium metabisulphite also has an antimicrobial action which is greatest at acid pH due to the increased presence of sulphur dioxide and sulphurous acid liberated by reaction between the metabisulphite and the acid. It may be used as a preservative in acidic solutions and syrups.
Sodium metabisulphite is used in the food industry as an antoxidant, antimicrobial preservative, and anti-browning agent. It is also used in wine-making as an antimicrobial preservative, antoxidant, clarifier, and equipment cleanser; for this purpose sodium metabisulphite is widely available as Campden Tablets.
At concentrations above about 500 ppm, sodium metabisulphite imparts a noticeable taste to preparations.
Other sulphites including potassium bisulphite, sodium bisulphite, potassium metabisulphite, and sodium sulphite (below) have been used similarly.

Confirmation of the previously allocated acceptable daily intake (ADI) for sulphur dioxide and sulphites of up to 700 µg per kg body-weight (expressed as sulphur dioxide). This ADI covered sodium and potassium metabisulphite, sodium sulphite, potassium and sodium bisulphite, and sodium thiosulphate but could not be extended to calcium metabisulphite as no specifications were available (Twenty-seventh Report of the Joint FAO/WHO Expert Committee on Food Additives, *Tech. Rep. Ser. Wld Hlth Org. No. 696*, 1983). However the ADI was extended to include potassium sulphite (Twenty-ninth Report of the Joint FAO/WHO Expert Committee on Food Additives, *Tech. Rep. Ser. Wld Hlth Org. No. 733*, 1986). A further review of this ADI gave particular consideration to sulphite-related adverse effects such as bronchoconstriction and anaphylactic-type reactions. The Committee noted that these sensitivity reactions to sulphiting agents had been life-threatening in some cases and that several deaths associated with sulphite-treated foods had been reported. While recognising the utility and versatility of sulphiting agents as food additives, they recommended that, where possible, suitable alternative methods of preservation should be encouraged, particularly when the use of sulphites might lead to high levels of acute exposure such as in the control of enzymatic browning of fresh salad vegetables. The estimated ADI for sulphur dioxide and sulphites was retained but the Committee recommended that the frequency of idiosyncratic adverse reactions and the relative toxicity of free and bound sulphur dioxide should be kept under review (Thirtieth Report of the Joint FAO/WHO Expert Committee on Food Additives, *Tech. Rep. Ser. Wld Hlth Org. No. 751*, 1987).
For the effect of sodium metabisulphite on adrenaline degradation, see under Adrenaline Acid Tartrate, p.1454.

6678-c

Anhydrous Sodium Sulphite *(BAN)*.

Exsiccated Sodium Sulphite; E221; Natrii Sulfis Siccatus; Natrii Sulphis; Sodium Sulfite; Sulfito Dissódico Sêco.
Na_2SO_3=126.0.

CAS — 7757-83-7; 10102-15-5 (heptahydrate).

Pharmacopoeias. In *Br., Fr., Jpn,* and *Span. Port.* includes the heptahydrate.

A white odourless or almost odourless crystalline powder. **Soluble** in water; practically insoluble in alcohol. **Store** in well-closed containers.

Sodium sulphite is an antoxidant and antimicrobial preservative with actions and uses similar to those of sodium metabisulphite (above); it may be preferred to sodium metabisulphite for alkaline preparations.

For the estimated acceptable daily intake of sulphur dioxide and sulphites including sodium sulphite, see under Sodium Metabisulphite, above.

6679-k

Sorbic Acid *(BAN, USAN)*.

Acidum Sorbicum; E200. Hexa-2,4-dienoic acid.
$C_6H_8O_2$=112.1.

CAS — 110-44-1; 22500-92-1.

Pharmacopoeias. In *Aust., Belg., Br., Cz.,* and *Jug.* Also in *U.S.N.F.* Some pharmacopoeias specify the (*E,E*)-hexa-2,4-dienoic acid.

A free-flowing, white or creamy-white, crystalline powder with a faint characteristic odour. *B.P.* solubilities are: slightly **soluble** in water and in fats and fatty oils; soluble 1 in 10 of alcohol and

1 in 20 of ether. *U.S.N.F.* solubilities are: soluble 1 in 1000 of water, 1 in 10 of alcohol, 1 in 8 of dehydrated alcohol, 1 in 15 of chloroform, 1 in 30 of ether, 1 in 8 of methyl alcohol, and 1 in 19 of propylene glycol. **Store** at a temperature not exceeding 15° in airtight containers. Protect from light.

Studies on the stability and antimicrobial effectiveness of sorbic acid solutions with respect to packaging and temperature: T. J. McCarthy, *Pharm. Weekbl. Ned.*, 1972, *107*, 1; T. J. McCarthy *et al.*, *Cosmet. Perfum.*, 1973, *88*, (May), 43.

Adverse Effects and Precautions

Sorbic acid can be irritant to the eyes and mucous membranes. It is a weak sensitiser but has occasionally been implicated as causing contact urticaria.

ALLERGY AND INTOLERANCE. A patient with psoriasis on her hands and feet developed erythema, soreness, and pruritus in these areas within 12 hours of applying Unguentum Merck Ointment. The only ingredient of this ointment to give an allergic type of reaction to patch tests was sorbic acid.— E. M. Saihan and R. R. M. Harman, *Br. J. Derm.*, 1978, *99*, 583.

The reaction of buccal mucosa to 20 minute patch tests with sorbic acid was studied in 11 subjects. Aqueous solutions of sorbic acid 0.1 and 1.0% elicited no mucosal reaction; a 5% solution caused slight erythema in 2 patients; a 10% solution resulted in erythema in all patients with a greyish-white macular mucosal reaction in 5 and slight signs of urticaria in 1. These findings supported the clinical impression that sorbic acid used as a preservative in relevant concentrations was not urticariogenic or otherwise harmful to the oral mucosa.— O. J. Clemmensen and M. Schiødt, *Contact Dermatitis*, 1982, *8*, 341.

Uses.

Sorbic acid has antibacterial and antifungal properties particularly against moulds and yeasts. As the most active form is the undissociated acid, it is more effective at a pH of 4 or below; it is relatively ineffective above about pH 6.5.

It is used as a preservative in pharmaceutical and cosmetic preparations such as ointments and creams at a usual concentration of 0.1 to 0.2%. It is also used in concentrations of up to 0.2% as a preservative in food.

Its salts, potassium sorbate (p.1362) and to a lesser extent calcium sorbate and sodium sorbate are commonly preferred because of their greater solubility in water.

Estimated sum acceptable daily intake for sorbic acid, calcium sorbate, and potassium sorbate: up to 25 mg per kg body-weight (expressed as sorbic acid).— Seventeenth Report of the Joint FAO/WHO Expert Committee on Food Additives, *Tech. Rep. Ser. Wld Hlth Org. No. 539*, 1974. Extended to cover sodium sorbate.— Twenty-ninth Report of the Joint FAO/WHO Expert Committee on Food Additives, *Tech. Rep. Ser. Wld Hlth Org. No. 733*, 1986.

ANTIMICROBIAL ACTIVITY. Study to determine the minimum inhibitory concentration of sorbic acid at different pH levels for various micro-organisms. Sensitivity to sorbic acid and the dependency on pH varied among the organisms tested. Nevertheless, for all the micro-organisms studied, dissociated acid had some antimicrobial effect and although this effect was much less than for undissociated acid, it became appreciable with increasing pH.— T. Eklund, *J. appl. Bact.*, 1983, *54*, 383.

Proprietary Names and Manufacturers

Sorbistat *(Pfizer, UK).*

6680-w

Sulphur Dioxide

E220; Sulfur Dioxide *(USAN)*.
SO_2=64.06.

CAS — 7446-09-5.

Pharmacopoeias. In *U.S.N.F.*

A colourless non-inflammable gas with a strong suffocating odour characteristic of burning sulphur. It condenses readily under pressure to a colourless liquid which boils at about −10° and has a wt per mL of about 1.5 g.

Soluble 36 in 1 of water and 114 in 1 of alcohol by vol. at 20° and normal pressure; soluble in chloroform and ether. **Store** in cylinders. It is usually packaged under pressure in liquid form.

Adverse Effects and Precautions

Sulphur dioxide gas is highly irritant to the eyes, skin, and mucous membranes. Inhalation results in irritation of the respiratory tract which may lead to bronchoconstriction and pulmonary oedema; very high concentrations may cause respiratory arrest and asphyxia. Contact with liquid sulphur dioxide results in acid burns.

Sulphiting agents containing active sulphur dioxide may cause allergic reactions including anaphylaxis, particularly in patients with asthma.

Treatment of foods with sulphur dioxide reduces their thiamine content.

In Great Britain the recommended exposure limits of sulphur dioxide are 2 ppm (long-term) and 5 ppm (short-term). In the US the permissible and recommended exposure limits are 13 mg per m^3 and 1.3 mg per m^3 respectively.

AIR POLLUTION. Assessment of the health effects of atmospheric sulphur oxides and particulate matter.— J. H. Ware *et al.*, *Environ. Health Perspect.*, 1981, *41*, 255.

A study of the long-term effects of chronic exposure to sulphur dioxide in employees of a sulphite pulp factory and paper mill concluded that sulphur dioxide and other irritating gases might contribute to the development of chronic bronchitis, particularly in smokers, but the disease was usually the less severe form, without chronic airways obstruction.— N. Stjernberg *et al.*, *Bull. int. Un. Tuberc.*, 1984, *59*, 43. See also N. Stjernberg *et al.*, *Eur. J. resp. Dis.*, 1985, *67*, 41.

ALLERGY AND INTOLERANCE. For reviews and reports of hypersensitivity reactions associated with sulphites including sulphur dioxide, see under Sodium Metabisulphite, p.1363.

Uses.

Sulphur dioxide has antoxidant and antimicrobial properties and is used as a preservative for food. Its sulphite salts have similar properties (see under Sodium Metabisulphite, p.1363).

Sulphur dioxide dissolves in water at low pH to yield sulphurous acid and bisulphite and sulphite ions; the antimicrobial activity of this solution is maximal at a pH of less than 4.

Sulphur dioxide has also been used as a fumigant and to disinfect equipment in the wine and food industries.

For the estimated acceptable daily intake of sulphur dioxide and sulphites, see under Sodium Metabisulphite, p.1363.

9873-x

Tertiary Butylhydroquinone

TBHQ. 2-*tert*-butylhydroquinone.
$C_{10}H_{14}O_2$=166.2.

Tertiary butylhydroquinone is an antoxidant used in foods.

Evidence that tertiary butylhydroquinone may have antimicrobial as well as antoxidant activity.— J. J. Zeelie and T. J. McCarthy, *Cosmet. Toilet.*, 1982, *97*, 61.

A temporary estimated acceptable daily intake for tertiary butylhydroquinone of up to 200 µg per kg body-weight was established.— Thirtieth Report of the Joint FAO/WHO Expert Committee on Food Additives, *Tech. Rep. Ser. Wld Hlth Org. No. 751*, 1987.

Proprietary Names and Manufacturers

Embanox 101 *(May & Baker, UK)*; Embanox TBHQ *(May & Baker, UK)*; Tenox 20 *(Eastman, UK)*; Tenox 20A *(Eastman, UK)*; Tenox TBHQ *(Eastman, UK)*.

The following names have been used for multi-ingredient preparations containing tertiary butylhydroquinone— Embanox 102 *(May & Baker, UK)*; Embanox 106 *(May & Baker, UK)*; Tenox 22 *(Eastman, UK)*; Tenox 26 *(Eastman, UK)*; Tenox 27 *(Eastman, UK)*.

Prostaglandins

8070-d

'Prostaglandin' was the name given by von Euler to a substance found in extracts and secretions from the human prostate gland and seminal vesicles which greatly lowered the blood pressure after injection into animals and stimulated the isolated intestine and uterus. There is now known to be an extensive family of prostaglandins and related compounds which are involved in many different biological functions. The prostaglandins, along with thromboxanes and leukotrienes are all derived from 20-carbon polyunsaturated fatty acids and are collectively termed eicosanoids. In man, the most common precursor is arachidonic acid (eicosatetraenoic acid) whereas eicosapentaenoic acid is a predominant precursor in fish and marine animals.

Arachidonic acid is released from cell-membrane phospholipids by the enzyme phospholipase A_2 and is then rapidly metabolised by two distinct pathways, one involving the enzyme cyclo-oxygenase (prostaglandin synthetase) and the other involving lipoxygenases. The prostaglandins, thromboxanes, and prostacyclin (sometimes collectively termed prostanoids) all contain ring structures and are products of arachidonic-acid oxidation by cyclo-oxygenase, an enzyme widely distributed in cell membranes. The leukotrienes are products of the lipoxygenase pathway (see below). The initial step in the cyclo-oxygenase pathway is the formation of cyclic endoperoxides prostaglandin G_2 (PGG_2) and prostaglandin H_2 (PGH_2). Prostaglandin H_2 is then converted to the primary prostaglandins prostaglandin D_2, prostaglandin E_2, and prostaglandin $F_{2\alpha}$, to thromboxane A_2 (TXA_2) via the enzyme thromboxane synthetase, or to prostacyclin (PGI_2) via the enzyme prostacyclin synthetase. These products are further metabolised and rapidly inactivated in the body. The secondary prostaglandins, prostaglandin A_2 (PGA_2), prostaglandin B_2 (PGB_2), and prostaglandin C_2 (PGC_2) are derived from prostaglandin E_2, but are formed during extraction and probably do not occur biologically.

The prostaglandins are all derivatives of the carbon skeleton 7-(2-octylcyclopentyl)heptanoic acid (also known as prostanoic acid). All natural prostaglandins have a double bond at position 1,2 and a hydroxyl group at position 3 of the octyl side-chain. Depending on the structure of the cyclopentane ring, the main series of prostaglandins are distinguished by the letters A, B, C, D, E, and F; the members of each series are distinguished by subscript numbers which indicate degrees of unsaturation in the side-chains—hence, those derived from eicosatrienoic acid(dihomo-γ-linolenic acid) have the subscript 1, those derived from arachidonic acid have the subscript 2, and those derived from eicosapentaenoic acid have the subscript 3, according to the degree of unsaturation of these precursors. In man, only prostaglandins of the '2' series appear to be of physiological importance. Thromboxane A_2 has an oxane rather than a cyclopentane ring; it is chemically unstable and breaks down to thromboxane B_2. Prostacyclin has a double-ring structure and breaks down to 6-keto-prostaglandin $F_{1\alpha}$.

Endogenous prostaglandins are autacoids; they can be formed by virtually all tissues and cells in response to a variety of stimuli, produce a wide range of effects, and are involved in the regulation of virtually all biological functions. Prostaglandins appear to act through various receptor-mediated mechanisms. Some of their effects are mediated within cells by activation or inhibition of adenylate cyclase and the regulation of cyclic adenosine monophosphate production. At one time prostaglandin E_2 and prostaglandin $F_{2\alpha}$ were thought to be of paramount importance, but with the discovery of thromboxane A_2, prostacyclin, and the leukotrienes it was realised that these primary prostaglandins belong to a large family of physiologically active eicosanoids. Thromboxane A_2 induces platelet aggregation and constricts arterial smooth muscle whereas prostacyclin causes vasodilatation and prevents platelet aggregation; the balance between these opposing actions has an important role in the regulation of intravascular platelet aggregation and thrombus formation. The leukotrienes are important mediators of inflammation.

The pharmacological properties of prostaglandins are wide-ranging and include contraction or relaxation of smooth muscle in the blood vessels, bronchi, uterus, and gastro-intestinal tract; inhibition of gastric acid secretion; and effects on platelet aggregation, the endocrine system, and metabolic processes.

Individual prostaglandins vary greatly in their activities and potencies; their actions also depend on the animal species and the tissues in which they are acting, and entirely opposite actions may be elicited with very small structural changes in the molecule. Some of the important effects of individual prostaglandins are: vasodilatation by prostaglandins of the E and A series; vasoconstriction by prostaglandin $F_{2\alpha}$ and prostaglandin D_2; bronchodilatation by prostaglandin E_5; bronchoconstriction by prostaglandin $F_{2\alpha}$ and prostaglandin D_2; uterine stimulation by prostaglandin E_2 and prostaglandin $F_{2\alpha}$; inhibition of gastric acid secretion by prostaglandin E_5 and prostaglandin A_5; and inhibition of platelet aggregation by prostaglandin E_1 and prostaglandin D_2.

Uses of prostaglandins. The diverse clinical applications of prostaglandins reflect their wide-ranging physiological and pharmacological properties. Synthetic analogues have been developed with the aim of obtaining compounds which are more stable, have a longer duration of action, and a more specific effect.

Prostaglandins used as uterine stimulants in obstetrics and gynaecology include: dinoprost (prostaglandin $F_{2\alpha}$)(p.1368) and its analogue carboprost (p.1367); dinoprostone (prostaglandin E_2) (p.1370) and its analogues meteneprost (p.1374) and sulprostone (p.1375); and gemeprost (p.1373), an analogue of prostaglandin E_1. Synthetic analogues of prostaglandin $F_{2\alpha}$ are used as luteolytic agents in veterinary medicine.

Prostaglandins used as vasodilators and inhibitors of platelet aggregation include: alprostadil (prostaglandin E_1) (p.1366) and epoprostenol (prostacyclin)(p.1371) and its analogues ciprostene (p.1367) and iloprost (p.1374).

Prostaglandins used as inhibitors of gastric acid secretion and to protect the gastro-intestinal mucosa include the prostaglandin E_1 analogue misoprostol (p.1374) and the prostaglandin E_2 analogues arbaprostil (p.1367) and enprostil (p.1370).

Inhibition of endogenous prostaglandins also has potential therapeutic applications. The mode of action and many of the adverse effects of anti-inflammatory analgesics such as aspirin or indomethacin have been found to depend on their inhibition of cyclo-oxygenase and hence of endogenous prostaglandin synthesis; they do not inhibit lipoxygenases and an increase in leukotriene synthesis has been suggested as a mechanism for aspirin-induced asthma. For the prophylaxis of thrombosis, attempts have been made to exploit their ability to inhibit thromboxane A_2 but avoid their associated ability to inhibit prostacyclin, with the aim of reducing inappropriate coagulation within vessel walls; specific thromboxane synthetase inhibitors such as dazoxiben are under study.

General reviews of endogenous prostaglandins: S. Moncada and J. R. Vane, *New Engl. J. Med.*, 1979, *300*, 1142 (arachidonic-acid metabolites and interactions between platelets and blood-vessel walls); M. A. Crawford, *Br. med. Bull.*, 1983, *39*, 210 (essential fatty acids and their prostanoid derivatives); Y. S. Bakhle, *ibid.*, 214 (synthesis and catabolism of cyclo-oxygenase products); G. J. Blackwell and R. J. Flower, *ibid.*, 260 (inhibition of phospholipase); G. A. Higgs and J. R. Vane, *ibid.*, 265 (cyclo-oxygenase and lipoxygenase inhibition and the potential of dual inhibitors); E. N. Wardle, *Br. J. Hosp. Med.*, 1985, *34*, 229 (structure and action); P. J. Barnes, *ibid.*, 339 (role in asthma); C. J. Hawkey and D. S. Rampton, *Gastroenterology*, 1985, *89*, 1162 (role in the gastro-intestinal mucosa); A. S. Nies, *Clin. Pharmac. Ther.*, 1986, *39*, 481 (control of the circulation); *Lancet*, 1986, *1*, 301 (role in the adult respiratory distress syndrome).

Proceedings of a symposium on arachidonic acid metabolism, the process of inflammation, and therapeutic implications.— *Drugs*, 1987, *33*, *Suppl.* 1, 1–66.

2932-v

Leukotrienes

Leukotrienes belong to the family of endogenous substances termed eicosanoids (see Prostaglandins, above). They are straight-chain derivatives of the oxidation of arachidonic acid by lipoxygenases. In the most important pathway, arachidonic acid is oxidised by 5-lipoxygenase to the hydroperoxide 5-hydroperoxyeicosatetraenoic acid (5-HPETE) which is then converted to 5-hydroxyeicosatetraenoic acid (5-HETE) or to leukotriene A_4 (LTA_4); leukotriene A_4 may be transformed to leukotriene B_4 (LTB_4) or to (leukotriene C_4 (LTC_4), and leukotriene C_4 to leukotriene D_4 (LTD_4), leukotriene E_4 (LTE_4), and leukotriene F_4 (LTF_4). Other lipoxygenases identified include 12-lipoxygenase and 15-lipoxygenase which form 12-hydroxyeicosatetraenoic acid (12-HETE) and 15-hydroxyeicosatetraenoic acid (15-HETE) respectively; 15-HETE is a major product of arachidonic-acid metabolism in the lung.

Leukotrienes may be synthesised from fatty acids other than arachidonic acid; those derived from eicosatrienoic acid have the subscript 3, those derived from arachidonic acid have the subscript 4, and those derived from eicosapentaenoic acid have the subscript 5. They were originally discovered in leucocytes, but synthesis has since been demonstrated in other cells and tissues including macrophages, mast cells in the lung, and vascular tissue.

Like prostaglandins, the leukotrienes are autacoids with potent local mediator actions. They have an important role in inflammatory and allergic processes and are involved in the pathophysiology of asthma. Leukotriene B_4 is a potent chemotactic agent which induces the migration of leucocytes. The slow-reacting substance of anaphylaxis (SRS-A) is now known to be a mixture of leukotriene C_4, leukotriene D_4, and leukotriene E_4, all of which are potent bronchoconstrictors. With increasing knowledge of the role of leukotrienes, specific antagonists or inhibitors of leukotriene synthesis are being sought for use in the treatment of asthma and inflammatory diseases. High doses of anti-inflammatory corticosteroids are known to interfere with the synthesis of prostaglandins and leukotrienes by inhibiting the release of arachidonic acid from phospholipids; other dual inhibitors such as BW-755C are under study.

General reviews of leukotrienes: G. W. Taylor and H. R. Morris, *Br. med. Bull.*, 1983, *39*, 219 (lipoxygenase pathways); M. A. Bray, *ibid.*, 249 (leukotriene B_4); P. J. Piper, *ibid.*, 255 (pharmacology); G. J. Blackwell and R.

J. Flower, *ibid.*, 260 (inhibition of phospholipase); G. A. Higgs and J. R. Vane, *ibid.*, 265 (cyclo-oxygenase and lipoxygenase inhibition and the potential of dual inhibitors); G. A. Higgs and S. Moncada, *Drugs*, 1985, *30*, 1 (pathophysiology and the potential for drug development); P. J. Barnes, *Br. J. Hosp. Med.*, 1985, *34*, 339 (role in asthma); N. Wardle, *ibid.*, 1986, *35*, 382 (pharmacology).

18611-g

Alfaprostol *(BAN, USAN, rINN).*
K-11941; Ro-22-9000. Methyl (*Z*)-7-{(1*R*,2*S*,3*R*,5*S*)-2-[(3*S*)-5-cyclohexyl-3-hydroxypent-1-ynyl]-3,5-dihydroxycyclopentyl}hept-5-enoate.
$C_{24}H_{38}O_5$=406.6.

CAS — 74176-31-1.

Alfaprostol is a synthetic analogue of dinoprost (prostaglandin $F_{2\alpha}$). It is used as a luteolytic agent in veterinary medicine.

Proprietary Veterinary Names and Manufacturers
Alfavet *(Roche, USA).*

8071-n

Alprostadil *(BAN, USAN, rINN).*

PGE$_1$; Prostaglandin E$_1$; U-10136. (*E*)-(8*R*,11*R*,12*R*,15*S*)-11,15-Dihydroxy-9-oxoprost-13-enoic acid; 7-{(1*R*,2*R*,3*R*)-3-Hydroxy-2-[(*E*)-(3*S*)-3-hydroxyoct-1-enyl]-5-oxocyclopentyl}heptanoic acid.
$C_{20}H_{34}O_5$=354.5.

CAS — 745-65-3.

NOTE. In *Martindale* the term alprostadil is used for the exogenous form and prostaglandin E$_1$ for the endogenous form.

Pharmacopoeias. In *U.S.*

A white to off-white crystalline powder. M.p. about 110°.**Soluble** in water; freely soluble in alcohol; soluble in acetone; very slightly soluble in chloroform and ether; slightly soluble in ethyl acetate.**Store** between 2° and 8° in airtight containers.

CAUTION. Great care should be taken to prevent inhaling particles of alprostadil and exposing the skin to it.

Adverse Effects and Precautions

The adverse effects reported most commonly in infants with congenital heart disease treated with alprostadil are apnoea, fever, flushing, hypotension, bradycardia, tachycardia, and convulsions. Other adverse effects reported include diarrhoea, oedema, cardiac arrest, hypokalaemia, disseminated intravascular coagulation, and cortical proliferation of the long bones.

Adverse effects reported in adults given alprostadil have included headache, flushing, hypotension, nausea, diarrhoea, and pain and inflammation at the infusion site.

Alprostadil should be avoided in neonates with hyaline membrane disease and should be used with caution in those with bleeding tendencies; blood pressure and respiratory status should be monitored during infusion.

A review of the incidence of side-effects in 492 infants with critical congenital heart disease treated with alprostadil at 56 centres in the *US* over a 3-year period. At least one intercurrent medical event was reported in 213 infants (43%) during therapy, but only 49% of these reactions were believed to be related to or probably related to alprostadil administration. *Cardiovascular events* (cutaneous vasodilatation or oedema, rhythm or conduction disturbances, and hypotension) occurred in 90 infants (18%) and were thought to be related to alprostadil in 54% of occurrences. Intra-aortic infusion of alprostadil, used more commonly in cyanotic infants, was associated with a significantly greater incidence of cutaneous dilatation than the intravenous route; although reversed by repositioning the catheter, intravenous infusion was considered preferable. Cardiovascular effects were more likely in infants of less than 2 kg birth-weight or when the duration of infusion exceeded 48 hours. *Central nervous system events* (seizure-like activity, temperature elevation, irritability, or lethargy) occurred in 81 infants (16%) and were more frequent when the duration of infusion exceeded 48 hours. *Respiratory depression* (apnoea or hypoventilation), the most worrying side-effect, occurred in 58 infants (12%) and was thought to be related to alprostadil in 68% of occurrences. It was significantly more common in cyanotic infants and those weighing less than 2 kg at birth and was the most common reason for discontinuing infusion of alprostadil. Assisted ventilation should be readily available before initiating therapy with alprostadil. *Metabolic abnormalities* (hypoglycaemia or hypocalcaemia) occurred in 12 infants. *Gastro-intestinal disturbances* also occurred in 12. Diarrhoea was the most common disturbance; necrotising enterocolitis and hyperbilirubinaemia were isolated occurrences. *Infections*(sepsis or wound infections) in 12 infants, *haematological abnormalities*(haemorrhage, disseminated intravascular coagulation, and thrombocytopenia) in 9, and *renal failure* or *insufficiency* in 9 were generally not considered to be related to alprostadil infusion. There was insufficient data to confirm earlier reports of histological changes in the ductus arteriosus wall (A.C. Gittenberger-De Groot *et al.*, *Br. Heart J.*, 1978, *40*, 215) and in the small pulmonary arteries (S.G. Haworth *et al.*, *ibid.*, 1980, *43*, 306).— A. B. Lewis *et al.*, *Circulation*, 1981, *64*, 893.

EFFECTS ON BONES. Bone lesions resembling cortical hyperostosis occurred in 2 infants following long-term therapy with alprostadil for cyanotic congenital heart disease.— K. Ueda *et al.*, *J. Pediat.*, 1980, *97*, 834. An infant who developed generalised exuberant periostitis after long-term alprostadil infusion prompted a retrospective review of 30 neonates treated with alprostadil. Radiographic signs of periosteal reactions were present in 5, including the index patient in whom reactions were first noted on the 50th day of treatment. However, even short courses of therapy could produce distinct signs of periostitis; 3 developed relatively mild periosteal changes in the ribs after infusions ranging from 9 to 205 hours and one had involvement of the left femur after infusion for 71 hours. Complete resolution had occurred in most of the bones 6 to 12 months later.— R. E. Ringel *et al.*, *J. Pediat.*, 1983, *103*, 251.

EFFECTS ON THE METABOLISM. Severe hyperglycaemia with apparent ketoacidosis occurred during infusion with alprostadil postoperatively in the infant of a diabetic mother. The manufacturers have received reports of hyperglycaemia associated with alprostadil in 5 infants, one of whom had a diabetic mother.— M. H. Cohen and M. R. Nihill, *Pediatrics*, 1983, *71*, 842 (for a report of hypoglycaemia, see above).

INFECTION. Four of 25 neonates with cyanotic congenital heart disease who received alprostadil developed a significant wound infection compared with none of 13 similar neonates not given alprostadil. All infants were on the same prophylactic antibiotic regimen.— W. H. Fleming *et al.*, *Chest*, 1984, *85*, 241.

Absorption and Fate

Following infusion alprostadil is rapidly metabolised during passage through the pulmonary circulation. Metabolites are excreted in the urine within about 24 hours.

Uses and Administration

Alprostadil is a prostaglandin which causes vasodilatation and prevents platelet aggregation. The endogenous substance is termed prostaglandin E$_1$. It is used to maintain the patency of the ductus arteriosus in neonates with congenital heart disease until surgery is possible. It is administered by continuous intravenous infusion beginning with doses of 100 nanograms per kg body-weight per minute; doses should be reduced as soon as possible. Some workers recommend a lower starting dose. Alprostadil has also been tried in peripheral vascular disease.

CARDIOVASCULAR DISORDERS. *Congenital heart disease.* The physiological role of prostaglandins in the foetal and neonatal circulation are discussed in reviews of ductus arteriosus-dependent congenital heart disease and its management (M.A. Heymann and R.I. Clyman, *Pharmacotherapy*, 1982, *2*, 148; E.D. Silove, *Archs Dis. Childh.*, 1986, *61*, 827). Prostaglandins, especially prostaglandin E$_2$, are probably involved in maintaining the ductus arteriosus in a dilated state during normal foetal life. Prostacyclin has also been shown to dilate the ductus, but is less active than prostaglandin E$_2$. At birth the placental source of prostaglandin E$_2$ is lost and the rise in blood-oxygen tension is thought to trigger closure of the ductus. However, in some conditions the oxygen stimulus does not seem to operate fully. In congenital right heart obstructive lesions the ductus arteriosus often closes despite severe hypoxaemia and prostaglandins of the E type have been used to maintain ductus patency prior to surgery. Conversely, the ductus may remain patent in premature infants despite normal blood-oxygen tension and inhibitors of prostaglandin synthesis, notably indomethacin, have been given to encourage ductus constriction.

Alprostadil by intra-arterial or intravenous infusion was generally beneficial in a multicentre study involving 492 infants with ductus arteriosus-dependent congenital heart disease (M.D. Freed *et al.*, *Circulation*, 1981, *64*, 899); 385 had diminished effective pulmonary flow due to cyanotic congenital heart disease, including pulmonary atresia, pulmonary stenosis, tricuspid atresia, and transposition of the great arteries, and the remainder had reduced systemic blood flow associated with aortic arch anomalies. In infants with cyanotic disease oxygenation improved dramatically in those younger than 4 days and with an initial PaO$_2$ of less than 30 mmHg. Alprostadil infusion was recommended for this group of infants, starting with 50 ng per kg body-weight per minute, preferably intravenously, and halving the dose once stable improvement is achieved; it should be used more cautiously in older infants and those with a PaO$_2$ greater than 30 mmHg. In infants with acyanotic disease age was not so critical, but time to maximal response ranged from 15 minutes to 11 hours compared to within 30 minutes for cyanotic infants.

Most reports have referred to infants given prostaglandins after establishing a diagnosis, but 52 neonates with suspected major ductus-dependent cardiac defects were given alprostadil into a peripheral vein (K.A. Hallidie-Smith, *Archs Dis. Childh.*, 1984, *59*, 1020) in order to establish a safe and effective regimen that could be used before diagnosis was confirmed. Doses of 5 to 10 ng per kg per minute were found to be effective and free from serious side-effects and it was suggested that treatment should begin with doses of 1 to 10 ng per kg per minute, increased if necessary once the infant has been assessed in a specialised unit.

Many reports have emphasised the use of infusions of alprostadil or dinoprostone for just a few hours prior to emergency surgery. However, long-term administration of dinoprostone by mouth to allow growth of the infants and their pulmonary arteries before surgery has been successful (E.D. Silove *et al.*, *Archs Dis. Childh.*, 1985, *60*, 1025; E.D. Silove, *ibid.*, 1986, *61*, 827).

Ischaemic heart disease. A review of the role of prostaglandins in ischaemic heart disease. Alprostadil has a similar haemodynamic profile to epoprostenol, but is a less potent platelet inhibitor. When given to patients with acute myocardial infarction haemodynamic effects have been similar to those following intravenous glyceryl trinitrate or nitroprusside therapy.— B. Pitt *et al.*, *Ann. intern. Med.*, 1983, *99*, 83.

Alprostadil infused into a central vein at a rate of 5 to 30 ng per kg body-weight per minute for 24 to 72 hours reduced the frequency and/or severity of episodes of rest angina in 16 of 19 patients with an unstable acute ischaemic syndrome.— R. J. Siegel *et al.*, *Am. Heart J.*, 1984, *108*, 863.

Peripheral vascular disease. In a discussion on prostaglandins in peripheral vascular disease (*Lancet*, 1983,*1*, 1199) it was noted that intra-arterial alprostadil had been of benefit, but epoprostenol was considered to be more convenient since, unlike alprostadil, it is not metabolised in the lung and can therefore be effective when given intravenously. Commenting on this Kyle and Hazleman (*ibid.*, *2*, 282) stressed that although 90% of alprostadil is inactivated on first passage through the pulmonary vascular bed it can, like epoprostenol, produce peripheral vasodilatation when administered intravenously. Appreciable symptomatic improvement occurred in 25 of 26 patients with severe Raynaud's phenomenon of varying aetiology given alprostadil by infusion into a central vein for 72 hours at a rate of 6 to 10 ng per kg body-weight per minute (P.C. Clifford *et al.*, *Br. med. J.*, 1980, *281*, 1031); 21 reported maintained improvement after 2 weeks. Subjective benefit was also claimed by 6 of 8 patients with Raynaud's phenomenon secondary to progressive systemic sclerosis given similar intravenous infusions of alprostadil (M.F.R. Martin and J.E. Tooke *ibid.*, 1982, *285*, 1688). However, no significant improvement was seen in double-blind studies comparing alprostadil by intravenous infusion with placebo in 30 patients with lower limb ischaemia due to atherosclerotic occlusive disease (G.S. Telles *et al.*, *Br. J. Surg.*, 1984, *71*, 506) and 55 patients with Raynaud's syndrome (J.S. Mohrland *et al.*, *Ann. rheum. Dis.*, 1985, *44*, 754).

RENAL DISORDERS. Renal function was improved by the intravenous infusion of alprostadil in 7 patients with chronic glomerulonephritis, one with mixed connective tissue disease (T. Niwa *et al.*, *Lancet*, 1982, *1*, 687), and one with rapidly progressive glomerulonephritis (T. Niwa *et al.*, *New Engl. J. Med.*, 1983, *308*, 969).

RESPIRATORY DISORDERS. Evidence that alprostadil may be a useful therapeutic adjunct in adult respiratory distress syndrome. When alprostadil was infused at a rate of up to 30 ng per kg body-weight per minute in surgical patients with severe adult respiratory distress syndrome vasodilatation occurred in the pulmonary and systemic circulations; pulmonary artery pressure and pulmonary vascular resistance were decreased and cardiac index, oxygen delivery, oxygen consumption, and subsequently PaO_2 were increased.— W. C. Shoemaker and P. L. Appel, *Surgery, St Louis*, 1986, *99*, 275. Further promising results in patients with adult respiratory distress syndrome given alprostadil for up to 7 days in a double-blind study. Alprostadil was infused through a central venous catheter or through the right atrial port of a pulmonary arterial catheter at a starting dose of 5 ng per kg per minute, gradually increased over 3 hours to 30 ng per kg per minute. Only 2 of 21 patients given alprostadil died with severe pulmonary failure compared with 9 of 20 patients given placebo. Survival at 30 days after the end of the infusion was significantly better in those patients who received alprostadil, although there was no significant improvement in overall survival.— J. W. Holcroft *et al.*, *Ann. Surg.*, 1986, *203*, 371.

Preparations

Alprostadil Injection *(U.S.P.)*

Proprietary Preparations

Prostin VR *(Upjohn, UK)*. *Injection*, for intravenous infusion, alprostadil 500 µg/mL, in dehydrated alcohol, in ampoules of 1 mL; to be diluted before use.

Proprietary Names and Manufacturers

Minprog *(Upjohn, Ger.)*; Prostavasin *(Schwarz, Ger.)*; Prostin VR *(Upjohn, Austral.; Upjohn, Canad.; Upjohn, S.Afr.; Upjohn, UK; Upjohn, USA)*; Prostine VR *(Upjohn, Fr.)*; Prostivas *(Upjohn, Swed.)*.

8072-h

Arbaprostil *(USAN, rINN)*.
15(*R*)-15-Methylprostaglandin E_2; 15-Me-PGE_2; Methyldinoprostone; U-42842. (5*Z*,13*E*)-(8*R*,11*R*,12*R*,15*R*)-11,15-Dihydroxy-15-methyl-9-oxoprosta-5,13-dienoic acid; (*Z*)-7-{(1*R*,2*R*,3*R*)-3-Hydroxy-2-[(*E*)-(3*R*)-3-hydroxy-3-methyloct-1-enyl]-5-oxocyclopentyl}hept-5-enoic acid.
$C_{21}H_{34}O_5$=366.5.

CAS — 55028-70-1.

8073-m

Arbaprostil Methyl *(rINNM)*.
U-38833. The methyl ester of arbaprostil.
$C_{22}H_{36}O_5$=380.5.

Arbaprostil, a synthetic analogue of dinoprostone (prostaglandin E_2), inhibits gastric acid secretion. It has actions and uses similar to those of misoprostol (p.1374) and has been given by mouth in the treatment of peptic ulcer. The methyl ester of arbaprostil has also been used.

GASTRO-INTESTINAL DISORDERS. An early study with arbaprostil methyl and 15(*S*)-15-methylprostaglandin E_2 methyl ester (U-35960) indicated that they inhibited gastric acid secretion and promoted healing of gastroduodenal ulcers when given by mouth (K. Gibiński *et al.*, *Gut*, 1977, *18*, 636); the 15(*S*)-isomer appeared to be more potent. The same workers (J. Rybicka and K. Gibiński, *Scand. J. Gastroenterol.*, 1978, *13*, 155) subsequently reported that arbaprostil methyl, the methyl ester of the 15(*S*)-isomer, and dimethyldinoprostone (16,16-dimethylprostaglandin E_2) accelerated the healing of duodenal ulcers, but not of gastric ulcers. In a study involving 173 patients (G. Vantrappen *et al.*, Gastroenterology, 1982, *83*, 357), duodenal ulcers were healed in 55 of 82 patients given arbaprostil 100 µg four times daily for 4 weeks and in 35 of 91 given placebo; diarrhoea occurred in 31 patients receiving arbaprostil. There is evidence that arbaprostil will protect the gastric mucosa against the erosive effects of aspirin (D.A. Gilbert *et al.*, *Gastroenterology*, 1984, *86*, 339), but acute bleeding from ulcerative lesions in the stomach or duodenum was not controlled by arbaprostil 50 µg by mouth every 6 hours for up to 7 days when compared with placebo in 81 patients (K. Lauritsen *et al.*, *Br. med. J.*, 1985, *291*, 1093).

For reviews on prostaglandin analogues in the treatment of peptic ulcer and discussion on their reputed cytoprotective properties, see Misoprostol, p.1374.

OBSTETRICS AND GYNAECOLOGY. References to the use of 15(*S*)-15-methylprostaglandin E_2 and its methyl ester for termination of pregnancy: S. M. Karim and S. S. Ratnam (letter), *Br. med. J.*, 1974, *4*, 161; W. E. Brenner *et al.*, *Fert. Steril.*, 1975, *26*, 369; S. M. M. Karim *et al.*, *Singapore J. Obstet. Gynaec.*, 1980, *11*, 7.

Proprietary Names and Manufacturers

Upjohn, USA.

8074-b

Carboprost *(BAN, USAN, rINN)*.
15(*S*)-15-Methylprostaglandin $F_{2\alpha}$; 15-Me-$PGF_{2\alpha}$; Methyldinoprost; U-32921. (5*Z*,13*E*)-(8*R*,9*S*,11*R*,12*R*-,15*S*)-9,11,15-Trihydroxy-15-methylprosta-5,13-dienoic acid; (*Z*)-7-{(1*R*,2*R*,3*R*,5*S*)-3,5-Dihydroxy-2-[(*E*)-(3*S*)-3-hydroxy-3-methyloct-1-enyl]cyclopentyl}hept-5-enoic acid.
$C_{21}H_{36}O_5$=368.5.

CAS — 35700-23-3.

8075-v

Carboprost Methyl *(BANM, USAN, rINNM)*.
U-36384. The methyl ester of carboprost.
$C_{22}H_{38}O_5$=382.5.

CAS — 35700-21-1.

8076-g

Carboprost Trometamol *(BANM, rINNM)*.
Carboprost Tromethamine *(USAN)*; U-32921E.
A compound of carboprost with trometamol in a ratio of 1:1.
$C_{21}H_{36}O_5,C_4H_{11}NO_3$=489.6.

CAS — 58551-69-2.

Pharmacopoeias. In *U.S.*

Carboprost trometamol 1.3 µg is approximately equivalent to 1 µg of carboprost. **Store** at −20° to −10°. Aqueous solutions for injection have a pH of 7.0 to 8.0; they should be stored at 2° to 8°.

CAUTION. Great care should be taken to prevent inhaling particles of carboprost trometamol and exposing the skin to it.

Adverse Effects and Precautions

As for Dinoprost, p.1368.

Uses and Administration

Carboprost is a synthetic 15-methyl analogue of dinoprost (prostaglandin $F_{2\alpha}$). It is a uterine stimulant with a more prolonged action than dinoprost; the presence of the methyl group delays inactivation by enzymic dehydrogenation.

Carboprost is used for the termination of pregnancy. It is administered intramuscularly as the trometamol salt and vaginally as the methyl ester. For the termination of midtrimester pregnancy (between the 13th and 20th weeks of gestation) the equivalent of 250 µg is given by intramuscular injection and repeated every 1½ to 3½ hours depending on the uterine response; if necessary the dose may be increased to 500 µg, but the total dose given should not exceed 12 mg of carboprost. If preferred a test dose of 100 µg may be given initially.

Carboprost methyl has been given as vaginal pessaries for menstrual induction and termination of pregnancy in the second trimester.

OBSTETRICS AND GYNAECOLOGY. *Postpartum haemorrhage.* Severe postpartum haemorrhage due to uterine atony was controlled successfully by carboprost in 44 of 51 patients unresponsive to conventional therapy with oxytocin, methylergometrine, and manual uterine massage. Carboprost 250 µg was generally injected intramuscularly and repeated at intervals of 1.5 hours or longer up to a maximum of 5 repeated injections; an average of 1.6 injections was required. Side-effects were infrequent and mild. Of 6 patients who received carboprost by intramyometrial injection, 2 responded to a single injection and 3 responded to a second injection.— R. H. Hayashi *et al.*, *Obstet. Gynec.*, 1984, *63*, 806.

Termination of pregnancy. Carboprost methyl given vaginally has been tried in a variety of dosage regimens for termination of pregnancy in the second trimester and menstrual induction in early pregnancy. Abortion occurred within 24 hours in 88.4% of patients at 13 to 20 weeks' gestation given vaginal pessaries containing carboprost methyl 1.5 mg every 3 hours for up to 24 hours; abortion was complete in 49.9% and the most common side-effects were vomiting and diarrhoea (M. Bygdeman *et al.*, *Contraception*, 1977, *16*, 175). Menstrual induction in early pregnancy has been achieved following administration of a single vaginal pessary containing 2, 2.5, or 3 mg of carboprost methyl (K. Green *et al.*, *ibid.*, 1978, *18*, 551); Spilman *et al.* (*ibid.*, 1980, *21*, 353) also reported a successful outcome in 56 of 80 women given a 3-mg pessary, but they suggested that a vaginal delivery system that releases the drug faster and more predictably is required. A controlled-release vaginal delivery system containing carboprost methyl has been used successfully for menses induction in patients with amenorrhoea of up to 49 days' duration (M. Bygdeman *et al.*, *ibid.*, 1983, *27*, 141) and they considered it to be superior to vaginal pessaries; in addition abortion was achieved in some patients in the second trimester of pregnancy. Carboprost 0.5 mg given in a vaginal pessary has also been effective in ripening the cervix prior to termination of pregnancy in the first trimester (F.Arias, *Am. J. Obstet. Gynec.*, 1984, *149*, 100).

Further references: G. Tsalacopoulos *et al.*, *S. Afr. med. J.*, 1982, *61*, 822 (intramuscular administration for termination of midtrimester pregnancy); *idem*, 825 (intramuscular or extra-amniotic administration for intra-uterine foetal death); *idem*, 828 (intramuscular route for missed abortion).

See also under Dinoprost, p.1369.

Preparations

Carboprost Tromethamine Injection *(U.S.P.)*. A sterile aqueous solution of carboprost trometamol.

Proprietary Names and Manufacturers

Prostin/15M *(Upjohn, Canad.; Upjohn, USA)*; Prostinfenem *(Upjohn, Swed.)*.

18972-p

Ciprostene Calcium *(USAN, pINNM)*.
9β-Methyl Carbacyclin Calcium; 9β-Methylcarbacyclin Calcium; U-61431F. Calcium (*Z*)-(3a*S*,5*R*,6*R*,6a*R*)-hexahydro-5-hydroxy-6-[(*E*)-(3*S*)-3-hydroxy-1-octenyl]-3a-methyl-$\Delta^2(1H)$,δ-pentalenevalerate.
$(C_{22}H_{35}O_4)_2Ca$=767.1.

CAS — 81845-44-5 (ciprostene); 81703-55-1 (ciprostene calcium).

Ciprostene, a vasodilator and platelet aggregation inhibitor, is a stable analogue of the prostaglandin epoprostenol (p.1371) and has similar actions and uses. The calcium salt has been given by intravenous infusion.

References: J. O'Grady *et al.*, *Br. J. clin. Pharmac.*, 1984, *18*, 921 (pharmacology of ciprostene compared with epoprostenol); R. D. Hughes *et al.*, *J. Pharm. Pharmac.*, 1986, *38*, 63 (potential of ciprostene to prevent platelet losses during charcoal haemoperfusion); O. I. Linet *et al.*, *J. clin. Pharmac.*, 1986, *26*, 131 (tolerance and pharmacology of ciprostene).

Proprietary Names and Manufacturers

Wellcome, UK; Upjohn, USA.

8077-q

Cloprostenol Sodium *(BANM, USAN, rINNM)*.
ICI-80996. Sodium (±)-(*Z*)-7-{(1*R*,2*R*,3*R*,5*S*)-2-[(*E*)-(3*R*)-4-(3-chlorophenoxy)-3-hydroxybut-1-enyl]-3,5-dihydroxycyclopentyl}hept-5-enoate.
$C_{22}H_{28}ClNaO_6$=446.9.

CAS — 40665-92-7 (cloprostenol); 55028-72-3 (sodium salt).

Pharmacopoeias. In *B.P. Vet.*

A white or almost white amorphous hygroscopic powder.

Freely **soluble** in water, alcohol, and methyl alcohol; practically insoluble in acetone. Solutions are **sterilised** by autoclaving. **Store** in airtight containers. Protect from light.

CAUTION. Cloprostenol sodium is extremely potent and extra-ordinary care should be taken in any procedure in which it is used.

Cloprostenol sodium is a synthetic analogue of dinoprost (prostaglandin $F_{2\alpha}$). It is used as a luteolytic agent in veterinary medicine.

Proprietary Veterinary Names and Manufacturers
Estrumate *(Coopers Animal Health, UK)*; Planate *(Coopers Animal Health, UK)*.

2931-b

Dinoprost *(BAN, USAN, rINN)*.

$PGF_{2\alpha}$; Prostaglandin $F_{2\alpha}$; U-14583. (5*Z*,13*E*)-(8*R*,9*S*,11*R*,12*R*,15*S*)-9,11,15-Trihydroxyprosta-5,13-dienoic acid; (*Z*)-7-{(1*R*,2*R*,3*R*,5*S*)-3,5-Dihydroxy-2-[(*E*)-(3*S*)-3-hydroxyoct-1-enyl]cyclopentyl}hept-5-enoic acid.
$C_{20}H_{34}O_5$=354.5.

CAS — 537-11-1; 551-11-1.

NOTE. In *Martindale* the term dinoprost is used for the exogenous form and prostaglandin $F_{2\alpha}$ for the endogenous form.

8081-m

Dinoprost Trometamol *(BANM, rINNM)*.

Dinoprost Tromethamine *(USAN)*; $PGF_{2\alpha}$ THAM; Prostaglandin $F_{2\alpha}$ Trometamol; U-14583E. A compound of dinoprost with trometamol in a ratio of 1:1.
$C_{20}H_{34}O_5,C_4H_{11}NO_3$=475.6.

CAS — 38562-01-5.

Pharmacopoeias. In *U.S.*

A white to off-white crystalline powder. Dinoprost trometamol 1.3 µg is approximately equivalent to 1 µg of dinoprost. Very **soluble** in water; slightly soluble in chloroform; freely soluble in dimethylformamide; soluble in methyl alcohol. Aqueous solutions for injection have a pH of 7.0 to 9.0. **Store** in airtight containers.

CAUTION. Great care should be taken to prevent inhaling particles of dinoprost trometamol and exposing the skin to it.

Adverse Effects

The incidence and severity of adverse reactions to dinoprost are dose-related and also depend to some extent on the route of administration; the intravenous route has been associated with a high incidence of adverse effects. Nausea, vomiting, and diarrhoea are common. Transient cardiovascular symptoms have included flushing, shivering, headache, dizziness, and hypotension; there have been rare reports of sudden cardiovascular collapse. Convulsions and EEG changes have also occurred rarely. Local tissue irritation and erythema may follow intravenous administration; the erythema disappears 2 to 5 hours after infusion. Temporary pyrexia and raised white cell count may occur but generally revert to normal after termination of the infusion. Local infection may follow intra- or extra-amniotic therapy. Excessive uterine activity may occur and there have been occasional reports of uterine rupture following the use of prostaglandins to terminate pregnancy or induce labour; foetal distress and, rarely, foetal death have occurred during the induction of labour.

Dinoprost can cause bronchoconstriction and bronchospasm with wheezing and dyspnoea has occurred, especially in asthmatic patients.

Side-effects were evaluated in 626 patients undergoing abortion (usually in the second trimester), using extra-amniotic or intra-amniotic dinoprost or dinoprostone, often with oxytocin. Vomiting occurred in 291, diarrhoea in 28, pyrexia in 34, transient hypotension (fall in systolic blood pressure of at least 20 mmHg) in 25, transient bronchospasm in 2 patients given extra-amniotic dinoprost, and blood loss exceeding 250 mL in 68 (38 lost more than 500 mL). There were no convulsions even though 8 patients were epileptics receiving anticonvulsant therapy. Three patients sustained lacerations to the cervix. Five patients complained of breast soreness or lactation; these symptoms may have been under-reported. Overall 14 patients were re-admitted; 13 because of excessive vaginal bleeding and 1 because of pelvic infection.— I. Z. MacKenzie *et al.*, *Br. med. J.*, 1974, *4*, 683.

EFFECTS ON THE BLOOD. In 12 patients in the second trimester of pregnancy, in whom abortion was induced by the extra-amniotic infusion of dinoprost, the prothrombin time was significantly decreased and the concentrations of factors V, VIII, and X were significantly increased. These coagulation changes were probably related to physiological changes occurring in the second trimester; in susceptible patients abortion after the first trimester might give rise to defective haemostasis or thrombo-embolism.— M. H. H. Badraoui *et al.*, *Br. med. J.*, 1973, *1*, 19. Coagulation changes in 29 women during dinoprost-induced abortion (intra- or extra-amniotic, intravenous, or vaginal) were less than those which occurred with hypertonic sodium chloride solution.— *idem*, *4*, 375. There were signs of disseminated intravascular coagulation in 9 women given dinoprostone intra-amniotically with hypertonic urea for second-trimester abortion, a less pronounced effect in 9 given dinoprostone with hypertonic glucose, and no signs of coagulation changes in 9 given dinoprostone alone.— I. Z. MacKenzie *et al.*, *Lancet*, 1975, *2*, 1066.

EFFECTS ON THE CARDIOVASCULAR SYSTEM. Sudden cardiovascular collapse and eventual death in 2 women following the use of dinoprost intra-amniotically to induce abortion at approximately 16 weeks' gestation. Burt *et al.* (*Obstet. Gynec.*, 1977, *50*, *Suppl.*, 45S) previously reported a serious cardiac arrhythmia associated with the intra-amniotic instillation of dinoprost, which they attributed to hypokalaemia. However, the aetiology of the collapse and arrhythmia in these 2 women is unclear. In the 9 known deaths following the use of dinoprost to induce abortion, sudden collapse within minutes of instillation is the only fatal cause to have occurred more than once.— W. Cates and H. V. F. Jordaan, *Am. J. Obstet. Gynec.*, 1979, *133*, 398.

Reports of severe cardiovascular reactions associated with the use of dinoprostone: J. P. Phelan *et al.*, *Am. J. Obstet. Gynec.*, 1978, *132*, 28 (dramatic pyrexial and cardiovascular reactions resembling endotoxic shock in 2 women given dinoprostone intravaginally to induce labour following intra-uterine foetal death); S. P. Patterson *et al.*, *Obstet. Gynec.*, 1979, *54*, 123 (fatal cardiac arrest about 25 days after dinoprostone intravaginally for late abortion following intra-uterine foetal death); I. T. Cameron and D. T. Baird (letter), *Lancet*, 1984, *2*, 1046 (sudden collapse following dinoprostone intra-amniotically for termination of pregnancy in the second trimester).

EFFECTS ON THE FOETUS. Intra-uterine foetal death occurred in 2 high-risk pregnancies following insertion into the extra-amniotic space of dinoprost 10 mg in Tylose gel to ripen the cervix.— M. A. Quinn and A. J. Murphy, *Br. J. Obstet. Gynaec.*, 1981, *88*, 650. A report of placental abruption and neonatal death following the administration of a 3 mg dinoprostone vaginal pessary for the induction of labour. No foetal deaths have been reported previously in 10 studies involving 2012 women given dinoprostone vaginally or extra-amniotically for the induction of labour.— K. Simmons and W. Savage, *ibid.*, 1984, *91*, 598.

A woman who failed to abort despite receiving carboprost intravaginally 7 weeks after conception gave birth at term to an infant with hydrocephalus and abnormal digits.— F. S. Collins and M. J. Mahoney, *J. Pediat.*, 1983, *102*, 620.

EFFECTS ON THE LIVER. A study involving 739 infants indicated that neonatal jaundice after labour induced or stimulated by dinoprostone or oxytocin is associated primarily with foetal maturity and not with the drugs used.— A. P. Lange *et al.*, *Lancet*, 1982, *1*, 991.

EFFECTS ON THE NERVOUS SYSTEM. Convulsions occurred in 5 of 320 women who were given dinoprost intra-amniotically for the termination of pregnancy during the second trimester. EEG changes were noted in 4 of 8 patients after dinoprost was administered.— R. C. Lyneham *et al.*, *Lancet*, 1973, *2*, 1003. An absence of convulsions in other large series of patients given dinoprost or dinoprostone.— I. Z. MacKenzie *et al.* (letter), *ibid.*, 1323; M. Thiery *et al.* (letter), *ibid.*, 1974, *1*, 218; I. S. Fraser and C. Gray (letter), *ibid.*, 360.

EFFECTS ON THE UTERUS. Uterine rupture has been reported following the termination of pregnancy with dinoprost given intra-amniotically (S.M.M. Karim and S.S. Ratnam, *Br. med. J.*, 1974, *4*, 161); dinoprostone given intra-amniotically (I.S. Fraser, *ibid.*, 404), intravenously (A.M.Smith, *ibid.*, 1975, *1*, 205), or extra-amniotically (A.I. Traub and J.W.K. Ritchie, *ibid.*, 1979, *2*, 496); and carboprost given intramuscularly (I. Vergote *et al.*, *Lancet*, 1982, *2*, 1402). Vergote *et al.* noted that uterine rupture was not always suspected, but should be considered if established uterine contractions disappear or there is vaginal blood loss without concomitant progressive dilatation. Rupture has also followed the use of dinoprostone pessaries for the induction of labour (P. Claman *et al.*, *Am. J. Obstet. Gynec.*, 1984, *150*, 889; F. Keller and T.H. Joyce, *Can. Anaesth. Soc. J.*, 1984, *31*, 80); rupture of a uterine scar occurred in 2 patients (D.R. Bromham and R.S. Anderson, *Lancet*, 1980, *2*, 485). Larsen *et al.* (*S. Afr. med. J.*, 1984, *65*, 615) have also reported complications following the use of dinoprostone to induce labour; one patient given dinoprostone by mouth developed severe postpartum haemorrhage due to uterine rupture and died and another given dinoprostone vaginally was found to have a ruptured uterus following delivery of a stillborn infant. They considered that induction of labour with dinoprostone was not safer than carefully controlled oxytocin infusion with amniotomy and recommended restricting the vaginal dose of dinoprostone in grand multiparas to 3 mg if the cervix is unripe, to 2 mg if the cervix is ripe, and advise that administration should not be repeated for at least 24 hours.

OVERDOSAGE. Severe adverse effects have been attributed to inappropriate systemic absorption of prostaglandins. Ross and Whitehouse (*Br. med. J.*, 1974, *1*, 642) reported rigors, vomiting, severe abdominal pain, and an intense desire to urinate and defaecate in 3 patients given dinoprostone intra-amniotically, together with urea in 2, for mid-trimester abortion; one patient had peripheral vasoconstriction and a rapid low-volume pulse, with hypotension, and another had peripheral cyanosis. Craft and Bowen-Simpkins (*ibid.*, *2*, 446) attributed these symptoms to a relatively large dose of prostaglandin rapidly reaching the systemic circulation, possibly as a result of displacement of the needle or cannula and Karim (*ibid.*, *3*, 347) suggested that prior administration of urea would increase the rate of absorption of prostaglandins from the amniotic cavity. In a further report (R. Brown, *ibid.*, *2*, 382), flushing, severe headache, and nausea immediately after a test dose of dinoprost 2.5 mg was also thought to be due to incorrect positioning of the needle in the amniotic cavity with consequent injection into the systemic circulation; Karim (*ibid.*, *3*, 347) suggested that at least part of the dose had been injected into the peritoneal cavity.

Severe reactions have also been reported with prostaglandins given to abort hydatidiform moles. A 20-year-old woman given 20 mg of dinoprostone by injection into the uterine cavity developed profound hypotension, bradycardia, and rigors, followed by nausea, vomiting, suprapubic pain, an increased pulse-rate, pyrexia, and generalised flushing (A.M. Smith, *ibid.*, *2*, 382). Karim (*ibid.*, *3*, 347) pointed out that because of the absence of foetal membranes in a molar pregnancy, intra-uterine administration was similar to extra-amniotic administration and the dose used had been 100 times higher than the usual extra-amniotic dose. However, in a similar patient (E.McNicol and H. Gray, *Br. J. Obstet. Gynaec.*, 1977, *84*, 229) 'extra-amniotic' instillation of dinoprostone 200 µg was followed immediately by nausea, retching, severe abdominal pain, dizziness, difficulty in breathing and the production of frothy blood-stained sputum, an imperceptible pulse, and hypotension; since there is no extra-amniotic space in a hydatidiform mole the dinoprostone had probably been injected directly into the maternal circulation.

Precautions

Dinoprost should not be given to patients in whom oxytocic drugs (see Oxytocin, p.1146) are generally contra-indicated, or where prolonged contractions of the uterus are considered inappropriate, as, for example, in patients with a history of Caesarean section or major uterine surgery, where major degrees of cephalopelvic disproportion may be present, where foetal malpresentation is present, where there is suspicion of foetal distress, where there is a history of difficult labour or traumatic delivery, in grand multiparae with 6 or more previous term pregnancies, or in those with a history of pelvic inflammatory disease.

Since prostaglandins enhance the effects of oxytocin use of the 2 agents together or in sequence should be carefully monitored. Dinoprost should be used with caution in patients with glaucoma or raised intra-ocular pressure, asthma or a history of asthma, epilepsy, or cardiovascular disease.

In the induction of labour cephalopelvic relationships should be carefully evaluated before use. During infusion uterine activity, foetal status, and the progress of cervical dilatation should be carefully monitored to detect adverse responses, such as hypertonus, sustained uterine contractions, or foetal distress. In patients with a history of hypertonic uterine contractility or tetanic uterine contractions, uterine activity and the state of the foetus should be continuously monitored throughout labour. Where high-tone myometrial contractions are sustained the possibility of uterine rupture should be considered.

In the therapeutic termination of pregnancy, foetal damage has been observed in cases of incomplete termination and the appropriate treatment for complete evacuation of the uterus should therefore be instituted whenever termination is incomplete. Dinoprost should not be used for termination in patients with pelvic infection, unless adequate treatment has already been started.

ADMINISTRATION. For the hazards of unintentional systemic absorption of prostaglandins following their intra-uterine administration for the termination of pregnancy and abortion of hydatidiform moles, see Overdosage in Adverse Effects.

EFFECTS ON THE FOETUS. Four of 9 patients who received dinoprost intravenously in early pregnancy did not abort and curettage specimens showed histological damage.— A. C. Wentz and G. S. Jones, *Fert. Steril.*, 1973, *24*, 569.

INTERACTIONS. Marked hypertension, vomiting, and severe dyspnoea occurred following the sequential administration of oxytocin, methylergometrine, and dinoprost within the space of 10 minutes to a woman with postpartum haemorrhage.— S. Cohen *et al.*, *N.Y. St. J. Med.*, 1983, *83*, 1060.

Uses and Administration

Dinoprost is a prostaglandin of the F series (see p.1365) with actions on smooth muscle; the endogenous substance is termed prostaglandin $F_{2\alpha}$ and is rapidly metabolised in the body. It induces contraction of uterine muscle at any stage of pregnancy and is reported to act predominantly as a vasoconstrictor on blood vessels and as a bronchoconstrictor on bronchial muscle. Dinoprost is used principally for the termination of pregnancy; it may also be used for missed abortion, hydatidiform mole, induction of labour, and foetal death *in utero*.

Dinoprost is usually administered intra-amniotically. It may be given intravenously, but this route has been associated with a high incidence of adverse effects and is generally only used for missed abortion or hydatidiform mole. Dinoprost is given as the trometamol salt, doses being expressed in terms of the equivalent amount of dinoprost. It should not be administered continuously for more than two days.

For the termination of pregnancy during the second trimester 40 mg of dinoprost is administered intra-amniotically by slowly injecting 8 mL of a solution containing 5 mg per mL into the amniotic sac.

Dinoprost has also been given by intravenous infusion for the termination of pregnancy, missed abortion, or hydatidiform mole, a solution containing 50 µg per mL of dinoprost being infused at a rate of 25 µg per minute for at least 30 minutes, then maintained or increased to 50 µg per minute according to response and maintained at this rate for at least 4 hours before increasing further.

For the induction of labour dinoprost has been given intravenously but is no longer recommended for routine use by most authorities. A suggested intravenous dosage regimen has been 2.5 µg per minute infused as a solution containing 15 µg per mL for at least 30 minutes and then maintained or increased according to the patient's response; in foetal death *in utero* higher doses may be required and an initial rate of 5 µg per minute has been used with increases at intervals of not less than 1 hour.

OBSTETRICS AND GYNAECOLOGY. Prostaglandins have a major role in reproduction, including the control of parturition, but of those occurring naturally only prostaglandin E_2 (PGE_2) and prostaglandin $F_{2\alpha}$ ($PGF_{2\alpha}$) are clinically important. They are strikingly uterotonic, PGE_2 being about five times more potent a stimulant of uterine contractions than $PGF_{2\alpha}$, and also soften and ripen the uterine cervix. Prostaglandins also have a possible role as luteolytic agents since they are known to inhibit the corpus luteum and prevent the production of progesterone in *animals*. Therapeutic uses include prelabour cervical priming as well as induction of labour, termination of first and second trimester pregnancy, and management of abnormal pregnancy. The prostaglandins were first used clinically by intravenous infusion, but this route has generally been superseded by oral, intramuscular, intra-uterine (extra-amniotic or intra-amniotic), and vaginal administration since it became apparent that intravenous administration caused unpleasant side-effects, notably vomiting and diarrhoea, especially in the high concentration needed for abortion.— M. P. Embrey, *Br. med. J.*, 1981, *283*, 1563.

Further reviews: S. M. M. Karim, *Ann. Acad. Med. Singapore*, 1982, *11*, 493.

Induction of labour. In 1981 Embrey (*Br. med. J.*, 1981, *283*, 1563) noted that in early studies prostaglandins given intravenously had been effective for the induction of labour, but no more so than oxytocin except when the cervix was unripe. Early fears that prostaglandins would produce hypertonus and foetal distress more often than oxytocin had not been clearly substantiated. Because of the frequency of gastro-intestinal side-effects with intravenous administration, oral, intra-uterine, and vaginal routes were investigated. Oral treatment was convenient, but generally less effective than other routes and again systemic absorption produced troublesome gastro-intestinal effects. More recently the ripening effect of prostaglandins, especially dinoprostone, on the cervix has been exploited. The prognosis in induced labour is governed mainly by the degree of ripeness of the cervix and Embrey considered that pre-induction ripening of the unfavourable cervix with dinoprostone administered vaginally was of established value, relatively safe, and associated with a low incidence of gastro-intestinal or thermogenic effects; he suggested that routine induction of labour with vaginal prostaglandins was perhaps more controversial although gaining in popularity. Since 1981 many studies have confirmed the value of dinoprostone administered vaginally for the induction of labour. Dinoprostone vaginal gel and pessaries for the induction of labour are now commercially available in many countries, including the *UK*, and are replacing intravenous oxytocin as the method of choice. A dinoprostone gel for intracervical rather than intravaginal application is also under study.

Termination of pregnancy. A summary from Sweden of clinical experience with prostaglandins for the termination of pregnancy. Vacuum aspiration is the most widely used method for termination in the *first trimester*. Cervical dilatation with prostaglandin analogues such as carboprost methyl, gemeprost, and meteneprost given vaginally or sulprostone given intramuscularly facilitates the procedure and reduces the risk of complications. For termination of very early pregnancy, vaginal or intramuscular administration of the latest generation of prostaglandin analogues has been shown to be as effective as vacuum aspiration if restricted to the first 3 weeks following the first missed menstrual period; gastro-intestinal side-effects are still a problem but less than with natural prostaglandins. Termination in the *second trimester* is generally associated with higher morbidity and mortality than in the first trimester. Non-surgical techniques used most routinely are the extra- or intra-amniotic administration of dinoprost and dinoprostone and the intra-amniotic administration of hypertonic sodium chloride injection. Approximately 90% of patients will abort in 20 to 24 hours when dinoprost 750 µg or dinoprostone 200 µg is injected extra-amniotically every 2 hours; the frequency of side-effects is low with occasional vomiting in about 25% and diarrhoea in 1 to 2%. Only dinoprost has been widely used intra-amniotically, usually in a dose of 25 mg repeated after 6 hours or as a single dose of 40 or 50 mg; success rates in large multicentre studies have ranged from 81.7 to 86.6% within 48 hours of the start of therapy. The frequency of side-effects is reported to be generally higher with intra-amniotic than with extra-amniotic administration. Some of the major complications associated with second trimester abortion are due to inadvertent intravenous injection during intra-amniotic administration. Prostaglandin analogues such as carboprost, sulprostone, and meteneprost can be given by the non-invasive vaginal or intramuscular routes for termination during the early and late parts of the second trimester.— M. Bygdeman, *Clin. Obstet. Gynec.*, 1984, *11*, 573.

A review from the *USA* of current methods of pregnancy termination. Pregnancies of different gestational ages require different termination techniques. These ages do not correspond with the traditional trimesters of pregnancy, but may be divided into 3 phases: early pregnancy (up to 49 days past the last menstrual period), from 8 to 15 weeks, and from 16 to 24 weeks. *Before 8 weeks' gestation* suction dilatation and curettage is the preferred method although a medical approach, possibly self-administered, is feasible. Prostaglandins are known to be effective abortifacients in early pregnancy but the naturally occurring prostaglandins, dinoprost (prostaglandin $F_{2\alpha}$) and dinoprostone (prostaglandin E_2), given intravenously or in vaginal pessaries are associated with too high a frequency of gastro-intestinal and other side-effects at the high doses required; injection of dinoprost 5 mg or dinoprostone 1.5 mg into the uterus will induce abortion with fewer side-effects but premedication is necessary. Prostaglandin analogues such as the methyl esters of arbaprostil, carboprost, and gemeprost were also effective by the intra-uterine route and required less premedication, but this route has largely been abandoned because of its invasive nature and because it is reported to be more painful than vaginal administration or vacuum aspiration. The F analogues are highly effective but are associated with a high frequency of gastro-intestinal side-effects when administered by the noninvasive vaginal and intramuscular routes. The E analogues produce fewer gastro-intestinal effects but have lacked stability. However, more stable E analogues such as sulprostone, gemeprost, and meteneprost have been shown to be very effective when given by intramuscular injection or as vaginal or cervical pessaries; drawbacks include the amount of bleeding, the necessity for analgesia, and fever.

From *8 to 15 weeks' gestation* suction dilatation and curettage or dilatation and evacuation is the unchallenged technique for termination of pregnancy in the *US*. Pre-operative ripening of the cervix with prostaglandin analogues might be worthwhile in selected patients.

There is considerable controversy over the best method of termination between the *16th and 24th week of gestation*. Techniques have included the use of hypertonic sodium chloride, prostaglandin, or urea-prostaglandin injections and of dilatation and evacuation. When prostaglandins are used the most frequent approach in the *USA* is the intra-amniotic injection of dinoprost 40 or 50 mg or 25 mg repeated 6 hours later. In Scandinavia, carboprost and analogues of dinoprostone have been used successfully by the intramuscular route, vaginally, or as an intracervical or extra-amniotic gel. Dinoprost and its analogues are best given by intra-amniotic injection because of the high frequency of gastro-intestinal effects. The E analogues are associated with fewer gastro-intestinal symptoms but hyperpyrexia is frequent. Prostaglandins used alone have several deficiencies including a high incidence of gastro-intestinal side-effects and a high failure rate and frequency of retained placenta. The instillation of hyperosmolar urea followed by dinoprost 5 mg acts more rapidly than prostaglandin alone, is more foetotoxic, and gastro-intestinal effects are less frequent although the incidence of incomplete abortion is still high. After 20 weeks' gestation, urea-prostaglandin is probably safer than dilatation and evacuation.— R. G. Castadot, *Fert. Steril.*, 1986, *45*, 5.

Some comparisons between different methods of second-trimester abortion: M. A. Rettenmaier and F. W. Hanson, *Surgery Gynec. Obstet.*, 1983, *156*, 585 (intra-amniotic dinoprost 40 mg or dinoprostone 20 mg as vaginal pessaries); S. S. Sørensen and P. Wolf, *Contraception*, 1984, *29*, 171 (intra-amniotic dinoprost or intracervical dinoprostone gel); M. E. Kafrissen *et al.*, *J. Am. med. Ass.*, 1984, *251*, 916 (intra-amniotic hyperosmolar urea and dinoprost or dilatation and evacuation).

The successful use of local dinoprost injection for the termination of ectopic pregnancy.— B. Lindblom *et al.*, *Lancet*, 1987, *1*, 776.

URINARY-TRACT DISORDERS. Both dinoprost and dinoprostone are known to contract the bladder (S.M.M. Karim, *Ann. Acad. Med. Singapore*, 1982, *11*, 493) and in preliminary studies beneficial results were achieved when dinoprostone (M.I. Bultitude *et al.*, *Br. J. Urol.*, 1976, *48*, 631) or dinoprost (S.S. Ratnam *et al.*, *Singapore J. Obstet. Gynaec.*, 1979, *10*, 23) was instilled into the bladder in women with chronic urinary retention or patients with acute postoperative or postpartum urinary retention, respectively. However, Delaere *et al.* (*Br. J. Urol.*, 1981, *53*, 306) found instillation of dinoprostone in doses of 0.5 to 10 mg or dinoprost in doses of 1 or 5 mg to be ineffective in 13 women with difficulty in micturition and Wagner *et al.* (*Am. J. Obstet. Gynec.*, 1985, *151*, 375) reported no benefit with dinoprostone 0.75, 1.5, or 2.25 mg instilled into the bladder in a double-blind placebo-controlled study in 28 women with postoperative urinary retention.

Preparations

Dinoprost Tromethamine Injection *(U.S.P.)*. A sterile aqueous solution of dinoprost trometamol.

Proprietary Preparations

Prostin F2 alpha *(Upjohn, UK)*. *Injection*, for intravenous infusion, dinoprost 5 mg (as trometamol salt)/mL, in ampoules of 1.5 and 5 mL; to be diluted before use. *Injection*, for intra-amniotic administration, dinoprost 5 mg (as trometamol salt)/mL, in ampoules of 4 and 8 mL.

Proprietary Names and Manufacturers

Amoglandin *(KabiVitrum, Denm.; KabiVitrum, Norw.; Kabi, Swed.)*; Minprostin $F_{2\alpha}$ *(Upjohn, Ger.)*; Prostalmon F *(Jpn)*; Prostamodin-F *(Jpn)*; Prostin *(Upjohn, Swed.)*; Prostin F2 alpha *(Upjohn, Ital.; Neth.; Upjohn, S.Afr.; Switz.; Upjohn, UK)*; Prostine F_2 Alpha *(Upjohn, Fr.)*.

8082-b

Dinoprostone *(BAN, USAN, rINN)*.

PGE_2; Prostaglandin E_2; U-12062. (5*Z*,13*E*)-(8*R*,11*R*,12*R*,15*S*)-11,15-Dihydroxy-9-oxoprosta-5,13-dienoic acid; (*Z*)-7-{(1*R*,2*R*,3*R*)-3-Hydroxy-2-[(*E*)-(3*S*)-3-hydroxyoct-1-enyl]-5-oxocyclopentyl}hept-5-enoic acid.

$C_{20}H_{32}O_5$=352.5.

CAS — 363-24-6.

NOTE. In *Martindale* the term dinoprostone is used for the exogenous form and prostaglandin E_2 for the endogenous form.

Store at 2° to 8°.

The extemporaneous preparation of dinoprostone vaginal gel using hydroxyethylcellulose gel as the vehicle.— L. J. Gauger (letter), *Am. J. Hosp. Pharm.*, 1984, *41*, 1761.

Details of the preparation and stability of wax based dinoprostone vaginal pessaries.— B. L. Goodwin *et al.*, *Pharm. J.*, 1986, *2*, 801.

Adverse Effects, and Precautions

As for Dinoprost, p.1368.

The extra-amniotic route should not be used in patients with cervicitis or vaginal infections. Vaginal preparations of dinoprostone should not be used in the induction of labour once the membranes are ruptured.

EFFECTS ON BONES. Reversible widening of cranial sutures occurred in 2 newborn infants given dinoprostone intravenously for 95 and 97 days in addition to the reversible periosteal reactions of the long bones and bone thickening previously described in infants given prostaglandins of the E series long-term.— H. Hoevels-Guerich *et al.*, *J. Pediat.*, 1984, *105*, 72.

Uses and Administration

Dinoprostone is a prostaglandin of the E series (see p.1365) with actions on smooth muscle; the endogenous substance is termed prostaglandin E_2 and is rapidly metabolised in the body. It induces contraction of uterine muscle at any stage of pregnancy and is reported to act predominantly as a vasodilator on blood vessels and as a bronchodilator on bronchial muscle. Dinoprostone is used principally in the induction of labour; it may also be used for the termination of pregnancy, missed abortion, hydatidiform mole, and foetal death *in utero*.

Dinoprostone is usually administered vaginally. It may also be given intravenously, extra-amniotically, or by mouth, but the intravenous route has been associated with a high incidence of adverse effects and is generally only used for missed abortion or hydatidiform mole; continuous administration for more than two days is not recommended.

In the induction of labour at term dinoprostone is administered vaginally to ripen the cervix before the membranes are ruptured. A dose of 1 mg is administered as vaginal gel followed, if necessary, by a further 1 or 2 mg after 6 hours; a total dose of 3 mg should not be exceeded. Alternatively, 3 mg is administered in a vaginal pessary followed, if necessary, by a further 3 mg after 6 to 8 hours; a total dose of 6 mg should not be exceeded. Dinoprostone may be given by mouth for the induction of labour in an initial dose of 0.5 mg, repeated hourly, and increased if necessary to 1 mg hourly until an adequate response is achieved; single doses of 1.5 mg should not be exceeded. It has been given intravenously for the induction of labour but is no longer recommended for routine use by most authorities. A suggested intravenous dosage regimen has been 250 nanograms of dinoprostone per minute infused as a solution containing 1.5 µg per mL for 30 minutes, the dose being subsequently maintained or increased according to the patient's response; in foetal death *in utero* higher doses may be required and an initial rate of 500 nanograms per minute has been used with increases at intervals of not less than 1 hour.

For the termination of pregnancy 1 mL of a solution containing 100 µg of dinoprostone per mL may be instilled extra-amniotically through a suitable Foley catheter, with subsequent doses of 1 or 2 mL given at intervals usually of 2 hours, according to response. Dinoprostone has also been given intravenously for the termination of pregnancy and for missed abortion or hydatidiform mole. A suggested dosage regimen is the intravenous infusion of a solution containing 5 µg per mL at a rate of 2.5 µg per minute for 30 minutes, then maintained or increased to 5 µg per minute; this rate should be maintained for at least 4 hours before making further increases.

In the *USA* dinoprostone pessaries are used for the termination of second trimester pregnancy, a dose of 20 mg being administered intravaginally and repeated every 3 to 5 hours according to response; a total dose of 240 mg should not be exceeded. Pessaries are also used in the *USA* in missed abortion, foetal death *in utero*, and benign hydatidiform mole.

CARDIOVASCULAR DISORDERS. *Congenital heart disease.* An evaluation of dinoprostone in the management of 62 infants with ductus-dependent congenital heart disease and recommendations on dosage and the method of administration. The short-term use of prostaglandins to maintain the patency of ductus arteriosus is well-established. Treatment for a longer period may facilitate later surgery by allowing growth of the infants and their pulmonary arteries and to this end oral administration of dinoprostone in an initial dose of 20 to 25 µg per kg body-weight hourly is recommended, decreasing the frequency of doses after the first week. Treatment is continued for up to 4 weeks initially and a decision then made whether to proceed with surgery or to plan a longer course of treatment to encourage further growth. When gastro-intestinal absorption is expected to be poor or when oral treatment is ineffective low doses of dinoprostone are given intravenously, beginning with the infusion of 0.003 µg per kg per minute; it is rarely necessary to increase the dose for more than a few hours and doses as high as 0.01 to 0.02 µg per kg per minute are exceptional.— E. D. Silove *et al.*, *Archs Dis. Childh.*, 1985, *60*, 1025.

For the role of prostaglandins in ductus arteriosus-dependent congenital heart disease, see Alprostadil, p.1366.

Peripheral vascular disease. Beneficial results with dinoprostone applied topically as a solution dispersed in hydrocolloid granules in 2 patients with chronic leg ulcers unresponsive to conventional treatment; one had an arterial ulcer, the other a venous ulcer. Local mechanisms, including vasodilatation, were thought to be responsible for the effect.— G. Eriksson *et al.* (letter), *Lancet*, 1986, *1*, 905.

GASTRO-INTESTINAL DISORDERS. Prostaglandins of the E series have been found to inhibit gastric acid secretion and to stabilise the gastric and duodenal mucosa. The naturally occurring prostaglandins are inactivated in the body too rapidly to be therapeutically useful in peptic ulcer disease and thus more stable synthetic analogues have been developed. These include the dinoprostone derivatives arbaprostil, enprostil, and trimoprostil and the alprostadil derivatives misoprostol and rioprostil.— S. J. Sontag, *Drugs*, 1986, *32*, 445.

For more details on the role of prostaglandins in peptic ulcer disease and discussion on their reputed cytoprotective properties, see Misoprostol, p.1374.

Dinoprostone 1 mg four times daily by mouth prevented faecal blood loss associated with aspirin ingestion in healthy subjects, indicating a protective effect on the gastric mucosa. However, the dose of dinoprostone given would be too large to be administered to women who might be pregnant.— M. M. Cohen *et al.*, *Gut*, 1980, *21*, 602.

Beneficial results with topical dinoprostone in 4 of 6 patients with chemotherapy-associated mucosal lesions. Five patients with ulcerations in the mouth and oropharynx chewed dinoprostone 250 µg three times daily; in the sixth, dinoprostone was applied to vaginal lesions. Prophylaxis with dinoprostone was effective in 2 of 3 further patients.— I. Kührer *et al.* (letter), *Lancet*, 1986, *1*, 623.

References to the gastro-intestinal effects of the dinoprostone analogue dimethyldinoprostone (16,16-dimethylprostaglandin E_2): P. Müller *et al.* (letter), *Lancet*, 1981, *1*, 333 (cytoprotective properties); H. G. Dammann *et al.* (letter), *Br. J. clin. Pharmac.*, 1982, *13*, 456 (inhibition of gastric acid secretion).

OBSTETRICS AND GYNAECOLOGY. See Dinoprost, p.1369.

URINARY-TRACT DISORDERS. Dinoprostone 750 µg in 200 mL of sodium chloride solution instilled into the bladder, left *in situ* for 4 hours, and repeated daily for 4 days successfully controlled severe cyclophosphamide-induced haemorrhagic cystitis in a bone-marrow transplant patient. Haematuria had persisted for 120 days despite treatment with multiple platelet transfusions, fresh frozen plasma, and tranexamic acid. It was suggested that smaller volumes should be instilled in future.— J. Mohiuddin *et al.* (letter), *Ann. intern. Med.*, 1984, *101*, 142.

For reference to the use of dinoprostone in urinary retention, see Dinoprost, p.1369.

Proprietary Preparations

Prepidil *(Upjohn, UK)*. *Gel*, dinoprostone 500 µg, in pre-filled syringes of 2.5 mL.

Prostin E2 *(Upjohn, UK)*. *Tablets*, dinoprostone 500 µg. *Injection*, for intravenous infusion, dinoprostone 1 mg/mL, in dehydrated alcohol, in ampoules of 0.75 mL; to be diluted before use. *Injection*, for intravenous infusion, dinoprostone 10 mg/mL, in dehydrated alcohol, in ampoules of 0.5 mL; to be diluted before use. *Injection*, for extra-amniotic administration, dinoprostone 10 mg/mL, in dehydrated alcohol, in ampoules of 0.5 mL; supplied with 50-mL vials of diluent. *Vaginal gel*, dinoprostone 1 mg in 3 g and 2 mg in 3 g. *Vaginal tablets*, dinoprostone 3 mg.

Proprietary Names and Manufacturers

Minprostin *(Denm.; Upjohn, Norw.; Upjohn, Swed.)*; Minprostin E_2 *(Upjohn, Ger.)*; Prepidil *(Upjohn, UK)*; Prostarmon-E *(Jpn)*; Prostin E2 *(Upjohn, Canad.; Neth.; Upjohn, S.Afr.; Upjohn, Switz.; Upjohn, UK)*; Prostine E_2 *(Upjohn, Fr.)*.

16628-f

Enprostil *(BAN, USAN, rINN)*.

RS-84135. Methyl (*E*)-(11*R*,15*R*)-11,15-dihydroxy-9-oxo-16-phenoxy-17,18,19,20-tetranorprosta-4,5,13-trienoate; Methyl 7-{(*E*)-(3*R**)-3-hydroxy-2-[(1*R**,2*R**,3*R**)-3-hydroxy-4-phenoxybut-1-enyl]-5-oxocyclopentyl}hepta-4,5-dienoate.

$C_{23}H_{28}O_6$=400.5.

CAS — 73121-56-9.

Enprostil, a synthetic analogue of dinoprostone (prostaglandin E_2), inhibits gastric acid secretion. It has actions and uses similar to those of misoprostol (p.1374) and has been given by mouth in the treatment of peptic ulcer.

A review of enprostil.— K. L. Goa and J. P. Monk, *Drugs*, 1987, *34*, 539.

GASTRO-INTESTINAL DISORDERS. As well as inhibiting gastric acid secretion enprostil, unlike misoprostol, is reported to inhibit gastrin release (V. Mahachai *et al.*, *Gastroenterology*, 1985, *89*, 555). It has a longer duration of action than misoprostol and has been given in doses of 35 μg twice daily by mouth in the treatment of duodenal and gastric ulcers. Enprostil appears to be no more effective than the histamine H_2-antagonists at healing ulcers and less effective at relieving pain. A summary of pooled European studies (L. Winters *et al.*, *Am. J. Med.*, 1986, *81, Suppl.* 2A, 69) concluded that enprostil was about as good as cimetidine at healing duodenal ulcers. It was less effective than ranitidine in a double-blind study involving 180 patients with duodenal ulcers (K. Lauritsen *et al.*, *Br. med. J.*, 1986, *292*, 864), but of similar efficacy in patients with gastric ulcers (H.-G. Dammann *et al.*, *Am. J. Med.*, 1986, *81, Suppl.* 2A, 80). Enprostil 70 μg at night was also less effective than ranitidine 300 mg at night in patients with duodenal ulcers (R.P. Walt *et al.*, *Gastroenterology*, 1986, *90*, 1683).

Enprostil has mucosal protective properties and was found to reduce aspirin-induced bleeding from the gastric mucosa (C.J. Hawkey *et al.*, *Gut*, 1985, *26*, A560), but cytoprotection alone as an ulcer-healing mechanism has not been demonstrated (S.J. Sontag, *Drugs*, 1986, *32*, 445). When compared with ranitidine 150 mg at bedtime, enprostil 35 μg also at bedtime was much less effective at preventing relapse of duodenal ulcer (K. Lauritsen *et al.*, *Br. med. J.*, 1987, *294*, 932); relapse rates with enprostil were comparable with those described after placebo, thus challenging the clinical role of any so called cytoprotective effect.

For reviews on prostaglandin analogues in the treatment of peptic ulcer and discussion on their reputed cytoprotective properties, see Misoprostol, p.1374.

Proprietary Names and Manufacturers

Gardrin *(Syntex, Mex.)*; Gardrine *(Syntex, Fr.)*.

8084-g

Epoprostenol *(USAN, rINN).*

PGI_2; PGX; Prostacyclin; Prostaglandin I_2; Prostaglandin X; U-53217. (5*Z*,13*E*)-(8*R*,9*S*,11*R*,12*R*,15*S*)-6,9-Epoxy-11,15-dihydroxyprosta-5,13-dienoic acid; (*Z*)-5-{(3a*R*,4*R*,5*R*,6a*S*)-5-Hydroxy-4-[(*E*)-(3*S*)-3-hydroxyoct-1-enyl]perhydrocyclopenta[*b*]furan-2-ylidene}valeric acid.

$C_{20}H_{32}O_5$=352.5.

CAS — 35121-78-9.

NOTE. In *Martindale* the term epoprostenol is used for the exogenous form and prostacyclin for the endogenous form.

8085-q

Epoprostenol Sodium *(BAN, USAN, rINNM).*

U-53217A.

$C_{20}H_{31}NaO_5$=374.5.

CAS — 61849-14-7.

Store at 2° to 8°. Protect from light.

STABILITY IN SOLUTION. Epoprostenol is unstable at physiological pH and solutions for infusion are prepared in an alkaline glycine buffer at pH 10.5. The half-life in aqueous solution of pH 7.4 has been reported to be less than 3 minutes at 37° (K.E.H. El Tahir *et al.*, *Clin. Sci.*, 1980, *59*, Sept., 28P), but increased stability has been reported in plasma, albumin, or whole blood and Mikhailidis *et al.* (*Lancet*, 1982, *2*, 767) suggested that it may be possible to infuse epoprostenol in these biological fluids at near physiological pH rather than in highly alkaline irritant solutions.

Adverse Effects and Precautions

The incidence of adverse reactions to epoprostenol is dose-related. Side-effects during intravenous infusion commonly include hypotension, increased heart-rate, flushing, and headache. Dosage should be reduced or the epoprostenol infusion stopped if excessive hypotension occurs. Bradycardia together with pallor, sweating, nausea, and abdominal discomfort may occur. Erythema over the intravenous infusion site has been noted. Other side-effects reported have included nausea and vomiting, jaw pain, hyperglycaemia, drowsiness, and chest pain.

Since epoprostenol is a potent vasodilator and inhibitor of platelet aggregation, care should be taken in patients receiving other vasodilators or anticoagulants concomitantly. The hypotensive effects of epoprostenol may be exacerbated by using acetate in dialysis fluids.

Adverse effects during 50 intravenous infusions of epoprostenol given to 24 healthy subjects for a maximum of 100 minutes were as follows: facial flushing and headache during all infusions in all subjects; erythema over the infusion site on 13 occasions in 9 subjects; 'vagal reflex' with bradycardia accompanied by pallor, sweating, nausea and sometimes abdominal discomfort on 7 occasions in 5 subjects; nausea on 1 occasion in 1 subject and abdominal discomfort on 5 occasions in 4 subjects, without bradycardia; chest pain or tightness on 2 occasions in 1 subject, and drowsiness on 2 occasions in 2 subjects. Restlessness or unease was also noted in some subjects but was not necessarily attributable to epoprostenol. A significant rise in pulse-rate and drop in diastolic blood pressure was found; some subjects were aware of the tachycardia. Ventricular ectopic beats were noted in 1 subject receiving epoprostenol 10 ng per kg body-weight per minute. Subjects varied in their susceptibility to epoprostenol but the same sequence of events was usually present. A change in pre-ejection period and facial flushing was often apparent at an infusion rate of 2 to 2.5 ng per kg per minute. A rise in heart-rate and change in other cardiovascular variables was present when the infusion rate had increased to 4 to 5 ng per kg per minute; headache, generally the dose-limiting factor, was usually present at this dose and increased as the dose was raised, as did the other effects. Erythema over the vein and 'vagal reflex' only appeared after at least 1 hour of infusion; 'vagal reflex' took only a few seconds to develop.

A review of the literature revealed that: flushing and headache have been consistently reported; bradycardia has occurred infrequently at lower as well as higher doses; a higher incidence of nausea, vomiting, and abdominal discomfort has been recorded in other studies; drowsiness and lassitude, as in the present report, have been infrequent complaints; a modest tachycardia and fall in diastolic pressure is usually produced, the hypotension which results from peripheral vasodilatation usually being asymptomatic. Additional adverse effects occasionally reported by other workers have included lightheadedness, blurred vision, sighing and yawning, slurred speech, pain in the limbs (with intra-arterial injections) and jaw, a paradoxical rise in blood pressure, bleeding, moderate hyperglycaemia in diabetic patients, sweating, hypotonia, anxiety, and a brisk diuresis; epoprostenol by inhalation has caused pharyngeal irritation and coughing.

The epoprostenol now available is probably twice as potent as that used some years ago. Although a maximum infusion rate of 10 ng per kg per minute for infusions lasting up to 60 minutes has been recommended, all the adverse effects in the 24 subjects occurred at a lower dose and in general a maximum of 4 ng per kg per minute is suggested for prolonged infusions. Careful attention to infusion technique is necessary and monitoring of the heart-rate is advisable in view of the suddenness with which the 'vagal reflex' can occur. Most of the adverse effects reported here have responded to a reduction in dosage.— H. Pickles and J. O'Grady, *Br. J. clin. Pharmac.*, 1982, *14*, 177.

EFFECTS ON THE BLOOD. Reports of rebound platelet activation during continuous epoprostenol infusion.— D. A. Yardumian and S. J. Machin (letter), *Lancet*, 1984, *1*, 1357; H. Sinzinger *et al.* (letter), *ibid.*, *2*, 759.

EFFECTS ON THE CARDIOVASCULAR SYSTEM. Evidence that epoprostenol and its analogue iloprost can induce myocardial ischaemia in patients with coronary artery disease.— R. Bugiardini *et al.*, *Clin. Pharmac. Ther.*, 1985, *38*, 101.

EFFECTS ON MENTAL STATE. Symptoms of depression were associated with intravenous epoprostenol therapy in 4 patients.— D. Ansell *et al.* (letter), *Lancet*, 1986, *2*, 509.

Absorption and Fate

Endogenous prostacyclin is a product of arachidonic acid metabolism with a very short half-life. Following intravenous infusion of epoprostenol the half-life is only about 3 minutes, epoprostenol being hydrolysed rapidly to the more stable but much less active 6-keto-prostaglandin $F_{1\alpha}$ (6-oxo-prostaglandin $F_{1\alpha}$). Unlike many other prostaglandins, epoprostenol is not inactivated in the pulmonary circulation.

References: B. Rosenkranz *et al.*, *Clin. Pharmac. Ther.*, 1981, *29*, 420 (metabolism).

Uses and Administration

Epoprostenol is a prostaglandin (see p.1365) which causes vasodilatation and prevents platelet aggregation. The endogenous substance is termed prostacyclin.

Epoprostenol is used as an anticoagulant during cardiopulmonary bypass, charcoal haemoperfusion, and haemodialysis. It has also been used in severe peripheral vascular disease and has been tried in a variety of other disorders including ischaemic heart disease, primary pulmonary hypertension, pre-eclampsia, stroke, and the platelet consumption syndromes thrombotic thrombocytopenic purpura and haemolytic-uraemic syndrome. However, epoprostenol is unstable in solution at physiological pH and also has a very short duration of action because of its rapid hydrolysis *in vivo*. It must therefore be administered by continuous infusion. More stable analogues under study include ciprostene (p.1367) and iloprost (p.1374).

It is given as the sodium salt and doses are expressed in terms of epoprostenol. Great care must be taken in preparing a suitably diluted solution for infusion and only glycine buffer, as supplied by the manufacturer, should be used to reconstitute epoprostenol.

In extracorporeal procedures epoprostenol is administered by continuous intravenous infusion or into the blood supplying the extracorporeal circulation. Recommended dosage schedules are: for cardiopulmonary bypass, 10 nanograms per kg body-weight per minute intravenously by central venous catheter after induction of anaesthesia, until the start of bypass, then 20 ng per kg per minute during bypass; for charcoal haemoperfusion, 2 to 16 ng per kg per minute intravenously before haemoperfusion, then 16 ng per kg per minute into the proximal line of the charcoal column during haemoperfusion; for renal dialysis, 5 ng per kg per minute intravenously before dialysis, then 5 ng per kg per minute into the arterial inlet of the dialyser during dialysis.

A review of the discovery, properties, and clinical applications of prostacyclin. Prostaglandin endoperoxides, isolated in the early 1970s by Samuelsson and others were found to be transformed by thromboxane synthetase in platelets to thromboxane A_2, which caused platelet aggregation and vascular contraction. In contrast, prostaglandin endoperoxides were transformed by blood vessel microsomes to prostacyclin, which had potent anti-aggregatory properties and relaxed vascular strips. It was suggested that a balance between the amounts of thromboxane A_2 formed by platelets and prostacyclin formed by blood vessel walls might be critical for thrombus formation and this concept is now well established. Prostacyclin is the main product of arachidonic acid in all vascular tissues so far tested, endothelial cells from vessel walls being the most active producers. It is a strong hypotensive agent through vasodilatation of all vascular beds studied, including the pulmonary and cerebral circulations, and is also the most potent endogenous inhibitor of platelet aggregation yet discovered. Inhibition of aggregation is achieved by stimulation of adenylate cyclase, leading to an increase in cyclic adenosine monophosphate (cAMP) levels in the platelets. By inhibiting several steps in the activation of the arachidonic acid metabolic cascade, prostacyclin exerts an overall control of platelet aggregability. Prostacyclin also increases cAMP levels in cells other than platelets and thus the prostacyclin/thromboxane A_2 system may have wider biological significance in cell regulation.— J. R. Vane, *Postgrad. med. J.*, 1983, *59*, 743. Endogenous prostacyclin and thromboxane A_2 now appear to be of more physiological and pathological importance than the more classical prostanoids prostaglandin E_2 and prostaglandin $F_{2\alpha}$. They have directly opposing pharmacological actions in many systems, such as on platelet function, vascular smooth muscle, bronchopulmonary function, and gastro-intestinal integrity. Thus prostanoid-mediated control of cellular and tissue function may reflect an interactive modulation between prostacyclin and thromboxane A_2 with imbalance resulting in dysfunction, for example in platelet and vascular disorders. Thromboxane A_2 has both bronchoconstrictor and pulmonary irritant actions and has brought about marked changes in respiratory function in experimental models; prostacyclin may oppose these effects on both the pulmonary vasculature and bronchial smooth muscle.

Thromboxane A_2 has induced marked renal vasoconstriction *in vitro* whereas renal vasodilatation and stimulation of the release of renin has followed the administration of epoprostenol [exogenous prostacyclin] in *animals*. In contrast to the pro-ulcerogenic actions of thromboxane A_2, epoprostenol and its analogues, like other prostaglandins, have potent gastro-intestinal anti-ulcer properties which can be disassociated from their gastric antisecretory properties. The term 'cytoprotection' has been used to describe this ability of exogenous prostaglandins to prevent gastro-intestinal damage; endogenous prostaglandins might have a similar protective role. Epoprostenol also has a cytoprotective effect against experimental damage in the gastric mucosa, myocardium, and liver whereas thromboxane A_2 has a cytolytic effect.— B. J. R. Whittle and S. Moncada, *Br. med. Bull.*, 1983, *39*, 232. Discussion on manipulation of the balance between thromboxane A_2 and prostacyclin in the treatment of thrombosis and other disorders. Possible approaches include the use of stable readily administered epoprostenol analogues, increasing the concentration of natural prostacyclin with prostacyclin releasers or inhibitors of its degradation, blocking thromboxane A_2 production with thromboxane synthase inhibitors such as dazoxiben, and blocking thromboxane A_2 receptors.— J. R. A. Mitchell, *ibid.*, 289.

Further reviews of epoprostenol and its clinical potential.— *Lancet*, 1982, *2*, 424; P. J. Lewis and C. T. Dollery, *Br. med. Bull.*, 1983, *39*, 281; J. R. A. Mitchell, *Br. med. J.*, 1983, *287*, 1824.

Studies on 6-keto-prostaglandin E_1 (6-oxo-prostaglandin E_1), a metabolite of endogenous prostacyclin: P. S. Wilsoncroft *et al.*, *J. Pharm. Pharmac.*, 1985, *37*, 139 (effect *in vitro* on platelet aggregation); I. Miyamori *et al.*, *Br. J. clin. Pharmac.*, 1985, *20*, 681 (effect *in vivo* on platelet aggregation and plasma renin).

BLOOD DISORDERS. *Thrombotic thrombocytopenic purpura* is characterised by thrombocytopenia, microangiopathic haemolytic anaemia, neurological abnormalities, fever, and renal disease. Platelet aggregation has a major role in the pathogenesis of thrombotic thrombocytopenic purpura and the related disorder, *haemolytic-uraemic syndrome*. Prostacyclin deficiency has been demonstated in both conditions, but results with epoprostenol have been variable. Intravenous infusion of epoprostenol was ineffective in 2 patients with thrombotic thrombocytopenic purpura refractory to standard therapy (G.T. Budd *et al.*, *Lancet*, 1980, *2*, 915; J.E. Johnson *et al.*, *J. Am. med. Ass.*, 1983, *250* 3089), but was associated with complete remission in 2 further patients (G.A. Fitzgerald *et al.*, *Ann. intern. Med.*, 1981, *95*, 319; C.D. Payton *et al.*, *Lancet*, 1985, *1*, 927).The patient treated successfully by Payton *et al.* responded dramatically to the intravenous infusion of epoprostenol gradually increased to 8 ng per kg body-weight per minute, continued for 7 days, and then given for a further 12 days at a dose of 4 ng per kg per minute for 8 hours a day; they suggested that epoprostenol should be started early, used in the maximum tolerable dose, and continued for as long as circulating platelet aggregates can be detected. A further patient with intractable thrombotic thrombocytopenic purpura responded to treatment with epoprostenol in association with nafazatrom, a stimulant of prostacyclin synthesis (S.T.S. Durrant *et al.*, *Lancet*, 1985, *2*, 842).

Prolonged epoprostenol infusion may have contributed to the recovery of a patient with post partum haemolytic-uraemic syndrome and evidence of prostacyclin deficiency (J. Webster *et al.*, *Br. med. J.*, 1980, *281*, 271) and 3 children with haemolytic-uraemic syndrome also responded to treatment with epoprostenol (T.J. Beattie *et al.*, *ibid.*, 1981, *283*, 470).

A 25-year-old woman with a history of recurrent deep venous thromboses and spontaneous abortions responded to treatment with epoprostenol infusion following life-threatening arterial *thrombosis* which occurred despite the administration of heparin. Evidence for deficient prostacyclin production was found.— J. G. Lanham *et al.*, *Br. med. J.*, 1986, *292*, 435.

CARDIOVASCULAR DISORDERS. The property of epoprostenol to inhibit platelet aggregation and dilate blood vessels has led to its evaluation in a number of conditions including myocardial ischaemia, stroke [see under Cerebrovascular Disorders], Raynaud's phenomenon, peripheral vascular disease, thrombotic thrombocytopenic purpura [see under Blood Disorders], and pre-eclampsia. Although there are grounds for cautious optimism in some of these conditions the only proven value of epoprostenol is in extracorporeal haemoperfusion systems [see under Extracorporeal Circulation]. The original potential of epoprostenol, or stable analogues, in atherosclerotic vascular disease remains under study and although the proposal that platelets might be involved in the development of atheroma has gone in and out of favour, the discovery of platelet-derived growth factor has suggested a new role for platelets in atherogenesis.— J. MacDermot, *Br. J. Hosp. Med.*, 1986, *35*, 289.

Congenital heart disease. Comment on the role of prostacyclin in the ductus arteriosus and pulmonary circulation of the foetus and neonate. Prostaglandin E_2 is functionally the most important prostaglandin formed in the ductus, but prostacyclin may contribute to ductus patency. Epoprostenol reduced pulmonary vascular resistance when given to an infant with refractory hypoxaemia secondary to pulmonary vasoconstriction (J.E. Lock *et al.*, *Lancet*, 1979, *1*, 1343) and might be of value in neonatal disorders with pulmonary hypertension.— F. Coceani *et al.*, *Eur. J. clin. Pharmac.*, 1980, *18*, 75.

For further reference to the role of prostaglandins in ductus arteriosus-dependent congenital heart disease, see Alprostadil, p.1366.

Hypertension in pregnancy. Haemolysis and thrombocytopenia with terminal disseminated intravascular coagulation are recognised features of pre-eclampsia and eclampsia and reflect a generalised disturbance of the clotting system. It has been suggested that an imbalance between thromboxane A_2 and prostacyclin might cause some arterial or platelet disorders including pre-eclampsia. However, the evidence for prostacyclin deficiency in pre-eclampsia relates more to the foetus and can explain the foetal but not the maternal complications of this disorder. There is also evidence for excess thromboxane production from the placenta, platelets, or both and the suggestion that changes in prostaglandin metabolism cause pre-eclamptic hypertension has also been made. An imbalance of vasoconstrictor and vasodilator prostaglandins, either circulating or in the arterial wall, might alter arterial tone in pre-eclampsia and, since the vasoconstricting factor might be thromboxane released by circulating platelets, intravenous epoprostenol and other anti-platelet agents, including aspirin and dazoxiben, have been used to prevent or treat pre-eclampsia. Results with aspirin have been most promising, although the case for its routine use has not yet been established.— *Lancet*, 1986, *1*, 18.

Epoprostenol given by intravenous infusion for 80 minutes in incremental doses up to 8 ng per kg body-weight per minute decreased blood pressure in 13 pregnant women with pre-eclampsia, but did not increase placental or umbilical blood flow. No changes in maternal or foetal pulse-rate or in uterine contractility were seen. Since foetal complications in pre-eclampsia are thought to be a result of the inadequacy of placental blood flow, epoprostenol does not appear to be specific therapy to increase placental or umbilical blood flow.— P. Jouppila *et al.*, *Am. J. Obstet. Gynec.*, 1985, *151*, 661.

Severe pregnancy-associated hypertension, refractory to conventional therapy, was controlled by the intravenous infusion of epoprostenol at doses of up to 1 to 6 ng per kg body-weight per minute for 5 hours to 7 days in 4 pregnant women. Blood pressure in a fifth patient was not reduced to normal following infusion of 2.5 ng per kg per minute for 11 days and increasing the dose resulted in vasodilator-related side-effects. There was no effect on uterine activity.— J. J. F. Belch *et al.*, *Clin. exp. Hypertens. B*, 1985, *B4*, 75. See also J. Fidler *et al.* (letter), *Lancet*, 1980, *2*, 31.

Ischaemic heart disease. A review of the role of prostaglandins in ischaemic heart disease. Although it is still uncertain whether an imbalance in the ratio of prostacyclin and thromboxane A_2 production, with resultant platelet aggregation and coronary vasoconstriction, is a primary or secondary event in the development of myocardial ischaemia and infarction, it seems likely that alterations of this balance may be important in preventing or limiting the extent of ischaemic injury and its consequences. Possible treatment strategies include the administration of epoprostenol or its stable substitutes, or alprostadil. Epoprostenol has proved to be a potent coronary vasodilator and inhibitor of platelet aggregation in normal subjects, but conflicting results have been reported following intravenous infusions in patients with angina pectoris and the situation is even less clear in those with acute myocardial infarction.— B. Pitt *et al.*, *Ann. intern. Med.*, 1983, *99*, 83. Increased biosynthesis of thromboxane A_2 and a compensatory increase in prostacyclin biosynthesis was noted during myocardial ischaemia in patients with unstable angina, suggesting that episodic platelet activation occurs. Increased biosynthesis of these eicosanoids was not seen at rest or during exercise-induced myocardial ischaemia in patients with stable coronary artery disease.— D. J. Fitzgerald *et al.*, *New Engl. J. Med.*, 1986, *315*, 983.

Intravenous infusion of epoprostenol 5 ng per kg body-weight per minute for 12 to 48 hours had a very favourable effect in 9 patients with unstable angina, but a dose of 5 to 10 ng per kg per minute offered no protection against anginal attacks precipitated by atrial pacing in any of 7 patients studied.— A. Szczeklik *et al.* (letter), *New Engl. J. Med.*, 1980, *303*, 881. The coronary and systemic effects of epoprostenol 2, 4, 6, and 8 ng per kg body-weight per minute in 10 male patients with coronary heart disease were similar to those produced by short-acting nitrates and, together with improved pacing time to angina, indicate an acute beneficial effect.— G. Bergman *et al.*, *Lancet*, 1981, *1*, 569. Only 1 of 9 patients suffering frequent anginal attacks benefited from intravenous epoprostenol.— S. Chierchia *et al.*, *Circulation*, 1982, *65*, 470. Lack of benefit in 4 of 5 patients with evolving myocardial infarction given intracoronary infusion of epoprostenol 8 to 20 ng per kg body-weight per minute.— R. Grose *et al.*, *Am. J. Cardiol.*, 1985, *55*, 1625. Lack of benefit, in a double-blind placebo-controlled study in 45 patients with acute myocardial infarction, with epoprostenol 1 to 5 ng per kg per minute given by intravenous infusion within 16 hours of the onset of symptoms.— F. J. Kiernan *et al.*, *Br. Heart J.*, 1986, *56*, 428.

Peripheral vascular disease. Striking clinical improvement was obtained in 5 patients with advanced arteriosclerosis obliterans of the lower limbs, following intra-arterial infusion of epoprostenol in an initial dose of 2 ng per kg body-weight per minute, increased at hourly intervals to 5 to 10 ng per kg per minute, and given for 72 hours.— A. Szczeklik *et al.*, *Lancet*, 1979, *1*, 1111.

Intermittent intravenous infusions of epoprostenol produced marked clinical improvement when compared with placebo in a double-blind study in patients with severe chronic Raynaud's syndrome. Seven patients received a 5-hour intravenous infusion of epoprostenol at a dose of 7.5 ng per kg body-weight per minute after the first hour; infusions were given weekly for 3 weeks. A further 7 patients received only buffer. Epoprostenol significantly decreased the frequency and duration of attacks and promoted healing of ischaemic skin lesions for up to 6 weeks after the last infusion. All patients receiving epoprostenol had facial flushing during infusion and 3 had headache, but none required a reduction in dosage. Cumulative experience in over 30 patients now indicates that a short course of epoprostenol is useful for up to 2 months in patients with severe Raynaud's syndrome.— J. J. F. Belch *et al.*, *Lancet*, 1983, *1*, 313. Epoprostenol also relieved ischaemic rest pain in a double-blind study in 28 patients with severe peripheral arterial disease. Rest pain was reduced in all of 15 patients 24 hours after the end of a 4-day intravenous infusion of epoprostenol, but in only 3 of 13 controls. Epoprostenol was given initially at a rate of 2.5 ng per kg body-weight per minute and increased over 4 hours to 10 ng per kg per minute. In some patients the effect of epoprostenol lasted for over a month; by 6 months the benefit was less pronounced.— J. J. F. Belch *et al.*, *ibid.*, 315. Comment on these encouraging results. The persistent effect of epoprostenol is surprising in view of the fact that its vasodilator action ceases within minutes of the termination of the infusion and its platelet-inhibiting effect lasts hours rather than days. Existing medical treatment for peripheral vascular disease is not very effective and, despite uncertainty over its mode of action, the possibility that patients might have known they were on active treatment because of side-effects such as facial flushing, and the fact that not all controlled trials have shown prolonged benefit, intravenous epoprostenol must be recommended for patients threatened by amputation. The development of orally active stable vasodilator prostaglandins should allow trials of prolonged treament in peripheral vascular disease.— *ibid.*, 1199.

Infusions of epoprostenol or the stable mimetic drug iloprost have been reported to improve the prognosis and symptoms in peripheral vascular disease caused by atherosclerosis. Epoprostenol and the orally active mimetic agent RS-93427-007 have now been found to inhibit both of the basic mechanisms of early atherogenesis. In studies *in vitro* they inhibited release of mitogens, including platelet-derived growth factor, from platelets and prevented accumulation of cholesteryl esters in macrophages. Thus, epoprostenol and its analogues may increase limb perfusion in atherosclerotic subjects by suppressing the underlying atherogenic process rather than by reversal of thrombosis or by vasodilatation. A cytoprotective effect might be involved since epoprostenol has effects that clearly outlast the presence of what is a short-lived unstable molecule.— A. L. Willis *et al.* (letter), *Lancet*, 1986, *2*, 682.

Further reports of beneficial results with intravenous infusions of epoprostenol in patients with peripheral vascular disease: H. Zygulska-Mach *et al.* (letter), *Lancet*, 1980, *2*, 1075 (in 2 of 3 patients with central retinal vein occlusion given 5 ng per kg body-weight per minute for 72 hours); P. M. Dowd *et al.*, *Br. J. Derm.*, 1982, *106*, 81 (in 21 of 24 patients with Raynaud's phenomenon due to systemic sclerosis given 2.5 to 10 ng per kg per minute for 72 hours); C. De San Lazaro *et al.*, *Archs Dis. Childh.*, 1985, *60*, 370 (in a child with severe familial peripheral vascular disease causing gangrene given 10 ng per kg per minute for 3 days and then 10 days); E. C. Burns *et al.*, *ibid.*, 537 (in 2 children with acute attacks of Raynaud's disease; one was subsequently maintained on transdermal viprostol); D. W. Denning *et al.* (letter), *Lancet*, 1986, *2*, 1401 (in 2 patients with severe gangrene as a complication of bacterial sepsis given epoprostenol and tissue plasminogen activator; one received 18 ng per kg per minute of epoprostenol for 7 days and the other 10 ng per kg per minute for 10 days); B. Leaker *et al.* (letter), *ibid.*, 1987, *1*, 156 (in a patient with severe gangrene, disseminated intravascular coagulation, and acute renal failure given epoprostenol 6 to 10 ng per kg per minute with an on/off regimen at 8-hourly intervals).

Pulmonary hypertension. A brief discussion on primary pulmonary hypertension and its management. Treatment aims to reduce the consequences of low cardiac output. Anticoagulants improve survival by preventing secondary thrombo-embolism whereas vasodilators relieve the symptoms by raising cardiac output and therefore oxygen tissue delivery. Patients who will benefit from vasodilator therapy can be identified by assessing their response to a titrated dose of intravenous epoprostenol during catheterisation. Those responding should be given anticoagulants and an oral vasodilator (hydralazine, captopril, or diltiazem) if they have clear ventilation and perfusion scans and a mixed venous oxygen saturation greater than 63%. Long-term infusion of epoprostenol can improve the quality of life in those responders with a mixed venous oxygen saturation of less than 63%; as epoprostenol inhibits platelet aggregation, anticoagulants are theoretically not needed.— T. Higenbottam, *Br. med. J.*, 1986, *293*, 1456. Critical comment. The acute response to epoprostenol has been found to be no better at predicting the degree of reversible vasoconstriction than the response to nifedipine, although it has the virtue of being immediately reversible in the event of an unfavourable response with a fall in systemic blood pressure. Oral nifedipine has been found as effective as intravenous epoprostenol in removing the reversible component of pulmonary hypertension and thus the long-term use of intravenous infusions of epoprostenol is considered unnecessary, complicated, dangerous, expensive, and of unproven benefit compared with oral vasodilator therapy.— C. M. Oakley and A. Rozkovec (letter), *ibid.*, 1987, *294*, 122.

Further reviews of primary pulmonary hypertension and its treatment, including the use of epoprostenol.— C. M. Oakley, *Br. Heart J.*, 1985, *53*, 1; *Lancet*, 1986, *1*, 1420; A. A. McLeod and D. E. Jewitt, *Drugs*, 1986, *31*, 177.

Continuous intravenous infusion, for over a year, of epoprostenol 20 ng per kg body-weight per minute enabled a 27-year-old woman, previously bed-bound with severe primary pulmonary hypertension and awaiting heart-lung transplantation, to live independently at home; there was no reversal of the disease process. Orally administered vasodilators had been discontinued because hydralazine caused syncope on exertion and nifedipine was ineffective.— T. Higenbottam *et al.*, *Lancet*, 1984, *1*, 1046.

Oxygenation was improved in 2 of 5 neonates with pulmonary hypertension given epoprostenol by intra-arterial infusion at doses of up to 4 and 10 ng per kg body-weight per minute respectively; pulmonary hypertension was idiopathic in one and associated with meconium aspiration in the other. Epoprostenol was of limited benefit in a futher neonate with meconium aspiration-associated pulmonary hypertension and of no benefit in the 2 with pulmonary hypoplasia.— P. Kääpä *et al.*, *J. Pediat.*, 1985, *107*, 951.

For further reference to the use of epoprostenol in neonatal disorders with pulmonary hypertension, see Congenital Heart Disease (above).

Vascular prosthetic grafts. Intermittent infusion of epoprostenol 3 ng per kg body-weight per minute for 6 hours daily for 5 days significantly decreased platelet deposition on synthetic carotid artery grafts, especially on new grafts; it remains to be established whether early and late graft patency will be improved.— H. Sinzinger *et al.* (letter), *Lancet*, 1984, *2*, 1212. See also H. Sinzinger *et al.* (letter), *ibid.*, 1983, *1*, 1275.

CEREBROVASCULAR DISORDERS. The role of prostaglandins in ischaemic brain damage is controversial (N.M. Dearden, *Lancet*, 1985, *2*, 255) and results with epoprostenol in patients with ischaemic stroke have been inconclusive. There was no evidence of improved mortality or morbidity in patients with acute cerebral infarction given epoprostenol 5 ng per kg body-weight per minute by intravenous infusion, when compared with placebo (J.F. Martin *et al.*, *New Engl. J. Med.*, 1985, *312*, 1642), and although some benefit was seen in a further study in patients with completed ischaemic stroke (J. Huczynski *et al.*, *Stroke*, 1985, *16*, 810) the results remained inconclusive.

EXTRACORPOREAL CIRCULATION. Epoprostenol is used to inhibit the platelet aggregation which results from blood in extracorporeal circulations, such as those used in haemodialysis, cardiopulmonary bypass, and haemoperfusion, coming into contact with artificial surfaces. This platelet aggregation can lead to thrombocytopenia and bleeding and the aggregates may block filters in the circuits; embolisation of aggregates may cause cerebral dysfunction after cardiopulmonary bypass. Although epoprostenol undoubtedly protects platelets from activation during extracorporeal circulation and also has a heparin-sparing effect, its routine use in such procedures, with the possible exception of charcoal haemoperfusion, has been questioned.

References: P. J. Lewis and C. T. Dollery, *Br. med. Bull.*, 1983, *39*, 281; M. J. Weston, *ibid.*, 285; *Drug & Ther. Bull.*, 1984, *22*, 101.

Cardiopulmonary bypass. The administration of epoprostenol preserved platelet number and function, reduced postoperative blood loss, and had a heparin-sparing effect in a double-blind placebo-controlled study in 23 patients undergoing open-heart surgery.— D. B. Longmore *et al.*, *Lancet*, 1981, *1*, 800.

Charcoal haemoperfusion. Infusion of epoprostenol allowed charcoal haemoperfusion to be carried out daily without significant platelet loss or other serious side-effects in the treatment of 76 patients with fulminant hepatic failure.— A. E. S. Gimson *et al.*, *Lancet*, 1982, *2*, 681. Correction to the dosage of epoprostenol.— S. L. Thomas (letter), *ibid.*, 885.

Haemodialysis. Epoprostenol has been used with heparin or as sole antithrombotic agent in patients with renal failure undergoing haemodialysis. When epoprostenol 5 ng per kg body-weight per minute was infused continuously in patients also receiving heparin (J.H. Turney *et al.*, *Lancet*, 1980, *2*, 219) platelets were protected and the biological activity of heparin was enhanced, suggesting that lower doses of heparin could be used and thus make dialysis safer, especially in patients at risk of bleeding. Epoprostenol has also been used successfully as sole antithrombotic agent (R.M. Zusman *et al.*, *New Engl. J. Med.*, 1981, *304*, 934; J.H. Turney *et al.*, *Lancet*, 1981, *1*, 1101) and was considered to have a role in patients at risk of bleeding with routine heparin anticoagulation. Zusman *et al.* found it necessary to reduce the infusion rate of epoprostenol from 4 ng per kg per minute to as little as 0.25 ng per kg per minute in some patients because of a fall in blood pressure, but Turney *et al.* (*Lancet*, 1981, *1*, 1101; J.H. Turney and M.J. Weston, *ibid.*, *2*, 693) had not encountered clinically significant hypotension. More recently, clotting in the extracorporeal circuit has been reported in patients given epoprostenol as sole antithrombotic treatment (F. Knudsen *et al.*, *Lancet*, 1984, *2*, 235; P.B. Rylance *et al.*, *ibid.*, 744). Although their experience indicates that many patients will dialyse successfully with epoprostenol alone, Rylance *et al.* suggest that the infusion of epoprostenol 5 ng per kg per minute, together with a small bolus dose of heparin (500 to 1000 units) at the start of dialysis and further bolus doses to maintain a small prolongation of activated whole-blood clotting-time, will permit safe haemodialysis, especially in the patient who is bleeding, by protecting platelets and preventing fibrin generation.

RESPIRATORY DISORDERS. Epoprostenol given by inhalation prevented bronchoconstriction induced by inhalation of a mist of distilled water and by exercise in asthmatic subjects, but did not have bronchodilator activity.— S. Bianco *et al.*, *IRCS Med. Sci.*, 1978, *6*, 256. It was ineffective in preventing bronchoconstriction induced by inhalation of a pneumoallergen.— *idem*, *Eur. J. resp. Dis.*, 1980, *61*, *Suppl.* 106, 81.

Proprietary Preparations

Flolan *(Wellcome, UK)*. *Infusion*, powder for reconstitution, epoprostenol 500 µg (as sodium salt), supplied with 50-mL vials of glycine buffer as diluent. Store at 2° to 8°; protect from light. Use reconstituted solutions within 12 hours.

8086-p

Fenprostalene *(BAN, USAN, rINN)*.
RS-84043. Methyl (±)-7-{(1*R*,2*R*,3*R*,5*S*)-3,5-dihydroxy-2-[(*E*)-(3*R*)-3-hydroxy-4-phenoxybut-1-enyl]cyclopentyl}hepta-4,5-dienoate.
$C_{23}H_{30}O_6$=402.5.

CAS — 69381-94-8.

Fenprostalene is a synthetic analogue of dinoprost (prostaglandin $F_{2\alpha}$). It is used as a luteolytic agent in veterinary medicine.

Proprietary Veterinary Names and Manufacturers
Synchrocept B *(Syntex, UK)*.

8087-s

Fluprostenol Sodium *(BANM, USAN, rINNM)*.
ICI-81008. Sodium (±)-(*Z*)-7-{(1*R*,2*R*,3*R*,5*S*)-3,5-dihydroxy-2-[(*E*)-(3*R*)-3-hydroxy-4-(3-trifluoromethylphenoxy)but-1-enyl]cyclopentyl}hept-5-enoate.
$C_{23}H_{28}F_3NaO_6$=480.5.

CAS — 40666-16-8 (fluprostenol); 55028-71-2 (sodium salt).

Pharmacopoeias. In *B.P. Vet.*

A white or almost white hygroscopic powder. Freely **soluble** in water, alcohol, and methyl alcohol; practically insoluble in acetone. Solutions are **sterilised** by autoclaving. **Store** in airtight containers. Protect from light.

CAUTION. Fluprostenol sodium is extremely potent and extra-ordinary care should be taken in any procedure in which it is used.

Fluprostenol sodium is a synthetic analogue of dinoprost (prostaglandin $F_{2\alpha}$). It has been used as a luteolytic agent in veterinary medicine.

Proprietary Veterinary Names and Manufacturers
Equimate *(ICI Pharmaceuticals, UK)*.

8088-w

Gemeprost *(BAN, USAN, rINN)*.

16,16-Dimethyl-*trans*-$\triangle^2$-prostaglandin E_1 methyl ester; ONO-802; SC-37681. Methyl (2*E*,13*E*)-(8*R*,11*R*,12*R*,15*R*)-11,15-dihydroxy-16,16-dimethyl-9-oxoprosta-2,13-dienoate; Methyl (*E*)-7-{(1*R*,2*R*,3*R*)-3-hydroxy-2-[(*E*)-(3*R*)-3-hydroxy-4,4-dimethyloct-1-enyl]-5-oxocyclopentyl}hept-2-enoate.
$C_{23}H_{38}O_5$=394.6.

CAS — 64318-79-2.

Store vaginal pessaries containing gemeprost below −10°.

Adverse Effects

Gemeprost is given vaginally as pessaries and systemic adverse effects such as nausea, vomiting, and diarrhoea are relatively mild. Other side-effects reported have included headache, muscle weakness, dizziness, flushing, chills, backache, dyspnoea, chest pain, palpitations, and mild pyrexia.

Precautions

Complete termination of pregnancy must be ensured in patients given gemeprost prior to evacuation of the uterus since its effects on the foetus are not known. Gemeprost should be used with caution in patients with obstructive airways disease, cardiovascular disease, raised intra-ocular pressure, cervicitis, or vaginitis.

Uses and Administration

Gemeprost is a synthetic analogue of alprostadil (prostaglandin E_1). It is a uterine stimulant, but is used mainly to soften and dilate the cervix prior to surgical procedures for the termination of pregnancy in the first trimester. A pessary containing gemeprost 1 mg is inserted into the vagina 3 hours before surgery. Gemeprost may also be used for termination of pregnancy in the second trimester when a 1-mg pessary is inserted every 3 hours to a maximum of 5 pessaries. Should this course be ineffective one further course may be given after an interval of 24 hours.

OBSTETRICS AND GYNAECOLOGY. *Termination of pregnancy.* Gemeprost 1-mg vaginal pessaries given every 3 hours up to a total of 5 doses were used successfully to terminate early pregnancy in women with less than 49 days of amenorrhoea (S.K. Smith and D.T. Baird, *Br. J. Obstet. Gynaec.*, 1980, *87*, 712) and were as effective as dinoprostone administered extra-amniotically for termination in early second trimester (12 to 16 weeks' gestation) (I.T. Cameron and D.T. Baird, *ibid.*, 1984, *91*, 1136). However, gemeprost pessaries are used principally to dilate the cervix, by insertion of a single 1-mg pessary, prior to vacuum aspiration for termination in the first trimester (P.R. Fisher and J.H. Taylor, *ibid.*, 1141; P. Kajanoja *et al.*, *Contraception*, 1984, *29*, 251; N.J. Christensen and M. Bygdeman, *ibid.*, 457).

See also under Termination of Pregnancy in Dinoprost (p.1369).

Proprietary Preparations

Cervagem *(May & Baker, UK)*. *Pessaries*, gemeprost 1 mg.

Proprietary Names and Manufacturers

Cervagem *(Rhone-Poulenc, Denm.*; *Leo Rhodia, Swed.*; *May & Baker, UK)*; Cervageme *(Bellon, Fr.)*.

16847-w

Iloprost *(rINN)*.

Ciloprost; ZK-36374. (*E*)-(3a*S*,4*R*,5*R*,6a*S*)-Hexahydro-5-hydroxy-4-[*E*)-(3*S*,4*RS*)-2-hydroxy-4-methyl-1-octen-6-ynyl]-Δ^2(1*H*),δ-pentalenevaleric acid.

$C_{22}H_{32}O_4$=360.5.

CAS — 73873-87-7.

Iloprost, a vasodilator and platelet aggregation inhibitor, is a stable analogue of the prostaglandin epoprostenol (p.1371) and has similar actions and uses. It has been given by intravenous infusion.

A study of the haemodynamic effects of the carbaprostacyclin analogue iloprost given by intravenous infusion for 3 days to 10 patients with advanced obliterative arterial disease of the lower extremities. Iloprost resembles epoprostenol in many respects, but it is more stable in solution, its storing and handling is less complex, and its plasma half-life is about 13 minutes compared to about 3 minutes for epoprostenol. The most prominent effects of iloprost were marked vasodilatation and decreased vascular resistance. Patients experienced the improved peripheral circulation as pleasant; the skin became warm and pain in the legs usually disappeared. At an infusion rate of 4 ng per kg body-weight per minute almost maximal haemodynamic reponses were achieved, but at higher doses all patients experienced headache, nausea, abdominal colic, or vomiting, to some extent. A dose of 1 to 2 ng per kg per minute was tolerated by all and appeared to be clinically feasible.— S. Kaukinen *et al.*, *Clin. Pharmac. Ther.*, 1984, *36*, 464.

Further references to iloprost: R. Bugiardini *et al.*, *Clin. Pharmac. Ther.*, 1985, *38*, 101 (haemodynamics and side-effects); R. Chiesa *et al.* (letter), *Lancet*, 1985, *2*, 95 (beneficial results in a diabetic patient with severe lower limb ischaemia); R. Bugiardini *et al.*, *Am. J. Cardiol.*, 1986, *58*, 453 (a reduction in platelet aggregation and increased exercise capacity in some patients with angina); J. W. Upward *et al.* (letter), *Br. J. clin. Pharmac.*, 1986, *21*, 241 (hypotension and other side-effects); P. C. Waller *et al.*, *ibid.*, 562P (lack of benefit in stable intermittent claudication).

Proprietary Names and Manufacturers

Schering, Ger.

8089-e

Luprostiol *(BAN, rINN)*.

(±)-(*Z*)-7-{(1*S*,2*R*,3*R*,5*S*)-2-[(2*S*)-3-(3-Chlorophenoxy)-2-hydroxypropylthio]-3,5-dihydroxycyclopentyl}hept-5-enoic acid.

$C_{21}H_{29}ClO_6S$=445.0.

CAS — 67110-79-6.

Luprostiol is a synthetic analogue of dinoprost (prostaglandin $F_{2\alpha}$). It is used as a luteolytic agent in veterinary medicine.

Proprietary Veterinary Names and Manufacturers

Prosolvin *(Intervet, UK)*.

8090-b

Meteneprost *(USAN, rINN)*.

9-Deoxo-16,16-dimethyl-9-methylene-prostaglandin E_2; U-46785. (5*Z*,13*E*)-(8*R*,11*R*,12*R*,15*R*)-11,15-Dihydroxy-16,16-dimethyl-9-methyleneprosta-5,13-dienoic acid; (*Z*)-7-{(1*R*,2*R*,3*R*)-3-Hydroxy-2-[(*E*)-(3*R*)-3-hydroxy-4,4-dimethyloct-1-enyl]-5-methylenecyclopentyl}hept-5-enoic acid.

$C_{23}H_{38}O_4$=378.6.

CAS — 61263-35-2.

Meteneprost is a synthetic derivative of dinoprostone (Prostaglandin E_2). It is a uterine stimulant and has been used for the termination of pregnancy.

OBSTETRICS AND GYNAECOLOGY. *Termination of pregnancy.* Meteneprost exhibits greater biological selectivity than dimethyldinoprostone, together with greatly enhanced chemical stability. Of 24 second-trimester patients, treated at 0 and 8 hours with one vaginal suppository containing meteneprost 75 mg, 20 aborted within 24 hours and one at 26 hours without further therapy. Eleven patients vomited during treatment and one had 2 episodes of diarrhoea.— M. Bygdeman *et al.* (letter), *Lancet*, 1979, *1*, 1136. Meteneprost is also effective for the termination of early pregnancy. A vaginal pessary containing 50 or 60 mg of meteneprost, repeated after 6 hours, and administered in hospital (18 patients) or self-administered at home (17) was as effective as vacuum aspiration (18) in terminating pregnancy in the 5th to 7th week; all patients aborted apart from one in the home treatment group. Those given meteneprost had a higher frequency of gastro-intestinal side-effects, a longer and heavier period of bleeding after treatment, and experienced more pain than those who underwent vacuum aspiration, but prostaglandin treatment in hospital or at home was well accepted by the majority of patients.— A. -S. Rosén *et al.*, *Contraception*, 1984, *29*, 423.

See also under Termination of Pregnancy in Dinoprost (p.1369).

Proprietary Names and Manufacturers

Upjohn, USA.

16898-r

Misoprostol *(BAN, USAN, rINN)*.

SC-29333. (±)-Methyl 7-{(1*R*,2*R*,3*R*)-3-hydroxy-2-[(*E*)-(4*RS*)-4-hydroxy-4-methyloct-1-enyl]-5-oxocyclopentyl}heptanoate; (±)-Methyl (13*E*)-11,16-dihydroxy-16-methyl-9-oxoprost-13-enoate.

$C_{22}H_{38}O_5$=382.5.

CAS — 59122-46-2.

Adverse Effects and Precautions

The commonest side-effect occurring with misoprostol is diarrhoea. Increased uterine contractility has been reported with misoprostol and it should not be given to pregnant women.

A summary of data on misoprostol presented to the FDA. During controlled studies the most common adverse effect was diarrhoea (8.2% compared with 3.1% for placebo); it was dose-related but usually mild, only 8 of 2003 subjects receiving misoprostol having withdrawn because of incapacitating diarrhoea. Headaches and abdominal discomfort were also reported. The effects of misoprostol on the uterus and the potential risks of uterine bleeding or abortion in pregnant women were of more concern. In nonpregnant women taking part in the controlled studies there were menstrual complaints in 15 of 410 (3.7%) receiving misoprostol compared with 2 of 115 (1.7%) given placebo. In a study in pregnant women who had elected to undergo first trimester abortion, all 6 who had a spontaneous expulsion of the uterine contents had received 1 or 2 doses of misoprostol 400 µg the previous evening, while none of those given placebo aborted spontaneously; overall 25 of the 56 women receiving misoprostol experienced uterine bleeding compared to only 2 of 55 on placebo.— J. H. Lewis, *Am. J. Gastroent.*, 1985, *80*, 743. See also R. L. Herting and C. H. Nissen, *Dig. Dis. Scis*, 1986, *31*, *Suppl.*, 47S.

Absorption and Fate

Misoprostol is reported to be rapidly absorbed and metabolised to its free acid following administration by mouth.

An overview of metabolism and pharmacokinetic studies with radioactively labelled misoprostol. Following administration by mouth misoprostol was so rapidly de-esterified to its free acid (SC-30695) that plasma concentrations could not be measured. The free acid was further metabolised to more polar compounds; the di-nor and tetra-nor (SC-41411) metabolites were found in urine. Additional metabolites identified were the prostaglandin F_1 analogue of SC-41411 and its ω-16-carboxylic acid derivative. Mean elimination half-lives for plasma total radioactivity were about 1.7 hours (fast phase) and 157 hours (slow phase); the slow phase was due to the long half-life of the tritiated water produced from the metabolism of misoprostol. The mean plasma elimination half-life of the free acid was 20.6 minutes. About 80% of total radioactivity recovered in the urine and faeces was eliminated within 24 hours of administration; twice the amount of free acid and its metabolites were excreted in the urine as in the faeces. The free acid was 81 to 88% bound to serum protein in young subjects and 81 to 89% bound in elderly subjects.— G. Schoenhard *et al.*, *Dig. Dis. Scis*, 1985, *30*, *Suppl.*, 126S.

Uses and Administration

Misoprostol is a synthetic analogue of alprostadil (prostaglandin E_1). It inhibits gastric acid secretion and has been given by mouth in doses of 200 µg four times daily in the treatment of duodenal and gastric ulcers. Misoprostol has also been used in conjunction with non-steroidal anti-inflammatory drugs for prophylaxis against NSAID-induced ulcers.

GASTRO-INTESTINAL DISORDERS. An extensive review of endogenous and exogenous prostaglandins and the gastro-intestinal tract, including their role in mucosal protection in ulcer healing, in diarrhoea, and in gastro-intestinal inflammation.— C. J. Hawkey and D. S. Rampton, *Gastroenterology*, 1985, *89*, 1162.

A review of prostaglandins in peptic ulcer disease. Naturally occurring prostaglandins of the E series inhibit gastric acid secretion, but their action is short-lived because of rapid inactivation *in vivo*. Synthetic analogues of alprostadil (prostaglandin E_1) and dinoprostone (prostaglandin E_2) have been developed which are resistant to normal enzymatic metabolism and inhibit gastric acid secretion when given by mouth. In addition to their acid-reducing abilities an independent 'cytoprotective' role for prostaglandins has been proposed since they were found to protect the *rat* gastric mucosa against macroscopic damage caused by acid, alcohol, bile acids, hypertonic saline, and boiling water (A. Robert, *Gastroenterology*, 1979, *77*, 761); in *rats* this protective action occurred at much lower doses than were required for gastric antisecretory activity. There has been much debate as to whether prostaglandins do truly protect cells, but although the terms 'cytoprotection' or 'mucosal protection' are not completely adequate, there is little doubt that pretreatment with prostaglandins offers protection to the gastric mucosa. However, for a compound to be considered 'cytoprotective' the effect must be independent of any effect on gastric acid secretion. Proposed mechanisms for this 'cytoprotective' effect have included strengthening of the gastric mucosal barrier with a reduction in H^+ back-diffusion, increased gastric and duodenal mucus secretion, increased gastric and duodenal bicarbonate secretion, and increased gastric mucosal blood flow. In view of the apparent role of prostaglandins in maintaining integrity of the gastro-intestinal mucosa, it has been proposed that peptic ulcer disease might be a prostaglandin deficiency state and that an imbalance between aggressive factors, such as acid, and defensive factors providing mucosal protection might be involved. There is some evidence that smoking, a major risk factor for peptic ulcer, adversely affects mucosal integrity by inhibiting endogenous production of mucosal prostaglandins.

The prostaglandin analogues studied most extensively are the alprostadil derivative misoprostol and the dinoprostone derivatives arbaprostil and enprostil. The results indicate that prostaglandins are effective in healing duodenal and gastric ulcers, but it appears that antisecretory doses are needed and 'cytoprotection' alone as an ulcer-healing mechanism has not been demonstrated with lower doses. Preliminary studies have indicated that the 'cytoprotective' properties of prostaglandin analogues might prevent gastroduodenal damage caused by aspirin and other non-steroidal anti-inflammatory drugs, but this awaits confirmation in larger controlled studies.— S. J. Sontag, *Drugs*, 1986, *32*, 445.

An evaluation of the current status of prostaglandin analogues in the treatment of peptic ulcer, in view of their properties of mucosal defence and acid inhibition. Misoprostol, enprostil, arbaprostil, and trimoprostil have been shown to be competent but not outstanding ulcer-healing drugs and to produce less symptomatic relief than cimetidine or ranitidine. The implication is that the cytoprotective properties demonstrated in *animals* play no part in ulcer healing and do not compensate for their relatively weak antisecretory activity. Antisecretory doses of prostaglandin analogues may also be necessary for effective protection against non-steroidal anti-inflammatory drugs. Thus, the evidence suggests that prostaglandin analogues currently available are not sufficiently effective at healing duodenal or gastric ulcers to justify their routine use in preference to H_2-receptor antagonists. The hope that relapse rates might be less after ulcer healing with prostaglandin analogues has not yet been substantiated.— C. J. Hawkey and R. P. Walt, *Lancet*, 1986, *2*, 1084.

A detailed review of misoprostol and its use in the treatment of peptic ulcer disease. Large well-controlled studies have shown that misoprostol is of value, especially in patients with duodenal ulcer, although it is no more effective than cimetidine at healing ulcers and is less effective at relieving pain. As with other available drug therapy, ulcer recurrence rate is unaffected by misoprostol; maintenance therapy has not yet been assessed. The usual dose of 200 µg four times daily has substantial antisecretory activity; 400 µg twice daily has also been effective. Lower doses of misoprostol, without antisecretory activity but reputedly with cytoprotective properties, have been of little benefit.

Mucosal protection against gastro-intestinal damage induced by aspirin has been demonstrated in healthy subjects given antisecretory doses of misoprostol, but results have been inconsistent at lower doses; antisecretory doses have also protected against alcohol-induced mucosal damage in healthy subjects. As yet there is little evidence to support claims that, because of its cytoprotective properties, misoprostol might be particularly effective in smokers and in protecting against ulcer development associated with non-steroidal anti-inflammatory drugs.— J. P. Monk and S. P. Clissold, *Drugs*, 1987, *33*, 1.

Further reviews: R. L. Herting and C. H. Nissen, *Dig. Dis. Scis*, 1986, *31, Suppl.*, 47S.

Studies with misoprostol in the treatment of duodenal ulcer: D. L. Brand *et al.*, *Dig. Dis. Scis*, 1985, *30, Suppl.*, 147S (misoprostol 50 or 200 µg four times daily compared with placebo); P. A. Nicholson, *Dig. Dis. Scis*, 1985, *30, Suppl.*, 171S (misoprostol 50 or 200 µg four times daily compared with cimetidine); P. Bright-Asare *et al.*, *Dig. Dis. Scis*, 1986, *31, Suppl.*, 63S (misoprostol 200 or 400 µg twice daily compared with placebo).

Studies with misoprostol in the treatment of gastric ulcer: D. Rachmilewitz *et al.*, *Dig. Dis. Scis*, 1986, *31, Suppl.*, 75S (misoprostol 50 or 200 µg four times daily compared with cimetidine).

Proceedings of a symposium on misoprostol in gastroenterology.— *Postgrad. med. J.*, 1988, *64, Suppl.* 1, 1–88.

Proprietary Preparations

Cytotec *(Searle, UK)*. *Tablets*, scored, misoprostol 200 µg.

Proprietary Names and Manufacturers

Cytotec *(Searle, Austral.; Searle, Canad.; Searle, Fr.; Searle, Ger.; Searle, Mex.; Searle, Switz.; Searle, UK)*.

8095-s

Prostalene *(BAN, USAN, pINN)*.

RS-9390. Methyl (±)-(13*E*)-(8*R*,9*S*,11*R*,12*R*)-9,11,15-trihydroxy-15-methylprosta-4,5,13-trienoate; Methyl (±)-7-{(1*R*,2*R*,3*R*,5*S*)-3,5-dihydroxy-2-[(*E*)-3-hydroxy-3-methyloct-1-enyl]cyclopentyl}hepta-4,5-dienoate.

$C_{22}H_{36}O_5$=380.5.

CAS — 54120-61-5.

Prostalene is a synthetic analogue of prostaglandin F_1. It is used as a luteolytic agent in veterinary medicine.

Proprietary Veterinary Names and Manufacturers

Synchrocept E *(Syntex, UK)*.

18675-f

Rioprostil *(BAN, USAN, rINN)*.

BAY-o-6893; ORF-15927; TR-4698. (*E*)-(2*R*,3*R*,4*R*)-4-Hydroxy-2-(7-hydroxyheptyl)-3-(4-hydroxy-4-methyloct-1-enyl)cyclopentanone.

$C_{21}H_{38}O_4$=354.5.

CAS — 77287-05-9.

Rioprostil, a synthetic analogue of alprostadil (prostaglandin E_1), inhibits gastric acid secretion. It has actions and uses similar to those of misoprostol (p.1374) and has been given by mouth in the treatment of peptic ulcer.

GASTROINTESTINAL DISORDERS. Aspirin-induced gastrointestinal blood loss was reduced by rioprostil 60, 120, or 300 µg four times daily by mouth in healthy subjects.— A. Cohen *et al.*, *J. clin. Pharmac.*, 1984, *24*, 401.

A single bedtime dose of rioprostil 600 µg for 4 weeks was successful in the treatment of acute duodenal ulcer and comparable with ranitidine 300 mg at night in promoting ulcer healing and pain relief in a double-blind study in 208 patients. Cumulative healing rates at 4 weeks were 84.4% for rioprostil and 89.9% for ranitidine. Diarrhoea seemed to be less of a problem with a single dose of rioprostil at night than it is with more frequent prostglandin administration; no patient on rioprostil suffered severe diarrhoea and abdominal pain.— H. G. Dammann *et al.* (letter), *Lancet*, 1986, *2*, 335. Comment on the impressive healing rate with rioprostil. This may not be explained completely on the basis of suppression of acidity, which again raises the issue of whether or not cytoprotection is of value in treating duodenal ulceration.— C. W. Howden (letter), *ibid.*, 686.

For reviews on prostaglandin analogues in the treatment of peptic ulcer and discussion on their reputed cytoprotective properties, see Misoprostol, p.1374.

Proprietary Names and Manufacturers

Bayer, Ger.

16980-z

Rosaprostol *(rINN)*.

9-Hydroxy-19,20-bis-nor-prostanoic Acid. 2-Hexyl-5-hydroxycyclopentaneheptanoic acid, mixture of (1*RS*,2*SR*,5*RS*) and (1*RS*,2*SR*,5*SR*) isomers.

$C_{18}H_{34}O_3$=298.5.

CAS — 56695-65-9.

Rosaprostol is a synthetic prostaglandin derivative which inhibits gastric acid secretion. It has actions and uses similar to those of misoprostol (p.1374) and has been given by mouth in the treatment of peptic ulcer.

GASTRO-INTESTINAL DISORDERS. Duodenal ulcers were completely healed in 12 of 20 patients given rosaprostol 500 mg four times daily by mouth for 6 weeks compared with 15 of 20 given cimetidine. Side-effects associated with rosaprostol were constipation in 3 patients, diarrhoea in 2, belching in 1, and headache in 1.— D. Foschi *et al.*, *Drugs exp. & clin. Res.*, 1984, *10*, 427.

For reviews on prostaglandin analogues in the treatment of peptic ulcer and discussion on their reputed cytoprotective properties, see Misoprostol, p.1374.

Proprietary Names and Manufacturers

Rosal *(Ibi, Ital.)*.

8096-w

Sulprostone *(USAN, rINN)*.

16-Phenoxy-ω-17,18,19,20-tetranor-prostaglandin E_2-methylsulfonylamide; CP-34089; SHB-286; ZK-57671. (*Z*)-7-{(1*R*,2*R*,3*R*)-3-Hydroxy-2-[(*E*)-(3*R*)-3-hydroxy-4-phenoxybut-1-enyl]-5-oxocyclopentyl]-*N*-(methylsulphonyl)}hept-5-enamide.

$C_{23}H_{31}NO_7S$=465.6.

CAS — 60325-46-4.

Sulprostone is a synthetic derivative of dinoprostone (prostaglandin E_2). It is a uterine stimulant and is used for the termination of pregnancy. Sulprostone has been given intravenously, intramuscularly, extra-amniotically, and vaginally.

OBSTETRICS AND GYNAECOLOGY. Distinct cervical dilatation was achieved in 20 of 69 nonpregnant women given sulprostone 500 µg intramuscularly in order to facilitate various intra-uterine manipulations; 31 of the women had slight dilatation and the remainder had none.— L. V. Rivero *et al.*, *Curr. ther. Res.*, 1984, *35*, 799.

Termination of pregnancy. Sulprostone has been used in a variety of ways for the termination of pregnancy in the first trimester. Complete abortion occurred in 76.6% of 77 women at 5 to 12 weeks' gestation given sulprostone 1 mg by intravenous infusion over 10 hours; adverse effects included uterine pain and nausea and vomiting (B. Schuessler *et al.*, *Contraception*, 1979, *19*, 29). Menstrual induction was achieved in 96% of 90 women following the intramuscular injection of sulprostone 500 µg, usually repeated after 4 hours; adverse effects included vomiting in 26%, diarrhoea in 10%, and endometritis in 2% (A.I. Csapo *et al.*, *Lancet*, 1980, *1*, 90). Sulprostone has also been used to dilate the cervix prior to vacuum aspiration. In a study involving 200 women in the 8th to 12th week of pregnancy (N.J. Christensen, *Contraception*, 1985, *32*, 359) 250 or 500 µg of sulprostone given intramuscularly 3 to 4 hours before surgery was equally effective in dilating the cervix and in controlling bleeding, but gastro-intestinal side-effects and painful uterine contractions were more frequent with the higher dose. Cervical priming has also been achieved by the intracervical application of gels containing 50 or 100 µg of sulprostone 6 to 8 hours before curettage (W. Rath *et al.*, *Contraception*, 1983, *28*, 209; W. Rath *et al.*, *ibid.*, 1985, *31*, 207).

Sulprostone has also been used for the termination of pregnancy in the second trimester, although results were judged to be poor in 70 women given 3 or 4 intramuscular injections of sulprostone 500 µg at 3-hourly intervals or 25, 50, or 100 µg given extra-amniotically (P. Fylling, *Contraception*, 1982, *26*, 279).

See also under Dinoprost, p.1369.

Proprietary Names and Manufacturers

Nalador *(Schering, Fr.; Schering, Ger.; Schering, Ital.; Schering, Switz.)*.

17016-h

Trimoprostil *(USAN, rINN)*.

Ro-21-6937/000. (*Z*)-7-{(1*R*,2*R*,3*R*)-2-[(*E*)-(3*R*)-3-Hydroxy-4,4-dimethyl-1-octenyl]-3-methyl-5-oxocyclopentyl}-5-heptenoic acid; (5*Z*,11α,13*E*,15*R*)-15-Hydroxy-11,16,16-trimethyl-9-oxoprosta-5,13-dien-1-oic acid.

$C_{23}H_{38}O_4$=378.6.

CAS — 69900-72-7.

Trimoprostil, a synthetic analogue of dinoprostone (prostaglandin E_2), inhibits gastric acid secretion. It has actions and uses similar to those of misoprostol (p.1374) and has been given by mouth in the treatment of peptic ulcer.

Pharmacokinetic studies of trimoprostil: R. J. Wills, *J. clin. Pharmac.*, 1984, *24*, 194 (influence of food on bioavailability); R. J. Wills *et al.*, *Clin. Pharmac. Ther.*, 1985, *37*, 113 (plasma concentrations and gastric acid inhibition in healthy subjects); R. J. Wills *et al.*, *J. clin. Pharmac.*, 1986, *26*, 48 (plasma concentrations and gastric acid inhibition in patients with duodenal ulcers).

GASTRO-INTESTINAL DISORDERS. Trimoprostil 750 µg four times daily by mouth was less effective than cimetidine in healing duodenal ulcers and relieving pain in a double-blind study in 60 patients. Of 30 patients given trimoprostil, 5 had to be withdrawn from the study because of continuing ulcer pain, nausea, and vomiting, and another patient defaulted.— K. D. Bardhan *et al.*, *Gut*, 1984, *25*, A580.

For reviews on prostaglandin analogues in the treatment of peptic ulcer and discussion on their reputed cytoprotective properties, see Misoprostol, p.1374.

Proprietary Names and Manufacturers

Roche, USA.

18694-h

Viprostol *(BAN, USAN, rINN)*.

CL-115347. Methyl (5*Z*,13*E*)-(11*R*,16*RS*)-7-[3-hydroxy-2-(4-hydroxy-4-vinyloct-1-enyl)-5-oxocyclopentyl]hept-5-enoate.

$C_{23}H_{36}O_5$=392.5.

CAS — 73647-73-1.

Viprostol is a synthetic analogue of dinoprostone (prostaglandin E_2). It is a vasodilator which is absorbed through the skin and has been applied topically in the treatment of peripheral vascular disease. It has also been tried in male-pattern baldness.

Beneficial results were achieved with viprostol administered transdermally for 6 weeks in 15 patients with Raynaud's phenomenon when compared with placebo in 14 similar patients. Viprostol 1 mg every 24 hours was administered as an ointment spread onto adhesive plaster delivering approximately 100 µg per cm^2 skin surface-area. The frequency and duration of attacks was still reduced 2 weeks after the cessation of treatment. There was a transient fall in systolic blood pressure after 2 weeks of treatment, but diastolic blood pressure remained unchanged. Vasodilatory side-effects occurred in 4 treated patients; flushing in 1 and headaches in 3. One patient had diarrhoea. Although it has been suggested that viprostol produces its benefit by both vasodilatory and antiplatelet effects, initial decreases in platelet aggregation were not maintained.— J. J. F. Belch *et al.*, *Lancet*, 1985, *1*, 1180. Transdermal viprostol was beneficial in 3 children with primary Raynaud's disease, 2 of whom were treated throughout the winter.— D. B. Dunger *et al.* (letter), *ibid.*, *2*, 50.

Proprietary Names and Manufacturers
Lederle, USA.

Radiopharmaceuticals

5850-b

Radioactive compounds are used in medicine as sources of radiation for radiotherapy and for diagnostic purposes. They have numerous uses in research and industry. These compounds may be considered as sealed radioactive sources that are bonded or encapsulated to prevent the escape of the radioactive material and are used as supplied.

Unsealed sources, on the other hand, are radioactive materials usually in liquid, particulate, or gaseous form that are removed from their containers for application. Radiopharmaceuticals come within this category.

The aim of this section is to provide background information on the radionuclides that are used mainly as radiopharmaceuticals. Care is required in the preparation, handling, use, and disposal of these compounds, they are thus best dealt with by those with suitable experience and training.

Atomic Stucture, Radioisotopes, and Radionuclides

An atom is composed of a central positively charged nucleus around which, and at relatively great distances away, negatively charged electrons revolve in orbits. The electrons are arranged round the atomic nucleus in a series of 'shells' in each of which is a limited number of orbits.

The nucleus consists of 2 main kinds of particles known as protons, each of unit positive charge, and neutrons, which are uncharged; the total number of these particles in the nucleus is known as the *mass number* .

Each electron carries a negative charge which is of the same size as the positive charge of the proton, so that in the neutral atom the number of electrons is equal to the number of protons in the nucleus.

The number of protons in the nucleus is known as the *atomic number*, which determines the number of electrons in the extranuclear structure. Thus all the atoms of a particular chemical element have the same atomic number. But while the number of protons (atomic number) in a given element is constant, the number of neutrons in the atoms, and thus their masses (mass numbers), may vary. These different forms of the same element are known as isotopes of the element and these isotopes differ in some of their physical properties.

Some isotopes may be stable, the differences between them arising solely from their difference in mass; others may be radioactive (*radioisotopes*), their nuclei changing spontaneously and emitting particles or electromagnetic waves, or both.

Most of the naturally occurring isotopes are stable, though there are a number which are unstable and therefore radioactive, for example, uranium-235. In addition, artificial radionuclides are prepared by converting stable nuclei into unstable forms and even naturally occurring radionuclides may be prepared by artificial means. Radionuclides may therefore not necessarily be radioisotopes.

The symbol used for a nuclide is a development of the chemical symbol for the atom, with the mass number as a superscript and the atomic number as a subscript; thus the symbols for the 3 hydrogen isotopes—common hydrogen, deuterium, and tritium—are ${}^{1}_{1}H$, ${}^{2}_{1}H$, and ${}^{3}_{1}H$, and the symbols for the 3 naturally occurring uranium isotopes are ${}^{234}_{92}U$, ${}^{235}_{92}U$, and ${}^{238}_{92}U$; as the atomic number can be inferred from the chemical symbol it is the usual practice to omit the subscript. It is also common practice to write out the full name of the element followed by the superscript, e.g. chromium-51 for ${}^{51}Cr$.

Emissions from Radioisotopes

The 3 main types of emission from radioactive substances are *alpha particles, beta particles,* and *gamma-rays*. Most sources emit more than one type of radiation.

Alpha particles are positively charged particles (helium nuclei), each consisting of 2 protons and 2 neutrons.

Beta particles (β^- or β^+) are identical with electrons or positrons but arise from the nucleus. They are emitted with great velocity and their energies are spread over a spectrum. Positrons are similar to electrons, having a similar mass but a positive charge.

Gamma-rays are electromagnetic radiations with a wavelength much shorter than those of light.

In certain cases, e.g. chromium-51, *electron capture* (EC) occurs, an electron from an inner shell being absorbed by the nucleus with the production of an *X-ray* characteristic of the daughter atom or emission of an *Auger electron.*

The type of emission from a radionuclide largely determines its usefulness in medicine. Those emitting α-particles are very little used partly because detection and measurement are difficult. Positron-emitters, such as carbon-11, nitrogen-13, and oxygen-15, have become more popular in recent years and are used in positron-emission tomography (PET) where the radiation is measured from within the body as opposed to computerised tomography when the energy is supplied from an external source. Gamma-ray emitting radionuclides are most accessible and are the most common radiation source in radiopharmaceuticals. Positrons on contact with matter release gamma rays.

The radiation data given under the radionuclides described in the following pages show the half-life, the energy of the radiation of particles in million electronvolts (MeV), and the percentage of total number of transformations which gives rise to the emission of the particular radiation. Since one transformation may give rise to more than one gamma-ray the percentages do not necessarily add up to 100%. X-rays, together with minor emissions, have been omitted unless they are a significant part of the total emission.

Decay of Radionuclides

A radionuclide will consist of unstable atoms which will at some time undergo an energy change with the emission of ionising radiation, those which are actually undergoing this change, and those which have undergone the change. In quantitative terms this transition occurs at a rate which is characteristic of the radionuclide and it is expressed as its half-life—the time required for the activity to fall by one-half. Many radionuclides have complex decay characteristics with several possible energies of emitted particles and radiation. Some radionuclides may be in an excited or metastable state denoted by the suffix m attached to the mass number (e.g. Technetium-99m) and undergo *isomeric transition* (IT) with the release of γ-rays.

The activity of radionuclides is measured in terms of the rate of transformation or disintegration. The unit is the becquerel (Bq)=1 transformation per second; the curie (Ci) was formerly used as the unit of activity; 1 $Ci=3.7\times10^{10}$ Bq.

Supply, Preparation, and Control of Radioactive Materials

A wide range of radionuclides and specially formulated radiopharmaceuticals is available from specialised manufacturers. However, there are national controls on the use, transport, storage, and disposal of such compounds. Authority and guidance should be sought from the relevant bodies and authorities before using such compounds. Some of the bodies involved include the International Commission on Radiological Protection, the World Health Organisation, and for the *UK*, the National Radiological Protection Board.

Generators are special features in the supply of radionuclides. They are receptacles containing a parent and daughter nuclide in equilibrium and from which the daughter nuclide which usually has a short half-life may be eluted. Generators are available for the production of indium-113m and technetium-99m. Generators are also available for some positron-emitters.

Storage conditions for radiopharmaceuticals should be such as to prevent the inadvertent emission of radioactivity as well as to meet the storage requirements for the pharmaceutical that has been labelled. Thus due account still has to be paid, for instance, to the effects of temperature and light. Radiopharmaceuticals are liable to decomposition by self-irradiation effects which may cause degradation of solvent, preservative, or other compounds. There can also be a continuous formation of oxidising and reducing chemical species arising from the effect of the radioactivity on any chemical substances present in the radiopharmaceutical, even in minute amounts.

Adverse Effects of Radionuclides

The internal irradiation of tissues following the administration of radionuclides carries similar dangers to exposure to ionising radiation from an external source, and local high irradiation doses may arise if these nuclides are specifically localised in a tissue. The most serious danger is genetic damage prior to and during the reproductive period. Tissues whose cells are in a continuous state of multiplication are particularly sensitive to the effects of radiation.

Untoward effects of exposure to the larger doses of irradiation include leucopenia, anaemia, inflammation of the skin, radiation sickness, and neoplasms.

In considering the effect of a given radionuclide it is usual to calculate the dose to the organ most critically affected, and also the dose to the whole body.

In considering the adverse effects of radiopharmaceuticals one should not forget the effects that might arise from the carrier or from contaminants.

General Uses of Radioactive Materials

Radiopharmaceuticals are used widely in many branches of medicine and surgery, mainly for the diagnosis and sometimes for the treatment of disease. They can offer facilities not provided by other diagnostic techniques such as contrast media, ultrasound, and computerised tomography or other external irradiation. Interesting developments have followed the tagging of monoclonal antibodies with radionuclides.

Many investigations involve the oral or parenteral administration of radionuclides or labelled compounds, and the subsequent measurement of radioactive concentrations in organs, tissues, blood, urine, or faeces. The quantities used are always the smallest which will give the desired accuracy of image or of measurement.

Radiological Terms Associated with Description of Radionuclides.

Alpha particles. Nuclei of helium atoms emitted by radioactive atomic nuclei.

Annihilation. The interaction and disappearance of a positive and a negative electron with the conversion of their energy into electromagnetic radiation.

Atomic number (Z). The number of protons in the atomic nucleus.

Auger effect. The emission of an electron from an atom due to the filling of a vacancy in an inner electron shell.

Becquerel (Bq). The SI unit of activity, defined as 1 transformation per second. The curie (below) was formerly used as the unit of activity. 1 Bq=2.7×10^{-11} Ci.

Beta particles. Electrons or positrons emitted by radioactive atomic nuclei.

Biological half-life. The time required for the amount of a particular substance to be halved by biological means, when the rate of removal is approximately exponential.

Carrier-free. A preparation in which substantially all the atoms of the activated element present are radioactive. Material of high specific activity is often loosely referred to as 'carrier-free'.

Curie (Ci). Now superseded as a unit of activity by the becquerel. A curie (Ci) represented 3.7×10^{10} transformations per second. 1 Ci=3.7×10^{10} Bq.

Daughter. Of a given nuclide, any nuclide that originates from it by radioactive decay.

Electron capture (EC). A mode of radioactivity decay involving the capture of an orbital electron by its nucleus.

Gamma-radiation. Electromagnetic radiation emitted in the process of a change in configuration of a nucleus or particle annihilation and having wavelengths shorter than those of X-rays.

Gray (Gy). The SI unit of absorbed dose, defined as 1 J per kg. The rad (below) was formerly used as the unit of absorbed dose. 1 Gy=100 rads.

Isomeric transition (IT). The decay of one isomer to another having a lower energy state. The transition is accompanied by the emission of gamma-radiation.

Isomers. Nuclides with the same mass number and atomic number but with nuclei having different energy states.

Isotopes. Nuclides with the same atomic number but different mass numbers.

MBq. Megabecquerel=10^6 Bq.

mCi. Millicurie=10^{-3} Ci.

Nuclide. A species of atom having a specific mass number, atomic number, and nuclear energy state.

Photon. A quantum of electromagnetic radiation.

Positron. A positive beta particle.

Rad (radiation absorbed dose).
Now superseded as a unit of absorbed dose by the gray. A rad is equal to 10^{-2} J per kg. The röntgen and the rad in soft tissue are approximately equivalent in magnitude for moderate energies. 1 rad=10^{-2} Gy.

Radioactive decay. The spontaneous change of a nucleus resulting in the emission of a particle or a photon.

Radioactivity. The property of certain nuclides of spontaneously emitting particles or photons or of undergoing spontaneous fission.

Radioisotope. An isotope that is radioactive.

Radionuclide. A nuclide that is radioactive.

Rem (röntgen-equivalent-man).
Now superseded as a unit of dose equivalent by the sievert (Sv). A rem is numerically equal to the absorbed dose in rads multiplied by the appropriate quality factor defining the biological effect and by any other modifying factors. The Sievert is the joule per kg ($J\ kg^{-1}$) equal to 100 rem.

Röntgen (R). A unit of exposure of X- or gamma-radiation, equal to 2.58×10^{-4} coulombs per kg in air superseded by the SI unit of exposure, the coulomb per kg ($C\ kg^{-1}$). 1 $C\ kg^{-1}$=3.876×10^3 R.

Sievert (Sv). The SI unit of dose equivalent numerically equal to the absorbed dose in grays multiplied by the appropriate quality factor defining the biological effect and by any other modifying factors expressed in J per kg.

Specific activity. The activity per unit mass of a material containing a radioactive substance.

X-rays. Electromagnetic radiation other than annihilation radiation originating in the extranuclear part of the atom and having wavelengths much shorter than those of visible light.

5852-g

Calcium-47 ($^{47}_{20}Ca$)

HALF-LIFE. 4.54 days

RADIATION EMITTED. β^- 0.69 (82%), 1.99 (17.9%) MeV; γ 0.489 (6.8%), 0.808 (6.8%), 1.297 (75.1%) MeV.

Calcium-47 is supplied as calcium chloride (^{47}Ca) in the form of an injection containing more than 3.7 megabecquerels (100 microcuries) per mg of calcium. This is injected intravenously in doses of 185 to 740 kBq (5 to 20 microcuries) for the investigation of calcium metabolism. It is of limited use in some aspects of calcium metabolism because its half-life is short in relation to the processes to be measured. Solutions of calcium chloride (^{47}Ca) are contaminated with small quantities of calcium-45 and scandium-47. The solution must therefore be used within a short time of receipt.
Calcium-45 is available for the investigation of calcium metabolism.
Calcium-46 has also been used as a urinary and faecal marker.

9907-j

Carbon-11 ($^{11}_{6}C$)

HALF-LIFE. 20.4 minutes

RADIATION EMITTED. β^+ 1.0 MeV

Carbon-11 is a positron-emitter which is used in positron-emission tomography.

5853-q

Carbon-14 ($^{14}_{6}C$)

HALF-LIFE. 5730 years

RADIATION EMITTED. β^- 0.156 (100%) MeV.

Many organic compounds labelled with carbon-14 are available but few are used *in vivo* except in research.

5854-p

Chromium-51 ($^{51}_{24}Cr$)

HALF-LIFE. 27.7 days

RADIATION EMITTED. EC (100%); γ 0.320 (9.9%) MeV; X-rays (vanadium) 0.005 to 0.006 (~22%) MeV.

Chromium-51 is usually supplied as sodium chromate (^{51}Cr) solutions or injections containing 3700 to 37 000 megabecquerels (100 to 1000 millicuries) per mg of chromium. *B.P.* and *Eur. P.* specify not less than 370 megabecquerels (10 millicuries) per mg of chromate ion and *U.S.P.* specifies not less than 370 megabecquerels (10 millicuries) per mg of sodium chromate at the end of the expiry period. Chromium-51 is also supplied as chromic chloride (^{51}Cr) injection, iso-osmotic with serum, containing 1850 to 37 000 megabecquerels (50 to 1000 millicuries) per mg of chromium, and as chromium (^{51}Cr) edetate injection, containing 37 to 74 megabecquerels (1 to 2 millicuries) per mg of chromium.
Chromium-51, as Sodium Chromate (^{51}Cr) Sterile Solution, is used to label red blood cells so that red-cell survival and red-cell volume can be measured. Chromium-51 activity in the faeces can be used to estimate gastro-intestinal blood losses. The usual dose is 0.74 to 3.7 megabecquerels (20 to 100 microcuries). Red blood cells labelled with chromium-51 and damaged by heat before reinjection have been used for spleen scanning.
As Chromium Edetate (^{51}Cr) Injection, chromium-51 is used in the determination of the glomerular filtration-rate. The usual dose is 1.295 to 11.1 MBq (35 to 300 microcuries) administered intravenously.
As chromic chloride (^{51}Cr) injection, chromium-51 is also administered intravenously in usual doses of 1.11 to 3.7 MBq (30 to 100 microcuries) for the determination of loss of serum protein into the gastro-intestinal tract.

Preparations
Chromium (^{51}Cr) Edetate Injection *(B.P., Eur. P.)*
Sodium Chromate Cr 51 Injection *(U.S.P.)*
Sodium Chromate (^{51}Cr) Sterile Solution *(B.P., Eur. P.)*

5855-s

Cobalt-57 ($^{57}_{27}Co$)

HALF-LIFE. 271 days

RADIATION EMITTED. EC (100%); γ 0.014 (9.5%), 0.122 (85.6%), 0.136 (10.7%), 0.570 (0.01%), 0.692 (0.16%) MeV; X-rays (iron) 0.006 to 0.007 (~56%) MeV.

Cobalt-57 is usually supplied as cyanocobalamin (^{57}Co) in the form of an aqueous solution containing 18.5 kilobecquerels (0.5 microcurie) per µg or more than 37 kilobecquerels (1 microcurie) per µg of cyanocobalamin. *U.S.P.* specifies not less than 18.5 kilobecquerels (0.5 microcurie) per µg of cyanocobalamin. It is also supplied as cyanocobalamin (^{57}Co) in the form of capsules containing 18.5 kilobecquerels (0.5 microcurie) per µg of cyanocobalamin. *U.S.P.* specifies not less than 18.5 kilobecquerels (0.5 microcurie) per µg of cyanocobalamin. Cobalt-57 is also supplied for *in vitro* diagnostic procedures as cyanocobalamin (^{57}Co) in the form of aqueous solutions containing 0.37 to 11.1 megabecquerels (10 to 300 microcuries) per µg of cyanocobalamin.
Cyanocobalamin (^{57}Co) is used for the measurement of absorption of vitamin B_{12} in the diagnosis of pernicious anaemia and other malabsorption syndromes in doses of 18.5 to 37 kBq (0.5 to 1 microcurie) by mouth. It is also used with cyanocobalamin (^{58}Co), see below.

Preparations
Cyanocobalamin (^{57}Co) Solution *(B.P., Eur. P.)*
Cyanocobalamin Co 57 Capsules *(U.S.P.)*
Cyanocobalamin Co 57 Oral Solution *(U.S.P.)*

5856-w

Cobalt-58 ($^{58}_{27}Co$)

HALF-LIFE. 70.8 days

RADIATION EMITTED. β^+ 0.475 (15%) MeV; EC (85%); γ 0.511 (from β^+), 0.811 (99.4%), 0.864 (0.7%), 1.675 (0.5%) MeV; X-rays (iron) 0.006 to 0.007 (~26%) MeV.

Cobalt-58 is usually supplied as cyanocobalamin (^{58}Co) in the form of an aqueous solution containing more than 37 kilobecquerels (1 microcurie) per µg of cyanocobalamin and is used for the measurement of absorption of vitamin B_{12} in the diagnosis of pernicious anaemia and other malabsorption syndromes.
The usual dose is 18.5 to 37 kBq (0.5 to 1 microcurie) by mouth.
The different energies of cobalt-57 and cobalt-58 facilitate separation of the isotopes in a mixture. Advantage is taken of this to differentiate between failure of absorption due to lack of intrinsic factor (pernicious anaemia) and that due to ileal malabsorption by the simultaneous administration of cyanocobalamin (^{58}Co) and cyanocobalamin (^{57}Co) bound to gastric juice. A dual isotope kit is available for this purpose.

Preparations
Cyanocobalamin (^{58}Co) Solution *(B.P., Eur. P.)*

5857-e

Cobalt-60 ($^{60}_{27}Co$)

HALF-LIFE. 5.27 years

RADIATION EMITTED. β^- 0.318 (99.9%), 1.491 (0.1%) MeV; γ 1.173 (99.86%), 1.333 (99.98%) MeV.

Cobalt-60 is used for radiotherapy in the form of alloys in large sealed sources.
It is also used as a radiation source for sterilisation by gamma-irradiation.
Cyanocobalamin (^{60}Co) has been used as a diagnostic aid in the detection of pernicious anaemia but, because of its long half-life, it has been superseded for this purpose by cyanocobalamin (^{58}Co) and cyanocobalamin (^{57}Co).

Preparations
Cyanocobalamin Co 60 Capsules *(U.S.P.)*
Cyanocobalamin Co 60 Oral Solution *(U.S.P.)*

2037-x

Erbium-169 ($^{169}_{68}$Er)

HALF-LIFE. 9.4 days

RADIATION EMITTED. β^- 0.343 (42%), 0.352 (58%) MeV.

Erbium-169 is supplied as erbium citrate (^{169}Er) in the form of an injectable suspension containing 37 to 1110 megabecquerels (1 to 30 millicuries) per mg of erbium. It is used in the treatment of arthritic conditions particularly of the small joints when it is injected intra-articularly.

19185-l

Fluorine-18 ($^{18}_{9}$F)

HALF-LIFE. 110 minutes

RADIATION EMITTED. β^+ 0.6 MeV.

Fluorine-18 is a positron-emitting radionuclide. Fluorine-18-labelled analogues of glucose, principally 2-fluoro-2-deoxy-D-glucose have been used clinically in the assessment of regional cerebral and myocardial metabolism and for the detection of tumours in the lungs and liver. Fluorine-18-labelled amino acids have also been used for pancreatic scintigraphy.

5858-l

Gallium-67 ($^{67}_{31}$Ga)

HALF-LIFE. 78.26 hours

RADIATION EMITTED. EC (100%); γ 0.091 (3.6%), 0.185 (23.5%), 0.209 (2.6%), 0.300 (16.7%), 0.394 (4.4%) MeV; X-rays (zinc) 0.008 to 0.010 (~43%) MeV. It also decays via zinc-67m [half-life: 9.2 microseconds. γ 0.093 (37.6%) MeV; X-rays (zinc) 0.008 to 0.010 (~13%) MeV].

Gallium-67 is supplied as gallium citrate (^{67}Ga) in the form of a carrier-free injection containing 74 megabecquerels (2 millicuries) per mL or 37 megabecquerels (1 millicurie) per mL. Gallium-67, in the form of the citrate, is concentrated in some tumours of the lymphatic system and other soft tissues, and is used in doses of 55.5 to 92.5 MBq (1.5 to 2.5 millicuries) for tumour visualisation by scanning techniques. Carcinoma of the lung may be diagnosed and staged with gallium-67.
Localisation has been reported in inflammatory lesions and gallium-67 has been used for the diagnosis of various infections, sarcoidosis, and other inflammatory lesions.

Preparations
Gallium (^{67}Ga) Citrate Injection *(B.P., Eur. P.)*
Gallium Citrate Ga 67 Injection *(U.S.P.)*

5859-y

Gold-198 ($^{198}_{79}$Au)

HALF-LIFE. 65 hours (2.7 days)

RADIATION EMITTED. β^- 0.29 (1.0%), 0.966 (98.9%) MeV; γ 0.412 (95.6%), 0.676 (0.8%), 1.088 (0.2%) MeV.

Gold-198 is supplied as sterile colloidal suspensions of metallic gold stabilised with gelatin and glucose for therapeutic or diagnostic use and containing 37 to 740 megabecquerels (1 to 20 millicuries) per mg of gold.
Gold-198, as Colloidal Gold (^{198}Au) Injection with most of the activity associated with particles of diameter 5 to 20 nm, has been used in the treatment of malignant ascites and malignant pleural effusion in doses of up to 7400 MBq (200 millicuries) by intrapleural or intraperitoneal injection. However, this form of therapy is less commonly used because the patient constitutes a radiation hazard and antineoplastic agents instilled similarly appear to be equally effective. It has also been used in the treatment of rheumatoid arthritis.
The above injection has also been given intravenously in doses of 0.37 to 7.4 MBq (10 to 200 microcuries) for the measurement of liver blood flow, in liver scanning, and for general investigations of the reticuloendothelial system. Since the gamma-ray energies are not particularly good for scanning and the radiation dose to the patient is relatively high, it has generally been superseded by more suitable agents such as technetium-99m-labelled compounds.
Gold-198 grains have been used for direct implantation into tissues for various therapeutic radiation therapies.

Preparations
Colloidal Gold (^{198}Au) Injection *(B.P., Eur. P.)*

5860-g

Indium-111 ($^{111}_{49}$In)

HALF-LIFE. 67 hours (2.8 days)

RADIATION EMITTED. EC (100%); γ 0.171 (90.9%), 0.245 (94.2%) MeV; X-rays (cadmium) 0.023 to 0.027 (~84%) MeV.

Indium-111 is supplied as a complex of indium (^{111}In) with bleomycin sulphate in the form of a carrier-free injection containing 40.7 MBq (1.1 millicuries) per mL. Indium-111 is also supplied as a complex of indium (^{111}In) with calcium trisodium pentetate (calcium DTPA) in the form of a carrier-free injection containing 24.05 megabecquerels (0.65 millicuries) per mL or 74 megabecquerels (2 millicuries) per mL. It is also available as a sterile carrier-free solution of indium chloride containing 148 megabecquerels (4 millicuries) per mL or 370 megabecquerels (10 millicuries) per mL and as a sterile, carrier-free solution of indium oxine complex containing 37 megabecquerels (1 millicurie) per mL.
Indium (^{111}In) bleomycin injection is used for the detection of tumours in doses of 74 to 185 MBq (2 to 5 millicuries) intravenously.
Indium-111 as indium (^{111}In) complexed with calcium trisodium pentetate is used in diagnostic scintigraphy in cerebrospinal fluid studies, cisternography, and ventriculography. The usual dose is 18.5 to 37 MBq (0.5 to 1 millicuries) administered by intrathecal, intracisternal, or intraventricular injection, or by injection into neurosurgical shunts. Indium-111 has also been used for the detection of tumours using monoclonal antibodies labelled with the indium-111-DTPA chelate.
Platelets labelled with indium-111-oxine have been used for the detection of thrombi and other haematological disorders and leucocytes and granulocytes similarly labelled have been used in the detection of abscesses, infectious diseases, inflammatory bowel disease, and transplant rejection.
Colloids have been prepared using indium chloride (^{111}In) solution and have been used for investigation of the lymphatic system.

Preparations
Indium In 111 Pentetate Injection *(U.S.P.)*

5861-q

Indium-113m ($^{113m}_{49}$In)

HALF-LIFE. 99.5 minutes

RADIATION EMITTED. IT (100%); γ 0.392 (64.9%) MeV; X-rays (indium) 0.024 to 0.028 (~24%) MeV.

Indium-113m is a daughter of tin-113 ($^{113}_{50}$Sn, half-life 115 days, γ- and X-radiation) and because of its short half-life is normally prepared just before use by elution from a sterile generator consisting of tin-113 adsorbed on an ion-exchange material contained in a column. Indium-113m is obtained by elution with a standardised dilute solution of hydrochloric acid. Columns containing 185, 370, 740, 1110, 1480, 1850, and 3700 megabecquerels (5, 10, 20, 30, 40, 50, and 100 millicuries) of tin-113 are available and they have a useful life of 6 months.
Radiopharmaceuticals of indium-113m are prepared shortly after elution to reduce loss by decay.
Indium-113m is used for labelling a variety of materials with differing physical properties suited to scanning procedures for various organs and tissues. The short half-life of indium-113m and its lack of β-emission allow large doses to be given with a small radiation dose to the patient. High count-rates for scanning are therefore achieved.
For lung scanning, indium-113m is incorporated into particulate matter of a suitable particle size. The usual dose is 37 to 74 MBq (1 to 2 millicuries).
A colloidal form of indium-113m can be prepared by adding pre-dispensed sterile reagents to the eluate from a generator. This colloid is taken up by the reticuloendothelial cells and is suitable for liver and spleen scanning. The usual dose for liver scanning is 37 to 148 MBq (1 to 4 millicuries).
An eluted ionic chloride which labels plasma transferrin is used for location of blood 'pools', such as in the placenta or heart. The usual dose in placentography is 9.25 to 37 MBq (0.25 to 1 millicuries) and in cardiac blood pool scintigraphy about 74 MBq (2 millicuries).
A chelate of indium-113m with pentetic acid is used for brain scanning and for renal-function studies. Doses of up to 370 MBq (10 millicuries) are used. This preparation has also been used for labelling liquids in the measurement of gastric emptying.

5862-p

Iodine-123 ($^{123}_{53}$I)

HALF-LIFE. 13.2 hours

RADIATION EMITTED. EC (100%); γ 0.159 (83.4%), 0.346 (0.10%), 0.440 (0.40%), 0.505 (0.30%), 0.529 (1.40%), 0.538 (0.40%) MeV; X-rays (tellurium) 0.027 to 0.032 (~87%) MeV.

Iodine-123 has similar adverse effects and precautions to iodine-131 (p.1380). Its principal uses are in thyroid scanning as sodium iodide (^{123} I). Sodium iodohippurate (^{123}I) injection is employed in tests of renal function.

Preparations
Iodohippurate Sodium I 123 Injection *(U.S.P.)*
Sodium Iodide I 123 Capsules *(U.S.P.)*
Sodium Iodide I 123 Solution *(U.S.P.)*
Sodium Iodide (^{123}I) Solution *(Eur. P.)*
Sodium Iodohippurate (^{123}I) Injection *(Eur. P.)*

5863-s

Iodine-125 ($^{125}_{53}$I)

HALF-LIFE. 60 days

RADIATION EMITTED. EC (100%); γ 0.035 (7%) MeV; X-rays (tellurium) 0.027 to 0.032 (138%) MeV.

Iodine-125 has similar adverse effects and precautions to iodine-131 (p.1380).
Iodine-125 is not very suitable for the external counting of radioactivity in the thyroid gland because its γ-energy is weak and tissue absorption is high. However, it is very suitable for assays *in vitro* and because it has a long half-life it is preferred as a label for many compounds. It is common practice to saturate the thyroid with non-radioactive iodine when uptake of radiation by the thyroid is not desired.
Iodine-125, as iodinated (^{125}I) human fibrinogen injection, is used in a dose of 3.7 MBq (100 microcuries) to demonstrate and locate deep vein thrombosis of the leg. Iodinated (^{125}I) fibrinogen has also been used in the measurement of fibrinogen metabolism in certain disturbances of blood coagulation.
The use of Iodinated (^{125}I) Albumin Injection is described under Iodine-131, p.1380.
Sodium iothalamate (^{125}I) injection is used in doses of 0.185 to 1.85 MBq (5 to 50 microcuries) intravenously in the determination of glomerular filtration-rate.
Sodium iodohippurate (^{125}I), specially purified to contain minimal amounts of free iodide, is given in doses of 0.185 to 1.85 MBq (5 to 50 microcuries) intravenously for the measurement of effective renal plasma flow and has also been used for renography.
Iodinated povidone (^{125}I) injection in doses of 185 to 925 kBq (5 to 25 microcuries) administered intravenously is used for the diagnosis of protein-losing gastrointestinal disorders and for permeability studies.
Iodine-125 may also be used as a solution of sodium iodide (^{125}I), in the diagnosis of thyroid disorders.
Iodinated (^{125}I) rose bengal sodium injection has been used intravenously for estimations of liver function.
Liothyronine (^{125}I) is available as a solution and as a kit for tests *in vitro* of thyroid function such as the liothyronine (T_3) uptake test. Thyroxine (^{125}I) is used similarly.
Many other compounds labelled with iodine-125 are

available for *in vitro* assays to detect and estimate drugs and hormones in body fluids.

Preparations

Iodinated (^{125}I) Albumin Injection *(B.P.)*. Iodinated (^{125}I) Human Albumin Injection

Iodinated I 125 Albumin Injection *(U.S.P.)*

Sodium Iodide (^{125}I) Solution *(Eur. P.)*

Sodium Iodide I 125 Capsules *(U.S.P.)*

Sodium Iodide I 125 Solution *(U.S.P.)*

5864-w

Iodine-131 ($^{131}_{53}$I)

HALF-LIFE. 8.04 days

RADIATION EMITTED. β^- 0.247 (1.8%), 0.304 (0.6%), 0.334 (7.2%), 0.606 (89.7%), 0.806 (0.7%) MeV; γ 0.08 (2.4%), 0.284 (5.9%), 0.364 (81.8%), 0.637 (7.2%), 0.723 (1.8%) MeV. 1.3% of iodine-131 decays via xenon-131m [half-life: 12 days. IT (100%); γ 0.164 (2%) MeV].

Adverse Effects

A small percentage of patients treated with iodine-131 for thyrotoxicosis become hypothyroid each year so that eventually most patients will require thyroid replacement therapy. Hypoparathyroidism has also been reported. Radiation thyroiditis with soreness may develop shortly after treatment. There may be severe and potentially dangerous swelling of the thyroid especially in patients with large goitres and this has on rare occasions produced asphyxiation. Leukaemia and carcinoma of the thyroid have occasionally been reported, particularly in young patients. However retrospective studies have shown no increased incidence in adults after iodine-131 treatment for thyrotoxicosis.

In the treatment of thyroid carcinoma, the larger doses of radioactive iodine sometimes cause nausea and vomiting a few days after ingestion, which may be due to gastritis as iodine-131 is also concentrated in gastric mucosa. Large doses depress the bone marrow. Chromosomal aberrations have been reported.

Reviews of the adverse effects of iodine-131 in the treatment of thyrotoxicosis: K. E. Halnan, *Br. med. J.*, 1983, *287*, 1821; G. D. Graham and K. D. Burman, *Ann. intern. Med.*, 1986, *105*, 900.

Precautions

The use of sodium iodide (^{131}I) is contra-indicated, even in diagnostic doses, during pregnancy and lactation. Sodium iodide (^{131}I) should not be given to patients with large toxic nodular goitres or to patients with severe thyrotoxic heart disease.

Many drugs have been reported to interfere with thyroid- or other organ-function studies and checks should be made on any treatment the patient might be receiving before any estimations are carried out.

The National Radiological Protection Board recommended regular thyroid monitoring as well as routine monitoring of skin and clothing for people working with radio-iodine. If an accident occurred thyroid uptake of radio-iodine could be blocked by giving 100 mg of stable iodine by mouth as sodium or potassium iodide or iodate. Spilled radio-iodine should be stabilised by treatment with excess sodium thiosulphate before decontamination.— *Lancet*, 1976, *1*, 133.

Uses and Administration

Iodine radioisotopes are mainly used in studies of thyroid function and in the treatment of thyrotoxicosis and some forms of thyroid carcinoma. They are also used for tests on the function of the heart, kidneys, and liver, and on fat absorption or protein loss from the gastro-intestinal tract. They can be incorporated into liothyronine and thyroxine, triglycerides and fatty acids, such as triolein and oleic acid, and proteins, such as iodinated human albumin, with varying degrees of stability and with little or no change in the biological activity of the labelled molecule.

It is common practice to saturate the thyroid with non-radioactive iodine when uptake of radiation by the thyroid is not desired.

USES OF IODINATED HUMAN ALBUMIN. Human albumin iodinated with iodine-125 or iodine-131 is employed, usually in doses of 37 to 185 kBq (1 to 5 microcuries), in the determination of the plasma volume and doses of up to 3.7 MBq (100 microcuries) are employed in other circulatory investigations. Human serum albumin iodinated with iodine-125 is often preferred for these measurements, as the dose to the patient is less than with iodine-131.

A form of iodinated (^{131}I) human albumin, in which the albumin is aggregated by denaturing, has been used by intravenous injection for lung scanning but has been largely superseded by other agents.

USES OF SODIUM IODIDE (^{131}I). Sodium Iodide (^{131}I) Solution is given by mouth in studies of thyroid function, particularly in measurements of the uptake of iodine by the thyroid, and in thyroid scanning. The usual dose is from 0.185 to 3.7 MBq (5 to 100 microcuries). It is also used in the treatment of thyrotoxicosis in doses of 185 to 555 MBq (5 to 15 millicuries), according to the dose regimen adopted. Doses of up to about 3700 MBq (100 millicuries) are employed in the treatment of malignant neoplasm of the thyroid.

Sodium iodide (^{131}I) capsules containing Sodium Iodide (^{131}I) Solution absorbed on an inert carrier are given by mouth in routine investigations of thyroid function; a colour code on the capsules identifies the activity on different days in relation to a standard.

Sodium Iodide (^{131}I) Injection is given intravenously in investigations of thyroid function, usually in a dose of 0.185 to 3.7 MBq (5 to 100 microcuries).

OTHER USES OF IODINE-131. Sodium Iodohippurate (^{131}I) Injection is used intravenously in renography in usual doses of 0.37 to 1.11 MBq (10 to 30 microcuries). A special grade of sodium iodohippurate (^{131}I) injection is available for the determination of effective renal plasma flow and is given in usual doses of 0.185 to 1.85 MBq (5 to 50 microcuries).

Rose bengal sodium (^{131}I) injection is given intravenously in tests of liver function. The usual dose is 185 to 925 kBq (5 to 25 microcuries) and for liver scintigraphy a dose of 5.55 to 11.1 MBq (150 to 300 microcuries) is employed.

An injection containing 6β-iodomethyl-19-norcholest-5(10)-en-3β-ol labelled with iodine-131 is available for adrenal scintigraphy and is given in usual doses of 18.5 to 37 MBq (0.5 to 1 millicurie) by slow intravenous injection.

Iodinated (^{131}I) povidone injection has been given intravenously as an aid to the diagnosis of protein-losing enteropathy.

Injections containing *m*-iodobenzylguanidine labelled with iodine-131 are available for the localisation and treatment of phaeochromocytoma and neuroblastoma.

Monoclonal antibodies labelled with iodine-131 are used for the detection of tumours.

Various solutions and test kits containing iodine-131 labelled compounds are also available for *in vitro* thyroid function studies.

PHAEOCHROMOCYTOMA. A review of the use of *m*-iodobenzylguanidine labelled with iodine-131 in the detection and treatment of phaeochromocytoma.— *Lancet*, 1984, *2*, 905.

THYROTOXICOSIS. A review of the use of iodine-131 in the treatment of thyrotoxicosis.— G. Hennemann *et al.*, *Lancet*, 1986, *1*, 1369.

Preparations

Iodinated I 131 Albumin Aggregated Injection *(U.S.P.)*. Macroaggregated Iodinated I 131 Serum Albumin

Iodinated I 131 Albumin Injection *(U.S.P.)*. Iodinated I 131 Serum Albumin; Radio-iodinated (^{131}I) Serum Albumin (Human)

Iodohippurate Sodium I 131 Injection *(U.S.P.)*

Rose Bengal Sodium I 131 Injection *(U.S.P.)*. Sodium Rose Bengal I 131 Injection

Sodium Iodide I 131 Capsules *(U.S.P.)*

Sodium Iodide (^{131}I) Solution *(B.P., Eur. P.)*

Sodium Iodide I 131 Solution *(U.S.P.)*

Sodium Iodohippurate (^{131}I) Injection *(B.P., Eur. P.)*

5866-l

Iron-59 ($^{59}_{26}$Fe)

HALF-LIFE. 44.6 days

RADIATION EMITTED. β^- 0.084 (0.1%), 0.132 (1.1%), 0.274 (45.8%), 0.467 (52.7%), 1.566 (0.3%) MeV; γ 0.143 (0.8%), 0.192 (2.8%), 0.335 (0.3%), 0.383 (0.02%), 1.099 (55.8%), 1.292 (43.8%), 1.482 (0.06%) MeV.

Iron-59 is supplied as ferric chloride (^{59}Fe) in the form of a solution containing 3.7 to 37 megabecquerels (0.1 to 1 millicurie) per mL. It is also supplied as ferric citrate (^{59}Fe) in the form of an injection, containing 111 to 2220 megabecquerels (3 to 60 millicuries) per mg of iron. *B.P.* specifies not less than 37 megabecquerels (1 millicurie) per mg of iron at the date stated on the label. Iron-59 is also supplied in the *USA* as ferrous citrate (^{59}Fe) injection and *U.S.P.* specifies the content as not less than 185 megabecquerels (5 millicuries) per mg of ferrous citrate on the date of manufacture.

Iron-59, in the form of ferric citrate (^{59}Fe) is used in the measurement of iron absorption and utilisation. It is given by intravenous injection in doses of 111 to 370 kBq (3 to 10 microcuries). Ferric chloride (^{59}Fe) is given as a solution for the same purpose.

Iron-59, in the form of ferrous citrate (^{59}Fe) is used for similar purposes in the *USA*.

Iron-59 has also been used in *in vitro* radioassay tests.

Preparations

Ferric Citrate (^{59}Fe) Injection *(B.P.)*

Ferrous Citrate Fe 59 Injection *(U.S.P.)*

18354-v

Krypton-81m ($^{81m}_{36}$Kr)

HALF-LIFE. 13 seconds

RADIATION EMITTED. γ 0.191 (96.5%) MeV.

Krypton-81m is a daughter of rubidium-81 ($^{81}_{37}$Rb; half-life 4.58 hours), and is prepared immediately before use by elution from a generator containing rubidium-81 adsorbed on a suitable ion-exchange column using humidified air or oxygen as the eluent. Krypton-81m is used as a gas in lung ventilation studies. Krypton-81m may also be eluted with water or aqueous solution and used by intravenous infusion in perfusion studies of the lung, heart, and brain.

Preparations

Krypton Kr 81m *(U.S.P.)*. A gas suitable for inhalation.

3878-d

Krypton-85 ($^{85}_{36}$Kr)

HALF-LIFE. 10.7 years

RADIATION EMITTED. β^- 0.173 (0.43%), 0.687 (99.57%) MeV; γ 0.514 (0.43%) MeV.

Krypton-85 is supplied in the form of an injection and has been used in circulation and respiratory studies.

Preparations

Krypton (^{85}Kr) Injection *(Eur. P.)*

5867-y

Mercury-197 ($^{197}_{80}$Hg)

HALF-LIFE. 64.1 hours

RADIATION EMITTED. EC (100%); γ 0.077 (18.9%), 0.191 (0.57%), 0.269 (0.05%) MeV; X-rays (gold) 0.067 to 0.080 (~73%) MeV.

Mercury-197 may be supplied as mercuric chloride (^{197}Hg) in the form of an injection containing 9250 to 37 000 megabecquerels (250 to 1000 millicuries) per mg of mercury. Mercury-197 was formerly available as an injection containing chlormerodrin (^{197}Hg), which was used in renal scanning and in brain scanning but mercury has been largely superseded by other agents, such as technetium-99m.

Preparations

Mercuric (^{197}Hg) Chloride Injection *(Eur. P.)*

5869-z

Phosphorus-32 ($^{32}_{15}$P)

HALF-LIFE. 14.3 days

RADIATION EMITTED. β^- 1.709 (100%) MeV.

Phosphorus-32 is supplied as sodium phosphate (^{32}P) in the form of an injection containing 111 to 259 megabecquerels (3 to 7 millicuries) per mg of phosphorus in phosphate buffer and also as an injection containing 740 megabecquerels (20 millicuries) per mg of phosphorus. *B.P.* specifies not less than 11.1 megabecquerels (300 microcuries) per mg of orthophosphate ion. Phosphorus-32 is also supplied as chromium hydroxide (^{32}P) in the form of a colloidal injection containing 37 to 185 megabecquerels (1 to 5 millicuries) per mg of chromium hydroxide.

Phosphorus-32, given intravenously as Sodium Phosphate (^{32}P) Injection is used extensively in the treatment of polycythaemia vera by intravenous injection; phosphorus-32 taken up by trabecular bone in close relation to the haemopoietic red bone marrow delivers a sufficient dose to reduce the production of red cells. The dosage varies according to the regimen adopted. A dose of up to 185 MBq (5 millicuries) may be given initially followed if necessary by increased doses at intervals of 3 months. Sodium phosphate (^{32}P) has also been given by mouth in doses of up to about 222 MBq (6 millicuries).

Sodium phosphate (^{32}P) is also employed in the diagnosis of malignant neoplasms especially those affecting the eye, brain, and skin.

Phosphorus-32 was formerly used in the palliative treatment of chronic myeloid leukaemia. It has also been tried in bone metastases.

Preparations

Chromic Phosphate P 32 Suspension *(U.S.P.)*
Sodium Phosphate (^{32}P) Injection *(B.P., Eur. P.)*
Sodium Phosphate P 32 Solution *(U.S.P.)*

5871-s

Potassium-42 ($^{42}_{19}$K)

HALF-LIFE. 12.36 hours

RADIATION EMITTED. β^- 1.683 (0.3%), 1.995 (17.6%), 3.520 (82%) MeV; γ 0.312 (0.3%), 0.900 (0.05%), 1.021 (0.02%), 1.525 (17.9%), 1.921 (0.04%), 2.424 (0.02%) MeV.

Potassium-42 is supplied as potassium chloride (^{42}K) in the form of an injection containing 592 kilobecquerels (16 microcuries) per mg of potassium.

Potassium-42, as potassium chloride (^{42}K), is given by mouth or intravenously to determine the body's total exchangeable potassium and potassium space. The usual dose is 2.59 to 5.55 MBq (70 to 150 microcuries); the higher doses in this range may be necessary if radionuclides such as sodium-24 are given for the simultaneous measurement of other mineral constituents in the body.

Potassium-43 which has a longer half-life (22 hours) has also been used to measure exchangeable potassium as well as for myocardial scanning.

3879-n

Rhenium-186 ($^{186}_{75}$Re)

HALF-LIFE. 90.6 hours

RADIATION EMITTED. β^- 0.940 (21.5%), 1.077 (71.6%) MeV; γ 0.123 (0.6%), 0.137 (9.4%) MeV; X-rays 0.058 to 0.074 (~9.4%) MeV.

Rhenium-186 is supplied as a suspension of colloidal rhenium-186 in the form of an injection containing 740 to 7400 megabecquerels (20 to 200 millicuries) per mg of rhenium for the treatment of arthritic joint conditions.

3880-k

Rubidium-86 ($^{86}_{37}$Rb)

HALF-LIFE. 18.6 days

RADIATION EMITTED. β^- 0.698 (8.7%), 1.774 (91.3%) MeV; γ 1.077 (8.7%) MeV.

Rubidium-86 is supplied as rubidium chloride (^{86}Rb) in the form of an injection containing 37 to 740 megabecquerels (1 to 20 millicuries) per mg of rubidium. It is used for the measurement of myocardial blood flow.

5872-w

Selenium-75 ($^{75}_{34}$Se)

HALF-LIFE. 119 days

RADIATION EMITTED. EC (100%); γ 0.066 (1.1%), 0.097 (2.9%), 0.121 (15.7%), 0.136 (54.0%), 0.199 (1.5%), 0.265 (56.9%), 0.280 (18.5%), 0.401 (11.7%) MeV; X-rays (arsenic) 0.010 to 0.012 (~50%) MeV. It also decays via arsenic-75m [half-life: 16.4 milliseconds. γ 0.024 (0.03%), 0.280 (5.4%), 0.304 (1.2%) MeV; X-rays (arsenic) 0.010 to 0.012 (~2.6%) MeV].

Selenium-75 is supplied as L-selenomethionine (^{75}Se) in the form of an injection containing 37 to 370 megabecquerels (1 to 10 millicuries) or 111 to 740 megabecquerels (3 to 20 millicuries) per mg of selenomethionine. *B.P.* specifies not less than 37 megabecquerels (1 millicurie) per mg of L-selenomethionine and *U.S.P.* specifies not less than 37 megabecquerels (1 millicurie) per mg of selenium at the time of manufacture. Selenium-75 is supplied as selenonorcholestenol (^{75}Se) {6β-[(methyl-[^{75}Se]seleno)methyl]-19-norcholest-5(10)-en-3β-ol} in the form of an injection containing 74 to 740 megabecquerels (2 to 20 millicuries) per mg of selenonorcholestenol. Selenium-75 is also supplied as capsules containing 37 kilobecquerels (1 microcurie) or 370 kilobecquerels (10 microcuries) of tauroselcholic acid.

When injected, methionine with selenium-75 introduced in place of sulphur apparently enters the same metabolic pathways as the unaltered amino acid. Selenomethionine (^{75}Se) is concentrated by the pancreas, by the parathyroid glands, and other organs. The usual dose for pancreas and parathyroid scanning is 7.4 to 11.1 MBq (200 to 300 microcuries) by intravenous injection. L-Selenomethionine (^{75}Se) has been used to locate malignant lymphomas.

Selenium-75 in the form of 6β-[(methyl[^{75}Se]-seleno)methyl]-19-norcholest-5(10)-en-3β-ol [selenonorcholestenol (^{75}Se)] is used in adrenal scintigraphy in usual doses of 7.4 MBq (200 microcuries).

Selenium-75 in the form of tauroselcholic acid (SeHCAT) is used in the measurement of bile acid absorption for the assessment of ileal function.

Preparations

L-Selenomethionine (^{75}Se) Injection *(B.P., Eur. P.)*
Selenomethionine Se 75 Injection *(U.S.P.)*

5873-e

Sodium-22 ($^{22}_{11}$Na)

HALF-LIFE. 2.6 years

RADIATION EMITTED. EC (9.46%); β^+ 0.546 (90.49%), 1.820 (0.05%) MeV; γ 0.511 (from β^+), 1.275 (99.95%) MeV.

Sodium-22 is supplied as sodium chloride (^{22}Na) in the form of an injection containing 925 kilobecquerels (25 microcuries) per mg of sodium.

Sodium chloride (^{22}Na) has been used as an alternative to sodium chloride (^{24}Na) in the determination of the body's exchangeable sodium and sodium space in doses of 111 to 740 kBq (3 to 20 microcuries).

5874-l

Sodium-24 ($^{24}_{11}$Na)

HALF-LIFE. 15.02 hours

RADIATION EMITTED. β^- 0.284 (0.08%), 1.392 (99.92%) MeV; γ 1.369 (100%), 2.754 (99.85%), 3.861 (0.08%) MeV.

Sodium-24 is supplied as sodium choride (^{24}Na) in the form of an injection containing 12.58 megabecquerels (340 microcuries) per mg of sodium.

Sodium-24, as sodium chloride (^{24}Na) injection, is given by mouth or intravenously to determine the body's total exchangeable sodium and sodium space. The usual dose is 0.185 to 3.7 MBq (5 to 100 microcuries).

5875-y

Strontium-85 ($^{85}_{38}$Sr)

HALF-LIFE. 64.8 days

RADIATION EMITTED. EC (100%); γ 0.36 (0.002%), 0.88 (0.01%) MeV; X-rays (rubidium) 0.013 to 0.015 (~60%) MeV. It also decays via rubidium-85m [half-life: 0.96 microseconds. γ 0.514 (99.2%) MeV].

Strontium-85 is supplied as strontium chloride (^{85}Sr) in the form of an injection containing 74 to 370 megabecquerels (2 to 10 millicuries) per mg of strontium.

Strontium isotopes are taken up by the bones and the major use of strontium-85 has been in bone scanning. The doses used range from 0.74 to 3.7 MBq (20 to 100 microcuries) by intravenous injection. The use of strontium isotopes for bone scanning, however, has in general declined.

3881-a

Strontium-89 ($^{89}_{38}$Sr)

HALF-LIFE. 50.5 days

RADIATION EMITTED. β^- 0.554 (0.01%), 1.463 (100%) MeV. It also decays via yttrium-89m [half-life: 16 seconds. γ 0.909 (0.01%) MeV].

Strontium-89 is supplied as strontium chloride (^{89}Sr) in the form of an injection containing 3.33 to 5.0 megabecquerels (90 to 135 microcuries) per mg of strontium. Strontium-89 is used for the palliation of pain in patients with bone metastases.

5877-z

Sulphur-35 ($^{35}_{16}$S)

HALF-LIFE. 87.4 days

RADIATION EMITTED. β^- 0.167 (100%) MeV.

Sulphur-35 is supplied as sodium sulphate (^{35}S) in the form of a carrier-free injection containing 37 to 185 megabecquerels (1 to 5 millicuries) per mL and is used for the estimation of the extracellular fluid volume. The usual dose is 3.7 MBq (100 microcuries) administered intravenously.

5878-c

Technetium-99m ($^{99m}_{43}Tc$)

HALF-LIFE. 6.02 hours

RADIATION EMITTED. IT (100%); γ 0.141 (88.5%), 0.143 (0.03%) MeV; decays to daughter technetium-99 [half-life: 2.13 × 10^5 years. β^- 0.293 (~100%) MeV].

Adverse Effects

Allergic reactions have been reported with technetium-99m preparations.

Uses and Administration

Technetium-99m is a daughter of molybdenum-99 ($^{99}_{42}Mo$, half-life 66.2 hours) and because of its short half-life is normally prepared just before use by elution from a sterile generator consisting of molybdenum-99 adsorbed on to alumina in a glass column. Technetium-99m as pertechnetate ($^{99m}TcO_4^-$) is obtained by elution with a sterile solution of sodium chloride. Radiopharmaceuticals of technetium-99m are prepared shortly after elution to reduce loss by decay.

Because it has a short half-life and can be administered in relatively large doses, and because the energy of its γ-emission is readily detected, technetium-99m is very widely used, either as the pertechnetate or in the form of various labelled compounds, particles, and colloids for scanning bone and organs such as the brain, liver, lung, spleen, and thyroid.

Provided that it is sterile, pertechnetate (^{99m}Tc) eluted from the generator may be injected intravenously for detecting and localising tumours and other pathological lesions in the brain. It may also be used to measure cerebral blood flow. Its effectiveness depends on the fact that after clearance from the blood very little technetium-99m is retained by healthy brain tissue. Potassium perchlorate is usually given about 1 hour before injection to prevent uptake in the thyroid or choroid plexus.

Pertechnetate (^{99m}Tc) is retained by thyroid cells and it is frequently used for thyroid scanning. It may also be used for scintigraphy of the salivary glands, stomach, heart, and joints.

Macroaggregates of human albumin labelled with technetium-99m [macrosalb (^{99m}Tc)] are used in lung scanning for the detection of abnormal lung perfusion patterns in usual doses of 37 to 111 MBq (1 to 3 millicuries); following the intravenous injection of a suspension of suitable particle size, usually 10 to 100 μm, the particles become trapped in the lung capillaries enabling ischaemic areas to be defined. Labelled albumin microspheres of particle size 10 to 40 μm are used similarly.

When technetium-99m bound to human serum albumin is administered intravenously it becomes evenly distributed in the circulation and highly vascular organs or pools of blood may be readily located. Such a preparation is used in localisation of the placenta and in examination of the heart.

Technetium-99m in the form of a colloid, such as sulphur, antimony sulphide, rhenium sulphide, or tin, is used for the examination of the liver, spleen, and bone marrow. A labelled preparation of calcium phytate is also used for similar purposes.

Technetium-99m complexes of iminodiacetic acid derivatives, such as *N*-[*N'*-(2,6-diethylphenyl)carbamoylmethyl]iminodiacetic acid (etifenin; EHIDA), are employed in the investigation of hepatic function and in the imaging of the hepatobiliary system. Technetium-99m-labelled pyridoxylidene glutamate has also been used for the examination of the gall-bladder.

Technetium-99m-labelled agents used in both brain and renal imaging are calcium gluconate and calcium trisodium pentetate (calcium DTPA). Usual doses employed for brain studies are 370 to 740 MBq (10 to 20 millicuries) and for kidney studies 74 to 740 MBq (2 to 20 millicuries). Other technetium-99m-labelled compounds are used in brain and kidney scanning; the succimer salt (technetium-99m DMSA) for instance has been used in kidney studies.

For bone scanning various labelled phosphate compounds may be used and include the methylene diphosphonate (medronate; MDP) and the pyrophosphate. Technetium-99m as the pyrophosphate is also used in similar doses in cardiac scintigraphy for the detection of myocardial infarction. Technetium-99m medronate and pyrophosphate are also used to label red blood cells for use in blood pool scintigraphy, cardiac scintigraphy, detection of gastro-intestinal bleeding, and testicular scintigraphy.

Many other technetium-99m-labelled compounds have been prepared and used in different clinical studies for the examination of different organs or systems. Like radio-iodine, technetium-99m in various forms has been used to detect deep-vein thrombosis of the legs. Use with other radionuclides includes subtraction scanning with thallium-201 to detect parathyroid tumours.

Preparations

Sodium Pertechnetate (^{99m}Tc) Injection (Fission) *(B.P., Eur. P.)*

Sodium Pertechnetate (^{99m}Tc) Injection (Non-Fission) *(B.P., Eur. P.)*

Sodium Pertechnetate Tc 99m Injection *(U.S.P.)*

Technetium (^{99m}Tc) Colloidal Rhenium Sulphide Injection *(Eur. P.)*

Technetium (^{99m}Tc) Colloidal Antimony Sulphide Injection *(B.P., Eur. P.)*

Technetium (^{99m}Tc) Colloidal Sulphur Injection *(B.P., Eur. P.)*

Technetium (^{99m}Tc) Macrosalb Injection *(B.P., Eur. P.)*

Technetium (^{99m}Tc) Microspheres Injection *(Eur. P.)*

Technetium (^{99m}Tc) Tin Pyrophosphate Injection *(B.P., Eur. P.)*

Technetium Tc 99m Albumin Aggregated Injection *(U.S.P.)*

Technetium Tc 99m Albumin Injection *(U.S.P.)*

Technetium Tc 99m Etidronate Injection *(U.S.P.)*

Technetium Tc 99m Ferpentetate Injection *(U.S.P.)*. Technetium Tc 99m Iron Ascorbate Pentetic Acid Complex Injection

Technetium Tc 99m Gluceptate Injection *(U.S.P.)*

Technetium Tc 99m Medronate Injection *(U.S.P.)*

Technetium Tc 99m Oxidronate Injection *(U.S.P.)*

Technetium Tc 99m Pentetate Injection *(U.S.P.)*

Technetium Tc 99m (Pyro- and trimeta-) Phosphates Injection *(U.S.P.)*

Technetium Tc 99m Pyrophosphate Injection *(U.S.P.)*

Technetium Tc 99m Succimer Injection *(U.S.P.)*

Technetium Tc 99m Sulfur Colloid Injection *(U.S.P.)*

5879-k

Thallium-201 ($^{201}_{81}Tl$)

HALF-LIFE. 73.1 hours

RADIATION EMITTED. EC (100%); γ 0.135 (2.7%), 0.166 (0.1%), 0.167 (10.0%) MeV; X-rays (mercury) 0.068 to 0.082 (95%) MeV.

Thallium-201 is supplied as thallous chloride (^{201}Tl) in the form of an injection containing more than 18 500 megabecquerels (500 millicuries) per mg of thallium or in the form of an injection containing 37 megabecquerels (1 millicurie) per mL. It is administered by intravenous injection for scanning the myocardium in the investigation of coronary artery disease, acute myocardial infarction, and for post-surgical assessment of coronary artery bypass graft patency.

Other uses include the localisation of parathyroid adenomas by thallium-201 and technetium-99m subtraction scanning.

Thallium-201 has also been used in brain scanning.

Preparations

Thallous (^{201}Tl) Chloride Injection *(Eur. P.)*

Thallous Chloride Tl 201 Injection *(U.S.P.)*

5881-e

Tritium (^3_1H). Hydrogen-3

HALF-LIFE. 12.3 years

RADIATION EMITTED. β^- 0.0186 (100%) MeV.

Tritium, in the form of tritiated water injection, has been used to determine the total body water by a dilution technique.

Various tritiated compounds are used for *in vitro* and *in vivo* estimations.

Preparations

Tritiated (^3H) Water Injection *(Eur. P.)*

5882-l

Xenon-133 ($^{133}_{54}Xe$)

HALF-LIFE. 5.25 days

RADIATION EMITTED. β^- 0.266 (0.9%), 0.346 (99.1%) MeV; γ 0.080 (0.4%), 0.081 (36.6%), 0.160 (0.05%) MeV; X-rays (caesium) 0.030 to 0.036 (~46%) MeV.

Xenon-133 is supplied in the form of an injection, in which the gas is dissolved in sodium chloride injection, containing 74 000 to 370 000 megabecquerels (2 to 10 curies) per cm^3 of xenon at standard temperature and pressure or in the form of an injection containing 3.7 to 555 megabecquerels (0.1 to 15 microcuries) per mL. Xenon-133 gas is available in glass ampoules for use by inhalation after mixing with air or oxygen. Xenon-133 gas is also available in vials, mixed with air to standard pressure, containing 74 to 1480 megabecquerels (2 to 40 millicuries) per mL.

Xenon-133 is an inert gas with relatively low solubility in plasma. It is administered, in the form of an injection in sodium chloride injection, for measurements of lung perfusion and regional blood flow. After intravenous injection, the gas is excreted promptly through the lungs.

Regional blood flow and other circulatory measurements of various regions including the brain, heart, and kidneys are carried out with xenon-133 administered intra-arterially or intravenously. Xenon-133 has also been used for the measurement of liver blood flow.

In the gaseous form, xenon-133 is mixed with air or oxygen in a bag or in a closed or open circuit spirometer. When the administration of gas is stopped, xenon-133 is excreted promptly and completely through the lungs.

Xenon-127 has also been used in ventilation studies.

Preparations

Xenon (^{133}Xe) Injection *(B.P., Eur. P.)*

Xenon Xe 133 *(U.S.P.)*. A gas suitable for inhalation.

Xenon Xe 133 Injection *(U.S.P.)*

5883-y

Yttrium-90 ($^{90}_{39}Y$)

HALF-LIFE. 64.1 hours

RADIATION EMITTED. β^- 2.274 (~99.98%) MeV.

Yttrium-90 is supplied as a suspension of colloidal yttrium (^{90}Y) silicate in aqueous solution containing 2 to 4 mg of sodium silicate per mL in the form of an injection containing 259 to 1295 megabecquerels (7 to 35 millicuries) per mg of yttrium. It is also supplied as a suspension of colloidal yttrium (^{90}Y) citrate in the form of an injection containing 37 to 370 megabecquerels (1 to 10 millicuries) per mg of yttrium.

Yttrium-90, in the form of a colloidal suspension of yttrium silicate (^{90}Y) is suitable for instillation into pleural or peritoneal cavities in the treatment of malignant pleural effusion or malignant ascites. Doses of 370 to 1480 MBq (10 to 40 millicuries) are infused after paracentesis. Other therapies are equally effective and are generally preferred. Yttrium-90 is also used in the treatment of arthritic conditions of joints, a dose of 185 MBq (5 millicuries) being appropriate for injection into the knee.

Yttrium-90 as yttrium oxide (^{90}Y) rods or grains have been used by implantation for the irradiation of the pituitary gland.

Sex Hormones

9020-r

The male and female sex organs, the adrenal cortex, and the placenta produce steroidal hormones which influence the development and maintenance of the structures directly and indirectly associated with reproduction.

The secretion of the sex hormones is controlled by the gonadotrophic hormones of the anterior lobe of the pituitary gland, but the level of secretion of the gonadotrophic hormones is in turn influenced by the hypothalamus as well as the concentration of circulating sex hormones. This section describes the natural sex hormones together with synthetic compounds that possess their actions.

Of the 3 principal types of hormones involved, the general properties of the *androgens* together with the closely related *anabolic steroids*, the *oestrogens*, and the *progestogens* are discussed in more detail below. Also included in this section are the *anti-androgens*, cyproterone acetate and flutamide, and certain compounds such as clomiphene citrate used in the treatment of female infertility. Hormonal contraception is described on p.1387.

SEX HORMONES IN ANIMAL FEEDS. Some sex hormones have been used as growth promoters in animal feeds. Because of the danger of residues of these substances being present in foods for human consumption, the use of androgenic, oestrogenic, or progestogenic compounds as growth promoters in animal feeds has been banned in many countries. In the *UK* the administration of natural or synthetic hormone growth promoters to animals is prohibited by The Medicines (Hormone Growth Promoters) (Prohibition of Use) Regulations 1986, SI 1986:No.1876; the use of these compounds, however, is still permitted in veterinary medicine for the therapeutic treatment or for the control of fertility and reproduction.

Some references to possible adverse effects in humans associated with the administration of hormonal growth promoters to animals: C. A. Sáenz de Rodríguez (letter), *New Engl. J. Med.*, 1984, *310*, 1741; A. Loizzo *et al.* (letter), *Lancet*, 1984, *1*, 1014; *ibid.*, 1986, *1*, 721; W. H. James (letter), *ibid.*, 1987, *1*, 216; R. J. Heitzman (letter), *ibid.*, 453; M. M. Lloyd *et al.* (letter), *ibid.*, 561; L. J. Kinlen (letter), *ibid.*, 629; E. S. Johnson (letter), *ibid.*, 814 and 994.

3875-x

Anabolic Steroids and Androgens

Although a few compounds are reported to possess either pure androgenic activity or pure anabolic activity most compounds exhibit dual activity with one type sometimes predominating. The general properties of the natural androgenic hormones and synthetic androgens and anabolic steroids are discussed below. Further details may be found in the individual monographs.

Adverse Effects

Both the natural and synthetic androgens may give rise to side-effects which can be related to their androgenic or anabolic activities. They include increase in nitrogen retention and skeletal weight, sodium and water retention, oedema, increased vascularity of the skin, hypercalcaemia, and increased growth of the bone. Large and repeated doses in early puberty may cause closure of the epiphyses and stop linear growth.

Abnormal liver function tests may occur and there have been reports of jaundice and cholestatic hepatitis. There have also been reports of hepatic tumours in patients who have received high doses over prolonged periods. These adverse hepatic effects have occurred primarily with the 17-α alkylated derivatives.

In men, large doses suppress spermatogenesis and cause degenerative changes in the seminiferous tubules. Excessive sexual stimulation or priapism is a sign of excessive dosage and may occur especially in elderly males.

Androgens may accelerate the growth of malignant neoplasms of the prostate.

In women, the inhibitory action of androgens on the activity of the anterior pituitary results in the suppression of ovarian activity and menstruation. Continued administration of large doses produces symptoms of virilism, such as male-pattern hirsutism, deepening of the voice, atrophy of the breasts and endometrial tissue, acne, and hypertrophy of the clitoris; libido is increased and lactation suppressed.

The anabolic steroids, because they generally retain some androgenic activity, share the adverse effects of the androgens described above, but generally their virilising effects, especially in women, are usually less.

EFFECTS ON THE ENDOCRINE SYSTEM. Mention of gynaecomastia being associated with the use of androgens.— H. E. Carlson, *New Engl. J. Med.*, 1980, *303*, 795.

EFFECTS ON MENTAL STATE. A report of psychotic episodes apparently associated with the use of anabolic steroids. One man had received methyltestosterone for idiopathic impotence and one man took methandrostenolone for body-building. An interview with 31 other anabolic steroid users recruited by advertising in gymnasia revealed that psychotic symptoms had been experienced by 3 and subthreshold psychotic symptoms by at least another 4. All these 7 experienced the symptoms only when taking orally active 17-alkylated steroids (methandienone, oxandrolone, and/or oxymetholone). It was also observed that 4 interviewees met criteria for manic episodes while taking anabolic steroids.— H. G. Pope and D. L. Katz (letter), *Lancet*, 1987, *1*, 863. Comment that further controlled studies are needed to clarify the relationship between exogenous androgen administration and psychiatric effects.— R. O'Carroll (letter), *ibid.*, 1212.

MALIGNANT NEOPLASMS. Results of a retrospective epidemiological study of deaths from hepatic angiosarcoma in the USA indicated that 4 of 168 were associated with long-term use of androgenic anabolic steroids (testosterone enanthate, fluoxymesterone, testosterone and methyltestosterone, and stanozolol having been administered to the 4 patients). Previously known causes (vinyl chloride, thorium dioxide, and inorganic arsenic) were associated with another 37.— H. Falk *et al.*, *Lancet*, 1979, *2*, 1120.

Primary hepatic malignancy developed in a young man after taking androgens to increase his skeletal muscle mass. During the previous 4 years he had used methandienone, oxandrolone, stanozolol, nandrolone decanoate, and methenolone.— W. L. Overly *et al.* (letter), *Ann. intern. Med.*, 1984, *100*, 158.

A report of an hepatic adenomata in a patient who had previously received androgenic therapy for 12 years. He had received either nandrolone phenpropionate or testosterone enanthate and had never received a 17-α alkylated compound. The development of hepatic tumours in patients receiving androgenic therapy has been well documented and the 17-α alkylated compounds have been invariably involved. This therefore appeared to be the first report associated with a non-17-α alkylated derivative.— D. Carrasco *et al.*, *Ann. intern. Med.*, 1984, *100*, 316.

Precautions

Androgens and anabolic steroids should be used cautiously in patients with cardiovascular disorders, renal or hepatic impairment, epilepsy, migraine, diabetes mellitus or other conditions which may be aggravated by the possible fluid retention or oedema caused. They should not be given to patients with hypercalcaemia. The use of the 17-α alkylated derivatives is probably best avoided altogether in patients with hepatic impairment because of the increased risk of hepatic adverse effects associated with these compounds.

In men, androgens and anabolic steroids should not be given to those with either carcinoma of the breast or prostate (although in women they have been used in the treatment of certain breast carcinomas).

Androgens and anabolic steroids should not be given during pregnancy because of the risk of virilisation of a female foetus. Similarly they should be avoided in women who are breast-feeding.

Androgens and anabolic steroids should be used with extreme care in children because of the masculinising effects and also because premature closure of the epiphyses may occur resulting in inhibited linear growth and small stature.

Uses and Administration

Testosterone is the main androgenic hormone formed in the interstitial (Leydig) cells of the testes under the control of the anterior lobe of the pituitary gland. It controls the development and maintenance of the male sex organs and the male secondary sex characteristics. A small proportion of the circulating testosterone is derived from the metabolism of less potent androgens secreted by the adrenal cortex and ovaries.

In underdeveloped or adolescent males, testosterone increases the size of the scrotum, phallus, seminal vesicles, and prostate; libido and sexual activity may also be increased.

Testosterone also produces systemic effects, such as increased retention of nitrogen, calcium, sodium, potassium, chloride, and phosphate. This leads to an increase in skeletal weight, water retention, and increased growth of bone. The skin becomes more vascular and erythropoiesis is increased.

Androgens, such as testosterone or its esters, may be used as replacement therapy in male hypogonadal disorders caused by either pituitary or testicular disorders or in hypogonadism following orchidectomy. In hypopituitarism androgens may be given to produce normal sexual development but do not lead to fertility. Although androgens have been tried in many cases of infertility or subfertilty in men they are of no value unless there is also a hypogonadal state.

They have also been used in adolescent males with delayed puberty but great care is necessary when using androgens for such conditions as bone growth may be inibited by the early fusion of the epiphyses.

In females androgens are occasionally used in the management of disseminated breast carcinoma but care should be taken to choose a compound with a lower masculinising effect; the synthetic compounds including some of the anabolic steroids are usually preferred for such purposes. In females they have also sometimes been used in conjunction with oestrogens in the management of certain postmenopausal disorders.

The androgens generally possess anabolic activity and were formerly used to increase weight in patients suffering from emaciation or debilitating diseases. The anabolic steroids, which generally also possess some androgenic activity, were developed in order to enhance the ability to build proteins and diminish the virilising and masculinising effects of the natural androgens. The anabolic steroids have again, like the androgens, been used in an attempt to produce weight gain in wasting diseases but generally have not proved totally successful. They may also be used in the treatment of certain aplastic anaemias. In females they have been used, like the androgens, in the management of disseminated breast cancer, and in certain postmenopausal disorders, particularly the prevention of osteoporosis (for further comments see under oestrogens, p.1386).

The anabolic steroids have been the subject of much misuse and abuse by athletes, sports persons, and body builders in an attempt to increase muscle mass and body-weight but such use cannot be justified.

BLOOD DISORDERS. A short comment that although androgens have formerly been recommended (*Lancet*, 1975, *1*, 959) to enhance erythropoietin production and to stimulate erythropoiesis in anaemia associated with renal failure they are now seldom used because of the side-effects.— *Lancet*, 1983, *1*, 965.

A report of the prophylactic treatment of haemophilia B Leyden with anabolic steroids. In an 8-year-old boy both testosterone undecanoate and ethyloestrenol increased factor IX to concentrations that were sufficient to prevent most haemorrhages but treatment with testosterone induced signs of masculinisation and an increased growth-rate that were considered unacceptable. Ethyloestrenol proved more acceptable and had been given without interruption for 12 months.— E. Briët *et al.*, *Ann. intern. Med.*, 1985, *103*, 225.

MALE FERTILITY. A review and discussion on the treatment of male infertility. Men with oligospermia can be divided into two major groups. In men with spermatogenic failure and elevated serum concentrations of FSH there is no known therapy. Several treatments, including the use of androgens, have been postulated for men with oligospermia and normal serum concentrations of LH, FSH, and testosterone, a condition often referred to as idiopathic oligospermia. Testosterone esters suppress LH and possibly FSH secretion when given intramuscularly in doses of 200 to 250 mg every 2 weeks and spermatogenesis is inhibited secondarily. Three months after therapy, gonadotrophin secretion will return and sperm concentrations may rebound to a higher level this being the premise for androgen-rebound therapy. However reports have shown only 28% of women whose partners had been so treated conceived and in another study pregnancy did not occur more frequently than in an untreated infertile group. Conversely androgens in low doses have also been used to stimulate spermatogenesis. Methyltestosterone 10 to 50 mg daily, mesterolone 50 to 75 mg daily, and fluoxymesterone 5 to 20 mg daily have all been used for periods of 3 months in an effort to increase sperm concentration or motility but results have varied. Although the germinal epithelium and epididymis may have been directly stimulated, the stimulation may suppress further gonadotrophin secretion and sperm production.— *Ann. intern. Med.*, 1985, *103*, 906.

A further review and discussion on male infertility. Androgens are used for replacement therapy in testosterone-deficient men with primary hypergonadotrophic hypogonadism but there is no evidence that androgen therapy, either supplementary or rebound, has a place in the treatment of subfertility. Although mesterolone, a synthetic androgen which has advantages in the fact that no hepatotoxicity has been observed and because it cannot be metabolised to oestrogen thus not inhibiting gonadotrophin secretion, has been reported in individual patients to improve sperm count motility no published studies have shown a convincing improvement in pregnancy-rates.— A. A. Templeton, *Prescribers' J.*, 1985, *25*, 91.

MALIGNANT NEOPLASMS. A brief comment that androgenic hormones have proved effective in the treatment of advanced breast cancer although the response-rate is probably lower than that for oestrogens. Most experience has been with testosterone propionate or fluoxymesterone.— R. Stuart-Harris, *Prescribers' J.*, 1984, *24*, 133.

3876-r

Oestrogens

The general properties of oestrogens, both natural and synthetic are discussed below. Further details may be found in the individual monographs.

Adverse Effects

Oestrogens give rise to side-effects which are related to their oestrogenic and their general metabolic effects.

There may be sodium retention and oedema, nitrogen retention and weight gain, tenderness of the breasts, gynaecomastia in the male, alterations in liver function, jaundice, depression, headache, and dizziness. Large doses may cause premature closure of the epiphyses. Hypercalcaemia has been reported especially when oestrogens are employed in metastatic malignant conditions. Most oestrogens produce dose-related nausea and vomiting. Skin reactions include chloasma, rashes, and urticaria. Erythema multiforme has been reported.

Unopposed oestrogen therapy stimulates endometrial growth and may cause endometrial proliferation. The risk of an increased incidence of endometrial hyperplasia and consequently carcinoma is now well-established. This association may be prevented if oestrogens are given cyclically with added progestogens (for further details see Uses and Administration, below). A role in precipitating other cancers such as breast or ovarian cancer is not established.

Oestrogens appear to have complex effects on the cardiovascular system. The larger doses that have been used for prostatic cancer in men or for suppressing lactation have been associated with an increased risk of thrombo-embolic events but this risk does not seem to occur in postmenopausal women receiving replacement therapy. For reports of vaginal adenocarcinoma in the offspring of women given oestrogenic substances during pregnancy, see stilboestrol, p.1413.

For the adverse effects of oestrogens used in oral contraceptives, see p.1387.

For a general review of the actions and uses of oestrogens, including adverse effects, see under Uses and Administration (below).

A review of the adverse effects resulting from the use of topical skin and hair cosmetics containing oestrogens. It is not known how many oestrogen-containing cosmetics are sold in the *USA* as no federal requirements for registration or sale exist. Even small amounts of oestrogens in cosmetics may cause precocious puberty in infants and children and gynaecomastia or postmenopausal bleeding in adults.— *Med. Lett.*, 1985, *27*, 54. A short comment that in the *UK* three oestrogens are allowed in cosmetic products; oestradiol and oestriol have no restriction on the amount present whereas oestrone is restricted to a maximum concentration of 0.004%. It is considered that the uncontrolled and possibly long-term use of oestrogen-containing cosmetics exposes women to an increased oestrogen load that is quite unjustified.— K. A. Winship, *Adverse Drug React. Ac. Pois. Rev.*, 1987, *6*, 37.

EFFECTS ON THE CARDIOVASCULAR SYSTEM. The effects of oestrogens on the cardiovascular system are complex and appear to be dependent not only upon the dose and duration of therapy employed, but upon the sex of the patient, and in females whether the woman is premenopausal or postmenopausal.

In men the administration of oestrogens for the management of prostatic carcinoma is generally accepted to carry an increased risk of cardiovascular adverse effects and has led to lower doses, particularly of stilboestrol, than those formerly employed being used in order to lessen this risk.

In premenopausal women taking oestrogens together with progestogens as oral contraceptives it is again generally accepted that the oestrogenic component is associated with a risk of cardiovascular hazards and this has partly led to the formulation of preparations with a lower oestrogen content (for further details see p.1387).

Conflicting results have been published concerning the possible role of oestrogens in cardiovascular disease in postmenopausal women. Several studies have indicated a protective role, rather than an adverse role, of oestrogens when given as replacement therapy. Bush *et al.* (*J. Am. med. Ass.*, 1983, *249*, 903), in a study involving 2269 women, found a significant negative association of oestrogen use with mortality and considered that some, but not all, of the lower risk of mortality could be accounted for by an increase in the concentrations of high-density lipoprotein cholesterol, a factor considered by some workers to be protective against myocardial infarction. Stampfer *et al.* (*New Engl. J. Med.*, 1985, *313*, 1044) during an observation of 32 317 postmenopausal women who were initially free of coronary disease found that 90 suffered either non-fatal myocardial infarctions or fatal coronary heart disease. Compared with the risk in women who had never used postmenopausal hormones the relative risk of coronary disease was calculated to be 0.3 in current users, and 0.5 in previous users, data which was considered to support the hypothesis that postmenopausal oestrogen therapy reduces the risk of severe coronary heart disease. In contrast to this study another published at the same time reported very different results. Wilson *et al.* (*New Engl. J. Med.*, 1985, *313*, 1038) studying the effect of postmenopausal oestrogen use on morbidity from cardiovascular disease in 1234 women found a 50% elevated risk of cardiovascular morbidity and more than a two-fold risk of cerebrovascular disease in women reporting oestrogen use. Several reasons for the discrepancy in findings between this study and previous studies were postulated but the authors did consider that the findings suggested that the potential adverse effects should be considered carefully before recommending the widespread use of oestrogen therapy in postmenopausal women. These 2 studies resulted in a considerable amount of correspondence and speculation (*New Engl. J. Med.*, 1986, *315*, 131-6; *ibid.*, 1987, *316*, 342-3; *ibid.*, 1274-5) with the matter not being entirely resolved. Following the studies of Stampfer *et al.* and Wilson *et al.* two subsequent studies were published firstly by Henderson *et al.* (*Am. J. Obstet. Gynec.*, 1986, *154*, 1181) and secondly by Colditz *et al.* (*New Engl. J. Med.*, 1987, *316*, 1105) both of which gave support to the view that oestrogens administered postmenopausally had a protective effect resulting in a decreased mortality-rate due to cardiovascular disease.

EFFECTS ON THE GALL-BLADDER. A brief discussion on the gallstone-producing capacity of oestrogens.— *Lancet*, 1977, *2*, 177. See also L. J. Bennion and S. M. Grundy, *New Engl. J. Med.*, 1978, *299*, 1221.

MALIGNANT NEOPLASMS. *Breast.* Although the use of unopposed oestrogen therapy is generally accepted to be associated with an increased risk of endometrial carcinoma, their role in the causation of breast carcinoma is far less clear.

Most reports involving pre-menopausal women have been in those given oestrogens together with progestogens as oral contraceptives (see p.1389) or in those formerly given stilboestrol during pregnancy to prevent abortion, a therapy no longer practised because of the adverse effects on the foetus. In a report by Bibbo *et al.* (*New Engl. J. Med.*, 1978, *298*, 763) no statistically significant difference in the incidence of breast cancer was found among a group of 693 women who had received stilboestrol during pregnancy 25 years earlier compared to a control group of 668 who had not. This finding was, however, criticised by Clark and Portier (*New Engl. J. Med.*, 1979, *300*, 263) on the basis that the study lacked the statistical power to reject the null hypothesis. In another study Greenberg *et al.* (*New Engl. J. Med.*, 1984, *311*, 1393) compared the incidence of breast cancer in 3033 women who had taken stilboestrol in pregnancy during the period 1940 to 1960 with the incidence in a comparable group of unexposed women. This study involved over 85 000 women-years of follow-up in each group and it was found that the incidence of breast cancer per 100 000 women-years was 134 in the exposed group and 93 in the unexposed group. The authors concluded that in those women given stilboestrol there was a moderately increased incidence of breast cancer but that some unrecognised concomitant of exposure could not be excluded as a possibility for the increase.

In a study in postmenopausal women who had used oestrogen replacement therapy Wingo *et al.* (*J. Am. med. Ass.*, 1987, *257*, 209) found that analysis of 1369 cases of recently diagnosed breast cancer and 1645 controls revealed that the overall risk of breast cancer did not appear to increase appreciably; this was in agreement with most other studies that had indicated that women who had ever used oestrogen replacement therapy did not have an increased risk. Caution in accepting this conclusion was urged by Lemon and Foley (*J. Am. med. Ass.*, 1987, *257*, 2165) who considered that a study with a longer follow-up was needed but in reply Wingo *et al.* (*ibid.*, 2166) still considered that any increased risk of breast cancer was unlikely to outweigh the benefits of oestrogen replacement therapy in postmenopausal women.

It should be noted that in postmenopausal women oestrogen therapy is sometimes used as part of the management of breast carcinoma (see below under Uses and Administration).

Endometrium. Studies demonstrating an increased incidence of endometrial hyperplasia and carcinoma in women receiving oestrogen therapy and also estimating the risk ratio: D. C. Smith *et al.*, *New Engl. J. Med.*, 1975, *293*, 1164; H. K. Ziel and W. D. Finkle, *ibid.*, 1167; R. D. Gambrell, *J. reprod. Med.*, 1977, *18*, 301; J. Gordon *et al.*, *New Engl. J. Med.*, 1977, *297*, 570; L. A. Gray *et al.*, *Obstet. Gynec.*, 1977, *49*, 385; T. W. McDonald *et al.*, *Am. J. Obstet. Gynec.*, 1977, *127*, 572; D. W. Sturdee *et al.*, *Br. med. J.*, 1978, *1*, 1575; C. M. F. Antunes *et al.*, *New Engl. J. Med.*, 1979, *300*, 9; H. Jick *et al.*, *ibid.*, 218; M. E. L. Paterson *et al.*, *Br. med. J.*, 1980, *280*, 822; I. Persson *et al.*, *Eur. J. clin. Pharmac.*, 1983, *25*, 625; S. Shapiro *et al.*, *New Engl. J. Med.*, 1985, *313*, 969.

PORPHYRIA. A report on porphyria cutanea tarda in 40 patients. Alcohol ingestion and the use of oestrogens were the most frequently associated aetiological factors.— M. E. Grossman *et al.*, *Am. J. Med.*, 1979, *67*, 277.

Precautions

The use of oestrogens is contra-indicated in patients with a family or personal history of malignant neoplastic disease of the breast or genital tract (unless indicated for the treatment of the neoplasm) and in those with previous thrombo-embolic disorders, cardiovascular disease, thrombophlebitis, undiagnosed vaginal bleeding, or endometriosis. Their use is also contra-indicated in patients with liver impairment.

Since oestrogens may cause fluid retention they should be used with care in patients with asthma, epilepsy, migraine, or heart or kidney disease. They should also be used with care in disorders such as otosclerosis which are known to be subject to deterioration during pregnancy. Oestrogens may precipitate porphyria in susceptible patients and may exacerbate diabetes mellitus.

Oestrogens have been reported to increase the plasma concentrations of cortisol- and thyroxine-binding globulin.

Oestrogens should be avoided in pregnant women since stilboestrol (see p.1413) has been implicated in the induction of tumours in female offspring and changes in male offspring.

See also contraceptives, p.1390.

SURGERY. A reminder that oestrogens used for the control of menopausal symptoms should be stopped for at least one month before surgical operations to reduce the risk of deep-vein thrombosis.— *Drug & Ther. Bull.*, 1984, *22*, 73.

Absorption and Fate

In general, oestrogens are readily absorbed from the gastro-intestinal tract and through the skin or mucous membranes. Metabolism is largely in the liver with some undergoing enterohepatic recycling. Excretion of the less active metabolites is in the urine. Oestrogens cross the placenta.

Uses and Administration

Of the naturally occurring oestrogenic hormones formed in the ovarian follicles under the influence of the pituitary, oestradiol is the most active. The development and maintenance of the female sex organs, the secondary sex characteristics, and the mammary glands are controlled as well as certain functions of the human uterus and accessory organs, particularly the proliferation of the endometrium, the development of the decidua, and the cyclic changes in the cervix and vagina. Low physiological amounts stimulate the gonadotrophic and lactogenic activities of the anterior pituitary, but large amounts depress these activities. In late pregnancy, oestradiol increases the spontaneous activity of the uterine muscle and its response to oxytocic drugs.

The additional activity of progesterone is essential for the complete biological function of the female sex organs.

The main therapeutic use of oestrogens is for replacement therapy in deficiency states and for the management of the menopausal syndrome.

Physiological replacement therapy may be necessary in conditions such as primary ovarian failure or primary amenorrhoea.

The menopausal and postmenopausal symptoms that are treated with oestrogens are the vasomotor symptoms such as hot flushes and vaginal or vulval atrophy. Oestrogens are also considered to be effective in the prophylaxis of postmenopausal osteoporosis. Various routes of administration for the different oestrogenic compounds are available inculding the oral route, intramuscular injections, subcutaneous implants, local applications for vulvovaginal use, and transdermal skin patches. If prolonged therapy (for more than 2 to 4 weeks) with an oestrogen by any route is envisaged in a woman with an intact uterus, it is generally considered that the oestrogen should be given on a cyclical basis for 3 weeks out of 4 with an added progestogen by mouth being given during the last 10 to 13 days of oestrogen administration. This will cause withdrawal bleeding, reverse the endometrial stimulation caused by oestrogens, and thus reduce the increased risk of endometrial hyperplasia and carcinoma associated with the use of unopposed oestrogen therapy.

Oestrogens may also be used for the treatment of malignant neoplasms of the prostate and of the breast of postmenopausal women. They have been used for the suppression of lactation but alternative methods, including the use of bromocriptine are now preferred.

Oestrogens such as ethinyloestradiol and mestranol are also used as the oestrogenic component of combined oral contraceptives (see p.1391).

A detailed and comprehensive review and discussion on the actions and uses of unopposed oestrogens. The naturally occurring ovarian steroids are oestriol, oestrone, and oestradiol (in ascending order of potency) and semi-synthetic oestrogens include ethinyloestradiol and the benzoate and dipropionate esters of oestradiol. Although a number of synthetic chemicals, including chlorotrianisene, dienoestrol, hexestrol, and stilboestrol, also possess marked oestrogenic activity little or no significant therapeutic advantage has been found in these compounds when compared with ethinyloestradiol.

In general, the adverse effects of oestrogens apply to all unopposed oestrogen preparations and are mainly related to their hormonal and general metabolic effects. One of the most serious effects is the development of cancers. The development of cancers or other disorders of the vagina and cervix in young women whose mothers had received stilboestrol during pregnancy led to the use of such preparations in pregnancy being discontinued. An increased incidence of various genito-urinary abnormalities in males similarly exposed has been reported although not all studies have confirmed this association. With regard to cancer of the uterus data from epidemiological studies indicate that the use of long-term unopposed oestrogen-replacement therapy by postmenopausal women with an intact uterus is strongly associated with the development of endometrial hyperplasia and carcinoma. The degree of risk is variously estimated to be increased by 2- to 15-fold and is also related to the duration of use and dosage. Benign and malignant liver tumours have occurred in women using oral contraceptives but further studies are needed to determine whether oestrogens alone play a major role in the development of such tumours. The other major concern of oestrogen therapy is cardiovascular hazards. The risks of venous thrombo-embolic disorders are now well recognised, although the position regarding arterial disorders, including coronary heart disease, is less clear-cut.

The uses of oestrogens can largely be put into 4 main groups: the management of the menopausal and postmenopausal syndrome; physiological replacement therapy in conditions such as ovarian dysgenesis and the premature menopause; the palliative treatment of prostatic cancer and of breast cancer in postmenopausal women; the inhibition or suppression of lactation.

The main proven benefit of oestrogen replacement therapy at and after the menopause is in the management of genital atrophy; there is no evidence at present to justify the use of oestrogens in the treatment of psychological problems. The advantage of continuing oestrogen therapy past the menopause is in the prevention of osteoporosis. Oestrogens for menopausal and postmenopausal disorders should be given on a cyclical basis for 3 weeks out of 4 and in women with an intact uterus should be given with an added progestogen for 10 to 13 days of each cycle to protect against endometrial hyperstimulation. In patients in whom oestrogens are contra-indicated a small dose of a progestogen daily continuously may be used for the prevention of osteoporosis though treatment is not as effective.

For replacement therapy in ovarian development failure oestrogens are only justified when given in as small a dose as possible and for as short a time as possible; ethinyloestradiol 1 µg daily for a period of months may be given and gradually increased to 20 µg daily when a progestogen should be added.

Oestrogens, particularly stilboestrol, have been widely used in postmenopausal breast cancer and in prostatic cancer with temporary disease regression occurring in approximately 30% and 80% of cases respectively. However other forms of therapy such as tamoxifen for the breast cancers and cyproterone acetate for the prostatic cancers have assumed increasing importance and luteinising-hormone-releasing-hormone analogues are being evaluated; such alternative forms of therapy could soon replace the use of oestrogens in this field.

Oestrogens have long been used for the inhibition or suppression of lactation but this is no longer considered to be an appropriate indication and cannot be justified because of the risk of venous thrombo-embolism.

Other miscellaneous conditions for which oestrogens have been used include acne, alopecia in women, premenstrual aphthous ulceration, dysmenorrhoea, dysfunctional uterine bleeding, hirsutism, and threatened or habitual abortion. In general, unopposed oestrogen therapy is no longer used for such conditions although some may be treated with oestrogens when combined with a progestogen. Oestrogens have occasionally been used to accelerate epiphyseal closure in tall girls with ethinyloestradiol 0.05 to 1 mg daily used cyclically with an added progestogen for 7 days being most commonly employed. Oestrogens are known to enhance coagulation and although there have been case reports of cessation of spontaneous or traumatic bleeding, most studies have failed to confirm this benefit. In general oestrogens are not considered to be of any benefit in the treatment of hyperlipidaemia but may have a limited therapeutic role in women with type III hyperlipoproteinaemia who cannot be controlled by other measures.

Regarding the choice of preparations for oestrogen therapy oral therapy is the preferred method because the action is rapid and treatment can be stopped promptly. Parenteral therapy has no advantages and is unsuitable for use for postmenopausal symptoms when cyclical therapy is desirable; it may, however, be appropriate for some patients with prostatic cancer should oestrogen therapy be chosen. Oestrogens are easily absorbed through the vaginal epithelium and continued use may lead to endometrial hyperplasia. It has therefore been suggested that if topical vaginal therapy is necessary for longer than 2 weeks an added progestogen by mouth should be given for 10 to 13 days of each cycle. Oestrogen implants have a duration of action generally of 6 to 12 months and again because of the risk of endometrial hyperplasia their use should be limited to women who are willing to take an oral progestogen as well or to women who have had a hysterectomy.— K. A. Winship, *Adverse Drug React. Ac. Pois. Rev.*, 1987, *6*, 37. For a shorter similar review, see *idem*, *Adverse Drug React. Bull.*, 1987, Oct. (No.126), 472.

GROWTH DISORDERS. A discussion on the effects of oestrogens on growth. Early researchers found that doses of oestrogens which greatly stimulated uterine growth also inhibited somatic growth and from this experience oestrogens, such as ethinyloestradiol in oral doses of over 200 µg daily, came to be used for the treatment of acromegaly and for the arrest of growth in tall girls. However, it has become apparent that treatment with physiologic doses causes growth stimulation, not inhibition, and such physiologic doses are used to promote growth in conditions such as female hypogonadism and Turner's syndrome. Thus, oestrogens clearly have biphasic effects on growth with stimulation occurring at low doses and inhibition at high doses.— R. L. Rosenfield, *New Engl. J. Med.*, 1983, *309*, 1120.

A preliminary study of the effect of oestrogen dosage on growth in Turner's syndrome. In 19 patients the ulnar growth rate was nearly doubled by the relatively low dose of ethinyloestradiol 100 ng per kg body-weight given daily for one month whereas doses of 400 and 800 ng per kg daily had no significant effect.— J. L. Ross *et al.*, *New Engl. J. Med.*, 1983, *309*, 1104.

HAEMORRHAGIC DISORDERS. References to the use of oestrogens in various haemorrhagic disorders: J. A. Kirchner, *New Engl. J. Med.*, 1982, *307*, 1126 (hereditary haemorrhagic telangiectasia); Y. K. Liu *et al.*, *Lancet*, 1984, *2*, 887 (uraemic bleeding); M. Livio *et al.*, *New Engl. J. Med.*, 1986, *315*, 731 (uraemic bleeding).

HYPERPARATHYROIDISM. A review and discussion concerning the role of oestrogen therapy for postmenopausal women with primary hyperparathyroidism. Oestrogens are an attractive form of therapy as they may ameliorate some consequences of the hyperparathyroidism as well as mitigate the osteoporosis but no study has yet been large enough or lasted long enough to give clear evidence of the balance between risk and benefit.— F. L. Coe *et al.*, *New Engl. J. Med.*, 1986, *314*, 1508.

Further reviews: *Lancet*, 1984, *2*, 727.

Some studies on the use of oestrogens in the treatment of postmenopausal women with hyperparathyroidism: R. Marcus *et al.*, *Ann. intern. Med.*, 1984, *100*, 633 (conjugated oestrogens); P. L. Selby and M. Peacock, *New Engl. J. Med.*, 1986, *314*, 1481 (ethinyloestradiol).

INHIBITION OF LACTATION. A recommendation for discontinuing the use of oestrogens for the inhibition or suppression of lactation.— S. J. Steele (letter), *Br. med. J.*, 1968, *4*, 578.

Oestrogens suppressed lactation but had many drawbacks—increase of lochial loss, precipitation of withdrawal bleeding, rebound lactation on withdrawal, and the risk of thrombosis. Oestrogens no longer had a place in the suppression of lactation.— *Br. med. J.*, 1977, *1*, 189.

LABOUR. A short review of some studies covering the use of oestrogens to produce cervical ripening in labour and concluding that there is no evidence to suggest that oestradiol is better than dinoprostone.— A. J. Gordon and A. A. Calder, *Br. J. Hosp. Med.*, 1983, *30*, 52.

MALIGNANT NEOPLASMS. *Breast.* Reviews of the use of hormonal therapy, including oestrogens, in the treatment of breast cancer. It has remained a poorly understood paradox that pre-menopausal patients may respond to oestrogen deprivation by oophorectomy while postmenopausal patients may respond to oestrogen supplementation. About 30% of postmenopausal women respond to oestrogen therapy. The mean duration of response is probably about one year but a few patients remain in remission for much longer periods.— R. Stuart-Harris, *Prescribers' J.*, 1984, *24*, 133; J. N. Ingle, *Mayo Clin. Proc.*, 1984, *59*, 232; M. J. Daly and M. G. Rowlands, *Pharm. J.*, 1986, *2*, 244 and 694.

Prostate. Oestrogens, but particularly stilboestrol, have been used in the management of prostatic carcinoma. The doses of stilboestrol formerly used were generally higher than those currently employed and were associated with adverse cardiovascular effects. Although some of the oestrogens are still used in the management of prostatic carcinoma suggestions have been made (J.C. Gingell, *Br. med. J.*, 1985, *291*, 1101; J. Waxman, *ibid.*, 1987, *295*, 1085) that the anti-androgens such as cyproterone or flutamide or the gonadotrophin hormone releasing analogues may prove to be valuable alternatives to orchidectomy or the use of oestrogens.

MENOPAUSAL DISORDERS. An evaluation and discussion concerning the current status of postmenopausal oestrogen therapy.— R. L. Young and J. W. Goldzieher, *Drugs*, 1987, *33*, 95.

Results of a study involving 102 postmenopausal women investigating a method for determining the optimal dosage of progestogen to be added to their oestrogen therapy. Regardless of the preparation and dosage of oestrogen and progestogen used, the mean day of onset of vaginal bleeding reflected the underlying endometrial histology. Bleeding on or before the tenth day after the addition of a progestogen was always associated with a wholly or predominantly proliferative endometrium whereas bleeding on or after the eleventh day was associated with either wholly or predominantly secretory endometrium or a lack of endometrial tissue. It was considered that the dose of progestogens should be adjusted with the aim of inducing a regular pattern of withdrawal bleeding on or after the eleventh day following the introduction of the progestogen to the cycle. Preliminary data had indicated that this could be achieved in most patients with norethisterone 0.35 to 1.05 mg daily.— M. L. Padwick *et al.*, *New Engl. J. Med.*, 1986, *315*, 930.

Some studies have shown implants combining oestrogen therapy (oestradiol) with testosterone to be beneficial in relieving menopausal symptoms in general (M. Brincat *et al.*, *Lancet*, 1984, *1*, 16) or specific symptoms such as depression (J.C. Montgomery *et al.*, *ibid.*, 1987, *1*, 297) or libido (H. Burger, *et al.*, *Br. med. J.*, 1987, *294*, 936). However these latter 2 studies have been criticised particularly on methodological problems (*Lancet*, 1987, *1*, 694-5 and 1038-9; *Br. med. J.*, 1987, *294*, 1417-8).

Osteoporosis. A consensus statement on the prophylaxis and treatment of osteoporosis released following a conference sponsored by the European Foundation for Osteoporosis and Bone Disease held in October 1987. Oestrogen therapy is currently the only well-established prophylactic measure that reduces the frequency of osteoporotic fractures in postmenopausal women. The minimal effective doses of oral short-acting oestrogens are 0.625 mg of conjugated oestrogens, 2 mg of oestradiol, and 25 µg of ethinyloestradiol. Oestradiol percutaneously also appears to prevent postmenopausal bone loss but the optimal dose remains to be defined; no convincing data are available on oestradiol transdermally. Oestrogens also reduce or eliminate menopausal symptoms such as hot flushes, episodic sweating, vaginal dryness, and urethral irritation. Unfavourable effects of oestrogen therapy include the well documented risk of an increased incidence of endometrial hyperplasia and cancer, the risk being related to the dose and duration of treatment. Well-designed epidemiological studies, however, do not suggest an overall increase in the risk of breast cancer and there is also evidence that oestrogen therapy may reduce the incidence of cardiovascular disease including coronary heart disease. The available evidence indicates that postmenopausal women identified to be at risk of developing osteoporosis should receive oestrogens provided there are no contra-indications to such therapy and that careful follow-up is ensured. In women with an intact uterus the concomitant use of cyclic or continuous progestogen therapy is recommended in order to control bleeding and to reduce the risk of endometrial cancer. Treatment should be started as soon as possible after the menopause and although the appropriate duration of treatment is unknown, at least 10 years appears to be reasonable.

Although anabolic steroids can increase bone mass in women with established osteoporosis, serious concerns remain about their safety, and the steroids currently available do not have a place in preventing osteoporosis in women.

Calcium in the diet does not substitute for oestrogen in preventing perimenopausal bone loss and its efficacy in preventing fracture is uncertain. However it seems prudent to recommend a calcium intake of about 1.5 g daily in postmenopausal women with established osteoporosis and women recognised to be at high risk of fracture.

The use of fluoride should be reserved for patients with severe vertebral osteoporosis. It should not be used in patients with predominantly cortical osteoporosis, and it does not have a place in the prophylaxis of bone loss. It has been suggested that doses of elemental fluoride of approximately 20 mg daily are effective but the optimum dose and duration of treatment are not yet known, although the duration should probably not exceed 5 years.

The use of vitamin D derivatives, other than in the treatment of co-existing vitamin D deficiency, is not recommended in postmenopausal osteoporosis. There is no evidence that vitamin D, its analogues, or metabolites decrease the rate of bone loss or fracture in the early postmenopausal period and there are conflicting and unresolved observations concerning its effect in established osteoporosis.

The use of calcitonin may be considered in the primary prevention of osteoporosis in women at high risk who are not candidates for oestrogen therapy, although its efficacy has not been extensively studied.— *Br. med. J.*, 1987, *295*, 914. Publication of this document resulted in several comments.

Nordin *et al.* (*Br. med. J.*, 1987, *295*, 1276) made the following comments: the minimum effective dose of ethinyloestradiol necessary to suppress bone resorption is 15 µg daily, not 25 µg daily, a recommendation which may cause a lot of over-prescribing; the use of oestrogens is overemphasised, it not being recognised that the protective effect is probably lost within a few years of stopping treatment; the section on anabolic steroids is also mistaken in its emphasis, particularly in relation to the side-effects which are made over grim; the sections on calcium and fluoride are ambiguous with the doses for calcium not being entirely clear; the section on vitamin D is positively misleading with no mention being made of calcium malabsorption, a common feature of established osteoporosis which responds dramatically to alfacalcidol or calcitriol and also no attempt is made to distinguish between the use of low dose calcitriol for correcting malabsorption which is almost certainly beneficial and high-dose treatment for stimulating bone turnover which is almost certainly harmful; above all the weakness of the report is the failure to identify which women should be given the oestrogen therapy so strongly advocated.

Kopera (*Br. med. J.*, 1987, *295*, 1277) considered also that the anabolic steroids had been too severely criticised and might result in them being avoided rather than used properly.

Reviews and discussions on the prevention and treatment of postmenopausal osteoporosis including the difficulty of accurately identifying women at risk of developing the disorder: P. C. MacDonald, *New Engl. J. Med.*, 1986, *315*, 959; F. M. Hall *et al.*, *ibid.*, 1987, *316*, 212; R. Smith, *Br. med. J.*, 1987, *294*, 329; *Drug & Ther. Bull.*, 1987, *25*, 33; *Med. Lett.*, 1987, *29*, 75; T. Smith, *Br. med. J.*, 1987, *295*, 872; *Lancet*, 1987, *2*, 833.

A report describing a possible method to predict which postmenopausal women are at risk of rapid bone loss and thus candidates for oestrogen replacement therapy.— C. Christiansen *et al.*, *Lancet*, 1987, *1*, 1105.

3877-f

Progestogens

The general properties of both natural and synthetic progestogens are described below. For further details see under the individual monographs.

Adverse Effects

Side-effects of progestogens may include gastro-intestinal disturbances, acne, fluid retention or oedema, weight gain, allergic skin rashes or urticaria, mental depression, breast changes including discomfort or occasionally gynaecomastia, changes in libido, and altered menstrual cycles or irregular menstrual bleeding. Alterations in liver-function tests have been reported and jaundice has been reported rarely.

Some progestogens when given during pregnancy have been reported to cause virilisation of a female foetus and this appears to have been associated with those progestogens with more pronounced androgenic activity; the natural progestogenic hormone, progesterone, does not appear to have been associated with such effects. Some progestogens, which were formerly used as hormonal diagnostic pregnancy tests have been associated with an increased incidence of congenital abnormalities. For the side-effects of progestogens when administered either alone or with oestrogens as contraceptives, see also under hormonal contraceptives, below.

ALLERGY. Progesterone dermatitis in 7 women possibly due to the earlier ingestion of progestogens.— R. Hart, *Archs Derm.*, 1977, *113*, 426.

PREGNANCY AND THE NEONATE. Mention of the widespread use of progestogens for hormonal support therapy in pregnant women in Hungary (A. Czeizel *et al.*, *Acta paediat. hung.*, 1983, *24*, 91) and a case-control study (A. Czeizel *et al.*, *Hum. Hered.*, 1979, *29*, 166) indicating a causal relationship between such treatment and hypospadias in their offspring.— A. Czeizel (letter), *Lancet*, 1985, *1*, 462. Comment that in British Columbia, an area where such hormonal treatment is much less used, no increase in the incidence of hypospadias over a 16-year period has been observed.— P. A. Baird (letter), *ibid.*, 1162.

A brief comment on the increasing incidence of hypospadias. Although there is some evidence that progestogens taken in early pregnancy may increase the risk of hypospadias, no risk factors have been clearly established. The matter appears to warrant a large prospective study.— *Lancet*, 1985, *1*, 1311.

Further studies failing to demonstrate any increased incidence of congenital abnormalities when progestogens were given during pregnancy: L. J. Resseguie *et al.*, *Fert. Steril.*, 1985, *43*, 514; J. A. Rock *et al.*, *ibid.*, *44*, 17.

Precautions

Progestogens should be used with caution in patients with cardiovascular, renal, or hepatic impairment, diabetes mellitus, asthma, epilepsy, migraine, or other conditions which may be aggravated by fluid retention. They should also be used with care in persons with a history of mental depression.

Progestogens should not be given to patients with undiagnosed vaginal bleeding, nor to those with a history of thrombo-embolic disorders. Unless progestogens are being used as part of the management of breast carcinoma they should not be given to patients with this condition.

Although progestogens have been given as hormonal support during early pregnancy such use is not now generally advised and many authorities now recommend that progestogens should not be used at all in early pregnancy.

For precautions to be observed when progestogens are used as contraceptives, see under hormonal contraceptives, below.

Progestogens had been reported to precipitate attacks of porphyria.— *Drug & Ther. Bull.*, 1976, *14*, 55.

Uses and Administration

Progesterone is the main hormone of the corpus luteum and the placenta. It acts on the endometrium by converting the proliferative phase induced by oestrogen to a secretory phase and preparing the uterus to receive the fertilised ovum. It also suppresses uterine motility and is responsible for the further development of the breasts.

Progesterone has a catabolic action and a slight rise in basal body temperature occurs during the secretory phase of menstruation. Progestogens may be used in many menstrual disorders and irregularities such as dysmenorrhoea and dysfunctional uterine bleeding. They may be given either alone for part of the menstrual cycle or in combination with oestrogens; combined oral contraceptives (see below) containing a progestogenic component may also be suitable for such purposes. Progestogens have also been used in the treatment of endometriosis. Progestogens have also been used for the management of the premenstrual syndrome but such a practice often arouses debate and controversy.

Progestogens are often used in combination with oestrogens in the management of postmenopausal disorders. The progestogenic component is added to reduce the increased risk of endometrial hyperplasia and carcinoma which occurs when unopposed long-term oestrogen therapy is employed. Progestogens have a lesser effect in preventing postmenopausal osteoporosis than oestrogens but may sometimes be used alone if the woman is considered to be at risk of developing osteoporosis and the use of oestrogens is contra-indicated.

Some progestogens, notably medroxyprogesterone and norethisterone, may be used as part of the management of certain breast or endometrial carcinomas.

Progestogens are frequently employed in hormonal contraceptive preparations. They may be given either alone, by mouth or as long-acting depot preparations intramuscularly, or combined with oestrogens orally. For further details see under hormonal contraceptives, below.

Progestogens have been widely advocated for either the prevention of habitual abortion or the treatment of threatened abortion but many authorities now consider that there is little evidence of any benefit from such a practice and recommend against the use of progestogens in early pregnancy.

Some progestogens were formerly used as hormonal pregnancy tests, the progestogens inducing withdrawal bleeding if the woman was not pregnant. Such tests are no longer used because of the associated incidence of congenital disorders in infants born to mothers who had used these tests.

A short review of the physiological action of progesterone and the pharmacological effects of some progestogens.— F. Neumann, *Postgrad. med. J.*, 1978, *54, Suppl.* 2, 11.

ACTION. Results of a placebo-controlled double-blind crossover study in 6 men and 4 postmenopausal women with mild to moderate hypotension given progesterone in doses increased to 300 mg twice daily by mouth indicated that progesterone had an antihypertensive action rather than a hypertensive action as previously thought. It was suggested that progesterone was a "protective" female hormone and that the low blood-progesterone concentrations present after the menopause could account for the finding that the prevalence of high blood pressure and incidence of cardiovascular disease in women tend to catch up with those in men. This property would recommend the use of natural progesterone in combined oral contraceptives instead of synthetic gestagens.— P. B. Rylance *et al., Br. med. J.*, 1985, *290*, 13. Comments, including the statement that it should be remembered that the terms progesterone and progestogen are not interchangeable.— I. Simpson (letter), *ibid.*, 557; K. Cleur (letter), *ibid.*, 558; J. W. W. Studd *et al., ibid.*

MENOPAUSAL DISORDERS. For the role of progestogens in the management of menopausal disorders, see under oestrogens (above).

PREMATURE LABOUR. In a review of normal and preterm labour Huszar and Naftolin (*New Engl. J. Med.*, 1984, *311*, 571) considered that although the use of progestogens in prevention of preterm labour had been advocated the efficacy of such an approach had not been proved. In a subsequent study Erny *et al.* (*Am. J. Obstet. Gynec.*, 1986, *154*, 525) studying 29 pregnant women at risk of premature labour found that the oral administration of progesterone decreased uterine activity more than did bed rest and a placebo. It was, however, concluded that the tocolytic effect of progesterone was not as intense or as rapid as that of the beta-sympathomimetics.

PREMENSTRUAL SYNDROME. Many reviews and studies with conflicting results and advice have been published regarding the use of progestogens in the management of the premenstrual syndrome. The syndrome itself is poorly defined and there is little evidence to support the hypothesis that it is caused by a progesterone deficiency. Symptoms associated with the premenstrual syndrome include headache, weight gain or oedema, painful breasts, and mental changes including irritability, anxiety, and depression. Most reviews on the subject have criticised the open nature of many of the studies and have concluded that there is no firm evidence or rationale for therapy with progestogens (P.M.S. O'Brien, *Drugs*, 1982, *24*, 140; *Lancet*, 1983, *2*, 950; *Med. Lett.*, 1984, *26*, 101; B.L. True *et al., Drug Intell. & clin. Pharm.*, 1985, *19*, 714; S.F. Panser *et al., Am. J. Obstet. Gynec.*, 1985, *153*, 599). Some recent studies (M.A. Richter *et al., Curr. ther. Res.*, 1984, *36*, 840; S. Maddocks *et al., Am. J. Obstet. Gynec.*, 1986, *154*, 573) have also failed to demonstrate any beneficial effect of progesterone when compared with a placebo although a beneficial effect has been reported in some studies (L. Dennerstein *et al., Br. med. J.*, 1985, *290*, 1617).

THREATENED ABORTION. Results of a survey concerning the reported management of threatened abortion by 1290 general practitioners in the *UK*. Based upon a 10% sample of the response, 14 of 104 respondents prescribed progestogens for threatened abortions and 90 never did so. The results suggested that less than half of those who did prescribe them actually believed that the chances of a normal pregnancy were increased. A comprehensive overview of controlled trials has provided no evidence that progestogens are useful in such circumstances but despite this many textbooks still recommend their use. It has been estimated that 3% of all progestogens prescribed in the *UK* are for threatened abortion and other surveys have suggested that in some countries up to 10% of pregnant women receive these drugs. It is the authors' strong belief that progestogens should not be prescribed in pregnancy except within the context of further randomised trials which should include only women whose pregnancies have been deemed to be viable on ultrasound examination.— C. Everett *et al., Br. med. J.*, 1987, *295*, 583.

9021-f

Hormonal Contraceptives

Hormonal contraceptives are only generally available for women although preparations for men are being evaluated. Many differing methods of non-hormonal contraception are available for both use by women and men and details on spermicides (see p.1245) and copper-containing intra-uterine devices (see p.1259) may be found in other sections of *Martindale*.

Adverse Effects

Many reports have been published of adverse effects associated with the use of oral contraceptives, the composition of which has changed with time.

Some side-effects are considered to result from the relative balance of oestrogenic and progestogenic effects of particular products and the incidence of side-effects may be reduced by a change to a different product.

There may be gastro-intestinal side-effects such as nausea or vomiting, chloasma and other skin or hair changes, headache, oedema, weight gain, and breast tenderness. Spotting, breakthrough bleeding, or amenorrhoea can occur during treatment and amenorrhoea may also occur when oral contraceptives are withdrawn. Intolerance to contact lenses has been reported. Some patients may experience depression and other mental changes.

There is an increased risk of thrombo-embolic and cardiovascular disease related, at least in part, to the oestrogen content of combined oral contraceptives; the dose of oestrogen is therefore seldom more than 50 µg daily. The increased mortality risk factor from thrombo-embolic disease is greatest with increased age and in cigarette smokers.

Hypertension is associated with combined oral contraceptives and there may be changes in carbohydrate and lipid metabolism. Liver function can be impaired, although jaundice is rare. There appears to be a marked increase (though the incidence is still very low) in the relative risk of benign liver tumours.

EFFECTS ON THE CARDIOVASCULAR SYSTEM. *Hypertension.* A study demonstrating significantly higher mean systolic and diastolic blood pressures in 222 women under the age of 35 years taking oral contraceptives compared to a control group of 176 women.— K. T. Khaw and W. S. Peart, *Br. med. J.*, 1982, *285*, 403.

A study of malignant hypertension in 34 women of child-bearing age (defined as 15 to 44 years of age). Eleven of the women were taking oral contraceptives at presentation and of these 6 were known to have had normal blood pressure immediately before starting to take oral contraceptives. Malignant hypertension developed in 4 women within 4 months after starting therapy and in the remaining 7 it developed after a period of 14 months to 8 years. With regard to the type of preparation used, 8 patients were taking a formulation containing 50 µg or more of oestrogen, 2 were taking 30 µg of oestrogen, and 1 a 20 µg preparation; apart from the oestrogen component preparations included four different progestogens. These 11 patients had less underlying renal disease and less renal failure than the group of 23 non-users and the ten-year survival was 90% and 50% respectively. These results suggested that oral contraceptives may be a common cause of malignant hypertension but providing therapy is stopped and underlying renal disease excluded the long-term prognosis for such patients is excellent.— K. G. Lim *et al., Br. med. J.*, 1987, *294*, 1057.

Further references to studies investigating the association of oral contraceptives with hypertension: C. C. Tsai *et al., Am. J. Obstet. Gynec.*, 1985, *151*, 28.

Myocardial infarction. A study in 5779 women aged 18 to 44 years on the relative impact of cigarette smoking and oral contraceptive use on health. Smoking, regardless of oral contraceptive use, was the major risk factor for myocardial infarction but combined smoking and oral contraceptive use was associated with an inordinate proportion of cases.— G. M. Goldbaum *et al., J. Am. med. Ass.*, 1987, *258*, 1339.

Some earlier studies reporting an increased risk of myocardial infarction with oral contraceptives: S. Shapiro *et al., Lancet*, 1979, *1*, 743; D. Slone *et al., New Engl. J. Med.*, 1981, *305*, 420.

See also under Effects on Serum Lipids (below).

Venous thrombo-embolism. A summary of the latest findings on oral contraceptives and venous thrombo-embolism from the Oxford Family Planning Association contraceptive study; previous findings had been reported in 1978. The report concerned 105 women suffering a first attack of venous thrombo-embolism unassociated with pregnancy or the puerperium.

In 71 women suffering thrombo-embolism unassociated with surgery a strong association between current oral contraceptive use and certain or probable thrombo-embolism (relative risk 7.2) was found; a weaker association with possible thrombo-embolism (relative risk 3.1) was observed; and little or no association with superficial venous thrombosis (relative risk 1.4). No significant association between risk and duration of use was found. In current users taking oral contraceptives containing 50 µg or more of oestrogen, 20 cases of certain or probable thrombo-embolism occurred during 32 082 woman-years of observation and in those using preparations of less than 50 µg of oestrogen 3 cases during 7606 woman-years of observation. The corresponding figures for possible thrombo-embolism were 9 and 0 cases respectively; possible thrombo-embolism also occurred in one patient receiving a progestogen-only oral contraceptive.

Analysis of the data on the 34 cases of postoperative thrombo-embolism showed that the incidence was almost twice as high in those using oral contraceptives during the month before surgery (12 of 1244) compared to those not doing so (22 of 4359), but this difference was not significant.

It was concluded that the results were in agreement with other major studies, namely that the association is strongest in a certain or probable diagnosis, is limited to current users, and is unrelated to duration of use. The findings were consistent with the view that the risk is lower with preparations containing less than 50 μg of oestrogen but the data were too few to actually confirm this.— M. Vessey *et al.*, *Br. med. J.*, 1986, *292*, 526. See also: A. Kierkegaard, *Contraception*, 1985, *31*, 29; S. P. Helmrich *et al.*, *Obstet. Gynec.*, 1987, *69*, 91.

Some earlier studies: *Lancet*, 1981, *1*, 541 (Royal College of General Practitioners' Oral Contraception Study).

EFFECTS ON THE CEREBROVASCULAR SYSTEM. A study of the incidence of stroke in 192 000 woman-years of observation in the Oxford Family Planning Association study revealed that for subarachnoid haemorrhage there was a strong association with hypertension or cigarette smoking but only a weak association with the use of oral contraceptives. For non-haemorrhagic stroke, however, there was little evidence of an association with hypertension or smoking but there was a significant association with current usage of oral contraceptives. No strokes had been observed in 9100 woman-years of observation in women taking products containing less than 50 μg of oestrogen.— M. P. Vessey *et al.*, *Br. med. J.*, 1984, *289*, 530. Earlier studies also demonstrating a small, but not significant, excess risk of subarachnoid haemorrhage in oral contraceptive users: W. H. W. Inman, *ibid.*, 1979, *2*, 1468; M. Thorogood *et al.*, *ibid.*, 1981, *283*, 762.

Individual reports of adverse cerebrovascular events associated with oral contraceptives: F. Montón *et al.*, *Postgrad. med. J.*, 1984, *60*, 426 (cerebral arterial occlusion and intracranial venous thrombosis); E. Chilvers and P. Rudge, *Br. med. J.*, 1986, *292*, 524 (cerebral venous thrombosis and subarachnoid haemorrhage).

See also under Effects on Serum Lipids (below).

EFFECTS ON THE EAR. In the Royal College of General Practitioners' study of oral contraception in the *UK*, by 1981 there had been 13 cases of newly occurring otosclerosis in each of the groups of oral contraceptive users (101 985 woman-years) and controls (146 534 woman-years); this showed a non-significant relative risk of 1.29. Although, by an analogy with pregnancy, it may be prudent to suppose that oral contraceptives could exacerbate pre-existing otosclerosis, the data do not support the view that the condition is associated with their use.— C. R. Kay and S. J. Wingrave, *Br. med. J.*, 1984, *288*, 1164.

EFFECTS ON THE ENDOCRINE SYSTEM. Hyperprolactinaemia may be the mechanism whereby oral contraceptives, when used infrequently and irregularly, result in a milky discharge from the nipple.— *Lancet*, 1983, *2*, 1405.

See also under Effects on Fertility, Effects on Glucose Tolerance, and Malignant Neoplasms (all below).

EFFECTS ON THE EYE. Mention that after the introduction of oral contraceptives a number of reports of ocular side-effects were published. Since then there has been an increasing awareness that many of the toxic effects originally described were not due to this group of drugs.— A. L. Crombie, *Prescribers' J.*, 1981, *21*, 222.

A further review mentioning various ocular side-effects reported to be associated with oral contraceptives.— M. A. Spiteri and D. G. James, *Postgrad. med. J.*, 1983, *59*, 343.

EFFECTS ON FERTILITY. Following the discontinuation of hormonal contraceptives some patients may experience amenorrhoea, anovulation, and infertility. This infertility, however, has been shown by most studies to be only temporary.

With regard to oral contraceptives data from the Oxford Family Planning Association study (*Br. J. Family Planning*, 1986, *11*, 120) have indicated that impairment of fertility was only very slight and short-lived in women who had previously had a baby. In nulliparous women aged 25 to 29 years impairment of fertility was more severe but the effect had almost entirely disappeared after 48 months. In the older, aged 30 to 34 years, nulliparous women there was even more impairment of fertility but this was not permanent as by 72 months after stopping oral contraceptive use the numbers of women who had not conceived were comparable to a group who had previously used non-hormonal methods of contraception.

With regard to injectable contraceptives, smaller studies have indicated again that there are no long-lasting effects on fertility (K. Fotherby *et al.*, *Contraception*, 1984, *29*, 447) but it has also been suggested that a return to ovulation occurs significantly earlier in prior norethisterone enanthate users than in medroxyprogesterone users (J. Garza-Flores *et al.*, *Contraception*, 1985, *31*, 361).

Infertility may also be related to the presence of pelvic inflammatory disease; for further details concerning the role of contraceptives see under Pelvic Inflammatory Disease (below).

EFFECTS ON THE GALL-BLADDER. Data from the Royal College of General Practitioners' Oral Contraception Study accumulated up to December 1979 no longer demonstrated an excess of total gall-bladder disease despite the indications of earlier data and other studies relating to short-term use.— S. J. Wingrave and C. R. Kay, *Lancet*, 1982, *2*, 957. In a comparison of 200 women with gall-stones and 234 hospital controls and 182 community controls the relative risk of developing gall-stones in women taking oral contraceptives exceeded unity only in women below the age of 30. There was similar age dependency between gall-stone disease and previous pregnancy.— R. K. R. Scragg *et al.*, *Br. med. J.*, 1984, *288*, 1795. A further study finding an increased relative risk of gall-bladder disease associated with oral contraceptives in young women (15 to 19 years of age) compared to older women (40 to 44 years of age). It was considered that the age difference may account for some of the previously conflicting reports and that although oral contraceptives are risk factors for gall-bladder disease, this risk was of sufficient magnitude to be of clinical importance only in younger women.— B. L. Strom *et al.*, *Clin. Pharmac. Ther.*, 1986, *39*, 335.

Further references: R. H. L. Down *et al.*, *Gut*, 1983, *24*, 253 (effect on bile lipid composition).

EFFECTS ON THE GASTRO-INTESTINAL TRACT. Oral contraceptive use before colonic Crohn's disease was significantly higher than before small-bowel Crohn's disease or ulcerative colitis. In 399 patients with Crohn's disease the colon was involved more than twice as often in women as in men. Oral contraceptive usage may predispose to a colitis that resembles colonic Crohn's disease.— J. M. Rhodes *et al.*, *Br. med. J.*, 1984, *288*, 595. An examination of the data on chronic inflammatory bowel disease obtained in the Oxford Family Planning Association contraceptive study revealed the following incidences of disease per 1000 woman-years of observation: ulcerative colitis, 0.26 in oral contraceptive users and 0.11 in non-users; Crohn's disease, 0.13 in users and 0.07 in non-users. The use of oral contraceptives was therefore more strongly associated with ulcerative colitis than with Crohn's disease although even that association fell short of conventional levels of significance. The suggestion that oral contraceptives have an aetiological role in chronic inflammatory bowel disease cannot yet be regarded as established.— M. Vessey *et al.*, *ibid.*, 1986, *292*, 1101. See also: J. H. Entrican and W. Sircus (letter), *ibid.*, 1464.

EFFECTS ON GLUCOSE TOLERANCE. A review and discussion on the effects of drugs on glucose tolerance. Early studies suggested that the prevalence of abnormal glucose tolerance in oral contraceptive users was increased from about 4% to 35% but subsequent studies produced conflicting results. Possible reasons for these discrepancies may include failure to discriminate between differing doses of oestrogen and between the differing types and doses of progestogen used in the preparation; it has been shown that the decrease in glucose tolerance is related not only to oestrogen doses greater than 75 μg daily but also to the type of progestogen. As most oral contraceptives used currently contain lower doses of oestrogen (about 30 to 50 μg daily) the important question is whether such low-dose preparations have deleterious effects. Levonorgestrel has been reported to be the most potent progestogen in decreasing glucose tolerance (J. A. Perlman *et al.*, *J. chron. Dis.*, 1985, *38*, 857) whereas preliminary results of another study have suggested that a combined oral contraceptive containing norethisterone does not result in a deterioration of glucose tolerance (V. Wynn, *Am. J. Obstet. Gynec.*, 1982, *142*, 739). It is therefore considered that preparations containing high doses of levonorgestrel should be prescribed for long-term use only after the most careful consideration, especially in patients with a past history of gestational diabetes or with impaired glucose tolerance.— R. Taylor, *Adverse Drug React. Bull.*, 1986, Dec., 452.

Further references to studies of the effects of oral contraceptives on glucose tolerance: T. J. Duffy and R. Ray, *Contraception*, 1984, *30*, 197.

EFFECTS ON MENTAL STATE. A review of drug-induced mental depression. As mood disturbance is common during the menstrual cycle and particularly in the premenstrual phase it is difficult to evaluate the possible association of depression with oral contraceptives. The evidence, however, suggests that the incidence is a little greater than with control subjects but it is still only 4 to 6%. Although oral contraceptives may lead to a functional deficiency of pyridoxine there is no evidence that this deficiency is a cause of depression or that concurrent use of pyridoxine lowers the incidence of depression.— P. J. Tyrer, *Prescribers' J.*, 1981, *21*, 237. A similar review commenting that oral contraceptives have too easily been implicated as causes of depression and that the association is, at best, controversial. In a number of surveys in which oral contraceptives have been compared with either placebo or an intra-uterine device no increase in depression or other nervous symptoms has been found.— D. J. King, *ibid.*, 1986, *26*, 50.

EFFECTS ON MUCOUS MEMBRANES. A short comment that oestrogen-containing contraceptives can occasionally induce a light brown pigmentation of the oral mucous membrane which is of little clinical relevance but should be distinguished from other conditions such as the pigmentation which occurs in Addison's disease or melanoma.— K. D. Hay and P. C. Reade, *Drugs*, 1983, *26*, 268.

EFFECTS ON THE MUSCULOSKELETAL SYSTEM. A brief comment that pain in the calves, occurring on walking but which subsides only very slowly on resting, has been described as an adverse effect of oral contraceptives and another syndrome characterised by myalgia, arthralgia, and swelling of the hands has also been attributed to their use. The myalgia may be caused by the mild fluid retention produced by the oral contraceptives.— D. M. Davies, *Adverse Drug React. Bull.*, 1985, Jun., 416.

Rheumatoid arthritis. While reviews (D.F. Hart, *Drugs*, 1984, *28*, 347) have commented on the rare reports of arthritis or arthropathies attributed to oral contraceptives some large studies have investigated the incidence of rheumatoid arthritis in oral contraceptive users. A negative association between the use of oral contraceptives and the development of rheumatoid arthritis has been reported in two studies (S.J. Wingrave and C.R. Kay, *Lancet*, 1978, *1*, 569; J.P. Vandenbroucke *et al.*, *ibid.*, 1982, *2*, 839) thus giving rise to the suggestion that oral contraceptive use may, in fact, have some sort of protective role. These findings were not, however, substantiated by other workers (A. Linos *et al.*, *Lancet*, 1983, *1*, 1299; D.J. del Junco *et al.*, *J. Am. med. Ass.*, 1985, *254*, 1938) who found no association, either beneficial or detrimental, between the use of oral contraceptives and the later development of rheumatoid arthritis. The publication of the findings of the studies gave rise to a variety of correspondence (*Lancet*, 1982, *2*, 1282; *ibid.*, 1983, *1*, 1437; *ibid.*, *2*, 228; *J. Am. med. Ass.*, 1986, *256*, 215) with no clear outcome as to whether there is a real protective role or not.

EFFECTS ON THE NERVOUS SYSTEM. Choreic involuntary movements have been described following the administration of oral contraceptives, although the disorder generally resolves within 2 months of discontinuing therapy.— R. J. M. Lane and P. A. Routledge, *Drugs*, 1983, *26*, 124. A report of Sydenham's chorea in a patient possibly associated with the use of a combined oral contraceptive.— W. B. Wadlington *et al.*, *Clin. Pediat.*, 1981, *20*, 804.

Although a number of different drugs have been suspected of causing the carpal tunnel syndrome, in the cases associated with the use of oral contraceptives it is thought that oedema, rather than a fibrotic reaction, was the cause of the symptoms.— *Adverse Drug React. Bull.*, 1985, Aug., 420.

EFFECTS ON THE PANCREAS. Reports of pancreatitis associated with the use of combined oral contraceptives: W. A. Parker, *Clin. Pharm.*, 1983, *2*, 75; P. M. Stuyt *et al.*, *Br. med. J.*, 1986, *293*, 734.

EFFECTS ON SERUM LIPIDS. Because oral contraceptives have been reported to be associated with an excess risk of various adverse cardiovascular and cerebrovascular events (see above) and because other epidemiological evidence suggests that the composition of blood lipids may be one of several factors involved in the aetiology of some of these disorders many workers have investigated the biochemical profiles in women taking various formulations of oral contraceptives. Results have often been contradictory and conflicting as oral contraceptives with very differing compositions in terms of oestrogenic and progestogenic content have been studied but in general terms there has been the suggestion that total serum concentrations of cholesterol and triglyceride are increased. For further details concerning the proposed role of the various serum lipids and subfractions in the aetiology of cardiovascular disease see under lipid regulating agents (p.1196).

Some references to studies investigating the effect of hormonal contraceptives on serum lipids: R. M. Krauss *et al.*, *Am. J. Obstet. Gynec.*, 1983, *145*, 446; R. P. Smith and R. Sizto, *Contraception*, 1983, *28*, 189; A. Sassolas *et al.*, *ibid.*, 357; S. O. Skouby *et al.*, *ibid.*, 489; P. Wahl *et al.*, *New Engl. J. Med.*, 1983, *308*, 862; I. F. Godsland and V. Wynn (letter), *Lancet*, 1984, *2*, 359; T. Kuusi *et al.* (letter), *ibid.*, 1163; I. F. Godsland and V. Wynn (letter), *ibid.*, 1406; W. Marz *et al.*, *Am. J. Obstet. Gynec.*, 1985, *153*, 287; U. J. Gaspard *et al.*,

Contraception, 1985, *31*, 395; J. P. Deslypere *et al.*, *ibid.*, 633; *ibid.*, *32*, 223; P. R. Baker *et al.*, *Gut*, 1985, *26*, A1127; P. V. Luoma *et al.*, *Eur. J. clin. Pharmac.*, 1987, *31*, 563.

EFFECTS ON THE SKIN. A mention that oral contraceptives may occasionally cause photosensitivity.— K. Stone, *Aust. J. Pharm.*, 1985, *66*, 415. A survey of people using UV-A sunbeds at commercial premises in the *UK* revealed that the prevelance of pruritus, nausea, and skin rashes as side-effects to the sunbeds was higher in women taking oral contraceptives than in women receiving no medication.— B. L. Diffey, *Br. J. Derm.*, 1986, *115*, 67.

See also under Malignant Neoplasms (below).

EFFECTS ON THE UTERUS. Data from the Oxford Family Planning Association study providing the first real evidence that the risk of developing uterine leiomyomas (uterine fibroids) is reduced by the use of oral contraceptives. The observed reduction in risk was approximately 17% with each five years of oral contraceptive use. Although it was difficult to interpret the results with regard to the types of oral contraceptives used, the data suggested that for a series of preparations all with ethinyloestradiol 50 µg and with varying amounts of norethisterone acetate, a greater protective effect occurred with the higher doses of the progestogen; none of the formulations with ethynodiol diacetate as the progestogen was associated with a decreased risk of fibroids. The investigation also examined the risks associated with other factors such as number of pregnancies, body-weight, and cigarette smoking and overall the risk factor appeared to be the same as that for endometrial carcinoma, namely unopposed oestrogen.— R. K. Ross *et al.*, *Br. med. J.*, 1986, *293*, 359. Comment on the possible flaw in the study in that in the *USA* the existence of uterine fibroids has been considered to be a contra-indication to the use of oral contraceptives.— H. Ratner (letter), *ibid.*, 1027. Reply that as far as the authors can ascertain the presence of fibroids has not been regarded as a contra-indication to oral contraceptive use in Great Britain so that the patient selection was not likely to be biased.— R. K. Ross *et al.* (letter), *ibid.*

See also under Malignant Neoplasms (below).

MALIGNANT NEOPLASMS. Concern has often been expressed as to whether the use of hormonal contraceptives by normally healthy women may either cause or increase the risk of developing malignant neoplasms. To investigate any possible link between such use and cancer, two main types of study have been employed by epidemiologists, namely the prospective study and the case-control study. Two large prospective studies in the *UK* are those of the Oxford Family Planning Association which is following about 17 000 women, recruited between 1969 and 1974, and using different types of both hormonal and non-hormonal contraceptives and The Royal College of General Practitioners Oral Contraceptive Study which is following about 23 000 women using oral contraceptives and a similar group of controls. In the *USA* a large case-control study is that of the Cancer and Steroid Hormone Study (CASH) of the Centers for Disease Control and the National Institute of Child Health and Human Development. This study identifies women with a particular form of disease and compares their current or past contraceptive use with control subjects. The WHO Collaborative Study of Neoplasia and Steroid Contraceptives is another large case-control study being performed, largely in developing countries, in order to determine whether either oral contraceptives or long-acting injectable contraceptives alter the risk of a woman developing malignant neoplasms. Many other studies, both prospective or case-control, have been or are being performed in other countries. Many factors have made direct comparison of results difficult and such factors include the type and composition of oral contraceptive used (which has changed over the years), the age of the patient, the age at which the contraceptives were first used, and the obstetric history of the patient. Overall, however, the evidence suggests that combined oral contraceptives, far from increasing the risk of endometrial and ovarian carcinoma, may actually exert a protective effect. With regard to carcinomas of the breast and cervix conflicting results have been published so that the effect of oral contraceptives still appears to remain uncertain. For further details concerning the effects on individual organs, see below.

Some general reviews on hormonal contraception and cancer: J. Drife and J. Guillebaud, *Br. J. Hosp. Med.*, 1986, *35*, 25; S. K. Khoo, *Med. J. Aust.*, 1986, *144*, 185.

Breast. The possibility that the use of oral contraceptives may increase the risk of breast cancer has aroused much controversy and reports have often been confusing and conflicting.

Although there had been earlier suggestions of an increased risk, together with those showing no association, publication in 1983 of a report by Pike *et al.* (*Lancet*, 1983, *2*, 926) from the *USA* caused great concern and controversy. This was a case-control study of 314 patients with breast cancer aged under 37 years at diagnosis and 314 matched controls. The findings were stated to suggest that long-term use before the age of 25 years of a product with a high progestogenic component was associated with an increased risk but that use of a product with a low progestogenic component altered the risk little or not at all. Many other workers commented on or criticised this report on several methodological grounds and also criticised the way in which progestogenic potency of the compounds had been calculated (*Lancet*, 1983, *2*, 1019; *ibid.*, 1145; *ibid.*, 1201; *ibid.*, 1414; *ibid.*, 1984, *1*, 389; *ibid.*, 791).

Publication, also in 1983, of preliminary results from a *UK* study by McPherson *et al.* (*Lancet*, 1983, *2*, 1414) failed to confirm a specific association of risk with use before the age of 25 years and it was believed by the authors of this report that any relationship of oral contraceptive use with breast cancer was more plausible if related to the period before a full-term pregnancy. Some support for the hypothesis that early use of oral contraceptives carried an increased risk was provided by Olsson *et al.* (*Lancet*, 1985, *1*, 748) who in a case-control study of 80 young Swedish women with breast cancer estimated that those who started using oral contraceptives at 20 to 24 years of age had three times the risk of developing breast cancer before 46 years of age when compared with non-users.

Several reports then followed which, overall, failed to show any significant association between oral contraceptive use and breast cancer. A prospective study by Lipnick *et al.* (*J. Am. med. Ass.*, 1986, *255*, 58) involving 121 964 nurses in the *USA* indicated that although there was a moderate increase in breast cancers among current users it was of borderline statistical significance and that the data when taken with the results of previous studies offered re-assuring evidence of no excess risk within a few years of cessation of use. A study from Australia by Ellery *et al.* (*Med. J. Aust.*, 1986, *144*, 173) and one from New Zealand by Paul *et al.* (*Br. med. J.*, 1986, *293*, 723) also failed to show any adverse effect of oral contraceptives. Both were again case-control studies of 141 and 433 women with breast cancer respectively along with control patients. The Australian study after adjustment for other risk factors estimated that the relative risk was 0.9 in women who had ever used an oral contraceptive and analysis in terms of duration of use and dosage provided no evidence of an increased risk. The New Zealand study found a very similar relative risk of 0.94 in women who had ever used oral contraceptives and anaylsis of these results by duration of use, age at first use, and time since first use showed no adverse effects. Particularly no increased risk was found in women who had used oral contraceptives, even for prolonged periods, before the age of 25 or before their first pregnancy. The largest case-control study is that of The Cancer and Steroid Hormone Study (CASH) in the *USA* and their report (*New Engl. J. Med.*, 1986, *315*, 405) also provided further support for the contention that oral-contraceptive use does not increase the risk of breast cancer. The study analysed data on 4711 women with breast cancer and reported a relative risk of 1.0 in users. Neither the type of oestrogen nor the type of progestogen was associated with an increased risk and similarly, duration of use and time since last use had no influence. Additionally no association between the use of oral contraceptives before a first term pregnancy and the risk of breast cancer was found.

In contrast to these studies essentially reporting no adverse outcome Meirik *et al.* (*Lancet*, 1986, *2*, 650) from a case-control study in Sweden and Norway found that information obtained from 422 patients with breast cancer and 722 controls revealed a significant association between total duration of oral contraceptive use and breast cancer risk. They found a relative risk of 2.2 after 12 years or more of use and an increased risk, of borderline significance, in women who had used oral contraceptives for more than 7 years before a first full-term pregnancy. In the following year McPherson *et al.* (*Br. J. Cancer.*, 1987, *56*, 653) reported their final findings from a case-control study of 1125 women with breast cancer and a similar group of controls. They confirmed their earlier suggestion that there may be a 2½-fold increase in the risk of breast cancer in women up to the age of 45 years who had taken oral contraceptives for 4 years or more before a first full-term pregnancy; no association was observed in women who had started to use oral contraceptives after their first pregnancy nor was there any association between past use and breast cancer in women aged 45 or more at the time of diagnosis of breast cancer.

Many commentators have speculated on possible reasons including type and formulation of preparations used, duration of use, age at first use, and obstetric history, for all these conflicting results but have generally agreed that further work is necessary before any final conculsions can be made. In response to all these studies the Committee on Safety of Medicines in the *UK* stated that the findings did not indicate the need to change the current advice regarding the use of the presently available oral contraceptive agents and the view remained that a product with the lowest suitable content of both oestrogen and progestogen should be used (*Br. med. J.*, 1987, *295*, 1418; *Lancet*, 1987, *2*, 1267; *Pharm. J.*, 1987, *2*, 640).

Experience relative to the use of medroxyprogesterone acetate as a long-acting injectable contraceptive is much less than that accumulated from oral contraceptive use but a study by Liang *et al.* (*J. Am. med. Ass.*, 1983, *249*, 2909) and preliminary evidence from the WHO Collaborative Study of Neoplasia and Steroid Contraceptives (*Bull. Wld Hlth Org.*, 1985, *63*, 513; *ibid.*, 1986, *64*, 375) have failed to indicate any increased risk, but the WHO study noted that the data were insufficient to assess any influence in long-term users or to assess the risk long after initial exposure.

Some reviews: K. McPherson and J. O. Drife, *Br. med. J.*, 1986, *293*, 709; *Lancet*, 1986, *2*, 665.

Cervix. It is often considered difficult to carry out satisfactory epidemiological studies on the relationship between hormonal contraceptives and cervical cancer because of the many known variables and factors which may influence the development of this type of neoplasm; sexual behaviour of both the woman and her partner are generally considered to be important as well as the use of other non-hormonal barrier methods of contraception which may offer some protection against cervical neoplasia.

Nevertheless, there have been some suggestions that the use of oral contraceptives may be associated with an increased risk. An analysis from the Oxford Family Planning Association study (M.P. Vessey *et al.*, *Lancet*, 1983, *2*, 930) showed that of 6838 women using oral contraceptives and 3154 using an intra-uterine device, all of the 13 cases of invasive cervical cancer found over a 10-year period occurred in the users of oral contraceptives; there was also a positive correlation between the risk of this condition and the duration of use. The incidence of carcinoma-in-situ and dysplasia was also higher in oral contraceptive users than IUD users but was not statistically significant. An attempt was also made to determine whether cervical neoplasia was associated with any particular type or formulation of oral contraceptive but no significant findings were obtained; it was, however, noted that there had been a high use of products containing 50 µg or more of oestrogen. The conclusion made from this data was that it offered considerable support to the view that long-term oral contraceptive use may increase the risk of cervical neoplasia but that it could not be certain that other factors may not also be involved. Several comments (*Lancet*, 1983, *2*, 1018; *ibid.*, 1146; *ibid.*, 1310; *ibid.*, 1358) were made in response to this publication and the many other factors influencing the development of cervical neoplasia were discussed with some correspondents agreeing and some disagreeing with the conclusions of the study. Preliminary results from another study, that of the WHO Collaborative Study of Neoplasia and Steroid Contraceptives (*Br. med. J.*, 1985, *290*, 961), also found, after adjustment for 23 potentially confounding variable factors, that the overall relative risk although increased (1.19) in women who had ever used oral contraceptives was of borderline significance; the risk did increase with duration of use (1.53 after 5 years). Again the findings were considered to support a causal interpretation but that the increased risk observed could also be due to other factors.

The WHO study also investigated any possible link between the use of medroxyprogesterone acetate as a long-acting injectable contraceptive and cervical neoplasia. The preliminary results and interim analyses (*Bull. Wld Hlth Org.*, 1985, *63*, 505; *ibid.*, 1986, *64*, 375) showed a small non-significant elevated risk, the magnitude of which was similar to the oral contraceptive users, and it was considered again that any causal association was still unresolved.

Endometrium. Long-term unopposed oestrogen therapy is generally accepted to carry an increased risk of endometrial hyperplasia and carcinoma but addition of progestogenic compounds to such therapy is also considered to negate or reduce this risk.

Many small studies have shown that combined oral contraceptives containing both oestrogens and progestogens are associated with a decreased risk of endometrial carcinoma and these findings have recently been con-

firmed in a large study. The Cancer and Steroid Hormone Study (CASH) in the *USA* (*J. Am. med. Ass.*, 1987, *257*, 796), studying 433 women with confirmed epithelial endometrial cancer and 3191 control women, found that women who had used combination oral contraceptives for at least 12 months had an adjusted risk of 0.6 relative to those women who had never used such contraceptives. The protective effect was found to persist for at least 15 years after the cessation of use. Examination of the most frequently used formulations revealed little difference.
No evidence of an increased risk of developing uterine cancer has been found in women receiving medroxyprogesterone acetate injections as a long-acting contraceptive (A.P. Liang, *J. Am. med. Ass.*, 1983, *249*, 2909; memorandum from a WHO meeting, *Bull. Wld Hlth Org.*, 1986, *64*, 375) but the WHO study did note that insufficient data had been accumulated to assess the risk in long-term users or the risk long after initial exposure.

Liver. Anecdotal case reports have described the occurrence of hepatocellular carcinoma in women receiving oral contraceptives but the association has often been controversial. Henderson *et al.* (*Br. J. Cancer*, 1983, *48*, 437) reported that women diagnosed with hepatocellular carcinoma in the *USA* had a greater use of oral contraceptives than matched controls and two case-control studies in the *UK* by Neuberger *et al.* (*Br. med. J.*, 1986, *292*, 1355) and by Forman *et al.* (*Br. med. J.*, 1986, *292*, 1357) also indicated an increased risk in oral contraceptive users. Neuberger *et al.* studied a series of 26 women with hepatocellular carcinoma and found that 18 had used oral contraceptives. Comparing this group with a group of 1333 control women they estimated that the use of oral contraceptives for up to 8 years had no increased relative risk but that prolonged use for longer than this time period was associated with a 4.4 fold greater risk. Forman *et al.* investigated the histories of use of oral contraceptives in all women in England and Wales certified as having died from primary liver cancer between the ages of 20 and 44 over the period 1979 to 1982. The results, after age-adjustment, again showed that use for more than 8 years was associated with a significantly increased risk (relative risk of 20.1). This study also demonstrated an increased risk for use of under 8 years duration but this was not significant. Both studies emphasised that hepatocellular carcinoma still remains an exceptionally rare disease in the *UK* and that further studies were therefore necessary, especially in countries which have a much higher incidence of the disease. Publication of these 2 studies produced correspondence (*Br. med. J.*, 1986, *292*, 1392; *ibid.*, 1667; *ibid.*, *293*, 204) and in general the view was held that in countries such as Western Europe and the *USA*, where the incidence of hepatocellular carcinoma is low, any possible adverse effects of oral contraceptives would be outweighed by the protective effect these agents have in reducing the risk of ovarian cancer.
Results from a WHO study (*Bull. Wld Hlth Org.*, 1986, *64*, 375) provided no evidence that use of medroxyprogesterone acetate as a long-acting injectable contraceptive altered the risk of developing liver cancer but the power of the study to detect any small alterations in risk was accepted to be low.

Ovary. Several case-control studies have previously indicated that the use of oral contraceptives may exert a protective effect against the development of ovarian cancer and recent findings from two large ongoing studies have been published to support this view.
The results from The Cancer and Steroid Hormone Study (CASH) in the *USA* (*New Engl. J. Med.*, 1987, *316*, 650), which investigated 492 women with epithelial ovarian cancer and 4228 controls, reported a relative risk of 0.6 in women who had ever used oral contraceptives compared with women who reported never having used them. The risk was also found to be lower with increasing duration of use and this was statistically significant. The most marked reduction in risk was in those women who had first used oral contraceptives at least 10 years before diagnosis or interview. A negative association was also apparent for any use of each of the most commonly reported combination oral contraceptives regardless of the type or amount of oestrogen or progestogen in the formulation. An assessment of any association with non-epithelial ovarian cancers could not be made because of the insufficient number of cases. The authors concluded that the use of oral contraceptives decreases the risk of epithelial ovarian cancer and estimated that in 1982, the last year of recruitment to the study, over 1700 cases of ovarian cancer were prevented in the *USA* by the use of these agents.
Similar results were reported in the same year from the Oxford Family Planning Association contraceptive study in the *UK* (M. Vessey *et al.*, *Br. med. J.*, 1987, *294*, 1518). Again a reduced incidence of epithelial carcinoma of the ovary was noted in women who had ever used oral contraceptives; the incidence was only 25% compared to the group of women who had never used them. There was no suggestion of any association between oral contraceptive use and benign teratoma and the incidence of cystadenoma did not approach significance.
Preliminary evidence also suggests that there is no increased risk of ovarian cancer in women receiving medroxyprogesterone acetate depot injections as a method of hormonal contraception (A.P. Liang *et al.*, *J. Am. med. Ass.*, 1983, *249*, 2909; memorandum from a WHO meeting, *Bull. Wld Hlth Org.*, 1986, *64*, 375). The WHO study did, however, note that the data was insufficient to assess the influence on risk among long-term users or risk after long-term exposure.

Skin. Although there have been some suggestions of a possible association between the use of oral contraceptives and the development of malignant melanoma (V. Beral *et al.*, *Br. J. Cancer*, 1977, *36*, 804; A.B. Lerner *et al.*, *New Engl. J. Med.*, 1979, *301*, 47; V. Beral *et al.*, *Br. J. Cancer*, 1984, *50*, 681) most studies, which involved anaylsis of relatively large numbers of women suffering from malignant melanoma, found no such association with either current or prior use of oral contraceptive preparations (R.G. Stevens *et al.*, *New Engl. J. Med.*, 1980, *302*, 966; C. Bain *et al.*, *J. Natl. Cancer Inst.*, 1982, *68*, 537; S.P. Helmrich *et al.*, *ibid.*, 1984, *72*, 617; A. Green and C. Bain, *Med. J. Aust.*, 1985, *142*, 446).

PELVIC INFLAMMATORY DISEASE. Concern over the widely disseminated generalisation that oral contraceptives protect against all forms of pelvic inflammatory disease led to an evaluation of the validity of this association by analysing published epidemiological evidence and reviewing relevant information from other disciplines. Most studies have been limited to hospitalised women who represent less than 25% of all cases of pelvic inflammatory disease and are likely to have relatively severe forms of the disease, and secondly have failed to distinguish between gonococcal and non-gonococcal disease. While oral contraceptives may provide some protection against gonococcal pelvic inflammatory disease, epidemiological and biological evidence suggests that infection with *Chlamydia trachomatis*, the leading cause of non-gonococcal disease, is enhanced by oral contraceptives; in 12 of the 14 epidemioligic studies a two- to three-fold increase in the prevalence of cervical *C. trachomatis* infection was demonstrated in oral contraceptive users. It was concluded that the suggestion that oral contraceptives protect against all forms of pelvic inflammatory disease was premature. It was also considered that any protection against clinically apparent pelvic inflammatory disease does not guarantee protection against tubal factor infertility.— A. E. Washington *et al.*, *J. Am. med. Ass.*, 1985, *253*, 2246. Comment.— S. A. Gall (letter), *ibid.*, 1986, *255*, 38. Reply.— A. E. Washington *et al.*, *ibid.*
A study on the relationship of tubal infertility to oral contraceptive use. Past contraceptive use was studied:- 283 nulliparous infertile women and in 3833 women at delivery. No association between past oral contraceptive use and tubal infertility was observed in cases with or without a history of pelvic inflammatory disease. It may, however, be misleading to group all oral contraceptive users into a single category since a considerable variation in risk by type of formulation was observed. Users of oestrogen-dominant oral contraceptives (containing 75 µg or more of oestrogen together with a progestogen with enhanced oestrogenic activity such as ethynodiol diacetate or norethisterone acetate) had an elevated risk for tubal infertility while users of low-oestrogen preparations (containing 50 µg or less of oestrogen together with norgestrel or norethisterone) had no increased risk. Age at first use of oral contraceptives also appeared to be a variable factor. Women who had first used a low-oestrogen preparation between the ages of 20 and 24 years had a decreased risk of tubal infertility, while women who had first used other types of formulations before the age of 20 years had a significantly elevated risk. Two experimental observations may be revelant to the apparent difference in risk with regard to the oestrogenic activity. Cervical mucus under the influence of oestrogens tends to be thin and clear with sperm penetration favoured and this may also favour bacterial ascent. Also, although progesterone appears to be necessary for the initiation of chlamydial infection, oestrogen may be more important in its spread. It was concluded that this study offers more reason for women to avoid oral contraceptives with a high oestrogenic content.— D. W. Cramer *et al.*, *J. Am. med. Ass.*, 1987, *257*, 2446.

PREGNANCY AND THE NEONATE. Experience with oral contraceptives during pregnancy is obviously very limited and has generally occurred either in patients experiencing contraceptive failure or in those starting to take oral contraceptives whilst not realising they were, in fact, pregnant.
In contrast to the numerous cases of congenital malformations reported after the use of sex hormones for hormonal pregnancy tests there have been only a few suggestions that continued administration of oral contraceptives during early pregnancy may result in congenital limb reduction deformities (D.T. Janerich *et al.*, *New Engl. J. Med.*, 1974, *291*, 697; J. McCredie *et al.*, *Lancet*, 1983, *2*, 623; A. Kricker *et al.*, *Am. J. Obstet. Gynec.*, 1986, *155*, 1072).
Many studies, however, have provided evidence that the use of oral contraceptives provided they are discontinued before conception has no association with congenital malformations or teratogenic effects (S.C. Robinson, *Am. J. Obstet. Gynec.*, 1971, *109*, 354; C.R. Kay, *Br. J. Obstet. Gynaec.*, 1976, *83*, 608; K. J. Rothman and C. Louik, *New Engl. J. Med.*, 1978, *299*, 522; M. Vessey *et al.*, *Br. J. Obstet Gynaec.*, 1979, *86*, 548; S. Linn *et al.*, *Am. J. Obstet. Gynec.*, 1983, *147*, 923; S. Magidor *et al.* *Contraception*, 1984, *29*, 203).

Precautions

Before hormonal contraceptives are given the woman should undergo an appropriate medical examination and her medical history should be carefully evaluated. Regular examination is recommended during use.
Combined oral contraceptives, phased oral contraceptives, or **sequential oral contraceptives**, having both an oestrogenic and progestogenic component, are contra-indicated in patients with recurrent cholestatic jaundice or markedly impaired liver function, porphyria, oestrogen-dependent neoplasms, previous thrombo-embolic disorders, cardiovascular disease and thrombophlebitis, severe migraine, Dubin-Johnson syndrome, Rotor syndrome, undiagnosed vaginal bleeding, possible pregnancy, sickle-cell anaemia, or a history during pregnancy of pruritus, herpes, deteriorating otosclerosis, or idiopathic jaundice. They should be administered with caution to women with a history of diabetes mellitus, hypertension, mental depression, asthma, epilepsy, migraine, cardiac or renal dysfunction, gall-bladder disease, or other conditions influenced by fluid retention. They should also be used with caution in cigarette-smokers and patients over the age of 35 years. Administration to those undergoing surgery or prolonged bed rest may increase the risk of thrombo-embolic episodes and it is generally recommended that use of such oral contraceptives should be discontinued 4 to 6 weeks before major elective surgery. In nursing mothers, lactation may be reduced and oestrogen may pass to the baby in small quantities in the milk. Increased concentrations of thyroxine-binding globulin, reflected in increased levels of protein-bound iodine, occur and while the thyroid state is generally unaffected, some tests of thyroid function give abnormal results. Cortisol-binding globulin may also be increased and some other laboratory test values may be affected.
There have been reports of pregnancy in women taking such oral contraceptives concomitantly with anti-epileptics (barbiturates, primidone, phenytoin, and carbamazepine), rifampicin, and other antibiotics such as ampicillin. There have been suggestions that other drugs may be involved; these include analgesics (aspirin, amidopyrine, phenazone, phenacetin, phenylbutazone, oxyphenbutazone), chloramphenicol, chlorpromazine, chlordiazepoxide, diazepam, dihydroergotamine, ethosuximide, isoniazid, meprobamate, neomycin, nitrofurantoin, phenoxymethylpenicillin, promethazine, sulphamethoxypyridazine.
Progestogen-only contraceptives, whether oral or injectable, may be used in women when oestrogenic-containing preparations are contra-indicated but certain contra-indications and precautions must still be observed. They are contra-indicated in patients with undiagnosed vaginal bleeding, possible pregnancy, a past ectopic pregnancy, history during pregnancy of pruritus, herpes, or idiopathic jaundice, hormone-dependent neoplasms, severe liver impairment, Dubin-Johnson syndrome and Rotor syndrome.

Some guidance on starting, stopping, or changing oral contraceptives.— *Drug & Ther. Bull.*, 1985, *23*, 37.

INTERACTIONS. A review of drug interactions causing inhibition of oral contraceptive efficacy. As the hormonal content of oral contraceptives has declined reports of menstrual irregularities and unintended pregnancies due to drug interactions have increased. A large number of drugs purportedly reduce the effect of oral contraceptives but sources of information do not usually differentiate between the interactions which are reasonably well-documented and those for which little clinical evidence exists.
Oral contraceptive failure has been reported in numerous cases during periods of concurrent *anti-epileptic therapy*. Taken together, the evidence strongly suggests that the enzyme-inducing anti-epileptics are capable of inhibiting oral contraceptive efficacy. In a patient receiving such anti-epileptics an oral contraceptive with an oestrogen content of 50 to 100 µg is generally adequate although an occasional patient may not be protected in this dosage range.
A variety of *antibiotics* have been reported to decrease oral contraceptive efficacy.
Although approximately 25 cases of unintended pregnancies have been reported in women receiving *ampicillin* the ability of ampicillin to inhibit oral contraceptive efficacy remains unproven. The data are consistent, however, with the supposition that efficacy is occasionally impaired and it would be prudent to use supplemental contraceptive methods during cycles in which ampicillin is used.
Menstrual irregularities have been reported in women receiving oral contraceptives and *griseofulvin* concurrently and more studies are needed to confirm the existence of the interaction and the mechanism of action involved. Additional contraceptive measures should be considered in women using the two drugs concurrently.
Rifampicin regularly results in menstrual irregularities and occasionally in unintended pregnancies in women receiving oral contraceptives. If the rifampicin therapy is short-term the addition of other forms of contraception is sufficient to prevent pregnancy or a preparation containing 50 to 100 µg of oestrogen may result in adequate conception control.
Several cases of unintended pregnancies have been reported following the use of *tetracyclines* and enough evidence for this interaction exists to warrant the addition of other forms of contraception.
With regard to other antimicrobials, in theory any one with significant effects on intestinal flora could affect contraceptive efficacy. Isolated cases of pregnancy have been reported following the use of *cephalosporins, chloramphenicol, dapsone, isoniazid, nitrofurantoin, sulphonamides*, and *co-trimoxazole* but it is impossible to determine which, if any, of these interactions is real. Until more is known it is recommended that supplementary contraception be used when any antibiotic is prescribed for women using oral contraceptives, especially if the oestrogen content is less than 50 µg.
Other drugs which have been reported to produce contraceptive failure include *antihistamines, analgesics*, and *tranquillisers*, but supporting evidence is lacking.— *Drug Interact. News.*, 1985, *5*, 7. Further reviews.— M. J. Brodie, *Prescribers' J.*, 1983, *23*, 140; P. F. D'Arcy, *Drug Intell. & clin. Pharm.*, 1986, *20*, 353. A short comment that oral contraceptives may, as well as being affected themselves by drug interactions, affect other drugs. Although the clinical relevance of many of these types of interactions has not been established surprisingly there has been a report of potentiation of the anticoagulant activity of nicoumalone.— G. P. Stoehr (letter), *Drug Intell. & clin. Pharm.*, 1986, *20*, 714.

Some references to an actual or potential decreased contraceptive efficacy associated with the concomitant administration of other drugs: M. Friedman *et al.*, *J. Obstet. Gynaecol.*, 1982, *2*, 195 (cephalexin; pregnancy); T. J. Silber, *J. adolesc. Health Care*, 1983, *4*, 287 (oxacillin; pregnancy); M. P. Diamond *et al.*, *Contraception*, 1985, *31*, 623 (anti-epileptics; menstrual irregularities); R. H. Mattson *et al.*, *J. Am. med. Ass.*, 1986, *256*, 238 (anti-epileptics; review).

Some references indicating no interaction of oral contraceptives with other drugs: D. J. Back *et al.*, *Br. J. clin. Pharmac.*, 1982, *14*, 43 (ampicillin); S. F. M. Grimmer *et al.*, *Contraception*, 1983, *28*, 53 (co-trimoxazole); P. Crawford *et al.*, *Br. J. clin. Pharmac.*, 1985, *20*, 288P (valproic acid).

Some references to the effect of oral contraceptives on other drugs: M. C. Mitchell *et al.*, *Clin. Pharmac. Ther.*, 1983, *34*, 48 (increased clearance of paracetamol); P. D. Kroboth *et al.*, *ibid.*, 1985, *38*, 525 (enhanced sensitivity to psychomotor effects of benzodiazepines); U. F. Legler and L. Z. Benet *ibid.*, 1986, *39*, 425 (decrease in prednisolone clearance); W. B. Ross *et al.*, (letter), *Lancet*, 1986, *1* 330 (increased cyclosporin concentrations); G. Deray *et al.* (letter), *ibid.*, 1987, *1* 158 (enhanced cyclosporin hepatotoxicity).

Reference to increased plasma concentrations of ethinyloestradiol in women given paracetamol.— S. M. Rogers *et al.*, *Br. J. clin. Pharmac.*, 1987, *23*, 721.

LUPUS ERYTHEMATOSUS. A short comment that despite there being occasional reports of lupus being exacerbated by oral contraceptives, the vast majority of patients with systemic lupus erythematosus experience no adverse effects, especially from low oestrogen preparations.— G. R. V. Hughes, *Prescribers' J.*, 1987, *27*, 1.

MIGRAINE. A brief review of the use of oral contraceptives in women with migraine. Patients with classical migraine should not take a combined oral contraceptive. Common migraine itself is not a contra-indication and some patients unpredictably experience fewer attacks when they start to take the contraceptive pill.— *Drug & Ther. Bull.*, 1987, *25*, 95.

SICKLE-CELL ANAEMIA. A brief comment on sickle-cell trait and sickle-cell disease and whether patients with such disorders may use oral contraceptives. In sickle-cell disease there is an increased risk of thrombosis; oral contraceptive use also carries an increased risk of thrombosis but it is by no means certain that the two risks are additive. Some manufacturers have specifically warned against their use in sickle-cell disease but it has also been considered (H.M.P. Freie, *Acta obstet. gynec. scand.*, 1983, *62*, 211) that there is no contra-indication to the use of low-dose combined preparations. Trials of the combined pill in sickle-cell disease are being planned but until the results are published it seems preferable to prescribe a progestogen-only pill. For sickle-cell trait there is no risk of thrombosis and no contra-indication to the use of a combined preparation. Many women with sickle-cell trait have, unnecessarily, been denied the use of oral contraceptives in the mistaken belief that what may have an adverse effect in sickle-cell disease may have a similar adverse outcome in the trait.— D. I. K. Evans, *Br. med. J.*, 1984, *289*, 425.

SURGERY. A review and discussion concerning whether oral contraceptives should be stopped pre-operatively. Case reports and epidemiological studies showing an increased risk of spontaneous deep-vein thrombosis and pulmonary embolism in young women taking oral contraceptives led to the widespread belief that oral contraceptives may predispose to deep-vein thrombosis postoperatively. Many women are currently advised not to take the combined oral contraceptive for 4 to 6 weeks before an elective operation and others are given prophylactic therapy if they are still taking the contraceptives at the time of the operation. The epidemiological studies have relied almost entirely on cases of venous thrombosis diagnosed clinically, a diagnosis that is subject to both false-positive and false-negative results even when made by experts. A report by Vessey *et al.* (*Br. med. J.*, 1986, *292*, 526) showed that the incidence of deep-vein thrombosis postoperatively in young women taking combined oral contraceptives was about twice that of women not taking contraceptives but the difference was not statistically significant. The authors have found only three studies of young women taking the pill in which iodine-125 fibrinogen scans were used to diagnose thrombosis postoperatively. The incidences were 4.6% in patients undergoing gynaecological operations (S.C. Tso *et al.*, *Br. J. Haemat.*, 1980, *46*, 603), 0% in patients undergoing abdominal operations (A. S. Gallus *et al.*, *Thromb. Res.*, 1984, *35*, 513), and 20% in patients undergoing emergency appendectomies (S. Sagar *et al.*, *Lancet*, 1976, *1*, 509). It was considered that the present evidence showed that the risk to young women of becoming pregnant from discontinuing oral contraceptives or of developing side-effects from prophylaxis may be greater than the risk of developing postoperative deep-vein thrombosis. There was an urgent need to define the true incidence of postoperative thrombosis so that a rational policy can be adopted. In the meantime it was considered that combined oral contraceptives should not be withheld from young women who require abdominal operations and that the routine use of prophylaxis in women on the pill is probably unnecessary, particularly if they have no other risk factors.— H. Sue-Ling and L. E. Hughes, *Br. med. J.*, 1988, *296*, 447. An earlier review advocating, if possible, discontinuation of combined oral contraceptives four weeks before major elective surgery.— J. Guillebaud, *Br. med. J.*, 1985, *291*, 498.

Uses and Administration

Of the varying hormonal contraceptives available for use by women **oral contraceptives** have been the most widely employed. *Combined oral contraceptives*, containing both an oestrogen and a progestogen in a fixed proportion, are the most effective type for general use. They are taken for 21 days (or occasionally 22 days) followed by an interval of 7 days (or 6 days) when menstrual bleeding will occur. A formulation containing the lowest dose of both oestrogen and progestogen compatible with good cycle control should be chosen. The oestrogen content of most preparations is currently in the range of 20 to 50 µg daily although higher doses were often formerly used; doses higher than 50 µg are not now generally employed but may be necessary in the occasional patient. Ethinyloestradiol and mestranol are the oestrogens typically used in such preparations. The progestogen component is represented by a wider variety of agents including desogestrel, ethynodiol diacetate, gestodene, levonorgestrel, lynoestrenol, norethisterone, norethisterone acetate, and norgestrel. When first starting combined oral contraceptives the first tablet may be taken on the first day of the menstrual cycle (the first day of bleeding) and additional contraceptive precautions are unnecessary; if first taken on the fifth day of the cycle, additional contraceptive precautions should be undertaken for 14 days. Additional precautions are also necessary if changing from a high-dose to a low-dose preparation. Meticulous regularity of dosage is essential and contraceptive protection may be lost if a dose is not taken at the proper time or is missed. These combined oral contraceptives appear to act by suppressing the mid-cycle peak of luteinising hormone and follicle-stimulating hormone, thereby inhibiting ovulation; both the oestrogen and progestogen constituents have this property. They also cause alterations to the endometrium and may prevent implantation and the progestogen component also produces thickening of the cervical mucus, rendering it hostile to sperm penetration. The combined oral contraceptives may also be used in some cases for menstrual irregularities.
Phased oral contraceptives also contain an oestrogen and progestogen but the amounts taken throughout the cycle are not constant; they are generally designed to mimic more closely the pattern of cyclic endogenous hormone secretion.
Sequential oral contraceptives consist of formulations where an oestrogen alone is taken for part of the cycle and an oestrogen together with a progestogen for the other part of the cycle. Preparations formerly used consisted of an oestrogen taken for about 15 days and the combination for about 7 days whereas the preparations used in some countries now generally consist of the oestrogen alone for 7 days with the oestrogen and progestogen for 15 days.
Progestogen-only oral contraceptives are suitable for women when an oestrogen component is contra-indicated. They are taken every day, with no interval during menstrual bleeding, but may be associated with a higher failure-rate than the combined preparations. Regularity in taking the doses is even more essential with this type of preparation. Commonly used progestogens include ethynodiol diacetate, levonorgestrel, and norethisterone.
Progestogens are also used alone as **injectable contraceptives**. Medroxyprogesterone acetate is given by intramuscular injection as a long-acting depot preparation in a dose of 150 mg to provide contraception for up to a 3-month period. Norethisterone enanthate is used similarly in a dose of 200 mg to provide protection for up to 2 months. Injectable contraceptives are usually used to provide short-term protection or are used in women unable to use other methods.
Implantable contraceptives containing a progestogen are also used. Levonorgestrel is used in the form of a subcutaneous implant; each implant contains 36 mg and is reported to release 30 µg

of levonorgestrel daily.

Progesterone-releasing intra-uterine devices have also been used in some countries.

Postcoital contraceptives have to be taken very shortly after an act of unprotected intercourse to be effective. They should only be used in emergencies and should not be used as a routine method of contraception. A preparation available for such use consists of tablets each containing ethinyloestradiol 50 µg and levonorgestrel 250 mg; 2 tablets should be taken within 72 hours and a further 2 tablets 12 hours later.

Many other methods of hormonal contraception for women have been investigated and include the use of vaginal devices which release progestogens.

Some general reviews and discussions concerning the use and choice of hormonal contraceptives: *Chronicle Wld Hlth Org.*, 1982, *36*, 179; A. D. Hofmann, *Bull. Wld Hlth Org.*, 1984, *62*, 331; *Drug & Ther. Bull.*, 1986, *24*, 73; *Pharm. J.*, 1986, *1*, 526; D. A. Grimes, *J. Am. med. Ass.*, 1986, *255*, 69; A. A. Kubba and J. Guillebaud, *Br. med. J.*, 1986, *293*, 1491; R. J. Pepperell, *Med. J. Aust.*, 1986, *144*, 169; K. Wellings, *Pharm. J.*, 1986, *1*, 525; J. Guillebaud, *Prescribers' J.*, 1987, *27*, (5), 1.

IMPLANTABLE CONTRACEPTIVES. A memorandum from a WHO meeting reviewing an implantable contraceptive containing levonorgestrel (Norplant). It was considered that this subdermal implant is a very efficient method of contraception, remaining effective for at least 5 years. The potential side-effects are minimised because only small amounts of levonorgestrel (about 30 µg daily) are released. The Norplant method of contraception was considered suitable for use in family planning programmes along with other currently available contraceptive preparations and devices.— *Bull. Wld Hlth Org.*, 1985, *63*, 485.

Some references to studies using levonorgestrel by subcutaneous implant for hormonal contraception: I. Sivin *et al.*, *Fert. Steril.*, 1983, *39*, 799; S. Roy *et al.*, *Am. J. Obstet. Gynec.*, 1984, *148*, 1006; M. M. Shaaban and M. Salah, *Contraception*, 1984, *29*, 335; D. N. Robertson *et al.*, *ibid.*, 1985, *31*, 351; P. Holma, *ibid.*, 231; G. Lopez *et al.*, *Obstet. Gynec.*, 1986, *68*, 204.

Some references to studies using norethisterone by subcutaneous implant for hormonal contraception: G. N. Gupta *et al.*, *Fert. Steril.*, 1984, *41*, 726; R. Rivera *et al.*, *ibid*, *42*, 228; G. N. Gupta *et al.*, *Contraception*, 1984, *30*, 239.

INJECTABLE CONTRACEPTIVES. A memorandum from a WHO meeting reviewing the use of medroxyprogesterone acetate and norethisterone enanthate as long-acting depot injectable contraceptives.— *Bull. Wld Hlth Org.*, 1982, *60*, 199. See also: G. Benagiano and F. M. Primiero, *Drugs*, 1983, *25*, 570.

Some references to studies on injectable contraceptives: H. K. Toppozada *et al.*, *Contraception*, 1983, *28*, 1 (medroxyprogesterone acetate and norethisterone enanthate); S. K. Banerjee *et al.*, *ibid.*, 1984, *30*, 561 (norethisterone enanthate); S. S. Rahman *et al.*, *Bull. Wld Hlth Org.*, 1985, *63*, 785 (norethisterone enanthate).

ORAL CONTRACEPTIVES. General reviews and discussions concerning the use and choice of oral contraceptives: M. L'E. Orme, *Br. J. clin. Pharmac.*, 1982, *14*, 31; J. Drife, *Br. med. J.*, 1983, *287*, 1397; *Drug & Ther. Bull.*, 1984, *22*, 69; *Can. med. Ass. J.*, 1985, *133*, 463; R. P. Shearman, *Med. J. Aust.*, 1986, *144*, 201.

Phased contraceptives. Reviews and discussions on some phased oral contraceptive preparations: *Med. Lett.*, 1982, *24*, 93; *ibid.*, 1984, *26*, 93; *ibid.*, 1985, *27*, 48; *Drug & Ther. Bull.*, 1985, *20*, 79.

Some references to studies using triphasic oral contraceptives: L. Carlborg, *Contraception*, 1983, *27*, 439; U. J. Gaspard *et al.*, *Curr. med. Res. Opinion*, 1983, *8*, 395; U. J. Gaspard *et al.*, *Contraception*, 1984, *29*, 305; M. Toews *et al.*, *Curr. ther. Res.*, 1987, *41*, 509.

Postcoital contraceptives. In a brief review, it was concluded that a preparation (PC4) containing ethinyloestradiol 50 µg and levonorgestrel 250 µg per tablet and given in a dose of 2 tablets within 72 hours of unprotected intercourse followed by a further 2 tablets exactly 12 hours later was effective for emergency postcoital contraception. It should not be used for routine contraception because it is less effective than conventional contraceptives and may cause more adverse effects.— *Drug & Ther. Bull.*, 1985, *23*, 97.

Further reviews on postcoital contraception: S. Rowlands, *Br. med. J.*, 1982, *285*, 322; *Lancet*, 1983, *1*, 855.

Some references to studies on postcoital contraception using total dosages of ethinyloestradiol 200 µg together with either levonorgestrel 1 mg or norgestrel 2 mg and given within 72 hours of intercourse: A. A. Yuzpe *et al.*, *Fert. Steril.*, 1982, *37*, 508; A. A. Kubba and J. Guillebaud, *Br. med. J.*, 1983, *287*, 1343; M. R. Van Santen and A. A. Haspels, *Contraception*, 1985, *31*, 275; *idem*, *Fert. Steril.*, 1985, *43*, 206.

Progestogen-only contraceptives. A study of women receiving progestogen-only oral contraceptives (ethynodiol diacetate, levonorgestrel, norethisterone).— M. C. Robertson, *Practitioner*, 1984, *228*, 435.

Proprietary Preparations of Combined Oral Contraceptives

Brevinor *(Syntex, UK)*. *Tablets*, 21-day calendar pack, norethisterone 500 µg, ethinyloestradiol 35 µg.

Conova 30 *(Gold Cross, UK)*. *Tablets*, 21-day calendar pack, ethynodiol diacetate 2 mg, ethinyloestradiol 30 µg.

Eugynon 30 *(Schering, UK)*. *Tablets*, 21-day calendar pack, levonorgestrel 250 µg, ethinyloestradiol 30 µg.

Eugynon 50 *(Schering, UK)*. *Tablets*, 21-day calendar pack, norgestrel 500 µg, ethinyloestradiol 50 µg.

Femodene *(Schering, UK)*. *Tablets*, 21-day calendar pack, gestodene 75 µg, ethinyloestradiol 30 µg.

Gynovlar 21 *(Schering, UK)*. *Tablets*, 21-day calendar pack, norethisterone acetate 3 mg, ethinyloestradiol 50 µg.

Loestrin 20 *(Parke, Davis, UK)*. *Tablets*, 21-day calendar pack, norethisterone acetate 1 mg, ethinyloestradiol 20 µg.

Loestrin 30 *(Parke, Davis, UK)*. *Tablets*, 21-day calendar pack, norethisterone acetate 1.5 mg, ethinyloestradiol 30 µg.

Marvelon *(Organon, UK)*. *Tablets*, 21-day calendar pack, desogestrel 150 µg, ethinyloestradiol 30 µg.

Mercilon *(Organon, UK)*. *Tablets*, 21-day calendar pack, ethinyloestradiol 20 µg, desogestrel 150 µg.

Microgynon 30 *(Schering, UK)*. *Tablets*, 21-day calendar pack, levonorgestrel 150 µg, ethinyloestradiol 30 µg.

Minilyn *(Organon, UK)*. *Tablets*, 22-day calendar pack, lynoestrenol 2.5 mg, ethinyloestradiol 50 µg.

Minovlar *(Schering, UK)*. *Tablets*, 21-day calendar pack, norethisterone acetate 1 mg, ethinyloestradiol 50 µg. *Tablets*, (Minovlar ED), 28-day calendar pack, as Minovlar but with 7 additional inactive tablets.

Minulet *(Wyeth, UK)*. *Tablets*, 21-day calendar pack, gestodene 75 µg, ethinyloestradiol 30 µg.

Neocon 1/35 *(Ortho-Cilag, UK)*. *Tablets*, 21-day calendar pack, norethisterone 1 mg, ethinyloestradiol 35 µg.

Norimin *(Syntex, UK)*. *Tablets*, 21-day calendar pack, norethisterone 1 mg, ethinyloestradiol 35 µg.

Norinyl-1 *(Syntex, UK)*. *Tablets*, 21-day calendar pack, norethisterone 1 mg, mestranol 50 µg.

Ortho-Novin 1/50 *(Ortho-Cilag, UK)*. *Tablets*, 21-day calendar pack, norethisterone 1 mg, mestranol 50 µg.

Ovran *(Wyeth, UK)*. *Tablets*, 21-day calendar pack, levonorgestrel 250 µg, ethinyloestradiol 50 µg.

Ovran 30 *(Wyeth, UK)*. *Tablets*, 21-day calendar pack, levonorgestrel 250 µg, ethinyloestradiol 30 µg.

Ovranette *(Wyeth, UK)*. *Tablets*, 21-day calendar pack, levonorgestrel 150 µg, ethinyloestradiol 30 µg.

Ovysmen 0.5/35 *(Ortho-Cilag, UK)*. *Tablets*, 21-day calendar pack, norethisterone 500 µg, ethinyloestradiol 35 µg.

Proprietary Preparations of Phased Oral Contraceptives

Binovum *(Ortho-Cilag, UK)*. *Tablets*, 21-day calendar pack: 7 tablets, norethisterone 500 µg, ethinyloestradiol 35 µg; 14 tablets norethisterone 1 mg, ethinyloestradiol 35 µg.

Logynon *(Schering, UK)*. *Tablets*, 21-day calendar pack: 6 tablets, levonorgestrel 50 µg, ethinyloestradiol 30 µg; 5 tablets, levonorgestrel 75 µg, ethinyloestradiol 40 µg; 10 tablets, levonorgestrel 125 µg, ethinyloestradiol 30 µg. *Tablets* (Logynon ED), 28-day calendar pack, as Logynon but with 7 additional inactive tablets.

Synphase *(Syntex, UK)*. *Tablets*, 21-day calendar pack: 7 tablets, norethisterone 500 µg, ethinyloestradiol 35 µg; 9 tablets, norethisterone 1 mg, ethinyloestradiol 35 µg; 5 tablets, norethisterone 500 µg, ethinyloestradiol 35 µg.

Trinordiol *(Wyeth, UK)*. *Tablets*, 21-day calendar pack: 6 tablets, levonorgestrel 50 µg, ethinyloestradiol 30 µg; 5 tablets, levonorgestrel 75 µg, ethinyloestradiol 40 µg; 10 tablets, levonorgestrel 125 µg, ethinyloestradiol 30 µg.

Trinovum *(Ortho-Cilag, UK)*. *Tablets*, 21-day calendar pack: 7 tablets, norethisterone 500 µg, ethinyloestradiol 35 µg; 7 tablets, norethisterone 750 µg, ethinyloestradiol 35 µg; 7 tablets, norethisterone 1 mg, ethinyloestradiol 35 µg.

Proprietary Preparations of Progestogen-only Oral Contraceptives

Femulen *(Gold Cross, UK)*. *Tablets*, 28-day calendar pack, ethynodiol diacetate 500 µg.

Micronor *(Ortho-Cilag, UK)*. *Tablets*, 28-day calendar pack, norethisterone 350 µg.

Microval *(Wyeth, UK)*. *Tablets*, 35-day calendar pack, levonorgestrel 30 µg.

Neogest *(Schering, UK)*. *Tablets*, 35-day calendar pack, levonorgestrel 37.5 µg (as norgestrel 75 µg).

Norgeston *(Schering, UK)*. *Tablets*, 35-day calendar pack, levonorgestrel 30 µg.

Noriday *(Syntex, UK)*. *Tablets*, 28-day calendar pack, norethisterone 350 µg.

Proprietary Preparations of Postcoital Oral Contraceptives

Schering PC4 *(Schering, UK)*. *Tablets*, 4 tablets, levonorgestrel 250 µg (as norgestrel 500 µg), ethinyloestradiol 50 µg. *Dose.* Two tablets up to a maximum of 72 hours after coitus, and 2 further tablets after 12 hours.

Proprietary Preparations of Injectable Contraceptives

Depo-Provera *(Upjohn, UK)*. *Injection*, medroxyprogesterone acetate 50 mg/mL, in vials of 1, 3, and 5 mL. *Dose.* 150 mg by deep intramuscular injection, repeated at 3-monthly intervals.

For details of other Depo-Provera preparations used for non-contraceptive purposes, see under medroxyprogesterone acetate (p.1402).

Noristerat *(Schering, UK)*. *Injection*, norethisterone enanthate 200 mg/mL, in ampoules of 1 mL. *Dose.* 200 mg by intramuscular injection, repeated once after 8 weeks.

Proprietary Names and Manufacturers of Combined Oral Contraceptives

Anacyclin *(Ciba, Ger.)*; Anacycline 101 *(Ciba, Switz.)*; Anovial *(Schering, Spain)*; Anovlar *(Schering, Arg.; Schering, Denm.; Schering, Ger.; Schering, Ital.; Schering, S.Afr.)*; Anovlar mite *(Schering, Swed.)*; Brevicon *(Astra-Syntex, Norw.; Syntex, USA)*; Brevicon 0.5/35 *(Syntex, Canad.; Syntex, Denm.)*; Brevicon 1/35 *(Syntex, Canad.)*; Brevinor *(Syntex, Austral.; Syntex, S.Afr.; Syntex, UK)*; Brevinor-1 *(Syntex, Austral.)*; Conceplan 21 *(Grünenthal, Ger.)*; Conceplan 21 mite *(Grünenthal, Ger.)*; Conlumin *(Syntex, Denm.; Astra-Syntex, Fin.; Astra-Syntex, Swed.)*; Conova 30 *(Searle, Belg.; Searle, Denm.; Searle, Neth.; Gold Cross, UK)*; Demulen *(Searle, S.Afr.)*; Demulen 1/35 *(Searle, USA)*; Demulen 1/50 *(Searle, USA)*; Demulen 30 *(Searle, Canad.)*; Demulen 50 *(Searle, Canad.)*; Duoluton *(Schering, Arg.)*; Econ *(Farmos, Denm.; Laakefarmos, Fin.)*; Econ mite *(Farmos, Denm.)*; Ediwal *(Schering, Ger.)*; Egogyn 30 *(Schering, Ital.)*; Elan *(Valeas, Ital.)*; Enovid 5 mg *(Searle, USA)*; Enovid-E *(Searle, USA)*; Etalontin *(Parke, Davis, Ger.; Parke, Davis, Switz.)*; Eugynon *(Schering, Arg.; Schering, Denm.; Schering, Ger.; Schering, Ital.; Schering, Norw.; Schering, S.Afr.; Schering, Spain; Schering, Switz.)*; Eugynon 30 *(Schering, UK)*; Eugynon 50 *(Schering, UK)*; Evanor-d *(Wyeth, Ital.)*; Evelea *(Elea, Arg.)*;

Femodene *(Schering, UK)*; Femovan *(Schering, Ger.)*; Follimin *(KabiVitrum, Norw.; Kabi, Swed.)*; Follinett *(Kabi, Swed.)*; Gentrol *(Wyeth, Denm.)*; Gestrol *(Samil, Ital.)*; Gynatrol *(Wyeth, Denm.)*; Gynovlane *(Schering, Fr.)*; Gynovlar *(Schering, Arg.; Schering, S.Afr.; Schering, UK)*; Levlen *(Berlex, USA)*; Lindiol 2.5 *(Organon, Arg.)*; Loestrin 1/20 *(Parke, Davis, USA)*; Loestrin 1.5/30 *(Parke, Davis, Canad.; Parke, Davis, USA)*; Loestrin 20 *(Parke, Davis, UK)*; Loestrin 30 *(Parke, Davis, UK)*; Lo/Ovral *(Wyeth, USA)*; Lyndiol *(Organon, Belg.; Organon, Denm.; Organon, Ger.; Organon, Neth.; Organon, Norw.; Organon, S.Afr.; Organon, Spain; Organon, Swed.; Organon, Switz.)*; Lyndiol E *(Ravasini, Ital.)*; Lyndiolett *(Organon, Fin.; Organon, Swed.)*; Lyn-ratiopharm *(Ratiopharm, Ger.)*; Marvelon *(Organon, Arg.; Organon, Belg.; Organon, Denm.; Organon, Fin.; Organon, Ger.; Organon, Neth.; Organon, Norw.; Organon, S.Afr.; Organon, Switz.; Organon, UK)*; Mercilon *(Organon, UK)*; Metrulen *(SPA, Ital.)*; Metrulen M *(Searle, Spain)*; Microdiol *(Organon, Spain)*; Microgyn *(Schering, Denm.)*; Microgynon *(Schering, Arg.; Schering, Austral.; Leiras, Fin.; Schering, Ger.; Schering, Ital.; Schering, Norw.; Schering, Spain)*; Microgynon 30 *(Schering, Belg.; Schering, Neth.; Schering, Switz.; Schering, UK)*; Micro-

gynon 50 *(Schering, Belg.; Schering, Neth.; Schering, Switz.)*; Mikro Plan *(DAK, Denm.)*; Milli Anovlar *(Schering, Fr.)*; Minestrin 1/20 *(Parke, Davis, Canad.)*; Mini Pregnon *(Nourypharma, Neth.)*; Minidril *(Wyeth-Byla, Fr.)*; Minifol *(Samil, Ital.)*; Miniluteolas *(Serono, Ital.)*; Minilyn *(Organon, UK)*; Ministat *(Organon, Belg.; Organon, Neth.)*; Minovlar *(Schering, Austral.; Schering, S.Afr.; Schering, UK)*; Min-Ovral *(Wyeth, Canad.)*; Minulet *(Wyeth, UK)*; Modicon *(Cilag, Austral.; Cilag, Neth.; Ortho Pharmaceutical, USA)*;
Neo Lyndiol *(Organon, Spain)*; Neo Norinyl *(Syntex-Latino, Spain)*; Neo Ovopausine *(Syntex-Latino, Spain)*; Neocon *(Cilag, Neth.)*; Neocon 1/35 *(Ortho-Cilag, UK)*; Neogentrol *(Wyeth, Denm.)*; Neo-Gentrol *(Wyeth, Fin.)*; Neogynon *(Schering, Arg.; Schering, Austral.; Schering, Belg.; Schering, Denm.; Schering, Ger.; Schering, Neth.; Schering, Switz.)*; Neogynona *(Schering, Spain)*; Neo-Primovlar *(Leiras, Fin.)*; Neorlest *(Parke, Davis, Ger.)*; Neo-Stediril *(Wyeth, Belg.; Wyeth, Ger.; Wyeth, Neth.; Wyeth, Switz.)*; Neovletta *(Schering, Swed.)*; Neovulen *(Searle, Denm.)*; Noracyclin *(Ciba, Ger.)*; Noracycline *(Ciba, Switz.)*; Nordette *(Wyeth, Arg.; Wyeth, Austral.; Wyeth, S.Afr.; Wyeth, USA)*; Nordiol *(Wyeth, Arg.; Wyeth, Austral.; Wyeth, S.Afr.)*; Norimin *(Syntex, UK)*; Norinyl-1 *(Syntex, Austral.; Syntex, S.Afr.; Syntex, UK)*; Norinyl 1/50 *(Syntex, Canad.)*; Norinyl 1+35 *(Syntex, USA)*; Norinyl 1+50 *(Syntex, USA)*; Norinyl 1+80 *(Syntex, USA)*; Norinyl 2 mg *(Syntex, USA)*; Norinyl-2 *(Syntex, Austral.)*; Norlestrin *(Parke, Davis, Arg.)*; Norlestrin 1/50 *(Parke, Davis, Canad.; Parke, Davis, USA)*; Norlestrin 2.5/50 *(Parke, Davis, Canad.; Parke, Davis, USA)*; Novogyn *(Schering, Ital.)*; Novostat *(Kabi, Spain)*;
Orlest *(Parke, Davis, Ger.; Parke, Davis, Switz.)*; Ortho 0.5/35 *(Ortho, Canad.)*; Ortho 1/35 *(Ortho, Canad.)*; Orthonett Novum *(Cilag-Chemie, Denm.; Cilag, Swed.)*; Ortho-Novin 1/50 *(Ortho-Cilag, UK)*; Ortho-Novum 1/35 *(Cilag, Fr.; Ortho Pharmaceutical, USA)*; Ortho-Novum 1/50 *(Cilag, Austral.; Cilag, Belg.; Ortho, Canad.; Cilag, Ger.; Cilag, Ital.; Cilag, Neth.; Cilag, Switz.; Ortho Pharmaceutical, USA)*; Ortho-Novum 1/80 *(Cilag, Belg.; Cilag, Ger.; Cilag, Switz.; Ortho Pharmaceutical, USA)*; Ortho-Novum 2 mg *(Cilag, Ger.; Cilag, Switz.; Ortho Pharmaceutical, USA)*; Ovamezzo *(CCD, Fr.)*; Ovariostat *(Organon, Fr.)*; Ovcon-35 *(Mead Johnson Laboratories, USA)*; Ovcon-50 *(Mead Johnson Laboratories, USA)*; Ovoplex *(Orfi, Spain)*; Ovoresta *(Organon, Ger.)*; Ovoresta micro *(Organon, Spain)*; Ovostat *(Organon, Belg.; Organon, Neth.; Organon, S.Afr.; Organon, Switz.)*; Ovostat micro *(Organon, Switz.)*; Ovral *(Wyeth, Arg.; Wyeth, Austral.; Wyeth, Canad.; Wyeth, S.Afr.; Wyeth, USA)*; Ovran *(Wyeth, UK)*; Ovran 30 *(Wyeth, UK)*; Ovranet *(Wyeth, Ital.)*; Ovranette *(Wyeth, UK)*; Ovulen *(Searle, Arg.; Searle, Ger.; Searle, S.Afr.; Searle, USA)*; Ovulen 0.5 *(Searle, Austral.; Searle, Switz.)*; Ovulen 0.5/50 *(Searle, Austral.)*; Ovulen 1 *(Searle, Austral.; Searle, Belg.; Searle, Switz.)*; Ovulen 1/50 *(Searle, Austral.)*; Ovulen 50 *(Searle, Belg.; Searle, Neth.; Searle, Switz.)*; Ovulen Novum *(Searle, Norw.)*; Ovysmen *(Cilag, Belg.; Cilag, Ital.)*; Ovysmen 0.5/35 *(Cilag, Ger.; Cilag, Switz.; Ortho-Cilag, UK)*; Ovysmen 1/35 *(Cilag, Ger.; Cilag, Switz.)*;
Plan mite *(DAK, Denm.)*; Planor *(Roussel, Fr.)*; Planum *(Manarini, Ital.)*; Practil *(Ravasini, Ital.)*; Prandiol *(Ferran, Spain)*; Pregnon *(Aaciphar, Belg.; Erco, Denm.; Nourypharma, Ger.; Nourypharma, Neth.)*; Profinix *(Schering, Spain)*; Regovar *(Recordati, Ital.)*; Regunon *(Schering, Swed.)*; Restovar *(Organon, Denm.; Organon, Fin.; Organon, Norw.; Organon, S.Afr.; Organon, Swed.)*; Stediril *(Wyeth, Belg.; Wyeth-Byla, Fr.; Wyeth, Ger.; Wyeth, Switz.)*; Stediril 30 *(Wyeth, Belg.; Wyeth, Ger.; Wyeth, Neth.; Wyeth, Switz.)*; Stediril-d *(Wyeth, Belg.; Wyeth, Ger.; Wyeth, Neth.; Wyeth, Switz.)*; Trentovlane *(Schering, Fr.)*; Varnoline *(Organon, Fr.)*; Yermonil *(Geigy, Ger.; Ciba, Switz.)*.

Proprietary Names and Manufacturers of Phased Oral Contraceptives

Adepal *(Wyeth-Byla, Fr.)*; Binordiol *(Wyeth, Belg.; Wyeth, Denm.; Wyeth, Fin.; Wyeth, Ital.; Wyeth, Neth.; Wyeth, Switz.)*; Binovum *(Cilag, Ital.; Cilag, Switz.; Ortho-Cilag, UK)*; Biphasil *(Wyeth, Austral.; Wyeth, S.Afr.)*; Bivlar *(Schering, Ital.)*; Fironetta *(Schering, Denm.)*; Gynophase *(Schering, Fr.)*; Logynon *(Schering, S.Afr.; Schering, UK)*; Miniphase *(Schering, Fr.)*; Neo-Eunomin *(Grünenthal, Ger.)*; Normovlar *(Schering, S.Afr.)*; Ortho 7/7/7 *(Ortho, Canad.)*; Ortho 10/11 *(Ortho, Canad.)*; Ortho-Novum 7/7/7 *(Ortho Pharmaceutical, USA)*; Ortho-Novum 10/11 *(Ortho Pharmaceutical, USA)*; Perikursal *(Wyeth, Ger.)*; Prolorfin *(Orfi, Spain)*; Sekvilar *(Leiras, Fin.)*; Sequilar *(Schering, Austral.; Schering, Belg.; Schering, Ger.; Schering, Neth.; Schering, Switz.)*; Sequilarum *(Schering, Denm.; Schering, Swed.)*; Sinovula *(Asche, Ger.)*; Synfase *(Astra-Syntex, Swed.)*; Synphase *(Syntex, UK)*; Synphasec *(Grünenthal, Ger.)*; Synphasic *(Syntex, Austral.)*;
Triagynon *(Schering, Spain)*; Triciclor *(Orfi, Spain)*; Tridestan *(Gador, Arg.)*; Triella *(Cilag, Fr.)*; Trigynon *(Schering, Belg.; Schering, Ital.; Schering, Neth.)*; Trikvilar *(Leiras, Fin.)*; Tri-Levlen *(Berlex, USA)*; Trinordiol *(Wyeth, Arg.; Wyeth, Belg.; Wyeth, Denm.; Wyeth, Fin.; Wyeth-Byla, Fr.; Wyeth, Ger.; Wyeth, Ital.; Wyeth, Neth.; KabiVitrum, Norw.; Kabi, Swed.; Wyeth, Switz.; Wyeth, UK)*; Tri-Norinyl *(Syntex, USA)*; Trinovum *(Cilag-Chemie, Denm.; Cilag, Ger.; Cilag, Ital.; Cilag, Neth.; Cilag, S.Afr.; Cilag, Swed.; Cilag, Switz.; Ortho-Cilag, UK)*; Trionetta *(Schering, Norw.; Schering, Swed.)*; Triphasil *(Wyeth, Austral.; Wyeth, Canad.; Wyeth, S.Afr.; Wyeth, USA)*; Triquilar *(Schering, Arg.; Schering, Austral.; Schering, Denm.; Schering, Ger.; Schering, Switz.)*; Tristep *(Asche, Ger.)*.

Proprietary Names and Manufacturers of Progestogen-only Oral Contraceptives

Conludag *(Astra-Syntex, Norw.)*; Exlutena *(Organon, Swed.)*; Exluton *(Organon, Arg.; Organon, Belg.; Organon, Fin.; Organon, Fr.; Organon, Neth.; Organon, S.Afr.)*; Exlutona *(Organon, Denm.; Organon, Ger.; Organon, Norw.; Organon, Switz.)*; Femulen *(Searle, S.Afr.; Gold Cross, UK)*; Follistrel *(Kabi, Swed.)*; Gesta Plan *(DAK, Denm.)*; Microlut *(Schering, Austral.; Schering, Belg.; Schering, Ger.; Schering, Ital.)*; Microluton *(Schering, Denm.; Leiras, Fin.; Schering, Norw.)*; Micronor *(Cilag, Austral.; Ortho, Canad.; Ortho-Cilag, UK; Ortho Pharmaceutical, USA)*; Micronovum *(Cilag, Ger.; Johnson & Johnson, S.Afr.; Cilag, Switz.)*; Microval *(Wyeth, Austral.; Wyeth, Belg.; Wyeth, Denm.; Wyeth, Fin.; Wyeth-Byla, Fr.; Wyeth, S.Afr.; Wyeth, UK)*; Mikro-30 *(Wyeth, Ger.)*; Milligynon *(Schering, Fr.)*; Minette *(Orion, Fin.)*; Mini-Pe *(Syntex, Denm.; Astra-Syntex, Swed.)*; Mini-Pill *(Astra-Syntex, Fin.)*; Neogest *(Schering, UK)*; Norgeston *(Schering, UK)*; Noriday *(Syntex, Austral.; Syntex, S.Afr.; Syntex, UK)*; Nor-QD *(Syntex, USA)*; Ogyline *(Roussel, Fr.)*; Ovrette *(Wyeth, USA)*.

Proprietary Names and Manufacturers of Sequential-type Oral Contraceptives

Eunomin *(Grünenthal, Ger.)*; Fysionorm *(Nourypharma, Ger.)*; Fysioquens *(Aaciphar, Belg.; Organon, Denm.; Organon, Fin.; Nourypharma, Neth.)*; Lyn-ratiopharm-Sequenz *(Ratiopharm, Ger.)*; Normophasic *(Nourypharma, Switz.)*; Ortho-Novum SQ *(Cilag, Belg.)*; Ovanon *(Aaciphar, Belg.; Organon, Fr.; Nourypharma, Ger.; Nourypharma, Neth.; Ercopharm, Switz.)*; Ovanon-E *(Organon, S.Afr.)*; Ovanone *(Erco, Denm.; Erco, Swed.)*; Ovidol *(Aaciphar, Belg.; Nourypharma, Neth.; Nourypharma, Switz.)*; Oviol *(Nourypharma, Ger.)*; Phasicon *(Organon, S.Afr.)*; Physiostat *(Organon, Fr.)*.

Proprietary Names and Manufacturers of Postcoital Oral Contraceptives

Schering PC4 *(Schering, UK)*; Tetragynon *(Schering, Switz.)*.

Proprietary Names and Manufacturers of Injectable Contraceptives

Atrimon *(Beta, Arg.)*; Damix *(Valles Mestre, Spain)*; Depo-Clinovir *(Upjohn, Ger.)*; Depo-Provera *(Upjohn, Belg.; Upjohn, Denm.; Upjohn, Fr.; Upjohn, Neth.; Upjohn, S.Afr.; Upjohn, Swed.; Upjohn, Switz.; Upjohn, UK)*; Noristerat *(Schering, Denm.; Schering, Fr.; Schering, Ger.; Schering, UK)*; Nur-Isterate *(Schering, S.Afr.)*; Perlutal *(Promeco, Arg.)*; Topasel *(Castejon, Spain)*.

Proprietary Names and Manufacturers of Progestogen-releasing Intra-uterine Devices

Biograviplan Progestasert *(Grünenthal, Ger.)*; Progestasert *(Recordati, Ital.; Polcrome, UK)*.

Proprietary Names and Manufacturers of Implantable Contraceptives

Norplant *(Leiras, Fin.; Leiras, Swed.)*.

9022-d

Algestone Acetophenide *(USAN, rINNM)*.

Alphasone Acetophenide; Dihydroxyprogesterone Acetophenide; SQ-15101. 16α, 17α-(1-Phenylethylidenedioxy)pregn-4-ene-3,20-dione.
$C_{29}H_{36}O_4$=448.6.

CAS — 595-77-7 (algestone); 24356-94-3 (acetophenide).

Algestone acetophenide is a progestogen with actions and uses similar to those described for the progestogens in general (see p.1386). It has been given by intramuscular injection in monthly doses of 150 mg in conjunction with oestradiol enanthate as a contraceptive.

Proprietary Names and Manufacturers

Neolutin Depositum *(Medici, Ital.)*.
The following names have been used for multi-ingredient preparations containing algestone acetophenide—Atrimon *(Beta, Arg.)*; Damix *(Valles Mestre, Spain)*; Perlutal *(Promeco, Arg.)*; Topasel *(Castejohn, Spain)*.

9023-n

Allyloestrenol *(BAN)*.

Allylestrenol *(rINN)*. 17α-Allylestr-4-en-17β-ol.
$C_{21}H_{32}O$=300.5.

CAS — 432-60-0.

Adverse Effects and Precautions

As for the progestogens in general, p.1386.

Uses and Administration

Allyloestrenol is a progestogen with actions and uses similar to those described for the progestogens in general (see p.1386). In threatened abortion suggested doses have been 5 mg three times daily by mouth for 5 to 7 days and in habitual abortion 5 to 10 mg daily.

Proprietary Preparations

Gestanin *(Organon, UK). Tablets*, allyloestrenol 5 mg.

Proprietary Names and Manufacturers

Gestanin *(Organon, Austral.; Organon, S.Afr.; Organon, UK)*; Gestanon *(Belg.; Organon, Ger.; Ravasini, Ital.; Jpn; Neth.; Organon, Spain; Organon, Switz.)*; Gestanyn *(Swed.)*.

9025-m

Benzestrol *(BAN, rINN)*.

Benzoestrol; Octoestrolum. 4,4′-(1,2-Diethyl-3-methyltrimethylene)diphenol.
$C_{20}H_{26}O_2$=298.4.

CAS — 85-95-0.

Pharmacopoeias. In *Rus.*

Benzestrol is a synthetic non-steroidal oestrogen structurally related to stilboestrol (p.1413). It possesses the general properties typical of oestrogens (see p.1384) and was formerly administered by mouth and by intramuscular injection.

For a general review covering the actions and uses of oestrogens, see p.1385.

12450-m

Boldenone Undecenoate *(BANM, rINNM)*.

Ba-29038; Boldenone Undecylenate *(USAN)*. 17β-Hydroxyandrosta-1,4-dien-3-one 17-(undec-10-enoate).
$C_{30}H_{44}O_3$=452.7.

CAS — 846-48-0 (boldenone); 13103-34-9 (undecenoate).

Boldenone undecenoate is an anabolic steroid used in veterinary practice.

Proprietary Veterinary Names and Manufacturers

Vebonol *(Ciba-Geigy Agrochemicals, UK)*.

12456-s

Broparestrol *(rINN)*.

α-Bromo-β-(4-ethylphenyl)stilbene.
$C_{22}H_{19}Br$=363.3.

CAS — 479-68-5.

Broparestrol is a synthetic oestrogen with the general properties described as for the oestrogens in general (see p.1384). Like many other oestrogens it has been given for the suppression of lactation and in neoplastic disease. It has also been used topically in acne and similar skin disorders.

Proprietary Names and Manufacturers

Acnestrol *(Scharper, Ital.)*; Longestrol *(Laroche Navarron, Fr.; Landerlan, Spain)*.

9026-b

Calusterone *(USAN, rINN).*
7β,17α-Dimethyltestosterone; NSC-88536; U-22550.
17β-Hydroxy-7β,17α-dimethylandrost-4-en-3-one.
$C_{21}H_{32}O_2$=316.5.

CAS — 17021-26-0.

Calusterone has properties similar to those of testosterone and has been used in the palliative treatment of breast cancer in postmenopausal women but is reported to have virilising effects. It has been given by mouth in doses of 50 mg three to six times daily.

Proprietary Names and Manufacturers
Methosarb *(Upjohn, USA).*

9027-v

Chlormadinone Acetate *(BANM, USAN, rINNM).*
6-Chloro-17-hydroxypregna-4,6-diene-3,20-dione acetate.
$C_{23}H_{29}ClO_4$=404.9.

CAS — 1961-77-9 (chlormadinone); 302-22-7 (acetate).

Pharmacopoeias. In *Fr.*

Adverse Effects and Precautions
As for the progestogens in general, p.1386.
Because the proportion of small nodules in the breast of beagle dogs was found to be increased by continuous doses of chlormadinone acetate, the manufacture of both 'sequential' and 'progestogen-only' oral contraceptive preparations containing chlormadinone acetate was suspended in 1970.

EFFECTS ON THE SKIN. A report of autoimmune dermatitis in one patient associated with chlormadinone acetate.— I. Katayama and K. Nishioka, *Br. J. Derm.*, 1985, *112*, 487.

MALIGNANT NEOPLASMS. Doses of chlormadinone acetate and megestrol acetate that were 25 times greater than the expected human dose induced mammary tumours in beagles. This was not considered to be a useful indication of carcinogenicity in women.— L. W. Nelson *et al.*, *J. Am. med. Ass.*, 1972, *219*, 1601.

Absorption and Fate
Chlormadinone acetate is readily absorbed from the gastro-intestinal tract. It is distributed in body fat from which it is slowly released.

Uses and Administration
Chlormadinone acetate is a progestogen with actions and uses similar to those described for the progestogens in general (see p.1386). It has been reported to have very slight oestrogenic activity. It is active by mouth and was formerly used with mestranol as a 'sequential' oral contraceptive and as a 'progestogen-only' oral contraceptive.

Proprietary Names and Manufacturers
Cero *(Arg.)*; Gestafortin *(E. Merck, Ger.)*; Lutéran *(Cassenne, Fr.)*; Menstridyl *(Syntex, Belg.)*; Progestormon *(Syntex-Latino, Spain)*; Traslan *(Gramon, Arg.).*

The following names have been used for multi-ingredient preparations containing chlormadinone acetate— Eunomin *(Grünenthal, Ger.)*; Neo-Eunomin *(Grünenthal, Ger.).*

9029-q

Chlorotrianisene *(BAN, USAN, rINN).*
Tri-*p*-anisylchloroethylene. Chlorotris(4-methoxyphenyl)ethylene.
$C_{23}H_{21}ClO_3$=380.9.

CAS — 569-57-3.

Pharmacopoeias. In *Br., Rus.,* and *U.S.*

Small white odourless crystals or crystalline powder. **Soluble** 1 in 4200 of water, 1 in 360 of alcohol and of methyl alcohol, 1 in 7 of acetone, 1 in 1.5 of chloroform, 1 in 28 of ether, and 1 in 100 of fixed oils; practically insoluble in 2,2,4-trimethylpentane. **Store** in airtight containers.

CAUTION. *Chlorotrianisene is a powerful oestrogen. Contact with the skin or inhalation should be avoided. Rubber gloves and a face mask should be worn when handling the powder.*

Adverse Effects and Precautions
As for the oestrogens in general, p.1384.

Uses and Administration
Chlorotrianisene is a synthetic non-steroidal oestrogen with actions and uses similar to those described for the oestrogens in general (see p.1385). It has a prolonged action.
Chlorotrianisene is given by mouth for the treatment of menopausal and postmenopausal symptoms in a dosage of 12 to 25 mg daily.
Chlorotrianisene has also been used, like many other oestrogens, in metastatic prostatic carcinoma and for the suppression of lactation.

For a general review covering the actions and uses of oestrogens, see p.1385.

Preparations
Chlorotrianisene Capsules *(B.P.).* A solution of chlorotrianisene in a suitable fixed oil, enclosed in capsules.
Chlorotrianisene Capsules *(U.S.P.)*
Chlorotrianisene Tablets *(B.P.)*

Proprietary Names and Manufacturers
Anisene *(Ital.)*; Clorotrisin *(Ital.)*; Hormonisene *(Arg.)*; Merbentul *(Merrell, Ger.)*; Tace *(Austral.; Belg.; Merrell Dow, Canad.; Merrell, Fr.; Ital.; S.Afr.; Merrell Dow, Spain; Merrell Dow, Switz.; Merrell, UK; Merrell Dow, USA)*; Triagen *(Ital.).*

9031-n

Clomiphene Citrate *(BANM, USAN).*

Chloramiphene Citrate; Clomifene Citrate *(rINNM)*; MRL-41; NSC-35770. A mixture of the *E* and *Z* isomers of 2-[4-(2-chloro-1,2-diphenylvinyl)phenoxy]triethylamine dihydrogen citrate.
$C_{26}H_{28}ClNO,C_6H_8O_7$=598.1.

CAS — 911-45-5 (clomiphene); 15690-57-0 (clomiphene, E); 15690-55-8 (clomiphene, Z); 50-41-9 (citrate); 7599-79-3 (citrate, E); 7619-53-6 (citrate, Z).

NOTE. Clomiphene may be separated into its *Z* and *E* isomers, zuclomiphene and enclomiphene.

Pharmacopoeias. In *Br., Braz., Egypt., It., Jpn, Nord.,* and *U.S.*

A white to pale yellow, odourless or almost odourless powder. It contains 30 to 50% of the *Z* isomer. Slightly **soluble** in water and chloroform; sparingly soluble in alcohol; freely soluble in methyl alcohol; practically insoluble in ether. **Protect** from light.

Adverse Effects
Side-effects with clomiphene citrate generally appear to be related to the dose employed. The commonest reported adverse effects are reversible ovarian enlargement, vasomotor flushes resembling menopausal symptoms, and abdominal or pelvic discomfort or pain sometimes with nausea or vomiting. Transient eye disturbances such as blurring of vision may occur and there have been rare reports of cataracts. Skin reactions such as allergic rashes and urticaria have occasionally been reported and slight alopecia has been reported rarely. Central nervous system disturbances have included dizziness, lightheadedness, or vertigo, insomnia, and depression. Abnormalities in liver function tests have sometimes been reported.
Following therapy with clomiphene citrate there is an increased risk of multiple births. Although there have been reports of congenital disorders such as neural tube defects or Down's syndrome in infants born to women treated with clomiphene the role of the drug in the causation of these defects has not been established and the incidence is reported to be similar to that in women with other types of infertility problems.

PREGNANCY AND THE NEONATE. Of 21 patients with tubal pregnancies, 3 had received clomiphene. Also 2 patients with hydatidiform mole were observed in a group of pregnant women who had been given clomiphene.— D. B. Weiss and Y. Aboulafia (letter), *Lancet*, 1975, *2*, 1094.

Effects on the foetus. Individual reports of congenital disorders after treatment of the mother with clomiphene: J. L. Dyson and H. G. Kohler (letter), *Lancet*, 1973, *1*, 1256 (anencephaly); B. Field and C. Kerr (letter), *ibid.*, 1974, *2*, 1511 (neural tube defects); P. Berman (letter), *ibid.*, 1975, *2*, 878 (multiple abnormalities); O. Ylikorkala (letter), *ibid.*, 1262 (multiple abnormalities); M. Singh *et al.*, *J. Pediat.*, 1978, *93*, 152 (neural tube defects); F. Halal *et al.*, *Can. med. Ass. J.*, 1980, *122*, 1159 (multiple abnormalities).

Precautions
Clomiphene citrate is contra-indicated in patients with liver disease or a history of liver dysfunction, endometrial carcinoma or ovarian cysts (other than polycystic ovary) and during pregnancy. Before starting treatment patients should be thoroughly examined to exclude liver disease, pituitary or ovarian failure, and neoplasms of the endometrium. The cause of infertility and any abnormal bleeding should be investigated. The patient should be warned of the possibility of multiple births, particularly if higher doses are used. The patient should also be instructed to report any abdominal or pelvic pain as this may indicate the presence or enlargement of ovarian cysts. Patients with polycystic ovaries undergoing therapy with clomiphene should receive the lowest doses possible to prevent any further enlargement or cyst formation. Prolonged courses of treatment are not recommended.

Absorption and Fate
Clomiphene citrate is absorbed from the gastro-intestinal tract and slowly excreted through the liver into the bile. The biological half-life is reported to be 5 days. Enterohepatic recirculation takes place.

Uses and Administration
Clomiphene is chemically related to chlorotrianisene. It stimulates the secretion of pituitary gonadotrophic hormones probably by blocking the effect of oestrogens at receptor sites in the hypothalamus and pituitary.
Clomiphene is used in the treatment of anovulatory infertility. Therapy with clomiphene will not be successful unless the woman, though anovulatory, is capable of ovulation and her partner is fertile. It is ineffective in primary pituitary or primary ovarian failure. The usual dose by mouth is 50 mg of the citrate daily for 5 days, starting on or about the 5th day of the menstrual cycle or at any time if there is amenorrhoea. If ovulation does not occur, a course of 100 mg daily for 5 days may be given. Differing recommendations have been made as to how many courses of therapy should be given and the maximum dose that may be administered. Some sources have stated that 3 courses of therapy are adequate to assess whether a response is obtainable while others have stated that up to 6 courses are permissible. Similarly the maximum dose has been stated to be either 100 or 200 mg daily for 5 days.
Clomiphene is also sometimes used in conjunction with gonadotrophins and in *in-vitro* fertilisation programmes.

FEMALE INFERTILITY. Reviews of the treatment of female infertility including the use of clomiphene citrate: *Med. Lett.*, 1985, *27*, 82; M. M. Quigley, *Drugs*, 1986, *32*, 169.

MALE INFERTILITY. A review and discussion on the management of male infertility. The use of clomiphene citrate in men remains controversial. Despite this, and despite the fact that it is not recommended for the use of male infertility in the *UK* it has been extensively prescribed. Dosage regimens varying from 50 to 400 mg daily have been given for periods of 2 to 12 months. However, none of the studies that have adhered to the rules governing clinical trials have been able to show a convincing increase in the pregnancy-rate over that which might have happened by chance.— A. A. Templeton, *Prescribers' J.*, 1985, *25*, 91. A similar view.— *Ann. intern. Med.*, 1985, *103*, 906.

Preparations
Clomiphene Citrate Tablets *(U.S.P.)*

Clomiphene Tablets *(B.P.)*. Tablets containing clomiphene citrate.

Proprietary Preparations

Clomid *(Merrell, UK)*. *Tablets*, clomiphene citrate 50 mg.

Serophene *(Serono, UK)*. *Tablets*, clomiphene citrate 50 mg.

Proprietary Names and Manufacturers

Clomid *(Merrell Dow, Austral.; Belg.; Merrell Dow, Canad.; Merrell, Fr.; Lepetit, Ital.; Neth.; Mer-National, S.Afr.; Merrell Dow, Switz.; Merrell, UK; Merrell Dow, USA)*; Clomivid *(Draco, Denm.; Draco, Norw.; Draco, Swed.)*; Clostilbegyt *(Hung.)*; Dyneric *(Merrell, Ger.)*; Genozym *(Arg.)*; Omifin *(Spain)*; Pergotime *(Serono, Denm.; Serono, Fr.; Serono, Ger.; Ika-Pharm, Swed.)*; Prolifen *(Chiesi, Ital.)*; Serophene *(Pharmascience, Canad.; Serono, S.Afr.; Serono, Switz.; Serono, UK; Serono, USA)*.

9032-h

Clostebol Acetate *(BAN, rINNM)*.

4-Chlorotestosterone Acetate; Chlortestosterone Acetate. 4-Chloro-3-oxoandrost-4-en-17β-yl acetate.

$C_{21}H_{29}ClO_3$=364.9.

CAS — 1093-58-9 (clostebol); 855-19-6 (acetate).

Pharmacopoeias. In *Roum.*

Clostebol acetate has anabolic properties and has been given in doses of 40 mg twice weekly by intramuscular injection. It has also been applied topically in dermatological and ophthalmological preparations.

Proprietary Names and Manufacturers

Alfa-Trofodermin *(Farmitalia, Ital.)*; Clostene *(SIFI, Ital.)*; Steranabol *(Farmitalia, Ger.; Farmitalia, Neth.)*.

NOTE. The name Steranabol has also been used to denote a preparation of oxabolone cypionate.

9033-m

Cyclofenil *(BAN, rINN)*.

F-6066; ICI-48213. 4,4'-(Cyclohexylidenemethylene)bis(phenyl acetate).

$C_{23}H_{24}O_4$=364.4.

CAS — 2624-43-3.

Pharmacopoeias. In *Nord.*

Adverse Effects and Precautions

Side-effects include gastro-intestinal effects and very occasionally hot flushes. Cholestatic jaundice has been reported and cyclofenil should not be given to patients with liver disorders.

A review of 30 patients with reversible hepatic reactions to cyclofenil.— R. Olsson *et al., Gut*, 1983, *24*, 260.

Uses and Administration

Cyclofenil is used in the treatment of anovulatory infertility. It appears to be less effective than clomiphene.

It is given by mouth in doses of 100 mg twice daily for 10 days of 3 cycles.

Proprietary Preparations

Rehibin *(Serono, UK)*. *Tablets*, scored, cyclofenil 100 mg.

Proprietary Names and Manufacturers

Ciclifen *(Arg.)*; Fertodur *(Schering, Ger.; Schering, Ital.; Schering, Switz.)*; Neoclym *(Poli, Ital.)*; Ondogyne *(Roussel, Fr.)*; Ondonid *(Austral.; Roussel, UK)*; Rehibin *(Serono, UK)*; Sexovid *(Denm.; Jpn; Norw.; Leo, Swed.)*; Yobel *(IBYS, Spain)*.

9034-b

Cyproterone Acetate *(BANM, USAN, rINNM)*.

SH-714. 6-Chloro-1β,2β-dihydro-17α-hydroxy-3'*H*-cyclopropa[1,2]pregna-1,4,6-triene-3,20-dione acetate.

$C_{24}H_{29}ClO_4$=416.9.

CAS — 2098-66-0 (cyproterone); 427-51-0 (acetate).

Pharmacopoeias. In *It.*

Adverse Effects

When given to males cyproterone inhibits spermatogenesis, reduces the volume of ejaculate, and causes infertility; these effects are slowly reversible. Abnormal spermatozoa may be produced. Gynaecomastia is common and permanent enlargement of the mammary glands may occur; galactorrhoea and benign nodules have been reported. There may be initial sedation and depressive mood changes. Patients may experience alterations in hair pattern, skin reactions, weight changes, headache, anaemia, gastro-intestinal disturbance, and vasomotor changes with fluctuations in blood pressure.

When given with ethinyloestradiol to women the adverse effects associated with oral contraceptives (see p.1387) may occur.

PREGNANCY AND THE NEONATE. Reports of aborted foetuses with no malformations or of healthy infants born to mothers who had inadvertently taken a combination of cyproterone acetate and ethinyloestradiol during the early stages of pregnancy.— B. N. Statham *et al.* (letter), *Br. J. Derm.*, 1985, *113*, 374; P. Bye (letter), *ibid.*, 1986, *114*, 516; T. Bergh and O. Bakos, *Br. med. J.*, 1987, *294*, 677.

Precautions

Unless indicated for use in prostatic carcinoma cyproterone is contra-indicated in patients with acute liver disorders or malignant or wasting diseases. It should not be given to patients with severe chronic depression or to those with a history of thrombo-embolic disorders. It may delay bone maturation and testicular development and so should not be given to immature youths.

It should be given with care to patients with chronic liver disease, and, since it can interfere with carbohydrate metabolism, to those with diabetes mellitus. Since anaemia has been observed blood estimations are recommended regularly during treatment. Alcohol is reported to reduce the effects of cyproterone acetate. Depression of adrenal function has been reported.

Patients should be advised that the initial sedative effects may interfere with driving and the operation of machinery.

When cyproterone is given in conjunction with ethinyloestradiol to women the precautions for oral contraceptives (see p.1390) should be observed.

Absorption and Fate

Cyproterone acetate is poorly absorbed from the gastro-intestinal tract. It is rapidly metabolised and slowly excreted in the faeces and urine.

In 2 men given cyproterone acetate 100 mg by mouth as a single dose, peak plasma concentrations of 100 to 150 ng per mL occurred 5 to 10 hours after administration. Absorption from the gastro-intestinal tract was poor and after 8 days 90% of the dose was eliminated in the faeces.— E. Gerhards *et al., Arzneimittel-Forsch.*, 1973, *23*, 1550.

Absorption and fate of cyproterone acetate in 16 healthy subjects after receiving very low doses by mouth or intramuscularly.— D. Jentsch *et al., Arzneimittel-Forsch.*, 1976, *26*, 914.

In 5 healthy men given cyproterone acetate 50 mg by mouth peak plasma concentrations of 265 to 332 ng per mL (mean 285 ng per mL) occurred 3 to 4 hours after administration.— M. Hümpel *et al., Arzneimittel-Forsch.*, 1978, *28*, 319.

Uses and Administration

Cyproterone acetate has anti-androgenic and some progestogenic properties.

It is used for the control of libido in severe hypersexuality or sexual deviation in adult males. The usual dose is 50 mg twice daily.

It is also used in males for the palliative treatment of prostatic carcinoma. The usual initial dose is 300 mg daily in 2 to 3 divided doses after meals and maintenance treatment is continued with doses of 200 to 300 mg daily.

Cyproterone acetate may be used in conjunction with ethinyloestradiol in females for the control of severe acne and idiopathic hirsutism. The usual doses are 2 mg of cyproterone acetate with 35 μg of ethinyloestradiol given daily for 21 days of each menstrual cycle.

HIDRADENITIS SUPPURATIVA. Reports of a beneficial response of female hidradenitis suppurativa, an androgen-dependent disorder of the skin and hair in the pubic and axillary regions, to cyproterone acetate with ethinyloestradiol: P. S. Mortimer *et al., Br. J. Derm.*, 1986, *115*, 263; R. S. Sawers *et al., ibid.*, 269; P. S. Mortimer *et al.* (letter), *Br. med. J.*, 1986, *292*, 961.

PROSTATIC CARCINOMA. Reviews on the treatment of prostatic carcinoma including the use of cyproterone acetate: D. Kirk, *Br. med. J.*, 1985, *290*, 875; *Drug & Ther. Bull.*, 1986, *24*, 85.

Significant reduction of troublesome hot flushes which occurred after orchidectomy for prostatic carcinoma was achieved in 12 men given cyproterone acetate 100 mg three times daily.— A. C. Eaton and N. McGuire, *Lancet*, 1983, *2*, 1336. A brief mention that a dose of only 50 mg of cyproterone acetate daily is usually sufficient to control such hot flushes.— J. C. Gingell, *Br. med. J.*, 1984, *288*, 709.

Reports and correspondence concerning the use of the anti-androgens cyproterone or flutamide to prevent disease flare in patients with prostatic carcinoma being treated with luteinising hormone-releasing hormones: F. Labrie *et al.* (letter), *Lancet*, 1984, *2*, 1090 (flutamide); J. G. M. Klign *et al.* (letter), *ibid.*, 1985, *2*, 493 (cyproterone); F. Labrie *et al.* (letter), *ibid.*, 1986, *1*, 48 (flutamide).

Proprietary Preparations

Androcur *(Schering, UK)*. *Tablets*, scored, cyproterone acetate 50 mg.

Cyprostat *(Schering, UK)*. *Tablets*, scored, cyproterone acetate 50 mg.

Dianette *(Schering, UK)*. *Tablets*, cyproterone acetate 2 mg, ethinyloestradiol 35 μg.

Proprietary Names and Manufacturers

Androcur *(Berlex, Canad.; Schering, Denm.; Schering, Fr.; Schering, Ger.; Schering, Ital.; Neth.; Schering AG, Norw.; Schering, Spain; Schering, Swed.; Schering, Switz.; Schering, UK)*; Cyprostat *(Schering, UK)*.

The following names have been used for multi-ingredient preparations containing cyproterone acetate— Diane *(Schering, Ger.; Schering, Ital.; Schering, Switz.; Schering, UK)*; Dianette*(Schering, UK)*.

9035-v

Danazol *(BAN, USAN, pINN)*.

Win-17757. 17α-Pregna-2,4-dien-20-yno[2,3-*d*]-isoxazol-17β-ol.

$C_{22}H_{27}NO_2$=337.5.

CAS — 17230-88-5.

Pharmacopoeias. In *U.S.*

A white or pale yellow crystalline powder. Practically **insoluble** in water and light petroleum; sparingly soluble in alcohol; freely soluble in chloroform, slightly soluble in ether; soluble in acetone. **Store** in airtight containers. Protect from light.

Adverse Effects

Side-effects reflecting inhibition of the pituitary-ovarian axis include amenorrhoea, hot flushes, sweating, changes (usually decrease) in breast size, changes in libido, and vaginitis.

Side-effects attributable to androgenic activity include acne, oily skin or hair, hirsutism, oedema, gain in weight, deepening of the voice, and occasionally clitoral hypertrophy.

Other side-effects include gastro-intestinal disturbances, headache, dizziness, tremor, depression, sleep disorders, muscle spasm or cramp, skin rash, hyperglucagonaemia, and occasionally elevation of liver-function test values.

EFFECTS ON THE LIVER. Danazol was associated with biochemical evidence of liver injury in 4 patients and with jaundice in one patient.— K. Pearson and H. J. Zimmerman (letter), *Lancet*, 1980, *1*, 645.

Further reports of danazol-induced liver disorders: T. Ohsawa and S. Iwashita (letter), *Drug Intell. & clin. Pharm.*, 1986, *20*, 889 (hepatitis); F. Boue *et al.*, (letter), *Ann. intern. Med.*, 1986, *105*, 139 (cholestatic hepatitis).

EFFECTS ON THE MUSCLES. Myalgia and elevated creatine phosphokinase concentrations occurred in a 40-year-old woman given danazol 200 mg two or three times daily to treat hereditary angioedema.— W. B. Spaulding (letter), *Ann. intern. Med.*, 1979, *90*, 854.

EFFECTS ON THE VOICE. A 27-year-old woman treated for 7 to 8 months with danazol 600 mg daily experienced voice changes (huskiness, voice weakness, lowering of pitch, loss of pitch control) which persisted 16 months after discontinuing treatment.— P. G. Wardle *et al.*, *Br. med. J.*, 1983, *287*, 946. See also: R. Epstein and M. Bridger (letter), *ibid.*, 1308.

PREGNANCY AND THE NEONATE. Reports of masculinisation of female infants born to mothers who had received danazol during pregnancy: R. W. Shaw and J. W. Farquhar, *Br. J. Obstet. Gynaec.*, 1984, *91*, 386; A. C. Kingsbury, *Med. J. Aust.*, 1985, *143*, 410.

Precautions

Danazol should be used with caution in conditions which may be adversely affected by fluid retention, such as cardiac and renal disorders and migraine. It should also be used with care in patients with hepatic disorders. It should not be given to patients with porphyria as it may enhance porphyrin metabolism.

Therapy with danazol may necessitate adjustment in the dosage of anti-epileptic medication and may also increase insulin resistance thus interfering with the control of diabetic patients. It may potentiate the action of anticoagulants and has been reported to increase serum-cyclosporin concentrations. The concurrent administration of oestrogens or progestogens, including oral contraceptives, may modify the action of danazol and non-hormonal contraceptives are preferred.

Danazol should not be given during pregnancy because of a possible androgenic effect on the foetus and should also not be given to breast-feeding mothers.

Absorption and Fate

Danazol is absorbed from the gastro-intestinal tract and metabolised in the liver. A half-life of about 4.5 hours has been reported. 2-Hydroxymethylethisterone and ethisterone have been identified in the urine.

Plasma concentrations of danazol.— J. G. Lloyd-Jones and T. Williams-Ross, *J. int. med. Res.*, 1977, *5*, *Suppl.* 3, 18.

Uses and Administration

Danazol suppresses the pituitary-ovarian axis by inhibiting pituitary output of gonadotrophins. It has some androgenic activity.

It is used in the treatment of endometriosis. The usual initial dose is 200 to 400 mg daily by mouth, in up to 4 divided doses, starting on the first day of the menstrual cycle (to exclude pregnancy); maintenance doses are in the range of 200 to 800 mg daily and may be given for up to 6 to 9 months.

Danazol is also used in the treatment of benign breast disorders initially in a dose of 300 mg daily in divided doses, subsequently adjusted according to response, and continued for 3 to 6 months. It may also be used in other breast disorders such as gynaecomastia and pubertal breast hypertrophy.

In primary menorrhagia and the premenstrual syndrome doses of 200 mg daily have been employed.

In primary constitutional precocious puberty 100 to 400 mg daily has been given according to the child's age and weight.

Danazol has also been found to be of value in the treatment of hereditary angioedema. Suggested initial doses have been in the range of 400 to 600 mg daily.

The actions and uses of danazol.— I. S. Fraser, *Scott. med. J.*, 1979, *24*, 147.

ANGIOEDEMA. In 9 patients with hereditary angioedema there were 44 attacks during 47 courses of treatment with placebo and 1 attack during 46 courses of treatment with danazol 200 mg three times daily given for 28 days or until an attack occurred. Depressed C1 esterase inhibitor activity was corrected. Side-effects were minimal—weight gain and amenorrhoea.— J. A. Gelfand *et al.*, *New Engl. J. Med.*, 1976, *295*, 1444.

Danazol 300 to 600 mg daily with a gap of 5 or 7 days every 7 days was effective in the treatment of 10 patients with hereditary angioedema.— A. Agostoni *et al.* (letter), *Lancet*, 1978, *1*, 453.

An 8-year-old boy with hereditary angioedema remained free from attacks on danazol 200 mg every other day.— G. Tappeiner *et al.*, *Br. J. Derm.*, 1979, *100*, 207.

Of 55 patients with hereditary angioedema 95% were free from attacks on danazol 600 mg daily, 88% on 400 mg daily, 68% on 300 mg daily, and 11% on 200 mg daily. Short-term prophylaxis before dental procedures was achieved with 600 mg daily for 10 days.— S. W. Hosea and M. M. Frank, *Drugs*, 1980, *19*, 370.

A 24-year-old woman with hereditary angioedema and a lupus erythematosus-like syndrome and a low level of C_1 esterase inhibitor obtained a clinical remission on administration of danazol.— R. Masse *et al.* (letter), *Lancet*, 1980, *2*, 651. A similar finding.— V. H. Donaldson and E. V. Hess (letter), *ibid.*, 1145.

Control of hereditary angioedema in 2 patients with danazol in doses gradually reduced to 200 mg three times a week or 300 mg weekly.— J. T. Macfarlane and D. Davies, *Br. med. J.*, 1981, *282*, 1275.

Further references: *Lancet*, 1979, *1*, 417; H. Hinter *et al.*, *Dt. med. Wschr.*, 1979, *104*, 1269; S. W. Hosea *et al.*, *Ann. intern. Med.*, 1980, *93*, 809; C. Rajagopal and J. R. Harper, *Archs Dis. Childh.*, 1981, *56*, 229.

BENIGN BREAST DISEASE. Of 58 women with benign breast disorders (mazoplasia, mastodynia, or fibrocystic disease) 44 were markedly improved after treatment with danazol 100 to 400 mg daily for 74 to 310 days. Objective evidence of improvement was seen in 16 of 19 patients subjected to mammography. Amenorrhoea occurred in half the patients treated; other side-effects were considered trivial.— R. H. Asch and R. B. Greenblatt, *Am. J. Obstet. Gynec.*, 1977, *127*, 130.

Relief of pain and tenderness and some reduction in nodularity in 18 women with fibrocystic disease of the breast given danazol 100 to 400 mg daily.— L. J. Humphrey and N. C. Estes, *Postgrad. med. J.*, 1979, *55*, *Suppl.* 5, 48. Relief of pain, discomfort, heaviness, and tenderness in 6 patients with cyclical breast pain, given danazol 400 mg daily.— R. E. Mansel *et al.*, *ibid.*, 61. A favourable report of the use of danazol 400 mg daily in 27 patients with chronic cystic mastopathy.— M. Dhout *et al.*, *ibid.*, 66.

Further references: N. H. Lauerson and K. H. Wilson, *Obstet. Gynec.*, 1976, *48*, 93; W. P. Blackmore, *Int. J. med. Res.*, 1977, *5*, *Suppl.* 3, 101; M. F. Aksu *et al.*, *J. reprod. Med.*, 1978, *21*, 181; J. D. Brookshaw, *Postgrad. med. J.*, 1979, *55*, *Suppl.* 5, 52; B. Greenblatt and I. Ben-Nun, *Drugs*, 1980, *19*, 349.

BLOOD DISORDERS. Although it has been reported that danazol increases plasma concentrations of factor VIII and factor IX and may therefore be beneficial in the treatment of haemophilia A or haemophilia B (Christmas disease) (H.R. Gralnick and M.E. Rick, *New Engl. J. Med.*, 1983, *308*, 1393; H.R. Gralnick *et al.*, *J. Am. med. Ass.*, 1985, *253*, 1151) other workers have failed to substantiate these results and indeed have sometimes suggested that danazol may even increase the frequency of bleeding in such patients (H.S. Garewal *et al.*, *J. Am. med. Ass.*, 1985, *253*, 1154; R. Ambriz *et al.*, *ibid.*, *254*, 754; C.K. Kasper and A.L. Boylen, *Blood*, 1985, *65*, 211; D.C. Heaton *et al.*, *N.Z. med. J.*, 1986, *99*, 185).

Treatment with danazol has, however, been reported to be beneficial in the treatment of idiopathic thrombocytopenic purpura resulting in increased platelet counts (Y.S. Ahn *et al.*, *New Engl. J. Med.*, 1983, *308*, 1396; M. Buelli *et al.*, *Acta haemat.*, 1985, *74*, 97; B.A. McVerry *et al.*, *Br. J. Haemat.*, 1985, *61*, 145). A study investigating the possible mode of action in this disorder (A.D. Schreiber *et al.*, *New Engl. J. Med.*, 1987, *316*, 503) indicated that danazol may mediate an effect by influencing the number of available binding sites for monomeric immunoglobulin G (Fc receptors) on monocytes.

Additionally there have been reports of response to danazol therapy in patients with auto-immune haemolytic anaemia (Y.S. Ahn *et al.*, *Ann. intern. Med.*, 1985, *102*, 298), myelodysplastic syndromes (D.B. Cines *et al.*, *Ann. intern. Med.*, 1985, *103*, 58; A. Kornberg *et al.*, *ibid.*, 1986, *104*, 445), and paroxysmal cold haemoglobinuria (M. A. Gertz, *Ann. intern. Med.*, 1987, *106*, 635).

ENDOMETRIOSIS. In 370 patients with endometriosis studied in 10 centres in the *USA* and treated with danazol 200 to 800 mg daily (usually 800 mg) for up to 7 months, dysmenorrhoea was relieved in 85 to 95%, pelvic pain in 70 to 89%, dyspareunia in 69 to 84%, and induration of the pouch of Douglas in 73 to 82%.— M. D. Young and W. P. Blackmore, *J. int. med. Res.*, 1977, *5*, *Suppl.* 3, 86.

Of 99 patients with endometriosis treated with danazol 200 mg four times daily for 3 to 18 months 39 had recurrence of symptoms when re-evaluated about 3 years after ceasing treatment. A pregnancy-rate of 46% was achieved in those desiring pregnancy or 72% if corrected to exclude those in whom an absolute sterility factor was involved. Four foetal deaths occurred in women who conceived within 3 cycles of discontinuing danazol; this might be due to endometrial thinning and abnormal placentation.— W. P. Dmowski and M. R. Cohen, *Am. J. Obstet. Gynec.*, 1978, *130*, 41.

Of 44 patients with endometriosis 7 required 600 mg daily of danazol for control; 27 were maintained on 400 mg daily, and 10 on 200 mg daily.— G. D. Ward, *Postgrad. med. J.*, 1979, *55*, *Suppl.* 5, 7. See also J. A. Chalmers and P. C. Shervington, *ibid.*, 44.

GYNAECOMASTIA. Danazol was given to 42 men or youths with gynaecomastia—idiopathic in 17, spironolactone-induced in 13, thyrotoxic in 1, and pubertal in 11. The dose for adults was 300 mg daily for 4 to 6 weeks, increased to 600 mg daily for 4 to 6 months, then 200 to 300 mg daily for 4 to 6 months. In adolescents the initial dose was 200 to 300 mg daily with a maintenance dose of 200 mg daily. Of the 42 patients 25 showed marked regression and 10 moderate regression.— R. Buckle, *Postgrad. med. J.*, 1979, *55*, *Suppl.* 5, 71. See also *idem*, *Drugs*, 1980, *19*, 356.

MENORRHAGIA. Reduction of blood loss in patients with menorrhagia treated with danazol 400 mg daily.— T. H. Chimbira *et al.*, *Br. J. Obstet. Gynaec.*, 1979, *86*, 46.

PRECOCIOUS PUBERTY. A favourable report on the use of danazol in 12 children (11 girls, 1 boy) with precocious puberty.— C. S. Smith and F. Harris, *Postgrad. med. J.*, 1979, *55*, *Suppl.* 5, 81.

PREMENSTRUAL SYNDROME. The possible value of danazol in the premenstrual syndrome.— J. Day, *Postgrad. med. J.*, 1979, *55*, *Suppl.* 5, 87.

Preparations

Danazol Capsules *(U.S.P.)*

Proprietary Preparations

Danol *(Winthrop, UK)*. *Capsules*, danazol 200 mg. *Capsules*, (Danol-½), danazol 100 mg.

Proprietary Names and Manufacturers

Cyclomen *(Winthrop, Canad.)*; Danatrol *(Belg.; Sterling Winthrop, Fr.; Maggioni-Winthrop, Ital.; Sterwin, Spain; Winthrop, Switz.)*; Danocrine *(Winthrop, Austral.; Winthrop, Denm.; Fin.; Winthrop, Norw.; Sterling-Winthrop, Swed.; Winthrop-Breon, USA)*; Danokrin *(Aust.)*; Danol *(Winthrop, UK)*; Ladogar *(Winthrop, S.Afr.)*; Winobanin *(Winthrop, Ger.)*.

12628-y

Delmadinone Acetate *(BANM, USAN, rINNM)*.
RS-1301. 6-Chloro-17α-hydroxypregna-1,4,6-triene-3,20-dione acetate.
$C_{23}H_{27}ClO_4$=402.9.

CAS — 15262-77-8 (delmadinone); 13698-49-2 (acetate).

Delmadinone acetate is a progestogen with anti-androgen and anti-oestrogen activity. It has been used as an anti-androgen in veterinary practice.

Proprietary Veterinary Names and Manufacturers
Tardak *(Syntex, UK)*.

12629-j

Demegestone *(rINN)*.
R-2453. 17α-Methyl-19-norpregna-4,9-diene-3,20-dione.
$C_{21}H_{28}O_2$=312.5.

CAS — 10116-22-0.

Adverse Effects and Precautions
As for the progestogens in general, p.1386.

Uses and Administration
Demegestone is a progestogen with actions and uses similar to those described for the progestogens in general (see p.1386). It has been given in doses of 0.5 to 2 mg daily by mouth.

Proprietary Names and Manufacturers
Lutionex *(Roussel, Fr.)*.

12633-w

Desogestrel *(BAN, rINN)*.

Org-2969. 13β-Ethyl-11-methylene-18,19-dinor-17α-pregn-4-en-20-yn-17β-ol.
$C_{22}H_{30}O$=310.5.

CAS — 54024-22-5.

Adverse Effects and Precautions
As for the progestogens in general, p.1386.
See also under hormonal contraceptives, p.1387.

Uses and Administration
Desogestrel is a progestogen with actions and uses similar to those described for the progestogens in general (see p.1386).
It is used as the progestogenic component of combined oral contraceptive preparations (see p.1391).

Proprietary contraceptive preparations containing desogestrel are described under the section on hormonal contraceptives (p.1392).

Proprietary Names and Manufacturers
The following names have been used for multi-ingredient preparations containing desogestrel—Marvelon *(Organon, Arg.; Organon, Belg.; Organon, Denm.; Organon, Fin.; Organon, Ger.; Organon, Neth.; Organon, Norw.; Organon, S.Afr.; Organon, Switz.; Organon, UK)*; Mercilon *(Organon, UK)*; Microdiol *(Organon, Spain)*; Ovidol *(Aaciphar, Belg.; Nourypharma, Neth.; Nourypharma, Switz.)*; Oviol *(Nourypharma, Ger.)*; Planum *(Menarini, Ital.)*; Practil *(Ravasini, Ital.)*; Varnoline *(Organon, Fr.)*.

9037-q

Dienoestrol *(BAN)*.

Dehydrostilbestrol; Dienestrol *(USAN, rINN)*; Dienestrolum; Dienoestrolum; Oestrodienolum. *(E,E)*-4,4′-[Di(ethylidene)ethylene]diphenol.
$C_{18}H_{18}O_2$=266.3.

CAS — 84-17-3; 13029-44-2 (E,E).

Pharmacopoeias. In *Arg., Aust., Br., Braz., Egypt., Eur., Fr., Ger., Hung., Ind., Int., It., Jug., Neth., Swiss, Turk.,*and *U.S.*
Aust. also includes dienoestrol diacetate, 3,4-bis(*p*-acetoxyphenyl)hexa-2,4-diene.

White or almost white, odourless, crystals or crystalline powder. Practically **insoluble** in water; soluble 1 in 8 of alcohol, 1 in 5 of acetone, and 1 in 15 of ether; soluble in methyl alcohol, propylene glycol, and solutions of alkali hydroxides; slightly soluble in chloroform. **Store** in well-closed containers and protect from light.

CAUTION. *Dienoestrol is a powerful oestrogen. Contact with the skin or inhalation should be avoided. Rubber gloves and a face mask should be worn when handling the powder.*

Adverse Effects and Precautions
As for the oestrogens in general, p.1384.

A 70-year-old man developed gynaecomastia while exposed to the vaginal dienoestrol cream used by his wife.— C. V. DiRaimondo *et al.* (letter), *New Engl. J. Med.*, 1980, *302*, 1089.

Uses and Administration
Dienoestrol is a synthetic non-steroidal oestrogen structurally related to stilboestrol (p.1413). It has actions and uses similar to those described for the oestrogens in general (see p.1385).
Dienoestrol is used as a cream containing 0.01 or 0.025% in the treatment of vaginal and vulval menopausal and post menopausal symptoms.

For a general review covering the actions and uses of oestrogens, see p.1385.

Preparations
Dienestrol Cream *(U.S.P.)*. Dienoestrol in a suitable water-miscible basis.

Proprietary Preparations
Dienoestrol Cream *(Ortho-Cilag, UK)*. *Vaginal cream*, dienoestrol 0.01%.
Hormofemin *(Medo, UK)*. *Vaginal cream*, dienoestrol 0.025%.

Proprietary Names and Manufacturers
Cycladiene *(Belg.; Bruneau, Fr.)*; Dienoestrol Cream *(Ortho-Cilag, UK)*; DV *(Merrell Dow, USA)*; Estraguard *(Reid-Provident, USA)*; Eufemine *(Belg.)*; Hormofemin *(Medo, UK)*; Klianyl Forte *(Lundbeck, Denm.)*; Sexadien *(Leo, Denm.)*; Sexadieno *(Spain)*.

9038-p

Dimethisterone *(BAN, USAN, rINN)*.
6α,21-Dimethylethisterone. 17β-Hydroxy-6α,21-dimethyl-17α-pregn-4-en-20-yn-3-one monohydrate.
$C_{23}H_{32}O_2,H_2O$=358.5.

CAS — 79-64-1 (anhydrous); 41354-30-7 (monohydrate).

Adverse Effects and Precautions
As for the progestogens in general, p.1386.
Pelvic pain resembling dysmenorrhoea, breast turgidity, nausea, and vertigo may occur with large doses.

Uses and Administration
Dimethisterone is a progestogen with actions and uses similar to those described for the progestogens in general (see p.1386). It is reported to have no significant oestrogenic or androgenic properties. It was formerly administered by mouth and was also formerly given as the progestogenic component of 'sequential' oral contraceptive preparations.

Proprietary Names and Manufacturers
Secrosteron *(Duncan, Flockhart, UK)*.

9039-s

Drostanolone Propionate *(BANM, rINNM)*.

Dromostanolone Propionate *(USAN)*. 17β-Hydroxy-2α-methyl-5α-androstan-3-one propionate.
$C_{23}H_{36}O_3$=360.5.

CAS — 58-19-5 (drostanolone); 521-12-0 (propionate).

Pharmacopoeias. In *Br.*

A white or almost white crystalline powder. Practically **insoluble** in water; soluble in alcohol, 1 in 2 of chloroform, and 1 in 20 of ether. **Protect** from light. Oily solutions for injections may be **sterilised** by dry heat.

Adverse Effects and Precautions
As for the androgens and anabolic steroids in general, p.1383.

Uses and Administration
Drostanolone has anabolic and androgenic properties.
Drostanolone propionate is given by intramuscular injection in an oily solution and has a prolonged duration of effect. It is used in the treatment of advanced malignant neoplasms of the breast in postmenopausal women. The usual dose is 100 mg three times weekly.

Preparations
Drostanolone Injection *(B.P.)*. Drostanolone Propionate Injection. A sterile solution of drostanolone propionate in a suitable fixed oil.

Proprietary Preparations
Masteril *(Syntex, UK)*. *Injection*, drostanolone propionate 100 mg/mL, in ampoules of 1 mL.

Proprietary Names and Manufacturers
Drolban *(USA)*; Masterid *(Grünenthal, Ger.; Switz.)*; Masteril *(Austral.; S.Afr.; Syntex, UK)*; Masteron *(Belg.; Recordati, Ital.; Neth.)*; Metormon *(Spain)*; Permastril *(Cassenne, Fr.)*.

9040-h

Dydrogesterone *(BAN, USAN, rINN)*.

6-Dehydro-9β,10α-progesterone; Dehydroprogesterone; Didrogesteron; Isopregnenone. 9β,10α-Pregna-4,6-diene-3,20-dione.
$C_{21}H_{28}O_2$=312.5.

CAS — 152-62-5.

Pharmacopoeias. In *Br.* and *U.S.*

A white to pale yellow odourless crystalline powder. Practically **insoluble** in water; soluble 1 in 40 to 52 of alcohol, 1 in 17 of acetone, 1 in 2 of chloroform, 1 in 140 to 200 of ether, 1 in 40 of methyl alcohol, and 1 in 180 of fixed oils. **Protect** from light.

Adverse Effects and Precautions
As for the progestogens in general, p.1386.
Dydrogesterone is reported not to produce virilisation of the foetus.

PORPHYRIA. Dydrogesterone was considered to be unsafe in patients with acute porphyria although there is conflicting experimental evidence on porphyrinogenicity.— M.R. Moore and K.E.L. McColl, *Porphyrias, Drug Lists*, Glasgow, Porphyria Research Unit, University of Glasgow, 1987.

PREGNANCY AND THE NEONATE. *Effects on the foetus.* Anomalies of the genito-urinary tract were found in a 4-month-old baby whose mother had taken dydrogesterone 20 mg daily from the 8th to 20th week of pregnancy and 10 mg daily from then until term. She had also been given hydroxyprogesterone hexanoate 250 mg by intramuscular injection weekly from the 8th to the 20th week.— I. F. Roberts and R. J. West (letter), *Lancet*, 1977, *2*, 982.

Absorption and Fate
Dydrogesterone is absorbed from the gastro-intestinal tract. Plasma concentrations fall rapidly and about half a dose is excreted in the urine, within 24 hours.

Uses and Administration
Dydrogesterone is a progestogen with actions and uses similar to those described for the progestogens in general (see p.1386). However, unlike progesterone, dydrogesterone does not induce an increase in temperature or inhibit ovulation and may be preferred to other progestational agents when a contraceptive effect is not required. It does not have oestrogenic or androgenic properties.
Dydrogesterone is given by mouth usually in a dose of 10 mg twice daily. In threatened abortion suggested doses have been 40 mg initially followed by 10 mg or more 8-hourly, continued for a week after symptoms cease. In habitual abortion suggested doses have been 10 mg twice daily.

Preparations
Dydrogesterone Tablets *(B.P.)*
Dydrogesterone Tablets *(U.S.P.)*

Proprietary Preparations
Duphaston *(Duphar, UK)*. *Tablets*, scored, dydrogesterone 10 mg.

Proprietary Names and Manufacturers
Dabrostan *(Jug.)*; Dufaston *(ISM, Ital.)*; Duphaston *(Cilag, Austral.; Belg.; Duphar, Fr.; Duphar, Ger.; Neth.; Duphar, S.Afr.; Kali-Farma, Spain; Ferrosan, Swed.; Duphar, Switz.; Duphar, UK; USA)*; Gynorest *(USA)*; Terolut *(Ferrosan, Denm.; Ferrosan, Fin.; Ferrosan, Norw.)*.

12693-f

Epimestrol *(BAN, USAN, rINN).*
NSC-55975; Org-817. 3-Methoxyestra-1,3,5(10)-triene-16α,17α-diol.
$C_{19}H_{26}O_3$=302.4.

CAS — 7004-98-0.

Epimestrol is the 3-methyl ether of the naturally occurring hormone 17-epioestriol. It is suggested for use in the treatment of female infertility due to anovulation and a variety of other disorders resulting from anovulation.

Proprietary Names and Manufacturers
Alene *(Organon, Spain)*; Stimovul *(Organon, Ger.; Ravasini, Ital.; Organon, Neth.).*

9041-m

Epioestriol *(BAN).*
16-Epioestriol; Epiestriol *(rINN).* Estra-1,3,5(10)-triene-3,16β,17β-triol.
$C_{18}H_{24}O_3$=288.4.

CAS — 547-81-9.

Epioestriol is a naturally occurring oestrogen, closely related chemically to oestriol (p.1408). It was formerly used by topical application in the treatment of acne.

Proprietary Names and Manufacturers
Actriol *(Organon, UK).*

12694-d

Epitiostanol *(rINN).*
10275-S. 2α,3α-Epithio-5α-androstan-17β-ol.
$C_{19}H_{30}OS$=306.5.

CAS — 2363-58-8.

Epitiostanol is reported to have anabolic activity. It has been used in various breast disorders including neoplasms of the breast.

Proprietary Names and Manufacturers
Thiodrol *(Shionogi, Jpn).*

18357-p

Equilin *(USAN).*
3-Hydroxyestra-1,3,5(10),7-tetraen-17-one.
$C_{18}H_{20}O_2$=268.4.

CAS — 474-86-2.

Pharmacopoeias. In *U.S.*

Store in airtight containers. Protect from light.

Equilin is an oestrogenic hormone and sodium equilin sulphate is one of the components of both conjugated and esterified oestrogens.

9042-b

Estropipate *(USAN).*

Piperazine Estrone Sulfate; Piperazine Oestrone Sulphate. Piperazine 17-oxo-estra-1,3,5(10)-trien-3-yl sulphate.
$C_4H_{10}N_2,C_{18}H_{22}O_5S$=436.6.

CAS — 7280-37-7.

Pharmacopoeias. In *U.S.*

A fine, white to yellowish-white, crystalline powder, odourless or with a slight odour. Very slightly **soluble** in water, alcohol, chloroform, and ether; soluble 1 in 500 of warm alcohol. **Store** in airtight containers.

Adverse Effects and Precautions
As for the oestrogens in general, p.1384.

Uses and Administration
Estropipate is a synthetic oestrogen conjugate with actions and uses similar to those described for the oestrogens in general (see p.1385). Its action is due to oestrone (p.1409) to which it is hydrolysed in the body.

Estropipate is given by mouth for the treatment of menopausal and postmenopausal symptoms; suggested doses have ranged from 0.75 to 6 mg daily. Estropipate is also used as a vaginal cream containing 0.15%.

For a general review covering the actions and uses of oestrogens, see p.1385.

Preparations
Estropipate Tablets *(U.S.P.)*
Estropipate Vaginal Cream *(U.S.P.)*

Proprietary Preparations
Harmogen *(Abbott, UK). Tablets,* scored, estropipate 1.5 mg.

Proprietary Names and Manufacturers
Harmogen *(Abbott, Switz.; Abbott, UK)*; Harmonet *(Denm.; Swed.)*; Ogen *(Abbott, Austral.; Abbott, Canad.; Abbott, USA)*; Sultrex *(Arg.).*

9043-v

Ethinyloestradiol *(BAN).*

Aethinyloestradiolum; Ethinyl Estradiol *(USAN)*; Ethinylestradiol *(rINN)*; Ethinylestradiolum; Etinilestradiol. 17α-Ethynylestra-1,3,5(10)-triene-3,17β-diol; 19-Nor-17α-pregna-1,3,5(10)-trien-20-yne-3,17β-diol.
$C_{20}H_{24}O_2$=296.4.

CAS — 57-63-6.

Pharmacopoeias. In *Arg., Aust., Br., Braz., Chin., Cz., Egypt., Eur., Fr., Ger., Ind., Int., It., Jpn, Jug., Neth., Nord., Port., Roum., Rus., Swiss, Turk.,* and *U.S.* Also in *B.P. Vet.*

A white to slightly yellowish-white, odourless, crystalline powder. *B.P.* **solubilities** are: practically insoluble in water; soluble 1 in 6 of alcohol; freely soluble in ether; sparingly soluble in chloroform; soluble in dilute solutions of alkali hydroxides. *U.S.P.* solubilities are: insoluble in water; soluble in alcohol, chloroform, ether, vegetable oils, and solutions of fixed alkali hydroxides. **Store** in non-metallic airtight containers. Protect from light.

CAUTION. *Ethinyloestradiol is a powerful oestrogen. Contact with the skin or inhalation should be avoided. Rubber gloves and a face mask should be worn when handling the powder.*

Adverse Effects and Precautions
As for the oestrogens in general, p.1384.
See also under hormonal contraceptives, p.1387.

EFFECTS ON THE SKIN. A 15-year-old girl developed erythema multiforme, the Stevens-Johnson syndrome, after taking a preparation containing ethinyloestradiol and megestrol acetate for 14 weeks. She had also taken ferrous succinate and aspirin.— J. O. O'Callaghan and G. Jones, *Med. J. Aust.*, 1972, *1*, 695.

HYPERCALCAEMIA. Two patients with metastatic breast cancer given ethinyloestradiol rapidly developed irreversible and fatal hypercalcaemia considered to be due to stimulation of osteolysis by the oestrogen.— M. Cornbleet *et al.*, *Br. med. J.*, 1977, *1*, 145.

INTERACTIONS. *Antituberculous agents.* Rifampicin increased the rate of hydroxylation of ethinyloestradiol *in vitro* and this might account for the decreased effectiveness of oral contraceptives in patients also taking rifampicin.— H. M. Bolt *et al.* (letter), *Lancet*, 1974, *1*, 1280.

Vitamins. In 5 volunteers mean plasma-ethinyloestradiol concentrations were increased by 16.3 and 47.6% six and 24 hours respectively after the ingestion of ascorbic acid 1 g.— D. J. Back *et al.*, *Br. med. J.*, 1981, *282*, 1516. Breakthrough bleeding possibly associated with withdrawal of high doses of vitamin C.— J. C. Morris *et al.* (letter), *ibid.*, *283*, 503. Evidence that the overall effect of a large vitamin C supplement is to convert a low-oestrogen oral contraceptive into a high-dose oral contraceptive.— M. H. Briggs (letter), *ibid.*, 1547.

Absorption and Fate
Ethinyloestradiol is rapidly and well absorbed from the gastro-intestinal tract but is subject to some first-pass metabolism in the gut-wall. Compared to many other oestrogens it is only slowly metabolised in the liver. Excretion is via the kidney with some appearing also in the faeces.

Studies on the metabolism of ethinyloestradiol in the gut wall.— D. J. Back *et al.*, *Br. J. clin. Pharmac.*, 1982, *13*, 325.

Uses and Administration
Ethinyloestradiol is a semi-synthetic oestrogen with actions and uses similar to those described for the oestrogens in general (see p.1385).

Ethinyloestradiol is frequently used as the oestrogenic component of combined oral contraceptive preparations (see p.1391).

In menopausal and postmenopausal symptoms, doses of 10 to 50 µg daily are given by mouth, usually on a cyclical basis and in conjunction with an added progestogen for part of the cycle.

For the treatment of primary amenorrhoea, 50 µg has been given up to three times daily for 14 consecutive days in every 4 weeks, followed by a progestogen for the next 14 days; an alternative schedule is to start with low doses of ethinyloestradiol alone gradually increasing to up to 50 µg daily when a progestogen should be added for the last 5 days of the cycle.

For the palliative treatment of malignant neoplasms of the prostate and of the breast in postmenopausal women doses of about 0.1 to 2 mg have been given daily.

Ethinyloestradiol is also given in conjunction with norethisterone acetate for disorders of menstruation.

Ethinyloestradiol has also been used, like many other oestrogens, for the suppression of lactation.

For a general review covering the actions and uses of oestrogens, see p.1385.

ACNE. For the use of cyproterone acetate with ethinyloestradiol in patients with acne, see cyproterone acetate, p.1395.

Preparations
Ethinyl Estradiol Tablets *(U.S.P.).* Tablets containing ethinyloestradiol.
Ethinyloestradiol Tablets *(B.P.)*

Further preparations containing ethinyloestradiol are listed under ethynodiol diacetate (p.1399), norethisterone and norethisterone acetate (p.1405), and norgestrel and levonorgestrel (p.1407).

Proprietary preparations containing ethinyloestradiol are described under cyproterone acetate (p.1395) and under norethisterone acetate (p.1406).

Proprietary contraceptive preparations containing ethinyloestradiol are described under the section on hormonal contraceptives (p.1392)

Proprietary Names and Manufacturers
Duramen *(Switz.)*; Edrol *(Austral.)*; Estigyn *(Glaxo, Austral.)*; Estinyl *(Schering, Canad.; Scherag, S.Afr.; Schering, USA)*; Eticyclin forte *(Switz.)*; Etifollin *(Nyco, Norw.)*; Etivex *(Leo, Swed.)*; Farmacyrol forte *(Ger.)*; Feminone *(Upjohn, USA)*; Gynolett *(Ger.)*; Linoral *(Organon, Swed.)*; Lynoral *(Austral.; Belg.; Ger.; Neth.; Switz.; Organon, UK)*; Pabendrol *(Paines & Byrne, UK)*; Primogyn C *(Schering, Austral.)*; Progynon C *(Schering, Ger.; Spain; Schering, Switz.)*; Progynon M *(Ger.; Spain).*

The following names have been used for multi-ingredient preparations containing ethinyloestradiol—Adepal *(Wyeth-Byla, Fr.)*; AlfamesE *(Kade, Ger.)*; Amenorone *(Roussel, UK)*; Anacyclin *(Ciba, Ger.)*; Anoryol *(Desbergers, Canad.)*; Anovial *(Schering, Spain)*; Anovlar *(Schering, Austral.; Schering, Denm.; Fr.; Schering, Ital.)*; Anovlar 21 *(Schering, Arg.; Schering, Ger.; Schering, S.Afr. Switz.; Schering, UK)*; Anovlar mite *(Schering, Swed.)*; Binordiol *(Wyeth, Belg.; Wyeth, Denm.; Wyeth, Fin.; Wyeth, Ital.; Wyeth, Neth.; Wyeth, Switz.)*; Binovum *(Cilag, Ital.; Cilag, Switz.; Ortho-Cilag, UK)*; Biphasil *(Wyeth, Austral.; Wyeth, S.Afr.)*; Bivlar *(Schering, Ital.)*; Brevicon *(Syntex, Canad.; Syntex, Denm.; Astra-Syntex, Norw.; Syntex, USA)*; Brevinor *(Syntex, Austral.; Syntex, S.Afr.; Syntex, UK)*; Cilest *(Cilag, Ger.)*; Climatone *(Paines & Byrne, UK)*; Conceplan 21 Mite *(Grünenthal, Ger.)*; Conova 30 *(Searle, Belg.; Searle, Denm.; Searle, Neth.; Gold Cross, UK)*; Controvlar *(Schering, UK)*; Demulen *(Searle, Canad.;*

Searle, S.Afr.; Searle, UK; Searle, USA); Diane *(Schering, Ger.; Schering, Ital.; Schering, Switz.; Schering, UK)*; Dianette *(Schering, UK)*; Duoluton *(Schering, Arg.; Schering, Austral.)*;
Econ *(Farmos, Denm.; Laakefarmos, Fin.)*; Econ mite *(Farmos, Denm.)*; Ediwal *(Schering, Ger.)*; Egogyn 30 *(Schering, Ital.)*; Etalontin *(Parke, Davis, Ger.; Parke, Davis, Switz.)*; Eugynon *(Schering, Arg.; Schering, Austral.; Belg.; Schering, Denm.; Schering, Ger.; Schering, Ital.; Neth.; Schering, Norw.; Schering, S.Afr.; Schering, Spain; Schering, Switz.)*; Eugynon 30 *(Schering, UK)*; Eugynon 50 *(Schering, UK)*; Evanor-d *(Wyeth, Ital.)*; Evelea *(Elea, Arg.)*; Femovan *(Schering, Ger.)*; Femodene *(Schering, UK)*; Fironetta *(Schering, Denm.)*; Follimin *(KabiVitrum, Norw.; Kabi, Swed.)*; Follinett *(Kabi, Swed.)*; Fysionorm *(Nourypharma, Ger.)*; Fysioquens *(Aaciphar, Belg.; Organon, Denm.; Organon, Fin.; Nourypharma, Neth.)*; Gentrol *(Wyeth, Denm.)*; Gestrol *(Samil, Ital.)*; Gynatrol *(Wyeth, Denm.)*; Gynophase *(Schering, Fr.)*; Gynovlane *(Schering, Fr.)*; Gynovlar *(Schering, Arg.; Schering, Austral.; Denm.)*; Gynovlar 21 *(Neth.; Schering, S.Afr.; Switz.; Schering, UK)*; Levlen *(Berlex, USA)*; Lindiol 2.5 *(Organon, Arg.)*; Loestrin *(Parke, Davis, UK)*; Loestrin 1/20 *(Parke, Davis, USA)*; Loestrin 1.5/30 *(Parke, Davis, Canad.; Parke, Davis, USA)*; Loestrin Fe *(Parke, Davis, USA)*; Logest 1/50 *(Canad.)*; Logest 1.5/30 *(Canad.)*; Logynon *(Schering, UK)*; Logynon ED *(Schering, S.Afr.; Schering, UK)*; Lo/Ovral *(Wyeth, USA)*; Lyndiol *(Belg.; Organon, Denm.; Organon, Ger.; Neth.; Organon, Norw.; Organon, S.Afr.; Organon, Swed.; Organon, Switz.)*; Lyndiol E *(Ravasini, Ital.)*; Lyndiolett *(Organon, Fin.; Organon, Swed.)*; Lynratiopharm *(Ratiopharm, Ger.)*; Lyn-ratiopharm-Sequenz *(Ratiopharm, Ger.)*;
Marvelon *(Organon, Arg.; Organon, Belg.; Organon, Denm.; Organon, Fin.; Organon, Ger.; Organon, Neth.; Organon, Norw.; Organon, S.Afr.; Organon, Switz.; Organon, UK)*; Menolet Sublets *(Marshall's Pharmaceuticals, UK)*; Menopax *(Nicholas, UK)*; Menopax Forte *(Nicholas, UK)*; Mepilin *(Allen & Hanburys, Canad.; Duncan, Flockhart, UK)*; Mepogen *(Faulding, Austral.)*; Mercilon *(Organon, UK)*; Microdiol *(Organon, Spain)*; Microgyn *(Schering, Denm.)*; Microgynon *(Schering, Arg.; Schering, Austral.; Leiras, Fin.; Schering, Ger.; Schering, Ital.; Schering, Norw.; Schering, Spain)*; Microgynon 30 *(Schering, Belg.; Schering, Neth.; Schering, Switz.; Schering, UK)*; Microgynon 50 *(Schering, Belg.; Schering, Neth.; Schering, Switz.)*; Microgynon ED *(Schering, Austral.)*; Mikro Plan *(DAK, Denm.)*; Milli Anovlar *(Schering, Fr.)*; Minestrin 1/20 *(Parke, Davis, Canad.)*; Mini Pregnon *(Nourypharma, Neth.)*; Minidril *(Wyeth-Byla, Fr.)*; Minifol *(Samil, Ital.)*; Miniluteolas *(Serono, Ital.)*; Minilyn *(Organon, UK)*; Miniphase *(Schering, Fr.)*; Ministat *(Organon, Belg.; Ital.; Organon, Neth.)*; Minovlar *(Schering, Austral.; Schering, UK)*; Minovlar ED *(Schering, Austral.; Schering, S.Afr.; Schering, UK)*; Min-Ovral *(Wyeth, Canad.)*; Minulet *(Wyeth, UK)*; Mixogen Tablets *(Organon, Austral.; Organon, UK)*; Modicon *(Cilag, Austral.; Cilag, Neth.; Ortho Pharmaceutical, USA)*;
Neo Lyndiol *(Organon, Spain)*; Neo Norinyl *(Syntex-Latino, Spain)*; Neo Ovopausine *(Syntex-Latino, Spain)*; Neocon *(Cilag, Austral.; Cilag, Neth.)*; Neocon 1/35 *(Ortho-Cilag, UK)*; Neo-Eunomin *(Grünenthal, Ger.)*; Neogentrol *(Wyeth, Denm.)*; Neo-Gentrol *(Wyeth, Fin.)*; Neogynon *(Schering, Arg.; Schering, Austral.; Schering, Belg.; Schering, Denm.; Schering, Ger.; Schering, Neth.; Schering, Switz.)*; Neogynona *(Schering, Spain)*; Neo-Mens *(Neolab, Canad.)*; Neo-Primovlar *(Leiras, Fin.)*; Neorlest *(Parke, Davis, Ger.)*; Neo-Stediril *(Wyeth, Belg.; Wyeth, Ger.; Wyeth, Neth.; Wyeth, Switz.)*; Neovlar *(Swed.)*; Neovletta *(Schering, Swed.)*; Neovulen *(Searle, Denm.)*; Nonovulet *(Denm.)*; Noracyclin *(Ciba, Ger.)*; Nordette *(Wyeth, Arg.; Wyeth, Austral.; Wyeth, S.Afr.; Wyeth, USA)*; Nordiol *(Wyeth, Arg.; Wyeth, Austral.; Wyeth, S.Afr.)*; Norimin *(Syntex, UK)*; Norinyl 1+35 *(Syntex, USA)*; Norlestrin *(Parke, Davis, Arg.; Parke, Davis, Austral.; Spain; Parke, Davis, UK)*; Norlestrin 1/50 *(Parke, Davis, Canad.; Parke, Davis, USA)*; Norlestrin 2.5/50 *(Parke, Davis, Canad.; Parke, Davis, USA)*; Norlestrin Fe *(Parke, Davis, USA)*; Normapause *(Negma, Fr.)*; Normophasic *(Nourypharma, Switz.)*; Normovlar *(Schering, S.Afr.)*; Novogyn *(Schering, Ital.)*; Novostat *(Kabi, Spain)*; Orlest *(Parke, Davis, Austral.; Parke, Davis, Ger.; Parke, Davis, Switz.; Parke, Davis, UK)*; Ortho 0.5/35 *(Ortho, Canad.)*; Ortho 10/11 *(Ortho, Canad.)*; Ortho 1/35 *(Ortho, Canad.)*; Ortho 7/7/7 *(Ortho, Canad.)*; Orthonett Novum *(Cilag-Chemie, Denm.; Cilag, Swed.)*; Ortho-Novum 1/35 *(Cilag, Fr.; Ortho Pharmaceutical, USA)*; Ortho-Novum 7/7/7 *(Ortho Pharmaceutical, USA)*; Ortho-Novum 10/11 *(Ortho Pharmaceutical, USA)*; Ovamezzo *(CCD, Fr.)*; Ovanon *(Aaciphar, Belg.; Organon, Fr.; Nourypharma, Ger.; Nourypharma, Neth.; Ercopharm, Switz.)*; Ovanon-E *(Organon, S.Afr.)*; Ovanone *(Erco, Denm.; Erco, Swed.)*; Ovariostat *(Organon, Fr.)*; Ovcon *(Mead Johnson Pharmaceutical, USA)*; Ovidol *(Aaciphar, Belg.; Nourypharma, Neth.; Nourypharma, Switz.)*; Oviol *(Nourypharma, Ger.)*; Ovoplex *(Orfi, Spain)*; Ovoresta *(Organon, Ger.; Organon, Spain)*; Ovostat *(Organon, Belg.; Organon, Neth.; Organon, S.Afr.; Organon, Switz.)*; Ovostat micro *(Organon, Switz.)*; Ovral *(Wyeth, Arg.; Wyeth, Austral.; Wyeth, Canad.; Wyeth, S.Afr.; Wyeth, USA)*; Ovran *(Wyeth, UK)*; Ovran 30 *(Wyeth, UK)*; Ovranet *(Wyeth, Ital.)*; Ovranette *(Wyeth, UK)*; Ovulen 0.5/50 *(Searle, Austral.)*; Ovulen 1/50 *(Searle, Austral.)*; Ovulen 50 *(Searle, Belg.; Searle, Neth.; Searle, Switz.; Gold Cross, UK)*; Ovulen Novum *(Searle. Norw.)*; Ovysmen *(Cilag, Belg.; Cilag, Ger.; Cilag, Ital.; Cilag, Switz.; Ortho-Cilag, UK)*;
Paralut Tablets *(Wallace Mfg Chem., UK)*; Perikursal *(Wyeth, Ger.)*; Phasicon *(Organon, S.Afr.)*; Physiostat *(Organon, Fr.)*; Piloval *(Apothekernes Laboratorium, Norw.; A.L., Swed.)*; Planor *(Roussel, Fr.)*; Planum *(Menarini, Ital.)*; Plex-Hormone Tablets *(Consolidated Chemicals, UK)*; Practil *(Ravasini, Ital.)*; Pregnon *(Aaciphar, Belg.; Erco, Denm.; Nourypharma, Ger.; Nourypharma, Neth.)*; Primodos *(Schering, UK)*; Primovlar *(Swed.)*; Profinix *(Schering, Spain)*; Progylut *(Schering, Fr.)*; Prolorfin *(Orfi, Spain)*; Rélovis *(Substantia, Fr.)*; Regunon *(Schering, Swed.)*; Restovar *(Organon, Denm.; Organon, Fin.; Organon, Norw.; Organon, S.Afr.; Organon, Swed.)*; Schering PC4 *(Schering, UK)*; Sekvilar *(Leiras, Fin.)*; Sequilar *(Schering, Austral.; Schering, Belg.; Schering, Ger.; Schering, Neth.; Schering, Switz.)*; Sequilarum *(Schering, Denm.; Schering, Swed.)*; Serial 28 *(BDH Pharmaceuticals, UK)*; Sinovula *(Asche, Ger.)*; Stediril *(Wyeth, Belg.; Wyeth-Byla, Fr.; Wyeth, Ger.; Wyeth, Switz.)*; Stediril 30 *(Wyeth, Belg.; Wyeth, Ger.; Wyeth, Neth.; Wyeth, Switz.)*; Stediril-d *(Wyeth, Belg.; Wyeth, Ger.; Wyeth, Neth.; Wyeth, Switz.)*; Synfase *(Astra-Syntex, Swed.)*; Synphase *(Syntex, UK)*; Synphasec *(Grünenthal, Ger.)*; Synphasic *(Syntex, Austral.; Syntex, Canad.)*;
Tetragynon *(Schering, Switz.)*; Trentovlane *(Schering, Fr.)*; Triagynon *(Schering, Spain)*; Triciclor *(Orfi, Spain)*; Triella *(Cilag, Fr.)*; Trigynon *(Schering, Belg.; Schering, Ital.; Schering, Neth.)*; Trikvilar *(Leiras, Fin.)*; Tri-Levlen *(Berlex, USA)*; Trimone Sublets *(Marshall's Pharmaceuticals, UK)*; Trinordiol *(Wyeth, Arg.; Wyeth, Belg.; Wyeth, Denm.; Wyeth, Fin.; Wyeth-Byla, Fr.; Wyeth, Ger.; Wyeth, Ital.; Wyeth, Neth.; KabiVitrum, Norw.; Kabi, Swed.; Wyeth, Switz.; Wyeth, UK)*; Tri-Norinyl *(Syntex, USA)*; Tri-Novum *(Cilag, Ital.)*; Trinovum *(Cilag-Chemie, Denm.; Cilag, Ger.; Cilag, Ital.; Cilag, Neth.; Johnson & Johnson, S.Afr.; Cilag, Swed.; Cilag, Switz.; Ortho-Cilag, UK)*; Trionetta *(Schering, Norw.; Schering, Swed.)*; Triphasil *(Wyeth, Austral.; Wyeth, Canad.; Wyeth, S.Afr.; Wyeth, USA)*; Triquilar *(Schering, Arg.; Schering, Austral.; Schering, Denm.; Schering, Ger.; Schering, Switz.)*; Tristep *(Asche, Ger.)*; Varnoline *(Organon, Fr.)*; Volidan *(Duncan, Flockhart, UK)*; Yermonil *(Geigy, Ger.; Ciba, Switz.)*.

9044-g

Ethisterone *(BAN, rINN)*.
Anhydrohydroxyprogesterone; Ethinyltestosterone; Ethisteronum; Praegnin; Pregneninolone; Pregnin. 17β-Hydroxy-17α-pregn-4-en-20-yn-3-one.
$C_{21}H_{28}O_2$=312.5.

CAS — 434-03-7.

Pharmacopoeias. In *Aust., Br., Egypt., Eur., Fr., Int., It., Jug., Mex., Neth., Nord., Rus., Swiss,* and *Turk.*

A white or almost white, odourless or almost odourless, crystalline powder. Practically **insoluble** in water; slightly soluble in alcohol and chloroform. **Store** in well-closed containers and protect from light.

Adverse Effects and Precautions
As for the progestogens in general, p.1386.
Androgenic side-effects may predominate.

Uses and Administration
Ethisterone is a progestogen with actions and uses similar to those described for the progestogens in general (see p.1386) but it also has oestrogenic and androgenic properties and the latter may limit its usefulness. It was formerly given by mouth.

Proprietary Names and Manufacturers
Etherone *(Austral.)*; Gestone-Oral *(Paines & Byrne, UK)*.

The following names have been used for multi-ingredient preparations containing ethisterone—Amenorone *(Roussel, UK)*; Neo-Mens *(Neolab, Canad.)*; Paralut Tablets *(Wallace Mfg Chem., UK)*; Trimone Sublets *(Marshall's Pharmaceuticals, UK)*.

9045-q

Ethyloestrenol *(BAN)*.
Ethylestrenol *(USAN, rINN)*. 17α-Ethylestr-4-en-17β-ol; 19-Nor-17α-pregn-4-en-17β-ol.
$C_{20}H_{32}O$=288.5.

CAS — 965-90-2.

Pharmacopoeias. In *Br.* and *Ind.* Also in *B.P. Vet.*

A white or almost white odourless crystalline powder. Practically **insoluble** in water; soluble 1 in 9 of alcohol, 1 in 2 of chloroform, and 1 in 6 of ether. **Store** at a temperature not exceeding 15°. Protect from light.

Adverse Effects and Precautions
As for the androgens and anabolic steroids in general, p.1383. Ethyloestrenol is reported, however, to have little androgenic effect at doses normally used. High doses produce progestational effects and nausea, vomiting, fluid retention, and amenorrhoea may occur. Ethyloestrenol should be used with care in patients with liver disorders.

INTERACTIONS. For the effect of ethyloestrenol on phenindione, see p.347.

Uses and Administration
Ethyloestrenol has anabolic properties and also has slight progestational activity but has little androgenic activity at doses normally used.
It has been given in doses of 2 to 4 mg daily by mouth.

Preparations

Ethyloestrenol Tablets *(B.P.)*

Proprietary Names and Manufacturers
Maxibolin *(Organon, Canad.; Organon, USA)*; Orabolin *(Organon, Austral.; Belg.; Organon, S.Afr.; Organon, UK)*; Orgabolin *(Fr.; Ravasini, Ital.; Neth.; Swed.)*.

9046-p

Ethynodiol Diacetate *(BANM, USAN)*.

Etynodiol Diacetate *(pINNM)*; SC-11800. 19-Nor-17α-pregn-4-en-20-yne-3β,17β-diol diacetate.
$C_{24}H_{32}O_4$=384.5.

CAS — 1231-93-2 (ethynodiol); 297-76-7 (diacetate).

Pharmacopoeias. In *Br., Braz.,* and *U.S.*

A white or almost white, odourless, crystalline powder. Very slightly **soluble** in water; soluble 1 in 15 of alcohol, 1 in 1 of chloroform, and 1 in 3.5 of ether; sparingly soluble in fixed oils. **Store** in well-closed containers and protect from light.

Adverse Effects and Precautions
As for the progestogens in general, p.1386.
See also hormonal contraceptives, p.1387.

PREGNANCY AND THE NEONATE. *Effects on the foetus.* Foetal adrenal cytomegaly in a 17-week-old foetus associated with the maternal ingestion of an oral contraceptive containing ethynodiol diacetate 2 mg and mestranol 100 μg from the sixth to the fourteenth week of pregnancy.— G. S. Gau and M. J. Bennett (letter), *J. clin. Path.*, 1979, *32*, 305.

Absorption and Fate
Ethynodiol diacetate is readily absorbed from the gastro-intestinal tract and rapidly metabolised, largely to norethisterone.

The metabolites of ethynodiol diacetate in human plasma.— C. E. Cook *et al.*, *J. Pharmac. exp. Ther.*, 1973, *185*, 696.

Uses and Administration
Ethynodiol diacetate is a progestogen with actions and uses similar to those described for the progestogens in general (see p.1386).
It is used as the progestogenic component of combined oral contraceptives and also alone as a progestogen-only type of oral contraceptive (see p.1391).

Preparations

Ethynodiol Diacetate and Ethinyl Estradiol Tablets *(U.S.P.)*. Tablets containing ethynodiol diacetate and ethinyloestradiol.

Ethynodiol Diacetate and Mestranol Tablets *(U.S.P.)*

Proprietary contraceptive preparations containing ethynodiol diacetate are described under the section on hormonal contraceptives (p.1392).

Proprietary Names and Manufacturers

Femulen *(Searle, S.Afr.; Gold Cross, UK)*; Luteonorm *(Serono, Ital.)*; Lutométrodiol *(Searle, Fr.)*.

The following names have been used for multi-ingredient preparations containing ethynodiol diacetate—AlfamesE *(Kade, Ger.)*; Anoryol *(Desbergers, Canad.)*; Conova 30 *(Searle, Belg.; Searle, Denm.; Searle, Neth.; Gold Cross, UK)*; Demulen *(Searle, Canad.; Searle, S.Afr.; Searle, UK; Searle, USA)*; Etinodiene *(Farmila, Ital.)*; Metrulen *(Canad.; SPA, Ital.; Searle, UK)*; Metrulen M *(Searle, Spain; Searle, UK)*; Miniluteolas *(Serono, Ital.)*; Neovulen *(Searle, Denm.)*; Ovulen *(Searle, Arg.; Searle, Austral.; Searle, Ger.; Searle, S.Afr.; Searle, UK; Searle, USA)*; Ovulen 0.5 *(Searle, Austral.; Searle, Canad.; Searle, Switz.)*; Ovulen 0.5/50 *(Searle, Austral.)*; Ovulen 1/50 *(Searle, Austral.)*; Ovulen 1 *(Searle, Austral.; Searle, Belg.; Searle, Canad.; Searle, Switz.)*; Ovulen 50 *(Searle, Belg.; Searle, Neth.; Searle, Switz.; Gold Cross, UK)*; Ovulen Novum *(Searle, Norw.)*; Prandiol *(Ferran, Spain)*; Soluna *(Elea, Arg.)*.

9049-e

Fluoxymesterone *(BAN, USAN, rINN)*.

NSC-12165. 9α-Fluoro-11β,17β-dihydroxy-17α-methylandrost-4-en-3-one.

$C_{20}H_{29}FO_3$=336.4.

CAS — 76-43-7.

Pharmacopoeias. In *Br., Egypt.*, and *U.S.*

A white or creamy-white, odourless, crystalline powder. Practically **insoluble** in water; soluble 1 in 70 of alcohol and 1 in 200 of chloroform. **Store** in well-closed containers and protect from light.

Adverse Effects and Precautions

As for the androgens and anabolic steroids in general, p.1383.

Fluoxymesterone, given for prolonged periods, may cause jaundice and is contra-indicated in patients with liver disturbances.

Uses and Administration

Fluoxymesterone has androgenic properties. It is effective when given by mouth and is more potent than methyltestosterone.

In the treatment of male hypogonadism, fluoxymesterone is usually given in a dosage of 5 to 20 mg daily. In the palliation of inoperable neoplasms of the breast in postmenopausal women, it is given in daily doses of up to 40 mg, in divided doses.

Fluoxymesterone has been administered for its anabolic effect but less virilising anabolic agents such as methandienone are usually preferred.

Preparations

Fluoxymesterone Tablets *(B.P.)*

Fluoxymesterone Tablets *(U.S.P.)*

Proprietary Names and Manufacturers

Android-F *(Brown, USA)*; Halotestin *(Upjohn, Austral.; Upjohn, Canad.; Upjohn, Denm.; Upjohn, Fr.; Upjohn, Ital.; Upjohn, Neth.; Upjohn, Norw.; Upjohn, S.Afr.; Upjohn, Swed.; Upjohn, USA)*; Oralsterone *(Bouty, Ital.)*; Oratestin *(Hoechst, Canad.)*; Ora-Testryl *(Squibb, USA)*; Testoral *(Midy, Ital.)*; Ultandren *(Ciba, Ger.; Ciba, Norw.; Ciba, Switz.; Ciba, UK)*.

9050-b

Flutamide *(BAN, USAN, rINN)*.

Sch-13521. α′,α′,α′-Trifluoro-4′-nitroisobutyro-*m*-toluidide.

$C_{11}H_{11}F_3N_2O_3$=276.2.

CAS — 13311-84-7.

Adverse Effects and Precautions

As for cyproterone acetate, p.1395.

Absorption and Fate

Flutamide is reported to be rapidly and completely metabolised with the major metabolite also possessing active anti-androgenic properties. The half-life of both flutamide and the major metabolite is about 5 to 6 hours. Excretion is predominantly in the urine with only minor amounts appearing in the faeces.

Uses and Administration

Flutamide has anti-androgenic properties and is used in the palliative treatment of prostatic carcinoma. The usual dose by mouth is 250 mg three times daily.

For references to the use of flutamide in prostatic carcinoma, see under cyproterone acetate (p.1395).

Proprietary Names and Manufacturers

Euflex *(Schering, Canad.; Schering, USA)*; Eulexin *(Schering Corp., Denm.; Essex, Ital.; Scherag, S.Afr.; Essex, Spain)*; Flucinome *(Essex, Switz.)*; Fugerel *(Essex, Ger.)*.

9051-v

Formebolone *(BAN, rINN)*.

Formyldienolone. 11α,17β-Dihydroxy-17β-methyl-3-oxoandrosta-1,4-diene-2-carbaldehyde.

$C_{21}H_{28}O_4$=344.5.

CAS — 2454-11-7.

Formebolone has anabolic properties and has been given in doses of 5 to 10 mg daily by mouth. It has also been given by intramuscular injection.

Proprietary Names and Manufacturers

Esiclene *(LPB, Ital.)*; Hubernol *(Hubber, Spain)*.

9052-g

Fosfestrol *(BAN, rINN)*.

Diethylstilbestrol Diphosphate *(USAN)*; Phosphoestrolum; Stilboestrol Diphosphate. (*E*)-αα′-Diethylstilbene-4,4′-diol bis(dihydrogen phosphate); (*E*)-4,4′-(1,2-Diethylvinylene)bis(phenyl dihydrogen phosphate).

$C_{18}H_{22}O_8P_2$=428.3.

CAS — 522-40-7.

Pharmacopoeias. In *Ind.* and *U.S.*

An off-white odourless crystalline powder. Sparingly **soluble** in water; soluble in alcohol and dilute alkalis. **Store** at a temperature not exceeding 21° in airtight containers.

9053-q

Fosfestrol Sodium *(BANM, rINNM)*.

$C_{18}H_{18}Na_4O_8P_2$=516.2.

CAS — 23519-26-8 (xNa).

Pharmacopoeias. In *Br.*, which specifies xH_2O. In *Cz.* under the title Diaethylstilboestrolum Solubile.

A white or almost white powder. Fosfestrol 100 mg is approximately equivalent to 121 mg of fosfestrol sodium. Freely **soluble** in water; practically insoluble in dehydrated alcohol and ether. **Store** in well-closed containers and protect from light.

Adverse Effects and Precautions

As for the oestrogens in general, p.1384.

Nausea and vomiting are common side-effects but may be less troublesome than with equivalent doses of stilboestrol. Following intravenous injection there may be temporary local pain in the perineal and sacral regions and at the site of bony metastases. Injections should be given slowly, with the patient lying down.

Uses and Administration

Fosfestrol (stilboestrol diphosphate) is stated to require dephosphorylation before it is active. Fosfestrol and its sodium salt are used in the treatment of malignant neoplasms of the prostate.

Tablets and injections of fosfestrol sodium are available in varying strengths in different countries and in addition doses are expressed in varying ways, either as fosfestrol or as fosfestrol sodium (the tetrasodium salt). Tablets of fosfestrol are also used.

In terms of fosfestrol sodium, initial therapy for the first 5 days generally may range from 550 or 600 mg to 1.1 or 1.2 g daily by intravenous infusion. In terms of fosfestrol, these doses range from 460 or 500 mg to 920 mg or 1 g. Maintenance may be with up to half these doses given one to four times a week. Maintenance may also be with oral therapy, daily doses ranging from 100 to 600 mg of either fosfestrol or fosfestrol sodium.

For a general review covering the actions and uses of oestrogens, see p.1385.

Preparations

Diethylstilbestrol Diphosphate Injection *(U.S.P.)*. A sterile buffered solution of fosfestrol 45 to 55 mg per mL.

Proprietary Preparations

Honvan *(Boehringer Ingelheim, UK)*. *Tablets*, fosfestrol sodium 100 mg.

Injection, fosfestrol sodium 55.2 mg/mL, in ampoules of 5 mL.

Proprietary Names and Manufacturers of Fosfestrol and Fosfestrol Sodium

Fosfostilben *(Arg.)*; Honvan *(Bristol-Myers, Austral.; Belg.; Asta, Denm.; Asta Pharma, Ger.; Schering, Ital.; Neth.; Asta, Norw.; Noristan, S.Afr.; Funk, Spain; Asta-Werke, Swed.; Degussa, Switz.; Boehringer Ingelheim, UK)*; Honvol *(Horner, Canad.)*; ST-52 *(Lucien, Fr.)*; Stilphostrol *(Miles Pharmaceuticals, USA)*.

9054-p

Furazabol *(pINN)*.

Androfurazanol. 17α-Methyl-5α-androstano[2,3-*c*]-[1,2,5]oxadiazol-17β-ol.

$C_{20}H_{30}N_2O_2$=330.5.

CAS — 1239-29-8.

Furazabol has anabolic properties and has been given by mouth in doses of up to 3 mg daily and intramuscularly in doses of about 25 mg once or twice weekly.

Proprietary Names and Manufacturers

Miotolon *(Daiichi, Jpn)*.

18649-x

Gestodene *(BAN, USAN, rINN)*.

SH-B-331. 13β-Ethyl-17β-hydroxy-18,19-dinor-17α-pregna-4,15-dien-20-yn-3-one.

$C_{21}H_{26}O_2$=310.4.

CAS — 60282-87-3.

Adverse Effects and Precautions

As for the progestogens in general, p.1386.

Uses and Administration

Gestodene is a progestogen with actions and uses similar to those described for the progestogens in general (see p.1386).

It is used as the progestogenic component of combined oral contraceptive preparations (see p.1387).

Proprietary contraceptive preparations containing gestodene are described under the section on hormonal contraceptives (p.1392)

Proprietary Names and Manufacturers

The following names have been used for multi-ingredient preparations containing gestodene—Femodene *(Schering, UK)*; Femovan *(Schering, Ger.)*; Minulet *(Wyeth, UK)*.

12782-d

Gestrinone *(USAN, rINN)*.

A-46745; R-2323; RU-2323. 13β-Ethyl-17β-hydroxy-18,19-dinor-17α-pregna-4,9,11-trien-20-yn-3-one.

$C_{21}H_{24}O_2$=308.4.

CAS — 16320-04-0; 40542-65-2.

Gestrinone is a progestogen with actions and uses similar to those described for the progestogens in general (see p.1386). It is used in the treatment of endometriosis in doses of 2.5 mg twice weekly by mouth.

Beneficial results with gestrinone 2.5 mg twice weekly in asymptomatic endometriosis in a study reported to be the first double-blind, randomised, placebo-controlled trial of any treatment of endometriosis. Since the usual course of the disease was an unpredictable deterioration it was recommended that treatment should be given to all patients.— E. J. Thomas and I. D. Cooke, *Br. med. J.*, 1987, *294*, 272. See also: *idem*, 1117.

Proprietary Names and Manufacturers
Tridomose *(Roussel, S.Afr.)*.

9055-s

Gestronol Hexanoate *(BANM)*.

Gestonorone Caproate *(USAN, rINN)*; SH-582. 17α-Hydroxy-19-norpregn-4-ene-3,20-dione hexanoate.

$C_{26}H_{38}O_4$=414.6.

CAS — 1253-28-7.

Adverse Effects and Precautions

As for the progestogens in general, p.1386.

Local reactions have occurred at the site of injection.

Uses and Administration

Gestronol hexanoate is a long-acting progestogen with actions and uses similar to those described for the progestogens in general (see p.1386).

It is given in an oily solution by intramuscular injection in doses of 200 to 400 mg every 5 to 7 days for the adjunctive treatment of endometrial carcinoma.

It has also been tried in the management of benign prostatic hypertrophy in doses of 200 mg weekly.

PROSTATIC HYPERTROPHY. Gestronol hexanoate was considered to be of no value in the management of benign prostatic hypertrophy.— *Drug & Ther. Bull.*, 1973, *11*, 75.

Beneficial results with gestronol hexanoate in mild to moderate benign prostatic hypertrophy.— O. Yoshida and K. Okada, *Curr. ther. Res.*, 1984, *35*, 139.

Proprietary Preparations

Depostat *(Schering, UK)*. *Injection*, gestronol hexanoate 100 mg/mL, in ampoules of 2 mL.

Proprietary Names and Manufacturers

Depostat *(Belg.; Schering, Fr.; Schering, Ger.; Schering, Ital.; Neth.; Norw.; Schering, Spain; Swed.; Schering, Switz.; Schering, UK)*; Primostat *(Arg.; S.Afr.)*.

9056-w

Hexestrol *(rINN)*.

Dihydrostilboestrol; Hexanoestrol; Hexoestrol; Synestrol; Synoestrol. *meso*-4,4′-(1,2-Diethylethylene)diphenol.

$C_{18}H_{22}O_2$=270.4.

CAS — 5635-50-7; 84-16-2 (meso).

Pharmacopoeias. In *Aust.*, *Egypt.*, and *Rus.*
Roum. includes Hexestrol Diacetate ($C_{22}H_{26}O_4$=354.4).

Hexestrol is a synthetic non-steroidal oestrogen structurally related to stilboestrol (p.1413). It possesses the general properties typical of oestrogens (see p.1384) and was formerly administered by mouth and by intramuscular injection.

For a general review covering the actions and uses of oestrogens, see p.1385.

Proprietary Names and Manufacturers

Cycloestrol *(Belg.)*; Hormoestrol *(Siegfried, Switz.)*; Neoestrolo *(De Angeli, Ital.)*; Sintestrol *(Abello, Spain)*.

12833-a

Hydroxyestrone Diacetate

16α-Hydroxyoestrone Diacetate. 3,16α-Dihydroxyestra-1,3,5(10)-trien-17-one diacetate.

$C_{22}H_{26}O_5$=370.4.

CAS — 566-76-7 (hydroxyestrone); 1247-71-8 (diacetate).

Hydroxyestrone diacetate has oestrogenic properties similar to those described for the oestrogens in general (see p.1384). It has been used by mouth in usual doses of 200 to 300 μg daily in vulvo-vaginal disorders.

Proprietary Names and Manufacturers

Colpoginon *(Boizot, Spain)*; Colpogynon *(Laboratories de l'Hepatrol, Switz.)*; Colpormon *(Millet, Arg.; Anphar-Rolland, Fr.)*; Hormobion *(Boizot, Spain)*.

9057-e

Hydroxyprogesterone Hexanoate *(BANM)*.

17-AHPC; Hydroxyprogesterone Caproate *(USAN, rINN)*. 3,20-Dioxopregn-4-en-17α-yl hexanoate.

$C_{27}H_{40}O_4$=428.6.

CAS — 68-96-2 (hydroxyprogesterone); 630-56-8 (hexanoate).

Pharmacopoeias. In *Br.*, *Chin.*, *Cz.*, and *U.S.*

A white or creamy-white crystalline powder, odourless or with a slight odour. Practically **insoluble** in water; soluble 1 in 10 of alcohol, 1 in 0.4 of chloroform, and 1 in 10 of ether; soluble in fixed oils and esters. **Protect** from light.

Oily solutions for injection are **sterilised** by dry heat.

Adverse Effects and Precautions

As for the progestogens in general, p.1386.

Cholestatic jaundice may occur in previously sensitised patients. There may be local reactions at the site of injection.

PREGNANCY AND THE NEONATE. *Effects on the foetus.* Tetralogy of Fallot in an infant born to a mother who had received hydroxyprogesterone during pregnancy.— O. P. Heinonen *et al.*, *New Engl. J. Med.*, 1977, *296*, 67.

Genito-urinary abnormalities in 2 infants born to women given hydroxyprogesterone hexanoate in pregnancy.— A. N. W. Evans *et al.*, *Practitioner*, 1980, *224*, 315.

Adrenocortical carcinoma in the infant daughter of a women who received hydroxyprogesterone during the first trimester of the pregnancy.— J. R. Mann *et al.*, *Lancet*, 1983, *2*, 580.

For a report of congenital hypospadias in an infant born to a mother who had received hydroxyprogesterone hexanoate during the first trimester of pregnancy, see norethisterone, p.1406.

For a report of abnormalities of the genito-urinary tract in an infant whose mother had taken dydrogesterone and hydroxyprogesterone hexanoate during early pregnancy, see dydrogesterone, p.1397.

Uses and Administration

Hydroxyprogesterone hexanoate is a progestogen with actions and uses similar to those described for the progestogens in general (see p.1386). In habitual abortion suggested doses have been 250 to 500 mg weekly by intramuscular injection.

Preparations

Hydroxyprogesterone Caproate Injection *(U.S.P.)*. A sterile solution of hydroxyprogesterone hexanoate in a suitable fixed oil.

Hydroxyprogesterone Injection *(B.P.)*. A sterile solution of hydroxyprogesterone hexanoate in a suitable ester, a suitable fixed oil, or any mixture of these. For intramuscular injection only.

Proprietary Preparations

Proluton Depot (formerly known as Primolut Depot) *(Schering, UK)*. *Injection*, hydroxyprogesterone hexanoate 250 mg/mL, in ampoules of 1 and 2 mL.

Proprietary Names and Manufacturers

Delalutin *(Squibb, Canad.; Squibb, USA)*; Hyproval PA *(Reid-Provident, USA)*; Idrogestene *(Ital.)*; Lentogest *(Samil, Ital.)*; Luteocrin depot *(Ital.)*; Pergestron *(Spain)*; Primolut Depot *(Schering, UK)*; Primolut-Depot *(Schering AG, Norw.; Schering, S.Afr.)*; Prodrox *(Legere, USA)*; Proge Depot *(Jpn)*; Progestérone-Retard Pharlon *(Schering, Fr.)*; Proluton Depot *(Arg.; Schering, Austral.; Belg.; Denm.; Schering, Ger.; Schering, Ital.; Neth.; Schering, Spain; Schering, Swed.; Schering, Switz.; Schering, UK)*; Relutin *(USA)*; Retar-Gen P *(Arg.)*.

9059-y

Lynoestrenol *(BAN)*.

Linestrenol; Lynenol; Lynestrenol *(USAN, rINN)*. 19-Nor-17α-pregn-4-en-20-yn-17β-ol.

$C_{20}H_{28}O$=284.4.

CAS — 52-76-6.

Pharmacopoeias. In *Br.*, *Eur.*, *Ind.*, and *Jug.*

A white or almost white, odourless, crystalline powder. Practically **insoluble** in water; soluble 1 in 15 of alcohol and of dehydrated alcohol, 1 in 12 of acetone, 1 in 8 of chloroform, and 1 in 12 of ether. **Store** in well-closed containers and protect from light.

Adverse Effects and Precautions

As for the progestogens in general, p.1386.

See also contraceptives, p.1387.

EFFECTS ON THE LIVER. Reports of jaundice or liver damage associated with lynoestrenol: G. Cullberg *et al.*, *Br. med. J.*, 1965, *1*, 695; B. A. Stoll *et al.*, *ibid.*, 1966, *1*, 960; E. T. Heath and D. R. McTaggart, *Med. J. Aust.*, 1967, *2*, 352.

Absorption and Fate

Lynoestrenol is absorbed from the gastro-intestinal tract.

The pharmacokinetics of lynoestrenol.— M. Humpel *et al.*, *Contraception*, 1977, *16*, 199.

Uses and Administration

Lynoestrenol is a progestogen with actions and uses similar to those described for the progestogens in general (see p.1386). It is used as the progestogenic component of some combined oral contraceptives (see p.1391).

Proprietary contraceptive preparations containing lynoestrenol are described under the section on hormonal contraceptives (p.1392)

Proprietary Names and Manufacturers

Exlutena *(Organon, Swed.)*; Exluton *(Organon, Arg.; Organon, Belg.; Organon, Fin.; Organon, Fr.; Organon, Neth.; Organon, S.Afr.)*; Exlutona *(Organon, Denm.; Organon, Ger.; Organon, Norw.; Organon, Switz.)*; Minette *(Orion, Fin.)*; Orgametril *(Belg.; Organon, Denm.; Organon, Fr.; Organon, Ger.; Neth.; Organon, Spain; Organon, Swed.; Organon, Switz.)*.

The following names have been used for multi-ingredient preparations containing lynoestrenol—Anacyclin *(Ciba, Ger.)*; Anacycline 101 *(Ciba, Switz.)*; Fysionorm *(Nourypharma, Ger.)*; Fysioquens *(Aaciphar, Belg.; Organon, Denm.; Organon, Fin.; Nourypharma, Neth.)*; Gestrol *(Samil, Ital.)*; Lindiol 2.5 *(Organon, Arg.)*; Lyndiol *(Belg.; Organon, Denm.; Organon, Ger.; Neth.; Organon, Norw.; Organon, S.Afr.; Organon, Spain; Organon, Swed.; Organon, Switz.)*; Lyndiol E *(Ravasini, Ital.)*; Lyndiolett *(Organon, Fin.; Organon, Swed.)*; Lyn-ratiopharm *(Ratiopharm, Ger.)*; Lyn-ratiopharm-Sequenz *(Ratiopharm, Ger.)*; Mini Pregnon *(Nourypharma, Neth.)*; Minifol *(Samil, Ital.)*; Minilyn *(Organon, UK)*; Ministat *(Organon, Belg.; Ital.; Organon, Neth.)*; Neo Lyndiol *(Organon, Spain)*; Nonovulet *(Denm.)*; Noracyclin *(Ciba, Ger.)*; Noracycline *(Ciba, Switz.)*; Normophasic *(Nourypharma, Switz.)*; Novostat *(Kabi, Spain)*; Orgaluton *(Neth.)*; Ovamezzo *(CCD, Fr.)*; Ovanon *(Aaciphar, Belg.; Organon, Fr.; Nourypharma, Ger.; Nourypharma, Neth.; Ercopharm, Switz.; Organon, UK)*; Ovanon-E *(Organon, S.Afr.)*; Ovanone *(Erco, Denm.; Erco, Swed.)*; Ovariostat *(Organon, Fr.)*; Ovoresta *(Organon, Ger.)*; Ovoresta micro *(Organon, Spain)*; Ovostat *(Organon, Belg.; Organon, Neth.; Organon, S.Afr.; Organon, Switz.)*; Ovostat micro *(Organon, Switz.)*; Phasicon *(Organon, S.Afr.)*; Physiostat *(Organon, Fr.)*; Pregnon *(Aaciphar, Belg.; Erco, Denm.; Nourypharma, Ger.; Nourypharma, Neth.)*; Restovar *(Organon, Denm.; Organon, Fin.: Organon, Norw.; Organon, S.Afr.; Organon, Swed.)*; Yermonil *(Geigy, Ger.; Ciba, Switz.)*.

12915-x

Mebolazine *(rINN)*.

3,3′-Azinobis(2α,17α-dimethyl-5α-androstan-17β-ol).

$C_{42}H_{68}N_2O_2$=633.0.

CAS — 3625-07-8.

Mebolazine has been used as an anabolic agent.

Proprietary Names and Manufacturers

Roxilon *(Lepetit, Spain)*.

9061-q

Medrogestone *(BAN, USAN, rINN).*
AY-62022; Metrogestone. 6,17α-Dimethylpregna-4,6-diene-3,20-dione.
$C_{23}H_{32}O_2$=340.5.

CAS — 977-79-7.

Adverse Effects and Precautions
As for the progestogens in general, p.1386.

Uses and Administration
Medrogestone is a progestogen with actions and uses similar to those described for the progestogens in general (see p.1386). It has been given in usual doses of 5 to 10 mg daily by mouth.

Proprietary Names and Manufacturers
Colpro *(Ayerst, Belg.; Ayerst, Neth.; Ayerst, S.Afr.; Inibsa, Spain; Ayerst, Switz.)*; Colprone *(Ayerst, Canad.; Ayerst, Fr.; Ayerst, Ital.)*; Prothil *(Kali-Chemie, Ger.)*.

9062-p

Medroxyprogesterone Acetate *(BANM, USAN, rINNM).*

Methylacetoxyprogesterone; Metipregnone. 6α-Methyl-3,20-dioxopregn-4-en-17α-yl acetate.
$C_{24}H_{34}O_4$=386.5.

CAS — 520-85-4 (medroxyprogesterone); 71-58-9 (acetate).

Pharmacopoeias. In *Br., Braz., Chin., It., Roum.,* and *U.S.* Also in *B.P. Vet.*

A white, or off-white odourless, crystalline powder. Practically **insoluble** in water; soluble 1 in 800 of alcohol, 1 in 50 of acetone, 1 in 10 of chloroform, and 1 in 60 of dioxan; slightly soluble in methyl alcohol and ether. **Store** in airtight containers. Protect from light.

Adverse Effects and Precautions
As for the progestogens in general, p.1386. See also under hormonal contraceptives, p.1387.

Absorption and Fate
Medroxyprogesterone is absorbed from the gastro-intestinal tract. It is hydroxylated in the liver.

PREGNANCY AND THE NEONATE. In 7 lactating women given medroxyprogesterone acetate 150 mg the concentration of medroxyprogesterone acetate in breast milk was broadly comparable to that in plasma.— B. N. Saxena *et al., Contraception,* 1977, *16,* 605.

Uses and Administration
Medroxyprogesterone acetate is a synthetic progestogen with actions and uses similar to those of the progestogens in general (see p.1386). It is active when given by mouth and may also be given by intramuscular injection in aqueous suspensions for prolonged action.

It is used for the treatment of functional uterine bleeding and secondary amenorrhoea in doses of 2.5 to 10 mg daily by mouth for 5 to 10 days starting on the assumed or calculated 16th to 21st day of the cycle.

It is given by intramuscular injection in the treatment of endometriosis when 50 mg may be given weekly or 100 mg every 2 weeks for 6 months or more.

Medroxyprogesterone acetate may also be used by mouth or by intramuscular injection in the palliative treatment of some hormone-dependent malignant neoplasms. In breast carcinoma recommended doses have ranged from 0.4 to 1.5 g daily by mouth and from 0.5 g twice weekly to 1 g daily by intramuscular injection. In endometrial and renal carcinoma recommended doses have ranged from 100 to 500 mg daily by mouth and from 0.4 to 1 g weekly by intramuscular injection. In prostatic carcinoma recommended doses have been 100 to 500 mg daily by mouth and 0.5 g weekly or twice weekly by intramuscular injection.

Medroxyprogesterone acetate is also given by intramuscular injection as a 'progestogen-only' contraceptive (see under hormonal contraceptives, p.1391).

BLOOD DISORDERS. An assessment of the haematological and clinical effects of medroxyprogesterone acetate in a 2-year study completed by 23 patients with homozygous sickle-cell disease revealed that painful crises were significantly less frequent during treatment phases with medroxyprogesterone than during placebo phases. Medroxyprogesterone acetate was given intramuscularly in a dose of 150 mg every 3 months.— K. de Ceulaer *et al., Lancet,* 1982, *2,* 229.

ENDOMETRIOSIS. A report of the successful use of medroxyprogesterone acetate intramuscularly every 2 weeks for 6 months to alleviate symptoms of endometriosis associated with massive ascites; the combination of ascites with endometriosis is rare and surgery is usually necessary.— V. Naraynsingh *et al., Postgrad. med. J.,* 1985, *61,* 539.

EPILEPSY. Significant reduction in the frequency of seizures was observed in 7 of 11 women with uncontrolled partial or absence seizures following the addition of medroxyprogesterone acetate orally to their existing anti-epiletic medication. These preliminary findings suggested further evaluation of medroxyprogesterone acetate for catamenial seizures was warranted.— R. H. Mattson *et al., Neurology,* 1984, *34,* 1255.

HIRSUTISM. Medroxyprogesterone acetate 100 mg was given intramuscularly every 15 days for 110 to 405 days to 24 hirsute women. Obvious diminution of hirsutism occurred in 23 patients whose improvement was maintained by continuing treatment with medroxyprogesterone by mouth.— R. F. Corrêa de Oliveira *et al., Ann. intern. Med.,* 1975, *83,* 817.

In a pilot study involving 26 women with hirsutism given medroxyprogesterone acetate the best clinical result was obtained in those given 100 mg by subcutaneous injection every 6 weeks; intramuscular injection of 150 mg every 6 weeks was less successful and topical application of an 0.2% ointment twice daily was the least successful.— J. B. Schmidt *et al., Br. J. Derm.,* 1985, *113,* 161.

MALIGNANT NEOPLASMS. *Breast.* A review of endocrine therapy in advanced breast cancer. There has been less clinical experience with progestogens than with oestrogens or androgens. Most experience with progestogens has been with medroxyprogesterone acetate, usually in doses of 100 to 300 mg daily by mouth although a study using very large doses of 1.5 g intramuscularly daily has claimed to show a response-rate of over 40%. This has stimulated further interest in the use of progestogens.— R. Stuart-Harris, *Prescribers' J.,* 1984, *24,* 133.

Complete or partial remissions in 19 of 44 patients with metastatic breast disease given high doses of medroxyprogesterone acetate (1.5 g daily by intramuscular injection in 2 divided doses for up to 30 days).— F. Pannuti *et al., Cancer Treat. Rep.,* 1978, *62,* 499.

An objective response was obtained in 7 of 26 patients with metastatic breast cancer after treatment with high-dose oral medroxyprogesterone acetate therapy (2 g daily for 30 days followed by 1 g daily for 60 days). It was believed that the optimal daily dose may be between 0.6 and 1.2 g but a randomised clinical study was needed.— A. Guarnieri *et al., Chemioterapia,* 1984, *3,* 320.

Further references: D. Hedley *et al., Aust. N.Z. J. Med.,* 1984, *14,* 251; M. Izuo *et al., Cancer,* 1985, *56,* 2576; F. Pannuti *et al., Chemioterapia,* 1986, *5,* 159.

RESPIRATORY DISORDERS. The use of medroxyprogesterone in 2 children with alveolar hypoventilation syndrome.— J. Milerad *et al., Archs Dis. Childh.,* 1985, *60,* 150.

Preparations
Medroxyprogesterone Acetate Tablets *(U.S.P.)*
Sterile Medroxyprogesterone Acetate Suspension *(U.S.P.)*

Proprietary Preparations
Depo-Provera *(Upjohn, UK). Injection,* medroxyprogesterone acetate 50 mg/mL, in vials of 1, 3, and 5 mL. *Injection,* medroxyprogesterone acetate 150 mg/mL, in vials of 3 mL.

Farlutal *(Farmitalia Carlo Erba, UK). Tablets,* scored, medroxyprogesterone acetate 100, 250, and 500 mg. *Injection,* medroxyprogesterone acetate 200 mg/mL, in vials of 2.5 and 5 mL.

Provera *(Upjohn, UK). Tablets,* scored, medroxyprogesterone acetate 5, 100, 200, and 400 mg. *Suspension,* medroxyprogesterone acetate 400 mg/5 mL.

Proprietary contraceptive preparations containing medroxyprogesterone acetate are described under the section on hormonal contraceptives (p.1392)

Proprietary Names and Manufacturers
Amen *(Carnrick, USA)*; Climateran *(Wasserman, Spain)*; Clinovir *(Upjohn, Denm.; Upjohn, Ger.)*; Curretab *(Reid-Rowell, USA)*; Dépo-Prodasone *(Upjohn, Fr.)*; Depo-Clinovir *(Upjohn, Ger.)*; Depo-Progevera *(Upjohn, Spain)*; Depo-Provera *(Arg.; Upjohn, Austral.; Belg.; Upjohn, Canad.; Upjohn, Denm.; Upjohn, Fr.; Upjohn, Ital.; Neth.; Upjohn, Norw.; Upjohn, S.Afr.; Upjohn, Swed.; Upjohn, Switz.; Upjohn, UK; Upjohn, USA)*; Farlutal *(Austral.; Belg.; Farmitalia, Denm.; Farmitalia Carlo Erba, Fr.; Farmitalia, Ger.; Farmitalia, Ital.; Neth.; Farmitalia, Norw.; Farmitalia, Spain; Farmitalia Carlo Erba, Swed.; Farmitalia Carlo Erba, Switz.; Farmitalia Carlo Erba, UK)*; Farlutale *(Arg.)*; Gestapuran *(Lövens, Swed.)*; G-Farlutal *(Farmitalia, Ger.)*; Luteocrin orale *(Ital.)*; Luteodione *(Ital.)*; Luteos *(Biopharma, Ital.)*; Lutoral *(Midy, Ital.)*; Metilgestene *(Ital.)*; Perlutex *(Leo, Denm.; Leo, Norw.)*; Piermap *(Pierrel, Ital.)*; Prodafem *(Upjohn, Switz.)*; Prodasone *(Upjohn, Fr.)*; Progevera *(Upjohn, Spain)*; Provera *(Upjohn, Austral.; Belg.; Upjohn, Canad.; Upjohn, Ital.; Neth.; Upjohn, Norw.; Upjohn, S.Afr.; Upjohn, Swed.; Upjohn, Switz.; Upjohn, UK; Upjohn, USA)*.

The following names have been used for multi-ingredient preparations containing medroxyprogesterone acetate— Esprogyn *(Metro Med, USA)*.

9063-s

Megestrol Acetate *(BANM, USAN, pINNM).*

BDH-1298; SC-10363. 6-Methyl-3,20-dioxopregna-4,6-dien-17α-yl acetate.
$C_{24}H_{32}O_4$=384.5.

CAS — 3562-63-8 (megestrol); 595-33-5 (acetate).

Pharmacopoeias. In *Br., Chin., Ind.,* and *U.S.* Also in *B.P. Vet.*

An odourless, white to creamy-white, crystalline powder. Practically **insoluble** in water; soluble 1 in 55 of alcohol, 1 in 0.8 of chloroform, and 1 in 130 of ether; soluble in acetone; slightly soluble in fixed oils. **Protect** from light.

Adverse Effects and Precautions
As for the progestogens in general, p.1386.

Because the proportion of tumours in the breasts of beagle *dogs* was found to be increased by megestrol acetate, the manufacture of 'combined' and 'sequential' oral contraceptives containing it was discontinued in Great Britain in 1975.

For reports and comments on breast neoplasms in beagle dogs, see chlormadinone acetate, p.1394.

Irreversible insulin-dependent diabetes mellitus developed in a middle-aged woman 6 weeks after starting treatment with megestrol acetate 40 mg four times daily.— J. C. Bottino and C. K. Tashima (letter), *Ann. intern. Med.,* 1976, *84,* 341.

Severe pain of the hands occurred in 4 women while taking megestrol acetate and melphalan; megestrol appeared to be responsible.— P. J. DiSaia and C. P. Morrow, *Am. J. Obstet. Gynec.,* 1977, *129,* 460.

PORPHYRIA. Megestrol acetate was considered to be unsafe in patients with acute porphyria because it has been shown to be porphyrinogenic in *animals* or *in-vitro* systems.— M.R. Moore and K.E.L. McColl, *Porphyrias, Drug Lists,* Glasgow, Porphyria Research Unit, University of Glasgow, 1987.

Absorption and Fate
Megestrol acetate is absorbed from the gastro-intestinal tract. It is excreted mainly in the urine, but also in the faeces, in the form of the glucuronides of its metabolites.

Uses and Administration
Megestrol acetate is a progestogen with actions and uses similar to those of the progestogens in general (see p.1386).

It is active when given by mouth and is used in the palliative treatment or as an adjunct to other therapy in endometrial carcinoma in doses of 40 to 320 mg daily in divided doses continued for at least 2 months, and in doses of 40 mg four times a day in breast cancer.

MALIGNANT NEOPLASMS. *Endometrium.* Long-term effect of megestrol acetate in the treatment of endometrial hyperplasia.— D. Gal *et al.*, *Am. J. Obstet. Gynec.*, 1983, *146*, 316.

Preparations

Megestrol Acetate Tablets *(U.S.P.)*

Proprietary Preparations

Megace *(Bristol-Myers Pharmaceuticals, UK). Tablets*, scored, megestrol acetate 40 and 160 mg.

Proprietary Names and Manufacturers

Megace *(Bristol, Canad.; Bristol-Myers Pharmaceuticals, UK; Bristol-Myers Oncology, USA)*; Megestat *(Bristol, Ger.; Bristol, Switz.)*; Niagestin *(Novo, Denm.; Novo, Ger.; Novo, Neth.; Novo, Norw.; Novo, Swed.; Novo, Switz.)*; Niagestine *(Novo, Belg.; Novo, Switz.)*; Pallace *(Bristol, USA)*.

The following names have been used for multi-ingredient preparations containing megestrol acetate—Serial 28 *(BDH Pharmaceuticals, UK)*; Volidan *(Duncan, Flockhart, UK)*.

12930-t

Mepitiostane *(rINN)*.

S-10364. 17β-(1-Methoxycyclopentyloxy)-2α,3α-epithio-5α-androstane.

$C_{25}H_{40}O_2S$=404.7.

CAS — 21362-69-6.

Mepitiostane has been used by mouth in various breast disorders including neoplasms of the breast.

Proprietary Names and Manufacturers

Thioderon *(Shionogi, Jpn)*.

9064-w

Mesterolone *(BAN, USAN, rINN)*.

SH-723. 17β-Hydroxy-1α-methyl-5α-androstan-3-one.

$C_{20}H_{32}O_2$=304.5.

CAS — 1424-00-6.

Pharmacopoeias. In *Nord.*

Adverse Effects and Precautions

As for the androgens in general (p.1383).

It is reported not to inhibit gonadotrophin secretion or spermatogenesis.

Uses and Administration

Mesterolone has androgenic properties but is reported to have less inhibitory effect on intrinsic testicular function than testosterone.

Mesterolone is used in the treatment of hypogonadism in initial doses of 75 to 100 mg daily followed by doses of 50 to 75 mg daily for maintenance. Doses of 100 mg daily are used in male infertility due to oligospermia.

Reviews of the actions and uses of mesterolone: P. Bye, *Postgrad. med. J.*, 1975, *51*, 215.

Proprietary Preparations

Pro-viron *(Schering, UK). Tablets*, scored, mesterolone 25 mg.

Proprietary Names and Manufacturers

Mestoranum *(Schering, Denm.; Schering AG, Norw.; Schering, Swed.)*; Proviron *(Arg.; Schering, Austral.; Belg.; Schering, Fr.; Schering, Ger.; Schering, Ital.; Neth.; Schering, S.Afr.; Schering, Spain; Schering, Switz.; Schering, UK)*.

9065-e

Mestranol *(BAN, USAN, rINN)*.

Compound 33355; EE3ME; Ethinyloestradiol-3-methyl Ether; Mestranolum. 3-Methoxy-19-nor-17α-pregna-1,3,5(10)-trien-20-yn-17β-ol.

$C_{21}H_{26}O_2$=310.4.

CAS — 72-33-3.

Pharmacopoeias. In *Br., Braz., Cz., Eur., Ind., Jug., Swiss,* and *U.S.*

A white to creamy-white, odourless, crystalline powder. Practically **insoluble** in water; soluble 1 in 44 of alcohol, 1 in 23 of acetone and of ether, 1 in 4.5 of chloroform, and 1 in 12 of dioxan; slightly soluble in methyl alcohol. **Protect** from light.

CAUTION. *Mestranol is a powerful oestrogen. Contact with the skin or inhalation should be avoided. Rubber gloves and a face mask should be worn when handling the powder.*

Adverse Effects and Precautions

As for the oestrogens in general, p.1384.

See also under contraceptives, p.1387.

ALLERGY. A 23-year-old woman who had taken an oral contraceptive containing mestranol and norethynodrel for six months developed, 2 years later, transient acute polyneuritis affecting the feet and ankles 3 days after starting another oral contraceptive containing mestranol; this possibly represented allergic sensitisation to mestranol.— I. Eibschitz and B. Sharf (letter), *Br. med. J.*, 1974, *1*, 198.

PORPHYRIA. Mestranol was considered to be unsafe in patients with acute porphyria because it has been shown to be porphyrinogenic in *animals* or *in-vitro* systems.— M.R. Moore and K.E.L. McColl, *Porphyrias, Drug Lists*, Glasgow, Porphyria Research Unit, University of Glasgow, 1987.

Absorption and Fate

Mestranol is readily absorbed from the gastro-intestinal tract. Compared to many others oestrogens it is only slowly metabolised in the liver. Excretion is via the kidney. The biological half-life is about 50 hours.

Uses and Administration

Mestranol is a synthetic oestrogen with actions and uses similar to those described for the oestrogens in general (see p.1385).

Mestranol is often used as the oestrogenic component of combined oral contraceptive preparations (see p.1391).

Mestranol is also used for the treatment of menopausal and postmenopausal disorders, a combination product with norethisterone as the added progestogen often being employed (see under Proprietary Preparations, below).

For a general review covering the actions and uses of oestrogens, see p.1385.

Preparations

Preparations containing mestranol are listed under ethynodiol diacetate (p.1399) and norethisterone (p.1406)

Proprietary Preparations

Syntex Menophase *(Syntex, UK). Tablets*, 28-day pack; 5 tablets, mestranol 12.5 µg; 8 tablets, mestranol 25 µg; 2 tablets, mestranol 50 µg; 3 tablets, mestranol 25 µg, norethisterone 1 mg; 6 tablets, mestranol 30 µg, norethisterone 1.5 mg; 4 tablets, mestranol 20 µg, norethisterone 750 µg. For menopausal symptoms.

Proprietary contraceptive preparations containing mestranol are described under the section on hormonal contraceptives (p.1392)

Proprietary Names and Manufacturers

The following names have been used for multi-ingredient preparations containing mestranol—Anacycline 101 *(Ciba, Switz.)*; Conceplan 21 *(Grünenthal, Ger.)*; Conlumin *(Syntex, Denm.; Astra-Syntex, Fin.; Astra-Syntex, Swed.)*; Conovid *(Searle, UK)*; Conovid-E *(Searle, Austral.; Searle, S.Afr.; Searle, UK)*; Elan *(Valeas, Ital.)*; Enavid *(Searle, Neth.; Searle, UK)*; Enavid-E *(Searle, Arg.; Searle, Neth.; Searle, UK)*; Enovid 5 mg *(Searle, USA)*; Enovid-E *(Searle, Canad.; Searle, USA)*; Etinodiene *(Farmila, Ital.)*; Eunomin *(Grünenthal, Ger.)*; Kontrazeptivum 63-ratiopharm *(Ratiopharm, Ger.)*; Lyndiol *(Organon, Spain)*; Metrulen *(Canad.; SPA, Ital.; Searle, UK)*; Metrulen M *(Searle, Spain; Searle, UK)*; Noracycline *(Ciba, Switz.)*; Norinyl *(Spain; Syntex, USA)*; Norinyl 1/28 *(Syntex, S.Afr.; Syntex, UK)*; Norinyl 1/50 *(Syntex, Canad.)*; Norinyl 1/80 *(Syntex, Canad.)*; Norinyl 2 mg *(Syntex, USA)*; Norinyl 1+50 *(Syntex, USA)*; Norinyl 1+80 *(Syntex, USA)*; Norinyl-1 *(Syntex, Austral.; Syntex, S.Afr.; Syntex, UK)*; Norinyl-2 *(Syntex, Austral.; Syntex, Canad.; Syntex, UK)*; Novinol *(Desbergers, Canad.)*; Orgaluton *(Neth.)*; Orthonett *(Norw.)*; Ortho-Novin 1/50 *(Ortho-Cilag, UK)*; Ortho-Novin 2 mg *(S.Afr.)*; Ortho-Novum 0.5 mg *(Ortho, Canad.)*; Ortho-Novum 1/50 *(Cilag, Austral.; Cilag, Belg.; Ortho, Canad.; Cilag, Ger.; Cilag, Ital.; Cilag, Neth.; Cilag, Switz.; Ortho Pharmaceutical, USA)*; Ortho-Novum 1/80 *(Cilag, Austral.; Belg.; Ortho, Canad.; Cilag, Ger.; Cilag, Switz.; Ortho Pharmaceutical, USA)*; Ortho-Novum 2 mg *(Ortho, Canad.; Cilag, Ger.; Cilag, Ital.; Cilag, Switz.; Ortho Pharmaceutical USA)*; Ortho-Novum SQ *(Cilag, Belg.)*; Ovanon *(Organon, UK)*; Ovarion *(Fher, Spain)*; Ovulen *(Searle, Arg.; Searle, Ger.; Searle, S.Afr.; Searle, UK; Searle, USA)*; Ovulen 0.5 *(Searle, Austral.; Searle, Canad.; Searle, Switz.)*; Ovulen 1 *(Searle, Austral.; Searle, Belg.; Searle, Canad.; Searle, Switz.)*; Ovulen Novum *(Vita, Spain)*; Plan mite *(DAK, Denm.)*; Prandiol *(Ferran, Spain)*; Program *(Ortho, Canad.)*; Regovar *(Recordati, Ital.)*; Syntex Menophase *(Syntex, UK)*; Tridestan *(Galor, Arg.)*.

9066-l

Methallenoestril *(BAN)*.

Methallenestril *(rINN)*; Methallenoestrol. 3-(6-Methoxy-2-naphthyl)-2,2-dimethylpentanoic acid.

$C_{18}H_{22}O_3$=286.4.

CAS — 517-18-0.

Adverse Effects and Precautions

As for the oestrogens in general, p.1384.

Uses and Administration

Methallenoestril is a synthetic non-steroidal oestrogen with actions and uses similar to those described for the oestrogens in general (see p.1385).

Methallenoestril may be given by mouth for the treatment of menopausal and postmenopausal symptoms in a usual dosage of 6 mg daily.

Methallenoestril has also been used, like many other oestrogens, in metastatic prostatic carcinoma.

For a general review covering the actions and uses of oestrogens, see p.1385.

Proprietary Names and Manufacturers

Geklimon *(GEA, Denm.)*; Vallestril *(Searle, Austral.; Searle, Canad.; Searle, Denm.; Searle, Norw.; Searle, Switz.; Searle, UK)*.

9067-y

Methandienone *(BAN)*.

Metandienone *(pINN)*; Methandrostenolone. 17β-Hydroxy-17α-methylandrosta-1,4-dien-3-one.

$C_{20}H_{28}O_2$=300.4.

CAS — 72-63-9.

Pharmacopoeias. In *Cz., Hung., Ind., Jug.,* and *Rus.*

Adverse Effects and Precautions

As for the androgens and anabolic steroids in general, p.1383.

Methandienone, given for prolonged periods, may cause jaundice and is contra-indicated in patients with liver disturbances.

Methandienone may enhance the effects of coumarin and indanedione anticoagulants.

EFFECTS ON THE LIVER. Carcinoma of the liver occurring in a patient given methandienone.— F. L. Johnson *et al.*, *Lancet*, 1972, *2*, 1273.

A benign liver adenoma developed in one patient after taking methandienone for 3 years.— L. Hernandez-Nieto *et al.*, *Cancer*, 1977, *40*, 1761.

Uses and Administration

Methandienone has anabolic properties that are more pronounced than its androgenic effects. It has little progestational activity.

Methandienone has been given by mouth in doses ranging from about 5 mg daily to about 2.5 mg every second or third day.

Proprietary Names and Manufacturers

Andoredan *(Jpn)*; Danabol *(Canad.)*; Dianabol *(Austral.; Belg.; Denm.; Fr.; Ger.; Spain; Swed.; Switz.; Ciba, UK; USA)*; Encephan *(Jpn)*; Lanabolin *(Switz.)*; Metabolina *(Ital.)*; Metanabol *(Pol.)*; Metastenol *(Farber-Ref, Ital.)*; Nerobol *(Hung.)*; Perbolin *(Ital.)*.

The following names have been used for multi-ingredient preparations containing methandienone— Metaboline *(Desbergers, Canad.)*.

9068-j

Methandriol *(rINN).*
Methylandrostenediol. 17α-Methylandrost-5-ene-3β,17β-diol.
$C_{20}H_{32}O_2$=304.5.

CAS — 521-10-8.

Pharmacopoeias. In *Cz., Rus.,* and *Turk.*

Methandriol has anabolic and androgenic properties and has been given by mouth in doses of 50 to 150 mg daily.

Proprietary Names and Manufacturers
Sinesex *(Ital.)*; Stenediol *(Organon, UK)*; Troformone *(Biomedica Foscama, Ital.).*

9069-z

Methenolone Acetate *(BANM, USAN).*
Metenolone Acetate *(rINNM)*; SH-567; SQ-16496.
17β-Hydroxy-1-methyl-5α-androst-1-en-3-one acetate.
$C_{22}H_{32}O_3$=344.5.

CAS — 153-00-4 (methenolone); 434-05-9 (acetate).

Pharmacopoeias. In *Jpn.*

9070-p

Methenolone Enanthate *(BANM, USAN).*
Metenolone Enantate *(rINNM)*; Metenolone Enanthate; Methenolone Oenanthate; NSC-64967; SH-601; SQ-16374. 17β-Hydroxy-1-methyl-5α-androst-1-en-3-one heptanoate.
$C_{27}H_{42}O_3$=414.6.

CAS — 303-42-4.

Pharmacopoeias. In *Jpn.*

Adverse Effects and Precautions
As for the androgens and anabolic steroids in general, p.1383.

Uses and Administration
Methenolone has androgenic and anabolic properties. It has been given by mouth as the acetate in doses of up to 20 mg daily and intramuscularly as the enanthate in doses of 100 mg every 2 to 4 weeks.

Proprietary Names and Manufacturers of Methenolone and its Esters
Primobolan *(Schering, Austral.; Schering, Belg.; Schering, Denm.; Schering, Fr.; Schering, Ger.; Schering AG, Norw.; Schering, S.Afr.; Schering, Spain; Schering, Swed.; Schering, Switz.; Schering, UK)*; Primobolan Depot *(Schering, Austral.; Schering, Belg.; Schering, Denm.; Schering, Fr.; Schering, Ger.; Schering, Ital.; Schering AG, Norw.; Schering, S.Afr.; Schering, Spain; Schering, Switz.; Schering, UK)*; Primobolan S *(Schering, Neth.; Schering, S.Afr.; Schering, Switz.)*; Primonabol *(Schering, Arg.).*

9071-s

Methyltestosterone *(BAN, USAN, rINN).*

Methyltestosteronum. 17β-Hydroxy-17α-methylandrost-4-en-3-one.
$C_{20}H_{30}O_2$=302.5.

CAS — 58-18-4.

Pharmacopoeias. In *Aust., Br., Braz., Chin., Cz., Egypt., Eur., Fr., Ger., Int., It., Jpn, Jug., Mex., Neth., Nord., Pol., Roum., Rus., Span., Swiss, Turk.,* and *U.S.* Also in *B.P. Vet.*

A white or slightly yellowish-white, odourless, slightly hygroscopic, crystalline powder. Practically **insoluble** in water; soluble 1 in 5 of alcohol, 1 in 10 of acetone, and 1 in 160 of arachis oil; freely soluble in chloroform and dioxan; soluble in methyl alcohol; sparingly soluble in vegetable oils; slightly soluble in ether. **Protect** from light.

Adverse Effects and Precautions
As for the androgens and anabolic steroids in general, p.1383.
Methyltestosterone and other androgens or anabolic steroids with a 17α-alkyl substituent can produce a cholestatic hepatitis with jaundice especially when given in large doses or for prolonged periods. Methyltestosterone is contra-indicated in patients with liver disturbances.

EFFECTS ON THE LIVER. Peliosis hepatis developed in 7 patients on androgenic-anabolic steroid therapy, usually for bone-marrow stimulation, for periods of 2 to 27 months. Hepatic injury was a contributory cause of death in each case.— S. A. Bagheri *et al., Ann. intern. Med.,* 1974, *81,* 610.

Elevated serum-aspartate-aminotransferase (SGOT) concentrations were found in 19 of 60 patients (42 female transexuals and 18 impotent males) who had been taking methyltestosterone 50 mg three times daily by mouth for between 2 weeks and 5 years. Liver scans in 52 patients showed abnormalities in 33. Liver biopsies from 11 patients showed histological changes in each specimen; there was evidence of early peliosis hepatis. One patient had a liver adenoma and one additional patient, not in the survey, had rupture of the liver and peliosis hepatis. The hepatotoxicity appeared to be related to the duration of methyltestosterone use.— D. Westaby *et al., Lancet,* 1977, *2,* 261. Follow-up of some of these patients suggested that the liver damage was reversible.— C. P. Lowdell and I. M. Murray-Lyon, *Br. med. J.,* 1985, *291,* 637.

Neoplasms. Case reports of hepatocellular carcinoma associated with methyltestosterone.— J. T. Henderson *et al.* (letter), *Lancet,* 1973, *1,* 934; G. C. Farrell *et al., Lancet,* 1975, *1,* 430; M. A. Goodman and A. M. J. Laden, *Med. J. Aust.,* 1977, *1,* 220.

Reports of other liver tumours.— P. R. Boyd and G. J. Mark, *Cancer,* 1977, *40,* 1765; G. B. Coombes *et al., Br. J. Surg.,* 1978, *65,* 869.

INTERACTIONS. For the effect of methyltestosterone on some other drugs see under cyclosporin (p.616) and amitriptyline hydrochloride (p.353).

Absorption and Fate
Methyltestosterone is absorbed from the gastro-intestinal tract and from the oral mucosa. It is more resistant to metabolism than testosterone.

Maximum serum concentrations of methyltestosterone of 24 to 39 ng per mL were reached within 1 to 2 hours of administration of a 10-mg tablet to 2 volunteers. The biological half-life was about 2.7 hours.— D. Alkalay *et al., J. pharm. Sci.,* 1972, *61,* 1746. See also D. Alkalay *et al., J. clin. Pharmac.,* 1973, *13,* 142.

Uses and Administration
Methyltestosterone has androgenic and anabolic properties. It is effective when given by mouth; its effect is increased about 2-fold when given sublingually. When given by mouth it has one-third to one-quarter of the androgenic activity of the same weight of testosterone propionate administered intramuscularly.
Suggested doses of methyltestosterone for androgen replacement therapy in the male have been 10 to 50 mg daily orally or 5 to 25 mg daily buccally. Suggested doses for use in metastatic breast carcinoma in postmenopausal women have been 50 to 200 mg daily orally or 25 to 100 mg daily buccally.

Preparations
Methyltestosterone Capsules *(U.S.P.)*
Methyltestosterone Tablets *(U.S.P.)*

Proprietary Names and Manufacturers
Android *(Brown, USA)*; Glosso-Stérandryl *(Roussel, Fr.)*; Mesteron *(Pol.)*; Metandren *(Ciba, Canad.; Ciba, USA)*; Neo-Hombreol *(Belg.; Neth.)*; Neohombreol M *(Swed.; USA)*; Orchisterone *(Ital.)*; Oreton Methyl *(Schering, USA)*; Perandren *(Austral.; Ciba, UK)*; Primotest *(Arlo, USA)*; Testin *(Norw.)*; Testomet *(Protea, Austral.)*; Testoviron *(Arg.; Austral.; Ital.; Spain; Switz.)*; Testovis *(SIT, Ital.)*; Testred *(ICN, USA)*; Virilon *(Star, USA)*; Virormone-Oral *(Paines & Byrne, UK).*

The following names have been used for multi-ingredient preparations containing methyltestosterone—Climatone *(Paines & Byrne, UK)*; Eldec *(Parke, Davis, Austral.)*; Estratest *(Reid-Rowell, USA)*; Mediatric *(Ayerst, USA)*; Menolet Sublets *(Marshall's Pharmaceuticals, UK)*; Menopax Forte *(Nicholas, UK)*; Mepilin *(Allen & Hanburys, Canad.; Duncan, Flockhart, UK)*; Mepogen *(Faulding, Austral.)*; Mixogen Tablets *(Organon, Austral.; Organon, UK)*; Plex-Hormone Tablets *(Consolidated Chemicals, UK)*; Potensan Forte *(Medo, UK)*; Premarin with Methyltestosterone *(Ayerst, USA)*; Trimone Sublets *(Marshall's Pharmaceuticals, UK)*; Tylosterone *(Lilly, USA).*

12957-q

Mibolerone *(BAN, USAN, rINN).*
NSC-72260; U-10997. 17β-Hydroxy-7α,17α-dimethylestr-4-en-3-one.
$C_{20}H_{30}O_2$=302.5.

CAS — 3704-09-4.

Mibolerone is an anabolic and androgenic agent which has been used in veterinary practice as a contraceptive for bitches.

12981-q

Moxestrol *(rINN).*
R-2858. 11β-Methoxy-19-nor-17α-pregna-1,3,5(10)-trien-20-yne-3,17-diol.
$C_{21}H_{26}O_3$=326.4.

CAS — 34816-55-2.

Adverse Effects and Precautions
As for the oestrogens in general, p.1384.

Uses and Administration
Moxestrol is a synthetic oestrogen with actions and uses similar to those described for the oestrogens in general (see p.1385).
Moxestrol is reported to have a prolonged duration of action and suggested doses for the treatment of menopausal and postmenopausal symptoms are 50 to 100 μg weekly by mouth.

For a general review covering the actions and uses of oestrogens, see p.1385.

Proprietary Names and Manufacturers
Surestryl *(Roussel, Fr.).*

9072-w

Nandrolone Cyclohexylpropionate *(BANM, rINNM).*

3-Oxoestr-4-en-17β-yl 3-cyclohexylpropionate.
$C_{27}H_{40}O_3$=412.6.

CAS — 434-22-0 (nandrolone); 912-57-2 (cyclohexylpropionate).

9073-e

Nandrolone Decanoate *(BANM, USAN, rINNM).*

Nortestosterone Decylate. 3-Oxoestr-4-en-17β-yl decanoate.
$C_{28}H_{44}O_3$=428.7.

CAS — 360-70-3.

Pharmacopoeias. In *Br., Ind.,* and *U.S.*

A white to creamy-white crystalline powder, odourless or with a faint characteristic odour. Practically **insoluble** in water; soluble 1 in 1 of alcohol; freely soluble in chloroform, ether, fixed oils, and esters; soluble in acetone. The *B.P.* specifies **storage** at 2° to 10° in an atmosphere of

nitrogen. The *U.S.P.* specifies storage at 2° to 8° in airtight containers. Protect from light.
Oily solutions for injection are **sterilised** by dry heat.

12997-z

Nandrolone Hemisuccinate *(BANM, rINNM).*

3-Oxoestr-4-en-17β-yl hydrogen succinate.
$C_{22}H_{30}O_5$=374.5.

CAS — 6785-62-2.

12998-c

Nandrolone Laurate *(BANM, rINNM).*

Nandrolone Dodecanoate. 3-Oxoestr-4-en-17β-yl dodecanoate.
$C_{30}H_{48}O_3$=456.7.

CAS — 26490-31-3.

Pharmacopoeias. In *B.P. Vet.*

A white to creamy-white crystalline powder with a faint characteristic odour. Practically **insoluble** in water; soluble 1 in 1 of alcohol; freely soluble in chloroform, ether, fixed oils, and esters of fatty acids. **Store** at 2° to 8°. Protect from light.

9074-l

Nandrolone Phenylpropionate *(BANM, rINNM).*

19-Norandrostenolone Phenylpropionate; Nandrolone Phenpropionate *(USAN)*; Nortestosterone Phenylpropionate. 3-Oxoestr-4-en-17β-yl 3-phenylpropionate.
$C_{27}H_{34}O_3$=406.6.

CAS — 62-90-8.

Pharmacopoeias. In *Br., Chin., Cz., Ind., Jug.,* and *U.S.* Also in *B.P. Vet.*

A white to creamy-white crystalline powder with a slight characteristic odour. *B.P.* **solubilities** are: practically insoluble in water; soluble 1 in 20 of alcohol. *U.S.P.* solubilities are: practically insoluble in water; soluble 1 in 2 of alcohol; soluble in chloroform, dioxan, and vegetable oils. **Store** in airtight containers. Protect from light.
Oily solutions for injection are **sterilised** by dry heat.

Adverse Effects and Precautions

As for the androgens and anabolic steroids in general, p.1383.

Intrahepatic cholestasis in a patient after receiving nandrolone cyclohexylpropionate.— V. G. Gil *et al.* (letter), *Ann. intern. Med.,* 1986, *104,* 135.

Uses and Administration

Nandrolone has anabolic and androgenic properties.
It is administered usually as the decanoate or phenylpropionate esters in the form of oily intramuscular injections.
Suggested doses of nandrolone decanoate and phenylpropionate are generally the same but the decanoate ester has a longer duration of action being given generally every 2 or 3 weeks whilst the phenylpropionate is usually given each week. Doses of 25 to 50 mg have been used as an anabolic after debilitating illness and doses of 50 mg have been suggested for use in postmenopausal osteoporosis and postmenopausal metastatic breast carcinoma.
Doses of between 50 and 200 mg weekly have been suggested for nandrolone decanoate in the treatment of anaemias.
Nandrolone cyclohexylpropionate and nandrolone laurate have been used in veterinary medicine.

MALE CONTRACEPTION. Five healthy men were given intramuscular injections of nandrolone hexyloxyphenylpropionate 100 mg weekly for 3 weeks followed by 200 mg weekly for a further 10 weeks. Azoospermia occurred 7 to 13 weeks after initiation of treatment and persisted for 4 to 14 weeks after the last injection. No serious side-effects were noted and it was concluded that nandrolone is an interesting candidate for further evaluation as an agent for male fertility control T. Schürmeyer *et al., Lancet,* 1984, *1,* 417.

Preparations of Nandrolone and its Esters

Nandrolone Decanoate Injection *(B.P.).* A sterile solution of nandrolone decanoate in ethyl oleate or other suitable ester, in a suitable fixed oil, or in a mixture of these. For intramuscular use only.

Nandrolone Decanoate Injection *(U.S.P.).* A sterile solution of nandrolone decanoate in sesame oil.

Nandrolone Phenpropionate Injection *(U.S.P.).* A sterile solution of nandrolone phenylpropionate in a suitable oil.

Nandrolone Phenylpropionate Injection *(B.P.).* A sterile solution of nandrolone phenylpropionate in ethyl oleate or other suitable ester, in a suitable fixed oil, or in a mixture of these. For intramuscular injection only.

Proprietary Preparations of Nandrolone and its Esters

Deca-Durabolin *(Organon, UK). Injection,* nandrolone decanoate 25 or 50 mg/mL, in ampoules of 1 mL or in Orgaject disposable syringes of 1 mL.

Deca-Durabolin 100 *(Organon, UK). Injection,* nandrolone decanoate 100 mg/mL, in ampoules of 1 mL.

Durabolin *(Organon, UK). Injection,* nandrolone phenylpropionate 25 mg/mL, in ampoules of 1 mL and Orgaject disposable syringes of 1 mL.
Injection, nandrolone phenylpropionate 50 mg/mL, in Orgaject disposable syringes of 1 mL.

Proprietary Names and Manufacturers of Nandrolone and its Esters

Activin *(Aristegui, Spain)*; Anabolicus *(Spain)*; Anabolin Dépôt *(Amino, Switz.)*; Anabolin LA-100 *(USA)*; Anador *(Logeais, Fr.)*; Anadur *(Belg.; Denm.; Pharmacia Arzneimittel, Ger.; Neth.; Mekos, Norw.; Leo, Swed.; Leo Suede, Switz.)*; Androlone *(Keene, USA)*; Androlone-D *(Keene, USA)*; Anticatabolin *(Nativelle, Ital.)*; Deca-Durabol *(Organon, Swed.)*; Deca-Durabolin *(Arg.; Organon, Austral.; Belg.; Organon, Canad.; Organon, Denm.; Organon, Fr.; Organon, Ger.; Ravasini, Ital.; Neth.; Organon, Norw.; Organon, S.Afr.; Organon, Switz.; Organon, UK; Organon, USA)*; Decadurabolin *(Organon, Spain)*; Durabolin *(Organon, Austral.; Belg.; Organon, Canad.; Organon, Denm.; Organon, Fr.; Ravasini, Ital.; Neth.; Organon, S.Afr.; Organon, Spain; Organon, Switz.; Organon, UK; Organon, USA)*; Dynabolon *(Théramex, Fr.; Crinos, Ital.)*; Fherbolico *(Fher, Spain)*; Hybolin Decanoate *(Hyrex, USA)*; Hybolin Improved *(Hyrex, USA)*; Kabolin *(Legere, USA)*; Kératyl *(Chauvin-Blache, Fr.)*; Menidrabol *(Menarini, Ital.)*; Methybol-Depot *(Switz.)*; Nandrolin *(Reid-Provident, USA)*; Neo-Durabolic *(Hauck, USA)*; Norandrol *(Ital.)*; Norandros *(Spain)*; Nortesto *(Ital.)*; Sintabolin *(Ital.)*; Stenabolin *(AFI, Ital.)*; Strabolene *(Isola-Ibi, Ital.)*; Superbolin *(Ital.)*.

3147-e

Nomegestrol Acetate *(rINNM).*

17-Hydroxy-6-methyl-19-norpregna-4,6-diene-3,20-dione acetate.
$C_{23}H_{30}O_4$=370.5.

CAS — 58691-88-6 (nomegestrol).

Adverse Effects and Precautions

As for the progestogens in general, p.1386.

Uses and Administration

Nomegestrol acetate is a progestogen with actions and uses similar to those described for the progestogens in general (see p.1386). It has been given in doses of 5 mg by mouth.

Proprietary Names and Manufacturers

Lutenyl *(Théramex, Fr.)*.

13030-j

Norclostebol Acetate *(rINNM).*

4-Chloro-3-oxoestr-4-en-17β-yl acetate.
$C_{20}H_{27}ClO_3$=350.9.

CAS — 13583-21-6 (norclostebol).

Norclostebol acetate has been used by intramuscular injection as an anabolic agent.

Proprietary Names and Manufacturers

Anabol 4-19 *(Piam, Ital.)*.

9075-y

Norethandrolone *(BAN, rINN).*

17β-Hydroxy-19-nor-17α-pregn-4-en-3-one.
$C_{20}H_{30}O_2$=302.5.

CAS — 52-78-8.

Pharmacopoeias. In *It.*

Adverse Effects

As for the androgens and anabolic steroids in general, p.1383.
Because of the progestational activity of norethandrolone, amenorrhoea and uterine bleeding may result when treatment is stopped. Jaundice may develop occasionally.

A 74-year-old man was given norethandrolone 30 mg daily for 6 months. He died in hepatic coma after severe alterations of liver function which autopsy showed to be due to intrahepatic cholestasis.— E. F. Gilbert *et al., J. Am. med. Ass.,* 1963, *185,* 538.

Precautions

As for the androgens and anabolic steroids in general, p.1383.
Norethandrolone should be used with caution in patients with impaired liver function.
It may enhance the effects of anticoagulants of the coumarin type.

Uses and Administration

Norethandrolone has anabolic and androgenic properties and also has moderate progestational activity.
Norethandrolone has been given by mouth in a dose of 10 to 30 mg daily.

Proprietary Names and Manufacturers

Nilevar *(Canad.; Searle, Fr.; Searle, UK)*.

9078-c

Norethisterone *(BAN, pINN).*

Ethinylnortestosterone; Norethindrone *(USAN)*; Norethisteronum; Noretisterone; Norpregneninolone. 17β-Hydroxy-19-nor-17α-pregn-4-en-20-yn-3-one.
$C_{20}H_{26}O_2$=298.4.

CAS — 68-22-4.

Pharmacopoeias. In *Br., Braz., Chin., Cz., Eur., It., Jpn, Swiss, Turk.,* and *U.S.*

A white or yellowish-white odourless crystalline powder. Practically **insoluble** in water; slightly to sparingly soluble in alcohol; soluble 1 in 30 of chloroform; soluble in dioxan; slightly soluble in ether. **Protect** from light.

9077-z

Norethisterone Acetate *(BANM, pINNM).*

Norethindrone Acetate *(USAN)*. 17β-Hydroxy-19-nor-17α-pregn-4-en-20-yn-3-one acetate.
$C_{22}H_{28}O_3$=340.5.

CAS — 51-98-9.

Pharmacopoeias. In *Br., Int., Jug.,* and *U.S.*

A white or creamy-white, odourless, crystalline powder. Practically **insoluble** in water; soluble 1 in 10 to 12.5 of alcohol, 1 in 4 of acetone, 1 in less than 1 of chloroform, 1 in 2 of dioxan, and 1 in 18 of ether. **Protect** from light.

9076-j

Norethisterone Enanthate *(BANM).*

Norethisterone Enantate *(pINNM)*; Norethisterone Heptanoate. 17β-Hydroxy-19-nor-17α-pregn-4-en-20-yn-3-one heptanoate.
$C_{27}H_{38}O_3$=410.6.

CAS — 3836-23-5.

Adverse Effects and Precautions

As for the progestogens in general, p.1386.
See also hormonal contraceptives, p.1387.

EFFECTS ON THE LIVER. There were 6 cases of jaundice among 107 patients with breast cancer treated with norethisterone acetate. The jaundice which was of an obstructive type was reversible when norethisterone was withdrawn.— A. O. Langlands and W. M. C. Martin (letter), *Lancet*, 1975, *1*, 584.

PREGNANCY AND THE NEONATE. The use of hormonal pregnancy tests appeared to be the only significant difference in drug treatment during pregnancy in women who gave birth to infants with meningomyelocele or hydrocephalus and those who gave birth to normal infants. Hormonal pregnancy tests, which usually contained either norethisterone acetate 10 mg and ethinyloestradiol 20 µg (Primodos) or ethisterone 50 mg and ethinyloestradiol 50 µg (Amenorone Forte), were taken by 19% of the mothers who gave birth to infants with congenital malformation and by 4% of those who gave birth to healthy infants.— I. Gal *et al.* (letter), *Nature*, 1967, *216*, 83.

Ectopic pregnancy. There were 4 ectopic pregnancies in 3 years in women using low-dose progestogen oral contraceptives (norethisterone 300 µg) for an estimated 1000 woman-years.— P. Liukko and R. Erkkola (letter), *Br. med. J.*, 1976, *2*, 1257. Further reports: J. Bonnar (letter), *Lancet*, 1974, *1*, 170; *idem* (letter), *Br. med. J.*, 1974, *1*, 287; K. M. Huntington (letter), *Lancet*, 1974, *1*, 360; R. Corcoran and R. Howard (letter), *Lancet*, 1977, *1*, 98.

Effects on the foetus. Thirty-five pregnant women, given norethisterone usually in doses of 10 to 40 mg daily to prevent threatened abortion, gave birth to female infants showing masculinisation as also did 1 woman who received norethynodrel. Similarly, an examination of paediatric records and other sources showed that ethisterone had, though less frequently and severely, also been associated with masculinisation of female infants born to mothers given it to avert abortion.— L. Wilkins, *J. Am. med. Ass.*, 1960, *172*, 1028.

Of 80 infants with congenital hypospadias 5 were born to mothers who had taken progestogens during the first trimester of pregnancy. A causal relationship was suspected. Two had received medroxyprogesterone and hydroxyprogesterone hexanoate respectively for threatened abortion, and 3 had received progestogens as pregnancy tests—norethisterone, norethisterone and ethinyloestradiol, and probably either norethisterone or medroxyprogesterone respectively.— D. Aarskog, *Acta paediat. scand.*, 1970, *Suppl.*, 203.

Absorption and Fate

Norethisterone is absorbed from the gastro-intestinal tract and its effects last for at least 24 hours. When injected, it is detectable in the plasma after 2 days and is not completely excreted in the urine after 5 days.

The pharmacokinetics of norethisterone and norethisterone acetate.— D. J. Back *et al.*, *Br. J. clin. Pharmac.*, 1977, *4*, 729P. See also D. J. Back *et al.*, *Clin. Pharmac. Ther.*, 1978, *24*, 439 and 448.

PREGNANCY AND THE NEONATE. In 5 lactating women taking norethisterone 350 µg daily the concentration of norethisterone in breast milk was about one-tenth of that in plasma.— B. N. Saxena *et al.*, *Contraception*, 1977, *16*, 605.

Uses and Administration

Norethisterone, norethisterone acetate, and norethisterone enanthate are progestogens with actions and uses similar to those of the progestogens in general (see p.1386). They also have weak oestrogenic and androgenic properties.

Norethisterone and norethisterone acetate may be used for the treatment of conditions such as abnormal uterine bleeding and endometriosis. In abnormal uterine bleeding, norethisterone is given in doses of 5 to 20 mg daily for 10 days and norethisterone acetate in doses of 2.5 to 10 mg daily. In endometriosis the dosage of norethisterone is 10 to 30 mg daily and of norethisterone acetate 5 to 15 mg daily.

Norethisterone and norethisterone acetate are both used as the progestogenic component of combined oral contraceptives (see p.1391). Norethisterone is also used as a progestogen-only type of oral contraceptive (see p.1391) and norethisterone enanthate is used as a long-acting injectable contraceptive (see p.1391).

In metastatic breast cancer doses of up to 60 mg daily of either norethisterone or norethisterone acetate have been suggested.

Norethisterone is also used as the added progestogen to oestrogenic therapy in menopausal disorders.

Preparations

Norethindrone Tablets *(U.S.P.)*. Tablets containing norethisterone.

Norethisterone Tablets *(B.P.)*

Norethindrone and Ethinyl Estradiol Tablets *(U.S.P.)*. Tablets containing norethisterone and ethinyloestradiol.

Norethindrone and Mestranol Tablets *(U.S.P.)*. Tablets containing norethisterone and mestranol.

Norethindrone Acetate Tablets *(U.S.P.)*. Tablets containing norethisterone acetate.

Norethindrone Acetate and Ethinyl Estradiol Tablets *(U.S.P.)*. Tablets containing norethisterone acetate and ethinyloestradiol.

Proprietary Preparations

Controvlar *(Schering, UK)*. *Tablets*, 21-day calendar pack, norethisterone acetate 3 mg, ethinyloestradiol 50 µg. For menstrual disorders.

Primolut N *(Schering, UK)*. *Tablets*, norethisterone 5 mg.

SH420 *(Schering, UK)*. *Tablets*, scored, norethisterone acetate 10 mg.

Utovlan *(Syntex, UK)*. *Tablets*, scored, norethisterone 5 mg.

Further proprietary preparations containing norethisterone are described under mestranol (p.1403) and containing norethisterone acetate under oestriol (p.1409).

Proprietary contraceptive preparations containing norethisterone, norethisterone acetate, or norethisterone enanthate, are described under the section on hormonal contraceptives (p.1392).

Proprietary Names and Manufacturers of Norethisterone and its Esters

Aygestin *(Ayerst, USA)*; Conludag *(Astra-Syntex, Norw.)*; Gesta Plan *(DAK, Denm.)*; Micronor *(Cilag, Austral.; Ortho, Canad.; Ortho-Cilag, UK; Ortho Pharmaceutical, USA)*; Micronovum *(Cilag, Ger.; Johnson & Johnson, S.Afr.; Cilag, Switz.)*; Milligynon *(Schering, Fr.)*; Mini-Pe *(Syntex, Denm.; Astra-Syntex, Swed.)*; Mini-Pill *(Astra-Syntex, Fin.)*; Norfor *(Smith Kline & French, Fr.)*; Norgestin *(Janus, Ital.)*; Noriday *(Syntex, Austral.; Syntex, S.Afr.; Syntex, UK)*; Noristerat *(Schering, Denm.; Schering, Fr.; Schering, Ger.; Schering, UK)*; Norlutate *(Parke, Davis, Canad.; Parke, Davis, USA)*; Norluten *(Smith Kline & French, Fr.)*; Norlutin *(Canad.; Parke, Davis, USA)*; Norlutin-A *(Parke, Davis, UK)*; Nor-QD *(Syntex, USA)*; Nur-Isterate *(Schering, S.Afr.)*; Primolut *(Schering, Denm.)*; Primolut N *(Schering, Austral.; Neth.; Schering AG, Norw.; Schering, S.Afr.; Schering, Switz.; Schering, UK)*; Primolut Nor *(Arg.; Schering, Austral.; Belg.; Schering, Fr.; Schering, Ger.; Schering, Ital.; Schering, Spain; Schering, Swed.; Schering, Switz.)*; Proluteasi *(Ital.)*; SH420 *(Schering, Austral.; Schering, S.Afr.; Schering, UK)*; Utovlan *(Syntex, UK)*.

The following names have been used for multi-ingredient preparations containing norethisterone and its esters—Anovial *(Schering, Spain)*; Anovlar *(Schering, Austral.; Schering, Denm.; Fr.; Schering, Ital.)*; Anovlar 21 *(Schering, Arg.; Schering, Ger.; Schering, S.Afr.; Switz.; Schering, UK)*; Anovlar mite *(Schering, Swed.)*; Binovum *(Cilag, Ital; Cilag, Switz.; Ortho-Cilag, UK)*; Brevicon *(Syntex, Canad.; Syntex, Denm.; Astra-Syntex, Norw.; Syntex, USA)*; Brevinor *(Syntex, Austral.; Syntex, S.Afr.; Syntex, UK)*; Conceplan 21 *(Grünenthal, Ger.)*; Conceplan 21 Mite *(Grünenthal, Ger.)*; Conlumin *(Syntex, Denm.; Astra-Syntex, Fin.; Astra-Syntex, Swed.)*; Controvlar *(Schering, UK)*; Econ *(Farmos, Denm.; Laakefarmos, Fin.)*; Econ mite *(Farmos, Fin.)*; Estrapak 50 *(Ciba, UK)*; Etalontin *(Parke, Davis, Ger.; Parke, Davis, Switz.)*; Gynophase *(Schering, Fr.)*; Gynovlane *(Schering, Fr.)*; Gynovlar *(Schering, Arg.; Schering, Austral.; Denm.)*; Gynovlar 21 *(Neth.; Schering, S.Afr.; Switz.; Schering, UK)*; Loestrin *(Parke, Davis, UK)*; Loestrin 1/20 *(Parke, Davis, USA)*; Loestrin 1.5/30 *(Parke, Davis, Canad.; Parke, Davis, USA)*; Loestrin Fe *(Parke, Davis, USA)*; Logest 1/50 *(Canad.)*; Logest 1.5/30 *(Canad.)*; Mikro Plan *(DAK, Denm.)*; Milli Anovlar *(Schering, Fr.)*; Minestrin 1/20 *(Parke, Davis, Canad.)*; Miniphase *(Schering, Fr.)*; Minovlar *(Schering, Austral.; Schering, UK)*; Minovlar ED *(Schering, Austral.; Schering, S.Afr.; Schering, UK)*; Modicon *(Cilag, Austral.; Cilag, Neth.; Ortho Pharmaceutical, USA)*; Neo Norinyl *(Syntex-Latino, Spain)*; Neo Ovopausine *(Syntex-Latino, Spain)*; Neocon *(Cilag, Austral.; Cilag, Neth.)*; Neocon 1/35 *(Ortho-Cilag, UK)*; Neorlest *(Parke, Davis, Ger.)*; Norimin *(Syntex, UK)*; Norinyl *(Spain; Syntex, USA)*; Norinyl 1+35 *(Syntex, USA)*; Norinyl 1/28 *(Syntex, S.Afr.; Syntex, UK)*; Norinyl 1/50 *(Syntex, Canad.)*; Norinyl 1+50 *(Syntex, USA)*; Norinyl 1/80 *(Syntex, Canad.)*; Norinyl 1+80 *(Syntex, USA)*; Norinyl 2 mg *(Syntex, USA)*; Norinyl-1 *(Syntex, Austral.; Syntex, S.Afr.; Syntex, UK)*; Norinyl-2 *(Syntex, Austral.; Syntex, Canad.; Syntex, UK)*; Norlestrin *(Parke, Davis, Arg.; Parke, Davis, Austral.; Spain; Parke, Davis, UK)*; Norlestrin 1/50 *(Parke, Davis, Canad.; Parke, Davis, USA)*; Norlestrin 2.5/50 *(Parke, Davis, Canad.; Parke, Davis, USA)*; Norlestrin Fe *(Parke, Davis, USA)*; Normapause *(Negma, Fr.)*;

Orlest *(Parke, Davis, Austral.; Parke, Davis, Ger.; Parke, Davis, Switz.; Parke, Davis, UK)*; Ortho 0.5/35 *(Ortho, Canad.)*; Ortho 10/11 *(Ortho, Canad.)*; Ortho 1/35 *(Ortho, Canad.)*; Ortho 7/7/7 *(Ortho, Canad.)*; Orthonett Novum *(Cilag-Chemie, Denm.; Cilag, Swed.)*; Ortho-Novin 1/50 *(Ortho-Cilag, UK)*; Ortho-Novin 2 mg *(S.Afr.)*; Ortho-Novum 1/35 *(Cilag, Fr.; Ortho Pharmaceutical, USA)*; Ortho-Novum 0.5 mg *(Ortho, Canad.)*; Ortho-Novum 1/50 *(Cilag, Austral.; Cilag, Belg.; Ortho, Canad.; Cilag, Ger.; Cilag, Ital.; Cilag, Neth.; Cilag, Switz.; Ortho Pharmaceutical, USA)*; Ortho-Novum 1/80 *(Cilag, Austral.; Belg.; Ortho, Canad.; Cilag, Ger.; Cilag, Switz.; Ortho Pharmaceutical, USA)*; Ortho-Novum 2 mg *(Ortho, Canad.; Cilag, Ger.; Cilag, Ital.; Cilag, Switz.; Ortho Pharmaceutical, USA)*; Ortho-Novum 7/7/7 *(Ortho Pharmaceutical, USA)*; Ortho-Novum 10/11 *(Ortho Pharmaceutical, USA)*; Ortho-Novum SQ *(Cilag, Belg.)*; Ovcon *(Mead Johnson Laboratories, USA)*; Ovysmen *(Cilag, Belg.; Cilag, Ger.; Cilag, Ital.; Cilag, Switz.; Ortho-Cilag, UK)*; Plan mite *(DAK, Denm.)*; Primodos *(Schering, UK)*; Profinix *(Schering, Spain)*; Program *(Ortho, Canad.)*; Progylut *(Schering, Fr.)*; Regovar *(Recordati, Ital.)*; Sinovula *(Asche, Ger.)*; Synfase *(Astra-Syntex, Swed.)*; Synphase *(Syntex, UK)*; Synphasec *(Grünenthal, Ger.)*; Synphasic *(Syntex, Austral.; Syntex, Canad.)*; Syntex Menophase *(Syntex, UK)*; Trentovlane *(Schering, Fr.)*; Triella *(Cilag, Fr.)*; Tri-Norinyl *(Syntex, USA)*; Trinovum *(Cilag-Chemie, Denm.; Cilag, Ger.; Cilag, Ital.; Cilag, Neth.; Johnson & Johnson, S.Afr.; Cilag, Swed.; Cilag, Switz.; Ortho-Cilag, UK)*; Tri-Novum *(Cilag, Ital.)*; Trisekvens *(Novo, Swed.)*; Trisequens *(Novo, Fr.; Novo, Switz.; Novo, UK)*.

9079-k

Norethynodrel *(BAN, USAN)*.

Noretynodrel *(rINN)*. 17β-Hydroxy-19-nor-17α-pregn-5(10)-en-20-yn-3-one.

$C_{20}H_{26}O_2$=298.4.

CAS — 68-23-5.

Pharmacopoeias. In *It.*, *Turk.*, and *U.S.*

A white or almost white, odourless, crystalline powder. The *U.S.P.* specifies not more than 2% of norethisterone. Practically **insoluble** in water; soluble 1 in 30 of alcohol, 1 in 7 of chloroform, and 1 in 60 of ether; soluble in acetone; very slightly soluble in light petroleum. **Protect** from light.

Adverse Effects and Precautions

As for the progestogens in general, p.1386.

Thrombo-embolic disorders have occurred following the use of norethynodrel.

See also hormonal contraceptives, p.1387.

PORPHYRIA. Norethynodrel was considered to be unsafe in patients with acute porphyria because it has been shown to be porphyrinogenic in *animals* or *in-vitro* systems.— M.R. Moore and K.E.L. McColl, *Porphyrias, Drug Lists*, Glasgow, Porphyria Research Unit, University of Glasgow, 1987.

Absorption and Fate

Norethynodrel is absorbed from the gastro-intestinal tract.

METABOLISM. Norethynodrel is rapidly metabolised, in part to norethisterone.— C. E. Cook *et al.*, *J. Pharmac. exp. Ther.*, 1972, *183*, 197.

Uses and Administration

Norethynodrel is a progestogen with actions and uses similar to those for the progestogens in general (see p.1386). The mestranol present in some commercial samples confers slight oestrogenic activity. It is active by mouth and is given in conjunction with an oestrogen such as mestranol.

Norethynodrel is sometimes used as the progestogenic component of combined oral contraceptives (see p.1391).

In the treatment of functional uterine bleeding

and other menstrual disorders, it is given in a dosage of 5 to 10 mg daily usually from the 5th to the 24th day of the cycle; 20 to 30 mg may be required for the initial control of bleeding. In the treatment of endometriosis the usual initial dose is 5 to 10 mg daily increased to 20 mg daily and maintained for at least 6 to 9 months. Doses of up to 40 mg may be given to control break-through bleeding.

Proprietary Names and Manufacturers

The following names have been used for multi-ingredient preparations containing norethynodrel—Conovid *(Searle, UK)*; Conovid-E *(Searle, Austral.; Searle, S.Afr.; Searle, UK)*; Elan *(Valeas, Ital.)*; Enavid *(Searle, Neth.; Searle, UK)*; Enavid-E *(Searle, Arg.; Searle, Neth.; Searle, UK)*; Enovid 5 mg *(Searle, USA)*; Enovid-E *(Searle, Canad.; Searle, USA)*; Kontrazeptivum 63-ratiopharm *(Ratiopharm, Ger.)*; Novinol *(Desbergers, Canad.)*; Ovarion *(Fher, Spain)*; Ovulen Novum *(Vita, Spain)*.

13031-z

Norgestimate *(BAN, USAN, rINN)*.

D-138; Dexnorgestrel Acetime; ORF-10131. 13β-Ethyl-3-hydroxyimino-18,19-dinor-17α-pregn-4-en-20-yn-17β-yl acetate.

$C_{23}H_{31}NO_3$=369.5.

CAS — 35189-28-7.

Norgestimate is a progestogen with actions and uses similar to those described for the progestogens in general (see p.1386).

Proprietary Names and Manufacturers

Ortho Pharmaceutical, USA.

The following names have been used for multi-ingredient preparations containing norgestimate— Cilest *(Cilag, Ger.)*.

9080-w

Norgestrel *(BAN, USAN, rINN)*.

dl-Norgestrel; DL-Norgestrel; Wy-3707. (±)-13-Ethyl-17β-hydroxy-18,19-dinor-17α-pregn-4-en-20-yn-3-one.

$C_{21}H_{28}O_2$=312.5.

CAS — 6533-00-2.

Pharmacopoeias. In *Chin., Nord.,* and *U.S.*

A white or practically white, practically odourless crystalline powder. Practically **insoluble** in water; sparingly soluble in alcohol; freely soluble in chloroform.

9081-e

Levonorgestrel *(BAN, USAN, rINN)*.

D-Norgestrel; Wy-5104. The (−)-isomer of norgestrel.

CAS — 797-63-7.

NOTE. The name Dexnorgestrel has been used.

Pharmacopoeias. In *Br., Nord.,* and *U.S.*

A white or almost white, odourless or almost odourless, crystalline powder. Practically **insoluble** in water; slightly soluble in alcohol, acetone, and ether; soluble 1 in 45 of chloroform. **Store** at a temperature not exceeding 15°. Protect from light.

Adverse Effects and Precautions

As for the progestogens in general, p.1386.

See also under hormonal contraceptives, p.1387.

EFFECTS ON THE SKIN. A sudden onset of moderate to severe papulopustular acne was noted in about 20 patients taking norgestrel in an oral contraceptive preparation, and was considered to be due to norgestrel being an androgen-dominant progestogen.— R. K. Woodward, *Archs Derm.*, 1974, *110*, 812.

PREGNANCY AND THE NEONATE. *Effects on the foetus.* A 23-year-old woman who had taken norgestrel and ethinyloestradiol for the first 3 months of pregnancy gave birth to an infant with a tracheo-oesophageal fistula.— O. Frost, *Br. med. J.*, 1976, *2*, 978.

Inoperable hepatoblastoma in a 7-month-old male infant might have been associated with ingestion of norgestrel 30 μg daily by the mother during the first 3 months of pregnancy.— J. Otten *et al.* (letter), *New Engl. J. Med.*, 1977, *297*, 222.

Absorption and Fate

Norgestrel and levonorgestrel are absorbed from the gastro-intestinal tract. Metabolites are excreted in the urine and faeces as glucuronide and sulphate conjugates.

PREGNANCY AND THE NEONATE. The concentration of D-norgestrel in milk was about 15% of that in plasma; it could not be detected in the milk of women taking only 30 μg daily.— S. Nilsson *et al.*, *Am. J. Obstet. Gynec.*, 1977, *129*, 178.

Uses and Administration

Norgestrel and levonorgestrel are progestogens with actions and uses similar to those described for the progestogens in general (see p.1386). They are more potent as inhibitors of ovulation than norethisterone and have androgenic activity. Levonorgestrel is the active isomer; norgestrel, the racemate, has therefore half the potency of levonorgestrel.

They are both used as the progestogenic component of combined oral contraceptives and are also used as progestogen-only types of oral contraceptives (see p.1391).

Either norgestrel or levonorgestrel are also used as the added progestogen to oestrogenic therapy in menopausal disorders.

Preparations

Levonorgestrel and Ethinyl Estradiol Tablets *(U.S.P.)*. Tablets containing levonorgestrel and ethinyloestradiol.

Norgestrel Tablets *(U.S.P.)*

Norgestrel and Ethinyl Estradiol Tablets *(U.S.P.)*. Tablets containing norgestrel and ethinyloestradiol.

Proprietary Preparations

Proprietary preparations containing norgestrel or levonorgestrel are described under conjugated oestrogens (p.1409) and under oestradiol valerate (p.1408).

Proprietary contraceptive preparations containing norgestrel or levonorgestrel are described under the section on hormonal contraceptives (p.1392)

Proprietary Names and Manufacturers of Norgestrel and Levonorgestrel

Follistrel *(Kabi, Swed.)*; Microlut *(Schering, Austral.; Schering, Belg.; Schering, Ger.; Schering, Ital.; Switz.)*; Microluton *(Schering, Denm.; Leiras, Fin.; Schering AG, Norw.; Swed.)*; Microval *(Wyeth, Austral.; Wyeth, Belg.; Wyeth, Denm.; Wyeth, Fin.; Wyeth-Byla, Fr.; Wyeth, S.Afr.; Wyeth, UK)*; Mikro-30 *(Wyeth, Ger.)*; Neogest *(Schering, UK)*; Norgeston *(Schering, UK)*; Norplant *(Leiras, Fin.; Leiras, Swed.)*; Ovrette *(Wyeth, USA)*.

The following names have been used for multi-ingredient preparations containing norgestrel and levonorgestrel—Adepal *(Wyeth-Byla, Fr.)*; Binordiol *(Wyeth, Belg.; Wyeth, Denm.; Wyeth, Fin.; Wyeth, Ital.; Wyeth, Neth.; Wyeth, Switz.)*; Biphasil *(Wyeth, Austral.; Wyeth, S.Afr.)*; Bivlar *(Schering, Ital.)*; Cyclo-Progynova *(Schering, UK)*; Duoluton *(Schering, Arg.; Schering, Austral.)*; Ediwal *(Schering, Ger.)*; Egogyn 30 *(Schering, Ital.)*; Eugynon *(Schering, Arg.; Schering, Austral.; Belg.; Schering, Denm.; Schering, Ger.; Schering, Ital.; Neth.; Schering, Norw.; Schering, S.Afr.; Schering, Spain; Schering, Switz.)*; Eugynon 30 *(Schering, UK)*; Eugynon 50 *(Schering, UK)*; Evanor-d *(Wyeth, Ital.)*; Evelea *(Elea, Arg.)*; Fironetta *(Schering, Denm.)*; Follimin *(KabiVitrum, Norw.; Kabi, Swed.)*; Follinett *(Kabi, Swed.)*; Gentrol *(Wyeth, Denm.)*; Gynatrol *(Wyeth, Denm.)*; Levlen *(Berlex, USA)*; Logynon *(Schering, UK)*; Logynon ED *(Schering, S.Afr.; Schering, UK)*; Lo/Ovral *(Wyeth, USA)*; Microgyn *(Schering, Denm.)*; Microgynon *(Schering, Arg.; Schering, Austral.; Leiras, Fin.; Schering, Ger.; Schering, Ital.; Schering, Norw.; Schering, Spain)*; Microgynon 30 *(Schering, Belg.; Schering, Neth.; Schering, Switz.; Schering, UK)*; Microgynon 50 *(Schering, Belg.; Schering, Neth.; Schering, Switz.)*; Microgynon ED *(Schering, Austral.)*; Minidril *(Wyeth-Byla, Fr.)*; Min-Ovral *(Wyeth, Canad.)*; Neogentrol *(Wyeth, Denm.)*; Neo-Gentrol *(Wyeth, Fin.)*; Neogynon *(Schering, Arg.; Schering, Austral.; Schering, Belg..; Schering, Denm.; Schering, Ger.; Schering, Neth.; Schering, Switz.)*; Neogynona *(Schering, Spain)*; Neo-Primovlar *(Leiras, Fin.)*; Neo-Stediril *(Wyeth, Belg.; Wyeth, Ger.; Wyeth, Neth.; Wyeth, Switz.)*; Neovlar *(Swed.)*; Neovletta *(Schering, Swed.)*; Nordette *(Wyeth, Arg.; Wyeth, Austral.; Wyeth, S.Afr.; Wyeth, USA)*; Nordiol *(Wyeth, Arg.; Wyeth, Austral.; Wyeth, S.Afr.)*; Normovlar *(Schering, S.Afr.)*; Novogyn *(Schering, Ital.)*; Ovoplex *(Orfi, Spain)*; Ovral *(Wyeth, Arg.; Wyeth, Austral.; Wyeth, Canad.; Wyeth, S.Afr.; Wyeth, USA)*; Ovran *(Wyeth, UK)*; Ovran 30 *(Wyeth, UK)*; Ovranet *(Wyeth, Ital.)*; Ovranette *(Wyeth, UK)*; Perikursal *(Wyeth, Ger.)*; Prempak *(Ayerst, UK)*; Prempak-C *(Ayerst, UK)*; Primovlar *(Swed.)*; Prolorfin *(Orfi, Spain)*; Regunon *(Schering, Swed.)*; Schering PC4 *(Schering, UK)*; Sekvilar *(Leiras, Fin.)*; Sequilar *(Schering, Austral.; Schering, Belg.; Schering, Ger.; Schering, Neth.; Schering, Switz.)*; Sequilarum *(Schering, Denm.; Schering, Swed.)*; Stediril *(Wyeth, Belg.; Wyeth-Byla, Fr.; Wyeth, Ger.; Wyeth, Switz.)*; Stediril 30 *(Wyeth, Belg.; Wyeth, Ger.; Wyeth, Neth.; Wyeth, Switz.)*; Stediril-d *(Wyeth, Belg.; Wyeth, Ger.; Wyeth, Neth.; Wyeth, Switz.)*; Tetragynon *(Schering, Switz.)*; Triagynon *(Schering, Spain)*; Triciclor *(Orfi, Spain)*; Tridestan *(Gador, Arg.)*; Trigynon *(Schering, Belg.; Schering, Ital.; Schering, Neth.)*; Trikvilar *(Leiras, Fin.)*; Tri-Levlen *(Berlex, USA)*; Trinordiol *(Wyeth, Arg.; Wyeth, Belg.; Wyeth, Denm.; Wyeth, Fin.; Wyeth-Byla, Fr.; Wyeth, Ger.; Wyeth, Ital.; Wyeth, Neth.; KabiVitrum, Norw.; Kabi, Swed.; Wyeth, Switz.; Wyeth, UK)*; Trionetta *(Schering, Norw.; Schering, Swed.)*; Triphasil *(Wyeth, Austral.; Wyeth, Canad.; Wyeth, S.Afr.; Wyeth, USA)*; Triquilar *(Schering, Arg.; Schering, Austral.; Schering, Denm.; Schering, Ger.; Schering, Switz.)*; Tristep *(Asche, Ger.)*.

13032-c

Norgestrienone *(rINN)*.

17β-Hydroxy-19-nor-17α-pregna-4,9,11-trien-20-yn-3-one.

$C_{20}H_{22}O_2$=294.4.

CAS — 848-21-5.

Adverse Effects and Precautions

As for the progestogens in general, p.1386.

Uses and Administration

Norgestrienone is a progestogen with actions and uses similar to those of the progestogens in general (see p.1386). It is used as the progestogenic component of some combined oral contraceptives and is also used as a progestogen-only type of oral contraceptive (see p.1391).

Proprietary Names and Manufacturers

Ogyline *(Roussel, Fr.)*.

The following names have been used for multi-ingredient preparations containing norgestrienone— Planor *(Roussel, Fr.)*.

9082-l

Normethandrone

Methylestrenolone; Methylnortestosterone; Normethandrolone. 17β-Hydroxy-17α-methylestr-4-en-3-one.

$C_{19}H_{28}O_2$=288.4.

CAS — 514-61-4.

Normethandrone has progestogenic properties (see p.1386) and has been given by mouth in doses of 5 mg daily.

Proprietary Names and Manufacturers

Orga-Steron *(Organon, Belg.; Organon, Neth.)*.

9083-y

Oestradiol *(BAN)*.

Beta-oestradiol; Dihydrofolliculine; Dihydrotheelin; Dihydroxyoestrin; Estradiol *(USAN, rINN)*. Estra-1,3,5(10)-triene-3,17β-diol.

$C_{18}H_{24}O_2$=272.4.

CAS — 50-28-2.

Pharmacopoeias. In *Aust., Fr., Mex., Span., Turk.,* and *U.S.*

White or creamy-white, odourless, hygroscopic crystals or crystalline powder. Practically **insoluble** in water; soluble 1 in 28 of alcohol, 1 in 435 of chloroform, and 1 in 150 of ether; soluble in acetone, dioxan, and solutions of fixed alkali hydroxides; sparingly soluble in vegetable oils. **Store** in airtight containers. Protect from light.

9084-j

Oestradiol Benzoate *(BANM)*.

Beta-estradiol Benzoate; Dihydroxyoestrin Monobenzoate; Estradiol Benzoate *(rINN)*; Estradioli Benzoas. Estra-1,3,5(10)-triene-3,17β-diol 3-benzoate.

$C_{25}H_{28}O_3$=376.5.

CAS — 50-50-0.

Pharmacopoeias. In *Arg., Aust., Belg., Br., Braz., Chin., Cz., Egypt., Eur., Fr., Ger., Hung., Ind., Int., It., Jpn, Jug., Mex., Neth., Nord., Pol., Port., Roum., Span., Swiss,* and *Turk.* Also in *B.P. Vet.*

Colourless crystals or a white or almost white

crystalline powder. Practically **insoluble** in water; slightly soluble in alcohol and fixed oils; soluble 1 in 50 of acetone. **Protect** from light. Oily solutions for injection are **sterilised** by dry heat.

9085-z

Oestradiol Cypionate *(BANM)*.

Estradiol Cipionate *(rINNM)*; Estradiol Cypionate *(USAN)*; Oestradiol Cyclopentylpropionate. Estra-1,3,5(10)-triene-3,17β-diol 17-(3-cyclopentylpropionate).
$C_{26}H_{36}O_3$=396.6.

CAS — 313-06-4.

Pharmacopoeias. In *Braz.* and *U.S.*

A white or practically white crystalline powder, odourless or with a slight odour. Practically **insoluble** in water; soluble 1 in 40 of alcohol, 1 in 7 of chloroform, and 1 in 2800 of ether; soluble in acetone and dioxan; sparingly soluble in vegetable oils. **Store** in airtight containers. Protect from light.

9086-c

Oestradiol Dipropionate *(BANM)*.

Dihydroxyoestrin Dipropionate; Estradiol Dipropionate *(rINNM)*. Estra-1,3,5(10)-triene-3,17β-diol dipropionate.
$C_{24}H_{32}O_4$=384.5.

CAS — 113-38-2.

Pharmacopoeias. In *Arg., Aust., Braz., Cz., Ind., Jug.,* and *Swiss. Hung.* includes oestradiol 17-monopropionate ($C_{21}H_{28}O_3$ = 328.5).

9087-k

Oestradiol Enanthate *(BANM)*.

Estradiol Enantate *(rINNM)*; Estradiol Enanthate *(USAN)*; Oestradiol 17-Heptanoate; SQ-16150. Estra-1,3,5(10)-triene-3,17β-diol 17-heptanoate.
$C_{25}H_{36}O_3$=384.6.

CAS — 4956-37-0.

13039-d

Oestradiol Hexahydrobenzoate *(BANM)*.

Estradiol Hexahydrobenzoate *(rINNM)*. Estra-1,3,5(10)-triene-3,17β-diol 17-cyclohexanecarboxylate.
$C_{25}H_{34}O_3$=382.5.

CAS — 15140-27-9.

9088-a

Oestradiol Undecanoate *(BANM)*.

Estradiol Undecylate *(USAN, rINN)*; SQ-9993. Estra-1,3,5(10)-triene-3,17β-diol 17-undecanoate.
$C_{29}H_{44}O_3$=440.7.

CAS — 3571-53-7; 33613-02-4.

9089-t

Oestradiol Valerate *(BANM)*.

Estradiol Valerate *(USAN, rINN)*. Estra-1,3,5(10)-triene-3,17β-diol 17-valerate.
$C_{23}H_{32}O_3$=356.5.

CAS — 979-32-8.

Pharmacopoeias. In *Chin.* and *U.S.*

A white crystalline powder which is odourless or has a faint fatty odour. Practically **insoluble** in water; soluble in benzyl benzoate, dioxan, methyl alcohol, and castor oil; sparingly soluble in arachis oil and sesame oil. **Store** in airtight containers. Protect from light.

Adverse Effects and Precautions

As for the oestrogens in general, p.1384.

Absorption and Fate

Oestradiol is absorbed from the gastro-intestinal tract and through the skin. It is partly bound (about 50%) to plasma proteins and is rapidly metabolised mainly in the liver to the less active oestriol and oestrone. It is excreted in the urine as sulphate and glucuronide esters together with a small proportion of unchanged oestradiol. Numerous other metabolites have been identified.

Uses and Administration

Oestradiol is a naturally occurring oestrogenic hormone with the actions and uses described for the oestrogens in general (see p.1385). Oestradiol and its semi-synthetic esters are primarily used in the treatment of menopausal and postmenopausal symptoms. For administration by mouth oestradiol or oestradiol valerate are normally employed; doses of 1 to 2 mg daily are given, usually on a cyclical basis and in conjunction with an added progestogen for part of the cycle. Oestradiol may also be applied locally and up to 4 g of a 0.01% vaginal cream may be used daily. Oestradiol may also be used topically as transdermal skin patches to provide a systemic effect; patches are available which release up to 100 µg of oestradiol daily although new patches are applied not daily, but usually every 3 to 4 days. In order to prolong the duration of action either subcutaneous implants of oestradiol or intramuscular injections of oestradiol esters may be employed. For subcutaneous implantation the dose of oestradiol is generally 25 to 100 mg with a new implant being administered after about 4 to 8 months. For intramuscular injection the benzoate or cypionate esters are normally used as oily solutions to provide a depot; the dose is generally 1 to 5 mg every 2 weeks. The dipropionate, enanthate, hexahydrobenzoate, and undecanoate esters have been used similarly as intramuscular injections.

Oestradiol has also been used, like many other oestrogens, in metastatic prostate cancer and breast cancer in postmenopausal women.

For a general review covering the actions and uses of oestrogens, see p.1385.

ADMINISTRATION. *Implants.* A study in 12 women who had had a total hysterectomy and bilateral salpingo-oophorectomy who received oestradiol 100 mg implants every 6 months to prevent a premature menopause showed striking variation in oestradiol concentrations. Concentrations 6 months after an implant ranged from 37 to 1869 pmol per litre despite the fact that all patients were of similar age and weight. It was considered that oestradiol concentrations should lie within the range of 200 to 800 pmol per litre and that after the first implant the concentration should be checked at intervals of 3 months until it drops below 200 pmol per litre when another implant should be inserted. Oestradiol implants should not be inserted at fixed times for several years without monitoring of concentrations.— R. R. Guirgis (letter), *Lancet*, 1987, *2*, 856.

Transdermally. A short review of transdermal oestrogen patches. The advantages claimed for the patch over oestradiol by mouth are that the oestradiol enters the blood directly, thus avoiding the gastro-intestinal effects, first-pass hepatic metabolism, and stimulation of hepatic enzymes, that the doses used are much lower, and that blood concentrations more closely resemble those found naturally before the menopause. The patches do appear to be as effective as much higher doses of oestrogens by mouth in treating postmenopausal vasomotor symptoms but whether they are safer remains to be determined.— *Med. Lett.*, 1986, *28*, 119.

Some studies and comments on transdermal oestradiol patches: R. J. Chetkowski *et al.*, *New Engl. J. Med.*, 1986, *314*, 1615; L. Lasagna and D. J. Greenblatt, *ibid.*, 1638; P. L. Selby and M. Peacock, *Br. med. J.*, 1986, *293*, 1337; J. C. Stevenson *et al.* (letter), *ibid.*, 1987, *294*, 181; M. Peacock and P. Selby (letter), *ibid.*, 440; M. I. Whitehead *et al.* (letter), *ibid.*, 769.

Preparations of Oestradiol and its Esters

Sterile Estradiol Suspension *(U.S.P.)*. A sterile suspension of oestradiol in water for injections.

Oestradiol Injection *(B.P.)*. Oestradiol Benzoate Injection. A sterile solution of oestradiol benzoate in ethyl oleate or other suitable ester, in a suitable fixed oil, or in any mixture of these. For intramuscular injection only.

Estradiol Cypionate Injection *(U.S.P.)*. A sterile solution of oestradiol cypionate in a suitable oil.

Estradiol Valerate Injection *(U.S.P.)*. A sterile solution of oestradiol valerate in a suitable vegetable oil.

Estradiol Pellets *(U.S.P.)*. Oestradiol compressed in the form of sterile pellets with no binder, diluent, or excipient.

Estradiol Tablets *(U.S.P.)*. Tablets containing oestradiol.

Estradiol Vaginal Cream *(U.S.P.)*. Vaginal cream containing oestradiol.

Proprietary Preparations of Oestradiol and its Esters

Benztrone *(Paines & Byrne, UK)*. *Injection*, oestradiol benzoate 1 mg/mL, in ampoules of 1 mL.
Injection, oestradiol benzoate 5 mg/mL, in ampoules of 1 mL.

Cyclo-Progynova *(Schering, UK)*. *Tablets* (Cyclo-Progynova 1 mg), 21-day calendar pack; 11 tablets, oestradiol valerate 1 mg; 10 tablets, oestradiol valerate 1 mg, levonorgestrel 250 µg.
Tablets (Cyclo-Progynova 2 mg), 21-day calendar pack; 11 tablets, oestradiol valerate 2 mg; 10 tablets, oestradiol valerate 2 mg, norgestrel 500 µg.
For menopausal symptoms.

Estraderm TTS *(Ciba, UK)*. *Patches*, transdermal drug-delivery system, oestradiol 2 mg (approximately 25 µg/patch absorbed in 24 hours), oestradiol 4 mg (approximately 50 µg/patch absorbed in 24 hours), and oestradiol 8 mg (approximately 100 µg/patch absorbed in 24 hours). *Administration.* One patch to be applied every 3 or 4 days.

Oestradiol Implants *(Organon, UK)*. *Implants*, oestradiol 25, 50, or 100 mg.

Progynova *(Schering, UK)*. *Tablets*, oestradiol valerate 1 and 2 mg.

Further proprietary preparations containing oestradiol are described under oestriol (p.1409).

Proprietary Names and Manufacturers of Oestradiol and its Esters

Benzo-Gynestryl-5 *(Arg.)*; Benzo-Gynoestryl *(Roussel, Fr.)*; Benztrone *(Samil, Ital.; Paines & Byrne, UK)*; Delestrogen *(Squibb, Canad.; Squibb, USA)*; Depo-Estradiol Cypionate *(Upjohn, USA)*; Depofemin *(Hoechst, Denm.)*; Dimenformon *(Belg.; Neth.)*; E-Cypionate *(Legere, USA)*; Estrace *(Bristol, Canad.; Mead Johnson Laboratories, USA)*; Estradep *(Millet, Arg.)*; Estraderm *(Ciba, USA)*; Estraderm TTS *(Geigy, Ger.; Ciba, Switz.; Ciba, UK)*; Etrosteron *(Gador, Arg.)*; Farmacyrol *(Ger.)*; Femogex *(Stickley, Canad.)*; Follicyclin *(Denm.)*; Gynécormone *(Fr.)*; Gynoestryl *(Fr.)*; Menaval *(Legere, USA)*; Neoginon Depositum *(Lusofarmaco, Ital.)*; Östrogynol sine *(Ger.)*; Oestradiol Implants *(Organon, UK)*; Oestramine *(Austral.)*; Oestrogel *(Besins-Iscovesco, Fr.)*; Ormogamma *(Ital.)*; Ovex *(Leo, Denm.)*; Ovocyclin *(Ciba-Geigy, Switz.)*; Ovocyclin M *(Ger.; Switz.)*; Ovolacer *(Spain)*; Pertradiol *(Spain)*; Primogyn Depot *(Schering, Austral.; Schering AG, Norw.; Schering, S.Afr.; Schering, UK)*; Progynon *(Arg.; Schering, Denm.; Ital.; Schering, Spain; Schering, Swed.; USA)*; Progynon B *(Schering, Ger.; Spain)*; Progynon B Oleoso *(Arg.; Schering, Ital.)*; Progynon Depot *(Arg.; Schering, Denm.; Schering, Ger.; Schering, Ital.; Schering, Neth.; Schering AG, Norw.; Swed.; Schering, Switz.)*; Progynon Retard *(Schering, Fr.)*; Progynova *(Arg.; Schering, Austral.; Belg.; Schering, Fr.; Schering, Ger.; Schering, Ital.; Neth.; Schering AG, Norw.; Schering, S.Afr.; Schering, Spain; Schering, Switz.; Schering, UK)*; Progynova 21 Mitis *(Belg.)*.

The following names have been used for multi-ingredient preparations containing oestradiol and its esters—Atrimon *(Beta, Arg.)*; Climacteron *(Frosst, Canad.)*; Cyclo-Progynova *(Schering, UK)*; Damix *(Valles Mestre, Spain)*; Deladumone *(Squibb, Canad.)*; Ditate-DS *(Savage, USA)*; Duogex *(Stickley, Canad.)*; Estrand *(Taro, Canad.)*; Estrapak 50 *(Ciba, UK)*; Hormonin *(Carnrick, UK)*; Mixogen Injection *(Organon, Austral.; Organon, UK)*; Neo-Pause *(Neolab, Canad.)*; Paralut Injection *(Wallace Mfg Chem., UK)*; Perlutal *(Promeco, Arg.)*; Plex-Hormone Injection *(Consolidated Chemicals, UK)*; Primodian Depot *(Schering, Austral.; Schering, Ital.)*; T-E Cypionate *(Legere, USA)*; Testaval *(Legere, USA)*; Topasel *(Castejon, Spain)*; Trisekvens *(Novo, Swed.)*; Trisequens *(Novo, Fr.; Novo, Switz.; Novo, UK)*.

9090-l

Oestriol

Estriol *(USAN)*; Theelol. Estra-1,3,5(10)-triene-3,16α,17β-triol.
$C_{18}H_{24}O_3$=288.4.

CAS — 50-27-1.

Pharmacopoeias. In *U.S.*

A white or practically white, odourless, crystalline powder. Practically **insoluble** in water; sparingly soluble in alcohol; soluble in acetone, chloroform, dioxan, ether, and vegetable oils. **Store** in airtight containers.

Adverse Effects and Precautions

As for the oestrogens in general, p.1384.

Uses and Administration

Oestriol is a naturally occurring oestrogenic hormone with actions and uses similar to those described for the oestrogens in general (see p.1385). It is claimed to have a selective action on the cervix and vagina and to have relatively little effect on the endometrium.

It is used for the treatment of menopausal and postmenopausal disorders. Doses by mouth have generally been up to about 500 µg daily and for topical vaginal therapy pessaries containing 500 µg or a 0.1% cream have been employed.

For a general review covering the actions and uses of oestrogens, see p.1385.

Proprietary Preparations

Hormonin *(Carnrick, UK). Tablets,* oestriol 270 µg, oestrone 1.4 mg, oestradiol 600 µg. For menopausal disorders.

Ortho-Gynest *(Ortho-Cilag, UK). Pessaries,* oestriol 500 µg.

Ovestin *(Organon, UK). Tablets,* oestriol 250 µg. *Vaginal cream,* oestriol 0.1%.

Trisequens *(Novo, UK). Tablets,* 28-day calendar pack; 12 tablets, oestriol 1 mg, oestradiol 2 mg; 10 tablets, oestriol 1 mg, oestradiol 2 mg, norethisterone acetate 1 mg; 6 tablets, oestriol 500 µg, oestradiol 1 mg. For menopausal symptoms.

Proprietary Names and Manufacturers

Aacifemine *(Belg.)*; Colpogyn *(Angelini, Ital.)*; Gynasan *(Bastian, Ger.)*; Holin *(Jpn)*; Hormomed *(Merckle, Ger.)*; Klimadoral *(Leo Suede, Switz.)*; Klimadurin *(Lundbeck, Denm.; Mekos, Norw.; Abello, Spain; Leo Suede, Switz.)*; Klimax-E *(Fink, Ger.)*; Oekolp *(Kade, Ger.)*; Oestrilir *(Ardeypharm, Ger.)*; Orgastyptin *(Organon, Ger.)*; Orgestriol *(Arg.)*; Ortho-Gynest *(Cilag, Ger.; Cilag, Switz.; Ortho-Cilag, UK)*; Ovesterin *(Organon, Norw.; Organon, Swed.)*; Ovestin *(Organon, Austral.; Belg.; Organon, Denm.; Organon, Fr.; Organon, Ger.; Ravasini, Ital.; Neth.; Organon, Switz.; Organon, UK)*; Ovestinon *(Organon, Spain)*; Ovo-Vinces *(Wolff, Ger.)*; Sinapause *(Organon, Arg.)*; Styptanon *(Belg.; Neth.; Organon, Switz.)*; Synapasa *(Erco, Denm.)*; Synapause *(Organon, Fr.; Nourypharma, Ger.; Neth.; Organon, S.Afr.; Organon, Spain; Nourypharma, Switz.)*; Triodurin *(Pharmacia Arzneimittel, Ger.; Swed.)*; Triovex *(Leo, Swed.)*.

The following names have been used for multi-ingredient preparations containing oestriol—Hormonin *(Carnrick, UK)*; Trisequens *(Novo, Fr.; Novo, Switz.; Novo, UK)*.

9091-y

Conjugated Oestrogens

Conjugated Estrogens *(USAN)*.

Pharmacopoeias. In *Braz.* and *U.S.*

A mixture of sodium oestrone sulphate and sodium equilin sulphate, derived wholly or in part from equine urine or synthetically from oestrone and equilin. It may contain other oestrogenic substances of the type excreted by pregnant mares. It contains 50 to 63% of sodium oestrone sulphate and 22.5 to 32.5% of sodium equilin sulphate.

If it is obtained from natural sources it is a buff-coloured amorphous powder which is odourless or has a slight characteristic odour; the synthetic form is a white to light buff-coloured crystalline or amorphous powder, odourless or with a slight odour. **Store** in airtight containers.

Adverse Effects and Precautions

As for the oestrogens in general, p.1384.

ALLERGY. A report of an anaphylactic reaction following the intravenous administration of conjugated oestrogens.— C. J. Searcy *et al., Clin. Pharm.,* 1987, *6,* 74.

EFFECTS ON THE CARDIOVASCULAR SYSTEM. In a collaborative study by the Coronary Drug Project Group, treatment of men with a previous myocardial infarction with conjugated oestrogens 2.5 mg daily was discontinued because of suggestions of adverse trends including a greater incidence of venous thrombo-embolism.— Coronary Drug Project Research Group, *J. Am. med. Ass.,* 1973, *226,* 652.

Transient episodes of imbalance and episodes of amaurosis fugax in a 52-year-old woman were considered due to emboli from her prosthetic heart valve, caused by conjugated oestrogens.— D. Pitcher and P. Curry, *Br. med. J.,* 1979, *2,* 244.

EFFECTS ON THE GALL BLADDER. Analysis of data obtained during the Coronary Drug Project indicated a significant increase in the development of gall-bladder disease among patients treated with conjugated oestrogens 2.5 and 5 mg daily, compared with those treated with placebo.— Coronary Drug Project Research Group, *New Engl. J. Med.,* 1977, *296,* 1185.

INTERACTIONS. A report of phenytoin diminishing the effect of conjugated oestrogens in a menopausal woman.— M. Notelovitz *et al.* (letter), *New Engl. J. Med.,* 1981, *304,* 788.

Absorption and Fate

Conjugated oestrogens are absorbed from the gastro-intestinal tract. Metabolism occurs primarily in the liver; there is some enterohepatic recycling.

Uses and Administration

Conjugated oestrogens have actions and uses similar to those described for the oestrogens in general (see p.1385).

In menopausal and postmenopausal symptoms, doses of 0.3 to 1.25 mg daily are given by mouth, usually on a cyclical basis and in conjunction with an added progestogen for part of the cycle. Topical vaginal therapy may also be used; up to 4 g of a 0.0625% cream may be employed daily.

Primary ovarian failure has been treated with doses of 1.25 mg daily and female hypogonadism with doses of up to 7.5 mg daily administered on a cyclical basis.

For the palliative treatment of prostatic carcinoma, a daily dose of 3.75 to 7.5 mg has been employed. A dose of 10 mg three times daily for at least 3 months has been used for breast carcinoma in postmenopausal women.

Abnormal uterine bleeding has been treated by giving 25 mg by intramuscular or intravenous injection repeated if required after 6 to 12 hours.

For a general review covering the actions and uses of oestrogens, see p.1385.

Preparations

Conjugated Estrogens Tablets *(U.S.P.).* Tablets containing conjugated oestrogens.

Proprietary Preparations

Premarin *(Ayerst, UK). Tablets,* conjugated oestrogens 0.625, 1.25, and 2.5 mg.
Vaginal cream, conjugated oestrogens 0.625 mg/g.

Prempak-C *(Ayerst, UK). Tablets* (Prempak-C 0.625), 28-day pack; 28 tablets, conjugated oestrogens 0.625 mg; 12 tablets, norgestrel 150 µg, to be taken additionally on days 17 to 28.
Tablets (Prempak-C 1.25), 28-day pack; 28 tablets, conjugated oestrogens 1.25 mg; 12 tablets, norgestrel 150 µg, to be taken additionally on days 17 to 28. For menopausal symptoms.

Proprietary Names and Manufacturers

Ayerogen *(Venez.)*; BayEstros *(Bay, USA)*; CES *(ICN, Canad.)*; Conestron *(Inibsa, Spain)*; Emopremarin *(Ayerst, Ital.)*; Equigyne *(Belg.; Fr.; Neth.)*; Equin *(Aldo, Spain)*; Equormon *(Biopharma, Ital.)*; Estrocon *(Savage, USA)*; Evoquin *(S.Afr.)*; Mepausial *(Medical, Spain)*; Neo-Menovar *(Arg.)*; Oestrilin *(Canad.)*; Oestro-Feminal *(Mack, Illert., Ger.; S.Afr.; Mack, Switz.)*; Oestropak *(S.Afr.)*; Prémauclair *(Ayerst, Fr.)*; Premarin *(Ayerst, Austral.; Ayerst, Canad.; Ayerst, Denm.; Ayerst, Fr.; Ayerst, Ital.; Ayerst, S.Afr.; Ayerst, Switz.; Ayerst, UK; Ayerst, USA)*; Presomen *(Kali-Chemie, Ger.)*; Promarit *(Ayerst, Swed.)*; Transannon *(Heyden, Ger.; Heyden, Switz.)*.

The following names have been used for multi-ingredient preparations containing conjugated oestrogens— Esprogyn *(Metro Med, USA)*; Mediatric *(Ayerst, USA)*; PMB *(Ayerst, USA)*; Premarin with Methyltestosterone *(Ayerst, USA)*; Prempak *(Ayerst, UK)*; Prempak-C *(Ayerst, UK)*.

10069-v

Esterified Oestrogens

Esterified Estrogens *(USAN)*.

Pharmacopoeias. In *U.S.*

A mixture of the sodium salts of the sulphate esters of the oestrogenic substances, principally oestrone. It contains 75 to 85% of sodium oestrone sulphate and 6 to 15% of sodium equilin sulphate, in such a proportion that the total of these two components is not less than 90%.

A white or buff-coloured amorphous powder which is odourless or has a slight characteristic odour. **Store** in airtight containers.

Adverse Effects and Precautions

As for the oestrogens in general, p.1384.

Uses and Administration

Esterified oestrogens have actions and uses similar to those described for the oestrogens in general (see p.1385). They are used for same purposes and in the same dosage by mouth as conjugated oestrogens (see above).

For a general review covering the actions and uses of oestrogens, see p.1385.

Preparations

Esterified Estrogens Tablets *(U.S.P.).* Tablets containing esterified oestrogens.

Proprietary Names and Manufacturers

Amnestrogen *(USA)*; Climestrone *(Canad.)*; Estratab *(Reid-Rowell, USA)*; Estromed *(Canad.)*; Evex *(Syntex, USA)*; Menest *(Beecham Laboratories, USA)*; Neo-Estrone *(Neolab, Canad.)*.

The following names have been used for multi-ingredient preparations containing esterified oestrogens— Estratest *(Reid-Rowell, USA)*; Menrium *(Roche, Canad.; Roche, USA)*.

9092-j

Oestrone *(BAN)*.

Estrone *(USAN, rINN)*; Folliculin; Ketohydroxyoestrin.
3-Hydroxyestra-1,3,5(10)-trien-17-one.
$C_{18}H_{22}O_2$=270.4.

CAS — 53-16-7.

Pharmacopoeias. In *Arg., Aust., Braz., Fr., Hung., It., Mex., Neth., Pol., Span., Turk.,* and *U.S.*

Odourless, small white crystals or white to creamy-white crystalline powder. Practically **insoluble** in water; soluble 1 in 250 of alcohol and 1 in 110 of chloroform at 15°; soluble 1 in 50 of boiling alcohol, 1 in 33 of boiling acetone, and 1 in 80 of boiling chloroform; soluble 1 in 50 of acetone at 50°; soluble in dioxan and vegetable oils; slightly soluble in solutions of fixed alkali hydroxides. **Store** in airtight containers. Protect from light.

Adverse Effects and Precautions

As for the oestrogens in general, p.1384.

Uses and Administration

Oestrone is a naturally occurring oestrogenic hormone with actions and uses similar to those described for the oestrogens in general (see p.1385).

Oestrone may be given by mouth, often as a combination product with other oestrogens, for the treatment of menopausal and postmenopausal symptoms; doses of 0.7 to 2.8 mg daily have been used in combination with other oestrogens. Oestrone has also been administered by intramuscular injection in oily solutions and aqueous suspensions.

For a general review covering the actions and uses of oestrogens, see p.1385.

Studies with ^{14}C-labelled oestrone indicated that oestrone undergoes enterohepatic recirculation, that it is metabolised in the liver and intestine and that excretion is mainly as metabolites via the urine. Metabolic clearance was estimated to be about 90 litres per m^2 body-surface daily.— L. A. Pagliaro *et al.*, *J. Am. pharm. Ass.*, 1977, *NS17*, 755.

Preparations

Estrone Injection *(U.S.P.)*. A sterile solution of oestrone in a suitable oil.

Sterile Estrone Suspension *(U.S.P.)*. A sterile suspension of oestrone in water for injections.

Proprietary Preparations

A proprietary preparation containing oestrone is described under oestriol (see p.1409).

Proprietary Names and Manufacturers

Cristallovar *(Ibi, Ital.; Panpharma, Switz.)*; Femogen *(Stickley, Canad.)*; Kolpon *(Organon, Austral.)*; Oestrilin *(Desbergers, Canad.)*.

The following names have been used for multi-ingredient preparations containing oestrone— Eldec *(Parke, Davis, Austral.)*; Hormonin *(Carnrick, UK)*.

13050-a

Oxabolone Cypionate

Oxabolone Cipionate *(rINN)*. 4,17β-Dihydroxyestr-4-en-3-one 17-(β-cyclopentylpropionate).

$C_{26}H_{38}O_4$=414.6.

CAS — 1254-35-9.

Oxabolone cypionate has anabolic properties and has been given by intramuscular injection in doses of 25 to 50 mg about every 7 to 10 days.

Proprietary Names and Manufacturers

Steranabol Depot *(Farmitalia, Ger.)*; Steranabol Ritardo *(Farmitalia, Ital.)*.

9093-z

Oxandrolone *(BAN, USAN, rINN)*.

17β-Hydroxy-17α-methyl-2-oxa-5α-androstan-3-one.

$C_{19}H_{30}O_3$=306.4.

CAS — 53-39-4.

Pharmacopoeias. In *U.S.*

A white odourless crystalline powder. **Soluble** 1 in 5200 of water, 1 in 57 of alcohol, 1 in 69 of acetone, 1 in less than 5 of chloroform, and 1 in 860 of ether. **Protect** from light.

Adverse Effects and Precautions

As for the androgens and anabolic steroids in general, p.1383.

Oxandrolone, given for long periods, may cause jaundice and is contra-indicated in patients with liver disturbances.

Absorption and Fate

Oxandrolone is rapidly absorbed from the gastro-intestinal tract. It is excreted mainly in the urine as metabolites and unchanged oxandrolone. A small amount is excreted in the faeces.

Investigations in 6 healthy male subjects demonstrated that following oral ingestion of oxandrolone 10 mg there was rapid absorption resulting in a maximum plasma concentration of 417 ng per mL between 30 and 90 minutes. Plasma concentrations then declined in 2 phases: from 90 minutes to 4 hours with a half-life of about 33 minutes; from 4 to 48 hours the half-life was about 9 hours. Only 2.8% of the dose was excreted in the faeces whereas 60.4% was excreted in the urine within 96 hours (43.6% in the first 24 hours). Unchanged oxandrolone in the urine accounted for 28.7% of the administered dose.— A. Karim *et al.*, *Clin. Pharmac. Ther.*, 1973, *14*, 862.

Uses and Administration

Oxandrolone has anabolic and androgenic properties and has been given in doses of 2.5 to 20 mg daily by mouth.

Twenty-four boys with constitutional delay of growth, associated with delayed puberty in 14, were treated with oxandrolone, 2.5 mg daily by mouth for 3 to 6 months. Four patients received a second course since height velocity was not maintained after the first course. Mean height velocity increased from 3.7 cm per year to 8.1 cm per year and was maintained at 7.4 cm per year during a mean period after stopping treatment of 0.45 years. No adverse effects were observed.— R. Stanhope and C. G. D. Brook, *Archs Dis. Childh.*, 1985, *60*, 379. Comment.— M. A. Preece (letter), *ibid.*, 783. Reply.— R. Stanhope *et al.*, *ibid.*, 784.

Preparations

Oxandrolone Tablets *(U.S.P.)*

Proprietary Names and Manufacturers

Anavar *(Searle, USA)*; Antitriol *(Spain)*; Lonavar *(Searle, Arg.; Searle, Austral.; Dainippon, Jpn)*.

9094-c

Oxymesterone *(BAN, rINN)*.

Methandrostenediolone. 4,17β-Dihydroxy-17α-methylandrost-4-en-3-one.

$C_{20}H_{30}O_3$=318.5.

CAS — 145-12-0.

Oxymesterone has anabolic and androgenic properties and has been given by mouth in doses of 10 to 40 mg daily.

Proprietary Names and Manufacturers

Anamidol *(Jpn)*; Balnimax *(Geve, Spain)*; Oranabol *(Spain)*; Oranabol 10 *(Farmitalia Carlo Erba, UK)*.

9095-k

Oxymetholone *(BAN, USAN, rINN)*.

17β-Hydroxy-2-hydroxymethylene-17α-methyl-5α-androstan-3-one.

$C_{21}H_{32}O_3$=332.5.

CAS — 434-07-1.

Pharmacopoeias. In *Br.*, *Jpn*, and *U.S.*

A white to creamy-white, odourless, crystalline powder. *B.P.* **solubilities** are: practically insoluble in water; soluble 1 in 50 of alcohol and 1 in 9 of chloroform; slightly soluble in ether. *U.S.P.* solubilities are: practically insoluble in water; soluble 1 in 40 of alcohol, 1 in 5 of chloroform, 1 in 82 of ether, and 1 in 14 of dioxan. **Protect** from light. Avoid contact with ferrous metals.

Adverse Effects

As for the androgens and anabolic steroids in general, p.1383.

Liver disturbances and jaundice are common with normal doses and hepatic neoplasms have also been reported. Oxymetholone is contra-indicated in patients with liver disturbances and it may enhance the actions of anticoagulants.

Toxic confusional state and choreiform movements in a 66-year-old man given oxymetholone.— A. Tilzey *et al.*, *Br. med. J.*, 1981, *283*, 349.

Pronounced hyperglucagonaemia in 6 patients treated with oxymetholone.— G. Williams *et al.*, *Br. med. J.*, 1986, *292*, 1637.

EFFECTS ON THE BLOOD. Leukaemia in 4 patients given oxymetholone for aplastic anaemia. A causal relationship had not been proved.— I. W. Delamore and C. G. Geary, *Br. med. J.*, 1971, *2*, 743. See also A. D. Ginsburg (letter), *Ann. intern. Med.*, 1973, *79*, 914. Of patients who present with aplastic anaemia 1 to 5% actually have leukaemia.— B. M. Camitta *et al.*, *New Engl. J. Med.*, 1982, *306*, 645.

EFFECTS ON THE LIVER. Peliosis hepatis associated with oxymetholone.— G. Groos *et al.* (letter), *Lancet*, 1974, *1*, 874; E. C. McDonald and C. E. Speicher, *J. Am. med. Ass.*, 1978, *240*, 243.

Reports of various liver tumours associated with oxymetholone: M. S. Bernstein *et al.*, *New Engl. J. Med.*, 1971, *284*, 1135; F. L. Johnson *et al.*, *Lancet*, 1972, *2*, 1273; G. C. Farrell *et al.*, *ibid.*, 1975, *1*, 430; P. P. Anthony (letter), *ibid.*, 685; M. Bruguera, *ibid.*, 1295; M. Lesna *et al.*, *ibid.*, 1976, *1*, 1124; S. T. Mokrohisky *et al.* (letter), *New Engl. J. Med.*, 1977, *296*, 1411.

Uses and Administration

Oxymetholone has anabolic and androgenic properties. It is used mainly in the treatment of anaemias such as aplastic anaemias.

The usual dosage is 1 to 5 mg per kg body-weight daily. Response may not be immediate and treatment for 3 to 6 months is suggested; maintenance dosage is often necessary. Up to 150 mg daily has been suggested as an adjunct to cytotoxic therapy and radiotherapy.

ANAEMIA. Only 5 of 21 patients with aplastic anaemia treated with oxymetholone 150 to 300 mg daily survived. One patient treated with fluoxymesterone died six months after the start of treatment. Few of the patients survived long enough to respond to oxymetholone.— S. Davis and A. D. Rubin, *Lancet*, 1972, *1*, 871.

Of 28 patients with aplastic anaemia treated with oxymetholone, 1 achieved a temporary complete remission and 10 achieved a partial response with appreciable improvement in the haemoglobin concentration and some increase in the white-cell count. Two patients who responded initially failed to respond when given oxymetholone again after brief withdrawal. Three patients developed leukaemia.— M. A. Mir and I. W. Delamore, *Postgrad. med. J.*, 1974, *50*, 166.

The survival rate in patients with aplastic anaemia treated with oxymetholone, with or without corticosteroids, was slightly but not significantly better than that earlier achieved with supportive therapy only.— M. A. Mir and C. G. Geary, *Postgrad. med. J.*, 1980, *56*, 322.

Further references: B. M. Camitta *et al.*, *Blood*, 1979, *53*, 504.

Preparations

Oxymetholone Tablets *(B.P.)*

Oxymetholone Tablets *(U.S.P.)*

Proprietary Preparations

Anapolon 50 *(Syntex, UK)*. *Tablets*, scored, oxymetholone 50 mg.

Proprietary Names and Manufacturers

Adroyd *(Parke, Davis, Austral.; Canad.; Neth.)*; Anadrol-50 *(Syntex, USA)*; Anadroyd *(Belg.)*; Anapolon *(Syntex, Austral.; Syntex, Canad.; Syntex, S.Afr.; Syntex, UK)*; Anasteron *(Syntex, Denm.; Astra-Syntex, Norw.; Syntex, Swed.)*; Anasteronal *(Spain)*; Nastenon *(Fr.)*; Oxitosona-50 *(Syntex-Latino, Spain)*; Pardroyd *(Parke, Davis, Ger.)*; Plenastril *(Grünenthal, Ger.; Grünenthal, Switz.)*; Synasteron *(Belg.)*; Zenalosyn *(Neth.)*.

9096-a

Pentagestrone Acetate *(rINNM)*.

3-Cyclopentyloxy-20-oxopregna-3,5-dien-17α-yl acetate.

$C_{28}H_{40}O_4$=440.6.

CAS — 7001-56-1 (pentagestrone); 1178-60-5 (acetate).

Uses and Administration

Pentagestrone acetate is a progestogen with actions and uses similar to those described for the progestogens in general (see p.1386).

Proprietary Names and Manufacturers

Gestovis *(Vister, Ital.)*.

9097-t

Polyestradiol Phosphate *(BAN, rINN)*.

Leo-114; Polyoestradiol Phosphate.

CAS — 28014-46-2.

A water-soluble polymeric ester of oestradiol and phosphoric acid with a molecular weight of about 26 000.

Adverse Effects and Precautions

As for the oestrogens in general, p.1384.

Uses and Administration

Polyestradiol phosphate, being a polymer of the

oestrogen oestradiol with phosphoric acid, has actions and uses similar to those described for the oestrogens in general (see p.1385).

Polyestradiol phosphate has a prolonged duration of action and may be administered by deep intramuscular injection in doses of 80 to 160 mg every 4 weeks for 2 to 3 months in the treatment of metastatic prostatic carcinoma. Doses of 40 to 80 mg every 4 weeks may be used for maintenance.

For a general review covering the actions and uses of oestrogens, see p.1385.

Proprietary Preparations

Estradurin *(Lundbeck, UK). Injection,* powder for reconstitution, polyestradiol phospate (with mepivacaine and nicotinamide) 40 and 80 mg.

Proprietary Names and Manufacturers

Estradurin *(Ayerst, Austral.; Lundbeck, Denm.; Pharmacia Arzneimittel, Ger.; Parke, Davis, Ital.; Neth.; S.Afr.; Abello, Spain; Lundbeck, UK; Ayerst, USA).*

9036-g

Prasterone *(rINN).*

Dehydroepiandrosterone; Dehydroisoandrosterone. 3β-Hydroxyandrost-5-en-17-one.

$C_{19}H_{28}O_2$=288.4.

CAS — 53-43-0.

Prasterone is a naturally occurring but relatively weak androgen. It has been given by intramuscular injection.

Proprietary Names and Manufacturers

17-Chetovis *(Vister, Ital.)*; Astenile *(Recordati, Ital.)*; Deandros *(Ital.)*; Diandrone *(Organon, UK)*; Mentalormon *(SIT, Ital.).*

9098-x

Progesterone *(BAN, USAN, rINN).*

Luteal Hormone; Luteine; NSC-9704; Pregnenedione; Progesteronum; Progestin. Pregn-4-ene-3,20-dione.

$C_{21}H_{30}O_2$=314.5.

CAS — 57-83-0.

Pharmacopoeias. In *Arg., Aust., Belg., Br., Braz., Chin., Cz., Egypt., Eur., Fr., Ger., Hung., Int., It., Jpn, Jug., Mex., Neth., Nord., Pol., Port., Roum., Rus., Span., Swiss, Turk.,* and *U.S.* Also in *B.P. Vet.*

Colourless crystals or a white or slightly yellowish-white, odourless, crystalline powder. *B.P.* **solubilities** are: practically insoluble in water; soluble 1 in 8 of alcohol and 1 in less than 1 of chloroform; sparingly soluble in acetone, dioxan, ether, and fatty oils. *U.S.P.* solubilities are: practically insoluble in water; soluble in alcohol, acetone, and dioxan; sparingly soluble in vegetable oils. **Store** in airtight containers. Protect from light. Oily solutions for injection are **sterilised** by dry heat.

Adverse Effects and Precautions

As for the progestogens in general, p.1386.

ALLERGY. A report of a patient with progesterone sensitivity causing recurrent anaphylaxis.— W. J. Meggs *et al., New Engl. J. Med.,* 1984, *311,* 1236.

PORPHYRIA. Progesterone was considered to be unsafe in patients with acute porphyria as it has been associated with acute attacks.— M.R. Moore and K.E.L. McColl, *Porphyrias, Drug Lists,* Glasgow, Porphyria Research Unit, University of Glasgow, 1987.

Absorption and Fate

Progesterone is absorbed from the gastro-intestinal tract; it has been believed that it is rapidly inactivated in the liver thus producing little biological effect when administered by mouth but some recent studies have suggested that it may in fact be active after oral administration. It is absorbed when administered buccally, rectally, or vaginally, and rapidly absorbed from the site of an oily intramuscular injection. The half-life in blood is only a few minutes. It is metabolised in the liver, about 12% to pregnanediol which is excreted in the urine conjugated with glucuronic acid.

In 5 postmenopausal women given progesterone 100 mg by mouth daily for 5 days peak concentrations were present 1 to 3 hours after the last dose. Among the metabolites the concentration of pregnanediol-3α-glucuronide was most elevated, that of 17-hydroxyprogesterone least elevated, and that of 20α-dihydroprogesterone was intermediate. The concentrations of oestradiol were not significantly affected. Progesterone by mouth might be of value when synthetic progestogens had caused adverse effects.— M. I. Whitehead *et al., Br. med. J.,* 1980, *280,* 825.

Uses and Administration

Progesterone is a natural progestogen with actions and uses similar to those described for the progestogens in general (see p.1386).

It is usually administered as an oily intramuscular injection or as pessaries or suppositories. In dysfunctional uterine bleeding 5 to 10 mg daily is normally given by intramuscular injection for about 5 to 10 days before the anticipated onset of menstruation. Intramuscular injection in doses of 10 to 20 mg twice weekly has also been used for habitual abortion. Intramuscular daily doses of 50 mg for nulliparous women and 100 mg for parous women have been used in the management of the premenstrual syndrome starting at about the twelfth day of the menstrual cycle and continuing until the onset of menstruation. Progesterone has also been given vaginally or rectally in doses of 200 mg daily to 400 mg twice daily in a similar schedule for the premenstrual syndrome.

Progesterone has also been incorporated into an intra-uterine device for female contraception.

Preparations

Progesterone Injection *(B.P.).* A sterile solution of progesterone in ethyl oleate or other suitable ester, in a suitable fixed oil, or in any mixture of these. For intramuscular injection only.

Progesterone Injection *(U.S.P.)*

Progesterone Intrauterine Contraceptive System *(U.S.P.)*

Sterile Progesterone Suspension *(U.S.P.)*

Proprietary Preparations

Cyclogest *(Cox, UK). Suppositories,* progesterone 200 or 400 mg; for rectal or vaginal use.

Gestone *(Paines & Byrne, UK). Injection,* progesterone 10 mg/mL, in ampoules of 1 mL.

Injection, progesterone 25 mg/mL, in ampoules of 1 mL.

Injection, progesterone 50 mg/mL, in ampoules of 1 and 2 mL.

Progesterone Implants *(Organon, UK). Implants,* progesterone 50 and 100 mg.

Proprietary Names and Manufacturers

BayProgest *(Bay, USA)*; Biograviplan Progestasert *(Grünenthal, Ger.)*; Colprosterone *(Inibsa, Spain)*; Corlutina *(Arg.)*; Cutifitol *(Llorente, Spain)*; Cyclogest *(Cox, UK)*; Gesterol *(Stickley, Canad.)*; Gesterol 50 *(Forest Pharmaceuticals, USA)*; Gestone *(Paines & Byrne, UK)*; Gestone *(Samil, Ital.)*; Lutocyclin *(Switz.)*; Lutogyl *(Fr.)*; Oophormin Luteum *(Jpn)*; Progelun *(Ital.)*; Progestasert *(Recordati, Ital.; NZ; Polcrome, UK; Alza, USA)*; Progesterone Implants *(Organon, UK)*; Progestilin *(Canad.)*; Progestin *(Austral.)*; Progestine *(Neth.)*; Progestogel *(Besins-Iscovesco, Fr.; Nourypharma, Ger.; Lusofarmaco, Ital.; Seid, Spain; Golaz, Switz.)*; Progestol *(Bruco, Ital.)*; Progestolo *(Ital.)*; Progestosol *(Besins-Iscovesco, Fr.; Seid, Spain; Besins-Iscovesco, Switz.)*; Proluton *(Arg.; Schering, Austral.; Schering, Ital.; Spain)*; Utrogestan *(Besins-Iscovesco, Fr.; Golaz, Switz.).*

The following names have been used for multi-ingredient preparations containing progesterone—Paralut Injection *(Wallace Mfg Chem., UK).*

3871-c

Promegestone *(rINN).*

17α-Methyl-17-propionylestra-4,9-dien-3-one.

$C_{22}H_{30}O_2$=326.5.

CAS — 34184-77-5.

Adverse Effects and Precautions

As for the progestogens in general, p.1386.

Uses and Administration

Promegestone is a progestogen with actions and uses similar to those described for the progestogens in general (see p.1386). It is given by mouth in doses of 125 to 500 μg daily.

Proprietary Names and Manufacturers

Surgestone *(Cassenne, Fr.).*

13176-s

Promestriene *(rINN).*

17β-Methoxy-3-propoxyestra-1,3,5(10)-triene.

$C_{22}H_{32}O_2$=328.5.

CAS — 39219-28-8.

Promestriene has been used topically in vulvo-vaginal conditions such as atrophic vaginitis and in seborrhoea.

Proprietary Names and Manufacturers

Colpotrofin *(Spain)*; Colpotrophine *(Théramex, Fr.; Biochimica, Switz.)*; Délipoderm *(Théramex, Fr.; Reig Jofré, Spain).*

9099-r

Promethoestrol Dipropionate *(BANM).*

Dimethylhexestrol Dipropionate; Methestrol Dipropionate *(rINNM)*; Methoestrol Dipropionate. 4,4′-(1,2-Diethylethylene)di(*o*-tolyl propionate).

$C_{26}H_{34}O_4$=410.6.

CAS — 130-73-4 (promethoestrol); 84-13-9 (dipropionate).

Promethoestrol dipropionate is a synthetic oestrogen with properties similar to those described for the oestrogens in general (see p.1384). It was formerly given by mouth.

For a general review covering the actions and uses of oestrogens, see p.1385.

Proprietary Names and Manufacturers

Meprane Dipropionate *(Reed & Carnrick, USA).*

13198-z

Quinbolone *(USAN, rINN).*

17β-(Cyclopent-1-enyloxy)androsta-1,4-dien-3-one.

$C_{24}H_{32}O_2$=352.5.

CAS — 2487-63-0.

Quinbolone has anabolic properties and has been given in doses of up to 30 mg daily by mouth.

9100-r

Quinestradol *(BAN, rINN).*

Oestriol 3-Cyclopentyl Ether. 3-Cyclopentyloxyestra-1,3,5(10)-triene-16α,17β-diol.

$C_{23}H_{32}O_3$=356.5.

CAS — 1169-79-5.

Adverse Effects and Precautions

As for the oestrogens in general, p.1384.

Uses and Administration

Quinestradol is a synthetic oestrogen with actions and uses similar to those described for the oestrogens in general (see p.1385). It is claimed to have relatively less activity on breast and endometrial tissue than on the vagina.

Quinestradol has been given by mouth for the treatment

of menopausal and postmenopausal symptoms in a dosage of 500 μg twice daily.

For a general review covering the actions and uses of oestrogens, see p.1385.

Proprietary Names and Manufacturers
Colpovis *(SIT, Ital.; S.Afr.)*; Colpovister *(Spain)*; Pentovis *(Warner, UK)*.

9101-f

Quinestrol *(BAN, USAN, rINN)*.
Ethinyloestradiol-3-cyclopentyl Ether; W-3566. 3-Cyclopentyloxy-19-nor-17α-pregna-1,3,5(10)-trien-20-yn-17β-ol.
$C_{25}H_{32}O_2$=364.5.

CAS — 152-43-2.

Pharmacopoeias. In *U.S.*

A white practically odourless powder. Practically **insoluble** in water; soluble in alcohol, chloroform, and ether.

Adverse Effects and Precautions
As for the oestrogens in general, p.1384.

ALLERGY. A 30-year-old woman developed an allergic reaction, with urticaria, slight dyspnoea, and oedema, following a single dose of quinestrol by mouth D. A. Aitken and E. G. Daw (letter), *Br. med. J.*, 1970, *2*, 177.

Absorption and Fate
Quinestrol is absorbed from the gastro-intestinal tract and is stored in body fat. It is slowly released over several days and metabolised to ethinyloestradiol which is excreted in the urine.

Uses and Administration
Quinestrol is a synthetic oestrogen with actions and uses similar to those described for the oestrogens in general (see p.1385). It has a prolonged duration of action.
Quinestrol is given by mouth for the treatment of menopausal and postmenopausal symptoms; the usual initial dose is 100 μg daily for 7 days followed by maintenance doses of 100 to 200 μg weekly.
Quinestrol has also been used, like many other oestrogens, for the suppression of lactation.

For a general review covering the actions and uses of oestrogen, see p.1385.

Preparations
Quinestrol Tablets *(U.S.P.)*

Proprietary Names and Manufacturers
Agalacto-Quilea *(Arg.)*; Basaquines *(Arg.)*; Eston *(Arg.)*; Estrovis *(Belg.; Gödecke, Ger.; Ital.; Neth.; Warner, S.Afr.; Warner, UK; Parke, Davis, USA)*; Qui-Lea *(Arg.)*.

The following names have been used for multi-ingredient preparations containing quinestrol—Soluna *(Elea, Arg.)*.

9102-d

Quingestanol Acetate *(BANM, USAN, rINNM)*.
W-4540. 3-(Cyclopentyloxy)-19-nor-17α-pregna-3,5-dien-20-yn-17-ol acetate.
$C_{27}H_{36}O_3$=408.6.

CAS — 10592-65-1 (quingestanol); 3000-39-3 (acetate).

Quingestanol acetate is a progestogen with actions and uses similar to those described for the progestogens in general (see p.1386).

Proprietary Names and Manufacturers
Demovis *(Vister, Ital.)*; Pilomin *(Apothekernes Laboratorium, Norw.; A.L., Swed.)*.

The following names have been used for multi-ingredient preparations containing quingestanol acetate— Piloval *(Apothekernes Laboratorium, Norw.; A.L., Swed.)*; Rélovis *(Substantia, Fr.)*.

9103-n

Stanolone *(BAN)*.
Androstanolone *(rINN)*; Dihydrotestosterone. 17β-Hydroxy-5α-androstan-3-one.
$C_{19}H_{30}O_2$=290.4.

CAS — 521-18-6.

Stanolone has anabolic and androgenic properties and has been given by mouth, preferably sublingually or sublabially in doses of 50 to 75 mg daily.

Proprietary Names and Manufacturers
Anabolex *(Samil, Ital.; Lloyd-Hamol, Reckitt & Colman Pharm., UK)*; Andractim *(Besins-Iscovesco, Fr.)*; Pesomax *(Boniscontro & Gazzone, Ital.)*.

9104-h

Stanozolol *(BAN, USAN, rINN)*.
Androstanazole; Methylstanazole; Win-14833. 17α-Methyl-2′*H*-5α-androst-2-eno[3,2-c]-pyrazol-17β-ol.
$C_{21}H_{32}N_2O$=328.5.

CAS — 10418-03-8.

Pharmacopoeias. In *Br., It.*, and *U.S.*

A white or almost white, odourless crystalline powder. There are 2 forms; needles melt at about 155° and prisms at about 235°. Practically **insoluble** in water; soluble 1 in 41 of alcohol, 1 in 74 of chloroform, and 1 in 370 of ether; soluble in dimethylformamide; slightly soluble in acetone and ethyl acetate. **Store** in airtight containers. Protect from light.

Adverse Effects and Precautions
As for the androgens and anabolic steroids in general, p.1383.
Stanozolol, given for prolonged periods, may cause jaundice and should be used with caution in patients with liver disturbances.

Masculinisation, characterised by loss of scalp hair, deepening of the voice, and hirsutism, in an elderly woman receiving stanozolol.— H. J. Dodd and I. Sarkany, *Br. med. J.*, 1985, *290*, 30.

EFFECTS ON THE LIVER. A 66-year-old man developed jaundice after treatment for 7 months with stanozolol 10 mg daily. The histological appearance of the liver suggested cholestatic jaundice of the hypersensitivity type. The condition regressed when stanozolol was withdrawn.— S. D. Slater *et al.*, *Postgrad. med. J.*, 1976, *52*, 229.

A further report of severe cholestatic jaundice in 3 patients associated with the use of stanozolol.— R. S. Evely *et al.*, *Br. med. J.*, 1987, *294*, 612.

INTERACTIONS. For the effect of stanozolol on some anticoagulants, see under warfarin sodium (p.347).

PORPHYRIA. A study in *rats* and in healthy men demonstrating that stanozolol has a porphyrinogenic effect.— G. G. Thompson *et al.*, *Eur. J. clin. Pharmac.*, 1984, *26*, 587.

Uses and Administration
Stanozolol has anabolic and androgenic properties. Suggested doses of stanozolol have been: for vascular disorders including the treatment of the complications of deep-vein thrombosis, prevention of deep-vein thrombosis, and the control of Raynaud's phenomenon in patients with systemic sclerosis, 10 mg daily by mouth; for hereditary angioedema 2.5 to 10 mg daily by mouth initially with reduced dosage for maintenance; for postmenopausal osteoporosis, 5 mg daily by mouth; for use as an anabolic following debilitating illness, 5 mg daily by mouth. Stanozolol has also been given by intramuscular injection in doses of 50 mg every 2 or 3 weeks.

ANGIOEDEMA. A 31-year-old man with a 13-year history of severe abdominal manifestations of angioedema and a 3-year history of cutaneous manifestations obtained complete relief of all abdominal and cutaneous symptoms following administration of stanozolol 5 mg twice daily.— D. J. Gould *et al.* (letter), *Lancet*, 1978, *1*, 770.

VASCULAR DISORDERS. A brief review of published clinical studies did not support the claims that stanozolol is beneficial in the prevention or treatment of venous ulceration.— *Drug & Ther. Bull.*, 1985, *23*, 91. Severe criticism and disagreement.— N. L. Browse and K. G. Burnand (letter), *Br. med. J.*, 1986, *292*, 825. Reply.— A. Herxheimer (letter), *ibid.*, 1014.

Preliminary observations showed that treatment for up to 2½ years with inositol nicotinate 1 g three times daily used alone or following treatment with stanozolol caused improvement in 16 patients with necrobiosis lipoidica and cleared 2 other patients; of 3 further patients given stanozolol alone, 1 found no effect and 2 some improvement.— E. L. Rhodes, *Br. J. Derm.*, 1976, *95*, 673. In 14 patients with long-standing liposclerosis of the leg, fibrinolytic activity was increased by treatment with stanozolol 5 mg twice daily; the mean area of liposclerosis was reduced by 73%, pain was reduced, the skin became softer, and pigmentation less obvious. Five patients had been cured and 9 continued to improve. Six patients suffered intermittent cramp and 3 recurrence of migraine.— N. L. Browse *et al.*, *Br. med. J.*, 1977, *2*, 434. In a double-blind crossover study in 34 legs of 23 patients with longstanding liposclerosis the mean area of healing under treatment with stanozolol 5 mg twice daily and elastic stockings was 155 mm^2 compared with 78 mm^2 under treatment with placebo and elastic stockings. While the difference was not statistically significant it was considered biologically important. Most patients considered they had improvement in respect of pain, heat, colour, and induration. Continued treatment had led to loss of induration and regression of pigmentation. Such treatment was considered useful in intractable cases.— K. Burnand *et al.*, *Br. med. J.*, 1980, *280*, 7. Criticism.— H. L. Muston (letter), *Br. med. J.*, 1980, *280*, 254.

Of 16 men with idiopathic recurrent superficial thrombophlebitis and who had on average one severe attack every 8 weeks for 7.7 years, 15 had evidence of decreased fibrinolytic activity. After treatment for 6 months with stanozolol 5 mg twice daily, thrombophlebitis had ceased in 13 patients and ceased in the remaining 3 after longer treatment. Thrombophlebitis had not recurred in 11 for a mean of 12.5 months (range 3 to 24 months).— P. E. M. Jarrett *et al.*, *Br. med. J.*, 1977, *1*, 933.

In 16 patients with severe Raynaud's syndrome and who had already undergone sympathectomy, hand blood flow, palm and index-finger temperature, and grip strength were significantly increased, and plasma-fibrinogen concentrations significantly decreased after treatment for 3 months with stanozolol 5 mg twice daily. Most patients experienced subjective improvement. Three-month courses of stanozolol, repeated after periods of 1 or 2 months, were recommended for patients in whom all other treatments had failed.— P. E. M. Jarrett *et al.*, *Br. med. J.*, 1978, *2*, 523.

Preparations
Stanozolol Tablets *(B.P.)*
Stanozolol Tablets *(U.S.P.)*

Proprietary Preparations
Stromba *(Sterling Research, UK)*. *Tablets*, scored, stanozolol 5 mg.
Injection, stanozolol 50 mg/mL, in ampoules of 1 mL.

Proprietary Names and Manufacturers
Anasyth *(Ital.)*; Stromba *(Aust.; Belg.; Winthrop, Denm.; Fin.; Fr.; Winthrop, Ger.; Neth.; Winthrop, Norw.; Sterling-Winthrop, Swed.; Winthrop, Switz.; Sterling Research, UK)*; Strombaject *(Belg.; Fr.; Winthrop, Ger.)*; Winstrol *(Winthrop, Canad.; Zambon, Ital.; S.Afr.; Zambon, Spain; Winthrop-Breon, USA)*.

13268-y

Stenbolone Acetate *(USAN, rINNM)*.
17β-Hydroxy-2-methyl-5α-androst-1-en-3-one acetate.
$C_{22}H_{32}O_3$=344.5.

CAS — 5197-58-0 (stenbolone); 1242-56-4 (acetate).

Stenbolone acetate has been used as an anabolic agent.

Proprietary Names and Manufacturers
Stenobolone *(Spain)*.

9106-b

Stilboestrol *(BAN).*

Diethylstilbestrol *(USAN, rINN)*; Diethylstilbestrolum; Diethylstilboestrol; NSC-3070. *(E)*-αβ-Diethylstilbene-4-4′-diol.

$C_{18}H_{20}O_2$=268.4.

CAS — 56-53-1.

Pharmacopoeias. In *Aust., Belg., Br., Chin., Cz., Egypt., Eur., Fr., Ger., Ind., Int., Jug., Mex., Neth., Nord., Port., Roum., Rus., Swiss, Turk.,* and *U.S.*

A white or almost white, odourless, crystalline powder. Practically **insoluble** in water; soluble 1 in 5 of alcohol, 1 in 3 of ether, 1 in 40 of arachis oil, and 1 in 90 of olive oil; slightly soluble in chloroform; soluble in fatty oils and aqueous solutions of alkali hydroxides. **Store** in airtight containers. Protect from light.

CAUTION. *Stilboestrol is a powerful oestrogen. Contact with the skin or inhalation should be avoided. Rubber gloves and a face mask should be worn when handling the powder.*

9105-m

Stilboestrol Dipropionate *(BANM).*

Diethylstilbestrol Dipropionate *(rINNM)*. *(E)*-αβ-Diethylstilbene-4,4′-diol dipropionate.

$C_{24}H_{28}O_4$=380.5.

CAS — 130-80-3.

Pharmacopoeias. In *Aust., Cz., Jug., Pol.,* and *Rus.*

Adverse Effects

As for the oestrogens in general, p.1384.

An increased incidence of changes in the cervix and vagina including adenosis and adenocarcinoma has been noted, particularly in the USA, in the postpubertal daughters of women who received stilboestrol or related substances during pregnancy. An increased incidence of abnormalities of the genital tract and of abnormal spermatozoa has been reported in males similarly exposed.

EFFECTS ON THE BLOOD. Severe bone-marrow changes occurred in a 71-year-old man given stilboestrol in a dose of 150 mg daily for 7 years.— A. L. Anderson and E. C. Lynch, *Archs intern. Med.*, 1980, *140*, 976.

MALIGNANT NEOPLASMS. Hepatic angiosarcoma developed in a 76-year-old man who had received stilboestrol 3 mg daily for 12 years.— C. Hoch-Ligeti, *J. Am. med. Ass.*, 1978, *240*, 1510. See also: J. J. Brooks, *J. Urol., Baltimore*, 1982, *128*, 1044 (hepatoma).

Renal carcinoma associated with the use of stilboestrol in 2 men.— I. Nissenkorn *et al., Br. J. Urol.*, 1979, *51*, 6.

See also below under Pregnancy and the Neonate.

PORPHYRIA. Porphyria cutanea tarda developed in 2 patients, each receiving stilboestrol 5 mg daily for prostatic carcinoma. Symptoms regressed on withdrawal of the stilboestrol.— J. T. Vail, *J. Am. med. Ass.*, 1967, *201*, 671.

PREGNANCY AND THE NEONATE. A review of vaginal adenosis and its association with maternal stilboestrol ingestion during pregnancy. The link between stilboestrol and particularly the benign changes in the vagina and cervix (adenosis) seems well established. The association between this drug and the development of genital malignancies is less clear, and the very low incidence in the prospective studies in the *USA* supports this concept. The size of the problem in the *UK* is small, but clinicians should be aware that it exists. Cases of vaginal adenosis in young women should be investigated and screened appropriately, and preferably referred to centres where colposcopic expertise is available. Treatment of simple vaginal adenosis should be avoided.— M. Emens, *Br. J. Hosp. Med.*, 1984, *31*, 42.

A controlled study was carried out on the female offspring, aged 18 years or older, of mothers who had received stilboestrol at some time during their pregnancy. Of the 110 exposed women, 22% had transverse fibrous ridges of the vagina and cervix, compared with none in the 82 controls; in 56% of the exposed, portions of the vaginal mucosa failed to stain with iodine compared with 1%; and in 35% of the exposed, vaginal adenosis was present compared with 1% in the controls. In an uncontrolled study of exposed females vaginal adenosis was more frequent in those whose mothers had taken stilboestrol early in pregnancy and was not detected at all in those where stilboestrol was started in the 18th week or later. There was also a lower incidence of vaginal adenosis in those offspring who had used oral contraceptives.— A. L. Herbst *et al., New Engl. J. Med.*, 1975, *292*, 334.

The Professional and Public Relations Committee of the DESAD (Diethylstilboestrol and Adenosis) Project of the Division of Cancer Control and Rehabilitation reported that of nearly 300 young females with clear-cell adenocarcinoma of the genital tract, more than 80% had been exposed *in utero* to stilboestrol-type hormones. Patients had been aged 7 to 28 years at the time of diagnosis. Doses and duration of treatment varied widely; 1.5 mg of stilboestrol daily throughout pregnancy or varying amounts for a week or more during the first trimester had shown an association. Vaginal adenosis, rare in unexposed young women, was present in about a third of those exposed in the first 4 months of pregnancy, and cervical ectropion in more than two-thirds.— *J. Am. med. Ass.*, 1976, *236*, 1107. Of 3339 women entered into the DESAD project 1340 were identified by review of their records and were considered the best population on which inferences of the effects of stilboestrol should be based; the incidence of vaginal epithelial changes was 34% in this group compared with 59 or 65% in referred (or similar) groups. From analysis of the data on 298 women for whom complete records were available, vaginal epithelial changes were most closely associated with early exposure to stilboestrol, with the total dose, and with the duration of exposure; their incidence decreased with age. No severe dysplasia or carcinoma was found in the record-review group; the risk of cancer in the first 25 years after exposure was small.— P. C. O'Brien *et al., Obstet. Gynec.*, 1979, *53*, 300. Preliminary findings on fertility and outcome of pregnancy in a subgroup of women enrolled in the DESAD Project; 618 women who had been exposed *in utero* to stilboestrol were compared with 618 control subjects. There was no difference in fertility between the 2 groups when measured in terms of pregnancies achieved. An increased risk of unfavourable outcome of pregnancy was seen in 220 women exposed prenatally to stilboestrol compared with 224 control subjects; the relative risk was 1.69. However, of the women who became pregnant, 81% of those exposed to stilboestrol and 95% of control subjects had at least one full-term live birth.— A. B. Barnes *et al., New Engl. J. Med.*, 1980, *302*, 609.

On the assumption that 1 to 10% of pregnant women in the USA were exposed to stilboestrol in 1951 to 1953 it was estimated that the risk of clear-cell adenocarcinoma of the vagina and cervix in offspring was 0.14 to 1.4 per thousand.— A. L. Herbst *et al., Am. J. Obstet. Gynec.*, 1977, *128*, 43.

Of 46 women with documented exposure *in utero* to stilboestrol and 14 with probable exposure 40 had radiological evidence of changes in the uterus; in 36 the cervix showed gross anatomic changes. Of 20 with a normal uterus 4 had gross abnormal changes in the cervix. It was too early to evaluate the clinical significance of the findings.— R. H. Kaufman *et al., Am. J. Obstet. Gynec.*, 1977, *128*, 51.

In 199 women with probable exposure *in utero* to stilboestrol (confirmed in 180) abnormalities of the vagina and/or cervix (assessed colposcopically) were present in 86.4%. Vaginal adenosis was present in 14.1% (or 45.2% if a more liberal definition of the vagina was used). Grade 1 cervical intra-epithelial neoplasia was present in 36 women and grade 3 neoplasia in 8; the risk of neoplasia in stilboestrol-exposed women was 4.4 to 13.3 times that in non-exposed women. There was no case of clear-cell adenocarcinoma.— W. C. Fowler and D. A. Edelman, *Obstet. Gynec.*, 1978, *51*, 459.

Development of clear-cell adenocarcinoma in a young woman after earlier negative examination emphasised the need for regular screening in women exposed *in utero* to stilboestrol.— B. Anderson *et al., Obstet. Gynec.*, 1979, *53*, 293.

A further report from the DESAD project. The incidence-rate for dysplasia and carcinoma *in situ* of the cervix and vagina was significantly higher in the women exposed to stilboestrol than in those not exposed in the matched control group.— S. J. Robboy *et al., J. Am. med. Ass.*, 1984, *252*, 2979. Criticism.— R. M. Richart (letter), *ibid.*, 1986, *255*, 36. Reply.— S. J. Robboy *et al.* (letter), *ibid.*, 37.

A review of 519 cases of clear-cell adenocarcinoma of the vagina and cervix revealed that in 60% of all cases the patient's mother had received stilboestrol during pregnancy. The risk that the clear-cell adenocarcinoma will develop in an exposed female from birth to the age of 34 years is 1 case per 1000 women. The rarity of the tumour suggests that stilboestrol is not a complete carcinogen but that some other factor is also involved.— S. Melnick *et al., New Engl. J. Med.*, 1987, *316*, 514.

Further references: K. L. Noller *et al., Am. J. Obstet. Gynec.*, 1983, *146*, 279; R. H. Kaufman *et al., ibid.*, 1986, *154*, 1312.

Effects on the male foetus. A report of hypogonadism and anosmia in a 17-year-old boy whose mother had taken stilboestrol during pregnancy.— D. Hoefnagel (letter), *Lancet*, 1976, *1*, 152.

Problems in passing urine and abnormalities of the penile urethra were significantly more common in young males exposed *in utero* to stilboestrol than in controls.— B. E. Henderson *et al., Pediatrics*, 1976, *58*, 505.

No cancer had been reported in the male offspring of women given synthetic hormones during pregnancy, but genital tract abnormalities (cysts of the epididymis, capsular induration, defective testicles) occurred in 41 of 163 exposed men compared with 11 of 168 controls. Sperm counts and motility were reduced.— *J. Am. med. Ass.*, 1977, *238*, 932.

In 308 males exposed *in utero* to stilboestrol the incidence of epididymal cysts was 20.8% compared with 4.9% in controls, and that of testicular hypoplasia was 8.4% compared with 1.9%. The incidence of severely pathological semen was increased.— W. B. Gill *et al., J. Urol., Baltimore*, 1979, *122*, 36.

A report of seminoma and epididymal cysts in a young man with known stilboestrol exposure *in utero*.— G. R. Conley *et al., J. Am. med. Ass.*, 1983, *249*, 1325.

A study involving 828 men exposed to stilboestrol *in utero* and 676 control men did not suggest that overall stilboestrol exposure resulted in an increased risk of genito-urinary abnormalities, infertility, or testicular cancer. Previously reported increased frequencies of these abnormalities may have resulted from a selection bias, from a difference in stilboestrol usage, or from both.— F. J. Leary *et al., J. Am. med. Ass.*, 1984, *252*, 2984.

Further references: M. D. Cosgrove *et al., J. Urol., Baltimore*, 1977, *117*, 220; W. B. Gill *et al., ibid.*, 477.

Precautions

As for the oestrogens in general, p.1385.

INTERACTIONS. A report of pseudocholinesterase deficiency and prolonged respiratory insufficiency after suxamethonium in a 78-year-old man. The deficiency appeared to be related to stilboestrol therapy; liver disease might have been a contributory factor.— T. L. Archer and E. C. Janowsky, *Anesth. Analg. curr. Res.*, 1978, *57*, 726.

Absorption and Fate

Stilboestrol is readily absorbed from the gastro-intestinal tract. It is slowly inactivated in the liver and excreted in the urine and faeces.

Uses and Administration

Stilboestrol is a non-steroidal synthetic oestrogen with actions and uses similar to those described for the oestrogens in general (see p.1385).

Stilboestrol is administered by mouth and has also been administered in pessaries.

Daily doses of 10 to 20 mg are used by mouth in the palliative treatment of malignant neoplasms of the breast. The usual dose in carcinoma of the prostate is 1 to 3 mg daily; higher doses were formerly given. Stilboestrol has been used as pessaries at a dose of up to 1 mg daily in the management of menopausal and postmenopausal vaginal disorders.

Stilboestrol has been given to *domestic animals* for growth-promoting purposes; this practice is controversial and in some countries has been banned.

For a general review covering the actions and uses of oestrogens, see p.1385.

Preparations

Diethylstilbestrol Injection *(U.S.P.)*. A sterile solution of stilboestrol in a suitable vegetable oil.

Diethylstilbestrol Suppositories *(U.S.P.)*. Suppositories [pessaries] containing stilboestrol.

Diethylstilbestrol Tablets *(U.S.P.)*. Tablets containing stilboestrol.

Stilboestrol Pessaries *(B.P.)*. Diethylstilbestrol Pessaries.

Stilboestrol Pessaries *(A.P.F.)*. Pessaries containing stilboestrol 500 μg.

Stilboestrol Tablets *(B.P.)*. Diethylstilbestrol Tablets

Proprietary Preparations

APS Stilboestrol *(Approved Prescription Services, UK)*. *Tablets*, stilboestrol 1 and 5 mg.

Tampovagan Stilboestrol and Lactic Acid *(Norgine, UK)*. *Pessaries*, stilboestrol 500 µg, lactic acid 5%.

Proprietary Names and Manufacturers of Stilboestrol and its Esters

APS Stilboestrol *(Approved Prescription Services, UK)*; Cyren-A *(Ger.)*; Desma *(USA)*; Dicorvin *(USA)*; Distilbene *(Belg.; Gerbiol, Fr.)*; Estilbin *(Denm.)*; Oestros *(Fuchs, Switz.)*; Oestrostilben *(Streuli, Switz.)*; Pabestrol *(Paines & Byrne, UK)*; Stibilium *(Canad.)*; Stilbocream *(Ford, Austral.)*; Stilbol *(Swed.)*.

The following names have been used for multi-ingredient preparations containing stilboestrol and its esters—Tampovagan Stilboestrol and Lactic Acid *(Norgine, Austral.; Norgine, UK)*; Tylosterone *(Lilly, USA)*.

9107-v

Testolactone *(USAN, rINN)*.

1-Dehydrotestololactone; NSC-23759; SQ-9538. D-Homo-17a-oxa-androsta-1,4-diene-3,17-dione.

$C_{19}H_{24}O_3$=300.4.

CAS — 968-93-4.

Pharmacopoeias. In *U.S.*

A white to off-white, practically odourless, crystalline powder.

Soluble 1 in 4050 of water; soluble in alcohol and chloroform; slightly soluble in benzyl alcohol; practically insoluble in ether and petroleum spirit. **Store** in airtight containers.

Testolactone is a derivative of testosterone (see below) and it has been used in the palliative treatment of malignant neoplasms of the breast in postmenopausal women. It has no significant androgenic activity.

The usual dose is 250 mg four times daily by mouth.

A report of encouraging results using testolactone in the treatment of 5 girls with precocious puberty due to the McCune-Albright syndrome. Testolactone was given by mouth in an initial dose of 20 mg per kg body-weight daily in four divided doses increased over 3 weeks to a maximum of 40 mg per kg daily. Testolactone blocked the synthesis of oestrogens by virtue of its being an aromatase inhibitor.— P. P. Feuillan *et al.*,, *New Engl. J. Med.*, 1986, *315*, 1115.

Preparations

Sterile Testolactone Suspension *(U.S.P.)*

Testolactone Tablets *(U.S.P.)*

Proprietary Names and Manufacturers

Fludestrin *(Heyden, Ger.)*; Teslac *(Byk Liprandi, Arg.; Squibb, Belg.; Squibb, Canad.; Squibb, Ital.; Squibb, USA)*.

9108-g

Testosterone *(BAN, USAN, rINN)*.

17β-Hydroxyandrost-4-en-3-one.

$C_{19}H_{28}O_2$=288.4.

CAS — 58-22-0.

Pharmacopoeias. In *Arg., Aust., Br., Braz., Mex., Roum., Span., Swiss,* and *U.S.* Also in *B.P. Vet.*

White or creamy-white, odourless or almost odourless, crystals or crystalline powder. Practically **insoluble** in water; soluble 1 in 5 of alcohol, 1 in 6 of dehydrated alcohol, 1 in 2 of chloroform, 1 in 100 of ether; slightly soluble in ethyl oleate; soluble in dioxan and vegetable oils. **Protect** from light.

9109-q

Testosterone Acetate *(BANM, rINNM)*.

3-Oxoandrost-4-en-17β-yl acetate.

$C_{21}H_{30}O_3$=330.5.

CAS — 1045-69-8.

Pharmacopoeias. In *Braz.* and *Fr.*

9110-d

Testosterone Cypionate *(BANM, USAN)*.

Testosterone Cipionate *(rINNM)*; Testosterone Cyclopentylpropionate. 3-Oxoandrost-4-en-17β-yl 3-cyclopentylpropionate.

$C_{27}H_{40}O_3$=412.6.

CAS — 58-20-8.

Pharmacopoeias. In *U.S.*

A white or creamy-white, crystalline powder, odourless or with a slight odour. Practically **insoluble** in water; freely soluble in alcohol, chloroform, dioxan, and ether; soluble in vegetable oils. **Protect** from light.

9111-n

Testosterone Decanoate *(BANM, rINNM)*.

3-Oxoandrost-4-en-17β-yl decanoate.

$C_{29}H_{46}O_3$=442.7.

CAS — 5721-91-5.

Pharmacopoeias. In *Br.*

White or creamy-white crystals or crystalline powder. Practically **insoluble** in water; very soluble in alcohol and chloroform. **Store** at a temperature not exceeding 15°. Protect from light.

9112-h

Testosterone Enanthate *(BANM, USAN)*.

Testosterone Enantate *(rINNM)*; Testosterone Heptanoate. 3-Oxoandrost-4-en-17β-yl heptanoate.

$C_{26}H_{40}O_3$=400.6.

CAS — 315-37-7.

Pharmacopoeias. In *Br., Braz., Jpn,* and *U.S.*

A white or creamy-white crystalline powder. It is odourless or has a faint odour characteristic of heptanoic acid. Practically **insoluble** in water; very soluble in ether; freely soluble in fatty oils. **Store** at a temperature not exceeding 15°. Protect from light.

9113-m

Testosterone Isocaproate *(BANM, rINNM)*.

Testosterone Isohexanoate. 3-Oxoandrost-4-en-17β-yl 4-methylpentanoate.

$C_{25}H_{38}O_3$=386.6.

CAS — 15262-86-9.

Pharmacopoeias. In *Br.*

White to creamy-white crystals or crystalline powder. Practically **insoluble** in water; very soluble in alcohol and chloroform. **Store** at a temperature not exceeding 15°. Protect from light.

9114-b

Testosterone Phenylpropionate *(BANM, rINNM)*.

3-Oxoandrost-4-en-17β-yl 3-phenylpropionate.

$C_{28}H_{36}O_3$=420.6.

CAS — 1255-49-8.

Pharmacopoeias. In *B.P. Vet.*

A white to almost white crystalline powder with a characteristic odour. Practically **insoluble** in water; soluble 1 in 40 of alcohol. **Protect** from light.

Oily solutions for injection are **sterilised** by dry heat.

9115-v

Testosterone Propionate *(BANM, USAN, rINNM)*.

NSC-9166; Testosteroni Propionas. 3-Oxoandrost-4-en-17β-yl propionate.

$C_{22}H_{32}O_3$=344.5.

CAS — 57-85-2.

Pharmacopoeias. In *Arg., Aust., Belg., Br., Braz., Chin., Cz., Egypt., Eur., Fr., Ger., Hung., Ind., Int., It., Jpn, Jug., Mex., Neth., Nord., Pol., Port., Roum., Rus., Span., Swiss, Turk.,* and *U.S.* Also in *B.P. Vet.*

A white or creamy-white odourless crystalline powder or colourless to white or creamy-white crystals. Practically **insoluble** in water; soluble 1 in 6 of alcohol and 1 in 4 of acetone; very soluble in chloroform; freely soluble in dioxan, ether, and methyl alcohol; soluble in vegetable oils. **Protect** from light.

Oily solutions for injection are **sterilised** by dry heat.

9116-g

Testosterone Undecanoate *(BANM, rINNM)*.

3-Oxoandrost-4-en-17β-yl undecanoate.

$C_{30}H_{48}O_3$=456.7.

Adverse Effects and Precautions

As for the androgens and anabolic steroids in general, p.1383.

EFFECTS ON THE CEREBROVASCULAR SYSTEM. A report of a cerebrovascular accident in a young man following the overzealous self-administration of testosterone enanthate intramuscularly for hypogonadism. It was noted that thrombo-embolic complications are not generally recognised as side-effects of androgen therapy although there is some experimental evidence that testosterone stimulates thrombus formation.— S. B. Nagelberg *et al.* (letter), *New Engl. J. Med.*, 1986, *314*, 649.

INTERACTIONS. For the effect of testosterone on warfarin, see p.347.

MALIGNANT NEOPLASMS. A report of carcinoma of the liver occurring in association with methyltestosterone given in conjunction with testosterone enanthate.— F. L. Johnson *et al.*, *Lancet*, 1972, *2*, 1273.

Concern about the possibility that the administration of testosterone esters for male contraception may after many years of use lead to an increase in the number of cases of prostate cancer or benign prostate hyperplasia.— A. V. Schally and A. M. Comaru-Schally (letter), *Lancet*, 1987, *1*, 448.

PREGNANCY AND THE NEONATE. A report of virilisation of a foetus born to a mother who had received methyltestosterone during pregnancy. At birth the infant was believed to be male with hypoplastic external genitalia but following surgery and raising the child as a female the patient completed a successful pregnancy in adult life.— J. Dewhurst and R. R. Gordon (letter), *Lancet*, 1984, *2*, 1461. A similar report following the use of testosterone in the mother during pregnancy.— E. Reschini *et al.* (letter), *ibid.*, 1985, *1*, 1226.

Absorption and Fate

Testosterone is absorbed from the gastro-intestinal tract, the skin, and the oral mucosa. It is largely metabolised in the liver to the weakly androgenic androsterone and inactive etiocholanolone which are excreted in the urine mainly as glucuronides and sulphates. Testosterone absorbed from the gastro-intestinal tract is almost completely metabolised in the liver before it reaches the systemic circulation. Testosterone is extensively bound to a plasma globulin that also binds oestradiol, and a small proportion is converted to oestrogenic derivatives in the body. Only about 2% of testosterone is unbound and the plasma half-life is about 10 to 20 minutes.

Testosterone is believed to be converted to the more active dihydrotestosterone in some target organs.

The active metabolite of testosterone in human skin during *in vitro* studies was considered to be 5α-dihydrotestosterone, produced together with androstenedione, androsterone, and other 17-oxosteroids.— J. B. Hay, *Br. J. Derm.*, 1977, *97*, 237.

Uses and Administration

Testosterone and its esters have the general properties of anabolic agents and androgens (see p.1383). For the treatment of male hypogonadism either testosterone or one of its esters may be employed. Testosterone is usually used as a subcutaneous implant in a dose of 200 to 600 mg; the duration of effect of such implants is up to about 8 months. The testosterone esters are usually formulated as oily solutions for intramuscular use to give a prolonged duration of action. Suggested doses for the various esters are; 50 to 400 mg every 2 to 4 weeks for the cypionate; 50 to 400 mg every 2 to 4 weeks for the enanthate; and 10 to 50 mg 2 to 3 times weekly for the propionate. The isocaproate, phenylpropionate, and propionate esters are also sometimes given in a combined intramuscular preparation. The undecanoate ester is given by mouth in a dose of up to 160 mg daily.

Testosterone esters have also been used in postmenopausal breast carcinoma and in some postmenopausal disorders such as osteoporosis.

Some of the esters are being investigated as male contraceptives.

DELAYED PUBERTY. A short report of the beneficial effect of testosterone enanthate 125 mg intramuscularly every month for 3 months in 33 boys with delayed puberty.— M. D. C. Donaldson and D. C. L. Savage, *Archs Dis. Childh.*, 1987, *62*, 647.

MALE HYPOGONADISM. A review of testosterone undecanoate by mouth for male hypogonadism.— *Drug & Ther. Bull.*, 1985, *23*, 7.

A report of the use of a transdermal delivery system for the administration of testosterone in the treatment of male hypogonadism.— M. Bals-Pratsch *et al.*, *Lancet*, 1986, *2*, 943.

MENOPAUSAL DISORDERS. For reference to the use of testosterone in conjunction with oestrogens for menopausal disorders, see under oestrogens, p.1386.

Preparations

Testosterone Implants *(B.P.)*

Testosterone Pellets *(U.S.P.)*

Sterile Testosterone Suspension *(U.S.P.)*

Testosterone Cypionate Injection *(U.S.P.)*. A sterile solution of testosterone cypionate in a suitable vegetable oil.

Testosterone Enanthate Injection *(U.S.P.)*. A sterile solution of testosterone enanthate in a suitable vegetable oil.

Testosterone Propionate Injection *(B.P.)*. A sterile solution of testosterone propionate in ethyl oleate or other suitable ester, in a suitable fixed oil, or in any mixture of these. For intramuscular injection only.

Testosterone Propionate Injection *(U.S.P.)*. A sterile solution of testosterone propionate in a suitable vegetable oil.

Proprietary Preparations

Primoteston Depot *(Schering, UK)*. *Injection*, testosterone enanthate 250 mg/mL, in ampoules of 1 mL.

Restandol *(Organon, UK)*. *Capsules*, testosterone undecanoate 40 mg.

Sustanon *(Organon, UK)*. *Injection* (Sustanon 100), testosterone propionate 20 mg, testosterone phenylpropionate 40 mg, testosterone isocaproate 40 mg/mL, in ampoules of 1 mL.
Injection (Sustanon 250), testosterone propionate 30 mg, testosterone phenylpropionate 60 mg, testosterone isocaproate 60 mg, testosterone decanoate 100 mg/mL, in ampoules of 1 mL.

Testosterone Implants *(Organon, UK)*. *Implants*, testosterone 100 or 200 mg.

Virormone *(Paines & Byrne, UK)*. *Injection*, testosterone propionate 25 mg/mL, in ampoules of 1 mL, and 50 mg/mL, in ampoules of 1 and 2 mL.

Proprietary Names and Manufacturers of Testosterone and its Esters

Andradurin *(Swed.)*; Andriol *(Organon, Austral.; Organon, Ger.; Ravasini, Ital.; Neth.; Organon, Switz.)*; Andromar Retard *(Marshall's Pharmaceuticals, UK)*; Andronaq *(Central Pharmaceuticals, USA)*; Andronate *(Pasadena Research Labs, USA)*; Androtardyl *(Schering, Fr.)*; Androxil *(Spain)*; Androxon *(Organon, Norw.)*; BayTestone *(Bay, USA)*; Benzotest *(Ital.)*; Biosterone *(Biopharm, S.Afr.)*; Cetovister *(Spain)*; Ciclosterone *(Farmigea, Ital.)*; Delatestryl *(Squibb, Canad.; Squibb, USA)*; Depo-Testosterone *(Upjohn, Canad.; Upjohn, USA)*; Depotrone *(Propan, S.Afr.)*; Durathate *(Hauck, USA)*; Enarmon Depot *(Jpn)*; Femalone 25 *(Marshall's Pharmaceuticals, UK)*; Framviron *(Oftalmiso, Spain)*; Hydrotest *(Ital.)*; Jectatest-LA *(Reid-Provident, USA)*; Lontanyl *(Roussel, Fr.)*; Malogen *(Stickley, Canad.)*; Malogen LA *(USA)*; Malogex *(Stickley, Canad.)*; Neo-Hombreol *(Neth.)*; Orchisterone *(Ital.)*; Oreton *(Schering, USA)*;
Pantestone *(Organon, Fr.)*; Perandren *(Switz.)*; Percutacrine Androgénique Forte *(Fr.)*; Primoteston Depot *(Schering, Austral.; Schering AG, Norw.; Schering, S.Afr.; Schering, UK)*; Rektandron *(Swed.)*; Restandol *(Organon, Denm.; Organon, UK)*; Retar-Gen A *(Temis-Lostalo, Arg.)*; Stérandryl *(Fr.)*; Sustanon *(Organon, Austral.)*; Sustanon 100 *(Organon, UK)*; Sustanon 250 *(Organon, UK)*; T-Cypionate *(Legere, USA)*; Tes. PP *(Organon, UK)*; Testate *(Savage, USA)*; Testex *(Leo, Spain)*; Testex Prolongatum *(Leo, Spain)*; Testinon Depot *(Jpn)*; Testo-Enant *(Geymonat, Ital.)*; Testone LA *(Ortega, USA)*; Testoral *(Austral.; Organon, S.Afr.)*; Testoral Sublings *(Organon, UK)*; Testosterone Implants *(Organon, S.Afr.; Organon, UK)*; Testostroval-PA *(Reid-Provident, USA)*; Testotets *(Pharmadrug, Ger.)*; Testoviron *(Arg.; Schering, Austral.; Schering, Ger.; Schering, Ital.; Spain; Schering, Swed.)*; Testoviron-Depot *(Belg.; Schering, Denm.; Schering, Ger.; Schering, Ital.; Schering, Spain; Schering, Swed.; Switz.)*; Testovis *(SIT, Ital.)*; Testred Cypionate *(ICN, USA)*; Triolandren *(Ciba, Denm.; Ciba, Norw.; Ciba, Swed.; Ciba, Switz.)*; Undestor *(Organon, Swed.)*; Virormone *(Ital.; Paines & Byrne, UK)*.

The following names have been used for multi-ingredient preparations containing testosterone and its esters— Climacteron *(Frosst, Canad.)*; Deladumone *(Squibb, Canad.)*; Ditate-DS *(Savage, USA)*; Duogex *(Stickley, Canad.)*; Estrand *(Taro, Canad.)*; Mixogen Injection *(Organon, Austral.; Organon, UK)*; Neo-Pause *(Neolab, Canad.)*; Plex-Hormone Injection *(Consolidated Chemicals, UK)*; Primodian Depot *(Schering, Austral.; Schering, Ital.)*; T-E Cypionate *(Legere, USA)*; Testaval *(Legere, USA)*.

13342-q

Tibolone *(BAN, USAN, rINN)*.

Org-OD-14. 17β-Hydroxy-7α-methyl-19-nor-17α-pregn-5(10)-en-20-yn-3-one.

$C_{21}H_{28}O_2$=312.5.

CAS — 5630-53-5.

Tibolone is reported to have androgenic, oestrogenic, and progestogenic properties and has been investigated for use in the treatment of menopausal and postmenopausal symptoms.

9117-q

Trenbolone Acetate *(BANM, USAN, rINNM)*.

Trienbolone Acetate. 17β-Hydroxyestra-4,9,11-trien-3-one acetate.

$C_{20}H_{24}O_3$=312.4.

CAS — 10161-33-8 (trenbolone); 10161-34-9 (acetate).

Trenbolone acetate is used as an anabolic agent in veterinary practice.

Proprietary Names and Manufacturers

Parabolan *(Negma, Fr.)*.

Proprietary Veterinary Names and Manufacturers

Finajet *(Hoechst Animal Health, UK)*; Finaplix *(Hoechst Animal Health, UK)*.

13367-c

Trengestone *(rINN)*.

Ro-4-8347. 6-Chloro-9β,10α-pregna-1,4,6-triene-3,20-dione.

$C_{21}H_{25}ClO_2$=344.9.

CAS — 5192-84-7.

Adverse Effects and Precautions

As for the progestogens in general, p.1386.

Uses and Administration

Trengestone is a progestogen with actions and uses similar to those described for the progestogens in general (see p.1386). It has been given in usual doses of 4 to 8 mg daily by mouth.

Proprietary Names and Manufacturers

Retroide *(Roche, Switz.)*.

14027-b

Zeranol *(BAN, USAN, rINN)*.

MK-188; P-1496; Zearalanol. (3*S*,7*X*)-3,4,5,6,7,8,9,10,11,12-Decahydro-7,14,16-trihydroxy-3-methyl-1*H*-2-benzoxacyclotetradecin-1-one.

$C_{18}H_{26}O_5$=322.4.

CAS — 26538-44-3.

Zeranol is an oestrogenic agent. It has also been used as a growth promoter in veterinary practice.

Proprietary Names and Manufacturers

Frideron *(Ital.)*; Ralone *(Ist. Chim. Inter., Ital.; Llorens, Spain)*.

Soaps and other Anionic Surfactants

6010-a

Soaps are the sodium or potassium salts of fatty acids or similar products formed by the saponification or neutralisation of fats or oils with organic or inorganic bases.

A *detergent* is any surface-active agent which concentrates at oil-water interfaces, and possesses emulsifying properties; thus it also possesses cleansing properties.

Anionic surfactants dissociate in aqueous solution to form an anion, which is responsible for the surface activity, and a cation which is devoid of surface-active properties. Anionic surfactants can be conveniently classified into several groups:

Alkali-metal and ammonium soaps which are the sodium, potassium, and ammonium salts of the higher fatty acids and are used mainly for their detergent properties; they are also used as solubilising agents in disinfectants.

Metallic soaps which are the calcium, zinc, magnesium, and aluminium salts of the higher fatty acids and produce water-in-oil emulsions; the soaps are often made by chemical reaction during the preparation of the emulsion.

Amine soaps are salts of amines, with fatty acids. Like the other soaps, they are suitable only for preparations intended for external use.

Alkyl sulphates or *sulphated fatty alcohols* are salts of the sulphuric acid esters of the higher fatty alcohols and are sometimes known incorrectly as 'sulphonated fatty alcohols'.

Sulphated fatty alcohols are widely used in industry and in the preparation of many 'soapless' washing powders and liquids for domestic use. They are very useful for cleansing glassware. Pharmaceutical applications include the preparation of 'soapless' shampoos, toilet and cosmetic preparations, toothpastes, and toothpowders. They are also employed as ingredients of insecticides and in fruit-washing solutions.

Alkyl ether sulphates are formed by the addition of a short macrogol chain to a fatty alcohol, followed by sulphation and neutralisation. They are similar in general properties to alkyl sulphates.

Proprietary preparations of alkyl ether sulphates are described under Sodium Lauryl Sulphate, p.1417.

Sulphated oils are prepared by treating fixed oils with sulphuric acid and neutralising with sodium hydroxide solution. They have similar properties to the sulphated fatty alcohols.

Many *sulphonated compounds* have been produced which possess surface-active properties and are used as detergents; they include alkyl sulphonates, alkyl aryl sulphonates, and amide sulphonates. Docusate sodium (p.1088), a sulphonated dibasic acid ester, is used in medicine and pharmacy.

Ampholytic surfactants are described below.

For the general properties of *cationic surfactants* see under Cetrimide, p.953.

For *nonionic surfactants* see p.1243.

Adverse Effects and Treatment

Anionic detergents may be irritant to the skin by removing natural oils and may produce redness, soreness, cracking and scaling and papular dermatitis. There may be some irritation of the eyes and mucous membranes. Ingestion of anionic detergents may cause gastro-intestinal irritation with nausea, diarrhoea, intestinal distension, and occasionally vomiting. Treatment is symptomatic.

A severe allergic reaction occurred in a 33-year-old pregnant woman soon after being given an enema consisting of a proprietary brand of soap flakes in about 2 pints of water. She developed swelling of the mouth, numbness in the limbs, tightness in the chest, bronchospasm, and generalised urticaria and subsequently collapsed and became unconscious. She soon recovered consciousness with oxygen therapy, adrenaline, and chlorpheniramine and delivered a baby without any further untoward effects.— D. Smith, *Br. med. J.*, 1967, *4*, 215.

Meningitis in 3 women who had received spinal anaesthesia was attributed to the use of detergent solution (Alconox) in the cleansing of syringes. Small amounts of residue were found in syringes subjected to the procedure. Alconox consisted of a blend of alkyl aryl sulphonates and fatty alcohol sulphates, with carbonates and complex phosphates.— R. B. Gibbons, *J. Am. med. Ass.*, 1969, *210*, 900.

A soap enema prepared inaccurately and containing perhaps 10 to 50 mL of concentrated soap solution in a litre produced inflammation of the colonic mucosa with hypotension, nausea and vomiting, and fever in a woman in active labour. The baby was stillborn. Such enemas were hazardous and of questionable value.— B. F. Pike *et al.*, *New Engl. J. Med.*, 1971, *285*, 217.

The anionic surfactants used in household detergents had moderate toxicity. The acute LD50 in *animals* ranged from 1 to 5 g per kg body-weight and the maximum safe amount that children could ingest had been estimated at 0.1 to 1 g per kg.— *Bull. Nat. Clearinghouse Poison Control Centers*, 1975, Jan.–Feb.,.

Evidence of a strong association between dysuria and the use of soap. Of 22 women with dysuria, who stopped (16) or reduced (6) their use of soap on the sexual organs, dysuria disappeared completely in 17; 4 of 6 whose use of soap was unchanged still had dysuria on follow-up.— U. Ravnskov (letter), *Lancet*, 1984, *1*, 1027.

A study involving *rats* suggested that the chronic ingestion of household detergents, such as may occur by using unrinsed eating-utensils, might predispose to chronic inflammatory and atrophic gut disease (L.A. Mercurius-Taylor *et al.*, *Gut*, 1982, *23*, A443; *idem*, *Br. J. ind. Med.*, 1984, *40*, 279). However, it was felt that the concentrations to which the *rats* were exposed were considerably higher than likely human exposure levels and no similar adverse effects had been observed during the many toxicity studies of detergents in current use (*Lancet*, 1984, *2*, 384).

6014-f

Soft Soap *(BAN)*.

Green Soap *(USAN)*; Jabon Blando; Medicinal Soft Soap; Potassium Soap; Sabão Mole; Sap. Moll.; Sapo Mollis.

Pharmacopoeias. In *Br.*, *Chin.*, *Egypt.*, *Port.*, *Span.*, and *U.S.*

Span. specifies linseed oil and potassium hydroxide; *Port.* specifies olive oil and potassium hydroxide; *U.S.P.* includes Green Soap from vegetable oils (excluding coconut oil and palm-kernel oil) and potassium hydroxide.

Prepared by the interaction of any suitable vegetable oil or oils, or their fatty acids, with potassium hydroxide or sodium hydroxide.

It is a yellowish-white to green or brown transparent, soft, unctuous substance with a slight characteristic odour, yielding not less than 44% of fatty acids. Chlorophyll or not more than 0.015% of a suitable green soap dye may be added to give a green colour.

Soluble in water and in alcohol. A 5% solution is alkaline to bromothymol blue. **Store** in well-closed containers.

Adverse Effects and Treatment

As for Soaps and other Anionic Surfactants, above.

Uses and Administration

Soft soap is used to remove incrustations in chronic scaly skin diseases such as psoriasis and to cleanse the scalp before the application of lotions. A solution in industrial methylated spirit, with the addition of solvent ether, is used to cleanse the skin. A solution of soft soap in warm water has been used as an enema to soften impacted faeces but should be avoided as it may inflame the colonic mucosa; deaths have occurred. Soap Liniment is a mild counter-irritant which is used in the treatment of sprains and bruises and to dilute more active liniments. Potash soap (linseed oil soap) has been used in the preparation of liquid soaps. Hard soap (castile soap) and curd soap were formerly used as pill excipients and hard soap was also formerly used in the preparation of plasters.

Preparations

Ethereal Soap Solution *(B.P.C. 1973)*. Liquor Saponis Aethereus; Liq. Sap. Aether.; Ether Soap; Solutio Saponis Aetherea. Prepared by mixing oleic acid 35 mL and alcohol (90%) (or industrial methylated spirit, suitably diluted) 15 mL and neutralising with a saturated solution of potassium hydroxide in water (1 in 1); the product is allowed to cool, lavender oil 0.21 mL is added, and the solution is diluted to 100 mL with solvent ether. Store in a cool place in airtight containers. This preparation is inflammable. Keep away from an open flame.

Soap Liniment *(B.P.C. 1973)*. Linimentum Saponis; Lin. Sap.; Opodeldoc. Oleic acid 4 g, potassium hydroxide solution 14 mL, alcohol (90%) (or industrial methylated spirit, suitably diluted) 70 mL, camphor 4 g, rosemary oil 1.5 mL, freshly boiled and cooled water to 100 mL. After preparation it should be allowed to stand for not less than 7 days and then filtered. pH 7.4 to 8.

A similar preparation is included in many pharmacopoeias.

Soap Solution Alcoholic *(A.P.F.)*. Spirit Shampoo. Soft soap 50 g, alcohol (90%) to 100 mL. Medicaments such as thymol 0.5% or coal tar solution 5% may be added.

Soap Spirit *(B.P.)*. Spiritus Saponatus; Spiritus Saponis; Sp. Sap. Soft soap 65% w/v in alcohol (90%) (or industrial methylated spirit, suitably diluted). Store at a temperature not exceeding 25°.

Green Soap Tincture *(U.S.P.)*. Green soap *U.S.P.* 65 g, lavender oil 2 mL, alcohol to 100 mL. pH 9.5 to 11.5. Store in airtight containers.

6015-d

Aluminium Monostearate

Aluminii Monostearas; Aluminum Monostearate *(USAN)*.

CAS — 7047-84-9 (monostearate).

Pharmacopoeias. In *Hung.*, *Int.*, and *Jpn.* Also in *U.S.N.F.*

A compound of aluminium with a mixture of solid organic acids obtained from fats and consisting mainly of variable proportions of aluminium monostearate and aluminium monopalmitate. Its aluminium content is equivalent to 14.5 to 16.5% of Al_2O_3.

It is a fine white to yellowish-white bulky powder with a faint characteristic odour. **Insoluble** in water, alcohol, and ether. **Store** in well-closed containers.

Aluminium monostearate forms gels with fixed or mineral oils when heated to about 60°; such gels are used to suspend medicaments in oily injections.

6031-d

Ampholytic Surfactants

An ampholytic (or amphoteric) surfactant possesses at least one anionic group and at least one cationic group in its molecule and can therefore have anionic, nonionic, or cationic properties depending on the pH. When the strength of the cationic portion of the molecule is equivalent to

that of the anionic portion the isoelectric point occurs at pH 7 and the molecule is said to be balanced. Ampholytic surfactants used include derivatives of long-chain *N*-substituted amino acids, and derivatives of imidazoline. Long-chain betaines are sometimes classed as ampholytic surfactants.
Ampholytic surfactants have the detergent properties of anionic surfactants and the disinfectant properties of cationic surfactants. Their activity depends on the pH of the media in which they are used. Compounds used include aminocarboxylic acids, aminopropionic acid derivatives, imidazoline derivatives, dodicin hydrochloride [dodecyldi (aminoethyl) glycine hydrochloride], and pendecamaine.
Ampholytic surfactants have been used generally for their disinfectant properties. Balanced ampholytic surfactants are reputed to be non-irritant to the eyes and skin and have therefore been used in baby shampoos.

Proprietary Names and Manufacturers
Amphionic 25B *(ABM Chemicals, UK)*; Crodateric *(Croda, UK)*; Cycloteric *(Witco, UK)*; Deriphats *(USA)*; Miranol *(Venture Chemicals, UK)*; Rewoteric *(Rewo, UK)*; Rexoteric *(Grace, UK)*; Tego *(Goldschmidt, UK)*; Tego Betain C *(Goldschmidt, UK)*; Tego Betain L7 *(Goldschmidt, UK)*; Tego MHG *(Goldschmidt, UK)*.

6016-n

Calcium Stearate *(USAN)*.

CAS — 1592-23-0 (stearate); 542-42-7 (palmitate).

Pharmacopoeias. In *Jpn.* Also in *U.S.N.F.*

A compound of calcium with a mixture of solid organic acids obtained from fats, consisting mainly of variable proportions of calcium stearate and calcium palmitate. It contains the equivalent of 9 to 10.5% of CaO.
A fine, white to yellowish-white, bulky, unctuous powder free from grittiness with a slight characteristic odour. **Insoluble** in water, alcohol, and ether. **Store** in well-closed containers.

Calcium stearate is added to granules as a lubricant in tablet-making.

6017-h

Sulphated Castor Oil
Ol. Ricin. Sulphat.; Oleum Ricini Sulphatum; Sulphonated Castor Oil.

Sulphated castor oil is a non-irritating detergent and wetting agent and may be used to cleanse the skin when soap is contra-indicated.
It was formerly used as an emulsifying agent.
It has also been used in the manufacture of soapless shampoos, liquid soaps, and deodorant sprays.
Turkey red oil (alizarine oil) is a commercial variety of sulphated castor oil used in the dyeing industry.

6022-f

Magnesium Stearate *(BAN, USAN)*.
572; Estearato de Magnésio; Mag. Stear.; Magnesii Stearas.

CAS — 557-04-0 (stearate); 2601-98-1 (palmitate).

Pharmacopoeias. In *Arg., Aust., Br., Braz., Chin., Cz., Eur., Fr., Ger., Hung., Ind., It., Jpn, Jug., Neth., Nord., Pol., Port., Roum.,* and *Swiss.* Also in *U.S.N.F.*

It consists chiefly of a mixture of magnesium stearate and magnesium palmitate and contains 3.8 to 5% of Mg. *U.S.N.F.* describes a compound of magnesium with a mixture of solid organic acids obtained from fats consisting chiefly of magnesium stearate and magnesium palmitate, containing the equivalent of 6.8 to 8% of MgO.
It is a fine, white, bulky, unctuous powder, free from grittiness, and odourless or with a faint odour of stearic acid. It adheres readily to the skin. Practically **insoluble** in water, alcohol, and ether. **Store** in well-closed containers.

Physical and chemical characteristics of some high purity magnesium stearate and palmitate powders.— T. A. Miller and P. York, *Int. J. Pharmaceut.*, 1985, *23*, 55.

Magnesium stearate is added as a lubricant to the granules in tablet-making and has been used as a dusting-powder.

6024-n

Sodium Lauryl Sulphate *(BAN)*.
Natrii Laurilsulfas; Natrium Lauryl Sulphuricum; Sod. Lauryl Sulph.; Sodium Laurilsulfate *(pINNM)*; Sodium Lauryl Sulfate *(USAN)*.

CAS — 151-21-3.

Pharmacopoeias. In *Aust., Belg., Br., Braz., Cz., Egypt., Eur., Fr., Hung., Ind., Jpn, Jug., Neth., Pol., Roum.,* and *Swiss.* Also in *U.S.N.F.*

A mixture of sodium alkyl sulphates, consisting mainly of sodium dodecyl sulphate, $C_{12}H_{25}O.SO_2.ONa$. *B.P.* specifies that the mixture contains not less than 85% of sodium alkyl sulphates and both *B.P.* and *U.S.N.F.* specify not more than a total of 8% of sodium chloride and sodium sulphate.
It is a white or pale yellow powder or crystals with a slight characteristic odour. **Soluble** 1 in 10 of water giving an opalescent solution; partly soluble in alcohol. **Store** in well-closed containers.

HYDROLYSIS. Practically no hydrolysis occurred in solutions of sodium lauryl sulphate at pH 4 and above. Below pH 2.5, hydrolysis to lauryl alcohol and sodium acid sulphate was accelerated; the rate of hydrolysis also varied with the temperature and the concentration.— R. R. Read and W. G. Fredell, *Drug Cosmet. Ind.*, 1959, *84*, 178.

Sodium lauryl sulphate is an anionic emulsifying agent. It is a detergent and wetting agent, effective in both acid and alkaline solution and in hard water. It is used in medicated shampoos and as a skin cleanser. It is used in the preparation of Emulsifying Wax (see p.1325). Sodium cetostearyl sulphate has been used for the same purposes as sodium lauryl sulphate.
Magnesium lauryl sulphate is used as a lubricant in tablets.

Reviews of the uses of sodium and other lauryl sulphates: E. S. Lower, *Mfg Chem.*, 1983, *54*, 63 and 79.

Proprietary Names and Manufacturers
Alquil Dermol *(Frumtost, Spain)*; Anticerumen *(Liade, Spain)*; Capillex *(Rougier, Canad.)*; Cycloryl *(Witco, UK)*; Empicols *(Albright & Wilson, Marchon Division, UK)*; Maprofix LK *(Onyx Chemical Co., USA)*; Neopon *(Witco, UK)*; Pentrones *(ABM Chemicals, UK)*; Rewopols *(Rewo, UK)*; Solumins *(ABM Chemicals, UK)*; Sulphonated Lorol *(Ronsheim & Moore, UK)*; Teepol *(Shell Chemicals, UK)*; Tersus *(Trans Canaderm, Canad.)*.

6025-h

Sodium Oleate

$C_{18}H_{33}NaO_2$=304.4.

CAS — 143-19-1.

Sodium oleate has been used as an ingredient in preparations for the symptomatic relief of haemorrhoids and pruritus ani.
Zinc oleate has been used in ointments for eczema.

Proprietary Preparations
Alcos-anal *(Norgine, UK). Ointment*, sodium oleate 10%, laureth '9' 2%, chlorothymol 0.1%.
Suppositories, sodium oleate 200 mg, laureth '9' 20 mg, chlorothymol 700 µg.

Proprietary Names and Manufacturers
The following names have been used for multi-ingredient preparations containing sodium oleate— Alcos-Anal *(Norgine, Austral.; Norgine, UK)*; Artéchol *(Anglo-French Laboratories, Canad.)*.

6026-m

Sodium Ricinoleate
Sodium Ricinate.

CAS — 5323-95-5.

Sodium ricinoleate possesses surface-active properties. It has been used in toothpastes. A 2% solution has been used as a sclerosing agent.

6027-b

Sodium Stearate *(USAN)*.
Estearato de Sodio. A mixture of sodium stearate, $C_{18}H_{35}NaO_2$, and sodium palmitate, $C_{16}H_{31}NaO_2$.

CAS — 822-16-2 (stearate); 408-35-5 (palmitate).

Pharmacopoeias. In *Belg., It., Port., Span.,* and *Swiss.* Also in *U.S.N.F.*

A mixture containing not less than 90% of sodium stearate and sodium palmitate; the content of sodium stearate is not less than 40% of the total. It contains small amounts of the sodium salts of other fatty acids.
A fine white powder, soapy to the touch, with a faint tallow-like odour. Slowly **soluble** in water and alcohol; readily soluble in hot water and hot alcohol. A solution in water is alkaline to phenolphthalein. **Store** in well-closed containers. Protect from light.

Sodium stearate is used in the preparation of vanishing creams. It is an ingredient of Glycerin Suppositories *U.S.P.*

6028-v

Sodium Tetradecyl Sulphate *(BAN, rINN)*.
Sodium 4-ethyl-1-isobutyloctyl sulphate.
$C_{14}H_{29}NaO_4S$=316.4.

CAS — 139-88-8.

Pharmacopoeias. Br. has a monograph for Sodium Tetradecyl Sulphate Concentrate.

Store the concentrate in a well-closed container at a temperature not exceeding 15°. Protect from light.

Adverse Effects and Precautions
The complications of injection sclerotherapy with sclerosants such as sodium tetradecyl sulphate are discussed under Ethanolamine, p.1569.

Uses and Administration
Sodium tetradecyl sulphate is an anionic surfactant. It has sclerosing properties and is used in the treatment of varicose veins.

A 3% buffered solution is used. A test dose of 0.5 mL of a 1% solution should be injected and the patient observed for several hours for any reaction before a larger injection is administered. Not more than 1 mL of a 3% solution should be injected at any one site and the total volume given at one session should not exceed 4 mL. Care is necessary to avoid injecting the solution outside the vein or sloughing may occur.

Sodium tetradecyl sulphate is also used in disinfectant solutions as a surfactant to increase the penetration of the disinfectant.

CYSTIC LESIONS. The sclerosing action of sodium tetradecyl sulphate had been used in the management of cystic lesions in the thyroid gland.— P. G. Walfish *et al.*, *Can. med. Ass. J.*, 1976, *115*, 35.

SCLEROTHERAPY. For a review of injection sclerotherapy in the management of varicose veins and oesophageal varices, including mention of sodium tetradecyl sulphate, see under Ethanolamine, p.1569.

Preparations

Sodium Tetradecyl Sulphate Injection *(B.P.)*. A solution of Sodium Tetradecyl Sulphate Concentrate *B.P.* in Water for Injections, sterilised by heating in an autoclave, and labelled for use only in the treatment of varicose veins. pH 7.5 to 7.9. Store at a temperature not exceeding 15° and protect from light.

Proprietary Preparations
STD *(STD Pharmaceutical Products, UK). Injection,* sodium tetradecyl sulphate 3%, benzyl alcohol 2%, buffered to pH 7.6, in ampoules of 1 mL and vials of 30 mL.

Proprietary Names and Manufacturers
Sotradecol *(Elkins-Sinn, USA)*; STD *(Faulding, Austral.; STD Pharmaceutical Products, UK)*; Trombovar *(Therapex, Canad.; Promedica, Fr.; Bouty, Ital.; Neth.; Globopharm, Switz.)*.

6030-f

Zinc Stearate *(BAN, USAN)*.

Zinc Stear; Zinci Stearas.

CAS — 557-05-1 (stearate); 4991-47-3 (palmitate).

Pharmacopoeias. In *Arg., Aust., Br., Eur., Fr., Ind., It., Neth., Pol., Swiss, Turk.*, and *U.S.*

It consists mainly of zinc stearate ($C_{36}H_{70}O_4Zn$ = 632.3) with a variable proportion of zinc palmitate ($C_{32}H_{62}O_4Zn$ = 576.2) and usually a small amount of zinc oleate. *B.P.* specifies 10 to 12% of zinc. *U.S.P.* specifies the equivalent of 12.5 to 14% of ZnO.

It is a light, white, amorphous powder, free from gritty particles, with a faint characteristic odour. Practically **insoluble** in water, alcohol, and ether. It is neutral to moistened litmus paper. **Store** in well-closed containers.

Zinc stearate is used as a soothing and protective application in the treatment of skin inflammation. It is used either alone or with other powders or in the form of a cream.

Zinc stearate is also added as a lubricant to the granules in tablet-making. Zinc stearate inhalation has caused fatal pneumonitis, particularly in infants.

In Great Britain the recommended exposure limits of zinc stearate total dust are 10 mg per m^3 (long-term); 20 mg per m^3 (short-term) and respirable dust 5 mg per m^3 (long-term).

6032-n

Some Proprietary Detergent Preparations

Adverse Effects and Treatment
As for Soaps and other Anionic Surfactants, p.1416.

Uses.
Proprietary detergent preparations may contain anionic surfactants such as alkyl sulphonates, alkyl aryl sulphonates, amide sulphonates, and alkyl sulphates, together with nonionic surfactants and mineral salts such as complex phosphates and sodium carbonates. They are used for domestic and industrial cleansing purposes.

Proprietary Names and Manufacturers
Alconox *(K & K-Greeff, UK)*; Decon 90 *(Decon Laboratories, UK)*; Dri-Decon *(Decon Laboratories, UK)*; Liqui-Nox *(Cambrian, UK)*; Neutrobrite *(Albright & Wilson, Eire)*; Pyroneg *(Diversey, UK)*; TAGG *(Eagle, Austral.)*.

Sodium Cromoglycate and related Anti-allergic Agents

7720-w

Sodium cromoglycate is an anti-allergic agent which is used prophylactically in allergic disorders including asthma and rhinitis. It is not absorbed from the gastro-intestinal tract and efforts have been made to find a similar substance which is absorbed when taken by mouth.

Ketotifen is an antihistamine which also has anti-allergic properties and is absorbed when taken by mouth. The use of other antihistamines in allergic conditions is described under Antihistamines, p.444.

A review of the actions of sodium cromoglycate and the prospects for the development of an orally-active cromoglycate-like drug. A very large number of compounds has been identified with similar actions to sodium cromoglycate *in vitro* and in animals, some of them proving many times more potent in their ability to prevent passive cutaneous anaphylaxis (PCA) in *rats*, but clinical information is scanty. Some reports of efficacy against antigen-induced bronchoconstriction have been published although exercise-induced asthma might have been a better predictor of efficacy. There have been fewer clinical studies of these drugs in chronic asthma, and the most notable feature of those that have been reported is the poor or absent efficacy. Of the four assumptions that underlie the search for cromoglycate-like drugs— that sodium cromoglycate is effective in asthma, that it is possible to develop more potent drugs capable of oral absorption, that its route of administration is inconvenient and not an essential quality of the drug, and that there exist *animal* or *in-vitro* models predictive of anti-asthma activity for this class of drugs— the first two are unequivocally established. The assumption that the oral route is to be preferred over inhalation is a contentious one, since the anti-allergic effect of such drugs may not be equated with the anti-asthma activity: it has been proposed that the critical events in the induction of bronchospasm by antigen take place at the mucosal surface, in which case inhalation would be the preferred route of administration and the only way in which adequate concentrations of cromoglycate-like drugs might be achieved in lung tissue to exert an anti-asthma effect. The assumption that *animal* or *in-vitro* models are predictive of this effect is also tenuous. Disappointing clinical results are most simply explained by the suggestion that research has focused on a property of sodium cromoglycate that is not predictive of its anti-asthma effects: sodium cromoglycate has been too readily accepted as acting in asthma by mast cell stabilisation when it clearly operates by some mechanism other than, or in addition to, this property, and at present we know of no model that will predict efficacy of cromoglycate-like drugs in asthma. It seems likely that prospects for an 'oral sodium cromoglycate' will remain poor until its mechanism of action has been identified.— T. C. Stokes and J. Morley, *Br. J. Dis. Chest*, 1981, *75*, 1.

A detailed review of the design and synthesis of pulmonary and anti-allergic drugs, including sodium cromoglycate and other chromones such as proxicromil, evicromil (FPL-52757), AA-344, and PRD-92; quinolones such as bufrolin; pyrimidones such as zaprinast and BL-5255; xanthones and related compounds such as tixanox (RS-7337), AH-7725, and doxantrazole; oxamates such as lodoxamide ethyl and lodoxamide trometamol; and other compounds such as nivimedone and tranilast. Though a large number of compounds such as these have appeared promising in preclinical *animal* studies, studies in humans have generally been disappointing and only one of the drugs mentioned, tranilast, has thus far appeared on the market. Part of the problem rests with the inadequacy of existing preclinical and clinical models, as well as the lack of information about action at the receptor level, but in spite of this there is reason for optimism that sodium cromoglycate is not unique and that improved drugs will be forthcoming.— J. P. Devlin and K. D. Hargrave, in *Pulmonary and Anti-allergic Drugs*, J.P. Devlin (Ed.), Chichester, John Wiley, 1985, p.191.

7721-e

Sodium Cromoglycate *(BANM).*

Cromolyn Sodium *(USAN)*; Disodium Cromoglycate; FPL-670; Natrii Cromoglicas; Sodium Cromoglicate *(rINNM)*. Disodium 4,4′-dioxo-5,5′-(2-hydroxytrimethylenedioxy)di(4*H*-chromene-2-carboxylate).

$C_{23}H_{14}Na_2O_{11}$=512.3.

CAS — 16110-51-3 (cromoglycic acid); 15826-37-6 (disodium salt).

Pharmacopoeias. In *Br., Chin., Eur., Ind., Jpn, Nord.,* and *U.S.*

A white, odourless, hygroscopic, crystalline powder, tasteless at first with a slightly bitter after-taste. **Soluble** 1 in 20 of water; practically insoluble in alcohol and chloroform. A solution in water has a pH of 4.0 to 7.0. **Store** in airtight containers. Protect from light.

Adverse Effects

Sodium cromoglycate is generally well tolerated and side-effects are often transient.

Inhalation of the dry powder may have a direct irritant effect with bronchospasm, wheezing, cough, nasal congestion, and irritation of the throat. Some of the irritant effects may be attributed to the powder rather than the drug itself. Nausea, vomiting, headache, dizziness, and joint pain and swelling have been reported. Other reactions, which have sometimes occurred after treatment for several weeks or months, include aggravation of existing asthma, urticaria, rashes, and pulmonary infiltrates with eosinophilia. Severe hypersensitivity reactions such as bronchospasm, laryngeal oedema, angioedema, and anaphylaxis have been reported rarely. Sodium cromoglycate may be inhaled with isoprenaline and for reference to the adverse effects associated with isoprenaline, see p.1466.

There may be transient irritation of the nasal mucosa, sneezing, and occasionally epistaxis following the intranasal use of sodium cromoglycate. Nausea, skin rashes, and joint pains have occurred when it is taken by mouth.

A study of the immunological components of hypersensitivity reactions to sodium cromoglycate. Of 6 asthmatic patients studied, 3 had acute reactions to sodium cromoglycate, occurring 1 to 6 weeks after therapy had begun, and consisting of generalised urticaria, oropharyngeal oedema, or anaphylaxis, immediately after inhaling a dose. Subacute reactions in the other 3, which were noted after therapy for 3 to 8 months, consisted of the insidious onset of polymyositis, myocardiopathy with pulmonary infiltrates and eosinophilia, and polymorphous skin eruptions with fever. Both types of reaction were associated with alterations in immunological parameters *in vitro*.— A. L. Sheffer *et al.*, *New Engl. J. Med.*, 1975, *293*, 1220. In a cooperative study, adverse reactions (excluding local irritation) occurred in only 8 of 375 asthmatic patients who had received sodium cromoglycate by inhalation for periods ranging from 2 days to 1 year. The reactions were: generalised dermatitis in 3 patients, facial dermatitis in 2, myositis in 2, and gastro-enteritis in 1. The dermatitis was usually pruritic. Reactions were reversible and all returned on rechallenge. An immunological basis for the adverse reactions could not be proved.— G. A. Settipane *et al.*, *J. Am. med. Ass.*, 1979, *241*, 811.

A report of anaphylactic shock in a 57-year-old patient, with severe bronchial asthma and no previous history of drug allergy, following a single dose of sodium cromoglycate. Symptoms, which developed within 20 minutes of administration, were generalised pruritus, joint pains, urticaria, severe bronchospasm, stridor, angioedema, severe nausea, paraesthesia, peripheral cyanosis, hypotension, and sinus tachycardia; the reaction was probably a type 1 hypersensitivity reaction.— S. Ahmad (letter), *Ann. intern. Med.*, 1983, *99*, 882.

Reports of adverse effects associated with the inhalation or insufflation of sodium cromoglycate: H. Löbel *et al.* (letter), *Lancet*, 1972, *2*, 1032 (pulmonary eosinophilia); L. W. Burgher *et al.*, *Chest*, 1974, *66*, 84 (pulmonary eosinophilia); U. K. Repo and P. Nieminen, *Scand. J. resp. Dis.*, 1976, *57*, 1 (pulmonary eosinophilia); I. C. Paterson *et al.*, *Br. med. J.*, 1976, *2*, 916 (exacerbation of asthma); E. E. Slater, *Chest*, 1978, *73*, 878 (peripheral eosinophilia and pericarditis with cardiac tamponade); R. H. Israel and J. Wood (letter), *J. Am. med. Ass.*, 1979, *242*, 2758 (oesophagitis); J. Serup, *Acta med. scand.*, 1979, *205*, 447 (exacerbation of asthma); *Med. J. Aust.*, 1979, *2*, 608 (ulceration in the mouth and pharynx, and possible oesophagitis, following nasal insufflation); H. V. Price (letter), *Lancet*, 1982, *2*, 606 (precipitation of asthma attacks in a child with α_1-antitrypsin deficiency); *Med. J. Aust.*, 1982, *1*, 522 (burning of eyes, facial rash, and periorbital oedema).

Reports of adverse effects associated with the oral administration of sodium cromoglycate: G. M. Fairris (letter), *Br. med. J.*, 1984, *289*, 470 (exacerbation of eczema).

EFFECTS ON THE EYES. Comment on an acute conjunctival reaction following the topical administration of sodium cromoglycate. The reaction was considered to be an anaphylactic type of response.— H. B. Ostler (letter), *Lancet*, 1982, *2*, 1287.

For a report of ocular stinging associated with the preservative used in sodium cromoglycate eye-drops, see Conjunctivitis in Uses, below.

Precautions

Sodium cromoglycate should not be given to patients with known hypersensitivity to it.

Because the action of sodium cromoglycate is prophylactic it is important that regular administration is maintained. It has no role in the treatment of acute asthmatic attacks or status asthmaticus. Withdrawal of sodium cromoglycate may lead to recurrence of the symptoms of asthma. Should withdrawal be necessary it has been suggested that the dose be reduced gradually over a period of one week. Patients in whom sodium cromoglycate therapy has permitted a reduction of corticosteroid dosage may require restoration of full steroid cover.

Systemic corticosteroid therapy that has been reduced or discontinued in asthmatic patients may need to be reinstated if symptoms increase, during periods of stress, or where airways obstruction impairs inhalation of sodium cromoglycate.

The precautions for isoprenaline (see p.1466) should be observed for patients using sodium cromoglycate with isoprenaline.

Absorption and Fate

Sodium cromoglycate is poorly absorbed from the gastro-intestinal tract. Following inhalation as a fine powder only about 8% of a dose is reported to be deposited in the lungs from where it is rapidly absorbed and excreted unchanged in the urine and bile. Less than 7% of an intranasal dose is absorbed. The majority of an inhaled or an intranasal dose is swallowed and excreted unchanged in the faeces.

Studies of the absorption and fate of sodium cromoglycate: G. F. Moss *et al.*, *Toxic. appl. Pharmac.*, 1971, *20*, 147 (fluorimetric and colorimetric studies after inhalation and oral administration); S. R. Walker *et al.*, *J. Pharm. Pharmac.*, 1972, *24*, 525 (fate of radiolabelled sodium cromoglycate following inhalation and oral or intravenous administration); B. Clark *et al.*, *J. Pharm. Pharmac.*, 1978, *30*, 386 (protein binding); R. W. Fuller and J. G. Collier, *J. Pharm. Pharmac.*, 1983, *35*, 289 (radioimmunoassay).

Uses and Administration

Sodium cromoglycate is used for the prevention of allergic reactions but its precise mode of action remains uncertain. It has no intrinsic antihistaminic or anti-inflammatory action and is generally considered to possess no bronchodilator activity (but see under Action, below).

It is used in the prophylactic treatment of asthma but does not affect an established asthmatic attack and thus it is not used for acute attacks including severe acute asthma or status asthmaticus. It may be possible to reduce or discontinue concomitant corticosteroid therapy once benefit with sodium cromoglycate has been established but the reduction in corticosteroid dosage must be gradual and carefully supervised; a reduction in the frequency of concomitant bronchodilator therapy may also be possible.

Sodium cromoglycate is also used prophylactically in the treatment of seasonal and perennial allergic rhinitis, and in the treatment of vernal keratoconjunctivitis and other allergic conditions of the eye.

It has been given by mouth for the prevention of food allergies.

Because of the prophylactic nature of its action the maintenance of regular dosage is important.

In asthma, sodium cromoglycate is administered as a dry powder or as a nebulised solution in a usual dose of 20 mg by inhalation 4 times daily; in some patients 20 mg may need to be given 6 to 8 times daily. Alternatively it may be inhaled from a metered aerosol. Aerosols are metered to provide 1 mg or 5 mg per inhalation; doses may consist of 2 mg or 10 mg four times daily, increased if necessary to 6 to 8 times daily. Once the condition is stabilised it may be possible to reduce the dosage. To prevent attacks of exercise-induced asthma, an additional dose may be inhaled up to 1 hour before exertion. Prophylaxis with sodium cromoglycate should be tried for several weeks before the benefits of treatment are assessed. Since inhalation of the dry powder may cause bronchospasm, isoprenaline has been inhaled concomitantly; however the use of a bronchodilator, such as salbutamol, inhaled a few minutes beforehand is preferable.

For allergic rhinitis, 10 mg of sodium cromoglycate as powder is given by nasal insufflation into each nostril up to 4 times daily or approximately 5 mg as a 2% or 4% solution is administered as drops or spray into each nostril up to 6 times daily. In ophthalmic conditions it is applied as drops of 2 or 4%, or as a 4% eye ointment.

In food allergy, sodium cromoglycate may be given by mouth in usual doses of 200 mg four times daily before meals either as capsules or as an oral solution prepared by dissolving the contents of the capsules in water; children over 2 years may be given 100 mg four times daily. If satisfactory control is not achieved within 2 to 3 weeks the dosage may be doubled, but should not exceed 40 mg per kg body-weight daily; a reduction in dosage may be possible once symptoms have been controlled.

ACTION. The precise mode of action of sodium cromoglycate remains uncertain. Mast-cell degranulation in target organs such as the bronchi, nasal mucosa, gastro-intestinal tract, or skin, has been widely assumed to be responsible for most of the common 'allergic' disorders in atopic subjects, and the hypothesis that sodium cromoglycate acts as a mast-cell stabiliser and inhibits the release from sensitised mast cells of histamine and other inflammatory mediators (including those leukotrienes formerly known as slow-reacting substance of anaphylaxis) has been promulgated as a result of indirect evidence and studies *in vitro*. However, there is no evidence that these properties are of clinical significance and the therapeutic effects of sodium cromoglycate cannot be explained on the basis of mast-cell stabilisation alone (*Br. med. J.*, 1981, *282*, 587). It has been pointed out that sodium cromoglycate has several properties that could account for its activity in asthma, such as phosphodiesterase inhibition, reduction of alpha-adrenoceptor density, suppression of the effects of platelet-activating factor, inhibition of IgE-dependent mediator secretion by cell types other than mast cells, and inhibition of neural transmission in vagal C fibres (P.J. Thompson *et al.*, *Lancet*, 1983, *2*, 848). Although sodium cromoglycate has been considered to be devoid of intrinsic bronchodilator activity some researchers (J.T.N. Chung and R.S. Jones, *Br. med. J.*, 1979, *2*, 1033; C.R. Horn *et al.*, *Br. J. clin. Pharmac.*, 1984, *18*, 798) have claimed that it may possess some bronchodilating action.

It has been proposed as a result of earlier findings that exacerbation of asthma symptoms is a consequence of the formation of platelet-activating factor (PAF; paf-acether) in the lung and that its inflammatory sequelae, including an effect of platelets or their products on airway smooth muscle, cause the characteristic bronchial hyperreactivity and induce hypertrophy of smooth muscle. The actions of sodium cromoglycate in asthma might be related to an effect on tissues responding to platelet-activating factor (J. Morley *et al.*, *Lancet*, 1984, *2*, 1142). However, some other researchers have found no evidence for an involvement of platelets in asthma (I.A. Greer *et al.*, *ibid.*, 1479; S.R. Durham *et al.*, *ibid.*, 1985, *2*, 36). Also, it has been pointed out that many inflammatory mediators may be implicated in asthma and explanations in terms of a single mediator or a single cell type are unlikely to result in useful therapy (P.J. Barnes, *Br. J. Hosp. Med.*, 1985, *34*, 339).

A hypothesis that axon reflexes are involved in the pathophysiology of asthma. Sodium cromoglycate might have an inhibitory effect by preventing the release of sensory neuropeptides.— P. J. Barnes, *Lancet*, 1986, *1*, 242.

ADMINISTRATION. Some children can use the Intal Spinhaler satisfactorily by the age of 3 but the majority obtain little benefit until they are 5 years old. For those unable to use the Spinhaler, sodium cromoglycate can be given as a nebulised solution delivered by a compressor/nebuliser system. Administration takes up to 10 minutes and must be repeated 3 to 4 times daily. When the child has troublesome coughing and wheezing further improvement can be achieved by adding 0.5 mL of 0.5% salbutamol respirator solution to the sodium cromoglycate.— A. D. Milner, *Prescribers' J.*, 1980, *20*, 33.

Sodium cromoglycate as a metered-dose pressurised aerosol is available as an alternative to inhalation of the dry powder in the management of asthma, and may be more convenient in that it does not have to be charged before each inhalation, but some patients, especially children, can use a dry-powder inhaler when they cannot manage metered-dose aerosols (*Drug & Ther. Bull.*, 1981, *19*, 41). The pressurised aerosol system was also considered to be quieter and less obtrusive than powder inhalation although the ten-fold difference in dose between the aerosol and the powder was questioned (*ibid.*, 1982, *20*, 27). Placebo-controlled studies have shown administration by pressurised aerosol to be effective in children aged 4 to 13 years (C. Geller-Bernstein and S. Levin, *Curr. ther. Res.*, 1983, *34*, 345) and in adults (D. Wheatley, *Curr. med. Res. Opinion*, 1983, *8*, 333; A.E. Rubin *et al.*, *ibid.*, 553). In a comparison with inhalation as dry powder Robson *et al.* (*Br. J. clin. Pharmac.*, 1981, *11*, 383) found 20 mg four times daily as dry powder to be more effective in preventing asthmatic symptoms than 2 mg four times daily from a pressurised aerosol in children aged 6 to 13 years; similarly, Bar-Yishay *et al.* (*Archs Dis. Childh.*, 1983, *58*, 624) found the aerosol to be less effective than the dry powder in protecting against exercise-induced asthma in children 9 to 14 years of age. However, sodium cromoglycate 2 mg from an aerosol was as effective as 20 mg inhaled as dry powder against bronchoconstriction stimulated by hyperventilation of cold air in adults (K.M. Latimer *et al.*, *Thorax*, 1984, *39*, 277).

ASTHMA. Guidelines for the general management of asthma. The decision to use regular treatment in patients with chronic asthma will depend on the frequency and severity of symptoms; when mild episodes of wheezing occur once or twice a month, inhalation of beta-stimulants to relieve the symptoms usually suffices. When attacks are more frequent, regular treatment with beta-stimulants, inhaled steroids, or sodium cromoglycate is necessary. When chronic symptoms persist despite appropriate inhaled treatment a short course of oral corticosteroids often produces improvement which can last for many months.— J. Rees, *Br. med. J.*, 1984, *288*, 1595. Sodium cromoglycate is used as the first line prophylactic agent after failure to control chronic asthma with occasional inhalation of a beta-agonist. Success is most likely in young atopic asthmatics, but may occur at all ages. Cromoglycate should not be dismissed as ineffective until it has been tried for at least 4 weeks , and it must be used regularly. Reflex bronchoconstriction due to irritant effects of the dry powder may be overcome by switching to the metered-dose aerosol or by inhalation of a beta-agonist beforehand: the use of compound preparations containing cromoglycate with isoprenaline is unsatisfactory, as patients tend to use the preparation inappropriately, for the immediate bronchodilator effect.— *idem*, 1819.

Asthma in children. A review of asthma in childhood. Infants under 18 months of age are relatively unresponsive to beta agonists, but inhaled ipratropium bromide for temporary relief or oral theophylline for continuing problems may be helpful. If further prophylaxis is needed regular nebulised cromoglycate may be effective. Over 18 months of age the beta agonists become more effective and over 4 years of age inhalation treatment becomes easier. Mild episodic asthma responds to beta agonists and more frequent attacks benefit from regular prophylaxis with slow-release theophylline preparations or inhaled sodium cromoglycate. Explanation of the correct use of sodium cromoglycate is important since many treatment failures are due to irregular use or inadequate technique. If the above treatment fails, inhaled corticosteroids are required.— J. Reiser, *Br. J. Hosp. Med.*, 1985, *33*, 196. See also J. Price, *Br. med. J.*, 1984, *288*, 1895.

Comparative studies of sodium cromoglycate with other agents in the management of childhood asthma.— G. Hambleton *et al.*, *Lancet*, 1977, *1*, 381 (with theophylline); A. T. Edmunds *et al.*, *Br. med. J.*, 1980, *281*, 842 (with slow-release aminophylline); R. L. Henry *et al.*, *Archs Dis. Childh.*, 1984, *59*, 54 (with ipratropium bromide).

See also Administration, above and Bronchitis, below.

Exercise-induced asthma. A brief review of the pathophysiology and management of exercise-induced asthma. Of the drugs which can be given before exercise to inhibit the symptoms, sodium cromoglycate or theophylline are less effective than inhaled sympathomimetics. Sodium cromoglycate is effective immediately after inhalation in the majority of children, but its effect largely wears off after about 2 to 3 hours.— S. Godfrey, *Archs Dis. Childh.*, 1983, *58*, 1.

Results of a study of the dose-response effect of sodium cromoglycate pressurised aerosol in patients with exercise-induced asthma showed that the optimum prophylactic dose varied between patients, but suggested that an aerosol supplying 5 mg in each inhalation would allow greater flexibility in adjusting dosage and frequency of administration.— W. M. Tullett *et al.*, *Thorax*, 1985, *40*, 41.

For a comparison of nebulised sodium cromoglycate and verapamil in the management of adults with exercise-induced asthma, see under Verapamil Hydrochloride, p.92.

Pregnancy and the neonate. A review of the management of asthma in pregnancy. For mild episodes of bronchospasm requiring drug therapy, and where theophylline or ephedrine cannot be tolerated, sodium cromoglycate can be considered.— P. A. Greenberger and R. Patterson, *New Engl. J. Med.*, 1985, *312*, 897.

BRONCHITIS. Response to treatment with nebulised sodium cromoglycate was found to be age-related in a crossover study in 44 children with recurrent or persistent wheezy bronchitis and a history of allergic symptoms. Sodium cromoglycate was superior to placebo in the 12- to 24-month age group, but not in those below 12 months of age. This age-related response might reflect differing aetiology. Most of the older group appeared to have early-onset asthma whereas in infants below 12 months wheezy bronchitis is frequently triggered by respiratory viral infections.— C. Geller-Bernstein and S. Levin, *Respiration*, 1982, *43*, 294.

CONJUNCTIVITIS. A detailed review of the use of sodium cromoglycate in allergic eye disease. Sodium cromoglycate eye-drops or eye ointment have been used primarily in the prophylaxis of allergic eye conditions involving type I (IgE-mediated) hypersensitivity reactions, such as hay-fever conjunctivitis, acute and chronic allergic conjunctivitis (caused by allergens other than pollens), and vernal keratoconjunctivitis. Ocular sodium cromoglycate has little or no effect on types II, III, and IV hypersensitivity reactions; however, it has proved useful in giant papillary conjunctivitis, which is associated with the use of contact lenses or ocular prostheses, and in which, despite many similarities to vernal keratoconjunctivitis, IgE concentrations may be normal. In open studies, good responses have been seen within 7 days of beginning treatment in patients with acute allergic or hay-fever conjunctivitis, but in more chronic forms of allergic conjunctivitis an effect may not be exerted for 10 to 14 days. Patients may be advised to initiate prophylactic treatment with ocular sodium cromoglycate some weeks before they are likely to encounter allergens which are known to precipate their ocular attacks. In those conditions in which it is effective, sodium cromoglycate may diminish the need for ophthalmic corticosteroid treatment, with its associated hazards; however, in combination with corticosteroids it has proved to be highly effective in treating acute exacerbations or severe chronic cases of these diseases. Although further trials are needed to establish clearly the comparative efficacy of ocular sodium cromoglycate and corticosteroids in type I allergic reactions, the safety profile of sodium cromoglycate may especially favour its use in chronic or recurrent allergic eye conditions throughout the duration of exposure to the offending allergens. When drug therapy is indicated in these type I allergic eye diseases, sodium cromoglycate should be considered as a first-line agent.— E. M. Sorkin and A. Ward, *Drugs*, 1986, *31*,

131. See also *Med. Lett.*, 1985, *27*, 7.

See also under Rhinitis, below.

A study involving 31 patients with hay-fever conjunctivitis was considered to demonstrate that ocular stinging with sodium cromoglycate eye-drops was mainly due to the phenethyl alcohol preservative, and that a newer formulation containing benzalkonium chloride as sole preservative was better tolerated, and as a result, more effective.— C. G. Inerfield *et al.*, *Practitioner*, 1984, *228*, 543.

FOOD ALLERGY. A review of the management of food allergy. Dietary elimination is the most effective, safest, and least expensive treatment of food allergy. In most instances, avoidance of the offending food or foods is feasible and results in a satisfactory control of symptoms, but pharmacological agents may be used for symptomatic or prophylactic relief. Oral sodium cromoglycate has shown promising results in the prophylaxis of food allergy, but because it is not absorbed to any degree it has proved much more effective in preventing symptoms in the gastro-intestinal tract than in remote organs. It is most effective when administered 30 to 60 minutes before food, usually in doses between 50 and 200 mg although doses up to 800 mg may sometimes be required; when high doses are required initially, the dose may be gradually reduced later to the smallest effective quantity. The effects usually last for a few hours.— S. L. Bahna, *Ann. Allergy*, 1984, *53*, 678.

In a placebo-controlled double-blind crossover study 14 of 20 subjects with food allergies obtained relief from both gastro-intestinal and systemic symptoms while taking sodium cromoglycate in doses of 50 or 100 mg in about 50 mL of warm water swilled around the mouth and swallowed half-an-hour before the 3 main meals and before bedtime. Four of the 14 patients, however, developed an adverse reaction to sodium cromoglycate (headaches in 2, insomnia in 1, and urticaria in 1). A further 3 of an initial 24 selected for the study also developed adverse reactions (headaches in 2 and rhinorrhoea in 1).— G. A. Vaz *et al.*, *Lancet*, 1978, *1*, 1066.

Sodium cromoglycate by mouth in a dose of 800 mg daily for a week or as a single 1-g dose before challenge, failed to protect 9 patients from asthma or urticaria, or both, induced by various foods or by aspirin. However in 4 of them sodium cromoglycate 40 mg by inhalation gave almost immediate protection against rapid asthmatic reactions to coconut, port, tartrazine, and Bacardi, respectively.— M. G. Harries *et al.*, *Clin. Allergy*, 1978, *8*, 423.

A significant protective effect on the symptoms of gastro-intestinal food allergy was shown when sodium cromoglycate was administered by mouth for 2 days prior to antigen ingestion in children with diarrhoea directly related to food proteins. It has not proved effective when given to symptomatic children taking antigen at the time therapy was initiated.— S. Kocoshis and J. D. Gryboski, *J. Am. med. Ass.*, 1979, *242*, 1169.

In a double-blind controlled study 8 of 20 patients who had suffered from persistent diarrhoea for periods ranging from 3 to 30 years noted significant improvement while taking sodium cromoglycate 800 mg daily by mouth. The results suggested that food allergy may be a contributory factor in diarrhoea of unknown aetiology.— T. D. Bolin, *Gut*, 1980, *21*, 848. Beneficial results with sodium cromoglycate 1.5 g daily by mouth for 8 weeks in patients with positive skin prick tests to food allergens and irritable bowel syndrome characterised by predominant diarrhoea.— G. F. Stefanini *et al.* (letter), *Lancet*, 1986, *1*, 207.

Studies suggesting that migraine may be a food-allergic disease and that oral sodium cromoglycate exerts a protective effect in some patients.— J. Monro *et al.*, *Lancet*, 1980, *2*, 1; J. Monro *et al.*, *ibid.*, 1984, *2*, 719. Severe criticism.— J. N. Blau (letter), *ibid.*, 926; J. M. S. Pearce (letter), *ibid.*

GASTRO-INTESTINAL DISORDERS. *Crohn's disease.* Sodium cromoglycate 800 mg daily by mouth was of no benefit in a controlled study of 25 patients with Crohn's disease whose sulphasalazine treatment had been stopped.— V. Binder *et al.*, *Gut*, 1981, *22*, 55.

Food allergy. See above.

Gastritis. In a study in patients with diffuse varioliform gastritis, an uncommon form of gastric mucosal inflammation in which type I hypersensitivity may play a role, sodium cromoglycate 200 or 400 mg daily by mouth for 28 days, resulted in significant clinical improvement compared with placebo.— C. André *et al.*, *Gut*, 1982, *23*, 348.

Ulcerative colitis and proctitis. Commenting on the management of symptomatic proctitis and distal ulcerative colitis, Allan (*Br. med. J.*, 1982, *284*, 70) noted that most patients respond rapidly to standard treatment, including sulphasalazine and corticosteroid retention enemas, and that the role of sodium cromoglycate seems limited. Although Mani *et al.* (*Lancet*, 1976, *1*, 439) reported beneficial results with oral sodium cromoglycate in a small study in 12 patients with ulcerative colitis, Binder *et al.* (*Gut*, 1981, *22*, 55) subsequently found sodium cromoglycate 800 mg daily by mouth to be no more effective than placebo in a study involving 141 similar patients. In comparative studies of the maintenance of remission in ulcerative colitis (M.W. Dronfield and M.J.S. Langman, *Gut*, 1978, *19*, 1136; C.P. Willoughby *et al.*, *Lancet*, 1979, *1*, 119) sodium cromoglycate proved much less effective than sulphasalazine, although Whorwell *et al.* (*Postgrad. med. J.*, 1981, *57*, 436) reported sodium cromoglycate to be more effective than placebo in preventing relapse. Allan notes, however, that there is general agreement that the addition of sodium cromoglycate to conventional treatment confers no benefit. More recently Grace *et al.* (*Gut*, 1984, *25*, A1156) have reported beneficial results with sodium cromoglycate retention enemas in patients with distal ulcerative colitis.

HAY FEVER. See Conjunctivitis, above, and Rhinitis, below.

MASTOCYTOSIS. In a double-blind crossover study involving 5 patients, sodium cromoglycate 100 mg four times daily by mouth relieved the symptoms of systemic mastocytosis in the skin, gastro-intestinal tract, and central nervous system when compared with placebo. Of the 4 who received a total of 18 courses of sodium cromoglycate, lasting from 1 to 10 months, marked improvement was seen in 3 but patients relapsed within 2 to 3 weeks of stopping treatment.— N. A. Soter *et al.*, *New Engl. J. Med.*, 1979, *301*, 465.

RHINITIS. A review of the treatment of rhinitis. Sodium cromoglycate is effective in both seasonal and perennial allergic rhinitis for the prevention of sneezing, rhinorrhoea, nasal itching, and, to a lesser extent, nasal congestion. However, the degree of improvement in nasal symptoms is modest and some patients get no symptomatic relief, perhaps in part because of poor compliance. Nasal polyps are not reduced in size, and there is no significant benefit in nonallergic eosinophilic rhinitis.— F. E. R. Simons and K. J. Simons, *Clin. Rev. Allergy*, 1984, *2*, 237.

A review of the management of hay fever. Patients only mildly affected, or severely affected on only a few days, need a preparation which gives immediate relief and can be used intermittently, but severely affected patients may need prophylaxis before the hay-fever season starts, as well as topical therapy throughout the season or even systemic treatment. Sodium cromoglycate is effective only if used prophylactically and should be applied at least 4 times a day. Nasal symptoms alone are best treated prophylactically with a topical corticosteroid or sodium cromoglycate as nasal insufflation, spray, or drops. If congestion impedes delivery of cromoglycate to the mucosa a topical sympathomimetic should be given immediately beforehand, preferably for no longer than a few days. Eye symptoms alone are treated with sodium cromoglycate eye-drops or, if intermittent, with antihistamine-decongestant drops. If symptoms occur in combination or are accompanied by itching of palate or ears, an oral antihistamine is more appropriate. Hyposensitisation or systemic corticosteroids need rarely be used.— *Drug & Ther. Bull.*, 1985, *23*, 25.

SKIN DISORDERS. Reports of the *topical application* of sodium cromoglycate in individual patients with a variety of skin disorders: G. Silverman (letter), *Br. med. J.*, 1973, *3*, 502 (application of insufflation capsule contents to allergic urticarial wheals); P. Lip (letter), *Med. J. Aust.*, 1978, *2*, 32 (powder from capsules emptied into chronic leg ulcers); K. M. De Cock and M. G. Thorne, *Br. J. Derm.*, 1980, *102*, 231 (2% solution applied topically in pyoderma gangrenosum).

Reports of sodium cromoglycate given *by mouth* to individual patients with various skin disorders: E. L. Rhodes, *Br. J. Derm.*, 1978, *99*, 581 (response in dermatitis herpetiformis); A. D. Ormerod and P. J. A. Holt, *Br. J. Derm.*, 1983, *108*, 723 (prevention of alcohol-induced urticaria); S. Hatty *et al.*, *Postgrad. med. J.*, 1983, *59*, 586 (lack of benefit from oral administration in severe exercise-induced urticaria and angioedema but response when given by insufflation); M. L. Wood and D. N. Slater (letter), *Lancet*, 1983, *2*, 282 (resolution of cutaneous manifestations of the hypereosinophilic syndrome); H. A. Jenkinson and K. W. Scott, *Br. J. Derm.*, 1984, *111*, *Suppl.* 26 99 (improvement in bullous urticaria pigmentosa).

Eczema. Contrary to previous anecdotal reports, sodium cromoglycate 100 mg four times daily by mouth was no more effective than placebo in a crossover study in 29 children with atopic eczema. The study was restricted to children who had already benefited from dietary avoidance of egg and milk.— D. J. Atherton *et al.*, *Br. J. Derm.*, 1982, *106*, 681. See also P. Graham *et al.*, *ibid.*, 1984, *110*, 457.

Variable results have been reported with sodium cromoglycate applied *topically* in atopic eczema. In a study in children Haider (*Br. med. J.*, 1977, *1*, 1570) found a 10% ointment applied twice daily to be more effective than placebo; pruritus was significantly reduced by week 4. However, no benefit was seen in a similar study (T. Thirumoorthy and M.W. Greaves, *ibid.*, 1978, *2*, 500) in adults and older children with more severe forms of atopic eczema. M. Ariyanayagam *et al.* (*Br. J. Derm.*, 1985, *112*, 343) noted some benefit with a 4% sodium cromoglycate cream, although a large placebo effect was seen in children and in general there was no benefit in severe eczema.

ULCER, APHTHOUS. Aphthous ulcers cleared in 2 patients when given sodium cromoglycate 2.5% in a toothpaste which they used three times daily.— M. Frost (letter), *Lancet*, 1973, *2*, 389. The presence of a soap was needed to allow adequate oral absorption of sodium cromoglycate.— *idem* (letter), *Br. dent. J.*, 1978, *144*, 269.

A crossover study in 27 patients with recurrent oral aphthae not associated with other disorders demonstrated no significant effect of sodium cromoglycate 4% as a toothpaste formulated with Tween 80, compared with placebo, when both were used twice daily for 12 weeks.— A. J. C. Potts *et al.*, *ibid.*, 1984, *156*, 250.

Preparations

Cromolyn Sodium for Inhalation *(U.S.P.)*. Hard gelatin capsules containing a mixture of equal parts of sodium cromoglycate and lactose.

Cromolyn Sodium Inhalation *(U.S.P.)*. A sterile solution of sodium cromoglycate.

Cromolyn Sodium Nasal Solution *(U.S.P.)*. A solution of sodium cromoglycate.

Cromolyn Sodium Ophthalmic Solution *(U.S.P.)*. A sterile solution of sodium cromoglycate.

Sodium Cromoglycate Insufflation *(B.P.)*. Hard gelatin capsules containing either sodium cromoglycate or sodium cromoglycate mixed with an approximately equal amount of lactose. The capsules are intended for use in an inhaler.

Proprietary Preparations

Intal *(Fisons, UK)*. *Inhaler*, aerosol, sodium cromoglycate 1 mg/metered inhalation.
Inhaler (Intal 5), aerosol, sodium cromoglycate 5 mg/metered inhalation.
Nebuliser solution, sodium cromoglycate 10 mg/mL, in ampoules of 2 mL.
Spincaps, inhalation cartridges, sodium cromoglycate 20 mg, for use in specially designed inhalers (Halermatic or Spinhaler).

Intal Compound *(Fisons, UK)*. *Spincaps*, inhalation cartridges, sodium cromoglycate 20 mg, isoprenaline sulphate 100 μg, for use in specially designed inhalers (Halermatic or Spinhaler).

Nalcrom *(Fisons, UK)*. *Capsules*, sodium cromoglycate 100 mg. To be swallowed whole, or the contents dissolved in water and sipped.

Opticrom *(Fisons, UK)*. *Eye-drops*, sodium cromoglycate 2%.
Eye ointment, sodium cromoglycate 4%.

Rynacrom *(Fisons, UK)*. *Insufflation cartridges*, sodium cromoglycate 10 mg, for use in a specially designed nasal insufflator.
Nasal drops, sodium cromoglycate 2%.
Nasal spray (formerly known as Rynacrom M), sodium cromoglycate 2% (approximately 2.6 mg/metered dose).

Rynacrom Compound *(Fisons, UK)*. *Nasal spray*, sodium cromoglycate 2%, xylometazoline hydrochloride 0.025% (sodium cromoglycate approximately 2.6 mg, xylometazoline hydrochloride approximately 32.5 μg/metered dose).

Proprietary Names and Manufacturers

Alercrom *(Arg.)*; Alerion *(Bouchara, Fr.)*; Allergocrom *(Ursapharm, Ger.)*; Colimune *(Fisons, Ger.)*; Cromantal *(Nuovo, Ital.)*; Cromo-Asma *(Aldo, Spain)*; Cromoptic *(Chauvin-Blache, Fr.)*; Cusicrom *(Cusi, Spain)*; Duracroman *(Durachemie, Ger.)*; Esirhinol *(Declimed, Ger.)*; Fivent *(Fisons, Canad.)*; Frenal *(ISF, Ital.; Sigma Tau, Spain)*; Gastrofrenal *(ISF, Ital.)*; Intal *(Arg.; Fisons, Austral.; Fisons, Canad.; Fisons, Ger.; Jpn; Searle, Spain; Fisons, Switz.; Fisons, UK; Fisons, USA)*; Lomudal *(Belg.; Fisons, Denm.; Fisons, Fr.; Fisons, Ital.; Neth.; Fisons, Norw.; Fisons, S.Afr.; Fisons, Swed.; Fisons, Switz.)*; Lomupren *(Fisons, Ger.)*; Lomusol *(Belg.; Fr.; Neth.; Fisons, UK)*; Lomuspray *(Fisons, Ital.)*; Nalcrom *(Fisons, Canad.; Fisons, Ital.; NZ; Fisons, S.Afr.; Fisons, Switz.; Fisons, UK)*; Nalcron

(Fisons, Fr.); Nasalcrom *(Fisons, USA)*; Nasmil *(Spain)*; Nebulasma *(Septa, Spain)*; Opticrom *(Fisons, Austral.; Fisons, Canad.; Fisons, Ger.; NZ; Fisons, Switz.; Fisons, UK; Fisons, USA)*; Opticron *(Fisons, Fr.)*; Rynacrom *(Fisons, Austral.; Belg.; Fisons, Canad.; Neth.; Fisons, S.Afr.; Fisons, UK)*; Sificrom *(SIFI, Ital.)*; Vividrin *(Mann, Ger.)*.

13170-m

Ambicromil *(BAN, rINN)*.
FPL-58668KC *(calcium salt)*; Probicromil. 4,6-Dioxo-10-propyl-4*H*,6*H*-pyrano[3,2-*g*]chromene-2,8-dicarboxylic acid.
$C_{17}H_{12}O_8$=344.3.

CAS — 58805-38-2 (ambicromil); 71144-97-3 (calcium salt).

NOTE. Probicromil Calcium is *USAN*.

Ambicromil has been investigated for the prophylaxis of allergic conditions.

Proprietary Names and Manufacturers
Fisons, UK.

7722-l

Bufrolin Sodium *(BANM, pINNM)*.
ICI-74917. Disodium 6-butyl-1,4,7,10-tetrahydro-4,10-dioxo-1,7-phenanthroline-2,8-dicarboxylate.
$C_{18}H_{14}N_2Na_2O_6$=400.3.

CAS — 54867-56-0 (bufrolin); 54545-84-5 (disodium salt).

Bufrolin sodium has an action on mast cells resembling that of sodium cromoglycate and has been administered by aerosol inhalation in the prophylactic treatment of asthma.

Proprietary Names and Manufacturers
ICI Pharmaceuticals, UK.

7723-y

Doxantrazole
3-(1*H*-Tetrazol-5-yl)-9*H*-thioxanthen-9-one 10,10-dioxide.
$C_{14}H_8N_4O_3S$=312.3.

CAS — 51762-95-9.

Preliminary studies indicated that doxantrazole had an action on mast cells resembling that of sodium cromoglycate and was effective by mouth, but benefit was not confirmed in subsequent clinical studies in asthmatics.

Proprietary Names and Manufacturers
Wellcome, UK.

7724-j

Ketotifen Fumarate *(BANM, USAN, rINNM)*.

HC-20511 *(ketotifen)*. 4-(1-Methylpiperidin-4-ylidene)-4*H*-benzo[4,5]cyclohepta-[1,2-*b*]-thiophen-10(9*H*)-one hydrogen fumarate.
$C_{19}H_{19}NOS,C_4H_4O_4$=425.5.

CAS — 34580-13-7 (ketotifen); 34580-14-8 (fumarate).

Ketotifen fumarate 1.38 mg is approximately equivalent to 1 mg of ketotifen. Readily **soluble** in water.

Adverse Effects, Treatment, and Precautions
As for the antihistamines in general, p.443.
Increased appetite and weight gain have been reported. A reversible fall in the platelet count has been observed in a few patients receiving ketotifen concomitantly with oral antidiabetic agents and it has been suggested that this combination should therefore be avoided.
For precautions to be observed in asthmatic patients, see sodium cromoglycate (p.1419).

Sedation, tiredness, weight gain, and dry mouth were the most common side-effects in postmarketing surveillance of ketotifen involving 19 252 patients, 8291 of whom were studied for 1 year. Other frequently reported side-effects, definitely or probably related to the drug, were dizziness, nausea, and headache; exacerbation of asthma, bronchospasm, and status asthmaticus occurred in some patients while receiving ketotifen.— W. P. Maclay *et al., Br. med. J.*, 1984, *288*, 911.

OVERDOSAGE. Eight patients aged 6 to 34 years took overdoses of ketotifen in doses stated to range from 10 to 120 mg. Plasma concentrations of ketotifen base in 4 patients were 5 to 122 ng per mL (therapeutic range 1 to 4 ng per mL). Symptoms included drowsiness, confusion, dyspnoea, bradycardia or tachycardia, disorientation, and convulsions. Gastric lavage was performed in 6, and all 8 recovered within 12 hours after supportive treatment.— D. B. Jefferys and G. N. Volans, *Br. med. J.*, 1981, *282*, 1755.

Absorption and Fate
Ketotifen fumarate is absorbed from the gastro-intestinal tract and, together with metabolites, is excreted in the urine and faeces.

Uses and Administration
Ketotifen has the properties of the antihistamines (p.444) in addition to actions on mast cells analogous to those of sodium cromoglycate. It is used in the prophylactic treatment of asthma and has also been given in the treatment of allergic conditions such as rhinitis and conjunctivitis.
Ketotifen fumarate is taken by mouth in doses equivalent to 1 mg of ketotifen twice daily with food, increased if necessary to the equivalent of 2 mg twice daily; children over 2 years may be given 1 mg twice daily.

A brief review of the actions and uses of ketotifen.— G. F. MacDonald, *Chest*, 1982, *82*, 30S.

ACTION. A review of the pharmacology of ketotifen and the conclusion that its anti-allergic action could be dissociated from, and was not dependent on, its antihistaminic properties. In addition to its antihistaminic action, inhibition of phosphodiesterases, blockade of calcium channels, inhibition of the release of the mixture of leukotrienes known as slow-reacting substance of anaphylaxis (SRS-A), and functional antagonism of the effects of SRS-A have been demonstrated, and there is now some evidence for an effect on beta$_2$-receptor mediated reactions.— C. Greenwood, *Chest*, 1982, *82*, 45S.

For discussion of the potential role of platelet-activating factor in asthma, including mention of the ability of ketotifen to inhibit the induction of platelet-dependent bronchoconstriction, see J. Morley *et al., Lancet*, 1984, *2*, 1142.

ASTHMA. Ketotifen has an action resembling that of sodium cromoglycate and can prevent attacks of allergic asthma, but only achieves its maximal effect after it has been taken for several weeks. Trials lasting 4 weeks or less have shown little benefit.— *Drug & Ther. Bull.*, 1980, *18*, 14. In postmarketing surveillance of ketotifen, 76% of 19 252 asthmatic patients considered the drug effective after treatment for 3 months.— W. P. Maclay *et al., Br. med. J.*, 1984, *288*, 911. Although the results of studies *in vitro* with ketotifen are impressive, and clinical studies have shown some protective effect, its place in the management of childhood asthma is still not clearly established.— J. Price, *ibid.*, 1895.

A crossover study in 43 patients with bronchial asthma showed no significant difference in effectiveness overall between ketotifen 1 mg twice daily by mouth and sodium cromoglycate 20 mg four times daily by inhalation, both for 12 weeks. Some individual patients appeared to do better on ketotifen and others on cromoglycate.— J. W. Paterson *et al., Eur. J. clin. Pharmac.*, 1983, *25*, 187.

RHINITIS. Comment that in hay fever ketotifen seems to be acting mainly as an antihistamine.— *Drug & Ther. Bull.*, 1985, *23*, 25.

Studies on the use of ketotifen in patients with allergic rhinitis: G. Melillo *et al., Curr. ther. Res.*, 1983, *34*, 350; O. Resta *et al., ibid.*, 1984, *35*, 235; L. Businco *et al., ibid.*, 239; D. Wheatley, *Practitioner*, 1984, *228*, 685.

SKIN DISORDERS. References to the use of ketotifen in urticaria: K. Kuokkanen, *Acta allerg.*, 1975, *30*, 73; *idem*, 1977, *32*, 316.

Proprietary Preparations
Zaditen *(Sandoz, UK)*. *Capsules*, ketotifen 1 mg (as fumarate).
Tablets, scored, ketotifen 1 mg (as fumarate).
Elixir, ketotifen 1 mg (as fumarate)/5 mL.

Proprietary Names and Manufacturers
Globofil *(Robert, Spain)*; Ketasma *(Lesvi, Spain)*; Totifen *(Master Pharma, Ital.)*; Zaditen *(Belg.; Sandoz, Fr.; Wander, Ger.; Sandoz, Ital.; Lux.; Neth.; Wander, S.Afr.; Wander, Switz.; Sandoz, UK)*; Zasten *(Sandoz, Spain)*.

12899-y

Lodoxamide *(BAN, rINN)*.
U-42585E *(lodoxamide trometamol)*; U-42718 *(lodoxamide ethyl)*. *N,N'*-(2-Chloro-5-cyano-*m*-phenylene)dioxamic acid.
$C_{11}H_6ClN_3O_6$=311.6.

CAS — 53882-12-5 (lodoxamide); 53882-13-6 (lodoxamide ethyl); 63610-09-3 (lodoxamide trometamol).

NOTE. Lodoxamide Ethyl and Lodoxamide Tromethamine are *USAN*.

Lodoxamide has an action on mast cells resembling that of sodium cromoglycate and has been given by mouth, generally as the ethyl ester, or by aerosol inhalation, generally as the trometamol salt, in studies of its prophylactic effect in the treatment of asthma.

In a study involving 13 patients with a history of allergic asthma lodoxamide ethyl in doses of 1 or 3 mg by mouth 30 minutes before antigen challenge gave significant protection against immediate bronchospasm, but 4 subsequently experienced a delayed asthmatic reaction after several hours. A dose of 300 µg gave no significant protection. Side-effects were frequent, the commonest being a generalised sensation of warmth, transient nausea, and diaphoresis; use of a 10 mg dose was stopped halfway through the study because of the incidence of side-effects.— R. L. Case *et al., J. Am. med. Ass.*, 1982, *247*, 661.

Lodoxamide trometamol 100 or 500 µg given 4 times daily by aerosol inhalation was of no benefit when compared with placebo in a 4-week double-blind study in 43 asthmatic patients, perhaps because longer term administration was necessary.— J. D. Wolfe *et al., J. Allergy & clin. Immunol.*, 1982, *69*, 153. Similar results from a study involving 68 patients with perennial allergic asthma given lodoxamide trometamol 250 µg four times daily by inhalation for 12 weeks, or placebo.— J. S. Mann *et al., ibid.*, 1985, *76*, 83.

Proprietary Names and Manufacturers
Upjohn, USA.

18666-r

Nedocromil Sodium *(BANM, USAN, rINNM)*.

FPL-59002 *(nedocromil)*; FPL-59002KC *(calcium salt)*; FPL-59002KP *(sodium salt)*. Disodium 9-ethyl-6,9-dihydro-4,6-dioxo-10-propyl-4*H*-pyrano-[3,2g]quinoline-2,8-dicarboxylate.
$C_{19}H_{15}NNa_2O_7$=415.3.

CAS — 69049-73-6 (nedocromil); 69049-74-7 (sodium salt).

NOTE. Nedocromil calcium is *USAN*.

Nedocromil sodium has an action on mast cells resembling that of sodium cromoglycate. It is given by inhalation in the prophylactic treatment of asthma in usual doses of 4 mg twice daily, increased to 4 mg four times daily where necessary.

A review of the pharmacodynamic and pharmacokinetic properties of nedocromil sodium, and its therapeutic efficacy in the treatment of reversible obstructive airways disease.— J. P. Gonzalez and R. N. Brogden, *Drugs*, 1987, *34*, 560.

Proprietary Preparations
Tilade *(Fisons, UK)*. *Inhaler*, aerosol, nedocromil sodium 2 mg/metered inhalation.

13137-h

Pirquinozol *(BAN, USAN, rINN).*
SQ-13847. 2-(Hydroxymethyl)pyrazolo[1,5-*c*]quinazolin-5(6*H*)-one.
$C_{11}H_9N_3O_2$=215.2.

CAS — 65950-99-4.

Pirquinozol has been reported to have anti-allergic activity.

Proprietary Names and Manufacturers
Squibb, UK.

13184-s

Proxicromil *(BAN, USAN, rINN).*
FPL-57787. 6,7,8,9-Tetrahydro-5-hydroxy-4-oxo-10-propyl-4*H*-benzo[*g*]chromene-2-carboxylic acid.
$C_{17}H_{18}O_5$=302.3.

CAS — 60400-92-2.

Proxicromil was under study as a prophylactic anti-allergic agent but study ceased because of toxicity in *animals.*

Proprietary Names and Manufacturers
Fisons, UK.

12988-j

Tranilast *(USAN, rINN).*
MK-341; N-5'. *N*-(3,4-Dimethoxycinnamoyl)anthranilic acid.
$C_{18}H_{17}NO_5$=327.3.

CAS — 53902-12-8.

Tranilast has an action on mast cells resembling that of sodium cromoglycate. It has been given by mouth in the prophylactic treatment of asthma.

A brief review of the actions and uses of tranilast. Preliminary studies of tranilast for the prophylactic treatment of asthma have been promising. Dosage is generally 100 mg three times daily by mouth in adults and 5 mg per kg body-weight daily in divided doses in children. Adverse reactions that may occur include anorexia, nausea, vomiting, abdominal pain, gastric discomfort, headache, drowsiness, insomnia, dizziness, malaise, and a decrease in the red blood cell count and haemoglobin; more rarely, palpitations, oedema, facial flushing, stomatitis, and occasional abnormalities of liver function may occur. Caution should be observed in patients with liver disorders.— *Drugs Today,* 1983, *19,* 486.

Further references: H. Azuma *et al., Br. J. Pharmac.,* 1976, *58,* 483; H. Shioda *et al., Allergy,* 1979, *34,* 213.

7725-z

Xanoxate Sodium *(USAN, rINNM).*
RS-6818; Sodium Xanoxate. Sodium 7-(1-methylethoxy)-9-oxo-9*H*-xanthene-2-carboxylate.
$C_{17}H_{13}NaO_5$=320.3.

CAS — 33459-27-7 (xanoxic acid); 41147-04-0 (sodium salt).

Xanoxate sodium has an action on mast cells resembling that of sodium cromoglycate and has been given by inhalation or by mouth in the prophylactic treatment of asthma.

Proprietary Names and Manufacturers
Syntex, USA.

14026-m

Zaprinast *(BAN, rINN).*
M&B-22948. 1,4-Dihydro-5-(2-propoxyphenyl)-1,2,3-triazolo[4,5-*d*]pyrimidin-7-one.
$C_{13}H_{13}N_5O_2$=271.3.

CAS — 37762-06-4.

Zaprinast has an action on mast cells resembling that of sodium cromoglycate and has been given by mouth for the prophylaxis of asthma.

References: R. M. Rudd *et al., Br. J. Dis. Chest,* 1983, *77,* 78.

Proprietary Names and Manufacturers
May & Baker, UK.

Solvents

6500-y

The solvents described in this section are those generally without specific therapeutic uses. Additional solvents used in pharmacy and described in other sections include alcohols, chlorinated hydrocarbons such as chloroform, and trichloroethylene, fixed oils, glycols, and paraffins.

Regulations governing the packaging and labelling of some of the solvents described in this section exist in certain countries including the *UK*. Some solvents are permitted for use in food; maximum concentrations are sometimes specified. Certain solvents are subject to abuse by inhalation and this has led to statutory controls over their supply.

An epidemiological review of deaths during 1971 to 1983 in the *UK* from the abuse of volatile substances; 282 deaths were detected and the number appeared to have increased during the most recent years, reaching 80 in 1983. Most deaths occurred in male subjects under 20 years of age. In 51% of cases death was attributed to the direct toxic effects of the solvent.— H. R. Anderson *et al.*, *Br. med. J.*, 1985, *290*, 304.

Further reviews and discussions of solvent abuse.— J. L. Herzberg and S. N. Wolkind, *Br. J. Hosp. Med.*, 1983, *29*, 72; D. V. Hamilton (letter), *ibid.*, 302; I. Sourindrhin, *Br. med. J.*, 1985, *290*, 94.

6501-j

Acetone *(BAN, USAN)*.

2-Propanone; Cetona; Dimethyl Ketone.
$CH_3.CO.CH_3$=58.08.

CAS — 67-64-1.

Pharmacopoeias. In *Arg., Aust., Br., Fr., Hung., Mex., Nord.,* and *Span.* Also in *U.S.N.F.*

A clear, colourless, volatile, mobile, inflammable liquid with a characteristic odour. *B.P.* specifies wt per mL 0.789 to 0.791 g *U.S.N.F.* specifies sp. gr. not more than 0.789. *B.P.* specifies a b.p. of 55.7° to 56.7°.

Miscible with water, alcohol, chloroform, ether, and most essential oils. A 50% solution in water is neutral to litmus. *B.P.* specifies **store** in well-closed containers at a temperature not exceeding 15°. *U.S.P.* specifies store in airtight containers.

Adverse Effects

Inhalation of acetone vapour causes excitement followed by CNS depression with headache, restlessness, and fatigue, leading to narcosis and unconsciousness at high concentrations. Vomiting and haematemesis may occur, and there is often a latent period of several hours. Hyperglycaemia has been reported after ingestion. The vapour is irritant to the eyes and respiratory tract in high concentrations.

Acetone is one of the solvents abused in 'glue-sniffing'.

In Great Britain the recommended exposure limits of acetone are 1000 ppm (long-term); 1250 ppm (short-term). In the *US* the permissible and recommended exposure limits are 2400 mg per m^3 and 590 mg per m^3 respectively.

Absorption and Fate

Acetone is absorbed through the lungs. It is mostly excreted unchanged through the lungs and in the urine.

Uses and Administration

Acetone is widely used as an industrial and pharmaceutical solvent; it is also used as a solvent in food processing. It is an ingredient of some skin preparations.

A suggestion that topical application of acetone might be useful in the dissolution of sea urchin spines.— J. S. Millar, *Br. med. J.*, 1984, *288*, 390.

6502-z

Acetonitrile

Ethanenitrile; Methyl Cyanide.
$CH_3.CN$=41.05.

CAS — 75-05-8.

A colourless liquid with an aromatic odour. Wt per mL about 0.79 g. B.p. about 81°.

Acetonitrile emits highly toxic fumes of hydrogen cyanide when heated to decomposition or when reacted with acids or oxidising agents.

Adverse Effects and Treatment

As for cyanides (see p.1350).

In Great Britain the recommended exposure limits of acetonitrile are 40 ppm (long-term); 60 ppm (short-term). In the *US* the permissible and recommended exposure limits are 70 mg per m^3 and 34 mg per m^3 respectively.

Uses and Administration

Acetonitrile is used as a pharmaceutical solvent.

6503-c

Amyl Acetate

A mixture of isomers, principally *iso-*, *sec-*, and *n*-amyl acetate. Amyl acetate used in pharmacy consists mainly of isoamyl acetate (3-methylbutyl acetate), perhaps with a small amount of the *sec*-isomer (2-methylbutyl acetate).
$C_7H_{14}O_2$=130.2.

CAS — 123-92-2 (iso-amyl acetate); 53496-15-4 (sec-amyl acetate); 628-63-7 (n-amyl acetate).

A colourless liquid with a sharp, fruity odour. Wt per mL about 0.87 g. B.p. about 140°.

Adverse Effects

Prolonged exposure to amyl acetate may produce headache, fatigue, and depression of the central nervous system. Irritation of the gastro-intestinal tract, respiratory tract, and eyes may also occur.

In Great Britain the recommended exposure limits are: *iso*-amyl acetate 100 ppm (long-term); 125 ppm (short-term); *n*-amyl acetate 100 ppm (long-term); 150 ppm (short-term); *sec*-amyl acetate 125 ppm (long-term); 150 ppm (short-term).

EFFECTS ON THE HEART. A 27-year-old man developed headache, nausea, and vomiting after using a paint containing amyl acetate as the solvent in an unventilated room. Some days later chest pain and dyspnoea developed; he was admitted to hospital 2 weeks after exposure with congestive heart failure which slowly responded to treatment.— P. L. Weissberg and I. D. Green, *Br. med. J.*, 1979, *2*, 1113.

Uses and Administration

Amyl acetate is used as an industrial solvent.

6504-k

Aniline

Phenylamine.
$C_6H_5.NH_2$=93.13.

CAS — 62-53-3.

A colourless or pale yellow oily liquid with a characteristic odour, readily darkening to brown on exposure to air and light. Wt per mL about 1.02 g. B.p. about 183°. **Store** in airtight containers. Protect from light.

Adverse Effects and Treatment

Inhalation, ingestion, or cutaneous absorption of aniline results in methaemoglobinaemia, with cyanosis, headache, weakness, stupor, and coma. Skin sensitisation, nausea, liver and kidney damage, and cardiac arrhythmias may occur. Haemolysis has been reported. Treatment may involve methylene blue, transfusions, or haemodialysis.

Bladder papillomas have been reported in workers previously exposed to aniline. Commercial aniline may be contaminated with β-naphthylamine, a potential carcinogen.

In Great Britain the recommended exposure limits of aniline are 2 ppm (long-term); 5 ppm (short-term); suitable precautions should be taken to prevent absorption through the skin.

Uses and Administration

Aniline has wide industrial applications. The use of aniline and its salts in cosmetics is prohibited by law in the *UK*.

6505-a

Benzene

Phenyl hydride.
C_6H_6=78.11.

CAS — 71-43-2.

NOTE. Benzene may be known as 'benzina', 'benzol', 'benzole', or 'benzolum'. However, 'benzol' is also used to describe a mixture of hydrocarbons and 'benzine' is used as a name for a commercial form of petroleum spirit.

Pharmacopoeias. In *Aust., Hung., Port.,* and *Span.*

A clear colourless inflammable liquid with a characteristic aromatic odour. Wt per mL about 0.88 g. B.p. about 80°.

Store in airtight containers.

Adverse Effects and Treatment

Symptoms of acute poisoning following inhalation or ingestion include initial excitement or euphoria followed by CNS depression with headache, dizziness, blurred vision, and ataxia, which in severe cases may progress to convulsions, coma, and death from respiratory failure. Other symptoms include nausea and irritation of the mucous membranes, ventricular arrhythmias may occur. Direct skin contact with liquid benzene may result in marked irritation, and dermatitis may develop on prolonged or repeated exposure.

Prolonged industrial exposure to benzene vapour has been associated with adverse effects on the gastro-intestinal tract and the CNS but in particular with marked effects on the bone marrow and blood, characterised by hypoplastic changes which may result in leucopenia, thrombocytopenia, and aplastic anaemia. Chromosome abnormalities have also been reported. These effects have been reported in workers exposed to relatively high concentrations of the vapour (around 200 ppm or more) but reduced red blood cell counts and anaemia have also been reported at lower concentrations. Early symptoms of chronic intoxication include headache, dizziness, irritability, fatigue, anorexia, pallor, and petechiae.

An association between chronic exposure to benzene and acute myelogenous leukaemia has been established.

Treatment consists of symptomatic and supportive measures. Gastric lavage may be performed for acute intoxication if the patient presents soon after ingestion but care must be taken to avoid aspiration. In chronic poisoning, repeated blood transfusions may be necessary. Adrenaline should be avoided because of the risk of precipitating cardiac arrhythmias.

In Great Britain the recommended exposure limit of benzene is 10 ppm (long-term). In the *US* the permissible and recommended exposure limits are 10 ppm and 1 ppm respectively.

Review of the toxicity of benzene.— R. J. Fielder, Benzene, *Health and Safety Executive, Toxicity Review 4*, London, HM Stationery Office, 1982.

CARCINOGENICITY. A retrospective mortality study of workers exposed to benzene between 1940 and 1950 showed a statistically significant increase in deaths due to leukaemia over that expected from *U.S.* death-rates standardised for sex, age, and calendar period.— R. A. Rinsky *et al.*, *Am. J. ind. Med.*, 1981, *2*, 217. See also P. F. Infante *et al.*, *Lancet*, 1977, *2*, 76.

Absorption and Fate

Benzene is absorbed by inhalation, and ingestion, but is not significantly absorbed through the skin. Some is excreted unchanged from the lungs; the remainder is either oxidised to phenol and related quinol compounds and excreted in the urine as conjugates of sulphuric or glucuronic acid, or retained in the body.

Uses and Administration

Benzene was formerly applied as a pediculicide. Its use as an industrial solvent is decreasing. The use of benzene in cosmetics is prohibited by law in the *UK*.

Benzene is not suitable for use as a food additive.— Twenty-third Report of Joint FAO/WHO Expert Committee on Food Additives, *Tech. Rep. Ser. Wld Hlth Org. No. 648*, 1980.

12482-e

Butyl Acetate
n-Butyl acetate.
$C_6H_{12}O_2$=116.2.

CAS — 123-86-4.

A colourless inflammable liquid with a strong fruity odour. Wt per mL about 0.88 g. B.p. about 126°. **Store** in airtight containers.

Butyl acetate has mild irritant and CNS depressant effects. It is used as an industrial solvent and as an extraction solvent in food processing.

In Great Britain the recommended exposure limits of butyl acetate are 150 ppm (long-term); 200 ppm (short-term).

16556-f

Butyl Alcohol *(USAN).*
n-Butanol; *n*-Butyl Alcohol. Butan-1-ol.
$C_4H_{10}O$=74.12.

CAS — 71-36-3.

Pharmacopoeias. In *U.S.N.F.*

A clear, colourless, mobile liquid with a characteristic odour. B.p. about 118°.

Soluble in water; miscible with alcohol, ether, and many other organic solvents.

Store in airtight containers at a temperature not exceeding 40°.

Adverse Effects

Butyl alcohol may cause irritation of the eyes, skin, and mucous membranes and mild CNS depression with headache, dizziness, and drowsiness.

In Great Britain the recommended exposure limit of butyl alcohol is 50 ppm; suitable precautions should be taken to prevent absorption through the skin.

Uses and Administration

Butyl alcohol is used as an industrial and pharmaceutical solvent.

12484-y

Butylamine
n-Butylamine.
$C_4H_{11}N$=73.1.

CAS — 109-73-9.

A colourless inflammable liquid with an ammoniacal odour. Wt per mL about 0.744 g. B.p. about 78°. **Store** in airtight containers.

Butylamine is used as a solvent; it is irritant.

In Great Britain the recommended exposure limit of butylamine is 5 ppm; suitable precautions should be taken to prevent absorption through the skin.

6506-t

Carbon Disulphide

Carbon Bisulphide; Carbonei Sulfidum; Carboneum Bisulfuratum; Carboneum Sulfuratum; Schwefelkohlenstoff.
CS_2=76.14.

CAS — 75-15-0.

Pharmacopoeias. In *Aust., Nord., Pol.,* and *Span.*

A clear, colourless, volatile, inflammable liquid with an unpleasant odour. Wt per mL about 1.26 g. B.p. about 46°.

Store in airtight containers.

The vapour mixed with air in the proportions of 1 to 50% is explosive, and can be ignited even by hot steam pipes.

Adverse Effects and Treatment

Carbon disulphide is irritant to the skin, mucous membranes, and the eye. Toxic effects may occur as a result of inhalation, ingestion, or absorption through the skin. Acute poisoning is uncommon but may result in dyspnoea, nausea, and excitement, followed by depression of the CNS with headache, dizziness, blurred vision, irritability, confusion, and in severe cases, delirium, hallucinations, stupor, coma, and death due to respiratory failure.

Chronic poisoning has been associated with exposure to carbon disulphide concentrations of 30 ppm or more for prolonged periods. It is characterised by peripheral neuropathies. Other symptoms include CNS effects such as headache, dizziness, fatigue, insomnia, tremor, emotional lability, depression, and psychosis; gastro-intestinal effects including anorexia and weight loss; and effects on the eye. Occupational exposure to carbon disulphide has been shown to be associated with an increased incidence of mortality from coronary heart disease. Atherosclerosis, encephalopathy, reduced serum-thyroxine concentrations, menstrual irregularities, an increased incidence of spontaneous abortions and premature births, loss of libido, and sperm abnormalities have also been reported.

Treatment consists of removal from exposure and general supportive and symptomatic measures. Peripheral neuropathies may be only slowly reversible.

In Great Britain the control exposure limit of carbon disulphide is 10 ppm (long-term); suitable precautions should be taken to prevent absorption through the skin. In the *US* the permissible and recommended exposure limits are 20 ppm (long-term) and 1 ppm (short-term).

Health risks of carbon disulphide and measures for avoiding them.— Carbon Disulphide, *Environmental Health Criteria No. 10*, Geneva, UN/WHO, 1978. See also: Recommended Health-based Limits in Occupational Exposure to Selected Organic Solvents, *Tech. Rep. Ser., Wld Hlth Org. No. 664*, 1981.

A brief discussion of the hazards of carbon disulphide.— *Lancet*, 1980, *2*, 1347.

Review of the toxicity of carbon disulphide.— R. J. Fielder and R. O. Shillaker, Carbon Disulphide, *Health and Safety Executive, Toxicity Review 3*, London, HM Stationery Office, 1981.

A report of adverse effects observed in 27 subjects following acute exposure to carbon disulphide.— D. A. Spyker *et al., J. Toxicol. clin. Toxicol.*, 1982, *19*, 87.

EFFECTS ON BLOOD SUGAR. A study showing decreased glucose tolerance in workers exposed to carbon disulphide compared with control subjects.— G. Franco *et al.* (letter), *Lancet*, 1978, *2*, 1208. See also V. Kujalová *et al.* (letter), *Lancet*, 1979, *1*, 664.

EFFECTS ON THE HEART. Two groups, each of 343 men, were studied; one group consisted of men who had been occupationally exposed to carbon disulphide for at least 5 of the last 25 years; the others had had no such exposure. The respective incidence of various events during a 5-year follow-up was: deaths from coronary heart disease, 14 and 3 men; non-fatal first myocardial infarctions, 11 and 4 men; a history of angina, 25 and 13%; prevalence of typical angina, 12 and 5%. Causes of death other than coronary heart disease were evenly distributed between the groups.— M. Tolonen *et al., Br. J. ind. Med.*, 1975, *32*, 1. After a further 3-year follow-up, at the start of which the exposure of workers to carbon disulphide was reduced and the atmospheric concentration lowered to 10 ppm, there was evidence of reduced mortality from heart disease amongst workers at risk.— M. Nurminen, *Int. J. Epidemiol.*, 1976, *5*, 179. Follow-up for a further 7 years indicated that the relative risk of mortality from cardiovascular disease in the exposed workers was reduced to that of the unexposed group during the period 1974 to 1982.— M. Nurminen and S. Hernberg, *Br. J. ind. Med.*, 1985, *42*, 32.

Further references: M. Tolonen *et al., Int. Archs occup. environ. Hlth*, 1976, *37*, 249; P. G. Vertin, *J. occup. Med.*, 1978, *20*, 346.

Absorption and Fate

Carbon disulphide is rapidly absorbed when inhaled and is also absorbed through intact skin. It is excreted unchanged through the lungs and in the urine as metabolites.

Uses and Administration

Carbon disulphide is used as an industrial solvent and has been used, in the vapour form, as an insecticide, and veterinary parasiticide. The use of carbon disulphide in cosmetics is prohibited by law in the *UK*.

767-z

Carbon Tetrachloride *(USAN).*
Tetrachloromethane.
CCl_4=153.8.

CAS — 56-23-5.

Pharmacopoeias. In *Arg., Belg., Cz., Fr., Hung., Mex., Nord., Pol., Span.,* and *Turk.* Also in *U.S.N.F.*

A clear, colourless, volatile liquid with a chloroform-like odour; it is non-inflammable but in contact with a flame it decomposes and gives rise to toxic products, including phosgene, with an acrid odour. Sp. gr. 1.588 to 1.590. B.p. 76° to 78°.

Practically **insoluble** in water; miscible with alcohol, chloroform, ether, light petroleum, and fixed and vegetable oils. It is slowly decomposed by light and by various metals if moisture is present. **Store** at a temperature not exceeding 30° in airtight containers. Protect from light.

CAUTION. Avoid contact with carbon tetrachloride; the vapour and liquid are poisonous. Care should be taken not to vaporise carbon tetrachloride in the presence of a flame because of the production of harmful gases, mainly phosgene.

Adverse Effects

Early symptoms of acute intoxication following ingestion, inhalation, or absorption of carbon tetrachloride through the skin are similar to those with other chlorinated hydrocarbons such as trichloroethane (p.1431) and include excitement and then depression of the CNS. However, carbon tetrachloride is much more toxic, especially to the liver and kidneys; highly reactive metabolites of carbon tetrachloride are thought to be responsible.

Even small amounts of carbon tetrachloride may cause drowsiness, giddiness, headache, mental confusion, nausea, and vomiting. Occasionally, more severe symptoms may follow 1 or 2 weeks later, especially cellular necrosis of the kidneys and liver with uraemia, oliguria, and convulsions. Central nervous system depression and respiratory failure may precede death. Adverse effects are more likely to occur in alcoholics.

Inhalation of concentrations of 1000 ppm of the vapour even for short periods may give rise to acute toxic reactions including dizziness, stupor, loss of consciousness, and cardiac arrhythmias, and may result in death from respiratory or cardiac failure. Exposure to high concentrations may also result in delayed systemic poisoning characterised by epigastric pain, vomiting, and albuminuria. Continued exposure to concentrations of even less than 100 ppm may give rise to chronic poisoning leading to acute nephritis, jaundice, toxic hepatitis, or aplastic anaemia.

Dependence on carbon tetrachloride has been reported.

In Great Britain the recommended exposure limits of carbon tetrachloride are 10 ppm (long-term); 20 ppm (short-term); suitable precautions should be taken to prevent absorption through the skin. In the *US* the permissible and recommended exposure limits are 10 ppm and 2 ppm respectively.

For toxicological data, see 1971 Evaluations of some Pesticide Residues in Food, *Pestic. Residue Ser. Wld Hlth Org. No. 1*, 1972.

Extrapyramidal symptoms responsive to levodopa occurred in a 40-year-old man exposed for about 3 months to carbon tetrachloride vapour.— E. Melamed and S. Lavy (letter), *Lancet*, 1977, *1*, 1015. A report of cerebellar dysfunction after acute carbon tetrachloride poisoning.— B. P. Johnson *et al.* (letter), *ibid.*, 1983, *2*, 968.

Acute renal failure in 3 patients following the topical application of a proprietary benzyl benzoate lotion containing 67% w/w of carbon tetrachloride as an excipient.— A. J. Perez *et al.* (letter), *Lancet*, 1987, *1*, 515.

Treatment of Adverse Effects

If carbon tetrachloride vapour has been inhaled remove the patient to the fresh air. Remove clothing contaminated by liquid and wash the skin. If it has been recently ingested the stomach should be emptied by aspiration and lavage.

The usual symptomatic and supportive measures should

be instituted. Hepatic and renal function should be monitored closely. Haemodialysis may be needed if renal function is impaired. Oils, fats, alcohol, and sympathomimetic agents should be avoided.
Acetylcysteine has been administered to patients recently exposed to carbon tetrachloride in an attempt to prevent or modify liver and kidney damage.

For the symptoms and treatment of poisoning with carbon tetrachloride, see *Poisonous Chemicals used on Farms and Gardens*, London, Department of Health and Social Security, 1969.

A 29-year-old man who had swallowed 100 mL of carbon tetrachloride in association with alcohol developed acute tubular necrosis and signs of hepatic impairment. He was successfully treated with haemodialysis for 11 of the next 15 days and total parenteral nutrition for 12 days; by 37 days after ingestion, recovery of renal and hepatic function was complete.— R. P. Fogel *et al.*, *Can. med. Ass. J.*, 1983, *128*, 560.

For reference to the use of acetylcysteine in the treatment of acute carbon tetrachloride poisoning, see acetylcysteine (p.904).

Absorption and Fate
Carbon tetrachloride is readily absorbed after inhalation. It is also absorbed from the gastro-intestinal tract and through the skin. Metabolism to reactive free radicals is thought to account for the hepatorenal toxicity of carbon tetrachloride.
Carbon tetrachloride is slowly excreted from the body via the lungs, urine, and faeces.

Uses and Administration
Carbon tetrachloride is employed in industry as a solvent and degreaser. It was formerly used in certain types of fire extinguisher and as an industrial and domestic dry cleaner but has been largely replaced for this purpose by less toxic substances. Carbon tetrachloride has also been used for the fumigation of cereals.
It should only be used under conditions of adequate ventilation.
Carbon tetrachloride was formerly given by mouth as an anthelmintic but it has been superseded by equally effective and less toxic agents.

6507-x

Cyclohexane

Hexahydrobenzene; Hexamethylene.
C_6H_{12}=84.2.

CAS — 110-82-7.

A colourless, inflammable liquid. Wt per mL about 0.78 g. B.p. about 81°. **Store** in airtight containers.

Adverse Effects
Cyclohexane may irritate mucous membranes, and may also have central nervous system effects.
In Great Britain the recommended exposure limits of cyclohexane are 300 ppm (long-term); 375 ppm (short-term).

Uses and Administration
Cyclohexane is used as an industrial solvent.

19073-b

Dichloropropane

Propylene Dichloride. 1,2-Dichloropropane.
$C_3H_6Cl_2$=113.0.

CAS — 78-87-5.

A colourless inflammable liquid. Wt per mL about 1.16 g. B.p. about 96°. **Store** in airtight containers.

Adverse Effects
Dichloropropane may cause irritation of the eyes, skin, and respiratory tract; high concentrations may result in CNS depression.

ABUSE. A report of acute renal failure, haemolytic anaemia, acute liver disease, and disseminated intravascular coagulation following intentional dichloropropane inhalation; the patient recovered following blood transfusions and haemodialysis.— F. Locatelli and C. Pozzi (letter), *Lancet*, 1983, *2*, 220.

Uses and Administration
Dichloropropane is used as an industrial solvent, dry cleaning agent, and agricultural defumigant.

6508-r

Diethyl Phthalate *(BAN, USAN)*.

Ethyl Phthalate. The diethyl ester of benzene-1,2-dicarboxylic acid.
$C_{12}H_{14}O_4$=222.2.

CAS — 84-66-2.

Pharmacopoeias. In *Br.* Also in *U.S.N.F.*

A clear, colourless or nearly colourless liquid; odourless or almost odourless. *B.P.* specifies wt per mL 1.115 to 1.119 g. *U.S.N.F.* specifies sp. gr. 1.118 to 1.122 at 20°. B.p. about 295°. Practically **insoluble** in water; miscible with alcohol, ether, and aromatic hydrocarbons.

Adverse Effects
Diethyl phthalate vapour is irritant to mucous membranes and, in high concentration, causes CNS depression.
In Great Britain the recommended exposure limits of diethyl phthalate are 5 mg per m^3 (long-term); 10 mg per m^3 (short-term).

Phthalate esters: the question of safety.— W. H. Lawrence, *Clin. Toxicol.*, 1978, *13*, 89.

Uses and Administration
Diethyl phthalate is used as a denaturant of alcohol, e.g. in surgical spirit, and as a solvent and plasticiser.

6509-f

Dimethyl Sulphoxide *(BAN)*.

Dimethyl Sulfoxide *(USAN, rINN)*; DMSO; Methyl Sulphoxide; SQ-9453.
C_2H_6OS=78.14.

CAS — 67-68-5.

Pharmacopoeias. In *Br.* and *U.S.*

A colourless hygroscopic liquid; odourless or almost odourless. F.p. not lower than 18.3°; b.p. about 189°. *B.P.* specifies wt per mL 1.099 to 1.101 g. *U.S.P.* specifies sp. gr. 1.095 to 1.097. **Miscible** with water with the evolution of heat, and with alcohol, ether, and most organic solvents; immiscible with paraffin hydrocarbons. **Store** in airtight containers out of contact with plastics. Protect from light and moisture.

Adverse Effects
High concentrations applied to the skin may cause burning discomfort, itching, erythema, and occasionally vesiculation—effects resulting from marked vasodilatation. Continued use may result in scaling, and dermatitis. Nausea, vomiting, abdominal cramps, chest pain, chills, drowsiness, headache, and hypersensitivity reactions have been reported following topical use. Administration of dimethyl sulphoxide by any route is followed by a garlic-like odour in the breath.
Intravascular haemolysis has been reported following intravenous administration. Local discomfort and spasm may occur when given by bladder instillation. When used as a penetrating basis for other drugs, dimethyl sulphoxide may enhance their toxic effects—see Precautions.

Human toxicology of dimethyl sulphoxide.— R. D. Brobyn, *Ann. N.Y. Acad. Sci.*, 1975, *243*, 497.

A review of the toxicology of dimethyl sulphoxide including its teratogenicity in *animals*.— C. C. Willhite and P. I. Katz, *J. appl. Toxicol.*, 1984, *4*, 155.

Skin irritation (as measured by changes in electrical impedance) in healthy subjects exposed to dimethyl sulphoxide increased with increasing concentrations. However, there was some evidence that repeated exposure results in adaptation and a lessening irritant effect.— K. E. Malten and J. den Arend, *Contact Dermatitis*, 1978, *4*, 80.

Dimethyl sulphoxide administered by intravenous infusion to 14 patients caused transient haemolysis and haemoglobinuria. Infusion strengths greater than 10% were associated with grossly discoloured urine but there was no evidence of kidney damage.— R. S. Muther and W. M. Bennett, *J. Am. med. Ass.*, 1980, *244*, 2081.

An elderly married couple developed raised liver and muscle enzyme concentrations, mild jaundice, and evidence of haemolysis after receiving dimethyl sulphoxide intravenously for painful arthritic knees. The husband never became seriously ill, but the wife developed acute renal tubular necrosis, deterioration in her level of consciousness and evidence of cerebral infarction. Efforts to remove dimethyl sulphoxide using peritoneal dialysis failed. It was considered that intravenous dimethyl sulphoxide was potentially dangerous and should not be used for the treatment of arthritis.— P. Yellowlees *et al.*, *Lancet*, 1980, *2*, 1004. Criticisms: L. J. Knott, *Kendall Arthritis Clinic* (letter), *ibid.*, 1299; M. H. van Rijswijk (letter), *ibid.*, 1981, *1*, 41; J. P. Griffin, *DHSS* (letter), *ibid;* J. C. de la Torre (letter), *ibid.*, 157. Reply, including the view that the adverse reaction was not due to enhancement of any drug action.— C. Greenfield (letter), *ibid.*, 276. A severe reaction after the infusion of dimethyl sulphoxide with cryopreserved bone marrow, but without signs of renal impairment. Reservations about the intravenous infusion of dimethyl sulphoxide merit further attention.— J. R. O'Donnell *et al.* (letter), *ibid.*, 498.

Precautions
When used as a penetrating basis for other drugs applied topically, dimethyl sulphoxide may enhance their toxic effects. High concentrations should not be applied to the eyes and should be applied with care around the eyes. Dimethyl sulphoxide should be avoided in patients with a history of eye disease or liver or renal impairment. During long-term treatment, ophthalmic, liver, and renal function should be assessed at about 6-monthly intervals. Bladder instillation may be harmful in patients with urinary tract malignancy because of vasodilatation.
It is suggested that it should not be used during pregnancy or in lactating mothers.

INTERACTIONS. Experience with dimethyl sulphoxide given by mouth and intravenously for amyloidosis, indicated that simultaneous treatment with anticoagulants, digoxin, non-steroidal anti-inflammatory drugs, corticosteroids, and cytostatics did not appear to provide special problems. A 39-year-old woman with renal failure did, however, react with severe hypotension to the administration of carbachol and a 28-year-old man acquired a transient paralytic ileus after the administration of hyoscine butylbromide.— M. H. van Rijswijk (letter), *Lancet*, 1981, *1*, 41.

Report of peripheral neuropathy following treatment with sulindac combined with surreptitious topical administration of dimethyl sulphoxide.— B. N. Swanson *et al.*, *Arthritis Rheum.*, 1983, *26*, 791.

Absorption and Fate
Dimethyl sulphoxide is readily absorbed by injection, by mouth, and through the skin. It is metabolised by oxidation to dimethyl sulphone and by reduction to dimethyl sulphide. Dimethyl sulphoxide and the sulphone metabolite are excreted in the urine and faeces. Dimethyl sulphide is excreted through the lungs and skin and is responsible for the characteristic odour from patients.

Uses and Administration
Dimethyl sulphoxide is a highly polar substance which has exceptional solvent properties for both organic and inorganic chemicals, and is widely used as an industrial solvent.
It has been reported to have a wide spectrum of pharmacological activity including membrane penetration, anti-inflammatory effects, local analgesia, weak bacteriostasis, diuresis, vasodilatation, and dissolution of collagen.
The principal therapeutic use of dimethyl sulphoxide is as a vehicle for drugs such as idoxuridine (see p.694); it aids penetration of the drug into the skin, and so may enhance the drug's effect. It is also used as a 50% aqueous solution for bladder instillation for the symptomatic relief of interstitial cystitis; doses of 50 mL are instilled and allowed to remain for 15 minutes. Treatment is repeated every 2 weeks initially. Dimethyl sulphoxide is also used to protect living cells during cold storage.
Dimethyl sulphoxide has been tried clinically for a wide range of indications including cutaneous and musculoskeletal disorders, but with little evidence of beneficial effects.
The use of dimethyl sulphoxide in cosmetic pro-

ducts is prohibited by law in the *UK*.
It is also used in veterinary medicine.

Reviews and discussions on the uses and adverse effects of dimethyl sulphoxide: *Med. Lett.*, 1980, *22*, 94; M. J. Finkel, *J. Am. med. Ass.*, 1980, *244*, 2767.

AMYLOIDOSIS. Following administration of dimethyl sulphoxide for more than a year, improvement in renal function and general condition was obtained in 2 patients with renal amyloidosis secondary to rheumatoid arthritis.— M. H. van Rijswijk *et al.* (letter), *Lancet*, 1979, *1*, 207.

A view that the beneficial effect of dimethyl sulphoxide on amyloidosis may be related, at least in part, to its ability to scavenge hydroxyl radicals.— D. Harman (letter), *Lancet*, 1980, *2*, 593.

Further references: *Lancet*, 1980, *1*, 1062; G. G. Glenner, *New Engl. J. Med.*, 1980, *302*, 1333.

CEREBRAL OEDEMA. Elevated intracranial pressure, unresponsive to treatment with barbiturates and diuretics, was reduced to normal in 7 patients after intravenous infusion of dimethyl sulphoxide 1 g per kg body-weight. The previously refractory pressure was easily controlled by further infusions of dimethyl sulphoxide.— F. T. Waller *et al.*, *Neurosurgery*, 1979, *5*, 383.

Results of a preliminary trial on the use of intravenous infusions of dimethyl sulphoxide for the treatment of intracranial hypertension. Although the raised intracranial pressure was initially well-controlled, problems with fluid overload and severe electrolyte disturbances occurred, and mechanical difficulties were encountered in the administration of dimethyl sulphoxide.— L. F. Marshall *et al.*, *Neurosurgery*, 1984, *14*, 659.

CRYOPROTECTION. A review of recent advances in cryobiology including the use of dimethyl sulphoxide as a cryoprotectant.— D. E. Pegg, *Practitioner*, 1978, *221*, 543.

Dimethyl sulphoxide 5% was used as a cryoprotective agent in the preparation of frozen blood platelets for subsequent transfusion in patients with leukaemia. There were no side-effects from the transfusion of small residual amounts of dimethyl sulphoxide.— C. A. Schiffer *et al.*, *New Engl. J. Med.*, 1978, *299*, 7.

CYSTITIS. A review of the use of dimethyl sulphoxide in a 50% aqueous solution for bladder instillation in the treatment of chronic interstitial cystitis concluded that it should be reserved for patients with severe symptoms who had not responded to other treatment.— *Med. Lett.*, 1978, *20*, 76.

Prospective study of the use of a 50% aqueous solution of dimethyl sulphoxide for bladder instillation in the treatment of suspected early interstitial cystitis; partial or complete symptomatic remissions were achieved in 19 of 20 patients.— J. E. Fowler, *Urology*, 1981, *18*, 21.

DIABETIC FOOT ULCER. Topical treatment with dimethyl sulphoxide solution resulted in complete healing of chronic resistant foot ulcers in 14 of 20 diabetic patients compared with only 2 of 20 patients treated conventionally; in addition partial improvement occurred in a further 4 of the dimethyl sulphoxide treated group.— M. Lishner *et al.*, *J. Am. Geriat. Soc.*, 1985, *33*, 41.

MUSCULOSKELETAL AND JOINT DISORDERS. Review of the use of dimethyl sulphoxide in rheumatic disorders.— J. M. Trice and R. S. Pinals, *Semin. Arthritis Rheum.*, 1985, *15*, 45.

SCLERODERMA. A double-blind trial in 84 patients with scleroderma compared the results of topical treatment of digital ulcers with 2% dimethyl sulphoxide, 70% dimethyl sulphoxide, or 0.85% saline; there were no statistically significant differences in efficacy among the three treatment groups. Adverse effects were most severe in the patients treated with 70% dimethyl sulphoxide and 29% of these patients were withdrawn because of severe skin reactions.— H. J. Williams *et al.*, *Arthritis Rheum.*, 1985, *28*, 308.

TISSUE NECROSIS. Possible beneficial effect of topical dimethyl sulphoxide after accidental subcutaneous daunorubicin extravasation.— H. J. Lawrence and S. H. Goodnight, *Ann. intern. Med.*, 1983, *98*, 1025.

Proprietary Preparations

Rimso-50 *(Research Industries Corp., USA: Britannia Pharmaceuticals, UK). Bladder instillation,* dimethyl sulphoxide 50%.

6510-z

Dimethylacetamide

Acetyldimethylamine; DMAC. *NN*-Dimethylacetamide.
C_4H_9NO=87.12.

CAS — 127-19-5.

A colourless liquid. B.p. about 165°. Wt per mL about 0.94 g. **Miscible** with water and most organic solvents.

Adverse Effects

As for Dimethylformamide (below); it may be less toxic than dimethylformamide.

In Great Britain the recommended exposure limits are 10 ppm (long-term); 15 ppm (short-term); suitable precautions should be taken to prevent absorption through the skin.

Animal studies on embryotoxic and teratogenic effects of dimethylacetamide.— J. Merkle and H. Zeller, *Arzneimittel-Forsch.*, 1980, *30*, 1557; E. F. Stula and W. C. Krauss, *Toxic. appl. Pharmac.*, 1977, *41*, 35; T. Kreybig *et al.*, *Arzneimittel-Forsch.*, 1969, *19*, 1073.

Uses and Administration

Dimethylacetamide is used as a solubilising agent and as a solvent in pharmaceutical products. It has been used as a cryoprotectant.

6511-c

Dimethylformamide

DMF. *NN*-Dimethylformamide.
C_3H_7NO=73.09.

CAS — 68-12-2.

A clear colourless liquid. B.p. about 153°. Wt per mL about 0.95 g.

Adverse Effects

Dimethylformamide may cause ocular irritation or damage, skin irritation, and nausea and vomiting. CNS effects have been reported including weakness and incoordination. Kidney and liver damage may occur. Loss of appetite and digestive disturbances have been reported in exposed industrial workers.

In Great Britain the recommended exposure limits are 10 ppm (long-term); 20 ppm (short-term); suitable precautions should be taken to prevent absorption through the skin.

Reports of disulfiram-like effects after alcohol consumption in workers exposed to dimethylformamide.— C. P. Chivers (letter), *Lancet*, 1978, *1*, 331; W. H. Lyle *et al.*, *Br. J. ind. Med.*, 1979, *36*, 63. Investigations in *rats* indicated that metabolic-acetaldehyde accumulation might be a factor in reports of intolerance to alcoholic beverages experienced by subjects following exposure to dimethylformamide; its metabolite methylformamide had similar effects.— G. K. Hanasono *et al.*, *Toxic. appl. Pharmac.*, 1977, *39*, 461.

Absorption and Fate

Dimethylformamide is absorbed after inhalation and through intact skin. It is metabolised to *N*-methylformamide and formamide and is mainly excreted in the urine as metabolites.

Uses and Administration

Dimethylformamide has been used as a solvent for various drugs. The use of dimethylformamide in cosmetics is prohibited by law in the *UK*.

6512-k

Dioxan

Diethylene Dioxide; Diethylene Ether; Dioxane. 1,4-Dioxane.
$C_4H_8O_2$=88.11.

CAS — 123-91-1.

NOTE. Do not confuse dioxan and dioxin (see p.1621).

A colourless inflammable liquid with an ethereal odour. B.p. about 101°. Wt per mL about 1.03 g. **Store** in airtight containers.

CAUTION. *It is dangerous to distil or evaporate dioxan unless precautions have been taken to remove explosive peroxides.*

Adverse Effects

Dioxan vapour is irritant to the nose and eyes. High concentrations may cause dyspnoea, nausea and vomiting, and depression of the CNS with headache, dizziness, drowsiness, and in severe cases unconsciousness. On repeated exposure, severe liver and kidney damage, including necrotic changes, can occur and may be fatal.

In Great Britain the recommended exposure limit of dioxan, technical grade, is 50 ppm (long-term); suitable precautions should be taken to prevent absorption through the skin. In the *US* the permissible and recommended exposure limits are 360 mg per m^3 and 3.6 mg per m^3 respectively.

Absorption and Fate

Dioxan is absorbed after inhalation and through the skin. It is metabolised by oxidation to β-hydroxyethoxy-acetic acid.

Uses and Administration

Dioxan is a chemical reagent and industrial solvent.
The use of dioxan in cosmetic products is prohibited by law in the *UK*.

6513-a

Solvent Ether *(BAN)*.

Aether Aethylicus; Aether Solvens; Diethyl Ether; Éther rectifié; Eter; Ether *(USAN)*; Ethyl Ether; Ethyl Oxide.
$(C_2H_5)_2O$=74.12.

CAS — 60-29-7.

NOTE. Solvent ether is not intended for anaesthesia; only ether of a suitable quality (see p.1116) should be so used.

Pharmacopoeias. In *Arg., Aust., Belg., Br., Cz., Egypt., Fr., Hung., Jpn, Jug., Mex., Nord., Pol., Port., Roum., Rus., Span.,* and *Turk. U.S.* has a monograph on Ether, with special storage requirements if for anaesthetic use.

Solvent ether is a colourless, transparent, very volatile, inflammable, very mobile liquid with a characteristic odour. It volatilises very quickly and by so doing reduces temperature. Though ether is one of the lightest of liquids, its vapour is very heavy, being 2½ times heavier than air. *B.P.* specifies wt per mL 0.714 to 0.718 g. *U.S.P.* specifies sp. gr. 0.713 to 0.716. B.p. 34° to 36°. *B.P.* **solubilities** are: soluble 1 in 15 of water; miscible with alcohol, chloroform, and fixed and volatile oils. *U.S.P.* solubilities are: soluble 1 in 12 of water; miscible with alcohol, chloroform, light petroleum and with fixed and volatile oils. *B.P.* specifies **store** in well-closed containers at a temperature not exceeding 15° and protect from light. *U.S.P.* specifies store in partly filled, tight, light-resistant containers at a temperature not exceeding 30°. If the containers are closed with corks these should be protected with metal foil. Protect from light.

CAUTION. *Ether is very volatile and inflammable and mixtures of its vapour with oxygen, nitrous oxide, or air at certain concentrations are explosive. It should not be used in the presence of an open flame or any electrical apparatus liable to produce a spark; precautions should be taken against the production of static electrical discharge. Explosive peroxides are generated by the atmospheric oxidation of solvent ether and it is dangerous to distil a sample which contains peroxides.*

Adverse Effects

As for Anaesthetic Ether, p.1116. Ingestion of 30 to 60 mL may be fatal.

In Great Britain the recommended exposure limits of ether are 400 ppm (long-term); 500 ppm (short-term).

A report of interstitial cystitis following attempted dissolution of a Foley catheter balloon with ether.— R. E. Nellans *et al.*, *J. Am. med. Ass.*, 1985, *254*, 530.

Uses and Administration

Solvent ether is widely used as a pharmaceutical

and industrial solvent, and is used as a solvent in food processing. It has been used for cleaning the skin before surgical operations and for removing adhesive plaster from the skin.

Some references to ether being ineffective in the topical treatment of herpes simplex infection.— L. Corey *et al.*, *New Engl. J. Med.*, 1978, *299*, 237; M. E. Guinan *et al.*, *J. Am. med. Ass.*, 1980, *243*, 1059.

6514-t

Ethyl Acetate *(USAN).*
Acetic Ether; Aethylis Acetas; Aethylium Aceticum.
$CH_3.CO.O.C_2H_5$=88.11.

CAS — 141-78-6.

Pharmacopoeias. In *Jug.* Also in *U.S.N.F.*

A colourless, transparent, inflammable liquid with a fragrant, refreshing, slightly acetous odour. Specific gravity 0.894 to 0.898. B.p. 76° to 77.5°. **Soluble** in water. **Store** at a temperature not exceeding 40° in airtight containers.

Adverse Effects
Ethyl acetate is irritant to mucous membranes. High concentrations may cause depression of the central nervous system.
In Great Britain the recommended exposure limit of ethyl acetate is 400 ppm (long-term).

Uses and Administration
Ethyl acetate has been used to flavour pharmaceutical preparations. It is largely employed in industry as a solvent and is used as an extraction solvent in food processing.

6516-r

Formamide
Carbamaldehyde; Methanamide.
CH_3NO=45.04.

CAS — 75-12-7.

A colourless, hygroscopic, oily liquid. B.p. 210°. Wt per mL, about 1.13 g.

Adverse Effects
Formamide is reported to be irritant to skin and mucous membranes.
In Great Britain the recommended exposure limits of formamide are 20 ppm (long-term); 30 ppm (short-term).

Uses and Administration
Formamide is used as a pharmaceutical solvent.

9935-a

Glycofurol
Glycofurol 75; Tetraglycol; Tetrahydrofurfuryl Alcohol Polyethylene Glycol Ether. α-(Tetrahydrofuranyl)-ω-hydroxypoly(oxyethylene).

CAS — 9004-76-6.

A clear, colourless, almost odourless liquid. Wt per mL about 1.08 g. **Incompatible** with oxidising agents. **Store** in airtight containers. Protect from light.

Glycofurol is used as a pharmaceutical solvent for injections.

9931-j

***n*-Hexane**

C_6H_{14}=86.18.

CAS — 110-54-3.

A colourless, inflammable, volatile liquid with a faint odour. Wt per mL about 0.66 g. B.p. about 69°. **Store** in airtight containers.

Adverse Effects
n-Hexane is irritant to the eyes, skin, and respiratory tract. Acute exposure may result in CNS depression with drowsiness, dizziness, weakness, blurred vision, and in severe cases unconsciousness. Chronic industrial exposure and solvent abuse have been associated with the development of peripheral neuropathies.
n-Hexane is one of the solvents abused in 'glue-sniffing'.
In Great Britain the recommended exposure limits of *n*-hexane are 100 ppm (long-term); 125 ppm (short-term). The recommended exposure limits of other hexane isomers are 500 ppm (long-term); 1000 ppm (short-term).

A review of the toxicity of *n*-hexane.— N. K. Jørgensen and K. H. Cohr, *Scand. J. Work Environ. & Hlth*, 1981, *7*, 157.

Reports of peripheral neuropathy associated with *n*-hexane.— G. Abbritti *et al.*, *Br. J. ind. Med.*, 1976, *33*, 92 (industrial exposure); J. Towfighi *et al.*, *Neurology*, 1976, *26*, 238 (abuse). See also *Lancet*, 1979, *2*, 942 (a brief discussion on the nature of the neuropathy); M. Tenenbein *et al.*, *Can. med. Ass. J.*, 1984, *131*, 1077 (abuse).

Uses and Administration
n-Hexane is widely used as an industrial solvent and is used as a solvent in glues.

6517-f

Kerosene
Kerosine; 'Paraffin'. A mixture of hydrocarbons, chiefly members of the alkane series distilled from petroleum.

CAS — 8008-20-6.

It is a colourless or pale yellow mobile oily liquid with a characteristic odour. B.p. 175° to 325°. Wt per mL about 0.8 g. An odourless grade is available. **Store** in airtight containers.

Adverse Effects
Ingestion of kerosene results in a burning sensation in the mouth and throat and gastro-intestinal disturbances; cough, dyspnoea, and transient cyanosis may occur and there may be depression of the central nervous system, with weakness, dizziness, drowsiness, confusion, incoordination, restlessness, convulsions, and coma. Cardiac arrhythmias have been reported. The chief danger is pneumonitis and attendant pulmonary complications resulting from the aspiration of kerosene. Spontaneous or induced vomiting increases the risk of aspiration.
Euphoria may follow inhalation. The course of poisoning from inhalation is similar to that following ingestion. Kerosene is a skin and eye irritant.
In the *US* the recommended exposure limit is 100 mg per m^3; suitable precautions should be taken to prevent absorption through the skin.

Epidermal necrolysis developed in a 12-year-old boy after wearing kerosene-soaked clothing.— R. L. Barnes and D. S. Wilkinson, *Br. med. J.*, 1973, *4*, 466.

ABUSE. Reports of patients who injected themselves intravenously with kerosene- or petroleum distillate-containing products.— D. O. Green, *Clin. Toxicol.*, 1977, *10*, 283; E. M. Neeld and M. C. Limacher, *Radiology*, 1978, *129*, 36.

A report of abscesses following repeated injections of kerosene.— E. Rubinstein *et al.* (letter), *Archs intern. Med.*, 1985, *145*, 371.

EFFECT ON BLOOD-LIPID CONCENTRATION. A report of hypolipidaemia following severe kerosene intoxication in 2 'fire-eaters'.— A. Basdevant and B. Guy-Grand (letter), *Lancet*, 1986, *2*, 526.

Treatment of Adverse Effects
Treatment of kerosene poisoning is supportive and symptomatic. Every precaution should be taken to avoid aspiration of kerosene into the lungs. Most authorities agree that emesis and gastric lavage should generally be avoided unless an additional toxin such as a pesticide has been ingested.

In a review of 950 children who had ingested products containing hydrocarbons it was reported that only 117 developed clinical or radiological evidence of pulmonary involvement. Induced vomiting or gastric lavage was carried out in 42 patients but was found to have no beneficial or adverse effects on the incidence of complications or duration of hospitalisation.— N. Anas *et al.*, *J. Am. med. Ass.*, 1981, *246*, 840.

Uses and Administration
Kerosene is used as a degreaser and cleaner and as an illuminating and fuel oil in kerosene ('paraffin') lamps and stoves. The odourless grade has been used as a solvent in the preparation of some insecticide sprays.

12943-n

2-Methoxyethanol
Ethylene Glycol Monomethyl Ether.
$C_3H_8O_2$=76.1.

CAS — 109-86-4.

A colourless liquid. Wt per mL about 0.96 g. B.p. about 125°.

Adverse Effects
2-Methoxyethanol is irritant to the eyes and mucous membranes. Ingestion may result in CNS depression with confusion, weakness, and in severe cases coma and death. Nausea, metabolic acidosis, and kidney damage may also occur. Prolonged industrial exposure has been associated with severe effects on the CNS characterised by headache, dizziness, lethargy, weakness, disorientation, mental changes, ataxia, tremor, and visual and auditory disturbances. Anaemia and weight loss have also been reported.
In Great Britain the control exposure limit of 2-methoxyethanol is 5 ppm (long-term); suitable precautions should be taken to prevent absorption through the skin. In the *US* the permissible exposure limit is 80 mg per m^3.

Report of embryotoxic effects caused by 2-methoxyethanol in *mice*.— K. Nagano *et al.*, *Toxicology*, 1981, *20*, 335.

Review of the toxicity of glycol ethers.— M. P. A. Illing and J. J. B. Tinkler, Glycol Ethers, *Health and Safety Executive*, *Toxicity Review 10*, London, HM Stationery Office, 1985.

Uses and Administration
2-Methoxyethanol is used as an industrial solvent.

556-b

Methyl Alcohol *(USAN).*
Methanol.
CH_3OH=32.04.

CAS — 67-56-1.

Pharmacopoeias. In *U.S.N.F.*

A clear, colourless, inflammable liquid with a characteristic odour. **Miscible** with water, alcohol, ether, and most other organic solvents. **Store** in a cool place in airtight containers.

Adverse Effects
Immediate signs of acute poisoning following ingestion of methyl alcohol resemble those of alcohol intoxication (see p.950), but characteristic symptoms develop after a latent period of up to 48 hours (usually 12 to 18 hours). There is severe abdominal pain, metabolic acidosis with rapid, shallow breathing, and visual disturbances which often proceed to irreversible blindness. Other symptoms include headache, nausea, vomiting, diarrhoea, weakness, vertigo, ataxia, mild tachycardia, confusion, dizziness, delirium, and coma which in severe cases may terminate in death due to respiratory failure or, rarely, to circulatory collapse. Mania and convulsions occasionally occur. Individual response to methyl alcohol varies widely. Ingestion of less than 30 mL is considered to be potentially fatal and as little as 10 mL has been reported to cause permanent blindness.
Absorption of methyl alcohol through the skin or inhalation of the vapour may also lead to toxic systemic effects.

In Great Britain the recommended exposure limits of methyl alcohol are 200 ppm (long-term); 250 ppm (short-term); suitable precautions should be taken to prevent absorption through the skin. In the *USA* the permissible and recommended exposure limits are 260 mg per m^3 and 262 mg per m^3 respectively.

A review of methyl alcohol and ethylene glycol poisonings and their respective treatments.— D. Jacobsen and K. E. McMartin, *Med. Toxicol.*, 1986, *1*, 309. See also *Lancet*, 1983, *1*, 910.

Treatment of Adverse Effects
Recent ingestion should be treated by gastric lavage with sodium bicarbonate solution 2 to 5%. The outstanding feature of methyl alcohol poisoning is acidosis, which should be immediately corrected with intravenous sodium bicarbonate. Alcohol, which delays the oxidation of methyl alcohol to its toxic metabolites, should be administered while the blood-methyl alcohol concentration is being determined. In order to attain the desired blood-alcohol concentration of 1 to 2 mg per mL, an oral dose of about 50 g (equivalent to 150 mL of 40% v/v alcohol) for an adult of around 70 kg body-weight has been suggested; the alcohol should be well diluted before administration. If required, an alcohol infusion may then be given for which the following doses have been used: 120 mL of 10% alcohol or 250 mL of 5% alcohol per hour. The infusion rate should be adjusted if necessary to maintain a blood-alcohol concentration of 1 to 2 mg per mL. For alcoholic patients or those with induced liver enzymes, the dose of alcohol should be increased accordingly. Suggested doses are 145 mL of 10% alcohol or 300 mL of 5% alcohol per hour.
Haemodialysis, or peritoneal dialysis if haemodialysis is unavailable, may be indicated if the response is unsatisfactory. Some sources recommend initiation of haemodialysis if the amount of methyl alcohol ingested exceeds 30 g (equivalent to about 40 mL), if the blood-methyl alcohol concentration is greater than 500 µg per mL, or if visual complications develop. If haemodialysis is used, a constant blood-alcohol concentration may be ensured either by increasing the alcohol infusion rate or by addition of alcohol to the dialysate fluid. Haemodialysis, together with the alcohol infusion should be continued until the concentration of methyl alcohol in the blood is reduced to around 200 to 300 µg per mL. Suitable supportive treatment should be carried out as required.

In 4 patients with methyl alcohol poisoning, serum-formate concentrations correlated more closely with their clinical condition than did methyl alcohol concentrations. It was suggested that measurement of serum-formate concentration may be a more useful guide for the initiation of haemodialysis.— J. D. Osterloh *et al.*, *Ann. intern. Med.*, 1986, *104*, 200.

Absorption and Fate
Methyl alcohol is readily absorbed from the gastro-intestinal tract and distributed throughout the body fluids. It may also be absorbed by inhalation or through large areas of skin. Oxidation by alcohol dehydrogenase with formation of formic acid and formaldehyde takes place mainly in the liver and kidney. These metabolites are thought to be largely responsible for the characteristic metabolic acidosis which occurs as a result of methyl alcohol poisoning. Metabolism is much slower than for ethyl alcohol, which competitively inhibits the metabolism of methyl alcohol. Oxidation and excretion may continue for several days after ingestion.

Uses and Administration
Methyl alcohol is widely used as a solvent. It is also used as 'wood naphtha' to denature alcohol in the preparation of industrial methylated spirits; wood naphtha contains methyl alcohol together with acetone and other impurities. Wood naphtha used in the *UK* in the preparation of industrial methylated spirits must contain not less than 72% v/v of methyl alcohol. In the *UK* the use of methyl alcohol in cosmetics is restricted by law.

6519-n

Methyl Chloride
Monochloromethane. Chloromethane.
CH_3Cl=50.49.
CAS — 74-87-3.

A colourless gas compressed to a colourless liquid with an ethereal odour. B.p. about −24°.

Adverse Effects and Treatment
Symptoms of methyl chloride intoxication often appear after a latent period of several hours and may include weakness, confusion, dizziness, drowsiness, fatigue, headache, visual disturbances, nausea, vomiting, abdominal pain, paraesthesias, mental changes, muscle dysfunction, convulsions, and coma. Kidney damage, acidosis, and jaundice may occasionally occur.
Treatment should be supportive and symptomatic.
In Great Britain the recommended exposure limits of methyl chloride are 50 ppm (long-term); 100 ppm (short-term). In the *US* the permissible exposure limit is 100 ppm.

A review of the toxicity of methyl chloride.— J. D. Repko and S. M. Lasley, *CRC crit. Rev. Toxicol.*, 1979, *6*, 283.

Reports of poisoning from methyl chloride.— H. C. Scharnweber *et al.*, *J. occup. Med.*, 1974, *16*, 112; L. Spevak *et al.*, *Br. J. ind. Med.*, 1976, *33*, 272.

Uses and Administration
Methyl chloride is used as an industrial solvent. It has been used as an aerosol propellent and refrigerant and was formerly used as a local anaesthetic.

16890-y

Methyl Ethyl Ketone
Ethyl Methyl Ketone; MEK. Butan-2-one.
C_4H_8O=72.11.
CAS — 78-93-3.

A colourless inflammable liquid with a characteristic odour. Wt per mL about 0.81 g. B.p. about 79° to 81°. **Store** in airtight containers.

Adverse Effects
Methyl ethyl ketone is irritant to the eyes, skin, and mucous membranes. Inhalation may result in mild CNS effects including headache and dizziness; nausea and vomiting may also occur.
Methyl ethyl ketone is one of the solvents abused in 'glue-sniffing'.
In Great Britain the recommended exposure limits of methyl ethyl ketone are 200 ppm (long-term); 300 ppm (short-term). In the *US* the permissible exposure limit is 590 mg per m^3.

A brief discussion of the hazards of methyl ethyl ketone including a suggestion that it speeded up the development of polyneuropathy in glue sniffers.— L. Magos, *Br. med. J.*, 1982, *285*, 551.

A report of unconsciousness, hypotension, and severe metabolic acidosis following ingestion of methyl ethyl ketone.— P. G. Kopelman and P. Y. Kalfayan, *Br. med. J.*, 1983, *286*, 21.

Uses and Administration
Methyl ethyl ketone is used as an industrial and pharmaceutical solvent and as an extraction solvent in food processing.

6520-k

Methyl Isobutyl Ketone *(USAN).*
Hexone; Isopropylacetone. 4-Methylpentan-2-one.
$C_6H_{12}O$=100.2.
CAS — 108-10-1.

Pharmacopoeias. In *U.S.N.F.*

A transparent, colourless, mobile, volatile liquid with a faint ketonic and camphoraceous odour. Sp. gr. not more than 0.799. B.p. 114° to 117°. Slightly **soluble** in water; miscible with alcohol and ether. **Store** in airtight containers.

Adverse Effects
Methyl isobutyl ketone may depress the central nervous system in high concentrations. The vapour is irritating to mucous membranes.
In Great Britain the recommended exposure limits of methyl isobutyl ketone are 50 ppm (long-term); 75 ppm (short-term); suitable precautions should be taken to prevent absorption through the skin. In the *US* the permissible and recommended exposure limits are 410 mg per m^3 and 200 mg per m^3 respectively.

EFFECTS ON THE NERVOUS SYSTEM. Report of peripheral neuropathies developing in 86 of 1157 workers following the replacement of methyl isobutyl ketone by methyl *n*-butyl ketone.— N. Allen *et al.*, *Archs Neurol., Chicago*, 1975, *32*, 209. See also *Lancet*, 1979, *2*, 942.

Uses and Administration
Methyl isobutyl ketone is used as an industrial solvent and has been used as an alcohol denaturant.

6521-a

Methylene Chloride *(USAN).*
Dichloromethane.
CH_2Cl_2=84.93.
CAS — 75-09-2.

Pharmacopoeias. In *U.S.N.F.*

A clear, colourless, mobile, volatile liquid with a chloroform-like odour. Sp. gr. 1.318 to 1.322. B.p. 39.5° to 40.5°. Its vapour is not explosive when mixed with air.
Store in airtight containers.

Adverse Effects and Treatment
Inhalation of methylene chloride vapour may cause headache and nausea; high concentrations depress the central nervous system. Pulmonary oedema may occur. Haemolysis has been reported. Significant exposure may result in raised blood concentrations of carboxyhaemoglobin and symptoms of carbon monoxide poisoning. Neurological symptoms, including paraesthesias, respiratory irritation, and gastro-intestinal disturbances have been reported following chronic exposure.
The liquid is irritant to the skin and high concentrations of the vapour are irritant to the eyes.
Treatment should be supportive and symptomatic.
In Great Britain the control exposure limit of methylene chloride is 100 ppm (long-term); the recommended short-term limit is 250 ppm. In the *US* the permissible and recommended exposure limits are 500 ppm and 75 ppm respectively.

The temporary estimated acceptable daily intake of methylene chloride given in the Twenty-third Report was withdrawn and it was recommended that the use of methylene chloride as an extraction solvent should be limited to ensure that its residues in food are as low as practicable.— Twenty-seventh Report of Joint FAO/WHO Expert Committee on Food Additives, *Tech. Rep. Ser. Wld Hlth Org. No. 696*, 1983.

Reviews of the toxicity of methylene chloride Methylene Chloride, *Environmental Health Criteria 32*, Geneva, Wld Hlth Org., 1984; H. P. A. Illing and R. O. Shillaker, Dichloromethane (Methylene Chloride), *Health and Safety Executive*, *Toxicity Review 12*, London, HM Stationery Office, 1985.

A 38-year-old man recovered after ingesting between 1 and 2 pints of a paint remover containing methylene chloride as the active ingredient (Nitromors). Initially he was comatose with haemolysis and acidosis. The onset of recovery was, however, rapid and induction of diuresis was considered to have played a particularly important role in preventing acute renal damage. A late effect was the development of jejunal ulceration and diverticula.— C. J. C. Roberts and F. P. F. Marshall, *Br. med. J.*, 1976, *1*, 20.

Rash, mental impairment, oedema, and temporary diabetes mellitus after exposure to a paint stripper containing methylene chloride.— N. A. Memon and A. R. Davidson, *Br. med. J.*, 1981, *282*, 1033. Personal experience of vomiting, anorexia, nausea, lassitude, urinary frequency and mental impairment lasting for up to 24 hours after exposure to a paint stripper containing methylene chloride.— B. Lee (letter), *ibid.*, 1321. Epidemiological studies showed that fears for a multisystem disorder arising from exposure to methylene chloride were unfounded.— B. A. Walker and P. L. Wyke (letter), *ibid.*, 2057.

Fatal exposure to methylene chloride vapour.— C. L. Winek *et al.*, *Forensic Sci. Int.*, 1981, *18*, 165.

EFFECTS ON THE BLOOD. Reports of raised blood-carboxyhaemoglobin concentrations following exposure to methylene chloride.— R. D. Stewart and C. L. Hake, *J. Am. med. Ass.*, 1976, *235*, 398; H. T. Benzon *et al.* (letter), *ibid.*, 1978, *239*, 2341; J. Fagin *et al.* (letter), *Br. med. J.*, 1980, *281*, 1461.

EFFECTS ON THE LIVER. A report of raised serum alanine aminotransferase values following accidental skin exposure to 10 to 15 litres of methylene chloride.— J. Puurunen and E. Sotaniemi (letter), *Lancet*, 1985, *1*, 822.

EFFECTS ON THE NERVOUS SYSTEM. A study comparing 29 workers occupationally exposed to methylene chloride in concentrations of 75 to 100 ppm with a non-exposed control group found no evidence of long-term neurological damage attributable to methylene chloride.— N. Cherry *et al.*, *Br. J. ind. Med.*, 1981, *38*, 351.

A report of delirium resulting from occupational methylene chloride exposure.— P. N. Tariot, *J. clin. Psychiat.*, 1983, *44*, 340.

EFFECTS ON THE SKIN. Report of second- and third-degree chemical burns following exposure to methylene chloride.— G. G. Wells and H. A. Waldron, *Br. J. ind. Med.*, 1984, *41*, 420.

Absorption and Fate

Methylene chloride is rapidly absorbed following inhalation and is also absorbed after ingestion and through intact skin. After inhalation it is partially metabolised to carbon dioxide and carbon monoxide and significant blood-carboxyhaemoglobin concentrations may be attained. Small amounts are excreted unchanged in the urine.

Uses and Administration

Methylene chloride is commonly used with other solvents in the pharmaceutical industry and is used as an extraction solvent in food processing. Its use in cosmetics is controlled in the *UK*.

Methylene chloride is widely used in paint strippers.

A mention of the experimental use of methylene chloride as an antisickling agent.— J. Dean and A. N. Schechter, *New Engl. J. Med.*, 1978, *299*, 863.

6518-d

Petroleum Spirit

Benzin; Benzinum Medicinale; Light Petroleum; Petroleum Benzin; Petroleum Ether; Solvent Hexane.

Pharmacopoeias. In *Arg.*, *Aust.*, *Ger.*, *Jpn*, *Jug.*, *Mex.*, *Nord.*, and *Pol.* Various boiling ranges are specified. *Swiss* describes Benzinum Medicinale, consisting mainly of hexane and heptane.

NOTE. The motor fuel termed 'petrol' in the *UK* and 'gasoline' in the *USA* is a mixture of volatile hydrocarbons of variable composition containing paraffins (alkanes), olefins (alkenes), cycloparaffins, and aromatic compounds.

A purified distillate of petroleum, consisting of a mixture of the lower members of the paraffin series of hydrocarbons. It is a colourless, transparent, very volatile, highly inflammable liquid with a characteristic odour. It is available in a variety of boiling ranges.

Practically **insoluble** in water; soluble in dehydrated alcohol; miscible with chloroform, ether, and most fixed and volatile oils. The vapour is explosive when mixed with air. **Store** in a cool place in airtight containers. Protect from light.

Adverse Effects and Treatment

As for Kerosene, p.1428. Petroleum spirit and petrol, being more volatile than kerosene, are more likely to be inhaled and to cause aspiration pneumonitis. The toxicity of petrol varies with its composition. Chemical burns have been reported following topical exposure to petrol.

Pneumonitis in a 22-year-old man who sucked about half a cup of petrol into his mouth during a siphoning procedure.— T. H. Lee and W. M. Seymour (letter), *Lancet*, 1979, *2*, 149.

ABUSE. A review of petrol (gasoline) sniffing.— A. Poklis and C. Burkett, *Clin. Toxicol.*, 1977, *11*, 35.

The relationship between gasoline sniffing, cardiac arrhythmias, and sudden death.— M. Bass (letter), *New Engl. J. Med.*, 1978, *299*, 203.

A review of petrol (gasoline) sniffing and lead encephalopathy.— C. A. Ross, *Can. med. Ass. J.*, 1982, *127*, 1195.

Petrol sniffing and a possible association with schizophrenia in a group of Pacific islands.— A. M. Daniels and R. W. Latcham (letter), *Lancet*, 1984, *1*, 389.

High blood and skeletal lead concentrations in Aboriginal petrol sniffers.— H. D. Eastwell, *Med. J. Aust.*, 1985, *143*, *Suppl* S63.

Report of petrol sniffing in young children.— C. S. Hornfeldt *et al.* (letter), *Clin. Pediat.*, 1986, *25*, 114.

CARCINOGENICITY. Occupational exposure to petroleum products or to their combustion products was significantly higher (36%) in 50 men with acute non-lymphocytic leukaemia than in controls (10%).— L. Brandt *et al.*, *Br. med. J.*, 1978, *1*, 553. Exposure to petroleum products seemed to be associated with normal chromosomes, in contrast to exposure to chemical solvents and insecticides.— F. Mitelman *et al.* (letter), *Lancet*, 1979, *2*, 1195.

Uses and Administration

Petroleum spirit is used as a solvent for fats and as an extraction solvent in food processing.

6522-t

Tetrachloroethane

Acetylene Tetrachloride. 1,1,2,2-Tetrachloroethane.

$C_2H_2Cl_4$=167.8.

CAS — 79-34-5.

A clear colourless liquid with a chloroform-like odour. B.p. about 146°. Wt per mL about 1.59 g.

Adverse Effects and Treatment

Tetrachloroethane is probably the most toxic of the chlorinated hydrocarbons. Poisoning can occur through percutaneous absorption as well as ingestion or inhalation. Adverse effects include mucosal irritation, gastro-intestinal disturbances, CNS depression, which may follow a latent period, haemolysis, and severe injury to liver and kidneys with jaundice, cirrhosis, liver necrosis, and oliguria. Treatment consists of supportive measures. Administration of acetylcysteine has been suggested to try to protect against liver damage.

In the *US* the permissible exposure limit is 35 mg per m^3; suitable precautions should be taken to prevent absorption through the skin.

Uses and Administration

Tetrachloroethane is used as an industrial solvent.

6523-x

Toluene

Methylbenzene; Toluol; Toluole.

C_7H_8=92.14.

CAS — 108-88-3.

A colourless, mobile, highly inflammable liquid with a characteristic odour. Wt per mL about 0.87 g. B.p. about 110°. **Store** in airtight containers.

Adverse Effects

Toluene has similar acute toxicity to Benzene, p.1424, but is a less serious industrial hazard. It is a common constituent of adhesives and is abused in glue-sniffing. Commercial toluene may contain benzene, and this may perhaps influence the pattern of adverse effects. Chronic toluene poisoning has been associated with nervous system disorders including muscle weakness, mental changes and encephalopathy.

In Great Britain the recommended exposure limits of toluene are 100 ppm (long-term); 150 ppm (short-term); suitable precautions should be taken to prevent absorption through the skin. In the *US* the permissible and recommended exposure limits are 200 ppm and 100 ppm respectively.

A review of the toxicology of toluene.— J. W. Hayden *et al.*, *Clin. Toxicol.*, 1977, *11*, 549. See also Recommended Health-based Limits in Occupational Exposure to Selected Organic Solvents, *Tech. Rep. Ser. Wld Hlth Org. No. 664*, 1981.

ABUSE. A severe renal tubular defect with metabolic acidosis, a normal 'anion gap', hyperchloraemia, and a high urinary pH was associated with toluene sniffing in 2 patients.— S. M. Taher *et al.*, *New Engl. J. Med.*, 1974, *290*, 765. Metabolic acidosis with a high 'anion gap' in 2 patients who had been sniffing toluene.— C. M. Fischman and J. R. Oster, *J. Am. med. Ass.*, 1979, *241*, 1713. See also *idem*, *242*, 1491.

Convulsions in 3 patients after sniffing glue containing toluene.— M. Helliwell and M. Murphy (letter), *Br. med. J.*, 1979, *1*, 1283.

A report of psychosis associated with toluene sniffing.— M. J. Tarsh, *J. Soc. occup. Med.*, 1979, *29*, 131.

Reversible renal damage in one patient associated with toluene sniffing.— A. M. Will and E. H. McLaren, *Br. med. J.*, 1981, *283*, 525. Progressive renal failure in another patient.— G. Venkataraman (letter), *ibid.*, 1467.

Acute encephalopathy due to toluene intoxication in 19 children.— M. D. King *et al.*, *Br. med. J.*, 1981, *283*, 663. Status epilepticus in one boy associated with toluene abuse.— C. Allister *et al.*, *ibid.*, 1156.

Syndromes of toluene sniffing in adults.— H. Z. Streicher *et al.*, *Ann. intern. Med.*, 1981, *94*, 758.

Multifocal central nervous system damage in 4 toluene abusers.— R. B. Lazar *et al.*, *Neurology*, 1983, *33*, 1337.

A report of sinus bradycardia in a patient admitted to hospital with muscle weakness, gastro-intestinal disturbances, and rhabdomyolysis from toluene inhalation.— C. -S. Zee-Cheng *et al.* (letter), *Ann. intern. Med.*, 1985, *103*, 482.

Reversible respiratory arrest following an acute episode of toluene inhalation in a 21-year-old chronic glue-sniffer.— S. L. Cronk *et al.* (letter), *Br. med. J.*, 1985, *290*, 897.

INTERACTIONS. Administration of alcohol was reported to decrease the total uptake of toluene in 11 subjects exposed to toluene vapour; the maximum blood-toluene concentration was however increased and the apparent clearance significantly decreased.— M. Wallén *et al.*, *Toxic. appl. Pharmac.*, 1984, *76*, 414.

PREGNANCY AND THE NEONATE. A child with nearly classic foetal alcohol syndrome was born to a woman whose major addiction was to solvents (primarily toluene). She had a 14-year history of daily solvent abuse and a 3-year history of alcohol intake of about a 6-pack of beer weekly.— C. Toutant and S. Lippmann (letter), *Lancet*, 1979, *1*, 1356.

Absorption and Fate

Toluene is absorbed by inhalation, ingestion, and to some extent through the skin. It is metabolised mainly by oxidation to benzoic acid which is excreted in the urine largely as the glycine conjugate hippuric acid; *o*-cresol is a minor urinary metabolite. Some unchanged toluene is excreted through the lungs.

Uses and Administration

Toluene is widely used as an industrial solvent.

6524-r

Trichloroethane

α-Trichloroethane; Methylchloroform. 1,1,1-Trichloroethane.

$C_2H_3Cl_3$=133.4.

CAS — 71-55-6.

A colourless liquid. Sp. gr. about 1.31. B.p about 74°. Practically **insoluble** in water; miscible with alcohol, ether and chloroform. Non-inflammable.

Adverse Effects

Acute intoxication with trichloroethane may result in initial excitement followed by depression of the central nervous system with dizziness, drowsiness, headache, lightheadedness, and ataxia. There may be liver and kidney impairment. Cardiac arrhythmias may develop. Fatalities have occurred following accidental exposure to high concentrations of trichloroethane in confined spaces.

Nausea, vomiting, and diarrhoea have been reported following ingestion. Trichloroethane is a mild eye and skin irritant.

In Great Britain the control exposure limits of trichloroethane are 350 ppm (long-term); 450 ppm (short-term). In the *US* the permissible and recommended exposure limits are 350 ppm.

A review of the toxicity of trichloroethane.— R. J. Fielder and S. J. Williams, 1,1,1-Trichloroethane, *Health and Safety Executive, Toxicity Review 9*, London, HM Stationery Office, 1984.

A report of 2 fatalities due to acute occupational exposure to trichloroethane.— R. R. Northfield, *J. Soc. occup. Med.*, 1981, *31*, 164.

During the period 1961 to 1980, 52 cases of industrial poisoning due to trichloroethane inhalation were reported to HM Factory Inspectorate. Unconsciousness was reported in 26 cases, including 2 fatalities, other CNS symptoms in 18, gastro-intestinal symptoms in 9, and respiratory symptoms in 11 subjects.— T. B. McCarthy and R. D. Jones, *Br. J. ind. Med.*, 1983, *40*, 450.

ABUSE. A report of the symptoms and management of trichloroethane intoxication in a 22-year-old girl who was already in end-stage renal failure due to Goodpasture's syndrome associated with a prolonged history of drug abuse which included the regular sniffing of various glues and organic solvents. Failure of renal transplantation led to a return of her solvent abuse and she inhaled 400 mL of Zoff in 36 hours. Her symptoms included persistent vomiting, extreme drowsiness and flaccidity as well as fresh bruising on her arms; she had depressed respiration and liver damage. Treatment was supportive and included lactulose, cimetidine and a high carbohydrate-low protein dietary regimen. Four hours after her last exposure to trichloroethane her regular haemodialysis was performed followed (because of initially suspected paracetamol ingestion, and also the ease of vascular access) by charcoal haemoperfusion. Clinical recovery was complete within 48 hours; by 96 hours, liver function had returned to base-line, and the trichloroethane had been completely eliminated.— A. W. Nathan and P. A. Toseland (letter), *Br. J. clin. Pharmac.*, 1979, *8*, 284.

Of 140 deaths associated with volatile substance abuse in the *UK* between 1971 and 1981, 20 were associated with abuse of trichloroethane.— H. R. Anderson *et al.*, *Hum. Toxicol.*, 1982, *1*, 207.

A report of 4 cases of sudden death in adolescents associated with inhalation of typewriter correction fluids containing trichloroethane.— G. S. King *et al.*, *J. Am. med. Ass.*, 1985, *253*, 1604.

EFFECTS ON THE KIDNEY. A report of Goodpasture's syndrome tentatively associated with exposure to methylene chloride and trichloroethane which was exacerbated after further inadvertent exposure to trichloroethane.— A. M. Keogh *et al.*, *Br. med. J.*, 1984, *288*, 188.

EFFECTS ON THE RESPIRATORY SYSTEM. A report of chest pain, dyspnoea, cough, and hypoxia following exposure to an aerosol waterproofing product containing trichloroethane and a surfactant.— O. F. Woo *et al.*, *J. Toxicol. clin. Toxicol.*, 1983, *20*, 333.

Absorption and Fate

Trichloroethane is absorbed after inhalation, ingestion, and through intact skin. Small amounts are metabolised to trichloroethanol and trichloroacetic acid and excreted in the urine, but it is largely excreted unchanged through the lungs over a period of days.

Uses and Administration

Trichloroethane has wide applications as a solvent. It is commonly used in dry cleaning, typewriter correction fluids, and as a solvent for plaster removal. Its use in cosmetics is controlled in the *UK*.

6525-f

White Spirit

A mixture of hydrocarbons to which a denaturant may be added.

A colourless liquid with a boiling range of 130° to 220°.

Adverse Effects, Treatment, and Precautions

As for Kerosene, p.1428.

In Great Britain the recommended exposure limits of white spirit are 100 ppm (long-term); 125 ppm (short-term).

Uses and Administration

White spirit is used as an industrial solvent.

6526-d

Xylene

Xylol; Xylole. A mixture of *o*-, *m*-, and *p*-dimethylbenzene in which the *m*-isomer predominates.

C_8H_{10}=106.2.

CAS — 1330-20-7; 108-38-3 (m-xylene); 95-47-6 (o-xylene); 106-42-3 (p-xylene).

Pharmacopoeias. In *Span.*

A colourless inflammable liquid. Wt per mL about 0.86 g. B.p. about 138° to 142°.

Solvent naphtha (Coal Tar Solvent Naphtha) consists chiefly of xylenes and trimethylbenzenes; various fractions are available. It should be distinguished from solvent mineral naphtha which is a petroleum product.

Adverse Effects

The toxicity of xylene is similar to that of benzene (p.1424) but is less marked.

Commercial xylene may contain benzene, and this may perhaps influence the pattern of adverse effects.

In Great Britain the recommended exposure limits of xylene are 100 ppm (long-term); 150 ppm (short-term); suitable precautions should be taken to prevent absorption through the skin. In the *US* the permissible and recommended exposure limits are 100 ppm.

For a review of health hazards and effects of occupational exposure to xylene see Recommended Health-based limits in Occupational Exposure to Selected Organic Solvents, *Tech. Rep. Ser. Wld Hlth Org. No. 664*, 1981.

Death of one man and prolonged unconsciousness in 2 others followed prolonged inhalation of fumes from paint in which xylene comprised more than 90% of the solvent. The 2 patients who subsequently recovered were unconscious for 15 and 18 hours respectively, and both patients had transient liver cell damage, and one had temporary impairment of renal function.— R. Morley *et al.*, *Br. med. J.*, 1970, *3*, 442.

Xylene-induced epilepsy following use of a xylene-based glue.— L. J. H. Arthur and D. A. Curnock (letter), *Br. med. J.*, 1982, *284*, 1787.

Absorption and Fate

Xylene is absorbed after inhalation, ingestion, and to some extent through the skin. It is metabolised by oxidation to the corresponding *o*-, *m*-, or *p*-toluic acids and excreted in the urine largely as the glycine conjugate, methylhippuric acid. It is partly excreted unchanged through the lungs.

Uses and Administration

Xylene is used as a solvent and as a clearing agent in microscopy. It is also used in preparations to dissolve ear wax.

Proprietary Names and Manufacturers

Cerulisina *(Bouty, Ital.)*; Cerulyse *(Chauvin-Blache, Fr.; Spain)*; Novo-Cérusol *(Novopharma, Switz.)*.

Stabilising and Suspending Agents

5400-n

The stabilising and suspending agents described in this section have the property of increasing the viscosity of water when dissolved or dispersed. The rheological properties of the dispersions can vary widely from thin liquids to thick gels.

As well as being used as thickening and suspending agents many are used in emulsions as stabilisers and in some cases as emulsifying agents. They therefore have wide applications both in pharmacy and in the food industry.

Some of the agents in this section are used in artificial saliva and artificial tear preparations which are used in conditions in which the normal secretion of saliva or tears respectively is reduced or absent. The agents most commonly used are carmellose sodium, hypromellose, methylcellulose, and povidone.

Some of the agents in this section are also used in the manufacture of tablets as disintegrants, binding and granulating agents and for film or enteric coating.

ARTIFICIAL SALIVA. For references to the use of carmellose and hypromellose in the treatment of dry mouth, see p.1433 and p.1435, respectively.

ARTIFICIAL TEARS. The use of artificial tear preparations in the treatment of dry eye.— *Drug & Ther. Bull.*, 1985, *23*, 81.

See also under Hydroxypropylcellulose, p.1435 and Polyvinyl Alcohol, p.1247.

5402-m

Acacia *(BAN, USAN).*

Acac.; Acaciae Gummi; E414; Gomme Arabique; Gomme de Sénégal; Gum Acacia; Gum Arabic; Gummi Africanum; Gummi Arabicum; Gummi Mimosae.

CAS — 9000-01-5.

Pharmacopoeias. In *Arg., Aust., Belg., Br., Cz., Egypt., Eur., Fr., Ger., Hung., Ind., Int., It., Jpn, Jug., Mex., Neth., Nord., Pol., Port., Roum., Span.,* and *Swiss.* Also in *U.S.N.F.* The *B.P.* also specifies powdered acacia; the *B.P.* and *Eur. P.* have monographs for spray-dried acacia. The *U.S.N.F.* monograph for acacia encompasses flake acacia, powdered acacia, granular acacia, and spray-dried acacia.

The air-dried gummy exudate from the stem and branches of *Acacia senegal* (Leguminosae) and other species of *Acacia* of African origin.

Almost odourless, white or yellowish-white to pale amber, brittle tears; it may also appear as a powder, granules or flakes.

Very slowly but almost completely **soluble** 1 in 2 of water leaving only a very small residue of vegetable particles; practically insoluble in alcohol and ether. **Incompatibilities** have been reported with a number of substances including: alcohol, amidopyrine, apomorphine, borax, cresol, ferric salts, lead subacetate, morphine, phenol, physostigmine, tannins, thymol, and vanillin. Acacia contains an oxidising enzyme which may affect preparations containing easily oxidised substances; the enzyme may be inactivated by heating at 100° for a short time. **Store** in airtight containers.

Adverse Effects

Hypersensitivity reactions have occurred rarely after inhalation or ingestion of acacia.

Three renal transplant recipients found to be hypersensitive to prednisone tablets had reacted to the tragacanth and acacia used in their manufacture. Their symptoms subsided when a formulation using methylcellulose was substituted.— D. Rubinger *et al.* (letter), *Lancet*, 1978, *2*, 689.

Uses and Administration

Acacia is used as a suspending and emulsifying agent and as a tablet binder. It is often used with tragacanth.

It is used in the food industry.

Sensitivity reactions occurred rarely after inhalation or ingestion of acacia. Its use in food was not limited but further information was required.— *Fd Add. Ser. Wld Hlth Org. No. 5*, 1974.

Preparations

Acacia Mucilage *(A.P.F.).* Acacia 40, benzoic acid solution 2.0, compound hydroxybenzoate solution 1.0, purified water 60.

Acacia Syrup *(U.S.N.F.).* Acacia 10 g, sodium benzoate 100 mg, vanilla tincture 0.5 mL, sucrose 80 g, water to 100 mL. Store at a temperature not exceeding 40° in airtight containers.

5403-b

Agar *(BAN, USAN).*

Agar-agar; Colle du Japon; E406; Gélose; Gelosa; Japanese Isinglass; Layor Carang.

CAS — 9002-18-0.

Pharmacopoeias. In *Arg., Aust., Br., Braz., Chin., Cz., Egypt., Eur., Fr., Hung., It., Jpn, Jug., Mex., Neth., Nord., Pol., Port., Span.,* and *Swiss.* Also in *U.S.N.F.* The *B.P.* and *U.S.N.F.* also specify powdered agar.

Polysaccharides obtained by extracting various species of Rhodophyceae algae. The *B.P.* specifies mainly those belonging to the genus *Gelidium*; the *U.S.N.F.* specifies *Gelidium cartilagineum, Gracilaria confervoides* and related red algae of this class.

Odourless or almost odourless, thin, colourless to yellow, translucent strips, flakes, or granules; tough when damp but becoming more brittle on drying. **Soluble** in boiling water to produce a clear solution that gels on cooling; practically insoluble in cold water. **Store** in well-closed containers.

Agar is used as a suspending or thickening agent in pharmacy and in the food industry. It has been used as a bulk laxative, since by taking up moisture it increases the volume of the faeces. For this purpose it has been taken in doses of 4 to 16 g once or twice daily.

The use of agar in food was limited only by good manufacturing practice. For background toxicological information, see *Fd Add. Ser. Wld Hlth Org. No. 5*, 1974.

A study in 80 premature infants given agar as a supplement to feeds indicated that it was of no value in the management of hyperbilirubinaemia in low birth-weight newborn infants.— C. Romagnoli *et al., Archs Dis. Childh.*, 1975, *50*, 202.

For a reference to a gel polymer of agar and acrylamide used as a nontextile wound dressing, see under Dermatological Agents p.929.

12341-r

Alginic Acid *(BAN, USAN).*

Acide Alginique; Acidum Alginicum; E400.

CAS — 9005-32-7.

Pharmacopoeias. In *Fr.* and *Nord.* Also in *U.S.N.F.*

A polyuronic acid composed of residues of D-mannuronic and L-guluronic acids extracted from algae belonging to the Phaeophyceae, mainly species of *Laminaria*. A white to yellowish-white, odourless or almost odourless, fibrous powder. Practically **insoluble** in water and organic solvents; soluble in alkaline solutions. A 3% dispersion in water has a pH of 1.5 to 3.5. **Store** in well-closed containers.

5459-x

Sodium Alginate *(USAN).*

Algin; E401; Sodium Polymannuronate.

CAS — 9005-38-3.

Pharmacopoeias. In *Aust., Fr.,* and *It.* Also in *U.S.N.F.* and *B.P.C. 1973.*

It consists chiefly of the sodium salt of alginic acid, a polyuronic acid composed of linked residues of βD-mannuronic acid, and is obtained from brown seaweeds.

A white or buff powder which is odourless or almost odourless.

Slowly **soluble** in water, forming a viscous colloidal solution; alginic acid is precipitated below pH 3. Practically insoluble in alcohol, chloroform, and ether, and in aqueous solutions containing more than 30% of alcohol.

Incompatibilities have been observed with acridine derivatives, crystal violet, phenylmercuric acetate and nitrate, calcium salts, alcohol in concentrations greater than 5%, and heavy metals. High concentrations of electrolytes cause an increase in viscosity until salting-out of sodium alginate occurs; salting-out occurs if more than 4% of sodium chloride is present. **Store** in airtight containers.

Sodium alginate is used as a suspending and thickening agent and in the preparation of water-miscible pastes, creams, and gels. Sodium alginate and alginic acid may be used as stabilisers for oil-in-water emulsions and as binding and disintegrating agents in tablets. They are widely used in the food industry.

They are used with an antacid in the management of gastro-oesophageal reflux.

Because of its property of instantaneous precipitation when brought into contact with free calcium ions, yielding calcium alginate, sodium alginate is employed as a haemostatic (see also Calcium Alginate, p.1132).

Estimated acceptable daily intake: up to 25 mg, as alginic acid, per kg body-weight.— Seventeenth Report of FAO/WHO Expert Committee on Food Additives, *Tech. Rep. Ser. Wld Hlth Org. No. 539*, 1974.

An alginate suspension has been shown to form a raft on the stomach contents (A.P. McKay *et al., Gut*, 1986, *27*, A609). This raft is claimed to impede gastro-oesophageal reflux though not alleviate symptoms of any reflux; a combination of alginate and antacid may provide symptomatic relief (M. Atkinson, *Prescriber's J.*, 1982, *22*, 129). There has been some argument about the benefits of alginates in reflux (*Lancet*, 1983, *1*, 1081; N.C. Varey *ibid.*, *2*, 103).

Proprietary Names and Manufacturers of Alginic Acid and its Salts

Alginade *(Kelco International, UK)*; Collatex A *(Kelco International, UK)*; Manucol *(Kelco International, UK)*; Manugel *(Kelco International, UK)*; Manutex *(Kelco International, UK)*; Sazio *(Zyma, Ital.)*.

The following names have been used for multi-ingredient preparations containing alginic acid and its salts—Algicon *(Rorer, Canad.; Rorer, UK)*; Antiflux *(Ayerst, Canad.)*; Gastrocote *(MCP Pharmaceuticals, UK)*; Gastron *(Winthrop, UK)*; Gavigrans *(Reckitt & Colman, Austral.)*; Gaviscon Granules *(Reckitt & Colman, Austral.)*; Gaviscon Infant Preparations *(Reckitt & Colman, Austral.; Reckitt & Colman Pharmaceuticals, UK)*; Gaviscon Liquid *(Reckitt & Colman, Austral.; Winthrop, Canad.; Reckitt & Colman Pharmaceuticals, UK)*; Gaviscon Tablets *(Reckitt & Colman, Austral.; Winthrop, Canad.; Reckitt & Colman Pharmaceuticals, UK)*; Meracote *(Merrell Dow, Austral.)*; Pyrogastrone Tablets *(Winthrop, UK)*; Topal *(ICI Pharmaceuticals, UK)*.

5405-g

Aluminium Magnesium Silicate *(BAN).*
Magnesium Aluminium Silicate; Magnesium Aluminum Silicate *(USAN)*; Saponite.

CAS — 1327-43-1; 12511-31-8.

Pharmacopoeias. In *Br.* Also in *U.S.N.F.*

A hydrated native colloidal saponite freed from gritty particles. It is an odourless or almost odourless, creamy-white powder or small flakes. Practically **insoluble** in water, but swells to form a colloidal dispersion; practically insoluble in organic solvents.
The *B.P.* specifies that a 4% dispersion in water has a pH of about 9.0.
The *U.S.N.F.* specifies that a 5% dispersion in water has a pH of 9.0 to 10.0, and also describes several types with varying ranges of aluminium:magnesium content and varying viscosity ranges for dispersions of approximately 5%.
Store in airtight containers.

Aluminium magnesium silicate has a variety of pharmaceutical uses, including use as a suspending and thickening agent, an emulsion stabiliser, and as a binder and disintegrating agent in tablets.
An artificial form of aluminium magnesium silicate hydrate known as almasilate (p.1074) is used as an antacid in doses of 1 g.

An evaluation of aluminium magnesium silicate as an alternative to tragacanth.— C. A. Farley and W. Lund, *Pharm. J.*, 1976, *1*, 562.

Proprietary Names and Manufacturers
Dianeusine *(Fr.)*; Sicco-Gynaedron *(Artesan, Ger.)*; Tri-Om *(Om, Switz.)*; Veegum *(Vanderbilt, USA: K & K-Greeff, UK).*

5407-p

Bentonite *(BAN, USAN).*
558; Bentonitum; Mineral Soap; Soap Clay; Wilkinite.

CAS — 1302-78-9.

Pharmacopoeias. In *Arg., Aust., Br., Cz., Egypt., Eur., Fr., Ger., Ind., It., Jpn, Neth.,* and *Swiss.* Also in *U.S.N.F. U.S.N.F.* also includes Purified Bentonite.

Native colloidal hydrated aluminium silicate consisting mainly of montmorillonite, $Al_2O_3,4SiO_2,H_2O$; it may also contain calcium, magnesium, and iron.
An odourless, hygroscopic, very fine, homogeneous, greyish-white powder with a yellowish tint.
Practically **insoluble** in water and in aqueous solutions, but swells into a homogeneous mass occupying about 12 times the volume of the dry powder. Practically insoluble, and does not swell, in organic solvents. The *U.S.N.F.* specifies that a 2% suspension in water has a pH of 9.5 to 10.5; a 5% suspension of purified bentonite has a pH of 9.0 to 10.0. **Store** in airtight containers.

Bentonite absorbs water readily to form sols or gels, depending on its concentration. It is used as a suspending and stabilising agent and as an adsorbent or clarifying agent.

Preparations
Bentonite Magma *(U.S.N.F.).* Bentonite 5% w/w in water.

5409-w

Carbomer *(BAN, rINN).*
Carbomer 934P *(USAN)*; Carboxypolymethylene; Carboxyvinyl Polymer.

CAS — 9003-01-4; 54182-57-9.

Pharmacopoeias. In *Br.* Also in *U.S.N.F.*

A synthetic high molecular weight polymer of acrylic acid cross-linked with allylsucrose and containing 56 to 68% of carboxylic acid groups, calculated as the dry substance.
A white, fluffy, acidic, hygroscopic powder with a slight characteristic odour. Neutralised with alkali hydroxides or amines, it is **soluble** in water, alcohol, and glycerol.
Store in airtight containers.

Carbomer is used as a suspending agent, a gel basis, an emulsifier, and a binding agent in tablets.

Studies on the rheological properties of Carbopol gels.— B. W. Barry and M. C. Meyer, *Int. J. Pharmaceut.*, 1979, *2*, 1 and 27.

There was an increase in gastric mucosal protection in the *rat* when carbomer 934P was given with carbenoxolone sodium; this has led to the combination being evaluated clinically in the treatment of gastritis.— P. W. Dettmar *et al.*, *Gut*, 1985, *26*, A1107.

Mucosal adhesive dosage forms were prepared for antineoplastic agents and triamcinoline acetonide using a combination of carbomer and hydroxypropylcellulose. A nasal mucosal dosage form of insulin that employed hydroxypropylcellulose was also being investigated.— T. Nagai and Y. Machida, *Pharm. Int.*, 1985, *6*, 196.

Proprietary Names and Manufacturers
Carbopol *(Goodrich, UK).*

5410-m

Carmellose Calcium *(rINNM).*
Calcium Carboxymethylcellulose; Carboxymethylcellulose Calcium *(USAN).*

CAS — 9050-04-8.

Pharmacopoeias. In *Jpn.* Also in *U.S.N.F.*

A white to yellowish-white hygroscopic powder. It swells in water to form a suspension; practically **insoluble** in acetone, alcohol, chloroform, and ether. A 1% suspension in water has a pH of 4.5 to 6.0. **Store** in airtight containers.

5411-b

Carmellose Sodium *(BAN, rINNM).*
Carboxymethylcellulose Sodium *(USAN)*; Cellulose Gum; CMC; E466; SCMC; Sodium Carboxymethylcellulose; Sodium Cellulose Glycollate.

CAS — 9004-32-4.

Pharmacopoeias. In *Arg., Aust., Br., Braz., Cz., Egypt., Eur., Fr., Hung., Ind., It., Jpn, Jug., Nord., Roum., Swiss,* and *U.S. U.S.N.F.* includes Croscarmellose Sodium, a cross-linked polymer of carmellose sodium, for use as a tablet disintegrant. *U.S.N.F.* also includes Carboxymethylcellulose Sodium 12.

The sodium salt of a polycarboxymethyl ether of cellulose. The *B.P.* specifies a sodium content of 6.5 to 10.8%, and the *U.S.P.* 6.5 to 9.5%, both calculated on the dry substance. Carboxymethylcellulose Sodium 12 *(U.S.N.F.)* has a sodium content of 10.5 to 12.0%, calculated on the dry substance. The degree of polymerisation affects the viscosity of solution.
Carmellose sodium is a white to cream-coloured, odourless or almost odourless, hygroscopic powder or granules. It loses not more than 10% of its weight on drying.
Easily **dispersed** in water forming colloidal solutions; practically insoluble in alcohol, ether, and most other organic solvents. The *B.P.* specifies that a 1% solution in water has a pH of 6.0 to 8.0; the *U.S.P.* specifies a pH range of 6.5 to 8.5.
Incompatibilities have been reported with strongly acidic solutions, with soluble salts of iron and some other metals, and with xanthan gum. **Store** in airtight containers.

Carmellose sodium is used as a suspending agent and as an emulsifying agent, it is used in the preparation of gels and is added in the proportions of about 1 part to 9 to microcrystalline cellulose to improve dispersion.
Carmellose sodium is an ingredient of protective preparations used in the fitting of ileostomy and colostomy appliances. It is also used for the mechanical protection of oral and perioral lesions, and has been used as a sialagogue in the management of dry mouth.
Carmellose sodium is widely used in the food industry.

Estimated acceptable daily intake: up to 25 mg per kg body-weight, as the sum of total modified celluloses. The figure may be exceeded for dietetic purposes.— Seventeenth Report of the FAO/WHO Expert Committee on Food Additives, *Tech. Rep. Ser. Wld Hlth Org. No. 539*, 1974.

DRY MOUTH. *Va-OraLube.* A saliva substitute solution developed specifically for use in patients receiving radiotherapy for malignancy of the head and neck. It is stated to contain potassium phosphates, potassium chloride, sodium chloride, magnesium chloride, calcium chloride, sodium fluoride (2 ppm of F), sorbitol, 'binder' [probably carmellose], flavouring, dye, preservative, and water. Specific gravity 1.0054. pH is 7.0. The viscosity and electrolyte concentration are adjusted to approximate whole saliva. The solution was used 1 to 8 times a day by 30 patients with dry mouth who were taking neuroleptics or tricyclic antidepressants. Relief of symptoms of dryness was immediate and complete following rinsing of the mouth with a small volume. The lubricant effect generally lasted from 1 to 3 hours.— W. E. Fann and I. L. Shannon, *Am. J. Psychiat.*, 1978, *135*, 251.
In a double-blind, crossover study a carmellose sodium-based saliva substitute was compared with a mouthwash containing glycerol and lemon for the management of dry mouth. The carmellose sodium preparation offered no significant advantage over the glycerol and lemon mouthwash but both preparations were preferred to water.— D. Wiesenfeld *et al.*, *Br. dent. J.*, 1983, *155*, 155.

Preparations
Carboxymethylcellulose Sodium Paste *(U.S.P.).* A paste containing carmellose sodium 16 to 17%. Store in well-closed containers at a temperature not exceeding 30°.
Carboxymethylcellulose Sodium Tablets *(U.S.P.).* Tablets containing carmellose sodium.

Proprietary Preparations
Orabase *(Squibb Surgicare, UK). Ointment,* carmellose sodium, pectin, and gelatin in Plastibase (a liquid paraffin-polyethylene basis). For protection of lesions of the mouth and skin.
Orahesive *(Squibb Surgicare, UK). Powder,* carmellose sodium, pectin, gelatin. For protection of lesions of the mouth and skin.
Stomahesive *(Squibb Surgicare, UK). Adhesive plasters,* carmellose sodium, gelatin, pectin, and polyisobutylene, with a polyethylene backing. For peristomal protection.
Varihesive *(Squibb Surgicare, UK). Paste,* carmellose sodium, gelatin, pectin, polyisobutylene. For leg ulcers and stoma care.

Proprietary Names and Manufacturers of Carmellose or its Salts
Blanose *(Aqualon, UK)*; Cekol *(Billerud, Swed. : Berol Kemi, UK)*; Courlose *(Courtaulds, UK)*; Eksplorationscreme *(DAK, Denm.)*; Glandosane *(Dylade, UK)*; Orora *(Belg.)*; Solvacton *(Arg.).*

The following names have been used for multi-ingredient preparations containing carmellose or its salts—Anorex-CCK *(Robertson/Taylor, USA)*; Orabase *(Squibb, Austral.; Squibb, Canad.; Squibb Surgicare, UK)*; Orahesive *(Squibb, Austral.; Squibb, Canad.; Squibb Surgicare, UK)*; Stomahesive *(Squibb Surgicare, UK)*; Varihesive *(Squibb Surgicare, UK).*

5412-v

Carrageenan *(USAN).*
Carrageenin; Carraghénates; Chondrus Extract; E407; Irish Moss Extract.

CAS — 9000-07-1 (carrageenan); 11114-20-8 (κ-carrageenan); 9064-57-7 (λ-carrageenan).

Pharmacopoeias. In *Fr.* Also in *U.S.N.F.*

The *U.S.N.F.* defines carrageenan as the hydrocolloid obtained by extraction with water or aqueous alkali from some members of the class Rhodophyceae (red seaweeds). It consists chiefly of a mixture of the ammonium, calcium, magnesium, potassium, and sodium esters of galactose and 3-6-anhydrogalactose copolymers. The prevalent copolymers in the hydrocolloids are κ-carrageenan, ι-carrageenan, and λ-carrageenan.
A white to yellowish or brown, coarse or fine, practically odourless powder. **Soluble** 1 in 30 of water at 80° forming a viscous clear or slightly opalescent solution. It disperses more readily if first mixed with alcohol, glycerol, or syrup.
Store in airtight containers in a cool place.

Carrageenan is used in pharmacy and the food industry as a suspending and gelling agent.
Chondrus was used similarly.
A degraded form of carrageenan used to be given in gastro-intestinal disorders but it was associated with lesions in *animals* and is no longer used.

After considering further *animal* data it was decided that an acceptable daily intake (ADI) of 'not specified' be allocated to refined non-degraded carrageenan. This means that on the basis of available data, the total daily intake of this form of carrageenan, arising from its use at the levels necessary to achieve the desired effect and from its acceptable background in food, does not represent a hazard to health. The establishment of an acceptable daily intake was not deemed necessary. The Committee was aware of the toxic effects associated with degraded carrageenan and of the use of 'semi-refined' carrageenan as a food in some countries; the ADI of 'not specified' did not apply to these forms of carrageenan. The ADI did, however, apply to furcellaran [a similar extract from Rhodophyceae] which is included in the specifications for food-grade carrageenan.— Twenty-eighth Report of the FAO/WHO Expert Committee on Food Additives, *Tech. Rep. Ser. Wld Hlth Org. No. 710,* 1984.

Proprietary Names and Manufacturers
Coréine *(Daniel-Brunet, Fr.)*; Gelcarin *(Honeywill & Stein, UK)*; Hydrogel *(Honeywill & Stein, UK)*; Seaspen *(Honeywill & Stein, UK)*; Viscarin *(Honeywill & Stein, UK)*.

5413-g

Cellacephate *(BAN)*.

CAP; Cellacefate *(pINN)*; Cellulose Acetate Phthalate *(USAN)*; Cellulosi Acetas Phtalas; Cellulosi Acetas Phthalas; Cellulosum Acetylphthalicum; Celophthalum.

CAS — 9004-38-0.

Pharmacopoeias. In *Aust., Br., Braz., Cz., Eur., Fr., Ger., Hung., Ind., It., Jpn, Neth., Nord.,* and *Swiss.* Also in *U.S.N.F.*

Cellulose in which some of the hydroxyl groups are acetylated and some are esterified by hydrogen phthaloyl groups.

A hygroscopic, white, free-flowing powder or colourless flakes, odourless or with a slight odour of acetic acid. The *B.P.* specifies 17 to 26% of acetyl groups and 30 to 40% of hydrogen phthaloyl groups, both calculated with reference to the anhydrous substance, and not more than 3% of free acid calculated as phthalic acid. The *U.S.N.F.* specifies 21.5 to 26.0% of acetyl groups and 30 to 36% of phthalyl groups, and not more than 6% of free acid.

The *B.P.* **solubilities** are: practically insoluble in water, alcohol, and chlorinated and non-chlorinated hydrocarbons; freely soluble in acetone; soluble in diethylene glycol, dioxan, and in dilute solutions of alkalis. **Store** in airtight containers and at a temperature between 8° and 15°.

Cellacephate is unaffected by immersion in acid media in the stomach but softens and swells in intestinal fluid. It is used as an enteric-coating material for tablets and capsules, usually with a plasticiser. Films of cellacephate are reported to be permeable to some ionic substances such as ammonium chloride and such substances require a sealing coat.

Proprietary Names and Manufacturers
Eastman, UK.

5415-p

Dispersible Cellulose *(BAN)*.

Microcrystalline Cellulose and Carboxymethylcellulose Sodium *(USAN)*.

Pharmacopoeias. In *Br.* Also in *U.S.N.F.*

An odourless white to off-white coarse to fine powder consisting of a colloid-forming attrited mixture of microcrystalline cellulose and carmellose sodium.

Dispersible in water, with swelling, to produce a white, opaque dispersion or gel; practically insoluble in organic solvents and dilute acids. A dispersion in water has a pH of 6 to 8. **Store** in a cool dry place in airtight containers and at a temperature between 8° and 15°.

Dispersible cellulose is used as a suspending agent.

References to dispersible cellulose as a suspending agent for the extemporaneous dispensing of liquids prepared from crushed tablets: B. A. Miller, *Pharm. J.,* 1983, *2,* 385; S. W. Bond and K. G. Hutchison (letter), *ibid.,* 630.

Proprietary Names and Manufacturers
Avicel RC.591 *(Honeywill & Stein, UK)*.

5414-q

Microcrystalline Cellulose *(BAN, USAN)*.

Cellulosa Microgranulare; Cellulose Gel; Crystalline Cellulose; E460.

CAS — 9004-34-6.

Pharmacopoeias. In *Br., Eur., Fr., Ind., It., Jpn,* and *Neth.* Also in *U.S.N.F.*

A fine, white or almost white, odourless or almost odourless, crystalline powder consisting of partially depolymerised cellulose, prepared from alpha-cellulose. Practically **insoluble** in water and in acids and most organic solvents. The *B.P.* specifies that the pH of the supernatant liquid of a 2% dispersion in water is 5.0 to 7.5. The *U.S.N.F.* specifies a pH range of 5.0 to 7.0 for the supernatant liquid of a 12.5% dispersion.

Store in well-closed containers.

There are 2 grades of microcrystalline cellulose for pharmaceutical use, a colloidal grade and a non-dispersible grade. The colloidal grade is used generally in conjunction with other cellulose derivatives such as carmellose sodium as a suspending agent. The non-dispersible grade is used in tabletting.

Degradation in the gastro-intestinal tract of a radiolabelled native cellulose.— J. Kelleher *et al., Gut,* 1984, *25,* 811. See also J. H. Cummings, *ibid.,* 805.

Proprietary Names and Manufacturers
Avicel *(Honeywill & Stein, UK)*; Emcocel *(Mendell, USA: Forum Chemicals, UK)*.

The following names have been used for multi-ingredient preparations containing microcrystalline cellulose— Nilstim *(De Witt, UK)*.

5416-s

Powdered Cellulose *(BAN, USAN)*.

Alpha Cellulose; Cellulose Powder; E460.

Pharmacopoeias. In *Br., Eur., Fr., Ger., It., Neth.,* and *Swiss.* Also in *U.S.N.F.*

A purified mechanically disintegrated cellulose prepared from wood (alpha) cellulose. It is a white or almost white, odourless, fine, granular, or fluffy powder.

Practically **insoluble** in water, dilute acids, and most organic solvents. The *U.S.N.F.* has slightly soluble in sodium hydroxide solution (1 in 20). The supernatant liquid of a 2 or 10% dispersion in water has a pH of 5.0 to 7.5. **Store** in well-closed containers.

Powdered cellulose is used in tabletting.

In Great Britain the recommended exposure limits of cellulose total dust are 10 mg per m^3 (long-term) and 20 mg per m^3 (short-term); for respirable dust the limit is 5 mg per m^3 (long-term).

Proprietary Names and Manufacturers
Elcema *(Degussa, UK)*; Unifiber *(Hickam, USA)*.

5417-w

Ceratonia

Carob Bean Gum; Carob Gum; Cerat.; Ceratonia Gum; E410; Gomme de Caroube; Locust Bean Gum.

CAS — 9000-40-2.

Pharmacopoeias. In *Fr.*

The endosperms separated from the seeds of the locust bean tree, *Ceratonia siliqua* (Leguminosae).

Ceratonia is now used as a thickening agent in the food industry and is employed in infant feeds for the control of diarrhoea and vomiting.

A temporary acceptable daily intake (ADI) of 'not specified' had been allocated in the 19th report of the Committee. A review of the considerable body of relevant toxicological data enabled the Committee to remove the temporary status of the ADI. The statement 'ADI not specified' means that on the basis of the available data, the total daily intake of the substance, arising from its use at the levels necessary to achieve the desired effect and from its acceptable background in food, does not represent a hazard to health. The establishment of an acceptable daily intake was not deemed necessary.— Twenty-fifth Report of the FAO/WHO Expert Committee on Food Additives, *Tech. Rep. Ser. Wld Hlth Org. No. 669,* 1981.

Proprietary Names and Manufacturers
Arobon *(Nestlé, Norw.; Nestlé, UK)*; Carobel *(Key, Austral.; Cow & Gate, UK)*; Nestargel *(Nestle, Switz.; Nestlé, UK)*.

5420-v

Dextrates *(USAN)*.

CAS — 39404-33-6.

Pharmacopoeias. In *U.S.N.F.*

A purified anhydrous or hydrated mixture of saccharides obtained by the controlled enzymatic hydrolysis of starch. Free-flowing, porous, white odourless spherical granules. Freely **soluble** in water (solubility increases in hot water); soluble in dilute acids and alkalis and in basic organic solvents; insoluble in common organic solvents. A 20% solution has a pH of 3.8 to 5.8. **Store** in well-closed containers in a cool dry place.

Dextrates is used as a tablet diluent.

Proprietary Names and Manufacturers
Emdex *(Mendell, USA: Forum Chemicals, UK)*.

5421-g

Ethylcellulose *(USAN)*.

E462.

CAS — 9004-57-3.

Pharmacopoeias. In *U.S.N.F.*

An ethyl ether of cellulose containing 44 to 51% of ethoxyl ($-OC_2H_5$) groups, calculated on the dried basis.

A free-flowing white to light tan powder. Its aqueous suspensions are neutral to litmus. Practically **insoluble** in water, glycerol, and propylene glycol. Ethylcellulose containing less than 46.5% of ethoxyl groups is freely soluble in chloroform, methyl acetate, and tetrahydrofuran, and in mixtures of aromatic hydrocarbons with alcohol; ethylcellulose containing not less than 46.5% of ethoxyl groups is freely soluble in alcohol, chloroform, ethyl acetate, methyl alcohol, and toluene. **Store** in well-closed containers.

Ethylcellulose is used as a binder in tablets and as a coating material for tablets, granules, and microcapsules. It is also used as a thickening agent.

Proprietary Names and Manufacturers
Aquacoat *(Honeywill & Stein, UK)*; Ethocel *(Merrell Dow, USA: K & K-Greeff, UK)*.

5429-j

Hydroxyethylcellulose *(BAN)*.

Hydroxyethyl Cellulose *(USAN)*.

CAS — 9004-62-0.

Pharmacopoeias. In *Br., Eur., Fr., Neth.,* and *Swiss.* Also in *U.S.N.F.*

A partially substituted 2-hydroxyethyl ether of cellulose. Various grades are available and are distinguished by appending a number indicative of the apparent viscosity of a 2% solution measured at 20°.

A white, yellowish-white, or greyish-white, practically odourless, hygroscopic powder or granules. **Soluble** in cold or hot water, forming colloidal solutions; practically insoluble in most organic solvents. A 1% solution in water has a pH of 5.5 to 8.5 (*B.P.*) or 6.0 to 8.5 (*U.S.P.*)

Store in well-closed containers.

Hydroxyethylcellulose is used as a thickener and stabiliser and is present in lubricant preparations, some of which are used in ocular disorders.

In a study assessing subject acceptance of various polymers as thickening agents for eye drops, hydroxyethylcellulose was reported to be the preferred polymer.— O. Dudinski *et al., Curr. ther. Res.,* 1983, *33,* 322.

A report on the use of sterile hydroxyethylcellulose gel (K-Y Lubricating Jelly) as the vehicle for extemporaneous preparation of dinoprostone vaginal gels.— L. J. Gauger (letter), *Am. J. Hosp. Pharm.*, 1984, *41*, 1761.

The use of hydroxyethylcellulose gel (K-Y Lubricating Jelly) in gonioscopy procedures.— H. K. Mehta, *Br. J. Ophthal.*, 1984, *68*, 765; L. Apt (letter), *ibid.*, *69*, 635.

Proprietary Names and Manufacturers

Cellobond HEC *(BP Chemicals, UK)*; Comfort Tears *(Barnes-Hind, USA)*; Gelaser *(Alcon, Switz.)*; K-Y Lubricating Jelly *(Johnson & Johnson, UK)*; Lyteers *(Barnes-Hind, USA)*; Natrosol *(Aqualon, UK)*; Neo-Tears *(Barnes-Hind, USA)*.

The following names have been used for multi-ingredient preparations containing hydroxyethylcellulose—Adsorbotear *(Alcon, Canad.; Alcon Laboratories, USA)*.

5430-q

Hydroxyethylmethylcellulose *(BAN)*.
HEMC; Hydroxyethyl Methylcellulose; Methylhydroxyethylcellulose.

CAS — 9032-42-2.

Pharmacopoeias. In *Br.*, *Eur.*, *Fr.*, *Neth.*, and *Swiss.*

A partially substituted ether of cellulose containing methoxyl and 2-hydroxyethyl groups. Various grades are available and are distinguished by appending a number indicative of the apparent viscosity of a 2% solution measured at 20°.

A white, yellowish-white, or greyish-white, practically odourless, hygroscopic powder or granules.

Practically **insoluble** in hot water, dehydrated alcohol, acetone, and ether; soluble in cold water forming a colloidal solution. A 1% solution has a pH of 5.5 to 8.0. **Store** in well-closed containers.

Hydroxyethylmethylcellulose is used similarly to the other cellulose derivatives as a pharmaceutical adjuvant.

5431-p

Hydroxypropylcellulose *(BAN)*.
E463; Hydroxypropyl Cellulose *(USAN)*.

CAS — 9004-64-2.

Pharmacopoeias. In *Br.*, *Eur.*, *Fr.*, *It.*, *Jpn*, *Neth.* and *Swiss.* Also in *U.S.N.F.* which specifies not more than 80.5% of hydroxypropoxy groups.

A partially substituted 2-hydroxypropyl ether of cellulose. Various grades are available and may be distinguished by appending a number indicative of the apparent viscosity of a 2% solution measured at 20°. The *U.S.N.F.* permits up to 0.6% of silica or other suitable anticaking agent.

A white or yellowish-white, practically odourless, hygroscopic granular solid or powder.

Soluble in cold water, alcohol, chloroform, and propylene glycol, forming colloidal solutions; practically insoluble in hot water. The *B.P.* also specifies soluble in methyl alcohol and that it dissolves in glacial acetic acid forming colloidal solutions; sparingly soluble or slightly soluble in acetone. A 1% solution in water has a pH of 5.0 to 8.5 (*B.P.*) or 5.0 to 8.0 (*U.S.N.F.*) **Store** in well-closed containers.

Adverse Effects

Hydroxypropylcellulose used as a solid ocular insert may result in blurred vision and ocular discomfort or irritation.

Uses and Administration

Hydroxypropylcellulose is used in the film coating of tablets, as a tablet excipient, as a thickener, and in microencapsulation. It is also used as a slow-release solid insert in the management of dry eye. Grades are available for use in the food industry.

Estimated acceptable daily intake: up to 25 mg per kg body-weight, as the sum of total modified celluloses. The figure may be exceeded for dietetic purposes.— Seventeenth Report of FAO/WHO Expert Committee on Food Additives, *Tech. Rep. Ser. Wld Hlth Org. No. 539*, 1974.

A slow-release artificial tear insert containing hydroxypropylcellulose was used in 11 patients with the practolol oculomucocutaneous syndrome. Two patients could not tolerate the inserts, 3 obtained greater cooling and soothing effect from instillation of their previous eye-drops, and one reported an increase in frequency of use of drops 1 week after starting to use the inserts. In the 5 patients who completed the study an objective and symptomatic improvement was noted and no serious adverse effects occurred.— P. Wright and R. Vogel, *Br. J. Ophthal.*, 1983, *67*, 393. For a reference to hydroxypropylcellulose being used in the preparation of adhesive mucosal forms of various drugs, see carbomer (p.1433).

Proprietary Names and Manufacturers

Klucel *(Aqualon, UK)*; Lacrisert *(Merck Sharp & Dohme, Canad.; Merck Sharp & Dohme, Denm.; Merck Sharp & Dohme, Norw.; MSD, Swed.; Merck Sharp & Dohme, USA)*.

5432-s

Hypromellose *(BAN, rINN)*.

E464; Hydroxypropyl Methylcellulose *(USAN)*; Hydroxypropylmethylcellulose; Methyl Hydroxypropyl Cellulose; Methylcellulose Propylene Glycol Ether; Methylhydroxypropylcellulose.

CAS — 8063-82-9; 9004-65-3.

Pharmacopoeias. In *Br.*, *Eur.*, *Fr.*, *It.*, *Jpn*, *Neth.*, *Swiss*, and *U.S.*

A mixed ether of cellulose containing a variable proportion of methoxyl and 2-hydroxypropoxyl groups. Several grades are available. In the *UK* these are distinguished by appending a number indicative of the apparent viscosity of a 2% solution measured at 20° (e.g. hypromellose 20, hypromellose 4500). In the *US* they are distinguished by appending a number in which the first 2 digits represent the approximate percentage composition of methoxyl groups, and the third and fourth digits the approximate percentage composition of hydroxypropoxyl groups. Hypromellose 1828, hypromellose 2208, hypromellose 2906, and hypromellose 2910 are described in the *U.S.P.*

A white, yellowish-white, or greyish-white, practically odourless, fibrous powder or granules.

Soluble in cold water, forming a colloidal solution; practically insoluble in hot water, dehydrated alcohol, chloroform, and ether. The *B.P.* also has practically insoluble in acetone. A 1% solution has a pH of 5.5 to 8.0. **Store** in well-closed containers.

5436-y

Hypromellose Phthalate *(BANM, rINNM)*.

Hydroxypropyl Methylcellulose Phthalate *(USAN)*; Methylhydroxypropylcellulose Phthalate.

Pharmacopoeias. In *Br.*, *Eur.*, *Fr.*, *Jpn*, *Neth.*, and *Swiss.* Also in *U.S.N.F.*

A cellulose with some of the hydroxyl groups in the form of the methyl ether, some in the form of the 2-hydroxypropyl ether, and some in the form of the phthalyl ester. Different grades in the *US* are distinguished by appending a number in which the first 2 digits represent the approximate percentage composition of the methoxyl groups, the next 2 digits the approximate percentage composition of hydroxypropoxyl groups, and the last 2 digits the approximate percentage composition of the phthalyl groups.

White to slightly off-white free-flowing flakes or a granular powder, odourless or with a slight acidic odour.

Practically **insoluble** in water and dehydrated alcohol, very slightly soluble in acetone, soluble in a mixture of equal volumes of acetone and methyl alcohol, and in a mixture of equal volumes of methyl alcohol and dichloromethane. **Store** in well-closed containers.

Hypromellose has properties similar to those of methylcellulose (p.1436). Since mucilages of hypromellose have greater clarity and fewer undispersed fibres are usually present, it is preferred to methylcellulose in the preparation of ophthalmic solutions; it prolongs the action of medicated eye-drops and is employed in alkaline eye-drops used as artificial tears to prevent damage to the cornea in patients with keratoconjunctivitis sicca or keratitis or during gonioscopy procedures. Hypromellose phthalate is used similarly. Hypromellose is also used to moisten hard contact lenses and to lubricate artificial eyes. Certain grades of hypromellose and hypromellose phthalate are used in the film-coating of tablets. Hypromellose is also used as a tablet binder.

Estimated acceptable daily intake: up to 25 mg per kg body-weight, as the sum of total modified celluloses. The figure may be exceeded for dietetic purposes.— Seventeenth Report of FAO/WHO Expert Committee on Food Additives, *Tech. Rep. Ser. Wld Hlth Org. No. 539*, 1974.

A solution of hypromellose, to the formula of Hypromellose Eye-drops and flavoured, was used as a rinse for dry mouth.— *Drug & Ther. Bull.*, 1975, *13*, 38. It is considered that the use of the eye-drops as a mouth-rinse intended to be swallowed is not desirable because of the unsuitability of the borax-boric acid buffer and the benzalkonium chloride for internal use.— Pharm. Soc. Lab. Rep. P/80/2, 1980.

Hypromellose in a physiological solvent was used to prevent damage to the corneal endothelium during implantation of an intra-ocular lens in over 400 operations. One drop of a hypromellose 1% solution was applied to the lens before insertion or alternatively the anterior chamber was filled with hypromellose 2% prior to implanting the lens. Hypromellose facilitated the operation and no ill-effects related to its use were seen.— P. U. Fechner and M. U. Fechner, *Br. J. Ophthal.*, 1983, *67*, 259.

In a study involving 24 patients with recurrent corneal erosions secondary to map-dot-fingerprint dystrophy, treatment with hypromellose eye-drops four times daily and simple eye ointment at night was more effective and accompanied by fewer complications than treatment with therapeutic contact lenses.— R. Williams and R. J. Buckley, *Br. J. Ophthal.*, 1985, *69*, 435.

SPERMICIDAL ACTIVITY. Aqueous solutions of hypromellose 1 to 3% caused immediate and permanent immobilisation of human spermatozoa *in vitro*. Neither storage for 2.5 years nor marked decreases in viscosity affected the potency of the hypromellose solutions.— K. Loewit, *Contraception*, 1977, *15*, 233.

Preparations

Artificial Saliva *(D.P.F.)*. Contains hypromellose '4500'. It may contain an antimicrobial preservative.

Hydroxypropyl Methylcellulose Ophthalmic Solution *(U.S.P.)*. A sterile solution of hypromellose. It may contain suitable antimicrobial, buffering, and stabilising agents. pH 6.0 to 7.8.

Hypromellose Eye Drops *(A.P.F.)*. Artificial-tears Solution. Hypromellose '4000/4500' 300 mg, sodium chloride 900 mg, benzalkonium chloride solution 0.02 mL, disodium edetate 50 mg, Water for Injections to 100 mL. Sterilised by autoclaving. Redisperse the hypromellose by shaking whilst cooling.

NOTE. The *A.P.F.* directs that when Methylcellulose Eye Drops are requested, Hypromellose Eye Drops should be supplied.

Hypromellose Eye-drops *(B.P.C. 1973)*. Alkaline Eye-drops; Artificial Tears; HPRM. Hypromellose '4000', '4500', or '5000' 300 mg, sodium chloride 450 mg, potassium chloride 370 mg, borax 190 mg, boric acid 190 mg, benzalkonium chloride solution 0.02 mL, water to 100 mL. Sterilise by autoclaving or maintaining at 98° to 100° for 30 minutes. Redisperse the coagulated hypromellose by shaking when cool. pH 8.4 to 8.6. When the solution is supplied for use in gonioscopy procedures, the concentration of hypromellose may be increased; a concentration of 0.7 to 1.5% may be suitable.

NOTE. The *B.P.C.1973* directs that when Methylcellulose Eye-drops are requested, Hypromellose Eye-drops should be supplied.

User comfort of Hypromellose Eye-drops was reported to be related to viscosity and it was suggested that the viscosity of the *B.P.C. 1973* preparation might be too low for optimum comfort since most patients preferred drops with a viscosity of 20 centistokes. Viscosity values for eye-drops using 0.3% hypromellose (the concentration in the *B.P.C. 1973* formulation) were 5.4 and 7.7 centistokes with the 4500 and 5000 grades respectively. Viscosity increased as the concentration of hypromellose increased and a concentration of 0.4 to 0.45% of hypromellose 5000 would produce eye-drops with a viscosity of 15 to 20 centistokes. However increasing the viscosity had been shown to reduce the activity of benzalkonium chloride and microbiological studies should be carried out.— Pharm. Soc. Lab. Rep. P/76/12, 1976.

Proprietary Preparations

BJ6 *(Macarthys, UK: Thornton & Ross, UK). Eye-drops*, hypromellose 0.25%.

Isopto Alkaline *(Alcon, UK). Eye-drops*, hypromellose 1%.

Isopto Plain *(Alcon, UK). Eye-drops*, hypromellose 0.5%.

Tears Naturale *(Alcon, UK). Eye-drops*, hypromellose 0.3%, dextran '70' 0.1%.

Proprietary Names and Manufacturers

BJ6 *(Macarthys, UK : Thornton & Ross, UK)*; Celacol HPM *(Courtaulds, UK)*; Gonak *(Akorn, USA)*; Goniosol *(Cooper, USA)*; Isopto Alkaline *(Alcon, UK)*; Isopto Plain *(Alcon, S.Afr.; Alcon, Swed.; Alcon, UK)*; Isopto Tears *(Alcon, Austral.; Belg.; Alcon, Canad.; Alcon, Switz.)*; Isopto-Alkaline *(S.Afr.)*; Isopto-Fluid *(Alcon, Ger.)*; Lacril *(Allergan, Austral.; Allergan, USA)*; Methocel *(Merrell Dow, USA : Colorcon, UK)*; Methopt *(Sigma, Austral.)*; Muro Tears *(Charton, Canad.; Bausch & Lomb, USA)*; Opti-Tears *(Alcon Laboratories, USA)*; Spersatear *(Restan, S.Afr.)*; Ultra Tears *(Alcon, Switz.)*; Viskose *(DAK, Denm.)*.

The following names have been used for multi-ingredient preparations containing hypromellose—Lubrifair Solution *(Pharmafair, USA)*; Murine *(Abbott, Austral.)*; Tears Naturale *(Alcon, Austral.; Alcon, Canad.; Alcon, UK; Alcon Laboratories, USA)*; Tears Renewed *(Akorn, USA)*.

NOTE. Preparations containing hypromellose as a pharmaceutical adjuvant are not included.

5441-w

Linseed *(BAN)*.

Flaxseed; Leinsamen; Lin; Linho; Lini Semina; Linum; Semen Lini; Semilla de Lino.

Pharmacopoeias. In *Aust., Belg., Br., Cz., Egypt., Eur., Fr., Ger., Hung., It., Neth., Nord., Pol., Port., Roum., Span.,* and *Swiss. Br.* also describes Powdered Linseed.

The dried ripe seeds of *Linum usitatissimum* (Linaceae). **Store** in well-closed containers. Protect from light.

Preparations of linseed have been administered for their demulcent action. Crushed linseed has been used as a poultice.

Linseed oil is described on p.1584.

5443-l

Magnesium Silicate *(USAN)*.

553(a) *(synthetic magnesium silicate)*.

CAS — 1343-88-0.

Pharmacopoeias. In *U.S.N.F.*

A compound of magnesium oxide and silicon dioxide. It is a fine white odourless powder free from grittiness. **Insoluble** in water, and in alcohol. It is readily decomposed by mineral acids. A 10% suspension in water has a pH of 7.0 to 10.8. **Store** in well-closed containers.

Magnesium silicate is used as an anticaking agent.

The temporary acceptable daily intake (ADI) of 'not specified' was extended for magnesium silicate. The Committee still awaited the results of short-term studies to determine whether the renal lesions reported with medicinal magnesium trisilicate might also be caused by ingestion of food-grade magnesium silicate Twenty-fourth Report of the FAO/WHO Expert Committee on Food Additives, *Tech. Rep. Ser. Wld Hlth Org. No. 653*, 1980.

Proprietary Names and Manufacturers

Bentone EW *(Steetley Berk, UK)*; Sepiolite *(Steetley Berk, UK)*.

5401-h

Methylcellulose *(BAN, USAN, rINN)*.

E461; Metilcelulosa.

CAS — 9004-67-5.

Pharmacopoeias. In *Arg., Aust., Br., Braz., Eur., Fr., Hung., It., Jpn, Jug., Neth., Roum., Span., Swiss,* and *U.S. Cz.* includes Methylcellulose 450. *U.S.* specifies 27.5 to 31.5% of methoxy groups.

A cellulose having some of the hydroxyl groups in the form of the methyl ether. It is a white, yellowish-white, or greyish-white, practically odourless, hygroscopic fibrous powder or granules.

B.P. **solubilities** are: practically insoluble in hot water, dehydrated alcohol, acetone, and ether; forms a colloidal solution in cold water. *U.S.P.* **solubilities** are: insoluble in alcohol, chloroform, and ether; soluble in glacial acetic acid and in a mixture of equal volumes of alcohol and chloroform; swells in water producing a clear to opalescent, viscous, colloidal suspension. A 1% solution in water has a pH of 5.5 to 8.0.

Incompatibilities have been reported with a number of compounds including chlorocresol, hydroxybenzoates, and phenol. Large amounts of electrolytes increase the viscosity of methylcellulose mucilages owing to salting-out of the methylcellulose; in very high concentrations of electrolytes, the methylcellulose may be completely precipitated.

Store in well-closed containers.

Various grades of methylcellulose are available and are distinguished by appending a number indicating the apparent viscosity of a 2% solution at 20°.

Adverse Effects

Large quantities of methylcellulose may temporarily increase flatulence and distension and there is a risk of intestinal obstruction. Oesophageal obstruction may occur if compounds like methylcellulose are swallowed dry.

Precautions

Methylcellulose and other bulk laxatives should not be given to patients with intestinal obstruction or conditions likely to lead to intestinal obstruction. They should be taken with sufficient fluid to prevent faecal impaction or oesophageal obstruction.

Bulk laxatives lower the transit time through the gut and could affect the absorption of other drugs.

Uses and Administration

Various grades of methylcellulose are used as emulsifying agents, as thickening agents for gels and creams, as dispersing and thickening agents in suspensions, as binding and disintegrating agents in tablets, and in tablet coating. A 0.5 to 1% solution of a high-viscosity grade has been used as a vehicle for eye-drops and as artificial tears and contact lens solution but hypromellose (see p.1435) is now generally preferred for this purpose.

Medium- or high-viscosity grades are used as bulk laxatives since by taking up moisture they increase the volume of the faeces and promote peristalsis. They are usually given in the form of granules or tablets, in a dosage of 1 to 6 g daily in divided doses taken with plenty of fluid. They are also given with a minimum amount of water, for the control of diarrhoea and in the management of ostomies and are also used in the management of diverticular disease and haemorrhoids. Methylcellulose has also been used to relieve hunger in the management of obesity but there is little evidence of efficacy. It has also been used as a sialogogue in the management of dry mouth.

Methylcellulose is employed in the food industry.

Estimated acceptable daily intake: up to 25 mg per kg body-weight, as the sum of total modified celluloses. The figure may be exceeded for dietetic purposes.—Seventeenth Report of FAO/WHO Expert Committee on Food Additives, *Tech. Rep. Ser. Wld Hlth Org. No. 539*, 1974.

Preparations

Methylcellulose Granules *(B.P.)*

Methylcellulose Mucilage *(A.P.F.)*. Mucil. Methylcellulos. Methylcellulose '20' 2, compound hydroxybenzoate solution 1, freshly boiled and cooled water to 100.

Methylcellulose Ophthalmic Solution *(U.S.P.)*. A sterile solution of methylcellulose. It may contain suitable antimicrobial, buffering, and stabilising agents.

Methylcellulose Oral Solution *(U.S.P.)*. A flavoured solution of methylcellulose, with alcohol 3.5 to 6.5%. Store at a temperature not exceeding 40° in airtight containers; avoid freezing. Protect from light.

Methylcellulose Tablets *(U.S.P.)*

Proprietary Preparations

Celevac *(Boehringer Ingelheim, UK). Tablets*, methylcellulose '450' 500 mg.
Granules, methylcellulose '450' 64%.

Cologel *(Lilly, UK). Liquid*, methylcellulose 9%.

Nilstim *(De Witt, UK). Tablets*, methylcellulose '2500' 400 mg, microcrystalline cellulose 220 mg.

Proprietary Names and Manufacturers

BFL *(Canad.)*; Celacol *(Courtaulds, UK)*; Celevac *(Boehringer Ingelheim, UK)*; Cellucon *(Medo, UK)*; Cellulone *(Comstock, Austral.)*; Citrucel *(Lakeside, USA)*; Cologel *(Lilly, UK)*; Lacril *(Allergan, Canad.)*; MC *(E-Z-EM, Canad.)*; Methocel A *(Merrell Dow, USA: Colorcon, UK)*; Murocel *(Charton, Canad.; Bausch & Lomb, USA)*; Viscosae *(Denm.)*.

The following names have been used for multi-ingredient preparations containing methylcellulose—Celluka *(Bio-Chemical Laboratory, Canad.)*; Merasyn *(Merrell Dow, Austral.)*; Nilstim *(De Witt, UK)*.

5447-c

Pectin *(USAN)*.

E440(a); E440(b) *(amidated pectin)*.

CAS — 9000-69-5.

Pharmacopoeias. In *Aust., Ind., Span.,* and *U.S.*

A purified carbohydrate product obtained from the dilute acid extract of the inner portion of the rind of citrus fruits or from apple pomace; it consists mainly of partially methoxylated polygalacturonic acids.

A coarse or fine, yellowish-white, almost odourless powder. Almost completely **soluble** 1 in 20 of water, forming a viscous, opalescent, colloidal solution which flows readily and is acid to litmus; practically insoluble in alcohol and other organic solvents. It dissolves more readily in water if first moistened with alcohol, glycerol, or syrup, or if mixed with 3 or more parts of sucrose. **Store** in airtight containers.

Apart from its commercial uses pectin has been given with kaolin in the treatment of diarrhoea but its value is doubtful.

It is used as a gelling agent in acid media. There has been considerable investigation on the possible effect of pectin on blood glucose and on blood lipids.

A group acceptable daily intake (ADI) of 'not specified' was established for pectins and amidated pectins. This means that on the basis of available data, the total daily intake of pectins or amidated pectins, singly or in combination, arising from use at the levels necessary to achieve the desired effect and from the acceptable background in food does not represent a hazard to health Twenty-fifth Report of the Joint FAO/WHO Expert Committee on Food Additives, *Tech. Rep. Ser. Wld Hlth Org. No. 669*, 1981.

Proprietary Names and Manufacturers

Sango-Stop *(Ger.)*; Ulcoseid *(Seid, Spain)*.

The following names have been used for multi-ingredient preparations containing pectin—ADM *(Wellcome, Austral.)*; Diaguard *(Nelson, Austral.)*; Diaguard Forte *(Nelson, Austral.)*; Diaguard Tablets *(Nelson, Austral.)*; Diarcalm *(McGloin, Austral.)*; Diareze *(Key, Austral.)*; Diban *(Robins, Canad.)*; Donnagel *(Robins, Austral.; Robins, Canad.)*; Donnagel with Neomycin *(Robins, Canad.; Robins, UK)*; Donnagel-MB *(Robins, Canad.)*; Donnagel-PG *(Robins, Canad.; Robins, USA)*; Glucomagma *(Drug Houses Austral., Austral.)*; Kao-Con *(Upjohn, Austral.; Upjohn, Canad.)*; Kaomagma with Pectin *(Wyeth, Austral.)*; Kaomycin *(Upjohn, Canad.)*; Kaopectate *(Upjohn, Austral.; Upjohn, Canad.)*; Maws KLN *(Ashe, UK)*; Parepectolin *(Rorer, USA)*; Pectokay *(Bowman, USA)*; Polymagma *(Wyeth, USA)*; Pomalin *(Winthrop, Canad.)*; Streptomagma *(Wyeth, Austral.)*.

5450-e

Povidone *(BAN, USAN)*.

Polyvidone *(pINN)*; Polyvidone-Excipient; Polyvidonum; Polyvinylpyrrolidone; PVP; Vinylpyrrolidinone Polymer.
$(C_6H_9NO)_n = 111.1 \times n$.

CAS — 9003-39-8.

Pharmacopoeias. In *Br., Cz., Fr., Hung., Ind., It., Roum.,* and *U.S.*
U.S.N.F. includes Crospovidone, a synthetic cross-linked homopolymer of povidone, that is insoluble in water and most organic solvents.

A mixture of essentially linear synthetic polymers of 1-vinylpyrrolidin-2-one of different chain lengths and molecular weights.
A fine white or very slightly cream-coloured, odourless or almost odourless, hygroscopic powder. **Soluble** in water, alcohol, and in chloroform; practically insoluble in ether. The *U.S.P.* specifies that a 5% solution in water has a pH of 3 to 7. The *B.P.* and *U.S.P.* state that the viscosity in aqueous solution, relative to water, is expressed as a K-value, ranging from 10 to 95 and that this K-value should be stated on the label.
Store in airtight containers.

Adverse Effects

Injection of povidone can lead to deposits in various tissues with consequent lesions and pain. There have been occasional reports of liver involvement.

A 54-year-old woman with diabetes insipidus received intramuscular injections of a depot preparation of posterior-pituitary lobe containing povidone for 13 years. During treatment abscesses and inflammatory reactions occurred at the site of injection with infiltrations and swellings developing in various muscle groups. Hepatomegaly and splenomegaly became predominant symptoms with pancytopenia and spontaneous fracture of several vertebrae also occurring.— J. M. Bert *et al., Sem. Hôp. Paris,* 1972, *48,* 1809.

A 54-year-old woman developed large foreign body granulomas in the breast and epigastric area after repeated injections of a depot preparation containing povidone, self-administered into the left breast. Povidone was identified in granulomatous tissue.— J. Gille and H. Brandau, *Geburtsh. Frauenheilk.,* 1975, *35,* 799.

Pseudotumours in the limbs of 2 patients contained foreign material which was probably associated with subcutaneous injections of a preparation containing procaine with povidone.— S. Soumerai, *J. med. Soc. New Jers.,* 1978, *75,* 407.

A report of periorbital swelling, necessitating plastic surgery, and rosacea in a patient associated with the repeated subcutaneous injection of a depot preparation containing povidone.— H. Mensing *et al., Z. Hautkrankheiten,* 1983, *59,* 1027.

Uses and Administration

Povidone is used as a suspending and dispersing agent and as a tablet binding, granulating, and coating agent. It is used as a carrier for iodine (see povidone-iodine, p.1187).
Povidone solutions may be used as artificial tears.
A grade of povidone suitable for parenteral administration has been used as a plasma expander but other compounds are now preferred.
An insoluble cross-linked form known as crospovidone is used as a tablet disintegrant.

Because of concern about the implications of accumulation of povidone in the cells of the reticuloendothelial system, the previous acceptable daily intake of up to 1 mg daily was withdrawn in the seventeenth report. Povidone was reconsidered in 2 further reports as well as in the current report in which a temporary acceptable daily intake of up to 25 mg per kg was set. Evidence was required from feeding studies in non-rodent species that the accumulation of povidone in cells of the reticuloendothelial system does not entail adverse effects. Studies with ^{14}C-labelled insoluble crospovidone showed almost complete lack of absorption. An acceptable daily intake "not specified" was allocated.— Twenty-seventh Report of the FAO/WHO Expert Committee on Food Additives, *Tech. Rep. Ser. Wld Hlth Org. No. 696,* 1983.

Proprietary Names and Manufacturers of Povidone and Crospovidone

Adsorbobase *(Alcon Laboratories, USA)*; Bolinan *(Hamilton, Austral.; Syntex, Fr.; Syntex, Switz.)*; Kollidon *(BASF, UK)*; Periston-N-Toxobin *(Ital.)*; Plasdone *(GAF, UK)*; Plasmoid *(Grifols, Spain)*; Plassint *(Ital.)*; Polyplasdone XL *(GAF, UK)*; Protagent *(Thilo, Ger.)*.

The following names have been used for multi-ingredient preparations containing povidone and crospovidone— Adsorbotear *(Alcon, Canad.; Alcon Laboratories, USA)*; Tears Plus *(Allergan, Canad.)*.

5451-l

Propylene Carbonate *(USAN)*.

4-Methyl-1,3-dioxolan-2-one.
$C_4H_6O_3 = 102.1$.

CAS — 108-32-7.

Pharmacopoeias. In *U.S.N.F.*

A clear colourless mobile liquid. Specific gravity 1.203 to 1.210. Freely **soluble** in water; miscible with alcohol and chloroform; practically insoluble in petroleum spirit. **Store** in airtight containers.

Propylene carbonate is used as a gelling agent.

5456-k

Purified Siliceous Earth *(USAN)*.

Diatomaceous Earth; Diatomite; Purified Infusorial Earth; Purified Kieselguhr; Terra Silicea Purificada.

Pharmacopoeias. In *U.S.N.F.*

An amorphous form of silicon dioxide consisting chiefly of frustules and fragments of diatoms purified by calcining.
A fine, white, light grey, or pale buff, gritty powder. Practically **insoluble** in water, acids, and in dilute solutions of alkali hydroxides. It absorbs about 4 times its weight of water without becoming fluid. **Store** in well-closed containers.

5455-c

Silicon Dioxide *(USAN)*.

Precipitated Silica; Silica Gel.
$SiO_2,xH_2O = 60.08$.

CAS — 63231-67-4; 7631-86-9.

Pharmacopoeias. In *U.S.N.F.*

The *U.S.N.F.* states that 'silicon dioxide is obtained by insolubilizing the dissolved silica in sodium silicate solution. Where obtained by the addition of sodium silicate to a mineral acid, the product is termed silica gel; where obtained by the destabilization of a solution of sodium silicate in such a manner as to yield very fine particles, the product is termed precipitated silica.'
A fine, white, odourless, hygroscopic, amorphous powder in which the diameter of the average particles ranges from 2 to 10 μm.
Practically **insoluble** in water, alcohol, and other organic solvents; soluble in hot solutions of alkali hydroxides. A 5% suspension in water has a pH of 4 to 8. **Store** in airtight containers.

5457-a

Colloidal Silicon Dioxide *(USAN)*.

Acidum Silicicum Colloidale; Colloidal Silica; Hochdisperses Silicumdioxid; Silice Precipitata.
$SiO_2 = 60.08$.

Pharmacopoeias. In *Aust., Br., Eur., Ger., Hung., It., Neth.,* and *Swiss.* Also in *U.S.N.F. Jpn* includes Light Anhydrous Silicic Acid.

A submicroscopic fumed silica, prepared by the vapour-phase hydrolysis of a silicon compound. It is a light, white, odourless, non-gritty powder; particle size about 15 nm.
Practically **insoluble** in water and acids, except hydrofluoric acid; soluble in hot solutions of alkali hydroxides. A 4% dispersion has a pH of 3.5 to 4.4. **Store** in well-closed containers.

Purified siliceous earth is used as a filtering medium and adsorbent. Silicon dioxide is used as a suspending agent and, as silica gel, as a desiccant.
Colloidal silicon dioxide is used as a suspending agent and thickener, as a stabiliser in emulsions, and as an anticaking agent and desiccant.
Silicon dioxide (Silicea) is used in homoeopathic medicine.
These forms of silica do not appear to be associated with silicosis; exposure limits have been set in Great Britain for amorphous and fused silica as well as natural diatomaceous earth.

The acceptable daily intake for man of silicon dioxide was only limited by good manufacturing practice.— Seventeenth Report of FAO/WHO Expert Committee on Food Additives, *Tech. Rep. Ser. Wld Hlth Org. No. 539,* 1974.

Proprietary Names and Manufacturers of Silica Preparations

Aerosil *(Degussa, UK)*; Dissolvurol *(Dissolvurol, Mon.)*; Entero-Teknosal *(Taco, Ger.)*; Sipernat *(Degussa, UK)*.

5458-t

Slippery Elm

Elm Bark; Slippery Elm Bark; Ulmus; Ulmus Fulva.

The dried inner bark of *Ulmus fulva* (=*U. rubra*) (Ulmaceae).

Slippery elm contains much mucilage and has been used as a demulcent.

5460-y

Sodium Starch Glycollate *(BAN)*.

Sodium Carboxymethyl Starch; Sodium Starch Glycolate *(USAN)*; Starch Sodium Glycollate.

CAS — 9063-38-1.

Pharmacopoeias. In *Br.* Also in *U.S.N.F.*

The sodium salt of a poly-α-glucopyranose in which some of the hydroxyl groups are in the form of the carboxymethyl ether.
A very fine, odourless, white or off-white, free-flowing powder. Practically **insoluble** in water and most organic solvents. A 2% **dispersion** in cold water settles, on standing, to give a highly hydrated layer. The *B.P.* specifies that a 2% dispersion in water has a pH of 5.5 to 7.5. The *U.S.N.F.* specifies that a 3.3% dispersion in water has a pH either between 3.0 and 5.0 or between 5.5 and 7.5. **Store** in well-closed containers. Protect from variations in temperature and humidity.

Sodium starch glycollate is used as a disintegrating agent in tablet manufacture.

Some references to sodium starch glycollate as a tablet disintegrant: E. Mendell, *Pharm. Acta Helv.,* 1974, *49,* 248; K. A. Khan and C. T. Rhodes, *J. pharm. Sci.,* 1975, *64,* 447; E. M. Rudnic *et al., Drug Dev. ind. Pharm.,* 1983, *9,* 303.

Some references to sodium starch glycollate being used as a suspending agent: C. A. Farley and W. Lund, *Pharm. J.,* 1976, *1,* 562; G. Smith and I. E. E. McIntosh (letter), *ibid.,* 1976, *2,* 42.

Proprietary Names and Manufacturers

Explotab *(Mendell, USA: Forum Chemicals, UK)*; Primojel *(Tunnel Avebe, UK)*.

5463-c

Tragacanth *(BAN, USAN)*.

E413; Goma Alcatira; Gomme Adragante; Gum Dragon; Gum Tragacanth; Trag.; Tragacantha; Tragacanto; Tragant.

CAS — 9000-65-1.

Pharmacopoeias. In *Arg., Aust., Belg., Br., Cz., Egypt., Eur., Fr., Ger., Hung., Ind., It., Jpn, Jug., Mex., Neth., Nord., Pol., Port., Roum., Span., Swiss,* and *Turk.* Also in *U.S.N.F.*

The dried gummy exudation flowing naturally or obtained by incision from the trunk and branches of *Astragalus gummifer* and some other Asiatic species of *Astragalus* (Leguminosae).

It occurs as thin, flattened, more or less curved, ribbon-like, white or pale yellow, somewhat translucent, horny odourless flakes. **Powdered Tragacanth**, which is specified in the *B.P.* and *U.S.N.F.*, is a white or yellowish-white odourless powder.

It forms a mucilaginous gel with a small amount of water. The *U.S.N.F.* identification is to add 1 g to 50 mL of water; it swells and forms a smooth, nearly uniform, stiff, opalescent mucilage, free from cellular fragments. **Store** in well-closed containers.

Adverse Effects

Allergic reactions, sometimes severe, have occurred rarely after the administration of tragacanth. Contact dermatitis has been reported following the external use of tragacanth.

Contact dermatitis in a 4-year-old boy, at the sites of ECG electrodes, was due to tragacanth in the electrode jelly.— R. J. Coskey, *Archs Derm.*, 1977, *113*, 839.

Three renal transplant recipients found to be hypersensitive to prednisone tablets had reacted to the tragacanth and acacia used in their manufacture. Their symptoms subsided when a formulation using methylcellulose was substituted.— D. Rubinger *et al.* (letter), *Lancet*, 1978, *2*, 689.

An immediate life-threatening allergic reaction in a 35-year-old woman was attributed to the tragacanth which was present in the beefburger she was eating.— D. Danoff *et al.* (letter), *New Engl. J. Med.*, 1978, *298*, 1095.

Uses and Administration

Tragacanth forms viscous solutions or gels with water, depending on the concentration. In dispensing aqueous preparations of tragacanth, the powdered tragacanth is first dispersed in a distributing agent, such as alcohol, to prevent agglomeration on the addition of water.

Tragacanth, in the form of Tragacanth Mucilage or Compound Tragacanth Powder, is widely used as a suspending agent. It is also used as an emulsifying agent and has been used in lozenges for its demulcent properties. It has long been used in the food industry.

The Expert Committee had reviewed tragacanth many times in the past but had not been able to establish an acceptable daily intake (ADI) because of insufficient toxicological data. However, in considering all the available information the Committee at this review established an ADI 'not specified'. This meant that on the basis of available data the total daily intake of tragacanth, arising from its use at the levels necessary to achieve the desired effect and from its acceptable background in food, does not represent a hazard to health. The establishment of an ADI in numerical form was not deemed necessary.— Twenty-ninth Report of the Joint FAO/WHO Expert Committee on Food Additives, *Tech. Rep. Ser. Wld Hlth Org. No. 723* 1986.

For the effect of tragacanth on postprandial blood-glucose concentrations, see D. J. A. Jenkins, *Br. med. J.*, 1978, *1*, 1392.

Preparations

Hydroxybenzoate Gel *(A.P.F.)*. Catheter Lubricant; Surgical Lubricant. Propyl hydroxybenzoate 30 mg, methyl hydroxybenzoate 70 mg, tragacanth 3 g, glycerol 25 mL, water to 100 g. Sterilised by autoclaving.

Phenylmercuric Nitrate Gel *(A.P.F.)*. Phenylmercuric Nitrate Glycanth. Phenylmercuric nitrate 10 mg, tragacanth 2.5 g, glycerol 25 mL, water to 100 g. Sterilised by maintaining at 98° to 100° for 30 minutes.

Tragacanth Mucilage *(A.P.F.)*. Tragacanth 1.25, alcohol (90%) 2.0, benzoic acid solution 2.0, compound hydroxybenzoate solution 1.0, purified water to 100.

Tragacanth Mucilage *(B.P.C. 1973)*. Tragacanth 1.25 g, alcohol (90%) 2.5 mL, chloroform water to 100 mL.

Tragacanth Powder Compound *(A.P.F.)*. Tragacanth 15, acacia 20, starch 20, and sucrose 45.

5465-a

Xanthan Gum *(USAN)*.

Corn Sugar Gum; E415; Polysaccharide B 1459; Xantham Gum.

CAS — 11138-66-2.

Pharmacopoeias. In *U.S.N.F.*

A gum produced by a pure-culture fermentation of a carbohydrate with *Xanthomonas campestris* and purified. It is the sodium, potassium, or calcium salt of a high molecular weight polysaccharide containing D-glucose, D-mannose, and D-glucuronic acid. It also contains not less than 1.5% of pyruvic acid.

A cream-coloured powder. **Soluble** in hot and cold water. A solution in water is neutral to litmus.

Incompatibilites with xanthan gum: C. V. Walker and J. I. Wells, *Int. J. Pharmaceut.*, 1982, *11*, 309 (carmellose sodium); J. L. Zatz *et al.*, *Drug Dev. ind. Pharm.*, 1986, *12*, 561 (dried aluminium hydroxide gel); G. Bumphrey, *Pharm. J.*, 1986, *2*, 665 (amitriptyline, tamoxifen, and verapamil); B. K. Evans and V. Fenton-May, *ibid.*, 736 (film-coated tablets).

Xanthan gum is used as a stabiliser, thickener, and emulsifier. It is also used in the food industry.

Estimated acceptable daily intake of xanthan gum: up to 10 mg per kg body-weight.— Twenty-ninth Report of the Joint FAO/WHO Expert Committee on Food Additives, *Tech. Rep. Ser. Wld Hlth Org. No. 733*, 1986.

DIABETES MELLITUS. The addition of xanthan gum 12 g daily, in the form of xanthan-containing muffins, to the diet of 9 recently diagnosed type 2 diabetics significantly lowered fasting serum-glucose concentrations within 3 weeks, with a further lowering in the second 3-week period. Postload serum-glucose concentrations were also lowered by prior feeding of xanthan gum.— O. Osilesi *et al.*, *Am. J. clin. Nutr.*, 1985, *42*, 597.

SUSPENDING AGENT. Suspensions of crushed tablets or insoluble powders made with xanthan gum were reported to be preferable to those made with tragacanth (G. Bumphrey, *Pharm.J.*, 1986, *2*, 665). The stability was generally good and only a small number of drugs had been found to be incompatible (amitriptyline, tamoxifen, and verapamil). The most commonly used suspensions were allopurinol 50 mg in 5 mL, diazepam 5 mg in 5 mL, and spironolactone 5 mg in 5 mL and these were stable for 12 weeks at room temperature, and were now prepared in batches. For extemporaneous dispensing, a 1% solution of xanthan gum with hydroxybenzoate, prepared in advance, was diluted to 0.5% with water when preparing the suspension.

Evans and Fenton-May (*ibid.*, 736) supported Bumphrey's report. They had also found xanthan gum to be a suitable suspending vehicle for delivering antispasmodics topically along the length of the oesophagus in patients with oesophageal spasm. Coagulation of the gum had been observed when it was used for suspensions of certain film-coated tablets.

Proprietary Names and Manufacturers

A6B569 *(Kelco International, UK)*; Keltrol *(Kelco International, UK)*; Kelzan *(Kelco International, UK)*.

Stimulants and Anorectics

1410-k

This section includes compounds used for their central stimulant, anorectic, or respiratory stimulant effects.
The use of central stimulants is now generally limited to narcolepsy and as an adjunct in the management of some hyperkinetic states in children. Their use for other indications has been discouraged, especially as these compounds are subject to abuse.
Strychnine is also included in this section, mainly because of its toxic central stimulant activity. Nux vomica is a source of strychnine, hence its inclusion in this section despite its use as a bitter to stimulate appetite.
Anorectic agents suppress appetite or the sensation of hunger. They have been used to increase weight loss in obese patients but their efficacy is limited and their central stimulant effects have been a problem. Anorectics, if used, are indicated only as an adjunct to dietary control in the short-term management of moderate to severe obesity and require close medical supervision.
Most respiratory stimulants have little use nowadays and can cause central stimulation in high doses.

12342-f

Almitrine Dimesylate *(BANM).*
Almitrine Dimesilate *(rINNM)*; S-2620 (almitrine).
NN'-Diallyl-6-[4-(4,4'-difluorobenzhydryl)piperazin-1-yl]-1,3,5-triazine-2,4-diyldiamine bis(methanesulphonate).
$C_{26}H_{29}F_2N_7,2CH_4SO_3=669.8$.

CAS — 27469-53-0 (almitrine).

Almitrine dimesylate is given by mouth as a respiratory stimulant in conditions such as chronic obstructive pulmonary disorders. Usual doses range from 50 to 100 mg daily and treatment may be intermittent. Higher doses have been given by injection. Almitrine dimesylate appears not to cause adverse central effects. There have been reports of peripheral neuropathy in patients taking almitrine dimesylate, although it has been pointed out that neuropathy is also associated with chronic obstructive pulmonary disorders.
It has also been given with raubasine.

Some case reports and discussions of peripheral neuropathy associated with almitrine dimesylate: F. Chedru *et al., Br. med. J.,* 1985, *290,* 896; R. Gherardi *et al., Lancet,* 1985, *1,* 1247; A. J. Suggett *et al.* (letter), *ibid., 2,* 830; F. Louarn and R. Gherardi (letter), *ibid.,* 1068; S. M. Alani *et al.* (letter), *ibid.,* 1251; N. Moore *et al.* (letter), *ibid.,* 1311.

Some references to almitrine dimesylate in the treatment of chronic obstructive pulmonary disorders: G. Huchon, *Postgrad. med. J.,* 1983, *59, Suppl.* 3, 66; R. C. Bell *et al., Ann. intern. Med.,* 1986, *105,* 342.

Proprietary Names and Manufacturers
Vectarion *(Eutherapie, Fr.; Itherapia, Ger.).*

The following names have been used for multi-ingredient preparations containing almitrine dimesylate— Duxil *(Servier, Fr.).*

12365-g

Aminorex *(BAN, USAN, rINN).*
Aminoxaphen; McN-742. 2-Amino-5-phenyl-2-oxazoline.
$C_9H_{10}N_2O=162.2$.

CAS — 2207-50-3.

Aminorex was used as an anorectic agent but was withdrawn because of its association with pulmonary hypertension which sometimes proved fatal.

1411-a

Amiphenazole Hydrochloride *(BANM, rINNM).*
Amiphenazole Chloride. 5-Phenylthiazole-2,4-diamine hydrochloride.
$C_9H_9N_3S,HCl=227.7$.

CAS — 490-55-1 (amiphenazole); 942-31-4 (hydrochloride).

Amiphenazole has similar actions to doxapram hydrochloride (p.1442) and was used as a respiratory stimulant in usual doses of 30 to 150 mg intramuscularly or intravenously.
Lichenoid reactions have been reported in addition to those reactions expected from its central activity.

Proprietary Names and Manufacturers
Daptazile *(Nicholas, Ger.)*; Daptazole *(Nicholas, Neth.; Nicholas, Switz.; Nicholas, UK).*

1412-t

Amphetamine
Amfetamine *(rINN)*; Anfetamina; Racemic Desoxynorephedrine.
$C_9H_{13}N=135.2$.

CAS — 300-62-9 (amphetamine); 139-10-6 (phosphate).

Pharmacopoeias. In *Arg., Belg., Braz.,* and *Turk. Hung.* specifies the phosphate.

A colourless, mobile, slowly volatile liquid with a slight characteristic odour of geranium leaves and an acrid taste.

1414-r

Amphetamine Sulphate *(BAN).*
Amfetamine Sulphate *(rINNM)*; Amphetamine Sulfate *(USAN)*; Amphetamini Sulfas; Phenaminum; Phenylaminopropanum Racemicum Sulfuricum. (±)-α-Methylphenethylamine sulphate.
$(C_9H_{13}N)_2,H_2SO_4=368.5$.

CAS — 60-13-9.

Pharmacopoeias. In *Arg., Aust., Belg., Br., Cz., Egypt., Eur., Fr., Ger., Int., It., Jug., Mex., Neth., Nord., Pol., Port., Roum., Rus., Span., Swiss, Turk.,* and *U.S.*

A white odourless crystalline powder. **Soluble** 1 in 9 of water; slightly soluble in alcohol; practically insoluble in ether. A solution in water has a pH of 5.0 to 6.0.

Amphetamine is an indirect-acting sympathomimetic agent with actions and uses similar to those of its isomer dexamphetamine (see p.1440); it has less central stimulant activity than dexamphetamine and more pronounced peripheral effects. Amphetamine sulphate is given by mouth in doses similar to those of dexamphetamine sulphate. The laevo isomer, levamphetamine was formerly used in a similar manner. Amphetamine, being volatile, was formerly employed by inhalation. Amphetamine has also been used as the aspartate and phosphate.

Preparations
Amphetamine Sulfate Tablets *(U.S.P.)*

Proprietary Names and Manufacturers of Amphetamine and its Salts
Amfetamin *(DAK, Denm.; NAF, Norw.)*; Benzedrine *(Smith Kline & French, USA)*; Centramina *(Miquel, Spain)*; Perduretas Anfetamina *(Medea, Spain)*; Simpatina *(Spain).*

The following names have been used for multi-ingredient preparations containing amphetamine and its salts— Biphetamine *(Pennwalt, USA)*; Durophet *(Riker, UK)*; Durophet-M *(Riker, UK)*; Obetrol *(Rexar, USA).*

1415-f

Amphetaminil
Amfetaminil *(rINN).* α-(α-Methylphenethylamino)-α-phenylacetonitrile.
$C_{17}H_{18}N_2=250.3$.

CAS — 17590-01-1.

Amphetaminil is given by mouth as a stimulant of the central nervous system.

Proprietary Names and Manufacturers
AN 1 *(Voigt, Ger.).*

1416-d

Bemegride *(BAN, rINN).*
Bemegridum. 3-Ethyl-3-methylglutarimide; 4-Ethyl-4-methylpiperidine-2,6-dione.
$C_8H_{13}NO_2=155.2$.

CAS — 64-65-3.

Pharmacopoeias. In *Int.* and *Rus.*

Bemegride has similar actions to doxapram hydrochloride (p.1442). It was formerly given intravenously as a respiratory stimulant in doses of up to 50 mg.

Bemegride was considered to be unsafe in patients with acute porphyria as it has been associated with acute attacks.— M.R. Moore and K.E.L. McColl, *Porphyrias, Drug Lists,* Glasgow, Porphyria Research Unit, University of Glasgow, 1987.

Proprietary Names and Manufacturers
Bemegrin *(Montedison, Arg.)*; Eukraton *(Nordmark, Ger.)*; Megimide *(Adcock Ingram, S.Afr.; Inibsa, Spain; Nicholas, UK).*

1471-q

Benzphetamine Hydrochloride *(BANM).*
Benzfetamine Hydrochloride *(rINNM).* (+)-*N*-Benzyl-*N*α-dimethylphenethylamine hydrochloride.
$C_{17}H_{21}N,HCl=275.8$.

CAS — 156-08-1 (benzphetamine); 5411-22-3 (hydrochloride).

Benzphetamine hydrochloride is a sympathomimetic agent with the actions of dexamphetamine (p.1440). It is used as an anorectic and is administered by mouth as an adjunct to dietary measures in the short-term treatment of moderate to severe obesity. The usual initial dose is 25 to 50 mg once daily, subsequently adjusted, according to requirements, to a dose of 25 to 50 mg once to three times daily.
Diabetic control should be monitored in patients given drugs such as benzphetamine hydrochloride for the control of obesity.

Proprietary Names and Manufacturers
Didrex *(Upjohn, UK; Upjohn, USA)*; Inapétyl *(Upjohn, Fr.).*

1472-p

Chlorphentermine Hydrochloride *(BANM, USAN, rINNM).*
S-62. 4-Chloro-αα-dimethylphenethylamine hydrochloride.
$C_{10}H_{14}ClN,HCl=220.1$.

CAS — 461-78-9 (chlorphentermine); 151-06-4 (hydrochloride).

Pharmacopoeias. In *Fr.*

Chlorphentermine hydrochloride is a sympathomimetic agent that has been used as an anorectic. It has similar actions to dexamphetamine (p.1440). It has been implicated in lipid storage disorders and pulmonary hypertension. Diabetic control should be monitored if used in the control of obesity.
Chlorphentermine has a long half-life; chlorphentermine hydrochloride was given in doses equivalent to 65 mg of chlorphentermine once daily.

Proprietary Names and Manufacturers
Apsedon *(Lensa, Spain)*; Desopimon *(EGIS, Hung.)*; Lucofen SA *(Warner, UK)*; Pre-Sate *(Warner, Austral.; Parke, Davis, Canad.; Warner, S.Afr.; Parke, Davis, USA).*

1473-s

Clobenzorex Hydrochloride *(rINNM).*
SD-271-12. (+)-*N*-(2-Chlorobenzyl)-α-methylphenethylamine hydrochloride.
$C_{16}H_{18}ClN,HCl = 296.2$.

CAS — 13364-32-4 (clobenzorex); 5843-53-8 (hydrochloride).

Clobenzorex hydrochloride is a sympathomimetic agent with the actions of dexamphetamine (below). It is used as an anorectic and is given by mouth as an adjunct to dietary measures in the short-term treatment of moderate to severe obesity. Usual doses consist of 30 mg twice daily before meals. Diabetic control should be monitored when clobenzorex is used in the control of obesity.

Proprietary Names and Manufacturers
Dinintel *(Diamant, Fr.)*; Finedal *(Llorente, Spain)*; Rexigen *(Bago, Arg.)*.

12587-x

Cloforex *(rINN).*
D-237. Ethyl (*p*-chloro-α,α-dimethylphenethyl)carbamate.
$C_{13}H_{18}ClNO_2 = 255.7$.

CAS — 14261-75-7.

Cloforex is an anorectic used as an adjunct to dietary measures in the short-term treatment of moderate to severe obesity. As with other anorectics diabetic control will need to be monitored.

Proprietary Names and Manufacturers
Lipociden *(Lesvi, Spain)*.

1474-w

Clortermine Hydrochloride *(USAN, rINNM).*
Su-10568. 2-Chloro-αα-dimethylphenethylamine hydrochloride.
$C_{10}H_{14}ClN,HCl = 220.1$.

CAS — 10389-73-8 (clortermine); 10389-72-7 (hydrochloride).

Clortermine hydrochloride, the ortho isomer of chlorphentermine hydrochloride, is a sympathomimetic agent with the actions of dexamphetamine (below) that has been used as an anorectic. It has been given in single daily doses of 50 mg by mouth as an adjunct to dietary measures in the short-term treatment of moderate to severe obesity.

Diabetic control should be monitored in patients given drugs such as clortermine hydrochloride for the control of obesity.

Proprietary Names and Manufacturers
Voranil *(USV Pharmaceutical Corp., USA)*.

12624-s

Deanol *(BAN).*
Démanol. 2-Dimethylaminoethanol.
$C_4H_{11}NO = 89.14$.

CAS — 108-01-0; 3342-61-8 (aceglumate); 968-46-7 (benzilate); 71-79-4 (benzilate hydrochloride).

NOTE. Deanol Aceglumate is pINN.

Deanol, a precursor of choline, may enhance central acetylcholine formation. It has been employed as a central stimulant and in the treatment of hyperactivity in children but its efficacy has not been substantiated. It has been tried in the treatment of dyskinesias and Alzheimer's disease.

It has been used as a variety of salts and esters including deanol aceglumate, deanol acetamidobenzoate, deanol cyclohexylpropionate (cyprodenate; cyprodemanol), deanol hemisuccinate, deanol phosphate, and deanol hydrogen tartrate. Deanol benzilate (deanol diphenylglycolate; benzacine) has been used to relieve the symptoms of rhinitis and as an antispasmodic.

Proprietary Names and Manufacturers of Deanol Esters and Salts
Actébral *(Laboratoires Biologiques de l'Île-de-France, Fr.; Boizot, Spain)*; Arinol *(Ital.)*; Asaletten *(Thilo, Ger.)*; Betoxin *(Nessa, Spain)*; Cervoxan *(SMB, Belg.)*; Clérégil *(Merck-Clévenot, Fr.; Merck-Clévenot, Switz.)*; Deaner *(Riker, Arg.; Riker, Austral.; Riker, Canad.; Riker, USA)*; Diforène *(Choay, Fr.)*; Endocaina *(Lafage, Arg.)*; Labotropin *(Labopharma, Ger.)*; Pabenol *(Gentili, Ital.)*; Panclar *(Astra, Arg.; Astra, Fr.; Made, Spain)*; Plenium *(Millet, Arg.)*; Risatarun *(Ravensberg, Ger.)*; Rischiaril *(Piam, Ital.)*; Tonibral *(Sobio, Fr.)*.

1419-m

Dexamphetamine Sulphate *(BANM).*

Dexamfetamine Sulphate *(pINNM)*; Dexamphetamini Sulfas; Dextro Amphetamine Sulphate; Dextroamphetamine Sulfate *(USAN)*. (*S*)-α-Methylphenethylammonium sulphate; (+)-α-Methylphenethylamine sulphate.
$(C_9H_{13}N)_2,H_2SO_4 = 368.5$.

CAS — 51-64-9 (dexamphetamine); 7528-00-9 (phosphate); 51-63-8 (sulphate).

Pharmacopoeias. In *Br., Fr., Int., Swiss,* and *U.S.*

A white or almost white, odourless or almost odourless, crystalline powder. **Soluble** 1 in 9 or 10 of water and 1 in 800 of alcohol; practically insoluble in ether. A 5% solution in water has a pH of 5.0 to 6.0. **Store** in well-closed containers.

Adverse Effects

The side-effects of dexamphetamine are commonly symptoms of overstimulation of the central nervous system and include insomnia, nervousness, restlessness, irritability, and euphoria that may be followed by fatigue and depression. There may be dryness of the mouth, anorexia, abdominal cramps and other gastro-intestinal disturbances, headache, dizziness, tremor, sweating, tachycardia, palpitations, increased blood pressure, difficulty in micturition, altered libido, and impotence. Psychotic reactions have occurred as has muscle damage with associated renal complications.

In acute overdosage, the adverse effects are accentuated and may be accompanied by hyperpyrexia, mydriasis, hyperreflexia, chest pain, cardiac arrhythmias, confusion, panic states, aggressive behaviour, hallucinations, delirium, convulsions, respiratory depression, coma, circulatory collapse, and death.

Individual patient response may vary widely and toxic manifestations may occur at relatively low doses.

Dependence. Tolerance can develop to some of dexamphetamine's central effects leading to increased doses and habituation. Abrupt cessation after prolonged treatment or abuse of amphetamines has been associated with fatigue, hyperphagia, and depression. However, it is generally accepted that the amphetamines are not associated with significant physical dependence.

Amphetamines are widely abused for their euphoriant effects and their use and distribution has been controlled by legislation in many countries. Abuse of amphetamines has resulted in bruxism, personality changes, compulsive and stereotyped behaviour, and may induce a toxic psychosis with auditory and visual hallucinations and paranoid delusions.

CARCINOGENICITY. Findings from an evaluation of the relationship of amphetamine exposure with malignant lymphoma by the Boston Collaborative Drug Surveillance Program did not lend support to the suggestion by Newell *et al.* (*J. natn. Cancer Inst.*, 1973, *51*, 1437) that amphetamine use was associated with increased risk of Hodgkin's disease.— *J. Am. med. Ass.*, 1974, *229*, 1462.

EFFECTS ON THE ENDOCRINE SYSTEM. Increased serum concentrations of thyroxine were associated with heavy amphetamine abuse in 4 psychiatric patients.— J. E. Morley *et al.*, *Ann. intern. Med.*, 1980, *93*, 707.

EFFECTS ON GROWTH. The Pediatric Subcommittee of the FDA Psychopharmacologic Drugs Advisory Committee reviewed the growth-suppressing effects of stimulant medication in hyperkinetic children. There was reasonable evidence that stimulant drugs, particularly in higher doses, moderately suppressed growth in weight and might have a minor suppressing effect on growth in stature. There were indications that some growth caught up during drug holidays, and that early growth suppression was not evident in adulthood. As most of the studies were in small groups of prepubescent children, the effects of treatment during pubescence and early adolescence were unknown and the risk of greater effects in a few children was unclear. Careful monitoring during treatment was recommended.— A. F. Roche *et al.*, *Pediatrics*, 1979, *63*, 847.

See also under Methylphenidate Hydrochloride, p.1445.

EFFECTS ON THE HEART. Reports of cardiomyopathy associated with dexamphetamine: H. J. Smith *et al.*, *Am. Heart J.*, 1976, *91*, 792 (prolonged intake of high doses of dexamphetamine); T. D. Call *et al.*, *Ann. intern. Med.*, 1982, *97*, 559 (intravenous amphetamine abuse).

EFFECTS ON MENTAL STATE. A review of the mechanisms underlying altered behaviour following administration of psychomotor stimulants such as cocaine and the amphetamines. Chronic use may result in adverse effects such as hallucinations, a delusional disorder resembling paranoid schizophrenia, stereotyped behaviour, and movement disorders. Although chronic intoxication was the most common precondition for psychosis, individual sensitivities were an important aspect of the drug reaction.— E. H. Ellinwood and M. M. Kilbey, *Biol. Psychiat.*, 1980, *15*, 749.

EFFECTS ON MUSCLE AND KIDNEY. Abuse of methylamphetamine intravenously has been associated with necrotizing angiitis by Citron *et al.* (*New Engl. J. Med.*, 1970, *283*, 1003). In addition, Kendrick *et al.* (*Ann. intern. Med.*, 1977, *86*, 381) described a syndrome characterised by circulatory collapse, fever, leukaemoid reaction, disseminated intravascular coagulation, and rhabdomyolysis with diffuse myalgias and muscle tenderness in 5 drug abusers who had administered amphetamines including phenmetrazine intravenously. Scandling and Spital (*Sth. med. J.*, 1982, *75*, 237) reported a 30-year-old man who had ingested 50 amphetamine sulphate tablets and developed rhabdomyolysis and myoglobinuric renal failure possibly secondary to a crush syndrome but in the absence of prolonged coma or other major myotoxic factors. In contrast, Foley *et al.* (*Sth. med. J.*, 1984, *77*, 258) reported a patient who developed acute interstitial nephritis and acute renal failure after oral amphetamine abuse without the associated factors of rhabdomyolysis, hyperpyrexia, or necrotizing angiitis.

EFFECTS ON THE NERVOUS SYSTEM. In a review of clinical reports, Shapiro and Shapiro (*Compreh. Psychiat.*, 1981, *22*, 265) concluded that there was virtually no evidence that central stimulants caused or provoked Tourette's syndrome and weak or inadequate evidence that clinically appropriate doses of central stimulants caused tics in previously asymptomatic patients or exacerbated pre-existing symptoms. However, they suggested that there was evidence that high or toxic doses might exacerbate or provoke tics in predisposed patients. However, Lowe *et al.* (*J. Am. med. Ass.*, 1982, *247*, 1729) reported on 15 children who developed Gilles de la Tourette's syndrome while receiving stimulant medication for attention deficit disorders; 13 of these children had either pre-existing tics or a family history of tics or of Tourette's syndrome. They considered that stimulant therapy for hyperactivity was contra-indicated in children with motor tics or diagnosed Tourette's syndrome and should be used with caution in children with a family history of these symptoms. In addition, they suggested that the development of motor tic symptoms in any child receiving stimulants should be a clear indication for immediate discontinuation to minimise the possibility of eliciting a full-blown Tourette's syndrome.

Cerebral haemorrhage. Reports of intracerebral haemorrhage associated with the use of amphetamines.— P. Delaney and M. Estes, *Neurology*, 1980, *30*, 1125; H. Harrington *et al.*, *Archs Neurol., Chicago*, 1983, *40*, 503; V. Salanova and R. Taubner, *Postgrad. med. J.*, 1984, *60*, 429.

PREGNANCY AND THE NEONATE. In a retrospective study by Nelson and Forfar (*Br. med. J.*, 1971, *1*, 523), dexamphetamine prescribed to mothers during pregnancy appeared to be associated with the occurrence of congenital abnormalities. In contrast, Milkovich and van den Berg (*Am. J. Obstet. Gynec.*, 1977, *129*, 637) found no difference in the incidence of severe congenital anomalies between 1 824 children of mothers prescribed amphetamines or phenmetrazine during pregnancy and 8 989 children of mothers who had not received these drugs. Though an excess of oral clefts was noted in the offspring of mothers prescribed amphetamines, there was no excess of congenital heart disease as previously suggested (J.J. Nora *et al.*, *Lancet*, 1970, *1*, 1290). Milkovich and van den Berg concluded that uncertainty still existed about the safe use of amphetamines and their congeners in pregnancy.

Treatment of Adverse Effects

In general the management of overdosage with amphetamines involves supportive and symptomatic therapy. Sedation is usually sufficient. Forced acid diuresis has been advocated to increase amphetamine excretion but should only be considered in severely poisoned patients and requires close supervision and monitoring.

Precautions

Dexamphetamine is contra-indicated in patients with cardiovascular disease including moderate to severe hypertension, hyperthyroidism, glaucoma, extrapyramidal disorders, hyperexcitability, or agitated states. It should be given with caution to patients with anorexia, insomnia, impaired kidney function, unstable personality, or a history of drug abuse. Height and weight in children should be monitored. Prolonged high doses may need gradual withdrawal as abrupt cessation may produce fatigue and mental depression. Central stimulants are likely to reduce the convulsive threshold. Caution is therefore advised when using them in patients with epilepsy.

Dexamphetamine is an indirect-acting sympathomimetic and may interact with a number of other drugs. It should not be given to patients being treated with a monoamine oxidase inhibitor or within 14 days of stopping such treatment. Dexamphetamine may also diminish the effects of guanethidine and similar antihypertensive agents and concurrent use should be avoided. The urinary excretion of amphetamines is reduced by urinary alkalinisers which may enhance or prolong their effects; excretion is increased by urinary acidifiers.

For precautions in Gilles de la Tourette's syndrome, see Effects on the nervous system, above.

INTERACTIONS. A review of laboratory data indicating the potential drug interactions of amphetamines.— E. H. Ellinwood *et al.*, *Ann. N.Y. Acad. Sci.*, 1976, *281*, 393.

Experience with 3 patients suggested that the effects of amphetamines were antagonised by lithium carbonate.— A. Flemenbaum, *Am. J. Psychiat.*, 1974, *131*, 820. Lithium and α-methyltyrosine may antagonise the euphoria and activation induced by amphetamines.— W. E. Bunney *et al.*, *Ann. intern. Med.*, 1977, *87*, 319.

PORPHYRIA. Amphetamines were considered to be unsafe in patients with acute porphyria although there is conflicting experimental evidence on porphyrinogenicity.— M.R. Moore and K.E.L. McColl, *Porphyrias, Drug Lists*, Glasgow, Porphyria Research Unit, University of Glasgow, 1987.

Absorption and Fate

Dexamphetamine is readily absorbed from the gastro-intestinal tract and is resistant to metabolism by monoamine oxidase. It is partly metabolised in the liver, but a considerable fraction may be excreted in the urine unchanged. Urinary elimination is pH-dependent and enhanced in acid urine.

PREGNANCY AND THE NEONATE. Evidence of excretion in breast milk in a 36-year-old nursing mother who received racemic amphetamine 5 mg four times daily for narcolepsy. The concentrations of amphetamine in breast milk were almost 3 times higher than in maternal plasma on the 10th day after delivery and the ratio increased to about 7 on the 42nd day. No untoward effects were noted in the infant at 24 months but, considering the possible effects of amphetamine on normal psychobehavioural development, it would seem prudent to abstain from long-term nursing during amphetamine treatment.— E. Steiner *et al.*, *Eur. J. clin. Pharmac.*, 1984, *27*, 123.

Uses and Administration

Dexamphetamine, the dextrorotatory isomer of amphetamine, is an indirect-acting sympathomimetic agent with alpha- and beta-adrenergic activity. It has a marked stimulant effect on the central nervous system, particularly the cerebral cortex.

Dexamphetamine sulphate is given by mouth. It is used clinically in the treatment of narcolepsy and has been advocated as an adjunct to psychological, educational, and social measures in the treatment of hyperkinetic states in children. It was formerly used as an anorectic agent in the short-term treatment of obesity. Amphetamines have also been used to overcome fatigue but such use is undesirable.

In the treatment of narcolepsy, the usual starting dose is 5 to 10 mg daily in divided doses, increased if necessary at weekly intervals to a maximum of 60 mg daily. In hyperkinetic states individualisation of treatment is especially important; children aged 6 years and over usually start with a dose of 5 mg once or twice daily, increased if necessary by 5 mg at weekly intervals to an upper limit of 20 mg daily, though older children might require up to 40 mg daily.

Dexamphetamine sulphate has been formulated as a sustained-release preparation; dexamphetamine has also been given as the phosphate, saccharate, tannate, and tartrate.

DEPRESSION. Dexamphetamine appeared to have little effect on depressive illness but might be appropriate for poorly motivated patients. However, the use of stimulant drugs in the aged had not been developed or adequately evaluated in general practice (A.N.G. Clark, *Practitioner*, 1978, *220*, 735). Although Ostow (*J. Am. med. Ass.*, 1983, *249*, 1825) supported the use of dexamphetamine and methylphenidate in the control of symptoms of depression, Jones (*ibid.*, *250*, 2286) considered that, while there was some evidence that stimulants of the central nervous system might be helpful in some depressive conditions, other studies had shown that many types of depressed patients did not experience any benefits over placebo. A retrospective survey by Woods *et al.* (*J. clin. Psychiat.*, 1986, *47*, 12) indicated that psychostimulants might be of value in a substantial proportion of depressed patients with medical illness. However the authors regarded their conclusions as tentative until confirmed by prospective studies.

Diagnostic use. There was preliminary evidence that in depressed patients, psychostimulant response might be a useful predictor of tricyclic antidepressant response. It was often the older patients with agitated depression in whom a rapid determination of the optimal antidepressant would be most desirable, but administration of an amphetamine test to agitated patients might give cause for concern. A test dose of dexamphetamine sulphate 10 mg was given to 2 patients with unipolar depression with agitation; both became more relaxed and pleasant. Depressed agitated patients might be suitable for a dexamphetamine test if not contra-indicated by medical problems and if started with low doses under supervised conditions. More controlled studies were required to determine if a dexamphetamine test was a clinically useful tool.— N. G. Ward and T. H. Lampe, *J. clin. Psychiat.*, 1982, *43*, 35.

NARCOLEPSY. Dexamphetamine, or alternatively methylphenidate, were considered to reduce the number of narcoleptic attacks but not the other features of the narcoleptic syndrome, including cataplexy, sleep paralysis, or hypnagogic hallucinations. These 3 symptoms might respond to tricyclic antidepressant drugs, of which clomipramine seemed the most effective.— *Lancet*, 1975, *1*, 845.

In a placebo-controlled study involving 20 patients with narcoleptic syndrome, dexamphetamine sulphate 10 mg daily, mazindol 4 mg daily, or fencamfamin hydrochloride 60 mg daily for 4 weeks reduced the reported frequency of sleep attacks by approximately half. A dose of dexamphetamine sulphate 30 mg daily was only slightly more effective than the lower dose of dexamphetamine sulphate 10 mg daily. No treatment significantly reduced the number of attacks of cataplexy.— J. Shindler *et al.*, *Br. med. J.*, 1985, *290*, 1167.

SENILITY. There was no convincing evidence that central nervous system stimulants were of any value in the treatment of memory lapses, difficulty in concentrating, mild depression, or other symptoms associated with senility.— *Med. Lett.*, 1978, *20*, 75.

Preparations

Dexamphetamine Tablets *(B.P.)*. Tablets containing dexamphetamine sulphate.

Dextroamphetamine Sulfate Capsules *(U.S.P.)*

Dextroamphetamine Sulfate Elixir *(U.S.P.)*

Dextroamphetamine Sulfate Tablets *(U.S.P.)*

Proprietary Preparations of Dexamphetamine and its Salts

Dexedrine *(Smith Kline & French, UK)*. *Tablets*, scored, dexamphetamine sulphate 5 mg.

Proprietary Names and Manufacturers of Dexamphetamine and its Salts

Afatin *(Spain)*; Amphaetex *(Switz.)*; Dexamed *(Medo, UK)*; Dexamin *(Switz.)*; Dexampex *(Lemmon, USA)*; Dexedrina *(Smith Kline & French, Spain)*; Dexedrine *(Belg.; Smith Kline & French, Canad.; Switz.; Smith Kline & French, UK; Smith Kline & French, USA)*; Ferndex *(Ferndale, USA)*; Maxiton *(Spain)*; Mephadexamin-R *(Switz.)*; Stil-2 *(Spain)*; Synatan *(Landerlan, Spain)*.

The following names have been used for multi-ingredient preparations containing dexamphetamine and its salts— Biphetamine *(Pennwalt, USA)*; Drinamyl *(Smith Kline & French, UK)*; Durophet *(Riker, UK)*; Durophet-M *(Riker, UK)*; Obetrol *(Rexar, USA)*; Steladex *(Smith Kline & French, UK)*.

18628-z

Dexfenfluramine Hydrochloride *(BANM, rINNM)*.

S-5614 *(base)*. *(S)*-*N*-Ethyl-α-methyl-3-trifluoromethylphenethylamine hydrochloride.

$C_{12}H_{16}F_3N,HCl = 267.7$.

CAS — 3239-45-0; 3239-44-9 (both dexfenfluramine).

Dexfenfluramine is the *S* isomer of fenfluramine (p.1443) and it is used similarly as the hydrochloride as an anorectic.

Doses of up to 15 mg of dexfenfluramine hydrochloride twice daily are given by mouth as an adjunct to dietary measures in the short-term treatment of moderate to severe obesity.

Diabetic control should be monitored in patients given drugs such as dexfenfluramine hydrochloride for the control of obesity.

Proprietary Names and Manufacturers

Isoméride *(Ardix, Fr.)*.

12648-k

Diethylaminoethanol

2-Diethylaminoethanol.

$C_6H_{15}NO = 117.2$.

CAS — 100-37-8.

Diethylaminoethanol is an analogue of deanol (p.1440) and has been used similarly as the malate. In Great Britain the recommended exposure limit of diethylaminoethanol is 10 ppm (long-term); suitable precautions should be taken to prevent absorption through the skin.

Proprietary Names and Manufacturers of Diethylaminoethanol and its Salts

Cérébrol *(Fr.)*.

1475-e

Diethylpropion Hydrochloride *(BANM, USAN)*.

Amfepramone Hydrochloride *(pINNM)*. *N*-(1-Benzoylethyl)-*NN*-diethylammonium chloride; 2-Diethylaminopropiophenone hydrochloride.

$C_{13}H_{19}NO,HCl = 241.8$.

CAS — 90-84-6 (diethylpropion); 134-80-5 (hydrochloride).

Pharmacopoeias. In *Br.* and *U.S.*

A white to off-white fine crystalline powder, odourless or with a slight characteristic odour. The *B.P.* and *U.S.P.* both permit the addition of tartaric acid as a stabilising agent. **Soluble** 1 in

0.5 of water, 1 in 3 of alcohol, and 1 in 3 of chloroform; practically insoluble in ether. **Store** in well-closed containers at a temperature not exceeding 25°. Protect from light.

Adverse Effects, Treatment, and Precautions

As for Dexamphetamine Sulphate, p.1440. Diabetic control should be monitored in patients given drugs such as diethylpropion hydrochloride for the control of obesity.

Diethylpropion hydrochloride is subject to abuse.

PORPHYRIA. Diethylpropion was considered to be unsafe in patients with acute porphyria because it has been shown to be porphyrinogenic in *animals* or *in-vitro* systems.— M.R. Moore and K.E.L. McColl, *Porphyrias, Drug Lists*, Glasgow, Porphyria Research Unit, University of Glasgow, 1987.

Absorption and Fate

Diethylpropion is readily absorbed from the gastro-intestinal tract. It is extensively metabolised in the liver and possibly the gastro-intestinal tract and is excreted in the urine.

Metabolism of diethylpropion in man involved routes of de-ethylation and reduction resulting in a complex mixture of active compounds with different physico-chemical properties and susceptibilities to metabolic processes, and further metabolism to inactive compounds. The rate of elimination of the drug and the ratio of metabolites excreted was dependent on urinary pH.— A. H. Beckett, *Curr. med. Res. Opinion*, 1979, *6, Suppl.* 1, 107.

Percutaneous absorption and metabolism of diethylpropion and some other aminopropiophenones.— S. L. Markantonis *et al.*, *J. Pharm. Pharmac.*, 1986, *38*, 515.

Uses and Administration

Diethylpropion hydrochloride is a sympathomimetic agent with the actions of dexamphetamine (p.1441). It is used as an anorectic and is administered by mouth as an adjunct to dietary measures in the short-term treatment of moderate to severe obesity.

The usual dose is 25 mg three times daily 1 hour before meals or 75 mg, as a sustained-release preparation, once daily in mid-morning. It may be given intermittently, a period of several week's treatment being followed by a similar period without treatment.

Its dimethyl analogue dimepropion hydrochloride was formerly used as an anorectic.

OBESITY. Diethylpropion, mazindol, and phentermine could be used intermittently in the treatment of obesity as this was as effective, cheaper, and presumably less likely to lead to drug abuse than continuous treatment. One regime was to give the active preparation for 4 weeks every second month.— S. M. Galloway *et al.*, *Postgrad. med. J.*, 1984, *60, Suppl.* 3, 19.

For a comparison of diethylpropion and phentermine in the treatment of obesity, see p.1447.

Preparations

Diethylpropion Hydrochloride Tablets *(U.S.P.)*

Proprietary Preparations

Apisate *(Wyeth, UK). Tablets*, sustained-release, diethylpropion hydrochloride 75 mg, thiamine hydrochloride 5 mg, riboflavine 4 mg, pyridoxine hydrochloride 2 mg, nicotinamide 30 mg.

Tenuate Dospan *(Merrell, UK). Tablets*, sustained-release, scored, diethylpropion hydrochloride 75 mg.

Proprietary Names and Manufacturers

Adiposan *(Switz.)*; Adipyn *(Switz.)*; Alipid *(Arg.)*; Anorex *(Crinex, Fr.)*; Apisate *(Wyeth, UK)*; Brendalit *(Arg.)*; Controlgras *(Arg.)*; Danylen *(Swed.)*; Delgamer *(Merrell Dow, Spain)*; Dietec *(Canad.)*; Dietil Retard *(Belg.)*; D.I.P. *(Canad.)*; Dobesin *(Denm.)*; Frekentine *(Neth.)*; Keramik *(Arg.)*; Lineal-Rivo *(Switz.)*; Linea-Valeas *(Valeas, Ital.)*; Lipomin *(Spain)*; Magrene *(Ital.)*; Menutil *(Belg.)*; Moderatan Diffucap *(Théranol, Fr.)*; Nobensine-75 *(Canad.)*; Nobesine *(Nadeau, Canad.)*; Nulobes *(Arg.)*; Prefamone *(Belg.; Dexo, Fr.; Dexo, Switz.)*; Propion *(Pro Doc, Canad.)*; Redicres *(Arg.)*; Regenon *(Belg.; Temmler, Denm.; Temmler, Ger.; Sorel, Ital.; Temmler, Switz.)*; Regenon retard *(Ger.; Temmler, Switz.)*; Regibon *(Canad.)*; Sinapet *(Arg.)*; Tenuate *(Merrell Dow, Austral.; Merrell Dow, Canad.; Merrell, Ger.; Merrell Dow, Switz.; Merrell, UK; Lakeside, USA)*; Tenuate Dospan *(Merrell Dow, Austral.; Belg.; Merrell, Fr.; Lepetit, Ital.; Mer-National, S.Afr.; Merrell, UK; Merrell Dow, USA)*; Tepanil *(Riker, USA)*.

1420-t

Dimefline Hydrochloride *(BANM, USAN, rINNM)*.

DW-62; Rec-7-0267. 8-Dimethylaminomethyl-7-methoxy-3-methyl-2-phenyl-4*H*-chromen-4-one hydrochloride.

$C_{20}H_{21}NO_3,HCl=359.9$.

CAS — 1165-48-6 (dimefline); 2740-04-7 (hydrochloride).

Dimefline hydrochloride has the actions of doxapram hydrochloride and is used similarly as a respiratory stimulant in usual doses of 8 to 12 mg 2 or 3 times daily by mouth, or 8 mg once or twice daily by intramuscular injection.

Proprietary Names and Manufacturers

Remeflin *(Recordati, Ital.; Jpn; Zambon, Spain; Recordati, Switz.)*; Remefline *(Recordati, Belg.)*.

12664-k

Dimorpholamine

NN'-Ethylenebis(*N*-butylmorpholine-4-carboxamide).

$C_{20}H_{38}N_4O_4=398.5$.

CAS — 119-48-2.

Pharmacopoeias. In *Jpn.*

Dimorpholamine is reported to be a cardiac and respiratory stimulant.

Proprietary Names and Manufacturers

Theraplina Theraplix *(Vaillant, Ital.)*.

1421-x

Doxapram Hydrochloride *(BANM, USAN, rINNM)*.

AHR-619. 1-Ethyl-4-(2-morpholinoethyl)-3,3-diphenylpyrrolidin-2-one hydrochloride monohydrate.

$C_{24}H_{30}N_2O_2,HCl,H_2O=433.0$.

CAS — 309-29-5 (doxapram); 113-07-5 (hydrochloride, anhydrous); 7081-53-0 (hydrochloride, monohydrate).

Pharmacopoeias. In *Br., Braz.,* and *U.S.* Also in *B.P. Vet.*

A white to off-white, odourless or almost odourless, crystalline powder. **Soluble** in water and in chloroform; sparingly soluble in alcohol; practically insoluble in ether. A 1% solution in water has a pH of 3.5 to 5.0. The *B.P.* injection is **sterilised** by autoclaving. The commercial injection is reported to be **incompatible** with alkaline solutions such as aminophylline, frusemide, or thiopentone sodium. **Store** in airtight containers.

Adverse Effects

As with other respiratory stimulants, there is a risk that doxapram will produce adverse effects due to general stimulation of the CNS.

Doxapram may produce dyspnoea and other respiratory problems such as coughing, bronchospasm, and laryngospasm. Muscle involvement may range from fasciculations to spasticity or seizures. Headache, dizziness, and confusion can occur as can hyperpyrexia or a sensation of warmth. There may be nausea, vomiting, diarrhoea, and problems with urination. Cardiovascular effects include alterations in blood pressure and various arrhythmias.

Thrombophlebitis may follow extravasation of doxapram during injection.

EFFECTS ON THE LIVER. Acute hepatic necrosis in one patient was attributed to a 24-hour infusion of doxapram. Liver function tests returned to normal over 3 weeks.— G. J. Fancourt *et al.*, *Postgrad. med. J.*, 1985, *61*, 833.

Precautions

Doxapram should be given cautiously to patients with heart diseases or obstructive airway disease; where these conditions are severe its use is contra-indicated. It should not be administered to patients with epilepsy or other convulsive disorders, cerebral oedema, cerebrovascular accident, status asthmaticus, severe hypertension, coronary artery disease, hyperthyroidism, or phaeochromocytoma.

Patients should be carefully supervised during administration of doxapram; special attention should be paid to changes in blood gas measurements.

The pressor effects of doxapram may be enhanced by sympathomimetic agents or monoamine oxidase inhibitors.

Intravenous injections of doxapram should be given slowly to minimise the the risk of haemolysis which had been found to occur *in vitro* when the drug was mixed with blood.— R. J. Trudnowski (letter), *Br. J. Anaesth.*, 1973, *45*, 303.

Absorption and Fate

Doxapram is rapidly metabolised after intravenous injection and metabolites are excreted in the urine. Some absorption has been demonstrated when doxapram is given by mouth.

References: R. H. Robson and L. F. Prescott, *Br. J. clin. Pharmac.*, 1979, *7*, 81; R. H. Robson *et al.*, *ibid.*, 1978, *5*, 363P.

Uses and Administration

Doxapram hydrochloride is a central and respiratory stimulant; it has a brief duration of action. It is used in the treatment of respiratory depression following anaesthesia, usually in a dose of 0.5 to 1.5 mg per kg body-weight intravenously. This dose may be repeated at hourly intervals. It may also be given by intravenous infusion, initially administered at a rate of 2 to 5 mg per minute and then reduced, according to the patient's response, to 1 to 3 mg per minute; a recommended maximum total dosage is 4 mg per kg.

Doxapram may be infused at a rate of 1.5 to 4.0 mg per minute in the treatment of acute respiratory failure.

ADMINISTRATION. Following a preliminary report (R.H. Robson and L.F. Prescott, *Br. J. clin. Pharmac.*, 1979, *7*, 81) showing that plasma-doxapram concentrations fall rapidly after intravenous bolus injections and after short-duration infusions and that steady-state concentrations are not achieved for many hours with a constant-rate infusion it was suggested that a variable-rate infusion may overcome these problems. In contrast to some recommendations that the dose be successively increased it is suggested that to achieve an early therapeutic effect the initial infusion-rate should be fast but thereafter reduced to avoid high steady-state concentrations.— J. A. Clements *et al.*, *Eur. J. clin. Pharmac.*, 1979, *16*, 411; *idem, J. Pharm. Pharmac.*, 1979, *31, Suppl.*, 41P.

ADMINISTRATION IN RENAL FAILURE. Despite renal failure and probable hypothyroidism a 65-year-old patient given doxapram 870 µg per kg body-weight in a 1-hour infusion appeared to distribute, metabolise, and excrete doxapram and one of its major metabolites AHR-5955 normally.— J. R. Baker *et al.* (letter), *Br. J. clin. Pharmac.*, 1981, *11*, 305.

RESPIRATORY STIMULATION. Some references to doxapram being used as a respiratory stimulant: P. K. Gupta and J. W. Dundee, *Anaesthesia*, 1974, *29*, 33 and 40 (reduction of respiratory depression induced by opioids for postoperative analgesia); T. H. Gawley *et al.*, *Br. med. J.*, 1976, *1*, 122 (postoperative with opioid analgesics); C. J. Allen and K. R. Gough, *ibid.*, 1983, *286*, 1181 (to aid recovery from deep diazepam sedation); C. J. Wells *et al.* (letter), *Lancet*, 1984, *1*, 739 (to counteract the respiratory depression from anaesthesia and opioid analgesics).

Apnoea of prematurity. Doxapram has been infused in doses of 2.5 mg per kg body-weight per hour to treat apnoea of prematurity where xanthines alone have proved ineffective (E. Sagi *et al.*, *Archs Dis. Childh.*, 1984, *59*, 281; F. Eyal *et al.*, *Pediatrics*, 1985, *75*, 709). However, adverse effects have been reported (P.R.F. Dear and D. Wheeler, *ibid.*, 903).

A lower dose of 250 µg per kg per hour has been shown to be effective (A. Bairam and P. Vert, *Lancet*, 1986, *1*, 793).

Preparations

Doxapram Hydrochloride Injection *(U.S.P.)*

Doxapram Injection *(B.P.)*. Doxapram Hydrochloride Injection. Store at a temperature not exceeding 25° and do not allow to freeze.

Proprietary Preparations

Dopram *(Robins, UK)*. *Intravenous infusion*, doxapram hydrochloride 2 mg/mL, in glucose intravenous infusion. *Injection*, doxapram hydrochloride 20 mg/mL, in ampoules of 5 mL.

Proprietary Names and Manufacturers

Docatone *(Rovi, Spain)*; Dopram *(Robins, Austral.*; *Robins, Canad.*; *Robins, Denm.*; *Martinet, Fr.*; *Brenner, Ger.*; *Jpn*; *Neth.*; *Robins, Norw.*; *NZ*; *Continental Ethicals, S.Afr.*; *Robins, Switz.*; *Robins, UK*; *Robins, USA)*; Doxapril *(Carlo Erba, Ital.)*.

1422-r

Ethamivan *(BAN, USAN)*.

Etamivan *(rINN)*; Vanillic Acid Diethylamide; Vanillic Diethylamide. *NN*-Diethylvanillamide.

$C_{12}H_{17}NO_3$=223.3.

CAS — 304-84-7.

Pharmacopoeias. In *Br.*

A white crystalline powder, odourless or almost odourless. M.p. 96° to 99°. **Soluble** 1 in 100 of water, 1 in 2 of alcohol, 1 in 3 of acetone, 1 in 1.5 of chloroform, and 1 in 50 of ether. A 1% solution in water has a pH of 5.5 to 7.0.

Ethamivan has similar actions to doxapram hydrochloride (p.1442) and is used similarly as a respiratory stimulant. It has been given intravenously to adults in doses ranging from 50 to 250 mg. An oral solution is available for infants and doses that have been given are: 12.5 mg for premature infants and 25 mg for full-term infants.

Preparations

Ethamivan Oral Solution *(B.P.)*. Ethamivan Solution. A solution containing ethamivan 5% and alcohol 25% in water. Store at a temperature not exceeding 15°. The solution should not be diluted; doses should be measured in a graduated pipette.

Proprietary Preparations

Clairvan *(Sinclair, UK)*. *Oral solution*, ethamivan 50 mg/mL, in alcohol(25%).
Injection, ethamivan 50 mg/mL, in ampoules of 2 mL.

Proprietary Names and Manufacturers

Clairvan *(Sinclair, UK)*; Corivanil *(Ital.)*; Romecor *(Ital.)*; Vallimida *(Spain)*; Vandid *(Austral.*; *S.Afr.*; *Switz.*; *Riker, UK)*.

12708-y

Ethylamphetamine Hydrochloride

Etilamfetamine Hydrochloride *(rINN)*. *N*-Ethyl-α-methylphenethylamine hydrochloride.

$C_{11}H_{17}N,HCl$=199.7.

CAS — 457-87-4 (ethylamphetamine); 1858-47-5 (hydrochloride).

Ethylamphetamine hydrochloride has been used as an anorectic agent.

Proprietary Names and Manufacturers

Apetinil *(Neth.)*; Apetinil-Depo *(Will-Pharma, Belg.*; *Syntex, Switz.)*.

1423-f

Fencamfamin Hydrochloride *(BANM, rINNM)*.

H-610. *N*-Ethyl-3-phenylbicyclo[2.2.1]hept-2-ylamine hydrochloride.

$C_{15}H_{21}N,HCl$=251.8.

CAS — 1209-98-9 (fencamfamin); 2240-14-4 (hydrochloride).

Fencamfamin hydrochloride is given by mouth as a stimulant of the central nervous system.

NARCOLEPSY. For a report of fencamfamin hydrochloride reducing the incidence of sleep attacks, see Dexamphetamine Sulphate, p.1441.

Proprietary Names and Manufacturers

The following names have been used for multi-ingredient preparations containing fencamfamin hydrochloride—Reactivan *(E. Merck, UK)*.

12738-t

Fenethylline Hydrochloride *(BANM, USAN)*.

7-Ethyltheophylline Amphetamine Hydrochloride; Amfetyline Hydrochloride; Fenetylline Hydrochloride *(rINNM)*; H-814; R-720-11. 7-[2-(α-Methylphenethylamino)ethyl]theophylline hydrochloride.

$C_{18}H_{23}N_5O_2,HCl$=377.9.

CAS — 3736-08-1 (fenethylline); 1892-80-4 (hydrochloride).

Fenethylline is a theophylline derivative of amphetamine with similar actions to those of dexamphetamine (p.1440). It has been used for its central stimulant effect. Fenethylline is subject to abuse.

Proprietary Names and Manufacturers

Captagon *(de Bournonville, Belg.*; *Promedica, Fr.*; *Asta Pharma, Ger.)*.

1478-j

Fenfluramine Hydrochloride *(BANM, USAN, rINNM)*.

S-768. *N*-Ethyl-α-methyl-3-trifluoromethylphenethylamine hydrochloride.

$C_{12}H_{16}F_3N,HCl$=267.7.

CAS — 458-24-2 (fenfluramine); 404-82-0 (hydrochloride).

NOTE. Dexfenfluramine is the *S* isomer.

Pharmacopoeias. In *Br.* and *Ind.*

A white odourless or almost odourless crystalline powder. **Soluble** 1 in 20 of water and 1 in 10 of alcohol and chloroform; practically insoluble in ether.

Adverse Effects and Treatment

Fenfluramine hydrochloride has similar adverse effects to Dexamphetamine Sulphate p.1440 except that at therapeutic doses it usually depresses rather than stimulates the central nervous system. Patients being treated with fenfluramine therefore tend to experience drowsiness rather than insomnia. High doses produce symptoms of overstimulation.

Treatment of adverse effects is similar to that for dexamphetamine.

In a double-blind placebo-controlled study of an extended-release preparation of fenfluramine 60 mg in 51 patients, the major adverse effects were drowsiness and dizziness. Complaints of fatigue, vivid dreams, diarrhoea, and dry mouth were also slightly greater in patients taking fenfluramine when compared to those on placebo but many of the adverse effects diminished rapidly.— M. Weintraub *et al.*, *Clin. Pharmac. Ther.*, 1983, *33*, 621.

ABUSE. The risk of drug abuse with fenfluramine, a non-stimulant anorectic, has been considered to be virtually non-existent (*Drug & Ther. Bull.*, 1982, *20*, 35). However, there have been reports of fenfluramine abuse involving large doses (A. Levin, *Postgrad. med. J.*, 1975, *51*, *Suppl.* 1, 186; H.P. Rosenvinge, *Br. med. J.*, 1975, *1*, 735; G.L. Dare and R.D. Goldney, *Med. J. Aust.*, 1976, *2*, 537). In the sample of young men surveyed by Levin (*loc. cit.*), single oral doses of fenfluramine 80 to 500 mg were used to elicit a psychotomimetic state consisting of euphoria, relaxation, and inane laughter, often accompanied by perceptual alterations, including visual hallucinations, alterations in sense of temperature, derealisation, and depersonalisation.

EFFECTS ON THE CARDIOVASCULAR SYSTEM. Reports of pulmonary hypertension associated with fenfluramine: J. G. Douglas *et al.*, *Br. med. J.*, 1981, *283*, 881; J. McMurray *et al.*, *ibid.*, 1986, *292*, 239.

EFFECTS ON SLEEP. Fenfluramine induced changes in dream pattern in 13 of 20 patients studied. Dreams were more frequent and vivid; the degree of change in sleep pattern was dose-related.— A. Mullen *et al.*, *Br. med. J.*, 1977, *1*, 70. See also A. Mullen and C. W. M. Wilson (letter), *Lancet*, 1974, *2*, 594.

OVERDOSAGE. In a review of 53 cases of fenfluramine poisoning, the most commonly observed symptoms were mydriasis, tachycardia, and facial flushing; additional signs included nystagmus, hypertonia, trismus, hyperreflexia, clonus, excitation, hyperthermia, and sweating; in severe intoxication coma and convulsions were frequently present. Onset was rapid and symptoms could persist for several days. Nine patients died following cardiac and respiratory arrest that occurred 1 to 4 hours after ingestion.— K. E. von Mühlendahl and E. G. Krienke, *Clin. Toxicol.*, 1979, *14*, 97.

Precautions

Fenfluramine hydrochloride should not be given to patients with glaucoma or a history of drug abuse or alcoholism. It should be given with caution to patients with cardiovascular disease including hypertension, epilepsy, or psychiatric illness. Patients with mental depression should be treated carefully; there may be mood changes during fenfluramine treatment, and abrupt cessation can produce severe depression. Withdrawal of fenfluramine may therefore need to be gradual. Patients should be advised that fenfluramine can cause drowsiness and that they should if affected not drive or operate machinery and should avoid alcoholic drink.

Fenfluramine hydrochloride should not be given to patients being treated with a monoamine oxidase inhibitor or within at least 14 days of stopping such treatment. As fenfluramine hydrochloride has some intrinsic hypoglycaemic activity it may potentiate the effects of antidiabetic drugs and diabetic control will need monitoring. Fenfluramine may also possess some hypotensive activity that may slightly enhance the effect of antihypertensives.

A 46-year-old woman with a history of minor epileptic disturbances and of a convulsion 5 months earlier showed bizarre behaviour with marked generalised EEG abnormalities 24 hours after abruptly stopping fenfluramine. Minor EEG changes in 2 of 18 obese patients, without epilepsy, after the abrupt withdrawal of fenfluramine were of uncertain significance. It was suggested that fenfluramine should not be used in obese epileptic patients, and should always be withdrawn gradually.— D. L. Davidson *et al.*, *Postgrad. med. J.*, 1975, *51*, *Suppl.* 1, 174.

INTERACTIONS. Possible interaction between fenfluramine and halothane anaesthesia resulting in cardiac arrest.— J. A. Bennett and R. J. Eltringham, *Anaesthesia*, 1977, *32*, 8. Despite severe criticism of the report it was still considered that potent anaesthetic agents should be administered with caution to patients taking fenfluramine.— A. P. Winnie (letter), *ibid.*, 1979, *34*, 79.

A schizophrenic man maintained on haloperidol decanoate became agitated and deluded after ingesting 3 fenfluramine tablets.— D. Murphy and J. Watters, *Br. med. J.*, 1986, *292*, 992. The *UK* manufacturers commented that by virtue of its pharmacological profile, fenfluramine is contraindicated in certain psychiatric states and in combination with some psychoactive substances including neuroleptics.— K. Watters and A. Le Ridant (letter), *ibid.*, 1465.

For the effect of fenfluramine on amitriptyline, see Amitriptyline Hydrochloride, p.353.

Absorption and Fate

Fenfluramine is readily absorbed from the gastro-intestinal tract. It is extensively metabolised and some metabolism has been reported to take place in the gastro-intestinal tract as well as the liver. Initial metabolism involves de-ethylation to active norfenfluramine. Excretion is via the urine in the form of unchanged drug and metabolites. The rate of excretion is influenced by urinary pH and urinary flow, being somewhat increased in acid urine.

Studies by Hossain and Campbell (*Postgrad. med. J.*, 1975, *51*, *Suppl.* 1, 178) and by Innes *et al.* (*Br. med. J.*, 1977, *2*, 1322) indicated a significant correlation between weight loss and plasma concentrations of fenfluramine and its active metabolite norfenfluramine. In contrast, Pietrusko *et al.* (*Int. J. Obes.*, 1982, *6*, 567) found no such correlation in a group of 36 obese women treated with fenfluramine and behaviour therapy.

Uses and Administration

Fenfluramine hydrochloride is used as an anorectic agent. It is given by mouth as an adjunct to dietary measures in the short-term treatment of moderate to severe obesity.

The usual initial dose is 20 mg twice or three times a day before meals, increased gradually after the first week as required to a usual maximum of 120 mg daily. Fenfluramine hydrochloride is also formulated as a sustained-release preparation which is given in a dose of 60 or 120 mg once daily. Fenfluramine treatment should be withdrawn gradually.

ACTION. Some references to the action of fenfluramine: S. Garattini *et al.*, *Curr. med. Res. Opinion*, 1979, *6*, *Suppl.* 1, 15 (action through the serotoninergic system); P. Turner, *ibid.*, 101 (peripheral action); P. Turner *et al.*, *Int. J. Obes.*, 1982, *6*, 411 (peripheral action on serotonin receptors); M. Horowitz *et al.*, *Br. J. clin. Pharmac.*, 1985, *19*, 849 (delayed gastric emptying).

AUTISM. Fenfluramine was administered to 3 young autistic boys with hyperserotoninaemia. Preliminary results showed that fenfluramine reduced blood serotonin concentrations and improved behaviour and cognitive function (E. Geller *et al.*, *New Engl. J. Med.*, 1982, *307*, 165). Controlled studies failed fully to support these results; although fenfluramine acted as a potent serotonin suppressor, clinical efficacy and blood-serotonin concentrations did not appear to be related, and fenfluramine did not improve intellectual function (G.J. August *et al.*, *J. nerv. ment. Dis.*, 1984, *172*, 604; H.H. Ho *et al.*, *J. Pediat.*, 1986, *108*, 465). Ho *et al.* found no consistent or uniform improvement in social responsiveness or cognitive ability in 7 autistic children during fenfluramine therapy and suggested that the main effect of the drug might be to improve attention rather than a direct effect on cognition or behaviour. Gualtieri (*J. Pediat.*, 1986, *108*, 417) considered that fenfluramine was not effective in the treatment of autism and might be neurotoxic; it should not be prescribed to autistic children. In a more recent placebo-controlled study Kohler *et al.* (*Br. med. J.*, 1987, *295*, 885) did not demonstrate any improvement in autistic symptoms with fenfluramine.

EPILEPSY. Fenfluramine was used to treat 3 patients with intractable self-induced photosensitive epilepsy. It seemed likely that fenfluramine reduced or suppressed a compulsive need for self-induction of seizures but a direct anti-epileptic mechanism could not be excluded.— J. Aicardi and H. Gastaut (letter), *New Engl. J. Med.*, 1985, *313*, 1419.

See also Precautions, above.

OBESITY. Results of a controlled study comparing behaviour therapy, pharmacotherapy with fenfluramine, and the two together in the treatment of obesity, indicated that addition of pharmacotherapy, although providing initially improved weight loss, apparently compromised the long-term effects of behaviour therapy. There was no evidence of the influence of fenfluramine on blood pressure that had sometimes been reported.— A. J. Stunkard *et al.*, *Lancet*, 1980, *2*, 1045. Of 42 obese women who had lost at least 6 kg body-weight during oral fenfluramine therapy, 21 were gradually transferred to a near-equivalent maintenance dose of fenfluramine in a sustained-release preparation and 21 were transferred to placebo. By 12 months, 13 of the patients on active drug had been withdrawn, 7 because of regained weight, whereas in the placebo group, 19 patients had been withdrawn because of weight gain. Short-term drug therapy might compromise the long-term effect of behavioural modification and could only be justified if there was a temporary need for weight loss. Longer term treatment with fenfluramine would maintain weight loss in some obese subjects but the possible hazards of prolonged treatment had to be more fully evaluated.— J. G. Douglas *et al.*, *ibid.*, 1983, *1*, 384.

Preparations

Fenfluramine Tablets *(B.P.)*

Proprietary Preparations

Ponderax *(Servier, UK)*. *Pacaps*, sustained-release capsules, fenfluramine hydrochloride 60 mg.

Proprietary Names and Manufacturers

Acino *(Arg.)*; Adipomin; Dima-fen *(Stroder, Ital.)*; Kataline *(Neth.)*; Obedrex; Pesos *(Valeas, Ital.)*; Ponderal *(Arg.; Belg.; Servier, Canad.; Benzon, Denm.; Biopharma, Fr.; Servier, Ital.; Neth.; Servier, Spain; Benzon, Swed.)*; Ponderax *(Servier, Austral.; Itherapia, Ger.; Servier, S.Afr.; Servier, UK)*; Pondimin *(Robins, Canad.; Robins, USA)*; Ponflural *(Servier, Switz.)*; Redufen *(S.Afr.)*.

1479-z

Fenproporex Hydrochloride *(rINNM)*.

N-2-Cyanoethylamphetamine Hydrochloride. (±)-3-(α-Methylphenethylamino)propionitrile hydrochloride.
$C_{12}H_{16}N_2,HCl=224.7$.

CAS — 15686-61-0 (fenproporex); 18305-29-8 (hydrochloride).

Pharmacopoeias. In *Braz.*

Fenproporex hydrochloride is a sympathomimetic agent with the actions of dexamphetamine (p.1440). It is used as an anorectic as an adjunct to dietary measures in the short-term treatment of moderate to severe obesity. Following administration by mouth it is reported to be metabolised to amphetamine. Fenproporex has also been given as the base or the diphenylacetate.

Doses of 20 mg as the base have been given daily by mouth in single or divided doses depending on the formulation.

Diabetic control should be monitored when fenproporex or its salts are used for the control of obesity.

Proprietary Names and Manufacturers of Fenproporex and its Salts

Antiobes Retard *(Frumtost, Spain)*; Appetitzügler *(Sagitta, Ger.)*; Dicel *(Lasa, Spain)*; Falagan *(Infar Nattermann, Spain)*; Gacilin *(Andromaco, Arg.)*; Grasmin *(Infale, Spain)*; Lineal *(Roussel, Arg.)*; Perphoxen *(Bottu, Switz.)*; Perphoxene *(Bottu, Belg.)*; Solvolip *(Knoll, Arg.)*; Tegisec *(Roussel, Spain)*.

1424-d

Flurothyl *(BAN, USAN)*.

Flurotyl *(rINN)*; Hexafluorodiethyl Ether; SKF-6539.
Bis(2,2,2-trifluoroethyl) ether.
$C_4H_4F_6O=182.1$.

CAS — 333-36-8.

Pharmacopoeias. In *U.S.*

A clear, colourless, volatile, inflammable liquid, with a pleasant mild ethereal odour. B.p. about 64°. Specific gravity 1.415 to 1.419. **Soluble** 1 in 500 of water; miscible with alcohol, ether, propylene glycol, and halogenated solvents. **Store** at a temperature not exceeding 40° in single-dose glass ampoules.

Flurothyl stimulates the central nervous system and induces convulsions. It was formerly used by inhalation or intravenous injection as an alternative to electro-convulsive therapy in the treatment of severe depression.

1426-h

Lobelia *(BAN)*.

Indian Tobacco; Lobelia Herb.

Pharmacopoeias. In *Aust., Belg., Br., Braz., Egypt., Fr., Pol., Port.,* and *Span. Br.* also describes Powdered Lobelia. *Chin.* specifies *Lobelia chinensis.*

The dried aerial parts of *Lobelia inflata* (Lobeliaceae) containing not less than 0.25% of total alkaloids calculated as lobeline.

1427-m

Lobeline Hydrochloride *(rINNM)*.

Alpha-lobeline Hydrochloride; Lobelini Hydrochloridum.
2-[6-(β-Hydroxyphenethyl)-1-methyl-2-piperidyl]acetophenone hydrochloride.
$C_{22}H_{27}NO_2,HCl=373.9$.

CAS — 90-69-7 (lobeline); 134-63-4 (hydrochloride).

Pharmacopoeias. In *Aust., Belg., Egypt., Int., It., Pol., Port., Span.,* and *Turk.*

1428-b

Lobeline Sulphate *(rINNM)*.

$(C_{22}H_{27}NO_2)_2,H_2SO_4=773.0$.

CAS — 134-64-5.

Adverse Effects

Side-effects of lobelia and lobeline include nausea and vomiting, diarrhoea, coughing, tremors, and dizziness. Symptoms of overdosage include profuse diaphoresis, paresis, tachycardia, hypothermia, hypotension, and coma: fatalities have occurred.

Uses and Administration

Lobeline, which chiefly accounts for the activity of lobelia, has peripheral and central effects similar to those of nicotine.

Lobelia has been incorporated in preparations aimed at relieving bronchial asthma and chronic bronchitis. Lobeline hydrochloride was formerly given intramuscularly as a respiratory stimulant. Lobeline, by mouth, as the hydrochloride or sulphate, has been used as a smoking deterrent.

Preparations of Lobelia and Lobeline Salts

Ethereal Lobelia Tincture *(B.P.C. 1973)*. 1 in 5; prepared by percolation with ether spirit and adjusted to contain 0.05 to 0.075% w/v of alkaloids calculated as lobeline. Store in a cool place in airtight containers.

Proprietary Names and Manufacturers of Lobelia and Lobeline Salts

Desista *(Cambridge Laboratories, Austral.)*; Habit-X *(Glenden, Switz.)*; Lobatox *(Sobio, Fr.)*; Lobidan *(Berk, S.Afr.; Doetsch, Grether, Switz.; Berk Pharmaceuticals, UK)*; Nicoban *(Honeyrose, UK)*; Nikoban *(USA)*; Refrane *(Lederle, Austral.)*; Smokeless *(Inibsa, Spain)*; Stopsmoke *(Landerlan, Spain)*; Test Sixty *(Ashe, UK)*; Unilobin *(Badische, Ger.)*.

1482-w

Mazindol *(BAN, USAN, rINN)*.

AN-448; SaH-42-548. 5-(4-Chlorophenyl)-2,5-dihydro-3*H*-imidazo[2,1-*a*]isoindol-5-ol.
$C_{16}H_{13}ClN_2O=284.7$.

CAS — 22232-71-9.

Pharmacopoeias. In *U.S.*

White to off-white, crystalline powder, having not more than a faint odour. **Insoluble** in water; slightly soluble in methyl alcohol and in chloroform. **Store** in airtight containers.

Adverse Effects, Treatment, and Precautions

As for Dexamphetamine Sulphate, p.1440. The possibility that dependence might develop should be borne in mind.

Diabetic control should be monitored in patients given drugs such as mazindol for the control of obesity. As drowsiness has occurred in some patients, it is recommended that patients taking mazindol should if affected not drive or operate machinery and should avoid alcoholic drink.

A study in 18 obese patients with maturity-onset diabetes concluded that mazindol was well tolerated by diabetics taking either oral hypoglycaemic drugs or insulin. However, insulin requirements needed assessing regularly as they could fluctuate with weight change.— M. Sanders and H. Breidahl, *Med. J. Aust.*, 1976, *2*, 576.

Report on 8 men who developed testicular pain after

taking mazindol.— J. McEwen and R. H. B. Meyboom, *Br. med. J.*, 1983, *287*, 1763.

INTERACTIONS. For the effect of mazindol on lithium carbonate, see p.368.

Absorption and Fate

Mazindol is absorbed from the gastro-intestinal tract and is excreted in the urine, partly unchanged and partly as metabolites.

Uses and Administration

Mazindol has the actions of dexamphetamine (p.1441). It is used as an anorectic and is given by mouth as an adjunct to dietary measures in the short-term treatment of obesity. The usual dose is 2 mg once daily or 1 mg three times a day.

NARCOLEPSY. Beneficial results in patients with narcolepsy receiving mazindol 3 to 8 mg daily for 1 year. Cataplexy and sleep paralysis did not respond.— J. D. Parkes and M. Schachter, *Acta neurol. scand.*, 1979, *60*, 250.

For a report of mazindol reducing the incidence of sleep attacks, see Dexamphetamine Sulphate, p.1441.

OBESITY. For a recommendation to use mazindol intermittently in the management of obesity, see Diethylpropion Hydrochloride, p.1442.

PARKINSONISM. Results indicated that mazindol, a blocker of dopamine and noradrenaline re-uptake, might be of benefit in patients with the less advanced stages of parkinsonism.— P. J. Delwaide *et al.*, *Archs Neurol., Chicago*, 1983, *40*, 788.

URINARY INCONTINENCE. In a double-blind placebo-controlled study of mazindol in the control of micturition, 17 of 25 patients with incontinence responded to mazindol 1 to 3 mg daily by mouth.— C. R. J. Woodhouse and R. C. Tiptaft, *Br. J. Urol.*, 1983, *55*, 636.

Preparations

Mazindol Tablets *(U.S.P.)*. Store at a temperature not exceeding 25° in airtight containers.

Proprietary Preparations

Teronac *(Sandoz, UK)*. *Tablets*, scored, mazindol 2 mg.

Proprietary Names and Manufacturers

Afilan *(Arg.)*; Dimagrir *(Arg.)*; Magrilan *(Arg.)*; Mazanor *(Wyeth, USA)*; Mazildene *(Ital.)*; Samonter *(Arg.)*; Sanorex *(Sandoz, Austral.; Sandoz, Canad.; Sandoz, USA)*; Teronac *(Wander, Ger.; Neth.; Wander, S.Afr.; Sandoz, Spain; Wander, Switz.; Sandoz, UK)*.

1483-e

Mefenorex Hydrochloride *(USAN, pINNM)*.

Ro-4-5282. *N*-(3-Chloropropyl)-α-methylphenethylamine hydrochloride.

$C_{12}H_{18}ClN,HCl=248.2$.

CAS — 17243-57-1 (mefenorex); 5586-87-8 (hydrochloride).

Mefenorex hydrochloride is a sympathomimetic agent with the actions of dexamphetamine (p.1440). It is used as an anorectic as an adjunct to dietary measures in the short-term treatment of moderate to severe obesity. The usual dose is the equivalent of 40 mg of mefenorex once or twice daily by mouth. Mefenorex is also administered as the base.

Diabetic control should be monitored in patients given mefenorex base or hydrochloride for the control of obesity.

Proprietary Names and Manufacturers

Doracil *(Gador, Arg.)*; Pondinil *(Roche, Belg.; Roche, Fr.; Roche, Spain; Sauter, Switz.)*; Pondinol *(Roche, Arg.)*; Rondimen *(Degussa, Ger.)*.

12922-t

Mefexamide *(USAN, rINN)*.

ANP-297; NP-297. *N*-(2-Diethylaminoethyl)-2-(4-methoxyphenoxy)acetamide.

$C_{15}H_{24}N_2O_3=280.4$.

CAS — 1227-61-8.

Mefexamide has been used as a central nervous system stimulant. Mefexamide hydrochloride has also been used.

Proprietary Names and Manufacturers

Méfexadyne *(Anphar-Rolland, Fr.)*; Perneuron *(Crinos, Ital.)*; Timodyne *(Montpellier, Arg.; Anphar-Rolland, Fr.; Max Ritter, Switz.)*.

12933-f

Metamivan

3-Ethoxy-*NN*-diethyl-4-hydroxybenzamide.

$C_{13}H_{19}NO_3=237.3$.

CAS — 13898-68-5.

Metamivan is an analogue of ethamivan (p.1443) and has been used similarly.

Proprietary Names and Manufacturers

Anacardiol *(Ibi, Ital.)*.

1431-f

Methylamphetamine Hydrochloride

d-Deoxyephedrine Hydrochloride; *d*-Desoxyephedrine Hydrochloride; Metamfetamine Hydrochloride *(rINNM)*; Methamphetamine Hydrochloride; Methamphetamini Hydrochloridum; Phenylmethylaminopropane Hydrochloride. (+)-*N*α-Dimethylphenethylamine hydrochloride.

$C_{10}H_{15}N,HCl=185.7$.

CAS — 537-46-2 (methylamphetamine); 51-57-0 (hydrochloride).

Pharmacopoeias. In *Aust., Braz., Ger., Ind., Int., Jpn, Swiss,* and *Turk.*

Methylamphetamine hydrochloride is an indirect-acting sympathomimetic agent with actions and uses similar to those of dexamphetamine sulphate (p.1440).

It is used in the treatment of hyperkinetic states in children aged 6 years and over; initial doses are 2.5 to 5.0 mg by mouth once or twice daily, increased if necessary by 5 mg at weekly intervals to the optimum effective dose, usually 20 to 25 mg daily. Methylamphetamine hydrochloride is also used in the management of obesity when it has been given in a dose of 2.5 to 5 mg before each meal. Alternatively 10 or 15 mg has been given as a sustained-release preparation once daily in the morning. Methylamphetamine hydrochloride has been given parenterally as a pressor agent.

Methylamphetamine, being volatile, was formerly employed by inhalation for the relief of nasal congestion.

Proprietary Names and Manufacturers

Desoxyn *(Abbott, USA)*; Methampex *(Lemmon, USA)*; Methedrine *(Wellcome, UK)*; Pervitin *(Trenker, Belg.; Temmler, Ger.; Temmler, Switz.)*.

The following names have been used for multi-ingredient preparations containing methylamphetamine hydrochloride—Mediatric *(Ayerst, USA)*; Phelantin *(Parke, Davis, Canad.)*.

1433-n

Methylphenidate Hydrochloride *(BANM, USAN, rINNM)*.

Methyl Phenidate Hydrochloride. Methyl α-phenyl-α-(2-piperidyl)acetate hydrochloride.

$C_{14}H_{19}NO_2,HCl=269.8$.

CAS — 113-45-1 (methylphenidate); 298-59-9 (hydrochloride).

Pharmacopoeias. In *Braz., Cz., Hung., Swiss,* and *U.S.*

Odourless fine white crystalline powder. Freely **soluble** in water and methyl alcohol; soluble in alcohol; slightly soluble in acetone and chloroform. Solutions in water are acid to litmus.

Adverse Effects and Treatment

As for Dexamphetamine Sulphate, p.1440. Allergic reactions have been reported.

ABUSE. Reports of adverse effects following the abuse of methylphenidate by injecting solutions of crushed tablets.— J. Wolf *et al.*, *Ann. intern. Med.*, 1978, *89*, 224; H. Schatz and M. Drake, *J. Am. med. Ass.*, 1979, *241*, 546.

ALLERGY. Allergic manifestations in 2 children treated with methylphenidate; one developed angioneurotic oedema and the other developed urticaria. Substitution with dexamphetamine in the first child produced an urticarial reaction.— J. Sverd *et al.*, *Pediatrics*, 1977, *59*, 115.

EFFECTS ON GROWTH. Methylphenidate resulted in significant decreases in weight percentiles and a progressive decrement in height percentiles that became significant after 2 years' treatment.— J. A. Mattes and R. Gittelman, *Archs gen. Psychiat.*, 1983, *40*, 317.

Results of a study on prolactin, growth hormone, and growth responses in 8 children treated with methylphenidate for one year suggested that moderate doses of methylphenidate might have a lower risk for long-term height suppression than dexamphetamine.— L. L. Greenhill *et al.*, *J. Am. Acad. child Psychiatry*, 1984, *23*, 58.

See also under Dexamphetamine Sulphate, p.1440.

EFFECTS ON THE HEART. Cardiomyopathic findings in a patient treated with methylphenidate for 4½ years.— V. W. Fischer and H. Barner (letter), *J. Am. med. Ass.*, 1977, *238*, 1497.

EFFECTS ON THE LIVER. Hepatotoxicity with elevated concentrations of serum aspartate aminotransferase (SGOT) and serum alanine aminotransferase (SGPT) in a 67-year-old woman was associated with the administration of methylphenidate hydrochloride 30 mg daily by mouth.— C. R. Goodman, *N.Y. St. J. Med.*, 1972, *72*, 2339. Methylphenidate-induced hepatocellular injury in a 19-year-old woman who developed jaundice, fever, and malaise after intravenous abuse of methylphenidate hydrochloride tablets.— H. Mehta *et al.*, *J. clin. Gastroenterol.*, 1984, *6*, 149.

EFFECTS ON THE NERVOUS SYSTEM. For a discussion on central stimulants provoking Gilles de la Tourette's syndrome, see Dexamphetamine Sulphate, p.1440.

Precautions

As for Dexamphetamine Sulphate p.1441.

INTERACTIONS. Methylphenidate, like dexamphetamine, interacts with a number of other drugs including those listed below. Information about these interactions may be found in the individual monographs: Phenylbutazone, Phenytoin Sodium, and tricyclic antidepressants (see under Amitriptyline Hydrochloride). There are conflicting reports of methylphenidate interacting with ethyl biscoumacetate, see under Warfarin.

Absorption and Fate

Methylphenidate is readily absorbed from the gastro-intestinal tract. It is rapidly metabolised and excreted in the urine. Urinary excretion is not pH dependent.

Studies in man indicated that methylphenidate hydrochloride was essentially completely and quickly absorbed when administered by mouth as shown by the pattern of urinary excretion and minimal faecal elimination. Methylphenidate was rapidly metabolised, and the main urinary metabolite was the de-esterified product, ritalinic acid.— B. A. Faraj *et al.*, *J. Pharmac. exp. Ther.*, 1974, *191*, 535.

There was no correlation between clinical response and serum concentrations of methylphenidate in hyperactive children.— C. T. Gualtieri *et al.*, *Ther. Drug Monit.*, 1984, *6*, 379.

Further references: B. L. Hungund *et al.*, *Br. J. clin. Pharmac.*, 1979, *8*, 571; E. Redalieu *et al.*, *Drug Metab. & Disposit.*, 1982, *10*, 708; W. Wargin *et al.*, *J. Pharmac. exp. Ther.*, 1983, *226*, 382.

See under Administration, below, for a report of food not impeding the absorption or metabolism of methylphenidate.

Uses and Administration

Methylphenidate hydrochloride is an indirect-acting sympathomimetic agent with actions and uses similar to Dexamphetamine Sulphate, p.1441. It is used in the treatment of narcolepsy and as an adjunct to psychological, educational, and social measures in the treatment of hyperkinetic states in children.

In the treatment of narcolepsy, the usual dose is 20 to 30 mg daily by mouth in divided doses, normally 30 to 45 minutes before meals, but the effective dose may range from 10 to 60 mg daily. In hyperkinetic states children aged 6 years and over usually start with a dose of 5 mg twice daily by mouth before breakfast and lunch, increased if necessary by 5 to 10 mg at weekly intervals to a maximum of 60 mg daily. Methylphenidate hydrochloride may be administered as a sustained-release preparation. It has also been given by injection.

ADMINISTRATION. In 7 hyperactive children, oral administration of methylphenidate with a meal did not impede the rate of absorption or metabolism compared with that following administration to children in a fasted state.These results questioned the practice of administering methylphenidate before meals.— Y. -P. M. Chan *et al.*, *Pediatrics*, 1983, *72*, 56.

HYPERKINETIC STATES. In 20 hyperactive children, learning performance showed a peak enhancement at a dosage of 300 µg per kg body-weight by mouth whereas social behaviour showed maximum improvement at 1 mg per kg.— R. L. Sprague and E. K. Sleator, *Science*, 1977, *198*, 1274. Results of a placebo-controlled study in 12 boys with attention deficit disorder indicated that methylphenidate produced some benefits, but each child showed a slightly different pattern of responses. The major effect appeared to be a decrease in impulsiveness. Benefits increased as the dose increased from 300 to 600 µg per kg body-weight.— M. M. Sebrechts *et al.*, *Pediatrics*, 1986, *77*, 222.

The efficacy of methylphenidate in the treatment of attention deficit disorder, residual type; was studied in 37 adult patients. A moderate-to-marked therapeutic response occurred in 21 patients while taking methylphenidate and in 4 while taking placebo.— P. H. Wender *et al.*, *Am. J. Psychiat.*, 1985, *142*, 547.

INVOLUNTARY VOCALISATION. Methylphenidate 90 mg daily in 3 divided doses was effective in controlling involuntary vocalisations including loud whining and inappropriate laughter in a patient with postencephalitic parkinsonism and pseudobulbar palsy.— J. Jankovic (letter), *New Engl. J. Med.*, 1985, *313*, 1478.

NARCOLEPSY. Methylphenidate was considered to be of benefit in the long-term treatment of 106 patients with narcolepsy.— Y. Honda *et al.*, *Curr. ther. Res.*, 1979, *25*, 288.

For a reference to methylphenidate reducing the number of narcoleptic attacks but not affecting other features of the narcoleptic syndrome, see Dexamphetamine Sulphate, p.1441.

POSTOPERATIVE TREMOR. Methylphenidate has been tried in the management of postoperative tremors but this use was not trouble-free. References: G. Brichard and M. Johnstone, *Br. J. Anaesth.*, 1970, *42*, 718; M. E. Dodson and J. M. Fryer, *ibid.*, 1980, *52*, 1265; A. Fassoulaki (letter), *ibid.*, 1981, *53*, 1365; M. E. Dodson, *Adverse Drug React. Bull.*, 1982, Oct., 352.

Preparations

Methylphenidate Hydrochloride Tablets *(U.S.P.)*. Store in airtight containers.

Methylphenidate Hydrochloride Extended-release Tablets *(U.S.P.)*

Proprietary Names and Manufacturers

Methidate *(Canad.)*; Rilatine *(Belg.)*; Ritalin *(Ciba, Austral.; Ciba, Canad.; Ciba, Denm.; Geigy, Ger.; Ciba, Ital.; Neth.; Ciba, Norw.; Ciba, S.Afr.; Ciba, UK; Ciba, USA)*; Ritaline *(Ciba, Switz.)*; Rubifen *(Rubio, Spain)*.

1434-h

Nikethamide *(BAN, rINN)*.

Diethylamide Nicotinic Acid; Nicethamidum; Nicotinoyldiaethylamidum; Nikethylamide. *NN*-Diethylnicotinamide; *NN*-Diethylpyridine-3-carboxamide.

$C_{10}H_{14}N_2O$=178.2.

CAS — 59-26-7.

Pharmacopoeias. In *Aust., Belg., Br., Chin., Cz., Eur., Fr., Ger., Hung., Ind., Int., Jug., Mex., Neth., Nord., Pol., Rus., Swiss*, and *Turk*.

A colourless or slightly yellow oily liquid or crystalline mass with a slight characteristic odour. **Miscible** with water, alcohol, chloroform, and ether. A 25% solution in water has a pH of 6.0 to 7.8. Injections are **sterilised** by autoclaving.

Nikethamide has similar actions to doxapram hydrochloride (p.1442) and has been advocated for the treatment of drug overdosage due to central nervous system depressants but is considered to be of no value for such purposes and may be dangerous. However, nikethamide may very occasionally be of emergency value as a respiratory stimulant prior to assisted respiration.

Nikethamide has been given in usual doses of 0.5 to 1 g intravenously. It has also been given by mouth and by subcutaneous or intramuscular injection.

Nikethamide was considered to be unsafe in patients with acute porphyria as it has been associated with acute attacks.— M.R. Moore and K.E.L. McColl, *Porphyrias, Drug Lists*, Glasgow, Porphyria Research Unit, University of Glasgow, 1987.

Preparations

Nikethamide Injection *(B.P.)*. A sterile 25% solution in Water for Injections.

Proprietary Names and Manufacturers

Cardamin *(Stotzer, Switz.)*; Cora Rapide *(Rapide, Spain)*; Coracanfor *(Spain)*; Coractiv N *(Phyteia, Switz.)*; Corafasa *(Sabater, Spain)*; Coramin *(Ciba, Ger.; Ciba, Switz.)*; Coramina *(Ciba, Arg.; Ciba, Spain)*; Coramine *(Ciba, Belg.; Ciba, Canad.; Ciba, Fr.; Ciba, Neth.; Ciba, Switz.; Ciba, UK; Ciba, USA)*; Corazon *(Grossmann, Switz.)*; Cormed *(Schwarzhaupt, Ger.)*; Juvacor *(Cambridge Laboratories, Austral.)*; Kardonyl *(Canad.)*; Nicaethacor *(Mepha, Switz.)*; Niketamid *(DAK, Denm.)*; Percoral *(Streuli, Switz.)*.

538-h

Nux Vomica *(BAN)*.

Brechnuss; Neuz Vómica; Noce Vomica; Noix Vomique; Strychni Semen.

CAS — 357-57-3 (brucine, anhydrous).

Pharmacopoeias. In *Arg., Aust., Belg., Chin., Cz., Egypt., Fr., Hung., Jpn, Mex., Pol., Port., Roum., Rus., Span.*, and *Swiss*.

Fr. also includes Powdered Nux Vomica.

Port. P. and *Span. P.* also include Ignatia from *Strychnos ignatii*.

Chin. P. also allows *S. pierriana*.

The dried ripe seeds of *Strychnos nux-vomica* (Loganiaceae).

Nux vomica has the actions of strychnine (p.1449). Extracts of nux vomica have been used in a number of preparations, some of which are described in *B.P.C. 1973*.

As well as containing strychnine, nux vomica contains brucine which has similar properties.

Nux vomica (Nux vom.) is used in homoeopathic medicine. Ignatia is also used in homoeopathic medicine where it is known as Ignatia amara.

1436-b

Pemoline *(BAN, USAN, rINN)*.

5-Phenylisohydantoin; LA-956. 2-Imino-5-phenyl-oxazolidin-4-one.

$C_9H_8N_2O_2$=176.2.

CAS — 2152-34-3 (pemoline); 68942-31-4 (hydrochloride); 18968-99-5 (magnesium pemoline).

Adverse Effects, Treatment, and Precautions

As for Dexamphetamine Sulphate, p.1440, though the effects of over-stimulation and sympathomimetic activity are considered to be less with pemoline. There have been reports of impaired liver function in patients taking pemoline; its use is contra-indicated in patients with liver disorders.

ABUSE. Paranoid psychosis was observed in a 38-year-old man taking pemoline 75 to 225 mg daily. The patient's compulsive use of the drug, development of tolerance, depressive withdrawal syndrome, and inability to abstain indicated dependence and it was evident that the patient was addicted to pemoline.— S. E. Polchert and R. M. Morse, *J. Am. med. Ass.*, 1985, *254*, 946.

EFFECTS ON GROWTH. Results of a study in 24 hyperkinetic children suggested that growth suppression was a potential side-effect of prolonged treatment with clinically effective doses of pemoline and that this effect might be dose-related.— L. C. Dickinson *et al.*, *J. Pediat.*, 1979, *94*, 538. See also under Dexamphetamine Sulphate, p.1440.

EFFECTS ON THE LIVER. Of children taking pemoline for hyperkinesis, 2% had elevated concentrations of serum aspartate aminotransferase (SGOT) and serum alanine aminotransferase (SGPT); the effect was stated to be transient and reversible.— *J. Am. med. Ass.*, 1975, *232*, 1204. Acute hepatitis associated with pemoline in a 10-year-old boy. Liver enzyme values fell to normal after withdrawal. Rechallenge with lower doses did not increase the enzyme values suggesting a toxic threshold. Close attention to hepatic function during the first few weeks of pemoline therapy was considered essential and it was recommended that serum enzymes should be measured at no less than every 2 weeks for the first 6 weeks and then every other month.— J. F. Patterson (letter), *Sth. med. J.*, 1984, *77*, 938.

EFFECTS ON THE NERVOUS SYSTEM. For a discussion on central stimulants provoking Gilles de la Tourette's syndrome, see Dexamphetamine Sulphate, p.1440.

EFFECTS ON THE PROSTATE. Experience in one patient suggested that pemoline might adversely affect the prostate or interfere with tests for prostatic acid phosphatase used in the diagnosis of carcinoma of the prostate.— W. Lindau and E. De Girolami (letter), *Lancet*, 1986, *1*, 738.

Absorption and Fate

Pemoline is readily absorbed from the gastro-intestinal tract. About 50% is bound to plasma protein. It is partially metabolised in the liver and excreted in the urine as unchanged pemoline and metabolites.

It has been suggested that magnesium hydroxide might increase the absorption of pemoline. Pemoline with magnesium hydroxide was known as magnesium pemoline.

References: N. Plotnikoff and P. Meekma, *J. pharm. Sci.*, 1967, *56*, 290 (*animal* study suggesting that magnesium hydroxide might increase the absorption of pemoline); N. P. E. Vermeulen *et al.*, *Br. J. clin. Pharmac.*, 1979, *8*, 459 (pharmacokinetics in adults); F. Sallee *et al.*, *Clin. Pharmac. Ther.*, 1985, *37*, 606 (pharmacokinetics in children); C. P. Collier *et al.*, *Clin. Pharmacokinet.*, 1985, *10*, 269 (pharmacokinetics in children).

Uses and Administration

Pemoline has similar actions to dexamphetamine (see p.1441) and is used similarly in the management of hyperkinetic states in children. In the *US* the initial dose by mouth in such children is 37.5 mg each morning, increased gradually at weekly intervals by 18.75 mg; the usual range is 56.25 to 75 mg daily and the maximum recommended daily dose is 112.5 mg. Lower doses have been used in the *UK*.

References to the use of pemoline: Y. Honda and Y. Hishikawa, *Curr. ther. Res.*, 1980, *27*, 429 (narcolepsy and daytime sleepiness); W. J. Newlands, *Practitioner*, 1980, *224*, 1199 (antihistamine-induced drowsiness).

Proprietary Preparations

Volital *(Laboratories for Applied Biology, UK)*. *Tablets*, scored, pemoline 20 mg.

Proprietary Names and Manufacturers

Cylert *(Abbott, Canad.; Abbott, UK; Abbott, USA)*; Deltamine *(Fr.)*; Dinergil *(Arg.)*; Dynalert *(Restan, S.Afr.)*; Hyton Asa *(Pharmacia, Denm.)*; Kethamed *(Medo, UK)*; Potensan Forte *(Medo, UK)*; Psicodelta *(Chiesi, Ital.)*; Ronyl *(Lipha, UK)*; Sigmadyn *(Lipha, Ital.)*; Sindromida *(Arg.)*; Stimul *(Ger.; Switz.)*; Tamilan *(Arg.)*; Tradon *(Beiersdorf, Ger.)*; Tropocer *(Spain)*; Volital *(Laboratories for Applied Biology, UK)*.

1437-v

Pentetrazol *(BAN, rINN)*.

1,5-Pentamethylenetetrazole; Corazol; Leptazol; Pentamethazol; Pentazol; Pentetrazolum; Pentylenetetrazol. 6,7,8,9-Tetrahydro-5*H*-tetrazoloazepine.

$C_6H_{10}N_4$=138.2.

CAS — 54-95-5.

Pharmacopoeias. In *Arg., Aust., Belg., Cz., Fr., Hung., Ind., Int., It., Jug., Mex., Neth., Nord., Pol., Port., Rus., Span.*, and *Turk*.

Pentetrazol is a central and respiratory stimulant similar to doxapram hydrochloride and was formerly used in respiratory depression. It has been given to the elderly to alleviate the symptoms of senility, but its value has not been substantiated.

Administration has been by mouth and by injection.

Pentetrazol was considered to be unsafe in patients with acute porphyria as it has been associated with acute attacks.— M.R. Moore and K.E.L. McColl, *Porphyrias, Drug Lists*, Glasgow, Porphyria Research Unit, University of Glasgow, 1987.

Proprietary Names and Manufacturers

Cardiazol *(Knoll, Ger.; Medinsa, Spain; Knoll, Switz.)*;

Cardiorapide *(Rapide, Spain)*; Metrazol *(Knoll, USA)*; Supergotal *(Wasserman, Spain)*.

1438-g

Phenatine
N-(α-Methylphenethyl)nicotinamide.
$C_{15}H_{16}N_2O$=240.3.

CAS — 139-68-4 (phenatine); 2964-23-0 (diphosphate).

Pharmacopoeias. In *Rus.* where the name phenatine is used for the diphosphate salt.

The diphosphate salt of phenatine has been used to stimulate the central nervous system in a similar way to dexamphetamine.

1485-y

Phenbutrazate Hydrochloride *(BANM).*
Fenbutrazate Hydrochloride *(rINNM)*; R-381. 2-(3-Methyl-2-phenylmorpholino)ethyl 2-phenylbutyrate hydrochloride.
$C_{23}H_{29}NO_3$,HCl=403.9.

CAS — 4378-36-3 (phenbutrazate); 6474-85-7 (hydrochloride).

Phenbutrazate hydrochloride has been used in conjunction with phenmetrazine theoclate as an anorectic agent.

Proprietary Names and Manufacturers
The following names have been used for multi-ingredient preparations containing phenbutrazate hydrochloride—Filon *(Berk Pharmaceuticals, UK)*.

1486-j

Phendimetrazine Tartrate *(BANM, USAN, rINNM).*

Phendimetrazine Acid Tartrate; Phendimetrazine Bitartrate. (+)-3,4-Dimethyl-2-phenylmorpholine hydrogen tartrate.
$C_{12}H_{17}NO,C_4H_6O_6$=341.4.

CAS — 634-03-7 (phendimetrazine); 7635-51-0 (hydrochloride); 50-58-8 (tartrate).

Pharmacopoeias. In *U.S.*

A white odourless crystalline powder. Freely **soluble** in water; sparingly soluble in warm alcohol; practically insoluble in acetone, chloroform, and ether. A 2.5% solution in water has a pH of 3.0 to 4.0. **Store** in airtight containers.

Adverse Effects, Treatment, and Precautions
As for Dexamphetamine Sulphate, p.1440. Diabetic control should be monitored in patients given drugs such as phendimetrazine tartrate for the control of obesity.

Absorption and Fate
Phendimetrazine tartrate is absorbed from the gastro-intestinal tract and is excreted in the urine, partly unchanged and partly as metabolites, including phenmetrazine.

Uses and Administration
Phendimetrazine tartrate is a sympathomimetic agent with the actions of dexamphetamine (p.1441). It is used as an anorectic and is administered by mouth as an adjunct to dietary measures in the short-term treatment of moderate to severe obesity.
The usual dose is 35 mg twice or three times daily 1 hour before meals, but doses should be individualised and in some cases 17.5 mg twice daily may be adequate; the dose should not exceed 70 mg three times daily. An alternative dose is 105 mg once daily in the morning as a sustained-release preparation. Phendimetrazine has also been used as the hydrochloride.

Preparations
Phendimetrazine Tartrate Capsules *(U.S.P.)*
Phendimetrazine Tartrate Tablets *(U.S.P.)*

Proprietary Names and Manufacturers of Phendimetrazine and its Salts
Adipost *(Ascher, USA)*; Anorex *(Dunhall, USA)*; Antapentan *(Gerot, Belg.; Gerot, Switz.)*; Bacarate *(Reid-Provident, USA)*; Bontril *(Carnrick, USA)*; Dyrexan-OD *(Trimen, USA)*; Hyrex-105 *(Hyrex, USA)*; Melfiat *(Reid-Rowell, USA)*; Obesan-X *(S.Afr.)*; Obex LA *(Rio, S.Afr.)*; Phenazine *(Legere, USA)*; Plegine *(Ayerst, Ital.; Ayerst, USA)*; Prelu-2 *(Boehringer Ingelheim, USA)*; PT-105 *(Legere, USA)*; Slyn-LL *(Edwards, USA)*; Statobex *(Lemmon, USA)*; Trimcaps *(Mayrand, USA)*; Trimstat *(Laser, USA)*; Trimtabs *(Mayrand, USA)*; Wehless *(Hauck, USA)*; X-Trozine *(Rexar, USA)*.

1487-z

Phenmetrazine Hydrochloride *(BANM, USAN, rINNM).*

Oxazimédrine. (±)-*trans*-3-Methyl-2-phenylmorpholine hydrochloride.
$C_{11}H_{15}NO$,HCl=213.7.

CAS — 134-49-6 (phenmetrazine); 1707-14-8 (hydrochloride); 13931-75-4 (theoclate).

Pharmacopoeias. In *U.S. Cz.* specifies the dextro isomer (Dexphenmetrazinium Chloratum).

A white to off-white odourless crystalline powder. **Soluble** 1 in 0.4 of water, 1 in 2 of alcohol, and 1 in 2 of chloroform. A 2.5% solution in water has a pH of 4.5 to 5.5. **Store** in airtight containers.

Adverse Effects, Treatment, and Precautions
As for Dexamphetamine Sulphate, p.1440. There are reports of phenmetrazine being abused. Diabetic control should be monitored in patients given drugs such as phenmetrazine hydrochloride for the control of obesity.

For a reference to the adverse effects on muscle and kidney following abuse of amphetamines including phenmetrazine, see Dexamphetamine Sulphate, p.1440.

Absorption and Fate
Phenmetrazine hydrochloride is readily absorbed from the gastro-intestinal tract.

Uses and Administration
Phenmetrazine hydrochloride is a sympathomimetic agent with the actions of dexamphetamine (p.1441). It is used as an anorectic and is administered by mouth as an adjunct to dietary measures in the short-term treatment of moderate to severe obesity.
The usual dose is 25 mg twice or three times daily 1 hour before meals or 75 mg once daily as a sustained-release preparation. Phenmetrazine has also been used as the theoclate.

A discussion on the benefit to risk ratio of phenmetrazine in the management of obesity concluded that it should not be prescribed; it had a history of extremely high abuse and a lower anorectic efficacy than the alternative drugs available which also had less abuse liability.— J. Mellar and L. E. Hollister, *Clin. Pharmac. Ther.*, 1982, *32*, 671.

Preparations
Phenmetrazine Hydrochloride Tablets *(U.S.P.)*

Proprietary Names and Manufacturers of Phenmetrazine and its Salts
Preludin *(Boehringer Ingelheim, UK; Boehringer Ingelheim, USA)*.

The following names have been used for multi-ingredient preparations containing phenmetrazine and its salts—Filon *(Berk Pharmaceuticals, UK)*.

1490-w

Phentermine *(BAN, USAN, rINN).*

αα-Dimethylphenethylamine.
$C_{10}H_{15}N$=149.2.

CAS — 122-09-8.

Pharmacopoeias. In *Fr.*

1489-k

Phentermine Hydrochloride *(BANM, USAN, rINNM).*

$C_{10}H_{15}N$,HCl=185.7.

CAS — 1197-21-3.

Pharmacopoeias. In *U.S.*

A white, odourless, hygroscopic, crystalline powder. Phentermine hydrochloride 1.24 mg is approximately equivalent to 1 mg of phentermine. **Soluble** in water, and in the lower alcohols; slightly soluble in chloroform; insoluble in ether. A 2% solution in water has a pH of 5.0 to 6.0. **Store** in airtight containers.

Adverse Effects, Treatment, and Precautions
As for Dexamphetamine Sulphate, p.1440. Diabetic control should be monitored in patients given phentermine or the hydrochloride for the control of obesity.

EFFECTS ON THE CARDIOVASCULAR SYSTEM. Pulmonary hypertension associated in one patient with the use of phentermine.— L. Heuer *et al.*, *Chir. Praxis*, 1978, *23*, 497.

Absorption and Fate
Phentermine is readily absorbed from the gastro-intestinal tract and is excreted in the urine, partly unchanged and partly as metabolites.

Uses and Administration
Phentermine is a sympathomimetic agent with the actions of dexamphetamine (p.1441). It is used as an anorectic and is administered by mouth as the base or hydrochloride as an adjunct to dietary measures in the short-term treatment of moderate to severe obesity.
The usual dose of phentermine is 15 to 30 mg once daily before breakfast; it is given as an ion-exchange resin complex that provides sustained-release. A suggested dose for phentermine hydrochloride is 8 mg three times daily before meals or 15 to 37.5 mg once daily in the morning.

OBESITY. Phentermine as a resin complex 15 to 60 mg (mean 36 mg) was administered to 50 women with refractory obesity as an adjunct to dietary restriction. The mean weight loss achieved by the 34 patients who completed the 20-week study was 6.7 kg but there was considerable individual variation and weight change ranged from a gain of 2.2 kg to a loss of 28.6 kg. Seven patients were withdrawn from the study because of side-effects, including 3 who complained of incapacitating headaches. There was no significant relationship between the plasma concentrations of phentermine and the daily dosage, weight loss, or side-effects. Although this study confirmed that phentermine could produce substantial weight loss, individual response could only be determined by clinical trial and as weight tended to be regained once drug therapy was discontinued, therapy could best be justified only if there was a clearly defined short-term need.— A. Douglas *et al.*, *Int. J. Obes.*, 1983, *7*, 591.

In a 12-week study involving 5 general practices, 99 obese patients on a calorie-restricted diet were given phentermine 30 mg daily before breakfast or diethylpropion 75 mg daily mid-morning. Weight loss was significantly greater in those treated with phentermine, the main difference occurring during the last 4-weeks of the study suggesting that tolerance may develop more readily to the anorectic effect of diethylpropion than to that of phentermine.— J. C. Vallé-Jones *et al.*, *Pharmatherapeutica*, 1983, *3*, 300.

For a recommendation to use phentermine intermittently in the management of obesity, see Diethylpropion Hydrochloride, p.1442.

Preparations

Phentermine Hydrochloride Capsules *(U.S.P.)*

Phentermine Hydrochloride Tablets *(U.S.P.)*

Proprietary Preparations of Phentermine and Phentermine Hydrochloride

Duromine *(Riker, UK). Capsules,* sustained-release, phentermine 15 and 30 mg (as an ion-exchange resin complex).

Ionamin *(Lipha, UK). Capsules,* sustained-release, phentermine 15 and 30 mg (as an ion-exchange resin complex).

Proprietary Names and Manufacturers of Phentermine and Phentermine Hydrochloride

Adipex Nouveau *(Gerot, Switz.)*; Adipex-P *(Lemmon, USA)*; Bellapront *(Boehringer, Arg.)*; Duromine *(Riker, Austral.; Riker, S.Afr.; Riker, UK)*; Fastin *(Beecham, Canad.; Beecham Laboratories, USA)*; Ionamin *(Pennwalt, Canad.; Lipha, UK; Pennwalt, USA)*; Ionamine *(Sodip, Switz.)*; Linyl *(Roussel, Fr.)*; Lipopill *(Roussel Maestretti, Ital.)*; Minobese Forte *(Restan, S.Afr.)*; Mirapront *(Novo, Denm.; Ital.; Neth.; Pfizer, Spain)*; Oby-Trim *(Rexar, USA)*; Omnibex *(Arg.)*; Panbesy *(Biothera-Asperal, Belg.)*; Phentermyl *(Switz.)*; Pronidin *(Trianon, Canad.)*; Span R/D *(Metro Med, USA)*; Teramine *(Legere, USA)*.

1439-q

Picrotoxin

Cocculin; Picrotoxinum.

$C_{30}H_{34}O_{13}$=602.6.

CAS — 124-87-8.

Pharmacopoeias. In *Arg., Int., Mex., Span.,* and *Turk.*

An active principle from the seeds of *Anamirta cocculus* (=*A. paniculata*) (Menispermaceae).

Picrotoxin has similar actions to doxapram hydrochloride and was formerly used as a respiratory stimulant.

1440-d

Pipradrol Hydrochloride *(BANM, rINNM).*

α-(2-Piperidyl)benzhydrol hydrochloride; αα-Diphenyl-α-(2-piperidyl)methanol hydrochloride.

$C_{18}H_{21}NO,HCl$=303.8.

CAS — 467-60-7 (pipradrol); 71-78-3 (hydrochloride).

Pipradrol hydrochloride was formerly used as a stimulant of the central nervous system.

Proprietary Names and Manufacturers

Detaril *(ISOM, Ital.)*; Meratran *(Merrell Dow, Austral.)*; Stimolag Fortis *(Lagap, Switz.)*.

The following names have been used for multi-ingredient preparations containing pipradrol hydrochloride— Alertonic *(Merrell Dow, Austral.; Merrell Dow, Canad.)*.

1441-n

Cropropamide *(BAN, pINN).*

NN-Dimethyl-2-(*N*-propylcrotonamido)butyramide.

$C_{13}H_{24}N_2O_2$=240.3.

CAS — 633-47-6.

1442-h

Crotethamide *(BAN).*

Crotetamide *(rINN)*. 2-(*N*-Ethylcrotonamido)-*NN*-dimethylbutyramide.

$C_{12}H_{22}N_2O_2$=226.3.

CAS — 6168-76-9.

1443-m

Prethcamide

G-5668. A mixture of equal parts by wt of cropropamide and crotethamide.

CAS — 8015-51-8.

Prethcamide has similar actions to doxapram hydrochloride (p.1442) and was formerly used as a respiratory stimulant.

Proprietary Names and Manufacturers of Prethcamide

Micoren *(Ger.; Ital.; Neth.; Switz.; Geigy, UK)*; Micorene *(Belg.)*.

1444-b

Prolintane Hydrochloride *(BANM, USAN, rINNM).*

SP-732. 1-(α-Propylphenethyl)pyrrolidine hydrochloride.

$C_{15}H_{23}N,HCl$=253.8.

CAS — 493-92-5 (prolintane); 1211-28-5 (hydrochloride).

Prolintane hydrochloride is claimed to be a mild stimulant of the central nervous system, and has similar actions to dexamphetamine (p.1440). It is available mainly in mixed preparations that also contain vitamin supplements. Doses may range from 5 to 10 mg twice daily by mouth.

Proprietary Preparations

Villescon *(Boehringer Ingelheim, UK). Tablets,* prolintane hydrochloride 10 mg, thiamine mononitrate 5 mg, riboflavine 3 mg, pyridoxine hydrochloride 1.5 mg, nicotinamide 15 mg, ascorbic acid 50 mg.

Oral liquid, prolintane hydrochloride 2.5 mg, thiamine hydrochloride 1.67 mg, riboflavine sodium phosphate 1.36 mg, pyridoxine hydrochloride 500 μg, nicotinamide 5 mg/5 mL.

Proprietary Names and Manufacturers

Promotil *(Boehringer Ingelheim, Fr.)*.

The following names have been used for multi-ingredient preparations containing prolintane hydrochloride— Catovit *(Boehringer Ingelheim, Austral.)*; Villescon *(Boehringer Ingelheim, UK)*.

1445-v

Propylhexedrine *(BAN, USAN, rINN).*

Propylhexed. (±)-2-Cyclohexyl-*N*,1-dimethylethylamine.

$C_{10}H_{21}N$=155.3.

CAS — 101-40-6; 3595-11-7(±).

Pharmacopoeias. In *Arg.* and *U.S.*

A clear colourless liquid with a characteristic amine-like odour. It slowly volatilises at room temperature and absorbs carbon dioxide from the air. B.p. about 205°.

Very slightly **soluble** in water; soluble 1 in 0.4 of alcohol, 1 in 0.2 of chloroform, and 1 in 0.1 of ether. Solutions in water are alkaline to litmus. **Store** in airtight containers.

1446-g

Propylhexedrine Hydrochloride *(BANM, rINNM).*

$C_{10}H_{21}N,HCl$=191.7.

CAS — 1007-33-6; 6192-95-6(±).

Adverse Effects, Treatment and Precautions

As for Dexamphetamine Sulphate (p.1440). It is subject to abuse. Excessive inhalation of propylhexedrine may cause stinging, rebound congestion, headache, and temporary enlargement of the nasal turbinates. Chronic rhinitis may follow prolonged use. Diabetic control should be monitored in patients given propylhexedrine hydrochloride for obesity.

ABUSE. Results of an examination of 9 deaths following abuse of propylhexedrine by intravenous route using a solution prepared from the cotton pledgets removed from inhalers. In 5 cases a combination of intimal and medial cellular proliferation had produced severe narrowing of pulmonary arterioles; 2 further patients had diffuse pulmonary fibrosis without obvious vascular changes, cardiomegaly being present in both these patients and in 4 of the previous 5. Seven of the 9 subjects had pulmonary foreign-body granulomas containing birefringent material. It was suspected that the mechanism of sudden unexpected death involved cardiac arrhythmias in association with pulmonary hypertension and cor pulmonale. Since the foreign-body granulomas were no different from those found in drug abusers in general they were not considered to be related to the vascular lesions. One death following ingestion of the pledget by mouth was also known.— L. White and V. J. M. DiMaio (letter), *New Engl. J. Med.,* 1977, *297,* 1071. See also R. J. Anderson *et al., Am. J. Med.,* 1979, *67,* 15.

Severe left ventricular failure in 4 men associated with chronic abuse of intravenous propylhexedrine C. H. Croft *et al., Ann. intern. Med.,* 1982, *97,* 560.

Pulmonary hypertension associated with chronic oral abuse of propylhexedrine hydrochloride in 1 patient.— J. Cameron *et al., Med. J. Aust.,* 1984, *140,* 595.

Uses and Administration

Propylhexedrine is a sympathomimetic agent with some of the actions of dexamphetamine (p.1441). It is used as an inhalant for nasal decongestion. Two inhalations through each nostril have been employed, repeated if necessary every one or two hours.

Propylhexedrine is also given as the hydrochloride in usual doses of 50 to 150 mg daily in divided doses by mouth as an anorectic agent in conjunction with dietary measures in the short-term treatment of moderate to severe obesity.

Preparations

Propylhexedrine Inhalant *(U.S.P.).* Cylindrical rolls of suitable fibrous material impregnated with propylhexedrine, usually with aromatics and contained in an inhaler. Store at a temperature not exceeding 40°.

Proprietary Names and Manufacturers of Propylhexedrine and its Salts

Benzedrex *(Smith Kline & French, Austral.; Smith Kline & French, Canad.; Smith Kline & French, S.Afr.; Smith Kline & French, UK)*; Eggobesin *(Eggochemia, Aust.)*; Eventin *(Schering, Austral.; Minden, Ger.; Knoll, S.Afr.; Knoll, Switz.)*; Eventine *(Knoll, Belg.)*.

13195-l

Pyrovalerone *(rINN).*
F-1983 *(hydrochloride).* 4′-Methyl-2-(pyrrolidin-1-yl)valerophenone.
$C_{16}H_{23}NO$=245.4.

CAS — 3563-49-3 (pyrovalerone); 1147-62-2 (hydrochloride).

NOTE. Pyrovalerone Hydrochloride is USAN.

Pyrovalerone was formerly used as a central stimulant; it has been subject to abuse.

542-r

Strychnine
Estricnina; Strychnina. Strychnidin-10-one.
$C_{21}H_{22}N_2O_2$=334.4.

CAS — 57-24-9.

Pharmacopoeias. In *Port.* and *Span.*

An alkaloid obtained from nux vomica and the seeds of other species of *Strychnos.*

543-f

Strychnine Hydrochloride
Strych. Hydrochlor.; Strychninae Hydrochloridum.
$C_{21}H_{22}N_2O_2,HCl,2H_2O$=406.9.

CAS — 1421-86-9 (anhydrous); 6101-04-8 (dihydrate).

Pharmacopoeias. In *Egypt.* Also in *B.P.C. 1973.*

Colourless crystals or white crystalline powder with a very bitter taste. **Soluble** 1 in 40 of water and 1 in 85 of alcohol; practically insoluble in ether.

544-d

Strychnine Nitrate
Azotato de Estricnina; Nitrato de Estricnina; Strychninae Nitras; Strychninum Nitricum.
$C_{21}H_{22}N_2O_2,HNO_3$=397.4.

CAS — 66-32-0.

Pharmacopoeias. In *Arg., Aust., Belg., Cz., Hung., Jug., Nord., Pol., Port., Rus., Span.,* and *Swiss.*

545-n

Strychnine Oxide Hydrochloride
Strychnine N^6-oxide hydrochloride.
$C_{21}H_{22}N_2O_3,HCl$=386.9.

CAS — 7248-28-4 (strychnine oxide).

546-h

Strychnine Sulphate
Strychninae Sulphas; Strychninum Sulfuricum; Sulfato de Estricnina.
$(C_{21}H_{22}N_2O_2)_2, H_2SO_4,5H_2O$=857.0.

CAS — 60-41-3 (anhydrous); 60491-10-3 (pentahydrate).

Pharmacopoeias. In *Arg., Fr., Mex., Port., Roum.,* and *Span.*

Adverse Effects
The symptoms of poisoning are mainly those arising from stimulation or rather reduction of the normal inhibition of the central nervous system. Early signs occurring within 15 to 30 minutes of ingestion include tremors, slight twitching, and stiffness of the face and legs. Painful convulsions develop and may be triggered by minor sensory stimuli; since consciousness is not impaired patients may be extremely distressed. The body becomes arched backwards in hyperextension with the arms and legs extended and the feet turned inward. The jaw is rigidly clamped and contraction of the facial muscles produces a characteristic grinning expression known as 'risus sardonicus'. The convulsions may recur repeatedly and are followed by a period of relaxation. Few patients survive more than 5 episodes of convulsions, death usually occurring due to respiratory arrest. Fatalities have occurred with doses of 10 mg or less. Secondary effects arising from the severe spasms include lactic acidosis, rhabdomyolysis, renal failure, and hyperthermia.
In Great Britain the recommended exposure limits of strychnine are 0.15 mg per m^3 (long-term); 0.45 mg per m^3 (short-term).
There are some indications that strychnine is subject to intentional abuse.

Some references to strychnine poisoning: W. G. O'Callaghan *et al., Br. med. J.,* 1982, *285,* 478; P. G. Blain *et al., J. Toxicol. clin. Toxicol.,* 1982, *19,* 215; R. E. Boyd *et al., Am. J. Med.,* 1983, *74,* 507.

Treatment of Adverse Effects
The main object of therapy in strychnine poisoning is the prompt prevention or control of convulsions and asphyxia. Patients should be given activated charcoal. Convulsions should be controlled or prevented by diazepam given intravenously in doses of up to 10 mg; several doses may be required usually up to a total dose of 30 mg. Should diazepam fail then muscle relaxants should be tried together with intubation and assisted respiration. Gastric lavage should only be carried out when the patient is no longer at risk from convulsions. All unnecessary external stimuli should be avoided and if possible the patient should be kept in a quiet darkened room. Patients should be monitored for any secondary effects from the convulsions so that appropriate symptomatic treatment can be given.

Uses and Administration
Strychnine competes with glycine which is an inhibitory neurotransmitter; it thus exerts a central stimulant effect through blocking an inhibitory activity.
Strychnine was formerly used as a bitter and analeptic and is now mainly used under strict control as a rodenticide, or as a fox or mole poison. It has been tried in the treatment of nonketotic hyperglycinaemia and of sleep apnoea.

NONKETOTIC HYPERGLYCINAEMIA. A 4-month-old child receiving sodium benzoate to treat nonketotic hyperglycinaemia had a beneficial response to concurrent administration of strychnine 100 µg per kg body-weight daily (in 4 divided doses) subsequently increased to 200 µg per kg daily which was aimed at counteracting the effects of high glycine concentrations within the CNS. This corroborated the result of R. Gitzelmann *et al.* (personal communication) in a similar patient.— L. T. Ch'ien *et al.* (letter), *New Engl. J. Med.,* 1978, *298,* 687. The dose of strychnine used in the treatment of nonketotic hyperglycinaemia was considered inadequate. A similar 6-month-old child has been given strychnine nitrate 300 µg per kg body-weight daily for 6 months, 700 µg per kg daily for 4 months, and 0.9 to 1.1 mg per kg daily since then, by mouth, in 4 divided doses. There have been no untoward side-effects and progress in the child's psychomotor development continues after taking strychnine for 18 months. In 2 similar patients treatment has been less successful.— R. Gitzelmann *et al.* (letter), *ibid.,* 1424.
Further references to strychnine in the treatment of nonketotic hyperglycinaemia: D. Arneson *et al., Pediatrics,* 1979, *63,* 369; K. D. MacDermot *et al., ibid.,* 1980, *65,* 61; K. Sankaran *et al., Clin. Pediat.,* 1982, *21,* 636.

SLEEP APNOEA. Strychnine 100 µg per kg body-weight administered during sleep through a nasogastric catheter ameliorated obstructive sleep apnoea in one patient on 2 occasions.— J. E. Remmers *et al., Sleep,* 1980, *3,* 447.

Proprietary Names and Manufacturers of Strychnine Salts
Movellan *(Asta, Ger.).*
The following names have been used for multi-ingredient preparations containing strychnine salts—Aneurone *(Philip Harris, UK)*; Aperient Dellipsoids D9 *(Pilsworth, UK)*; Nerve Dellipsoids D16 *(Pilsworth, UK)*; Neuro Phosphates *(Smith Kline & French, UK)*; Potensan *(Medo, UK)*; Potensan Forte *(Medo, UK)*; Tonic Dellipsoids D 2 *(Pilsworth, UK)*; Viraxatone *(Faulding, Austral.).*

1432-d

Tenamfetamine *(rINN).*
MDA; Methylenedioxyamphetamine; SKF-5. α-Methyl-3,4-methylenedioxyphenethylamine.
$C_{10}H_{13}NO_2$=179.2.

CAS — 4764-17-4; 51497-09-7.

Tenamfetamine is an amphetamine compound with hallucinogenic effects; it has been subject to abuse and dependence. A number of similar amphetamine compounds are known because of their abuse and include: brolamfetamine (2,5-dimethyoxy-4-bromoamphetamine or DOB), methyoxyamphetamine, methylenedioxymethamphetamine (MDMA), and 2,5-dimethyoxy-4-methylamphetamine (DOM or STP).
Tenamfetamine is chemically related to mescaline and amphetamine and has been widely abused under such names as Mellow Drug of America, Love Drug, Love Pill, or MDA.— K. K. Midha *et al., J. pharm. Sci.,* 1976, *65,* 188.

12766-d

Tiflorex *(rINN).*
Flutiorex *(racemic mixture).* (+)-*N*-Ethyl-α-methyl-*m*-(trifluoromethylthio)phenethylamine.
$C_{12}H_{16}F_3NS$=263.3.

CAS — 59173-25-0 (flutiorex); 53993-67-2 (tiflorex).

Tiflorex has been investigated as an anorectic.

References: J. F. Giudicelli *et al., Br. J. clin. Pharmac.,* 1976, *3,* 113; *idem, Eur. J. clin. Pharmac.,* 1976, *10,* 325; T. Silverstone *et al., Br. J. clin. Pharmac.,* 1979, *7,* 353.

Sunscreen Agents

9300-g

Exposure to strong sunlight can cause erythema and sunburn. Immediate tanning may occur resulting from the oxidation of melanin precursors in the uppermost layers of the skin. There may also be a delayed and indirect pigmentation due to the formation of new melanin. The ability of an individual to form a tan is genetically predetermined. Melanin provides some protection against further exposure, but the main protection is provided by thickening of the corneous layer. Excessive and prolonged exposure to intense sunlight may lead to degenerative changes in the skin (premature ageing of the skin) and some skin cancers. Ultraviolet light of wavelengths 320 to 400 nm (UVA) produces immediate direct tanning of the skin with little erythema. Ultraviolet light of wavelengths 290 to 320 nm (UVB) is about 1000 times stronger than UVA in producing erythema and is that part of the sun's spectrum that is responsible for producing sunburn. UVB also produces tanning by indirect pigmentation. The earth's surface is usually screened, by the ozone layer, from ultraviolet light of wavelengths 200 to 290 nm (UVC). However artificial sources such as bactericidal lamps and industrial welding arcs can emit UVC radiation which produces erythema without tanning. Reflected ultraviolet light from snow, white sand, or water adds to direct irradiation. A sunscreen agent that provides protection against UVB light only, will usually be suitable for healthy persons who merely wish to prevent sunburn. An agent that gives protection against both UVB and UVA light will usually be necessary in patients being treated with photosensitising drugs or in patients with diseases such as lupus erythematosus, polymorphic light eruptions, certain porphyrias, solar urticaria, and xeroderma pigmentosum, that are characterised by photosensitive reactions or are exacerbated by light. In many of these cases the photosensitivity is particularly associated with the longer UVA wavelengths. Medical personnel exposed to ultraviolet bactericidal lamps may also need an agent which provides protection against the whole of the UV spectrum.

Sunscreen agents are of 2 types, chemical agents that because of their chromophore groups absorb a particular range of wavelengths within the UV spectrum and physical agents that are opaque and reflect most UV radiation. Compounds used as chemical sunscreens include the aminobenzoates (see below), benzophenones (see p.1452), camphor derivatives (see p.1451), cinnamates (see p.1451), salicylates (see p.1451), and anthranilates. Benzophenones and anthranilates absorb both UVA and UVB light whereas the other compounds absorb only UVB light. Physical sunscreens include titanium dioxide (see p.935) and zinc oxide (see p.936). Other agents used as physical sunscreens include calcium carbonate, kaolin, magnesium oxide, red veterinary petroleum, and talc. Powders may be dusted onto the skin or applied in an aqueous or oily basis but these types of sunscreens are usually cosmetically unappealing.

The efficacy of a particular sunscreen preparation is often expressed as its sun protection factor (SPF). This is a ratio of the time required for irradiation to produce minimal perceptible erythema (minimal erythemal dose; MED) with the skin protected with the suncreen compared to the MED without protection. The scale ranges from SPF2, representing minimal protection from sunburn, but permitting suntanning to SPF15, representing maximum protection against sunburn with no permitted tanning.

Photosensitisation may occur with chemical agents, and skin irritation has also been reported. Sunscreen agents in highly alcoholic vehicles should not be used on patients with inflamed skin.

In Great Britain and the EEC various legislative documents list permitted and provisionally permitted UV filters for use in cosmetics together with their maximum concentrations.

Several other agents including betacarotene (see p.1257) and psoralens (see Methoxsalen, p.926), which are neither chemical nor physical sunscreens, have been used to increase tolerance to sunlight in various diseases characterised by photosensitivity. Dihydroxyacetone and lawsone (see p.919 and p.1451) when employed together appear to provide some protection against UV light although neither are effective when used alone.

Reviews and discussions on sunscreen agents: R. Roelandts *et al.*, *Int. J. Derm.*, 1983, *22*, 247; A. Watson, *Aust. J. Derm.*, 1983, *24*, 17; *Med. Lett.*, 1984, *26*, 56; S. Edwards, *Can. pharm. J.*, 1984, *117*, 223; *idem*, 259; R. Marks, *Prescribers' J.*, 1984, *24*, 32; G. M. Murphy and J. L. M. Hawk, *Pharm. J.*, 1984, *2*, 43.

A study in 6 patients with severe chronic actinic dermatitis and exhibiting broad action-spectrum photosensitivity indicated the importance of using a sunscreen which protects against UVA as well as UVB radiation. The authors note that the measured SPF of a preparation is usally based on UVB radiation and often does not relate to UVA radiation to which these patients are also susceptible.— B. L. Diffey and P. M. Farr, *Br. J. Derm.*, 1985, *112*, 83. A discussion on the reliability of sun protection factors.— P. M. Farr and B. L. Diffey, *ibid.*, 113.

ADVERSE EFFECTS. Of 23 patients with reactions to various sunscreen preparations 13 had a pre-existing chronic light-sensitive disorder which was exacerbated by the use of such agents. Patch and photopatch testing demonstrated the existence of plain contact allergy or photocontact allergy only to the following drugs: aminobenzoic acid, 6 and 5 patients respectively; glyceryl aminobenzoate, 1 patient for each category; padimate, 1 patient for each category; padimate O, 2 and 0 patients respectively; cinoxate, 1 and 2 patients respectively; and oxybenzone, 0 and 3 patients respectively.— P. Thune, *Photodermatol.*, 1984, *1*, 5.

7871-h

Aminobenzoic Acid *(BAN, USAN).*

Amben; PAB; PABA; Pabacidum; Para-aminobenzoic Acid; Vitamin H'. 4-Aminobenzoic acid.

$C_7H_7NO_2$=137.1.

CAS — 150-13-0.

Pharmacopoeias. In *Br., Braz., Cz., Pol., Roum., Span., Swiss,* and *U.S.*

White or slightly yellow odourless or almost odourless crystals or crystalline powder. It gradually darkens on exposure to air and light.

Slightly **soluble** in water and in chloroform; sparingly soluble in ether; soluble 1 in 8 of alcohol. *U.S.P.* states freely soluble while *B.P.* states dissolves in solutions of alkali hydroxides and carbonates. **Incompatible** with ferric salts and oxidising agents. **Store** in airtight containers. Protect from light.

Adverse Effects

Contact and photocontact allergic dermatitis has been reported following the topical administration of aminobenzoate sunscreen agents.

Facial irritation following the use of an alcoholic-based sunscreen containing 2 esters of aminobenzoic acid.— J. A. Parrish *et al.* (letter), *Archs Derm.*, 1975, *111*, 525.

A case of allergic contact photodermatitis to aminobenzoic acid in an alcohol base. Although patch tests with aminobenzoic acid in a soft paraffin basis have been recommended, photopatch tests in this patient demonstrated photosensitisation to aminobenzoic acid in an alcoholic base only, and it was therefore emphasised that the selection of an appropriate vehicle for such tests is an important consideration.— C. G. T. Mathias *et al.*, *Archs Derm.*, 1978, *114*, 1665. A similar report of allergic contact photodermatitis caused by aminobenzoic acid.— J. Marmelzat and M. J. Rapaport, *Contact Dermatitis*, 1980, *6*, 230.

Contact and photocontact allergic dermatitis from aminobenzoic acid in a 6-year-old girl with xeroderma pigmentosum; the photoallergic reaction was found to be much stronger after exposure to wavelengths within the UVA range than to those within the UVB range. Photosensitisation to UVA light could not be induced in albino *guinea-pigs* and it was concluded that although aminobenzoic acid appeared to be a very weak photosensitiser in normal subjects it may induce photoallergy when applied to diseased or damaged skin such as that in xeroderma pigmentosum.— T. Horio and T. Higuchi, *Dermatologica*, 1978, *156*, 124.

Development of vitiligo in sun-exposed areas in a 40-year-old woman and her 13-year-old daughter following self-administration of aminobenzoic acid by mouth.— C. G. Hughes (letter), *J. Am. Acad. Derm.*, 1983, *9*, 770. See also under Precautions (below).

For a further report of allergic and photoallergic reactions to aminobenzoic acid, see above.

Precautions

Aminobenzoate sunscreen agents should not be used by patients with previous experience of photosensitive or allergic reactions to chemically-related drugs such as sulphonamides, thiazide diuretics, and certain local anaesthetics, particularly benzocaine.

Aminobenzoic acid may stain clothing.

Comment that the use of orally-administered aminobenzoic acid in the prevention of phototoxic reactions should be discouraged as side-effects have been demonstrated and the benefits are unproven.— S. Worobec and A. LaChine (letter), *J. Am. med. Ass.*, 1984, *251*, 2348.

Absorption and Fate

If administered by mouth, aminobenzoic acid is absorbed from the gastro-intestinal tract. It is metabolised in the liver and excreted in the urine as unchanged drug and metabolites.

Uses and Administration

Aminobenzoic acid has sometimes been included as a member of the vitamin-B group, but deficiency of aminobenzoic acid in man or animals has not been demonstrated.

Aminobenzoic acid is used by topical application as a sunscreen agent; a concentration of 5% is commonly used. Aminobenzoic acid and its derivatives effectively absorb light throughout the UVB range but absorb little or no UVA light. Aminobenzoate sunscreen agents, therefore, may be used to prevent sunburn but are unlikely to prevent drug-related or other photosensitive reactions associated with UVA light; combination with a benzophenone, however, may give some added protection against such photosensitive disorders.

The PABA or BTPABA test is used to assess pancreatic function by measuring concentrations of aminobenzoic acid and metabolites in urine following the administration of bentiromide, a synthetic peptide derivative of aminobenzoic acid.

The efficacy of aminobenzoic acid in an alcoholic solution was greater than that of several other sunscreen agents tested (glyceryl aminobenzoate, padimate, homosalate, and some benzophenones) with protection remaining during sweating; immersion in water, however, caused a serious loss of protection. Aminobenzoic acid appeared to diffuse into the horny layer of the skin and significant protection remained for 3 days after a single application of a 5% preparation. Alcohol 50% or 60% was more effective than a number of other bases. Application of 5% alcoholic solutions once daily for 30 days did not give rise to cutaneous or systemic toxic symptoms. Aminobenzoic acid had no protective effect when given by mouth.— I. Willis and A. M. Kligman, *Archs Derm.*, 1970, *102*, 405. See also M. A. Pathak *et al.*, *New Engl. J. Med.*, 1969, *280*, 1459.

Preparations

Aminobenzoic Acid Gel *(U.S.P.)*

Aminobenzoic Acid Lotion *(B.P.).* Contains aminobenzoic acid 5% and alcohol (or industrial methylated spirit) 60%.

Aminobenzoic Acid Topical Solution *(U.S.P.).* Contains aminobenzoic acid 4.5 to 5.5% and alcohol 65 to 75%.

Proprietary Names and Manufacturers

Hachemina *(Medea, Spain)*; Hill-Shade *(Hill, USA)*; Pabagel *(Canad.)*; Pabanol *(Elder, Canad.)*; Pabina *(SCS, S.Afr.)*; Paraminan *(Gallier, Fr.)*; RVPaba *(Elder, Canad.; Elder, USA)*.

The following names have been used for multi-ingredient preparations containing aminobenzoic acid—Presun 15

Lotion *(Westwood, Canad.; Westwood, USA)*; Spectraban 15 *(Stiefel, S.Afr.; Stiefel, UK)*.

9302-p

Cinoxate *(USAN, rINN)*.
2-Ethoxyethyl *p*-methoxycinnamate.
$C_{14}H_{18}O_4$=250.3.

CAS — 104-28-9.

Pharmacopoeias. In *U.S.*

A slightly yellow, practically odourless, viscous liquid. Very slightly **soluble** in water; slightly soluble in glycerol; soluble in propylene glycol; miscible with alcohol and vegetable oils. **Store** in airtight containers. Protect from light.

Cinoxate, a substituted cinnamate, is used as a sunscreen agent by topical application; concentrations of up to 5% may be used. Cinnamate sunscreen agents effectively absorb light throughout the UVB range but absorb little or no UVA light and may therefore be used to prevent sunburn but are unlikely to prevent drug-related or other photosensitive reactions associated with UVA light. Combination with a benzophenone, however, may give some added protection against such photosensitive disorders.

Cinnamates may occasionally produce photosensitivity reactions.

Two patients developed acute inflammatory photosensitive reactions following local application of sunscreen preparations containing cinoxate; tests suggested that the reactions were of a direct phototoxicity type rather than a photoallergy.— M. G. Davies *et al.*, *Contact Dermatitis*, 1982, *8*, 190.

Further references to adverse effects: T. F. Goodman (letter), *Archs Derm.*, 1970, *102*, 563 (photocontact dermatitis).

For a further report of allergic and photoallergic reactions to cinoxate, see p.1450.

Preparations

Cinoxate Lotion *(U.S.P.)*

Proprietary Names and Manufacturers
Giv-Tan F *(Givaudan, USA)*; Sundare *(Cooper Dermatology, USA)*.

The following names have been used for multi-ingredient preparations containing cinoxate— RVPaque *(Elder, USA)*.

9303-s

Dioxybenzone *(USAN, rINN)*.
Benzophenone-8. 2,2′-Dihydroxy-4-methoxybenzophenone.
$C_{14}H_{12}O_4$=244.2.

CAS — 131-53-3.

Pharmacopoeias. In *U.S.*

An off-white to yellow powder. It congeals at not less than 68°. Practically **insoluble** in water; freely soluble in alcohol and toluene. **Store** in airtight containers. Protect from light.

Dioxybenzone, a substituted benzophenone, is a sunscreen agent similar to oxybenzone (p.1452). It is effective against UVB and some UVA light.

A report of contact dermatitis in a 46-year-old man after the use of a sunscreen preparation containing dioxybenzone and oxybenzone. Patch testing indicated sensitivity to dioxybenzone with a weak positive reaction to oxybenzone.— R. J. Pariser, *Contact Dermatitis*, 1977, *3*, 172.

Preparations

Dioxybenzone and Oxybenzone Cream *(U.S.P.)*. Dioxybenzone and oxybenzone, 2.7 to 3.3% of each.

Proprietary Names and Manufacturers
The following names have been used for multi-ingredient preparations containing dioxybenzone—Solaquin Cream *(Elder, Canad.)*; Solaquin Forte Cream *(Elder, Canad.; Elder, USA)*; Solaquin Forte Gel *(Elder, USA)*; Solbar Plus 15 *(Person & Covey, USA)*.

9324-j

Ethylhexyl *p*-Methoxycinnamate
Octyl methoxycinnamate. 2-Ethylhexyl-*p*-methoxycinnamate.
$C_{18}H_{26}O_3$=290.4.

Ethylhexyl *p*-methoxycinnamate, a substituted cinnamate, is a sunscreen agent similar to cinoxate, (above), and is effective against UVB light. It is used topically in concentrations of up to 5%.

Proprietary Preparations

Coppertone Ultrashade 23 *(Plough, UK)*. *Lotion*, ethylhexyl *p*-methoxycinnamate 7.5%, oxybenzone 3%, padimate O 2.5%.

RoC Total Sunblock Cream 15A + B (colourless or tinted) *(Roc, UK)*. *Cream*, ethylhexyl *p*-methoxycinnamate 7%, zinc oxide.

Proprietary Names and Manufacturers
Sola Stick Broad Spectrum *(Hamilton, Austral.)*; UV Sun Block *(Austral.)*; UV Sun Filter *(Austral.)*.

The following names have been used for multi-ingredient preparations containing ethylhexyl *p*-methoxycinnamate—Coppertone Ultrashade 23 *(Plough, UK)*; Piz Buin *(Greiter, Switz. : Ciba Consumer, UK)*; RoC Total Sunblock *(Roc, UK)*; Solar Block Sunstick *(Rosken, Austral.)*; Solbar PF 15 *(Person & Covey, USA)*; Uval Improved *(Dorsey Laboratories, USA)*; Uvistat Aqua Factor 10 *(Windsor, UK)*; Uvistat Sunscreen Factor 10 *(Windsor, UK)*; Uvistik *(Dalcross, Austral.)*.

9305-e

Glyceryl Aminobenzoate
Glyceryl PABA. Glyceryl 1-(4-aminobenzoate).
$C_{10}H_{13}NO_4$=211.2.

CAS — 136-44-7.

Adverse Effects and Precautions
As for Aminobenzoic Acid, p.1450.

In 20 patients previously proven to be patch-test reactive to benzocaine 5%, positive patch tests to 2 commercial samples of glyceryl aminobenzoate containing 0.3 or 0.001% of benzocaine were obtained in 11 and 0 patients respectively. The results indicated that these patients were reacting to the free benzocaine in the preparation rather than to glyceryl aminobenzoate itself.— N. Hjorth *et al.*, *Contact Dermatitis*, 1978, *4*, 46.

For a report of allergic and photoallergic reactions to glyceryl aminobenzoate, see p.1450.

Uses and Administration
Glyceryl aminobenzoate is a sunscreen agent similar to aminobenzoic acid, (p.1450). It is effective against UVB light. It is used topically in concentrations of up to 5%.

For a comparison of the efficacy of glyceryl aminobenzoate with that of aminobenzoic acid, see Aminobenzoic Acid, p.1450.

Proprietary Names and Manufacturers
Escalol 106 *(Van Dyk, USA)*; Nipa GMPA *(Nipa, UK)*.

9306-l

Homosalate *(USAN, rINN)*.
Homomenthyl Salicylate. 3,3,5-Trimethylcyclohexyl salicylate.
$C_{16}H_{22}O_3$=262.3.

CAS — 118-56-9.

Homosalate is a substituted salicylate used by topical application as a sunscreen agent; concentrations of up to 10% are employed. Salicylates effectively absorb light throughout the UVB range but absorb little or no UVA light. Salicylate sunscreen agents, therefore, may be used to prevent sunburn but are unlikely to prevent drug-related or other photosensitive reactions associated with UVA light; combination with a benzophenone, however, may give some added protection.
Salicylates may occasionally produce photosensitive reactions.

A report of 2 patients who developed contact dermatitis to homosalate.— R. L. Rietschel and C. W. Lewis, *Archs Derm.*, 1978, *114*, 442.

For a comparison of the efficacy of homosalate with that of aminobenzoic acid, see Aminobenzoic Acid, p.1450.

Proprietary Names and Manufacturers
Heliophan *(Greeff, USA)*.
The following names have been used for multi-ingredient preparations containing homosalate— Antiviray *(Bush Boake Allen, UK)*.

9307-y

Lawsone
2-Hydroxy-1,4-naphthoquinone.
$C_{10}H_6O_3$=174.2.

CAS — 83-72-7.

Lawsone is a dye present in henna, the leaves of *Lawsonia* spp., and may also be prepared synthetically.

Lawsone has been used with dihydroxyacetone in sunscreen preparations. There appears to be no evidence that it has any sunscreening properties when used alone.

9327-k

3-(4-Methylbenzylidene)bornan-2-one
3-(4-Methylbenzylidene)camphor.
$C_{18}H_{22}O$=254.4.

CAS — 36861-47-9.

3-(4-Methylbenzylidene)bornan-2-one is a camphor derivative used as a sunscreen agent. It is used topically in concentrations of up to 6%.

Allergic contact dermatitis from 3-(4-methylbenzylidene)bornan-2-one developed in a 17-year-old patient.— W. Hunloh and G. Goerz, *Contact Dermatitis*, 1983, *9*, 333.

Proprietary Names and Manufacturers
Eusolex 6300 *(E. Merck, UK)*.

The following names have been used for multi-ingredient preparations containing 3-(4-methylbenzylidene)bornan-2-one—Delial 10 *(Bayer, UK)*.

18316-f

5-Methyl-2-phenylbenzoxazole
2-Phenyl-5-methylbenzoxazole.
$C_{14}H_{11}NO$=209.2.

CAS — 7420-86-2.

5-Methyl-2-phenylbenzoxazole is used topically as a sunscreen agent in concentrations of up to 4%.

A report of contact dermatitis to 5-methyl-2-phenylbenzoxazole [an ingredient of Delial Factor 10].— N. -J. Mørk and J. Austad, *Contact Dermatitis*, 1984, *10*, 122.

Proprietary Names and Manufacturers
The following names have been used for multi-ingredient preparations containing 5-methyl-2-phenylbenzoxazole—Delial 10 *(Bayer, UK)*.

9310-p

Mexenone *(BAN, pINN)*.
Benzophenone-10. 2-Hydroxy-4-methoxy-4′-methylbenzophenone.
$C_{15}H_{14}O_3$=242.3.

CAS — 1641-17-4.

Pharmacopoeias. In *Br.*

A pale yellow odourless or almost odourless crystalline powder. Practically **insoluble** in water; soluble 1 in 70 of alcohol and 1 in 7 of acetone.

Mexenone, a substituted benzophenone, is a sunscreen agent similar to oxybenzone (p.1452). It is effective against UVB and some UVA light. It is used topically in concentrations of up to 4%.

Preparations

Mexenone Cream *(B.P.)*

Proprietary Preparations

Uvistat *(Windsor, UK)*. *Cream* (Uvistat Sunscreen Factor 10), mexenone 4%, Parsol Mcx [ethylhexyl *p*-methoxycinnamate] 7.5%.

Cream (Uvistat Aqua Factor 10), mexenone 4%, Parsol Mcx [ethylhexyl *p*-methoxycinnamate] 7.5% in water resistant basis.
Cream (Uvistat Sun Cream Factor 4), mexenone 4%.
Lipstick (Uvistat-L Factor 5), mexenone 4%.

Proprietary Names and Manufacturers
Uvicone *(Austral.)*; Uvistat *(Boehringer Ingelheim, Austral.)*; Uvistat Sun Cream Factor 4 *(Windsor, UK)*; Uvistat-L Factor 5 *(Windsor, UK)*.

The following names have been used for multi-ingredient preparations containing mexenone— Uvistat Aqua Factor 10 *(Windsor, UK)*; Uvistat Sunscreen Factor 10 *(Windsor, UK)*; Uvistat-L *(Boehringer Ingelheim, Austral.)*.

9312-w

Oxybenzone *(USAN, rINN)*.
Benzophenone-3. 2-Hydroxy-4-methoxybenzophenone.
$C_{14}H_{12}O_3$=228.2.

CAS — 131-57-7.

Pharmacopoeias. In *U.S.*

A white to off-white powder. It congeals at not less than 62°. Practically **insoluble** in water; freely soluble in alcohol and toluene. **Store** in airtight containers. Protect from light.

Oxybenzone is a substituted benzophenone used by topical application as a sunscreen agent in concentrations of up to 10%. Benzophenones effectively absorb light throughout the UVB range (wavelengths 290 to 320 nm) and also absorb some UVA light with wavelengths of 320 to about 360 nm and some UVC light with wavelengths of about 250 nm to 290 nm. Benzophenones, therefore, may be used to prevent sunburn and may also provide some protection against drug-related or other photosensitive reactions associated with UVA light.

Contact and photocontact allergic dermatitis has occasionally been reported following the topical administration of benzophenone sunscreen agents.

Allergic contact dermatitis in one patient attributed to dioxybenzone and oxybenzone.— G. Thompson *et al.*, *Archs Derm.*, 1977, *113*, 1252.

For a report of photoallergic reactions to oxybenzone, see p.1450.

For a comparison of the efficacy of some benzophenones with that of aminobenzoic acid, see Aminobenzoic Acid, p.1450.

Proprietary Preparations

Coppertone Sunblock Milk (formerly known as Coppertone Supershade 15) *(Plough, UK)*. *Lotion*, padimate O 7%, oxybenzone 3%.

Piz Buin *(Greiter, Switz.: Ciba Consumer, UK)*. *Cream* (Factor 6), ethylhexyl *p*-methoxycinnamate 4.1%, oxybenzone 1.3%.
Cream (Factor 8), ethylhexyl *p*-methoxycinnamate 4.8%, oxybenzone 1.7%.
Cream (Factor 12), ethylhexyl *p*-methoxycinnamate 4.8%, oxybenzone 2.2%, talc 4.5%, zinc oxide 4.5%.
Lipstick (Factor 8), ethylhexyl *p*-methoxycinnamate 4.8%, oxybenzone 2.2%.

Proprietary Names and Manufacturers
The following names have been used for multi-ingredient preparations containing oxybenzone—Blistik Medicated Lip Balm *(Key, Austral.)*; Block-Aid *(Elder, Canad.)*; Coppertone Sunblock Milk *(Plough, UK)*; Coppertone Supershade 15 *(Plough, UK)*; Coppertone Ultrashade 23 *(Plough, UK)*; Episun *(Schering, Canad.)*; Esoterica Facial *(Lentheric Morny, UK)*; Esoterica Fortified *(USV, Austral.; Lentheric Morny, UK)*; Pabafilm 10 *(Alcon, Austral.; Alcon, Canad.)*; Pabafilm 15 *(Alcon, Austral.; Alcon, Canad.)*; Paba-Tan-12 *(Ayerst, Canad.)*; Paba-Tan-21 *(Ayerst, Canad.)*; Piz Buin *(Greiter, Switz. : Ciba Consumer, UK)*; Presun 15 Cream and Lotion *(Westwood, Canad.; Westwood, USA)*; Presun 8 *(Westwood, Canad.; Westwood, USA)*; Solaquin Cream *(Elder, Canad.)*; Solaquin-Forte Cream *(Elder, USA)*; Solar Block Lotion and Sunstick *(Rosken, Austral.)*; Solbar PF 15 *(Person & Covey, USA)*; Solbar Plus 15 *(Person & Covey, USA)*; Total Eclipse *(Dorsey Laboratories, USA)*; Ultrastop SPF15 *(Canderm, Canad.)*; Uval Improved *(Dorsey Laboratories, USA)*.

9313-e

Padimate *(BAN, rINN)*.
Amyl Dimethylaminobenzoate; Isoamyl Dimethylaminobenzoate; Padimate A *(USAN)*. A mixture of pentyl, isopentyl, and 2-methylbutyl 4-dimethylaminobenzoates.
$C_{14}H_{21}NO_2$=235.3.

CAS — 14779-78-3.

Adverse Effects and Precautions
As for Aminobenzoic Acid, p.1450.

Using a newly developed procedure, phototoxicity to padimate, a substance previously considered to be non-photosensitising, was demonstrated in healthy subjects. It was considered that phototoxic reactions to padimate may occur but since the reactions might be indistinguishable from sunburn, users might conclude that the sunscreen was ineffective.— K. H. Kaidbey and A. M. Kligman, *Archs Derm.*, 1978, *114*, 547.

For a further report of allergic and photoallergic reactions to padimate, see p.1450.

Uses and Administration
Padimate, a substituted aminobenzoate, is a sunscreen agent similar to aminobenzoic acid (p.1450), and is effective against UVB light. It is used topically in concentrations of up to 5%.

For a comparison of the efficacy of padimate with that of aminobenzoic acid, see Aminobenzoic Acid, p.1450.

Proprietary Names and Manufacturers
Escalol 506 *(Van Dyk, USA : Black, UK)*; Lipguard Gel *(Nelson, Austral.)*; Pabafilm *(Alcon, Austral.; USA)*; Spectraban 4 *(Stiefel, Ger.; S. Afr.)*; Uvosan *(Prosana, Austral.)*.

The following names have been used for multi-ingredient preparations containing padimate—Spectraban 15 *(Stiefel, S.Afr.)*.

9314-l

Padimate O *(USAN)*.
Octyl dimethyl PABA. 2-Ethylhexyl 4-(dimethylamino)benzoate.
$C_{17}H_{27}NO_2$=277.4.

CAS — 21245-02-3.

Adverse Effects and Precautions
As for Aminobenzoic Acid, p.1450.

A case of photocontact allergy to padimate O following its use over a period of 2 months.— P. Weller and S. Freeman, *Aust. J. Derm.*, 1984, *25*, 73.

For a further report of allergic reactions to padimate O, see p.1450.

Uses and Administration
Padimate O, a substituted aminobenzoate, is a sunscreen agent similar to aminobenzoic acid (p.1450) and is effective against UVB light. It is used topically in concentrations of up to 8%.

Proprietary Preparations
Spectraban *(Stiefel, UK)*. *Lotion* (Spectraban 4), padimate O 3.2%, in alcohol.
Lotion (Spectraban 15), padimate O 3.2%, aminobenzoic acid 5%, in alcohol.

Proprietary Names and Manufacturers
Chap Stick *(Robins Consumer Products, UK)*; Chapstick *(Robins, Austral.)*; Escalol 507 *(Van Dyk, USA : Black, UK)*; Lip-Sed Jel *(Rosken, Austral.)*; Lip-Sed Stick *(Rosken, Austral.)*; Pabafilm 5 *(Alcon, Canad.)*; Paba-Tan *(Ayerst, Canad.)*; Phiasol *(Robins, Austral.)*; Presun 4 *(Westwood, Canad.; Westwood, USA)*; Spectraban 4 *(Stiefel, UK)*.

The following names have been used for multi-ingredient preparations containing padimate O—Banquin *(Kramer, USA)*; Blistik Medicated Lip Balm *(Key, Austral.)*; Coppertone Sunblock Milk *(Plough, UK)*; Coppertone Supershade 15 *(Plough, UK)*; Coppertone Ultrashade 23 *(Plough, UK)*; Episun *(Schering, Canad.)*; Esoterica Facial *(Lentheric Morny, UK)*; Esoterica Fortified *(USV, Austral.; Lentheric Morny, UK)*; Herpecin-L *(Campbell, USA)*; Pabafilm 10 *(Alcon, Austral.; Alcon, Canad.)*; Pabafilm 15 *(Alcon, Austral.; Alcon, Canad.)*; Paba-Tan-12 *(Ayerst, Canad.)*; Paba-Tan-21 *(Ayerst, Canad.)*; Presun 15 Cream and Lotion *(Westwood, Canad.; Westwood, USA)*; Presun 8 *(Westwood, Canad.; Westwood, USA)*; Solar Block Lotion *(Rosken, Austral.)*; Solbar Plus 15 *(Person & Covey, USA)*; Spectraban 15 *(Stiefel, UK)*; Total Eclipse *(Dorsey Laboratories, USA)*; Ultrastop SPF15 *(Canderm, Canad.)*; Uvistat-L *(Boehringer Ingelheim, Austral.)*.

9329-t

2-Phenyl-1*H*-benzimidazole-5-sulphonic Acid

$C_{13}H_{10}N_2O_3S$=274.3.

CAS — 27503-81-7.

2-Phenyl-1*H*-benzimidazole-5-sulphonic acid is used as a sunscreen agent in concentrations of up to 8%.

Proprietary Names and Manufacturers
Eusolex 232 *(E. Merck, UK)*.

The following names have been used for multi-ingredient preparations containing 2-phenyl-1*H*-benzimidazole-5-sulphonic acid— Delial 10 *(Bayer, UK)*.

9316-j

Sulisobenzone *(USAN, rINN)*.
Benzophenone-4. 5-Benzoyl-4-hydroxy-2-methoxybenzenesulphonic acid.
$C_{14}H_{12}O_6S$=308.3.

CAS — 4065-45-6.

Sulisobenzone, a substituted benzophenone, is a sunscreen agent similar to oxybenzone (above). It is effective against UVB and some UVA light. It is used topically in concentrations of up to 5%.

A report of both immediate urticaria and delayed contact sensitivity to sulisobenzone being used by a 54-year-old black male for broad-spectrum light sensitivity.— D. L. Ramsay *et al.*, *Archs Derm.*, 1972, *105*, 906.

Proprietary Names and Manufacturers
Cyasorb UV 284 *(Cyanamid, UK)*; Uval *(Dorsey Laboratories, USA)*; Uvinul MS-40 *(BASF, UK)*.

Sympathomimetics

2040-z

This section includes those agents that have actions similar to those that follow stimulation of postganglionic sympathetic or adrenergic nerves.

Adverse Effects of Sympathomimetics

Sympathomimetics may produce a wide range of adverse effects, most of which mimic the results of excessive stimulation of the sympathetic nervous system. These effects are mediated via the various types of adrenergic receptor, and the adverse effects of an individual drug depend to some extent upon its relative agonist activity on these different types of receptor at a given dose.

Central effects of sympathomimetic agents include fear, anxiety, restlessness, tremor, insomnia, confusion, irritability, weakness, and psychotic states. Appetite may be reduced, and nausea and vomiting may occur.

Effects on the cardiovascular system are complex: stimulation of alpha-adrenergic receptors produces vasoconstriction, sometimes sufficiently severe to produce gangrene when infiltrated into the digits, with resultant hypertension; the rise in blood pressure may produce cerebral haemorrhage and pulmonary oedema. There may also be a reflex bradycardia, but stimulation of β_1-adrenergic receptors of the heart may produce tachycardia and cardiac arryhthmias, anginal pain, palpitations, and cardiac arrest; hypotension with dizziness and fainting, and flushing, may occur. An increased incidence of sudden death, perhaps as a result of the induction of ventricular arrhythmias, has been associated with the excessive use of sympathomimetic agents in aerosol form; although the association has been questioned by some authorities, it is important to avoid excessive doses.

Other effects that may occur with sympathomimetic agents include difficulty in micturition and urinary retention, dyspnoea, altered metabolism including disturbances of glucose metabolism, sweating, and hypersalivation. Headache is also common.

Extravasation of parenterally-administered catecholamines may result in tissue necrosis and sloughing. Myocardial and arterial necrosis have been reported in some patients given prolonged infusions of noradrenaline.

SUDDEN DEATH. Between 1961 and 1966, rapid growth in the sales of pressurised aerosols of sympathomimetics in England and Wales corresponded with an increase in mortality due to asthma. The increase was greatest in children aged 10 to 14 years. Since March 1967, there had been a sharp fall in deaths due to asthma, together with a reduction in the use of pressurised aerosols.— W. H. W. Inman and A. M. Adelstein, *Lancet*, 1969, *2*, 279. See also H. E. Lewis (letter), *ibid.*, 799; *ibid.*, 800. For a similar report for Eire, see W. D. Linehan (letter), *Br. med. J.*, 1969, *4*, 172.

Comment on the surge in asthma fatalities that occurred in the 1960s and the growing realisation that pressurised aerosols were probably not the main culprit.— *Lancet*, 1979, *2*, 337. Strong disagreement with the view that the evidence is declining that pressurised aerosols were reponsible for the epidemic of asthma deaths in the 1960s.— P. D. Stolley and R. Schinnar (letter), *ibid.*, 897. Overuse of isoprenaline aerosols results in tolerance, not toxicity and the conclusion from this and other data can only be that the rise and fall of asthma mortality has a multifactorial aetiology which is only partly known.— H. Herxheimer (letter), *ibid.*, 1084. Following a general alert and warning on aerosol canisters, asthma mortality quickly declined to its former level.— A. M. Adelstein (letter), *Lancet*, 1979, *2*, 1247.

Early information from the British Thoracic Association's confidential enquiry into asthma deaths has indicated that, in general, patients die from asthma rather than from its treatment. When excessive use of bronchodilators does occasionally coincide with asthma death, it is likely that this indicates the need for further treatment by other drugs such as corticosteroids and is not itself the cause of death.— C. J. Stewart *et al.* (letter), *Lancet*, 1981, *2*, 747. Further comment. In contrast to suggestions that excessive treatment is implicated in asthma deaths, treatment in most fatal attacks in the British Thoracic Association study had been inadequate. Both doctors and patients underestimated the severity of the attacks, and doctors appeared reluctant to prescribe corticosteroids for severe asthmatic episodes. About a quarter of the deaths occurred less than an hour after the start of an exacerbation; patients showing such rapid deterioration were particularly vulnerable, and if rapid deterioration had been observed in the past, patients should have suitable treatment available at home and have access to immediate further help.— J. Rees, *Br. med. J.*, 1984, *288*, 1441.

Precautions for Sympathomimetics

Sympathomimetic agents should be used with caution in patients who may be hypersusceptible to their effects, particularly those with hyperthyroidism. Great care is also needed in patients with cardiovascular disease such as ischaemic heart disease; arrhythmia or tachycardia; occlusive vascular disorders, including arteriosclerosis; hypertension; or aneurysms. Anginal pain may be precipitated in patients with angina pectoris. Excessive administration to the nasal mucosa may produce rebound congestion and rhinorrhoea.

Care is also required when sympathomimetics are given to patients with diabetes mellitus or closed-angle glaucoma.

Tolerance may develop in asthmatic patients given sympathomimetics for their bronchodilator effects; if tolerance occurs and the patient's condition worsens, alternative or additional therapy should be instituted. The dose of the sympathomimetic should not be increased in such cases.

Sympathomimetics should be avoided or used with caution in patients undergoing anaesthesia with cyclopropane, halothane, or other halogenated anaesthetics, as they may induce ventricular fibrillation. An increased risk of arrhythmias may also occur if sympathomimetic agents are given to patients receiving cardiac glycosides, quinidine, or tricyclic antidepressants.

Many sympathomimetics interact with monoamine oxidase inhibitors, and should not be given to patients receiving such treatment or within 14 days of its termination (see phenelzine sulphate, p.378).

Reversal of the action of many antihypertensive agents occurs in patients given sympathomimetics and therefore special care is advisable in patients receiving antihypertensive therapy. Interactions of sympathomimetic agents with alpha- and beta-blocking drugs may be complex.

Action and Use of Sympathomimetics

Sympathomimetic agents mimic the actions produced by stimulation of postganglionic sympathetic or adrenergic nerves, including stimulation of the heart and central nervous system, vasoconstriction of blood vessels supplying skin and mucous membranes, dilatation of the bronchi and of blood vessels supplying skeletal muscle, and modulation of metabolism. Within the body 3 catecholamine sympathetic agents occur: noradrenaline, which is the endogenous neurotransmitter at postganglionic sympathetic nerves and within the central nervous system; adrenaline, with predominantly metabolic functions; and dopamine, which is predominantly a central neurotransmitter.

Sympathomimetic agents differ in their actions according to the receptors at which they act. The basic subdivision, first postulated by R.P. Ahlquist (*Am. J. Physiol.*, 1948, *153*, 586) is into alpha- and beta-adrenergic receptors. These may be further categorised into:

α_1 receptors, which are predominantly located at postsynaptic sites on smooth muscle and glands, and which are involved in the vasoconstrictor actions of sympathomimetics;

α_2 receptors, believed to exist on presynaptic nerve terminals, are thought to be involved in feedback inhibition of neurotransmitter release and may be responsible for the inhibition of intestinal activity seen with alpha-adrenergic agonists;

β_1 receptors, which are involved in the effects of sympathomimetics on the heart;

β_2 receptors, which amongst other effects, mediate bronchodilatation.

Adrenergic receptors in the CNS remain largely unclassified at present; dopamine acts at specific dopaminergic receptors within the CNS, and possibly at some peripheral sites.

Sympathomimetic agents may act directly upon the adrenergic receptor, or indirectly, acting by the release of stored noradrenaline from nerve endings; many, such as ephedrine, possess a mixture of direct and indirect actions.

Sympathomimetic agents possess a wide variety of uses. Many, such as ephedrine, salbutamol, and terbutaline, have been used for their bronchodilator properties in the treatment of asthma and similar respiratory disorders, either by mouth or more commonly by inhalation.

Other agents have been used for their effects on the cardiovascular system in the treatment of heart block, heart failure or shock; or in the treatment of nasal congestion. Agents such as ritodrine, salbutamol, or terbutaline have also been employed in the prevention of premature labour.

Other sympathomimetics used for their central stimulant and anoretic effects may be found under Stimulants and Anorectics, p.1439.

2041-c

Adrenaline *(BAN)*.

Epinefrina; Epinephrine *(USAN, rINN)*; Epinephrinum; Epirenamine; Levorenin; Suprarenin.

(−)-1-(3,4-Dihydroxyphenyl)-2-methylaminoethanol.

$C_9H_{13}NO_3$=183.2.

CAS — 51-43-4.

Pharmacopoeias. In *Arg., Belg., Br., Braz., Chin., Egypt., Hung., Ind., Int., It., Jpn, Mex., Neth., Nord., Pol., Port., Roum., Span., Turk.*, and *U.S. U.S.* also includes Racepinephrine, which is the racemic substance, and Racepinephrine Hydrochloride.

Adrenaline is an active principle of the medulla of the adrenal gland. It may be obtained from the adrenal glands of certain mammals or it may be prepared synthetically. Endogenous adrenaline and the monograph substance are the laevo isomer.

A white or creamy-white, odourless, crystalline powder or granules. It darkens in colour on exposure to air and light.

Sparingly **soluble** in water; practically insoluble in alcohol, chloroform, ether, and fixed and volatile oils. Adrenaline dissolves in solutions of mineral acids and in solutions of sodium or potassium hydroxide, but not in solutions of ammonia or of the alkali carbonates. Solutions in water are alkaline to litmus. It is unstable in neutral or alkaline solution which rapidly becomes red on exposure to air. **Store** in airtight containers, preferably in which the air has been replaced by nitrogen. Protect from light.

2042-k

Adrenaline Acid Tartrate *(BAN)*.

Adrenaline Bitartrate; Adrenaline Tartrate; Adrenalini Bitartras; Adrenalinii Tartras; Adrenalinium Hydrogentartaricum; Epinephrine Bitartrate *(USAN, rINNM)*; Epinephrine Hydrogen Tartrate; Epirenamine Bitartrate.

$C_9H_{13}NO_3,C_4H_6O_6$=333.3.

CAS — 51-42-3.

Pharmacopoeias. In *Aust., Belg., Br., Braz., Cz., Egypt., Eur., Fr., Ger., Ind., Int., It., Jug., Neth., Nord., Rus., Swiss, Turk.*, and *U.S.* Also in *B.P.Vet.*

A white to greyish-white or light brownish-grey, odourless, crystalline powder. It slowly darkens on exposure to air and light. Adrenaline acid tartrate 1.8 mg is approximately equivalent to 1 mg of adrenaline.

Soluble 1 in 3 of water; slightly soluble in alcohol; practically insoluble in chloroform and ether. The *B.P.* injection has a pH of 2.8 to 3.6 and is **sterilised** by autoclaving. Aqueous solutions have their optimum stability at about pH 3.6.

Store in airtight containers, preferably in a vacuum-sealed tube or in an atmosphere of inert gas. Protect from light.

STABILITY. A solution of adrenaline 0.1% (as acid tartrate) and sodium metabisulphite 0.1% with a pH of 3.6 in full 2-mL ampoules was sterilised by autoclaving. Bio-assay showed little loss of potency after storage for 6 years at room temperature in the dark. Over the same period slightly greater losses occurred at pH 3.0 and 4.2.— G. B. West, *J. Pharm. Pharmac.*, 1950, *2*, 864.

Degradation of adrenaline solutions stored in an oxygen-free atmosphere proceeded at a faster rate in the presence of sodium metabisulphite than in its absence probably due to the formation of an addition compound.— L. C. Schroeter *et al.*, *J. Am. pharm. Ass., scient. Edn*, 1958, *47*, 723. See also T. Higuchi and L. C. Schroeter, *ibid.*, 1959, *48*, 535. It was postulated that boric acid stabilised adrenaline against degradation by sodium metabisulphite in an oxygen-free atmosphere, and that this was due to chelation of the adrenaline by the boric acid; the degree of chelation and the consequent stability of the adrenaline increased with rise of pH. If, however, a solution of adrenaline with sodium metabisulphite was exposed to atmospheric oxygen, oxidation was not prevented by the addition of boric acid. At a pH above 4.5 the metabisulphite was oxidised even in the dark; after this oxidation was complete the adrenaline was stable for several days, if kept in the dark, but quickly started to oxidise with the development of a red colour on exposure to light.— S. Riegelman and E. Z. Fischer, *J. pharm. Sci.*, 1962, *51*, 206 and 210.

The stability during storage of adrenaline injection 1 in 10 000 was investigated. Solutions were prepared to the following formulas: (1) adrenaline acid tartrate 18 mg, sodium metabisulphite 100 mg, sodium chloride 800 mg, Water for Injections to 100 mL (pH 4.15); (2) as formula 1, but with the addition of 50 mg of tartaric acid. Both solutions were autoclaved at 115° for 30 minutes. The percentage losses after autoclaving, after 2 weeks' and after 5 weeks' storage at 37° were respectively 1.3, 3.9, and 6% for formula 1, and 0.4, 2.8, and 5.6% for formula 2.— Pharm. Soc. Lab. Rep. No. 21, 1964.

Adrenaline injection 0.1% (pH 3.6), containing adrenaline acid tartrate 0.182%, sodium chloride 0.8%, sodium metabisulphite 0.05%, and Water for Injections to 100 mL (K. Backe-Hansen *et al.*, *J. Pharm. Pharmac.*, 1963, *15*, 804), and sterilised by autoclaving at 120° for 20 minutes showed no decrease in biological activity after storage for 5 years in the dark at 4°. Non-stabilised injections (pH 3) had lost about 10% activity.— K. Backe-Hansen *et al.*, *Acta pharm. suec.*, 1966, *3*, 269.

The shelf-life of 1 and 2% lignocaine hydrochloride injections containing adrenaline 0.001%, sodium metabisulphite 0.05%, methyl hydroxybenzoate 0.1%, 0.03M acetate buffer to pH 4.0 or 4.4, and sodium chloride sufficient to produce an iso-osmotic solution was studied by accelerated storage tests. It was estimated that adrenaline would lose 15% of its potency anaerobically at pH 4.4 in 15 months at 30°, 11 years at 15°, and 31 years at 8°. As *U.S.P.* injections could have a pH of up to 5.5, injections should be stored in a cold place and the upper limit of pH should be 4.4.— B. R. Hajratwala, *Drug Dev. ind. Pharm.*, 1977, *3*, 65. See also *idem*, *J. pharm. Sci.*, 1975, *64*, 45.

A study of the effect of anaerobic processing and varying concentrations of sodium metabisulphite on the stability of Adrenaline Injection (*B.P. 1980*). [The *B.P. 1988* does not specify sodium metabisulphite in Adrenaline Injection]. Samples of 0.1% adrenaline injection were prepared from adrenaline acid tartrate, to contain 0.001%, 0.005%, 0.01%, 0.05%, and 0.1% sodium metabisulphite, or none at all; samples were prepared both in air and under nitrogen and the pH was adjusted to 3.6. When prepared in air, minimum degradation, as assessed by high-performance liquid chromatography, was observed over 2 months after storage at 35° in samples containing 0.005 and 0.01% metabisulphite. These were the only samples that remained colourless, the others turning pink and developing black particles; however, even at these concentrations there was a substantial fall in pH and a loss of adrenaline of about 6 to 8%. Visible degradation of injections prepared under nitrogen occurred only in the absence of metabisulphite or at its lowest concentration. However, at the highest concentrations of sodium metabisulphite increased degradation of adrenaline occurred due to sulphonation; the optimum stability was achieved with 0.005% metabisulphite. It was concluded that 0.005% sodium metabisulphite would be the optimum concentration where exclusion of air during processing can be guaranteed; the inclusion of 0.1%, as specified by the *B.P. 1980* may be a reasonable compromise if manufacture and filling are not adequately controlled to exclude air, but degradation of adrenaline to the inactive sulphonate will still lead to an inconveniently short shelf-life.— J. B. Taylor *et al.*, *Pharm. J.*, 1984, *1*, 646.

Adverse Effects

For adverse effects of sympathomimetics, see p.1453.

Melanin-like deposits in the cornea and conjunctiva may follow the use of eye-drops of adrenaline and have also caused obstruction of the naso-lachrymal ducts. Repeated ocular administration of adrenaline may cause oedema, hyperaemia, and inflammation of the eyes.

Inhalation of adrenaline may cause epigastric pain and the mouth and throat should be rinsed with water after inhaling.

Adrenaline eye-drops may, rarely, cause faintness, trembling, sweating, headache, and hypertension. Adrenaline can be absorbed from the eye in amounts large enough to react with MAOIs and cause hypertensive crisis.— *Med. Lett.*, 1982, *24*, 53. See also C. R. Kerr, *Br. J. Ophthal.*, 1982, *66*, 109. and under Effects on the Eyes, below.

EFFECTS ON ELECTROLYTES. Adrenaline appears to produce hypokalaemia via a specific action on β_2-adrenergic receptors and may be responsible physiologically for the hypokalaemia associated with myocardial infarction.— M. J. Brown *et al.*, *New Engl. J. Med.*, 1983, *309*, 1414. Comment on the role of the sympathetic nervous system in potassium regulation.— F. H. Epstein and R. M. Rosa, *ibid.*, 1450. Criticism.— S. G. Ball *et al.* (letter), *ibid.*, 1984, *310*, 1330.

EFFECTS ON THE EYES. During 4 years, 15 patients showed reactions to adrenaline eye-drops, usually 2% of the hydrochloride or acid tartrate, while some used 1% epinephryl borate. Blurring and distortion of vision were followed by decreased visual acuity, and by the appearance of oedema and sometimes haemorrhage in the macular region. A few patients developed cysts near the fovea. These effects appeared within a few weeks of, or several months after, commencement of therapy and were usually reversible. All except 1 of the patients were aphakic (devoid of lens). In a study of 200 consecutive patients receiving adrenaline therapy, 23 were aphakic, and 7 experienced these reactions to adrenaline.— A. E. Kolker and B. Becker, *Archs Ophthal., N.Y.*, 1968, *79*, 552.

EFFECTS ON THE HEART. A report of severe myocardial ischaemia following injection of adrenaline 300 µg intravenously, rather than subcutaneously, to combat anaphylaxis.— A. Horak *et al.*, *Br. med. J.*, 1983, *286*, 519. See also E. M. Barach *et al.*, *J. Am. med. Ass.*, 1984, *251*, 2118.

EFFECTS ON THE SALIVARY GLANDS. Non-inflammatory enlargement of salivary glands (termed sialosis) is sometimes encountered in asthmatic patients having sustained treatment with sympathomimetic drugs.— D. K. Mason and M. M. Ferguson, *Practitioner*, 1978, *221*, 571.

ISCHAEMIA. Extravasation of adrenaline or noradrenaline can cause intense local vasoconstriction with ischaemia of the skin leading to necrosis.— N. R. Gaze, *Lancet*, 1978, *2*, 417.

Gas gangrene associated with intramuscular injection. A fatal occurrence of gas gangrene after the intramuscular injection of adrenaline in oil in the left buttock.— R. Van Hook and A. G. Vandevelde (letter), *Ann. intern. Med.*, 1975, *83*, 669. Further references: W. B. Maguire and N. F. Langley, *Med. J. Aust.*, 1967, *1*, 973; P. W. Harvey and G. V. Purnell, *Br. med. J.*, 1968, *1*, 744; H. Gaylis (letter), *ibid.*, 1968, *3*, 59.

Topical application. Severe skin necrosis and cellulitis in 1 patient were attributed to vasoconstriction following liberal application of a cream containing adrenaline 0.02%.— R. M. Antrum and J. B. Kersley, *Br. J. clin. Pract.*, 1984, *38*, 191.

OVERDOSAGE. A report of inadvertent administration to a 13-month-old infant of a solution containing racemic adrenaline meant for nebulisation. The infant received approximately 327 µg per kg body-weight of *l*-adrenaline intravenously. Marked pallor, pulselessness, and profound bradycardia ensued, but the child responded to cardiopulmonary resuscitation and was subsequently discharged with no evidence of long-term sequelae.— S. C. Kurachek and M. A. Rockoff, *J. Am. med. Ass.*, 1985, *253*, 1441.

PREGNANCY AND THE NEONATE. A recurring medication error which mimicked an epidemic of neonatal sepsis involved the inadvertent substitution of inhalant adrenaline for vitamin E given to neonates via a nasogastric tube as a nutritional supplement. Six babies were affected, and required mechanical ventilation for progressive respiratory insufficiency. One of the 6 died, and was found at autopsy to have extensive necrosis of the gut mucosa, but the remaining infants subsequently recovered.— S. L. Solomon *et al.*, *New Engl. J. Med.*, 1984, *310*, 166.

A report of tachycardia and acute heart failure in 4 neonates following application of a sponge soaked in adrenaline 0.1% solution to stop bleeding after ritual circumcision. The use of topical adrenaline after circumcision should be prohibited.— A. Mor *et al.*, *Archs Dis. Childh.*, 1987, *62*, 80.

Treatment of Adverse Effects

Because of the short duration of the adverse effects of adrenaline, due to inactivation in the body, treatment of severe toxic reactions in hypersensitive patients or after overdose is primarily supportive. Prompt injection of a rapidly-acting alpha-adrenergic blocking agent, such as phentolamine, followed by a beta blocker such as propranolol, has been tried to counteract the pressor and arrhythmogenic effect of adrenaline; rapidly-acting vasodilators such as glyceryl trinitrate have also been used.

Precautions

For precautions necessary with sympathomimetics, see p.1453.

Discussion of drug-induced staining of soft-contact lenses. Adrenochrome staining of contact lenses of patients using adrenaline eye-drops has been reported. Melanin deposits may also become locked into the lens; such deposits may be broken down by hydrogen peroxide but in practice the lens is usually discarded. Patients prescribed drugs likely to cause this problem should be given appropriate warning.— D. V. Ingram, *Br. med. J.*, 1986, *292*, 1619.

INTERACTIONS. A review of the factors and interactions affecting the use of vasoconstrictors in local anaesthetics. There is no special risk in patients on *monoamine oxidase inhibitors*, since inactivation depends chiefly on uptake into nerves and tissues and not upon metabolism; patients taking these drugs have a normal response to intravenous doses of adrenaline and noradrenaline, though they are at risk from a pressor crisis if noradrenaline-releasing agents, such as tyramine are used. Drugs that blockade adrenergic neurones increase sensitivity to circulating catecholamines several-fold, as do the *tricyclic antidepressants* such as imipramine, which block the uptake of adrenaline and noradrenaline into nerves; in each case enhancement of the effect of the catecholamines is likely to be important only if a dose is injected intravenously.— *Br. med. J.*, 1970, *4*, 633.

Anaesthetic agents. Sensitisation of the myocardium to β-adrenergic stimulation caused by some anaesthetics was of clinical importance when adrenaline was injected into an operation area to reduce bleeding. It had been considered that adrenaline could not be given when the patient had been anaesthetised with cyclopropane, halothane, or similar anaesthetics. However, it was now evident that adrenaline could safely be used so long as the dose was small and other factors likely to increase the irritability of the myocardium, such as carbon-dioxide retention, hypoxia, or the simultaneous use of cocaine were avoided. The conclusions of R.L. Katz and G.J. Katz (*Br. J. Anaesth.*, 1966, *38*, 712) were that provided the solution of adrenaline was not stronger than 1 in 100 000 and that the rate of injection did not exceed 10 mL per 10 minutes or 30 mL an hour no serious results should ensue under halothane or trichloroethylene anaesthesia. The technique should not be used with cyclopropane. Where a high risk of intravascular injection occurred, such as in the sub-occipital area, the neck, the broad ligaments of the uterus, and in the erectile tissue of the external genitalia in both sexes, a vasoconstrictor drug which would not produce arrhythmias, such as felypressin, might be valuable.— *Lancet*, 1967, *1*, 484. Cyclopropane could also be used although the risk of arrhythmias was higher than with halothane or trichloroethylene.— R. L. Katz and R. A. Epstein, *Anesthesiology*, 1968, *29*, 763.

In 19 patients undergoing cataract removal under halothane anaesthesia, with lignocaine used to provide topical anaesthesia of the larynx, adrenaline 0.4 to 68 μg per kg body-weight by intra-ocular injection did not increase the incidence of cardiac arrhythmias compared with a control group.— R. B. Smith *et al.*, *Br. J. Anaesth.*, 1972, *44*, 1314.

Beta blockers. A review of the effects of beta blockers on adrenaline. Patients given adrenaline while receiving non-selective beta blockers such as propranolol develop elevated blood pressure due to alpha-mediated vasoconstriction, followed by reflex bradycardia, and occasionally arrhythmias; the bronchodilator effects of adrenaline are also inhibited. In contrast, cardioselective beta blockers such as metoprolol, which act preferentially at $beta_1$ adrenergic receptors, do not prevent adrenaline-induced vasodilation via $beta_2$ receptors, and in consequence blood pressure and heart-rate change only minimally. Low doses of cardioselective beta blockers do not appear to interfere with adrenaline-induced bronchodilation, although the effect of larger doses is uncertain.— *Drug Interact. News.*, 1983, *3*, 41 and 48.

A report of 6 cases of a potentially fatal interaction between adrenaline, as a component of a local anaesthetic solution, and propranolol. The interaction was characterised by marked hypertension followed by reflex bradycardia. This sequence of events may ultimately lead to cardiac arrest or hypertensive stroke.— C. A. Foster and S. J. Aston, *Plastic reconstr. Surg.*, 1983, *72*, 74.

A further report of a severe hypertensive reaction in a patient who had been receiving propranolol and who was given a subcutaneous injection of adrenaline for a presumed anaphylactic reaction.— T. V. Whelan (letter), *Ann. intern. Med.*, 1987, *106*, 327.

Calcium-channel blockers. For reference to the interaction of adrenaline with verapamil, see under Verapamil, p.90.

Diuretics. Pretreatment with a thiazide diuretic, bendrofluazide, increased the hypokalaemia induced by infusion of adrenaline in 6 healthy subjects.— A. D. Struthers *et al.*, *Lancet*, 1983, *1*, 1358.

Local anaesthetics. Results in *animals* suggesting that lignocaine may antagonise the vasoconstrictor actions of adrenaline.— S. Pateromichelakis and J. P. Rood, *Br. J. Anaesth.*, 1986, *58*, 649.

Absorption and Fate

As a result of enzymatic degradation in the gut and first-pass metabolism in the liver, adrenaline is almost totally inactive when given by mouth. It acts rapidly following subcutaneous or intramuscular injection, although absorption is slowed by local vasoconstriction (it can be hastened by massaging the injection site).

Most adrenaline that is either injected into the body or released into the circulation from the adrenal medulla, is very rapidly inactivated by processes which include uptake into adrenergic neurones, diffusion, and enzymatic degradation in the liver and body tissues. One of the enzymes responsible for the chemical inactivation of this exogenous or hormonal adrenaline is catechol-*O*-methyltransferase (COMT), the other is monoamine oxidase (MAO). In general, adrenaline is methylated to metanephrine by COMT followed by oxidative deamination by MAO to 4-hydroxy-3-methoxymandelic acid (formerly termed vanillylmandelic acid; VMA), or oxidatively deaminated by MAO to 3,4-dihydroxymandelic acid which, in turn, is methylated by COMT, once again to 4-hydroxy-3-methoxymandelic acid; the metabolites are excreted in the urine mainly as their glucuronide and ethereal sulphate conjugates.

The ability of catechol-*O*-methyltransferase to effect introduction of a methyl group is an important step in the chemical inactivation of adrenaline and similar catecholamines (in particular, noradrenaline). It means that the termination of the pharmacological response of catecholamines is not simply dependent upon monoamine oxidase. In its role of neurotransmitter intraneuronal catecholamine (mainly noradrenaline) is, however, enzymatically regulated by monoamine oxidase.

Adrenaline crosses the placenta to enter foetal circulation.

PROTEIN BINDING. A brief review of studies on the binding of catecholamines to plasma proteins.— J. J. Vallner, *J. pharm. Sci.*, 1977, *66*, 447.

Uses and Administration

Adrenaline is an active principle of the adrenal medulla which is used as a direct-acting sympathomimetic agent. It has a somewhat more marked effect on beta-adrenoceptors than on alpha-adrenoceptors, and this property explains many aspects of its pharmacology; in addition, its actions vary considerably according to the dose given, and the consequent reflex compensating responses of the body.

In practice, major effects of adrenaline include increased speed and force of cardiac contraction (with lower doses this causes increased systolic pressure yet reduced diastolic pressure since overall peripheral resistance is lowered, but with higher doses both systolic and diastolic pressure are increased as stimulation of peripheral alpha-receptors increases peripheral resistance); blood flow to skeletal muscle is increased (reduced with higher doses); metabolic effects include increased glucose output as well as markedly increased oxygen consumption; blood flow in the kidneys, mucosa, and skin is reduced; there is little direct effect on cerebral blood flow.

Aqueous solutions of adrenaline are usually prepared using the acid tartrate or the hydrochloride but the dosage is generally stated in terms of the equivalent content of adrenaline. In general, aqueous injections have an adrenaline content equivalent to 1 in 1000 (1 mg per mL).

Adrenaline relaxes the bronchial musculature and has been injected subcutaneously to relieve bronchial spasm in acute attacks of bronchial asthma. The adult dose is 0.2 to 0.5 mL of a 1 in 1000 aqueous solution (200 to 500 μg); children should receive 0.01 mL (10 μg) per kg body-weight to a maximum total dose of 0.5 mL (500 μg). Benefit usually occurs within minutes but if the dose fails to control the attack, it may be repeated at 15- to 20-minute intervals for 2 doses, then subsequently every 4 hours if needed. The attack is more effectively treated with small doses of adrenaline at first than with larger doses at the peak. Tolerance or refractoriness may develop, particularly in patients with acute severe asthma. For prolonged control of asthmatic attacks adrenaline has been given by subcutaneous injection of a 1 in 200 aqueous suspension; an oily suspension has also been given intramuscularly. Such injections have been associated with tissue necrosis owing to their prolonged vasoconstrictor properties and, in particular, the oily injections have been associated with gas gangrene (see under Adverse Effects, above). The use of sympathomimetics with an intrinsically prolonged duration of action is accordingly preferable to such slow-release preparations of adrenaline.

Aqueous solutions with an adrenaline content equivalent to 1 in 100 have been used by inhalation as a spray to alleviate asthmatic spasms; these solutions must never be confused with the weaker strength used for injection. Pressurised aerosols delivering metered doses of adrenaline acid tartrate equivalent to approximately 160 μg of adrenaline are more convenient; the recommended adult dosage is 1 to 3 metered doses repeated, if necessary, after 30 minutes up to a maximum of 8 metered doses in 24 hours. If more than 1 metered dose is inhaled at a time, at least 1 or 2 minutes should elapse between any 2 inhalations. Overuse of such preparations may be dangerous (see Adverse Effects of Sympathomimetics on p.1453). It is therefore essential to instruct the patients in the correct use of such preparations; if relief is not obtained the dose should not be increased and alternate therapy should be given. Swallowing adrenaline may cause some epigastric pain and it is advisable to rinse the mouth and throat with water after using the inhalation.

In general, the use of adrenaline in asthma has been superseded by $beta_2$-selective sympathomimetic agents, such as salbutamol (p.1482) which can alleviate bronchospasm with fewer effects on the heart.

Subcutaneous or, preferably, intramuscular injection of 0.2 to 0.5 mL (200 to 500 μg) of adrenaline (1 in 1000) gives symptomatic relief in acute allergy and may be life-saving in anaphylactic shock. Up to 1 mL (1 mg) may be given, and more than one dose may be required (for further details see under Allergy and Anaphylaxis, below).

Subcutaneous or intramuscular adrenaline is similarly indicated for cardiovascular resuscitation procedures. Although very hazardous, in extreme emergencies a dilute solution of adrenaline may be given by very slow intravenous injection; in some circumstances intracardiac injection may be required (for further details see under Cardiac Resuscitation, below). Endotracheal administration has also been tried.

Adrenaline was formerly given intramuscularly in the emergency treatment of hypoglycaemia, but treatment with glucose or glucagon is generally preferred.

Adrenaline is frequently added to local anaesthetics, such as lignocaine hydrochloride (p.1220), and procaine hydrochloride (p.1226), to retard diffusion and limit absorption, to prolong the duration of effect, and to lessen the danger of toxicity. A concentration of 1 in 200 000 (5 μg per mL) is usually effective for infiltration injections; as little as 1 in 500 000 may be adequate though in some preparations 1 in 50 000 continues to be available. Even the 1 in 200 000 concentration should not be used for digits, ears, nose, penis, or scrotum owing to the risk of ischaemic tissue necrosis. Adrenaline has also been added to injections for spinal anaesthesia to delay absorption and prolong the effect but its use is not recommended because of the danger of reducing the blood supply to the cord. For further details of the appropriate concentrations and doses of adrenaline in local anaesthetic preparations see under Local Anaesthetics, p.1205.

Adrenaline constricts arterioles and capillaries and causes blanching when applied locally to mucous membranes and exposed tissues. It is used as an aqueous solution in strengths up to a 1 in 1000 dilution to check capillary bleeding, epistaxis, and bleeding from superficial wounds and abrasions, but it does not stop internal haemorrhage. It is usually applied as a spray or on pledgets of cotton wool or gauze. It may also be used as a 1 in 200 000 to 1 in 80 000 solution during surgical operations, especially on the eye, ear, nose, throat, or larynx to produce ischaemia of the operative field but this may make tying off of bleeding points difficult.

In ophthalmology, adrenaline in strengths up to 1 in 1000 is used to reduce conjunctival congestion, and 1 in 100 is used to reduce intra-ocular pressure in simple glaucoma. It is a poor mydriatic.

Adrenaline was formerly incorporated in creams used in the treatment of rheumatic and muscular disorders, and in rectal preparations used in the treatment of haemorrhoids.

In the *UK*, the use of adrenaline in cosmetics is prohibited.

ALLERGY AND ANAPHYLAXIS. Comment on the causes, symptoms, and management of anaphylactic shock and the key role of adrenaline. As soon as the reaction is recognised 0.5 to 1 mg (0.5 to 1 mL of so-called 1:1000) should be injected intramuscularly (not subcutaneously because absorption is too slow, especially in the presence of shock). A slow intravenous injection of a histamine H_1-receptor antagonist, such as chlorpheniramine 10 to 20 mg, should be given immediately after the intramuscular adrenaline and repeated over the subsequent 24 to 48 hours to prevent relapse. Although histamine H_1-receptor antagonists are particularly effective in the management of angio-oedema, pruritus, and urticaria, they remain second-line treatment. Local injection of adrenaline into the site of antigen administration is beneficial only in the early stages of the reaction. Intravenous corticosteroids have little place in the immediate management of anaphylaxis, since their beneficial effects are delayed for several hours but in severely ill patients early administration may help prevent deterioration after the primary treatment has been given. Continuing deterioration with circulatory collapse, bronchospasm, or laryngeal oedema requires further treatment including intravenous fluids, intravenous aminophylline, a nebulised β_2-agonist (such as salbutamol or terbutaline), oxygen, assisted respiration (if necessary), and possibly, emergency tracheostomy. If electrolyte solutions are used for volume replacement large amounts may be necessary because it has been reported that the plasma loss in severe anaphylactic shock may constitute 20 to 40% of the plasma volume. Colloid solutions, such as plasma protein fraction or dextran are theoretically preferable, but they may themselves release histamine, although in severe anaphylaxis intracellular stores of histamine are likely to have been depleted.— *Br. med. J.*, 1981, *282*, 1011.

Further reviews of anaphylaxis and its management: R. C. Godfrey, *Prescribers' J.*, 1981, *21*, 215; J. J. Fath and F. B. Cerra, *Drug Intell. & clin. Pharm.*, 1984, *18*, 14.

A report of myocardial ischaemia following the intravenous use of adrenaline in a patient with anaphylactic shock following a bee-sting, and discussion of the use of adrenaline by the intravenous route for anaphylaxis.— E. M. Barach *et al.*, *J. Am. med. Ass.*, 1984, *251*, 2118. Comment, and a reminder that adrenaline alone is not adequate in the management of anaphylaxis. Fluid replacement, and maintenance of an airway, are important.— M. J. Bennett and C. A. Hirshman (letter), *ibid.*, 1985, *253*, 510. The intravenous administration of adrenaline is a hazardous procedure rarely warranted in anaphylactic reactions. Subcutaneous or intramuscular adrenaline can achieve the same results without the hazards. If intravenous adrenaline is required it should be given slowly and in high dilution. While the authors fully support the use of adrenaline in anaphylaxis, care is needed in the route of administration.— P. Roberts-Thomson *et al.* (letter), *Med. J. Aust.*, 1985, *142*, 708. Agreement. Intravenous adrenaline should be reserved for patients who are not responding to other intensive measures— including intramuscular adrenaline where, if reasonable circulation is present, absorption is rapid. However, if the patient has associated venous or arterial circulatory failure there is little point in giving adrenaline even by the intravenous route; here an intracardiac dose of 50 to 100 µg of a 1 in 10 000 dilution is more likely to revive a moribund patient. The management of severe anaphylaxis is still poor in many areas. The basic treatment is essentially to overcome shock and laryngeal or bronchial obstruction by ensuring a good airway, giving adrenaline and 100% oxygen, and maintaining an adequate circulation. Other drugs, such as antihistamines, aminophylline, or corticosteroids should be regarded as second-line therapy.— R. M. Ford (letter), *ibid.*, *143*, 319.

For information on desensitisation procedures for allergic subjects, see Allergens and Specific Desensitisation, p.464.

Urticaria. A discussion of urticaria, angioedema, and their treatment. Subcutaneous adrenaline is usually the drug of choice for severe acute urticaria, generally in a dose of 300 µg as a 1 in 1000 dilution. Small children may be given 10 µg per kg body-weight. If necessary, such doses may be repeated once or twice at intervals of 15 minutes or longer. However, only in rare cases of unusually severe acute urticaria is it necessary to have adrenaline immediately available for injection. In patients with the more usual mild to moderate, recurrent or chronic urticaria, antihistamines are the drugs of first choice.— K. P. Mathews, *Drugs*, 1985, *30*, 552. See also R. H. Champion, *Br. med. J.*, 1973, *4*, 730.

ASTHMA. A discussion on the avoidance of asthma fatalities with emphasis on the importance of the prompt treatment of severe acute asthma. Concerning the choice of a bronchodilator drug, there seems to be no place for subcutaneous adrenaline.— *Br. med. J.*, 1978, *1*, 873. A defence of the use of subcutaneous adrenaline in asthma, and the view that it still remains an effective first-line drug for the hospital management of the young acute asthmatic.— T. Waterston (letter), *ibid.*, 1350.

A comparison of subcutaneous adrenaline 10 µg per kg body-weight and nebulised salbutamol 100 µg per kg, each in 20 patients, in the treatment of acute asthma in children. Both groups had significant improvement in indexes of pulmonary function following treatment but adverse effects were seen in 10 of the 20 children given adrenaline, compared with none of those given salbutamol. Nebulised salbutamol, rather than adrenaline, is recommended as the drug of choice in children with acute asthma.— A. B. Becker *et al.*, *J. Pediat.*, 1983, *102*, 465.

A double-blind study comparing subcutaneous adrenaline and nebulised orciprenaline in the management of acute asthma. Patients were randomly assigned to receive adrenaline 300 µg subcutaneously, repeated after 20 minutes if necessary to a total dose of 900 µg, or 0.3mL of a 5% orciprenaline solution via a nebuliser; there were 20 patients in each group. Both groups showed a significant increase in peak expiratory flow rate following treatment, and there was no significant difference between groups; neither drug appeared effective in patients whose baseline peak expiratory flow rate was less than 30% of predicted value (implying severe airflow restriction). Although both drugs were associated with equal improvement in pulmonary function there was a slight but significant increase in blood pressure in patients receiving adrenaline, which was not seen in those given orciprenaline.— R. M. Elenbaas *et al.*, *Drug Intell. & clin. Pharm.*, 1985, *19*, 567.

See also under Pregnancy and the Neonate, below.

BLEEDING. Gauze soaked with 0.1 mL of Moffat's solution (cocaine 30 mg per mL and adrenaline 250 µg per mL) was being tried, together with infiltration of the palate with lignocaine 0.5% and adrenaline 1:200 000, to reduce blood loss in cleft palate surgery in children.— F. J. M. Walters, *Postgrad. med. J.*, 1983, *59*, 611.

The use of endoscopic injection of 0.5 mL aliquots of 1:10 000 adrenaline to stop bleeding from peptic ulcers.— J. W. C. Leung and S. C. S. Chung, *Gut*, 1985, *26*, A1136. Further references: S. C. S. Chung *et al.*, *Br. med. J.*, 1988, *296*, 1631.

CARDIAC RESUSCITATION. Updated standards and guidelines from the 1985 National Conference on Cardiopulmonary Resuscitation and Emergency Cardiac Care. The early establishment of a reliable intravenous route for the administration of necessary drugs and fluids is essential; however initial defibrillation attempts should not be delayed for placement of an intravenous line. If an endotracheal tube is in place and there is delay in gaining venous access adrenaline, lignocaine, and atropine can be administered endotracheally. Drugs used in cardiac life support are oxygen; intravenous fluids; morphine sulphate; lignocaine, procainamide, beta-blockers, atropine, isoprenaline or verapamil for control of heart rate and rhythm; adrenaline, noradrenaline, dopamine, dobutamine, amrinone, cardiac glycosides, glyceryl trinitrate, sodium nitroprusside, sodium bicarbonate, and diuretics, to improve cardiac output and blood pressure. Adrenaline is beneficial in cardiac arrest, primarily because of its alpha-agonist properties; the value and safety of beta-mediated effects remains controversial. The recommended dose is 0.5 to 1 mg, given intravenously as 5 to 10 mL of a 1:10 000 solution; doses may be given every 5 minutes during the resuscitation effort. Adrenaline may be given via an endotracheal tube prior to establishing venous access in a dose of 1 mg, as 10 mL of a 1:10 000 solution. Intracardiac injection is only used if other routes are persistently inaccessible; this is because of the risk of coronary artery laceration, cardiac tamponade, and pneumothorax. Intracardiac injections also cause interruption of external chest compressions and ventilation. Adrenaline can also be used as a pressor agent via continuous infusion, although it is not a first line agent. 1 mg of the hydrochloride can be added to 250 mL of 5% glucose in water and an infusion started at a rate of 1 µg per minute and titrated to effect. In children the recommended resuscitation dose is 10 µg per kg given intravenously as a 1 in 10 000 solution. It is also useful as an infusion to treat hypotension or poor perfusion after restoration of spontaneous circulation following cardiac arrest, or in inadequate circulatory function unresponsive to fluids. Infusion is begun at a rate of 0.1 µg per kg per minute and titrated up to 1 µg per kg per minute according to effect.— American Heart Association and the National Academy of Sciences–National Research Council, *J. Am. med. Ass.*, 1986, *255*, 2905. A postmortem study of intracardiac injection sites in 18 patients who died after unsuccessful cardiopulmonary resuscitation found that the heart was entered only in 13 patients and of the 46 transthoracic injections carried out, only 5 entered the left ventricle, assumed to be the optimum site. This represents a very poor success rate and the value of the technique remains debatable, despite studies such as that of R. Davison *et al.* (*J. Am. med. Ass.*, 1980, *244*, 1110) which have shown that in expert hands the complications can be minimised and rapid access to the circulation achieved.— H. I. Sabin *et al.*, *Lancet*, 1983, *2*, 1054. Comment on the dangers of transthoracic injection. Central venous catheters can safely deliver intended intracardiac medication.— J. J. Steinberg (letter), *ibid.*, 1984, *1*, 218.

A study suggesting that endotracheal administration of adrenaline is not reliable in the management of patients presenting to accident and emergency departments with cardiac arrest.— D. N. Quinton *et al.*, *Lancet*, 1987, *1*, 828. Comment. The above study compared the same dose of adrenaline given intravenously and endotracheally. In view of the fact that bioavailability of drugs given by the endotracheal route cannot be 100% the United Kingdom Resuscitation Council recommends using twice the usual adult dose of adrenaline, i.e. 20 mL of 1 in 10 000, for endotracheal use.— B. Marchant, *ibid.*, 1098.

The early use of 10 mL of 1 in 10 000 adrenaline, given intravenously or transbronchially in routine resuscitation from ventricular fibrillation after failure of defibrillation, was associated with a significant reduction in initial survival when compared with previous experience with a dose of 2 to 5 mL.— T. H. Marwick *et al.*, *Lancet*, 1988, *2*, 66. These results could be interpreted as showing a lack of effect with either dose.— N. A. Paradis and C. G. Brown (letter), *ibid.*, 749.

MALARIA. Mention of the use of subcutaneous adrenaline, 1 mL of 1:1000 solution [1 mg], prior to administration of quinine for cerebral malaria.— I. Patrick (letter), *Br. med. J.*, 1982, *284*, 1954. Severe criticism of such a use.— N. J. White and D. A. Warrell (letter), *ibid.*, *285*, 439. Further criticism. The use of adrenaline was first advocated in the 1930's when it was proposed that constriction of the spleen squeezed the parasites out of that organ. But the early benefits reported then in Italy and Greece have not been confirmed by subsequent researchers, including the author.— L. J. Bruce-Chwatt (letter), *ibid.*, 653.

OCULAR DISORDERS. Adrenaline increases outflow through the trabecular meshwork and may reduce production of aqueous humour. Adrenaline drops may be employed alone in early cases of open-angle glaucoma. They produce pupillary dilation which will be advantageous in elderly patients with central lens opacities. Combinations of adrenaline and guanethidine are more effective than adrenaline alone but may produce more severe local side-effects. Adrenaline will also have an additive effect with pilocarpine but not, in most cases, with timolol. Adrenaline eye-drops are contra-indicated in closed-angle glaucoma.— R. A. Hitchings, *Prescribers' J.*, 1983, *23*, 106.

PREGNANCY AND THE NEONATE. The view that subcutaneous adrenaline is the drug of choice for acute episodes of bronchospasm in pregnant asthmatics: it is quickly metabolised and has not been associated with long-term sequelae. Other beta-agonists, such as terbutaline, orciprenaline, and salbutamol may be safe for the emergency treatment of asthma during pregnancy but published data confirming this are lacking.— P. A. Greenberger and R. Patterson, *New Engl. J. Med.*, 1985, *312*, 897.

Preparations

Adrenaline Eye Drops Strong *(A.P.F.).* Contain adrenaline 1%.

Adrenaline Injection *(B.P.).* Adrenaline Tartrate Injection. Contains the equivalent of adrenaline 0.1% as the acid tartrate; potency is expressed as adrenaline 1 in 1000.

Adrenaline Solution *(B.P.).* Adrenaline Tartrate Solution. Contains the equivalent of 0.1% adrenaline (adrenaline 1 in 1000) as the acid tartrate. Store in well-filled, well-closed containers.

NOTE. The *B.P.* states that when a solution of Adrenaline Hydrochloride is prescribed or demanded, Adrenaline Solution may be dispensed or supplied.

Epinephrine Bitartrate Inhalation Aerosol *(U.S.P.).* An aerosol spray in a pressurised container containing a fine suspension of adrenaline acid tartrate in propellents. Store in containers with metered-dose valves and oral inhalation actuators. Protect from light.

Epinephrine Bitartrate for Ophthalmic Solution *(U.S.P.).* A sterile dry mixture of adrenaline acid tartrate and suitable antoxidants, prepared by freeze-drying. The solution is prepared by the addition of diluent before use. Potency is expressed in terms of the equivalent amount of adrenaline.

Epinephrine Bitartrate Ophthalmic Solution *(U.S.P.).* A sterile, buffered, aqueous solution containing adrenaline acid tartrate. Potency is expressed in terms of the equivalent amount of adrenaline. pH 3.0 to 3.8. Store in small well-filled airtight containers. Protect from light.

It should not be used if it is brown or contains a precipitate.

Epinephrine Inhalation Aerosol *(U.S.P.)*. An aerosol spray in a pressurised container containing a solution of adrenaline in propellents and alcohol prepared with the aid of mineral acid. Store in containers with metered-dose valves and oral inhalation actuators. Protect from light.

Epinephrine Inhalation Solution *(U.S.P.)*. A solution of adrenaline 0.9 to 1.15% in water, prepared with the aid of hydrochloric acid. Store in small well-filled airtight containers. Protect from light. It should not be used if it is brown or contains a precipitate.

Epinephrine Injection *(U.S.P.)*. A sterile solution of adrenaline in Water for Injections prepared with the aid of hydrochloric acid. pH 2.2 to 5.0. Protect from light. It should not be used if it is brown or contains a precipitate.

Epinephrine Nasal Solution *(U.S.P.)*. A solution of adrenaline 0.09 to 0.115% in water, prepared with the aid of hydrochloric acid. Store in small well-filled airtight containers. Protect from light. It should not be used if it is brown or contains a precipitate.

Epinephrine Ophthalmic Solution *(U.S.P.)*. A sterile aqueous solution of adrenaline prepared with the aid of hydrochloric acid; pH 2.2 to 4.5. Store in airtight containers. Protect from light. It should not be used if it is brown or contains a precipitate.

Epinephryl Borate Ophthalmic Solution *(U.S.P.)*. A sterile aqueous solution containing adrenaline as a borate complex (known as epinephryl borate, $C_9H_{12}BNO_4$ = 209.0). pH 5.5 to 7.6. Potency is expressed in terms of the equivalent amount of adrenaline. Store in small well-filled airtight containers. Protect from light. It should not be used if it is brown or contains a precipitate.

Neutral Adrenaline Eye-drops *(B.P.C. 1973)*. ADN. A sterile solution containing adrenaline 1% in a borate buffer solution adjusted to pH 7.4 (limits: 7.2 to 7.6) with sodium hydroxide in containers in which the air has been replaced with nitrogen or other inert gas. Store in a cool place. Protect from light.

Racepinephrine Inhalation Solution *(U.S.P.)*. An aqueous solution of racemic adrenaline, prepared with the aid of hydrochloric acid, or of racemic adrenaline hydrochloride. Store in airtight containers and avoid freezing. Protect from light. It should not be used if it is brown or contains a precipitate.

Sterile Epinephrine Oil Suspension *(U.S.P.)*. A sterile suspension of adrenaline, 1.8 to 2.4 mg per mL, in a suitable vegetable oil. Protect from light.

Zinc and Adrenaline Eye Drops *(A.P.F.)*. BZA Eye Drops. Adrenaline solution 10 mL, zinc sulphate 250 mg, boric acid 1.5 g, sodium metabisulphite 50 mg, chlorbutol 500 mg, glycerol 1 mL, Water for Injections to 100 mL. Sterilise by autoclaving. Protect from light.

For preparations of local anaesthetics with adrenaline see the appropriate monographs under Local Anaesthetics, p.1205.

Proprietary Preparations

Brovon *(Napp, UK)*. *Inhalant solution*, adrenaline 0.5% (as hydrochloride), atropine methonitrate 0.14%, papaverine hydrochloride 0.88%.

Epifrin *(Allergan, UK)*. *Eye-drops*, adrenaline 1.0% (as hydrochloride).

Eppy *(Smith & Nephew Pharmaceuticals, UK)*. *Eye-drops*, adrenaline 1%.

Isopto Epinal *(Alcon, UK)*. *Eye-drops*, adrenaline 0.5 or 1% (as the borate complex).

Medihaler-Epi *(Riker, UK)*. *Inhaler*, aerosol, adrenaline acid tartrate 280 μg/metered dose.

Min-I-Jet Adrenaline *(IMS, UK)*. *Injection*, adrenaline 1 in 1000 [1 mg (as hydrochloride)/mL], in single-use prefilled syringes of 0.5 and 1 mL.
Injection, adrenaline 1 in 10 000 [100 μg (as hydrochloride)/mL], in single-use prefilled syringes of 3 and 10 mL.

Riddobron *(Seaford, UK)*. *Inhalant solution*, adrenaline hydrochloride 0.5%, atropine methylnitrate 0.14%, papaverine hydrochloride 0.88%.

Rybarvin *(Rybar, UK)*. *Inhalant solution*, adrenaline 0.4%, atropine methonitrate 0.1%, papaverine hydrochloride 0.08%, benzocaine 0.08%.

Simplene *(Smith & Nephew Pharmaceuticals, UK)*. *Eye-drops*, adrenaline 0.5 and 1.0%.

Proprietary Names and Manufacturers of Adrenaline, Adrenaline Acid Tartrate, or a related compound

Adrenalin Isopto *(Alcon, Denm.)*; Adrenalin-Medihaler *(Riker, Denm.; Kettelhack Riker, Ger.; Riker, Norw.; Riker, Swed.)*; Adrenapax *(Sinclair, UK)*; Ana-Kit *(Miles Laboratories, USA)*; Anaphylaxie-Besteck *(Tropon, Ger.)*; Bronkaid Mistometer *(Winthrop, Canad.)*; Dysne-Inhal *(Rougier, Canad.)*; Dyspne-Inhal *(Augot, Fr.; Ital.; Switz.)*; E1 *(USA)*; E2 *(USA)*; Epifrin *(Allergan, Austral.; Belg.; Allergan, Canad.; Allergan, S.Afr.; Switz.; Allergan, UK; Allergan, USA)*; Epifrina *(Arg.)*; Epiglaufrin *(Allergan, Ger.)*; Epinal *(Alcon, Austral.; Alcon, Canad.; S.Afr.)*; Epipen *(Center Laboratories, USA)*; Epirest *(Neth.)*; Epitrate *(Canad.; S.Afr.; Ayerst, USA)*; Eppy *(Pharmacia, Denm.; Merck Sharp & Dohme, Ital.; Dulcis, Mon.; Smith & Nephew, S.Afr.; Pharmacia, Swed.; Smith & Nephew Pharmaceuticals, UK)*; Eppy N *(Barnes-Hind, Austral.; Barnes-Hind, Canad.; Barnes-Hind, Switz.)*; Glaucon *(Alcon, Austral.; Alcon, Canad.; Switz.; Alcon Laboratories, USA)*; Glaufrin *(Allergan, Swed.)*; Glauposine *(P.O.S., Fr.; Switz.)*; Glycirenan *(Atmos, Ger.)*; Hektalin *(Denm.)*; Isopto Epinal *(Neth.; Alcon, Norw.; Alcon, Spain; Alcon, Swed.; Alcon, Switz.; Alcon, UK)*; Levocon *(Alcon, Norw.)*; Liadren *(Allergan, Ital.)*; Lloyd's Cream with Adrenaline *(Howard Lloyd, UK)*; Lyophrin *(Alcon, UK)*; Medihaler-Epi *(Riker, Austral.; Riker, Canad.; Riker, S.Afr.; Riker, UK; Riker, USA)*; Micronefrin *(Austral.; S.Afr.; Bird, USA)*; Min-I-Jet Adrenaline *(IMS, UK)*; Primatene Mist *(Whitehall, USA)*; Simplene *(Smith & Nephew, S.Afr.; Smith & Nephew Pharmaceuticals, UK)*; Suprarenin *(Hoechst, Ger.)*; Sus-Phrine *(Berlex, Canad.; Forest Pharmaceuticals, USA)*; Vaponefrin *(Rorer, Canad.; Fisons, Norw.; Fisons, USA)*.

The following names have been used for multi-ingredient preparations containing adrenaline, adrenaline acid tartrate, or a related compound—Asma-Vydrin *(Lipomed, UK)*; BayCaine-E *(Bay, USA)*; Brovon *(Napp, UK)*; Brovon Pressurised Inhalant *(Napp, UK)*; Citanest Forte *(Astra, Canad.)*; Citanest with Adrenaline *(Astra, Austral.; Astra, UK)*; Cremor Urical Co. *(Sinclair, UK)*; Drenalgin *(Lloyds Pharmaceuticals, Reckitt & Colman Pharm., UK)*; Duranest with Adrenaline *(Astra, Austral.; Astra, USA)*; E-Carpine *(Alcon, Austral.)*; E-Pilo *(Coopervision, Canad.; Coopervision, USA)*; Ganda *(Smith & Nephew Pharmaceuticals, UK)*; Lidocaton *(Pharmaton, Switz.; Claudius Ash, UK)*; Lignostab-A *(Boots, UK)*; Marcain with Adrenaline *(Astra, UK)*; Marcaine with Adrenaline *(Astra, Austral.; Cook-Waite, USA; Winthrop-Breon, USA)*; Nurocain *(Astra, Austral.)*; Octocaine with Epinephrine *(Canad.)*; Rectinol *(G.P. Laboratories, Austral.)*; Riddobron Inhalant *(Seaford, UK)*; Riddofan *(Seaford, UK)*; Riddovydrin Inhalant *(Seaford, UK)*; Rybarex *(Rybar, UK)*; Rybarvin *(Rybar, UK)*; Sensorcaine with Adrenaline *(Astra, USA)*; Silbe *(Berk Pharmaceuticals, UK)*; Ultracaine D-S *(Hoechst, Canad.)*; URA *(Protea, Austral.)*; Welder's Flash Drops *(Industrial Pharmaceutical, UK)*; Xylocaine with Adrenaline *(Astra, Austral.; Astra, UK; Astra, USA)*; Xylotox 2% E.80 *(Pharmaceutical Mfg, UK)*.

12353-h

Amezinium Methylsulphate

Amezinium Metilsulfate *(rINN)*. 4-Amino-6-methoxy-1-phenylpyridazinium methylsulphate.
$C_{12}H_{15}N_3O_5S$=313.3.

CAS — 30578-37-1.

Adverse Effects and Precautions

For the adverse effects of sympathomimetic agents, and precautions to be observed, see p.1453.

Uses and Administration

Amezinium methylsulphate is a sympathomimetic agent which has been used in the treatment of hypotension.

Proprietary Names and Manufacturers

Regulton *(Nordmark, Ger.; Knoll, Switz.)*; Supratonin *(Grünenthal, Ger.)*.

2044-t

Angiotensin Amide *(BAN, USAN)*.

Angiotensinamide *(rINN)*; NSC-107678. Asn-Arg-Val-Tyr-Val-His-Pro-Phe; [1-Asparagine, 5-valine]-angiotensin II.
$C_{49}H_{70}N_{14}O_{11}$=1031.2.

CAS — 11128-99-7 (angiotensin II); 53-73-6 (amide).

The manufacturers (*Ciba*) state that angiotensin amide is incompatible with blood or serum.

Adverse Effects

Rapid infusion of angiotensin amide may readily cause very severe hypertension; bradycardia and ventricular arrhythmias may occur rarely.

A fatality arising from acute hypertension has been reported in a healthy volunteer given a prolonged intravenous infusion of angiotensin.— C. T. Dollery, *Prescribers' J.*, 1977, *17*, 126.

Precautions

Angiotensin amide should not be given to patients being treated with a monoamine oxidase inhibitor or within 14 days of stopping such treatment (see Precautions for Phenelzine Sulphate p.378). It should be given with caution to patients with cardiovascular disease or cardiac insufficiency.

Absorption and Fate

Angiotensin amide is rapidly inactivated in the tissues and circulation by peptidases. When given by intravenous injection it has a duration of action of only a few minutes.

Uses and Administration

Angiotensin amide is a pressor agent related to the naturally occurring peptide angiotensin II. It increases the peripheral resistance mainly in cutaneous, splanchnic, and renal blood vessels and acts both directly and via the sympathetic nervous system. The increased blood pressure is accompanied by a reflex reduction in heart-rate, and cardiac output may also be reduced.
Angiotensin amide has been used in the treatment of states of collapse and shock, but it has not achieved general acceptance as a satisfactory alternative to sympathomimetic agents.
Angiotensin amide has been used (with due caution) to restore blood pressure in hypotensive crises during anaesthesia with chloroform, cyclopropane, halothane, and other halogenated anaesthetics.
It is given by continuous intravenous infusion usually in a concentration of 10 mg per litre of sodium chloride injection, glucose injection, or other suitable diluent, at a usual rate varying between 3 and 10 μg per minute according to the blood pressure response. Blood pressure must be monitored continuously during the infusion. Once the patient's condition improves the dosage should be reduced gradually before withdrawal.
Infusions of angiotensin amide were formerly advocated to treat the adverse effects of an overdose of an angiotensin-converting enzyme inhibitor such as enalapril.

Reference to the use of angiotensin to produce a selective increase in blood flow to tumour tissue and thus maximise local delivery of chemotherapy in patients with malignant melanoma.— H. Takematsu *et al.*, *Br. J. Derm.*, 1985, *113*, 463.

SHOCK. In 12 patients in shock the effect of angiotensin was compared with noradrenaline and metaraminol. It was found that there was significantly lower cardiac output and urine flow and a disproportionate increase of peripheral vascular resistance when angiotensin was employed and the rationale for its use in the treatment of shock was questioned.— V. N. Udhoji and M. H. Weil, *New Engl. J. Med.*, 1964, *270*, 501.

Proprietary Names and Manufacturers

Hypertensin *(Ciba, Austral.; Ciba, Ger.; Ciba, UK)*; Hypertensine *(Ciba, Switz.)*.

12447-p

Bitolterol Mesylate *(BANM, USAN)*.

Bitolterol Mesilate *(rINNM)*; Win-32784. 4-[2-(*tert*-Butylamino)-1-hydroxyethyl]-*o*-phenylene di(*p*-toluate) methanesulphonate.
$C_{28}H_{31}NO_5,CH_4O_3S$=557.7.

CAS — 30392-40-6 (bitolterol); 30392-41-7 (mesylate).

Adverse Effects and Precautions

For the adverse effects of sympathomimetic agents, and precautions to be observed, see p.1453.

Uses and Administration
Bitolterol is a direct-acting sympathomimetic agent with actions similar to those of salbutamol (p.1482). It is hydrolysed by esterases in tissue and plasma to the active form colterol. It is used as a long-acting bronchodilator. It is given by inhalation via a metered-dose aerosol supplying 370 μg of bitolterol mesylate per inhalation; usual doses of 2 inhalations (740 μg) three times daily have been given.

A brief review of the use of bitolterol in the management of asthma and bronchospasm. Bitolterol is an inactive prodrug that is hydrolysed to produce colterol, an active catecholamine. The hydrolysing esterases required for this process are found in higher concentrations in the lungs than in the heart, favouring bronchodilator over cardiovascular effects. Available data are conflicting over whether bitolterol has a longer duration of action than drugs such as salbutamol.— *Med. Lett.*, 1985, *27*, 46.

Further reviews of bitolterol: S. B. Walker *et al.*, *Pharmacotherapy*, 1985, *5*, 127.

Proprietary Names and Manufacturers
Tornalate *(Winthrop-Breon, USA)*.

2045-x

Butethamate Citrate *(BANM)*.

Butetamate Citrate *(rINNM)*. 2-Diethylaminoethyl 2-phenylbutyrate citrate.
$C_{16}H_{25}NO_2,C_6H_8O_7$=455.5.

CAS — 14007-64-8 (butethamate); 13900-12-4 (citrate).

Uses and Administration
Butethamate citrate is reported to be an antispasmodic and bronchodilator and has been used in mixtures with sympathomimetics for the symptomatic treatment of asthma and bronchitis.

Proprietary Names and Manufacturers
The following names have been used for multi-ingredient preparations containing butethamate citrate— CAM *(Rybar, UK)*.

12480-s

Butopamine *(USAN, rINN)*.

LY-131126. *(R)*-4-Hydroxy-α-{[*(R)*-3-(4-hydroxyphenyl)-1-methylpropyl]aminomethyl}benzyl alcohol.
$C_{18}H_{23}NO_3$=301.4.

CAS — 66734-12-1.

Butopamine is structurally related to dobutamine (p.1459) and is reported to have inotropic effects on the heart.

References: M. J. Thompson *et al.*, *Clin. Pharmac. Ther.*, 1980, *28*, 324.

Proprietary Names and Manufacturers
Lilly, USA.

2046-r

Carbuterol Hydrochloride *(BANM, USAN, rINNM)*.

SKF-40383-A. [5-(2-*tert*-Butylamino-1-hydroxyethyl)-2-hydroxyphenyl]urea hydrochloride.
$C_{13}H_{21}N_3O_3,HCl$=303.8.

CAS — 34866-47-2 (carbuterol); 34866-46-1 (hydrochloride).

Carbuterol hydrochloride is a direct-acting sympathomimetic agent with general properties similar to those of salbutamol (p.1480). It has been used as a bronchodilator in doses of 1 to 3 mg three or four times daily by mouth, or by inhalation in doses of 100 to 200 μg at intervals of not less than 3 hours.

Proprietary Names and Manufacturers
Bronsecur *(Parke, Davis, Ital.; Warner, S.Afr.)*; Dilabron *(Warner, S.Afr.)*; Pirem *(Sasse, Ger.)*; Rispran *(Smith Kline & French, Spain)*.

16579-g

Cinnamedrine Hydrochloride *(rINNM)*.

N-Cinnamylephedrine Hydrochloride. α-{1-[Methyl(3-phenyl-2-propenyl)amino]ethyl}benzenemethanol hydrochloride.
$C_{19}H_{23}NO,HCl$=317.9.

CAS — 90-86-8.

NOTE. Cinnamedrine is *USAN*.

Adverse Effects and Precautions
For the adverse effects of sympathomimetic agents, and precautions to be observed see p.1453.

Uses and Administration
Cinnamedrine hydrochloride is reported to have sympathomimetic actions resembling those of ephedrine (p.1462) but less effect on the central nervous system. It has been used in combination with analgesics in the symptomatic relief of dysmenorrhoea.

Proprietary Names and Manufacturers
The following names have been used for multi-ingredient preparations containing cinnamedrine hydrochloride— Midol *(Nyal, Austral.; Sterling, Canad.; Glenbrook, USA)*.

2047-f

Clenbuterol Hydrochloride *(BANM, rINNM)*.

NAB-365. 1-(4-Amino-3,5-dichlorophenyl)-2-*tert*-butylaminoethanol hydrochloride.
$C_{12}H_{18}Cl_2N_2O,HCl$=313.7.

CAS — 37148-27-9 (clenbuterol); 21898-19-1 (hydrochloride).

Adverse Effects, Treatment, and Precautions
As for Salbutamol, p.1480.

Some conflicting reports on the incidence of side-effects, such as anxiety, agitation, and muscle tremor in patients receiving clenbuterol: P. L. Kamburoff *et al.*, *Br. J. clin. Pharmac.*, 1977, *4*, 67; C. Mazzola and C. Vibelli, *Curr. ther. Res.*, 1978, *23*, 231; T. L. Whitsett *et al.*, *Clin. Pharmac. Ther.*, 1980, *27*, 294.

In a comparison of the pulmonary, cardiac, and neuromuscular effects of clenbuterol and terbutaline, although both drugs were found to produce tremor, higher doses of 60 or 80 μg of clenbuterol were associated with an increased incidence of headache, nervousness, and light-headedness.— T. L. Whitsett *et al.*, *Br. J. clin. Pharmac.*, 1981, *12*, 195.

Uses and Administration
Clenbuterol hydrochloride is a direct-acting sympathomimetic agent with general properties similar to those of salbutamol (p.1482). It is used as a bronchodilator in the management of asthma and obstructive lung disease in doses of 20 to 40 μg twice daily by mouth. It has also been given by inhalation.

Clenbuterol 20 or 40 μg given twice daily by mouth was as effective as salbutamol 2 or 4 mg three times daily in a crossover study in 21 patients with chronic obstructive lung disease (asthma or bronchitis) who also continued regular therapy with theophylline, corticosteroids, or inhaled bronchodilators. The higher doses did not produce a significantly greater benefit. The main side-effects with both drugs were tremor and palpitations, which were greater at higher doses. As basic therapy for this group of patients clenbuterol 20 μg twice daily would seem adequate as part of a long-term regimen.— B. Blom-Bülow *et al.*, *Curr. ther. Res.*, 1985, *37*, 51.

PREGNANCY AND THE NEONATE. Clenbuterol 40, 60, or 100 μg by mouth, or 60 μg intravenously caused a significant decrease in frequency and amplitude of uterine contractions in 20 of 26 women who experienced uterine hyperactivity during labour. Onset of action was 47 minutes after an oral dose and about 3 minutes after an intravenous dose; the duration of action was about 2 hours. There were no significant adverse effects on mothers or offspring. In a further 21 women with signs of imminent premature labour clenbuterol 40 μg every 12 hours by mouth initially, subsequently reduced to 40 μg daily, maintained uterine relaxation for a mean of 63 days; only 3 patients delivered prematurely. There were no adverse effects on foetal heart-rate or Apgar score; 2 babies had transient respiratory distress syndrome. Adverse effects in the mothers included tremor, nervousness, and palpitations.— V. Zahn and G. Krumbachner, *J. perinat. Med.*, 1981, *9*, 96.

Proprietary Names and Manufacturers
Broncodil *(Von Boch, Ital.)*; Clenasma *(Biomedica Foscama, Ital.)*; Clenbutol *(Scharper, Ital.)*; Contrasmina *(Lifepharma, Ital.)*; Monores *(Valeas, Ital.)*; Prontovent *(Salus, Ital.)*; Spiropent *(Thomae, Ger.; De Angeli, Ital.; Castejon, Spain)*.

2048-d

Clorprenaline Hydrochloride *(BANM, USAN, rINNM)*.

Chlorprenaline Hydrochloride; Isoprophenamine Hydrochloride. 1-(2-Chlorophenyl)-2-isopropylaminoethanol hydrochloride monohydrate.
$C_{11}H_{16}ClNO,HCl,H_2O$=268.2.

CAS — 3811-25-4 (clorprenaline); 6933-90-0 (hydrochloride, anhydrous); 5588-22-7 (hydrochloride, monohydrate).

Clorprenaline hydrochloride is a sympathomimetic agent with general properties similar to those of isoprenaline (p.1466) which has been used as a bronchodilator.

Proprietary Names and Manufacturers
Asthone *(Jpn)*; Bazarl *(Jpn)*; Broncon *(Jpn)*; Cosmoline *(Jpn)*; Effectol *(Jpn)*; Kalutein *(Jpn)*; Pentadoll *(Jpn)*; Restanolon *(Jpn)*.

The following names have been used for multi-ingredient preparations containing clorprenaline hydrochloride— Vortel *(Lilly, UK)*.

2049-n

Coumazoline Hydrochloride *(rINNM)*.

L-5818. 2-(2-Ethylbenzofuran-3-ylmethyl)-2-imidazoline hydrochloride.
$C_{14}H_{16}N_2O,HCl$=264.8.

CAS — 37681-00-8 (coumazoline).

Coumazoline hydrochloride is a sympathomimetic agent used topically as a nasal vasoconstrictor.

Proprietary Names and Manufacturers
Galenyl *(Labaz, Belg.)*; Gayenil *(Labaz, Spain)*.

2050-k

Cyclopentamine Hydrochloride *(BANM, USAN, rINNM)*.

Cyclopentadrin Hydrochloride. 2-Cyclopentyl-1,*N*-dimethylethylamine hydrochloride.
$C_9H_{19}N,HCl$=177.7.

CAS — 102-45-4 (cyclopentamine); 3459-06-1 (hydrochloride).

Pharmacopoeias. In *U.S.*

A white crystalline powder with a slight characteristic odour. **Soluble** 1 in 1 of water, 1 in 2 of alcohol, and 1 in 1 of chloroform; slightly soluble in ether. A 1% solution in water has a pH of about 6. **Store** in airtight containers.

Cyclopentamine hydrochloride is a sympathomimetic agent which was formerly used as a nasal decongestant.

Preparations
Cyclopentamine Hydrochloride Nasal Solution *(U.S.P.)*

Proprietary Names and Manufacturers
The following names have been used for multi-ingredient preparations containing cyclopentamine hydrochloride— Aerolone Compound *(Lilly, Canad.)*; Co-Pyronil *(Lilly, UK)*; Hista-Clopane *(Lilly, USA)*.

2051-a

Dimetofrine Hydrochloride *(rINNM)*.

Dimetophrine Hydrochloride. 1-(4-Hydroxy-3,5-dimethoxyphenyl)-2-methylaminoethanol hydrochloride.
$C_{11}H_{17}NO_4,HCl$=263.7.

CAS — 22950-29-4 (dimetofrine); 22775-12-8 (hydrochloride).

Dimetofrine hydrochloride is a sympathomimetic agent which has been used by mouth or intravenously for the treatment of hypotension.

References to the use of dimetofrine in hypotension: V. Baldrighi *et al.*, *Curr. med. Res. Opinion*, 1984, *9*, 78;

U. Marini *et al.*, *ibid.*, 265; V. Marsoni, *ibid.*, 1985, *9*, 578.

Proprietary Names and Manufacturers
Dovida *(Zambeletti, Spain)*; Pressamina *(Zambeletti, Ital.)*; Superten *(Beta, Arg.)*.

12670-z

Dipivefrine Hydrochloride *(BANM, rINNM)*.

Dipivalyl Adrenaline Hydrochloride; Dipivalyl Epinephrine Hydrochloride; Dipivefrin Hydrochloride *(USAN)*; DPE. (*RS*)-4-(1-Hydroxy-2-methylaminoethyl)-*o*-phenylene dipivalate hydrochloride.
$C_{19}H_{29}NO_5,HCl = 387.9$.

CAS — 52365-63-6 (dipivefrine); 64019-93-8 (hydrochloride).

Pharmacopoeias. In *U.S.*

White crystals or crystalline powder, with a faint odour. Very **soluble** in water. The *U.S.P.* ophthalmic solution has a pH of between 2.5 and 3.5. **Store** in airtight containers. The ophthalmic solution should be protected from light.

Dipivefrine is an ester and prodrug of adrenaline (p.1453). A 0.1% solution of the hydrochloride is applied to the eye in the treatment of open-angle glaucoma.

A review of the use of dipivefrine in glaucoma. Dipivefrine 0.1% lowers intra-ocular pressure in patients with glaucoma and ocular hypertension as effectively as adrenaline 1%. It is not known whether dipivefrine has fewer systemic or local adverse effects at equipotent doses, but otherwise it does not appear to have any advantages over the standard adrenaline drops.— *Drug & Ther. Bull.*, 1985, *23*, 27. Despite representations from the manufacturers *(Allergan)* that dipivefrine causes fewer unwanted effects there seems no reason to change this conclusion.— J. Collier (letter), *Pharm. J.*, 1985, *1*, 777.

Proprietary Preparations

Propine *(Allergan, UK)*. *Eye-drops*, dipivefrine hydrochloride 0.1%.

Proprietary Names and Manufacturers
d Epifrin *(Allergan, Ger.)*; Diopine *(Spain)*; Glaucothil *(Thilo, Ger.)*; Glaudrops *(Cusi, Spain)*; Propine *(Allergan, Austral.*; *Allergan, Canad.*; *Allergan, Denm.*; *Allergan, Ital.*; *Allergan, UK)*.

2052-t

Dobutamine Hydrochloride *(BANM, USAN, rINNM)*.

46236; Compound 81929 *(dobutamine)*. (±)-4-{2-[3-(4-Hydroxyphenyl)-1-methylpropylamino]-ethyl}pyrocatechol hydrochloride; (±)-4-{2-[3-(4-Hydroxyphenyl)-1-methylpropylamino]ethyl-}benzene-1,2-diol hydrochloride.
$C_{18}H_{23}NO_3,HCl = 337.8$.

CAS — 34368-04-2 (dobutamine); 49745-95-1 (hydrochloride).

Pharmacopoeias. In *U.S.*

Store at 15° to 30° in airtight containers.

Dobutamine was stable for at least 48 hours when diluted at a concentration of 1 mg per mL in glucose injection, sodium chloride injection, lactated Ringer's injection, and 5% glucose and 0.45% sodium chloride injection.— H. L. Kirschenbaum *et al.*, *Am. J. Hosp. Pharm.*, 1982, *39*, 1923. Dobutamine hydrochloride was not stable when added to 5% sodium bicarbonate injection, in which a precipitate formed within 3 hours of storage at 25°. There was a loss of nearly 50% of the original drug concentration of approximately 1 mg per mL on storage of the mixture for 48 hours. However, visual inspection suggested that dobutamine hydrochloride 0.1% was compatible for 24 hours when mixed with dopamine hydrochloride, heparin sodium, lignocaine hydrochloride, or procainamide hydrochloride in either glucose or sodium chloride injection. Similar mixtures with aminophylline, frusemide, or phenytoin sodium became cloudy or produced a precipitate while there were colour changes in mixtures with bretylium, calcium chloride, calcium gluconate, digoxin, insulin, magnesium sulphate, or potassium chloride.— H. L. Kirschenbaum *et al.*, *ibid.*, 1983, *40*, 1690.

Dobutamine hydrochloride was visually compatible with most of 29 injectable drugs added in 5-mL aliquots to a solution in glucose injection or sodium chloride injection. Precipitates were noted with bumetanide, calcium gluconate, or insulin. Precipitation was also seen, as expected, on mixing dobutamine with alkaline preparations such as aminophylline, frusemide, and sodium bicarbonate solutions, and with diazepam and phenytoin injections which are relative insoluble in various fluids.— G. R. Hasegawa and J. F. Eder, *Am. J. Hosp. Pharm.*, 1984, *41*, 949. Although the previous study demonstrated no precipitation with dobutamine hydrochloride and heparin sodium, which is in agreement with the findings of Kirschenbaum *et al.* (see above), the manufacturers *(Lilly)* state that such a mixture is incompatible, and on repetition of this portion of the study using different lots of drugs dobutamine and heparin yielded a precipitate when diluted in glucose injection but not in sodium chloride injection. In view of the unpredictable nature of precipitate formation dobutamine hydrochloride and heparin sodium should not be mixed or infused through the same intravenous line.— *idem*, 2588.

Adverse Effects

For adverse effects of sympathomimetics see p.1453.

Dobutamine acts primarily on $beta_1$ receptors, and may produce hypertension, tachycardia, and ectopic heart-beats.

The most serious adverse effect of all the sympathomimetic amines is the precipitation of arrhythmias; it is claimed that dobutamine causes a lower incidence of arrhythmias compared with isoprenaline and dopamine. If rapid ventricular rates occur in the presence of obstructive coronary artery disease, ischaemia can be induced or worsened. Dobutamine may cause a marked increase in heart-rate or systolic blood pressure. Approximately 10% of patients in clinical studies have had rate increases of 30 beats per minute or more, and about 7.5% have had an increase of systolic blood pressure of 50 mmHg or higher. Reduction of dosage usually reverses these effects promptly. Because dobutamine facilitates atrioventricular conduction, patients with atrial fibrillation may be at risk of developing a rapid ventricular response. Other side-effects reported in 1 to 3% of patients include nausea, headache, anginal pain, palpitation, and shortness of breath. No abnormal laboratory values have been attributable to dobutamine, and infusions of up to 72 hours have revealed no adverse effects other than those seen with shorter infusions.— E. H. Sonnenblick *et al.*, *New Engl. J. Med.*, 1979, *300*, 17.

A report of troublesome pruritus of the scalp associated with dobutamine infusion.— C. S. McCauley and M. S. Blumenthal (letter), *Ann. intern. Med.*, 1986, *105*, 966.

Treatment of Adverse Effects

Since the half-life of dobutamine is only about 2 minutes most adverse effects can be corrected by discontinuing or reducing the rate of infusion.

Precautions

For precautions with sympathomimetics, see p.1453.

Dobutamine hydrochloride should be avoided or only used with great caution in patients with marked obstruction of cardiac ejection, such as with idiopathic hypertrophic subaortic stenosis. It may exacerbate pre-existing tachycardia and hypertension; patients with atrial fibrillation should be given a cardiac glycoside before dobutamine treatment to reduce the risk of enhanced atrio-ventricular conduction leading to ventricular fibrillation. Hypovolaemia should be corrected before treatment.

Although it is less likely than adrenaline to produce ventricular arrhythmias, dobutamine should be avoided or only used with extreme caution during anaesthesia with cyclopropane, halothane, and other halogenated anaesthetics. The inotropic effects of dobutamine on the heart are reversed by concomitant administration of beta-blockers. Dobutamine may be ineffective or may have a slight vasoconstricting effect in patients who have recently received beta-adrenoceptor blocking agents.

Absorption and Fate

For a brief outline of the absorption and fate of a catecholamine, see Adrenaline, p.1455.

Like adrenaline, dobutamine is inactive when given by mouth, and it is rapidly inactivated in the body by similar processes.

A study of the pharmacokinetics of dobutamine in 7 patients with severe heart failure. The elimination half-life after intravenous infusion was less than 3 minutes. From the limited data available the volume of distribution of dobutamine appeared to be related to the extent of oedema.— R. E. Kates and C. V. Leier, *Clin. Pharmac. Ther.*, 1978, *24*, 537.

Further references: D. W. McKennon and R. E. Kates, *J. pharm. Sci.*, 1978, *67*, 1756 (plasma concentrations).

Uses and Administration

Dobutamine is a sympathomimetic agent with direct effects on $beta_1$-adrenergic receptors, which confer upon it a prominent inotropic action on the heart. Dobutamine differs from dopamine in not having the specific dopaminergic properties of dopamine which induce renal mesenteric vasodilatation; however it has some alpha and $beta_2$-agonist properties. It is reported not to have indirect sympathomimetic effects. Like dopamine, the inotropic action of dobutamine on the heart is associated with less cardiac-accelerating effect than that of isoprenaline.

Dobutamine is used as the hydrochloride in the management of congestive heart failure associated with organic heart disease, cardiogenic or septic shock, myocardial infarction, and cardiac surgery. It is administered as a dilute solution, in glucose injection, sodium chloride injection, or sodium lactate injection, by intravenous infusion. The usual rate is 2.5 to 10 μg per kg body-weight per minute, according to the patient's heart-rate, blood pressure, cardiac output, and urine output. Up to 40 μg per kg per minute may occasionally be required. It has been recommended that treatment with dobutamine should be discontinued gradually.

A review of dobutamine.— C. V. Leier and D. V. Unverferth, *Ann. intern. Med.*, 1983, *99*, 490.

ACTION. Recent *animal* studies show that the ability of dobutamine to stimulate $alpha_1$- and $beta_2$-adrenergic receptors appears to be as great as its $beta_1$-stimulant properties, and it has been proposed that the inotropic action results from a combination of alpha-stimulant activity on myocardial $alpha_1$ receptors, a property residing mainly in the (−)-enantiomer, with $beta_1$ stimulation by the (+)-enantiomer; peripherally, alpha-mediated vasoconstriction would be opposed by the $beta_2$-agonist properties of the (+)-enantiomer, resulting in the net inotropic action with relatively little effect on blood pressure seen with the racemic mixture used clinically.— R. R. Ruffolo (letter), *Ann. intern. Med.*, 1984, *100*, 313.

CARDIAC DISORDERS. Updated standards and guidelines from the 1985 National Conference on Cardiopulmonary Resuscitation and Emergency Cardiac Care. Dobutamine hydrochloride is a potent inotropic agent useful in the treatment of heart failure. It increases myocardial contractility and it frequently induces reflex peripheral vasodilation. It may be used synergistically with sodium nitroprusside. The usual dosage range is 2.5 to 10 μg per kg body-weight per minute; doses greater than 20 μg per kg per minute often produce considerable increases in heart rate (greater than 10%) which may induce or exacerbate myocardial ischaemia. Experience with dobutamine in children is limited but it does improve myocardial function in the child with diminished cardiac output and is indicated in children with poor myocardial function.— American Heart Association and the National Academy of Sciences–National Research Council., *J. Am. med. Ass.*, 1986, *255*, 2905. An earlier review of developments in cardiac drug therapy. For acute severe heart failure, such as cardiogenic shock associated with acute myocardial infarction dobutamine may be given combined with dopamine, both in low doses such as 7.5 μg per kg per minute of each. Conditioning with weekly infusions of dobutamine may potentially improve the capacity for physiological inotropic responses in outpatients.— L. H. Opie, *Lancet*, 1984, *1*, 496.

The management of congestive heart failure in patients with acute myocardial infarction. Dobutamine and dopamine are the agents of choice for inotropic support. Dobutamine reduces left-ventricular filling pressure and is useful for increasing cardiac output in patients with pulmonary congestion. Increased cardiac work is balanced by increased coronary blood flow following dobutamine treatment, and it does not appear to increase infarct size, although doses should be tailored to avoid excessive increases in heart rate, which *animal* studies suggest may exacerbate ischaemia. Direct measurement of cardiac output is required to accurately assess the haemodynamic response to dobutamine. Dopamine is indicated where hypotension requiring vasoconstriction is predominant. Its pressor effect is more marked than dobutamine. Dobutamine and dopamine have been used in combination in patients with cardiogenic shock.— R. Genton and A. S. Jaffe, *J. Am. med. Ass.*, 1986, *256*, 2556.

A discussion of positive inotropic therapy in chronic congestive heart failure. Such therapy rests upon a number of assumptions, the first of which, that a contractile reserve exists in these patients that may be tapped by an inotropic agent, has been shown to be true. However, the second assumption, that haemodynamic improvement is sustained, cannot be unreservedly accepted. The effects of beta-adrenergic stimulants such as dopamine and dobutamine have been shown to attenuate over time. This is attributed to down regulation of numbers and stimulatory activity of the beta-receptors. There is also no certainty that functional capacity can be improved (the third assumption) by sympathomimetics such as dopamine or dobutamine, or by other types of inotropic agent. The fourth assumption is that patients will feel better with inotropic therapy: symptomatic improvement with dobutamine has been attributed to a 'conditioning' effect on the cardiovascular system. Finally, it is assumed that inotropic agents do not have a deleterious effect on the heart: studies with dobutamine have conflicted as to whether dobutamine exacerbates myocardial ischaemic injury. Although new inotropic therapy offers exciting potential the available data do not recommend it as a form of therapy until the above assumptions are shown to be true.— B. F. Uretsky, *Postgrad. med. J.*, 1986, *62*, 585.

A review of the use of intermittent infusions of dobutamine in congestive heart failure. Continuing clinical and haemodynamic improvement of congestive heart failure has been noted for weeks to months after discontinuation of infusions of dobutamine. Studies in groups of patients given intermittent weekly infusions, a schedule adopted because of the development of tolerance to the drug's effects with prolonged infusions, have demonstrated increased exercise tolerance and improved functional capacity. The mechanism by which these improvements occur is not known but has been suggested to be a result of a myocardial conditioning effect similar to that resulting from exercise. Although intermittent dobutamine may be a therapeutic option in severe refractory congestive heart failure, further studies are required to determine the long-term benefits, if any, and the most appropriate dosage regimen.— V. F. Mauro and L. S. Mauro, *Drug Intell. & clin. Pharm.*, 1986, *20*, 919. See also R. L. Thomas *et al.*, *Pharmacotherapy*, 1987, *7*, 47.

Dobutamine was given in doses up to 15 µg per kg per minute as a 48-hour infusion every week to outpatients with intractable congestive heart failure. The drug was administered via a portable infusion pump and infusions were carried out at home. Therapy for between 3 and 24 months resulted in an improvement in New York Heart Association functional class in 10 of 11 patients; the mean improvement was 1.2 grades. However, it was uncertain whether survival was enhanced by therapy: 8 of the 11 patients died during the study. There were 9 infectious episodes associated with the venous catheter but only 1 patient developed bacteraemia. An improvement in functional capacity that permits patients to ambulate when they were previously disabled by congestive symptoms should be considered a worthwhile therapeutic goal: further investigation of the effect of long-term dobutamine on survival seems warranted.— D. S. Roffman *et al.*, *Clin. Pharm.*, 1985, *4*, 195.

A study in 13 patients with severe congestive heart failure concluded that intermittent ambulatory dopamine infusions did not improve survival and only partially improved symptoms. There was an improvement in functional class in 7 patients, but only 3 patients were still alive after 6 months, 2 of whom had also been receiving amiodarone.— M. J. Krell *et al.*, *Am. Heart J.*, 1986, *112*, 787.

Shock. References to the use of dobutamine in the treatment of shock: R. A. Eskridge, *Drug Intell. & clin. Pharm.*, 1983, *17*, 92 (in the later stages of septic shock); A. P. Rae and I. Hutton, *Br. J. Anaesth.*, 1986, *58*, 151 (cardiogenic shock); I. M. Ledingham and G. Ramsay, *ibid.*, 169 (mention of use with dopamine in hypovolaemic shock refractory to fluid replacement); K. Balakumaran and P. G. Hugenholtz, *Drugs*, 1986, *32*, 372 (cardiogenic shock).

Preparations

Dobutamine Hydrochloride for Injection *(U.S.P.)*. A sterile mixture of dobutamine hydrochloride with suitable diluents. Potency is expressed in terms of the equivalent amount of dobutamine.

Proprietary Preparations

Dobutrex *(Lilly, UK)*. *Infusion*, powder for reconstitution, dobutamine hydrochloride equivalent to dobutamine 250 mg.
Infusion, dobutamine hydrochloride equivalent to dobutamine 12.5 mg/mL, in vials of 20mL.

Proprietary Names and Manufacturers

Dobutrex *(Lilly, Austral.; Lilly, Canad.; Lilly, Denm.; Lilly, Fr.; Lilly, Ger.; Neth.; Lilly, Norw.; Lilly, S.Afr.; Lilly, Spain; Lilly, Swed.; Lilly, Switz.; Lilly, UK; Lilly, USA)*.

2053-x

Dopamine Hydrochloride *(BANM, USAN, rINNM)*.

3-Hydroxytyramine Hydrochloride; ASL-279.
4-(2-Aminoethyl)pyrocatechol hydrochloride; 4-(2-Aminoethyl)benzene-1,2-diol hydrochloride.
$C_8H_{11}NO_2,HCl=189.6$.

CAS — 51-61-6 (dopamine); 62-31-7 (hydrochloride).

Pharmacopoeias. In *Br.*, *Chin.*, *It.*, and *U.S.*

A white or almost white, odourless or almost odourless crystalline powder. Freely **soluble** in water, in methyl alcohol, and in solutions of alkali hydroxides; sparingly soluble in alcohol; practically insoluble in ether and in chloroform. The *B.P.* states that the pH of a 4% solution containing 1% sodium metabisulphite is 2.5 to 5.5; the *U.S.P.* gives the pH of a 4% solution as between 3.0 and 5.5. **Store** in airtight containers. Protect from light.

Dopamine hydrochloride was stable for 48 hours at 25° in 8 intravenous fluids of pH 5.4 to 6.85. It was incompatible with sodium bicarbonate and the solution became pink in colour.— L. A. Gardella *et al.*, *Am. J. Hosp. Pharm.*, 1975, *32*, 575. Dopamine hydrochloride in glucose injection was physically incompatible (precipitate) with amphotericin; with ampicillin sodium a pink colour appeared 3 hours after admixture; dopamine potency was maintained for 24 hours in the presence of benzylpenicillin potassium, cephalothin sodium, and gentamicin sulphate but the antibiotic potencies were not maintained beyond 6 hours.— *idem*, 1976, *33*, 537. Evidence (that has been confirmed) of a much lower loss of gentamicin.— S. S. Chrai *et al.* (letter), *ibid.*, 1977, *34*, 348. Dopamine hydrochloride in glucose injection was physically compatible for 24 hours, unprotected from light, with heparin sodium, lignocaine hydrochloride, neutral cephalothin sodium, oxacillin sodium, gentamicin sulphate, methylprednisolone sodium succinate, hydrocortisone sodium succinate, potassium chloride, calcium chloride, or calcium gluceptate.— L. A. Gardella *et al.*, *Am. J. Hosp. Pharm.*, 1978, *35*, 581.

Adverse Effects

For the adverse effects of sympathomimetics see p.1453.

Other side-effects that have been occasionally associated with dopamine infusion, include bradycardia and aberrant conduction, and piloerection; raised BUN has also been reported.

A report of fixed dilated pupils due to the administration of high doses of dopamine hydrochloride.— G. L. Ong and H. A. Bruning, *Crit. Care Med.*, 1981, *9*, 658.

ISCHAEMIA AND GANGRENE. Cyanosis, progressing to gangrene, developed in the feet and toes of a 51-year-old man during a 2-day infusion of dopamine 10 µg per kg body-weight per minute after a mitral valve replacement operation. He had previously suffered 3 episodes of frost-bite in his feet. It was suggested that dopamine should be used with caution in elderly patients with pre-existing vascular damage.— C. S. Alexander *et al.*, *New Engl. J. Med.*, 1975, *293*, 591. Massive local arterial and venous vasoconstriction followed infiltration of dopamine from an infusion into the dorsum of the left hand using a 21-gauge scalp-vein needle. There was no response to local injection of phentolamine or systemic injection of papaverine and the patient required partial amputation of the index finger and debridement followed by skin grafting of the entire dorsum of the left hand. Administration of dopamine had since been allowed only through indwelling venous catheters.— R. S. Boltax *et al.* (letter), *ibid.*, 1977, *296*, 823.

A 58-year-old woman with mild diabetes was treated for cardiogenic shock with dopamine hydrochloride. Gangrenous changes followed initial dopamine therapy and administration of very high doses of dopamine led to rapid progression of these changes.— N. K. Julka and J. R. Nora (letter), *J. Am. med. Ass.*, 1976, *235*, 2812.

Infusion of dopamine 7 µg per kg body-weight per minute via a peripheral vein of the left foot was effective in combating progressive hypotension in a neonate with sepsis, but discoloration of the foot developed after 28 hours and progressed despite discontinuing the infusion. The toes became black, shrivelled, and cracked and 4 toes eventually self-amputated due to progressive dry gangrene.— J. C. Maggi *et al.*, *J. Pediat.*, 1982, *100*, 323.

Treatment of Adverse Effects

Since the half-life of dopamine is only about 2 minutes most adverse effects can be corrected by discontinuing or reducing the rate of infusion. If these measures fail excessive vasoconstriction and hypertension may be treated with an alpha-adrenoceptor blocking agent such as 5 to 10 mg of phentolamine mesylate intravenously, repeated as necessary.

Relief from tissue necrosis and pain may be given by immediate infiltration with phentolamine.

A report of the use of 2% glyceryl trinitrate ointment, applied locally as a thin film, to improve capillary blood flow in 2 patients with dopamine-induced ischaemia of the toes.— N. M. Gibbs and T. E. Oh, *Lancet*, 1983, *2*, 290. Agreement. The author's own findings in over 200 patients support those of Gibbs and Oh, and the following method is suggested in all shocked patients who are at risk of peripheral ischaemia and reduced organ perfusion. The toe temperature should be continuously monitored, whether or not the patient is receiving dopamine at the time, and if it falls below 25° glyceryl trinitrate ointment is applied to the warmest area of the skin (usually the chest or abdominal wall), rather than directly to the periphery which appears to be less effective. The dose is increased hourly until the toe temperature is above 30° and then repeated hourly until shock has resolved—in practice, the ointment is used for 24 hours. If the toe temperature falls below 25° on withdrawal of the ointment the process is repeated until the temperature can be maintained without ointment. If there is no response to 8 inches of ointment an intravenous infusion of glyceryl trinitrate may be used.— J. Coakley (letter), *ibid.*, 633.

Precautions

For precautions with sympathomimetic agents see p.1453.

Although it is less likely than adrenaline to produce ventricular arrhythmias, dopamine should be avoided or only used with extreme caution during anaesthesia with cyclopropane, halothane, and other halogenated anaesthetics.

Following a report in 1976 to the FDA by R.P. Rapp of hypotension in patients given phenytoin in addition to dopamine infusion R.D. Smith and T.E. Lomas (*Toxic. appl. Pharmac.*, 1978, *45*, 665) studied the potential interaction, and found that dopamine given by intravenous infusion concomitantly with phenytoin infusion to *dogs*, did not alter the CNS effects of phenytoin nor result in hypotension and cardiovascular collapse. Large doses of phenytoin alone, had a reproducible hypotensive effect which was reduced by dopamine, suggesting a possible supportive role in phenytoin-induced hypotension.

Fatal paradoxical hypotension in a man given *tolazoline* in addition to dopamine.— G. C. Carlon, *Chest*, 1979, *76*, 336.

For a report of gangrene associated with the use of dopamine after ergometrine administration see Ergometrine Maleate, p.1054.

Dopamine produced a lesser increase in cardiac output

for a given dose in 6 patients with ischaemic heart disease, compared with 6 healthy subjects, and was associated in the former group with an increase in end-diastolic and end-systolic volume, with no overall improvement in left ventricular function. This deleterious effect of dopamine on myocardial function, despite apparent clinical improvement, is compatible with the development of acute myocardial ischaemia.— R. W. Kerwin *et al*, *Br. J. clin. Pharmac.*, 1985, *20*, 269P.

Absorption and Fate

For a brief outline of the absorption and fate of a catecholamine, see Adrenaline, p.1455.

The vasoconstrictor properties of dopamine preclude its administration by subcutaneous or intramuscular administration. Like adrenaline it is inactive when given by mouth, and it is rapidly inactivated in the body by similar processes, with a half-life of about 2 minutes. Dopamine is a metabolic precursor of noradrenaline and a proportion is excreted as the metabolic products of noradrenaline. Nevertheless, the majority appears to be directly metabolised into dopamine-related metabolic products.

Uses and Administration

The catecholamine, dopamine, is a sympathomimetic agent with both direct and indirect effects. It is formed in the body by the decarboxylation of levodopa, and is both a neurotransmitter in its own right (notably in the brain) and a precursor of noradrenaline. Dopamine differs from adrenaline and noradrenaline in dilating renal and mesenteric blood vessels and increasing urine output, apparently by a specific dopaminergic mechanism. This effect is predominant at low infusion-rates (about 2 μg per kg body-weight per minute); at slightly higher infusion-rates (up to about 10 μg per kg per minute) it also stimulates $beta_1$-adrenergic receptors in the myocardium. The inotropic action of dopamine on the heart is associated with less cardiac-accelerating effect, and a lower incidence of arrhythmias, than that of isoprenaline. In the treatment of shock this dual action of dopamine has the advantage that it can correct haemodynamic imbalance by exerting an inotropic effect on the heart, without undue tachycardia, and at the same time improve renal perfusion. However, at larger doses dopamine also exerts alpha-stimulant effects, notably vasoconstriction; when high doses are given this may ultimately prevail over the renal vasodilatation.

Concentrations of dopamine are reduced in the brains of patients with Parkinson's disease; increased brain-dopamine concentrations are accordingly beneficial in this condition. In practice, as dopamine is not active by mouth and does not readily cross the blood-brain barrier, its precursor, levodopa (p.1018) is given for treatment.

Dopamine also inhibits release of prolactin from the anterior pituary (see Prolactin, p.1145).

Dopamine is used as the hydrochloride in the treatment of shock unresponsive to replacement of fluid loss and especially where renal function is impaired. It is used to correct haemodynamic imbalances associated with myocardial infarction, trauma, septic shock, and cardiac surgery; it is also used in the management of congestive heart failure. It is administered as a dilute solution, in glucose injection, sodium chloride injection, or other suitable diluents, by intravenous infusion. The initial rate is 2 to 5 μg per kg body-weight per minute, gradually increased by 5 to 10 μg per kg per minute according to the patient's blood pressure, cardiac output, and urine output. Up to 20 to 50 μg per kg per minute may be required in seriously ill patients; higher doses have been given. A reduction in urine flow, without hypotension, may indicate a need to reduce the dose. To avoid tissue necrosis dopamine is best administered into a large vein high up in a limb, preferably the arm. It has been recommended that on gradual discontinuation of dopamine care should be taken to avoid undue hypotension associated with very low dosage levels where vasodilatation could predominate.

ADMINISTRATION. A recommendation to calculate an individual concentration of dopamine so that 1 μg per kg body-weight per minute is equivalent to 1 drop per minute. Thus, with a drip set delivering 60 drops per mL, the amount of dopamine in mg in 100 mL of infusion must be 6 times the patient's weight in kg. The method may be adapted for other drip sets by ensuring that the dopamine content of each drop in μg is the same numerically as the patient's weight in kg, when the same drop-to-dose relationship will apply. Children or infants may require double or fourfold concentration to reduce fluid input, but the essential simplicity remains.— J. M. Chapman and J. R. Davies (letter), *Br. med. J.*, 1978, *2*, 437. A similar recommendation.— J. M. Nappi (letter), *Am. J. Hosp. Pharm.*, 1979, *36*, 881.

The use of a dopamine infusion into the tibial bone-marrow to treat severe hypotension following cardiac arrest in a child in whom intravenous access was difficult.— R. A. Berg, *Am. J. Dis. Child.*, 1984, *138*, 810.

Results in 14 critically-ill neonates given stepwise infusions of dopamine, at an initial dose of 1 to 2 μg per kg per minute, for cardiovascular compromise suggested that the minimum effective dose to produce an increase in mean blood pressure was only 0.5 to 1 μg per kg per minute, while that to produce an increase in systolic blood pressure was 1 to 2 μg per kg per minute; doses of 2 to 3 μg per kg per minute were required to produce an increase in heart-rate. These trends were seen irrespective of birthweight or gestational age. Administration of dopamine by sequential increase in rate from lower doses than are commonly recommended may produce positive inotropic responses without undesirable tachycardia and arrhythmias.— J. F. Padbury *et al.*, *J. Pediat.*, 1987, *110*, 293.

BLEEDING. A report of the successful use of a regional intra-arterial infusion of dopamine in 4 patients for the management of traumatic haemorrhage. In one patient with a fracture of the right pubic bone, noradrenaline controlled the haemorrhage, but caused anuria. The noradrenaline was stopped and dopamine 7.5 μg per kg body-weight per minute was infused into the right hypogastric artery. Haemostasis was maintained and renal function returned. The infusion was tapered over 14 hours and the patient made an uneventful recovery.— H. J. Mud and H. A. Bruining (letter), *New Engl. J. Med.*, 1980, *303*, 754.

CARDIAC DISORDERS. Updated standards and guidelines from the 1985 National Conference on Cardiopulmonary Resuscitation and Emergency Cardiac Care. Dopamine is one of the drugs used to improve cardiac output and blood pressure in advanced cardiac life-support in the context of conditions such as shock and heart failure. It is available only for intravenous use, the initial rate of infusion being 2 to 5 μg per kg per minute; the infusion is subsequently titrated to effect. To obtain the optimal effect, haemodynamic monitoring is required. On terminating therapy it should be tapered gradually rather than being abruptly discontinued. Its inotropic actions, which include an indirect component due to the release of stored noradrenaline from cardiac sympathetic nerves may be reduced in chronic congestive heart failure where noradrenaline stores are depleted, or in infants in whom sympathetic innervation of the myocardium is incomplete. Infusions of over 20 μg per kg per minute may result in excessive vasoconstriction; if further inotropic support is needed once this dose is reached either adrenaline or dobutamine should be considered.— American Heart Association and the National Academy of Sciences–National Research Council, *J. Am. med. Ass.*, 1986, *255*, 2905. Correction.— *ibid.*, *256*, 1727.

For mentions of the use of dopamine in congestive heart failure see under Dobutamine Hydrochloride, p.1459.

Shock. A review of *cardiogenic shock*. Haemodynamics and renal function can be improved in the pump failure patient by infusion of dopamine, but at doses greater than 10 μg per kg per minute increases in heart rate and, more importantly, systemic vascular resistance, occur. The effects of inotropic agents on myocardial metabolism and oxygen usage must also be considered, and dopamine increases myocardial oxygen consumption which may lead to extension of the size of the infarct.— A. P. Rae and I. Hutton, *Br. J. Anaesth.*, 1986, *58*, 151. See also C. E. Handler, *Postgrad. med. J.*, 1985, *61*, 705.

In patients with *hypovolaemic shock* in whom restoration of blood volume and red-cell mass fails to restore cardiac output pharmacological assistance may be required, most commonly with an inotropic agent. Dopamine has proved attractive for its effects on both cardiac and urinary output. If administered by intravenous infusion at a rate that keeps systolic arterial pressure from rising above 80 to 100 mmHg, dopamine will normally induce a gratifying diuresis. If the rate is increased arrhythmias may occur. The risk of intrapulmonary shunting should be noted, and the fact that toxic effects increase with the passage of time. One manoeuvre which is gaining popularity is to use dopamine by low-dose infusion during the early stages of resuscitation to maintain renal perfusion and, if cardiac output requires to be augmented, either to increase the dose of dopamine, or to add dobutamine which has less marked effects on heart-rate and excitability.— I. M. Ledingham and G. Ramsay, *Br. J. Anaesth.*, 1986, *58*, 169.

Dopamine is perhaps the most commonly used vasopressor and inotropic agent in *septic shock*. Its dose-dependent actions allow selection of haemodynamic effects to meet the patient's needs. Dilation of the renal, mesenteric, and splanchnic vasculature at low doses is useful in the phase of septic shock where blood flow to the bowel and kidneys is somewhat compromised but the heart is performing effective pumping action, whereas the more pronounced inotropic action at moderate doses can be helpful when the heart needs inotropic assistance to maintain blood pressure. The vasoconstriction at higher doses may sometimes be necessary to maintain adequate arterial pressures but blood flow to vital organs such as the bowel and kidneys may be compromised.— R. A. Eskridge, *Drug Intell. & clin. Pharm.*, 1983, *17*, 92.

RENAL DISORDERS. Infusion of low doses of dopamine hydrochloride (1 μg per kg body-weight per minute) significantly increased urine output in early oliguric acute tubular necrosis in 11 patients. It was concluded that infusion of low doses of dopamine is worthy of further trial in oliguric states.— I. S. Henderson *et al.*, *Lancet*, 1980, *2*, 827. Comments on the role of the frusemide which was also given.— G. Graziani *et al.* (letter), *ibid.*, 1301; C. Brun-Buisson and J. R. Le Gall (letter), *ibid.* Similar findings using a dose of 2 μg per kg per minute. Irrespective of the primary pathology, continuous infusion of dopamine has been found to promote a diuresis, reducing dialysis requirements and simplifying management. The use of dopamine has been extended to prophylaxis in high-risk patients. Thus, a low-dose infusion of dopamine is started in all patients with acute pancreatitis, bacterial toxaemia, haemorrhagic shock, and severe trauma requiring admission to the intensive care unit. As yet there is insufficient data for statistical analysis, but acute renal failure seems to have been averted in some patients.— A. R. Luksza and S. T. Atherton (letter), *ibid.*, 1036. A further study in 24 oliguric patients unresponsive to infusions of mannitol and frusemide. Patients were given dopamine 1 to 3 μg per kg per minute and frusemide 30 to 50 mg per hour, intravenously, for up to 24 hours. Diuresis improved in 19 patients from an initial mean of 11.2 mL per hour to 85.1 mL per hour, with a concomitant rise in natriuresis and a fall in plasma creatinine concentrations. Five patients did not respond; therapy had not been instituted until more than 24 hours after the onset of oliguria in these patients, in contrast to those who responded, all of whom began therapy within 24 hours of oliguria. The combination of low-dose dopamine and high-dose frusemide seems able to combat acute renal failure in oliguric patients when therapy is commenced soon after the onset of symptoms.— G. Graziani *et al.*, *Nephron*, 1984, *37*, 39.

Comment on the possible relationship between changes in the treatment of poor cardiac performance and circulatory failure, including the use of dopamine, and the decline in cases of oliguria in patients with acute renal failure.— B. D. Myers and S. M. Moran, *New Engl. J. Med.*, 1986, *314*, 97.

Preparations

Dopamine Hydrochloride and Dextrose Injection *(U.S.P.)*. A sterile solution of dopamine hydrochloride and glucose in water for injections. pH between 2.5 and 4.5. It should not be used if darker than slightly yellow or otherwise discoloured.

Dopamine Hydrochloride Injection *(U.S.P.)*. It has a pH of 2.5 to 5.0. The injection should be diluted before use and should not be used if it is darker than slightly yellow or otherwise discoloured.

Dopamine Intravenous Infusion *(B.P.)*. Dopamine Hydrochloride Intravenous Infusion. A sterile solution containing dopamine hydrochloride 800 mg in 500 mL, prepared immediately before use by diluting Strong Sterile Dopamine Solution with a suitable diluent.

Strong Sterile Dopamine Solution *(B.P.)*. Strong Sterile Dopamine Hydrochloride Solution. It is sterilised by filtration, and has a pH of 2.5 to 5.5. It should be diluted before use with a non-alkaline diluent.

Proprietary Preparations

Intropin *(American Hospital Supply, UK). Concentrate for intravenous infusion,* dopamine hydrochloride 40 mg/mL, in ampoules or pre-filled syringes of 5 mL, and 160 mg/mL, in ampoules of 5 mL.

Select-A-Jet Dopamine Hydrochloride Injection *(IMS, UK). Concentrate for intravenous infusion,* dopamine hydrochloride 40 mg/mL, in cartridge assemblies containing 5, 10, and 20 mL.

Proprietary Names and Manufacturers

Aprical-Dopamina *(Farmasimes, Spain)*; Dopastat *(Parke, Davis, USA)*; Dopmin *(Erco, Denm.)*; Dynatra *(Belg.)*; Giludop *(Giulini, Denm.; Kali-Chemie, Swed.)*; Hettytropin *(Arg.)*; Inotropin *(Arg.)*; Inovan *(Jpn)*; Intropin *(Boots, Austral.; Du Pont, Canad.; Neth.; Boots, S.Afr.; American Critical Care, Swed.; American Hospital Supply, UK; American Critical Care, USA)*; Revimine *(USV, Austral.; Rorer, Canad.)*; Revivan *(Simes, Ital.)*; Select-A-Jet Dopamine Hydrochloride *(IMS, UK)*.

18632-e

Dopexamine Hydrochloride *(BANM, USAN, rINNM).*

FPL-60278 (dopexamine); FPL-60278AR. 4-{2-[6-(Phenethylamino)hexylamino]ethyl}pyrocatechol dihydrochloride.

$C_{22}H_{32}N_2O_2,2HCl=429.4$.

CAS — 86197-47-9 (dopexamine); 86484-91-5 (hydrochloride).

Adverse Effects and Precautions

For the adverse effects of sympathomimetic agents, and precautions to be observed, see p.1453.

Uses and Administration

Dopexamine hydrochloride is a derivative of dopamine (p.1460) which has been investigated for its peripheral vasodilator and inotropic effects in the management of heart failure.

References: B. E. Jaski *et al., Br. J. clin. Pharmac.,* 1986, *21,* 393; F. Magrini *et al., Eur. J. clin. Pharmac.,* 1987, *32,* 1.

Proprietary Names and Manufacturers

Fisons, UK.

2054-r

Ephedra

Ma-huang.

Pharmacopoeias. In *Chin.* and *Jpn.*

Ephedra consists of the dried young branches of *Ephedra sinica, E. equisetina,* and *E. gerardiana* (including *E. nebrodensis*) (Ephedraceae), containing not less than 1.25% of alkaloids, calculated as ephedrine. (*Jpn P.* specifies not less than 0.6%). *Chin.P.* also includes Radix Ephedrae, prepared from the roots of *E.sinica* or *E.intermedia.*

The action of ephedra is due to the presence of ephedrine and pseudoephedrine. It has been used chiefly as a source of the alkaloids.

Comment on the abuse of 'Ma-Huang Incense'.— R. K. Siegel (letter), *New Engl. J. Med.,* 1980, *302,* 817.

2055-f

Ephedrine *(BAN, USAN).*

Hydrated Ephedrine; Efedrina; Ephedrina; (−)-Ephedrine; Ephedrine Hemihydrate; Ephedrinum; Ephedrinum Hemihydricum. (1*R*,2*S*)-2-Methylamino-1-phenylpropan-1-ol hemihydrate.

$C_{10}H_{15}NO,\frac{1}{2}H_2O=174.2$

CAS — 50906-05-3 (hemihydrate).

Pharmacopoeias. In *Aust., Belg., Br., Eur., Fr., Ger., It., Neth.,* and *Swiss. Braz., Ind., Mex.,* and *U.S.* specify anhydrous or hemihydrate.

An alkaloid obtained from species of *Ephedra,* or prepared synthetically. Colourless crystals or white crystalline powder. The m.p. varies according to the moisture content; the *B.P.* specifies that the undried substance melts at about 42°.

B.P. **solubilities** are: soluble in water; very soluble in alcohol; freely soluble in ether. *U.S.P.* solubilities are: soluble 1 in 20 of water and 1 in 0.2 of alcohol; soluble in chloroform and ether; moderately and slowly soluble in liquid paraffin, the solution becoming turbid if the water content exceeds 1%. Ephedrine decomposes on exposure to light. **Store** at a temperature not exceeding 8° in airtight containers. Protect from light.

2056-d

Anhydrous Ephedrine

Efedrina; Ephed. Anhydros.; Ephedrine; Ephedrinum Anhydricum. The anhydrous alkaloid prepared by vacuum distillation of the hydrate.

CAS — 299-42-3.

Pharmacopoeias. In *Arg., Aust., Br., Eur., Fr., Ger., It., Neth., Span.,* and *Swiss. Braz., Ind., Mex.,* and *U.S.* specify anhydrous or hemihydrate.

Colourless crystals or white crystalline powder. M.p. about 36°.

Soluble in water and in chloroform; very soluble in alcohol; freely soluble in ether. Ephedrine decomposes on exposure to light. **Store** at a temperature not exceeding 8° in airtight containers. Protect from light.

2057-n

Ephedrine Hydrochloride *(BANM, USAN).*

Ephedrinae Hydrochloridum; Ephedrine Chloride; Ephedrini Hydrochloridum; Ephedrinium Chloratum; *l*-Ephedrinum Hydrochloricum.

$C_{10}H_{15}NO,HCl=201.7$.

CAS — 50-98-6.

Pharmacopoeias. In *Arg., Aust., Belg., Br., Braz., Chin., Cz., Eur., Egypt., Fr., Ger., Ind., Int., It., Jpn, Jug., Mex., Neth., Nord., Pol., Port., Roum., Rus., Span., Swiss, Turk.,* and *U.S. Hung. P.* includes only the racemic form (racephedrine hydrochloride).

Odourless colourless crystals or white crystalline powder.

The *B.P.* states that it is **soluble** 1 in 4 of water, and 1 in 17 of alcohol; very slightly soluble in chloroform; practically insoluble in ether. The *U.S.P.* has soluble 1 in 3 of water and 1 in 14 of alcohol. It is affected by light. **Store** in well-closed containers. Protect from light.

2058-h

Ephedrine Sulphate *(BANM).*

Ephedrine Sulfate *(USAN).*

$(C_{10}H_{15}NO)_2,H_2SO_4=428.5$.

CAS — 134-72-5.

Pharmacopoeias. In *Arg., Braz.,* and *U.S.*

Fine white odourless crystals or powder. It darkens on exposure to light. **Soluble** 1 in 1.3 of water and 1 in 90 of alcohol. **Store** in well-closed containers. Protect from light.

Adverse Effects

For the adverse effects of sympathomimetics see p.1453.

Injection of ephedrine during labour can cause foetal tachycardia.

Paranoid psychosis, delusions, and hallucinations may also follow ephedrine overdosage. Prolonged administration has no cumulative effect, but tolerance with dependence has been reported.

In hypersensitive patients local application of the drug may cause a contact dermatitis.

OVERDOSAGE. A 15-year-old girl took about 30 tablets of Franol. Four hours later she was found to be flushed, sweating, and vomiting profusely. Her heart-rate was 140 per minute. The main effect was apparently due to the ephedrine content of the tablets and bore some similarity to the symptoms and signs of diabetic precoma. The effects persisted for about 18 hours and then gradually subsided.— P. E. M. Jarrett (letter), *Lancet,* 1966, *2,* 1190.

Symptoms of cardiomyopathy, with clinical, haemodynamic, and ECG features resembling those of phaeochromocytoma, occurred in a 34-year-old man after chronic excessive intake of ephedrine. Symptoms slowly regressed after prolonged bed rest.— W. Van Mieghem *et al., Br. med. J.,* 1978, *1,* 816.

Precautions

For precautions necessary with sympathomimetics see p.1453. In patients with prostatic enlargement, ephedrine may increase difficulty with micturition.

Due to its stimulant effects on the central nervous system ephedrine should not usually be given after about 4 pm. Children, however, are reportedly less susceptible to this stimulant effect.

The vasoconstrictor effects of drugs such as ephedrine applied topically as a nasal spray or drops in sinusitis or head colds may cause local ischaemia or eventually exacerbate rather than relieve the nasal symptoms.— R. Lancaster, *Prescribers' J.,* 1983, *23,* 47.

PREGNANCY AND THE NEONATE. Ephedrine and pseudoephedrine are present in breast-milk in sufficient concentration to be harmful to the baby, and are contra-indicated in women who are breast-feeding.— P. C. Rubin, *Br. med. J.,* 1986, *293,* 1415.

TACHYPHYLAXIS. A report of tolerance to ephedrine developing in a 12-year-old boy on 3 occasions within only a few days of starting therapy for bronchospasm.— P. Rangsithienchai and R. W. Newcomb (letter), *J. Am. med. Ass.,* 1978, *240,* 20.

Absorption and Fate

Ephedrine is readily and completely absorbed from the gastro-intestinal tract. It is resistant to metabolism by monoamine oxidase and is largely excreted unchanged in the urine, together with small amounts of metabolites produced by hepatic metabolism. Ephedrine has been variously reported to have a plasma half-life ranging from 3 to 6 hours depending on urinary pH; elimination is enhanced and half-life accordingly shorter in acid urine.

The absorption, metabolism, and excretion of ephedrine, norephedrine, and methylephedrine under constant acidic urine control.— G. R. Wilkinson and A. H. Beckett, *J. pharm. Sci.,* 1968, *57,* 1933. See also *idem, J. Pharmac. exp. Ther.,* 1968, *162,* 139. Urinary excretion of ephedrine in healthy subjects without pH control of urine.— P. G. Welling *et al., J. pharm. Sci.,* 1971, *60,* 1629. Metabolism of ephedrine in healthy subjects.— P. S. Sever *et al., Eur. J. clin. Pharmac.,* 1975, *9,* 193. Pharmacokinetics of ephedrine in asthmatic subjects.— M. E. Pickup *et al., Br. J. clin. Pharmac.,* 1976, *3,* 123. Absorption and excretion of ephedrine in one healthy subject.— K. K. Midha *et al., J. pharm. Sci.,* 1979, *68,* 557.

Uses and Administration

Ephedrine is a sympathomimetic agent with direct and indirect effects on adrenergic receptors. It has alpha- and beta-adrenergic activity and has pronounced stimulating effects on the central nervous system. It has a more prolonged though less potent action than adrenaline. In therapeutic doses it raises the blood pressure by increasing cardiac output and also by inducing peripheral vasoconstriction. Tachycardia may occur but is less frequent than with adrenaline. Ephedrine also causes bronchodilatation, reduces intestinal tone and motility, relaxes the bladder wall while contracting the sphincter muscle but relaxes the detrusor muscle of the bladder and usually reduces the activity of the uterus. It has a stimulant action on the respiratory centre. It dilates the pupil but does not affect the light reflexes. After ephedrine has been used for a short while, tachyphylaxis may develop.

Ephedrine hydrochloride or sulphate, in doses of 15 to 60 mg by mouth 3 or 4 times a day, may be used to prevent bronchial spasm in asthma, but the more beta$_2$-selective sympathomimetic bronchodilating agents, such as salbutamol (p.1482) are now preferred. Similar doses have been given by subcutaneous or intramuscular injection. A suggested dose for children is 500 μg per kg body-weight three or four times daily.

Ephedrine salts are occasionally used in the treatment of narcolepsy, and, (usually as an adjunct to neostigmine), were formerly used in the management of myasthenia gravis; doses of up to 60 mg have been given at night for enuresis.

Ephedrine salts have been given by subcutaneous or intramuscular injection to combat a fall in blood pressure during spinal anaesthesia. Ephedrine is of little value in hypotensive crises due to shock, circulatory collapse, or haemorrhage. It is no longer generally advocated for orthostatic hypotension.

Ephedrine salts have been used, either alone or in conjunction with other agents, in the symptomatic relief of nasal congestion associated with the common cold, hay-fever, or rhinitis or sinusitis. However, the continued use of nasal decongestants is liable to aggravate the condition and may lead to rebound congestion and drug-induced rhinitis. Nasal drops or sprays usually containing 0.5% are used; a 0.25% or 0.5% strength is used for infants and young children.

For preparing solutions in oil, anhydrous ephedrine was formerly preferred but oily sprays and nasal drops should no longer be used since they reduce ciliary activity and may cause lipoid pneumonia.

Ephedrine eye-drops have been used as a mydriatic; accommodation is not significantly affected and ephedrine does not cause increased intra-ocular pressure. The effect lasts several hours. Ephedrine is often ineffective in the presence of inflammation and also in highly pigmented eyes.

Ephedrine has also been given as the camsylate.

In the *UK* the use of ephedrine or its salts in cosmetics is prohibited.

ALLERGY AND ANAPHYLAXIS. Addition of ephedrine 25 mg by mouth to a pre-treatment regimen of prednisone and diphenhydramine was more effective than the same regimen alone in preventing allergic reactions to radiographic contrast media in high-risk patients.— P. A. Greenberger *et al., J. Allergy & clin. Immunol.*, 1984, *74*, 540.

ASTHMA. A recommendation that non-selective oral bronchodilator drugs such as ephedrine should not be used for bronchodilatation.— A. B. X. Breslin, *Drugs*, 1979, *18*, 103.

See also under Pregnancy and the Neonate, below.

HICCUP. Twelve patients who developed hiccup during anaesthesia and surgery were treated successfully with an intravenous injection of ephedrine 5 mg (eleven cases) or 10 mg (one case). Nine of the patients had previously proved refractory to other attempts to alleviate the spasms. No adverse haemodynamic changes were seen in these patients.— Y. Z. Sohn *et al., Can. Anaesth. Soc. J.*, 1978, *25*, 431.

HYPOTENSION. Ephedrine in doses of 30 mg abolished the postural symptoms in 4 patients with orthostatic hypotension but also produced recumbent hypertension. The long-term use of ephedrine for this condition was considered hazardous.— B. Davies *et al., Lancet*, 1978, *1*, 172. Administration of ephedrine in association with propranolol had no beneficial effect in 4 patients with idiopathic orthostatic hypotension (Shy-Drager syndrome) and 1 with orthostatic hypotension believed to be of different origin.— M. S. Kochar and H. D. Itskovitz, *ibid.*, 1011.

MYASTHENIA GRAVIS. The beneficial effect of ephedrine in myasthenia gravis has long been recognised, though the response is rarely striking. A dose of 30 mg three times daily should be tried if the response to anticholinesterase agents is inadequate.— C. W. H. Havard, *Br. med. J.*, 1977, *2*, 1008.

OEDEMA. Ephedrine, in doses of 30 mg three or four times daily was given to 3 insulin-dependent diabetics who had severe neuropathy associated with intractable oedema of the feet and lower legs; a fourth, similar patient was given 60 mg three times daily. Ephedrine produced a rapid decrease in weight and a diminution of oedema. Sodium excretion was also increased and peripheral diastolic flow was reduced. No side effects were noted and there was no significant change in blood pressure in any of the patients, including one with a history of hypertension. All 4 patients have continued on ephedrine for 12 to 15 months, and the effects have been sustained with no sign of tachyphylaxis, perhaps because patients with autonomic neuropathy have depleted catecholamine stores and ephedrine is probably acting mainly as a direct-acting sympathomimetic.— M. E. Edmonds *et al., Lancet*, 1983, *1*, 548.

PREGNANCY AND THE NEONATE. A review of the management of asthma during pregnancy. Ephedrine, and theophylline and its derivatives, are not thought to be teratogenic and one or both may be administered for mild episodes of bronchospasm requiring drug therapy.— P. A. Greenberger and R. Patterson, *New Engl. J. Med.*, 1985, *312*, 897. Comments, and criticism of the use of combination preparations in the management of asthma.— K. M. Altenburger (letter), *ibid.*, *313*, 517.

See also under Asthma, above.

SYNCOPE. A report of a favourable response to ephedrine 25 mg four times daily and fludrocortisone 100 µg daily in a patient with vasodepressor carotid sinus syncope.— T. Rentmeester *et al., Br. med. J.*, 1984, *289*, 720.

Preparations of Ephedrine and its Salts

Ephedrine Elixir *(B.P.)*. Ephedrine Hydrochloride Elixir; Ephedrine Oral Solution. Contains ephedrine hydrochloride 0.3% in a suitable flavoured vehicle containing 12% of alcohol.

Ephedrine Hydrochloride Tablets *(B.P.)*

Ephedrine Instillation *(A.P.F.)*. Ephedrine Nasal Drops; Ephedrine Nasal Spray. Contains ephedrine hydrochloride 1%.

Ephedrine Nasal Drops *(B.P.C. 1973)*. Contain ephedrine hydrochloride 0.5%.

Ephedrine Sulfate Capsules *(U.S.P.)*. Capsules containing ephedrine sulphate.

Ephedrine Sulfate and Phenobarbital Capsules *(U.S.P.)*. Capsules containing ephedrine sulphate and phenobarbitone.

Ephedrine Sulfate Injection *(U.S.P.)*. A sterile solution of ephedrine sulphate in Water for Injections. pH 4.5 to 7.0.

Ephedrine Sulfate Nasal Solution *(U.S.P.)*. A solution containing ephedrine sulphate. Store in airtight containers.

Ephedrine Sulfate Syrup *(U.S.P.)*. Contains ephedrine sulphate 18 to 22 mg in each 5 mL. Store at a temperature not exceeding 40° in airtight containers.

Ephedrine Sulfate Tablets *(U.S.P.)*. Contain ephedrine sulphate.

Proprietary Preparations of Ephedrine and its Salts

CAM (Children's Antispasmodic Mixture) *(Rybar, UK)*. *Mixture*, ephedrine hydrochloride 4 mg, butethamate citrate 4 mg/5 mL. For asthma and bronchitis. *Dose.* 20 mL three to four times daily. Children, up to 2 years, 2.5 mL three times daily; 3 to 4 years, 5 mL; over 4 years, 10 mL.

Expurhin Paediatric Decongestant *(Galen, UK)*. *Paediatric linctus*, ephedrine hydrochloride 4 mg, chlorpheniramine maleate 1 mg, menthol 1.1 mg/5 mL.

Franol (known in some countries as Franyl) *(Winthrop, UK)*. *Tablets*, ephedrine hydrochloride 11 mg, theophylline 120 mg. For asthma and bronchitis. *Dose.* 1 tablet 3 times daily; children, one-third to one-half the adult dose. NOTE. These tablets were reformulated to exclude phenobarbitone.

Franol Plus *(Winthrop, UK)*. *Tablets*, ephedrine sulphate 15 mg, theophylline 120 mg. For asthma and bronchitis. *Dose.* 1 tablet three times daily and 1 at bedtime where there are nocturnal asthma attacks; children, one-third to one-half the adult dose. NOTE. These tablets were reformulated to exclude phenobarbitone and thenyldiamine hydrochloride.

Tedral *(Parke, Davis, UK)*. *Tablets*, ephedrine hydrochloride 24 mg, theophylline 120 mg.

Elixir, ephedrine hydrochloride 6 mg, theophylline 30 mg/5 mL. *Dose.* 1 tablet or 20 mL of elixir every 4 hours after food.

Proprietary Names and Manufacturers of Ephedrine and its Salts

Ectasule Minus *(Fleming, USA)*; Efed II Yellow *(Alto, USA)*; Efetonina *(Bracco, Ital.)*; Ephedral *(Belg.)*; Ephetonin *(E. Merck, Ger.)*; Fedrine *(USV, Austral.)*; Minims Ephedrine Hydrochloride *(Smith & Nephew Pharmaceuticals, UK)*; Rhino-Vaccin *(Rodeca, Canad.)*; Rino Pumilene *(Montefarmaco, Ital.)*; Roter *(Neth.)*; Spaneph *(Smith Kline & French, UK)*; Stopasthme *(Granions, Mon.)*.

The following names have been used for multi-ingredient preparations containing ephedrine and its salts—Amesec *(Lilly, Austral.; Lilly, Canad.; Lilly, UK)*; Argotone *(Riker, Austral.; Lipha, UK)*; Asmal *(Norton, UK)*; Asmapax *(Nicholas, UK)*; Asthma Dellipsoids D17 *(Pilsworth, UK)*; Auralgicin *(Fisons, UK)*; Breezeazy *(Cambridge Laboratories, Austral.)*; Bronchial Dellipsoids D15 *(Pilsworth, UK)*; Bronchotone *(Rorer, UK)*; Bronkolixir *(Winthrop-Breon, USA)*; Bronkotabs *(Winthrop-Breon, USA)*; CAM *(Rybar, UK)*; Davenol *(Wyeth, UK)*; Dolvan *(Norma, UK)*; Elixir Sibec *(Vestric, UK)*; Ephedramine *(Drug Houses Austral., Austral.)*; Ephedrine and Amytal *(Lilly, USA)*; Ephedrine and Seconal Sodium *(Lilly, USA)*; Expansyl *(Smith Kline & French, UK)*; Expurhin *(Galen, UK)*; Falcodyl *(Norton, UK)*; Flavelix *(Pharmax, UK)*; Franol *(Winthrop, UK)*; Franol Plus *(Winthrop, UK)*; Franyl; Haymine *(Pharmax, UK)*; Hemocane *(Key, Austral.)*; Histadyl EC *(Lilly, UK)*; Iodo-Ephedrine *(Philip Harris, UK)*; Iso-Bronchisan *(Berk Pharmaceuticals, UK)*; Isuprel Compound Elixir *(Winthrop, Canad.; Breon, USA : Winthrop-Breon, USA)*; Lotussin *(Searle, UK)*;

Marax *(Roerig, USA)*; Medicone Derma-HC *(Medicone, USA)*; Mudrane *(Poythress, USA)*; Mudrane GG *(Poythress, USA)*; Mudrane GG Elixir *(Poythress, USA)*; Nomaze *(Fisons, UK)*; Noradran *(Norma, UK)*; Norgotin *(Norgine, UK)*; Nyquil *(Richardson-Vicks, Canad.)*; Omni-Tuss *(Pennwalt, Canad.)*; Paranorm *(Wallace Mfg Chem., UK)*; Paspat *(Luitpold, Austral.)*; Pazo *(Bristol-Myers Products, USA)*; PEM *(Loveridge, UK)*; Phensedyl *(May & Baker, UK)*; Pholdrine *(Austral.)*; Phyldrox *(Carlton Laboratories, UK)*; Priatan *(Schering, Austral.)*; Primatene *(Whitehall, USA)*; Primatene M *(Whitehall, USA)*; Primatene P *(Whitehall, USA)*; Quadrinal *(Knoll, USA)*; Quelidrine *(Abbott, USA)*; Quiactin Mixture *(Merrell Dow, Austral.)*; Quibron Plus *(Mead Johnson Laboratories, USA)*; Rectinol *(G.P. Laboratories, Austral.)*; Rhinamid *(Bailly, Fr. : Bengué, UK)*; Riddobron Tablets *(Seaford, UK)*; Riddofan *(Seaford, UK)*; Rubelix *(Pharmax, UK)*; Rynatuss *(Wallace, USA)*; Taumasthman *(Wallace Mfg Chem., UK)*; Tedral *(Parke, Davis, Canad.; Parke, Davis, UK; Parke, Davis, USA)*; Tedral Expectorant *(Warner, UK)*; Tedral SA *(Warner, UK)*; Tedral-25 *(Parke, Davis, USA)*; T.E.H. *(Geneva, USA)*; T-E-P *(Schein, USA)*; T.E.P. *(Geneva, USA)*; Terra-Bron *(Pfizer, UK)*; Theozine *(Schein, USA)*; Valledrine *(May & Baker, Austral.; May & Baker, UK)*; Wyanoids *(Wyeth, USA)*.

2059-m

Etafedrine Hydrochloride *(BANM, USAN, rINNM)*.

Ethylephedrine Hydrochloride. (−)-2-(Ethylmethylamino)-1-phenylpropan-1-ol hydrochloride.

$C_{12}H_{19}NO,HCl = 229.7$.

CAS — 48141-64-6 (etafedrine); 5591-29-7 (hydrochloride).

Etafedrine hydrochloride is a sympathomimetic agent with an action similar to that of ephedrine (p.1462) but reportedly fewer cardiovascular effects. It has been used in the management of bronchospasm.

Proprietary Names and Manufacturers

The following names have been used for multi-ingredient preparations containing etafedrine hydrochloride— Calmydone *(Technilab, Canad.)*; Mercodol with Decapryn *(Dow, Canad.)*; Nethaprin Dospan *(Merrell, UK)*; Nethaprin Expectorant *(Merrell, UK)*; Quiactin Linctus *(Merrell Dow, Austral.)*.

2060-t

Ethylnoradrenaline Hydrochloride

Ethylnorepinephrine Hydrochloride *(USAN)*. 2-Amino-1-(3,4-dihydroxyphenyl)butan-1-ol hydrochloride.

$C_{10}H_{15}NO_3,HCl = 233.7$.

CAS — 536-24-3 (ethylnoradrenaline); 3198-07-0 (hydrochloride).

Pharmacopoeias. In *U.S.*

A white or almost white crystalline powder; it darkens on exposure to light. **Soluble** in water and in alcohol; practically insoluble in ether. **Store** in well-closed containers. Protect from light.

Ethylnoradrenaline is a sympathomimetic agent with predominantly beta-adrenergic activity. Its actions are similar to those of isoprenaline (p.1466) but it is reportedly less potent. Ethylnoradrenaline hydrochloride is usually given by subcutaneous or intramuscular injection in doses of 1 to 2 mg for its bronchodilator action in bronchial asthma.

Preparations

Ethylnorepinephrine Hydrochloride Injection *(U.S.P.)*. A sterile solution of ethylnoradrenaline hydrochloride in Water for Injections. pH 2.5 to 5.0. It should not be used if it is brown or contains a deposit.

Proprietary Names and Manufacturers

Bronkephrine *(Winthrop, Austral.; Winthrop-Breon, USA)*.

2061-x

Etilefrine Hydrochloride *(rINNM).*
Ethyladrianol Hydrochloride; Ethylnorphenylephrine Hydrochloride; M-I-36. 2-Ethylamino-1-(3-hydroxyphenyl)ethanol hydrochloride.
$C_{10}H_{15}NO_2,HCl=217.7$.

CAS — 709-55-7 (etilefrine); 943-17-9 (hydrochloride).

Pharmacopoeias. In *Jpn.*

Etilefrine hydrochloride is a sympathomimetic agent which has been used for the treatment of hypotension. The pivalate ester of etilefrine hydrochloride has also been investigated.

Proprietary Names and Manufacturers
Cardiosimpal *(Inibsa, Spain)*; Circupon *(Tropon, Ger.; Medichemie, Switz.)*; Confidol *(Pharmasal, Ger.)*; Effoless *(Jpn)*; Effortil *(Boehringer Sohn, Arg.; Boehringer Ingelheim, Belg.; Abbott, Denm.; Boehringer Ingelheim, Denm.; Boehringer Ingelheim, Fr.; Boehringer Ingelheim, Ger.; Boehringer Ingelheim, Ital.; Boehringer Ingelheim, Neth.; Boehringer Ingelheim, Norw.; Boehringer Ingelheim, S.Afr.; Boehringer Ingelheim, Swed.; Boehringer Ingelheim, Switz.)*; Efortil *(Fher, Spain)*; Eti-Puren *(Klinge-Nattermann, Ger.)*; Presotona *(Erco, Denm.)*; Pressoton *(Erco, Swed.)*; Sanlephrin *(Jpn)*; Tensio Retard *(Trenker, Belg.)*; Tensofar *(Alet, Arg.)*; Tonus-forte-Tablinen *(Beiersdorf, Ger.)*.

2063-f

Fenoterol Hydrobromide *(BANM, rINNM).*

TH-1165a. 1-(3,5-Dihydroxyphenyl)-2-(4-hydroxy-α-methylphenethylamino)ethanol hydrobromide.
$C_{17}H_{21}NO_4,HBr=384.3$.

CAS — 13392-18-2 (fenoterol); 1944-12-3 (hydrobromide).

NOTE. Fenoterol is *USAN*.

Pharmacopoeias. In *Br.*

A white crystalline powder. **Soluble** in water and in alcohol; practically insoluble in chloroform and in ether. A 4% solution in water has a pH of 4.2 to 5.2.

Store in well-closed containers. Protect from light.

Adverse Effects

For the adverse effects of sympathomimetic agents, see p.1453.

EFFECTS ON ELECTROLYTES. Plasma potassium concentrations decreased significantly in 12 healthy subjects who inhaled fenoterol compared with a further 4 who received placebo; the mean fall was greater in subjects given larger doses. Patients receiving high doses of beta$_2$-agonists by inhalation may be at increased risk of cardiac arrhythmias because of this pronounced fall in plasma potassium.— J. R. E. Haalboom *et al.*, *Lancet*, 1985, *1*, 1125. Comment. The effect appears to be more pronounced than that seen previously with salbutamol. Hypokalaemia induced by these agents may be exacerbated by theophylline.— S. R. Smith *et al.* (letter), *ibid.*, 1394. Doubts as to the clinical relevance of the findings and reminders of the dangers of inadequate treatment in acute asthma: K. E. Berkin *et al.* (letter), *ibid;* R. M. Cayton (letter), *ibid.*, 1395.

EFFECTS ON THE HEART. Angina pectoris associated with the use of a fenoterol inhaler.— *Med. J. Aust.*, 1979, *2*, 92.

Precautions

For precautions necessary with sympathomimetics see p.1453.

For reference to pulmonary oedema developing when fenoterol was given for premature labour, see under Salbutamol, p.1481.

Absorption and Fate

Fenoterol is incompletely absorbed from the gastro-intestinal tract and is also subject to extensive first-pass metabolism by sulphate conjugation. It is excreted in the urine and bile almost entirely as the inactive sulphate conjugate.

A study of the pharmacokinetics of fenoterol after administration to *animals* and man. Fenoterol was readily absorbed from the gastro-intestinal tract; the half-life in man was estimated as 6 to 7 hours.— K. L. Rominger and W. Pollmann, *Arzneimittel-Forsch.*, 1972, *22*, 1190.

Uses and Administration

Fenoterol hydrobromide is a direct-acting sympathomimetic agent with actions and uses similar to those of salbutamol (p.1482).

In the treatment of bronchial asthma fenoterol hydrobromide is used by inhalation in a dose of 1 or 2 inhalations of 200 µg, delivering at the mouthpiece 180 µg, three times daily; up to 2 inhalations (400 µg, delivering at the mouthpiece 360 µg) may be used every 4 hours if necessary. It may also be given as a nebulised solution, in doses of 0.5 to 2.5 mg inhaled up to 4 times daily; higher doses have been given. A suggested dose for children is 1 inhalation of 180 µg three times daily, increased to a maximum of every 4 hours if necessary, or up to 1 mg as a nebulised solution up to 3 times daily.

Fenoterol is also used similarly to salbutamol in the management of premature labour.

ADMINISTRATION. Administration of fenoterol as a dry powder inhalation to children.— V. Graff-Lonnevig, *Allergy*, 1982, *37*, 609. Fenoterol was equally effective administered via a metered-dose inhaler or a dry powder inhaler in a crossover study in 20 asthmatic patients. Dry powder inhalation may be a useful alternative in patients who have difficulty using the metered-dose inhaler.— K. Kiviranta, *ibid.*, 1985, *40*, 305. See also A. Lahdensuo *et al.*, *Eur. J. resp. Dis.*, 1986, *68*, 332.

In a double-blind crossover study in 10 asthmatics fenoterol 800 µg intranasally or 400 µg by mouth both produced a significant improvement in respiratory function compared with placebo. For patients experiencing attacks of extreme bronchoconstriction severely reducing their ventilation one of these alternative routes may be of value.— S. Groth *et al.*, *J. Allergy & clin. Immunol.*, 1984, *74*, 536.

Pharmacokinetic variability may partly explain some of the differences in the apparent efficacy of fenoterol when administered buccally to patients with asthma in various studies, although the extent to which these studies were properly controlled must also have influenced the results. Shore *et al.* (*S. Afr. med. J.*, 1976, *50*, 1362) demonstrated bronchodilation in an uncontrolled study using buccal fenoterol, but in other studies the effect was either less than that of inhaled fenoterol (D. Rodenstein *et al.*, *Br. J. Dis. Chest*, 1982, *76*, 365) or barely distinguishable from that of placebo (R.E. Ruffin *et al.*, *Chest*, 1978, *74*, 256).— *Lancet*, 1987, *1*, 666.

ASTHMA. Comparisons of fenoterol with other agents in the management of asthma: P. Chervinsky, *Ann. Allergy*, 1978, *40*, 189 (with terbutaline: similar responses); B. J. Gray *et al.*, *Br. J. Dis. Chest*, 1982, *76*, 341 (a longer and more specific action with terbutaline than fenoterol); B. Hockley and N. M. Johnson, *Postgrad. med. J.*, 1983, *59*, 504 (greater bronchodilation and duration of action than equal doses of salbutamol); M. I. Asher and C. Dunn, *Aust. paediat. J.*, 1985, *21*, 119 (no significant difference between fenoterol and salbutamol in asthmatic children); D. Bellamy and A. Penketh, *Postgrad. med. J.*, 1987, *63*, 459 (salbutamol as effective as fenoterol in 8 asthmatics, and had fewer side-effects).

Results suggesting that fenoterol combined with ipratropium bromide might be more effective than salbutamol as a bronchodilator in asthmatic patients: K. C. Flint *et al.*, *Postgrad. med. J.*, 1983, *59*, 724.

Fenoterol hydrobromide 200 µg plus ipratropium bromide 80 µg did not produce significantly greater bronchodilation than fenoterol hydrobromide 200 or 400 µg alone in a single-dose crossover study in 9 patients.— P. Lawford and K. N. V. Palmer, *Postgrad. med. J.*, 1983, *59*, 28.

A brief review of the use of ipratropium bromide and fenoterol hydrobromide as a combined preparation. Such a preparation has only a slight statistical advantage over a beta$_2$-stimulant alone, and cannot be considered a first-line treatment for bronchoconstriction.— *Drug & Ther. Bull.*, 1985, *23*, 3.

See also under Ipratropium Bromide, p.537.

PREGNANCY AND THE NEONATE. References to the use of fenoterol in premature labour: C. Lecart *et al.*, *Acta ther.*, 1981, *7*, 197; S. N. Caritis, *Drugs*, 1983, *26*, 243.

For a comparison of fenoterol with ritodrine in the management of premature labour see Ritodrine Hydrochloride, p.1480.

Proprietary Preparations

Berotec *(Boehringer Ingelheim, UK). Inhaler*, aerosol, fenoterol hydrobromide 180 µg/metered inhalation. *Nebuliser solution*, fenoterol hydrobromide 5 mg/mL.

Duovent *(Boehringer Ingelheim, UK). Inhaler*, aerosol, fenoterol hydrobromide 90 µg, ipratropium bromide 36 µg/metered inhalation.

Proprietary Names and Manufacturers

Berotec *(Arg.; Boehringer Ingelheim, Austral.; Belg.; Boehringer Ingelheim, Canad.; Boehringer Ingelheim, Denm.; Boehringer Ingelheim, Fr.; Boehringer Ingelheim, Ger.; Neth.; Boehringer Ingelheim, Norw.; Boehringer Ingelheim, S.Afr.; Fher, Spain; Boehringer Ingelheim, Swed.; Boehringer Ingelheim, Switz.; WB Pharmaceuticals, UK: Boehringer Ingelheim, UK)*; Dosberotec *(Boehringer Ingelheim, Ital.)*; Partusisten *(Arg.; Belg.; Boehringer Ingelheim, Ger.; Neth.; NZ; S.Afr.; Boehringer Ingelheim, Switz.)*.

2064-d

Fenoxazoline Hydrochloride *(rINNM).*
2-(2-Isopropylphenoxymethyl)-2-imidazoline hydrochloride.
$C_{13}H_{18}N_2O,HCl=254.8$.

CAS — 4846-91-7 (fenoxazoline); 21370-21-8 (hydrochloride).

A 0.05 or 0.1% solution of fenoxazoline hydrochloride has been applied to the nasal mucosa as a nasal decongestant.

Proprietary Names and Manufacturers
Aturgyl *(Dausse, Fr.)*; Nebulicina *(Castejon, Spain)*; Snup *(Karlspharma, Ger.)*.

2065-n

Hexoprenaline Hydrochloride *(BANM, rINNM).*
ST-1512. *NN′*-Hexamethylenebis[4-(2-amino-1-hydroxyethyl)pyrocatechol] dihydrochloride; *NN′*-Hexamethylenebis[2-amino-1-(3,4-dihydroxyphenyl)ethanol] dihydrochloride.
$C_{22}H_{32}N_2O_6,2HCl=493.4$.

CAS — 3215-70-1 (hexoprenaline); 4323-43-7 (hydrochloride).

2066-h

Hexoprenaline Sulphate *(BANM, rINNM).*

$C_{22}H_{32}N_2O_6,H_2SO_4=518.6$.

CAS — 32266-10-7.

Adverse Effects and Precautions
For the adverse effects of sympathomimetics, and precautions to be observed, see p.1453.

A report of atrial fibrillation following the use of hexoprenaline for premature labour.— M. C. Frederiksen *et al.*, *Am. J. Obstet. Gynec.*, 1982, *145*, 108.

Uses and Administration
Hexoprenaline is a direct-acting sympathomimetic agent with general properties similar to those of salbutamol (p.1480). The sulphate has been used as a bronchodilator in doses of 250 to 500 µg three times daily by mouth. It has also been given in doses of 200 µg by inhalation.

A study of the dose-response relationship to hexoprenaline 2.5 µg intravenously given every 15 minutes, to a total cumulative dose of 15 µg, in 8 asthmatics and 7 patients with chronic obstructive pulmonary disease compared to 5 healthy subjects. Hexoprenaline produced a dose-related increase in heart-rate in all 3 groups without significantly increasing mean arterial blood pressure. Hexoprenaline caused a significant dose-related improvement in pulmonary function in all patients, which was greatest in those with asthma. There was no such significant improvement among the healthy subjects.— M. S. Lin *et al.*, *Curr. ther. Res.*, 1987, *41*, 380.

PREGNANCY AND THE NEONATE. A favourable report of the use of bolus injections of hexoprenaline 10 µg to improve the foetal heart-rate in labour in 6 patients.— J. Lipshitz, *Am. J. Obstet. Gynec.*, 1977, *129*, 31. Studies suggesting that the metabolic effects produced by an infusion of hexoprenaline 10 µg in women in the third trimester of pregnancy would be beneficial to the foetus, especially in cases of acute foetal distress.— J. Lipshitz *et al.*, *ibid.*, 1978, *130*, 761. For criticisms of recommendations that a similar beta-adrenoceptor stimulant, ritodrine, should be used for the treatment of foetal distress, see *Drug & Ther. Bull.*, 1975, *13*, 26. See also *ibid.*, 1978, *16*, 83.

A study of the effects of hexoprenaline given together with metoprolol in the treatment of preterm labour.— U. Siekmann *et al.*, *Arzneimittel-Forsch.*, 1984, *34*, 1025. See also J. Lipshitz E. M. Lipshitz, *Obstet. Gynec.*, 1984, *63*, 396.

Proprietary Names and Manufacturers of Hexoprenaline Salts

Bronalin *(Byk Liprandi, Arg.)*; Etoscol *(Byk Gulden, Ger.; Jpn)*; Gynipral *(Chemie-Linz, Switz.)*; Ipradol *(Chemie-Linz, Aust.; Rosco, Denm.; Continental Ethicals, S.Afr.; Lacer, Spain)*; Leanol *(Jpn)*.

2067-m

Hydroxyamphetamine Hydrobromide *(BANM, USAN)*.

Bromhidrato de Hidroxianfetamina; Hydroxyamfetamine Hydrobromide *(rINNM)*; Oxamphetamine Hydrobromide. (±)-4-(2-Aminopropyl)phenol hydrobromide.
$C_9H_{13}NO,HBr=232.1$.

CAS — 103-86-6 (hydroxyamphetamine); 1518-86-1 (hydroxyamphetamine, ±); 306-21-8 (hydrobromide); 140-36-3 (hydrobromide, ±).

Pharmacopoeias. In *Arg.* and *U.S.*

A white crystalline powder. Freely **soluble** in water and in alcohol; slightly soluble in chloroform; practically insoluble in ether. Solutions in water have a pH of about 5. **Store** in well-closed containers. Protect from light.

Adverse Effects and Precautions

For the adverse effects of sympathomimetics, and precautions to be observed, see p.1453.

Uses and Administration

Hydroxyamphetamine hydrobromide is a sympathomimetic agent with an action similar to that of ephedrine (p.1462), but it has little or no stimulant effect on the central nervous system. It was formerly used as a pressor agent and in the management of some cardiac disorders.

In ophthalmology, hydroxyamphetamine hydrobromide is used in a 1% solution as a mydriatic and in the diagnosis of Horner's syndrome.

Preparations

Hydroxyamphetamine Hydrobromide Ophthalmic Solution *(U.S.P.)*. pH 4.2 to 6.0.

Proprietary Names and Manufacturers

Paredrine *(Smith Kline & French, USA)*.

The following names have been used for multi-ingredient preparations containing hydroxyamphetamine hydrobromide—Sulfex *(Smith Kline & French, UK)*; Vasocort *(Smith Kline & French, UK)*.

2068-b

Hydroxyephedrine

p-Hydroxyephedrine; Methylsynephrine; Oxyephedrine. 1-(4-Hydroxyphenyl)-2-methylaminopropan-1-ol.
$C_{10}H_{15}NO_2=181.2$.

CAS — 365-26-4.

Hydroxyephedrine is a sympathomimetic agent with an action similar to that of ephedrine (p.1462). Its salts have been used in antitussive preparations.

Proprietary Names and Manufacturers

The following names have been used for multi-ingredient preparations containing hydroxyephedrine— Cophylac *(Hoechst, Canad.)*; Cophylac Expectorant *(Hoechst, Canad.)*; Ticarda *(Hoechst, Austral.)*.

12838-d

Ibopamine Hydrochloride *(BANM, rINNM)*.

SB-7505 *(ibopamine)*; SKF-100168 *(ibopamine)*. 4-(2-Methylaminoethyl)-*o*-phenylene di-isobutyrate hydrochloride.
$C_{17}H_{25}NO_4,HCl=343.9$.

CAS — 66195-31-1 (ibopamine).

NOTE. Ibopamine is *USAN*.

Adverse Effects and Precautions

For the adverse effects of sympathomimetic agents, and precautions to be observed, see p.1453.

Uses and Administration

Ibopamine hydrochloride is a peripheral dopamine agonist with inotropic effects which increases renal blood flow. It is used in the management of congestive heart failure in usual doses of 50 to 100 mg by mouth two or three times daily.

The effects of ibopamine on cardiovascular and renal function in 8 healthy subjects.— J. -H. Ren *et al.*, *Curr. ther. Res.*, 1983, *34*, 667.

Ibopamine 100 to 200 mg (1.2 to 3.3 mg per kg body-weight) as a single dose by mouth significantly improved cardiac performance in 10 patients with severe congestive heart failure. The maximum haemodynamic effect occurred on average after 180 minutes and its effects were still measurable 5 hours after the dose. Heart rate and arterial blood pressure were not affected.— P. Ghirardi *et al.*, *Br. J. clin. Pharmac.*, 1985, *19*, 613.

Further references to ibopamine in heart failure: J. Col *et al.*, *Eur. J. clin. Pharmac.*, 1983, *24*, 297 (promising preliminary results in severe congestive heart failure); N. Marchionni *et al.*, *J. clin. Pharmac.*, 1986, *26*, 74 (in congestive heart failure refractory to cardiac glycosides, diuretics, and captopril); A. Banassi *et al.*, *Arzneimittel-Forsch.*, 1986, *36*, 390 (cardiomyopathy and heart failure); A. Avanzini *et al.*, *ibid.*, 394 (congestive heart failure); V. Ferrarri *et al.*, *ibid.*, 398 (beneficial results in combination therapy of congestive heart failure); A. Galassi *et al.*, *Curr. ther. Res.*, 1986, *40*, 337 (improvement in heart failure in 19 patients with pacemakers).

RENAL DISORDERS. A preliminary study in 6 patients with chronic renal failure and 6 healthy controls demonstrated an increase in creatinine clearance and diuresis in both groups following ibopamine 50 mg twice daily for a week.— S. Stefoni *et al.*, *Br. J. clin. Pharmac.*, 1981, *1*, 69. Ibopamine 150 mg had no effect on renal function in 10 healthy subjects; in a further six given 600 mg there was a similar lack of response.— J. N. Harvey *et al.*, *ibid.*, 1984, *17*, 671.

Proprietary Names and Manufacturers

Inopamil *(Simes, Ital.)*; Scandine *(Zambon, Ital.)*.

2069-v

Ibuterol Hydrochloride *(rINNM)*.

KWD-2058. 2-*tert*-Butylamino-1-(3,5-di-isobutyryloxyphenyl)ethanol hydrochloride; 5-(2-*tert*-Butylamino-1-hydroxyethyl)-*m*-phenylene di-isobutyrate hydrochloride.
$C_{20}H_{31}NO_5,HCl=401.9$.

CAS — 53034-85-8 (ibuterol); 61435-51-6 (hydrochloride).

Ibuterol is an inactive ester of terbutaline (p.1483). After absorption into the body it is hydrolysed into terbutaline. It has been given as a bronchodilator by mouth as the hydrochloride in doses of 2 and 4 mg.

The short duration of action following ibuterol administration appears to demand 5 times daily dosage in order to maintain an adequate serum concentration of active terbutaline during the 24-hour period.— Y. Hörnblad *et al.*, *Eur. J. clin. Pharmac.*, 1976, *10*, 9.

12848-h

Indanazoline *(rINN)*.

2-(Indan-4-ylamino)-2-imidazoline.
$C_{12}H_{15}N_3=201.3$.

CAS — 40507-78-6.

Indanazoline is a sympathomimetic related to naphazoline (p.1470) which has been used as a spray or drops for the relief of nasal catarrh.

Proprietary Names and Manufacturers

Farial *(Nordmark, Ger.)*.

2070-r

Isoetharine Hydrochloride *(BANM, USAN)*.

Etyprenaline Hydrochloride; Isoetarine Hydrochloride *(rINNM)*; *N*-Isopropylethylnoradrenaline Hydrochloride. 1-(3,4-Dihydroxyphenyl)-2-isopropylaminobutan-1-ol hydrochloride.
$C_{13}H_{21}NO_3,HCl=275.8$.

CAS — 530-08-5 (isoetharine); 50-96-4 (hydrochloride).

Pharmacopoeias. In *U.S.*

A white to off-white odourless crystalline solid. **Soluble** in water; sparingly soluble in alcohol; practically insoluble in ether. A 1% solution in water has a pH of 4.0 to 5.6. **Store** in airtight containers.

2071-f

Isoetharine Mesylate *(BANM, USAN)*.

Isoetarine Mesilate *(rINNM)*; Isoetharine Methanesulphonate; *N*-Isopropylethylnoradrenaline Mesylate; Win-3406 *(isoetharine)*.
$C_{13}H_{21}NO_3,CH_4O_3S=335.4$.

CAS — 7279-75-6.

Pharmacopoeias. In *U.S.*

White or almost white odourless crystals. Freely **soluble** in water; soluble in alcohol; practically insoluble in acetone and ether. A 1% solution in water has a pH of 4.5 to 5.5. **Store** in airtight containers.

Adverse Effects and Precautions

For the adverse effects of sympathomimetic agents, and precautions to be observed, see p.1453.

Paradoxical bronchoconstriction in an asthmatic patient following the use of nebulised isoetharine appeared to be caused by sodium bisulfite present as a preservative.— J. W. Koepke *et al.*, *J. Am. med. Ass.*, 1984, *251*, 2982.

ABNORMAL COLORATION. Pink sputum mimicking haemoptysis occurred in many patients using isoetharine inhalation solution and could be alarming. The effect appeared to be due to oxidation of the drug when the preparation's antioxidant was diluted by water and sputum.— P. L. Hooper *et al.* (letter), *New Engl. J. Med.*, 1983, *308*, 1602.

Uses and Administration

Isoetharine is a sympathomimetic agent with predominantly beta-adrenergic activity. Its actions are reportedly similar to those of isoprenaline (p.1467) but it has less beta$_1$-stimulant effect. It is used as a bronchodilator in asthma and chronic bronchitis. It is given by inhalation, as a nebulised solution of the hydrochloride in strengths up to 1%, or as an aerosol inhalation of the mesylate; it may also be given by mouth as the hydrochloride in usual doses of 10 or 20 mg three or four times daily as a sustained-release tablet.

Preparations of Isoetharine Salts

Isoetharine Inhalation Solution *(U.S.P.)*. Isoetharine Hydrochloride Inhalation. A solution of isoetharine hydrochloride in water. May contain sodium chloride. pH 2.5 to 5.5. Store in small well-filled airtight containers. Protect from light.

Isoetharine Mesylate Inhalation Aerosol *(U.S.P.)*. Contains a solution of isoetharine mesylate in alcohol, in an inert propellent basis. Store in small containers with metered-dose valves and oral inhalation actuators. Protect from light.

Proprietary Preparations of Isoetharine Salts

Bronchilator *(Sterling Research, UK)*. *Inhaler*, aerosol, isoetharine mesylate 350 µg, phenylephrine hydrochloride 70 µg/metered inhalation.

Numotac *(Riker, UK)*. *Tablets*, sustained-release, isoetharine hydrochloride 10 mg.

Proprietary Names and Manufacturers of Isoetharine Salts

Asthmalitan *(Kettelhack Riker, Ger.)*; Bronkometer *(Winthrop-Breon, USA)*; Bronkosol *(Winthrop-Breon, USA)*; Numotac *(Belg.; Riker, Denm.; Neth.; Norw.; Riker, UK)*.

2072-d

Isometheptene Hydrochloride *(BANM, rINNM).*

1,5,*N*-Trimethylhex-4-enylamine hydrochloride; 1,5-Dimethylhept-4-enyl(methyl)amine hydrochloride.

$C_9H_{19}N,HCl=177.7$.

CAS — 503-01-5 (isometheptene); 6168-86-1 (hydrochloride).

2073-n

Isometheptene Mucate *(BANM, rINNM).*

Isometheptene galactarate.

$(C_9H_{19}N)_2,C_6H_{10}O_8=492.7$.

CAS — 7492-31-1.

Adverse Effects and Precautions

For the adverse effects of sympathomimetic agents, and precautions to be observed, see p.1453.

PORPHYRIA. Isometheptene mucate was considered to be unsafe in patients with acute porphyria because it has been shown to be porphyrinogenic in *animals* or *in vitro* systems.— M.R. Moore and K.E.L. McColl, *Porphyrias, Drug Lists*, Glasgow, Porphyria Research Unit, University of Glasgow, 1987.

Uses and Administration

Isometheptene is an indirect adrenergic agent which has been given as the hydrochloride and as the mucate. It is given for a vasoconstrictor effect in migraine.

In the *UK*, the use of isometheptene and its salts in cosmetics is prohibited.

Proprietary Preparations

Midrid *(Carnrick, UK). Capsules*, isometheptene mucate 65 mg, paracetamol 325 mg. *Dose.* For migraine headaches, 2 capsules initially, followed by 1 capsule every hour up to a maximum of 5 capsules in 12 hours; for tension headaches, 2 capsules initially, followed by 1 or 2 capsules every 4 hours up to a maximum of 8 capsules per day.

NOTE. These capsules were reformulated to exclude dichloralphenazone.

Proprietary Names and Manufacturers

Octinum *(Knoll, Ital.; Knoll, Switz.).*

The following names have been used for multi-ingredient preparations containing isometheptene mucate— Midrid *(Carnrick, UK)*; Midrin *(Carnrick, USA)*; Migralam *(Bart, USA).*

2074-h

Isoprenaline Hydrochloride *(BANM, rINNM).*

Isopropylarterenol Hydrochloride; Isopropylnoradrenaline Hydrochloride; Isoproterenol Hydrochloride *(USAN)*. 1-(3,4-Dihydroxyphenyl)-2-isopropylaminoethanol hydrochloride.

$C_{11}H_{17}NO_3,HCl=247.7$.

CAS — 7683-59-2 (isoprenaline); 51-30-9 (hydrochloride).

Pharmacopoeias. In *Arg., Br., Braz., Chin., Hung., Ind., Int., It., Jpn, Roum., Turk.,* and *U.S.*

A white or almost white, odourless or almost odourless, crystalline powder. It gradually darkens on exposure to air and light. The *B.P.* states that it is very **soluble** in water; soluble 1 in 55 of alcohol; insoluble in chloroform and ether. *U.S.P.* solubilities are 1 in 3 of water and 1 in 50 of alcohol. A 1% solution in water has a pH of about 5. The *B.P.* injection is **sterilised** by filtration. Solutions become pink to brownish-pink on standing exposed to air and almost immediately so when made alkaline. **Store** in airtight containers. Protect from light.

2075-m

Isoprenaline Sulphate *(BANM, rINNM).*

Isopropylarterenol Sulphate; Isopropylnoradrenaline Sulphate; Isoproterenol Sulfate *(USAN).*

$(C_{11}H_{17}NO_3)_2,H_2SO_4,2H_2O=556.6$.

CAS — 299-95-6 (anhydrous); 6700-39-6 (dihydrate).

Pharmacopoeias. In *Aust., Br., Cz., Fr., Ger., Ind., Int., It., Jug., Neth., Nord., Pol., Swiss, Turk.,* and *U.S.*

A white or almost white, odourless crystalline powder. It gradually darkens on exposure to light and air. Isoprenaline sulphate 1.32 mg is approximately equivalent to 1 mg of isoprenaline or to 1.17 mg of the hydrochloride. **Soluble** 1 in 4 of water; slightly soluble in alcohol; practically insoluble in chloroform and ether. A 5% solution in water has a pH of 4.3 to 5.5. Solutions become pink to brownish-pink on standing exposed to air, and almost immediately so when made alkaline. **Store** in airtight containers. Protect from light.

STABILITY. The addition of sodium metabisulphite 0.1% reduced the discoloration and deposition of particles in an injection containing isoprenaline sulphate 0.02% in water, water adjusted to pH 3 with hydrochloric acid, or in McIlvaine's citrate-phosphate buffer solution pH 3. Solutions made using the buffer were more stable than those adjusted with acid. Autoclaving a solution adjusted with hydrochloric acid to pH 3 led to a 30% loss of potency. If sodium metabisulphite or McIlvaine's buffer solution was used the loss was about 7%. During storage, solutions sterilised by filtration lost no potency at 0° to 4°, about 2 to 10% at 25° over 24 weeks, and 5 to 23% at 37° over 8 weeks. A 0.02% injection of isoprenaline sulphate containing sodium metabisulphite 0.1%, buffered to pH 3 and sterilised by filtration, could be expected to maintain its appearance and potency for up to 6 months when stored in a refrigerator.— Pharm. Soc. Lab. Rep. P/77/2, 1977.

Addition of disodium edetate 0.01% to isoprenaline hydrochloride 0.02% and 0.1% injections, either alone or in combination with ascorbic acid 0.1%, was effective in stabilising the injection during autoclaving and subsequent storage for 1 year at 5 or 25°. Stability was greatest when pH of the injection was adjusted to 2.8, and was greater using the mixture with ascorbic acid than with disodium edetate alone. Storage under nitrogen did not appear to influence the extent of degradation in these solutions.— G. Smith *et al., J. clin. Hosp. Pharm.*, 1984, *9*, 209.

Adverse Effects

For the adverse effects of sympathomimetic agents, see p.1453.

Prolonged use of isoprenaline may lead to resistance, and eventual deterioration, with hypoxia in asthmatic patients.

Prolonged use of isoprenaline tablets sublingually has been reported to cause severe damage to the teeth.

BRONCHOSPASM. Twelve of 41 patients with intractable asthma who were known not to be isoprenaline abusers developed paradoxical bronchospasm after inhalation of isoprenaline. They had not used isoprenaline aerosol for a year prior to evaluation. Furthermore, they consistently showed the expected bronchodilatory response when repeatedly challenged with terbutaline aerosol.— J. Trantlein *et al., Chest*, 1976, *70*, 711. Discussion on the possible reason for such a paradoxical response (including a possible reaction to the aerosol propellent), and comments on the need for further information.— J. W. Jenne and T. W. Chick, *ibid.*, 691.

EFFECTS ON THE HEART. The cardiac effect of repeated inhaled doses of isoprenaline was studied in 18 patients with moderate to severe asthma. Only 1 patient experienced a significant increase in heart-rate immediately after a therapeutic dose of isoprenaline. Arrhythmias did not develop even after repeated inhalations every 5 to 20 minutes.— C. Shim and M. H. Williams, *Ann. intern. Med.*, 1975, *83*, 208.

A review of patient records revealed 8 cases of documented isoprenaline cardiotoxicity at therapeutic dosages. Two patients developed acute myocardial infarction; a 3-year-old child developed reversible subendocardial ischaemia on receiving an isoprenaline infusion following cardiac surgery; and 5 patients with bronchial asthma demonstrated periods of transient myocardial ischaemia.— T. Winsor *et al., Am. Heart J.*, 1975, *89*, 814.

EFFECTS ON SALIVARY GLANDS. Salivary-gland enlargement resembling mumps has been associated with the administration of isoprenaline.— K. D. Hay and P. C. Reade, *Drugs*, 1983, *26*, 268.

EFFECTS ON THE TEETH. A 12-year-old girl, who had been taking isoprenaline sulphate tablets sublingually for 6 years, developed discoloration and destruction of her permanent incisor and canine teeth. They were discoloured a chalky-white with a loss of the natural enamel translucency. Similar results were obtained with experimental teeth when they were immersed for 2 weeks in a solution of isoprenaline sulphate.— J. S. Ball (letter), *Br. med. J.*, 1965, *1*, 1189.

OVERDOSAGE. A 64-year-old patient who had been taking up to 260 mg of isoprenaline daily as sublingual tablets for bronchitis developed tremors, incoordination, a disturbing sleep pattern, and deep ulceration of the tongue. When isoprenaline was withdrawn the patient improved and after 4 weeks the ulcer had healed.— R. D. Brown and G. Bolas, *Br. dent. J.*, 1973, *134*, 336.

For controversy surrounding the role of overuse of isoprenaline aerosols and sudden death in asthmatics, see Sudden Death, under Adverse Effects of Sympathomimetics, p.1453.

Treatment of Adverse Effects

Most toxic effects of isoprenaline subside rapidly when treatment is stopped. Tachycardia and cardiac arrhythmias induced by isoprenaline may be diminished by propranolol but it must not be given to asthmatics because of the risk of increasing bronchoconstriction. Cautious use of a cardioselective beta-adrenoceptor blocking agent may be indicated in asthmatic patients.

Precautions

For precautions with sympathomimetic agents, see p.1453.

Isoprenaline should never be given at the same time as adrenaline but may be used alternately. Isoprenaline may be used simultaneously with phenylephrine.

The saliva or sputum of patients using isoprenaline inhalations may be coloured pink or red.

INTERACTIONS. Concomitant administration with isoprenaline of drugs, such as salicylamide, which are themselves extensively conjugated with sulphate, could increase the pharmacological effects of isoprenaline. Conjugation of isoprenaline in the gut wall could be decreased by salicylamide, thus increasing the amount of pharmacologically active isoprenaline absorbed.— M. E. Conolly *et al., Br. J. Pharmac.*, 1972, *46*, 458. See also C. F. George *et al., J. Pharm. Pharmac.*, 1974, *26*, 265.

Antidepressants. In 4 volunteers pretreated with phenelzine or tranylcypromine for 7 days, the pressor effects of isoprenaline were not enhanced and isoprenaline-induced tachycardia was significantly reduced. Imipramine increased isoprenaline-induced tachycardia two-fold in one of the subjects.— A. J. Boakes *et al., Br. med. J.*, 1973, *1*, 311.

Absorption and Fate

As a result of sulphate conjugation in the gut, isoprenaline is considerably less active following administration by mouth than following parenteral administration. It is absorbed through the oral mucosa and is accordingly given sublingually, but absorption by this route remains very erratic. This explains the wide difference between oral and parenteral doses of isoprenaline.

Isoprenaline in the body is resistant to metabolism by monoamine oxidase, but is metabolised by catechol-*O*-methyltransferase in the liver, lungs, and other tissues, this metabolite being subsequently conjugated before excretion in the urine. Whereas the sulphate conjugate of isoprenaline is inactive the methylated metabolite exhibits weak activity.

Following intravenous injection isoprenaline has a plasma half-life of about one to several minutes according to whether the rate of injection is rapid or slow; it is almost entirely excreted in the urine as unchanged drug and metabolites within 24 hours. A much slower onset of action and a more extended initial half-life has been demonstrated following oral administration. Isoprenaline is reported to have a duration of action of up to about 2 hours after inhalation; it has been demonstrated that a large proportion of an inhaled dose is swallowed.

References to studies on the absorption and fate of isoprenaline: E. W. Blackwell *et al., Br. J. Pharmac.*, 1970, *39*, 194P (metabolism following inhalation); C. T. Dollery *et al.*, *Ann. N.Y. Acad. Sci.*, 1971, *179*, 108 (metabolism following inhalation); M. E. Conolly *et al.*, *Br. J. Pharmac.*, 1972, *46*, 458 (metabolism in dogs and man); E. W. Blackwell *et al.*, *Br. J. Pharmac.*, 1974, *50*, 587 (metabolism in the lungs); C. F. George *et al.*, *J. Pharm. Pharmac.*, 1974, *26*, 265 (metabolism in the intestine); D. Kadar *et al.*, *Clin. Pharmac. Ther.*, 1974, *16*, 789 (metabolic studies in brain-damaged children); J. G. Kelly and D. G. McDevitt, *Br. J. clin. Pharmac.*, 1977, *4*, 628P; *idem*, 1978, *6*, 123 (plasma-protein binding studies).

Uses and Administration

Isoprenaline is a sympathomimetic agent which acts almost exclusively on beta-adrenergic receptors. It stimulates the central nervous system. It has a powerful stimulating action on the heart and increases cardiac output, excitability, and rate; it also causes peripheral vasodilatation and produces a fall in diastolic blood pressure and usually maintains or slightly increases systolic blood pressure.

It is used for its powerful bronchodilator effects in the symptomatic relief of bronchial asthma although the beta$_2$-selective sympathomimetic agents, such as salbutamol are now generally preferred. Resistance to isoprenaline may develop and it is dangerous in the presence of hypoxia.

It is also used in the treatment of bradycardia in patients with heart block, as a stimulant following cardiac arrest, and to control attacks of Stokes-Adams syndrome. In cardiogenic and endotoxic shock, isoprenaline has been used to treat patients who have failed to respond to replacement of electrolyte and water deficiencies.

Isoprenaline is usually administered sublingually or by inhalation, as the hydrochloride or sulphate, for its bronchodilator effects. Pressurised aerosols containing isoprenaline and delivering metered doses of 80 micrograms of the sulphate are a commonly used form of inhaler. The hydrochloride is also used. The recommended adult dosage is 1 to 3 inhalations of 80 µg repeated, if necessary, after not less than 30 minutes up to a maximum of 8 inhalations in 24 hours. If more than 1 inhalation is taken at a time, at least 1 minute should elapse between any 2 inhalations. A stronger aerosol inhaler which delivers metered doses of 400 µg is also available in Great Britain. In the 1960s overuse of pressurised aerosol inhalers was an associated factor in an increase in sudden deaths among asthmatic patients (see under Adverse Effects of Sympathomimetic Agents, p.1453). It is therefore essential to instruct the patients in the correct use of such preparations. If relief is not obtained the dose should not be increased and alternative therapy should be given.

Solutions containing up to 1% or more of isoprenaline sulphate or hydrochloride have been inhaled in the form of a fine mist using a non-metallic nebuliser, and the very finely powdered solid has also been inhaled.

Isoprenaline has been given by sublingual administration in the management of bronchospasm as the hydrochloride or the sulphate in usual doses of 10 to 20 mg three times daily. The tablets were allowed to dissolve under the tongue without being sucked and as little saliva as possible was swallowed. It was recommended that isoprenaline should not be given more than four times daily by this route, and an interval of not less than 3 hours should be allowed between doses. A suggested dose for children was 5 to 10 mg sublingually three times daily.

Doses of 10 to 30 mg have been administered sublingually 4 to 6 times daily to prevent cardiac stand-still in patients with a hyperactive carotid sinus reflex or in the treatment of heart block.

Sustained-release tablets of isoprenaline hydrochloride have been administered by mouth (*not* sublingually) in a dose of 30 mg three times daily increased until the heart is sufficiently accelerated: the daily dose may range from 90 to 840 mg daily, divided into a dosage frequency which may vary from every 2 to every 8 hours.

Isoprenaline, usually as 5 or 10 mg of the sulphate has also been given by the rectal route for cardiac disorders.

Isoprenaline has also been given cautiously under ECG control, usually as a solution of the hydrochloride containing 1 mg in 500 mL of glucose injection by slow intravenous infusion in the treatment of heart block, cardiogenic and endotoxic shock, and as a test of cardiac function. Concentrations of up to 10 mg in 500 mL have been used where limitation of volume is essential. The infusion-rate should provide 0.5 to 10 µg per minute, according to the patient's need; up to 40 µg per minute may be required for monitoring patients with heart block. It has been given subcutaneously or intramuscularly in doses of 200 µg (as 1 mL of a 0.02% solution). In emergencies it may be given by slow intravenous injection of 10 to 60 µg as 0.5 to 3 mL of a 0.002% solution. Intracardiac injections of 20 µg as a 0.02% solution (0.1 mL) have been used.

In the *UK* the use of isoprenaline in cosmetics is prohibited.

ASTHMA AND BRONCHITIS. Because they have a short duration of action and cause marked tachycardia inhalers containing isoprenaline are not recommended in asthma, a selective beta$_2$-agonist being preferred. Combined preparations of isoprenaline and sodium cromoglycate should also be avoided owing to the dangers of inappropriate use.— M. F. Muers, *Prescribers' J.*, 1983, *23*, 32.

CARDIAC DISORDERS. Updated standards and guidelines from the 1985 National Conference on Cardiopulmonary Resuscitation and Emergency Cardiac Care. Isoprenaline has potent inotropic and chronotropic properties that generally result in an increase in cardiac output and increased myocardial work, exacerbating ischaemia and arrhythmia in patients with ischaemic heart disease. The only indication for isoprenaline in acute cardiac life support is the immediate temporary control of significant bradycardia refractory to atropine, in a patient with a pulse. The use of the drug is a temporary measure until pacemaker therapy can be initiated. The recommended infusion rate is 2 to 10 µg per minute titrated according to the heart rate and rhythm response. In children the recommended infusion rate is 0.1 to 1 µg per kg body-weight per minute, but adrenaline may be preferred. Isoprenaline is *not* indicated in patients with cardiac arrest.— American Heart Association and the National Academy of Sciences—National Research Council, *J. Am. med. Ass.*, 1986, *255*, 2905.

Heart block and Stokes-Adams syndrome. Linenthal and Zoll (*Circulation*, 1963, *27*, 5) reported that attacks of **Stokes-Adams syndrome** could be successfully treated with intravenous infusions of isoprenaline or adrenaline at rates of 4 to 8 µg per minute although occasionally higher rates might be necessary. Dack (*Am. Heart J.*, 1963, *66*, 579) recommended injection of isoprenaline 200 µg or Adrenaline Injection 0.5 mL for immediate resuscitative measures, followed by intracardiac injection of isoprenaline or adrenaline 100 µg in 10 mL of Water for Injections if this was unsuccessful; an infusion of isoprenaline or adrenaline, 2 mg in a litre of glucose injection, should then be given at a rate of 4 µg per minute or more according to the ventricle-rate; after stabilisation of the cardiac rhythm the infusion could be gradually reduced and replaced by intermittent intramuscular injections of isoprenaline 200 µg or adrenaline 500 µg, supplemented by isoprenaline orally.

Similar therapy using weaker solutions and slower infusion-rates was recommended for Stokes-Adams syndrome precipitated by ventricular tachycardia or fibrillation.

Isoprenaline as sustained-action tablets was recommended for long-term maintenance therapy in chronic **atrioventricular block**, side-effects being less evident than with sublingual treatment. Because of the risk of prolonged periods of arrhythmias precipitated by sustained-action isoprenaline an initial course of isoprenaline sublingually or intravenously was advocated by Bluestone and Harris (*Lancet*, 1965, *1*, 1299), and Redwood (*Br. med. J.*, 1968, *1*, 419) stated that the development of cardiac arrhythmias following a brief intravenous infusion of isoprenaline, 10 to 20 µg per minute, indicated when treatment with isoprenaline by mouth could be dangerous. Isoprenaline by intravenous route was more reliable than oral or sublingual administration for stimulating the higher pacemaker centres but constant ECG monitoring was needed to detect isoprenaline-induced ectopic tachycardia (R.M. Stanzler, *New Engl. J. Med.*, 1966, *274*, 1307).

Despite well-documented reports of the value of long-acting isoprenaline hydrochloride tablets in carefully selected patients with chronic heart-block (D. Redwood, *Br. med. J.*, 1969, *1*, 26) it has been suggested that the mortality-rate remained lower in patients with endocardial pacing (M.E. Scott *et al.*, *Lancet*, 1967, *2*, 1382). However, transvenous pacing is now the treatment of choice for those patients with atrioventricular block requiring treatment (A.P. Rae and I. Hutton, *Br. J. Anaesth.*, 1986, *58*, 151), but an isoprenaline infusion may 'buy time' until a pacemaker is inserted.

Myocardial infarction. A review of the role of inotropic agents and infarct size. Isoprenaline is traditionally used to treat 2 specific complications of acute myocardial infarction: cardiogenic shock and bradycardia. In fact, its use in pump failure syndromes in acute myocardial infarction appears to be contra-indicated. Nor is it the treatment of choice to accelerate cardiac-rate when asymptomatic bradycardia complicates acute myocardial infarction. However, if atropine is ineffective and pacemaker therapy either unavailable or must be delayed, isoprenaline should not be withheld if it reverses bradycardia-induced hypotension, since the unequivocal risks of sustained hypotension far outweigh those of any potential extension of infarct size.— M. Lesch, *Am. J. Cardiol.*, 1976, *37*, 508.

Torsades de pointes. Treatment of torsades de pointes is directed towards shortening the Q-T interval. Anti-arrhythmic drug therapy is withheld and hypokalaemia is corrected. The tachycardia can be terminated and suppressed by an intravenous infusion of isoprenaline, but transvenous pacing is the treatment of choice.— A. P. Rae and I. Hutton, *Br. J. Anaesth.*, 1986, *58*, 151.

DIAGNOSTIC USE. A comparison of 2 isoprenaline sensitivity tests used to assess beta-adrenergic receptors.— J. M. O. Arnold and D. G. McDevitt, *Br. J. clin. Pharmac.*, 1982, *14*, 581P. See also *idem*, 1984, *18*, 145; *idem*, 1985, *19*, 114.

Cardiac disorders. Infusion of isoprenaline 1 to 2 µg per minute as a solution containing 2 µg per mL in glucose solution was comparable to a treadmill exercise test in causing S-T depression of the ischaemic type, predictive of the presence of coronary artery disease. In 35 patients about to undergo coronary arteriography correct predictions were made in 71 and 68% respectively of the patients.— D. T. Combs and C. M. Martin, *Am. Heart J.*, 1974, *87*, 711. Exercise studies remain the method of choice for the complete evaluation of patients with aortic or pulmonary stenosis.— N. J. Truccone *et al.*, *Circulation*, 1977, *56*, 79.

A review of sick sinus syndrome. Isoprenaline has been used in the diagnosis of the syndrome: administration of isoprenaline should result in an increase in sinus rate if the sino-atrial node function is normal. However, this is a difficult test to assess as normal values are not clear.— D. S. Reid, *Br. J. Hosp. Med.*, 1984, *31*, 341.

DIALYSIS. Reference to the use of isoprenaline to enhance peritoneal clearance in peritoneal dialysis.— D. K. Scott and D. E. Roberts, *Pharm. J.*, 1985, *1*, 592.

OCULAR DISORDERS. A report of permanent visual impairment in 2 patients, associated with severe attacks of migraine. In a further 4 patients transient visual loss associated with attacks of migraine was alleviated by prompt inhalation of isoprenaline. Prophylactic inhalation of isoprenaline by migraine patients with visual symptoms may prevent transient visual loss, and possibly avoid permanent visual impairment.— M. J. Kupersmith *et al.*, *Stroke*, 1979, *10*, 299.

PULMONARY HYPERTENSION. A patient with primary pulmonary hypertension obtained a sustained beneficial response to administration of isoprenaline 20 mg sublingually every 2 hours with supplementary doses as needed; there were no unpleasant side-effects.— U. R. Shettigar *et al.*, *New Engl. J. Med.*, 1976, *295*, 1414. Marked symptomatic improvement was achieved in a 32-year-old woman with primary pulmonary hypertension by the administration of isoprenaline sublingually, taken to the limit of tolerance. Sudden death occurred after her condition had remained stable for about 2 years on isoprenaline 5 to 7.5 mg every 2 hours.— J. A. Pantano (letter), *New Engl. J. Med.*, 1980, *302*, 919. Isoprenaline caused exacerbation in a 46-year-old man; amelioration by isoprenaline is the exception not the rule, and monitoring of the pulmonary vascular pressures is mandatory to avoid aggravating the condition.— M. J. Belman *et al.* (letter), *ibid.*, 1978, *298*, 51. Reply.— H. N. Hultgren and U. R. Shettigar (letter), *ibid.*, 52.

Further references: D. A. Pietro *et al.*, *New Engl. J. Med.*, 1984, *310*, 1032; R. A. Hogan (letter), *ibid.*,

1984, *311*, 538; M. Packer, *Ann. intern. Med.*, 1985, *103*, 258; A. A. McLeod and D. E. Jewitt, *Drugs*, 1986, *31*, 177; *Lancet*, 1986, *1*, 1420.

Preparations of Isoprenaline Salts

Isoprenaline Aerosol Inhalation *(B.P.C. 1973)*. An aerosol spray in a pressurised container containing a fine suspension of isoprenaline sulphate in a suitable mixture of aerosol propellents. Each metered dose delivers 80 μg of isoprenaline sulphate to the patient. Store in a cool place.

Isoproterenol Hydrochloride and Phenylephrine Bitartrate Inhalation Aerosol *(U.S.P.)*. An aerosol spray in a pressurised container containing a microfine suspension of isoprenaline hydrochloride and phenylephrine acid tartrate ($C_9H_{13}NO_2,C_4H_6O_6$ = 317.3) in suitable propellents. Store in small containers with metered-dose valves and oral inhalation actuators.

Isoproterenol Hydrochloride Inhalation Aerosol *(U.S.P.)*. An aerosol spray in a pressurised container containing a solution of isoprenaline hydrochloride in alcohol in an inert propellent vehicle. Store in small containers with metered-dose valves and oral inhalation actuators.

Isoprenaline Injection *(B.P.)*. Isoprenaline Hydrochloride Injection. pH 2.5 to 3.0. Store in a cool place.

Isoproterenol Hydrochloride Injection *(U.S.P.)*. A sterile solution of isoprenaline hydrochloride in Water for Injections. pH 2.5 to 4.5. It should not be used if it is pinkish to brownish in colour or contains a precipitate.

Isoproterenol Hydrochloride Tablets *(U.S.P.)*. Tablets containing isoprenaline hydrochloride. Store in well-closed containers.

Isoproterenol Inhalation Solution *(U.S.P.)*. Isoproterenol Hydrochloride Inhalation. A solution of isoprenaline hydrochloride in water. It may contain sodium chloride. It should not be used if it is pinkish or brown in colour or contains a precipitate. pH 2.5 to 4.5. Store in small well-filled airtight containers.

Isoproterenol Sulfate Inhalation Aerosol *(U.S.P.)*. Isoproterenol Sulfate Aerosol. A suspension of microfine isoprenaline sulphate in fluorochlorohydrocarbon propellents in a pressurised container. Potency is expressed in terms of anhydrous isoprenaline sulphate. Store in small containers with metered-dose valves and oral inhalation actuators.

Isoproterenol Sulfate Inhalation Solution *(U.S.P.)*. A solution of isoprenaline sulphate in water. It may contain sodium chloride. Potency is expressed in terms of anhydrous isoprenaline sulphate. It should not be used if it is brown in colour or contains a precipitate. Store in small well-filled airtight containers.

Strong Isoprenaline Aerosol Inhalation *(B.P.C. 1973)*. An aerosol spray in a pressurised container containing a fine suspension of isoprenaline sulphate in a suitable mixture of aerosol propellents. Each metered dose delivers 400 μg of isoprenaline sulphate to the patient. Store in a cool place.

CAUTION. This preparation is approximately 5 times as strong as Isoprenaline Aerosol Inhalation (*B.P.C. 1973*).

Proprietary Preparations

Duo-Autohaler *(Riker, UK)*. *Inhaler*, breath-actuated aerosol, isoprenaline hydrochloride 160 μg, phenylephrine acid tartrate 240 μg/metered inhalation.

Iso-Autohaler *(Riker, UK)*. *Inhaler*, breath-actuated aerosol, isoprenaline sulphate 80 μg/metered inhalation.

Isuprel *(Winthrop, UK)*. *Injection*, isoprenaline hydrochloride 200 μg/mL, in ampoules of 1 and 5 mL.

Medihaler Iso *(Riker, UK)*. *Inhaler*, aerosol, isoprenaline sulphate 80 μg/metered inhalation.

Medihaler Iso Forte *(Riker, UK)*. *Inhaler*, aerosol, isoprenaline sulphate 400 μg/metered inhalation.

Medihaler-duo *(Riker, UK)*. *Inhaler*, aerosol, isoprenaline hydrochloride 160 μg, phenylephrine acid tartrate 240 μg/metered inhalation.

Min-I-Jet Isoprenaline Hydrochloride Injection *(IMS, UK)*. *Injection*, isoprenaline hydrochloride 20 μg/mL, in vials of 10 mL.

Saventrine *(Pharmax, UK)*. *Tablets*, sustained-release, isoprenaline hydrochloride 30 mg.
Injection, isoprenaline hydrochloride 1 mg/mL, in ampoules of 2 mL.

Proprietary Names and Manufacturers of Isoprenaline Salts

Aerolone *(Lilly, USA)*; Aleudrin *(Boehringer Ingelheim, Ital.; Neth.; Switz.; Lipomed, UK)*; Aleudrina *(Boehringer Ingelheim, Spain)*; Aleudrine *(Belg.; Fr.)*; Aludrin *(Boehringer Ingelheim, Ger.)*; Bellasthman Medihaler *(Kettelhack Riker, Ger.)*; Ingelan *(Boehringer Ingelheim, Ger.)*; Iso-Autohaler *(Austral.; Riker, UK)*; Isomenyl *(Jpn)*; Isoprenalin-Medihaler *(Riker, Denm.; Riker, Swed.)*; Isopropydrin *(Swed.)*; Isuprel *(Winthrop, Austral.; Belg.; Winthrop, Canad.; Sterling Winthrop, Fr.; Winthrop, S.Afr.; Winthrop, Switz.; Winthrop, UK; Winthrop-Breon, USA)*; Lomupren *(Fisons, UK)*; Medihaler Iso *(Riker, Austral.; Belg.; Riker, Canad.; Neth.; Riker, S.Afr.; Riker 3M, Switz.; Riker, UK; Riker, USA)*; Meterdos *(Inibsa, Spain)*; Min-I-Jet Isoprenaline Hydrochloride *(IMS, UK)*; Mistaprel *(Swed.)*; Norisodrine *(S.Afr.; Abbott, USA)*; Prenomiser *(Fisons, UK)*; Proterenal *(Arg.)*; Proternol *(Belg.; Switz.; USA)*; Saventrine *(Protea, Austral.; Pharmax, Norw.; Pharmax, S.Afr.; Switz.; Pharmax, UK)*; Select-A-Jet Isoprenaline Hydrochloride *(IMS, UK)*; Suscardia *(Switz.)*; Vapo-Iso *(Fisons, USA)*.

The following names have been used for multi-ingredient preparations containing isoprenaline salts—Aerolone Compound *(Lilly, Canad.)*; Brontisol *(Brocades, UK)*; Duo-Autohaler *(Riker, UK)*; Duo-Medihaler *(Riker, Canad.; Riker, USA)*; Intal Compound *(Fisons, UK)*; Iso-Bronchisan *(Berk Pharmaceuticals, UK)*; Isuprel Compound Elixir *(Winthrop, Canad.; Winthrop-Breon, USA)*; Isuprel-Neo *(Winthrop, Canad.)*; Medihaler-duo *(Riker, UK)*; Norisodrine With Calcium Iodide Syrup *(Abbott, USA)*; PIB *(Napp, UK)*; Prenomiser Plus *(Fisons, UK)*; Riddobron Tablets *(Seaford, UK)*.

2076-b

Levonordefrin *(USAN)*.

l-3,4-Dihydroxynorephedrine; *l*-Nordefrin. (−)-2-Amino-1-(3,4-dihydroxyphenyl)propan-1-ol.
$C_9H_{13}NO_3$=183.2.

CAS — 829-74-3 (levonordefrin); 6539-57-7 (nordefrin); 138-61-4 (nordefrin hydrochloride).

Pharmacopoeias. In *U.S. Aust., Cz.*, and *Pol.* include Nordefrin Hydrochloride, which is the salt of the racemic substance.

A white to buff-coloured, odourless, crystalline powder. Practically **insoluble** in water; slightly soluble in alcohol, acetone, chloroform, and ether; freely soluble in aqueous solutions of mineral acids.

Levonordefrin is a sympathomimetic which has been used as a vasoconstrictor in dentistry in a concentration of 1 in 20 000 in solutions of local anaesthetics.

Proprietary Names and Manufacturers

The following names have been used for multi-ingredient preparations containing levonordefrin— Carbocaine with Neo-Cobefrin *(Cook-Waite, USA)*.

2077-v

Mephentermine *(BAN, rINN)*.

Nαα-Trimethylphenethylamine.
$C_{11}H_{17}N$=163.3.

CAS — 100-92-5.

2078-g

Mephentermine Sulphate *(BANM, rINNM)*.

Sulfato de Mefentermina; Mephentermine Sulfate *(USAN)*; Mephentermini Sulfas; Mephetedrine Sulphate.
Nαα-Trimethylphenethylamine sulphate dihydrate.
$(C_{11}H_{17}N)_2,H_2SO_4,2H_2O$=460.6.

CAS — 1212-72-2 (anhydrous); 6190-60-9 (dihydrate).

Pharmacopoeias. In *Arg., Chin., Int., Ind.*, and *Turk. U.S.* has anhydrous or $2H_2O$.

White odourless crystals or crystalline powder. Mephentermine base 15 mg is approximately equivalent to 21 mg of mephentermine sulphate. **Soluble** 1 in 18 of water and 1 in 220 of alcohol; practically insoluble in chloroform and ether. Solutions in water have a pH of about 6. The *U.S.P.* injection has a pH of 4.0 to 6.5. **Store** in well-closed containers. Protect from light.

Adverse Effects, Treatment, and Precautions

For the adverse effects of sympathomimetic agents, and precautions to be observed, see p.1453. Mephentermine may produce CNS stimulation, especially in overdosage: anxiety, drowsiness, incoherence, and convulsions have been reported.

Although the central stimulant effects of mephentermine are much less than those of amphetamine its use may lead to dependence of the amphetamine type.

The hypertensive effects of mephentermine may be treated with an alpha-adrenergic blocking agent such as phentolamine mesylate.

ABUSE. Paranoid hallucinations, which seemed to be identical to amphetamine psychosis or acute paranoid schizophrenia, occurred in 3 patients after abuse of mephentermine aerosols.— B. M. Angrist *et al.*, *Am. J. Psychiat.*, 1970, *126*, 1315.

Absorption and Fate

Mephentermine acts in about 10 minutes following intramuscular injection and has a duration of action of up to about 4 hours; it acts almost immediately following intravenous injection with a duration of action of about 30 minutes. It is rapidly metabolised in the body by demethylation; hydroxylation may follow. It is excreted as unchanged drug and metabolites in the urine; excretion is more rapid in acidic urine.

Uses and Administration

Mephentermine sulphate is a sympathomimetic agent with mainly indirect effects on adrenergic receptors. It has alpha- and beta-adrenergic activity, and a slight stimulating effect on the central nervous system.

Mephentermine sulphate has been used to maintain blood pressure in hypotensive states, for example following spinal anaesthesia. Doses of the equivalent of 15 to 60 mg of mephentermine base have been given by slow intravenous injection, or 15 to 30 mg intramuscularly. It has also been given by intravenous infusion of 600 mg in 500 mL of glucose injection at a rate sufficient to maintain blood pressure.

Mephentermine sulphate was also formerly given by mouth for its mood-elevating effects. A 0.5% solution of mephentermine sulphate was applied locally as a nasal decongestant.

Preparations

Mephentermine Sulfate Injection *(U.S.P.)*. A sterile solution of mephentermine sulphate in Water for Injections. Potency is expressed in terms of the equivalent amount of mephentermine.

Proprietary Names and Manufacturers

Mephine *(Wyeth, UK)*; Wyamine *(Wyeth, Belg.; Wyeth, Neth.; Wyeth, USA)*.

2079-q

Metaraminol Tartrate *(BANM, rINNM)*.

Hydroxynorephedrine Bitartrate; Metaradrine Bitartrate; Metaraminol Acid Tartrate; Metaraminol Bitartrate *(USAN)*. (−)-2-Amino-1-(3-hydroxyphenyl)propan-1-ol hydrogen tartrate.
$C_9H_{13}NO_2,C_4H_6O_6$=317.3.

CAS — 54-49-9 (metaraminol); 33402-03-8 (tartrate).

Pharmacopoeias. In *Br., Braz., Chin., Nord., Turk.*, and *U.S.*

An odourless, or almost odourless, white, crystalline powder. Metaraminol tartrate 9.5 mg is approximately equivalent to 5 mg of metaraminol. **Soluble** 1 in 3 of water and 1 in 100 of alcohol; practically insoluble in chloroform and ether. A 5% solution in water has a pH of 3.2 to 3.5; the *B.P.* and *U.S.P.* injections have a pH of 3.2 to 4.5. The *B.P.* injection is **sterilised** by filtration. **Store** in airtight containers.

INCOMPATIBILITY. Metaraminol 20 mg was 'physically incompatible' with fibrinogen 200 mg, thiopentone sodium 250 mg, or warfarin sodium 10 mg in 100 mL of glucose injection.— R. D. Dunworth and F. R. Kenna, *Am. J. Hosp. Pharm.*, 1965, *22*, 190. There was loss of clarity when intravenous solutions of metaraminol tartrate were mixed with those of benzylpenicillin, hydrocortisone sodium succinate, methicillin sodium, or phenytoin sodium, or (in glucose injection) thiopentone sodium or warfarin sodium.— J. A. Patel and G. L. Phillips, *ibid.*, 1966, *23*, 409. See also R. Misgen, *ibid.*, 1965, *22*, 92. Nitrofurantoin sodium in glucose injection was incompatible with metaraminol tartrate; the pH fell to 7.2 and a brown precipitate was formed.— M. Edward, *ibid.*, 1967, *24*, 440. A report of compatibility for 24 hours.— E. A. Parker, *ibid.*, 1970, *27*, 672. A haze developed over 3 hours when metaraminol tartrate 200 mg per litre was mixed with amphotericin 200 mg per litre in glucose injection; a crystalline precipitate occurred with sulphadiazine sodium 4 g per litre in glucose injection or sodium chloride injection.— B. B. Riley, *J. Hosp. Pharm.*, 1970, *28*, 228. Metaraminol tartrate was physically incompatible with methylprednisolone sodium succinate, hydrocortisone sodium succinate, prednisolone sodium phosphate, and dexamethasone sodium phosphate in sodium chloride injection and glucose injection. However, metaraminol appeared to be compatible with hydrocortisone and hydrocortisone 21-phosphate.— F. E. Turner and J. C. King, *Am. J. Hosp. Pharm.*, 1973, *30*, 128.

STABILITY. Metaraminol tartrate 100 mg per litre had good chemical and biological stability in intravenous fluids at pH 3.75 to 6.25 for up to 48 hours at room temperature.— E. A. Parker, *Am. J. Hosp. Pharm.*, 1967, *24*, 425. Metaraminol tartrate was stable under the following conditions for at least 48 hours at concentrations commonly used in intravenous fluids at pH values from 2.1 to 9.9; in conjunction with hydrocortisone sodium succinate; in conjunction with glucose 5% in sodium chloride injection; and in conjunction with both hydrocortisone sodium succinate and glucose 5% in sodium chloride injection.— R. W. Anderson and C. J. Latiolais, *ibid.*, 1970, *27*, 540.

Adverse Effects, Treatment, and Precautions

For the adverse effects of sympathomimetic agents, and precautions to be observed, see p.1453.

After metaraminol has been infused for some time, tachyphylaxis may lead to recurrent hypotension; it has been suggested that an infusion of noradrenaline may restore responsiveness.

Tissue necrosis can occur as a result of accidental extravasation during intravenous injection.

The hypertensive effects of metaraminol may be treated with an alpha-adrenoceptor blocking agent such as phentolamine mesylate.

Absorption and Fate

Metaraminol is absorbed when taken by mouth but considerably greater amounts are necessary to equal the effects of intramuscular or intravenous injections. It acts about 10 minutes after intramuscular injection with a duration of action of about 1 hour. Effects are seen 1 to 2 minutes after intravenous injection with a duration of action of about 20 minutes.

Uses and Administration

Metaraminol tartrate is a sympathomimetic agent with direct and indirect effects on adrenergic receptors. It has alpha- and beta-adrenergic activity, the former being predominant. Metaraminol increases cardiac output, peripheral resistance, and blood pressure. Coronary blood flow is increased and the heart-rate slowed. In doses equivalent to metaraminol 2 to 10 mg by intramuscular injection, metaraminol tartrate is used for its pressor action in hypotensive states, e.g. following surgical operation or spinal anaesthesia. As the maximum effects are not immediately apparent, at least 10 minutes should elapse before repeating a dose and the possibility of a cumulative effect should be borne in mind. An intravenous infusion of 15 to 100 mg per 500 mL of glucose injection or sodium chloride injection may also be used for maintaining the blood pressure. In an emergency a dose of 0.5 to 5 mg may be given by direct intravenous injection.

Suggested doses for children are the equivalent of 100 µg per kg body-weight by intramuscular injection, the equivalent of 400 µg per kg by intravenous infusion at a rate determined by the blood pressure, or the equivalent of 10 µg per kg by intravenous injection.

Metaraminol has also been given by subcutaneous injection but such administration increases the risk of local tissue necrosis and sloughing.

ADMINISTRATION. Reference to the successful endotracheal administration of the equivalent of metaraminol 5 to 10 mg in cardiopulmonary resuscitation.— C. L. Raehl, *Clin. Pharm.*, 1986, *5*, 572.

CARDIAC DISORDERS. Patients with paroxysmal supraventricular tachycardia but without organic heart disease had been treated for some years with carotid sinus pressure, or, if necessary, 5 mg of metaraminol given subcutaneously. If the paroxysms continued for more than 20 minutes, 2 mg made up to 2 mL with the patient's venous blood was slowly injected intravenously while monitoring the heart beat for conversion to sinus rhythm. In cases where this failed, sedation and digitalis were given.— D. Bowers (letter), *Can. med. Ass. J.*, 1968, *99*, 868.

DIAGNOSIS AND TESTING. The use of metaraminol as a provocative test in the diagnosis of familial Mediterranean fever. All of 21 patients with familial Mediterranean fever developed symptoms within 48 hours of intravenous infusion of metaraminol 10 mg in 500 mL of sodium chloride injection, whereas none of 21 control subjects did so.— M. H. Barakat *et al.*, *Lancet*, 1984, *1*, 656. Comment. Diagnostic difficulty is usually restricted to those rare cases with few symptoms and no family history, and the value of the metaraminol provocation test should be assessed in such patients. The drug is not a harmless one, and should not be used unless absolutely necessary.— D. Cattan *et al.*, (letter), *ibid.*, 1130. Reply.— M. H. Barakat *et al.* (letter), *ibid.*, *2*, 41.

PRIAPISM. A report of the use of metaraminol to treat drug-induced priapism in 5 patients. Treatment consisted of withdrawing 20 to 70 mL of blood from one of the corpora cavernosa, injection of 0.8 to 3 mg of metaraminol, and massage of the penis for 30 seconds to distribute the drug. Definite improvement was seen after between 7 and 40 minutes in most cases. The treatment appears worth a trial in other forms of priapism. A dose of 2 mg may be effective, and can be repeated if necessary an hour later.— G. S. Brindley (letter), *Lancet*, 1984, *2*, 220. Further references: A. Stanners and D. Colin-Jones (letter), *ibid.*, 978 (use in priapism associated with chronic myeloid leukaemia); J. Lindoro *et al.* (letter), *ibid.*, 1348 (the importance of rapid surgery if other measures, such as metaraminol, fail); B. Branger *et al.* (letter), *ibid.*, 1985, *1*, 641 (use in haemodialysis-associated priapism).

Preparations

Metaraminol Bitartrate Injection *(U.S.P.)*. A sterile solution of metaraminol tartrate in Water for Injections. It contains the equivalent of 9 to 11 mg of metaraminol per mL. Protect from light.

Metaraminol Injection *(B.P.)*. Metaraminol Tartrate Injection. Potency is expressed in terms of the equivalent amount of metaraminol. Protect from light.

Proprietary Preparations

Aramine *(Merck Sharp & Dohme, UK)*. *Injection*, metaraminol tartrate equivalent to metaraminol 10 mg/mL, in ampoules of 1 mL.

Proprietary Names and Manufacturers

Aramine *(Merck Sharp & Dohme, Austral.; Belg.; Canad.; Denm.; Merck Sharp & Dohme-Chibret, Fr.; Merck Sharp & Dohme, Norw.; Swed.; Merck Sharp & Dohme, UK; Merck Sharp & Dohme, USA)*; Araminum *(Merck Sharp & Dohme, Ger.)*; Levicor *(Bioindustria, Ital.)*; Select-A-Jet Metaraminol *(IMS, UK)*.

2080-d

Methoxamine Hydrochloride *(BANM, USAN, rINNM)*.

Methoxamedrine Hydrochloride. 2-Amino-1-(2,5-dimethoxyphenyl)propan-1-ol hydrochloride.

$C_{11}H_{17}NO_3$,HCl=247.7.

CAS — 390-28-3 (methoxamine); 61-16-5 (hydrochloride).

Pharmacopoeias. In *Br.*, *Chin.*, *Int.*, *Nord.*, and *U.S.*

Colourless or white plate-like crystals or white crystalline powder; odourless or almost odourless.

Soluble 1 in 2.5 of water and 1 in 12 of alcohol; very slightly soluble in chloroform and ether. A 2% solution in water has a pH of 4 to 6; the *U.S.P.* injection has a pH of 3 to 5. The *B.P.* injection is **sterilised** by autoclaving. **Store** in well-closed containers. Protect from light.

Adverse Effects, Treatment, and Precautions

For the adverse effects of sympathomimetic agents, and precautions to be observed, see p.1453.

Methoxamine may also induce a desire to micturate and a pilomotor reaction (goose flesh). The hypertensive effects of methoxamine may be treated with an alpha-adrenoceptor blocking agent such as phentolamine mesylate.

Absorption and Fate

Methoxamine acts about 1 to 2 minutes after intravenous injection and within about 15 to 20 minutes of intramuscular injection; in the latter case its effects last for about 1½ hours.

Uses and Administration

Methoxamine hydrochloride is a sympathomimetic agent with mainly direct effects on adrenergic receptors. It has alpha-adrenergic activity entirely; beta-adrenergic activity is not demonstrable and beta-adrenoceptor blockade has been postulated.

Methoxamine hydrochloride causes prolonged peripheral vasoconstriction and consequently a rise in arterial blood pressure. It has little effect on the heart, though reflex bradycardia may occur. It has a marked pilomotor effect but does not stimulate the central nervous system or cause bronchodilatation. It markedly reduces blood flow to the kidney.

In usual doses of 10 to 15 mg intramuscularly (range 5 to 20 mg), methoxamine hydrochloride is used for its pressor action in hypotensive states, notably in general or spinal anaesthesia; it may be used in patients who have received cyclopropane or halothane anaesthesia. As the maximum effects are not immediately apparent, about 15 minutes should elapse before repeating a dose. In an emergency 3 to 5 mg may be given by slow intravenous injection. In children, doses of 250 µg per kg body-weight intramuscularly, or 80 µg per kg by slow intravenous injection have been suggested.

Methoxamine hydrochloride may be given for paroxysmal supraventricular tachycardia in doses of 10 mg intravenously.

Preparations

Methoxamine Hydrochloride Injection *(U.S.P.)*

Methoxamine Injection *(B.P.)*. Contains methoxamine hydrochloride 2%.

Proprietary Preparations

Vasoxine *(Calmic, UK)*. *Injection*, methoxamine hydrochloride 20 mg/mL, in ampoules of 1 mL.

Proprietary Names and Manufacturers

Idasal *(Gayoso Wellcome, Spain)*; Vasoxine *(Wellcome, Ital.; Calmic, UK)*; Vasoxyl *(Wellcome, Canad.; Wellcome, USA)*; Vasylox *(Wellcome, Austral.; Wellcome, UK)*.

The following names have been used for multi-ingredient preparations containing methoxamine hydrochloride— Vasylox Plus *(Wellcome, Austral.)*.

2081-n

Methoxyphenamine Hydrochloride *(BANM, USAN, rINNM)*.

Methoxiphenadrin Hydrochloride; Mexyphamine Hydrochloride. 2-Methoxy-*N*α-dimethylphenethylamine hydrochloride.

$C_{11}H_{17}NO$,HCl=215.7.

CAS — 93-30-1 (methoxyphenamine); 5588-10-3 (hydrochloride).

Pharmacopoeias. In *U.S.*

White or off-white crystals or powder with a faint characteristic odour. Freely **soluble** in water, alcohol, and chloroform; slightly soluble in ether. **Store** in airtight containers. Protect from light.

Adverse Effects and Precautions

For the adverse effects of sympathomimetic agents, and precautions to be observed, see p.1453.

Uses and Administration

Methoxyphenamine hydrochloride is a sympathomimetic agent which has been given as a bronchodilator in doses of 50 to 100 mg by mouth every 4 hours.

Proprietary Names and Manufacturers
Asmi *(Denm.)*; Euspirol *(AFOM, Ital.)*; Metasma *(Ital.)*; Mimexina *(Ital.)*; Orthoxine *(Austral.; Belg.; S.Afr.; Upjohn, UK)*; Oxynarin *(Jpn)*; Proasma *(Ital.)*.

The following names have been used for multi-ingredient preparations containing methoxyphenamine hydrochloride— Orthoxicol *(Upjohn, Austral.; Upjohn, UK)*.

2083-m

Methylephedrine Hydrochloride *(BANM)*.

l-N-Methylephedrine Hydrochloride; *l*-Methylephedrine Hydrochloride. (1*RS*,2*RS*)-2-Dimethylamino-1-phenylpropan-1-ol hydrochloride.
$C_{11}H_{17}NO,HCl=215.7$.

CAS — 552-79-4 (methylephedrine, −); 1201-56-5 (methylephedrine, ±); 38455-90-2 (hydrochloride, −); 942-46-1; 18760-80-0 (both hydrochloride, ±).

Pharmacopoeias. Jpn includes the (±)-form, *dl*-Methylephedrine Hydrochloride.

Methylephedrine hydrochloride is a sympathomimetic agent which has been used as a bronchodilator.
Methylephedrine has also been given as the camsylate.

Proprietary Names and Manufacturers
Metheph *(Napp, UK)*; Tybraïne *(Cooper, Switz.)*.

The following names have been used for multi-ingredient preparations containing methylephedrine hydrochloride—Daribiol *(Cambridge Laboratories, Austral.)*; Pholcomed Expectorant *(Medo, UK)*; Pulmodrine Expectorant *(Medo, UK)*; Riddovydrin Capsules, Elixir, and Suppositories *(Seaford, UK)*.

NOTE. The name Pulmodrine Expectorant has also been used to denote the preparation now known in the UK as Pholcomed Expectorant.

12959-s

Midodrine Hydrochloride *(BANM, USAN, rINNM)*.

ST-1085. 2-Amino-*N*-(β-hydroxy-2,5-dimethoxyphenethyl)acetamide hydrochloride; (*RS*)-*N'*-(β-Hydroxy-2,5-dimethoxyphenethyl)glycinamide hydrochloride.
$C_{12}H_{18}N_2O_4,HCl=290.7$.

CAS — 42794-76-3 (midodrine); 3092-17-9 (hydrochloride).

Adverse Effects and Precautions
For the adverse effects of sympathomimetic agents, and precautions to be observed, see p.1453.

Uses and Administration
Midodrine hydrochloride is a direct-acting sympathomimetic agent which reportedly has prolonged alpha-adrenergic activity; the active moiety is stated to be its major metabolite, ST-1059. It is used in the treatment of hypotension in usual doses of 5 mg twice daily by mouth. It has also been given by injection.

Use in incontinence.— D. Jonas, *J. Urol., Baltimore*, 1977, *118*, 980.

Use in idiopathic orthostatic hypotension and Shy-Drager syndrome.— A. Schirger *et al., Mayo Clin. Proc.*, 1981, *56*, 429.

Pharmacodynamics of midodrine in patients with orthostatic hypotension.— P. K. Zachariah, *Clin. Pharmac. Ther.*, 1986, *39*, 586.

Proprietary Names and Manufacturers
Gutron *(Chemie-Linz, Aust.; Hormonchemie, Ger.; Guidotti, Ital.; Chemie-Linz, Switz.)*.

2085-v

Naphazoline Hydrochloride *(BANM, USAN, rINNM)*.

Cloridrato de Nafazolina; Naphtazolini Hydrochloridum. 2-(1-Naphthylmethyl)-2-imidazoline hydrochloride.
$C_{14}H_{14}N_2,HCl=246.7$.

CAS — 835-31-4 (naphazoline); 550-99-2 (hydrochloride).

Pharmacopoeias. In *Arg., Aust., Belg., Braz., Jpn, Nord., Port., Roum.,* and *U.S.*

A white or almost white, odourless, crystalline powder. Freely **soluble** in water and in alcohol; very slightly soluble in chloroform; practically insoluble in ether. A 1% solution in water has a pH of 5.0 to 6.6. The *U.S.P.* ophthalmic solution has a pH of 5.5 to 7.0. **Store** in airtight containers. Protect from light.

2086-g

Naphazoline Nitrate *(BANM, rINNM)*.

Nafazolina Nitrato; Naphazolini Nitras; Naphazolinium Nitricum; Naphthizinum *(Rus.P.)*. 2-(1-Naphthylmethyl)-2-imidazoline nitrate.
$C_{14}H_{14}N_2,HNO_3=273.3$.

CAS — 5144-52-5.

Pharmacopoeias. In *Aust., Br., Cz., Egypt., Eur., Fr., It., Jpn, Jug., Neth., Rus.,* and *Swiss.*

A white or almost white, odourless or almost odourless, crystalline powder. **Soluble** 1 in 36 of water and 1 in 16 of alcohol; very slightly soluble in chloroform; practically insoluble in ether. A 1% solution in water has a pH of 5.0 to 6.5. **Store** in well-closed containers. Protect from light.

Naphazoline is reported to be incompatible with aluminium and should not be used in aluminium-containing containers.

Adverse Effects, Treatment, and Precautions
For the adverse effects of sympathomimetic agents, and precautions to be observed, see p.1453.

After local use of naphazoline transient irritation may occur. Nausea and headache have been reported. Overdosage or accidental administration by mouth may cause depression of the central nervous system with marked reduction of body temperature and symptoms of bradycardia, sweating, drowsiness, and coma, particularly in children; it should be used with great caution, if at all, in infants and young children. Hypertension may be followed by rebound hypotension. Treatment of side-effects is symptomatic.

Reference to the adverse effects associated with the imidazoline derivatives naphazoline, xylometazoline, oxymetazoline, and antazoline.— S. Chaplin, *Adverse Drug React. Bull.*, 1984, Aug., 396.

Absorption and Fate
Systemic absorption has been reported following topical application of solutions of naphazoline. It is not used systemically, but it is readily absorbed from the gastro-intestinal tract.

Uses and Administration
Naphazoline is a sympathomimetic agent with marked alpha-adrenergic activity. It is a vasoconstrictor with a rapid and prolonged action in reducing swelling and congestion when applied to mucous membranes. Rebound congestion and rhinorrhoea may occur after frequent or prolonged use. It is used for the symptomatic relief of rhinitis and sinusitis. Nasal drops or spray are used as a 0.05% aqueous solution of the hydrochloride or nitrate, 2 drops being instilled in each nostril not more often than every 3 hours.

A 0.1% solution has been instilled into the eye as a conjunctival decongestant.

In the *UK* the use of naphazoline and its salts in cosmetics is prohibited.

Preparations of Naphazoline Salts

Naphazoline Hydrochloride Nasal Solution *(U.S.P.)*

Naphazoline Hydrochloride Ophthalmic Solution *(U.S.P.)*

Proprietary Names and Manufacturers of Naphazoline Salts
Ak-Con *(Akorn, Canad.)*; Albalon *(Allergan, Austral.; Allergan, Canad.; Bournonville, Neth.; Allergan, S.Afr.)*; Allerest Eye Drops *(Pharmacraft, USA)*; Clear Eyes *(Abbott, Austral.; Ross, USA)*; Clera *(Person & Covey, USA)*; Col Alfa *(Rovi, Spain)*; Colirio Alfa *(Rovi, Spain)*; Dazolin *(Roux-Ocefa, Arg.)*; Degest 2 *(Barnes-Hind, Canad.)*; Desamin Same *(Savoma, Ital.)*; Imidazyl *(Allergan, Ital.)*; Imizol *(Farmigea, Ital.)*; Naftazolina *(Bruschettini, Ital.)*; Naphcon *(Alcon, Canad.; Alcon Laboratories, USA)*; Nasal Yer *(Yer, Spain)*; Opcon *(Charton, Canad.)*; Optazine *(Lederle, Austral.)*; Otrivin *(Ciba, Spain)*; Privin *(Ciba, Denm.; Ciba, Ger.; Ciba, Switz.)*; Privina *(Ciba, Arg.; Ciba, Ital.; Ciba, Spain)*; Privine *(Ciba, Austral.; Ciba, Belg.; Ciba-Geigy, Canad.; Ciba, Neth.; Ciba, Switz.; Ciba, UK; Ciba, USA)*; Ran *(Corvi, Ital.)*; Rhino-Mex *(Charton, Canad.)*; Rhinospray *(Spain)*; Rimidol *(Leo, Swed.)*; Rinazina *(Maggioni-Winthrop, Ital.; Maggioni, Switz.)*; Rinoftal *(Istituto Wassermann, Ital.)*; Vasocon *(Coopervision, Canad.; Cooper, Ger.; Coopervision, USA)*; Vasoconstrictor *(Pensa, Spain)*; Vistalbalon *(Allergan, Ger.)*; Zolina *(Llorens, Spain)*.

The following names have been used for multi-ingredient preparations containing naphazoline salts—4-Way Nasal Spray *(Bristol-Myers Products, USA)*; Albalon A Liquifilm *(Allergan, Austral.; Allergan, Canad.)*; Antistine-Privine *(Zyma, Austral.)*; Antistin-Privine *(Ciba Consumer, UK)*; Naphcon-A *(Alcon, Canad.; Alcon Laboratories, USA)*; Nomaze *(Fisons, UK)*; Opcon-A *(Charton, Canad.)*; Vasocon-A *(Coopervision, Canad.; CooperVision, UK)*; Zincfrin-A *(Alcon, Canad.)*.

2087-q

Noradrenaline Acid Tartrate *(BANM)*.

Arterenol Acid Tartrate; *l*-Arterenol Bitartrate; *l*-Norepinephrine Bitartrate; Levarterenol Acid Tartrate; Levarterenol Bitartrate; Levarterenoli Bitartras; Noradren. Tart.; Noradrenaline Bitartrate; Noradrenaline Tartrate; Noradrenalini Tartras; Norepinephrine Bitartrate *(USAN, rINNM)*. (*R*)-2-Amino-1-(3,4-dihydroxyphenyl)ethanol hydrogen tartrate monohydrate.
$C_8H_{11}NO_3,C_4H_6O_6,H_2O=337.3$.

CAS — 51-41-2 (noradrenaline); 51-40-1 (acid tartrate, anhydrous); 69815-49-2 (acid tartrate, monohydrate).

Pharmacopoeias. In *Arg., Aust., Br., Braz., Chin., Egypt., Eur., Fr., Ger., Hung., Ind., Int., It., Jug., Neth., Nord., Pol., Roum., Rus., Swiss, Turk.,* and *U.S.* Also in *B.P.Vet. Ger.* also includes the hydrochloride. *Cz.* and *Fr.* include the base (Noradrenalinum). *Jpn* includes the base in the racemic form (Norepinephrinum; Norepirenamine).

A white or faintly grey, odourless, crystalline powder. M.p. 98° to 104°. It darkens on exposure to air and light. Noradrenaline acid tartrate 2 micrograms is approximately equivalent to 1 microgram of noradrenaline. **Soluble** 1 in 2.5 of water and 1 in 300 of alcohol; practically insoluble in chloroform and ether. Solutions in water have a pH of about 3.5; the *U.S.P.* injection has a pH between 3.0 and 4.5, the *B.P.* solution a pH of 3.0 to 4.6. The *B.P.* solution is **sterilised** by autoclaving. **Store** in airtight containers, or preferably, in a sealed tube under vacuum or an inert gas. Protect from light.

INCOMPATIBILITY. There was loss of clarity when intravenous solutions of noradrenaline acid tartrate were mixed with those of amylobarbitone sodium, chlorpheniramine maleate, chlorothiazide sodium, nitrofurantoin sodium, novobiocin sodium, pentobarbitone sodium, phenobarbitone sodium, phenytoin sodium, quinalbarbitone sodium, sodium bicarbonate, sodium iodide, streptomycin sulphate, sulphadiazine sodium, sulphafurazole diethanolamine, or thiopentone sodium.— J. A. Patel and G. L. Phillips, *Am. J. Hosp. Pharm.*, 1966, *23*, 409. Noradrenaline acid tartrate is incompatible with cephalothin.— B. Flouvat and P. Lechat, *Thérapie*, 1974, *29*, 337. Solutions of noradrenaline acid tartrate lost 15% of their potency in 4 hours when mixed with solutions of cefapirin sodium.— V. K. Prasad *et al., Curr. ther. Res.*, 1974, *16*, 540.

STABILITY OF SOLUTIONS. Solutions of noradrenaline acid tartrate (pH 3.6) with sodium metabisulphite 0.1%, enclosed in well-filled ampoules, could be sterilised by autoclaving at 115° for 30 minutes with negligible loss of activity. Dilutions of these solutions in 5% glucose solutions, distilled water, or plasma, might be stored at room temperature for up to 24 hours with little loss of activity; these dilutions were more stable than those in saline solution or blood.— G. B. West, *J. Pharm. Pharmac.*, 1952, *4*, 560. Less oxidation and racemisation of noradrenaline occurred in injection solutions when air was replaced by carbon dioxide. Autoclaving did not cause significant degradation immediately or on storage if air was excluded.— P. Buri *et al.*, *Pharm. Acta Helv.*, 1969, *44*, 764. See also U. Kesselring and L. Kapétanidis, *ibid.*, 1966, *41*, 428.

Intravenous solutions of noradrenaline should be diluted with glucose injection or 5% glucose in sodium chloride injection to minimise oxidation.— J. M. Meisler and M. W. Skolaut, *Am. J. Hosp. Pharm.*, 1966, *23*, 557. At a room temperature of 29° to 30.5°, noradrenaline acid tartrate, 4 mg per 540 mL, was found to be stable for 4 hours in solutions of glucose 5% in water or glucose 5% in normal saline but there was significant loss of activity of noradrenaline in solutions of normal saline.— C. W. Ogle (letter), *Br. med. J.*, 1968, *2*, 490. Noradrenaline acid tartrate was stable for about 24 hours in glucose injection at pH 3.6 to 6.0— E. A. Parker, *Am. J. Hosp. Pharm.*, 1975, *32*, 214. The stability of noradrenaline in physiological saline solutions.— I. E. Hughes and J. A. Smith, *J. Pharm. Pharmac.*, 1978, *30*, 124.

Adverse Effects

For the adverse effects of sympathomimetic agents, see p.1453.

Noradrenaline acid tartrate is a severe tissue irritant and only very dilute solutions may be injected. The needle must be inserted well into the vein and extravasation must be avoided, otherwise severe phlebitis and sloughing may occur.

The Committee on the Safety of Medicines had received 11 reports of severe occipital headache, with fatal cerebral haemorrhage in 1 patient, in dental patients who had injections of lignocaine 2% with noradrenaline 1 in 25 000 (Xylestesin). Similar symptoms occurred in a patient given butanilicaine and procaine with noradrenaline 1 in 25 000 (Hostacain NOR). The effects of these preparations were compared in 35 dental patients with lignocaine with adrenaline or noradrenaline 1 in 80 000 and prilocaine with felypressin 0.03 units per mL. Noradrenaline 1 in 25 000 produced increases of 21 to 92% in the blood pressure and its use at this strength could not be justified. Of the patients in the 11 original case reports, 1 was taking desipramine, 1 nortriptyline, and 1 might have been taking desipramine or protriptyline; these antidepressants could have enhanced the pressor effects. Felypressin was the vasoconstrictor of choice in such patients.— A. J. Boakes *et al.*, *Br. dent. J.*, 1972, *133*, 137. A discussion of the hazards and precautions to be taken when vasoconstrictors are used in conjunction with local anaesthetics.— *Lancet*, 1972, *2*, 584. Comment.— F. Reynolds (letter), *ibid.*, 764 and 834.

Treatment of Adverse Effects

The hypertensive effects of noradrenaline may be treated with an alpha-adrenoceptor blocking agent such as phentolamine mesylate. Relief from tissue necrosis and pain may be given by immediate infiltration with phentolamine and local anaesthetics, and by the application of hot packs.

Any ischaemic areas should be infiltrated subcutaneously with 5 to 10 mL of saline solution containing 2.5 mg of phentolamine hydrochloride and 300 units of hyaluronidase. For areas larger than 30 cm^2 half the area should be infiltrated and the other half infiltrated 30 minutes later. The phentolamine infiltration was used 26 times in 20 patients and in no case was there any systemic manifestation due to the phentolamine and in none of the patients did a slough occur.— A. S. Close, *J. Am. med. Ass.*, 1959, *170*, 1916. Extravasation of noradrenaline into the dorsum of the hand in 2 patients produced uncontrollable oedema with venous occlusion of the hands and ischaemic necrosis of the fingers. Both patients later died. Phentolamine injected locally within 12 hours after extravasation of noradrenaline prevented tissue necrosis. Between 12 and 18 hours after extravasation its effect was less predictable, and after 18 hours it was of no value.— P. M. Weeks, *J. Am. med. Ass.*, 1966, *196*, 288.

Precautions

For the precautions to be observed with sympathomimetic agents, see p.1453.

In late pregnancy noradrenaline provokes uterine contractions which can result in foetal asphyxia.

INTERACTIONS. When given 1 hour before noradrenaline acid tartrate in *rats*, *chlorpheniramine hydrochloride*, *tripelennamine hydrochloride*, and *desipramine*, but not mepyramine, significantly increased the toxicity of noradrenaline. Some antihistamines blocked the uptake of catecholamines by peripheral tissues and enhanced the toxicity of exogenous noradrenaline.— A. Jori (letter), *J. Pharm. Pharmac.*, 1966, *18*, 824. Studies *in vitro* of the nerve uptake of noradrenaline demonstrated an inhibition by *imipramine, desipramine, amitriptyline, nortriptyline,* and *chlorpromazine*. Studies *in vivo* showed that the pressor effects of tyramine were blocked by chlorpromazine, desipramine, and nortriptyline.— D. Tuck *et al.* (letter), *Lancet*, 1972, *2*, 492.

Administration of noradrenaline concurrently with *guanethidine* or *bethanidine* was not advisable since both depleted the adrenergic nerves of noradrenaline, thus enhancing the effect of exogenous noradrenaline.— A. Herxheimer, *Prescribers' J.*, 1969, *9*, 62.

Studies of the effect of noradrenaline on *beta-blockade* alone and in the presence of *atropine*.— D. A. Richards *et al.*, *Br. J. clin. Pharmac.*, 1979, *7*, 429P.

For the effect of *monoamine oxidase inhibitors* and *tricyclic antidepressants* on noradrenaline in local anaesthetics, see Adrenaline, p.1454.

Absorption and Fate

For a brief outline of the absorption and fate of a catecholamine, see Adrenaline, p.1455.

Noradrenaline cannot be given by subcutaneous or intramuscular injection owing to its powerful vasoconstrictor properties. Like adrenaline it is inactive when given by mouth, and it is rapidly inactivated in the body by similar processes. Only small amounts of noradrenaline are excreted unchanged in the urine of healthy subjects.

An account of the catabolism of catecholamines and a review of studies.— D. F. Sharman, *Br. med. Bull.*, 1973, *29*, 110. Biochemical aspects of monoamine oxidase.— K. F. Tipton, *ibid.*, 116. Mechanisms involved in the release of noradrenaline from sympathetic nerves.— A. D. Smith, *ibid.*, 123. Catecholamine uptake processes.— L. L. Iversen, *ibid.*, 130. Uptake of noradrenaline by smooth muscle.— J. S. Gillespie, *ibid.*, 136. Factors affecting plasma-noradrenaline concentrations, including various neurological disorders, such as the Shy-Drager syndrome.— I. J. Kopin *et al.*, *Ann. intern. Med.*, 1978, *88*, 671. Kinetics of infused noradrenaline in healthy subjects.— G. A. FitzGerald *et al.*, *Clin. Pharmac. Ther.*, 1979, *26*, 669. Discrepancies between plasma concentrations of noradrenaline determined by radioenzymatic assay, which measures free noradrenaline, and by radioimmunoassay, which measures both free and conjugated noradrenaline.— D. C. Aron *et al.* (letter), *Ann. intern. Med.*, 1983, *98*, 1023.

Uses and Administration

The catecholamine, noradrenaline, is a direct-acting sympathomimetic agent with pronounced effects on alpha-adrenergic receptors and less marked effects on beta-adrenergic receptors. It is a neurotransmitter, stored in granules in nerve axons, which is released at the terminations of post-ganglionic adrenergic nerve fibres when they are stimulated; some is also present in the adrenal medulla from which it is liberated together with adrenaline. A major effect of noradrenaline is to raise systolic and diastolic blood pressure (which is accompanied by reflex slowing of the heart-rate). This is a result of its alpha-stimulant effects which cause vasoconstriction, with reduced blood flow in the kidneys, liver, skin, and usually skeletal muscle. The pregnant uterus also contracts; high doses liberate glucose from the liver and have other hormonal effects similar to those of adrenaline. There is little stimulation of the central nervous system. Beta-stimulant effects of noradrenaline have a positive inotropic action on the heart, but there is little bronchodilator effect.

Noradrenaline may be used in concentrations of 1 in 100 000 to 1 in 50 000 to diminish the absorption and localise the effects of local anaesthetics. Locally applied solutions have also been used to control bleeding.

Noradrenaline has been used in the treatment of hypotensive states in which the blood volume is adequate, such as after the removal of a phaeochromocytoma, and in myocardial infarction. To avoid tissue necrosis it is best administered through a fine catheter into a large vein high up in a limb, preferably the arm; some sources have suggested that addition of phentolamine 5 to 10 mg to the infusion may prevent sloughing without affecting the vasopressor action.

Noradrenaline acid tartrate is usually administered by intravenous infusion as a solution containing 8 µg, equivalent to 4 µg of the base, per mL of glucose injection or sodium chloride and glucose injection; it is less stable in plasma, blood, or sodium chloride injection. This solution is usually given initially at a rate of 2 to 3 mL per minute and adjusted according to the response so as to maintain the desired blood pressure, the blood pressure being initially recorded every 2 minutes, and the rate of infusion being continuously monitored. The average maintenance dose is 0.5 to 1 mL per minute, but there is a wide variation. According to the patient's fluid requirements the concentration of the infusion may need increasing or decreasing. On some occasions the infusion may be continued for days; it must not be stopped suddenly but should be gradually withdrawn to guard against disastrous falls in blood pressure.

A rapid intravenous or intracardiac injection of 100 to 150 µg of the acid tartrate (50 to 75 µg of base) as 0.5 to 0.75 mL of a solution containing noradrenaline acid tartrate 200 µg per mL has been suggested as an adjunct in the treatment of cardiac arrest.

In the *UK* the use of noradrenaline acid tartrate in cosmetics is prohibited.

CARDIOVASCULAR DISORDERS. Updated standards and guidelines from the 1985 National Conference on Cardiopulmonary Resuscitation and Emergency Cardiac Care. Noradrenaline is indicated in patients with severe hypotension and a low total peripheral resistance, to whom it is administered by intravenous infusion, but it is contra-indicated in hypovolaemia. Myocardial oxygen requirement may be increased, and it must be used with caution in patients with ischaemic heart disease. Standard blood pressure measurements may be falsely low when high doses of a vasoconstrictor such as noradrenaline are used, and intra-arterial pressure monitoring may be necessary for accurate determination of response.— American Heart Association and the National Academy of Sciences –National Research Council., *J. Am. med. Ass.*, 1986, *255*, 2905.

The observation that the renal circulation in patients with acute renal failure is unresponsive to noradrenaline makes the use of this drug an attractive choice for the treatment of recurrent, dialysis-related hypotensive episodes in patients with acute renal failure. It seems likely that under these circumstances noradrenaline can be used without fear of inducing renal vasoconstriction and thereby worsening hypoperfusion; renal perfusion will probably increase with increased perfusion pressure.— B. D. Myers and S. M. Moran, *New Engl. J. Med.*, 1986, *314*, 97.

Shock. A review of the management of septic shock. Noradrenaline is used less in septic shock since the introduction of dopamine, and its use is usually limited to final attempts to maintain blood pressure in patients with severe shock.— R. A. Eskridge, *Drug Intell. & clin. Pharm.*, 1983, *17*, 92.

Sympathomimetic inotropes may improve circulatory haemodynamics in cardiogenic shock in the short term but long-term survival is rarely improved. Noradrenaline, like other sympathomimetics may damage the heart due to the ischaemia resulting from increased afterload, and is in addition arrhythmogenic and decreases renal blood flow. These disadvantages usually offset any gains from an increased systolic blood pressure although it may have a place in a severely hypotensive patient who has not responded to either dopamine or dobutamine.— C. E. Handler, *Postgrad. med. J.*, 1985, *61*, 705.

GASTRO-INTESTINAL DISORDERS. Massive upper gastro-intestinal haemorrhage occurring in 12 patients with advanced malignant disease was controlled by noradrenaline acid tartrate in 11. In 11 patients noradrenaline was administered by naso-gastric tube as a 0.008% solution in iso-osmotic saline and in 1 patient by intraperitoneal infusion of a 0.0016% solution in iso-osmotic saline. Intraperitoneal administration of noradrenaline led to transient rise in blood pressure.— H. O. Douglass, *J. Am. med. Ass.*, 1974, *230*, 1653.

A 59-year-old man with a history of chronic alcohol and analgesic abuse developed severe gastric bleeding from a 1-cm longitudinal Mallory-Weiss mucosal laceration just below the cardio-oesophageal junction. He required 7 units of whole blood, and gastric lavage with 500 mL of cold normal saline containing noradrenaline 1 mg failed to arrest the bleeding. Noradrenaline 1 mg in 10 mL of physiological saline was then applied directly on the lesion, the mucosa around the lesion blanched and oozing ceased immediately. No further haematemesis or passage of fresh blood per rectum occurred and repeat endoscopy before discharge demonstrated complete healing of the lesion.— D. Curran *et al.* (letter), *Lancet*, 1980, *1*, 538.

A reminder that the medical treatment of acute non-variceal upper gastro-intestinal bleeding is based on empirical and anecdotal evidence. Some 80 to 90% of patients with upper gastro-intestinal haemorrhage stop bleeding spontaneously and there have been no controlled studies of the effectiveness of local measures such as lavage with ice water, saline, or noradrenaline.— D. E. Larson and M. B. Farnell, *Mayo Clin. Proc.*, 1983, *58*, 371.

Preparations

Noradrenaline Injection *(B.P.)*. Noradrenaline Acid Tartrate Injection. A sterile solution of noradrenaline acid tartrate, prepared immediately before use by diluting Strong Sterile Noradrenaline Solution to 250 times its volume with Sodium Chloride and Glucose Intravenous Infusion or Glucose Intravenous Infusion. It contains 8 µg of noradrenaline acid tartrate, equivalent to approximately 4 µg of noradrenaline, in 1 mL.

Norepinephrine Bitartrate Injection *(U.S.P.)*. A sterile solution of noradrenaline acid tartrate in Water for Injections. Potency is expressed in terms of the equivalent amount of noradrenaline. It should not be used if the solution is brown or contains a precipitate.

Strong Sterile Noradrenaline Solution *(B.P.)*. An isotonic solution containing noradrenaline acid tartrate 0.2%. It must be diluted before administration. It should not be used if it is brown in colour.

Proprietary Preparations

Levophed *(Winthrop, UK)*. *Solution*, concentrate for intravenous infusion, noradrenaline acid tartrate 2 mg (equivalent to noradrenaline 1 mg)/mL, in ampoules of 2 and 4 mL.

Injection (Levophed Special), noradrenaline acid tartrate 200 µg (equivalent to noradrenaline 100 µg)/mL, in ampoules of 2 mL.

Proprietary Names and Manufacturers

Adrenor *(Llorens, Spain)*; Arterenol *(Hoechst, Ger.)*; Levophed *(Winthrop, Austral.*; *Belg.*; *Winthrop, Canad.*; *Denm.*; *Winthrop, Fr.*; *Winthrop, UK*; *Winthrop-Breon, USA)*; Noradrec *(Recordati, Ital.)*; Reargon *(Spain)*.

The following names have been used for multi-ingredient preparations containing noradrenaline acid tartrate— Hostacain NOR; Lignostab-N *(Boots, UK)*.

2089-s

Norfenefrine Hydrochloride *(rINNM)*.

m-Norsynephrine Hydrochloride; Norphenylephrine Hydrochloride; WV-569. 2-Amino-1-(3-hydroxyphenyl)ethanol hydrochloride.

$C_8H_{11}NO_2,HCl = 189.6$.

CAS — 536-21-0 (norfenefrine); 15308-34-6 (hydrochloride).

NOTE. *m*-Octopamine has been used as a synonym for norfenefrine. Care should be taken to avoid confusion between the 2 compounds.

Norfenefrine hydrochloride is a sympathomimetic agent with predominantly alpha-adrenergic activity, which is used in the treatment of hypotension. Doses of 3 to 9 mg by mouth have been given 3 times daily; doses of 15 or 45 mg have been given three times daily as controlled-release tablets. Norfenefrine has also been given by injection.

The bioavailability of norfenefrine in man, related to its metabolism.— J. H. Hengstmann *et al.*, *Eur. J. clin. Pharmac.*, 1975, *8*, 33.

Reference to the use of norfenefrine in orthostatic essential hypotension.— K. A. Raij, *Br. J. clin. Pract.*, 1983, *37*, 289.

Proprietary Names and Manufacturers

Coritat *(Jpn)*; Energona *(Maurer, Ger.)*; Esbuphon *(Schaper & Brümmer, Ger.)*; Euro-cir *(Ital.)*; Molycor *(Mepha, Switz.)*; Nevadral *(Pharmacia, Swed.)*; Norenol *(Spain)*; Normetolo *(Selvi, Ital.)*; Novadral *(Parke, Davis, Arg.*; *Pharmacia, Denm.*; *Gödecke, Ger.*; *Warner-Lambert, Switz.)*; Stagural *(Stada, Ger.)*; Tonolift *(Jpn)*; Vingsal *(Stroschein, Ger.)*; Zondel *(Jpn)*.

2090-h

Octopamine *(rINN)*.

β,4-Dihydroxyphenethylamine; *p*-Hydroxymandelamine; *p*-Norsynephrine; ND-50; Noroxedrine. 2-Amino-1-(4-hydroxyphenyl)ethanol.

$C_8H_{11}NO_2 = 153.2$.

CAS — 104-14-3.

NOTE. *m*-Octopamine has been used as a synonym for norfenefrine. Care should be taken to avoid confusion between the 2 compounds.

Octopamine is a sympathomimetic agent with predominantly alpha-adrenergic activity. It has been used as the hydrochloride or the tartrate in the treatment of hypotension.

Reference to octopamine as a false neurotransmitter possibly associated with neurotoxic effects in hepatic encephalopathy.— C. L. Fraser and A. I. Arieff, *New Engl. J. Med.*, 1985, *313*, 865.

Proprietary Names and Manufacturers

Norden *(Byk Gulden, Ital.)*; Norfen *(Jpn)*; Norphen *(Byk Gulden, Ger.*; *Byk Gulden, Switz.)*.

2091-m

Orciprenaline Sulphate *(BANM, rINNM)*.

Metaproterenol Sulfate *(USAN)*; Metaproterenol Sulphate; Th-152. 1-(3,5-Dihydroxyphenyl)-2-isopropylaminoethanol sulphate; *N*-Isopropyl-*N*(*β*,3,5-trihydroxyphenethyl)ammonium sulphate.

$(C_{11}H_{17}NO_3)_2,H_2SO_4 = 520.6$.

CAS — 586-06-1 (orciprenaline); 5874-97-5 (sulphate).

Pharmacopoeias. In *Br.*, *Cz.*, *Jug.*, and *U.S.*

A white to off-white odourless or almost odourless crystalline powder The *B.P.* states that it contains up to 6% of water and methyl alcohol of crystallisation of which not more than 2% is water.

Soluble 1 in 2 of water, 1 in 1 of alcohol; practically insoluble in chloroform and ether. A 10% solution in water has a pH of 4.0 to 5.5. The *B.P.* injection has a pH of 3 to 4, while the *U.S.P.* inhalation solution has a pH between 2.8 and 4.0

The *B.P.* injection is **sterilised** by autoclaving. **Store** in airtight containers. Protect from light.

Adverse Effects and Precautions

For the adverse effects of sympathomimetic agents, and precautions to be observed, see p.1453.

Orciprenaline acts mainly on beta$_2$-adrenergic receptors but is less selective than salbutamol.

Adverse effects were not severe after inhalations or oral doses of up to 100 mg daily of orciprenaline sulphate. Above this dose adverse effects were frequent, continuous, and severe; trembling and palpitations were common. Three patients receiving 120 mg daily had a rise of systolic blood pressure; in 2 of these patients the rise occurred once only and in the third a rise of 30 mmHg systolic persisted for 48 hours and then settled spontaneously while treatment was continued.— G. Edwards, *Br. med. J.*, 1964, *1*, 1015. Muscular cramps that had occurred in about 8% of patients receiving orciprenaline disappeared when potassium was given concomitantly. Extrasystoles or tachycardia and severe headaches which occurred as side-effects of treatment with orciprenaline were also found to decrease or disappear in patients who were given potassium supplements.— L. Lotzof (letter), *Med. J. Aust.*, 1968, *1*, 1105.

Comment on the availability, for a brief period only, of orciprenaline inhalers over-the-counter in the *US*, and a reminder, with reference to events in the *UK* and Australia, of the hazards of self-medication.— L. Hendeles and M. Weinberger, *New Engl. J. Med.*, 1984, *310*, 207.

Absorption and Fate

Following oral administration orciprenaline is absorbed from the gastro-intestinal tract and undergoes extensive first-pass metabolism; about 40% of an oral dose is reported to reach the circulation unchanged. It is excreted in the urine primarily as glucuronide conjugates.

Pharmacokinetics of orciprenaline after administration in sustained-release form.— H. J. Gilfrich *et al.*, *Arzneimittel-Forsch.*, 1979, *29*, 967.

A study of the bioavailability of orciprenaline sulphate as a 10 mg tablet in 6 healthy subjects, compared with an oral solution of the deuterated analogue given simultaneously. The tablet formulation had a relative bioavailability of 92% compared with solution; peak plasma concentrations of 2.2 to 13 ng per mL were achieved at between 0.75 and 3 hours after administration, and the mean terminal half-life was calculated to be 2.1 hours.— F. Hatch *et al.*, *J. pharm. Sci.*, 1986, *75*, 886.

Uses and Administration

Orciprenaline sulphate is a direct-acting sympathomimetic agent with actions and uses similar to those of salbutamol (p.1482).

In the treatment of bronchial asthma it is given by mouth in a dose of 20 mg four times daily. A suggested dose for children is: up to 1 year, 5 to 10 mg three times daily; 1 to 3 years, 5 to 10 mg four times daily; 3 to 12 years, 10 mg four times daily to 20 mg three times daily.

Orciprenaline sulphate may be inhaled in 5% solution from a hand nebuliser, the usual adult dose being 10 inhalations; if the solution is used with any other nebulising device the usual adult dose is 0.3 mL of a 5% solution diluted with 2.5 mL of sterile water or physiological saline. Adequate oxygenation is necessary to avoid hypoxaemia. Pressurised aerosols providing 750 µg in each metered dose, delivering at the mouthpiece 670 µg, are the usual method of inhalation. The usual adult dosage is 1 or 2 inhalations, repeated, if required, usually after 3 to 4 hours, but in any case after not less than 30 minutes, to a maximum of 12 inhalations in 24 hours.

In the treatment of severe forms of bronchospasm orciprenaline sulphate 500 µg may be given by intramuscular injection; the injection may be repeated if necessary after 30 minutes. Adequate oxygenation is necessary to avoid hypoxaemia. A suggested dose by intramuscular injection for children aged less than 6 years is 250 µg.

Orciprenaline has also been used similarly to salbutamol as an intravenous infusion in the management of premature labour.

In a comparison of the cardiovascular effects of various intravenous doses of orciprenaline and isoprenaline in 3 healthy men, isoprenaline was found to be between 10 and 40 times as potent as orciprenaline. Both drugs increased the heart-rate and forearm blood flow and acted by stimulating *β*-adrenergic receptors.— R. G. Shanks *et al.*, *Br. med. J.*, 1967, *1*, 610.

ASTHMA. Results of a double-blind study completed by 17 asthma patients confirmed the impression that orciprenaline is far better tolerated following inhalation of the aerosol than following administration of the tablets.— C. Shim and M. H. Williams, *Ann. intern. Med.*, 1980, *93*, 428.

A double-blind crossover study in 20 asthmatic patients who received either orciprenaline 1.3 mg alone, via a metered dose inhaler, or the same dose combined with either 10 or 20 mg of orciprenaline by mouth, or else 20 mg by mouth alone. Measures of pulmonary function were more significantly improved in those regimens providing orciprenaline by inhalation than when given by mouth alone, but were significantly greater following 20 mg by mouth plus 1.3 mg by inhalation than after 1.3 mg by inhalation. Side-effects, including tachycardia and raised systolic blood pressure, were more prominent after regimens with an oral component. Inhaled orciprenaline appears to be preferable to oral in the treatment of moderately severe airways obstruction, but addition of oral orciprenaline may improve the response.— G. P. Maguire and C. Emirgil, *Am. J. med. Sci.*, 1986, *291*, 168.

For a comparison of nebulised orciprenaline with subcutaneous adrenaline in the management of acute asthma, see Adrenaline Acid Tartrate, p.1456.

Preparations

Metaproterenol Sulfate Inhalation Aerosol *(U.S.P.)*. An aerosol spray in a pressurised container containing a microfine suspension of orciprenaline sulphate in propellents. Store in containers with metered-dose valves and oral inhalation actuators.

Metaproterenol Sulfate Inhalation Solution *(U.S.P.)*. A solution of orciprenaline sulphate in water. It may contain sodium chloride. It should be stored in small, well-filled airtight containers and should not be used if it is brown or contains a precipitate.

Metaproterenol Sulfate Syrup *(U.S.P.)*. Contains orciprenaline sulphate. When mixed with 4 times its volume of water it has a pH between 2.5 and 4.0.

Metaproterenol Sulfate Tablets *(U.S.P.)*. Contain orciprenaline sulphate.

Orciprenaline Aerosol Inhalation *(B.P.C. 1973)*. An aerosol spray in a pressurised canister containing a fine suspension of orciprenaline sulphate in a suitable mixture of aerosol propellents. Store in a cool place.

Orciprenaline Elixir *(B.P.C. 1973)*. Orciprenaline Sulphate Elixir; Orciprenaline Syrup. A solution of orciprenaline sulphate in a suitable flavoured vehicle. Store in a cool place. Protect from light.

Orciprenaline Injection *(B.P.)*. Contains orciprenaline sulphate.

Orciprenaline Tablets *(B.P.)*. Contain orciprenaline sulphate.

Proprietary Preparations

Alupent *(Boehringer Ingelheim, UK)*. *Tablets*, orciprenaline sulphate 20 mg.
Syrup, orciprenaline sulphate 10 mg/5 mL.
Inhaler, aerosol, orciprenaline sulphate 670 µg/metered inhalation.

Proprietary Names and Manufacturers

Alupent *(Arg.; Boehringer Ingelheim, Austral.; Belg.; Boehringer Ingelheim, Canad.; Denm.; Boehringer Ingelheim, Fr.; Boehringer Ingelheim, Ger.; Boehringer Ingelheim, Ital.; Neth.; Boehringer Ingelheim, Norw.; Boehringer Ingelheim, S.Afr.; Boehringer Ingelheim, Spain; Boehringer Ingelheim, Swed.; Boehringer Ingelheim, Switz.; Boehringer Ingelheim, UK; Boehringer Ingelheim, USA)*; Auramide *(Lennon, S.Afr.)*; Dosalupent *(Ital.)*; Metaprel *(Sandoz, USA)*; Novasmasol *(Zambeletti, Ital.)*.

2092-b

Oxedrine Tartrate *(BANM)*.

Aetaphen. Tartrat.; Aethaphenum Tartaricum; Oxedrini Tartras; Oxyphenylmethylaminoethanol Tartrate; Sinefrina Tartrato; Synephrine Tartrate. Bis[(*βRS*)-β,4-dihydroxyphenethyl-*N*-methylammonium]tartrate; (±)-1-(4-Hydroxyphenyl)-2-methylaminoethanol tartrate.
$(C_9H_{13}NO_2)_2,C_4H_6O_6=484.5$.

CAS — 94-07-5 (oxedrine); 16589-24-5 (tartrate); 67-04-9 (tartrate, ±).

NOTE. *m*-Synephrine has been used as a synonym for phenylephrine. Care should be taken to avoid confusion between the 2 compounds.

Pharmacopoeias. In *Aust., Fr., It., Jug., Neth., Nord.,* and *Swiss.*
Sympaethaminum (*Hung.*) is the base.

Oxedrine is a sympathomimetic agent which has been given as the tartrate in hypotensive states in doses of about 100 mg three times daily by mouth; it has also been given by subcutaneous, intramuscular, or intravenous injection in doses of 60 to 120 mg.
It has been used in eye-drops as an ocular decongestant.

Proprietary Names and Manufacturers

Cardiodinamin *(Ital.)*; Chibro-Bora *(Chibret, Ger.)*; Dulcidrine *(Fr.)*; Simpadren *(Arg.)*; Sympacor *(Switz.)*; Sympalept *(Switz.)*; Sympatol *(Belg.; Boehringer Ingelheim, Ger.; Boehringer Ingelheim, Ital.; Boehringer Ingelheim, Switz.; Lipomed, UK)*.

13063-d

Oxidopamine *(USAN, rINN)*.

6-Hydroxydopamine. 5-(2-Aminoethyl)benzene-1,2,4-triol.
$C_8H_{11}NO_3=169.2$.

CAS — 1199-18-4.

Oxidopamine has been used by subconjunctival injection to produce chemical sympathectomy in glaucoma.

Oxidopamine 1 to 5 mg in 0.5 mL of 0.005M ascorbic acid solution, buffered to pH 6 with sodium ascorbate, injected subconjunctivally lowered intra-ocular pressure within 3 hours in 9 of 11 glaucomatous eyes resistant to other medication. Topical application of adrenaline 1% eye-drops four times daily maintained the reduction in intra-ocular pressure for up to 3 months. A further injection of oxidopamine produced a similar response.— J. G. Diamond, *Archs Ophthal., N.Y.*, 1976, *94*, 41.

In patients with primary open angle glaucoma, refractory to other therapy, 63 eyes of 61 subjects were given a 0.2 mL subconjunctival injection of 2% oxidopamine. Adrenaline eye-drops were used by all patients up to 48 to 72 hours before injection and were re-instituted 48 hours after the injection. A significant decrease in mean ocular tension was seen after treatment: 10 eyes showed no significant decrease in ocular tension; 40 eyes showed a significant decrease for 12 weeks, and 21 eyes were controlled for 20 weeks. The fellow control eyes, showed a slight, but non-significant, decrease in ocular tension.— E. Talusan *et al.*, *Am. J. Ophthal.*, 1981, *92*, 792.

NEUROBLASTOMA. For reference to the use of oxidopamine in purging bone-marrow for autologous transfusion in patients with neuroblastoma see Choice of Antineoplastic Agent, p.593.

Proprietary Names and Manufacturers

Cooper, USA.

2093-v

Oxymetazoline Hydrochloride *(BANM, USAN, rINNM)*.

H990; Sch-9384. 2-(4-*tert*-Butyl-3-hydroxy-2,6-dimethylbenzyl)-2-imidazoline hydrochloride; 6-*tert*-Butyl-3-(2-imidazolin-2-ylmethyl)2,4-xylenol hydrochloride.
$C_{16}H_{24}N_2O,HCl=296.8$.

CAS — 1491-59-4 (oxymetazoline); 2315-02-8 (hydrochloride).

Pharmacopoeias. In *Braz.* and *U.S.*

A white or almost white, hygroscopic, crystalline powder. **Soluble** 1 in 6.7 of water and 1 in 3.6 of alcohol; practically insoluble in chloroform and ether. A 5% solution in water has a pH of 4.0 to 6.5. **Store** in airtight containers.

Adverse Effects and Precautions

For the adverse effects of sympathomimetic agents, and precautions to be observed, see p.1453.
Oxymetazoline may occasionally cause local stinging or burning, sneezing, and dryness of the mouth and throat. Prolonged use may cause rebound congestion and drug-induced rhinitis.

Bradycardia, postural hypotension, dizziness, and weakness in a patient with cerebellar degeneration and peripheral neuropathy due to prior alcohol abuse were sufficiently severe for the patient to be considered for a cardiac pacemaker but were found to be associated with the use of an oxymetazoline nasal spray. Within 24 hours of discontinuing its use the patient was much improved and subsequently had no further symptoms. Cerebellar degeneration and peripheral neuropathy may have predisposed this patient to a more profound response to the drug's effects.— F. Glazener *et al.* (letter), *New Engl. J. Med.*, 1983, *309*, 731.

An account of 6 young children with various CNS reactions to oxymetazoline nose-drops or spray, reported during the period 1968-82, to the Swedish Adverse Drug Reactions Advisory Committee and the Drug Information Centre of Huddinge University Hospital. The doses used were apparently normal in all but one child who received about 2 to 3 times the recommended dose. The incidence of CNS reactions to oxymetazoline is unknown but adverse effects are probably rare. However, they should be borne in mind especially when prescribing nose-drops to infants and small children. There should be a note of caution about overdoses on the label or package inserts.— P. Söderman *et al.* (letter), *Lancet*, 1984, *1*, 573. Comment. The manufacturers' literature does not support the use of oxymetazoline in children under 2 years of age.— H. I. Silverman (letter), *ibid.*, *2*, 347. Reply.— B. -E. Wiholm (letter), *ibid.*

PORPHYRIA. Oxymetazoline was considered to be unsafe in patients with acute porphyria because it has been shown to be porphyrinogenic in *animals* or *in vitro* systems.— M.R. Moore and K.E.L. McColl, *Porphyrias, Drug Lists*, Glasgow, Porphyria Research Unit, University of Glasgow, 1987.

Uses and Administration

Oxymetazoline hydrochloride is a direct sympathomimetic agent which is used in 0.05% solution as a vasoconstrictor to relieve nasal congestion. It acts within a few minutes and the effect lasts for several hours.

Preparations

Oxymetazoline Hydrochloride Nasal Solution *(U.S.P.)*

Proprietary Preparations

Afrazine *(Kirby-Warrick, UK)*. *Nasal drops*, oxymetazoline hydrochloride 0.05%.
Paediatric nasal drops, oxymetazoline hydrochloride 0.025%.
Nasal spray, oxymetazoline hydrochloride 0.05%.

Proprietary Names and Manufacturers

4-Way Long Acting Nasal Spray *(Bristol-Myers Products, USA)*; Afrazine *(Kirby-Warrick, UK)*; Afrin *(Scherag, S.Afr.; Schering, USA)*; Coldrex Nasal Spray *(Nyal, Austral.)*; Dristan Long Lasting Nasal Spray *(Whitehall, USA)*; Dristan Nasal Mist *(Whitehall, UK)*; Drixin *(Schering Corp., Denm.)*; Drixine *(Essex, Austral.; Scherag, S.Afr.)*; Drixoral Nasal Spray *(Schering, Canad.)*; Durazol *(Austral.)*; Hazol *(Austral.)*; Iliadin *(Austral.; E. Merck, Denm.; E. Merck, Norw.; Merck, S.Afr.; E. Merck, Swed.)*; Iliadine *(Merck-Clévenot, Fr.)*; Iliadin-Mini *(E. Merck, UK)*; Lidil *(Arg.)*; Nafrine *(Schering, Canad.)*; Nasivin *(E. Merck, Ger.; Ital.; Neth.)*; Nasivine *(E. Merck, Switz.)*; Nasofarma *(Igoda, Spain)*; Neo-Synephrine 12 Hour *(Winthrop-Breon, USA)*; Nesivine *(Belg.)*; Nezeril *(Draco, Denm.; Draco, Swed.)*; Nostrilla *(Boehringer Ingelheim, USA)*; NTZ *(Winthrop-Breon, USA)*; Ocuclear *(Schering, Canad.)*; Respibien *(Cinfa, Spain)*; Respir *(Essex, Spain)*; Rhinolitan *(Kettelhack Riker, Ger.)*; Rhinox *(NAF, Norw.)*; Rinofol *(Hosbon, Spain)*; Sinarest 12 Hour *(Pharmacraft, USA)*; Sinex Long-Acting *(Richardson-Vicks, USA)*; Utabon *(Uriach, Spain)*; Vistoxyn *(Allergan, Ger.)*; Zolin *(ACO, Swed.)*.

2094-g

Phenylephrine Hydrochloride *(BANM, USAN, rINNM)*.

Fenilefrina Cloridrato; *m*-Synephrine Hydrochloride; Mesatonum; Metaoxedrini Chloridum; Néosynéphrine Chlorhydrate; Phenylephrinium Chloratum. (*S*)-1-(3-Hydroxyphenyl)-2-methylaminoethanol hydrochloride.
$C_9H_{13}NO_2,HCl=203.7$.

CAS — 59-42-7 (phenylephrine); 61-76-7 (hydrochloride).

NOTE. Synephrine has been used as a synonym for oxedrine. Care should be taken to avoid confusion between the 2 compounds.

Pharmacopoeias. In *Br., Braz., Chin., Egypt., Ind., It., Jpn, Jug., Neth., Nord., Port., Rus., Swiss, Turk.,* and *U.S.*

White or almost white, odourless or almost odourless, crystalline powder. **Soluble** 1 in 2 of water, 1 in 4 of alcohol, and 1 in 2 of glycerol. The *B.P.* injection has a pH of 4.5 to 6.5; the *U.S.P.* specifies a pH between 3.0 and 6.5.
The *B.P.* injection is **sterilised** by filtration. **Store** in airtight containers. Protect from light.

INCOMPATIBILITY. Particulate matter was observed within 2 hours when 1 mL of commercial phenylephrine hydrochloride injection was mixed with 5 mL of sterile water and 1 mL of commercial phenytoin sodium injection.— R. Misgen, *Am. J. Hosp. Pharm.*, 1965, *22*, 92. See also J. A. Patel and G. L. Phillips, *Am. J. Hosp. Pharm.*, 1966, *23*, 409.

STABILITY OF SOLUTIONS. No detectable loss occurred in a solution at pH 2 kept at 97° for longer than 10 days, but a rise in pH, particularly above pH 9, accelerated decomposition.— H. A. M. El-Shibini *et al.*, *Arzneimittel-Forsch.*, 1969, *19*, 676. See also *idem*, 1613. Yellow discoloration of phenylephrine solutions was an indication of appreciable degradation. Metals, especially copper, when present in 10 ppm concentration, accelerated degradation, though calcium had no influence and magnesium increased stability. Heavy metals might combine with phenylephrine to yield auto-oxidisable complexes. This could be prevented by adding edetic acid 500 µg per mL.— *idem*, 828.

Phenylephrine hydrochloride 250 mg was stable for 84 days at up to 60° in Water for Injections 100 mL; in sodium chloride injection 100 mL; with chloramphenicol succinate 50 mg in sodium chloride injection 100 mL; with chloramphenicol succinate 50 mg in glucose injection 100 mL (pH 6); and with potassium chloride 4 mmol (4 mEq) in glucose injection 100 mL. With chloramphenicol succinate 50 mg and sodium bicarbonate 750 mg in glucose injection 100 mL (pH 8.2), phenylephrine hydrochloride was stable for 84 days only when stored at 22° and unstable at higher temperatures.— C. R. Weber and V. D. Gupta, *J. Hosp. Pharm.*, 1970, *28*, 200.

Adverse Effects

For the adverse effects of sympathomimetic agents, see p.1453.

Phenylephrine hydrochloride is irritant and may cause local discomfort at the site of application; extravasation of the injection may even cause local tissue necrosis.

EFFECTS ON THE CARDIOVASCULAR SYSTEM. When 1 drop of a 10% solution of phenylephrine eye-drops was instilled into the eyes of low birth-weight infants, their systolic and diastolic pressures were increased considerably. This effect lasted for 70 minutes or more and could be hazardous if a left-to-right shunt existed. It was suggested that the 10% solution should be replaced by a 2.5% solution, not only in neonates but in all other patients.— V. Borromeo-McGrail *et al.*, *Pediatrics*, 1973, *51*, 1032. See also *Br. med. J.*, 1974, *1*, 2. One drop of phenylephrine 10% eye-drops instilled into each eye of an infant produced acute pulmonary oedema with associated hypertension.— T. G. Matthews *et al.* (letter), *Lancet*, 1977, *2*, 827.

An 8-year-old boy who received 14 to 18 mg of phenylephrine as eye-drops to stop excessive bleeding developed severe hypertension, and ventricular arrhythmias which were eventually controlled with lignocaine administered intravenously. Absorption from mucosal surfaces was almost as rapid as with intravenous administration and thus the amount of phenylephrine administered was an overdose.— R. W. Vaughan, *Anesth. Analg. curr. Res.*, 1973, *52*, 161.

Persistent hypertension in a 7.5-week-old infant with a respiratory infection was associated with the use during the previous 7 days of phenylephrine in nasal drops together with a preparation containing pseudoephedrine given 4 times daily by mouth.— R. Saken *et al.*, *J. Pediat.*, 1979, *95*, 1077.

Data on 32 patients who suffered systemic reactions possibly associated with phenylephrine given by topical application of 10% eye-drops, or on a cotton pledget, by subconjunctival injection, or by irrigation of the lachrymal sac. Of 15 patients with myocardial infarct (9 of whom had a previous history of cardiovascular disease), 11 died; 7 additional patients required cardiopulmonary resuscitation for cardiac arrhythmia or cardiac arrests; the remainder of the adverse reactions were severe increase of systemic blood pressure, tachycardia, and reflex bradycardia. The following guidelines are suggested for the clinical use of phenylephrine: use 10% phenylephrine with caution in patients with known cardiac disease, hypertension, aneurysms, and advanced arteriosclerosis; only use the 2.5% solutions in infants and the elderly; the use of 10% phenylephrine to irrigate, with a conjunctival pledget, or injected subconjunctivally should be discouraged; only one application is allowable per hour to each eye; contra-indicated in patients taking monoamine oxidase inhibitors and tricyclic antidepressants; be aware that pressor effects and tachycardia can be induced in the atropinised patient.— F. T. Fraunfelder and A. F. Scafidi, *Am. J. Ophthal.*, 1978, *85*, 447. Results of a prospective double-blind study indicated that the incidence of severe hypertensive response to topically administered ocular 10% phenylephrine is very low.— M. M. Brown *et al.*, *Archs Ophthal., N.Y.*, 1980, *98*, 487. See also V. Kumer *et al.*, *Am. J. Ophthal.*, 1985, *99*, 180.

EFFECTS ON MENTAL FUNCTION. A report of the development of hallucinations and paranoid delusions in a patient following excessive use of a nasal spray containing phenylephrine 0.5%. The patient, who had used such sprays for 13 years, experienced choking sensations when the drug was withdrawn but subsequently recovered.— S. S. Snow *et al.*, *Br. J. Psychiat.*, 1980, *136*, 297. See also B. G. H. Waters and Y. D. Lapierre, *Am. J. Psychiat.*, 1981, *38*, 837 (mania following high doses by mouth).

Precautions

For the precautions that should be observed with sympathomimetic agents, see p.1453.

Phenylephrine eye-drops should be avoided or only used with extreme caution in infants since they can have powerful systemic effects (see under Adverse Effects, above).

Excessive use of phenylephrine nasal drops can lead to rebound congestion. Phenylephrine is less liable than adrenaline and noradrenaline to induce fibrillation if used as a pressor agent during anaesthesia with chloroform, cyclopropane, halothane, and trichloroethylene; nevertheless, caution is necessary.

INTERACTIONS. A 46-year-old man taking *debrisoquine* 20 mg thrice daily for hypertension with satisfactory control was given phenylephrine 50 mg by mouth. Marked hypertension occurred which was reduced by phentolamine.— J. Aminu *et al.* (letter), *Lancet*, 1970, *2*, 935. Investigations in 4 healthy subjects indicated that the hypertensive effect of phenylephrine could be markedly enhanced by administration of *debrisoquine*.— W. Allum *et al.*, *Br. J. clin. Pharmac.*, 1974, *1*, 51.

In 4 volunteers pretreated with *imipramine*, 25 mg three times daily for 5 days, the pressor effect of phenylephrine was enhanced by a factor of 2 to 3, that of adrenaline by a factor of 2 to 4, and that of noradrenaline by a factor of 4 to 8, with no significant difference in the response to isoprenaline. All 4 subjects experienced cardiac arrhythmias when given adrenaline. Felypressin might be a more suitable vasoconstrictor for use in patients taking tricyclic antidepressants. When they were pretreated with monoamine oxidase inhibitors (phenelzine 15 mg three times daily or tranylcypromine 10 mg three times daily) for 7 days the pressor effect of *phenylephrine* was significantly enhanced but there was no significant change in the response to *adrenaline*, *noradrenaline*, or *isoprenaline*. Isoprenaline-induced tachycardia was significantly reduced. It was unlikely that patients taking monoamine oxidase inhibitors would be seriously at risk if given noradrenaline in local anaesthetic solutions.— A. J. Boakes *et al.*, *Br. med. J.*, 1973, *1*, 311. The finding that imipramine enhanced the pressor effects of sympathomimetic agents to a greater degree than did monoamine oxidase inhibitors was at variance with clinical experience.— G. G. Wallis (letter), *ibid.*, 549.

A study indicating that pre-operative phenylephrine eye-drops can be hazardous in patients with sympathetic denervation such as those with long-standing insulin-dependent diabetes or hypertensive patients receiving *reserpine* or *guanethidine*.— J. M. Kim *et al.*, *Am. J. Ophthal.*, 1978, *85*, 862.

A report of a fatality occurring in a 49-year-old woman with asymptomatic hypertension on a regimen of hydrochlorothiazide 50 mg twice daily and propranolol hydrochloride 40 mg four times daily following the instillation of one drop of 10% phenylephrine hydrochloride solution in each eye during an ophthalmological examination.— E. Cass *et al.*, *Can. med. Ass. J.*, 1979, *120*, 1261.

Absorption and Fate

Phenylephrine has reduced bioavailability from the gastro-intestinal tract owing to irregular absorption and first-pass metabolism by monoamine oxidase in the gut and liver. When injected intramuscularly it takes 10 to 15 minutes to act and subcutaneous and intramuscular injections are effective for about an hour. Intravenous injections are effective for about 20 minutes.

Uses and Administration

Phenylephrine hydrochloride is a sympathomimetic agent with mainly direct effects on adrenergic receptors. It has predominantly alpha-adrenergic activity and is without significant stimulating effects on the central nervous system at usual doses. Its pressor activity is weaker than that of noradrenaline (see p.1471) but of longer duration. After injection it produces peripheral vasoconstriction and increased arterial pressure; it also causes reflex bradycardia. It reduces blood flow to the skin and to the kidneys.

Phenylephrine hydrochloride has been used in the treatment of hypotensive states, e.g. circulatory failure, spinal anaesthesia, or drug-induced hypotension, including that following the use of chlorpromazine and other phenothiazines. It has been administered in a dose of 2 to 5 mg subcutaneously or intramuscularly with further doses of 1 to 10 mg if necessary, according to response or in a dose of 100 to 500 µg by slow intravenous injection as a 0.1% solution, repeated as necessary after at least 15 minutes. Alternatively, 10 mg in 500 mL of glucose injection or sodium chloride injection has been infused intravenously, initially at a rate of up to 180 µg per minute, reduced, according to the response, to 30 to 60 µg per minute.

A suggested dose for children is 100 µg per kg body-weight, subcutaneously or intramuscularly.

Phenylephrine hydrochloride has been given by intravenous injection to stop paroxysmal supraventricular tachycardia but other agents may be preferred. The initial dose is usually not greater than 500 µg given as a 0.1% solution with subsequent doses gradually increased up to 1 mg if necessary.

Phenylephrine has been used as an ingredient of combination aerosol inhalers to prolong the bronchodilator effects of isoprenaline. Metered-dose inhalers providing 240 µg of phenylephrine acid tartrate and 160 µg of isoprenaline hydrochloride per dose are available.

Phenylephrine hydrochloride has been used in a concentration of 1 in 20 000 as a vasoconstrictor with local anaesthetics.

Locally, phenylephrine hydrochloride is used as a nasal decongestant in rhinitis and sinusitis. For this purpose 2 to 3 drops of a 0.25 to 0.5% solution may be instilled into each nostril every 3 to 4 hours. It may cause local irritation; overuse causes rebound congestion. It may also be given by mouth in preparations for the relief of nasal congestion; doses of 10 mg three or four times daily have been given.

In ophthalmology, phenylephrine hydrochloride is employed as a mydriatic and conjunctival decongestant as a 0.1% to 10% solution. The effect lasts several hours. Solutions stronger than 2% may cause intense irritation and a local anaesthetic other than butacaine (which is incompatible) should be added to these. In open-angle glaucoma phenylephrine is sometimes used to lower intra-ocular pressure temporarily. Owing to the risk of systemic effects the 10% strength is contra-indicated in infants and in patients with aneurysms or other risk factors such as hypertension or coronary heart disease.

ANAESTHESIA. In a study in 65 patients undergoing spinal anaesthesia with lignocaine 62.5 mg in 7.5% glucose, 25 received lignocaine alone, 21 received lignocaine with phenylephrine 2 mg and 19 lignocaine with phenylephrine 5 mg. The mean level of anaesthesia achieved did not differ between the groups but the mean time for regression of anaesthesia to the T12 dermatome was 109 minutes in the first group compared with 130 minutes in the second and 162 minutes in the third. These regression times were all significantly different: clinically useful prolongation of sensory analgesia may be obtained by the addition of phenylephrine to lignocaine during spinal anaesthesia.— G. T. Vaida *et al.*, *Anesth. Analg.*, 1986, *65*, 781.

CARDIAC DISORDERS. Phenylephrine terminated ventricular tachycardia in 12 of 13 patients. In 4 patients extensively studied doses of 0.4 to 1 mg were required. The required dose was reduced by a factor of at least 2 when edrophonium hydrochloride 10 to 20 mg was first given; the required dose was increased by a similar factor when atropine 2.4 mg was first given. Carotid sinus massage alone did not break ventricular tachycardia but was effective after edrophonium in doses of 15 or 20 mg. A vagal mechanism was considered to be involved.— M. B. Waxman and R. W. Wald, *Circulation*, 1977, *56*, 385.

HYPOTENSION. Phenylephrine in doses of 30 mg abolished the postural symptoms in 4 patients with orthostatic hypotension but also produced recumbent hypertension. The long-term use of phenylephrine for this condition is considered hazardous.— B. Davies *et al., Lancet*, 1978, *1*, 172.

OCULAR DISORDERS. A discussion of drugs used to dilate the pupil for examination of the fundus. Tropicamide 0.5% eye-drops are almost ideal in terms of their onset and duration of action but their action may be supplemented by phenylephrine 10% to produce a wide mydriasis. Phenylephrine may also be used alone and works moderately well, with an effect in about 20 minutes. In patients in whom a predisposition to glaucoma is suspected, one pupil only should be dilated with phenylephrine 10% and its effects reversed with thymoxamine 0.5%, leaving examination of the other eye to a subsequent visit.— C. I. Phillips, *Br. med. J.*, 1984, *288*, 1779. Comment. Phenylephrine has only achieved about 10% of its mydriatic effect after 20 minutes, and is a much slower mydriatic than tropicamide, the time to maximum effect having been reported as 70 and 39 minutes respectively. However, a combination of the two agents provides excellent response in patients with diabetic retinopathy, who are notoriously resistant to conventional regimens: such patients are especially sensitive to topical phenylephrine because of pupillary sympathetic neuropathy.— S. E. Smith and S. A. Smith (letter), *ibid.*, *289*, 111. See also M. J. E. Huber *et al., Br. J. Ophthal.*, 1985, *69*, 425.

RETROGRADE EJACULATION. A satisfactory result was achieved in 1 of 6 young men with retrograde ejaculation treated with intravenous phenylephrine. Findings in the other 5, who had a predominant disorder of emission and therefore diminished sperm counts in the postcoital urine, indicated that restitution of vas deferens function cannot be achieved pharmacologically.— K. Stockamp *et al., Fert. Steril.*, 1974, *25*, 817.

Preparations

Phenylephrine Eye-drops *(B.P.C. 1973)*. PHNL. Contain phenylephrine hydrochloride 10%. Sterilised by filtration.

Phenylephrine Eye-drops Strong *(A.P.F.)*. Gutt. Phenylephrin. Fort. Contain phenylephrine hydrochloride 10%. Sterilised by autoclaving.

Phenylephrine Eye-drops Weak *(A.P.F.)*. Gutt. Phenylephrin. Contain phenylephrine hydrochloride 0.125% Sterilised by autoclaving.

Phenylephrine Injection *(B.P.)*. Phenylephrine Hydrochloride Injection. Contains phenylephrine hydrochloride.

Phenylephrine Hydrochloride Injection *(U.S.P.)*. A sterile solution of phenylephrine hydrochloride in Water for Injections.

Phenylephrine Hydrochloride Nasal Jelly *(U.S.P.)*

Phenylephrine Hydrochloride Nasal Solution *(U.S.P.)*

Phenylephrine Hydrochloride Ophthalmic Solution *(U.S.P.)*. A sterile aqueous solution of phenylephrine hydrochloride. pH 4 to 7.5 (buffered); 3 to 4.5 (unbuffered).

Phenylephrine Instillation *(A.P.F.)*. Phenylephrine Nasal Drops; Phenylephrine Nasal Spray. Contain phenylephrine hydrochloride 0.25%. Store in small, well-filled, airtight containers.

Phenylephrine Instillation Strong *(A.P.F.)*. Strong Phenylephrine Nasal Drops; Strong Phenylephrine Nasal Spray. Contains phenylephrine hydrochloride 1%. Store in small, well-filled, airtight containers.

Proprietary Preparations

Hayphryn *(Winthrop, UK)*. *Nasal spray*, phenylephrine hydrochloride 0.5%, thenyldiamine hydrochloride 0.1%.

Isopto Frin *(Alcon, UK)*. *Eye-drops*, phenylephrine hydrochloride 0.12%, hypromellose 0.5%.

Minims Phenylephrine Hydrochloride *(Smith & Nephew Pharmaceuticals, UK)*. *Eye-drops*, phenylephrine hydrochloride 2.5 and 10%, in single-use disposable applicators.

Neophryn *(Winthrop, UK)*. *Nasal drops*, phenylephrine hydrochloride 0.25%.
Nasal spray, phenylephrine hydrochloride 0.5%.

Uniflu *(Unigreg, UK)*. *Tablets*, composite pack, comprising:
Uniflu tablets, phenylephrine hydrochloride 10 mg, caffeine 30 mg, codeine phosphate 10 mg, diphenhydramine hydrochloride 15 mg, paracetamol 500 mg;
Gregovite C tablets, ascorbic acid 300 mg. For colds and influenza. *Dose.* 1 of each every 4 hours.

Vibrocil *(Zyma, UK)*. *Nasal drops*, phenylephrine 0.25%, dimethindene maleate 0.025%, neomycin sulphate 0.35%.
Nasal gel, phenylephrine 0.25%, dimethindene maleate 0.025%, neomycin sulphate 0.35%.
Nasal spray, phenylephrine 0.25%, dimethindene maleate 0.025%, neomycin sulphate 0.35%.

Proprietary Names and Manufacturers of Phenylephrine Salts

Adrianol *(Boehringer Ingelheim, Ital.)*; Ak-Dilate *(Akorn, Canad.)*; Allerest Nasal *(Pharmacraft, USA)*; Analux *(Cusi, Spain)*; Boraline *(Neth.)*; Col Liquipom Constrictor *(Iquinosa, Spain)*; Fenilfar *(Ital.)*; Fenox *(Boots, Austral.)*; I-Care *(Austral.)*; Isonefrine *(Allergan, Ital.)*; Isophrin *(USA)*; Isopto Frin *(Alcon, Austral.; Canad.; Alcon, UK)*; Isopto Phenylephrine *(Austral.)*; Isopto-Frin *(S.Afr.; Alcon, Switz.)*; Isotropina *(Ital.)*; Metaoxedrin Minims *(Smith & Nephew, Norw.)*; Minims Phenylephrine Hydrochloride *(Smith & Nephew, Austral.; Smith & Nephew, S.Afr.; Smith & Nephew Pharmaceuticals, UK)*; Mistol Mist *(Austral.)*; Mydfrin *(Alcon, Canad.; Alcon Laboratories, USA)*; Narex *(Norton, UK)*; Nasalmed *(Vernleigh, S.Afr.)*; Neophryn *(Winthrop, UK)*; Neosinefrina *(Spain)*; Neosyn *(Swed.)*; Neo-Synephrine *(Winthrop, Austral.; Wellcome, Canad.; Winthrop, Ger.; Maggioni-Winthrop, Ital.; Winthrop, Switz.; Winthrop-Breon, USA)*; Neosynephrine *(Winthrop, Denm.; Boehringer Ingelheim, Fr.; Sterling-Winthrop, Swed.)*; Nostril *(Boehringer Ingelheim, USA)*; Optistin *(Allergan, Ital.)*; Optocrymal *(Canad.)*; Poen-Efrina *(Arg.)*; Prefrin *(Allergan, Canad.; Allergan, S.Afr.; Allergan, UK)*; Pulverizador Nasal *(Collado, Spain)*; Relief Eye Drops *(Allergan, USA)*; Rinex *(Belg.)*; Sinarest Nasal *(Pharmacraft, USA)*; Soothe *(Canad.)*; Visadron *(Belg.; Basotherm, Ger.; Boehringer Ingelheim, Ital.; Neth.; Boehringer Ingelheim, Spain)*; Visopt *(Sigma, Austral.)*; Vistosan *(Allergan, Ger.)*.

The following names have been used for multi-ingredient preparations containing phenylephrine salts—4-Way Nasal Spray *(Bristol-Myers Products, USA)*; Ak-Vernacon *(Akorn, Canad.)*; Albatussin *(Bart, USA)*; Atrohist *(Adams, USA)*; Benatuss *(Parke, Davis, Austral.)*; Benyphed *(Parke, Davis, Austral.)*; Betnovate Compound Suppositories *(Glaxo, UK)*; Betnovate Rectal *(Glaxo, UK)*; Biohisdex DHC *(Everest, Canad.)*; Biohisdex DM *(Everest, Canad.)*; Biohisdine *(Everest, Canad.)*; Biohisdine DHC *(Everest, Canad.)*; Biohisdine DM *(Everest, Canad.)*; Biomydrin *(Warner, UK)*; Blephamide *(Allergan, Austral.; Allergan, Canad.)*; BPP *(Gen, Canad.)*; Brocon *(Forest Laboratories, USA)*; Bromphen Compound *(Schein, USA)*; Bronchilator *(Sterling Research, UK)*; Cerose-DM *(Wyeth, USA)*; Chemhisdex C *(Clark, Canad.)*; Chemhisdex-DHC *(Clark, Canad.)*; Chemhisdex-DHC-Expectorant *(Clark, Canad.)*; Chemhisdex-DM *(Clark, Canad.)*; Chemhisdine-DHC-Child *(Clark, Canad.)*; Chemhisdine-DHC-Expectorant *(Clark, Canad.)*; Chemhisdine-DM *(Clark, Canad.)*; Citra Forte Capsules *(Boyle, USA)*; Codalin *(Clark, Canad.)*; Codimal DH *(Central Pharmaceuticals, USA)*; Codimal DM *(Central Pharmaceuticals, USA)*; Codimal PH *(Central Pharmaceuticals, USA)*; Comhist *(Norwich Eaton, USA)*; Conar-A *(Beecham Laboratories, USA)*; Congespirin *(Bristol-Myers Products, USA)*; Congespirin Aspirin Free *(Bristol-Myers Products, USA)*; Coristex-DH *(Technilab, Canad.)*; Coristine-DH *(Technilab, Canad.)*; Coryban-D Cough Syrup *(Pfipharmecs, USA)*; Dallergy *(Laser, USA)*; Dallergy-D Syrup *(Laser, USA)*; Deconsal *(Adams, USA)*; Decotan *(Gen, Canad.)*; Demazin Repetabs *(Schering, USA)*; Demazin Syrup *(Schering, Austral.; Schering, USA)*; Dexylets *(Parke, Davis, UK)*; Dimetane Expectorant *(Robins, Canad.)*; Dimetane Expectorant-C *(Robins, Canad.)*; Dimetane Expectorant-DC *(Robins, Canad.)*; Dimetapp *(Robins, Austral.; Robins, Canad.)*; Dimetapp Elixir-Plus *(Robins, Canad.)*; Dimetapp-A *(Robins, Canad.)*; Dimetapp-C *(Robins, Canad.)*; Dimetapp-DM *(Robins, Canad.)*; Dimotane Expectorant *(Robins, UK)*; Dimotane Expectorant DC *(Robins, UK)*; Dimotapp *(Robins, UK)*; Dimotapp P *(Robins, UK)*; Donatussin DC *(Laser, USA)*; Donatussin Drops *(Laser, USA)*; Dristan Advanced Formula *(Whitehall, Canad.; Whitehall, USA)*; Dristan Decongestant Tablets with Antihistamine *(Whitehall, UK)*; Dristan Nasal Spray *(Whitehall, USA)*; Drixine Cough Expectorant *(Essex, Austral.)*; Duo-Autohaler *(Riker, UK)*; Duo-Medihaler *(Riker, Canad.; Riker, USA)*; Dura-Gest *(Dura, USA)*; Dura-Tap/PD *(Dura, USA)*; Dura-Vent/DA *(Dura, USA)*; ENT Syrup *(Springbok, USA)*; ENT Tablets *(Springbok, USA)*; Entex *(Norwich Eaton, USA)*; E-Tapp *(Edwards, USA)*; Extendryl *(Fleming, USA)*; Exyphen *(Norton, UK)*; Hayphryn *(Winthrop, UK)*; Hemorex *(Winthrop, Austral.)*; Histalet Forte *(Reid-Rowell, USA)*; Histamic *(Metro Med, USA)*; Histaspan-D *(USV Pharmaceutical Corp., USA)*; Histaspan-P *(Rorer, Canad.)*; Histaspan-Plus *(USV Pharmaceutical Corp., USA)*; Histor-D *(Hauck, USA)*; Hycomine *(Du Pont, Austral.; Du Pont, Canad.)*; Hycomine Compound *(Du Pont, USA)*;
Isuprel-Neo *(Winthrop, Canad.)*; Korigesic *(Trimen, USA)*; Medihaler-duo *(Riker, UK)*; Naldecon *(Bristol, USA)*; Neo-Synephrine Antihistamine Cold Tablets *(Winthrop, Austral.)*; Neo-Synephrine Cold Tablets *(Winthrop, Austral.)*; Neo-Synephrine Linctus *(Winthrop, Austral.)*; Neo-Tuss *(Neolab, Canad.)*; Nethaprin Dospan *(Merrell, UK)*; Novahistex C *(Dow, Canad.)*; Novahistex DH *(Dow, Canad.)*; Novahistex DM *(Dow, Canad.)*; Novahistex Expectorant *(Dow, Canad.)*; Novahistine DH *(Dow, Canad.)*; Novahistine DM *(Dow, Canad.)*; NTZ *(Winthrop, Austral.)*; NTZ Superinone *(Winthrop, Austral.)*; Papzans Modified *(Bowman, USA)*; Pediacof *(Winthrop-Breon, USA)*; Phenephrin *(Nelson, Austral.)*; Phenergan VC *(Wyeth, USA)*; Phenergan VC Expectorant *(Rhône-Poulenc, Canad.)*; Phenergan VC Expectorant with Codeine *(Rhône-Poulenc, Canad.)*; Phenergan VC with Codeine *(Wyeth, USA)*; Phenyltrope *(Akorn, Canad.)*; Prednefrin *(Allergan, Austral.)*; Prefrin Liquifilm *(Allergan, Austral.; Allergan, USA)*; Prefrin-A *(Allergan, Canad.; Allergan, USA)*; Prefrin-Z *(Allergan, Austral.)*; Prometh VC *(National Pharm., USA)*; Protid *(Lasalle, USA)*; Pulmorphan *(Riva, Canad.)*; P-V-Tussin Syrup *(Reid-Provident, USA)*;
Quadrahist *(Schein, USA)*; Quelidrine *(Abbott, USA)*; Ru-Tuss Liquid *(Boots, USA)*; Ru-Tuss Plain *(Boots, USA)*; Ru-Tuss Tablets *(Boots, USA)*; Ru-Tuss with Hydrocodone *(Boots, USA)*; Rymed-Jr. *(Edwards, USA)*; Rynatan *(Wallace, USA)*; Rynatuss *(Wallace, USA)*; Sequels *(Lederle, USA)*; Singlet *(Lakeside, USA)*; Sinovan Timed *(Drug Industries, USA)*; Sinuzets *(Boots, Austral.)*; Soframycin Nebuliser *(Roussel, Austral.; Roussel, UK)*; S-T Decongest *(Scot-Tussin, USA)*; S-T Forte *(Scot-Tussin, USA)*; Tamine *(Geneva, USA)*; T-Dry *(T.E. Williams, USA)*; Thenfacol *(Winthrop, Austral.)*; Tonolift *(Drug Houses Austral., Austral.)*; Tussar DM *(USV Pharmaceutical Corp., USA)*; Tussirex *(Scot-Tussin, USA)*; Tympagesic *(Adria, USA)*; Uniflu *(Unigreg, UK)*; Vasocort *(Smith Kline & French, UK)*; Vasosulf *(Coopervision, Canad.; Coopervision, USA)*; Vibrocil *(Zyma, UK)*; Zincfrin *(Alcon, Austral.; Alcon, Canad.; Alcon, UK)*.

2095-q

Phenylpropanolamine Hydrochloride

(BANM, USAN).

Cloridrato de Fenilpropanolamine; *dl*-Norephedrine Hydrochloride; Mydriatin. (1*RS*,2*SR*)-2-Amino-1-phenylpropan-1-ol hydrochloride. $C_9H_{13}NO,HCl = 187.7$.

CAS — 14838-15-4 (phenylpropanolamine); 154-41-6 (hydrochloride).

Pharmacopoeias. In *Br.*, *Braz.*, and *U.S.*

A white to creamy-white crystalline powder, odourless or with a slight aromatic odour.

The *B.P.* states that it is **soluble** 1 in 2.5 of water, 1 in 9 of alcohol; practically insoluble in chloroform and ether; *U.S.P.* solubilities are 1 in 1.1 of water and 1 in 7.4 of alcohol. A 3% solution in water has a pH of 4.5 to 6.0 (*B.P.*) or 4.2 to 5.5 (*U.S.P.*). **Store** in airtight containers. Protect from light.

Adverse Effects and Precautions

For the adverse effects of sympathomimetic agents, and precautions to be observed, see p.1453.

Severe hypertensive episodes have followed phenylpropanolamine ingestion.

Comment on the potentially fatal side-effects of phenylpropanolamine.— S. M. Mueller (letter), *New Engl. J. Med.*, 1983, *308*, 653. Comment by a manufacturer. The reports cited need to be put into perspective. Properly manufactured and marketed phenylpropanolamine products, taken as directed, have had an excellent safety record.— M. B. Saltzman (letter), *ibid.*, 1984, *310*, 395. Reply. The overall picture is alarming. A total of 1053 emergency room admissions due to ingestion of over-the-counter phenylpropanolamine diet aids were reported to the *US* Drug Abuse Warning Network last year; 54% of those asked admitted to abusing the preparation with suicidal intent. Phenylpropanolamine is a drug of abuse, and in view of the lack of efficacy of such drugs in obesity the author remains unconvinced that the risk justifies the benefit. However, nasal decongestants, which generally contain lower doses of phenylpropanolamine, may be associated with a lesser risk.— S. M. Mueller (letter), *ibid.*

ABUSE. See above, and under Effects on Mental Function (below).

EFFECTS ON THE KIDNEYS. A report of acute interstitial nephritis in a young woman who had taken an appetite suppressant containing phenylpropanolamine (Fullstop) over the previous 3 weeks. She had also taken 2 or 3 tablets containing aspirin 325 mg, and paracetamol 650 mg.— W. M. Bennett (letter), *Lancet*, 1979, *2*, 42.

A report of 2 cases of acute renal failure and rhabdomyolysis in patients who had taken phenylpropanolamine.— R. D. Swenson *et al.*, *J. Am. med. Ass.*, 1982, *248*, 1216.

EFFECTS ON MENTAL FUNCTION. During 1979 the Swedish Adverse Drug Reaction Committee received several reports of psychic disturbances during treatment with phenylpropanolamine. Of 61 cases reported, 48 were in children aged 0 to 15 years. The dominant symptoms were restlessness, irritability, aggression (especially in younger children), and sleep disturbances. Five cases of psychotic episodes have also been reported. These included 2 boys aged 3 and 8 years who were confused and unable to recognise their parents a few hours after taking phenylpropanolamine (Rinexin, *Leo*); a 4-year-old girl who had episodes of visual hallucinosis and a grand-mal seizure after phenylpropanolamine in association with the antihistamine, brompheniramine (Lunerin, *Draco*); a 25-year-old woman who became increasingly excited and lacking in concentration with sleep/wakefulness disturbances during treatment with phenylpropanolamine (Monydrin, *Draco*), after 9 days experiencing vivid paranoid misconceptions and episodic muscular twitchings in the legs, her symptoms disappearing within 24 hours of stopping the drug; and a 17-year-old who was admitted to mental hospital on 3 occasions with signs and symptoms of acute mania-like psychosis with excessive motor excitement, aggressive behaviour, and elevated mood with uncontrollable thought and speech, and hallucinosis and confusion on the third admission, who on recovery was found to have taken large quantities of phenylpropanolamine (Rinexin) and brompheniramine (Rinomar, *Leo*) before each episode.— G. Norvenius *et al.* (letter), *Lancet*, 1979, *2*, 1367. While adverse effects are not unlikely after the use of virtually any drug in the susceptible patient no adverse effects have been described in patients young or old from the use of phenylpropanolamine alone used in the correct dose.— H. I. Silverman (letter), *Lancet*, 1984, *2*, 347. The Swedish Adverse Drug Reactions Advisory Committee has on file 118 reports at the time of writing, representing probable or possible adverse reactions to single ingredient phenylpropanolamine. The most common symptoms are mental disturbances (62), skin reactions (27), neurological disorders (16), and micturition problems (11). Of the cases of mental disturbance 36 were in patients aged up to 14 years; 20 of the 36 had received a higher-than-recommended dose of whom 6 had also received other preparations. However this left 16 reported cases of children with psychiatric reactions to phenylpropanolamine in recommended doses. Psychiatric symptoms were most often excitation with disturbed sleep, sometimes with agitation or confusion.— B. -E. Wiholm (letter), *ibid.*

A report of 7 cases of central nervous system reactions (anxiety, agitation, hallucinations, dizziness) following single doses of phenylpropanolamine 50 or 70 mg, alone or combined with caffeine. All patients also had tachypnoea and tachycardia. Symptoms resolved in 6 in 2 to 4 hours; one patient had to be hospitalised for acute psychosis that resolved only after several days.— A. J. Dietz, *J. Am. med. Ass.*, 1981, *245*, 601.

Reference to the abuse of phenylpropanolamine-containing products as CNS stimulants and amphetamine substitutes.— P. S. Jordan (letter), *Am. J. Hosp. Pharm.*, 1981, *38*, 29. See also A. Blum, *J. Am. med. Ass.*, 1981, *245*, 1346.

HYPERTENSION. All of 37 healthy normotensive young adults had a rise in blood pressure within an hour of taking a capsule of an anorectic preparation containing phenylpropanolamine 85 mg (Trimolets); in 12 of the 37, peak supine diastolic blood pressures of 100 mmHg or more were recorded compared with 1 of 35 similar subjects who took matching placebo. Three of the 12 subjects required antihypertensive therapy. Symptoms reported by the subjects receiving phenylpropanolamine were: tingling feelings in head (6); dizziness which was not postural (5); postural dizziness (4); palpitations (5); headache (6); chest tightness (3); rash (3); tremor (2); nausea (2); lassitude (1); tinnitus (1); 'hot feeling' (1); 17 of those receiving active drug did not report symptoms. One subject in the placebo group reported nausea. Because of these blood pressure effects, study of Trimolets was discontinued and a preparation containing less phenylpropanolamine was investigated instead (capsules of Contac 500, which contain phenylpropanolamine 50 mg and belladonna alkaloids 250 µg). In 34 subjects who took one Contac 500 capsule there was a small mean rise in blood pressure, and 4 developed supine diastolic blood pressures of 100 mmHg or more, compared with none of 35 who took matching placebo. No subjects in either group reported symptoms. These results indicate that the availability of high-dose phenylpropanolamine-containing preparations without medical advice is potentially hazardous. Although the second preparation produced far less dramatic effects, it would also be likely to induce dangerous degrees of hypertension if more than one capsule were taken.— J. D. Horowitz *et al.*, *Lancet*, 1980, *1*, 60. Hypertensive episodes appear to be more likely with preparations containing phenylpropanolamine in the free form rather than in the slow-release form.— M. F. Cuthbert (letter), *Lancet*, 1980, *1*, 367. A vigorous defence of the safety of phenylpropanolamine by a manufacturer. It was difficult to reconcile the results of Horowitz *et al.* with clinical experience in normotensive subjects.— M. B. Saltzman (letter), *Lancet*, 1982, *1*, 1242.

A review of the toxicity of over-the-counter stimulants, including phenylpropanolamine. The most common and important adverse effect of phenylpropanolamine is hypertension. At doses of up to 50 mg the drug increases blood pressure only minimally in healthy normotensive subjects but it has a low therapeutic index and may produce severe or even life-threatening hypertension at less than 3 times the recommended maximum dose for *US* over-the-counter products of 37.5 mg. Hypertension from phenylpropanolamine alone is usually accompanied by a reflex bradycardia that may help to limit it, but drugs that abolish this effect, such as atropine, or that can accelerate heart-rate, such as caffeine, may exacerbate the hypertensive effect.— P. Pentel, *J. Am. med. Ass.*, 1984, *252*, 1898. Severe criticism. Phenylpropanolamine is a safe drug associated with a low incidence of adverse reactions.— L. Lasagna, *ibid.*, 1985, *253*, 2491. Reply. The observation that recommended doses of phenylpropanolamine are usually safe is correct. However, the salient point is that the drug has a very low therapeutic index. Recent reports of fatal intracerebral haemorrhage, hypertensive encephalopathy, ventricular arrhythmias, and myocardial injury illustrate the potential toxicity of the drug.— P. Pentel (letter), *ibid.*, 2492.

A report of stroke, not related to hypertension, associated with excessive phenylpropanolamine intake, as diet pills, in 2 patients.— D. A. Johnson *et al.* (letter), *Lancet*, 1983, *2*, 970. A Boston Collaborative Drug Surveillance Program review of the experience of Group Health Cooperative of Puget Sound indicating that the risk of cerebral haemorrhage requiring hospital admission and attributable to taking phenylpropanolamine-containing cough and cold remedies, if present at all, is very small; this conclusion was not affected by changing the assumption of the risk period from 30 to 90 days after the prescription was dispensed.— H. Jick *et al.*, *Lancet*, 1984, *1*, 1017.

Studies suggesting that phenylpropanolamine has no adverse effect on blood pressure in healthy subjects: M. B. Saltzman *et al.*, *Drug Intell. & clin. Pharm.*, 1983, *17*, 746 (75 mg daily by mouth, in divided doses or as a single sustained-release dose). Correction.— *ibid.*, *18*, 532; R. P. Goodman *et al.*, *Clin. Pharmac. Ther.*, 1986, *40*, 144 (75 mg as a sustained-release preparation). See also R. E. Noble (letter), *Lancet*, 1982, *1*, 1419.

A study of the use of propranolol to reverse the hypertensive effects of phenylpropanolamine in 6 healthy subjects.— P. R. Pentel *et al.*, *Clin. Pharmac. Ther.*, 1985, *37*, 488. Criticism of the experimental design.— J. P. Morgan (letter), *ibid.*, 1986, *39*, 102.

In view of reports that doses of phenylpropanolamine higher than 75 mg may cause serious elevations in blood pressure the FDA would not permit phenylpropanolamine to be marketed at a dosage level higher than 75 mg daily, pending a review of the findings.— *FDA Consumer*, 1984, (Feb.), 29. In the *UK* phenylpropanolamine hydrochloride was now only available without prescription in oral preparations with a maximum strength of 25 mg (or 50 mg for controlled release capsules) and a maximum daily dose of 100 mg.— *Pharm. J.*, 1986, *1*, 452.

INTERACTIONS. Phenylpropanolamine 50 mg by mouth in 3 healthy men produced a rise of 18 to 26 mmHg in systolic blood pressure, but this dose in a slow-release form with an atropine-like compound had no significant effect. After tranylcypromine 30 mg daily had been taken for 20 to 30 days, phenylpropanolamine 50 mg caused a rapid and potentially dangerous rise of blood pressure with an associated bradycardia and intense throbbing headache. Phentolamine was used to lower the blood pressure. When a capsule containing phenylpropanolamine 50 mg and isopropamide 2.5 mg in a slow-release form was taken after tranylcypromine, a gradual rise of blood pressure to 150 to 160 mmHg systolic and 95 to 100 mmHg diastolic occurred over 90 minutes and fell after 2 hours. Severe hypertensive episodes were more likely to occur when preparations containing phenylpropanolamine in a free form rather than slow-release form were taken by patients receiving monoamine oxidase inhibitors.— M. F. Cuthbert *et al.*, *Br. med. J.*, 1969, *1*, 404.

Severe headache, visions of coloured lights, tightness of the chest, and heart pounding were reported by a patient who had taken phenylpropanolamine 64 mg after eating a meal which included cheese. His blood pressure was 180/110 mmHg after 20 minutes but fell rapidly towards normal.— G. J. Gibson and D. A. Warrell (letter), *Lancet*, 1972, *2*, 492.

A 27-year-old woman with schizophrenia and T-wave abnormality of the heart, who had responded to thioridazine 100 mg daily with procyclidine 2.5 mg twice daily, died from ventricular fibrillation within 2 hours of taking a single dose of a preparation reported to contain chlorpheniramine maleate 4 mg with phenylpropanolamine hydrochloride 50 mg (Contac C), concurrently with thioridazine.— G. Chouinard *et al.*, *Can. med. Ass. J.*, 1978, *119*, 729.

A 27-year-old woman who had been taking D-phenylpropanolamine [sic.] 85 mg daily for some months, experienced severe hypertension when she also took indomethacin 25 mg. In a placebo-controlled challenge neither drug alone caused any significant rise in blood pressure, but administration of phenylpropanolamine followed 40 minutes later by indomethacin, caused very severe hypertension within half an hour. Administration of diazepam caused sedation without affecting the blood pressure, whereas phentolamine rapidly reduced it. It was considered that the inhibition of prostaglandin by indomethacin might have caused enhancement of the sympathomimetic effect of phenylpropanolamine.— K. Y. Lee *et al.*, *Lancet*, 1979, *1*, 1110. See also *idem* (letter), *Med. J. Aust.*, 1979, *1*, 525.

For the effect of phenylpropanolamine on antihypertensive therapy, see Methyldopa, p.489.

Absorption and Fate

Phenylpropanolamine is readily and completely absorbed from the gastro-intestinal tract, peak plasma concentrations being achieved about an hour or two after oral administration. It is excreted largely unchanged in the urine.

About 94% of a 25-mg dose of radioactive phenylpropanolamine was excreted in the urine in 24 hours; nearly 90% of the dose was excreted unchanged. Of 1 to 7% of the dose which was metabolised at least one-third was metabolised to hippuric acid.— J. E. Sinsheimer *et al.*, *Biochem. Soc. Trans.*, 1973, *1*, 1160.

Uses and Administration

Phenylpropanolamine hydrochloride is a largely indirect-acting sympathomimetic agent with an action similar to that of ephedrine (p.1462) but less active as a central nervous stimulant. It is given in usual doses of 25 mg three or four times daily for the symptomatic relief of nasal congestion. Sustained-release preparations are given in doses of 50 mg every 12 hours in conjunction with an antihistamine.

It has also been given to control urinary incontinence, and has been advocated for appetite reduction. Phenylpropanolamine polistirex (a phenylpropanolamine and sulphonated diethenylbenzene-ethenylbenzene copolymer complex) is also used.

OBESITY. Evidence of the effectiveness of phenylpropanolamine as an aid in weight reduction is limited; the magnitude of any weight loss is small, and it is maintained only as long as drug use is continued. Long term effectiveness has not been demonstrated.— *Med. Lett.*, 1984, *26*, 55.

RETROGRADE EJACULATION. Reports of the use of preparations containing phenylpropanolamine to correct retrograde ejaculation: B. H. Stewart and J. A. Bergant, *Fert. Steril.*, 1974, *25*, 1073; S. Thiagarajah *et al.*, *ibid.*, 1978, *30*, 96.

URINARY INCONTINENCE. A review of the treatment of incontinence in the elderly. Stress incontinence is usually treated with pelvic floor exercises, sometimes with local or topical oestrogens, but if not contra-indicated by other medical conditions treatment with an alpha-adrenergic agonist such as phenylpropanolamine 50 to 100 mg daily in divided doses may be added, and is often beneficial.— N. M. Resnick and S. V. Yalla, *New Engl. J. Med.*, 1985, *313*, 800. See also S. A. Awad *et al.*, *Br. J. Urol.*, 1978, *50*, 332; P. H. L. Worth, *Practitioner*, 1979, *223*, 325; M. E. Williams and F. C. Pannill, *Ann. intern. Med.*, 1982, *97*, 895; P. A. L. Haber, *ibid.*, 1986, *104*, 429.

Proprietary Preparations

Eskornade *(Smith Kline & French, UK)*. *Spansules*, sustained-release capsules, phenylpropanolamine hydrochloride 50 mg, diphenylpyraline hydrochloride 5 mg. *Syrup*, phenylpropanolamine hydrochloride 12.5 mg, diphenylpyraline hydrochloride 1.5 mg/5 mL.

Procol *(Menley & James, UK)*. *Capsules*, sustained-release, phenylpropanolamine hydrochloride 50 mg.

Rinurel *(Parke, Davis, UK)*. *Tablets*, phenylpropanolamine hydrochloride 25 mg, paracetamol 300 mg, phenyltoloxamine citrate 22 mg. *Linctus*, phenylpropanolamine hydrochloride 12.5 mg, paracetamol 150 mg, phenyltoloxamine citrate 11 mg, pholcodine 5 mg/5 mL.

Triogesic *(Intercare, UK)*. *Tablets*, scored, phenylpropanolamine hydrochloride 12.5 mg, paracetamol 500 mg. *Elixir*, phenylpropanolamine hydrochloride 3 mg, paracetamol 125 mg, alcohol 0.5 mL/5 mL.

Triominic *(Intercare, UK)*. *Tablets*, phenylpropanolamine hydrochloride 25 mg, pheniramine maleate 25 mg. *Syrup*, phenylpropanolamine hydrochloride 12.5 mg, pheniramine maleate 12.5 mg/5 mL.

Proprietary Names and Manufacturers of Phenylpropanolamine Salts

Acutrim *(Ciba, USA)*; Coldecon *(Canad.)*; Control *(Thompson, USA)*; Dexatrim *(Sauter, Switz.*; *Thompson, USA)*; Efed II Yellow *(Alto, USA)*; Fugoa *(Scheurich, Ger.)*; Help *(Verex, USA)*; Kontexin *(Leo Suede, Switz.)*; Monydrin *(Draco, Norw.*; *Draco, Swed.)*; Procol *(Menley & James, UK)*; Prolamine *(Thompson, USA)*; Propadrine *(Merck Sharp & Dohme, USA)*; Propagest *(Carnrick, USA)*; Rhindecon *(McGregor, USA)*; Rinexin *(Mekos, Norw.*; *Leo, Swed.)*; Tepanil *(Austral.)*.

The following names have been used for multi-ingredient preparations containing phenylpropanolamine salts—4-Way Tablets *(Bristol-Myers Products, USA)*; Alka-Seltzer Plus *(Miles Laboratories, USA)*; Allerest *(Pharmacraft, USA)*; Aller-eze Plus *(Intercare, UK)*; Appedrine *(Thompson, USA)*; Asbron *(Anca, Canad.)*; Bayer Cough Syrup *(Glenbrook, USA)*; Benylin Day and Night Cold Treatment *(Warner-Lambert, UK)*; Biphetap *(USA)*; BPP *(Gen, Canad.)*; Brocon *(Forest Laboratories, USA)*; Bromphen Compound *(Schein, USA)*; Bromphen DC *(Schein, USA)*; Caldomine-DH *(Technilab, Canad.)*; CAM Decongestant *(Rybar, UK)*; Codimal Expectorant *(Central Pharmaceuticals, USA)*; Cold Factor 12 *(Pharmacraft, USA)*; Coldex *(Gen, Canad.)*; Comtrex *(Bristol-Myers Products, USA)*; Conex *(Forest Pharmaceuticals, USA)*; Conex with Codeine *(Forest Pharmaceuticals, USA)*; Congesprin *(Bristol-Myers Products, USA)*; Coricidin D *(Schering, Canad.)*; Corsym *(Pennwalt, Canad.*; *Pennwalt, USA)*; Coryban-D *(Pfipharmecs, USA)*; CoTylenol, Children's *(McNeil Consumer, USA)*; Cremacoat *(Richardson-Vicks, Canad.)*;
Dehist *(Forest Pharmaceuticals, USA)*; Dexatrim 15 *(Thompson, USA)*; Dexatrim Extra Strength *(Thompson, USA)*; Dexatrim Maximum Strength *(Thompson, USA)*; Dieutrim *(Legere, USA)*; Dimetane Expectorant *(Robins, Canad.)*; Dimetane Expectorant-C *(Robins, Canad.)*; Dimetane Expectorant-DC *(Robins, Canad.)*; Dimetane-DC *(Robins, USA)*; Dimetapp *(Robins, Austral.*; *Robins, Canad.*; *Robins, USA)*; Dimetapp Elixir-Plus *(Robins, Austral.)*; Dimetapp-A *(Robins, Canad.)*; Dimetapp-C *(Robins, Canad.)*; Dimetapp-DM *(Robins, Canad.)*; Dimotane Expectorant *(Robins, UK)*; Dimotane Expectorant DC *(Robins, UK)*; Dimotapp *(Robins, UK)*; Dimotapp P *(Robins, UK)*; Dorcol *(Ancalab, Canad.)*; Dorcol Paediatric *(Dorsey Laboratories, USA)*; Drize *(Ascher, USA)*; Dura-Gest *(Dura, USA)*; Dura-Tap/PD *(Dura, USA)*; Dura-Vent *(Dura, USA)*; Dura-Vent/A *(Dura, USA)*;
ENT Syrup *(Springbok, USA)*; ENT Tablets *(Springbok, USA)*; Entex *(Norwich Eaton, USA)*; Entex LA *(Norwich-Eaton, Canad.*; *Norwich Eaton, USA)*; Eskornade *(Smith Kline & French, Austral.*; *Smith Kline & French, UK)*; E-Tapp *(Edwards, USA)*; Exyphen *(Norton, UK)*; Fiogesic *(Sandoz, USA)*; Fullstop; Head & Chest *(Richardson-Vicks, USA)*; Histalet Forte *(Reid-Rowell, USA)*; Histamic *(Metro Med, USA)*; Hycomine *(Du Pont, USA)*; Korigesic *(Trimen, USA)*; Kronohist *(Ferndale, USA)*; Myphetapp *(Bay, USA)*; Naldecon *(Bristol, USA)*; Naldecon-CX *(Bristol, USA)*; Naldecon-DX *(Bristol, USA)*; Naldecon-EX *(Bristol, USA)*; Neo-Diophen *(Hamilton, Austral.)*; Neo-Nasol *(Neolab, Canad.)*; Nezcaam *(Rybar, UK)*; Nolamine *(Carnrick, USA)*; Ornade *(Smith Kline & French, Canad.*; *Smith Kline & French, USA)*; Ornade Expectorant *(Smith Kline & French, Canad.)*; Ornade-DM *(Smith Kline & French, Canad.)*; Phenate *(Mallard, USA)*; Pholcolix *(Parke, Davis, UK)*; Poly-Histine CS *(Bock, USA)*; Poly-Histine DM *(Bock, USA)*; Poly-Histine Expectorant Plain *(Bock, USA)*; Poly-Histine Expectorant with Codeine *(Bock, USA)*; Poly-Histine-D *(Bock, USA)*; Quadrahist *(Schein, USA)*;
Resaid *(Geneva, USA)*; Rescaps-D *(Geneva, USA)*; Rhinolar *(McGregor, USA)*; Rhinolar-EX *(McGregor, USA)*; Rinurel Linctus *(Warner, UK)*; Rinurel Tablets *(Warner, UK)*; Robitussin-CF *(Robins, Canad.*; *Robins, USA)*; Ru-Tuss II *(Boots, USA)*; Ru-Tuss Tablets *(Boots, USA)*; Ru-Tuss with Hydrocodone *(Boots, USA)*; Rymed-Jr. *(Edwards, USA)*; Sequels *(Lederle, USA)*; Sinarest *(Pharmacraft, USA)*; Sinubid *(Parke, Davis, USA)*; Sinulin *(Carnrick, USA)*; Sinutab *(Warner-Lambert, UK)*; Sinutab SA *(Parke, Davis, Canad.)*; Sinutab with Codeine *(Warner, Austral.)*; S-T Decongest *(Scot-Tussin, USA)*; S-T Forte *(Scot-Tussin, USA)*; Symptrol *(Saron, USA)*;
Tamine *(Geneva, USA)*; Tavist-D *(Sandoz, USA)*; T-Dry *(T.E. Williams, USA)*; Totolin *(Galen, UK)*; Triaminic Preparations *(Ancalab, Canad.*; *Dorsey Laboratories, USA)*; Triaminicin *(Ancalab, Canad.*; *Dorsey Laboratories, USA)*; Triaminicol *(Dorsey Laboratories, USA)*; Triaminicol DM *(Ancalab, Canad.)*; Trind *(Mead Johnson Nutritional, USA)*; Triogesic *(Sandoz, Austral.*; *Intercare, UK)*; Triominic *(Sandoz, Austral.*; *Intercare, UK)*; Triotussic *(Beecham Research, UK)*; Trisulfaminic *(Ancalab, Canad.)*; Tuss-Ade *(Schein, USA)*; Tussaminic C *(Ancalab, Canad.)*; Tussaminic DH *(Ancalab, Canad.)*; Tuss-Ornade *(Smith Kline & French, Canad.*; *Smith Kline & French, USA)*; Vicks Formula 44D *(Richardson-Vicks, Canad.)*.

3776-k

Pirbuterol Acetate *(BANM, USAN, rINNM)*.

CP-24314-14. 2-*tert*-Butylamino-1-(5-hydroxy-6-hydroxymethyl-2-pyridyl)ethanol acetate.
$C_{12}H_{20}N_2O_3,C_2H_4O_2=300.4$.

CAS — 38677-81-5 (pirbuterol); 65652-44-0 (acetate).

13127-d

Pirbuterol Hydrochloride *(BANM, USAN, rINNM)*.

CP-24314-1; Pyrbuterol Hydrochloride. 2-*tert*-Butylamino-1-(5-hydroxy-6-hydroxymethyl-2-pyridyl)ethanol dihydrochloride.
$C_{12}H_{20}N_2O_3,2HCl=313.2$.

CAS — 38029-10-6.

Adverse Effects and Precautions

For the adverse effects of sympathomimetic agents, and precautions to be observed, see p.1453.

Uses and Administration

Pirbuterol is a direct-acting sympathomimetic agent with actions and uses similar to those of salbutamol (p.1482). It is used in the management of asthma and bronchospasm; doses of 10 or 15 mg have been given 3 or 4 times daily by mouth as the hydrochloride. It has also been given by inhalation as the acetate in doses of 400 µg three or four times daily. A suggested dose in children aged 6 to 12 years is 7.5 mg as the hydrochloride by mouth 3 or 4 times daily.

A detailed review of pirbuterol.— D. M. Richards and R. N. Brogden, *Drugs*, 1985, *30*, 6. An earlier review.— *Drug & Ther. Bull.*, 1984, *22*, 70.

CARDIOVASCULAR DISORDERS. Discussion of the use of beta-agonists in heart failure. Much attention has been focussed on pirbuterol, which can cause a substantial rise in cardiac output, due principally to a reduction in peripheral vascular resistance but which may also have a small direct inotropic effect. Pirbuterol also reduces pulmonary vascular resistance in patients with chronic air-flow obstruction and cor pulmonale but this benefit may be offset by worsened hypoxaemia. As with all forms of beta-agonist therapy for heart failure responses to pirbuterol vary greatly between patients. Long-term studies will be needed before this or similar agents can be advocated for routine maintenance therapy in heart failure.— *Lancet*, 1983, *2*, 1063. See also K. T. Weber *et al.*, *Drugs*, 1987, *33*, 503.

The haemodynamic effects of pirbuterol in hypoxic cor pulmonale.— W. MacNee *et al.*, *Br. med. J.*, 1983, *287*, 1169. Criticism of the methodology of the study.— D. W. Green (letter), *ibid.*, 1984, *288*, 233. Reply.— W. MacNee *et al.* (letter), *ibid.*,.

Criticism of marketing claims made for pirbuterol. The effects of pirbuterol on pulmonary circulation and right-ventricular function are not unique, and it should not be prescribed in the belief that it has properties not shared by other selective beta$_2$-adrenergic agonists.— G. K. Crompton and I. W. B. Grant (letter), *Lancet*, 1984, *1*, 795.

Proprietary Preparations

Exirel *(Pfizer, UK)*. *Capsules*, pirbuterol 10 and 15 mg (as hydrochloride).
Syrup, pirbuterol 7.5 mg (as hydrochloride)/5 mL.
Inhaler, aerosol, pirbuterol 200 µg (as acetate)/metered inhalation.

Proprietary Names and Manufacturers

Epital *(DAK, Denm.)*; Exirel *(Pfizer, UK*; *Pfizer, USA)*.

15332-r

Prednazoline *(rINN)*.

Prednisolone-fenoxazoline Compound. 11β,17α,21-Trihydroxypregna-1,4-diene-3,20-dione 21-(dihydrogen phosphate) compound with 2-(2-isopropylphenoxymethyl)-2-imidazoline.
$C_{22}H_{29}O_8P,C_{13}H_{18}N_2O=670.7$.

CAS — 6693-90-9.

Prednazoline has the general properties of prednisolone (see p.899) and of fenoxazoline (see p.1464) and has been used locally in the treatment of pharyngitis, rhinitis, and sinusitis.

Proprietary Names and Manufacturers

Déturgylone *(Dausse, Fr.)*.

13164-v

Prenalterol Hydrochloride *(BANM, USAN, rINNM)*.

C-50005/A-Ba (racemate); CGP-7760-B; H133/22; H-80/62 (racemate). (*S*)-1-(4-Hydroxyphenoxy)-3-isopropylaminopropan-2-ol hydrochloride.
$C_{12}H_{19}NO_3,HCl=261.8$.

CAS — 57526-81-5 (prenalterol); 61260-05-7 (hydrochloride).

Adverse Effects and Precautions

For the adverse effects of sympathomimetic agents, and precautions to be observed, see p.1453.

Uses and Administration

Prenalterol hydrochloride is a sympathomimetic agent with stimulant effects on beta$_1$-adrenoceptors. It has an inotropic action on the heart with relatively little chronotropic effect. Prenalterol hydrochloride has been used in the treatment of heart failure associated with myocardial infarction or open-heart surgery or shock. A suggested dose was 0.5 mg per minute by slow intravenous

infusion to a total of not more than 20 mg.
It was also promoted for the reversal of beta-blockade.

Proprietary Names and Manufacturers
Hyprenan *(Hässle, Denm.; Hässle, Norw.; Hässle, Swed.; Astra, UK)*; Varbian *(Ciba, UK)*.

13171-b

Procaterol Hydrochloride *(BANM, USAN, rINNM)*.
CI-888; OPC-2009. (±)-*erythro*-8-Hydroxy-5-(1-hydroxy-2-isopropylaminobutyl)quinolin-2(1*H*)-one hydrochloride.
$C_{16}H_{22}N_2O_3,HCl=326.8$.

CAS — 72332-33-3 (procaterol); 59828-07-8 (hydrochloride).

NOTE. The commercial substance is the hemihydrate ($C_{16}H_{22}N_2O_3,HCl,½H_2O$ = 335.8).

Adverse Effects and Precautions
For the adverse effects of sympathomimetic agents, and precautions to be observed, see p.1453.

Uses and Administration
Procaterol hydrochloride is a direct-acting sympathomimetic agent with actions and uses similar to those of salbutamol (p.1482). It has been given by mouth in doses of 50 or 100 µg for its bronchodilator properties.

A study of the bronchodilator effects of procaterol in patients with reversible airways obstruction.— C. L. Zanetti *et al., J. clin. Pharmac.*, 1982, *22*, 250.

A comparative study of the effects of procaterol 50 and 100 µg as a single dose by mouth with salbutamol 4 mg by mouth in 24 asthmatic patients. Bronchodilator response was similar with both doses of procaterol to that seen with salbutamol, and there were no significant differences in the adverse effects.— M. J. Crowe *et al., Br. J. clin. Pharmac.*, 1985, *19*, 787.

Proprietary Names and Manufacturers
Masacin *(Boehringer Biochemia, Ital.)*; Normalin *(Noristan, S.Afr.)*; Onsukil *(Grünenthal, Ger.; Miquel, Spain)*; Procadil *(Recordati, Ital.)*; Promaxol *(Esteve, Spain)*.

2097-s

Protokylol Hydrochloride *(BANM, rINNM)*.
JB-251; Protochylol Hydrochloride. 1-(3,4-Dihydroxyphenyl)-2-(α-methyl-3,4-methylenedioxyphenethylamino)ethanol hydrochloride.
$C_{18}H_{21}NO_5,HCl=367.8$.

CAS — 136-70-9 (protokylol); 136-69-6 (hydrochloride).

Adverse Effects and Precautions
For the adverse effects of sympathomimetic agents, and precautions to be observed, see p.1453.

Uses and Administration
Protokylol hydrochloride is a sympathomimetic agent with predominantly beta-adrenergic activity and actions and uses similar to those of isoprenaline (p.1467). It has been given by mouth as a bronchodilator in doses of 2 to 4 mg four times daily.

Proprietary Names and Manufacturers
Asmetil *(Benvegna, Ital.)*; Beres *(Simes, Ital.)*; Palison *(Farmasimes, Spain)*; Ventaire *(Marion Laboratories, USA)*.

2098-w

Pseudoephedrine Hydrochloride *(BANM, USAN, rINNM)*.

d-Isoephedrine Hydrochloride; *d*-Ψ-Ephedrine Hydrochloride. (+)-(1*S*,2*S*)-2-Methylamino-1-phenylpropan-1-ol hydrochloride; (α*R*,β*R*)-β-Hydroxy-α-methylphenethyl-*N*-methylammonium chloride.
$C_{10}H_{15}NO,HCl=201.7$.

CAS — 90-82-4 (pseudoephedrine); 345-78-8 (hydrochloride).

Pharmacopoeias. In *Br.* and *U.S.*

The hydrochloride of an alkaloid obtained from *Ephedra* spp. White or off-white crystals or powder, with a faint characteristic odour.

B.P. **solubilities** are: 1 in 1.6 of water, 1 in 4 of alcohol, and 1 in 60 of chloroform. The *U.S.P.* has: 1 in 0.5 of water, 1 in about 4 of alcohol and 1 in 91 of chloroform; very slightly soluble in ether. A 5% solution in water has a pH of 4.6 to 6.0. **Store** in airtight containers. Protect from light.

2099-e

Pseudoephedrine Sulphate *(BANM, rINNM)*.

Pseudoephedrine Sulfate *(USAN)*; Sch-4855.
$(C_{10}H_{15}NO)_2,H_2SO_4=428.5$.

CAS — 7460-12-0.

Pharmacopoeias. In *U.S.*

White odourless crystals or crystalline powder. Freely **soluble** in alcohol. A 5% solution in water has a pH of 5.0 to 6.5. **Store** in airtight containers. Protect from light.

Adverse Effects and Precautions
For the adverse effects of sympathomimetic agents, and precautions to be observed, see p.1453.

In 34 healthy males given pseudoephedrine 120 or 150 mg, as a sustained-release preparation, twice daily for 7 days mean plasma concentrations were about 450 and 510 ng per mL respectively. Side-effects (dry mouth, anorexia, insomnia, anxiety, tension, restlessness, tachycardia, palpitations) were common; there was some evidence of tachyphylaxis.— J. Dickerson *et al., Eur. J. clin. Pharmac.*, 1978, *14*, 253.

There were no hospitalisations that could be attributed to pseudoephedrine in a follow-up study carried out by the Boston Collaborative Drug Surveillance Program among over 100 000 patients who took the drug.— M. Porta *et al., Ann. Allergy*, 1986, *57*, 340.

EFFECTS ON THE HEART. Asymptomatic multifocal ventricular premature contractions in a pilot were attributed to the pseudoephedrine in Actifed, of which he had taken 2 tablets every 4 hours day and night for several days.— C. E. Billings *et al., Aerospace Med.*, 1974, *45*, 551.

In a study in 6 healthy subjects there was a significant increase in the incidence of sinus arrhythmia after exercise following an oral dose of 120 mg of pseudoephedrine hydrochloride, but not after 60 mg. Blood pressure appeared to be unaffected by the drug.— T. P. Bright *et al., J. clin. Pharmac.*, 1981, *21*, 488.

EFFECTS ON MENTAL FUNCTION. Reports of adverse mental effects associated with a preparation containing pseudoephedrine and triprolidine (Actifed): K. M. Leighton, *Br. med. J.*, 1982, *284*, 789 (paranoid psychosis following prolonged abuse); R. J. Sankey *et al., ibid.*, 1984, *288*, 1369 (visual hallucinations in children given recommended doses of Actifed); M. A. Stokes (letter), *ibid.*, 1540 (nightmares in a 3-year-old child). Although visual hallucinations and dystonic reactions may be rare side-effects of decongestant antihistamine mixtures the widespread prescribing of these drugs should be more seriously questioned.— J. Bain (letter), *ibid.*, 1688.

INTERACTIONS. The absorption rate of pseudoephedrine hydrochloride was increased by the concomitant administration of aluminium hydroxide mixture.— R. L. Lucarotti *et al., J. pharm. Sci.*, 1972, *61*, 903.

Absorption and Fate
Pseudoephedrine is absorbed from the gastro-intestinal tract. It is resistant to metabolism by monoamine oxidase and is largely excreted unchanged in the urine together with small amounts of its hepatic metabolite. It has a half-life of several hours; elimination is enhanced and half-life accordingly shorter in acid urine.

The plasma half-lives in 3 subjects given pseudoephedrine 180 mg by mouth were 5.2, 7.6, and 8 hours when their urinary pH was between 5.6 and 6. When the pH was increased to 8 the plasma half-lives lengthened to 9.2, 16, and 15 hours and when the pH was reduced the half-lives shortened.— R. G. Kuntzman *et al., Clin. Pharmac. Ther.*, 1971, *12*, 62. Pseudoephedrine has been shown to accumulate to toxic concentrations in children with renal tubular acidosis, in whom a persistently alkaline urine favoured passive reabsorption of the drug.— D. C. Brater, *Drugs*, 1980, *19*, 31. See also D. C. Brater *et al., Clin. Pharmac. Ther.*, 1980, *28*, 690.

Under steady-state conditions in 5 healthy subjects given pseudoephedrine hydrochloride 120 mg with chlorpheniramine maleate 8 mg as a sustained-release preparation twice daily for 8 days 91% of a pseudoephedrine dose administered was excreted unchanged in the urine between successive doses.— C. M. Lai *et al., J. pharm. Sci.*, 1979, *68*, 1243. See also D. M. Baaske *et al., J. pharm. Sci.*, 1979, *68*, 1472; A. Yacobi *et al., ibid.*, 1980, *69*, 1077.

PREGNANCY AND THE NEONATE. A study of concentrations of pseudoephedrine and triprolidine in plasma and breast milk of 3 lactating mothers for up to 48 hours after ingestion of a preparation containing pseudoephedrine hydrochloride 60 mg with triprolidine hydrochloride 2.5 mg. Concentrations of pseudoephedrine in milk were consistently higher than in plasma; the half-life in both fluids was between 4.2 and 7 hours. Assuming a generous milk secretion of 500 mL over 12 hours it was calculated that the excreted dose was the equivalent of 250 to 330 µg of pseudoephedrine base, or 0.5 to 0.7% of the dose ingested by the mothers, In contrast to pseudoephedrine, triprolidine did not appear to be concentrated in breast milk.— J. W. A. Findley *et al., Br. J. clin. Pharmac.*, 1984, *18*, 901. See also M. S. Meskin and E. J. Lien, *J. clin. Hosp. Pharm.*, 1985, *10*, 269.

Uses and Administration
Pseudoephedrine is a stereoisomer of ephedrine (p.1462) and has a similar action, but has been stated to have less pressor activity and central nervous system effects. The hydrochloride is used as a decongestant, usually in doses of 60 mg three or four times daily. Sustained-release preparations are given in a usual dose of 120 mg every 12 hours. Pseudoephedrine sulphate is also used. A suggested dose of pseudoephedrine hydrochloride or sulphate for children is 1 mg per kg body-weight 4 times daily. Pseudoephedrine polistirex (a pseudoephedrine and sulphonated diethenylbenzene-ethenylbenzene copolymer complex) is also used.

ASTHMA. The bronchodilator effect of pseudoephedrine was less than half that of ephedrine in 9 patients with reversible airways obstruction.— C. D. M. Drew *et al., Br. J. clin. Pharmac.*, 1978, *6*, 221.

ENT DISORDERS. A double-blind study involving 466 adults indicating that pseudoephedrine alone or in combination with triprolidine relieved symptoms of the common cold.— C. E. Bye *et al., Br. med. J.*, 1980, *281*, 189.

In a multicentre study in general practice involving 189 children pseudoephedrine 30 mg twice daily or triprolidine 2.5 mg twice daily, given for 8 weeks, were not more effective than placebo in relieving the symptoms of otitis media, or in preventing recurrence.— D. J. G. Bain, *Br. med. J.*, 1983, *287*, 654.

For a lack of beneficial effect of combined pseudoephedrine and chlorpheniramine in children with otitis media, see under Chlorpheniramine Maleate, p.448.

Preparations

Pseudoephedrine and Codeine Mixture *(A.P.F.)*. Pseudoephedrine hydrochloride 30 mg, codeine phosphate 10 mg, tolu syrup 1 mL, concentrated anise water 0.25 mL, concentrated chloroform water 0.25 mL or compound hydroxybenzoate solution 0.1 mL, purified water to 10 mL.

Pseudoephedrine Hydrochloride Syrup *(U.S.P.)*

Pseudoephedrine Hydrochloride Tablets *(U.S.P.)*

Proprietary Preparations

Actifed *(Wellcome, UK)*. Also known as **Sudafed Plus** *(Calmic, UK)*. *Tablets*, scored, pseudoephedrine hydrochloride 60 mg, triprolidine hydrochloride 2.5 mg.
Syrup, pseudoephedrine hydrochloride 30 mg, triprolidine hydrochloride 1.25 mg/5 mL.

Actifed Compound *(Wellcome, UK)*. *Linctus*, pseudoephedrine hydrochloride 30 mg, triprolidine hydrochloride 1.25 mg, dextromethorphan hydrobromide 10 mg/5 mL.

Actifed Expectorant *(Wellcome, UK)*. *Syrup*, pseudoephedrine hydrochloride 30 mg, guaiphenesin 100 mg, triprolidine hydrochloride 1.25 mg/5 mL.

Galpseud *(Galen, UK)*. *Tablets*, pseudoephedrine hydrochloride 60 mg.
Linctus, pseudoephedrine hydrochloride 30 mg/5 mL.

Sudafed *(Calmic, UK)*. *Tablets*, pseudoephedrine hydrochloride 60 mg.
Elixir, pseudoephedrine hydrochloride 30 mg/5 mL.

Sudafed Expectorant *(Calmic, UK). Syrup*, pseudoephedrine hydrochloride 30 mg, guaiphenesin 100 mg/5 mL.

Sudafed SA *(Calmic, UK). Capsules*, sustained-release, pseudoephedrine hydrochloride 120 mg.

Sudafed-Co *(Calmic, UK). Tablets*, scored, pseudoephedrine hydrochloride 60 mg, paracetamol 500 mg.

Proprietary Names and Manufacturers of Pseudoephedrine Salts

Afrinol *(Schering, USA)*; D-Feda *(USA)*; Dorcol Children's Decongestant *(Dorsey Laboratories, USA)*; Drixora *(Essex, Austral.; Scherag, S.Afr.)*; Eltor *(Dow, Canad.)*; Galpseud *(Galen, UK)*; Isofedrin *(Braz.)*; Narixan *(Ciba, Ital.)*; Novafed *(Merrell Dow, USA)*; Otrinol *(Ciba, Switz.)*; Pediacare Infant Drops *(McNeil Consumer, USA)*; Pseudofrin *(Trianon, Canad.)*; Robidrine *(Robins, Canad.)*; Sudafed *(Wellcome, Austral.; Wellcome, Canad.; Wellcome, Ital.; Wellcome, S.Afr.; Calmic, UK; Wellcome, USA)*; Sudafed SA *(Calmic, UK)*.

The following names have been used for multi-ingredient preparations containing pseudoephedrine salts—Actifed *(Wellcome, Austral.; Wellcome, Canad.; Wellcome, UK; Wellcome, USA)*; Actifed Compound *(Wellcome, UK)*; Actifed DM *(Wellcome, Canad.)*; Actifed Expectorant *(Wellcome, UK)*; Actifed with Codeine *(Wellcome, USA)*; Actifed-A *(Wellcome, Canad.)*; Actifed-C *(Wellcome, USA)*; Actifed-CC *(Wellcome, Austral.)*; Alpha-Phed *(Metro Med, USA)*; Ambenyl-D *(Forest Pharmaceuticals, USA)*; Anafed *(Everett, USA)*; Anamine *(Mayrand, USA)*; Benadryl Cold and Flu Tablets *(Parke, Davis, Austral.)*; Benadryl Decongestant *(Parke, Davis, USA)*; Benafed *(Parke, Davis, UK)*; Benylin Decongestant *(Parke, Davis, Canad.; Warner-Lambert, UK)*; Benylin Mentholated *(Warner-Lambert, UK)*; Benylin-DM-D *(Parke, Davis, Canad.)*; Beta-Phed *(Metro Med, USA)*; Brexin EX *(Savage, USA)*; Brexin LA *(Savage, USA)*; Bromfed *(Muro, USA)*; Bromfed-PD *(Muro, USA)*; Bromphen Expectorant *(Schein, USA)*;

Capedrin *(Key, Austral.)*; Cardec DM *(Schein, USA)*; Chlorafed *(Hauck, USA)*; Chlor-Trimeton Decongestant *(Schering, USA)*; Chlor-Tripolon Decongestant *(Schering, Canad.)*; CoActifed *(Wellcome, Canad.)*; CoActifed Expectorant *(Wellcome, Canad.)*; Codimal-L.A. *(Central Pharmaceuticals, USA)*; Codral Cold Tablets *(Wellcome, Austral.)*; Codral Flu And Cold Tablets *(Wellcome, Austral.)*; Codral Linctus *(Wellcome, Austral.)*; Cold War *(Key, Austral.)*; Congess *(Fleming, USA)*; Congestac *(Menley & James, USA)*; Congesteze *(Kirby-Warrick, UK)*; Contac *(Allergan, Austral.)*; Co-Pyronil *(Dista, USA)*; Cotaminol *(Gen, Canad.)*; Cotrol-D *(Beecham Laboratories, USA)*; CoTylenol *(McNeil Consumer, USA)*; Cremacoat 3 *(Richardson-Vicks, USA)*; Cremacoat 4 *(Richardson-Vicks, USA)*; Dallergy-D Capsules *(Laser, USA)*; Dallergy-JR *(Laser, USA)*; Deconamine *(Berlex, USA)*; Demazin Repetabs *(Schering, Austral.)*; Demazin Tablets *(Schering, Austral.)*; Deproist with Codeine *(Geneva, USA)*; Detussin *(USA)*; Detussin Expectorant *(USA)*; Dimedrine *(Robins, Canad.)*; Dimetane-DX *(Robins, USA)*; Dimotane CO *(Robins, UK)*; Dimotane Plus *(Robins, UK)*; Dimotane Plus LA *(Robins, UK)*; Dimotane with Codeine *(Robins, UK)*; Disobrom *(Geneva, USA)*; Disophrol *(Schering, USA)*; Dorcol Children's Cold Formula *(Dorsey Laboratories, USA)*; Dorcol Children's Cough Syrup *(Dorsey Laboratories, USA)*; Drixoral *(Schering, Canad.; Schering, USA)*; Drixtab *(Schering, Canad.)*;

Eltor AF *(Dow, Canad.)*; Emprazil *(Calmic, UK)*; Entuss-D *(Hauck, USA)*; Expulin *(Galen, UK)*; Ex-Span *(Rotex, USA)*; Extil Compound *(Evans Medical, UK)*; Fabahistin Plus *(Bayer, Austral.)*; Fedahist *(Kremers-Urban, USA)*; Fedahist Expectorant *(Kremers-Urban, USA)*; Fedrazil *(Wellcome, USA)*; Guaifed *(Muro, USA)*; Guaifed-PD *(Muro, USA)*; Halin *(Nicholas, UK)*; Histalet *(Reid-Rowell, USA)*; Histalet DM *(Reid-Rowell, USA)*; Histalet X *(Reid-Rowell, USA)*; Isoclor *(Fisons, USA)*; Kronofed-A *(Ferndale, USA)*; Linctifed *(Wellcome, UK)*; Novafed A *(Merrell Dow, USA)*; Novahistex Cold Capsules *(Dow, Canad.)*; Novahistine DH *(Lakeside, USA)*; Novahistine DMX *(Lakeside, USA)*; Novahistine Expectorant *(Lakeside, USA)*; Nucofed *(Beecham Laboratories, USA)*; Nucofed Expectorant *(Beecham Laboratories, USA)*; Nucosef *(Beecham, Austral.)*; Orthoxicol Cold & Flu Caps *(Upjohn, Austral.)*; Paragesic *(Sandoz, UK)*; Pediacare-2 *(McNeil Consumer, USA)*; Pediacare-3 *(McNeil Consumer, USA)*; Pharma-Col *(Rosken, Austral.)*; Phenergan-D *(Wyeth, USA)*; Phensedyl *(May & Baker, Austral.)*; Poly-Histine-DX *(Bock, USA)*; Probahist Capsules *(Legere, USA)*; Promatussin *(Wyeth, Canad.)*; Promist HD *(Russ, USA)*; Promist LA *(Russ, USA)*; Pseudo-Bid *(Holloway, USA)*; Pseudo-Hist *(Holloway, USA)*; Pseudo-Hist Expectorant *(Holloway, USA)*;

Respaire *(Laser, USA)*; Robitussin Plus *(Robins, UK)*; Robitussin-DAC *(Robins, USA)*; Robitussin-PE *(Robins, Canad.; Robins, USA)*; Robitussin-PS *(Robins, Austral.)*; Rondec *(Ross, USA)*; Rondec-DM *(Ross, USA)*; Ru-Tuss Expectorant *(Boots, USA)*; Rymed *(Edwards, USA)*; Rymed-TR *(Edwards, USA)*; Rynofen *(Charton, Canad.)*; Sancos Co *(Sandoz, UK)*; Sigma Relief *(Sigma, Austral.)*; Sigma Relief Cold Tablets *(Sigma, Austral.)*; Sigma Relief Junior *(Sigma, Austral.)*; Sine-Aid *(McNeil Consumer, USA)*; Sinitol *(Nicholas, UK)*; Sinufed *(Hauck, USA)*; Sinutab Preparations *(Warner, Austral.; Parke, Davis, Canad.)*; Sinuzets *(Boots, Austral.)*; Sudafed DM *(Wellcome, Canad.)*; Sudafed Expectorant *(Wellcome, Canad.; Calmic, UK)*; Sudafed Plus *(Calmic, UK; Wellcome, USA)*; Sudafed-Co *(Calmic, UK)*; Sudelix Junior *(Wellcome, Austral.)*;

Teldrin Capsules *(Menley & James, USA)*; T-Moist *(T.E. Williams, USA)*; Triafed *(Schein, USA)*; Triafed-C *(Schein, USA)*; Trifed *(Geneva, USA)*; Trinalin *(Schering, Canad.; Schering, USA)*; Trinex *(Mastar, USA)*; Triocos *(Sandoz, UK)*; Triolinctus *(Sandoz, UK)*; Triolix *(Drug Houses Austral., Austral.)*; Tuscodin Cold Capsules *(Schering, Austral.)*; Tussafed *(Everett, USA)*; Tusselix *(Key, Austral.)*; Tussend *(Merrell Dow, USA)*; Tussend Expectorant *(Merrell Dow, USA)*; Tylenol Sinus Medication *(McNeil, Canad.; McNeil Consumer, USA)*; Ursinus *(Dorsey Laboratories, USA)*; Vasofrinic *(Trianon, Canad.)*; Vasofrinic DH *(Trianon, Canad.)*; Vasofrinic Plus *(Trianon, Canad.)*; Zephrex *(Bock, USA)*; Zephrex-LA *(Bock, USA)*.

2101-l

Reproterol Hydrochloride *(BANM, USAN, rINNM)*. D-1959 *(reproterol)*; W-2946M. 7-{3-[(3,5,β-Trihydroxyphenethyl)amino]propyl}theophylline hydrochloride.

$C_{18}H_{23}N_5O_5,HCl = 425.9$.

CAS — 54063-54-6 (reproterol); 13055-82-8 (hydrochloride).

Reproterol hydrochloride is a direct-acting sympathomimetic agent with general properties similar to those of salbutamol (p.1480). It is given as a bronchodilator, by mouth, in doses of 10 to 20 mg three times daily, or by inhalation, in doses of 0.5 to 1 mg, at intervals of 3 to 6 hours if required. It has also been given by injection.

CARDIAC DISORDERS. Evidence that reproterol may be a useful drug in refractory chronic heart failure.— E. Pretolani *et al.* (letter), *Lancet*, 1984, *1*, 170.

Proprietary Preparations

Bronchodil *(Schering, UK). Tablets*, scored, reproterol hydrochloride 20 mg.
Elixir, reproterol hydrochloride 10 mg/5 mL.
Inhaler, aerosol, reproterol hydrochloride 500 µg/metered inhalation.
Respirator solution, reproterol hydrochloride 10 mg/mL.

Proprietary Names and Manufacturers

Asmaterolo *(Lusofarmaco, Ital.)*; Bronchodil *(Schering, UK)*; Bronchospasmin *(Degussa, Ger.)*; Broncospasmin *(Farmades, Ital.; Igoda, Spain)*; Epiferol *(Juventus, Spain)*; Gensasmol *(Morgens, Spain)*; Reprol *(Selvi, Ital.)*; Sanasma *(Serpero, Ital.)*; Teofluid *(Carulla Vekar, Spain)*.

2102-y

Rimiterol Hydrobromide *(BANM, USAN, rINNM)*.

R-798; WG-253. *erythro*-3,4-Dihydroxy-α-(2-piperidyl)benzyl alcohol hydrobromide; *erythro*-(3,4-Dihydroxyphenyl) (2-piperidyl)methanol hydrobromide.

$C_{12}H_{17}NO_3,HBr = 304.2$.

CAS — 32953-89-2 (rimiterol); 31842-61-2 (hydrobromide).

Adverse Effects and Precautions

For the adverse effects of sympathomimetic agents, and precautions to be observed, see p.1453.

A study of the metabolic and cardiovascular side-effects of salbutamol and rimiterol in healthy subjects.— P. J. Phillips *et al.*, *Br. J. clin. Pharmac.*, 1980, *9*, 483.

Absorption and Fate

Rimiterol is readily absorbed from the gastro-intestinal tract. It is subject not only to extensive first-pass metabolism by sulphate and glucuronide conjugation, but also to metabolism by catechol-*O*-methyltransferase and therefore has a very short plasma half-life of less than 5 minutes. Rimiterol also appears to be metabolised by catechol-*O*-methyltransferase in the lungs. It is excreted in both the urine and the bile.

In studies in 4 subjects rimiterol had 18 to 80 times less chronotropic action on the heart than isoprenaline. Its half-life after intravenous injection was similar to that of isoprenaline. Urinary excretion included unchanged drug, glucuronide, and 3-*O*-methyl derivatives. Mean faecal excretion over 72 hours was about 45%.— J. P. Griffin *et al.*, *Clin. Trials J.*, 1973, *10*, (1), 13.

Difference in the pattern of 3-*O*-methylation and conjugation of rimiterol following administration by mouth and by inhalation.— M. E. Evans *et al.*, *Br. J. Pharmac.*, 1973, *49*, 153P. Evidence that rimiterol might be partially metabolised in the lung.— G. M. Shenfield *et al.*, *Br. J. clin. Pharmac.*, 1976, *3*, 583.

Uses and Administration

Rimiterol hydrobromide is a direct-acting sympathomimetic agent with general properties similar to those of salbutamol (p.1482).

In the treatment of bronchial asthma it is given as an aerosol in a dose of 1 to 3 inhalations of 200 µg; if more than 1 inhalation is taken at a time, at least 1 minute should elapse between any 2 inhalations. This treatment dose should not be repeated in less than 30 minutes. No more than 8 treatments should be taken in any 24-hour period.

Where a beta$_2$-adrenergic stimulant is prescribed for reversible obstructive airways disease longer acting drugs such as salbutamol are generally preferred to rimiterol.— G. K. Crompton, *Prescribers' J.*, 1982, *22*, 104.

CARDIAC DISORDERS. The cardiovascular effects of infusions of rimiterol and isoprenaline were compared in patients with suspected coronary artery disease. Rimiterol 100 to 200 ng per kg body-weight per minute for 10 minutes was given by intravenous infusion to 10 patients. Isoprenaline 5 to 50 ng per kg per minute was infused into 5 similar patients to produce changes in cardiac output similar to those seen with rimiterol. Both drugs produced significant dose-related increases in cardiac output accompanied by similar increases in heart-rate and myocardial oxygen consumption. Isoprenaline produced greater increases in coronary sinus flow. Unlike isoprenaline, rimiterol did not cause direct coronary vasodilatation and might be preferable to isoprenaline in the treatment of patients with left ventricular failure when there was regional myocardial ischaemia.— J. D. Stephens *et al.*, *Br. J. clin. Pharmac.*, 1978, *6*, 163.

Proprietary Preparations

Pulmadil *(Riker, UK). Inhaler*, aerosol, rimiterol hydrobromide 200 µg/metered dose.
Inhaler (Pulmadil Auto), breath-actuated aerosol, rimiterol hydrobromide 200 µg/metered dose.

Proprietary Names and Manufacturers

Asmaten *(Arg.)*; Pulmadil *(Riker, Austral.; Belg.; Riker, Denm.; Neth.; Riker, Norw.; NZ; Riker, S.Afr.; Riker, Swed.; Switz.; Riker, UK)*.

2103-j

Ritodrine Hydrochloride *(BANM, USAN, rINNM)*.

DU-21220 *(ritodrine)*. *erythro*-2-(4-Hydroxyphenethylamino)-1-(4-hydroxyphenyl)propan-1-ol hydrochloride.

$C_{17}H_{21}NO_3,HCl = 323.8$.

CAS — 26652-09-5 (ritodrine); 23239-51-2 (hydrochloride).

Pharmacopoeias. In *U.S.*

White, or nearly white, odourless or practically odourless crystalline powder. Freely **soluble** in

water and in alcohol; soluble in propyl alcohol; practically insoluble in ether. A 2% solution has a pH between 4.5 and 6.0; the *U.S.P.* injection has a pH between 4.8 and 5.5.
Store in airtight containers at a temperature below 30°.

Adverse Effects and Precautions

For the adverse effects of sympathomimetic agents, and precautions to be observed, see p.1453.

EFFECTS ON BODY TEMPERATURE. A report of fever associated with administration of ritodrine.— G. D. Hankins and K. J. Leveno, *Am. J. Obstet. Gynec.*, 1983, *146*, 110.

EFFECTS ON THE HEART. Supraventricular tachycardia developed in a 23-year-old heroin addict given ritodrine for premature labour. Ritodrine must be given with care, if at all, to patients addicted to narcotics.— B. J. Fink and T. Weber, *Acta obstet. gynec. scand.*, 1981, *60*, 521. A further report of maternal supraventricular tachycardia following ritodrine administration.— J. J. Kjer and K. H. Pedersen, *ibid.*, 1982, *61*, 281. Tachycardia occurred in both mother and neonate following maternal administration of ritodrine. The mother developed pulmonary oedema and myocardial ischaemia following delivery, which was by caesarean section. Episodes of paroxysmal supraventricular tachycardia in the child were treated with digoxin. Both mother and child subsequently recovered.— P. Brosset *et al.* (letter), *Lancet*, 1982, *1*, 1468. See also M. C. Hermansen and G. L. Johnson, *Am. J. Obstet. Gynec.*, 1984, *149*, 798 (neonatal supraventricular tachycardia).

Sinus bradycardia following withdrawal of ritodrine in a patient who had been receiving the drug for placenta praevia.— H. Dean *et al.*, *J. Am. med. Ass.*, 1982, *247*, 1810.

Reports of myocardial ischaemia in women given intravenous ritodrine for premature labour: D. Michalak *et al.*, *Am. J. Obstet. Gynec.*, 1983, *146*, 861; I. Ben-Shlomo *et al.* (letter), *Lancet*, 1986, *2*, 917.

EFFECTS ON METABOLISM. Adverse metabolic effects of ritodrine.— W. N. Spellacy *et al.*, *Am. J. Obstet. Gynec.*, 1978, *131*, 637 (hyperglycaemia); S. R. Richards *et al.*, *ibid.*, 1983, *146*, 1 (raised blood-lactate concentrations).

PULMONARY OEDEMA. Eleven hours after delivery, a 24-year-old woman who had received ritodrine, indomethacin, and betamethasone for premature labour, developed acute pulmonary oedema. Patients receiving such therapy should be monitored not only during treatment but for at least 24 hours after it stops.— D. J. Tinga and J. G. Aarnoudse (letter), *Lancet*, 1979, *1*, 1026. A further case in a pre-eclamptic patient.— N. Gleicher *et al.* (letter), *New Engl. J. Med.*, 1982, *306*, 174.

See also under Salbutamol Sulphate, p.1481.

Absorption and Fate

Ritodrine is rapidly absorbed from the gastro-intestinal tract but is subject to fairly extensive first-pass metabolism; about 30% of an oral dose is bioavailable. It is metabolised in the liver and excreted in urine as unchanged drug and metabolites. About 90% of a dose is reported to be excreted within 24 hours. It crosses the placenta.

A study of the pharmacokinetics of ritodrine in healthy subjects following administration by intravenous infusion, intramuscularly, and by mouth; and a comparison of the pharmacokinetics of ritodrine with those of fenoterol, salbutamol, and terbutaline. Following oral administration the bioavailability of ritodrine was 30% indicating a first-pass effect. The dominant half-life after intramuscular injection was 2 hours while in the oral study half-lives of 1.3 hours and 20 hours were discernible. The half-life of salbutamol is about the same as that of ritodrine and the half-life of terbutaline seems to be slightly longer. Studies in women given ritodrine to arrest preterm labour indicated that ritodrine crosses the placental barrier and enters the foetal circulation.— R. Gandar *et al.*, *Eur. J. clin. Pharmac.*, 1980, *17*, 117.

Further references.— C. Romanini *et al.*, *Pharmatherapeutica*, 1977, *1*, 546 (transplacental diffusion); A. S. Gross and K. F. Brown, *Eur. J. clin. Pharmac.*, 1985, *28*, 479 (protein binding).

Uses and Administration

Ritodrine hydrochloride is a direct-acting sympathomimetic agent with general properties similar to those of salbutamol (p.1482). It is given by intravenous infusion to arrest premature labour; infusion rates are usually 150 to 350 µg per minute, as a solution containing 300 µg per mL, according to the patient's response. The recommended initial rate of infusion is 50 µg per minute increased at intervals of 10 minutes by 50-µg increments until there is evidence of patient response. The infusion should be continued for 12 to 48 hours after the contractions have stopped; where intravenous infusion is inappropriate 10 mg may be given intramuscularly every 3 to 8 hours and continued for 12 to 48 hours after the contractions have stopped. The maternal pulse should be monitored throughout the infusion and the rate adjusted to avoid a maternal heart-rate of more than 140 beats per minute. Ritodrine hydrochloride may subsequently be given by mouth in an initial dose of 10 mg every 2 hours followed by 10 to 20 mg every 4 to 6 hours according to the patient's response; the first dose is given 30 minutes before the end of the infusion. The total daily dose by mouth should not exceed 120 mg.

Ritodrine hydrochloride has also been given intravenously to the mother as an emergency means of alleviating foetal asphyxia while other procedures are being arranged.

A comparison of ritodrine with fenoterol in the management of premature labour.— J. Gerris *et al.*, *Eur. J. clin. Pharmac.*, 1980, 18, 443.

FOETAL DISTRESS. A report of the use of ritodrine by infusion in a case of severe foetal distress occurring during labour. Propranolol was given to the mother after delivery to slow her increased heart-rate.— A. Schoenfeld *et al.*, *Br. J. Anaesth.*, 1978, *50*, 969. Criticism of recommendations that ritodrine should be used for the treatment of foetal distress.— *Drug & Ther. Bull.*, 1975, *13*, 26. See also *ibid.*, 1978, *16*, 83.

PEMPHIGOID. Bullous pemphigoid in a patient with AIDS-related complex, in whom corticosteroid treatment was thought to pose an unacceptable risk, was successfully treated with ritodrine at an average daily dosage of 40 mg.— P. M. Levy *et al.* (letter), *Br. J. Derm.*, 1986, *114*, 635. Ritodrine had also proven beneficial in a patient with herpes gestationis. Further evaluation of the clinical and pharmacological effect of ritodrine in pemphigoid and other bullous diseases is called for.— K. MacDonald and E. J. Raffle (letter), *ibid.*, 636.

Preparations

Ritodrine Hydrochloride Injection *(U.S.P.)*

Ritodrine Hydrochloride Tablets *(U.S.P.)*

Proprietary Preparations

Yutopar *(Duphar, UK). Tablets*, scored, ritodrine hydrochloride 10 mg.
Injection, ritodrine hydrochloride 10 mg/mL, in ampoules of 5 mL.

Proprietary Names and Manufacturers

Miolene *(Lusofarmaco, Ital.)*; Pre-Par *(Aust.; Belg.; Duphar, Fr.; Duphar, Ger.; Ind.; Ital.; Jug.; Neth.; Kali-Farma, Spain)*; Utopar *(Ferrosan, Denm.; Iceland; Ferrosan, Norw.; Swed.)*; Yutopar *(Cilag, Austral.; Bristol, Canad.; Berlimed, S.Afr.; Duphar, UK; Astra, USA)*.

2104-z

Salbutamol *(BAN, rINN)*.

AH-3365; Albuterol *(USAN)*; Sch-13949W. 2-*tert*-Butylamino-1-(4-hydroxy-3-hydroxymethylphenyl)ethanol.
$C_{13}H_{21}NO_3$=239.3.
CAS — 18559-94-9.

Pharmacopoeias. In *Br., Cz., Eur., It.,* and *U.S.*

A white or almost white, crystalline powder. **Soluble** 1 in 70 of water and 1 in 25 of alcohol; slightly soluble in ether. **Store** in well-closed containers. Protect from light.

2105-c

Salbutamol Sulphate *(BANM, rINNM)*.

Albuterol Sulfate *(USAN)*; Salbutamol Hemisulphate.
$C_{13}H_{21}NO_3,\frac{1}{2}H_2SO_4$=288.4.
CAS — 51022-70-9.

Pharmacopoeias. In *Br., Chin., Ind., Jpn,* and *U.S.*

A white or almost white odourless or almost odourless powder. Salbutamol sulphate 1.2 mg is approximately equivalent to 1 mg of salbutamol. **Soluble** 1 in 4 of water; slightly soluble in alcohol, chloroform, and ether. The *B.P.* injection has a pH of 3.4 to 5.0, and is sterilised by autoclaving. **Store** in well-closed containers. Protect from light.

STABILITY. The stability of salbutamol sulphate in aqueous phosphate buffers decreased with increase in pH above 6.9. In glucose solution 5%, salbutamol was more stable and lost 10% potency in about 19.9 weeks at 50°.— B. P. Wall and V. B. Sunderland, *Aust. J. Hosp. Pharm.*, 1976, *6*, 156.

Adverse Effects

For the adverse effects of sympathomimetic agents see p.1453.

Salbutamol may cause fine tremor of skeletal muscle (particularly the hands), palpitations, and muscle cramps. Slight tachycardia, tenseness, headaches, and peripheral vasodilatation have been reported after large doses.

The high doses of salbutamol used intravenously to delay premature labour have been associated with nausea and vomiting, and with adverse cardiac and metabolic effects.

A report on the nature and incidence of side-effects of salbutamol in 50 patients with chronic airflow obstruction who had been taking 4 mg three times daily for a year. The incidence of side-effects was: finger tremor 42%, palpitation 20%, muscle cramp 46%, and other symptoms 6%. Although finger tremor and palpitation are well recognised, muscle cramp is not; patients should be warned of this possibility. In view of this rather high incidence of side-effects when salbutamol is taken by mouth, it should be used by inhalation whenever possible.— K. N. V. Palmer (letter), *Br. med. J.*, 1978, *2*, 833.

ABUSE. Acute atypical psychosis in a 51-year-old woman was attributed to the excessive use of salbutamol; she had been taking 30 to 40 mg daily and using at least 12 inhalations daily for 10 days before admission to hospital. The patient claimed that salbutamol made her bright, alert, and forgetful of her anxieties.— L. Gluckman, *N.Z. med. J.*, 1974, *80*, 411, per *Practitioner*, 1975, *214*, 600.

Fears that adolescent asthmatics are abusing salbutamol by inhalation. This abuse appears to be spreading to non-asthmatic teenagers.— P. O. Brennan (letter), *Lancet*, 1983, *2*, 1030.

A report of the abuse of salbutamol and beclomethasone inhalers by a teenage asthmatic; the entire contents of a canister were inhaled at one time. Most probably the patient was dependent upon the fluorinated hydrocarbons used as the propellent of the aerosols. Less severe forms of abuse may be common among younger asthmatics.— P. J. Thompson *et al.*, *Br. med. J.*, 1983, *287*, 1515. Agreement, and a report of 5 further cases. Some of the effects attributed to salbutamol inhalers may in fact be due to the salbutamol content.— P. O. Brennan (letter), *ibid.*, 1877. Further reports: H. Wickramasinghe and H. J. Liebeschuetz (letter), *ibid.*; J. M. Raine (letter), *ibid.*, 1984, *288*, 241. Comment by the manufacturer. The balance of evidence indicates that fluorocarbons rather than salbutamol are responsible for the stimulatory effects on the central nervous system. A change to inhalation capsules is recommended where abuse of aerosols is suspected.— I. M. Slessor (letter), *Br. med. J.*, 485.

CARCINOGENICITY. A statement from the manufacturers attempting to put into perspective findings that long-term administration of very high doses of salbutamol has been associated with the development of benign mesovarian leiomyomas in some species of *rats*, who are known to respond aberrantly to beta-stimulants. There is no evidence that salbutamol is carcinogenic in any species, and much evidence that it is unlikely to be so.— D. Poynter *et al.* (letter), *Br. med. J.*, 1978, *1*, 46. Reply.— M. J. Finkel, *US Food and Drug Administration* (letter), *ibid.*, 649.

EFFECTS ON ELECTROLYTES. Since hypokalaemia had been reported following the inhalation or intravenous administration of salbutamol plasma-potassium concentrations were studied in 6 healthy subjects and 16 patients given salbutamol by mouth. The healthy subjects received single doses of 4 mg and the patients 5-day courses of 6 to 16 mg daily. There was no significant hypokalaemic effect and digitalised patients were not considered to be at special risk from salbutamol by mouth.— S. P. Deacon (letter), *Lancet*, 1976, *1*, 1302.

Preliminary results from a study in 6 healthy subjects suggested that a 5 mg dose of nebulised salbutamol produced a maximum fall in serum potassium of 0.5 μmol per mL 40 minutes after administration. This treatment is often used in patients with acute exacerbations of chronic bronchitis who may well be taking diuretics and digoxin for co-existent ischaemic heart disease; any worsening of pre-existing diuretic-induced hypokalaemia by $beta_2$-agonists may expose them to an increased risk of arrhythmias. There may be a case for checking serum potassium in such patients before starting treatment with $beta_2$-agonists, and for exercising caution with regard to dose.— S. R. Smith and M. J. Kendall (letter), *Lancet*, 1983, *2*, 218.

For further studies of the effect of a $beta_2$-agonist on plasma potassium concentrations, and the view that physicians should not be deterred from prescribing adequate doses of such agents, see under Fenoterol Hydrobromide, p.1464.

A study of the mechanism by which salbutamol induces hypokalaemia. Results suggested that salbutamol-induced hypokalaemia was not the result of $beta_2$-adrenergic-receptor induced insulin release but was consistent with stimulation of a $beta_2$ receptor linked to a membrane-bound Na^+/K^+ ATPase.— K. F. Whyte *et al.*, *Br. J. clin. Pharmac.*, 1987, *23*, 65.

EFFECTS ON THE HEART. Following intravenous infusion of salbutamol 10 μg per minute in a placebo-controlled study of 7 healthy subjects the ventilatory response to carbon dioxide was increased in both hypoxia and hyperoxia; a pronounced increase in heart-rate occurred which was more marked when hypoxia was associated with hypercapnia; a pronounced fall in plasma-potassium concentration occurred with a concomitant rise in plasma-glucose and serum-insulin concentrations. It was suggested that if salbutamol was infused intravenously in the management of severe asthma both the plasma potassium and the ECG should be carefully monitored as there might be a predisposition to cardiac arrhythmias.— A. G. Leitch *et al.*, *Br. med. J.*, 1976, *1*, 365. Comment on tachycardia associated with the intravenous administration of salbutamol and the view that it should be administered intravenously slowly over at least 5 minutes.— A. J. Johnson *et al.* (letter), *ibid.*, 1977, *1*, 772.

Evidence that salbutamol aerosol causes a tachycardia due to the inhaled rather than the swallowed fraction.— J. G. Collier *et al.* (letter), *Br. J. clin. Pharmac.*, 1980, *9*, 273. Studies indicating a lack of adverse effects on the heart from inhaled salbutamol: N. A. Martelli *et al.*, *Chest*, 1986, *89*, 192; J. J. Gilmartin *et al.*, *Thorax*, 1986, *41*, 331.

Five of 16 asthmatic patients experienced enhanced or additional cardiac arrhythmias while taking salbutamol sustained-release tablets in a single-blind crossover study; 3 also experienced arrhythmias while taking sustained-release tablets of terbutaline. The clinical significance of the arrhythmias was not clear.— A. H. Al-Hillawi *et al.*, *Br. med. J.*, 1984, *288*, 367. Comment.— P. Harrison (letter), *ibid.*, 863. Reply and further data.— A. H. Al-Hillawi (letter), *ibid.*

EFFECTS ON MENTAL FUNCTION. A brief report of visual hallucinations lasting for an hour following administration of nebulised salbutamol to an elderly patient. The manufacturers were aware of 3 cases of hallucinations in children given oral salbutamol but no such reaction had been previously reported in adults given recommended doses.— P. B. Khanna and R. Davies, *Br. med. J.*, 1986, *292*, 1430.

EFFECTS ON METABOLISM. Salbutamol sulphate given as a bolus intravenous injection of 50 to 150 μg in 9 volunteers increased heart-rate, stimulated the release of free fatty acids and insulin, produced a moderate rise in plasma-lactate concentrations, and a small increase in plasma-glucose concentrations. Growth-hormone concentrations were not affected. Pretreatment with the β_1-adrenergic blocker practolol reduced or abolished these changes except for release of free fatty acids.— R. Goldberg *et al.*, *Postgrad. med. J.*, 1975, *51*, 53. Salbutamol 150 ng per kg body-weight per minute given as an intravenous infusion for 60 minutes increased the heart-rate, release of insulin, and reduced the serum concentration of potassium in 4 healthy subjects. Serum-potassium concentrations should be monitored when salbutamol is administered since the hypokalaemic effect produced could provoke cardiac dysrhythmias particularly in patients receiving digoxin.— N. Berend and G. E. Marlin, *Br. J. clin. Pharmac.*, 1978, *5*, 207. There were no significant changes in the plasma concentrations of non-esterified fatty acids, triglyceride, glucose, insulin, or hydrocortisone in 7 of 8 patients with asthma or chronic bronchitis, up to 4 hours after they inhaled salbutamol 5 mg by intermittent positive-pressure ventilation. Plasma concentrations of insulin were elevated up to 4 hours after inhalation in the eighth patient.— S. M. Bateman *et al.*, *Br. J. clin. Pharmac.*, 1978, *5*, 127.

OVERDOSAGE. A 44-year-old asthmatic woman with depressive symptoms swallowed 100 salbutamol tablets 2 mg. When admitted to hospital 2 hours 45 minutes later there was peripheral vasodilatation, increased pulse-rate, sinus tachycardia, and agitation with increased irritability of skeletal muscle. An insignificant amount of salbutamol was recovered following gastric lavage. The patient was managed successfully with practolol, propranolol, and diazepam.— G. W. Morrison and M. J. B. Farebrother (letter), *Lancet*, 1973, *2*, 681.

In 40 patients who had taken overdoses of salbutamol (5 to 100 mg in those under 10 years; 14 to 240 mg in older patients) symptoms included muscle tremor, flushing, agitation, palpitations, sinus tachycardia, and hypokalaemia. No patient developed convulsions or ventricular arrhythmias. Treatment included gastric lavage or emesis in 20, and the use of beta-adrenoceptor blocking agents, usually propranolol, in 10, though propranolol was probably not necessary.— J. G. Prior *et al.*, *Br. med. J.*, 1981, *282*, 1932.

Hypokalaemia associated with salbutamol overdosage.— I. A. D. O'Brien *et al.*, *Br. med. J.*, 1981, *282*, 1515. Hypokalaemia and hyperglycaemia following an overdose of salbutamol in an adolescent were reversed by intravenous administration of propranolol.— J. M. C. Connell *et al.*, *Br. med. J.*, 1982, *285*, 779.

PREGNANCY AND THE NEONATE. Profuse uterine bleeding has been reported by P.S. Vinall and D.M. Jenkins (*Lancet*, 1977, *2*, 1355) following uterine evacuation in an asthmatic woman who inhaled salbutamol prior to the termination of her 13-week pregnancy. Most adverse effects associated with salbutamol in pregnancy relate, however, to the cardiovascular and metabolic effects of the very high doses given by intravenous infusion in attempts to delay premature labour. Thus, M.I. Whitehead *et al.* (*Lancet*, 1979, *2*, 904) have reported myocardial ischaemia on stopping an infusion, and W.C. Chew and L.C. Lew (*Lancet*, 1979, *2*, 1383) have reported unifocal ventricular ectopics associated with the hypokalaemic response to intravenous salbutamol. A further report by M.I. Whitehead *et al.* (*Br. med. J.*, 1980, *280*, 1221) concerning congestive heart failure in a hypertensive woman aroused controversy surrounding the management of such patients, including comment on the possible enhancement of the adverse effects of salbutamol by ergometrine (see P.A. Poole-Wilson, *Br. med. J.*, 1980, *281*, 226; A.J. Fogarty, *ibid.*; P.D.O. Davies, *ibid.*; M. Robertson and A.E. Davies, *ibid.*, 227; P. Crowley, *ibid.*; M.I. Whitehead *et al.*, *ibid.*). Metabolic acidosis following salbutamol infusions in diabetic women has been reported by M.G. Chapman (*Br. med. J.*, 1977, *1*, 639) and D.J.B. Thomas *et al.* (*Br. med. J.*, 1977, *2*, 438). That this problem is a particular hazard in diabetic women, particularly those given corticosteroids to promote foetal surfactant production, has subsequently been emphasised by a study by A.S. Gündoğdu *et al.* (*Lancet*, 1979, *2*, 1317).

PULMONARY OEDEMA. A review of pulmonary oedema associated with $beta_2$-selective sympathomimetic treatment of premature labour. Of 73 cases reviewed only some are reported in detail in the literature; these involve terbutaline (24 cases), ritodrine (11), isoxsuprine (4), salbutamol (2), and fenoterol (4); most of the residual cases implicate fenoterol. Reports involve oral, subcutaneous, and intravenous administration of these drugs and no correlation is obvious with total dose administered or infusion rate. Certain factors appear to be associated with increased risk of developing pulmonary oedema, namely twin pregnancy, the concomitant use of corticosteroids, positive fluid balance, a maternal pulse rate sustained above 140 per minute for prolonged periods, and the use of general anaesthesia. The pathogenesis of the syndrome appears to be multifactorial, but a direct toxic effect on the heart cannot be excluded. If detected early, pulmonary oedema is usually adequately and completely treated by cessation of $beta_2$-agonist therapy, oxygen administration, and diuretics. The more fulminant form, which has characteristics of adult respiratory distress syndrome is more common after general anaesthesia and requires sophisticated ventilatory support and invasive haemodynamic monitoring. Treatment with $beta_2$-agonists should be restricted to centres where facilities for maternal resuscitation exist.— F. Hawker, *Anaesth. & intensive Care*, 1984, *12*, 143.

URINARY RETENTION. Beta-receptor stimulants such as salbutamol and terbutaline are unlikely to produce urinary retention when administered by inhalation, but may do so when given by mouth or intravenously.— P. Turner, *Prescribers' J.*, 1978, *18*, 94.

Precautions

For precautions that should be observed with sympathomimetic agents see p.1453.

Salbutamol is not indicated for the prevention of premature labour associated with toxaemia of pregnancy or antepartum haemorrhage, nor should it be used for threatened abortion during the first and second trimesters of pregnancy.

Adverse metabolic effects of high doses of salbutamol may be exacerbated by concomitant administration of high doses of corticosteroids; patients should therefore be monitored carefully when the 2 forms of therapy are used together. Propranolol and other beta-adrenoceptor blocking agents antagonise the effects of salbutamol. Hypokalaemia associated with high doses of salbutamol may result in increased susceptibility to digitalis-induced cardiac arrhythmias. The effects of salbutamol may be enhanced by concomitant administration of aminophylline or other xanthines.

A warning that home nebulising units for salbutamol administration to asthmatic children may lead to delay in seeking help when needed.— A. W. Lillington *et al.* (letter), *Lancet*, 1983, *2*, 1032. Further references: *ibid.*, 1984, *2*, 789; J. A. Kuzemko (letter), *ibid.*, 1985, *1*, 49; B. G. Loftus and J. F. Price (letter), *ibid.*, 393.

A reminder that nebulisation with air may aggravate hypoxaemia in patients with severe chronic lung disease.— H. Cass *et al.* (letter), *Br. med. J.*, 1984, *288*, 1009. If patients are very hypoxic it is perhaps wise to use oxygen to drive the nebuliser but only for the shortest possible period; patients with carbon dioxide retention should be watched carefully as oxygen-driven nebulisers cause a rise in carbon dioxide pressure.— K. A. Gunawardena *et al.* (letter), *ibid.*, 1237.

INTERACTIONS. Comment on the risks of combined therapy with beta-adrenergic agonists and methylxanthines in asthma.— J. D. Wilson and D. C. Sutherland (letter), *New Engl. J. Med.*, 1982, *307*, 1707. Criticism. The authors have frequently prescribed salbutamol and high-dose sustained-release theophylline for the treatment of asthmatic children and believe such therapy to be highly successful and safe.— A. F. Isles and C. J. L. Newth (letter), *ibid.*, 1983, *309*, 432. Comment. It is conceivable that in the dosages used in asthma adverse effects with this drug combination may not normally pose a great threat but until such information can be unequivocally provided clinicians would do well to heed the warnings about concomitant use of beta-adrenergic agonists and methylxanthines, and to exercise appropriate caution.— D. Lehr and G. Guideri (letter), *ibid.*, 1581.

A study suggesting that *nifedipine* can prolong the bronchodilator action of salbutamol.— A. M. L. Lever *et al.*, *Thorax*, 1984, *39*, 576. Results in 15 asthmatics failed to demonstrate any potentiation of the effects of salbutamol by nifedipine.— M. Molho *et al.*, *Chest*, 1987, *91*, 667.

TOLERANCE. In healthy subjects specific airway conductance was progressively reduced when salbutamol up to 400 μg four times daily was inhaled over 4 to 5 weeks. Hydrocortisone 200 mg intravenously or aminophylline restored the response.— A. E. Tattersfield and S. T. Holgate (letter), *Lancet*, 1976, *1*, 422. See also S. T. Holgate *et al.*, *Lancet*, 1977, *2*, 375; *idem*, *Clin. Sci.*, 1980, *59*, 155.

Absorption and Fate

Salbutamol is readily absorbed from the gastro-intestinal tract. It is subject to first-pass metabolism in the liver; about a half is excreted in the urine as an inactive sulphate conjugate, following oral administration (the rest being unchanged salbutamol), whereas rather less is excreted as the conjugate following intravenous administration. Salbutamol does not appear to be metabolised in the lung, therefore its behaviour following inhalation depends upon the delivery method used, which determines the proportion of inhaled salbutamol relative to the proportion inadvertently swallowed.

The plasma half-life of salbutamol has been estimated to range from about 2 to as much as 7 hours. In general the shorter values have followed intravenous administration, the intermediate values oral administration, and the longer values aerosol inhalation. It has been suggested that the slightly extended half-life following inhalation may reflect slow removal of active drug from the lungs.

Tritiated salbutamol given by mouth in a dose of 4 or 8 mg to 6 patients with asthma was well absorbed giving peak plasma concentrations within 3 hours and up to 78% being excreted in the urine within 24 hours. Measurements in 4 patients showed that 1.2 to 7% was excreted in the faeces. When given by aerosol to another 6 asthmatic patients in doses estimated at 40 to 100 μg, peak plasma concentrations were obtained at 3 to 5 hours; up to 89.6% was excreted in the urine within 24 hours, and in 2 patients 10.2 and 12% of the dose was recovered from the faeces. In both groups just under half the dose was excreted in the urine as a metabolite at the same rate as salbutamol. There was an increase in the 1-second forced expiratory volume (FEV_1) in both groups but this correlated with the dose only in those given salbutamol by mouth. In 5 of the 6 given salbutamol by inhalation, the maximum increase in FEV_1 occurred within 15 minutes, indicating a local effect.— S. W. Walker *et al.*, *Clin. Pharmac. Ther.*, 1972, *13*, 861.

A study of salbutamol pharmacokinetics following intravenous and oral doses in 10 healthy subjects. Mean elimination half-life following a 2-hour intravenous infusion was 3.9 hours; volume of distribution was fairly large at 156 litres, indicating extensive extravascular uptake. Urinary excretion of both unchanged salbutamol (64% of the dose) and the sulphate conjugate (12%) was complete after 24 hours. Following oral administration the systemic availability of salbutamol was 50%; significantly less was excreted as unchanged drug (32%) and more as the sulphate conjugate (48%) compared to the intravenous route, presumably representing first-pass conjugation in the gut wall.— D. J. Morgan *et al.*, *Br. J. clin. Pharmac.*, 1986, *22*, 587.

Further references to the absorption and fate of salbutamol: G. L. Snider and R. Laguarda, *J. Am. med. Ass.*, 1972, *221*, 682 (duration of action of the aerosol); G. M. Shenfield *et al.*, *Br. J. clin. Pharmac.*, 1974, *1*, 295 (influence of delivery method on the absorption and metabolism of salbutamol); M. R. Hetzel and T. J. H. Clark, *Br. med. J.*, 1976, *2*, 919 (comparison of intravenous and aerosol routes); S. P. Deacon (letter), *Br. med. J.*, 1976, *2*, 1134; *idem*, 1977, *1*, 639 (comments on the metabolism following oral, intravenous, and aerosol administration); G. M. Shenfield *et al.*, *Br. J. clin. Pharmac.*, 1976, *3*, 583 (salbutamol and absorption in the lung); C. Lin *et al.*, *Drug Metab. & Dispos.*, 1977, *5*, 234 (isolation and identification of the major metabolite).

Uses and Administration

Salbutamol is a direct-acting sympathomimetic agent with predominantly beta-adrenergic activity and a selective action on $beta_2$ receptors. It is used as a bronchodilator. It has more prolonged actions than isoprenaline and also, as a predominantly $beta_2$-receptor stimulant, has a more selective action, its bronchodilating action being relatively more prominent than its effect on the heart. Such $beta_2$-adrenoceptor stimulants are preferred to isoprenaline for the management of asthma.

Salbutamol is used as the base in aerosol inhalers and as the sulphate in other preparations and its dosage is expressed in terms of salbutamol base.

In the treatment of bronchial asthma it is given by mouth in a dose of 2 to 4 mg three or four times daily; some patients may require doses of up to 8 mg. Elderly patients should be given the lower doses initially. A dose of 1 to 2 mg three or four times daily is suggested for children aged 2 to 6 years or 2 mg for older children.

Salbutamol is given as an aerosol for the chronic management or prophylactic therapy of bronchial asthma, in a dose of 2 inhalations of 100 μg of salbutamol 3 or 4 times daily; for the relief of acute bronchospasm or for managing intermittent episodes of asthma 1 or 2 inhalations of 100 μg may be administered as a single dose when required (the bronchodilator effects last at least 4 hours). Exercise-induced bronchospasm may be prevented by 2 inhalations of 100 μg before exertion. Children should be given 1 inhalation of 100 μg of salbutamol 3 or 4 times daily for routine maintenance or prophylactic therapy, increased to 2 inhalations if necessary. Worsening asthma should not be treated by increased doses of salbutamol (see Precautions with Sympathomimetic Agents, p.1453).

Although salbutamol is generally inhaled in aerosol form, inhalation capsules of salbutamol sulphate are available for patients who experience difficulty in using the aerosol. Owing to differences in the relative bioavailability to the lungs of the 2 preparations a 200 μg dose (expressed in terms of salbutamol) from an inhalation capsule is approximately equivalent in activity to a 100-μg dose from an aerosol and the recommended doses are therefore twice those suggested for the aerosol.

In more severe or unresponsive asthma salbutamol sulphate has also been given via a nebuliser in doses of 2.5 to 5 mg of salbutamol as a solution containing the equivalent of 1 mg of salbutamol, as the sulphate, per mL. Treatment may be repeated up to 4 times daily.

Salbutamol may be used together with other forms of therapy (see Corticosteroids, p.876), in the treatment of acute severe asthma or other forms of severe bronchospasm. 2 mL of salbutamol sulphate solution containing the equivalent of salbutamol 0.5% (10 mg) may be inhaled up to 4 times daily as a mist in oxygen-enriched air through an intermittent positive-pressure ventilator over a period of about 3 minutes; similarly a 0.005 to 0.01% solution in sterile water may be administered as a mist by means of an intermittent positive-pressure ventilator at the rate of 1 to 2 mg of salbutamol per hour. Adequate oxygenation is essential to avoid hypoxaemia. Alternatively, salbutamol may be given in a dose of 500 μg by subcutaneous or intramuscular injection repeated every 4 hours as required, or by slow intravenous injection of 250 μg as a solution containing 50 μg per mL. It may also be given as a solution containing 5 mg in 500 mL (10 μg per mL) in infusions such as sodium chloride and glucose intravenous infusion. The infusion rate should provide 3 to 20 μg per minute according to the patient's need; higher dosages have been used in patients with respiratory failure.

Infusions containing 5 mg in 500 mL (10 μg per mL) are also given to arrest premature labour (but see Precautions); infusion rates are usually 10 to 45 μg per minute, according to the patient's response. The recommended initial rate of infusion is 10 μg per minute increased at intervals of 10 minutes until there is evidence of patient response as shown by reduction in strength, frequency, or duration of contractions; the rate is then increased slowly until contractions cease. The infusion should be maintained at the rate at which contractions cease for one hour, then reduced by decrements of 50% at intervals of 6 hours. The maternal pulse should be monitored throughout the infusion and the rate adjusted to avoid a maternal heart-rate of more than 140 beats per minute. Salbutamol may subsequently be given by mouth in a dose of 4 mg three or four times daily.

As an alternative procedure, or to counteract inadvertent overdosage with oxytocic drugs, salbutamol may be given as a single injection by slow intravenous or intramuscular injection of 100 to 250 μg, repeated according to the patient's response.

In *dogs* and *guinea-pigs* (−)-salbutamol was much more potent than (+)-salbutamol on beta-adrenergic receptors. Both (−)- and (+)-salbutamol showed high selectivity for beta-adrenergic receptors in bronchial muscle compared to cardiac muscle, in this way resembling racemic salbutamol.— R. T. Brittain *et al.*, *Br. J. Pharmac.*, 1973, *48*, 144.

ASTHMA. In the management of asthma, salbutamol and similar $beta_2$-selective sympathomimetic agents have the great advantage over isoprenaline, of a pronounced effect on bronchospasm at doses which have little effect on the heart. Furthermore, inhalation of salbutamol appears to provide an even more specific effect on bronchospasm than administration by mouth. The route of choice for the prophylactic and therapeutic management of bronchial spasms has therefore become inhalation of the aerosol preparation. A large number of children and some adults, however, are unable to use aerosol inhalations in the manner necessary to provide an adequate dose to the lungs and, although tachycardia is not a significant feature of standard oral doses of salbutamol, the incidence of other side-effects, such as muscle tremor and palpitations, may be higher. For such patients, an inhalation-activated device which provides salbutamol in the form of a powder mixed with lactose, has been developed; alternatively they will require administration of salbutamol by mouth.

The hospital patient with severe asthma requiring emergency supportive respiratory care until corticosteroid therapy has taken effect may also be unable to respond to inhaled salbutamol, probably owing to factors such as mucous plugs in the lungs. Since adverse cardiovascular effects, notably tachycardia, can occur following parenteral administration of salbutamol, several delivery methods have been studied which supply moist inhalations of salbutamol to enhance penetration in the lungs. In general, the parenteral route may be necessary for the acute emergency, but once the patient can cough and produce sputum moist inhalation methods are preferred.

General reviews of the treatment of asthma: T. J. H. Clark, *Postgrad. med. J.*, 1983, *59*, *Suppl.* 3, 54; I. D. Green, *J. clin. Hosp. Pharm.*, 1984, *9*, 1; J. Rees, *Br. med. J.*, 1984, *288*, 1595; M. R. Hetzel, *Postgrad. med. J.*, 1984, *60*, 201; R. M. Cherniack, *Chest*, 1985, *87*, *Suppl.*, 94S.

A review of the management of *acute asthma*. In the *UK* most respiratory physicians would probably start treatment, in a patient ill enough to require admission to hospital, with oxygen by high-concentration mask, hydrocortisone 200 mg intravenously every 4 or 6 hours, and a nebulised $beta_2$-agonist. Nebulised $beta_2$-agonists seem to be the bronchodilator of choice: salbutamol or terbutaline 2.5 mg is adequate for most patients and less likely to cause side-effects than higher doses. Administration via a jet nebuliser is very satisfactory and the addition of intermittent positive pressure breathing confers no advantage. The intravenous route may be necessary for patients unable to use or respond to nebulised $beta_2$-agonists although most workers comparing the nebulised and intravenous routes have found in favour of the nebulised drug. When an intravenous drug is needed there seems to be little to choose between aminophylline and a $beta_2$-agonist. Although the evidence is conflicting both seem to be of similar bronchodilating efficacy but the risks may be higher with aminophylline. For patients who do not respond adequately to oxygen, corticosteroids, and a $beta_2$-agonist, the main therapeutic options are to add nebulised ipratropium bromide or intravenous aminophylline to the nebulised $beta_2$-agonist. Ipratropium bromide may give useful additional bronchodilation, but should be given with or after the $beta_2$-agonist to offset any small risk of paradoxical bronchoconstriction. In patients with very severe asthma who may respond less well to a $beta_2$-agonist, and in whom the alternative may be mechanical ventilation, it seems reasonable to try the addition of intravenous aminophylline, although any benefit is likely to be small and side-effects should be anticipated. In patients with less severe acute asthma, addition of a theophylline is more likely to increase side-effects than airway calibre.— *Lancet*, 1986, *1*, 131.

Further references to the management of acute severe asthma: *Lancet*, 1982, *2*, 420; J. Rees, *Br. med. J.*, 1984, *288*, 1747; M. E. Tatham and A. R. Gellert, *Postgrad. med. J.*, 1985, *61*, 599.

The treatment of *chronic asthma*. The mainstay of treatment in mild intermittent asthma is one of the selective $beta_2$-agonists taken by inhalation. Their onset of action is fast, and salbutamol, terbutaline, and fenoterol have an effect lasting for 4 to 6 hours. If more than occasional doses are required their regular use should be considered, with additional symptomatic use as necessary. The dose needed varies between patients, and it makes little sense rigidly to restrict the daily dose to 2 puffs four times daily. A maximum daily dose of perhaps 20 inhalations should be established so that the patient can seek help if he feels he needs to exceed this dose. Patients should be taught to monitor their inhaler dose and understand that if this increases or its effects get less these are danger signals indicating deterioration in asthmatic control and the need for further treatment.— J. Rees, *Br. med. J.*, 1984, *288*, 1819.

Asthma in children. A review of asthma in childhood. Infants under 18 months of age are relatively unresponsive to beta agonists, but inhaled ipratropium bromide for temporary relief or oral theophylline for continuing problems may be helpful. If further prophylaxis is needed regular nebulised cromoglycate may be effective. Over 18 months of age the beta agonists become more effective and over 4 years of age inhalation treatment becomes easier. Mild episodic asthma responds to beta agonists and more frequent attacks benefit from regular prophylaxis with slow-release theophylline preparations or inhaled sodium cromoglycate.— J. Reiser, *Br. J. Hosp. Med.*, 1985, *33*, 196. See also J. Price, *Br. med. J.*, 1984, *288*, 1895; P. D. Phelan, *Med. J. Aust.*, 1985, *143*, 455.

A number of drugs can inhibit exercise-induced asthma in children if given before exercise, but by far the most effective is an inhaled beta$_2$-agonist such as 2 puffs of salbutamol or terbutaline, taken between 5 and 10 minutes before exercise. It has been suggested that oral sympathomimetic agents may be ineffective in preventing exercise-induced asthma, but it is chiefly a problem in older children, who can generally be taught to use an aerosol inhaler successfully. Any child on regular maintenance treatment with sodium cromoglycate, theophylline, or inhaled corticosteroids may still need to take an additional aerosol sympathomimetic if exercise-induced asthma remains troublesome.— S. Godfrey, *Archs Dis. Childh.*, 1983, *58*, 1.

BRONCHITIS AND BRONCHIOLITIS. For a study indicating an apparent lack of value for nebulised salbutamol in infants with acute bronchiolitis, see under Ipratropium Bromide, p.538.

CARDIAC DISORDERS. In 11 patients with acute myocardial infarction complicated by left ventricular failure the infusion of salbutamol 10, 20, or 40 µg per minute increased cardiac output while the mean systemic arterial pressure fell slightly; heart-rate increased by only 10 beats per minute. While salbutamol increases cardiac output in patients in whom poor perfusion is the most important haemodynamic disturbance, it fails to reduce left ventricular filling pressure and cannot be recommended for patients with pulmonary oedema after acute infarction.— A. D. Timmis *et al.*, *Br. med. J.*, 1979, *2*, 1101. See also M. B. Fowler *et al.*, *Br. med. J.*, 1980, *280*, 435 (comparison with sodium nitroprusside); A. D. Timmis *et al.*, *Br. med. J.*, 1981, *282*, 7 (comparison with dopamine).

EPIGLOTTITIS, LARYNGITIS, AND CROUP. There was a higher rate of recovery from pertussis in children given erythromycin plus salbutamol than in those given erythromycin and a placebo.— D. Pavesio and A. Ponzone (letter), *Lancet*, 1977, *1*, 150.

In an uncontrolled study in 4 infants with severe pertussis, salbutamol 300 to 500 µg per kg body-weight daily, divided into 3 doses given by mouth, reduced the frequency and duration of whooping but not of coughing episodes. Salbutamol may be of benefit in children with pertussis but should be reserved for the most severe cases until optimum dosage and duration of therapy can be determined.— H. Peltola and K. Michelsson, *Lancet*, 1982, *1*, 310. Further reports of benefit.— A. Brunskill and D. Langdon (letter), *ibid.*, 1986, *2*, 282; A. Y. -C. Tam and C. -Y. Yeung, *Archs Dis. Childh.*, 1986, *61*, 600.

Salbutamol had no significant effects on the course or severity of whooping cough in a double-blind study in 9 children.— I. Krantz *et al.*, *Pediatr. infect. Dis.*, 1985, *4*, 638.

HYPERKALAEMIA. Salbutamol in 2 inhalations of 200 µg every 15 minutes for up to 1 hour successfully controlled hyperkalaemic paralysis in 13 patients. It had insufficient effect in another patient.— P. Wang and T. Clausen, *Lancet*, 1976, *1*, 221. See also C. Busche (letter), *ibid.*, 1983, *2*, 797 (nebulised salbutamol in drug-induced hyperkalaemia).

OCULAR DISORDERS. One instillation of a solution of salbutamol sulphate 4.8% (equivalent to salbutamol 4%) lowered intra-ocular pressure in 15 glaucomatous patients. In a further study with 4 patients the fall in pressure was equivalent to that produced by adrenaline 1%. However, with a twice daily instillation intolerable hyperaemia with irritation developed in about half the patients.— G. D. Paterson and G. Paterson, *Br. J. Ophthal.*, 1972, *56*, 288. See also R. L. Coakes and P. B. Siah, *ibid.*, 1984, *68*, 393 (the effects of salbutamol eye-drops on aqueous humour dynamics).

PREGNANCY AND THE NEONATE. *Premature labour.* A very large number of studies have been carried out into the efficacy of salbutamol and similar beta$_2$-selective adrenoceptor stimulants, particularly fenoterol and ritodrine, for the prevention of premature labour. In a review of 18 of these E. Hemminki and B. Starfield (*Br. J. Obstet. Gynec.*, 1978, *85*, 411) found few that did not contain any methodological drawbacks: only 5 were therapeutic rather than prophylactic studies, and in only 2 of these was the active drug more effective than placebo, moreover, a favourable effect in terms of foetal outcome was found in only one. Nevertheless, in what Hemminki and Starfield considered to be one of the more satisfactory studies, A. Wesselius-de Casparis *et al.* (*Br. med. J.*, 1971, *3*, 144) did find a postponement of preterm labour in 80% of patients receiving ritodrine compared with 48% in the placebo group.

Preterm delivery is responsible for about 7% of all births but accounts for 75% of perinatal mortality. Although many drugs have been claimed to suppress premature labour the tacit assumption that this is necessarily beneficial should not go unquestioned: it has been suggested that only 10% of patients in early or suspected premature labour can even theoretically profit from tocolytic agents. It is therefore unsurprising that the incidence of infants with birth weight of less than 2.5 kg is unchanged over the past 3 decades, with or without tocolytic agents, and it must be concluded that these drugs are generally overused.— F. Hawker, *Anaesth. & intensive Care*, 1984, *12*, 143.

For adverse effects associated with the use of salbutamol in premature labour, see under Adverse Effects (above).

PROCTALGIA FUGAX. A report of the value of inhaled salbutamol in the relief of proctalgia fugax.— J. E. Wright (letter), *Lancet*, 1985, *2*, 659.

SKIN DISORDERS. In a double-blind placebo-controlled study, the effects of topical and oral salbutamol were evaluated in 21 patients with atopic dermatitis. Salbutamol ointment therapy resulted in a reduction in the score for redness, but there was no marked clinical improvement in any of the treatment groups.— C. B. Archer and D. M. MacDonald, *Br. J. Derm.*, 1986, *115*, *Suppl.* 30, 33.

Preparations

Salbutamol Aerosol Inhalation *(B.P.C. 1973).* An aerosol spray in a pressurised canister containing a fine suspension of salbutamol in a suitable mixture of aerosol propellents. Store in a cool place.

Salbutamol Injection *(B.P.).* Salbutamol Sulphate Injection. Potency is expressed in terms of the equivalent amount of salbutamol.

Salbutamol Tablets *(B.P.).* Tablets containing salbutamol sulphate. Potency is expressed in terms of the equivalent amount of salbutamol.

Proprietary Preparations

Aerolin *(Riker, UK). Inhaler*, aerosol, salbutamol 100 µg (as sulphate)/metered dose.
Inhaler (Aerolin Auto), breath-actuated aerosol, salbutamol 100 µg (as sulphate)/metered dose.

Asmaven *(Approved Prescription Services, UK). Tablets*, salbutamol 2 and 4 mg (as sulphate).
Inhaler, aerosol, salbutamol 100 µg/metered inhalation.

Cobutolin *(Cox, UK). Tablets*, salbutamol 2 and 4 mg (as sulphate).
Inhaler, aerosol, salbutamol 100 µg/metered inhalation.

Salbulin *(Riker, UK). Tablets*, salbutamol 2 and 4 mg (as sulphate).
Inhaler, aerosol, salbutamol 100 µg/metered inhalation.

Ventide *(Allen & Hanburys, UK). Inhaler*, aerosol, salbutamol 100 µg, beclomethasone dipropionate 50 µg/metered inhalation.
Rotacaps, inhalation cartridges, salbutamol 400 µg (as sulphate), beclomethasone dipropionate 200 µg.
Paediatric Rotacaps, inhalation cartridges, salbutamol 200 µg (as sulphate), beclomethasone dipropionate 100 µg.

Ventodisks *(Allen & Hanburys, UK). Discs*, salbutamol 200 and 400 µg (as sulphate)/dose. For use in a specially designed inhaler (Diskhaler).

Ventolin *(Allen & Hanburys, UK). Tablets*, salbutamol 2 and 4 mg (as sulphate).
Spandets, sustained-release tablets, salbutamol 8 mg (as sulphate).
Syrup, salbutamol 2 mg (as sulphate)/5 mL.
Injection, salbutamol 50 µg (as sulphate)/mL, in ampoules of 5 mL and 500 µg (as sulphate)/mL, in ampoules of 1 mL.
Concentrate for intravenous infusion, salbutamol 1 mg (as sulphate)/mL, in ampoules of 5 mL.
Inhaler, aerosol, salbutamol 100 µg/metered inhalation.
Respirator solution, salbutamol 5 mg (as sulphate)/mL.
Nebules, respirator solution, salbutamol 1 and 2 mg (as sulphate)/mL, in ampoules of 2.5 mL.
Rotacaps, inhalation cartridges, salbutamol 200 and 400 µg (as sulphate), for use in a specially designed inhaler (Rotahaler).
NOTE. The availability of salbutamol to the lungs depends upon the formulation used; Ventolin Inhaler and Ventolin Rotacaps differ in this respect. For further details see under Uses (above).

Volmax *(Duncan, Flockhart, UK). Tablets*, sustained-release, salbutamol 4 mg and 8 mg (as sulphate).

Proprietary Names and Manufacturers

Aerolin *(Riker, UK)*; Asmatol *(Arg.)*; Asmaven *(Approved Prescription Services, UK)*; Asmidon *(Jpn)*; Broncho-Spray *(Klinge, Ger.)*; Broncovaleas *(Valeas, Ital.)*; Buto-Asma *(Aldo, Spain)*; Cobutolin *(Cox, UK)*; Novosalmol *(Novopharm, Canad.)*; Proventil *(Schering, USA)*; Respolin *(Riker, Austral.)*; Salbulin *(Riker, Denm.; Riker, UK)*; Salbutan *(Ital.)*; Salbuvent *(Nyco, Denm.; Nyco, Norw.; Nycomed, Swed.)*; Sultanol *(Glaxo, Ger.; Jpn)*; Venetlin *(Jpn)*; Venteze *(Lennon, S.Afr.)*; Ventodisks *(Allen & Hanburys, UK)*; Ventolin *(Arg.; Glaxo, Austral.; Belg.; Allen & Hanburys, Canad.; Glaxo, Ital.; Neth.; Allen & Hanburys, S.Afr.; Glaxo, Spain; Glaxo, Switz.; Allen & Hanburys, UK; Glaxo, USA)*; Ventoline *(Glaxo, Denm.; Glaxo, Fr.; Glaxo, Norw.; Glaxo, Swed.)*; Volmax *(Duncan, Flockhart, UK)*.

2106-k

Salmefamol *(BAN, rINN).*

AH-3923. 1-(4-Hydroxy-3-hydroxymethylphenyl)-2-(4-methoxy-α-methylphenethylamino)ethanol.
$C_{19}H_{25}NO_4$=331.4.

CAS — 18910-65-1.

Salmefamol is a direct-acting sympathomimetic agent with general properties similar to those of salbutamol (p.1480). It has been given for the relief of bronchospasm in doses of 100 to 200 µg by inhalation and 1 to 2 mg by mouth.

Proprietary Names and Manufacturers
Glaxo, UK.

13303-d

Tefazoline *(rINN).*

Tenaphtoxaline. 2-(5,6,7,8-Tetrahydro-1-naphthylmethyl)-2-imidazoline.
$C_{14}H_{18}N_2$=214.3.

CAS — 1082-56-0.

Tefazoline is a sympathomimetic agent related to naphazoline (p.1470), which has been used as a nasal decongestant.

Proprietary Names and Manufacturers
Tenaphto *(UPB, Belg.)*.

2107-a

Terbutaline Sulphate *(BANM, rINNM).*

KWD-2019; Terbutaline Sulfate *(USAN)*; Terbutalini Sulphas. 2-*tert*-Butylamino-1-(3,5-dihydroxyphenyl)ethanol sulphate.
$(C_{12}H_{19}NO_3)_2,H_2SO_4$=548.7.

CAS — 23031-25-6 (terbutaline); 23031-32-5 (sulphate).

Pharmacopoeias. In *Br.*, *Jpn*, *Nord.*, and *U.S.*

A white to greyish-white odourless or almost odourless crystalline powder.
Soluble 1 in 4 of water; slightly soluble in alcohol and in methyl alcohol; practically insoluble in chloroform and ether. The *U.S.P.* injection has a pH of 3 to 5. **Store** at 15° to 30° in well-closed containers. Protect from light.

Terbutaline sulphate was very stable to oxidative degradation in solution at pH 5.— L. -Å. Svensson, *Acta pharm. suec.*, 1972, *9*, 141.

Adverse Effects

For the adverse effects of sympathomimetic agents see p.1453.

Ten asthmatic patients received terbutaline 250 µg subcutaneously, 5 mg by mouth, and 10 mg by mouth, on separate days. In a dose of 10 mg, terbutaline caused a disproportionate increase in heart-rate compared with the small ventilatory advantage over a 5-mg dose. Side-effects were slight and included tremor and, in 3 patients, prolonged sleep.— B. J. Freedman, *Br. med. J.*, 1971, *1*, 633. In 16 patients with reversible airway disease, administration of terbutaline sulphate 500 µg three times daily by inhalation was associated with a high incidence of side-effects—headache (9), nervousness (9), dizziness (8), pounding in chest (5), nausea (5), somnolence (5), diarrhoea (4), flushing (4), insomnia (3), tremors (3), sweating (3), and constipation (1).— J. Trautlein *et al.*, *J. clin. Pharmac.*, 1977, *17*, 76. A report in 1 patient of muscle twitching and cramp associated with the use of terbutaline sulphate 5 mg three times daily.— S. Zelman (letter), *J. Am. med. Ass.*, 1978, *239*, 930.

BRONCHOSPASM. Paradoxical bronchoconstriction occurred on 2 occasions 4 or 5 hours after ingestion of terbutaline 2.5 mg by mouth by an asthmatic patient. The bronchospasm was successfully treated with orciprenaline sulphate by intravenous infusion. The long time-lag between ingestion of the drug and symptoms suggests that the reaction may have been due to a metabolite of terbutaline.— H. Drexel *et al.* (letter), *Lancet*, 1982, *2*, 446.

EFFECTS ON THE HEART. A report of ventricular arrhythmias in a man with coronary heart disease, following oral administration of terbutaline sulphate 5 mg by mouth.— E. L. Kinney (letter), *J. Am. med. Ass.*, 1978, *240*, 2247.

For a report of arrhythmias following administration of salbutamol or terbutaline see under Salbutamol Sulphate, p.1481.

EFFECTS ON THE NERVOUS SYSTEM. A report of seizures in a 7-year-old child previously maintained on high-dose terbutaline 1 mg per kg body-weight daily, when the drug was re-introduced after a 4-day abstinence. The patient suffered 2 more seizures following ingestion of 7.5-mg doses.— R. Friedman *et al.*, *Am. J. Dis. Child.*, 1982, *136*, 1091.

HYPOTENSION. For a report of severe hypotension following the use of terbutaline in quadriplegic patients see under Precautions, below.

OVERDOSAGE. Tremor and tachycardia persisted for 24 hours after a 77-year-old man had taken an overdose of 20 tablets of terbutaline 2.5 mg and 9 tablets of flurazepam 15 mg.— I. Gomolin and J. A. Ingelfinger (letter), *New Engl. J. Med.*, 1979, *300*, 143.

Lactic acidosis, high plasma-glucose concentrations, and hypokalaemia occurred in a 28-year-old woman who took an overdose of terbutaline 225 mg, together with clomipramine, oxazepam, chloral hydrate, and wine.— M. Fahlén and L. Lapidus (letter), *Br. med. J.*, 1980, *281*, 390.

In an attempt to arrest premature labour a 35-year-old insulin-dependent diabetic woman was given an intravenous infusion of terbutaline 250 µg hourly for 12 hours, during which time her heart-rate varied between 90 to 114 beats per minute. Her terbutaline was then changed to the subcutaneous route and an hour later she was inadvertently given 2.5 mg, instead of 250 µg, subcutaneously. Ten minutes later non-radiating substernal chest pressure developed with a tachycardia of 150 beats per minute. ECG changes were noted and she was admitted to coronary care to rule out a myocardial infarction. She was given no medication except insulin and her cardiac course remained essentially benign. The tachycardia resolved after 10 hours and the cardiac enzymes over 2 days were essentially normal; the ECG reverted to normal over these 2 days. The terbutaline was not successful in preventing an abortion.— R. D. Brandstetter and V. Gotz (letter), *Lancet*, 1980, *1*, 485. The potentially dangerous cardiac effects could have been treated with a beta-adrenoceptor antagonist, such as propranolol.— R. J. Walden (letter), *ibid.*, 709. A further report of the inadvertent administration of terbutaline sulphate 2.5 mg subcutaneously instead of 250 µg.— C. Lawyer and A. Pond (letter), *New Engl. J. Med.*, 1977, *296*, 821.

PULMONARY OEDEMA. For a review of pulmonary oedema in women given beta$_2$-agonists, including terbutaline, for premature labour, see under Salbutamol Sulphate, p.1481.

Precautions

For the precautions to be observed with sympathomimetic agents, see p.1453.

Results of a comparative study of the effects of age on cardiovascular responses to terbutaline showed that whereas diastolic pressure fell in both groups, in 8 patients aged 18 to 25 years terbutaline infusion produced an increase in systolic pressure, but in 8 subjects aged 68 to 83 years there was a significant fall in systolic pressure. Heart rate was increased significantly less in older than in younger subjects. The results suggest that there is an age-related impairment in beta$_1$-adrenergic receptor sensitivity. The systemic use of beta-adrenergic receptor agonists may produce undesirable haemodynamic effects in the elderly.— M. J. Kendall *et al.*, *Br. J. clin. Pharmac.*, 1982, *14*, 821.

A report of severe hypotension in 2 patients with quadriplegia given terbutaline 500 µg subcutaneously for respiratory disorders. Indiscriminate use of beta$_2$-agonists such as terbutaline should be avoided in quadriplegic patients because of the potential for the development of life-threatening hypotension.— S. K. Pingleton *et al.*, *Am. Rev. resp. Dis.*, 1982, *126*, 723.

INTERACTIONS. The metabolic and cardiovascular responses to terbutaline infusion were significantly enhanced following administration of theophylline in a study in 7 healthy subjects; in particular the fall in serum potassium was greater when both drugs were given. Careful monitoring of serum potassium would seem justified if theophylline and beta$_2$-agonists are given together.— S. R. Smith and M. J. Kendall, *Br. J. clin. Pharmac.*, 1986, *21*, 451. See also J. J. Coleman *et al.*, *Chest*, 1986, *90*, 45.

Absorption and Fate

Terbutaline is incompletely absorbed from the gastro-intestinal tract and is also subject to fairly extensive first-pass metabolism by sulphate (and some glucuronide) conjugation in the liver and possibly the gut wall. It is accordingly excreted in the urine partly as the inactive conjugates and partly as unchanged terbutaline, the ratio depending upon whether it was given by mouth or parenterally.

In 7 hypertensive subjects the metabolism of radioactive terbutaline was dependent on the route of administration. After intravenous dosing unchanged drug accounted for most of the radioactivity in plasma. More than 80% of the dose was excreted in urine, mainly (68%) as terbutaline with only 14% as the sulphate conjugate; only 2 to 3% of the dose was excreted in faeces. After dosing by mouth an average of 47% of the radioactivity was recovered in faeces as unchanged drug indicating that terbutaline was incompletely absorbed; less than 15% of the plasma radioactivity was unchanged terbutaline and 70% of the radioactivity excreted in urine was a conjugate of terbutaline.— D. S. Davies *et al.*, *Br. J. clin. Pharmac.*, 1974, *1*, 129.

A study of terbutaline pharmacokinetics in 5 asthmatic children following high and low doses of terbutaline. Patients received either 75 or 250 µg of terbutaline per kg body-weight, by mouth, up to a maximum dose, in the latter case, of 5 mg. Although both doses resulted in improved peak expiratory flow-rate this was significant only after the higher dose which produced a steady increase in plasma terbutaline concentrations, peaking at 2 hours after ingestion. In contrast, plasma concentrations after the lower dose were more variable.— R. Dinwiddie *et al.*, *Archs Dis. Childh.*, 1983, *58*, 223. Comment. There is a marked individual variation in response to terbutaline, and high doses, in excess of 100 µg per kg have been shown to produce side-effects without concomitant improvement in pulmonary function.— I. Blumenthal (letter), *ibid.*, 663. Reply and disagreement. It is the authors' experience that children are generally more tolerant of this drug, and that higher proportionate doses are often required for therapeutic effect. However, it is agreed that individual variation may occur with any drug: the dosage should be tailored to the patient and the response to treatment. Furthermore, as previously stated, a dose of 5 mg should not be exceeded.— R. Dinwiddie (letter), *ibid.*

Uses and Administration

Terbutaline sulphate is a direct-acting sympathomimetic agent with actions and uses similar to those of salbutamol (p.1482).

In the treatment of bronchial asthma terbutaline sulphate is given by mouth in a dose of 5 mg two or three times daily; for children aged 3 to 7 years a dose of 0.75 to 1.5 mg three times daily is suggested, or 1.5 to 3 mg for older children.

Terbutaline sulphate may also be used as an aerosol in a dose of 1 or 2 inhalations of 250 µg about every 4 hours as required, to a maximum of 8 inhalations in 24 hours; a short interval is recommended between inhalations.

In the treatment of severe forms of bronchospasm terbutaline sulphate 250 µg may be given by subcutaneous, intramuscular, or slow intravenous injection up to 4 times daily; if required the dose may be doubled. Adequate oxygenation is necessary to avoid hypoxaemia. A suggested dose by injection for children aged 2 to 15 years is 10 µg per kg body-weight to a maximum total dose of 300 µg.

Terbutaline sulphate may also be given by intravenous infusion, as a solution containing 3 to 5 µg per mL in sodium chloride or glucose injection, at a rate of 0.5 to 1 mL per minute.

Recommended doses of terbutaline sulphate by inhalation as a mist depend on the ventilator machine used, and include 2 to 5 mg, or in severe cases up to 10 mg, in a volume of about 3 to 5 mL; alternatively dilution to a 0.01% solution in a sterile solution of sodium chloride 0.9% is recommended for chronic administration at a rate of 1 to 2 mg per hour.

Infusions containing 5 mg in 1 litre (5 µg per mL) have been given to arrest premature labour. The recommended initial rate of infusion is 10 µg per minute increased by 5 µg per minute at intervals of 10 minutes until contractions stop. Rates in excess of 25 µg per minute should be avoided. The maternal pulse should be monitored throughout the infusion and adjusted to avoid a maternal heart-rate of more than 135 beats per minute. Once contractions cease the dose may be decreased by 5 µg per minute at 30 minute intervals to the lowest maintenance dose that produces continued suppression of contractions. Subsequently, subcutaneous doses of 250 µg four times daily may be given for 3 days, during which period oral maintenance therapy with 5 mg three times daily should be started and continued until the 37th week of pregnancy.

ADMINISTRATION. For controversy over the appropriate dosage of terbutaline in children see under Absorption and Fate, above.

ADMINISTRATION IN RENAL FAILURE. Terbutaline could be given in usual doses by mouth to patients with renal failure. It could be given in usual doses intravenously or subcutaneously in patients with a glomerular filtration-rate of more than 50 mL per minute, but doses should be reduced to half in those with a glomerular filtration-rate of 10 to 50 mL per minute, and it should be avoided intravenously in those with a glomerular filtration-rate of less than 10 mL per minute.— W. M. Bennett *et al.*, *Am. J. Kidney Dis.*, 1983, *3*, 155.

ALLERGY. Beneficial results in patients with chronic urticaria following administration of terbutaline 1.25 mg three times daily.— B. Kennes *et al.*, *Clin. Allergy*, 1977, *7*, 35. Benefit in conjunction with ketotifen.— E. M. Saihan, *Br. J. Derm.*, 1981, *104*, 205.

Terbutaline sulphate 2.5 mg three times daily by mouth significantly reduced the incidence of coughing in a double-blind crossover study in 30 patients with chronic allergic cough unresponsive to other measures. Nine patients failed to respond until given prednisolone 15 to 30 mg daily for 3 weeks; terbutaline then maintained them free of cough.— R. Ellul-Micallef, *Br. med. J.*, 1983, *287*, 940.

For reviews of the use of beta$_2$ selective sympathomimetics in the management of asthma, including reference to the use of terbutaline, see under Salbutamol Sulphate, p.1482.

CARDIOVASCULAR DISORDERS. Results in 8 patients with severe refractory heart failure suggesting that terbutaline 0.3 µg per kg body-weight per minute by intravenous infusion might prove to be a useful agent in the acute management of heart failure.— R. Y. C. Wang *et al.*, *Am. Heart J.*, 1982, *104*, 1016. See also *idem*, *J. clin. Pharmac.*, 1983, *23*, 362. Further references to the use of terbutaline in cardiovascular disorders: *idem*, 355 (cardiogenic shock).

Terbutaline 2.5 mg four times daily by mouth for 2 weeks produced a significant increase in concentrations of high-density lipoprotein in the serum of 15 healthy subjects. However the value of such a terbutaline-induced rise in high-density lipoprotein concentration in conferring a decreased risk of coronary artery disease is conjectural, and the possibility of detrimental effects on the cardiovascular system exists.— P. L. Hooper *et al.*, *New Engl. J. Med.*, 1981, *305*, 1455.

PREGNANCY AND THE NEONATE. *Premature labour.* For comments on the efficacy of beta$_2$-selective adrenoceptor stimulants in the prevention of premature labour, see Salbutamol, p.1483.

Further references to the use of terbutaline in the management of preterm labour: I. Ingemarsson and B. Bengtsson, *Obstet. Gynec.*, 1985, *66*, 176 (good results in a retrospective review of 330 cases); M. H. Beall *et al.*, *Am. J. Obstet. Gynec.*, 1985, *153*, 854 (greater incidence of side-effects with terbutaline in a comparative study with ritodrine and magnesium sulphate); S. Kullander and L. Svanberg, *Acta obstet. gynec. scand.*, 1985, *64*, 613 (good results with vaginal application as a gel and in a vaginal ring); A. F. Kaul *et al.*, *Drug Intell. & clin. Pharm.*, 1985, *19*, 369 (use with nifedipine).

Preparations

Terbutaline Sulfate Injection *(U.S.P.)*. A sterile solution of terbutaline sulphate in Water for Injections. It should not be used if it is discolored.

Terbutaline Sulfate Tablets *(U.S.P.)*. Contain terbutaline sulphate.

Terbutaline Tablets *(B.P.)*. Terbutaline Sulphate Tablets

Proprietary Preparations

Bricanyl *(Astra, UK)*. *Tablets*, scored, terbutaline sulphate 5 mg.
Tablets (Bricanyl SA), sustained-release, terbutaline sulphate 7.5 mg.
Syrup, terbutaline sulphate 1.5 mg/5 mL.
Injection, terbutaline sulphate 500 μg per mL, in ampoules of 1 mL.
Inhaler, aerosol, terbutaline sulphate 250 μg/metered inhalation, also available with extended mouthpiece (Bricanyl Spacer Inhaler), or with plastic cone extension (Bricanyl Nebuhaler).
Inhaler (Bricanyl Turbohaler), terbutaline sulphate 500 μg/metered inhalation.
Respirator solution, terbutaline sulphate 2.5 mg/mL, in ampoules of 2 mL, or 10 mg/mL in bottles of 10 mL.

Bricanyl Compound *(Astra, UK)*. *Tablets*, terbutaline sulphate 2.5 mg, guaiphenesin 100 mg.

Bricanyl Expectorant *(Astra, UK)*. *Solution*, terbutaline sulphate 1.5 mg, guaiphenesin 66.5 mg/5 mL.

Monovent *(Lagap, UK)*. *Tablets*, scored, terbutaline sulphate 5 mg.
Tablets (Monovent SA), sustained-release, terbutaline sulphate 7.5 mg.
Syrup, terbutaline sulphate 1.5 mg/5 mL.

Proprietary Names and Manufacturers

Brethaire *(Geigy, USA)*; Brethine *(Geigy, USA)*; Bricanyl *(Arg.; Astra, Austral.; Belg.; Astra, Canad.; Draco, Denm.; Astra, Fr.; Astra, Ger.; Neth.; Draco, Norw.; Astra, S.Afr.; Draco, Swed.; Switz.; Astra, UK; Merrell Dow, USA)*; Bristurin *(Jpn)*; Feevone *(Austral.)*; Filair *(Riker, UK)*; Monovent *(Lagap, UK)*; Terbasmin *(Farmitalia, Ital.; Ifesa, Spain)*.

2108-t

Tetrahydrozoline Hydrochloride *(BANM, USAN)*.

Cloridrato de Tetrizolina; Tetryzoline Hydrochloride *(rINNM)*. 2-(1,2,3,4-Tetrahydro-1-naphthyl)-2-imidazoline hydrochloride.
$C_{13}H_{16}N_2,HCl = 236.7$.

CAS — 84-22-0 (tetrahydrozoline); 522-48-5 (hydrochloride).

Pharmacopoeias. In *Braz.* and *U.S.*

A white odourless solid. **Soluble** 1 in 3.5 of water and 1 in 7.5 of alcohol; very slightly soluble in chloroform; practically insoluble in ether. The *U.S.P.* nasal solution has a pH of between 5.3 and 6.5, and the ophthalmic solution a pH between 5.8 and 6.5. **Store** in airtight containers.

Adverse Effects and Precautions

As for Naphazoline, p.1470.

Absorption and Fate

Systemic absorption may follow topical administration of solutions of tetrahydrozoline. It is not used systemically, but it is readily absorbed from the gastro-intestinal tract.

Uses and Administration

Tetrahydrozoline hydrochloride is a sympathomimetic agent with alpha-adrenergic activity. It has actions and uses similar to those of naphazoline (p.1470). Nasal drops are used as a 0.1% solution, 2 to 4 drops being instilled in each nostril not more often than every 3 hours for the symptomatic relief of rhinitis and sinusitis. Children aged 2 to 6 years of age may be given 2 to 3 drops of a 0.05% solution instilled in each nostril not more often than every 3 hours.

Solutions containing 0.05% are used as a conjunctival decongestant.

Preparations

Tetrahydrozoline Hydrochloride Nasal Solution *(U.S.P.)*

Tetrahydrozoline Hydrochloride Ophthalmic Solution *(U.S.P.)*

Proprietary Names and Manufacturers

Cleer *(Mack, Illert., Ger.)*; Collyrium *(Wyeth, Canad.)*; Collyrium 2 *(Wyeth, USA)*; Constrilia *(P.O.S., Fr.)*; Demetil *(Farmila, Ital.)*; Ischemol *(Farmila, Ital.)*; Murine *(Abbott, Switz.)*; Murine Plus *(Abbott, Austral.; Ross, USA)*; Nasan *(Beecham-Wülfing, Ger.)*; Octilia *(SIFI, Ital.)*; Rhinopront *(Mack, Illert., Ger.)*; Soothe *(Alcon, Austral.)*; Stilla *(Angelini, Ital.)*; Tyzanol *(Pfizer, Norw.)*; Tyzine *(G.P. Laboratories, Austral.; Roerig, Belg.; Pfizer, Denm.; Pfizer, Ger.; Pfizer, S.Afr.; Pfizer, Spain; Pfizer, Switz.; Key, USA)*; Vasorinil *(Farmila, Ital.)*; Visina *(Pfizer, Spain)*; Visine *(G.P. Laboratories, Austral.; Pfizer, Ital.; Pfizer, Switz.; Unicliffe, UK; Leeming, USA)*; Visumetilen *(LOA, Arg.)*; Yxin *(Pfizer, Ger.)*.

The following names have been used for multi-ingredient preparations containing tetrahydrozoline hydrochloride— Visine A.C. *(Leeming, USA)*; Visine Plus *(G.P. Laboratories, Austral.)*.

2109-x

Tramazoline Hydrochloride *(BANM, USAN, rINNM)*.

2-(5,6,7,8-Tetrahydro-1-naphthylamino)-2-imidazoline hydrochloride.
$C_{13}H_{17}N_3,HCl = 251.8$.

CAS — 1082-57-1 (tramazoline); 3715-90-0 (hydrochloride).

Tramazoline hydrochloride is a nasal decongestant similar to naphazoline (p.1470). It has been given as a metered-dose nasal spray in doses of 120 μg into each nostril 3 or 4 times daily. In the treatment of allergic rhinitis it has also been given with dexamethasone and neomycin.

ENT DISORDERS. In 88 of 93 patients undergoing nasal surgery the use of a nasal spray containing tramazoline, dexamethasone isonicotinate, and neomycin sulphate (Tobispray) was a very good alternative to nasal packing.— L. W. Wing, *Med. J. Aust.*, 1977, *1*, 752. See also D. A. Sykes *et al.*, *Lancet*, 1986, *2*, 359 (dexamethasone and tramazoline alone or with neomycin in mucopurulent rhinosinusitis).

Proprietary Preparations

Dexa-Rhinaspray *(Boehringer Ingelheim, UK)*. *Nasal spray*, aerosol, tramazoline hydrochloride 120 μg, dexamethasone isonicotinate 20 μg, neomycin sulphate 100 μg/metered dose. *Dose.* 1 metered dose in each nostril up to 6 times daily.

Proprietary Names and Manufacturers

Biciron *(Basotherm, Ger.)*; Ellatun *(Basotherm, Ger.)*; Rhinaspray *(Boehringer Ingelheim, Austral.)*; Rhinogutt *(Ger.; Neth.)*; Rhinospray *(Belg.; Thomae, Ger.; Neth.; Boehringer Ingelheim, Spain)*; Rinogutt *(Boehringer Ingelheim, Ital.)*; Spray-Tish *(Boehringer Ingelheim, Austral.)*.

The following names have been used for multi-ingredient preparations containing tramazoline hydrochloride— Dexa-Rhinaspray *(Boehringer Ingelheim, UK)*; Tobispray *(Boehringer Ingelheim, Austral.)*.

2110-y

Tretoquinol Hydrochloride *(pINNM)*.

AQ-110; Ro-07-5965; Trimethoquinol Hydrochloride; Trimetoquinol Hydrochloride. (−)-1,2,3,4-Tetrahydro-1-(3,4,5-trimethoxybenzyl)isoquinoline-6,7-diol hydrochloride monohydrate.
$C_{19}H_{23}NO_5,HCl,H_2O = 399.9$.

CAS — 30418-38-3 (tretoquinol); 18559-59-6 (hydrochloride, anhydrous).

Pharmacopoeias. In *Jpn.*

Tretoquinol is reported to be a direct-acting sympathomimetic agent with general properties similar to those of salbutamol (p.1480). It has been given by mouth in doses of up to 6 mg three times daily. It has also been given by inhalation and by injection.

Proprietary Names and Manufacturers

Antene *(Syntex-Latino, Spain)*; Inolin *(Tanabe, Jpn; Neth.; Tanabe, Switz.)*; Vems *(Searle, Ital.)*.

2111-j

Tuaminoheptane *(BAN, USAN, rINN)*.

1-Methylhexylamine.
$C_7H_{17}N = 115.2$.

CAS — 123-82-0.

Pharmacopoeias. In *U.S.*

A colourless or pale yellow volatile liquid with an amine-like odour. It absorbs carbon dioxide on exposure to air, forming a white precipitate of tuaminoheptane carbonate. Specific gravity 0.760 to 0.763. **Soluble** 1 in 100 of water, 1 in 25 of alcohol, and 1 in 20 of chloroform; freely soluble in ether. **Store** in a cool place in airtight containers.

2112-z

Tuaminoheptane Sulphate *(BANM, rINNM)*.

$(C_7H_{17}N)_2,H_2SO_4 = 328.5$.

CAS — 6411-75-2.

Adverse Effects and Precautions

For the adverse effects of sympathomimetic agents, and precautions to be observed, see p.1453.

Uses and Administration

Tuaminoheptane is a volatile sympathomimetic agent which has been used for the symptomatic relief of nasal congestion. A solution of the sulphate has been used similarly.

Preparations

Tuaminoheptane Inhalant *(U.S.P.)*. Cylindrical rolls of suitable fibrous material impregnated with tuaminoheptane (as the carbonate), usually with aromatics, and contained in a suitable inhaler. Store at a temperature not exceeding 40° in airtight containers.

Proprietary Names and Manufacturers

Heptedrine *(Bellon, Belg.)*; Tuamine Sulfate *(Lilly, NZ)*.

17020-r

Tulobuterol Hydrochloride *(BANM, rINNM)*.

C-78. 2-*tert*-Butylamino-1-*o*-chlorophenylethanol hydrochloride.
$C_{12}H_{18}ClNO,HCl = 264.2$.

CAS — 41570-61-0 (tulobuterol).

Adverse Effects and Precautions

For the adverse effects of sympathomimetic agents, and precautions to be observed, see p.1453.

Uses and Administration

Tulobuterol is a direct-acting sympathomimetic with actions similar to those of salbutamol (p.1482). It has been used for its bronchodilator properties in total doses of 2 to 6 mg daily, given in divided doses by mouth. It has also been investigated by inhalation.

References: K. R. Patel, *Br. J. clin. Pharmac.*, 1985, *20*, 717 (comparison of bronchodilator effects of tulobuterol and salbutamol by inhalation); *idem*, *21*, 234 (protective effect in exercise-induced asthma); M. A. T. Javier and M. L. Noche, *J. int. med. Res.*, 1986, *14*, 228 (by mouth in childhood asthma); L. F. Chasseaud and S. G. Wood, *ibid.*, 223 (pharmacokinetics after oral doses).

Proprietary Names and Manufacturers
Atenos *(UCB, Ger.)*; Brelomax *(Abbott, Ger.; Abbott, Philipp.)*; Bremax *(Abbott, Philipp.)*.

2113-c

Tymazoline Hydrochloride *(BANM).*

2-Thymyloxymethyl-2-imidazoline Hydrochloride. 2-(2-Isopropyl-5-methylphenoxymethyl)-2-imidazoline hydrochloride.

$C_{14}H_{20}N_2O,HCl=268.8$.

CAS — 24243-97-8 (tymazoline); 28120-03-8 (hydrochloride).

Tymazoline hydrochloride is a sympathomimetic agent related to naphazoline (p.1470). A solution containing 0.05% is used as a nasal decongestant.

Proprietary Names and Manufacturers
Pernazène *(Robert et Carrière, Fr.)*.

17031-n

Xamoterol *(BAN, USAN, rINN).*

ICI-118587. *N*-[2-[2-Hydroxy-3-(4-hydroxyphenoxy)propylamino]ethyl]morpholine-4-carboxamide.

$C_{16}H_{25}N_3O_5=339.4$.

CAS — 81801-12-9 (xamoterol); 73210-73-8 (fumarate).

Xamoterol is a beta$_1$-adrenoceptor partial agonist used in the treatment of chronic heart failure. The recommended dose for adults is xamoterol 200 mg (as the fumarate) twice daily by mouth.

References: G. D. Johnston, *Br. med. J.*, 1985, *290*, 803; J. W. J. Lammers *et al.*, *Br. J. clin. Pharmac.*, 1986, *22*, 595; F. L. Tseu *et al.*, *Br. Heart J.*, 1986, *56*, 469; I. F. Goldenberg, *J. Am. med. Ass.*, 1987, *258*, 493; H. Yamashita *et al.* (letter), *Lancet*, 1987, *1*, 1431; The German and Austrian Xamoterol Study Group, *ibid.*, 1988, *1*, 489; H. Pouleur and M. F. Rousseau (letter), *ibid.*, 877; D. P. Nicholls and J. S. Elborn (letter), *ibid;* G. Kaufmann (letter), *ibid;* K. v. Olshausen (letter), *ibid.*, 1162; R. Blackwood and H. F. Marlow, *J. Am. Coll. Cardiol.*, 1988, *11*, 143A.

Proprietary Preparations
Corwin *(Stuart, UK)*. *Tablets*, xamoterol 200 mg (as fumarate).

2114-k

Xylometazoline Hydrochloride *(BANM, USAN, rINNM).*

2-(4-*tert*-Butyl-2,6-dimethylbenzyl)-2-imidazoline hydrochloride.

$C_{16}H_{24}N_2,HCl=280.8$.

CAS — 526-36-3 (xylometazoline); 1218-35-5 (hydrochloride).

Pharmacopoeias. In *Br.* and *U.S.*

A white to off-white odourless or almost odourless crystalline powder. The *B.P.* states that it is **soluble** 1 in 12 of water, 1 in 4 of alcohol, and 1 in 25 of chloroform; practically insoluble in ether. The *U.S.P.* has: soluble 1 in 35 of water. A 5% solution in water has a pH of 5.0 to 6.6. The *B.P.* nasal drops have a pH of 5.0 to 6.6, the *U.S.P.* preparation a pH of between 5.0 and 7.5. **Store** in airtight containers. Protect from light.

Adverse Effects and Precautions
As for Naphazoline, p.1470.

Uses and Administration
Xylometazoline hydrochloride is a sympathomimetic agent with actions and uses similar to those of naphazoline (p.1470). It is a vasoconstrictor with a rapid and prolonged action and is used in 0.1% solution two or three times daily for the relief of nasal congestion caused by rhinitis and sinusitis; 2 or 3 drops of the solution or 1 or 2 applications of spray are used in each nostril. A 0.05% solution is used once or twice daily for children less than 12 years of age; 1 or 2 drops of the solution are used in each nostril.

A 0.05% solution has been instilled into the eye as a conjunctival decongestant.

Preparations
Xylometazoline Nasal Drops *(B.P.)*. Xylometazoline Hydrochloride Nasal Drops
Xylometazoline Hydrochloride Nasal Solution *(U.S.P.)*

Proprietary Preparations
Otrivine *(Ciba, UK)*. *Nasal drops*, xylometazoline hydrochloride 0.1%.
Paediatric nasal drops, xylometazoline hydrochloride 0.05%.
Nasal spray, xylometazoline hydrochloride 0.1%.
Otrivine-Antistin (also known as Otrivine Hay Fever Formula) *(Ciba, UK)*. *Nasal drops*, xylometazoline hydrochloride 0.05%, antazoline sulphate 0.5%.
Nasal spray, xylometazoline hydrochloride 0.05%, antazoline sulphate 0.5%.
Otrivine-Antistin Eye Drops *(Zyma, UK)*. *Eye-drops*, xylometazoline hydrochloride 0.05%, antazoline sulphate 0.5%.

Proprietary Names and Manufacturers
4-Way Long Acting Nasal Spray *(Bristol-Myers Products, USA)*; Balkis *(Dolorgiet, Ger.)*; Nasengel *(Ratiopharm, Ger.)*; Nasenspray *(Ratiopharm, Ger.)*; Nasentropfen *(Ratiopharm, Ger.)*; Neo-Synephrine II *(Winthrop-Breon, USA)*; Olynth *(Adenylchemie, Ger.)*; Otriven *(Ciba, Ger.; Dispersa, Ger.)*; Otrivin *(Ciba, Austral.; Zyma, Austral.; Ciba-Geigy, Canad.; Ciba, Denm.; Ciba, Ital.; Neth.; Ciba, Norw.; Ciba, S.Afr.; Ciba, Spain; Ciba, Swed.; Geigy, USA)*; Otrivina *(Arg.)*; Otrivine *(Belg.; Ciba, Switz.; Ciba, UK)*; Otrix *(Austral.)*; Sinex Long-Acting *(Richardson-Vicks, USA)*; Sinutab Sinus Spray *(Parke, Davis, Canad.; Warner, S.Afr.)*; Xymelin *(DAK, Denm.)*.

The following names have been used for multi-ingredient preparations containing xylometazoline hydrochloride—Otrivin Hay-Fever Formula *(Ciba-Geigy, Canad.)*; Otrivine Hay Fever Formula *(Ciba, UK)*; Otrivine-Antistin *(Ciba, UK; Zyma, UK)*; Rynacrom Compound *(Fisons, UK)*.

Thyroid Agents

9000-k

The main hormonal activity of the normal thyroid gland is dependent upon the production of L-thyroxine (T_4) and L-tri-iodothyronine (T_3) and their production is dependent on the gland having an adequate supply of iodine. Dietary iodine, as iodide, is actively trapped by the follicular cells of the gland and converted to an oxidised form of iodine. Iodination of L-tyrosine residues present in the glycoprotein thyroglobulin then takes place to form L-mono-iodotyrosine (MIT) and L-di-iodotyrosine (DIT) and coupling of these iodotyrosines yields either L-tri-iodothyronine or L-thyroxine. The hormones are then stored, joined to thyroglobulin, in the follicular colloid and their release into the circulation is mediated by the action of lysozymes.

The thyroid hormones circulate in the blood almost entirely bound to plasma proteins. Only about 0.05% of thyroxine and 0.5% of tri-iodothyronine exist in the free unbound state.

Although both thyroxine and tri-iodothyronine are produced by the thyroid gland, thyroxine is produced in much larger quantities. The daily production by the normal gland is reported to be 70 to 90 µg of thyroxine and 15 to 30 µg of tri-iodothyronine. About 35% of the thyroxine produced is de-iodinated in peripheral tissues to yield tri-iodothyronine and some is converted to the inactive reverse tri-iodothyronine (rT_3). Thus a large proportion of the circulating tri-iodothyronine is produced from the peripheral conversion of thyroxine and not by direct glandular secretion. Tri-iodothyronine, and not thyroxine, is now considered to be the major pharmacologically active hormone.

The synthesis and secretion of thyroid hormones is regulated by complex feedback mechanisms. The thyroid gland is stimulated into production by the action of thyroid-stimulating hormone (TSH) produced in the anterior pituitary, the release of which is controlled by thyrotrophin-releasing hormone (TRH) from the hypothalamus and probably by other mechanisms. The thyroid hormones circulating in the blood act as feedback inhibitors of the secretion of both TSH and TRH. Thus when concentrations in blood are increased the secretion of both TSH and TRH will be suppressed and conversely when decreased the secretions will be stimulated.

Thyroid hormones influence most bodily functions but principally affect growth, development, and metabolic processes. Deficiency of thyroid hormones results in hypothyroidism and excess in hyperthyroidism.

Values applicable to normal thyroid physiology may be altered in various disease states, in pregnancy, and by the administration of drugs and this should be borne in mind when performing thyroid function tests.

When used exogenously L-tri-iodothyronine is known as liothyronine, thyroid-stimulating hormone as thyrotrophin, and thyroid-releasing hormone as protirelin.

ACTION. Reviews and discussions of the mechanism of action of thyroid hormones at the cellular and nuclear level.— K. Sterling, *New Engl. J. Med.*, 1979, *300*, 117; *idem*, 173; J. H. Oppenheimer, *Ann. intern. Med.*, 1985, *102*, 374.

Feedback regulation of thyroid-stimulating hormone secretion by thyroid hormones.— P. R. Larsen, *New Engl. J. Med.*, 1982, *306*, 23.

Uses and Administration

Thyroid agents are used for replacement therapy in thyroid-deficiency states such as hypothyroidism. They have also been used in certain forms of thyroiditis.

Preparations of natural origin derived from the thyroid gland of animals include thyroid and thyroglobulin and synthetic agents include thyroxine sodium and liothyronine sodium. Thyroxine sodium is usually the drug of preference for routine management.

The following equivalencies of the thyroid agents based on clinical response have been suggested: thyroxine sodium 100 µg or less; liothyronine sodium 20 to 25 µg; thyroglobulin 60 to 65 mg; and thyroid 60 to 65 mg.

HYPOTHYROIDISM. Reviews and discussions on the management of thyroid disorders, including hypothyroidism. — I. R. McDougall, *J. clin. Pharmac.*, 1981, *21*, 365; R. Wilkinson, *Prescribers' J.*, 1984, *24*, 97.

Pregnancy and the neonate. Reviews and discussions on the management of thyroid disorders in pregnancy, including hypothyroidism.— I. Ramsay, Thyroid Disease in *Medical Disorders in Obstetric Practice*, M. de Swiet (Ed.), London, Blackwell Scientific Publications, 1984, p.385; Z. M. van der Spuy and H. S. Jacobs, *Postgrad. med. J.*, 1984, *60*, 245.

9006-d

Liothyronine Sodium *(BANM, USAN, rINNM).*

3,5,3′-Tri-iodo-L-thyronine Sodium; Liothyronine Sod.; Liothyroninum Natricum; L-Tri-iodothyronine Sodium; Sodium Liothyronine. Sodium 4-*O*-(4-hydroxy-3-iodophenyl)-3,5-di-iodo-L-tyrosinate.

$C_{15}H_{11}I_3NNaO_4$=673.0.

CAS — 6893-02-3 (liothyronine); 55-06-1 (sodium salt).

NOTE. The abbreviation T_3 is often used for tri-iodothyronine in medical and biochemical reports.

Pharmacopoeias. In *Br.*, *Braz.*, *Egypt.*, *Int.*, *It.*, *Jpn*, *Nord.*, *Turk.*, and *U.S.* Also in *B.P. Vet.*

Cz. includes liothyronine. *Hung.* has liothyronine hydrochloride.

A white to buff-coloured odourless solid or a light tan-coloured odourless crystalline powder. Each g represents about 1.49 mmol of sodium. Liothyronine sodium 10.3 µg is approximately equivalent to 10 µg of liothyronine. Very slightly **soluble** to practically insoluble in water; practically insoluble in chloroform, ether, and most other organic solvents; slightly soluble in alcohol; soluble in solutions of alkali hydroxides. A solution in a mixture of hydrochloric acid and alcohol is dextrorotatory. **Store** in airtight containers. Protect from light.

Adverse Effects, Treatment, and Precautions

As for Thyroxine Sodium, p.1488. However, greater caution is required with liothyronine sodium because of its higher potency and more rapid onset of action.

OVERDOSAGE. An hour after taking 80 tablets of liothyronine 20 µg (total dose 1.6 mg), 40 tablets of brompheniramine (total dose 480 mg), and 20 tablets of clomipramine (total dose 200 mg), a 30-year-old woman arrived at hospital mentally confused but with no other signs of intoxication. Gastric lavage was performed and she was transferred to an intensive care unit, where 4 to 5 hours later she developed tachycardia (sinus rhythm 110 beats per minute) and started sweating but retained normal body temperature. Over the next 12 hours these symptoms disappeared, she became mentally orientated, and could be referred to her psychiatrist for further care. Although the laboratory findings indicated that the liothyronine overdosage had pronounced metabolic effects on thyroid hormone homoeostasis the patient had only moderate clinical signs of thyrotoxicosis, owing to the rapid clearance of liothyronine from the vascular compartment.— P. A. Dahlberg *et al.* (letter), *Lancet*, 1979, *2*, 700.

Absorption and Fate

Liothyronine sodium is almost completely absorbed from the gastro-intestinal tract. It is less readily bound to plasma proteins than thyroxine and about 0.5% exists in the unbound form. The half-life in blood of liothyronine is about 1 to 2 days in euthyroidism.

Thyroid hormones do not readily cross the placenta (see p.1489).

Uses and Administration

Liothyronine sodium is sometimes used in the treatment of thyroid-deficiency states when a rapid effect is necessary but thyroxine sodium is usually considered to be the drug of choice for routine replacement therapy. The onset of action of liothyronine is rapid, developing within a few hours of administration, and the peak therapeutic effect may be achieved after 24 to 72 hours; the duration of action is reported to be between 24 and 72 hours. Liothyronine is usually administered in 2 or 3 divided doses daily. Doses in the UK are expressed in terms of liothyronine sodium while doses in the USA are expressed in terms of liothyronine.

In hypothyroidism the initial adult dose is usually 10 to 20 or 25 µg daily by mouth increased by increments of 10 to 25 µg every 1 to 2 weeks until the thyroid deficiency is corrected. The adult maintenance dose may be between 25 and 100 µg daily. In elderly patients, in those with cardiac insufficiency, or in those with severe long-standing hypothyroidism the initial dose should usually be reduced and the increments may be smaller.

In myxoedemic coma liothyronine sodium is usually given intravenously although administration via a stomach tube has been employed. A suggested dose to be given via a stomach tube is 60 µg initially followed by 20 µg every 8 hours. For intravenous administration 5 to 20 µg by slow injection may be given initially and repeated, if necessary, usually at 12-hourly intervals; the minimum interval between doses is 4 hours. Some authorities have advocated an initial dose of 50 µg intravenously followed by further injections of 25 µg every 8 hours until improvement occurs. The dosage may then be reduced to 25 µg intravenously twice daily.

Liothyronine may also be used in the diagnosis of thyrotoxicosis in adults. Radio-iodine uptake tests are performed before and after the administration of liothyronine sodium 80 µg daily in 3 or 4 divided doses for 7 or 8 days. In patients with hyperthyroidism the uptake of radio-iodine by the thyroid gland will not be substantially affected while in the euthyroid patient the uptake will be suppressed.

Liothyronine sodium has also been used as an adjunct in hyperthyroidism as part of the block-replacement regimen. A suggested dose to be given in conjunction with carbimazole is 80 µg daily.

ADJUNCT IN HYPERTHYROIDISM. For comments on the use of thyroid hormones as part of the block-replacement regimen in the treatment of hyperthyroidism, including the treatment in pregnancy, see p.683.

DEPRESSION. Liothyronine 25 µg given daily for 2 weeks in a controlled study of euthyroid depressed patients enhanced the antidepressant activity of imipramine 150 mg daily.— A. Coppen *et al.*, *Archs gen. Psychiat.*, 1972, *26*, 234. Liothyronine in doses of 20 and 40 µg significantly enhanced the antidepressant effect of amitriptyline in a controlled study of 52 patients. This effect was more pronounced with the higher dose and in women.— D. Wheatley, *Archs gen. Psychiat.*, 1972, *26*, 229. In 33 depressed women resistant to treatment with amitriptyline in doses of up to 200 mg daily, liothyronine was given in addition in doses of 20 to 40 µg daily, resulting in improvement in 23 after 7 days; the remaining 10 did not respond. In a further 16 amitriptyline-resistant women the dose of amitriptyline was increased to 300 to 350 mg daily, and produced an improvement in 4 cases. Dysphoria and anxiety in 1 patient given liothyronine led to discontinuation. It was suggested that liothyronine is effective in patients with subclinical hypothyroidism, which contributes to depression; patients in this group had T_3 and T_4 values in the low normal range.— C. M. Banki, *Eur. J. clin. Pharmac.*, 1977, *11*, 311. The view that depression and other non-thyroidal disorders should not be treated with thyroid hormones unless there is a proved thyroid deficiency.— I. R. McDougall, *J. clin. Pharmac.*, 1981, *21*, 365. In 12 patients with depression who had gained no response or only a partial response to amitriptyline or imipramine given for periods of between 26 and 112 days the addition of liothyronine 25 or 50 µg daily to therapy produced improvement in 9.— F. K. Goodwin *et al.*, *Am. J. Psychiat.*, 1982, *139*, 34.

HYPOTHYROIDISM. For comments regarding the choice of thyroid hormones for replacement therapy in hypothyroidism, see Thyroxine Sodium, p.1490.

Administration with thyroxine. For the administration of liothyronine sodium together with thyroxine sodium, see Thyroxine Sodium, p.1490.

Induced hypothyroidism. For reference to the use of liothyronine for hypothyroidism in patients following treatment for thyroid carcinoma, see Thyroxine Sodium, p.1490.

Myxoedemic coma. Initial treatment for patients in myxoedemic coma should be with liothyronine sodium 10 to 20 µg given by intravenous injection, followed by up to 50 µg daily given by intravenous injection in small doses at 6-hourly intervals or by slow intravenous infusion.— G. A. Smart, *Prescribers' J.*, 1972, *12*, 112.

The successful use of liothyronine given intravenously to 5 patients with myxoedemic coma. The dose of liothyronine given during the first 24 hours varied from 10 to 50 µg; the total amount given intravenously ranged from 30 to 240 µg.— A. A. Khaleeli, *Postgrad. med. J.*, 1978, *54*, 825.

OBESITY. A brief review of the use of thyroid hormones for obesity. Liothyronine or thyroxine should be used in physiological replacement doses only for obese patients in whom hypothyroidism can be documented clearly by clinical and laboratory criteria.— R. S. Rivlin, *New Engl. J. Med.*, 1975, *292*, 26. A similar view stating that obesity and other non-thyroidal disorders should not be treated with thyroid hormones unless there is a proved thyroid deficiency.— I. R. McDougall, *J. clin. Pharmac.*, 1981, *21*, 365.

A double-blind study comparing the weight loss of obese patients given a very-low-calorie liquid dietary regimen together with liothyronine sodium 20 µg thrice daily, and that of similar patients given the dietary regimen and placebo tablets. Results broadly supported other views that there are some obese patients, albeit a small proportion of the total, who become metabolically adapted to low-calorie diets. In such patients small doses of liothyronine and a very low-calorie formula diet may be effective, although further studies are needed to determine whether protein supplements would be necessary for long-term nitrogen balance.— R. Moore *et al.*, *Lancet*, 1980, *1*, 223. Comments and criticisms.— W. H. Taylor (letter), *ibid.*, 652; G. C. Schussler (letter), *ibid.* Reply.— R. Moore *et al.* (letter), *ibid.*

For a report of hypothyroidism following the withdrawal of liothyronine used to treat simple obesity, and a recommendation to avoid thyroid hormones for this purpose, see Thyroxine Sodium, p.1491.

Preparations

Liothyronine Sodium Tablets *(U.S.P.)*. Tablets containing liothyronine sodium. Potency is expressed in terms of the equivalent amount of liothyronine.

Liothyronine Tablets *(B.P.)*. L-Tri-iodothyronine Sodium Tablets. Tablets containing liothyronine sodium.

Liotrix Tablets *(U.S.P.)*. Tablets containing thyroxine sodium and liothyronine sodium.

Proprietary Preparations

Tertroxin *(Glaxo, UK)*. *Tablets*, scored, liothyronine sodium 20 µg.

Triiodothyronine Injection *(Glaxo, UK)*. *Injection*, powder for reconstitution, liothyronine sodium 20 µg (with dextran).

Proprietary Names and Manufacturers

3-I-T-Bowers *(Arg.)*; Cynomel *(Merrell, Fr.; Smith Kline & French, Switz.)*; Cytomel *(Belg.; Smith Kline & French, Canad.; Neth.; Smith Kline & French, USA)*; Halotri *(Spain)*; J-Tiron *(Ital.)*; Linomel *(Arg.)*; Ro-Thyronine *(USA)*; Tertroxin *(Glaxo, Austral.; Glaxo, Denm.; Glaxo, S.Afr.; Glaxo, UK)*; Thybon *(Hoechst, Ger.)*; Thyrotardin *(Henning Berlin, Ger.)*; Tironina *(Spain)*; Ti-Tre *(Glaxo, Ital.)*; Trithyrone *(Fr.)*.

The following names have been used for multi-ingredient preparations containing liothyronine sodium— Euthroid *(Parke, Davis, USA)*; Thyrolar *(Rorer, Canad.; USV Pharmaceutical Corp., USA)*.

9007-n

Thyroglobulin *(USAN, rINN)*.

CAS — 9010-34-8.

Pharmacopoeias. In *U.S.*

Thyroglobulin *(U.S.P.)* is an extract obtained by the fractionation of thyroid glands from the hog, *Sus scrofa* (Suidae). On hydrolysis it yields not less than 90% and not more than 110% of the labelled amounts of thyroxine and liothyronine. It is free from iodine in inorganic form or in any combination other than that peculiar to thyroglobulin. It loses not more than 5% of its weight on drying. It may contain a suitable diluent such as glucose, lactose, sodium chloride, starch, or sucrose.

A cream- to tan-coloured free-flowing powder with a slight characteristic odour. Practically **insoluble** in water, alcohol, chloroform, carbon tetrachloride, dimethylformamide, and hydrochloric acid. **Store** in airtight containers.

Adverse Effects, Treatment, and Precautions

As for Thyroxine Sodium, p.1488.

Uses and Administration

Thyroglobulin has been administered to provide the effects of thyroxine and of liothyronine which are the active principles.

It has been used in the treatment of adult hypothyroidism in an initial daily dose by mouth of 16 to 32 mg gradually increased up to a maintenance dose usually between 32 and 200 mg daily.

Preparations

Thyroglobulin Tablets *(U.S.P.)*. Tablets containing not less than 90% and not more than 110% of the labelled amounts of thyroxine and liothyronine, the labelled amounts being 36 µg of thyroxine and 12 µg of liothyronine for each 65 mg of the labelled content of thyroglobulin.

Proprietary Names and Manufacturers

Proloid *(Belg.; Parke, Davis, Canad.; Warner, S.Afr.; Parke, Davis, USA)*; Proloide *(Parke, Davis, Arg.; Parke, Davis, Spain)*.

9001-a

Thyroid *(USAN)*.

Dry Thyroid; Getrocknete Schilddrüse; Thyreoidin; Thyroid Extract; Thyroid Gland; Thyroidea; Thyroideum Siccum; Tiroide Secca.

Pharmacopoeias. In *Arg., Aust., Braz., Chin., Egypt., Fr., Hung., Ind., Int., Jpn, Mex., Pol., Port., Rus., Span., Turk.,* and *U.S.*

Thyroid *(U.S.P.)* is the cleaned, dried, and powdered thyroid gland, previously deprived of connective tissue and fat, obtained from domesticated animals used for food by man. On hydrolysis it yields not less than 90% and not more than 110% each of the labelled amounts of thyroxine and liothyronine calculated on the dried basis. It is free from iodine in inorganic form or in any combination other than that peculiar to the thyroid gland. It loses not more than 6% of its weight on drying. It may contain a suitable diluent such as glucose, lactose, sodium chloride, starch, or sucrose.

A yellowish to buff-coloured amorphous powder with a slight characteristic meat-like odour and a saline taste. **Store** in airtight containers.

Adverse Effects, Treatment, and Precautions

As for Thyroxine Sodium, p.1488.

Uses and Administration

Thyroid has been administered to provide the effects of thyroxine and of liothyronine which are the active principles.

It has been used in the treatment of adult hypothyroidism in an initial daily dose by mouth of 15 mg gradually increased up to a maintenance dose usually between 60 and 180 mg daily.

Thyroid has sometimes been given as enteric-coated tablets.

HYPOTHYROIDISM. For comments regarding the choice of thyroid hormones for replacement therapy in hypothyroidism, see Thyroxine Sodium, p.1490.

Preparations

Thyroid Tablets *(U.S.P.)*. Tablets containing not less than 85% and not more than 115% of the labelled amount of thyroxine and not less than 90% and not more than 110% of the labelled amount of liothyronine, the labelled amounts being 38 µg of thyroxine and 9 µg of liothyronine for each 65 mg of the labelled content of thyroid.

Proprietary Names and Manufacturers

Armour Thyroid *(USV Pharmaceutical Corp., USA)*; Cinetic *(IRBI, Ital.)*; S-P-T *(Fleming, USA)*; Thyranon *(Organon, Belg.; Organon, Neth.; Organon, Spain; Organon, Swed.)*; Thyrar *(USV Pharmaceutical Corp., USA)*; Thyreoid *(Kali-Chemie, Ger.)*; Thyroboline *(Choay, Fr.)*; Thyrocrine *(Lemmon, USA)*; Thyroïdine *(Labaz, Fr.)*; Tiroides *(Leo, Spain)*.

The following names have been used for multi-ingredient preparations containing thyroid— Thyropit *(Medo, UK)*.

9008-h

Thyroxine Sodium *(BAN)*.

3,5,3′,5′-Tetra-iodo-L-thyronine Sodium; Levothyroxine Sodium *(USAN, rINN)*; Levothyroxinnatrium; Levothyroxinum Natricum; L-Thyroxine Sodium; Thyroxine Sod.; Thyroxinum Natricum; Tirossina; Tiroxina Sodica. Sodium 4-*O*-(4-hydroxy-3,5-di-iodophenyl)-3,5-di-iodo-L-tyrosinate hydrate.

$C_{15}H_{10}I_4NNaO_4,xH_2O=798.9$.

CAS — 51-48-9 (L-thyroxine); 55-03-8 (sodium salt, anhydrous); 25416-65-3 (sodium salt, hydrate).

NOTE. The abbreviation T_4 is often used for thyroxine in medical and biochemical reports.

Pharmacopoeias. In *Br., Braz., Egypt., Eur., Fr., Ger., Ind., It., Jpn, Neth., Nord., Swiss, Turk.,* and *U.S. Ind., Int., and Jug.* specify the pentahydrate. *Arg.* includes a monograph on DL-thyroxine sodium . *Aust.* and *Mex.* include monographs on DL-thyroxine. Also in *B.P. Vet.*

An odourless almost white to pale brownish-yellow, tasteless, hygroscopic, amorphous or crystalline powder. It may assume a slight pink colour on exposure to light. The *U.S.P.* states that it may be obtained from the thyroid gland of domesticated animals used for food by man or be prepared synthetically. Each g of anhydrous thyroxine sodium represents about 1.25 mmol of sodium.

The *B.P.* specifies 6 to 12% loss of weight on drying; the *U.S.P.* specifies not more than 11%.

Very slightly **soluble** in water (the solubility decreasing as the pH falls); slightly soluble in alcohol; practically insoluble in acetone, chloroform, and ether; soluble in solutions of alkali hydroxides and in hot solutions of alkali carbonates. A saturated solution in water has a pH of about 8.9. The *B.P.* and *Eur.P.* state that a solution in a mixture of hydrochloric acid and alcohol is dextrorotatory. The *U.S.P.* states that a solution in a mixture of sodium hydroxide and alcohol is laevorotatory. **Store** in airtight containers. Protect from light.

Adverse Effects

The adverse effects of thyroid hormones are generally associated with excessive dosage and correspond to the symptoms of hyperthyroidism. The effects may include tachycardia, palpitations, anginal pain, cardiac arrhythmias, headache, nervousness, excitability, restlessness, insomnia, cramps in skeletal muscle, muscular weakness, tremors, sweating, flushing, intolerance to heat, fever, diarrhoea, vomiting, and excessive loss of weight. Symptoms may not appear until several days after the administration of thyroxine. All these reactions usually disappear on reduction of dosage or temporary withdrawal of treatment.

Cardiac disease may be exacerbated by the administration of thyroid hormones resulting in severe angina pectoris, myocardial infarction, or sudden cardiac death.

Gross overdosage has been reported to result in a clinical state resembling thyroid storm, and in collapse and coma.

ABUSE. Features suggestive of hyperthyroidism in 4 patients were due to the surreptitious ingestion of thyroxine-containing preparations.— R. F. Harvey, *Br. med. J.*, 1973, *2*, 35.

Thyrotoxicosis factitia, due to surreptitious ingestion of thyroid hormones, in 6 women and its diagnosis.— S. Mariotti *et al.*, *New Engl. J. Med.*, 1982, *307*, 410.

See also under Effects on muscles (below).

CARCINOGENICITY. An association between the use of thyroid hormones and an increased risk of breast cancer in women was proposed by C.C. Kapdi and J.N. Wolfe (*J. Am. med. Ass.*, 1976, *236*, 1124). A further analysis by P. Mustacchi and F. Greenspan (*J. Am. med. Ass.*, 1977, *237*, 1446) of the data from the same group of patients did not confirm such an association nor did later studies by R.B. Wallace *et al.* (*J. Am. med. Ass.*, 1978, *239*, 958), S. Shapiro *et al.* (*J. Am. med. Ass.*, 1980, *244*, 1685), and D.A. Hoffman *et al.* (*J. Am. med. Ass.*, 1984, *251*, 616).

EFFECTS ON BONES AND JOINTS. A report of slipped capital femoral epiphysis in a child during treatment with thyroxine for hypothyroidism. Slipping occurred after a period of rapid growth in response to therapy.— A. B. Zubrow *et al.*, *J. Bone Jt Surg.*, 1978, *60*, 256.

EFFECTS ON FERTILITY. A report of infertility in 2 women with iatrogenic thyrotoxicosis receiving thyroid and thyroxine respectively. Shortly after restoration to the euthyroid state both patients became pregnant.— S. S. Stoffer, *Fert. Steril.*, 1978, *29*, 468.

EFFECTS ON THE LIVER. Evidence from a study involving 8 patients with primary atrophic or Hashimoto's hypothyroidism receiving thyroxine replacement therapy that abnormally raised free thyroxine values may be accompanied by subclinical liver damage as assessed by plasma values of glutathione S-transferase. This suggested that hepatic function should be assessed periodically in patients receiving thyroxine.— G. J. Beckett *et al.*, *Br. med. J.*, 1985, *291*, 427. Comment.— P. Daggett (letter), *ibid.*, 823. Reply that studies have been extended to over 100 patients receiving thyroxine replacement therapy with findings that 20% have abnormal liver function tests. The authors were not aware, however, of patients receiving conventional doses of thyroxine in whom overt liver disease, attributable to the treatment, had developed.— G. J. Beckett and A. D. Toft (letter), *ibid.*

EFFECTS ON MUSCLES. A report of periodic paralysis developing in 3 patients who took thyroid hormones in an attempt to lose weight. Two patients were taking excessive doses of thyroid but the third, of Japanese origin, was taking thyroxine 100 µg with liothyronine 25 µg daily. It was suggested that this patient had the same defect that is responsible for periodic paralysis in endogenous thyrotoxicosis, a trait that is most common in oriental males.— R. B. Layzer and E. Goldfield, *Neurology*, 1974, *24*, 949.

Mention that thyroid hormones may occasionally induce or exacerbate a pre-existing myasthenic syndrome.— F. L. Mastaglia, *Drugs*, 1982, *24*, 304. See also.— R. J. M. Lane and P. A. Routledge, *ibid.*, 1983, *26*, 124.

EFFECTS ON THE NERVOUS SYSTEM. A report of the development of pseudotumour cerebri (benign intracranial hypertension) in 2 children shortly after the initiation of thyroxine therapy for hypothyroidism.— C. Van Dop *et al.*, *New Engl. J. Med.*, 1983, *308*, 1076. Further reports.— R. McVie (letter), *ibid.*, *309*, 731 (one child); L. C. Hymes *et al.* (letter), *ibid.*, 732 (one child).

EFFECTS ON RESPIRATION. Difficulty in breathing in one patient associated with the administration of thyroxine; serum-thyroxine concentrations were in excess of 250 nmol per mL.— M. Partridge, *Br. J. Hosp. Med.*, 1984, *31*, 288.

OVERDOSAGE. An increase in heart-rate to 104 beats per minute for a few hours was the only side-effect noted after a patient accidentally took 2 mg of thyroxine sodium instead of 200 µg on 2 successive days.— *J. Am. med. Ass.*, 1966, *197*, 379.

A woman with hypothyroidism took 10 mg of thyroxine, and vomited 2 hours later. When examined 12 hours later she was still clinically euthyroid. By the fifth day she was thyrotoxic. Propranolol hydrochloride was given from day 6 to day 16. Clinical symptoms of hypothyroidism developed on day 29 and the patient resumed thyroxine therapy.— S. E. Von Hofe and R. L. Young, *J. Am. med. Ass.*, 1977, *237*, 1361.

See also under Effects on muscles (above).

PREGNANCY AND THE NEONATE. Of 50 282 children born to mothers monitored by the Collaborative Perinatal Project 537 were found to have been exposed to thyroid or thyroxine, and possibly other drugs, at some time during the first 4 months of pregnancy. An association between exposure to these agents and cardiac malformations was detected.— O. P. Heinonen *et al.*, *Birth Defects and Drugs in Pregnancy*, Littleton MA, Publishing Sciences Group, 1977, p.388.

A study of the drug histories (in the trimester before the last menstrual period, and in the first trimester of pregnancy) of the mothers of 764 infants born with anomalies of the CNS and 764 controls did not reveal any statistically significant risk with regard to the use of thyroid hormones.— K. A. Winship *et al.*, *Archs Dis. Childh.*, 1984, *59*, 1052.

Treatment of Adverse Effects

In acute overdosage empty the stomach by aspiration and lavage or by emesis; further treatment is symptomatic. The appearance of symptoms due to thyroxine may be delayed.

Following an overdose with thyroxine (estimated intake 5 to 10 mg) a young man was treated with intravenous fluids, propranolol, gastric lavage, charcoal, and plasmaphaeresis. The amount of thyroxine calculated to have been removed by plasmaphaeresis was only 6 to 12% of that ingested, the half-life was calculated to be 2 days (usual 6 to 7 days). Because of the rapid clearance and the remarkable efficacy of medical treatment for thyrotoxicosis, it was concluded that plasmaphaeresis was appropriate in the treatment of thyroxine overdose only in life-threatening conditions.— M. E. May *et al.*, *J. Toxicol. clin. Toxicol.*, 1983, *20*, 517.

A report of thyroxine overdosage and its treatment in 2 children with a review of 9 published cases of acute overdosage with thyroid preparations. It was believed that charcoal haemoperfusion is ineffective in removing thyroid hormones and that, if the clinical situation warrants attempts to remove them, exchange transfusion should be used.— L. M. Lehrner and M. R. Weir, *Pediatrics*, 1984, *73*, 313.

Precautions

Thyroid hormones should be used with caution in patients with cardiovascular disorders including angina pectoris, arteriosclerosis, coronary artery disease, hypertension, and myocardial infarction, and in the elderly. A patient with prolonged myxoedema should be restored to normality only gradually. Patients with panhypopituitarism or other disorders predisposing to adrenal insufficiency should first be treated with corticosteroids to prevent precipitation of acute adrenocortical insufficiency.

The effect of anticoagulants may be enhanced by the concomitant administration of thyroid hormones and liothyronine has been reported to enhance the effects of tricyclic antidepressants. Diabetic patients receiving thyroid hormones should be monitored for increased requirements of insulin or oral hypoglycaemic agents. If thyroxine therapy is initiated in digitalised patients, the dose of digitalis may require adjustment.

EFFECTS ON THE HEART. Aldosterone excretion rates and plasma-aldosterone concentrations were monitored in 10 patients being treated with incremental doses of thyroxine for myxoedema. At a dose of 200 µg, thyroxine precipitated heart failure in 2 patients, both of whose plasma-aldosterone concentrations had risen abnormally. The heart failure resolved on reduction of the dose. One of the mechanisms of heart failure in myxoedematous patients treated rapidly with thyroxine might be induction of aldosterone with consequent salt and water retention.— P. Marks *et al.*, *Lancet*, 1978, *2*, 1277. See also K. Ølgaard and K. Borup (letter), *ibid.*, 1979, *1*, 218. Sodium retention in hypothyroid patients receiving thyroxine may have a second mechanism as well as aldosterone induction. On theoretical grounds spironolactone might be useful to reduce the risk of cardiac failure.— G. Huston (letter), *ibid.*, 387.

INTERACTIONS. *Barbiturates*. An 80-year-old woman who had been taking thyroxine 300 µg daily and 2 capsules of Tuinal (each containing quinalbarbitone sodium 100 mg and amylobarbitone sodium 100 mg), for many years, became thyrotoxic on halving her nightly dose of Tuinal. She recovered after discontinuation of her thyroxine for a week and restarting at a dose of 150 µg daily. She appears to have been euthyroid on a supranormal dose of thyroxine owing to lowering of her circulating thyroid-hormone concentrations by barbiturates.— B. I. Hoffbrand (letter), *Lancet*, 1979, *2*, 903.

Beta-blockers. Studies in healthy subjects receiving thyroxine and propranolol suggested that propranolol impairs de-iodination of iodothyronines resulting in decreased serum concentrations of tri-iodothyronine and increased serum concentrations of reverse tri-iodothyronine; the serum-thyroxine concentrations were not affected. It was suggested that any changes of serum concentration of tri-iodothyronine in patients receiving propranolol should be interpreted with caution.— J. B. Chambers *et al.*, *J. clin. Pharmac.*, 1982, *22*, 110. A study on thyroid hormone changes in 40 patients with acute myocardial infarction. The magnitude of the fall in tri-iodothyronine plasma-concentrations, and the concomitant rise in plasma concentration of 3,3′,5′-tri-iodothyronine [reverse tri-iodothyronine], was directly correlated with the severity of the infarction. Beta-blockade with alprenolol 200 mg twice daily for five days following admission did not demonstrate any significant effect on thyroid hormone levels in 19 of the patients compared with placebo in the remaining 21, implying that alprenolol can be given in acute myocardial infarction without any additional disturbance of the physiologically-active thyroid hormones.— F. Pedersen *et al.*, *Eur. J. clin. Pharmac.*, 1984, *26*, 669.

Cholestyramine. Studies in 5 healthy subjects indicated that cholestyramine interferes with the absorption of thyroxine, that this is greatest when the two drugs are given simultaneously, and that it can be reduced by allowing about 5 hours to elapse before giving the second of the two drugs.— R. C. Northcutt *et al.*, *J. Am. med. Ass.*, 1969, *208*, 1857. See also *ibid.*, 1898.

Ketamine. Marked hypertension and tachycardia in 2 patients undergoing ketamine anaesthesia possibly due to an interaction between ketamine and thyroxine which both patients were receiving.— J. A. Kaplan and L. H. Cooperman, *Anesthesiology*, 1971, *35*, 229.

Phenytoin. Cardiac complications developed in one patient when phenytoin was added to treatment with quinidine sulphate and thyroxine sodium. Phenytoin should be given with caution to patients receiving thyroid replacement therapy because it displaced bound thyroxine from plasma protein.— M. Fulop *et al.*, *J. Am. med. Ass.*, 1966, *196*, 454. Two cogent criticisms.— S. Farzan and H. L. Gasper (letters), *ibid.*, *197*, 63.

A report of a young woman receiving long-term thyroxine replacement therapy who developed clinical hypothyroidism following the addition of phenytoin to her medication; the symptoms of hypothyroidism improved following an increase in the dosage of thyroxine and continuation of phenytoin.— J. L. Blackshear *et al.*, *Ann. intern. Med.*, 1983, *99*, 341.

Tricyclic antidepressants. A 61-year-old woman taking thyroxine developed supraventricular fibrillation or tachycardia on 3 occasions when imipramine was added to her treatment.— K. B. Ramanathan and C. Davidson, *Br. med. J.*, 1975, *1*, 661.

For reports of liothyronine enhancing the antidepressant effect of tricyclic antidepressants, see p.1487.

Absorption and Fate

Thyroxine sodium is incompletely and variably absorbed from the gastro-intestinal tract, especially when taken with food. It is almost completely bound to plasma proteins, only about 0.05% existing as free unbound thyroxine. Most of the binding is to thyroxine-binding globulin (TBG) (about 80%); lesser amounts are bound to thyroxine-binding pre-albumin (TBPA) or to albumin. Its half-life in blood is about 6 to 7 days in euthyroidism, about 9 to 10 days in hypothyroidism, and about 3 to 4 days in hyperthyroidism. Thyroxine is de-iodinated to tri-iodothyronine as well as inactive reverse tri-iodothyronine in peripheral tissues. Some thyroxine is also metabolised in the liver and excreted in the bile.

Thyroid hormones do not readily cross the placenta and replacement therapy in hypothyroid women should not normally be discontinued during pregnancy. Minimal amounts of thyroid hormones are reported to be excreted in breast milk.

ABSORPTION. Malabsorption of thyroxine had been described in coeliac disease.— *Drug & Ther. Bull.*, 1976, *14*, 57.

BIOAVAILABILITY. References to the differing bioavailability and potency of commercially available preparations of thyroxine in the USA.— A. Ramos-Gabatin *et al.*, *J. Am. med. Ass.*, 1982, *247*, 203; S. S. Stoffer and W. E. Szpunar, *ibid.*, 1984, *251*, 635; C. T. Sawin *et al.*, *Ann. intern. Med.*, 1984, *100*, 641; J. V. Hennessey and L. Wartofsky (letter), *ibid.*, *101*, 140; S. S. Stoffer (letter), *ibid;* J. I. Hamburger (letter), *ibid; Med. Lett.*, 1984, *26*, 41.

PREGNANCY AND THE NEONATE. *Excretion in breast milk.* Thyroxine was not considered to enter milk in significant concentrations.— R. L. Savage, *Adverse Drug React. Bull.*, 1976, (Dec.), 212. Endogenous thyroxine may be secreted into milk in amounts sufficient to mask signs of hypothyroidism in the suckling baby.— *Br. med. J.*, 1977, *2*, 1589. Following childbirth there is no contra-indication to breast feeding just because the mother is taking thyroxine. Usually the dose of thyroxine will need to be reduced post partum because of the loss of weight.— I. Ramsay, Thyroid Disease, in *Medical Disorders in Obstetric Practice*, M. de Swiet (Ed.), London, Blackwell Scientific Publications, 1984, p.385.

Uses and Administration

Thyroxine sodium is employed in the treatment of thyroid-deficiency states. Because of its long half-life the peak therapeutic effect with regular oral administration may not be achieved for 1 to 2 weeks and the duration of action after withdrawal is estimated to be between 1 and 3 weeks. A single daily dose is usually satisfactory and because of its irregular absorption thyroxine sodium is best taken on an empty stomach.

In hypothyroidism the initial adult dose of thyroxine sodium is 50 or 100 µg daily by mouth increased by increments of 50 µg every 2 to 4 weeks until the thyroid deficiency is corrected, usually with a dose of 200 µg or less. The adult maintenance dose is commonly between 100 and 200 µg daily. In elderly patients, in those with cardiac insufficiency, or in those with severe hypothyroidism of long-standing the initial dose should usually be reduced to 12.5 to 25 µg daily, followed by increments of 25 to 50 µg at 2-to 4-week intervals.

In myxoedemic coma, where a rapid response is required, thyroxine sodium may be given intravenously. In the absence of cardiac disease, a suggested dose is 200 to 500 µg (2 to 5 mL of a solution containing 100 µg per mL) initially, followed on the next day by 100 to 300 µg if there is no evidence of improvement. Thereafter smaller doses may be given until the patient can tolerate administration by mouth.

Thyroxine sodium is also used in the treatment of congenital hypothyroidism. Suggested daily doses by mouth are: 0 to 6 months, 25 to 50 µg (8 to 10 µg per kg body-weight); 6 to 12 months, 50 to 75 µg (6 to 8 µg per kg); 1 to 5 years, 75 to 100 µg (5 to 6 µg per kg); 6 to 12 years, 100 to 150 µg (4 to 5 µg per kg); over 12 years, 150 to 200 µg (2 to 3 µg per kg).

Thyroxine sodium is also used to treat hypothyroidism occurring in patients after therapy for hyperthyroidism or thyroid cancer and has been used as an adjunct in hyperthyroidism as part of the block-replacement regimen.

ADJUNCT IN HYPERTHYROIDISM. For comments on the use of thyroid hormones as part of the block-replacement regimen in the treatment of hyperthyroidism, including the treatment in pregnancy, see p.683.

HYPOTHYROIDISM. Comment, based on clinical experience and studies, that the use of thyroid extract for the treatment of hypothyroidism should be abandoned.— W. van't Hoff *et al.* (letter), *Br. med. J.*, 1978, *2*, 200; I. M. Jackson and W. E. Cobb, *Am. J. Med.*, 1978, *64*, 284; R. Penny and S. D. Frasier, *Am. J. Dis. Child.*, 1980, *134*, 16.

Comment that thyroxine is the drug of choice for routine thyroid replacement therapy.— *Med. Lett.*, 1977, *19*, 50; I. R. McDougall, *J. clin. Pharmac.*, 1981, *21*, 365; R. Wilkinson, *Prescribers' J.*, 1984, *24*, 97. See also under Induced hypothyroidism (below).

In recent years many studies have been published regarding the appropriate dose of thyroxine (as the sodium salt) to be given as replacement therapy to hypothyroid patients and the relevant methods for monitoring the response in such patients. D. Evered *et al.* (*Br. med. J.*, 1973, *3*, 131) reported that in 22 patients with untreated symptomatic hypothyroidism adequate control, as assessed by clinical response and reduction of serum-TSH concentrations to normal, was achieved with daily doses of thyroxine 100 µg in 13, with 150 µg in 6, and with 200 µg in 3. They concluded that the results strongly supported the view that the then conventional doses of thyroxine of 200 to 400 µg daily often induced a mild state of hyperthyroidism which could not be detected by clinical methods alone; they also considered that it was not possible to be certain whether this mild state of hyperthyroidism was detrimental to the patient. Likewise, in a similar study involving 44 patients, J.M. Stock *et al.* (*New Engl. J. Med.*, 1974, *290*, 529) found that 89% of the patients required doses of thyroxine between 100 and 200 µg daily. Following this, an analysis published in 1980 by the Scottish Automated Follow-up Register Group (*Br. med. J.*, 1980, *281*, 969), of the prescribing patterns and problems of thyroxine replacement therapy showed that many patients were still receiving more than the replacement doses suggested by the previous studies to be optimal for suppressing serum-TSH concentrations. However it still remained to be shown whether these patients did have persisting biochemical or other evidence of hyperthyroidism and what effect "overtreatment" had on long-term morbidity and mortality. C.J. Pearce and R.L. Himsworth (*Br. med. J.*, 1984, *288*, 693) then conducted a study of the total and free concentrations of thyroxine and tri-iodothyronine in 122 clinically euthyroid patients stabilised on thyroxine (daily doses of 100 µg in 18, 150 µg in 29, 200 µg in 72, and 300 µg in 3). This revealed that in 52 the free thyroxine was raised while in only 8 was the free tri-iodothyronine raised. They considered that although physiological measurements could show evidence of overexposure to thyroid hormones there were no deleterious biological consequences of the lack of fine tuning of dosage. Commenting on this work J.H. Marigold *et al.* (*Br. med. J.*, 1984, *289*, 699) recommended that in addition to clinical examination, serum concentrations of TSH and free tri-iodothyronine should be estimated in patients on long-term thyroxine therapy, especially in the elderly. In contradiction to the work of Pearce and Himsworth is a report by P.E. Jennings *et al.* (*Br. med. J.*, 1984, *289*, 1645) of 15 patients with primary hypothyroidism receiving thyroxine 100 to 200 µg daily. These patients had raised concentrations of free thyroxine, total thyroxine, and reverse tri-iodothyronine with normal values of free and total tri-iodothyronine; this suggested that raised serum-thyroxine concentrations were often associated with tissue thyrotoxicosis as assessed by cardiovascular and pituitary responses. Jennings *et al.* concluded that a raised circulating thyroxine value might be indicative of tissue thyrotoxicosis and should prompt the lowering of the dose. This work was, however, criticised by J.A. Franklyn and M.C. Sheppard (*Br. med. J.*, 1985, *290*, 393) who felt that on the basis of the evidence presented a reduction in the dosage of thyroxine in all patients with a total or free thyroxine measurement above the normal range was not justified. A reduction might be more sensibly confined to patients in whom a high serum concentration of tri-iodothyronine was documented in addition to a high serum-thyroxine concentration in the presence of clinical signs or symptoms of thyrotoxicosis. However, W.D. Fraser *et al.* (*Br. med. J.*, 1985, *290*, 394) stated that in their experience measurement of tri-iodothyronine was of little value. In another study of 38 clinically euthyroid patients receiving thyroxine 75 to 200 µg daily for primary hypothyroidism and of 6 receiving 100 to 200 µg daily after ablative radio-iodine therapy for thyroid carcinoma, R.J. Mardell *et al.* (*Br. med. J.*, 1985, *290*, 355) confirmed that thyroxine treatment might result in raised concentrations of free thyroxine accompanied by normal concentrations of free tri-iodothyronine. The suggestion was made again that these patients had received too much thyroxine and were subclinically hyperthyroid. G.J. Beckett *et al.* (*Br. med. J.*, 1985, *291*, 427) in a study involving 8 patients with primary atrophic or Hashimoto's hypothyroidism receiving thyroxine 100 to 200 µg daily found that during therapy 3 patients had abnormally raised free thyroxine concentrations but of these only one had an abnormally raised total thyroxine value; free and total tri-iodothyronine concentrations were within the normal range for all 8 patients. In all 3 patients with raised free thyroxine values abnormally high plasma values of glutathione S-transferase (an indicator of hepatocellular damage) were also detected suggesting that administration of thyroxine in doses which result in raised plasma concentrations of free thyroxine may produce subclinical liver damage. They concluded that patients should be monitored by the measurement of free, not total, hormone concentrations, and that in those in whom the free thyroxine value was raised the dose of thyroxine should be reduced.

Administration in cardiac disorders and the elderly. A study in 23 elderly and 44 younger adult patients with primary hypothyroidism revealed that the average replacement dose of thyroxine in the older group was 118 µg daily and was significantly less than that of 158 µg daily required by the younger group; the difference remained significant when defined by body-weight (1.86 µg per kg daily and 2.06 µg per kg daily respectively).— R. L. Rosenbaum and U. S. Barzel, *Ann. intern. Med.*, 1982, *96*, 53.

Whilst full thyroxine replacement dosage can often be administered from the initiation of treatment without untoward effects, in severely hypothyroid patients, in the elderly, or in individuals with heart disease it is wise to build up the dose gradually. Initially thyroxine [sodium] 25 to 50 µg daily is given increasing by 25 to 50 µg at 2 to 4 week intervals until a full replacement dose is reached. The replacement dose of thyroxine is usually between 100 and 200 µg daily.— R. Wilkinson, *Prescribers' J.*, 1984, *24*, 97.

Administration with liothyronine. In a comparison of thyroxine sodium with a combined preparation of thyroxine sodium and liothyronine sodium in 87 hypothyroid patients, thyroxine alone was preferred because side-effects occurred less frequently.— R. N. Smith *et al.*, *Br. med. J.*, 1970, *4*, 145.

A view that there is no justification for the use of tablets containing both thyroxine and liothyronine.— R. Wilkinson, *Prescribers' J.*, 1984, *24*, 97.

Congenital hypothyroidism. The presence of endemic goitre due to iodine deficiency has a deleterious effect on the outcome of pregnancy. In mothers who are euthyroid the iodine deficiency during the first three months of pregnancy may lead to failure of proper development of the fetal central nervous system so that the baby is born with neurological cretinism. The baby is usually euthyroid, more often than not has a goitre, but is suffering from mental retardation, deafness, and spasticity. This type of cretinism, which is due to iodine deficiency and not fetal hypothyroidism, does not respond to any form of treatment. When iodine deficiency leads to fetal hypothyroidism in the second and third trimesters of pregnancy, the baby is born as a hypothyroid cretin. The baby is lethargic, has a large tongue, a hoarse cry, dry coarse skin, a pot belly, and sometimes an umbilical hernia. Neonatal jaundice may be prolonged, the infant feeds badly, is constipated, and has weak muscles; goitre is rarely present. This type of cretinism responds to thyroid hormone replacement, the efficacy of which is directly related to how soon after birth it is started.— I. Ramsay, Thyroid Disease in *Medical Disorders in Obstetric Practice*, M. de Swiet (Ed.), London, Blackwell Scientific Publications, 1984, p.385.

A review and discussion regarding the screening and treatment of congenital hypothyroidism. It has been recognised for many years that thyroxine replacement therapy is very effective at reversing the symptoms of congenital hypothyroidism but it is less well known that as a result of thyroxine deficiency in the neonatal period many hypothyroid children suffer long-term neurological problems which do not respond so readily to treatment; probably the most devastating of these problems for the child is mental retardation. The recognition that mental retardation in congenital hypothyroidism is largely preventable along with recent technical advances has been a great spur to the widespread introduction of neonatal screening for congenital hypothyroidism. During 1982 all areas of the United Kingdom will be screened and a central register has been established to evaluate the results. The benefits of screening may be reduced by inadequate treatment, so attention now needs to be focussed on giving the children optimal replacement therapy; it is important that the dose should be related to the child's age and weight and that regular biochemical monitoring be undertaken. A suitable daily dose of thyroxine [sodium] is: 0 to 6 months, 25 to 50 µg (8 to 10 µg per kg body-weight); 6 to 12 months, 50 to 75 µg (6 to 8 µg per kg); 1 to 5 years, 75 to 100 µg (5 to 6 µg per kg); 6 to 12 years, 100 to 150 µg (4 to 5 µg per kg); over 12 years, 150 to 200 µg (2 to 3 µg per kg). The treatment of congenital hypothyroidism is not particularly complicated but does require close supervision, particularly during infancy, as the long-term implications are so important. With a combination of early diagnosis by screening and good subsequent management, the potentially damaging effects of pre-natal hypothyroidism should be almost entirely preventable.— J. A. Hulse, *Pharm. J.*, 1982, *228*, 644.

In a study of 141 hypothyroid children to provide retrospective control data for a neonatal screening programme for congenital hypothyroidism, the best intellectual prognosis was for those children diagnosed and starting treatment before 6 weeks of age. Of the 6 children so diagnosed none was mentally retarded compared with 75% of those diagnosed between 6 and 9 months.— J. A. Hulse, *Archs Dis. Childh.*, 1984, *59*, 23.

Induced hypothyroidism. In most clinical situations thyroxine is the preferred form of replacement. Liothyronine has a role in patients who are athyreotic [hypothyroid] after treatment for thyroid carcinoma and who undergo whole-body radio-iodine scans to detect metastases. In these patients it is necessary to discontinue the hormone therapy prior to the diagnostic scan; liothyronine, because of its shorter half-life, need only be stopped for 2 to 3 weeks, whereas thyroxine has to be stopped for 4 to 6 weeks. Liothyronine is given in doses of 20 to 25 µg three times daily. Even in this situation the author prefers thyroxine because of the smoother status of the patient on treatment.— I. R. McDougall, *J. clin. Pharmac.*, 1981, *21*, 365.

Pregnancy and the neonate. The use of thyroxine in the intra-uterine treatment of a hypothyroid foetus whose mother had inadvertently received iodine-131 during the thirteenth week of pregnancy. The mother was severely myxoedematous at the twenty-fourth week of pregnancy and received liothyronine 100 µg daily by mouth. In addition, because of the high risk of foetal hypothyroidism and because of the limited placental transfer of iodothyronines, transabdominal transuterine injections of thyroxine sodium 120 µg were given into the buttock of the foetus beginning at 32 weeks; four such injections were given at 2-week intervals, the last being 2 weeks before parturition. The infant, who showed no signs of cretinism, received thyroxine 50 µg daily starting immediately after birth but testing at 3 years suggested mild developmental retardation.— A. J. Van Herle *et al.*, *J. clin. Endocr. Metab.*, 1975, *40*, 474. A favourable report of the intra-amniotic injection of thyroxine 500 µg weekly for about 6 weeks to counter possible hypothyroidism in the foetus; the mother had inadvertently been given iodine-131 during pregnancy.— E. S. Lightner *et al.*, *Am. J. Obstet. Gynec.*, 1977, *127*, 487.

Once hypothyroidism has been diagnosed in the pregnant woman treatment should be instituted without delay. So long as the woman has no evidence of disease, replacement therapy can be instituted rapidly. Thyroxine [sodium] can be given in an initial dose of 100 µg every morning for a week and then adjusted according to the patient's weight; a replacement dose of 2 µg per kg body-weight provides a rough guide. It is wise to check the hormone concentrations monthly during the rest of pregnancy, because as the patient gains more weight, the dosage of thyroxine may need to be increased.— I. Ramsay, Thyroid Disease, in *Medical Disorders in Obstetric Practice*, M. de Swiet (Ed.), London, Blackwell Scientific Publications, 1984, p.385. See also.— Z. M. van der Spuy and H. S. Jacobs, *Postgrad. med. J.*, 1984, *60*, 245.

OBESITY. A brief review of the use of thyroid hormones as therapy for obesity. Liothyronine or thyroxine should be used in physiological replacement doses only for obese patients in whom hypothyroidism can be documented clearly by clinical and laboratory criteria.— R. S. Rivlin, *New Engl. J. Med.*, 1975, *292*, 26. A similar view stating that obesity, and other non-thyroidal disorders should not be treated with thyroid hormones unless there is a proven thyroid deficiency.— I. R. McDougall, *J. clin. Pharmac.*, 1981, *21*, 365.

A report of hypothyroidism developing in 5 patients following the withdrawal of thyroxine or liothyronine which had been used for the management of simple obesity; all patients had been clinically euthyroid at the start of treatment. Since the administration of exogenous thyroxine and liothyronine is of debatable value in the treatment of simple obesity and the incidence of subclinical auto-immune thyroiditis relatively common, the use of this treatment should be reconsidered.— A. Dornhorst *et al.* (letter), *Lancet*, 1981, *1*, 52.

Preparations

Levothyroxine Sodium Tablets *(U.S.P.)*

Thyroxine Tablets *(B.P.)*. Thyroxine Sodium Tablets; L-Thyroxine Sodium Tablets

Proprietary Preparations

Eltroxin *(Glaxo, UK)*. *Tablets*, scored, thyroxine sodium 50 µg.
Tablets, thyroxine sodium 100 µg. Potency is expressed in terms of anhydrous thyroxine sodium.

Proprietary Names and Manufacturers

Cytolen *(USA)*; Eferox *(Efeka, Ger.)*; Elthyrone *(Belg.)*; Eltroxin *(Austral.; Glaxo, Canad.; Glaxo, Denm.; Glaxo, S.Afr.; Glaxo, Switz.; Glaxo, UK)*; Euthyrox *(Belg.; E. Merck, Ger.)*; Eutirox *(Bracco, Ital.)*; Levaxin *(Nycomed, Swed.)*; Levoid *(USA)*; Levothroid *(Armour, Spain; Rorer, USA)*; Levothyroid *(USA)*; Levothyrox *(Merck-Clévenot, Fr.)*; Levotirox *(IRBI, Ital.)*; Oroxine *(Wellcome, Austral.)*; Percutacrine Thyroxinique *(Besins-Iscovesco, Fr.)*; Ro-Thyroxine *(USA)*; Synthroid *(Flint, Canad.; Flint, USA)*; Thevier *(Glaxo, Ger.)*; Thyrax *(Organon, Spain)*; Thyroxinal *(Fawns & McAllan, Austral.)*.

The following names have been used for multi-ingredient preparations containing thyroxine sodium— Euthroid *(Parke, Davis, USA)*; Thyrolar *(Rorer, Canad.; USV Pharmaceutical Corp., USA)*.

Vasodilators

9200-h

The vasodilators described in this section are mainly those used for angina pectoris or for cerebral or peripheral vascular disorders.

Vasodilators used in the management of angina pectoris include the nitrates and the calcium-channel blocking agents. The nitrates were formerly regarded as *coronary* vasodilators, but their primary mode of action is now considered to be a reduction of oxygen demand due to venodilatation. The calcium-channel blocking agents have coronary and peripheral vasodilatory activity. For further details, see Glyceryl Trinitrate, p.1501 and Nifedipine, p.1511.

Cerebral and *peripheral* vasodilators fall primarily into 3 main groups: (1) alpha-adrenoceptor blocking agents; (2) smooth muscle relaxants; and (3) those that act by simulating the effects of beta-adrenoceptor stimulation. Some agents were originally regarded as vasodilators but are now thought to act by reducing the viscosity of the blood or by altering tissue metabolism.

Other drugs that have been used in peripheral vascular and cerebral disorders include co-dergocrine mesylate (see p.1051), histamine (see p.941), acetylcholine (see p.1328), epoprostenol (see p.1371), and nicotinic acid (see p.1269). Many antihypertensive agents have powerful peripheral vasodilator effects and are described under Antihypertensive Agents, p.466.

CARDIAC DISORDERS. *Angina pectoris.* Reviews of the use of vasodilators in angina pectoris: D. Maclean and J. Feely, *Br. med. J.*, 1983, *286*, 1127; H. N. Hultgren *et al.*, *J. Am. med. Ass.*, 1985, *253*, 2555.

Heart failure. Discussion of the use of vasodilators in heart failure.— *Lancet*, 1987, *2*, 311. See also R. Genton and A. S. Jaffe, *J. Am. med. Ass.*, 1986, *256*, 2556.

PERIPHERAL VASCULAR AND CEREBRAL DISORDERS. Vasodilators are widely used for treating Raynaud's phenomenon, chronic occlusive arterial disease of the leg and cerebral vascular disorders. There is little sound rationale or proof of efficacy for the use of vasodilators in these disorders, especially since there may be structural changes in the affected arteries which make them resistant to vasodilatation. Vasodilators may in fact decrease the blood flow to ischaemic regions by 'stealing' blood into other regions. Any organic mental impairment in the elderly is often inappropriately described as a cerebral vascular disorder and assessment of drug treatment in demented patients is difficult.— G. D. O. Lowe, *Br. med. J.*, 1983, *286*, 1262.

Cerebrovascular disorders. A review summarising the pathophysiology of cerebrovascular disease and dementia and the pharmacology of cerebral vasodilators, including their use in these disorders. Cerebral vasodilators must be regarded as contra-indicated in all patients with acute stroke and may sometimes be harmful in chronic cerebrovascular disease in view of their intracerebral-steal effect.— P. Cook and I. James, *New Engl. J. Med.*, 1981, *305*, 1508 and 1560.

A discussion of the drug treatment of dementia. Pathological findings in patients with dementia call into question the use of cerebral metabolic enhancers and centrally active vasodilators. While there is no evidence of clinical benefit from the use of centrally acting vasodilators, some agents with a secondary action of enhancing cerebral metabolism, for example co-dergocrine mesylate, have been reported to improve behaviour and cognition. Other drugs that have been investigated include the opiate antagonist naloxone, the 'nootropic' drugs, for example piracetam, and cholinergic enhancers including lecithin, choline, and physostigmine. At present, even those agents which have shown some consistent improvements seem to offer neither sufficiently practical nor sufficiently sustained benefits to justify their general use outside a research setting.— J. Byrne and T. Arie, *Br. med. J.*, 1985, *290*, 1845.

Further reviews and discussions of the use of vasodilators in cerebral disorders: C. F. George and M. R. P. Hall, *Prescribers' J.*, 1981, *21*, 272 (dementia); A. Spagnoli and G. Tognoni, *Drugs*, 1983, *26*, 44 (cerebral disease); D. J. Thomas, *Br. med. J.*, 1984, *288*, 2 (stroke); L. E. Hollister, *Drugs*, 1985, *29*, 483 (Alzheimer's disease).

Peripheral vascular disorders. A review of the non-surgical management of peripheral vascular disease. There is little evidence that vasodilators have much to offer.— C. A. C. Clyne, *Br. med. J.*, 1980, *281*, 794.

Vasodilator drugs offer no benefits in theory or practice in the treatment of claudication, although those that have an effect on tissue metabolism or blood viscosity, for example naftidrofuryl or oxpentifylline, may merit a trial in selected patients with severe symptoms.— C. V. Ruckley, *Br. med. J.*, 1986, *292*, 970. See also: A. Marston, *Prescribers' J.*, 1981, *21*, 233; P. A. Blombery, *Drugs*, 1987, *34*, 404.

9201-m

Adenosine Phosphate *(BAN, USAN, rINN).*

5′-Adenylic Acid; A-5MP; Adenosine 5′-Monophosphate; Adenosine-5′-(dihydrogen phosphate); Adenosine-5′-phosphoric Acid; AMP; Monophosadénine; Muscle Adenylic Acid; NSC-20264. 6-Amino-9-β-D-ribofuranosylpurine 5′-(dihydrogen phosphate).

$C_{10}H_{14}N_5O_7P$=347.2.

CAS — 61-19-8.

Adenosine phosphate has a number of actions and has been used as a vasodilator in the treatment of complications of varicose ulcers. It has been given in usual doses of 80 to 120 mg daily by mouth or up to 100 mg daily by intramuscular injections. It has also been given for pruritus, multiple sclerosis, bursitis and tendinitis.

Adenosine base is under study as an anti-arrhythmic agent (see p.70).

Adenosine phosphate 160 to 200 mg daily for at least 4 weeks was effective in controlling all the symptoms of porphyria cutanea tarda, apart from the hypersensitivity of the skin to slight injuries, in 19 of 21 patients. The improvement lasted for several years in about half the group. Relapses responded to further treatment.— A. Gajdos (letter), *Lancet*, 1974, *1*, 163.

HERPES INFECTIONS. In an open study involving 130 patients, adenosine phosphate 1.5 to 2.0 mg per kg body-weight by intramuscular injection on alternate days for 12 to 15 injections was found to reduce the discomfort, malaise, and pain of herpes zoster infections, and to produce rapid drying and desquamation of lesions with no evidence of post-herpetic neuralgia during a 2-year follow-up (S.H. Sklar and J.S. Wigand, *Br.J. Derm.*, 1981, *104*, 351). Subsequently, similar results were obtained from a double-blind study (S.H. Sklar *et al.*, *J. Am. med. Ass.*, 1985, *253*, 1427), although only 32 patients were involved. It was also shown that adenosine phosphate treatment reduced viral shedding and cleared the virus faster than placebo. Sherlock and Corey (*ibid.*, 1444) expressed concern over the small number of patients in the study, the comparability of the treatment groups, and over the potential toxicity of adenosine phosphate which could affect most tissues and the immune, vascular, neural, and endocrine systems. It was generally agreed (S.H. Sklar *et al.*, *ibid.*, *254*, 912) that further studies were necessary.

Proprietary Names and Manufacturers

Adenyl *(Ayerst, Fr.; Auclair, Switz.; Lipha, UK)*; Cobalasine *(Keene, USA)*; My-B-Den *(Dome, USA)*.

9203-v

Adenosine Triphosphate

5′-Adenyldiphosphoric Acid; Adenosine 5′-Triphosphate; Adenylpyrophosphoric Acid; ATP; Triphosadénine. Adenosine 5′-(tetrahydrogen triphosphate).

$C_{10}H_{16}N_5O_{13}P_3$=507.2.

CAS — 56-65-5.

Pharmacopoeias. Cz. includes the disodium salt under the title Natrium Adenosintriphosphoricum $C_{10}H_{14}N_5Na_2O_{13}P_3$=551.1

Adenosine triphosphate is a nucleotide constituent of animal cells with a fundamental role in biological energy transformations, being concerned with the storage and release of energy; it is converted to adenosine diphosphate, release of energy occurring during the process. Its administration has been claimed to improve peripheral and cardiac circulation and muscular power. It has been given in the treatment of a variety of rheumatic conditions and has been used in the treatment of coronary insufficiency and supraventricular tachycardia.

Adenosine base is under study as an anti-arrhythmic agent (see p.70).

A study in 10 patients suggesting that adenosine triphosphate may be effective in the treatment of paroxysmal supraventricular tachycardia.— D. Saito *et al.*, *Br. Heart J.*, 1986, *55*, 291.

Proprietary Names and Manufacturers

Adenotriphos *(Austral.; Lipha, UK)*; Atepodin *(Medix, Spain)*; Atriphos *(Hung.; Biochimica, Switz.)*; Estriadin *(Spain)*; Nucleocardyl *(Spain)*; Striadyne *(Belg.; Ayerst, Fr.)*; Striadyne forte *(Switz.)*; Triadenyl ATP *(Ger.)*; Triadesin-A *(Jpn)*; Trinosin *(Jpn)*.

18613-p

Amlodipine *(BAN, rINN).*

UK-48340-11 (maleate). 3-Ethyl 5-methyl 2-(2-aminoethoxymethyl)-4-(2-chlorophenyl)-1,4-dihydro-6-methylpyridine-3,5-dicarboxylate.

$C_{20}H_{25}ClN_2O_5$=408.9.

CAS — 88150-42-9 (amlodipine); 88150-47-4 (maleate).

NOTE. Amlodipine Maleate is *USAN*.

Amlodipine is a calcium-channel blocking agent with vasodilatory activity and actions similar to those of nifedipine (p.1511).

The minimum, effective, intravenous dose of amlodipine that produced haemodynamic effects in patients with coronary artery disease was 10 mg.— M. A. Frais *et al.*, *Br. J. clin. Pharmac.*, 1986, *22*, 232P.

Amlodipine, 2.5 mg or 10 mg daily, appeared to improve exercise time in a study of 35 male patients with chronic stable angina pectoris.— N. C. Jackson *et al.*, *Br. J. clin. Pharmac.*, 1985, *20*, 248P.

ABSORPTION AND FATE. Amlodipine was rapidly absorbed after oral administration with peak plasma amlodipine concentrations occurring at a mean of 7.8 hours. Availability following a single oral dose was between 52 and 88%, which is higher than that found with other calcium-channel blockers. The half-life was 35.7 ± 6.1 hours following a single oral dose, and 44.7 ± 8.6 hours after repeated daily dosing for 14 days. Steady-state plasma concentrations were apparently reached by the seventh dose and the small degree of fluctuation between peak and trough amlodipine concentrations was considered to favour a uniform response in patients.— J. K. Faulkner *et al.*, *Br. J. clin. Pharmac.*, 1986, *22*, 21.

Proprietary Names and Manufacturers

Pfizer, USA.

9205-q

Amyl Nitrite *(USAN).*

Amylis Nitris; Amylium Nitrosum; Azotito de Amilo; Isoamyl Nitrite; Isopentyl Nitrite; Nitrito de Amilo; Pentanolis Nitris.

$C_5H_{11}NO_2$=117.1.

Pharmacopoeias. In *Arg., Aust., Belg., Cz., Egypt., Hung., Int., It., Jpn, Jug., Mex., Nord., Pol., Port., Rus., Span., Turk.*, and *U.S.* Also in *B.P.C. 1973.*

A clear, yellow, volatile, inflammable liquid with a fragrant odour. B.p. 96°. It consists of the nitrites of 3-methylbutan-1-ol, $(CH_3)_2CH,CH_2,CH_2OH$, and 2-methylbutan-1-ol, $CH_3,CH_2,CH(CH_3),CH_2OH$, with other nitrites of the homologous series. The *U.S.P.* specifies a mixture of the nitrite esters of 3-methylbutan-1-ol and 2-methylbutan-1-ol, with not less than 85% and not more than 103% of $C_5H_{11}NO_2$.

Practically **insoluble** in water; miscible with alcohol, and ether. It is volatile even at low temperatures and is liable to decompose with evolution of nitrogen, particularly if it has become acid in reaction. **Store** in a cool place in airtight containers. Protect from light.

CAUTION. *Amyl nitrite is very inflammable and must not be used where it may be ignited.*

Adverse Effects, Treatment, and Precautions

As for Glyceryl Trinitrate, p.1500.

ABUSE. Comment on volatile nitrites being abused, in the belief that they expand creativity, stimulate music appreciation, promote a sense of abandon in dancing, and intensify sexual experience.— L. T. Sigell *et al.*, *Am. J. Psychiat.*, 1978, *135*, 1216.

Inhalation of amyl, butyl, or isobutyl nitrite has caused headache, tachycardia, syncope, acute psychosis, increased intra-ocular pressure, transient hemiparesis, methaemoglobinaemia, coma, and, rarely, sudden death.— *Med. Lett.*, 1987, *29*, 83.

The social use of amyl nitrite and other inhaled nitrites is widespread, particularly among the homosexual population (*Med. J. Aust.*, 1981, *1*, 273; T.J. McManus *et al.*, *Lancet*, 1982, *1*, 503; R.W. Wood, *New Engl. J. Med.*, 1982, *306*, 932; G.R. Newell *et al.*, *Pharmacotherapy*, 1984, *4*, 284). Amyl nitrite abuse has been implicated as a possible contributory factor in the development of opportunistic infections and Kaposi's sarcoma in homosexual men with immunodeficiency syndrome (R.O. Brennan and D.T. Durack, *Lancet*, 1981, *2*, 1338; J.J. Goedert, *et al.*, *ibid.*, 1982, *1*, 412; M. Marmor, *et al.*, *ibid.*, 1083; U. Mathur-Wagh, *et al.*, *ibid.*, 1984, *1*, 1033). However, these observations were not confirmed by Jaffe, *et al.*, (*Ann. intern. Med.*, 1983, *99*, 145) who found that nitrite abuse was not strongly associated with an increased risk of disease, and Durack (*New Engl. J. Med.*, 1981, *305*, 1465) speculated that amyl nitrite users tended to have more sexual partners than non users, and so were at higher risk of immunosuppression. Cohen (*Br. J. Hosp. Med.*, 1984, *31*, 250) believed that amyl nitrite could no longer be regarded as a major risk factor, although Mathur-Wagh (*New Engl. J. Med.*, 1985, *313*, 1542) concluded that nitrite inhalants could be a cofactor in the development of Kaposi's sarcoma.

EFFECTS ON THE BLOOD. Heinz body haemolytic anaemia was reported in 2 patients after abuse of amyl and butyl nitrite for protracted periods.— K. R. Romeril and A. J. Concannon, *Med. J. Aust.*, 1981, *1*, 302.

Methaemoglobinaemia was reported in a patient who had ingested 10 mL of amyl nitrite in an unsuccessful suicide attempt.— J. P. Laaban *et al.* (letter), *Ann. intern. Med.*, 1985, *103*, 804.

Methaemoglobin involving 23 to 73% of total haemoglobin was reported in 5 patients who ingested alkyl nitrites including amyl, butyl, and isobutyl nitrites. Other major clinical manifestations of nitrite poisoning that have been reported include unconsciousness, stupor, tachycardia, cyanosis, hypotension, and tachypnoea.— J. Osterloh and K. Olson, *Ann. intern. Med.*, 1986, *104*, 727.

Uses and Administration

Amyl nitrite is rapidly absorbed on inhalation when it has an action similar to that of glyceryl trinitrate (p.1501).

It is employed by repeated inhalations in the immediate treatment of the conscious patient with definite cyanide poisoning to induce the formation of methaemoglobin which combines with the cyanide to form non-toxic cyanmethaemoglobin. The inhalations are given for up to 30 seconds every 2 or 3 minutes. Up to 6 ampoules have been used.

It is seldom used in the treatment of acute attacks of angina pectoris, but doses of 0.12 to 0.3 mL by inhalation are usually effective within 30 seconds; the duration of action is about 5 minutes.

A review of the use of aids to cardiac auscultation including amyl nitrite. Amyl nitrite has been used in the differential diagnosis of cardiac murmurs. It was concluded that the usefulness of these aids was generally limited by a lack of sensitivity and specificity.— A. Rothman and A. L. Goldberger, *Ann. intern. Med.*, 1983, *99*, 346.

SULPHIDE POISONING. For reference to the use of amyl nitrite in the management of hydrogen sulphide poisoning, see Hydrogen Sulphide, p.1070.

Preparations

Amyl Nitrite Inhalant *(U.S.P.)*. Crushable glass capsules containing amyl nitrite *U.S.P.*

Amyl Nitrite Vitrellae *(B.P.C. 1973)*. Amyl nitrite in crushable glass capsules. To be crushed between finger and thumb, and the vapour inhaled.

Proprietary Names and Manufacturers

Amyl Nitrite Aspirols *(Lilly, USA)*; Amyl Nitrite Vaporole *(Wellcome, USA)*; Nitrit *(DAK, Denm.)*.

12409-h

Azaclorzine Hydrochloride *(USAN, rINNM)*.

AY-25239; Nonachlazine; Nonakhlazine. 2-Chloro-10-[3-(perhydropyrrolo[1,2-*a*]pyrazin-2-yl)propionyl]phenothiazine dihydrochloride.

$C_{22}H_{24}ClN_3OS,2HCl=486.9$.

CAS — 49864-70-2 (azaclorzine); 49780-10-1 (hydrochloride).

Azaclorzine hydrochloride is a phenothiazine derivative that has been used as a coronary vasodilator.

Proprietary Names and Manufacturers

Ayerst, USA.

9206-p

Azapetine Phosphate *(BANM)*.

Azepine Phosphate; Ro-2-3248. 6-Allyl-6,7-dihydro-5*H*-dibenz[*c,e*]azepine dihydrogen phosphate.

$C_{17}H_{17}N,H_3PO_4=333.3$.

CAS — 146-36-1 (azapetine); 130-83-6 (phosphate).

Azapetine is a vasodilator with alpha-adrenoceptor blocking activity.

It has been used in doses equivalent to 25 to 75 mg of azapetine 3 times daily in the treatment of peripheral vascular disorders.

Proprietary Names and Manufacturers

Ilidar *(Roche, Belg.; Roche, Ger.; Roche, Swed.; Roche, Switz.)*.

9207-s

Bamethan Sulphate *(BANM, rINNM)*.

Bamethan Sulfate *(USAN)*. 2-Butylamino-1-(4-hydroxyphenyl)ethanol sulphate.

$(C_{12}H_{19}NO_2)_2,H_2SO_4=516.6$.

CAS — 3703-79-5 (bamethan); 5716-20-1 (sulphate).

Adverse Effects

Bamethan sulphate may cause dizziness and other signs of hypotension, facial flushing, and tachycardia.

Precautions

Bamethan sulphate should be given with caution to patients with angina pectoris and is contra-indicated in recent myocardial infarction.

Uses and Administration

Bamethan sulphate is a peripheral vasodilator which acts on vascular smooth muscle. It is used in the treatment of peripheral vascular disorders in usual doses of 25 mg four times daily.

Proprietary Names and Manufacturers of Bamethan Salts

Angiolast *(Manetti Roberts, Ital.)*; Patol *(Jpn)*; Rotesar *(Arg.)*; Simpelate *(Jpn)*; Taivin *(Ferrer, Spain)*; Vasculat *(Arg.; Belg.; Boehringer Ingelheim, Fr.; Boehringer Ingelheim, Ger.; Boehringer Ingelheim, Ital.; Neth.; Boehringer Ingelheim, S.Afr.; Boehringer Ingelheim, Spain; Boehringer Ingelheim, Switz.)*; Vasculit *(Boehringer Ingelheim, UK)*.

9208-w

Bencyclane Fumarate *(rINNM)*.

Bencyclane Hydrogen Fumarate. 3-(1-Benzylcycloheptyloxy)-*NN*-dimethylpropylamine hydrogen fumarate.

$C_{19}H_{31}NO,C_4H_4O_4=405.5$.

CAS — 2179-37-5 (bencyclane); 14286-84-1 (fumarate).

Bencyclane fumarate is a vasodilator that has been given in the treatment of peripheral and cerebral vascular disorders in usual doses of 100 to 200 mg three times a day by mouth or 50 mg by intramuscular, intravenous, or intra-arterial injection.

Proprietary Names and Manufacturers of Bencyclane Salts

Angiociclan *(Ravasini, Ital.)*; Benciclan *(Pan Química Farmac., Spain)*; Bioarterol *(Unifa, Arg.)*; Desoblit *(Elmu, Spain)*; Dilangio *(Montpellier, Arg.; Andreu, Spain)*; Fludilat *(Organon, Arg.; Organon, Fr.; Thiemann, Ger.; Thiemann, Switz.)*; Flussema *(Italfarmaco, Switz.)*; Fluxema *(Italfarmaco, Ital.; Rovi, Spain)*; Halidor *(EGIS, Hung.; Jpn)*; Inphos *(Arg.)*; Vasodarkey *(Cuatrecasas-Darkey, Spain)*.

9210-b

Benfurodil Hemisuccinate *(rINN)*.

CB-4091. 1-[5-(2,5-Dihydro-5-oxo-3-furyl)-3-methylbenzofuran-2-yl]ethyl hydrogen succinate.

$C_{19}H_{18}O_7=358.3$.

CAS — 3447-95-8.

Benfurodil hemisuccinate is a vasodilator used in the treatment of peripheral and coronary vascular disease. It is given in doses of about 50 mg six times daily by mouth or 200 to 500 mg daily by intramuscular or intravenous injection.

Proprietary Names and Manufacturers

Clinodilat *(Liade, Spain)*; Eucilat *(Clin-Comar-Byla, Fr.)*.

9211-v

Benziodarone *(BAN, rINN)*.

L-2329. 2-Ethylbenzofuran-3-yl 4-hydroxy-3,5-di-iodophenyl ketone.

$C_{17}H_{12}I_2O_3=518.1$.

CAS — 68-90-6.

Benziodarone is a vasodilator which has been used in the prophylaxis of angina pectoris and after myocardial infarction.

Benziodarone has also been given to diminish uricaemia in gout. Doses of 100 to 200 mg daily have been recommended.

Benziodarone has been associated with jaundice and thyroid disorders.

Proprietary Names and Manufacturers

Ampliacor *(RBS Pharma, Ital.)*; Amplivix *(Labaz, Belg.; Labaz, Fr.; Sigmatau, Ital.; Labaz, Neth.; Labaz, Switz.)*; Becumaron *(Arg.)*; Coronal *(Crinos, Ital.)*; Dilacoron *(Ital.)*; Dilafurane *(Labaz, Spain)*; Plexocardio *(Benvegna, Ital.)*; Uricor *(Ravizza, Ital.)*.

12435-b

Bepridil Hydrochloride *(BANM, USAN, rINNM)*.

CERM-1978; Org-5730. *N*-(3-Isobutoxy-2-pyrrolidin-1-ylpropyl)-*N*-phenylbenzylamine hydrochloride monohydrate.

$C_{24}H_{34}N_2O,HCl,H_2O=421.0$.

CAS — 64706-54-3; 49571-04-2 (both bepridil); 64616-81-5 (hydrochloride, anhydrous); 74764-40-2 (hydrochloride, monohydrate).

Bepridil hydrochloride is a calcium-channel blocking agent with properties similar to Nifedipine p.1509. It has been used in angina pectoris in doses of 100 mg three times daily after food.

Because of torsades de pointes occurring in some patients given bepridil, reduced doses are recommended in elderly patients. Use is not recommended in patients at risk because of other cardiac arrhythmias.

A review of the pharmacology and clinical efficacy of bepridil. Bepridil is a calcium-channel blocking agent with anti-anginal activity and anti-arrhythmic activity characteristic of classes I and IV, with some class III activity. In clinical studies bepridil has generally been well tolerated, with adverse effects mainly affecting the gastro-intestinal tract and the central nervous system, although torsades de pointes has been reported. Bepridil has an elimination half-life of 1 to 5 days and is effective when administered once daily.— J. S. Alpert *et al.*, *Pharmatherapeutica*, 1985, *4*, 195. See also.— E. N. Prystowsky, *Am. J. Cardiol.*, 1985, *55*, 59C; S. F. Flaim and D. M. Cummings, *Curr. ther. Res.*, 1986, *39*, 568; F. P. Zeller and S. A. Spinler, *Drug Intell. & clin. Pharm.*, 1987, *21*, 487.

Reports of clinical studies of bepridil: W. Shapiro *et al.*, *Am. J. Cardiol.*, 1985, *55*, 36C (angina pectoris); A. P. Rae *et al.*, *Br. J. clin. Pharmac.*, 1985, *19*, 343 (angina pectoris); P. F. Nestico *et al.*, *Am. J. Cardiol.*, 1986, *58*, 1001 (arrhythmias).

An antisickling effect of bepridil was demonstrated *in vitro*. This effect, coupled with the vascular effects of bepridil, suggests that bepridil might have a use in vaso-occlusive crises in patients with sickle-cell anaemia.— M. P. Reilly and T. Asakura (letter), *Lancet*, 1986, *1*, 848.

ADVERSE EFFECTS. Reports of cardiac arrhythmias including torsades de pointes occurring in patients taking bepridil.— J. F. Leclercq *et al.*, *Archs Mal. Coeur*, 1983, *76*, 341. See also A. Chabanier *et al.* (letter), *Thérapie*, 1983, *38*, 702.

Proprietary Names and Manufacturers

Bepadil *(Wallace, USA)*; Cordium *(Riom, Fr.)*; Cruor *(Volpino, Arg.)*; Vascor *(McNeil Pharmaceutical, USA)*.

9213-q

Betahistine Hydrochloride *(USAN, rINNM)*.

Betahistine Dihydrochloride *(BANM)*; PT-9. *N*-Methyl-2-(2-pyridyl)ethylamine dihydrochloride.

$C_8H_{12}N_2,2HCl=209.1$.

CAS — 5638-76-6 (betahistine); 5579-84-0 (hydrochloride).

Adverse Effects

Gastro-intestinal disturbances, headache, and skin rashes have been reported.

Precautions

Betahistine hydrochloride should be given with care to patients with asthma, peptic ulcer or a history of peptic ulcer. It should not be given to patients with phaeochromocytoma. It has been suggested that it should not be given concomitantly with antihistamines.

Absorption and Fate

Betahistine hydrochloride is readily absorbed from the gastro-intestinal tract. It is converted to 2 metabolites and peak concentrations in blood of the 2 metabolites are achieved within 3 to 5 hours. Most of a dose is excreted in the urine, in the form of the metabolites, in about 3 days.

Uses and Administration

Betahistine hydrochloride is an analogue of histamine and is claimed to improve the microcirculation. It is used to reduce the symptoms of Ménière's disease. The usual initial dose is 8 to 16 mg three times daily taken preferably with meals; maintenance doses of up to 48 mg daily have been recommended.

MÉNIÈRE'S DISEASE. Reports and studies of betahistine hyrochloride in Ménière's disease: I. J. C. Frew and G. N. Menon, *Postgrad. med. J.*, 1976, *52*, 501; T. J. Wilmot and G. N. Menon, *J. Lar. Otol.*, 1976, *90*, 833; *Drug & Ther. Bull.*, 1981, *19*, 17; G. B. Brookes, *Drugs*, 1983, *25*, 77; A. Wright, *Br. J. Hosp. Med.*, 1985, *34*, 366.

Proprietary Preparations

Serc *(Duphar, UK)*. *Tablets*, betahistine hydrochloride 8 mg.

Proprietary Names and Manufacturers

Aequamen *(Promonta, Ger.)*; Betaserc *(Belg.; Cyp.; Denm.; Egypt; Fin.; Greece; Neth.; Kali-Farma, Spain; Duphar, Switz.)*; Deanosart *(Jpn)*; Extovyl *(Merrell, Fr.)*; Fidium *(Fides, Spain)*; Hainimeru *(Jpn)*; Medan *(Jpn)*; Meginalisk *(Jpn)*; Melopat *(Pharmasal, Ger.)*; Meniace *(Jpn)*; Menietol *(Jpn)*; Menitazine *(Jpn)*; Meotels *(Jpn)*; Merislon *(Jpn)*; Microser *(Formenti, Ital.)*; Pyritylulon *(Jpn)*; Remark *(Jpn)*; Ribrain *(Searle, Ger.)*; Riptonin *(Jpn)*; Serc *(Fisons, Austral.; Unimed, Canad.; Duphar, Fr.; Unimed, S.Afr.; Duphar, UK)*; Sinmenier *(Spain)*; Suzotolon *(Jpn)*; Tenyl-D *(Jpn)*; Urutal *(Jug.)*; Vasomotal *(Duphar, Ger.)*.

12465-w

Buflomedil Hydrochloride *(BANM, rINNM)*.

LL-1656. 2′,4′,6′-Trimethoxy-4-(pyrrolidin-1-yl)butyrophenone hydrochloride.

$C_{17}H_{25}NO_4,HCl=343.8$.

CAS — 55837-25-7 (buflomedil); 35543-24-9 (hydrochloride).

Adverse Effects

Buflomedil has been reported to cause gastro-intestinal disturbances, headache, hypotension, and paraesthesia. Overdosage may produce severe hypotension, tachycardia, and convulsions.

Encephalopathy with myoclonic movements of the limbs and tongue was associated with excessive doses of buflomedil in an 80-year-old patient. Symptoms disappeared within 36 hours of stopping treatment.— R. Treves and R. Desproges-Gotteron (letter), *Presse méd.*, 1983, *12*, 645.

Report of convulsions in 2 patients associated with buflomedil overdosage. Impaired renal function, low body-weight, and concomitant administration of other agents which predispose to epilepsy were considered to be contributory factors.— M. Otmane-Telba *et al.* (letter), *Presse méd.*, 1985, *14*, 286.

Uses and Administration

Buflomedil hydrochloride is a vasodilator that has been used in the treatment of peripheral arterial diseases including intermittent claudication. It is given by mouth in usual doses of 450 mg daily, or by intramuscular or slow intravenous injection in doses of 100 mg daily.

A review of the vasoactive drug, buflomedil hydrochloride. Buflomedil hydrochloride produces a number of pharmacological effects including nonspecific inhibition of alpha-adrenoceptors in vascular smooth muscle, inhibition of platelet aggregation, improved erythrocyte deformability, nonspecific calcium antagonistic activity, and oxygen-sparing activity. It has been studied in the treatment of peripheral and cerebrovascular disorders, in which its main beneficial property seems to be an improvement in the nutritional blood flow in ischaemic tissues without the production of systemic effects. Buflomedil hydrochloride is absorbed from the gastro-intestinal tract, with a reported bioavailability of between 50 and 80%. It is mainly excreted in the urine, with a total body clearance of 15.7 to 38.3 litres per hour. The mean elimination half-life has been reported to be between 1.5 and 4.3 hours. There is evidence to suggest that elimination may be impaired in patients with renal or hepatic failure, although dosage adjustments are probably only necessary in patients with liver disease since buflomedil is eliminated mainly via metabolic pathways.

A small number of placebo-controlled and comparative studies of buflomedil have shown some modest benefit in peripheral vascular disorders. In patients with cerebrovascular disease, buflomedil alleviates many signs and symptoms associated with the impairment of cognitive and psychomotor function but the clinical usefulness in individual patients remains to be determined. Encouraging preliminary results have also been obtained in studies of buflomedil in patients with Raynaud's phenomenon, diabetic retinopathy, frostbite, algodystrophies, and cochlear-vestibular disorders. It was considered that further well-designed placebo-controlled studies of long duration were required to define the place of buflomedil in therapy S. P. Clissold *et al.*, *Drugs*, 1987, *33*, 430.

A study of the metabolic effects of buflomedil in relation to the vasodilatory activity and the effect on the rheology of blood.— F. Briguglio *et al.*, *J. int. med. Res.*, 1985, *13*, 131.

Further studies into the effects of buflomedil on erythrocyte deformability.— M. Guerrini *et al.*, *J. int. med. Res.*, 1982, *10*, 387; S. Coccheri *et al.*, *ibid.*, 394; M. A. Perego *et al.*, *Curr. med. Res. Opinion*, 1982, *8*, 178; G. Leonardo *et al.*, *Curr. ther. Res.*, 1984, *36*, 1016.

CEREBROVASCULAR DISORDERS. Buflomedil was reported to be as effective as or more effective than dihydrogenated ergot alkaloids in a study of patients with senile dementia associated with cerebrovascular insufficiency.— W. Jansen *et al.*, *J. int. med. Res.*, 1985, *13*, 48.

PERIPHERAL VASCULAR DISORDERS. Studies of the use of buflomedil in peripheral arterial disorders.— S. Forconi *et al.*, *J. int. med. Res.*, 1984, *12*, 188; G. Trübestein *et al.*, *Angiology*, 1984, *35*, 500; E. Mozzi *et al.*, *J. int. med. Res.*, 1985, *13*, 317; F. Briguglio *et al.*, *ibid.*, 1986, 14, 115.

Proprietary Names and Manufacturers

Bufedil *(Abbott, Ger.)*; Bufene *(Ist. Chim. Inter., Ital.)*; Buflan *(Pierrel, Ital.)*; Defluina *(Nattermann, Ger.)*; Flomed *(Pulitzer, Ital.)*; Fonzylane *(Lafon, Fr.)*; Hemoflux *(Sifarma, Ital.)*; Irrodan *(Biomedica Foscama, Ital.)*; Lofton *(Abbott, Spain)*; Loftyl *(Abbott, Ital.; Abbott, Switz.)*; Sinoxis *(Hosbon, Spain)*.

9214-p

Buphenine Hydrochloride *(BANM, rINNM)*.

Nylidrin Hydrochloride *(USAN)*; Nylidrinium Chloride. 1-(4-Hydroxyphenyl)-2-(1-methyl-3-phenylpropylamino)propan-1-ol hydrochloride.

$C_{19}H_{25}NO_2,HCl=335.9$.

CAS — 447-41-6 (buphenine); 849-55-8 (hydrochloride).

An odourless, white, crystalline powder. **Soluble** 1 in 65 of water and 1 in 40 of alcohol; slightly soluble in chloroform and ether. A 1% solution in water has a pH of 4.5 to 6.5. **Store** in airtight containers.

Adverse Effects

Buphenine hydrochloride may cause nausea and vomiting, hypotension, flushing, headache, trembling, nervousness, weakness, dizziness, and palpitations. Anaemia has been reported. Chest pain, blurred vision, and a metallic taste may occur at high doses.

Precautions

Buphenine hydrochloride is contra-indicated in patients with myocardial infarction, hyperthyroidism, paroxysmal tachycardia, or severe angina pectoris. It should be used with caution in patients with peptic ulcers, tachyarrhythmias, or uncompensated congestive heart failure.

Uses and Administration

Buphenine is a peripheral vasodilator which produces beta-adrenoceptor stimulation and has a direct action on the arteries and arterioles of the skeletal muscles. It also produces positive inotropic effects.

Buphenine has been used in the treatment of peripheral vascular disease.

It has also been used in the treatment of circulatory disorders of the internal ear.

The usual dose of buphenine hydrochloride is 3 to 12 mg by mouth three or four times daily.

CEREBROVASCULAR DISORDERS. Although buphenine may cause cerebral vasodilatation, this is offset by a fall in blood pressure. Most studies have found either no change or a decrease in cerebral blood flow after short-term administration. One uncontrolled study showed an increase in cerebral blood flow and oxygen consumption in patients with cerebrovascular disease who were treated for 2 to 6 weeks with buphenine, but no adequately controlled trials in cerebrovascular disease have been reported.— P. Cook and I. James, *New Engl. J. Med.*, 1981, *305*, 1560.

PERIPHERAL VASCULAR DISEASE. A review of vasodilator drugs in peripheral vascular disease concluded that there was no indication for the use of buphenine.— J. D. Coffman, *New Engl. J. Med.*, 1979, *300*, 713.

Preparations

Nylidrin Hydrochloride Injection *(U.S.P.)*. A sterile solution of buphenine hydrochloride in Water for Injections.

Nylidrin Hydrochloride Tablets *(U.S.P.)*. Tablets containing buphenine hydrochloride.

Proprietary Names and Manufacturers

Arlibide *(Arg.)*; Arlidin *(Rorer, Canad.; USV Pharmaceutical Corp., USA)*; Bufedon *(Cedona, Neth.)*; Diatolil *(Fardi, Spain)*; Dilatol *(Tropon, Ger.; Vesta, S.Afr.)*; Dilydrin *(Medichemie, Switz.)*; Dilydrine Retard *(Medichemie, Switz.)*; Opino *(Bayropharm, Ital.)*; Penitardon *(Rorer, Ger.)*; Perdilatal Forte *(Smith & Nephew Pharmaceuticals, UK)*; Pervadil *(ICN, Canad.)*; Tocodilydrin *(Swiss-Pharma, Ger.)*; Tocodrine *(Medichemie, Switz.)*.

9215-s

Butalamine Hydrochloride *(BANM, rINNM).*
LA-1221. *NN*-Dibutyl-*N'*-(3-phenyl-1,2,4-oxadiazol-5-yl)ethylenediamine hydrochloride.
$C_{18}H_{28}N_4O,HCl = 352.9$.

CAS — 22131-35-7 (butalamine); 56974-46-0 (hydrochloride).

Butalamine hydrochloride is a vasodilator which has been given in the treatment of peripheral and cerebral vascular disorders in a usual dose of 80 to 160 mg daily.

Proprietary Names and Manufacturers
Adrevil *(Zyma, Ger.)*; Hemotrope *(Andromaco, Arg.)*; Surem *(CEPA, Spain)*; Surheme *(Aron, Fr.; Lipha, Ital.).*

18887-e

Butoprozine Hydrochloride *(USAN, rINNM).*
L-9394. {4-[3-(dibutylamino)-propoxy]phenyl}(2-ethyl-3-indolizinyl)-methanone monohydrochloride.
$C_{28}H_{38}N_2O_2,HCl = 471.1$.

CAS — 62134-34-3; 62228-20-0 (butoprozine).

Butoprozine is reported to have anti-anginal and anti-arrhythmic activity.

References: A. Waleffe *et al., Br. Heart J.*, 1979, *41*, 89.

Proprietary Names and Manufacturers
Labaz, Fr.

12520-n

Capobenic Acid *(USAN, rINN).*
C-3. 6-(3,4,5-Trimethoxybenzamido)hexanoic acid.
$C_{16}H_{23}NO_6 = 325.4$.

CAS — 21434-91-3; 27276-25-1 (capobenate sodium).

Capobenic acid is a coronary vasodilator that has been used in the prevention and treatment of myocardial infarction and myocardial ischaemia.

Proprietary Names and Manufacturers of Capobenic Acid and its Salts
Capben *(Schwarz, Ital.)*; Cardiobiol *(Spain)*; Cardiobiomar *(Spain)*; C-Tre *(Ital.)*; Kelevitol *(Migra, Arg.)*; Miocorden *(Lafarquim, Spain)*; Paracordial *(IBYS, Spain)*; Pectoris *(Llorens, Spain)*; Trifartine *(Phoenix, Arg.).*

9217-e

Cetiedil Citrate *(USAN, rINNM).*
2-(Perhydroazepin-1-yl)ethyl α-cyclohexyl-α-(3-thienyl)acetate dihydrogen citrate monohydrate.
$C_{20}H_{31}NO_2S,C_6H_8O_7,H_2O = 559.7$.

CAS — 14176-10-4 (cetiedil); 16286-69-4 (citrate, anhydrous).

Cetiedil citrate is a vasodilator that has been given in the treatment of peripheral vascular disorders. It is also reported to have an antisickling effect and has been used in sickle-cell crises.

Study of the blood concentrations, metabolism, and excretion of cetiedil.— A. M. Soeterboek *et al., Eur. J. clin. Pharmac.*, 1977, *12*, 205.

The administration of cetiedil by intravenous infusion to 10 healthy subjects elicited atropine-like adverse effects on salivation, bronchomotor tone, and visual accommodation. The incidence and duration of the adverse effects diminished with repeated infusions, indicating the development of tolerance.— G. P. Lewis and Y. W. Cho, *J. clin. Pharmac.*, 1982, *22*, 243.

SICKLE-CELL ANAEMIA. A review of the treatment of sickle-cell disease, including the actions and effectiveness of cetiedil.— Y. W. Cho and D. M. Aviado, *J. clin. Pharmac.*, 1982, *22*, 1.

Reports and studies of the use of cetiedil in sickle-cell crisis.— R. Cabannes *et al., Clin. Trials J.*, 1983, *20*, 207; L. J. Benjamin *et al., Blood*, 1986, *67*, 1442; E. P. Orringer *et al., Clin. Pharmac. Ther.*, 1986, *39*, 276.

Proprietary Names and Manufacturers
Celsis *(McNeil Pharmaceutical, USA)*; Huberdilat *(Hubber, Spain)*; Stratene *(Innothéra, Fr.; Sigmatau, Ital.)*; Vasocet *(Cipharm, Fr.).*

9218-l

Chromonar Hydrochloride *(USAN).*
A27053; AG-3; Carbocromen Hydrochloride *(rINNM)*; Cassella-4489. Ethyl 3-(2-diethylaminoethyl)-4-methylcoumarin-7-yloxyacetate hydrochloride.
$C_{20}H_{27}NO_5,HCl = 397.9$.

CAS — 804-10-4 (chromonar); 655-35-6 (hydrochloride).

Chromonar hydrochloride is a vasodilator that has been used in the prophylaxis of angina pectoris.

Absorption, blood concentrations, and excretion of chromonar.— Y. C. Martin and R. G. Wiegand, *J. pharm. Sci.*, 1970, *59*, 1313.

CARDIAC DISORDERS. A multicentre double-blind crossover study of 187 patients with angina pectoris who received chromonar for 8 weeks (79 patients) or 12 weeks (108 patients) at a dosage of 150 mg three times daily (73 patients) or 225 mg three times daily (114 patients) demonstrated significant prevention of anginal attacks by the lower dose, and improvement in attack-rate and glyceryl trinitrate requirement by the higher dose although the higher dose failed to show any advantage over placebo when the glyceryl trinitrate requirement was considered alone.— R. J. Bing *et al., Clin. Pharmac. Ther.*, 1974, *16*, 4.

Proprietary Names and Manufacturers
Antiangor *(ISM, Ital.)*; Cardiocap *(Miba, Ital.)*; Cromene *(Scharper, Ital.)*; Intensacrom *(Spain)*; Intensaïne *(Cassella-Riedel, Switz.)*; Intensain *(CCP, Belg.; Diamant, Fr.; Cassella-Riedel, Ger.; Pierrel, Ital.; Pierrel Hospital, Ital.; Jpn; Boehringer Mannheim, S. Afr.; Normon, Spain).*

12566-z

Ciclonicate *(rINN).*
Cyclonicate. *trans*-3,3,5-Trimethylcyclohexyl nicotinate.
$C_{15}H_{21}NO_2 = 247.3$.

CAS — 53449-58-4.

Ciclonicate is a vasodilator and is used in cerebral and peripheral vascular disorders.

References: G. Tiberio *et al., Curr. ther. Res.*, 1983, *34*, 365; J. Latorre *et al., ibid.*, 1984, *36*, 970.

Proprietary Names and Manufacturers
Bled *(Poli, Ital.)*; Cortofludan *(Knoll, Switz.)*; Euronicato *(Castejon, Spain)*; Vasociclate *(Alter, Spain).*

9219-y

Cinepazet Maleate *(BANM, USAN, pINNM).*
Cinepazic Acid Ethyl Ester Maleate. Ethyl 4-(3,4,5-trimethoxycinnamoyl)piperazin-1-ylacetate hydrogen maleate.
$C_{20}H_{28}N_2O_6,C_4H_4O_4 = 508.5$.

CAS — 23887-41-4 (cinepazet); 50679-07-7 (maleate).

Cinepazet maleate is a coronary and peripheral vasodilator that has been used in the treatment of angina pectoris.

Absorption and fate of cinepazet in man. Most of a dose given by mouth was eliminated within 24 hours, mostly in the urine. The major metabolite was cinepazic acid.— L. F. Chasseaud *et al., Arzneimittel-Forsch.*, 1972, *22*, 2003.

Proprietary Names and Manufacturers
Vascoril *(Delalande, Belg.; Delalande, Fr.; Delalande, Ital.; Delalande, Switz.).*

9220-g

Cinepazide Maleate *(BANM, rINNM).*
MD-67350. 1-(Pyrrolidin-1-ylcarbonylmethyl)-4-(3,4,5-trimethoxycinnamoyl)piperazine hydrogen maleate.
$C_{22}H_{31}N_3O_5,C_4H_4O_4 = 533.6$.

CAS — 23887-46-9 (cinepazide); 26328-04-1 (maleate).

Cinepazide maleate is a vasodilator which has been used in peripheral vascular disorders.

Proprietary Names and Manufacturers
Arteripax *(Rocador, Spain)*; Vasodistal *(Delalande, Fr.; Delalande, Ital.; Delalande, Switz.)*; Vasolande *(Frumtost, Spain).*

12573-j

Cinpropazide
Cinpropazine *(rINN)*. *N*-Isopropyl-2-[4-(3,4,5-trimethoxycinnamoyl)piperazin-1-yl]acetamide.
$C_{21}H_{31}N_3O_5 = 405.5$.

CAS — 23887-47-0.

Cinpropazide is reported to be a coronary vasodilator.

Proprietary Names and Manufacturers
Delalande, Fr.

9221-q

Cloridarol *(rINN).*
Clobenfurol. α-(Benzofuran-2-yl)-α-(4-chlorophenyl)methanol.
$C_{15}H_{11}ClO_2 = 258.7$.

CAS — 3611-72-1.

Cloridarol is a coronary vasodilator that has been given in the prevention and treatment of coronary insufficiency.

Proprietary Names and Manufacturers
Cordium *(Serono, Arg.)*; Menacor *(Menarini, Ital.)*; Menoxicor *(Menarini, Spain).*

9222-p

Cyclandelate *(BAN, rINN).*
BS-572. 3,3,5-Trimethylcyclohexyl mandelate.
$C_{17}H_{24}O_3 = 276.4$.

CAS — 456-59-7.

Adverse Effects
Nausea, gastro-intestinal distress, or flushing may follow high doses of cyclandelate.
Other adverse effects reported include tingling, tachycardia, sweating, dizziness, and headache.

Precautions
Cyclandelate is contra-indicated in the acute phase of a cerebrovascular accident. It should be used with caution in patients with severe obliterative coronary artery disease or cerebrovascular disease.

Uses and Administration
Cyclandelate is a vasodilator used in the treatment of cerebrovascular and peripheral vascular disorders. It is given in a dosage of up to 1.6 g daily in divided doses although a daily dose of 400 to 800 mg may be adequate.

In 1983 a symposium sponsored by the manufacturer was held (*Br. J. clin. Pract.*, 1984, *38*, *Suppl.* 34) to discuss the mode of action and clinical effects of cyclandelate. A review of the published literature (C.B. Blakemore, *ibid.*, 3) had shown that cyclandelate had produced clinically beneficial responses in both cerebral and peripheral vascular disorders. A series of *in vitro* and *in vivo* studies supported some of the mechanisms of action proposed by Timmerman (*ibid.*, 10) including selective phosphodiesterase inhibition (W.E. van den Hoven, *et al., ibid.*, 20), and inhibition of aldose reductase (*idem.*, 31). Among the actions demonstrated were preservation of erythrocyte deformability (*idem.*, 26), inhibition of platelet aggregation (W.E. van den Hoven and D.W.R.

Hall, *ibid.*, 34), inhibition of atherosclerosis (A. Middleton *et al.*, *ibid.*, 39), and inhibition of endogenous cholesterol synthesis (B. Middleton *et al.*, *ibid.*, 43). Preliminary clinical studies indicated beneficial effects in a variety of cerebrovascular disorders (K. Schaffler, *ibid.*, 51; M. Le Poncin-Lafitte, *ibid.*, 58; M.G. Albizzati *et al.*, *ibid.*, 69) and on diabetic peripheral neuropathy (N. Canal *et al.*, *ibid.*, 62).
However, no direct evidence of a calcium modifying effect as the main mechanism of action was available. This was supplied at a subsequent symposium in 1986 (*Drugs*, 1987, *33*, *Suppl.* 2). Calcium entry blockade was considered to be the mechanism responsible for the improvement in the rheological properties of blood caused by cyclandelate (H. Timmerman, *ibid.*, 1). Another mechanism of action, inhibition of the hepatic microsomal enzyme acetyl coenzyme A: cholesterol acyl transferase (ACAT), was shown to be responsible for the inhibition of cholesterol esterification (B. Middleton *et al.*, *ibid.*, 75). Cyclandelate compared favourably with flunarizine (M.G. Albizzati *et al.*, *ibid.*, 90; G. Nappi *et al.*, *ibid.*, 103) in mild cerebrovascular dementia and migraine prophylaxis, and preliminary results from a number of open multi-centre studies in general practice were reported. Encouraging results in diabetic neuropathy were also reported (I.H. De Leeuw *et al.*, *ibid.*, 125).
In his closing remarks O'Brien (*ibid.*, 140) commented that it would now be necessary to establish a link between the pharmacological studies and clinical observations.

Proprietary Preparations

Cyclobral *(Norgine, UK). Capsules*, cyclandelate 400 mg.

Cyclospasmol *(Brocades, UK). Capsules*, cyclandelate 400 mg.
Tablets, cyclandelate 400 mg.
Suspension, powder for reconstitution, cyclandelate 400 mg/5 mL when reconstituted with water.

Proprietary Names and Manufacturers

Arto-Espasmol *(Spain)*; Ciclospasmol *(Brocades, Ital.)*; Cyclergine *(Valpan, Fr.)*; Cyclobral *(Norgine, UK)*; Cyclomandol *(Gist-Brocades, Swed.)*; Cyclospasmol *(Astra, Austral.; Belg.; Wyeth, Canad.; Gist-Brocades, Denm.; Beytout, Fr.; Neth.; Norw.; Brocades, S.Afr.; Gist-Brocades, Switz.; Brocades, UK; Wyeth, USA)*; Cyvaso *(Reid-Provident, USA)*; Natil *(Kettelhack Riker, Ger.)*; Novodil *(Chauvin-Blache, Fr.)*; Spasmocyclon *(Kettelhack Riker, Ger.)*; Vasodyl *(Morrith, Spain)*.

19036-f

Darodipine *(USAN, rINN)*.

Dazodipine; PY-108-068. Diethyl 4-(4-benzofurazanyl)-1,4-dihydro-2,6-dimethylpyridine-3,5-dicarboxylate.
$C_{19}H_{21}N_3O_5$=371.4.

CAS — 72803-02-2.

Darodipine is a calcium-channel blocking agent with vasodilatory properties similar to Nifedipine, see p.1511.

Darodipine 75 mg or 150 mg daily was effective in increasing exercise tolerance in 19 patients with stable angina.— M. J. O'Hara, *et al.*, *Br. J. clin. Pharmac.*, 1984, *17*, 210P.

Beneficial effects were reported in 12 patients with angina pectoris treated with darodipine. Darodipine also reduced mean diastolic and systolic blood pressure without a substantial effect on heart rate.— M. de Buitleir and D. M. Krikler, *Br. J. clin. Pharmac.*, 1984, *17*, 636P.

Further references: M. de Buitleir *et al.*, *Am. J. Cardiol.*, 1986, *57*, 15; S. R. Olive *et al.*, *Chest*, 1986, *90*, 208.

Proprietary Names and Manufacturers
Sandoz, UK; Sandoz, USA.

9223-s

Di-isopropylammonium Dichloroacetate

Di-isopropylamine Dichloroacetate; Di-isopropylamine Dichloroethanoate; DIPA-DCA.
$C_8H_{17}Cl_2NO_2$=230.1.

CAS — 660-27-5.

Di-isopropylammonium dichloroacetate is a vasodilator which has been given in the treatment of peripheral and cerebral vascular disorders. It may account for any activity of some forms of pangamic acid (p.1598).

A review of the pharmacology and therapeutic effects of di-isopropylammonium dichloroacetate.— P. W. Stacpoole, *J. clin. Pharmac.*, 1969, *9*, 282.

Proprietary Names and Manufacturers
B-15 *(APS, Ger.)*; Cubisol *(Piam, Ital.)*; Dedyl *(Difrex, Austral.; Houdé, Fr.)*; Diedi *(Belg.; Seber, Spain)*; Kalodil *(Fidia, Ital.)*; Neovascoril *(Ital.)*; Nutricor *(Llorens, Spain)*; Oxypangam *(Beiersdorf, Ger.)*; Vasculene *(Von Boch, Ital.)*.

9224-w

Dilazep Hydrochloride *(rINNM)*.

Asta C-4898. Perhydro-1,4-diazepin-1,4-diylbis(trimethylene 3,4,5-trimethoxybenzoate) dihydrochloride.
$C_{31}H_{44}N_2O_{10},2HCl$=677.6.

CAS — 35898-87-4 (dilazep); 20153-98-4 (hydrochloride).

Dilazep hydrochloride is a vasodilator that has been given in the treatment of coronary insufficiency and angina pectoris.

For a series of papers on the pharmacology and use of dilazep in ischaemic heart disease, see *Arzneimittel-Forsch.*, 1974, *24*, 1851 to 1926.

The effects of dilazep on blood platelet aggregation.— F. Kuzuya, *Arzneimittel-Forsch.*, 1979, *29*, 539.

Clinical evaluation of the anti-anginal activity of dilazep in two different formulations.— A. M. Tomasi *et al.*, *Curr. ther. Res.*, 1983, *34*, 567.

Proprietary Names and Manufacturers
Coratoline *(Prodes, Spain)*; Cormelian *(Asta, Ger.; Schering, Ital.; Roche, Spain)*; Demicardio *(Valles Mestre, Spain)*; Komerian *(Jpn)*; Labitan *(Labinca, Arg.)*.

9225-e

Diltiazem Hydrochloride *(BANM, USAN, rINNM)*.

CRD-401; Latiazem Hydrochloride. *cis*-(+)-3-Acetoxy-5-(2-dimethylaminoethyl)-2,3-dihydro-2-(4-methoxyphenyl)-1,5-benzothiazepin-4(5*H*)-one hydrochloride.
$C_{22}H_{26}N_2O_4S,HCl$=451.0.

CAS — 42399-41-7 (diltiazem); 33286-22-5 (hydrochloride).

Pharmacopoeias. In *Jpn.*

Adverse Effects and Precautions

Treatment with diltiazem is generally well tolerated. Adverse effects associated with a depression of cardiac conduction include atrioventricular block, bradycardia, and, rarely, sinus arrest. Patients with sick sinus syndrome, pre-existing atrioventricular block, or bradycardia, or those taking beta-blocking agents or digitalis may be at particular risk of developing these reactions. Diltiazem can also cause headache, ankle oedema, hypotension, and flushing. Diltiazem should be administered with caution to patients with pre-existing hypotension and probably also to those with impaired left ventricular function due to the potential negative inotropic properties of diltiazem. Diltiazem may also cause nausea and gastro-intestinal discomfort. There have been reports of hyperactivity sometimes with associated psychiatric symptoms. Gynaecomastia has also been reported.

Diltiazem has been shown to cause teratogenicity in *animal* studies.
Treatment should commence with reduced doses in elderly patients and in patients with impaired liver or kidney function.

Reports to the Committee on Safety of Medicines during 1985 indicate that diltiazem has been associated with severe skin reactions including exfoliative dermatitis and epidermal necrolysis, hypotension, and a single case of agranulocytosis.— *Br. med. J.*, 1986, *293*, 688.

EFFECTS ON CARBOHYDRATE METABOLISM. Blood-glucose concentrations and insulin requirements rose in a diabetic patient during treatment with diltiazem.— H. A. Pershadsingh and N. Grant (letter), *J. Am. med. Ass.*, 1987, *257*, 930.

EFFECTS ON THE HEART. Prolonged atrioventricular conduction occurred in 4 patients taking diltiazem, 3 of whom were concurrently taking beta blockers.— K. F. Hossack (letter), *New Engl. J. Med.*, 1982, *307*, 953.

Atrioventricular dissociation and sinus arrest was associated with the administration of diltiazem in 3 patients.— T. Ishikawa *et al.* (letter), *New Engl. J. Med.*, 1983, *309*, 1124.

Withdrawal. Withdrawal of diltiazem over a 4-day period from a patient with stable angina pectoris was followed by recurrence of anginal attacks. Ambulatory ECG monitoring confirmed worsening myocardial ischaemia that responded to re-introduction of diltiazem. Two further patients experienced similar withdrawal effect.— V. Bala Subramanian *et al.*, *Br. med. J.*, 1983, *286*, 520.

Severe coronary vasospasm occurred after withdrawal of diltiazem from 2 patients and of nifedipine from 2 patients prior to coronary revascularisation. Myocardial infarction occurred in 2 of these patients, in 1 case fatal. Treatment with glyceryl trinitrate and nifedipine successfully reversed the ischaemic process in the remaining 2 patients.— R. M. Engelman *et al.*, *Ann. thorac. Surg.*, 1984, *37*, 469.

EFFECTS ON THE KIDNEY. Diltiazem was the most likely cause of acute renal failure in a 77-year-old patient.— P. M. ter Wee *et al.* (letter), *Lancet*, 1984, *2*, 1337. Comment that the only mechanism by which diltiazem could have induced acute renal failure would be by allergic interstitial nephritis.— V. Achenbach *et al.* (letter), *ibid.*, 1985, *1*, 176.

EFFECTS ON NERVOUS SYSTEM. Akathisia occurred in a 62-year-old patient one day after starting treatment with diltiazem. Symptoms disappeared when treatment was withdrawn and recurred on rechallenge after the third dose of diltiazem.— M. B. Jacobs, *Ann. intern. Med.*, 1983, *99*, 794.

A report of restlessness with associated mania in a 56-year-old patient taking diltiazem.— D. D. Brink (letter), *ibid.*, 1984, *100*, 459.

INTERACTIONS. Cimetidine administration caused increases in plasma-diltiazem concentrations and in plasma-deacetyldiltiazem concentrations in 6 subjects given a single dose of diltiazem 60 mg by mouth. Ranitidine produced a similar, though less marked effect.— L. C. Winship *et al.*, *Pharmacotherapy*, 1985, *5*, 16.

For reports of a potentially beneficial interaction between diltiazem and cyclosporin, see under Uses, below.

For a report of diltiazem administration precipitating carbamazepine toxicity, see under Carbamazepine, p.401.

For a discussion of interactions between digoxin and calcium-channel blocking agents including diltiazem, see p.828.

PORPHYRIA. Diltiazem was considered to be unsafe in patients with acute porphyria because it has been shown to be porphyrinogenic in *animals* or *in vitro* systems.— M.R. Moore and K.E.L. McColl, *Porphyrias, Drug Lists*, Glasgow, Porphyria Research Unit, University of Glasgow, 1987.

OVERDOSAGE. A 58-year-old patient who took approximately 10.8 g of diltiazem developed hypotension and complete heart block. Dopamine, isoprenaline, and calcium chloride were required to maintain the blood pressure. The ECG reverted to sinus rhythm after 31 hours. The plasma-diltiazem concentration was 1670 ng per mL 43 hours after ingestion and fell to 12.1 ng per mL over a further 55.5 hours with an elimination half-life of 7.9 hours.— N. Malcolm *et al.* (letter), *Drug Intell. & clin. Pharm.*, 1986, *20*, 888.

PREGNANCY AND THE NEONATE. Diltiazem has been detected in the breast milk, see below.

Absorption and Fate

Diltiazem is rapidly and almost completely

absorbed from the gastro-intestinal tract following oral administration, but undergoes extensive first-pass hepatic metabolism. The bioavailability has been reported to be about 40%, although there is considerable inter-individual variation in plasma concentrations. Diltiazem is about 80% bound to plasma proteins. It is extensively metabolised in the liver; one of the metabolites, desacetyl diltiazem has been reported to have 25 to 50% of the activity of the parent compound. The half-life is reported to be about 3 to 4 hours. Approximately 60% of the dose is excreted in the bile and 35 to 40% in the urine, 2 to 4% as unchanged diltiazem.

A review of diltiazem including details of the pharmacokinetics.— M. Chaffman and R. N. Brogden, *Drugs*, 1985, *29*, 387.

EFFECTS OF RENAL FAILURE. The pharmacokinetics of diltiazem and its major metabolite desacetyl diltiazem in patients with severely impaired renal function were similar to those in patients with normal renal function.— N. Pozet *et al.*, *Eur. J. clin. Pharmac.*, 1983, *24*, 635.

PREGNANCY AND THE NEONATE. Concentrations of diltiazem were almost the same in serum and breast milk from a woman receiving diltiazem 60 mg four times daily by mouth. The results show that diltiazem is freely diffusible in human milk, and it should not be given to nursing women until more information becomes available concerning its safety in infants.— M. Okada *et al.* (letter), *New Engl. J. Med.*, 1985, *312*, 992.

Uses and Administration

Diltiazem hydrochloride is a calcium-channel blocking agent with properties similar to nifedipine (p.1511). It is a peripheral and coronary vasodilator with some negative inotropic activity. Unlike nifedipine, diltiazem inhibits cardiac conduction particularly at the sino-atrial and atrioventricular nodes. Diltiazem is used in the management of classical and vasospastic angina pectoris and has also been used in the treatment of essential hypertension.

The usual dose is 60 mg three times daily by mouth, although in the *USA*, the recommended starting dose is 30 mg four times a day increasing at 1- to 2-day intervals. There is considerable variation in dosage requirements with some patients requiring up to 360 mg daily. Doses of 480 mg daily have been given in unstable angina. Lower doses may be required in elderly patients and in those with impaired renal or hepatic function; the dose should not be increased if the heart rate drops to less than 50 beats a minute.

A detailed review of diltiazem including pharmacodynamics, pharmacokinetics, adverse effects, and therapeutic uses. Diltiazem appears to be an effective agent for the treatment of variant angina due to coronary artery spasm. Substantial efficacy has been demonstrated in the prophylaxis of stable exertional angina and unstable angina. Diltiazem has shown some efficacy in the treatment of mild to moderate hypertension and in the control or prophylaxis of supraventricular tachyarrhythmias, although the exact role of diltiazem in these conditions remains to be defined. Comparative studies between diltiazem and nifedipine or verapamil have been limited, but diltiazem appears to be of similar efficacy to these drugs in the treatment of angina pectoris while causing somewhat less frequent or severe adverse effects.— M. Chaffman and R. N. Brogden, *Drugs*, 1985, *29*, 387.

A review of the haemodynamic effects of diltiazem in patients with coronary artery disease. Diltiazem, nifedipine, and verapamil display major differences in potency and tissue specificity both in isolated tissue preparations and in the clinical setting. The haemodynamic and electrophysiological effects of diltiazem appear to resemble those of verapamil more than those of nifedipine. It inhibits sino-atrial and atrioventricular nodal function in clinically employed doses. The effects on sino-atrial function are more pronounced than those observed after verapamil. Diltiazem causes a decrease in the rate-pressure product indicating that decreased oxygen demand is a likely mechanism of action in relieving angina pectoris. Like verapamil, but unlike nifedipine, diltiazem does not appear to cause significant increases in coronary blood flow. The negative inotropic effect of diltiazem is presumably counteracted by afterload reduction.— A. L. Soward *et al.*, *Drugs*, 1986, *32*, 66. See also M. J. Kendall and J. V. Okopski, *J. clin. Hosp. Pharm.*, 1986, *11*, 159.

ASTHMA. A review of the use of calcium-channel blocking agents in asthma. Studies have indicated that inhaled diltiazem has no clinically important effect on exercise-induced bronchospasm in asthmatics although oral diltiazem was found to have a modest protective effect. Oral diltiazem had little or no effect against histamine- or methacholine-induced bronchospasm.— K. L. Massey and L. Hendeles, *Drug Intell. & clin. Pharm.*, 1987, *21*, 505.

Studies of the use of diltiazem in asthma: H. Magnussen *et al.*, *Thorax*, 1984, *39*, 579; J. Lichey *et al*, *Respiration*, 1986, *50*, 44.

For reviews and reports of the use of calcium-channel blocking drugs in asthma, see under Nifedipine, p.1511.

CARDIAC DISORDERS. For a discussion of the uses of calcium-channel blocking agents in heart disease, see under Nifedipine, p.1511.

Angina Pectoris. The results of a postmarketing study involving 3913 Japanese patients treated with diltiazem for up to 360 days indicated that diltiazem was effective for the long-term treatment of ischaemic heart disease and produced an overall frequency of adverse effects of 1.8%. Diltiazem appeared to be safe and possibly beneficial in patients with heart failure. No deleterious effects on cardiac conduction were found in 205 patients receiving beta-blocking agents concomitantly, or in 238 patients receiving concomitant digitalis glycosides.— B. F. McGraw *et al.*, *Pharmacotherapy*, 1982, *2*, 156.

Diltiazem 180 mg daily and amiodarone 400 mg daily had similar anti-anginal efficacy and were somewhat more effective than sublingual glyceryl trinitrate.— J. P. Lesbre and J. P. Eloy, *Drugs*, 1985, *29*, *Suppl.* 3, 31.

Diltiazem 360 mg daily by mouth in combination with propranolol improved exercise capacity and reduced symptoms in a study involving 24 patients with angina pectoris compared with therapy with either drug alone, or with diltiazem 240 mg daily plus propranolol. There was no increase in adverse effects nor deterioration of left ventricular function.— D. P. Humen *et al.*, *J. Am. Coll. Cardiol.*, 1986, *7*, 329.

A study of the haemodynamics of intravenous diltiazem in 12 patients with chronic stable angina. The results suggested that intravenous diltiazem could be of use in acute vasospastic episodes.— B. Silke *et al.*, *Br. J. clin. Pharmac.*, 1987, *23*, 165.

Myocardial infarction. A study involving 576 patients found that treatment with diltiazem for up to 14 days had a protective effect against re-infarction and refractory angina in patients recovering from acute non-Q-wave or subendocardial infarction.— R. S. Gibson *et al.*, *New Engl. J. Med.*, 1986, *315*, 423. Criticism of the statistical analysis used and the study design.— R. A. Reeves (letter), *ibid.*, 1987, *316*, 220. The multicenter diltiazem postinfarction trial research group found no overall effect of diltiazem on cumulative mortality or cardiac events in a study involving 2466 patients with a previous infarction.— *New Engl. J. Med.*, 1988, *319*, 385.

HYPERTENSION. Diltiazem exerted a hypotensive effect similar to that induced by metoprolol in a double-blind study of 20 patients with mild to moderate hypertension.— B. Trimarco *et al.*, *J. clin. Pharmac.*, 1984, *24*, 218.

The antihypertensive effect of sustained-release diltiazem 240 to 360 mg daily was found to be similar to that of hydrochlorothiazide 50 mg daily in a double-blind multicentre study involving 207 patients with mild to moderate hypertension. Hydrochlorothiazide 100 mg daily produced greater reductions in systolic blood pressure than either dose of diltiazem. About 56% of patients who did not respond to either drug taken alone responded to the two drugs taken in association.— W. H. Frishman *et al.*, *Am. J. Cardiol.*, 1987, *59*, 615.

Further studies of the antihypertensive action of diltiazem.— W. H. Frishman *et al.*, *Am. J. Cardiol.*, 1985, *56*, 92H; P. E. Pool *et al.*, *ibid.*, 1986, *57*, 212; K. Yamauchi *et al.*, *ibid.*, 1986, *57*, 609; E. F. Valdés *et al.*, *Curr. ther. Res.*, 1987, *41*, 318.

MIGRAINE. Beneficial effect with diltiazem in refractory migraine after 8 weeks of treatment in a group of 9 patients who had previously been treated unsuccessfully with nadolol.— R. Smith and A. Schwartz (letter), *New Engl. J. Med.*, 1984, *310*, 1327.

PERIPHERAL VASCULAR DISORDERS. Reports of studies of diltiazem in the treatment of Raynaud's phenomenon.— A. Kahan *et al.*, *Ann. rheum. Dis.*, 1985, *44*, 30; A. Rhedda *et al.*, *J. Rheumatol.*, 1985, *12*, 724.

PROCTALGIA FUGAX. Beneficial response to diltiazem in a patient with proctalgia fugax.— J. Boquet *et al.* (letter), *Lancet*, 1986, *1*, 1493. The resting pressure of the internal anal sphincter decreased by a mean of 20.6% in all but 1 of 13 patients treated with diltiazem 60 mg by mouth. This ability to relax smooth muscle could account for the effect of diltiazem in proctalgia fugax.— P. Jonard and B. Essamri (letter), *ibid.*, 1987, *1*, 754.

RENAL TRANSPLANTATION. Beneficial effects on graft function of diltiazem treatment of donor and recipient in kidney transplant patients.— K. Wagner and H. -H. Neumayer (letter), *Lancet*, 1985, *2*, 1355. Improved graft function was maintained after 6 months in 20 patients treated with diltiazem compared with 22 controls. Increased trough plasma concentrations of cyclosporin in diltiazem-treated patients enabled a reduction in cyclosporin dosage by about one third.— H. -H. Neumayer and K. Wagner (letter), *ibid.*, 1986, *2*, 523.

TARDIVE DYSKINESIA. Diltiazem in doses of up to 360 mg daily was associated with immediate clinical improvement in 3 patients with tardive dyskinesia.— J. L. Ross *et al.* (letter), *Lancet*, 1987, *1*, 268.

Proprietary Preparations

Britiazim *(Thames, UK). Tablets*, modified-release, diltiazem hydrochloride 60 mg.

Calcicard *(Riker, UK). Tablets*, modified release, diltiazem hydrochloride 60 mg.

Tildiem *(Lorex, UK). Tablets*, modified-release diltiazem hydrochloride 60 mg.

Proprietary Names and Manufacturers

Acalix *(Roemmers, Arg.)*; Altiazem *(Lusofarmaco, Ital.)*; Angizem *(Inverni della Beffa, Ital.)*; Britiazim *(Thames, UK)*; Calcicard *(Riker, UK)*; Cardizem *(Nordic, Canad.*; *Ferrosan, Denm.*; *Ferrosan, Swed.*; *Marion Laboratories, USA)*; Diladel *(Delalande, Ital.)*; Dilzem *(Gödecke, Ger.*; *Warner-Lambert, Switz.)*; Dilzene *(Sigmatau, Ital.)*; Dinisor *(Parke, Davis, Spain)*; Hart *(Syncro, Arg.)*; Herbesser *(High Noon, Pakistan)*; Incoril *(Bago, Arg.)*; Masdil *(Esteve, Spain)*; Presokin *(Sintyal, Arg.)*; Tilazem *(Parke, Davis, Arg.*; *Parke, Davis, S.Afr.)*; Tildiem *(Dausse, Fr.*; *Lirca, Ital.*; *Lorex, UK)*; Zilden *(Schiapparelli, Ital.)*.

9226-l

Dipyridamole *(BAN, USAN, rINN)*.

RA-8. 2,2′,2″,2‴-[(4,8-Dipiperidinopyrimido-[5,4-*d*]pyrimidine-2,6-diyl)dinitrilo]tetraethanol.
$C_{24}H_{40}N_8O_4$=504.6.

CAS — 58-32-2.

Pharmacopoeias. In *Br.*, *Fr.*, and *U.S.*

An odourless or almost odourless, intensely yellow, crystalline powder or needles. *B.P.* **solubilities** are: practically insoluble in water; freely soluble in chloroform; soluble in alcohol. *U.S.P.* solubilities are: slightly soluble in water; very soluble in chloroform, in alcohol, and in methyl alcohol; very slightly soluble in acetone and in ethyl acetate. **Store** in airtight containers. Protect from light.

Adverse Effects and Treatment

Gastric disturbances, including nausea, vomiting, and diarrhoea, headache, dizziness, faintness, facial flushing, and skin rash may occur after administration of dipyridamole. The adverse effects are generally dose-related. Rapid intravenous injection or excessive doses of dipyridamole may cause a lowering of blood pressure. Dipyridamole can also induce angina in some patients. Coronary vasodilatation may be reversed with aminophylline.

Symptoms of thrombotic thrombocytopenic purpura developed in a patient taking dipyridamole and digoxin.— J. R. Lindquist and R. P. George (letter), *J. Am. med. Ass.*, 1981, *246*, 2577.

A report of a disagreeable taste associated with other gastro-intestinal symptoms occurring in one patient taking dipyridamole. Two similar cases had been reported to the C.S.M.— J. M. T. Willoughby, *Adverse Drug React. Bull.*, 1983, Jun., 368.

Transient myocardial ischaemia occurred in 4 patients with unstable angina and multivessel coronary artery disease during oral treatment with dipyridamole.— T. N. Keltz *et al.*, *J. Am. med. Ass.*, 1987, *257*, 1515. Comment that other larger studies have shown that the incidence of severe myocardial ischaemic episodes after dipyridamole is low.— A. Ranhosky (letter), *ibid.*, *258*, 203.

Precautions

Dipyridamole should be given with care to patients with hypotension and should not be given to patients with haemodynamic instability following myocardial infarction. Administration with anticoagulant agents may result in excessive bleeding even when prothrombin times are maintained within the therapeutic range.

INTERACTIONS. In 24 patients with glomerulonephritis who were stabilised on either warfarin or phenindione, dipyridamole in doses up to 400 mg daily did not affect prothrombin activity. Evidence of bleeding occurred in 3 patients during dipyridamole therapy. It was recommended that when dipyridamole was used the prothrombin activity should be maintained at the upper end of the therapeutic range in order to avoid possible bleeding complications due to the slight anticoagulant activity of dipyridamole.— S. Kalowski and P. Kincaid-Smith, *Med. J. Aust.*, 1973, *2*, 164.

INTERFERENCE WITH DIAGNOSTIC TESTS. Serum from a patient taking dipyridamole gave very high readings when lipoproteins were being measured by nephelometry. Dipyridamole imparts a yellowish-blue fluorescence to solutions and could interfere in other laboratory tests involving fluorescence or nephelometry measurements.— K. Wiener (letter), *Lancet*, 1981, *2*, 634.

PREGNANCY AND THE NEONATE. A young woman with a prosthetic heart valve was successfully managed throughout pregnancy with the aid of dipyridamole and delivered a healthy infant.— R. Ahmad *et al.* (letter), *Lancet*, 1976, *2*, 1414. See also Y. Biale *et al.* (letter), *Lancet*, 1977, *1*, 907.

Absorption and Fate

Dipyridamole is absorbed from the gastro-intestinal tract. It is metabolised in the liver and is mainly excreted in the bile. Excretion may be delayed by enterohepatic recirculation. A small amount is excreted in the urine as glucuronide.

Following intravenous administration of dipyridamole to 6 healthy subjects the concentration-time curve followed a tri-exponential decline with a final elimination half-life of 11.6 hours. The plasma half-life following oral administration was 11.4 hours. Plasma-dipyridamole concentrations rose between 6 and 10 hours after administration in the female subjects in the study, possibly due to enterohepatic recirculation: the average amount of the dose apparently recycled was 16%. The bioavailability following oral administration ranged from 27 to 59%, with peak plasma concentrations delayed for 2 to 2.5 hours after dosing.— C. Mahony *et al.*, *Clin. Pharmac. Ther.*, 1982, *31*, 330.

In a study of 20 patients receiving dipyridamole by 2 different dosage regimens it was found that a regimen of 75 mg twice a day did not result in lower trough plasma concentrations than a regimen of 50 mg three times a day. The study also revealed considerable inter-patient variation of about 7-fold in peak dipyridamole concentrations and about 15-fold in trough concentrations during chronic dosing. The plasma half-life was found to be about 12 hours.— C. Mahony *et al.*, *J. clin. Pharmac.*, 1983, *23*, 123.

Uses and Administration

Dipyridamole has antithrombotic activity and is used in conditions where modification of platelet function may be beneficial. For this purpose the usual dose is 100 mg four times daily before food increased if necessary, to 600 mg daily often in conjunction with aspirin or an anticoagulant.

It has also been used as a vasodilator in the long-term management of chronic angina pectoris in usual doses of 50 mg three times daily. It has also been given by slow intravenous injection as an adjunct to thallium-201 myocardial scanning.

A review of actions, pharmacokinetics, and clinical efficacy of dipyridamole. The effects of dipyridamole on platelet function have not been completely described. The *in vitro* and *ex vivo* tests used to assess antiplatelet activity may not mirror *in vivo* events adequately. Studies suggest that dipyridamole does not affect platelet adhesion, but inhibition of platelet aggregation has been demonstrated *ex vivo*. Dipyridamole has been shown to correct shortened platelet survival.

Dipyridamole is thought to exert its major anti-aggregatory action by interacting with thromboxane A_2 and prostacycline. Dipyridamole inhibits phosphodiesterase activity, thereby increasing the intracellular concentration of cyclic AMP and potentiating the effect of prostacycline. Dipyridamole may also have an effect on blood vessel endothelialisation and development of atherosclerotic lesions, although results of studies are conflicting.— M. P. Rivey *et al.*, *Drug Intell. & clin. Pharm.*, 1984, *18*, 869. A further review of dipyridamole: G. A. FitzGerald, *New Engl. J. Med.*, 1987, *316*, 1247.

Inhibition of platelet aggregation by aspirin was shown to be enhanced by dipyridamole when studied in whole blood. The potentiation may be the consequence of the two drugs working through different mechanisms: dipyridamole by inhibiting erythrocyte-adenosine uptake and thus leading to a stimulation of adenylate cyclase and aspirin by blocking synthesis of thromboxane A_2 or other mechanisms.— P. Gresele *et al.* (letter), *Lancet*, 1985, *1*, 937.

Evidence to suggest that dipyridamole increases red cell deformability.— S. O. Sowemimo-Coker *et al.*, *Br. J. clin. Pharmac.*, 1983, *16*, 423.

A sharp decline in lymphocyte response to mitogens occurred after 3 and 6 days of dipyridamole treatment, although no reduction in lymphocyte response was evident in patients treated for 1 year.— I. Melamed *et al.*, *Eur. J. clin. Pharmac.*, 1985, *28*, 263.

Further references to the action of dipyridamole on platelets: S. Moncada and R. Korbut, *Lancet*, 1978, *1*, 1286; D. F. Horrobin *et al.* (letter), *ibid.*, *2*, 270; L. C. Best *et al.* (letter), *ibid.*, 846; G. Masotti *et al.* (letter), *Lancet*, 1979, *1*, 1412; G. Di Minno *et al.* (letter), *ibid.*, 1979, *2*, 701; G. de Gaetano *et al.*, *Lancet*, 1982, *2*, 974.

DIAGNOSTIC USE. A study in 12 patients comparing dipyridamole 300 mg by mouth with 40 mg intravenously in thallium-201 myocardial imaging. It was concluded that oral dipyridamole is at least as effective as intravenous dipyridamole in thallium-201 myocardial imaging, and that the technique is safe, easy to perform, and suitable for out-patient use. One patient developed angina and ST-segment depression after oral dipyridamole, which was abolished by aminophylline 50 mg intravenously.— P. Walker *et al.*, *Clin. Sci.*, 1980, *59*, 5P.

Dipyridamole-thallium-201 scintigraphy appeared to be relatively safe in patients recovering from acute myocardial infarction. The use of dipyridamole permits an evaluation of myocardial function during maximal coronary perfusion that appears to be more sensitive in predicting subsequent ischaemic cardiac symptoms than sub-maximal exercise testing.— J. A. Leppo *et al.*, *New Engl. J. Med.*, 1984, *310*, 1014.

Further references to the use of dipyridamole-thallium imaging.— C. A. Boucher *et al.*, *New Engl. J. Med.*, 1985, *312*, 389; P. F. Pasternack and A. M. Imparato (letter), *ibid.*, 1641; R. W. McIntyre and K. D. Knopes (letter), *ibid*; K. A. Eagle *et al.*, *J. Am. med. Ass.*, 1987, *257*, 2185; R. M. Meyer (letter), *ibid.*, *258*, 1171; B. Kleinman and T. C. Smith (letter), *ibid.*

MELANOMA. A report of encouraging survival-rates with dipyridamole 100 mg three times daily in 39 patients with Clark's level III or IV melanomas.— E. L. Rhodes *et al.* (letter), *Lancet*, 1985, *1*, 693.

PREGNANCY AND THE NEONATE. For discussion on the use of antiplatelet therapy in the prevention of pre-eclampsia, see under Aspirin, p.7. See also.— P. Capetta *et al.* (letter), *Lancet*, 1986, *1*, 919.

See also under Precautions, above.

RENAL TRANSPLANTS. In a controlled study of 54 patients who had received primary renal allografts, the use of dipyridamole 100 to 400 mg daily with phenindione or warfarin sodium was associated with a significant improvement in the histological appearance of the glomeruli and blood vessels.— T. H. Mathew *et al.*, *Lancet*, 1974, *1*, 1307.

THROMBOEMBOLIC DISORDERS. *Cardiac disorders*. The use of anti-platelet therapy to prevent thromboembolism following heart valve replacement, to improve coronary vein graft patency, and to prevent relapse after myocardial infarction is discussed under Aspirin p.6 —See also under Anticoagulants, p.338. Studies on the effectiveness of dipyridamole in combination with aspirin or with warfarin in these indications have been generally encouraging, although the effectiveness of dipyridamole alone is controversial. See J. Webster, *Br. J. Hosp. Med.*, 1983, *30*, 45; *Drug & Ther. Bull.*, 1984, *22*, 25; J. R. Hampton, *Br. med. J.*, 1985, *290*, 414; *Clin. Pharm.*, 1986, *5*, 439.

Cerebrovascular disorders. The results of the AICLA, (Accidents, Ischémiques Cérébraux Liés à l'Athérosclerose) study involving 604 patients indicated that dipyridamole 225 mg with aspirin 1 g daily by mouth was no better than aspirin alone in the secondary prevention of atherothrombotic cerebral infarction.— M. G. Bousser *et al.*, *Stroke*, 1983, *14*, 5. Results of the Persantin Aspirin Trial in 890 patients indicated that the addition of dipyridamole 300 mg to aspirin 1300 mg daily contributed nothing to the effectiveness of aspirin alone in patients with a history of transient ischaemic attacks.— The American-Canadian Co-operative Study Group, *ibid.*, 1985, *16*, 406.

Dipyridamole, alone or with aspirin, was considered to have little to offer in the treatment of transient cerebral ischaemia.— C. Warlow, *Drugs*, 1985, *29*, 474.

For discussions on the use of antiplatelet therapy in cerebrovascular disorders, see under Aspirin, p.6.

Homocystinaemia. It was reported by L.A. Harker *et al.* (*New Engl. J. Med.*, 1974, *291*, 537) that 4 patients with homocystinaemia due to cystathionine synthase deficiency manifested a shortened platelet survival *in vivo*, and that this platelet survival could be increased nearly to normal by treatment with dipyridamole and aspirin. Treatment with dipyridamole 100 mg and aspirin 1 g daily appeared to be associated with an abolition of subsequent vascular occlusive or thrombo-embolic events in their patients. The shortening of platelet survival was not confirmed by E.R. Uhlemann *et al.* (*New Engl. J. Med.*, 1976, *295*, 1283) in 6 patients, but nevertheless they elected to prescribe long-term dipyridamole and aspirin for patients with homocystinaemia in the hope that the regimen might be of benefit. Experience with a 13-year-old boy who developed bilateral pulmonary emboli following appendicectomy, despite treatment with dipyridamole and aspirin from the third postoperative day, however, has prompted these workers to raise the need for a controlled clinical study (see J. D. Schulman *et al.*, *New Engl. J. Med.*, 1978, *299*, 661).

Peripheral vascular disorders. A study of 199 patients with peripheral occlusive arteriosclerosis over 2 years indicated that treatment with dipyridamole 75 mg and aspirin 330 mg three times daily was superior to aspirin alone in slowing the course of the disease.— H. Hess *et al.*, *Lancet*, 1985, *1*, 415.

For references to the use of antiplatelet therapy including dipyridamole in necrobiotic diabetic skin lesions and membranoproliferative glomerulonephritis, see under Aspirin, p.7.

Thrombocythaemia. Comment on the excellent clinical response of patients with essential thrombocythaemia, to antiplatelet drugs, and the view that in its milder forms the diagnosis may often be overlooked. In 19 of 35 patients given enteric-coated aspirin 325 mg and dipyridamole 100 mg, both three times daily, there was complete disappearance of pain and gangrene with healing of previous gangrenous changes within 4 to 6 weeks of starting therapy. Five patients relapsed on withdrawal of aspirin and dipyridamole, but again responded when therapy was reintroduced.— W. Morris-Jones and F. E. Preston (letter), *Br. med. J.*, 1981, *282*, 317.

Preparations

Dipyridamole Tablets *(B.P.)*
Dipyridamole Tablets *(U.S.P.)*

Proprietary Preparations

Persantin *(Boehringer Ingelheim, UK). Tablets*, dipyridamole 25 mg and 100 mg.

Proprietary Names and Manufacturers

Anginal *(Jpn)*; Cleridium *(Marcofina, Fr.)*; Coribon *(Radiumfarma, Ital.)*; Coronarine *(Negma, Fr.)*; Corosan *(Farmacologico Milanese, Ital.)*; Coroxin *(Malesci, Ital.)*; Dipramol *(Protea, Austral.)*; Dipyrida *(Ger.)*; Functiocardon *(Ger.)*; Maxicardil *(Northia, Arg.)*; Miosen *(Davur, Spain)*; Natyl *(Fr.; Nativelle, Switz.)*; Novodil *(OFF, Ital.)*; Péridamol *(Boehringer Ingelheim, Fr.)*; Perkod *(Biogalenique, Fr.)*; Persantin *(Boehringer Sohn, Arg.; Boehringer Ingelheim, Austral.; Boehringer Ingelheim, Denm.; Thomae, Ger.; Boehringer Ingelheim, Ital.; Neth.; Boehringer Ingelheim, Norw.; Boehringer Ingelheim, S.Afr.; Boehringer Ingelheim, Spain; Boehringer Ingelheim, Swed.; Switz.; Boehringer Ingelheim, UK)*; Persantine *(Belg.; Boehringer Ingelheim, Canad.; Boehringer Ingelheim, Fr.; Boehringer Ingelheim, Switz.; Boehringer Ingelheim, USA)*; Plato *(Lennon, S.Afr.)*; Prandiol *(Bottu, Fr.)*; SK-Dipyridamole *(Smith Kline & French, USA)*; Stenocardil *(Ital.)*; Stenocor *(Lagap, Ital.)*; Stimolcardio *(Panthox & Burck, Ital.)*; Trancocard *(Benvegna, Ital.)*; Viscor *(Ital Suisse, Ital.)*.

The following names have been used for multi-ingredient preparations containing dipyridamole— Asasantine *(Boehringer Ingelheim, Canad.)*.

9227-y

Efloxate *(rINN).*
7-(Carbethoxymethoxy)flavone; 7-Ethyloxyacetate Flavone; Efloxatum; Ethyl Flavone-7-oxyacetate; Flavone-7-ethyloxyacetate; Rec 1/0185. Ethyl 4-oxo-2-phenyl-4*H*-chromen-7-yloxyacetate.
$C_{19}H_{16}O_5$=324.3.

CAS — 119-41-5.

Efloxate is a vasodilator that has been used in the treatment of angina pectoris and coronary insufficiency.

Proprietary Names and Manufacturers
Dilatan Kore *(Lenza, Ital.)*; Recordil *(Recordati, Belg.; Méram, Fr.; Recordati, Ital.)*; Recordil LA *(Recordati, Switz.)*.

9229-z

Erythrityl Tetranitrate *(USAN).*
Eritrityl Tetranitrate; Erythritol Tetranitrate; Erythrol Nitrate or Tetranitrate; Nitroerythrite; Nitroerythrol; Tetranitrol. Butane-1,2,3,4-tetrol tetranitrate.
$C_4H_6(O.NO_2)_4$=302.1.

CAS — 7297-25-8.

Pharmacopoeias. Diluted Erythrityl Tetranitrate is included in *Aust.* (25% in lactose), *Nord.* (10% in lactose), and *U.S.* (in lactose or other suitable inert excipient; the strength is not specified).

Diluted Erythrityl Tetranitrate is a mixture of erythrityl tetranitrate and lactose, the latter being added to minimise the risk of explosion.
It is a white powder with a slight odour of nitric oxides. **Store** at a temperature not exceeding 40° in airtight containers.

CAUTION. Erythrityl Tetranitrate can be exploded by percussion or excessive heat.

Erythrityl tetranitrate is a vasodilator with general properties similar to glyceryl trinitrate (p.1500). When administered sublingually or buccally its effects are evident within 5 minutes and when swallowed within 30 minutes.
Erythrityl tetranitrate is used for the prophylaxis of angina pectoris. The usual dose is 5 to 10 mg sublingually or by mouth three or four times daily, increased as necessary up to not more than 100 mg daily.

Preparations
Erythrityl Tetranitrate Tablets *(U.S.P.)*. Tablets containing diluted erythrityl tetranitrate *U.S.P.*

Proprietary Names and Manufacturers
Cardilate *(Wellcome, Austral.; Wellcome, Canad.; Wellcome, Ital.; Wellcome, USA)*; Cardiwell *(Wellcome, Fr.)*.

9230-p

Etafenone Hydrochloride *(rINNM).*
LG-11457. 2′-(2-Diethylaminoethoxy)-3-phenylpropiophenone hydrochloride.
$C_{21}H_{27}NO_2$,HCl=361.9.

CAS — 90-54-0 (etafenone); 2192-21-4 (hydrochloride).

Etafenone hydrochloride has been used in the treatment of angina pectoris and coronary insufficiency.

Proprietary Names and Manufacturers
Asamedel *(Jpn)*; Baxacor *(Helopharm, Ger.; Schering, Ital.)*; Cardilicor *(Jpn)*; Corodilan *(Jpn)*; Corofenon *(Jpn)*; Coronabason *(Jpn)*; Dialicor *(Guidotti, Ital.; Jpn)*; Esanthin-S *(Jpn)*; Etafenarin *(Jpn)*; Hypochit *(Jpn)*; Pagano *(Helopharm, Ger.)*; Perucor *(Carulla Vekar, Spain)*; Relicor *(Davur, Spain)*.

16801-t

Felodipine *(BAN, USAN, rINN).*
Felodipin; H-154/82. Ethyl methyl 4-(2,3-dichlorophenyl)-1,4-dihydro-2,6-dimethylpyridine-3,5-dicarboxylate.
$C_{18}H_{19}Cl_2NO_4$=384.3.

CAS — 72509-76-3.

Felodipine is a calcium-channel blocking agent with vasodilating properties similar to Nifedipine, p.1511. It has been investigated for the treatment of hypertension.

A review of the actions and clinical uses of felodipine.— D. D. Freedman and D. D. Waters, *Drugs*, 1987, *34*, 578.

Haemodynamic effects of felodipine in healthy subjects.— G. Johnsson *et al.*, *Eur. J. clin. Pharmac.*, 1983, *24*, 49.

Felodipine, 5 mg twice daily increased as necessary to a maximum dose of 20 mg twice daily reduced the blood pressure more effectively than hydralazine in a study involving 101 hypertensive patients. All patients were concurrently treated with atenolol and chlorthalidone. Adverse effects associated with felodipine therapy included ankle swelling and flushing.— Cooperative Study Group, *Br. J. clin. Pharmac.*, 1986, *21*, 621.

Persistent reduction of blood pressure without a consistent change in heart rate was found after 8 weeks of felodipine treatment in 10 patients with essential hypertension. Plasma-renin activity was found to be increased with a concomitant increase in urinary aldosterone excretion.— P. L. Katzman *et al.*, *Br. J. clin. Pharmac.*, 1986, *21*, 633.

Further references to the haemodynamic effects of felodipine: H. Emanuelsson *et al.*, *Eur. J. clin. Pharmac.*, 1985, *28*, 489; O. K. Andersson *et al.*, *Drugs*, 1985, *29*, *Suppl.* 2, 102; P. Collste *et al.*, *ibid.*, 124; R. Fagard *et al.*, *Eur. J. clin. Pharmac.*, 1987, *32*, 71.

ABSORPTION AND FATE. Felodipine was rapidly absorbed after oral administration to 8 healthy subjects, but presystemic elimination reduced the bioavailability to 10 to 25%. Peak plasma concentrations varied from 38 to 125 nmol per litre and were achieved between 30 and 90 minutes after administration. Between 62 and 78% of an intravenous radiolabelled dose was recovered from the urine during the first 72 hours after dosing; the corresponding urinary recovery after oral dosing was 54 to 65% as metabolites. Approximately 10% of the administered dose was excreted in the faeces.— B. Edgar *et al.*, *Clin. Pharmac. Ther.*, 1985, *38*, 205.

Proprietary Names and Manufacturers
Astra, UK.

9232-w

Fenalcomine Hydrochloride *(rINNM).*
1-{4-[2-(α-Methylphenethylamino)ethoxy]phenyl-}propan-1-ol hydrochloride.
$C_{20}H_{27}NO_2$,HCl=349.9.

CAS — 34616-39-2 (fenalcomine); 34535-83-6 (hydrochloride).

Fenalcomine hydrochloride has been given in the treatment of angina pectoris.

Proprietary Names and Manufacturers
Cordoxène *(Laroche Navarron, Fr.)*; Oxileina *(Funk, Spain)*.

9233-e

Fendiline Hydrochloride *(pINNM).*
N-(2-Benzhydrylethyl)-α-methylbenzylamine hydrochloride.
$C_{23}H_{25}N$,HCl=351.9.

CAS — 13042-18-7 (fendiline); 13636-18-5 (hydrochloride).

Fendiline hydrochloride is a vasodilator that has been used in the treatment of coronary heart disease.

Proprietary Names and Manufacturers
Cordan *(Ibi, Ital.)*; Difmecor *(UCM-Difme, Ital.)*; Fendilar *(SPA, Ital.)*; Olbiacor *(Salus, Ital.)*; Sensit *(Thiemann, Ger.; Organon, Spain; Thiemann, Switz.)*; Sensit-F *(Ravasini, Ital.)*.

16804-f

Fenoxedil *(rINN).*
2-(*p*-Butoxyphenoxy)-*N*-(2,5-diethoxyphenyl)-*N*-[2-(diethylamino)ethyl]acetamide.
$C_{28}H_{42}N_2O_5$=486.6.

CAS — 54063-40-0.

Fenoxedil is a vasodilator that has been used in the treatment of peripheral and cerebral vascular disorders.

Proprietary Names and Manufacturers
Suplexedil *(Anphar-Rolland, Fr.)*.

9234-l

Gapicomine Citrate *(rINNM).*
4,4′-(Iminodimethylene)dipyridine dihydrogen citrate.
$C_{12}H_{13}N_3$,$C_6H_8O_7$=391.4.

CAS — 1539-39-5 (gapicomine); 24631-38-7 (citrate).

Gapicomine citrate is a vasodilator which has been used in ischaemic coronary disorders.

Proprietary Names and Manufacturers
Bicordin *(Polfa, Pol.)*.

9237-z

Glyceryl Trinitrate

Glonoin; Nitroglycerin; Nitroglycerol; Trinitrin; Trinitroglycerin. Propane-1,2,3-triol trinitrate.
$C_3H_5(O.NO_2)_3$=227.1.

CAS — 55-63-0.

Pharmacopoeias. Br. includes Concentrated Glyceryl Trinitrate Solution which contains between 9 and 11% glyceryl trinitrate in alcohol. *U.S.* includes Diluted Nitroglycerin which usually contains 10% glyceryl trinitrate in specified diluents. *Nord.* includes a similar solution.
Arg., Aust., Belg., Chin., Cz., Egypt., Hung., It., Mex., Pol., Port., Rus., and *Span.* include a 1% solution.

A white to pale yellow, thick, inflammable, explosive liquid. Slightly **soluble** in water; soluble in methyl alcohol, in alcohol, in carbon disulphide, in acetone, in chloroform, in ether, and in glacial acetic acid.
Concentrated Glyceryl Trinitrate Solution *B.P.* is a 9 to 11% solution of glyceryl trinitrate in alcohol (96%). **Miscible** with acetone and ether.
Diluted Nitroglycerin *U.S.P.* is a mixture of glyceryl trinitrate with lactose, glucose, alcohol, propylene glycol, or other suitable inert excipient. It usually contains approximately 10% of glyceryl trinitrate. Solutions in either alcohol or propylene glycol are clear, colourless, or pale yellow liquids. Dilution of 1% alcoholic solutions of glyceryl trinitrate with an equal volume of water produces a clear solution; dilution with twice its volume of water produces a turbid mixture from which glyceryl trinitrate deposits on standing; careless handling can then lead to explosion. Glyceryl trinitrate is saponified by strong alkalis. **Store** in a cool place in airtight containers. Protect from light.

CAUTION.*Undiluted glyceryl trinitrate can be exploded by percussion or excessive heat and only exceedingly small amounts should be isolated. In solution it is dangerous if spilled and allowed to evaporate; it may be rendered harmless by strong alkalis.*

A review of the pharmaceutical considerations of glyceryl trinitrate including the compatibility and stability of tablets, ointments, intravenous admixtures, and compatibility with intravenous giving sets and containers.— A. Yacobi *et al.*, *Drug Intell. & clin. Pharm.*, 1983, *17*, 255.

A review of the development and pharmacokinetics of various dosage administration systems designed to overcome some of the problems inherent in conventional formulations of organic nitrates.— U. E. Jonsson, *Drugs*, 1987, *33*, *Suppl.* 4, 23.

INCOMPATIBILITY. No evidence of physical incompatibility or loss of concentration was observed in admixtures of glyceryl trinitrate and lignocaine injections stored at room temperature for 48 hours. However, administration of both drugs from a single container was not recommended, and the manufacturer recommends that admixtures of glyceryl trinitrate and lignocaine should be avoided.— A. Sanburg and J. P. O'Shea (letter), *Med. J. Aust.*, 1984, *140*, 723.

There was no evidence of instability or incompatibility in admixtures of glyceryl trinitrate 100 μg per mL and dobutamine 500 μg per mL stored at 4° or 25° for 24 hours.— M. Thompson *et al.*, *Am. J. Hosp. Pharm.*, 1985, *42*, 361.

Further references to the compatibility of glyceryl trinitrate injection: K. J. Klamerus *et al.*, *Am. J. Hosp. Pharm.*, 1984, *41*, 303; A. S. Alam (letter), *ibid.*, 1518.

STABILITY. Many studies have demonstrated that glyceryl trinitrate tablets are very unstable and subject to considerable loss of potency in contact with packaging components such as adhesive labels, cotton and rayon fillers, and plastic bottles and caps, but V.A. Russell *et al.* (*Pharm. J.*, 1973, *2*, 466) found that mannitol-based tablets stored at 25° in glass containers sealed with foil-lined screw caps and opened 4 times daily to simulate use still had 90.9% of their activity after 35 days. For further reports and studies on the instability and deterioration of glyceryl trinitrate tablets, see M. O'Hanrahan *et al.*, *Br. med. J.*, 1982, *284*, 1183; J. Marty *et al.*, *Aust. N.Z. J. Med.*, 1983, *13*, 147; K. Hackett (letter), *Pharm. J.*, 1983, *230*, 482; W. C. Crabbs *et al.*, *Am. J. Hosp. Pharm.*, 1983, *40*, 2170.

The effect of glyceryl trinitrate-soluble additives on the stability of moulded glyceryl trinitrate tablets. Additives which lowered the vapour pressure of glyceryl trinitrate tended to increase the stability of glyceryl trinitrate tablets stored in glass bottles.— M. J. Pikal *et al.*, *J. pharm. Sci.*, 1984, *73*, 1608.

The Council of the Pharmaceutical Society of Great Britain recommends that glyceryl trinitrate tablets *B.P.* should be labelled with an indication that they should be discarded after eight weeks in use. The recommendation applies both to dispensed tablets and to tablets sold over the counter. Pharmacists are reminded that glyceryl trinitrate tablets should be dispensed only in glass containers sealed with a foil lined cap and containing no cotton wool wadding.— *Pharm. J.*, 1986, *237*, 270.

A study indicating that the usefulness of subjective indicators of potency following the administration of sublingual glyceryl trinitrate such as local burning sensations were of limited value.— G. R. Hasegawa and S. S. Gubin (letter), *New Engl. J. Med.*, 1987, *316*, 947.

The loss of glyceryl trinitrate from solution by adsorption or absorption into the plastic of intravenous administration sets has been recognised for some years. Crouthamel *et al.* (*New Engl. J. Med.*, 1978, *299*, 262) showed that within 2 hours there was a 50% loss of potency of glyceryl trinitrate solutions in plastic (Travenol Viaflex) bags and also showed a reduction in potency during flow through polyvinyl plastic giving sets. Adsorption by plastic infusion bags, burettes, and tubing was confirmed by Roberts *et al.* (*J. Pharm. Pharmac.*, 1980, *32*, 237) who showed that the extent of loss was proportional to the area of contact per unit volume and the flow rate through the system. Studies by Yliruusi *et al.* (*Am. J. Hosp. Pharm.*, 1982, *39*, 1018), Jacobi *et al.* (*ibid.*, 1983, *40*, 1980), Hola (*ibid.*, 1984, *41*, 142), and Schaber *et al.* (*Drug Intell. & clin. Pharm.*, 1985, *19*, 572) have shown that loss is greater from polyvinyl chloride (PVC) and silicone rubber than from glass or polyethylene. Adsorption of glyceryl trinitrate onto polyolefin containers was found to be negligible by Kowaluk *et al.* (*Am. J. Hosp. Pharm.*, 1983, *40*, 118) and Wagenknecht *et al.* (*ibid.*, 1984, *41*, 1807). Baaske *et al.* (*ibid.*, 1980, *37*, 201) found a loss of 55% of glyceryl trinitrate from 250 mL of solution passed through a cellulose triacetate filter (Gelman GA), 5% from a cellulose acetate/nitrate filter (Millipore GS), and 2% from a Gelman Tuffryn filter. Adsorption onto treated or untreated cellulose ester inline filters of less than 6% was considered by Kanke *et al.* (*ibid.*, 1983, *40*, 1323) to be of little clinical importance.

Nix *et al.* (*ibid.*, 1984, *41*, 1835) attempted to presaturate PVC giving sets prior to administration but found that this only led to a greater variation in the amount of glyceryl trinitrate delivered over a 24-hour period. Administration sets developed for use with glyceryl trinitrate injection have been shown to reduce loss compared with conventional giving sets in studies by Baaske *et al.* (*ibid.*, 1982, *39*, 121) and Lee and Fenton-May (*Pharm. J.*, 1984, *233*, 425). However Pendleton and Wellman (*Am. J. Hosp. Pharm.*, 1982, *39*, 1145) and St. Peter and Cochran (*ibid.*, 1328) have highlighted the problems of using such giving sets with volumetric pumps that normally have some PVC components.

Adverse Effects

Glyceryl trinitrate may cause flushing of the face, dizziness, tachycardia, and throbbing headache. Large doses cause vomiting, restlessness, hypotension, syncope, and rarely cyanosis, and methaemoglobinaemia; coldness of the skin, impairment of respiration, and bradycardia may ensue.

Chronic nitroglycerin poisoning may occur in industry but tolerance develops when nitroglycerin is regularly handled and nitrate dependence can lead to severe withdrawal symptoms in subjects abruptly removed from chronic exposure. Loss of such tolerance is rapid and may cause poisoning on re-exposure. Tolerance may occur during clinical use of preparations that produce sustained plasma concentrations, but this has not been observed consistently. Prolonged contact on the skin can cause contact dermatitis and rashes.

In Great Britain the recommended exposure limit of glyceryl trinitrate is 0.2 ppm; suitable precautions should be taken to prevent absorption through the skin. In the US the permissible and recommended exposure limits are 2 mg per m^3 and 0.1 mg per m^3 respectively.

Weakness, low blood pressure, and a feeling of warmth occurred in an 81-year-old patient who used glyceryl trinitrate plasters prescribed for chest pain to treat backache.— D. T. Nash (letter), *New Engl. J. Med.*, 1984, *310*, 658.

Headache, lightheadedness, and syncope occurred in an 81-year-old woman who inadvertently used glyceryl trinitrate ointment in mistake for toothpaste.— J. H. O'Keefe *et al.* (letter), *New Engl. J. Med.*, 1986, *315*, 1030.

ABUSE. For comment on the abuse of volatile nitrites, see under Amyl Nitrite, p.1493.

ALLERGY. Allergic reactions to glyceryl trinitrate ointment occurred in 5 male patients.— P. A. N. Chandraratna and R. E. O'Dell, *Curr. ther. Res.*, 1979, *25*, 481.

Report of allergic contact dermatitis caused by glyceryl trinitrate ointment in 1 patient confirmed by patch testing.— W. F. Sausker and F. D. Frederick (letter), *J. Am. med. Ass.*, 1978, *239*, 1743.

EFFECTS ON THE HEART. Paradoxical angina occurred after injection of glyceryl trinitrate into the left coronary artery in 1 patient.— A. A. Bove and R. E. Vlietstra (letter), *New Engl. J. Med.*, 1982, *306*, 484.

Complete heart block after sublingual administration of glyceryl trinitrate in a patient with no evidence of cardiac ischaemia or underlying heart disease.— L. Lancaster and P. E. Fenster, *Chest*, 1983, *84*, 111.

Asystole occurred following the administration of glyceryl trinitrate 0.3 mg sublingually to a 33-year-old patient.— E. A. Ong *et al.* (letter), *Archs intern. Med.*, 1985, *145*, 954.

INTRAVENOUS ADMINISTRATION. Some commercial formulations of glyceryl trinitrate for intravenous use contain substantial quantities of alcohol in the solvent. There have been several reports of alcohol intoxication occurring in patients during high-dose intravenous glyceryl trinitrate infusion. Blood-alcohol concentrations of 0.21 and 1.78 mg per mL were reported in 2 patients treated with an infusion of glyceryl trinitrate 2 mg per minute (T.L. Shook *et al.*, *Ann. intern. Med.*, 1984, *101*, 498) and of 1.78 mg per mL in a patient treated with glyceryl trinitrate 1.5 mg per minute (T.J. Daly *et al.*, *New Engl. J. Med.*, 1984, *310*, 1123). It was calculated that these infusion rates delivered 20.7 and 12.6 mL of alcohol per hour respectively from the preparations used. Korn and Comer (*Ann. intern. Med.*, 1985, *102*, 274) reported ethanol intoxication in a further patient with a blood-alcohol concentration of 2.67 mg per mL during an infusion of glyceryl trinitrate 2 mg per minute and suggested that adsorption of glyceryl trinitrate onto the PVC tubing may have increased the dose requirement and thus the amount of alcohol given.

Wernicke's encephalopathy which developed in a patient during glyceryl trinitrate infusion was attributed to both the alcohol and the propylene glycol in the solvent (J. Shorey *et al.*, *ibid.*, 1984, *101*, 500). Glucose in the diluent could also have been a contributory factor. However, the diagnosis of Wernicke's encephalopathy was questioned by Ohar *et al.* (*ibid.*, *102*, 558) who attributed the neurological abnormalities seen in a similar patient to elevated intracranial pressure caused by the glyceryl trinitrate itself.

OVERDOSAGE. Methaemoglobinaemia in an 80-year-old man was believed to have been induced by an overdose of glyceryl trinitrate. He had taken 100 tablets of glyceryl trinitrate 400 μg during the 36 hours before admission to hospital.— J. B. Marshall and R. E. Ecklund (letter), *J. Am. med. Ass.*, 1980, *244*, 330.

A report of severe hyperosmolality, lactic acidosis, central nervous system depression, and haemolysis in a 72-year-old woman with impaired renal function who received large amounts of propylene glycol intravenously as a solvent for infusions of glyceryl trinitrate. She was treated with haemodialysis, and hypertonic saline was administered to prevent a sudden drop in osmolality. It was considered that the haemolysis probably occurred because red blood cells and propylene glycol 50% solution were administered through the same intravenous line.— H. Demey *et al.* (letter), *Lancet*, 1984, *1*, 1360.

Treatment of Adverse Effects

Syncope and hypotension should be treated by keeping the patient in a recumbent position with the head lowered. The administration of oxygen, with assisted respiration may be necessary in severe poisoning. If methaemoglobinaemia occurs give methylene blue 1 mg per kg body-weight by slow intravenous injection. The circulation may be maintained with infusions of plasma or suitable electrolyte solutions. In the case of severe poisoning with oral tablets the stomach should be emptied by gastric aspiration or lavage.

Precautions

Glyceryl trinitrate should not be used in patients with marked anaemia or with raised intracranial pressure due to head trauma or cerebral haemorrhage. Nitrates may increase intra-ocular pressure in patients with closed-angle glaucoma but the clinical significance of this effect is uncertain. Intravenous administration of glyceryl trinitrate is contra-indicated in patients with constrictive pericarditis, severe hypotension, or uncorrected hypovolaemia, and should be used with caution in patients with severely impaired renal or hepatic function. Some effects of glyceryl trinitrate are enhanced by alcohol.

An explosion occurred during defibrillation in a patient with a glyceryl trinitrate transdermal patch on the left side of the chest. There was no visible injury to the patient. Subsequent studies suggested that this was caused by an electrical arc between the defibrillator paddle and the aluminium backing of the patch rather than explosion of the glyceryl trinitrate.— J. C. Babka (letter), *New Engl. J. Med.*, 1983, *309*, 379.

INTERACTIONS. A patient developed resistance to the effects of heparin on 2 occasions during intravenous administration of glyceryl trinitrate. The interaction could not be attributed to propylene glycol in the solvent, since resistance also occurred during administration of a formulation of glyceryl trinitrate without propylene glycol.— M. A. Habbab and J. I. Haft (letter), *Ann. intern. Med.*, 1986, *105*, 305.

Delayed dissolution of glyceryl trinitrate tablets in patients with dry mouths has been reported by Robbins (*New Engl. J. Med.*, 1983, *309* ,985) in a patient taking imipramine and by Kimchi (*ibid.*, 1984, *310*, 1122) in a patient treated with atropine. Kimchi suggested the use of the lingual spray rather than a sublingual tablet to overcome the problem, while Rasler (*ibid*, 1986, *314*, 181) suggested applying 1 mL of saline under the tongue to aid dissolution of the tablet.

TOLERANCE. A review of the development of tolerance to glyceryl trinitrate associated with transdermal administration. The failure of patients to respond to nitrates may have several explanations: inadequate nitrate plasma and tissue concentrations due to low doses or poor absorption or both; the development of nitrate tolerance causing attenuation or complete loss of vasodilatation after an inital response; or true nitrate resistance in patients with therapeutic plasma-nitrate concentrations. Sustained-release preparations of glyceryl trinitrate and other nitrates that release the drug continuously over 24 hours appear to induce the rapid development of partial or complete tachyphylaxis or tolerance to nitrates within 12 to 24 hours after acute dosing which is not associated with inadequate plasma concentrations. Experiments have indicated that vascular responsiveness to nitrates can be restored by a nitrate-free interval, and it may be possible to maintain responsiveness to nitrates by applying transdermal formulations for only part of each day.— J. Abrams, *Ann. intern. Med.*, 1986, *104*, 424 and 897. See also A. G. Kriegman (letter), *ibid.*, 1987, *106*, 325; J. Abrams (letter), *ibid.*

Studies and discussions of haemodynamic and biochemical aspects of nitrate tolerance: L. Erhardt, *Drugs*, 1987, *33*, *Suppl.* 4, 55; K. L. Axelsson and J. Ahlner, *ibid.*,

63; M. Packer *et al., New Engl. J. Med.*, 1987, *317*, 799; D. C. May *et al., ibid.*, 805.

Absorption and Fate

Glyceryl trinitrate is rapidly absorbed from the oral mucosa, but rapidly metabolised so that it only has a brief duration of action.

Glyceryl trinitrate is also well absorbed from the gastro-intestinal tract, but owing to extensive first-pass metabolism in the liver its bioavailability is reduced. In view of its short plasma half-life of 1 to 4 minutes various long-acting formulations are available for oral administration.

Glyceryl trinitrate is also absorbed through the skin from an ointment basis and transdermal delivery systems.

Glyceryl trinitrate is metabolised by hydrolysis to dinitrates and the mononitrate.

A review of the clinical pharmacokinetics of glyceryl trinitrate following the use of systemic and topical preparations. Measuring the plasma concentration of glyceryl trinitrate accurately is difficult, and assay difficulties, together with differences in study design, are probably responsible for some of the discrepancies between published results. However, important inter- and intra-individual variability of plasma concentrations has been found; this could be related to degradation in red blood cells leading to very high and largely extrahepatic clearance; plasma clearance values reported vary from 216 to 3270 litres per hour. It has not been possible to find a relationship between the plasma concentrations of glyceryl trinitrate and the clinical effect.— M. G. Bogaert, *Clin. Pharmacokinet.*, 1987, *12*, 1.

BIOAVAILABILITY. Application of glyceryl trinitrate ointment 2% to the chest or flank in amounts containing 12.5 to 25 mg to 9 patients and 50 mg to 5 patients with congestive heart failure produced mean plasma concentrations of glyceryl trinitrate 1 hour after application of 3.1 ng per mL and 8.9 ng per mL respectively and these concentrations were maintained for a further 3 hours. An unexpected finding was that although plasma concentrations decreased substantially following removal of the ointment, glyceryl trinitrate was still detectable in the plasma 30 minutes thereafter suggesting that a depot for glyceryl trinitrate exists in the skin after percutaneous application. It was concluded that glyceryl trinitrate ointment provides therapeutic concentrations that are associated with substantial haemodynamic benefit in selected patients with heart failure but in those in whom an attenuated response is found during intravenous infusion large doses of ointment are unlikely to be beneficial.— P. W. Armstrong *et al., Am. J. Cardiol.*, 1980, *46*, 670.

A study of the effect on plasma-glyceryl trinitrate concentrations of the area to which 2% glyceryl trinitrate ointment is applied. Plasma concentrations following application to an area of 100 cm^2 were at least double those obtained following an application of the same quantity of glyceryl trinitrate ointment to an area of 25 cm^2. It was also found that doubling the dose applied to a 100 cm^2 area increased the 0 to 90-minute area under the curve by only 76% but caused a 3.5-fold increase in the 90-minute plasma concentration.— S. Sved *et al., J. pharm. Sci.*, 1981, *70*, 1368. See also P. R. Imhof *et al., Eur. J. clin. Pharmac.*, 1984, *27*, 7.

A study involving 5 healthy subjects indicated a bioavailability of less than 1% following administration by mouth of glyceryl trinitrate capsule and oral solution. However, the weakly pharmacologically active dinitrate metabolites reached relatively high concentrations after oral glyceryl trinitrate administration and it was suggested that these metabolites may be responsible for the activity of oral glyceryl trinitrate.— P. K. Noonan and L. Z. Benet, *J. pharm. Sci.*, 1986, *75*, 241.

Uses and Administration

Glyceryl trinitrate relaxes smooth muscle, including vascular muscle, and reduces the blood pressure. It is believed that its anti-anginal effect mainly depends on reducing myocardial oxygen demand by means of peripheral vasodilatation. This causes decreased venous tone resulting in a reduction in preload and decreased arterial resistance resulting in a reduction in afterload. The effect of glyceryl trinitrate in relaxing coronary vessels may be the predominant mechanism in vasospastic or Prinzmetals angina.

The effect of glyceryl trinitrate sublingually occurs within 2 to 3 minutes and its action lasts for about 30 to 60 minutes. Tolerance may develop with regular use but withdrawal for a short period may re-establish the original sensitivity.

Glyceryl trinitrate is used as a vasodilator in the prophylaxis and treatment of angina pectoris.

Glyceryl trinitrate solution is usually administered as tablets which should be allowed to dissolve in the mouth. The usual dose in the *UK* is the equivalent of 0.5 to 1 mg of glyceryl trinitrate when required: in the *USA* the recommended dose is 0.15 to 0.6 mg repeated not more than 3 times in 15 minutes. A lingual spray is also available. For prophylaxis of angina, glyceryl trinitrate may be given as sustained-release oral tablets or capsules in a usual dose of 2.5 to 12.8 mg two or three times daily, although doses of up to 26 mg four times a day have been reported. Glyceryl trinitrate may also be given in a transdermal formulation as an ointment or adhesive patch. Sustained-release buccal tablets produce a rapid effect which persists for 3 to 5 hours or for as long as the tablet is retained in the buccal cavity. The usual dose is 1 to 3 mg every 3 to 8 hours or as required. This dose form is also used for congestive heart failure when 5 mg or occasionally 10 mg is given three times daily. A dose of 5 mg is used in acute heart failure and is repeated as required.

Glyceryl trinitrate may also be given by intravenous infusion for the treatment of angina pectoris not responsive to recommended doses of organic nitrates and/or beta blockers, of congestive heart failure associated with acute myocardial infarction, for the control of peri-operative hypertension, and for the production of controlled hypotension for certain surgical procedures. The injection should be diluted before use in accordance with the manufacturers directions. The usual initial dose for angina is 10 µg per minute increasing gradually until a response is obtained or adverse haemodynamic effects occur. Initial doses of 20 to 25 µg per minute may be required during surgery or for the treatment of congestive heart failure following myocardial infarction.

A review of organic nitrates.— J. Abrams, *Drugs*, 1987, *34*, 391.

ADMINISTRATION. The metered buccal aerosol preparation of glyceryl trinitrate is stable for 3 years and may be more convenient than sublingual tablets for patients who need infrequent doses.

For prolonged prophylaxis, isosorbide dinitrate is the most widely used nitrate. Glyceryl trinitrate may be given as a sustained-release buccal tablet or a transdermal patch, both of which are acceptable to many patients, but the messy nitrate ointment is unsuitable for long-term use.— *Drug & Ther. Bull.*, 1984, *22*, 77.

Buccal and sublingual administration. Glyceryl trinitrate 800 µg by lingual spray produced a less pronounced haemodynamic response than glyceryl trinitrate 500 µg by sublingual tablets. This unexpected result was attributed to shaking the canister before use which produced bubbles which impeded delivery of the active drug.— M. Heber *et al., Br. med. J.*, 1984, *289*, 1269.

A brief review of glyceryl trinitrate lingual spray.— *Med. Lett.*, 1986, *28*, 59 and 90. See also M. J. Vandenburg *et al., Br. J. clin. Pract.*, 1986, *40*, 524.

Parenteral administration. A review of the pharmacological properties and therapeutic efficacy of intravenous glyceryl trinitrate.— E. M. Sorkin *et al., Drugs*, 1984, *27*, 45.

Transdermal administration. A review on glyceryl trinitrate ointment.— U. Elkayam and W. S. Aronow, *Drugs*, 1982, *23*, 165.

Local application of glyceryl trinitrate 1 to 2 mg as ointment was found to be a useful aid to venepuncture in a study of 50 patients undergoing surgery.— J. F. Hecker *et al., Lancet*, 1983, *1*, 332. See also M. Lohmann *et al., ibid.*, 1984, *1*, 1416; S. C. Parakh and A. Patwari, *Br. J. Anaesth.*, 1986, *58*, 822.

Local topical application of glyceryl trinitrate to skin adjacent to intravenous infusion sites decreased the frequency of infusion failure due to extravasation or phlebitis.— A. Wright *et al., Lancet*, 1985, *2*, 1148.

Transdermal administration of glyceryl trinitrate was initially developed to overcome the substantial first-pass metabolism which has been shown after oral administration. Transdermal patches have advantages over glyceryl trinitrate ointment of improved patient acceptability, and accuracy and consistency of dosing. However, there has been considerable controversy over the efficacy and duration of action of transdermal glyceryl trinitrate patches. The Medical Letter, reviewing the situation in 1984 (*Med. Lett.*, 1984, *26*, 59), concluded that even fairly high doses of transdermal glyceryl trinitrate appeared to be less effective than sublingual glyceryl trinitrate. Conner and Gelman (*Drug Intell. & clin. Pharm.*, 1984, *18*, 889) commented that, despite the popularity and extensive use of glyceryl trinitrate patches, there were surprisingly few adequate clinical studies demonstrating persistence of anti-anginal effects for 24 hours. Further concern was expressed over the low plasma concentrations achieved as compared with conventional dosing, and the possibility of tolerance or tachyphylaxis occurring in the presence of prolonged steady-state nitrate-plasma concentrations compared with intermittent dosing. Significant haemodynamic benefit had been observed for 24 hours, however, in patients with congestive heart failure using transdermal doses of 30 to 40 mg. Determination of the duration of anti-anginal action was hampered by the absence of exercise testing between 8 and 24 hours after administration in most reported trials (E.A. Forrence and J.K. Elenbaas, *ibid.*, 1985, *19*, 587). A similar conclusion was drawn by Parker (*Ann. intern. Med.*, 1985, *102*, 548) who also considered the apparent development of tolerance to be a particular problem. There is evidence to suggest that tolerance to glyceryl trinitrate is due to a reduction in tissue responsiveness rather than to increased drug elimination (S.H. Curry, *Clin. Pharm.*, 1985, *4*, 453), and also that tolerance is more likely to develop with the demonstrably constant plasma concentrations produced by transdermal patches than with intermittent transdermal or sublingual dosing. The need for 24-hour therapy of angina was questioned and it was suggested that tolerance may by overcome by applying the patch for only 8 to 16 hours each day. Further scepticism about the efficacy of transdermal glyceryl trinitrate administration has been expressed in subsequent reviews (*Lancet*, 1985, *2*, 594; *Drug & Ther. Bull.*, 1986, *24*, 5; A. Desilvio and M.P. Barlattani, *Br. med. J.*, 1987, *295*, 1163), although Weber (*Am. Heart J.*, 1986, *112*, 238) considered that, despite the variability in response, a clinical improvement could be expected in 80 to 90% of patients with coronary artery disease.

CARDIAC DISORDERS. *Angina pectoris.* Review of the use of nitrates in angina pectoris. Patients who have predictable angina often find it more effective to take sublingual glyceryl trinitrate just before exertion, rather than to wait for the pain to begin. The tablets may be taken as often as necessary without loss of effect. Headache is the most common adverse effect and is sometimes severe enough to preclude use of the drug. It may be reduced by spitting out the remains of the tablet once the chest pain is relieved. Postural hypotension or syncope may also occur, and the patient should be advised to sit down when they take a tablet.— C. Wren, *Prescribers' J.*, 1983, *23*, 93.

A discussion on nitrates and angina. The exact mechanism by which nitrates relieve angina probably varies from patient to patient: in those with typical angina of effort the dominant lesions are likely to be fixed coronary artery stenoses, whereas in those with unstable angina, with variant angina, or with early acute myocardial infaction, large-vessel spasm may be of major importance. The mode of action of nitrates in chronic stable angina remains an open question but in patients with vasospastic angina, many of whom have quite normal coronary arteries on angiography, the response to nitrates clearly owes much to direct coronary vasodilatation.— *Lancet*, 1984, *1*, 998.

A discussion of the selection of optimal drug therapy for patients with angina pectoris. Initial treatment may consist of nitrates or beta blockers, either alone or in combination. Calcium-channel blockers may also be used: verapamil or diltiazem are tolerated better than nifedipine when used in combination with a nitrate. However, the use of several anti-anginal drugs in combination may be harmful to some patients.— C. Shub *et al., Mayo Clin. Proc.*, 1985, *60*, 539.

Further references to the actions and uses of nitrates in angina pectoris: J. D. Horowitz and P. J. Henry, *Med. J. Aust.*, 1987, *146*, 93; J. O. Parker, *New Engl. J. Med.*, 1987, *316*, 1635.

Myocardial infarction. Comment on the role of glyceryl trinitrate in myocardial infarction. Although glyceryl trinitrate was formerly shunned in acute myocardial infarction, it may indeed be beneficial. Since the hazard of hypotension induced by glyceryl trinitrate cannot be dismissed the possibility of counteracting a fall in blood pressure with phenylephrine or, in selected patients, avoiding it by direct intracoronary administration of glyceryl trinitrate should be considered.— E. Braunwald, *New Engl. J. Med.*, 1978, *299*, 1301. Comment on the potential hazard of injecting commercial preparations of glyceryl trinitrate containing propylene glycol directly into coronary arteries.— M. L. S. Cuddy *et al.* (letter), *New Engl. J. Med.*, 1981, *305*, 1651.

A review of the use of nitrate vasodilators in acute myocardial infarction. Nitrate vasodilators appear to have beneficial effects on short- and long-term indices of the extent of infarction as well as beneficial effects on left ventricular function and ventricular arrhythmias after infarction. However more information is needed to determine which patients may obtain the greatest benefit, and there is a need for larger and better-controlled studies.— M. A. Stratton, *Clin. Pharm.*, 1984, *3*, 32.

An overview of 10 randomised studies involving about 2000 patients of intravenous nitrate treatment in acute myocardial infarction indicated that treatment reduced mortality by between one-sixth and one-half in patients at relatively high risk of death, including many with heart failure. The greatest reduction in mortality occurred during the first week or so of follow-up, with a non-significant further reduction after this period, suggesting that early benefit was not rapidly lost.— S. Yusuf *et al.*, *Lancet*, 1988, *1*, 1088.

Ten patients with acute myocardial infarction were given glyceryl trinitrate by intravenous infusion sufficient to reduce the arterial pressure by about 20 mmHg for 60 minutes. Left ventricular filling pressure was reduced and the magnitude of the ST-segment elevation decreased when compared with 7 controls. However the subsequent infusion of phenylephrine caused an increase in the magnitude of the ST-segment elevation and in left ventricular filling pressure. It was considered that the addition of phenylephrine to glyceryl trinitrate therapy was not beneficial to patients with acute myocardial infarction.— P. C. Come *et al.*, *New Engl. J. Med.*, 1975, *293*, 1003. A similar study indicating an additional benefit with phenylephrine only in patients without left-ventricular failure.— J. S. Borer *et al.*, *ibid.*, 1008.

Initial favourable results on the extent of necrosis had been obtained following infusion of glyceryl trinitrate in patients with acute myocardial infarction.— J. P. Derrida *et al.* (letter), *New Engl. J. Med.*, 1977, *297*, 336.

CONTROLLED HYPOTENSION. Glyceryl trinitrate given by intravenous infusion successfully induced rapid, stable, and reversible hypotension to around 50 mm Hg in 19 out of 30 patients undergoing surgery for intracranial aneurysm. Hypotension was achieved 4 to 5 minutes after the start of the infusion and maintained for about 30 minutes. In 9 of the remaining 11 patients, the desired hypotensive effect was achieved by the addition of sodium nitroprusside 0.5 to 2 µg per kg body-weight per minute by intravenous infusion.— M. Guggiari *et al.*, *Br. J. Anaesth.*, 1985, *57*, 142.

Glyceryl trinitrate and nifedipine were both found to be effective in the control of arterial pressure during coronary artery surgery in patients with good left ventricular function. Verapamil was not recommended.— H. B. van Wezel *et al.*, *Br. J. Anaesth.*, 1986, *58*, 267.

Further references to the use of glyceryl trinitrate in cardiovascular surgery: W. Hess *et al.*, *Br. J. Anaesth.*, 1979, *51*, 1063; S. C. Balderman and J. Aldridge, *J. clin. Pharmac.*, 1986, *26*, 175.

GALL STONES. Endoscopic removal of bile stones was facilitated by glyceryl trinitrate 1.2 to 3.6 mg applied to the tongue. Glyceryl trinitrate 1.2 mg was shown to relax the sphincter of Oddi to approximately 30% of its normal pressure.— M. Staritz *et al.* (letter), *Lancet*, 1984, *1*, 956.

OESOPHAGEAL DISORDERS. Glyceryl trinitrate 400 µg sublingually may be effective in the treatment of oesophageal spasm. Long-acting oral nitrates singly or in combination with nifedipine or propantheline bromide can be used for prophylaxis if pain occurs frequently.— M. Traube and R. W. McCallum, *Drugs*, 1985, *30*, 66.

PERIPHERAL VASCULAR DISORDERS. Reports of beneficial effects of glyceryl trinitrate applied topically in the treatment of Raynaud's disease.— A. G. Franks, *Lancet*, 1982, *1*, 76; J. S. Coppock *et al.*, *Postgrad. med. J.*, 1986, *62*, 15.

Local percutaneous treatment with glyceryl trinitrate was used successfully to alleviate the ischaemic pain in a patient with 'burning feet' syndrome.— G. B. H. Lewis (letter), *Med. J. Aust.*, 1987, *146*, 56.

PULMONARY HYPERTENSION. A brief review of the use of glyceryl trinitrate in pulmonary hypertension. Glyceryl trinitrate produces pulmonary vasodilatation in doses which exert minimal effects on systemic arterial resistance. Several studies have shown an increase in cardiac output, and a reduction in mean pulmonary artery pressure and pulmonary vascular resistance during glyceryl trinitrate therapy. However, if the decrease in pulmonary vascular resistance that can be achieved by drug therapy is limited by irreversible structural changes in the lung parenchyma, the venodilator effects of glyceryl trinitrate may be sufficiently marked to produce a decline in cardiac output.— M. Packer, *Ann. intern. Med.*, 1985, *103*, 258.

Preparations

Glyceryl Trinitrate Tablets *(B.P.)*. Trinitrin Tablets; Nitroglycerin Tablets. Tablets containing glyceryl trinitrate in a basis of mannitol. They should be protected from light and stored at a temperature not exceeding 25° in a glass container closed by means of a screw closure lined with aluminium or tin foil; additional packing that absorbs glyceryl trinitrate should be avoided. Glyceryl trinitrate tablets should be issued for patients in containers of not more than 100 tablets. The tablets should be allowed to dissolve slowly in the mouth.

Nitroglycerin Tablets *(U.S.P.)*. Tablets containing glyceryl trinitrate. Store at 15° to 30° in airtight containers, preferably of glass, containing not more than 100 tablets. For sublingual use.

Proprietary Preparations

Coro-Nitro *(MCP Pharmaceuticals, UK)*. *Buccal spray*, aerosol, glyceryl trinitrate 400 µg/metered dose.

Deponit *(Sanol Schwarz, UK)*. *Patches* (Deponit 5), transdermal drug-delivery system, glyceryl trinitrate 16 mg, approximately 5 mg/patch absorbed in 24 hours. *Patches* (Deponit 10), transdermal drug-delivery system, glyceryl trinitrate 32 mg, approximately 10 mg/patch absorbed in 24 hours. *Administration.* One patch to be applied daily.

GTN 300 *(Martindale Pharmaceuticals, UK)*. *Tablets*, sublingual, glyceryl trinitrate 300 µg.

Nitrocine *(Sanol Schwarz, UK)*. *Injection*, glyceryl trinitrate 1 mg/mL, in a vehicle containing no alcohol or potassium in ampoules of 10 mL and in bottles of 50 mL.

NOTE. Glass or polyethylene infusion apparatus is preferable; loss of drug can occur if PVC apparatus is used.

Nitrocontin continus (formerly known as Nitrolan) *(Napp, UK)*. *Tablets*, sustained-release, glyceryl trinitrate 2.6 and 6.4 mg.

Nitrolingual *(Lipha, UK)*. *Buccal spray*, aerosol, glyceryl trinitrate 400 µg/metered dose.

NOTE. The spray should not be inhaled.

Nitronal *(Lipha, UK)*. *Injection*, glyceryl trinitrate 1 mg/mL, in a vehicle containing no alcohol, potassium, or propylene glycol, in ampoules of 5 and 25 mL and in vials of 50 mL.

NOTE. Glass or polyethylene infusion apparatus is preferable; loss of drug can occur if PVC apparatus is used.

Percutol *(Rorer, UK)*. *Ointment*, glyceryl trinitrate 2%. One inch of ointment contains glyceryl trinitrate 16.64 mg. *Administration.* ½ to 2 inches at each application; not to be rubbed in.

Suscard *(Pharmax, UK)*. *Tablets*, buccal, sustained-release, glyceryl trinitrate 1, 2, 3, and 5 mg. *Administration.* Not to be chewed, swallowed whole, or used sublingually.

Sustac *(Pharmax, UK)*. *Tablets*, sustained-release, glyceryl trinitrate 2.6, 6.4 and 10.0 mg.

NOTE. The name Sustac is also applied to Carbenoxolone Sodium, see p.1081.

Transiderm-Nitro *(Ciba, UK)*. *Patches* (Transiderm-Nitro 5), transdermal drug-delivery system, glyceryl trinitrate 25 mg, approximately 5 mg/patch absorbed in 24 hours.

Patches (Transiderm-Nitro 10), transdermal drug-delivery system, glyceryl trinitrate 50 mg, approximately 10 mg/patch absorbed in 24 hours.

Administration. One patch to be applied every 24 hours; patch-free intervals may be required.

Tridil *(American Hospital Supply, UK)*. *Injection*, glyceryl trinitrate 0.5 mg/mL, in a vehicle containing alcohol 10%, in ampoules of 10 mL, and 5 mg/mL, in a vehicle containing alcohol 30% and propylene glycol 30%, in ampoules of 10 mL.

NOTE. Glass or polyethylene infusion apparatus is preferable; loss of drug can occur if PVC apparatus is used.

Proprietary Names and Manufacturers

A 12 *(Belg.)*; Aldonitrin *(Aldo, Spain)*; Anginine *(Wellcome, Austral.)*; Angiospray *(UCB, Ital.)*; Angiplex *(Roussel, Norw.; Leiras, Swed.)*; Angised *(Wellcome, S.Afr.)*; Angitrine *(Pech, Fr.)*; Aquo-Trinitrosan *(E. Merck, Ger.)*; Cardabid *(Saron, USA)*; Colenitral *(Seid, Spain)*; Corditrine *(Specia, Fr.)*; Coro-Nitro *(Kettelhack Riker, Ger.; MCP Pharmaceuticals, UK)*; Deponit *(Schwarz, Ger.; Cedona, Neth.; Schwarz, Switz.; Sanol Schwarz, UK; Wyeth, USA)*; Ecardial *(Andromaco, Arg.)*; Enetege *(Fada, Arg.)*; Glucor nitro *(Ger.)*; Gilustenon *(Giulini, Ger.)*; GTN 300 *(Martindale Pharmaceuticals, UK)*; Klavikordal *(Ger.; US Ethicals, USA)*; Lenitral *(Besins-Iscovesco, Fr.)*; Lentonitrina *(Pierrel, Ital.; Spain)*; Maycor Nitrospray *(Parke, Davis, Ger.)*;

Natirose *(Nativelle, Fr.)*; Natispray *(Nativelle, Fr.)*; Niong *(US-Ethicals, Switz.; US Ethicals, USA)*; Nitora *(USA)*; Nitracut *(Switz.)*; Nitradisc *(Searle, Austral.; Searle, Denm.; Searle, Ger.; Searle, Norw.; Searle, S.Afr.)*; Nitrangin *(Ger.)*; Nitriderm TTS *(Geigy, Fr.)*; Nitro Mack *(Mack, Illert., Ger.; Spain; Mack, Switz.)*; Nitro Retard *(Ital.)*; Nitrobaat *(Belg.; Neth.)*; Nitro-Bid *(Protea, Austral.; Roussel, Canad.; Marion Laboratories, USA)*; Nitrochron Retard *(Switz.)*; Nitrocine *(Sanol Schwarz, UK)*; Nitrocontin Continus *(Napp, UK)*; Nitrocor *(Recordati, Ital.)*; Nitro-Corangin *(Ciba, Ger.)*; Nitroderm TTS *(Ciba, Arg.; Ciba, Ger.; Geigy, Ital.; Ciba, S.Afr.; Ciba, Spain; Ciba, Switz.)*; Nitrodisc *(Searle, Arg.; Searle, USA)*; Nitro-Dur *(Essex, Arg.; Sigmatau, Ital.; Key, USA)*; Nitro-Dur II *(Key, USA)*; Nitrofortin *(Plantorgan, Ger.)*; Nitrogard *(Syntex, Canad.; Parke, Davis, USA)*; Nitro-gesanit *(Rorer, Ger.)*; Nitroglin *(Stadapharm, Ger.)*; Nitroglyn *(Ital.; Kabi, Swed.; Key, USA)*; Nitrol *(Rorer, Canad.; Adria, USA)*; Nitrolate *(Roche, Austral.)*; Nitro-lent *(Switz.)*; Nitrolin *(Schein, USA)*; Nitrolingual *(Szama, Arg.; Belg.; Rorer, Canad.; Pohl, Denm.; Pohl, Ger.; Neth.; Pohl, Norw.; Pohl-Boskamp, Swed.; Pohl-Boskamp, Switz.; Lipha, UK; Rorer, USA)*; Nitromex *(Dumex, Denm.; Dumex, Norw.; Dumex, Swed.)*; Nitromint *(Switz.)*; Nitronal *(Pohl, Ger.; Pohl-Boskamp, S.Afr.; Pohl-Boskamp, Switz.; Lipha, UK)*; Nitronet *(US Ethicals, USA)*; Nitrong *(Belg.; Rhône-Poulenc, Canad.; Ethicals, Denm.; Manetti Roberts, Ital.; Neth.; US Ethicals, Norw.; May & Baker, S.Afr.; Ethicals, Swed.; Wharton, USA)*; Nitroperlinit *(RAN, Ger.)*; Nitroprol *(Belg.)*; Nitroprontan *(Boehringer, Arg.)*; Nitroran *(Switz.)*; Nitrorectal *(Pohl, Ger.)*; Nitroretard *(Dumex, Norw.; Dumex, Swed.)*; Nitro-SA *(USA)*; Nitrospan *(USV Pharmaceutical Corp., USA)*; Nitrostabilin *(Allen & Hanburys, Canad.)*; Nitrostat *(Parke, Davis, Canad.; Substantia, Neth.; Parke, Davis, USA)*; Nitrotard *(Inibsa, Spain)*; Nitrovas *(USA)*; Nitrozel LP *(Spain)*; Nitrozell *(Byk Gulden, Ger.; Neth.)*; NTS *(Bolar, USA)*; Nysconitrine Forte *(Belg.)*;

Percutol *(Rorer, UK)*; Perlinganit *(Schwarz, Ger.; Schwarz, Switz.)*; Solinitrina *(Infale, Spain)*; Susadrin *(Merrell Dow, USA)*; Suscard *(Pierrel, Ital.; Hässle, Swed.; Pharmax, UK)*; Sustac *(Austral.; Forest, Denm.; Neth.; Pharmax, UK)*; Sustac-Retard *(Ger.)*; Topi-Nitro *(Key, Denm.; Smith Kline & French, Norw.)*; Transderm-Nitro *(Ciba, USA)*; Transiderm-Nitro *(Ciba, Austral.; Ciba, Denm.; Geigy, Neth.; Ciba, Norw.; Ciba, Swed.; Ciba, UK)*; Trates *(Reid-Provident, USA)*; Tridil *(Boots, Austral.; Du Pont, Canad.; Boots, S.Afr.; American Hospital Supply, UK; American Critical Care, USA)*; Trinalgon *(Belg.)*; Trinitran *(Bottu, Fr.)*; Trinitrina *(Carlo Erba, Ital.)*; Trinitrine *(Sodip, Switz.)*; Trinitrosan *(E. Merck, Ger.)*; Venitrin *(Simes, Ital.)*; Vernies *(Parke, Davis, Spain)*.

The following names have been used for multi-ingredient preparations containing glyceryl trinitrate— Cardiac Dellipsoids D 18 *(Pilsworth, UK)*; Hypotensive Dellipsoids D 8 *(Pilsworth, UK)*; Natirose *(Lipomed, UK)*.

9238-c

Hepronicate *(rINN)*.

Heptylidynetris(methylene nicotinate).

$C_{28}H_{31}N_3O_6$=505.6.

CAS — 7237-81-2.

Hepronicate is a vasodilator that has been given in the treatment of peripheral vascular disorders.

Proprietary Names and Manufacturers

Malgerin *(Tanabe, Jpn)*; Megrin *(Yoshitomi, Jpn)*.

9239-k

Hexobendine Hydrochloride *(BANM, rINNM).*
ST-7090. *NN'*-Ethylenebis(3-methylaminopropyl 3,4,5-trimethoxybenzoate) dihydrochloride.
$C_{30}H_{44}N_2O_{10},2HCl=665.6$.

CAS — 54-03-5 (hexobendine); 50-62-4 (hydrochloride).

NOTE. Hexobendine is *USAN.*

Hexobendine hydrochloride is a vasodilator that has been given in the treatment of coronary insufficiency and angina pectoris.

Proprietary Names and Manufacturers
Flussicor *(Ital.)*; Reoxyl *(Hormonchemie, Ger.)*; Ustimon *(Chemie-Linz, Aust.*; *Merck-Clévenot, Fr.*; *Petersen, S.Afr.*; *Lacer, Spain*; *Chemie-Linz, Switz.)*;
Manufacturers also include—*Merrell Dow, USA.*

9241-e

Ifenprodil Tartrate *(rINNM).*
RC-61-91. (±)-2-(4-Benzylpiperidino)-1-(4-hydroxyphenyl)propan-1-ol tartrate.
$(C_{21}H_{27}NO_2)_2,C_4H_6O_6=801.0$.

CAS — 23210-56-2 (ifenprodil); 23210-58-4 (tartrate).

Ifenprodil tartrate is a vasodilator, with alpha-adrenoceptor blocking properties, that has been given in peripheral and cerebral vascular disorders.

A beneficial effect on some parameters following intravenous administration of ifenprodil tartrate to patients with intermittent claudication.— M. O. Spach and J. Schwartz, *Thérapie*, 1977, *32*, 301.

Proprietary Names and Manufacturers
Dilvax *(Promeco, Arg.)*; Serocral *(Jpn)*; Vadilex *(Robert et Carrière, Fr.*; *Promesa, Spain).*

9242-l

Imolamine Hydrochloride *(BANM, rINNM).*
LA-1211. 2-(5-Imino-3-phenyl-1,2,4-oxadiazolin-4-yl)triethylamine hydrochloride.
$C_{14}H_{20}N_4O,HCl=296.8$.

CAS — 318-23-0 (imolamine); 15823-89-9 (hydrochloride).

Imolamine hydrochloride is a vasodilator that has been used in the treatment of angina pectoris.

Proprietary Names and Manufacturers
Coremax *(Ciba, Arg.*; *Zyma, Spain)*; Irrigor *(Anphar-Rolland, Fr.*; *Karlspharma, Ger.*; *Lipha, Ital.*; *Heineking, Switz.).*

9243-y

Inositol Nicotinate *(BAN, rINN).*
Inositol Niacinate *(USAN)*; Win-9154. *meso*-Inositol hexanicotinate.
$C_{42}H_{30}N_6O_{12}=810.7$.

CAS — 6556-11-2.

Pharmacopoeias. In *Br.*

A white or almost white odourless or almost odourless powder. Practically **insoluble** in water, in alcohol, in acetone, and in ether; sparingly soluble in chloroform. It dissolves in dilute mineral acids. **Store** in well-closed containers.

Inositol nicotinate is a vasodilator and is believed to be slowly hydrolysed to nicotinic acid. It is given in the treatment of peripheral vascular disorders and in conditions arising from arterial insufficiency such as intermittent claudication and peripheral arteriosclerosis.
Treatment is usually started with 1.5 g daily and increased, if necessary, to 3 to 4 g daily in divided doses. Initial doses of 3 g daily have been used in arterial insufficiency.
Inositol nicotinate is claimed to have a fibrinolytic effect and to reduce hypercholesterolaemia.

PERIPHERAL VASCULAR DISORDERS. References: E. F. J. Ring *et al., J. int. med. Res.*, 1981, *9*, 393 (Raynaud's syndrome); R. Murphy, *Clin. Trials J.*, 1985, *22*, 521 (Raynaud's syndrome); J. O'Hara, *J. int. med. Res.*, 1985, *13*, 322 (intermittent claudication).

Preparations
Inositol Nicotinate Tablets *(B.P.)*

Proprietary Preparations
Hexopal *(Winthrop, UK). Tablets*, scored, inositol nicotinate 500 mg.
Suspension, inositol nicotinate 1 g/5 mL.
Hexopal Forte *(Winthrop, UK). Tablets*, scored, inositol nicotinate 750 mg.

Proprietary Names and Manufacturers
Dilcit *(Denm.*; *Swed.)*; Dilexpal *(Sterling Winthrop, Fr.)*; Esantene *(Ital.)*; Evicyl *(Arg.)*; Hämovannad *(Bastian, Ger.)*; Hexanicit *(Astra, Denm.*; *Astra, Ger.*; *Norw.*; *Astra, Swed.*; *Switz.)*; Hexopal *(Winthrop, UK)*; Linodil *(Winthrop, Canad.)*; Palohex *(Belg.*; *Neth.)*; Vasodil *(Austral.).*

9245-z

Isosorbide Dinitrate

ISDN; Sorbide Nitrate. 1,4:3,6-Dianhydro-D-glucitol 2,5-dinitrate.
$C_6H_8N_2O_8=236.1$.

CAS — 87-33-2.

Pharmacopoeias. In *Chin., It.*, and *Jpn.*
Br., Braz., Ind., and *U.S.* include Diluted Isosorbide Dinitrate.

A white crystalline powder. Very slightly **soluble** in water; sparingly soluble in alcohol; very soluble in acetone; freely soluble in chloroform.
Diluted Isosorbide Dinitrate is a mixture of isosorbide dinitrate (usually 20 to 50%) with lactose, mannitol, or other suitable inert excipients, the latter being added to minimise the risk of explosion. It may contain up to 1% of a suitable stabiliser such as ammonium phosphate. **Store** in airtight containers at a temperature not exceeding 15°. Protect from light.

CAUTION. Isosorbide dinitrate may explode if subjected to percussion or excessive heat.

The loss of isosorbide dinitrate from solution during infusion was found to be 30% with conventional plastic intravenous infusion sets but negligible when polyolefin or glass delivery systems were used.— E. A. Kowaluk *et al., Am. J. Hosp. Pharm.*, 1983, *40*, 118. See also P. A. Cossum and M. S. Roberts, *Eur. J. clin. Pharmac.*, 1981, *19*, 181.

Adverse Effects, Treatment, and Precautions

As for Glyceryl Trinitrate, p.1500.

Halitosis had occurred in several patients taking isosorbide dinitrate sublingually.— D. Bauman (letter), *J. Am. med. Ass.*, 1975, *234*, 482.

A severe continuous unilateral headache with an oculosympathetic paresis on the same side was associated with isosorbide dinitrate therapy in a 54-year-old man.— R. A. Mueller and O. Meienberg (letter), *New Engl. J. Med.*, 1983, *308*, 458.

EFFECTS ON THE BLOOD. Haemolysis occurred in 2 patients with glucose-6-phosphate dehydrogenase deficiency during treatment with isosorbide dinitrate.— D. Aderka *et al.* (letter), *Acta haemat.*, 1983, *69*, 63.

EFFECTS ON THE PERIPHERAL CIRCULATION. Reports of ankle oedema associated with isosorbide dinitrate therapy.— J. C. Rodger, *Br. med. J.*, 1981, *283*, 1365.

INTERACTIONS. The effectiveness of sublingual isosorbide dinitrate was reduced in a patient taking disopyramide. The interaction was considered to be due to diminished salivary secretions caused by the antimuscarinic action of disopyramide which inhibited the dissolution of the sublingual isosorbide dinitrate tablet.— M. A. Barletta and H. Eisen (letter), *Drug Intell. & clin. Pharm.*, 1985, *19*, 764.

For further discussion of delayed dissolution of sublingual tablets see Glyceryl Trinitrate, Precautions p.1500.

Absorption and Fate

Like glyceryl trinitrate, isosorbide dinitrate is readily absorbed from the oral mucosa. Isosorbide dinitrate is also readily absorbed following administration by mouth and undergoes extensive first-pass metabolism, mainly in the liver. The major metabolites of isosorbide dinitrate, isosorbide 2-mononitrate and isosorbide 5-mononitrate both possess vasodilatory activity and may contribute to the activity of the parent compound. After sublingual administration, isosorbide dinitrate has a plasma half-life of 45 to 60 minutes. In view of its short plasma half-life various long-acting formulations are available for oral administration.
Isosorbide dinitrate is also absorbed through the skin from an ointment basis.

Isosorbide dinitrate 10 mg four times daily initially, increased gradually to 360 to 720 mg daily in divided doses for about 1 to 8 weeks was well-tolerated in 7 patients with angina pectoris. Prolonged high plasma concentrations of isosorbide dinitrate and higher concentrations of its metabolites isosorbide 2-mononitrate (up to 5-fold higher) and isosorbide 5-mononitrate (up to 30-fold higher) were achieved although there was considerable individual variation. It was considered that high plasma concentrations were attained because the high chronic doses of isosorbide dinitrate had saturated the intrahepatic biotransformation process.— S. J. Shane *et al., Br. J. clin. Pharmac.*, 1978, *6*, 37.

Following administration of isosorbide dinitrate 5 mg sublingually the half-life of isosorbide dinitrate was about 28 minutes, while those of the metabolites isosorbide 2-mononitrate and isosorbide 5-mononitrate were 1.7 and 7.6 hours respectively. No correlation was found between plasma concentrations of isosorbide dinitrate or its metabolites and the haemodynamic activity as measured by digital plethysmography.— S. Spörl-Radun *et al., Eur. J. clin. Pharmac.*, 1980, *18*, 237.

The plasma half-life of isosorbide dinitrate ranged from 4.3 to 11.2 hours in 6 patients with coronary artery disease after chronic oral administration.— H. -L. Fung and J. O. Parker, *Br. J. clin. Pharmac.*, 1983, *15*, 746.

The bioavailability of isosorbide dinitrate after sublingual administration to 6 patients with coronary artery disease was incomplete and variable with a range of 19 to 93%, possibly due either to presystemic metabolism by the sublingual mucosa or hepatic first-pass metabolism after partial swallowing of the dose.— R. A. Morrison *et al., Clin. Pharmac. Ther.*, 1983, *33*, 747.

It was considered that the measurement of isosorbide dinitrate in saliva could not be used to monitor therapy in individual patients, although saliva concentrations of isosorbide mononitrate probably gave a more reliable reflection of plasma-isosorbide mononitrate concentrations.— I. W. Taylor *et al., Br. J. clin. Pharmac.*, 1984, *17*, 585.

The terminal elimination half-life of isosorbide dinitrate was 54.7 minutes following intravenous injection, 48.8 minutes following sublingual administration, and 47.7 minutes following oral administration. Total plasma clearance was 136 litres per hour. Isosorbide dinitrate bioavailability was about 29% after oral or sublingual dosing.— P. Straehl and R. L. Galeazzi, *Clin. Pharmac. Ther.*, 1985, *38*, 140.

Further references: Y. Santoni *et al., J. Pharmacokinet. Biopharm.*, 1986, *14*, 1; U. Abshagen *et al., Eur. J. clin. Pharmac.*, 1985, *27*, 637.

Uses and Administration

Isosorbide dinitrate is a vasodilator with general properties similar to those of glyceryl trinitrate (p.1501). Isosorbide dinitrate is suitable for oral as well as sublingual administration. In view of its brief plasma half-life preparations of isosorbide dinitrate for oral administration are available in sustained-release form. When administered sublingually its effects begin within about 5 minutes and last for about 2 hours; when swallowed its effects are evident after about 30 minutes and last for about 5 hours.
It is used prophylactically in the treatment of angina pectoris in oral doses of 5 to 20 mg three or four times daily according to the patient's needs or the equivalent dose in a sustained-release formulation. Increases in dosage should be gradual to avoid side-effects. Up to 240 mg daily in divided doses may be necessary. For acute attacks the usual dose is 2.5 to 10 mg sublingually. Isosorbide dinitrate may also be used in similar doses as adjunctive therapy in congestive heart failure.
Isosorbide dinitrate may also be given by intravenous infusion as a solution usually containing about 100 to 200 μg per mL in sodium chloride injection (0.9%) or glucose injection (5.0%). For unresponsive congestive cardiac failure or severe or unstable angina a recommended

starting dose is 2 mg per hour increased if necessary to 7 mg per hour; doses of up to 10 mg per hour may be necessary in some patients.

Isosorbide dinitrate has also been applied topically.

A review of the pharmacological properties and therapeutic use of isosorbide dinitrate.— U. Elkayam and W. S. Aronow, *Drugs*, 1982, *23*, 165.

A review of therapy with organic and inorganic nitrates including a discussion of the routes of administration of isosorbide dinitrate.— J. Abrams, *Drugs*, 1987, *34*, 391.

A preliminary report of experience with isosorbide dinitrate cream.— B. Cheadle *et al.* (letter), *Br. med. J.*, 1981, *283*, 1549.

CARDIAC DISORDERS. *Angina pectoris.* Reports and studies on the use of isosorbide dinitrate in angina pectoris: C. E. Handler and I. D. Sullivan, *Int. J. Cardiol.*, 1985, *7*, 149; C. E. Rackley, *Am. Heart J.*, 1985, *110*, 269; C. R. Conti *et al.*, *ibid.*, 251; J. O. Parker *et al.*, *Am. J. Cardiol.*, 1985, *56*, 724; P. Rizzon *et al.*, *Eur. Heart J.*, 1986, *7*, 67; D. P. Nicholls *et al.*, *Br. J. clin. Pharmac.*, 1986, *22*, 15; M. Äärynen and K. Soininen, *J. int. med. Res.*, 1986, *14*, 303; J. O. Parker *et al.*, *New Engl. J. Med.*, 1987, *316*, 1440.

Heart Failure. In patients with acute heart failure following acute myocardial infarction isosorbide dinitrate intravenously produced a more rapid and effective reduction in pulmonary vascular pressure than frusemide intravenously, and also produced more favourable haemodynamic changes.— G. I. C. Nelson *et al.*, *Lancet*, 1983, *1*, 730. Comments.— C. D. Burgess (letter), *ibid.*, 1108; O. Bertel *et al.* (letter), *ibid.*, 1109.

A review of the vasodilator drugs including nitrates used in the treatment of chronic congestive heart failure. Vasodilator therapy was considered to be useful in patients who have symptoms of congestive heart failure despite treatment with digitalis or diuretics. Sustained improvement in haemodynamics and exercise tolerance has been demonstrated with isosorbide dinitrate, although an effect on survival has not been determined.— *Med. Lett.*, 1984, *26*, 115.

A review of the treatment of heart failure, including the use of isosorbide dinitrate. It was concluded that, on the basis of available data, nitrates have not been shown to improve quality of life and could not be recommended as routine, long-term therapy for patients with heart failure.— G. H. Guyatt, *Drugs*, 1986, *32*, 538.

Results of a study involving 642 male patients with symptomatic chronic congestive heart failure treated with digoxin and diuretics indicated that the addition of isosorbide dinitrate and hydralazine could have a favourable effect on left ventricular function and mortality.— J. N. Cohn *et al.*, *New Engl. J. Med.*, 1986, *314*, 1547. Discussion of the influence of possible differences in baseline variables between patients in different treatment groups on the outcome of the trial.— C. P. Taliercio (letter), *ibid.*, *315*, 1227; O. Bertel (letter), *ibid*; R. H. Falk (letter), *ibid.* Reply.— J. N. Cohn and D. G. Archibald (letter), *ibid.*, 1228.

Myocardial infarction. A study in 45 patients in the early stages of acute myocardial infarction indicated that intracoronary therapy with isosorbide dinitrate and streptokinase may increase the rate of coronary recanalisation.— D. Hackett *et al.*, *New Engl. J. Med.*, 1987, *317*, 1055.

OESOPHAGEAL DISORDERS. A review of the treatment of oesophageal motility disorders. In patients with achalasia, who are unfit or unwilling to undergo surgery, isosorbide dinitrate 5 mg sublingually 15 minutes before meals or 10 mg orally 30 to 60 minutes before meals may be tried. Isosorbide dinitrate may also be useful in patients with diffuse oesophageal spasm.— *Drug & Ther. Bull.*, 1984, *22*, 17. See also M. Traube and R. W. McCallum, *Drugs*, 1985, *30*, 66.

PORTAL HYPERTENSION. A brief review of the use of isosorbide dinitrate and other nitrates in the treatment of portal hypertension. Nitrates have been used alone and in combination with vasopressin therapy.— W. G. Rector, *Ann. intern. Med.*, 1986, *105*, 96.

Further references.— J. G. Freeman *et al.*, *Br. med. J.*, 1985, *291*, 561; J. Dawson *et al.*, *Gut*, 1985, *26*, 843.

PULMONARY HYPERTENSION. Isosorbide dinitrate, in doses of 25 to 40 mg, may be useful in reducing pulmonary hypertension in patients with chronic obstructive pulmonary disease.— D. T. Danahy *et al.*, *Clin. Pharmac. Ther.*, 1979, *25*, 541. See also J. B. Hermiller *et al.*, *Ann. intern. Med.*, 1982, *97*, 480.

Preparations

Isosorbide Dinitrate Chewable Tablets *(U.S.P.)*

Isosorbide Dinitrate Extended-release Capsules *(U.S.P.)*

Isosorbide Dinitrate Extended-release Tablets *(U.S.P.)*

Isosorbide Dinitrate Sublingual Tablets *(U.S.P.)*

Isosorbide Dinitrate Tablets *(B.P.).* Sorbide Nitrate Tablets. Contain diluted isosorbide dinitrate.

Isosorbide Dinitrate Tablets *(U.S.P.)*

Proprietary Preparations

Cedocard *(Tillotts, UK). Tablets* (Cedocard-5), oral and sublingual, scored, isosorbide dinitrate 5 mg.
Tablets (Cedocard-10), scored, isosorbide dinitrate 10 mg.
Tablets (Cedocard-20), scored, isosorbide dinitrate 20 mg.
Tablets, (Cedocard-40), scored, isosorbide dinitrate 40 mg.
Injection, isosorbide dinitrate 1 mg/mL, in ampoules of 10 mL and bottles of 50 and 100 mL. Normally diluted before use.

NOTE. Glass or polyethylene infusion apparatus is preferable; loss of drug can occur if PVC apparatus is used.

Cedocard Retard *(Tillotts, UK). Tablets,* (Cedocard Retard-20), sustained-release, scored, isosorbide dinitrate 20 mg.
Tablets, (Cedocard Retard-40), sustained-release, scored, isosorbide dinitrate 40 mg.

Isoket *(Sanol Schwarz, UK). Tablets* (Isoket 5), oral and sublingual, isosorbide dinitrate 5 mg.
Tablets (Isoket 10), oral and sublingual, isosorbide dinitrate 10 mg.
Tablets (Isoket 20), oral and sublingual, isosorbide dinitrate 20 mg.
Concentrate for intravenous infusion, (Isoket 0.1%), isosorbide dinitrate 1 mg/mL, in ampoules of 10 mL and bottles of 50 and 100 mL. Dilute before use.

NOTE. Glass or polyethylene infusion apparatus is preferable; loss of drug can occur if PVC apparatus is used.

Isoket Retard *(Sanol Schwarz, UK). Tablets,* (Isoket Retard 20), sustained-release, scored, isosorbide dinitrate 20 mg.
Tablets, (Isoket Retard 40), sustained-release, scored, isosorbide dinitrate 40 mg.

Isordil *(Ayerst, UK). Tablets,* scored, isosorbide dinitrate 10 and 30 mg.
Tablets, sublingual, isosorbide dinitrate 5 mg.

Isordil Tembids *(Ayerst, UK). Capsules,* sustained-release, isosorbide dinitrate 40 mg.

Soni-Slo *(Lipha, UK). Capsules,* sustained-release, isosorbide dinitrate 20 and 40 mg.

Sorbichew (formerly known as Sorbitrate Chewable) *(Stuart, UK). Tablets,* chewable, scored, isosorbide dinitrate 5 mg.

Sorbid *(Stuart, UK). Capsules,* (Sorbid-20 SA), sustained-release, isosorbide dinitrate 20 mg.
Capsules, (Sorbid-40 SA), sustained-release, isosorbide dinitrate 40 mg.

Sorbitrate *(Stuart, UK). Tablets,* scored, isosorbide dinitrate 10 and 20 mg.

Vascardin *(Nicholas, UK). Tablets,* oral and sublingual, scored, isosorbide dinitrate 10 mg.
Tablets, scored, isosorbide dinitrate 30 mg.

Proprietary Names and Manufacturers

Acordin *(Mepha, Switz.)*; Apo-ISDN *(Apotex, Canad.)*; Cardio *(Nicholas, Ger.)*; Cardopax *(Erco, Denm.)*; Carvasin *(Austral.*; *Ayerst, Ital.)*; Cedocard *(Belg.*; *Neth.*; *S.Afr.*; *Switz.*; *Tillotts, UK)*; Conducil *(Casasco, Arg.)*; Coronex *(Ayerst, Canad.)*; Corosorbide *(Arg.)*; Corovliss *(Boehringer Mannheim, Ger.)*; Dilatrate-SR *(Reed & Carnrick, USA)*; Directan *(Jpn)*; Disorlon *(Nativelle, Fr.)*; Duranitrat *(Durachemie, Ger.)*; EureCor *(Kade, Ger.)*; Isdin *(Medice, Ger.)*; Iso Mack *(Mack, Illert., Ger.*; *Swisspharm, S.Afr.*; *Mack, Switz.)*; Iso-Bid *(Geriatric Pharm. Corp., USA)*; Isochron *(Forest Laboratories, USA)*; Iso-D *(USA)*; Isoforce *(RAN, Ger.)*; Isoket *(Schering, Arg.*; *Schwarz, Ger.*; *Lacer, Spain*; *Schwarz, Switz.*; *Sanol Schwarz, UK)*; Iso-Puren *(Klinge-Nattermann, Ger.)*; Isorbid *(Mex.)*; Isordil *(Ayerst, Arg.*; *Ayerst, Austral.*; *Belg.*; *Wyeth, Canad.*; *Ayerst, S.Afr.*; *Inibsa, Spain*; *Ayerst, Switz.*; *Ayerst, UK*; *Wyeth, USA)*; Isostenase *(Azuchemie, Ger.)*; Isotrate *(Parke, Davis, Austral.*; *Hauck, USA)*; Langoran *(Merrell, Fr.)*; Maycor *(Arg.*; *Parke, Davis, Ger.*; *Parke, Davis, Spain)*; Myorexon *(Switz.)*; Nitro *(Ger.)*; Nitrol *(Jpn)*; Nitrosorbide *(Lusofarmaco, Ital.)*; Nitrosorbon *(Pohl, Ger.)*; Nitro-Tablinen *(Beiersdorf, Ger.)*; Novosorbide *(Novopharm, Canad.)*; Rifloc *(Merrell, Ger.)*; Risordan *(Théraplix, Fr.)*; Sigillum *(Arg.)*; Soni-Slo *(Lipha, UK)*; Sorate *(Trimen, USA)*; Sorbangil *(KabiVitrum, Norw.*; *Kabi, Swed.)*; Sorbichew *(Stuart, UK)*; Sorbid *(Stuart, UK)*; Sorbide *(Mayrand, USA)*; Sorbidilat *(Belg.*; *Fresenius, Ger.*; *Astra, Switz.)*; Sorbitrate *(I.C.I.-Pharma, Fr.*; *Stuart, UK*; *Stuart Pharmaceuticals, USA)*; Sorquad *(Reid-Provident, USA)*; Surantol *(Arg.)*; TD Spray *(Mack, Illert., Ger.)*; Vascardin *(Nicholas, UK)*; Vasodilat *(Arg.)*; Vasotrate *(USA)*; Vermicet *(Winthrop, Ger.)*.

15336-h

Isosorbide Mononitrate *(BAN, rINN).*

BM-22.145; IS-5-MN; Isosorbide-5-mononitrate.
1,4:3,6-Dianhydro-D-glucitol 5-nitrate.
$C_6H_9NO_6$=191.1.

CAS — 16051-77-7.

Adverse Effects, Treatment, and Precautions

As for Glyceryl Trinitrate, p.1500.

Absorption and Fate

Isosorbide mononitrate is readily absorbed from the gastro-intestinal tract following oral administration. Unlike isosorbide dinitrate, isosorbide mononitrate does not undergo first-pass hepatic metabolism and is eliminated more slowly.

Isosorbide mononitrate is rapidly absorbed following oral administration and the maximum plasma concentration is reached after about 1 hour. The plasma half-life has been reported as 4.0 to 4.9 hours (U. Abshagen and S. Spörl-Radun, *Eur. J. clin. Pharmac.*, 1981, *19*, 423; T. Taylor, *et al.*, *Biopharm. Drug Disposit.*, 1981, *2*, 255).

For reports of the plasma concentration and half-life of isosorbide mononitrate following isosorbide dinitrate administration, see Isosorbide Dinitrate, Absorption and Fate p.1503.

Uses and Administration

Isosorbide mononitrate is an active metabolite of the vasodilator isosorbide dinitrate and is used prophylactically in the treatment of angina pectoris and chronic congestive heart failure. The usual oral dose is 20 mg two or three times daily, although maintenance doses ranging from 20 to 120 mg daily have been given.

A brief review. Available clinical data do not seem to justify the claim of greater efficacy, longer action, or fewer adverse effects of isosorbide mononitrate over sustained-release isosorbide dinitrate.— *Drug & Ther. Bull.*, 1984, *22*, 7.

CARDIAC DISORDERS. Studies of the use of isosorbide mononitrate in angina pectoris: H. J. Überbacher *et al.*, *Pharmatherapeutica*, 1983, *3*, 331; G. Müller *et al.*, *Klin. Wschr.*, 1983, *61*, 409; R. S. Kohli *et al.*, *Am. J. Cardiol.*, 1986, *58*, 727; G. Nyberg *et al.*, *Eur. Heart J.*, 1986, *7*, 835; A. Reale *et al.*, *Curr. ther. Res.*, 1986, *39*, 912; G. Koch *et al.*, *ibid.*, 1987, *41*, 454; U. Thadani *et al.*, *Clin. Pharmac. Ther.*, 1987, *42*, 58.

Evidence of tolerance to the effects of isosorbide mononitrate was seen during chronic dosing with a sustained-release preparation in a study involving 9 patients with angina pectoris.— U. Thadani *et al.*, *Am. J. Cardiol.*, 1987, *59*, 756. There was no indication of the development of tolerance to the anti-anginal effects of isosorbide mononitrate following treatment with isosorbide mononitrate 60 mg daily in a sustained-release formulation.— M. Meffert and I. -M. Paeckelmann, *Drugs*, 1987, *33*, *Suppl.* 4, 104. Similar results with sustained-release isosorbide mononitrate used concomitantly with beta blockers. It was suggested that tolerance was avoided because plasma concentrations fall to a low level for a period during the day when this formulation is given once daily.— A. Uusitalo, *ibid.*, 111.

Proprietary Preparations

Elantan *(Sanol Schwarz, UK). Capsules* (Elantan LA50), sustained-release, isosorbide mononitrate 50 mg.
Tablets (Elantan 20), scored, isosorbide mononitrate 20 mg.
Tablets (Elantan 40), scored, isosorbide mononitrate 40 mg.

Imdur *(Astra, UK). Tablets,* sustained-release, scored, isosorbide mononitrate 60 mg.

Ismo *(MCP Pharmaceuticals, UK). Tablets,* isosorbide mononitrate 10, 20, and 40 mg.
Starter Pack, 8 tablets, isosorbide mononitrate 10 mg in a calendar pack; 60 tablets, isosorbide mononitrate 20 mg.

Monit *(Stuart, UK). Tablets,* scored, isosorbide mononitrate 20 mg.

Monit LS *(Stuart, UK). Tablets,* isosorbide mononitrate 10 mg.

Mono-Cedocard *(Tillotts, UK). Tablets,* (Mono-Cedocard-10), scored, isosorbide mononitrate 10 mg.

Tablets, (Mono-Cedocard-20), scored, isosorbide mononitrate 20 mg.

Tablets, (Mono-Cedocard-40), scored, isosorbide mononitrate 40 mg.

Proprietary Names and Manufacturers

Coleb *(Astra, Ger.)*; Conpin *(TAD, Ger.)*; Corangin *(Ciba, Ger.)*; Coronur *(Boehringer Mannheim, Spain)*; Duramonitat *(Durachemie, Ger.)*; Elantan *(Schwarz, Ger.; Schwarz, Switz.; Sanol Schwarz, UK)*; Imdur *(Hässle, Denm.; Astra, UK)*; Ismo *(Boehringer, Arg.; Erco, Denm.; Boehringer Mannheim, Ger.; Boehringer Biochemia, Ital.; Boehringer Mannheim, Norw.; Boehringer Mannheim, S.Afr.; Boehringer Mannheim, Swed.; Boehringer Mannheim, Switz.; MCP Pharmaceuticals, UK)*; Medocor *(Roemmers, Arg.)*; Monocinque *(Lusofarmaco, Ital.)*; Monicor *(P.F.M., Fr.)*; Monit *(Stuart, UK)*; Monit-Puren *(Klinge-Nattermann, Ger.)*; Mono Mack *(Mack, Illert., Ger.)*; Mono-Cedocard *(Tillotts, UK)*; Monoclair *(Hennig, Ger.)*; Monoket *(Chiesi, Ital.; Ferrosan, Swed.)*; Monopur *(Pohl, Ger.)*; Monosorb *(Unicet, Fr.)*; Monostenase *(Azuchemie, Ger.)*; Mono-Wolff *(Wolff, Ger.)*; Olicard *(Giulini, Ger.)*; Uniket *(Lacer, Spain)*.

9246-c

Isoxsuprine Hydrochloride *(BANM, USAN, rINNM).*

Caa-40; Phenoxyisopropylnorsuprifen. 1-(4-Hydroxyphenyl)-2-(1-methyl-2-phenoxyethylamino)propan-1-ol hydrochloride.

$C_{18}H_{23}NO_3,HCl=337.8.$

CAS — 395-28-8 (isoxsuprine); 579-56-6 (hydrochloride).

Pharmacopoeias. In *Br., Ind.,* and *U.S.*

A white or almost white odourless or almost odourless crystalline powder. **Soluble** 1 in 500 of water, 1 in 100 of alcohol and dilute sodium hydroxide solution, and 1 in 2500 of dilute hydrochloric acid; practically insoluble in chloroform and ether. A 1% solution in water has a pH of 4.5 to 6.0. **Store** in airtight containers. Solutions are **sterilised** by autoclaving.

Adverse Effects

Isoxsuprine may cause transient flushing and gastro-intestinal disturbances. Larger doses cause tachycardia and hypotension. A slight increase in the rate of the foetal heart-beat has been noted when isoxsuprine has been given by intravenous infusion during the late stages of pregnancy. Rarely, severe skin rashes have been associated with its administration. Maternal pulmonary oedema has been reported following intravenous administration in premature labour.

ALLERGY. A report of allergic dermatitis in 2 women given isoxsuprine for premature labour. The eruption was pruritic and papular in both women.— J. J. Horowitz and R. K. Creasy, *Am. J. Obstet. Gynec.*, 1978, *131*, 225.

PREGNANCY AND THE NEONATE. In a study involving 40 neonates whose mothers had received isoxsuprine within 24 hours of delivery and 40 matched controls, ileus was found to be more common in the isoxsuprine group than in the controls. The isoxsuprine group was subdivided according to concentrations found in the cord blood and the incidence of respiratory distress syndrome was minimal in the group with absent or low drug values but rose to surpass the control group as the isoxsuprine concentration exceeded 10 ng per mL; likewise the incidence of hypocalcaemia and hypotension rose progressively with increasing concentrations. The cord concentrations correlated inversely with the drug-free interval before delivery and it was suggested that with frequent assessment of uterine response it should be possible to avoid delivering infants at a time when they have high plasma-isoxsuprine concentrations.— J. E. Brazy *et al., J. Pediat.*, 1981, *98*, 146.

In a study of the association between ruptured membranes, beta-adrenergic therapy and respiratory distress syndrome, it was found that both therapy with isoxsuprine and premature rupture of membranes were individually associated with a lowered incidence of respiratory distress syndrome, but when present together they resulted in an increased risk of respiratory distress syndrome. It was suggested that therapy with beta-adrenergic agents including isoxsuprine should be restricted to patients with intact membranes.— L. B. Curet *et al., Am. J. Obstet. Gynec.*, 1984, *148*, 263.

Pulmonary oedema. Report of 6 patients who developed symptoms of pulmonary oedema during isoxsuprine therapy for premature labour. It was suggested that pulmonary complications may be reduced by careful attention to fluid balance.— D. A. Nagey and M. C. Crenshaw, *Obstet. Gynec.*, 1982, *59, Suppl.*, 38S.

Pulmonary oedema occurred in 7 patients who received treatment with intravenous isoxsuprine for premature labour. A further 1276 patients who received intravenous isoxsuprine did not develop pulmonary oedema. It was suggested that caution should be exercised when doses in excess of 0.5 mg per minute and treatment for longer than 48 hours are required. Treatment of pulmonary symptoms with oxygen, diuretics, and digoxin was considered effective.— C. Nimrod *et al., Am. J. Obstet. Gynec.*, 1984, *148*, 625.

Precautions

Isoxsuprine is contra-indicated following recent arterial haemorrhage. It should not be administered parenterally to patients with hypotension, known heart disease, severe anaemia, or tachycardia.

It should not be given where there is premature detachment of the placenta or immediately post partum.

In premature labour patients should be maintained in the lateral position during infusion.

For reports of the effect of isoxsuprine following administration during labour, see under Adverse Effects, above.

Absorption and Fate

Isoxsuprine hydrochloride is well absorbed from the gastro-intestinal tract. The maximum concentration in the circulation occurs about 1 hour after administration by mouth or intramuscular injection, and is maintained for about 3 hours. A plasma half-life of 1.5 hours has been reported. Isoxsuprine is in part conjugated in the blood and is excreted in the urine. Faecal excretion is insignificant.

Uses and Administration

Isoxsuprine is a vasodilator that produces the effects of beta-adrenoceptor stimulation and alpha-adrenoceptor antagonism, the former effect predominating. It also causes direct relaxation of vascular and uterine smooth muscle. Its dilating action is greater on the arteries supplying skeletal muscles than on those supplying skin. Isoxsuprine also produces positive inotropic effects.

Isoxsuprine hydrochloride is used in the treatment of cerebral and peripheral vascular disease in doses of up to 20 mg four times daily by mouth, or by intramuscular injection in doses of up to 10 mg four times daily. Isoxsuprine hydrochloride may also be given by intravenous infusion as a solution containing 200 µg per mL in 5% glucose infusion. A twice-daily dose of 300 µg (1.5 mL) per minute for a maximum of 67 minutes has been recommended.

Isoxsuprine hydrochloride is also used to arrest premature labour. It is given initially by intravenous infusion; a solution containing 100 mg in 500 mL of glucose injection (5%) is infused at the rate of 1 to 1.5 mL per minute (200 to 300 µg per minute) increased, according to the patient's response, to 2.5 mL per minute (500 µg per minute) with regular monitoring of blood pressure and maternal and foetal heart-rates, and continued until control is established. Subsequent treatment consists of intramuscular injections of 10 mg every 3 hours for 24 hours, every 4 to 6 hours for a further 48 hours, and then 20 mg by mouth 4 times daily.

CEREBROVASCULAR DISORDERS. A review of the use of cerebral vasodilators, including isoxsuprine. Two out of 3 double-blind studies reported some improvement in cognitive function in patients with cerebrovascular disease or dementia, but no practical benefit was demonstrated.— P. Cook and I. James, *New Engl. J. Med.*, 1981, *305*, 1560.

PERIPHERAL VASCULAR DISORDERS. Results of studies do not support the use of isoxsuprine in obstructive arterial disease; since it is not a cutaneous vasodilator, it should not be used in vasospastic disease.— J. D. Coffman, *New Engl. J. Med.*, 1979, *300*, 713.

In an open study of 51 patients with intermittent claudication treated for 3 months with sustained-release isoxsuprine, there was subjective improvement in 25 patients and objective improvement in 26 patients out of 36 patients who completed the study: 6 patients were withdrawn from the study because of adverse effects, and 2 were withdrawn due to lack of effect. Twenty-three patients took other medication concomitantly during the study period.— W. Mackenzie and S. Wonnacott, *Br. J. clin. Pract.*, 1985, *39*, 30.

PREGNANCY AND THE NEONATE. *Premature labour.* A review of the management of premature labour, including the use of isoxsuprine. Isoxsuprine may be administered by mouth, or by intravenous or intramuscular injection. Dosage regimens vary widely. Two controlled studies have indicated that isoxsuprine is more effective than placebo in prolonging pregnancy. Other uncontrolled studies have also suggested that isoxsuprine is a potent inhibitor of labour.

Drug concentrations in foetal plasma were reported to be 90% of those in the mother. The likelihood and severity of adverse effects in the mother appear to be related to the dosage and duration of treatment. The half-life of isoxsuprine in neonates was 1.7 to 8.0 hours, with the longer half-lives occurring in younger infants. The incidence of hypotension and hypocalcaemia in infants was 89 and 100% respectively when the concentration in cord blood exceeded 10 ng per mL.— S. N. Caritis, *Drugs*, 1983, *26*, 243. See also *Drug & Ther. Bull.*, 1980, *18*, 34.

Report of the use of isoxsuprine in premature labour and the effect on the foetus in 70 patients. In patients with intact membranes, therapeutic outcome was influenced by the status of the cervix at the initiation of isoxsuprine therapy: prolongation of pregnancy for more than 7 days occurred in 77% of women with 50% cervical effacement or less and 3 cm dilatation or less. Foetal tachycardia, maternal hypotension, and maternal tachycardia were generally seen with infusion rates of more than 0.25 mg per minute. The isoxsuprine concentration in cord blood averaged 90% of the maternal concentration at delivery. Adverse foetal effects were uncommon with cord blood concentrations of less than 2 ng per mL, which occurred after a drug-free interval of more than 5 hours following intravenous administration or in patients who were exposed only to oral therapy in the 12 hours before delivery.— J. E. Brazy *et al., Obstet. Gynec.*, 1981, *58*, 297.

In a study to assess the development of 20 very-low-birth-weight infants born within 24 hours of attempting to arrest premature labour with isoxsuprine, the outcome at 2 years of age was similar to that of a matched group of preterm infants without isoxsuprine exposure.— J. E. Brazy *et al., J. Pediat.*, 1983, *102*, 611.

See also under Salbutamol, p.1483.

For references to possible complications of isoxsuprine therapy during premature labour see under Adverse Effects, above.

Preparations

Isoxsuprine Hydrochloride Injection *(U.S.P.)*

Isoxsuprine Hydrochloride Tablets *(U.S.P.)*

Isoxsuprine Injection *(B.P.).* Isoxsuprine Hydrochloride Injection

Isoxsuprine Tablets *(B.P.).* Isoxsuprine Hydrochloride Tablets

Proprietary Preparations

Duvadilan *(Duphar, UK).*

Injection, isoxsuprine hydrochloride 5 mg/mL, in ampoules of 2 mL.

Proprietary Names and Manufacturers

Cardilan *(Norw.)*; Defencin CP *(Bristol-Myers Pharmaceuticals, UK)*; Duvadilan *(Arg.; Cilag, Austral.; Belg.; Duphar, Fr.; Duphar, Ger.; ISM, Ital.; Neth.; S.Afr.; Kali-Farma, Spain; Ferrosan, Swed.; Switz.; Duphar, UK)*; Duvadilan Retard *(Duphar, UK)*; Fenam *(ISM, Ital.)*; Isokulin *(Jpn)*; Largiven *(Bristol Italiana Sud, Ital.)*; Suprilent *(Switz.)*; Synzedrin *(Jpn)*; Vahodilan *(Jpn)*; Vascuprin *(Ital.)*; Vasodilan *(Bristol, Canad.; Mead Johnson Pharmaceutical, USA)*; Vasodilene

(Chiesi, Ital.); Vasoplex *(Ger.)*; Vasosuprina *(Lusofarmaco, Ital.)*; Vasotran *(Bristol-Myers Pharmaceuticals, UK)*; Xuprin *(Aust.)*.

19367-a

Isradipine *(BAN, rINN)*.
Isrodipine; PN-200-110. Isopropyl methyl-4-(4-benzofurazanyl)-1,4-dihydro-2,6-dimethyl-3,5-pyridinedicarboxylate.
$C_{19}H_{21}N_3O_5$=371.4.

CAS — 75695-93-1.

Isradipine is a calcium-channel blocking agent with properties similar to Nifedipine, p.1511. It has been tried in the treatment of hypertension and angina pectoris.

References: C. E. Handler and E. Sowton, *Eur. J. clin. Pharmac.*, 1984, *27*, 415; E. B. Nelson *et al.*, *Clin. Pharmac. Ther.*, 1986, *40*, 694; L. Hansson and B. Dahlof, *Am. J. Cardiol.*, 1987, *59*, 137B; B. P. Hamilton, *ibid.*, 141B; F. L. S. Tse and J. M. Jaffe, *Eur. J. clin. Pharmac.*, 1987, *32*, 361.

Proprietary Names and Manufacturers
Sandoz, Switz.; Sandoz, USA.

9247-k

Itramin Tosylate *(BAN)*.
Itramin Tosilate *(rINN)*. 2-Aminoethyl nitrate toluene-4-sulphonate.
$C_2H_6N_2O_3,C_7H_8O_3S$=278.3.

CAS — 646-02-6 (itramin); 13445-63-1 (tosylate).

Itramin tosylate is a vasodilator formerly used in the treatment of angina pectoris.

Proprietary Names and Manufacturers
Cardisan *(Takeda, Jpn)*; Nilatil *(Pharmacia, Swed.)*.

9248-a

Kallidinogenase *(BAN, rINN)*.
Callicrein; Kalléone; Kallikrein.

CAS — 9001-01-8.

An enzyme isolated from the pancreas and urine of mammals.

The properties and assay methods of kallidinogenase.— Kallikrein, in *Pharmaceutical Enzymes*, R. Ruyssen and A. Lauwers (Ed.), Gent, E. Story-Scientia, 1978, p. 145.

Kallidinogenase converts the kinin, kallidin, from kininogen. It has vasodilating properties and has been used in the treatment of peripheral vascular disorders. It has also been tried in the treatment of male infertility.

A discussion of the treatment of male fertility disturbances, including the use of kallidinogenase.— W. -B. Schill and M. Michalopoulos, *Drugs*, 1984, *28*, 263.

Proprietary Names and Manufacturers
Bioactin *(Jpn)*; Depot-Padutin *(Bayer, Denm.)*; Glumorin *(Bayer, UK)*; Onokrein-P *(Jpn)*; Padukrein *(Bayropharm, Ger.)*; Padutin *(Bayer, Denm.; Bayropharm, Ger.)*; Padutina Depot *(Bayer, Spain)*; Padutine-Dépot *(Bayer, Belg.)*; Prokrein *(Jpn)*.

9249-t

Khellin *(rINN)*.
Khelline; Khellinum; Visammin. 4,9-Dimethoxy-7-methyl-5*H*-furo[3,2-*g*]chromen-5-one.
$C_{14}H_{12}O_5$=260.2.

CAS — 82-02-0.

Pharmacopoeias. In *Aust.*, *Egypt.*, and *Rus. Egypt.*, *Fr.*, *Ger.*, and *Pol.* also include Ammi Visnaga Fruit.

Khellin is obtained by extraction from the dried ripe fruit of ammi visnaga (Umbelliferae) or by synthesis.

Khellin is a coronary vasodilator and also has bronchodilatory action. It has been employed in the treatment of angina pectoris, and in the treatment of asthma. Doses of 40 mg have been given two to four times daily by mouth; 50 mg has been given one to four times daily by intramuscular injection.

CARDIAC DISORDERS. A discussion on abandoned treatments for angina pectoris, including khellin, which is now believed to have no specific physiological efficacy yet was formerly found to be effective and was used extensively.— H. Benson and D. P. McCallie, *New Engl. J. Med.*, 1979, *300*, 1424.

Proprietary Names and Manufacturers of Khellin and Ammi Visnaga Fruit
Aspas *(Biochimica Zanardi, Ital.)*; Kelicorin *(Infale, Spain)*; Kellina *(UCB, Ital.)*; Kellosal *(Biosint, Ital.)*; Visnacorin *(Infale, Spain)*.

9250-l

Lidoflazine *(BAN, USAN, rINN)*.
McN-JR-7904; Ordiflazine; R-7904. 4-[3-(4,4′-Difluorobenzhydryl)propyl]piperazin-1-ylaceto-2′,6′-xylidide.
$C_{30}H_{35}F_2N_3O$=491.6.

CAS — 3416-26-0.

Adverse Effects
Side-effects associated with lidoflazine include gastro-intestinal upset, transient dizziness, tinnitus and headache. Lidoflazine may also cause or aggravate ventricular arrhythmias.

Uses and Administration
Lidoflazine is used for the long-term management of angina pectoris. It has calcium-channel blocking properties (see under Nifedipine p.1511). A recommended dosage schedule is 60 to 120 mg daily initially for the first week, increased at weekly intervals to 120 mg three times daily.

Comment on the different action of drugs given the general description of calcium antagonists, and the view that they should be subdivided into 4 or more classes according to their principal therapeutic effects; lidoflazine inhibits excess ingress of calcium into cells deprived of oxygen without affecting calcium homoeostasis in the well-oxygenated cell.— A. L. Macnair and H. A. Waldron (letter), *Br. med. J.*, 1981, *282*, 400.

For further comments on the mode of action of calcium-channel blockers, see under Nifedipine, p.1511.

CARDIAC DISORDERS. A review of the use of lidoflazine in the treatment of angina pectoris. Published studies suggest that lidoflazine has an anti-anginal effect comparable to that seen with beta-blockers. Lidoflazine has some calcium-channel blocking activity that appears to be confined to smooth muscle. There is no direct evidence of an effect on the cardiac conduction system, although the Q-T interval is prolonged. The mechanism of action in angina pectoris remains obscure.
There is a delay in the onset of anti-anginal activity of 4 to 6 weeks, and maximal benefit is not reached until several months of treatment. Lidoflazine should not be given to patients with severe ischaemia and only with caution to those taking beta-blockers, digoxin or potassium-depleting diuretics. The delay in onset of activity makes it unacceptable as first-line treatment of angina, and its use is restricted to patients with mild ischaemia in whom conventional drug therapy is inadequate.— *Drug & Ther. Bull.*, 1983, *21*, 27.

Proprietary Preparations
Clinium *(Janssen, UK)*. *Tablets*, lidoflazine 120 mg.

Proprietary Names and Manufacturers
Clavidene *(Corvi, Ital.)*; Clinium *(Arg.; Belg.; Janssen, Fr.; Janssen, Ger.; Ital.; Neth.; Janssen, S.Afr.; Janssen, UK)*; Corflazine *(Syntex, Fr.)*; Klinium *(Esteve, Spain)*.

9251-y

Mannityl Hexanitrate
Mannitol Hexanitrate *(rINN)*; Nitromannite; Nitromannitol.
$C_6H_8(O.NO_2)_6$=452.2.

CAS — 15825-70-4.

Mannityl hexanitrate has general properties similar to those of glyceryl trinitrate (p.1499) and has been used in the prophylaxis of angina pectoris.

Proprietary Names and Manufacturers
Moloid *(Südmedica, Ger.)*; Nitranitrol *(Merrell Dow, USA)*.

12916-r

Mecinarone *(rINN)*.
1-[6-(2-Dimethylaminoethoxy)-4,7-dimethoxybenzofuran-5-yl]-3-(4-methoxyphenyl)prop-2-en-1-one.
$C_{24}H_{27}NO_6$=425.5.

CAS — 26225-59-2.

Mecinarone is reported to be a vasodilator.

Proprietary Names and Manufacturers
Delalande, Fr.

9253-z

Methyl Nicotinate
Methyl pyridine-3-carboxylate.
$C_7H_7NO_2$=137.1.

CAS — 93-60-7.

Pharmacopoeias. In *Br.*

White or almost white crystals or crystalline powder with a characteristic odour; m.p. 40° to 42°. **Soluble** 1 in 0.7 of water and of alcohol, 1 in 0.4 of chloroform, and 1 in 1 of ether.
Store in well-closed containers.

Methyl nicotinate, usually in a concentration of 1 to 2%, is used in ointments and creams for topical application as a rubefacient for the relief of pain in muscular rheumatism, lumbago, and fibrositis.
Other nicotinates, including benzyl nicotinate, butoxyethyl nicotinate, ethyl nicotinate, hexyl nicotinate, and thurfyl nicotinate, are used in a similar way.

Proprietary Preparations containing Nicotinates
Algipan *(Wyeth, UK)*. *Cream*, methyl nicotinate 1%, glycol salicylate 10%, capsicum oleoresin 0.1%.
Topical spray (Algipan Pain Relieving Spray), aerosol, methyl nicotinate 1.5%, glycol salicylate 10%.
Bayolin *(Bayer, UK)*. *Cream*, benzyl nicotinate 2.5%, glycol salicylate 10%, heparinoid 'Bayer' equivalent to heparin 50 units/g.
Cremalgin *(Berk Pharmaceuticals, UK)*. *Cream*, methyl nicotinate 1%, glycol salicylate 10%, capsicum oleoresin 0.1%.
Finalgon *(Boehringer Ingelheim, UK)*. *Ointment*,butoxyethyl nicotinate 2.5%, nonivamide 0.4%.
Transvasin *(Lloyd-Hamol, Reckitt & Colman Pharm., UK)*. *Cream*, ethyl nicotinate 2%, hexyl nicotinate 2%, thurfyl salicylate 14%, benzocaine 2%.

Proprietary Names and Manufacturers of Nicotinates
Rubriment *(Ger.)*; Trafuril *(Fr.; Switz.; Ciba, UK)*.

The following names have been used for multi-ingredient preparations containing nicotinates—Algipan *(Wyeth, UK)*; Bayolin *(Bayer, UK)*; Biogesic *(Everest, Canad.)*; Cremalgex *(Norton, UK)*; Cremalgin *(Berk Pharmaceuticals, UK)*; Crematherm *(Sinclair, UK)*; Decontractyl-Baume *(Anglo-French Laboratories, Canad.)*; Dubam *(Norma, UK)*; Finalgon *(Boehringer Ingelheim, Austral.; Boehringer Ingelheim, Canad.; Boehringer Ingelheim, UK)*; Transvasin *(Reckitt & Colman, Austral.; Lloyd-Hamol, Reckitt & Colman Pharm., UK)*.

12971-v

Molsidomine *(BAN, USAN, rINN)*.
CAS-276; Morsydomine; SIN-10. *N*-Ethoxycarbonyl-3-morpholinosydnonimine.
$C_9H_{14}N_4O_4$=242.2.

CAS — 25717-80-0.

Molsidomine is a vasodilator that has been used in the treatment and prophylaxis of angina pectoris.

A study of the pharmacodynamics and pharmacokinetics of molsidomine in 8 healthy subjects.— R. Bergstrand *et al.*, *Eur. J. clin. Pharmac.*, 1984, *27*, 203. See also K. R. Karsch *et al.*, *Eur. J. clin. Pharmac.*, 1978, *13*, 241.

CARDIAC DISORDERS. Molsidomine was effective in reducing systolic, diastolic, and mean blood pressure in a study involving 38 hypertensive patients. The clinical effect was found to persist for at least 6 hours due to the formation of long-acting metabolites.— J. Milei *et al.*, *Eur. J. clin. Pharmac.*, 1980, *18*, 231.

A study of the acute haemodynamic and clinical efficacy of molsidomine in 27 patients with angina pectoris indicated that molsidomine has a similar action to glyceryl trinitrate but a longer duration of anti-anginal activity.— P. A. Majid *et al.*, *New Engl. J. Med.*, 1980, *302*, 1.

A double-blind crossover study in 30 patients with stable angina pectoris indicated that molsidomine 2 mg in association with penbutolol 40 mg was superior to penbutolol alone in preventing effort-induced angina.— A. E. Balestrini *et al.*, *Eur. J. clin. Pharmac.*, 1984, *27*, 1. A double-blind study in 31 patients with chronic, stable angina pectoris which had not responded to treatment with a beta blocker indicated that treatment with molsidomine 4 mg daily in association with metoprolol 200 mg daily was well tolerated, but clinical response was not substantially greater than with metoprolol alone.— J. P. van Mantgem *et al.*, *Eur. J. clin. Pharmac.*, 1985, *28*, 109.

Beneficial haemodynamic effects of molsidomine in pump failure complicating acute myocardial infarction.— S. Drajer *et al.*, *Eur. J. clin. Pharmac.*, 1984, *27*, 419.

Proprietary Names and Manufacturers
Corangor *(Berenguer-Beneyto, Spain)*; Corvasal *(Hoechst, Fr.)*; Corvaton *(Cassella-Riedel, Ger.*; *Hoechst, Switz.)*; Duracoron *(Durachemie, Ger.)*; Molsidain *(Hoechst, Spain)*; Molsidaine *(Hoechst, Arg.)*; Molsidolat *(Hoechst, Ital.)*; Molsiton *(Edmond Pharma, Ital.)*; Morial *(Jpn)*.

9256-a

Naftidrofuryl Oxalate *(BANM, rINNM)*.

EU-1806; LS-121; Nafronyl Oxalate *(USAN)*. 2-Diethylaminoethyl 3-(1-naphthyl)-2-tetrahydrofurfurylpropionate hydrogen oxalate.
$C_{24}H_{33}NO_3,C_2H_2O_4$=473.6.

CAS — 31329-57-4 (naftidrofuryl); 3200-06-4 (oxalate).

Adverse Effects and Precautions

Naftidrofuryl oxalate may cause nausea and epigastric pain. Convulsions may occur at high doses, and have also been reported following administration via the coronary artery.

Naftidrofuryl should not be administered by injection to patients with atrioventricular block, and should be given with care to patients with severe cardiac insufficiency or conduction disorders. Depression of cardiac conduction may occur following overdosage.

Oesophageal ulceration in a patient attributed to the taking of naftidrofuryl capsules without an adequate accompanying amount of fluid.— E. C. McCloy and S. Kane (letter), *Br. med. J.*, 1981, *282*, 1703.

Severe hepatitis was associated with naftidrofuryl therapy in a 60-year-old patient. Liver function tests had returned to normal one year after naftidrofuryl was discontinued.— J. S. de Caestecker and R. C. Heading, *Postgrad. med. J.*, 1986, *62*, 309.

Thrombophlebitis following intravenous infusion of naftidrofuryl 200 mg in 200 mL of sodium chloride or glucose injection occurred at 10 out of 13 injection sites in 7 consecutive patients (C.R.J. Woodhouse and D.G.A. Eadie, *Br. med. J.*, 1977, *1*, 1320). It was suggested by Charlesworth (*ibid.*, 1537), Gann (*ibid.*, 1598), Chamberlain (*ibid.*, *2*, 121), and Morris-Jones (*ibid.*) that this problem could be overcome by using 500 mL of diluent. However, thrombo-embolism was not considered by MacLellan (*ibid.*, 267) or Standing *et al.*, (*ibid.*, 895) to be a problem particularly associated with naftidrofuryl infusions, and a survey of 13 centres in Germany by Heidrich (*ibid.*, 1978, *1*, 618) did not confirm a high incidence of thrombophlebitis associated with naftidrofuryl infusion.

Uses and Administration

Naftidrofuryl oxalate is used in the treatment of peripheral and cerebral vascular disorders. It is claimed to enhance cellular oxidative capacity and to be a spasmolytic.

The usual dose for cerebrovascular disorders is 100 mg three times daily by mouth. The usual dose for peripheral vascular disorders is 100 to 200 mg three times daily. Rest pain, gross ischaemia, and incipient gangrene may initially be treated for 7 to 10 days with 200 mg twice daily by intravenous or intra-arterial infusion over a minimum of 90 minutes in 250 to 500 mL of sodium chloride injection (0.9%), glucose injection (5%), or dextran 40 intravenous infusion, together with oral therapy. Oral therapy is then continued for a minimum of 3 months.

A review of naftidrofuryl.— *Drug & Ther. Bull.*, 1988, *26*, 25.

It is possible that stimulation of cellular metabolism with naftidrofuryl could be used to improve the nitrogen balance in the post-operative period. Naftidrofuryl administered twice daily by intravenous infusion was found by Burns *et al.* (*Br. med. J.*, 1981, *283*, 7) to reduce postoperative nitrogen losses in a study involving 34 patients. Postoperative urea clearance was not affected, thus excluding an effect on renal function. It was suggested that naftidrofuryl might improve cellular metabolism either by an effect on the tricarboxylic-acid cycle or by an insulin-like action. However, Jackson *et al.* (*ibid.*, 1984, *289*, 581) were not able to show any nitrogen-sparing effect in a similar study. Inglis *et al.* (*ibid.*, 1002) reported a small but statistically insignificant reduction in nitrogen excretion which reached significance on the second day of the study in patients undergoing cholecystectomy, and no significant reduction in nitrogen excretion in patients following major surgery.

CEREBROVASCULAR DISORDERS. A review of drugs used in senile dementia. Several studies have suggested that naftidrofuryl improves memory and behaviour, but further studies are needed to establish whether it improves activities of daily living.— *Br. med. J.*, 1979, *2*, 511. A similar view and the warning that all cerebral vasodilator therapy must be regarded as contra-indicated in patients with acute stroke and may sometimes be harmful in patients with chronic cerebrovascular disease.— P. Cook and I. James, *New Engl. J. Med.*, 1981, *305*, 1508 and 1560.

A review of drugs used in cerebrovascular disorders, including naftidrofuryl. Many clinical studies of naftidrofuryl in chronic cerebral insufficiency have involved ill-defined diagnostic and admission criteria and mean follow-up periods of 2 to 3 months. Some studies have had high drop-out rates. Results have been generally inconclusive.— A. Spagnoli and G. Tognoni, *Drugs*, 1983, *26*, 44.

Stroke. Double-blind placebo-controlled study of naftidrofuryl in 91 patients with acute stroke. The extent of recovery was greater following 12 weeks of treatment with naftidrofuryl and patients were able to leave hospital on average 25 days sooner than patients taking placebo.— A. K. Admami, *Br. med. J.*, 1978, *2*, 1678. Criticisms of admission criteria and trial design led to the conclusion that the benefit of naftidrofuryl in stroke had not been demonstrated.— T. Steiner *et al.* (letter), *ibid.*, 1979, *1*, 412.

Topical application of naftidrofuryl (as Praxilene Forte 200 mg in 10 mL) on the superficial temporal artery when performing extracranial/intracranial anastomosis for cerebral revascularisation has been found to be a useful means of increasing the diameter of the vessel and increasing the blood flow.— C. M. Bannister (letter), *Lancet*, 1980, *2*, 372.

PERIPHERAL VASCULAR DISORDERS. A brief discussion on the actions and uses of naftidrofuryl oxalate in peripheral vascular disorders.— *Drug & Ther. Bull.*, 1979, *17*, 83.

Beneficial response to naftidrofuryl was reported in a study of 37 patients with severe peripheral vascular disease.— S. E. Meehan *et al.*, *Angiology*, 1982, *33*, 625.

Proprietary Preparations

Praxilene *(Lipha, UK)*. *Capsules*, naftidrofuryl oxalate 100 mg.

Praxilene Forte *(Lipha, UK)*. *Concentrate for intravenous infusion*, naftidrofuryl oxalate 20 mg/mL, in ampoules of 10 mL. Dilute before use.

Proprietary Names and Manufacturers

Citoxid *(Arg.)*; Di-actane *(Roland-Marie, Fr.)*; Dusodril *(Lipha, Ger.)*; Gevatran *(Anphar-Rolland, Fr.)*; Iridus *(Arg.)*; Naftilux *(Lucien, Fr.)*; Nafti-Ratiopharm *(Ratiopharm, Ger.)*; Praxilene *(Belg.*; *Oberval, Fr.*; *Formenti, Ital.*; *Faes, Spain*; *Lipha, Switz.*; *Lipha, UK)*.

9257-t

Nicametate Citrate *(BANM, rINNM)*.

Diethylaminoethyl Nicotinate Citrate; Nicametate Dihydrogen Citrate. 2-Diethylaminoethyl nicotinate dihydrogen citrate.
$C_{12}H_{18}N_2O_2,C_6H_8O_7$=414.4.

CAS — 3099-52-3 (nicametate); 1641-74-3 (citrate).

Nicametate citrate is a vasodilator with general properties similar to those of nicotinic acid (see p.1268), to which it is slowly hydrolysed. It is given for the treatment of peripheral vascular disorders and cerebral insufficiency.

Proprietary Names and Manufacturers
Euclidan *(Millot-Solac, Fr.*; *Crinos, Ital.*; *Solac, Switz.)*; Nicopile *(Jpn)*.

13008-c

Nicardipine Hydrochloride *(BANM, USAN, rINNM)*.

RS-69216; RS-69216-XX-07-0; YC-93. 2-(*N*-Methylbenzylamino)ethyl methyl 1,4-dihydro-2,6-dimethyl-4-(3-nitrophenyl)pyridine-3,5-dicarboxylate hydrochloride.
$C_{26}H_{29}N_3O_6$,HCl=516.0.

CAS — 55985-32-5 (nicardipine); 54527-84-3 (hydrochloride).

Adverse Effects and Precautions

As for Nifedipine, p.1509. Nicardipine should be used with caution in patients with impaired liver function or reduced hepatic blood flow. Nicardipine should be discontinued if ischaemic chest pain occurs following administration.

In a study of 91 patients with stable essential hypertension treated with oral nicardipine, 49 patients experienced a total of 96 adverse reactions, mostly occurring in the first 3 months of treatment. The most frequently reported problems were peripheral oedema and headaches. Others included dyspepsia, dizziness, skin rash and vasodilatation.— S. H. Taylor *et al.*, *Br. J. clin. Pharmac.*, 1985, *20*, 139S.

Absorption and Fate

Nicardipine is rapidly absorbed from the gastro-intestinal tract but is subject to saturable first-pass hepatic metabolism. Bioavailability of about 35% has been reported following a 30 mg dose at steady state. There is considerable interindividual variation in plasma-nicardipine concentrations. Steady-state plasma concentrations are achieved after about 3 days dosing. Nicardipine is reported to be about 97% bound to plasma proteins and to have a half-life of about 7 to 12 hours. Nicardipine is extensively metabolised in the liver and is excreted in the urine and faeces, mainly as inactive metabolites.

Study of the pharmacokinetics of nicardipine in healthy subjects. Following oral administration, maximum nicardipine-plasma concentrations were achieved between 20 minutes and 2 hours. Bioavailability was found to increase over the first 7 days of multiple oral dosing. This was thought to be due in part to saturation or equilibration of pre-systemic elimination processes. Bioavailability was also found to increase disproportionately with dose, being approximately 15% at a 10 mg dose and approximately 45% at a 40 mg dose. Less interindividual variation was seen after intravenous than after oral administration. After intravenous administration, plasma clearance values were of the same order as hepatic blood flow.— D. J. M. Graham *et al.*, *Postgrad. med. J.*, 1984, *60*, *Suppl.* 4, 7. Following administration of a single oral dose of radiolabelled nicardipine, 60% of excreted ^{14}C was recovered in the urine. The metabolism of nicardipine was shown to be rapid and extensive. No nicardipine was excreted unchanged in the urine; the major metabolic products in the urine were conjugates of the alcohol metabolite. Administration of nicardipine with food appeared to reduce the bioavailability and delay the achievement of peak plasma concentrations of nicardipine.— D. J. M. Graham *et al.*, *Br. J. clin. Pharmac.*, 1985, *20*, 23S.

Uses and Administration

Nicardipine hydrochloride is a calcium-channel blocking agent with actions and uses similar to nifedipine (p.1511). It is used in the management of patients with chronic stable angina and for the treatment of mild to moderate hypertension.

An initial dose of nicardipine 20 mg by mouth three times a day is recommended. The dose may be increased at intervals of 3 days until the required effect is achieved. The effective dose range is between 60 and 120 mg per day, the usual dose being 30 mg three times a day. It has also been given by intravenous injection.

A review of nicardipine. Nicardipine is a calcium-channel blocking agent which has potent coronary and peripheral arterial dilator properties. It causes improvement in oxygen supply and reduction in systemic vascular resistance.
Clinical studies have shown nicardipine to be as effective as nifedipine in the treatment of chronic stable angina pectoris and it may have an advantage in not depressing cardiac conduction or left ventricular function even in patients with compromised cardiac pumping ability. Nicardipine may also be effective in the treatment of angina at rest due to coronary artery spasm. It also appears to be useful in the treatment of mild to moderate hypertension, either alone or in combination with other antihypertensive drugs. Unlike other vasodilators used in hypertension it does not produce fluid retention or weight gain. Encouraging preliminary results have also been obtained in studies of nicardipine in congestive heart failure and cerebrovascular disease.
Nicardipine appears to be effective and well tolerated in the treatment of angina pectoris and hypertension, although more long-term comparative studies are needed to define its place in therapy.— E. M. Sorkin and S. P. Clissold, *Drugs*, 1987, *33*, 296. See also D. D. Freedman and D. D. Waters, *ibid.*, *34*, 578.
Nicardipine was found to have similar haemodynamic effects to nifedipine in a study in 16 healthy subjects.— A. Iliopoulou *et al.*, *Br. J. clin. Pharmac.*, 1983, *15*, 59.
Nicardipine was shown to reduce systemic vascular resistance and blood pressure with a resultant reduction in left ventricular afterload and associated increases in cardiac output and stroke volume in patients with severe coronary heart disease. The expected reduction in cardiac work due to the reduction in left ventricular afterload was partially offset by reflex tachycardia. There was no direct evidence of cardiac depression.— B. Silke *et al.*, *Br. J. clin. Pharmac.*, 1984, *18*, 717.
Intravenous infusion of nicardipine 1 mg per hour and 5 mg per hour for 3 hours resulted in a small increase in cerebral blood flow in 12 healthy subjects. Changes in blood pressure and heart rate were only seen at the higher dose.— I. Savage and I. James, *Br. J. clin. Pharmac.*, 1986, *21*, 591P.
Further references to the clinical pharmacology of nicardipine: *Br. J. clin. Pharmac.*, 1986, *22*, *Suppl.* 3, 193S to 236S.

CARDIAC DISORDERS. *Angina pectoris.* Nicardipine was shown to be comparable in efficacy to nifedipine in the treatment of chronic stable angina.— N. S. Khurmi *et al.*, *J. Am. Coll. Cardiol.*, 1984, *4*, 908.
Nicardipine was found to be effective and well tolerated in the treatment of patients with vasospastic angina.— C. J. Pepine and J. S. Gelman, *Br. J. clin. Pharmac.*, 1985, *20*, 187S.
Sustained subjective and objective benefits from nicardipine therapy were seen for a period of up to 1 year in patients with chronic stable angina, and adverse effects were minor and well tolerated. Abrupt withdrawal of nicardipine resulted in a rapid return of original symptoms without further deterioration from the baseline status.— M. Gheorghiade *et al.*, *Br. J. clin. Pharmac.*, 1985, *20*, 195S.
Nicardipine was found to be less effective than verapamil in treating stable angina in a study involving 20 patients.— E. A. Rodrigues *et al.*, *Br. J. clin. Pharmac.*, 1986, *21*, 593P.
Further references to the use of nicardipine in angina pectoris.— S. Scheidt *et al.*, *Br. J. clin. Pharmac.*, 1985, *20*, 178S; D. McGill *et al.*, *Am. J. Cardiol.*, 1986, *57*, 39; *Br. J. clin. Pharmac.*, 1986, *22*, *Suppl.* 3, 307S to 350S.

HYPERTENSION. Nicardipine administered in combination with atenolol was shown to be effective in lowering blood pressure in a study involving 20 hypertensive patients. The incidence of adverse effects was low.— R. Kolloch *et al.*, *Br. J. clin. Pharmac.*, 1985, *20*, 130S.
Nicardipine compared favourably with hydrochlorothiazide in the control of mild to moderate hypertension in 65 patients.— G. Creytens and A. Saelen, *Br. J. clin. Pract.*, 1986, *40*, 518.
Further references to the use of nicardipine in hypertension.— M. Bellet *et al.*, *J. cardiovasc. Pharmac.*, 1985, *7*, 1149; J. Asplund, *Br. J. clin. Pharmac.*, 1985, *20*, 120S; *Br. J. clin. Pharmac.*, 1986, *22*, *Suppl.* 3, 237S to 306S; C. Armstrong *et al.*, *Postgrad. med. J.*, 1987, *63*, 463; K. A. Conrad *et al.*, *Clin. Pharmac. Ther.*, 1987, *42*, 113.

Proprietary Preparations
Cardene *(Syntex, UK). Capsules*, nicardipine hydrochloride 20 and 30 mg.

Proprietary Names and Manufacturers
Angioflebil *(Infale, Spain)*; Cardene *(Syntex, UK)*; Dagan *(Zambeletti, Spain)*; Flusemide *(Roger, Spain)*; Lecibral *(Nezel, Spain)*; Lincil *(Funk, Spain)*; Loxen *(Sandoz, Fr.)*; Nerdipina *(Ferrer, Spain)*; Nicardal *(Italfarmaco, Ital.)*; Nicodel *(Mitsui, Jpn)*; Nimicor *(Formenti, Ital.)*; Perdipina *(Sandoz, Ital.)*; Perdipine *(Yamanouchi, Jpn)*; Ranvil *(Gentili, Ital.)*; Rycarden *(Syntex, Denm.)*; Vasodin *(Istituto Wassermann, Ital.)*; Vasonase *(Syntex-Latino, Spain)*; Vatrasin *(Aristegui, Spain)*.

9258-x

Niceritrol *(BAN, rINN).*

Pentaerythritol tetranicotinate; 2,2-Bis(hydroxymethyl)propane-1,3-diol tetranicotinate.
$C_{29}H_{24}N_4O_8$=556.5.

CAS — 5868-05-3.

NOTE. The synonym PETN has been applied to both niceritrol and pentaerythritol tetranitrate.

Niceritrol, an ester of pentaerythritol and nicotinic acid, is a vasodilator with general properties similar to those of nicotinic acid (see p.1268), to which it is slowly hydrolysed. It is used in the treatment of peripheral and coronary vascular disorders. It is also used as a hypolipidaemic agent.

A brief discussion of niceritrol alone and in conjunction with clofibrate in the treatment of type IIa and IIb hyperlipoproteinaemia.— L. Orö *et al.*, *Postgrad. med. J.*, 1975, *51*, *Suppl.* 8, 76.

Proprietary Names and Manufacturers
Bufor *(Astra, Denm.)*; Perycit *(Tosi, Ital.; Inibsa, Spain; Astra, Swed.; Bofors, Switz.)*.

9259-r

Nicofuranose *(BAN, rINN).*

ES-304; Tetranicotinoylfructofuranose; Tetranicotinoylfructose. β-D-Fructofuranose 1,3,4,6-tetranicotinate.
$C_{30}H_{24}N_4O_{10}$=600.5.

CAS — 15351-13-0.

Nicofuranose is a vasodilator with general properties similar to those of nicotinic acid (see p.1268), to which it is slowly hydrolysed. It is given in the treatment of peripheral vascular disorders in a usual dosage of 500 mg three times daily but doses of 0.75 to 1 g three times daily may be given.
Similar doses have been given to lower blood-cholesterol concentrations.

Proprietary Preparations
Bradilan *(Napp, UK). Tablets*, enteric-coated, nicofuranose 250 mg.

Proprietary Names and Manufacturers
Bradilan *(Ger.; Ital.; S.Afr.; Napp, UK)*; Buclidan *(Spain)*; Vasperdil *(Switz.)*.

13010-w

Nicofurate *(rINN).*

1-(4-Methoxycarbonyl-5-methyl-2-furyl)butane-1,2,3,4-tetrayl tetranicotinate.
$C_{35}H_{28}N_4O_{11}$=680.6.

CAS — 4397-91-5.

Nicofurate has the general properties of nicotinic acid (see p.1268) and has been used as a vasodilator and in lipid disorders.

Proprietary Names and Manufacturers
Arteriolase *(Bago, Arg.)*.

9260-j

Nicomethanol Nicotinate

3-Pyridylmethyl nicotinate.
$C_{12}H_{10}N_2O_2$=214.2.

CAS — 49673-77-0.

Nicomethanol nicotinate is a vasodilator that has been given in the treatment of peripheral and cerebral vascular disorders.

Proprietary Names and Manufacturers
Nicodue *(SIT, Ital.)*.

16912-m

Nicorandil *(USAN, rINN).*

SG-75. *N*-[2-(nitroxy)ethyl]-3-pyridinecarboxamide.
$C_8H_9N_3O_4$=211.2.

CAS — 65141-46-0.

Nicorandil is reported to have vasodilatory activity and has been used in the treatment of angina pectoris.

References: G. G. Belz *et al.*, *Eur. J. clin. Pharmac.*, 1984, *26*, 681; M. Kinoshita *et al.*, *Am. J. Cardiol.*, 1986, *58*, 733; N. Hayata *et al.*, *Am. Heart J.*, 1986, *112*, 1245.

Proprietary Names and Manufacturers
Sigmart *(Chugai, Jpn)*;
Manufacturers also include—*Upjohn, USA*.

9261-z

Nicotinyl Alcohol *(BAN, USAN).*

3-Hydroxymethylpyridine; 3-Pyridinemethanol; β-Pyridylcarbinol; Nicotinic Alcohol; NU-2121; Ro-1-5155. 3-Pyridylmethanol.
C_6H_7NO=109.1.

CAS — 100-55-0.

9262-c

Nicotinyl Alcohol Tartrate *(BANM).*

Nicotinyl Tartrate. 3-Pyridylmethanol hydrogen tartrate.
$C_6H_7NO,C_4H_6O_6$=259.2.

CAS — 6164-87-0.

Pharmacopoeias. In *Br.*

A white or almost white odourless or almost odourless crystalline powder. Nicotinyl alcohol tartrate 2.4 g is approximately equivalent to 1 g of nicotinyl alcohol. Freely **soluble** in water; slightly soluble in alcohol; practically insoluble in chloroform and in ether. A 5% solution in water has a pH of 2.8 to 3.7.

Adverse Effects and Precautions
Nicotinyl alcohol may cause flushing of the skin of the face and neck, dizziness, faintness, nausea and vomiting, and hypotension. These effects tend to be dose-related. Skin rashes and urticaria have been reported. Glucose tolerance may be impaired particularly at higher doses, and abnormal liver function tests indicating hepatotoxicity have been reported when high doses are used for long periods.
Nicotinyl alcohol and nicotinyl alcohol tartrate should be used with care in diabetic or pre-diabetic patients.

Uses and Administration
Nicotinyl alcohol is a vasodilator with general properties similar to those of nicotinic acid (see p.1269), to which it is partly hydrolysed.
Nicotinyl alcohol or its tartrate is given by mouth in the treatment of peripheral vascular disorders in usual doses equivalent to 25 to 50 mg of nicotinyl alcohol 4 times daily or as a sustained-release preparation in doses of 150 to 300 mg of nicotinyl alcohol twice daily.
It has also been given to lower blood-cholesterol concentrations and for the treatment of Ménière's disease. Doses of 0.9 to 1.8 g daily have been recommended for the treatment of hypercholesterolaemia.

Study of the effect of nicotinyl alcohol on lipids and lipoproteins, in primary hyperlipoproteinaemia Type IIa.— V. Hutt *et al.*, *Arzneimittel-Forsch.*, 1983, *33*, 1682.

Preparations
Nicotinyl Alcohol Tablets *(B.P.).* Contain nicotinyl alcohol tartrate.

Proprietary Preparations of Nicotinyl Alcohol and its Tartrate

Ronicol *(Roche, UK). Tablets,* scored, nicotinyl alcohol 25 mg (as nicotinyl alcohol tartrate).

Ronicol Timespan *(Roche, UK). Tablets,* sustained-release, nicotinyl alcohol 150 mg (as nicotinyl alcohol tartrate).

Proprietary Names and Manufacturers of Nicotinyl Alcohol and its Tartrate

Pyridylcarbinol *(Ratiopharm, Ger.)*; Riko *(Kettelhack Riker, Ger.)*; Roniacol *(Arg.; Roche, Canad.; USA)*; Ronicol *(Roche, Austral.; Roche, Denm.; Fr.; Roche, Ger.; Roche, Ital.; Neth.; Roche, Norw.; Roche, S.Afr.; Roche, Spain; Roche, Swed.; Roche, Switz.; Roche, UK)*; Selcarbinol *(Sella, Ital.)*; Tebarcon *(Kanoldt, Ger.)*.

9263-k

Nifedipine *(BAN, USAN, rINN).*

Bay-a-1040; Nifedipinum. Dimethyl 1,4-dihydro-2,6-dimethyl-4-(2-nitrophenyl)pyridine-3,5-dicarboxylate.

$C_{17}H_{18}N_2O_6$=346.3.

CAS — 21829-25-4.

Pharmacopoeias. In *Jpn* and *U.S.*

A yellow powder. Practically **insoluble** in water; soluble 1 in 10 of acetone. **Store** in airtight containers. Protect from light.

In a study of the stability of nifedipine in an electrolyte solution used to induce cardioplegia, it was found that nifedipine degraded more rapidly at 25° than at 4°. However, even when protected from light and refrigerated, nifedipine concentrations declined to approximately 90% of their original value within 6 hours of preparation. In view of the prolonged nature of cardiac surgery requiring cardioplegia it was recommended that solutions containing nifedipine should be prepared immediately before surgery.— M. B. Bottorff *et al., Am. J. Hosp. Pharm.*, 1984, *41,* 2068.

Adverse Effects

The most common adverse effects of nifedipine are associated with the vasodilatory action, such as dizziness, flushing, headache, hypotension, and peripheral oedema. A paradoxical increase in ischaemic chest pain may occur at the start of treatment. There have been reports of abnormalities in liver function due to hypersensitivity reactions, and gingival hyperplasia has been reported. Overdosage with nifedipine may be associated with bradycardia and hypotension.

Review of the adverse effects of calcium antagonists.— J. G. Lewis, *Drugs*, 1983, *25,* 196.

ALLERGY. See under Effects on the Liver, below.

EFFECTS ON THE BLOOD. Agranulocytosis in a 73-year-old patient was believed to be associated with nifedipine therapy, although the patient was also taking chloral hydrate which has been reported to cause leukopenia.— A. J. Voth and R. H. Turner (letter), *Ann. intern. Med.*, 1983, *99,* 882.

EFFECTS ON CARBOHYDRATE METABOLISM. The effects of nifedipine on glucose tolerance are conflicting. A report by Bhatnagar *et al.* (*Br. med. J.*, 1984, *289,* 19) of deterioration of diabetes in 1 patient and the development of diabetes in another patient associated with nifedipine treatment prompted a report of the development of diabetes in 3 out of 235 patients within 3 weeks of receiving nifedipine 40 mg daily (A.V. Zezulka *et al., ibid.*, 437). These authors also found a small but significant increase in non-fasting blood glucose in 117 paired measurements taken before and during nifedipine therapy. An earlier study by Giugliano *et al.* (*Eur. J. clin. Pharmac.*, 1980, *18,* 395) had found that nifedipine administration to 10 patients with impaired glucose tolerance had resulted in a further reduction of both insulin secretion and glucose tolerance. In 10 patients with normal glucose tolerance, nifedipine administration resulted in reduced insulin response in the first 60 minutes but improved glucose tolerance. Charles *et al.* (*Br. med. J.*, 1981, *283,* 19) found significant increases in plasma-glucose concentrations after glucose-tolerance tests in 6 healthy subjects who had received nifedipine 60 mg daily for 3 days. However, these results were not confirmed by Harrower and Donnelly (*ibid.*, 796), Greenwood (*ibid.*, 1982, *284,* 50), Abadie and Passa (*ibid.*, 1984, *289,* 438), Dante (*Ann. intern. Med.*, 1985, *104,* 125), or Whitcroft *et al.* (*Br. J. clin. Pharmac.*, 1986, *22,* 208P), all of whom found no change in glucose tolerance in either diabetic or non-diabetic patients taking nifedipine 20 to 40 mg daily.

Review of the effects of calcium-channel blockers on glycaemic control. It was concluded that for non-diabetic patients there was no consistent evidence that glucose tolerance is adversely affected in the short- or long-term by normal therapeutic doses of calcium-channel blockers, although further information is required. In diabetic patients there is evidence to suggest that verapamil may improve glucose tolerance. The evidence that nifedipine may be associated with glucose intolerance in some circumstances is inconclusive. In addition, studies must consider the risk of spontaneous development of diabetes mellitus and the hyperglycaemic effects of other antihypertensive drugs.— M. J. Kendall *et al., J. clin. Hosp. Pharm.*, 1986, *11,* 175.

See also under Precautions, below.

EFFECTS ON THE CEREBROVASCULAR SYSTEM. A report of cerebral ischaemia in 2 elderly patients given nifedipine.— E. Nobile-Orazio and R. Sterzi, *Br. med. J.*, 1981, *283,* 948.

See also under Effects on Mental Function, below.

EFFECTS ON THE ENDOCRINE SYSTEM. *Gynaecomastia.* Unilateral gynaecomastia developed in 3 men 4, 6, and 26 weeks after starting nifedipine therapy.— C. A. C. Clyne (letter), *Br. med. J.*, 1986, *292,* 380.

EFFECTS ON THE EYE. Transient unilateral retinal ischaemia with loss of vision was associated in one patient with a 20-mg dose of nifedipine. The symptoms recurred on challenge. The patient had previously taken nifedipine 10 mg four times daily without adverse effects.— S. Pitlik *et al., Br. med. J.*, 1983, *287,* 1845.

Severe periorbital oedema accompanied by facial flushing, paraesthesia, headache, and dizziness occurred in a 54-year-old patient after the first dose of nifedipine. Symptoms lasted for 6 hours and recurred after 2 subsequent doses.— P. H. Silverstone (letter), *Br. med. J.*, 1984, *288,* 1654. Report of similar cases.— K. Tordjman *et al., Am. J. Cardiol.*, 1985, *55,* 1445.

Nifedipine was considered to be a possible risk factor for cataract; 9 out of 300 (3%) patients with cataract had taken nifedipine compared to 7 out of 607 (1.2%) controls (R. van Heyningen and J.J. Harding, *Lancet*, 1986, *1,* 1111). The significance of the risk associated with nifedipine was difficult to assess. Five of the 9 had angina and 8 of the 9 hypertension and these latter disorders might have been responsible for the cataracts rather than the nifedipine (*idem, 2,* 283).

EFFECTS ON THE HEART. Complete heart block occurred one week after starting treatment with nifedipine, 5 mg three times daily in a patient who had previously developed heart block during treatment with verapamil. Sinus rhythm was restored 1 week after nifedipine was stopped.— D. A. Chopra and R. T. Maxwell, *Br. med. J.*, 1984, *288,* 760.

Sudden circulatory collapse 2 to 4 hours after routine coronary bypass surgery in 4 patients being treated with nifedipine. Three patients recovered after treatment with large doses of calcium chloride and a continuous infusion of adrenaline. The fourth patient died. No similar collapses occurred when treatment with calcium-channel blockers was interrupted for at least 48 hours before surgery.— J. J. Goiti (letter), *Br. med. J.*, 1985, *291,* 1505.

Ischaemic chest pain. Three patients experienced severe chest pain, simulating angina pectoris or myocardial infarction and lasting 0.5 to 2 hours, after taking nifedipine.— A. G. Jariwalla and E. G. Anderson, *Br. med. J.*, 1978, *1,* 1181.

Myocardial ischaemia was possibly precipitated by the initial administration of nifedipine in 3 patients with unstable angina.— S. T. B. Sia *et al., Med. J. Aust.*, 1985, *142,* 48. A similar report in 3 patients receiving sublingual nifedipine for severe hypertension.— J. J. O'Mailia *et al., Ann. intern. Med.*, 1987, *107,* 185.

Anginal chest pain associated with a fall in arterial blood pressure and increased heart rate occurred in 10 patients within 20 to 30 minutes of taking nifedipine 20 to 30 mg by mouth. Patients were taking nifedipine 80 to 120 mg daily in conjunction with nitrates and, in 7 cases, beta-blockers for the treatment of refractory angina pectoris. Symptoms improved when the dose of nifedipine was reduced, or a calcium-channel blocker with a less pronounced peripheral vasodilatory effect was substituted.— W. E. Boden *et al., J. Am. med. Ass.*, 1985, *253,* 1131.

Withdrawal. The reappearance of symptoms effectively suppressed by treatment could be misinterpreted as a rebound phenomenon due to withdrawal of calcium-channel blockers.— J. Nehring and A. J. Camm (letter), *Br. med. J.*, 1983, *286,* 1057. Exacerbation of coronary ischaemia and thrombosis of arteriovenous graft could have resulted from withdrawal of nifedipine in 1 patient.— M. Mysliwiec *et al.* (letter), *ibid.*, 1898. Eight patients with well-controlled vasospastic angina experienced a marked increase in frequency and duration of anginal episodes following involuntary cessation of nifedipine therapy.— J. Lette *et al., Can. med. Ass. J.*, 1984, *130,* 1169.

EFFECTS ON THE KIDNEY. Four patients with underlying mild to moderate renal insufficiency demonstrated reversible deterioration in renal function without any appreciable accompanying decline in systemic arterial blood pressure while receiving nifedipine. It was suggested that either an alteration in intrarenal haemodynamics or inhibition of synthesis of vasodilatory prostaglandins could have been responsible.— J. R. Diamond *et al., Am. J. Med.*, 1984, *77,* 905.

Excessive diuresis occurred in a patient taking nifedipine 30 mg daily. It was suggested that diuresis might be due to an increased renal blood flow resulting from dilatation of the renal arteries.— D. Antonelli *et al.* (letter), *Br. med. J.*, 1984, *288,* 760.

Nifedipine was identified as the cause of nocturia in 9 patients referred for prostatic surgery. Nocturia ceased in 6 patients and improved considerably in 3 when nifedipine treatment was discontinued.— G. Williams and R. M. Donaldson (letter), *Lancet*, 1986, *1,* 738.

EFFECTS ON THE LIVER. Hepatitis developed in a 69-year-old man after 10 days' therapy with nifedipine 40 mg daily for severe stable angina. The clinical features, immunological studies, and a later positive challenge test indicated a hypersensitive mechanism.— H. H. Rotmensch *et al., Br. med. J.*, 1980, *281,* 976. A similar case.— A. R. Davidson (letter), *ibid.*, 1354.

Abnormal liver function in 2 patients was associated with the use of nifedipine. In both cases liver function returned to normal after withdrawal of the drug. Evidence suggested that the toxic effect on the liver was due to hypersensitivity.— M. Abramson and G. O. Littlejohn, *Med. J. Aust.*, 1985, *142,* 47.

EFFECTS ON THE MENSTRUAL CYCLE. Menorrhagia in 2 women possibly associated with nifedipine therapy.— J. C. Rodger and T. C. Torrance (letter), *Lancet*, 1983, *2,* 460. Irregular menstrual cycle with heavy bleeding occurred in 1 patient during treatment with nifedipine.— G. Singh *et al.* (letter), *ibid.*, 1022.

EFFECTS ON MENTAL FUNCTION. Insomnia, hyperexcitability, pacing, agitation, and depression were associated with nifedipine therapy in a 62-year-old patient. The symptoms disappeared within 2 days of withdrawal of nifedipine.— S. Ahmad (letter), *J. Am. Geriat. Soc.*, 1984, *32,* 408.

Nifedipine can also cause cerebral ischaemia; see under Effects on the Cerebrovascular System.

EFFECTS ON THE MOUTH. *Gingival hyperplasia.* Gingival hyperplasia in 5 patients associated with the administration of nifedipine.— Y. Ramon *et al., Int. J. Cardiol.*, 1984, *5,* 195.

Further reports of nifedipine-induced gingival hyperplasia.— E. E. van der Wall *et al., Oral Surg.*, 1985, *60,* 38; P. L. Bencini *et al., Acta derm.-vener., Stockh.*, 1985, *65,* 362; C. M. Jones (letter), *Br. dent. J.*, 1986, *160,* 416.

Parotitis. Acute swelling of the parotid glands occurred in a patient after sublingual administration of nifedipine.— X. Bosch *et al.* (letter), *Lancet*, 1986, *2,* 467.

EFFECTS ON THE MUSCLES. Severe muscle cramps in 3 patients taking nifedipine; the condition recurred in 2 when given challenge doses.— S. Keidar *et al., Br. med. J.*, 1982, *285,* 1241. A further case in which the cramps were associated with paraesthesia.— J. B. Macdonald (letter), *ibid.*, 1744.

EFFECTS ON THE NERVOUS SYSTEM. Myoclonic dystonia occurred in a 35-year-old patient during treatment with nifedipine 20 mg twice daily. Nifedipine was withdrawn and symptoms disappeared after 24 hours.— A. de Medina *et al., Ann. intern. Med.*, 1985, *104,* 125.

Tremor. A 46-year-old man experienced fine tremor, particularly of the upper limbs, while taking nifedipine 30 mg daily. When the dose was increased to 60 mg daily he experienced chest pain after most doses; the pain ceased when nifedipine was withdrawn.— C. Rodger and A. Stewart (letter), *Br. med. J.*, 1978, *1,* 1619.

EFFECTS ON THE PERIPHERAL CIRCULATION. Severe pain, oedema, erythematous rash, and a burning sensation in all 4 limbs occurred several hours after the first dose of nifedipine in a 57-year-old woman. Symptoms recurred after the next dose.— Z. Grunwald, *Drug Intell. & clin. Pharm.*, 1982, *16*, 492.

An erythromelalgia-like eruption occurred in a 44-year-old patient 8 weeks after starting therapy with nifedipine. Symptoms included severe burning pain and swelling in the feet and lower legs, which were fiery red, tender, and warm to the touch. Symptoms resolved in 2 days when nifedipine was discontinued.— J. R. Fisher *et al.* (letter), *Ann. intern. Med.*, 1983, *98*, 671. A similar report.— G. J. Brodmerkel (letter), *ibid.*, *99*, 415.

EFFECTS ON THE RESPIRATORY SYSTEM. A report of nifedipine precipitating acute pulmonary oedema in a 71-year-old man with symptoms of severe angina pectoris and a clinical diagnosis of moderate aortic valve stenosis and probable coronary artery disease. The patient had taken two 10-mg doses.— D. J. Gillmer and P. Kark, *Br. med. J.*, 1980, *280*, 1420.

Pulmonary oedema occurred on 2 occasions in an 81-year-old patient with aortic stenosis when nifedipine was administered.— D. Aderka and J. Pinkhas, *Br. med. J.*, 1984, *289*, 1272. A further report.— A. K. Batra *et al.*, *Respiration*, 1985, *47*, 161.

EFFECTS ON THE SKIN. *Photosensitivity*. Severe, blistering skin eruptions occurred on areas exposed to light in 2 patients taking nifedipine.— S. E. Thomas *et al.*, *Br. med. J.*, 1986, *292*, 992.

EFFECTS ON TASTE PERCEPTION. Distortion of taste and smell was encountered in 2 patients taking nifedipine. Symptoms disappeared when nifedipine was discontinued.— J. L. Levenson and K. Kennedy (letter), *Ann. intern. Med.*, 1985, *102*, 135.

Treatment of Adverse Effects

In overdosage by mouth the stomach should be emptied by aspiration and lavage. Hypotension may be treated by placing the patient in the supine position with the feet raised; standard measures, such as atropine for bradycardia and noradrenaline for hypotension, have been suggested if necessary. It also has been suggested that calcium gluconate combined with metaraminol may be of benefit.

Precautions

Nifedipine should be used with caution in patients with hypotension and in patients whose cardiac reserve is poor. In patients with severe aortic stenosis nifedipine may increase the risk of developing heart failure.

Nifedipine may enhance the antihypertensive effects of beta-adrenoceptor blocking agents although the combination is generally well tolerated. The use of nifedipine in diabetic patients may require adjustment of their control.

Nifedipine should be discontinued in patients who experience ischaemic pain following its administration.

A review of anaesthesia and hypertension including a discussion of problems in the management of patients treated with calcium-channel blocking agents. Pre-existing therapy with nifedipine, while adequate to maintain everyday control of hypertension does not preclude the tachycardia or hypertensive responses associated with adrenergic stimulation during or after anaesthesia.— C. Prys-Roberts, *Br. J. Anaesth.*, 1984, *56*, 711.

Dietary sodium restriction was found to cause a reduction in the blood pressure of hypertensive patients unless they were taking calcium-channel blocking agents. Patients taking calcium-channel blockers differed in their response from other patients in that the blood pressure did not fall and supine diastolic blood pressure rose.— T. Morgan *et al.* (letter), *Lancet*, 1986, *1*, 793.

A comment that blood pressure should be reduced slowly and gradually in patients with malignant hypertension by using smaller doses of nifedipine than normally recommended (R. Ahmad, *Br. med. J.*, 1985, *290*, 1592). It was suggested that the apparent acute renal impairment reported in such a patient by Spencer *et al.* (*ibid.*, 1112) could have been due to the administration of a high initial dose of nifedipine 20 mg.

For a report concerning lower dosage requirements for nifedipine in patients with liver cirrhosis due to altered pharmacokinetics see under Absorption and Fate, below.

For reports of the use of nifedipine during pregnancy, see under Uses, below.

INTERACTIONS. A review of drug interactions involving calcium-channel blocking agents. Most patients receiving concurrent therapy with calcium-channel blockers and beta-blockers do not manifest important adverse interactions. However, patients with certain predisposing factors appear to be at greater risk of developing adverse effects due to the combination. Such factors probably include pre-existing impaired left ventricular function, cardiac arrhythmia, aortic stenosis, large doses or intravenous administration of either or both drugs, and possibly therapy with agents that decrease alpha-adrenergic vasomotor tone, such as methyldopa.

Experience indicates that combined therapy with digitalis and calcium-channel blockers is generally well tolerated. However, patients should be monitored for an increase in serum-digoxin concentrations. Nifedipine is less likely than verapamil to have an additive depressant effect on cardiac conduction.

Nifedipine and verapamil appear to have complex actions on carbohydrate metabolism.— *Drug Interact. News.*, 1982, *2*, 27.

Anti-arrhythmic agents. For the effect of nifedipine on *quinidine* serum concentrations, see Quinidine Sulphate, p.86.

Antidiabetic agents and glucose metabolism. A review of the effects of nifedipine and other calcium-channel blockers on glycaemic control and hypoglycaemic agents. Results of studies in healthy subjects have been contradictory, and nifedipine appears to have no consistent effect on glucose tolerance in subjects without diabetes. In patients with non-insulin-dependent diabetes results are equally divergent, with glucose tolerance being either decreased or unchanged. It was concluded that chronic administration of nifedipine to diabetic patients will not cause a predictable change in glucose tolerance.— *Drug Interact. News.*, 1985, *5*, 27.

See also under Adverse Effects, above.

Anti-epileptics. For reports of an interaction between nifedipine and *phenytoin* see under Phenytoin Sodium, p.409.

Beta-blockers. Two patients developed heart failure when nifedipine was given in addition to beta-blockers.— C. J. Anastassiades, *Br. med. J.*, 1980, *281*, 1251. See also R. H. Robson and M. C. Vishwanath, *ibid.*, 1982, *284*, 104; C. Anastassiades (letter), *ibid.*, 506.

A report of severe hypotension in a patient with hypertension and angina taking atenolol when nifedipine was added to his treatment. When atenolol was withdrawn he developed unstable angina. In such situations the nifedipine should be withdrawn.— L. H. Opie and D. A. White, *Br. med. J.*, 1980, *281*, 1462. See also J. S. Staffurth and P. Emery (letter), *ibid.*, *282*, 225.

In a study in 12 healthy subjects given nifedipine and propranolol there was evidence that the kinetics of both drugs were altered when they were given concomitantly. Steady-state plasma concentrations of propranolol were decreased by approximately 40% immediately after nifedipine administration, and steady-state concentrations of nifedipine were increased by approximately 50% following propranolol administration although in each case the unbound fraction was unchanged. The interaction was attributed to transient changes in liver blood flow. The ultimate effect depended upon the relative doses and routes of administration of the drugs.— C. H. Kleinbloesem *et al.*, *Br. J. clin. Pharmac.*, 1985, *19*, 537P.

For the use of nifedipine in association with beta-adrenoceptor blocking agents, see under Hypertension, below.

Digitalis glycosides. For the effect of nifedipine on digoxin, see Digoxin, p.828.

Histamine H_2 antagonists. Pharmacokinetic studies by Kirch *et al.* (*Dt. med. Wschr.*, 1983, *108*, 1757), Renwick *et al.* (*Eur. J. clin. Pharmac.* 1987, *32*, 351), and Smith *et al.* (*Br. J. clin. Pharmac.*, 1987, *23*, 311) have indicated that concurrent administration of nifedipine and cimetidine can increase the bioavailability of nifedipine; Renwick *et al.*, and Smith *et al.* showed an increase in the area under the plasma concentration-time curve of between 77 and 92%. Kirch *et al.* also showed a potentiation of the hypotensive effect of nifedipine by cimetidine in 7 hypertensive patients. The mechanism of the interaction was thought to be due to inhibition of the cytochrome P-450 system by cimetidine and thus inhibition of the metabolism of nifedipine.

Ranitidine was found to have little effect on the pharmacokinetics of nifedipine, although Kirch *et al.* (*Clin. Pharmac. Ther.*,, 1985, *37* 204) were able to show an increase in the bioavailability of nifedipine during ranitidine administration. It was concluded that ranitidine may be a more appropriate choice in patients who require an H_2-antagonist while taking nifedipine.

Tobacco smoking. In a study of the effects of cigarette smoking and the treatment of angina with nifedipine, propranolol, or atenolol, smoking was shown to have direct and adverse effects on the heart and to interfere with the efficacy of all 3 anti-anginal agents, with nifedipine being the most affected.— J. Deanfield *et al.*, *New Engl. J. Med.*, 1984, *310*, 951.

PORPHYRIA. Nifedipine was considered to be unsafe in patients with acute porphyria because it has been shown to be porphyrinogenic in *animals* or *in vitro* systems.— M.R. Moore and K.E.L. McColl, *Porphyrias, Drug Lists*, Glasgow, Porphyria Research Unit, University of Glasgow, 1987.

Absorption and Fate

Nifedipine is rapidly and almost completely absorbed from the gastro-intestinal tract, although the bioavailability after oral administration is reported to be between 45 and 75%. Following administration by mouth peak blood concentrations are reported to occur after 30 to 120 minutes with a half-life of 2 to 5 hours.

Nifedipine is about 92 to 98% bound to plasma proteins. It is extensively metabolised in the liver and 70 to 80% is excreted in the urine mainly as inactive metabolites.

A review of the pharmacokinetics of nifedipine. Studies of the pharmacokinetics of nifedipine have been complicated by the difficulty in preparing a stable intravenous formulation and the problems in developing a sufficiently sensitive and specific method of analysis. Nearly 100% of an oral dose of nifedipine is absorbed in the small intestine although the bioavailability from capsules is 45 to 68%. The rate of absorption from both oral and sublingual capsules varies widely among individuals: there has been a report that high plasma-nifedipine concentrations are achieved more rapidly if the capsule is bitten and swallowed than from standard oral and sublingual administration. The absorption of nifedipine from tablets is slower than from capsules, with maximum plasma concentrations occurring at 1.6 to 4.2 hours compared with 0.5 to 2.17 hours, and absorption may still be occurring at 24 to 32 hours after administration.

Nifedipine undergoes almost complete hepatic oxidation to 3 pharmacologically inactive metabolites which are excreted in the urine. It has been reported that following oral administration 30 to 40% of the amount absorbed is metabolised during the first pass through the liver. The elimination half-life of nifedipine is apparently dependent upon the dosage form in which it is administered, with half-lives of 6 to 11 hours, 2 to 3.4 hours, and 1.3 to 1.8 hours measured after oral tablet, oral capsule, and intravenous administration respectively. The total systemic clearance of nifedipine from plasma ranges from 27 to about 66 litres per hour. Renal impairment does not substantially alter nifedipine pharmacokinetics.— E. M. Sorkin *et al.*, *Drugs*, 1985, *30*, 182. See also H. Echizen and M. Eichelbaum, *Clin. Pharmacokinet.*, 1986, *11*, 425.

The pharmacokinetics of sustained-release nifedipine during chronic dosing appeared to be similar to those derived from single-dose studies.— N. M. G. Debbas *et al.*, *Br. J. clin. Pharmac.*, 1986, *21*, 385.

ABSORPTION. A single-dose study in 10 patients with myocardial infarction indicated that the maximum plasma-nifedipine concentration was reduced and delayed when nifedipine was administered after a meal compared with administration 30 minutes before a meal. Haemodynamic measurements indicated that adverse vasodilatory effects related to high plasma concentrations might be reduced by administering nifedipine after food.— K. Hirasawa *et al.*, *Eur. J. clin. Pharmac.*, 1985, *28*, 105. See also V. Challenor *et al.*, *Br. J. clin. Pharmac.*, 1986, *22*, 565.

EFFECTS OF HEPATIC FAILURE. The pharmacokinetics of nifedipine were found to be considerably altered in 7 patients with liver cirrhosis. Systemic plasma clearance was substantially reduced and the elimination half-life was considerably longer than in healthy subjects. In addition, systemic availability of oral nifedipine was much higher in patients with cirrhosis and was complete in 3 patients with surgical portacaval shunt. Patients with liver cirrhosis seemed to be more sensitive to the effects of nifedipine on diastolic blood pressure and heart rate, and this could be explained by the higher free drug concentrations observed. It was concluded that lower doses of nifedipine may be required in patients with liver cirrhosis, and the patient's response should be closely monitored.— C. H. Kleinbloesem *et al.*, *Clin. Pharmac. Ther.*, 1986, *40*, 21.

EFFECTS OF RENAL FAILURE. Haemodialysis was not found to affect the pharmacokinetics of nifedipine in a study involving 10 patients. There was considerable interindividual variation in plasma concentrations, half-life, and clearance. It was suggested that the variability in hepatic extraction might be related to hepatic blood flow modifications as frequently observed in patients with kidney disease.— H. Martre *et al.*, *Br. J. clin. Pharmac.*, 1985, *20*, 155. See also.— C. H. Kleinbloesem *et al.*, *Clin. Pharmacokinet.*, 1986, *11*, 316.

Uses and Administration

Nifedipine is a calcium-channel blocking agent. Calcium-channel blockers, also known as calcium antagonists, calcium entry blockers, and slow-channel blockers, inhibit the cellular influx of calcium which is responsible for maintenance of the plateau phase of the action potential. Thus calcium-channel blockers primarily affect tissues in which depolarisation is dependent upon calcium rather than sodium influx, and these include vascular smooth muscle, myocardial cells, and cells within the sino-atrial (SA) and atrioventricular (AV) nodes. The main actions of the calcium-channel blockers include dilatation of coronary and peripheral arteries and arterioles, a negative inotropic action, reduction of heart rate, and slowing of AV conduction. The effects of individual agents are modified by their selectivity of action at different tissue sites and by baroreceptor reflexes. Thus nifedipine, unlike verapamil or diltiazem, has little or no action at the SA or AV nodes, and negative inotropic activity is rarely seen at therapeutic doses. Administration of nifedipine results primarily in vasodilatation, with reduced peripheral resistance, blood pressure, and afterload, increased coronary blood flow, and a reflex increase in heart rate. This in turn results in an increase in myocardial oxygen supply and cardiac output. Nifedipine has no anti-arrhythmic activity.

Nifedipine is used in the treatment and prophylaxis of angina pectoris particularly when a vasospastic element is present, and in the treatment of hypertension and Raynaud's syndrome.

The usual oral dose is 10 mg three times daily taken during or after meals increased, if necessary, to 20 mg three times daily. A maximum daily dose of 180 mg has been recommended. A recommended initial dose for elderly patients or those on concomitant medication is 5 mg three times daily.

It may also be administered sublingually or buccally by directing the patient to bite the capsule for a more rapid effect. Nifedipine may be given as a sustained-release tablet in a dose of 10 to 40 mg twice daily in hypertension. Nifedipine may also be given concomitantly with beta blockers in the treatment of angina or hypertension and with nitrates in angina.

Nifedipine may be administered by injection via a coronary catheter for the treatment of coronary spasm during coronary angiography and balloon angioplasty in a usual dose of 100 to 200 µg injected over 90 to 120 seconds. The maximum recommended total dose is 1200 µg within a 3-hour period. Blood pressure and heart rate should be monitored carefully.

Reviews of the mechanisms of action of calcium-channel blocking agents and their therapeutic applications: E. Braunwald, *New Engl. J. Med.*, 1982, *307*, 1618; T. T. Zsotér and J. G. Church, *Drugs*, 1983, *25*, 93; S. H. Snyder and I. J. Reynolds, *New Engl. J. Med.*, 1985, *313*, 995; J. Ferlinz, *Ann. intern. Med.*, 1986, *105*, 714 (and *ibid.*, 1987, *106*, 174).

General reviews of the properties and uses of calcium-channel blockers: A. Dodek and J. Ruedy, *Can. med. Ass. J.*, 1983, *128*, 911; *Drug & Ther. Bull.*, 1984, *22*, 65; A. L. Soward *et al.*, *Drugs*, 1986, *32*, 66.

Reviews of pharmacodynamic, pharmacokinetic, and therapeutic effects of nifedipine.— E. M. Sorkin *et al.*, *Drugs*, 1985, *30*, 182.

The negative inotropic effect of nifedipine may be seen in patients when reflex sympathetic mechanisms are impaired as by simultaneous therapy with beta-blocking drugs.— D. J. Sheridan *et al.* (letter), *New Engl. J. Med.*, 1982, *307*, 1026.

There has been some evidence *in vitro* to suggest that nifedipine has some alpha-adrenergic blocking activity in addition to its calcium-channel blocking activity (W.G. Strickland *et al.*, *New Engl. J. Med.*, 1982, *307*, 757), but this was not confirmed by Murphy and Brown (*Br. J. clin. Pharmac.*, 1984, *17*, 189P) in a study in 6 healthy subjects.

ACTIONS ON BLOOD CELLS. Nifedipine was shown to reduce calcium-dependent platelet aggregation moderately and prolong bleeding time by 12%.— J. Dale *et al.*, *Am. Heart J.*, 1983, *105*, 103.

Results of a study suggesting that improvement in the deformability of red blood cells by nifedipine could contribute to the therapeutic effects in myocardial ischaemia.— D. G. Waller *et al.*, *Br. J. clin. Pharmac.*, 1984, *17*, 133.

The decrease in the platelet aggregation ability and in the thromboxane B_2 concentration due to treatment with nifedipine in hypertensive patients suggested that nifedipine may be beneficial in various cardiovascular disorders with platelet involvement.— S. Uehara *et al.*, *Arzneimittel-Forsch.*, 1986, *36*, 1687.

ASTHMA. Calcium-channel blocking drugs are an important contribution to the therapy of patients with angina and concomitant reactive airway disease because they do not exacerbate airflow obstruction in such susceptible patients. Furthermore, they inhibit bronchoconstriction induced in asthmatic patients by a variety of stimuli, including exercise, histamine, methacholine, and allergens to a limited extent. Early clinical trials of these drugs in ambulatory asthmatic patients have shown little if any therapeutic benefit, but results must be considered preliminary in view of the nature of the short-term, small-scale studies performed to date. However, they do serve as a powerful probe into the role of calcium in airway physiology and in the pathophysiologic features of asthma.— C. H. Fanta, *Am. J. Cardiol.*, 1985, *55*, 202B.

There has been great interest in the potential use of calcium-channel blockers in the treatment of asthma because calcium is crucial for airway smooth muscle contraction, degranulation of mast cells, and secretion of mucus. However, clinical studies with currently available calcium-channel blockers have failed to show any clinically significant effect on resting bronchial tone in asthma patients, although there is evidence that beta-adrenoceptor stimulation and calcium-channel blockade have a synergistic relaxing effect on bronchial smooth muscle. Calcium-channel blockade usually has a protective effect on bronchoconstriction provoked by exercise, cold, histamine, and leukotriene. The main therapeutic application of calcium-channel blockers in asthmatics remains in the treatment of concomitant angina pectoris or hypertension.— C. -G. Löfdahl and P. J. Barnes, *Eur. J. resp. Dis.*, 1985, *67*, 233.

A review of calcium-channel blockers in the management of asthma. Most studies to date have demonstrated that calcium-channel blockers have only a modest effect on airway smooth muscle contraction. Until the results of clinical studies become available it would seem reasonable to use a calcium-channel blocker for the treatment of hypertension or angina in patients with airway obstruction in whom beta blockers are contra-indicated.— K. L. Massey and L. Hendeles, *Drug Intell. & clin. Pharm.*, 1987, *21*, 505.

Studies of the use of nifedipine and other calcium-channel blockers in asthma: D. O. Williams *et al.*, *Br. med. J.*, 1981, *283*, 348; K. R. Patel and M. Al-Shamma, *ibid.*, 1982, *284*, 1916; S. Malik and M. F. Sudlow (letter), *ibid.*, *285*, 292; N. Nair *et al.*, *Chest*, 1984, *86*, 515; G. Ozenne *et al.*, *Eur. J. resp. Dis.*, 1985, *67*, 238; G. Moscato *et al.*, *Ann. Allergy*, 1986, *56*, 145; R. S. Schwartzstein and C. H. Fanta, *Am. Rev. resp. Dis.*, 1986, *134*, 262; C. Spedini and C. Lombardi, *Eur. J. clin. Pharmac.*, 1986, *31*, 105.

CARDIAC DISORDERS. A review of the uses of calcium-channel blocking agents in heart disease. Calcium-channel blocking agents differ from each other in their chemical structure, their mechanism of action at a cellular level, and their pharmacological effects.

The main indication for calcium-channel blocking agents is *chronic stable angina*. Although it is claimed that the beneficial effect in stable angina is gained through an increase in coronary blood flow, a more likely mechanism of action is a reduction in myocardial oxygen consumption. There may also be an effect on myocardial cells.

The beneficial effects appear to be sustained with long-term therapy. The first treatment in patients with angina pectoris should be with a short-acting nitrate. Next, beta blockade remains the prophylactic treatment of choice. In patients unable to tolerate beta blockade or in whom its use is contra-indicated, treatment with verapamil or diltiazem appears to be an effective alternative; nifedipine should be used alone with caution in stable angina since response is variable and angina is increased in some patients. Nifedipine is safe and effective when added to the treatment of a patient whose symptoms persist despite administration of an adequate dose of a beta-blocking agent. If this combination does not provide adequate relief then beta blockade combined with verapamil or diltiazem may be more effective, but patients should be monitored carefully for adverse effects due to depression of cardiac conduction. Beneficial response to calcium-channel blockers has also been reported in patients with angina associated with coronary artery spasm.

Calcium-channel blocking agents have proved extremely effective in the treatment of *unstable angina*, providing valuable symptomatic relief, and, when added to conventional anti-anginal treatment they reduce the incidence of sudden death, myocardial infarction, and the need for coronary artery surgery. Diltiazem or verapamil may be preferable to nifedipine for use as the sole agent in unstable angina because of the increased risk of adverse effects with nifedipine.

Nifedipine is simple, safe, and effective in the management of hypertensive emergencies and as a third-line agent in the treatment of *hypertension*. Diltiazem and verapamil are also effective. Verapamil and diltiazem also impair atrioventricular and sino-atrial conduction and are effective in the management of certain nodal and supraventricular *arrhythmias*.

The experience of calcium-channel blocking agents so far indicates that they are safe and effective in many cardiovascular disorders.— J. Kenny, *Br. med. J.*, 1985, *291*, 1150.

Angina pectoris. For prophylaxis of variant or Prinzmetal's angina the calcium-channel blockers have been found effective and superior to nitrates, with nifedipine and diltiazem being slightly better than verapamil. Most patients who do not respond to one agent will respond to another agent, to a combination of a nitrate and a calcium-channel blocker, or to the co-administration of two calcium-channel blockers. In the treatment of unstable angina, nifedipine may be administered with a beta-blocking agent, but administration with a nitrate may accentuate adverse vasodilatory effects. Diltiazem has been given safely with propranolol although the effect on the atrioventricular node may be additive, and adverse effects are less of a problem when diltiazem is given with a nitrate. Nifedipine appears to be preferable to diltiazem in patients with adverse cardiac effects from propranolol, while in patients with adverse effects from nitrates, diltiazem seems preferable to nifedipine.— R. Zelis, *New Engl. J. Med.*, 1982, *306*, 926.

Calcium-channel blockers are effective in the management of patients with stable angina when used alone or in combination with beta-blockers. They are also useful for the treatment of unstable angina, but beta-blockers remain the first-line drugs of choice. Nifedipine should only be given to patients with unstable angina with a beta-blocker since the increase in heart-rate may increase ischaemia. Diltiazem is of value in the treatment of coronary spasm (Prinzmetal's syndrome) and thus may be useful in patients with unstable angina where spasm may be part of the mechanism of ischaemic pain. Verapamil may also be useful but should be used with caution in patients with left ventricular dysfunction.— H. N. Hultgren *et al.*, *J. Am. med. Ass.*, 1985, *253*, 2555. See also P. Théroux *et al.*, *Drugs*, 1983, *25*, 178.

In a study in 10 patients with stable exertional angina pectoris response to nifedipine was highly variable; some patients showing improvement at intermediate doses deteriorated with larger doses. Dose titration was therefore considered essential.— J. Deanfield *et al.*, *Br. med. J.*, 1983, *286*, 1467.

Clinical studies of nifedipine in angina pectoris: G. Gerstenblith *et al.*, *New Engl. J. Med.*, 1982, *306*, 885 (unstable angina); R. L. Feldman *et al.* (letter), *ibid.*, *307*, 627 (unstable angina); J. E. Muller *et al.*, *Circulation*, 1984, *69*, 728 (in combination with a beta blocker); C. R. Conti *et al.*, *Am. Heart J.*, 1985, *110*, 251 (in combination with isosorbide dinitrate); G. W. Vetrovec and V. E. Parker, *Am. J. Med.*, 1986, *81*, *Suppl.* 4A, 20 (alone or with beta blockers in stable angina); I. M. Findlay *et al.*, *Br. Heart J.*, 1986, *55*, 240 (in combination with atenolol); E. E. van der Wall *et al.*, *Am. J. Cardiol.*, 1986, *57*, 1029 (unstable angina); P. Rizzon *et al.*, *Eur. Heart J.*, 1986, *7*, 67 (unstable angina).

Cardiomyopathy. Nifedipine improved diastolic compliance and systolic performance, and relieved dyspnoea and chest pain in a 54-year-old woman with severe hypertrophic cardiomyopathy.— B. H. Lorell *et al.*, *New Engl. J. Med.*, 1980, *303*, 801.

The results of a study of the acute effects of a single dose of nifedipine administered to 15 patients with hypertrophic cardiomyopathy suggested an improvement in diastolic function and in left ventricular distensibility. The reasons for the improvement in the diastolic function were thought to be altered left ventricular loading associated with vasodilatation, reduction of subendothelial left ventricular ischaemia, and a direct effect on the myocardium associated with myocardial calcium availability.— B. H. Lorell *et al.*, *Postgrad. med. J.*, 1985, *61*, 1117.

Further references to beneficial effects in hypertrophic cardiomyopathy: W. J. Paulus *et al.*, *J. Am. Coll. Cardiol.*, 1983, *2*, 879; H. R. Figulla *et al.*, *Dt. med. Wschr.*, 1986, *111*, 11.

Heart failure. A review of the use of calcium-channel blocking agents in chronic heart failure. Patients with chronic heart failure often have either ischaemic heart disease, hypertension, or long-standing chest disease with pulmonary hypertension as a major underlying cause of their heart disease. Calcium-channel blocking agents have the potential to ameliorate these underlying disorders and also to correct the disturbed haemodynamic state which occurs in cardiac failure. Encouraging results of acute haemodynamic studies of nifedipine have suggested that nifedipine may reduce afterload and preload. Chronic studies have yielded conflicting results, but these studies are difficult to perform and interpret since patients are usually elderly and on other medication. Verapamil has been used to treat heart failure but care is needed when establishing the dose since the negative inotropic effect may be detrimental. Verapamil may be beneficial in suppressing arrhythmias that may be responsible for sudden death in these patients.

Calcium-channel blocking agents are potentially useful in the treatment of heart failure but their place in management has yet to be determined.— M. J. Kendall *et al.*, *Postgrad. med. J.*, 1986, *62*, 713. See also: S. Charlap and W. H. Frishman, *Int. J. Cardiol.*, 1984, *6*, 665; W. S. Colucci *et al.*, *Am. J. Med.*, 1985, *78*, *Suppl.* 2B, 9.

Myocardial infarction. In a study involving 171 patients with threatened myocardial infarction, treatment with nifedipine did not alter the incidence of progression to infarction, infarct size, or 6-month mortality compared with placebo. There was a statistically significant increase in 2-week mortality in patients treated with nifedipine.— J. E. Muller *et al.*, *Circulation*, 1984, *69*, 740. Similar results from a study involving 227 patients.— P. A. Sirnes *et al.*, *ibid.*, *70*, 638. Similar results from the Trent study involving 4491 patients. Mortality at 1 month was similar for patients taking nifedipine or placebo.— R. G. Wilcox *et al.*, *Br. med. J.*, 1986, *293*, 1204.

CARDIOVASCULAR SURGERY. Beneficial effects on haemodynamic performance were reported in 170 high-risk patients undergoing open heart surgery treated with nifedipine in the cardioplegic solution compared with 35 patients who received cardioplegic solution alone. There was also a reduction in the incidence of acute low cardiac output and related deaths with nifedipine.— R. E. Clark *et al.*, *Ann. thorac. Surg.*, 1983, *36*, 654.

For a report of the stability of nifedipine in cardioplegic solutions, see above.

Arterial blood pressure was well controlled by both nifedipine and glyceryl trinitrate given by intravenous infusion to 23 patients undergoing coronary artery surgery. Increases in coronary sinus blood flow and oxygen consumption were observed in patients treated with nifedipine. Although the increase in coronary sinus blood flow was anticipated, the increase in oxygen consumption remained unexplained.— H. B. van Wezel *et al.*, *Br. J. Anaesth.*, 1986, *58*, 125P. See also H. B. van Wezel *et al.*, *ibid.*, 267.

DYSMENORRHOEA. In 10 women with severe primary dysmenorrhoea given nifedipine 20 to 40 mg by mouth on the first menstrual day, pain relief occurred within 10 to 30 minutes of administration.— K. -E. Andersson and U. Ulmsten, *Br. J. Obstet. Gynaec.*, 1978, *85*, 142.

HICCUPS. Intractable hiccups unresponsive to conventional treatment resolved completely with nifedipine 20 mg every 8 hours in 1 patient.— P. Mukhopadhyay *et al.* (letter), *New Engl. J. Med.*, 1986, *314*, 1256.

HYPERTENSION. A review of the use of calcium-channel blocking agents in the treatment of hypertension. The calcium-channel blockers are potent vasodilators that can reduce the elevated peripheral vascular resistance which is the primary haemodynamic derangement in hypertension. Most of the studies reviewed show that these drugs are effective antihypertensive agents without producing excessive blood pressure reduction or postural symptoms, but long-term studies are needed to confirm their efficacy and safety as monotherapy. Calcium-channel blockers offer useful alternative antihypertensive therapy in the elderly, in patients with low renin activity, concurrent ischaemic heart disease, supraventricular arrhythmias, bronchospastic disease, peripheral vascular disease, or diabetes mellitus. They may be used as first-line therapy in patients with contra-indications to beta-blockers or diuretics.

In hypertensive crisis or severe hypertension, nifedipine has been shown to produce a very rapid reduction in blood pressure ranging from 20 to 36% in mean arterial pressure at approximately 15 to 30 minutes after nifedipine 10 mg sublingually or 1 hour after 10 to 20 mg orally. Most studies indicate that the degree of blood pressure reduction is related to the magnitude of the systolic and diastolic pressures prior to nifedipine treatment, but not related to the age of the patient.

In short-term studies in mild to moderate hypertension with nifedipine 30 to 60 mg daily, a 14 to 21% reduction in mean arterial pressure has been reported. There was a wide range in the duration of blood pressure reduction between 2 and 8 hours, with most studies using a 6-hourly dosing regimen. Combination treatment with other antihypertensive agents has also been found to be effective, and adverse effects associated with nifedipine therapy have been reduced. Verapamil and diltiazem have also been shown to have an antihypertensive effect, although experience with diltiazem is limited. In long-term management verapamil and diltiazem have fewer adverse effects than nifedipine. In patients with heart failure, nifedipine and diltiazem are preferable to verapamil.— Y. W. F. Lam *et al.*, *Drug Intell. & clin. Pharm.*, 1986, *20*, 187. See also: L. H. Opie, *Lancet*, 1984, *1*, 496; E. M. Sorkin *et al.*, *Drugs*, 1985, *30*, 182.

Studies of the use of nifedipine in hypertension: S. Dean and M. J. Kendall, *Eur. J. clin. Pharmac.*, 1983, *24*, 1 (in difficult to control hypertension); O. de Divitiis *et al.*, *Arzneimittel-Forsch.*, 1984, *34*, 710 (in comparison and combined with acebutolol); B. D. Given *et al.*, *Archs intern. Med.*, 1985, *145*, 281 (in patients with hypertension and congestive heart failure); G. Masotti *et al.*, *J. clin. Pharmac.*, 1985, *25*, 27 (using sublingual administration); J. Moreira *et al.*, *Nephron*, 1985, *41*, 314 (in patients with hypertension and renal disease); W. B. White *et al.*, *Clin. Pharmac. Ther.*, 1986, *39*, 43 (in combination with captopril); A. R. Daniels and L. H. Opie, *Am. J. Cardiol.*, 1986, *57*, 965 (in combination with atenolol in mild to moderate hypertension); A. A. Jennings *et al.*, *Am. Heart J.*, 1986, *111*, 557 (in severe or refractory hypertension); L. E. Ramsay *et al.*, *Postgrad. med. J.*, 1987, *63*, 99 (compared with hydralazine and prazosin as third-line management); P. H. Winocour *et al.*, *Br. J. clin. Pract.*, 1987, *41*, 772 (in insulin-dependent diabetic hypertensive patients); G. Macdonald and P. B. St Leger, *ibid.*, 659 (hypotensive effect in patients up to 70 years).

Hypertensive crisis. Nifedipine 20 mg sublingually successfully reduced systolic and diastolic blood pressures in 26 of 30 patients with hypertensive crisis. Adverse effects were observed in 4 patients: brief flushing in 2, urticaria in 1, and decrease in systolic pressure of 100 mmHg in 1. A brief, minor increase in heart-rate was observed in 2 patients.— R. Erbel *et al.*, *Postgrad. med. J.*, 1983, *59*, *Suppl.* 3, 134.

Nifedipine 10 to 20 mg orally reduced systolic and diastolic blood pressure in 25 patients with very high blood pressure requiring emergency reduction. Increases in heart-rate were inversely related to age. No serious adverse effects were observed. Measurement of cerebral blood flow after nifedipine showed an increase in 4 out of 5 patients.— O. Bertel *et al.*, *Br. med. J.*, 1983, *286*, 19.

Nifedipine reduced blood pressure acutely and safely in 44 out of 45 patients with severe or apparently refractory hypertension. The antihypertensive effect was maintained for up to 24 months when added to existing therapy. Adverse effects included headache in 1 patient, mild dizziness in 3, transient palpitations in 1, and facial flushing in 1.— L. H. Opie and A. Jennings (letter), *Lancet*, 1985, *2*, 555.

A review of the use of nifedipine and other calcium-channel blocking agents in hypertensive emergencies.— R. H. Ferguson and P. H. Vlasses, *J. Am. med. Ass.*, 1986, *255*, 1607.

Further references: J. I. Haft and W. E. Litterer, *Archs intern. Med.*, 1984, *144*, 2357.

MIGRAINE. Nifedipine was found to be effective in reducing the frequency and severity of migraine associated with Raynaud's phenomenon (A. Kahan *et al.*, *New Engl. J. Med.*, 1983, *308*, 1102) and in patients with systemic lupus erythematosus (F.W. Miller and T.J. Santoro, *ibid.*, 1984, *311*, 921). However, headache severity and duration were reported to be worsened by nifedipine in a study of 6 patients with classic migraine (R. Kanter *et al.*, *Cephalalgia*, 1985, *5*, *Suppl.* 3, 148).

OESOPHAGEAL DISORDERS. A review of the treatment of oesophageal motility disorders. Dilatation or cardiomyotomy was considered to be the treatment of choice in achalasia but treatment with isosorbide dinitrate or nifedipine sublingually might be tried in mildly affected patients. Drug treatment should also be tried in diffuse oesophageal spasm.— *Drug & Ther. Bull.*, 1984, *22*, 17. A further review. Nifedipine 10 to 30 mg sublingually 30 minutes before meals was recommended for the medical treatment of achalasia. Some beneficial results have also been obtained with nifedipine in diffuse oesophageal spasm and 'nutcracker' oesophagus.— M. Traube and R. W. McCallum, *Drugs*, 1985, *30*, 66.

In clinical studies involving 29 patients with achalasia given nifedipine 10 to 20 mg sublingually 15 to 30 minutes before each meal and up to a maximum of 60 mg daily, responses were classified as excellent or good in 21, moderate in 5, and poor in 3.— M. Bortolotti and G. Labo, *Gastroenterology*, 1981, *80*, 39.

Radionuclide studies in 15 patients with achalasia showed that nifedipine was less effective than isosorbide dinitrate in improving dysphagia. Seven patients failed to respond to treatment with either drug.— M. Gelfond *et al.*, *Gastroenterology*, 1982, *83*, 963.

Beneficial effects of nifedipine 10 mg half-an-hour before meals in 1 patient with diffuse oesophageal spasm.— S. M. Nasrallah (letter), *Lancet*, 1982, *2*, 1285.

Nifedipine 20 mg sublingually decreased the lower oesophageal sphincter pressure by approximately 30% in 20 patients with achalasia. In patients with high-amplitude peristaltic oesophageal contractions ('nutcracker' oesophagus) the same dose of nifedipine orally decreased lower oesophageal sphincter pressure and contraction amplitude.— M. Traube *et al.*, *J. Am. med. Ass.*, 1984, *252*, 1733. A similar observation in 14 patients and comment on the differences between the action of nifedipine on the oesophagus in achalasia and 'nutcracker' oesophagus.— F. J. Roman *et al.* (letter), *ibid.*, 1985, *253*, 2046.

Symptomatic relief of radiotherapy-induced oesophagitis with nifedipine was reported in 3 patients.— E. Finkelstein (letter), *Lancet*, 1986, *1*, 1205.

Further references to nifedipine in oesophageal disorders: J. E. Richter *et al.*, *Gastroenterology*, 1985, *89*, 549; S. M. Nasrallah *et al.*, *Sth. med. J.*, 1985, *78*, 312; E. Thomas *et al.*, *ibid.*, 1986, *79*, 847.

PERIPHERAL VASCULAR DISORDERS. A review of the clinical use of calcium-channel blockers in cerebral and peripheral vascular disorders.— K. J. Tietze *et al.*, *Drugs*, 1987, *32*, 531.

Successful treatment of a diabetic ulcer with nifedipine 10 mg four times daily.— R. J. Lazarus *et al.* (letter), *Ann. intern. Med.*, 1983, *98*, 414. See also T. Y. Woo *et al.*, *Int. J. Derm.*, 1984, *23*, 678.

In 7 out of 10 patients with severe idiopathic perniosis (chilblains), established lesions resolved within 7 to 10 days of starting treatment with nifedipine 60 mg daily as a sustained-release tablet, and no new lesions developed during treatment. Chilblains recurred in 5 patients within 1 week when placebo was substituted.— P. M. Dowd *et al.*, *Br. med. J.*, 1986, *293*, 923.

Raynaud's syndrome. A review of the treatment of Raynaud's phenomenon. There have been numerous reports of favourable clinical responses to oral nifedipine 20 to 80 mg per day in primary and secondary Raynaud's phenomenon in placebo-controlled studies substantiated by objective measurements of blood flow. Therapeutic benefit has been seen in about 60% of patients treated with nifedipine. The most common adverse effects were flushing, light-headedness, and ankle swelling; they tended to be dose-related and might disappear with continued therapy. Adverse effects were reported to be less marked with sustained-release preparations.— P. M. Dowd, *Br. J. Derm.*, 1986, *114*, 527. See also: S. Roath, *Br. med. J.*, 1986, *293*, 88; C. M. Black, *Prescribers' J.*, 1987, *27*, 6.

The effect of nifedipine on cold-induced digital vasospasm was substantial and treatment was beneficial in all but 1 of 8 patients with disabling Raynaud's phenomenon. The effect was dose-dependent.— H. Nilsson *et al.*, *Acta med. scand.*, 1984, *215*, 135.

In a double-blind study in 16 patients with Raynaud's disease, significant increases in digital blood flow and skin temperature were observed 2 hours after acute dosing with nifedipine 20 mg and after chronic dosing with nifedipine for 14 days. The number, duration, and severity of attacks were decreased following nifedipine compared with placebo.— M. B. Finch *et al.*, *Br. J. clin. Pharmac.*, 1986, *21*, 100P.

Further references to nifedipine in Raynaud's syndrome: C. D. Smith and R. J. R. McKendry, *Lancet*, 1982, *2*, 1299; M. H. A. Rustin *et al.* (letter), *ibid.*, 1983, *1*, 130; S. J. Hawkins *et al.*, *Rheumatol. Int.*, 1986, *6*, 85; C. J. White *et al.*, *Am. J. Med.*, 1986, *80*, 623; J. Sarkozi *et al.*, *J. Rheumatol.*, 1986, *13*, 331.

PHAEOCHROMOCYTOMA. A patient with a noradrenaline-secreting phaeochromocytoma experienced great improvement in cardiovascular symptoms during treatment with nifedipine (D. Serfas *et al.*, *Lancet*, 1983, *2*, 711). Symptomatic relief was associated with a pronounced decline in elevated urinary noradrenaline concentrations and it was suggested that nifedipine could interfere with the release of noradrenaline from phaeochromocytoma tissue. However, Lenders *et al.* (*Br. med. J.*, 1985, *290*, 1624) reported studies in a patient with phaeochromocytoma in which they showed very high-plasma concentrations of noradrenaline despite abolition of the associated increase in blood pressure by nifedipine. This suggested that nifedipine was interfering with the action of noradrenaline by acting directly on the vascular smooth muscle. A similar result was obtained by Favre and Vallotton (*Ann. intern. Med.*, 1985, *104*, 125).

PREGNANCY AND THE NEONATE. Labour was successfully postponed in a patient treated with nifedipine 20 mg three times a day and terbutaline 5 mg 4-hourly by mouth. Terbutaline 0.25 mg up to 4 times a day by subcutaneous injection was also occasionally necessary. Nifedipine was administered from the 26th week of pregnancy for 55 days. A normal, healthy infant was delivered in the 36th week of pregnancy.— A. F. Kaul *et al.*, *Drug Intell. & clin. Pharm.*, 1985, *19*, 369.

Nifedipine 30 mg initially then 20 mg every 8 hours by mouth was found to be more effective in suppressing premature labour than ritodrine given intravenously or no treatment.— M. D. Read and D. E. Wellby, *Br. J. Obstet. Gynaec.*, 1986, *93*, 933.

PULMONARY HYPERTENSION. Results from studies involving 13 patients with acute respiratory failure given nifedipine 20 mg sublingually indicated that nifedipine vasodilates pulmonary vessels constricted by hypoxia, without deleterious effects on arterial oxygenation.— G. Simonneau *et al.*, *New Engl. J. Med.*, 1981, *304*, 1582.

Two out of 6 patients with chronic obstructive pulmonary disease and secondary pulmonary hypertension responded well to treatment with nifedipine (N. Kastanos *et al.*, *New Engl. J. Med.*, 1982, *307*, 1215). In contrast nifedipine reduced cardiac output and oxygen delivery in 2 patients with a more severe degree of airflow obstruction. This was thought to be related to the combination of advanced fixed vascular disease and decreased end-diastolic pressure in the right ventricle caused by nifedipine, but Packer *et al.* (*ibid.*) suggested that these effects might have been the result of a direct negative inotropic effect on right ventricular systolic function.

Results of a study in 9 patients with primary pulmonary hypertension. Nifedipine treatment decreased total pulmonary resistance and increased both cardiac output and stroke volume. Right ventricular function also improved after sublingual treatment. Markedly elevated pulmonary arterial pressure occurred in 1 patient after a single sublingual dose and it was considered that continued treatment with nifedipine would be unwise. Of 6 patients treated with nifedipine orally for 4 to 14 months, 5 patients maintained haemodynamic improvement. Nifedipine was considered to be a potentially useful agent in the management of some patients with primary pulmonary hypertension.— L. J. Rubin *et al.*, *Ann. intern. Med.*, 1983, *99*, 433.

One patient became dyspnoeic after nifedipine treatment despite apparently beneficial haemodynamic changes. This suggested that nifedipine might increase the physiologic shunt through the lungs by preferentially vasodilating relatively under ventilated hypoxic regions in certain patients with primary pulmonary hypertension. Measurement of arterial blood gases is necessary to find this effect.— R. C. Krol *et al.* (letter), *Ann. intern. Med.*, 1984, *100*, 163.

A discussion of the drug treatment of primary pulmonary hypertension. Nifedipine produced beneficial haemodynamic effects in 4 patients. However, 1 patient with thrombo-embolic pulmonary hypertension did not respond to oral therapy and developed severe fluid retention which was unresponsive to treatment. Haemodynamic and symptomatic benefit was maintained in 3 patients with continued treatment for 1 year. While these results and those of other investigators are encouraging, it was considered that invasive investigation was essential when using nifedipine in the treatment of primary pulmonary hypertension.— A. A. McLeod and D. E. Jewitt, *Drugs*, 1986, *31*, 177.

Nifedipine relieved symptoms of high-altitude pulmonary oedema sufficiently to allow safe descent from a mountain. It was suggested that nifedipine may provide simple emergency treatment when oxygenation and evacuation is not possible.— O. Oelz (letter), *J. Am. med. Ass.*, 1987, *257*, 780.

URINARY-TRACT DISORDERS. Administration of a single dose of nifedipine 10 to 30 mg by mouth had an inhibiting effect on the detrusor contractions in 10 women with urge incontinence; following treatment with nifedipine 10 to 20 mg twice daily for 1 week all patients reported subjective improvement.— T. Rud *et al.*, *Urol. int.*, 1979, *34*, 421.

A report of rapid pain relief with nifedipine 10 mg in 2 patients with ureteral colic (W. Carrol, *Ann. intern. Med.*, 1985, *102*, 864) has not been confirmed by subsequent prospective studies (M. McCormack *et al.*, *ibid.*, *104*, 590; S. Viskin *et al.*, *ibid.*, *105*, 142; L. Coppens and F. Lustman, *ibid.*, 967).

URTICARIA PIGMENTOSA. Nifedipine 10 mg three times a day was used successfully to suppress the symptoms of urticaria pigmentosa in 1 patient.— J. A. Fairley *et al.*, *J. Am. Acad. Derm.*, 1984, *11*, 740.

Preparations

Nifedipine Capsules *(U.S.P.)*

Proprietary Preparations

Adalat *(Bayer, UK). Capsules* (Adalat 5), buccal or oral, nifedipine 5 mg.

Capsules, buccal or oral, nifedipine 10 mg. For buccal administration, the capsule should be bitten and the liquid contents retained in the mouth.

Adalat IC *(Bayer, UK). Injection*, nifedipine 100 µg/mL, in pre-filled syringes of 2 mL.

Adalat retard *(Bayer, UK). Tablets*, sustained-release, nifedipine 20 mg.

Tablets (Adalat retard 10), sustained-release, nifedipine 10 mg.

Symptomatic hypotension necessitating admission to hospital occurred in a patient who had been given Adalat 10 mg capsules and instructed to take 2 capsules twice daily when nifedipine 20 mg tablets (Adalat 20) had been prescribed. It was suggested that the problem could be overcome by indicating the different pharmacokinetic properties of the tablet in the proprietary name.— S. N. Hunyor and D. Moes (letter), *Med. J. Aust.*, 1987, *146*, 228.

Proprietary Names and Manufacturers

Adalat *(Bayer, Arg.; Bayer, Austral.; Belg.; Miles, Canad.; Bayer, Denm.; Bayer, Ger.; Bayer, Ital.; Jpn; Bayer, Norw.; Bayer, S.Afr.; Bayer, Spain; Bayer, Swed.; Bayer, Switz.; Bayer, UK; Miles Pharmaceuticals, USA)*; Adalate *(Bayer, Fr.)*; Anifed *(Zoja, Ital.)*; Aprical *(Rentschler, Ger.)*; Citilat *(CT, Ital.)*; Coral *(Tosi, Ital.)*; Cordicant *(Mundipharma, Ger.)*; Cordilan *(Andreu, Spain)*; Corotrend *(Siegfried, Ger.; Sigamed, Switz.)*; Dilcor *(Boi, Spain)*; Duranifin *(Durachemie, Ger.)*; Fedipina *(Bonomelli, Ital.)*; Hinoxon *(Celtia, Arg.)*; Nifecor *(Kettelhack Riker, Ger.)*; Nifedicor *(Schiapparelli, Ital.)*; Nifedin *(Benedetti, Ital.)*; Nifedipat *(Azuchemie, Ger.)*; Nifedipina Retard *(Volpino, Arg.)*; Nifelat *(Sidus, Arg.; Remedica, Cyprus)*; Nifenitron *(Quesada, Arg.)*; Nife-Puren *(Klinge-Nattermann, Ger.)*; Nifical *(Beiersdorf, Ger.)*; Pidilat *(Giulini, Ger.)*; Procardia *(Pfizer, USA)*; Tibricol *(Pfizer, Arg.)*.

The following names have been used for multi-ingredient preparations containing nifedipine— Beta-Adalat *(Bayer, UK)*; Nif-Ten *(ICI, Ger.)*; Tenif *(Stuart, UK)*.

NOTE. The name Adalat is used in some countries to denote the tablet formulation known in the UK as Adalat Retard which produces delayed absorption compared with the liquid-filled capsule.

16913-b

Niludipine *(BAN).*

Bay-a-7168. Bis(2-propoxyethyl)1,4-dihydro-2,6-dimethyl-4-(3-nitrophenyl)pyridine-3,5-dicarboxylate.

$C_{25}H_{34}N_2O_8$=490.6.

CAS — 22609-73-0.

Niludipine is a calcium-channel blocking agent with vasodilatory properties.

References: K. Ogawa *et al.*, *Arzneimittel-Forsch.*, 1982, *32*, 542; K. Aoki and K. Sato, *ibid.*, 1141; H. Yasuda *et al.*, *ibid.*, 1984, *34*, 614; E. Kusano *et al.*, *ibid.*, 624.

Proprietary Names and Manufacturers
Bayer, Switz.

16914-v

Nimodipine *(BAN, USAN).*

Bay-e-9736. Isopropyl 2-methoxyethyl 1,4-dihydro-2,6-dimethyl-4-(3-nitrophenyl)pyridine-3,5-dicarboxylate.

$C_{21}H_{26}N_2O_7$=418.4.

CAS — 66085-59-4.

Nimodipine is a calcium-channel blocker primarily used for its cerebral vasodilatory effect. It has been used for neurological deficits following cerebral ischaemia and in migraine. For the treatment of ischaemic neurological deficits caused by arterial spasm following subarachnoid haemorrhage, nimodipine is administered via a by-pass into a running intravenous infusion of a suitable solution using an infusion pump via a central catheter. The recommended dose is nimodipine 1 mg per hour for 2 hours, then 2 mg per hour provided no severe decrease in blood pressure is observed. The starting dose should be reduced to 0.5 mg or less per hour in patients weighing less than 70 kg or with unstable blood pressure.

A review of the actions and applications of calcium-channel blockers including nimodipine.— D. D. Freedman and D. D. Waters, *Drugs*, 1987, *34*, 578.

A study to assess the effectiveness of nimodipine in preventing or altering the severity of ischaemic neurological deficits due to spasm. Results suggested that patients who are essentially neurologically normal after a subarachnoid haemorrhage from an aneurysm may benefit from oral administration of nimodipine for 3 weeks after the haemorrhage.— G. S. Allen *et al.*, *New Engl. J. Med.*, 1983, *308*, 619. Comments on the design of the trial, diagnostic criteria, and outcome.— M. Vermeulen *et al.* (letter), *ibid.*, *309*, 437.

Reviews of brain ischaemia and ischaemic stroke including comments on the use of calcium-channel blockers.— N. M. Dearden, *Lancet*, 1985, *2*, 255; P. Sandercock, *Br. med. J.*, 1987, *295*, 1224. Studies into the use of nimodipine in brain ischaemia: H. J. Gelmers, *Am. J. Cardiol.*, 1985, *55*, 144B (in stroke); G. S. Allen, *ibid.*, 149B (after subarachnoid haemorrhage); L. M. Auer *et al.*, *Acta neurochir.*, 1986, *82*, 7 (after subarachnoid haemorrhage).

Reports of beneficial effects of nimodipine in reducing ischaemic damage in the brain due to subarachnoid haemorrhage and stroke. The view that nimodipine acts primarily as a vasodilator may be an oversimplification. The action may also depend on blocking a calcium-ion dependent 'cascade' of biochemical processes leading to cell damage, on improving cell energy production, and on preventing a calcium-induced decrease in red blood cell deformability.— *Pharm. J.*, 1987, *1*, 475.

CARDIAC DISORDERS. The safety and efficacy of nimodipine in cardiopulmonary resuscitation after cardiac arrest due to ventricular fibrillation was studied. The treatment was well tolerated, and results suggested that nimodipine might increase the number of survivors.— R. O. Roine *et al.*, *Br. med. J.*, 1987, *294*, 20.

MIGRAINE. A review of the use of calcium-channel blockers in vascular headaches. Nimodipine is more selective for cephalic blood vessels than either verapamil or nifedipine, and also produces less serious adverse effects. Double-blind studies report that 80 to 90% of patients with vascular headaches benefit from nimodipine treatment. Nimodipine has been found to be effective in classical and complicated migraine, and cluster headaches, and gives partial or complete relief of both prodromal and headache symptoms. Calcium-channel blockers are less effective in common migraine, with improvement in about half to two-thirds of patients. After starting treatment, there is a delay of 10 to 14 days before relief from prodromes begins and decreases in headache frequency and severity are often delayed for 2 to 4 weeks.— J. S. Meyer, *Ann. intern. Med.*, 1985, *102*, 395. Clinical studies into the use of nimodipine in migraine: H. J. Gelmers, *Headache*, 1983, *23*, 106; H. Havanka-Kanniainen *et al.*, *Cephalalgia*, 1985, *5*, 39; K. Jensen *et al.*, *ibid.*, 125.

Proprietary Preparations

Nimotop *(Bayer, UK). Intravenous infusion*, nimodipine 200 µg/mL, in vials of 50 mL.

Proprietary Names and Manufacturers

Nimotop *(Bayer, Denm.; Bayer, Ger.; Bayer, UK; Miles Pharmaceuticals, USA)*.

13022-j

Nisoldipine *(BAN, USAN, rINN).*
Bay-k-5552. Isobutyl methyl 1,4-dihydro-2,6-dimethyl-4-(2-nitrophenyl)pyridine-3,5-dicarboxylate.
$C_{20}H_{24}N_2O_6$=388.4.

CAS — 63675-72-9.

Nisoldipine is a calcium-channel blocking agent with properties similar to those of nifedipine p.1509.

A review of the actions and clinical uses of nisoldipine.— D. D. Freedman and D. D. Waters, *Drugs*, 1987, *34*, 578.

The haemodynamic effects of nisoldipine were investigated in 16 patients with stable coronary artery disease. At rest and during exercise nisoldipine resulted in reduced systemic vascular resistance and mean arterial pressure, and increased heart rate, cardiac and stroke volume indices. The results suggested that nisoldipine improved cardiac pumping function in patients with severe but clinically stable angina pectoris. There was no evidence of cardiac depression.— B. Silke *et al., Br. J. clin. Pharmac.*, 1985, *20*, 675.

In normotensive subjects, nisoldipine caused a significant fall in systolic blood pressure. Antihypertensive efficacy was also demonstrated in 8 patients with essential hypertension treated with nisoldipine 10 mg twice daily for 4 weeks. Adverse effects included headache, facial flushing, and mild ankle oedema F. Pasanisi *et al., Eur. J. clin. Pharmac.*, 1985, *29*, 21.

Results of a study involving 15 patients suggested that nisoldipine is safe and effective in the treatment of exercise-induced angina pectoris. Nisoldipine appears to act by reducing myocardial oxygen demand at rest and during exercise. A dose of 20 mg daily, given in two doses appears to be beneficial in a majority of patients.— L. M. Lopez *et al., Am. Heart J.*, 1985, *110*, 991.

A single dose of nisoldipine in patients with coronary artery disease had a predominantly peripheral effect without impairment of cardiac contractility. There was also evidence to suggest an effect on myocardial oxygen supply.— F. Tartagni *et al., Arzneimittel-Forsch.*, 1986, *36*, 1528.

Further references: J. Lam *et al., J. Am. Coll. Cardiol.*, 1985, *6*, 447 (in angina pectoris); H. Suryapranata *et al., Aust. N.Z. J. Med.*, 1985, *15*, 685 (haemodynamics); P. A. Crean *et al., Am. Heart J.*, 1987, *113*, 261 (in comparison with nifedipine in angina pectoris).

WITHDRAWAL SYMPTOMS. Abrupt withdrawal of nisoldipine from 15 patients with stable angina pectoris after 6 weeks of therapy resulted in severe unstable angina in 2 patients and acute myocardial infarction in 1 patient. It was postulated that the withdrawal effect could be due to an increase in sensitivity of vascular α_2 adrenoceptors to circulating adrenaline.— J. Mehta and L. M. Lopez, *Am. J. Cardiol.*, 1986, *58*, 242.

Proprietary Names and Manufacturers
Bayer, Ger.; Bayer, UK.

16915-g

Nitrendipine *(BAN, USAN, rINN).*
Bay-e-5009. Ethyl methyl 1,4-dihydro-2,6-dimethyl-4-(3-nitrophenyl)pyridine-3,5-dicarboxylate.
$C_{18}H_{20}N_2O_6$=360.4.

CAS — 39562-70-4.

Nitrendipine is a calcium-channel blocking agent with properties similar to nifedipine (p.1509). It is used in the treatment of hypertension; a dose of 20 mg daily has been recommended.

Nitrendipine is a calcium-channel blocking agent with predominantly peripheral rather than coronary vasodilating properties. It does not alter cardiac conduction unlike verapamil, diltiazem, and nifedipine. It has been shown to reduce both systolic and diastolic blood pressure to within normal limits in 45 to 86% of patients with mild to moderate hypertension, but there is evidence to suggest that it has less hypotensive activity in normotensive subjects. The antihypertensive effect appears to be sustained during long-term therapy, although further clinical studies are required. The response rates can be increased by the addition of a beta-blocker or a diuretic. There is also evidence to suggest that nitrendipine in combination with captopril may provide a useful alternative treatment in hypertensive patients unresponsive to conventional therapy.
Although nitrendipine produces significant reduction in systemic vascular resistance, alterations in cardiac output and decreases in left ventricular filling pressure have not been consistently observed and are probably not significant during long-term use. Some reduction in left ventricular hypertrophy has been observed, particularly in elderly patients, although there was no apparent correlation with blood pressure reduction. Nitrendipine produces an increase in heart rate in both normotensive and hypertensive patients, but this effect is not sustained during prolonged use. No changes in renal blood flow, renovascular resistance, or glomerular filtration-rate have been seen in patients or in healthy subjects. There is evidence to suggest an initial increase in plasma renin activity, but this effect may diminish with prolonged treatment. There is also a short-term increase in sodium and water excretion. No effects have been seen on plasma glucose or lipid concentrations.
Pharmacokinetic studies have shown that about 80% of the oral dose is absorbed with peak blood concentrations at 1 to 2 hours, but bioavailability is relatively low and variable. Nitrendipine is extensively metabolised in the liver. Less than 0.1% of an oral dose appears unchanged in the urine, while about 77% of the dose is recovered from the urine and about 8% from the faeces as inactive metabolites within 96 hours of an oral dose. The total clearance from the plasma is about 81 to 87 litres per hour. Plasma concentrations and elimination half-life have been shown to be raised in patients with hepatic disease, and plasma concentrations are also elevated in the elderly. The effect of renal disease on the pharmacokinetics of nitrendipine is minimal.
Commonly reported adverse effects of nitrendipine include headache, flushing, ankle oedema, and palpitations. Although the incidence of adverse effects has been reported to be about 40%, they are generally mild and disappear on continued treatment, and have accounted for the withdrawal of nitrendipine in 5 to 10% of patients. Dizziness, allergy, polyuria, and fatigue have also been reported and there have been a few cases of increases in serum alkaline phosphatase.
The usual initial dose in mild to moderate hypertension is 5 to 20 mg once daily in the morning, preferably with or after food, increasing to 5 to 20 mg once or twice daily as necessary. The elderly may respond to lower daily doses of 5 to 10 mg.— K. L. Goa and E. M. Sorkin, *Drugs*, 1987, *33*, 123. See also D. D. Freedman and D. D. Waters, *ibid.*, *34*, 578.

An inverse correlation was found between age and the reduction in diastolic blood pressure produced by nitrendipine. It was suggested that this could be related to the natriuretic effect seen during prolonged treatment.— L. A. Ferrara *et al., Eur. J. clin. Pharmac.*, 1985, *28*, 473.

Bioavailability of nitrendipine was significantly increased and the elimination half-life was prolonged in patients with liver disease.— W. Kirch *et al., J. clin. Pharmac.*, 1985, *25*, 455.

In a study in 19 hypertensive patients, peak plasma-nitrendipine concentrations occurred 1 to 2 hours after oral administration, and peak blood pressure reductions occurred 4 hours after the last dose and were associated with an increase in heart rate. Nitrendipine produced a hypotensive effect similar to propranolol, but also increased plasma-renin activity after exertion. Nitrendipine did not cause the unwanted metabolic effects seen with propranolol.— B. F. Johnson *et al., Clin. Pharmac. Ther.*, 1986, *39*, 389.

A preliminary study of nitrendipine in early pregnancy suggesting that nitrendipine could be useful in the treatment of pregnancy-induced hypertension although further studies will be necessary.— M. R. Lawrence and F. B. Pipkin, *Br. J. clin. Pharmac.*, 1987, *23*, 683.

Clinical studies of the effect of nitrendipine in hypertension: T. C. Fagan *et al., J. cardiovasc. Pharmac.*, 1984, *Suppl.* 7, 1109; L. A. Ferrara *et al., Clin. Pharmac. Ther.*, 1985, *38*, 434; M. De Kock *et al., Eur. Heart J.*, 1986, *7*, 792; B. M. Massie *et al., Am. J. Cardiol.*, 1986, *58*, 16D; F. G. McMahon, *ibid.*, 8D; J. R. M'Buyamba-Kabangu *et al., Clin. Pharmac. Ther.*, 1987, *41*, 45.

Proprietary Names and Manufacturers
Bayotensin *(Bayropharm, Ger.)*; Baypress *(Bayer, Denm.; Bayer, Switz.; Miles Pharmaceuticals, USA).*

9265-t

Nonivamide *(rINN).*
N-Vanillylnonamide.
$C_{17}H_{27}NO_3$=293.4.

CAS — 2444-46-4.

Nonivamide is a topical vasodilator. It is used, in a concentration of 0.4%, in rubefacient ointments.

Proprietary Names and Manufacturers
Rheumaplast *(Ger.).*

The following names have been used for multi-ingredient preparations containing nonivamide—Finalgon *(Boehringer Ingelheim, Austral.; Boehringer Ingelheim, Canad.; Boehringer Ingelheim, UK).*

9267-r

Oxpentifylline *(BAN).*

BL-191; Pentoxifylline *(USAN, rINN).* 3,7-Dimethyl-1-(5-oxohexyl)xanthine.
$C_{13}H_{18}N_4O_3$=278.3.

CAS — 6493-05-6.

Adverse Effects

Oxpentifylline can cause nausea, gastro-intestinal disturbances, dizziness, and headache. Flushing, angina, and palpitations may also occur. There have been occasional reports of cardiac arrhythmias, hepatitis, jaundice, and blood dyscrasias.
Overdosage with oxpentifylline may be associated with fever, faintness, flushing, hypotension, drowsiness, agitation, and seizures.

Severe contact dermatitis occurred under a leather watch strap in a patient while taking oxpentifylline. The skin reaction cleared when oxpentifylline was stopped and recurred when oxpentifylline treatment was restarted.— P. R. Kumar (letter), *Br. med. J.*, 1986, *293*, 1103.

OVERDOSAGE. A 22-year-old woman who took oxpentifylline 4 to 6 g with suicidal intent experienced severe bradycardia and first- and second-degree atrioventricular block; other side-effects included nausea, vomiting, abdominal cramps, hypokalaemia, excitation, and insomnia. She recovered after intensive supportive and symptomatic treatment.— I. J. Sznajder *et al., Br. med. J.*, 1984, *288*, 26.

Precautions

Oxpentifylline should be avoided in patients intolerant to xanthine derivatives. It should be used with caution in patients with severe coronary artery disease or hypotension; oxpentifylline may potentiate the effect of antihypertensive agents. High parenteral doses of oxpentifylline may enhance the hypoglycaemic action of insulin in diabetic patients.
In patients with a creatinine clearance of less than 10 mL per minute, it may be necessary to adjust the dose of oxpentifylline to avoid accumulation.

PREGNANCY AND THE NEONATE. For reference to the excretion of oxpentifylline in breast milk see below.

Absorption and Fate

Oxpentifylline is readily absorbed from the gastro-intestinal tract but undergoes extensive first-pass hepatic metabolism; several metabolites have been identified. The terminal half-life of oxpentifylline is related to the dosage and is reported to be 0.4 to 0.8 hours: the half-life of the metabolites is 1.0 to 1.6 hours. In 24 hours about 94% of a dose is recovered in the urine mainly as metabolites and less than 4% in the faeces. The bioavailability is increased and the rate of excretion is decreased in elderly patients.

References: H. -J. Hinze *et al., Arzneimittel-Forsch.*, 1972, *22*, 1144; H. -J. Hinze, *ibid.*, 1492; H. J. Hinze *et al., Pharmatherapeutica*, 1976, *1*, 160; R. V. Smith *et al., J. pharm. Sci.*, 1986, *75*, 47; A. Ward and S. P. Clissold, *Drugs*, 1987, *34*, 50.

PREGNANCY AND THE NEONATE. Oxpentifylline and its metabolites were detectable in the breast milk of 5 mothers following administration of oxpentifylline

400 mg.— F. R. Witter and R. V. Smith, *Am. J. Obstet. Gynec.*, 1985, *151*, 1094.

Uses and Administration

Oxpentifylline reduces blood viscosity probably by effects on erythrocyte deformability, platelet adhesion, and platelet aggregation. It is also claimed to improve oxygenation of ischaemic tissues. Oxpentifylline is used mainly in the treatment of peripheral vascular disorders including intermittent claudication. The usual dose is 400 mg three times daily by mouth in a sustained-release formulation, reducing to 400 mg twice daily if adverse effects are troublesome. Doses should be taken with meals to reduce gastro-intestinal disturbances. Oxpentifylline may also be given by intravenous or intra-arterial infusion. Oxpentifylline has also been used in cerebrovascular disorders.

A review of the pharmacodynamic properties and therapeutic efficacy of oxpentifylline.— A. Ward and S. P. Clissold, *Drugs*, 1987, *34*, 50.

Results of a study suggesting that in addition to increasing the filterability of red blood cells, oxpentifylline also decreases the adherence of red blood cells to endothelial cells.— S. O. Sowemimo-Coker and P. Turner, *Eur. J. clin. Pharmac.*, 1985, *29*, 55.

CEREBROVASCULAR DISORDERS. A review of the drugs used in the treatment of cerebrovascular disorders, including oxpentifylline. Beneficial responses in clinical symptoms in patients with cerebrovascular insufficiency have been demonstrated in 3 double-blind placebo-controlled studies.— A. Spagnoli and G. Tognoni, *Drugs*, 1983, *26*, 44.

A study involving 66 patients (E. Herskovits *et al.*, *Lancet*, 1981, *1*, 966) indicated that oxpentifylline was beneficial in reducing the incidence of recurrence of transient ischaemic attacks compared with treatment with dipyridamole in association with aspirin. However, the inclusion criteria of patients were criticised by Gawel *et al.* (*ibid.*, 1266) and Warlow and Peto (*ibid.*, 1103) pointed out an error in the calculation of statistical significance. Both correspondents also commented on the small number of patients included in the study.

Further references to the use of oxpentifylline in cerebrovascular disorders: D. Harwart, *Curr. med. Res. Opinion*, 1979, *6*, 73; A. Hartmann, *ibid.*, 1985, *9*, 475; E. Herskovits *et al.*, *Eur. Neurol.*, 1985, *24*, 73.

INFERTILITY. Some improvement in sperm count and motility with oxpentifylline 1.2 g daily in a study involving 22 infertile men. Three pregnancies had resulted at 5 months.— P. Marrama *et al.*, *Andrologia*, 1985, *17*, 612. Treatment with oxpentifylline for 6 months did not significantly increase sperm concentration or sperm motility in 11 patients with oligospermia.— C. Wang *et al.*, *Fert. Steril.*, 1983, *40*, 358.

PERIPHERAL VASCULAR DISORDERS. Review of the clinical pharmacology of oxpentifylline in the treatment of intermittent claudication. Results of studies in Europe and the United States have shown improvements in the signs and symptoms of claudication after oral oxpentifylline treatment.— H. R. Dettelbach and D. M. Aviado, *J. clin. Pharmac.*, 1985, *25*, 8. See also D. E. Baker and R. K. Campbell, *Drug Intell. & clin. Pharm.*, 1985, *19*, 345.

Further reviews of the use of oxpentifylline in intermittent claudication: *Med. Lett.*, 1984, *26*, 103; D. M. Aviado and J. M. Porter, *Pharmacotherapy*, 1984, *4*, 297; J. A. Spittell, *Ann. intern. Med.*, 1985, *102*, 126.

Proprietary Preparations

Trental *(Hoechst, UK). Tablets* (Trental 400), sustained-release, oxpentifylline 400 mg.

Proprietary Names and Manufacturers

Azutrentat *(Azuchemie, Ger.)*; Claudicat *(Promonta, Ger.)*; Durapental *(Durachemie, Ger.)*; Hemovas *(Robert, Spain)*; Pento-Puren *(Klinge-Nattermann, Ger.)*; Rentylin *(Rentschler, Ger.)*; Tarontal *(Greece)*; Terental *(Mex.)*; Torental *(Hoechst, Fr.; Mor.; Tun.)*; Trental *(Arg.; Hoechst, Austral.; Hoechst, Canad.; Albert-Roussel, Ger.; Albert-Farma, Ital.; Jpn; Noristan, S.Afr.; Hoechst, Switz.; Hoechst, UK; Hoechst, USA)*.

9268-f

Oxyfedrine Hydrochloride *(BANM, rINNM)*.

D-563; Oxifedrini Chloridum. L-3-(β-Hydroxy-α-methylphenethylamino)-3′-methoxypropiophenone hydrochloride.

$C_{19}H_{23}NO_3,HCl=349.9$.

CAS — 15687-41-9 (oxyfedrine); 16777-42-7 (hydrochloride).

Pharmacopoeias. In *Nord.*

Adverse Effects

Oxyfedrine administration has been associated with reversible loss of taste sensation.

A study indicating that usual therapeutic doses of oxyfedrine strongly interfere with colour vision.— J. Laroche and C. Laroche, *Annls pharm. fr.*, 1977, *35*, 173.

Absorption and Fate

Oxyfedrine hydrochloride is absorbed from the gastro-intestinal tract. It is reported to be metabolised to phenylpropanolamine.

Uses and Administration

Oxyfedrine hydrochloride is used in the treatment of angina pectoris. It is given in usual doses of 8 to 16 mg three times daily. It may also be given by slow intravenous injection.

Comment on the anti-anginal properties of oxyfedrine despite properties which could be classified as those of a beta-adrenoceptor agonist.— *Lancet*, 1981, *1*, 25. Oxyfedrine is not simply a beta-adrenoceptor agonist; it is a partial agonist at these receptors and could be accurately described as a beta-adrenoceptor blocking drug with marked intrinsic sympathomimetic activity. Other properties, however, including a combination of myocardial stimulation with peripheral venodilatation may adequately explain its beneficial effects.— J. R. Parratt (letter), *ibid.*, 441. Further discussion of the mode of action of oxyfedrine.— J. R. Parratt and J. E. MacKenzie (letter), *Br. J. clin. Pharmac.*, 1981, *11*, 307.

CARDIAC DISORDERS. Indication that oxyfedrine has a beneficial effect in angina pectoris comparable to that of propranolol.— J. Whittington and E. B. Raftery, *Br. J. clin. Pharmac.*, 1980, *10*, 439.

Further studies of oxyfedrine in angina pectoris: L. Fananapazir and C. Bray, *Br. J. clin. Pharmac.*, 1985, *20*, 405.

Proprietary Names and Manufacturers

Ildamen *(Homburg, Belg.; Asta Pharma, Ger.; Farmades, Ital.; Homburg, Neth.; Lacer, Spain; Treupha, Switz.)*; Modacor *(Houdé, Fr.)*.

9270-c

Pentaerythritol Tetranitrate *(BAN, USAN)*.

Erynite; Nitropentaerythrol; Nitropenthrite; Pentaerithrityl Tetranitrate *(rINN)*; Pentaerythritolum Tetranitricum; Pentaerythrityl Tetranitrate; Pentanitrol. 2,2-Bis(hydroxymethyl)propane-1,3-diol tetranitrate.

$C_5H_8N_4O_{12}=316.1$.

CAS — 78-11-5.

Pharmacopoeias. In *Cz.*

Aust., Braz., and *U.S.* also include Diluted Pentaerythritol Tetranitrate as does *B.P.C. 1973.*

A white crystalline powder. Practically **insoluble** in water; slightly soluble in alcohol and in ether; soluble in acetone.

Diluted Pentaerythritol Tetranitrate is a mixture of pentaerythritol tetranitrate with lactose, mannitol, or other suitable inert excipients, the latter being added to minimise the risk of explosion. **Store** in a cool place in airtight containers. Protect from light.

CAUTION. Pentaerythritol Tetranitrate can be exploded by percussion or excessive heat.

Adverse Effects, Treatment, and Precautions

As for Glyceryl Trinitrate, p.1500. In Great Britain the recommended exposure limits of pentaerythritol total dust are 10 mg per m^3 (long-term) and 20 mg per m^3 (short-term). The long-term exposure limit for respirable dust is 5 mg per m^3.

EFFECTS ON THE SKIN. A 63-year-old man who had taken pentaerythritol tetranitrate and glyceryl trinitrate for 8 years developed extensive erythroderma due to the drugs. The condition regressed when the drugs were withdrawn but re-appeared after separate challenge doses of each drug.— F. P. Ryan, *Br. J. Derm.*, 1972, *87*, 498.

Uses and Administration

Pentaerythritol tetranitrate is a vasodilator with general properties similar to those of glyceryl trinitrate (p.1501) but its duration of action is more prolonged. Its effect begins in 20 minutes to 1 hour and lasts about 5 hours.

It is used prophylactically in the treatment of angina pectoris, usually in doses of 10 to 40 mg three or four times daily before meals; doses of up to 160 to 180 mg daily are normally used, although doses of up to 240 mg daily have been recommended. It is also given as sustained-release preparations.

Pentaerythritol trinitrate, an active metabolite of pentaerythritol tetranitrate, has also been used clinically under the name pentrinitrol.

CARDIAC DISORDERS. Data indicating that in congestive heart failure pentaerythritol tetranitrate may have a beneficial effect on preload and afterload lasting 5 hours or more.— F. G. Shellock *et al.*, *Clin. Pharmac. Ther.*, 1980, *28*, 436.

Preparations

Pentaerythritol Tetranitrate Tablets *(B.P.)*. Pentaerythritol Tablets

Pentaerythritol Tetranitrate Tablets *(U.S.P.)*

Proprietary Preparations

Cardiacap *(Consolidated Chemicals, UK). Capsules*, sustained-release, pentaerythritol tetranitrate 30 mg.

Mycardol (known in some countries as Mycartal) *(Winthrop, UK). Tablets*, scored, pentaerythritol tetranitrate 30 mg.

Proprietary Names and Manufacturers of Pentaerythritol Nitrates

Antime *(USA)*; Cardiacap *(Consolidated Chemicals, UK)*; Cordilate *(Vernleigh, S.Afr.)*; Dilcoran *(Gödecke, Ger.; Switz.)*; Duotrate *(Marion Laboratories, USA)*; El-Petn *(USA)*; Lentrat *(Switz.)*; Metranil *(USA)*; Mycardol *(Austral.; Winthrop, UK)*; Mycartal; Niscodil *(Cilag, Ital.)*; Nitrodex *(Dexo, Fr.; Dexo, Switz.)*; Nitropent *(ACO, Swed.)*; Penritol *(Austral.)*; Pentafin *(USA)*; Pentanitrine *(Fr.)*; Pentral *(Concept Pharmaceuticals, UK)*; Pentral 80 *(S.Afr.)*; Pentrit *(Neth.)*; Pentrite *(Adroka, Switz.)*; Pentritol *(USV Pharmaceutical Corp., USA)*; Pentryate *(USA)*; Peritrate *(Arg.; Warner, Austral.; Belg.; Parke, Davis, Canad.; Substantia, Fr.; Parke, Davis, Ital.; Neth.; Warner, S.Afr.; Parke, Davis, Spain; Parke, Davis, UK; Parke, Davis, USA)*; Petrin (pentrinitrol) *(Parke, Davis, USA)*; Quintrate *(USA)*; Terpate *(USA)*; Tranite *(USA)*; Vasolate *(USA)*.

The following names have been used for multi-ingredient preparations containing pentaerythritol nitrates— Pentoxylon *(Riker, UK)*; Pentrium *(Roche, Canad.; Roche, UK)*.

9272-a

Perhexiline Maleate *(BANM, USAN, rINNM)*.

WSM-3978G. 2-(2,2-Dicyclohexylethyl)piperidine hydrogen maleate.

$C_{19}H_{35}N,C_4H_4O_4=393.6$.

CAS — 6621-47-2 (perhexiline); 6724-53-4 (maleate).

Adverse Effects

Perhexiline occasionally produces severe adverse effects including peripheral neuropathy affecting all 4 limbs with associated papilloedema, severe and occasionally fatal hepatic toxicity, and metabolic abnormalities with marked weight loss, hypertriglyceridaemia, and profound hypoglycaemia.

Transient or dose-related adverse effects which may occur particularly at the beginning of treatment include dizziness, unsteadiness, headache, nausea, vomiting, and other gastro-intestinal disturbances, ataxia, moderate hypoglycaemia, alterations in the electrocardiogram, and liver enzyme, bilirubin, and plasma lipid abnormalities. Weakness, anxiety, tremors, syncope, changes in libido, paraesthesias, genito-urinary symptoms, flushing and sweating, visual disturbances, extrapyramidal symptoms, and skin rash and urticaria have also been reported.

Comment on peripheral neuropathy associated with perhexiline therapy. Symptomatic neuropathy occurs in about 0.1% of treated patients, but subclinical disorders have been found in as many as two-thirds of patients studied electrophysiologically. Sensory symptoms, including muscle pain and tenderness, are usually prominent, appearing as early as three weeks after treatment begins, and may be followed by severe weakness of distal and even of proximal muscle groups. In most cases symptoms have occurred only after several months of treatment with daily doses of 200 to 300 mg of the drug. Papilloedema, dysgeusia, deafness, cerebellar signs, autonomic disorders, and raised concentrations of protein in cerebrospinal fluid have been reported. Histological studies of peripheral-nerve biopsy specimens have shown prominent segmental demyelination with associated axonal degeneration, and membranous and paracrystalline inclusions in Schwann cells and endothelial cells. Biochemical studies have shown an increased ganglioside content in peripheral nerve. Complete recovery usually occurs within several months of stopping treatment.— Z. Argov and F. L. Mastaglia, *Br. med. J.*, 1979, *1*, 663.

The pathological process in perhexiline-induced peripheral neuropathy is mainly segmental demyelination, possibly due to interference with glycolipid metabolism. Electrophysiological evidence of neuropathy may be present in over 60% of cases, although frank neuropathy is less common and develops only after months of treatment on doses up to 300 mg daily. Painful paraesthesiae are common in the early stages but later, weakness may be severe. Central nervous system involvement with intracranial hypertension and cranial neuropathies may develop. Recovery is generally complete several months after perhexiline withdrawal, but painful paraesthesiae may persist.— R. J. M. Lane and P. A. Routledge, *Drugs*, 1983, *26*, 124.

Report of raised intracranial pressure in 3 patients who had each been taking perhexiline for at least 10 months. Papilloedema improved in each case when perhexiline was stopped, but one patient showed a permanent impairment of visual acuity.— W. P. Stephens *et al.*, *Br. med. J.*, 1978, *1*, 21. Chronic papilloedema in a 62-year-old patient who had been taking perhexiline maleate 200 mg daily for 8 months resulted in a long-standing and probably permanent visual defect.— J. M. Gibson *et al.*, *Br. J. Ophthal.*, 1984, *68*, 553.

A study indicating that the development of neuropathy in patients receiving perhexiline may be linked with impaired oxidative metabolism. Routine determination of drug oxidation phenotype using debrisoquine might be of predictive value in determining perhexiline dosage and controlling its neurotoxicity.— R. R. Shah *et al.*, *Br. med. J.*, 1982, *284*, 295. Genetically determined impairment of oxidation capacity was found in 3 out of 4 patients with perhexiline-induced hepatic injury using debrisoquine phenotyping. Impaired oxidation capacity was found in 8.6% of 70 patients with chronic liver disease not taking perhexiline.— M. Y. Morgan *et al.*, *Gut*, 1984, *25*, 1057.

For references to discussions of the usefulness of determining oxidation phenotype status in patients taking perhexiline, see below under Absorption and Fate.

Precautions

In view of severe toxicity associated with perhexiline it should only be used in patients who have not responded to other anti-anginal agents.

It is contra-indicated in patients with impaired hepatic or renal function. The safety and efficacy of perhexiline in the acute stage of myocardial infarction has not been established. Perhexiline should be administered with caution to diabetic patients.

During treatment with perhexiline it is recommended that the patient should be examined for the signs and symptoms of peripheral neuropathy, papilloedema, hepatic toxicity, hypoglycaemia, and loss of weight and that treatment should be discontinued should any of these occur. It is recommended that serum-perhexiline concentrations should be monitored regularly; serum concentrations of perhexiline maleate should not exceed 2 μg per mL.

Perhexiline may produce or exacerbate ventricular conduction disorders.

Absorption and Fate

Perhexiline is absorbed from the gastro-intestinal tract. It is metabolised in the liver and excreted as the parent drug and its metabolites in the bile and urine. Metabolism of perhexiline is genetically determined, and accumulation of the drug may occur in poor hydroxylators. The half-life varies considerably between individuals; it is generally 2 to 6 days, but may be more than 30 days in some cases.

The absorption, excretion, and metabolism of perhexiline maleate.— G. J. Wright *et al.*, *Postgrad. med. J.*, 1973, *49*, (Apr.), *Suppl.*, 8.

A rapid method for the determination of perhexiline in serum using gas-liquid chromatography.— J. D. H. Cooper and D. C. Turnell, *Ann. clin. Biochem.*, 1980, *17*, 155.

A study of the metabolism of the stereoisomers of perhexiline maleate in 8 healthy subjects indicated that there were significant differences in metabolism depending on oxidation phenotype and that metabolism of perhexiline displays a high degree of stereospecificity with the (−)-isomer having the greater rate of metabolic clearance.— N. S. Oates *et al.*, *Br. J. clin. Pharmac.*, 1984, *18*, 307P.

Discussions of oxidation polymorphism suggesting that determination of debrisoquine-oxidation status could be useful in reducing the incidence of adverse effects in patients treated with perhexiline.— J. R. Idle and R. L. Smith (letter), *Br. J. clin. Pharmac.*, 1984, *17*, 492; *Lancet*, 1984, *1*, 1337; R. G. Cooper and D. A. P. Evans (letter), *ibid.*, *2*, 227.

For references to a possible link between oxidation phenotype and adverse effects of perhexiline, see under Adverse Effects, above.

Uses and Administration

Perhexiline maleate may be used in the prophylaxis of severe angina pectoris in patients who have not responded to other anti-anginal agents. Its mode of action is complex but may be partly due to calcium antagonism. The usual initial dose is 100 to 200 mg daily in 2 divided doses adjusted at intervals of 2 to 4 weeks according to the response of the patient; it is generally recommended not to administer more than 300 mg daily although doses of 400 mg daily have been necessary in some patients.

CARDIAC DISORDERS. A review of drugs and the heart, including perhexiline, which has complex actions, with both anti-anginal and anti-arrhythmic activities. Although perhexiline has been designated as a calcium antagonist, additional quinidine-like and mild diuretic properties make the true classification difficult; it also differs from other calcium antagonists in lacking an acute effect against Prinzmetal's angina. Experimentally, there is a nitrate-like effect with redistribution of blood flow to the endocardial zones. Perhexiline has been used as an anti-anginal agent when beta-blockade and nitrates fail, but in view of the very serious side-effects now recognised, other calcium antagonists should be tried first.— L. H. Opie, *Lancet*, 1980, *1*, 806.

Anti-arrhythmic action and The Puzzle of Perhexiline, E.M. Vaughan Williams, London, Academic Press, 1980.

Proprietary Names and Manufacturers

Corzepin *(Prodes, Spain)*; Daprin *(Gramon, Arg.)*; Pexid *(Merrell Dow, Austral.*; *Belg.*; *Merrell, Fr.*; *Merrell, Ger.*; *Ital.*; *Mer-National, S.Afr.*; *Spain*; *Merrell Dow, Switz.*; *Merrell, UK*; *Merrell Dow, USA)*.

9274-x

Pipratecol *(rINN)*.

711-SE. 1-(3,4-Dihydroxyphenyl)-2-[4-(2-methoxyphenyl)piperazin-1-yl]ethanol.

$C_{19}H_{24}N_2O_4$=344.4.

CAS — 15534-05-1.

Pipratecol is a peripheral vasodilator that has been given in conjunction with raubasine (p.1517) in the treatment of cerebrovascular disorders.

Proprietary Names and Manufacturers

The following names have been used for multi-ingredient preparations containing pipratecol— Hydrosarpan 711 *(Servier, Fr.)*.

9275-r

Prenylamine Lactate *(BANM, rINNM)*.

B-436 *(prenylamine)*; Hoechst 12512; Prenylamini Lactas. *N*-(2-Benzhydrylethyl)-α-methylphenethylamine lactate.

$C_{24}H_{27}N,C_3H_6O_3$=419.6.

CAS — 69-43-2 (lactate); 390-64-7 (prenylamine).

NOTE. Prenylamine is *USAN*.

Pharmacopoeias. In *Br.*, *Cz.*, *Jpn*, and *Roum.*

A white, odourless or almost odourless, crystalline powder. Prenylamine lactate 76.4 mg is approximately equivalent to 60 mg of prenylamine. Very slightly **soluble** in water and in ether; soluble 1 in 5 of alcohol, and 1 in 2 of chloroform. **Store** in well-closed containers. Protect from light.

Adverse Effects

Prenylamine may cause sedation and gastro-intestinal disturbances including nausea, vomiting, and diarrhoea. Skin reactions, extrapyramidal symptoms, and intention tremor have been reported. Ventricular arrhythmias and ECG abnormalties have also been reported. Overdosage may cause hypotension, tachycardia, acute myocardial depression, and possibly convulsions.

EFFECTS ON THE HEART. Ventricular tachycardia and syncope associated with prolongation of the Q-T interval occurred in 2 elderly women taking prenylamine. The ECG should be checked every 3 months in patients taking prenylamine.— R. Puritz *et al.*, *Br. med. J.*, 1977, *2*, 608. Comment.— W. Bogie (letter), *ibid.*, 829.

A study indicating significant prolongation of the Q-T interval in patients with angina pectoris given prenylamine. The Q-T interval returned to normal on withdrawal of prenylamine and no serious problems were encountered.— D. Oakley *et al.*, *Postgrad. med. J.*, 1980, *56*, 753.

A case of prenylamine toxicity possibly showing the *torsades de pointes* phenomenon in a patient with a prolonged Q-T interval and sinus rhythm.— C. I. Meanock and M. I. M. Noble, *Postgrad. med. J.*, 1981, *57*, 381. A further report of torsades de pointes occurring in 1 patient taking prenylamine.— A. G. Fraser and S. Ikram (letter), *Lancet*, 1986, *2*, 572. Comment.— R. Mohr, *ibid.*, 1218.

EFFECTS ON THE LIVER. A patient taking prenylamine 240 mg daily developed nausea and raised SGOT values which returned to normal when the dose was reduced to 180 mg daily.— N. Cardoe, *Br. J. clin. Pract.*, 1968, *22*, 299.

EFFECTS ON THE NERVOUS SYSTEM. Drug-induced parkinsonism was reported in 3 patients taking prenylamine. The tremor and akinesia were considered to be related to the amphetamine- and reserpine-like properties of prenylamine.— M. Gonce and P. Meyer, *Br. med. J.*, 1984, *288*, 1048.

Precautions

Prenylamine should not be given to patients with severe uncompensated heart failure, defects of cardiac conduction, or with severe hepatic or renal impairment.

Prenylamine should not be administered concurrently with beta-adrenoceptor blocking agents or other drugs with negative inotropic activity. It should be given only with care to patients taking antihypertensive agents, the dose of which may need to be reduced, or to patients receiving drugs liable to produce hypokalaemia.

INTERACTIONS. Ventricular tachycardia occurred after the intravenous injection of sodium iothalamate in a patient taking prenylamine.— J. S. Duncan and L. E. Ramsay, *Postgrad. med. J.*, 1985, *61*, 415.

Uses and Administration

Prenylamine is used prophylactically in the treatment of angina pectoris. It depletes myocardial catecholamine stores and has some calcium-channel blocking activity. The usual initial dosage of prenylamine lactate is the equivalent of 180 mg of prenylamine daily in 3 divided doses, increased to 300 mg daily if necessary, and reduced after a few weeks to the lowest effective maintenance dose.

A review of the use of prenylamine in angina pectoris. It was concluded that prenylamine has no significant advantages over other anti-anginal drugs, and is more hazardous.— *Drug & Ther. Bull.*, 1987, *25*, 59.

Study suggesting that prenylamine has similar anti-anginal activity to penbutolol.— L. C. Slegers *et al.*, *J. int. med. Res.*, 1985, *13*, 229.

Preparations

Prenylamine Tablets *(B.P.)*. Prenylamine Lactate

Tablets. Potency is expressed in terms of the equivalent amount of prenylamine.

Proprietary Names and Manufacturers
Angormin *(Unifa, Arg.)*; Angorsan *(Isola-Ibi, Ital.)*; Bismetin *(Jpn)*; Carditin-same *(Savoma, Ital.)*; Crepasin *(Jpn)*; Daxauten *(Kettelhack Riker, Ger.)*; Epocol *(Jpn)*; Eucardion *(Ital.)*; Herzcon *(Jpn)*; Hostaginan *(Arg.; Belg.)*; Incoran *(ITA, Ital.)*; Lactamine *(Jpn)*; NP 30 *(Jpn)*; Nyuple *(Jpn)*; Onlemin *(Jpn)*; Piboril *(Arg.)*; Reocorin *(Ital.)*; Sedolatan *(Hoechst, Swed.)*; Segontin *(Hoechst, Austral.; Hoechst, Canad.; Hoechst, Denm.; Albert-Roussel, Ger.; Hoechst, Ital.; S.Afr.; Switz.)*; Segontine *(Hoechst, Fr.; Hoechst, Switz.)*; Synadrin *(Neth.; Norw.; Hoechst, Spain; Hoechst, UK)*; Wasangor *(IFI, Ital.)*.

9276-f

Propatylnitrate *(BAN, rINN).*
ETTN; Ettriol Trinitrate; Propatyl Nitrate *(USAN)*; Trinettriol; Win-9317. 2-Ethyl-2-hydroxymethylpropane-1,3-diol trinitrate.
$C_6H_{11}N_3O_9$=269.2.

CAS — 2921-92-8.

Propatylnitrate is a vasodilator with general properties similar to those of glyceryl trinitrate (p.1499). It has been given by mouth in usual doses of 10 mg three times daily for the prophylaxis of angina pectoris and in doses of 10 mg sublingually for acute attacks.

Proprietary Names and Manufacturers
Etrynit *(Astra, Denm.; Inibsa, Spain; Astra, Swed.; Sterling, USA)*; Gina *(Winthrop, UK)*; Vasangor *(Winthrop, Belg.)*.

9277-d

Raubasine
Ajmalicine; Alkaloid F; δ-Yohimbine. Methyl 16,17-didehydro-19α-methyl-18-oxayohimban-16-carboxylate.
$C_{21}H_{24}N_2O_3$=352.4.

CAS — 483-04-5.

Raubasine is an alkaloid obtained from *Vinca rosea, Catharanthus roseus* (Apocynaceae) and *Rauwolfia serpentina* (Apocynaceae).

Raubasine is related chemically to reserpine (see p.498) but has less antihypertensive activity. It has been given in peripheral and cerebral vascular disorders.

Absorption and excretion of raubasine in healthy subjects.— A. Marzo *et al., Arzneimittel-Forsch.*, 1977, *27*, 2343.

Proprietary Names and Manufacturers
Circolene *(Inverni della Beffa, Ital.)*; Hydrosarpan *(Eutherapie, Belg.; Servier, Canad.; Servier, Fr.; Servier, Switz.)*; Isoarteril *(Isola-Ibi, Ital.)*; Lamuran *(Boehringer, Arg.; Galenus Mannheim, Ger.; Boehringer Biochemia, Ital.; Boehringer Mannheim, Switz.)*; Loparol *(Boehringer Mannheim, Spain)*; Melanex *(Boehringer Mannheim, S.Afr.)*; Perife *(Savio, Ital.)*; Raubasil *(Biochimica Zanardi, Ital.)*; Sarpan *(Farge, Ital.)*.

The following names have been used for multi-ingredient preparations containing raubasine— Duxil *(Servier, Fr.)*; Hydrosarpan 711 *(Servier, Fr.)*.

9278-n

Suloctidil *(BAN, USAN, rINN).*
CP-556S. 1-(4-Isopropylthiophenyl)-2-octylaminopropan-1-ol.
$C_{20}H_{35}NOS$=337.6.

CAS — 54063-56-8.

Adverse Effects
Suloctidil has been associated with hepatotoxicity; some deaths have been reported.

Elevated liver enzymes were found in 3 of 20 patients taking suloctidil 400 mg three times daily by mouth. Liver enzyme values reverted to normal within 2 months after suloctidil was withdrawn.— J. A. Schouten and R. F. Westerman, *Eur. J. clin. Pharmac.*, 1982, *22*, 559.

Uses and Administration
Suloctidil is a vasodilator that has been used in the treatment of peripheral and cerebral vascular disorders.

Proprietary Names and Manufacturers
Locton *(Lepetit, Ital.)*; Sulocton *(Continental Pharma, Belg.; Continental Pharma, Switz.)*.

13302-f

Teasuprine
Isoxsuprine Theophylline-7-acetate; TI-72. 1-(4-Hydroxyphenyl)-2-(1-methyl-2-phenoxyethylamino)propan-1-ol theophyllin-7-ylacetate.
$C_{27}H_{33}N_5O_7$=539.6.

CAS — 60640-79-1.

Teasuprine is a peripheral vasodilator. It is given by mouth in a usual dose of 40 mg three times a day in the treatment of peripheral and cerebral vascular disorders.

Proprietary Names and Manufacturers
Angiclan *(Juste, Spain)*.

13304-n

Tenitramine
NNN'N'-Tetrakis(2-hydroxyethyl)ethylenediamine tetranitrate (ester).
$C_{10}H_{20}N_6O_{12}$=416.3.

CAS — 21946-79-2.

Tenitramine is a vasodilator with general properties similar to those of glyceryl trinitrate (p.1499). It has been used for the prophylaxis and treatment of angina pectoris and as an adjunct in other cardiac disorders.

References: M. Romano *et al., Curr. ther. Res.*, 1984, *36*, 171; C. Indolfi *et al., ibid.*, 1986, *40*, 953.

Proprietary Names and Manufacturers
Tenitran *(Elea, Arg.; Bioindustria, Ital.; Roger, Spain)*.

9280-a

Thymoxamine Hydrochloride *(BANM).*

Moxisilita Clorhidrato; Moxisylyte Hydrochloride *(rINNM)*. 4-(2-Dimethylaminoethoxy)-5-isopropyl-2-methylphenyl acetate hydrochloride.
$C_{16}H_{25}NO_3$,HCl=315.8.

CAS — 54-32-0 (thymoxamine); 964-52-3 (hydrochloride).

Pharmacopoeias. In *Br.*

A white odourless or almost odourless crystalline powder. Thymoxamine hydrochloride 45.2 mg is approximately equivalent to 40 mg of thymoxamine. **Soluble** 1 in 2.5 of water, 1 in 11 of alcohol, and 1 in 3 of chloroform; practically insoluble in ether and petroleum spirit. A 5% solution in water has a pH of 4.5 to 5.5. **Protect** from light.

Adverse Effects
Thymoxamine hydrochloride may cause nausea, diarrhoea, headache, vertigo, and flushing of the skin. Overdosage may cause hypotension.
Transient ptosis may occur occasionally following ophthalmic application.

Treatment of Adverse Effects
As for Tolazoline Hydrochloride, p.1518.

Precautions
Thymoxamine hydrochloride should be given with care to patients with angina pectoris, recent mycocardial infarction, or diabetes mellitus.
Thymoxamine may enhance the effects of antihypertensive agents and the hypotensive effect of thymoxamine may be enhanced by tricyclic antidepressants.

Uses and Administration
Thymoxamine is an alpha-adrenoceptor blocking agent which is used for the treatment of peripheral vascular disorders.

The usual dose is the equivalent of 40 mg of thymoxamine four times daily. It is also given intravenously in a dose of 100 µg per kg bodyweight, which may be given 4 times daily, or by intravenous infusion using 30 mg in 500 mL of sodium chloride infusion (0.9%) every 6 hours. A single dose of 5 mg may be given intra-arterially into the distal end of an artery to reduce vasospasm after arterial surgery or before the withdrawal of a cardiac catheter. Thymoxamine is also used locally in the eye to reverse the mydriasis caused by phenylephrine and other sympathomimetic agents.

OPHTHALMIC USE. In 12 healthy subjects thymoxamine eye-drops 0.1% completely reversed the mydriasis produced by ephedrine 5% but incompletely reversed that caused by homatropine 0.5% or by ephedrine and homatropine. A small reduction in accommodation produced by ephedrine was reversed by thymoxamine but the greater reduction in accommodation produced by homatropine was only partially reversed.— S. Small *et al., Br. J. Ophthal.*, 1976, *60*, 132.

Thymoxamine caused incomplete reversal of mydriasis produced by tropicamide; 0.2% solutions of thymoxamine were tolerated in the eye but did not appear to be more effective than 0.1% solutions.— G. L. Mayer *et al., Curr. med. Res. Opinion*, 1977, *4*, 660.

Thymoxamine 0.5% eye-drops selectively eliminate sympathetic stimulation only of the eye, thus providing a precise way to reverse the effect of phenylephrine.— C. I. Phillips, *Br. med. J.*, 1984, *288*, 1779.

PERIPHERAL VASCULAR DISORDERS. Reports and studies on the use of thymoxamine in peripheral vascular disorders: S. S. Rose, *Br. J. clin. Pract.*, 1979, *33*, 223; G. V. Jaffe and J. J. Grimshaw, *Br. J. clin. Pract.*, 1980, *34*, 343; M. Aylward *et al., Curr. med. Res. Opinion*, 1982, *8*, 158.

TREMOR. Single intravenous doses of thymoxamine have been shown to reduce essential tremor, possibly by a central effect. Clinical studies of oral alpha-adrenergic blockers are required before the usefulness of this group of drugs in essential tremor can be assessed.— L. J. Findley, *Br. J. Hosp. Med.*, 1986, *35*, 388. See also B. Abila *et al., Br. J. clin. Pharmac.*, 1984, *18*, 282P.

Preparations

Thymoxamine Tablets *(B.P.)*. Tablets containing thymoxamine hydrochloride. Potency is expressed in terms of the equivalent amount of thymoxamine.

Proprietary Preparations

Minims Thymoxamine Hydrochloride *(Smith & Nephew Pharmaceuticals, UK). Eye-drops*, thymoxamine hydrochloride 0.5%, in single-use disposable applicators.
NOTE. The code THY is permitted in Great Britain for single-dose eye-drops of thymoxamine.

Opilon *(Parke, Davis, UK). Tablets*, scored, thymoxamine 40 mg (as hydrochloride).

Proprietary Names and Manufacturers
Apifor *(Parke, Davis, Spain)*; Arlitene *(Chinoin, Ital.)*; Carlytene *(Dedieu, Fr.)*; Minims Thymoxamine Hydrochloride *(Smith & Nephew Pharmaceuticals, UK)*; Opilon *(Ital.; Warner, S.Afr.; Parke, Davis, UK)*; Valyten *(Landerlan, Spain)*; Vasoklin *(Ger.)*.

13338-e

Tiapamil *(BAN, rINN).*
Ditian Tetraoxide; Ro-11-1781; Verocainine. *N*-(3,4-Dimethoxyphenethyl)-3-[2-(3,4-dimethoxyphenyl)-1,3-dithian-2-yl]-*N*-methylpropylamine 1,1,3,3-tetraoxide.
$C_{26}H_{37}NO_8S_2$=555.7.

CAS — 57010-31-8; 87434-83-1 (hydrochloride).

NOTE. Tiapamil Hydrochloride is *USAN*.

Tiapamil is a calcium antagonist with vasodilator properties that has been used in cardiac disorders and hypertension.

Tiapamil 450 mg by mouth reduced both diastolic and systolic blood pressure in 10 elderly hypertensive patients without an accompanying variation in heart rate. The hypotensive effect lasted for 10 to 12 hours.— P. Balansard *et al., Br. J. clin. Pharmac.*, 1984, *18*, 823.

A study of the pharmacokinetic and haemodynamic effects of tiapamil in 16 patients with coronary artery disease or chronic ischaemic heart disease. There was evidence that tiapamil might undergo saturable intestinal wall metabolism or saturable hepatic elimination.

Tiapamil reduced the rate-pressure product, an index of myocardial oxygen requirements, despite increasing exercise tolerance. It was concluded that oral tiapamil therapy was not associated with signs of a depressant action on haemodynamic variables and that the intrinsic negative inotropic effect of tiapamil was probably outweighed by the tendency to enhance peripheral vasodilatation.— M. Eckert *et al.*, *J. clin. Pharmac.*, 1984, *24*, 165.

The anti-anginal effect of a single oral dose of tiapamil 600 mg lasted under 3 hours in a study of 10 patients.— M. B. Maltz *et al.*, *Eur. J. clin. Pharmac.*, 1987, *32*, 339.

Further references to the clinical use of tiapamil: H. G. Eichler *et al.*, *Circulation*, 1985, *71*, 779 (after myocardial infarction); J. P. Fauchier *et al.*, *Eur. Heart J.*, 1985, *6*, 525 (atrioventricular node re-entry tachycardias); M. Caruana *et al.*, *J. cardiovasc. Pharmac.*, 1986, *8*, 1074 (hypertension); T. L. Storm *et al.*, *J. clin. Pharmac.*, 1987, *27*, 18 (hypertension).

Proprietary Names and Manufacturers
Roche, UK.

13353-w

Tipropidil Hydrochloride *(USAN, rINNM).*
MJ-12880-1. 1-[4-(Isopropylthio)phenoxy]-3-octylaminopropan-2-ol hydrochloride.
$C_{20}H_{35}NO_2S,HCl=390.0$.

CAS — 70895-45-3 (tipropidil); 70895-39-5 (hydrochloride).

Tipropidil hydrochloride is reported to have vasodilator activity.

Proprietary Names and Manufacturers
Bristol, USA; Mead Johnson Pharmaceutical, USA.

9281-t

Tolazoline Hydrochloride *(BANM, USAN, rINNM).*

Benzazoline Hydrochloride; Tolazol. Hydrochlor.; Tolazolinium Chloratum. 2-Benzyl-2-imidazoline hydrochloride.
$C_{10}H_{12}N_2,HCl=196.7$.

CAS — 59-98-3 (tolazoline); 59-97-2 (hydrochloride).

Pharmacopoeias. In *Arg., Aust., Braz., Cz., Hung., It., Jug., Nord., Pol., Roum.,* and *U.S.*

A white to off-white crystalline powder. **Soluble** 1 in less than 1 of water, 1 in 2 of alcohol, and 1 in 3 of chloroform; practically insoluble in ether. The *U.S.P.* injection has a pH of 3.0 to 4.0. **Store** in well-closed containers.

Adverse Effects

Common side-effects of tolazoline hydrochloride include pilo-erection, headache, flushing, tachycardia, cardiac arrhythmias, tingling, chilliness, shivering, sweating, nausea, vomiting, diarrhoea, and epigastric pain. Orthostatic hypotension or marked hypertension may occur, especially with large doses. Tolazoline has been implicated as a precipitating factor in myocardial infarction. Intra-arterial injection may be followed by a burning sensation in the limb. Administration of tolazoline has been associated with exacerbation of peptic ulcer and gastric haemorrhage. Oliguria, haematuria, thrombocytopenia and other blood dyscrasias have been reported.

PREGNANCY AND THE NEONATE. Hypochloraemic metabolic alkalosis in an infant with respiratory distress was apparently related to gastric hypersecretion following infusion of tolazoline.— J. M. Adams *et al.*, *Pediatrics*, 1980, *65*, 298.

The combination of severe hypoxaemia and the use of tolazoline in the newborn infant whose systemic arterial blood pressure is inadequately controlled, may predispose to hypotension and acute renal failure. Two infants in whom this combination of circumstances occurred required peritoneal dialysis before return of renal function.— R. S. Trompeter *et al.* (letter), *Lancet*, 1981, *1*, 1219.

A report of duodenal perforation associated with the use of tolazoline for pulmonary hypertension in a neonate.— R. G. Wilson *et al.*, *Archs Dis. Childh.*, 1985, *60*, 878. See also M. Matsuo *et al.* (letter), *J. Pediat.*, 1982, *100*, 1005.

Further reports of gastro-intestinal haemorrhage in patients treated with tolazoline.— R. G. Dillard, *Clin. Pediat.*, 1982, *21*, 761.

Treatment of Adverse Effects

In severe overdosage by mouth the stomach should be emptied by aspiration and lavage. Hypotension is probably best treated by keeping the patient recumbent with the head lowered. If necessary the circulation may be maintained by infusion of suitable electrolyte solutions. Hypotension may be treated with ephedrine. Adrenaline is not suitable for the reversal of hypotension induced by alpha-adrenoceptor blocking agents since it may exacerbate the hypotension by stimulating beta-receptors.

Precautions

Tolazoline hydrochloride should not be given to patients with coronary artery disease, hypotension, or after cerebrovascular accident. Since tolazoline hydrochloride stimulates gastric secretion of hydrochloric acid, it should not be used in the presence of peptic ulceration. Tolazoline should be used with caution in patients with mitral stenosis when given parenterally.
Tolazoline may cause a disulfiram-like reaction if given with alcohol.

For the effect of tolazoline on dopamine, see Dopamine Hydrochloride, p.1460.

Absorption and Fate

Tolazoline hydrochloride is absorbed from the gastro-intestinal tract. It is more rapidly absorbed after intramuscular injection, producing the maximum effects after 30 to 60 minutes. A plasma half-life in neonates of 3 to 10 hours has been reported. Tolazoline hydrochloride is rapidly excreted in the urine, largely unchanged.

Uses and Administration

Tolazoline hydrochloride is a vasodilator which has a direct dilator action on the peripheral blood vessels. It has some alpha-adrenoceptor blocking activity and also stimulates smooth muscle in the gastro-intestinal tract, increases gastro-intestinal secretion, and has a stimulant effect on the heart.
Tolazoline is used to reduce pulmonary artery pressure in persistent pulmonary hypertension in newborn infants with persistent foetal circulation. The usual dose is 1 to 2 mg per kg body-weight over 10 minutes by intravenous infusion followed by 1 to 2 mg per kg per hour thereafter.
Tolazoline has been used in the treatment of peripheral vascular disorders in doses of 25 to 50 mg four times daily by mouth.
Tolazoline hydrochloride has been given in doses of up to 50 mg by subcutaneous, intramuscular, intravenous, or slow intra-arterial injection.
Tolazoline has also been used as a 10% solution as eye-drops in the treatment of ophthalmic conditions.

PERIPHERAL VASCULAR DISORDERS. A review of drugs, including tolazoline, used in the management of peripheral vascular disease. In the author's clinical experience, tolazoline has not been of benefit in obstructive vascular disease, but in association with other agents, is occasionally useful in patients with Raynaud's phenomenon.— J. D. Coffman, *New Engl. J. Med.*, 1979, *300*, 713.

PREGNANCY AND THE NEONATE. *Diaphragmatic hernia.* Tolazoline was used as a pulmonary vasodilator to reverse right-to-left shunting of blood in 4 infants with congenital diaphragmatic hernias.— E. Sumner and J. D. Frank, *Archs Dis. Childh.*, 1981, *56*, 350.

Persistent foetal circulation syndrome. Tolazoline 500 µg per kg body-weight by intravenous injection followed by 500 µg per kg per hour by continuous infusion was suggested for the treatment of persistent foetal circulation syndrome of the newborn.— P. Monin *et al.*, *Eur. J. clin. Pharmac.*, 1987, *31*, 569.

Respiratory distress syndrome. Tolazoline hydrochloride 1 to 2 mg per kg body-weight injected intravenously or via the umbilical artery produced clinical improvement in 10 of 20 preterm infants with severe hyaline membrane disease. Renal failure occurred in one infant and 2 suffered irritability associated with blood-stained cerebrospinal fluid.— N. McIntosh and R. O. Walters, *Archs Dis. Childh.*, 1979, *54*, 105. See also B. W. Goetzman *et al.*, *J. Pediat.*, 1976, *89*, 617.

PULMONARY HYPERTENSION. A patient with primary pulmonary hypertension obtained a beneficial response to tolazoline hydrochloride 50 mg but the therapy could not be tolerated owing to nausea and vomiting.— U. R. Shettigar *et al.*, *New Engl. J. Med.*, 1976, *295*, 1414.

A brief review of the use of tolazoline in primary pulmonary hypertension. Tolazoline has been used to produce pulmonary vasodilatation, but studies have failed to confirm a reduction in pulmonary vascular resistance after intravenous or oral administration. Successful use of tolazoline in the acute management of persistent foetal circulation indicates that it may be lifesaving in this situation.— M. D. McGoon and R. E. Vlietstra, *Mayo Clin. Proc.*, 1984, *59*, 672.

For reports of adverse effects of tolazoline in neonates and infants, see above.

Preparations

Tolazoline Hydrochloride Injection *(U.S.P.)*
Tolazoline Hydrochloride Tablets *(U.S.P.)*

Proprietary Names and Manufacturers
Dilazol *(Switz.)*; Priscol *(Ciba, Austral.; Dispersa, Ger.; Spain; Dispersa, Switz.; Ciba, UK)*; Priscoline *(Ciba, Canad.; Ciba, USA)*; Zoline *(Protea, Austral.)*.

13360-s

Tolmesoxide *(BAN, rINN).*
RX-71107. 4,5-Dimethoxy-*o*-tolyl methyl sulphoxide.
$C_{10}H_{14}O_3S=214.3$.

CAS — 38452-29-8.

Tolmesoxide is reported to have vasodilator activity and has been tried in congestive heart failure and hypertension.

Investigation of the actions of tolmesoxide in healthy subjects.— J. A. Buylla *et al.*, *Br. J. clin. Pharmac.*, 1979, *8*, 402P.

Tolmesoxide produced beneficial haemodynamic effects in 8 patients with refractory congestive heart failure lasting 1 to 2 hours after intravenous administration without an accompanying fall in systemic arterial pressure.— P. Lauwers and J. G. Nievel, *Eur. J. clin. Pharmac.*, 1982, *21*, 473.

Report of a dose-ranging study in 4 patients with essential hypertension. The effective hypotensive dose of tolmesoxide was found to range from 200 to 600 mg producing a maximum effect at 3 to 4 hours and a duration of up to 12 hours. The hypotensive effect was associated with an increase in heart rate. Symptoms of postural hypotension occurred in 1 patient.— C. P. O'Boyle *et al.*, *Eur. J. clin. Pharmac.*, 1982, *23*, 93.

Proprietary Names and Manufacturers
Reckitt & Colman Pharmaceuticals, UK.

13366-z

Trapidil *(rINN).*

AR-12008. 7-Diethylamino-5-methyl-1,2,4-triazolo[1,5-*a*]pyrimidine.
$C_{10}H_{15}N_5=205.3$.

CAS — 15421-84-8.

Trapidil is reported to be a coronary vasodilator.

References to the actions and uses of trapidil: M. Di Donato *et al.*, *Arzneimittel-Forsch.*, 1985, *35*, 1295; S. Bongrani *et al.*, *Br. J. clin. Pharmac.*, 1986, *21*, 105P; J. Sasaki *et al.*, *Curr. ther. Res.*, 1986, *40*, 619.

Proprietary Names and Manufacturers
Locorunal; Rocornal.

9282-x

Trimetazidine Hydrochloride *(BANM, rINNM).*
Trimetazine Hydrochloride. 1-(2,3,4-Trimethoxybenzyl)piperazine dihydrochloride.
$C_{14}H_{22}N_2O_3,2HCl$=339.3.

CAS — 5011-34-7 (trimetazidine); 13171-25-0 (hydrochloride).

Trimetazidine hydrochloride is a vasodilator that has been used prophylactically in the treatment of angina pectoris and in Ménière's disease.

Proprietary Names and Manufacturers
Cartoma *(Jpn)*; Idaptan *(Servier, Spain)*; Vastarel *(Biopharma, Fr.; Servier, UK)*; Vastazin *(Jpn)*.

9283-r

Trolnitrate Phosphate *(BAN, rINN).*
Aminotrate Phosphate; Nitranolum; Triethanolamine Trinitrate Diphosphate. Nitrilotrisethylene trinitrate diphosphate.
$C_6H_{12}N_4O_9,2H_3PO_4$=480.2.

CAS — 7077-34-1 (trolnitrate); 588-42-1 (phosphate).

Pharmacopoeias. In *Rus. Cz.* includes Trolnitratium Diphosphoricum cum Saccharo Lactis, containing trolnitrate phosphate 25% in lactose.

Trolnitrate phosphate is a vasodilator with general properties similar to those of glyceryl trinitrate (see p.1499). It has been used for the prophylaxis of angina pectoris in usual doses of 2 to 4 mg three or four times daily. Doses of up to 40 mg daily have been employed.

Proprietary Names and Manufacturers
Angitrit *(Leo, Belg.; Leo, Denm.; Nordmark, Ger.; Leo, Neth.)*; Metamine *(Pfizer, USA)*; Nitretamin *(Squibb, USA)*; Nitroduran *(Lövens, Swed.)*; Praenitron *(Pfizer, Austral.)*.

9284-f

Visnadine *(BAN, rINN).*
10-Acetoxy-9,10-dihydro-8,8-dimethyl-2-oxo-2*H*,8*H*-pyrano[2,3-*f*]chromen-9-yl 2-methylbutyrate.
$C_{21}H_{24}O_7$=388.4.

CAS — 477-32-7.

Visnadine is a vasodilator obtained from ammi visnaga fruit that has been used in the treatment of coronary insufficiency.

Proprietary Names and Manufacturers
Carduben *(Madaus, Ger.)*; Vibeline *(Bellon, Fr.; Promesa, Spain)*; Visnamine *(Chinoin, Ital.)*.

9285-d

Xanthinol Nicotinate *(BANM).*
SK-331A; Xanthinol Niacinate *(USAN)*; Xantinol Nicotinate *(rINN)*. 7-{2-Hydroxy-3-[(2-hydroxyethyl)methylamino]propyl}theophylline nicotinate.
$C_{13}H_{21}N_5O_4,C_6H_5NO_2$=434.5.

CAS — 2530-97-4 (xanthinol); 437-74-1 (nicotinate).

Pharmacopoeias. In *Cz.*

Xanthinol nicotinate is a vasodilator that has been given in the treatment of peripheral and cerebral vascular disorders. It has also been given in hyperlipidaemias. Doses of up to 1.5 g daily or more have been given by mouth. It has also been given by intramuscular or slow intravenous injection in doses of 900 mg or more daily.

Proprietary Names and Manufacturers
Adrogeron Retard *(Adroka, Switz.)*; Angioamin *(Dompè, Ital.)*; Complamex *(Gemini, UK)*; Complamin *(Wulfing, Belg.; Beecham, Canad.; Tika, Denm.; Beecham-Wülfing, Ger.; Italchimici, Ital.; Bencard, Neth.; Tika, Norw.; Adcock Ingram, S.Afr.; Tika, Swed.; Beecham, Switz.)*; Complamina *(Raffo, Arg.)*; Complamine *(Latéma, Fr.)*; Emodinamin *(Sigurtà, Ital.)*; Landrina *(Landerlan, Spain)*; Vasoprin *(Alfa Farmaceutici, Ital.)*; Vedrin *(Polifarma, Ital.)*.

Water

7700-g

Water

Aqua; Aqua Communis; Aqua Fontana; Aqua Potabilis; Eau Potable; Wasser.
H_2O=18.015.

CAS — 7732-18-5.

In *Martindale,* as in the *B.P.* the term 'water' used without qualification in formulas refers to suitable potable water freshly drawn direct from the public supply and suitable for drinking or, if this is not available, freshly boiled and cooled Purified Water; this may be called Water for Preparations as it is in the *B.N.F.*

Potable water is derived mainly from surface sources such as lakes, rivers, and streams, and from underground sources such as wells and springs. In emergencies it may be obtained directly from the sea either by distillation or by demineralisation with ion-exchange materials. The chemical composition of potable water is variable and the nature and concentration of the impurities in it depend upon the source from which it is drawn. However, potable water must be both palatable and safe to drink.

There are international standards for the quality of water intended for human consumption. Toxic substances such as arsenic, barium, cadmium, chromium, copper, cyanide, lead, and selenium may constitute a danger to health if present in drinking water in excess of the recommended concentrations. Water-borne infections are also a hazard.

Fluoride is regarded as an essential constituent of drinking water but may endanger health if present in excess—see Sodium Fluoride, p.1615. Ingestion of water containing 45 mg or more per litre of nitrates may cause methaemoglobinaemia in infants.

The use of tap water containing metal ions (such as aluminium, copper, and lead), fluoride, or chloramine, for dialysis may be hazardous.

A hard water contains soluble calcium and magnesium salts, which cause the precipitation of soap and prevent its lathering and form scale and sludge in boilers, water pipes, and autoclaves. Temporary hardness in water is due to the presence of bicarbonates which are converted to insoluble carbonates on heating. Permanent hardness is due to dissolved chlorides, nitrates, and sulphates, which do not form a precipitate on heating. The presence or absence of such salts can play a part in cardiovascular health.

Without further purification, potable water may be unsuitable for certain pharmaceutical purposes. For example, the concentration of calcium present in water affects the sol viscosities and gel strengths of alginate and pectin dispersions, the colour of some mixtures may be affected by the pH of the water employed, and precipitates may be formed when hard water is used. In such instances, purified water should always be used. Most pharmacopoeias include monographs on various preparations of water, such as water for injection or injections. Potable water should not be used when such preparations of water are specified.

Excessive ingestion of water can lead to water intoxication with disturbances of the electrolyte balance.

7701-q

Purified Water

Aqua Purificata.

Pharmacopoeias. In *Arg., Aust., Br., Chin., Cz., Egypt., Eur., Fr., Ger., Hung., Ind., Int., It., Jpn, Jug., Mex., Neth., Nord., Pol., Port., Roum., Rus., Span., Swiss, Turk.*, and *U.S.*

Also in *B.P. Vet.* Some pharmacopoeias only include distilled water or have additional monographs for distilled water.

A clear, colourless, odourless, and tasteless liquid prepared from suitable potable water either by distillation, by treatment with ion-exchange materials, by reverse osmosis, or by any other suitable method. *U.S.P.* specifies pH 5 to 7. **Store** in airtight containers which do not alter the properties of the water.

The *B.P.* directs that when Distilled Water is prescribed or demanded Purified Water be dispensed or supplied.

Purified Water is unsuitable for preparing injections; for this purpose Water for Injections must be used.

PREPARATION BY DEIONISATION. By passing potable water through columns of anionic and cationic ion-exchange resins, ionisable substances can be removed, producing a water of high specific resistance. Colloidal and non-ionisable impurities such as pyrogens may not be removed by this process.

PREPARATION BY DISTILLATION. In this process water is separated as vapour from non-volatile impurities and is subsequently condensed. In practice, non-volatile impurities may be carried into the distillate by entrainment unless a suitable baffle is fitted to the still.

7702-p

Water for Injections

Aq. pro Inj.; Aqua ad Iniectabilia; Aqua ad Injectionem; Aqua Injectabilis; Aqua pro Injectione; Aqua pro Injectionibus; Eau pour Préparations Injectables; Wasser für Injektionszwecke; Water for Injection.

Pharmacopoeias. In *Arg., Aust., Belg., Br., Chin., Cz., Egypt., Eur., Fr., Ger., Hung., Ind., Int., It., Jpn, Jug., Mex., Neth., Nord., Pol., Port., Rus., Span., Swiss, Turk.*, and *U.S.* Also in *B.P. Vet.*

U.S.P. also includes Sterile Water for Injection, Sterile Water for Inhalation, Sterile Water for Irrigation, and Bacteriostatic Water for Injection.

Water for Injections (*B.P.*) is sterilised distilled water free from pyrogens; it is prepared by distillation of potable water, purified water, or distilled water from a neutral glass, quartz, or suitable metal still fitted with an efficient device for preventing the entrainment of droplets; the first portion of the distillate is discarded and the remainder collected in a suitable container and sterilised by autoclaving.

Water for Injection (*U.S.P.*) is water purified by distillation or by reverse osmosis and contains no added substance. It is intended for use as a solvent in parenteral solutions which are to be sterilised after preparation. Sterile Water for Injection (*U.S.P.*) is the subject of a separate monograph.

When Water for Injections free from carbon dioxide or dissolved air is required for a preparation, the distillate, freshly prepared as above, is boiled for at least 10 minutes with as little exposure to air as possible, cooled, distributed into the final containers, and sterilised by autoclaving. It is used for the preparation of solutions of the soluble salts of weakly acidic substances, since the slight acidity due to dissolved carbon dioxide might cause the formation of a precipitate.

Xanthines

620-t

The principal xanthines (or methylxanthines) used in medicine are caffeine and theophylline. This group of drugs is of value for its effects on bronchial smooth muscle, the central nervous system, and the myocardium.
Caffeine and its salts are the most active in stimulating the central nervous system and are principally used for this purpose, as in the treatment of apnoea.
The bronchodilator effects of such drugs as theophylline and aminophylline are of value in asthma, both prophylactically and in the treatment of acute attacks. Their benefit in chronic obstructive lung diseases is less certain.
The chief usefulness of the xanthines in cardiac conditions is in paroxysmal dyspnoea associated with left heart failure in asthmatics or bronchitics, and for this aminophylline has been employed.
Because some theophylline compounds such as aminophylline are highly alkaline and cause gastro-intestinal irritation, they are not well tolerated. Attempts to overcome this have included modification of tablet formulation or the use of less alkaline salts of theophylline, such as choline theophyllinate or derivatives which do not liberate theophylline in the body such as diprophylline. Because of the short serum half-life of theophylline, sustained-release preparations are now widely used.
Tolerance to some of the effects of the xanthines, particularly the diuretic effect, may readily develop.
Beverages containing xanthines are very widely used and include coffee, tea, cocoa, and cola drinks.
The xanthine derivative oxpentifylline is described in the section on Vasodilators.

627-m

Acepifylline *(BAN).*
Acefylline Piperazine *(rINN)*; Piperazine Theophylline Ethanoate. Piperazine bis(theophyllin-7-ylacetate) (1:1).
$(C_9H_{10}N_4O_4)_2,C_4H_{10}N_2$=562.5.

CAS — 18833-13-1; 18428-63-2.

Acepifylline is a theophylline derivative which is used similarly to theophylline (see p.1532), but it is reported to be better tolerated by mouth. Acepifylline is poorly absorbed from the gastro-intestinal tract and it does not liberate theophylline in the body.
Acepifylline has been given by mouth in doses of up to 3 g daily. It has also been given by rectum as suppositories, or by intramuscular or slow intravenous injection.

A study involving healthy subjects and one patient, indicated that following intravenous administration acepifylline is completely eliminated by the kidneys within 4 hours, and that following administration by mouth absorption is very poor. No theophylline or other xanthine derivatives were detected in serum or urine.— J. Zuidema and F. W. H. M. Merkus (letter), *Lancet*, 1978, *1*, 1318.

Proprietary Names and Manufacturers
Dynaphylline *(Canad.)*; Etafillina *(Delalande, Ital.)*; Etaphylline *(Difrex, Austral.; Fr.; Neth.; Delalande, Switz.)*; Etaphylline simple *(Belg.)*; Etophylate *(Delandale, UK)*; Minophylline *(Egypt)*.

The following names have been used for multi-ingredient preparations containing acepifylline— Heptonal *(Delandale, UK)*.

3873-a

Aminophylline *(BAN, USAN, pINN).*

Aminofilina; Aminophyllinum; Euphyllinum; Metaphyllin; Theophyllaminum; Theophylline and Ethylenediamine; Theophylline Ethylenediamine Compound; Theophyllinum et Ethylenediaminum.
A mixture of theophylline and ethylenediamine, its composition approximately corresponding to the formula.
$(C_7H_8N_4O_2)_2,C_2H_4(NH_2)_2$=420.4.

CAS — 317-34-0 (anhydrous).

Pharmacopoeias. In *Aust., Br., Egypt., Eur., Fr., Int., Neth.,* and *Swiss. U.S.* allows anhydrous or up to 2 molecules of water of hydration.

White or slightly yellowish granules or powder, odourless or with a faintly ammoniacal odour. It is a stable mixture or combination containing between 84.0% and 87.4% of anhydrous theophylline and 13.5 to 15% of ethylenediamine.
Soluble 1 in 5 of water but the addition of ethylenediamine may be necessary to give complete solution (the solution may become cloudy in the presence of carbon dioxide); practically insoluble in dehydrated alcohol and in ether. Solutions are **sterilised** by autoclaving, exposure to carbon dioxide and contact with metal being avoided throughout.
In moist air it gradually loses ethylenediamine and absorbs carbon dioxide with the liberation of theophylline. **Store** in well-filled airtight containers. Protect from light.
Incompatibility has been reported with acids, bleomycin sulphate, chlorpromazine hydrochloride, clindamycin phosphate, corticotrophin, dimenhydrinate, doxorubicin, erythromycin gluceptate, hydralazine hydrochloride, hydroxyzine hydrochloride, opioid analgesics, oxytetracycline hydrochloride, phenytoin sodium, procaine hydrochloride, prochlorperazine salts, promazine hydrochloride, promethazine hydrochloride, sulphafurazole diethanolamine, and vancomycin hydrochloride; with lactose, a yellow or brown colour develops on standing; in the presence of copper, solutions develop a blue colour.
Occasional incompatibility has occurred with cefapirin sodium depending on the strength and composition of the vehicle.

628-b

Aminophylline Hydrate *(BAN, USAN, pINNM).*

$(C_7H_8N_4O_2)_2,C_2H_4(NH_2)_2,2H_2O$=456.5.

CAS — 49746-06-7 (dihydrate).

Pharmacopoeias. In *Arg., Aust., Belg., Br., Braz., Chin., Cz., Eur., Fr., Ger., Ind., It., Jpn, Jug., Mex., Neth., Pol., Port., Roum., Rus., Span., Swiss,* and *Turk. U.S.* allows anhydrous or up to 2 molecules of water of hydration.

A white or slightly yellowish powder or granular powder. It is odourless or has a slight ammoniacal odour. **Soluble** 1 in 5 of water and the solution may become cloudy due to the presence of carbon dioxide; practically insoluble in dehydrated alcohol and in ether. **Store** in well-filled airtight containers. Protect from light. **Incompatibilities** as for aminophylline, above.

The osmolality of small-volume intravenous admixtures, including aminophylline in sodium chloride injection (0.9%) and glucose injection (5%).— D. P. Wermeling *et al., Am. J. Hosp. Pharm.*, 1985, *42*, 1739.

INCOMPATIBILITY. The addition of aminophylline to glucose injection raised the pH by over 4 units to pH 7.7 to 10.45, so that insulin, which is inactivated above pH 7.5, was incompatible, as was erythromycin gluceptate. Tetracycline hydrochloride lowered the pH to 3.6 to 4 rendering the aminophylline less stable. A mixture of benzylpenicillin and aminophylline in glucose injection was initially compatible but on standing for 12 hours the pH fell from 8.2 to 6 with the risk of theophylline precipitation.— M. Edward, *Am. J. Hosp. Pharm.*, 1967, *24*, 440.

Precipitation was observed when dobutamine was mixed with aminophylline in solution.— G. R. Hasegawa and J. F. Eder, *Am. J. Hosp. Pharm.*, 1984, *41*, 949.

Aminophylline is visually incompatible with amiodarone hydrochloride injection.— G. R. Hasegawa and J. F. Eder, *Am. J. Hosp. Pharm.*, 1984, *41*, 1379.

RELEASE FROM SUPPOSITORIES. Aminophylline suppositories: *in vitro* dissolution and bioavailability in man.— J. B. Taylor and D. E. Simpkins, *Pharm. J.*, 1981, *2*, 601. Further references: F. Newwald and P. Ackad, *Am. J. Hosp. Pharm.*, 1966, *23*, 347; J. M. Plaxco *et al., J. pharm. Sci.*, 1967, *56*, 809; J. M. Plaxco and F. Foreman, *ibid.*, 1968, *57*, 698.

STABILITY. Aminophylline, about 450 mg per litre, was stable for up to 2 days at 25° in glucose injection over a pH range of 3.5 to 8.6.— E. A. Parker, *Am. J. Hosp. Pharm.*, 1970, *27*, 67. See also S. Boddapati *et al., ibid.*, 1982, *39*, 108.

The stability of aminophylline in parenteral nutrition solutions.— P. W. Niemiec *et al., Am. J. Hosp. Pharm.*, 1983, *40*, 428. See also B. Kirk and J. M. Sprake, *Br. J. intraven. Ther.*, 1982, *3*, (Nov.), 4.

Adverse Effects, Treatment, and Precautions
As for Theophylline (see p.1526).

For mention of cross sensitisation to ethylenediamine and to antihistamines, see Ethylenediamine p.1569.

Uses and Administration
Aminophylline has the actions and uses of theophylline (see p.1532), but is used when greater solubility in water is required, particularly in injectable preparations.
In the treatment of acute severe asthma aminophylline is administered intravenously. To reduce adverse effects, the rate of intravenous administration of aminophylline should not exceed 25 mg per minute. In patients who have not been taking aminophylline or theophylline, aminophylline is given in a loading dose of 5 to 6 mg per kg body-weight by slow intravenous injection, usually over 20 to 30 minutes. In patients who have been receiving aminophylline or theophylline, ideally the serum-theophylline concentration should be measured before administering a loading dose. The loading dose can then be determined on the basis that aminophylline 600 µg per kg lean body-weight can be expected to increase the serum-theophylline concentration by approximately 1 µg per mL, and a serum concentration of 10 to 20 µg per mL is required. In an emergency where the serum-theophylline concentration is not available, a loading dose of 2.5 to 3.0 mg per kg may be given and is unlikely to be dangerous in patients not exhibiting theophylline toxicity. If necessary, a maintenance dose may be given by slow intravenous infusion after the loading dose. In the *UK* the following aminophylline intravenous infusion maintenance doses are suggested: children aged 6 months to 9 years 1.0 mg per kg body-weight hourly; children aged 10 to 16 years 800 µg per kg hourly; adults 500 µg per kg hourly. In the *US* the following aminophylline intravenous maintenance doses are suggested, the dose being reduced after 12 hours: children aged 6 months to 9 years 1.2 mg per kg body-weight hourly, reduced to 1.0 mg per kg hourly; children aged 9 to 16 years and adult smokers 1.0 mg per kg hourly, reduced to 800 µg per kg hourly; non-smoking adults 700 µg per kg hourly, reduced to 500 µg per kg hourly; older patients or patients with cor pulmonale 600 µg per kg hourly, reduced to 300 µg per kg hourly; and in patients with congestive heart failure or liver disease 500 µg per kg hourly, reduced to 100 to 200 µg per kg hourly. Serum-theophylline concentration measurement is recommended, and maintenance doses should be reduced if serum concentrations exceed 20 µg per mL or the patient experiences

toxicity.
In the treatment of acute bronchospasm which does not require intravenous therapy, aminophylline may be given by mouth in the form of conventional tablets and capsules, or liquid preparations; sustained-release preparations are not suitable. Doses used have generally ranged from 100 to 300 mg three or four times daily after food.
In the treatment or prevention of chronic bronchospasm aminophylline may also be given by mouth as conventional or as sustained-release preparations. Doses of sustained-release aminophylline have generally ranged from 225 to 700 mg once or twice daily in adults. Children have been given sustained-release aminophylline 12-hourly in doses of 6 mg per kg body-weight, increased after 1 week to 12 mg per kg. Since aminophylline and aminophylline hydrate contain approximately 86 and 79% of anhydrous theophylline respectively, the doses of aminophylline by mouth can be calculated more accurately using the guidelines described under theophylline (p.1532).
Aminophylline has also been given rectally as an enema or suppositories in doses of 255 to 720 mg daily. Children have been given aminophylline by suppository in the following doses once or twice daily: age up to 1 year 12.5 to 25 mg; 1 to 5 years 50 to 100 mg; 6 to 12 years 100 to 200 mg. Suppositories of aminophylline have generally been replaced by sustained-release theophylline preparations which give a more predictable response without the hazard of proctitis.

Preparations

Aminophylline Enema *(U.S.P.)*. An aqueous solution of aminophylline prepared with the aid of ethylenediamine. Potency is expressed in terms of anhydrous theophylline. pH 9 to 9.5. It contains 218 to 267 mg of ethylenediamine per g of anhydrous theophylline but no other substance may be added to adjust the pH.

Aminophylline Injection *(B.P.)*. Contains aminophylline or aminophylline hydrate. It may be prepared using ethylenediamine and theophylline or theophylline hydrate. Ethylenediamine in excess to that required for the formation of aminophylline may be added but the total amount of ethylenediamine should not exceed 0.295 g for each g of anhydrous theophylline. Potency is expressed in terms of the equivalent amount of aminophylline. pH 8.8 to 10.0. Do not allow to come into contact with metals.

Aminophylline Injection *(U.S.P.)*. A sterile solution of aminophylline in Water for Injection, or a sterile solution of theophylline in Water for Injection prepared with the aid of ethylenediamine. It contains, in each mL, an amount of aminophylline equivalent to 18.35 to 21.12 mg of anhydrous theophylline. pH 8.6 to 9.0. It contains 166 to 192 mg of ethylenediamine per g of anhydrous theophylline but no other substance may be added to adjust the pH. It must not be used if crystals have separated.

Aminophylline Suppositories *(B.P.)*.

Aminophylline Suppositories *(U.S.P.)*. Potency is expressed in terms of anhydrous theophylline. Store at a temperature not exceeding 8° in well-closed containers.

Aminophylline Tablets *(B.P.)*

Aminophylline Tablets *(U.S.P.)*. Potency is expressed in terms of anhydrous theophylline.

Proprietary Preparations

Phyllocontin *(Napp, UK)*. *Tablets*, sustained-release, aminophylline 225 mg.
Tablets (Phyllocontin Forte), sustained-release, aminophylline 350 mg.
Tablets (Phyllocontin Paediatric), sustained-release, aminophylline 100 mg.

Theodrox *(Riker, UK)*. *Tablets*, aminophylline 195 mg, dried aluminium hydroxide gel 260 mg.

Proprietary Names and Manufacturers of Aminophylline
Afonilum *(Minden, Ger.)*; Aminocont *(Pharmacia, Swed.)*; Aminodur *(Berlex, USA)*; Aminomal *(Malesci, Ital.)*; Aminophyl *(Canad.)*; Aminophyllin *(Nyco, Norw.; Searle, USA)*; Androphyllin *(Austral.)*; Cardophyllin *(Fisons, UK)*; Cardophyllin *(Hamilton, Austral.)*; Carine *(Austral.)*; Corophyllin *(Beecham, Canad.)*; Corphyllamin *(Switz.)*; Duraphyllin *(Durachemie, Ger.)*; Escophyllin *(Switz.)*; Escophylline *(Streuli, Switz.)*; Eufilina *(Elmu, Spain)*; Euphyllin *(Lundbeck, Denm.; Byk Gulden, Ger.; Neth.; Lundbeck, Norw.; Byk Gulden, S.Afr.; Byk Gulden, Switz.)*; Euphyllina *(Byk Gulden, Ital.)*; Fergupirina *(Bauxili, Spain)*; Godafilin *(Spain)*; Inophyline *(Millot-Solac, Fr.)*; Lixaminol *(Ferndale, USA)*; Mini-lix *(USA)*; Palaron *(Fisons, Canad.)*; Peterphyllin *(Lennon, S.Afr.)*; Phyldrox Suppositories *(Carlton Laboratories, UK)*; Phyllocontin *(Purdue Frederick, Canad.; Pharmacia, Denm.; Mundipharma, S.Afr.; Napp, UK; Purdue Frederick, USA)*; Phyllotemp *(Mundipharma, Ger.; Mundipharma, Switz.)*; Planphylline *(Plantier, Fr.)*; Rectalad-Aminophylline *(USA)*; Tefamin *(Recordati, Ital.)*; Teofylamin *(DAK, Denm.)*; Teofyllamin *(NAF, Norw.; ACO, Swed.)*; Variaphylline L.A. *(Switz.)*; Vernaphyllin *(Vernleigh, S.Afr.)*.

The following names have been used for multi-ingredient preparations containing aminophylline—Amesec *(Lilly, Austral.; Lilly, Canad.; Lilly, UK)*; Breezeazy *(Cambridge Laboratories, Austral.)*; Mudrane *(Poythress, USA)*; Mudrane GG Tablets *(Poythress, USA)*; Mudrane GG-2 *(Poythress, USA)*; Mudrane-2 *(Poythress, USA)*; Riddovydrin Capsules and Suppositories *(Riddell, UK)*; Theodrox *(Riker, UK)*.

629-v

Bamifylline Hydrochloride *(BANM, USAN, rINNM)*.
AC-3810; CB-8102. 8-Benzyl-7-[2-(*N*-ethyl-*N*-2-hydroxyethylamino)ethyl]theophylline hydrochloride.
$C_{20}H_{27}N_5O_3,HCl=421.9$.

CAS — 2016-63-9 (bamifylline); 20684-06-4 (hydrochloride).

Bamifylline is a theophylline derivative which is used for the same purposes as theophylline (see p.1532), but it is reported to be better tolerated by mouth. It is readily absorbed from the gastro-intestinal tract and does not liberate theophylline in the body. It has been given in doses of up to 1.8 g daily by mouth. It has also been given as suppositories, or by intramuscular or slow intravenous injection.

Proprietary Names and Manufacturers
Bamifix *(Chiesi, Ital.)*; Trentadil *(Christiaens, Belg.; Spret-Mauchant, Fr.; Fresenius, Ger.; Padro, Spain; Schwarz, Switz.; Armour, UK)*.

630-r

Bufylline *(BAN)*.
Ambuphylline *(USAN)*; Theophylline-aminoisobutanol. 2-Amino-2-methylpropan-1-ol theophyllinate.
$C_{11}H_{19}N_5O_3=269.3$.

CAS — 5634-34-4.

Bufylline is a theophylline derivative which has been used for the same purposes as theophylline (see p.1532).

Proprietary Names and Manufacturers
Buthoid *(Merrell Dow, Canad.)*; Dilcovit *(OFF, Ital.)*.

The following names have been used for multi-ingredient preparations containing bufylline— Nethaprin Dospan *(Merrell, UK)*; Nethaprin Expectorant *(Merrell, UK)*.

621-x

Caffeine *(BAN, USAN)*.

Anhydrous Caffeine; Caféine; Coffeinum; Guaranine; Methyltheobromine; Théine. 1,3,7-Trimethylpurine-2,6(3*H*,1*H*)-dione; 1,3,7-Trimethylxanthine; 7-Methyltheophylline.
$C_8H_{10}N_4O_2=194.2$.

CAS — 58-08-2.

Pharmacopoeias. In *Arg., Aust., Belg., Br., Braz., Chin., Cz., Egypt., Eur., Fr., Ger., Hung., Ind., Int., It., Jpn, Jug., Mex., Neth., Nord., Pol., Port., Roum., Rus., Span., Swiss, Turk.*, and *U.S.*.

Odourless silky white crystals, usually matted together, or a white crystalline powder. It sublimes readily.
B.P. **solubilities** are: soluble 1 in 60 of water; freely soluble in boiling water and in chloroform; slightly soluble in alcohol and in ether. It dissolves in concentrated solutions of alkali benzoates or salicylates. *U.S.P.* solubilities are: sparingly soluble in water and in alcohol; freely soluble in chloroform; slightly soluble in ether. Solutions in water are neutral to litmus. **Store** in well-closed containers.

626-h

Caffeine Citrate *(BANM)*.

Caffein. Cit.; Citrated Caffeine; Coffeinum Citricum.
$C_8H_{10}N_4O_2,C_6H_8O_7=386.3$.

CAS — 69-22-7.

Pharmacopoeias. In *Aust., Hung., Roum.*, and *Span.*

622-r

Caffeine Hydrate

Caffeine Monohydrate; Coffeinum Monohydricum.
$C_8H_{10}N_4O_2,H_2O=212.2$.

CAS — 5743-12-4.

Pharmacopoeias. In *Aust., Br., Chin., Egypt., Eur., Fr., Ind., Int., It., Jug., Neth., Swiss*, and *U.S.*

Odourless silky white crystals, usually matted together, or a white crystalline powder. It effloresces in air and sublimes readily.
B.P. **solubilities** are: soluble 1 in 60 of water; freely soluble in boiling water and in chloroform; slightly soluble in alcohol and in ether. It dissolves in concentrated solutions of alkali benzoates or salicylates. *U.S.P.* solubilities are: soluble 1 in 50 of water, 1 in 75 of alcohol, 1 in 6 of chloroform, and 1 in 600 of ether. Solutions in water are neutral to litmus. **Store** in airtight containers.

STABILITY. The stability of citrated caffeine solutions for injectable and enteral use.— M. G. Eisenberg and N. Kang, *Am. J. Hosp. Pharm.*, 1984, *41*, 2405.

Adverse Effects, Treatment, and Precautions

As for theophylline (see p.1526). See also under Xanthine-containing Beverages, p.1535. The fatal dose of caffeine is probably about 10 g.

Reports and reviews of caffeine toxicity: P. B. Kulkarni and R. D. Dorand, *Pediatrics*, 1979, *64*, 254 (neonatal toxicity); W. Banner and P. A. Czajka, *Am. J. Dis. Child.*, 1980, *134*, 495 (neonatal toxicity); P. M. Zimmerman *et al.*, *Ann. emerg. Med.*, 1985, *14*, 1227 (acute poisoning); R. R. Dalvi, *Vet. hum. Toxicol.*, 1986, *28*, 144 (a review).

For reviews of caffeine toxicity resulting from the ingestion of xanthine-containing beverages, see under Adverse Effects in Xanthine-containing Beverages, p.1535.

INTERACTIONS, DRUGS. Caffeine reduces plasma flow in the liver and may therefore prolong the half-life and increase steady-state concentrations of hepatically eliminated drugs.— J. Onrot *et al.*, *Clin. Pharmac. Ther.*, 1986, *40*, 506.

Alcohol. In a study of 8 healthy subjects given alcohol by mouth in a dose of 2.2 mL per kg body-weight, caffeine 150 mg by mouth did not antagonise the central effects of alcohol and, instead, potentiated the detrimental effect on reaction time.— D. J. Oborne and Y. Rogers, *Aviat. Space & Environ. Med.*, 1983, *54*, 528.

Allopurinol. In a study in 2 healthy subjects, the plasma half-life of caffeine was essentially unchanged by 7 days' treatment with allopurinol 300 mg or 600 mg daily by mouth. However, allopurinol caused a specific, dose-dependent inhibition of the conversion of 1-methylxanthine to 1-methyluric acid.— D. M. Grant *et al.*, *Br. J. clin. Pharmac.*, 1986, *21*, 454.

Anti-arrhythmics. In 7 healthy subjects, mexiletine in a single dose of 200 mg reduced the elimination of caffeine by 30 to 50%. Lignocaine, flecainide, and tocainide had no effect on caffeine elimination.— R. Joeres and E. Richter (letter), *New Engl. J. Med.*, 1987, *317*, 117.

For the effect of verapamil on caffeine, see Verapamil, p.90.

Antibiotics. Caffeine elimination half-life was increased and clearance decreased by the concomitant administration of ciprofloxacin and enoxacin; ofloxacin did not affect these parameters.— W. Stille *et al.*, *J. antimicrob. Chemother.*, 1987, *20*, 729.

H_2 antagonist antihistamines. Cimetidine 1 g daily by mouth significantly reduced the systemic clearance of caffeine and prolonged its elimination half-life in 5 healthy subjects. Although the steady-state plasma-caffeine concentration would increase by approximately 70%, it was thought unlikely that this would produce adverse clinical effects.— L. J. Broughton and H. J. Rogers, *Br. J. clin. Pharmac.*, 1981, *12*, 155.

Idrocilamide. In 4 healthy subjects, idrocilamide inhibited the biotransformation of caffeine and increased its half-life 9 times. Partial or total avoidance of caffeine-containing products was recommended when idrocilamide was being taken.— J. L. Brazier *et al.*, *Eur. J. clin. Pharmac.*, 1980, *17*, 37.

Sex hormones. Reference to oral contraceptives impairing the elimination of caffeine.— R. V. Patwardhan *et al.*, *J. Lab. clin. Med.*, 1980, *95*, 603. See also D. R. Abernethy and E. L. Todd, *Eur. J. clin. Pharmac.*, 1985, *28*, 425.

Smoking. Tobacco smoking enhanced the clearance of caffeine.— G. W. Dawson and R. E. Vestal, *Pharmac. Ther.*, 1981, *15*, 207.

PREGNANCY AND THE NEONATE. For a comment on the inadvisability of using caffeine and sodium benzoate injection in neonates, see under Benzoic Acid, p.1355.

For a report of increased gastro-oesophageal reflux in neonates receiving caffeine, see Reflux Oesophagitis under Precautions in Theophylline Hydrate, p.1530.

Lactation. For studies examining the transfer of caffeine into breast milk and its consequences see under Absorption and Fate, below.

SPORT. The International Olympic Committee has banned the use of large amounts of caffeine by athletes. Smaller amounts, compatible with a moderate intake of coffee or soft drinks, are permitted (*Med. Lett.*, 1984, *26*, 65); the maximum permissible caffeine concentration in urine is 12 µg per mL (*Drug & Ther. Bull.*, 1987, *25*, 55).

Absorption and Fate

Caffeine is absorbed readily after oral, rectal, or parenteral administration and is widely distributed throughout the body. It is also absorbed through the skin. Caffeine passes readily into the central nervous system and into saliva; low concentrations are also present in breast milk. Caffeine crosses the placenta.

In adults, caffeine is metabolised almost completely via oxidation, demethylation, and acetylation, and is excreted in the urine as 1-methyluric acid, 1-methylxanthine, 7-methylxanthine, 1,7-dimethylxanthine (paraxanthine), 5-acetylamino-6-formylamino-3-methyluracil (AFMU), and other metabolites with only about 1% unchanged. Neonates have a greatly reduced capacity to metabolise caffeine and it is largely excreted unchanged in the urine until hepatic metabolism becomes significantly developed, usually by 3 to 6 months of age. Elimination half-lives are approximately 3 to 5 hours in adults and 36 to 144 hours in neonates.

Reviews of the pharmacokinetics of caffeine: R. Newton *et al.*, *Eur. J. clin. Pharmac.*, 1981, *21*, 45 (salivary pharmacokinetics); R. Gorodischer and M. Karplus, *ibid.*, 1982, *22*, 47 (neonates); M. Bonati *et al.*, *Clin. Pharmac. Ther.*, 1982, *32*, 98 (adults); D. D. Tang-Liu *et al.*, *J. Pharmac. exp. Ther.*, 1983, *224*, 180 (adults); A. Lelo *et al.*, *Br. J. clin. Pharmac.*, 1986, *22*, 183 (adults).

DISTRIBUTION. The therapeutic range for caffeine in neonates is not well defined. The minimal effective serum concentration may be as low as 3 µg per mL, but a concentration of about 8 µg per mL is recommended as the lower end of the therapeutic range. Ventilatory response has been reported to plateau at serum concentrations of 20 µg per mL and many centres take an upper limit based around that value, but neurological and cardiovascular toxicity has been reported to occur only at concentrations above 50 µg per mL.— C. Edwards, *Pharm. J.*, 1986, *2*, 128.

METABOLISM AND EXCRETION. Four- to five-fold differences in plasma half-lives of caffeine are common among healthy people. The plasma half-life of caffeine is decreased by smoking and other liver-enzyme inducing agents, and is increased by liver disease such as cirrhosis and viral hepatitis (W. Kalow, *Arzneimittel-Forsch.*, 1985, *35*, 319), pregnancy (R. Knutti *et al.*, *Eur. J. clin. Pharmac.*, 1981, *21*, 121), and the use of oral contraceptives (D.R. Abernethy and E.L. Todd, *ibid.*, 1985, *28*, 425). The plasma half-life of caffeine is not affected by old age (J. Blanchard and S.J. Sawers, *J. Pharmacokinet. Biopharm.*, 1983, *11*, 109) or obesity (D.R. Abernethy *et al.*, *Br. J. clin. Pharmac.*, 1985, *20*, 61).

Reviews of the metabolism and metabolites of caffeine: D. M. Grant *et al.*, *Clin. Pharmac. Ther.*, 1983, *33*, 355 and 591; W. W. Weber and D. W. Hein, *Pharmac. Rev.*, 1985, *37*, 25; J. Blanchard *et al.*, *Br. J. clin. Pharmac.*, 1985, *19*, 225.

PREGNANCY AND THE NEONATE. The mean half-life of caffeine in pregnant women was 8.3 hours compared with a mean of 3.4 hours in 9 male and 11 non-pregnant females. In most cases, the half-lives returned to normal values within one month of delivery (R. Knutti *et al.*, *Eur. J. clin. Pharmac.*, 1981, *21*, 121). There was a significant decrease in the production of 1-methyl metabolites of caffeine in 15 pregnant women compared with 9 non-pregnant women. It has been suggested that this might be due to hormonal influences on the hepatic caffeine metabolising enzymes (N.R. Scott *et al.*, *Br. J. clin. Pharmac.*, 1986, *22*, 475).

Lactation. Studies examining the transfer of caffeine into breast milk after doses of 36 to 335 mg of caffeine by mouth have recorded peak maternal plasma concentrations of 2.4 to 4.7 µg per mL, peak maternal saliva concentrations of 1.1 to 9.2 µg per mL, and peak breast-milk concentrations of 1.3 to 7.2 µg per mL. At these concentrations in breast milk, the calculated daily caffeine ingestion by breast-fed infants ranged from 1.3 to 3.1 mg, which was not thought to present a hazard, although irritability and a poor sleeping pattern have been reported (E.E. Tyrala and W.E. Dodson, *Archs Dis. Childh.*, 1979, *54*, 787; R. Hildebrandt *et al.*, *Br. J. clin. Pharmac.*, 1983, *15*, 612P; R. Sagraves *et al.*, *Drug Intell. & clin. Pharm.*, 1984, *18*, 507; C.M. Berlin *et al.*, *Pediatrics*, 1984, *73*, 59).

Uses and Administration

Caffeine is a central nervous system stimulant. It inhibits the enzyme phosphodiesterase and has an antagonistic effect at central adenosine receptors. Its action on the central nervous system is mainly on the higher centres and it produces a condition of wakefulness and increased mental activity. It may stimulate the respiratory centre, increasing the rate and depth of respiration. Its stimulant action on the medullary vasomotor centre and its positive inotropic action on the myocardium are compensated by its peripheral vasodilator effect on the arterioles, so that the blood pressure usually remains unchanged. Caffeine facilitates the performance of muscular work and increases the total work which can be performed by a muscle. The diuretic action of caffeine is weaker than that of theophylline.

Caffeine increases the absorption of ergotamine and is sometimes given with ergotamine in the treatment of migraine.

Caffeine is administered in powder or tablets in doses of 100 to 300 mg. It is frequently included in analgesic preparations with aspirin or codeine. Caffeine citrate has been used similarly. Caffeine and sodium benzoate, caffeine and sodium iodide (iodocaffeine), and caffeine and sodium salicylate are all readily soluble in water and have been used for the administration of caffeine by injection, as has caffeine citrate.

Beverages of coffee, tea, and cola provide active doses of caffeine.

A review of the actions and uses of caffeine.— P. W. Curatolo and D. Robertson, *Ann. intern. Med.*, 1983, *98*, 641.

ASTHMA. The bronchodilator effect of caffeine has been found to be about 40% of that of an equivalent molar dose of theophylline (H. Gong *et al.*, *Chest*, 1986, *89*, 335). In 8 asthmatic patients of mean age 65 years, caffeine 5 mg per kg body-weight by mouth was significantly more effective than placebo in improving pulmonary function (M. Bukowskyj and K. Nakatsu, *Am. Rev. resp. Dis.*, 1987, *135*, 173), and in 23 asthmatics aged 8 to 18 years, anhydrous caffeine 10 mg per kg body-weight and theophylline 5 mg per kg, both given by mouth, did not differ significantly in their bronchodilating effects (A.B. Becker *et al.*, *New Engl. J. Med.*, 1984, *310*, 743). Neither Becker *et al.* (1984) nor Bukowskyj and Nakatsu (1987) advocated the routine use of caffeine as a bronchodilator although Becker *et al.* suggested that it might be of value for temporary use when prescribed anti-asthma medications were not readily available.

DERMATITIS. In a double-blind study in 28 patients with atopic dermatitis the application for 3 weeks of a 30% caffeine cream produced significantly greater benefit (in terms of erythema, scaling, lichenification, oozing, and excoriation) than a placebo. It was considered that caffeine increased the concentrations of cyclic AMP in the skin.— R. J. Kaplan *et al.* (letter), *Archs Derm.*, 1977, *113*, 107. See also *idem*, 1978, *114*, 60 (combined use with topical hydrocortisone).

DIAGNOSIS AND TESTING. Calculation of the urinary molar ratio of the caffeine metabolites 5-acetylamino-6-formylamino-3-methyluracil to 1-methylxanthine from a single urine sample obtained 2 to 6 hours after caffeine ingestion allowed the determination of acetylator phenotype.— D. M. Grant *et al.*, *Br. J. clin. Pharmac.*, 1984, *17*, 459. See also R. B. Rankin *et al.*, *J. clin. Pharm. Ther.*, 1987, *12*, 47.

ECT. In 6 patients whose seizure duration was declining despite maximal ECT stimulation, the use of caffeine 250 to 750 mg, given by intravenous injection over 60 seconds as caffeine and sodium benzoate, resulted in lengthening of seizures by an average of 107% and clinical improvement of depression— P. E. Hinkle *et al.*, *Am. J. Psychiat.*, 1987, *144*, 1143.

HYPERKINETIC STATES. Early reports and some studies suggested that caffeine might be useful in the treatment of children with hyperkinetic states (minimal brain dysfunction) (R.C. Schnackenberg, *Am. J. Psychiat.*, 1973, *130*, 796; D.H.P. Harvey and R.W. Marsh, *Develop. Med. Child Neurol.*, 1978, *20*, 81; C.C. Reichard and S.T. Elder, *Am. J. Psychiat.*, 1977, *134*, 144). However, other studies have shown no difference between caffeine and placebo and that caffeine is inferior to methylphenidate or dexamphetamine (R.D. Huestis *et al.*, *Am. J. Psychiat.*, 1975, *132*, 868; C.K. Conners, *Int. J. Mental Hlth*, 1975, *4*, 132; B.D. Garfinkel *et al.*, *Am. J. Psychiat.*, 1975, *132*, 723; L.E. Arnold *et al.*, *Archs gen. Psychiat.*, 1978, *35*, 463; P. Firestone *et al.*, *J. Am. Acad. Child Psychiat.*, 1978, *17*, 445).

ORTHOSTATIC HYPOTENSION. In a study of 12 patients with orthostatic hypotension due to autonomic failure, acute administration of caffeine 250 mg by mouth following 3 days of abstinence from methylxanthine ingestion led to a significant increase in blood pressure. The authors now advised patients with autonomic failure and postprandial hypotension to drink 2 cups of coffee (approximately 200 to 250 mg of caffeine) with breakfast and to abstain for the rest of the day, to try and prevent tolerance (J. Onrot *et al.*, *New Engl. J. Med.*, 1985, *313*, 549). Of 5 patients with autonomic neuropathy, caffeine 250 mg was effective or partially effective in 3 at preventing postprandial hypotension, but in combination with dihydroergotamine, all 5 responded (R.D. Hoeldtke *et al.*, *Ann. intern. Med.*, 1986, *105*, 168).

PAIN. Although some studies have found no benefit from the use of caffeine as an analgesic adjuvant (L. Winter *et al.*, *Curr. ther. Res.*, 1983, *33*, 115), a review of 30 studies involving more than 10 000 patients concluded that to obtain the same response from an analgesic without caffeine required an analgesic dose approximately 40% greater than one with caffeine. It was speculated that caffeine doses studied previously were too low (E.M. Laska *et al.*, *J. Am. med. Ass.*, 1984, *251*, 1711). There were criticisms regarding the methodology of this review and the clinical significance of the results (A.R. Temple and J.G. Pigeon, *ibid.*, 1985, *253*, 779), but other studies have also shown an additive effect with caffeine (S.A. Cooper *et al.*, *Clin. Pharmac. Ther.*, 1984, *35*, 232; A. Rubin and L. Winter, *J. int. med. Res.*, 1984, *12*, 338).

Headache. Fourteen of 18 patients with postdural puncture headaches experienced relief after one or 2 doses of caffeine sodium benzoate 500 mg given intravenously over one hour.— A. P. Jarvis *et al.* (letter), *Anesth. Analg.*, 1986, *65*, 316.

PREGNANCY AND THE NEONATE. *Neonatal apnoea.* In cases of infantile apnoea, caffeine citrate has been given intravenously or by mouth in a loading dose of 20 mg per kg body-weight, followed 2 to 3 days later by maintenance doses of 5 to 10 mg per kg given once or twice daily (J.V. Aranda *et al.*, *J. Pediat.*, 1977, *90*, 467). It has been shown to increase ventilation, tidal volume, and mean inspiratory flow (J.V. Aranda *et al.*, *ibid*., 1983, *103*, 975), resulting in a reduction in the number of apnoeic attacks (J.V. Aranda *et al.*, 1977; I. Murat *et al.*, *ibid*., 1981, *99*, 984; M. Anwar *et al.*, *Archs Dis. Childh*., 1986, *61*, 891). A maintenance dose of 3 mg per kg daily has also been tried, but was less effective in decreasing apnoeic attacks, although there were fewer gastro-intestinal adverse effects (E. Autret *et al.*, *Thérapie*, 1985, *40*, 235). For the low doses of caffeine required for neonates, caffeine itself can be dissolved in water by using a water bath (P. Frauch and M.J. van Pernis, *Am. J. Hosp. Pharm*., 1984, *41*, 2590). Advantages of using caffeine instead of theophylline to treat infantile apnoea include the wider therapeutic index of caffeine, once daily dosing with caffeine, compared with every 6 to 12 hours for theophylline, and the fact that caffeine levels need only be measured weekly compared with every day or two for theophylline (D.N. Spierer and E.A. Koyama, *Drug Intell. & clin. Pharm*., 1985, *19*, 763).

For the risks associated with the use of caffeine and sodium benzoate injection in neonates, see under Benzoic Acid, p.1355.

RHINITIS. A report of relief of symptoms of allergic rhinitis following a dose of caffeine approximately 140 mg by mouth.— P. Shapiro (letter), *Lancet*, 1982, *1*, 793.

SPERM MOTILITY. There have been reports that caffeine added to semen *in vitro* increases the percentage, quality, and duration of action of the spermatozoa, but other studies have failed to confirm this. Moussa (*Fert. Steril*., 1983, *39*, 845) found that low doses of caffeine increased the percentage of motile sperm, but had no effect on sperm velocity, while very high doses caused complete immobilisation. Suggestions that caffeine causes damage to sperm have not been confirmed, and an improvement in sperm fertilising capacity has been suggested.— J. O. Drife, *Drugs*, 1987, *33*, 610.

Preparations

Caffeine Iodide Elixir *(B.P.C. 1973)*. Caffeine 150 mg, sodium iodide 450 mg, liquorice liquid extract 0.3 mL, chloroform 0.01 mL decoction prepared from a sufficient quantity of recently ground roasted coffee of commerce and water to 5 mL.

The liability of Caffeine Iodide Elixir to spoilage.— T. R. R. Kurup and L. S. C. Wan, *Pharm. J*., 1986, *2*, 761.

Caffeine and Sodium Benzoate Injection *(U.S.P.)*. A sterile solution in Water for Injections; pH 6.5 to 8.5.

Proprietary Names and Manufacturers of Caffeine and its Salts

Efed II Black *(Alto, USA)*; No Doz *(Key, Austral.; Bristol-Myers Products, USA)*; Percoffedrinol *(Passauer, Ger.)*; Percutafeine *(Pierre Fabre, Fr.)*.

The following names have been used for multi-ingredient preparations containing caffeine or its salts—282 Mep *(Frosst, Canad.)*; 217 Tablets *(Frosst, Canad.)*; 222 Tablets *(Frosst, Canad.)*; 282 Tablets *(Frosst, Canad.)*; 292 Tablets *(Frosst, Canad.)*; 293 Tablets *(Frosst, Canad.)*; 692 Tablets *(Frosst, Canad.)*; A.C. & C. *(Pharmascience, Canad.)*; Achrocidin *(Lederle, Canad.)*; Alpha-Phed *(Metro Med, USA)*; Amaphen *(Trimen, USA)*; Amaphen with Codeine *(Trimen, USA)*; Anacin *(Whitehall, USA)*; Anacin with Codeine *(Whitehall, Canad.)*; Analgesic Dellipsoids D6 *(Pilsworth, UK)*; Ancasal *(Anca, Canad.)*; Aneurone *(Philip Harris, UK)*; Anoquan *(Mallard, USA)*; Antoin *(Cox, UK)*; Atasol-15 *(Horner, Canad.)*; Atasol-30 *(Horner, Canad.)*; Atasol-8 *(Horner, Canad.)*; B-A-C *(Mayrand, USA)*; B-A-C 3 *(Mayrand, USA)*; Beta-Phed *(Metro Med, USA)*; Bronchial Dellipsoids D15 *(Pilsworth, UK)*; C-2 *(Wampole, Canad.)*; Cafadol *(Typharm, UK)*; Cafergot *(Sandoz, Austral.; Sandoz, Canad.; Sandoz, UK; Sandoz, USA)*; Cafergot P-B *(Sandoz, USA)*; Cafergot-PB *(Sandoz, Austral.; Sandoz, Canad.)*; Cafetrate-PB *(Schein, USA)*; Cardiac Dellipsoids D18 *(Pilsworth, UK)*; Citra Forte Capsules *(Boyle, USA)*; Codalan *(Lannett, USA)*; Coda-Med *(Dep, UK)*; Codamin *(Clark, Canad.)*; Codaminophen *(Clark, Canad.)*; Compal *(Reid-Rowell, USA)*; Coricidin with Codeine *(Schering, Canad.)*; Coryban-D *(Pfipharmecs, USA)*;

D & M Tablets *(Cambridge Laboratories, Austral.)*; Damason-P *(Mason, USA)*; Darvon Compound *(Lilly, USA)*; Darvon-N Compound *(Lilly, Canad.)*; Dasikon *(Beecham Laboratories, USA)*; Dasin *(Beecham Laboratories, USA)*; Dexkaf *(Nelson, Austral.)*; Dia-Gesic *(Central Pharmaceuticals, USA)*; Dolene Compound-65 *(Lederle, USA)*; Doloxene Compound *(Lilly, UK)*; Dolvan *(Norma, UK)*; Dristan Advanced Formula *(Whitehall, Canad.)*; Dristan Decongestant Tablets with Antihistamine *(Whitehall, UK)*; Drixine Cough Suppressant *(Essex, Austral.)*; Effergot *(Wander, UK)*; Effico *(Pharmax, UK)*; Elixir Sibec *(Vestric, UK)*; Ergodryl *(Parke, Davis, Austral.; Parke, Davis, Canad.; Parke, Davis, UK)*; Esgic *(Forest Pharmaceuticals, USA)*; Eupinal *(Cuxson, Gerrard, UK)*; Eupnine Vernade *(Wilcox, UK)*; Excedrin *(Bristol-Myers Products, USA)*; Exdol *(Frosst, Canad.)*; Fioricet *(Sandoz, USA)*; Fiorinal *(Sandoz, Canad.; Sandoz, USA)*; Fiorinal with Codeine *(Sandoz, USA)*; Fiorinal-C *(Sandoz, Canad.)*; G-1 Capsules *(Hauck, USA)*; Glykola *(Sinclair, UK)*; Hycomine Compound *(Du Pont, USA)*; Hyco-Pap *(Lasalle, USA)*; Hypon *(Calmic, UK)*; Iodo-Ephedrine *(Philip Harris, UK)*; Juvatral *(Cambridge Laboratories, Austral.)*; Korigesic *(Trimen, USA)*; Labiton *(Laboratories for Applied Biology, UK)*; Lenoltec with Codeine *(Technilab, Canad.)*; Medigesic Plus *(US Pharmaceutical, USA)*; Midol *(Sterling, Canad.; Glenbrook, USA)*; Migral *(Wellcome, Austral.)*; Migralam *(Bart, USA)*; Migril *(Wellcome, UK)*; Myolgin *(Cox, UK)*; Norgesic *(Riker, Canad.; Riker, USA)*; Novogesic *(Novopharm, Canad.)*; Orgraine *(Organon, UK)*; P-A-C *(Upjohn, USA)*; Pacaps *(Lasalle, USA)*; Paragesic *(Sandoz, UK)*; Parahypon *(Calmic, UK)*; Paralgin *(Norton, UK)*; Para-seltzer *(Sandoz, UK)*; Pardale *(Martindale Pharmaceuticals, UK)*; Paxidal *(Wallace Mfg Chem., UK)*; Pharmidone *(Farmitalia Carlo Erba, UK)*; Pneumogeine *(Gamaprod, Austral.)*; Propain *(Panpharma, UK)*; Repan *(Everett, USA)*;

Saleto *(Mallard, USA)*; Solpadeine *(Sterling Research, UK)*; Supac *(Mission Pharmacal, USA)*; Synalgos-DC *(Wyeth, USA)*; Syndol *(Merrell, UK)*; Talwin Compound *(Winthrop, Canad.)*; Tecnal *(Technilab, Canad.)*; Tecnal C *(Technilab, Canad.)*; T-Gesic *(T.E. Williams, USA)*; Travacalm *(Hamilton, Austral.)*; Triad *(UAD, USA)*; Triaminicin *(Ancalab, Canad.)*; Tropinal *(Hamilton, Austral.)*; Tussirex *(Scot-Tussin, USA)*; Two-Dyne *(Hyrex, USA)*; Tylenol No. 1 *(McNeil, Canad.)*; Uniflu *(Unigreg, UK)*; Unigesic *(Unimed, UK)*; Vanquish *(Glenbrook, USA)*; Vasobral *(Logeais, Fr.)*; Vibrona *(Vine Products, UK)*; Vikonon *(Savoy Laboratories, UK)*; Wigraine *(Organon, Canad.; Organon, USA)*; Wigraine-PB *(Organon, USA)*.

631-f

Choline Theophyllinate *(BAN, rINN)*.

Choline Theoph.; Oxtriphylline *(USAN)*; Theophylline Cholinate.

$C_{12}H_{21}N_5O_3$=283.3.

CAS — 4499-40-5.

Pharmacopoeias. In *Br*., *Chin*., and *U.S.*

A white crystalline powder, odourless or with a faint amine-like odour. Choline theophyllinate 1.57 g is approximately equivalent in theophylline content to 1 g of theophylline. Very **soluble** in water; soluble 1 in 10 of alcohol; very slightly soluble in chloroform and ether. A 1% solution in water has a pH of about 10.3. **Store** at a temperature not exceeding 25° in airtight containers. Protect from light.

Adverse Effects, Treatment, and Precautions

As for theophylline (p.1526).

Absorption and Fate

Choline theophyllinate is readily absorbed from the gastro-intestinal tract and liberates theophylline in the body.

Studies on the serum-theophylline concentrations and clinical response after oral administration of sustained-release choline theophyllinate preparations to asthmatics: C. Legris *et al.*, *Curr. ther. Res*., 1985, *37*, 103; S. J. Berg *et al.*, *Br. J. clin. Pharmac*., 1985, *20*, 89; S. G. Hibberd *et al.*, *ibid*., 1986, *22*, 337; R. Boileau and J. J. Brossard, *Curr. ther. Res*., 1986, *39*, 319.

Uses and Administration

Choline theophyllinate is a theophylline salt which is used for the same purposes as theophylline (see p.1532), but it is reported to be better tolerated by mouth. The usual dosage for adults is 100 to 400 mg four times daily by mouth; it should be taken during or after a meal to reduce gastro-intestinal side-effects. The dosage for children aged 3 to 6 years is 62.5 to 125 mg three times daily and for children aged over 6 years, 300 to 400 mg daily in divided doses. Choline theophyllinate is also given by mouth as a sustained-release tablet in usual adult doses of 424 mg in the morning and 848 mg at night.

ADMINISTRATION. Results from 90 patients with chronic airway obstruction suggested that an 8-hour dosage regimen may be adequate for choline theophyllinate.— F. Morell *et al.* (letter), *Drug Intell. & clin. Pharm*., 1983, *17*, 133.

ASTHMA. In a study of 9 patients with nocturnal asthma the administration of sustained-release choline theophyllinate 1.272 g daily in divided doses prevented overnight bronchoconstriction but impaired the quality of sleep.— G. B. Rhind *et al.*, *Br. med. J*., 1985, *291*, 1605. See also J. M. Mungavin and J. Simpson-Laing, *Clin. Trials J*., 1984, *21*, 80.

Preparations

Choline Theophyllinate Tablets *(B.P.)*

Oxtriphylline Elixir *(U.S.P.)*. An elixir containing choline theophyllinate, with alcohol 18 to 22%. pH 8 to 9.

Oxtriphylline Tablets *(U.S.P.)*. Tablets containing choline theophyllinate; they may be partially enteric-coated.

Proprietary Preparations

Choledyl *(Parke, Davis, UK)*. *Syrup*, choline theophyllinate 62.5 mg/5 mL.
Tablets, choline theophyllinate 100 and 200 mg.

Choledyl Syrup (*UK*) contains sugar which could cause extensive and severe dental caries in young children needing long-term treatment (*Drug & Ther. Bull*., 1983, *21*, 56), but does not contain allergenic colouring agents to which asthmatic children may be sensitive (D.W. Denning and R. Vijeratnam, *Lancet*, 1985, *1*, 461).

Sabidal SR *(Zyma, UK)*. *Tablets*, sustained-release, choline theophyllinate 424 mg (equivalent to theophylline 270 mg).

Proprietary Names and Manufacturers

Brondecon-PD *(Parke, Davis, Austral.)*; Choledyl *(Warner, Austral.; Parke, Davis, Canad.; Denm.; Norw.; Warner, S.Afr.; Parke, Davis, Spain; Parke, Davis, UK; Parke, Davis, USA)*; Cholegyl *(Neth.)*; Chophyllin *(Ferraton, Denm.)*; Dilasmyl *(Neth.)*; Euspirax *(Asche, Ger.)*; Novotriphyl *(Novopharm, Canad.)*; Rouphylline *(Rougier, Canad.)*; Sabidal *(Zyma, Denm.)*; Sabidal Retention Enema *(Zyma, UK)*; Sabidal SR *(Zyma, UK)*; Sclerofillina *(Ital.)*; Teocolina *(Nessa, Spain)*; Teofilcolina *(Salfa, Ital.)*; Teovent *(Ferrosan, Norw.; Ferrosan, Swed.)*; Theocoline *(Jpn)*; Theophyl-Choline *(Perkins, Ital.)*; Theophylline Choline *(Canad.)*.

The following names have been used for multi-ingredient preparations containing choline theophyllinate— Brondecon *(Parke, Davis, USA)*; Brondecon Expectorant *(Warner, Austral.)*; Choledyl Expectorant *(Parke, Davis, Canad.)*.

633-n

Diprophylline *(BAN, rINN)*.

Dihydroxypropyltheophyllinum; Diprophyllinum; Dyphylline *(USAN)*; Glyphyllinum; Hyphylline.
7-(2,3-Dihydroxypropyl)-1,3-dimethylxanthine; 7-(2,3-Dihydroxypropyl)theophylline.

$C_{10}H_{14}N_4O_4$=254.2.

CAS — 479-18-5.

Pharmacopoeias. In *Aust*., *Br*., *Chin*., *Eur*., *Fr*., *Ger*., *Neth*., *Nord*., *Rus*., *Swiss*, and *U.S.*

A white odourless amorphous or crystalline powder. Freely **soluble** in water; slightly soluble in alcohol and in chloroform; practically insoluble in ether. A 1% solution in water has a pH of 5.0 to 7.5. **Store** in airtight containers. Protect from light.

Adverse Effects, Treatment, and Precautions

Diprophylline may cause less nausea and gastric irritation than aminophylline. The intramuscular injection is claimed to be almost painless. Diprophylline should be administered with caution to patients with renal failure since it is excreted renally.

INTERACTIONS. The extremely rapid clearance of diprophylline was inhibited by probenecid in 5 healthy subjects.— D. C. May and C. H. Jarboe (letter), *New Engl. J. Med.*, 1981, *304*, 791. See also: D. C. May and C. H. Jarboe, *Clin. Pharmac. Ther.*, 1983, *33*, 822; M. Acara *et al.*, *J. Pharm. Pharmac.*, 1987, *39*, 526.

Absorption and Fate

Diprophylline is rapidly absorbed from the gastro-intestinal tract and from the site of intramuscular injections. Diprophylline does not liberate theophylline in the body and is largely excreted unchanged in the urine with an elimination half-life of approximately 2 hours.

The bioavailability of diprophylline preparations: K. J. Simons *et al.*, *J. clin. Pharmac.*, 1977, *17*, 237; J. J. Stablein *et al.*, *Eur. J. clin. Pharmac.*, 1983, *25*, 281; A. B. Straughn *et al.*, *J. pharm. Sci.*, 1985, *74*, 335.

PREGNANCY AND THE NEONATE. In a study of 20 lactating women given diprophylline by intramuscular injection, diprophylline was found to concentrate in breast milk, with a milk to serum concentration ratio of approximately 2. However, it was felt that the quantity of diprophylline a breast-feeding infant would ingest was unlikely to produce any pharmacological action unless the child was very sensitive.— C. H. Jarboe *et al.*, *J. clin. Pharmac.*, 1981, *21*, 405.

Uses and Administration

Diprophylline is a theophylline derivative which is used similarly to theophylline (see p.1532), but it is better tolerated by mouth and by intramuscular injection. The bronchodilating potency of diprophylline is only 10 to 20% that of theophylline.

The usual dose of diprophylline by mouth is 15 mg per kg body-weight every 6 hours. It may also be given intramuscularly in an initial dose of 500 mg followed by 250 to 500 mg every 2 to 6 hours to a maximum of 15 mg per kg body-weight every 6 hours.

The nicotinate of diprophylline, diniprofylline, has also been used.

In a double-blind study of 20 patients with exercise-induced bronchospasm, improvements in measurements of lung function after diprophylline in doses of 15 and 20 mg per kg body-weight by mouth were one third to one half those obtained after theophylline 6 mg per kg by mouth. Tremor was twice as common with theophylline. It was felt that further evaluations to elucidate optimal dosage were needed.— C. T. Furukawa *et al.*, *J. clin. Pharmac.*, 1983, *23*, 414.

Preparations

Dyphylline Elixir *(U.S.P.)*. Contains diprophylline and alcohol.

Dyphylline Injection *(U.S.P.)*. Contains diprophylline. Store at a temperature above 15°, but avoid excessive heat. Protect from light. Do not use if crystals have separated.

Dyphylline Tablets *(U.S.P.)*

Proprietary Names and Manufacturers

Aerophylline *(Canad.)*; Airet *(USA)*; Asthmolysin *(Kade, Ger.)*; Astmamasitt *(Jpn)*; Brosema *(Legere, USA)*; Dicoryllin *(Switz.)*; Difilina *(Liade, Spain)*; Difillin *(Lisapharma, Ital.)*; Dilin *(Canad.; Hauck, USA)*; Dilor *(Savage, USA)*; Droxine *(Shear/Kershman, USA)*; Dyflex *(Econo Med, USA)*; Emfabid *(USA)*; Glyfyllin *(DAK, Denm.)*; Katasma *(Bruschettini, Ital.)*; Lancephylline *(Lancet, UK)*; Lufyllin *(Wallace, USA)*; Neophyllin M *(Jpn)*; Neothylline *(Lemmon, USA)*; Neo-Vasophylline *(Neth.)*; Neutrafillina *(Roussel Maestretti, Ital.)*; Neutraphylline *(Belg.; Houdé, Fr.; Cox, UK)*; Neutroxantina *(Ralay, Spain)*; Prophyllen *(Switz.)*; Protophylline *(Rougier, Canad.)*; Silbephylline *(S.Afr.; Berk Pharmaceuticals, UK)*; Synthophylline *(Switz.)*; Thylline *(Schein, USA)*.

The following names have been used for multi-ingredient preparations containing diprophylline— Dilor-G *(Savage, USA)*; Emfaseem *(Saron, USA)*; Lufyllin-GG *(Wallace, USA)*; Noradran *(Norma, UK)*; Oxycap *(Hyrex, USA)*; Tedral Expectorant *(Warner, UK)*; Thylline-GG *(Schein, USA)*.

16624-a

Enprofylline *(USAN, rINN)*.

3-Propylxanthine; D-4028. 3,7-Dihydro-3-propyl-1*H*-purine-2,6-dione.

$C_8H_{10}N_4O_2$=194.2.

CAS — 41078-02-8.

Enprofylline is a theophylline derivative which is well absorbed from the gastro-intestinal tract. It does not liberate theophylline in the body and is largely excreted unchanged in the urine. Enprofylline has been used for the relief of bronchospasm in asthmatic patients, and is reported to have a bronchodilating potency about 5 times that of theophylline.

References to the cardiovascular effects of enprofylline: T. B. Conradson, *Eur. J. clin. Pharmac.*, 1984, *27*, 319; M. Esquivel *et al.*, *Clin. Pharmac. Ther.*, 1986, *39*, 395.

References to the pharmacokinetics of enprofylline: E. Lunnell *et al.*, *Acta pharmac. tox.*, 1983, *53*, 205 (pharmacokinetics and adverse effects in healthy subjects); O. Borgå *et al.*, *Clin. Pharmac. Ther.*, 1983, *34*, 799 (pharmacokinetics in healthy subjects); K. Tegnér *et al.*, *Eur. J. clin. Pharmac.*, 1983, *25*, 703 (plasma protein binding); L. C. Laursen *et al.*, *Br. J. clin. Pharmac.*, 1984, *18*, 591 (serum concentrations); E. Lunnell *et al.*, *Eur. J. clin. Pharmac.*, 1984, *27*, 329 (gastro-intestinal absorption); L. C. Laursen *et al.*, *ibid.*, 1985, *29*, 115 (pharmacokinetics in patients requiring high or low doses of theophylline); E. Lunnell and O. Borgå, *ibid.*, 1987, *32*, 67 (pharmacokinetics in healthy, elderly subjects); C. Hultqvist and O. Borgå, *ibid.*, 533 (pharmacokinetics in children).

References to the use of enprofylline in asthma and obstructive airways disease: L. C. Laursen *et al.*, *Eur. J. clin. Pharmac.*, 1983, *24*, 323 (intravenous administration); L. C. Laursen *et al.*, *ibid.*, 1984, *26*, 707 (comparison with theophylline, oral administration); E. Lunell *et al.*, *Eur. J. resp. Dis.*, 1984, *65*, 28 (comparison with placebo, intravenous administration); L. C. Laursen *et al.*, *ibid.*, 504 (comparison with theophylline, oral sustained-release administration); L. C. Laursen *et al.*, *Allergy*, 1985, *40*, 506 (comparison with theophylline in exercise-induced asthma, intravenous administration); L. C. Laursen *et al.*, *Respiration*, 1986, *50*, 57 (comparison with theophylline, oral administration); J. Boe *et al.*, *Ann. Allergy*, 1987, *59*, 155 (comparison with theophylline in acute asthma, intravenous administration); J. B. Rasmussen and E. Lunell, *Eur. J. clin. Pharmac.*, 1987, *32*, 23 (combination therapy with terbutaline, intravenous administration).

Proprietary Names and Manufacturers

Astra, Swed.

634-h

Etamiphylline Camsylate *(BANM)*.

Diétamiphylline Camphosulfonate; Etamiphyllin Camsilate *(rINNM)*; Etamphyllin Camsylate. 7-(2-Diethylaminoethyl)-1,3-dimethylxanthine camphor-10-sulphonate; 7-(2-Diethylaminoethyl)theophylline camphor-10-sulphonate.

$C_{23}H_{37}N_5O_6S$=511.6.

CAS — 314-35-2 (etamiphylline); 19326-29-5 (camsylate).

Pharmacopoeias. In *Br.* Also in *B.P. Vet.*

A white or almost white powder with a faint camphoraceous odour. Very **soluble** in water; soluble in alcohol and in chloroform; very slightly soluble in ether. A 10% solution in water has a pH of 3.9 to 5.4. Solutions are **sterilised** by heating in an autoclave. **Store** in well-closed containers.

Etamiphylline camsylate is a theophylline derivative which is used similarly to theophylline (see p.1532), but it is reported to be better tolerated by mouth. Etamiphylline does not liberate theophylline in the body.

Etamiphylline is given by mouth in doses of 100 to 300 mg three or four times daily after meals, by intramuscular injection in doses of 700 mg three or four times daily, or by slow intravenous injection in doses of 350 mg, repeated as required. It is given by rectum once or twice daily as suppositories containing 500 mg.

Etamiphylline has also been used as the hydrochloride and the methiodide.

From a study of 27 asthmatic children given etamiphylline or theophylline 6.96 mg per kg body-weight, or placebo by mouth, it was concluded that the bronchodilator effect of oral etamiphylline is weaker than that of theophylline, possibly in part due to its poor bioavailability. Theophylline was considered the only xanthine clinically useful for the oral treatment of bronchial asthma.— C. Vazquez *et al.* (letter), *Lancet*, 1984, *1*, 914. Data from an earlier double-blind placebo-controlled study in 13 asthmatic patients given a dose of etamiphylline 100 mg by mouth also contained no evidence of a bronchodilatory effect and no human pharmacokinetic data were available.— G. J. Addis (letter), *ibid.*, 1083.

Preparations

Etamiphylline Injection *(B.P.)*. Etamiphylline Camsylate Injection

Etamiphylline Suppositories *(B.P.)*. Etamiphylline Camsylate Suppositories

Proprietary Names and Manufacturers of Etamiphylline Salts

Boifilina *(Boi, Spain)*; Camphophyline *(Fr.)*; Iodafilina *(Boi, Spain)*; Iodaphyline *(Millot-Solac, Fr.)*; Millophyline *(Martindale Pharmaceuticals, UK)*; Solufilina *(Boi, Spain)*.

635-m

Etofylline *(BAN, rINN)*.

Aethophyllinum; Etofyllinum; Hydroxyaethyltheophyllinum; Hydroxyéthylthéophylline; Oxyetophylline. 7-(2-Hydroxyethyl)-1,3-dimethylxanthine; 7-(2-Hydroxyethyl)theophylline.

$C_9H_{12}N_4O_3$=224.2.

CAS — 519-37-9.

Pharmacopoeias. In *Aust., Br., Cz., Eur., Fr., Ger., Ind., Neth.,* and *Swiss.*

A white crystalline powder.

Soluble in water; slightly soluble in alcohol; sparingly soluble in chloroform; practically insoluble in ether. **Store** in well-closed containers and protect from light.

Etofylline is a theophylline derivative and is used in doses ranging up to 0.5 g daily for the same purposes as theophylline (see p.1532). It does not liberate theophylline in the body. It is given by mouth and by intramuscular injection and has also been given by slow intravenous injection. It may be given by rectum as suppositories.

Proprietary Names and Manufacturers of Etophylline and its Salts

Bio-Phyllin *(Bio-Chemical Laboratory, Canad.)*; De-Oxin *(Berenguer-Beneyto, Spain)*; Dilaphyllin *(Streuli, Switz.)*; Hesotin *(Lannacher, Denm.; Malesci, Ital.)*; Oxyphylline *(Amido, Fr.)*; Theostat *(MPS Lab., S.Afr.)*.

636-b

Heptaminol Acephyllinate

Acéfyllinate d'Heptaminol; Heptaminol Theophylline Ethanoate; Heptaminol Theophylline-7-acetate. The 6-amino-2-methylheptan-2-ol salt of theophyllin-7-ylacetic acid.

$C_8H_{19}NO,C_9H_{10}N_4O_4$=383.4.

CAS — 5152-72-7; 10075-18-0.

Heptaminol acephyllinate is a theophylline derivative with uses similar to those of theophylline (see p.1532). Heptaminol acephyllinate is poorly absorbed from the gastro-intestinal tract and does not liberate theophylline in the body. It has been administered by mouth in doses of up to 3 g daily. It has also been given by intramuscular or slow intravenous injection.

Proprietary Names and Manufacturers

Cariamyl *(Carrion, Fr.; Clin-Midy, Spain; Delalande, Switz.)*; Corophylline *(Fisons, Fr.)*; Funesil *(Spain)*; Theo-Heptylon *(Delalande, Ger.)*.

13117-r

Pimefylline Nicotinate *(rINNM).*
7-[2-(3-Pyridylmethylamino)ethyl]theophylline pyridine-3-carboxylate.
$C_{15}H_{18}N_6O_2,C_6H_4NO_2$=436.5.

CAS — 10001-43-1 (pimefylline); 10058-07-8 (nicotinate).

Pimefylline nicotinate has been used in the treatment of cardiovascular disorders.

Proprietary Names and Manufacturers
Teonicon *(Neopharmed, Ital.).*

13183-p

Protheobromine *(rINN).*
3,7-Dihydro-1-(2-hydroxypropyl)-3,7-dimethylpurine-2,6(1*H*)-dione.
$C_{10}H_{14}N_4O_3$=238.2.

CAS — 50-39-5.

Protheobromine is a derivative of theobromine and has been used for its diuretic and vasodilating properties.

Proprietary Names and Manufacturers
Idromin *(Arnaldi, Ital.)*; Tebe *(Simes, Ital.)*; Tebesimes *(Farmasimes, Spain)*; Teocorin *(Ital.)*; Thebes *(Sintesa, Belg.).*

640-d

Proxyphylline *(BAN, rINN).*
Proxyphyllinum. 7-(2-Hydroxypropyl)-1,3-dimethylxanthine; 7-(2-Hydroxypropyl)theophylline.
$C_{10}H_{14}N_4O_3$=238.2.

CAS — 603-00-9.

Pharmacopoeias. In *Aust., Br., Eur., Fr., Ger., Neth., Nord.*, and *Swiss.*

A white crystalline powder. Very **soluble** in water; soluble in alcohol; freely soluble in chloroform; slightly soluble in ether. **Store** in well-closed containers. Protect from light.

Proxyphylline is a theophylline derivative which is used similarly to theophylline (see p.1532), but it is reported to be better tolerated by mouth. Proxyphylline is readily absorbed from the gastro-intestinal tract and it does not liberate theophylline in the body. The usual dose by mouth is 300 mg three times daily but larger doses may be given. It has been given by intramuscular or slow intravenous injection in doses of 300 to 400 mg and is given rectally as suppositories containing 500 mg.

ABSORPTION AND FATE. The biological half-life of proxyphylline was reported to be 4.3 hours.— W. A. Ritschel, *Drug Intell. & clin. Pharm.*, 1970, *4*, 332.

In healthy volunteers a mean peak plasma concentration of about 7 µg per mL was obtained about 30 minutes after a 300 mg dose by mouth. After 400 mg thrice daily for 5 days the mean peak plasma concentration was 18 µg per mL. About 25% of a given dose was excreted unchanged in the urine; the excretion half-life was about 6.5 hours (range 4.8 to 9.2).— C. Graffner *et al., Acta pharm. suec.*, 1973, *10*, 425.

The elimination of proxyphylline and its metabolites.— K. Selvig, *Br. J. clin. Pharmac.*, 1982, *14*, 608P.

ASTHMA. Proxyphylline 300 mg by mouth was no more effective than a placebo in reducing asthmatic airway obstruction in 12 patients.— K. N. V. Palmer *et al.* (letter), *Br. med. J.*, 1971, *1*, 727.

In a double-blind, placebo-controlled study in 10 asthmatic patients given sustained-release theophylline 400 mg twice daily by mouth or sustained-release proxyphylline 1200 mg twice daily by mouth, there were no significant differences between the treatments with regard to asthmatic symptoms, need for additional medication, or incidence and intensity of side-effects.— H. Mosbech *et al., Pharmatherapeutica*, 1984, *3*, 626.

Proprietary Names and Manufacturers
Brontyl 300 *(Lloyd-Hamol, Reckitt & Colman Pharm., UK)*; Monophyllin *(Norw.)*; Neofyllin *(Pharmacia, Denm.)*; Pantafillina *(Ceccarelli, Ital.)*; Proxy-Retardoral *(Artesan, Ger.)*; Purophyllin *(Siegfried, Switz.)*; Spantin *(Pharmacia, Ger.)*; Spasmolysin *(Kade, Ger.)*; Thean *(Lagap, UK)*; Theon *(Draco, Swed.).*

641-n

Pyridofylline *(rINN).*
Pyridophylline; Pyridoxine *O*-(Theophyllin-7-ylethyl)sulphate. 3-Hydroxy-4,5-bis(hydroxymethyl)-2-methylpyridine 2-(theophyllin-7-yl)ethyl sulphate.
$C_{17}H_{23}N_5O_9S$=473.5.

CAS — 53403-97-7.

Pyridofylline is a theophylline derivative which has been used for purposes similar to those of theophylline (see p.1532).

Proprietary Names and Manufacturers
Athérophylline *(Merrell, Fr.).*

13293-j

Suxamidofylline
7-[2-(3-Diethylcarbamoylpropionyloxy)ethyl]theophylline.
$C_{17}H_{25}N_5O_5$=379.4.

CAS — 12712-75-3.

Suxamidofylline is a derivative of theophylline which has been used similarly to theophylline (see p.1532).

Proprietary Names and Manufacturers
Argecor *(Farge, Ital.)*; Cardiodest *(Biotrading, Ital.).*

643-m

Theobromine *(BAN).*
Santheose; Theobrominum. 3,7-Dihydro-3,7-dimethylpurine-2,6(1*H*)-dione; 3,7-Dimethylxanthine.
$C_7H_8N_4O_2$=180.2.

CAS — 83-67-0.

Pharmacopoeias. In *Arg., Aust., Belg., Br., Braz., Cz., Egypt., Eur., Fr., Ger., Hung., Jug., Mex., Neth., Pol., Port., Roum., Rus., Span.*, and *Swiss.*

A white odourless powder.
Very slightly **soluble** in water, in alcohol, and in chloroform; practically insoluble in ether; slightly soluble in aqueous ammonia. It dissolves in dilute solutions of alkali hydroxides and in mineral acids.

Theobromine has the general properties of the other xanthines (see p.1521). It has a weaker diuretic activity than theophylline and is also a less powerful stimulant of smooth muscle. It has practically no stimulant effect on the central nervous system. Large doses can cause nausea and vomiting. Theobromine was formerly used as a diuretic and in the treatment of angina pectoris and hypertension, but more effective treatment is now available. Theobromine and calcium salicylate (theosalicin), theobromine and sodium acetate, and theobromine and sodium salicylate (themisalum, theobromsal) have all been used similarly to theobromine.
Theobromine is the chief xanthine in the beverage cocoa which may contain more than 200 mg per cup. It is also present in tea and chocolate. Theobroma oil may contain up to 2% theobromine.

ABSORPTION AND FATE. The pharmacokinetics and metabolic disposition of theobromine.— S. M. Tarka *et al., Clin. Pharmac. Ther.*, 1983, *34*, 546.

ASTHMA. In a double-blind study 21 asthmatic patients were given theobromine 10 mg per kg body-weight or theophylline 5 mg per kg by mouth. Both treatments significantly improved lung function, but there was no significant difference between treatments. It was recommended that patients avoid the ingestion of theobromine during investigations of bronchodilators and that people who regularly ingest large amounts of theobromine in chocolate or cocoa should be excluded from long-term clinical studies of anti-asthmatic medications.— F. E. R. Simons *et al., J. Allergy & clin. Immunol.*, 1985, *76*, 703.

PREGNANCY AND THE NEONATE. It was reported that theobromine passed into the breast milk of 6 nursing mothers who had eaten 4 ounces of chocolate containing about 240 mg of theobromine.— B. H. Resman *et al.*, Seventy-eighth Annual Meeting of the American Society for Clinical Pharmacology and Therapeutics,, per *Clin. Pharmac. Ther.*, 1977, *21*, 115. See also *idem, J. Pediat.*, 1977, *91*, 477.

Proprietary Names and Manufacturers
Théosalvose *(Techni-Pharma, Mon.).*

The following names have been used for multi-ingredient preparations containing theobromine—Hypotensive Dellipsoids D 8 *(Pilsworth, UK)*; Riddospas *(Riddell, UK)*; Riddovydrin Elixir *(Riddell, UK)*; Seominal *(Winthrop, UK)*; Theogardenal *(May & Baker, UK)*; Theominal *(Winthrop, UK).*

647-q

Theophylline *(BAN, USAN).*

Anhydrous Theophylline; Teofilina; Theophyll.; Theophyllinum. 3,7-Dihydro-1,3-dimethylpurine-2,6(1*H*)-dione; 1,3-Dimethylxanthine.
$C_7H_8N_4O_2$=180.2.

CAS — 58-55-9.

Pharmacopoeias. In *Aust., Br., Egypt., Eur., Fr., Ger., Hung., Ind., Int., It., Jpn, Neth., Pol., Swiss, Turk.*, and *U.S.*

A white odourless crystalline powder.
B.P. **solubilities** are: soluble 1 in 80 of alcohol; slightly soluble in water and in chloroform; very slightly soluble in ether. Dissolves in solutions of alkali hydroxides, in aqueous ammonia, and in mineral acids. *U.S.P.* solubilities are: slightly soluble in water, more soluble in hot water; sparingly soluble in alcohol, in chloroform, and in ether; freely soluble in solutions of alkali hydroxides, and in ammonia. **Store** in well-closed containers.

648-p

Theophylline Hydrate *(BAN).*

Theophylline *(USAN)*; Theophylline Monohydrate; Theophyllinum Monohydricum.
$C_7H_8N_4O_2,H_2O$=198.2.

CAS — 5967-84-0.

Pharmacopoeias. In *Arg., Aust., Belg., Br., Braz., Chin., Cz., Egypt., Eur., Fr., Ger., Ind., It., Jug., Mex., Neth., Nord., Pol., Roum., Rus., Span., Swiss, Turk.*, and *U.S.*

Store in well-closed containers.

SOLUBILITY. The solubility of theophylline at 25° increased from 8 mg per mL in water to 8.3 mg per mL in 30% w/w sucrose solution. A further increase in sucrose concentration to that of syrup decreased the solubility to 6.2 mg per mL.— A. N. Paruta and B. B. Sheth, *J. pharm. Sci.*, 1966, *55*, 896.

STABILITY. The stability of theophylline in polypropylene and glass containers.— J. M. Christensen *et al., Am. J. Hosp. Pharm.*, 1983, *40*, 612 and 1663.

Adverse Effects

The side-effects commonly encountered with theophylline and its derivatives irrespective of the route of administration, are gastro-intestinal irritation and stimulation of the central nervous system.
Theophylline may cause nausea, vomiting, abdominal pain, gastro-intestinal bleeding, insomnia, headache, anxiety, restlessness, vertigo, and palpitations. Severe overdosage or idiosyncrasy may also lead to maniacal behaviour, diuresis and repeated vomiting with extreme thirst, tremor, delirium, hyperthermia, tachycardia, tachypnoea, electrolyte disturbances, convulsions, and death. Convulsions may not be preceded by milder symptoms of toxicity. Hypotension may follow intravenous injection, particularly if the injection is too rapid, and sudden deaths have been reported. Proctitis may follow repeated administration of aminophylline suppositories and intramuscular injections are painful, the pain lasting several hours.
Plasma concentrations of theophylline greater than 20 µg per mL are considered to be toxic.

For correlation of theophylline serum concentrations with adverse effects, see Serum Concentrations under Absorption and Fate, below.

ALLERGY. In the past 20 years, 31% of adverse reactions to aminophylline reported to the Committee on Safety of Medicines were of cutaneous or allergic origin compared with 12% with theophylline (*Lancet*, 1984, *2*, 1192). Aminophylline given intravenously or applied topically produces both immediate and delayed hypersensitivity reactions, but such reactions are much less frequent when aminophylline is given by mouth (C. Boroda and A.J. Miller, *ibid.*, 1985, *1* 289). Delayed-type hypersensitivity reactions to aminophylline are due to the ethylenediamine component; there are no reports of delayed-type hypersensitivity reactions to anhydrous theophylline. However, a proportion of immediate-type reactions are due to theophylline alone (W.R.G. Gibb, *ibid.*, 49).

Reports of allergic reactions to aminophylline or theophylline: D. Wong *et al.*, *J. Allergy & clin. Immunol.*, 1971, *48*, 165; A. E. Fishman, *Ann. Allergy*, 1974, *33*, 161; B. H. Booth *et al.*, *ibid.*, 1979, *43*, 289; C. Hardy *et al.*, *Br. med. J.*, 1983, *286*, 2051; Z. Mohsenifar *et al.*, *Ann. Allergy*, 1982, *49*, 281; D. W. Nierenberg and F. S. Glazener, *West. J. Med.*, 1982, *137*, 328; S. Mendel *et al.*, *Clin. Pharm.*, 1985, *4*, 334.

EFFECTS ON THE BREAST. Gynaecomastia occurred in a 61-year-old man after one to two months of oral theophylline therapy and resolved within one month of discontinuation.— K. R. Dardick, *J. fam. Pract.*, 1984, *18*, 141.

EFFECTS ON THE GASTRO-INTESTINAL TRACT. *Necrotising enterocolitis.* For a study suggesting that theophylline does not contribute to the development of neonatal necrotising enterocolitis, see under Pregnancy and the neonate, below.

Oesophageal ulceration. Oesophageal erosion and ulceration have been reported in patients taking theophylline (R.W. Enzenauer *et al.*, *New Engl. J. Med.*, 1984, *310*, 261) and aminophylline tablets (J.L. Stoller, *Lancet*, 1985, *2*, 328) at bedtime and without any accompanying fluid.

EFFECTS ON THE HEART. *Arrhythmias.* Theophylline can precipitate sinus tachycardia, atrial, and ventricular premature contractions at therapeutic serum theophylline concentrations (G.W. Josephson *et al.*, *Chest*, 1980, *78*, 429) and in overdose (A. Greenberg *et al.*, *Am. J. Med.*, 1984, *76*, 854). Multifocal atrial tachycardia has also been associated with both theophylline overdose (A. Greenberg *et al.*, 1984) and serum theophylline concentrations within the generally accepted range of 10 to 20 µg per mL (J.H. Levine *et al.*, *Lancet*, 1985, *1*, 12). Combined oral administration of theophylline with beta adrenoceptor stimulants does not increase the incidence of arrhythmias compared with the administration of theophylline alone (J.J. Coleman *et al.*, *Chest*, 1986, *90*, 45; T.-B. Conradson *et al.*, *ibid.*, 1987, *91*, 5).

Myocarditis. Theophylline could cause toxic myocarditis.— *Lancet*, 1985, *2*, 1165.

EFFECTS ON MENTAL FUNCTION. *Depression.* Paradoxical depression associated with the use of theophylline in 2 patients.— M. B. Murphy *et al.*, *Br. med. J.*, 1980, *281*, 1322.

Learning and behaviour problems. Studies in children suggest that theophylline therapy may be associated with learning and behaviour problems (C.T. Furukawa *et al.*, *Lancet*, 1984, *1*, 621), particularly in those with lower intelligence quotients (C. Springer *et al.*, *J. Allergy & clin. Immunol.*, 1985, *76*, 64). Depression induced by theophylline has been proposed as an explanation for these observations (R.A. Brumback *et al.*, *Lancet*, 1984, *1*, 958).

For reports of aminophylline and theophylline overdosage causing behaviour disorders and symptoms simulating dementia in the elderly, see under Overdosage, below.

EFFECTS ON THE NERVOUS SYSTEM. *Convulsions.* Generalised convulsions occurred in 8 patients, 4 of whom died, whilst receiving aminophylline intravenously in a mean dose of 34 mg per kg body-weight daily. This effect was correlated with a mean serum-theophylline concentration of 53 µg per mL. Four further patients with less serious side-effects had a mean serum-theophylline concentration of 35 µg per mL compared with a mean of 19 µg per mL in 15 patients with no side-effects. Hepatic dysfunction in 11 of the 12 patients with side-effects and high doses contributed to the high serum-theophylline concentrations.— C. W. Zwillich *et al.*, *Ann. intern. Med.*, 1975, *82*, 784. See also M. H. Jacobs and R. M. Senior, *Am. Rev. resp. Dis.*, 1974, *110*, 342; P. R. Yarnell and N. -S. Chu, *Neurology*, 1975, *25*, 819.

The Boston Collaborative Drug Surveillance Program reported that drug-induced convulsions occurred in 2 of 2870 patients given aminophylline.— J. Porter and H. Jick, *Lancet*, 1977, *1*, 587.

Spasticity. A patient with an ischaemic cerebrovascular accident experienced notable exacerbation of spasticity and pain in his hemiplegic limbs within 36 hours of commencing theophylline therapy. Restitution of limb motion and resolution of pain occurred within 48 hours of discontinuing theophylline.— J. E. Clark and J. K. Devenport, *J. Am. med. Ass.*, 1983, *250*, 485.

Speech disturbances. A report of stammering in a 4-year-old boy undergoing oral treatment with theophylline.— M. M. McCarthy (letter), *Pediatrics*, 1981, *68*, 749.

EFFECTS ON SERUM ELECTROLYTE AND GLUCOSE HOMOEOSTASIS. In a study of 7 patients with chronic obstructive pulmonary disease given an intravenous infusion of theophylline to produce a mean plasma-theophylline concentration of 12.5 µg per mL, mean plasma-potassium concentration fell from a pre-infusion level of 3.88 mmol per litre to 3.58 mmol per litre one hour after the infusion. Potassium concentrations 2 and 4 hours after infusion were still below pre-infusion levels and 4 patients became hypokalaemic (plasma potassium below 3.40 mmol per litre). Plasma-phosphate and plasma-sodium concentrations also fell after the infusion, but magnesium and calcium concentrations did not change significantly.— F. A. Zantvoort *et al.*, *Ann. intern. Med.*, 1986, *104*, 134.

For reports of hypokalaemia, hypophosphataemia, hypercalcaemia, hyperglycaemia, and metabolic acidosis following theophylline overdose, see under Overdosage, below.

For a report of hyperglycaemia in neonates following therapeutic doses of aminophylline and theophylline, see under Pregnancy and the Neonate, below.

Hyperuricaemia. In a study of 112 asthmatic patients receiving sustained-release theophylline 200 to 400 mg 12-hourly, there was a significant correlation of serum-uric-acid concentrations and serum-theophylline concentrations.— Y. Morita *et al.*, *J. Allergy & clin. Immunol.*, 1984, *74*, 707.

Lactic acidosis. Lactic acidosis occurred in a 22-year-old woman treated with intravenous theophylline, inhaled orciprenaline, and intravenous methylprednisolone sodium succinate. It was suggested that theophylline could potentiate the lactate-producing effects of beta-adrenergic agents by raising intracellular cyclic AMP levels through phosphodiesterase inhibition.— G. L. Braden *et al.*, *New Engl. J. Med.*, 1985, *313*, 890.

EFFECTS ON THE SKIN. For reports of cutaneous allergic reactions to theophylline and aminophylline, see under Allergy, above.

EFFECTS ON THE URINARY TRACT. Theophylline was associated with urinary retention in 2 middle-aged men with evidence of prostatic enlargement.— G. R. Owens and R. Tannenbaum (letter), *Ann. intern. Med.*, 1981, *94*, 212. See also: M. Prakash and J. D. Washburne (letter), *ibid.*, 823; S. N. Hassan (letter), *Sth. med. J.*, 1983, *76*, 408.

Renal failure. For a report of rhabdomyolysis-induced acute renal failure occurring after aminophylline overdose, see under Overdosage, below.

OVERDOSAGE. Reviews of the clinical features of theophylline overdosage: A. Greenberg *et al.*, *Am. J. Med.*, 1984, *76*, 854; D. A. R. Boldy *et al.*, *J. clin. Hosp. Pharm.*, 1984, *9*, 147; *Lancet*, 1985, *1*, 146; J. A. Vale, *Prescribers' J.*, 1986, *26*, 107; P. Gaudreault and J. Guay, *Med. Toxicol.*, 1986, *1*, 169.

Episodic, bizarre behaviour was the principal manifestation of theophylline toxicity in a 58-year-old woman.— W. G. Wasser *et al.*, *Ann. intern. Med.*, 1981, *95*, 191.

Three elderly women who had taken excessive amounts of aminophylline had symptoms simulating dementia.— I. Drummond, *Br. med. J.*, 1982, *285*, 779.

In a 53-year-old man, fatal theophylline overdose simulated the clinical picture of acute pancreatitis and produced appreciably raised serum amylase activity, although the pancreas was normal at necropsy.— T. H. S. Burgan *et al.*, *Br. med. J.*, 1982, *284*, 939.

Massive overdoses of sustained-release aminophylline and salbutamol together had no important cardiac effects in a 26-year-old man.— K. F. Whyte and G. J. Addis (letter), *Lancet*, 1983, *2*, 618.

A marked, transient hypokalaemia is a frequent complication of theophylline poisoning and may be a major factor in the genesis of dysrhythmias and possibly of convulsions. Observations indicated that urinary excretion of potassium is not increased in theophylline poisoning and that theophylline probably causes the redistribution of potassium into cells at the expense of the extracellular pool.— B. M. Buckley *et al.* (letter), *Lancet*, 1983, *2*, 618.

In a retrospective analysis of 22 cases of theophylline poisoning hypokalaemia, hyperglycaemia, and leucocytosis were frequent findings, and respiratory alkalosis, hypophosphataemia, and hypomagnesaemia were also common.— K. W. Hall *et al.*, *Ann. intern. Med.*, 1984, *101*, 457.

Rhabdomyolysis-induced acute renal failure with profound hypocalcaemia occurred in a 19-year-old woman after an overdose of oral aminophylline (J.B. Macdonald *et al.*, *Lancet*, 1985, *1*, 932). Similar cases suggested that theophylline-induced hypokalaemia and generalised convulsions were important in the pathogenesis of the observed rhabdomyolysis (K.W. Rumpf *et al.*, *ibid.*, 1451; K.B. Modi *et al.*, *ibid.*, *2*, 160).

Hypokalaemia, hypophosphataemia, hyperglycaemia, metabolic acidosis, and hypotension associated with serum-theophylline concentrations of 43.9 to 175 µg per mL were observed in a 16-year-old girl after ingesting 12 g of a sustained-release theophylline preparation. These findings and data from *animal* studies suggested that theophylline toxicity may be mediated by the beta-adrenergic system.— T. Kearney *et al.*, *Ann. intern. Med.*, 1985, *102*, 766. A similar case.— D. C. Pagniez *et al.* (letter), *ibid.*, 1986, *104*, 284.

Eleven of 60 patients hospitalised with theophylline toxicity had hypercalcaemia. Serum-calcium concentrations returned to normal as theophylline concentrations fell to therapeutic or subtherapeutic levels. A significant increase in serum calcium associated with therapeutic serum-theophylline concentrations in normal volunteers was reversed by propranolol.— M. L. McPherson *et al.*, *Ann. intern. Med.*, 1986, *105*, 52.

For the use of beta-adrenoceptor blocking agents in the management of theophylline toxicity, see under Treatment of Adverse Effects, below.

A 64-year-old woman who died following an overdose of sustained-release aminophylline tablets despite gastric lavage was found at necropsy to have a pale, compacted mass of tablets in the stomach containing the equivalent of 3.3 g of theophylline. Such bezoar formation may explain why side-effects of poisoning may suddenly appear some hours after ingestion and why a secondary rise in theophylline concentration occurs.— M. Coupe, *Hum. Toxicol.*, 1986, *5*, 341.

For recommendations to use endoscopy to remove bezoars following overdosage with sustained-release aminophylline or theophylline tablets, see under Treatment of Adverse Effects, below.

PREGNANCY AND THE NEONATE. For a report suggesting that theophylline is not teratogenic, see Pregnancy and the Neonate under Uses and Administration, below.

For reports of irritability and other symptoms occurring in neonates and breast-fed infants whose mothers were taking aminophylline or theophylline, see Pregnancy and the Neonate under Absorption and Fate, below.

Hyperglycaemia. In 29 preterm infants, mean plasma-glucose concentrations were significantly higher after treatment with intravenous aminophylline and oral theophylline than in those not treated. Two of 15 treated infants developed clinically significant hyperglycaemia and glycosuria.— G. Srinivasan *et al.*, *J. Pediat.*, 1983, *103*, 473.

Necrotising enterocolitis. Although there have been reports of necrotising enterocolitis in neonates associated with oral theophylline and aminophylline administration (M.J. Robinson *et al.*, *Archs Dis. Childh.*, 1980, *55*, 494; A.J. Williams, *ibid.*, 973), a study of 275 infants concluded that theophylline did not significantly contribute to its development (J.M. Davis *et al.*, *J. Pediat.*, 1986, *109*, 344). It has been suggested that the high osmolality of liquid feeds and drugs including oral theophylline preparations may be involved in the aetiology of necrotising enterocolitis (M. Watkinson *et al.*, *Pharm. J.*, 1987, *2*, 488).

Reflux oesophagitis. For a report of increased gastro-oesophageal reflux in infants receiving theophylline, see Pregnancy and the Neonate under Precautions, below.

Withdrawal syndromes. Episodes of apnoea occurred 28 hours after birth in a neonate whose mother had taken aminophylline and theophylline throughout pregnancy. Administration of theophylline to the infant resulted in resolution of apnoea, and treatment was discontinued after 4 months.— D. A. Horowitz and W. Jablonski, *Am. J. Dis. Child.*, 1982, *136*, 73.

Treatment of Adverse Effects

After theophylline or aminophylline overdosage by mouth the stomach should be emptied by emesis, or gastric aspiration and lavage; enemas may be used for overdosage by rectum. Activated charcoal should be given by mouth; repeated doses have been recommended. A saline laxative may also be given, especially if slow-release preparations have been taken. Metabolic abnormalities, particularly hypokalaemia, should be corrected and convulsions controlled by the intravenous administration of diazepam. Charcoal haemoperfusion and haemodialysis are effective if the above measures fail.

Reviews of the treatment of theophylline overdose: A. Greenberg *et al.*, *Am. J. Med.*, 1984, *76*, 854; D. A. R. Boldy *et al.*, *J. clin. Hosp. Pharm.*, 1984, *9*, 147; *Lancet*, 1985, *1*, 146; J. A. Vale, *Prescribers' J.*, 1986, *26*, 107; P. Gaudreault and J. Guay, *Med. Toxicol.*, 1986, *1*, 169.

Every theophylline overdose should be regarded as potentially fatal and all patients should be closely monitored. Serial plasma-theophylline concentrations provide much more information than a single value. The concentrations may rise up to 24 hours after an overdose so an early low value may be misleading. The vast majority of theophylline overdoses will respond to supportive measures. Prompt correction of any hypokalaemia will usually be the most aggressive treatment required. The commonly associated sinus tachycardia rarely requires treatment. Non-selective beta-blockers may be helpful in non-asthmatic patients in counteracting the cardiovascular and metabolic toxicity in theophylline overdose, but should not be given to asthmatics. Verapamil has been used effectively for supraventricular tachycardias after theophylline overdose. Active elimination procedures should be reserved for patients who have not responded to supportive measures.— T. Mant *et al.*, *Br. med. J.*, 1984, *289*, 1133.

Gastric lavage or emesis should be performed if more than 2.5 g of theophylline has been ingested (or over 500 mg for small children) within the previous 4 hours (or 8 hours if a delayed release preparation has been taken).— J. Henry and G. Volans, *Br. med. J.*, 1984, *289*, 304.

ACTIVATED CHARCOAL. Oral activated charcoal has been shown to reduce the gastro-intestinal absorption of aminophylline (P.J. Neuvonen *et al.*, *Eur. J. clin. Pharmac.*, 1983, *24*, 557), and repeated oral doses of activated charcoal enhance the non-renal clearance, and decrease the serum half-life of theophylline (W.G. Berlinger *et al.*, *Clin. Pharmac. Ther.*, 1983, *33*, 351; C.K. Mahutte *et al.*, *Am. Rev. resp. Dis.*, 1983, *128*, 820; L. Radomski *et al.*, *Clin. Pharmac. Ther.*, 1984, *35*, 402). The decrease in theophylline serum half-life is affected by the activated charcoal dosage regimen used (G.D. Park *et al.*, *ibid.*, 1983, *34*, 663) and the surface area of the activated charcoal (G.D. Park *et al.*, *J. Clin. Pharmac.*, 1984, *24*, 289). Work in *animals* has suggested that although the serum half-life of theophylline is decreased, the time for serum-theophylline concentrations to fall below toxic levels is not affected (R.E. Brashear and G.R. Aronoff, *ibid.*, 1985, *25*, 460), but nonetheless, in cases of overdosage with oral theophylline preparations the use of repeated oral activated charcoal has resulted in a reduction of serum-theophylline concentrations and resolution of signs of toxicity (C.K. Mahutte *et al.*, 1983; L. Radomski *et al.*, 1984; A.N. Laggner *et al.*, *Br. med. J.*, 1984, *288*, 1497; P. Gal *et al.*, *J. Am. med. Ass.*, 1984, *251*, 3130). The use of repeated oral doses of activated charcoal for theophylline poisoning has been suggested where haemoperfusion is unavailable (P. Gal *et al.*, 1984; K.F. Whyte and G.J. Addis, *Br. med. J.*, 1984, *288*, 1835) since activated charcoal is as, or more, effective than haemodialysis and, in some cases, has given clearances approaching those obtained with haemoperfusion (A. Heath and K. Knudsen, *Med. Toxicol.*, 1987, *2*, 294). However, administration of activated charcoal may be difficult in severely poisoned patients because of persistent centrally-induced vomiting which can seldom be ameliorated even by substantial doses of anti-emetics (J.A. Vale, *Prescribers' J.*, 1986, *26*, 107). Ranitidine and droperidol have been used successfully to control theophylline-induced vomiting, allowing the use of activated charcoal (Y. Amitai *et al.*, *Ann. intern. Med.*, 1986, *105*, 386). The addition of sorbitol to an oral regimen of multiple doses of activated charcoal decreased serum-theophylline concentrations to a greater extent than did the activated charcoal alone (M.J. Goldberg *et al.*, *Clin. Pharmac. Ther.*, 1987, *41*, 108).

BETA ADRENOCEPTOR BLOCKING AGENTS. Propranolol has been used as an anti-arrhythmic in theophylline overdosage (A. Greenberg *et al.*, *Am. J. Med.*, 1984, *76*, 854). During the infusion of propranolol in 2 non-asthmatic patients with hyperglycaemia, hypokalaemia, tachycardia, and hypotension following theophylline overdose, plasma glucose fell, plasma potassium increased, the pulse rate fell, and blood pressure rose. It was suggested that beta-adrenergic blockade may be of benefit in the management of the metabolic changes of theophylline poisoning, especially in the non-asthmatic patient, and possibly also in the asthmatic patient with severe hypokalaemia or cardiac arrhythmias if mechanical ventilation was available (T.E. Kearney *et al.*, *Ann. intern. Med.*, 1985, *102*, 766; D.N. Amin and J.A. Henry, *Lancet*, 1985, *1*, 520). Farrar and Dunn (*ibid.*, 983) suggested that since propranolol reduced the clearance of theophylline, a water-soluble, non-selective beta-blocker, such as sotalol or nadolol, may be more appropriate.

For reports of propranolol decreasing the clearance of theophylline, see Interactions under Precautions, below.

ENDOSCOPY. Worsening symptoms of toxicity and a rising serum-theophylline concentration occuring in an 18-year-old woman after an overdose of sustained-release theophylline tablets did not respond to gastric lavage and oral activated charcoal. Endoscopy revealed a friable bolus of congealed tablets in the stomach, and endoscopic removal of this bezoar, followed by irrigation of the stomach and the administration of mannitol 1% solution by mouth resulted in abatement of symptoms and a fall in serum-theophylline concentration. An intragastric aggregation of sustained-release tablets with gradual leaching of active drug may delay absorption and prolong the duration of toxicity.— J. -M. Cereda *et al.*, *Br. med. J.*, 1986, *293*, 1143. Bezoar formation by agents such as sustained-release theophylline taken in overdose is more common than generally realised. Of 11 patients admitted with a theophylline overdose, one vomited a bezoar, 2 had bezoars removed at gastroscopy, and one was found to have a bezoar at necropsy. Gastroscopy should be performed early in patients with clinical and laboratory evidence of serious poisoning, particularly if there are signs of serious poisoning.— W. D. F. Smith (letter), *ibid.*, 1987, *294*, 125. The administration of intravenous propranolol after overdose of a sustained-release theophylline preparation may make subsequent endoscopy a lot less hazardous. Endoscopy might be inappropriate or unsafe in patients taking theophylline for reversible airways obstruction when ingestion of only a small amount of the drug had caused severe symptoms. Propranolol administration may benefit these patients despite the risk of bronchospasm.— T. M. E. Davis and J. Nicholls (letter), *ibid.*

H_2 ANTAGONIST ANTIHISTAMINES. Gastro-intestinal haemorrhage may follow theophylline-induced peptic ulceration and for this reason H_2 receptor antagonists have sometimes been used prophylactically though efficacy is unproven. Cimetidine inhibits theophylline metabolism, increasing toxicity and hence ranitidine is indicated.— J. A. Vale, *Prescribers' J.*, 1986, *26*, 107.

HAEMODIALYSIS AND HAEMOPERFUSION. A review of extracorporeal theophylline removal techniques. Neither peritoneal dialysis nor exchange transfusion produced a significant increase in the total body clearance of theophylline, whereas haemodialysis could be expected to double clearance, and haemoperfusion results in 4- to 6-fold increases in clearance. Charcoal haemoperfusion should be considered if the plasma-theophylline concentration exceeds 100 μg per mL in an acute intoxication, or 60 μg per mL in chronic overdose (40 μg per mL if there is significant respiratory or heart failure, or liver disease), or if there is intractable vomiting, arrhythmias, or seizures. In most patients a 4-hour haemoperfusion allows significant clinical improvement, but treatment should continue until plasma concentrations are below 15 μg per mL. Plasma concentrations should be followed at least every 4 hours for the first 12 hours post-perfusion, as rebound increases have been noted on terminating perfusion. Haemodialysis may rarely be an alternative if haemoperfusion is not available, or in series with haemoperfusion if significant rhabdomyolysis is present.— A. Heath and K. Knudsen, *Med. Toxicol.*, 1987, *2*, 294.

Reports of the successful use of charcoal haemoperfusion: S. M. Ehlers *et al.*, *J. Am. med. Ass.*, 1978, *240*, 474; M. E. Russo, *New Engl. J. Med.*, 1979, *300*, 24; D. B. Jefferys *et al.*, *Br. med. J.*, 1980, *280*, 1167; S. Sahney *et al.*, *Pediatrics*, 1983, *71*, 615; R. G. van Kesteren *et al.*, *Hum. Toxicol.*, 1985, *4*, 127.

Precautions

Theophylline or aminophylline should be given with caution to patients with peptic ulceration, hyperthyroidism, hypertension, cardiac arrhythmias, or other cardiovascular disease, as these conditions may be exacerbated. Theophylline or aminophylline should also be given with caution to patients with congestive heart failure, hepatic dysfunction or chronic alcoholism, acute febrile illness, severe hypoxia, cor pulmonale, acute pulmonary oedema, or other chronic lung disease, and to neonates and the elderly, since in all of these circumstances theophylline clearance may be decreased, resulting in increases in serum-theophylline concentrations and serum half-life (see under Absorption and Fate, below).

The bronchodilator and toxic effects of theophylline or aminophylline and sympathomimetics or other xanthines are additive. Concomitant use with other xanthine medications should be avoided; if intravenous aminophylline is to be given, serum-theophylline concentrations should be measured first where possible.

Interaction with allopurinol, cimetidine, influenza vaccine, propranolol, erythromycin, and some other macrolides may result in decreased hepatic theophylline clearance and increased serum half-life, necessitating dosage reduction. Phenytoin and some other anticonvulsants, and cigarette smoking may increase theophylline clearance, necessitating an increase in dose or dosing frequency (see under Absorption and Fate, and also under Interactions, below).

Intravenous injections of theophylline or aminophylline must be administered very slowly to prevent dangerous central nervous system and cardiovascular side-effects resulting from the direct stimulant effect.

In view of the many factors affecting theophylline clearance, serum concentration monitoring is recommended to ensure concentrations are within the therapeutic range.

Patients should not be transferred from one sustained-release theophylline or aminophylline preparation to another without measuring serum-theophylline concentrations and clinical assessment because of bioavailability differences.

ECT. A 71-year-old woman with no history of seizures and with a serum-theophylline concentration slightly above the normal range (22.6 μg per mL) developed status epilepticus during electroconvulsive therapy.— S. G. Peters *et al.*, *Mayo Clin. Proc.*, 1984, *59*, 568.

INTERACTIONS, DRUGS. Reviews of drug interactions with theophylline and their mechanisms: J. H. G. Jonkman and R. A. Upton, *Clin. Pharmacokinet.*, 1984, *9*, 309; *Drug Interact. News.*, 1985, *5*, 41; H. W. Kelly, *ibid.*, 1986, *6*, 45.

Theophylline reduces liver plasma flow and may therefore prolong the half-life and increase steady-state levels of hepatically eliminated drugs.— J. Onrot *et al.*, *Clin. Pharmac. Ther.*, 1986, *40*, 506.

Antacids. Increases of up to 25% in peak serum-theophylline concentrations have been reported during concomitant oral administration of antacids (L.J. Darzentas *et al.*, *Drug Intell. & clin. Pharm.*, 1983, *17*, 555; K.I. Myhre and R.A. Walstad, *Br. J. clin. Pharmac.*, 1983, *15*, 683). The total absorption of theophylline does not seem to be affected (L.A. Arnold *et al.*, *Am. J. Hosp. Pharm.*, 1979, *36*, 1059; L. Shargel *et al.*, *J. Pharm. Sci.*, 1981, *70*, 599). In a study of asthmatic patients treated with oral theophylline or aminophylline, an intensive antacid regimen had no effect on steady-state bioavailability (R.C. Reed and H.J. Schwartz, *J. Pharmacokinet. Biopharm.*, 1984, *12*, 315).

Antibiotics. Some studies have found that erythromycin decreases the clearance of theophylline due to inhibition of its hepatic metabolism, resulting in increases of 30 to 100% in serum-theophylline concentrations and 21 to 56% prolongation of serum half-life (L.H. Cummins *et al.*, *Pediatrics*, 1977, *59*, 144; B.J.M. Zarowitz *et al.*, *Clin. Pharmac. Ther.*, 1981, *29*, 601; K.W. Renton *et al.*, *ibid.*, *30*, 422; D.C. May *et al.*, *J. clin. Pharmac.*, 1982, *22*, 125). Some have detected no interaction (M.S. Maddux *et al.*, *Chest*, 1982, *81*, 563; R. Hildebrandt *et al.*, *Eur. J. clin. Pharmac.*, 1984, *26*, 485), possibly due to the confounding effects of duration of erythromycin therapy, cigarette smoking, interpatient variability, erythromycin salt used, and age of patients (*Drug Interact. News.*, 1983, *3*, 13). It has also been noted that the serum concentrations and bioavailability of erythromycin may be reduced by theophylline (A. Iliopoulou *et al.*, *Br. J. clin. Pharmac.*, 1982, *14*, 495; O. Paulsen *et al.*, *Eur. J. clin. Pharmac.*, 1987, *32*, 493). An arbitary decrease in theophylline dose may not be justified for all patients receiving erythromycin, since many do not exhibit the interaction (T.M. Ludden, *Clin. Pharmacokinet.*, 1985, *10*, 63). The clearance of theophylline is also markedly decreased by the concomitant administration of triacetyloleandomycin (M. Weinberger *et al.*, *J. Allergy & clin. Immunol.*, 1977, *59*, 228; J.L. Brazier *et al.*, *Thérapie*, 1980, *35*, 545; J. Lavarenne *et al.*, *ibid.*, 1981, *36*, 451), but there have been reports that the pharmacokinetics of theophylline do not seem to be significantly altered by josamycin (J.L. Brazier *et al.*, 1980; F. Ruff *et al.*, *Nouv. Presse Méd.*, 1981, *10*,

175), midecamycin (J. Lavarenne *et al.*, 1981; N. Principi *et al.*, *Eur. J. clin. Pharmac.*, 1987, *31*, 701), or rokitamycin (T. Ishioka, *Acta ther.*, 1987, *13*, 17).

Serious nausea and vomiting, tachycardia, and headache, associated with unexpectedly high serum-theophylline concentrations, occurred after the administration of enoxacin by mouth to patients receiving theophylline (W.J.A. Wijnands *et al.*, *Lancet*, 1984, *2*, 108). Enoxacin markedly inhibits the metabolic clearance of theophylline, prolongs its serum half-life, and increases its serum concentrations. To avoid toxicity, a 40% reduction of theophylline dosage before starting enoxacin therapy is recommended (W.J.A. Wijnands *et al.*, *Br. J. clin. Pharmac.*, 1985, *20*, 583). Ciprofloxacin, ofloxacin, and pefloxacin also inhibit the metabolic clearance of theophylline, but to a lesser extent than enoxacin (*idem*, 1986, *22*, 677; D.E. Nix *et al.*, *J. antimicrob. Chemother.*, 1987, *19*, 263; S.L. Gregoire *et al.*, *Antimicrob. Ag. Chemother.*, 1987, *31*, 375). While there have been reports of no clinical toxicity (F.P.V. Maesen *et al.*, *Lancet*, 1984, *2*, 530; S.L. Gregoire *et al.*, 1987), the CSM in the *UK* had by April 1988 received 8 reports of clinically important interactions between theophylline and ciprofloxacin including one death in a patient with a plasma theophylline concentration of 188 μmol per litre (*Br. med. J.*, 1988, *296*, 1131). It could not be predicted which patients would suffer an interaction and it was suggested that ciprofloxacin should not normally be used in patients taking theophylline. Norfloxacin has been reported not to affect the disposition of theophylline in healthy subjects (M. Sano *et al.*, *Eur. J. clin. Pharmac.*, 1987, *32*, 431).

Rifampicin 600 mg daily by mouth for 6 to 14 days has been shown to increase plasma-theophylline clearance by 25 to 82% due to enhancement of hepatic theophylline metabolism. This increase in clearance is sufficient to cause clinical effects in some patients (A.B. Straughn *et al.*, *Ther. Drug Monit.*, 1984, *6*, 153; R.A. Robson *et al.*, *Br. J. clin. Pharmac.*, 1984, *18*, 445; E.G. Boyce *et al.*, *J. clin. Pharmac.*, 1986, *26*, 696), including children (D.R. Brocks *et al.*, *Clin. Pharm.*, 1986, *5*, 602).

Although tetracycline may weakly inhibit theophylline clearance in non-smoking adults with chronic obstructive airways disease (V.P. Gotz and G.G. Ryerson, *Drug Intell. & clin. Pharm.*, 1986, *20*, 694), doxycycline has been reported not to have any significant effect on theophylline pharmacokinetics in healthy subjects (J.H.G. Jonkman *et al.*, *Ther. Drug Monit.*, 1985, *7*, 92).

There have been reports of no significant effect on the pharmacokinetics of theophylline by amoxycillin (J.H.G. Jonkman *et al.*, *Br. J. clin. Pharmac.*, 1985, *19*, 99), cefaclor (J.H.G. Jonkman *et al.*, *Int. J. clin. Pharmac. Ther. Toxic.*, 1986, *24*, 88), co-trimoxazole (J.H.G. Jonkman *et al.*, *J. Pharm. Sci.*, 1985, *74*, 1103), or metronidazole (D.P. Reitberg *et al.*, *Clin. Pharm.*, 1983, *2*, 441).

Anti-epileptics. Phenytoin markedly decreases the serum half-life and increases the clearance of theophylline, probably due to hepatic enzyme induction, at therapeutic serum-phenytoin concentrations (J.-F. Marquis *et al.*, *New Engl. J. Med.*, 1982, *307*, 1189; R.C. Reed and H.J. Schwartz, *ibid.*, 1983, *308*, 724; S.J. Sklar and J.C. Wagner, *Drug Intell. & clin. Pharm.*, 1985, *19*, 34) at subtherapeutic phenytoin concentrations (R.C. Reed and H.J. Schwartz, 1983; M. Miller *et al.*, *Clin. Pharmac. Ther.*, 1984, *35*, 666), and even in heavy smokers (R.C. Reed and H.J. Schwartz, 1983). A preliminary report suggested that the serum concentration of phenytoin may be decreased simultaneously (J.W. Taylor *et al.*, *Drug Intell. & clin. Pharm.*, 1980, *14*, 638), perhaps due to reduced phenytoin absorption (L. Hendeles *et al.*, *J. Allergy & clin. Immunol.*, 1979, *63*, 156). The interaction between phenytoin and theophylline has been reported to occur within 5 to 14 days of commencing concomitant therapy, increases in theophylline clearance have ranged from 45 to 350%, and reductions in serum half-life have ranged from 25 to 70% of initial values (M. Miller *et al.*, 1984; S.J. Sklar and J.C. Wagner, 1985).

Carbamazepine has also been observed to increase theophylline elimination. In one patient, theophylline serum half-life was decreased by approximately 24 to 60%, and clearance was increased by about 35 to 100% when carbamazepine was given concomitantly (R.C. Reed and H.J. Schwartz, 1983). In an 11-year-old girl theophylline-serum half-life was almost halved after 3 weeks of concurrent carbamazepine therapy (K.R. Rosenberry *et al.*, *J. Pediat.*, 1983, *102*, 472).

Although phenobarbitone was not found to have a significant effect on the pharmacokinetics of theophylline given intravenously (K.M. Piafsky *et al.*, *Clin. Pharmac. Ther.*, 1977, *22*, 336), enhanced theophylline clearance has been seen in patients after longer periods of treatment with phenobarbitone (R.A. Landay *et al.*, *J. Allergy & clin. Immunol.*, 1978, *62*, 27; W.J. Jusko *et al.*, *J. Pharm. Sci.*, 1979, *68*, 1358; C.L. Saccar *et al.*, *J. Allergy & clin. Immunol.*, 1985, *75*, 716). The magnitude of the changes in theophylline elimination appears to be smaller with phenobarbitone than phenytoin, and it seems likely that only an occasional patient would require increased theophylline dosage (*Drug Interact. News.*, 1982, *2*, 45). Pentobarbitone in high doses has also been reported to increase theophylline metabolism (G.A. Gibson *et al.*, *Ther. Drug Monit.*, 1985, *7*, 181).

Antigout agents. Evidence that on long-term administration, allopurinol inhibits theophylline metabolism.— R. L. Manfredi and E. S. Vesell, *Clin. Pharmac. Ther.*, 1981, *29*, 224.

A study indicating that probenecid has no significant effect on the hepatic metabolism or total body clearance of theophylline.— T. W. D. Chen and T. F. Patton, *Drug Intell. & clin. Pharm.*, 1983, *17*, 465.

In 6 healthy volunteers sulphinpyrazone 800 mg daily for 7 days increased total plasma theophylline clearance by 22%, due to the selective induction of a group of cytochrome P-450 enzymes.— D. J. Birkett *et al.*, *Br. J. clin. Pharmac.*, 1983, *15*, 567.

Antineoplastic agents. For reference to a possible interaction between theophylline and lomustine, see Lomustine, p.633.

Arbaprostil. In a study of 7 healthy subjects, the administration of arbaprostil 200 μg daily for 7 days had no effect on the hepatic metabolism or pharmacokinetics of theophylline.— S. B. Reele *et al.* (letter), *Br. J. clin. Pharmac.*, 1986, *21*, 239.

Benzodiazepines. Aminophylline given intravenously in doses of 1.0 to 5.6 mg per kg body-weight, resulting in serum-theophylline concentrations below the therapeutic range for bronchodilatation, has resulted in rapid reversal of sedation induced by diazepam (J.A. Stirt, *Anesth. Analg.*, 1981, *60*, 767; S.B. Arvidsson *et al.*, *Lancet*, 1982, *2*, 1467) and lorazepam (M.A. Wangler and D.S. Kilpatrick, *Anesth. Analg.*, 1985, *64*, 834), but was not effective in antagonising sedation induced by midazolam (H.M.L. Mathews *et al.*, *Br. J. Anaesth.*, 1986, *58*, 1333P).

Beta adrenoceptor blocking agents. Propranolol reduced theophylline clearance by 36% in healthy subjects given aminophylline intravenously. Metoprolol did not reduce clearance in the group as a whole, but a reduction was noted in some smokers whose theophylline clearance was initially high (K.A. Conrad and D.W. Nyman, *Clin. Pharmac. Ther.*, 1980, *28*, 463). Propranolol is thought to exert a dose-dependent selective inhibitory effect on the separate forms of cytochrome P-450 involved in theophylline demethylation and 8-hydroxylation (J.O. Miners *et al.*, *Br. J. clin. Pharmac.*, 1985 *20*, 219).

Beta adrenoceptor stimulants. See under Sympathomimetic Agents, below.

Caffeine. Removal of methylxanthines from the diet in 4 adults led to faster elimination and more extensive metabolism of theophylline (T.J. Monks *et al.*, *Clin. Pharmac. Ther.*, 1979, *26*, 513). However, the addition of extra caffeine to the diet did not alter the disposition of theophylline (W.J. Jusko *et al.*, *J. Pharm. Sci.*, 1979, *68*, 1358; T.J. Monks *et al.*, *Biopharm. Drug Disposit.*, 1981, *2*, 31). Even if a slight kinetic interaction between caffeine and theophylline does exist, its clinical importance is probably limited because most patients do not abruptly change the caffeine content of their diet (J.H.G. Jonkman and R.A. Upton, *Clin. Pharmacokinet.*, 1984, *9*, 309).

Calcium-channel blockers. Symptoms of theophylline toxicity, associated with a serum-theophylline concentration above the therapeutic range, occurred in a 76-year-old woman taking theophylline after 6 days of therapy with verapamil. Symptoms subsided when theophylline was discontinued (T.G. Burnakis *et al.*, *Clin. Pharm.*, 1983, *2*, 458). In a study of healthy subjects chronic oral dosing with nifedipine increased the volume of distribution for theophylline and reduced serum-theophylline concentrations. Theophylline clearance, bioavailability, and elimination half-life were not significantly altered (S.H.D. Jackson *et al.*, *Br. J. clin. Pharmac.*, 1986, *21*, 389). However, in 2 patients, increased serum-theophylline concentrations have been reported after the addition of nifedipine (S.J. Parrillo and M. Venditto, *Ann. emerg. Med.*, 1984, *13*, 216; C.S. Harrod, *Ann. intern. Med.*, 1987, *106*, 480), and 2 further studies (14 and 30 days of concomitant treatment) have concluded that combined therapy with nifedipine and theophylline is safe (M. Garty *et al.*, *Clin. Pharmac. Ther.*, 1986, *40*, 195; C. Spedini and C. Lombardi, *Eur. J. clin. Pharmac.*, 1986, *31*,105).

Contraceptives, oral. Oral contraceptives have been reported to decrease the clearance of theophylline by about 30%, and serum concentrations may be increased (K.M. Tornatore *et al.*, *Eur. J. clin. Pharmac.*, 1982, *23*, 129; M.J. Gardner *et al.*, *Br. J. clin. Pharmac.*, 1983, *16*, 271; R.K. Roberts *et al.*, *J. Lab. clin. Med.*, 1983, *101*, 821).

Corticosteroids. In 3 patients with status asthmaticus given aminophylline intravenously, serum-theophylline concentrations rose rapidly from the therapeutic range to between 40 and 50 μg per mL when hydrocortisone was given intravenously (N. Buchanan *et al.*, *S. Afr. med. J.*, 1979, *56*, 1147). In 11 patients with chronic obstructive airways disease, medroxyprogesterone acetate by mouth had no significant effect on theophylline disposition (V.P. Gotz *et al.*, *J. clin. Pharmac.*, 1983, *23*, 281) and in studies in healthy subjects, no significant changes in serum-theophylline concentrations were noted after the concomitant administration of hydrocortisone, methylprednisolone (D.C. Leavengood *et al.*, *Ann. Allergy*, 1983, *50*, 249), or prednisone (J.L. Anderson *et al.*, *Clin. Pharm.*, 1984, *3*, 187). In pre-term neonates, exposure to betamethasone *in utero* stimulated the hepatic metabolism of theophylline (E. Jager-Roman *et al.*, *Develop. Pharmac. Ther.*, 1982, *5*, 127; J. Baird-Lambert *et al.*, *ibid.*, 1984, *7*, 239), but it is not possible to apply these findings to adults with fully functioning hepatic drug-metabolising enzymes (*Drug Interact. News.*, 1984, *4*, 17).

Frusemide. Although increased mean serum-theophylline concentrations were noted in 10 patients receiving continuous intravenous aminophylline infusions after intravenous injection of frusemide (P.F. Conlon *et al.*, *Am. J. Hosp. Pharm.*, 1981, *38*, 1345), decreased theophylline concentrations were noted in 4 neonates receiving oral or intravenous theophylline when given frusemide. Serum-theophylline concentrations returned to normal when frusemide and theophylline were given more than 2 hours apart (J.W. Toback and M.E. Gilman, *Pediatrics*, 1983, *71*, 140). In 8 patients with chronic stable asthma, mean peak serum-theophylline concentrations were reduced from 12.14 μg per mL with placebo to 7.16 μg per mL when frusemide was given. Reduced concentrations were noted for up to 6 hours after frusemide administration (G. Carpentiere *et al.*, *Ann. intern. Med.*, 1985, *103*, 957).

H_2 antagonist antihistamines. Cimetidine inhibits the oxidative metabolism of theophylline, reducing its clearance by 25 to 33% and prolonging its serum half-life (J.E. Jackson *et al.*, *Pharmacologist*, 1980, *22*, 231; J.H. Bauman *et al.*, *Ann. Allergy*, 1982, *48*, 100; R.E. Vestal *et al.*, *Br. J. clin. Pharmac.*, 1983, *15*, 411; R.K. Roberts *et al.*, *Med. J. Aust.*, 1984, *140*, 279). This inhibition of theophylline metabolism may be enhanced by liver disease (R. Gugler *et al.*, *Klin. Wschr.*, 1984, *62*, 1126) but may be partially antagonised by smoking (J.J. Grygiel *et al.*, *Eur. J. clin. Pharmac.*, 1984, *26*, 335). Studies have suggested that ranitidine does not significantly inhibit theophylline metabolism (J.R. Powell *et al.*, *Clin. Pharmac. Ther.*, 1982, *31*, 261; K.J. Breen *et al.*, *ibid.*, 297; R. Dal Negro *et al.*, *Int. J. clin. Pharmac. Ther. Toxic.*, 1984, *22*, 221; J.S. Seggev *et al.*, *Archs intern. Med.*, 1987, *147*, 179), although there have been occasional reports of theophylline toxicity after concomitant ranitidine therapy (E. Fernandes and F.M. Melewicz, *Ann. intern. Med.*, 1984, *100*, 459; M.E. Gardner and G.W. Sikorski, *ibid.*, 1985, *102*, 559). A study using very high doses of ranitidine (1200 or 4200 mg daily) did not detect any effect on theophylline metabolism (H.W. Kelly *et al.*, *Clin. Pharmac. Ther.*, 1986, *39*, 577). There has been a report of famotidine not interfering with theophylline disposition (A.N. Chremos *et al.*, *Clin. Pharmac. Ther.*, 1986, *39*, 187).

Interferon. After a single injection of recombinant human interferon-alfa theophylline clearance was reduced by 33 to 81%, resulting in a 1.5 to 6-fold increase in theophylline elimination half-life, in 5 patients with stable chronic active hepatitis B and 3 of 4 healthy controls. The remaining control showed no change in theophylline clearance. A selective inhibitory effect of interferon on the cytochrome P-450 isozymes involved in theophylline metabolism was suggested.— S. J. Williams *et al.*, *Lancet*, 1987, *2*, 939.

Ketoconazole. There have been reports that ketoconazole does not appear significantly to alter the pharmacokinetics of theophylline (M.W. Brown *et al.*, *Clin. Pharmac. Ther.*, 1985, *37*, 290; J.J. Heusner *et al.*, *Drug Intell. & clin. Pharm.*, 1987, *21*, 514).

Ketotifen. Theophylline attenuated the central sedative effects of ketotifen in 12 healthy volunteers, but ketotifen did not affect the disposition of theophylline in this study (M. Matejcek *et al.*, *Int. J. clin. Pharmac. Ther. Toxic.*, 1985, *23*, 258) or in a study of 6 asthmatic children (M. Garty *et al.*, *Eur. J. clin. Pharmac.*, 1987, *32*, 187).

Lithium. For the effect of theophylline on lithium, see Lithium Carbonate, p.368.

Nicotine. Although tobacco smoking enhances the metabolism of theophylline (see under Absorption and Fate, p.1532), nicotine administered in the form of a chewing gum had no effect on theophylline clearance in one study (B. L. Lee *et al.*, *Ann. intern. Med.*, 1987, *106*, 553).

Protirelin. The thyrotrophin response to thyrotrophin-releasing hormone is enhanced by theophylline.— P. H. Baylis, *Adverse Drug React. Bull.*, 1986, (Feb.), 432.

Sympathomimetic agents. In adults, theophylline pharmacokinetics are reported not to be affected by concomitant therapy with orciprenaline (K.A. Conrad and J.R. Woodworth, *Br. J. clin. Pharmac.*, 1981, *12*, 756) or terbutaline (J. Snidow *et al.*, *Eur. J. clin. Pharmac.*, 1987, *32*, 191), but in children increased theophylline clearance has been reported after the concurrent use of isoprenaline (M.P. Hemstreet *et al.*, *J. Allergy & clin. Immunol.*, 1982, *69*, 360) or terbutaline (Y. Danziger *et al.*, *Clin. Pharmac. Ther.*, 1985, *37*, 469). When given concurrently with theophylline, there is potentiation of the side-effects of terbutaline including hypokalaemia, hyperglycaemia, tachycardia, hypertension (S.R. Smith and M.J. Kendall, *Br. J. clin. Pharmac.*, 1986, *21*, 451), and tremor (A.P.H. van der Vet *et al.*, *Int. J. clin. Pharmac. Ther. Toxic.*, 1986, *24*, 569).

For a report suggesting that theophylline could potentiate the lactate-producing effects of beta-adrenoceptor stimulants, see under Adverse Effects, above.

For reports that the combined oral administration of theophylline with beta-adrenoceptor stimulants did not increase the incidence of cardiac arrhythmias compared to the administration of theophylline alone, even in overdosage, see also under Adverse Effects, above.

See also Combination Therapy with Beta-Adrenoceptor Stimulants under Uses and Administration, below.

Thiabendazole. An elderly man receiving aminophylline by infusion suffered severe nausea, lethargy, and general malaise, associated with a rise in serum-theophylline concentration from 21 to 46 μg per mL, when he was given thiabendazole.— A. M. Sugar *et al.*, *Am. Rev. resp. Dis.*, 1980, *122*, 501.

Ticlopidine. Theophylline elimination half-life was increased, and plasma clearance was decreased in 10 healthy subjects after the administration of ticlopidine 500 mg daily by mouth for 10 days.— A. Colli *et al.*, *Clin. Pharmac. Ther.*, 1987, *41*, 358.

Vaccines. Transient inhibition of the hepatic metabolism of theophylline, possibly secondary to interferon production, resulting in increased theophylline serum half-lives and concentrations has been reported after BCG vaccination (J.D. Gray *et al.*, *Br. J. clin. Pharmac.*, 1983, *16*, 735) and influenza vaccination (K.W. Renton *et al.*, *Can. med. Ass. J.*, 1980, *123*, 288; S. Walker *et al.*, *ibid.*, 1981, *125*, 243). Other studies have not been able to confirm the interaction with influenza vaccine (R.S. Goldstein *et al.*, *ibid.*, 1982, *126*, 470; R.G. Fischer *et al.*, *ibid.*, 1312; L. Britton and F.L. Ruben, *ibid.*, 1375; P.A. Patriarca *et al.*, *New Engl. J. Med.*, 1983, *308*, 1601). The differing findings may be due to differences in patients and healthy subjects studied, to drugs, to smoking (*Drug Interact. News.*, 1984, *4*, 21), and most importantly, to differences in vaccine; purified subvirion vaccines which do not induce interferon production have been reported not to alter theophylline metabolism (B.M. Stults and P.A. Hashisaki, *West. J. Med.*, 1983, *139*, 651; P.A. Winstanley *et al.*, *Br. J. clin. Pharmac.*, 1985, *19*, 569P).

See also Pulmonary Disease under Absorption and Fate, below, and Interferon, above.

Vidarabine. Serum theophylline concentrations increased from within the therapeutic range to 24 μg per mL in a 62-year-old woman after 4 days of concomitant treatment with vidarabine 400 mg daily; theophylline half-life increased to 24 hours from 9 hours. Inhibition of xanthine oxidase by a vidarabine metabolite was suspected.— R. Gannon *et al.* (letter), *Ann. intern. Med.*, 1984, *101*, 148.

INTERACTIONS, ASSAYS. In a review of drug interferences in therapeutic drug monitoring, the following drugs were reported to interfere with the assay of theophylline by high pressure liquid chromatography: acetazolamide, caffeine, some cephalosporins and penicillins, chloramphenicol, dimenhydrinate, diprophylline, paracetamol, procainamide, salicylates, some sulphonamides, theobromine, and trisulphapyrimidines (S. Yosselson-Superstine, *Clin. Pharmacokinet.*, 1984, *9*, 67). Metronidazole was also found to cause interference (D. Garfinkel *et al.*, *Ann. intern. Med.*, 1987, *106*, 171). Measurement of plasma-theophylline concentrations by spectrophotometric methods, such as that of Schack and Waxler (*J. Pharmac. exp. Ther.*, 1949, *97*, 283) had been reported to be affected by the presence of allopurinol, barbiturates, caffeine, carbamazepine, cephazolin, chlordiazepoxide, dicoumarol, diprophylline, frusemide, gentamicin, hydrochlorothiazide, hydroxyzine, methyclothiazide, morphine, nitrofurantoin, oxazepam, oxyphenbutazone, paracetamol, phenacetin, phenylbutazone, phenytoin, probenecid, procainamide, salicylates, some sulphonamides, tetracycline, theobromine, thiamine, thiopentone, and warfarin (S. Yosselson-Superstine, 1984). Enzyme immunoassay techniques are more specific (M. Weinberger, *Lancet*, 1978, *2*, 789); it is reported that only caffeine and theobromine interfere with substrate-labelled fluorescent immunoassays (S. Yosselson-Superstine, 1984).

Oxypentifylline and its principal metabolite are reported not to interfere with theophylline determination by fluorescence immunoassay, enzyme immunoassay, or high-performance liquid chromatography techniques.— D. M. Cummings *et al.*, *Am. J. Hosp. Pharm.*, 1985, *42*, 2717.

PORPHYRIA. Theophylline was considered to be unsafe in patients with acute porphyria as it has been associated with acute attacks.— M.R. Moore and K.E.L. McColl, *Porphyrias, Drug Lists*, Glasgow, Porphyria Research Unit, University of Glasgow, 1987.

PREGNANCY AND THE NEONATE. Theophylline was not considered to be teratogenic.— F. J. Stanley and C. Bower, *Med. J. Aust.*, 1986, *145*, 596.

For further references to the use of theophylline in pregnancy, see under Uses and Administration, below.

For a report of increased gastro-oesophageal reflux in neonates receiving theophylline or caffeine, see under Reflux Oesophagitis, below.

For reports of alterations in maternal theophylline clearance during pregnancy and recommendations for serum concentration measurements, see under Absorption and Fate, below.

REFLUX OESOPHAGITIS. Theophylline drugs and β_2-stimulants have a relaxing influence on the lower oesophageal sphincter and may therefore provoke nocturnal asthma due to gastro-oesophageal reflux.— U. Bengtsson *et al.* (letter), *Lancet*, 1985, *1*, 1501.

Episodes of gastro-oesophageal reflux increased in 12 of 18 and 15 of 30 infants receiving theophylline and caffeine respectively. The increases were independent of plasma-xanthine concentrations (within or below the therapeutic range).— Y. Vandenplas *et al.*, *Pediatrics*, 1986, *77*, 807.

SURGERY. The patient can take his usual dose of bronchodilators on the day of operation. An additional dose of aminophylline can be given by rectum with the premedication. Any tachycardia produced is usually less hazardous than bronchospasm.— *Drug & Ther. Bull.*, 1984, *22*, 73.

WITHDRAWAL SYNDROMES. For a report of apnoea occurring in a neonate whose mother had taken aminophylline and theophylline throughout pregnancy, and which resolved on theophylline administration, see under Pregnancy and the Neonate, in Adverse Effects, above.

Absorption and Fate

Theophylline is rapidly and completely absorbed from liquid preparations, capsules, and uncoated tablets. The rate, but not the extent of absorption is decreased by food. Absorption is slower and may be incomplete from sustained-release and enteric-coated preparations. Rectal absorption is rapid from enemas, but may be slow and erratic from suppositories. Peak serum-theophylline concentrations occur 1 to 2 hours after ingestion of liquid preparations, capsules, and uncoated tablets, and between 4 and 12 hours after ingestion of sustained-release preparations.

Theophylline is approximately 60% bound to plasma proteins, but in neonates or adults with liver disease, binding is reduced to 30 to 40%. Optimum therapeutic serum concentrations range from 10 to 20 μg per mL (55 to 110 μmol per litre).

Theophylline is metabolised in the liver to 1,3-dimethyluric acid, 1-methyluric acid, and 3-methylxanthine. These metabolites are excreted in the urine. In adults, about 10% of a dose of theophylline is excreted unchanged in the urine, but in neonates around 50% is excreted unchanged, and a large proportion is excreted as caffeine. Considerable inter-individual differences in the rate of hepatic metabolism of theophylline result in large variations in clearance, serum concentrations, and half-lives. Hepatic metabolism is further affected by factors such as age, smoking, disease, diet, and drug interactions. The serum half-life of theophylline in an otherwise healthy, non-smoking asthmatic adult is 7 to 9 hours, in children 3 to 5 hours, in cigarette smokers 4 to 5 hours, and in premature infants or patients with lung disease, cardiac failure, or liver disease, over 24 hours.

Theophylline crosses the placenta; it also enters breast milk.

In a comparative study in healthy subjects, almost identical serum concentration-time curves were obtained for theophylline and aminophylline after both oral and intravenous administration. It was concluded that ethylenediamine did not influence the overall pharmacokinetics or the binding of theophylline to serum proteins.— A. Aslaksen *et al.*, *Br. J. clin. Pharmac.*, 1981, *11*, 269.

Further studies demonstrating a lack of effect of ethylenediamine on theophylline pharmacokinetics: J. Caldwell and I. A. Cotgreave, *Br. J. clin. Pharmac.*, 1982, *14*, 610P; I. A. Cotgreave and J. Caldwell, *J. Pharm. Pharmac.*, 1983, *35*, 378; *idem*, 1985, *37*, 618; J. Caldwell *et al.*, *Br. J. clin. Pharmac.*, 1986, *22*, 351.

ABSORPTION. Studies of the absorption characteristics and bioavailability of sustained-release theophylline preparations in asthmatics: J. R. Haltom and S. J. Szefler, *J. Pediat.*, 1985, *107*, 805; R. J. Rogers *et al.*, *ibid.*, *106*, 496; A. Boner *et al.*, *Drug Intell. & clin. Pharm.*, 1987, *21*, 221. See also M. M. Weinberger, *Pharmacotherapy*, 1984, *4*, 181.

Cystic fibrosis. In a study of 16 patients with cystic fibrosis it was concluded that theophylline malabsorption is significant in certain of these patients and may be related to age and weight.— M. V. Miles and G. R. Cutter, *Clin. Pharmac. Ther.*, 1984, *35*, 259.

Diurnal variation. Higher peak serum concentrations are achieved more quickly when a dose of oral theophylline is given in the morning than when a similar dose is given at night (L.J. Lesko *et al.*, *J. Pharm. Sci.*, 1980, *69*, 358; P.J. Thompson *et al.*, *Br. J. clin. Pharmac.*, 1981, *12*, 443; P.H. Scott *et al.*, *J. Pediat.*, 1981, *99*, 476; W.R. Primrose, *Lancet*, 1983, *1*, 927; J.H.G. Jonkman and W.J.V. van der Boon, *ibid.*, 1278; D.R. Taylor *et al.*, *Br. J. clin. Pharmac.*, 1984, *18*, 27). When sustained-release preparations are given 12-hourly, this diurnal variation can result in higher pre-dose serum-theophylline concentrations in the morning than in the evening (P.H. Scott *et al.*, 1981; J.H.G. Jonkman and W.J.V. van der Boon, 1983), which could have important consequences when adjusting doses. The most widely accepted explanation for the circadian variation in theophylline phamacokinetics is slower absorption at night (P.J. Thompson *et al.*, 1981; P.H. Scott *et al.*, 1981; K.P. Coulthard *et al.*, *Eur. J. clin. Pharmac.*, 1983, *25*, 667; D.R. Taylor *et al.*, *Br. J. clin. Pharmac.*, 1983, *16*, 413; *idem*, 1984, *18*, 27), since no diurnal variation in metabolic clearance has been observed (K.P. Coulthard *et al.*, 1983; D.R. Taylor *et al.*, 1983; M.V. St.-Pierre *et al.*, *Clin. Pharmac. Ther.*, 1985, *38*, 89). Resorption of theophylline from the bladder (J.H. Wood and L.K. Garrettson, *Lancet*, 1983, *2*, 570) and the effects of supine posture (J. Warren, *ibid.*, 850; J.B. Warren *et al.*, *Br. J. clin. Pharmac.*, 1983, *16*, 405; J.B. Warren *et al.*, *ibid.*, 1985, *19*, 707) have also been suggested as contributory factors, although night-workers still exhibit slower theophylline absorption at night (S. DeCourt *et al.*, *ibid.*, 1982, *13*, 567). In another study changing the times of dosing from 11am and 11pm to 5am and 5pm respectively abolished circadian variation in trough serum-theophylline concentrations (S.H.D. Jackson *et al.*, *ibid.*, 1984, *17*, 777).

Effects of food. The effects of food on theophylline absorption from sustained-release oral preparations is variable. Some workers have found that administration after meals is followed by decreases in theophylline absorption rate, peak serum concentrations, and/or bioavailability compared with administration in the fasting state (S. Pedersen, *Br. J. clin. Pharmac.*, 1981, *12*, 904; S. Pedersen and J. Møller-Petersen, *Pediatrics*, 1984, *74*, 534). Others have noted a rapid increase in the rate and/or extent of absorption following meals ('dose-dumping'), especially meals with a high fat content (L. Hendeles *et al.*, *Lancet*, 1984, *2*, 1471; A. Karim *et al.*, *Clin. Pharmac. Ther.*, 1985, *38*, 642). Food reduced the rate but not the extent of absorption of theophylline from an aqueous solution of choline theophyllinate (J.H.G. Jonkman *et al.*, *Eur. J. clin. Pharmac.*, 1985, *28*, 225).

Percutaneous absorption. Therapeutic serum-theophylline concentrations (over 4 μg per mL) were achieved in

11 of 13 infants, who had not previously received the drug, after the application under occlusion of a gel containing theophylline sodium glycinate 0.25 mL (equivalent to anhydrous theophylline 17 mg) to a small area of abdominal skin. In 12 studies in infants previously receiving aminophylline, serum-theophyline concentrations were maintained for up to 70 hours. As the infants' postnatal age increased there was a significant decline in the amount of theophylline absorbed in the first 24 hours after application, but satisfactory serum concentrations were achieved in infants up to 20 days of age.— N. J. Evans *et al.*, *J. Pediat.*, 1985, *107*, 307. See also N. J. Evans *et al.*, *J. Pharm. Pharmac.*, 1984, *36*, *Suppl.*, 10P.

Rectal absorption. The administration of theophylline suppositories to young asthmatic children resulted in a variable bioavailability (mean 80%) and a mean absorption half-life of 43 minutes. In contrast, theophylline enemas had an average bioavailability of 100% and a mean absorption half-life of 5.5 minutes. Administration of an enema (theophylline 6 to 8 mg per kg bodyweight) three times daily produced continuous therapeutic serum concentrations of theophylline. Constant serum-theophylline concentrations have also been obtained in healthy subjects by the continuous rectal infusion of a solution using an osmotic delivery system. The plasma concentration profile was not influenced by renewing the delivery system or by defaecation.— A. G. De Boer *et al.*, *Br. J. Anaesth.*, 1984, *56*, 69.

DISTRIBUTION. Studies examining serum-theophylline concentrations during the chronic administration of various sustained-release preparations in patients with obstructive airways disease: H. W. Kelly and S. Murphy, *Pediatrics*, 1980, *66*, 97; M. Weinberger *et al.*, *J. Pediat.*, 1981, *99*, 145; D. R. Taylor *et al.* (letter), *Br. J. clin. Pharmac.*, 1982, *13*, 569; S. H. D. Jackson and J. M. Wright, *Eur. J. clin. Pharmac.*, 1983, *24*, 205; M. A. Butcher *et al.*, *Aust. J. Hosp. Pharm.*, 1984, *14*, 121; P. E. Williams *et al.*, *Br. J. clin. Pharmac.*, 1986, *22*, 383.

Protein binding. Albumin is the major plasma binding protein for theophylline, binding is pH-dependent, and the percentage of theophylline bound at physiological pH is reported to range from about 35 to 45% (D. Buss *et al.*, *Br. J. clin. Pharmac.*, 1983, *15*, 399; O. Brørs *et al.*, *ibid.*, 393). Some studies have found the plasma protein binding of theophylline to be concentration dependent (J.A. Fleetham *et al.*, *Thorax*, 1981, *36*, 382; L. Shaw *et al.*, *Clin. Pharmac. Ther.*, 1982, *32*, 490; U. Gundert Remy *et al.*, *Br. J. clin. Pharmac.*, 1983, *16*, 573), but others have not confirmed this (D. Buss *et al.*, 1983; C. Knott *et al.*, *Br. J. clin. Pharmac.*, 1984, *17*, 9; D.C. Buss *et al.*, *ibid.*, 1985, *19*, 529). There appears to be little variation in plasma protein binding between healthy subjects and patients with obstructive airways disease (P. Ebden *et al.*, *Thorax*, 1984, *39*, 352), but in patients with hypoalbuminaemia due to renal failure, binding is reduced (D. Leopold *et al.*, *Br. J. clin. Pharmac.*, 1985, *19*, 823).

Salivary concentrations. The use of salivary concentrations for monitoring theophylline dosage requirements has been suggested (M.G. Horning *et al.*, *Clin. Chem.*, 1977, *23*, 157; F. Plasvic *et al.*, *Br. J. clin. Pharmac.*, 1981, *11*, 533), but poor correlation between salivary- and serum-theophylline concentrations, and errors in serum concentration predictions have been reported (D.L. Uden *et al.*, *Ther. Drug Monit.*, 1981, *3*, 143; J. Culig *et al.*, *Br. J. clin. Pharmac.*, 1982, *13*, 243; A.H. Jackson *et al.*, *ibid.*, 1983, *15*, 407). Salivary sampling may be useful in children, as there appears to be a better correlation between salivary- and serum-theophylline concentrations (S.J. Goldsworthy and M. Kemp, *ibid.*, 1981, *11*, 434P; N. Krivoy *et al.*, *Pharmatherapeutica*, 1985, *4*, 285), but in older patients it is felt that the technique is only useful to assess compliance (M.E. Gardiner *et al.*, *Aust. J. Hosp. Pharm.*, 1986, *16*, 4).

Serum concentrations. A therapeutic serum-concentration range of 10 to 20 µg per mL (55 to 110 µmol per litre) has been suggested for theophylline (K.M. Piafsky and R.I. Ogilvie, *New Engl. J. Med.*, 1975, *292*, 1218), since the degree of bronchodilatation is approximately proportional to the logarithm of serum-theophylline concentrations in this range (P.A. Mitenko and R.I. Ogilvie, *ibid.*, 1973, *289*, 600). The optimal serum-theophylline concentration required depends upon the severity of the airways obstruction. For moderately severe asthma, serum concentrations between 10 and 15 µg per mL are usually adequate (F. Ruff *et al.*, *Revue fr. mal. Resp.*, 1980, *8*, 21), whilst for severe chronic asthma concentrations of 10 to 20 µg per mL are needed (G. Hambleton *et al.*, *Lancet*, 1977, *1*, 381; P.W. Trembath *et al.*, *J. int. med. Res.*, 1979, *7*, *Suppl.* 1, 4). However, side-effects become more common at serum-theophylline concentrations exceeding 9 µg per mL (L.E. Ramsay *et al.*, *Br. J. clin. Pharmac.*, 1980, *10*, 101), with nausea becoming more frequent at serum concentrations of 15 µg per mL and over, cardiac arrhythmias occurring more often at serum concentrations over 20 µg per mL, and convulsions occurring particularly over 40 µg per mL (R.I. Ogilvie *Clin. Pharmacokinet.*, 1978, *3*, 267), with a mortality of up to 50% (C.W. Zwillich *et al.*, *Ann. intern. Med.*, 1975, *82*, 784; R.I. Ogilivie, 1978; A.A. Woodcock *et al.*, *Lancet*, 1983, *2*, 610).

Some premature apnoeic babies have been reported to benefit from serum-theophylline concentrations of 1 to 2 µg per mL (M.J. Boutroy *et al.*, *J. Pediat.*, 1979, *94*, 996), but the lower limit is usually set at about 5 µg per mL (C. Edwards, *Pharm. J.*, 1986, *2*, 128). Tachycardia has been noted with serum-theophylline concentrations of 13 µg per mL (D.C. Shannon *et al.*, *Pediatrics*, 1975, *55*, 589), but does not usually occur until a concentration of about 20 µg per mL is reached (J.V. Aranda *et al.*, *New Engl. J. Med.*, 1976, *295*, 413; A.L. Neese and L.F. Soyka, *Clin. Pharmac. Ther.*, 1977, *21*, 633). A working therapeutic range of 5 to 15 µg per mL is generally used (C. Edwards, 1986).

METABOLISM AND EXCRETION. The serum concentration of theophylline reflects its rate of hepatic metabolism as only small amounts are excreted unchanged. Theophylline is metabolised by hydroxylation and demethylation to 1,3-dimethyluric acid (40 to 50%), 3-methylxanthine (10 to 15%), 1-methyluric acid (10 to 15%) and smaller amounts of 1-methylxanthine. The remainder is excreted unchanged (J.J. Grygiel *et al.*, *Clin. Pharmac. Ther.*, 1979, *26*, 660; J.H.G. Jonkman *et al.*, *Eur. J. clin. Pharmac.*, 1981, *20*, 435; D.D. Tang-Lui *et al.*, *Clin. Pharmac. Ther.*, 1982, *31*, 358). Elderly patients excrete a significantly higher fraction of a dose of theophylline as 1-methyluric acid and a lower fraction as theophylline (E.J. Antal *et al.*, *Br. J. clin. Pharmac.*, 1981, *12*, 637). In premature neonates, the absence of oxidative metabolic pathways unmasks the methylation of theophylline to caffeine. About 30 to 50% of a dose of theophylline may be metabolised in this way, and a large proportion of theophylline is excreted unchanged. In adults the caffeine produced from the metabolism of theophylline is very rapidly metabolised itself (C. Bory *et al.*, *J. Pediat.*, 1979, *94*, 988; M.J. Boutroy *et al.*, *ibid.*, 996; K.-Y. Tserng *et al.*, *Clin. Pharmac. Ther.*, 1983, *33*, 522).

The clearance of theophylline from the body by metabolism and excretion varies widely between individuals. It is reported to be affected by age, cardiac, hepatic, and pulmonary disease, diet, dosage regimen, pregnancy, smoking (see below), and interaction with other drugs (see Interactions under Precautions, above). Theophylline clearance is also reported to be decreased by exercise (F. Schlaeffer *et al.*, *Respiration*, 1984, *45*, 438) and severe hypothyroidism (C.F. Seifert *et al.*, *Drug Intell. & clin. Pharm.*, 1987, *21*, 442) and increased in severe psoriasis (D.P. West *et al.*, *Drug Intell. & clin. Pharm.*, 1984, *18*, 494). Factors found not to affect theophylline clearance include renal failure (L.A. Bauer *et al.*, *J. clin. Pharmac.*, 1982, *22*, 65), obesity (R.L. Slaughter and R.A. Lane, *Drug Intell. & clin. Pharm.*, 1983, *17*, 274), and malnutrition (M. Eriksson *et al.*, *Eur. J. clin. Pharmac.*, 1983, *24*, 89).

Age. From approximately one year of age until adolescence, children have a rapid theophylline clearance (E.J. Ginchansky and M.W. Weinberger, *J. Pediat.*, 1977, *91*, 655; D.E. Zaske *et al.*, *J. Am. med. Ass.*, 1977, *237*, 1453). Premature infants under one year of age have a slower clearance (J.V. Aranda *et al.*, *New Engl. J. Med.*, 1976, *295*, 413; E.G. Nassif *et al.*, *J. Pediat.*, 1981, *98*, 158) due to immature metabolic pathways (J.J. Grygiel and D.J. Birkett, *Clin. Pharmac. Ther.*, 1980, *28*, 456; K.-Y. Tserng *et al.*, *ibid.*, 1981, *29*, 594), although clearance is more rapid on the first day of life in premature neonates (I.L. Stile *et al.*, *Clin. Ther.*, 1986, *8*, 336). The rapid childhood clearance values decline towards adult values in the late teenage years (R.I. Ogilvie, *Clin. Pharmacokinet.*, 1978, *3*, 267). Some studies have demonstrated a progressive decline in clearance throughout adult years (W.J. Jusko *et al.*, *J. Pharm. Sci.*, 1979, *68*, 1358; W.C. Randolph *et al.*, *Br. J. clin. Pharmac.*, 1986, *22*, 603) whereas others have not (J.K. Wiffen *et al.*, *ibid.*, 1984, *17*, 219P). Similarly, some studies have noted a decreased clearance in the elderly (E.J. Antal *et al.*, *ibid.*, 1981, *12*, 637) but others have found no change, especially in elderly smokers (B. Cusack *et al.*, *Br. J. clin. Pharmac.*, 1980, *10*, 109; L.A. Bauer and R.A. Blouin, *Clin. Pharmacokinet.*, 1981, *6*, 469; R.W. Fox *et al.*, *Clin. Pharmac. Ther.*, 1983, *34*, 60).

Cardiac disease. Decreased theophylline clearance has been reported in patients with acute pulmonary oedema (K.M. Piafsky *et al.*, *Clin. Pharmac. Ther.*, 1977, *21*, 310), cor pulmonale (N. Vicuna *et al.*, *Br. J. clin. Pharmac.*, 1979, *7*, 33), and congestive heart failure (M.W. Weinberger *et al.*, *J. Am. med. Ass.*, 1976, *235*, 2110; J.W. Jenne *et al.*, *Am. J. Hosp. Pharm.*, 1977, *34*,, 408; W.J. Jusko *et al.*, *Ann. intern. Med.*, 1977, *86*, 400). Mild congestive heart failure may not affect theophylline clearance (W.J. Jusko *et al.*, *J. Pharm. Sci.*, 1979, *68*, 1358), but resolution of congestive heart failure has resulted in improvement in theophylline clearance (J.R. Powell *et al.*, *Am. Rev. resp. Dis.*, 1978, *118*, 229). The decrease in theophylline clearance in congestive heart failure has been attributed to decreased liver blood flow, liver hypoxia, or passive congestion of the liver (S. Vozeh *et al.*, *J. Am. med. Ass.*, 1978, *240*, 1882).

Diet. A diet high in protein and low in carbohydrate has been reported to increase theophylline clearance, and *vice versa.* It was suggested that the increased protein intake induces hepatic drug-metabolising enzymes whereas carbohydrates may inhibit them (A. Kappas *et al.*, *Clin. Pharmac. Ther.*, 1976, *20*, 643; C.H. Feldman *et al.*, *Pediatrics*, 1980, *66*, 956; C.H. Feldman *et al.*, *Ther. Drug Monit.*, 1982, *4*, 69; D. Juan *et al.*, *Clin. Pharmac. Ther.*, 1986, *40*, 187), although one study suggested greater effects on the absorption and distribution of theophylline (P.J. Thompson *et al.*, *Br. J. clin. Pharmac.*, 1983, *16*, 267). The consumption of methylxanthines, particularly caffeine, in the diet has been shown to decrease theophylline clearance (J. Caldwell *et al.*, *Br. J. clin. Pharmac.*, 1977, *4*, 637P).

See also Caffeine in Interactions, under Precautions, above. Food may also affect the absorption of theophylline; see under Absorption, above.

Dosage regimen. There is evidence that the elimination of theophylline is dose-dependent and that at high serum concentrations, a small change in dose could cause a disproportionate increase in serum-theophylline concentration, due to a reduction in clearance (M. Weinberger and E.J. Ginchansky, *J. Pediat.*, 1977, *91*, 820; D.D. Tang-Lui *et al.*, *Clin. Pharmac. Ther.*, 1982, *31*, 358; M.A. Butcher *et al.*, *Br. J. clin. Pharmac.*, 1982, *13*, 241). However, there is debate as to whether this effect is clinically significant when serum-theophylline concentrations are within the therapeutic range (G.H. Koëter *et al.*, *Br. J. clin. Pharmac.*, 1981, *12*, 647; V. Rovei *et al.*, *ibid.*, 1982, *14*, 769; U. Gundert-Remy *et al.*, *Eur. J. clin. Pharmac.*, 1983, *24*, 71; P.J. Brown *et al.*, *ibid.*, 525; G. Milavetz and M. Weinberger, *Pharmacotherapy*, 1984, *4*, 216). It has also been suggested that repeated oral dosing of theophylline might result in a decrease of clearance compared with pre-treatment values (H. Efthimiou *et al.*, *Br. J. clin. Pharmac.*, 1984, *17*, 525). The disparate data on dose-dependent elimination have been explained in terms of Michaelis-Menten kinetics (J.G. Wagner, *Clin. Pharmacokinet.*, 1985, *10*, 432).

Hepatic disease. Theophylline clearance may be markedly reduced in patients with hepatic disease, especially cirrhosis (K.M. Piafsky *et al.*, *New Engl. J. Med.*, 1977, *296*, 1495; A. Mangione *et al.*, *Chest*, 1978, *73*, 616) and, to a lesser extent, acute hepatitis (A.H. Staib *et al.*, *Int. J. clin. Pharmac. Ther. Toxic.*, 1980, *18*, 500; R.A. Feinstein and M.V. Miles, *Clin. Pediat.*, 1985, *24*, 357). Since changes in liver blood flow have little effect on theophylline clearance, (low hepatic extraction ratio) the effect of hepatic disease is probably due to altered hepatocellular function (R.I. Ogilvie, *Clin. Pharmacokinet.*, 1978, *3*, 267).

Pregnancy. For studies describing the effects of pregnancy on maternal theophylline pharmacokinetics, see under Pregnancy and the Neonate, below.

Pulmonary disease. Reduced theophylline clearance has been noted in patients with hypoxia (S. Vozeh *et al.*, *J. Am. med. Ass.*, 1978, *240*, 1882), acute respiratory failure (A. Durocher *et al.*, *Rev. Méd. Interne*, 1982, *3*, 361), chronic obstructive lung disease, pneumonia (M. Weinberger *et al.*, *J. Am. med. Ass.*, 1976, *235*, 2110; J.R. Powell *et al.*, *Am. Rev. resp. Dis.*, 1978, *118*, 229), and acute viral respiratory illness (K.C. Chang *et al.*, *Lancet*, 1978, *1*, 1132; J.A. Fleetham *et al.*, *ibid.*, *2*, 898; C.J. Clark and G. Boyd, *ibid.*, 1979, *1*, 492; M.J. Kraemer *et al.*, *Pediatrics*, 1982, *69*, 476). It has been suggested that rather than infection resulting in decreased theophylline clearance, a sub-population of patients may react to infections with alterations in hepatic metabolism, and then develop theophylline toxicity (M. Bukowskyj *et al.*, *Ann. intern. Med.*, 1984, *101*, 63). Influenza vaccination has also been reported to reduce theophylline clearance (see Interactions under Precautions, above). Increased theophylline clearance has been noted in patients with cystic fibrosis (A. Isles *et al.*, *Am. Rev. resp. Dis.*, 1983, *127*, 417; C. Saccar *et al.*, *J. clin. Pharmac.*, 1985, *25*, 468), although others have found clearance values similar to those in normal and asthmatic children (J.W. Georgitis *et al.*, *Ann. Allergy*, 1982, *48*, 175).

Smoking. Cigarette smoking increases theophylline clearance by as much as 66% and shortens its serum half-life, probably due to hepatic enzyme induction by components of tobacco smoke (S.N. Hunt *et al.*, *Clin. Pharmac. Ther.*, 1976, *19*, 546; W.J. Jusko *et al.*, *ibid.*, 1978, *24*, 406; J.J. Grygiel and D.J. Birkett, *ibid.*, 1981, *30*, 491). The inductive effect of smoking may override factors that tend to decrease theophylline clearance, such as congestive heart failure (B. Cusack *et al.*, *Br. J. clin. Pharmac.*, 1980, *10*, 109) and old age (P.W. Trembath *et al.*, *Hum. Toxicol.*, 1986, *5*, 265). The duration of enzyme induction after stopping smoking is uncertain; theophylline clearance decreased by 38% after one week of abstinence from smoking in one study (B.L. Lee *et al.*, *Ann. intern. Med.*, 1987, *106*, 553), whilst others have found changes in clearance persisting for at least 3 months (S.N. Hunt *et al.*, 1976). Tobacco chewing has also been reported to increase theophylline clearance (R. Rockwood and N. Henann, *Drug Intell. & clin. Pharm.*, 1986, *20*, 624).

PREGNANCY AND THE NEONATE. An increase in the volume of distribution of theophylline, a decrease in its plasma-protein binding, and a continuing decrease in its clearance throughout pregnancy have been noted in some patients, especially during the later part of pregnancy, necessitating dosage reduction to avoid toxicity (B.L. Carter *et al.*, *Obstet. Gynec.*, 1986, *68*, 555; M.C. Frederiksen *et al.*, *Clin. Pharmac. Ther.*, 1986, *40*, 321; M.J. Gardner *et al.*, *Eur. J. clin. Pharmac.*, 1987, *31*, 289). Some studies have found that after delivery there is a return of clearance values to those existing before pregnancy (B.L. Carter *et al.*, 1986), whilst others have not (M.J. Gardner *et al.*, 1987). One study demonstrated an increase in renal clearance accompanying decreased hepatic clearance, but it could not be determined if this compensatory increase would prevent an increase in unbound serum-theophylline concentrations (M.C. Frederiksen *et al.*, 1986). Other studies have noted an increase in theophylline clearance during pregnancy (R. Romero *et al.*, *Am. J. Perinatol.*, 1983, *1*, 31; P.C. Rubin, *Br. med. J.*, 1986, *293*, 1415). It was recommended that serum concentrations are measured at monthly intervals throughout pregnancy and again one and four weeks after delivery (P.C. Rubin, 1986).

In a study of 12 neonates whose mothers received various theophylline preparations throughout their pregnancies maternal, cord, and neonatal heelstick theophylline concentrations were not notably different, and ranged from 2.3 to 19.6 µg per mL. Transient jitteriness was seen in 2 neonates and tachycardia in one, at cord theophylline concentrations of 11.7 to 17 µg per mL. There were no instances of vomiting, seizure, arrhythmias, diarrhoea, or feeding disturbances which had been reported previously.— E. Labovitz and S. Spector, *J. Am. med. Ass.*, 1982, *247*, 786.

Lactation. Irritability occurred in a breast-fed infant when the mother took aminophylline 200 mg every 6 hours. In 5 nursing mothers given aminophylline the ratio of milk concentration of theophylline to serum concentration was about 0.7.— A. M. Yurchak and W. J. Jusko, *Pediatrics*, 1976, *57*, 518. See also G. P. Stec *et al.*, *Clin. Pharmac. Ther.*, 1980, *28*, 404.

Uses and Administration

Theophylline relaxes smooth muscle, relieves bronchospasm, and has a stimulant effect on respiration. It stimulates the myocardium and central nervous system, decreases peripheral resistance and venous pressure, and causes diuresis. It is still not clear how theophylline exerts these effects. Inhibition of phosphodiesterase with a resulting increase in intracellular cyclic adenosine monophosphate (cyclic AMP) does occur, but not apparently at concentrations normally used for clinical effect. Other proposed mechanisms of action include adenosine receptor antagonism, prostaglandin antagonism, and effects on intracellular calcium, but these actions also appear to occur only with high doses.

The main indication for theophylline is the relief of bronchospasm in asthma, bronchitis, emphysema, and acute respiratory infections. Theophylline is also used to relieve apnoea. It was formerly used in the treatment of congestive heart failure, angina pectoris, and for its diuretic action, but more effective agents are now available.

Theophylline is available in oral dosage forms intended for administration every 4 to 6 hours. It is also available in a range of sustained-release oral preparations that only need to be administered once or twice daily. Dose forms are also available for rectal and for intravenous administration.

Optimum therapeutic serum concentrations of theophylline are considered to range from 10 to 20 µg per mL and toxic effects are more common above 20 µg per mL (see under Absorption and Fate, above).

In the treatment of acute severe asthma theophylline is administered intravenously usually as aminophylline (see p.1521). To reduce adverse effects, the rate of intravenous administration of theophylline should not exceed 20 mg per minute. In patients who have not been taking theophylline or aminophylline, theophylline is given in a loading dose of 5 mg per kg body-weight by slow intravenous injection, usually over 20 to 30 minutes. In patients who have been receiving theophylline or aminophylline, ideally the serum-theophylline concentration should be measured before administering a loading dose. The loading dose can then be determined on the basis that theophylline 500 µg per kg lean body-weight can be expected to increase the serum-theophylline concentration by approximately 1 µg per mL, and a serum concentration of 10 to 20 µg per mL is required. In an emergency where the serum-theophylline concentration is not available, a loading dose of 2.5 mg per kg may be given and is unlikely to be dangerous in patients not exhibiting theophylline toxicity. If necessary, a maintenance infusion may be given after the loading dose. In the *US* the following theophylline intravenous maintenance doses are suggested, the dose being reduced after 12 hours: children aged 6 months to 9 years 950 µg per kg body-weight hourly, reduced to 790 µg per kg hourly; children aged 9 to 16 years and adult smokers 790 µg per kg hourly, reduced to 630 µg per kg hourly; non-smoking adults 550 µg per kg hourly, reduced to 390 µg per kg hourly; older patients or patients with cor pulmonale 470 µg per kg hourly, reduced to 240 µg per kg hourly; and in patients with congestive heart failure or liver disease 390 µg per kg hourly reduced to 80 to 160 µg per kg hourly. These doses should be reduced if serum concentrations exceed 20 µg per mL or the patient experiences toxicity.

In the treatment of acute bronchospasm which does not require intravenous therapy, theophylline may be given by mouth in the form of conventional tablets and capsules, or liquid preparations; sustained-release preparations are not suitable. In patients who have not been taking theophylline or aminophylline, theophylline may be given by mouth in similar loading doses to those used for intravenous treatment. Maintenance treatment is then given after the loading dose. In the *UK* preparations are available that can provide 60 to 250 mg up to four times daily. In the *US* the following theophylline oral maintenance doses are suggested: children aged 6 months to 9 years 4 mg per kg body-weight every 4 to 6 hours; children aged 9 to 16 years and adult smokers 3 mg per kg 4 to 6 hourly; non-smoking adults 3 mg per kg 6 to 8 hourly; older patients or patients with cor pulmonale 2 mg per kg 6 to 8 hourly; and in patients with congestive heart failure or liver disease 1 to 2 mg per kg 8 to 12 hourly. Doses higher than these should not be administered without serum-theophylline concentration measurements, and even at these doses, measurement is recommended.

In the treatment or prevention of chronic bronchospasm theophylline may be given by mouth as conventional tablets and capsules, liquid preparations, or sustained-release preparations. However, sustained-release preparations are more commonly used as they reduce the need for frequent dosing, especially in patients with a rapid theophylline clearance. In the *UK* conventional dose forms are given in doses ranging from 60 to 250 mg up to four times daily depending on age and response. Adult doses of sustained-release theophylline of 175 to 500 mg 12-hourly or 600 to 900 mg daily are used, depending upon the formulation. Reduced doses similar to those listed below are used for children.

In the *US* the following theophylline oral doses are suggested: adults and children over 1 year of age 16 mg per kg body-weight daily or 400 mg daily, whichever is the smaller, in divided doses where appropriate. If tolerated, the dose should then be increased in increments of approximately 25% at 2- to 3-day intervals until the following maximum daily doses are reached, which are the highest recommended without serum-theophylline concentration measurement: children aged 1 to 9 years 24 mg per kg body-weight; children aged 9 to 12 years 20 mg per kg; children aged 12 to 16 years 18 mg per kg; patients aged 16 years and above 13 mg per kg or 900 mg, whichever is the smaller. If toxicity is experienced at these doses, or higher doses are to be given, serum-theophylline concentration should be measured and final dosage adjustments based upon the results and the patient's clinical state. In all cases, serum-theophylline concentration should be rechecked at 6-to 12-monthly intervals. Also retitration of dosage is required if the patient is changed from one sustained-released preparation to another.

Theophylline monoethanolamine (theophylline olamine), theophylline calcium salicylate, theophylline and sodium acetate, (theophylline sodium acetate), theophylline sodium glycinate (theophylline sodium aminoacetate), and theophylline calcium glycinate have all been used similarly to theophylline.

Reviews of the actions and uses of theophylline and aminophylline: D. C. Flenley, *Postgrad. med. J.*, 1983, *59*, 1; L. Hendeles and M. Weinberger, *Pharmacotherapy*, 1983, *3*, 2; M. Bukowskyj *et al.*, *Ann. intern. Med.*, 1984, *101*, 63; P. J. Barnes, *Prescribers' J.*, 1986, *26*, 26.

ADMINISTRATION. Theophylline dosage prediction from serum concentrations obtained after a test dose given intravenously or by mouth, or at steady-state: R. W. Fitzpatrick, *Pharm. J.*, 1983, *2*, 384 (adults); D. R. Taylor *et al.*, *Br. J. clin. Pharmac.*, 1983, *15*, 689 (adults); *idem*, *16*, 511 (adults, oral test dose); D. T. Beswick *et al.*, *ibid.*, 1984, *18*, 298P (children); T. G. Wells *et al.*, *Ther. Drug Monit.*, 1984, *6*, 402 (children, Chiou and Vozeh methods); M. H. Johnson and W. S. Burkle, *Clin. Pharm.*, 1984, *3*, 174 (adults, Chiou method); M. J. Haumschild and J. E. Murphy, *ibid.*, 1985, *4*, 59 (adults, condition correction factors); M. E. Burton *et al.*, *Clin. Pharmacokinet.*, 1985, *10*, 1 (comparison of algorithms, pharmacokinetic, and Bayesian methods); H. Chrystyn *et al.*, *Pharm. J.*, 1985, *2*, 596 (adults, Bayesian analysis); K. A. Rodvold *et al.*, *Clin. Pharm.*, 1986, *5*, 403 (accuracy of Chiou and Bayesian methods, and standardised guidelines).

Administration in children. A 3-year-old asthmatic girl treated with an intravenous loading dose of aminophylline 6 mg per kg body-weight followed by a maintenance infusion of 1 mg per kg per hour required two further bolus doses of 3 mg per kg and an increase in the maintenance infusion rate to 1.5 mg per kg per hour to control her symptoms and give a serum-theophylline concentration within the therapeutic range. Some children require large doses to achieve a satisfactory serum concentration and clinical response.— D. W. Denning *et al.* (letter), *Lancet*, 1984, *1*, 223.

Administration in neonates. The following theophylline dosage guidelines for infants under one year of age have been suggested by the FDA: loading dose, when clinically indicated: 1 mg per kg body-weight for each 2 µg per mL desired increase in the serum-theophylline concentration. Initial maintenance doses: preterm infants up to 40 weeks postconception age (gestational age at birth plus postnatal age), 1 mg per kg every 12 hours; term infants (either at birth or 40 weeks postconception) up to 4 weeks postnatal, 1 to 2 mg per kg every 12 hours; infants aged 4 to 8 weeks, 1 to 2 mg per kg every 8 hours; infants aged over 8 weeks, 1 to 3 mg per kg every six hours. The final maintenance dose and dosage interval should be guided by serum-theophylline concentrations obtained after steady-state has been achieved.

Serum concentrations should be kept below 20 µg per mL for infants and 10 µg per mL for neonates.— *FDA Drug Bull.*, 1985, *15*, 16.

Administration in obesity. Data suggesting that the difference in volume of distribution for theophylline based on ideal body-weight and total body-weight increases as the degree of obesity increases. Hence the conflicting recommendations of the studies in which loading doses were calculated using ideal or total body-weight may be because the clinical importance of this difference is apparent only in morbidly obese patients.— N. Visram *et al.* (letter), *Clin. Pharm.*, 1987, *6*, 188.

ADMINISTRATION IN RENAL FAILURE. Theophylline can be given in usual doses to patients with renal failure. Concentrations are affected by haemodialysis or peritoneal dialysis.— W. M. Bennett *et al.*, *Am. J. Kidney Dis.*, 1983, *3*, 155.

In a study of 3 patients undergoing peritoneal dialysis after the administration of theophylline, the average values for clearance, elimination half-life, and percentage of dose recovered were 9.5 mL per minute, 5.5 hours, and 3.2% respectively. In 4 patients undergoing haemodialysis, the corresponding values were 84.8 mL per minute, 2.5 hours, and 40%. It was concluded that haemodialysis would be preferable to peritoneal dialysis for theophylline detoxification, but in uraemic patients requiring theophylline therapy, peritoneal dialysis may be preferred.— C. -S. C. Lee *et al.*, *J. clin. Pharmac.*, 1983, *23*, 274. See also J. R. Anderson *et al.*, *ibid.*, 428 (haemodialysis).

APNOEA. For the use of theophylline and aminophylline in neonatal apnoea, see under Pregnancy and the Neonate, below.

ASTHMA. Reviews on the use of theophylline and aminophylline in asthma: L. Hendeles and M. Weinberger, *Pharmac. Ther.*, 1983, *18*, 91; J. W. Jenne, *Clin. chest Med.*, 1984, *5*, 645; J. W. Paterson and R. A. Tarala, *Med. J. Aust.*, 1985, *143*, 390 and 453; *Med. Lett.*, 1987, *29*, 11; A. S. Rebuck and K. R. Chapman, *Can. med. Ass. J.*, 1987, *136*, 483.

Acute severe asthma. In the *UK* the treatment of patients with acute asthma severe enough to warrant hospital admission is usually started with oxygen, intravenous hydrocortisone, and a nebulised beta-2 selective stimulant. For those not responding to a nebulised bronchodilator, or those unable to use a nebuliser, the intravenous route may be necessary. Aminophylline and beta-2 selective stimulants are both effective when given intravenously and there seems little to choose between them in terms of bronchodilating efficacy although the risks may be higher with intravenous aminophylline. Also the risk with aminophylline is higher if it is given to patients on oral theophylline but most ill-effects probably result from over-rapid administration. For patients not responding adequately to oxygen, steroids, and a nebulised or intravenous beta-2 selective stimulant, the main therapeutic options are to add nebulised ipratropium bromide or intravenous aminophylline to the nebulised beta-2 selective stimulant. However, studies have found that the addition of intravenous aminophylline to nebulised salbutamol or inhaled isoprenaline did not enhance bronchodilatation, though tachycardia and other side-effects were increased (S.J. Williams *et al.*, *Br. med. J.*, 1975, *2*, 685; C.H. Fanta *et al.*, *Am. J. Med.*, 1982, *72*, 416), and the addition of intravenous aminophylline to inhaled orciprenaline made no difference to the rate of recovery of patients in a third study (D. Siegel *et al.*, *Am. Rev. resp. Dis.*, 1985, *132*, 283). However, patients with very severe asthma may respond less well to a nebulised beta-2 selective stimulant and may possibly show some response to aminophylline. Since the alternative may be mechanical ventilation it is reasonable to try the addition of intravenous aminophylline although any benefit is likely to be small and side-effects need to be anticipated.— *Lancet*, 1986, *1*, 131. See also: P. D. Phelan, *Med. J. Aust.*, 1985, *143*, 455 (acute asthma in children). Corrections regarding doses: J. W. Cox (letter), *ibid.*, 1986, *144*, 111; P. D. Phelan (letter), *ibid.*

To avoid the risk of toxicity in patients with acute severe asthma who have received xanthine therapy within the previous 24 hours and where serum-theophylline concentrations cannot be measured promptly, it has been suggested that the intravenous loading dose of aminophylline is omitted and treatment commenced with a maintenance dose infusion (P.J. Thompson and J.G. Hay, *Lancet*, 1982, *2*, 1228; D.J. O'Donoghue, *Br. med. J.*, 1983, *286*, 1053; J.R. Eason and M.R. Partridge, *Lancet*, 1983, *2*, 850; M.F. Stewart *et al.*, *Br. med. J.*, 1984, *288*, 450; M.C. Bateson, *Lancet*, 1986, *1*, 617). However, others have suggested that due to poor compliance, many patients will have subtherapeutic serum-theophylline concentrations and that to achieve rapid relief a bolus intravenous dose of aminophylline is necessary, with treatment based on repeated measurements of serum concentrations (S.P. Conway *et al.*, *Br. med. J.*, 1984, *288*, 715; C.S. Munro and K. Prowse, *ibid.*, *289*, 354; R. Feinmann *et al.*, *ibid.*, 767).

Childhood asthma. Orally administered beta-2 selective stimulants are usually considered the drugs of choice in the treatment of asthma in young children, but if side-effects are troublesome or the wheeze is not well controlled, theophylline should be added, preferably in combination. Generally, wheezing in infants under the age of 12 months responds neither to beta-2 selective stimulants nor to theophylline, irrespective of the route of administration, but there are exceptions, and a trial is often worthwhile. By the age of 12 to 18 months, wheezing in most children will respond to orally administered bronchodilator drugs.— C. M. Mellis, *Med. J. Aust.*, 1984, *141*, 167.

Children with moderate or severe asthma need drugs which prevent wheezing. Cromoglycate and slow-release theophyllines are equally effective, and there is no added benefit from giving both together. Inhaled steroids are more powerful prophylactic agents than either inhaled cromoglycate or oral theophylline. Steroids potentiate the effect of bronchodilators and children on inhaled steroids benefit from the concurrent use of either continuous beta adrenoceptor stimulants or oral theophylline.— J. Price, *Br. med. J.*, 1984, *288*, 1895.

For further references on the combined use of sodium cromoglycate with theophylline and corticosteroids with theophylline, see below.

Guidelines for the use of theophylline in children with asthma.— Allergy Section, Canadian Paediatric Society, *Can. med. Ass. J.*, 1985, *132*, 1011.

Combination therapy with beta-adrenoceptor stimulants. Some studies in chronic asthmatics have found that the addition of a beta-adrenoceptor stimulant to theophylline or aminophylline treatment, or *vice versa*, results in further bronchodilatation, and that the maximal bronchodilatation obtained with either agent singly can be obtained with lower doses of the 2 agents used in combination, sometimes reducing side-effects (J.D. Wolfe *et al.*, *New Engl. J. Med.*, 1978, *298*, 363; G. Lönnerholm *et al.*, *Br. med. J.*, 1981, *282*, 1029; K. Svedmyr, *Eur. J. resp. Dis.*, 1981, *62*, *Suppl.* 116, 1; J.J. Klein *et al.*, *Am. Rev. resp. Dis.*, 1983, *127*, 413; L.C. Laursen *et al.*, *Eur. J. resp. Dis.*, 1985, *66*, 82). However, other studies, particularly in patients with acute asthmatic attacks, have found little or no additional benefit from combined therapy (P.A. Eggleston *et al.*, *Chest*, 1981, *79*, 399; P.D.J. Handslip *et al.*, *Thorax*, 1981, *36*, 741; D. Siegel *et al.*, *Am. Rev. resp. Dis.*, 1985, *132*, 283; C.H. Fanta *et al.*, *Am. J. Med.*, 1986, *80*, 5). The discrepancy in findings has been attributed to the variability of airflow limitation in asthma (D.C. Flenley, *Postgrad. Med. J.*, 1983, *59*, 1). It was suggested that the combined use of theophylline or aminophylline with beta-adrenoceptor stimulants had caused an increase in deaths in asthmatics in New Zealand due to cardiovascular side-effects (J.D. Wilson *et al.*, *Lancet*, 1981, *1*, 1235; R.T. Jackson *et al.*, *Br. med. J.*, 1982, *285*, 771) and the FDA issued a caution concerning possible deleterious side-effects with the concomitant use of methylxanthines and beta-adrenoceptor stimulants (*FDA Drug Bull.*, 1981, *11*, 19). However, the temporal association between mortality and sales of drugs in New Zealand, Australia, and the *UK* suggested that direct drug toxicity is unlikely (G. Keating *et al.*, *Br. med. J.*, 1984, *289*, 348). Underuse of oral corticosteroids and overdependence on corticosteroid aerosols was implicated as a more important cause of asthma deaths (I.W.B. Grant, *Br. med. J.*, 1983, *286*, 374).

For reports suggesting that the combined oral administration of theophylline with beta-adrenoceptor stimulants does not increase the incidence of cardiac arrhythmias compared with administration of theophylline alone, even in overdose, see under Adverse Effects, above.

Combination therapy with hydroxyzine. The addition of hydroxyzine therapy to theophylline in patients with chronic asthma produced further improvements in lung function and reduced gastric irritation due to theophylline (K. Alanko and K. Sahlström, *Ann. clin. Res.*, 1983, *15*, 10; A. Lahdensuo and A. Jukkara, *ibid.*, 1986, *18*, 199).

Comparison with ketotifen. Eighteen children aged 1.5 to 6 years with severe asthma requiring prophylaxis were treated for 6 weeks in a double-blind study with ketotifen, 250 or 500 µg twice daily, placebo, or sustained-release theophylline at a dose adjusted to maintain optimum serum concentrations. Asthma symptom scores from the last 4 weeks of each treatment period showed a significant reduction in total symptoms with theophylline but not with ketotifen. Peak flow rates measured in 12 children were significantly improved by theophylline compared with ketotifen or placebo.— D. Stratton *et al.*, *Br. J. Dis. Chest*, 1984, *78*, 163.

Comparison with sodium cromoglycate. Theophylline given by mouth as choline theophyllinate was as effective as nebulised sodium cromoglycate in reducing sleep disturbance, cough, and wheeze in 16 children under 5 years of age (J. Glass *et al.*, *Archs Dis. Childh.*, 1981, *56*, 648). Similar symptomatic relief was obtained in 40 children aged 5 to 15 years and treated as above, but fewer side-effects were associated with sodium cromoglycate therapy (C.T. Furukawa *et al.*, *Pediatrics*, 1984, *74*, 453). It was considered that a patient inadequately controlled on sodium cromoglycate might gain some additional benefit from concomitant therapy with theophylline, but not *vice versa*, and there was no indication for the routine use of both drugs together (G. Hambleton *et al.*, *Lancet*, 1977, *1*, 381).

Exercise-induced asthma. The protective effects of theophylline in exercise-induced asthma are less than those of the sympathomimetics and are dose-dependent. Theophylline is not suitable for the prevention of exercise-induced asthma on an as-required-basis, and children on regular maintenance treatment with theophylline may still need inhaled sympathomimetics.— S. Godfrey, *Archs Dis. Childh.*, 1983, *58*, 1.

Inhalational theophylline therapy. In a study of 8 patients with severe asthma, theophylline 10 mg per mL, glycine theophyllinate 50 mg per mL, aminophylline 50 mg per mL, and diprophylline 125 mg per mL were effective bronchodilators when administered by inhalation after nebulisation, but were unpalatable and considerably less potent than inhaled salbutamol 200 µg.— M. J. Cushley and S. T. Holgate, *Thorax*, 1983, *38*, 223. See also P. J. Thompson *et al.*, *Br. J. clin. Pharmac.*, 1982, *14*, 463.

Nocturnal asthma. Sustained-release preparations of theophylline or aminophylline given at night to produce therapeutic serum-theophylline concentrations over the following 10 to 12 hours seem to be the most effective treatment for nocturnal asthma and early morning wheeze or 'morning-dipping' (P.J. Barnes *et al.*, *Lancet*, 1982, *1*, 299; F. Manresa *et al.*, *ibid.*, 1984, *2*, 52; P.D.O. Davies *et al.*, *Br. J. clin. Pharmac.*, 1984, *17*, 335; R. Walker *et al.*, *Pharm. J.*, 1987, *2*, R16).

For reports of diurnal variation in theophylline pharmacokinetics, see under Absorption and Fate, above.

Oral sustained-release therapy. The short and unpredictable half-life of theophylline, resulting from its rapid absorption and variable clearance, has led to the introduction of sustained-release preparations which may be given 12-hourly or once daily (*Drug & Ther. Bull.*, 1985, *23*, 33). Some sustained-release preparations have been shown to be more effective in controlling bronchospasm than conventional preparations (R. Andrasch and M. Schmitz-Schumann, *Pharmatherapeutica*, 1984, *3*, 668) and they may decrease the need for additional bronchodilators (P.J. Barnes *et al.*, *Lancet*, 1982, *1*, 299) and improve patient compliance (J.K. Wiffen and S.H.D. Jackson, *J. R. Soc. Med.*, 1983, *76*, 917). However, it has been reported that adverse effects may persist for longer (*Med. Lett.*, 1981, *23*, 97), and that children and adult smokers who metabolise theophylline the most rapidly may require 8-hourly administration of sustained-release preparations intended for twice-daily dosage (M. Weinberger and L. Hendeles, *New Engl. J. Med.*, 1983, *308*, 760). Some sustained-release preparations for once-daily administration appear to be as effective as those given 12-hourly (R.J. Dockhorn *et al.*, *Ann. Allergy*, 1985, *55*, 658; W.W. Arkinstall *et al.*, *Am. Rev. resp. Dis.*, 1987, *135*, 316), and may improve nocturnal symptoms (P.W. Welsh *et al.*, *Am. J. Med.*, 1986, *80*, 1098; S. Levene and S. McKenzie, *Br. J. Dis. Chest*, 1986, *80*, 66).

CARDIAC ARRHYTHMIAS. The successful use of oral theophylline to prevent recurrent symptomatic bradyarrhythmias in 6 of 8 adolescents and young adults.— D. G. Benditt *et al.*, *Am. J. Cardiol.*, 1983, *52*, 1223.

CHRONIC OBSTRUCTIVE AIRWAYS DISEASE. In addition to its bronchodilating activity, theophylline may also increase diaphragmatic contractility (M.A. Aubier *et al.*, *New Engl. J. Med.*, 1981, *305*, 249), suppress diaphragmatic fatigue (D. Murciano *et al.*, *ibid.*, 1984, *311*, 349), and produce a modest improvement in cardiac performance in patients with chronic obstructive airways diseases such as chronic bronchitis and emphysema (R.A. Matthay *et al.*, *Am. Heart J.*, 1982, *104*, 1022). Some studies have demonstrated an improvement in lung function and exercise tolerance in such patients following theophylline or aminophylline administration (C.R. McGavin *et al.*, *Br. med. J.*, 1976, *1*, 822; M.L. Eaton *et al.*, *Ann. intern. Med.*, 1980, *92*, 758; A.G. Leitch *et al.*, *Thorax*, 1981, *36*, 787; R.M. Nietrzeba *et* al., *Bull. Eur. Physiopathol. Respir.*, 1984, *20*, 361; W.V. Evans, *Br. J. clin. Pract.*, 1986, *40*, 245). Other studies have found no worthwhile benefit (P.F. Jenkins *et al.*, *Br. J. Dis. Chest*, 1982, *76*, 57; M.L. Eaton *et al.*, *Chest*, 1982, *82*, 538; W.V. Evans, *Br. med. J.*, 1984, *289*, 1649; K.L. Rice *et al.*, *Ann. intern. Med.*, 1987, *107*, 305). It has been suggested that theophylline should be tried only if symptoms of chronic obstructive bronchitis persist after the use of optimum doses of inhaled bronchodilators (G.M. Cochrane, *Br. med. J.*, 1984, *289*, 1643), whereas others have suggested the combined use of theophylline and inhaled bronchodilators (D.G. McDevitt, *ibid.*, 1985, *290*, 466). The addition of inhaled antimuscarinic agents (P.M. Passamonte and A.J. Martinez, *Chest*, 1984, *85*, 610) or beta-2 selective stimulants (D.R. Taylor *et al*, *Am. Rev. resp. Dis.*, 1985, *131*, 747; G.H. Guyatt *et al.*, *ibid.*, 1987, *135*, 1069) to theophylline therapy in patients with chronic obstructive airways disease has resulted in a further increase in lung function, and the combination of theophylline, inhaled antimuscarinic agent, and inhaled beta-2 selective stimulant was more effective than theophylline with either an inhaled antimuscarinic agent or beta-2 selective stimulant (N. Krivoy *et al.*, *Postgrad. med. J.*, 1987, *63*, *Suppl.* 1, 21a).

HEART FAILURE. Theophylline administered as choline theophyllinate 600 mg by mouth to 9 patients with chronic left ventricular failure due to myocardial dysfunction, and refractory to diuretics, increased cardiac index in 7 patients. Lack of response was due to poor absorption in one and extensive myocardial hypokinesia in the other. Mean stroke volume index and systemic arterial pressure increased and left ventricular filling pressure and right atrial pressure fell in all patients.— S. Al-Damluji *et al.*, *Postgrad. med. J.*, 1982, *58*, 216.

IMMUNOSUPPRESSANT ACTION. In a prospective study, the addition of aminophylline 900 mg daily by mouth to conventional immunosuppressive therapy of azathioprine plus prednisolone improved the 6-month graft survival from 50 to 72.7% in patients receiving cadaveric renal transplants.— P. J. Guillou *et al.*, *Transplantn Proc.*, 1984, *16*, 1218.

PAIN. *Headache.* Theophylline was significantly more effective than placebo in relieving headache following lumbar puncture in a double-blind study in 11 patients.— T. J. Feuerstein and A. Zeides, *Klin. Wschr.*, 1986, *64*, 216.

Renal colic. In a preliminary study, aminophylline given by slow intravenous injection relieved the pain caused by the passage of ureter stones in 5 of 6 patients. Pain relief lasted for 30 minutes; additional drug treatment was required within 30 minutes to 2.5 hours after aminophylline.— K. Katevuo *et al.*, *Int. J. clin. Pharmac. Ther. Toxic.*, 1981, *19*, 512.

PREGNANCY AND THE NEONATE. The most commonly used and best studied bronchodilator in pregnancy is oral theophylline. Theophylline readily crosses the placenta, but neonates seem to tolerate theophylline concentrations within the usual therapeutic range without serious side-effects. No dysmorphogenic effects have been attributed to theophylline or aminophylline.— H. Mawhinney and S. L. Spector, *Drugs*, 1986, *32*, 178. See also: A. M. Weinstein *et al.*, *J. Am. med. Ass.*, 1979, *241*, 1161; P. A. Greenberger and R. Patterson, *New Engl. J. Med.*, 1985, *312*, 897.

For reports of alterations in maternal theophylline clearance during pregnancy, see Pregnancy and the Neonate under Absorption and Fate, above.

Neonatal apnoea. Theophylline and aminophylline have been used successfully to prevent or decrease the frequency of apnoeic attacks in premature infants (J.A. Kuzemo and J. Paala, *Archs Dis. Childh.*, 1973, *48*, 404; M.J. Boutroy *et al.*, *Lancet*, 1978, *1*, 1257; R.A.K. Jones and E. Baillie, *Archs Dis. Childh.*, 1979, *54*, 190; J.-L. Brazier *et al.*, *ibid.*, 194; A.J. Lyon and N. McIntosh, *ibid.*, 1985, *60*, 38), and may be more effective than continuous positive airways pressure treatment in very immature infants (R.A.K. Jones, *ibid.*, 1982, *57*, 761).

Neonatal respiratory distress syndrome. Aminophylline has been used successfully to facilitate weaning of infants with respiratory distress syndrome or hyaline membrane disease from mechanical ventilation (P.A. Barr, *Archs Dis. Childh.*, 1978, *53*, 598; N.V. Erkan *et al.*, *ibid.*, 1979, *54*, 81; C. Castalos *et al.*, *ibid.*, 404; M.C. Harris *et al.*, *J. Pediat.*, 1983, *103*, 303).

Aminophylline given *ante partum* to women at risk of premature delivery has reduced the incidence of neonatal respiratory distress syndrome (E. Hadjigeorgiou *et al.*, *Am. J. Obstet. Gynec.*, 1979, *135*, 257) and has been reported to be as effective as the *ante partum* administration of betamethasone (B. Granati *et al.*, *Pediat. Pharmacol.*, 1984, *4*, 21). However, the administration of aminophylline to premature neonates did not significantly alter the course and outcome of respiratory distress syndrome (T. Hegyi *et al.*, *Clin. Ther.*, 1986, *8*, 439).

RHINITIS. In a placebo-controlled crossover study of 10 patients with pollen-induced rhinitis, theophylline given as a 400-mg sustained-release tablet twice daily for 7 days was significantly more effective than placebo in reducing sneezing and the concentrations of histamine and other mediators in nasal secretions.— R. M. Naclerio *et al.*, *J. Allergy & clin. Immunol.*, 1986, *78*, 874.

SLEEP DISORDERS. Theophylline has not been shown to be of long-term benefit in obstructive sleep apnoea.— P. D. Bull, *Practitioner*, 1987, *231*, 1182.

Preparations

Theophylline Capsules *(U.S.P.)*. Potency is expressed in terms of anhydrous theophylline.

Theophylline, Ephedrine Hydrochloride, and Phenobarbital Tablets *(U.S.P.)*. Contain theophylline, ephedrine hydrochloride, and phenobarbitone. The potency of theophylline is expressed in terms of anhydrous theophylline. Store in airtight containers.

Theophylline and Guaifenesin Capsules *(U.S.P.)*. Contain theophylline and guaiphenesin. The potency of theophylline is expressed in terms of anhydrous theophylline. Store in airtight containers.

Theophylline and Guaifenesin Oral Solution *(U.S.P.)*. Contains theophylline and guaiphenesin. The potency of theophylline is expressed in terms of anhydrous theophylline. Store in airtight containers.

Theophylline Sodium Glycinate Elixir *(U.S.P.)*. Contains alcohol 17 to 23%. pH 8.7 to 9.1. Store in airtight containers.

Theophylline Sodium Glycinate Tablets *(U.S.P.)*

Theophylline Tablets *(U.S.P.)*. Potency is expressed in terms of anhydrous theophylline.

Proprietary Preparations

Biophylline *(Delandale, UK)*. *Syrup*, theophylline hydrate 125 mg/5 mL (as theophylline sodium glycinate).

Labophylline *(Laboratories for Applied Biology, UK)*. *Injection*, anhydrous theophylline 20 mg/mL, lysine 12.2 mg/mL, in ampoules of 10 mL.

Lasma *(Pharmax, UK)*. *Tablets*, sustained-release, scored, anhydrous theophylline 300 mg.

Nuelin *(Riker, UK)*. *Liquid*, theophylline hydrate 60 mg/5 mL (as theophylline sodium glycinate). *Tablets*, microcrystalline anhydrous theophylline, 125 mg.
Tablets (Nuelin SA), sustained-release, anhydrous theophylline 175 mg.
Tablets (Nuelin SA-250), sustained-release, anhydrous theophylline 250 mg.

Nuelin liquid (*UK*) contains sugar which could cause extensive and severe dental caries in young children needing long-term treatment (*Drug & Ther. Bull.*, 1983, *21*, 56). Nuelin formulations (*UK*) do not contain allergenic colouring agents to which asthmatic children may be sensitive (D.W. Denning and R. Vijeratnam, *Lancet*, 1985, *1*, 461).

Pro-Vent *(Calmic, UK)*. *Capsules*, sustained-release, anhydrous theophylline 300 mg.

Slo-Phyllin *(Lipha, UK)*. *Capsules*, anhydrous theophylline 60 mg, 125 mg, and 250 mg in sustained-release pellets, which may be administered in food.

Theo-Dur *(Astra, UK)*. *Tablets*, scored, sustained-release, anhydrous theophylline 200 mg and 300 mg.

Theo-Dur tablets (*UK*) do not contain allergenic colouring agents to which asthmatic children may be sensitive.— D. W. Denning and R. Vijeratnam (letter), *Lancet*, 1985, *1*, 461.

Uniphyllin Continus *(Napp, UK)*. *Tablets*, sustained-release, scored, anhydrous theophylline 200, 300, and 400 mg.

Uniphyllin 200 mg tablets (*UK*) do not contain allergenic colouring agents to which asthmatic children may be sensitive.— *Lancet*, 1985, *1*, 754.

Proprietary Names and Manufacturers of Theophylline or Theophylline Compounds

Accurbron *(Merrell Dow, USA)*; Aerobin *(Schwabe-Farmasan, Ger.)*; Aerolate *(Fleming, USA)*; Afonilum *(Minden, Ger.)*; Aminomal *(Malesci, Ital.)*; Aminomed *(Medo, UK)*; Aquaphyllin *(Ferndale, USA)*; Armophylline *(Rorer, Fr.)*; Asmafil *(Ital.)*; Asperal-T *(Belg.)*; Asthmophylline *(Canad.)*; Bilordyl *(Fisons, Ger.)*; Biophylline *(Delandale, UK)*; Bronchoparat *(Klinge, Ger.)*; Bronchoretard *(Klinge, Ger.)*; Bronkodyl *(Winthrop-Breon, USA)*; Cetraphylline *(Unicet, Fr.)*; Constant-T *(Geigy, USA)*; Cronasma *(Farmitalia, Ger.)*; Diffumal *(Malesci, Ital.)*; Dilatrane *(Fisons, Fr.)*; Duraphyl *(Forest Pharmaceuticals, USA)*; Duraphyllin *(Durachemie, Ger.)*; Elixicon *(Berlex, USA)*; Elixomin *(USA)*; Elixophyllin *(Schering, Austral.; Berlex, Canad.; Forest Pharmaceuticals, USA)*; Elixophylline *(Schering, Switz.)*; Englate *(Nicholas, UK)*; Euphyllina Rilcon *(Byk Gulden, Ital.)*; Euphylline *(Valpan, Fr.)*; Godafilin *(Igoda, Spain)*; Inophyline *(Millot-Solac, Fr.)*; Labid *(Norwich Eaton, USA)*; Labophylline *(Laboratories for Applied Biology, UK)*; Lasma *(Pharmax, UK)*; Lodrane *(Poythress, USA)*; Micro-Phyllin *(Script Intal, S.Afr.)*; Monotheamin *(Lilly, UK)*; Nuelin *(Riker, Austral.; Riker, Denm.; Riker, Norw.; Riker, S.Afr.; Riker, UK)*; Oxyphyllin *(Draco, Swed.)*; Paidomal *(Malesci, Ital.)*; Physpan *(Savage, USA)*; Pro-Vent *(Calmic, UK)*; Pulm *(Saron, USA)*; Pulmidur *(Astra, Ger.)*; Pulmophylline *(Riva, Canad.)*; Pulmo-Timelets *(Temmler, Denm.; Temmler, Ger.)*; Quibron-T *(Bristol, Canad.; Bristol, USA)*; Respbid *(Boehringer Ingelheim, Canad.; Boehringer Ingelheim, USA)*; Rona-Phyllin *(Lipha, UK)*; Slo-Bid *(Rorer, USA)*; Slo-Phyllin *(Rorer, Ital.; Lipha, UK; Rorer, USA)*; Sodiphylline *(Sodip, Switz.)*; Solosin *(Cassella-Riedel, Ger.)*; Somofillina *(Fisons, Ital.)*; Somophyllin *(Fisons, Austral.; Fisons, Canad.; Fisons, Denm.; Fisons, S.Afr.; Fisons, USA)*; Somophylline *(Fisons, Switz.)*; Sustaire *(Pfizer, USA)*; Synophylate *(Central Pharmaceuticals, USA)*; Tagilen *(Mepha, Switz.)*; Techniphylline *(Techni-Pharma, Mon.)*; Tefamin *(Recordati, Ital.)*; Teoclasma *(Ital.)*; Teofyllin *(DAK, Denm.; Nyco, Norw.)*; Teoglicina *(FAMA, Ital.)*; Teolixir Normal *(Spain)*; Teonova *(Corvi, Ital.)*; Theo-24 *(Searle, USA)*; Theobid *(Glaxo, USA)*; Theocap *(USA)*; Theoclear *(Central Pharmaceuticals, USA)*; Theocontin *(Napp, UK)*; Theocot T.D. *(USA)*; Theocyne *(Canad.)*; Theo-Dur *(Astra, Austral.; Astra, Canad.; Draco, Denm.; Recordati, Ital.; Draco, Norw.; Antibioticos, Spain; Draco, Swed.; Astra, Switz.; Astra, UK; Key, USA)*; Theodur *(Astra, S.Afr.)*; Theofrenon *(Hefa-Frenon, Ger.)*; Theograd *(Abbott, UK)*; Theolair *(Belg.; Riker, Canad.; Riker, Fr.; Kettelhack Riker, Ger.; Selvi, Ital.; Neth.; Abello, Spain; Swed.; Riker 3M, Switz.; Riker, USA)*; Theolixir *(Canad.)*; Theon *(Bock, USA)*; Theopexine *(Synthelabo, Fr.)*; Theophyl *(Canad.; McNeil Pharmaceutical, USA)*; Theosol *(Martindale Pharmaceuticals, UK)*; Theospan *(Laser, USA)*; Theospirex *(Krewel, Ger.)*; Theostat *(Sinbio, Fr.; Laser, USA)*; Theovent *(Schering, USA)*; Unifyl *(Mundipharma, Switz.)*; Uniphyl *(Purdue Frederick, USA)*; Uniphyllin *(Mundipharma, Ger.; Napp, UK)*; Unixan *(Pharmacia, Denm.)*; Vent-retard *(Boi, Spain)*; Xantivent *(Essex, Switz.)*.

The following names have been used for multi-ingredient preparations containing theophylline or theophylline compounds—Acet-Am *(Organon, Canad.)*; Asbron *(Anca, Canad.)*; Asbron G *(Sandoz, USA)*; Asmapax *(Nicholas, UK)*; Bronkolixir *(Winthrop-Breon, USA)*; Bronkotabs *(Winthrop-Breon, USA)*; Eclabron *(Wharton, USA)*; Elixophyllin-GG *(Forest Pharmaceuticals, USA)*; Elixophyllin-KI *(Schering, Austral.; Berlex, Canad.; Forest Pharmaceuticals, USA)*; Entair *(Duncan, Flockhart, UK)*; Franol *(Winthrop, UK)*; Franol Expect *(Winthrop, UK)*; Franol Plus *(Winthrop, UK)*; Franyl; IDM *(Rougier, Canad.)*; IDM-Expectorant *(Rougier, Canad.)*; Iso-Bronchisan *(Berk Pharmaceuticals, UK)*; Isuprel Compound Elixir *(Winthrop, Canad.; Breon, USA; Winthrop-Breon, USA)*; Marax *(Roerig, USA)*; Mudrane GG Elixir *(Poythress, USA)*; Phyldrox *(Carlton Laboratories, UK)*; Pneumogeine *(Gamaprod, Austral.)*; Priatan *(Schering, Austral.)*; Primatene M *(Whitehall, USA)*; Primatene P *(Whitehall, USA)*; Quadrinal *(Knoll, USA)*; Quibron *(Astra, Austral.; Bristol, USA)*; Quibron Plus *(Mead Johnson Laboratories, USA)*; Riddospas *(Riddell, UK)*; Slo-phyllin GG *(Rorer, USA)*; Synophylate-GG *(Central Pharmaceuticals, USA)*; Tancolin *(Ashe, UK)*; Tedral *(Parke, Davis, Canad.; Parke, Davis, UK; Parke, Davis, USA)*; Tedral SA *(Warner, UK)*; Tedral-25 *(Parke, Davis, USA)*; T.E.H. *(Geneva, USA)*; T-E-P *(Schein, USA)*; T.E.P. *(Geneva, USA)*; Theolair-Plus *(Riker, USA)*; Theonar *(MCP Pharmaceuticals, UK)*; Theo-Organidin *(Horner, Canad.; Wallace, USA)*; Theozine *(Schein, USA)*.

3874-t

Xanthine-containing Beverages

Evaluations of the caffeine content of various foods, beverages, and drugs: *FDA Consumer*, 1984, (Mar.), 14.

European Economic Community regulations direct that the term 'decaffeinated' relates to coffee extracts the anhydrous caffeine content of which does not exceed 0.3% by weight of its coffee-based dry matter content.— *Off. J. E.E.C.*, 1977, *20*, L172, 20.

Adverse Effects

The adverse effects of xanthine-containing beverages are largely due to their caffeine, theophylline, and theobromine content and are described under theophylline (see p.1526). Common side-effects are sleeplessness, anxiety, tremor, palpitations, and withdrawal headache.

Reviews of caffeine toxicity resulting from the ingestion of xanthine-containing beverages: J. E. James and K. P. Stirling, *Br. J. Addict.*, 1983, *78*, 251; *J. Am. med. Ass.*, 1984, *252*, 803; P. J. Abbott, *Med. J. Aust.*, 1986, *145*, 518.

Comment on the adverse effects associated with coffee drinking.— *Lancet*, 1981, *1*, 256.

A report of 2 deaths associated with the use of coffee enemas.— J. W. Eisele and D. T. Reay, *J. Am. med. Ass.*, 1980, *244*, 1608.

EFFECTS ON THE BREAST. Three case-controlled studies have found no association between benign breast disease in women and coffee or tea consumption or methylxanthine intake (D.H. Lawson *et al.*, *Sugery, St. Louis*, 1981, *90*, 801; J. Marshall *et al.*, *Am. J. publ. Hlth*, 1982, *72*, 610; F. Lubin *et al.*, *J. Am. med. Ass.*, 1985, *253*, 2388), but 2 similar studies have demonstrated an increased risk (C.A. Boyle *et al.*, *J. natn. Cancer Inst.*, 1984, *72*, 1015; C. La Vecchia *et al.*, *ibid.*, 1985, *74*, 995). The discrepancy in findings was attributed to such studies failing to find an association if all individuals are not equally susceptible to developing a disease, and double-blind controlled challenge studies were recommended (M.F. Jacobson and B.F. Liebman, *J. Am. med. Ass.*, 1986, *255*, 1438). It was felt that sensitive benign breast disease would resolve after complete methylxanthine abstention (J.P. Minton, *ibid.*, 1985, *254*, 2408).

For reports suggesting that there is not a causal relationship between coffee intake and breast cancer, see under Malignant Neoplasms, below.

EFFECTS ON THE CARDIOVASCULAR SYSTEM. *Arrhythmias.* Seven healthy subjects and 12 patients with heart disease were given either coffee 200 mL (containing caffeine 200 mg) by mouth, or caffeine citrate 200 mg intravenously and monitored for cardiac arrhythmias after atrial pacing. Sustained atrial tachyarrhythmias developed in 3 of 5 patients receiving coffee, and 2 of 7 patients and 3 of 7 controls receiving caffeine citrate. Nonsustained ventricular tachycardia developed in one patient receiving coffee and one receiving caffeine citrate. The effects of caffeine and coffee were not significantly different (D.J. Dobmeyer *et al.*, *New Engl. J. Med.*, 1983, *308*, 814; S.F. Schaal, *ibid.*, *309*, 559).

Ischaemic heart disease. Reports from the Boston Collaborative Drug Surveillance Program (*Lancet*, 1972, *2*, 1278; *New Engl. J. Med.*, 1973, *289*, 63) and others (D.A. Snowdon *et al.*, *Prev. Med.*, 1984, *13*, 490; A.Z. LaCroix *et al.*, *New Engl. J. Med.*, 1986, *315*, 977) have suggested an association between coronary heart disease, acute myocardial infarction, and coffee consumption. This has not been confirmed by studies taking other risk factors into account (A.L. Klatsky *et al.*, *J. Am. med. Ass.*, 1973, *226*, 540; T.R. Dawber *et al.*, *New Engl. J. Med.*, 1974, *291*, 871; C.H. Hennekens *et al.*, *ibid.*, 1976, *294*, 633; K. Yano *et al.*, *ibid.*, 1977, *297*, 405; C.A. Bertrand *et al.*, *ibid.*, 1978, *299*, 315 and 726; S. Heyden *et al.*, *Archs intern. Med.*, 1978, *138*, 1472; K. Yano *et al.*, *New Engl. J. Med.*, 1987, *316*, 946).

Hypertension. Coffee drinking has been shown to cause an acute transient increase in blood pressure in healthy subjects who do not normally ingest methylxanthines (D. Robertson *et al.*, *J. clin. Invest.*, 1981, *67*, 1111; P. Smits *et al.*, *Am. J. Cardiol.*, 1985, *56*, 958), as well as in untreated and thiazide-treated mild hypertensives (S. Freestone and L.E. Ramsay, *Br. J. clin. Pharmac.*, 1981, *11*, 428P). This increase in blood pressure is not seen after drinking decaffeinated coffee, suggesting that it is mainly due to caffeine (P. Smits *et al.*, *ibid.*, 1985, *19*, 852), and decreases as consumption of coffee is continued, possibly due to adaptation (D. Robertson *et al.*, 1981; H.P.T. Ammon *et al.*, *Br. J. clin. Pharmac.*, 1983, *15*, 701). The long-term administration of caffeine to borderline hypertensives did not result in a sustained significant increase in blood pressure (D. Robertson *et al.*, *Am. J. Med.*, 1984, *77*, 54).

EFFECTS ON THE GASTRO-INTESTINAL TRACT. Heartburn was the major gastro-intestinal symptom associated with drinking coffee in a study of 31 subjects with a history of these symptoms. The heartburn appeared to be associated with lower oesophageal sphincter dysfunction and gastro-oesophageal reflux rather than gastric hypersecretion although symptoms could be modified by a reduction in acid secretion. Intrinsic harmful components in coffee do not appear to be responsible.— S. Cohen, *New Engl. J. Med.*, 1980, *303*, 122.

EFFECTS ON IRON ABSORPTION. Tea produced a 41 to 95% inhibition of iron absorption; the effect was apparently specific for non-haem iron and could be especially useful in the management of patients with thalassaemia intermedia who might absorb large amounts of dietary iron.— P. A. de Alarcon *et al.*, *New Engl. J. Med.*, 1979, *300*, 5.

In 37 iron-replete subjects, a cup of filter coffee taken simultaneously with, or one hour after, a meal reduced non-haem iron absorption by an average of 39%. When no food was present, coffee reduced iron absorption by 70%.— T. A. Morck *et al.*, *Am. J. clin. Nutr.*, 1983, *37*, 416.

EFFECTS ON THE LIVER. A woman who had been eating 227 g of tea every 3 to 4 days for about 5 years developed liver dysfunction. Splenomegaly and ascites resolved when she ceased eating tea but liver fibrosis was still present 15 years later. The liver dysfunction could have been due to the tannin content of tea.— K. J. Murphy, *Med. J. Aust.*, 1975, *2*, 428.

Veno-occlusive disease of the liver in a young woman was attributed to the consumption of large quantities of maté tea over a number of years.— J. O'D. McGee *et al.*, *J. clin. Path.*, 1976, *29*, 788.

A few days after hospital admission for severe abdominal symptoms hepatic coma developed in a 35-year-old black, diabetic, alcoholic, male, associated with caffeine accumulation following ingestion of 7 cups of coffee (totalling about 800 mg of caffeine) daily.— B. E. Statland *et al.* (letter), *New Engl. J. Med.*, 1976, *295*, 110.

EFFECTS ON SERUM LIPIDS. Several studies have noted a positive association between coffee drinking and increased serum-cholesterol concentrations (D.S. Thelle *et al.*, *New Engl. J. Med.*, 1983, *308*, 1454; E. Arnesen *et al.*, *Br. med. J.*, 1984, *288*, 1960; P.T. Williams *et al.*, *J. Am. med. Ass.*, 1985, *253*, 1407; A.L. Klatsky *et al.*, *Am. J. Cardiol.*, 1985, *22*, 577; S.M. Haffner *et al.*, *Am. J. Epidem.*, 1985, *122*, 1; J.D. Curb *et al.*, *ibid.*, 1986, *123*, 648) and in a group of hypercholesterolaemic men, abstention from coffee drinking resulted in a significant fall in serum-cholesterol concentrations (O.H. Førde *et al.*, *Br. med. J.*, 1985, *290*, 893). Others have found no association between coffee drinking and increased serum-cholesterol concentrations (A. Hofman *et al.*, *New Engl. J. Med.*, 1983, *309*, 1248; M.G. Kovar *et al.*, *ibid.*, 1249; R.B. Shekelle *et al.*, *ibid.*; P.I. Hershberg, *J. Am. med. Ass.*, 1985, *254*, 2737), or have noted a positive association only in young people (L. Arab *et al.*, *New Engl. J. Med.*, 1983, *309*, 1250) or in women (M. Shirlow and C. Mathers, *ibid.*; S. Mathias *et al.*, *Am. J. Epidem.*, 1985, *121*, 896). Attempts to explain these discrepancies have cited differences in diet (I.A. Ockene *et al.*, *New. Engl. J. Med.*, 1983, *309*, 1248; I.E. Roeckel, *ibid.*), stress (G. Modest, *ibid.*; P.J. Rosch, *J. Am. med. Ass.*, 1985, *254*, 2738), the quantity of coffee consumed (M.G. Kovar *et al.*, 1983; L. Arab *et al.*, 1983), or the method of brewing the coffee (M.G. Kovar *et al.*, 1983; R.B. Shekelle *et al.*, 1983).

MALIGNANT NEOPLASMS. A study of 1013 patients found an unexpected positive association between coffee or tea consumption and pancreatic cancer (B. MacMahon *et al.*, *New Engl. J. Med.*, 1981, *304*, 630) and some later studies have also tentatively suggested such an association (A. Nomura *et al.*, *Lancet*, 1981, *2*, 415; C.-C. Hsieh *et al.*, *New Engl. J. Med.*, 1986, *315*, 587; F. Clavel *et al.*, *ibid.*, 1987, *316*, 483). However, others have not been able to confirm these findings (H. Jick and B.J. Dinan, *Lancet*, 1981, *2*, 92; I. Heuch *et al.*, *Br. J. Cancer*, 1983, *48*, 637; E.L. Wynder *et al.*, *Cancer Res.*, 1983, *43*, 3900; L.J. Kinlen and K. McPherson, *Br. J. Cancer*, 1984, *49*, 93; M.A. Bernarde and W. Weiss, *Br. med. J.*, 1982, *284*, 400; L. Kinlen *et al.*, *Lancet*, 1984, *1*, 282), or have found an exposure-response relationship only in certain groups: in women (E.B. Gold *et al.*, *Cancer*, 1985, *55*, 460), in men (T.M. Mack *et al.*, *J. natn. Cancer Inst.*, 1986, *76*, 49), or in women consuming decaffeinated coffee (R.S. Lin and I.I. Kessler, *J. Am. med. Ass.*, 1981, *245*, 147). It was suggested that the positive association between coffee consumption and pancreatic cancer may be due to increased coffee intake resulting from thirst caused by the cancer (L. Kinlen *et al.*, 1984); this explanation was partly supported by the data of Nomura *et al.* (*Lancet*, 1984 *1*, 917), but refuted by the work of Heuch *et al.* (*ibid.*, 1985, *1*, 339). A possible association between the use of methylxanthine bronchodilators and pancreatic cancer was also postulated (C.D. Robinette, *ibid.*, 1981, *2*, 754), but was not supported by the data of Kummet *et al.* (*ibid.*, 1983, *2*, 231).

Suggestions that coffee drinking is involved in the aetiology of bladder and renal cancer (P. Cole, *ibid.*, 1971, *1*, 1335; R. Schmauz and P. Cole, *J. natn. Cancer Inst.*, 1974, *52*, 1431; D.H. Shennan, *Br. J. Cancer*, 1973, *28*, 473) have not been confirmed (R.W. Morgan and M.G. Jain, *Can. med. Ass. J.*, 1974, *111*, 1067; B. Armstrong *et al.*, *Br. J. Cancer*, 1976, *33*, 127).

Evidence suggests that there is not a causal relationship between coffee intake and breast cancer and that caffeine may have antineoplastic effects (P. Dews *et al.*, *Food Chem. Toxicol.*, 1984, *22*, 163; F. Lubin, *et al.*, *J. natn. Cancer Inst.*, 1985, *74*, 569; J. Pozner *et al.*, *J. Am. med. Ass.*, 1986, *255*, 748).

PREGNANCY AND THE NEONATE. Reports of low-birth weight and birth defects associated with a high maternal caffeine intake (as coffee) during pregnancy (G. Mau and P. Netter, *Geburtsh. Frauenheilk.*, 1974, *34*, 1018; P.S. Weathersbee *et al.*, *Postgrad. Med.*, 1977, *62*, 64; I. Borlée *et al.*, *Louvain Méd.*, 1978, *97*, 279) prompted the *US* Food and Drug Administration in 1980 to advise pregnant women to limit their caffeine intake (J.E. Goyen, *FDA News Release*, 1980, *P80-36*, 3). However, several large studies have since found no association between birth defects and coffee consumption during pregnancy (L. Rosenberg *et al.*, *J. Am. med. Ass.*, 1982, *247*, 1429; S. Linn *et al.*, *New Engl. J. Med.*, 1982, *306*, 141; K. Kurppa *et al.*, *ibid.*, 1548), but a cohort study of 3135 pregnant women did find an association between 'moderate to heavy' caffeine consumption during pregnancy and late spontaneous abortion (W. Srisuphan and M.B. Bracken *Am. J. Obstet. Gynec.*, 1986, *154*, 14).

Uses and Administration

Xanthine-containing beverages including chocolate, coffee, cocoa, cola, maté, and tea are widely consumed, mainly for their mild stimulant effect.

Coffee is the kernel of the dried ripe seeds of *Coffea arabica*, *C. liberica*, *C. canephora* (robusta coffee), and other species of *Coffee* (Rubiaceae), roasted until it acquires a deep brown colour and a pleasant characteristic aroma. It contains about 1 to 2% of caffeine. Coffee has been used in the form of an infusion or decoction as a stimulant and as a flavouring agent in some pharmaceutical preparations.

A decoction is used as a beverage containing up to about 100 mg of caffeine per 100 mL (see p.1523). Preparations of instant coffee may contain up to 40% less caffeine while decaffeinated preparations may contain only about 3 mg per 100 mL.

Kola (cola, cola seeds, kola nuts) is the dried cotyledons of *Cola nitida* and *C. acuminata* (Sterculiaceae), containing about 1.5 to 2.5% of caffeine and traces of theobromine. Kola is used in the preparation of cola drinks which may contain up to 20 mg of caffeine per 100 mL. Kola has been used to treat migraine in homoeopathic medicine.

Maté (Paraguay Tea) is the dried leaves of *Ilex paraguensis* (Aquifoliaceae), containing 0.2 to 2% of caffeine. Maté is less astringent than tea and is extensively used as a beverage in South America.

Tea (thea, chá, thé, tee) is the prepared young leaves and leaf-buds of *Camellia sinensis* (=*C. thea*) (Theaceae). It contains 1 to 4% of caffeine and 7 to 15% of tannin. Tea is used in an infusion as a beverage containing up to about 60 mg of caffeine per 100 mL.

ASTHMA. For a report suggesting that coffee could be used as a bronchodilator when other anti-asthmatic medications are unavailable, see under caffeine hydrate (p.1523).

ORTHOSTATIC HYPOTENSION. For the use of coffee in the management of autonomic failure with postprandial hypotension, see under caffeine hydrate (p.1523).

SPERMICIDE. All samples of Coca-Cola tested markedly reduced sperm motility. The effectiveness of Coca-Cola as a spermicide had been attributed to its acidic pH. However, although the pH values of the formulations tested did not differ significantly, the spermicidal effect did vary and a component of the formulation was suggested as a cofactor. Coca-Cola products were not recommended for post coital contraception.— S. A. Umpierre *et al.* (letter), *New Engl. J. Med.*, 1985, *313*, 1351.

THALASSAEMIAS. For a report suggesting that the inhibition of iron absorption by tea may be useful in the management of patients with thalassaemia intermedia, see Effects on Iron Absorption under Adverse Effects, above.

Part 2

Supplementary Drugs and Other Substances

1891-b

A-56268

TE-031.

A macrolide antibiotic under investigation.

References: N. -X. Chin *et al.*, *Antimicrob. Ag. Chemother.*, 1987, *31*, 463; W. R. Bowie *et al.*, *ibid.*, 470; S. Floyd-Reising *et al.*, *ibid.*, 640; R. N. Jones and A. L. Barry (letter), *J. antimicrob. Chemother.*, 1987, *19*, 841.

12303-z

Abrus

Abrus Seed; Indian Liquorice; Jequirity Bean; Jumble Beads; Prayer Beads; Rosary Beans.

CAS — 1393-62-0 (abrin).

The seeds of *Abrus precatorius* (Leguminosae), one of whose constituents is abrin.

Abrin is considered responsible for the toxic effects of abrus seeds. Deaths of children have occurred from eating one or more seeds. Toxic effects include gastro-enteritis, haemorrhages, necrosis of the liver and kidneys, agglutination and haemolysis of the red blood cells, and convulsions. Treatment is symptomatic.

Inhibition of tumour growth in *animals* by abrin, a protein isolated from *Abrus precatorius*.— J. Lin *et al.* (letter), *Nature*, 1970, *227*, 292.

Studies in *animals* have demonstrated the potential value of toxins, including abrin, linked to monoclonal antibodies in drug-targetting against tumour cells.— K. Sikora *et al.*, *Br. med. Bull.*, 1984, *40*, 233.

521-c

Absinthium

Absinthii Herba; Assenzio; Losna; Pelin; Wermutkraut; Wormwood.

CAS — 546-80-5 (α-thujone); 471-15-8 (β-thujone).

Pharmacopoeias. In *Aust.*, *Cz.*, *Fr.*, *Ger.*, *Hung.*, *Jug.*, *Pol.*, *Roum.*, and *Swiss.*

The fresh or dried leaves and flowering tops of wormwood, *Artemisia absinthium* (Compositae). Thujone, related to camphor, is the major constituent of the essential oil derived from absinthium.

Absinthium has been used as a bitter. It is also used in small quantities as a flavouring agent in alcoholic beverages. Habitual use or large doses cause absinthism, which is characterised by restlessness, vomiting, vertigo, tremors, and convulsions. It is considered in some countries not to be safe for use in foods, beverages, or drugs.

Thujone was the active principle of *Artemisia absinthium* and was derived from the essential oil absinthol. Its structure was compared to that of tetrahydrocannabinol. It was postulated that thujone and THC interacted with a common receptor in the CNS.— J. del Castillo *et al.* (letter), *Nature*, 1975, *253*, 365.

2545-k

Aceclofenac *(rINN).*

[*o*-(2,6-Dichloroanilino)phenyl]acetate glycolic acid ester.

$C_{16}H_{13}Cl_2NO_4$=354.2.

CAS — 89796-99-6.

Aceclofenac is under investigation as an analgesic and anti-inflammatory agent.

Proprietary Names and Manufacturers

Tresquim *(Prodes, Spain).*

12306-a

Aceglutamide *(rINN).*

N^2-Acetyl-L-glutamine; 2-Acetylamino-L-glutaramic acid.

$C_7H_{12}N_2O_4$=188.2.

CAS — 2490-97-3.

Aceglutamide has been given in an attempt to improve memory and concentration.

1306-k

Glacial Acetic Acid *(BAN, USAN).*

Acide Acetique Cristallisable; Concentrated Acetic Acid; E260 *(acetic acid)*; Eisessig; Etanoico; Ethanoic Acid; Glac. Acet. Acid; Konzentrierte Essigsäure.

$C_2H_4O_2$=60.05.

CAS — 64-19-7.

Pharmacopoeias. In *Arg.*, *Br.*, *Chin.*, *Fr.*, *Egypt.*, *Ger.*, and *Jpn*; also in *B.P. Vet.*; in *Aust.*, *Belg.*, *Hung.*, *Jug.*, *Pol.*, and *Roum.* (all not less then 96%); in *Nord.* (not less than 96.5%); in *Cz.*, *It.*, *Port.*, *Span.*, and *Swiss* (not less than 98%); in *Mex.* and *U.S.* (both not less than 99.5%). The title Acidum Aceticum is used in *Arg.*, *Belg.*, *Mex.*, *Pol.*, *Port.*, *Roum.*, and *Span.*

A translucent crystalline mass or a clear colourless liquid with a pungent odour. B.p. about 117 to 118°. F.p. not lower than 14.8°.

Miscible with water, alcohol, chloroform, glycerol, and most fixed and volatile oils. **Store** in airtight containers.

1305-c

Acetic Acid *(BAN, USAN).*

NOTE. The nomenclature of acetic acid often leads to confusion as to whether concentrations are expressed as percentages of glacial acetic acid ($C_2H_4O_2$) or of this diluted form. In *Martindale*, the percentage figures given against acetic acid represent the amount of $C_2H_4O_2$.

Pharmacopoeias. In *Br.* (33%), *Aust.* (33.7 to 35.5%), *Chin.* (36 to 37%), *Egypt.* (32 to 34%), *Jpn* (30 to 32%), and *Pol.* (30%). In the following under the title or synonym Acidum Aceticum Dilutum: *Belg.*, *Jug.*, *Pol.*, *Roum.*, *Swiss* (all 30%), *Hung.* (20%), and *Span.* (36%). Also in *U.S.N.F.* (36 to 37%).

The following pharmacopoeias include weaker solutions under the titles or synonyms Dilute Acetic Acid or Diluted Acetic Acid: *Br.*, *Cz.*, *Egypt.*, and *U.S.N.F.* (all 6%), *Aust.* (11.5 to 12.2%), *Fr.*, *It.*, and *Port.* (10%).

A clear colourless liquid with a pungent odour. **Miscible** with water, alcohol, and glycerol. **Store** in airtight containers.

Adverse Effects and Treatment

Glacial acetic acid can produce similar adverse effects to the mineral acids as described under hydrochloric acid (p.1578); it is considered to be less corrosive. Treatment of adverse effects is as for hydrochloric acid (p.1578). In Great Britain the recommended exposure limits of acetic acid are 10 ppm (long-term); 15 ppm (short-term).

Allergy to acetic acid in one patient.— B. Przybilla and J. Ring (letter), *Lancet*, 1983, *1*, 483.

Glacial acetic acid was used in error instead of acetic acid 5% in a colposcopy clinic. The 4 or 5 patients who received the wrong acid were kept in hospital overnight and discharged the following morning having suffered no detectable harm.— *Pharm. J.*, 1987, *1*, 129.

Uses and Administration

Glacial acetic acid has been used as an escharotic. Diluted forms have been used among other things as an expectorant, antibacterial (it is reported to be effective against bacteria of the *Haemophilus* and *Pseudomonas* spp.), antifungal, and antiprotozoal in vaginal gels and douches, irrigations, or eardrops, as a spermicide, astringent lotion, and as a treatment for certain jellyfish stings.

A solution containing 4% w/v $C_2H_4O_2$ is known as artificial vinegar or non-brewed condiment. Vinegar is a product of fermentation.

COLPOSCOPY. The use of a 2 to 3% solution of acetic acid with acetylcysteine to clean the cervix and remove cervical mucus before colposcopy.— A. D. Martins, *Eur. J. resp. Dis.*, 1980, *61*, *Suppl.* 111, 172.

JELLY-FISH STING. References to the use of vinegar or weak solutions of acetic acid in the treatment of potentially fatal jelly-fish stings including a reference to certain species where the risk is increased by application of acetic acid due to the further discharge rather than inactivation of nematocysts: R. J. Hartwick *et al.*, *Med. J. Aust.*, 1980, *1*, 15; P. J. Fenner *et al.*, *ibid.*, 1985, *143*, 550; P. J. Fenner and P. F. Fitzpatrick (letter), *ibid.*, 1986, *145*, 174.

STOMA CARE. Crystalline phosphatic deposits that build up on the stoma of a urostomy can be dissolved by dabbing vinegar onto the stoma. A few drops of vinegar into the appliance will reduce the odour of stale urine.— J. C. Smith *et al.*, *Prescribers' J.*, 1983, *23*, 21.

Preparations

Acetic Acid Ear Drops *(A.P.F.).* Acetic acid (33 per cent) 3 mL, freshly boiled and cooled water to 100 mL.

Acetic Acid Irrigation *(A.P.F.).* Acetic acid (33 per cent) 6 mL, Water for Injections to 100 mL. Sterilised by autoclaving.

Acetic Acid Irrigation *(U.S.P.).* A sterile solution of glacial acetic acid 0.2375 to 0.2625% w/v in Water for Injections. pH 2.8 to 3.4.
For bladder irrigation.

Acetic Acid Otic Solution *(U.S.P.).* A solution of glacial acetic acid in a suitable nonaqueous solvent. pH 2.0 to 4.0 when diluted with an equal volume of water.

Proprietary Preparations

Aci-jel *(Ortho-Cilag, UK). Vaginal jelly,* glacial acetic acid 0.92% w/w buffered to pH 4.

Proprietary Names and Manufacturers

Aci-jel *(Cilag, Austral.; Ortho, Canad.;Ortho-Cilag, UK; Ortho Pharmaceutical, USA)*; Aquaear *(Robins, Austral.)*; Vosol *(Carter-Wallace, Austral.)*; VoSoL *(Wallace, USA).*

The following names have been used for multi-ingredient preparations containing acetic acid—Aerosporin *(Wellcome, Austral.)*; Fungi-Nail *(Kramer, USA)*; Otipyrin *(Kramer, USA)*; Phytex *(Drug Houses Austral., Austral.)*; Tridesilon Otic *(Miles Pharmaceuticals, USA)*; VoSoL HC *(Horner, Canad.; Wallace, USA)*.

12310-j

Acetohydroxamic Acid *(USAN, rINN)*.

AHA; *N*-Acetyl Hydroxyacetamide.
$C_2H_5NO_2$=75.07.

CAS — 546-88-3.

Pharmacopoeias. In *U.S.*

Colourless or white granules or powder. Freely **soluble** in water; practically insoluble in acetone and in alcohol. **Store** in airtight containers.

Adverse Effects and Precautions

Phlebitis, thrombo-embolism, haemolytic anaemia, and iron-deficiency anaemia have occurred in patients treated with acetohydroxamic acid. Other adverse effects associated with its use include headache, gastro-intestinal disturbances, alopecia, rash, trembling, and mental symptoms including anxiety and depression. Blood counts and renal function should be monitored during treatment. Patients with acute renal failure should not be given acetohydroxamic acid. Acetohydroxamic acid chelates iron administered orally, resulting in reduced absorption of both.

Studies in *animals* indicate that acetohydroxamic acid is teratogenic.

In a long-term study of 76 patients undergoing treatment for recalcitrant renal stones with acetohydroxamic acid adverse effects included mild headache during the first few days of treatment (in 75% of patients), gastro-intestinal disturbances (50%), and anaemia (20%). One patient developed pulmonary emboli.— D. P. Griffith, *et al., Wld J. Urol.*, 1983, *1*, 170.

Absorption and Fate

Acetohydroxamic acid is absorbed from the gastro-intestinal tract with peak serum concentrations being reached within 1 hour. The plasma half-life of acetohydroxamic acid is reported to be up to 10 hours in patients with normal renal function; it may be prolonged in patients with impaired renal function. Acetohydroxamic acid is partially metabolised in the liver but about two-thirds of a dose may be excreted unchanged in the urine, and it is the unchanged form that is pharmacologically active.

References: S. Feldman *et al., Investve Urol.*, 1978, *15*, 498; L. Putcha *et al., Eur. J. clin. Pharmac.*, 1985, *28*, 439.

Uses and Administration

Acetohydroxamic acid acts by inhibiting bacterial urease, thus decreasing urinary ammonia concentration and alkalinity. It is used in the prophylaxis of renal calculi formed as a result of bacterial urease and can be used as an adjunct in the treatment of chronic urinary-tract infection due to urease-splitting bacteria. Acetohydroxamic acid is usually given in a dose of 250 mg three or four times a day, up to a maximum of 1.5 g daily. Children have been given 10 mg per kg body-weight daily.

RENAL CALCULI. A brief review of the use of acetohydroxamic acid in the management of infection-induced renal calculi.— D. P. Griffith, *Kidney Int.*, 1982, *21*, 422.

A study of the urinary saturation in 10 patients receiving acetohydroxamic acid for renal calculi. Reductions in urinary pH and ammonia concentrations were observed; changes in urinary saturation were small; urinary excretion of magnesium and phosphate was increased.— R. G. Burr and I. Nuseibeh, *Br. J. Urol.*, 1983, *55*, 162.

A double-blind study of acetohydroxamic acid in struvite nephrolithiasis. Acetohydroxamic acid reduced growth of stones in 18 out of 18 patients taking acetohydroxamic acid. None of the treated group experienced a doubling of stone area or development of a new stone compared with 18 of 19 patients given placebo. Two patients taking acetohydroxamic acid withdrew from the study and 7 required a reduction in dosage because of adverse effects.— J. J. Williams *et al., New Engl. J. Med.*, 1984, *311*, 760. See also L. H. Smith, *ibid.*, 792.

Further references: A. Martelli *et al., Urology*, 1981, *17*, 320; J. S. Rodman *et al., ibid.*, 1983, *22*, 410.

Preparations

Acetohydroxamic Acid Tablets *(U.S.P.)*

Proprietary Names and Manufacturers

Lithostat *(Mission Pharmacal, USA)*; Uronefrex *(Ferrer, Spain)*.

3931-l

Acetoxolone

3-(Acetyloxy)-11-oxoolean-12-en-29-oic acid.
$C_{32}H_{48}O_5$=512.7.

CAS — 6277-14-1.

Acetoxolone is a derivative of carbenoxolone. The aluminium salt has been given by mouth for peptic ulcers.

Proprietary Names and Manufacturers

Oriens *(Inverni della Beffa, Ital.)*.

3015-f

Acetylcarnitine Hydrochloride

L-Acetylcarnitine Hydrochloride; ST-200. (3-Carboxy-2-hydroxypropyl)trimethylammonium acetate (ester) chloride.
$C_9H_{17}NO_4$,HCl=239.7.

CAS — 5080-50-2; 3040-38-8 (hydroxide, inner salt).

Acetylcarnitine hydrochloride acts on the central nervous system and has been described as a 'nootropic' or 'cognition adjuvant'. It has been tried in the treatment of senile dementia.

References: E. Bonavita, *Int. J. clin. Pharmac. Ther. Toxic.*, 1986, *24*, 511.

Proprietary Names and Manufacturers

Branigen *(Glaxo, Ital.)*.

12313-k

Acetylleucine *(rINN)*.

Acetyl-DL-leucine; RP-7542. *N*-Acetyl-DL-leucine.
$C_8H_{15}NO_3$=173.2.

CAS — 99-15-0.

Acetylleucine has been used in the treatment of vertigo in doses of up to 2 g daily by mouth in divided doses. The ethanolamine derivative has been given by slow intravenous injection in doses of up to 1 g daily.

Proprietary Names and Manufacturers

Tanganil *(Specia, Fr.)*.

2247-q

Acid Fuchsine

Acid Magenta; Acid Roseine; Acid Rubine; CI Acid Violet 19; Colour Index No. 42685. The disodium or diammonium salt of the trisulphonic acid of magenta.

Acid fuchsine is used as a microscopic stain and a pH indicator.

18714-y

Acifran *(USAN, rINN)*.

AY-25712. (±)-4,5-Dihydro-5-methyl-4-oxo-5-phenyl-2-furoic acid.
$C_{12}H_{10}O_4$=218.2.

CAS — 72420-38-3.

A hypolipidaemic agent under investigation.

References: D. B. Hunninghake *et al., Clin. Pharmac. Ther.*, 1985, *38*, 313.

Proprietary Names and Manufacturers

Reductol *(Ayerst, USA)*.

12319-d

Aclatonium Napadisylate *(BAN)*.

Aclatonium Napadisilate *(rINN)*; Celatonium Napadisilate; Choline Naphthalene-1,5-Disulphonate (2:1) Dilactate Diacetate. 2-(2-Acetoxypropionyloxy)ethyltrimethylammonium naphthalene-1,5-disulphonate (2:1).
$2C_{10}H_{20}NO_4,C_{10}H_6O_6S_2$=722.8.

CAS — 55077-30-0.

An antispasmodic agent that has been tried in gastro-intestinal disorders.

Proprietary Names and Manufacturers

Toyama, Jpn.

1947-b

Aconiazide *(rINN)*.

α-Isonicotinylhydrazone *o*-tolyloxyacetic acid.
$C_{15}H_{13}N_3O_4$=299.3.

CAS — 13410-86-1.

An antituberculous agent under investigation.

12320-c

Aconite

Acetylbenzoylaconine *(aconitine)*; Aconit.; Aconit Napel; Aconite Root; Aconiti Tuber; Monkshood Root; Radix Aconiti; Wolfsbane Root. 8-Acetoxy-3,11,18-trihydroxy-16-ethyl-1,6,19-trimethoxy-4-methoxymethylaconitan-10-yl benzoate *(aconitine)*.
$C_{34}H_{47}NO_{11}$ (aconitine)=645.7 (aconitine).

CAS — 8063-12-5 (aconite); 302-27-2 (aconitine).

NOTE. Aconitine is *USAN*.

Wolfsbane is also used as a common name for arnica flower.

Pharmacopoeias. In *Arg., Belg., Braz., Cz., Fr., Egypt., Mex., Port., Roum.,* and *Span.* Also in *B.P.C. 1973. Arg., Aust., Port.,* and *Span.* also include aconitine.

The dried root of *Aconitum napellus* agg. (Ranunculaceae). The *B.P.C. 1973* specifies not less than 0.5% of alkaloids, calculated as aconitine, and the minimum content specified by pharmacopoeias varies between 0.15 and 0.8%.

Adverse Effects

Aconite has variable effects on the heart leading to heart failure. It also affects the central nervous system.

Symptoms of aconite poisoning may appear almost immediately and are rarely delayed beyond an hour; in fatal poisoning death usually occurs within 6 hours, although with larger doses it may be instantaneous.

Moderately toxic doses produce a tingling of the tongue, mouth, stomach, and skin (this is the most important diagnostic feature) followed by numbness and anaesthesia. Other symptoms include gastro-intestinal disturbances; irregular pulse; difficult respiration; cold, clammy, and livid skin; muscular weakness, incoordination, and vertigo.

Treatment of aconite poisoning is symptomatic; atropine sulphate may be given in severe cases.

Uses and Administration

Aconite should not be used internally because of its low therapeutic index and variable potency.

Aconite liniments were formerly used extensively in the treatment of neuralgia, sciatica, and rheumatism. However, sufficient aconitine may be absorbed through the skin to cause serious poisoning; liniments should never be applied to wounds or abraded surfaces.

A preparation of aconite is used in homoeopathic medicine.

18717-c

Acridine Orange

3,6-Bis(dimethylamino)acridine.
$C_{17}H_{19}N_3$=265.4.

CAS — 494-38-2.

Acridine orange is a dye with antiseptic properties. It has been used as a diagnostic stain in microbiology.

18718-k

Acrihellin *(rINN).*

D-12316. 3-O-(3-Methyl-2-butenoyl)3,5,14-trihydroxy-19-oxo-20,22-bufadienolide.
$C_{29}H_{38}O_7$=498.6.

CAS — 67696-82-6.

A positive inotropic drug under investigation.

References: C. Achenbach *et al., Arzneimittel-Forsch.*, 1983, *33*, 1425.

12322-a

Acrolein

Acraldehyde; Acrylaldehyde; Acrylic Aldehyde. Prop-2-enal.
C_3H_4O=56.1.

CAS — 107-02-8.

Acrolein is irritant to the skin and may cause vesiculation. The vapour causes lachrymation and nasal irritation. Inhalation may cause pulmonary oedema, nephritis, or pneumonia. It has various industrial uses.
In Great Britain the recommended exposure limits of acrolein are 0.1 ppm (long-term); 0.3 ppm (short-term).

A review.— C. Izard and C. Libermann, *Mutat. Res.*, 1978, *47*, 115.

12324-x

Acrylamide

Propenamide.
C_3H_5NO=71.1.

CAS — 79-06-1.

Acrylamide is highly toxic and irritant; it can be absorbed through unbroken skin. Symptoms of poisoning include sweating hands and peripheral neuropathies with numbness, paraesthesias and weakness, especially associated with the lower limbs.
Acrylamide has various industrial applications, including use as a plasticiser and a waterproof 'chemical grout'.
In Great Britain the recommended exposure limits of acrylamide are 0.3 mg per m^3 (long-term); 0.6 mg per m^3 (short-term); suitable precautions should be taken to prevent absorption through the skin. In the *US* the permissible and recommended exposure limits are 0.3 mg per m^3.

Reports of neuropathies associated with exposure to acrylamide: R. B. Auld and S. F. Bedwell, *Can. med. Ass. J.*, 1967, *96*, 652; H. Igisu, *J. Neurol. Neurosurg. Psychiat.*, 1975, *38*, 581; C. M. Kesson *et al., Postgrad. med. J.*, 1977, *53*, 16.

A review of a wound dressing (Geliperm) comprising a gel made by polymerising acrylamide with agar.— J. A. Myers, *Pharm. J.*, 1983, *1*, 263. Comments: S. Thomas (letter,), *ibid.*, 275; M. Seabright and G. F. Batstone (letter), *ibid.*, 448.

12325-r

Adenine *(USAN).*

Vitamin B_4. 6-Aminopurine; 1,6-Dihydro-6-iminopurine.
$C_5H_5N_5$=135.1.

CAS — 73-24-5.

Pharmacopoeias. In *U.S.*

Adenine is a constituent of coenzymes and nucleic acids.
Adenine has been used to extend the storage life of Blood (see p.813).
It has also been given for the management of white blood-cell disorders.

Striking improvement in megaloblastic anaemia in a 9-year-old boy with Lesch-Nyhan syndrome following treatment with adenine in divided doses of up to 1.5 g daily. Hyperuricaemia resulting from degradation of adenine was corrected by allopurinol.— S. P. M. van der Zee *et al.* (letter), *Lancet*, 1968, *1*, 1427.

A review of toxicological and pharmacological aspects, in *animals* and man, of the use of adenine to improve preservation of red blood cells. The only toxic effect of purified adenine appears to result from deposition of the metabolite 2,8-dioxyadenine in the kidney tubules, although this does not lead to chronic disease and tubular function is re-established after discontinuation of the drug. Up to 15 mg per kg body-weight may be given without crystal deposition occurring. The toxicity of adenine in patients with chronic liver and kidney dysfunction has not been studied and the effects, if any, of the 8-oxyadenine intermediate are not known.— W. L. Warner, *Transfusion, Philad.*, 1977, *17*, 326.

Proprietary Names and Manufacturers
B4 Hemosan *(Pons, Spain)*; Biadenina *(Biagini, Ital.)*; Leuco-4 *(Pharmascience, Fr.)*.

3226-w

Adenosine Deaminase

An endogenous enzyme which converts adenosine to inosine. A macrogol-modified form (PEG-adenosine deaminase; PEG-ADA) has been used in the treatment of adenosine deaminase deficiency.

References: M. S. Hershfield *et al., New Engl. J. Med.*, 1987, *316*, 589.

12326-f

S-Adenosyl-L-methionine

Methioninyl adenylate; SAMe. (S)-5′-[(3-Amino-3-carboxypropyl)methylsulphonio]-5′-deoxyadenosine hydroxide, inner salt.
$C_{15}H_{22}N_6O_5S$=398.4.

CAS — 29908-03-0.

S-Adenosyl-L-methionine, the active derivative of methionine, has been studied for the treatment of hepatic disorders. It has also been investigated for the treatment of depression.

The mean terminal half-life of *S*-adenosyl-L-methionine following intravenous doses of 100 mg and 500 mg to 6 healthy subjects was 81 minutes and 101 minutes respectively. Disappearance from plasma mainly occurred within 4 hours of administration; data obtained suggested that body accumulation of the drug is unlikely at these doses.— P. Giulidori *et al., Eur. J. clin. Pharmac.*, 1984, *27*, 119.

A report of the reduction of erythrocyte macrocytosis in chronic alcoholics with liver damage following the administration of *S*-adenosyl-L-methionine.— R. Turpini *et al., Curr. ther. Res.*, 1987, *41*, 38.

Successful treatment of porphyria cutanea tarda in 2 children with a combination of low-dose chloroquine and *S*-adenosyl-L-methionine by mouth.— A. M. D. C. Batlle *et al., Br. J. Derm.*, 1987, *116*, 407.

ARTHRITIS. In a double-blind randomised multicentre study administration of *S*-adenosyl-L-methionine 400 mg three times daily gave favourable results in 75 patients with osteoarthritis of hip or knee joints or both. Comparison with 75 patients given ibuprofen in the same dosage demonstrated no significant differences in efficacy. Side-effects developed in 5 patients receiving *S*-adenosyl-L-methionine and in 16 of those receiving ibuprofen.— R. Marcolongo *et al., Curr. ther. Res.*, 1985, *37*, 82.

DEPRESSION. A double-blind study in 36 patients with depression indicated that *S*-adenosyl-L-methionine could have potential use as an antidepressant.— D. De Leo, *Curr. ther. Res.*, 1987, *41*, 865. Further studies: M. W. P. Carney *et al.* (letter), *Lancet*, 1983, *1*, 820; I. Caruso *et al.* (letter), *ibid.*, 1984, *1*, 904; T. Bottiglieri *et al.* (letter), *ibid.*, *2*, 224.

Proprietary Names and Manufacturers
S-Amet *(Castejon, Spain)*; Samyr *(Bioresearch, Ital.)*.

18725-c

Adimolol *(rINN).*

Imidolol; MEN-935. (±)-1-(3-{[2-Hydroxy-3-(1-naphthyloxy)propyl]amino}-3-methylbutyl)-2-benzimidazolinone.
$C_{25}H_{29}N_3O_3$=419.5.

CAS — 75708-29-1 (hydrochloride); 78459-19-5.

A long-acting beta blocker under investigation.

References: J. G. Riddell *et al., Br. J. clin. Pharmac.*, 1985, *19*, 405; H. L. Elliott *et al., ibid.*, 1986, *22*, 235P; H. L. Elliott *et al., ibid.*, 1987, *23*, 511.

12328-n

Adipic Acid

355; Hexanedioic Acid.
$C_6H_{10}O_4$=146.1.

CAS — 124-04-9.

Adipic acid is used as an acidulating agent in foods.

Estimated acceptable daily intake of free acid, potassium, sodium, and ammonium salts: up to 5 mg per kg body-weight.— Twenty-first Report of the Joint FAO/WHO Expert Committee on Food Additives, *Tech. Rep. Ser. Wld Hlth Org. No. 617*, 1978.

3018-h

Adrafinil *(rINN).*

CRL-40048. 2-[(Diphenylmethyl)sulfinyl]acetohydroxamic acid.
$C_{15}H_{15}NO_3S$=289.4.

CAS — 63547-13-7.

An alpha-adrenergic agonist used as a CNS stimulant.

Proprietary Names and Manufacturers
Olmifon *(Lafon, Fr.)*.

12329-h

Aesculus

Aesculus hippocastanum; Horse-chestnut.

CAS — 6805-41-0 (aescin); 11072-93-8 (β-aescin); 531-75-9 (esculoside, anhydrous).

Pharmacopoeias. Ger. and *Span.* describe the seeds and *Port.* describes the bark and seeds of *Aesculus hippocastanum. Fr.* includes esculoside in the sesquihydrate form.

The horse-chestnut, *Aesculus hippocastanum* (Hippocastanaceae) contains several active principles including esculoside (aesculin or esculin; 6-β-D-glucopyranosyloxy-7-hydroxycoumarin, $C_{15}H_{16}O_9$ = 340.3) and aescin (escin), which is a mixture of saponins.

Aesculus hippocastanum and other species of horse-chestnut may be poisonous.
β-Aescin has been used in the prevention and treatment of various peripheral vascular disorders. It has been given by mouth, by intravenous injection (in the form of sodium aescinate), and applied topically. It has also been administered intravenously in the prevention and treatment of post-operative oedema. The maximum dose for intravenous administration in adults for such conditions has been stated to be 20 mg daily; acute renal failure has been reported in patients given higher doses, sometimes in conjunction with other nephrotoxic drugs.
Esculoside is an ingredient of some suppositories used for the treatment of haemorrhoids.

There have been reports of poisoning in children from eating the seeds, or drinking infusions made from the leaves and twigs of horse-chestnut trees. The toxic substance is considered to be esculoside. Symptoms of poisoning were muscle twitching, weakness, lack of coordination, dilated pupils, vomiting, diarrhoea, paralysis, and stupor.— M. Nagy, *J. Am. med. Ass.*, 1973, *226*,

213.
A pseudolupus syndrome which occurred in 15 patients was associated with the use of a preparation containing an aesculus extract, phenopyrazone (a pyrazolone derivative), and various cardiac glycosides (Venocuran).— P. J. Grob *et al.*, *Lancet*, 1975, *2*, 144.

A report of the incidence of acute renal failure in patients following cardiac surgery and implicating high-dose intravenous aescin therapy. In 70 patients receiving a mean maximum daily dose of 340 µg per kg body-weight no alteration of renal function was observed; in 16 receiving 360 µg per kg mild renal impairment was observed; and in 40 receiving 510 µg per kg acute renal failure developed.— K. Hellberg *et al.*, *Thoraxchirurgie*, 1975, *23*, 396.

Proprietary Names and Manufacturers of Aesculus and its Active Principles
Escina Ausonia *(Farma-Lepori, Spain)*; Femirosine *(Jpn)*; Feparil *(Madaus Cerafarm, Spain)*; Marro-Dausse *(Charton, Canad.)*; Reparil *(Bellon, Fr.; Madaus, Ger.; Ibi, Ital.; Madaus, S.Afr.; Madaus, Switz.)*; Tochief *(Jpn)*; Venostasin *(Klinge, Ger.; Klinge, Switz.)*.

12330-a

Aflatoxins

CAS — 1162-65-8 (aflatoxin B_1); 7220-81-7 (aflatoxin B_2); 1165-39-5 (aflatoxin G_1); 7241-98-7 (aflatoxin G_2).

Aflatoxins are toxic metabolites produced by many strains of *Aspergillus flavus*, growing on many vegetable foods, notably peanuts. A number of forms, including aflatoxins B_1, B_2, G_1, G_2, and M_1 have been identified.

Aflatoxins have been implicated in liver cancer. Aflatoxin B_1 is reported to be one of the most potent carcinogens known in *animals*.

CONTAMINATION. Findings of aflatoxin B_1, in *Aspergillus* mould extracts used for injection immunotherapy (hyposensitisation).— M. S. Legator *et al.* (letter), *Lancet*, 1983, *2*, 915. Lack of confirmation. It was concluded that mould extracts do not pose an aflatoxin risk to patients being treated by injection immunotherapy.— J. C. Petricciani (letter), *ibid.*, 1984, *1*, 171.

KWASHIORKOR. Findings in a study of 252 Sudanese children suggesting that children with kwashiorkor had a greater exposure to aflatoxins, or possibly that the disease caused impairment of ability to transport and excrete aflatoxins.— R. G. Hendrickse *et al.*, *Br. med. J.*, 1982, *285*, 843. See also R. G. Hendrickse, *Trans. R. Soc. trop. Med. Hyg.*, 1984, *78*, 427. The view that aflatoxins are unlikely to be the primary cause of kwashiorkor development although reduced metabolism of aflatoxins by the malnourished liver may play a role.— *Lancet*, 1984, *2*, 1133.

LIVER CANCER. Discussion of the hypothesis that the role of aflatoxins in the development of hepatocellular cancer may be primarily mediated by immunosuppression, leading to increased chronic hepatitis B virus infection, rather than being a direct carcinogenic effect.— L. I. Lutwick, *Lancet*, 1979, *1*, 755.

Further references to liver cancer and the potential causal role of aflatoxins, alone or in combination with other factors: C. A. Linsell and F. G. Peers, *Trans. R. Soc. trop. Med. Hyg.*, 1977, *71*, 471; R. M. Willis *et al.* (letter), *Lancet*, 1980, *1*, 1198; P. Cook-Mozaffari and S. Van Rensburg, *Br. med. Bull.*, 1984, *40*, 342; C. O. Enwonwu, *Lancet*, 1984, *2*, 956.

REYE'S SYNDROME. Aflatoxin B_1 was found in the blood of 2 children with Reye's syndrome (characterised by acute encephalopathy and fatty degeneration of the viscera) during the acute phase of the disease.— G. R. Hogan *et al.* (letter), *Lancet*, 1978, *1*, 561.

Comparison of aflatoxin concentrations in serum and urine of 17 patients with Reye's syndrome and in 48 controls revealed no evidence that patients had been exposed to aflatoxin at a greater rate than controls, although it was recognised that these measurements reflected only recent exposure, rather than chronic ingestion which might be more important in the aetiology of the disease. Nonetheless, 23% of all subjects had evidence of recent exposure to aflatoxins, a fact which may be of significance for public health.— D. B. Nelson *et al.*, *Pediatrics*, 1980, *66*, 865.

18737-x

Alacepril *(rINN)*.

DU-1219. *N*-{1-[(*S*)-3-Mercapto-2-methylpropionyl]-L-prolyl}-3-phenyl-L-alanine acetate (ester).
$C_{20}H_{26}N_2O_5S$=406.5.

CAS — 74258-86-9.

An angiotensin-converting enzyme inhibitor similar to captopril and used in the treatment of hypertension.

References: K. Onoyama *et al.*, *Clin. Pharmac. Ther.*, 1985, *38*, 462; K. Onoyama *et al.*, *Curr. ther. Res.*, 1986, *40*, 543; T. Ogihara *et al.*, *ibid.*, 1987, *41*, 492; T. Ogihara *et al.*, *ibid.*, *42*, 324.

Proprietary Names and Manufacturers
Cetapril *(Dainippon, Jpn)*.

3021-x

Alexidine *(USAN, rINN)*.

Compound 904; Win-21904. 1,1′-Hexamethylenebis[5-(2-ethylhexyl)biguanide].
$C_{26}H_{56}N_{10}$=508.8.

CAS — 22573-93-9.

A bisbiguanide disinfectant similar to chlorhexidine.

References: J. Chawner *et al.*, *J. Pharm. Pharmac.*, 1986, *38*, *Suppl.*, 110P.

12026-w

Alfalfa

The plant *Medicago sativa* (Leguminosae) which is cultivated as an animal feedstuff.

The seeds and sprouts of alfalfa contain canavanine (2-amino-4-(guanidinooxy)butyric acid), a toxic amino acid structurally related to arginine; content is reported to represent about 1.5% of the dry weight. A syndrome resembling systemic lupus erythematosus has been recorded in *monkeys* fed alfalfa.

References: M. R. Malinow *et al.* (letter), *Lancet*, 1981, *1*, 615 (pancytopenia); M. R. Malinow *et al.*, *Science*, 1982, *216*, 415 (systemic lupus erythematosus in *monkeys*); J. L. Roberts and J. A. Hayashi (letter), *New Engl. J. Med.*, 1983, *308*, 1361 (reactivation of systemic lupus in 2 patients).

18612-q

Alfuzosin *(BAN, rINN)*.

SL-77499-10. *N*-{3-[4-Amino-6,7-dimethoxyquinazolin-2-yl(methyl)amino]propyl}tetrahydro-2-furamide.
$C_{19}H_{27}N_5O_4$=389.5.

CAS — 81403-80-7; 81403-68-1 (hydrochloride).

NOTE. Alfuzosin Hydrochloride is *USAN*.

An alpha-adrenoceptor blocking agent which has been tried similarly to prazosin in the treatment of hypertension and benign prostatic hypertrophy.

References: J. W. A. Ramsay *et al.*, *Br. J. Urol.*, 1985, *57*, 657; I. B. Davies *et al.*, *Br. J. clin. Pharmac.*, 1986, *22*, 231.

Proprietary Names and Manufacturers
Synthelabo, Fr.

18738-r

Alibendol *(rINN)*.

5-Allyl-*N*-(2-hydroxyethyl)-3-methoxysalicylamide.
$C_{13}H_{17}NO_4$=251.3.

CAS — 26750-81-2.

A choleretic used in the treatment of gastro-intestinal disorders.

Proprietary Names and Manufacturers
Cebera *(Bouchara, Fr.)*.

7352-h

Almond Oil *(BAN, USAN)*.

Aceite de Almendra; Expressed Almond Oil; Huile d'Amande; Mandelöl; Ol. Amygdal.; Oleum Amygdalae; Sweet Almond Oil.

CAS — 8007-69-0.

Pharmacopoeias. In *Arg.*, *Belg.*, *Br.*, *Egypt.*, *Eur.*, *Fr.*, *Neth.*, *Port.*, *Rus.*, *Span.*, and *Swiss* which specify *Prunus dulcis* var. *dulcis* or var. *amara*. or in some cases from a mixture of the two varieties. *It.* and *Mex.* specify oil from *Prunus dulcis* var. *dulcis*. *Aust.* specifies oil from *Prunus dulcis* var. *amara* or var. *communis* (=var. *sativa*). *U.S.N.F.* specifies oil from varieties of *Prunus dulcis*.
Fr. also specifies Huile de Noyaux, an oil obtained from various species of *Prunus*.

A pale yellow oil with a slight characteristic odour and a bland nutty taste, consisting of glycerides chiefly of oleic acid, with smaller amounts of linoleic and palmitic acids. It is expressed, without the application of heat, from the seeds of the bitter or the sweet almond, *Prunus dulcis (Prunus amygdalus; Amygdalus communis)* var. *amara* or var. *dulcis* (Rosaceae).
Slightly **soluble** in alcohol; miscible with chloroform, ether, and petroleum spirit. **Store** in a cool place in well-filled airtight containers. Protect from light.

Almond oil has nutritive and demulcent properties. It is also applied as an emollient for chapped hands. It is sometimes used in the preparation of cold creams, hair preparations, and other toilet articles. It is also employed as a vehicle in some injections.

3928-k

Alpha Fetoprotein

α-Fetoprotein.

Units
100 000 units of human alpha fetoprotein are contained in 139.91 mg of freeze-dried cord serum in one ampoule of the first International Standard Preparation (1975).

Uses and Administration
Alpha fetoprotein (AFP) is an alpha globulin of similar molecular weight to albumin. The concentration in foetal serum exceeds that of maternal serum and amniotic fluid. In the second trimester of pregnancy AFP concentrations in maternal serum are elevated in relation to non-pregnant concentrations.
Screening of AFP concentrations in maternal serum and amniotic fluid has been used for the diagnosis of neural tube defects associated with anencephaly and spina bifida.
Elevated concentrations of alpha fetoprotein have also been used as a marker or diagnostic test for testicular carcinoma.

16516-j

Alpha$_1$ Antitrypsin

Alpha$_1$ Proteinase Inhibitor.

An endogenous elastase inhibitor which prevents destruction of lung tissue by neutrophil elastase. Alpha$_1$ antitrypsin is prepared from pooled plasma and is given by intravenous infusion for replacement therapy in patients with emphysema who have congenital alpha$_1$ antitrypsin deficiency.

References: A. B. Cohen, *New Engl. J. Med.*, 1986, *314*, 778; M. D. Wewers *et al.*, *ibid.*, 1987, *316*, 1055; *Med. Lett.*, 1988, *30*, 29.

Proprietary Names and Manufacturers
Prolastin *(Cutter, USA)*.

5404-v

Althaea

Alteia; Alth.; Eibischwurzel; Marshmallow; Marshmallow Root; Racine de Guimauve; Raiz de Altea.

Pharmacopoeias. In *Aust., Belg., Cz., Fr., Ger., Hung., Jug., Mex., Pol., Port., Roum., Rus., Span.,* and *Swiss.* Althaea Leaf is included in *Aust., Belg., Cz., Fr., Hung., Jug., Pol.,* and *Roum.,* and Althaea Flower in *Belg.* and *Fr.*

The dried peeled root of *Althaea officinalis* (Malvaceae).

Althaea is demulcent and emollient and was formerly used for irritation and inflammation of the mucous membranes of the mouth and pharynx. It has also been used in traditional remedies for gastro-intestinal disturbances.

5261-g

Aluminium

Aluminum; E173.
Al=26.98154.

CAS — 7429-90-5.

A malleable and ductile soft silvery-white metal, becoming coated with a thin layer of oxide.

Incompatibilities have been reported between aluminium in injection equipment and metronidazole (K.H. Schell and J. R. Copeland, *Am. J. Hosp. Pharm.*, 1985, *42*, 1040; B.J. Struthers and R.J. Parr, *ibid.*, 2660) and between aluminium and various antineoplastic agents including cisplatin, daunorubicin, and doxorubicin (R.D. Bohart and G. Ogawa, *Cancer Treat. Rep.*, 1979, *63*, 2117; W.A. Gardiner, *Am. J. Hosp. Pharm.*, 1981, *38*, 1276; M.J. Williamson *et al.*, *ibid.*, 1983, *40*, 214; G.S. Ogawa, *ibid.*, 1985, *42*, 1042). The suitability of aluminium caps for sugar-containing liquids has been questioned. Abrasion of the aluminium caps by sugar from Ceporex Syrup has resulted in the formation of a black slime (L.J. Tressler, *Pharm. J.*, 1985, *2*, 99).

5262-q

Aluminium Powder

Pharmacopoeias. In *Arg.* and *Br.*

Aluminium powder is an odourless or almost odourless, silvery-grey powder. It consists mainly of metallic aluminium in very small flakes, usually with an appreciable quantity of aluminium oxide. It is lubricated with stearic acid to protect the metal from oxidation.

Practically **insoluble** in water and alcohol; very soluble, with evolution of hydrogen, in dilute acids and solutions of alkali hydroxides. **Store** in well-closed containers.

WARNING. *Aluminium powder has been used for the illicit preparation of explosives or fireworks; care is required with its supply.*

Adverse Effects

Aluminium toxicity is well recognised in patients with renal impairment. Patients undergoing dialysis have experienced encephalopathy, osteodystrophy, and anaemia associated with an aluminium salt taken as a phosphate binder or with aluminium present in the water supply. As a result, other phosphate binders are now used in dialysis patients; for a discussion of this topic see under aluminium hydroxide (p.1076); also the concentration of aluminium in dialysis fluid has been limited to not more than 10 μg per litre.

Aluminium toxicity has followed the administration of parenteral fluids and infant feeds with a high concentration of aluminium.

Aluminium toxicity may be treated by removal of the aluminium with desferrioxamine (p.838).

In Great Britain the recommended exposure limits of aluminium metal and aluminium oxide are 10 mg per m^3 (long-term); 20 mg per m^3 (short-term); the recommended exposure limit of soluble aluminium salts is 2 mg per m^3 (long-term).

The adverse effects of aluminium salts are described under aluminium hydroxide (p.1075).

Some references to aluminium toxicity arising from aluminium in infant feeds or parenteral fluids: M. Freundlich *et al.*, *Lancet*, 1985, *2*, 527 (infant feeds); D. S. Milliner *et al.*, *New Engl. J. Med.*, 1985, *312*, 165 (albumin solutions); A. B. Sedman *et al.*, *ibid.*, 1337 (parenteral nutrition in premature infants); M. McGraw *et al.* (letter), *Lancet*, 1986, *1*, 157 and 380 (parenteral and oral infant feeds); J. C. K. Wells (letter), *ibid.*, 380 (human milk); R. Weintraub *et al.*, *Archs Dis. Childh.*, 1986, *61*, 914 (infant feeds).

ALZHEIMER'S DISEASE. Conjecture on aluminium being implicated in Alzheimer's disease: *Lancet*, 1985, *1*, 616; R. H. Wheater, *J. Am. med. Ass.*, 1985, *253*, 2288; R. G. King and H. J. Worland (letter), *Med. J. Aust.*, 1985, *142*, 352; J. M. Candy *et al.*, *Lancet*, 1986, *1*, 354.

DIALYSIS. Some references to aluminium toxicity in dialysis patients: A. C. Alfrey *et al.*, *New Engl. J. Med.*, 1976, *294*, 184; I. S. Parkinson *et al.*, *Lancet*, 1979, *1*, 406; J. B. Cannata *et al.*, *ibid.*, 1983, *1*, 50; M. R. Wills and J. Savory, *ibid.*, 1983, *2*, 29; S. P. Andreoli *et al.*, *New Engl. J. Med.*, 1984, *310*, 1079; A. C. Alfrey, *ibid.*, 1113.

Uses and Administration

Aluminium is used in packaging and in injection equipment. The foil is also used as a dressing and for insulation.

Aluminium powder alone and in paste form with zinc oxide has been used as a dressing.

Astringent aluminium salts are used as antiperspirants. Aluminium hydroxide is used as an antacid.

The use of aluminium metal as a silvering decoration for certain items of confectionery was not considered to present a health hazard. Exposure levels of aluminium from food, drink, cooking utensils, and drugs were not available.— Twenty-second Report of Joint FAO/WHO Expert Committee on Food Additives, *Tech. Rep. Ser. Wld Hlth Org. No. 631*, 1978.

Preparations

Compound Aluminium Paste *(B.P.)*. Baltimore Paste. A paste containing aluminium powder 20%w/w and zinc oxide 40%w/w in a suitable hydrophobic liquid basis. For extemporaneous preparations the following formula may be used: aluminium powder 2, zinc oxide 4, and liquid paraffin 4, by wt.

9518-n

Basic Aluminium Carbonate

Pharmacopoeias. U.S. has a monograph for Basic Aluminum Carbonate Gel.

A combination of aluminium hydroxide and aluminium carbonate.

Basic aluminium carbonate gel is used as an antacid and as a phosphate-binder.

Preparations

Dried Basic Aluminum Carbonate Gel Capsules *(U.S.P.)*. Store in well-closed containers.

Dried Basic Aluminum Carbonate Gel Tablets *(U.S.P.)*. Store in well-closed containers.

Proprietary Names and Manufacturers

Basaljel *(USA)*.

12347-b

Aluminium Lactate

Tris(lactato)aluminium.
$C_9H_{15}AlO_9$=294.2.

CAS — 537-02-0; 18917-91-4.

Aluminium lactate is used in the local treatment of various disorders of the mouth.

Proprietary Names and Manufacturers

Aluctyl *(Roussel, Arg.; Brocades, Ital.; Liberman, Spain)*.

5226-m

Alverine Citrate *(BANM, USAN, pINNM)*.

Dipropyline Citrate; Phenpropamine Citrate.
N-Ethyl-3,3′-diphenyldipropylamine citrate.
$C_{20}H_{27}N,C_6H_8O_7$=473.6.

CAS — 150-59-4 (alverine); 5560-59-8 (citrate).

Alverine is an antispasmodic with actions similar to those of papaverine (p.1598). It is given by mouth as the citrate in doses of 60 to 120 mg (approximately equivalent to 40 to 80 mg of alverine), by suppository as alverine in doses of 80 mg, and by intramuscular or slow intravenous injection as the tartrate in doses equivalent to 40 mg of alverine.

Proprietary Preparations

Spasmonal *(Norgine, UK). Capsules*, alverine citrate 60 mg.

Proprietary Names and Manufacturers of Alverine or its Salts

Profenil Faible *(Canad.)*; Spasmavérine *(Bellon, Fr.; Switz.)*; Spasmonal *(Norgine, UK)*.

The following names have been used for multi-ingredient preparations containing alverine or its salts—Normacol Antispasmodic *(Norgine, Austral.; Norgine, UK)*.

16051-x

Amantanium Bromide *(rINN)*.

CR-898. Decyl(2-hydroxyethyl)dimethylammonium bromide 1-adamantanecarboxylate.
$C_{25}H_{46}BrNO_2$=472.5.

CAS — 58158-77-3.

A quaternary ammonium disinfectant.

Proprietary Names and Manufacturers

Amantol *(Rottapharm, Ital.)*.

5227-b

Ambucetamide *(BAN, rINN)*.

A-16. 2-Dibutylamino-2-(4-methoxyphenyl)acetamide.
$C_{17}H_{28}N_2O_2$=292.4.

CAS — 519-88-0.

Ambucetamide is used as an antispasmodic and is given in doses of 100 to 200 mg three times daily with paracetamol for the relief of dysmenorrhoea.

Proprietary Preparations

Femerital *(MCP Pharmaceuticals, UK). Tablets*, scored, ambucetamide 100 mg, paracetamol 250 mg.

12356-v

Amikhelline Hydrochloride *(rINNM)*.

9-(2-Diethylaminoethoxy)-4-hydroxy-7-methyl-5*H*-furo[3,2-*g*][1]benzopyran-5-one hydrochloride.
$C_{18}H_{21}NO_5,HCl$=367.8.

CAS — 4439-67-2 (amikhelline); 40709-23-7 (hydrochloride).

Amikhelline is used as an antispasmodic.

Proprietary Names and Manufacturers

Nokhel *(Promesa, Spain)*.

12359-p

Aminobutyric Acid

GABA; Gamma-aminobutyric Acid; Piperidic Acid. 4-Aminobutyric acid.
$C_4H_9NO_2$=103.1.

CAS — 56-12-2.

Aminobutyric acid is a principal inhibitory neurotransmitter in the CNS. It has been claimed to be of value in cerebral disorders and to have an antihypertensive effect.

Over a period of 2 months 7 patients with Huntington's chorea were treated with aminobutyric acid starting at a dose of 1 g and increasing to 12 to 32 g daily. Two patients gained improvement of function and a decrease in choreiform movements and a third patient showed moderate improvement.— R. Fisher *et al.* (letter), *Lancet*, 1974, *1*, 506.

Proprietary Names and Manufacturers
Gabob *(Jpn)*; Gamarex *(Ital.)*; Gamibetal *(Ono, Jpn)*; Gammalon *(Daiichi, Jpn)*; Kolpo *(Jpn)*; Mielogen *(Made, Spain)*; Sedanfactor *(IBE, Spain)*.

12360-n

Aminohydroxybutyric Acid

4-Amino-3-hydroxybutyric acid.
$C_4H_9NO_3$=119.1.

CAS — 352-21-6.

Aminohydroxybutyric acid has been claimed to be of value in neurological disorders and to have cerebral vasodilating properties.

Proprietary Names and Manufacturers
Aminoxan *(Kaken, Jpn)*; Bogil *(Llorente, Spain)*; Gabimex *(Gramon, Arg.)*; Gabob *(Jpn)*; Gabomade *(Knoll-Made, Spain)*; Gaboneuril *(Spain)*; Gaboril *(Seber, Spain)*; Gamibetal *(SIT, Ital.; Ono, Jpn; Ibsa, Switz.)*.

12364-v

4-Aminopyridine

$C_5H_6N_2$=94.1.

CAS — 504-24-5.

4-Aminopyridine is reported to reverse the effects of non-depolarising muscle relaxants and to have analeptic effects. Improvement of myasthenia gravis has been reported. Aminopyridine hydrochloride and aminopyridine sulphate have been used.

References: W. C. Bowman *et al.*, *J. Pharm. Pharmac.*, 1977, *29*, 616; H. Lundh *et al.*, *J. Neurol. Neurosurg. Psychiat.*, 1977, *40*, 1109; S. Agoston *et al.*, *Br. J. Anaesth.*, 1978, *50*, 383; H. Lundh *et al.*, *J. Neurol. Neurosurg. Psychiat.*, 1979, *42*, 171; S. Agoston *et al.*, *Br. J. Anaesth.*, 1980, *52*, 367; J. Evenhuis *et al.*, *ibid.*, 1981, *53*, 567.

Proprietary Names and Manufacturers
Pymadin.

1207-j

Amiprilose Hydrochloride *(USAN, pINNM)*.

SM-1213; Therafectin. 3-*O*-[3-(Dimethylamino)propyl]-1,2-*O*-isopropylidene-α-D-glucofuranose hydrochloride.
$C_{14}H_{27}NO_6$,HCl=341.8.

CAS — 56824-20-5 (amiprilose); 60414-06-4 (hydrochloride).

An immunomodulator under investigation. It has been tried in the treatment of rheumatoid arthritis.

References: S. J. Hopkins, *Drugs of the Future*, 1985, *10*, 301; J. A. M. Goldsmith *et al.*, *J. Immunopharmac.*, 1986, *3*, 1; K. E. MacLaughlin *et al.*, *Arthritis Rheum.*, 1986, *29*, *Suppl.*, S29; *Clin. Pharmac. Ther.*, 1987, *41*, 596.

Proprietary Names and Manufacturers
Greenwich Pharmaceuticals, USA.

2893-j

Amlexanox *(rINN)*.

2-Amino-7-isopropyl-5-oxo-5*H*-[1]benzopyrano-[2,3-*b*]pyridine-3-carboxylic acid.
$C_{16}H_{14}N_2O_4$=298.3.

CAS — 68302-57-8.

An anti-allergic drug used in the treatment of asthma and allergic rhinitis.

Proprietary Names and Manufacturers
Solfa *(Takeda, Jpn)*.

201-d

Strong Ammonia Solution

Ammoniaca; Ammoniacum; Ammoniaque Officinale; Liquor Ammoniae Fortis; Solutio Ammoniaci Concentrata; Stronger Ammonia Water; Stronger Ammonium Hydroxide Solution.

CAS — 7664-41-7 (NH_3).

NOTE. The food additive number 527 is used for ammonium hydroxide

Pharmacopoeias. In *Arg.* (31 to 33.5%), *Aust.* (24 to 26%), *Belg.* (16 to 17%), *Br.*, *Chin.* (25 to 28%), *Egypt.* (27 to 30%), *Fr.* (not less than 20%), *Hung.* (22 to 30%), *It.*, and *Mex.* (both with 27 to 30%), *Nord.* (23 to 26%), *Port.* (20 to 22%), and *Span.* (20.18%). Also in *U.S.N.F.* which has 27 to 31%.

A clear colourless liquid with a strongly pungent characteristic odour, containing 27 to 30% w/w of NH_3. '0.880 ammonia' contains about 35% w/w.

Store at a temperature not exceeding 20° in airtight containers.

CAUTION. *Strong Ammonia Solution should be handled with great care because of the caustic nature of the solution and the irritating properties of the vapour. Cool the container well before opening and avoid inhalation of the vapour.*

202-n

Dilute Ammonia Solution

Ammonia Water; Ammoniaque Officinale Diluée; Ammonium Hydricum Solutum; Diluted Ammonium Hydroxide Solution; Liquor Ammoniae; Liquor Ammoniae Dilutus.

Pharmacopoeias. In *Arg.*, *Br.*, *Chin.*, *Cz.*, *Egypt.*, *Hung.*, *Jpn*, *Pol.*, *Roum.*, and *Swiss* (all about 10%); in *Aust.* (10.2 to 11%), in *Mex.* (9 to 10%), and in *Port.* (10 to 11%).

Prepared by diluting Strong Ammonia Solution with freshly boiled and cooled Purified Water. It contains 9.5 to 10.5% w/w of NH_3. **Store** at a temperature not exceeding 20° in well-closed containers.

NOTE. The *B.P.* directs that when Ammonia Solution is prescribed or demanded, Dilute Ammonia Solution shall be dispensed or supplied.

Adverse Effects

Ingestion of strong solutions of ammonia causes severe pain in the mouth, throat, and gastro-intestinal tract, with cough, vomiting, and shock. Burns to the oesophagus and stomach may result in perforation. Stricture formation usually in the oesophagus can occur weeks or months later. Ingestion may also cause oedema of the respiratory tract and pneumonitis, though this may not develop for a few hours.

Inhalation of ammonia vapour causes sneezing and coughing and in high concentration causes pulmonary oedema. Asphyxia has been reported following oedema or spasm of the glottis. Ammonia vapour is irritant to the eyes and causes weeping; there may be conjunctival swelling and temporary blindness. Strong solutions on the conjunctiva cause a severe reaction with conjunctival oedema, corneal damage, and acute glaucoma. Late complications include closed-angle glaucoma, opaque corneal scars, atrophy of the iris, and formation of cataracts. Ammonia burns have resulted from treating insect bites and stings with the strong solution, and even with the dilute solution, especially if a dressing is subsequently applied.

In Great Britain the recommended exposure limits of ammonia (NH_3) are 25 ppm (long-term); 35 ppm (short-term). In the *USA* the permissible and recommended exposure limits are 35 mg per m^3 and 34.8 mg per m^3 respectively.

A 5-year follow-up study in a patient whose persistent airflow obstruction was caused by accidental inhalation of concentrated ammonia fumes.— K. E. Flury *et al.*, *Mayo Clin. Proc.*, 1983, *58*, 389.

Treatment of Adverse Effects

Ingestion should not be treated by lavage or emesis. Give copious drinks of water and follow this with demulcents. Appropriate measures should be taken to alleviate pain, shock and pulmonary oedema, and maintain an airway.

Contaminated skin and eyes should be flooded immediately with water and the washing continued for at least 15 minutes. Any affected clothing should be removed while flooding is being carried out. Pain in affected eyes may be relieved by the instillation of local anaesthetic eye-drops.

Uses and Administration

Dilute solutions of ammonia have been used as reflex stimulants either as smelling salts or solutions for oral administration. They have also been used as rubefacients and counter-irritants and to neutralise insect stings. Users should always be aware of the irritant properties of ammonia.

Hartshorn and Oil was sometimes used as a name for an ammonia liniment. Household ammonia and cloudy ammonia have been used as names for cleaning preparations of ammonia with oleic acid or soap respectively.

In the *UK* the use of ammonia in cosmetics is prohibited by law.

STINGS. Bathers who were stung after intercepting an armada of Portuguese men-of-war (*Physalia physalis*) were rapidly and effectively relieved of discomfort, paresis, irritation, and other symptoms by the application of aromatic ammonia spirit compresses.— I. G. Frohman (letter), *J. Am. med. Ass.*, 1966, *197*, 733.

Preparations

Aromatic Ammonia Solution *(B.P.)*. Ammonia Solution Aromatic *(A.P.F.)*; Sal Volatile Solution. Ammonium bicarbonate, strong ammonia solution, oils of lemon and nutmeg, alcohol (90%), and water. Store at a temperature not exceeding 25°. *Dose.* 1 to 5 mL diluted with water.

Aromatic Ammonia Solution *B.P.* was not adequately preserved against microbial spoilage as determined by the *B.P.* challenge test.— T. R. R. Kurup and L. S. C. Wan, *Pharm. J.*, 1986, *2*, 761.

Aromatic Ammonia Spirit *(B.P.)*. Sal Volatile Spirit. Ammonium bicarbonate dissolved in a mixture of strong ammonia solution with a distillate of lemon oil, nutmeg oil, alcohol, and water.

Aromatic Ammonia Spirit *(U.S.P.)*. Prepared by dissolving oils of lemon, lavender, and nutmeg in alcohol, adding a solution of ammonium carbonate and strong ammonia solution, and filtering after 24 hours. Store in airtight containers. Protect from light.

19210-x

Ammonium Lactate

$C_3H_9NO_3$=107.1.

CAS — 52003-58-4.

A humectant applied as a lotion in the treatment of dry scaly conditions of the skin including ichthyosis vulgaris.

Proprietary Names and Manufacturers
Lac-Hydrin *(Westwood, USA)*.

12368-s

Ammonium Persulphate

Ammonium Peroxydisulphate.
$(NH_4)_2S_2O_8$=228.2.

CAS — 7727-54-0.

Ammonium persulphate is a powerful oxidising agent which has been used in photography and various industrial processes. Strong solutions are irritant to the skin.

12369-w

Ammonium Phosphate *(USAN).*
545 *(ammonium polyphosphates)*; Diammonium Hydrogen Phosphate; Dibasic Ammonium Phosphate. Diammonium hydrogen orthophosphate.
$(NH_4)_2HPO_4$=132.1.

CAS — 7783-28-0.

Pharmacopoeias. In *U.S.N.F.*

A 1% solution in water has a pH of 7.6 to 8.2. **Incompatible** with alkalis, ferric salts, and salts of heavy metals. **Store** in airtight containers.

Ammonium phosphate was formerly used as a diuretic. It may be used as a buffering agent in pharmaceutical preparations.
Ammonium biphosphate (monobasic ammonium phosphate; $(NH_4)H_2PO_4$ = 115.0) has been used to acidify urine.

Proprietary Names and Manufacturers of Ammonium Phosphate or Ammonium Biphosphate
The following names have been used for multi-ingredient preparations containing ammonium phosphate or ammonium biphosphate— pHos-pHaid *(Guardian, Canad.; Guardian, USA)*.

16505-e

Amnion
Human extra-embryonic foetal membranes comprising an inner amniotic membrane and an outer membrane, the chorion. Amnion has been used as a dressing for raw wounds including chronic ulcers and burns.

References: *Lancet*, 1984, *1*, 719; A. D. Redmond (letter), *ibid.*, 902; T. J. Egan and J. O'Driscoll (letter), *ibid.*, 1024.

Proprietary Names and Manufacturers
Amniex *(Mastelli, Ital.)*.

2836-v

Amorolfine *(rINN).*
(±)-*cis*-2,6-Dimethyl-4-[2-methyl-3-(*p-tert*-pentylphenyl)propyl]morpholine.
$C_{21}H_{35}NO$=317.5.

CAS — 78613-35-1.

A topical antifungal drug under investigation.

Proprietary Names and Manufacturers
Roche, *Switz.*

18755-f

Amosulalol *(rINN).*
YM-09538. (±)-5-(1-Hydroxy-2-{[2-(*o*-methoxyphenoxy)ethyl]amino}ethyl)-*o*-toluenesulfonamide.
$C_{18}H_{24}N_2O_5S$=380.5.

CAS — 85320-68-9.

An antihypertensive agent with alpha and beta blocking properties.

References: *Drugs of the Future*, 1984, *9*, 557; *ibid.*, 1985, *10*, 582; *ibid.*, 1986, *11*, 610.

Proprietary Names and Manufacturers
Yamanouchi, Jpn.

16508-j

Amyl Salicylate
Isoamyl Salicylate; Isopentyl Salicylate. 3-Methylbutyl 2-hydroxybenzoate.
$C_{12}H_{16}O_3$=208.3.

CAS — 87-20-7.

Amyl salicylate is used in perfumery and has also been applied topically similarly to methyl salicylate (p.27) for its analgesic and anti-inflammatory actions.

12375-p

Anagrelide Hydrochloride *(USAN, rINNM).*
BL-4162A. 6,7-Dichloro-1,5-dihydroimidazo-[2,1-*b*]quinazolin-2(3*H*)-one hydrochloride.
$C_{10}H_7Cl_2N_3O,HCl$=292.6.

CAS — 68475-42-3 (anagrelide); 58579-51-4 (hydrochloride).

Anagrelide is reported to be an inhibitor of platelet aggregation.

References: R. C. Gaver *et al.*, *Clin. Pharmac. Ther.*, 1981, *29*, 381 (disposition and metabolism); M. N. Silverstein *et al.*, *New Engl. J. Med.*, 1988, *318*, 1292 (use in thrombocytosis in doses of 1 to 4 mg daily by mouth).

Proprietary Names and Manufacturers
Bristol, USA.

18757-n

Anaxirone *(rINN).*
NSC-332488; Triglycidylurazol. Tris(2,3-epoxypropyl)bicarbamimide.
$C_{11}H_{15}N_3O_5$=269.3.

CAS — 77658-97-0.

An antineoplastic agent.

References: *Drugs of the Future*, 1984, *9*, 209; *ibid.*, 1985, *10*, 266; *ibid.*, 1986, *11*, 210.

522-k

Andrographis
Kalmegh; Kirayat.

CAS — 5508-58-7 (andrographolide).

Pharmacopoeias. In *Chin.*

The dried entire plant or the dried leaves and tender shoots of *Andrographis paniculata* (Acanthaceae).

Andrographis has been used in Asia as a bitter and as a folk medicine for a variety of disorders.

3703-d

Anethole Trithione
SKF-1717; Trithioparamethoxyphenylpropene. 5-(4-Methoxyphenyl)-3*H*-1,2-dithiole-3-thione.
$C_{10}H_8OS_3$=240.4.

CAS — 532-11-6 (trithione).

NOTE. Distinguish from Anethole p.1060.

Anethole trithione is used as a choleretic. The usual dose is 50 mg daily in divided doses, before meals; children, 12.5 to 25 mg. It is also used in salivary insufficiency in doses of 25 mg three times daily. Anethole trithione may cause discoloration of the urine.

Proprietary Names and Manufacturers
Felviten *(Grünenthal, Ger.)*; Mucinol *(Plantorgan, Ger.)*; Sialor *(Charton, Canad.)*; Sonicur *(Kali-Farma, Spain)*; Sufralem *(Landerlan, Spain)*; Sulfarlem *(Latema, Belg.; Charton, Canad.; Latéma, Fr.; Farmades, Ital.; Ethimed, S.Afr.; Latéma, Switz.)*.

3328-c

Anipamil *(rINN).*
2-{3-[(*m*-Methoxyphenethyl)methylamino]-propyl}-2-(*m*-methoxyphenyl)-tetradecanenitrile.
$C_{34}H_{52}N_2O_2$=520.8.

CAS — 83200-10-6.

A calcium-channel blocker derived from verapamil.

References: *Drugs of the Future*, 1986, *11*, 171.

Proprietary Names and Manufacturers
Knoll, Ger.

16511-s

Aniracetam *(USAN, rINN).*
Ro-13-5057. 1-(4-Methoxybenzoyl)-2-pyrrolidinone.
$C_{12}H_{13}NO_3$=219.2.

CAS — 72432-10-1.

Aniracetam is a nootropic drug (see Piracetam, p.1602) which has been tried in dementia in the elderly.

2549-r

Anirolac *(USAN, pINN).*
RS-37326. (±)-5-*p*-Anisoyl-2,3-dihydro-1*H*-pyrrolizine-1-carboxylic acid.
$C_{16}H_{15}NO_4$=285.3.

CAS — 66635-85-6.

An analgesic with anti-inflammatory activity.

References: *Drugs of the Future*, 1986, *11*, 449; S. S. Bloomfield *et al.*, *Clin. Pharmac. Ther.*, 1987, *42*, 89.

Proprietary Names and Manufacturers
Syntex, USA.

18767-m

Antineoplaston A10
3-Phenylacetylamino-2,6-piperidinedione.
$C_{13}H_{14}N_2O_3$=246.3.

One of a group of peptides isolated from blood and urine and under investigation for the treatment of cancer.

References: S. R. Burzynski *et al.*, *Drugs exp. & clin. Res.*, 1984, *10*, 891;, *idem*, 611; S. R. Burzynski and E. Kubove, *ibid.*, 1986, *12*, *Suppl.* 1, 47.

12386-e

Apis mellifera
The honey bee.

A preparation containing the venom of *Apis mellifera* is used in homoeopathic medicine where it is known as Apis mellifica or Apis mel.

For reference to the use of whole body extracts or venom from *Hymenoptera* spp. in desensitisation procedures in allergic subjects see under Allergens and Specific Desensitisation, p.464.

There have been a number of anecdotal reports of successful treatment of chronic inflammatory disease such as arthritis with bee venom. Studies *in vitro* have shown that bee venom has anti-inflammatory activity similar to that of cyclophosphamide. Mellitin appears to be the active constituent, and seems to act by interfering with superoxide radical production from human leukocytes. Further studies are warranted to investigate the potential of this property *in vivo*.— S. D. Somerfield, *N.Z. med. J.*, 1986, *99*, 281.

3917-j

Apraclonidine Hydrochloride *(USAN).*
AL-02145; Aplonidine Hydrochloride. 2-[(4-Amino-2,6-dichlorophenyl)imino]imidazolidine hydrochloride; 2,6-Dichloro-N^1-2-imidazolidinylidene-1,4-benzenediamine hydrochloride.
$C_9H_{10}Cl_2N_4,HCl$=281.6.

CAS — 73218-79-8.

Apraclonidine eye-drops are used to control or prevent elevations in intra-ocular pressure following ophthalmological surgery.

Proprietary Names and Manufacturers
Iopidine *(Alcon Laboratories, USA)*.

7353-m

Arachis Oil *(BAN).*
Earth-nut Oil; Erdnussöl; Ground-nut Oil; Huile d'Arachide; Nut Oil; Óleo de Amendoim; Ol. Arach.; Oleum Arachidis; Oleum Arachis; Peanut Oil *(USAN)*.

CAS — 8002-03-7.

Pharmacopoeias. In *Arg., Aust., Belg., Br., Cz., Egypt., Eur., Fr., Ger., Ind., Int., It., Jpn, Mex., Neth., Nord., Pol., Port.,* and *Swiss.* In *B.P. Vet.* Also in *U.S.N.F.* (Peanut Oil) which specifies oil from the seed kernels of one or more of the cultivated varieties of *A. hypogaea.*

The refined fixed oil obtained from the seeds of *Arachis hypogaea* (Leguminosae). It is a pale yellow oil with a faint nutty odour and a bland nutty taste consisting of glycerides, chiefly of oleic and linoleic acids, with smaller amounts of other acids.

Very slightly **soluble** in alcohol; miscible with carbon disulphide, chloroform, ether, and petroleum spirit. **Store** at a temperature not exceeding 40° in well-filled airtight containers. Protect from light.

Emulsions containing arachis oil are used in nutrition. Arachis oil is given as an enema for softening impacted faeces. It has been used in drops for softening ear wax.

Hydrogenated arachis oil has been used in the preparation of ointments.

Proprietary Preparations

Calogen *(Scientific Hospital Supplies, UK). Emulsion,* arachis oil 50% in water. A dietary supplement of high energy value but low electrolyte content (provides 18.8 MJ per litre, with sodium 9 mmol and potassium 5 mmol).

NOTE The terms LCT Emulsion and Long Chain Triglyceride Emulsion are also applied to this preparation.

Fletchers' Arachis Oil Retention Enema *(Pharmax, UK). Enema,* arachis oil 130 mL, in a plastic bag fitted with a rectal tube.

Hydromol *(Quinoderm, UK). Cream,* arachis oil 10%, isopropyl myristate 5%, liquid paraffin 10%, sodium pidolate 2.5%, sodium lactate 1% in an emollient base.

Oilatum Cream *(Stiefel, UK). Cream,* arachis oil 21%, povidone 1%, in an oil-in-water emulsion basis.

Oilatum Soap *(Stiefel, UK). Skin cleanser,* unsaponified arachis oil 7.5%.

Proprietary Names and Manufacturers

Calogen *(Sharpe, Austral.; Scientific Hospital Supplies, UK)*; Fletchers' Arachis Oil Retention Enema *(Pharmax, UK)*; Oilatum Bar *(Stiefel, Austral.)*; Oilatum Cream *(Stiefel, UK)*; Oilatum Soap *(Stiefel, S.Afr.; Stiefel, UK)*; Olie *(DAK, Denm.)*; X-Vac *(Forrest, Austral. : Schering, UK)*.

19453-c

Argatroban *(pINN)*.

MD-805. (2*R*,4*R*)-4-Methyl-1-[(*S*)-N^2-{[(*RS*)-1,2,3,4-tetrahydro-3-methyl-8-quinolyl]sulfonyl}arginyl]pipecolic acid.

$C_{23}H_{36}N_6O_5S$=508.6.

CAS — 74863-84-6.

A synthetic thrombin inhibitor under investigation as an anticoagulant.

Proprietary Names and Manufacturers

Mitsubishi, Jpn.

18775-m

Arildone *(USAN, pINN)*.

Win-38020. 4-[6-(2-Chloro-4-methoxyphenoxy)hexyl]3,5-heptanedione.

$C_{20}H_{29}ClO_4$=368.9.

CAS — 56219-57-9.

An antiviral agent under investigation. It has been applied topically.

References to antiviral activity of arildone: M. F. Kuhrt *et al., Antimicrob. Ag. Chemother.,* 1979, *15,* 813; M. A. McKinlay *et al., ibid.,* 1982, *22,* 1022; M. P. Langford *et al., ibid.,* 1985, *28,* 578.

References to the topical use of arildone: D. J. Jeffries and A. S. Tyms (letter), *Lancet,* 1983, *1,* 1214; J. A. Bosso *et al., J. clin. Pharmac.,* 1985, *25,* 95; J. M. Douglas *et al., Antimicrob. Ag. Chemother.,* 1986, *29,* 464.

12396-y

Arsenic Trioxide

Acidum Arsenicosum Anhydricum; Arseni Trioxydum; Arsenic; Arsenicum Album; Arsenious Acid; Arsenous Oxide; White Arsenic.

As_2O_3=197.8.

CAS — 1327-53-3 (arsenic trioxide); 7784-45-4 (arsenic triiodide).

Pharmacopoeias. In *Arg., Hung., Jpn, Jug., Mex., Pol., Port., Rus., Span.,* and *Turk. Port.* also includes Arsenic triiodide (AsI_3 = 455.6).

A heavy white powder or irregular lumps with a vitreous fracture and often containing both transparent and opaque varieties.

Adverse Effects

The symptoms of acute poisoning due to arsenic usually occur within one hour of ingestion but may be delayed for up to 12 hours, especially in the presence of food. Symptoms initially consist of burning lips, constriction of the throat, dysphagia, followed by severe gastric pain, vomiting, and profuse watery or bloody diarrhoea resembling cholera. Patients often develop an intense thirst and muscle cramps. Oliguria with proteinuria, sometimes leading to anuria, usually develops. Cardiac arrhythmias may also occur. If dehydration is severe, patients may experience symptoms of shock sometimes followed by convulsions, coma, and finally death. From 120 to 300 mg of arsenic trioxide may be fatal depending on the physical form and the rate of absorption. In the absence of adequate treatment death can occur within one hour but a period of 24 hours is more usual. Patients who survive the initial effects of arsenic trioxide may develop severe peripheral neuropathies and encephalopathy. Other effects following acute poisoning resemble those seen in chronic poisoning. Pulmonary oedema, dyspnoea, cough, and cyanosis may also occur if arsenic is inhaled.

Early signs of chronic poisoning often include anorexia, mild nausea and vomiting, diarrhoea or constipation, and muscle aching and weakness. Characteristic signs include oedema, especially of the face and eyelids, skin pigmentation, especially of the eyelids, neck, nipples, and axillae, hyperkeratosis, vitiligo, dermatitis, dry skin, and alopecia. The breath and perspiration may have an odour of garlic. Patients may also experience excessive salivation, sweating, and lachrymation, pruritus, sore mouth and throat, and inflammation of the conjunctiva and nasal mucosa resembling coryza. Characteristic deposits of arsenic may appear in the nails 6 weeks after absorption. Obstructive jaundice may occur as a result of hepatomegaly and cirrhosis may eventually develop. Proteinuria, haematuria, and anuria may occur secondary to renal damage. In advanced poisoning neurological effects are prominent. Encephalopathy has been reported but peripheral neuropathies are more common. There is both sensory and motor involvement and patients may at first experience paraesthesia, and numbness and burning in the extremities, but eventually muscular atrophy and paralysis occur. The legs are usually more affected than the arms. Arsenic is toxic to the bone marrow and produces a wide range of blood disorders including leucopenia, thrombocytopenia, and various anaemias.

Chronic exposure to arsenic has been associated with neoplasms of the skin, lungs, and liver and possibly other organs.

In Great Britain the control exposure limit of arsenic and arsenic compounds (except arsine and lead arsenate) is 200 µg per m^3 as As (long-term). In the *US* the permissible and recommended exposure limits for inorganic arsenic are 10 µg and 2 µg per m^3 respectively.

A review of arsenic.— Arsenic, *Environmental Health Criteria 18,* Geneva, Wld Hlth Org., 1981.

The provisional maximum tolerable daily intake for ingested inorganic arsenic was 2 µg per kg body-weight; no figure could be arrived at for organic arsenicals in foods.— Twenty-seventh Report of Joint FAO/WHO Expert Committee on Food Additives, *Tech. Rep. Ser. Wld Hlth Org. No. 696,* 1983.

EFFECTS ON THE BLOOD. Aplastic anaemia and eventually acute myelogenous leukaemia developed in a 67-year-old man in association with the extensive use of arsenical pesticides.— C. R. Kjeldsberg and H. P. Ward, *Ann. intern. Med.,* 1972, *77,* 935.

EFFECT ON THE IMMUNE SYSTEM. A report of angioimmunoblastic lymphadenopathy associated with chronic arsenic ingestion in a 64-year-old man following regular use of an asthma remedy containing arsenic trioxide.— K. Offit and N. T. Macris (letter), *Lancet,* 1985, *1,* 220.

EFFECTS ON THE LIVER. Non-cirrhotic portal hypertension occurred in 2 men as a result of chronic treatment with Fowler's solution (Arsenical Solution *B.P.C. 1963*), it was suggested that arsenic damaged the intrahepatic portal veins.— J. S. Morris *et al., Gut,* 1973, *14,* 821.

Treatment of Adverse Effects

Acute poisoning due to the ingestion of arsenic compounds should be treated by immediate gastric aspiration and lavage or the induction of emesis if the patient has not already vomited. Activated charcoal may be of use to reduce absorption. Chelation therapy with intramuscular dimercaprol should be started immediately the cause of poisoning is suspected (see Dimercaprol, p.840, for details of dosage). Prompt treatment is necessary to prevent or reduce the severity of neuropathy. It has been suggested that administration of dimercaprol should continue until abdominal symptoms subside and the gut is clear of ingested arsenic. Oral treatment with penicillamine may then be substituted for dimercaprol (see Penicillamine, p.849, for details of dosage). A second course of treatment with penicillamine may be required if symptoms recur. Intravenous replacement of fluids and electrolytes should be undertaken as necessary to correct dehydration and electrolyte imbalance and to prevent shock. Morphine has been suggested for the control of severe abdominal pain but care should be taken that this does not lead to colonic retention of arsenic compounds.

If renal failure occurs haemodialysis may be required to remove any absorbed or chelated arsenic. Exchange blood transfusion may be required for severe liver damage.

Dimercaprol may also be used in the treatment of chronic poisoning, but penicillamine may be preferred.

Absorption and Fate

Water-soluble arsenic acids and their salts are more rapidly absorbed from the gastro-intestinal tract than poorly soluble arsenicals such as arsenic trioxide. The absorption of arsenic trioxide is dependent upon the physical form of the compound and coarsely powdered material may be eliminated in the faeces before significant dissolution and absorption can occur.

Once absorbed arsenic is stored mainly in the liver, kidney, and lung, with smaller amounts in the muscles and nervous tissue. About two weeks after ingestion, arsenic is deposited in the hair and nails and remains fixed to the keratin for years. It is also deposited in the bones and teeth.

Although pentavalent arsenic is reduced to some degree *in vivo* to the more toxic trivalent form, trivalent arsenic is slowly and extensively oxidised to pentavalent arsenic. Both forms are methylated to relatively non-toxic derivatives and excreted in the urine mainly as dimethylarsinic acid with smaller amounts appearing as monomethylarsonic acid and inorganic arsenic compounds. Although 50% of a dose may be eliminated in the urine within 3 days small amounts may continue to be excreted for several weeks after a single dose. Less significant amounts of arsenic are excreted in the faeces and sweat and via the lungs and skin. It is also excreted in breast milk and readily crosses the placenta.

Uses and Administration

The therapeutic use of inorganic arsenical preparations is no longer recommended. Arsenic trioxide and arsenic triiodide were formerly used internally as solutions or externally as ointments in the treatment of various skin diseases.

Externally, arsenic trioxide has a caustic action. Arsenic trioxide is used in homoeopathic medicine and in certain Asian herbal remedies.

Arsenic trioxide has been widely employed as a constituent of weedkillers and sheepdips and as a rodenticide.

12397-j

Arsine

Arsenic Trihydride; Hydrogen Arsenide.
AsH_3=77.9.

CAS — 7784-42-1.

Arsine is highly toxic. It causes severe haemolysis which may result in acute renal failure. Exposure to as little as 3 ppm may cause symptoms, after a latent period of 2 to 24 hours, including headache, fever, dyspnoea, tachycardia, abdominal pain, nausea, vomiting, anorexia, jaundice, haemolytic anaemia, haematuria, oliguria, and anuria. Treatment involves exchange transfusions and haemodialysis; dimercaprol has been used but may not be effective. See also under Arsenic Trioxide, above.

In Great Britain the recommended exposure limit of arsine is 0.05 ppm (long-term). In the *US* the permissible and recommended exposure limits are 0.2 mg per m^3 and 0.002 mg per m^3 respectively.

A review of arsine poisoning.— B. A. Fowler and J. B. Weissberg, *New Engl. J. Med.*, 1974, *291*, 1171.

Reports of arsine poisoning.— S. P. Wilkinson *et al.*, *Br. med. J.*, 1975, *3*, 559; E. Rathus *et al.*, *Med. J. Aust.*, 1979, *1*, 163; P. L. Williams *et al.*, *Am. ind. Hyg. Assoc. J.*, 1981, *42*, 911.

The importance of exchange transfusions in severe cases of arsine poisoning.— C. S. Hesdorffer *et al.*, *Br. J. ind. Med.*, 1986, *43*, 353.

272-z

Asafetida

Asant; Devil's Dung; Gum Asafetida.

CAS — 9000-04-8.

Pharmacopoeias. In *Port.* and *Span.*

An oleo-gum-resin obtained from various species of *Ferula* (Umbelliferae).

Asafetida has been used as a carminative and antispasmodic. It was also formerly used as an expectorant.

A report of methaemoglobinaemia associated with the administration of asafetida to a 5-week-old infant for the treatment of colic. Laboratory investigations demonstrated an oxidising effect of asafetida on foetal haemoglobin but not on adult haemoglobin.— K. J. Kelly *et al.*, *Pediatrics*, 1984, *73*, 717.

12401-k

Asarabacca

Rhizoma Asari; Wild Nard; Hazelwort.

The dried rhizome, roots, and leaves of *Asarum europaeum* (Aristolochiaceae).

Asarabacca is an ingredient of snuffs. It is also an irritant emetic and has been used in rodent poisons. Asarabacca has been used in homeopathic medicine.

12402-a

Asbestos

The name asbestos is applied to several naturally occurring and widely distributed fibrous mineral silicates of the serpentine and amphibole groups. They include amosite (brown asbestos), anthophyllite, chrysotile (white asbestos), and crocidolite (blue asbestos).

Asbestos has properties of heat resistance, insulation, and reinforcement and has been used extensively for heat or electrical insulation, fire protection, in friction materials, and in the construction industry in a wide variety of materials including cement, pipes, and tiles.

When inhaled asbestos fibres can cause asbestosis (pulmonary fibrosis), lung cancer, and mesothelioma of the pleura and peritoneum. Mesothelioma has been reported in persons exposed to relatively small amounts of asbestos after a latent period of more than 20 years. Occupational exposure has sometimes been associated with an increased incidence of gastro-intestinal, laryngeal, and other cancers. Some types of asbestos are more hazardous than others; crocidolite (a member of the amphibole group) is considered to be the most dangerous and is no longer used in Great Britain. Occupational exposure to asbestos dust is now rigorously controlled.

3930-e

Atrial Natriuretic Peptides

Atrial natriuretic peptides are endogenous substances with diuretic and natriuretic activity secreted by the heart. The active peptide has also been called atriopeptin, auriculin, or cardionatrin and is the 28-membered carboxy terminus of a precursor containing 126 amino acid residues and stored in the heart. Atrial peptides have been synthesised. The name anaritide has been applied to an atrial natriuretic peptide with the structure *N*-L-arginyl-[8-L-methionine-21a-L-phenylalanine-21b-L-arginine-21c-L-tyrosine]-atriopeptin-21.

Atrial natriuretic peptide appears to be closely involved in fluid and electrolyte homoeostasis and in the regulation of blood pressure, together with other complex systems such as the renin-angiotensin-aldosterone cascade. Its physiological and pathological role and potential clinical applications are under intensive investigation. Human atrial natriuretic peptide and available synthetic analogues have a short half-life and also have to be given parenterally. Long-acting analogues, particularly if stable when given by mouth would greatly increase the therapeutic potential.

Reviews: *Lancet*, 1986, *2*, 371; P. Needleman and J. E. Greenwald, *New Engl. J. Med.*, 1986, *314*, 828; G. Thibault *et al.*, *Drugs*, 1986, *31*, 369; D. R. J. Singer, *Postgrad. med. J.*, 1987, *63*, 1.

Studies of the haemodynamic effects of atrial natriuretic peptide in patients with congestive heart failure: I. G. Crozier *et al.*, *Lancet*, 1986, *2*, 1242 (synthetic analogue [Ileu-ANP]); H. Saito *et al.*, *Clin. Pharmac. Ther.*, 1987, *42*, 142 ([α-human atrial natriuretic peptide] or [α-hANP]).

12408-n

Avena

Aven; Oats; Cultivated White Oats; Oatmeal.

The grain of *Avena sativa* (Gramineae).

Avena is reputed to have antidepressant activity; an extract or tincture has been claimed to be of value in the treatment of drug dependence.

A colloidal fraction extracted from avena has been used in the preparation of emollient dermatological preparations.

Avenin, a protein present in oats, might be harmful to patients with coeliac disease.

Variable reports of the effects of avena on nicotine and morphine dependence: C. L. Anand (letter), *Nature*, 1971, *233*, 496; *idem* (letter), *Br. med. J.*, 1971, *3*, 640; C. G. Le Fevre (letter), *Med. J. Aust.*, 1972, *1*, 140; C. Bye *et al.* (letter), *Nature*, 1974, *252*, 580; J. W. Gabrynowicz (letter), *Med. J. Aust.*, 1974, *2*, 306; J. Connor *et al.*, *J. Pharm. Pharmac.*, 1975, *27*, 92.

Proprietary Preparations

Aveeno Colloidal *(Oral-B, UK). Bath additive*, colloidal oat fraction 100%.

Aveeno Oilated *(Oral-B, UK). Bath additive*, colloidal oat fraction 41%, liquid paraffin 35%.

Aveenobar *(Oral-B, UK). Skin cleanser*, colloidal oat fraction 52.6%, isopropyl myristate 3%, lanolin derivative 0.9%, in a soapless basis.

Aveenobar Oilated *(Oral-B, UK). Skin cleanser*, colloidal oat fraction 30%, vegetable oils 23%, lanolin derivative 1%, in a soapless basis.

Proprietary Names and Manufacturers

Aveeno *(Oral-B, Austral.; Johnson, Canad.; Rydelle, USA)*; Aveeno Colloidal *(Oral-B, UK)*; Aveeno Oilated *(Oral-B, UK)*; Aveenobar *(Oral-B, Austral.; Oral-B, UK)*; Aveenobar Oilated *(Oral-B, UK)*; Aveenoderm *(Sodip, Switz.)*.

523-a

Azadirachta

Margosa; Neem.

The dried stem bark, root bark, and leaves of *Azadirachta indica* (=*Melia azadirachta*) (Meliaceae).

Azadirachta has been used as a bitter. It is widely used in Asia and has been reported to have insecticidal and spermicidal properties.

Severe poisoning in Indian children given margosa oil as a remedy for minor ailments.— D. Sinniah and G. Baskaran, *Lancet*, 1981, *1*, 487.

Proprietary Preparations

Silvose *(Keimdiät, Ger.: Thomson & Joseph, UK)*. An extract from the bark of azadirachta. It is claimed to reduce dental caries and inflammation of the mouth when used as an ingredient in dental preparations.

18795-q

Azepexole *(BAN, rINN).*

BHT-933 (dihydrochloride). 6-Ethyl-5,6,7,8-tetrahydro-4*H*-oxazolo[4,5-*d*]azepin-2-ylamine.
$C_9H_{15}N_3O$=181.2.

CAS — 36067-73-9.

A selective alpha agonist with antihypertensive activity of the clonidine type. It also has anti-tussive activity.

References: L. Benedikter *et al.*, *Eur. J. clin. Pharmac.*, 1981, *20*, 321; J. B. S. Redpath and B. J. Pleuvry, *Br. J. clin. Pharmac.*, 1981, *12*, 901; B. J. Pleuvry and J. B. S. Redpath, *ibid.*, 1982, *14*, 559; D. W. G. Harron *et al.*, *ibid.*, 1985, *20*, 431; J. K. van Brummelen *et al.*, *Eur. J. clin. Pharmac.*, 1987, *32*, 115.

3467-b

Azithromycin *(BAN, pINN).*

CP-62993.
(2*R*,3*S*,4*R*,5*R*,8*R*,10*R*,11*R*,12*S*,13*S*,14*R*)-13-[(2,6-Dideoxy-3-*C*-methyl-3-*O*-methyl-α-L-*ribo*-hexopyranosyl)oxy]-2-ethyl-3,4,10-trihydroxy-3,5,6,8,10,12,14-heptamethyl-11-{[3,4,6-trideoxy-3-(dimethylamino)-β-D-*xylo*-hexopyranosyl]-oxy}-1-oxa-6-azacyclopentadecan-15-one.
$C_{38}H_{72}N_2O_{12}$=749.0.

CAS — 83905-01-5.

A macrolide antibiotic under investigation.

References: S. C. Aronoff *et al.* (letter), *J. antimicrob. Chemother.*, 1987, *19*, 275.

Proprietary Names and Manufacturers

Pfizer, USA.

18825-x

Bambuterol *(rINN).*

KWD-2183. (±)-5-[2-*tert*-Butylamino)-1-hydroxyethyl]-*m*-phenylene bis(dimethylcarbamate).

$C_{18}H_{29}N_3O_5$=367.4.

CAS — 81732-65-2; 81732-46-9 (monohydrochloride).

A sympathomimetic agent with bronchodilator activity. It is a pro-drug of terbutaline.

References: B. K. Pedersen *et al., Eur. J. clin. Pharmac.*, 1985, *29,* 425.

Proprietary Names and Manufacturers
Astra, Swed.

5263-p

Barium

Ba=137.33.

CAS — 7440-39-3.

A soft highly reactive silvery-white metal.

Adverse Effects and Treatment
The symptoms of barium poisoning from soluble barium salts arise from stimulation of all forms of muscle and include vomiting, colic, diarrhoea, hypertension, convulsive tremors, and muscular paralysis. Hypokalaemia is common. Death from cardiac or respiratory failure may occur within one to many hours.
In Great Britain the recommended exposure limit of soluble barium compounds (as Ba) is 0.5 mg per m^3 (long-term).
For the hazards of inhaling barium sulphate, see p.862.
Treatment of poisoning with soluble barium salts may involve emptying the stomach by emesis or lavage. A saline laxative such as magnesium or sodium sulphate may be given and has the added advantage of converting any barium to insoluble barium sulphate. Hypokalaemia should be corrected. Excretion may be increased by diuresis.

Of over 100 patients who ate sausage contaminated with barium carbonate 19 required hospital admission. Symptoms included: diarrhoea, vomiting, general weakness, dryness of the mouth, paralysis, tightness in the throat, dysarthria, and headaches; other symptoms were muscle twitching, testicular tenderness, urinary retention, and gastro-intestinal haemorrhage. Two severely affected patients had hypokalaemia with associated ECG changes.— Z. Lewi and Y. Bar-Khayim, *Lancet,* 1964, *2,* 342. Two severely affected patients suffered flaccid paralysis in all 4 extremities, associated with hypokalaemia. One recovered dramatically after intravenous injection of potassium chloride; the other responded initially but subsequently died, post-mortem examination revealing haemorrhagic gastritis and duodenitis, cardiac haemorrhage, and pulmonary oedema.— D. Diengott *et al., ibid.,* 343.

Acute renal failure associated with barium chloride poisoning.— S. F. Wetherill *et al., Ann. intern. Med.,* 1981, *95,* 187.

A 26-year-old man ingested a facial depilatory (Magic Shave), containing 15.8 g of barium sulphide. Despite ipecacuanha-induced vomiting he developed progressive paralysis after 3 hours. He was treated with oxygen, assisted respiration, sodium bicarbonate intravenously, magnesium sulphate by nasogastric tube, gastric lavage, diuresis (infusing a total of 6.5 litres of sodium chloride injection over 19 hours, augmented by frusemide 40 mg intravenously initially and repeated thrice over the 19 hours), and correction of profound hypokalaemia, a total of 260 mmol (260 mEq) of potassium being given over 19 hours. Correction of the hypokalaemia, diuresis, and assisted respiration were considered to have contributed greatly to his survival, the diuresis being considered as indispensable as the potassium.— D. B. Gould *et al., Archs intern. Med.,* 1973, *132,* 891.

A rapid severe fall in plasma-potassium concentrations was associated with barium poisoning. One patient who had taken a large dose of barium chloride was successfully treated with sodium sulphate 30 g by mouth and 30 g intravenously to precipitate the barium, potassium infusions, artificial respiration, and sodium bicarbonate. An infusion of 25 mmol of potassium appeared to be sufficient to balance the hypokalaemic action of the absorbed barium that had not been precipitated. An immediate bolus injection of 50 to 75 mmol might be given in severe cases.— J. Berning (letter), *Lancet,* 1975, *1,* 110. Following the ingestion of barium carbonate 40 g a 39-year-old subject developed muscle weakness and hypokalaemia as well as colicky abdominal pain, diarrhoea, and vomiting. Despite the administration of potassium, muscle weakness increased and the degree of weakness correlated with the plasma concentration of barium and not potassium. Renal insufficiency which resolved on day 6 might have been due to precipitation of barium suphate in renal tubules; this suggests that sulphate such as magnesium sulphate given intravenously should be avoided in the treatment of barium poisoning.— D. M. Phelan *et al., Br. med. J.,* 1984, *289,* 882.

Uses and Administration
The soluble barium salts are not used in therapeutics but are widely used in industry. Barium sulphide has been used as a depilatory and barium carbonate was used as a rodenticide. The insoluble barium sulphate (p.862) is used as a contrast medium.

203-h

Barium Hydroxide Lime *(USAN).*

A mixture of barium hydroxide octahydrate [$Ba(OH)_2,8H_2O$=315.5] and calcium hydroxide; it may also contain potassium hydroxide.

CAS — 17194-00-2 (barium hydroxide, anhydrous); 12230-71-6 (barium hydroxide, octahydrate).

Pharmacopoeias. In *U.S.*

White or greyish-white granules, or coloured with an indicator to show when absorptive power is exhausted. It absorbs not less than 19% of its weight of carbon dioxide. **Store** in airtight containers.

Barium hydroxide lime is used similarly to soda lime to absorb carbon dioxide in closed-circuit anaesthetic apparatus. Barium hydroxide lime contains a soluble form of barium and is toxic if swallowed.

12420-x

Bearberry

Bärentraubenblätter; Bearberry Leaves; Busserole; Ptarmiganberry Leaves; Uva Ursi.

Pharmacopoeias. In *Aust., Belg., Cz., Egypt., Ger., Hung., Jpn, Jug., Pol., Port., Rus.,* and *Swiss.*

The dried leaves of the bearberry, *Arctostaphylos uva-ursi* (Ericaceae).

Bearberry has been reported to be a diuretic and astringent and was used in the treatment of urethritis and cystitis. It is an ingredient of domestic anti-inflammatory remedies. Bearberry contains arbutin which is hydrolysed to hydroquinone (p.922).

12432-n

Benzarone *(USAN, rINN).*

L-2197. 2-Ethylbenzofuran-3-yl 4-hydroxyphenyl ketone.

$C_{17}H_{14}O_3$=266.3.

CAS — 1477-19-6.

Benzarone has been given by mouth and applied topically in the treatment of various peripheral vascular disorders.

Pharmacology of benzarone in *cats.*— E. Betz and W. Eitel, *Arzneimittel-Forsch.,* 1978, *28,* 626.

Proprietary Names and Manufacturers
Fragivix *(Labaz, Belg.; Labaz, Fr.; Sanol, Ger.; Sigmatau, Ital.; Labaz, Spain; Schwarz, Switz.);* Vasoc *(Lindopharm, Ger.);* Venagil *(Logifarm, Ital.).*

12434-m

Benzyl Isothiocyanate

Benzyl Mustard Oil; Benzylsenföl; Oleum Tropaeoli.

C_8H_7NS=149.2.

CAS — 622-78-6.

Pharmacopoeias. In *Fr.,* which also includes Capucine (*Tropaeolum majus*).

An oil obtained from Capuchin cress, *Tropaeolum majus* (Tropaeolaceae).

Benzyl isothiocyanate has been given as an antibacterial agent.

Proprietary Names and Manufacturers
Tromacaps *(Madaus, Ger.; Madaus, Switz.).*

524-t

Berberine

5,6-Dihydro-9,10-dimethoxybenzo[*g*]-1,3-benzodioxolo[5,6-*a*]quinolizinium.

$C_{20}H_{18}NO_4$=336.4.

CAS — 2086-83-1 (berberine); 633-66-9 (sulphate).

Pharmacopoeias. Chin., Ind., and *Jpn* include berberine chloride. *Jpn* also includes berberine tannate.

A quaternary alkaloid present in hydrastis, in various species of *Berberis,* and in many other plants.

Berberine has been used as a bitter. It possesses antimicrobial activity and has been tried in a number of infections including cutaneous leishmaniasis and cholera.
Both the sulphate and the chloride have been used.

Berberine has been reported to have a broad spectrum of activity against some bacteria, including *Vibrio cholerae,* shigella, pseudomonas, proteus, and *Escherichia coli,* fungi, and protozoa such as *Entamoeba histolytica,* trichomonas, giardia and leishmania. However, a study involving berberine, tetracycline and placebo in patients with watery diarrhoea did not appear to demonstrate a vibrostatic effect for berberine. The only improvements with berberine were a reduction in the volume of stools and in faecal concentration of cyclic adenosine monophosphate in those patients with cholera. Patients did less well on tetracycline and berberine than on tetracycline alone which might indicate antimicrobial antagonism.— Khin-Maung-U *et al., Br. med. J.,* 1985, *291,* 1601.

Experience in 5 patients with refractory congestive heart failure demonstrated improved left ventricular performance after berberine infusion.— P. R. Maroko and W. Ruzyllo, *Circulation,* 1983, *68, Suppl.* 3, III-374.

18723-j

Bermoprofen *(rINN).*

AD-1590. (±)-10,11-Dihydro-α,8-dimethyl-11-oxodibenz[*b,f*]oxepin-2-acetic acid.

$C_{18}H_{16}O_4$=296.3.

CAS — 72619-34-2.

A non-steroidal anti-inflammatory drug under investigation.

References: H. Nakamura *et al., J. Pharm. Pharmac.,* 1984, *36,* 182; H. Nakamura *et al., ibid.,* 1985, *37,* 894.

1303-j

Betaine Hydrochloride *(USAN).*

Trimethylglycine Hydrochloride. (Carboxymethyl)trimethylammonium hydroxide inner salt hydrochloride.

$C_5H_{11}NO_2,HCl$=153.6.

CAS — 107-43-7 (betaine); 590-46-5 (hydro-

chloride).

Pharmacopoeias. In *Aust., Hung., Jug., Port.,* and *U.S.*

A 25% solution has a pH of 0.8 to 1.2.
Store in well-closed containers.

Betaine hydrochloride has been given as a source of hydrochloric acid in the treatment of hypochlorhydria. A wide variety of betaine salts have been used in various countries, mainly for gastro-intestinal disturbances.

References to betaine being used in homocystinuria: L. A. Smolin *et al., J. Pediat.,* 1981, *99,* 467; D. E. L. Wilcken *et al., New Engl. J. Med.,* 1983, *309,* 448.

Proprietary Names and Manufacturers of Betaine Salts
Somatyl *(Anphar-Rolland, Fr.; Prophin, Ital.).*

The following names have been used for multi-ingredient preparations containing betaine salts—Acidol Pepsin *(Sterling Research, UK)*; Acidol-Pepsin *(Winthrop, Austral.)*; Kloref *(Cox, UK)*; Kloref-S *(Cox, UK).*

5267-l

Bibrocathol *(rINN).*

Bibrocathin; Bibrokatol; Bismuth Tetrabrompyrocatechinate; Tetrabromopyrocatechol Bismuth. 4,5,6,7-Tetrabromo-2-hydroxy-1,3,2-benzodioxabismole.
$C_6HBiBr_4O_3$=649.7.

CAS — 6915-57-7.

Pharmacopoeias. In *Nord.*

Practically **insoluble** in water.

Bibrocathol is a bismuth-containing compound that has been applied as an eye ointment in the treatment of blepharitis.

Proprietary Names and Manufacturers
Noviform *(Dispersa, Ger.; Meda, Swed.; Dispersa, Switz.)*; Noviforme *(Novopharma, Switz.)*; Posiformin *(Ursapharm, Ger.).*

16535-k

Biclotymol *(rINN).*

Biclothymol. 2,2'-Methylenebis(6-chlorothymole).
$C_{21}H_{26}Cl_2O_2$=381.3.

CAS — 15686-33-6.

An antiseptic which has been used in mouth and throat infections.

Proprietary Names and Manufacturers
Hexaspray *(Doms, Fr.).*

5229-g

Bietamiverine Hydrochloride *(rINNM).*

Dietamiverine Dihydrochloride. 2-Diethylaminoethyl-2-phenyl-1-piperidinoacetate dihydrochloride.
$C_{19}H_{30}N_2O_2$,2HCl=391.4.

CAS — 479-81-2 (bietamiverine); 2691-46-5 (hydrochloride).

Bietamiverine hydrochloride is used as an antispasmodic in doses of up to 200 mg daily.

Proprietary Names and Manufacturers
Fine-Dol *(Isola-Ibi, Ital.)*; Novosparol *(Prophin, Ital.)*; Spasmisolvina *(Dessy, Ital.).*

1962-m

Bifemelane *(rINN).*

N-Methyl-4-[(α-phenyl-*o*-tolyl)oxy]butylamine.
$C_{18}H_{23}NO$=269.4.

CAS — 90293-01-9.

A nootropic or cognition adjuvant for use in the treatment of senile dementia.

Proprietary Names and Manufacturers
Celeport *(Eisai, Jpn).*

998-q

Bile Acids and Salts

CAS — 81-25-4 (cholic acid); 8008-63-7 (ox bile extract); 11006-55-6 (sodium tauroglycocholate).

Pharmacopoeias. Aust. includes cholic acid. *Arg., Mex., Port.,* and *Span.* include fresh ox bile.

The principal primary bile acids, cholic acid and chenodeoxycholic acid (see p.1555), are produced in the liver from cholesterol and are conjugated with glycine or taurine to give glycocholic acid, taurocholic acid, glycochenodeoxycholic acid, and taurochenodeoxycholic acid before being secreted into the bile. Secondary bile acids are formed in the colon by bacterial deconjugation and 7α-dehydroxylation of cholic acid and chenodeoxycholic acid producing deoxycholic acid and lithocholic acid respectively, and are partially reabsorbed and conjugated. The sodium and potassium salts of the conjugated acids are referred to as the bile salts. Ursodeoxycholic acid (see p.1627) is a minor bile acid in man. Dehydrocholic acid (see p.1563) is a semi-synthetic bile acid.

Bile acids are choleretic agents. Chenodeoxycholic acid and ursodeoxycholic acid decrease the cholesterol content of bile and are used in the treatment of cholesterol-rich gall-stones. Bile salts are amphiphilic and are important for the emulsification of cholesterol and other lipids in bile, and also for the emulsification of dietary fats. Preparations containing bile salts have been used to assist the emulsification of fats and absorption of fat-soluble vitamins in conditions in which there is a deficiency of bile in the gastro-intestinal tract. Ox bile has also been used in the treatment of chronic constipation.

Proprietary Names and Manufacturers
Desicol *(Austral.)*; Felkreon *(Ger.).*

The following names have been used for multi-ingredient preparations containing bile acids and salts—Artéchol *(Anglo-French Laboratories, Canad.)*; Bilogene *(Bio-Chemical Laboratory, Canad.)*; Bilron *(Lilly, Canad.)*; Combizym Co. *(Luitpold, Austral.)*; Combizym Compositum *(Panpharma, UK)*; Cotazym B *(Organon, Austral.; Organon, Canad.; Organon, UK)*; Digepepsin *(Ram, USA)*; Donnazyme *(Robins, Canad.; Robins, USA)*; Entozyme *(Robins, Canad.; Robins, USA)*; Enzobile *(Mallard, USA)*; Enzypan *(Norgine, UK; Norgine, USA)*; Kanulase *(Dorsey Laboratories, USA)*; Karbokoff *(Arlo, USA)*; Opobyl *(Bengué, UK).*

18843-f

Binedaline *(rINN).*

Binodaline; Scha-1659; Sgd-20578; Sgd-Scha-1059. 1-[[2-(Dimethylamino)ethyl]methylamino]-3-phenylindole.
$C_{19}H_{23}N_3$=293.4.

CAS — 60662-16-0.

An antidepressant under investigation.

References: F. Faltus and F. C. Geerling, *Neuropsychobiology,* 1984, *12,* 34; P. H. Joubert *et al., Eur. J. clin. Pharmac.,* 1985, *27,* 667; J. Longmore *et al., Br. J. clin. Pharmac.,* 1985, *19,* 295.

Proprietary Names and Manufacturers
Siegfried, Switz.

3028-b

Biostim

RU-41740.

A glycoprotein with immunomodulating activity isolated from *Klebsiella pneumoniae.*

References: J. Bonde *et al., Eur. J. resp. Dis.,* 1986, *69,* 235; M. L. Profeta *et al.* (letter), *Lancet,* 1987, *1,* 973.

3368-n

Biriperone *(rINN).*

Centbutindole. (±)-4'-Fluoro-4-(3,4,6,7,12,12a-hexahydropyrazino[1',2':1,6]pyrido[3,4-*b*]indol-2(1*H*)-yl)butyrophenone.
$C_{24}H_{26}FN_3O$=391.5.

CAS — 41510-23-0.

A neuroleptic introduced in India.

18846-h

Bisantrene Hydrochloride *(USAN, rINNM).*

ADAH(bisantrene); ADC(bisantrene); CL-216942. 9,10-Anthracenedicarboxaldehyde bis(2-imidazolin-2-ylhydrazone) dihydrochloride.
$C_{22}H_{22}N_8$,2HCl=471.4.

CAS — 71439-68-4; 78186-34-2 (bisantrene).

An antineoplastic agent under investigation.

References: G. Powis and J. S. Kovach, *Cancer Res.,* 1983, *43,* 925; H. Y. Yap *et al., ibid.,* 1402.

Proprietary Names and Manufacturers
Lederle, USA.

5265-w

Bismuth

Bi=208.9804.

CAS — 7440-69-9.

A silvery-white crystalline brittle metal with a pinkish tinge.

Adverse Effects
The effects of acute bismuth intoxication include gastro-intestinal disturbances, skin reactions, and discoloration of mucous membranes; a characteristic blue line may appear on the gums. There may be renal failure and liver damage. These effects do not appear to be common with insoluble salts used for limited periods.

Reversible encephalopathy has been a problem in some countries, notably France and Australia, and is not necessarily associated with heavy or prolonged use of bismuth salts; bone and joint disorders have occurred and have sometimes been associated with the encephalopathy. These effects have led to restrictions on the use of bismuth salts.

Bismuth salts taken by mouth can produce black coloration of the faeces.

A detailed review of the toxicity of bismuth salts.— K. A. Winship, *Adverse Drug React. Ac. Pois. Rev.,* 1983, *2,* 103.

Adverse reactions reported to the Australian Drug Evaluation Committee by patients with colostomies and ileostomies taking bismuth subgallate by mouth were: an unwell feeling, lack of energy, peculiar sensation in the fingers and toes, and after a period of months or years, deterioration of mental ability, loss of concentration, impaired ability to read and write, and muscle twitching. Patients might become bedridden, incontinent, confused, and disorientated. In all patients full recovery occurred within a few weeks of discontinuing bismuth subgallate therapy.— A. W. Morrow (letter), *Med. J. Aust.,* 1973, *1,* 912.

An epidemiological study of intoxication by bismuth salts in France. Of 294 patients identified, 16 had died. It was considered that this was not a usual toxicological occurrence but might be associated with a bacterial factor which could convert the ingested bismuth salt into a more toxic form.— G. Martin-Bouyer, *Thérapie,* 1976, *31,* 683.

Some recent reports of encephalopathy in patients taking bismuth preparations: G. J. Hasking and J. M. Duggan (letter), *Med. J. Aust.,* 1982, *2,* 167; J. P. Stahl *et al.* (letter), *Nouv. Presse méd.,* 1982, *11,* 3856.

Absorption and Fate
Soluble bismuth salts are absorbed from the gastro-intestinal tract; excretion in the urine is rapid. They are also excreted in the saliva. The more insoluble bismuth salts are only slightly

absorbed. Absorbed bismuth salts are excreted mainly in the urine, but some bismuth is retained in the bones and tissues. Bismuth can cross the placenta.

Uses and Administration of Bismuth Salts
Bismuth and certain of its salts were formerly given mainly by injection, alone or with other agents, in the treatment of syphilis but were superseded by antibiotic therapy.
Some insoluble salts of bismuth have been given by mouth for their supposed antacid action and for their mildly astringent action in diarrhoea. Bismuth salicylate (p.1078) is still used in the treatment of diarrhoea, presumably because of its astringent action. Tripotassium dicitratobismuthate (p.1111) is used in the management of peptic ulcers.
Certain insoluble salts of bismuth have been applied topically in dusting powders and in ointments or suppositories for haemorrhoids but there is little confirmation of their value.

A method of preparation of bismuth phosphate injection to be used in the treatment of renal cysts according to a report by Zachrisson (*Acta radiol., Diagnosis*, 1982 *23*, Fasc 3A, 209).— M. R. Riley and R. Parkinson (letter), *Pharm. J.*, 1985, *1*, 808.

12445-g

Bismuth Dipropylacetate

Bismuth Valproate. Bismuth tris(2-propylvalerate).
$C_{24}H_{45}BiO_6$=638.6.

Bismuth dipropylacetate is available as suppositories in some countries for the treatment of minor infections.

Proprietary Names and Manufacturers
Birectal *(Labaz, Fr.)*; Neo-Laryngobis *(Bio-Chemical Laboratory, Canad.)*; Suppangin *(Südmedica, Ger.)*.

5271-p

Bismuth Oxide

Bismuth Trioxide.
Bi_2O_3=466.0.

CAS — 1304-76-3.

Practically **insoluble** in water.

Bismuth oxide has been used in ointments for ano-rectal disorders.

Proprietary Preparations
Anugesic-HC *(Parke, Davis, UK)). Cream*, bismuth oxide 0.875%, resorcinol 0.875%, Peru balsam 1.85%, zinc oxide 12.35%, benzyl benzoate 1.2%, pramoxine hydrochloride 1%, hydrocortisone acetate 0.5%.
For Anugesic-HC Suppositories, see below.
Anusol *(Warner-Lambert, UK). Cream*, bismuth oxide 2.14%, Peru balsam 1.8%, zinc oxide 10.75%.
For other Anusol Preparations, see below.

Proprietary Names and Manufacturers
The following names have been used for multi-ingredient preparations containing bismuth oxide— Anugesic-HC *(Parke, Davis, UK)*; Anusol *(Warner-Lambert, UK)*; Hemocane *(Intercare, UK)*.

18850-r

Bismuth Phosphate

$BiPO_4$=304.0.

CAS — 10049-01-1.

Pharmacopoeias. In *Fr.*

Bismuth phosphate has been used as an antacid.

Reference to bismuth phosphate injection for the treatment of renal cysts and a method of preparing the injection: M. R. Riley and R. Parkinson (letter), *Pharm. J.*, 1985, *1*, 808.

Proprietary Names and Manufacturers
Bismugel *(Bioterax, Spain)*.

5279-c

Bismuth Subcarbonate *(BAN)*.

Basic Bismuth Carbonate; Basisches Wismutkarbonat; Bism. Carb.; Bismuth Carbonate; Bismuth Oxycarbonate; Bismuthi Subcarbonas; Bismutylum Carbonicum; Carbonato de Bismutila.

CAS — 5892-10-4 (anhydrous); 5798-45-8 (hemihydrate).

Pharmacopoeias. In *Arg., Aust., Belg., Br., Chin., Cz., Egypt., Eur., Fr., Ger., Int., It., Jug., Mex., Neth., Nord., Pol., Port., Roum., Span.*, and *Turk.*

A white or almost white odourless powder.
Practically **insoluble** in water, alcohol, and ether; soluble in mineral acids with effervescence. **Protect** from light.

Bismuth subcarbonate has been given as an antacid. When given as a compound powder with other antacids, doses of bismuth subcarbonate have ranged from 125 to 625 mg.

5280-s

Bismuth Subgallate *(BAN)*.

Basic Bismuth Gallate; Basisches Wismutgallat; Bism. Subgall.; Bismuth Oxygallate.

CAS — 99-26-3.

Pharmacopoeias. In *Arg., Belg., Fr., Ger., Hung., Jpn, Jug., Neth., Pol., Port., Roum., Rus., Span.*, and *Turk.*

Bismuth subgallate has been employed as a dusting-powder in some skin disorders, and as suppositories in the treatment of haemorrhoids. It was formerly given for its supposed astringent properties in the treatment of diarrhoea, dysentery, and ulcerative colitis, in doses of 0.6 to 2 g. It has been administered by mouth to help control the odour and consistency of stool in patients with a colostomy or ileostomy. See also Uses and Administration of Bismuth Salts, above.

Proprietary Preparations
Anugesic-HC *(Parke, Davis, UK). Suppositories*, bismuth subgallate 59 mg, bismuth oxide 24 mg, Peru balsam 49 mg, zinc oxide 296 mg, benzyl benzoate 33 mg, pramoxine hydrochloride 27 mg, hydrocortisone acetate 5 mg. For Anugesic-HC Cream, see above.
Anusol *(Warner-Lambert, UK). Ointment*, bismuth subgallate 2.25%, bismuth oxide 0.875%, Peru balsam 1.875%, zinc oxide 10.75%.
Suppositories, bismuth subgallate 59 mg, bismuth oxide 24 mg, Peru balsam 49 mg, zinc oxide 296 mg. For Anusol Cream, see above.
Anusol-HC *(Parke, Davis, UK). Ointment*, bismuth subgallate 2.25%, bismuth oxide 0.875%, Peru balsam 1.875%, zinc oxide 10.75%, hydrocortisone acetate 0.25%, benzyl benzoate 1.25%, resorcinol 0.875%.
Suppositories, bismuth subgallate 59 mg, bismuth oxide 24 mg, Peru balsam 49 mg, zinc oxide 296 mg, hydrocortisone acetate 10 mg, benzyl benzoate 33 mg, resorcinol 24 mg.
Bismodyne *(Loveridge, UK). Ointment*, bismuth subgallate 2%, hexachlorophane 0.5%, lignocaine 0.5%, zinc oxide 7.5%.
Suppositories, bismuth subgallate 150 mg, hexachlorophane 2.5 mg, lignocaine 10 mg, zinc oxide 120 mg.

Proprietary Names and Manufacturers
Dermatol *(Chinosolfabrik, Ger.)*.

The following names have been used for multi-ingredient preparations containing bismuth subgallate—Anugesic-HC *(Parke, Davis, UK)*; Anusol *(Warner-Lambert, UK; Parke, Davis, USA)*; Anusol HC *(Warner, Austral.)*; Anusol-HC *(Parke, Davis, UK; Parke, Davis, USA)*; Bismodyne *(Loveridge, UK)*; Hedal HC *(Arlo, USA)*; Nupercainal Suppositories *(Ciba-Geigy, Canad.; Ciba, USA)*.

5281-w

Bismuth Subnitrate *(USAN)*.

Basic Bismuth Nitrate; Basisches Wismutnitrat; Bism. Subnit.; Bismuth Hydroxide Nitrate Oxide; Bismuth (Nitrate Basique de) Lourd; Bismuth Oxynitrate; Bismuthi Subnitras; Bismuthyl Nitrate; Magistery of Bismuth; Nitrato de Bismutilo; Subazotato de Bismuto; White Bismuth.

CAS — 1304-85-4.

Pharmacopoeias. In *Arg., Aust., Cz., Fr., Hung., Int., Jpn, Jug., Mex., Pol., Port., Roum., Rus., Span., Turk.*, and *U.S.* Also in *B.P.C. 1973. Fr.* also includes Bismuth (Nitrate Basique de) Léger (Bismuthi Subnitras Levis) which is described as a variable mixture of bismuth hydroxide, carbonate, and subnitrate.

Bismuth Subnitrate *(U.S.P.)* contains not less than 79% of Bi_2O_3 calculated on the dried basis. It is a white slightly hygroscopic powder. Practically **insoluble** in water and in alcohol; readily soluble in nitric and hydrochloric acids. **Store** in well-closed containers.

Bismuth subnitrate has been used as an antacid; doses of 300 to 600 mg have been employed. It has been used in the form of Bismuth Subnitrate and Iodoform Paste (BIPP) as a wound dressing (see Iodoform p.1186).
There is a risk of the nitrate being reduced to nitrite with the development of methaemoglobinaemia.

Preparations
Bismuth Subnitrate and Iodoform Paste. BIPP. See under Iodoform, p.1186.
Milk of Bismuth *(U.S.P.)*. A mixture prepared from bismuth subnitrate 8 g, nitric acid 12mL ammonium carbonate 1 g, and water to 100 mL. Strong ammonia solution is used in the preparation. It contains bismuth hydroxide and bismuth subcarbonate in suspension. Store in airtight containers. Protect from freezing.

Proprietary Preparations
Roter *(Roterpharma, UK). Tablets*, bismuth subnitrate 300 mg, light magnesium carbonate 400 mg, sodium bicarbonate 200 mg, frangula bark 25 mg. NOTE. The name Roter is also applied to a preparation of ephedrine.

References: R. Sezer *et al., Br. J. clin. Pract.*, 1975, *29*, 227; D. Carr-Locke and A. B. Wicks, *ibid.*, 1986, *40*, 373.

Proprietary Names and Manufacturers
Bismufilm *(Liade, Spain)*.

The following names have been used for multi-ingredient preparations containing bismuth subnitrate—Caved-S *(Muir & Neil, Austral.)*; Pepsillide *(Cambridge Laboratories, Austral.)*; Pep-Uls-Ade *(Cambridge Laboratories, Austral.)*; Roter *(Four Macs, Austral.; Anglo-French Laboratories, Canad.; Roterpharma, UK)*.

12449-w

Black Nightshade

Morelle Noire.

The leaves and flowering tops of the black or garden nightshade, *Solanum nigrum* (Solanaceae). It contains solanine and its allied alkaloids.

Black nightshade is distributed throughout most of the world as a weed of cultivation. It appears to have little medicinal value but was used in liniments, poultices, and decoctions for external application. Ingestion can cause typical antimuscarinic effects that may require treatment as described under Atropine, p.523.

261-l

Borax *(BAN)*.

E241; Natrii Tetraboras; Natrium Boricum; Purified Borax; Sodium Biborate or Pyroborate; Sodium Borate *(USAN)*; Sodium Tetraborate.
$Na_2B_4O_7,10H_2O$=381.4.

CAS — 1330-43-4; 61028-24-8 (both anhydrous); 1303-96-4 (decahydrate).

Pharmacopoeias. In *Arg., Aust., Belg., Br., Braz., Chin., Cz., Egypt., Eur., Fr., Ger., Hung., Int., It., Jpn, Jug., Mex., Neth., Nord., Pol., Port., Rus., Span., Swiss*, and *Turk.* Also in *U.S.N.F.*

Odourless transparent colourless crystals, crystalline masses, or white crystalline powder. It effloresces in dry air.
Soluble 1 in 20 of water, 1 in less than 1 of boiling water and 1 in 1 of glycerol; practically insoluble in alcohol. A 4% solution in water has

a pH of 9.0 to 9.6.
For a warning on the supply of preparations of borax see under boric acid, below. **Store** in a cool place in airtight containers.

260-e

Boric Acid *(BAN, USAN).*

Acidum Boricum; Boracic Acid; Borsäure; E240; Orthoboric Acid; Sal Sedativa de Homberg.
H_3BO_3=61.83.

CAS — 10043-35-3.

Pharmacopoeias. In *Arg., Aust., Belg., Br., Chin., Cz., Egypt., Eur., Fr., Ger., Hung., Ind., It., Jpn, Jug., Mex., Neth., Nord., Pol., Port., Rus., Span., Swiss,* and *Turk.* Also in *U.S.N.F.* and *B.P. Vet.*

Odourless colourless brilliant plates, or white crystals, somewhat pearly lustrous scales, or white crystalline powder, unctuous to the touch. It volatilises in steam. When heated to 100° it loses water and is slowly converted into metaboric acid (HBO_2); tetraboric acid ($H_2B_4O_7$) is formed at 140° and boron trioxide (B_2O_3) at higher temperatures. **Soluble** 1 in 20 of water, 1 in 3.6 of boiling water, 1 in 16 of alcohol, and 1 in 4 of glycerol (85%). **Store** in well-closed containers.

CAUTION. *Pharmacists are advised not to sell boric acid as such for use as a dusting-powder. Dusting-powders containing more than 5% of boric acid should be labelled: 'not to be applied to raw or weeping surfaces'. Pharmacists are also advised not to supply Borax Glycerin or Honey of Borax, even with an appropriate warning, because of the hazards associated with the use of these preparations in infants.*

Adverse Effects and Treatment

The main symptoms of acute boric acid poisoning are vomiting and diarrhoea, an erythematous rash followed by desquamation, and stimulation of the central nervous system followed by depression. There may be convulsions and changes in body temperature. There may also be renal damage. Death, resulting from circulatory collapse and shock, may occur within 3 to 5 days.
The slow excretion of boric acid can lead to cumulative toxicity during repeated use. Symptoms of chronic intoxication include anorexia, debility, confusion, dermatitis, menstrual disorders, anaemia, convulsions, and alopecia.
Fatalities have occurred most frequently in young children after the accidental ingestion of solutions of boric acid or after the application of boric acid powder to abraded skin. The concentration of boric acid in talcs and products for oral hygiene is limited in the *UK* to 5 and 0.5% respectively and talcs must be labelled 'not to be used on children less than 3 years old'. In the *UK* the concentration of boric acid in other cosmetic products is limited to 3%. Topical preparations of boric acid should not be applied to extensive areas of abraded or damaged skin.
Deaths have resulted from absorption following lavage of body cavities with solutions of boric acid, and this practice is no longer recommended.
Inhaled boric acid and borax are pulmonary irritants. In Great Britain the recommended exposure limit of disodium tetraborate anhydrous and pentahydrate is 1 mg per m^3 (long-term) and for the decahydrate, 5 mg per m^3 (long-term).
Treatment of poisoning is symptomatic. Exchange transfusions, peritoneal dialysis, or haemodialysis may be of value.

References to estimates of fatal doses of boric acid and its salts: C. Potter, *J. Am. med. Ass.*, 1921, *76*, 378 (30 to 45 g of borax in an adult); W. D. McNally and C. A. Rust, *ibid.*, 1928, *90*, 382 (15 to 30 g of boric acid or borax in adults; 1 to 6 g in infants).

Skin manifestations in acute boric acid poisoning.— B. M. Schillinger *et al.*, *J. Am. Acad. Derm.*, 1982, *7*, 667.

A report of seizures in 7 infants induced by chronic boric acid ingestion. All the infants had regularly been given soothers dipped in a proprietary borax and honey mixture.— K. O'Sullivan and M. Taylor, *Archs Dis. Childh.*, 1983, *58*, 737.

Absorption and Fate

Boric acid is absorbed from the gastro-intestinal tract, from damaged skin, from wounds, and from mucous membranes. It does not readily penetrate intact skin. About 50% of the amount absorbed is excreted in the urine within 12 hours; the remainder is probably excreted over 3 to 7 days.

Uses and Administration

Boric acid possesses weak bacteriostatic and fungistatic properties; it has been superseded by more effective and less toxic disinfectants.
Boric acid is used, usually with borax, as a buffer and antimicrobial in eye-drops and was formerly used as a soluble lubricant in solution-tablets. Boric acid and borax are not used internally.
The use of boric acid in cosmetics and toiletries is restricted under the Cosmetic Products Regulations 1984 (SI 1984: No. 1260).
Borax (sodium borate, sodium biborate, sodium pyroborate, or sodium tetraborate) is used similarly to boric acid and has also been used externally as a mild astringent and as an emulsifier in creams. Borax Glycerin and Honey of Borax were formerly used as paints for the throat, tongue, and mouth, but should not be used due to the risk of toxicity.

For formulas of borate buffers from pH 6.77 to 10.8, see G. E. Schumacher, *Am. J. Hosp. Pharm.*, 1966, *23*, 628.

It was concluded by the cosmetic ingredient review expert panel of the Cosmetic Toiletry and Fragrance Association that sodium borate and boric acid in concentrations less than or equal to 5% are safe as cosmetic ingredients when used as recommended. However, cosmetic formulations containing free sodium borate or boric acid at this concentration should not be used on infant or injured skin.— Final Report on the Safety Assessment of Sodium Borate and Boric Acid, *J. Am. Coll. Toxicol.*, 1983, *2*, 87.

Antimicrobial activity of borate-buffered solutions.— R. D. Houlsby *et al.*, *Antimicrob. Ag. Chemother.*, 1986, *29*, 803.

TRACHOMA. A study involving 175 children with ocular trachoma treated with ophthalmic ointments of tetracycline 1%, erythromycin 0.5%, or boric acid 5% twice daily for 5 consecutive days each month for a total of 6 months showed that antibiotic therapy was only marginally more effective than boric acid and that this slight clinical difference was no longer apparent 6 months after the end of treatment.— C. R. Dawson *et al.*, *Bull. Wld Hlth Org.*, 1981, *59*, 91.

URINE PRESERVATION. Boric acid 1.8% equivalent to 500 mg of powdered boric acid per 28 mL bottle, was found to be a suitable preservative for urine samples in transit requiring bacteriological examination. A concentration of 1.8% prevented multiplication of micro-organisms present in urine, though with occasional strains of *Proteus* and *Klebsiella* boric acid appeared to cause a reduction in the number of organisms. By keeping the urine acid, boric acid prevented dissolution of pus cells.— I. A. Porter and J. Brodie, *Br. med. J.*, 1969, *2*, 353. Boric acid appeared to be useful for the preservation of urine specimens but more fundamental work was required before boric acid could be recommended for routine use.— H. H. Johnston *et al.*, in The Bacteriological Examination of Urine: Report of a Workshop on Needs and Methods, *Public Health Laboratory Service Monograph Series No. 10*, P.D. Meers (Ed.), London, HM Stationery Office, 1978.

Proprietary Names and Manufacturers of Boric Acid or Borax

Boroformol *(Ingram & Bell, Canad.)*; Borsyre viskos *(DAK, Denm.)*; Komex *(Barnes-Hind, Canad.)*.

The following names have been used for multi-ingredient preparations containing boric acid or borax—Anusol HC *(Warner, Austral.)*; Egosol-BS *(Ego, Austral.)*; Normol *(Alcon, Austral.)*; Perborate *(Squibb, Canad.)*; Phytex *(Pharmax, UK)*.

18860-d

Botulinum A Toxin

A neurotoxin produced by *Clostridium botulinum*. It causes irreversible neuromuscular blockade and injection into a muscle results in flaccid paralysis the extent and duration of which is dependent on the dose. Botulinum A toxin has been given by local injection in the treatment of disorders of ocular muscle including blepharospasm and strabismus. It has also been tried in various neuromuscular disorders of the head and neck.

Brief reviews of botulinum A toxin for the treatment of ocular muscle disorders: *Lancet*, 1986, *1*, 76; J. S. Elston (letter), *ibid.*, 265; J. G. Spector and R. M. Burde (letter), *ibid.*, 855; *Med. Lett.*, 1987, *29*, 101.

Use in the treatment of blepharospasm: J. S. Elston and R. W. R. Russell, *Br. med. J.*, 1985, *290*, 1857; J. S. Elston, *Br. J. Ophthal.*, 1987, *71*, 664.

Use in the treatment of strabismus: J. S. Elston *et al.*, *Br. J. Ophthal.*, 1985, *69*, 718; J. S. Elston and J. P. Lee, *ibid.*, 891.

Use in the treatment of spasmodic torticollis: J. K. Tsui *et al.*, *Lancet*, 1986, *2*, 245.

Use in treatment of anismus in intractable constipation.— R. I. Hallan *et al.*, *Lancet*, 1988, *2*, 714.

3380-x

Bovine Surfactant

'Surfactant TA'.

Bovine surfactant has been investigated in the treatment of hyaline membrane disease.

References: T. N. K. Raju *et al.*, *Lancet*, 1987, *1*, 651; C. Morley (letter), *ibid.*, 1040; S. M. Gore (letter), *ibid;* T. N. Raju *et al.* (letter), *ibid.*, 1041; B. Lachmann (letter), *ibid.*, 1375.

Proprietary Names and Manufacturers

Tanabe, Jpn.

12451-b

Bradykinin

BRS-640; Kallidin-9.
$C_{50}H_{73}N_{15}O_{11}$=1060.2.

CAS — 58-82-2.

Bradykinin is a potent vasoactive nonapeptide. Physiologically, it is formed by the action of proteolytic enzymes (kallikreins) on a plasma globulin (kininogen). It is rapidly inactivated by peptidases. Its main pharmacological effects are smooth muscle stimulation, vasodilatation, increase in capillary permeability, production of oedema, and production of pain.

The pharmacology of bradykinin and related polypeptides.— H. P. J. Bennett and C. McMartin, *Pharmac. Rev.*, 1978, *30*, 247; D. Regoli and J. Barabe, *ibid.*, 1980, *32*, 1; H. S. Margolius, *Ann. Rev. Physiol.*, 1984, *46*, 309.

A study reporting the presence of kinins in nasal secretions following immunological challenge in allergic volunteers. Kinins may contribute to the symptomatology of the allergic reaction.— D. Proud *et al.*, *J. clin. Invest.*, 1983, *72*, 1678.

1739-t

Brequinar *(pINN).*

DuP-785; NSC-368390. 6-Fluoro-2-(2′-fluoro-4-biphenylyl)-3-methyl-4-quinolinecarboxylic acid.
$C_{23}H_{15}F_2NO_2$=375.4.

CAS — 96187-53-0.

An antineoplastic agent under investigation.

18866-g

BRL-26830A

BRL-26830.

$C_{19}H_{23}NO_3.0.5C_4H_4O_4$=909.8.

CAS — 87857-42-9.

BRL-26830A is a beta-adrenoceptor agonist under investigation for its hypoglycaemic and anti-obesity activity.

Proprietary Names and Manufacturers
Beecham Research, UK.

12452-v

Brocresine *(BAN, USAN, rINN).*

CL-54998; NSD-1055. α-Amino-oxy-6-bromo-*m*-cresol.

$C_7H_8BrNO_2$=218.1.

CAS — 555-65-7.

Brocresine is claimed to be a histidine decarboxylase inhibitor. It has been tried in pruritus, chronic urticaria, and parkinsonism.

References: *J. Am. med. Ass.*, 1968, *205* (Aug. 26), A27 (pruritus); M. W. Greaves, *Br. J. Derm.*, 1971, *85*, 467 (urticaria); P. M. Howse and W. B. Matthews, *J. Neurol. Neurosurg. Psychiat.*, 1973, *36*, 27 (parkinsonism).

1022-v

Bromine

Bromum.

Br_2=159.8.

CAS — 7726-95-6.

A dark reddish-brown, heavy, mobile liquid which gives off intensely irritating brown fumes.

Adverse Effects

Bromine is intensely irritating and corrosive to mucous membranes and, even in dilute solution, may cause fatal gastro-enteritis if swallowed. Contact with the skin can produce severe burns and inhalation of the vapour causes violent irritation of the respiratory tract and pulmonary oedema. In Great Britain the recommended exposure limits of bromine are 0.1 ppm (long-term); 0.3 ppm (short-term).

Treatment of Adverse Effects

Milk, white of egg, and starch mucilage, taken as soon as possible, have been recommended. If bromine vapour has been inhaled, give assisted respiration, if necessary, and oxygen. Splashes on the skin and eyes should be immediately washed off; washing under running water should continue for at least 15 minutes.

Uses and Administration

Bromine is used, in the form of an adduct with a quaternary ammonium compound in the treatment of plantar warts.

Proprietary Preparations

Callusolve *(Dermal Laboratories, UK). Paint*, benzalkonium chloride-bromine adduct 25%. For warts, particularly plantar and mosaic warts.

12460-v

Bryonia

The root of *Bryonia alba* (Cucurbitaceae).

Bryonia is used in homoeopathic medicine.

12461-g

Buchu

Bucco; Buchu Leaves; Diosma; Folia Bucco.

CAS — 68650-46-4 (buchu oil).

Pharmacopoeias. In *Egypt* and *Fr.*

The dried leaves of 'short' or 'round' buchu, *Agathosma betulina* (=*Barosma betulina*) (Rutaceae).

Buchu is a weak diuretic and urinary antiseptic and was formerly administered as an infusion in mixtures for urinary-tract infections.

5012-l

Bufotenine

5-Hydroxy-*NN*-dimethyltryptamine; *NN*-Dimethylserotonin; Mappine. 3-(2-Dimethylaminoethyl)indol-5-ol.

$C_{12}H_{16}N_2O$=204.3.

CAS — 487-93-4.

An indole alkaloid obtained from the seeds and leaves of *Piptadenia peregrina* from which the hallucinogenic snuff, cohoba is prepared, and *P. macrocarpa* (Mimosaceae). It was first isolated from the skin glands of toads (*Bufo* spp.) and has also been isolated from species of *Amanita* (Agaricaceae).

Bufotenine has serotonergic activity and is reported to have hallucinogenic properties. It has no therapeutic use.

Cohoba Snuff. A hallucinogenic snuff prepared from the seeds and leaves of *Piptadenia peregrina*. The plant has been found to contain bufotenine, dimethyltryptamine, *N*-methyltryptamine, and 5-methoxy-*NN*-dimethyltryptamine.— A. Hofmann, *Indian J. Pharm.*, 1963, *25*, 245. See also *Pharm. J.*, 1957, *2*, 420.

12473-w

Butaverine Hydrochloride *(rINNM).*

Butyl 3-phenyl-3-piperidinopropionate hydrochloride.

$C_{18}H_{27}NO_2,HCl$=325.9.

CAS — 55837-14-4 (butaverine).

Butaverine hydrochloride has been used as an antispasmodic.

Proprietary Names and Manufacturers
Espasmo Gemora *(Prodes, Spain).*

12474-e

Butazopyridine

2,6-Diamino-6′-butoxy-3,3′-azopyridine.

$C_{14}H_{18}N_6O$=286.3.

Butazopyridine has been used in the treatment of biliary and urinary disorders.

Proprietary Names and Manufacturers
Neotropina *(Schering, Ital.).*

12478-z

Butixirate *(USAN, rINN).*

MG-5771. The *trans*-4-phenylcyclohexylamine salt of 2-(biphenyl-4-yl)butyric acid.

$C_{16}H_{16}O_2,C_{12}H_{17}N$=415.6.

CAS — 19992-80-4.

Butixirate has been applied topically in a variety of inflammatory and oedematous disorders.

Proprietary Names and Manufacturers
Flectar *(Maggioni-Winthrop, Ital.).*

12483-l

Butyl Nitrite

$C_4H_9NO_2$=103.1.

Butyl nitrite is not used medicinally but is inhaled for its vasodilating and related effects. The association of this use with Kaposi's sarcoma is a subject of debate, see amyl nitrite (p.1493).

19217-b

BW-12C

5-(2-Formyl-3-hydroxyphenoxy)pentaenoic acid.

An anti-sickling drug under investigation for the treatment of sickle-cell disease.

References: P. Fitzharris *et al.*, *Br. J. clin. Pharmac.*, 1985, *19*, 471; A. J. Keidan *et al.*, *Lancet*, 1986, *1*, 831.

Proprietary Names and Manufacturers
Wellcome, UK.

1596-x

Cadmium

Cd=112.41.

CAS — 7440-43-9.

Cadmium is employed in a wide range of manufacturing processes and cadmium poisoning presents a recognised industrial hazard. Inhalation of cadmium fume during welding procedures may not produce symptoms until 4 to 10 hours have passed and these symptoms include respiratory distress leading to pulmonary oedema; kidney toxicity is also a feature of cadmium poisoning. Ingestion of cadmium or its salts has the additional hazard of severe gastro-intestinal effects.

In Great Britain the control exposure limit of cadmium and cadmium compounds (as Cd) is 0.05 mg per m^3 (long term). The control exposure limit for cadmium oxide fume (as Cd) is 0.05 mg per m^3 (long-term and short-term). The recommended exposure limits for cadmium sulphide pigments (as Cd) are 0.05 mg per m^3 (long-term); 0.2 mg per m^3 (short-term). In the *US* the permissible exposure limit for cadmium dust is 0.2 mg per m^3.

Cadmium sulphide has been used topically in some countries for the treatment of some skin conditions.

Some reviews on the toxicity of cadmium and its intake from occupational exposure or from foods.— Report of a WHO Study Group on Recommended Health-Based Limits in Occupational Exposure to Heavy Metals, *Tech. Rep. Ser. Wld Hlth Org. No. 647*, 1980; Cadmium and its Compounds, *Toxicity Review 7*, Health and Safety Executive, London, HM Stationery Office, 1983; Survey of Cadmium in Food, *First Supplementary Report, Food Surveillance Paper No.12, Minist. Agric. Fish. Fd*, London, HM Stationery Office, 1983; H. G. Gorchev and C. F. Jelinek, *Bull. Wld Hlth Org.*, 1985, *63*, 945.

Some recent reports of cadmium fatalities: A. Taylor *et al.*, *Br. med. J.*, 1984, *288*, 1270 (Smelting); H. M. Buckler *et al.*, *ibid.*, 1986, *292*, 1559 (self-poisoning by ingestion of cadmium chloride).

MALIGNANT NEOPLASMS. An increased incidence of cancer of the prostate has been reported (M.D. Kipling and J.A.H. Waterhouse, *Lancet*, 1967, *1*, 730), but has not been confirmed (B.G. Armstrong and G. Kazantzis, *ibid.*, 1983, *1*, 1425; T. Sorahan and J.A.H. Waterhouse, *ibid.*, 1985, *1*, 459). A view has been expressed that there may be an association between cadmium exposure and lung cancer (*Lancet*, 1986, *2*, 931), although as already observed by Armstrong and Kazantzis (1983) when commenting on an increased incidence of lung cancer in a low-exposure group, observations on this type of cancer are difficult to interpret because of exposure to other hazards such as smoking.

Proprietary Names and Manufacturers of Cadmium Salts
Biocadmio *(Uriach, Spain)*; Buginol *(GEA, Denm.).*

15308-r

Cafaminol *(rINN).*

7-Methyl-8-(2-hydroxy-*N*-methylethylamino)theophylline.

$C_{11}H_{17}N_5O_3$=267.3.

CAS — 30924-31-3.

Cafaminol has been used by mouth to relieve nasal congestion.

Proprietary Names and Manufacturers
Rhinoptil *(Promonta, Ger.).*

12500-x

Cafedrine Hydrochloride *(BANM, pINNM).*

H-8351; Kafedrin Hydrochloride. 7-[2-(β-Hydroxy-α-methylphenethylamino)ethyl]theophylline hydrochloride.

$C_{18}H_{23}N_5O_3$,HCl=393.9.

CAS — 58166-83-9 (cafedrine).

Cafedrine hydrochloride is a theophylline derivative which has been used in the treatment of hypotension.

Proprietary Names and Manufacturers
Akrinor *(Farmades, Ital.).*

525-x

Calamus

Acore Vrai; Calamus Rhizome; Kalmus; Sweet Flag Root.

CAS — 8015-79-0 (calamus oil).

Pharmacopoeias. In *Aust., Hung., Jug., Pol., Rus.,* and *Swiss.*
Pol. also includes the volatile oil.

The dried rhizome of the sweet flag, *Acorus calamus* (Araceae).

Calamus has been used as a bitter and carminative. In the *U.S.* the FDA has prohibited marketing calamus as a food or food additive; the oil (Jammu variety) is reported to be a carcinogen.

12504-n

Calcium Bromolactobionate

Calcium bromide lactobionate hexahydrate.

$Ca(C_{12}H_{21}O_{12})_2,CaBr_2,6H_2O$=1062.6.

CAS — 33659-28-8 (anhydrous).

Calcium bromolactobionate has sedative properties. The use of bromides is generally deprecated.

Proprietary Names and Manufacturers
Calcibromin *(Astra, Arg.)*; Calcibronat *(Sandoz, Arg.; Sandoz-Wander, Belg.; Sandoz, Fr.; Sandoz, Ger.; Sandoz, Ital.; Sandoz, Spain; Sandoz, Switz.).*

12506-m

Calcium Dobesilate *(rINN).*

205E; Calcii Dobesilas; Calcium Doxybenzylate. Calcium 2,5-dihydroxybenzenesulphonate.

$C_{12}H_{10}CaO_{10}S_2$=418.4.

CAS — 88-46-0 (dobesilic acid); 20123-80-2 (calcium salt).

Calcium dobesilate is claimed to reduce capillary permeability and has been used in diabetic retinopathy and other vascular disorders. Gastro-intestinal disturbances have occurred occasionally.

The metabolism and pharmacokinetics of calcium dobesilate in man.— A. Benakis *et al., Thérapie,* 1974, *29,* 211.

In a double-blind study, calcium dobesilate had a very slight inhibitory effect on the deterioration of diabetic retinopathy.— P. G. Binkhorst and O. P. Van Bijsterveld, *Curr. ther. Res.,* 1976, *20,* 283.

Proprietary Names and Manufacturers
Dexium *(Delalande, Ger.)*; Dobesifar *(Farmila, Ital.)*; Doxium *(Alcon, Arg.; Delalande, Belg.; Carrion, Fr.; Biogal, Hung.; Delalande, Ital.; Johnson & Johnson, S.Afr.; Esteve, Spain; Om, Switz.).*

12507-b

Calcium Fluoride

CaF_2=78.07.

CAS — 7789-75-5.

Pharmacopoeias. In *Fr.*

Calcium fluoride is used similarly to sodium fluoride for the prevention of dental caries.
Native calcium fluoride (Calcarea Fluorica; Calc. Fluor) is used in homoeopathic medicine.

12509-g

Calcium Hopantenate *(rINNM).*

Calcium Homopantothenate. The hemihydrate of the calcium salt of D(+)-4-(2,4-dihydroxy-3,3-dimethylbutyramido)butyric acid.

$Ca(C_{10}H_{18}NO_5)_2,½H_2O$=513.6.

CAS — 17097-76-6 (anhydrous); 18679-90-8 (hopantenic acid).

Calcium hopantenate is a homologue of pantothenic acid (p.1270) and has been tried in the treatment of various behavioural and extrapyramidal disorders.

Proprietary Names and Manufacturers
Hopate *(Tanabe, Jpn).*

204-m

Calcium Hydroxide *(BAN, USAN).*

526; Calcium Hydrate; Slaked Lime.

$Ca(OH)_2$=74.09.

CAS — 1305-62-0.

Pharmacopoeias. In *Br., Egypt., Ind., It., Jpn, Mex., Nord.,* and *U.S.*

A soft white powder with a slightly bitter alkaline taste.
B.P. **solubilities** are: almost entirely soluble 1 in 600 of water; soluble in aqueous solutions of glycerol and of sugars. *U.S.P.* solubilities are: soluble 1 in 630 of water, and 1 in 1300 of boiling water; soluble in glycerol and in syrup; insoluble in alcohol. A solution in water is alkaline to phenolphthalein and readily absorbs carbon dioxide.
Store in airtight containers.
Calcium hydroxide is a weak alkali. It is used in the form of Calcium Hydroxide Solution (lime water) in some skin lotions and oily preparations to form calcium soaps of fatty acids which produce water-in-oil emulsions.
Calcium hydroxide pastes are used in dentistry.
A paste made from a mixture of calcium hydroxide and potassium hydroxide and known as Vienna paste was used as an escharotic. (Soda lime is a mixture of calcium hydroxide and potassium hydroxide and or sodium hydroxide).
In Great Britain the recommended exposure limit of calcium hydroxide is 5 mg per m³ (long-term).

A review of the use of calcium hydroxide in root canal therapy.— D. M. Martin and H. S. M. Crabb, *Br. dent. J.,* 1977, *142,* 277.

Preparations

Calcium Hydroxide Solution *(B.P., A.P.F.).* Liquor Calcii Hydroxidi; Lime Water; Liquor Calcis; Aqua Calcariae; Eau de Chaux; Kalkwasser. A clear colourless liquid containing not less than 0.15% of $Ca(OH)_2$. It absorbs carbon dioxide from the air, a film of calcium carbonate forming on the surface. Store in well-filled, well-closed containers.

Calcium Hydroxide Topical Solution *(U.S.P.).* A solution containing, in each 100 mL, not less than 140 mg of $Ca(OH)_2$. Store in well-filled airtight containers.

12510-f

Calcium Oxide

529; Calcium Oxydatum; Calx; Calx Usta; Chaux Vive; Gebrannter Kalk; Lime *(USAN)*; Quicklime.

CaO=56.08.

CAS — 1305-78-8.

Pharmacopoeias. In *Arg., Belg., Hung., Jpn, Jug., Nord., Pol., Port., Span., Swiss,* and *U.S.*

Hard, odourless, white or greyish-white masses, granules, or powder. When it is moistened with water a reaction occurs, heat being evolved and calcium hydroxide formed. Slightly **soluble** in water, very slightly soluble in boiling water. **Store** in airtight containers.

Adverse Effects and Treatment
Calcium oxide may cause burns on contact with moist skin and mucous membranes; it is particularly irritant to the eyes. Washing or flooding of affected areas may need to be prolonged. Pneumonitis may follow inhalation.
In Great Britain the recommended exposure limit of calcium oxide is 2 mg per m³ (long-term).

Uses and Administration
Calcium oxide has been used in various dermatological preparations. With sulphur it forms sulphurated lime (p.933). A paste made from a mixture of calcium oxide and sodium hydroxide and known as London paste was used as an escharotic.

For the use of disodium edetate in treatment of lime burns of the eye, see p.841.

1163-a

Calcium Saccharate *(USAN, rINN).*

Calcii Saccharas; Calcium D-Saccharate. Calcium D-glucarate tetrahydrate.

$C_6H_8CaO_8,4H_2O$=320.3.

CAS — 5793-88-4 (anhydrous); 5793-89-5 (tetrahydrate).

Pharmacopoeias. In *Int., Nord., Turk.,* and *U.S.* which specifies the tetrahydrate.

A white, odourless, crystalline powder. Each g represents approximately 3.1 mmol of calcium. Calcium saccharate 8 g is approximately equivalent to 1 g of calcium.
Very slightly **soluble** in cold water; slightly soluble in boiling water; very slightly soluble in alcohol; practically insoluble in chloroform and ether; soluble in dilute mineral acids and in solutions of calcium gluconate. **Store** in well-closed containers.

Calcium saccharate is employed as a stabilising agent in solutions of calcium gluconate for injection.

12512-n

Calcium Sucrose Phosphate

A mixture having the approximate empirical formula of the calcium salt of a monophosphate ester of sucrose.

$C_{12}H_{21}CaO_{14}P,2H_2O$=496.4.

CAS — 12676-30-1; 25584-76-3 (both anhydrous).

Calcium sucrose phosphate has been used in the prevention of dental caries.

12513-h

Calcium Sulfexanoate

The calcium salt of 2,2′-dithiodi(hexanoic acid).

$C_{12}H_{20}CaO_4S_2$=332.5.

CAS — 22414-93-3.

Calcium sulfexanoate has been used in the treatment of hepatic disorders.

Proprietary Names and Manufacturers
Lepexal *(Berna, Ital.)*; Lipexal *(Berna, Spain)*.

1165-x

Calcium Sulphate

516; Calcium Sulfate *(USAN)*; Gypsum *(dihydrate)*.
$CaSO_4$=136.1.

CAS — 7778-18-9 (anhydrous); 10101-41-4 (dihydrate).

Pharmacopoeias. In *U.S.N.F.* which specifies the dihydrate or the anhydrous material. Also in *Fr.* and *Jpn* which specify the dihydrate.

A white to yellowish-white odourless fine powder. **Soluble** 1 in 375 of water and 1 in 485 of boiling water.

Calcium sulphate is used as an excipient for the preparation of tablets or capsules. In Great Britain the recommended exposure limits of calcium sulphate are 10 mg per m^3 (long-term) for total dust; 5 mg per m^3 (long-term) for respirable dust.

1166-r

Dried Calcium Sulphate

Calcii Sulfas Hemihydricus; Calcined Gypsum; Calcium Sulfuricum ad Usum Chirurgicum; Calcium Sulphuricum Ustum; Exsiccated Calcium Sulphate; Gebrannter Gips; Gêsso; Gypsum Siccatum; Plâtre Cuit; Plaster of Paris; Sulphate of Lime; Yeso Blanco.
$CaSO_4,\frac{1}{2}H_2O$=145.1.

CAS — 7778-18-9 (anhydrous); 10034-76-1; 26499-65-0 (both hemihydrate).

Pharmacopoeias. In *Arg., Aust., Br., Cz., Ger., Hung., Ind., Jpn, Jug., Mex., Pol., Port., Span.,* and *Swiss.*

A white or almost white, odourless or almost odourless hygroscopic powder. The *B.P.* permits the presence of suitable setting accelerators or decelerators. Slightly **soluble** in water; more soluble in dilute mineral acids; practically insoluble in alcohol. **Store** in well-closed containers.

Dried calcium sulphate is used for the preparation of Plaster of Paris Bandage which is used for the immobilisation of limbs and fractures. It is also employed for making dental casts. In Great Britain the recommended exposure limits of dried calcium sulphate are 10 mg per m^3 (long-term) for total dust; 5 mg per m^3 (long-term) for respirable dust.

An account of an outbreak of plaster-associated pseudomonas infection. Since the outbreak, plaster casts have been made up with sterile water in an autoclaved stainless-steel bowl, and no further plaster-related wound infections had been observed.— E. T. Houang *et al.* (letter), *Lancet*, 1981, *1*, 728. See also E. G. Dowsett (letter), *ibid.*, 954.

Preparations
Plaster of Paris Bandage *(B.P.)*. P.O.P. Bandage

Proprietary Names and Manufacturers
Cellona *(Athrodax, UK)*; Gypsona *(Smith & Nephew, UK)*; Orthoflex *(Johnson & Johnson Orthopaedic, UK)*.

1167-f

Calcium Tetrahydrogen Phosphate

Acid Calcium Phosphate; Calcium Dihydrogenphosphoricum; E341; Monobasic Calcium Phosphate; Monocalcium Phosphate. Calcium tetrahydrogen diorthophosphate monohydrate.
$CaH_4(PO_4)_2,H_2O$=252.1.

CAS — 7758-23-8 (anhydrous).

Pharmacopoeias. In *Arg., Belg., Jpn,* and *Span.* In *Port.* with $2H_2O$.

Calcium tetrahydrogen phosphate is used in fertilisers. It is also used as an antoxidant in baking powders and flours.

526-r

Calumba

Calumba Root; Colombo.

Pharmacopoeias. In *Jpn, Port.,* and *Span.*

The dried root of *Jateorhiza palmata* (=*J. columba*) (Menispermaceae).

Calumba has been used as a bitter and as a flavouring agent.

3922-e

Camostat Mesylate

Camostat Mesilate *(pINNM)*; FOY-305. *N,N*-Dimethylcarbamoylmethyl 4-(4-guanidinobenzoyloxy)phenylacetate mesylate.
$C_{20}H_{22}N_4O_5,CH_4O_3S$=494.5.

CAS — 59721-29-8; 59721-28-7 (camostat).

Camostat is an enzyme inhibitor under investigation in the treatment of pancreatitis.

Proprietary Names and Manufacturers
Ono, Jpn.

263-j

Camphor *(BAN, USAN).*

2-Camphanone; Alcanfor; Cânfora; Camph.; Camphora; Camphre Droit (natural); Camphre du Japon (natural); Kamfer. Bornan-2-one; 1,7,7-Trimethylbicyclo[2.2.1]heptan-2-one.
$C_{10}H_{16}O$=152.2.

CAS — 76-22-2; 464-49-3 (+); 464-48-2 (−); 21368-68-3 (±).

Pharmacopoeias. In *Arg., Aust., Belg., Br., Braz., Chin., Cz., Egypt., Fr., Ger., Hung., Int., It., Jpn, Jug., Mex., Nord., Pol., Port., Roum., Rus., Span., Swiss, Turk.,* and *U.S.*; some only describe natural camphor and some only synthetic camphor; *Aust., Belg.,* and *Jpn* have separate monographs for natural and synthetic camphor.

Camphor is a ketone obtained from *Cinnamomum camphora* (Lauraceae) and purified by sublimation, or it may be prepared synthetically. The natural product is dextrorotatory and the synthetic product is optically inactive.

Colourless transparent or white crystals, crystalline masses, blocks, or powdery masses known as 'flowers of camphor', with a penetrating characteristic aromatic odour.

Soluble 1 in 800 of water, 1 in 1 of alcohol, and 1 in 1 of ether; the *B.P.* specifies 1 in 0.25 and the *U.S.P.* specifies 1 in 0.5 of chloroform; freely soluble in fixed and volatile oils. **Store** at a temperature not exceeding 25° in airtight containers.

A liquid or soft mass is formed when camphor is triturated with chloral hydrate, menthol, phenol, and many other substances. Camphor is readily powdered by triturating with a few drops of alcohol, ether, or chloroform. It slowly volatilises at ordinary temperatures.

Adverse Effects
Poisoning usually occurs from administration of camphorated oil (camphor liniment) to children in mistake for castor oil. The symptoms include nausea, vomiting, colic, headache, dizziness, a feeling of warmth, delirium, muscle twitching, epileptiform convulsions, depression of the central nervous system, and coma. Breathing is difficult and the breath has a characteristic odour; anuria may occur. Death from respiratory failure is rare though fatalities in children have been recorded from 1 g. There have been reports of instant collapse in infants following the local application of camphor to their nostrils.

In Great Britain the recommended exposure limits of synthetic camphor are 2 ppm (long-term) and 3 ppm (short-term).

Treatment of Adverse Effects
Empty the stomach by gastric lavage and aspiration. Administer a saline laxative by mouth, such as sodium sulphate, 30 g in 250 mL of water or a dilute solution of sodium phosphate. Convulsions may be controlled by the slow intravenous administration of diazepam 5 to 10 mg or, if necessary, a short-acting barbiturate such as thiopentone sodium. Haemodialysis with a lipid dialysate has been employed; the use of haemoperfusion however has been criticised.

Precautions
It is dangerous to place camphor, for instance as an ointment, into the nostrils of an infant. A small quantity applied in this way may cause immediate collapse.

Absorption and Fate
Camphor is readily absorbed from all administration sites. It is hydroxylated in the liver to yield hydroxycamphor metabolites which are then conjugated with glucuronic acid and excreted in the urine. Camphor crosses the placenta.

Uses and Administration
Applied externally, camphor acts as a rubefacient and mild analgesic and is employed in liniments as a counter-irritant in fibrositis, neuralgia, and similar conditions. The use of camphor liniment (camphorated oil) is discouraged because of its potential toxicity. It has now been withdrawn from the market in both the *UK* and the *US*.

Taken internally camphor has irritant and carminative properties and has been used as a mild expectorant and to relieve griping. Camphor was formerly administered as a solution in oil by subcutaneous or intramuscular injection as a circulatory and respiratory stimulant, however parenteral administration of camphor is particularly hazardous.

Camphor-related monoterpene compounds have been used in the treatment of urolithiasis, renal disorders, and urinary-tract infections, and also with menthol in combination with chenodeoxycholic acid as adjunct therapy for the dispersal of bile duct stones.

It has been recommended by the Committee on the Review of Medicines that camphor should not be included in products intended for the treatment of hepatic and biliary disorders, gall stones, colic, renal disorders, urinary tract infections, or ureteral stones.— *Pharm. J.*, 1984, *1*, 792.

Preparations
Camphor Linctus Compound *(A.P.F.)*. Camphor spirit compound 1 mL, glycerol 1.5 mL, tolu syrup to 5 mL.

Camphor Liniment *(B.P. 1973)*. Camph. Lin.; Camphorated Oil. Camphor 20% w/w in arachis oil.

Camphor Spirit *(U.S.P.)*. Contains camphor 10 g, alcohol to 100 mL.

Camphor Spirit Compound *(A.P.F.)*. Camphor 300 mg, benzoic acid 500 mg, anise oil 0.3 mL, alcohol (60%) to 100 mL.

Concentrated Camphor Water *(B.P.)*. Camphor 4 g, alcohol (90%) 60 mL, water to 100 mL.

Proprietary Preparations
Baby Chest Rub *(Cupal, UK)*. Camphor 5%, turpentine oil 5%, menthol 2%, eucalyptus oil 2%, cedar wood oil 0.5%, nutmeg oil 0.1%, thyme oil 0.1%.

Boots Vapour Rub *(Boots, UK)*. Camphor 6%, turpentine oil 4%, eucalyptus oil 1.5%, menthol 1%, thymol 0.1%, pumilio pine oil 0.4%.

George's Vapour Rub *(Thomas, UK)*. Camphor 6%, menthol 3%, eucalyptus oil 3%, oil of rosemary 1%, oil of nutmeg 0.5% , oil of thyme 0.5%, turpentine oil 7%, methyl salicylate 2%.

Mentholatum Nasal Inhaler *(Mentholatum, UK)*. Camphor 270 mg, menthol 270 mg, methyl salicylate 74 mg, eucalyptus oil 34 mg, pumilio pine oil 27 mg.

Mentholatum Vapour Rub *(Mentholatum, UK)*. Camphor 10%, menthol 1.66%, eucalyptus oil 0.66%, pumilio pine oil 0.66%, methyl salicylate 0.66%.

Pernomol *(Laboratories for Applied Biology, UK)*. *Paint*, camphor 10%, chlorbutol 2%, phenol 0.95%, tannic acid 2.2%, spirit soap 34%. For chilblains.

Snufflebabe *(Pickles, UK)*. Camphor 3.5%, menthol 1.5%, pine oil 0.5%, cedar oil 0.25%, thyme oil 0.5%, cajuput oil 1%.

Vapex Inhalant *(Kerfoot, UK)*. Menthol 18.0%, linalyl acetate 0.65%, eucalyptus oil 4.80%, lavender oil 4.40%, bornyl acetate 0.40%, essential oil of camphor 1.40%, alcohol (72%) 70.00%.

Vicks Inhaler *(Richardson-Vicks, UK)*. Menthol 125 mg, camphor 50 mg, methyl salicylate 5 mg, oil of pine needles 10 mg.

Vicks VapoRub *(Richardson-Vicks, UK)*. Camphor 5.25%, menthol 2.82%, turpentine oil 4.77%, eucalyptus oil 1.35%, nutmeg oil 0.48%, cedar wood oil 0.45%, thymol 0.1%, white soft paraffin to 100%.

Proprietary Names and Manufacturers

Camphor is an ingredient of many cough and cold remedies.

Proprietary Preparations Containing Related Substances

Rowachol *(Tillotts, UK)*. *Capsules*, enteric-coated, menthol 32 mg, menthone ($C_{10}H_{18}O$ = 154.3) 6 mg, pinene ($C_{10}H_{16}$ = 136.2) 17 mg, borneol ($C_{10}H_{18}O$ = 154.3) 5 mg, camphene ($C_{10}H_{16}$ = 136.2) 5 mg, cineole 2 mg in olive oil. *Liquid*, borneol 50 mg, camphene 50 mg, cineole 20 mg, menthol 320 mg, menthone 60 mg, pinene 170 mg/g in olive oil.

An adjunct for the dispersal of gall-stones.

Rowatinex *(Tillotts, UK)*. *Liquid*, pinene 31%, camphene 15%, borneol 10%, anethole 4%, fenchone 4%, and cineole 3%, in olive oil.

Capsules, enteric-coated, each containing 0.1 mL of Rowatinex liquid.

For the treatment of urinary stones.

12514-m

Camphoscapine

Noscapine Camsylate, Noscapine camphor-10-sulphonate.

$C_{22}H_{23}NO_7,C_{10}H_{16}O_4S$=645.7.

CAS — 25333-79-3.

Camphoscapine is used for the relief of cough.

Proprietary Names and Manufacturers

Tulisan *(Logeais, Fr.)*.

The following names have been used for multi-ingredient preparations containing camphoscapine—Broncho-Tulisan Eucalyptol *(Logeais, Fr.)*; Gripposan *(Midyfarm, Fr.)*.

5230-f

Camylofin Hydrochloride *(rINNM)*.

Acamylophenine Hydrochloride; Camylofin Dihydrochloride. Isopentyl 2-(2-diethylaminoethylamino)-2-phenylacetate dihydrochloride.

$C_{19}H_{32}N_2O_2$,2HCl=393.4.

CAS — 54-30-8 (camylofin); 5892-41-1 (hydrochloride).

Camylofin hydrochloride is used as an antispasmodic in doses of 50 to 100 mg two to three times daily. It is also used as camylofin bis(noramidopyrine mesylate).

Proprietary Names and Manufacturers

Avacan *(Asta, Denm.; Asta, Ger.; Schering, Ital.; Asta, Neth.; Noristan, S.Afr.)*.

842-w

Cannabis

Cáñamo Indiano; Cannab.; Cannabis Indica; Chanvre; Ganja; Guaza; Hanfkraut; Indian Hemp.

CAS — 8063-14-7.

Pharmacopoeias. In *Chin.*, *Port.*, and *Span.*

The dried flowering or fruiting tops of the pistillate plant of *Cannabis sativa* (Cannabinaceae). In the *UK* cannabis is defined by law as any part of any plant of the genus *Cannabis*. *Marihuana* usually refers to a mixture of the leaves and flowering tops. *Bhang, dagga, ganja, kif,* and *maconha* are commonly used in various countries to describe similar preparations. *Hashish* and *charas* are names often applied to the resin, although in some countries *hashish* is applied to any cannabis preparation.

A series of cannabinoids has been extracted from the drug, the most important being Δ^9-tetrahydrocannabinol (dronabinol), Δ^8-tetrahydrocannabinol, Δ^9-tetrahydrocannabinolic acid, cannabinol, and cannabidiol. Cannabinol and cannabidiol may be present in large amounts but have little activity. The amount of Δ^9-tetrahydrocannabinol may average 1, 3, and 5% in marihuana, ganja, and hashish respectively.

Synonyms and approximate synonyms for cannabis included: Ait makhlif, Aliamba, Anassa, Anhascha, Assyuni, Bambalacha, Bambia, Bangi-Aku, Bango, Bangue, Bhang, Bhangaku, Canapa, Cangonha, Canhama, Cannacoro, Can-Yac, Caroçuda, Chur ganja, Chutras, Chutsao, Da-boa, Dacha, Dagga, Darakte-Bang, Diamba, Dirijo, Djamba, Djoma, Dokka, Donajuanita, Dormilona, Durijo, Elva, Erva maligna, Erva do norte, Esrar, Fêmea, Fininha, Finote, Fokkra, Fumo brabo, Fumo de caboclo, Gandia, Ganga, Ganja, Ganjila, Gnaoui, Gongo, Gozah, Grahni Sherdool, Greefe, Grifa, Guabza, Guaza, Gunjah, Gunza, Hamp, Haouzi, Hen-Nab, Hursini, Hashish, Igbo, Indische-hennepkruid, Indisk hampa, Intianhamppu, Intsangu, Isangu, Janjah, Jatiphaladya churna, Jea, Juana, Kanab, Karpura rasa, Khanh-Chha, Khanje, Kif, Kif tami, Kinnab, Liamba, Lianda, Maconha, Maconia, Madi, Magiyam, Makhlif, Malva, Maraguango, Marajuana, Marigongo, Marihuana, Mariquita, Maruamba, Matekwane, Mbanje, Meconha, Misari, Mnoana, Momea, Mota, Mulatinha, Mundyadi vatika, Namba, Nsangu, Nwonkaka, Peinka, Penek, Penka, Pito, Pot, Pretinha, Rafe, Rafi, Rafo, Riamba, Rongony, Rora, Rosa Maria, Sabsi, Sadda, Siddhi, Soñadora, Soussi, Subji, Summitates cannabis, Suruma, Tahgalim, Takrouri, Tedrika, Teloeut, Teriaki, Tronadora, Umya, Urumogi, Wee, Wewe, Yamba, Yoruba, Zacate chino, Zerouali, and Ziele konopi indyjskich.

Synonyms and approximate synonyms for cannabis resin included: Bheng, Charas, Charris, Chira, Churrus, Chus, Garaouich, Garawiche, Garoarsch, Gauja, Hachiche, Hascisc, Hashish, Hasis, Hasji's, Hasjisj, Haszysz, Haxixe, Heloua, Kamonga, Malak, Manzul, Momeka, N'rama, and Sighirma.— *Multilingual List of Narcotic Drugs Under International Control*, New York, United Nations, 1968.

Dependence

It has been reported that the prolonged heavy use of cannabis could lead to tolerance and psychic dependence but that physical dependence had not been demonstrated. There have been occasional reports of non-specific symptoms such as anorexia, anxiety, insomnia, irritability, restlessness, sweating, headache, and mild gastro-intestinal upsets occurring when cannabis is withdrawn.

There is a positive relationship between the use of cannabis and other drugs of abuse but the role of cannabis, if any, in the progression to these drugs is still not clear.

Adverse Effects

Nausea and vomiting may be the first effects of cannabis taken by mouth. The most frequent physical effects of cannabis intoxication are an increase in heart-rate with alterations in blood-pressure, injected conjunctival vessels, and deterioration in motor coordination. The psychological effects include elation, distortion of time and space, irritability, and disturbances of memory and judgement. Anxiety or panic reactions may occur, particularly in inexperienced users. Psychotic episodes of a paranoid or schizophrenic nature, and usually acute, have occurred in subjects taking cannabis, especially in large doses.

Some brief reviews of the adverse effects of cannabis: A. M. Nicholi, *New Engl. J. Med.*, 1983, *308*, 925; G. G. Nahas, *Med. J. Aust.*, 1986, *145*, 82.

EFFECTS ON THE ENDOCRINE SYSTEM. Gynaecomastia occurred in 3 young male patients, intensive smokers of cannabis, one for 6 years and another for 2 years. Tests were performed to rule out other possible causes of gynaecomastia. The chemical similarities of tetrahydrocannabinol and oestradiol were noted.— J. Harmon and M. A. Aliapoulios (letter), *New Engl. J. Med.*, 1972, *287*, 936.

Gynaecomastia in 3 men aged 21 to 30, may have been associated with chronic cannabis smoking. Plasma-prolactin concentrations were raised in all 3, compared with age-matched controls.— S. O. Olusi (letter), *Lancet*, 1980, *1*, 255.

EFFECTS ON MENTAL STATE. A review of 79 patients admitted to hospital for treatment of the toxic effects of cannabis showed that the most serious acute syndrome was a toxic confusional psychosis, possibly with disorientation and hallucinations. Lesser symptoms included increasing apprehension, anxiety, tremors, and vomiting.— A. A. Baker and E. G. Lucas, *Lancet*, 1969, *1*, 148.

A discussion of mental disturbances provoked by cannabis.— *Br. med. J.*, 1976, *2*, 1092.

Further references to psychosis associated with cannabis: D. Rottanburg *et al.*, *Lancet*, 1982, *2*, 1364; M. W. P. Carney *et al.*, *Br. med. J.*, 1984, *288*, 1047; S. Andréasson *et al.*, *Lancet*, 1987, *2*, 1483.

EFFECTS ON MOTOR PERFORMANCE. Simulated car driving tests were carried out on 8 subjects while under the influence of cannabis, alcohol, or placebo. Both alcohol and cannabis increased the brake time and start time. The effect produced by 70 g of alcohol was equivalent to that produced by the oral ingestion of 300 to 400 mg of cannabis resin containing about 4% of Δ^9-tetrahydrocannabinol.— O. J. Rafaelsen *et al.*, *Science*, 1973, *179*, 920.

In a double-blind trial there was an increase in major errors committed by pilots in flight simulation situations after smoking cannabis (6.3 mg of Δ^9-tetrahydrocannabinol) compared with placebo.— M. P. Meacham *et al.* (letter), *J. Am. med. Ass.*, 1974, *230*, 1258.

A report of a fatal motor accident in which cannabis was at least a contributory factor.— D. Teale and V. Marks, *Lancet*, 1976, *1*, 884.

PREGNANCY AND THE NEONATE. A brief review of the effect of foetal drug exposure to cannabis concluding that the available reports are too limited to formulate firm conclusions. However, limited data do suggest that the offspring of regular users may suffer from increased tremors and startles and altered visual responsiveness in the initial newborn period but that these problems appear to resolve by one month of age.— P. Gal and M. K. Sharpless, *Drug Intell. & clin. Pharm.*, 1984, *18*, 186. See also: C. S. Conner, *ibid.*, 233.

Treatment of Adverse Effects

Mild panic reactions do not usually require specific therapy; reassurance is generally sufficient. If acute psychotic or paranoid reactions occur, chlorpromazine or possibly diazepam may be necessary.

Precautions

Cannabis has been reported to affect driving. Cannabis and alcohol have additive effects; interactions might be expected between cannabis and a wide range of drugs.

INTERACTIONS. A brief review of interactions between cannabis and other drugs. Antimuscarinic agents, including tricyclic antidepressants, may produce additive increases in heart-rate whereas conversely propranolol tends to attenuate cannabis-induced tachycardia. Limited evidence indicates that a combination of disulfiram and cannabis may produce a hypomanic state.— *Drug Interact. News.*, 1984, *4*, 5.

Alcohol. Tetrahydrocannabinol and alcohol had an additive effect and significantly decreased perception and cognitive and motor functions in 12 healthy subjects.— G. B. Chesher *et al.*, *Med. J. Aust.*, 1976, *2*, 159.

Anaesthetics and analgesics. The sedation and respiratory depression caused by oxymorphone was increased by tetrahydrocannabinol, and accompanied by significant tachycardia. Pentobarbitone alone had no significant cardiovascular or respiratory effects, but addition of tetrahydrocannabinol produced severe psychological effects including hallucinations and anxiety in most subjects. These interactions could be significant in anaesthetising regular marihuana users.— R. E. Johnstone *et al.*, *Anesthesiology*, 1975, *42*, 674.

Antidepressants. Marked sinus tachycardia resulting from the synergistic effects of cannabis and nortriptyline.— J. R. Hillard and W. V. R. Vieweg, *Am. J. Psychiat.*, 1983, *140*, 626.

Disulfiram. A hypomanic-like reaction in a patient simultaneously taking disulfiram and cannabis.— R. B. Lacoursiere and R. Swatek, *Am. J. Psychiat.*, 1983, *140*, 243.

INTERFERENCE WITH DIAGNOSTIC TESTS. A spurious rise in chorionic gonadotrophin concentrations was seen in 2 patients with testicular cancer who smoked marihuana. Since raised chorionic gonadotrophin concentrations are used as tumour markers, false-positive results may lead to unnecessary treatment.— M. B. Garnick (letter), *New Engl. J. Med.*, 1980, *303*, 1177.

Absorption and Fate

The active principles of cannabis are absorbed from the gastro-intestinal tract and the lungs.

About 50% of the Δ^9-tetrahydrocannabinol available in cannabis is present in the smoke inhaled from a whole cannabis cigarette. This produces an effect almost immediately, reaches a peak in 20 to 30 minutes, and is dissipated in about 3 to 4 hours. When cannabis is taken by mouth absorption may be slow and irregular. Effects are not seen for 30 minutes to 1 hour and persist for about 8 hours.

Tetrahydrocannabinol is lipophilic and becomes widely distributed in the body. It is extensively metabolised, primarily in the liver, to the active 11-hydroxy derivative; both are extensively bound to plasma proteins. It is excreted in the urine and faeces, sometimes over prolonged periods. Excretion may be more rapid in chronic users.

Uses and Administration

Cannabis was formerly employed as a sedative or narcotic.

Although cannabis itself is no longer or rarely used as a therapeutic agent, the main active constituent Δ^9-tetrahydrocannabinol (dronabinol, see p.1090) and a synthetic cannabinol (nabilone, see p.1101) are used as anti-emetics in patients receiving cancer chemotherapy; they are also being investigated for a number of other potential therapeutic uses.

12517-g

Cantharides

Blistering Beetle; Cantharis; Insectes Coléoptères Hétéromères; Lytta; Méloides; Russian Flies; Spanish Fly.

Pharmacopoeias. In *Hung.*, *Nord.*, and *Port.*

The dried beetle *Cantharis vesicatoria* (=*Lytta vesicatoria*) (Meloidae) or other spp., containing not less than 0.6% of cantharidin. Cantharides having an ammoniacal odour should not be used.

Adverse Effects

Following ingestion of cantharides there is burning pain in the throat and stomach, with difficulty in swallowing; nausea, vomiting, haematemesis, abdominal pain, bloody diarrhoea, and tenesmus; renal pain, frequent micturition, haematuria, uraemia; severe hypotension and circulatory failure. Toxic effects have been produced by 600 mg, and death by 1.5 to 3 g, though recovery has occurred from much larger doses.

Treatment of Adverse Effects

Empty the stomach by inducing emesis or by aspiration and lavage; activated charcoal has been recommended; give demulcent drinks freely (but *not* oils or fats) and morphine for pain; hot applications to the abdomen may relieve the pain. The circulation should be maintained by the intravenous infusion of plasma or of suitable electrolyte solutions.

Uses and Administration

Preparations of cantharides have been employed externally as rubefacients, counter-irritants, and vesicants. They should not be taken internally or applied over large surfaces owing to the risk of absorption. The use of cantharides in cosmetic products is prohibited in the *UK* by law.

Cantharides is used in homoeopathic medicine.

12518-q

Cantharidin

Hexahydro-3aα,7aα-dimethyl-4β,7β-epoxyisobenzofuran-1,3-dione.

$C_{10}H_{12}O_4$=196.2.

CAS — 56-25-7.

Pharmacopoeias. In *Span.*

Cantharidin is obtained from cantharides (see above) or mylabris (see p.1593).

Cantharidin was formerly used as a counter-irritant and vesicant and was usually preferred to cantharides since the strength of preparations could be more readily controlled. Preparations of cantharidin were used in hair lotions for their rubefacient action. Cantharidin in flexible collodion has been applied for the removal of warts. It has also been used in veterinary medicine. Owing to the high toxicity of cantharidin it is recommended that preparations containing it should not be used medicinally. Adverse effects and treatment are those described for Cantharides (see above). The fatal dose is less than 60 mg.

Proprietary Names and Manufacturers

Canthacur *(Pharmascience, Canad.)*; Cantharone *(Dormer, Canad.; Seres, USA)*; Verr-Canth *(C & M, USA)*.

The following names have been used for multi-ingredient preparations containing cantharidin— Canthacur-PS *(Pharmascience, Canad.)*; Cantharone Plus *(Dormer, Canad.; Seres, USA)*; Verrusol *(C & M, USA)*.

3410-w

Carbetimer *(USAN, pINN).*

N-137. Maleic anhydride polymer with ethylene, reaction product with ammonia.

CAS — 82230-03-3.

An antineoplastic agent under investigation.

Proprietary Names and Manufacturers

Monsanto, USA.

3042-h

Carbocalcitonin

A synthetic derivative of eel calcitonin (elcatonin).

References: A. Caniggia, *Clin. Trials J.*, 1986, *23*, *Suppl.* 1; M. Piolini *et al.*, *Curr. ther. Res.*, 1986, *39*, 940.

12527-p

Carnauba Wax *(BAN, USAN).*

903; Caranda Wax; Cera Coperniciae.

Pharmacopoeias. In *Br.* Also in *U.S.N.F.*

It is obtained from the leaves of the Brazilian wax palm, *Copernicia cerifera* (Palmae).

Light brown to pale yellow moderately coarse powder, or flakes or irregular lumps, with a characteristic bland odour free from rancidity. Sp. gr. about 0.99. The *B.P.* states that it has a melting point of 78° to 85°; the *U.S.N.F.* gives a range of 81° to 86°. Practically **insoluble** in water; slightly soluble in boiling alcohol; soluble in warm chloroform and in warm toluene.

Carnauba wax is used in pharmacy as a tablet-coating and tablet-polishing agent. Various types and grades are used industrially in the manufacture of polishes. Its use is also permitted in certain foods.

12529-w

Caroverine Hydrochloride *(pINNM).*

1-(2-Diethylaminoethyl)-1,2-dihydro-3-(4-methoxybenzyl)quinoxalin-2-one hydrochloride.

$C_{22}H_{27}N_3O_2$,HCl=401.9.

CAS — 23465-76-1 (caroverine).

Caroverine hydrochloride is used as an antispasmodic. Doses of 40 mg have been given by mouth or injection up to three times daily.

Proprietary Names and Manufacturers

Espasmofibra *(Faes, Spain)*; Spasmium *(Medichemie, Switz.)*.

18917-n

Carvedilol *(BAN, rINN).*

BM-14190. 1-Carbazol-4-yloxy-3-[2-(2-methoxyphenoxy)ethylamino]propan-2-ol.

$C_{24}H_{26}N_2O_4$=406.5.

CAS — 72956-09-3.

A beta blocker with vasodilating properties under investigation in the treatment of angina and hypertension.

References to the pharmacology of carvedilol: R. Eggertsen *et al.*, *Eur. J. clin. Pharmac.*, 1984, *27*, 19; B. Tomlinson *et al.*, *Br. J. clin. Pharmac.*, 1986, *21*, 581P; E. v. Möllendorff *et al.*, *Clin. Pharmac. Ther.*, 1986, *39*, 677; L. X. Cubeddu *et al.*, *ibid.*, 1987, *41*, 31.

Use in angina: J. C. Kaski *et al.*, *Am. J. Cardiol.*, 1985, *56*, 35; E. A. Rodrigues *et al.*, *ibid.*, 1986, *58*, 916; A. Lahiri *et al.*, *ibid.*, 1987, *59*, 769.

Use in hypertension: R. Eggersten *et al.*, *Acta med. scand.*, 1985, *Suppl.* 693, 115; M. E. Heber *et al.*, *Am. J. Cardiol.*, 1987, *59*, 400.

Proprietary Names and Manufacturers

MCP Pharmaceuticals, UK.

7355-v

Castor Oil *(BAN, USAN).*

Aceite de Ricino; Huile de Ricin; Ol. Ricin.; Oleum Ricini; Ricini Oleum; Rizinusöl.

CAS — 8001-79-4.

Pharmacopoeias. In *Arg.*, *Aust.*, *Belg.*, *Br.*, *Chin.*, *Cz.*, *Egypt.*, *Eur.*, *Fr.*, *Ger.*, *Hung.*, *Ind.*, *Int.*, *It.*, *Jpn*, *Jug.*, *Mex.*, *Neth.*, *Nord.*, *Pol.*, *Port.*, *Roum.*, *Rus.*, *Span.*, *Swiss*, *Turk.*, and *U.S.* Also in *B.P. Vet.* *U.S.N.F.* also includes hydrogenated castor oil.

The fixed oil expressed, without the application of heat, from the seeds of *Ricinus communis* (Euphorbiaceae), containing about 80% of the triglyceride of ricinoleic acid. It is a nearly colourless or slightly yellow transparent viscid oil with a slight odour and taste which is bland at first, but afterwards slightly acrid.

Soluble 1 in 2.5 of alcohol; miscible with dehydrated alcohol, chloroform, ether, carbon disulphide, and glacial acetic acid; slightly soluble in petroleum spirit. **Store** at a temperature not exceeding 45° in well-filled airtight containers. Protect from light. Castor oil intended for use in the manufacture of a parenteral dosage form

should be kept in a glass container.
When castor oil is intended for parenteral administration it must contain no added antoxidant. When, for other purposes, such addition is authorised, the name and quantity of the added antoxidant is stated on the label.

Adverse Effects
The administration of castor oil by mouth, particularly in large doses, may produce nausea, vomiting, colic, and severe purgation.
The seeds of *Ricinus communis* contain a toxic protein, ricin (see p.1610). Allergic reactions have been reported in subjects handling the seeds.

Precautions
Castor oil should be used with caution during pregnancy or menstruation. It should not be used when abdominal pain, intestinal obstruction, nausea, or vomiting is present.
Castor oil may inhibit the absorption of fat-soluble vitamins.

Uses and Administration
Castor oil has been used for its laxative action, but other agents are now generally preferred.
Castor oil is a soothing application to the conjunctiva and allays irritation due to foreign bodies in the eye, and it has been employed for making solutions of alkaloidal bases for ophthalmic purposes.
Castor oil is used externally for its emollient effect and is employed in such preparations as Zinc and Castor Oil Ointment. Castor oil may be employed as the solvent in some injections.
Hydrogenated castor oil is used as a stiffening agent.

Preparations
Aromatic Castor Oil *(U.S.P.)*. Cinnamon oil *(U.S.N.F.)* 0.3 mL, clove oil 0.1 mL, saccharin 50 mg, vanillin 100 mg, alcohol 3 mL, castor oil to 100 mL. Store in airtight containers.
Castor Oil Capsules *(U.S.P.)*
Castor Oil Emulsion *(U.S.P.)*

Proprietary Preparations
Minims Castor Oil *(Smith & Nephew Pharmaceuticals, UK)*. *Eye-drops*, castor oil in single-dose disposable applicators.
NOTE. The code CAS OIL is permitted in Great Britain for single-dose eye-drops of castor oil.

Proprietary Names and Manufacturers
Laxopol *(Pohl, Ger.)*; Minims Castor Oil *(Smith & Nephew, Austral.; Smith & Nephew, S.Afr.; Smith & Nephew Pharmaceuticals, UK)*; Neoloid *(Lederle, Canad.; Lederle, USA)*; Ricifruit *(Sabex, Canad.)*; Unisoil *(Therapex, Canad.)*; Wonderolie *(Neth.)*.

12537-w

Catha

Abyssinian, African, or Arabian Tea; Kat; Kath; Khat; Miraa.

CAS — 71031-15-7 (cathinone).

The leaves of *Catha edulis* (Celastraceae), containing cathine (see below), cathinone ($C_9H_{11}NO$ = 149.2), celastrin, choline, tannins, and inorganic salts.

Catha is used for its stimulant properties among some cultures of Africa and the Middle East, usually by chewing the leaves. Its effects are reported to resemble those of the amphetamines (see p.1440), and are thought to be largely due to the content of cathinone. Dependence and psychotic reactions have been reported.

References to the pharmacology of catha: P. Kalix, *Gen. Pharmacol.*, 1984, *15*, 179; P. Kalix and I. Khan, *Bull. Wld Hlth Org.*, 1984, *62*, 681; P. Kalix and O. Braenden, *Pharmac. Rev.*, 1985, *37*, 149.

Further references: S. P. Gough and I. B. Cookson (letter), *Lancet*, 1984, *1*, 455 (catha-induced psychosis); J. Mayberry *et al.* (letter), *ibid* (use among immigrants in Wales); J. P. Roper, *Br. J. Ophthal.*, 1986, *70*, 779 (bilateral optic atrophy associated with catha chewing); A. J. Goudie (letter), *Lancet*, 1987, *2*, 1340 (comment on the high abuse potential of cathinone); P. H. Drake (letter), *ibid.*, 1988, *1*, 532 (adverse clinical effects of catha chewing).

Metabolism of cathinone to norephedrine and cathine.— R. Brenneisen *et al.*, *J. Pharm. Pharmac.*, 1986, *38*, 298.

12538-e

Cathine *(pINN)*.

(+)-Norpseudoephedrine. *threo*-2-Amino-1-phenylpropan-1-ol.
$C_9H_{13}NO$=151.2.

CAS — 492-39-7; 36393-56-3.

Cathine is a constituent of catha (above) and has been used as an anorectic agent.

The chemistry and pharmacology of cathine.— R. A. Heacock and J. E. Forrest, *Can. J. pharm. Sci.*, 1974, *9*, 64.

Cathine was excreted unchanged in the urine 30 to 50 minutes after ingestion of the synthetic drug, about 40% being recovered in the urine within 6 hours. Trace amounts were detected 24 hours later.— C. K. Maitai and G. M. Mugera, *J. pharm. Sci.*, 1975, *64*, 702.
Cathine 60 mg by mouth produced a mean peak plasma concentration in 6 healthy subjects of 200 ng per mL after 1.3 hours. Cathine could not be detected in the plasma after 24 hours.— F. Frosch, *Arzneimittel-Forsch.*, 1977, *27*, 665. The bioavailability of cathine from capsules or sustained-release dragees.— *idem*, 1076.

A report of rhabdomyolysis and acute renal failure following overdosage with a preparation containing cathine.— K. W. Rumpf *et al.*, *J. Am. med. Ass.*, 1983, *250*, 2112.

Proprietary Names and Manufacturers
Adiposetten *(Reiss, Ger.)*; Amorphan *(Heumann, Ger.)*; Appetrol *(Restan, S.Afr.)*; Dietene *(Bartiss, S.Afr.)*; Miniscap *(Cooper, Switz.)*; Minusin Depot *(Otto Jann, Switz.)*; Mirapront N *(Mack, Illert., Ger.)*; Neo-Soldana *(Girol, Switz.)*; Nobese *(Restan, S.Afr.)*; Reduform *(Para-Pharma, Switz.)*; Thinz *(Lennon, S.Afr.)*.

527-f

Centaury

Centaurii Minoris Herba; Petite Centaurée; Tausendgüldenkraut.

Pharmacopoeias. In *Aust., Cz., Fr., Ger., Hung., Jug., Pol., Roum., Span.,* and *Swiss.*

The dried flowering tops of the common centaury, *Centaurium minus*(=*C. umbellatum; Erythraea centaurium*), and other species of *Centaurium* (Gentianaceae).

Centaury is used as a bitter.

12549-j

Cerium Oxalate

CAS — 139-42-4 (cerous oxalate, anhydrous).

Pharmacopoeias. In *Aust.*

A white or pinkish, granular, odourless, tasteless powder consisting of about 50% of cerous oxalate, $(C_2O_4)_3Ce_2,10H_2O$=724.5, with the oxalates of numerous other rare earths, especially lanthanum, praseodymium, and neodymium. Practically **insoluble** in water; soluble in warm dilute acids.

Cerium oxalate has been used as an anti-emetic.

Proprietary Names and Manufacturers
Novonausin *(Camps, Spain)*.

12550-q

Cerous Nitrate

Cerium Nitrate.
$Ce(NO_3)_3$=326.1.

CAS — 10108-73-3.

Cerous nitrate has been used topically in the treatment of burns.

References: W. W. Monafo *et al.*, *Archs Surg.*, 1978, *113*, 397.

The antibacterial activity of cerous nitrate *in vitro*.— R. M. E. Richards and V. Magan, *J. Pharm. Pharmac.*, 1979, *31*, *Suppl.*, 33P.

16572-f

Cetamolol Hydrochloride *(USAN, pINNM)*.

AI-27303. (±)-2-[*o*-[3-(*tert*-Butylamino)-2-hydroxypropoxy]phenoxy]-*N*-methylacetamide monohydrochloride.
$C_{16}H_{26}N_2O_4$,HCl=346.9.

CAS — 77590-95-5; 34919-98-7 (cetamolol).

A cardioselective beta blocker under investigation.

References: M. A. Klausner *et al.*, *Curr. ther. Res.*, 1984, *36*, 379; J. Coelho *et al.*, *Br. J. clin. Pharmac.*, 1985, *19*, 411; W. B. White *et al.*, *Clin. Pharmac. Ther.*, 1986, *39*, 664; R. S. Perry, *Drugs Today*, 1986, *22*, 379.

Proprietary Names and Manufacturers
Ayerst, USA.

18617-l

Cetirizine Hydrochloride *(BANM, USAN, rINNM)*.

P-071; ucb-P071. The dihydrochloride of 2-[4-(4-chlorobenzhydryl)piperazin-1-yl]ethoxyacetic acid.
$C_{21}H_{25}ClN_2O_3$,2HCl=461.8.

CAS —83881-52-1 (hydrochloride); 83881-51-0 (cetirizine).

An antihistamine given by mouth in the treatment of various allergic disorders. It is given in single daily doses of 10 mg.

References: A. Brik *et al.*, *J. Allergy & clin. Immunol.*, 1987, *80*, 51.

Proprietary Names and Manufacturers
Zirtek *(Allen & Hanburys, UK)*; Zyrtec *(UCB, Belg.)*.

3706-m

Chenodeoxycholic Acid *(BAN, rINN)*.

CDCA; Chenic Acid; Chenodiol *(USAN)*.
3α,7α-Dihydroxy-5β-cholan-24-oic acid.
$C_{24}H_{40}O_4$=392.6.

CAS — 474-25-9.

Pharmacopoeias. In *Fr.*

Adverse Effects
Chenodeoxycholic acid may cause diarrhoea and pruritus. A transient rise in liver-function test values has been reported.

EFFECTS ON THE LIVER. In healthy persons and patients with gall-stones given chenodeoxycholic acid about 20% of lithocholate (the main bacterial metabolite and probably responsible for the reported liver damage in *animals*) was absorbed from the colon and then conjugated and sulphated to substances rapidly excreted in the faeces. A defective sulphation of lithocholate in the *rhesus monkey* had recently been reported. This difference in metabolism provided a simple explanation for the consistent toxicity of chenodeoxycholic acid in the *monkey* and its apparent safety in man.— R. N. Allan *et al.*, *Gut*, 1976, *17*, 405 and 413. A factor reducing the toxic potential of chenodeoxycholic acid was the epimerisation to ursodeoxycholic acid, which was not a preferred precursor for lithocholic acid.— *Lancet*, 1978, *1*, 805.

PREGNANCY AND THE NEONATE. The offspring of *monkeys* given chenodeoxycholic acid during pregnancy had congenital hepatic, renal, and adrenal abnormalities.— R. Heywood *et al.* (letter), *Lancet*, 1973, *2*, 1021. A report of species difference between *monkey* and man in the metabolism of chenodeoxycholic acid.— R. N. Allan *et al.*, *Gut*, 1976, *17*, 405 and 413.

Precautions

Chenodeoxycholic acid should not be administered to patients with chronic liver disease, severe renal impairment, peptic ulcers, or inflammatory diseases of the small intestine and colon. It has been recommended that since oral contraceptives may increase the lithogenicity of bile other methods of contraception should be used by women receiving chenodeoxycholic acid.

PREGNANCY AND THE NEONATE. See above under Adverse Effects.

Absorption and Fate

Chenodeoxycholic acid is absorbed from the gastro-intestinal tract and undergoes first-pass metabolism and enterohepatic recycling. It is partly conjugated in the liver before being excreted into the bile and under the influence of intestinal bacteria the free and conjugated forms undergo 7α-dehydroxylation to lithocholic acid some of which is excreted directly in the faeces and the rest absorbed mainly to be conjugated and sulphated by the liver. The sulphated compounds being water-soluble are then excreted in the faeces. Chenodeoxycholic acid also undergoes epimerisation to ursodeoxycholic acid.

Uses and Administration

Chenodeoxycholic acid is a naturally occurring bile acid (see p.1547). When given by mouth it reduces the ratio of cholesterol to bile salts plus phospholipids in bile and so causes desaturation of cholesterol-saturated bile; the exact mechanism of action has not been fully elucidated. It is used for the dissolution of cholesterol-rich gall-stones in patients with a functioning gall-bladder. It is considered to be ineffective against calcified or pigment-containing stones or in those patients with a non-functioning gall-bladder. The usual dose is 10 to 17.5 mg per kg body-weight daily in divided doses; obese patients may require doses of up to 20 mg per kg daily. The duration of treatment, which may be for up to 2 years, and efficacy appear to be correlated with the size of the stone. It has been recommended that treatment continues for up to 6 months after dissolution.

CEREBROTENDINOUS XANTHOMATOSIS. Beneficial results with chenodeoxycholic acid therapy in some patients with cerebrotendinous xanthomatosis (presence of tendon xanthomas and excessive accumulation of cholestanol in the central nervous system).— V. M. Berginer *et al.*, *New Engl. J. Med.*, 1984, *311*, 1649. Comment.— S. M. Grundy, *ibid.*, 1694.

Further reference.— G. Salen *et al.*, *New Engl. J. Med.*, 1987, *316*, 1233.

GALL-STONES. Reviews of the use of chenodeoxycholic acid in the management of gall-stones.— I. A. D. Bouchier, *Br. med. J.*, 1983, *286*, 778; *Pharm. J.*, 1984, *1*, 245.

Two doses of chenodeoxycholic acid, 750 mg daily and 375 mg daily and a placebo were compared in The National Cooperative Gallstone Study. Treatment was for 2 years and covered 916 patients with radiolucent gall-stones. The 750-mg dose provided complete dissolution in 13.5% of patients compared with 5.2% for the 375-mg dose and 0.8% for placebo. Thin patients or those with small gall-stones or serum-cholesterol concentrations of 2.27 mg or more per mL appeared to respond best. However, biliary symptoms and the need for surgery were not diminished, diarrhoea was frequent, hepatic dysfunction occurred, causing 3% of patients to withdraw, and there was an increase in serum concentrations of total and low-density lipoprotein cholesterol.— L. J. Schoenfield *et al.*, *Ann. intern. Med.*, 1981, *95*, 257. Follow-up of 48 patients with confirmed complete dissolution of gall-stones indicated that continued treatment with chenodeoxycholic acid 375 mg daily for 2 to 4.5 years was no more effective than placebo in preventing the recurrence of gall-stone formation.— J. W. Marks *et al.*, *Ann. intern. Med.*, 1984, *100*, 376. Further study involving patients who had had partial dissolution of gall-stones after the original 2 years of chenodeoxycholic acid treatment showed that continued treatment for a further period of up to 2 years with the same doses of 750 mg or 375 mg resulted in complete dissolution in 23% and 16% respectively. The reason for the resistance in patients who had already shown a response was unclear.— J. W. Marks *et al.*, *ibid.*, 382. Comments on the National Cooperative Gallstone Study including criticisms of the low doses employed.— M. C. Bateson, *Br. med. J.*, 1982, *284*, 1; R. H. Palmer and M. C. Carey, *New Engl. J. Med.*, 1982, *306*, 1171; R. H. Palmer, *Ann. intern. Med.*, 1984, *100*, 450.

Proprietary Preparations

Chendol *(CP Pharmaceuticals, UK)*. *Capsules*, chenodeoxycholic acid 125 mg.

Tablets, scored, chenodeoxycholic acid 250 mg.

Chenofalk *(Thames, UK)*. *Capsules*, chenodeoxycholic acid 250 mg.

Proprietary Names and Manufacturers

Calcolise *(Berenguer-Beneyto, Spain)*; Carbilcolina *(Spain)*; Chénodex *(Houdé, Fr.)*; Chelobil *(Oftalmiso, Spain)*; Chemicolina *(Spain)*; Chendal *(Denm.)*; Chendol *(Weddel, Austral.; Port.; Spain; CP Pharmaceuticals, UK)*; Chenix *(Reid-Rowell, USA)*; Cheno-Caps *(Neth.)*; Chenocedon *(Tillotts, UK)*; Chenocol *(Caber, Ital.)*; Chenocolic *(Torlan, Spain)*; Chenodecil *(Spain)*; Chenofalk *(Arg.; Aust.; Belg.; Chile; Falk, Ger.; Hong Kong; Also, Ital.; Kuwait; Mex.; Neth.; Peru; Philipp.; Switz.; Taiwan; Thai.; Thames, UK)*; Chenolith *(Belg.)*; Chenomas *(Spain)*; Chenossil *(Gipharmex, Ital.)*; Cholanorm *(Grünenthal, Ger.)*; Fluibil *(Zambon, Ital.)*; Hekbilin *(Hek, Ger.)*; Hepanem *(Chile)*; Kebilis *(Belg.)*; Quenobilan *(Estedi, Spain)*; Ulmenid *(Switz.)*.

18953-v

Chloroacetamide

Chloracetamide. 2-Chloroacetamide.

C_2H_4ClNO=93.51.

CAS — 79-07-2.

A preservative which has been used in topical pharmaceutical preparations and cosmetics. Chloroacetamide also has molluscicidal activity.

It is a sensitiser and has caused dermatitis.

Contact allergy associated with chloroacetamide.— S. E. Koch *et al.*, *Archs Derm.*, 1985, *121*, 172.

12553-w

Chloroacetophenone

CN; Phenacyl Chloride. 2-Chloroacetophenone.

C_8H_7ClO=154.6.

CAS — 532-27-4.

NOTE. The name mace is applied to solutions of chloroacetophenone.

Chloroacetophenone is a lachrymatory which is irritant to the skin and eyes. It has been used in a riot-control gas.

In Great Britain the recommended exposure limit of chloroacetophenone is 0.05 ppm (long-term).

Recommended treatment of exposure to chloroacetophenone included neutralisation by washing the skin with sodium bicarbonate solution and the instillation of boric acid solution into the eyes.— H. W. Jolly and C. L. Carpenter (letter), *J. Am. med. Ass.*, 1968, *203*, 808.

In a comparative study of chloroacetophenone and CS gas applied under a 4-cm diameter watch glass for a period of 1 hour to the skin of healthy subjects, chloroacetophenone was shown to present a far greater cutaneous hazard than CS gas. The reactions were more severe when it was applied moist. Treatment was not considered necessary in the subjects studied, but in the case of extreme irritation, the use of calamine cream with antihistamine therapy at night to aid sleep was recommended. The blisters would resolve spontaneously.— P. Holland and R. G. White, *Br. J. Derm.*, 1972, *86*, 150.

12555-l

Chloroplatinic Acid

Kloroplatinasyra. Hexachloroplatinic acid hexahydrate.

$H_2PtCl_6,6H_2O$=517.9.

CAS — 16941-12-1 (anhydrous); 18497-13-7 (hexahydrate).

Pharmacopoeias. In *Nord.*

Aqueous solutions of platinic chloride ($PtCl_4$=336.9) are used in corneal tattooing solutions.

A review of sensitivity to platinum compounds.— G. M. Levene, *Br. J. Derm.*, 1971, *85*, 590.

Platinum nephrotoxicity.— N. E. Madias and J. T. Harrington, *Am. J. Med.*, 1978, *65*, 307.

Occupational inhalation allergy in workers in the platinum- associated industry.— G. Schultze-Werninghaus *et al.*, *Dt. med. Wschr.*, 1978, *103*, 972.

12557-j

Cholesteryl Benzoate

Cholesterol Benzoate. Cholest-5-en-3β-yl benzoate.

$C_{34}H_{50}O_2$=490.8.

CAS — 604-32-0.

Cholesteryl benzoate is an ingredient in dermatological preparations.

12558-z

Chondroitin Sulphate A

CSA.

CAS — 24967-93-9.

An acid mucopolysaccharide which is a constituent of most mammalian cartilaginous tissues.

Chondroitin sulphate A has been given to patients with ischaemic heart disease and has also been used in osteoporosis and related disorders. A medium containing chondroitin sulphate A has been used to preserve corneas for transplantation.

Preparations containing chondroitin sulphate A have also been used as adjuncts to ocular surgery.

In a study of 46 elderly patients with atherosclerosis, 60 mg per kg body-weight daily of chondroitin sulphate A or placebo were given by mouth for 6 to 64 months. Serum cholesterol and triglyceride concentrations were reduced and clotting time was prolonged in the treated group although there was evidence of tolerance developing on long-term treatment in some patients.— K. Nakazawa and K. Murata, *J. int. med. Res.*, 1978, *6*, 217.

Further references: L. M. Morrison, *J. Am. Geriat. Soc.*, 1968, *16*, 779; *idem*, *J. Am. Geriat. Soc.*, 1969, *17*, 913; L. M. Morrison *et al.*, *J. Am. med. Ass.*, 1969, *208*, 1474; *ibid.*, *209*, 352.

References to the use of chondroitin sulphate A in media for corneal preservation: R. L. Lindstrom *et al.*, *Br. J. Ophthal.*, 1986, *70*, 47; M. Busin *et al.*, *ibid.*, 860; K. Tamaki, *ibid.*, 1987, *71*, 570.

Proprietary Names and Manufacturers

Condrofer *(Selvi, Ital.)*; Falenol *(Iquinosa, Spain)*; Lacrypos *(P.O.S., Fr.)*; Structum *(U.R.P.A.C., Fr.; Smith Kline & French, Switz.)*; Turkadon *(Iquinosa, Spain)*.

The following names have been used for multi-ingredient preparations containing chondroitin sulphate a— Viscoat *(Cilco, USA)*.

12559-c

Chrome Alum

Chromium Potassium Sulphate.

$KCr(SO_4)_2,12H_2O$=499.4.

CAS — 10141-00-1 (anhydrous).

Chrome alum is used in tanning, as a mordant in dyeing, and for hardening gelatin in photographic materials. It has been used as a sclerosant in medicine.

Proprietary Names and Manufacturers
Sclérémo *(Bouteille, Fr.)*.

12560-s

Chromium Trichloride

Chromic Chloride *(USAN)*.
$CrCl_3$=158.4.

CAS — 10025-73-7 (anhydrous); 10060-12-5 (hexahydrate).

Pharmacopoeias. U.S. has a monograph for the hexahydrate.

Chromium is an essential trace element involved in carbohydrate metabolism and chromium trichloride has been given as a chromium supplement.

In Great Britain the recommended exposure limit of chromium (III) compounds is 0.5 mg per m^3 (long-term).

For a comprehensive review of chromium deficiency, metabolism, human requirements, and toxicity, see Report of a WHO Expert Group on Trace Elements in Human Nutrition, *Tech. Rep. Ser. Wld Hlth Org. No. 532,* 1973, 20. See also A. S. Prasad, *Trace Elements and Iron in Human Metabolism,* Chichester, John Wiley, 1978.

The administration of supplementary chromium (as trichloride) 150 µg daily for 2 months resulted in the normalisation of impaired glucose tolerance in 4 of 8 nondiabetic subjects and some benefit in most of the others.— *J. Am. med. Ass.,* 1968, *206,* 36. Criticisms of the use of chromium trichloride in diabetes.— A. Wise (letter), *ibid.,* 1978, *240,* 2045.

Further references: W. H. Glinsmann and W. Mertz, *Metabolism,* 1966, *15,* 510; W. H. Glinsmann *et al., Science,* 1966, *152,* 1243; R. A. Levine *et al., Metabolism,* 1968, *17,* 114; R. A. Anderson *et al., ibid.,* 1987, *36,* 351.

Preparations

Chromic Chloride Injection *(U.S.P.)*. A sterile solution of chromium trichloride hexahydrate in Water for Injections. pH between 1.5 and 2.5.

Proprietary Names and Manufacturers
Chrometrace *(Armour, USA)*.

12561-w

Chromocarb Diethylamine

The diethylamine salt of 4-oxo-4*H*-1-benzopyran-2-carboxylic acid.
$C_{14}H_{17}O_4N$=263.3.

CAS — 4940-39-0 (chromocarb).

NOTE. Chromocarb is *rINN.*

Chromocarb diethylamine is used for its reputed effect on capillary fragility.

Proprietary Names and Manufacturers
Angiophtal *(Merck Sharp & Dohme-Chibret, Fr.)*; Campel *(Farmitalia Carlo Erba, Fr.)*; Fludarène *(Egic, Fr.)*; Fludarene *(Merck Sharp & Dohme, Ital.)*; Vitarel *(Davur, Spain)*.

12562-e

Chrysoidine Hydrochloride Citrate

4-Phenylazobenzene-1,3-diamine hydrochloride citrate; Azobenzene-2,4-diamine hydrochloride citrate.
$C_{12}H_{12}N_4,HCl,C_6H_8O_7$=440.8.

CAS — 532-82-1 (hydrochloride); 5909-04-6 (xHCl, citrate).

Chrysoidine hydrochloride citrate has been used as an antimicrobial agent. It has also been used as a dye but has been associated with tumours of the bladder. In the *UK* its use in cosmetic products is controlled by law.

Mention that the development of tumours of the urinary bladder in 3 anglers was possibly associated with the use of chrysoidine hydrochloride (chrysoidine Y; CI Basic Orange 2; Colour Index No. 11270) for colouring the maggots used as bait.— C. E. Searle and J. Teale (letter), *Lancet,* 1982, *1,* 564. See also.— *idem,* 1984, *1,* 563. Comment that chrysoidine dyes have been manufactured and used in industry for 100 years and there is no evidence that these dyes have presented an increased cancer risk to man. Anglers are, however, unable or unwilling to handle dyestuffs in a way which avoids unnecessary contamination.— A. J. Hinton (letter), *ibid.,* 1179. A report of transitional cell carcinoma of the bladder in 2 brothers. Both were heavy smokers and anglers, always using dyed maggots for bait and favouring the bronze (chrysoidine stained) variety. Their hands used to become stained with the dye, taking several days to wear off, and in winter when the maggots became cold and sluggish the men often put them into their mouths to warm them. It was concluded that smoking and prolonged heavy exposure to chrysoidine dye were the two factors most likely to have led to the development of the tumours.— G. M. Sole, *Br. med. J.,* 1984, *289,* 1043. A further report of 2 young men with transitional cell carcinoma both whom were again anglers who had used bronze maggots.— J. A. Massey *et al.* (letter), *ibid.,* 1451. A study indicating that coarse fishing is a risk factor for urothelial cancer and that duration of use of maggots stained with chrysoidine dyes was the most important predictor of risk. Although the National Federation of Anglers had banned the use of dyed maggots they were still extensively used outside official meetings. The effects of adding dyes to reservoirs storing drinking water is of concern.— G. Sole and T. Sorahan, *Lancet,* 1985, *1,* 1477.

Proprietary Names and Manufacturers
Azoangin *(Ger.)*; Azohel *(Ger.)*.

18965-s

Ciamexon *(BAN, rINN).*

BM-41332; Ciamexone. (*RS*)-1-(2-Methoxy-6-methyl-3-pyridylmethyl)aziridine-2-carbonitrile.
$C_{11}H_{13}N_3O$=203.2.

CAS — 75985-31-8.

An immunomodulator under investigation in the treatment of auto-immune disorders.

References: K. H. Usadel *et al.* (letter), *Lancet,* 1986, *2,* 567 (diabetes mellitus); U. Bicker and K. H. Usadel, *Klin. Wschr.,* 1986, *64,* 1261 (diabetes mellitus; rheumatoid arthritis).

Proprietary Names and Manufacturers
Boehringer Mannheim, Ger.

18966-w

Cianergoline *(rINN).*

(*α-RS*)-*α*-Cyano-6-methylergoline-8*β*-propionamide.
$C_{19}H_{22}N_4O$=322.4.

CAS — 74627-35-3.

Cianergoline, an ergoline derivative, is a dopaminergic agonist reported to have predominantly cardiovascular effects. It is under investigation as an antihypertensive agent.

References: G. Bise *et al., Eur. J. clin. Pharmac.,* 1985, *29,* 25.

Proprietary Names and Manufacturers
Farmitalia, Ital.

12563-l

Cianidanol *(rINN).*

(+)-Catechol; (+)-Cyanidanol-3; Dexcyanidanol. *trans*-2-(3,4-Dihydroxyphenyl)-3,4-dihydro-2*H*-1-benzopyran-3,5,7-triol.
$C_{15}H_{14}O_6$=290.3.

CAS — 154-23-4.

NOTE. The name cianidol has been used for this compound.

Cianidanol has been used in the treatment of hepatic disorders. Its use has been associated with severe haemolytic anaemia; fatalities have been reported.

Proprietary Names and Manufacturers
Ausoliver *(Ausonia, Ital.)*; Catergen *(Zyma, Ger.; Zyma, Ital.; Zyma, Switz.)*; Drenoliver *(Janus, Ital.)*.

3932-y

Ciclomethasone

RIB-222. (11*β*,16*β*)-21-[({4-[(Acetylamino)methyl]cyclohexyl}carbonyl)oxy]-9-chloro-11, 17-dihydroxy-16-methylpregna-1,4-diene-3,20-dione.
$C_{32}H_{44}ClNO_7$=590.2.

CAS — 67372-50-3.

Ciclomethasone is a glucocorticoid which has been applied topically in allergic and inflammatory skin disorders. It has also been given by inhalation in asthmatic conditions.

Proprietary Names and Manufacturers
Cycloderm *(Rottapharm, Ital.)*; Telocort *(Rottapharm, Ital.)*.

3428-x

Ciclotropium Bromide *(rINN).*

Cyclotropium Bromide. (8*r*)-3*α*-Hydroxy-8-isopropyl-1*αH*,5*αH*-tropanium bromide, *α*-phenylcyclopentane-acetate.
$C_{24}H_{36}BrNO_2$=450.5.

CAS — 85166-20-7.

Ciclotropium bromide is a quaternary ammonium antimuscarinic agent. It has been reported to delay gastric emptying.

References: G. Stacher *et al., Gut,* 1984, *25,* 485.

Proprietary Names and Manufacturers
Helopharm, Ger.

12569-a

Cicloxilic Acid *(rINN).*

cis-2-Hydroxy-2-phenylcyclohexanecarboxylic acid.
$C_{13}H_{16}O_3$=220.3.

CAS — 57808-63-6.

Cicloxilic acid has been used in the treatment of hepatic disorders.

Studies, including *animal* studies, on cicloxilic acid.— *Arzneimittel-Forsch.,* 1978, *28,* 1205–52.

Reduction of cholesterol supersaturation of gall-bladder bile.— M. Zuin *et al., Arzneimittel-Forsch.,* 1979, *29,* 837.

Use in chronic alcoholics.— S. Geminiani *et al., Farmaco, Edn prat.,* 1979, *34,* 449.

Further reference.— C. T. Degna *et al., Curr. med. Res. Opinion,* 1983, *8,* 472.

Proprietary Names and Manufacturers
Plecton *(Guidotti, Ital.)*.

1980-v

Cicloxolone *(BAN, rINN).*

BX-363A (disodium salt). 3*β*-[(*Z*)-2-Carboxycyclohexylcarbonyloxy]-11-oxo-18*β*-olean-12-en-30-oic acid.
$C_{38}H_{56}O_7$=624.9.

CAS — 52247-86-6.

Cicloxolone was initially under investigation for the treatment of gastric ulcers, similarly to carbenoxolone. More recently it has been tried by topical application in the treatment of herpes genitalis.

References: G. W. Csonka and D. A. Tyrrell, *Br. J. vener. Dis.,* 1984, *60,* 178; P. Sacra *et al., Br. J. Pharmac.,* 1986, *87, Suppl.,* 9P.

1981-g

Cilostazol *(pINN).*

OPC-13013. 6-[4-(1-Cyclohexyl-1*H*-tetrazol-5-yl)butoxy]-3,4-dihydrocarbostyril.
$C_{20}H_{27}N_5O_2$=369.5.

CAS — 73963-72-1.

It is used as an anticoagulant.

Proprietary Names and Manufacturers
Pletaal *(Otsuka, Jpn)*.

1702-g

Cimetropium Bromide *(rINN).*

DA-3177; Hyoscine-*N*-(cyclopropylmethyl) Bromide. 8-(Cyclopropylmethyl)-6β,7β-epoxy-3α-hydroxy-1αH,5αH-tropanium bromide, (−)-(*S*)-tropate.

$C_{21}H_{28}BrNO_4$=438.4.

CAS — 51598-60-8.

An antimuscarinic agent used in the treatment of gastro-intestinal and genito-urinary disorders.

References: F. Parente *et al.*, *J. int. med. Res.*, 1985, *13*, 332; C. Scarpignato and G. Bianchi Porro, *Int. J. clin. Pharmacol. Res.*, 1985, *5*, 467; A. Ferrari *et al.*, *Clin. Ther.*, 1986, *8*, 320.

Proprietary Names and Manufacturers
Alginor *(De Angeli, Ital.).*

12570-e

Cimicifuga

Black Cohosh. The roots of *Cimicifuga racemosa* (Ranunculaceae).

Pharmacopoeias. Chin. includes the rhizome of *C. heracleifolia, C. dahurica*, and *C. foetida. Jpn* includes the rhizome of *C. simplex* (=*C. foetida*) and other spp.

Cimicifuga is used in homoeopathic medicine where it is known as Actaea racemosa or Actaea rac.

18970-g

Cimoxatone *(rINN).*

MD-780515. α-{*p*-[5-(Methoxymethyl)-2-oxo-3-oxazolidinyl]phenoxy}-*m*-tolunitrile.

$C_{19}H_{18}N_2O_4$=338.4.

CAS — 73815-11-9.

Cimoxatone is a type A monoamine oxidase inhibitor under investigation as an antidepressant.

References: C. T. Dollery *et al.*, *Clin. Pharmac. Ther.*, 1983, *34*, 651; V. Rovei *et al.*, *Int. J. clin. Pharmac. Ther. Toxic.*, 1984, *22*, 56; *Drugs of the Future*, 1984, *9*, 412; *ibid.*, 1985, *10*, 500; *ibid.*, 1986, *11*, 505; N. Garrick *et al.*, *Clin. Pharmac. Ther.*, 1984, *35*, 243.

3711-d

Cinametic Acid *(rINN).*

Acidum Cinameticum. 4-(2-Hydroxyethoxy)-3-methoxycinnamic acid.

$C_{12}H_{14}O_5$=238.2.

CAS — 35703-32-3.

Cinametic acid is a choleretic. It has been given in doses of 500 to 750 mg daily.

Proprietary Names and Manufacturers
Transoddi *(Millet, Arg.; Anphar-Rolland, Fr.).*

529-n

Cinchona Bark *(BAN).*

Chinae Cortex; Chinarinde; Cinchona; Cinchonae Cortex; Cinchonae Succirubrae Cortex; Jesuit's Bark; Peruvian Bark; Quina; Quina Vermelha; Quinquina Rouge; Quinquinas; Red Cinchona Bark.

Pharmacopoeias. In *Aust., Belg., Br., Braz., Cz., Egypt., Eur., Fr., Ger., Hung., It., Jpn, Mex., Neth., Nord., Pol., Port., Roum., Span.*, and *Swiss. Arg.* specifies *C. calisaya. Braz.* also includes *C. calisaya* (Quina Amarela). Some pharmacopoeias also permit other species of Cinchona. *Br.* also includes Powdered Cinchona Bark.

The dried bark of *Cinchona pubescens* (=*Cinchona succirubra*) or of its varieties or hybrids, containing not less than 6.5% of total alkaloids, of which not less than 30% and not more than 60% consists of quinine-type alkaloids. **Store** in a well-closed container. Protect from light.

Cinchona bark is a bitter.

As its alkaloids are of the quinine group it may cause similar adverse effects to quinine.

Cinchonine possesses antimalarial activity.

12576-k

Citicoline *(pINN).*

CDP-Choline; Citidoline; Cytidine Diphosphate Choline. Choline cytidine-5′-pyrophosphate.

$C_{14}H_{26}N_4O_{11}P_2$=488.3.

CAS — 987-78-0.

Citicoline is a derivative of choline and cytidine involved in the biosynthesis of lecithin. It is claimed to increase blood flow and oxygen consumption in the brain and has been given by injection in the treatment of cerebrovascular disorders.

References: F. Salvadorini *et al.*, *Curr. ther. Res.*, 1975, *18*, 513 (use in depression); F. Boismare *et al.*, *Thérapie*, 1977, *32*, 345 (*animal* study); G. Palma *et al.*, *Curr. ther. Res.*, 1979, *26*, 1 (use in cardiac arrhythmias); A. Moglia *et al.*, *ibid.*, 1984, *36*, 309 (in cerebrovascular disease).

See also A. Spagnoli and G. Tognoni, *Drugs*, 1983, *26*, 44.

Proprietary Names and Manufacturers
Alaton *(Zambon, Ital.)*; Alfatidina *(Carol, Spain)*; Brassel *(Schiapparelli, Ital.)*; Cereb *(Jpn)*; Cidifos *(Neopharmed, Ital.)*; Cidilin *(Errekappa, Ital.)*; Colite *(Jpn)*; Corenalin *(Jpn)*; Cyscholin *(Jpn)*; Difosfocin *(Magis, Ital.)*; Encelin *(Crosara, Ital.)*; Ensign *(Jpn)*; Gerolin *(CT, Ital.)*; Haocolin *(Jpn)*; Hornkest *(Jpn)*; Logan *(Ist. Chim. Inter., Ital.)*; Neucolis *(Jpn)*; Neurodynamicum *(Faes, Spain)*; Neuroton *(Nuovo, Ital.)*; Nicholin *(Cyanamid, Ital.; Jpn)*; Nicolsint *(Von Boch, Ital.)*; Numatol *(Spyfarma, Spain)*; Recognan *(Jpn)*; Rexort *(Takeda, Fr.)*; Sauran *(Abello, Spain)*; Sinkron *(Ripari-Gero, Ital.)*; Sintoclar *(Pulitzer, Ital.)*; Somazina *(Ferrer, Spain)*; Suncholin *(Jpn).*

12577-a

Citiolone *(rINN).*

BO-714. *N*-(Perhydro-2-oxo-3-thienyl)acetamide.

$C_6H_9NO_2S$=159.2.

CAS — 1195-16-0.

Citiolone has been used in the treatment of hepatic disorders.

Proprietary Names and Manufacturers
Citiolase *(Roussel Maestretti, Ital.)*; Mucorex *(Berenguer-Beneyto, Spain)*; Sitilon *(Roussel, Arg.)*; Thioxidrène *(Bottu, Fr.).*

2732-x

Citrated Calcium Carbimide

Citrated Calcium Cyanamide. A mixture of 1 part by weight of highly purified calcium carbimide ($CCaN_2$ = 80.10) and 2 parts by weight of citric acid.

CAS — 156-62-7 (calcium carbimide); 8013-88-5 (citrated).

NOTE. Calcium Carbimide is rINN.

Calcium carbimide has actions and uses similar to those of disulfiram (see p.1565). The citrated form has been used as an adjunct in the treatment of chronic alcoholism in doses of 50 mg once or twice daily by mouth.

A comparative review of the alcohol deterrents calcium carbimide and disulfiram. Both drugs inhibit aldehyde dehydrogenase to produce raised acetaldehyde concentrations in the blood, and the ensuing adverse reaction, when alcohol is consumed during treatment. However, in *animals* inhibition with calcium carbimide is reported to be maximal 1 to 2 hours after administration and aldehyde dehydrogenase activity restored to 80% of control activity within 24 hours, whereas disulfiram inhibition develops slowly over 12 hours and is irreversible with restoration of activity dependent on synthesis of new enzyme over several days. It has been assumed that calcium carbimide produces a less intense interaction with alcohol than disulfiram, but appreciable cardiovascular changes have been observed. Behavioural and some other effects associated with disulfiram have been attributed to its inhibition of dopamine-β-hydroxylase; calcium carbimide does not inhibit this enzyme. There is little reliable toxicological information on calcium carbimide, but there have been reports of neuropathy, effects on the liver, and antithyroid effects (in *animals*). Calcium carbimide has been reported not to affect blood concentrations of phenytoin when given concomitantly.— J. E. Peachey *et al.*, *J. clin. Psychopharmacol.*, 1981, *1*, 21. See also E. M. Sellers *et al.*, *New Engl. J. Med.*, 1981, *305*, 1255; J. E. Peachey and C. A. Naranjo, *Drugs*, 1984, *27*, 171.

Little is known about the disposition and pharmacokinetics of calcium carbimide.— J. F. Brien and C. W. Loomis, *Drug Metab. Rev.*, 1983, *14*, 113.

Calcium carbimide 50 mg twice daily produced a reaction to a challenge dose of alcohol in an alcoholic who had failed to react while on disulfiram 600 mg daily.— C. Brewer (letter), *Lancet*, 1984, *2*, 171.

Adverse effects. Peripheral neuropathy attributed to citrated calcium carbimide.— T. M. Reilly (letter), *Lancet*, 1976, *1*, 911.

A preliminary report of distinctive hepatic lesions, characterised by inclusions in the hepatocytes, in chronic alcoholics treated with cyanamide or disulfiram.— J. J. Vázquez and S. Cervera (letter), *Lancet*, 1980, *1*, 361. Liver biopsies from 39 patients who had received cyanamide for 2 months to 7 years, displayed characteristic cytoplasmic inclusion bodies in the liver cells, fibrosis, and disruption of the parenchymal-connective tissue interface. There was a clear correlation between the duration of treatment and the stage of the hepatic lesion. None of the patients had evidence of alcoholic liver disease.— A. Moreno *et al.*, *Liver*, 1984, *4*, 15.

Potentially dangerous cardiovascular changes during the carbimide-alcohol reaction.— J. E. Peachey *et al.*, *Clin. Pharmac. Ther.*, 1981, *29*, 40; M. Kupari *et al.*, *J. Toxicol. clin. Toxicol.*, 1982, *19*, 79.

Proprietary Names and Manufacturers
Abstem *(Lederle, UK)*; Colme *(Lasa, Spain)*; Dipsan *(Lederle, Austral.; Lederle, Denm.; Neth.; Lederle, S.Afr.; Lederle, Swed.; Switz.)*; Temposil *(Lederle, Canad.).*

1307-a

Anhydrous Citric Acid *(BAN).*

Acidum Citricum; Citric Acid *(USAN)*; Citronensäure; E330. 2-Hydroxypropane-1,2,3-tricarboxylic acid.

$C_6H_8O_7$=192.1.

CAS — 77-92-9.

NOTE. Anhydrous citric acid was formerly known as citric acid.

Pharmacopoeias. In *Br., Eur., Fr., Ger., Ind., It., Jpn, Jug., Neth., Nord., Swiss*, and *U.S.*

Odourless or almost odourless, colourless crystals or white crystalline powder.

Soluble 1 in 1 of water and 1 in 1.5 of alcohol; sparingly soluble in ether. **Store** in airtight containers.

1308-t

Citric Acid Monohydrate *(BAN).*

Acido del Limón; Acidum Citricum Monohydricum; Citric Acid *(USAN)*; Hydrous Citric Acid.

$C_6H_8O_7,H_2O$=210.1.

CAS — 5949-29-1.

Pharmacopoeias. In *Arg., Aust., Belg., Br., Chin., Cz., Egypt., Eur., Fr., Ger., Hung., Ind., It., Jpn, Jug., Mex., Neth., Nord., Pol., Port., Roum., Span., Swiss, Turk.*, and *U.S.*

Odourless or almost odourless, efflorescent, colourless crystals or white crystalline powder.

Soluble 1 in less than 1 of water and 1 in 1.5 of alcohol; sparingly soluble in ether. **Store** in airtight containers.

Adverse Effects

Citric acid ingested frequently or in large quantities may cause erosion of the teeth and have a local irritant action.

Citric acid used as a sialogogue interferes with an enzyme assay for anticonvulsants.— R. D. Paton and R. W. Logan (letter), *Lancet*, 1986, *2*, 1340. Using smaller amounts of citric acid and a different form of the enzyme assay, there was no interference.— C. Knott and F. Reynolds (letter), *ibid.*, 1987, *1*, 97.

Uses and Administration

Citric acid is used in effervescing mixtures; citric acid monohydrate is used in the preparation of effervescent granules.

Citric acid monohydrate is used as a synergist to enhance the effectiveness of antoxidants.

Preparations containing citric acid are used to dissolve renal calculi, often in combination with a magnesium salt to minimise urinary tract irritation.

RENAL CALCULUS. Discussions on the use of preparations containing citric acid to dissolve renal calculi: D. Rennie, *New Engl. J. Med.*, 1979, *300*, 361; *Br. med. J.*, 1979, *1*, 1746.

New renal stones were completely dissolved in 4 of 6 patients suffering from recurrent stones composed of struvite ($MgNH_4PO_4$) or apatite ($CaPO_4$) or both, by irrigation with Hemiacidrin, a mixture of citric and gluconic acids, magnesium hydroxycarbonate, magnesium acid citrate, and calcium carbonate (Renacidin), through percutaneous nephrostomy tubes. Partial dissolution was achieved in the other 2 patients. Perfusion of up to 120 mL of Hemiacidrin per hour for 7 to 30 days provided continuous lavage of the surface of the stones. Less than 10 days' perfusion was necessary in 4 kidneys. On several occasions irrigation had to be stopped temporarily because of flank pain and low-grade fever. Calcium oxalate stones, the most common type of calculi, are insoluble in Hemiacidrin.— S. P. Dretler *et al.*, *New Engl. J. Med.*, 1979, *300*, 341. Criticism.— M. I. Resnick and W. H. Boyce (letter), *ibid.*, 1488. Reply.— S. P. Dretler *et al.* (letter), *ibid.*

See also I. M. Thompson and R. V. Mora, *J. Urol., Baltimore*, 1984, *132*, 741.

Further references: H. J. Suby and F. Albright, *New Engl. J. Med.*, 1943, *228*, 81 (use of Suby's G solution also known as Solution G); K. Somasundaram and H. B. Eckstein, *Br. med. J.*, 1966, *2*, 91.

USE OF DISINFECTANTS ON FARMS. In Great Britain, citric acid 1 in 500 of water is an approved disinfectant for foot-and-mouth disease.

Preparations

Citric Acid, Magnesium Oxide, and Sodium Carbonate Irrigation *(U.S.P.)*. Sterile. Store in single-dose containers. pH 3.8 to 4.2.

Proprietary Preparations

Renacidin *(Guardian, USA: Farillon, UK)*. *Bladder irrigation*, anhydrous citric acid 156 to 171 g, gluconic acid 21 to 30 g, with magnesium and calcium salts to 300 g. For use, as a 10% solution, to prevent calcification of indwelling urethral catheters and to promote the dissolution of renal calculi.

A method for the preparation and sterilisation of Renacidin irrigation using microporous membrane filtration.— D. W. Newton *et al.*, *Am. J. Hosp. Pharm.*, 1984, *41*, 121. Sterilisation of Renacidin irrigation in polypropylene containers by heating in an autoclave.— G. J. Sewell and B. Venables (letter), *ibid.*, 1985, *42*, 537.

Uro-Tainer Solution R *(Vifor, Switz.: CliniMed, UK)*. *Solution*, sterile, citric acid 6%, light magnesium carbonate 2.8%, gluconolactone 0.6%, in single-use disposable sachets of 100 mL. For flushing of indwelling urinary catheters.

Uro-Tainer Suby G *(Vifor, Switz.: CliniMed, UK)*. *Solution*, sterile, citric acid 3.23%, light magnesium oxide 0.38%, sodium bicarbonate 0.7%, in single-use disposable sachets of 100 mL. For flushing of indwelling urinary catheters.

Proprietary Names and Manufacturers of Anhydrous or Hydrated Citric Acid

The following names have been used for multi-ingredient preparations containing anhydrous or hydrated citric acid— Bicitra *(Willen, USA)*; Citrocarbonate *(Upjohn, Canad.)*; Polycitra *(Willen, USA)*; Polycitra-K *(Willen, USA)*; Renacidin *(Guardian, USA : Farillon, UK)*.

1982-q

Clobenoside *(pINN)*.

Ethyl 5,6-bis-*O*-(*p*-chlorobenzyl)-3-*O*-propyl-D-glucofuranoside.

$C_{25}H_{32}Cl_2O_6$=499.4.

CAS — 29899-95-4.

Clobenoside is a vasoprotective agent used topically and by mouth.

Proprietary Names and Manufacturers

Zyma, Switz.

12586-t

Clofoctol *(rINN)*.

2-(2,4-Dichlorobenzyl)-4-(1,1,3,3-tetramethylbutyl)phenol.

$C_{21}H_{26}Cl_2O$=365.3.

CAS — 37693-01-9.

Clofoctol is an antimicrobial compound administered as suppositories for respiratory infections.

Proprietary Names and Manufacturers

Gramplus *(Chiesi, Ital.)*; Octofene *(Debat, Fr.; Scharper, Ital.)*.

1985-w

Cloximate *(rINN)*.

DU-22599. 2-(Dimethylamino)ethyl (*E*)-{[(*p*-chloro-α-methylbenzylidene)amino]oxy}acetate.

$C_{14}H_{19}ClN_2O_3$=298.8.

CAS — 58832-68-1.

Cloximate has analgesic and anti-inflammatory properties.

15330-t

Cloxyquin *(USAN)*.

Cloxiquine *(rINN)*. 5-Chloroquinolin-8-ol.

C_9H_6ClNO=179.6.

CAS — 130-16-5.

Cloxyquin is an antimicrobial agent which has been used topically in mycotic infections. It is a component of halquinol, p.665.

Proprietary Names and Manufacturers

Chlorisept *(Chinosolfabrik, Ger.)*.

12596-r

Clupadonic Acid

Docosa-7,10,13,16,19-pentaenoic acid.

$C_{22}H_{34}O_2$=330.5.

CAS — 2234-74-4.

An active principle of cod-liver oil.

Proprietary Names and Manufacturers

Clupadene *(Ital.)*; Clupanina *(Arnaldi, Ital.)*.

530-k

Cnicus Benedictus

Blessed Thistle; Carbenia benedicta; Cardo Santo; Carduus Benedictus; Chardon Bénit; Holy Thistle; Kardobenediktenkraut.

CAS — 24394-09-0 (cnicin).

Pharmacopoeias. In *Aust., Hung.*, and *Span.*

The flowering tops of *Cnicus benedictus* (=*Carbenia benedicta; Carduus benedictus*) (Compositae).

Cnicus benedictus has been used as a bitter.

12597-f

Cobalt Chloride

Cobaltous Chloride.

$CoCl_2,6H_2O$=237.9.

CAS — 7646-79-9 (anhydrous).

Pharmacopoeias. In *Aust., Fr.*, and *Nord.*

Adverse Effects

Reactions to cobalt have included anorexia, nausea and vomiting, diarrhoea, precordial pain, cardiomyopathy, flushing of the face and extremities, skin rashes, tinnitus, temporary nerve deafness, renal injury, diffuse thyroid enlargement, and hypothyroidism. Cobalt induces severe nausea and vomiting in patients with pernicious anaemia. In large doses it may reduce the production of erythrocytes.

In Great Britain the recommended exposure limit of cobalt compounds, as cobalt, is 0.1 mg per m^3 (long-term).

A report of increased concentrations of cobalt in the blood and urine of patients with cobalt-containing metallic hip replacements.— R. F. Coleman *et al.*, *Br. med. J.*, 1973, *1*, 527.

ALLERGY. Of 1205 persons with dermatitis or eczema submitted to patch testing with 2% aqueous solution of cobalt chloride, 12.3% gave a positive reaction.— E. Rudzki and D. Kleniewska, *Br. J. Derm.*, 1970, *83*, 543.

Of 4000 patients subjected to patch testing in 5 European clinics 7.4% of males and 6.6% of females showed positive reactions to cobalt chloride 2% in soft paraffin.— H. Bandmann *et al.*, *Archs Derm.*, 1972, *106*, 335.

For reports and comments on cobalt sensitivity in patients with cobalt-containing hip prostheses, see M. W. Elves *et al.*, *Br. med. J.*, 1975, *4*, 376; G. K. McKee (letter), *ibid.*, 646; D. A. Jones and K. Lucas (letter), *ibid.*, 647; D. A. Jones *et al.*, *J. Bone Jt Surg.*, 1975, *57B*, 289.

Further references: N. K. Veien and K. Kaaber, *Contact Dermatitis*, 1979, *5*, 371.

EFFECTS ON THE HEART. Autopsy on 4 patients with renal failure indicated that cobalt might be a prime cause of uraemic cardiomyopathy.— K. Pehrsson and L.-E. Lins (letter), *Lancet*, 1978, *2*, 51.

A report of cobalt cardiomyopathy in a 17-year-old girl on maintenance haemodialysis, who had been given cobalt chloride 25 mg twice daily for about 9 months.— I. H. Manifold *et al.*, *Br. med. J.*, 1978, *2*, 1609.

Fatal myocardial disease associated with industrial exposure to powdered cobalt.— A. Kennedy *et al.*, *Lancet*, 1981, *1*, 412.

Uses and Administration

Cobalt chloride, when administered to both normal and anaemic subjects, produces reticulocytosis and a rise in the erythrocyte count. This property suggested its use in the treatment of certain types of anaemia, but its general therapeutic use is, however, unjustified and not without danger.

In veterinary medicine, cobalt chloride has been given as a dietary supplement to ruminants.

For a review of cobalt deficiency and toxic effects, see Report of a WHO Expert Group on Trace Elements in Human Nutrition, *Tech. Rep. Ser. Wld Hlth Org. No. 532*, 1973, 29. See also E. J. Underwood, *Nutr. Rev.*, 1975, *33*, 65.

12598-d

Cobalt Oxide *(BAN)*

Tricobalt Tetroxide. It consists of cobalt (II, III) oxide (tricobalt tetroxide) with a small proportion of cobalt (III) oxide (dicobalt trioxide).

Co_3O_4=240.8.

CAS — 1308-06-1.

Pharmacopoeias. In *B.P. Vet.*

A black odourless powder. Practically **insoluble** in water; freely soluble in mineral acids and in solutions of the alkali hydroxides.

Cobalt oxide is used in veterinary practice for the prevention of cobalt deficiency in ruminants. The sulphate has been used similarly.

7357-q

Fractionated Coconut Oil *(BAN).*

Thin Vegetable Oil.

Pharmacopoeias. In *Br. Ger.* has a similar preparation (Triglycerida mediocatenalia) obtained from vegetable oils.

It is prepared from the fixed oil obtained from the dried solid part of the endosperm of the coconut, the fruit of *Cocos nucifera* (Palmae), by hydrolysis, fractionation of the liberated fatty acids and re-esterification. It consists of a mixture of triglycerides containing only short- and medium-chain saturated fatty acids, mainly octanoic and decanoic acids.

It is a clear pale yellow odourless or almost odourless liquid with a characteristic taste. It solidifies at about 0°, and has a low viscosity even at temperatures near its solidification point. Practically **insoluble** in water; miscible with alcohol, chloroform, and ether. **Store** at a temperature not exceeding 25° in well-filled containers. Protect from light.

NOTE. Coconut oil is described in the section on Paraffins and Similar Bases, p.1324.

Fractionated coconut oil has been used as a basis for the preparation of oral suspensions of drugs unstable in aqueous media.

Fractionated coconut oil is used as a source of medium-chain triglycerides. Diets based on medium-chain triglycerides are used in conditions associated with malabsorption of fat, such as cystic fibrosis, enteritis, and steatorrhoea, and following intestinal resection. Medium-chain triglycerides are more readily hydrolysed than long-chain triglycerides and are not dependent upon biliary or pancreatic secretions for absorption from the gastro-intestinal tract. They provide 35 kJ (8.3 kcal) per g. Preparations containing fractionated coconut oil and used in modified diets are described on p.1289.

12604-v

Coenzyme A

CoA; CoASH. 5′-*O*-{3-Hydroxy-3-[2-(2-mercaptoethylcarbamoyl)ethylcarbamoyl]-2,2-dimethylpropyl}adenosine-3′-dihydrogenphosphate-5′-trihydrogendiphosphate.

$C_{21}H_{36}N_7O_{16}P_3S$=767.5.

CAS — 85-61-0.

Formed from adenosine triphosphate, cysteine, and pantothenic acid, coenzyme A is involved in the body in many physiological roles, including the formation of citrate, the oxidation of pyruvate, the oxidation and synthesis of fatty acids, the synthesis of triglycerides, cholesterol, and phospholipids, and the acetylation of amines, choline, and glucosamine. It has been given by injection in a variety of metabolic disorders and for protection against irradiation. Coenzyme A is contra-indicated in acute myocardial infarction.

The administration of coenzyme A was associated with a delay in the progression of muscular dystrophy.— H. Radu (letter), *Lancet*, 1973, *2*, 576.

Proprietary Names and Manufacturers

Aluzime *(Alter, Spain)*; Co-A *(Millot-Solac, Fr.; Morrith, Spain)*; Coalip *(ISF, Ital.)*.

12605-g

Cogalactoisomerase Sodium

UDPG; Uridine-5′-diphosphoglucose Sodium.

$C_{15}H_{22}N_2Na_2O_{17}P_2,3H_2O$=664.3.

CAS — 133-89-1 (cogalactoisomerase).

Cogalactoisomerase is used in various hepatic disorders. It is used as the disodium salt.

Proprietary Names and Manufacturers

Anatox *(Lagap, Ital.)*; Antitoxicum *(Biopharma, Ital.)*; Atoxepan *(Dukron, Ital.)*; Bivitox *(Terapeutico M.R., Ital.)*; Detoxasi *(Miba, Ital.)*; Encrevar *(Ital.)*; Eparasi *(Ital.)*; Epatoxil *(Tosi-Novara, Ital.)*; Evident *(FIRMA, Ital.)*; Gilasi *(Ital.)*; Glucodin *(Ital.)*; Glucoepasi *(Inverni della Beffa, Ital.)*; Glucuril *(Ital.)*; Liotoxid *(Recordati, Ital.)*; Liverasi *(Francia Farm., Ital.)*; Netox *(Vita, Ital.)*; Novatox *(Pulitzer, Ital.)*; Toxalen *(Lifepharma, Ital.)*; Toxepasi *(Boehringer Biochemia, Ital.; IBYS, Spain)*; Toxizim *(Ital.)*; Udepasi *(Aandersen, Ital.)*; Udetox *(San Carlo, Ital.)*; Udicit *(CT, Ital.)*; Udifos *(Ausonia, Ital.)*; Urepasina *(Radiumfarma, Ital.)*; Uridasi *(Coli, Ital.)*; Zimeton *(Ital Suisse, Ital.)*.

16542-c

Colforsin *(USAN, rINN).*

Boforsin; Forscolin; Forskolin; HL-362; L-75-1362B. (3*R*,4a*R*,5*S*,6*S*,6a*S*,10*S*,10a*R*,10b*S*)-Dodecahydro-5,6,10,10b-tetrahydroxy-3,4a,7,7,10a-pentamethyl-3-vinyl-1*H*-naphtho[2,1-*b*]pyran-1-one, 5-acetate.

$C_{22}H_{34}O_7$=410.5.

CAS — 66575-29-9.

Colforsin is an adenylate cyclase stimulator under investigation for use topically in glaucoma and intravenously in congestive heart failure.

References: E. Lindner *et al., Arzneimittel-Forsch.*, 1978, *28*, 284; J. Caprioli and M. Sears, *Lancet*, 1983, *1*, 958; I. W. Rodger and M. Shahid, *Br. J. Pharmac.*, 1984, *81*, 151; E. Lindner and H. Metzger, *Arzneimittel-Forsch.*, 1983, *33*, 1436; J. Lichey *et al.* (letter), *Lancet*, 1984, *2*, 167; *Drugs of the Future*, 1984, *9*, 66; *ibid.*, 1985, *10*, 72; *ibid.*, 1986, *11*, 59; M. Aviram *et al., Br. J. clin. Pharmac.*, 1985, *19*, 715; W. Kramer *et al., Arzneimittel-Forsch.*, 1987, *37*, 364.

15335-n

Collagen

A fibrous protein component of mammalian connective tissue making up almost one third of the total body protein.

Collagen, processed in a variety of ways, has been used in surgery as a haemostatic and as a repair and suture material. For cosmetic purposes it has been injected into the dermis to correct scars and other contour deformities of the skin.

Reference: C. K. Varnavides *et al., Br. J. Derm.*, 1987, *116*, 199 (collagen injection for acne scars).

Proprietary Preparations

Colgen *(Thames, UK). Powder, dressing,* non-denatured collagen. For use as a haemostatic.

Lyodura *(Davis & Geck, UK). Transplant material,* mesh-like texture of collagenous fibres developed from homologous human dura mater cerebri. For repair of lesions and reinforcement of body tissue.

Tutoplast Dura *(E. Merck, UK). Transplant material,* absorbable collagen from dehydrated human dura mater. For repair or closure of body tissue.

Zyderm *(Kirby-Warrick, UK). Zyderm Test Collagen implant,* highly purified bovine dermal collagen 35 mg/mL with lignocaine 0.3%, in syringes containing 0.1 mL. For sensitivity testing.
Zyderm I Collagen implant, highly purified bovine dermal collagen 35 mg/mL with lignocaine 0.3%, in syringes containing 1 mL. For correction of contour deformities of the skin.
Zyderm II Collagen implant, highly purified bovine dermal collagen 65 mg/mL with lignocaine 0.3%, in syringes containing 0.75 mL. For correction of contour deformities of the skin.

Proprietary Names and Manufacturers

Avitene *(Alcon PR, USA)*; Colgen *(Thames, UK)*; Collafilm *(Merck-Clévenot, Fr.)*; Instat *(Johnson & Johnson, USA)*; Lyodura *(Davis & Geck, UK)*; Pangen *(Holphar, Ger.)*; Pon-Emo *(Vectem, Spain)*; Tutoplast Dura *(E. Merck, UK)*; Zyderm *(Essex, Austral.; Kirby-Warrick, UK)*.

18987-z

Colony Stimulating Factors

Colony stimulating factors which promote the proliferation and differentiation of haematopoietic precursors are under investigation as immunoregulating agents as an adjunct in cancer therapy.

References: G. Morstyn *et al., Lancet*, 1988, *1*, 667; M. A. Socinski *et al., ibid.*, 1194; J. L. Gabrilove *et al., New Engl. J. Med.*, 1988, *318*, 1414.

276-t

Colophony *(BAN).*

Coloph.; Colophane; Colophonium; Resin; Resina Pini; Resina Terebinthinae; Rosin *(USAN).*

CAS — 8050-09-7.

Pharmacopoeias. In *Aust., Br., Egypt., Jpn, Nord., Pol., Port., Span., Swiss,* and *U.S.*

The residue left after distilling the volatile oil from the oleoresin obtained from various species of *Pinus* (Pinaceae). Translucent, pale yellow or brownish-yellow, angular, brittle, readily fusible, glassy masses, with a faint terebinthinate odour. Practically **insoluble** in water; soluble in alcohol, carbon disulphide, chloroform, ether, some fixed and volatile oils, glacial acetic acid, and dilute solutions of alkali hydroxides; partly soluble in petroleum spirit. It should be **stored** in well-closed containers, preferably in the unground condition.

Colophony is an ingredient of some collodions and plaster-masses and it was formerly extensively used as an ingredient of ointments, as dressings for blisters, and wounds, and as an application for indolent ulcers and boils. Skin sensitisation and allergic respiratory symptoms have been reported.

12607-p

Comfrey

Comfrey Root; Symphytum. The dried root and rhizome of *Symphytum officinale* (Boraginaceae). It contains about 0.7% of allantoin, large quantities of mucilage, and some tannin.

Pharmacopoeias. In *Pol.*

Comfrey was formerly used as an application to wounds and ulcers to stimulate healing and was also given internally for gastric ulcers. The healing action of comfrey has been attributed to the presence of allantoin (see p.916).

There has been considerable debate as to the potential hepatotoxicity and carcinogenicity of ingested comfrey preparations due to their content of pyrrolizidine alkaloids.

Results indicating that contrary to some claims comfrey leaves are not a source of vitamin B_{12}.— R. W. Payne and B. F. Savage (letter), *Br. med. J.*, 1977, *2*, 458.

Comment on the potential carcinogenicity of comfrey. Liver tumours have been reported in *rats* fed on diets containing high doses of comfrey.— *Br. med. J.*, 1979, *1*, 598.

Work carried out by the Toxicology Unit of the MRC Laboratories has demonstrated toxic pyrrolizidine alkaloids in comfrey. The alkaloid concentrations are highest in small, young leaves, especially early in the season; large, mature leaves carry the lowest concentrations of toxic alkaloids. Moreover, protein extracted from comfrey should not be harmful. The external use of comfrey preparations should not be hazardous since the alkaloids are converted to toxic metabolites by liver enzymes.— A. R. Mattocks (letter), *Lancet*, 1980, *2*, 1136. Comment on comfrey and liver damage, and the recommendation that its use should be discouraged.— J. N. Roitman (letter), *ibid.*, 1981, *1*, 944. Comfrey toxicity in perspective.— C. Anderson (letter), *ibid.*, 1424.

Further references: D. Wiesner, *Aust. J. Pharm.*, 1984, *65*, 959 (review of comfrey toxicity); C. F. M. Weston *et al.*, *Br. med. J.*, 1987, *295*, 183 (veno-occlusive liver disease attributed to comfrey).

531-a

Condurango

Condurango Bark; Eagle-vine Bark.

CAS — 1401-98-5 (condurangin).

Pharmacopoeias. In *Aust.*, *Belg.*, *Jpn*, *Port.*, *Span.*, and *Swiss.*

The dried stem-bark of *Marsdenia condurango* (=*Gonolobus condurango*) (Asclepiadaceae).

Condurango has been used as a bitter.

7358-p

Cottonseed Oil *(USAN)*.

Aceite de Algodon; Cotton Oil; Ol. Gossyp. Sem.; Oléo de Algodoeiro; Oleum Gossypii Seminis.

CAS — 8001-29-4.

Pharmacopoeias. In *Arg.*, *Egypt.*, and *Mex.* Also in *U.S.N.F.*

The refined fixed oil obtained by expression or solvent extraction from the seeds of the cotton plant, *Gossypium hirsutum*, and other cultivated species of *Gossypium* (Malvaceae).

It is a pale yellow odourless or nearly odourless oil with a bland taste.

Slightly **soluble** in alcohol; miscible with carbon disulphide, chloroform, ether, and petroleum spirit. **Store** at a temperature not exceeding 40° in well-filled airtight containers. Protect from light. At temperatures below 10° particles of solid fat may separate from the oil and at temperatures between 0° and −5° it congeals.

Cottonseed oil emulsions have been given as a source of energy or when a nitrogen-free diet was required. It is used as an oily vehicle.

An extract of cottonseed oil, gossypol (p.1576), has been tried as an antifertility agent in males.

Proprietary Names and Manufacturers

Neo-Cholex *(Horner, Canad.)*.

2388-x

Coumarin

1,2-Benzopyrone; Cumarin; Tonka Bean Camphor. *2H*-1-Benzopyran-2-one.

$C_9H_6O_2$=146.1.

CAS — 91-64-5.

Coumarin is the odorous principle of Tonka seed (Tonka or Tonquin bean); it may be prepared synthetically.

Coumarin is used as a fixative in perfumery. It has been used as a flavouring agent to mask unpleasant odours but because of its toxicity this use is now considered undesirable and it is no longer used as a food additive. It is reported to be an immunostimulant and has been tried in the treatment of malignant neoplasms.

Coumarin is reported to be a macrophage stimulant and has been tried with cimetidine in the treatment of melanoma and other tumours. References: R. D. Thornes *et al.* (letter), *Lancet*, 1982, *2*, 328; R. D. Thornes and G. Lynch (letter), *New Engl. J. Med.*, 1983, *308*, 591; M. E. Marshall *et al.*, *J. clin. Oncol.*, 1987, *5*, 862.

19000-w

Coumermycin *(USAN, pINN)*.

5-Methylpyrrole-2-carboxylic acid, diester with 3,3′-[(3-methylpyrrole-2,4-diyl)bis(carbonylimino)]bis{4-hydroxy-8-methyl-7-[(tetrahydro-3,4-dihydroxy-5-methoxy-6,6-dimethylpyran-2-yl)oxy]-coumarin}.

$C_{55}H_{59}N_5O_{20}$=1110.1.

CAS — 4434-05-3.

Coumermycin is an antibiotic reported to be active *in vitro* against methicillin-resistant *Staphylococcus aureus.*

Some references to coumermycin's antibacterial activity: D. C. Hooper *et al.*, *Antimicrob. Ag. Chemother.*, 1982, *22*, 662; H. C. Neu *et al.*, *ibid.*, 1984, *25*, 687; M. E. Gombert and T. M. Aulicino, *ibid.*, *26*, 933; O. E. Varnier *et al.*, *J. antimicrob. Chemother.*, 1984, *14*, 139; K. E. Aldridge *et al.*, *Antimicrob. Ag. Chemother.*, 1985, *28*, 634; B. R. Meyers *et al.*, *ibid.*, 706; D. E. Taylor *et al.*, *ibid.*, 708; M. G. Thomas and S. D. R. Lang (letter), *J. antimicrob. Chemother.*, 1985, *16*, 675; H. Hof, *J. Infect.*, 1986, *13*, 17; M. G. Thomas and S. D. R. Lang, *J. antimicrob. Chemother.*, 1986, *18*, 171; M. N. Guillemin *et al.*, *Antimicrob. Ag. Chemother.*, 1986, *29*, 608; C. M. Perronne *et al.*, *ibid.*, 1987, *31*, 539; P. Van der Auwera and P. Joly, *J. antimicrob. Chemother.*, 1987, *19*, 313.

12615-p

CR Gas

EA-3547. Dibenz[*b,f*][1,4]oxazepine.

$C_{13}H_9NO$=195.2.

CAS — 257-07-8.

A riot-control gas with properties similar to those of CS gas (see below). CR gas is reported not to be hydrolysed by water and therefore to be capable of use in water cannons.

12616-s

Creatinolfosfate Sodium *(rINNM)*.

The sodium salt of 1-(2-hydroxyethyl)-1-methylguanidine *O*-phosphate.

$C_4H_{11}N_3NaO_4P$=219.1.

CAS — 6903-79-3 (creatinolfosfate).

Creatinolfosfate is used as an adjuvant in the treatment of cardiac disorders.

For a series of papers, see *Arzneimittel-Forsch.*, 1979, *29*, 1445–94.

Further reference: M. Knippel *et al.*, *Curr. ther. Res.*, 1985, *37*, 369.

Proprietary Names and Manufacturers

Aplodan *(Simes, Ital.)*; Dragosil *(Farmasimes, Spain)*; Gipron *(Serpero, Ital.)*.

1983-p

Croconazole *(rINN)*.

710674-S; Cloconazole. 1-(1-{*o*-[(*m*-Chlorobenzyl)oxy]phenyl}vinyl)imidazole.

$C_{18}H_{15}ClN_2O$=310.8.

CAS — 77175-51-0.

Croconazole is used topically as an antifungal agent.

References: *Drugs Today*, 1986, *22*, 427.

Proprietary Names and Manufacturers

Shionogi, Jpn.

3034-h

Cromakalim *(BAN, pINN)*.

BRL-34915. (±)-*trans*-3,4-Dihydro-3-hydroxy-2,2-dimethyl-4-(2-oxopyrrolidin-1-yl)-*2H*-chromene-6-carbonitrile.

$C_{16}H_{18}N_2O_3$=286.3.

CAS — 94470-67-4.

Cromakalim is a potassium channel activator under investigation as an antihypertensive agent.

The cardiovascular effects of cromakalim.— J. S. Fox *et al.*, *Br. J. clin. Pharmac.*, 1987, *23*, 600P.

12021-v

Crotalaria

Liver damage has been reported following the ingestion of *Crotalaria* spp. used for their alleged medicinal properties.

References: *Br. med. J.*, 1979, *1*, 574; R. G. Penn, *Adverse Drug React. Bull.*, 1983, Oct., 376.

12618-e

CS Gas

α-(*o*-Chlorobenzylidene)malononitrile.

$C_{10}H_5ClN_2$=188.6.

CAS — 2698-41-1.

CS gas has been used as a riot-control gas.

Its toxic effects include irritation of the eyes and nose, with copious lachrymation and rhinorrhoea; a burning sensation of the mouth and throat; pain in the chest, with difficulty in breathing; coughing; an increase in salivation; and retching and vomiting. These effects usually disappear a few minutes after exposure ends. The effects of pre-existing disease of the chest may be exacerbated. Erythema and blistering of the skin may occur.

Exposed persons should be removed from the contaminated area. Treatment is symptomatic. Contaminated skin should be washed with soap and water. If contamination of the eyes has been severe they should be irrigated with physiological saline or water and amethocaine instilled to relieve pain.

Application of CS gas 20 to 30 mg under a watch glass on the skin of healthy men for a period of 1 hour produced faint erythema and transient irritation. The erythema faded over a period of 1 to 2 days leaving no residual pigmentation or blanching of the skin; there was no irritation or pruritus during the stage of erythema, and no vesication occurred. When the material was moistened the reactions were slightly more severe and occurred with quantities of 10 mg.— P. Holland and R. G. White, *Br. J. Derm.*, 1972, *86*, 150.

A discussion of the possible carcinogenicity of CS gas.— *Br. med. J.*, 1973, *1*, 129.

CS gas, administered by inhalation to *rats* and *rabbits*, and by intraperitoneal injection to *rats*, was not teratogenic.— D. E. Upshall, *Toxic. appl. Pharmac.*, 1973, *24*, 45.

Further references: *Report of the Enquiry into the Medical and Toxicological aspects of CS*, Part 1, London, HM Stationery Office, 1969; *ibid.*, Part 2, London, HM Stationery Office, 1971; G. R. N. Jones, *Nature*, 1972, *235*, 257; S. Park and S. T. Giammona, *Am. J. Dis. Child.*, 1972, *123*, 245; L. Leadbeater, *Toxic. appl. Pharmac.*, 1973, *25*, 101.

532-t

Cusparia

Angostura Bark; Carony Bark; Cusparia Bark.

The bark of *Galipea officinalis* (Rutaceae).

Cusparia has been used as a bitter.

It should be noted that 'Angostura Bitters' (*Dr. J.G.B. Siegert & Sons Ltd*) contain gentian and various aromatic ingredients but no cusparia; they are named after the town in which they were first made.

12619-l

Cyanoacrylate Adhesives

CAS — 1069-55-2 (bucrylate); 6606-65-1 (enbucrilate); 137-05-3 (mecrylate).

A number of cyanoacrylate compounds have been used as surgical tissue adhesives. They include bucrylate (isobutyl 2-cyanoacrylate, $C_8H_{11}NO_2$=153.2), enbucrilate (butyl 2-cyanoacrylate,$C_8H_{11}NO_2$=153.2), and mecrylate (methyl 2-cyanoacrylate, $C_5H_5NO_2$=111.1).

Bucrylate has been tried in occlusive therapy and mecrylate has been used to produce female steri-

lisation by occluding the fallopian tubes.
The manufacturers of a cyanoacrylate adhesive have stated that accidental spilling of cyanoacrylates on skin, mucous membranes, or eyes causes no permanent damage and surgery should never be necessary to separate accidentally bonded skin. In the event of accidental skin adhesion they recommend that the bonded surfaces should be immersed in warm soapy water, the surfaces peeled or rolled apart with the aid of a spatula, and the adhesive removed from the skin with soap and water; attempts should not be made to pull the surfaces apart. Eyelids stuck together or bonded to the eyeball should be washed thoroughly with warm water and a gauze patch applied; the eye will open without further action in 1 to 4 days. Manipulative attempts to open the eyes should not be made. Although cyanoacrylate introduced into the eyes may cause double vision and lachrymation they state that there is no residual damage. If lips are accidentally stuck together plenty of warm water should be applied and maximum wetting and pressure from saliva inside the mouth encouraged. Lips should be peeled or rolled apart and not pulled. Adhesive introduced into the mouth solidifies and adheres, but saliva will lift the adhesive in ½ to 2 days. Care should be taken to avoid choking.
Heat is evolved on solidification of cyanoacrylate and in rare cases may cause burns.

Management of 3 patients with accidentally bonded digits and one with adhesive in the eye.— A. K. Maitra, *Br. J. clin. Pract.*, 1984, *38*, 284.

Accidental instillation of Super Glue into the eye in mistake for eye-drops.— S. J. Morgan and N. J. Astbury, *Br. med. J.*, 1984, *289*, 226.

Dermatitis due to a cyanoacrylate adhesive.— E. D. Shelley and W. B. Shelley, *J. Am. med. Ass.*, 1984, *252*, 2455.

Asthma and rhinitis associated with the use of cyanoacrylate adhesives on model aircraft.— S. K. Kopp *et al.*, *Ann. intern. Med.*, 1985, *102*, 613.

USES. The use of enbucrilate as an adjunct in some types of retinal detachment surgery.— L. Regenbogen *et al.*, *Br. J. Ophthal.*, 1976, *60*, 561.

The successful removal of a stone from the oesophagus using Loctite Super Glue 3.— D. S. Macpherson and R. Wyatt, *Br. med. J.*, 1978, *2*, 476.

Complete pain relief was obtained in 3 of 6 patients with chronic alcoholic pancreatitis, following ductal obstruction by low-pressure injection of a rapid-setting cyanoacrylate glue into the pancreatic duct. The patients were given pancreatic supplements by mouth.— J. M. Little *et al.* (preliminary communication), *Lancet*, 1979, *2*, 557. Encouraging results with similar glues.— W. Rosch and C. Gebhardt (letter), *ibid.*, 1131; W. Land and H. Weitz (letter), *ibid.*

Use of bucrylate to embolise intracranial arteriovenous malformations.— H. V. Vinters *et al.*, *New Engl. J. Med.*, 1986, *314*, 477.

3712-n

Cyclobutyrol Sodium *(rINNM)*.

Sodium 2-(1-hydroxycyclohexyl)butyrate.
$C_{10}H_{17}NaO_3$=208.2.

CAS — 512-16-3 (cyclobutyrol); 1130-23-0 (sodium salt).

Cyclobutyrol sodium is a choleretic. It has been given in doses of 0.5 to 2 g daily, by mouth, in divided doses with meals and in doses of 500 mg intramuscularly or intravenously daily or on alternate days to a total dose of 3 g in 12 days.

Proprietary Names and Manufacturers
Bis-bil *(Isola-Ibi, Ital.)*; Cytinium *(Roques, Fr.)*; Epa-Bon *(Sifarma, Ital.)*; Hebucol *(Belg.; Logeais, Fr.; Logeais, Switz.)*; Lipotrin *(Jpn)*; Secrobil *(Ital.)*; Tri-bil *(Biologici Italia, Ital.)*; Tribilina *(Farge, Ital.)*.

16595-g

Cyclodextrins

Cyclodextrins (α-cyclodextrin, β-cyclodextrin, and γ-cyclodextrin) are produced by the enzymatic degradation of starch and have been used as carrier molecules for drug delivery systems.

References: J. S. Pagington, *Chem. in Br.*, 1987, *23*, 455; *Pharm. J.*, 1987, *2*, 377.

18624-e

Cycloprolol *(BAN)*.

Cicloprolol *(pINN)*; SL-75177-10 (hydrochloride). 1-{4-[2-(Cyclopropylmethoxy)ethoxy]phenoxy}-3-(isopropylamino)propan-2-ol.
$C_{18}H_{29}NO_4$=323.4.

CAS — 63659-12-1 (cycloprolol); 63686-79-3 (hydrochloride.

NOTE. Cycloprolol Hydrochloride is *USAN*.

Cycloprolol has been reported to have both beta-blocking activity and beta-agonist activity.

References: P. M. McCaffrey *et al.*, *Br. J. clin. Pharmac.*, 1987, *23*, 601P; B. Silke *et al.*, *ibid.*, 602P.

3713-h

Cyclovalone *(rINN)*.

Divanillidenecyclohexanone. 2,6-Divanillylidenecyclohexanone.
$C_{22}H_{22}O_5$=366.4.

CAS — 579-23-7.

Cyclovalone is a choleretic. It has been given in doses of 300 to 900 mg daily in divided doses.

Proprietary Names and Manufacturers
Vanidene *(Belgana, Belg.)*; Vanilon *(Uquifa, Spain)*; Vanilone *(Nicholas, Fr.)*.

3714-m

Cynara

Alcachôfra; Artichaut; Artichoke Leaf.

Pharmacopoeias. In *Braz.*, *Fr.*, and *Roum.*

The leaves of the globe artichoke, *Cynara scolymus* (Compositae).

NOTE. The Jerusalem artichoke is *Helianthus tuberosus* (Compositae).

Cynara is reputed to have diuretic and choleretic properties.

Proprietary Names and Manufacturers
Chophytol *(Rosa-Phytopharma, Fr.; CT, Ital.)*.

The following names have been used for multi-ingredient preparations containing cynara— Artéchol *(Anglo-French Laboratories, Canad.)*; Bilogene *(Bio-Chemical Laboratory, Canad.)*; Hepax *(Sabex, Canad.)*.

3715-b

Cynarine

1,5-Dicaffeoylquinic Acid; Cynarin. 1-Carboxy-4,5-dihydroxy-1,3-cyclohexylene bis(3,4-dihydroxycinnamate).
$C_{25}H_{24}O_{12}$=516.5.

CAS — 1182-34-9; 1884-24-8.

Cynarine is an active ingredient of cynara (see above). It is used as a choleretic in doses of 200 to 250 mg three times daily. It is also used for the treatment of hyperlipidaemia and hypercholesteraemia and has been given in doses of 500 mg twice daily initially followed by 250 mg twice daily for maintenance therapy.

References: M. Montini *et al.*, *Arzneimittel-Forsch.*, 1975, *25*, 1311; W. H. Hammerl *et al.*, *Wien. med. Wschr.*, 1973, *123*, 601.

Proprietary Names and Manufacturers
Cinarcaf *(Ital.)*; Listrocol *(Farmitalia, Ger.)*.

12622-q

Cytochrome C

A haemoprotein occurring in the body and involved in electron and hydrogen transport in biological oxidation processes.

CAS — 9007-43-6.

Pharmacopoeias. Chin. includes Cytochrome C Solution and preparations for injection.

Cytochrome C has been given intravenously in various hypoxic conditions.
Earlier encouraging results with cytochrome C have not been substantiated in subsequent *animal* studies on the treatment of poisoning with *Amanita phalloides* .

Proprietary Names and Manufacturers
Biocytmet *(Biosedra, Arg.)*; Cytochrom C-Uvocal *(Mulli, Ger.)*; Cyto-Mack *(Szama, Arg.; Mack, Switz.)*.

19035-r

Dapiprazole *(rINN)*.

5,6,7,8-Tetrahydro-3-[2-(4-*o*-tolyl-1-piperazinyl)ethyl]-*s*-triazolo[4,3-*a*]pyridine.
$C_{19}H_{27}N_5$=325.5.

CAS — 72822-12-9.

An alpha-adrenoceptor blocking agent administered as eye-drops in the treatment of glaucoma. Dapiprazole may also have antipsychotic activity.

References: L. Bonomi *et al.*, *Curr. ther. Res.*, 1983, *34*, 469; B. Catanese *et al.*, *Boll. chim.-farm.*, 1984, *123*, 27S.

Proprietary Names and Manufacturers
Glamidolo *(Angelini, Ital.)*.

16600-w

Dazmegrel *(BAN, USAN, rINN)*.

UK-38485. 3-(3-Imidazol-1-ylmethyl-2-methylindol-1-yl)propionic acid.
$C_{16}H_{17}N_3O_2$=283.3.

CAS — 76894-77-4.

Dazmegrel is a thromboxane synthetase inhibitor with antithrombotic activity.

References: A. H. Barnett *et al.*, *Lancet*, 1984, *1*, 1322; M. H. A. Rustin *et al.*, *Eur. J. clin. Pharmac.*, 1984, *27*, 61; R. P. Walt *et al.*, *Gut*, 1987, *28*, 541.

Proprietary Names and Manufacturers
Pfizer, USA.

16613-z

Dazoxiben *(BAN, pINN)*.

UK-37248. 4-(2-Imidazol-1-ylethoxy)benzoic acid.
$C_{12}H_{12}N_2O_3$=232.2.

CAS — 78218-09-4; 74226-22-5 (hydrochloride).

NOTE. Dazoxiben Hydrochloride is *USAN*.

Dazoxiben is a thromboxane synthetase inhibitor with antiplatelet activity and is under investigation in a similar variety of disorders to those in which aspirin has been employed as an anti-platelet agent.

A series of papers on dazoxiben including some pharmacological and clinical studies in man.— *Br. J. clin. Pharmac.*, 1983, *15*, *Suppl.* 1, 1S–140S.

Some references to clinical studies with dazoxiben: S. R. Reuben *et al.*, *Br. J. clin. Pharmac.*, 1983, *15*, 83S (no benefit in chronic stable angina); J. J. F. Belch *et al.*, *ibid.*, 113S (improvement in Raynaud's syndrome); T.

Hendra *et al.* (letter), *Lancet*, 1983, *1*, 1041 (no benefit in stable angina); W. H. Ettinger *et al.*, *Am. J. Med.*, 1984, *77*, 451 (no benefit in Raynaud's phenomenon); R. Malamet *et al.*, *ibid.*, 1985, *78*, 602 (no benefit in Raynaud's phenomenon); R. Joseph *et al.*, *Headache*, 1985, *25*, 204 (improvement in migraine).

19045-d

Deazauridine

3-Deazauridine; NSC-126849; WR-199830.

Deazauridine is under investigation as an antineoplastic agent.

References: *Drugs of the Future*, 1986, *11*, 886.

18626-y

Defibrotide *(BAN, rINN).*

Polydeoxyribonucleotides from bovine lung or other mammalian organs with molecular weight between 15 000 and 30 000.

An antithrombotic and fibrinolytic agent.

References: V. Bonomini *et al.*, *Nephron*, 1984, *37*, 144; V. Bonomini *et al.*, *ibid.*, 1985, *40*, 195.

Proprietary Names and Manufacturers
Noravid *(Roussel Maestretti, Ital.)*; Prociclide *(Crinos, Ital.)*.

3716-v

Dehydrocholic Acid *(BAN, USAN, rINN).*

Chologon; Triketocholanic Acid. 3,7,12-Trioxo-5β-cholan-24-oic acid.
$C_{24}H_{34}O_5$=402.5.

CAS — 81-23-2.

Pharmacopoeias. In *Aust.*, *Cz.*, *Hung.*, *It.*, *Jpn*, *Jug.*, *Mex.*, *Pol.*, *Rus.*, and *U.S. Braz.* includes Sodium Dehydrocholate.

A white fluffy odourless powder with a bitter taste. Practically **insoluble** in water; soluble 1 in 100 of alcohol and 1 in 35 of chloroform; soluble 1 in 130 of acetone, 1 in 135 of acetic acid and ethyl acetate, and 1 in 2200 of ether at 15°; solutions in alcohol and chloroform are usually slightly turbid; soluble in glacial acetic acid and in solutions of alkali hydroxides and carbonates.

Dehydrocholic acid is a semi-synthetic bile acid (see p.1547) which increases the volume and water content of the bile without appreciably altering the content of bile acids. It has been used to improve biliary drainage and has also been given for the temporary relief of constipation. Doses of up to 750 mg three times daily by mouth have been employed.
Sodium dehydrocholate has been used by slow intravenous injection.
Dehydrocholic acid is contra-indicated in complete mechanical biliary obstruction and in severe hepatitis.

Preparations

Dehydrocholate Sodium Injection *(U.S.P.).* Usually prepared by neutralising dehydrocholic acid. pH 8.5 to 9.5. Protect from light.

Dehydrocholic Acid Tablets *(U.S.P.)*

Proprietary Names and Manufacturers of Dehydrocholic Acid and Sodium Dehydrocholate
Biochol *(Jpn)*; Bio-Cholin *(Canad.)*; Chetocolina *(Ital.)*; Cholan-DH *(Pennwalt, USA)*; Cholan-HMB *(Pennwalt, USA)*; Choleubil *(Ibsa, Switz.)*; Cholypyl *(Canad.)*; Decholin *(Canad.*; *Cassella-Riedel, Ger.*; *Ital.*; *Switz.*; *Miles Pharmaceuticals, USA)*; Dehidrocolin *(Spain)*; Dehydrocholin *(Duncan, Flockhart, UK)*; Deidrocolico *(Ital.)*; Deidrocolit *(Ital.)*; Deidrosan *(Ital.)*; Dicolan *(Biologici Italia, Ital.)*; Didrocolo *(Recofarma, Ital.)*; Dycholium *(Rhône-Poulenc, Canad.*; *Théraplix, Fr.)*; Hepahydrin *(Great Southern, USA)*; Idrocrine *(Canad.)*; Medichol *(Medic, Canad.)*; Neocholan *(Merrell Dow, USA)*.

The following names have been used for multi-ingredient preparations containing dehydrocholic acid and sodium dehydrocholate— Bilax *(Drug Industries, USA)*; Cholibile *(Bio-Chemical Laboratory, Canad.)*; Neolax *(Central Pharmaceuticals, USA)*; Sarolax *(Saron, USA)*; Trilax *(Drug Industries, USA)*.

3933-j

Demexiptiline Hydrochloride *(rINNM).*

LM-2909. *O*-[2-(methylamino)ethyl]oxime-5*H*-dibenzo[*a*,*d*]cyclohepten-5-one hydrochloride.
$C_{18}H_{19}N_2OCl$=313.9.

CAS — 24701-51-7 (demexiptiline).

Demexiptiline hydrochloride is a tricyclic antidepressant.

Proprietary Names and Manufacturers
Deparon *(Aron, Fr.)*.

533-x

Denatonium Benzoate *(BAN, USAN, rINN).*

NSC-157658. Benzyldiethyl(2,6-xylylcarbamoylmethyl)ammonium benzoate monohydrate.
$C_{28}H_{34}N_2O_3,H_2O$=464.6.

CAS — 3734-33-6(anhydrous); 86398-53-0(monohydrate).

Pharmacopoeias. In *U.S.N.F.*

A white odourless crystalline powder with an intensely bitter taste. **Soluble** 1 in 20 of water, 1 in about 2 of alcohol, and 1 in about 3 of chloroform; very slightly soluble in ether. A 3% solution in water has a pH of 6.5 to 7.5. **Store** in airtight containers.

Denatonium benzoate is used where an intensely bitter taste is required for medicinal or industrial purposes and as a partial denaturant for alcohol in toilet preparations.

Proprietary Names and Manufacturers
Bitrex *(Macfarlan Smith, UK)*.

19049-b

Denopamine *(rINN).*

TA-064. (−)-(*R*)-α-{[(3,4-Dimethoxyphenethyl)amino]methyl}-*p*-hydroxybenzyl alcohol.
$C_{18}H_{23}NO_4$=317.4.

CAS — 71771-90-9.

Denopamine is a beta$_1$-agonist under investigation for the treatment of heart failure.

References: J. Thormann *et al.*, *Am. Heart J.*, 1985, *110*, 426.

12631-p

2-Deoxy-D-glucose

$C_6H_{12}O_5$=164.2.

CAS — 154-17-6.

2-Deoxy-D-glucose has been tried topically as an antiviral agent.

Report of the successful treatment of human genital herpes infections with 2-deoxy-D-glucose.— H. A. Blough and R. L. Giuntoli, *J. Am. med. Ass.*, 1979, *241*, 2798. Criticism.— L. Corey and K. K. Holmes (letter), *ibid.*, *243*, 29. See also *ibid.*, 1980, *244*, 2022.

A study of the antiviral mechanism of action of 2-deoxy-D-glucose.— J. G. Spivack *et al.*, *Virology*, 1982, *123*, 123.

12632-s

Deoxyribonucleic Acid

ADN; Animal Nucleic Acid; Desoxypentose Nucleic Acid; Desoxyribonucleic Acid; Desoxyribose Nucleic Acid; DNA; Thymus Nucleic Acid.

Pharmacopoeias. In *Fr.*

A nucleotide polymer, and 1 of the 2 distinct varieties of nucleic acid (see p.1596). It is found in the cell nuclei of living tissues.

Several proprietary preparations of deoxyribonucleic acid are marketed in some countries and are advocated for a variety of asthenic and convalescent conditions.

For the use of deoxyribonucleic acid by intradermal injection in the diagnosis of systemic lupus erythematosus, see R. O. Ores and E. H. Mandel, *Br. J. Derm.*, 1971, *84*, 217.

A review of the use of deoxyribonucleic acid as a carrier for antineoplastic agents.— A. Trouet *et al.*, Desoxyribonucleic Acid as Carrier of Antitumour Drugs, in *Drug Carriers in Biology and Medicine*, G. Gregoriadis (Ed.), London, Academic Press, 1979, pp. 87–105.

Proprietary Names and Manufacturers
A.D.N. *(Biostabilex, Fr.*; *Mayoly-Spindler, Fr.)*; Desoxiribon *(Craveri, Arg.)*; Eucytol *(Mayoly-Spindler, Fr.*; *Mayoly-Spindler, Switz.)*; Nuclifort *(Mayoly-Spindler, Fr.)*.

7869-p

Dexpanthenol *(BAN, USAN, rINN).*

Dextro-Pantothenyl Alcohol; Pantothenol. (*R*)-2,4-Dihydroxy-*N*-(3-hydroxypropyl)-3,3-dimethylbutyramide.
$C_9H_{19}NO_4$=205.3.

CAS — 81-13-0.

Pharmacopoeias. In *Aust.*, *Ind.*, *Nord.*, and *U.S. U.S.* also includes a racemic mixture under the title Panthenol.

A clear, odourless, hygroscopic, viscous liquid with a slight characteristic odour.
Freely **soluble** in water, alcohol, methyl alcohol, and propylene glycol; soluble in chloroform and ether; slightly soluble in glycerol. Some crystallisation may occur on standing. **Store** in airtight containers.

Adverse Effects and Precautions
There have been a few reports of allergic reactions associated with the administration of dexpanthenol although these have not been confirmed. Dexpanthenol is contra-indicated in haemophiliacs and in patients with ileus due to mechanical obstruction.

Uses and Administration
Dexpanthenol is the alcoholic analogue of pantothenic acid (p.1270). It has been given intramuscularly in doses of 250 to 500 mg to prevent or control gastro-intestinal atony but its value has not been established. It has also been given by slow intravenous infusion.
Dexpanthenol has been used topically as an ointment, cream, or solution, usually in a strength of 2%, for the treatment of various minor skin disorders.

Preparations

Dexpanthenol Preparation *(U.S.P.).* Contains dexpanthenol with pantolactone 2.7 to 4.2%.

Proprietary Names and Manufacturers
Bepanten *(Roche, Ital.)*; Bepanthen *(Roche, Austral.*; *Roche, Denm.*; *Roche, Ger.*; *Roche, Neth.*; *Roche, Swed.*; *Roche, Switz.)*; Bepanthene *(Roche, Belg.*; *Roche, Fr.*; *Roche, Spain*; *Roche, Switz.)*; Bepantol *(Roche, S.Afr.)*; Cutemul *(Pharmasal, Ger.)*; Dexol *(Legere, USA)*; Ilopan *(Adria, USA)*; Motilyn *(Abbott, Canad.)*; Panthoderm *(Arg.*; *USV, Canad.*; *USV Pharmaceutical Corp., USA)*; Panthogenat *(Azuchemie, Ger.)*; Thenalton *(Fulton, Ital.)*; Urupan *(Merckle, Ger.)*.

The following names have been used for multi-ingredient preparations containing dexpanthenol— Aquasol A Cream *(Rorer, Canad.)*; Dorbanate Liquid *(Riker, Austral.)*.

4810-e

Dextran Sulphate

Dextran Sulphate Sodium. The sodium salt of sulphuric acid esters of dextran.

CAS — 9042-14-2.

Dextran sulphate has been used similarly to heparin as an anticoagulant. Doses were expressed in units, 10 of which were considered to be approximately equivalent to 1 mg. Recent investigations of dextran sulphate have involved its antiviral activity.

Hydrogenated dextran sulphate has been used as an anti-ulcer agent.

Dextran sulphate potassium has been used as a hypolipidaemic.

In vitro studies on thrombin activity showed that dextran sulphates with a high molecular weight and high sulphur content inhibit thrombin activity directly and do not act via antithrombin III unlike heparin which may depend upon the presence of this factor to exert its anticoagulant effects.— K. Suzuki and S. Hashimoto, *J. clin. Path.*, 1979, *32*, 439.

Dextran sulphate possessed antiviral activity against HIV and displayed synergy with zidovudine *in vitro*: R. Ueno and S. Kuno (letter), *Lancet*, 1987, *1*, 1379; M. C. Berenbaum (letter), *ibid.*, *2*, 461; R. Ueno and S. Kuno (letter), *ibid.*, 796.

Proprietary Names and Manufacturers

Dextrarine *(Belg.; Egic, Switz.)*; Lipemol *(Rocador, Spain)*; MDS *(Jpn)*.

19066-v

Diaziquone *(USAN, pINN)*.

Aziridinylbenzoquinone; AZQ; CI-904; NSC-182986. Diethyl 2,5-bis-(1-aziridinyl)-3,6-dioxo-1,4-cyclohexadiene-1,4-dicarbamate.

$C_{16}H_{20}N_4O_6=364.4$.

CAS — 57998-68-2.

Diaziquone is under investigation as an antineoplastic agent.

References: G. A. Curt *et al.*, *Cancer Res.*, 1983, *43*, 6102; T. C. C. Tan, *ibid.*, 1984, *44*, 831; S. Zimm *et al.*, *ibid.*, 1698.

19071-h

Dichloroflavan

BW-683C. 4′,6-Dichloroflavan.

$C_{15}H_{12}Cl_2O=279.2$.

Dichloroflavan is under investigation as an antiviral agent against rhinoviruses.

Studies on the mode of action of dichloroflavan: M. Tisdale and J. W. T. Selway, *J. antimicrob. Chemother.*, 1984, *14*, *Suppl.* A, 97; Y. Ninomiya *et al.*, *Antimicrob. Ag. Chemother.*, 1985, *27*, 595. Failure of orally administered dichloroflavan to protect against experimentally induced rhinovirus infection in healthy subjects.— R. J. Phillpotts *et al.*, *Arch. Virol.*, 1983, *75*, 115.

205-b

Diethanolamine *(USAN)*.

Diaethanolamin; Diolamine *(pINN)*. Bis(2-hydroxyethyl)amine; 2,2′-Iminobisethanol.

$C_4H_{11}NO_2=105.1$.

CAS — 111-42-2.

Pharmacopoeias. In *Jug.* Also in *U.S.N.F.*, which specifies a mixture of ethanolamines consisting largely of diethanolamine.

White or clear, colourless crystals, deliquescing in moist air, or colourless liquid. **Miscible** with water, alcohol, acetone, chloroform, and glycerol; slightly soluble to insoluble in ether, and petroleum spirit. **Store** in airtight containers. Protect from light.

Diethanolamine is an organic base which is used as an emulsifying and dispersing agent.

It is used to solubilise, by the formation of the diethanolamine salt, fusidic acid. It has been used for the preparation of salts of iodinated organic acids used as contrast media. It may be irritating to the skin and mucous membranes.

19232-m

Difloxacin *(pINN)*.

A-56619 (hydrochloride); Abbott-56619 (hydrochloride). 6-Fluoro-1-(*p*-fluorophenyl)-1,4-dihydro-7-(4-methyl-1-piperazinyl)-4-oxo-3-quinolinecarboxylic acid.

$C_{21}H_{19}F_2N_3O_3=418.4$.

CAS — 98106-17-3; 91296-86-5 (hydrochloride).

NOTE. Difloxacin Hydrochloride is *USAN*.

Difloxacin is a fluorinated 4-quinolone antibacterial agent.

References: S. M. Smith, *Antimicrob. Ag. Chemother.*, 1986, *29*, 325 (*in vitro* activity against methicillin-resistant *Staphylococcus aureus*); G. R. Granneman *et al.*, *ibid.*, *30*, 689 (pharmacokinetics in healthy subjects); A. King and I. Phillips, *J. antimicrob. Chemother.*, 1986, *18*, *Suppl.* D, 1 (*in-vitro* activity); M. B. Bansal and H. Thadepalli, *Antimicrob. Ag. Chemother.*, 1987, *31*, 619 (*in-vitro* activity against clinical anaerobes).

12654-z

Dihydroxydibutylether

Hydroxybutyloxide. 4,4′-Oxybis(butan-2-ol).

$C_8H_{18}O_3=162.2$.

CAS — 821-33-0.

Dihydroxydibutylether is a choleretic agent.

Biliary secretion was increased by dihydroxydibutylether 300 to 750 mg by mouth.— F. Fici *et al.*, *Curr. ther. Res.*, 1976, *20*, 772.

Proprietary Names and Manufacturers

Boutybil *(Bouty, Ital.)*; Cistoquine *(Casasco, Arg.)*; Colenormol *(Beta, Ital.)*; Dis-Cinil *(Lusofarmaco, Ital.)*; Diskin *(Benedetti, Ital.)*; Dyskinébyl *(Zyma, Fr.)*; Dyskinebyl *(CCP, Belg.)*; Kinepar *(Berenguer-Beneyto, Spain)*; Liver-Chol *(Radiumfarma, Ital.)*.

19233-b

DL-*threo*-3,4-Dihydroxyphenylserine

DL-DOPS; DL-threo-DOPS; DOPS.

DL-*threo*-3,4-Dihydroxyphenylserine is a precursor of noradrenaline and is under investigation as an antiparkinsonian agent and in the treatment of orthostatic hypotension.

References: N. Ogawa *et al.*, *J. Med.*, 1985, *16*, 525 (benefit in parkinsonism); I. Biaggioni and D. Robertson, *Lancet*, 1987, *2*, 1170 (benefit in orthostatic hypotension); A. J. Man in't Veld *et al.*, *ibid.*, 1172 (benefit in orthostatic hypotension).

12655-c

Diiodhydrin

Iodazone; Iothion. 1,3-Di-iodopropan-2-ol.

$C_3H_6I_2O=311.9$.

CAS — 534-08-7.

NOTE. Distinguish iodazone from iodazine.

Diiodhydrin is an organic iodine-containing material for topical use; it is reported to have antibacterial properties.

Proprietary Names and Manufacturers

Glico-Iodazol *(Zambeletti, Ital.)*; Iodazol *(Zambeletti, Ital.)*.

3719-p

Di-isopromine Hydrochloride *(rINNM)*.

NN-Di-isopropyl-3,3-diphenylpropylamine hydrochloride.

$C_{21}H_{29}N,HCl=331.9$.

CAS — 5966-41-6 (di-isopromine); 24358-65-4 (hydrochloride).

Di-isopromine hydrochloride is an antispasmodic and choleretic used with sorbitol in gastro-intestinal disorders. It has been given in doses of 2 to 3 mg three times daily before meals.

Proprietary Names and Manufacturers

The following names have been used for multi-ingredient preparations containing di-isopromine hydrochloride—Agofell *(Janssen, Ger.; Janssen, S.Afr.)*; Bilagol *(Leo, Swed.)*; Do-Bil *(Dompè, Ital.)*; Galbil *(Janssen, Denm.)*; Mégabyl *(Janssen, Fr.)*.

206-v

Diisopropanolamine *(USAN)*.

1,1′-Iminobis(propan-2-ol).

$C_6H_{15}NO_2=133.2$.

CAS — 110-97-4.

Pharmacopoeias. In *U.S.N.F.*, which specifies a mixture of isopropanolamines consisting largely of diisopropanolamine.

Store in airtight containers. Protect from light.

Diisopropanolamine is an organic base which is used as a neutralising agent in cosmetics and toiletries.

18629-c

Dilevalol *(BAN, pINN)*.

R,R-Labetalol; Sch-19927 (hydrochloride). 5-{(*R*)-1-Hydroxy-2-[(*R*)-1-methyl-3-phenylpropylamino-]ethyl}salicylamide.

$C_{19}H_{24}N_2O_3=328.4$.

CAS — 75659-07-3; 75659-08-4 (hydrochloride).

NOTE. Dilevalol Hydrochloride is *USAN*.

Dilevalol is a beta-adrenoceptor blocking agent.

References: J. Soberman *et al.*, *J. clin. Hypertens.*, 1987, *3*, 271.

3720-n

Dimecrotic Acid *(rINN)*.

2,4-Dimethoxy-β-methylcinnamic acid.

$C_{12}H_{14}O_4=222.2$.

CAS — 7706-67-4.

Dimecrotic acid is a choleretic used as the magnesium salt ($C_{24}H_{26}MgO_8=466.8$). It has been given in doses of 50 mg three or four times daily with meals.

Proprietary Names and Manufacturers

Fisiobil *(Salvat, Spain)*; Hépadial *(Biocodex, Fr.)*.

3851-l

Dimethylhydroxypyridone

1,2-Dimethyl-3-hydroxypyrid-4-one.

$C_7H_9NO_2=139.2$.

Dimethylhydroxypyridone is an orally active iron chelator.

Effective use of dimethylhydroxypyridone in patients with iron overload (myelodysplasia or thalassaemia).— G. J. Kontoghiorghes *et al.*, *Br. med. J.*, 1987, *295*, 1509.

12659-x

3,5-Dimethyl-3′-isopropyl-L-thyronine

L-2-Amino-3-[4-(4-hydroxy-3-isopropylphenoxy)-3,5-dimethylphenyl]propionic acid.

$C_{20}H_{25}NO_4=343.4$.

3,5-Dimethyl-3′-isopropyl-L-thyronine is a thyroid hormone analogue.

A study in *rats* on the possible role of the thyroid hormone analogues 3,5-dimethyl-3′-isopropyl-L-thyronine (DIMIT), 3,5-di-iodo-3′-isopropyl-L-thyronine (DIIT), and 3,5-di-iodo-3′-*sec*-butyl-L-thyronine (DISBT) in the prevention of foetal goitre *in utero*.— F. Comite *et al.*, *Endocrinology*, 1978, *102*, 1670.

Further references: I. J. Chopra, *New Engl. J. Med.*, 1976, *295*, 335.

12660-y

Dimethylphenyliminothiazolidine Hydrorhodanide

CI-098. (−)-2-Imino-3,4-dimethyl-5-phenylthiazolidine thiocyanate.

$C_{11}H_{14}N_2S,HCNS=265.4$.

CAS — 14007-67-1 (dimethylphenyliminothiazolidine).

Dimethylphenyliminothiazolidine hydrorhodanide has been used in the treatment of various respiratory disorders. The hydrochloride and theophylline-7-acetate have also been used.

Proprietary Names and Manufacturers

The following names have been used for multi-ingredient preparations containing dimethylphenyliminothiazolidine hydrorhodanide— Priatan *(Schering, Austral.)*.

5013-y

Dimethyltryptamine

DMT; N,N-Dimethyltryptamine. 3-(2-Dimethylaminoethyl)indole.

$C_{12}H_{16}N_2=188.3$.

CAS — 61-50-7.

An active principle obtained from the seeds and leaves of *Piptadenia peregrina* (Mimosaceae) from which the hallucinogenic snuff cohoba is prepared and other South American plants.

Dimethyltryptamine produces hallucinogenic and sympathomimetic effects which are similar to those of lysergide (see p.1584), but of shorter duration. It has no therapeutic use. It is inactive when taken by mouth. Diethyltryptamine (DET) and dipropyltryptamine (DPT) are related synthetic hallucinogens with longer action but less potent than dimethyltryptamine.

References: A. Hofmann, *Indian J. Pharm.*, 1963, *25*, 245; D. R. Rubin (letter), *J. Am. med. Ass.*, 1967, *201*, 143; J. R. Unwin, *Can. med. Ass. J.*, 1968, *98*, 402.

12663-c

Dimophebumine Hydrochloride

Sp-281; Vetrabutin Hydrochloride. 1-(3,4-Dimethoxyphenyl)-*NN*-dimethyl-4-phenylbutylamine hydrochloride.

$C_{20}H_{27}NO_2,HCl=349.9$.

CAS — 3735-45-3 (dimophebumine).

Dimophebumine hydrochloride is a uterine relaxant which has been used to facilitate parturition.

Proprietary Names and Manufacturers

Monzal *(Thomae, Ger.)*.

Proprietary Veterinary Names and Manufacturers

Monzaldon *(Boehringer Ingelheim, UK)*.

5231-d

Dimoxyline Phosphate *(rINNM)*.

Dioxyline Phosphate; LO-8146. 1-(4-Ethoxy-3-methoxybenzyl)-6,7-dimethoxy-3-methylisoquinoline dihydrogen phosphate.

$C_{22}H_{25}NO_4,H_3PO_4=465.4$.

CAS — 147-27-3 (dimoxyline); 5667-46-9 (phosphate).

Dimoxyline phosphate is a synthetic analogue of papaverine (see p.1598). It has been given in doses of up to 600 mg daily by mouth as an antispasmodic mainly in ischaemia.

Proprietary Names and Manufacturers

Paveril *(Lilly, USA)*; Paverona *(Lilly, Ital.)*.

12667-x

Diosmin *(pINN)*.

Barosmin; Buchu Resin; Diosmetin 7-Rutinoside. 3′,5,7-Trihydroxy-4′-methoxyflavone 7-[6-*O*-(6-deoxy-α-L-mannopyranosyl)-β-D-glucopyranoside].

$C_{28}H_{32}O_{15}=608.6$.

CAS — 520-27-4.

Diosmin is a bioflavonoid which has been used similarly to rutin (see p.1610) in the treatment of venous disorders.

Proprietary Names and Manufacturers

Arvenum *(Stroder, Ital.)*; Daflon *(Servier, Fr.; Servier, Ital.; Servier, Spain; Servier, Switz.)*; Diosmil *(Bellon, Fr.)*; Diosminil *(Faes, Spain)*; Diovenor *(Innothéra, Fr.)*; Flebosmil *(Bouchara, Fr.)*; Flebosten *(Bonomelli, Ital.)*; Flebotropin *(Bago, Arg.)*; Insuven *(Berenguer-Beneyto, Spain)*; Tovene *(Kali-Chemie, Ger.)*; Ven-detrex *(Zyma, Switz.)*; Venosmine *(Geymonat, Ital.)*.

3923-l

Diprafenone *(rINN)*.

(±)-2′-[2-Hydroxy-3-(*tert*-pentylamino)propoxy]-3-phenylpropiophenone.

$C_{23}H_{31}NO_3=369.5$.

CAS — 81447-80-5; 86342-43-0 (hydrochloride).

Diprafenone is under investigation as an anti-arrhythmic agent.

Proprietary Names and Manufacturers

Helopharm, Ger.

12675-x

Disodium Guanylate

627; Disodium Guanosine-5′-monophosphate; Sodium 5′-Guanylate. Guanosine 5′-(disodium phosphate).

$C_{10}H_{12}N_5Na_2O_8P,xH_2O=407.2$.

CAS — 5550-12-9 (anhydrous).

Disodium guanylate has been used as a flavour enhancer in foods. The term sodium 5′-ribonucleotide has been used to refer to a mixture of disodium guanylate and disodium inosinate (see below).

12676-r

Disodium Inosinate

631; Disodium Inosine-5′-monophosphate; Sodium 5′-Inosinate. Inosine 5′-(disodium phosphate).

$C_{10}H_{11}N_4Na_2O_8P,xH_2O=392.2$.

CAS — 4691-65-0 (anhydrous).

Disodium inosinate has been used as a flavour enhancer in foods.

Proprietary Names and Manufacturers

Catacol *(P.O.S., Fr.; Alcon, Switz.)*.

2544-c

Disodium Oxidronate

HMDP (oxidronic acid); Oxidronate Disodium; Oxidronate Sodium; Sodium Oxidronate *(BANM)*. Disodium (hydroxymethylene)diphosphonate.

$CH_4Na_2O_7P_2=236.0$.

CAS — 14255-61-9; 15468-10-7 (oxidronic acid).

NOTE. Oxidronic Acid is *USAN* and *pINN*.

Disodium oxidronate is a biphosphonate similar to disodium etidronate.

2731-t

Disulfiram *(BAN, USAN, rINN)*.

Disulfiramum; Éthyldithiourame; TTD. Tetraethylthiuram disulphide; Bis(diethylthiocarbamoyl) disulfide.

$C_{10}H_{20}N_2S_4=296.5$.

CAS — 97-77-8.

Pharmacopoeias. In *Aust., Br., Fr., Cz., Hung., Jug., Roum., Swiss*, and *U.S.*

A white or almost white, odourless or almost odourless powder. *B.P.* **solubilities** are: practically insoluble in water; soluble 1 in 65 of alcohol, 1 in 2 of chloroform, and 1 in 20 of ether. *U.S.P.* solubilities are: very slightly soluble in water; soluble 1 in 30 of alcohol and 1 in 15 of ether; soluble in acetone, carbon disulphide, and chloroform. **Store** in airtight containers. Protect from light.

STABILITY. Studies on the stability of disulfiram preparations: V. D. Gupta, *Am. J. Hosp. Pharm.*, 1981, *38*, 363 (aqueous suspensions); M. Phillips *et al.*, *ibid.*, 1985, *42*, 343 (gamma-irradiated disulfiram for injection).

Adverse Effects

Drowsiness and fatigue are common during initial treatment with disulfiram. Other side-effects reported include a garlic-like or metallic after-taste, gastro-intestinal upsets, body odour, bad breath, headache, impotence, and allergic contact dermatitis. Peripheral and optic neuropathies, psychotic reactions, and hepatotoxicity may occur.

Disulfiram-alcohol reaction. The use of disulfiram in the management of alcoholism is based on the extremely unpleasant, but generally self-limiting, systemic effects which occur when a patient receiving the drug ingests alcohol. These effects begin with flushing of the face and, as vasodilatation spreads, throbbing in the head and neck and a pulsating headache may develop. Respiratory difficulties, nausea, copious vomiting, sweating, thirst, chest pain, tachycardia, palpitations, marked hypotension, giddiness, weakness, blurred vision, and confusion may follow. The intensity and duration of symptoms is very variable and even small quantities of alcohol may result in alarming reactions. In addition to the above effects, reactions have included respiratory depression, cardiovascular collapse, cardiac arrhythmias, myocardial infarction, acute congestive heart failure, unconsciousness, convulsions, and sudden death. Severe reactions require intensive supportive therapy; the intravenous administration of ascorbic acid, iron salts, or antihistamines has been suggested but no benefit has been established.

Comparison of the reported neurotoxic effects of disulfiram with those of its major metabolites suggested that carbon disulphide was responsible for the behavioural and neurological side-effects of disulfiram. Disulfiram, carbon disulphide, and another metabolite, diethyldithiocarbamate, have all been reported to inhibit dopamine-β-hydroxylase *in vitro* and *in vivo* in *animals*.— J. M. Rainey, *Am. J. Psychiat.*, 1977, *134*, 371. Behavioural toxicity might be the result of altered catecholamine concentrations in the brain, since disulfiram and its metabolite diethyldithiocarbamate have been reported to inhibit dopamine-β-hydroxylase, thus increasing dopamine and reducing noradrenaline concentrations in the brain and other tissues.— E. M. Sellers *et al.*, *New Engl. J. Med.*, 1981, *305*, 1255. Instances of behavioural toxicity are given under Overdosage and Effects on the nervous system, below.

Numerous side-effects, including tiredness, sleepiness, dizziness, sexual problems, poor memory, headache, unpleasant taste, bad breath and body odour, gastro-intestinal disturbances, and rash have been reported with disulfiram, but they could also be interpreted as symptoms of long-standing alcohol abuse. Side-effects were reassessed in a double-blind multicentre study completed by 158 alcoholics. Patients received either disulfiram 200 mg daily or placebo for 6 weeks and were questioned weekly about 27 expected and non-expected symptoms. There was no significant difference in side-effects between disulfiram and placebo except that sexual problems were over-represented in the placebo group.— J. K. Christensen *et al.*, *Acta psychiat. scand.*, 1984, *69*, 265.

EFFECTS ON THE BLOOD. There were isolated reports of blood dyscrasias associated with disulfiram in the 1960s. The US manufacturer recommends that blood counts should be performed every 6 months during treatment.

EFFECTS ON THE CARDIOVASCULAR SYSTEM. An alcoholic

with liver damage developed marked but reversible hypertension after receiving disulfiram 125 mg daily for over 6 months.— L. Volicer and K. L. Nelson, *Archs intern. Med.*, 1984, *144*, 1294.

EFFECTS ON THE JOINTS. A 49-year-old man developed painful swelling of the wrists and knees accompanied by carpal tunnel syndrome after taking disulfiram 250 mg daily by mouth for 2 months. Another patient complained of joint pains after 6 weeks of disulfiram therapy. Symptoms were reversible in both patients.— J. F. Howard, *Arthritis Rheum.*, 1982, *25*, 1494.

EFFECTS ON THE LIVER. Six patients developed signs of liver damage 3 to 25 weeks after starting to take disulfiram. All developed coma and 5 died. A causal relationship was confirmed by challenge test in the surviving patient.— L. Ranek and P. B. Andreasen, *Br. med. J.*, 1977, *2*, 94.

A 32-year-old woman who had been taking disulfiram 400 mg every second day for 2 months presented with small acneform eruptions on her legs and later developed a liver hypersensitivity reaction accompanied by extrahepatic allergic manifestations of rash, fever, and eosinophilia. Previous reports of disulfiram-induced liver damage were reviewed and jaundice appeared to be one of the commonest clinical signs whereas extrahepatic manifestations were infrequent. It was concluded that either disulfiram-related hepatic disease was extremely rare or had been overlooked because of the high prevalence of alcoholic liver disease in patients given disulfiram.— L. Nässberger, *Postgrad. med. J.*, 1984, *60*, 639.

Further references to disulfiram and liver damage: E. B. Keeffe and F. W. Smith, *J. Am. med. Ass.*, 1974, *230*, 435; H. J. Eisen and A. L. Ginsberg (letter), *Ann. intern. Med.*, 1975, *83*, 673; S. J. Morris *et al.*, *Gastroenterology*, 1978, *75*, 100.

For reference to a characteristic hepatic lesion in some patients taking disulfiram, see Citrated Calcium Carbimide, p.1558.

EFFECTS ON METABOLISM. *Acetonaemia.* Disulfiram 400 mg, administered on 2 consecutive days to 6 healthy subjects abstaining from alcohol, produced a marked and rapid rise in blood-acetone concentrations. Since the effect appeared to be independent of any increase in other ketone bodies, the origin of the acetone was unknown.— A. Stowell *et al.* (letter), *Lancet*, 1983, *1*, 882.

Hypercholesterolaemia. Chronic exposure to carbon disulphide, a metabolite of disulfiram, has been reported to cause an increase in serum-cholesterol concentrations and an increased prevalence of arteriosclerotic cardiovascular disease. Disulfiram 500 mg daily for 3 weeks in 6 alcoholics was associated with an increase in serum-cholesterol concentrations whereas 250 mg daily in a further 8 patients was not, but the fall in concentrations associated with abstinence from alcohol did not occur.— L. F. Major and P. F. Goyer, *Ann. intern. Med.*, 1978, *88*, 53.

EFFECTS ON THE NERVOUS SYSTEM. Case reports and a discussion on disulfiram-induced encephalopathy. A 2% incidence of reversible toxic encephalopathy has been reported in patients receiving disulfiram (S.T. Knee and J. Razani, *Am. J. Psychiat.*, 1974, *131*, 1281). Onset varies from days to months following the start of therapy and early signs include impaired concentration, memory deficits, anxiety, depression, and somnolence. Confusion and disorientation follow, often accompanied by paranoid delusions and sometimes hallucinations. Other symptoms may include ataxia, loss of fine motor coordination, slurred speech, and intention tremor. There are conflicting opinions on whether this psychosis is a toxic reaction to disulfiram or a response to abstinence from alcohol, but the authors suspect that most cases represent a toxic encephalopathy. Of the 2 cases reported, toxicity appeared in one patient 16 months after starting treatment with disulfiram 250 mg daily; he returned to normal within 5 days of disulfiram withdrawal. The second patient became depressed, withdrawn, and confused immediately after starting disulfiram 500 mg daily; toxic psychosis evolved in association with a generalised tonic-clonic seizure, but recovery was complete 4 weeks after disulfiram was stopped.— J. R. Hotson and J. W. Langston, *Archs Neurol., Chicago*, 1976, *33*, 141.

Peripheral neuropathy. A report of peripheral neuropathy associated with disulfiram in 4 patients and reference to 25 reported cases. Onset of neuropathy varied from days to months after starting disulfiram treatment and could develop with doses of 250 or 500 mg daily. The most common symptom reported was pins and needles, but numbness, pain/burning, and weakness were frequently described; usually both muscle weakness and sensory loss were noted. Optic atrophy has also been described. Although there might be some improvement immediately after disulfiram withdrawal, the neurological deficit only improved slowly and symptoms might persist for as long as 2 years.— C. P. Watson *et al.*, *Can. med. Ass. J.*, 1980, *123*, 123.

OVERDOSAGE. A 31-year-old man was suspected of having taken 30 tablets of disulfiram 250 mg. He was agitated, suspicious, and frightened and became delirious, somnolent, and catatonic. These symptoms, together with acetone on his breath and in his urine, leucocytosis, and an abnormal EEG were consistent with previous reports of disulfiram poisoning. Measurement of plasma concentrations of disulfiram and its metabolites confirmed the overdosage. Treatment was symptomatic and the patient had recovered completely by day 7.— V. Kirubakaran *et al.*, *Am. J. Psychiat.*, 1983, *140*, 1513.

A report of disulfiram intoxication in a 6-year-old boy who recovered after receiving disulfiram 250 mg four times daily to a total of 13 doses. Of 6 previous reports one child died and 3 had moderate or severe brain damage. The syndrome of disulfiram intoxication in children is distinct from the disulfiram-alcohol interaction or acute disulfiram intoxication in adults. It is characterised by lethargy or somnolence, weakness, hypotonia, and vomiting, beginning approximately 12 hours after ingestion and progressing to stupor or coma. Dehydration, moderate tachycardia, and marked tachypnoea occur frequently, muscle tone is greatly decreased, and deep-tendon reflexes may be weak or absent.— W. E. Benitz and D. S. Tatro, *J. Pediat.*, 1984, *105*, 487.

PREGNANCY AND THE NEONATE. A report of 2 infants with severe limb-reduction anomalies whose mothers had taken disulfiram during pregnancy. Only 2 similar cases had previously been reported.— A. H. Nora *et al.* (letter), *Lancet*, 1977, *2*, 664.

Precautions

Disulfiram is contra-indicated in the presence of cardiovascular disease or psychosis and should not be given to patients known to be hypersensitive to it or to other thiuram compounds, such as those used in rubber vulcanisation or pesticides. It should be used with caution in the presence of diabetes mellitus, epilepsy, impaired hepatic or renal function, respiratory disorders, cerebral damage, or hypothyroidism, especially in view of the risk of disulfiram-alcohol reactions occurring. Caution is advised when administering disulfiram to drug addicts. It is probably best avoided in pregnancy.

Disulfiram should not be given until at least 12 hours after the last ingestion of alcohol. Patients beginning therapy should be fully aware of the disulfiram-alcohol reaction and should be warned to avoid alcohol in any form, including alcohol-containing medicines and alcohol-based topical preparations. Reactions to alcohol may occur as long as 2 weeks after the cessation of disulfiram.

Several drug interactions have been reported with disulfiram and it should be used with especial care in patients receiving other medication. Disulfiram inhibits hepatic enzymes and may interfere with the metabolism of other drugs taken at the same time. It enhances the effects of phenytoin and coumarin anticoagulants and their dosage may need to be reduced. Toxic reactions have occurred following the concomitant administration of disulfiram and isoniazid or metronidazole. Disulfiram may potentiate the action of paraldehyde by inhibition of acetaldehyde metabolism and these drugs should not be given concomitantly.

The US manufacturers have recommended that regular blood counts and liver function tests should be performed during long-term therapy.

INTERACTIONS. The potential of disulfiram to impair drug metabolism was demonstrated by Vesell *et al.* (*Clin. Pharmac. Ther.*, 1971, *12*, 785) who found that it prolonged the plasma half-life of phenazone, probably by inhibiting the hepatic microsomal mixed function oxidases. They also suggested that disulfiram alters catecholamine metabolism since urinary excretion of vanilmandelic acid (VMA) was significantly reduced and that of homovanillic acid (HVA) was increased.

Although *chlorpromazine* was once given to reduce the nausea and vomiting associated with the disulfiram-alcohol reaction (J.F. Cummins and D.G. Friend, *Am. J. med. Sci.*, 1954, *227*, 561), Kwentus and Major (*J. Stud. Alcohol*, 1979, *40*, 428) considered that phenothiazine anti-emetics such as chlorpromazine might increase hypotension because of their α-adrenoceptor blocking activity and should therefore be contra-indicated. Sellers *et al.* (*New Engl. J. Med.*, 1981, *305*, 1255) also noted that clinically serious pharmacodynamic interactions could be anticipated during the disulfiram-alcohol reaction in patients taking other drugs that impair blood pressure regulation, such as α- and β-adrenoceptor blocking agents and vasodilators. MacCallum (*Lancet*, 1969, *1*, 313) reported that *amitriptyline* appeared to enhance the disulfiram-alcohol reaction. Sellers *et al.* pointed out the potential for serious interactions during the disulfiram-alcohol reaction with drugs having CNS actions mediated by noradrenaline or dopamine, such as tricyclic antidepressants and phenothiazines, or those inhibiting the same enzymes as disulfiram, such as *monoamine oxidase inhibitors*. Conversely, *diazepam* was reported by MacCallum to reduce the intensity of the disulfiram-alcohol reaction.

Reports of the effects of disulfiram on the following drugs may be found in their respective monographs: Amitriptyline Hydrochloride, Cannabis, Diazepam, Ethylene Dibromide, Isoniazid, Metronidazole, Paraldehyde, Perphenazine, Phenytoin Sodium, and Warfarin Sodium.

Absorption and Fate

Disulfiram is absorbed from the gastro-intestinal tract and is rapidly reduced to diethyldithiocarbamate, principally by the glutathione reductase system in the erythrocytes; reduction may also occur in the liver. Diethyldithiocarbamate is metabolised in the liver to its glucuronide and methyl ester and to diethylamine, carbon disulphide, and sulphate ions. Metabolites are excreted primarily in the urine; carbon disulphide is exhaled in the breath.

A review of the disposition and pharmacokinetics of disulfiram.— J. F. Brien and C. W. Loomis, *Drug Metab. Rev.*, 1983, *14*, 113. For the metabolic fate of disulfiram, see also D. I. Eneanya *et al.*, *Annu. Rev. Pharmacol. Toxicol.*, 1981, *21*, 575.

There was marked intersubject variability in plasma concentrations of disulfiram and its metabolites in a study of 15 male alcoholics given single 250-mg doses of disulfiram by mouth and repeated dosing with 250 mg daily for 12 days. Variability might result from the marked lipid solubility of disulfiram, differences in plasma protein binding, or enterohepatic cycling. Average times to reach peak plasma concentrations after single or repeated doses were 8 to 10 hours for disulfiram, diethyldithiocarbamate, diethyldithiocarbamate-methyl ester, and diethylamine, and for carbon disulphide in breath; peak plasma concentrations of carbon disulphide occurred after 5 to 6 hours. Plasma concentrations of disulfiram were negligible within 48 hours of a dose although concentrations of some metabolites were still raised. In urine, 1.7 and 8.3% of a disulfiram dose was eliminated as diethyldithiocarbamate-glucuronide in the 24 hours after a single and repeated dose, while diethylamine accounted for 1.6 and 5.7%, respectively. In the 24 hours after a single and repeated dose 22.4 and 31.3%, respectively, was eliminated as carbon disulphide in the breath.— M. D. Faiman *et al.*, *Clin. Pharmac. Ther.*, 1984, *36*, 520.

Uses and Administration

Disulfiram is used as an adjunct in the treatment of chronic alcoholism. It is not a cure and the treatment is likely to be of little value unless it is undertaken with the willing cooperation of the patient and is employed in conjunction with supportive psychotherapy.

Disulfiram inhibits aldehyde dehydrogenase, the enzyme responsible for the oxidation of acetaldehyde, a metabolite of alcohol. The resulting accumulation of acetaldehyde in the blood is widely believed to be responsible for many of the unpleasant symptoms of the disulfiram-alcohol reaction which occur when alcohol is taken, even in small quantities, after the administration of disulfiram (see Adverse Effects, above). Symptoms can arise within 10 minutes of the ingestion of alcohol and last from half an hour in mild cases to several hours in severe cases. It is advisable to carry out the initial treatment in hospital where the patient can be kept under close supervision.

Disulfiram is given by mouth. A suggested dose is 800 mg, taken as a single dose, on the first day of treatment, reduced by 200 mg daily to a maintenance dose which is usually 100 to 200 mg daily. In the US, where doses above 500 mg daily are not recommended, an initial dose of 500 mg daily for 1 to 2 weeks is suggested, followed by a maintenance dose of 250 mg daily or within the range of 125 to 500 mg daily.

A test dose of alcohol has been given under close supervision when the patient is receiving maintenance doses of disulfiram, in order to demonstrate the nature of the disulfiram-alcohol reaction. However, many authorities consider that an explicit description of the reaction is sufficient.

Disulfiram implants have been used in an attempt to overcome problems of patient compliance.

ACTION. Inhibition of aldehyde dehydrogenase by disulfiram and the consequent raised blood concentrations of acetaldehyde when alcohol is consumed during treatment has been studied in *animals*. Inhibition develops slowly over 12 hours and is irreversible, with restoration of activity dependent on synthesis of new enzyme over several days.— J. E. Peachey *et al., J. clin. Psychopharmacol.*, 1981, *1*, 21.

ALCOHOLISM. General reviews on disulfiram and other drugs in the treatment of alcoholism.— E. M. Sellers *et al., New Engl. J. Med.*, 1981, *305*, 1255; J. E. Peachey and C. A. Naranjo, *Drugs*, 1984, *27*, 171.

Reviews of disulfiram.— T. J. Haley, *Drug Metab. Rev.*, 1979, *9*, 319; J. Kwentus and L. F. Major, *J. Stud. Alcohol*, 1979, *40*, 428; D. I. Eneanya *et al., Annu. Rev. Pharmacol. Toxicol.*, 1981, *21*, 575.

Proceedings of a symposium on disulfiram in the treatment of alcohol dependence.— *Br. J. clin. Pract.*, 1984, *38, Suppl.* 36, 1-37.

A discussion on the use of disulfiram in alcoholism with emphasis on the importance of correct dosage and adequate supervision and its relatively low toxicity when compared with unchecked alcohol abuse. About 50% of patients may experience little or no reaction on disulfiram 200 mg daily, whereas 500 mg daily will produce a more impressive disulfiram-alcohol reaction in about 75% of patients. Some may need even higher doses and a few can drink even on 1 g daily or more. However, for patients who do not risk drinking, 200 mg daily or less is adequate, providing supervision and compliance are good. The prolonged action of disulfiram permits administration twice or three times weekly with appropriate dosage adjustment. The traditional loading dose is considered unnecessary.— C. Brewer, *Br. J. Hosp. Med.*, 1986, *35*, 116.

Results of a 1-year study in 128 alcoholics indicated that the threat of the disulfiram-alcohol reaction is as important in preventing drinking as the pharmacological action of the drug. Similar results were achieved in those who were told that they were receiving disulfiram, regardless of whether they had been assigned to a dose of 250 mg daily or a pharmacologically inactive dose of 1 mg daily; 20 of 86 patients receiving either dose of disulfiram were completely abstinent compared with only 5 of 42 who knew they were receiving placebo.— R. K. Fuller and H. P. Roth, *Ann. intern. Med.*, 1979, *90*, 901.

A study in non-alcoholic subjects supporting the claim that several small alcoholic drinks taken slowly over a few hours can diminish the intensity of the disulfiram-alcohol reaction. The effect was more pronounced for calcium carbimide than for disulfiram. It was suggested that in man disulfiram might not produce a completely irreversible inhibition of aldehyde dehydrogenase.— J. E. Peachey *et al.* (letter), *Lancet*, 1981, *1*, 943. A suggestion that rapid regeneration of aldehyde dehydrogenase in the liver might be responsible.— M. Phillips (letter), *ibid.*, *2*, 210.

Implants. Disulfiram implants have been used in alcoholics but there has been uncertainty as to the pharmacological effectiveness of such treatment. Malcolm and Madden (*Br. J. Psychiat.*, 1973, *123*, 41) reported beneficial results when they implanted ten 100-mg implant tablets, but subsequently concluded (M.T. Malcolm *et al., ibid.*, 1974, *125*, 485) that the deterrent effect was psychological rather than pharmacological. Kline and Kingstone (*Can. med. Ass. J.*, 1977, *116*, 1382) came to a similar conclusion and Bergström *et al.* (*Lancet*, 1982, *1*, 49) found little evidence of a reaction when patients with disulfiram implants were challenged with alcohol. In a study in 120 alcoholics given subcutaneous implants of 0.8, 1.2, or 1.6 g of disulfiram, Wilson *et al.* (*J. clin. Psychiat.*, 1984, *45*, 242) found that drinking behaviour was reduced in all groups, but there was no dose-response relationship; they acknowledged that a psychological deterrent component might outweigh any pharmacological deterrent effect.

NICKEL DERMATITIS. Some benefit was noted with disulfiram given by mouth in doses gradually increased to 100 mg twice daily in a double-blind placebo-controlled study involving 24 patients with nickel dermatitis. Two patients given disulfiram showed signs of hepatic toxicity. [Diethyldithiocarbamate, a metabolite of disulfiram, is a nickel-chelating agent].— K. Kaaber *et al., Contact Dermatitis*, 1983, *9*, 297.

Preparations

Disulfiram Tablets *(B.P.)*

Disulfiram Tablets *(U.S.P.)*

Proprietary Preparations

Antabuse 200 *(CP Pharmaceuticals, UK). Tablets*, scored, disulfiram 200 mg.

Proprietary Names and Manufacturers

Abstensyl *(Arg.)*; Abstinyl *(Switz.)*; Antabus *(Dumex, Denm.; Tosse, Ger.; Neth.; Dumex, Norw.; Abello, Spain; Dumex, Swed.; Dumex, Switz.)*; Antabuse *(Cilag, Austral.; Belg.; Ayerst, Canad.; Crinos, Ital.; MPS Lab., S.Afr.; CP Pharmaceuticals, UK; Ayerst, USA)*; Antietil *(Ital.)*; Antivitium *(Reder, Spain)*; Aversan *(Norw.)*; Espéral *(Millot-Solac, Fr.)*; Etiltox *(Candioli, Ital.)*; Refusal *(Neth.)*; Ro-Sulfiram-500 *(USA)*.

1737-k

Doxofylline *(pINN)*.

7-(1,3-Dioxolan-2-ylmethyl)theophylline.

$C_{11}H_{14}N_4O_4=266.3$.

CAS — 69975-86-6.

Doxofylline is a xanthine used in respiratory disorders such as bronchial asthma.

Proprietary Names and Manufacturers

Ansimar *(ABC, Ital.)*.

2852-v

Draquinolol *(rINN)*.

H-I-42-BS. 3-[*p*-[3-(*tert*-butylamino)-2-hydroxypropoxy]phenyl]-7-methoxy-2-methylisocarbostyril.

$C_{24}H_{30}N_2O_4=410.5$.

CAS — 67793-71-9.

Draquinolol is a cardioselective beta-adrenoceptor blocking agent.

References: T. H. Pringle *et al., Br. J. clin. Pharmac.*, 1987, *23*, 411.

12681-a

Drosera

Droserae Herba; Herba Rorellae; Rorela; Ros Solis; Sundew.

Pharmacopoeias. In *Belg.* and *Span.*

The air-dried entire plant *Drosera rotundifolia* (Droseraceae).

Preparations of drosera have been used for its reputed value in respiratory disorders but is of doubtful value.

It has been used in homoeopathic medicine.

12682-t

Drotaverine *(rINN)*.

1-(3,4-Diethoxybenzylidene)-6,7-diethoxy-1,2,3,4-tetrahydroisoquinoline.

$C_{24}H_{31}NO_4=397.5$.

CAS — 14009-24-6.

Drotaverine has been used as an antispasmodic.

Proprietary Names and Manufacturers

Deprolen *(Temis-Lostalo, Arg.)*; No-Spa *(Chinoin, Hung.)*; Nospasin *(Phoenix, Arg.)*.

12684-r

Dulcamara

Bittersweet; Douce-Amère; Dulcamarae Caulis; Woody Nightshade.

The dried stems and branches of *Solanum dulcamara* (Solanaceae).

Dulcamara was formerly a popular remedy for chronic rheumatism and skin eruptions and was administered as an infusion.

All parts of the plant are poisonous due to the presence of solanaceous alkaloids. The berries have caused poisoning in children. Adverse effects are treated as described under Atropine, p.523.

3898-b

Eledoisin *(pINN)*.

ELD-950. 5-Oxo-Pro-Pro-Ser-Lys-Asp-Ala-Phe-Ile-Gly-Leu-Met-NH_2.

$C_{54}H_{85}N_{13}O_{15}S=1188.4$.

CAS — 69-25-0.

Eledoisin is a peptide extracted from the posterior salivary glands of certain small octopi (*Eledone* spp., Mollusca), or obtained by synthesis. Its actions resemble those of substance P; it is a potent vasodilator and increases capillary permeability.

The methyl ester has been given as eye-drops containing 0.04%, instilled 3 times daily, as a stimulant of lachrymal secretion in keratoconjunctivitis sicca, Sjögren's syndrome and other dry eye conditions.

The trifluoroacetate has also reportedly been used.

Reference: Y. Kamikawa and Y. Shimo, *Br. J. Pharmac.*, 1984, *81*, 143.

Proprietary Names and Manufacturers

Eloisin *(Farmitalia, Spain)*.

18634-y

Elliptinium Acetate *(BAN, rINN)*.

9-Hydroxy-2,5,11-trimethyl-6*H*,2H^+-pyrido-[4,3*b*]carbazolium acetate.

$C_{20}H_{20}N_2O_3=336.4$.

CAS — 58337-35-2.

An antineoplastic agent.

Proprietary Names and Manufacturers

Celiptium *(Pasteur Vaccins, Fr.)*.

19128-m

Elmustine *(rINN)*.

HECNU; NSC-29485. 1-(2-Chloroethyl)-3-(2-hydroxyethyl)-1-nitrosourea.

$C_5H_{10}ClN_3O_3=195.6$.

CAS — 60784-46-5.

Elmustine is under investigation as an antineoplastic agent.

References: *Drugs of the Future*, 1984, *9*, 18; *ibid.*, 1985, *10*, 76.

18830-k

Emiglitate *(BAN, rINN)*.

Bay-o-1248. Ethyl 4-(2-[(2*R*,3*R*,4*R*,5*S*)-3,4,5-trihydroxy-2-(hydroxymethyl)piperidino]-ethoxy)benzoate.

$C_{17}H_{25}NO_7=355.4$.

CAS — 80879-63-6.

Emiglitate is an alpha-glucosidase inhibitor under investigation as an adjunct in the management of diabetes mellitus.

References: R. H. Taylor *et al., Gut*, 1984, *25*, A1155; G. Dimitriadis *et al., Klin. Wschr.*, 1986, *64*, 405; M.

A. K. Omar *et al.*, *S. Afr. med. J.*, 1987, *71*, 422; R. H. Taylor *et al.*, *Gut*, 1986, *27*, 1471.

16621-z

Enisoprost *(USAN, rINN).*

SC-34301. (±)-Methyl (*Z*)-7-{(1*R*,2*R*,3*R*)-3-hydroxy-2-[(*E*)-(4*RS*)-4-hydroxy-4-methyl-1-octenyl]-5-oxocyclopentyl}-4-heptenoate.
$C_{22}H_{36}O_5$=380.5.
CAS — 81026-63-3.

Enisoprost is a prostaglandin analogue under investigation for the treatment of peptic ulcer.

3541-r

Entsufon Sodium *(USAN, rINNM).*

2-[2-[2-[*p*-1,3,3-Tetramethylbutylphenoxy]ethoxy]ethoxy]-ethanesulfonate.
$C_{20}H_{33}NaO_6S$=424.5.
CAS — 2917-94-4 (entsufon sodium); 55837-16-6 (entsufon).

A detergent used for cleansing the skin.

Proprietary Names and Manufacturers
pHisoCare *(Sterling, Canad.)*; pHisoDerm *(Sterling, Canad.)*.

The following names have been used for multi-ingredient preparations containing entsufon— pHisoDan *(Sterling, Canad.)*; pHisodan *(Winthrop, Austral.)*.

18637-c

Epanolol *(BAN, rINN).*

ICI-141292. (*RS*)-*N*-[2-(3-*o*-Cyanophenoxy-2-hydroxypropylamino)ethyl]-2-(4-hydroxyphenyl)acetamide.
$C_{20}H_{23}N_3O_4$=369.4.
CAS — 86880-51-5.

Epanolol is reported to be a cardioselective beta-adrenoceptor blocking agent with selective $beta_1$-agonist activity also.

References: B. Dahlöf *et al.*, *Br. J. clin. Pharmac.*, 1984, *18*, 831; J. D. Harry *et al.*, *Br. J. clin. Pharmac.*, 1984, *18*, 291P; P. Lund-Johansen *et al.*, *Acta med. scand.*, 1985, *Suppl.* 693, 121; T. H. Pringle *et al.*, *Br. J. clin. Pharmac.*, 1985, *19*, 137P; S. Groth *et al.*, *Eur. J. clin. Pharmac.*, 1986, *30*, 653; T. H. Pringle *et al.*, *Br. J. clin. Pharmac.*, 1986, *21*, 249; J. Bonde *et al.*, *ibid.*, 1987, *23*, 35; G. M. Berkenboom *et al.*, *Cardiology*, 1987, *74*, 43.

16629-d

Eperisone *(pINN).*

4′-Ethyl-2-methyl-3-piperidinopropiophenone.
$C_{17}H_{25}NO$=259.4.
CAS — 64840-90-0.

Eperisone is used by mouth in the form of the hydrochloride as a muscle relaxant in cerebrovascular disorders.

Proprietary Names and Manufacturers
Myonal *(Eisai, Jpn)*.

12695-n

Epomediol

1,8-Epoxy-4-isopropyl-1-methylcylohexane-2,6-diol.
$C_{10}H_{18}O_3$=186.3.

Epomediol is used in the treatment of hepatic disorders.

References: L. Capurso *et al.*, *J. int. med. Res.*, 1987, *15*, 134.

Proprietary Names and Manufacturers
Clesidren *(Corvi, Ital.)*.

19144-m

Epostane *(BAN, USAN, rINN).*

Win-32729. 4α,5α-Epoxy-3,17β-dihydroxy-4β,17α-dimethyl-5α-androst-2-ene-2-carbonitrile.
$C_{22}H_{31}NO_3$=357.5.
CAS — 80471-63-2.

Epostane has antiprogestogenic activity and has been investigated for use as an abortifacient in conjunction with prostaglandins and as a uterine stimulant for the induction of labour.

References: Z. M. van der Spuy *et al.*, *Clin. Endocr.*, 1983, *19*, 521; N. S. Pattison *et al.*, *Fert. Steril.*, 1984, *42*, 875; M. A. Webster *et al.*, *Br. J. Obstet. Gynaec.*, 1985, *92*, 963; M. J. Crooij *et al.*, *New Engl. J. Med.*, 1988, *319*, 813.

16633-t

Eproxindine *(rINN).*

(±)-*N*-[3-(Diethylamino)-2-hydroxypropyl]-3-methoxy-1-phenylindole-2-carboxamide.
$C_{23}H_{29}N_3O_3$=395.5.
CAS — 83200-08-2.

Eproxindine is an anti-arrhythmic agent.

A report of sudden cardiorespiratory arrest and death in an apparently healthy subject shortly after receiving eproxindine 400 mg by intravenous infusion during the course of a clinical study. He was subsequently found to have received a depot injection of flupenthixol the previous day. Displacement of flupenthixol from its plasma binding sites by eproxindine may have been responsible.— A. Darragh *et al.*, *Lancet*, 1985, *1*, 93. Comments: J. M. Simister and A. Jorgensen (letter), *ibid.*, 343; A. Darragh *et al.* (letter), *ibid.*, 756.

12697-m

Eprozinol Hydrochloride *(rINNM).*

3-[4-(β-Methoxyphenethyl)piperazin-1-yl]-1-phenylpropan-1-ol dihydrochloride.
$C_{22}H_{30}N_2O_2$,2HCl=427.4.
CAS — 32665-36-4 (eprozinol).

Eprozinol hydrochloride inhibits bronchoconstriction and has been used in the treatment of asthmatic and bronchitic disorders. It also has a sedative action. It is given by mouth in doses of 50 mg three times daily.

Proprietary Names and Manufacturers
Alecor *(Andromaco, Arg.)*; Asmisul *(Inibsa, Spain)*; Brovel *(Lepetit, Ital.)*; Eupnéron *(Lyocentre, Fr.)*.

12699-v

Equisetum

Herba Equiseti; Horsetail; Schachtelhalmkraut.

Pharmacopoeias. In *Aust.*, *Cz.*, *Ger.*, *Hung.*, *Pol.*, *Roum.*, and *Swiss. Arg.* specifies *E. giganteum.*

The dried sterile green stems of the common horsetail, *Equisetum arvense* (Equisetaceae).

Equisetum has been used in the treatment of genito-urinary and respiratory disorders.

Alkaloids present in equisetum of British origin included nicotine and palustrine.— J. D. Phillipson and C. Melville, *J. Pharm. Pharmac.*, 1960, *12*, 506.

16635-r

Erythropoietin

Erythropoietin is a hormone produced in the kidney and excreted in the urine. It is a glycosylated polypeptide of molecular weight about 30 000. Erythropoietin produced by recombinant DNA technology is used clinically.

Units

10 units of erythropoietin, human, urinary, for bioassay are contained in approximately 2 mg of freeze-dried extract of human urine, with 3 mg of sodium chloride in one ampoule of the second International Reference Preparation (1970).

Uses and Administration

Erythropoietin is the major hormonal regulator of red blood cell production and is produced principally in the kidney and excreted in the urine. Erythropoietin concentrations are low in patients with certain renal disorders and erythropoietin produced by recombinant DNA technology has been shown to be effective in correcting the anaemia associated with end-stage renal disease in patients maintained on haemodialysis. It is usually given intravenously, often three times weekly after the end of haemodialysis. The subcutaneous route is being investigated.

A review of erythropoietin. Clinical studies have shown the effectiveness of erythropoietin made by recombinant DNA technology in correcting the anaemia of end-stage renal disease in patients maintained by haemodialysis. Although several factors contribute to the aetiology of the anaemia, including blood loss associated with dialysis, the main cause is inadequate production of erythropoietin from still unidentified sites in the kidney. From the trials reported so far, there seem to be few adverse effects although hypertension and its complications may develop or increase. In most reports erythropoietin has been given intravenously three times weekly, but other parenteral routes and less frequent administration are under study and are likely to be satisfactory. The dose for treatment is usually 75 to 450 units per kg bodyweight weekly.

Erythropoietin has also been studied in other conditions. The anaemias of chronic disorders (including rheumatoid arthritis and neoplastic disease) are possible candidates and more speculative uses include the anaemia of prematurity, replacement of homologous transfusion after surgery, stimulation of the production of foetal haemoglobin in sickle-cell anaemia, and provocation of bone marrow regeneration in hypoplastic anaemias.— P. M. Cotes, *Br. med. J.*, 1988, *296*, 805.

Further reviews and discussions on erythropoietin: *Lancet*, 1987, *1*, 781; *ibid.*, *2*, 1371; A. E. G. Raine, *ibid.*, 1988, *1*, 97; G. Remuzzi, *ibid.*, 1205.

Reports of a beneficial response to erythropoietin in patients with anaemia associated with renal disease: C. G. Winearls *et al.*, *Lancet*, 1986, *2*, 1175; J. W. Eschbach *et al.*, *New Engl. J. Med.*, 1987, *316*, 73; S. Casati *et al.*, *Br. med. J.*, 1987, *295*, 1017; M. Moia *et al.*, *Lancet*, 1987, *2*, 1227.

19145-b

Esaprazole *(rINN).*

Hexaprazole. *N*-Cyclohexyl-1-piperazineacetamide.
$C_{12}H_{23}N_3O$=225.3.
CAS — 64204-55-3.

Esaprazole is under investigation for the treatment of peptic ulcers.

References: L. Capurso *et al.*, *Clin. Trials J.*, 1986, *23*, 293; M. Lazzaroni *et al.*, *Curr. ther. Res.*, 1987, *41*, 290; P. R. Dal Monte *et al.*, *Drugs exp. & clin. Res.*, 1987, *13*, 305.

1798-q

Etanidazole *(pINN).*

NSC-301467; SR-2508. *N*-(2-Hydroxyethyl)-2-nitroimidazole-1-acetamide.
$C_7H_{10}N_4O_4$=214.2.
CAS — 22668-01-5.

Etanidazole is a radiosensitiser under investigation as an adjunct to radiotherapy in the treatment of cancer.

207-g

Ethanolamine *(BAN).*

Aethanolaminum; Monoethanolamine *(USAN)*; Olamine *(pINN)*. 2-Hydroxyethylamine; 2-Aminoethanol.
C_2H_7NO=61.08.
CAS — 141-43-5.

NOTE. Monoethanolamine Oleate is *rINN.*

Pharmacopoeias. In *Aust.* and *Br.* Also in *U.S.N.F.*

A clear colourless or pale yellow moderately viscous liquid with an ammoniacal odour. It is alkaline to litmus.

Miscible with water, alcohol, acetone, chloroform, and glycerol; it is immiscible with petroleum spirit and fixed oils but it will dissolve many essential oils. *B.P.* has slightly soluble in ether while *U.S.N.F.* has immiscible with ether. **Store** in airtight containers. Protect from light.

Adverse Effects

Ethanolamine is irritant to skin and mucous membranes. Hypersensitivity reactions have been reported after the use of ethanolamine oleate.

In Great Britain the recommended exposure limits of ethanolamine are 3 ppm (long-term); 6 ppm (short-term).

NEPHROTOXICITY. Acute renal failure, which cleared spontaneously within 3 weeks, occurred in 2 obese women given sclerosing injections of 15 to 20 mL of a solution containing ethanolamine oleate 5% and benzyl alcohol 2%.— T. J. B. Maling and M. J. Cretney, *N.Z. med. J.*, 1975, *82*, 269.

Uses and Administration

Ethanolamine, combined with oleic acid, is used as a sclerosing agent in the injection treatment of varicose veins and oesophageal varices. It is administered usually intravenously as Ethanolamine Oleate Injection in a dose of 0.5 to 1.5 mL into each vein to be treated. The treatment is repeated at intervals until the varices have been completely occluded.

SCLEROTHERAPY. Sclerosants are used in the management of varicosities including varicose veins and oesophageal varices when their capacity to damage veins is apparently put to good use. The mechanisms by which injection sclerotherapy works are not completely understood but are thought to involve damage to the intima, intraluminal thrombosis, and intravascular fibrous organisation. Sclerosants used include: ethanolamine oleate 5%, laureth 9 (p.1244), sodium tetradecyl sulphate 3% (p.1417), and sodium morrhuate 5% (p.1591). Complications of sclerotherapy vary due to significant differences in technique, the skill and experience of the endoscopist, the cause of the liver disease underlying the oesophageal varices, and the clinical state of the patient. There may be: tachycardia, aspiration pneumonia, pleural effusions, and oesophageal disturbances including ulceration, necrosis, stenosis or stricture, and perforation. Direct intravariceal injection of sclerosant is less likely to cause local necrosis, ulcer or stricture formation than paravariceal injection. Patients with bleeding oesophageal varices should have their haemorrhage controlled before being given the sclerosant, usually in several injections into or sometimes around the varix, using an endoscope for guidance. The amount injected is usually 6 to 8 mL per varix, in volumes of not more than 2 mL per injection. Alternative treatment includes surgery, vasopressin, propranolol, or somatostatin. Balloon tamponade may be useful before or after the sclerotherapy. Sclerotherapy has also been used in the treatment of recurrent fluid accumulation in various cysts and hydrocele.

It is generally accepted that sclerotherapy is useful in the management of patients who have bled from oesophageal varices and there are reports of this technique being as good as vasopressin with tamponade (A.W. Larson *et al.*, 1986, *255*, 497) or surgical shunting (J. P. Cello *et al.*, *New Engl. J. Med.*, 1986, *316*, 11). However, there are conflicting reports or studies about its value in improving survival (B.R.D. Macdougall *et al.*, *Lancet*, 1982, *1*, 124; D. Westaby *et al.*, *Gut*, 1983, *24*, A971; J. Terblanche *et al.*, *Lancet*, 1983, *2*, 1328; Copenhagen Esophageal Varices Sclerotherapy Project, *New Engl. J. Med.*, 1984, *311*, 1594) or as effective prophylaxis against variceal haemorrhage (L. Witzel *et al.*, *Lancet*, 1985, *1*, 773; A.K. Burroughs and G. Hamilton, *ibid.*, 1105). Studies tend to concentrate on the technique rather than the type of sclerosant. However, Rose and Smith (*Gut*, 1985, *26*, A1105) found ethanolamine oleate and sodium tetradecyl sulphate to be equally effective and Jourdan and McColl (*Br. J. clin. Pract.*, 1983, *37*, 325) expressed a preference for ethanolamine oleate as the larger volume injected provided a useful margin of safety.

For reference to the use of sclerotherapy in the management of malignant effusions, see p.588.

Preparations

Ethanolamine Oleate Injection *(B.P.)*. A sterile aqueous solution containing ethanolamine oleate 5% prepared by the interaction of ethanolamine and oleic acid. Sterilised by autoclaving. pH 8 to 9. Protect from light.

Proprietary Names and Manufacturers of Ethanolamine Oleate

Ethamolin *(Austral.)*; Etolein *(Swed.)*; Fosfor *(Liberman, Spain)*; Manufacturers also include—*Evans Medical, UK; Macarthys, UK.*

5232-n

Ethaverine Hydrochloride *(rINNM)*.

1-(3,4-Diethoxybenzyl)-6,7-diethoxyisoquinoline hydrochloride.

$C_{24}H_{29}NO_4,HCl = 432.0$.

CAS — 486-47-5 (ethaverine); 985-13-7 (hydrochloride).

Ethaverine is the tetraethoxy analogue of papaverine (see p.1598) and is used similarly as an antispasmodic in usual doses of 100 to 200 mg three times daily by mouth. It has been used at higher doses as an anti-arrhythmic.

In 14 healthy subjects, the mean terminal elimination half-life of ethaverine was 3.3 hours.— M. C. Meyer *et al.*, *Biopharm. Drug Disposit.*, 1983, *4*, 401.

Proprietary Names and Manufacturers

Cardiostron *(Solco, Ger.)*; Cebral *(Kenwood, USA)*; Circubid *(Merchant, USA)*; Eta-Lent *(Roger, USA)*; Etaverina *(Biologici Italia, Ital.)*; Ethaquin *(Ascher, USA)*; Ethatab *(Glaxo, USA)*; Ethavex *(Econo Med, USA)*; Isovex *(US Pharmaceutical, USA)*; Laverin *(Lemmon, USA)*; Pasmol *(Ram, USA)*; Pavaspan *(Jamieson-McKames, USA)*; Plaquivérine *(Monal, Fr.)*.

The following names have been used for multi-ingredient preparations containing ethaverine hydrochloride—Espasmotex *(Arlo, USA)*.

17040-h

Ethiofos *(USAN)*.

Gammaphos; NSC-296961; WR-2721. *S*-[2-[(3-Aminopropyl)amino]ethyl] dihydrogen phosphorothioate.

$C_5H_{15}N_2O_3PS = 214.2$.

CAS — 20537-88-6 (ethiofos); 63717-27-1 (monohydrate).

NOTE. The name Amifostine is *rINN* for the monohydrate.

Ethiofos has been investigated as a radioprotective agent and to reduce alkylating antineoplastic toxicity; the monohydrate (amifostine) has similar properties. Ethiofos has also been tried in the management of hyperparathyroidism and to reduce sputum viscosity in conditions such as cystic fibrosis.

References: N. F. Tabachnik *et al.*, *J. Pharmac. exp. Ther.*, 1980, *214*, 246 (in cystic fibrosis); D. J. Glover *et al.*, *Ann. intern. Med.*, 1985, *103*, 55 (hypercalcaemia); M. Morita *et al.*, *ibid.*, 961 (primary hyperparathyroidism); D. Glover *et al.*, *J. clin. Oncol.*, 1986, *4*, 584 (protection against cyclophosphamide-induced haematological toxicity).

7359-s

Ethyl Oleate *(BAN, USAN)*.

Aethylis Oleas; Ethylis Oleas.

$C_{20}H_{38}O_2 = 310.5$.

CAS — 111-62-6.

Pharmacopoeias. In *Br., Egypt., Fr., Ind., Int.,* and *It.* Also in *U.S.N.F.*

An almost colourless or pale yellow oily mobile liquid with a slight but not rancid odour and with a taste somewhat resembling that of olive oil. It consists of the ethyl esters of oleic acid and related high molecular weight fatty acids. Practically **insoluble** in water; miscible with alcohol, chloroform, ether, fixed oils, liquid paraffin, and most other organic solvents. Ethyl oleate dissolves some types of rubber and causes others to swell. It oxidises on exposure to air; the air in partially filled containers should be replaced by nitrogen or other suitable inert gas. **Store** in a cool place in small well-filled airtight containers or in an atmosphere of nitrogen. Protect from light.

Ethyl oleate is used as a vehicle in oily injections and liniments.

Ethyl oleate used as the vehicle in calciferol injection manufactured by *Evans, UK* reacted with the plastic in disposable syringes making it difficult to expel the contents of the syringe.— K. G. Halsall (letter), *Pharm. J.*, 1985, *2*, 99.

2393-k

Ethyl Vanillin *(USAN)*.

3-Ethoxy-4-hydroxybenzaldehyde.

$C_9H_{10}O_3 = 166.2$.

CAS — 121-32-4.

Pharmacopoeias. In *Fr.* Also in *U.S.N.F.*

Fine white or slightly yellowish crystals with a vanilla-like odour and taste.

Soluble 1 in 100 of water at 50°; soluble 1 in 2 of alcohol; freely soluble in chloroform, ether, and solutions of alkali hydroxides. **Store** in airtight containers. Protect from light.

Ethyl vanillin is used as a flavouring agent and in perfumery to impart the odour and taste of vanilla.

Estimated acceptable daily intake: up to 10 mg per kg body-weight.— Eleventh Report of the Joint FAO/WHO Expert Committee on Food Additives, *Tech. Rep. Ser. Wld Hlth Org. No. 383*, 1968.

208-q

Ethylenediamine *(BAN, USAN)*.

$C_2H_8N_2 = 60.10$.

CAS — 107-15-3 (anhydrous); 6780-13-8 (monohydrate).

Pharmacopoeias. In *Br., Jpn,* and *U.S.*
Aust., Br., Egypt., Hung., Ind., Int., Nord., and *Turk.* include the hydrate.

A clear, colourless or slightly yellow, strongly alkaline liquid with an ammoniacal odour. It absorbs carbon dioxide from the air. **Miscible** with water and alcohol. **Store** in airtight glass containers. Protect from light.

Adverse Effects

Ethylenediamine is irritant to the skin and to mucous membranes, and contact dermatitis has been reported from the use of preparations containing ethylenediamine. Concentrated solutions cause skin burns. Headache, dizziness, shortness of breath, nausea, and vomiting have also been reported following exposure to fumes. Ethylenediamine splashed onto the skin or eyes should be removed by flooding with water for a prolonged period.

In Great Britain the recommended exposure limit of ethylenediamine is 10 ppm (long-term).

A review of allergy to ethylenediamine and aminophylline.— *Lancet*, 1984, *2*, 1192.

Precautions

Skin reactions may occur in patients given aminophylline after they have become sensitised to ethylenediamine. Cross-sensitivity with edetic acid and with some antihistamines has been reported.

A 37-year-old man with a contact allergy to ethylenediamine (obtained from applications of Tri-Adcortyl cream) developed a cross-sensitivity reaction on 3 occasions to piperazine.— S. Wright and R. R. M. Harman, *Br. med. J.*, 1983, *287*, 463.

Uses and Administration

Ethylenediamine or ethylenediamine hydrate is

used in the manufacture of aminophylline or aminophylline hydrate.

12712-s

Etifelmine *(rINN).*

2-Diphenylmethylenebutylamine.
$C_{17}H_{19}N=237.3$.

CAS — 341-00-4.

Etifelmine hydrochloride has been used for the treatment of hypotension. A mixture of the hydrochloride and nicotinate is similarly used.

Proprietary Names and Manufacturers
Gilutensin *(Giulini, Ger.)*; Tensinase-D *(Jpn).*

19158-s

Etifoxine *(rINN).*

Hoe-36801. 6-Chloro-4-methyl-4-phenyl-3,1-benzoxazin-2-yl(ethyl)amine.
$C_{17}H_{17}ClN_2O=300.8$.

CAS — 21715-46-8.

An anxiolytic. It is given as the hydrochloride.

Proprietary Names and Manufacturers
Stresam *(Marcofina, Fr.).*

9808-e

Evening Primrose Oil

A fixed oil obtained from the seeds of *Oenothera biennis* or other spp. (Onagraceae) and containing linoleic acid with some γ-linolenic acid.

Linoleic and γ-linolenic acid act as prostaglandin precursors. Evening primrose oil, which contains these acids, has been investigated in a variety of disorders including atopic eczema, multiple sclerosis, and the premenstrual syndrome.

A brief review of the activity of evening primrose oil.— A. J. Barber, *Pharm. J.*, 1988, *1*, 723.

DIABETIC NEUROPATHY. Improvement in diabetic neuropathy with evening primrose oil.— G. A. Jamal *et al.* (letter), *Lancet*, 1986, *1*, 1098.

ECZEMA. Improvement in atopic eczema with evening primrose oil.— C. R. Lovell *et al.* (letter), *Lancet*, 1981, *1*, 278; S. Wright and J. L. Burton, *ibid.*, 1982, *2*, 1120; M. Schalin-Karrila *et al.*, *Br. J. Derm.*, 1987, *117*, 11.

No improvement in eczema or in ichthyosis vulgaris.— R. J. G. Chalmers and S. Shuster (letter), *Lancet*, 1983, *1*, 236.

MALIGNANT NEOPLASMS. No benefit from evening primrose oil in colorectal cancer in a controlled study.— M. B. McIllmurray and W. Turkie, *Br. med. J.*, 1987, *294*, 1260.

Subjective improvement in a variety of tumours in an open study of evening primrose oil.— C. F. Van der Merwe *et al.*, *Br. J. clin. Pract.*, 1987, *41*, 907.

MULTIPLE SCLEROSIS. Dietary supplementation with linoleic acid (around 20 g daily) might slow the progression of disability in patients with minimum disability. This view was supported by an analysis by Dworkin *et al.* (*Neurology*, 1984, *34*, 1441) of 3 studies of supplementation.— *Drug & Ther. Bull.*, 1986, *24*, 41.

PREMENSTRUAL TENSION. Brief discussion of evening primrose oil producing improvement in the premenstrual syndrome in a review of the treatment of this syndrome.— P. M. S. O'Brien, *Drugs*, 1982, *24*, 140.

Improvement in cyclical breast mastalgia with evening primrose oil amongst other compounds. None produced any benefit in noncyclical mastalgia.— J. K. Pye *et al.*, *Lancet*, 1985, *2*, 373.

Proprietary Preparations

Efamol *(Britannia Health, UK). Capsules* (Efamol 250), evening primrose oil 250 mg, vitamin E 5 mg.
Capsules (Efamol 500), evening primrose oil 500 mg, vitamin E 10 mg. This is reported to provide 45 mg of γ-linolenic acid. Also available as a composite pack (Efamol PMP) containing Efamol 500 capsules and Efavite tablets (see under Proprietary Multivitamin and Mineral Preparations, p.1291).
Oil, evening primrose oil 250 mg/5 drops, in a dropper bottle.

Efamol Marine *(Britannia Health, UK). Capsules*, evening primrose oil 430 mg, marine fish oil 107 mg, vitamin E 10 mg.

Efamol Plus *(Britannia Health, UK). Capsules*, evening primrose oil 250 mg, linseed oil 50 mg, safflower oil 200 mg, vitamin E 10 mg.

EPOC *(Evening Primrose Oil Co., UK). Capsules*, evening primrose oil 250 and 500 mg, stated to contain γ-linolenic acid 10/11%.
Capsules, evening primrose oil 400 mg, marine fish oil 100 mg, vitamin E 10 mg.
Oil, evening primrose oil in a dropper bottle.

Epogam *(Scotia, UK). Capsules*, evening primrose oil providing γ-linolenic acid 40 mg, vitamin E 10 mg.

Gammaoil Premium *(Quest, UK). Capsules*, evening primrose oil 500 mg, vitamin E 10 mg. This is reported to provide 50 mg of γ-linolenic acid.

Naudicelle (known in some countries as Preglandin) *(Bio-Oil Research, UK). Capsules*, evening primrose oil 552 mg, mixed tocopherols 4 mg. This is reported to provide 50 mg of γ-linolenic acid.

Naudicelle Plus *(Bio-Oil Research, UK). Capsules*, evening primrose oil 440 mg, marine oil 110 mg, vitamin E 10 mg. This is reported to provide 40 mg of γ-linolenic acid.

Super Gammaoil Marine *(Quest, UK). Capsules*, evening primrose oil and borage blend 500 mg, fish lipid concentrate 250 mg, vitamin E 15 mg. This is reported to provide 80 mg of γ-linolenic acid.

3929-a

Exifone *(rINN).*

2,3,3′,4,4′,5′-Hexahydroxybenzophenone.
$C_{13}H_{10}O_7=278.2$.

CAS — 52479-85-3.

A nootropic used in the treatment of cognitive memory problems in the elderly.

Proprietary Names and Manufacturers
Adlone *(Pharmascience, Fr.).*

12726-z

Exiproben Sodium *(rINNM).*

DCH-21. Sodium 2-(3-hexyloxy-2-hydroxypropoxy)benzoate.
$C_{16}H_{23}NaO_5=318.3$.

CAS — 26281-69-6 (exiproben); 3478-44-2 (sodium salt).

Exiproben sodium is a choleretic which has been used in the treatment of hepatic disorders.

Proprietary Names and Manufacturers
Droctil *(Geigy, Ital.)*; Etopalin *(Geigy, Arg.).*

16800-a

Febuprol *(rINN).*

1-Butoxy-3-phenoxy-2-propanol.
$C_{13}H_{20}O_3=224.3$.

CAS — 3102-00-9.

A choleretic used in the treatment of biliary-tract disorders.

Proprietary Names and Manufacturers
Valbil *(Röhm, Ger.).*

2491-t

Felbinac *(BAN, rINN).*

CL-83544. Biphenyl-4-ylacetic acid.
$C_{14}H_{12}O_2=212.2$.

CAS — 5728-52-9.

Felbinac has been applied for its anti-inflammatory and analgesic properties.

Proprietary Names and Manufacturers
Traxam *(Lederle, UK).*

12730-e

Fenaftic Acid

1-Diethylcarbamoyl-1,2,3,4,5,6,7,8-octahydro-6,6-dimethyl-8-oxo-3-phenyl-2-naphthoic acid.
$C_{24}H_{31}NO_4=397.5$.

CAS — 27736-80-7.

Fenaftic acid has been claimed to increase bile secretion and to improve its composition. It has been given in illness involving hepatobiliary insufficiency or dysfunction.

12731-l

Fenalamide *(USAN, pINN).*

Ethyl *N*-(2-diethylaminoethyl)-2-ethyl-2-phenylmalonamate.
$C_{19}H_{30}N_2O_3=334.5$.

CAS — 4551-59-1.

Fenalamide has been used as an antispasmodic.

Proprietary Names and Manufacturers
The following names have been used for multi-ingredient preparations containing fenalamide—Diarstop *(Schering, Ital.)*; Spasen *(FIRMA, Ital.)*; Spasmamide *(Schering, Ital.).*

12735-c

Fencibutirol *(USAN, rINN).*

Mg-4833. 2-(1-Hydroxy-4-phenylcyclohexyl)butyric acid.
$C_{16}H_{22}O_3=262.3$.

CAS — 5977-10-6.

Fencibutirol is a choleretic which has been used in the treatment of hepatic disorders.

Proprietary Names and Manufacturers
Hepasil *(Edmond Pharma, Ital.)*; Verecol *(Maggioni-Winthrop, Ital.)*; Verecolene *(Maggioni-Winthrop, Ital.).*

12736-k

Fenclonine *(USAN, rINN).*

CP-10188; NSC-77370; Parachlorophenylalanine; DL-*p*-Chlorophenylalanine. 2-Amino-3-(4-chlorophenyl)propionic acid.
$C_9H_{10}ClNO_2=199.6$.

CAS — 7424-00-2.

Fenclonine is an inhibitor of the biosynthesis of serotonin. It has been given to patients with carcinoid syndrome and some relief of symptoms, especially of diarrhoea, has been reported. Hypothermia has been reported during treatment with fenclonine. Bone marrow depression may also occur. Doses of 500 mg four times daily have been used; higher doses have been reported to produce psychic side-effects.

References: K. Engelman *et al.*, *New Engl. J. Med.*, 1967, *277*, 1103; M. Shani and C. Sheba, *Br. med. J.*, 1970, *4*, 784; A. B. Vaidya and R. J. Levine, *New Engl. J. Med.*, 1971, *284*, 255; P. N. Maton *et al.*, *Br. med. J.*, 1983, *287*, 932 and 1664; B. Clarke and H. J. F. Hodgson, *Br. J. Hosp. Med.*, 1986, *35*, 146.

Proprietary Names and Manufacturers
Pfizer, USA.

19169-l

Fenflumizole *(rINN).*

A-214; Fenflumizol. 2-(2,4-Difluorophenyl)-4,5-bis(*p*-methoxyphenyl)imidazole.
$C_{23}H_{18}F_2N_2O_2=392.4$.

CAS — 73445-46-2.

Fenflumizole has been investigated for its anti-inflammatory and platelet anti-aggregatory properties.

References: E. Vinge *et al.*, *Eur. J. clin. Pharmac.*, 1984, *26*, 711; P. Grande *et al.*, *ibid.*, 27, 169; C. Midskov *et al.*, *Acta pharmac. tox.*, 1984, *54*, 408; K. Christensen, *Scand. J. Rheumatol.*, 1986, *15*, 80; A.

-M. Grauholt *et al., Eur. J. clin. Pharmac.*, 1987, *31*, 547.

Proprietary Names and Manufacturers
Dumex, *Denm.*

3722-m

Fenipentol *(rINN).*

1-Phenylpentan-1-ol; α-Butylbenzyl alcohol.
$C_{11}H_{16}O=164.2$.

CAS — 583-03-9.

Pharmacopoeias. In *Cz.*

Fenipentol is a choleretic. It has been given in doses of 100 to 200 mg two or three times daily before meals.

Proprietary Names and Manufacturers
Kol *(Mitim, Ital.)*; Pancoral *(Jpn)*; Pentabil *(OFF, Ital.)*; Sapem *(Craveri, Arg.)*.

16803-r

Fenoldopam *(BAN, rINN).*

SKF-82526; SKF-82526-J (mesylate). 6-Chloro-2,3,4,5-tetrahydro-1-*p*-hydroxyphenyl-1*H*-3-benzazepine-7,8-diol.
$C_{16}H_{16}ClNO_3=305.8$.

CAS — 67227-56-9 (fenoldopam); 67227-57-0 (mesylate).

NOTE. Fenoldopam Mesylate is *USAN*.

Fenoldopam has dopamine agonist and vasodilator properties and has been tried in the treatment of hypertension. The mesylate has also been investigated.

References: R. M. Stote *et al., Clin. Pharmac. Ther.*, 1983, *34*, 309; J. N. Harvey *et al., Br. J. clin. Pharmac.*, 1985, *19*, 21; *idem*, *21*, 53; N. L. Allison *et al., Clin. Pharmac. Ther.*, 1987, *41*, 282; Z. Glück *et al., Hypertension*, 1987, *10*, 43.

12019-e

Fenoverine *(rINN).*

10-[(4-Piperonyl-1-piperazinyl)acetyl]phenothiazine.
$C_{26}H_{25}N_3O_3S=459.6$.

CAS — 37561-27-6.

Fenoverine is used as an antispasmodic in doses of 300 to 600 mg daily by mouth.

Proprietary Names and Manufacturers
Procalma *(Arg.)*; Spasmopriv *(Vaillant-Defresne, Fr.)*.

12741-j

Fenozolone *(rINN).*

LD-3394; Phenozolone. 2-Ethylamino-5-phenyl-2-oxazolin-4-one.
$C_{11}H_{12}N_2O_2=204.2$.

CAS — 15302-16-6.

Fenozolone is a psychostimulant which has been used in the treatment of memory disorders and other symptoms of intellectual impairment.

Proprietary Names and Manufacturers
Ordinator *(Sintyal, Arg.; Dausse, Fr.)*.

12746-t

Fenspiride Hydrochloride *(USAN, rINNM).*

Decaspiride; JP-428; NAT-333; NDR-5998A. 8-Phenethyl-1-oxa-3,8-diazaspiro[4.5]decan-2-one hydrochloride.
$C_{15}H_{20}N_2O_2,HCl=296.8$.

CAS — 5053-06-5 (fenspiride); 5053-08-7 (hydrochloride).

Fenspiride is reported to have bronchodilator and anti-inflammatory properties. It has been given in asthma and other respiratory disorders in a dose of 80 mg two to three times daily.

References: *J. Am. med. Ass.*, 1969, *209*, 1615; H. Brems *et al., Ars Med., Liesthal*, 1984, *39*, 55.

Proprietary Names and Manufacturers
Abronquil *(S. Chobet, Arg.)*; Decaspir *(Pulitzer, Ital.)*; De-pulmin *(Smaller, Spain)*; Espiran *(ICT-Lodi, Ital.)*; Fendel *(Sidus, Arg.)*; Fenspir *(Ibirn, Ital.)*; Fluiden *(Lafare, Ital.)*; Pneumorel *(Eutherapie, Belg.; Biopharma, Fr.; Stroder, Ital.)*; Respiride *(Schiapparelli, Ital.)*; Tegencia *(Elmu, Spain)*; Viarespan *(Spain)*.

12748-r

Fenugreek

Bockshornsame; Faenum-Graecum; Semen Foenugraeci; Semen Trigonellae.

Pharmacopoeias. In *Aust., Chin.,* and *Pol.*

The dried seeds of *Trigonella foenumgraecum* (Leguminosae), containing not less than 30% of water-soluble extractive.

Fenugreek has been used chiefly in veterinary medicine as an aromatic. It has also been used as an appetite stimulant.

Studies of the steroidal sapogenin yield of fenugreek.— R. Hardman and F. R. Y. Fazli, *Planta med.*, 1972, *21*, 322.

A report of 'maple-syrup' urine odour due to the ingestion of fenugreek.— G. B. Bartley *et al.* (letter), *New Engl. J. Med.*, 1981, *305*, 467.

Further references to the effects of fenugreek: J. Mishkinsky *et al.* (letter), *Lancet*, 1967, *2*, 1311.

Proprietary Names and Manufacturers
Fénugrène *(Lemoine, Fr.)*.

3934-z

Ferritin

Ferritin is the major iron storage protein of vertebrates found mainly in the liver, spleen, and bone marrow and consisting of a soluble protein shell (apoferritin) with a core of ferric hydroxyphosphate complex.

Ferritin has been given by mouth as a source of iron in various anaemias.

References: M. Layrisse *et al., Curr. ther. Res.*, 1986, *40*, 248.

16808-m

Feverfew

The leaves of the plant *Tanacetum parthenium* (*Chrysanthemum parthenium*) (Compositae).

Adverse Effects

Mouth ulceration and soreness have been reported following ingestion of feverfew, and may be due to sensitisation; contact dermatitis has been reported.

Uses and Administration

Feverfew has been used in the prophylactic treatment of migraine and has also been tried in inflammatory conditions including arthritis. Its effects have been attributed to the plant's content of sesquiterpene lactones, notably parthenolide.

Evidence from a double-blind study in 17 patients that feverfew, as standardised capsules of the freeze-dried powdered leaf, was superior to placebo in preventing or ameliorating migraine attacks.— E. S. Johnson *et al., Br. med. J.*, 1985, *291*, 569. Similar results.— J. J. Murphy *et al., Lancet*, 1988, *2*, 189.

Further references to the actions and uses of feverfew: A. N. Makheja and J. M. Bailey, *Lancet*, 1981, *2*, 1054; M. J. Biggs *et al.* (letter), *ibid.*, 1982, *2*, 776; S. Heptinstall *et al., ibid.*, 1985, *1*, 1071; *ibid.*, 1084; W. A. Groenewegen and S. Heptinstall (letter), *ibid.*, 1986, *1*, 44; R. G. Warren, *Aust. J. Pharm.*, 1986, *67*, 475; L. A. J. O'Neill *et al., Br. J. clin. Pharmac.*, 1987, *23*, 81; C. A. Baldwin *et al., Pharm. J.*, 1987, *2*, 237.

Proprietary Names and Manufacturers
Lomigran *(Booker Health, UK)*.

16809-b

Fibronectin

Cold-insoluble Globulin.

A polypeptide found in plasma and elsewhere, with a molecular weight of about 450 000.

Fibronectin has a variety of roles in the body which are not fully elucidated but which include attachment of cells to the extracellular matrix. Infusion of fibronectin or fibronectin-rich plasma has been tried in patients with sepsis and infection, and in severe malnutrition. Eye-drops of fibronectin have been used in the treatment of corneal erosions.

References to the use of fibronectin: L. D. Grouse, *J. Am. med. Ass.*, 1980, *244*, 173; *Lancet*, 1983, *1*, 106; B. J. Boughton *et al.* (letter), *ibid.*, 121; T. Nishida *et al.* (letter), *ibid.*, *2*, 521; J. Fredell *et al.* (letter), *ibid.*, 1987, *2*, 962.

12751-c

Fipexide Hydrochloride *(rINNM).*

BP-662. 1-(4-Chlorophenoxyacetyl)-4-piperonylpiperazine hydrochloride.
$C_{20}H_{21}ClN_2O_4,HCl=425.3$.

CAS — 34161-24-5 (fipexide); 34161-23-4 (hydrochloride).

Fipexide hydrochloride is a stimulant of the central nervous system and has been used in the treatment of depression and memory defects.

References: E. Rolandi *et al., Br. J. clin. Pharmac.*, 1984, *18*, 236; R. Bompani and G. Scali, *Curr. med. Res. Opinion*, 1986, *10*, 99.

Proprietary Names and Manufacturers
Attentil *(Ravizza, Ital.)*; Fipexium *(Rocador, Spain)*; Vigilor *(Bouchard, Fr.; Lusofarmaco, Ital.)*.

12752-k

Flavodate Sodium *(rINNM).*

Flavodate Disodium. Disodium (4-oxo-2-phenyl-4*H*-chromene-5,7-diyldioxy)diacetate.
$C_{19}H_{12}Na_2O_8=414.3$.

CAS — 37470-13-6 (flavodic acid); 13358-62-8 (disodium salt).

Flavodate sodium is stated to increase the resistance of capillaries and to reduce their permeability. It has been given in vascular disorders.

References: C. Schmidt *et al., Thérapie*, 1985, *40*, 221.

Proprietary Names and Manufacturers
Comparison *(Casasco, Arg.)*; Intercyton *(Millot-Solac, Fr.; Semar, Spain)*; Pericel *(Lirca, Ital.)*.

5233-h

Flavoxate Hydrochloride *(BANM, USAN, rINNM).*

DW-61; Rec-7-0040. 2-Piperidinoethyl 3-methyl-4-oxo-2-phenyl-4*H*-chromene-8-carboxylate hydrochloride.
$C_{24}H_{25}NO_4,HCl=427.9$.

CAS — 15301-69-6 (flavoxate); 3717-88-2 (hydrochloride).

Adverse Effects

Flavoxate hydrochloride causes adverse antimuscarinic effects including increased intra-ocular pressure. There may be gastro-intestinal disturbances and hypersensitivity reactions. Other adverse effects include headache, sedation, vertigo, and confusion. Leucopenia has been reported rarely.

Precautions

Flavoxate hydrochloride should not be used in patients with gastro-intestinal haemorrhage or at risk from its antimuscarinic effects (see p.523).

Absorption and Fate

It has been reported that 10 to 30% of a dose of

flavoxate hydrochloride given by mouth is excreted in the urine within 6 hours.

Uses and Administration

Flavoxate hydrochloride is an antispasmodic with some structural similarity to propantheline. It is used for the symptomatic relief of some disorders of the lower urinary tract and for the relief of vesico-urethral spasms resulting from instrumentation or surgery in doses of 100 to 200 mg by mouth three or four times daily.

Whilst Stanton (*J. Urol., Baltimore*, 1973, *110*, 529) found that flavoxate produced greater improvement than emepronium bromide, both given in doses of 200 mg three times daily by mouth, in 38 patients with incontinence of various aetiologies, Briggs *et al.* (*ibid.*, 1980, *123*, 665) found no consistent drug effect detectable in 6 elderly patients with incontinence due to uninhibited detrusor contractions given flavoxate 100 mg by intravenous injection followed by 200 mg by mouth 4 times daily. Also, Meyhoff *et al.* (*Br. J. Urol.*, 1983, *55*, 34) found that in 19 women with urge incontinence, neither flavoxate nor emepronium were significantly superior to placebo.

For a study demonstrating that neither flavoxate nor emepronium were significantly superior to placebo in women with urge incontinence, see under Emepronium Carrageenate, p.531.

Proprietary Preparations

Urispas *(Syntex, UK)*. *Tablets*, flavoxate hydrochloride 100 mg.

Proprietary Names and Manufacturers

Bradalone *(Jpn)*; Genurin *(Cusi, Spain)*; Genurin Semplice *(Recordati, Ital.)*; Spasuret *(Farmitalia, Ger.)*; Urispadol *(Pharmacia, Denm.; Pharmacia, Norw.)*; Urispas *(Protea, Austral.; Pharmascience, Canad.; Neth.; Syntex, S.Afr.; Galenica, Switz.; Syntex, UK; Smith Kline & French, USA)*.

2953-w

Fleroxacin *(USAN, rINN)*.

AM-833; Ro-23-6240/000. 6,8-Difluoro-1-(2-fluoroethyl)-1,4-dihydro-7-(4-methyl-1-piperazinyl)-4-oxo-3-quinolinecarboxylic acid.

$C_{17}H_{18}F_3N_3O_3$=369.3.

CAS — 79660-72-3.

Fleroxacin is a fluorinated 4-quinolone antimicrobial agent that has been investigated in the management of bacterial infections.

References: N. -X. Chin *et al.*, *Antimicrob. Ag. Chemother.*, 1986, *29*, 675; K. Hirai *et al.*, *ibid.*, 1059; R. Wise *et al.*, *ibid.*, 1987, *31*, 161; C. S. F. Easmon *et al.*, *J. antimicrob. Chemother.*, 1987, *19*, 761; L. Verbist, *ibid.*, *20*, 363; P. Hohl *et al.*, *ibid.*, 373.

Proprietary Names and Manufacturers

Roche, USA.

18708-z

Flestolol *(rINN)*.

ACC-9089. (±)-[2-[(2,3-Dihydroxypropyl)amino]-2-methylpropyl]urea 3-*o*-fluorobenzoate.

$C_{15}H_{22}FN_3O_4$=327.4.

CAS — 87721-62-8 (flestolol); 88844-73-9 (sulphate).

NOTE. Flestolol Sulfate is *USAN*.

Flestolol is a short-acting beta blocker which is reported to have an elimination half-life of about 6 to 10 minutes following intravenous administration. It has been given as the sulphate.

References: R. Achari *et al.*, *Br. J. clin. Pharmac.*, 1985, *20*, 691; P. Turlapaty *et al.*, *Clin. Pharmac. Ther.*, 1986, *39*, 543; S. D. Barton *et al.*, *J. clin. Pharmac.*, 1986, *26*, *Suppl.* A, A36; C. D. Swerdlow *et al.*, *Am. Heart J.*, 1986, *111*, 49.

5234-m

Flopropione *(rINN)*.

Fluropropiofenone; Phloropropiophenone; RP-13907. 2′,4′,6′-Trihydroxypropiophenone.

$C_9H_{10}O_4$=182.2.

CAS — 2295-58-1.

Flopropione is used as an antispasmodic in doses of 40 mg given three to four times daily by mouth.

Proprietary Names and Manufacturers

Bilup *(Jpn)*; Compacsul *(Jpn)*; Cospanon *(Jpn)*; Cospuron *(Jpn)*; Ecapron *(Jpn)*; Ephtanon *(Jpn)*; Flopion *(Jpn)*; Floveton *(Jpn)*; Gallepronin *(Jpn)*; Gasstenon *(Jpn)*; Labrodax *(Rhodia, Arg.; Belg.)*; Mirulevatin *(Jpn)*; Nichipanon *(Jpn)*; Padeskin *(Jpn)*; Pasmus *(Jpn)*; Pellegal *(Jpn)*; Sartiron *(Jpn)*; Spasmoril *(Jpn)*; Supanate *(Jpn)*; Toriphenon *(Jpn)*; Trytalon *(Jpn)*; Tuflit *(Jpn)*.

3723-b

Florantyrone *(BAN, rINN)*.

4-(Fluoranthen-8-yl)-4-oxobutyric acid.

$C_{20}H_{14}O_3$=302.3.

CAS — 519-95-9.

Florantyrone is a choleretic. Doses of 0.75 to 1 g daily have been given.

References: J. R. Kirkpatrick *et al.*, *Gut*, 1974, *15*, 830.

Proprietary Names and Manufacturers

Bilyn *(Janus, Ital.)*; Cistoplex *(Borromeo, Ital.)*; Idroepar *(Ital.)*; Zanchol *(Searle, Arg.; Searle, Belg.)*.

19184-e

Flumecinol *(rINN)*.

RGH-3332. α-Ethyl-3-(trifluoromethyl)benzhydrol.

$C_{16}H_{15}F_3O$=280.3.

CAS — 56430-99-0.

Flumecinol has been used in the treatment of infant jaundice.

Proprietary Names and Manufacturers

Zixoryn *(Hung.)*.

9048-w

Flumedroxone Acetate *(BANM, rINNM)*.

6α-Trifluoromethyl-17α-acetoxyprogesterone; WG-537. 3,20-Dioxo-6α-trifluoromethylpregn-4-en-17α-yl acetate.

$C_{24}H_{31}F_3O_4$=440.5.

CAS — 15687-21-5 (flumedroxone); 987-18-8 (acetate).

Flumedroxone acetate is a derivative of progesterone that is reported to possess no anabolic, androgenic, oestrogenic, or progestogenic activity. It has been used in the treatment of migraine in doses of 10 to 20 mg daily by mouth.

Proprietary Names and Manufacturers

Demigrana *(Lövens, Swed.)*.

16814-n

Fluperlapine *(rINN)*.

NB-106689. 3-Fluoro-6-(4-methyl-1-piperazinyl)morphanthridine.

$C_{19}H_{20}FN_3$=309.4.

CAS — 67121-76-0.

Fluperlapine is a neuroleptic related to clozapine (p.727) which has been tried in the treatment of schizophrenia.

References: M. Matejcek *et al.*, *Arzneimittel-Forsch.*, 1984, *34*, 114; B. Muller-Oerlinghausen, *ibid.*, 131; B. Woggon *et al.*, *Neuropsychobiology*, 1984, *11*, 116.

Proprietary Names and Manufacturers

Sandoz, Switz.

18646-k

Fluticasone *(BAN, rINN)*.

CCI-18781 (propionate). *S*-(Fluoromethyl) 6α,9-difluoro-11β,17-dihydroxy-16α-methyl-3-oxoandrosta-1,4-diene-17β-carbothioate.

$C_{22}H_{27}F_3O_4S$=444.5.

CAS — 90566-53-3 (fluticasone); 80474-14-2 (propionate).

NOTE. Fluticasone Propionate is *USAN*.

Fluticasone is a corticosteroid that has been investigated as a topical anti-inflammatory agent; it is also reportedly under investigation by inhalation in the management of asthma.

Proprietary Names and Manufacturers

Glaxo, UK.

1309-x

Formic Acid

Ameisensäure; Aminic Acid; E236; E237 *(*sodium formate*)*; E238 *(*calcium formate*)*.

CH_2O_2=46.03.

CAS — 64-18-6.

Pharmacopoeias. In *Aust.* and *Pol.*

Formic acid resembles acetic acid in its actions but is more irritating and pungent. The acid and its sodium and calcium salts are used as preservatives in food. Solutions containing about 60% formic acid are marketed for the removal of lime scales from kettles.

In Great Britain the recommended exposure limit of formic acid is 5 ppm.

Estimated acceptable daily intake: up to 3 mg per kg body-weight.— Seventeenth Report of the Joint FAO/WHO Expert Committee on Food Additives, *Tech. Rep. Ser. Wld Hlth Org. No. 539*, 1974. Ethyl formate could be included in the acceptable daily intake for formic acid.— Twenty-third Report of Joint FAO/WHO Expert Committee on Food Additives, *Tech. Rep. Ser. Wld Hlth Org. No. 648*, 1980.

A report of 3 patients who swallowed descaling agents containing 40 or 55% formic acid. The major complications included the local effects on the oropharynx, oesophagus, and stomach, metabolic acidosis, derangement of blood-clotting mechanisms with intravascular coagulation or haemolysis, and the acute onset of respiratory and renal failure. All 3 patients died between 5 to 14 days after admission to hospital.— R. B. Naik *et al.*, *Postgrad. med. J.*, 1980, *56*, 451.

A report of 53 cases of formic acid ingestion in India. Treatment was symptomatic.— N. Rajan *et al.*, *Postgrad. med. J.*, 1985, *61*, 35.

19193-l

Formoterol *(rINN)*.

BD-40A. (±)-2′-Hydroxy-5′-[(*RS*)-1-hydroxy-2-[[(*RS*)-*p*-methoxy-α-methylphenethyl]amino]ethyl] formanilide.

$C_{19}H_{24}N_2O_4$=344.4.

CAS — 73573-87-2.

Formoterol is a selective $beta_2$ adrenoceptor agonist which has been given as the fumarate for its bronchodilator properties.

Proprietary Names and Manufacturers

Atock *(Yamanouchi, Jpn)*.

3794-t

Fosfocreatinine *(rINN)*.

(1-Methyl-4-oxo-2-imidazolidinylidene)phosphoramidic acid.

$C_4H_8N_3O_4P$=193.1.

CAS — 5786-71-0.

Fosfocreatinine has been used in cardiovascular disorders. It has been given as the disodium salt.

Proprietary Names and Manufacturers

Creatergyl *(Midy, Ital.)*.

12771-x

Fosforylcholine

Phosphorylcholine. (2-Hydroxyethyl)trimethylammonium chloride dihydrogen phosphate.

$C_5H_{15}ClNO_4P$=219.6.

CAS — 107-73-3.

Fosforylcholine has been used in the treatment of hepatic disorders. The calcium salt has been used as a source of calcium and phosphorus.

Proprietary Names and Manufacturers of Calcium or Magnesium Fosforylcholine

Arenzil *(San Carlo, Ital.)*; Bifos *(Salus, Ital.)*; Colincalcium *(Farmacologico Milanese, Ital.)*; Colinef *(Brocchieri, Ital.)*; Contrasthen *(Müller/Göppingen, Ger.)*; Epafosforil *(Coli, Ital.)*; Epaspes *(Nuovo, Ital.)*; Fisiocolina *(IBIS, Ital.)*; Fosfocolina *(Azienda Farm., Ital.)*; Héparexine *(Astra, Fr.)*; Isocolin *(Isola-Ibi, Ital.)*; Tonepar *(Molteni, Ital.)*.

965-r

Fosinopril *(pINN)*.

SQ-28555. (4*S*)-4-Cyclohexyl-1-[[[(*RS*)-1-hydroxy-2-methylpropoxy](4-phenylbutyl)-phosphinyl]acetyl]-L-proline propionate.

$C_{30}H_{46}NO_7P$=563.7.

CAS — 97825-24-6.

NOTE. Fosinopril Sodium is *USAN*.

Fosinopril is an angiotensin-converting enzyme inhibitor that has been investigated as an antihypertensive agent.

19201-t

Fostedil *(USAN, rINN)*.

A-53986; Abbott-53986; KB-944. Diethyl (*p*-2-benzothiazolylbenzyl)phosphonate.

$C_{18}H_{20}NO_3PS$=361.4.

CAS — 75889-62-2.

Fostedil is reported to possess vasodilator and calcium-channel blocking activity.

Proprietary Names and Manufacturers

Abbott, USA.

19203-r

FPL-52694

[5-(2-Hydroxypropoxyl)-8-propyl-4-oxo-4*H*-benzopyran-2-carboxylate sodium.

$C_{16}H_{17}O_6Na$=328.3.

FPL-52694 is reported to have mast-cell stabilising actions and has been investigated for its ability to reduce gastric acid secretion as a potential agent in the management of peptic ulcer.

Reference: H. J. Reimann *et al., Gut,* 1984, *25,* 1221.

1310-y

Fumaric Acid *(USAN)*.

297; Allomalenic Acid; Boletic Acid. *trans*-Butenedioic acid.

$C_2H_2(CO_2H)_2$=116.1.

CAS — 110-17-8.

Pharmacopoeias. In *U.S.N.F.*

White odourless granules or crystalline powder. Slightly **soluble** in water and ether; soluble in alcohol; very slightly soluble in chloroform. **Store** in well-closed containers.

Fumaric acid is used as an acidifier and flavouring agent in foods.

Estimated acceptable daily intake: up to 6 mg per kg body-weight.— Eighteenth Report of the FAO/WHO Expert Committee on Food Additives, *Tech. Rep. Ser. Wld Hlth Org. No. 557,* 1974.

12777-m

Gabexate Mesylate

Gabexate Mesilate *(rINNM)*. Ethyl 4-(6-guanidinohexanoyloxy)benzoate methanesulphonate.

$C_{16}H_{23}N_3O_4,CH_4SO_3$=417.5.

CAS — 39492-01-8 (gabexate); 56974-61-9 (mesylate).

Gabexate mesylate is a proteolytic enzyme inhibitor used in the treatment of pancreatitis and as an anticoagulant for haemodialysis.

References: N. T. Richards and M. A. Mansell, *Br. J. Hosp. Med.,* 1986, *35,* 190; E. Menegatti *et al., J. pharm. Sci.,* 1986, *75,* 1171.

Proprietary Names and Manufacturers

Foy *(Ono, Jpn)*.

16820-f

Gangliosides

Gangliosides are endogenous substances present in mammalian cell membranes, especially in the cortex of the brain. They are glycosphingolipids composed of a hydrophilic oligosaccharide chain, characterised by sialic acid residues, attached to a lipophilic moiety. The four major gangliosides found in the mammalian brain are referred to as G_{M1}, G_{D1a}, G_{D1b}, and G_{T1b} and a preparation containing these four gangliosides has been given by intramuscular injection in the treatment of peripheral neuropathies. A monoganglioside preparation containing monosialoganglioside (G_{M1}) has been used in the treatment of cerebrovascular disorders. A synthetic monosialoganglioside siagoside (AGF_2) is also under investigation.

A detailed review of gangliosides and their use in the treatment of peripheral neuropathies.— J. C. Samson, *Drugs Today,* 1986, *22,* 73.

References: R. Y. Huaman *et al., Curr. ther. Res.,* 1986, *40,* 29 (Bell's palsy).

Proprietary Names and Manufacturers

Biosinax *(Rorer, Ital.)*; Cronassial *(Madaus, Ger.*; *Fidia, Ital.)*; Sygen *(Fidia, Ital.)*.

2014-y

Garlic

Ajo; Allium.

CAS — 8008-99-9 (extract); 8000-78-0 (oil).

Pharmacopoeias. In *Span.*

The fresh bulb of *Allium sativum* (Liliaceae).

Garlic has traditionally been reported to have expectorant, diaphoretic, disinfectant, and diuretic properties, and was formerly used in the treatment of pulmonary conditions such as tuberculosis. More recently, it has been investigated for its antimicrobial and lipid-lowering properties.

There have been some reports of contact dermatitis associated with garlic.

Evidence of a platelet aggregation inhibitor in garlic.— T. Ariga *et al.* (letter), *Lancet,* 1981, *1,* 150. See also D. J. Boullin (letter), *ibid.,* 776.

HYPERLIPIDAEMIA. In an open study involving 20 hypercholesteraemic patients, cholesterol, triglyceride, and high-density lipoprotein concentrations decreased to a greater extent after 4 weeks' treatment with garlic powder by mouth in association with a hypocaloric diet compared with treatment by diet alone.— E. Ernst *et al.* (letter), *Br. med. J.,* 1985, *291,* 139.

In 2 double-blind studies involving 34 and 51 patients with primary hyperlipoproteinaemia, the administration of dried garlic in the form of sugar-coated tablets failed to produce a significant effect on blood lipids, apolipoproteins or blood coagulation parameters.— C. Luley *et al., Arzneimittel-Forsch.,* 1986, *36,* 766.

INFECTION. Studies *in vitro* have shown garlic extract, probably consisting principally of allicin, to possess antifungal (Y. Yamada and K. Azuma, *Antimicrob. Ag. Chemother.,* 1977, *11,* 743), antitubercular (E.C. Delaha and V.F. Garagusi, *ibid.,* 1985, *27,* 485), and antiviral (Y. Tsai *et al., Planta med.,* 1985 (Oct.), 460) activity. Favourable results have been reported with garlic given intramuscularly or intravenously, and also, in most cases by mouth in the treatment of 16 patients with cryptococcal meningitis (*Chin. med. J.,* 1980, *93,* 123). In a study in 5 healthy subjects given a single dose of garlic extract by mouth, however, antifungal activity was not detected in urine, and was only detected in serum 30 and 60 minutes after administration (N. Caporaso *et al., Antimicrob. Ag. Chemother.,* 1983, *23,* 700). The authors considered that garlic would only be of limited value in the treatment of human fungal infections.

12781-f

Gelsemium

Gelsemium Root; Jessamine; Yellow Jasmine Root. The dried rhizome and roots of *Gelsemium sempervirens* (Loganiaceae) containing not less than 0.32% of total alkaloids, calculated as gelsemine ($C_{20}H_{22}N_2O_2$ = 322.4).

CAS — 509-15-9 (gelsemine).

Adverse Effects

These include giddiness, ptosis, double vision, dilated pupils, weakness, and respiratory depression. They may be delayed for some hours and may result from quite small doses of gelsemium. Fatal doses cause slowing and arrest of the respiration.

Treatment of Adverse Effects

After ingestion of gelsemium, empty the stomach by inducing emesis or by aspiration and lavage; give atropine by subcutaneous injection; assisted respiration may be necessary.

Uses and Administration

Gelsemium depresses the central nervous system and has been used mainly in neuralgic conditions, particularly trigeminal neuralgia and migraine. It has usually been employed as the tincture given in mixtures with bromides or other sedatives. Gelsemium is used in homoeopathic medicine.

Preparations

Compound Gelsemium and Hyoscyamus Mixture *(B.P.C. 1973)*. Gelsemium tincture 0.3 mL, potassium bromide 500 mg, hyoscyamus tincture 1 mL, double-strength chloroform water 5 mL, water to 10 mL. It should be recently prepared. *Dose.* 10 to 20 mL.

Gelsemium Tincture *(B.P.C. 1973)*. Tinct. Gelsem. Prepared from gelsemium by percolation with alcohol (60%) and adjusted to contain 0.030 to 0.034% w/v of total alkaloids, calculated as gelsemine. *Dose.* 0.3 to 1 mL.

Gowers' Mixture. A mixture containing gelsemium and used in the treatment of migraine. Various formulas have been used. They usually contained a bromide and strychnine as well as gelsemium tincture.

3927-c

Genetically Derived Compounds

Many protein compounds now in clinical use or under investigation are produced through genetic technology. One technique involves recombinant deoxyribonucleic acid (DNA) in which the gene or DNA fragment for a particular protein is isolated using a relevant enzyme and is introduced into a selected cell to stimulate production of the required protein. Quantities of the protein can then be obtained through cell culture. Some of the proteins produced by this technology include alteplase (p.1042), erythropoietin (p.1568), insulin (p.391), interferons (p.696), interleukins (p.632), various hormones (p.1135), and vaccines (p.1155).

Monoclonal antibodies (MAbs) are produced by the fusion of two cell types to produce a clone that in turn produces an antibody. Such antibodies once harvested have wide ranging applications in cancer therapy, delivery systems, and diagnosis. A monoclonal antibody known as muromonab-CD3 (p.645) is being used to treat acute allograft rejection in kidney transplants. Others such as campath-1 are being investigated as aids to bone-marrow transplantation. Monoclonal antibodies are employed in pregnancy tests (p.944) and are being investigated in the diagnosis of foetal disturbances. Other investigations include rheumatoid arthritis, the identification of infective agents, and the treatment of infections; one antibody, for example, is being studied for use in endotoxic shock resulting from Gram-negative bacteraemia.

References: A. E. H. Emery, *An Introduction to Recombinant DNA*, Chichester, Wiley, 1984; N. H. Carey, *Br. med. J.*, 1987, *295*, 907.

534-r

Gentian *(BAN).*

Enzianwurzel; Gentian Root; Gentiana; Gentianae Radix; Genziana; Raiz de Genciana.

Pharmacopoeias. In *Arg., Aust., Br., Cz., Egypt., Eur., Fr., Ger., Hung., It., Jpn, Jug., Neth., Nord., Pol., Port., Roum., Span.,* and *Swiss. Br.* also includes Powdered Gentian.

Aust., Cz., and *Hung.* allow also other species of *Gentiana.*

Jpn includes also Japanese Gentian, from *G. scabra. Chin.* specifies *G. scabra* and other species.

The dried underground organs of*Gentiana lutea* (Gentianaceae), yielding not less than 33% of water-soluble extractive. **Store** in well-closed containers. Protect from light.

Uses and Administration

Gentian is used as a bitter. An alcoholic infusion of gentian, bitter-orange peel, and lemon peel has been used as an ingredient in a number of bitter mixtures some of which are described in *B.P.C. 1973.*

Preparations

Acid Gentian Mixture *(B.P.C. 1973).* Concentrated compound gentian infusion 1 mL, dilute hydrochloric acid 0.5 mL, double-strength chloroform water 5 mL, water to 10 mL. It should be recently prepared.
Dose. 10 to 20 mL.

Alkaline Gentian Mixture *(B.P.).* Concentrated compound gentian infusion 1 mL, sodium bicarbonate 500 mg, double-strength chloroform water 5 mL, water to 10 mL. It should be recently prepared.
A.P.F. (Gentian Mixture Alkaline) has a similar formula with concentrated chloroform water or compound hydroxybenzoate solution.
Dose. 10 mL.

Compound Gentian Infusion *(B.P.).* Co. Gent. Inf. Concentrated compound gentian infusion 10 mL, water to 100 mL. It should be used within 12 hours of preparation.
Dose. 15 to 40 mL.

Concentrated Compound Gentian Infusion *(B.P.).* Conc. Co. Gent. Inf. Prepared by macerating gentian, dried bitter-orange peel, and dried lemon peel, about 1 in 10 of each, with alcohol (25%).
Dose. 1.5 to 4 mL.

Proprietary Names and Manufacturers

The following names have been used for multi-ingredient preparations containing gentian—Aneurone *(Philip Harris, UK)*; Effico *(Pharmax, UK)*; Glykola Infans *(Sinclair, UK).*

3272-c

Gentisic Acid Ethanolamide *(USAN).*

2,5-Dihydroxybenzoic acid ethanolamide.
$C_9H_{11}NO_4$=197.2.

Pharmacopoeias. In *U.S.N.F.*

A white to tan powder. Sparingly **soluble** in water; freely soluble in acetone, in alcohol, and in methyl alcohol; very slightly soluble in ether; practically insoluble in chloroform. **Store** in well-closed containers.

Gentisic acid ethanolamide is used as a complexing agent in the manufacture of pharmaceutical preparations.

19247-w

Gepirone *(pINN).*

BMY-13805; MJ-13805-1. 3,3-Dimethyl-*N*-{4-[4-(2-pyrimidinyl)-1-piperazinyl]butyl-}glutarimide.
$C_{19}H_{29}N_5O_2$=359.5.

CAS — 83928-76-1 (gepirone); 83928-66-9 (hydrochloride).

NOTE. Gepirone Hydrochloride is *USAN.*

Gepirone is under investigation as an anti-depressant and anxiolytic agent.

References: *Drugs of the Future,* 1985, *10,* 456; *ibid.,* 1986, *11,* 519; I. Csanalosi *et al., J. clin. Psychopharmacol.,* 1987, *7,* 31; J. Amsterdam *et al., Curr. ther. Res.,* 1987, *41,* 185.

12784-h

Ginseng

Ginseng Radix; Ninjin; Panax; Pannag. The dried root of *Panax ginseng* (= *P. schinseng*) (Araliaceae). Other varieties of ginseng include *Panax quinquefolium* (North America) and *P. pseudoginseng.* The Russian pharmacopoeia includes a monograph on the root of *Panax ginseng,* however, the root commonly known as Siberian or Russian ginseng belongs to the same family, Araliaceae, but is an entirely different plant, *Eleutherococcus senticosis.*

Pharmacopoeias. In *Aust., Chin., Jpn, Rus.,* and *Swiss. Chin.* also includes Radix Notoginseng from *P. notoginseng,* Rhizoma Panacis Japonica from *P. japonicus,* and Rhizoma Panacis Majoris from *P. japonicus* var. *major* and *P. japonicus* var. *bipinnatifidus.* Red Ginseng *(Jpn P.)* is the dried root of *P. ginseng* which has been steamed.

Ginseng contains complex mixtures of saponins termed ginsenosides or panaxosides. At least 13 saponins have been isolated from extracts of *P. ginseng* roots.

Studies in *animals* have demonstrated that ginseng has a wide range of pharmacological activities but their possible clinical significance has not been fully investigated by controlled studies in man although large scale studies have been carried out in the USSR on *Eleutherococcus.* Ginseng has been claimed to enhance the natural resistance and recuperative power of the body and to have both stimulant and sedative activity. Its toxicity appears to be low. It is available commercially as roots, powdered roots, tablets, capsules, teas, oils, or extracts.

For reviews of ginseng, see F. Sandberg, *Planta med.,* 1973, *24,* 392; W. E. Court, *Pharm. J.,* 1975, *1,* 180; J. D. Phillipson and L. A. Anderson, *Pharm. J.,* 1984, *1,* 161; C. A. Baldwin *et al., ibid.,* 1986, *2,* 583.

Effect of a standardised ginseng extract on psychomotor performance.— L. D'Angelo *et al., J. Ethnopharmacol.,* 1986, *16,* 15.

ADVERSE EFFECTS. A 2-year study of ginseng in 133 subjects who had used a wide variety of commercial preparations including roots, capsules, tablets, teas, extracts, cigarettes, chewing gum, and candies. The majority of preparations were taken by mouth but a few subjects had experimented with intranasal or parenteral routes and topical preparations had also been used. The stimulant effects of ginseng were confirmed but there was also a high incidence of side-effects including morning diarrhoea (47 subjects), skin eruptions (33), sleeplessness (26), nervousness (25), hypertension (22), euphoria (18), and oedema (14). The 'ginseng abuse syndrome' defined as hypertension together with nervousness, sleeplessness, skin eruptions, and morning diarrhoea was experienced by 14 subjects who took ginseng by mouth in an average daily dose of 3 g. Abrupt withdrawal precipitated hypotension, weakness, and tremor in one user. About 50% of the subjects had discontinued the use of ginseng within 2 years.— R. K. Siegel, *J. Am. med. Ass.,* 1979, *241,* 1614. Comment.— R. K. Siegel (letter), *ibid.,* 1980, *243,* 32.

Oestrogenic effects. A 70-year-old woman developed swollen tender breasts with diffuse nodularity on 3 occasions after taking ginseng.— B. V. Palmer (letter), *Br. med. J.,* 1978, *1,* 1284. See also O. M. Koriech, *ibid.,* 1556; M. N. G. Dukes (letter), *ibid.,* 1621.

A report of an oestrogen-like effect on the vaginal epithelium in a 62-year-old woman taking ginseng.— R. Punnonen and R. Lukola, *Br. med. J.,* 1980, *281,* 1110. See also E. M. Greenspan (letter), *J. Am. med. Ass.,* 1983, *249,* 2018 (vaginal bleeding).

Proprietary Names and Manufacturers

Bio-Star *(Novag, Spain)*; Ginsana *(Weimer, Ger.; Swisspharm, S.Afr.; GPL, Switz.).*

3905-w

Glicofosfopeptical

Fosfoglicopeptical.

Glicofosfopeptical is reported to possess immunostimulant properties and has been given in doses of 500 mg by mouth three times daily.

Proprietary Names and Manufacturers

Inmunoferon *(Andromaco, Spain).*

7711-s

Glucagon *(BAN, USAN, rINN).*

HGF. A polypeptide hormone derived from beef or pork pancreas. His-Ser-Gln-Gly-Thr-Phe-Thr-Ser-Asp-Tyr-Ser-Lys-Tyr-Leu-Asp-Ser-Arg-Arg-Ala-Gln-Asp-Phe-Val-Gln-Trp-Leu-Met-Asn-Thr.
$C_{153}H_{225}N_{43}O_{49}S$=3482.8.

CAS — 16941-32-5.

Pharmacopoeias. In *Br., Egypt.,*and *U.S.*

A white or faintly coloured, almost odourless, fine crystalline powder. Practically **insoluble** in water; soluble in dilute alkalis and acids; practically insoluble in most organic solvents. **Store** at 2° to 8° in airtight containers. The *U.S.P.* recommends storage under nitrogen.

Glucagon is administered by injection as a sterile solution of glucagon hydrochloride which has a pH of 2.5 to 4.0.

One unit of glucagon is approximately equivalent to 1 mg.

Units

1.49 units of glucagon, porcine for bioassay, are contained in approximately 1.5 mg of freeze-dried porcine glucagon, with lactose 5 mg and sodium chloride, in one ampoule of the first International Standard Preparation (1973).

1.49 units of glucagon, porcine for immunoassay, are contained in approximately 1.5 mg of freeze-dried porcine glucagon, with lactose 5 mg and sodium chloride, in one ampoule of the first International Reference Preparation (1974).

Adverse Effects

Nausea and vomiting may occur following administration of glucagon. Hypersensitivity reactions and hypokalaemia have also been reported.

Development of erythema multiforme in one patient following administration of glucagon 100 µg intravenously.— S. L. Edell, *Am. J. Roentg.,* 1980, *134,* 385.

Precautions

Glucagon should be administered with caution to patients with insulinoma or phaeochromocytoma as it may induce hypoglycaemia due to its insulin-releasing effect or marked hypertension due to subsequent catecholamine release. Caution is also required when it is being employed as a diagnostic aid in diabetic patients.

Glucagon is not effective in patients with marked depletion of liver glycogen stores, as in starvation, adrenal insufficiency, or chronic hypoglycaemia.

For a report of high doses of glucagon enhancing the anticoagulant effect of warfarin, see Warfarin Sodium, p.347.

Absorption and Fate

Glucagon has a plasma half-life of about 3 to 6 minutes. It is inactivated in the liver, kidneys, and plasma.

A study in 19 fasting patients undergoing myelography demonstrated that glucagon was present in CSF at an average of 28% of the concentration in serum. The expected ratio would be 10% if glucagon reached the CSF only through simple diffusion, and it is possible that glucagon, like insulin, is actively transported from blood into CSF.— J. L. Graner and C. Abraira (letter), *New Engl. J. Med.*, 1985, *312*, 994.

Uses and Administration

Glucagon is a polypeptide hormone which is produced by the alpha cells of the pancreatic islets of Langerhans. It is a *hyperglycaemic* agent which mobilises glucose by activating hepatic glycogenolysis. It can to a lesser extent stimulate the secretion of pancreatic insulin. Glucagon is administered as glucagon hydrochloride; doses are usually expressed as glucagon.

Glucagon is used in the treatment of insulin-induced hypoglycaemia when administration of glucose intravenously is not possible (see p.393). It is given by subcutaneous, intramuscular, or intravenous injection in a dose of 0.5 to 1 unit, repeated if necessary after 20 minutes.

As glucagon reduces the motility of the gastro-intestinal tract it is used as a diagnostic aid in gastro-intestinal radiological examinations. The route of administration is dependent upon the diagnostic procedure. A dose of 1 to 2 units administered intramuscularly has an onset of action of 4 to 14 minutes and a duration of effect of 10 to 40 minutes; 0.2 to 2 units given intravenously produces an effect within one minute that lasts for 9 to 25 minutes.

Glucagon possesses positive cardiac inotropic activity but is not generally considered a suitable agent for heart failure. However, as it can bypass blocked beta receptors, it is used in the treatment of beta-blocker overdosage, see p.801.

A detailed review of the pharmacology of glucagon.— A. E. Farah, *Pharmac. Rev.*, 1983, *35*, 181.

A brief report on glucagon stopping continuous hiccups. Glucagon was tried because of its dilating effect on Oddi's sphincter.— A. M. N. Gardner, *Br. med. J.*, 1985, *290*, 822.

A 75-year-old man who was being treated with atenolol developed anaphylactoid hypotension following injection of the radiocontrast dye meglumine diatrizoate. Adrenaline failed to produce a sustained increase in blood pressure, but administration of glucagon intravenously led to reversal of the hypotension.— G. P. Zaloga *et al.*, *Ann. intern. Med.*, 1986, *105*, 65.

ADMINISTRATION. In 7 healthy subjects glucagon given as nasal drops increased blood-glucose concentrations.— A. E. Pontiroli *et al.*, *Br. med. J.*, 1983, *287*, 462.

DIAGNOSIS AND TESTING. *Insulinoma.* A report on the use of glucagon in the diagnosis of insulinoma.— D. Kumar *et al.*, *Ann. intern. Med.*, 1974, *80*, 697.

Liver function. An assessment of the value of glucagon as a screening test for hepatic glycogen storage disease.— D. B. Dunger and J. V. Leonard, *Archs Dis. Childh.*, 1982, *57*, 384. Use of glucagon in the differential diagnosis of obstructive and hepatocellular jaundice.— D. A. Berstock *et al.*, *Postgrad. med. J.*, 1982, *58*, 485.

Phaeochromocytoma. In a review of the diagnosis, localisation, and management of phaeochromocytoma, the glucagon stimulation test was reported to be widely used. The suggested dose of glucagon for this purpose was 1 to 2 mg intravenously after determination of the patient's pressor response to a cold pressor test. A positive glucagon test required a clear increase (at least threefold or over 2 ng per mL [11.82 pmol per mL]) in plasma catecholamines, 1 to 3 minutes after drug administration. A simultaneous increase in blood pressure of at least 20/15 mm Hg above the pressor response to a cold pressor test was said to be desirable but not essential.— E. L. Bravo and R. W. Gifford, *New Engl. J. Med.*, 1984, *311*, 1298. See also.— Y. Miura *et al.* (letter), *ibid.*, 676.

The basis of false-positive glucagon tests for phaeochromocytoma.— O. Kuchel *et al.*, *Clin. Pharmac. Ther.*, 1981, *29*, 687.

Pituitary function. References to the use of glucagon in stimulatory tests in the investigation of growth hormone deficiency: R. D. G. Milner and E. C. Burns, *Archs Dis. Childh.*, 1982, *57*, 944 (intramuscular glucagon test); M. Colle *et al.*, *ibid.*, 1984, *59*, 670 (glucagon with betaxolol or propranolol); C. F. Abboud, *Mayo Clin. Proc.*, 1986, *61*, 35 (glucagon with propranolol); *Lancet*, 1986, *1*, 839 (subcutaneous glucagon test).

EFFECTS ON THE HEART. Glucagon has undergone extensive investigation as an alternative to beta-adrenergic agonists in the treatment of heart failure because of its ability to produce a positive inotropic effect by stimulating myocardial glucagon receptors. However, glucagon has not been useful clinically as a positive inotropic agent because of its low potency, high incidence of adverse gastro-intestinal effects, and rapid selective loss of inotropic effects.— W. S. Colucci *et al.*, *New Engl. J. Med.*, 1986, *314*, 290.

GASTRO-INTESTINAL DISORDERS. Glucagon has been used in several studies to treat various painful gastro-intestinal disorders associated with spasm. Daniel *et al.* (*Br. med. J.*, 1974, *3*, 720) reported quicker symptomatic relief of acute diverticulitis in patients treated with glucagon compared with those who had been treated with analgesics or antispasmodics. A review by Glauser *et al.*, (*J. Am. Coll. emergency Physns*, 1979, *8*, 228) described relief of acute oesophageal food obstruction following glucagon therapy. In another study glucagon significantly relieved pain and tenderness in 21 patients with biliary tract disease compared with 22 patients treated with placebo (M.J. Stower *et al.*, *Br. J. Surg.*, 1982, *69*, 591). Franken *et al.*, however, (*Radiology*, 1983, *146*, 687) failed to show any advantage of glucagon over placebo in the hydrostatic reduction of ileocolic intussusception in a study of 30 children, and Webb *et al.* (*Med. J. Aust.*, 1986, *144*, 124) concluded that glucagon was ineffective in the management of ureteric colic in a casualty department.

HYPOGLYCAEMIA. Successful long-term treatment of persistent hypoglycaemia with intramuscular zinc glucagon in 2 children who could not be managed by frequent feeding. Zinc glucagon was preferred to diazoxide due to the side-effects of the latter.— L. Kollée and L. Monnens (letter), *Lancet*, 1978, *1*, 668. See also L. A. Kollée *et al.*, *Archs Dis. Childh.*, 1978, *53*, 422.

LIVER FAILURE. For a report on the use of glucagon with insulin in the treatment of severe liver failure, see under insulin (p.396).

PANCREATITIS. Although an early report (J.R. Condon *et al.*, *Br. med. J.*, 1972, *1*, 376) suggested a beneficial role of glucagon in acute pancreatitis, a later MRC Multicentre Study (*Lancet*, 1977, *2*, 632; *Gut*, 1980, *21*, 334) and other studies (H.K. Dürr *et al.*, *Gut*, 1978, *19*, 175; A. Olazabal and R. Fuller, *Gastroenterology*, 1978, *74*, 489; H.T. Debas, *Can. J. Surg.*, 1980, *23*, 578) showed glucagon to be ineffective.

Preparations

Glucagon for Injection *(U.S.P.)*. A sterile mixture of glucagon hydrochloride with 1 or more suitable dry diluents; when dissolved in the sterile solvent provided it forms a clear solution.

Glucagon Injection *(B.P.)*. A sterile solution of glucagon with hydrochloric acid and lactose, prepared by dissolving the contents of a sealed container in a suitable solvent.

Proprietary Preparations

Glucagon Lilly *(Lilly, UK)*. *Injection,* powder for reconstitution, glucagon 1 unit (as hydrochloride), supplied with diluent.

Glucagon Novo *(Novo, UK)*. *Injection,* powder for reconstitution, glucagon 1 unit (as hydrochloride), supplied with diluent and a disposable syringe.
Injection, powder for reconstitution, glucagon 10 units (as hydrochloride), supplied with diluent.

16823-h

Glucomannan

Glucomannan, a powdered extract from the tubers of *Amorphophallus konjac*, has been promoted as an anorectic agent but there is no evidence to substantiate such a claim; it is claimed to act by being a bulking agent, absorbing liquid in the gastro-intestinal tract.

Possible similarity to guar gum in diabetes mellitus.— K. Doi (letter), *Lancet*, 1979, *1*, 987.

A brief discussion on glucomannan and comment that though the flower of *A. konjac* is a wondrous sight, its odour is extremely noxious resembling that of decomposing flesh. Devil's Tongue and Skunk Lilly seem appropriate common names.— *FDA Consumer*, 1984, (Feb.), 31.

Oesophageal obstruction associated with glucomannan.— D. Henry *et al.*, *Br. med. J.*, 1986, *292*, 591.

12790-d

Glucosamine *(USAN, pINN)*.

Chitosamine; NSC-758. 2-Amino-2-deoxy-β-D-glucopyranose.

$C_6H_{13}NO_5$=179.2.

CAS — 3416-24-8.

Glucosamine is found in chitin, mucoproteins, and mucopolysaccharides; it is isolated from chitin or prepared synthetically.

Glucosamine sulphate and hydriodide have been given in the treatment of rheumatic disorders. The hydrochloride has also been used.

References: A. Drovanti *et al.*, *Clin. Ther.*, 1980, *3*, 260; G. Crolle and E. D'Este, *Curr. med. Res. Opinion*, 1980, *7*, 104; J. M. Pujalte *et al.*, *ibid.*, 110; E. D'Ambrosio *et al.*, *Pharmatherapeutica*, 1981, *2*, 504; Y. Vajaradul, *Clin. Ther.*, 1981, *3*, 336; A. L. Vaz, *Curr. med. Res. Opinion*, 1982, *8*, 145.

Proprietary Names and Manufacturers

Adaxil *(Spedrog-Caillon, Arg.)*; Anartril *(Farma-Lepori, Spain)*; Arthryl *(Synlab, Fr.)*; Dona *(Opfermann, Ger.; Rottapharm, Ital.)*; Viartril *(Rottapharm, Ital.)*.

12792-h

Gluten

A mixture of 2 proteins, gliadin and glutenin, present in wheat flour and to a lesser extent in barley, oats, and rye. Gliadin is a prolamine, one of the 2 chief groups of plant proteins, and glutenin belongs to the other main group termed glutelins.

CAS — 8002-80-0.

Gluten is of medicinal and pharmaceutical interest in that patients with coeliac disease (non-tropical sprue; primary malabsorption syndrome; idiopathic steatorrhoea; gluten-induced enteropathy) are sensitive to the gliadin fraction of gluten contained in the normal diet. Claims that only the α-gliadin fraction is toxic have not been substantiated. Treatment consists of the use of gluten-free diets; wheat products are particularly to be avoided. Rye, which contains a small amount of gluten, and barley and oats, which contain the prolamines hordein and avenin respectively, should also be excluded from the diet of patients with coeliac disease.

A gluten-free diet may also be beneficial in patients with dermatitis herpetiformis.

A warning that some prescription medicines contained gluten and should be avoided by patients on a gluten-free diet. They included Dimotane LA, Dimotapp LA, Donnatal LA, Fybranta, Nardil, Natirose, Nulacin, Saroten, and Veracolate.— *Br. med. J.*, 1976, *2*, 185.

Juvela and Rite Diet gluten-free bread mixes contain acceptably low concentrations of gliadin and may be recommended for patients with coeliac disease.— P. J. Ciclitira *et al.*, *Br. med. J.*, 1984, *289*, 83. Diarrhoea occurred in 3 out of 10 coeliac patients when gluten-free bread based on wheat starch (Juvela) was added to their diet. Gluten-free products based on wheat starch should be considered as a possible cause of persistent symptoms in some treated coeliac patients.— P. J. Ciclitira *et al.*, *Gut*, 1985, *26*, A556.

Further references to the gluten content of pharmaceutical products and 'gluten-free' foods: G. B. Olson and G. R. Gallo, *Am. J. Hosp. Pharm.*, 1983, *40*, 121; *idem* (letter), 1308; D. G. Patel *et al.*, *Can. med. Ass. J.*, 1985, *133*, 114; C. Krogh (letter), *ibid.*, 636; R. G. Challen and R. M. O'Shannassy, *Med. J. Aust.*, 1987, *146*, 91.

A report of a child who was sensitive to wheat and who responded to a gluten-free dietary regimen yet who did not suffer from coeliac disease. She was considered to have a hereditary genetic disposition.— A. Jonas (letter), *Lancet*, 1978, *2*, 1047.

In patients with severe recurrent oral ulceration, the introduction of a gluten-free diet produced complete remission of the ulceration in 2 of 3 patients with raised α-gliadin antibodies. Dietary assessment showed non-compliance in the third patient. Gluten-free diets produced no clinical improvement in 2 patients with oral ulceration but negative α-gliadin antibodies.— C. O'Mahony *et al.*, *Gut*, 1985, *26*, A1137.

Good response to a gluten-free diet in a child with a 3-year history of idiopathic pulmonary haemosiderosis and evidence of gluten enteropathy.— R. Reading *et al.*, *Archs Dis. Childh.*, 1987, *62*, 513.

COELIAC DISEASE. A brief review of coeliac disease.— M. Shiner, *Postgrad. med. J.*, 1984, *60*, 773.

A study of 52 children with coeliac disease found that failure to comply with a gluten-free diet during childhood results in decreased adult stature and in persisting active enteropathy.— J. Colaco *et al.*, *Archs Dis. Childh.*, 1987, *62*, 706.

In a series of 202 patients with coeliac disease, 37 of the 97 deaths between 1941 and 1975 had been caused by malignant disease, particularly reticulum cell sarcoma and gastro-intestinal cancer. A gluten-free diet did not appear to protect against malignant complications but a longer follow-up would be needed.— G. K. T. Holmes *et al.*, *Gut*, 1976, *17*, 612.

Advice that children with coeliac disease must adhere to a gluten-free diet indefinitely.— A. S. McNeish, *Archs Dis. Childh.*, 1980, *55*, 110.

DERMATITIS HERPETIFORMIS. Comment on dermatitis herpetiformis and its association with gluten-sensitive enteropathy (coeliac disease).— *Lancet*, 1978, *2*, 458.

Reports on the beneficial effect of a gluten-free diet in patients with dermatitis herpetiformis.— L. Fry *et al.*, *Lancet*, 1973, *1*, 288; T. Reunala *et al.*, *Br. J. Derm.*, 1977, *97*, 473; C. I. Harrington and N. W. Read, *Br. med. J.*, 1977, *1*, 872; K. Ljunghall and U. M. Tjernlund (letter), *Lancet*, 1978, *2*, 1003; D. J. Gawkrodger and R. StC. Barnetson (letter), *Lancet*, 1982, *2*, 987; L. Fry *et al.*, *Br. J. Derm.*, 1982, *107*, 631; D. J. Hogan (letter), *Can. med. Ass. J.*, 1983, *128*, 512; *ibid.*, 1145; D. J. Gawkrodger *et al.*, *Gut*, 1984, *25*, 151; T. Reunala *et al.*, *Archs Dis. Childh.*, 1984, *59*, 517.

Gluten challenge has confirmed that dermatitis herpetiformis is gluten-dependent: J. N. Leonard *et al.*, *Br. J. Derm.*, 1982, *107 Suppl.* 22, 27; I. Kósnai *et al.*, *Gut*, 1986, *27*, 1464; J. Leonard *et al.*, *New Engl. J. Med.*, 1983, *308*, 816.

SCHIZOPHRENIA. In a double-blind study in 14 patients with schizophrenia on constant antipsychotic therapy, there was deterioration of their condition when challenged with wheat gluten.— M. M. Singh and S. R. Kay, *Science*, 1976, *191*, 401. Comments.— *Lancet*, 1976, *1*, 844; *ibid.*, 1983, *1*, 744.

Preparations

For some gluten-free dietary preparations, see p.1289.

1935-d

Glycerophosphoric Acid

Glycerylphosphoric Acid; Monoglycerylphosphoric Acid.

$C_3H_9O_6P$=172.1.

CAS — 27082-31-1; 57-03-4 (α); 17181-54-3 (β); 5746-57-6 (L-α); 1509-81-5 (DL-α).

Glycerophosphoric acid and various glycerophosphates have been used in tonics. They were once considered as a suitable means of providing phosphorus. Calcium and magnesium glycerophosphates are described in the Electrolytes section as they may be considered as a source of calcium and magnesium respectively.

Proprietary Preparations containing Glycerophosphates

Glykola *(Sinclair, UK). Elixir*, calcium glycerophosphate 30 mg, caffeine 20 mg, kola liquid extract 0.12 mL, chloroform spirit 0.12 mL, alcohol (90%) 0.5 mL, ferric chloride solution 0.01 mL/5 mL. *Dose.* 5 to 10 mL three times daily after meals.

Glykola Infans *(Sinclair, UK). Elixir*, manganese glycerophosphate 10 mg, kola liquid extract 0.066 mL, compound gentian infusion 1 mL, citric acid monohydrate 40 mg, and ferric chloride solution 0.016 mL/5 mL. *Dose.* 2.5 to 5 mL diluted with a little water.

Metatone *(Parke, Davis, UK). Mixture*, calcium glycerophosphate 45.6 mg, potassium glycerophosphate 45.6 mg, sodium glycerophosphate 22.8 mg, manganese glycerophosphate 5.7 mg, thiamine hydrochloride 500 µg/5 mL. (Suggested diluent water). *Dose.* 5 to 10 mL, preferably diluted, two or three times daily.

Verdiviton *(Squibb, UK). Elixir*, calcium glycerophosphate 110 mg, sodium glycerophosphate 80 mg, potassium glycerophosphate 20 mg, manganese glycerophosphate 10 mg, thiamine mononitrate 2 mg, riboflavine 1 mg, pyridoxine hydrochloride 500 µg, nicotinamide 15 mg, dexpanthenol 1 mg, cyanocobalamin 15 µg, alcohol (17%)/15 mL. *Dose.* Adults, 15 mL three times daily.

Proprietary Names and Manufacturers of Glycerophosphates

Phosthenine *(Cortunon, Canad.)*.

The following names have been used for multi-ingredient preparations containing glycerophosphates—Biotone *(Biorex, UK)*; Calsotone *(Southon-Horton, UK)*; Glykola *(Sinclair, UK)*; Glykola Infans *(Sinclair, UK)*; Glytona *(Philip Harris, UK)*; Ironorm *(Wallace Mfg Chem., UK)*; Labiton *(Laboratories for Applied Biology, UK)*; Metatone *(Warner-Lambert, UK)*; Minadex *(Seven Seas, UK)*; Neuro Phosphates *(Smith Kline & French, UK)*; Tonivitan A & D *(Medo, UK)*; Tonivitan B *(Medo, UK)*; Valonorm *(Wallace Mfg Chem., UK)*; Verdiviton *(Squibb, UK)*; Vibrona *(Vine Products, UK)*; Vikonon *(Savoy Laboratories, UK)*; Viraxatone *(Faulding, Austral.)*; Virvina *(Merck Sharp & Dohme, UK)*.

5292-y

Gold

E175.

Au=196.9665.

CAS — 7440-57-5.

A bright-yellow, malleable, and ductile metal; the finely divided powder may be black, ruby, or purple.

Adverse Effects

The main use of metallic gold in health care is now in dentistry. In therapeutics, gold is used in the form of compounds such as auranofin (p.8) aurothioglucose (p.8), and sodium aurothiomalate (p.40). The radionuclide gold-198 is described under the section on radiopharmaceuticals p.1379. There have been rare reports of allergic reactions to metallic gold.

ALLERGY. Some references to gold allergy: S. Comaish, *Archs Derm.*, 1969, *99*, 720; H. Petros and A. L. MacMillan, *Br. J. Derm.*, 1973, *88*, 505; E. Young, *Dermatologica*, 1974, *149*, 294.

12798-p

Gossypol

2,2′-Bis(1,6,7-trihydroxy-3-methyl-5-isopropylnaphthalene-8-carboxaldehyde).

$C_{30}H_{30}O_8$=518.6.

CAS — 303-45-7.

Gossypol is an ingredient extracted from cottonseed oil.

Gossypol has been studied, especially in China, as a male contraceptive.

Side-effects have included weakness, changes in appetite, gastro-intestinal effects, and some loss of libido. Hypokalaemia has occurred.

Some references to gossypol as a male contraceptive: *Lancet*, 1984, *1*, 1108; G. M. H. Waites, *Bull. Wld Hlth Org.*, 1986, *64*, 151.

3149-y

GR-38032F

Ondansetron Hydrochloride *(BANM, pINNM)*.

1,2,3,9-Tetrahydro-3-[(2-methylimidazol-1-yl)methyl]-9-methyl-4*H*-carbazol-4-one hydrochloride dihydrate.

$C_{18}H_{19}N_3O,HCl,2H_2O$=365.9.

CAS — 103639-04-9; 99614-02-5 (ondansetron).

GR-38032F is a serotonin antagonist highly selective against 5-HT_3 receptors. It is under investigation as an anti-emetic and is also reported to have anxiolytic and neuroleptic properties.

Prevention of emesis by GR-38032F in patients receiving cytotoxic drugs.— D. Cunningham *et al.*, *Lancet*, 1987, *1*, 1461. Comment.— *ibid.*, 1470.

Proprietary Names and Manufacturers

Glaxo, *UK*.

12983-s

Green-lipped Mussel

An extract from the green-lipped mussel *Perna canaliculata* (Mytilidae), stated to contain amino acids, fats, carbohydrates, and minerals, is promoted for the treatment of rheumatic disorders.

In a double-blind crossover study completed by 26 patients treatment of rheumatoid arthritis for 4 weeks with Seatone was no more effective than a placebo.— E. C. Huskisson *et al.*, *Br. med. J.*, 1981, *282*, 1358.

Other adverse comment: *Br. med. J.*, 1978, *2*, 49; M. J. Ahern *et al.*, *Med. J. Aust.*, 1980, *2*, 151; P. M. Brooks (letter), *ibid.*, 158; *Lancet*, 1981, *1*, 85.

A favourable report from a homoeopathic hospital.— R. G. Gibson and S. L. M. Gibson (letter), *Lancet*, 1981, *1*, 439.

Proprietary Names and Manufacturers

Seatex *(English Grains, UK)*; Seatone *(Booker Health, UK)*.

12801-w

Guacetisal *(rINN)*.

Acetylsalicylic Acid Guaiacol Ester. 2-Methoxyphenyl 2-acetoxybenzoate.

$C_{16}H_{14}O_5$=286.3.

CAS — 55482-89-8.

Guacetisal has been given by mouth and as suppositories for painful respiratory disorders.

Proprietary Names and Manufacturers

Balsacetil *(Janus, Ital.)*; Broncaspin *(Sigurtà, Ital.)*; Guaiaspir *(Lampugnani, Ital.)*; Guajabronc *(Isnardi, Ital.)*; Prontomucil *(Francia Farm., Ital.)*.

1611-m

Guaiazulene

1,4-Dimethyl-7-isopropylazulene.

$C_{15}H_{18}$=198.3.

CAS — 489-84-9.

Guaiazulene has been reported to have anti-allergic, anti-inflammatory, antipyretic, and antileprotic properties.

Proprietary Names and Manufacturers

AZ8 Beris *(Weimer, Ger.)*; Azuleno Ralay *(Ralay, Spain)*; Azulon *(Homburg, Ger.; Rorer, Ital.)*; Gastrozulen *(Szama, Arg.)*; Szamazulen *(Szama, Arg.)*.

12809-a

Gutta Percha *(USAN)*.

Gummi Plasticum; Gutt. Perch.

Pharmacopoeias. In *Span.* and *U.S.*

The coagulated, dried, purified latex of trees of the genera *Palaquium* and *Payena* and most commonly *Palaquium gutta* (Sapotaceae).

It occurs in lumps or blocks with a slight characteristic odour and is of a brown or greyish-brown to greyish-white colour externally and reddish-yellow or reddish-grey internally with a laminated or fibrous appearance; it is flexible, but only slightly elastic. Practically **insoluble** in water; partly soluble in carbon disulphide and turpentine oil; about 90% soluble in chloroform. **Store** under water in well-closed containers. Protect from light.

Gutta percha has been used in various dressings. In dentistry, gutta percha has been used as a filling material and as the basis of compounds for taking dental impressions.

2164-b

Haem Arginate

Haem arginate is used in the treatment of acute hepatic porphyria.

References: P. Mustajoki *et al.*, *Br. med. J.*, 1986, *293*, 538; V. Kordac and P. Martasek (letter), *ibid.*, 1098; A. Herrick *et al.*, *Lancet*, 1987, *2*, 1178.

12810-e

Haematin

Haemin; Hematin; Hemin.

Haematin, an enzyme inhibitor derived from red blood cells, is used intravenously for the amelioration of acute intermittent porphyria associated with the menstrual cycle in patients unresponsive to other therapy. It is given in a dose of 1 to 4 mg per kg body-weight daily for 3 to 14 days as an intravenous infusion over 10 to 15 minutes.

A brief review of the use of haematin administered intravenously for the treatment of acute intermittent porphyria.— *Med. Lett.*, 1984, *26*, 42.

Proprietary Names and Manufacturers
Panhematin *(Abbott, USA)*.

12811-l

Haematoporphyrin

A red pigment free from iron obtained from haematin.
$C_{34}H_{38}N_4O_6$=598.7.

CAS — 14459-29-1.

Haematoporphyrin has been used in the treatment of mental depression; it has been given by mouth and by intramuscular injection.

Some references to the use of haematoporphyrin derivatives as photosensitisers in the photochemotherapy of cancer: I. J. Forbes, *Med. J. Aust.*, 1984, *140*, 94; H. van den Bergh, *Chem. in Br.*, 1986, May, 430.

Proprietary Names and Manufacturers
Ematodyn *(Ital.)*; Hémédonine *(Laboratoires de l'Hémédonine, Fr.)*; Porfidyna *(Spain)*; Porphyrin *(Zilliken, Ital.)*; Pyrocal *(Mulli, Ger.)*.

5015-z

Harmaline

3,4-Dihydroharmine.
$C_{13}H_{14}N_2O$=214.3.

CAS — 304-21-2.

An alkaloid obtained from peganum, the dried seeds of *Peganum harmala* (Zygophyllaceae). It has also been found together with harmine in the South American hallucinogenic drink 'caapi'.

5016-c

Harmine

7-Methoxy-1-methyl-9*H*-pyrido[3,4-*b*]indole.
$C_{13}H_{12}N_2O$=212.3.

CAS — 442-51-3.

An alkaloid obtained from peganum, the dried seeds of *Peganum harmala* (Zygophyllaceae).
Harmine is identical with an alkaloid known as banisterine or telepathine obtained from *Banisteria caapi* (Malpighiaceae) and with the alkaloid, yageine, from *Haemadictyon amazonicum* (Apocynaceae).

A hallucinogenic drink which is known in the Western Amazonian regions as 'caapi' (Brazil and Colombia), 'Yagé' (Colombia), and 'ayahuasca' (Ecuador, Peru, and Bolivia), is made basically from the same or closely related plants of the family Malpighiaceae. The main active principles are harmine and harmaline. It has no therapeutic use.

References: A. Hofmann, *Indian J. Pharm.*, 1963, *25*, 245; D. H. Aarons *et al.*, *J. pharm. Sci.*, 1977, *66*, 1244.

12819-x

Heptaminol Hydrochloride

RP-2831. 6-Amino-2-methylheptan-2-ol hydrochloride.
$C_8H_{19}NO,HCl$=181.7.

CAS — 372-66-7 (heptaminol); 543-15-7 (hydrochloride).

Heptaminol hydrochloride is a cardiac stimulant and vasodilator and has been given in the treatment of cardiovascular disorders.

Proprietary Names and Manufacturers
Altocor *(Coop. Farm., Ital.)*; Arcor *(Manetti Roberts, Ital.)*; Coreptil *(Delalande, Ital.)*; Cortensor *(Wander, Switz.)*; Delmiton *(Rhodia, Arg.)*; Eoden *(Woelm, Ger.; Spain)*; Hept-a-myl *(Delalande, Belg.; Delalande, Fr.; Delalande, Switz.)*; Heptylon *(Delalande, Ger.)*; Myolytril *(Dorsch, Ger.)*.

The following names have been used for multi-ingredient preparations containing heptaminol hydrochloride— Heptonal *(Delandale, UK)*.

12820-y

Herniaria

Bruchkraut; Herba Herniariae; Herniary; Rupture-wort.

Pharmacopoeias. In *Aust.*, *Hung.*, *Jug.*, and *Pol.*

The dried leaves and flowering tops of various species of rupture-wort, chiefly *Herniaria glabra* and *H. hirsuta* (Caryophyllaceae).

Herniaria has astringent and diuretic properties and has been given by mouth, usually as an infusion, in bladder affections.

Eight saponins were isolated and identified in *Herniaria glabra*. Hydrolysis produced sugars and 7 aglycones.— T. Kartnig and O. Wegschaider, *Planta med.*, 1972, *21*, 144.

12821-j

Hesperidin

5-Hydroxy-2-(3-hydroxy-4-methoxyphenyl)-4-oxo-4*H*-chromen-7-yl rutinoside.
$C_{28}H_{34}O_{15}$=610.6.

CAS — 520-26-3.

A flavonoid isolated from the rind of certain citrus fruits.

12822-z

Hesperidin Methyl Chalcone

CAS — 24292-52-2.

Hesperidin and hesperidin methyl chalcone are flavonoids which have been used in the treatment of capillary fragility.

Proprietary Names and Manufacturers
The following names have been used for multi-ingredient preparations containing a hesperidin complex—Mevanin-C *(Beutlich, USA)*; Peridin-C *(Hamilton, Austral.; Beutlich, USA)*; Varicyl *(Nadeau, Canad.)*.
Hesperidin methyl chalcone is also an ingredient of a number of multivitamin and mineral preparations listed on p.1292.

12551-p

Hetaflur *(BAN, USAN, rINN)*.

Cetylamine Hydrofluoride; GA-242; SKF-2208.
Hexadecylamine hydrofluoride.
$C_{16}H_{35}N,HF$=261.5.

CAS — 143-27-1 (hexadecylamine); 3151-59-5 (hydrofluoride).

Hetaflur is used as an additive to toothpaste for the prevention of caries.

12824-k

Hexacyprone Calcium *(rINNM)*.

Calcium 3-(1-benzyl-2-oxocyclohexyl)propionate.
$(C_{16}H_{19}O_3)_2Ca$=558.7.

CAS — 892-01-3 (hexacyprone); 3837-23-8 (calcium salt).

Hexacyprone calcium is a choleretic which has been used in the treatment of hepatic disorders.

Proprietary Names and Manufacturers
Epadren *(Vister, Ital.)*.

12828-r

Hydrastine Hydrochloride

6,7-Dimethoxy-3-(5,6,7,8-tetrahydro-6-methyl-1,3-dioxolo[4,5-*g*]isoquinolin-5-yl)isobenzofuran-1(3*H*)-one hydrochloride.
$C_{21}H_{21}NO_6,HCl$=419.9.

CAS — 118-08-1 (hydrastine); 5936-28-7 (hydrochloride).

Pharmacopoeias. In *Span.*

The hydrochloride of an alkaloid obtained from *Hydrastis canadensis* (Ranunculaceae).

Hydrastine hydrochloride has been reputed to cause uterine contractions and arrest uterine haemorrhage but it is of doubtful value. It has also been used in gastro-intestinal disorders. Toxic doses are reported to cause strychnine-like convulsions and relaxation of the gut.

12830-z

Hydrastis

Golden Seal; Hidraste; Hydrast.; Idraste; Yellow Root.

Pharmacopoeias. In *Arg.*, *Belg.*, *Braz.*, *Egypt.*, *Fr.*, *Mex.*, *Port.*, *Roum.*, and *Span.*

The dried rhizome and roots of golden seal, *Hydrastis canadensis* (Ranunculaceae), containing not less than 1.5% of hydrastine; it also contains the alkaloids berberine and canadine.
The content of hydrastine specified in pharmacopoeias varies from 1.5% to not less than 2.5%.

Hydrastis was formerly used to check excessive uterine haemorrhage.

12831-c

Hydrazine Sulphate

$H_6N_2O_4S$=130.1.

CAS — 302-01-2 (hydrazine); 10034-93-2 (sulphate).

Hydrazine sulphate is employed in various industrial processes. It is used in the preparation of hydrazine hydrate which is applied after a solution of platinic chloride for corneal tattooing (see Chloroplatinic Acid, p.1556).

An account of the successful treatment of industrial hydrazine poisoning with pyridoxine.— J. K. Kirklin *et al.*, *New Engl. J. Med.*, 1976, *294*, 938.

A report of fatal choroidal melanoma in a worker who had been exposed to hydrazine for 6 years.— D. M. Albert and C. A. Puliafito (letter), *New Engl. J. Med.*, 1977, *296*, 634.

The use of hydrazine sulphate by a laboratory worker was associated with the development of a syndrome similar to systemic lupus erythematosus.— P. J. Durant and R. A. Harris (letter), *New Engl. J. Med.*, 1980, *303*, 584.

A discussion of hydrazine sulphate as an antineoplastic agent.— W. Regelson, *J. Am. med. Ass.*, 1980, *243*, 337.

Successful treatment of hydrazine intoxication with pyridoxine 10 g by intravenous injection. The patient subsequently developed peripheral neuropathy which was considered due to the pyridoxine therapy and resolved spontaneously over the subsequent six months.— Y. Harati and E. Niakan (letter), *Ann. intern. Med.*, 1986,

104, 728.

Hydrazine sulphate, 60 mg three times daily, produced beneficial metabolic changes in a double-blind study of 12 malnourished patients with lung cancer.— J. A. Tayek *et al., Lancet,* 1987, *2,* 241.

1301-l

Hydrochloric Acid *(BAN, USAN).*

507; Acidum Hydrochloricum; Acidum Hydrochloricum Concentratum; Concentrated Hydrochloric Acid; Salzsäure.

HCl=36.46.

CAS — 7647-01-0.

Pharmacopoeias. In *Arg., Aust., Belg., Br., Chin., Egypt., Eur., Fr., Ger., Ind., Int., It., Jpn, Mex., Neth., Nord., Port., Roum., Span., Swiss,* and *Turk.*; also in *B.P. Vet.* (all specify approximately 35 to 39% w/w). *U.S.N.F.* specifies 36.5 to 38.0% w/w. The following specify 25%: *Cz., Jug.,* and *Rus. Swiss* also has Acidum Hydrochloricum 25%. *Aust.* also has Acidum Hydrochloricum (19 to 21%). *Hung.* has Acidum Hydrochloricum Concentratissimum (36 to 39%) and Acidum Hydrochloricum Concentratum (25%). The impure acid of commerce is known as Spirits of Salt and as Muriatic Acid.

A clear colourless fuming aqueous solution of hydrogen chloride with a pungent odour, **Store** below 30° in airtight containers of glass or other inert material.

1302-y

Dilute Hydrochloric Acid *(BAN).*

Acidum Hydrochloricum Dilutum; Diluted Hydrochloric Acid *(USAN)*; Verdünnte Salzsäure.

Pharmacopoeias. In *Arg., Aust., Belg., Br., Chin., Egypt., Eur., Fr., Ger., Hung., Ind., Int., It., Jpn, Jug., Mex., Neth., Pol., Roum., Span., Swiss,* and *Turk.* (all approximately 9.5 to 10.5% w/w); in *Cz.* (11% w/w) and in *Rus.* (8.3% w/w). Also in *U.S.N.F.* (9.5 to 10.5% w/v).

The *B.P.* specifies 9.5 to 10.5% w/w of HCl prepared by mixing hydrochloric acid 274 g with water 726 g. The *U.S.N.F.* specifies 9.5 to 10.5% w/v prepared by mixing hydrochloric acid 226 mL with sufficient water to make 1000 mL. **Store** below 30° in airtight containers of glass or other inert material.

Adverse Effects

Hydrochloric acid is highly irritant and corrosive. Ingestion causes severe pain. There may be violent vomiting, haematemesis, and a rapid fall in blood pressure. The oesophagus may or may not be involved. Ulceration may lead to perforation and patients can suffer strictures and pyloric stenosis. Acids can produce intravascular coagulation and haemolysis.

In Great Britain the recommended exposure limit of hydrogen chloride is 5 ppm.

Chlorine and Hydrogen Chloride, *Environmental Health Criteria 21,* Geneva, *Wld Hlth Org.,* 1982.

Treatment of Adverse Effects

Aspiration and lavage or emetics must *not* be used. Emergency measures should consist of diluting the acid and relieving pain. Large amounts of water or milk should be drunk instantly for dilution. Symptoms should be treated symptomatically. Opioid analgesia may be required. Some authorities consider intubation to be worthwhile, others view it as dangerous. Surgical intervention may be required. While there is little evidence to support the value of corticosteroids in preventing stricture formation, some authorities consider that they are worth trying.

Acid burns of the skin should be flooded immediately with water and the washing should be copious and prolonged. Any affected clothing should be removed while flooding is being carried out. For burns in the eye, the lids should be kept open and the eye flushed with a steady stream of water. A few drops of a local anaesthetic solution will relieve lid spasm and facilitate irrigation.

Uses and Administration

Hydrochloric acid is an escharotic. It has been used medicinally in the diluted form for the treatment of achlorhydria. It has also been given intravenously in the management of metabolic alkalosis. When taken orally, it should be sipped through a straw to protect the teeth.

ALKALOSIS. Some references to hydrochloric acid being administered parenterally for alkalosis: G. M. Abouna *et al., Surgery, St Louis,* 1974, *75,* 194; L. I. G. Worthley, *Br. J. Anaesth.,* 1977, *49,* 811; W. J. Martin and G. R. Matzke, *Clin. Pharm.,* 1982, *1,* 42; O. H. Knutsen, *Lancet,* 1983, *1,* 953.

DIAGNOSTIC USE. In 48 patients with symptoms of reflux oesophagitis, the results of an acid perfusion test were significantly related to the symptom pattern and to endoscopic abnormality, but not to radiological evidence of reflux. In the acid perfusion test 0.15 M sodium chloride solution was perfused into the oesophagus at the rate of 10 mL per minute for 10 minutes, followed by 0.1 M hydrochloric acid at the same rate for 15 minutes or until typical symptoms were produced; the rate of perfusion was increased to 20 mL per minute for a further 15 minutes before the result was considered negative. After relief of symptoms by the perfusion of 0.1 M sodium bicarbonate the test was repeated for confirmation. The acid perfusion test was considered to be a useful procedure in patients with symptoms that were difficult to assess. A clear positive result would strongly support the diagnosis of reflux oesophagitis.— G. E. Sladen *et al., Br. med. J.,* 1975, *1,* 71.

A discussion of the diagnostic use of the acid perfusion test in angina and oesophageal disease.— *Lancet,* 1986, *1,* 191.

1311-j

Hydrofluoric Acid

Fluohydric Acid; Fluoric Acid.

HF=20.01.

CAS — 7664-39-3.

A solution of hydrogen fluoride in water. Various strengths are used. It attacks glass strongly.

Adverse Effects

As for Hydrochloric Acid (above). Although the corrosive effects of hydrofluoric acid tend to predominate absorption may produce systemic fluoride poisoning described under Sodium Fluoride, p.1615.

The pain from contact with weak solutions may be delayed, so that the patient does not know he has been burned until some hours later, when the area begins to smart; intense pain then sets in and this may persist for several days. Destruction of tissue proceeds under the toughened coagulated skin, so that the ulcers extend deeply, heal slowly, and leave a scar.

The fumes of hydrofluoric acid are highly irritant.

In Great Britain the recommended exposure limits of hydrogen fluoride (as F) are 3 ppm (long-term); 6 ppm (short-term). In the *US* the permissible and recommended exposure limits are 2.5 mg F per m^3.

Treatment of Adverse Effects

For the treatment of hydrofluoric acid burns in the eye, immediate and prolonged flooding of the eye with water is recommended.

Skin burns should be washed by prolonged flooding with cold water, after which magnesium oxide paste (heavy magnesium oxide 1, glycerol 1.5 or 2) or a gel of calcium gluconate is applied; large amounts may be required. Soaking in iced water after the initial washing has been found to be effective.

Hydrofluoric acid passes through finger- and toe-nails without causing any apparent damage; nails will therefore have to be removed to be able to treat the underlying tissues.

References to the treatment of hydrofluoric acid burns: T. D. Browne, *J. Soc. occup. Med.,* 1974, *24,* 80; P. B. Tepperman (letter), *J. occup. Med.,* 1982, *24,* 79; W. R. Lee, *Br. med. J.,* 1985, *290,* 375; K. C. Judkins (letter), *ibid.,* 713; J. R. B. Cooper (letter), *ibid;* R. C. Goodfellow (letter), *ibid.,* 937.

5901-f

Hydrogen Peroxide Solution (3 per cent) *(BAN).*

Dilute Hydrogen Peroxide Solution; Hydrogen Peroxide Solution (10-volume); Hydrogen Peroxide Topical Solution *(USAN)*; Hydrogenii Peroxidum Dilutum.

CAS — 7722-84-1 (H_2O_2).

Pharmacopoeias. In *Arg., Aust., Belg., Br., Chin., Cz., Egypt., Fr., Ger., Hung., It., Jpn, Jug., Mex., Neth., Nord., Pol., Port., Roum., Rus., Span., Swiss,* and *U.S. Turk.* specifies 3 to 3.5% w/v.

An aqueous solution containing 2.5 to 3.5% w/w of H_2O_2 (= 34.01) corresponding to about 10 times its volume of available oxygen. It may contain a suitable stabilising agent. The *U.S.P.* permits up to 0.05% of a suitable preservative or preservatives.

A clear, colourless liquid; odourless or having an odour resembling ozone. It decomposes in contact with oxidisable organic matter and with certain metals, and also if allowed to become alkaline.

Incompatible with reducing agents, including organic matter and oxidisable substances, and with alkalis, iodides, permanganates, and other stronger oxidising agents. Its decomposition is increased by metallic salts, light, agitation, and heat, as well as by metals. It is comparatively stable in the presence of a slight excess of acid. **Store** in airtight containers at 15° to 30°. Solutions not containing a stabiliser should be stored at a temperature not exceeding 15°. It should not be stored for long periods. Protect from light.

5902-d

Hydrogen Peroxide Solution (6 per cent) *(BAN).*

Hydrog. Preox. Soln; Hydrogen Dioxide Solution; Hydrogen Peroxide Solution; Hydrogen Peroxide Solution (20-volume); Liq. Hydrog. Perox.; Liquor Hydrogenii Peroxidi; Oxydol; Solución de Bióxido de Hidrogeno; Soluté Officinal d'Eau Oxygénée; Wasserstoffsuperoxydlösung.

Pharmacopoeias. In *Br.* and *Ind.*

An aqueous solution containing 5 to 7% w/v of H_2O_2 corresponding to about 20 times its volume of available oxygen. It may contain a suitable stabilising agent.

A clear, colourless liquid. It decomposes rapidly in contact with oxidisable organic matter and with certain metals, and also if allowed to become alkaline.

Incompatibility and **Storage.** As for Hydrogen Peroxide Solution (3 per cent) (above).

NOTE. The *B.P.* directs that when Hydrogen Peroxide is prescribed or demanded, Hydrogen Peroxide Solution (6 per cent) be dispensed or supplied.

5903-n

Hydrogen Peroxide Solution (27 per cent) *(BAN).*

Hydrogenii Peroxidum; Hydrogenii Peroxidum 27 per centum; Perossido D'Idrogeno Soluzione; Solutio Hydrogenii Peroxydati; Strong Hydrog. Perox. Soln; Strong Hydrogen Peroxide Solution.

Pharmacopoeias. In *Aust., Br., Eur., It., Neth., Swiss,* and *Turk.*

An aqueous solution containing 26 to 28% w/w of H_2O_2, corresponding to about 90 times its volume of available oxygen. It may contain a suitable stabilising agent.

A clear, colourless liquid. It decomposes vigorously in contact with oxidisable organic matter and with certain metals, and also if allowed to

become alkaline.
Incompatibility and **Storage.** As for Hydrogen Peroxide Solution (3 per cent) (above). Strong solutions of hydrogen peroxide are more stable than the weaker solutions.

5904-h

Hydrogen Peroxide Solution (30 per cent) *(BAN).*

Hydrogen Peroxide Solution (100-volume); Hydrogenii Peroxidum 30 per centum.

Pharmacopoeias. In *Arg., Aust., Belg., Br., Egypt., Eur., Fr., Ger., It., Neth., Nord., Pol., Roum., Span.,* and *Swiss. Cz.* specifies 28 to 32%, *Hung.* 27.5 to 32%, and *Jug.* 28 to 31%. *U.S.* specifies Hydrogen Peroxide Concentrate 29 to 32%.

An aqueous solution containing 29 to 31% w/w of H_2O_2, corresponding to about 100 times its volume of available oxygen. It may contain a suitable stabilising agent. The *U.S.P.* permits up to 0.05% of a suitable preservative or preservatives.
A clear, colourless liquid. It decomposes vigorously in contact with oxidisable organic matter and with certain metals and also if allowed to become alkaline.
Other industrial strengths of hydrogen peroxide solution are manufactured, including 35% w/w, 50% w/w, and 85% w/w.
Incompatibility as for Hydrogen Peroxide Solution (3 per cent). **Store** in partially-filled containers having a small vent in the closure, at a temperature of 8 to 15°. Protect from light.

Adverse Effects and Precautions
Strong solutions of hydrogen peroxide produce irritating 'burns' on the skin and mucous membranes with a white eschar, but the pain disappears in about an hour. Continued use of hydrogen peroxide as a mouth-wash may cause reversible hypertrophy of the papillae of the tongue.
It is dangerous to inject or instil hydrogen peroxide into closed body cavities from which the released oxygen has no free exit. Colonic lavage with solutions of hydrogen peroxide as weak as 0.75% has been followed by gas embolism and by gangrene of the intestine.
In Great Britain the recommended exposure limits of hydrogen peroxide are 1 ppm (long-term); 2 ppm (short-term).
There are restrictions in a number of countries on the concentration of hydrogen peroxide allowed in cosmetics.

One case of oxygen embolus and another of surgical emphysema following injection of hydrogen peroxide for wound and abscess cleaning illustrating the hazards of irrigation under pressure or into enclosed body cavities.— J. W. Sleigh and S. P. K. Linter, *Br. med. J.*, 1985, *291*, 1706.

Uses and Administration
Hydrogen peroxide is used as a disinfectant and deodorant. It owes its action to its ready release of oxygen when applied to tissues, but the effect lasts only as long as the oxygen is being released and is of short duration; in addition the antimicrobial effect of the liberated oxygen is reduced in the presence of organic matter.
Hydrogen peroxide is used to cleanse wounds and ulcers in concentrations of up to 6%. Injection into closed body cavities is dangerous (see above). Adhering and blood-soaked dressings may be released by the application of a solution of hydrogen peroxide.
A 1.5% solution of hydrogen peroxide has been used as a mouth-wash in the treatment of acute stomatitis and as a deodorant gargle. In dentistry, hydrogen peroxide has been used to clean septic sockets and root canals.
Hydrogen peroxide ear-drops have been used for the removal of wax. Such ear-drops were prepared by diluting a 6% solution of hydrogen peroxide with 3 parts of water preferably just before use.
For bleaching hair and delicate fabrics hydrogen peroxide 6% should be neutralised or rendered faintly alkaline and diluted with an equal volume of water. In some countries cosmetic product regulations limit the concentration of hydrogen peroxide in hair care products to 12%.
Strong solutions (27 per cent and 30 per cent) of hydrogen peroxide are used for the preparation of weaker solutions.
Hydrogen peroxide and other peroxides have many industrial uses as bleaching and oxidising agents.

In a study involving 49 patients with denture-induced stomatitis a peroxide denture cleaner was found to be no more effective than a placebo cleaning regimen in preventing candidial repopulation of denture or mucosa, or in reducing mucosal inflammation.— D. M. Walker *et al., Br. dent. J.*, 1981, *151*, 416.

Preparations
Hydrogen Peroxide Ear Drops *(A.P.F.)*

Proprietary Preparations
Hioxyl *(Quinoderm, UK). Cream,* hydrogen peroxide (stabilised), 1.5%.

Proprietary Names and Manufacturers
Brintoverilte *(DAK, Denm.)*; Caroxin *(Ferrosan, Denm.)*; Genoxide *(Interox, UK)*; Hioxyl *(Quinoderm, UK)*; Oxydol *(Petri, Denm.)*; Oxysept System *(Allergan, Austral.)*; Peroxyl *(Colgate-Hoyt, USA)*.

19307-g

4-Hydroxyandrostenedione

4-OHA; 4-OHAD. 4-Hydroxyandrost-4-ene-3,17-dione.
$C_{19}H_{26}O_3$=302.4.

4-Hydroxyandrostenedione is an inhibitor of the aromatase (oestrogen synthetase) system and is under investigation for the endocrine therapy of breast cancer.

References: R. C. Coombes *et al., Lancet*, 1984, *2*, 1237; M. J. Daly and M. G. Rowlands, *Pharm. J.*, 1986, *2*, 694.

12835-x

Hydroxymethylnicotinamide

N-Hydroxymethylnicotinamide; Nicotinylmethylamide. *N*-Hydroxymethylpyridine-3-carboxamide.
$C_7H_8N_2O_2$=152.2.

CAS — 3569-99-1.

Hydroxymethylnicotinamide is a cholagogue and has been used in the treatment of various disorders of the gall-bladder.

Proprietary Names and Manufacturers
Bilamid *(Cilag, Ger.; Bracco, Ital.; Cilag, Switz.)*; Bilamide *(Cilag-Chemie, Belg.)*; Biloide *(Labatec-Pharma, Switz.)*.

1614-g

Hydroxyquinoline Sulphate

Chinosolum; Oxichinolini Sulfas; Oxine Sulphate; Oxyquinol; Oxyquinoline Sulfate *(USAN)*; Sulfate d'Orthoxyquinoléine. Quinolin-8-ol sulphate; 8-Quinolinol sulphate.
$(C_9H_7NO)_2,H_2SO_4$=388.4.

CAS — 148-24-3 (hydroxyquinoline); 134-31-6 (sulphate).

Pharmacopoeias. In *Belg.* and *Rus. Fr., Nord.,* and *Swiss* specify monohydrate. Also in *U.S.N.F.*

A yellow powder. M.p. about 185°.
Very **soluble** in water; slightly soluble in alcohol; freely soluble in methyl alcohol; practically insoluble in acetone and ether. **Store** in well-closed containers.

Hydroxyquinoline sulphate has properties similar to those of potassium hydroxyquinoline sulphate (see p.1606) and has been used similarly in the topical treatment of skin infections.
It has been used for preserving syrups and has also been used as an antoxidant synergist since it forms complexes with some heavy metals and thus inhibits catalysis of oxidation by them.
The use of hydroxyquinoline sulphate in cosmetics and toiletries is controlled.

Proprietary Names and Manufacturers of Hydroxyquinoline Sulphate or another Salt of Hydroxyquinoline
Chinosol *(Chinosol, Denm.; Chinosolfabrik, Ger.)*; Oxykin *(DAK, Denm.)*; Semori *(Luitpold, Ger.; Luitpold, Switz.)*; Sérorhinol *(Goupil, Fr.)*; Superol *(Neth.; Superol, S.Afr.)*; Trimo-San *(Milex-Budlong, Canad.)*; Triva Douche Powder *(Boyle, USA)*.
The following names have been used for multi-ingredient preparations containing hydroxyquinoline sulphate or another salt of hydroxyquinoline—Aci-jel *(Cilag, Austral.; Ortho, Canad.; Ortho Pharmaceutical, USA)*; Benzease *(Bolton, Canad.)*; Chinosol *(Chinosolfabrik, Switz.)*; Dermacide *(Sabex, Canad.)*; Dermoplast *(Ayerst, Austral.; Ayerst, Canad.; Torbet Laboratories, UK)*; Medicone Derma-HC *(Medicone, USA)*; Quinoderm *(Quinoderm, UK)*; Quinoderm with Hydrocortisone *(Quinoderm, UK)*; Quinoped *(Quinoderm, UK)*; Rectal Medicone-HC *(Medicone, USA)*; Triva Jel *(Boyle, USA)*.

3725-g

Hymecromone *(USAN, rINN).*

Imecromone; LM-94. 7-Hydroxy-4-methylcoumarin.
$C_{10}H_8O_3$=176.2.

CAS — 90-33-5.

Hymecromone is a choleretic and biliary antispasmodic. Diarrhoea may occasionally occur. It has been given in doses of 400 mg three times daily before meals. It has also been given by slow intravenous injection as an adjunct to diagnostic procedures.

Proprietary Names and Manufacturers
Bicolic *(Unifa, Arg.)*; Bilicanta *(Boehringer Mannheim, Spain)*; Cantabilin *(Formenti, Ital.)*; Cantabiline *(Lipha, Belg.; Médicia, Fr.)*; Cholonerton *(Dolorgiet, Ger.)*; Cholspasmin *(Lipha, Ger.)*; Cumarote-C *(Jpn)*; Eurogale *(Spain)*; Himecol *(Jpn)*; Medilla *(Omega, Arg.)*.

12837-f

Hypoglycin A

L-2-Amino-3-(2-methylenecyclopropyl)propionic acid.
$C_7H_{11}NO_2$=141.2.

CAS — 156-56-9.

A toxic substance present in the arillus of unripe akee, the fruit of *Blighia sapida* (Sapindaceae).

Hypoglycin A is responsible for Jamaican vomiting sickness, with symptoms of acute and severe vomiting, hypoglycaemia, CNS depression, convulsions, and coma, frequently fatal.

Glycine might be useful in the treatment of poisoning by the unripe fruits of the Jamaican ackee [akee].— H. S. A. Sherratt and S. S. Al-Bassam (letter), *Lancet*, 1976, *2*, 1243. See also K. Tanaka (letter), *ibid.*, 1977, *1*, 370; H. S. A. Sherratt and S. S. Al-Bassam (letter), *ibid.*, 604.
Further references: R. Haeckel, *Germ. Med.*, 1972, *2*, 69; K. Tanaka *et al., New Engl. J. Med.*, 1976, *295*, 461; R. Bressler, *ibid.*, 500; D. Billington *et al., ibid.*, 1482.

1936-n

Hypophosphorous Acid *(USAN).*

Acidum Hypophosphorosum; Phosphinic Acid.
H_3PO_2=66.0.

CAS — 6303-21-5; 14332-09-3.

Pharmacopoeias. In *U.S.N.F.*

A colourless or slightly yellow odourless liquid, containing 30 to 32% of H_3PO_2. **Store** in airtight containers.

Hypophosphorous acid is used as an antoxidant. Hypophosphates were used in tonics; like the glycerophosphates they are not a suitable source of phosphorus.

19328-e

ICI-118551

erythro-DL-1(7-Methylindan-4-yloxy)-3-isopropylaminobutan-2-ol.
$C_{17}H_{27}NO_2$=277.4.

CAS — 72795-19-8; 75179-54-3 (hydrochloride).

A beta blocker with selective beta$_2$ activity under investigation in the treatment of anxiety, migraine, and essential tremor.

References: J. Huttunen *et al.* (letter), *Lancet*, 1984, *1*, 857; D. Jefferson *et al.*, *Br. J. clin. Pharmac.*, 1985, *20*, 244P; N. M. Devaney *et al.*, *ibid.*, 1986, *21*, 597P.

3089-k

ICS-205930

ICS-205-930. 3α-Tropanyl 1*H*-indole-3-carboxylic acid ester; 1*H*-indole-3-carboxylic acid 8-methyl-8-azabicyclo [3.2.1]oct-3-yl ester.
$C_{17}H_{20}N_2O_2$=284.4.

CAS — 89565-68-4.

ICS-205930 is a serotonin antagonist highly selective against 5-HT$_3$ receptors. It is under investigation as an anti-emetic and in the treatment of migraine.

Beneficial results with ICS-205930 in the prevention of emesis induced by cancer chemotherapy.— U. Leibundgut and I. Lancranjan (letter), *Lancet*, 1987, *1*, 1198. Comment.— *ibid.*, 1470.

Remission of symptoms in carcinoid syndrome with ICS-205930.— J. V. Anderson *et al.*, *Br. med. J.*, 1987, *294*, 1129. An adverse reaction in one of the patients.— M. Coupe (letter), *Lancet*, 1987, *1*, 1494.

Proprietary Names and Manufacturers
Sandoz, Switz.

3906-e

Imidazole Ketoglutarate

Imidazole 2-Oxoglutarate; Imidazole α-Ketoglutarate; Imidazole Cetoglutarate.

Imidazole ketoglutarate is used in the treatment of bone demineralisation and other disorders of calcium metabolism; it is also used for its reported effects on platelet aggregation in the treatment of thrombotic disorders. Doses have ranged from 1.6 to 4.8 g daily by mouth.

Proprietary Names and Manufacturers
Retencal *(UCB, Spain).*

12845-f

Impromidine Hydrochloride *(BANM, USAN, rINNM).*

SK&F-92676-A$_3$. 1-(3-Imidazol-4-ylpropyl)-3-[2-(5-methylimidazol-4-ylmethylthio)ethyl]guanidine trihydrochloride.
$C_{14}H_{23}N_7S,3HCl$=430.8.

CAS — 55273-05-7 (impromidine); 65573-02-6 (hydrochloride).

Impromidine hydrochloride is a histamine H$_2$ agonist, with potential use in the study of gastric secretion.

References:. W. L. Burland *et al.*, *Br. J. clin. Pharmac.*, 1979, *7*, 421P; U. Bangerter *et al.*, *Gut*, 1979, *20*, A938; R. H. Hunt *et al.*, *Gastroenterology*, 1980, *78*, 505; R. H. McIsaac *et al.*, *Gut*, 1981, *22*, 529.

Proprietary Names and Manufacturers
Smith Kline & French, UK.

19345-l

Inhibin

Inhibin is a glycoprotein secreted by the testes and ovaries which has been investigated as a potential contraceptive in both men and women, because of its ability to suppress secretion of follicle-stimulating hormone by the pituitary.

Isolation and synthesis of a human seminal plasma peptide with inhibin-like activity.— K. Ramasharma *et al.*, *Science*, 1984, *223*, 1199.

12852-r

Inosine *(rINN).*

Hypoxanthine Riboside. 6,9-Dihydro-9-β-D-ribofuranosyl-1*H*-purin-6-one.
$C_{10}H_{12}N_4O_5$=268.2.

CAS — 58-63-9.

Inosine has been used in the treatment of cardiac insufficiency and other cardiac disorders.

The successful use of inosine for perfusing the kidney during conservative renal surgery in 5 patients.— J. E. A. Wickham *et al.*, *Br. med. J.*, 1978, *2*, 173.

Proprietary Names and Manufacturers
Correctol *(P.O.S., Fr.)*; Inosipsina *(Zilliken, Ital.)*; Oxiamin *(Made, Spain)*; Tebertin *(Berenguer-Beneyto, Spain)*; Trophicardyl *(Innothéra, Fr.).*

16853-p

Interleukin-1

Catabolin; Endogenous Pyrogen; Haematopoietin-1; IL-1; Leucocyte Endogenous Mediator; Lymphocyte Activating Factor.

A protein produced by monocytes and a variety of other cell types *in vivo* and which may also be produced by recombinant DNA technology.

Interleukin-1 is one of a number of polypeptides produced by lymphocytes, monocytes, and other cells which are involved in the complex hormonal regulation of immune response, and which are known collectively as cytokines. The term lymphokines has also been used to describe these compounds but is more properly restricted to products of the various lymphocyte subsets, such as interleukin-2 (see p.632).

It has been suggested that it may be of value in a wide variety of conditions including rheumatoid arthritis, and burn and wound healing; as a radioprotective agent in patients receiving radiotherapy; and as an adjuvant to enhance the response to vaccines.

Other cytokines, including interleukin-3, -4, -4A, and -5 are under investigation.

References: C. A. Dinarello, *New Engl. J. Med.*, 1984, *311*, 1413; *Lancet*, 1985, *2*, 536; D. W. Horohov and J. P. Siegel, *Drugs*, 1987, *33*, 289; M. E. J. Billingham, *Br. med. Bull.*, 1987, *43*, 350.

Proprietary Names and Manufacturers
Syntex, USA.

18652-z

Iopronic Acid *(BAN, USAN, rINN).*

B-11420; SQ-21983. (±)-2-[2-(3-Acetamido-2,4,6-triiodophenoxy)ethoxymethyl]butyric acid.
$C_{15}H_{18}I_3NO_5$=673.0.

CAS — 37723-78-7.

A contrast medium given by mouth for visualisation of the biliary tract.

Proprietary Names and Manufacturers
Bilimiro *(Byk Gulden, Ger.).*

3807-p

Iotrolan *(BAN, USAN, rINN).*

Iotrol; Iotrolum; ZK-39482. *N,N′,N″,N‴*-Tetrakis(2,3-dihydroxy-1-hydroxymethylpropyl)-2,2′,4,4′,6,6′-hexaiodo-5,5′-(*N,N′*-dimethylmalonyldiimino)di-isophthalamide.
$C_{37}H_{48}I_6N_6O_{18}$=1626.2.

CAS — 79770-24-4.

Iotrolan is a radio-opaque contrast medium.

18654-k

Ipsalazide *(BAN, USAN).*

BX-650A *(sodium salt).* 4′-(3-Carboxy-4-hydroxyphenylazo)hippuric acid.
$C_{16}H_{13}N_3O_6$=343.3.

CAS — 80573-03-1.

Ipsalazide is an analogue of sulphasalazine which has been tried in the treatment of ulcerative colitis.

References: R. P. Chan *et al.*, *Dig. Dis. Scis*, 1983, *28*, 609; *Lancet*, 1987, *1*, 1299.

Proprietary Names and Manufacturers
Biorex, UK.

19357-c

Isaxonine Phosphate *(rINNM).*

2-(Isopropylamino)pyrimidine phosphate.
$C_7H_{14}N_3O_4P$=235.2.

CAS — 4214-72-6 (isaxonine).

Isaxonine has been reported to promote nerve growth and has been used as the phosphate in the treatment of peripheral neuropathies.

Its use has been associated with the development of toxic hepatitis.

Proprietary Names and Manufacturers
Nerfactor *(IPSEN, Fr.).*

16863-w

Isofezolac *(rINN).*

LM-22102. 1,3,4-Triphenylpyrazole-5-acetic acid.
$C_{23}H_{18}N_2O_2$=354.4.

CAS — 50270-33-2.

Isofezolac has anti-inflammatory activity.

References: E. Cullen, *J. pharm. Sci.*, 1984, *73*, 579 (comment on anti-inflammatory activity compared with indomethacin); A. Bannier *et al.*, *Eur. J. clin. Pharmac.*, 1985, *28*, 433 (effect of probenecid on isofezolac pharmacokinetics).

2547-t

Isospaglumic Acid *(rINN).*

Spaglumic Acid. *N*-(*N*-Acetyl-L-α-aspartyl)-L-glutamic acid.
$C_{11}H_{16}N_2O_8$=304.3.

CAS — 3106-85-2.

Isospaglumic acid is used topically as the magnesium salt in allergic eye conditions.

Proprietary Names and Manufacturers
Naaxia *(Dispersa, Ger.; Dispersa, Switz.).*

1339-m

Itazigrel *(USAN, rINN).*

U-53059. 4,5-bis(*p*-Methoxyphenyl)-2-(trifluoromethyl)thiazole.
$C_{18}H_{14}F_3NO_2S$=365.4.

CAS — 70529-35-0.

Itazigrel is under investigation for its platelet anti-aggregatory and antithrombotic effects.

Proprietary Names and Manufacturers
Upjohn, USA.

1456-p

Ivoqualine *(rINN).*

PK-5078; Viqualine. 6-Methoxy-4-[3-[(3*S*,4*R*)-3-vinyl-4-piperidyl]propyl]quinoline.
$C_{20}H_{26}N_2O$=310.4.

CAS — 72714-75-1.

Ivoqualine is an antidepressant.

References: M. Kenny *et al.*, *Eur. J. clin. Pharmac.*, 1983, *25*, 23; *Drugs of the Future*, 1984, *9*, 434 and 481; *ibid.*, 1985, *10*, 533; *ibid.*, 1986, *11*, 537.

12875-v

Jojoba Oil

An oil derived from the desert plant *Simmondsia californica*.

CAS — 61789-91-1.

It is proposed as a substitute for sperm whale oil.

References: *Drug Cosmet. Ind.*, 1980, *127* (Aug.), 14; *ibid.*, (Sept.), 60.

12878-p

Kava

Kava-Kava.

CAS — 500-64-1 (kawain); 495-85-2 (methysticin); 500-62-9 (yangonin).

The rhizome of *Piper methysticum* (Piperaceae), a shrub indigenous to islands of the South Pacific. It contains pyrones including kawain, methysticin, and yangonin.

Kava has been used to produce an intoxicating beverage used for recreational purposes and during convalescence in the South Pacific. It is reported to have skeletal muscle relaxing and anaesthetic properties. It has been given in some anxiety- and stress-related disorders. It was formerly used as an antiseptic and diuretic in inflammatory conditions of the genito-urinary tract in the form of a liquid extract.

A patient who drank a tea made from kava 5 to 6 times daily for 6 months experienced a chronic intoxicated feeling, ataxia, loss of appetite, diarrhoea, and skin reactions. Also his skin was yellow which might have been due to deposition of kava pyrones in the keratin. Use of the tea was discontinued and most symptoms had disappeared when he was examined 12 months later.— R. K. Siegel, *J. Am. med. Ass.*, 1976, *236*, 473.

A discussion of kava.— *Lancet*, 1988, *2*, 258.

Proprietary Names and Manufacturers

Neuronika *(Klinge, Ger.)*.

12879-s

Keracyanin *(rINN)*.

3-[6-*O*-(α-L-Rhamnopyranosyl)-β-D-glucopyranosyloxy]-3′,4′,5,7-tetrahydroxyflavylium chloride.
$C_{27}H_{31}ClO_{15}$=631.0.

CAS — 18719-76-1.

Keracyanin is claimed to improve visual adaptation to darkness.

Proprietary Names and Manufacturers

Meralop *(Merck Sharp & Dohme, Ital.; Cusi, Spain)*.

16867-j

Ketorolac Trometamol *(BANM, rINNM)*.

Ketorolac Tromethamine *(USAN)*; RS-37619-00-31-3. Trometamol salt of (±)-5-benzoyl-2,3-dihydro-1*H*-pyrrolizine-1-carboxylic acid.
$C_{19}H_{24}N_2O_6$=376.4.

CAS — 74103-06-3 (ketorolac); 74103-07-4 (trometamol).

Ketorolac trometamol is an analgesic.

References: S. S. Bloomfield *et al.*, *Clin. Pharmac. Ther.*, 1984, *35*, 228; J. Yee *et al.*, *ibid.*, 285; H. J. McQuay *et al.*, *ibid.*, 1986, *39*, 89; W. J. Honig and J. Van Ochten, *J. clin. Pharmac.*, 1986, *26*, 700; D. A. O'Hara *et al.*, *Clin. Pharmac. Ther.*, 1987, *41*, 556.

Proprietary Names and Manufacturers

Syntex, USA.

12883-v

Kinkéliba

Combreti Folium. The dried leaves of *Combretum micranthum* (=*C. altum; C. raimbaultii*) (Combretaceae), a shrub indigenous to West Africa.

Pharmacopoeias. In *Fr.* and *Span.*

Kinkéliba has been used as a liquid extract or tincture and is reputed to be of value in blackwater and other fevers.

A decoction of *Combretum mucronatum* root was apparently successful in the treatment of guinea-worm infection.— *Chronicle Wld Hlth Org.*, 1977, *31*, 428.

12884-g

Krebiozen

CAS — 9008-19-9.

Krebiozen is the name of a preparation that received much publicity, particularly in the USA, as a 'cancer cure'. It was stated to be obtained from the blood of horses previously injected with an extract of *Actinomyces bovis*.
The claims made for Krebiozen were never scientifically substantiated and, in 1966, the US Food and Drugs Administration pronounced it to be totally discredited.

12886-p

Laburnum

Golden Chain; Golden Rain. *Laburnum anagyroides* (= *L. vulgare; Cytisus laburnum*) (Leguminosae).

All parts of laburnum are toxic. The toxic principle is cytisine which has actions similar to nicotine.

A report of laburnum poisoning in 10 children.— R. G. Mitchell, *Lancet*, 1951, *2*, 57.

Comments on the incidence of laburnum poisoning in children and the suggestion that in general it is not as dangerous as has been thought.— R. M. Forrester, *Lancet*, 1979, *1*, 1073; J. M. Morfitt (letter), *ibid.*, 1195; K. C. Chin and T. J. Beattie (letter), *ibid.*, 1299; A. Bramley and R. Goulding, *Br. med. J.*, 1981, *283*, 1220.

2495-d

Lacidipine *(BAN, rINN)*.

GR-43659X. Diethyl 4-{2-[(*tert*-butoxycarbonyl)-vinyl]phenyl}-1,4-dihydro-2,6-dimethylpyridine-3,5-dicarboxylate.
$C_{26}H_{33}NO_6$=455.6.

CAS — 103890-78-4.

Lacidipine is a calcium-channel blocking agent under investigation for the treatment of hypertension.

Proprietary Names and Manufacturers

Glaxo, UK.

1312-z

Lactic Acid *(BAN, USAN)*.

Acidum Lacticum; E270; E326 (potassium lactate); Milchsäure. 2-Hydroxypropionic acid.
$C_3H_6O_3$=90.08.

CAS — 50-21-5; 79-33-4 (+); 10326-41-7 (−); 598-82-3 (±).

Pharmacopoeias. In *Arg., Aust., Belg., Br., Braz., Chin., Cz., Egypt., Eur., Fr., Ger., Hung., Ind., Int., It., Jpn, Jug., Mex., Neth., Nord., Pol., Port., Roum., Span., Swiss, Turk.,* and *U.S.*

A colourless or slightly yellow, viscous hygroscopic liquid, which is odourless or almost odourless.
The *B.P.* specifies a mixture of lactic acid, its condensation products such as lactoyl-lactic acid and other polylactic acids, and water. In most cases lactic acid is in the form of the racemate (*RS*-lactic acid), but in some cases the (+)-(*S*)-isomer is predominant. It contains the equivalent of 88 to 92% w/w of $C_3H_6O_3$.

The *U.S.P.* specifies a mixture of lactic acid and lactic acid lactate equivalent to 85 to 90% w/w of $C_3H_6O_3$. Lactic acid prepared by fermentation of sugars is laevorotatory; that prepared synthetically is racemic
Miscible with water, alcohol, and ether; immiscible with chloroform. **Store** in airtight containers.

Adverse Effects and Treatment

As for hydrochloric acid (p.1578), although it is less corrosive.

There was evidence that neonates had difficulty in metabolising D-(−)-lactic acid and this isomer and the racemate should not be used in foods for infants less than 3 months old.— Seventeenth Report of the FAO/WHO Expert Committee on Food Additives, *Tech. Rep. Ser. Wld Hlth Org. No. 539*, 1974.

Uses and Administration

Lactic acid has actions similar to those of acetic acid (p.1537). It is used in the preparation of lactate injections to provide a source of bicarbonate for the treatment of metabolic acidosis. Vaginal dose forms are used in the treatment of leucorrhoea. It is also employed in the treatment of warts.
Lactic acid is also used as a food preservative.

A study of 389 patients in 2 centres showed that the application of a mixture of salicylic acid 1 part and lactic acid 1 part in flexible collodion 4 parts (SAL paint) was as effective as that of liquid nitrogen or of a combination of both in the treatment of hard warts. The percentage cures were 67, 69, and 78 respectively and the differences were not statistically significant. No recurrences were reported 6 months after treatment with SAL paint in 46 of 50 patients in a general practice. Other studies indicated that SAL paint cured 45% of patients with mosaic plantar warts and it was no less effective than preparations containing fluorouracil 5%, idoxuridine 5%, a 10% buffered solution of glutaraldehyde, or a paint prepared to contain 40% of an adduct of benzalkonium chloride and bromine (Callusolve 40).— M. H. Bunney *et al.*, *Br. J. Derm.*, 1976, *94*, 667.

In a double-blind study, 60 patients with moderate to severe xerosis were treated for 21 days with either a neutralised 12% lactate lotion, a 5% lactic acid lotion, or a nonlactated emollient lotion. All 3 preparations significantly reduced the severity scores of xerosis, but 2 weeks after treatment was discontinued, the patients receiving the 12% lactate lotion had significantly greater reductions in the severity scores.— M. V. Dahl and A. C. Dahl, *Archs Derm.*, 1983, *119*, 27.

In 48 women with bacterial vaginosis, 7 days treatment with metronidazole 500 mg twice daily by mouth or daily vaginal application of lactate gel 5 mL significantly reduced the prevalence of anaerobes, with no significant difference between the treatment groups. No adverse effects were associated with lactate gel therapy.— B. Andersch *et al.*, *Gynec. Obstet. Invest.*, 1986, *21*, 19.

Preparations

Lactic Acid Pessaries *(B.P.)*. Similar pessaries are included in the *A.P.F.*

Lactic and Salicylic Acid Paint *(A.P.F.)*. See under salicylic acid (p.931).

Proprietary Names and Manufacturers

Lachydrin *(Westwood, Canad.)*; Lacta-Gynecogel *(Therapeutica, Belg.)*; pHygiene *(Alcon, Canad.)*; Tampovagan *(Winthrop, Ger.; Norgine, UK)*; Tonsillosan *(Spitzner, Ger.)*; Vagoclyss *(Wiedenmann, Switz.)*.

The following names have been used for multi-ingredient preparations containing lactic acid—Cornkil *(Rosken, Austral.)*; Cuplex *(Smith & Nephew Pharmaceuticals, UK)*; Duofilm *(Stiefel, Austral.; Stiefel, Canad.; Stiefel, UK; Stiefel, USA)*; Duoplant *(Stiefel, Canad.)*; Lactacyd *(Rhône-Poulenc, Canad.)*; Lacticare *(Stiefel, Austral.; Stiefel, Canad.; Stiefel, UK)*; Lacticare-HC *(Stiefel, USA)*; P&S *(Baker/Cummins, USA)*; Salactic *(Pedinol, USA)*; Salactol *(Dermal Laboratories, UK)*; SLT *(C & M, USA)*; Tampovagan Stilboestrol and Lactic Acid *(Norgine, Austral.; Norgine, UK)*; Variclene *(Dermal Laboratories, UK)*; Viranol *(American Dermal, USA)*; Wartkil *(Rosken, Austral.)*; Wart-Off *(Nelson, Austral.)*.

1313-c

Lactic-acid-producing Organisms

Lactic-acid-producing organisms were introduced as a therapeutic agent by Metchnikoff with the idea of acidifying the intestinal contents and thus preventing the growth of putrefactive organisms. The organism chosen by him for this purpose was *Lactobacillus bulgaricus*, which occurs in naturally soured milk, but many workers found it difficult to produce a growth of this organism in the intestines and preferred *L. acidophilus* which is an inhabitant of the human intestine. Yogurt is a common preparation of lactic-acid-producing organisms.

Lactobacillus preparations have been used in the treatment of vaginal and gastro-intestinal disorders but evidence to support this use is limited.

A vaccine from strains of lactobacillus found in women with trichomoniasis has been used in the prophylaxis of recurrent trichomoniasis.

References to the use of lactic-acid-producing organisms: M. S. Oh *et al.*, *New Engl. J. Med.*, 1979, *301*, 249 (severe metabolic acidosis and neurological manifestations in a man with short-bowel syndrome); V. P. Gotz *et al.*, *Am. J. Hosp. Pharm.*, 1979, *36*, 754 (reduction of the severity and duration of diarrhoea caused by ampicillin therapy); M. L. Clements *et al.*, *Prog. food nutr. Sci.*, 1983, *7*, 29 (reduction of the severity and duration of diarrhoea caused by neomycin therapy); R. L. Yost and V. P. Gotz, *Antimicrob. Ag. Chemother.*, 1985, *28*, 727 (no effect on the bioavailability of oral ampicillin by the concomitant administration of a lactobacillus preparation); S. L. Gorbach *et al.* (letter), *Lancet*, 1987, *2*, 1519 (successful treatment of relapsing *Clostridium difficile* colitis with lactobacillus).

Proprietary Names and Manufacturers

Acidofilofago *(Arg.)*; Antibiophilus *(Lyocentre, Fr.)*; Bacid *(Rorer, Canad.; Fisons, USA)*; Bioflorin *(Gipharmex, Ital.; Giuliani, Switz.)*; DōFus *(USA)*; Doderlein Med *(Med Fabrik, Ger.)*; Electrolactil *(Electrolactil, Spain)*; Endogen HS 15 *(Panthox & Burck, Ital.)*; Enpac *(Muir & Neil, Austral.; Switz.; Aplin & Barrett, UK)*; Entero Vacuna *(Arg.)*; Ferlactis *(Panthox & Burck, Ital.)*; Fermalac *(Rougier, Canad.)*; Fermenturto-Lio *(Teknofarma, Ital.)*; Ginatren *(LPB, Ital.)*; Gynatren *(Cabot, UK)*; Lacteol *(Lacteol du Dr Boucard, Fr.; Ramon Sala, Spain; Uhlmann-Eyraud, Switz.)*; Lactinex *(Hynson, Westcott & Dunning, Canad.; Hynson, Westcott & Dunning, USA)*; Lactipan *(Ibi, Ital.)*; Lacto Lemos *(Arg.)*; Lacto Level *(Spain)*; Lactobacillus Acidophilus Capsules *(Vitaplex, Austral.)*; Lactoferment *(Zyma, Switz.)*; Lactofilus *(Llorente, Spain)*; Lactoliofil *(Abello, Spain)*; Lactomicina *(Medici Domus, Ital.)*; Lactophilus *(Arg.)*; Lactum *(Bicther, Spain)*; Novaflor *(USA)*; Paraghurt *(Leo, Denm.)*; Proflor *(Bouchard, Fr.)*; Sisu-Dophilus *(Sisu, Canad.)*; SolcoTrichovac *(Solco, Switz.)*; Tapo *(Switz.)*; Uniflor *(Key, Austral.; Aplin & Barrett, UK)*; Vagiflor *(Asche, Ger.)*; Ventrux Acido *(Switz.)*; Vigardyne *(Milo, Spain)*.

The following names have been used for multi-ingredient preparations containing lactic-acid-producing organisms—Flar *(Consolidated Chemicals, UK)*.

19392-t

Lactitol

Lactitol is an intense and bulk sweetener and also has laxative properties. It is a disaccharide analogue of lactulose (see p.1092) and is used similarly in the treatment of hepatic encephalopathy. Lactitol has been reported to be more palatable than lactulose, more convenient to use since it is available as a powder rather than a liquid, and equally effective.

References: P. L. Lanthier and M. Y. Morgan, *Gut*, 1985, *26*, 415; K. Hawley and M. Y. Morgan, *ibid.*, 1986, *27*, A1266; D. H. Patil *et al.*, *ibid.*, 1987, *28*, 255; *Lancet*, 1987, *2*, 81; A. C. Douwes *et al.* (letter), *ibid.*, 688; O. M. Wrong and A. J. Vince (letter), *ibid.*, 1280.

Proprietary Names and Manufacturers

Importal *(Zyma, Switz.)*.

3907-l

Lactomicin

Gamma-lactomicin.

Lactomicin is described as a protein supplement and co-adjuvant in the treatment of bacterial and viral infections; it has also been advocated in the treatment of hepatitis and other liver disorders.

Proprietary Names and Manufacturers

Gamma-Lactomicina *(Euroulta, Spain)*.

12887-s

Laetrile

The term laetrile is used for a product consisting chiefly of amygdalin, which is the major cyanogenic glycoside of apricot kernels. Amygdalin is *R*-α-cyanobenzyl-6-*O*-β-D-glucopyranosyl-β-D-glucopyranoside, ($C_{20}H_{27}NO_{11}$=457.4). Laetrile is also used as a term for *R*-α-cyanobenzyl-6-*O*-β-D-glucopyranosiduronic acid ($C_{14}H_{15}NO_7$=309.3), which has also been referred to as mandelonitrile-β-glucuronide, 1-mandelonitrile-β-glucuronic acid, D-mandelonitrile-β-D-glucuronic acid, *R*-mandelonitrile-β-glucuronic acid, (−)-mandelonitrile-β-glucuronoside, and other names.

CAS — 1332-94-1 (laetrile); 29883-15-6 (amygdalin).

Laetrile is a controversial 'cancer' treatment; it has been postulated that amygdalin is preferentially hydrolysed in cancer cells by β-glucosidases to yield benzaldehyde and hydrogen cyanide in sufficient quantities to kill malignant cells. Available evidence indicates that amygdalin is not absorbed from the gastro-intestinal tract, and that both normal and malignant cells contain only traces of β-glucosidases. Laetrile has been claimed to be 'vitamin B_{17}', the deficiency of which is said to result in cancer; there is no evidence for accepting this view and laetrile is of no known value in human nutrition.

There have been several reports of cyanide poisoning and other adverse reactions associated with the use of laetrile, especially when taken by mouth.

A review of the sources, chemistry, metabolism, claims for efficacy, and toxicity of laetrile.— R. F. Chandler *et al.*, *Pharm. J.*, 1984, *1*, 330.

In a retrospective analysis by the National Cancer Institute of cancer patients who were thought to have shown objective benefit from laetrile, 6 of 67 evaluable patients were judged to have complete or partial responses.— N. M. Ellison *et al.*, *New Engl. J. Med.*, 1978, *299*, 549.

One hundred and seventy-eight patients with advanced cancer, but in good general condition, were given laetrile in doses typical of those which had been promoted, in association with vitamins, pancreatic enzymes, and a 'metabolic diet'. Of the 175 evaluable patients 79% had progression of disease at 2 months and 91% had progression at 3 months; only one patient had a transient partial response. Of the 178 patients 152 had died; the median survival for all patients was 4.8 months. Laetrile is of no substantive value in cancer; further investigation or clinical use is not justified.— C. G. Moertel *et al.*, *New Engl. J. Med.*, 1982, *306*, 201. See also A. S. Relman, *ibid.*, 236.

FORMULATION. Pharmaceutical assessment of tablets and an injectable product containing laetrile indicated that both forms were substandard by *US* criteria for manufactured pharmaceutical products. More than 20 samples of the injection were found to contain microbial contamination, and other samples were found to be pyrogenic. All samples were found to be chemically subpotent, mislabelled, and of poor manufacturing quality; the products were considered to be unfit for use in man.— J. P. Davignon *et al.*, *Cancer Treat. Rep.*, 1978, *62*, 99.

TOXICITY. A review of cyanide poisoning and other adverse reactions associated with laetrile. Some 37 poisonings and 17 deaths, mostly from the ingestion of apricot or other fruit kernels, had been recorded. Cyanide release from amygdalin is known to occur in the presence of hydrolysing β-glucosidase enzymes which are present in some raw fruits and vegetables including lettuce, mushrooms, certain fresh fruits, green peppers, celery, and sweet almonds; ingestion of any of these uncooked foods with amygdalin can produce cyanide poisoning. Other adverse reactions reported with laetrile include hypotension, haemoglobinuria, gastro-intestinal haemorrhage, vomiting, headache, diarrhoea, fever, rash, and muscular weakness. It is advised that physicians with patients using laetrile should watch for signs and symptoms of acute and chronic cyanide intoxication and be prepared to administer emergency treatment. Patients who use laetrile should be warned against taking the parenteral preparation by mouth since the high concentration can be rapidly fatal.— *FDA Drug Bull.*, 1977, *7*, 26.

A report of uncomplicated pregnancy and delivery at term of an infant to a woman taking laetrile during the third trimester.— R. G. Peterson and B. H. Rumack, *Clin. Toxicol.*, 1979, *15*, 181.

Individual reports of adverse reactions and cyanide poisoning in patients using laetrile: J. R. Humbert *et al.* (letter), *J. Am. med. Ass.*, 1977, *238*, 482; F. P. Smith *et al.* (letter), *ibid.*, 1361; *idem*, *Cancer Treat. Rep.*, 1978, *62*, 169; D. M. Maxwell (letter), *Can. med. Ass. J.*, 1978, *119*, 18; L. Sadoff *et al.*, *J. Am. med. Ass.*, 1978, *239*, 1532; J. A. Ortega and J. E. Creek, *J. Pediat.*, 1978, *93*, 1059; J. H. Carter and P. Goldman (letter), *ibid.*, *94*, 1018; K. T. Braico *et al.*, *New Engl. J. Med.*, 1979, *300*, 238; D. L. Morse *et al.* (letter), *ibid.*, 1979, *301*, 892; M. J. Rubino and F. Davidoff (letter), *J. Am. med. Ass.*, 1979, *241*, 359; C. G. Moertel *et al.*, *ibid.*, 1981, *245*, 591; K. B. Liegner *et al.*, *J. Am. med. Ass.*, 1981, *246*, 2841; U. P. Kalyanaraman *et al.*, *Cancer*, 1983, *51*, 2126.

12888-w

Laminaria Stalks

Stipites Laminariae; Styli Laminariae; Thallus Eckloniae; Thallus Laminariae.

Pharmacopoeias. In *Arg.*, *Chin.*, *Port.*, and *Span.*

The dried stalks of the seaweeds *Laminaria cloustoni*, *L. digitata*, and possibly other species of *Laminaria*.

Laminaria stalks swell in water to about 6 times their volume and have been used surgically to dilate cavities. For this purpose they are usually made into either solid or hollow cylinders ('laminaria tents') from 50 to 75 mm long and 8 to 12 mm wide. They have been supplied singly in sealed tubes after being sterilised by alcohol vapour in an autoclave at 120° for 50 minutes.

References to the use of laminaria for the induction of abortion: J. H. Duenhoelter *et al.*, *Obstet. Gynec.*, 1976, *47*, 469; J. H. Strauss *et al.*, *Am. J. Obstet. Gynec.*, 1979, *134*, 260; M. Hachamovitch *et al.*, *ibid.*, *135*, 327; K. Edström, *Bull. Wld Hlth Org.*, 1979, *57*, 481; K. F. Schulz *et al.*, *Lancet*, 1983, *1*, 1182; A. Jonasson *et al.*, *Curr. ther. Res.*, 1984, *35*, 793; A. Jonasson *et al.*, *ibid.*, *36*, 851.

12889-e

Lappa

Bardanae Radix; Bardane (Grande); Burdock; Burdock Root.

Pharmacopoeias. In *Chin.*, *Fr.*, and *Span. Fr. P.* also describes the leaves.

The dried root of the great burdock, *Arctium lappa* (= *A. majus*), and other species of *Arctium* (Compositae).

Lappa was formerly used in the form of a decoction as a diuretic and diaphoretic but there is little evidence of its efficacy.

A report of symptoms of antimuscarinic poisoning in a 26-year-old woman who had taken burdock root tea contaminated with atropine.— P. D. Bryson *et al.*, *J. Am. med. Ass.*, 1978, *239*, 2157. See also *idem* (letter), *240*, 1586; F. F. Hyde (letter), *Pharm. J.*, 1978, *2*, 204.

5298-t

Lead

Pb=207.2.

CAS — 7439-92-1.

A grey, malleable and ductile metal.

Adverse Effects

Lead poisoning may be due to inorganic or organic lead and may be acute or more often chronic. It has followed exposure to a wide range of compounds and objects from which lead may be absorbed following ingestion or inhalation. Some of those incriminated include paint, pottery glazes, petrol and poteen, cosmetics, herbal or folk remedies, newsprint, and even bullets. Children are often the victims of accidental poisoning. Symptoms of poisoning with inorganic lead include anorexia, colic, vomiting, anaemia, peripheral neuropathy, and encephalopathy with convulsions and coma. There may be kidney damage and impairment of mental function.

Organic lead poisoning produces mainly CNS symptoms; there can be gastro-intestinal and cardiovascular effects, and renal and hepatic damage.

In Great Britain the control exposure limits of lead in air are: except tetraethyl lead, 0.15 mg (as Pb) per m^3 (long-term); for tetraethyl lead 0.10 mg (as Pb) per m^3 (long-term). A repeat blood-lead concentration in excess of 0.7 μg per mL means that the subject has to be suspended from work. In the *US* the permissible and recommended exposure limits for inorganic lead are 0.05 mg per m^3 and less than 0.1 mg per m^3 respectively.

Recommended Health-Based Limits in Occupational Exposure to Heavy Metals, Report of a WHO Study Group, *Tech. Rep. Ser. Wld Hlth Org. No. 647*, 1980.

See also under Lead in Food, below.

A review of lead intoxication.— L. S. Ibels and C. A. Pollock, *Med. Toxicol.*, 1986, *1*, 387.

Acute lead intoxication following the intravenous injection of lead acetate.— F. Sixel-Dietrich *et al., Hum. Toxicol.*, 1985, *4*, 301.

Lead in Food

There are controls on the amount of lead in food. In Great Britain the amount is generally restricted to a maximum of 1 ppm with the exception of foods specially prepared for infants and children, where the limit is 0.2 ppm.

References: Survey of Lead in Food: Second Supplementary Report, *Food Surveillance Paper No. 10, Minist. Agric. Fish. Fd*, London, HM Stationery Office, 1982.

Provisional maximum tolerable weekly intake of lead: adults, 3 mg per person or 50 μg per kg body-weight; children and infants, 25 μg per kg.— Thirtieth Report of the Joint FAO/WHO Expert Committee on Food Additives, *Tech. Rep. Ser. Wld Hlth Org. No. 751*, 1987.

Treatment of Adverse Effects

Treatment is aimed at controlling symptoms and reducing the concentration of lead in the body. Chelating agents are usually given in acute poisoning with inorganic lead. The agents that are used include: sodium calciumedetate (see p.852) in conjunction with dimercaprol (see p.840). Succimer (p.855) is also used. Follow-up treatment has been given with penicillamine (see p.849).

A brief discussion of the treatment of lead poisoning in children. A blood-lead concentration of 0.2 to 0.3 μg per mL probably indicates some degree of overexposure; when it exceeds 0.7 μg per mL it is agreed that treatment is required. What measures to take when the concentration is between 0.3 and 0.7 μg per mL is subject to dispute.

With long-term exposure lead accumulates in bone and only that released into the blood can be removed by chelation. Acute short-term exposure can produce high concentrations in soft tissue but stores are less so chelation is more effective.— *Lancet*, 1984, *1*, 1278.

Absorption and Fate

Lead is absorbed from the gastro-intestinal tract. Lead is also absorbed by the lungs from dust particles.

Inorganic lead is not absorbed through intact skin, but organic lead compounds may be absorbed rapidly.

Lead is distributed in the soft tissues, with higher concentrations in the liver and kidneys. In the blood it is associated with the erythrocytes. Over a period of time lead accumulates in the body and is deposited in calcified bone, hair, and teeth. Lead crosses the placental barrier. It is excreted in the faeces, urine, in sweat, and in milk.

Uses and Administration

Lead compounds were formerly employed as astringents, but the medicinal use of preparations containing lead is no longer recommended. The lead salts or compounds that have been used have included lead acetate (for lead lotion, still known sometimes as lotio plumbi), lead carbonate, lead monoxide, and lead oleate (for lead plaster-mass).

596-l

Lecithin *(USAN)*.

E322.

CAS — 8002-43-5.

Pharmacopoeias. In *Aust.* and in *U.S.N.F. Port.* and *Span.* include Egg Lecithin or Ovolecithin.

A phospholipid composed of a complex mixture of acetone-insoluble phosphatidyl esters (phosphatides) which consist chiefly of phosphatidyl choline, phosphatidyl ethanolamine, phosphatidyl serine, and phosphatidyl inositol, combined with various amounts of other substances such as triglycerides, fatty acids, and carbohydrates, as separated from the crude vegetable oil source.

The consistency of both natural grades and refined grades of lecithin may vary from plastic to fluid, depending upon the content of free fatty acid and oil, and upon the presence or absence of other diluents. Its colour varies from light yellow to brown, depending on the source, on crop variations, and on whether it is bleached or unbleached.

It is odourless or has a characteristic, slight nut-like odour. It is partially **soluble** in water, but readily hydrates to form emulsions. The oil-free phosphatides are soluble in fatty acids, but are practically insoluble in fixed oils. When all phosphatide fractions are present, lecithin is partially soluble in alcohol and practically insoluble in acetone.

Lecithin is an emulsifying and stabilising agent used in both the pharmaceutical and the food industries. It has been used as a pulmonary surfactant in the treatment of neonatal respiratory distress syndrome.

Lecithin has also been used as a source of choline in the treatment of dementia and in various extrapyramidal disorders.

ALZHEIMER'S DISEASE. For reference to the use of lecithin as a source of choline in the treatment of Alzheimer's disease, see under Choline Chloride, p.1258.

EXTRAPYRAMIDAL DISORDERS. Lecithin, in daily doses of 3.6 to 49 g, reduced abnormal movements in 2 patients with tardive dyskinesia, produced only mild improvement in 3 patients with Huntington's chorea, no improvement in 6 patients with spastic spinocerebellar degeneration, and significant improvement in 10 patients with Friedreich's ataxia.— A. Barbeau (letter), *New Engl. J. Med.*, 1978, *299*, 200. A 12-week double-blind crossover study in 12 patients with Friedreich's ataxia failed to show any benefit from treatment with lecithin 25 g daily.— B. Pentland *et al., Br. med. J.*, 1981, *282*, 1197.

Gilles de la Tourette syndrome. In a controlled study of 6 patients with Gilles de la Tourette's syndrome, treatment with lecithin up to 45 g daily for up to 4 weeks induced a variety of individual responses but there was no discernable benefit for the group as a whole.— R. J. Polinsky *et al.* (letter), *New Engl. J. Med.*, 1980, *302*, 1310.

Tardive dyskinesia. Reduction of tardive dyskinesia accompanied by a significant rise in serum-choline concentrations in 3 patients following administration of lecithin 60 to 80 g daily, or 40 g of partially purified lecithin.— J. H. Growdon *et al.* (letter), *New Engl. J. Med.*, 1978, *298*, 1029. Criticism.— S. Fahn (letter), *ibid.*, *299*, 202.

See also under Choline Chloride, p.1258.

RESPIRATORY DISTRESS SYNDROME. A review of the use of surfactant therapy to treat and prevent neonatal respiratory distress syndrome. Substances which have been administered include a mixture of human surfactant phospholipids extracted from amniotic fluid, cow or other animal lung wastes, sometimes supplemented with synthetic phospholipids, and completely synthetic phospholipids, either pure dipalmitoyl phosphatidyl choline or a combination of this and phosphatidyl glycerol. The effectiveness of these substances in reducing the surface tension of lung fluids has been challenged. Most workers have flushed a saline suspension of their surfactant into the intubated lungs, others have used dry powdered surfactant. A provisional verdict is that exogenous surfactants do have some beneficial effect when given to preterm infants. The action of natural surfactants on respiratory variables such as oxygenation is faster and more pronounced than artificial surfactants but they are very expensive to extract and prepare. The future of surfactant therapy may lie in the production of a widely available synthetic third-generation surfactant mixture with physical properties closer to those of the real thing and cheap enough for widespread multicentre trials and therapeutic application.— *Lancet*, 1985, *2*, 867. See also C. J. Morley, *Archs Dis. Childh.*, 1983, *58*, 321.

Studies of surfactant therapy in the management of respiratory distress syndrome: H. L. Halliday *et al., Lancet*, 1984, *1*, 476 (artificial surfactant composed of dipalmitoyl phosphatidyl choline and phosphatidyl glycerol in suspension). Comments.— R. J. Davies and C. J. Morley (letter), *ibid.*, 954; D. Stowens (letter), *ibid.*, 955; B. Granati *et al.* (letter), *ibid.*; A. Wilkinson *et al., ibid.*, 1985, *2*, 287 (dry powdered artificial surfactant composed of dipalmitoyl phosphatidyl choline and phosphatidyl glycerol); T. A. Merritt *et al., New Engl. J. Med.*, 1986, *315*, 785 (human surfactant isolated from amniotic fluid); T. N. K. Raju *et al., Lancet*, 1987, *1*, 651 (reconstituted bovine surfactant). Comments and criticism.— C. Morley (letter), *ibid.*, 1040; S. M. Gore (letter), *ibid.*. Reply.— T. N. K. Raju *et al.* (letter), *ibid.*, 1041. Further comment.— B. Lachmann (letter), *ibid.*, 1375. Reply.— T. N. K. Raju (letter), *ibid.*

A report of a multicentre randomised study involving 308 evaluable infants delivered at 25 to 29 weeks' gestation; 159 infants received 100 mg of protein-free artificial surfactant (artificial lung expanding compound) composed of dipalmitoyl phosphatidyl choline and phosphatidyl glycerol as a cold saline crystalline suspension and administered at birth into the pharynx, and 149 infants received 1 mL of saline. Up to 3 or more endotracheal doses were given if the baby was intubated within 24 hours. Treatment with artificial surfactant reduced neonatal mortality in the first 28 days from 27 to 14%, mortality while in the neonatal unit from 30 to 19%, and incidence of parenchymal brain haemorrhage from 24 to 16%. Respiratory distress did not occur in 36% of surfactant-treated babies as compared to 25% of controls and the surfactant-treated babies required less respiratory support. Artificial surfactant had no effect on the incidence of pneumothoraces, pulmonary interstitial emphysema, patent ductus arteriosus, or postnatal infections, and had no serious side-effects.—The Ten Centre Study Group, *Br. med. J.*, 1987, *1*, 991.

Proprietary Names and Manufacturers

Buerlecithin *(Roland, Ger.)*; Foslip *(Pharmainvesti, Spain)*; Lecithin-1200 *(Gisand, Switz.)*.

The following names have been used for multi-ingredient preparations containing lecithin—Complex-15 *(Dormer, Canad.)*; Lipex *(Advanced Medical Nutrition, USA)*; Prehensol *(Dermal Laboratories, UK)*.

19404-q

Lentinan

LC-33.

A glucan extracted from the mushroom *Lentinus edodes*.

Lentinan appears to act as an immunostimulant.

References: T. Aoki *et al.* (letter), *Lancet*, 1984, *2*, 936; *Drugs Today*, 1986, *22*, 257; I. F. Cook, *Aust. J. Hosp. Pharm.*, 1987, *16*, 191.

Proprietary Names and Manufacturers
Ajinomoto, Jpn.

12894-p

Leucocianidol *(pINN)*.

2-(3,4-Dihydroxyphenyl)chroman-3,4,5,7-tetrol.
$C_{15}H_{14}O_7$=306.3.

CAS — 480-17-1.

Leucocianidol has been used for its reputed beneficial effects on capillary circulation.

Proprietary Names and Manufacturers
Flavan *(Leurquin, Fr.)*; Okavena *(Rovi, Spain)*; Résivit *(Oberlin, Fr.)*.

18660-z

Levocabastine *(BAN, rINN)*.

R-50547 (hydrochloride). (−)-*trans*-1-(*cis*-4-Cyano-4-*p*-fluorophenylcyclohexyl)-3-methyl-4-phenylpiperidine-4-carboxylic acid.
$C_{26}H_{29}FN_2O_2$=420.5.

CAS — 79516-68-0 (levocabastine); 79547-78-7 (hydrochloride); 79449-98-2 (cabastine).

NOTE. Levocabastine Hydrochloride is *USAN*. Cabastine is *rINN*.

Levocabastine is a histamine H_1 antagonist which has been used topically in the treatment of allergic conjunctivitis and allergic rhinitis.

References: U. Pipkorn *et al.*, *Allergy*, 1985, *40*, 491; M. Kolly and A. Pécoud, *Br. J. clin. Pharmac.*, 1986, *22*, 389.

12897-e

Lignin

A polymer occurring in plant fibrous tissue.

CAS — 9005-53-2.

Lignin has been reported to adsorb bile salts and acids and has been used in the treatment of diarrhoea.

References: L. C. Hillman *et al.*, *Gut*, 1986, *27*, 29.

2957-j

Limaprost *(rINN)*.

(*E*)-7-[(1*R*,2*R*,3*R*)-3-Hydroxy-2-[(*E*)-(3*S*,5*S*)-3-hydroxy-5-methyl-1-nonenyl]-5-oxocyclopentyl]-2-heptenoic acid compound with α-cyclodextrin.
$C_{22}H_{36}O_5$=380.5.

CAS — 88852-12-4.

Limaprost is a prostaglandin analogue.

Proprietary Names and Manufacturers
Ono, Jpn.

7360-h

Linseed Oil

Aceite de Linaza; Flaxseed Oil; Huile de Lin; Leinöl; Oleum Lini.

CAS — 8001-26-1.

Pharmacopoeias. In *Arg.*, *Aust.*, *Cz.*, *Egypt.*, *Hung.*, *Jug.*, *Nord.*, *Pol.*, *Port.*, *Roum.*, *Span.*, and *Swiss.* Also in *B.P. Vet. Br.* and *Eur.* include linseed. *Br.* also includes powdered linseed.

The fixed oil expressed from the ripe seeds of linseed, *Linum usitatissimum* (Linaceae).

Slightly **soluble** in alcohol; miscible with chloroform, ether, and petroleum spirit. **Store** in well-filled well-closed containers.

Linseed oil is used in veterinary medicine as a purgative for horses and cattle. It is no longer used as such in man, but linseed is sometimes employed as a demulcent and crushed linseed as a poultice (see p.1436).

Boiled linseed oil ('boiled oil') is linseed oil heated with litharge, manganese resinate, or other driers, to a temperature of about 150° so that metallic salts of the fatty acids are formed and cause the oil to dry more rapidly. It must not be used for medicinal purposes.

16879-a

Lobenzarit *(rINN)*.

CCA. 4-Chloro-2,2′-iminodibenzoate.
$C_{14}H_{10}ClNO_4$=291.7.

CAS — 63329-53-3 (lobenzarit); 64808-48-6 (disodium).

NOTE. Lobenzarit Sodium is *USAN*.

Lobenzarit is used in rheumatoid arthritis. It is reported to be an immunomodulator without non-steroidal analgesic or anti-inflammatory activity.

References: Y. Shiokawa *et al.*, *J. Rheumatol.*, 1984, *11*, 615.

Proprietary Names and Manufacturers
Carfenil *(Chugai, Jpn)*.

719-q

Lonapalene *(USAN, rINN)*.

RS-43179. 6-Chloro-2,3-dimethoxy-1,4-naphthalenediol diacetate.
$C_{16}H_{15}ClO_6$=338.7.

CAS — 91431-42-4.

Lonapalene has been applied topically for the treatment of psoriasis.

References: A. Lassus and S. Forsstrom, *Br. J. Derm.*, 1985, *113*, 103.

Proprietary Names and Manufacturers
Syntex, USA.

19416-e

Lonidamine *(rINN)*.

AF-1890; Diclondazolic Acid. 1-(2,4-Dichlorobenzyl)-1*H*-indazole-3-carboxylic acid.
$C_{15}H_{10}Cl_2N_2O_2$=394.4.

CAS — 50264-69-2.

An antineoplastic agent given by mouth.

18661-c

Loratadine *(BAN, USAN, rINN)*.

Sch-29851. Ethyl 4-(8-chloro-5,6-dihydro-11*H*-benzo[5,6]cyclohepta[1,2-*b*]pyridin-11-ylidene)piperidine-1-carboxylate.
$C_{22}H_{23}ClN_2O_2$=382.9.

CAS — 79794-75-5.

Loratadine is an antihistamine used in the treatment of allergic rhinitis in doses given once daily.

References: R. L. Batenhorst *et al.*, *Drug Intell. & clin. Pharm.*, 1984, *18*, 505; R. L. Batenhorst *et al.*, *Eur. J. clin. Pharmac.*, 1986, *31*, 247; G. Bruttmann and P. Pedrali, *J. int. med. Res.*, 1987, *15*, 63; R. J. Dockhorn *et al.*, *Ann. Allergy*, 1987, *58*, 407; C. M. Bradley and A. N. Nicholson, *Eur. J. clin. Pharmac.*, 1987, *32*, 419; C. M. Bradley and A. N. Nicholson, *Br. J. clin. Pharmac.*, 1987, *23*, 637P.

Proprietary Names and Manufacturers
Claritin *(Schering, Belg.)*.

19418-y

Losulazine Hydrochloride *(USAN, rINNM)*.

U-54669F. 1-[(*p*-Fluorophenyl)sulfonyl]-4-(*p*-{[7-(trifluoromethyl)-4-quinolyl]amino}benzoyl)-piperazine monohydrochloride.
$C_{27}H_{22}F_4N_4O_3S,HCl$=595.0.

CAS —81435-67-8.

Losulazine hydrochloride is an antihypertensive agent under investigation.

References: R. Gore *et al.*, *Clin. Pharmac. Ther.*, 1985, *38*, 195.

Proprietary Names and Manufacturers
Upjohn, USA.

19415-w

Loxoprofen *(rINN)*.

CS-600. (±)-*p*-[(2-Oxocyclopentyl)methyl]hydratropic acid.
$C_{15}H_{18}O_3$=246.3.

CAS — 68767-14-6.

Loxoprofen is an anti-inflammatory analgesic drug.

Proprietary Names and Manufacturers
Loxonin *(Sankyo, Jpn)*.

5011-e

Lysergide *(BAN, rINN)*.

LSD; LSD-25; Lysergic Acid Diethylamide. (+)-*NN*-Diethyl-D-lysergamide; (6a*R*,9*R*)-*NN*-Diethyl-4,6,6a,7,8,9-hexahydro-7-methylindolo-[4,3-*fg*]quinoline-9-carboxamide.
$C_{20}H_{25}N_3O$=323.4.

CAS — 50-37-3.

Adverse Effects

There is considerable variation in individual reaction to lysergide. Disorders of visual perception are among the first and most constant reactions to lysergide. Subjects may be hypersensitive to sound. Extreme alterations of mood, depression, distortion of body image, depersonalisation, disorders of thought and time sense, and synaesthesias may be experienced. Anxiety, often amounting to panic, may occur (a 'bad trip'). A prolonged toxic psychosis may be induced. The effects of lysergide may recur months after ingestion of lysergide; the recurrence or 'flashback' may be spontaneous or induced by alcohol, other drugs, stress, or fatigue.

The subjective effects of lysergide may be preceded or accompanied by somatic effects which are mainly sympathomimetic in nature and include mydriasis, tremor, hyperreflexia, hyperthermia, piloerection, and ataxia. There may be nausea and vomiting and variable effects on heart-rate and blood pressure. Derangement of blood clotting mechanisms has been described. There is no evidence of fatal reactions to lysergide in man, although accidental deaths, suicides, and homicides have occurred during lysergide intoxication.

Tolerance develops to the effects of lysergide after several days and may be lost over a similar period. There is cross-tolerance between lysergide, mescaline, and psilocybin and psilocin, but not to amphetamine or to cannabis.

Physical dependence on lysergide does not seem to occur.

A brief review of psychotic states induced by hallucinogenic drugs such as lysergide.— D. J. King, *Prescribers' J.*, 1986, *26*, 50.

CHROMOSOMAL ABERRATIONS. Lysergide has been reported to increase chromosomal abnormalities *in vitro* in cell culture (M.M. Cohen *et al.*, *Science*, 1967, *155*, 1417).

Studies of chromosomal damage in man following ingestion of lysergide have yielded contradictory results. In some studies a significant increase in chromosomal abnormalities has been reported in patients who had taken lysergide (S. Irwin and J. Egozcue, *Science*, 1967, *157*, 313; J. Nielsen *et al.*, *Br. med. J.*, 1968, *2*, 801; J. Nielsen *et al.* (letter), *Nature*, 1968, *218*, 488; J. Nielsen *et al.*, *Br. med. J.*, 1969, *3*, 634). Other studies have indicated that lysergide had no significant effect on chromosomal abnormalities (J.-H. Tijo *et al.*, *J. Am. med. Ass.*, 1969, *210*, 849; J.M. Aase *et al.*, *Lancet*, 1970, *2*, 100; K.W. Dumars, *Pediatrics*, 1971, *47*, 1037;

J.T. Robinson *et al.*, *Br. J. Psychiat.*, 1974, *125*, 238). Reviews of the effects of lysergide on chromosomes (N.I. Dishotsky *et al.*, *Science*, 1971, *172*, 431; P.J. Balson, *Adverse Drug React. Bull.*, 1972, Dec. 116; S.Y. Long, *Teratology*, 1972, *6*, 75; H. Tuchmann-Duplessis, *Monographs on Drugs, Vol. 2, Drug Effects on the Fetus*, G.S. Avery (Ed.), London, Adis, 1975, p. 158) have concluded that chromosomal damage *in vivo* cannot be attributed to lysergide and that claims for teratogenic, mutagenic, or carcinogenic action of lysergide have not been substantiated.

PREGNANCY AND THE NEONATE. The frequency of spontaneous abortions (15%) and premature births (7%) in 121 pregnancies following infrequent low doses of medically administered lysergide were within the normal ranges. The incidence of spontaneous abortions (37%) was above average for 27 pregnancies where lysergide was taken under both medical and non-medical conditions. In both groups there were more abortions when the mother or mother and father received lysergide than when only the father received lysergide. Congenital abnormalities were reported in 14 infants and some of these were minor. In all 14 lysergide was limited to medical use and the dosage range was 75 to 250 µg.— W. H. McGlothlin *et al.*, *J. Am. med. Ass.*, 1970, *212*, 1483.

There was no strong evidence of dysmorphogenic action by lysergide in *animals* or man.— H. Tuchmann-Duplessis, *Monographs on Drugs, Vol. 2, Drug Effects on the Fetus*, G.S. Avery (Ed.), London, Adis, 1975, p. 158. See also J. L. Schardein, *Drugs as Teratogens*, Cleveland, CRC, 1976, p. 129.

Ocular malformations in infants associated with maternal ingestion of lysergide during pregnancy.— C. C. Chan *et al.*, *Archs Ophthal., N.Y.*, 1978, *96*, 282.

Further reports of congenital abnormalities associated with lysergide: C. B. Jacobson and C. M. Berlin, *J. Am. med. Ass.*, 1972, *222*, 1367; B. Bogdanoff *et al.*, *Am. J. Dis. Child.*, 1972, *123*, 145; D. J. Apple and T. O. Bennett, *Archs Ophthal., N.Y.*, 1974, *92*, 301.

See also under Chromosomal Aberrations.

PSYCHOSIS. In studies on 19 patients who were admitted to mental hospitals with psychoses resulting from ingestion of lysergide, it was found that 6 had become psychotic after a single dose, although in 2 the onset of symptoms was delayed; of the other patients, 2 had become psychotic after 2 and 6 doses respectively and 11 were long-term users. Common symptoms included thought disorders, auditory hallucinations, disturbed behaviour, and paranoid delusions. Although similar to schizophrenia, detailed study revealed diagnostic differences. Chlorpromazine combined with ECT was the treatment of choice. Because of the danger of recurrent visual disturbances, patients should be warned not to drive.— K. Dewhurst and J. A. Hatrick, *Practitioner*, 1972, *209*, 327.

Treatment of Adverse Effects

The acute panic reaction is usually treated by keeping the patient in a calm supportive environment and giving frequent reassurance. Benzodiazepines may be useful, but phenothiazines should be avoided if it is possible that amphetamine-like agents have been used. Phenothiazines may be useful in lysergide-induced psychosis.

Discussion of the treatment of acute drug abuse reactions, including lysergide.— *Med. Lett.*, 1987, *29*, 83.

Precautions

The effects of lysergide may be enhanced by reserpine.

A report of chlorpromazine inducing psychosis in patients who had received lysergide.— C. J. Schwartz, *Can. med. Ass. J.*, 1971, *105*, 241.

Absorption and Fate

Lysergide is readily absorbed from the gastro-intestinal tract. It is metabolised in the liver and is excreted in the bile.

Uses and Administration

Lysergide has a doubtful therapeutic role and was formerly used mainly as an adjunct to psychotherapy although its use has now been abandoned. The effects of a dose may last for about 12 hours. It has been widely used as a drug of abuse for its hallucinogenic and psychedelic properties.

A discussion of drug dependence and its management including abuse of lysergide.— B. Davies, *Pharm. J.*, 1986, *2*, 525.

19438-k

Mabuterol *(rINN)*.

4-Amino-α-[(*tert*-butylamino)methyl]-3-chloro-5-trifluoromethyl)benzyl alcohol.

$C_{13}H_{18}ClF_3N_2O$=310.7.

CAS — 56341-08-3.

Mabuterol is a sympathomimetic agent under investigation as a bronchodilator.

References: T. W. Guentert *et al.*, *Arzneimittel-Forsch.*, 1984, *34*, 1691; W. T. Ulmer *et al.*, *ibid.*, 1697; Y. Kawakami, *ibid.*, 1699.

Proprietary Names and Manufacturers

Broncholin *(Kaken, Jpn)*.

18785-v

Mafosfamide *(rINN)*.

(±)-2-[[2-[Bis(2-chloroethyl)amino]tetrahydro-2*H*-1,3,2-oxazaphosphorin-4-yl]thio]ethanesulphonic acid *P-cis* oxide.

$C_9H_{19}Cl_2N_2O_5PS_2$=401.3.

CAS — 88859-04-5.

Mafosfamide is a derivative of cyclophosphamide (p.610) which is reported to have a similar spectrum of activity but is reported not to induce urotoxicity. It has been used to treat bone marrow for transplantation.

Proprietary Names and Manufacturers

Asta, Ger..

12908-r

Magnesium Ferulate

Magnesium 4-hydroxy-3-methoxycinnamate.

$(C_{10}H_9O_4)_2Mg$=410.7.

CAS — 32179-46-7.

Magnesium ferulate has been used as a choleretic agent.

Proprietary Names and Manufacturers

Fruchol *(Boehringer Ingelheim, Fr.)*.

12910-z

Magnesium Glutamate Hydrobromide

Magnesium α-Aminoglutarate Hydrobromide; Magnesium Bromoglutamate.

$(C_5H_8NO_4)_2Mg,HBr$=397.5.

Magnesium glutamate hydrobromide has been used as a sedative and hypnotic in the treatment of insomnia, neuroses, and behavioural disorders.

Proprietary Names and Manufacturers

Bromolate *(Austral.)*; Hyposed *(Nelson, Austral.)*; Psicosoma *(Trommsdorff, Ger.*; *Ferrer, Spain)*; Psycho-Soma *(Austral.*; *Boots-Dacour, Fr.)*; Psychoverlan *(Verla, Ger.)*.

5906-b

Magnesium Peroxide

Magnesium Perhydrolum.

CAS — 1335-26-8; 14452-57-4.

Pharmacopoeias. In *Arg., Aust., Cz., Fr., Ger., Hung., Neth., Port., Roum., Rus., Span.,* and *Swiss,* most of which specify about 25% of MgO_2 (6.5% available oxygen).

Magnesium peroxide is used as a deodorant and disinfectant. It has also been given for dyspepsia.

Proprietary Names and Manufacturers

Ozovit *(Pascoe, Ger.)*.

7361-m

Maize Oil

Corn Oil *(USAN)*; Huile de Maïs; Ol. Mayd.; Oleum Maydis.

CAS — 8001-30-7.

Pharmacopoeias. In *Cz., Egypt., Fr.,* and *Jpn.* Also in *U.S.N.F.*

The refined fixed oil obtained from the embryos of maize, *Zea mays* (Gramineae). It is a clear light yellow oil with a faint characteristic odour and taste.

Slightly **soluble** in alcohol; miscible with chloroform, ether, and petroleum spirit. **Store** at a temperature not exceeding 40° in airtight containers. Protect from light.

Maize oil has a high content of unsaturated acids and has been given instead of oils and fats with high concentrations of saturated acids in patients with hypercholesterolaemia. It is also used as an oily vehicle.

1314-k

Maleic Acid *(BAN)*.

Toxilic Acid. *cis*-Butenedioic acid.

$C_2H_2(CO_2H)_2$=116.1.

CAS — 110-16-7.

Pharmacopoeias. In *Br., Eur., Fr., Neth.,* and *Swiss.*

A white odourless crystalline powder. **Soluble** 1 in 1.5 of water and 1 in 2 of alcohol; sparingly soluble in ether. **Store** in well-closed glass containers. Protect from light.

Maleic acid is used in the preparation of Ergometrine Injection *B.P.* and Ergometrine and Oxytocin Injection *B.P.*

1315-a

Malic Acid *(USAN)*.

296 (DL-malic acid or L-malic acid); Apple Acid; Hydroxysuccinic Acid. Hydroxybutanedioic acid.

$C_4H_6O_5$=134.1.

CAS — 6915-15-7; 636-61-3 (+); 97-67-6 (−); 617-48-1 (±).

Pharmacopoeias. In *U.S.N.F.*

An acid present in apples, pears, and many other fruits. It occurs as a white or practically white crystalline powder or granules. Very **soluble** in water; freely soluble in alcohol. **Store** in well-closed containers.

The action of malic acid is similar to that of tartaric acid and it has been used in effervescent saline preparations. It is a permitted food additive and is also used as a sialogogue.

Proprietary Names and Manufacturers

The following names have been used for multi-ingredient preparations containing malic acid—Aserbine *(Bencard, UK)*; Malatex *(Norton, UK)*; Salivix *(Thames, UK)*.

17039-s

Malotilate *(rINN)*.

Diisopropyl 1,3-dithiole-$\Delta^{2,\alpha}$-malonate.

$C_{12}H_{16}O_4S_2$=288.4.

CAS — 59937-28-9.

Malotilate is reported to possess hepato-protective properties. It has been given by mouth to improve liver function, especially in hepatic sclerosis.

12913-a

Mammalian Tissue Extracts

Many medicinal preparations with definite pharmacological activity and valid clinical uses are of mammalian or similar origin and are described under their appropriate monographs—for exam-

ple, calcitonin, corticotrophin, hydrocortisone (cortisol), some enzymes, heparin, insulin, parathyroid, pituitary hormones, some sex hormones, thyroid.
Traditionally many other preparations of similar origin have been promoted for a wide variety of disorders. Evidence of pharmacological activity is often lacking, and many have fallen into disuse.

Proprietary Names and Manufacturers
H. 11 Extract *(Standard Laboratories, UK)*; Raveron *(LPB, Ital.; Robapharm, Switz.: Welbeck, UK)*; Recosen *(Berna, Spain; Robapharm, Switz.: Welbeck, UK)*.

280-z

Mastic

Almáciga; Mastiche; Mastix.

CAS — 61789-92-2.

Pharmacopoeias. In *Aust., Port., Span.,* and *Swiss.*

A resinous exudation from certain forms or varieties of *Pistacia lentiscus* (Anacardiaceae).

Solutions of mastic in alcohol, chloroform, or ether have been used, applied on cotton wool, as temporary fillings for carious teeth. Compound Mastic Paint was formerly used as a protective covering for wounds and to hold gauze in position.

1429-v

Meclofenoxate Hydrochloride *(BANM, rINNM).*

Centrophenoxine Hydrochloride; Clofenoxine Hydrochloride; Clophenoxate Hydrochloride; Deanol 4-Chlorophenoxyacetate Hydrochloride; Meclofenoxane Hydrochloride. 2-Dimethylaminoethyl 4-chlorophenoxyacetate hydrochloride.
$C_{12}H_{16}ClNO_3,HCl=294.2$.

CAS — 51-68-3 (meclofenoxate); 3685-84-5 (hydrochloride).

Pharmacopoeias. In *Cz.* and *Roum.*

Meclofenoxate hydrochloride has been claimed to aid cellular metabolism in the presence of diminished oxygen concentrations. It has been given mainly for mental changes in the elderly or following strokes.

Proprietary Names and Manufacturers
Helfergin *(Promonta, Ger.)*; Lucidril *(Montpellier, Arg.; Austral.; Anphar-Rolland, Fr.; Bracco, Ital.; ICN, Neth.; Adcock Ingram, S.Afr.; Max Ritter, Switz.; Reckitt & Colman Pharmaceuticals, UK)*; Luncidril *(Uquifa, Spain)*; Lutiaron *(Jpn)*; Ropoxyl *(Jpn)*.

12919-n

Mecrifurone Hydrochloride

9-[(2-Diethylamino)ethoxy]-7-methyl-5-oxo-5*H*-furo[3,2-g][1]benzopyran-4-yl 3-(3-pyridyl)prop-2-enoate hydrochloride.
$C_{26}H_{26}N_2O_6,HCl=499.0$.

CAS — 23845-79-6 (mecrifurone); 23829-65-4 (hydrochloride).

Mecrifurone has been used for the prevention and treatment of angina pectoris and related disorders.

Proprietary Names and Manufacturers
Coronplat *(Fisons, Ital.)*.

209-p

Meglumine *(BAN, USAN, rINN).*

N-Methylglucamine; 1-Methylamino-1-deoxy-D-glucitol.
$C_7H_{17}NO_5=195.2$.

CAS — 6284-40-8.

Pharmacopoeias. In *Br., Braz., Chin., Cz., Jpn, Jug., Nord.,* and *U.S.*

A white to faintly yellowish microcrystalline powder or crystals, odourless or with a slight odour. *B.P.* **solubilities** are: soluble 1 in 1 of water; slightly soluble in alcohol; practically insoluble in chloroform and ether. **Store** in well-closed containers.

Meglumine is an organic base used for the preparation of salts of iodinated organic acids used as contrast media.

12924-r

Melatonin

N-Acetyl-5-methoxytryptamine. *N*-[2-(5-Methoxyindol-3-yl)ethyl]acetamide.

$C_{13}H_{16}N_2O_2=232.3$.

CAS — 73-31-4.

Melatonin is a hormone produced in the pineal gland. Results mainly from *animal* studies indicate that melatonin increases the concentration of aminobutyric acid and serotonin in the midbrain and hypothalamus and enhances the activity of pyridoxal-kinase, an enzyme involved in the synthesis of aminobutyric acid, dopamine, and serotonin. Melatonin is involved in the inhibition of gonadal development and in the control of oestrus; there appears to be a diurnal rhythm of melatonin secretion.

A hypothesis that the pineal gland may play a role in the aetiology of breast cancer and that melatonin might suppress induction of breast cancer.— M. Cohen *et al.*, *Lancet*, 1978, *2*, 814. Comment and disagreement.— E. Tapp (letter), *ibid.*, 1001; R. A. Karmali *et al.* (letter), *ibid.*, 1002; H. -O. Adami *et al.* (letter), *ibid.*, 1312; M. Cohen *et al.* (letter), *ibid.*, 1381.

A study of the plasma concentrations of melatonin in healthy subjects following oral administration.— M. Aldhous *et al.*, *Br. J. clin. Pharmac.*, 1985, *19*, 517.

A discussion of the role of melatonin in mammalian reproduction.— L. Tamarkin *et al.*, *Science*, 1985, *227*, 714.

A discussion of the action of melatonin in jet lag and its place in treatment: *Lancet*, 1986, *2*, 493. See also.— J. Arendt and V. Marks (letter), *Lancet*, 1986, *2*, 698.

A report of an improvement in the sleep-wake cycle and a greatly enhanced sense of well-being in a blind man with a disturbed sleep-wake cycle following treatment with melatonin by mouth.— J. Arendt *et al.* (letter), *Lancet*, 1988, *1*, 772.

12926-d

Memotine Hydrochloride *(USAN, pINNM).*

UK-2371. 3,4-Dihydro-1-[(4-methoxyphenoxy)methyl]isoquinoline hydrochloride.
$C_{17}H_{17}NO_2,HCl=303.8$.

CAS — 18429-69-1 (memotine); 10540-97-3 (hydrochloride).

Memotine is an antiviral agent which has been tried in the prophylaxis of influenza.

Proprietary Names and Manufacturers
Pfizer, USA.

12927-n

Menbutone *(BAN, rINN).*

SC-1749 *(menbutone sodium)*. 4-(4-Methoxy-1-naphthyl)-4-oxobutyric acid.
$C_{15}H_{14}O_4=258.3$.

CAS — 3562-99-0.

Menbutone has been used as a choleretic agent. The magnesium salt has been similarly used.

Proprietary Names and Manufacturers
Hepalande *(Delalande, Ger.)*; Icteryl *(Delalande, Belg.; Delalande, Fr.)*; Sintobilina *(Azienda Farm., Ital.)*.

19470-k

Menogaril *(USAN, rINN).*

NSC-269148; 7-Omen; U-52047.
(2*R**,3*S**,4*R**,5*R**,6*R**,11*R**,13*R**)-4-(Dimethylamino)-3,4,5,6,11,12,13,14-octahydro-3,5,8,10,13-pentahydroxy-11-methoxy-6,13-dimethyl-2,6-epoxy-2*H*-naphthaceno[1,2-*b*]oxocin-9,16-dione.
$C_{28}H_{31}NO_{10}=541.6$.

CAS — 71628-96-1.

Menogaril is an antineoplastic agent under investigation.

Proprietary Names and Manufacturers
Tomosar *(Upjohn, USA)*.

266-k

Menthol *(BAN, USAN).*

Mentol. *p*-Menthan-3-ol; 2-Isopropyl-5-methylcyclohexanol.
$C_{10}H_{20}O=156.3$.

CAS — 89-78-1; 1490-04-6; 15356-60-2 (+); 2216-51-5 (−); 15356-70-4 (±).

Pharmacopoeias. In *Arg., Aust., Belg., Br., Braz., Chin., Cz., Egypt., Fr., Ger., Hung., Ind., It., Jpn, Jug., Mex., Nord., Pol., Port., Roum., Rus., Span., Swiss, Turk.,* and *U.S. Aust., Fr., Ger.,* and *Jpn* have separate monographs for laevo-menthol and racemic menthol.

Natural laevo-menthol obtained from the volatile oils of various species of *Mentha* (Labiatae) or synthetic laevo-menthol or racemic menthol.
It occurs as colourless, acicular or prismatic crystals or crystalline powder with a penetrating odour resembling that of peppermint. M.p. of natural or synthetic (−)-menthol 41° to 44°. F.p. of (±)-menthol 27° to 28°, rising on prolonged stirring to 30° to 32°.
Slightly **soluble** in water; very soluble in alcohol, chloroform, and ether; freely soluble in liquid paraffin and in fixed and volatile oils. A 5% solution in alcohol is neutral to litmus. **Store** at a temperature not exceeding 25° in airtight containers.
A liquid or soft mass is formed when menthol is triturated with camphor, chloral hydrate, phenol, and many other substances.

Adverse Effects

Menthol may give rise to hypersensitivity reactions including contact dermatitis. There have been reports of apnoea and instant collapse in infants following the local application of menthol to their nostrils. The fatal dose in man has been estimated to be about 2 g.

A woman who smoked 80 mentholated cigarettes daily for 3 months developed insomnia, unsteady gait, thick speech, tremor of the hands, mental confusion, depression, vomiting, and cramp in the legs. Her heart-rate was 44 per minute. The symptoms disappeared when menthol was withheld. Test dosage with 65 mg of menthol thrice daily produced bradycardia and evidence of toxicity after 7 days.— E. Luke (letter), *Lancet*, 1962, *1*, 110.

Ataxia, confusion, euphoria, nystagmus, and diplopia developed in a 13-year-old boy following the inhalation of 5 mL of Olbas oil instead of the recommended few drops. It was considered probable that the menthol in the preparation was responsible for the symptoms; the amount of menthol inhaled was approximately 200 mg.— N. M. O'Mullane *et al.* (letter), *Lancet*, 1982, *1*, 1121.

Treatment of Adverse Effects and Precautions

As for Camphor, p.1552.

Absorption and Fate

After absorption, menthol is excreted in the urine and bile as a glucuronide.

Uses and Administration

Menthol is chiefly used to relieve symptoms of bronchitis, sinusitis, and similar conditions. For this purpose it may be used as an inhalation, usually with benzoin, as pastilles, or as an ointment with camphor and eucalyptus oil for application to the chest or nostrils (but see Adverse Effects above).

When applied to the skin menthol dilates the blood vessels, causing a sensation of coldness followed by an analgesic effect. It relieves itching and is used in creams, lotions, or ointments in pruritus and urticaria.

In small doses by mouth menthol has a carminative action.

Estimated acceptable daily intake: up to 200 µg per kg body-weight. Further information was required from toxicity, carcinogenicity, and metabolic studies.— Twentieth Report of the Joint FAO/WHO Expert Committee on Food Additives, *Tech. Rep. Ser. Wld Hlth Org. No. 599*, 1976.

EFFECTS ON THE COLON. For reference to the muscle relaxant activity of menthol, the major constituent of peppermint oil, on the gastro-intestinal tract, see under Peppermint Oil, p.1066.

Preparations

Benzoin and Menthol Inhalation *(A.P.F.)*. menthol 2, compound benzoin tincture to 100.

Menthol Inhalation *(A.P.F.)*. Menthol 2, alcohol (90%) to 100.

Menthol and Benzoin Inhalation *(B.P.)*. Menthol 2 g, benzoin inhalation to 100 mL.

Menthol and Pine Inhalation *(A.P.F.)*. Menthol 2, pumilio pine oil 5, alcohol (90%) to 100. Melaleuca oil may be substituted for pumilio pine oil.

Tetracaine and Menthol Ointment *(U.S.P.)*. See under Amethocaine, p.1208.

Proprietary Preparations

Karvol *(Crookes Laboratories, UK). Inhalation capsules*, menthol 35.9 mg, with chlorbutol, cinnamon oil, pine oil, terpineol, and thymol. For congestion in the upper respiratory tract. The contents of a capsule should be expressed into a handkerchief, or into 500 mL of hot, not boiling, water, and the vapour inhaled freely.

Olbas *(Lane, UK). Oil*, cajuput oil 18.5%, clove oil 0.1%, eucalyptus oil 35.45%, juniper berry oil 2.7%, menthol 4.1%, peppermint oil 35.45%, wintergreen oil 3.7%. *Pastilles*, eucalyptus oil 1.16%, peppermint oil 1.12%, menthol 0.1%, juniper berry oil 0.067%, wintergreen oil 0.047%, clove oil 0.0025%.

Proprietary Names and Manufacturers

Menthol is an ingredient of many cough, cold, cooling, and traditional remedies.

537-n

Menyanthes

Bitterklee; Bogbean; Buckbean; Folia Trifoli Fibrini; Marsh Trefoil; Trèfle d'Eau.

Pharmacopoeias. In *Aust.*, *Cz.*, *Hung.*, *Pol.*, and *Rus.*

The dried leaves of the buckbean, *Menyanthes trifoliata* (Menyanthaceae).

Menyanthes has been used as a bitter. It is also used in folk medicine.

12931-x

Mepixanox *(rINN)*.

Mepixantone. 3-Methoxy-4-piperidinomethyl-9*H*-xanthen-9-one.

$C_{20}H_{21}NO_3$=323.4.

CAS — 17854-59-0.

Mepixanox has been used as a respiratory analeptic.

Proprietary Names and Manufacturers

Pimexone *(Formenti, Ital.)*.

5307-b

Mercuric Chloride

Bicloruro de Mercurio; Cloreto Mercúrico; Corrosive Sublimate; Hydrarg. Perchlor.; Hydrargyri Dichloridum; Hydrargyri Perchloridum; Hydrargyrum Bichloratum; Mercuric Chlor.; Mercurique (Chlorure); Mercury Bichloride; Mercury Perchloride; Quecksilberchlorid.

$HgCl_2$=271.5.

CAS — 7487-94-7.

Pharmacopoeias. In *Arg.*, *Aust.*, *Belg.*, *Braz.*, *Cz.*, *Eur.*, *Fr.*, *Ger.*, *Jpn*, *Jug.*, *Mex.*, *Neth.*, *Nord.*, *Pol.*, *Port.*, *Rus.*, *Span.*, *Swiss*, and *Turk.* Also in *B.P.C. 1973.*

A heavy, colourless or white, odourless, crystalline powder or crystalline masses. **Soluble** 1 in 15 of water, 1 in 3 of alcohol, 1 in 25 of ether, and 1 in 15 of glycerol. A solution in water is acid to litmus. **Incompatible** with alkalis, alkaloids (especially if iodides are present), lead acetate, silver nitrate, proteins, and vegetable astringents. Solutions made with tap water may yield a slight deposit on standing. **Protect** from light.

NOTE. Solutions of mercuric chloride for external use should be coloured with indigo carmine as a safety precaution. When dispensing mercuric chloride, steel instruments such as spatulas must not be used, and surgical instruments must not be put into solutions of mercuric chloride. Solutions of mercuric chloride and other mercurials should not be allowed to come into contact with aluminium, for instance in screw caps or collapsible tubes.

The use of mercuric chloride as an antibacterial substance is limited by its toxicity, its precipitating action on proteins, its irritant action on raw surfaces, its corrosive action on metals, and by the fact that its activity is greatly reduced in the presence of excreta or body fluids.

Details of the adverse effects of mercury compounds are provided below under Mercury.

No signs of mercurialism occurred in 6 patients following the use of about 1 litre of a 0.2% solution of mercuric chloride to wash out the rectal stump and a further 300 mL to mop out the lumen of the colon and other tissues (these being dried up before the abdomen was closed) to prevent implantation of cancer cells during surgery for adenocarcinoma of the rectum. In 1 patient a maximum urinary concentration of 232 µg of mercury per litre followed the treatment.— H. B. Devlin (letter), *Br. med. J.*, 1967, *3*, 679. Because of the danger of renal tubular damage, illustrated by a case report, it was recommended that mercuric chloride solution should not be used as an irrigating agent in the peritoneal cavity.— J. C. Gingell *et al.* (letter), *ibid.*, 867. A patient sustained a superficial chemical burn due to interaction between mercuric chloride solution (used to reduce exfoliated malignant cells during rectal surgery) and an aluminium diathermy plate electrode beneath the patient.— A. G. Nash (letter), *ibid.*, 1973, *4*, 783.

Some reports of poisoning with mercuric chloride: T. Stack *et al.*, *Br. med. J.*, 1983, *287*, 1513 (ingestion by a child; mild renal failure); D. P. Worth *et al.*, *Postgrad. med. J.*, 1984, *60*, 636 (ingestion of a moss killer containing mercuric chloride and mercurous chloride; acute renal failure); T. Laundy *et al.*, *Br. med. J.*, 1984, *289*, 96 (use for intraperitoneal lavage; acute renal failure and death).

5311-d

Yellow Mercuric Oxide

Gelbes Quecksilberoxyd; Hydrargyri Oxidum Flavum; Hydrargyri Oxydum Flavum; Mercurique (Oxyde) Jaune; Oxido Amarillo de Mercurio; Yellow Precipitate.

HgO=216.6.

CAS — 21908-53-2.

Pharmacopoeias. In *Arg.*, *Aust.*, *Belg.*, *Cz.*, *Egypt.*, *Fr.*, *Hung.*, *Int.*, *It.*, *Jug.*, *Mex.*, *Pol.*, *Port.*, *Roum.*, *Rus.*, and *Span.* Also in *B.P.C. 1973.*

Yellow mercuric oxide has been used in eye ointments for the local treatment of minor infections including the eradication of crab lice from the eyelashes. Absorption can occur and produce the adverse effects of inorganic mercury (below). Golden eye ointment was a preparation of yellow mercuric oxide.

Proprietary Names and Manufacturers

Gul-øjenslave *(DAK, Denm.)*; Ophtosept *(Winzer, Ger.)*; Poenhidrargil *(Poen, Arg.)*.

5314-m

Mercurous Chloride

Calomel; Calomelanos; Cloreto Mercuroso; Hydrarg. Subchlor.; Hydrargyri Subchloridum; Hydrargyrosi Chloridum; Hydrargyrum Chloratum (Mite); Mercureux (Chlorure); Mercurius Dulcis; Mercury Monochloride; Mercury Subchloride; Mild Mercurous Chloride; Protocloruro de Mercurio; Quecksilberchlorür.

HgCl=236.0.

CAS — 7546-30-7 (HgCl); 10112-91-1 (Hg_2Cl_2).

Pharmacopoeias. In *Arg.*, *Aust.*, *Belg.*, *Chin.*, *Fr.*, *Hung.*, *Mex.*, *Nord.*, *Pol.*, *Port.*, and *Span.*

Several pharmacopoeias include also precipitated mercurous chloride (hydrargyri subchloridum praecipitatum), a white amorphous powder, to which the synonym 'white precipitate' (praecipitatum album) is given by some pharmacopoeias. White precipitate has also been used as a name for ammoniated mercury.

Mercurous chloride was formerly given as a laxative and was applied topically as an antibacterial. It was one of the mercury compounds employed in the management of syphylis in the pre-antibiotic era.

The mercurous form of mercury does not possess the corrosive properties of the mercuric form and is not absorbed to any great extent. However, the mercurous form can be converted to the mercuric with consequent toxicity as described under mercury (below).

5306-m

Mercury

Hydrarg.; Hydrargyrum; Hydrargyrum Depuratum; Mercure; Mercurio; Quecksilber; Quicksilver.

Hg=200.59.

CAS — 7439-97-6.

Pharmacopoeias. In *Aust.*, *Belg.*, *Fr.*, *Hung.*, *Mex.*, *Pol.*, *Port.*, and *Span.*

A shining, silvery white, very mobile liquid, easily divisible into globules, which readily volatilises on heating.

Adverse Effects

Liquid mercury if ingested is poorly absorbed and, unless there is aspiration or pre-existing gastro-intestinal disorders, is not considered to be a severe toxicological hazard.

The greatest dangers from liquid mercury arise from the inhalation of mercury vapour. On acute exposure, it can cause various gastro-intestinal effects including nausea, vomiting, and diarrhoea; more importantly it is toxic to the respiratory system and this effect can be fatal. Some CNS involvement has also been reported. Liquid mercury is not without its dangers when injected and there have been a number of reports of accidental or intentional parenteral administration. Inorganic salts such as mercuric chloride are corrosive when ingested causing severe nausea, vomiting, pain, bloody diarrhoea, and necrosis. The kidney is also involved and tubular necrosis may develop. Mercurous salts are considered to be less hazardous, but the mercurous form can be converted to the mercuric.

Chronic mercury poisoning may result from inhalation of mercury vapour, skin contact with mercury or mercury compounds, or ingestion of mercury salts over prolonged periods. It is characterised by tremor, motor and sensory disturbances, mental deterioration, gastro-intestinal symptoms, dermatitis, kidney damage, salivation, and loosening of teeth. A blue line may be present on the gums.

Poisoning with mercury or inorganic mercury salts has arisen from a variety of sources such as batteries, cosmetics (although use in cosmetics is generally restricted by law, apart from some carefully defined exceptions for some organomercurial preservatives) dental materials, medical equipment, and jewellery manufacture. Barometers, sphygmomanometers, and thermometers are still sources of liquid mercury.

The syndrome of acrodynia (pink disease), with symptoms of sweat, rash, oedema of the extremities, photophobia, wasting, weakness, tachycardia, and diminished reflexes, occurred in children given mercury in teething powders or in ointments or dusting powders. Such preparations have long since been withdrawn from use. However, the syndrome is still a feature of mercury poisoning from other sources.

Organic mercurial compounds produce similar toxic effects to inorganic compounds, but they have a more selective action on the CNS that has proved difficult to treat. The degree of toxicity varies with the different groups of organic mercurials; those used as preservatives or disinfectants being less toxic than the ethyl or methyl compounds that are not used pharmaceutically or clinically. Methylmercury is notorious for its toxicity; there have been cases of foetal neurotoxicity during outbreaks of methylmercury poisoning. There is little difference between acute and chronic poisoning with organic mercurials.

Hypersensitivity to mercury and mercurial compounds has been reported.

Mercurialentis has been reported in patients treated with eye-drops containing an organomercurial preservative.

In Great Britain the recommended exposure limits of mercury and mercury compounds except mercury alkyls are 0.05 mg (as Hg) per m^3 (long-term) and 0.15 mg (as Hg) per m^3 (short-term). The recommended exposure limits of mercury alkyls are 0.01 mg (as Hg) per m^3 (long-term) and 0.03 mg (as Hg) per m^3 (short-term). Suitable precautions should be taken to prevent absorption of mercury alkyls through the skin. In the *US* the permissible and recommended exposure limits for inorganic mercury are 0.1 mg per m^3 and 0.05 mg per m^3 respectively.

SPILLAGE. A discussion of the problems of dealing with mercury spillage.— *Lancet*, 1975, *1*, 1021. See also: D. Anderton, *Pharm. J.*, 1986, *2*, 294; C. Washington (letter), *ibid.*, 384.

Mercury in Food

Mercury is widely distributed in nature in both the inorganic and organic forms. Methylmercury can be produced from inorganic mercury through microbial action and foods such as fish may have a high concentration of methylmercury. Organic mercury is used as a seed dressing and though not intended for consumption such seeds, through error, do sometimes enter the food chain.

Provisional tolerable weekly intake of mercury for man: up to 300 µg per person or 5 µg per kg body-weight. Not more than 200 µg per person or 3.3 µg per kg should be present as methylmercury expressed as mercury.— Sixteenth Report of FAO/WHO Expert Committee on Food Additives, *Tech. Rep. Ser. Wld Hlth Org. No. 505*, 1972.

It was estimated from a total diet study that the dietary intake of mercury from food and beverages in the *UK* was between 2 and 3 µg per day of which about 1 µg per day comes from fish. Individuals consuming large quantities of fish on a regular basis might exceed recommended provisional tolerable weekly intakes for mercury and methylmercury.— Survey of Mercury in Food: Second Supplementary Report, *Food Surveillance Paper No. 17, Minist. Agric. Fish. Fd*, London, HM Stationery Office, 1987.

Treatment of Adverse Effects

Ingestion of liquid mercury seldom requires active treatment. Acute poisoning due to other inorganic mercury sources should be treated if appropriate by immediate gastric aspiration and lavage; a 5% solution of sodium formaldehyde sulphoxylate may be used with the aim of converting the mercuric form to the mercurous. Alternatively a lavage solution of raw egg white may be used. Large quantities of milk or charcoal may also be given. Dimercaprol (see p.840) therapy should be started immediately. Other chelating agents that may be used include penicillamine (see p.849), acetylpenicillamine (p.835), and succimer (p.855).

Some centres institute haemodialysis at the beginning of treatment; others wait until renal failure develops when either haemodialysis or peritoneal dialysis is used.

Symptomatic measures should be used to alleviate the potentially wide range of toxic effects. Mercurials on the skin should be removed by copious washing with soap and water.

Poisoning due to organic mercury is difficult to treat. The same measures as above should be adopted, except that it is recommended by some that dimercaprol should not be used since *animal* evidence indicates that it may increase the brain concentrations of mercury. An additional measure that has been tried is the administration of a resin complex to prevent the reabsorption of mercury from the bile.

Absorption and Fate

There is little absorption of mercury from globules in the gastro-intestinal tract. The main hazard of liquid mercury is from absorption following inhalation of mercury vapour; this mercury is widely distributed before being oxidised to the mercuric form. Concentrations can be detected in the brain.

Soluble inorganic mercuric salts are readily absorbed from the gastro-intestinal tract and can also be absorbed through the skin. The mercury is distributed throughout the soft tissues with high concentrations in the kidneys; it is mainly excreted in the urine and through the colon. It may take years to eliminate mercury from the brain; elimination from other tissues may take several months.

Alkyl mercury compounds are also readily absorbed from both the gastro-intestinal and the respiratory tracts. They are widely distributed and can produce high concentrations in the brain. Alkyl mercury is excreted in urine and in the faeces with extensive enterohepatic recycling. The biological half-life varies but is longer than that of inorganic mercury.

Organic mercury, and to some extent inorganic mercury, diffuse across the placenta and are excreted in breast milk.

Uses and Administration

The hazards associated with mercury generally outweigh any therapeutic benefit and its clinical use has largely been abandoned. The use of mercurial diuretics such as mersalyl (see p.997) has generally been superseded by other diuretics. Ointments containing mercurials, such as ammoniated mercury (see p.926) have also generally been replaced by less toxic preparations. Mercurials were formerly used as spermicides.

The ionisable mercury salts and certain organic compounds of mercury have been used as disinfectants, and some mercury salts are effective parasiticides and fungicides. The organic mercurials are also used as preservatives and have been used for sterilisation of solutions by heating with a bactericide.

A nitrated oxide of mercury (Mercurius Solubilis; Merc. Sol.) is used in homoeopathic medicine.

5017-k

Mescaline

3,4,5-Trimethoxyphenethylamine.

$C_{11}H_{17}NO_3$=211.3.

CAS — 54-04-6.

An alkaloid obtained from the cactus *Lophophora williamsii* (=*Anhalonium williamsii*=*A. lewinii*) (Cactaceae), which grows in the northern regions of Mexico. The cactus is known in those areas by the Aztec name 'peyote' or 'peyotl' and dried slices of the cactus are called 'mescal buttons'. Both Mexican and North American Indians have used peyotl in religious ceremonies on account of its hallucinogenic activity.

Mescaline produces hallucinogenic and sympathomimetic effects similar to those produced by lysergide (see p.1584), but it is less potent. Its effects last for up to 12 hours. It has no therapeutic use.

Effects of mescaline in man.— A. Hofmann, *Indian J. Pharm.*, 1963, *25*, 254.

Pharmacological studies of mescaline *in vitro*.— E. Clemente and V. de P. Lynch, *J. pharm. Sci.*, 1968, *57*, 72.

A detailed review of the chemistry, biogenesis, and biological effects of 42 constituents of peyote.— G. J. Kapadia and M. B. E. Fayez, *J. pharm. Sci.*, 1970, *59*, 1699.

An investigation of the use of peyote among Navajo Indians.— R. L. Bergman, *Am. J. Psychiat.*, 1971, *128*, 695.

A study of 57 Huichol Indians with an individual and cultural tradition of peyote ingestion and 60 controls indicated that ingestion of peyote was not associated with abnormalities in lymphocyte chromosomes.— D. L. Dorrance *et al.*, *J. Am. med. Ass.*, 1975, *234*, 299. See also *ibid.*, 313.

3935-c

Mesoglycan

A mucopolysaccharide complex extracted from calf aorta.

Mesoglycan has antithrombotic, antiplatelet, and hypolipidaemic properties and has been given by mouth and intramuscular injection in atherosclerotic conditions and hyperlipidaemias.

References: P. Saba *et al.*, *Curr. ther. Res.*, 1986, *40*, 761.

Proprietary Names and Manufacturers

Perclar *(Parke, Davis, Ital.)*; Prisma *(Mediolanum, Ital.)*.

3936-k

Metapramine Hydrochloride *(rINNM)*.

10,11-Dihydro-*N*,5-dimethyl-5*H*-dibenz[*b,f*]azepin-10-amine hydrochloride.

$C_{16}H_{19}N_2Cl$=273.8.

CAS — 21730-16-5 (metapramine).

Metapramine hydrochloride is a tricyclic antidepressant that has been given by injection. The fumarate has been given by mouth.

Proprietary Names and Manufacturers

Timaxel *(Specia, Fr.)*.

12934-d

Metescufylline *(rINN)*.

7-(2-Diethylaminoethyl)theophylline (7-hydroxy-4-methylcoumarin-6-yloxy)acetate.

$C_{25}H_{31}N_5O_8$=529.5.

CAS — 15518-82-8.

Metescufylline has been used for its reputed effect on capillary circulation.

Proprietary Names and Manufacturers

Veinartan *(Millot-Solac, Fr.)*; Venarterin *(Boi, Spain)*.

12935-n

Methallibure *(BAN, USAN).*

AY-61122; ICI-33828; Metallibure; NSC-69536. 1-Methyl-6-(1-methylallyl)-2,5-dithiobiurea.
$C_7H_{14}N_4S_2$=218.3.

CAS — 926-93-2.

Methallibure has the property of reversibly inhibiting certain hypothalamic and anterior pituitary functions. It has been used in veterinary medicine.

5318-q

Methargen

Disilver(I) 3,3′-methylenebis(naphthalene-2-sulphonate).
$C_{21}H_{14}Ag_2O_6S_2$=642.2.

CAS — 53370-43-7.

Methargen is a silver compound that has been used as a disinfectant.

12937-m

Methicotinium Iodide

3-Methoxycarbonyl-1-methylpyridinium iodide.
$C_8H_{10}INO_2$=279.1.

CAS — 4685-10-3.

Methicotinium iodide has been used in the treatment of hypertension and arteriosclerosis.

Proprietary Names and Manufacturers
Iodonicot *(Ital.).*

12938-b

Methindizate Hydrochloride *(BANM).*

Metindizate Hydrochloride *(rINNM).* 2-(1-Methylperhydroindol-3-yl)ethyl benzilate hydrochloride.
$C_{25}H_{31}NO_3,HCl$=430.0.

CAS — 15687-33-9 (methindizate).

Methindizate hydrochloride is an antispasmodic used in veterinary medicine.

12939-v

Methiosulfonium Chloride

Methylmethionine Sulfonium Chloride; Vitamin U. (3-Amino-3-carboxypropyl)dimethylsulphonium chloride.
$C_6H_{14}ClNO_2S$=199.7.

CAS — 1115-84-0.

Methiosulfonium chloride has been used for its reputed protective effect on the liver and gastro-intestinal mucosa.

Proprietary Names and Manufacturers
Cabagin-U *(Jpn)*; Epadyn-U *(Ital.).*

12940-r

Methiosulfonium Iodide

Methylmethionine Sulfonium Iodide. (3-Amino-3-carboxypropyl)dimethylsulphonium iodide.
$C_6H_{14}INO_2S$=291.1.

CAS — 3493-11-6.

Methiosulfonium iodide has been used in rheumatic and other disorders.

Proprietary Names and Manufacturers
Lobarthrose *(Opodex, Fr.).*

12951-n

Methyl Fluorosulphate

Methyl Fluorosulphonate.
$CH_3O.SO_2F$=114.1.

Methyl fluorosulphate has been used as a laboratory methylating agent. Pulmonary oedema has occurred after inhalation, and concern has been expressed concerning possible carcinogenicity.

19482-r

Methyl *tert*-Butyl Ether

Methyl Terbutyl Ether; Methyl Tertiary Butyl Ether. 2-Methoxy-2-methylpropane.
$C_5H_{12}O$=88.15.

CAS — 1634-04-4.

Methyl *tert*-butyl ether is a solvent. It is being investigated for the rapid dissolution of cholesterol gall-stones.

A preliminary report on the use of methyl *tert*-butyl ether for the rapid dissolution of cholesterol gall-stones in 2 patients.— M. J. Allen *et al., New Engl. J. Med.*, 1985, *312*, 217. See also R. A. F. Gonzaga *et al.* (letter), *ibid., 313,* 385; F. J. Thaler (letter), *ibid.,*; T. Sauerbruch *et al.* (letter), *ibid.,*; J. L. Thistle *et al.* (letter), *ibid.*, 386; E. vanSonnenberg *et al., Am. J. Roentg.*, 1986, *146*, 865.

9254-c

Methylchromone *(BAN, rINN).*

3-Methyl-4*H*-chromen-4-one.
$C_{10}H_8O_2$=160.2.

CAS — 85-90-5.

Methylchromone is a spasmolytic which has been given in the treatment of angina pectoris and as an antispasmodic for the relief of biliary, hepatic or renal spasm.

Proprietary Names and Manufacturers
Cromonalgina *(Ceccarelli, Ital.)*; Diacromone *(Millot-Solac, Fr.).*

12948-g

Methylheptaminol Hydrochloride

2-Methyl-6-methylaminoheptan-2-ol hydrochloride.
$C_9H_{21}NO,HCl$=195.7.

Methylheptaminol hydrochloride has been used in the treatment of cardiac insufficiency.

Proprietary Names and Manufacturers
Corsanil *(SIT, Ital.)*; Eptaminal *(Ital.).*

12949-q

Methylhydroxyquinoline Methylsulphate

1-Methyl-8-hydroxyquinolinium methyl sulphate.
$C_{10}H_{10}NO,CH_3O_4S$=271.3.

Methylhydroxyquinoline methylsulphate has been used as eye-drops in a variety of conditions.

Proprietary Names and Manufacturers
Chibro-Uvélina *(Merck Sharp & Dohme, Spain)*; Chibro-Uvelin *(Chibret, Ger.)*; Chibro-Uveline *(UPB, Belg.)*; Uveline *(Merck Sharp & Dohme-Chibret, Fr.; Chibret, Switz.).*

12950-d

Methylmethacrylate

Methyl 2-methylacrylate; Methyl 2-methylpropenoate.
$C_5H_8O_2$=100.1.

CAS — 80-62-6.

Pharmacopoeias. Fr. includes a methacrylic acid ester copolymer. *U.S.N.F.* includes Methacrylic Acid Copolymer.

Adverse Effects
Methylmethacrylate monomer vapour may irritate the respiratory tract, eyes, and skin. Cases of occupational asthma have been reported. Contact dermatitis, dizziness, nausea and vomiting may also occur. Methylmethacrylate monomer may be harmful to the liver. It acts as a peripheral vasodilator and has caused hypotension and, rarely, cardiac arrest and death when absorbed during the use of polymethylmethacrylate (PMMA) as a bone cement during orthopaedic surgery.
Other adverse effects associated with the use of polymethylmethacrylate as a bone cement include thrombophlebitis, pulmonary embolism, haemorrhage, haematoma, short-term irregularities in cardiac conduction, and cerebrovascular accident.
In Great Britain the recommended exposure limit of methylmethacrylate is 100 ppm (long-term); 125 ppm (short-term).

Uses and Administration
Methylmethacrylate forms the basis of acrylic bone cements used in orthopaedic surgery. A liquid consisting chiefly of methylmethacrylate monomer with a polymerisation initiator is mixed with a powder consisting of polymethylmethacrylate (PMMA) or a methylmethacrylate ester copolymer. Barium sulphate or zirconium dioxide may be added as a contrast medium. The reaction is exothermic. Beads of polymethylmethacrylate containing gentamicin have been implanted in the prophylaxis and treatment of bone infections and some soft-tissue infections. A bone cement containing gentamicin is also available.
Polymethylmethacrylate has also been used as a material for intra-ocular lenses, for denture bases, as a cement for dental prostheses, and in composite resins for dental restoration.
Methacrylate polymers are used in pharmaceutical technology.

Proprietary Names and Manufacturers of Bone Cements
Antibiotic Simplex Radiopaque *(Howmedica, UK)*; CMW *(CMW Laboratories, UK)*; Implast *(Beiersdorf, Ger.)*; Palacos *(Schering Corp., Denm.)*; Palacos LV with Gentamicin *(Kirby-Warrick, UK)*; Palacos R *(E. Merck, Ger.; Essex, Switz.; Kirby-Warrick, UK)*; Palacos R with Gentamicin *(Kirby-Warrick, UK)*; Palacos-R with Garamycin *(Essex, Austral.)*; Surgical Simplex P *(Howmedica, UK).*

3727-p

Metochalcone *(rINN).*

CB1314; Methochalcone; Trimethoxychalcone. 2′,4,4′-Trimethoxychalcone.
$C_{18}H_{18}O_4$=298.3.

CAS — 18493-30-6.

Metochalcone is a choleretic. It has been given in doses of 1 to 2 g daily in divided doses with meals.

Proprietary Names and Manufacturers
Agobilex *(Ital.)*; Auxibilina *(Granata, Ital.)*; Chemicol *(Beta, Ital.)*; Cholesteril *(Tosi-Novara, Ital.)*; Choligen *(Ital Suisse, Ital.)*; Colazid *(Ital.)*; Colerex *(Tiber, Ital.)*; Megalip *(Biotrading, Ital.)*; Solvocolo *(Farmacologico Milanese, Ital.)*; Spechol *(Molteni, Ital.)*; Trimecolo *(Ital.)*; Vésidryl *(Clin-Comar-Byla, Fr.).*

2753-h

Mexiprostil *(rINN).*

Methyl (1*R*,2*R*,3*R*)-3-hydroxy-2-[(*E*)-(3*R*)-3-hydroxy-4-methoxy-4-methyloctyl]-5-oxocyclopentaneheptanoate.
$C_{23}H_{40}O_6$=412.6.

CAS — 88980-20-5.

Mexiprostil is a prostaglandin analogue reported to inhibit gastric acid secretion.

3694-z

Midaglizole *(rINN).*

(±)-2-[α-(2-Imidazolin-2-ylmethyl)benzyl]pyridine.
$C_{16}H_{17}N_3$=251.3.

CAS — 66529-17-7.

Midaglizole is under investigation as a hypoglycaemic agent. A proposed mode of action is stimulation of insulin secretion by antagonism of alpha$_2$-adrenoceptors.

Proprietary Names and Manufacturers
Daiichi, Jpn.

19513-l

Midalcipran *(pINN).*

F-2207. (±)-*cis*-2-(Aminomethyl)-*N,N*-diethyl-1-phenylcyclopropanecarboxamide.
$C_{15}H_{22}N_2O$=246.4.

CAS — 92623-85-3.

Midalcipran is an antidepressant under investigation.

References: C. Serre *et al.*, *Curr. ther. Res.*, 1986, *39*, 156.

Proprietary Names and Manufacturers
Pierre Fabre, Fr.

2815-d

Midazogrel *(rINN).*

(±)-1-[(*E*)-3-(benzyloxy)-1-octenyl]imidazole.
$C_{18}H_{24}N_2O$=284.4.

CAS — 80614-27-3.

Midazogrel is claimed to be a thromboxane synthetase inhibitor and to have potential value as an antithrombotic agent.

19516-z

Mifepristone *(rINN).*

RU-38486; RU-486. 11β-[*p*-(Dimethylamino)phenyl]-17-β-hydroxy-17-(1-propynyl)estra-4,9-dien-3-one.
$C_{29}H_{35}NO_2$=429.6.

CAS — 84371-65-3.

Mifepristone has antiprogestogenic activity. It has been given by mouth for the termination of early pregnancies and its efficacy has been shown to be increased when given in combination with a prostaglandin.

A review of mifepristone. Mifepristone binds strongly to progesterone and glucocorticoid receptors, weakly to androgen receptors, but has no anti-oestrogenic or anti-mineralocorticoid activity. Although its property of binding to glucocorticoid receptors, thereby enhancing the secretion of corticotrophin and cortisol, has proved useful for the treatment of Cushing's syndrome, the major clinical application has been as an antifertility agent by antagonising the action of progesterone.
Mifepristone inhibits ovulation when given in the late follicular phase of the menstrual cycle but this action has yet to be explored as a potential contraceptive.
In very early pregnancy (around the time of expected menstrual bleeding) mifepristone will provoke bleeding although preliminary studies suggest that the pregnancy will continue in about 20% of cases. Clearly, therefore, mifepristone is unacceptable as a 'contranidatory agent' in its present dosage regimen, even if the ethical and legal issues were to be resolved.
The widest application is likely to be as a medical abortifacient in early pregnancy. Mifepristone has been given by mouth in doses of 0.2 to 1 g in women with up to 9 weeks' amenorrhoea but subsequent surgical evacuation was necessary in about 30% of patients. However, it has proved more effective when used in combination with a prostaglandin and large multicentre studies of such a combination are being coordinated by the World Health Organization. Studies are also being performed to determine the efficacy of mifepristone in inducing cervical dilatation before termination of pregnancy in the second trimester.— *Lancet*, 1987, *2*, 1308. See also.— B. Couzinet and G. Schaison, *Drugs*, 1988, *35*, 187.

Some references to the use of mifepristone for the termination of pregnancy: L. Kovacs *et al.*, *Contraception*, 1984, *29*, 399 (early pregnancy); H. A. M. Vervest and A. A. Haspels, *Fert. Steril.*, 1985, *44*, 627 (early pregnancy); B. Couzinet *et al.*, *New Engl. J. Med.*, 1986, *315*, 1565 (early pregnancy); D. R. Urquhart and A. A. Templeton (letter), *Lancet*, 1987, *2*, 1405 (second trimester); M. W. Rodger and D. T. Baird, *ibid.*, 1415 (early pregnancy; with prostaglandins).

Proprietary Names and Manufacturers
Mifegyne *(Roussel, Fr.).*

18829-n

Miglitol *(BAN, pINN).*

Bay-m-1099. (2*R*,3*R*,4*R*,5*S*)-1-(2-Hydroxyethyl)-2-(hydroxymethyl)piperidine-3,4,5-triol.
$C_8H_{17}NO_5$=207.2.

CAS — 72432-03-2.

Miglitol is an alpha-glucosidase inhibitor under investigation as an adjunct in the management of diabetes mellitus.

References: R. H. Taylor *et al.*, *Gut*, 1984, *25*, A1155; P. H. Joubert *et al.*, *Eur. J. clin. Pharmac.*, 1985, *28*, 705; N. Katsilambros *et al.*, *Arzneimittel-Forsch.*, 1986, *36*, 1136; G. Dimitriadis *et al.*, *Klin. Wschr.*, 1986, *64*, 405; R. H. Taylor *et al.*, *Gut*, 1986, *27*, 1471; *Drugs of the Future*, 1986, *11*, 1039; *ibid.*, 1987, *12*, 1160; F. P. Kennedy and J. E. Gerich, *Clin. Pharmac. Ther.*, 1987, *42*, 455; P. H. Joubert *et al.*, *Eur. J. clin. Pharmac.*, 1987, *31*, 723.

Proprietary Names and Manufacturers
Bayer, Ger.

2185-s

Milacemide Hydrochloride *(USAN, rINNM).*

CP-1552S. 2-(Pentylamino)acetamide monohydrochloride.
$C_7H_{16}N_2O,HCl$=180.7.

CAS — 76990-56-2 (milacemide); 76990-85-7 (hydrochloride).

Milacemide hydrochloride is an anti-epileptic agent under investigation.

References: M. A. Houtkooper *et al.*, *Epilepsia*, 1986, *27*, 255.

12744-k

Milverine Hydrochloride *(pINNM).*

Fenpyramine Hydrochloride. 3,3-Diphenyl-*N*-(4-pyridyl)propylamine hydrochloride.
$C_{20}H_{20}N_2,HCl$=324.9.

CAS — 29769-70-8; 75437-14-8 (milverine).

Milverine hydrochloride has been used as an antispasmodic.

Proprietary Names and Manufacturers
Fenprin *(Rhone-Poulenc, Ital.).*

The following names have been used for multi-ingredient preparations containing milverine hydrochloride— Fenprinax *(RBS Pharma, Ital.).*

18663-a

Minocromil *(BAN, USAN, rINN).*

FPL-59360. 6-Methylamino-4-oxo-10-propyl-4*H*-pyrano[3,2-g]quinoline-2,8-dicarboxylic acid.
$C_{18}H_{16}N_2O_6$=356.3.

CAS — 85118-44-1 (minocromil); 75452-62-9 (sodium salt).

Minocromil is an anti-allergic drug similar to sodium cromoglycate.

References: J. A. Roberts and N. C. Thomson, *Clin. Allergy*, 1985, *15*, 377; U. G. Svendsen *et al.*, *Allergy*, 1985, *40*, 458.

Proprietary Names and Manufacturers
Fisons, UK.

18664-t

Mioflazine *(BAN, rINN).*

R-51469 (hydrochloride). 1-[4,4-Bis(4-fluorophenyl)butyl]-4-(2,6-dichlorophenylcarbamoylmethyl)piperazine-2-carboxamide.
$C_{29}H_{30}Cl_2F_2N_4O_2$=575.5.

CAS — 79467-23-5 (mioflazine); 79467-24-6 (hydrochloride).

NOTE. Mioflazine Hydrochloride is *USAN.*

Mioflazine is a calcium-channel blocking agent with vasodilatory activity.

Proprietary Names and Manufacturers
Janssen, Belg.

12965-q

Miracle Fruit

The fruit of *Synsepalum dulcificum* (=*Richardella dulcifica*) (Sapotaceae).

Miracle fruit contains a glycoprotein 'miraculin' with no apparent taste of its own but able to make sour substances taste sweet and to improve the flavour of foods. Its activity is reduced by heating.

885-r

Mistletoe

Gui; Tallo de muérdago; Visci Caulis; Viscum.

Pharmacopoeias. In *Fr.* and *Span.*

The dried, evergreen, dioecious semi-parasite, *Viscum album* (Loranthaceae), which grows on the branches of deciduous trees, chiefly apple, poplar, and plum. It occurs as a mixture of broken stems and leaves and occasional fruits.

Mistletoe has a vasodilator action and has been used for lowering blood pressure. Its action was reported usually to be delayed with a maximum effect reached 3 to 4 days after the commencement of treatment. It has also been used in hysteria and chorea and was reputed to be of use as an antineoplastic agent. Ingestion of the berries and other parts has been reported to cause nausea, vomiting, diarrhoea, and bradycardia.

A review of mistletoe.— L. A. Anderson and J. D. Phillipson, *Pharm. J.*, 1982, *2*, 437. See also R. A. Locock, *Can. pharm. J.*, 1986, *119*, 125.
Hepatitis due to the ingestion of a herbal remedy containing mistletoe.— J. Harvey and D. G. Colin-Jones, *Br. med. J.*, 1981, *282*, 186. Comments: F. Fletcher Hyde (letter), *ibid.*, 739; N. R. Farnsworth and W. D. Loub (letter), *ibid.*, *283*, 1058; D. G. Colin-Jones and J. Harvey (letter), *ibid.*, 1982, *284*, 744.

Proprietary Names and Manufacturers
Helixor *(Helixor, Ger.)*; Iscador *(Weleda, Ger.; Society for Cancer Research, Switz.: Weleda, UK)*; Mistel *(Curarina, Ger.)*; Plenosol *(Madaus, Ger.)*; Viscysat *(Ysatfabrik, Ger.).*

16899-f

Mitozolomide *(BAN, rINN).*

46241-RP; Azolastone; CCRG-81010; M&B-39565. 3-(2-Chloroethyl)-3,4-dihydro-4-oxoimidazo[5,1-*d*]-1,2,3,5-tetrazine-8-carboxamide.
$C_7H_7ClN_6O_2$=242.6.

CAS — 85622-95-3.

Mitozolomide is an antineoplastic agent under investigation.

Proprietary Names and Manufacturers
May & Baker, UK.

16900-f

Mizoribine *(rINN).*

5-Hydroxy-1-β-D-ribofuranosylimidazole-4-carboxamide.
$C_9H_{13}N_3O_6$=259.2.

CAS — 50924-49-7.

Mizoribine is an immunosuppressant agent which has been investigated in the management of kidney transplant patients. It has also been tried in the treatment of uveitis.

19528-t

MN-1695

2,4-Diamino-6-(2,5-dichlorophenyl)-*S*-triazine maleate.
$C_9H_7Cl_2N_5.C_4H_4O_4$=372.2.

CAS — 57381-26-7.

MN-1695 is under investigation as an anti-ulcer compound.

References: M. Nakashima *et al.*, *Arzneimittel-Forsch.*, 1984, *34*, 492; *Drugs of the Future*, 1984, *9*, 470; *ibid.*, 1985, *10*, 513.

Proprietary Names and Manufacturers
Gaslon *(Nippon Shinyaku, Jpn)*.

2963-l

Modafinil *(rINN)*.

2-[(Diphenylmethyl)sulfinyl]acetamide.
$C_{15}H_{15}NO_2S$=273.4.

CAS — 68693-11-8.

Modafinil is under investigation as a CNS stimulant.

Proprietary Names and Manufacturers
Lafon, Fr.

2964-y

Mometasone *(BAN, pINN)*.

Sch-32088. 9α,21-Dichloro-11β,17-dihydroxy-16α-methylpregna-1,4-diene-3,20-dione.
$C_{22}H_{28}Cl_2O_4$=427.4.

CAS — 105102-22-5.

NOTE. Mometasone Furoate is *USAN*.

Mometasone is a corticosteroid used topically in skin disorders as the furoate in a concentration of 0.1% as a cream or ointment.

References: *Med. Lett.*, 1987, *29*, 96.

Proprietary Names and Manufacturers of Mometasone and its Esters
Elocon *(Schering, USA)*.

12974-p

Monoacetin

Acetin; Monacetin. Glyceryl monoacetate.
$C_5H_{10}O_4$=134.1.

CAS — 26446-35-5.

Monoacetin has been suggested for use in the treatment of sodium fluoroacetate poisoning (see p.1354). It has also been used as a solvent.

The Food Additives and Contaminants Committee recommended that the mono-, di-, and tri-acetates of glycerol be temporarily permitted for use as solvents in food. Further studies on hydrolysis and toxicity were required.— *Report on the Review of Solvents in Food*, FAC/REP/25, Ministry of Agriculture, Fisheries and Food, London, HM Stationery Office, 1978.

1316-t

Monochloroacetic Acid

Chloroacetic Acid.
$CH_2Cl.CO_2H$=94.5.

CAS — 79-11-8.

Monochloroacetic acid has been used as an escharotic for plantar and mosaic warts.

12794-b

Mono-octanoin

A mixture of glycerol esters, principally Glyceryl Mono-octanoate, ($C_{11}H_{22}O_4$ = 218.3).

CAS — 26402-26-6 (glyceryl mono-octanoate).

Adverse Effects and Precautions

Abdominal pain, nausea, vomiting, and diarrhoea may occur particularly if mono-octanoin is infused rapidly: it has been recommended that perfusion pressure should not exceed 15cm of water. Irritation of the gastric and duodenal mucosa has been reported. Acidosis may occur, particularly in patients with impaired hepatic function. Mono-octanoin should not be administered to patients with impaired hepatic function.

Side-effects occurred in 67% of 343 patients treated with mono-octanoin perfusion, with multiple side-effects in 41%. Abdominal pain was the most common adverse effect occurring in 40% of patients. Nausea, vomiting, and diarrhoea were usually dose related, occurring in 25%, 15%, and 16% of patients respectively. Fever, attributed to cholangitis, was noted in 18 patients (5%). Severe side-effects occurred in 12 patients and included life-threatening haemorrhage from duodenal ulceration, acute pancreatitis, obstructive jaundice, acute pulmonary oedema, anaphylaxis, septicaemia, and leucopenia. A patient with cirrhosis developed acidosis and encephalopathic signs.— K. R. Palmer and A. F. Hofmann, *Gut*, 1986, *27*, 196.

Uses and Administration

Mono-octanoin is used to dissolve cholesterol gallstones retained following cholecystectomy. It is administered by continuous perfusion through a catheter inserted directly into the common bile duct at a rate of 3 to 5 mL per hour at a pressure of 10 cm of water. Perfusion may be suspended during meals. The solution should be warmed prior to perfusion, and the temperature should not fall below 18° during administration. Treatment is continued for 7 to 21 days. If no reduction in the size of the stones is detectable after 7 to 10 days of treatment, further treatment is unlikely to be effective.

Reviews of the use of mono-octanoin: M. A. Abate and T. L. Moore, *Drug Intell. & clin. Pharm.*, 1985, *19*, 708; *Med. Lett.*, 1987, *29*, 52.

An uncontrolled study of 343 patients with retained radiolucent gall stones in the bile duct. Mono-octanoin perfusion resulted in complete disappearance of stones in 25.6% of patients, and also in a further 8.5% of patients who received mono-octanoin as an adjunct to other forms of therapy. Partial success, defined by a reduction in size of the stones, was reported in another 20% of patients. Mono-octanoin had no effect on stone size and numbers in 36.2% of patients, and mono-octanoin was stopped in 9.3% of patients because of side-effects.— K. R. Palmer and A. F. Hofmann, *Gut*, 1986, *27*, 196.

Proprietary Names and Manufacturers
Capmul 8210; Moctanin *(Ethitek, USA: Lagap, UK)*.

19532-z

Mopidralazine *(rINN)*.

MDL-899. 4-{6-[(2,5-Dimethylpyrrol-1-yl)amino]-3-pyridazinyl}morpholine.
$C_{14}H_{19}N_5O$=273.3.

CAS — 75841-82-6.

An antihypertensive agent under investigation.

References: H. L. Elliott *et al.*, *J. cardiovasc. Pharmac.*, 1985, *7*, 948.

1317-x

Morrhuic Acid

Adverse Effects

Severe allergic reactions have occurred following administration of sodium morrhuate injection.

Uses and Administration

Morrhuic acid is used in the preparation of sodium morrhuate injection. Doses of 0.5 to 5 mL of a 5% solution of sodium morrhuate have been given as a sclerosing agent in the treatment of varicose veins but the sensitivity of the patient should be tested with a small preliminary dose. Details of sclerotherapy are provided on p.1569.

Acute respiratory failure after sodium morrhuate oesophageal sclerotherapy.— P. Monroe *et al.*, *Gastroenterology*, 1983, *85*, 693.

Little delivery of sodium morrhuate to the lung during endoscopic variceal sclerotherapy.— A. F. Connors *et al.*, *Ann. intern. Med.*, 1986, *105*, 539.

Preparations

Morrhuate Sodium Injection *(U.S.P.)*. A sterile solution of the sodium salts of the fatty acids of cod-liver oil containing 46.5 to 53.5 mg of sodium morrhuate in each mL. It may contain up to 0.5% of a suitable antimicrobial agent and not more than 3% of ethyl or benzyl alcohol. Solid matter may form on standing; the injection must not be used if such solid does not dissolve completely on warming.

Proprietary Names and Manufacturers
Scleromate *(Palisades, USA)*.

5237-g

Moxaverine Hydrochloride *(BANM, rINNM)*.

Meteverinum Hydrochloride. 1-Benzyl-3-ethyl-6,7-dimethoxyisoquinoline hydrochloride.
$C_{20}H_{21}NO_2$,HCl=343.9.

CAS — 10539-19-2 (moxaverine); 1163-37-7 (hydrochloride).

Moxaverine hydrochloride has a similar structure to papaverine (see p.1598) and has been given by mouth and injection as an antispasmodic in conditions such as ischaemia. The base is also used as an antispasmodic.

Proprietary Names and Manufacturers
Eupavérine *(E. Merck, Switz.)*; Eupaverin *(E. Merck, Ger.; E. Merck, Neth.; E. Merck, Swed.)*; Eupaverina *(Bracco, Ital.; Igoda, Spain)*; Kollateral *(Ursapharm, Ger.)*.

19534-k

Moxonidine *(rINN)*.

BDF-5895; BE-5895. 4-Chloro-5-(2-imidazolin-2-ylamino)-6-methoxy-2-methylpyrimidine.
$C_9H_{12}ClN_5O$=241.7.

CAS — 75438-57-2.

An antihypertensive agent under investigation.

References: V. Plänitz, *Eur. J. clin. Pharmac.*, 1984, *27*, 147; M. Frisk-Holmberg and V. Plänitz, *Curr. ther. Res.*, 1987, *42*, 138.

Proprietary Names and Manufacturers
Beiersdorf, Ger.

12350-f

Mushrooms

CAS — 23109-05-9 (α-amanitin); 21150-22-1 (β-amanitin); 21150-23-2 (γ-amanitin); 58919-61-2 (coprine); 16568-02-8 (gyromitrin); 2552-55-8 (ibotenic acid); 60-34-4 (methylhydrazine); 300-54-9 (muscarine); 2763-96-4 (muscimol); 37338-80-0 (orellanine); 17466-45-4 (phalloidin); 28227-92-1 (phalloin); 39412-56-1 (phallolysin).

Mushrooms can be classified into 8 groups according to their principal toxins and toxic effects:

Group I. Most deaths due to mushroom poisoning follow the ingestion of mushrooms containing cyclopeptides and among these mushrooms *Amanita phalloides* or 'death cap' has been reported to be responsible for 90% of all mushroom fatalities. The cyclopeptides are a group of heat-stable cyclic polypeptides with molecular weights ranging from 800 to 1100 and include the amatoxins (α-,β-, γ-amanitin) and phallotoxins (phalloidin, phaloin, phallolysin). Other mushrooms containing cyclopeptides include *A. verna* ('deadly agaric', fool's mushroom), *A. virosa*, and *A. bisporigera* (known as the 'destroying angel'), and *Galerina autumnalis, G. marginata*, and *G. venenata*.

Group II. Although *A. muscaria* ('fly agaric') and *A. pantherina* ('panther cap') may contain small amounts of muscarine, the antimuscarinic effects of the hallucinogenic agent muscimol and the insecticidal agent ibotenic acid usually predominate.

Group III. Many species of *Gyromitra* contain toxins known as gyromitrins that decompose to release methylhydrazine (monomethylhydrazine; MMH) an inhibitor of the coenzyme pyridoxal phosphate.

Group IV. Mushrooms whose principal toxin is muscarine include many of the *Clitocybe* and *Inocybe* spp. *A. muscaria* and *A. pantherina* (see above) may also contain small amounts.
Group V. Coprinus atramentarius ('ink cap') contains the compound coprine, one of whose metabolites is an inhibitor of acetaldehyde dehydrogenase and it may therefore produce 'disulfiram-like' symptoms after drinking alcohol.
Group VI. Mushrooms which may contain the hallucinogenic indoles psilocin and psilocybin include species of *Psilocybe*, *Panaeolus*, *Gymnopilus*, *Stropharia*, and *Conocybe*.
Group VII. Many mushrooms which only act as gastro-intestinal irritants and do not produce systemic effects are included in this group.
Group VIII. A further group has sometimes been used to classify some species of *Cortinarius* that contain a renal toxin whose exact nature remains to be determined. It is thought by some to be orellanine.

Adverse Effects
The clinical course of poisoning due to mushrooms containing cyclopeptides may be divided into three phases. Initial symptoms may occur 4 to 24 hours after ingestion and usually consist of gastro-intestinal effects such as abdominal pain, nausea, severe vomiting, and profuse diarrhoea similar to that in cholera. The patient may then appear to recover and be symptom-free for 2 to 3 days, but liver-enzyme values may be increasing. Following this phase, the more serious toxic effects of the amatoxins become apparent and there are signs of liver, renal, cardiac, and CNS toxicity. Symptoms include jaundice, oliguria, anuria, hypoglycaemia, coagulopathies, circulatory collapse, convulsions, and coma. The mortality-rate is high in this phase with death usually being due to liver failure following hepatic necrosis. Up to 90% of untreated patients may die, though the rate may be as low as 15 to 30% following treatment.
The adverse effects of mushrooms containing ibotenic acid and muscimol usually occur within 2 hours of ingestion. Symptoms may include, ataxia, euphoria, delirium, and hallucinations associated with other antimuscarinic effects. Fatalities are rare.
Patients who have ingested mushrooms containing gyromitrins usually develop symptoms of poisoning within 6 to 24 hours. These consist initially of nausea, vomiting, abdominal pain, and muscle cramps, headache, dizziness and fatigue. Delirium, convulsions, coma, methaemoglobinaemia and haemolysis may also occur. Occasionally jaundice and hepatic necrosis may lead to hepatic failure and death. Up to 40% of patients may die.
Symptoms typical of 'cholinergic crisis' (see neostigmine methylsulphate, p.1332) may appear about 30 minutes to 2 hours after ingestion of mushrooms containing muscarine. These may include bradycardia, bronchospasm, salivation, perspiration, lachrymation, rhinorrhoea, involuntary urination and defaecation, and diarrhoea. Miosis, hypotension, and cardiac arrhythmias may also occur. Rarely death may follow due to cardiac arrest or respiratory-tract obstruction.
Since one of the metabolites of coprine is an acetaldehyde dehydrogenase inhibitor, drinking alcohol, even up to several days after ingestion of mushrooms containing this compound, will produce symptoms similar to those of the 'disulfiram-alcohol' interaction (see disulfiram p.1565). Fatalities are rare.
The adverse effects of ingestion of mushrooms containing psilocin and psilocybin are similar to those described under lysergide (p.1584). Symptoms usually occur within about 30 minutes to 2 hours. Fatalities are rare.
There may be a delay of as long as 14 to 20 days before symptoms of poisoning due to *Cortinarius* appear. Patients will develop an intense thirst. Other symptoms usually include nausea, vomiting, diarrhoea, and anorexia. Muscle aching and spasms and a feeling of coldness may also occur. In severe cases renal failure may lead to death. It has been reported that up to 15% of patients may die.

PREGNANCY AND THE NEONATE. α-Amanitine does not appear to cross the placental barrier, even during the acute phase of intoxication.— F. Belliardo *et al.* (letter), *Lancet*, 1983, *1*, 1381.

Treatment of Adverse Effects
As there are no specific antidotes for the majority of cases of mushroom poisoning, treatment consists primarily of symptomatic and supportive measures. The stomach should be emptied by inducing emesis or by gastric aspiration and lavage if the patient has not already vomited spontaneously. However, if the onset of symptoms is delayed this is unlikely to be productive. Activated charcoal may be of use in binding toxins in the gastro-intestinal tract. Determining the interval between ingestion and the onset of symptoms may help to identify the type of mushrooms ingested. If possible specimens of the mushrooms or a sample of the stomach contents should be sent to an expert mycologist for identification. Particular attention should be paid to intravenous replacement of fluids and electrolytes especially if vomiting and diarrhoea are severe. If the ingestion of hepatotoxic or nephrotoxic mushrooms is suspected liver and renal function should be monitored. Although there is little evidence of efficacy, exchange transfusions, haemodialysis, or charcoal haemoperfusion may be of value to remove amatoxins. The removal of bile via a duodenal tube left *in situ* has been suggested to reduce enterohepatic circulation of amatoxins. Forced diuresis has also been advocated by some for amatoxin poisoning.
Since some mushrooms contain a wide range of toxins and patients may have ingested more than one species, specific therapy should only be instituted following positive identification.
Group I. There is little clinical evidence to support the efficacy of specific agents used in the treatment of cyclopeptide poisoning. A variety of agents including benzylpenicillin and sulphamethoxazole have been used in an attempt to increase the excretion of the amatoxins by displacing them from their plasma-binding sites. Thioctic acid, and silymarin or silybin (silibinin) have been administered to try to protect the liver against the hepatotoxic effects of the amatoxins but their use remains controversial. A radioimmunoassay for the detection of amatoxins is available in some countries to confirm a diagnosis of cyclopeptide poisoning.
Group II. Specific treatment is usually only required if symptoms are severe. Physostigmine should only be used if definite antimuscarinic symptoms are present. As mushrooms containing ibotenic acid and muscimol may also contain small amounts of muscarine, atropine may be required to control muscarinic symptoms.
Group III. Pyridoxine hydrochloride 25 mg per kg body-weight given as an intravenous infusion and repeated as required has been recommended as specific therapy to overcome the inhibition of pyridoxal phosphate by methylhydrazine. However, concern has been expressed that the use of such large doses of pyridoxine can itself produce adverse neurological effects. Methylene blue may be required if methaemoglobinaemia is severe.
Group IV. Atropine sulphate may be required to control the symptoms of muscarine poisoning but it should only be used if definite muscarinic symptoms are present.
Group V. There is no specific treatment for the 'disulfiram-alcohol' reaction except for the maintenance of blood pressure.
Group VI. If symptoms are severe some patients may require sedation with diazepam.

AMANITA PHALLOIDES. The use of specific antidotes in the treatment of poisoning due to *Amanita phalloides* remains controversial. Agents such as benzylpenicillin, sulphamethoxazole, thioctic acid, cytochrome C, ascorbic acid, insulin, growth hormone, silymarin or silybin, and corticosteroids have all been used or suggested. However, at present there is little clinical evidence to support their use. Olson *et al.* (*West J. Med.*, 1982, *137*, 282) reported that mortality due to ingestion of *A. phalloides* had been less than 15% in patients treated with supportive care alone and felt that the use of specific antidotes such as thioctic acid, benzylpenicillin, and corticosteroids was not supported by clinical evidence. They and others (G. L. Floersheim *J. Am. med. Ass.*, 1985, *253*, 3252) considered that mortality-rates of 50 to 90% quoted for amatoxin poisoning were erroneously high and that this would be likely to be misleading in the assessment of the efficacy of specific antidotes. Although agreeing that efficacy had not been proved in controlled studies Hanrahan and Gordon (*ibid.*, 1984, *251*, 1057; *ibid.*, 1985, *253*, 3131) considered that a favourable risk-benefit ratio supported the use of thioctic acid, benzylpenicillin, and corticosteroids until their efficacy was confirmed or disproved. Floersheim considered that it was unrealistic to call for controlled studies in the treatment of amatoxin poisoning and had conducted a retrospective study of 205 treated patients (*Schweiz. med. Wschr.*, 1982, *112*, 1164). Results indicated that the survival-rate was highest in patients who had received benzylpenicillin, hyperbaric oxygen, or benzylpenicillin with silybin. The use of thioctic acid, sulphamethoxazole, trometamol and sodium bicarbonate, plasma expanders, exchange transfusions, and haemodialysis had been more common in patients who did not survive and corticosteroids failed to show any beneficial effects. It was later suggested that thioctic acid and corticosteroids should no longer be used. Hruby *et al.* (*Hum. Toxicol.*, 1983, *2*, 183) also found in a retrospective study involving 18 patients that silybin given in conjunction with conventional therapy was effective in preventing severe liver damage if administered within 48 hours of mushroom ingestion.

12982-p

Musk

Almíscar; Deer Musk; Mosc.; Moschus. The dried secretions from the preputial follicles of the musk deer, *Moschus moschiferus* (Cervidae).

CAS — 8001-04-5 (musk); 541-91-3 (muskone).

Pharmacopoeias. In *Chin.*, *Jpn*, and *Port.*

Musk is used as a fragrance and fixative in perfumery.
A series of nitrated tertiary butyl toluenes or xylenes, or related compounds, are used as artificial musks. Musk ambrette, a synthetic nitromusk compound, has been reported to cause contact dermatitis and photosensitivity.

Reports of adverse effects following the use of toiletries containing musk ambrette: C. A. Ramsay, *Br. J. Derm.*, 1984, *111*, 423 (contact photosensitivity); F. Wojnarowska and C. D. Calnan, *ibid.*, 1986, *114*, 667 (contact and photocontact allergy).

12984-w

Mycophenolic Acid *(USAN, rINN).*

Lilly-68618; NSC-129185. An antimicrobial substance produced by the growth of *Penicillium stoloniferum*. (*E*)-6-(1,3-Dihydro-4-hydroxy-6-methoxy-7-methyl-3-oxoisobenzofuran-5-yl)-4-methylhex-4-enoic acid.
$C_{17}H_{20}O_6$=320.3.

CAS — 24280-93-1.

Mycophenolic acid is an antimetabolite which interferes with the synthesis of nucleic acids. It has been used in the treatment of psoriasis. Antitumour activity in *animals* has not generally been substantiated in clinical studies.

References to the use of mycophenolic acid in psoriasis: *J. Am. med. Ass.*, 1974, *227*, 606; E. J. Van Scott, *ibid.*, 1976, *235*, 197; R. Marinari *et al.*, *Archs Derm.*, 1977, *113*, 930.

Proprietary Names and Manufacturers
Leo, Denm.; ICI Pharmaceuticals, UK; Lilly, USA.

15302-z

Mylabris

Chinese Blistering Beetle; Chinese Cantharides; Indian Blistering Beetle; Mylab. The dried beetles *Mylabris sidae (=M. phalerata), M. cichorii*, and *M. pustulata* (Meloidae), containing not less than 1% of cantharidin.

Pharmacopoeias. In *Chin.*

Mylabris has been used as a source of cantharidin and as a substitute for cantharides in the East.

281-c

Myrrh

Gum Myrrh; Myrrha.

CAS — 9000-45-7.

Pharmacopoeias. In *Aust., Belg., Cz., Ger., Port., Span.*, and *Swiss.* Also in *B.P.C. 1973.*

An oleo-gum-resin obtained from the stem of *Commiphora molmol* and possibly other species of *Commiphora* (Burseraceae).

Myrrh is astringent to mucous membranes; the tincture is used in mouth-washes and gargles for ulcers in the mouth and pharynx. It has been used internally as a carminative.

Preparations

Myrrh Tincture *(B.P.C. 1973).* Prepared by macerating myrrh 1 in 5 of alcohol (90%). *Dose.* 2.5 to 5 mL.

12987-y

Myrtillus

Baccae Myrtilli; Bilberry; Blaeberry; Heidelbeere; Huckleberry; Hurtleberry; Myrtilli Fructus; Whortleberry. The dried fruits of *Vaccinium myrtillus* (Ericaceae).

Pharmacopoeias. In *Aust., Pol.*, and *Swiss.*

Myrtillus has diuretic and astringent properties. It has been used for ophthalmic and circulatory disorders.

Proprietary Names and Manufacturers

Alcodin *(Farmila, Ital.)*; Antocin *(Allergan, Ital.)*; Difrarel *(Merck Sharp & Dohme, Spain)*; Largitor *(Rhone, Spain)*; Purpuralin *(Alcon, Arg.)*; Retinol *(INTES, Ital.)*; Tegens *(Inverni della Beffa, Ital.).*

12991-s

Nadide *(BAN, USAN, rINN).*

Codehydrogenase I; Coenzyme I; Co-I; Diphosphopyridine Nucleotide; DPN; NAD; Nicotinamide Adenine Dinucleotide; NSC-20272. Nadide is a naturally occurring coenzyme substance. 1-(3-Carbamoylpyridinio)-β-D-ribofuranoside 5-(adenosine-5′-pyrophosphate).

$C_{21}H_{27}N_7O_{14}P_2$=663.4.

CAS — 53-84-9.

Nadide is a naturally occurring coenzyme which has been claimed to be of value in the treatment of alcohol and opioid addiction.

Proprietary Names and Manufacturers

D.P.N. *(Covan, S.Afr.)*; Nad-Medical *(Medical, Spain)*; Nicodrasi *(Bruco, Ital.).*

1775-d

Nafamostat *(pINN).*

6-Amidino-2-naphthyl *p*-guanidinobenzoate.

$C_{19}H_{17}N_5O_2$=347.4.

CAS — 81525-10-2.

Nafamostat is a proteolytic enzyme inhibitor. It has been used as the mesylate in the treatment of acute pancreatitis.

Proprietary Names and Manufacturers

Futhan *(Torii, Jpn).*

12993-e

Nafazatrom *(BAN, pINN).*

Bay-g-6575. 3-Methyl-1-[2-(2-naphthyloxy)ethyl]-5-pyrazolone.

$C_{16}H_{16}N_2O_2$=268.3.

CAS — 59040-30-1.

Nafazatrom has been claimed to enhance the synthesis of prostacyclin (see p.1371) and thus inhibit platelet aggregation and have an antithrombotic effect.

References on the actions and uses of nafazatrom: J. Vermylen *et al., Lancet,* 1979, *1,* 518 (pharmacological action); M. G. Elder and L. Myatt (letter), *ibid.,* 1984, *1,* 1350 (successful pregnancy after administration to a woman with a history of recurrent abortions); S. T. S. Durrant *et al.* (letter), *ibid.,* 1985, *2,* 842 (in combination with epoprostenol in the treatment of thrombocytopenic purpura); J. A. Copplestone *et al.* (letter), *ibid.,* 1986, *1,* 498 (in combination with dipyridamole in the treatment of thrombocytopenic purpura).

Proprietary Names and Manufacturers

Bayer, UK.

19553-x

Nafimidone *(rINN).*

2-Imidazol-1-yl-2′-acetonaphthone.

$C_{15}H_{12}N_2O$=236.3.

CAS — 64212-22-2.

NOTE. Nafimidone Hydrochloride is *USAN.*

An anti-epileptic drug under investigation.

References: D. M. Treiman *et al., Epilepsia,* 1985, *26,* 607; D. M. Treiman and S. Gunawan, *Clin. Pharmacokinet.,* 1987, *12,* 433.

Proprietary Names and Manufacturers

Syntex, USA.

12994-l

Nafiverine Hydrochloride *(rINNM).*

DA-914 (base). *NN′*-Bis{2-[2-(1-naphthyl)propionyloxy]ethyl}piperazine dihydrochloride.

$C_{34}H_{38}N_2O_4$,2HCl=611.6.

CAS — 5061-22-3 (nafiverine).

Nafiverine hydrochloride has been used as an antispasmodic. The dimesylate has also been used.

Proprietary Names and Manufacturers

Naftidan *(De Angeli, Ital.).*

15301-j

Neoarsphenamine *(rINN).*

'914'; NAB; Neoarsaminol; Neoarsenobenzol; Neoarsphenaminum; Neoarsphenolamine; Neosalvarsan; Novarsenobenzene; Novarsenol.

CAS — 457-60-3.

Pharmacopoeias. In *Belg., Fr., Int., Mex., Pol., Port., Rus.,* and *Span. Jpn* includes Neoarsphenamine Sodium for Injection.

Neoarsphenamine has been used topically in the treatment of oral infections, including Vincent's angina.

Arsenicals such as neoarsphenamine, arsphenamine, and sulpharsphenamine were formerly used in the treatment of syphilis.

Proprietary Names and Manufacturers

Collunovar *(Dexo, Fr.).*

13002-w

Neodymium Sulfisonicotinate

Neodymium 3-sulphoisonicotinate octahydrate.

$C_{18}H_9N_3Nd_2O_{15}S_3$,$8H_2O$=1036.1.

CAS — 13957-51-2 (anhydrous).

Neodymium sulfisonicotinate has been used for the prophylaxis and treatment of thrombo-embolic disorders.

Proprietary Names and Manufacturers

Isothrodym *(Mulli, Ger.).*

19564-d

Nesosteine *(rINN).*

o-(3-Thiazolidinylcarbonyl)benzoic acid.

$C_{11}H_{11}NO_3S$=237.3.

CAS — 84233-61-4.

A mucolytic which has been tried in patients with bronchitis.

References: J. Siquet, *Acta ther.,* 1985, *11,* 61; P. Mbuyamba, *Int. J. clin. Pharmacol. Res.,* 1986, *6,* 119; P. C. Braga *et al., J. int. med. Res.,* 1987, *15,* 57.

Proprietary Names and Manufacturers

Corvi, Ital.

13005-y

Neutral Red

CI Basic Red 5; Colour Index No. 50040; Neutral Red Chloride; Nuclear Fast Red; Toluylene Red. 3-Amino-7-dimethylamino-2-methylphenazine hydrochloride.

$C_{15}H_{16}N_4$,HCl=288.8.

CAS — 553-24-2.

Neutral red is a photoactive dye that has been tried in the treatment of recurrent herpes simplex infections. Some viruses can incorporate such dyes which attach to viral guanosine and subsequent exposure to light in the presence of oxygen causes breakage of DNA and RNA strands. Photodynamic inactivation by application of a 0.1% solution of neutral red followed by exposure to light has met with limited success; there is some evidence for the potential carcinogenicity of inactivated herpes simplex viruses. Allergic contact dermatitis has also been reported.

Neutral red is also used as a stain in microscopy.

References: T. D. Felber *et al., J. Am. med. Ass.,* 1973, *223,* 289; *Med. Lett.,* 1974, *16,* 112; T. D. Felber, *J. Am. med. Ass.,* 1975, *231,* 79; M. G. Myers *et al., New Engl. J. Med.,* 1975, *293,* 945; A. P. C. H. Roome *et al., Br. J. vener. Dis.,* 1975, *51,* 130; E. G. Friedrich *et al., Obstet. Gynec.,* 1976, *48,* 564; R. S. Berger and C. M. Papa, *J. Am. med. Ass.,* 1977, *238,* 133; A. W. Kopf *et al.* (letter), *ibid.,* 1978, *239,* 615; B. E. Juel-Jensen, *Practitioner,* 1979, *222,* 745.

Reference to the use of neutral red to estimate gastric mucosal blood flow.— S. E. Knight and R. L. McIsaac, *J. Physiol.,* 1977, *272,* 62P.

Neutral red uptake by macrophages in amniotic fluid could be used in the prenatal diagnosis of neural-tube defects.— K. Polgár *et al.* (letter), *New Engl. J. Med.,* 1984, *310,* 1463.

3938-t

Nicofetamide

C-1065. *N*-(1,2-Diphenylethyl)-3-pyridinecarboxamide.

$C_{20}H_{18}N_2O$=302.4.

CAS — 553-06-0.

Nicofetamide is an antispasmodic used in a variety of gastro-intestinal disorders.

Proprietary Names and Manufacturers

Lyspamin *(Bracco, Ital.).*

15303-c

Nicotine

(*S*)-3-(1-Methylpyrrolidin-2-yl)pyridine.
$C_{10}H_{14}N_2$=162.2.

CAS — 54-11-5.

NOTE. Nicotine Polacrilex (a complex of nicotine with a methacrylic acid polymer) is *USAN*.

A liquid alkaloid obtained from the dried leaves of the tobacco plant, *Nicotiana tabacum* and related species (Solanaceae). Tobacco leaves contain 0.5 to 8% of nicotine combined as malate or citrate.

Adverse Effects and Treatment

Nicotine is a highly toxic substance and in acute poisoning death may occur within a few minutes due to respiratory failure arising from paralysis of the muscles of respiration. The fatal dose of nicotine for an adult is from 30 to 60 mg.

Less severe poisoning causes burning of the mouth and throat, nausea and salivation, abdominal pain, vomiting, diarrhoea, dizziness, mental confusion, headache, disturbed hearing and vision, dyspnoea, faintness, convulsions, sweating, and prostration. Transient cardiac standstill or paroxysmal atrial fibrillation may occur.

Nicotine is rapidly absorbed through the skin or by inhalation and most cases of nicotine poisoning are due to careless handling when it is employed as a horticultural insecticide.

Prompt treatment of nicotine poisoning is essential. If contact was with the skin, remove contaminated clothing and wash the skin thoroughly with cold water without rubbing. If the patient has swallowed nicotine, induce emesis if there are no convulsions and the respiration is normal. Wash out the stomach. A suspension of activated charcoal may be left in the stomach. Diazepam, or if necessary a short-acting barbiturate should be given intravenously to control convulsions. Assisted respiration may be required.

A case report of a patient who developed nicotine poisoning after cutaneous application of nicotine sulphate. Measurement of nicotine and metabolite concentrations in the blood demonstrated prolonged absorption of nicotine despite vigorous skin decontamination, suggesting that the skin may be a reservoir for slow release of nicotine into the circulation. Despite extraordinarily high levels of nicotine, the patient had full resolution of signs and symptoms of intoxication, indicating rapid and profound development of tolerance.— N. L. Benowitz *et al., Clin. Pharmac. Ther.*, 1987, *42*, 119.

ADVERSE EFFECTS OF TOBACCO PRODUCTS. The effects of nicotine in relation to the smoking of tobacco and the tar and nicotine content of cigarettes: *Br. med. J.*, 1968, *1*, 73; R. Kumar *et al., Clin. Pharmac. Ther.*, 1977, *21*, 520; *Drug & Ther. Bull.*, 1978, *16*, 17; M. Lader, *Br. J. clin. Pharmac.*, 1978, *5*, 289; J. C. Robinson *et al., Can. med. Ass. J.*, 1980, *123*, 889; L. T. Kozlowski, *J. Am. med. Ass.*, 1981, *245*, 158; M. Kanzler *et al., Clin. Pharmac. Ther.*, 1983, *34*, 408.

A study of nicotine consumption by smokers of low-tar cigarettes.— N. L. Benowitz *et al., New Engl. J. Med.*, 1983, *309*, 139. Comment.— C. Lenfant, *ibid.*, 181. See also R. V. Ebert *et al., J. Am. med. Ass.*, 1983, *250*, 2840.

Action. Pharmacological effects of nicotine and smoking: P. E. Cryer *et al., New Engl. J. Med.*, 1976, *295*, 573; R. J. Lefkowitz, *ibid.*, 615 (noradrenaline release); D. K. Chattopadhyay *et al., Gut*, 1977, *18*, 833 (reduced lower oesophageal sphincter pressure); W. W. Winternitz and D. Quillen, *J. clin. Pharmac.*, 1977, *17*, 389 (plasma cortisol and growth hormone concentrations); J. L. Nadler *et al., Lancet*, 1983, *1*, 1248; A. Hofstetter *et al., New Engl. J. Med.*, 1986, *314*, 79.

Carcinogenicity. A review of the health effects and control of smoking including discussions on lung cancer, cancer of the larynx, oral cancer, carcinoma of the oesophagus, cancer of the bladder and pancreas.— J. E. Fielding, *New Engl. J. Med.*, 1985, *313*, 491.

Smoking as a risk factor in cervical neoplasia.— D. Hellberg *et al.* (letter), *Lancet*, 1983, *2*, 1497. See also E. Trevathan *et al., J. Am. med. Ass.*, 1983, *250*, 499; I. M. Sasson *et al.* (letter), *New Engl. J. Med.*, 1985, *312*, 315.

For reference to the carcinogenic potential of oral tobacco products see under Smokeless Tobacco, below.

Effects on the cardiovascular system. Results of the Walnut Creek Contraceptive Drug Study involving 17 939 women enrolled between 1969 and 1971 and during which 16 759 women were followed for an average of 6.5 years, indicated that the risk of subarachnoid haemorrhage in smokers was 5.7 times that of non-smokers, and of current oral contraceptive users 6.5 times that of non-users. The relative risk estimate for the association of smoking and current oral contraceptive use was 21.9.— D. B. Petitti and J. Wingerd, *Lancet*, 1978, *2*, 234.

Some studies linking smoking and cardiovascular disorders: P. J. A. Griffin *et al., Br. med. J.*, 1983, *286*, 685 (arteriovenous fistula); D. W. Kaufman *et al., New Engl. J. Med.*, 1983, *308*, 409 (myocardial infarction); J. P. Nicholson *et al., Lancet*, 1983, *2*, 765 (renal arterial stenosis); A. J. Hartz *et al., New Engl. J. Med.*, 1984, *311*, 1201 (cardiomyopathy); C. L. Jajich *et al., J. Am. med. Ass.*, 1984, *252*, 2831 (fatal coronary heart disease); R. L. Rogers *et al., ibid.*, 1985, *253*, 2970 (reduced cerebral perfusion); L. Rosenberg *et al., ibid.*, 2965 (myocardial infarction in women); L. Rosenberg *et al., New Engl. J. Med.*, 1985, *313*, 1511 (decreasing risk of myocardial infarction on stopping smoking); A. P. Hallstrom *et al., ibid.*, 1986, *314*, 271 (recurrent cardiac arrest); R. D. Abbott *et al., ibid.*, *315*, 717 (stroke); G. M. FitzGibbon *et al., Can. med. Ass. J.*, 1987, *136*, 45 (atherosclerosis of coronary bypass grafts).

For a study of trends in major risk factors for coronary heart disease in the *UK*, including cigarette smoking, see D. Simpson, *Postgrad. med. J.*, 1984, *60*, 20.

Effects on the gastro-intestinal tract. A study of 100 patients demonstrating an almost invariable concurrence of tobacco consumption and acute ulcerative gingivitis.— M. J. Kowolik and T. Nisbet, *Br. dent. J.*, 1983, *154*, 241.

Of 1217 outpatients who underwent upper gastro-intestinal endoscopy over an 18-month period, 624 were current smokers, 248 ex-smokers, and 345 non-smokers. Gastric ulcers occurred in 11.9% of smokers and 7.7% of ex-smokers, compared with 4.6% of non-smokers. Duodenal ulcers occurred in 12.8% of smokers, 6.8% of ex-smokers, and 6.1% of non-smokers. There was a dose-response effect between the number of cigarettes smoked and duodenal and gastric ulceration. Gastric cancer was also more frequent in smokers than non-smokers, but macroscopic oesophagitis less frequent. The results confirm the association between smoking and peptic ulcer.— C. C. Ainley *et al., Gut*, 1986, *27*, 648.

Effects on sexual function. References to sperm abnormalities and cigarette smoking: H. J. Evans *et al., Lancet*, 1981, *1*, 627; E. M. Berry (letter), *ibid.*, 1159.

Reduced female fertility associated with cigarette smoking.— D. D. Baird and A. J. Wilcox, *J. Am. med. Ass.*, 1985, *253*, 2979.

Passive smoking. Some references to the hazards from passive smoking: I. B. Tager *et al., New Engl. J. Med.*, 1983, *309*, 699; *Med. J. Aust.*, 1986, *145*, 404; D. T. Wigle *et al., Can. med. Ass. J.*, 1987, *136*, 945.

Pregnancy and the neonate. A discussion of foetal growth retardation associated with maternal smoking ('foetal tobacco syndrome'), and the association with an increased risk of abruptio placentae, bleeding during pregnancy, premature delivery, foetal deaths, neonatal mortality, and sudden infant death syndrome. Children of cigarette smokers may show deficits in growth, intellectual and emotional development, and behaviour.— P. Nieburg *et al., J. Am. med. Ass.*, 1985, *253*, 2998.

Further references to the effects of smoking on the foetus and neonate: M. Sexton and J. R. Hebel, *J. Am. med. Ass.*, 1984, *251*, 911; D. H. Rubin, *Lancet*, 1986, *2*, 415; P. H. Shiono, *J. Am. med. Ass.*, 1986, *255*, 82; M. Stjernfeldt *et al., Lancet*, 1986, *1*, 1350; M. Stjernfeldt *et al.* (letter), *ibid.*, *2*, 687; B. Taylor and J. Wadsworth, *Archs Dis. Childh.*, 1987, *62*, 786.

Smokeless tobacco. A discussion of a symposium on the health implications of smokeless tobacco.

Smokeless tobacco includes chewing tobacco and snuff. In chewing tobacco a portion is either chewed or held in place in the cheek or lower lip. In some countries including the *UK*, dry snuff is sniffed through the nose, but in the *US*, both dry and moist snuff are taken in the mouth or 'dipped'. A small amount, a 'pinch', is held in place between the lip or cheek and the gum. With the apparent resurgence in the use of smokeless tobacco, evidence is inconclusive concerning the increased risk of oral cancer, although, in studies in North Carolina, white women who used snuff had an increased risk of oral and pharyngeal cancer.

The epidemiologic evidence linking cancer of the mouth to the use of snuff is strong. In India, where use of chewing tobacco with betel nut is widespread, oral cancer is the primary cancer killer.

With regard to peridontal disease, the evidence presented did not show an association with gingivitis or dental caries. Several reports, however, have associated the use of snuff with the presence of leukoplakia.

The use of smokeless tobacco appears to produce the same functional relationships between drug administration and measures of dependence potential as seen with other drugs of dependence.— D. B. Nash, *Ann. intern. Med.*, 1986, *104*, 436. See also.— S. Davis and R. K. Severson (letter), *Lancet*, 1987, *2*, 910.

Further discussions on the health effects of smokeless tobacco: *J. Am. med. Ass.*, 1986, *255*, 1038; *ibid.*, 1045; G. N. Connolly *et al., New Engl. J. Med.*, 1986, *314*, 1020; C. E. Koop, *ibid.*, 1042; *Lancet*, 1986, *2*, 198; D. F. N. Harrison, *Br. med. J.*, 1986, *293*, 405.

A report of hypercholesterolaemia after administration of nicotine chewing gum.— J. C. Dousset *et al.* (letter), *Lancet*, 1986, *2*, 1393.

INTERACTIONS. The effect of tobacco smoking on drug metabolism.— A. P. Alvares, *Clin. Pharmacokinet.*, 1978, *3*, 462. See also.— K. Vähäkangas *et al., Clin. Pharmac. Ther.*, 1983, *33*, 375.

PHARMACOKINETICS. A review of the clinical pharmacokinetics of nicotine.— C. K. Svensson, *Clin. Pharmacokinet.*, 1987, *12*, 30.

A study of the absorption and metabolism of nicotine from cigarettes by 8 healthy men, 3 of whom were non-smokers. All the smokers who inhaled had an increase in their heart-rate proportional to the blood-concentrations of nicotine; blood pressure also rose but the correlation was not so clear. The results of the study supported the view that many smokers smoke to dose themselves with nicotine.— A. K. Armitage *et al., Br. med. J.*, 1975, *4*, 313. Estimation of urinary excretion of cotinine (a major metabolite of nicotine) may provide a useful index of smoking habits.— S. Matsukura *et al., Clin. Pharmac. Ther.*, 1979, *25*, 555. See also.— N. J. Wald *et al.* (letter), *Lancet*, 1984, *1*, 230; A. Woodward *et al.* (letter), *ibid.*, *2*, 935.

Pharmacokinetic studies of plasma nicotine levels produced by nicotine chewing gum: E. McKendree *et al., J. Am. med. Ass.*, 1982, *248*, 865; R. V. Ebert *et al., Clin. Pharmac. Ther.*, 1984, *35*, 495.

A study of the disposition and effects of the major metabolite of nicotine, cotinine, following intravenous administration as the fumarate.— N. L. Benowitz *et al., Clin. Pharmac. Ther.*, 1983, *34*, 604.

Buccal absorption of nicotine from smokeless tobacco sachets.— M. A. H. Russell *et al., Lancet*, 1985, *2*, 1370.

Lactation. Concentrations of nicotine and cotinine in the serum and milk of nursing smokers indicated that mothers should attempt to prolong the time between the last cigarette smoked and breast feeding in order to minimise exposure of the infant.— W. Luck and H. Nau, *Br. J. clin. Pharmac.*, 1984, *18*, 9.

Uses and Administration

Nicotine has no therapeutic uses but is of considerable pharmacological interest. The main physiological action is paralysis of all autonomic ganglia, preceded by stimulation. Centrally, small doses cause respiratory stimulation, while larger doses produce convulsions of the medullary type and cause arrest of respiration. The effects on skeletal muscle are similar to those on ganglia.

Nicotine has been used as a horticultural insecticide either as a vapour or as a spray.

Precautions should be taken when using these sprays to avoid inhalation or contact with the skin.

A chewing gum containing nicotine has been used as an aid to giving up smoking.

Mention of immediate symptomatic cure of refractory granular proctitis of 3 years' standing following treatment with a nicotine chewing gum (Nicorette) 2 mg three times daily.— W. J. Trowell, *Br. med. J.*, 1982, *285*, 1359.

A small study of nicotine chewing gum 4 mg in 10 patients with dysmenorrhoea showed that all experienced some relief of symptoms.— J. M. McGarry (letter), *Lancet*, 1983, *2*, 1498.

Nicotine chewing gum produced symptomatic relief in a patient with severe hemidystonia; the patient had previously obtained relief by smoking cigarettes.— A. J. Lees (letter), *Lancet*, 1984, *2*, 871.

SMOKING. A meta-analysis of 14 randomised controlled

studies that evaluated the efficacy of nicotine chewing gum in stopping patients smoking. The combined success rates in specialised cessation clinics were significantly higher with nicotine gum (27%) than with placebo gum (18%) at 6 months, falling to 23% and 13% respectively at 12 months. In contrast, success rates in general medical practices are similar with nicotine gum (11.4%) and with placebo gum (11.7%) at 6 months although success-rates were higher with nicotine gum when compared with patients given no placebo. The data suggest that proper use of nicotine gum in specialised clinics will increase the rate of stopping patients smoking. The use of the gum in general medical practices is questionable.— W. Lam *et al.*, *Lancet*, 1987, *2*, 27. Comment on the validity of the conclusions.— G. A. Colditz *et al.* (letter), *ibid.*, 458.

Other routes. Nicotine 2 mg administered intranasally to 3 healthy subjects as a 2% aqueous thickened solution was better absorbed than the same dose given as chewing gum. This method may be useful for denture-wearers or dyspeptic patients wishing to give up smoking.— M. A. H. Russell *et al.*, *Br. med. J.*, 1983, *286*, 683.

A double-blind study in 10 cigarette smokers suggesting that transdermal nicotine may enhance success in smoking cessation by preventing the rise in cigarette craving usually observed after cessation. Transdermal nicotine may be preferable to other routes of nicotine administration because of the relative absence of adverse side-effects.— J. E. Rose *et al.*, *Clin. Pharmac. Ther.*, 1985, *38*, 450.

Proprietary Preparations

Nicorette *(Lundbeck, UK). Chewing gum,* nicotine 2 and 4 mg (as resin complex).

Proprietary Names and Manufacturers

Nicoret *(Ciba, Fr.)*; Nicorette *(Glaxo, Austral.*; *Merrell Dow, Canad.*; *Lundbeck, Denm.*; *Boehringer Mannheim, Ger.*; *Serono, Ital.*; *MPS Lab., S.Afr.*; *Leo, Swed.*; *Leo Suede, Switz.*; *Lundbeck, UK*; *Lakeside, USA)*.

19568-b

Nifalatide

BW-942C. L-Tyrosyl-D-methionylglycyl-4-nitrophenylalanyl-L-prolinamide *S*-oxide.
$C_{30}H_{39}N_7O_9S$=673.7.

CAS — 73385-60-1; 98311-64-9 (hydrochloride).

Nifalatide is a pentapeptide enkephalin analogue under investigation for its antidiarrhoeal activity.

References: C. D. Ericsson *et al.*, *Antimicrob. Ag. Chemother.*, 1986, *29*, 1040; J. Ryan *et al.*, *Clin. Pharmac. Ther.*, 1986, *39*, 40; *Drugs of the Future*, 1986, *11*, 657; B. A. Boucher *et al.*, *J. clin. Pharmac.*, 1987, *27*, 151.

Proprietary Names and Manufacturers

Wellcome, UK.

13014-j

Nifuroxazide *(rINN).*

2′-(5-Nitrofurfurylidene)-4-hydroxybenzohydrazide.
$C_{12}H_9N_3O_5$=275.2.

CAS — 965-52-6.

Pharmacopoeias. In *Fr.*

Nifuroxazide is an antibacterial agent that has been used in the treatment of colitis and diarrhoea. It is poorly absorbed from the gastro-intestinal tract.

Proprietary Names and Manufacturers

Ambatrol *(Smith Kline & French, Fr.)*; Antinal *(Roques, Fr.*; *Interdelta, Switz.)*; Bacifurane *(Méram, Fr.)*; Ercefuryl *(Belg.*; *Robert et Carrière, Fr.*; *Promesa, Spain)*; Panfurex *(Crinex, Fr.)*; Pentofuryl *(Karlspharma, Ger.)*.

2968-k

Nilutamide *(rINN).*

5,5-Dimethyl-3-(α,α,α-trifluoro-4-nitro-*m*-tolyl)-hydantoin.
$C_{12}H_{10}F_3N_3O_4$=317.2.

CAS — 63612-50-0.

Nilutamide has anti-androgenic properties and is used similarly to flutamide in the treatment of prostatic carcinoma.

Use of nilutamide in advanced prostatic carcinoma.— F. Labrie *et al.* (letter), *Lancet*, 1984, *2*, 1090.

Reversible visual disturbances associated with the use of nilutamide.— C. Harnois *et al.*, *Br. J. Ophthal.*, 1986, *70*, 471. Comment.— J. M. Brisset *et al.* (letter), *ibid.*, 1987, *71*, 639.

Proprietary Names and Manufacturers

Anandron *(Cassenne, Fr.)*.

2192-p

Nilvadipine *(USAN, rINN).*

FK-235; FR-34235; SKF-102362; SK&F-102,362. 5-Isopropyl 3-methyl 2-cyano-1,4-dihydro-6-methyl-4-(*m*-nitrophenyl)-3,5-pyridinedicarboxylate.
$C_{19}H_{19}N_3O_6$=385.4.

CAS — 75530-68-6.

A calcium-channel blocking agent which has been tried in the treatment of hypertension.

2874-e

Niperotidine *(rINN).*

N-[2-[[5-[(Dimethylamino)methyl]furfuryl]thio]-ethyl]-2-nitro-*N′*-piperonyl-1,1-ethenediamine.
$C_{20}H_{26}N_4O_5S$=434.5.

CAS — 84845-75-0.

It is given by mouth in the treatment of peptic ulcer and other gastro-intestinal disorders associated with hyperacidity.

Proprietary Names and Manufacturers

Gafir *(Ausonia, Ital.)*.

19579-q

Nipradilol *(rINN).*

K-351; Nipradolol. 8-[2-Hydroxy-3-(isopropylamino)propoxy]-3-chromanol, 3-nitrate.
$C_{15}H_{22}N_2O_6$=326.3.

CAS — 81486-22-8.

An antihypertensive with beta-adrenoceptor blocking activity.

References: N. Nikamura *et al.*, *Curr. ther. Res.*, 1985, *37*, 853.

13023-z

Nitrefazole *(BAN, rINN).*

EMD-15700. 2-Methyl-4-nitro-1-(4-nitrophenyl)imidazole.
$C_{10}H_8N_4O_4$=248.2.

CAS — 21721-92-6.

Nitrefazole has been used in the treatment of alcoholism but has been withdrawn in certain countries because of its potential for inducing serious adverse effects.

Proprietary Names and Manufacturers

E. Merck, UK.

1318-r

Nitric Acid *(BAN, USAN).*

Aqua Fortis; Azotic Acid; Nit. Acid; Salpetersäure.
HNO_3=63.01.

CAS — 7697-37-2.

Pharmacopoeias. In *Br.* and *Mex.* (both approximately 70%). In *Belg.* (64 to 66%), *Egypt.* (65 to 71%), *Port.* (not less than 63%), and *Span.* (63.64%). *Aust.* has Acidum Nitricum Concentratum (64.3 to 66.4%) and Acidum Nitricum (31.1 to 32.2%). Also in *U.S.N.F.* (69 to 71%).

A clear, colourless or almost colourless, fuming liquid, with a characteristic irritating odour. **Store** in airtight containers.

Adverse Effects and Treatment

As for Hydrochloric Acid, p.1578.

There may be methaemoglobinaemia. Nitric acid stains the skin yellow.

In Great Britain the recommended exposure limits of nitric acid are 2 ppm (long-term); 4 ppm (short-term). In the *US* the permissible and recommended exposure limits are 5 mg per m^3.

A case of pneumonitis due to inhalation of nitrogen dioxide released during the cleaning of coins with nitric acid.— K. Sriskandan and K. W. Pettingale, *Postgrad. med. J.*, 1985, *61*, 819.

Uses and Administration

Nitric Acid has a powerful corrosive action and has been used to remove warts, but it should be applied with caution.

The use of nitric acid (6 to 7N) with organic acids for the removal of skin tumours such that the mummified tissue is capable of being examined histologically.— M. Weiner *et al.*, *Clin. Pharmac. Ther.*, 1983, *33*, 77.

13025-k

Nitrobenzene

Nitrobenzol; Oil of Mirbane.
$C_6H_5NO_2$=123.1.

CAS — 98-95-3.

A pale yellow liquid with an almond-like odour.

Adverse Effects

Nitrobenzene is highly toxic and the ingestion of 1 g may be fatal. Toxic effects from ingestion are usually delayed for several hours and may include nausea, prostration, burning headache, methaemoglobinaemia with cyanosis, haemolytic anaemia, vomiting (with characteristic odour), convulsions, and coma, ending in death after a few hours. Poisoning may also occur from absorption through the skin, or by inhalation.

In Great Britain recommended exposure limits of nitrobenzene are 1 ppm (long-term); 2 ppm (short-term); suitable precautions should be taken to prevent absorption through the skin.

Treatment of Adverse Effects

After ingestion of nitrobenzene the stomach should be emptied by emesis or lavage. Methaemoglobinaemia may be treated with methylene blue. Blood transfusions or haemodialysis may be necessary. Oxygen should be given if cyanosis is severe.

If the skin or eyes are splashed with nitrobenzene contaminated clothing should be removed immediately and the affected areas washed with running water for at least 15 minutes.

Uses.

Nitrobenzene is used in the manufacture of aniline, as a preservative in polishes, and in perfumery and soaps.

13028-x

Nitrovin Hydrochloride *(BANM).*

CL-48401. Bis[2-(5-nitro-2-furyl)vinyl]methylenehydrazinoformamidine hydrochloride; 1,5-Bis(5-nitro-2-furyl)penta-1,4-dien-3-one amidinohydrazone hydrochloride.
$C_{14}H_{12}N_6O_6$,HCl=396.7.

CAS — 804-36-4 (nitrovin); 2315-20-0 (hydrochloride).

Nitrovin hydrochloride is used as a food additive in veterinary practice to promote growth.

Proprietary Veterinary Names and Manufacturers

Payzone *(Cyanamid, UK)*; Pentazone *(Cheminex, UK)*.

19584-b

Nizofenone *(rINN).*

Y-9179. 2′-Chloro-2-[2-[(diethylamino)methyl]-imidazol-1-yl]-5-nitrobenzophenone.

$C_{21}H_{21}ClN_4O_3$=412.9.

CAS — 54533-85-6.

A nootropic or cognition adjuvant under investigation.

Proprietary Names and Manufacturers
Yoshitomi, Jpn.

3146-w

Nocloprost *(rINN).*

(*Z*)-7-[(1*R*,2*R*,3*R*,5*R*)-5-Chloro-3-hydroxy-2-[(*E*)-(3*R*)-3-hydroxy-4,4-dimethyl-1-octenyl]-cyclopentyl]-5-heptenoic acid.

$C_{22}H_{37}ClO_4$=401.0.

CAS — 79360-43-3.

A synthetic prostaglandin reported to inhibit gastric acid secretion.

Proprietary Names and Manufacturers
Schering, Ger.

19591-m

Nosantine *(BAN, pINN).*

NPT-15392. *Erythro*-9-[1-(1-hydroxyethyl)heptyl]hypoxanthine.

$C_{14}H_{22}N_4O_2$=278.4.

CAS — 76600-30-1.

Nosantine is under investigation as an immunomodulator.

Proprietary Names and Manufacturers
Newport, USA.

15306-t

Nucleic Acid

Acide Zymonucléique; Acidum Nucleicum; Nucleinic Acid.

Pharmacopoeias. In *Port.* and *Span.*

A complex mixture of phosphorus-containing organic acids present in living cells.

Nucleic acids are of 2 types, ribonucleic acids (RNA) (see p.1610) and deoxyribonucleic acids (DNA) (see p.1563). They are composed of chains of nucleotides (phosphate esters of purine or pyrimidine bases and pentose sugars).

Since the administration of nucleic acid gives rise to a marked temporary leucocytosis (usually preceded by a short period of leucopenia) it was formerly given in the treatment of a variety of bacterial infections in the hope of enhancing the natural defence mechanisms. Its therapeutic value, however, was never established.

13037-r

Octaverine Hydrochloride *(BANM, rINNM).*

6,7-Dimethoxy-1-(3,4,5-triethoxyphenyl)isoquinoline hydrochloride.

$C_{23}H_{27}NO_5$,HCl=433.9.

CAS — 549-68-8 (octaverine); 6775-26-4 (hydrochloride).

Octaverine hydrochloride has been used as an antispasmodic.

19599-e

Octenidine Hydrochloride *(BANM, USAN, rINNM).*

Win-41464 (octenidine); Win-41464-2; Win-41464-6 (octenidine saccharin). 1,1′,4,4′-Tetrahydro-*N*,*N*′-dioctyl-1,1′-decamethylenedi-(4-pyridylideneamine) dihydrochloride.

$C_{36}H_{62}N_4$,2HCl=623.8.

CAS — 71251-02-0 (octenidine); 70775-75-6 (hydrochloride).

Octenidine hydrochloride is an antimicrobial agent under investigation for topical use.

Activity of octenidine *in vitro* compared with chlorhexidine: A. M. Slee and J. R. O'Connor, *Antimicrob. Ag. Chemother.*, 1983, *23*, 379; D. M. Sedlock and D. M. Bailey, *Antimicrob. Ag. Chemother.*, 1985, *28*, 786.

Proprietary Names and Manufacturers
Sterling Research, UK.

2496-n

Olaflur *(BAN, USAN, rINN).*

GA-297; SKF-38095. 2,2′-(3-[*N*-(2-Hydroxyethyl)octadecylamino]propylimino)diethanol dihydrofluoride.

$C_{27}H_{60}F_2N_2O_3$=498.8.

CAS — 17671-49-7 (base); 6818-37-7 (dihydrofluoride).

Olaflur is used in the prevention of dental caries.

16936-e

Olaquindox *(BAN, rINN).*

Bay Va-9391. 2-(2-Hydroxyethylcarbamoyl)-3-methylquinoxaline 1,4-dioxide.

$C_{12}H_{13}N_3O_4$=263.3.

CAS — 23696-28-8.

Olaquindox is an antibacterial agent added to animal feedstuffs as a growth promoter.

1319-f

Oleic Acid *(BAN, USAN).*

Acidum Oleicum; Ölsäure.

CAS — 112-80-1 ($C_{18}H_{34}O_2$).

Pharmacopoeias. In *Arg., Aust., Br., Braz., Egypt., Hung., Ind., Mex., Pol., Span.,* and *Swiss.* Also in *U.S.N.F.* and *B.P. Vet.*

A colourless to pale brown oily liquid with a characteristic lard-like odour. On exposure to air it darkens in colour and the odour becomes more pronounced.

It consists chiefly of (*Z*)-octadec-9-enoic acid [$CH_3.(CH_2)_7.CH:CH.(CH_2)_7.CO_2H$ = 282.5] and also contains some stearic and palmitic acids, with traces of iron. Congealing point about 4° to 10°.

Practically **insoluble** in water; very soluble in alcohol, chloroform, ether, petroleum spirit, and fixed and volatile oils. **Store** in well-filled airtight containers. Protect from light.

Oleic acid forms soaps with alkaline substances and has been reported to assist the absorption by the skin of a number of drugs. It must not be used in eye ointments.

Oleic acid and oleyl alcohol each enhanced the penetration of acyclovir in propylene glycol across human skin *in vitro*.— E. R. Cooper *et al.*, *J. pharm. Sci.*, 1985, *74*, 688.

The enhancement in *dogs* of the oral bioavailability of cinnarizine in oleic acid.— T. Tokumura *et al.*, *J. pharm. Sci.*, 1987, *76*, 286.

Proprietary Names and Manufacturers
Priolene 6986 *(Unichema, UK).*

7363-v

Olive Oil *(BAN, USAN).*

Azeite; Oleum Olivae.

CAS — 8001-25-0.

Pharmacopoeias. In *Arg., Aust., Belg., Br., Cz., Egypt., Eur., Fr., Ger., It., Jpn, Jug., Mex., Port., Span., Swiss,* and *Turk.* Also in *U.S.N.F. Fr.* also includes olive leaves.

The fixed oil expressed from the ripe fruits of *Olea europaea* (Oleaceae). It is a pale yellow or light greenish-yellow oil with a slight characteristic odour and taste and a faintly acrid after-taste. At low temperatures it may be solid or partly solid.

Practically **insoluble** in alcohol; miscible with carbon disulphide, chloroform, ether, and petroleum spirit. **Store** at a temperature not exceeding 40° in well-filled airtight containers. Olive oil intended for use in the preparation of a parenteral dosage form should be kept in a glass container.

Internally, olive oil is nutrient, demulcent, and mildly laxative. It may also be given by rectal injection (100 to 500 mL warmed to about 32°) to soften impacted faeces. Olive oil in the form of an emulsion has been given as part of a nitrogen-free diet.

Externally, olive oil is emollient and soothing to inflamed surfaces, and is employed to soften the skin and crusts in eczema and psoriasis, and as a lubricant for massage. It is used to soften ear wax.

Olive oil is used in the preparation of liniments, ointments, plasters, and soaps; it is also used as a vehicle for oily suspensions for injection.

5018-a

Ololiuqui

CAS — 2889-26-1 (isoergine); 478-94-4 (ergine); 2390-99-0 (chanoclavine); 548-43-6 (elymoclavine); 602-85-7 (lysergol).

The seeds of *Rivea corymbosa* or *Ipomoea tricolor* (=*I. violacea*) both convolvulaceous plants similar to the common 'morning glory', *Ipomoea purpurea*. The brown seeds of *R. corymbosa* are known as 'badoh' and the black seeds of *I. tricolor* as 'badoh negro', the former containing 0.01% of alkaloid and the latter 0.05%.

Ololiuqui has hallucinogenic properties and is considered to be sacred by some Mexican Indians. Alkaloidal fractions contain at least 5 closely related individual components, viz. D-isolysergic acid amide (isoergine), D-lysergic acid amide (ergine), chanoclavine, elymoclavine, and lysergol.

The name 'ololiuqui' has been erroneously applied to seeds of *Datura metel* (Solanaceae).

Pharmacology of ololiuqui.— A. Hofmann, *Indian J. Pharm.*, 1963, *25*, 245.

Reports of adverse effects following ingestion of morning glory seeds.— A. L. Ingram, *J. Am. med. Ass.*, 1964, *190*, 1133; P. J. Fink *et al.*, *Archs gen. Psychiat.*, 1966, *15*, 209.

Following press reports in 1966 that 'morning glory' seeds were being purchased and used for their hallucinogenic properties, an investigation initiated in the laboratories of the Pharmaceutical Society of Great Britain showed that of the many species sold by seedsmen under the name 'morning glory', only those of *Ipomoea violacea* contained lysergic acid derivatives and presumably had hallucinogenic properties.— K. R. Capper, Lysergic Acid Derivatives in Morning Glory Seeds, *The Pharmacological and Epidemiological Aspects of Adolescent Drug Dependence*, C.W.M. Wilson, Oxford, Pergamon Press, 1968.

13040-c

Onion

The bulb of *Allium cepa* (Liliaceae).

Onion has been reported to reduce platelet aggregation and to enhance fibrinolysis.

References: I. S. Menon (letter), *Br. med. J.*, 1970, *2*, 421; K. I. Baghurst *et al.* (letter), *Lancet*, 1977, *1*, 101; C. Phillips and N. L. Poyser (letter), *Lancet*, 1978, *1*, 1051; T. H. Maugh, *Science*, 1979, *204*, 293; D. B. Louria *et al.*, *Curr. ther. Res.*, 1985, *37*, 127.

13041-k

Ononis

Arrête-Boeuf; Hauhechelwurzel; Racine de Bugrane; Radix Ononidis; Restharrow Root. The dried roots of *Ononis spinosa* (Leguminosae), containing saponins.

Pharmacopoeias. In *Aust.*, *Cz.*, *Hung.*, *Jug.*, and *Pol.*

Ononis has been used as a diuretic.

13042-a

Orazamide *(rINN)*.

AICA; Aica Orotate; Oroxamide. 5-Aminoimidazole-4-carboxamide orotate dihydrate.
$C_9H_{10}N_6O_5,2H_2O$=318.2.

CAS — 2574-78-9 (anhydrous); 60104-30-5 (dihydrate).

Orazamide has been used in the treatment of liver disorders.

Proprietary Names and Manufacturers
Aica-Hepat *(Montpellier, Arg.)*; Aicamin *(Labaz, Belg.*; *Crinos, Ital.*; *Fujisawa, Jpn*; *Made, Spain)*; Aïcamine *(Labaz, Fr.)* Aicorat *(Mack, Illert., Ger.)*.

2971-l

Ornoprostil *(rINN)*.

OU-1308. Methyl (−)-(1*R*,2*R*,3*R*)-3-hydroxy-2[(*E*)-(3*S*,5*S*)-3-hydroxy-5-methyl-1-nonenyl]-ϵ,5-dioxocyclopentanehептanoate.
$C_{23}H_{38}O_6$=410.6.

CAS — 70667-26-4.

Ornoprostil is a synthetic prostaglandin analogue used in the treatment of peptic ulcer.

Proprietary Names and Manufacturers
Ono, Jpn.

13045-r

Orotic Acid *(pINN)*.

Whey Factor; Animal Galactose Factor; Uracil-6-carboxylic Acid. 1,2,3,6-Tetrahydro-2,6-dioxopyrimidine-4-carboxylic acid monohydrate.
$C_5H_4N_2O_4,H_2O$=174.1.

CAS — 65-86-1 (anhydrous); 50887-69-9 (monohydrate).

Orotic acid occurs naturally in the body; it is found in milk. It is an intermediate in the biosynthesis of pyrimidine nucleotides which in turn are involved in the synthesis of DNA and RNA. Orotic acid and its lysine, magnesium, and potassium salts have been used in the treatment of hyperuricaemia and hypercholesterolaemia and in liver disorders. Calcium and magnesium orotate have been used as a mineral source.

References on the use of orotic acid: G. D. Kersley, *Ann. rheum. Dis.*, 1966, *25*, 353 (gout); *Br. med. J.*, 1972, *2*, 62 (to lower bilirubin concentrations in premature and full-term infants); P. J. Collipp, *Curr. ther. Res.*, 1987, *41*, 135 (degenerative retinal diseases).

Proprietary Names and Manufacturers
Calora *(Miller, USA)*; Crataron *(Spain)*; Dioron *(Belg.)*; Lactinium *(Roland, Ger.)*; Lysortine *(Théraplix, Fr.)*; Magora *(Miller, USA)*; Oroturic *(Grémy-Longuet, Fr.)*.

13046-f

Oryzanol

Gamma Oryzanol; γ-Oryzanol; γ-OZ. A substance extracted from rice bran oil and rice embryo bud oil. Triacontanyl 3-(4-hydroxy-3-methoxyphenyl)prop-2-enoate.
$C_{40}H_{58}O_4$=602.9.

CAS — 11042-64-1.

Oryzanol has been used in autonomic and endocrine disturbances.

Proprietary Names and Manufacturers
Caclate *(Jpn)*; Gammariza *(Jpn)*; Gammatsul *(Jpn)*; Guntrin *(Jpn)*; Hi-Z *(Jpn)*; Maintenan *(Jpn)*; Oliver *(Jpn)*; Thiaminogen *(Jpn)*.

3729-w

Osalmid *(rINN)*.

L-1718; Oxaphenamide. 4′-Hydroxysalicylanilide.
$C_{13}H_{11}NO_3$=229.2.

CAS — 526-18-1.

Pharmacopoeias. In *Rus.*

Osalmid is a choleretic. It has been given in doses of 500 mg to 1.5 g daily in divided doses.

Proprietary Names and Manufacturers
Bichol *(Jpn)*; Bilecoll *(Jpn)*; Cholatin *(Jpn)*; Coypanon *(Jpn)*; Driol *(Labaz, Belg.*; *Labaz, Switz.)*; Galerite *(Jpn)*; Gallocol *(Jpn)*; Isechol *(Jpn)*; Loibnal *(Jpn)*; Marionchol *(Jpn)*; Neodekoll *(Jpn)*; Sawacol *(Jpn)*; Shikichol *(Jpn)*; Taichol *(Jpn)*; Tanjuron *(Jpn)*; Yoshichol *(Jpn)*.

13047-d

Osmium Tetroxide

Osmic Acid.
OsO_4=254.2.

CAS — 20816-12-0.

CAUTION. *Osmium tetroxide solution and its fumes are corrosive to the eyes, mucous membranes, and skin.*

Osmium tetroxide is an oxidising agent. It has been given by intra-articular injection in rheumatic disorders of the knee, however, local pain, fever, and effusions have been associated with its use.

In Great Britain the recommended exposure limits of osmium tetroxide (as Os) are 0.0002 ppm (long-term) and 0.0006 ppm (short-term).

References: M. Nissilä, *Scand. J. Rheumatol.*, 1979, *Suppl.* 29;; H. Sheppeard and D. J. Ward, *Rheumatol. Rehabil.*, 1980, *19*, 25.

2293-y

Ostomy Deodorants

Atmocol *(Thackray, UK)*. A deodorant spray for use with colostomies and ileostomies.

Chironair Odour Control Liquid *(Downs, UK)*. A deodorant for use with colostomies and ileostomies.

Nilodor *(Loxley, UK)*. A deodorant liquid for use with colostomies and ileostomies.

No-Roma *(Salt, UK)*. A deodorant liquid for use with colostomies and ileostomies.

Ostobon *(Coloplast, UK)*. A deodorant powder for use with ostomies.

Translet Plus One (formerly known as Ostomy Plus One) *(Franklin Medical, UK)*. A deodorant liquid for use with colostomies and ileostomies.

Translet Plus Two (formerly known as Ostomy Plus Two) *(Franklin Medical, UK)*. A deodorant liquid for use with colostomies and ileostomies.

13249-w

Otimerate Sodium *(rINN)*.

Sodium 2-Ethylmercurithiobenzoxazole-5-carboxylate.
$C_{10}H_8HgNNaO_3S$=445.8.

CAS — 16509-11-8.

Otimerate sodium has bacteriostatic and antifungal properties. A 0.02% solution is used for the storage of bone for transplantation.

Proprietary Names and Manufacturers
Cialit *(Hoechst, UK)*.

13051-t

Oxaceprol *(rINN)*.

Acetylhydroxyproline; C061. (−)-1-Acetyl-4-hydroxy-L-proline.
$C_7H_{11}NO_4$=173.2.

CAS — 33996-33-7.

Oxaceprol is reported to affect connective-tissue metabolism and has been used in dermatology, to promote wound healing, and in rheumatic disorders. It has been used in doses of up to 600 mg daily by mouth. Adverse effects have included gastric pain, nausea, diarrhoea, dizziness, headache, and skin rashes.

Proprietary Names and Manufacturers
AHP *(Chephasaar, Ger.)*; Jonctum *(Lepetit, Fr.*; *Merrell, Ital.*; *Inibsa, Spain)*; Tejuntivo *(Iquinosa, Spain)*.

2295-z

Oxaflozane *(rINN)*.

1766-Cerm; CERM-1766.
4-Isopropyl-2-(α,α,α-trifluoro-*m*-tolyl)morpholine.
$C_{14}H_{18}F_3NO$=273.3.

CAS — 26629-87-8.

Oxaflozane is an antidepressant given by mouth as the hydrochloride.

References: E. Aguglia, *Acta ther.*, 1986, *12*, 259; F. Scavuzzo *et al.*, *ibid.*, 1987, *13*, 93.

Proprietary Names and Manufacturers
Conflictan *(Sarbach, Fr.)*.

1320-z

Oxalic Acid

$HO_2C.CO_2H,2H_2O$=126.1.

CAS — 144-62-7 (anhydrous); 6153-56-6 (dihydrate).

Adverse Effects
In dilute solution oxalic acid and its salts are toxic owing to withdrawal of ionisable calcium from the blood and tissues. Strong solutions of the acid are corrosive. In acute poisoning from ingestion there is local irritation and corrosion of the mouth, oesophagus, and stomach, with pain and vomiting, followed shortly by muscular tremors, convulsions, and collapse. Death may occur within a few minutes. After apparent recovery acute renal failure may occur from blocking of the renal tubules by calcium oxalate crystals.

In Great Britain the recommended exposure limits of oxalic acid are 1 mg per m^3 (long-term); 2 mg per m^3 (short-term).

A 16-year-old girl was accidentally given 1.2 g of sodium oxalate intravenously. She died after 5 minutes, but the heart function was restored by cardiac massage and maintained for 4 days without restoration of consciousness. Postmortem examination showed tubular necrosis of the kidneys, with calcium oxalate crystals in the lumen and epithelium of the tubules. Ganglion cells throughout the central nervous system were necrosed. This finding was attributed to blocking of glycogenolysis by the oxalate.— I. Dvořáčková, *Arch. Tox.*, 1966, *22*, 63.

Treatment of Adverse Effects
Give a dilute solution of any soluble calcium salt to precipitate the oxalate and if mucosal corrosion has not occurred carefully empty the stomach by aspiration and lavage using large quantities of diluted lime water or dilute solutions of other calcium salts. It is advisable to leave about 100 mL of the solution in the stomach. Calcium gluconate injection 10% should be given intravenously in doses of 10 to 20 mL to prevent tetany. If renal function is not impaired, 4 to 5 litres of fluid should be given daily to prevent crystalluria.

Uses.
Oxalic acid has varied industrial uses.

The administration by mouth of sodium oxalate and the measurement of urinary oxalate excretion as a screening test for steatorrhoea.— D. S. Rampton *et al.*, *Br. med. J.*, 1984, *288*, 1419 and 1728. See also *idem*, *Gut*, 1979, *20*, 1089.

13059-b

Oxetorone Fumarate *(USAN, rINNM).*
L-6257. 3-(6,12-Dihydrobenzofuro[3,2-*c*][1]benzoxepin-6-ylidene)-*NN*-dimethylpropylamine hydrogen fumarate.
$C_{21}H_{21}NO_2,C_4H_4O_4$=435.5.

CAS — 26020-55-3 (oxetorone); 34522-46-8 (fumarate).

Oxetorone fumarate has been used in the treatment of migraine in doses of up to 180 mg daily by mouth. Oxetorone is reported to have induced hyperplastic changes in breast tissue and the uterine endometrium of *rodents*. It is not recommended for use in young girls and pregnant women.

Proprietary Names and Manufacturers
Nocertone *(Armstrong, Arg.; Labaz, Belg.; Labaz, Fr.; Labaz, Ger.; Labaz, Spain; Labaz, Switz.).*

13061-r

Oxfenicine *(BAN, USAN, rINN).*
UK-25842. L-2-(4-Hydroxyphenyl)glycine.
$C_8H_9NO_3$=167.2.

CAS — 32462-30-9.

Oxfenicine is reported to have potential application in the treatment of ischaemic heart disease.

Proprietary Names and Manufacturers
Pfizer, UK.

2876-y

Oxindanac *(rINN).*
(±)-5-Benzoyl-6-hydroxy-1-indancarboxylic acid.
$C_{17}H_{14}O_4$=282.3.

CAS — 68548-99-2.

Oxindanac is a non-steroidal anti-inflammatory drug under investigation.

Proprietary Names and Manufacturers
Ciba-Geigy, Switz.

16922-v

Oxiracetam *(rINN).*
ISF-2522. 4-Hydroxy-2-oxo-1-pyrrolidineacetamide.
$C_6H_{10}N_2O_3$=158.2.

CAS — 62613-82-5.

Oxiracetam is chemically related to piracetam and has a similar nootropic action on the central nervous system. It has been used in organic brain syndromes and dementia in the elderly.

References: T. M. Itil *et al.*, *Drug Dev. Res.*, 1982, *2*, 447; *Drug & Ther. Bull.*, 1984, *22*, 98; E. Ferrero, *Curr. ther. Res.*, 1984, *36*, 298; E. Perucca *et al.*, *Eur. J. Drug Metab. Pharmacokinet.*, 1984, *9*, 267; E. Perucca *et al.*, *Br. J. clin. Pharmac.*, 1985, *19*, 577P; B. Saletu *et al.*, *Neuropsychobiology*, 1985, *13*, 44; A. Moglia *et al.*, *Clin. Neuropharmacol.*, 1986, *9*, *Suppl.* 3, 573; G. Spignoli and G. Pepeu, *Eur. J. clin. Pharmac.*, 1986, *126*, 253; M. Guazzelli *et al.*, *Curr. ther. Res.*, 1987, *41*, 234.

Proprietary Names and Manufacturers
Neupan *(Smith Kline & French, Ital.)*; Neuromet *(ISF, Ital.).*

13069-g

Oxybromonaftoic Acid
4-Bromo-3-hydroxy-2-naphthoic acid.
$C_{11}H_7BrO_3$=267.1.

CAS — 2208-15-3.

Oxybromonaftoic acid has been used in hepatic disorders.

Proprietary Names and Manufacturers
Naftocol *(Panthox & Burck, Ital.).*

19602-y

Ozagrel *(rINN).*
OKY-046 (hydrochloride). (*E*)-*p*-(imidazol-1-ylmethyl)cinnamic acid.
$C_{13}H_{12}N_2O_2$=228.2.

CAS — 82571-53-7.

Ozagrel is reported to be a thromboxane synthetase inhibitor under investigation as an anticoagulant.

References: *Drugs of the Future*, 1985, *10*, 343; *ibid.*, 1986, *11*, 339; *ibid.*, 1987, *12*, 405; K. Nagatsuka *et al.*, *Stroke*, 1985, *16*, 806; Y. Yui *et al.*, *J. Am. Coll. Cardiol.*, 1986, *7*, 25; M. Fujimura *et al.*, *Thorax*, 1986, *41*, 955.

Proprietary Names and Manufacturers
Kissei, Jpn; Ono, Jpn.

13073-h

Pamabrom *(USAN).*
2-Amino-2-methylpropan-1-ol 8-bromotheophyllinate.
$C_4H_{11}NO,C_7H_7BrN_4O_2$=348.2.

CAS — 606-04-2.

Pamabrom is a mild diuretic which has been used for the relief of premenstrual tension.

Proprietary Names and Manufacturers
The following names have been used for multi-ingredient preparations containing pamabrom— Midol PMS *(Sterling, Canad.; Glenbrook, USA).*

13074-m

Pangamic Acid

A substance isolated from apricot kernels and rice bran was termed pangamic acid and has also been described as 'vitamin B_{15}'. Although pangamic acid has been identified by some sources as gluconic acid 6-bis(*N*-di-isopropylamino)acetate, there is much uncertainty about the identity of products sold in health food stores as 'vitamin B_{15}', pangamic acid, or calcium pangamate and different brands have been reported to have completely different compositions.

Claims for the activity of pangamic acid as a promoter of tissue oxygenation and its alleged value in numerous disorders have not been substantiated. There is no evidence that pangamic acid is a vitamin.

References: *Med. Lett.*, 1978, *20*, 44; *J. Am. med. Ass.*, 1980, *243*, 2473.

Proprietary Names and Manufacturers
B-15 Naturtabs *(Cantassium Co., UK)*; Plentine *(Wasserman, Spain).*

5224-n

Papaverine Hydrochloride *(BANM, USAN).*
Papaverini Hydrochloridum; Papaverinii Chloridum; Papaverinium Chloride. 6,7-Dimethoxy-1-(3,4-dimethoxybenzyl)isoquinoline hydrochloride.
$C_{20}H_{21}NO_4,HCl$=375.9.

CAS — 58-74-2 (papaverine); 63817-84-5 (cromesilate); 61-25-6 (hydrochloride); 39024-96-9 (monophosadenine); 32808-09-6 (sulphate, anhydrous).

Pharmacopoeias. In *Arg., Aust., Belg., Br., Braz., Chin., Cz., Egypt., Eur., Fr., Ger., Hung., Int., It., Jpn, Jug., Mex., Neth., Nord., Pol., Port., Roum., Rus., Span., Swiss, Turk.,* and *U.S.*

Odourless white or almost white crystals or crystalline powder.
Soluble 1 in 30 to 40 of water and 1 in 120 of alcohol; soluble in chloroform; practically insoluble in ether. A 2% solution in water has a pH of 3 to 4. **Incompatible** with bromides, iodine and iodides, alkalis, and tannins. Precipitation may occur when Papaverine Hydrochloride Injection is added to Lactated Ringer's Injection. **Store** in airtight containers. Protect from light.

Adverse Effects and Precautions
Side-effects of papaverine include gastro-intestinal disturbance, flushing of the face, headache, malaise, drowsiness, skin rash, sweating, and vertigo. Jaundice, eosinophilia, and signs of altered liver function may occur due to hypersensitivity.
Papaverine should be used with caution intravenously since it can cause cardiac arrhythmias; a slow rate of injection is recommended. Intravenous injection is contra-indicated in patients with complete atrioventricular block. Papaverine should be used with caution in patients with glaucoma or depressed myocardial function.

For a report of papaverine decreasing the effectiveness of levodopa, see Levodopa, p.1017.

Absorption and Fate
The biological half-life of papaverine given by mouth is reported to be between one and two hours, but there is wide inter-individual variation.

Most of a dose is metabolised in the liver and excreted in the urine, almost entirely as demethylated glucuronide-conjugated phenolic metabolites.

Evidence in 5 patients that the elimination half-life of papaverine is significantly prolonged in cardiopulmonary bypass.— W. G. Kramer and A. Romagnoli, *Eur. J. clin. Pharmac.*, 1984, *27*, 127.

Uses and Administration
Papaverine inhibits phosphodiesterase and relaxes smooth muscle directly. It has been given with the intention of relieving ischaemia and the symptoms of senile dementia; it is also present in some cough preparations. However, there is little evidence to justify its clinical use in these conditions.
Papaverine has usually been given by mouth as the hydrochloride in doses of up to 600 mg daily. Sustained-release preparations have been used. It has also been given by injection using the intra-arterial, intramuscular, or intravenous routes (but see Adverse Effects and Precautions). The codecarboxylate, cromesilate, hydrobromide, monophosadenine, phenylglycolate, sulphate, and teprosilate have also been used.

IMPOTENCE. The intracavernous injection of papaverine 80 mg produced improvement in organic but not nonorganic impotence.— R. Virag (letter), *Lancet*, 1982, *2*, 938. A report of further experience with papaverine and proposals for guidelines for the pharmacological treatment and self-treatment of impotence.— *idem* (letter), 1985, *1*, 519. Intracavernous injection of papaverine 30 mg together with phentolamine 1 mg resulted in a good response for up to 1 month in patients with organic impotence and for up to 4 months in patients with psychogenic impotence. Some patients were successfully practising home self-injection.— E. A. Kiely *et al.* (letter), *Br. med. J.*, 1986, *292*, 1137. Criticism regarding diagnostic criteria.— K. Desai and J. C. Gingell (letter), *ibid.*, 1335. Further references: A. A. Sidi *et al.*, *J. Urol. Baltimore*, 1986, *135*, 704; G. Williams *et al.*, *Br. med. J.*, 1987, *295*, 595.

Preparations

Papaverine Hydrochloride Injection *(U.S.P.)*

Papaverine Hydrochloride Tablets *(U.S.P.)*

Proprietary Names and Manufacturers of Papaverine Hydrochloride and some other Papaverine Compounds

Albatran *(Beaufour, Fr.)*; Artegodan *(Artesan, Ger.)*; Cerebid *(Saron, USA)*; Cerespan *(USV Pharmaceutical Corp., USA)*; Dicertan *(Sarget, Fr.)*; Dilaspan *(Parkdale, USA)*; Dipav *(Lemmon, USA)*; Dylate *(Elder, USA)*; Kaldil *(Bruneau, Fr.)*; Kavrin *(Hyrex, USA)*; Maspaver *(Juste, Spain)*; Myobid *(Laser, USA)*; Opdensit *(Stroschein, Ger.)*; Optenyl *(Stroschein, Ger.)*; P-200 *(Boots, USA)*; Pameion *(Simes, Ital.)*; Panergon *(Mack, Illert., Ger.; Mack, Switz.)*; Papaverlumin Fuerte *(Spain)*; Pava-2 Caps *(General Pharm. Prods, USA)*; Pavabid *(Marion Laboratories, USA)*; Pavacap *(Reid-Provident, USA)*; Pavacen *(Central Pharmaceuticals, USA)*; Pavakey *(Key, USA)*; Pavased *(Mallard, USA)*; Pavatran *(Mayrand, USA)*; Pavatym *(Everett, USA)*; Pava-Wol *(Wolins, USA)*; Paveron *(Karlspharma, Ger.)*; Pavine TD *(Lexalabs, USA)*; Permavérine *(Armstrong, Arg.; Robert et Carrière, Fr.)*; Qua-Bid *(Quaker, USA)*; Sustaverine *(ICN, USA)*; Sustein *(Inibsa, Spain)*; Therapav *(Berlex, USA)*; Vasal *(Reid-Provident, USA)*; Vasocap *(Keene, USA)*; Vaso-Pav *(UAD, USA)*; Vasospan *(Ulmer, USA)*.

The following names have been used for multi-ingredient preparations containing papaverine hydrochloride and some other papaverine compounds—Actonorm *(Wallace Mfg Chem., UK)*; APP Stomach Preparations *(Consolidated Chemicals, UK)*; Asma-Vydrin *(Lipomed, UK)*; Bepro *(Wallace Mfg Chem., UK)*; Brovon *(Napp, UK)*; Copavin *(Lilly, USA)*; Cyclopane *(Alcon, Austral.)*; Migranol *(Alcon, Austral.)*; Pavacol-D *(Boehringer Ingelheim, UK)*; Pholcomed *(Medo, UK)*; Riddobron Inhalant *(Seaford, UK)*; Riddofan *(Seaford, UK)*; Riddovydrin Inhalant *(Seaford, UK)*; Rybarvin *(Rybar, UK)*.

13077-g

Papaveroline Meglumine *(BANM, rINNM)*.

The *N*-methylglucamine salt of 1-(3,4-dihydroxybenzyl)isoquinoline-6,7-diol.

$C_{16}H_{13}NO_4,C_7H_{17}NO_5=478.5$.

CAS — 574-77-6 (papaveroline).

Papaveroline meglumine has been used in the treatment of circulatory disorders in doses of up to 600 mg daily by mouth. The sulphonate has also been used.

Proprietary Names and Manufacturers

Modus *(Scharper, Ital.)*.

13083-b

Paroxypropione *(rINN)*.

B-360; H-365; NSC-2834. 4′-Hydroxypropiophenone.

$C_9H_{10}O_2=150.2$.

CAS — 70-70-2.

Paroxypropione is a pituitary gonadotrophic hormone inhibitor which has been used for the control of pituitary hyperactivity.

Proprietary Names and Manufacturers

Frenantol *(UPB, Belg.; Anglo-French Laboratories, Canad.; Laroche Navarron, Fr.)*; Frenantole *(Landerlan, Spain)*; Frenormon Fuerte *(Medea, Spain)*; Possipione *(Recordati, Ital.)*.

13086-q

Passion Flower

Grenadille; May-pop; Pasionari; Passiflora.

CAS — 486-84-0 (harman).

Pharmacopoeias. In *Egypt.*, *Fr.*, *Span.*, and *Swiss. Braz.* includes the leaves of *P. alata*, (Maracujá).

The dried flowering and fruiting tops of *Passiflora incarnata* (Passifloraceae). *Swiss P.* specifies not less than 0.3% of flavonoids calculated as hyperoside ($C_{21}H_{20}O_{12}$).

Passion flower is reputed to have antispasmodic and sedative properties. It has been used as a liquid extract and as a tincture.

A brief review.— J. D. Phillipson and L. A. Anderson, *Pharm. J.*, 1984, *2*, 80.

18950-h

Pentopril *(rINN)*.

CGS-13945. Ethyl $(\alpha R,\gamma R,2S)$-2-carboxy-α,γ-dimethyl-δ-oxo-1-indolinevalerate.

$C_{18}H_{23}NO_5=333.4$.

CAS — 82924-03-6.

Pentopril is an angiotensin-converting enzyme inhibitor under investigation in the treatment of hypertension.

References: M. D. Schaller *et al.*, *Curr. ther. Res.*, 1985, *37*, 843; A. Rakhit *et al.*, *J. clin. Pharmac.*, 1985, *25*, 424; A. Rakhit *et al.*, *ibid.*, 1986, *26*, 156.

Proprietary Names and Manufacturers

Ciba-Geigy, Switz.

3160-p

Peptide T

Peptide T is an octapeptide segment of the envelope glycoprotein of human immunodeficiency virus under investigation for the treatment of AIDS.

References: L. Wetterberg *et al.* (letter), *Lancet*, 1987, *1*, 159; J. Sodroski *et al.* (letter), *ibid.*, 1428; M. R. Ruff *et al.* (letter), *ibid.*, *2*, 751.

7364-g

Persic Oil *(USAN)*.

Peach or Apricot Kernel Oil; Oleum Persicorum.

CAS — 8002-78-6.

Pharmacopoeias. In *Rus.* Also in *U.S.N.F.*
Jpn and *Chin.* include Peach Kernel (Persicae Semen) and also Apricot Kernel (Armeniacae Semen).

The fixed oil expressed from the kernels of varieties of *Prunus persica*(peach) or *P. armeniaca* (apricot) (Rosaceae). It is a clear, colourless or pale straw-coloured, almost odourless oil with a bland taste. Slightly **soluble** in alcohol; miscible with chloroform, ether, and petroleum spirit. **Store** in airtight containers.

Persic oil closely resembles almond oil in its general characteristics and is used as an oily vehicle.

282-k

Peru Balsam

Bals. Peruv.; Baume du Pérou; Baume du San Salvador; Peruvian Balsam.

CAS — 8007-00-9.

Pharmacopoeias. In *Arg.*, *Aust.*, *Belg.*, *Cz.*, *Fr.*, *Ger.*, *Hung.*, *Jug.*, *Mex.*, *Nord.*, *Pol.*, *Port.*, *Roum.*, *Span.*, and *Swiss.* Also in *B.P.C. 1973.*

A balsam exuded from the trunk of *Myroxylon balsamum* var. *pereirae* (Leguminosae).

Peru balsam has a very mild antiseptic action by virtue of its content of cinnamic and benzoic acids. Diluted with an equal part of castor oil, it has been used as an application to bedsores and chronic ulcers; as an ointment (12.5% in Simple Ointment) it has been used in the treatment of eczema and pruritus. It is an ingredient of some rectal suppositories used for the symptomatic relief of haemorrhoids.

Peru balsam was formerly used in the treatment of scabies.

Skin sensitisation has been reported.

Proprietary Names and Manufacturers

Branolind *(Hartmann, Ger.)*; Dera *(Ingram & Bell, Canad.)*; Linitul *(Bama, Spain)*; Tulle Gras Lumiere *(Hefa-Frenon, Ger.)*.

The following names have been used for multi-ingredient preparations containing peru balsam—Anugesic-HC *(Parke, Davis, UK)*; Anusol *(Warner, Austral.; Warner-Lambert, UK; Parke, Davis, USA)*; Anusol-HC *(Warner, Austral.; Parke, Davis, UK; Parke, Davis, USA)*; Granulex *(Hickam, USA)*; Rectal Medicone-HC *(Medicone, USA)*; Stimuzyme Plus *(National Dermaceutical, USA)*; Wyanoids *(Wyeth, USA)*.

13098-e

Peruvoside

A glycoside obtained from *Thevetia neriifolia* (Apocynaceae), related to thevetin A.

$C_{30}H_{44}O_9=548.7$.

CAS — 1182-87-2.

Peruvoside has been used in congestive heart failure.

References: M. L. Bhatia *et al.*, *Br. med. J.*, 1970, *3*, 740; G. Lohmöller and H. Lydtin, *Arzneimittel-Forsch.*, 1971, *21*, 1567.

Proprietary Names and Manufacturers

Encordin *(E. Merck, Ger.)*; Largitor *(Inverni della Beffa, Ital.)*; Nerial *(Simes, Ital.)*; Perusid *(Malesci, Ital.)*.

13100-l

Phencyclidine Hydrochloride *(BANM, USAN, rINNM)*.

CI-395; CN-25253-2; GP-121; NSC-40902; PCP. 1-(1-Phenylcyclohexyl)piperidine hydrochloride.

$C_{17}H_{25}N,HCl=279.9$.

CAS — 77-10-1 (phencyclidine); 956-90-1 (hydrochloride).

NOTE. The name PCP has also been used as a synonym for pentachlorophenol.

Adverse Effects

Phencyclidine can induce a psychosis clinically indistinguishable from schizophrenia. Deaths have resulted from its illicit use. Adverse effects reported include bizarre and violent behaviour, hallucinations, agitation, catatonic rigidity, disorientation, incoordination, nystagmus, hypersalivation, vomiting, convulsions, numbness, hypertension, and tachycardia, rhabdomyolysis leading to renal failure, and occasionally, malignant hyperpyrexia.

Treatment of the adverse effects of phencyclidine is symptomatic; if agitated the patient should be kept quiet in a darkened room, and diazepam given if necessary. Acidification of the urine increases the rate of excretion of phencyclidine. Haloperidol or a similar butyrophenone may be preferable to chlorpromazine in the management of psychotic symptoms.

ABUSE. Street names for phencyclidine used illicitly have included: angel dust, angel hair, angel mist, crystal, cyclone, dust, elephant tranquilliser, embalming fluid, goon, hog, horse tranquilliser, killer weed, KW, mint weed, mist, monkey dust, peace pills, peace weed, rocket fuel, scuffle, sheets, super weed, surfer, and T.

Phencyclidine was a major component of street drug preparations. In liquid form it was sprayed on marihuana, parsley, oregano, or other plant leaves and sold as 'angel dust'. In powder form it was marketed as phencyclidine or 'peace pills'. It was frequently sold as lysergide, mescaline, psilocybin, cocaine, 3,4-methylenedioxyamphetamine (MDA), tetrahydrocannabinol and other drugs, or it might be mixed with these agents. Many unrecognised toxic reactions secondary to sympathomimetic anaesthetic abuse were occurring and phencyclidine, a major drug of abuse, was a member of this group.— J. M. Rainey and M. K. Crowder, *J. Am. med. Ass.*, 1974, *230*, 824. When used illicitly phencyclidine has been sniffed, injected, eaten, or smoked. Many analogues have been synthesised and at least 6 are sold illicitly in the U.S.— *Br. med. J.*, 1980, *281*, 1511.

Uses and Administration
Phencyclidine is related chemically to ketamine (p.1120) and is a potent analgesic and anaesthetic. It was formerly given intravenously to produce an amnesic trance-like state, with analgesia, but severe adverse effects, especially postoperative psychoses, precluded its use. It was formerly used in veterinary medicine as an immobilising agent and is widely used in some countries as a hallucinogenic drug of abuse (see above).
A number of analogues of phencyclidine have been similarly abused and include PHP (1-(1-phenylcyclohexyl)pyrrolidine), PCC (1-piperidinocyclohexanecarbonitrile), PCE (*N*-ethyl-1-phenylcyclohexylamine), and TCP (1-[1-(2-thienyl)cyclohexyl]piperidine).

15300-y

Phenylhydrazine Hydrochloride

Hydrazinobenzene Hydrochloride.
$C_6H_5.NH.NH_2,HCl=144.6$.

CAS — 100-63-0 (phenylhydrazine); 59-88-1 (hydrochloride).

Phenylhydrazine has a specific effect in destroying erythrocytes. Patients with glucose-6-phosphate dehydrogenase deficiency are particularly susceptible to its action and its use is best avoided in these subjects. It was formerly used in the treatment of polycythaemia vera but it has been replaced by more effective and less toxic medicaments. Phenylhydrazine may be absorbed from the skin.
In Great Britain the recommended exposure limits of phenylhydrazine are 5 ppm (long-term); 10 ppm (short-term); suitable precautions should be taken to prevent absorption through the skin. In the *US* the permissible and recommended exposure limits are 22 mg per m^3 and 0.6 mg per m^3 respectively.

Phenylhydrazine was considered to be unsafe in patients with acute porphyria because it has been shown to be porphyrinogenic in *animals* or *in vitro* systems.— M.R. Moore and K.E.L. McColl, *Porphyrias, Drug Lists*, Glasgow, Porphyria Research Unit, University of Glasgow, 1987.

3737-w

Phenylpropanol

α-Hydroxypropylbenzene; Ethyl Phenyl Carbinol; SH-261. 1-Phenylpropan-1-ol; α-Ethylbenzyl alcohol.
$C_9H_{12}O=136.2$.

CAS — 93-54-9.

Phenylpropanol is a choleretic. The usual dose is 100 to 200 mg.

Proprietary Names and Manufacturers
Bilergon *(Ital.)*; Ejibil *(Sopar, Belg.)*; Eufepar *(Arnaldi, Ital.)*; Felicur *(Schering, Arg.; Schering, Austral.; Asche, Ger.)*.

13104-c

Phloroglucinol

Phloroglucin. Benzene-1,3,5-triol.
$C_6H_6O_3=126.1$.

CAS — 108-73-6.

Phloroglucinol is used as an antispasmodic in doses of 480 mg daily by mouth, 450 mg daily rectally or 120 mg daily by intravenous or intramuscular injection. Phloroglucinol is used in combination with trimethylphloroglucinol in some preparations.

Proprietary Names and Manufacturers
Dilospan S *(Nippon Roussel, Jpn)*; Spasfon-Lyoc *(Lafon, Fr.)*.

13105-k

Phosgene

Carbonyl Chloride; Chloroformyl Chloride.
$COCl_2=98.92$.

CAS — 75-44-5.

Adverse Effects
Poisoning may occur from industrial use or from the generation of phosgene from chlorinated compounds such as chloroform or carbon tetrachloride in the presence of heat. Symptoms of poisoning, which may be delayed for up to 24 hours, include burning of the eyes and throat, cough, dyspnoea, cyanosis, and pulmonary congestion and oedema. Exposure to 50 ppm may be rapidly fatal. Massive exposure may cause intravascular haemolysis, thrombus formation, and immediate death. In Great Britain the recommended exposure limit of phosgene is 0.1 ppm (long-term). In the *US* the permissible and recommended exposure limits are 0.4 mg per m^3.

Treatment of Adverse Effects
After inhalation of phosgene or absorption from the skin, treatment consists of complete rest and the administration of oxygen. The mouth, eyes, nose, and skin should be irrigated with water; a 1% solution of sodium bicarbonate has also been advocated. Corticosteroids may reduce tissue damage. Further treatment is symptomatic.

Uses
Phosgene is used in the chemical industry. It has been used as a war gas.

3918-z

Phosphatidylserine

Phosphatidylserine has been tried in the treatment of organic psychiatric syndromes. It is under investigation as a cognitive adjuvant.

References: C. Villardita *et al.*, *Clin. Trials J.*, 1987, *24*, 84.

Proprietary Names and Manufacturers
Bros *(Fidia, Ital.)*.

1321-c

Phosphoric Acid *(BAN, USAN)*.

Acido Fosfórico; Acidum Phosphoricum Concentratum; Concentrated Phosphoric Acid; E338; Orthophosphoric Acid; Phosph. Acid; Phosphorsäure.
$H_3PO_4=98.00$.

CAS — 7664-38-2.

Pharmacopoeias. In *Arg.* (approximately 87 to 90%); in *Aust., Hung., Mex., Port.,* and *Span.* (approximately 85 to 88%); in *Belg., Br., Eur., Fr., It., Neth.,* and *Swiss* (84 to 90%); in *Egypt., Ger.,* and *Ind.* (85 to 90%); and in *Roum.* (50%). Also in *U.S.N.F.* (85 to 88%).

Odourless, clear, colourless, corrosive, syrupy liquid.
Miscible with water or alcohol. When stored at a low temperature it may solidify, forming a mass of colourless crystals which do not melt until the temperature reaches 28°. **Store** in airtight glass containers.

1322-k

Dilute Phosphoric Acid *(BAN)*.

Acidum Phosphoricum Dilutum; Diluted Phosphoric Acid *(USAN)*.

Pharmacopoeias. In *Arg., Aust., Belg., Br., Egypt., Eur., Fr., Ger., It., Neth., Pol., Roum., Span.,* and *Swiss.* Also in *U.S.N.F.*

Dilute Phosphoric Acid *B.P.* may be prepared by mixing phosphoric acid 115 g with water 885 g. Diluted Phosphoric Acid *U.S.N.F.* may be prepared by mixing phosphoric acid 69 mL with water to 1000 mL. **Store** in airtight containers.

Adverse Effects and Treatment
As for Hydrochloric Acid, p.1578.
In Great Britain the recommended exposure limits of phosphoric acid are 1 mg per m^3 (long-term); 3 mg per m^3 (short-term).

A report of severe postoperative ulceration and sequestration following restorative dental treatment with an acid-etch composite technique under local anaesthetic. The white sloughing ulcer corresponded in proportion to the cotton wool roll used in moisture control and it was possible that amounts of etchant phosphoric acid were absorbed into the cotton wool roll and held in contact with the already desiccated tissues. Superimposition of infecting bacteria may also have contributed to the ulceration and subsequent tissue loss.— D. L. Gutteridge, *Br. dent. J.*, 1984, *156*, 403.

Uses and Administration
Phosphoric acid has industrial uses. Dilute phosphoric acid has been used well diluted in bitter preparations.

The maximum tolerable daily intake of phosphates and polyphosphates (applied to the sum of phosphates naturally present in food and in food additives), expressed as phosphorus, was 70 mg per kg body-weight for diets nutritionally adequate in calcium. The aluminium-containing phosphates were considered separately.— Twenty-sixth Report of the FAO/WHO Expert Committee on Food Additives, *Tech. Rep. Ser. Wld Hlth Org. No. 683*, 1982.

USE OF DISINFECTANTS ON FARMS. In Great Britain, a technical grade of orthophosphoric acid 1 in 330 of water is an approved disinfectant for foot-and-mouth disease.

Proprietary Names and Manufacturers
The following names have been used for multi-ingredient preparations containing dilute phosphoric acid—Anvatrol *(Nelson, Austral.)*; Emetrol *(Boots, Austral.; Rorer, Canad.; Radiol, UK; Adria, USA)*.

13106-a

Phosphorus

Yellow Phosphorus; Fósforo.
$P=30.97376$.

CAS — 7723-14-0.

Pharmacopoeias. In *Port.* and *Span.*

It is unstable in air and should be **stored** under water.

WARNING.*Phosphorus has been used for the illicit preparation of explosives or fireworks; care is required with its supply.*

Adverse Effects
Symptoms of acute poisoning by phosphorus, a general protoplasmic poison, may include an odour of garlic in the breath, burning pain in the abdomen, intense thirst, nausea, vomiting, profuse diarrhoea, renal disorders, hypoprothrombinaemia and haemorrhage, delirium, convulsions, and coma. After a period usually of between 1 and 2 days there may be a remission of symptoms followed by jaundice, hepatic failure, peripheral circulatory collapse, prostration, coma, and death.

The fatal dose is about 100 mg, though it may be as low as 50 mg; a dose of 15 mg may be severely toxic.
Symptoms of chronic poisoning are very slow in onset and are associated with lowered resistance to infection and defective tissue repair. They include periostitis and necrosis of the upper and lower jaw ('phossy jaw').
Externally, phosphorus causes severe burns to the skin.
In Great Britain the recommended exposure limits of yellow phosphorus are 0.1 mg per m^3 (long-term); 0.3 mg per m^3 (short-term).

Three cases of acute phosphorus poisoning in children after accidental ingestion of unknown amounts of rat poisons.— F. A. Simon and L. K. Pickering, *J. Am. med. Ass.*, 1976, *235*, 1343.

For a reference to 3 cases of haemolytic anaemia following phosphorus burn injuries, see J. V. Dacie and S. M. Worrledge, *Prog. Hemat.*, 1969, *6*, 82.

Treatment of Adverse Effects

After ingestion of phosphorus the stomach should be washed out with copious amounts of water; a 1 in 5000 solution of potassium permanganate (very pale pink) or a 1 in 1000 solution of copper sulphate have also been advocated.

Liquid paraffin may be introduced into the stomach following lavage and left there. The use of digestible fats and oils should be avoided. Solutions of glucose should be given intravenously to correct dehydration and the circulation should be maintained by intravenous infusions of plasma or of suitable electrolyte solutions.

Treat for liver damage with a high-carbohydrate diet. Phytomenadione should be given intravenously and repeated according to the prothrombin time. Injections of hydrocortisone have been suggested for severe liver failure; exchange blood transfusions have also been suggested. Peritoneal dialysis or haemodialysis may be required for renal failure. Treat burns by irrigation with water and then large quantities of a 1% copper sulphate solution; sodium bicarbonate solution has also been used.

Uses and Administration

Elemental phosphorus is no longer used in medicine. Inorganic phosphates are given in deficiency states and bone diseases. Phosphorus has been used in the manufacture of rat poisons.

It is used in homoeopathic medicine.

Phosphorus in a 1 to 2% paste had been used as a cockroach poison and rodenticide. Because of the risk of fire, phosphorus should never be mixed with bait but should be mixed with substances containing liquids, such as molasses, fat, or water. However, it was recommended that phosphorus should no longer be used on account of its toxicity; 15 mg could be severely toxic and 50 mg fatal. Other more effective rodenticides were available.— Safe Use of Pesticides, Twentieth Report of the WHO Expert Committee on Insecticides, *Tech. Rep. Ser. Wld Hlth Org. No. 513*, 1973.

13109-r

Physalis

Alkekengi; Bladder Cherry; Chinese Lantern; Ground Cherry; Strawberry Tomato; Winter Cherry.

The berries of ***Physalis alkekengi*** (Solanaceae), reputed to have diuretic properties.

Cape gooseberry is the edible fruit of ***P. peruviana.***

Investigation of the potential antineoplastic constituents of Physalis in *mice*.— K. Dornberger, *Pharmazie*, 1986, *41*, 265.

13110-j

Phytohaemagglutinin

PHA; Phytohemagglutin.

CAS — 9008-97-3.

Phytohaemagglutinin is one of a group of proteins termed lectins that are reported to agglutinate cells by binding to specific carbohydrate residues. It is a complex mucoprotein extract from the seeds of the bean, ***Phaseolus vulgaris***, and certain other plants. It consists of at least 3 factors which, respectively, cause haemagglutination, serum-protein precipitation, and the stimulation of mitosis in white blood cells and has been found to stimulate the production of an interferon-like substance by human leucocytes ***in vitro***. The blastogenic response of lymphocytes to phytohaemagglutinin has been used extensively as a measure of immunocompetence and may be of value in detecting and monitoring malignant disease.

It has been tried in the treatment of aplastic anaemia but results have been equivocal.

A finding of cancer-specific changes in lymphocytes after stimulation with phytohaemagglutinin.— J. A. V. Pritchard *et al.*, *ibid.*, 1978, *2*, 1275.

An evaluation of phytohaemagglutinin as a diagnostic agent for sarcoidosis.— R. J. Bonforte *et al.* (letter), *Lancet*, 1972, *1*, 958.

Further references: J. Pepys, *Br. J. Hosp. Med.*, 1984, *32*, 120; D. H. Crawford, *ibid.*, 112; *Br. med. J.*, 1985, *290*, 584.

19656-b

Picartamide *(rINN)*.

RP-40749. (±)-Tetrahydro-*N*-methyl-2-(2-pyridyl)thio-2-thiophenecarboxamide.

$C_{11}H_{14}N_2S_2$=238.4.

CAS — 76732-75-7.

Picartamide inhibits gastric secretion and is under investigation for the treatment of peptic ulcers.

References: Y. Minaire *et al.* (letter), *Lancet*, 1982, *1*, 1179; Y. Minaire *et al.*, *Drugs exp. & clin. Res.*, 1983, *9*, 935; P. J. Malè *et al.*, *Gut*, 1984, *25*, A564; G. F. Nelis (letter), *Lancet*, 1984, *1*, 803; G. F. Nelis *et al.*, *Gut*, 1985, *26*, A1119; P. J. Malè *et al.*, *ibid.*, 1986, *27*, 423.

19658-g

Picenadol Hydrochloride *(USAN, rINNM)*.

LY-136595((-)-isomer); LY-136596((+)-isomer); LY-150720. (±)-*trans-m*-(1,3-Dimethyl-4-propyl-4-piperidyl)phenol hydrochloride.

$C_{16}H_{25}NO,HCl$=283.8.

CAS — 74685-16-8 (hydrochloride); 79201-85-7 (picenadol).

Picenadol hydrochloride is an opioid analgesic under investigation.

References: D. M. Sherline, *Am. J. Obstet. Gynec.*, 1983, *147*, 404.

Proprietary Names and Manufacturers

Lilly, USA.

19659-q

Picibanil

OK-432.

Picibanil which is derived from ***Streptococcus pyogenes*** is an immunomodulator employed in the treatment of malignant neoplasms and viral infections.

References to picibanil in hepatitis B: F. Ichida *et al.*, *J. int. med. Res.*, 1985, *13*, 59.

References to picibanil in malignant neoplasms: *Lancet*, 1983, *1*, 1258; M. Kato *et al.* (letter), *ibid.*, 1985, *2*, 270.

Proprietary Names and Manufacturers

Chugai, Jpn.

3939-x

Picotamide

4-Methoxy-*N*,*N*′-bis(3-pyridinylmethyl)-1,3-benzenedicarboxamide.

$C_{21}H_{20}N_4O_3$=376.4.

CAS — 32828-81-2; 86247-87-2 (tartrate).

Picotamide is an anticoagulant and fibrinolytic given by mouth in thrombo-embolic and atherosclerotic disorders.

Proprietary Names and Manufacturers

Plactidil *(Samil, Ital.)*.

2498-m

Picumast *(BAN, pINN)*.

BM-15100 (hydrochloride). 7-[3-(4-*p*-Chlorobenzylpiperazin-1-yl)propoxy]-3,4-dimethylcoumarin.

$C_{25}H_{29}ClN_2O_3$=441.0.

CAS — 39577-19-0; 39577-20-3 (hydrochloride).

Picumast is under investigation as an anti-allergic compound.

References: E. S. K. Assem and E. K. S. Chong, *Br. J. Pharmac.*, 1976, *57*, 437P; E. Gonsior *et al.*, *Int. J. clin. Pharmac. Biopharm.*, 1979, *17*, 283.

Proprietary Names and Manufacturers

Boehringer Mannheim, Ger.; MCP Pharmaceuticals, UK.

19663-m

Pimobendan *(rINN)*.

UD-CG-115-BS. 4,5-Dihydro-6-[2-(*p*-methyoxyphenyl)-5-benzimidazolyl]-5-methyl-3(2*H*)-pyridazinone.

$C_{19}H_{18}N_4O_2$=334.4.

CAS — 74150-27-9.

Pimobendan is a positive inotropic agent under investigation.

References: J. C. A. von Meel, *Arzneimittel-Forsch.*, 1985, *35*, 284; H. Maier-Lenz *et al.*, *J. clin. Pharmac.*, 1985, *25*, 455.

Proprietary Names and Manufacturers

Boehringer Ingelheim, Ger.

510-y

Pimonidazole *(BAN, rINN)*.

Ro-03-8799; Ro-03-8799-001 (hydrochloride). 1-(2-Nitroimidazol-1-yl)-3-piperidinopropan-2-ol.

$C_{11}H_{18}N_4O_3$=254.3.

CAS — 70132-50-2 (pimonidazole); 70132-51-3 (hydrochloride).

Pimonidazole is a hypoxic cell radiosensitiser under investigation as an adjunct to cancer chemotherapy.

References: J. G. Allen *et al.*, *Eur. J. clin. Pharmac.*, 1984, *27*, 483.

Proprietary Names and Manufacturers

Roche, Switz.

13119-d

Pinaverium Bromide *(rINN)*.

4-(6-Bromoveratryl)-4-{2-[2-(10-norpinan-2-yl)ethoxy]ethyl}morpholinium bromide.

$C_{26}H_{41}Br_2NO_4$=591.4.

CAS — 59995-65-2 (pinaverium); 53251-94-8 (bromide).

Pinaverium bromide is used as an antispasmodic in doses of 50 mg by mouth three times daily.

Studies ***in vitro*** have concluded that the inhibitory action of pinaverium bromide on smooth muscle contraction at low concentrations was due to an interaction with calcium channels (A. Baumgartner *et al.*, *Br. J. Pharmac.*, 1985, *86*, 89; F. Wuytack *et al.*, *Eur. J. Pharmac.*, 1985, *114*, 85).

Two patients experienced heartburn and dysphagia after taking pinaverium bromide by mouth between meals; endoscopy revealed acute oesophageal ulceration which healed on discontinuation of treatment. The manufacturers recommendation to take pinaverium bromide during meals was emphasised.— J. -M. André *et al.*, *Acta endosc.*, 1980, *10*, 289.

Pinaverium bromide might interfere with the absorption of drugs from the small bowel. However, it was not found to affect the activity of digoxin, digitoxin, heparin, nicoumalone, sulphonylurea hypoglycaemics, or insulin.— C. Devred *et al.*, *Curr. med. Res. Opinion*, 1986, *10*, 1.

For a report of the use of pinaverium bromide in irritable bowel syndrome, see Domperidone, p.1089.

Proprietary Names and Manufacturers
Dicetel *(Charton, Canad.; Latéma, Fr.; Farmades, Ital.; Kali-Chemie, Switz.)*; Eldicet *(Kali-Farma, Spain)*.

19665-v

Pipequaline *(rINN)*.

2-Phenyl-4-[2-(4-piperidyl)ethyl]quinoline.
$C_{22}H_{24}N_2$=316.4.

CAS — 77472-98-1.

Pipequaline is an anxiolytic agent under investigation.

References: J. A. Poggioli *et al., Curr. ther. Res.*, 1985, *38*, 423.

Proprietary Names and Manufacturers
Pharmuka, Fr.

19666-g

Piperaquine Phosphate

$C_{29}H_{32}Cl_2N_6.4H_3PO_4.4H_2O$=999.6.

Pharmacopoeias. In *Chin.*

Piperaquine, which is reported to be 1,3-bis[1-(7-chloro-4-quinolyl)-4-piperazinyl]propane, and hydroxypiperaquine have antimalarial activity.

References: L. Chen *et al., Chin. med. J.*, 1982, *95*, 281; W. B. Guan *et al., J. Parasitol. parasit. Dis.*, 1983, *1*, 88.

13121-k

Piperazine Camsylate

Piperazine di(camphor-10-sulphonate).
$C_4H_{10}N_2,(C_{10}H_{16}O_4S)_2$=550.7.

CAS — 27016-31-5.

Piperazine camsylate has been used for its reputed stimulant effect on the cardiovascular and respiratory systems.

Proprietary Names and Manufacturers
Solucamphre *(Delalande, Fr.; Delalande, Switz.)*.

5240-n

Pipoxolan Hydrochloride *(BANM, USAN, pINNM)*.

5,5-Diphenyl-2-(2-piperidinoethyl)-1,3-dioxolan-4-one hydrochloride.
$C_{22}H_{25}NO_3,HCl$=387.9.

CAS — 23744-24-3 (pipoxolan); 18174-58-8 (hydrochloride).

Pipoxolan hydrochloride is used as an antispasmodic in doses of 10 to 30 mg two or three times daily by mouth or rectum.

Proprietary Names and Manufacturers
Paraespas *(Ima, Arg.)*; Rocofin *(Alter, Spain)*; Rowapraxin *(Sanico, Belg.; Rowa-Wagner, Ger.; Rowa, S.Afr.)*.

3738-e

Piprozolin *(USAN, rINN)*.

Gö-919; W-3699. Ethyl (3-ethyl-4-oxo-5-piperidinothiazolidin-2-ylidene)acetate.
$C_{14}H_{22}N_2O_3S$=298.4.

CAS — 17243-64-0.

Piprozolin is a choleretic. It has been given in doses of 100 to 200 mg three times daily.

References: K. -O. Vollmer *et al., Arzneimittel-Forsch.*, 1977, *27*, 502; V. Gladigau and I. Ehret, *ibid.*, 512; E. Schleicher, *Arzneimittel-Forsch.*, 1977, *27*, 520.

Proprietary Names and Manufacturers
Probilin *(Gödecke, Ger.; Parke, Davis, Ital.; Parke, Davis, Spain)*; Prozobil *(Morgens, Spain)*; Secrebil *(Isnardi, Ital.)*.

13124-x

Piracetam *(BAN, USAN, rINN)*.

CI-871; Pyrrolidone Acetamide; UCB-6215. 2-(2-Oxopyrrolidin-1-yl)acetamide.
$C_6H_{10}N_2O_2$=142.2.

CAS — 7491-74-9.

Piracetam acts on the central nervous system and has been described as a 'nootropic' although its mode of action is not certain. It is said to protect the cerebral cortex against hypoxia and has been used following trauma or surgery and in a variety of disorders including alcoholism, vertigo, senile dementia, cerebrovascular accidents, and behavioural disorders in children. Piracetam has been given by mouth in doses of 800 mg three times daily. In severe disorders it has been given by intramuscular or intravenous injection.
Piracetam has also been tried in the treatment of sickle-cell anaemia.

A report of basic toxicological studies on piracetam.— M. Giurgea, *Farmaco, Edn prat.*, 1977, *32*, 47.

After administration by mouth to 6 fasting subjects, piracetam 800 mg gave peak plasma concentrations of about 15 to 19 µg per mL in about 30 minutes and declined with a half-life of about 5 to 6 hours. Elimination after intravenous injection was similar.— J. G. Gobert and E. L. Baltès, *Farmaco, Edn prat.*, 1977, *32*, 83.

Prothrombin time was increased in a patient stabilised on warfarin when treatment with piracetam was started.— H. Y. M. Pan and R. P. Ng, *Eur. J. clin. Pharmac.*, 1983, *24*, 711.

EFFECTS ON THE BLOOD. *Sickle-cell anaemia.* A report of piracetam inhibiting and reversing sickling *in vitro* and producing beneficial effects in 12 patients. The dose in a crisis was 80 mg per kg body-weight in 300 mL of glucose injection infused every 8 hours for 3 days. Maintenance was with 1 g intramuscularly daily for 6 months then 1.2 g every 8 hours by mouth. Maintenance in children was with 600 mg three times daily by mouth.— J. T. de Araujo and G. S. Nero (letter), *Lancet*, 1977, *2*, 411.

Further reports of *in-vivo* and *in-vitro* studies of piracetam in sickle-cell anaemia: G. O. S. de Melo, *Lancet*, 1976, *2*, 1139; R. M. Nalbandian *et al.* (letter), *ibid.*, 1978, *2*, 570; F. F. Costa *et al.* (letter), *ibid.*, 1979, *2*, 1302; I. M. Franklin (letter), *ibid.*, 1980, *1*, 767.

NEUROLOGICAL DISORDERS. A review of the treatment of memory loss in geriatric patients. Piracetam has been studied widely with contradictory results. Some investigators believe it shows promise as a cerebral stimulant in elderly subjects with mild to moderate cognitive impairment while other researchers found no significant results when using it in geriatric patients. Studies show that lower doses are best for long-term treatment: higher doses produce a rapid effect but are accompanied by a number of adverse effects including overstimulation, sleep disturbances, and dizziness. Piracetam is devoid of any sedative, analgesic, analeptic, neuroleptic, tranquillising, or autonomic effects. Some beneficial effects have been observed with the use of piracetam used in association with choline or lecithin in patients with Alzheimer's disease.— V. J. Galizia, *Drug Intell. & clin. Pharm.*, 1984, *18*, 784.

The use of piracetam in Alzheimer's disease has been reviewed by Hollister (*Drugs*, 1985, *29*, 483) who concluded that it produced a beneficial effect similar to that produced by co-dergocrine mesylate, and also by Kendall *et al.* (*J. clin. Hosp. Pharm.*, 1985, *10*, 327) who concluded that clinical studies had not shown evidence of convincing therapeutic efficacy. Hollander (*Br. med. Bull.*, 1986, *42*, 97) summarised the results of studies of the use of piracetam in association with lecithin, and concluded that this combination may have some beneficial effect in a subgroup of patients with Alzheimer's disease in whom the degenerative process has spared some quantity of functionally intact cholinergic neurones.

Further reviews and discussions of the use of piracetam in cerebrovascular and cognitive disorders: A. Spagnoli and G. Tognoni, *Drugs*, 1983, *26*, 44; *Drug & Ther. Bull.*, 1984, *22*, 98.

Piracetam 10 g daily was well accepted in a controlled study of 100 patients and was considered to improve the level of consciousness postoperatively.— A. E. Richardson and F. J. Bereen (preliminary communication), *Lancet*, 1977, *2*, 1110.

In a double-blind crossover study of 16 epileptic patients with learning difficulties, aged between 8 and 20 years, treatment with piracetam 1.2 to 2.4 g daily in divided doses, depending on body-weight, resulted in significant improvements in alertness, some aspects of visual perception, and achievement at school. The patients recovered more rapidly and were less confused following seizures.— P. S. Kunneke and G. M. Malan, *Br. J. clin. Pract.*, 1979, *33*, 266.

Report of beneficial response of vertigo to piracetam treatment.— W. J. Oosterveld, *Arzneimittel-Forsch.*, 1980, *30*, 1947.

Piracetam 4 g intravenously reduced extrapyramidal symptoms, particularly akathisia, induced by neuroleptic therapy in a cross-over, placebo-controlled study in 40 patients.— J. Kabes *et al., Int. Pharmacopsychiat.*, 1982, *17*, 185.

A favourable effect of piracetam 9 g daily by intravenous injection was observed in a double-blind cross-over study in 24 patients with alcoholic psychosis.— V. Skondia and J. Kabes, *J. int. med. Res.*, 1985, *13*, 185.

Further reports of the use of piracetam in alcoholic patients: S. J. Dencker *et al., J. int. med. Res.*, 1978, *6*, 395.

Improvement in reading speed and beneficial effect on short-term memory were observed following piracetam therapy in a study involving 240 dyslexic children.— M. di Ianni *et al., J. clin. Psychopharmacol.*, 1985, *5*, 272.

Proprietary Names and Manufacturers
Avigilen *(Efeka, Ger.)*; Cerebroforte *(Azuchemie, Ger.)*; Cerebropan *(ISM, Ital.)*; Cerebrosteril *(Fresenius, Ger.)*; Cetam *(Formenti, Ital.)*; Ciclocetam *(Spain)*; Ciclofalina *(Almirall, Spain)*; Cuxabrain *(TAD, Ger.)*; Durapitrop *(Durachemie, Ger.)*; Encefalux *(Geve, Spain)*; Encetrop *(Siegfried, Ger.)*; Gabacet *(Carrion, Fr.)*; Genogris *(Vita, Spain)*; Gericetam *(Level, Spain)*; Huberdasen *(Hubber, Spain)*; Idéaxan *(Millot-Solac, Fr.)*; Memo-Puren *(Klinge-Nattermann, Ger.)*; Merapiran *(Finadiet, Arg.)*; Neuronova *(Valles Mestre, Spain)*; Noostan *(Rhodia, Arg.)*; Nootrop *(UCB, Ger.)*; Noo-Tropicon *(Sidus, Arg.)*; Nootropil *(UCB, Belg.; UCB, Ital.; UCB, Neth.; UCB, S.Afr.; UCB, Spain; UCB, Switz.)*; Nootropyl *(UCB, Fr.)*; Normabrain *(Cassella-Riedel, Ger.)*; Norzetam *(Albert-Farma, Ital.)*; Novocetam *(Beiersdorf, Ger.)*; Pirroxil *(SIT, Ital.)*; Psycoton *(Esseti, Ital.)*; Stimucortex *(Kali-Farma, Spain)*; Tonibral *(Bago, Arg.)*.

2917-g

Pirarubicin *(rINN)*.

Theprubicin; THP-ADM; THP-doxorubicin. (8*S*,10*S*)-10-{[3-Amino-2,3,6-trideoxy-4-*O*-(tetrahydro-2*H*-pyran-2-yl)-α-L-*lyxo*-hexopyranosyl]-oxy}-8-glycoloyl-7,8,9,10-tetrahydro-6,8,11-trihydroxy-1-methoxy-5,12-naphthacenedione.
$C_{32}H_{37}NO_{12}$=627.6.

CAS — 72496-41-4.

Pirarubicin is an antineoplastic agent under investigation.

Proprietary Names and Manufacturers
Meiji, Jpn.

13131-t

Pirenoxine Sodium *(rINNM)*.

Catalin Sodium; Pirfenoxone Sodium. Sodium 1-hydroxy-5-oxo-5*H*-pyrido[3,2-*a*]phenoxazine-3-carboxylate.
$C_{16}H_7N_2NaO_5$=330.2.

CAS — 1043-21-6 (pirenoxine); 51410-30-1 (sodium salt).

Pirenoxine sodium has been used in the treatment of cataracts, usually as eye-drops.

References: A. Pirie and R. van Heyningen (letter), *Lancet*, 1974, *2*, 169; H. Maclean *et al.* (letter), *ibid.*, 895.

Proprietary Names and Manufacturers
Catalin *(Senju, Jpn)*; Clarvisan *(Allergan, Ital.; Abello, Spain)*; Clarvisor *(Thilo, Ger.)*.

13132-x

Pirglutargine

Arginine Pidolate; Arginine Pyroglutamate. L-Arginine DL-pyroglutamate.

$C_{11}H_{21}N_5O_5$=303.3.

CAS — 64855-91-0.

Pirglutargine has been used for its reputed cerebral stimulant effect.

Proprietary Names and Manufacturers

Adiuvant *(Manetti Roberts, Ital.).*

13133-r

Piridoxilate *(BAN, rINN).*

Pyridoxine α_5-Hemiacetal Glyoxylate; Pyridoxylate. The reciprocal salt of 2-(5-hydroxy-4-hydroxymethyl-6-methyl-3-pyridylmethoxy)glycolic acid with 2-[4,5-bis(hydroxymethyl)-2-methyl-3-pyridyloxy]glycolic acid (1:1).

$C_{10}H_{13}NO_6,C_{10}H_{13}NO_6$=486.4.

CAS — 24340-35-0.

Piridoxilate is claimed to increase tissue oxygenation. It has been used in the treatment of circulatory insufficiency, including peripheral, cerebral, and coronary disorders.

A report of nephrolithiasis in 2 patients on long-term treatment with piridoxilate. The stones were composed of calcium oxalate.— M. Daudon *et al.* (letter), *Lancet*, 1985, *1*, 1338.

Proprietary Names and Manufacturers

Glyo-6 *(Houdé, Fr.; Dieckmann, Ger.; Roussel Maestretti, Ital.)*; Venartan *(Fidia, Ital.).*

18947-q

Pirmagrel *(USAN, rINN).*

CGS-13080. Imidazo[1,5-*a*]pyridine-5-hexanoic acid.

$C_{13}H_{16}N_2O_2$=232.3.

CAS — 85691-74-3.

Pirmagrel is a thromboxane synthetase inhibitor under investigation in thrombotic or ischaemic disorders.

References: M. W. McNab *et al., J. clin. Pharmac.*, 1984, *24*, 76; A. M. Lefer, *Drugs of the Future*, 1984, *9*, 437; *ibid.*, 1986, *11*, 504.

Proprietary Names and Manufacturers

Ciba-Geigy, Switz.

5241-h

Pitofenone Hydrochloride *(rINNM).*

Methyl 2-[4-(2-piperidinoethoxy)benzoyl]benzoate hydrochloride.

$C_{22}H_{25}NO_4$,HCl=403.9.

CAS — 54063-52-4 (pitofenone).

Pitofenone hydrochloride is used as an antispasmodic; it has been given by mouth, rectally, or by intramuscular or slow intravenous injection.

190-y

Pivopril *(USAN, rINN).*

Pivalopril; REV-3659-(S); RHC-3659-(S); RHC-3659-S; USV-3659-(S). (−)-(*S*)-*N*-Cyclopentyl-*N*-(3-mercapto-2-methylpropionyl)glycine 2,2-dimethylthiopropionate.

$C_{16}H_{27}NO_4S$=329.5.

CAS — 81045-50-3.

Pivopril is an ACE inhibitor under investigation in hypertension.

References: M. Burnier *et al., Br. J. clin. Pharmac.*, 1981, *12*, 893; *Drugs of the Future*, 1986, *11*, 116.

Proprietary Names and Manufacturers

USV Pharmaceutical Corp., USA.

13140-x

Plasminogen

CAS — 9001-91-6.

Plasminogen is the specific substance derived from plasma which, when activated to plasmin by streptokinase, has the property of lysing fibrinogen, fibrin, and some other proteins.

Plasminogen is being investigated as a thrombolytic agent.

Proprietary Names and Manufacturers

Green Cross Corp., Jpn.

13141-r

Plastics

Pharmacopoeias. Many pharmacopoeias include standards for plastic containers and closures.

Adverse Effects

Plastic materials used in medicine and pharmacy may give rise to various adverse effects, either by direct contact of the plastic with tissues or by indirect contact as when a solution stored in a plastic container, such as a disposable syringe, is injected. Adverse effects may also arise among workers through handling the materials or by inhaling fumes during manufacture.

Pure polymeric plastics appear to be of low toxicity, but some monomers and substances added during manufacture to impart specific physical properties are toxic. These additives include plasticisers added to reduce brittleness, ultraviolet-ray absorbers to prevent degradation by light, and antioxidants and lubricants which are sometimes needed for satisfactory processing. The monomer residues and additives can leach out from the finished plastic materials and have been the main cause of the adverse effects that have been reported though carcinogenic effects have been produced by prolonged implantation of some pure plastics. The adverse effects produced are diverse, depending upon the nature of the plastic and the toxicity of the additives as well as upon the site and duration of contact; they include haemolysis of blood cells, thrombosis, sensitisation reactions, precancerous changes, and local tissue necrosis. Silicone particles have been shed from dialysis tubing resulting in hypersplenism, pancytopenia, and occasionally in the production of a granulomatous hepatitis.

See also under Vinyl Chloride, p.1629, Methylmethacrylate, p.1589, and Polytef, p.1604.

Trimellitic anhydride (TMA), used in the manufacture of plastics, epoxy resins, and paints can cause asthma and rhinitis, a late respiratory systemic syndrome, 'pulmonary disease-anaemia syndrome', and an irritant syndrome.

In Great Britain the recommended exposure limit of trimellitic anhydride is 0.04 mg per m^3 (long-term).

APPARATUS AND CONTAINERS. Chlormethiazole, diazepam, glyceryl trinitrate, hydralazine hydrochloride, insulin, isosorbide dinitrate, some phenothiazines, thiopentone sodium, vitamin A acetate, and warfarin sodium can be lost from infusion solutions in clinically significant amounts due to sorption to polyvinyl chloride giving sets and containers. Negligible sorption of many of these agents to polyethylene/polypropylene apparatus, and reduced sorption to polybutadiene/methacrylate butadiene stearate giving sets has been shown.

Bacterial adherence to plastics has been studied. Polytetrafluoroethylene had the lowest ability to attract bacteria, it was easy to wash, and no bacteria remained attached after washing. Polyethylene had the highest affinity for the bacteria tested.

Plasticisers. The plasticiser bis-(2-ethylhexyl)phthalate (di(2-ethylhexyl)phthalate) has been shown to leach from polyvinyl chloride containers and apparatus including blood bags and haemodialysis tubing. Leaching depends upon the hydropholicity of the solution in contact with the plastic and is greater with fat emulsions and blood than aqueous solutions. Long-term effects are unknown. The *Eur. P.* states that materials based on plasticised polyvinyl chloride for containers for human blood and blood components may not contain more than 40% of bis(2-ethylhexyl)phthalate.

In Great Britain the recommended exposure limits of bis(2-ethylhexyl)phthalate are 5 mg per m^3 (long-term) and 10 mg per m^3 (short-term). In the *US* the permissible exposure limit is 5 mg per m^3.

CONTACT LENSES. Hydrophilic plastics used for many soft contact lenses will selectively bind certain preservatives and could then be a source of irritation. Thiomersal is usually satisfactory. Chlorhexidine acetate is satisfactory in some cases, while phenylmercuric acetate or nitrate is usually satisfactory but is not recommended for long-term treatment. Benzalkonium chloride is unsuitable in all cases.

Loss of antibacterial preservatives from contact lens solutions stored in some types of plastic containers has occurred.

Topical fluorescein, Rose Bengal, and adrenaline have been reported to spoil hydrophilic contact lenses. Unless eye-drops are specifically indicated as safe to use with hydrophilic contact lenses, the lenses should be removed before instillation and not worn during the period of treatment.

Drugs excreted in the tears, such as rifampicin and sulphasalazine, may discolour soft contact lenses.

2366-j

Plaunotol *(rINN).*

CS-684. (2*Z*,6*E*)-2-[(3*E*)-4,8-Dimethyl-3,7-nonadienyl]-6-methyl-2,6-octadiene-1,8-diol.

$C_{20}H_{34}O_2$=306.5.

CAS — 64218-02-6.

Plaunotol has been used in the treatment of peptic ulcer.

Proprietary Names and Manufacturers

Kelnac *(Sankyo, Jpn).*

5006-j

Polacrilin Potassium *(USAN, rINNM).*

Polacrilinum Kalii.

CAS — 54182-62-6; 50602-21-6 (both used for polacrilin).

Pharmacopoeias. In *U.S.N.F.*

The potassium salt of a carboxylic cation-exchange resin prepared from methacrylic acid and divinylbenzene. An odourless or almost odourless, white to off-white, free-flowing powder. Practically **insoluble** in water and in most liquids.

Polacrilin potassium is used as a tablet disintegrant.

13143-d

Poly A.poly U

Polyadenylic-polyuridylic Acid.

CAS — 24936-38-7.

Poly A.poly U is a double-stranded polyribonucleotide comprising polyadenylic and polyuridylic acids, and is believed to be a stimulant of the immune system. It has been studied as an adjuvant in the management of operable solid tumours.

In a randomised study of 300 women with operable breast cancer treated with surgery followed, if axillary nodes were involved, by radiotherapy, 155 received poly A.poly U 30 mg intravenously weekly for 6 weeks while 145 received control injections of sodium chloride (0.9%). A significant increase in the overall 5-year survival was noted in the group given poly A.poly U and 'relapse-free' survival in patients with node involvement was particularly increased.— J. Lacour *et al., Lancet*, 1980, *2*, 161. At follow-up after a mean of 87 months the overall survival rate after surgery for breast cancer was significantly greater in patients who received poly A.poly U. In patients without lymph node involvement there was no difference in survival, but in those with lymph node involvement (up to 3 affected nodes) the survival-rate was significantly greater. Interferon and natural killer cell activity are possibly involved in the action of poly A.poly U.— *idem, Br. med. J.*, 1984, *288*, 589. Comment.— M. Baum and R. A'Hern, *ibid.*, 1009.

Further references: J. Lacour, *J. biol. Response Mod.*,

1985, *4*, 538; A. G. Hovanessian *et al.*, *Cancer*, 1985, *15*, 357; J. K. Youn *et al.*, *Int. J. Immunopharmacol.*, 1987, *9*, 313.

13144-n

Poly I.poly C

Polyinosinic-polycytidylic Acid.

CAS — 24939-03-5.

Poly I.poly C is a synthetic double-stranded polyribonucleotide complex of equimolar concentrations of polyinosinic and polycytidylic acids.

Poly I.poly C and the complex of poly I.poly C stabilised with poly-L-lysine in carboxymethylcellulose [poly(ICLC)] have been found to induce the production of interferon.

A review of interferons and interferon inducers.— R. B. Pollard, *Drugs*, 1982, *23*, 37.

Side-effects reported with poly I.poly C have included nausea, vomiting, and fever.— R. B. Pollard, *Drugs*, 1982, *23*, 37.

Fever was observed in 7 patients with malignant brain tumours given poly(ICLC) intravenously. Other adverse effects included modest hypotension, leucopenia, and transient elevation of liver enzymes.— O. Nakamura *et al.*, *J. Interferon Res.*, 1982, *2*, 1.

ACTION. Poly(ICLC) had antiviral activity against hepatitis B virus infection in *chimpanzees*.— R. H. Purcell *et al.*, *Lancet*, 1976, *2*, 757.

Poly I.poly C inhibited strains of herpes simplex virus isolated from patients with herpetic keratitis.— O. Smetana *et al.*, *Antimicrob. Ag. Chemother.*, 1977, *11*, 797.

The successful use of poly I.poly C with a single dose of human diploid rabies vaccine for the protection of rhesus *monkeys* from lethal doses of rabies virus.— G. M. Baer *et al.*, *Bull. Wld Hlth Org.*, 1979, *57*, 807.

The production *in vitro* of interferon through induction by poly I.poly C or by a complex of poly I.poly C and a dextran was enhanced from 10 to 100 times by pretreatment of cells with amphotericin or other polyene macrolides.— E. C. Borden *et al.*, *Antimicrob. Ag. Chemother.*, 1978, *13*, 159. See also E. C. Borden *et al.*, *ibid.*, 1979, *16*, 203.

CANCER. Clinical studies of poly I.poly C or poly(ICLC) in cancer patients: R. A. Robinson *et al.*, *J. natn. Cancer Inst.*, 1976, *57*, 599; A. S. Levine *et al.*, *Cancer Res.*, 1979, *39*, 1645; B. C. Lampkin *et al.*, *Cancer Res.*, 1985, *45*, 5904; R. L. Theriault *et al.*, *Cancer Treat. Rep.*, 1986, *70*, 1341; M. J. Droiler, *J. Urol., Baltimore*, 1987, *137*, 202.

MULTIPLE SCLEROSIS. References to the use of poly I.poly C to treat patients with multiple sclerosis: D. E. McFarlin *et al.*, *J. biol. Response Mod.*, 1985, *4*, 544; C. T. Bever *et al.*, *Neurology*, 1986, *36*, 494.

VIRAL INFECTIONS. An evaluation of poly I.poly C as an interferon inducer in viral respiratory diseases. A small but definite reduction in symptoms of upper respiratory tract illness had been associated with intranasal administration of poly I.poly C.— D. A. Hill *et al.*, *J. Am. med. Ass.*, 1972, *219*, 1179.

In a double-blind study of 24 children with cancer and herpes zoster the topical application to the herpes lesions of poly I.poly C in varying strengths was of no benefit.— S. Feldman *et al.*, *Antimicrob. Ag. Chemother.*, 1975, *8*, 289.

In a double-blind placebo-controlled study of 57 patients poly(ICLC) applied topically was of no benefit in the treatment of recurrent genital herpes simplex virus infection.— L. R. Crane *et al.*, *Antimicrob. Ag. Chemother.*, 1982, *21*, 481.

Beneficial results with poly(ICLC) in 2 children with recurrent laryngeal papillomatosis; continued administration appeared to be necessary.— B. G. Leventhal *et al.*, *J. Pediat.*, 1981, *99*, 614. Poly(ICLC) is a potent pyrogen and the recession of the tumours could have been due to the effect of hyperthermia.— R. M. Roberts (letter), *ibid.*, 1982, *101*, 158. Reply.— B. G. Leventhal (letter), *ibid.*, 159.

3940-y

Polyethylene Excipient *(USAN)*.

Pharmacopoeias. In *U.S.N.F.*

A homopolymer produced by the direct polymerisation of ethylene. Polyethylene excipient is a white, translucent, partially crystalline and partially amorphous resin. Available in various grades and types, differing from one another in molecular weight, molecular weight distribution, degree of chain branching, and extent of crystallinity. **Soluble** in hot benzene; insoluble in water. **Store** in well-closed containers.

Polyethylene excipient is used as a viscosity-modifying agent in pharmaceutical preparations.

3271-z

Polyethylene Oxide *(USAN)*.

Pharmacopoeias. In *U.S.N.F.*

A nonionic homopolymer of ethylene oxide, represented by the formula $(OCH_2CH_2)n$, in which *n* represents the average number of oxyethylene groups (about 2000 to over 100 000). It is obtainable in several grades, varying in viscosity profile. It may contain not more than 3% of silicon dioxide. All molecular weight grades are powdered or granular solids. **Soluble** in water; freely soluble in acetonitrile, in ethylene dichloride, in trichloroethylene, and in methylene chloride; insoluble in aliphatic hydrocarbons, in ethylene glycol, in diethylene glycol, and in glycerol. **Store** in airtight containers. Protect from light.

Polyethylene oxide is used as a tablet binder and viscosity-modifying agent in pharmaceutical preparations.

13146-m

Polyhexanide *(BAN)*.

ICI-9073; Polihexanide *(rINN)*. Poly(1-hexamethylenebiguanide hydrochloride).

$(C_8H_{17}N_5,HCl)_n$=219.7×*n*.

CAS — 28757-48-4.

Polyhexanide is an antibacterial agent which has been used in contact lens solutions and in veterinary preparations.

13147-b

Polyphloretin Phosphate

PPP. A mixture of phosphorylated phloretin polymers.

CAS — 9014-72-6.

Polyphloretin phosphate is an inhibitor of alkaline phosphatase, hyaluronidase, and prostaglandins. It is also reported to reduce the permeability of serous membranes and to diminish serous exudates.

3850-e

Polysaccharide-K

PSK; PS-K.

A protein-bound polysaccharide isolated from a fungus and claimed to have immunostimulant and antineoplastic properties.

References: S. Tsukagoshi *et al.*, *Cancer Treat. Rev.*, 1984, *11*, 131.

Proprietary Names and Manufacturers

Krestin *(Sankyo, Jpn)*.

13150-f

Polytef *(USAN)*.

Politef *(pINN)*; PTFE. Poly(tetrafluoroethylene). $(C_2F_4)_n$.

CAS — 9002-84-0.

Polytef has numerous industrial applications. As 'Teflon' it is used on 'non-stick' cooking utensils.

A paste of polytef has been used for a variety of purposes including the treatment of aphonia, for replacement grafts in vascular surgery, and in the correction of vesicoureteric reflux.

References: *Br. med. J.*, 1980, *281*, 1615 (aphonia); H. C. Stansel *et al.*, *Archs Surg.*, 1979, *114*, 1291 (vascular surgery); I. G. Kidson, *Br. J. Hosp. Med.*, 1983, *30*, 248 (vascular surgery); J. W. Polley *et al.*, *Plastic reconstr. Surg.*, 1987, *79*, 39 (orbital floor reconstruction); C. C. Schulman *et al.*, *Br. med. J.*, 1984, *288*, 192 (urinary stress incontinence); B. O'Donnell and P. Puri, *ibid.*, 1986, *293*, 1404 (vesicoureteric reflux).

283-a

Polyvinox *(BAN)*.

Polyvinylbutyl Ether; Vinylinum. Poly(1-butoxyethylene).

$C_{16}H_{34}O_3,(C_6H_{12}O)_n$=2000 (approx.).

CAS — 25232-87-5.

Pharmacopoeias. In *Rus.*

Polyvinox is a synthetic resin, developed as a substitute for Peru balsam. It is used by external application undiluted, as an oily solution, or as an ointment, in the treatment of wounds and burns and various skin diseases. Polyvinox has also been administered by mouth in the treatment of gastric and duodenal ulcers, gastritis, and colitis.

Proprietary Names and Manufacturers

Shostakovsky Balsam *(Leopold Charles, UK)*.

7365-q

Poppy-seed Oil

Huile d'Oeillette; Maw Oil; Oleum Papaveris; Oleum Papaveris Seminis.

CAS — 8002-11-7.

The fixed oil expressed from the ripe seeds of the opium poppy, *Papaver somniferum* (Papaveraceae).

Poppy-seed oil is used as a substitute for olive oil for culinary and pharmaceutical purposes. It is also used in the preparation of Iodised Oil Fluid Injection. Commercial grades are used in making soaps, paints, and varnishes.

13151-d

Porcine Skin

Sterile denatured lyophilised skin, of porcine origin, consisting of the dermal and/or epidermal layers.

Porcine skin is used as a temporary dressing in burns, ulcers, and other injuries associated with skin loss. The rationale is to prevent fluid and heat loss, to reduce infection, to protect exposed structures, to reduce pain, and to prepare the site for grafting.

The material is reconstituted by immersion in sterile water or suitable saline solution using strict aseptic technique. Bovine skin is similarly used.

References: A. M. Yiacoumettis, *Br. J. clin. Pract.*, 1979, *33*, 99.

Porcine dermis was found to be a very suitable alternative to autogenous split skin mucosal or dermal grafts for the repair of defects in the mucous membrane created by surgery.— R. Mitchell, *Br. dent. J.*, 1983, *155*, 346. Critical comment.— R. Hopkins (letter), *ibid.*, 1984, *156*, 4. Reply.— R. Mitchell (letter), *ibid.*, 5. Further comment.— A. A. Quayle (letter), *ibid.*

In a randomised study involving 47 patients, pinch skin grafting achieved more rapid healing of venous ulcers than dressings with porcine dermis.— K. R. Poskitt *et al.*, *Br. med. J.*, 1987, *294*, 674.

See also G. Eriksson *et al.*, *Curr. ther. Res.*, 1984, *35*, 678.

Proprietary Preparations

Armoderm *(Armour, UK)*. A temporary biological dressing consisting of sterilised freeze-dried porcine skin. For topical application to burns and varicose ulcers, after reconstitution in a sterile, balanced electrolyte solution.

Corethium 1 *(Johnson & Johnson, UK)*. A temporary biological dressing consisting of sterilised freeze-dried porcine skin. For topical application to burns, after reconstitution in sodium chloride injection or Ringer's solution. Also available glutaraldehyde-treated for use in oral surgery. **Corethium 2.** A similar temporary dressing consisting of porcine dermis. For application to varicose ulcers and similar skin conditions. **Corethium 3.** A similar temporary dressing consisting of bovine dermis. For application to burns and skin donor sites.

Fascia Lata *(Ethicon, UK).* Sterilised strips of bovine connective tissue obtained from below the hide. A substitute for human fascia lata for use in surgery.

Zenoderm Corium Implant *(Ethicon, UK).* A sterile material prepared from porcine dermis by enzyme treatment and glutaraldehyde-crosslinking. For use by surgical implantation as a supporting tissue.

7872-m

Potassium Aminobenzoate

Aminobenzoate Potassium *(USAN).* Potassium 4-aminobenzoate.

$C_7H_6KNO_2$=175.2.

CAS — 138-84-1.

Pharmacopoeias. In *U.S.*

A 5% solution in water has a pH of 8 to 9. **Store** in airtight containers.

Adverse Effects and Precautions

Anorexia, nausea, fever, and skin rash have been reported.

Potassium aminobenzoate should be given with caution to patients with renal impairment. It should not be given concomitantly with sulphonamides.

Uses and Administration

Potassium aminobenzoate has been used in the treatment of various disorders associated with excessive fibrosis, such as scleroderma and Peyronie's disease. The usual dose is 3 g four times daily by mouth.

The non-surgical treatment of Peyronie's disease remains empirical and controversial; the value of any adjuvant treatment is inconclusive.— J. C. Gingell (letter), *Br. med. J.*, 1984, *289*, 1068.

Preparations

Aminobenzoate Potassium Capsules *(U.S.P.)*

Aminobenzoate Potassium for Oral Solution *(U.S.P.).* pH of a 10% solution 7 to 9.

Aminobenzoate Potassium Tablets *(U.S.P.)*

Proprietary Preparations

Potaba *(Glenwood, UK). Capsules,* potassium aminobenzoate 500 mg.

Powder, (envules), potassium aminobenzoate 3 g/sachet. *Tablets,* potassium aminobenzoate 500 mg.

Proprietary Names and Manufacturers of Potassium Aminobenzoate or another salt of Aminobenzoic Acid

Epiteliplast *(Llorens, Spain)*; Epitelizante Vit H1 *(Llorens, Spain)*; Fibroderm *(Torlan, Spain)*; Potaba *(Cambridge Laboratories, Austral.*; *Glenwood, Canad.*; *Glenwood, Switz.*; *Glenwood, UK*; *Glenwood, USA).*

The following names have been used for multi-ingredient preparations containing potassium aminobenzoate or another salt of aminobenzoic acid—Pabalate *(Robins, USA).*

13152-n

Potassium Borotartrate

Potassium Sodium Borotartrate; Soluble Cream of Tartar.

Potassium borotartrate is reported to have similar properties to those of bromides. It has been used in nervous disorders and is used in photography as a retarder for alkaline developers. The toxic effects of chronic boron poisoning have been reported following the use of potassium borotartrate internally (see under Boric Acid, p.1549).

Proprietary Names and Manufacturers

Neurobore *(Bouteille, Fr.).*

13153-h

Potassium Bromate

924.

$KBrO_3$=167.0.

CAS — 7758-01-2.

Adverse Effects

Ingestion of potassium bromate is followed by nausea, vomiting, severe abdominal pain, and diarrhoea. The patient becomes apathetic but very irritable; loss of consciousness, central nervous depression, and loss of tendon reflexes ensue, but convulsions may occur. Methaemoglobinaemia may occur. Kidney damage, with albuminuria and oliguria or anuria may arise. Respiration becomes shallow and rapid, the heart-rate increases, and the blood pressure falls. Body temperature is lowered. Hepatitis, pulmonary oedema, and toxic myocarditis have been reported. Death from renal failure may occur within 1 to 2 weeks.

Reports of potassium bromate poisoning: A. H. Paul, *N.Z. med. J.*, 1966, *65*, 33 (contaminated sugar); T. H. Stewart *et al.*, *S. Afr. med. J.*, 1969, *43*, 200 (excessive amount used as a flour improver); B. L. Warshaw *et al.*, *Pediatrics*, 1985, *76*, 975 (hair permanent wave preparations).

Treatment of Adverse Effects

After the ingestion of potassium bromate the stomach should be emptied by aspiration and lavage and demulcent drinks such as milk given. Pain is relieved by the injection of pethidine. An intravenous infusion of 100 to 500 mL of a 1% sodium thiosulphate solution or intravenous injection of 10 to 50 mL of a 10% solution has been recommended. If vomiting is protracted, fluid intake should be maintained with copious drinks or the intravenous infusion of glucose injection. Oxygen may be indicated and if methaemoglobinaemia is severe exchange transfusion with whole blood may be necessary; the use of methylene blue should be avoided since it may enhance the toxicity of bromate.

The prompt use of haemodialysis or peritoneal dialysis has been suggested.

Uses.

Potassium bromate is an oxidising agent. It has no therapeutic uses but it has been widely used in home permanent-wave sets as the 'neutraliser' of thioglycollate hair-waving lotions. It is also used as a flour-maturing agent.

1026-s

Potassium Bromide *(BAN).*

Brometo de Potássio; Bromure de Potassium; Kalii Bromidum; Kalium Bromatum; Pot. Brom.; Potassii Bromidum.

KBr=119.0.

CAS — 7758-02-3.

Pharmacopoeias. In *Arg., Aust., Belg., Br., Chin., Cz., Egypt., Eur., Fr., Ger., Hung., Ind., Int., Jpn, Jug., Mex., Neth., Nord., Pol., Port., Roum., Rus., Span., Swiss,* and *Turk.*

Odourless colourless crystals or white crystalline powder. Each g represents 8.4 mmol of potassium and of bromide.

Freely **soluble** in water and in glycerol; slightly soluble in alcohol.

Adverse Effects

During prolonged administration bromide accumulation may occur giving rise to bromide intoxication or bromism. Symptoms include nausea and vomiting, slurred speech, memory impairment, drowsiness, irritability, ataxia, tremors, hallucinations, mania, stupor, coma, and other manifestations of central nervous system depression. Skin rashes of various types may occur. Death after acute poisoning appears to be rare as vomiting follows the ingestion of large doses.

There have been reports of neonatal bromide intoxication and growth retardation associated with maternal bromide ingestion during pregnancy. Symptoms of bromide intoxication have also been reported in breast-fed infants whose mothers were taking bromides.

Toxic effects may occur when bromide concentrations in blood are greater than 600 mg per litre (7.5 mmol per litre). A toxic concentration can be reached very rapidly if the intake of chloride is reduced.

Treatment of Adverse Effects

In acute poisoning the stomach should be emptied by aspiration and lavage and sodium chloride should be given by intravenous infusion. Glucose has also been administered and frusemide may be given to aid diuresis. In chronic poisoning, bromide administration is stopped, sodium chloride or ammonium chloride, up to 2 to 3 g three or four times daily, may be given by mouth with adequate amounts of fluid. Diuretics are of value. In severe cases of bromide intoxication or when the usual treatments cannot be used, haemodialysis may be of value.

Absorption and Fate

Bromides replace chloride in extracellular body fluids and have a half-life in the body of about 12 days. They may be detected in the milk of nursing mothers and in the foetus.

Uses and Administration

Bromides depress the central nervous system. Potassium bromide was formerly used as a sedative and anticonvulsant but has been replaced by more effective less toxic agents. Ammonium, calcium, sodium, and strontium bromide were used similarly, as were bromoform and dilute hydrobromic acid.

211-h

Potassium Hydroxide *(BAN, USAN).*

525; Ätzkali; Caustic Potash; Kalii Hydroxydum; Kalium Hydroxydatum; Potash Lye.

KOH=56.11.

CAS — 1310-58-3.

Pharmacopoeias. In *Aust., Br., Egypt., Hung., Int., Jpn, Jug., Mex., Nord., Port., Span., Swiss,* and *Turk.* Also in *B.P. Vet.* and *U.S.N.F.*

Dry, white or almost white deliquescent sticks, pellets, flakes, or fused masses. It is strongly alkaline and corrosive, and rapidly destroys tissues. It rapidly absorbs moisture and carbon dioxide.

Soluble or almost completely soluble 1 in 1 of water, and 1 in 3 of alcohol; very soluble in boiling alcohol or dehydrated alcohol. *U.S.N.F.* also has soluble in 2.5 of glycerol. **Store** in airtight containers.

Adverse Effects

The ingestion of caustic alkalis causes immediate burning pain in the mouth, throat, substernal region, and epigastrium, and the lining membranes become swollen and detached. There is dysphagia, hypersalivation, vomiting with the vomitus becoming blood-stained, diarrhoea, and shock. In severe cases, asphyxia due to oedema of the glottis, circulatory failure, oesophageal or gastric perforation, peritonitis, or pneumonia may occur. Stricture of the oesophagus can develop weeks or months later.

Caustic alkalis on contact with the eyes cause conjunctival oedema and corneal destruction.

In Great Britain the recommended exposure limit of potassium hydroxide is 2 mg per m^3.

Treatment of Adverse Effects

Ingestion should not be treated by lavage or emesis. Give copious drinks of water and follow this with demulcents. Maintain an airway and alleviate shock and pain.

Contaminated skin and eyes should be flooded immediately with water and the washing continued for about 30 minutes. Any affected clothing should be removed while flooding is being carried out. Pain in affected eyes may be relieved by instillation of local anaesthetic eye-drops.

Uses and Administration

Potassium hydroxide is a powerful caustic which has been used to remove warts. A 2.5% solution in glycerol has been used as a cuticle solvent. An escharotic preparation of potassium hydroxide and calcium hydroxide was known as Vienna paste.

In the *UK* the use of potassium hydroxide in cosmetics is prohibited by law.

Application of potassium hydroxide 1% reduced subsequent development of dithranol inflammation without loss of its therapeutic effect on psoriasis.— C. M. Lawrence *et al.*, *Br. J. Derm.*, 1987, *116*, 171.

Preparations

Potassium Hydroxide Solution *(B.P.)*. Potash Solution. An aqueous solution containing 4.9 to 5.1% w/v of total alkali, calculated as KOH. Store in well-closed containers of lead-free glass or of a suitable plastic.

Proprietary Names and Manufacturers

Cerumenol *(Jorba, Spain)*; Kuson *(Vera, Spain)*.

1630-g

Potassium Hydroxyquinoline Sulphate

Oxyquinol Potassium; Potassii Hydroxyquinolini Sulphas; Potassium Oxyquinoline Sulphate. An equimolecular mixture of potassium sulphate and quinolin-8-ol sulphate, containing the equivalent of 50% of quinolin-8-ol.

Pharmacopoeias. In *Aust.* and *Br.*

A pale yellow odourless or almost odourless microcrystalline powder. It partly liquefies at 172° to 184°. Freely **soluble** in water; insoluble in ether. **Incompatible** with many metallic salts.

Potassium hydroxyquinoline sulphate has antibacterial, antifungal, and deodorant properties and is used, often in conjunction with benzoyl peroxide, in the local treatment of fungal infections, minor bacterial infections, and acne.

Preparations

Potassium Hydroxyquinoline Sulphate and Benzoyl Peroxide Cream *(B.P.)*.

Proprietary Preparations

Quinoderm *(Quinoderm, UK)*. *Cream*, benzoyl peroxide 5% or 10%, potassium hydroxyquinoline sulphate 0.5%. *Lotio-gel*, benzoyl peroxide 5% or 10%, potassium hydroxyquinoline sulphate 0.5%. For acne.

Quinoderm with Hydrocortisone *(Quinoderm, UK)*. *Cream*, benzoyl peroxide 10%, potassium hydroxyquinoline sulphate 0.5%, hydrocortisone 1%. For acne.

Quinoped *(Quinoderm, UK)*. *Cream*, benzoyl peroxide 5%, potassium hydroxyquinoline sulphate 0.5%. For athlete's foot and related fungal infections.

Proprietary Names and Manufacturers

Vasinvas *(Bucca, Spain)*.

The following names have been used for multi-ingredient preparations containing potassium hydroxyquinoline sulphate—Quinocort *(Quinoderm, UK)*; Quinoderm *(Quinoderm, UK)*; Quinoderm with Hydrocortisone *(Quinoderm, UK)*; Quinoped *(Quinoderm, UK)*.

1182-r

Potassium Metaphosphate *(USAN)*.

E450(c); Potassium Kurrol's Salt; Potassium Polymetaphosphate.

$(KPO_3)_x$.

CAS — 7790-53-6.

Pharmacopoeias. In *U.S.N.F.*

A straight-chain polyphosphate, having a high degree of polymerisation, containing the equivalent of about 59 to 61% of P_2O_5.

It is a white odourless powder. Practically **insoluble** in water; soluble in dilute solutions of sodium salts.

Potassium metaphosphate is used as a buffering agent.

13155-b

Potassium Nitrate *(BAN)*.

Azotato de Potássio; E252; Kalii Nitras; Kalium Nitricum; Nitre; Saltpetre.

KNO_3=101.1.

CAS — 7757-79-1.

Pharmacopoeias. In *Arg.*, *Aust.*, *Br.*, *Braz.*, *Cz.*, *Fr.*, *Hung.*, *Jug.*, *Nord.*, *Pol.*, *Port.*, *Span.*, and *Swiss.*

Colourless crystals or a white crystalline powder. **Soluble** 1 in 3.3 of water.

WARNING. *Potassium nitrate has been used for the illicit preparation of explosives or fireworks; care is required with its supply.*

Adverse Effects

After ingestion of potassium nitrate gastro-enteritis, with severe abdominal pain, vomiting, vertigo, headache, flushing of the skin, irregular pulse, cyanosis, convulsions, and collapse may occur. The toxic dose varies greatly; 15 g may prove fatal but much larger doses have been taken without serious effects.

Potassium nitrate may be reduced to nitrite in the gastro-intestinal tract by the action of bacteria and ingestion can therefore cause methaemoglobinaemia. Poisoning has frequently been reported in infants given water from wells contaminated with nitrates. For reference to nitrites as precursors of nitrosamines and the potential role of nitrosamines as carcinogens, see p.854.

Toxicological information on potassium and sodium nitrates in food. The safe upper limit for nitrate in the drinking water of infants was probably 10 to 20 ppm.— *Fd Add. Ser. Wld Hlth Org. No. 5*, 1974.

Nitrates might be found in water and they were present in high concentrations in foods such as beets, spinach, carrots, and cabbages; conversion of nitrates to nitrites (which could cause methaemoglobinaemia) was enhanced when nitrate-containing foods spoiled. The lower stomach acidity of infants under 4 months of age might permit growth of bacteria capable of reducing nitrates to nitrites; deaths had occurred as a result of giving infants water with a high nitrate content and toxicity had also occurred in infants after nitrate was reduced to nitrite when jars of baby food were left open or cooked vegetables were kept at room temperature for some time. Although nitrates and nitrites were effective food preservatives they could lead to the formation of nitrosamines which might be carcinogenic in man.— *Med. Lett.*, 1974, *16*, 75.

Report of a WHO meeting on the health hazards from nitrates in drinking water.— *Environmental Health*, Copenhagen, WHO Regional Office for Europe, 1985.

EFFECTS ON THE BLOOD. A report of severe methaemoglobinaemia in 3 workers (fatal in one) following absorption of sodium and potassium nitrate through burnt skin areas after an industrial accident.— J. C. Harris *et al.*, *J. Am. med. Ass.*, 1979, *242*, 2869.

Absorption and Fate

Nitrates are readily absorbed from the gastro-intestinal tract and are rapidly excreted almost entirely unchanged in the urine; a small amount may be reduced to nitrite (but see Adverse Effects, above). Their excretion is similar to that of chloride ions.

Uses and Administration

Potassium nitrate, when taken by mouth in dilute solution, acts as a diuretic and it was formerly used for this purpose. It has been included in 'asthma powders' to assist combustion. It is used as a preservative in foods.

In Great Britain potassium nitrate is permitted as a preservative at a concentration of not more than 50 ppm, of which not more than 5 ppm may be potassium nitrite (both expressed as the sodium salt) in certain types of cheese and limits of not more than 150 to 500 ppm of potassium nitrate, of which not more than 50 to 200 ppm respectively may be potassium nitrite (both expressed as the sodium salt) in cured meats including cured meat products. The Regulations also prohibit the sale of any food specially prepared for babies or young children if it has in it or on it any added potassium nitrate or potassium nitrite.

Potassium nitrate has also been tried in the management of dentine hypersensitivity.

Estimated acceptable daily intake of nitrates: up to 500 μg per kg body-weight. No change was made from the Seventeenth Report [however, in that report an intake of up to *5 mg* per kg was given].— Twenty-third Report of Joint FAO/WHO Expert Committee on Food Additives, *Tech. Rep. Ser. Wld Hlth Org. No. 648*, 1980. Nitrate should on no account be added to baby foods.— *Fd Add. Ser. Wld Hlth Org. No. 5*, 1974.

DENTAL DISORDERS. In a study involving 76 patients with dentine hypersensitivity a toothpaste containing potassium nitrate and monofluorophosphate was at least as effective as a nicomethanol hydrofluoride toothpaste in relieving symptoms.— C. Lecointre *et al.*, *J. int. med. Res.*, 1986, *14*, 217.

13156-v

Potassium Nitrite

E249.

KNO_2=85.10.

CAS — 7758-09-0.

A white crystalline deliquescent powder. **Soluble** in water; practically insoluble in alcohol. A 5% solution has a pH of 6 to 9. **Store** in airtight containers.

Potassium nitrite has the pharmacological effects of the other nitrites (see Sodium Nitrite, p.854). It is used as a preservative in foods.

Food for babies less than 6 months of age should not contain added nitrites.— Twentieth Report of the Joint FAO/WHO Expert Committee on Food Additives, *Tech. Rep. Ser. Wld Hlth Org. No. 599*, 1976. Estimated acceptable daily intake of nitrites: up to 20 μg per kg body-weight. No change was made from the acceptable daily intake provided in the Seventeenth Report [however, in that report an intake of up to *200 μg* per kg was given].— Twenty-third Report of Joint FAO/WHO Expert Committee on Food Additives, *Tech. Rep. Ser. Wld Hlth Org. No. 648*, 1980.

5907-v

Potassium Permanganate *(BAN, USAN)*.

Kalii Permanganas; Kalium Hypermanganicum; Kalium Permanganicum; Pot. Permang.

$KMnO_4$=158.0.

CAS — 7722-64-7.

Pharmacopoeias. In *Arg.*, *Aust.*, *Belg.*, *Br.*, *Braz.*, *Chin.*, *Cz.*, *Egypt.*, *Eur.*, *Fr.*, *Ger.*, *Hung.*, *Ind.*, *It.*, *Jpn*, *Jug.*, *Mex.*, *Neth.*, *Nord.*, *Pol.*, *Port.*, *Roum.*, *Rus.*, *Span.*, *Swiss*, *Turk.*, and *U.S.*

Odourless dark purple or almost black crystals or granular powder, almost opaque by transmitted light and with a blue metallic lustre by reflected light. It decomposes, with a risk of explosion, in contact with certain organic substances.

Soluble 1 in 16 of water and 1 in 3.5 of boiling water giving purple solutions. An acidified solution in water is readily reduced by hydrogen peroxide, by easily oxidisable substances, and by organic matter. **Incompatible** with iodides, reducing agents, and most organic substances. **Store** in well-closed containers.

Adverse Effects

The crystals and concentrated solutions of potassium permanganate are caustic and even fairly dilute solutions are irritant to tissues. Repeated use of dilute solutions may cause corrosive burns.

Symptoms of poisoning following ingestion of potassium permanganate include nausea, vomiting of a brownish coloured material, corrosion, oedema, and brown coloration of the buccal mucosa, liver and kidney damage, and cardiovascular depression. The fatal dose is probably about 10 g and death may occur up to 1 month from the time of poisoning.

The insertion into the vagina of potassium permanganate in the form of tablets, crystals, or a douche, for its supposed abortifacient action, causes corrosive burns, severe vaginal haemorrhage, and perforation of the vaginal wall, leading to peritonitis. Vascular collapse may occur.

Potassium permanganate has been used for the illicit preparation of explosives or fireworks; care is required with its supply.

Methaemoglobinaemia in 2 patients associated with potassium permanganate ingestion.— M. C. Mahomedy *et al.*, *Anaesthesia*, 1975, *30*, 190.

Oesophageal stricture following ingestion of potassium permanganate.— R. Kochhar *et al.*, *Hum. Toxicol.*, 1986, *5*, 393.

Corrosive burns to the mouth, oesophagus, and trachea in a 3-year-old child who had swallowed between 5 and 10 g of potassium permanganate.— T. Southwood *et al.*, *Med. J. Aust.*, 1987, *146*, 639.

Treatment of Adverse Effects

Poisoning from the ingestion of potassium permanganate should be treated immediately with milk to delay absorption. The circulation should be maintained with infusions of plasma or suitable electrolyte solutions, but care is necessary as anuria may occur. Burns and ulcers of the mucous membranes should be treated by repeated copious washing with water.

The brown stain caused by solutions can be removed from the skin by oxalic or by sulphurous acid.

Uses and Administration

Potassium permanganate possesses oxidising properties which in turn confer disinfectant and deodorising properties. It is also astringent. Though bactericidal *in vitro* its clinical value as a bactericide is minimised by its rapid reduction in the presence of body fluids.

Solutions are used as cleansing applications to ulcers or abscesses and as wet dressings and in baths in eczematous conditions and acute dermatoses especially where there is secondary infection. The usual concentration is 1 in 10 000 (0.01%). Solutions have also been used in bromhidrosis, in mycotic infections such as athlete's foot, and in poison ivy dermatitis.

A 0.02% solution in water has been employed as a stomach wash-out in the treatment of poisoning by morphine, opium, and strychnine; its use should be followed by evacuation of the stomach. It is of no value in poisoning by atropine, cocaine, or the barbiturates.

Preparations

Potassium Permanganate Tablets for Topical Solution *(U.S.P.)*. Store in airtight containers.

Proprietary Preparations

Permitabs *(Bioglan, UK)*. *Solution tablets*, potassium permanganate 400 mg.

Proprietary Names and Manufacturers

Permantasico *(Brum, Spain)*; Permitabs *(Bioglan, UK)*.

13159-p

Potassium Selenate

K_2SeO_4=221.2.

CAS — 7790-59-2.

Pharmacopoeias. In *B.P. Vet.*

Colourless odourless crystals or a white crystalline powder. **Soluble** 1 in 1 of water.

Potassium selenate is used in veterinary practice in conjunction with vitamin E in the treatment of nutritional muscular dystrophy (white muscle disease, stiff lamb disease) in calves and lambs.

16967-a

Pramiracetam Sulphate *(rINNM)*.

Amacetam Sulphate; CI-879; Pramiracetam Sulfate *(USAN)*. *N*-[2-(Diisopropylamino)ethyl]-2-oxo-1-pyrrolidineacetamide sulphate.

$C_{14}H_{27}N_3O_2,H_2SO_4$=305.9.

CAS — 72869-16-0 (sulphate); 68497-62-1 (pramiracetam).

Pramiracetam sulphate is chemically related to piracetam and has a similar nootropic action on the central nervous system. It has been tried in dementia in the elderly.

J. Roland *et al.*, *Psychopharmac. Bull.*, 1983, *19*, 726; T. Chang *et al.*, *J. clin. Pharmac.*, 1985, *25*, 291; R. Dejong, *Curr. ther. Res.*, 1987, *41*, 254.

Proprietary Names and Manufacturers

Parke, Davis, USA.

5242-m

Pramiverine Hydrochloride *(BANM, rINNM)*.

EMD-9806 (pramiverine); HSP-2986 (pramiverine). *N*-Isopropyl-4,4-diphenylcyclohexylamine hydrochloride.

$C_{21}H_{27}N,HCl$=329.9.

CAS — 14334-40-8 (pramiverine); 14334-41-9 (hydrochloride).

Pramiverine hydrochloride is used as an antispasmodic in doses of up to 8 mg daily by mouth. It is also given rectally and by intramuscular or slow intravenous injection.

Proprietary Names and Manufacturers

Monoverin *(Igoda, Spain)*; Raptalgin *(Merck, Arg.)*; Sistalgin *(Cascan, Ger.*; *Bracco, Ital.)*.

232-q

Preclamol *(rINN)*.

3-(3-Hydroxyphenyl)-*N*-n-propylpiperidine; 3-PPP. (−)-(*S*)-*m*-(1-Propyl-3-piperidyl)phenol.

$C_{14}H_{21}NO$=219.3.

CAS — 85966-89-8.

Preclamol is a mixed dopamine agonist/antagonist under investigation.

18674-r

Premazepam *(BAN, rINN)*.

DL-181; DL-181-IT; L-12181; MDL-181. 1,2,3,7-Tetrahydro-6,7-dimethyl-5-phenylpyrrolo-[3,4-*e*][1,4]diazepin-4-one.

$C_{15}H_{15}N_3O$=253.3.

CAS — 57435-86-6.

Premazepam is an anxiolytic agent under investigation.

References: S. Golombok and M. Lader, *Br. J. clin. Pharmac.*, 1984, *18*, 127; B. Vitiello *et al.*, *Int. J. clin. Pharmac. Ther. Toxic.*, 1984, *22*, 273.

Proprietary Names and Manufacturers

Lepetit, Ital.

13169-w

Proadifen Hydrochloride *(USAN, rINNM)*.

NSC-39690; Propyladiphenine Hydrochloride; RP-5171; SKF-525A. 2-Diethylaminoethyl 2,2-diphenylvalerate hydrochloride.

$C_{23}H_{31}NO_2,HCl$=390.0.

CAS — 302-33-0 (proadifen); 62-68-0 (hydrochloride).

Proadifen has been found to enhance the effects of a large number of drugs. It may act by inhibiting drug metabolism.

References: G. V. Rossi, *J. pharm. Sci.*, 1963, *52*, 819; W. R. Ravis and S. Feldman, *ibid.*, 1979, *68*, 945; O. Pelkonen *et al.*, *Br. J. clin. Pharmac.*, 1985, *19*, 59.

Proprietary Names and Manufacturers

Smith Kline & French, USA.

13172-v

Procodazole *(rINN)*.

3-(Benzimidazol-2-yl)propionic acid.

$C_{10}H_{10}N_2O_2$=190.2.

CAS — 23249-97-0.

Procodazole is reported to have immunostimulant properties.

Proprietary Names and Manufacturers

Estimulocel *(Lafarquim, Spain)*.

13175-p

Prolonium Iodide *(rINN)*.

NN-(2-Hydroxytrimethylene)bis(trimethylammonium) di-iodide.

$C_9H_{24}I_2N_2O$=430.1.

CAS — 123-47-7.

Prolonium iodide has been used in the management of hyperthyroidism.

Proprietary Names and Manufacturers

Endo-Iodo *(Ital.)*; Endojodin *(Bayer, Ger.)*; Intrajodina *(Gentili, Ital.)*; Iodopropano *(Ital.)*; Iorganisan *(Santos, Spain)*; Soluyodina *(Spain)*; Yodofasa *(Lifasa, Spain)*.

3926-z

Propenidazole *(rINN)*.

Ethyl *trans*-α-acetyl-1-methyl-5-nitroimidazole-2-acrylate.

$C_{11}H_{13}N_3O_5$=267.2.

CAS — 76448-31-2.

Propenidazole is used for protozoal and fungal infections of the genito-urinary tract. It has been given by mouth or by the vaginal route.

Proprietary Names and Manufacturers

Naska *(Lifepharma, Ital.)*.

18363-g

Propylene Glycol Diacetate *(USAN)*.

Propanediol diacetate.

$C_7H_{12}O_4$=160.2.

CAS — 623-84-7 (1,2-isomer); 628-66-0 (1,3-isomer).

Pharmacopoeias. In *U.S.N.F.*

A clear, colourless liquid with a mild, fruity odour. **Soluble** in water. A 5% solution has a pH of 4 to 6. **Store** in airtight containers and avoid contact with metals.

Propylene glycol diacetate is stated to be an emulsifying and/or solubilising agent, and a solvent.

Estimated acceptable daily intake of 1,2-propylene glycol acetate: up to 25 mg, as propylene glycol, per kg body-weight.— Twenty-fifth Report of the FAO/WHO Expert Committee on Food Additives, *Tech. Rep. Ser. Wld Hlth Org. No. 669*, 1981.

13179-l

Proquamezine Fumarate *(BANM)*.

Aminopromazine Fumarate *(rINNM)*; Bayer-A-124; RP-3828; Tetrameprozine Fumarate. *NNN′N′*-Tetramethyl-3-(phenothiazin-10-yl)propane-1,2-diamine fumarate; Tetramethyl(1-phenothiazin-10-

ylmethylethylene)diamine fumarate.
$(C_{19}H_{25}N_3S)_2,C_4H_4O_4=771.1$.

CAS — 58-37-7 (proquamezine); 3688-62-8 (fumarate).

Proquamezine fumarate is a phenothiazine derivative with antispasmodic properties and is used in veterinary medicine.

Proprietary Veterinary Names and Manufacturers
Myspamol *(May & Baker, UK).*

5243-b

Proxazole Citrate *(USAN, rINNM).*

AF-634; PZ-17105. *NN*-Diethyl-2-[3-(α-ethylbenzyl)-1,2,4-oxadiazol-5-yl]ethylamine dihydrogen citrate.
$C_{17}H_{25}N_3O,C_6H_8O_7=479.5$.

CAS — 5696-09-3 (proxazole); 132-35-4 (citrate).

Proxazole citrate has actions similar to papaverine (see p.1598). It has been given as an antispasmodic in doses of 100 to 200 mg three times daily by mouth. It has also been given rectally and by injection.

Proprietary Names and Manufacturers
Recidol *(Lampugnani, Ital.)*; Solacil *(Finadiet, Arg.)*; Toness *(Angelini, Ital.; Farma-Lepori, Spain).*

3740-v

Prozapine Hydrochloride *(rINNM).*

Hexadiphane Hydrochloride. 1-(3,3-Diphenylpropyl)cyclohexamethyleneimine hydrochloride.
$C_{21}H_{27}N,HCl=329.9$.

CAS — 3426-08-2 (prozapine); 13657-24-4 (hydrochloride).

Prozapine hydrochloride is an antispasmodic used with sorbitol in gastro-intestinal disorders. It has been given in doses of 2 to 6 mg daily taken in water before meals.

Proprietary Names and Manufacturers
Norbiline *(Fournier Frères, Fr.; Semar, Spain).*

5019-t

Psilocin

4-Hydroxy-*NN*-dimethyltryptamine; Psilocyn. 3-(2-Dimethylaminoethyl)indol-4-ol.
$C_{12}H_{16}N_2O=204.3$.

CAS — 520-53-6.

An indole alkaloid obtained from the sacred Mexican mushroom (Teonanácatl), *Psilocybe mexicana* (Agaricaceae).

5020-l

Psilocybin *(BAN).*

4-Phosphoryloxy-*NN*-dimethyltryptamine; CY-39; Psilocybine *(rINN).* 3-(2-Dimethylaminoethyl)indol-4-yl dihydrogen phosphate.
$C_{12}H_{17}N_2O_4P=284.3$.

CAS — 520-52-5.

The main indole alkaloid present in the sacred Mexican mushroom (Teonanácatl), *Psilocybe mexicana* (Agaricaceae). Psilocybin is also present in other species of mushrooms including *Stropharia cubensis* and *Conocybe* spp.

Psilocybin has hallucinogenic and sympathomimetic properties similar to those of lysergide (p.1584). It is less potent than lysergide and its hallucinogenic effects last for up to 6 hours. There is evidence to suggest that psilocybin is converted to the active form psilocin in the body. It has no therapeutic use.

Effects of psilocybin on mental state.— A. Hofmann, *Indian J. Pharm.*, 1963, *25*, 245. See also R. Ružičková *et al.*, *Čslká Psychiat.*, 1967, *63*, 158; R. Fischer *et al.* (letter), *Nature*, 1968, *218*, 296; C. Hyde *et al.*, *Br. J. Psychiat.*, 1978, *132*, 602; C. Benjamin, *Br. med. J.*, 1979, *1*, 1319.

Psilocybin was identified in mushrooms of the *Gymnopilus* spp. Poisoning had occurred in 2 individuals after ingestion of *Gymnopilus validipes*.— G. M. Hatfield *et al.*, *Lloydia*, 1978, *41*, 140.

The clinical toxicology of *Psilocybe semilanceata* (magic mushroom; liberty cap): N. R. Peden *et al.*, *Postgrad. med. J.*, 1981, *57*, 543; A. D. Harries and V. Evans, *ibid.*, 571.

Discussion of the increase in abuse of 'magic mushrooms' (*Psilocybe semilanceata*) in Glasgow.— R. E. Young *et al.*, *Lancet*, 1982, *1*, 213.

Hepatic and renal impairment followed intravenous injection of an extract of *Psilocybe* mushrooms in 2 men.— G. Sivyer and L. Dorrington (letter), *Med. J. Aust.*, 1984, *140*, 182.

13187-l

Pulsatilla

Meadow Anemone. The whole plant of *Pulsatilla nigricans* (Ranunculaceae).

CAS — 62887-80-3.

Pulsatilla is used in homoeopathic medicine.

13188-y

Punarnava

Punarnaba. The fresh or dried plant *Boerhaavia diffusa* (= *B. repens*) (Nyctaginaceae), containing an alkaloid, punarnavine.

Punarnava has been used in India as a diuretic, usually in the form of a liquid extract.

13189-j

Pyran Copolymer

DIVEMA; NSC-46015C. An anionic copolymer of divinyl ether and maleic anhydride, with an average molecular weight of 17 000.

CAS — 27100-68-1.

Pyran copolymer has been reported to have antiviral activity and to induce the production of interferon in man.

References: T. C. Merigan and W. Regelson, *New Engl. J. Med.*, 1967, *277*, 1283; T. J. Leavitt *et al.*, *Am. J. Dis. Child.*, 1971, *121*, 43.

13191-p

Pyridinolcarbamate

Pyricarbate *(rINN).* Pyridine-2,6-diylbis(methylene *N*-methylcarbamate).
$C_{11}H_{15}N_3O_4=253.3$.

CAS — 1882-26-4.

Pyridinolcarbamate has been reported to be a bradykinin antagonist and has been claimed to have beneficial effects in the treatment of the complications of atherosclerosis. Adverse effects have included gastro-intestinal disturbances and liver damage.

References to the use of pyridinolcarbamate in atherosclerosis and related disorders: T. Shimamoto *et al.*, *Am. Heart J.*, 1970, *79*, 5; H. Yamazaki *et al.*, *ibid.*, 640; T. G. Judge, *Practitioner*, 1974, *213*, 10; L. Hunyi, *Therapia hung.*, 1976, *24*, 67.

Pharmacokinetic studies of pyridinolcarbamate: R. Mallein *et al.*, *Thérapie*, 1973, *28*, 115; R. Mallein *et al.*, *ibid.*, 129; J. Sassard *et al.*, *J. pharm. Sci.*, 1979, *68*, 1190.

Platelet hyper-aggregation was reduced in patients with damaged blood vessel walls receiving pyridinolcarbamate.— R. J. Prost-Djovakovic *et al.*, *Thérapie*, 1975, *30*, 429. See also A. Girolami *et al.*, *Arzneimittel-Forsch.*, 1977, *27*, 1202.

Reports of liver damage associated with the use of pyridinolcarbamate.— *Jpn med. Gaz.*, 1976, *13* (Sept. 20), 8; M. Biour *et al.*, *Thérapie*, 1984, *39*, 531.

Proprietary Names and Manufacturers
Acesterol *(Spain)*; Anginin *(Teva, Israel; Banyu, Jpn)*; Angio-Reder *(Spain)*; Angioxil *(FIRMA, Ital.)*; Angioxine *(Roussel, Fr.)*; Aterofal *(Nativelle, Ital.)*; Ateroqraso *(Spain)*; Aterollano *(Spain)*; Ateronova *(Spain)*; Aterosan *(Aandersen, Ital.)*; Atover *(Recordati, Ital.)*; Atrombogen *(Migra, Arg.)*; Carbatona *(Spain)*; Cicloven *(AGIPS, Ital.)*; Colesterinex *(Prodes, Spain; Galenica, Switz.)*; Dual-Xol *(Spain)*; Duaxol *(Argentia, Arg.)*; Duvaline *(Almirall, Spain)*; Esterbiol *(Inexfa, Spain)*; Exibral *(Bago, Arg.)*; Foslip Vascular *(Pharmainvesti, Spain)*; Gasparol *(Spain)*; Hematinol *(Septa, Spain)*; Idobernal *(Spain)*; Katrombin *(Spain)*; Movecil *(Carlo Erba, Ital.)*; Plavolex *(Spain)*; Prodectin *(Gedeon Richter, Hung.)*; Ravenil *(Caber, Ital.)*; Tripsix *(Arg.)*; Vasagin *(Salus, Ital.)*; Vasapril *(Ital.)*; Vasmol *(Sabater, Spain)*; Vasocil *(Aesculapius, Ital.)*; Vasovérine *(Biochimica, Switz.)*; Veranterol *(Spain).*

13192-s

Pyrisuccideanol Maleate

Pirisudanol Maleate *(rINNM).* Pyrisuccideanol is the succinic acid ester of pyridoxine (see p.1270) and of deanol (see p.1440). 2-Dimethylaminoethyl 5-hydroxy-4-hydroxymethyl-6-methyl-3-pyridylmethyl succinate maleate.
$C_{16}H_{24}N_2O_6,(C_4H_4O_4)_2=572.5$.

CAS — 33605-94-6 (pyrisuccideanol); 53659-00-0 (maleate).

Pyrisuccideanol has been reported to have antidepressant activity and has been used as the maleate in the treatment of cerebrovascular and similar disorders.

Proprietary Names and Manufacturers
Mentis *(Menarini, Ital.; Menarini, Spain)*; Mentium *(Guidotti, Ital.)*; Nadex *(Zyma, Switz.)*; Pridana *(Frumtost, Spain)*; Stivane *(Beaufour, Fr.; IBYS, Spain).*

13194-e

Pyritinol Hydrochloride *(BANM, rINNM).*

Pyrithioxine Hydrochloride. 3,3′-Dithiodimethylenebis(5-hydroxy-6-methyl-4-pyridylmethanol) dihydrochloride monohydrate.
$C_{16}H_{20}N_2O_4S_2,2HCl,H_2O=459.4$.

CAS — 1098-97-1 (pyritinol); 10049-83-9 (hydrochloride, anhydrous).

Pyritinol hydrochloride is claimed to promote the uptake of glucose by the brain and is used in the treatment of various cerebrovascular and mental disorders. It is given by mouth in doses of up to 600 mg daily; it is also given by intravenous infusion in doses of 200 to 400 mg daily.

Pyritinol is also given as an alternative to penicillamine in rheumatoid arthritis.

Review of the mechanism of action of pyritinol.— K. J. Martin, *J. int. med. Res.*, 1983, *11*, 55.

A review of the treatment of senile dementia with various drugs, including pyritinol.— J. A. Yesavage *et al.*, *Archs gen. Psychiat.*, 1979, *36*, 220.

Patients with organic brain disorders based on disturbed cerebral glucose metabolism improved after treatment with pyritinol hydrochloride 900 mg by mouth or 1 g by intravenous infusion daily for an average of 3 weeks.— S. Hoyer *et al.*, *Arzneimittel-Forsch.*, 1977, *27*, 671.

References to the cerebral effects of pyritinol hydrochloride and it use in various cerebral vascular disorders: E. Stoica *et al.*, *Eur. Neurol.*, 1972, *7*, 348 (cerebral infarct); C. Fehling-Joss, *Clin. Trials J.*, 1974, *11*, 123 (dyslexia); G. Logue *et al.*, *S. Afr. med. J.*, 1974, *48*, 2245 (behavioural disorders in children); D. J. L. O'Kelly, *J. int. med. Res.*, 1975, *3*, 323 (chronic alcoholism); J. Glatzel, *Medsche Klin.*, 1976, *71*, 1958 (various psychopathological syndromes); Z. Bystřický *et al.*, *Medsche Welt, Stuttg.*, 1977, *28*, 643 (brain contusion); W. Hamouz, *Pharmatherapeutica*, 1977, *1*, 398 (senile dementia); H. Herrschaft, *Münch. med. Wschr.*, 1978, *120*, 1263 (acute cerebral ischaemia); Y. Tazaki *et al.*, *J. int. med. Res.*, 1980, *8*, 118 (various cerebrovascular disorders).

Proprietary Names and Manufacturers
Biocefalin *(Ital.)*; Bonifen *(Igoda, Spain)*; Cefalogen *(Hammer Pharma, Ital.)*; Cerebropirina *(Ital.)*; Cerebrotrofina *(Nuovo, Ital.)*; Cervitalin *(Savoma, Ital.)*; Divalvon-D *(Jpn)*; Enbol *(Jpn)*; Encebrovit *(Ital.)*; Encefabol *(Bracco, Ital.)*; Encefort *(Ital.)*; Encephabol *(Merck, Aust.; Merck, Belg.; Merck-Clévenot, Fr.; E. Merck, Ger.; E. Merck, Neth.; Merck, S.Afr.; E. Merck, Switz.)*; Encerebron *(Pulitzer, Ital.)*; Epocan

(Merck, Arg.); Fulneurina *(Fulton, Ital.)*; Leonar *(Kalopharma, Ital.)*; Life *(Ital.)*; Maind *(Also, Ital.)*; Musa *(Ital.)*; Neuroxin *(Jpn)*; Piritiomin *(Jpn)*; Scintidin *(Ital.)*; Tonobrein *(CT, Ital.)*; Tonomentis *(Ital.)*.

539-m

Quassia

Bitter Wood; Leño de Cuasia; Quassia Wood; Quassiae Lignum; Quassiaholz.

CAS — 76-78-8 (quassin); 76-77-7 (neoquassin).

Pharmacopoeias. In *Egypt.*, *Fr.*, *Mex.*, *Port.*, and *Span.* All allow Jamaican or Surinam quassia. Also in *B.P.C. 1973* which specifies Jamaican quassia.

The dried stem wood of Jamaica quassia, *Picrasma excelsa* (=*Aeschrion excelsa; Picraena excelsa*) (Simaroubaceae) or of Surinam quassia, *Quassia amara* (Simaroubaceae).

Quassia has been used as a bitter. It was formerly given as an enema for the expulsion of threadworms and was applied for pediculosis. Extracts of quassia or preparations containing its alkaloid quassin are used to denature alcohol.

Proprietary Names and Manufacturers
Quassin Solution 'B' *(Bush Boake Allen, UK)*.

13201-k

Quinine and Urea Hydrochloride

Carbamidated Quinine Dihydrochloride; Chininum Dihydrochloricum Carbamidatum; Urea-Quinine.
$C_{20}H_{24}N_2O_2,CH_4N_2O,2HCl,5H_2O=547.5$.

CAS — 549-52-0 (anhydrous).

Pharmacopoeias. In *Arg.*, *Mex.*, and *Port.*

Quinine and urea hydrochloride was formerly used as a local anaesthetic, especially following rectal operations. It has also been administered intramuscularly for the therapeutic actions of quinine.

13202-a

Quinine Ascorbate *(USAN)*.

Quinine Biascorbate. A compound (2 : 1) of ascorbic acid with quinine.
$C_{20}H_{24}N_2O_2, 2C_6H_8O_6=676.7$.

CAS — 146-40-7.

Quinine ascorbate has been used as a smoking deterrent.

5244-v

Racefemine Fumarate *(rINNM)*.

CB-3697 *(racefemine)*. (±)-α-Methyl-*N*-(1-methyl-2-phenoxyethyl)phenethylamine hydrogen fumarate.
$C_{18}H_{23}NO,C_4H_4O_4=385.5$.

CAS — 22232-57-1 (racefemine); 1590-35-8 (fumarate).

Racefemine fumarate is used as a uterine relaxant in doses of up to 200 mg daily, by mouth. The dextrorotatory isomer, dextrofemine, is used intravenously in doses of up to 50 mg.

Proprietary Names and Manufacturers
Dysmalgine *(Clin Midy, Fr.)*.

7366-p

Rape Oil

Colza Oil; Oleum Rapae; Rapeseed Oil.

CAS — 8002-13-9.

Pharmacopoeias. In *Jpn* and *Pol.*

The fixed oil expressed from the seeds of *Brassica napus* (*Brassica campestris*) var. *oleifera* and certain other species of *Brassica* (Cruciferae).

Rape oil has been used in liniments in place of olive oil. It is used in some countries as an edible oil but the erucic acid ($C_{22}H_{42}O_2=338.6$) content of the oil has been implicated in muscle damage. The erucic acid content of oils and fats intended for human consumption and of foodstuffs containing oil or fat is subject to legal control. Contaminated rape oil was the cause of the toxic oil syndrome that affected thousands of Spanish citizens following its distribution in early 1981.

A discussion of the potential cardiotoxicity of rape oil in view of its use as a substitute for olive oil.— *Lancet*, 1974, *2*, 1359.

Some references to discussions and investigations of the toxic oil syndrome: J. M. Tabuenca, *Lancet*, 1981, *2*, 567; Toxic Epidemic Syndrome Study Group, *ibid.*, 1982, *2*, 697; *ibid.*, 1983, *1*, 1257; E. M. Kilbourne, *New Engl. J. Med.*, 1983, *309*, 1408; *Toxic Oil Syndrome*: Mass Food Poisoning in Spain, Report on a WHO Meeting, Copenhagen, Wld Hlth Org., 1984.

13207-d

Raspberry Leaf

Rubi Idaei Folium. The dried leaflets of *Rubus idaeus* (Rosaceae).

Raspberry leaf contains a principle, readily extracted with hot water, which relaxes the smooth muscle of the uterus and intestine of some *animals*.
Raspberry 'tea' has been a traditional remedy for painful and profuse menstruation and for use before and during confinement. The infusion has also been used as an astringent gargle.

1515-m

Recainam *(BAN, rINN)*.

Wy-42362. 1-[3-(Isopropylamino)propyl]-3-(2,6-xylyl)urea.
$C_{15}H_{25}N_3O=263.4$.

CAS — 74738-24-2; 74752-07-1 (hydrochloride); 74752-08-2 (tosylate).

NOTE. Recainam Hydrochloride and Recainam Tosylate are *USAN*.

Recainam is an anti-arrhythmic agent under investigation.

References: J. L. Bergey *et al.*, *Arzneimittel-Forsch.*, 1983, *33*, 1258; *Drugs of the Future*, 1984, *9*, 38; M. I. Anastasiou-Nana *et al.*, *J. Am. Coll. Cardiol.*, 1986, *8*, 427; J. L. Anderson *et al.*, *Am. J. Cardiol.*, 1987, *60*, 281.

Proprietary Names and Manufacturers
Wyeth, USA.

13208-n

Relaxin

A polypeptide hormone extracted from the corpus luteum of the ovaries of pregnant sows. It is reported to be related structurally to insulin and has a molecular weight of about 6000.

CAS — 9002-69-1.

Relaxin acts on connective tissue, including collagen, and causes relaxation of the pubic symphysis and softening of the uterine cervix. In many *animal* species it appears to play a major part in cervical ripening before parturition; significant species difference is shown. Relaxin is secreted by the human corpus luteum during pregnancy and is thought to interact with other reproductive hormones. Early clinical studies with impure extracts given parenterally or orally produced conflicting results. More recently a purified porcine relaxin preparation, used intravaginally in obstetric patients, induced cervical changes in the majority of patients.

A brief review of relaxin. Although the function of human relaxin is obscure, it is known to enhance the secretion of collagenase and plasminogen activator from dispersed amnion and chorion cell cultures *in vitro*; this indicates the possible local action of relaxin in collagen degradation in foetal membranes leading to their eventual rupture at parturition. Placental relaxin may act locally to bring about separation of the placenta from the uterus at birth.— *Lancet*, 1986, *1*, 1365. See also.— H. M. Schmeck, *Med. J. Aust.*, 1984, *141*, 666.

A radioimmunoassay for relaxin using a synthetic analogue of human relaxin. Modifications of this assay permit measurement of relaxin in pregnancy.— L. W. Eddie *et al.*, *Lancet*, 1986, *1*, 1344. Serum-relaxin concentrations during pregnancy.— A. H. MacLennan *et al.*, *ibid.*, 1986, *2*, 241. There may be a relationship between high serum-relaxin concentrations and pelvic pain and joint laxity during pregnancy.— A. H. MacLennan *et al.*, *ibid.*, 243.

In a double-blind study 30 women were given 2 mg of intravaginal purified porcine relaxin in a viscous gel on the evening before surgical induction of labour, while 30 similar women received the gel alone. Ten of the 30 women given relaxin went into labour before the proposed induction whereas none of the 30 control women did so. Twenty-five of the 30 women treated with relaxin had improved cervical scores after treatment and significantly fewer required intravenous oxytocin than those in the control group. No side-effects were experienced by the patients receiving relaxin and no neonatal complications were recorded. Relaxin 2 mg intravaginally appears to be at least as safe and effective as dinoprost 25 mg intravaginally and, in this study, labour was significantly shorter than in the control group.— A. H. MacLennan *et al.*, *Lancet*, 1980, *1*, 220. Similar findings in two randomised double-blind studies in 49 women in which relaxin 2 or 4 mg was applied to the cervix during induction of labour; it appeared to be of benefit in ripening the cervix and may be useful in pregnancies in which foetal stress occurs.— M. I. Evans *et al.*, *Am. J. Obstet. Gynec.*, 1983, *147*, 410.

497-s

Remoxipride *(BAN, USAN, rINN)*.

A-33547; FLA-731. (*S*)-3-Bromo-*N*-(1-ethylpyrrolidin-2-ylmethyl)-2,6-dimethoxylbenzamide.
$C_{16}H_{23}BrN_2O_3=371.3$.

CAS — 80125-14-0 (remoxipride); 82935-42-0 (hydrochloride).

Remoxipride, a substituted benzamide, is a specific dopamine (DA_2) antagonist under investigation as a neuroleptic.

References: M. -I. Nilsson *et al.*, *Clin. Pharmac. Ther.*, 1984, *35*, 263; R. G. McCreadie *et al.*, *Acta psychiat. scand.*, 1985, *72*, 139; A. L. Laursen and J. Gerlach, *ibid.*, 1986, *73*, 17; M. Nicklasson *et al.*, *Pharmazeut. Ind.*, 1985, *47*, 986.

Proprietary Names and Manufacturers
Astra, Swed.

3921-w

Rhamnose

L-Rhamnose. 6-Deoxy-L-mannose.
$C_6H_{12}O_5=164.2$.

Rhamnose is a monosaccharide used to assess intestinal permeability.

References: I. A. Santana *et al.*, *Gut*, 1984, *25*, A546; *Lancet*, 1985, *1*, 256; G. R. Struthers *et al.* (letter), *ibid.*, 587; D. J. Penny *et al.*, *Archs Dis. Childh.*, 1986, *61*, 1127.

13210-a

Rhus

Sumach Berries. The dried fruits of the smooth or Pennsylvanian sumach, *Rhus glabra* (Anacardiaceae).

Rhus has astringent and reputed diuretic properties. Poison ivy (*Rhus radicans*) and poison oak (*R. toxicodendron*), species growing in the USA, contain irritant poisons producing severe contact dermatitis. Extracts of poison ivy and poison oak have been used for the prophylaxis of poison ivy dermatitis but their effectiveness has not been proved.
Poison oak is used in homoeopathic medicine.

Five patients who were exquisitely sensitive to *Rhus* antigen developed a generalised eczematous dermatitis after eating large amounts of unroasted cashew nuts.— J. H. Ratner *et al.*, *Archs Derm.*, 1974, *110*, 921.

15326-d

Ribonucleic Acid

ARN; Plant Nucleic Acid; Ribose Nucleic Acid; RNA; Yeast Nucleic Acid. A nucleotide polymer, and 1 of the 2 distinct varieties of nucleic acid (see p.1596). It is found in the cytoplasm and in small amounts in the cell nuclei of living tissues. It can be extracted from beer or bread yeast.

Pharmacopoeias. In *Fr.*

Ribonucleic acid has been tried in the treatment of mental retardation and to improve memory in senile dementia and proprietary preparations containing various salts of ribonucleic acid have been advocated for a variety of asthenic and convalescent conditions.

Immune RNA (extracted from the spleens and lymph nodes of immunised animals) has been tried in the immunotherapy of hepatitis and cancer.

Reviews of pharmacological treatments of dementia including the effects of ribonucleic acid on memory.— M. D. Kopelman and W. A. Lishman, *Br. med. Bull.*, 1986, *42*, 101.

Ribonucleic acid was considered to be obsolete in the treatment of Alzheimer's disease.— L. E. Hollister, *Drugs*, 1985, *29*, 483.

13213-r

Ricin

A highly toxic lectin present in castor seeds, the seeds of *Ricinus communis* (Euphorbiaceae).

CAS — 9009-86-3.

NOTE. The title ricin is used for the castor seed in *Fr. P.*

Ricin is extremely toxic and the fatal dose by intravenous injection in experimental *animals* has been reported to be as low as 300 ng per kg body-weight. It has been investigated for use in chemical warfare. Ricin conjugated with monoclonal or polyclonal antibodies is being studied in the treatment of cancers.

Ingestion of 5 castor seeds in a child and 20 in an adult has proved fatal; signs and symptoms of poisoning are similar to those described for Abrus seeds (p.1537). After expression of the oil from castor seed (see p.1554), the ricin remains in the seed cake or 'pomace', which is subjected to steam treatment to destroy the ricin. The detoxified pomace is used as a fertiliser.

A review of the literature on ricin poisoning and a report of an extensive investigation of ricin poisoning in port workers while handling cargoes of castor pomace that had not been subjected to heat treatment.— W. C. Cooper *et al.*, *Am. ind. Hyg. Assoc. J.*, 1964, *25*, 431.

Inhibition of tumour growth in *animals* by ricin.— J. Lin *et al.*, *Nature*, 1970, *227*, 292.

A 57-year-old man suffered acute ricin intoxication after chewing a single castor bean. For a brief period he felt a sensation of burning in the mouth and throat, then collapsed and was in shock when admitted to hospital. He recovered in 2½ hours after symptomatic treatment with adrenaline, calcium, metaraminol, and infusions of electrolyte solutions and dextran 40.— J. Kingma, *Ned. Tijdschr. Geneesk.*, 1971, *115*, (July 10).

A discussion of the toxic effects of ricin and of its use for political assassination.— B. Knight, *Br. med. J.*, 1979, *1*, 350.

Review of tumor imaging and drug targeting including the use of 'immunotoxins' in the destruction of cancer cells. Studies in cell cultures of conjugates made from toxins such as abrin and ricin, linked to a monoclonal or polyclonal antibody, have shown them to be powerful cytotoxic agents for cells possessing appropriate antigens. However, lack of complete specificity has proved a problem and these conjugates have been highly toxic to *animals*. Modification of the immunotoxins by linking the isolated A chain of the toxin to an antibody in an attempt to increase specificity without reducing toxicity to cancer cells is currently being investigated.— K. Sikora *et al.*, *Br. med. Bull.*, 1984, *40*, 233. See also W. Cushley, *Pharm. Int.*, 1985, *6*, 33.

An immunotoxin of ricin A chain conjugated to thyroglobulin selectively suppressed the thyroglobulin autoantibody response of lymphocytes from patients with Hashimoto's thyroiditis.— D. P. Rennie *et al.*, *Lancet*, 1983, *2*, 1338.

1323-a

Ricinoleic Acid

A mixture of fatty acids obtained by the hydrolysis of castor oil.

Ricinoleic acid has been used with nonoxinols as a spermicide in some proprietary contraceptive creams and jellies.

Proprietary Names and Manufacturers
The following names have been used for multi-ingredient preparations containing ricinoleic acid— Aci-jel *(Cilag, Austral.; Ortho, Canad.; Ortho Pharmaceutical, USA)*.

18677-n

Ritanserin *(BAN, USAN, rINN)*.

R-55667. 6-{2-[4-(4,4′-Difluorobenzhydrylidene)piperidino]ethyl}-7-methyl[1,3]thiazolo[3,2-*a*]pyrimidin-5-one.

$C_{27}H_{25}F_2N_3OS=477.6$.

CAS — 87051-43-2.

Ritanserin is a serotonin antagonist under investigation in the treatment of anxiety and extrapyramidal disorders.

C. Korstanje *et al.*, *J. Pharm. Pharmac.*, 1986, *38*, 374; J. M. Van Nueten *et al.*, *Drug Dev. Res.*, 1986, *8*, 187; T. F. Meert, *ibid.*, 197; G. Bersani *et al.*, *Curr. ther. Res.*, 1986, *40*, 492; A. Maertens de Noordhout and P. J. Delwaide, *Clin. Neuropharmacol.*, 1986, *9*, 480; *Drugs of the Future*, 1986, *11*, 391; J. A. Barone *et al.*, *Drug Intell. & clin. Pharm.*, 1986, *20*, 770; J. Hildebrand and F. Delecluse, *Curr. ther. Res.*, 1987, *41*, 298; A. C. Declerck *et al.*, *ibid.*, 427; G. M. Bressa *et al.*, *Int. J. clin. Pharmacol. Res.*, 1987, *7*, 111.

Proprietary Names and Manufacturers
Janssen, Belg.

13217-h

Rociverine *(rINN)*.

LG-30158. 2-Diethylamino-1-methylethyl *cis*-1-hydroxy(bicyclohexyl)-2-carboxylate.

$C_{20}H_{37}NO_3=339.5$.

CAS — 53716-44-2.

Rociverine has been used as an antispasmodic.

Rociverine 20 mg three times daily by mouth was found to be successful in relieving symptoms in a double-blind placebo-controlled study in 90 patients with irritable bowel syndrome.— O. Ghidini *et al.*, *Curr. ther. Res.*, 1986, *39*, 541.

Proprietary Names and Manufacturers
Rilaten *(Guidotti, Ital.)*.

13220-x

Roxarsone *(BAN, USAN, rINN)*.

NSC-2101. 4-Hydroxy-3-nitrophenylarsonic acid.

$C_6H_6AsNO_6=263.0$.

CAS — 121-19-7.

Roxarsone is used as a growth promoter in animal feeds. The monosodium salt has also been used for the control of swine dysentery.

Proprietary Names and Manufacturers
Salsbury, UK.

13221-r

Royal Jelly

Queen Bee Jelly. A milky-white viscid secretion from the salivary glands of the worker hive bee, *Apis mellifera* (Apidae); it is essential for the development of queen bees.

Royal jelly has been used as a general 'tonic', to ward off the effects of old age, and to ease sufferers from chronic degenerative diseases, but of the many and diverse claims made for the therapeutic value of the jelly, none has been substantiated.

Royal jelly is also incorporated in some cosmetic preparations for its supposed beneficial effect on skin tissue.

Proprietary Names and Manufacturers
Apiserum *(Sidel, Fr.)*; Apistonico Real *(Sur De Espana, Spain)*.

716-b

RS-86

Spiro-(1-methyl-4-piperidyl)-*N*-ethyl succinimide hydrobromide.

$C_{11}H_{18}N_2O_2,HBr=291.2$.

RS-86 is a muscarinic agent under investigation in Alzheimer's disease.

References: *Am. J. Hosp. Pharm.*, 1963, *20*, 294; M. Berger *et al.* (letter), *Lancet*, 1985, *1*, 1385; E. Hollander *et al.*, *Br. med. Bull.*, 1986, *42*, 97; *Drugs of the Future*, 1986, *11*, 276; E. Hollander *et al.*, *Biol. Psychiat.*, 1987, *22*, 1067.

Proprietary Names and Manufacturers
Sandoz, Switz.

3913-w

Ruscogenin

(25*R*)-Spirost-5-ene-1β,3β-diol.

$C_{27}H_{42}O_4=430.6$.

CAS — 472-11-7.

A sapogenin obtained from butcher's broom, *Ruscus aculeatus* (Liliaceae).

Ruscogenin is chemically related to diosgenin and has been applied in the local treatment of haemorrhoids as rectal ointment or suppositories.

Proprietary Names and Manufacturers
Hemodren Simple *(Llorens, Spain)*; Ruscorectal *(Juste, Spain)*.

15304-k

Rutin

Rutoside *(rINN)*. A greenish-yellow microcrystalline powder obtained from buckwheat, *Fagopyrum esculentum* (Polygonaceae), or from other sources which include the flower buds of the Chinese pagoda-tree, *Sophora japonica*, and the leaves of several species of *Eucalyptus*. 2-(3,4-Dihydroxyphenyl)-3,5,7-trihydroxy-4-oxo-4*H*-chromen-3-yl rutinoside trihydrate.

$C_{27}H_{30}O_{16},3H_2O=664.6$.

CAS — 153-18-4 (anhydrous).

Pharmacopoeias. In *Aust., Belg., Braz., Egypt., Fr., Ger., Hung., Pol., Roum., Rus.,* and *Swiss.*

Rutin or rutin-like moieties were possibly contained in a tobacco glycoprotein, with allergenic and thrombogenic potential, present in cured tobacco leaves or cigarette smoke condensates.— *J. Am. med. Ass.*, 1978, *239*, 1476.

Rutin has been used in the treatment of disease states characterised by capillary bleeding associated with increased capillary fragility but evidence of its value is inconclusive.

Proprietary Names and Manufacturers
Birutan *(E. Merck, Ger.)*; Lifaton-P *(Lifasa, Spain)*; Neorutin *(Neomed, Switz.)*; Pecitrol *(Ferran, Spain)*; Permol *(Spain)*; Rutinion *(Rhein-Pharma, Ger.)*; Vasoforte *(Voigt, Ger.)*; Vasorutina *(Angelini, Ital.)*.

18680-t

Salmeterol *(BAN, rINN)*.

GR-33343X; Salmaterol. (*RS*)-5-{1-Hydroxy-2-[6-(4-phenylbutoxy)hexylamino]ethyl}salicyl alcohol.

$C_{25}H_{37}NO_4$=415.6.

CAS — 89365-50-4.

Salmeterol is a β_2 agonist under investigation as a bronchodilator.

Proprietary Names and Manufacturers
Glaxo, UK.

739-e

Sanguinaria

Bloodroot; Red Puccoon; Sanguinaria canadensis; Sanguinarine canadensis; Sanguinaris canadensis. The dried rhizome of *Sanguinaria canadensis* (Papaveraceae).

Sanguinarine, an alkaloid extracted from *Sanguinaria canadensis*, is used as an antiplaque agent in toothpaste and mouthwash preparations. Sanguinaria was formerly used as an expectorant but fell into disuse because of its toxicity (see *Martindale 25th Edn*, p.691). Sanguinaria has also been classified by the FDA as a herb that is unsafe for use in foods, beverages, or drugs.

References: R. T. Boulware *et al.*, *J. Soc. cosmet. Chem.*, 1985, *36*, 297; J. L. Dzink and S. S. Socransky, *Antimicrob. Ag. Chemother.*, 1985, *27*, 663.

2408-p

Sarsaparilla

Salsaparilha; Salsepareille; Sarsa; Sarsaparilla Root; Smilacis Rhizoma.

Pharmacopoeias. In *Belg., Chin., Jpn,* and *Port. Chin.* and *Jpn* specify *Smilax glabra.*

The dried root of various species of *Smilax* (Liliaceae).

Sarsaparilla, usually in the form of a decoction or extract, has been used as a vehicle and flavouring agent for medicaments. It is also an ingredient of herbal preparations.

Proprietary Names and Manufacturers
Sarsapsor *(Ysatfabrik, Ger.).*

746-w

Saxitoxin

Saxitoxin is a neurotoxin associated with paralytic shellfish poisoning. It is an endotoxin produced by *Gonyaulax tamarensis* present in infected molluscs.

References: B.W. Halstead and E.J. Schantz, *Paralytic Shellfish Poisoning*, Geneva, Wld Hlth Org., 1984.

13224-n

Scoparium

Broom Tops; Genêt; Genêt à Balai; Planta Genista; Scoparii Cacumina. The dried tops of broom, *Sarothamnus scoparius* (=*Cytisus scoparius*) (Leguminosae).

Pharmacopoeias. In *Fr.*

Scoparium is a mild diuretic and has been administered as a decoction or infusion. It has oxytoxic properties and should be avoided in pregnancy.

Scoparium is included in a list of herbs that have been officially designated by the Food and Drugs Administration of the *USA* as unsafe for foods, beverages and drugs.— *Am. Pharm.*, 1984, *NS24*, (Mar.), 20.

13225-h

Sebacic Acid

Decanedioic acid; Octane-1,8-dicarboxylic acid.

$C_{10}H_{18}O_4$=202.3.

CAS — 111-20-6.

Sebacic acid is an emollient included in preparations used to protect damaged skin.

Diisopropyl sebacate ($C_{16}H_{30}O_4$ = 286.4) is used as a skin moisturising agent.

Proprietary Names and Manufacturers
Domol *(Miles, Canad.; Miles Pharmaceuticals, USA).*

13226-m

Seclazone *(USAN, rINN).*

W-2354. 7-Chloro-3,3a-dihydro-2*H*,9*H*-isoxazolo[3,2-*b*][1,3]benzoxazin-9-one.

$C_{10}H_8ClNO_3$=225.6.

CAS — 29050-11-1.

Seclazone is an anti-inflammatory compound with uricosuric properties.

References: A. Jain and H. Hoyt, *Clin. Pharmac. Ther.*, 1972, *13*, 141; J. Edelson *et al.*, *J. pharm. Sci.*, 1973, *62*, 229; N. B. Banerjee *et al.*, *Toxic. appl. Pharmac.*, 1973, *25*, 444.

3941-j

Selenious Acid *(USAN).*

Monohydrated selenium dioxide.

H_2SeO_3=129.0.

CAS — 7783-00-8.

Pharmacopoeias. In *U.S.*

Store in airtight containers.

Selenious acid is used as a source of selenium, especially for patients with deficiency states following prolonged parenteral nutrition.

Preparations
Selenious Acid Injection *(U.S.P.).* pH 1.8 to 2.4.

13229-g

Senecio

Many species of the genus *Senecio* (Compositae), which includes the ragworts and groundsels, are poisonous and have been found to contain pyrrolizidine alkaloids which produce hepatic necrosis. The ragwort, *S. jacobaea*, which is abundant throughout the British Isles, is poisonous to livestock when eaten in quantity.

The ragwort and, in the USA, the golden ragwort, *Senecio aureus*, in the form of extracts have been used as emmenagogues but are of doubtful value. Ragwort, in the form of a decoction or ointment, has also been applied externally to aid wound healing.

Two alkaloids, senecionine and senecionine *N*-oxide were isolated from *Senecio triangularis*, growing in Colorado, USA. They inhibited growth of a carcinosarcoma in *mice* and this could be an explanation for the ancient use of *Senecio* spp. in the treatment of cancer.— S. M. Kupchan and M. I. Suffness (letter), *J. pharm. Sci.*, 1967, *56*, 541.

TOXICITY. An extensive review of the toxicity of pyrrolizidine alkaloids present in *Senecio* spp. and other plants.— E. K. McLean, *Pharmac. Rev.*, 1970, *22*, 429.

A report of liver damage and death associated with a herbal tea (Gordolobos) prepared from *Senecio longilobus* in Arizona, USA.— R. Huxtable, *J. Am. med. Ass.*, 1977, *238*, 1233. See also A. E. Stillman *et al.*, *Gastroenterology*, 1977, *73*, 349; A. E. Stillman *et al.*, *Morb. Mortal.*, 1977, *26*, 257. Further references to the hepatotoxic effects of *Senecio* spp. including veno-occlusive disease associated with ingestion of pyrrolizidine alkaloids: R. G. Penn, *Adverse Drug React. Bull.*, 1983, Oct., 376; *Lancet*, 1984, *1*, 201; C. R. Kumana *et al.*, *Gut*, 1985, *26*, 101.

The oral administration of ragwort, which contained 6 pyrrolizidine alkaloids, to *rats* produced hypertensive pulmonary vascular disease.— J. M. Kay *et al.*, *Thorax*, 1971, *26*, 262.

13230-f

Sepia

The dried inky secretion of the cuttle fish.

Sepia is used in homoeopathic medicine.

15305-a

Serotonin

5-HT; 5-Hydroxytryptamine; Enteramine. Serotonin is widely distributed in the body; it also occurs in stinging nettles (*Urtica dioica*), bananas, and other fruit, and in the stings of wasps and scorpions. 3-(2-Aminoethyl)-1*H*-indol-5-ol.

$C_{10}H_{12}N_2O$=176.2.

CAS — 50-67-9.

Serotonin is released by tryptaminergic neurones in the central nervous system, where it is believed to act as a neurotransmitter, and to be involved in the transmission of nervous impulses and in the control of the tone of the viscera. Serotonin is stored and synthesised mainly in enterochromaffin cells and in neurones and is also stored in blood platelets. It is considered to be implicated in causing the vascular headache of migraine; support for this view has been gained by the relief often obtained from the use of serotonin antagonists, such as methysergide and cyproheptadine. Serotonin has been suggested for use in the treatment of depression but as it does not pass the blood-brain barrier adequately, its precursor oxitriptan (5-hydroxytryptophan—see p.376) has been used.

Cardiac lesions have been found in patients with carcinoid tumours producing excessive amounts of serotonin, and endomyocardial fibrosis has been reported prevalent amongst Nigerians eating large quantities of serotonin-rich matoke bananas. Teratogenic effects have been found in *animals* given large amounts of serotonin.

A review of the origin, distribution in the body, physiological effects, and clinical and pharmacological aspects of serotonin.— A. Sirek and O. V. Sirek, *Can. med. Ass. J.*, 1970, *102*, 846. See also G. Bignami, *A. Rev. Pharmac. Toxic.*, 1976, *16*, 329; A. R. Green and D. G. Grahame-Smith, *Nature*, 1976, *260*, 487.

Two distinct types of serotonin receptor have been identified: 5-HT_1 receptors which may be involved with the influence of serotonin-like agents on adenylate cyclase, and 5-HT_2 receptors which may be associated with behavioural effects of serotonin. Both receptor types differentially regulate contractions of blood vessels.— S. H. Snyder, *Science*, 1984, *224*, 22.

Review of the actions of serotonin on the cardiovascular system.— D. S. Houston and P. M. Vanhoutte, *Drugs*, 1986, *31*, 149. See also *Serotonin and the Cardiovascular System*, P.M. Vanhoutte (Ed.), New York, Raven Press, 1985.

A discussion on serotonin and psychiatric illness.— *Lancet*, 1981, *2*, 788.

A review of monoamine research in depression including details of studies on serotonin.— H. M. van Praag, *Lancet*, 1982, *2*, 1259.

The behavioural effects of nutrients, including those effects due to food-related changes in brain serotonin concentrations.— R. J. Wurtman, *Lancet*, 1983, *1*, 1145 and 1396.

Biochemical studies of serotonin have suggested that it may play a role in hyperactivity in children (M. Coleman, *J. Pediat.*, 1971, *78*, 985), nasal allergy (Y.A. Habib *et al.*, *Acta allerg.*, 1971, *26*, 39), muscular dystrophy (D.L. Murphy, *Archs Neurol., Chicago*, 1973, *28*, 239), scleroderma and Raynaud's phenomenon (R.K. Winkelmann *et al.*, *Br. J. Derm.*, 1976, *95*, 51), conflict behaviour (N.C. Tye *et al.*, *Nature*, 1977, *268*, 741; C. Braestrup and M. Nielsen, *Lancet*, 1982, *2*, 1030), autism (*Br. med. J.*, 1978, *1*, 1651), and in suicidal depression (M. Stanley and J.J. Mann, *Lancet*, 1983, *1*, 214; G.P. Reynolds, *ibid.*, *2*, 977). Further studies are required to assess the clinical significance of serotonin in these conditions.

Serotonin competitively inhibited cholinesterase *in vitro*.— Y. S. Mohammed *et al.*, *Arzneimittel-Forsch.*, 1975, *25*, 1714.

Serotonin creatinine sulphate was the form of serotonin available for research and clinical use. Vertigo and tachycardia had followed rapid intravenous injection. There was no evidence that it was effective as a haemostatic.— M. Verstraete, *Haemostatic Drugs*, The Hague, Martinus Nijhoff, 1977, p. 68.

Myopathy thought to be secondary to muscle ischaemia was caused experimentally by serotonin alone or in combination with imipramine. It has also been shown to cause muscle necrosis experimentally.— F. L. Mastaglia, *Drugs*, 1982, *24*, 304.

Serotonin-induced platelet aggregation as an index of depression.— D. T. Healy *et al.*, *Br. J. clin. Pharmac.*, 1984, *17*, 202P. Serotonin-induced platelet aggregation responses in patients treated with neuroleptic drugs.— M. W. Orr *et al.*, *Br. J. clin. Pharmac.*, 1981, *11*, 255. See also J. M. Knox *et al.*, *ibid.*, 261.

In *animal* studies serotonin administered intraperitoneally was found to accelerate peritoneal drug transport.— D. K. Scott and D. E. Roberts, *Pharm. J.*, 1985, *1*, 592.

541-x

Serpentary

Texan or Virginian Snakeroot; Serpentaria; Serpentary Rhizome.

NOTE. Snakeroot is also used as a common name to describe poisonous *Eupatorium* spp.

Pharmacopoeias. In *Chin.* which allows various species of *Aristolochia.*

Preparations of serpentary have been employed as bitters. Its active ingredient is aristolochic acid and this and its sodium salt have been tried in a number of inflammatory disorders, mainly in folk medicine. However there is concern over its use since aristolochic acid has been reported to be carcinogenic in animals.

7368-w

Sesame Oil *(BAN, USAN).*

Benne Oil; Gingelly Oil; Oleum Sesami; Teel Oil.

CAS — 8008-74-0.

Pharmacopoeias. In *Aust., Belg., Br., Chin., Egypt., Eur., Fr., Ger., Int., Jpn, Mex., Neth.,* and *Swiss.* Also in *U.S.N.F.*.

The fixed oil obtained from the ripe seeds of *Sesamum indicum* (Pedaliaceae) by expression or extraction and subsequent refining. It is a pale yellow oil almost odourless and with a bland taste. It solidifies to a buttery mass at about −4°.

Practically **insoluble** in alcohol; miscible with carbon disulphide, chloroform, ether, and petroleum spirit. **Store** at a temperature not exceeding 40° in well-filled airtight containers. Protect from light. Sesame oil intended for use in the manufacture of a parenteral dosage form should be stored in a glass container.

Sesame oil has been used instead of olive oil in the preparation of liniments, plasters, ointments, and soaps. Because it is relatively stable, it is a useful solvent for certain steroids and other oil-soluble drugs administered in oily solution in capsules or in oily injections. Hypersensitivity reactions have been observed.

Acute polyneuropathy associated with the ingestion of sesame oil (gingili oil; jinjili oil) contaminated with tricresyl phosphates.— N. Senanayake and J. Jeyaratnam, *Lancet*, 1981, *1*, 88.

926-j

Sfericase

AI-794.

Sfericase is a proteolytic enzyme from *Bacillus sphaericus* under investigation as a mucolytic.

References: K. Yoshida, *Int. J. clin. Pharmac.*, 1983, *21*, 439; K. Itoh *et al.*, *Int. J. clin. Pharmac. Ther. Toxic.*, 1984, *22*, 32; Y. Miyoshi *et al.*, *ibid.*, 73.

285-x

Shellac *(USAN).*

904; Lacca; Lacca in Tabulis.

CAS — 9000-59-3.

Pharmacopoeias. In *Fr., Ind.,* and *Span. Jpn* includes Purified Shellac and White Shellac (Bleached). Also in *U.S.N.F.*

Shellac is obtained by purification of the resinous secretion of the insect *Laccifer lacca* Kerr (Coccidae). The *U.S.N.F.* describes 4 grades: Orange Shellac is produced by filtration in the molten state or by a hot solvent process, or both; removal of the wax produces Dewaxed Orange Shellac which may be lighter in colour; Regular Bleached (White) Shellac is prepared by dissolving the secretion in aqueous sodium carbonate, bleaching with hypochlorite, and precipitating with sulphuric acid; removal of the wax by filtration during the process produces Refined Bleached Shellac.

Insoluble in water; very slowly soluble in alcohol 85% to 95% (w/w); soluble in ether, 13% to 15%, and in aqueous solutions of ethanolamines, alkalis, and borax. **Store** in well-closed containers preferably at a temperature not exceeding 8°.

Shellac is used as an enteric coating for pills and tablets, but disintegration time has been reported to increase markedly on storage. Bleached shellac, in alcoholic solution, is used as a hair lacquer.

Preparations

Pharmaceutical Glaze *(U.S.N.F.).* A denatured solution containing 20 to 57% of anhydrous shellac, prepared with alcohol (95%) or dehydrated alcohol; it may contain waxes and titanium dioxide as an opaquing agent. Store at a temperature not exceeding 40° (preferably below 25°) in lined metal or plastic airtight containers.

273-c

Siam Benzoin

Benzoe Tonkinensis.

CAS — 9000-72-0.

Pharmacopoeias. In *Aust., Chin., Fr., Ger., It., Neth., Span.,* and *Swiss.* Also in many pharmacopoeias under the title benzoin and should not be confused with Sumatra Benzoin. *U.S.* allows both Siam benzoin and Sumatra benzoin under the title Benzoin.

A balsamic resin from *Styrax tonkinensis* (Styracaceae) and containing not more than 10% of alcohol (90%)-insoluble matter.

Yellowish-brown to rusty brown compressed pebble-like tears with an agreeable, balsamic, vanilla-like odour. The tears are separate or very slightly agglutinated, milky white on fracture, and hard and brittle at ordinary temperatures, but softened by heat. **Store** in well-closed containers.

Siam benzoin has been used similarly to Sumatra benzoin (p.1620). It has also been used as a preservative and was formerly used in the preparation of benzoinated lard.

5316-v

Silver

E174.

Ag=107.868.

CAS — 7440-22-4.

Pharmacopoeias. In *Swiss.*

A pure white, malleable and ductile metal.

Silver possesses antibacterial properties and is used topically either as the metal or as silver salts. Silver is used as a food colour for some types of confectionery. It is not absorbed to any great extent and the main problem associated with the metal is argyria, a general grey discoloration. In Great Britain the recommended exposure limit of silver is 0.1 mg per m^3 (long-term).

A report of reversible neuropathy associated with the absorption of silver from an arthroplasty cement.— H. Vik *et al.* (letter), *Lancet*, 1985, *1*, 872.

Coating catheters with silver reduced the incidence of catheter-associated bacteriuria.— T. Lundeberg (letter), *Lancet*, 1986, *2*, 1031.

5319-p

Silver Acetate

Argenti Acetas.

CH_3COOAg=166.9.

CAS — 563-63-3.

Pharmacopoeias. In *Aust.* and *Hung.*

Silver acetate has been used similarly to silver nitrate as a disinfectant. It has also been used in antismoking tablets.

5321-h

Silver Nitrate *(BAN, USAN).*

Argenti Nitras; Nitrato de Plata; Nitrato de Prata.

$AgNO_3$=169.9.

CAS — 7761-88-8.

Pharmacopoeias. In *Arg., Aust., Belg., Br., Cz., Egypt., Eur., Fr., Ger., Hung., Ind., Int., It., Jpn, Jug., Mex., Neth., Nord., Pol., Port., Roum., Rus., Span., Swiss, Turk.,* and *U.S.*

Colourless or white transparent crystals or crystalline odourless powder. On exposure to air or light in the presence of organic matter, silver nitrate becomes grey or greyish-black.

Soluble 1 in 0.5 of water, and 1 in 27 of alcohol; its solubility is increased in boiling water or alcohol.

Silver nitrate is **incompatible** with a range of substances. Although it is unlikely that there will be a need to add any of the interacting substances to silver nitrate solutions considering its current uses, pharmacists should be aware of the potential for incompatibility. **Store** in airtight non-metallic containers. Protect from light.

The reported yellow-brown discoloration of samples of silver nitrate bladder irrigation (1 in 10 000) probably arose from the reaction of the silver nitrate with alkali released from the glass bottle which appeared to be soda-glass.— Pharm. Soc. Lab. Rep. P/80/6, 1980.

Adverse Effects

Symptoms of poisoning stem from the corrosive action of silver nitrate and include pain in the mouth, sialorrhoea, diarrhoea, vomiting, coma, and convulsions.

A short lived minor conjunctivitis is common in infants given silver nitrate eye drops; repeated use or the use of high concentrations produces severe damage and even blindness. Chronic application to mucous surfaces or open wounds leads to argyria, which though difficult to treat is considered to be mainly a cosmetic hazard, see under Silver (above).

Absorption of the nitrate and reduction to nitrite may cause methaemoglobinaemia. There is also a risk of electrolyte disturbances.

Treatment of these adverse effects is symptomatic.

In Great Britain the recommended exposure limits of soluble silver compounds (as Ag) are 0.01 mg per m^3 (long-term); 0.03 mg per m^3 (short-term).

Silver nitrate from a stick containing 75% was applied to the eyes of a newborn infant instead of a 1% solution. After 1 hour there was a thick purulent secretion, the eyelids were red and oedematous, and the conjunctiva markedly injected. The corneas had a blue-grey bedewed appearance with areas of corneal opacification. After treatment by lavage and topical application of antibiotics and homatropine 2% there was a marked improvement and after 1 week topical application of corticosteroids was started. Residual damage was limited to slight corneal opacity.— A. Hornblass (letter), *J. Am. med. Ass.*, 1975, *231*, 245.

Absorption and Fate

Silver nitrate is not readily absorbed.

Uses and Administration

Silver nitrate possesses disinfectant properties and is used in many countries as a 1% solution for the prophylaxis of ophthalmia neonatorum when 2 drops are instilled into each conjunctival sac of the neonate. However, as it is not effective against chlamydia and can cause irritation, other agents are often used.

In stick form it has been used as a caustic to destroy warts and other small skin growths. Compresses soaked in a 0.5% solution of silver nitrate have been applied to severe burns to reduce infection. Solutions have also been used as topical disinfectants and astringents in other conditions.

Silver nitrate (Argentum Nitricum; Argent. Nit.) is used in homoeopathic medicine. It is also used in cosmetics to dye eyebrows and eye lashes.

CYSTITIS. Comment on silver nitrate irrigation having limited value in the management of haemorrhagic cystitis after radiotherapy.— *Lancet*, 1987, *1*, 304.

PREGNANCY AND THE NEONATE. Some references and reviews on the suppression of neonatal ophthalmia and covering the role of silver nitrate: *Can. med. Ass. J.*, 1983, *129*, 554; E. M. Zola, *Drug Intell. & clin. Pharm.*, 1984, *18*, 692; G. Schneider, *Can. med. Ass. J.*, 1984, *131*, 193; *Lancet*, 1984, *2*, 1375; F. P. Galega *et al.*, *Bull. Wld Hlth Org.*, 1984, *62*, 95; J. D. Oriel, *J. antimicrob. Chemother.*, 1984, *14*, 209; M. Laga *et al.*, *Lancet*, 1986, *2*, 1145.

Preparations

Silver Nitrate Ophthalmic Solution *(U.S.P.)*. A solution of silver nitrate 0.95 to 1.05% in an aqueous medium. pH 4.5 to 6.0. It may contain sodium acetate as a buffer. Store in inert collapsible capsules or in other suitable single-dose containers.

Toughened Silver Nitrate *(U.S.P.)*. Contains not less than 94.5% of $AgNO_3$, the remainder consisting of silver chloride.

Proprietary Names and Manufacturers

Argenpal *(Andalucia, Spain)*; Helvedstensstifter *(Braun, Denm.)*; Lapis *(DAK, Denm.)*; Mova Nitrat *(Lindopharm, Ger.)*; Pluralane *(Ardeypharm, Ger.)*.

5322-m

Silver Protein

Albumosesilber; Argentoproteinum; Argentum Proteinicum; Protargolum; Proteinato de Plata; Proteinato de Prata; Strong Protargin; Strong Protein Silver; Strong Silver Protein.

CAS — 9015-51-4; 9007-35-6 (colloidal silver).

NOTE. Synonyms for mild silver protein include: Argentoproteinum Mite; Argentum Vitellinicum; Mild Protargin; Mild Silver Proteinate; Silver Nucleinate; Silver Vitellin; Vitelinato de Plata and Vitelinato de Prata.

Pharmacopoeias. In *Arg., Aust., Belg., Cz., Fr., Hung., Int., It., Jpn, Pol., Port., Roum., Span.,* and *Turk.* Many of these pharmacopoeias include monographs on mild silver protein as well as on colloidal silver.

Silver protein solutions have antibacterial properties, due to the presence of low concentrations of ionised silver, and have been used as eye-drops. The mild form of silver protein is considered to be less irritating, but less active; it is used in nasal solutions.

Colloidal silver which is also a preparation of silver in combination with protein has also been used topically for its antibacterial activity.

Proprietary Names and Manufacturers of Various Silver Protein Preparations

Argincolor *(Fr.)*; Argirol *(Spain)*; Argyn *(USA)*; Argyrol *(Coopervision, USA)*; Néo-Collargol *(Martinet, Fr.)*; Stillargol *(Mayoly-Spindler, Fr.)*; Vitargénol *(Fr.)*.

The following names have been used for multi-ingredient preparations containing various silver protein preparations— Argotone *(Riker, Austral.; Lipha, UK)*.

13236-v

Silymarin

The active principle from the fruit of *Silybum marianum (=Carduus marianus)* (Compositae). The principal component is the flavonoid silibinin (silybin). 3,5,7-Trihydroxy-2[3-(4-hydroxy-3-methoxyphenyl)-2-(hydroxymethyl)-1,4-benzodioxan-6-yl]-4-chromanone (silibinin).

$C_{25}H_{22}O_{10}$=482.4.

CAS — 65666-07-1 (silymarin); 22888-70-6 (silibinin).

Pharmacopoeias. Ger. includes Milk Thistle Fruit, the ripe liberated fruit of *Silybum marianum* containing not less than 1% of silymarin calculated as silibinin.

Silymarin has been used for the treatment of hepatic disorders. Silymarin and disodium silibinin dihemisuccinate have been tried in *Amanita phalloides* poisoning. Silymarin is poorly water-soluble and has been given by mouth; disodium silibinin dihemisuccinate is water-soluble and has been given by intravenous injection.

Liver function in patients with chronic hepatitis and cholangitis improved after 3 months' therapy with silymarin.— G. Poser, *Arzneimittel-Forsch.*, 1971, *21*, 1209.

Silymarin 420 mg daily was given to 375 patients with cirrhosis. Of 20 followed up for 6 to 36 months 10 were definitely improved and 4 had deteriorated.— I. Benda and W. Zenz, *Wien. med. Wschr.*, 1973, *123*, 512.

The chemistry and active constituents of *Silybum marianum*.— H. Wagner *et al.*, *Arzneimittel-Forsch.*, 1974, *24*, 466; G. Halbach and W. Trost, *ibid.*, 866; I. Morelli; *Boll. chim.-farm.*, 1978, *117*, 258.

A dimer of silibinin had 10 times the activity of silibinin.— G. Vogel and W. Trost, *Arzneimittel-Forsch.*, 1975, *25*, 392.

Review of studies in *animals* and humans of the use of silymarin in the treatment of liver damage due to poisoning with *Amanita phalloides*.— D. Lorenz, *Dte Arzt*, 1982, *79*, 43. See also G. Vogel, The Anti-Amanita Effect of Silymarin, in *Amanita Toxins and Poisoning*, H. Faulstich *et al.* (Eds), Baden-Baden, Verlag Gerhard Witzstrock, 1980, p. 180.

Further references to the use of silymarin in hepatic disorders: S. Cavalieri, *Gazz. med. ital.*, 1974, *133*, 628 (oral silymarin in acute hepatitis); K. Hruby *et al.*, *Hum. Toxicol.*, 1983, *2*, 183 (intravenous silibinin in *Amanita phalloides* poisoning); H. A. Salmi and S. Sarna, *Scand. J. Gastroenterol.*, 1982, *17*, 517 (oral silymarin in acute and subacute liver disease).

For further references to the use of silymarin or silibinin in the treatment of *Amanita phalloides* poisoning, see p.1592.

A commercial preparation of silymarin (Legalon) enhanced the activity of the mixed function oxidation system in *rats* but did not prevent carbon tetrachloride-induced depression of the system. In human subjects the half-life of phenazone and phenylbutazone was not altered by silymarin and it was doubtful whether silymarin had a hepatic protective role in man.— H. W. Leber and S. Knauff, *Arzneimittel-Forsch.*, 1976, *26*, 1603.

In *rats* and humans silymarin administration markedly affected biliary lipid composition. In humans silymarin reduced biliary-cholesterol concentration with a resultant decrease in the cholesterol saturation of the bile.— L. Okolicsanyi *et al.*, *Drugs*, 1986, *31*, 430.

Proprietary Names and Manufacturers

Cardomarin *(Cheminova, Spain)*; Ciscolex *(Arg.)*; Cordomarin *(Spain)*; Cronol *(Spain)*; Dorogan *(Kairon, Spain)*; DuraSilymarin *(Durachemie, Ger.)*; Emil *(Spain)*; Enterohepat *(Arg.)*; Epacardo *(Savio, Ital.)*; Eparfit *(Spain)*; Eparsil *(Pulitzer, Ital.)*; Escarmine *(Spain)*; Halodren *(Spain)*; Hepadestal *(Krugmann, Ger.)*; Hepagerina *(Spain)*; Hepalar *(Spain)*; Hepallolina *(Spain)*; Hepato-Framan *(Oftalmiso, Spain)*; Laragon *(Roemmers, Arg.)*; Lecemin *(Spain)*; Legalon *(Madaus, Belg.; Bellon, Fr.; Madaus, Ger.; Ibi, Ital.; Madaus Cerafarm, Spain; Madaus, Switz.)*; Pluropon *(Spain)*; Sematron *(Spain)*; Silarine *(Vir, Spain)*; Silepar *(Ibirn, Ital.)*; Silgen *(Spain)*; Silibancol *(IBYS, Spain)*; Siliklari *(Clariana, Spain)*; Silimarina *(Medical, Spain)*; Silimazu *(Mazuelos, Spain)*; Silirex *(Lampugnani, Ital.)*; Silliver *(Abbott, Ital.)*.

932-l

Sinefungin *(USAN).*

Compound 57926. 6,9-Diamino-1-(6-amino-9*H*-purin-9-yl)-1,5,6,7,8,9,-hexadeoxy-β-D-*ribo*-decofuranuronic acid.

$C_{15}H_{23}N_7O_5$=381.4.

CAS — 58944-73-3.

Sinefungin is an antiprotozoal agent that has been produced from *Streptomyces griseolus*. There are reports of activity against *Leishmania* spp., *Plasmodium falciparum*, trypanosomes, and *Trichomonas vaginalis*. It has also been reported to possess antifungal activity.

References to the *in-vitro* and *in-vivo* activity of sinefungin against various organisms: W. Trager *et al.*, *Expl Parasit.*, 1980, *50*, 83 (*Plasmodium falciparum*); J. P. Nadler *et al.*, *Trans. R. Soc. trop. Med. Hyg.*, 1982, *76*, 285 (*Trypanosoma cruzi*); D. K. Dube *et al.*, *Am. J. trop. Med. Hyg.*, 1983, *32*, 31 (*Trypanosoma* spp.); A. Ferrante *et al.*, *Trans. R. Soc. trop. Med. Hyg.*, 1984, *78*, 837 (*Entamoeba histolytica*); R. A. Neal *et al.*, *ibid.*, 1985, *79*, 122 (*Leishmania donovani*); P. Paolantonacci *et al.*, *Antimicrob. Ag. Chemother.*, 1985, *28*, 528 (*Leishmania* spp.); K.-W. Thong and G. H. Coombs, *J. antimicrob. Chemother.*, 1987, *19*, 429 (*Trichomonas vaginalis*).

Proprietary Names and Manufacturers

Lilly, USA.

13238-q

Sitogluside *(USAN, rINN).*

AW-10; BSSG; EU-4906; WA-184. 3β-(β-D-Glucopyranosyloxy)stigmast-5-ene.

$C_{35}H_{60}O_6$=576.9.

CAS — 474-58-8.

Sitogluside is reported to have activity against prostatic hypertrophy.

Proprietary Names and Manufacturers

Norwich Eaton, USA.

1796-v

Sizofiran *(pINN).*

Schizophyllan. Poly[3→-(*O*-β-D-glucopyranosyl-(1→3)-*O*-[β-D-glucopyranosyl-(1→6)]-*O*-β-D-glucopyranosyl-(1→3)-*O*-β-D-glucopyranosyl)-→1].

$(C_{24}H_{40}O_{20})_n$.

CAS — 9050-67-3.

Sizofiran is reported to have immunomodulating activity and has been given in conjunction with other treatment in malignant neoplasms.

References: *Drugs of the Future*, 1986, *11*, 716; *Drugs Today*, 1987, *23*, 72.

Proprietary Names and Manufacturers

Kaken, Jpn.

212-m

Soda Lime *(BAN, USAN).*

Cal Sodada; Calcaria absorbens; Calcaria Compositio; Calx Sodica; Chaux Sodée.

CAS — 8006-28-8.

Pharmacopoeias. In *Arg., Br., Fr., Mex., Pol.,* and *Swiss.* Also in *U.S.N.F.*

The *B.P.* specifies a mixture of sodium hydroxide, or sodium hydroxide and potassium hydroxide, with calcium hydroxide. The *U.S.N.F* specifies a mixture of calcium hydroxide with sodium or potassium hydroxide or both.

White or greyish-white granules, or coloured with an indicator to show when absorptive power is exhausted. Soda lime absorbs about 20% of its weight of carbon dioxide. Partially **soluble** in water; almost completely soluble in 1M acetic acid. **Incompatible** with trichloroethylene. **Store** in airtight containers.

Soda lime is used to absorb carbon dioxide for instance in closed-circuit anaesthetic apparatus and in determining the basal metabolic rate. Limits are specified for particle size, and particles should be free from dust.

Soda lime must not be used with trichloroethylene, since this is decomposed by warm alkali into dichloroacetylene which is very toxic and gives rise to lesions of the nervous system.

13242-m

Sodium Arsenate

Natrium Arsenicicum; Sodium Arseniate.
$Na_2HAsO_4,7H_2O=312.0$.

CAS — 7778-43-0 (anhydrous); 10048-95-0 (heptahydrate).

Pharmacopoeias. In *Belg., Fr., Pol., Port., Rus.,* and *Swiss.*

Sodium arsenate was formerly used in the treatment of chronic skin diseases, in parasitic diseases of the blood, and in some forms of anaemia. It has the adverse effects of Arsenic Trioxide, p.1544.

13245-g

Sodium Cacodylate

Sod. Cacodyl.; Sodium Dimethylarsonate. Sodium dimethylarsinate trihydrate.
$C_2H_6AsNaO_2,3H_2O=214.0$.

CAS — 75-60-5 (cacodylic acid); 124-65-2 (sodium salt, anhydrous); 6131-99-3 (sodium salt, trihydrate); 5968-84-3 (ferric salt).

Pharmacopoeias. In *Mex., Port.,* and *Span. Span.* also includes ferric cacodylate.

The effects of sodium cacodylate are essentially those of the inorganic arsenic to which it is partly reduced in the body. It was formerly used, usually by subcutaneous injection, for the same purposes as arsenic trioxide. It has the adverse effects of Arsenic Trioxide, p.1544. Sodium cacodylate is more toxic when given by mouth than when injected because of the rapid release of inorganic arsenic by gastric juice; it imparts a strong garlic-like odour to the breath, urine, and perspiration, particularly when taken by mouth, due to the release of cacodylic oxide.

Ferric cacodylate (iron cacodylate; ferric dimethylarsinate), strychnine cacodylate, and sodium cacodylate were once popular ingredients of proprietary injections advocated for their stimulant effects in debilitated conditions.

213-b

Sodium Carbonate Anhydrous

500; Cenizas de Soda; Exsiccated Sodium Carbonate; Natrium Carbonicum Calcinatum; Natrium Carbonicum Siccatum; Sodium Carbonate *(USAN)*.
$Na_2CO_3=106.0$.

CAS — 497-19-8.

Pharmacopoeias. In *Arg., Fr., Hung., Jpn, Jug., Pol.,* and *Port.*

NOTE. Sodium Carbonate (*U.S.N.F.*) is anhydrous or the monohydrate.

Colourless crystals, or white, crystalline powder or granules. **Soluble** 1 in 3 of water and 1 in 1.8 of boiling water. **Store** in well-closed containers.

214-v

Sodium Carbonate Decahydrate *(BAN)*.

500; Cristales de Sosa; Natrii Carbonas; Natrii Carbonas Decahydricus; Natrium Carbonicum Crystallisatum.
$Na_2CO_3,10H_2O=286.1$.

CAS — 6132-02-1.

NOTE. Washing soda is a synonym for the technical grade of sodium carbonate decahydrate.

Pharmacopoeias. In *Arg., Aust., Belg., Br., Eur., Fr., Ger., Hung., It., Jpn, Jug., Neth., Nord., Pol., Span.,* and *Swiss.*

Odourless, colourless, efflorescent, transparent crystals or white crystalline powder. **Soluble** 1 in 2 of water; practically insoluble in alcohol. **Store** in well-closed containers.

215-g

Sodium Carbonate Monohydrate *(BAN)*.

500; Natrii Carbonas Monohydricus; Sodium Carbonate *(USAN)*.
$Na_2CO_3,H_2O=124.0$.

CAS — 5968-11-6.

Pharmacopoeias. In *Aust., Belg., Br., Braz., Eur., Fr., Ger., It., Neth.,* and *Swiss.*

NOTE. Sodium Carbonate (*U.S.N.F.*) is the anhydrous or the monohydrate.

Odourless, colourless crystals or white crystalline powder or granules. It is stable in air under ordinary conditions but effloresces when exposed to dry air above 50°; at 100° it becomes anhydrous.**Soluble** 1 in 3 of water and 1 in 1.8 of boiling water; practically insoluble in alcohol. **Store** in well-closed containers.

Anhydrous sodium carbonate and the monohydrate are used as reagents. The decahydrate has been used in alkaline baths and in Great Britain is an approved disinfectant for foot-and-mouth disease. Sodium carbonate in its anhydrous or hydrated form is also used as a water softener.

13246-q

Sodium Cyanate

NaCNO=65.01.

CAS — 917-61-3.

Adverse Effects

Peripheral neuropathies, gastro-intestinal effects, fatigue, and drowsiness have been reported with sodium cyanate.

EFFECTS ON THE EYE. Bilateral cataracts occurred in 2 patients receiving sodium cyanate. There was spontaneous regression in 1 patient when sodium cyanate was withdrawn.— D. H. Nicholson *et al., Archs Ophthal., N.Y.,* 1976, *94,* 927.

Uses and Administration

Sodium cyanate is an antisickling agent which causes carbamoylation of the terminal valine residues of haemoglobin and increases its oxygen affinity.

Preliminary clinical studies were encouraging when sodium cyanate was given by mouth to patients with sickle-cell disease but a subsequent controlled study demonstrated no beneficial effect and increasing evidence of unacceptable toxicity. There have been some encouraging results using extracorporeal treatment in which cyanate is added to blood previously withdrawn from the patient and then returned to the body.

13247-p

Sodium Dichloroacetate

DCA.
$C_2HCl_2NaO_2=150.9$.

CAS — 2156-56-1; 79-43-6 (dichloroacetic acid).

Sodium dichloroacetate activates pyruvate dehydrogenase. It has been tried in the treatment of lactic acidosis, including that caused by phenformin, but its use has been suspended by some workers because of toxicity in *animals* and a report of polyneuropathy in clinical studies.

The biological disposition of sodium dichloroacetate after intravenous administration.— G. Lukas *et al., J. pharm. Sci.,* 1980, *69,* 419.

ADVERSE EFFECTS. The chronic oral administration of dichloroacetate has been suspended because of adverse effects in *animals* and a polyneuropathy which developed in a patient given dichloroacetate for 16 weeks.— P. W. Stacpoole *et al.* (letter), *New Engl. J. Med.,* 1979, *300,* 372.

Mention of the mutagenicity of dichloroacetate.— V. Herbert *et al.* (letter), *New Engl. J. Med.,* 1979, *300,* 625.

LACTIC ACIDOSIS. Results demonstrating that dichloroacetate can have positive metabolic and haemodynamic effects in patients with lactic acidosis. Thirteen patients with lactic acidosis from various causes, treated unsuccessfully with sodium bicarbonate, were given sodium dichloroacetate by intravenous infusion. Of 11 evaluable patients (the other 2 also received sodium bicarbonate) 7 had an unequivocal metabolic response to therapy with a mean decrease in arterial blood-lactate concentration of 80%, a mean increase in arterial blood-bicarbonate concentration of 50%, and a raising of mean arterial pH to normal. Metabolic acidaemia, present initially in 6 of the 7, improved or completely resolved. All 4 patients who received dichloroacetate in a dose of 50 mg per kg body-weight had a metabolic response, compared with only 3 of 7 who received 35 mg per kg. All of the patients were hypotensive and an unexpected finding in 10 of the 13 was an increase in arterial systolic blood pressure, ranging from 10 to 40 mmHg, during dichloroacetate administration and lasting for several minutes to several hours. This rise in systolic pressure was accompanied by a mean increase in cardiac output of 21% in 4 patients monitored. There was no evidence of serious toxicity from dichloroacetate. Despite a marked improvement in overall morbidity with dichloroacetate, only one patient survived their underlying disease.— P. W. Stacpoole *et al., New Engl. J. Med.,* 1983, *309,* 390. Comment.— J.-L. Vincent (letter), *ibid.,* 1984, *310,* 320. Reply.— P. W. Stacpoole *et al.* (letter), *ibid.*

Further references to the use of dichloroacetate in the treatment of lactic acidosis: P. G. Wells *et al., Diabetologia,* 1980, *19,* 109; R. D. Cohen and H. F. Woods, *Diabetes,* 1983, *32,* 181; *Lancet,* 1983, *2,* 1288.

13248-s

Sodium Dithionite

Sodium Hydrosulphite; Sodium Sulphoxylate.
$Na_2S_2O_4=174.1$, or $Na_2S_2O_4,2H_2O = 210.1$.

CAS — 7775-14-6 (anhydrous).

NOTE. The name sodium hydrosulfite is also applied to $NaHSO_2 = 88.06$.

Sodium dithionite may be used in the form of a simple urine test in the detection of paraquat poisoning. A 0.25% solution has been used to remove phenazopyridine stains. It is irritant to the skin.

7733-z

Sodium Fluoride *(BAN, USAN)*.

Natrii Fluoridum; Natrium Fluoratum.
NaF=41.99.

CAS — 7681-49-4.

Pharmacopoeias. In *Arg., Br., Braz., Cz., Egypt., Eur., Hung., It., Jug., Nord., Pol., Roum., Swiss,* and *U.S.*

A white odourless powder or colourless crystals. Sodium fluoride 2.2 mg is approximately equivalent to 1 mg of fluoride. Each g provides approximately 23.8 mmol of sodium and fluoride. **Soluble** 1 in 25 of water; practically insoluble in alcohol. **Store** in well-closed containers. *U.S.P.* preparations should be stored in airtight containers; plastic containers should be used for Sodium Fluoride Oral Solution *U.S.P.* having a pH below 7.5 and for preparations also containing phosphoric acid.

Adverse Effects and Treatment

In the controlled amounts recommended for fluoridation of drinking water and at the recommended doses employed in dentistry for caries prophylaxis, sodium fluoride has not been shown to have significant side-effects.

In acute poisoning, sodium fluoride taken by mouth is corrosive, forming hydrofluoric acid in the stomach which can cause a variety of local effects. Sodium fluoride may also produce metabolic and electrolyte disturbances, including hypocalcaemia. Systemic effects include tremors, hyperreflexia, paraesthesia, tetany, convulsions, cardiac arrythmias, shock, respiratory arrest, and cardiac failure. Death may occur within 2 to 4 hours. Although there is much interindividual variation, a single oral dose of 5 to 10 g of sodium fluoride would be considered lethal in an untreated adult by most authorities. However, dangerous poisoning has been reported after oral doses of less than 1 g.

Treatment of acute poisoning involves gastric lavage with lime water or a weak solution of another calcium salt to precipitate fluoride, maintenance of high urine output, slow intravenous injections of calcium gluconate 10% for tetany, and symptomatic and supportive measures. Aluminium hydroxide administered after gastric lavage may reduce fluoride absorption. Haemodialysis may be considered.

Chronic fluoride poisoning may result in skeletal fluorosis manifestations of which include increased density and coarsened trabeculation of bone and calcification in ligaments, tendons, and muscle insertions. Clinical signs are joint pain, stiffness, limited movement, and in severe cases, crippling deformities. Prolonged excessive intake by children during the period of tooth development before eruption can result in dental fluorosis characterised by mottled enamel. At fluoride concentrations in drinking water of 1 to 2 ppm dental fluorosis is mild with white opaque flecks on the teeth. At higher concentrations, enamel defects become more severe with brown to black staining and the teeth have a pitted corroded appearance.

The fluoridation of water has been a subject of considerable controversy. Suggestions that it increases the incidence of thyroid disorders, chromosome aberrations, and cancer have not been substantiated.

In Great Britain the recommended exposure limit of fluoride (as fluorine) is 2.5 mg per m^3 (long-term). In the *US* the permissible and recommended exposure limits are 2.5 mg per m^3.

For a review of the toxic effects of fluoride salts, see Fluorine and Fluorides, *Environmental Health Criteria 36*, Geneva, World Health Organization, 1984, p.72.

ALLERGY. Contrasting opinions on the evidence for fluoride allergy.— D. Jackson (letter), *Br. dent. J.*, 1984, *156*, 430; R. V. Mummery (letter), *ibid.*, *157*, 48; I. P. D. Stocker (letter), *ibid.*, 188.

CARCINOGENICITY. Based on comparisons of cancer mortality rates for communities residing in fluoridated and non-fluoridated cities, Yiamouyiannis and Burk (*Fluoride*, 1977, *10*, 102) alleged that artificial fluoridation of water might be associated with an increased risk of cancer. Re-examination of their data by others failed to confirm this relationship nor did further studies in a number of countries (J. Clemmesen, *Bull. Wld Hlth Org.*, 1983, *61*, 871). In Great Britain, the Working Party on Fluoridation of Water and Cancer (*Fluoridation of Water and Cancer: A Review of the Epidemiological Evidence*, London, HM Stationery Office, 1985) found nothing which could lead them to conclude that either fluoride occurring naturally in water, or fluoride added to water supplies, was capable of inducing cancer, or of increasing the mortality from cancer. In this respect, fluoridation of drinking water was considered safe.

EFFECTS ON THE KIDNEY. Nephrotoxicity has been associated with high plasma concentrations of fluoride during anaesthesia with fluorine-containing anaesthetic agents such as methoxyflurane, enflurane, and isoflurane. Further information is contained within those monographs.

FLUOROSIS. A discussion of chronic fluorosis. In temperate climates, teeth seemed not to be affected if fluoride concentrations in drinking water were not greatly above 1 ppm; fluorosis affecting bone would not be detectable until concentrations at least exceeded 4 ppm.— *Br. med. J.*, 1981, *282*, 253.

OVERDOSAGE. Reviews and comments on acute fluoride toxicity.— *Fluoride*, 1979, *12*, 55; A. J. Duxbury *et al.*, *Br. dent. J.*, 1982, *153*, 64; R. J. Andlaw (letter), *ibid.*, 285; P. A. Monsour *et al.*, *Med. J. Aust.*, 1984, *141*, 503.

Fluoride is removed from plasma by dialysis *in vitro*; clinical improvement has been reported with haemodialysis for fluoride poisoning but the course of the poisoning is usually too rapid to achieve significant clinical benefit.— J. F. Winchester *et al.*, *Trans. Am. Soc. artif. internal Organs*, 1977, *23*, 762.

PREGNANCY AND THE NEONATE. Bacteriological and *animal* studies carried out under the auspices of the National Institutes of Health, USA indicated that fluorides did not increase chromosomal aberration and were not considered to be mutagenic.— *Br. dent. J.*, 1977, *143*, 325. See also: H. L. Needleman *et al.*, *New Engl. J. Med.*, 1974, *291*, 821 (no association with Down's Syndrome); J. D. Erickson, *Teratology*, 1980, *21*, 177 (another survey revealing no association).

Precautions

When considering fluoride supplementation, allowance should be made for fluorides ingested from other sources; fluoride supplements in children are not generally recommended when the fluoride content of drinking water is over 0.7 ppm (see also Uses, below). Care should be taken to prevent children swallowing excessive fluoride after topical application to teeth.

Patients with impaired renal function may be particularly susceptible to fluorosis. Regular dialysis with fluoridated water may result in additional fluoride absorption; a maximum concentration of 0.2 ppm of fluoride in the dialysate has been recommended. Dialysis patients not using deionised water are at risk from changes in the fluoride content of the water supply.

Concern regarding the possible ingestion by children of excessive fluoride from fluoridated dentifrices.— T. B. Dowell, *Br. dent. J.*, 1981, *150*, 247; S. A. Williams and C. G. Fairpo (letter), *ibid.*, 339; K. W. Stephen (letter), *ibid.*, 1984, *156*, 274. Recommendation that when fluoride supplements are used for pre-school children, then the quantity of fluoridated toothpaste should be limited to approximately 0.3 g, the size of a small pea.— T. B. Dowell and S. Joyston-Bechal, *ibid.*, 1981, *150*, 273.

In a study of 13 young adults, the mean quantities of fluoride presumed ingested following a topical application of acidulated sodium fluoride gel to the teeth ranged from 1.27 to 23.19 mg. As excessive fluoride ingestion might therefore occur, care should be exercised, especially in children; home care gel treatments should be discouraged.— D. R. McCall *et al.*, *Br. dent. J.*, 1983, *155*, 333. Fluoride varnishes might be preferable to gels as topical application was probably less haphazard, but care was still needed especially in younger children to avoid fluoride overdosage.— J. F. Roberts and P. Longhurst, *ibid.*, 1987, *162*, 463.

RENAL FAILURE. A decrease in the urinary excretion of fluoride with progressive renal impairment and a simultaneous increase in plasma-fluoride concentrations has been demonstrated in patients with chronic renal insufficiency (H. Spencer *et al.*, *Archs intern. Med.*, 1980, *140*, 1331; H.H. Schiffl and U. Binswanger, *Nephron*, 1980, *26*, 69). Parsons *et al.* (*Br. med. J.*, 1975, *1*, 128) and Schiffl and Binswanger (1980) estimated that such patients continued to excrete normal dietary loads of fluoride until the creatinine clearance decreased below 16 and 25 mL per minute respectively. Reduced fluoride excretion may result in excessive accumulation of fluoride in bone and skeletal fluorosis has occasionally been reported in patients with impaired renal function exposed to high concentrations of fluoride in water (L.I. Juncos and J.V. Donadio, *J. Am. med. Ass.*, 1972, *222*, 783) or receiving high doses of sodium fluoride for the treatment of osteoporosis (J.C. Gerster *et al.*, *Br. med. J.*, 1983, *287*, 723).

Absorption and Fate

Sodium fluoride and other soluble fluorides are readily absorbed from the gastro-intestinal tract. Absorption may be reduced by calcium, magnesium, and aluminium salts. Inhaled fluorides are absorbed through the lungs.

Fluoride is deposited predominantly in the bones and teeth; with a raised intake of fluoride, about one-half is retained.

Fluoride is principally excreted in the urine but small amounts may also be excreted in faeces and sweat. It diffuses across the placenta and is present in saliva, nails, and hair. There is some evidence of diffusion into milk.

The pharmacokinetics of sodium fluoride after single and multiple doses was studied in 8 healthy subjects. The concentration of fluoride in plasma and in saliva showed a fairly constant relationship.— J. Ekstrand *et al.*, *Eur. J. clin. Pharmac.*, 1977, *12*, 311.

Simultaneous administration with milk and dairy products reduced the bioavailability of sodium fluoride tablets.— J. Ekstrand and M. Ehrnebo, *Eur. J. clin. Pharmac.*, 1979, *16*, 211.

Results of single dose studies in 5 healthy subjects given sodium fluoride by mouth indicated that the renal clearance of fluoride was pH-dependent and enhanced under alkaline conditions.— J. Ekstrand *et al.*, *Eur. J. clin. Pharmac.*, 1980, *18*, 189. See also J. Ekstrand *et al.*, *Acta pharmac. tox.*, 1982, *50*, 321.

PREGNANCY AND THE NEONATE. Poor transfer of fluoride from plasma to breast milk in 5 mothers given 1.5 mg of fluoride as a single oral dose of sodium fluoride.— J. Ekstrand *et al.*, *Br. med. J.*, 1981, *283*, 761. Because of conflicting results at higher doses, further studies were required.— K. D. Moudgil (letter), *ibid.*, 1982, *284*, 200.

Uses and Administration

Sodium fluoride is used as an adjunct to diet and oral hygiene for the prevention of dental caries. It may render the enamel of teeth more resistant to acid, promote remineralisation, or reduce microbial acid production.

Fluoride may be administered through fluoridation of the public water supply to achieve a usual fluoride concentration of 1 ppm in temperate regions. The concentration may vary from 0.6 to 1.2 ppm depending on the climatic temperature with the lower concentrations being used in hotter regions where more water is likely to be consumed.

Alternatively, sodium fluoride may be administered as an oral supplement. The optimum daily dosage remains under discussion, but should be adjusted for the fluoride content of the drinking water, for fluorides ingested from other sources such as the diet, and for the age of the child. Where the drinking water contains less than 0.3 ppm of fluoride, children aged 2 weeks to 2 years may be given sodium fluoride 0.55 mg (equivalent to 0.25 mg of fluoride), although many authorities now recommend that fluoride supplements should not be given until 6 months of age; children aged 2 to 4 years may be given 1.1 mg (equivalent to 0.5 mg of fluoride); children older than 4 years may be given 2.2 mg (equivalent to 1 mg of fluoride). When drinking water contains 0.3 to 0.7 ppm of fluoride, no additional fluoride should be given to children less than 2 years of age and for older children the above doses should be halved. If the water contains more than 0.7 ppm of fluoride, supplementation is not recommended. Tablets should be sucked or chewed before swallowing since the topical action of fluoride on enamel and plaque is considered to be more important than the systemic effect. The value of giving fluoride during pregnancy, to benefit the child, is not established. Dental benefits from the use of dietary fluoride supplements by adults are unsubstantiated.

After tooth eruption, local applications are effective. Daily mouth-rinses of sodium fluoride 0.05% or weekly to monthly mouth-rinses of sodium fluoride 0.2% may be used but are not recommended for children aged under 6 years. Fluoridated dentifrices are now widely available. Sodium fluoride has also been applied topically as a varnish or 2% solution under professional supervision, usually at 6 to 12 monthly intervals. Alternatively, sodium fluoride solutions or gels acidified with phosphoric acid and commonly known as acidulated phosphate fluoride preparations may be used. These preparations are considered to increase the fluoride uptake by the enamel and protect the enamel from demineralisation. For maximum benefit, eating, drinking, or rinsing should be avoided for at least 30 minutes after topical application.

A paste consisting of equal parts of sodium fluoride, kaolin, and glycerol has been proposed for the treatment of hypersensitive dentine.

In the *UK*, the Cosmetic Products Regulations limit the concentration of total fluorine in oral hygiene products to a maximum concentration of 0.15%.

Sodium fluoride has been given to increase bone density and relieve bone pain in patients with various metabolic and neoplastic bone diseases including osteoporosis but many consider this use still to be experimental.

Sodium fluoride like some other fluoride compounds has also been used in rodenticides and insecticides. Other fluoride compounds used in oral hygiene products and dentifrices include aluminium fluoride, ammonium fluoride, calcium fluoride (p.1551), hetaflur (p.1577), nicomethanol hydrofluoride, olaflur (p.1596), potassium fluoride, sodium monofluorophosphate (p.1617), sodium silicofluoride (p.1618), and stannous fluoride (p.1619). Fluorides used in the fluoridation of water supplies include, in addition to sodium fluoride, sodium silicofluoride (p.1618).

ADMINISTRATION IN RENAL FAILURE. For references to the possible excessive accumulation of fluoride in patients with impaired renal function and precautions on the use of fluoridated water for dialysis, see under Precautions, above.

BLOOD PRESERVATIVE. In a concentration of 1%, sodium fluoride was considered the most efficient and suitable preservative for postmortem blood samples in preventing the generation of alcohol.— V. D. Plueckhahn and B. Ballard, *Med. J. Aust.*, 1968, *1*, 939.

DENTAL PROPHYLAXIS. A review of the mechanisms of action of fluoride in the prevention of dental caries.— R. S. Levine, *Br. dent. J.*, 1976, *140*, 9.

Reviews on the use and benefits of fluorides in the prevention of dental caries: H. S. Horowitz, *Br. dent. J.*, 1980, *149*, 311; *Drug & Ther. Bull.*, 1981, *19*, 81; G. B. Winter, *Archs Dis. Childh.*, 1983, *58*, 485; Prevention methods and programmes for oral diseases, *Tech. Rep. Ser. Wld Hlth Org. No. 713*, 1984.

Discussions and recommendations on the optimum dosage schedule for fluoride supplementation by mouth with reference to the risk of dental fluorosis and the variations in total fluoride intake from water, diet, and fluoridated dentifrices: *Pediatrics*, 1979, *63*, 150; T. B. Dowell and S. Joyston-Bechal, *Br. dent. J.*, 1981, *150*, 273; K. W. Stephen (letter), *ibid.*, *151*, 40; J. F. Neville (letter), *ibid.*, 41; K. W. Stephen (letter), *ibid.*, 1982, *153*, 390. See also under Precautions, above.

Results of a study demonstrated that the bactericidal activity of fluoride was increased as the pH was decreased. Five commercially available acidulated fluoride gels with pH's of 3.5 to 4.5 and fluoride concentrations ranging from 5.0 to 12.3 mg per mL failed to exert a bactericidal effect *in vitro* on *Streptococcus mutans*. In contrast, fluoride gels with a pH of either 2.0 or 2.5 were bactericidal at fluoride concentrations of approximately 1.1 and 12.0 mg per mL respectively.— P. W. Caufield and Y. Wannemuehler, *Antimicrob. Ag. Chemother.*, 1984, *26*, 807.

Dentifrices. In a double-blind study, the use of dentifrices containing 0.76% sodium monofluorophosphate with 0.10% sodium fluoride (total fluoride concentration 1450 ppm) every day for 3 years reduced the incidence of dental caries in 403 children (initially aged 11 to 12 years) by up to 27% when compared with 202 similar children who had used a non-fluoride dentifrice; a greater reduction was demonstrated in teeth erupting during the study. Results of the study also indicated that the addition of 0.10% sodium fluoride to a dentifrice containing 0.76% sodium monofluorophosphate enhanced its effectiveness.— H. C. Hodge *et al.*, *Br. dent. J.*, 1980, *149*, 201.

Review of the clinical efficacy of toothpastes containing sodium fluoride, sodium monofluorophosphate, and stannous fluoride. Recommendations included the use of effective fluoride toothpastes in public health programmes and further studies on formulation and efficacy.— *Bull. Wld Hlth Org.*, 1982, *60*, 633.

Evidence suggested that fluoride toothpastes had been the main factor in the reduction of caries in Britain, where only about 10% of the population received fluoridated water.— G. N. Jenkins, *Br. med. J.*, 1985, *291*, 1297. Criticism.— D. Jackson (letter), *ibid.*, 1650.

Fluoridation of drinking water. After an extensive review, the Royal College of Physicians concluded that fluoride, naturally present or added to drinking water at a concentration of approximately 1 mg per litre over the years of tooth formation, substantially reduced dental caries throughout life. In a temperate climate the consumption of water containing 1 mg per litre was safe irrespective of the hardness of the water. By comparison the use of systemic fluoride supplements such as tablets, drops, and fluoridated salt had not been shown to be as effective on a community basis. Fluoridation had negligible effects on the environment.— *Fluoride, Teeth and Health.* A Report and Summary on Fluoride and its Effect on Teeth and Health, Royal College of Physicians of London, Pitman Medical Publishing, 1976.

The results of a study in Welsh children indicated that the addition of fluorides to drinking water inhibited approximal caries more than occlusal caries. Overall there were over 50% fewer caries in 5-year-old children from an area fluoridated since 1955 than from a non-fluoridated area. At 15 years of age this difference was 42%. Consistently more teeth were missing because of caries in the non-fluoridated area, and at age 5 the number of extracted carious teeth in this area was approximately four times that in the fluoridated area.— D. Jackson *et al.*, *Br. dent. J.*, 1985, *158*, 45. Further studies.— J. L. Hardwick *et al.*, *ibid.*, 1982, *153*, 217; A. D. French *et al.*, *ibid.*, 1984, *156*, 54; G. Bradnock *et al.*, *ibid.*, 127; J. J. Murray *et al.*, *ibid.*, 255.

For the effect of the fluoridation of drinking water on bone fragility, see under Osteoporosis, below.

MULTIPLE MYELOMA. Sodium fluoride 100 to 200 mg daily has been used in patients with multiple myeloma to strengthen the skeleton and relieve bone pain but without conclusive benefit. References: P. Cohen, *J. Am. med. Ass.*, 1966, *198*, 583; J. B. Harley *et al.*, *New Engl. J. Med.*, 1972, *286*, 1283; R. A. Kyle *et al.*, *New Engl. J. Med.*, 1975, *293*, 1334.

OSTEOPOROSIS. The aim of fluoride treatment in osteoporosis is to improve bone strength by inducing subclinical fluorosis. The predominant effect of fluoride on the skeleton is to stimulate osteoblasts; osteoid is laid down but unless calcium supplements are provided, osteomalacia may develop. At the recommended daily dose of sodium fluoride 60 to 75 mg, about one-third to one-half of patients experience side-effects. Rheumatic symptoms are most common such as synovitis, plantar fasciitis, bone pain, and arthralgia; gastro-intestinal effects may be reduced if the fluoride is taken with meals. Carefully controlled studies are still required to access the value of this treatment.— *Lancet*, 1984, *1*, 547. Further reviews and discussions on fluoride in the treatment of osteoporosis.— D. D. Bikle, *Ann. intern. Med.*, 1983, *98*, 1013; A. St J. Dixon, *Br. med. J.*, 1983, *286*, 999; B. L. Riggs and L. J. Melton, *New Engl. J. Med.*, 1986, *314*, 1676.

Thirty-six patients with osteoporosis, treated initially with sodium fluoride 40 to 65 mg daily, calcium supplements and, usually, vitamin D were followed for up to 6 years. Of the 51 new vertebral fractures, 23 occurred in the first year of treatment; patients with X-ray evidence of fluoride changes in the vertebrae had a lower incidence of fractures. Eight patients withdrew because of adverse effects. The regimen should continue to be experimental.— B. L. Riggs *et al.*, *J. Am. med. Ass.*, 1980, *243*, 446. The occurrence of vertebral fractures was observed in patients with postmenopausal osteoporosis receiving placebo, conventional therapy (calcium alone, or with oestrogen, vitamin D, or oestrogen and vitamin D), or sodium fluoride and conventional therapy. The combination of calcium, oestrogen, and fluoride was the most effective. Optimism was expressed for the efficacy of sodium fluoride in combination with conventional therapy in the treatment of postmenopausal osteoporosis but a substantial minority did not respond to any therapy.— *idem*, *New Engl. J. Med.*, 1982, *306*, 446.

In a comparison of two communities, a lower incidence of bone fragility (measured as femoral-neck fractures) appeared to be associated with fluoridation of the drinking water to a concentration of 1 ppm.— O. Simonen and O. Laitinen, *Lancet*, 1985, *2*, 432. Criticism.— P. R. N. Sutton (letter), *Med. J. Aust.*, 1986, *144*, 277.

Sodium fluoride with calcium and alfacalcidol was of benefit in treating 2 children with severe corticosteroid-induced osteoporosis.— F. Rejou *et al.*, *Archs Dis. Childh.*, 1986, *61*, 1230.

OTOSCLEROSIS. In a double-blind, placebo-controlled study, treatment for 12 to 24 months with sodium fluoride 40 mg daily, calcium gluconate, and vitamin D, appeared to be of some benefit in approximately 20% of patients with otospongiosis by preventing further deterioration of hearing.— P. Bretlau *et al.*, *Ann. Otol. Rhinol. Lar.*, 1985, *94*, 103.

Preparations

Sodium Fluoride and Phosphoric Acid Gel *(U.S.P.)*

Sodium Fluoride and Phosphoric Acid Topical Solution *(U.S.P.)*

Sodium Fluoride Oral Solution *(U.S.P.)*

Sodium Fluoride Tablets *(U.S.P.)*. Tablets that are to be chewed may be labelled as Sodium Fluoride Chewable Tablets.

Proprietary Preparations

Duraphat *(Woelm, Ger.: Glover, UK)*. *Varnish*, sodium fluoride 50 mg/mL.

En-De-Kay *(Stafford-Miller, UK)*. *Tablets* (En-De-Kay Fluotabs Additive Free), sodium fluoride 0.55 mg. *Tablets* (En-De-Kay Fluotabs 2-4 Years), scored, sodium fluoride 1.1 mg. *Tablets* (En-De-Kay Fluotabs 4+ Years), scored, sodium fluoride 2.2 mg. *Oral drops* (En-De-Kay Fluodrops), sodium fluoride 0.55 mg/0.15 mL. *Mouth-wash* (En-De-Kay Fluorinse), sodium fluoride 2%. *Oral gel* (En-De-Kay Fluogel), acidulated sodium fluoride containing fluoride ion 1.23%.

Fluor-a-day Lac *(Dental Health Promotion, UK)*. *Tablets*, scored, sodium fluoride 2.2 mg.

Fluorigard (formerly known as Luride) *(Hoyt, UK)*. *Tablets*, sodium fluoride 1.1 and 2.2 mg. *Oral drops*, sodium fluoride 275 µg/drop. *Mouth-wash*, sodium fluoride 0.05%.

Fluorigard Weekly (formerly known as Point-Two) *(Hoyt, UK)*. *Mouth-wash*, sodium fluoride 0.2%.

Zymafluor *(Zyma, UK)*. *Tablets*, sodium fluoride 0.55 and 2.2 mg.

Proprietary Names and Manufacturers

AFI-Fluor *(Nyco, Norw.)*; Carident *(Norw.)*; Chemifluor *(Winthrop, Ger.)*; Denta-Mint Fluoride Mouthwash *(Orapharm, Austral.)*; Duraphat *(Woelm, Denm.; Woelm, Ger.: Glover, UK; Woelm, Norw.; Woelm-Pharma, Swed.)*; En-De-Kay Fluodrops *(Stafford-Miller, UK)*; En-De-Kay Fluogel *(Stafford-Miller, UK)*; En-De-Kay Fluorinse *(Stafford-Miller, UK)*; En-De-Kay Fluotabs *(Stafford-Miller, UK)*; Floran *(Austral.)*; Flozenges *(Oral-B, Canad.)*; Fludent *(A.L., Swed.)*; Fluogum *(Goupil, Fr.)*; Fluomin *(Ferrosan, Denm.)*; Fluor *(Belg.; DAK, Denm.; Monal, Fr.; Collett, Norw.; Nyco, Norw.)*; Fluor Oligosol *(Fr.)*; Fluor-a-day *(Pharmascience, Canad.)*; Fluor-a-day Lac *(Dental Health Promotion, UK)*; Fluoretten *(Albert-Roussel, Ger.)*; Fluorigard *(Hoyt, UK; Colgate-Hoyt, USA)*; Fluor-In *(Goupil, Fr.)*; Fluorinse *(Canad.)*; Fluoritab *(Fluoritab, USA)*; Fluoron *(Stickley, Canad.)*; Fluoros *(Biotherax, Ger.)*; Fluortannkrem *(Norw.)*; Fluotic *(Nordic, Canad.)*; Flura-tabs *(Fawns & McAllan, Austral.)*; Flurets *(Oral-B, Austral.)*; Flurexal *(Zyma, Switz.)*; Flux *(Apothekernes Laboratorium, Norw.)*; F-Tabs *(Denta-Health, Austral.)*; Hifluor *(Protea, Austral.; Glaxo, UK)*; Karidium *(Prof. Pharm. Corp., Canad.)*; Luride *(Hoyt, UK; Colgate-Hoyt, USA)*; Odontocromil Pasta *(Spain)*; Oligosol F *(Labcatal, Switz.)*; Orofluor *(Orapharm, Austral.)*; Oro-Naf *(Stickley, Canad.)*; Ossin *(Grünenthal, Ger.; Grünenthal, Switz.)*; Osteofluor *(Merck-Clévenot, Fr.)*; Osteopor-F *(Hausmann, Switz.)*; Pediaflor *(Ross, USA)*; Pedi-Dent *(Stanley, Canad.)*; Pharma-Fluor *(Neth.)*; Phos-Flur *(Hoyt, UK; Colgate-Hoyt, USA)*; Point-Two *(Hoyt, UK; Colgate-Hoyt, USA)*; Prevident *(Colgate-Hoyt, USA)*; Solu-Flur *(Stickley, Canad.)*; Thera-Flur *(Colgate-Hoyt, USA)*; Thera-flur-N *(Colgate-Hoyt, USA)*; Zymafluor *(Belg.; Zyma, Fr.; Zyma, Ger.; Zyma, Ital.; Neth.; Zyma, S.Afr.; Zyma, Switz.; Zyma, UK)*.

3942-z

Sodium Gluconate *(USAN)*.

Monosodium D-gluconate.
$C_6H_{11}NaO_7$=218.1.

CAS — 527-07-1.

Pharmacopoeias. In *U.S.*

Store in well-closed containers.

Gluconates act as acceptors of hydrogen ions produced by metabolic processes and are an indirect source of bicarbonate ions.

13251-b

Sodium Hyaluronate

The sodium salt of a high-viscosity mucopolysaccharide of high molecular weight.

CAS — 9004-61-9 (hyaluronic acid); 9067-32-7 (sodium salt).

The manufacturers state that solutions of sodium hyaluronate for injection which are stored at 2 to 8° and protected from light have a shelf-life of 3 years; they may be stored at room temperature for up to 4 weeks.

Adverse Effects

There have been reports of a transient rise in intra-ocular pressure following the administration of sodium hyaluronate into the eye. There have also been occasional reports of hypersensitivity.

Intra-ocular pressures increased during the first 2 days postoperatively in patients receiving sodium hyaluronate or sodium hyaluronate plus acetazolamide to reform the anterior chamber after cataract surgery, compared with those receiving air.— M. S. Passo *et al.*, *Br. J. Ophthal.*, 1985, *69*, 572.

Uses and Administration

Hyaluronic acid is widely distributed in body tissues and intracellular fluids including the aqueous and vitreous humour.
A viscous solution of sodium hyaluronate is used during surgical procedures on the eye. Introduction of the solution into the anterior or posterior chamber via a fine cannula or needle allows tissues to be separated during surgery and protects them from trauma.
Hyaluronic acid and sodium hyaluronate, administered as intra-articular injections, have been tried in the treatment of arthritis.

DRY EYE. In a study in 10 patients with dry eye topical application of a solution containing unpreserved sodium hyaluronate (0.1%) led to an increase in tear film stability compared with sodium chloride solution (0.9%) with the stabilising effect lasting for at least 40 minutes. The symptoms of burning and grittiness were also alleviated.— L. S. Mengher *et al.*, *Br. J. Ophthal.*, 1986, *70*, 442.

OSTEOARTHRITIS. Reports of beneficial results with intra-articular hyaluronic acid and sodium hyaluronate in the treatment of osteoarthritis of the knee: A. Bragantini *et al.*, *Clin. Trials J.*, 1987, *24*, 333 (hyaluronic acid); G. Grecomoro *et al.*, *Pharmatherapeutica*, 1987, *5*, 137 (sodium hyaluronate).

SURGICAL PROCEDURES INVOLVING THE EYE. In a study of 29 eyes undergoing trabeculectomy, the injection of sodium hyaluronate into the anterior chamber after the trabeculectomy had no advantage over trabeculectomy alone in preventing shallowing of the anterior chamber or hypotonia in the early postoperative period.— S. O. Hung, *Br. J. Ophthal.*, 1985, *69*, 46.
Prevention of scleral or corneal collapse during eye surgery by sodium hyaluronate.— S. P. B. Percival, *Br. J. Ophthal.*, 1985, *69*, 99.
In a study involving 45 patients undergoing cataract extraction, the increase in corneal thickness, an indicator of endothelial damage, was less in patients receiving sodium hyaluronate to reform the anterior chamber following cataract extraction and prior to lens implantation, than in those who had plain cataract extraction with or without lens implantation.— J. S. H. Jacob, *Br. J. Ophthal.*, 1985, *69*, 567.
In a study involving 10 patients undergoing cataract surgery the instillation of hyaluronidase following that of sodium hyaluronate led to a reduction in postoperative ocular hypertension.— I. G. Calder and V. H. Smith, *Br. J. Ophthal.*, 1986, *70*, 418.
The successful use of sodium hyaluronate in the evacuation of traumatic hyphaema.— R. S. Bartholomew, *Br. J. Ophthal.*, 1987, *71*, 27.

Proprietary Preparations

Healonid *(Pharmacia, UK)*. *Injection*, sodium hyaluronate 10 mg (obtained from avian tissue), sodium chloride 8.5 mg, sodium phosphate dihydrate 280 µg, and sodium acid phosphate monohydrate 40 µg/mL in single-use disposable syringes of 0.5 and 0.75 mL.

Proprietary Names and Manufacturers

Amvisc *(Precision-Cosmet, USA)*; ARTZ *(Kaken, Jpn)*; Connettivina *(Kreussler, Ger.; Fidia, Ital.)*; Healon *(Pharmacia, Austral.; Pharmacia, Canad.; Pharmacia, Denm.; Pharmacia, Ger.; Pharmacia, Norw.; MPS Lab., S.Afr.; Pharmacia, Swed.; Pharmacia, Switz.; Pharmacia, USA)*; Healonid *(Pharmacia, Fr.; Pharmacia, UK)*; Hyalgan *(Fidia, Ital.)*; Ial *(Fidia, Ital.)*; Opegan *(Santen, Jpn)*; Pandermin *(Vinas, Spain)*.

The following names have been used for multi-ingredient preparations containing sodium hyaluronate— Viscoat *(Cilco, USA)*.

13252-v

Sodium Hydrogen Sulphate

Sodium Acid Sulphate; Sodium Bisulphate.
$NaHSO_4,H_2O$=138.1.

CAS — 7681-38-1 (anhydrous); 10034-88-5 (monohydrate).

Sodium hydrogen sulphate is used for preparing effervescing baths.

216-q

Sodium Hydroxide *(BAN, USAN)*.

524; Ätznatron; Caustic Soda; Natrium Hydricum; Natrium Hydroxydatum; Soda Lye.
NaOH=40.00.

CAS — 1310-73-2.

Pharmacopoeias. In *Aust., Br., Chin., Egypt., Hung., Ind., Jpn, Jug., Mex., Nord., Port., Span., Swiss,* and *Turk.* Also in *B.P. Vet.* and *U.S.N.F.*

Dry, very deliquescent, white or almost white sticks, pellets, spherical particles, fused masses, or scales. It is hard and brittle and shows a crystalline fracture. Strongly alkaline and corrosive, and rapidly destroys organic tissues. When exposed to air it rapidly absorbs moisture and carbon dioxide.
Completely or almost completely **soluble** 1 in 1 of water; very soluble in alcohol. **Store** in airtight containers.

Adverse Effects

The ingestion of caustic alkalis causes immediate burning pain in the mouth, throat, substernal region, and epigastrium, and the lining membranes become swollen and detached. There is dysphagia, hypersalivation, vomiting with the vomitus becoming blood-stained, diarrhoea, and shock. In severe cases, asphyxia due to oedema of the glottis, circulatory failure, oesophageal or gastric perforation, peritonitis, or pneumonia may occur. Stricture of the oesophagus can develop weeks or months later.
Caustic alkalis on contact with the eyes cause conjunctival oedema and corneal destruction.
In Great Britain the recommended exposure limit of sodium hydroxide is 2 mg per m^3 (short-term and long-term). In the *USA* the permissible and recommended exposure limits are 2 mg per m^3.

Treatment of Adverse Effects

Ingestion should not be treated by lavage or emesis. Give copious drinks of water and follow this with demulcents. Maintain an airway and alleviate shock and pain.
Contaminated skin and eyes should be flooded immediately with water and the washing continued for about 30 minutes. Any affected clothing should be removed while flooding is being carried out. Pain in affected eyes may be relieved by instillation of local anaesthetic eye-drops.

Uses and Administration

Sodium hydroxide is a powerful caustic. A 2.5% solution in glycerol has been used as a cuticle solvent. An escharotic preparation of sodium hydroxide and calcium oxide was known as London paste. It is also used for adjusting the pH of solutions. In Great Britain, a 1% aqueous solution is an approved disinfectant for swine vesicular disease.
In the *UK* the use of sodium hydroxide in cosmetics is prohibited by law.

VIRUS DISINFECTION. When autoclaving is impractical, exposure to 1N sodium hydroxide for one hour has been found to be effective in the decontamination of Creutzfeldt-Jakob virus. Contaminated skin could be disinfected with little hazard by 5 to 10 minutes of exposure to 1N sodium hydroxide, followed by extensive washing with water.— P. Brown *et al.* (letter), *New Engl. J. Med.*, 1984, *310*, 727.

13253-g

Sodium Methylarsinate

Natrium Methylarsonicum; Sodium Metharsinite. Disodium methylarsonate hexahydrate.
$CH_3AsNa_2O_3,6H_2O$=292.0.

CAS — 5967-62-4.

Pharmacopoeias. In *Fr., Port.,* and *Span.*

Sodium methylarsinate has the actions and uses of sodium cacodylate but was stated not to impart the garlic odour to the breath characteristic of the cacodylates.

Proprietary Names and Manufacturers

Arsozon *(Takeda, Jpn)*; Disomear *(Jpn)*.

7735-k

Sodium Monofluorophosphate *(USAN)*.

MFP Sodium; Natrii Monofluorophosphas; Sodium Fluorophosphate. Disodium phosphorofluoridate.
Na_2PO_3F=143.9.

CAS — 10163-15-2.

Pharmacopoeias. In *Nord.* and *U.S.*

A white to slightly grey odourless powder. Freely **soluble** in water. A 2% solution in water has a pH of 6.5 to 8.0.

Sodium monofluorophosphate has similar actions to sodium fluoride (p.1615) and is used similarly in toothpastes for the prevention of dental caries.

In the *UK*, the Cosmetic Products Regulations limit the concentration of total fluorine in oral hygiene products to a maximum concentration of 0.15%. Other monofluorophosphate salts permitted for use in oral hygiene products and dentifrices include ammonium monofluorophosphate, calcium monofluorophosphate, and potassium monofluorophosphate.

For references to the use of sodium monofluorophosphate in dentifrices, see under Sodium Fluoride, p.1616.

13254-q

Sodium Nitrate

E251; Natrii Nitras; Natrium Nitricum.
$NaNO_3$=84.99.

CAS — 7631-99-4.

NOTE. Crude sodium nitrate is known as Chile Saltpetre.

Pharmacopoeias. In *Fr.*

WARNING. *Sodium nitrate has been used for the illicit preparation of explosives or fireworks; care is required with its supply.*

Sodium nitrate has similar properties to potassium nitrate. In Great Britain sodium nitrate is permitted as a preservative in certain types of cheese at a concentration of not more than

50 ppm, of which not more than 5 ppm may be sodium nitrite. It is also permitted in cured meats including cured meat products at limits of not more than 150 to 500 ppm of sodium nitrate, of which not more than 50 to 200 ppm respectively may be sodium nitrite. The sale of any food specially prepared for babies or young children is prohibited if it has in it or on it any added sodium nitrate or sodium nitrite.
Crude sodium nitrate is used as a fertiliser.

Estimated acceptable daily intake of nitrates: up to 500 µg per kg body-weight. No change was made from the Seventeenth Report [however, in that report an intake of up to 5 mg per kg was given].— Twenty-third Report of Joint FAO/WHO Expert Committee on Food Additives, *Tech. Rep. Ser. Wld Hlth Org. No. 648*, 1980. Nitrate should on no account be added to baby foods.— *Fd Add. Ser. Wld Hlth Org. No. 5*, 1974.

5908-g

Sodium Perborate *(BAN)*.

Natrii Perboras; Sod. Perbor.
$NaBO_2,H_2O_2,3H_2O$=153.9.

CAS — 7632-04-4 (anhydrous); 10042-94-1 (hydrate).

Pharmacopoeias. In *Br., Fr., Port.*, and *Span.*

Odourless or almost odourless, colourless prismatic crystals or a white powder, stable in crystalline form
Soluble 1 in 40 of water, with some decomposition. **Store** in airtight containers.

Adverse Effects

Frequent use of tooth-powders containing sodium perborate may cause blistering and oedema. Hypertrophy of the papillae of the tongue has also been reported.
The effects of swallowed sodium perborate are similar to those of boric acid (see p.1549).

Uses and Administration

Sodium perborate is a mild disinfectant and deodorant. It readily releases oxygen in contact with oxidisable matter and has been used in aqueous solutions for purposes similar to weak solutions of hydrogen peroxide. Vincent's infection may be treated by the application of a paste made with water or glycerol; the paste is retained in the mouth for 5 minutes and then rinsed out.
Sodium perborate has also been used, with calcium carbonate, as a tooth-powder. A 2% solution freshly prepared is used as a mouth-wash.
The less soluble $NaBO_2,H_2O_2$ known as sodium perborate monohydrate is used similarly.

A study of the absorption of boron after use of sodium perborate mouthwash [Bocosept] indicated that there was little risk of boron poisoning. Blood concentrations of boron did not exceed 320 ng per mL. Boron did not appear to be absorbed by the oral mucosa but was probably absorbed from the intestine after ingestion of residual amounts from the mouth.— L. Edwall *et al., Eur. J. clin. Pharmac.*, 1979, *15*, 417. See also H. Dill *et al., Int. J. clin. Pharmac. Biopharm.*, 1977, *15*, 16.

Proprietary Preparations

Bocasan *(Oral-B, UK). Mouth-wash*, powder for solution, sodium perborate monohydrate 68.635%.

Proprietary Names and Manufacturers

Amosan *(Oral-B, Austral.; Oral-B, Canad.)*; Bocasan *(Oral-B, UK)*; Bocosept; Kavosan.
The following names have been used for multi-ingredient preparations containing sodium perborate—Perborate *(Squibb, Canad.)*.

16986-r

Sodium Phenylacetate

$C_8H_7NaO_2$=158.1.

Sodium phenylacetate is used with sodium benzoate in hyperammonaemia in patients with enzymatic deficiencies in the urea cycle.

References: M. Bor *et al., Archs Dis. Childh.*, 1984, *59*, 1183; M. Msall *et al., New Engl. J. Med.*, 1984, *310*, 1500; S. W. Brusilow *et al., New Engl. J. Med.*, 1984, *310*, 1630; A. J. Watson *et al., Lancet*, 1985, *2*, 1271. Correction.— *ibid.*, 1986, *1*, 112.

Proprietary Names and Manufacturers

The following names have been used for multi-ingredient preparations containing sodium phenylacetate— Ucephan *(McGaw, USA)*.

13256-s

Sodium Pidolate

NaPCA; Sodium Pyroglutamate; Sodium Pyrrolidone Carboxylate. Sodium 5-oxopyrrolidine-2-carboxylate.
$C_5H_6NNaO_3$=151.1.

CAS — 28874-51-3.

Sodium pidolate is used as a humectant. It is applied topically as a cream or lotion in the treatment of dry skin disorders.

Proprietary Preparations

Humiderm *(BritCair, UK). Cream*, sodium pidolate 5%.
Lacticare *(Stiefel, UK). Lotion*, sodium pidolate 2.5%, lactic acid 5% in an oil-in-water basis.

Proprietary Names and Manufacturers

Ajidew A-100 *(Ajinomoto, Jpn: K & K-Greeff, UK)*; Ajidew N-50 *(Ajinomoto, Jpn: K & K-Greeff, UK)*; Humiderm *(BritCair, UK)*; Medicreme *(Pharma-Medica, Denm.)*.
The following names have been used for multi-ingredient preparations containing sodium pidolate—Lacticare *(Stiefel, Austral.; Stiefel, Canad.; Stiefel, UK)*; Lacticare-HC *(Stiefel, USA)*.

1640-p

Sodium Polymetaphosphate

E450(c) *(sodium polyphosphates)*.

CAS — 50813-16-6.

NOTE. Sodium Hexametaphosphate has been used as a synonym for this substance, but it exists in much higher degrees of polymerisation.

Pharmacopoeias. In *B.P.C. 1973.*

Sodium polymetaphosphate has been used as a 5% dusting-powder in hyperhidrosis and bromidrosis, and as a prophylactic against athlete's foot.

Sodium polymetaphosphate combines with calcium and magnesium ions to form complex soluble compounds and is used as a water softener. Added to water (1 ppm) in which instruments are boiled, it prevents rusting and deposition of a film if the solution is first made slightly alkaline with sodium carbonate. It is used in the food industry as a stabiliser.
Similar compounds, of slightly varying composition, and described as Sodium Metaphosphate are used in the food industry as emulsifying agents and chelating agents.

Estimated acceptable daily dietary intake: up to 70 mg as phosphorus per kg body-weight.— Seventh Report of FAO/WHO Expert Committee on Food Additives, *Tech. Rep. Ser. Wld Hlth Org. No. 281*, 1964.

Proprietary Names and Manufacturers

Calgon *(Benckiser, UK)*.

13260-v

Sodium Silicate

Soluble Glass; Water Glass.

CAS — 1344-09-8.

Concentrated aqueous solutions of sodium silicate are commercially available and have many industrial uses. The solutions vary in composition, viscosity, and density; the greater the ratio of Na_2O to SiO_2 the more tacky and alkaline the solution. A solution has been used, similarly to Plaster of Paris, for making fixed dressings for fractures.

7736-a

Sodium Silicofluoride

Sodium Fluorosilicate; Sodium Fluosilicate; Sodium Hexafluorosilicate.
Na_2SiF_6=188.1.

CAS — 16893-85-9.

Sodium silicofluoride has the actions of sodium fluoride (p.1615) and is used in controlled amounts for the fluoridation of drinking water. It has also been considered for inclusion in oral hygiene products; in the *UK* the maximum concentration of total fluorine allowed in such products is 0.15%.
Other silicofluoride (fluorosilicate) salts permitted for use in oral hygiene products include ammonium silicofluoride, magnesium silicofluoride, and potassium silicofluoride.
Sodium silicofluoride has also been used in insecticides.

16988-d

Sodium Thiosalicylate

$C_7H_5O_2NaS$=176.2.

Sodium thiosalicylate is an analgesic which is under investigation for its anti-inflammatory effects.

Proprietary Names and Manufacturers

Reocyl *(Bart, USA)*.

13264-s

Sparteine Sulphate *(rINNM)*.

l-Sparteine Sulphate; (−)-Sparteine Sulphate; Spart. Sulph.; Sparteine Sulfate *(USAN)*; Sparteinum Sulfuricum; Sulfato de Esparteina. Dodecahydro-7,14-methano-2*H*,6*H*-dipyrido[1,2-*a*:1′,2′-*e*][1,5]diazocine sulphate pentahydrate.
$C_{15}H_{26}N_2,H_2SO_4,5H_2O$=422.5.

CAS — 90-39-1 (sparteine); 299-39-8 (sulphate, anhydrous); 6160-12-9 (sulphate, pentahydrate).

Pharmacopoeias. In *Arg., Belg., Fr., Port., Roum.*, and *Span.*

Sparteine sulphate is a salt of the dibasic alkaloid, sparteine, obtained from scoparium, *Sarothamnus scoparius (=Cytisus scoparius)* (Leguminosae).

Sparteine sulphate has been reported to lessen the irritability and conductivity of cardiac muscle and has been used in the treatment of cardiac arrhythmias. Small doses stimulate and large doses paralyse the autonomic ganglia. Peripherally, it has a fairly strong curare-like action, arresting respiration by paralysing the phrenic endings.
Sparteine camsylate has also been used.

Proprietary Names and Manufacturers

Depasan *(Giulini, Ger.)*; Spartopan *(Paillusseau, Fr.)*.
The following names have been used for multi-ingredient preparations containing sparteine sulphate— Sedol *(Rhône-Poulenc, Canad.)*.

3919-c

Squaric Acid Dibutylester

Quadratic Acid Dibutylester. The dibutyl ester of 3,4-dihydroxy-3-cyclobutene-1,2-dione.
$C_{12}H_{18}O_4$=226.3.

CAS — 2892-51-5 (squaric acid).

Squaric acid dibutylester is under investigation in the treatment of alopecia.

References: R. J. Caserio, *Archs Derm.*, 1987, *123*, 1036.

7737-t

Stannous Fluoride *(USAN).*

Stannosi Fluoridum. Tin fluoride.
SnF_2=156.7.

CAS — 7783-47-3.

Pharmacopoeias. In *Nord.* and *U.S.*

A white crystalline powder with a bitter saline taste. Freely **soluble** in water; practically insoluble in alcohol, chloroform, and ether. A 0.4% freshly prepared solution in water has a pH of 2.8 to 3.5. Aqueous solutions decompose within a few hours with the formation of a white precipitate; they slowly attack glass. Preparations are stored in well-closed containers.

Stannous fluoride has similar actions to sodium fluoride (p.1615) and is used for the prophylaxis of dental caries. It may be applied to the teeth, under professional supervision, as a 5% gel or a freshly prepared 8% aqueous solution at intervals of 6 to 12 months. Gels containing concentrations of stannous fluoride 0.4% are available for daily use. Stannous fluoride has also been used in dentifrices and mouth rinses.

Stannous fluoride has been reported to have an unpleasant taste and to increase teeth discoloration.

In the *UK*, the Cosmetic Products Regulations limit the concentration of total fluorine in oral hygiene products to a maximum concentration of 0.15%.

For the use of stannous fluoride in dentifrices, see under Sodium Fluoride, p.1616.

Preparations

Stannous Fluoride Gel *(U.S.P.)*

Proprietary Preparations

Omnigel *(CTS Dental, UK). Oral gel,* stannous fluoride 0.4%.

Proprietary Names and Manufacturers

Floran *(Austral.)*; Gel-Kam *(Scherer, USA)*; Gelstan *(Stickley, Canad.)*; Omnigel *(CTS Dental, UK)*; Orostan *(Orapharm, Austral.)*.

3920-s

Starch Blockers

Inhibitors of alpha-amylase such as phaseolamin and tendamistat (HOE-467) are termed starch blockers and have been proposed as dietary aids; the principle behind this being that they would inhibit the absorption of starch. Various studies have shown that these compounds have no effect on calorie absorption (G.W. Bo-Linn *et al.*, *New Engl. J. Med.*, 1982, *307*, 1413; J.S. Garrow *et al.*, *Lancet*, 1983, *1*, 60). Other studies demonstrating that a blocking effect is dependent on the dose and coincidental administration with the carbohydrate (B.H. Meyer *et al.*, *Lancet*, 1983, *1*, 934; B.H. Meyer *et al.*, *Br. J. clin. Pharmac.*, 1983, *16*, 145) have been criticised (R.H. Taylor and H.M. Barker, *Lancet*, 1983, *1*, 1228). Commentaries have also pointed to the unlikely benefit from starch blockers as dietary aids to slimming (*Lancet*, 1983, *1*, 569; R.G. Penn, *Adverse Drug React. Bull.*, 1983, *Oct.*, 376). One manufacturer has stated that the role if any for alpha-amylase inhibitors is as an adjunct to the treatment of diabetes mellitus (K.E. Draeger *et al.*, *Lancet*, 1983, *1*, 354) and such a use is also proposed by others (P. Layer *et al.*, *Mayo Clin. Proc.*, 1986, *61*, 442; M. Boivin *et al.*, *ibid.*, 1987, *62*, 249). This concept of inhibiting carbohydrate absorption in diabetes mellitus is employed with alpha-glucosidase inhibitors such as acarbose (p.386), emiglitate (p.1567), and miglitol (p.1590). A recognised adverse effect of acarbose is flatulence arising from bacterial activity on undigested carbohydrate in the colon. One wonders if starch blockers are used as aids to slimming, whether the pleasures of eating what you like then blocking the carbohydrate absorption are worth the discomfort and social problems of increased flatulence.

13267-l

Statolon *(USAN).*

NSC-71901; Vistatolon *(rINN)*. An antiviral substance derived from *Penicillium stoloniferum*. The active constituent is a polyanionic polysaccharide.

CAS — 11006-77-2.

Statolon has been shown to induce the production of interferon by *animal* cells.

Proprietary Names and Manufacturers

Lilly, USA.

1324-t

Stearic Acid *(USAN).*

570; Acido Esteárico; Octadecanoic Acid; Stearinsäure.

CAS — 57-11-4 (stearic acid); 57-10-3 (palmitic acid).

Pharmacopoeias. In *Arg., Aust., Belg., Braz., Chin., Cz., Egypt., Fr., Hung., Ind., It., Jpn, Jug., Nord., Pol., Port., Roum., Span.,* and *Swiss.* Also in *U.S.N.F.*
U.S.N.F. also includes Purified Stearic Acid containing not less than 90% stearic acid and not less than 96% of stearic and palmitic acids. Congealing point 66° to 69°.

White, or yellowish, glossy crystalline solid or powder, with a slight odour suggesting tallow, consisting of a mixture of fatty acids, chiefly stearic and palmitic acids. *U.S.N.F.* specifies not less than 40% of stearic acid ($C_{18}H_{36}O_2$), not less than 40% of palmitic acid ($C_{16}H_{32}O_2$), and not less than 90% of stearic and palmitic acids. Congealing point not below 54°. It is sometimes wrongly called 'stearine' in commerce.

Practically **insoluble** in water; soluble 1 in 20 of alcohol, 1 in 2 of chloroform, and 1 in 3 of ether.

Store in well-closed containers.

Stearic acid is used as a lubricant in making tablets and capsules. It is also used as an emulsifying and solubilising agent.

Proprietary Names and Manufacturers

Emersol 132 *(USA)*; Pristerene 4900 *(Unichema, UK)*; Pristerene 4901 *(Unichema, UK)*; Pristerene 4968 *(Unichema, UK)*.

286-r

Storax *(BAN, USAN).*

Balsamum Styrax Liquidus; Estoraque Líquido; Liquid Storax; Styrax.

CAS — 8023-62-9.

Pharmacopoeias. In *Chin.* and *Egypt. Port.* and *Span.* specify crude storax.
Storax *U.S.P.* is crude storax from *L. orientalis* (Levant storax) or *L. styraciflua* (American storax).

The balsam obtained from the trunk of *Liquidambar orientalis* (Hamamelidaceae). It is a semiliquid grey to greyish-brown opaque mass with a characteristic odour.

Insoluble in water; soluble in warm alcohol (90%) (usually incompletely), carbon disulphide, and acetone; partly soluble in ether. **Store** in well-closed containers.

Storax has actions similar to those of Peru balsam (p.1599). Purified storax or prepared storax was formerly applied as an ointment in the treatment of parasitic skin diseases. It is an ingredient of Compound Benzoin Tincture and of Benzoin Inhalation. Skin sensitisation has been reported.

13270-q

Strontium Chloride

$SrCl_2,6H_2O$=266.6.

CAS — 10476-85-4 (anhydrous).

Strontium chloride is used as a 10% toothpaste for the relief of dental hypersensitivity.

985-h

Suanzaorentang

Ziziphus Soup.

Suanzaorentang is an ancient Chinese remedy for anxiety and insomnia. It contains five herbs: suanzaoren (*Zizyphus spinosus* of the Rhamnaceae), fuling (*Poria cocos* of the Polyporaceae), gancao (*Glycyrrhiza uralensis* of the Leguminosae), zhimu (*Anemarrhena asphodeloides* of the Liliaceae), and chuanxiong (*Ligusticum chuanxiong* of the Umbelliferae).

References: H. -C. Chen and M. -T. Hsieh, *Clin. Ther.*, 1985, *7*, 334; *Drugs of the Future*, 1986, *11*, 674.

13271-p

Succinimide

Butanimide. Pyrrolidine-2,5-dione.
$C_4H_5NO_2$=99.09.

CAS — 123-56-8.

Succinimide has been claimed to inhibit the formation of oxalic acid calculi in the kidney and to reduce hyperoxaluria.

Proprietary Names and Manufacturers

Orotric *(Vita, Spain)*; Succinimide-Sauba *(Sauba, Fr.)*.

13273-w

Sucrose Octa-acetate

Sucrose Octaacetate *(USAN)*
$C_{28}H_{38}O_{19}$=678.6.

CAS — 126-14-7.

Pharmacopoeias. In *U.S.N.F.*

A white, practically odourless, hygroscopic powder with an intensely bitter taste. **Soluble** 1 in 1100 of water, 1 in 11 of alcohol, 1 in 0.3 of acetone, and 1 in 0.5 of toluene; soluble in ether; very soluble in chloroform and methyl alcohol. **Store** in airtight containers.

Sucrose octa-acetate is used as an alcohol denaturant (see methylated spirits, p.965).

3943-c

Sulfenazone

Sulfamazone. α-{*p*-[(6-Methoxy-3-pyridazinyl)sulfamoyl]anilino}-2,3-dimethyl-5-oxo-1-phenyl-3-pyrazoline-4-methanesulphonic acid.
$C_{22}H_{24}O_7N_6S_2$=548.6.

CAS — 65761-24-2; 13061-27-3 (sodium salt).

Sulfenazone is an antibacterial agent which has been given as the sodium salt, by mouth or rectally, in infections of the upper respiratory tract.

Proprietary Names and Manufacturers

Marespin *(Gentili, Ital.)*.

18855-m

Sulotroban *(rINN).*

BM-13177. [*p*-(2-Benzenesulfonamidoethyl)-phenoxy]acetic acid.
$C_{16}H_{17}NO_5S$=335.4.

CAS — 72131-33-0.

Sulotroban is a thromboxane A_2 antagonist under investigation as an antithrombotic agent.

References: P. Gresele *et al.*, *Lancet*, 1984, *1*, 991; H. Patscheke *et al.*, *Clin. Pharmac. Ther.*, 1986, *39*, 145.

Proprietary Names and Manufacturers
Boehringer Mannheim, Ger.

1325-x

Sulphuric Acid *(BAN).*

513; Acid. Sulph. Conc.; Oil of Vitriol; Schwefelsäure; Sulfuric Acid *(USAN)*.
H_2SO_4=98.07.

CAS — 7664-93-9.

Pharmacopoeias. In *Aust.* (Acidum Sulfuricum Concentratum), *Br.*, *Egypt.*, *Nord.*, *Port.*, and *Span.* Also in *U.S.N.F.*

A colourless corrosive liquid of oily consistence. **Miscible** with water and with alcohol. Much heat is evolved when sulphuric acid is added to water. Concentrated oil of vitriol of commerce, 'COV', contains about 95 to 98% w/w, and brown oil of vitriol, 'BOV', contains 75 to 85% w/w of H_2SO_4. Nordhausen or fuming sulphuric acid, 'Oleum', is sulphuric acid containing SO_3; battery or accumulator acid is sulphuric acid diluted with distilled water to a specific gravity of 1.2 to 1.26. **Store** in airtight containers.

CAUTION. *When sulphuric acid is mixed with other liquids, it should always be added slowly, with constant stirring, to the diluent.*

1326-r

Dilute Sulphuric Acid *(BAN).*

Acid. Sulph. Dil.; Verdünnte Schwefelsäure.

Pharmacopoeias. In *Br.*, *Egypt.*, and *Span.* (all approximately 10%); in *Aust.* (9.1 to 9.4%) and in *Pol.* (16%).

Adverse Effects and Treatment
As for Hydrochloric Acid, p.1578.
In Great Britain the recommended exposure limit of sulphuric acid is 1 mg per m^3 (long-term). In the *US* the permissible and recommended exposure limits are 1 mg per m^3.

Uses and Administration
Dilute sulphuric acid has been used as an astringent in diarrhoea and it has occasionally been prescribed in mixtures with vegetable bitters to stimulate appetite.

18686-h

Sumacetamol *(BAN, rINN).*

SUR-2647. 4-Acetamidophenyl *N*-acetyl-DL-methionate.
$C_{15}H_{20}N_2O_4S$=324.4.

CAS — 69217-67-0.

Sumacetamol is a methionine ester of paracetamol and has been tried in combination with free paracetamol for the treatment of swelling and pain following oral surgery.

References: L. A. Skoglund and P. Skjelbred, *Eur. J. clin. Pharmac.*, 1984, *26*, 573; L. A. Skoglund, *ibid.*, 1986, *31*, 45.

Proprietary Names and Manufacturers
Winthrop, UK.

274-k

Sumatra Benzoin *(BAN).*

Benjoim; Benzoë; Benzoin; Gum Benjamin; Gum Benzoin.

CAS — 9000-73-1; 9000-05-9 (the first of these numbers is stated to apply to Sumatra benzoin and the second to benzoin).

Pharmacopoeias. In *Br.*, *Jpn*, and *Port.* In *Arg.*, *Belg.*, *Hung.*, *Ind.*, *Mex.*, and *U.S.*, all of which allow both Siam benzoin and Sumatra benzoin.

A balsamic resin from the incised stem of *Styrax benzoin* and of *S. paralleloneurus*. It contains not less than 25% of total balsamic acids, calculated as cinnamic acid and with reference to the dried material, and not more than 20% of alcohol (90%)-insoluble matter.
Hard brittle masses of whitish tears embedded in a greyish-brown to reddish-brown translucent matrix, or cream-coloured to rusty brown tears; it has an agreeable balsamic odour. **Store** in well-closed containers at a temperature not exceeding 25°. Protect from light.

Sumatra benzoin is an ingredient of inhalations which are used in the treatment of catarrh of the upper respiratory tract. Sumatra benzoin is also used in topical preparations for its antiseptic and protective properties. Skin sensitisation has been reported.

Preparations

Benzoin Inhalation *(B.P.).* Vap. Benzoin. Prepared by macerating Sumatra benzoin 10 g and prepared storax 5 g with alcohol (or industrial methylated spirit) to 100 mL.
5 mL is added to about 500 mL of hot, not boiling, water and the vapour inhaled.

Benzoin Tincture *(B.P.C. 1973).* Simple Benzoin Tincture. Sumatra benzoin 1 in 10, prepared by maceration with alcohol (90%). It has occasionally been administered internally in chronic bronchitis. *Dose.* 2.5 to 5 mL. Similar tinctures are included in several other pharmacopoeias.

Compound Benzoin Tincture *(B.P.).* Co. Benz. Tinct.; Tinct. Benz. Co.; Friars' Balsam. Prepared by macerating sumatra benzoin 10%, prepared storax 10%, and aloes 2% with alcohol (90%).

Compound Benzoin Tincture *(U.S.P.).* Prepared by macerating Siam benzoin or Sumatra benzoin 10%, storax *U.S.P.* 8%, tolu balsam 4%, and aloes 2% with alcohol. Store at a temperature not exceeding 40° in airtight containers. Protect from light.

Proprietary Preparations

Rikospray Balsam *(Riker, UK). Dressing*, aerosol spray, soluble benzoin solids 9% (equivalent to benzoin 12.5%), prepared storax 2.5% with solvent and propellent. For application to the skin under adhesive plaster dressings in colostomy and ileostomy hygiene, for the prevention of bedsores, and for the treatment of cracked nipples and skin fissures.

3945-a

Sumatriptan *(BAN).*

GR-43175X. 3-(2-Dimethylaminoethyl)indol-5-yl-*N*-methylmethanesulphonamide.
$C_{14}H_{21}N_3O_2S$=295.4.

CAS — 103628-46-2; 103628-47-3 (hemisuccinate); 103628-48-4 (succinate).

A selective ($5HT_1$) serotonin agonist under investigation in the treatment of migraine.

Proprietary Names and Manufacturers.
Glaxo, UK.

7370-b

Sunflower Oil

Huile de Tournesol; Oleum Helianthi; Sunflowerseed Oil.

CAS — 8001-21-6.

Pharmacopoeias. In *Cz.*, *Egypt.*, *Fr.*, *Hung.*, and *Roum.*

The fixed oil expressed from the fruits (achenes) of the sunflower, *Helianthus annuus* (Compositae).

Sunflower oil is used in some countries as a salad oil and margarine oil and as a substitute for olive and arachis oils in pharmaceutical preparations.

MULTIPLE SCLEROSIS. In a double-blind study in 75 patients with multiple sclerosis there was no significant difference in the number of relapses in 36 given two 30-mL doses daily for 2 years of a 50% emulsion of sunflower oil (each 30 mL providing 8.6 g of linoleic acid) and 39 given similar doses of a control emulsion of olive oil, but the severity and duration of relapses was significantly reduced. Platelet adhesiveness was not affected.— J. H. D. Millar *et al.*, *Br. med. J.*, 1973, *1*, 765. A discussion of factors which might affect results.— E. J. Field and B. K. Shenton (letter), *ibid.*, 1975, *1*, 456.

POLYNEURITIS. Recovery in 2 children with idiopathic polyneuritis (Guillain-Barré syndrome) of 6 and 12 months duration respectively was virtually complete after treatment with a diet containing 30 mL of sunflower oil daily; one child also received 1.5 mL of wheat-germ oil daily. Both children had been treated with no success with prednisolone and one also with cyclophosphamide. A diet with a high content of polyunsaturated fatty acid might be of use in long-term disability after idiopathic polyneuritis and in other autoimmune diseases.— B. D. Bower and E. A. Newsholme, *Lancet*, 1978, *1*, 583.

13290-e

Surgibone *(USAN).*

Sterile heterogeneous bone and cartilage for surgical use, obtained from young calves and bovine embryos and subjected to special processing which reduces the antigenicity.

Surgibone has been used for grafting procedures in orthopaedic and reconstructive surgery.

13296-k

Tamitinol *(BAN, rINN).*

4-(Ethylaminomethyl)-2-methyl-5-(methylthiomethyl)pyridin-3-ol.
$C_{11}H_{18}N_2OS$=226.3.

CAS — 59429-50-4.

Tamitinol has been investigated for possible use in the organic brain syndrome and behavioural disorders in children but research appears to have been discontinued.

Proprietary Names and Manufacturers
E. Merck, UK.

547-m

Taraxacum

Dandelion Root; Löwenzahnwurzel; Pissenlit; Taraxacum Root.

Pharmacopoeias. In *Aust.*, *Hung.*, and *Pol. Chin.* and *Cz.* specify Taraxacum Herb from other species of *Taraxacum*.

The fresh or dried root of the common dandelion, *Taraxacum officinale* (Compositae).

Taraxacum has been used as a bitter and as a mild laxative.

1327-f

Tartaric Acid *(BAN, USAN).*

353 (metatartaric acid); Acidum Tartaricum; E334; Tart. Acid; Tartrique (Acide); Weinsäure. (+)-L-Tartaric acid; (+)-L-2,3-Dihydroxybutanedioic acid.
$C_4H_6O_6$=150.1.

CAS — 87-69-4.

Pharmacopoeias. In *Arg.*, *Aust.*, *Belg.*, *Br.*, *Braz.*, *Cz.*, *Egypt.*, *Eur.*, *Fr.*, *Ger.*, *Hung.*, *Ind.*, *Int.*, *It.*, *Jpn*, *Jug.*, *Mex.*, *Neth.*, *Nord.*, *Pol.*, *Port.*, *Roum.*, *Span.*, *Swiss*, and *Turk.* Also in *U.S.N.F.*

Odourless, colourless crystals or a white or almost white crystalline powder.
Soluble in less than 1 of water, 1 in 2.5 of alcohol, 1 in 250 of ether, and 1 in 1.7 of methyl alcohol. **Store** in well-closed containers.

Adverse Effects
Strong solutions of tartaric acid are mildly irritant and if ingested undiluted may cause gastro-enteritis.

Absorption and Fate
Tartaric acid is absorbed from the gastro-intestinal tract but up to 80% of an ingested dose is probably destroyed by micro-organisms in the lumen of the intestine before absorption occurs. Absorbed tartaric acid is excreted unchanged in the urine.

Uses and Administration
Tartaric acid is used in the preparation of effer-

vescent powders, granules, and tablets, as an ingredient of cooling drinks, and as a saline purgative. If not neutralised, it must be taken well diluted. Tartaric acid is used in wine as a de-acidifying agent to assist in the removal of excess malic acid by forming an insoluble double salt with calcium carbonate.

Estimated acceptable daily intake: up to 30 mg per kg body-weight.— Seventeenth Report of the FAO/WHO Expert Committee on Food Additives, *Tech. Rep. Ser. Wld Hlth Org. No. 539*, 1974. The existing specifications were confirmed.— Twenty-first Report of the Joint FAO/WHO Expert Committee on Food Additives, *Tech. Rep. Ser. Wld Hlth Org. No. 617*, 1978.

The use of metatartaric acid is permitted in wine under the Miscellaneous Additives in Food Regulations 1980 (SI 1980: No. 1834) for England and Wales and the Miscellaneous Additives in Food (Scotland) Regulations 1980 [SI 1980: No. 1889 (S. 176)]. Metatartaric acid is defined as consisting chiefly of a mixture of polyesters obtained by the controlled dehydration of L-(+)-tartaric acid, together with unchanged L-(+)-tartaric acid.

Proprietary Names and Manufacturers
The following names have been used for multi-ingredient preparations containing tartaric acid—Baritop *(Concept Pharmaceuticals, UK)*; Baros *(Mallinckrodt, Canad.)*; Concept Effervescent Granules *(Concept Pharmaceuticals, UK)*; Unik-Zoru *(Therapex, Canad.)*.

13299-x

Taurine *(pINN)*.

2-Aminoethanesulphonic acid.
$C_2H_7NO_3S$=125.1.
CAS — 107-35-7.

Bile acids are conjugated in the body with glycine or with taurine.

Taurine has been used as an adjunct in the treatment of hypercholesterolaemia and in cardiovascular disorders.

Proprietary Names and Manufacturers
O-Due *(Nativelle, Ital.)*.

17001-a

Taurolidine *(BAN, rINN)*.

Taurolin. 4,4′-Methylenebis(perhydro-1,2,4-thiadiazine 1,1-dioxide).
$C_7H_{16}N_4O_4S_2$=284.4.
CAS — 19388-87-5.

Taurolidine is a broad-spectrum antimicrobial agent which is thought to act by releasing formaldehyde. It has been administered intraperitoneally or by instillation into the bladder.

References: M. K. Browne *et al., Surgery Gynec. Obstet.*, 1978, *146*, 721; M. K. Browne, *Pharmatherapeutica*, 1981, *2*, 517; B. I. Knight *et al., Br. J. clin. Pharmac.*, 1981, *12*, 695; F. Erb *et al., Eur. J. Drug Metab. Pharmacokinet.*, 1983, *8*, 163; D. S. Jones *et al., J. Pharm. Pharmac.*, 1986, *38, Suppl.*, 39P.

13301-r

TCDD

2,3,7,8-Tetrachlorodibenzo-*p*-dioxin.
$C_{12}H_4Cl_4O_2$=322.0.
CAS — 1746-01-6.

NOTE. The name Dioxin is often used for TCDD, and has also been applied to dimethoxane.

TCDD is a by-product in the manufacture of trichlorophenol and a contaminant of the herbicide trichlorophenoxyacetic acid (see p.1354). It has been incriminated as causing chloracne (a severe and persistent acne caused by chlorinated compounds), liver and kidney damage, hirsutism, and personality changes. It is a potent teratogen in *animals*. It is an inducer of the enzyme aryl hydrocarbon hydroxylase which is implicated in carcinogenesis. Conflicting evidence has occurred concerning the effects on the long-term health of military personnel exposed to a TCDD-contaminated herbicide (Agent Orange) used as a defoliant during the Vietnam conflict. Other chlorinated dibenzodioxins, sometimes called dioxins, have similar but lower toxicity.

3637-g

Telenzepine *(rINN)*.

4,9-Dihydro-3-methyl-[(4-methyl-1-piperazinyl)acetyl]-10*H*-thieno[3,4-*b*][1,5]-benzodiazepin-10-one.
$C_{19}H_{22}N_4O_2S$=370.5.
CAS — 80880-90-6.

Telenzepine is reported to have antimuscarinic properties and has been investigated for its ability to reduce gastric acid secretion as a potential agent in the management of peptic ulcer.

W. Londong *et al., Gut*, 1987, *28*, 888.

18690-r

Temelastine *(BAN, USAN, rINN)*.

SKF-93944. 2-[4-(5-Bromo-3-methyl-2-pyridyl)butylamino]-5-(6-methyl-3-pyridylmethyl)pyrimidin-4-(1*H*)-one.
$C_{21}H_{24}BrN_5O$=442.4.
CAS — 86181-42-4.

Temelastine is an antihistamine under investigation. It is reported not to penetrate the central nervous system.

References: M. Boyce, *Br. J. clin. Pharmac.*, 1984, *18*, 277P; F. Alexander *et al., J. int. med. Res.*, 1986, *14*, 200; L. Shall *et al., Br. J. Derm.*, 1987, *116*, 434.

13309-g

Terizidone *(rINN)*.

B-2360. 4,4′-[*p*-Phenylenebis(methyleneamino)]-bis(isoxazolidin-3-one).
$C_{14}H_{14}N_4O_4$=302.3.
CAS — 25683-71-0.

Terizidone has been used in the treatment of tuberculosis and infections of the urinary tract.

Proprietary Names and Manufacturers
Terivalidin *(SCS, S.Afr.; Vinas, Spain)*; Urovalidin *(Bracco, Ital.)*.

1145-c

Tetrachlorodecaoxide

TCDO; Tetrachlorodecaoxygen Anion Complex.
Cl_4O_{10}=301.8.

Tetrachlorodecaoxide is a water-soluble anion complex containing oxygen in a chlorite matrix. Active oxygen is only released in the presence of biological material. It is applied as a solution for the stimulation of wound healing.

References: J. Hinz *et al.* (letter), *Lancet*, 1984, *2*, 630; J. Hinz *et al., ibid.*, 1986, *1*, 825; *ibid.*, 1168 (correction); *Drugs Today*, 1986, *22*, 8.

Proprietary Names and Manufacturers
Oxoferin *(Ger.)*.

13312-n

Tetrahydrobiopterin

2-Amino-5,6,7,8-tetrahydro-6-(1,2-dihydroxypropyl)pteridin-4(3*H*)-one.
$C_9H_{15}N_5O_3$=241.2.
CAS — 17528-72-2.

An atypical phenylketonuria has been described, attributed to deficiency of tetrahydrobiopterin; there have been reports of response to tetrahydrobiopterin.

There have also been reports of a response to tetrahydrobiopterin in certain patients with endogenous depression.

13313-h

Tetramethylammonium Iodide

$C_4H_{12}IN$=201.0.
CAS — 75-58-1.

Tetramethylammonium iodide is a quaternary ammonium ganglion-blocking agent which has been used as an antihypertensive and antispasmodic agent. It has also been used as a disinfectant.

Proprietary Names and Manufacturers
Artilacer *(Lacer, Spain)*; Banikol *(Techni-Pharma, Mon.)*.

13316-v

Thalidomide *(BAN, USAN, rINN)*.

K-17. 2-Phthalimidoglutarimide.
$C_{13}H_{10}N_2O_4$=258.2.
CAS — 50-35-1.

Adverse Effects

Thalidomide, a non-barbiturate hypnotic, was generally withdrawn from the world market in the early 1960s after it was discovered that it produced teratogenic effects when administered to women in early pregnancy. These effects involved mainly malformations of the limbs and defects of the ears, eyes, and internal organs. Further abnormalities and problems, including effects on the CNS, continue to appear in affected individuals.

The other major adverse effect due to thalidomide is peripheral neuropathies which can be severe and irreversible. Other effects have included somnolence, constipation, peripheral oedema, dryness of the mouth and nasal mucosa, and erythema of the face or other rashes.

NEUROPATHY. For reference to peripheral neuropathies, see under Uses, below.

Precautions

Thalidomide should not be used in women of child-bearing potential.

A reminder that rifampicin impairs the effectiveness of oral contraceptives. The consequences of this could be disastrous in a lepromatous woman of child-bearing age receiving thalidomide to control a prolonged and severe lepra reaction.— W. H. Jopling and J. H. S. Pettit (letter), *Lepr. Rev.*, 1979, *50*, 331.

Potentially neurotoxic drugs and alcohol should be avoided during thalidomide therapy.— J. Knop *et al., Br. J. Derm.*, 1983, *108*, 461.

Uses and Administration

Thalidomide has been shown to have immunosuppressive activity. It is effective in the control of type 2 (erythema nodosum leprosum) lepra reactions (see p.552) and is usually given in doses of up to 400 mg daily reduced over a period of about 2 weeks to a maintenance dose of 50 to 100 mg. It is of no value in type 1 lepra reactions.

Because of its immunosuppressive activity thalidomide has been tried in a wide range of conditions whose aetiology may involve the immune system.

Following the discovery that thalidomide was effective in the treatment of erythema nodosum leprosum it has been tried in a wide range of apparently unrelated conditions presumably on the basis of its effect on the immune system. Few controlled studies have been carried out but it appears to be effective in some conditions that are often poorly controlled or refractory to standard therapies including: prurigo nodularis (R.K. Winkleman *et al., Acta derm.-vener., Stockh.*, 1984, *64*, 412), actinic prurigo (C.R. Lovell *et al., Br. J. Derm.*, 1983, *108*, 467), chronic discoid lupus erythematosus (J. Knop *et al., Br. J. Derm.*, 1983, *108*, 461), aphthosis (D. Grinspan, *J. Am. Acad. Derm.*, 1985, *12*, 85), orogenital ulceration (J.S. Jenkins *et al., Lancet*, 1984, *2*, 1424) and Behçet's syndrome (T. Saylan and I. Saltik, *Archs Derm.*, 1982, *118*, 536). Its use often facilitates the discontinuation of cortiscosteroid therapy or permits a reduction in the dosage required.

There have also been isolated reports of beneficial effects in ulcerative colitis (M.F.R. Waters *et al.*, *Br. med. J.*, 1979, *1*, 792), Weber-Christian disease (J. Eravelly and M.F.R. Waters, *Lancet*, 1977, *1*, 251), erythema multiforme (F.A. Bahmer *et al.*, *Acta derm.-vener., Stockh.*, 1982, *62*, 449), pyoderma gangrenosum (P.Y. Venencie and J.H. Saurat, *Annls Pédiat., Paris*, 1982, *29*, 67), postherpetic neuralgia (B. Juel-Jensen per R.L. Barnhill and A.C. McDougall, *J. Am. Acad. Derm.*, 1982, *7*, 317), Jessner-Kanof disease (lymphocytic infiltration of the skin) (G. Moulin *et al.*, *Annls Derm. Vener.*, 1983, *110*, 611), sarcoidosis (H. Barriere, *Presse méd.*, 1983, *12*, 963), rheumatoid arthritis (O. Gutiérrez-Rodríguez, *Arthritis Rheum.*, 1984, *27*, 1118), and for acute graft-versus-host disease after bone-marrow transplantation (S.H. Lim *et al.*, *Lancet*, 1988, *1*, 117; J.-H. Saurat *et al.*, *ibid.*, 359).

However, concern has been expressed not only about its teratogenic risk but also about the risk of patients developing potentially severe and irreversible neuropathy in diseases requiring long-term therapy. Although Grosshans and Illy (*Int. J. Derm.*, 1984, *23*, 598) consider that symptoms are not proportional to the duration of treatment nor to the doses used Wulff *et al.* (*Br. J. Derm.*, 1985, *112*, 475) recommended that thalidomide should only be used for short-term treatment after finding that neuropathy had developed in all of 8 patients who had received thalidomide for prurigo nodularis or aphthous stomatitis for 1 to 6 years. Since others had also found a high incidence of peripheral neuropathy in prurigo, Aronson *et al.* (*Archs. Derm.*, 1984, *120*, 1466) suggested that this may have been related to the disease itself. Similar rates have not generally been reported following the use of thalidomide in other conditions and Knop *et al.* (see above) considered that the incidence of 25% they found in patients treated for discoid lupus erythematosus may have been related to the large doses used. However, even the generally-held opinion that neuropathy does not develop in lepromatous patients receiving thalidomide for lepra reactions has been challenged by Crawford (*Lancet*, 1985, *2*, 331).

Futher references.— *Lancet*, 1985, *2*, 80.

Proprietary Names and Manufacturers

FUNED, Braz.; Interbras, Braz.; Grünenthal, Ger.

15328-h

Thallium Acetate

Thallous Acetate.

$C_2H_3O_2Tl$=263.4.

CAS — 563-68-8.

Adverse Effects

Thallium salts are toxic when inhaled, ingested, or absorbed through the skin. Symptoms of poisoning may appear within 12 to 24 hours of a single toxic dose and include severe abdominal pain, vomiting, diarrhoea, gastro-intestinal haemorrhage, and in severe cases tremors, delirium, convulsions, paralysis, and coma, leading to death in 1 to 2 days. However, the acute reaction may subside to be followed within about 10 days by the development of polyneuritis, psychosis, delirium, convulsions, and other signs of encephalopathy, tachycardia, hypertension, skin eruptions, and hepatorenal injury. Alopecia occurs within 15 to 20 days. Death may result from respiratory failure.

Smaller repeated doses are also toxic, with symptoms appearing over several weeks.

In Great Britain, the recommended exposure limit of soluble thallium compounds, as Tl, is 0.1 mg per m^3 (long-term). Suitable precautions should be taken to prevent absorption through the skin. Legislation in the *UK* prohibits the use of thallium compounds in cosmetic products.

The *minimum lethal dose* in an adult is about 800 mg of thallium sulphate, i.e. 12 mg per kg body-weight.— R. Hausman and W. J. Wilson, *J. forens. Sci.*, 1964, *9*, 72.

In view of the toxicity of thallium sulphate to man and other *animals* it was recommended that it should not be used as a rodenticide.— Safe Use of Pesticides, Twentieth Report of the WHO Expert Committee on Insecticides, *Tech. Rep. Ser. Wld Hlth Org. No. 513*, 1973.

Treatment of Adverse Effects

After the acute ingestion of thallium the stomach should be emptied by emesis or lavage and a saline purgative such as sodium sulphate may be given. Intensive supportive therapy is necessary. Various methods have been employed in an attempt to increase the faecal and urinary excretion of thallium. A suspension of activated charcoal has been given to reduce intestinal absorption but is less successful than Prussian blue administered by duodenal tube. Systemic chelating agents have been tried but are of doubtful value and potentially dangerous. The administration of potassium chloride by mouth may mobilise thallium from the tissues but is also hazardous; signs of poisoning may be transiently aggravated and there may be interference with the exchange of potassium ions from Prussian blue for thallium ions in the gut.

Haemoperfusion is reported to be effective in eliminating absorbed thallium; haemodialysis combined with forced diuresis has been reported to give better results.

Uses and Administration

Thallium acetate was formerly used by mouth for depilation in ringworm and as an ingredient of depilatory creams but owing to numerous fatalities following both systemic and local treatments it is no longer used for such purposes. However, it is used in industry and is therefore still a hazard.

13319-p

Thenoic Acid

α-Thiophenic Acid; Tenoic Acid. Thiophene-2-carboxylic acid.

$C_5H_4O_2S$=128.1.

CAS — 527-72-0.

Thenoic acid is an antimicrobial agent which has been administered by mouth, rectally, or as nasal drops as the sodium salt ($C_5H_3NaO_2S$ = 150.1) and by mouth as the lithium salt ($C_5H_3LiO_2S$ = 134.1), in the treatment of respiratory-tract infections.

Proprietary Names and Manufacturers

Soufrane *(Roland-Marie, Fr.)*; Thiophéol *(Biogalenique, Fr.)*; Thiopon *(Amido, Fr.)*; Trophires *(Semar, Spain)*.

2412-b

Prepared Theobroma

Cocoa *(USAN)*; Cacao or Cocoa Powder; Non-alkalised Cocoa Powder; Prep. Theobrom.; Theobroma Praeparata.

Pharmacopoeias. Nord. includes Cacao which contains 20 to 24% fat. *U.S.N.F.* includes Cocoa (Cacao. Also in *B.P.C. 1973.*

The roasted seed of theobroma, *Theobroma cacao* (Sterculiaceae) deprived of most of the shell, pressed to remove a portion of its fat, and finely ground. **Store** in well-closed containers.

Prepared theobroma is used as a flavoured basis for tablets and lozenges.

Preparations

Cocoa Syrup *(U.S.N.F.)*. Cocoa 18 g, sucrose 60 g, liquid glucose 18 g, glycerol 5 mL, sodium chloride 200 mg, vanillin 20 mg, sodium benzoate 100 mg, water to 100 mL. Boiled for 3 minutes. Store at a temperature not exceeding 40° in airtight containers.

NOTE. Cocoa containing not more than 12% of non-volatile ether-soluble extractive will yield a syrup having a minimum tendency to separate. 'Breakfast cocoa' contains over 22% of 'fat'.

Chocolate. Pasta Cacao; Pasta Theobromatis; Theobroma Saccharata. Cocoa nibs finely ground and mixed with powdered sugar and a proportion of cocoa fat, with the addition of a small amount of vanillin or other flavouring. After incorporation of the ingredients, the mixture is subjected to hot milling and then poured into moulds. It contains about 28 to 38% of fat and about 40 to 60% of sugar.

Chocolate powder is sometimes used in the preparation of tablets and lozenges.

13320-n

Theobromine Magnesium Oleate

Magnesium 3,7-dimethylxanthine oleate. The magnesium double salt of theobromine ($C_7H_8N_4O_2$) and oleic acid ($C_{18}H_{34}O_2$).

CAS — 6767-73-3.

Theobromine magnesium oleate has been given by mouth in the treatment of arteriosclerosis and peripheral vascular disease. Transient flushing and pruritus have been reported.

Proprietary Names and Manufacturers

Athemol *(Glaxo, USA)*.

13325-g

Thioctic Acid

Lipoic Acid. 5-(1,2-Dithiolan-3-yl)valeric acid.

$C_8H_{14}O_2S_2$=206.3.

CAS — 62-46-4.

Thioctic acid, its sodium salt, and its amide have been tried in the treatment of liver dysfunction; it has also been tried in subacute necrotising encephalopathy. Beneficial results have been claimed in amanitin poisoning following ingestion of the mushroom *Amanita phalloides*, but its use is controversial (see under Mushrooms, p.1592).

Proprietary Names and Manufacturers

Biletan *(Gador, Arg.)*; Lipoamid *(Fuso, Jpn)*; Lipoamin *(Sawai, Jpn)*; Thioami *(Hokuriku, Jpn)*; Thioctacid *(Asta Pharma, Ger.)*; Thioctan *(Katwijk, Neth.)*; Tioctan *(Fujisawa, S.Afr.)*; Tioctidasi *(ISI, Ital.)*; Tioctinessa *(Nessa, Spain)*.

13330-m

Thiram *(USAN, pINN)*.

NSC-1771; SQ-1489; TMT; TMTD. Tetramethylthiuram disulphide.

$C_6H_{12}N_2S_4$=240.4.

CAS — 137-26-8.

Thiram is the methyl analogue of disulfiram (p.1565) and has antibacterial and antifungal activity. It has been used as a fungicide in agriculture, and in industry as a rubber accelerator. Thiram is irritant to mucous membranes and skin.

In Great Britain the recommended exposure limits of thiram are 5 mg per m^3 (long-term) and 10 mg per m^3 (short-term).

13332-v

Thorium Dioxide

Thorium Oxide.

ThO_2=264.0.

CAS — 1314-20-1.

Colloidal solutions of thorium dioxide were formerly used as X-ray contrast media for examination of the liver and spleen, for arteriography, and occasionally for outlining the cerebral ventricles. Its elimination is very slow and incomplete. It accumulates in the reticulo-endothelial system, especially in the liver and spleen. As it is radioactive (half-life: 1.41 × 10^{10} years), this accumulation is dangerous and there is strong evidence that the ensuing prolonged exposure to its radiation is a contributing factor in the development of malignant diseases and blood disorders often 20 to 30 years after its administration.

Discussion of the toxicity of thorium dioxide.— *Lancet*, 1977, *1*, 1297.

Of 1107 patients given thorium dioxide between 1930 and 1952 primarily for the radiological visualisation of blood vessels, 699 had died and 408 were alive up to the end of 1963. The long-term sequelae were shown, statistically, to include local granulomas in 81, cirrhosis of the liver in 42, fatal blood disorders in 16, and haemangioendotheliomas occurring in 22 and virtually thorium-dioxide specific. It was considered that the use of thorium dioxide was never justified in patients with a life expectation of more than 2 years.— J. da Silva Horta *et al.*, *Lancet*, 1965, *2*, 201.

Brief case histories of 6 patients seen between 1967 and 1975, who had received thorium dioxide many years earlier. Complications included leukaemia, aplastic anaemia, tumours, and, in all patients, hyposplenism. The literature was reviewed and included 61 cases of leukaemia and 40 cases of marrow failure, almost all of which were attributed to thorium dioxide; liver cirrhosis or fibrosis and splenic atrophy were common.— S. A. N. Johnson *et al.*, *Q. J. Med.*, 1977, *46*, 259.

Proprietary Names and Manufacturers
Thorotrast.

13333-g

Thuja

The fresh leaves and twigs of *Thuja occidentalis* (Coniferae).

Thuja is used in homoeopathic medicine.

13335-p

Thymus Hormones

CAS — 69521-94-4 (thymosin α_1); 60529-76-2 (thymopoietin); 63340-72-7 (thymic humoral factor).

The thymus gland controls the development of T-lymphocytes and thereby plays a central role in cell-mediated immunity and the regulation of immune responses. It secretes hormones although the multiplicity of factors isolated has led to some confusion. Several polypeptides characterised in the thymus or serum are able to induce lymphocyte differentiation *in vitro* and *in vivo*. They include: thymosin fraction 5, a crude thymus gland extract; thymosin α_1, a component of fraction 5 which has been synthesised; thymic humoral factor (THF), isolated from crude thymic extract dialysate; nonathymulin (thymulin, serum thymic factor, Facteur Thymique Serique, FTS), a synthetic nonapeptide; thymomodulin, a partially purified extract from calf thymus; thymopoetin, a polypeptide of known amino acid sequence; thymopentin (thymopoetin pentapeptide, TP-5), a fragment of thymopoetin with 5 amino acids; and thymostimulin (TP-1), extracted from calf thymus.

Various preparations, including crude extracts from calf thymus gland, thymosin fraction 5, and thymosin α_1 have been tried as immunostimulants in immunodeficiency disorders and as an adjunct in the treatment of malignant disease.

Thymus hormones have been tried in the treatment of numerous conditions including congenital thymic insufficiency, sarcoidosis, malignant neoplasms, viral infections, AIDS, and after bone-marrow transplantation; any condition where they might possibly have been expected to help. The various extracts and peptides are reported to be relatively harmless, with only a few adverse reactions reported, mostly allergic reactions to calf thymus extracts in association with pre-existing bovine protein allergy.— *Lancet*, 1983, *1*, 1309.

Findings which indicate that measurement of thymic hormones in serum might be used to assess the competence of the immune system.— E. M. Hersh *et al.* (letter), *New Engl. J. Med.*, 1983, *308*, 45.

ARTHRITIS. Reports of the use of thymus hormones in the treatment of rheumatoid arthritis: M. G. Malaise *et al.*, *Lancet*, 1985, *1*, 832 (thymopentin by slow intravenous injection better than placebo); E. M. Veys *et al.*, *J. Rheumatol.*, 1984, *11*, 462 (failure of subcutaneous or intravenous thymopentin to demonstrate a beneficial effect); B. Amor *et al.*, *Ann. rheum. Dis.*, 1987, *46*, 549 (favourable response with subcutaneous nonathymulin compared with placebo).

IMMUNODEFICIENCY DISORDERS. Reports of the use of thymus hormones in the treatment of immunodeficiency disorders: P. Bordigoni *et al.*, *Lancet*, 1982, *2*, 293 (improvement in cell-mediated-immunity tests and reduction of infection with intravenous nonathymulin in immunodeficient children); F. Aiuti *et al.*, *ibid.*, 1983, *1*, 551 (mixed responses with intramuscular thymopentin in infants and children with primary immunodeficiencies); E. G. Davies *et al.* (letter), *New Engl. J. Med.*, 1983, *309*, 493 (unsuccessful results with subcutaneous thymopentin and intramuscular thymostimulin in children with histiocytosis); F. Mascart-Lemone *et al.* (letter), *Lancet*, 1983, *2*, 735 (some benefit with intravenous thymopentin in 3 patients with the acquired immune deficiency sydrome (AIDS)).

VIRAL INFECTIONS. Reports of the use of thymus hormones in the treatment of viral infections: F. Aiuti *et al.*, *Int. J. clin. Pharmac. Ther. Toxic.*, 1983, *21*, 81 (fever recurrences with thymostimulin compared to placebo in patients with recurrent herpes simplex labialis); K. Záruba *et al.* (letter), *Lancet*, 1983, *2*, 1245 (preliminary results indicating that thymopentin may be a useful adjuvant treatment in non- or hypo-responders to hepatitis B vaccination).

Proprietary Names and Manufacturers
Leucotrofina *(Ellem, Ital.)*; Sintomodulina *(Italfarmaco, Ital.)*; Timunox *(Cilag, Ger.*; *Cilag, Ital.)*.

13337-w

Tiamulin Fumarate *(BANM, USAN, rINNM)*.

81723-hfu; SQ-14055; SQ-22947. 11-Hydroxy-6,7,10,12-tetramethyl-1-oxo-10-vinylperhydro-3a,7-pentanoinden-8-yl (2-diethylaminoethylthio)acetate hydrogen fumarate.
$C_{28}H_{47}NO_4S,C_4H_4O_4$=609.8.

CAS — 55297-95-5 (tiamulin); 555297-96-6 (fumarate).

Tiamulin fumarate has been used in the treatment of dysentery in *pigs*.

Proprietary Veterinary Names and Manufacturers
Dynamutilin *(Squibb, UK)*.

1259-m

Tibalosin *(rINN)*.

CP-1068S; Tibalosine. (±)-*erythro*-2,3-Dihydro-α-{1-[(4-phenylbutyl)amino]ethyl}benzo[*b*]thiophene-5-methanol.
$C_{21}H_{27}NOS$=341.5.

CAS — 63996-84-9.

Tibalosin is an alpha-adrenoceptor blocking agent under investigation as an antihypertensive agent.

References: J. Staessen *et al.*, *Clin. Pharmac. Ther.*, 1983, *33*, 556; U. Staessen *et al.*, *Archs int. Pharmacodyn. Thér.*, 1986, *279*, 162.

13341-g

Tibezonium Iodide *(rINN)*.

Rec-15/0691. Diethylmethyl{2-[4-(4-phenylthiophenyl)-3*H*-1,5-benzodiazepin-2-ylthio]ethyl}ammonium iodide.
$C_{28}H_{32}IN_3S_2$=601.6.

CAS — 54663-47-7.

Tibezonium iodide has been used in the treatment of infections of the mouth and throat.

Proprietary Names and Manufacturers
Antoral *(Recordati, Ital.)*.

13343-p

Ticlopidine Hydrochloride *(USAN, rINNM)*.

5-(2-Chlorobenzyl)-4,5,6,7-tetrahydrothieno[3,2-*c*]pyridine hydrochloride.
$C_{14}H_{14}ClNS,HCl$=300.2.

CAS — 55142-85-3 (ticlopidine); 53885-35-1 (hydrochloride).

Adverse Effects and Precautions

Gastro-intestinal disturbances and skin rashes are the most commonly reported side-effects associated with ticlopidine therapy. Blood dyscrasias, particularly serious in elderly patients, have also occurred. There have been reports of vertigo and occasional reports of cholestatic jaundice.

Ticlopidine should not be administered to patients with haemorrhagic diathesis, gastro-intestinal ulcers, or severe liver dysfunction. It should not be given to patients receiving aspirin, anticoagulants, or corticosteroids.

Uses and Administration

Ticlopidine is an inhibitor of platelet aggregation. It has been given in the treatment of atherosclerotic disease and intermittent claudication in doses of 250 mg once or twice daily by mouth, with meals. Regular haematological monitoring has been recommended.

A detailed review of the pharmacokinetics, pharmacodynamics, and clinical use of ticlopidine in the treatment of platelet-dependent disease states.— E. Saltiel and A. Ward, *Drugs*, 1987, *34*, 222.

Further references: K. M. Fox *et al.*, *Lancet*, 1982, *2*, 727; C. Warlow, *Drugs*, 1985, *29*, 474; G. de Gaetano *et al.*, *ibid.*, 1986, *31*, 517.

Proprietary Names and Manufacturers
Anagregal *(Gentili, Ital.)*; Aplaquette *(Alfa Farmaceutici, Ital.)*; Opteron *(Coop. Farm., Ital.)*; Ticlid *(Millot-Solac, Fr.*; *Labaz, Neth.)*; Ticlodone *(Crinos, Ital.*; *Fher, Spain)*; Ticlosan *(Von Boch, Ital.)*; Tiklid *(Midy, Ital.*; *Labaz, Spain)*; Tiklyd *(Labaz, Ger.)*.

13345-w

Tilorone Hydrochloride *(USAN, rINNM)*.

NSC-143969. 2,7-Bis(2-diethylaminoethoxy)fluoren-9-one dihydrochloride.
$C_{25}H_{34}N_2O_3,2HCl$=483.5.

CAS — 27591-97-5 (tilorone); 27591-69-1 (hydrochloride).

Tilorone hydrochloride is an antiviral agent active by mouth. It has been reported to induce interferon production in *mice*.

ADVERSE EFFECTS. Significant retinopathy had been reported in 2 patients receiving long-term treatment with tilorone hydrochloride by mouth (J.N. Weiss *et al.*, *Am. J. Ophthal.*, 1980, *90*, 846).— R. B. Pollard, *Drugs*, 1982, *23*, 37.

USES AND ADMINISTRATION. Lack of benefit with tilorone in amyotrophic lateral sclerosis.— W. H. Olson *et al.*, *Neurology, Minneap.*, 1978, *28*, 1293.

Results indicating that tilorone hydrochloride may be of some use in the treatment of certain early T-cell lymphomas but it appears to be of no benefit in advanced disease.— C. P. Crotty and R. K. Winkelmann, *J. Am. Acad. Derm.*, 1982, *7*, 468.

Proprietary Names and Manufacturers
Merrell Dow, USA.

1262-r

Timegadine *(rINN)*.

SR-1368. 1-Cyclohexyl-2-(2-methyl-4-quinolyl)-3-(2-thiazolyl)guanidine.
$C_{20}H_{23}N_5S$=365.5.

CAS — 71079-19-1.

Timegadine is a non-steroidal anti-inflammatory agent under investigation.

References: S. George *et al.*, *Br. J. clin. Pharmac.*, 1983, *15*, 495 (effect of food on absorption); *idem*, 1984, *18*, 785 (protein binding); M. O'Sullivan *et al.*, *Clin. Rheumatol.*, 1985, *4*, 362 (use in rheumatoid arthritis).

Proprietary Names and Manufacturers
Leo, Denm.

3749-j

Timonacic *(rINN)*.

ATC; NSC-25855; Thioproline. Thiazolidine-4-carboxylic acid.
$C_4H_7NO_2S$=133.2.

CAS — 444-27-9.

NOTE. The name ATC has also been used for a

combination of paracetamol and trichloroethanol (4-acetamidophenyl 2,2,2-trichloroethyl carbonate).

Pharmacopoeias. In *Cz.*

Timonacic is used as an adjuvant in the treatment of acute and chronic hepatic disorders. It has been given in doses of 200 mg two or three times daily initially, followed by 100 mg twice daily for maintenance treatment. It has also been used as an adjuvant to the treatment of psoriasis and acne.

A report of beneficial results, with no side-effects, following administration of the sodium salt of timonacic to patients with advanced cancer. A mild antitumour effect was noted with a dose of timonacic, 5 mg per kg body-weight daily intravenously or by mouth; definite activity was noted with 20 mg per kg intravenously for 5 days every 3 weeks, with complete remission in 2 patients when this was increased to 40 mg per kg. A regimen of 40 mg per kg intravenously daily appeared to be the most effective, with complete clinical remission 1 month after therapy began in all of 4 patients, which had so far lasted for 1 to over 2.5 months, no patient having discontinued therapy.— A. Brugarolas and M. Gosalvez, *Lancet*, 1980, *1*, 68. A warning concerning the toxicity of timonacic. Overdosage induces status epilepticus and coma within 15 minutes to an hour of ingestion. The toxic dose is especially low in young children whose blood-brain barrier is less effective, and seizures may occur with doses of 30 mg per kg body-weight and are always reported with more than 50 mg per kg; in adults seizures have been recorded with 60 mg per kg. These neurological disturbances are associated with initial transient hypoglycaemia followed by longer-lasting hyperglycaemia, and sometimes with hyperthermia. Seizures are readily controlled with diazepam, but EEG disturbances may persist for several weeks or even months. There have also been a number of cases of auditory sequelae (deafness or hypacusia).— R. Garnier *et al.* (letter), *ibid.*, 365. Toxicological studies on the sodium salt have indicated that the oral form of timonacic is more toxic than the intravenous form. Possibly it is hydrolysed in the stomach to yield cysteine and formaldehyde. Following intravenous injection it is rapidly eliminated unchanged in the urine which is why it is proposed to administer it to cancer patients at a dosage of 40 mg per kg body-weight daily by injection (in divided doses every six hours).— M. Gosálvez (letter), *ibid.*, 597. In a study of 5 patients timonacic had no beneficial effect on the tumours, and all patients showed progressive disease while on treatment. Three patients had somnolence and mild confusion one week after starting treatment, and one of these subsequently had frank psychosis with paranoid delusions.— A. P. Sappino and I. E. Smith (letter), *ibid.*, 1980, *2*, 417. Further evidence that timonacic is toxic to the CNS and a report that it also disturbs renal function. Lack of therapeutic effect was noted.— S. Nasca *et al.* (letter), *ibid.*, 1981, *1*, 778.

Further comments on the possible anti-tumour action of timonacic.— T. F. Slater (letter), *Lancet*, 1980, *1*, 597; *ibid.*, 1983, *1*, 799; M. Gosalvez (letter), *ibid.*, 1108.

Proprietary Names and Manufacturers
Detoxepa *(Ayerst, Ital.)*; Héparégène *(Syntex, Switz.)*; Hepacitol *(Andromaco, Spain)*; Hepalidine *(Riker, Arg.; Riker, Fr.)*; Heparegen *(Gramon, Arg.; Syntex, Switz.)*; Livercrom *(Elmu, Spain)*; Sulfile *(Poli, Ital.)*; Tiazolidin *(UCM-Difme, Ital.)*.

5326-q

Tin

Sn=118.69.

CAS — 7440-31-5.

A bright white malleable but not very ductile, metal.

Owing to their low solubility tin and tin oxide are very poorly absorbed from the gastro-intestinal tract and are not toxic. Chronic inhalation causes a benign form of pneumoconiosis.

Organic compounds of tin are highly toxic and cause severe neurological damage associated with oedema of the white matter of the brain. Treatment has been symptomatic. Contamination of the skin with organic tin compounds can cause severe burning.

In Great Britain the recommended exposure limits of inorganic tin compounds, except stannic hydride (SnH_4), are 2 mg (as Sn) per m^3 (long-term) and 4 mg (as Sn) per m^3 (short-term); for organic tin compounds, except cyhexatin, the limits are 0.1 mg (as Sn) per m^3 (long-term) and 0.2 mg (as Sn) per m^3 (short-term). Suitable precautions should be taken to prevent absorption of organic tin compounds through the skin. In the US the permissible and recommended exposure limits of organotin compounds are 0.1 mg tin per m^3.

Tin and tin oxide have been given in the treatment of boils but there is little evidence of effectiveness; they were also formerly used in some countries for the treatment of tapeworm. Organic tin compounds, especially tributyltin oxide (TBTO) are used as molluscicides.

A review of tin deficiency and toxic effects.— Report of a WHO Expert Group on Trace Elements in Human Nutrition, *Tech. Rep. Ser. Wld Hlth Org., No. 532*, 1973, 38.

Tin and Organotin Compounds, *Environmental Health Criteria 15*, Geneva, Wld Hlth Org., 1980.

Excess amounts of tin in food, which tend to arise from tin-coated cans, produce gastric irritation and the threshold for this effect appears to occur with concentrations of about 200 mg of tin per kg of food. Consumers should be advised not to store food in open tin-coated cans. A provisional maximum tolerable daily intake of 2 mg per kg body-weight was allocated. This includes the food additive use of stannous chloride.— Twenty-sixth Report of Joint FAO/WHO Expert Committee on Food Additives, *Tech. Rep. Ser. Wld Hlth Org. No. 683*, 1982.

PREGNANCY AND THE NEONATE. Congenital malformations in 3 infants were associated with the administration of preparations containing tin and tin oxide to the mothers during pregnancy.— A. Notter *et al.*, *Bull. Féd. Socs Gynéc. Obstét. Lang. fr.*, 1968, *20*, *Suppl.*, 319.

13349-j

Tiopronin *(rINN).*

Thiopronine. *N*-(2-Mercaptopropionyl)glycine.
$C_5H_9NO_3S$=163.2.

CAS — 1953-02-2.

Adverse Effects

Tiopronin has similar adverse effects to those of penicillamine (p.847); pemphigus, proteinuria, nephrotic syndrome, and hepatic disorders have been reported.

A 38-year-old woman with cystinuria developed myopathy (quadriceps pain, swelling, and weakness) 7 days after starting treatment with tiopronin 600 mg daily.— D. S. M. Hales *et al.*, *Br. med. J.*, 1982, *285*, 939. Criticism.— M. A. Mansell (letter), *ibid.*, 1356.

Of 180 patients on long-term tiopronin therapy for rheumatoid arthritis, 3 developed skin lesions resembling pemphigus which improved when the drug was discontinued.— F. Trotta *et al.*, *Scand. J. Rheumatol.*, 1984, *13*, 93.

Uses and Administration

Tiopronin is a sulphydryl compound with properties similar to those of penicillamine (p.849). It may be given orally or by intramuscular or intravenous injection. It has been used in the treatment of hepatic and skin disorders and in cystinuria.

CHRONIC HEPATITIS. In a 12-week study involving 165 patients with chronic hepatitis, the administration of tiopronin 600 mg daily by mouth in divided doses was associated with an improvement in liver function tests regardless of the histological stage of the disease or HBsAg status.— F. Ichida *et al.*, *J. int. med. Res.*, 1982, *10*, 325.

CYSTINURIA. In a multicentre study, 66 patients with cystine nephrolithiasis were treated with tiopronin in doses of up to 2 g daily (mean 1.193 g); ongoing alkali therapy was continued and the same dietary and fluid regimens were maintained. Tiopronin significantly reduced urinary-cystine concentrations and the new stone formation rate. The adverse effects of tiopronin and penicillamine were compared in 49 patients who had been treated with penicillamine before starting the study. Both drugs had similar side-effects; 41 patients had side-effects to penicillamine of which 34 required cessation of drug therapy and 37 patients had side-effects to tiopronin of which 15 required drug withdrawal. However of the 34 patients who had to stop penicillamine therapy because of adverse effects, 22 were able to continue treatment with tiopronin. Of the 17 patients without a history of penicillamine therapy, 11 had adverse effects to tiopronin and 1 discontinued treatment because of proteinuria.— C. Y. C. Pak *et al.*, *J. Urol., Baltimore*, 1986, *136*, 1003.

Further references to tiopronin in cystinuria: J. Thomas *et al.*, *Thérapie*, 1976, *31*, 623; A. Berio (letter), *Archs Dis. Childh.*, 1980, *55*, 743.

EPILEPSY. The addition of tiopronin 200 mg three times daily to the anticonvulsant drug therapy of a 28-year-old man with uncontrolled epilepsy resulted in a disappearance of attacks and enabled a reduction of the doses of the regular anticonvulsive drugs. It was not, however, possible to reduce the dosage of tiopronin.— G. A. Rose (letter), *Lancet*, 1986, *1*, 452.

LEAD POISONING. Parenteral administration of tiopronin (30 g over a period of 10 days) to 27 men with symptoms of chronic lead poisoning had a beneficial effect on the biochemical indices of lead poisoning. The mechanism of action was not clear.— F. Candura *et al.* (letter), *Lancet*, 1979, *1*, 330.

MUCOLYTIC ACTIVITY. Studies on the mucolytic activity of tiopronin.— D. Costantini *et al.*, *Curr. ther. Res.*, 1982, *31*, 714; L. Carratù *et al.*, *ibid.*, *32*, 529; P. C. Braga *et al.*, *ibid.*, 1984, *36*, 921.

Proprietary Names and Manufacturers
Capen *(Phoenix, Arg.)*; Captimer *(Fresenius, Ger.)*; Epatiol *(Medici, Ital.)*; Mucolysin *(Proter, Ital.; Interdelta, Switz.)*; Sutilan *(Cusi, Spain)*; Thiola *(Sidus, Arg.; Coop. Farm., Ital.; Jpn; Multipharmax, Switz.)*; Thiosol *(Coop. Farm., Ital.)*; Tioglis *(Logifarm, Ital.)*; Vincol *(Reig Jofré, Spain)*.

1276-b

Tiquizium Bromide *(pINN).*

HSR-902. *trans*-3-(Di-2-thienylmethylene)octahydro-5-methyl-2*H*-quinolizinium bromide.
$C_{19}H_{24}BrNS_2$=410.4.

CAS — 71731-58-3.

Tiquizium bromide is used as an antispasmodic in gastro-intestinal disorders.

References: *Drugs Today*, 1985, *21*, 73.

Proprietary Names and Manufacturers
Thiaton *(Jpn)*.

9009-m

Tiratricol *(rINN).*

Triac; Triiodothyroacetic Acid. [4-(4-Hydroxy-3-iodophenoxy)-3,5-di-iodophenyl]acetic acid.
$C_{14}H_9I_3O_4$=621.9.

CAS — 51-24-1.

NOTE. The name Triac has also been applied to the diethanolamine salt of tiratricol and the name Tri-ac has been used to denote a preparation containing ethyl lactate and zinc sulphate.

Uses and Administration

Tiratricol, which is chemically similar to the thyroid hormones, has been suggested for use in obesity.

Proprietary Names and Manufacturers
Téatrois *(Théranol, Fr.)*; Triacana *(Ana, Fr.)*.

17012-r

Tiropramide *(rINN).*

DL-α-Benzamido-*p*-[2-(diethylamino)ethoxy]-*N*,*N*-dipropylhydrocinnamamide.
$C_{28}H_{41}N_3O_3$=467.7.

CAS — 55837-29-1.

Tiropramide is used as an antispasmodic in the treatment of biliary and gastro-intestinal disorders. It has been given as the hydrochloride.

References: E. Trabuccni *et al.*, *Pharmatherapeutica*, 1986, *4*, 541.

Proprietary Names and Manufacturers
Alfospas *(Rottapharm, Ital.)*; Maiorad *(Merck Sharp & Dohme, Ital.)*.

13355-l

Titanium

Ti=47.90.

CAS — 7440-32-6.

Titanium plate has been used in the repair of skull damage.

For the use of titanium in cranioplasty, see D. S. Gordon and G. A. S. Blair, *Br. med. J.*, 1974, *2*, 478; G. A. S. Blair *et al.*, *ibid.*, 1976, *2*, 907.

An evaluation of titanium cones for use as a root filling material.— J. J. Messing, *Br. dent. J.*, 1980, *148*, 41.

7900-j

Tocopherylquinone

α-Tocopherylquinone; α-Tocoquinone; Tocoferylchinonum. 2-(3-Hydroxy-3,7,11,15-tetramethylhexadecyl)-3,5,6-trimethyl-1,4-benzoquinone.
$C_{29}H_{50}O_3$=446.7.

CAS — 7559-04-8.

Tocopherylquinone is a vitamin E substance which has been used in a variety of conditions including hypertension and disorders of muscle and skin.

A report of the use of tocopherylquinone in the treatment of ulcerative colitis.— J. D. Bennet, *Gut*, 1986, *27*, 695. Comment.— E. Guthy (letter), *ibid.*, 1400.

Proprietary Names and Manufacturers
Eutrophyl *(Riker, Fr.)*; Ipotensil *(Tosi-Novara, Ital.)*; Tensiopress *(Biosint, Ital.)*; Trimina *(Ital.)*; Vitapressina *(Coli, Ital.)*.

13359-c

Toldimfos *(BAN, rINN).*

(4-Dimethylamino-*o*-tolyl)phosphinic acid.
$C_9H_{14}NO_2P$=199.2.

CAS — 57808-64-7; 5787-63-3 (sodium salt).

Toldimfos is a phosphorus source used in veterinary medicine.

Proprietary Veterinary Names and Manufacturers
Foston *(Hoechst, UK)*.

13362-e

Tolynol

1-(*p*-Tolyl)ethanol; *p*,α-Dimethylbenzyl alcohol.
$C_9H_{12}O$=136.2.

CAS — 536-50-5.

Tolynol has been used as a choleretic in the treatment of hepatic disorders.

Proprietary Names and Manufacturers
Curcumyl *(SMB, Belg.)*; Norbilan *(Face, Ital.)*.

2830-f

Toremifene *(BAN, rINN).*

FC-1157a. (*Z*)-2-[4-(4-Chloro-1,2-diphenylbut-1-enyl)phenoxy]ethyldimethylamine.
$C_{26}H_{28}ClNO$=406.0.

CAS — 89778-26-7.

Toremifene is an anti-oestrogen under investigation in malignant neoplasms of the breast.

A brief review of toremifene.— *Drugs of the Future*, 1986, *11*, 398; *ibid.*, 1987, *12*, 513.

A patient with multiple desmoid tumours, classified as fibromatoses, responded on different occasions to tamoxifen and to toremifene.— A. J. Wilson *et al.* (letter), *Lancet*, 1987, *1*, 508.

Some breast tumour shrinkage with toremifene in women who had disease progression while on tamoxifen.— S. R. Ebbs *et al.* (letter), *Lancet*, 1987, *2*, 621.

Proprietary Names and Manufacturers
Laakefarmos, Fin.

3924-y

Transcainide *(USAN, rINN).*

R-54718. (±)-*trans*-4-(Dimethylamino)-1-(2-hydroxycyclohexyl)-2′,6′-isonipectoxylidide
$C_{22}H_{35}N_3O_2$=373.5.

CAS — 88296-62-2.

Transcainide is an anti-arrhythmic agent under investigation.

References; R. Stroobandt *et al.*, *Eur. J. clin. Pharmac.*, 1987, *32*, 449.

Proprietary Names and Manufacturers
Janssen, Belg.

13365-j

Transfer Factor

A peptide constituent of dialysable leucocyte extracts.

Transfer factor can passively transfer cell-mediated immunity from a sensitised donor to a non-sensitised recipient. It is prepared from the leucocytes of the donor, whose sensitivity may have been demonstrated by skin tests.

Transfer factor has been suggested for use in infections due to bacteria, fungi, and viruses, inflammatory disorders, immunodeficiency diseases, leprosy, and malignancies.

Reviews concerning transfer factor: A. M. Attallah *et al.*, *Pharmac. Ther.*, 1983, *19*, 435; J. Gibson *et al.*, *Clin. Immunol. Allergy*, 1983, *3*, 331; H. H. Fudenberg, *Proc. Soc. exp. Biol. Med.*, 1985, *178*, 327; K. Y. Tsang and H. H. Fudenberg, *Springer Semin. Immunopathol.*, 1986, *9*, 19.

The results of a randomised double-blind placebo-controlled study in 61 children with acute lymphocytic leukaemia confirmed those of previous studies and demonstrated the efficacy of transfer factor in preventing varicella-zoster infection in susceptible subjects. Patients were given dialysable transfer factor by subcutaneous injection in doses of 1×10^8 lymphocyte equivalents per 7 kg of body-weight or placebo and have been followed-up for 12 to 30 months so far. Of the 31 children exposed to chicken-pox during the study, 14 became clinically infected and all but one of these were in the placebo group. Long-term follow-up is necessary before protection can be considered absolute.— R. W. Steele *et al.*, *New Engl. J. Med.*, 1980, *303*, 355. Comments.— C. H. Kirkpatrick, *ibid.*, 390.

In a double-blind placebo-controlled study the clinical state of 29 patients with multiple sclerosis of varying severity given transfer factor was compared with that of 29 carefully matched patients given placebo. The transfer factor was obtained from a pool of 20 spouses sharing the same house as an affected patient. Although the transfer factor did not significantly improve the clinical state of multiple sclerosis patients, the rate of progression in those with mild to moderate disease activity was slowed. The benefit of treatment with transfer factor was not apparent until 18 months to 2 years after its commencement. The findings justify long-term studies with transfer factor and comparison of transfer factor with other immunopotentiating agents, such as interferon.— A. Basten *et al.*, *Lancet*, 1980, *2*, 931. Comment.— *ibid.*, 953. A very important difference between the immunosuppressant approach to multiple sclerosis and attempts to stimulate the immune system with transfer factor is that immunosuppression is hazardous whereas transfer factor is at least safe.— H. Valdimarsson (letter), *ibid.*, 1191. Criticisms of the designation double-blind to the immunosuppressant regimen.— E. H. Jellinek (letter), *ibid.*, 1192; G. S. Plaut (letter), *ibid.*

Conversion of leprolin and early lepromin reactions was achieved by 2 injections of transfer factor made of lymphocytes from lepromin-positive tuberculoid leprosy patients. However, the late reaction to lepromin remained unchanged. The importance of the degree of sensitivity of the cell donor was demonstrated, and a booster dose was also found to be useful.— S. -H. Han *et al.*, *Chin. J. Microbiol. Immunol.*, 1980, *13*, 1.

A preliminary communication of a study in 9 patients with acquired immunodeficiency syndrome (AIDS). Administration of 4 weekly doses of transfer factor from patients with lymphadenopathy and antibodies to HIV resulted in a transient immune reconstitution, diminishing 5 weeks after the last transfer factor treatment.— J. T. Carey *et al.*, *J. Am. med. Ass.*, 1987, *257*, 651.

13369-a

Trepibutone *(rINN).*

AA-149; Trepionate. 3-(2,4,5-Triethoxybenzoyl)propionic acid.
$C_{16}H_{22}O_6$=310.3.

CAS — 41826-92-0.

Trepibutone is reported to have spasmolytic and choleretic activity.

Proprietary Names and Manufacturers
Supacal *(Jpn)*.

13374-z

Tribenoside *(USAN, rINN).*

21401-Ba; Ba-21401. Ethyl 3,5,6-tri-*O*-benzyl-D-glucofuranoside.
$C_{29}H_{34}O_6$=478.6.

CAS — 10310-32-4.

Tribenoside has been used in inflammatory and varicose disorders of the veins.

References: A. Sioufi and F. Pommier, *J. pharm. Sci.*, 1980, *69*, 167.

Proprietary Names and Manufacturers
Alven *(FIRMA, Ital.)*; Flebosan *(Dukron, Ital.)*; Glyvenol *(Ciba, Arg.*; *Ciba, Belg.*; *Ciba, Fr.*; *Ciba, Ger.*; *Ciba, Ital.*; *Ciba, Spain*; *Ciba, Switz.)*; Hemocuron *(Takeda, Jpn)*; Venalisin *(AGIPS, Ital.)*; Venex *(Recordati, Ital.)*; Venodin *(Tosi-Novara, Ital.)*.

13375-c

Tricaprylin

Caprylic Acid Triglyceride; Glycerin Tricaprylate. Glyceryl trioctanoate; Propane-1,2,3-triyl trioctanoate.
$C_{27}H_{50}O_6$=470.7.

CAS — 538-23-8.

Tricaprylin has the general properties of the medium-chain triglycerides (see under Fractionated Coconut Oil, p.1560) and has been similarly used.

Proprietary Names and Manufacturers
Mac-Eight *(Ono, Jpn)*.

13376-k

Tricarbaurinium

Aluminon. The triammonium salt of 3-(3,3′-dicarboxy-4,4′-dihydroxybenzhydrylidene)-6-oxocyclohexa-1,4-diene-1-carboxylic acid.
$C_{22}H_{23}N_3O_9$=473.4.

CAS — 569-58-4.

Tricarbaurinium has been used topically in the treatment of mouth disorders.

A histochemical method employing tricarbaurinium has been used in patients with dialytic bone disease to detect aluminium in undecalcified sections of bone biopsy specimens.— J. Denton *et al.*, *J. clin. Path.*, 1984, *37*, 136.

Proprietary Names and Manufacturers
Lysofon *(Lafon, Fr.)*.

1328-d

Trichloroacetic Acid *(BAN, USAN).*

Acidum Trichloraceticum; Trichloracetic Acid; Trichloressigsäure; Trichloroacet. Acid.
$CCl_3.CO_2H$=163.4.

CAS — 76-03-9.

Pharmacopoeias. In *Aust.*, *Egypt.*, *Fr.*, *Hung.*, *Neth.*, *Nord.*, *Pol.*, *Port.*, *Span.*, and *U.S.*

Colourless, deliquescent crystals with a slight characteristic odour. **Soluble** 1 in 0.1 of water; soluble in alcohol and ether. **Store** at 15° to 30° in airtight containers.

Adverse Effects and Treatment

As for Hydrochloric Acid, p.1578.

In Great Britain the recommended exposure limit of trichloroacetic acid is 1 ppm (long-term).

Uses and Administration

Trichloroacetic acid is caustic and astringent. It is used as a quick escharotic for warts. It is applied as a strong solution, prepared by adding 10% by weight of water; the surrounding parts are usually protected.

WARTS. For a study comparing podophyllin with a combination of podophyllin and trichloracetic acid in anogenital warts, see Podophyllum (p.929).

218-s

Triethanolamine *(BAN)*.

Trolamine *(USAN, pINN)*.

CAS — 102-71-6 (triethanolamine).

Pharmacopoeias. In *Aust., Br., Braz., Cz., Egypt., Fr., Hung., It., Jpn, Jug., Mex., Neth., Pol.,* and *Swiss.* Also in *U.S.N.F.*

A variable mixture of bases containing mainly 2,2′,2″-nitrilotriethanol, $(CH_2OH.CH_2)_3N$, together with 2,2′-iminobisethanol and smaller amounts of 2-aminoethanol. The *B.P.* specifies not less than 80% of nitrilotriethanol, and the *U.S.N.F.* specifies 99 to 107.4% of alkanolamines calculated on the anhydrous basis as triethanolamine.

It is a clear, colourless or pale yellow, viscous, hygroscopic liquid; odourless or with a slight ammoniacal odour.

Miscible with water and alcohol; soluble in chloroform; slightly soluble in ether. A 10% solution in water is strongly alkaline to litmus. **Store** in airtight containers. Protect from light.

Adverse Effects

It may be irritating to the skin and mucous membranes. Contact dermatitis has been reported following the use of ear-drops containing triethanolamine polypeptide oleate-condensate.

Uses and Administration

Triethanolamine is used combined with fatty acids such as stearic and oleic acids as an emulsifier.

Ear-drops containing triethanolamine polypeptide oleate-condensate 10% are used for the removal of impacted ear wax.

Topical analgesic preparations of triethanolamine combined with salicylic acid have also been used.

Proprietary Names and Manufacturers of Triethanolamine Compounds

Cerumenex *(Purdue Frederick, Canad.; Ethimed, S.Afr.; Purdue Frederick, USA)*; Seratyl *(Rougier, Canad.)*; Xerumenex *(Napp, UK)*.

1288-p

Triletide *(rINN)*.

Z-420; ZAMI-420. Methyl *N*-[*N*-(*N*-acetyl-3-phenyl-L-alanyl)-3-phenyl-L-alanyl]-L-histidine.

$C_{27}H_{31}N_5O_5$=505.6.

CAS — 62087-96-1.

Triletide is an inhibitor of thromboxane A_2 under investigation for the treatment of peptic ulcers.

A brief review of triletide.— *Drugs of the Future*, 1984, *9*, 281; *ibid.*, 1985, *10*, 354.

A series of studies on triletide in gastric and duodenal ulcers including one on its pharmacokinetics: *Pharmatherapeutica*, 1985, *4*, 146-194.

Proprietary Names and Manufacturers

Zambeletti, Ital.

13380-y

Trilostane *(BAN, USAN, pINN)*.

Win-24540. 4α,5α-Epoxy-17β-hydroxy-3-oxoandrostane-2α-carbonitrile.

$C_{20}H_{27}NO_3$=329.4.

CAS — 13647-35-3.

Adverse Effects

Side-effects reported with high doses of trilostane have included flushing, nausea, vomiting, diarrhoea, rhinorrhoea, and oedema of the palate.

A report of an addisonian crisis in a 57-year-old woman receiving trilostane 240 mg four times daily. The possibility of severe inhibition of the synthesis of cortisol with trilostane should be borne in mind when treating patients with Cushing's syndrome.— P. D. Ward *et al.* (letter), *Lancet*, 1981, *2*, 1178.

Ingestion of trilostane 3.6 g by a 29-year-old woman had no apparent adverse endocrine effects. Nevertheless, after overdosage, plasma-potassium concentrations and blood pressure should be monitored. The drug has a very high LD50 in *animals*.— N. Barnes and N. Thomas, *Br. med. J.*, 1983, *286*, 1784.

Precautions

Trilostane is contra-indicated in pregnancy and should be used with caution in patients with renal or hepatic dysfunction. Circulating corticosteroids and blood electrolytes should be monitored. During severe stress, the drug may have to be discontinued and corticosteroid supplements may be required.

Trilostane may interfere with the activity of oral contraceptives. Hyperkalaemia may occur if trilostane is given concurrently with potassium-sparing diuretics.

A preliminary report of trilostane interference with fluorimetric steroid assays.— D. Mattingly and C. Tyler (letter), *Lancet*, 1981, *1*, 561. Comment.— G. H. Beastall *et al.* (letter), *ibid.*, 727.

Marked depression of plasma-testosterone concentrations in a man given trilostane for recurrent Cushing's syndrome.— P. E. Belchetz *et al.* (letter), *Lancet*, 1981, *1*, 897.

Uses and Administration

Trilostane is an adrenocortical suppressant which inhibits the enzyme system essential for the production of glucocorticoids and mineralocorticoids. It is used in the treatment of Cushing's syndrome and primary aldosteronism.

The usual dose is 60 mg by mouth four times daily for at least 3 days and then adjusted, according to the patient's response, within the range of 120 to 480 mg daily. Doses of 960 mg daily have been given.

An evaluation of trilostane.— *Drug & Ther. Bull.*, 1982, *20*, 7.

Trilostane in the treatment of advanced breast cancer.— C. G. Beardwell *et al.*, *Cancer Chemother. Pharmac.*, 1983, *10*, 158.

A review of the use of trilostane for the treatment of Cushing's syndrome.— *Med. Lett.*, 1985, *27*, 87.

Proprietary Preparations

Modrenal *(Sterling Research, UK). Capsules,* trilostane 60 mg.

Proprietary Names and Manufacturers

Modrenal *(Winthrop, Denm.; Sterling Research, UK)*.

13381-j

Trimebutine Maleate *(BANM, rINNM)*.

2-Dimethylamino-2-phenylbutyl 3,4,5-trimethoxybenzoate hydrogen maleate.

$C_{22}H_{29}NO_5,C_4H_4O_4$=503.5.

CAS — 39133-31-8 (trimebutine); 34140-59-5 (maleate).

Trimebutine maleate has antispasmodic properties and has been used in the treatment of gastro-intestinal disorders.

In an 8-week double-blind study in 20 patients with irritable bowel syndrome, trimebutine 200 mg three times daily was more effective than placebo in relieving symptoms.— M. G. Moshal and M. Herron, *J. int. med. Res.*, 1979, *7*, 231.

Further references: O. Ghidini *et al.*, *Curr. ther. Res.*, 1986, *39*, 541 (comparison with rociverine).

Proprietary Names and Manufacturers

Debridat *(Armstrong, Arg.; Jouveinal, Fr.; Sigmatau, Ital.)*; Foldox *(Sidus, Arg.)*; Kalius *(Panthox & Burck, Ital.)*; Miopropan *(Bernabó, Arg.)*; Modulase *(IRBI, Ital.)*; Modulon *(Jouveinal, Canad.)*; Polibutin *(Juste, Spain)*; Spabucol *(Lagap, Ital.)*; Trimedat *(Lifepharma, Ital.)*.

5246-q

Trospium Chloride *(rINN)*.

3α-Benziloyloxynortropane-8-spiro-1′-pyrrolidinium chloride.

$C_{25}H_{30}ClNO_3$=428.0.

CAS — 10405-02-4.

Trospium chloride is used as an antispasmodic in doses of up to 10 mg three times daily, and 200 µg by intramuscular or slow intravenous injection as a single dose. It is also given rectally.

Proprietary Names and Manufacturers

Spasmex *(Pfleger, Ger.)*.

13386-t

Troxerutin *(BAN, rINN)*.

THR; Trioxyethylrutin; Z-6000. 3′,4′,7-Tris[*O*-(2-hydroxyethyl)]rutin; 5-Hydroxy-7-(2-hydroxyethoxy)-2-[3,4-bis(2-hydroxyethoxy)phenyl]-4-oxo-4*H*-chromen-3-yl rutinoside.

$C_{33}H_{42}O_{19}$=742.7.

CAS — 7085-55-4.

The principal component of a mixture, commonly called trihydroxyethylrutoside, which contains also the mono-, di-, and tetra-derivatives. The term oxerutins is applied to a mixture of 5 different hydroxyethylrutosides, not less than 45% of which is troxerutin.

Adverse Effects

Side-effects reported include gastro-intestinal disturbances, flushing, and headache.

Uses and Administration

Troxerutin is a flavonoid derivative thought to improve capillary function by reducing abnormal leakage. It has been given to relieve capillary impairment and venous insufficiency of the lower limbs, and for haemorrhoids. The usual oral dose is 750 mg to 1 g of oxerutins (containing at least 45% troxerutin) daily at mealtimes. Dosage may be reduced as improvement occurs.

Proprietary Preparations

Paroven *(Zyma, UK). Capsules,* oxerutins 250 mg.

Proprietary Names and Manufacturers

Flebil *(Molteni, Ital.)*; Paroven *(Zyma, Austral.; Zyma, S.Afr.; Zyma, UK)*; Pherarutin *(Kanoldt, Ger.)*; Posorutin *(Ursapharm, Ger.)*; Pur-Rutin *(Chassot, Switz.)*; Relvène *(Pharmascience, Fr.)*; Rutilémone *(Fr.)*; Varemoid *(Zyma, Austral.; Zyma, UK)*; Varemoïd *(Zyma, S.Afr.; Zyma, Switz.)*; Veinamitol *(Negma, Fr.)*; Veno SL *(Ursapharm, Ger.)*; Venolen *(Farmacologico Milanese, Ital.)*; Venoruton *(Arg.; Belg.; Zyma, Denm.; Zyma, Ger.; Zyma, Ital.; Neth.; Frumtost, Spain; Zyma, Switz.)*.

1329-n

Tuftsin

N^2-[1-(N^2-L-threonyl-L-lysyl)-L-prolyl]-L-arginine.

$C_{21}H_{40}N_8O_6$=500.6.

CAS — 9063-57-4.

Tuftsin is a naturally occurring tetrapeptide and is under investigation as the acetate for its immunostimulating activity.

A review of tuftsin: *Drugs of the Future*, 1984, *9*, 532; *ibid.*, 1985, *10*, 609; *ibid.*, 1986, *11*, 632; *ibid.*, 1987, *12*, 737.

1331-a

Tumour Necrosis Factor

Tumour necrosis factor (TNF) is one of the polypeptide inflammatory mediators which have been termed collectively cytokines (produced by various cell types) or lymphokines (produced by lymphocytes). Tumour necrosis factor is produced mainly by macrophages and lymphocytes. Two forms have been identified and appear to have identical biological properties: TNFα or cachectin, which is produced by macrophages, and TNFβ or lymphotoxin, which is produced by lymphocytes.

The antitumour effects of tumour necrosis factor *in vitro* and in *animals* have prompted investigation of recombinant TNFα in the treatment of cancer although, since tumour necrosis factor is also a mediator of cachexia and the manifestations of endotoxic shock, there has been concern about possible toxicity.

References: M. E. J. Billingham, *Br. med. Bull.*, 1987, *43*, 350; D. W. Horohov and J. P. Siegel, *Drugs*, 1987, *33*, 289; E. J. Ziegler, *New Engl. J. Med.*, 1988, *318*, 1533.

13387-x

Tyformin *(BAN)*.

Augmentin; HL-523 *(hydrochloride)*; Tiformin *(rINN)*. 4-Guanidinobutyramide.
$C_5H_{12}N_4O$=144.2.

CAS — 4210-97-3.

NOTE. A preparation containing amoxycillin and potassium clavulanate is marketed under the name Augmentin (see p.115).

Tyformin has been found to lower the blood concentration of urea when given to patients with uraemic diabetes.

16531-y

Ubenimex *(rINN)*.

NK-421. (−)-*N*-[(2*S*,3*R*)-3-Amino-2-hydroxy-4-phenylbutyryl]-L-leucine.
$C_{16}H_{24}N_2O_4$=308.4.

CAS — 58970-76-6.

Ubenimex is an immunostimulant being used in the management of patients with malignant neoplasms.

A review of ubenimex: *Drugs of the Future*, 1981, *6*, 604; *ibid.*, 1982, *7*, 760; *ibid.*, 1983, *8*, 882; *ibid.*, 1984, *9*, 778; *ibid.*, 1985, *10*, 859; *ibid.*, 1986, *11*, 878; *ibid.*, 1987, *12*, 1001.

Proprietary Names and Manufacturers
Nippon Kayaku, Jpn.

14000-c

Ubidecarenone *(rINN)*.

Coenzyme Q10; Ubiquinone-10. 2-Deca(3-methylbut-2-enylene)-5,6-dimethoxy-3-methyl-*p*-benzoquinone.
$C_{59}H_{90}O_4$=863.4.

CAS — 303-98-0.

M.p. about 48°.

Ubidecarenone is a naturally occurring coenzyme involved in electron transport in the mitochondria. It is claimed to be involved in the metabolism of cardiac muscle and in high doses has protected *animals* from isoprenaline-induced myocardial damage. It has been used, in conjunction with standard treatment, in mild or moderate congestive heart failure.

Ubidecarenone has also been tried in conditions associated with coenzyme deficiency.

References to the use of ubidecarenone in the treatment of cardiac disease: A. Cascone *et al.*, *Boll. chim.-Farm.*, 1984, *123*, 55S (congestive heart failure); B. D'Agnolo, *ibid.*, 1985, *124*, 7S (congestive heart failure); M. Gini *et al.*, *ibid.*, 21S (chronic bronchopulmonary disease or pulmonary cardiopathy); A. Cascone *et al.*, *ibid.*, 43S (congestive heart failure).

Proprietary Names and Manufacturers
Caomet *(Simes, Ital.)*; Decarene *(Recordati, Ital.)*; Decorenone *(Lifepharma, Ital.)*; Inokiten *(Jpn)*; Iuvacor *(Inverni della Beffa, Ital.)*; Mitocor *(Zambon, Ital.)*; Neuquinone *(Jpn)*; Roburis *(Ripari-Gero, Ital.)*; Ube-Q *(Jpn)*; Ubifactor *(IFI, Ital.)*; Ubimaior *(Master Pharma, Ital.)*; Ubione *(Prodes, Spain)*; Ubiten *(Italfarmaco, Ital.)*.

2998-d

Ulinastatin *(rINN)*.

Ulinastatin is a glycoprotein proteolytic enzyme inhibitor isolated from human urine. It has been given by injection in acute pancreatitis and in acute circulatory insufficiency.

Reported adverse effects include irritation at the site of injection, diarrhoea, raised transaminase values, and granulocytopenia.

Proprietary Names and Manufacturers
Miracrid *(Jpn)*.

14003-t

Urazamide

5-Aminoimidazole-4-carboxamide ureidosuccinate.
$C_9H_{14}N_6O_6$=302.2.

Urazamide has been used in the treatment of hepatic disorders.

Proprietary Names and Manufacturers
Aicase *(FIRMA, Ital.)*; Carbaica *(Selvi, Ital.)*; Colahepat Plus *(Ima, Arg.)*.

5910-d

Urea Hydrogen Peroxide

Carbamide Peroxide *(USAN)*; Hydroperite; Urea Peroxide.
$NH_2.CO.NH_2,H_2O_2$=94.07.

CAS — 124-43-6.

Pharmacopoeias. In *Hung.*

Urea hydrogen peroxide consists of hydrogen peroxide and urea in equimolecular proportions. It is used for the extemporaneous preparation of hydrogen peroxide. It has been employed for infections of the ear, mouth, and skin and for softening ear wax.

Preparations

Carbamide Peroxide Topical Solution *(U.S.P.)*. Carbamide Peroxide Solution. A solution of urea hydrogen peroxide in anhydrous glycerol. pH 4.0 to 7.5. Store at a temperature not exceeding 40° in airtight containers. Protect from light.

Proprietary Preparations

Exterol *(Dermal Laboratories, UK)*. *Ear-drops*, urea hydrogen peroxide 5% in glycerol.

Proprietary Names and Manufacturers
Caroxin *(Nyco, Norw.)*; Debrox *(Canad.; Marion Laboratories, USA)*; Ear Drops *(Pharmafair, USA)*; Exterol *(Dermal Laboratories, UK)*; Gly-Oxide *(Canad.; Marion Laboratories, USA)*; Lapural *(Laporte, UK)*; Proxigel *(Reed & Carnrick, USA)*.

The following names have been used for multi-ingredient preparations containing urea hydrogen peroxide—Murine Ear Drops *(Ross, USA)*.

14004-x

Uridine

Uracil Riboside. 1-β-D-Ribofuranosyluracil; 1-β-D-Ribofuranosylpyrimidine-2,4(1*H*,3*H*)-dione.
$C_9H_{12}N_2O_6$=244.2.

CAS — 58-96-8.

Uridine is one of the four nucleosides present in ribonucleic acid.

Haematological remission was induced when uridine was given to a 17-month-old boy with refractory megaloblastic anaemia associated with hereditary orotic aciduria.— D. M. O. Becroft and L. I. Phillips, *Br. med. J.*, 1965, *1*, 547. The patient now aged 21 years was considered to be the longest-surviving patient with hereditary orotic aciduria. He has been treated with uridine from the age of 17 months. In recent years his usual dose has been uridine 3 g daily by mouth.— D. M. O. Becroft *et al.* (letter), *New Engl. J. Med.*, 1984, *310*, 1333.

Further reference to the use of uridine in 2 siblings with cellular immune deficiency associated with hereditary orotic aciduria.— R. Girot *et al.*, *New Engl. J. Med.*, 1983, *308*, 700.

For studies indicating that addition of uridine rendered media containing thymine suitable for trimethoprim sensitivity testing, see S. G. B. Amyes and J. T. Smith, *J. antimicrob. Chemother.*, 1978, *4*, 415 and 421.

14005-r

Uridine Triphosphate

Uridine Triphosphoric Acid; UTP. Uridine 5′-(tetrahydrogen triphosphate).
$C_9H_{15}N_2O_{15}P_3$=484.1.

CAS — 63-39-8.

Uridine triphosphate has been claimed to be of value in muscular atrophy and muscular weakness.

Proprietary Names and Manufacturers
Fosforudin *(Francia Farm., Ital.)*; Miocuril *(Terapeutico M.R., Ital.)*; Miosprint *(Biosint, Ital.)*; Uteplex *(Ayerst, Belg.; Ayerst, Fr.; Auclair, Switz.; Lipha, UK)*; Utipina *(Arg.)*.

3753-w

Ursodeoxycholic Acid *(BAN, rINN)*.

UDCA; Ursodesoxycholic Acid. 3α,7β-Dihydroxy-5β-cholan-24-oic acid.
$C_{24}H_{40}O_4$=392.6.

CAS — 128-13-2.

Pharmacopoeias. In *Fr.* and *Jpn.*

Adverse Effects and Precautions

As for Chenodeoxycholic Acid, p.1555, but diarrhoea is reported to occur less frequently.

Absorption and Fate

Ursodeoxycholic acid is absorbed from the gastro-intestinal tract and undergoes enterohepatic recycling. In comparison with chenodeoxycholic acid, less ursodeoxycholic acid undergoes bacterial degradation to lithocholic acid.

Uses and Administration

Ursodeoxycholic acid is the 7β-epimer of chenodeoxycholic acid and is used similarly for the dissolution of cholesterol-rich gall-stones in patients with functioning gall-bladders. The usual dose is 8 to 12 mg per kg body-weight daily in 2 divided doses; obese patients may require up to 15 mg per kg daily.

Reviews of the use of ursodeoxycholic acid in the management of gall-stones.— I. A. D. Bouchier, *Br. med. J.*, 1983, *286*, 778; *Pharm. J.*, 1984, *1*, 245; M. C. Bateson, *Br. med. J.*, 1984, *289*, 1163; A. Ward *et al.*, *Drugs*, 1984, *27*, 95.

The use of ursodeoxycholic acid in primary biliary cirrhosis.— R. Poupon *et al.*, *Lancet*, 1987, *1*, 834. Comments.— A. F. Hofmann and H. Popper (letter), *ibid.*, *2*, 398; U. Leuschner and W. Kurtz, *ibid.*, 508.

The use of ursodeoxycholic acid in dyspeptic disorders associated with dysfunction of the hepatobiliary tract, with or without gallstones.— G. Mautone *et al.*, *Curr. ther. Res.*, 1986, *40*, 239.

Proprietary Preparations

Destolit *(Merrell, UK)*. *Tablets*, scored, ursodeoxycholic acid 150 mg.

Ursofalk *(Thames, UK)*. *Capsules*, ursodeoxycholic acid 250 mg.

Proprietary Names and Manufacturers
Arsacol *(Arsac, Fr.)*; Cholit-Ursan *(Fresenius, Ger.)*; Delursan *(Houdé, Fr.)*; Destolit *(Lepetit, Fr.; Merrell, UK)*; De-ursil *(Giuliani, Switz.)*; Deursil *(Gipharmex, Ital.)*; Litanin *(Pharmainvesti, Spain)*; Litocure *(Jorba,

Spain); Litursol *(Istituto Wassermann, Ital.)*; Lyeton *(Von Boch, Ital.)*; Peptarom *(Fresenius, Ger.)*; Ursacol *(Zambon, Ital.)*; Ursilon *(Logifarm, Ital.)*; Urso *(Jpn; Landerlan, Spain)*; Urso Vinas *(Vinas, Spain)*; Ursobil *(ABC, Ital.)*; Ursobilane *(Estedi, Spain)*; Ursochol *(Inpharzam, Ger.; Neth.; Zambon, Spain; Inpharzam, Switz.)*; Ursofalk *(Falk, Ger.; Falk, Switz.; Thames, UK)*; Ursoflor *(Locatelli, Ital.)*; Ursolisin *(Magis, Ital.)*; Ursolite *(Vita, Spain)*; Ursolvan *(Robert et Carrière, Fr.)*; Urson *(Ripari-Gero, Ital.)*; Ursotan *(Noristan, S.Afr.)*.

14006-f

Usnea barbata

Usnea barbata is a lichen.

CAS — 125-46-2 (usnic acid).

Usnea barbata contains usnic acid which is reported to have antimicrobial activity.

Proprietary Preparations

Omnigran *(Keimdiät, Ger.: Thomson & Joseph, UK)*. Ground lichen, *Usnea barbata*. For use in pharmaceutical and cosmetic preparations.

Usnagran-A *(Keimdiät, Ger.: Thomson & Joseph, UK)*. An alcoholic extract of lichen, *Usnea barbata*. For use in pharmaceutical and cosmetic preparations. **Usnagran-T**. Contains the fat-soluble and water-soluble constituents of lichen. For use in pharmaceutical and cosmetic preparations. **Usnagran-TP**. A 1% solution of Usnagran-T in propylene glycol.

Proprietary Names and Manufacturers

Granobil *(Ger.)*; Omnigran *(Keimdiät, Ger.: Thomson & Joseph, UK)*; Usnagran-A *(Keimdiät, Ger.: Thomson & Joseph, UK)*; Usnagran-T *(Keimdiät, Ger.: Thomson & Joseph, UK)*; Usnagran-TP *(Keimdiät, Ger.: Thomson & Joseph, UK)*.

14008-n

Valepotriates

Epoxy-iridoid esters, isolated from valerian.

CAS — 18296-45-2 (didrovaltrate); 18296-44-1 (valtrate); 25161-41-5 (acevaltrate).

NOTE. Valtrate is *pINN*.

They include *didrovaltrate* (6-acetoxy-1,4a,5,6,7,7a-hexahydro-1-isovaleryloxy-4-isovaleryloxymethylcyclopenta[*c*]pyran-7-spiro-2′-oxiran, $C_{22}H_{32}O_8$=424.5), *valtrate* (4-acetoxymethyl-1,6-di-isovaleryloxy-1,6,7,7a-tetrahydrocyclopenta[*c*]pyran-7-spiro-2′-oxiran, $C_{22}H_{30}O_8$=422.5), and *acevaltrate* (4-acetoxymethyl-(1 or 6)-3-(acetoxy-3-methylbutyryloxy)-1,6,7,7a-tetrahydro-(6 or 1)-isovaleryloxycyclopenta[*c*]pyran-7-spiro-2′-oxiran, $C_{24}H_{32}O_{10}$=480.5). On prolonged storage and drying they are hydrolysed to yield isovaleric acid.

A mixture stated to contain didrovaltrate, valtrate, and acevaltrate has been used as a sedative.

Proprietary Names and Manufacturers

Baldrisedon *(Scheurich, Ger.)*; Nervipan *(Medopharm, Ger.; Gazzoni, Ital.)*; Orasedon *(Oramon, Ger.)*; Valmane *(Kali-Chemie, Ger.; Kali-Chemie, Neth.; Ethimed, S.Afr.; Kali-Farma, Spain)*.

14009-h

Valerian *(BAN)*.

Baldrianwurzel; Valer; Valerian Rhizome; Valerian Root; Valerianae Radix.

CAS — 8057-49-6 (valerian extract).

Pharmacopoeias. In *Arg., Aust., Belg., Br., Cz., Egypt., Eur., Fr., Ger., Hung., It., Jug., Neth., Nord., Pol., Port., Roum., Rus., Span.,* and *Swiss. Br.* also describes Powdered Valerian.

Egypt. has valerian from *V. wallichii* (Indian Valerian). *Jpn* has Japanese Valerian from *V. fauriei* or allied plants; it also describes Powdered Japanese Valerian.

The subterranean organs, including the rhizome, root, and stolon of *Valeriana officinalis* (Valerianaceae), dried below 40°. It has a characteristic odour resembling that of valeric acid and camphor, and a sweet taste with a spicy bitter after-taste. **Store** in a well-closed container. Protect from light.

Valerian has been used as an extract, infusion, or tincture, often in conjunction with bromides, chloral hydrate, and phenobarbitone, in the treatment of hysteria and other nervous conditions. It has also been used as a carminative.

NOTE. The odour of valerian may be removed from a scale pan or from the hands by rubbing with sodium bicarbonate.

Proprietary Names and Manufacturers

Baldrian-Dispert *(Kali-Chemie, Denm.)*; Baldrisedon *(Switz.)*; Recvalysat *(Ysatfabrik, Ger.)*; Val Uno *(Edmond Pharma, Ital.)*; Valdispert *(Kali-Chemie, Ger.; Neth.)*; Zirkulin *(Roha, Ger.)*.

The following names have been used for multi-ingredient preparations containing valerian— Climacteric Dellipsoids D19 *(Pilsworth, UK)*; Macro-AntiStress *(Macro Vitamin, Austral.)*; Nerve Dellipsoids D16 *(Pilsworth, UK)*; Sedative Tonic Dellipsoids D14 *(Pilsworth, UK)*.

14010-a

Valeric Acid

Acido Delfinico; Acido Focénico; Baldriansäure; Valerianic Acid.

$C_5H_{10}O_2$=102.1.

CAS — 109-52-4.

Pharmacopoeias. In *Port.* and *Span. Span. P.* specifies a mixture of 2 isomers of valeric acid.

Valeric acid was formerly used in the treatment of hysteria and other nervous conditions.

Various salts of valeric acid have been used similarly to valerian and to valeric acid.

2416-p

Vanilla

Baunilha; Vainilla; Vanilla Beans; Vanilla Pods.

Pharmacopoeias. In *Arg., Fr., Mex.,* and *Port.* Also in *U.S.N.F.*

The cured, fully grown, unripe fruit of Madagascar, Mexican, or Bourbon vanilla, *Vanilla planifolia*, or of Tahiti vanilla, *V. tahitensis* (Orchidaceae). Its odour and flavour are not entirely due to vanillin but depend on the presence of other aromatic substances. **Store** at a temperature not exceeding 8° in airtight containers; vanilla which has become brittle should not be used.

Vanilla is used as a flavouring agent and in perfumery.

Preparations

Vanilla Tincture *(U.S.N.F.)*. 1 in 10; prepared by maceration and percolation with diluted alcohol and containing 20% w/v of sucrose. Store at a temperature not exceeding 40° in airtight containers. Protect from light.

2417-s

Vanillin *(BAN)*.

Vainillina; Vanillic Aldehyde. 4-Hydroxy-3-methoxybenzaldehyde.

$C_8H_8O_3$=152.1.

CAS — 121-33-5.

Pharmacopoeias. In *Arg., Aust., Belg., Br., Egypt., Fr., Ger., Hung., Ind., Jug., Mex., Nord., Port., Span.,* and *Swiss.* Also in *U.S.N.F.*

White or slightly yellow crystalline needles or powder with an odour and taste of vanilla. It can be extracted from vanilla or prepared synthetically. M.p. 81° to 83°.

Soluble 1 in 100 of water at 20°, 1 in 20 of water at 80°, 1 in 20 of glycerol; soluble in alcohol, chloroform, and ether, in fixed and volatile oils, and in solutions of alkali hydroxides. A saturated solution in water is acid to litmus. **Store** in airtight containers. Protect from light.

Vanillin is used as a flavouring agent and in perfumery.

Estimated acceptable daily intake: up to 10 mg per kg body-weight.— Eleventh Report of the Joint FAO/WHO Expert Committee on Food Additives, *Tech. Rep. Ser. Wld Hlth Org. No. 383*, 1968.

7371-v

Hydrogenated Vegetable Oil *(USAN)*.

Pharmacopoeias. In *U.S.N.F. Jpn* includes a hydrogenated oil of fish, animal, or vegetable origin.

Refined, bleached, hydrogenated, and deodorised vegetable oil stearins consisting mainly of the triglycerides of stearic and palmitic acids. It is a fine white powder at room temperature. M.p. 61° to 66°.

Practically **insoluble** in water; soluble in chloroform, petroleum spirit, and hot isopropyl alcohol. **Store** in a cool place in airtight containers.

Hydrogenated vegetable oil is used as a tablet lubricant.

14013-r

Veratrine

CAS — 8051-02-3 (mixture).

NOTE. Veratrine should be distinguished from protoveratrines obtained from veratrum.

Pharmacopoeias. In *Pol., Port.,* and *Span.*

A mixture of alkaloids from sabadilla.

Adverse Effects, Treatment, and Precautions

Veratrine resembles aconite (p.1538) in its action on the peripheral nerve endings and poisoning should be treated similarly. It is an intense local irritant and has a powerful direct stimulating action on all muscle tissues. *It has a violent irritant action on mucous membranes, even in minute doses, and must be handled with great care.* Internally, it causes violent vomiting, purging, an intense burning sensation in the mouth and throat, and general muscular weakness.

Uses and Administration

Veratrine should not be used internally. It was formerly applied externally for its analgesic properties and as a parasiticide, especially for head lice, but even when used in this way there is danger of systemic poisoning from absorption. The use of veratrine, its salts, and galenical preparations in cosmetic products is prohibited in the *UK* by law.

1450-h

Vibunazole

Bay-N-7133. α-[(4-Chlorophenoxy)methyl]-α-(1,1-dimethylethyl)-1*H*-1,2,4-triazole-1-ethanol.

$C_{15}H_{20}ClN_3O_2$=309.8.

CAS — 80456-55-9.

Vibunazole is under study as an antifungal agent.

Discussions on vibunazole: *Drugs of the Future*, 1984, *9*, 404 and 405; *ibid.*, 1987, *12*, 613 (this lists intervening updates).

Some references to the antifungal activity of vibunazole: H. Yamaguchi *et al.*, *J. antimicrob. Chemother.*, 1983, *11*, 135; J. D. Sobel and G. Muller, *Antimicrob. Ag. Chemother.*, 1983, *24*, 434; M. Plempel, *J. antimicrob. Chemother.*, 1984, *13*, 447; F. C. Odds *et al.*, *ibid.*, *14*, 105; P. D. Hoeprich and J. M. Merry, *Antimicrob. Ag. Chemother.*, 1984, *25*, 339; E. Stevens D. A. Lefler, *J. antimicrob. Chemother.*, 1985, *15*, 69. The pharmacokinetics of vibunazole.— C. van Gulpen *et al.*, *J. antimicrob. Chemother.*, 1985, *16*, 75.

Proprietary Names and Manufacturers
Bayer, Ger.

14014-f

Vinburnine *(rINN).*

3α,16α-Eburnamonine; CH-846; (−)-Eburnamonine; Vincamone. (3α,16α)-Eburnamenin-14(15*H*)-one.

$C_{19}H_{22}N_2O$=294.4.

CAS — 4880-88-0.

Vinburnine is used in conditions associated with cerebral circulatory insufficiency.

A critical review of drugs, including vinburnine, used in cerebrovascular disorders.— A. Spagnoli and G. Tognoni, *Drugs*, 1983, *26*, 44.

Proprietary Names and Manufacturers
Cervoxan *(Sobio, Fr.; Beecham, Spain)*; Eburnal *(Chiesi, Ital.)*; Eburnoxin *(Ifesa, Spain)*; Eubran *(ICT-Lodi, Ital.)*; Luvenil *(Ellem, Ital.)*; Scleramin *(Ibirn, Ital.)*; Tensiplex *(Francia Farm., Ital.)*.

14015-d

Vincamine *(BAN, rINN).*

An alkaloid obtained from *Vinca minor* (Apocynaceae). Methyl (3α,16α)-14,15-dihydro-14β-hydroxyeburnamenine-14-carboxylate.

$C_{21}H_{26}N_2O_3$=354.4.

CAS — 1617-90-9.

Pharmacopoeias. In *Fr.*

Vincamine is claimed to increase cerebral circulation and utilisation of oxygen and has been used in a variety of cerebral disorders. It has been given by mouth in doses of 40 to 80 mg daily and has also been administered intramuscularly and by intravenous infusion. Vincamine may have adverse effects on the cardiovascular system and care should be taken in patients with hypertension or cardiac dysfunction.

Vincamine salts including vincamine hydrochloride and vincamine tartrate have also been used.

A critical review of drugs, including vincamine, used in cerebrovascular disorders.— A. Spagnoli and G. Tognoni, *Drugs*, 1983, *26*, 44.

References to clinical studies of vincamine: P. Foltyn, *Arzneimittel-Forsch.*, 1978, *28*, 90 (psychiatric disturbances in the elderly); W. J. Dekoninck *et al.*, *ibid.*, 1654 (acute stroke); P. Mikus, *ibid.*, 2165 (cerebrovascular insufficiency); E. Thiery *et al.*, *ibid.*, 1979, *29*, 571 (acute stroke); E. Sinforiani *et al.*, *Clin. Trials J.*, 1984, *21*, 1 (use of vincamine teprosilate in cerebrovascular disorders).

Proprietary Names and Manufacturers of Vincamine and its Salts
Aethroma-30 *(Mepha, Switz.)*; Alfavinca *(Carol, Spain)*; Anasclerol *(ICT-Lodi, Ital.)*; Angiopac *(UCB, Ger.)*; Artensen *(Cusi, Spain)*; Arteriovinca *(Farma-Lepori, Spain)*; Asnai *(Spain)*; Atervit *(Arg.)*; Ausomina *(Ausonia, Ital.)*; Branex *(Galepharma, Spain)*; Cétal Retard *(Warner-Lambert, Switz.)*; Centractiva *(Spain)*; Cerebramina *(Benvegna, Ital.)*; Cerebroxine *(Belg.)*; Ceredilan *(Spain)*; Cetal *(Parke, Davis, Ger.)*; Cetovinca *(Elmu, Spain)*; Devincan *(Hung.)*; Dilar *(ISOM, Ital.)*; Dilarterial *(Llorente, Spain)*; Domeni *(Tafir, Spain)*; Encevin *(Caber, Ital.)*; Equipur *(Medipharma, Ger.)*; Esberidin *(Schaper & Brümmer, Ger.)*; Gibivi *(Ital.)*; Horusvin *(Spain)*; Novicet *(Ger.)*; Nuclesil *(Cheminova, Spain)*; Ocu-Vinc *(Alcon, Ger.)*; Oxicebral *(Pfizer, Spain)*; Oxovinca *(Schering, Fr.)*; Oxygeron *(Syntex, Switz.)*; Perphal *(Fr.)*; Pervincamin *(Karlspharma, Ger.)*; Pervincamina *(Schering, Ital.)*; Pervincamine *(Belg.; Dausse, Fr.; Synthelabo, Switz.)*; Pervone *(Switz.)*; Sostenil *(Arg.)*; Tefavinca *(Bohm, Spain)*; Teproside *(Malesci, Ital.)*; Tonifor *(Switz.)*; Tripervan *(Bellon, Fr.)*; Vadicate *(Bicther, Spain)*; Vasculogène *(Pharma 2000, Fr.)*; Vasonett *(INTES, Ital.)*; Vinca *(Belg.; Millot-Solac, Fr.; Ital.; Switz.)*; Vinca minor *(Hausmann, Switz.)*; Vincabiomar *(Spain)*; Vincabrain *(Bouchara, Fr.; Bouchara, Switz.)*; Vincacen *(Centrum, Spain)*; Vincadar *(Roussel Maestretti, Ital.; Roussel, Spain)*; Vinca-Dil *(Lepetit, Ital.)*; Vincafarm *(Radiumfarma, Ital.)*; Vincafolina *(Lampugnani, Ital.)*; Vincafor Retard *(Midy, Fr.)*; Vincagalup *(Spain)*; VincaHexal *(Ger.)*; Vincalen *(FIRMA, Ital.)*; Vincalex *(Arg.)*; Vincalvar *(Oftalmiso, Spain)*; Vincamed *(Belg.)*; Vincamidol *(Magis, Ital.)*; Vincaminol *(Alacan, Spain)*; Vincane *(Frumtost, Spain)*; Vincapan *(Arg.)*; Vincapront *(Mack, Illert., Ger.; Mack, Switz.)*; Vinca-ri *(Nativelle, Ital.)*; Vincasaunier *(Fr.)*; Vinca-treis *(Ecobi, Ital.)*; Vincavix *(Llorens, Spain)*; Vincimax *(Robert et Carrière, Fr.)*; Vinodrel *(Arg.)*; Vinsal *(Salus, Ital.)*; Visal *(Simes, Ital.)*; Vitren *(Kairon, Spain)*; Vraap *(Inverni della Beffa, Ital.)*.

14016-n

Vinpocetine *(USAN, rINN).*

AY-27255; Ethyl Apovincaminate; Ethyl Apovincaminoate; RGH-4405. Ethyl (3α,16α)-eburnamenine-14-carboxylate.

$C_{22}H_{26}N_2O_2$=350.5.

CAS — 42971-09-5.

Vinpocetine has been used in cognitive disorders and dementias.

For a series of papers on *animal* and clinical studies with vinpocetine, see *Arzneimittel-Forsch.*, 1976, *26*, 1907–1989.

Pharmacokinetics.— L. Vereczkey *et al.*, *Arzneimittel-Forsch.*, 1979, *29*, 957.

References to the use of vinpocetine in cerebrovascular and cognitive disorders: E. Manconi *et al.*, *Curr. ther. Res.*, 1986, *40*, 702.

Proprietary Names and Manufacturers
Cavinton *(Gedeon Richter, Hung.)*.

14017-h

Vinyl Chloride

VCM; Vinyl Chloride Monomer. Chloroethylene.

C_2H_3Cl=62.50.

CAS — 75-01-4.

Vinyl chloride is used in the manufacture of polyvinyl chloride (PVC) and other vinyl polymers. Occupational exposure to vinyl chloride in polymerisation plants has been associated with acro-osteolysis, especially in the terminal phalanges of the fingers, a condition resembling Raynaud's phenomenon, and sclerodermatous skin changes; liver damage and hepatic angiosarcoma; splenomegaly; thrombocytopenia; impaired respiratory function; and chromosomal abnormalities.

As a result of these toxic effects the use of vinyl chloride as an aerosol propellent and in cosmetics has been banned in many countries and efforts are being made to limit the amount of vinyl chloride present in food packaging materials.

See also under Plastics, p.1603.

In Great Britain the control limit for occupational exposure to vinyl chloride vapour in air is an annual control limit of 3 ppm for vinyl chloride manufacturing and polymerisation plants. The annual control limit is supplemented by an 8-hour time-weighted average control limit of 7 ppm for personal exposure provided that the annual control limit is not exceeded. In the *US* the permissible exposure limit is 1 ppm.

A detailed review of the chemistry, biotransformation, toxicology, and carcinogenicity of vinyl chloride. An increase in reported cases of vinyl chloride-induced liver malfunction, angiosarcoma, Raynaud's syndrome, scleroderma, and acro-osteolysis should be expected in the near future due to past exposures; the exposure of the general population to vinyl chloride-propelled aerosols and household products might contribute to these disease states. Occupational exposures would probably decrease as vinyl chloride-polyvinyl chloride plants met the new exposure limit of 1 ppm.— T. J. Haley, *J. Toxic. environ. Hlth*, 1975, *1*, 47.

A symposium reviewing the British experience of the environmental, epidemiological, and pathological effects of exposure to vinyl chloride arising during the course of polymerisation to polyvinyl chloride.— *Proc. R. Soc. Med.*, 1976, *69*, 275–310.

The FDA proposed to ban certain food packaging material made from vinyl chloride since it was found that residual vinyl chloride gas trapped in polyvinyl chloride could migrate into food.— *FDA Consumer*, 1976, (Dec.–Jan.), 5.

Further references: C. M. Black *et al.*, *Lancet*, 1983, *1*, 53; R. Spirtas *et al.* (letter), *ibid.*, *2*, 456; D. Forman *et al.*, *Br. J. ind. Med.*, 1985, *42*, 750.

PREGNANCY AND THE NEONATE. The incidence of foetal deaths was significantly increased in wives whose husbands were occupationally exposed to vinyl chloride.— P. F. Infante *et al.*, *Lancet*, 1976, *1*, 734.

Following exposure to vinyl chloride no teratogenic response was noted in *mice, rats,* or *rabbits*.— J. A. John *et al.*, *Toxic. appl. Pharmac.*, 1977, *39*, 497.

14019-b

Viquidil Hydrochloride *(rINNM).*

LM-192; Mequiverine Hydrochloride; Quinicine Hydrochloride. 1-(6-Methoxy-4-quinolyl)-3-(3-vinyl-4-piperidyl)propan-1-one hydrochloride.

$C_{20}H_{24}N_2O_2,HCl$=360.9.

CAS — 84-55-9 (viquidil); 52211-63-9 (hydrochloride).

Viquidil has been claimed to reduce arterial spasm, to increase cerebral blood flow, and to facilitate oxygen utilisation. It has been used in various cerebral disorders.

Effect on blood platelets *in vitro*.— C. Lecrubier *et al.*, *Arzneimittel-Forsch.*, 1972, *22*, 1334.

Effect on cerebral circulation.— B. Hünermann *et al.*, *Arzneimittel-Forsch.*, 1973, *23*, 1074.

Proprietary Names and Manufacturers
Desclidium *(Ima, Arg.; Rhone-Poulenc, Belg.; Spret-Mauchant, Fr.; Rhône-Poulenc, Ger.; Rorer, Ital.; Spain; Rhone-Poulenc, Switz.)*; Permiran *(Laphal, Fr.)*; Vasexten *(Bernabó, Arg.)*.

2418-w

Wild Cherry Bark

Prunus Serotina; Virginian Prune; Virginian Prune Bark; Wild Black Cherry Bark; Wild Cherry.

The dried bark of the wild or black cherry, *Prunus serotina* (Rosaceae), known in commerce as Thin Natural Wild Cherry Bark, containing not less than 10% of water-soluble extractive. It has a slight odour and an astringent, aromatic, bitter taste, recalling that of bitter almonds. It contains (+)-mandelonitrile glucoside (prunasin) and an enzyme system, which interact in the presence of water yielding benzaldehyde, hydrocyanic acid, and glucose.

Wild cherry bark, in the form of the syrup, has been used in the treatment of cough but it has little therapeutic value. It has also been used as a flavouring agent.

14020-x

Xantofyl Palmitate *(rINN).*

Heleniene; Xanthophyl Dipalmitate. β,ε-Carotene-3,3′-diyl dipalmitate.

$C_{72}H_{116}O_4$=1045.7.

CAS — 547-17-1.

Xantofyl palmitate has been used by mouth in the treatment of some visual disturbances.

Proprietary Names and Manufacturers
Adaptinol *(Bayer, Fr.; Bayropharm, Ital.)*.

14022-f

Xibornol *(BAN, rINN).*

1-BX; 1-HP; CP-3-H. 6-(Isoborn-2-yl)-3,4-xylenol; 6-[(1*R*,2*S*,4*S*)-Born-2-yl]-3,4-xylenol.
$C_{18}H_{26}O$=258.4.

CAS — 13741-18-9; 38237-68-2.

Xibornol is an antimicrobial agent which has been used in the treatment of infections of the respiratory tract.

Proprietary Names and Manufacturers
Bracen *(Zyma, Ital.)*; Nanbacine *(Pharmuka, Fr.)*; Xibor *(Benedetti, Ital.)*.

14023-d

Xylazine *(BAN, pINN).*

BAY-Va-1470. *N*-(5,6-Dihydro-4*H*-1,3-thiazin-2-yl)-2,6-xylidine.
$C_{12}H_{16}N_2S$=220.3.

CAS — 7361-61-7 (xylazine); 23076-35-9 (hydrochloride).

NOTE. Xylazine Hydrochloride is *USAN*.

Xylazine is a sedative, analgesic, and muscle relaxant used in veterinary medicine.

The varying pharmacological effects of xylazine in animals.— P. Simon *et al.*, *Thérapie*, 1973, *28*, 735.

A report of an overdosage with xylazine in man.— S. G. Carruthers *et al.*, *Clin. Toxicol.*, 1979, *15*, 281.

Severe bradycardia was associated with abuse of xylazine by a 39-year-old veterinary surgeon's wife.— S. Lewis *et al.*, *Br. med. J.*, 1983, *287*, 1369.

Proprietary Veterinary Names and Manufacturers
Rompun *(Bayer Agrochem, UK)*.

14024-n

Yohimbine Hydrochloride *(rINNM).*

Aphrodine Hydrochloride; Chlorhydrate de Québrachine; Corynine Hydrochloride. The hydrochloride of the principal alkaloid of the bark of the yohimbe tree, *Pausinystalia yohimbe* (= *Corynanthe yohimbi*) (Rubiaceae). Methyl 17α-hydroxy-yohimban-16α-carboxylate hydrochloride.
$C_{21}H_{26}N_2O_3$,HCl=390.9.

CAS — 146-48-5 (yohimbine); 65-19-0 (hydrochloride).

Pharmacopoeias. In *Aust.*, *Cz.*, *Fr.*, and *Span.*

Yohimbine produces an α_2-adrenoceptor block of short duration. It produces an antidiuretic action, increases in heart rate and blood pressure, and orthostatic hypotension. It has been reported to cause anxiety and manic reactions. It has been used for its alleged aphrodisiac properties but convincing evidence of such an effect is lacking. It is contra-indicated in renal or hepatic disease.

Yohimbine is an α_2-selective adrenoceptor antagonist that enhances noradrenaline efflux without blocking postsynaptic vascular α_1 receptors.— B. B. Hoffman and R. J. Lefkowitz, *New Engl. J. Med.*, 1980, *302*, 1390.

A review of the use of yohimbine in impotence.— *Lancet*, 1986, *2*, 1194.

Four of 6 impotent diabetics with incapacitating paraesthesia of the lower limbs noted prompt relief of paraesthesia after taking yohimbine 6 mg thrice daily by mouth. Paraesthesia recurred when treatment was interrupted.— A. Morales *et al.* (letter), *New Engl. J. Med.*, 1981, *305*, 1221.

A report of favourable effects with yohimbine in a double-blind placebo-controlled study of patients with clomipramine-induced orthostatic hypotension.— Y. Lecrubier *et al.* (letter), *Br. J. clin. Pharmac.*, 1981, *12*, 90.

Yohimbine produced beneficial responses in 46% of 48 patients with psychogenic impotence.— K. Reid *et al.*, *Lancet*, 1987, *2*, 421. Comments: M. L. Robinson (letter), *ibid.*, 1088; F. Abajo *et al.* (letter), *ibid.* Reply.— K. Reid (letter), *ibid.*

Proprietary Names and Manufacturers
Yocon *(Palisades, USA)*; Yohimex *(Kramer, USA)*.

The following names have been used for multi-ingredient preparations containing yohimbine hydrochloride— Potensan *(Medo, UK)*; Potensan Forte *(Medo, UK)*; Vikonon *(Savoy Laboratories, UK)*.

18696-b

Zaltidine *(BAN, rINN).*

CP-57361-01 (hydrochloride). [4-(2-Methyl-1*H*-imidazol-4-yl)thiazol-2-yl]guanidine.
$C_8H_{10}N_6S$=295.2.

CAS — 85604-00-8 (zaltidine); 90274-23-0 (hydrochloride).

NOTE. Zaltidine hydrochloride is *USAN*.

Zaltidine is a histamine H_2-antagonist reported to have a prolonged action.

References: G. Laferla *et al.*, *Br. J. clin. Pharmac.*, 1986, *22*, 395.

Proprietary Names and Manufacturers
Pfizer, UK.

14025-h

Zanthoxylum Fruit

Prickly Ash Berries. The pericarp of the ripe fruit of *Zanthoxylum piperitum* (= *Xanthoxylum piperitum*) (Rutaceae) or other species of *Zanthoxylum*.

Pharmacopoeias. In *Chin.* and *Jpn* which also includes Powdered Zanthoxylum Fruit.

It contains about 3.3% v/w of essential oil. It is an ingredient of Bitter Tincture (*Jpn P.*).

Zanthoxylum *B.P.C. 1934* (Toothache Bark; Xanthoxylum) is the dried bark of the northern prickly ash, *Z. americanum*, or the southern prickly ash, *Z. clavaherculis*.

Zanthoxylum fruit has carminative properties and has been used for rheumatic disorders.

Brief review of the pharmacognosy and properties of zanthoxylum fruit. Zanthoxylum contains toxic alkaloids and should not be recommended for use.— J. D. Phillipson and L. A. Anderson, *Pharm. J.*, 1984, *2*, 111.

Mention of possible carcinogenic effects of zanthoxylum fruit.— *Drug & Ther. Bull.*, 1986, *24*, 97. See also E. J. Shellard, *Pharm. J.*, 1986, *2*, 495.

3925-j

Zein *(USAN).*

Pharmacopoeias. In *U.S.N.F.*

A prolamine derived from corn, *Zea mays* (Gramineae). A white to yellow powder. **Insoluble** in water and in acetone; readily soluble in acetone-water mixtures (acetone 60 to 80% w/v); soluble in aqueous alcohols, in glycols, and in aqueous alkaline solutions of pH 11.5 and above; insoluble in all anhydrous alcohols except methyl alcohol. **Store** in airtight containers.

Zein is used as a coating agent for pharmaceutical preparations and foodstuffs. It has been used as a substitute for shellac.

17034-b

Zetidoline *(BAN, rINN).*

DL-308-IT (hydrochloride); L-9308 (hydrochloride); MDL-308 (hydrochloride). 1-(3-Chlorophenyl)-3-[2-(3,3-dimethylazetidin-1-yl)ethyl]-2-imidazolidone.
$C_{16}H_{22}ClN_3O$=307.8.

CAS — 51940-78-4 (zetidoline); 74315-62-1 (hydrochloride).

Zetidoline is under investigation as a neuroleptic.

References: *Drugs of the Future*, 1981, *6*, 162; *ibid.*, 1982, *7*, 218; *ibid.*, 1983, *8*, 287; *ibid.*, 1984, *9*, 236; *ibid.*, 1985, *10*, 266; *ibid.*, 1986, *11*, 248; T. Silverstone *et al.*, *Br. J. Psychiat.*, 1984, *145*, 294.

1587-t

Zidometacin *(USAN, rINN).*

P-74180. 1-(*p*-Azidobenzoyl)-5-methoxy-2-methylindole-3-acetic acid.
$C_{19}H_{16}N_4O_4$=364.4.

CAS — 62851-43-8.

Zidometacin or zidometacin sodium is under investigation as an anti-inflammatory agent.

References: *Drugs of the Future*, 1979, *4*, 839; *ibid.*, 1981, *6*, 742; *ibid.*, 1982, *7*, 851; L. Friez, *Acta ther.*, 1985, *11*, 109; D. Cerri *et al.*, *Boll. chim.-farm.*, 1984, *123*, 47S; G. Bonardi *et al.*, *Int. J. clin. Pharmacol. Res.*, 1984, *4*, 419; H. Bröll *et al.*, *ibid.*, 1986, *6*, 489.

Proprietary Names and Manufacturers
Pierrel, Ital.

5328-s

Zinc Acetate *(USAN).*

$(CH_3.CO_2)_2Zn,2H_2O$=219.5.

CAS — 557-34-6 (anhydrous); 5970-45-6 (dihydrate).

NOTE. Zinc Acetate, Basic is *rINN*.

Pharmacopoeias. In *U.S.*

White crystals or granules with a faint acetous odour. It effloresces slightly. **Soluble** 1 in 2.5 of water and 1 in 30 of alcohol. A 5% solution in water has a pH of 6.0 to 8.0.
Store in airtight containers.

Dilute solutions of zinc acetate have been used as eye lotions or eye-drops in the treatment of conjunctivitis. It is used in zinc-eugenol dental cements to accelerate setting.

5912-h

Zinc Peroxide

CAS — 1314-22-3.

Pharmacopoeias. In *Arg.*, *Fr.*, *Port.*, and *Span.* (all not less than 35%).

A mixture of zinc peroxide, zinc oxide, and zinc hydroxide.

The action of zinc peroxide is similar to that of hydrogen peroxide. Applied locally it has been used for disinfecting, deodorising, and promoting the healing of burns, wounds and various ulcers and lesions. It has been used as a bleaching agent in dental practice.

Proprietary Names and Manufacturers
Neo-Derm *(Desbergers, Canad.)*.

1667-t

Zolpidem *(BAN, rINN).*

SL-800750; SL-800750-23N (tartrate). *N,N*-Dimethyl-2-(6-methyl-2-*p*-tolylimidazo[1,2-*a*]-pyridin-3-yl)acetamide.
$C_{19}H_{21}N_3O$=307.4.

CAS — 82626-48-0 (zolpidem); 99294-93-6 (tartrate).

NOTE. Zolpidem Tartate is *USAN*.

Zolpidem is a hypnotic. It is available as the tartrate in tablets of 10 mg.

References: A. N. Nicholson and P. A. Pascoe, *Br. J. clin. Pharmac.*, 1986, *21*, 205; J. N. Cashman *et al.*, *ibid.*, 1987, *24*, 85.

Proprietary Names and Manufacturers
Stilnox *(Synthelabo, Fr.)*.

1668-x

Zonisamide *(BAN, USAN, rINN).*
AD-810; CI-912; PD-110843. 1-(1,2-Benzoxazol-3-yl)methanesulphonamide.
$C_8H_8N_2O_3S$=212.2.

CAS — 68291-97-4.

Zonisamide is an antiepileptic agent under investigation.

References: *Drugs of the Future,* 1980, *5,* 387; *ibid.,* 1987, *12,* 827 (this lists intervening updates); J. C. Sackellares *et al., Epilepsia,* 1985, *26,* 206; A. J. Wilensky *et al., ibid.,* 212; C. Berent *et al., ibid.,* 1987, *28,* 61; A. Shimizu *et al., Curr. ther. Res.,* 1987, *42,* 147.

Proprietary Names and Manufacturers
Warner-Lambert, UK; Parke, Davis, USA.

Part 3

Formulas of British Proprietary Medicines

Proprietary medicines that are primarily intended for supply against prescriptions written by medical practitioners for individual patients are described in Parts 1 and 2 of Martindale.

'Counter' Proprietaries

The formulas given in the following list are for proprietary medicines available in Great Britain and advertised for over-the-counter sale to the public. The list is not exhaustive. Herbal remedies have been excluded as have toiletries such as 'medicated' shampoos and toothpastes. No sharp distinction can be drawn between proprietary medicines in this list and those described in Parts 1 and 2 of this volume, as some of the medicines in this list may be prescribed, just as some of the medicines in Parts 1 and 2 of *Martindale* may lawfully be supplied to the public without a prescription.

Many of these preparations have a 'licence of right' and remain to be examined by the Committee on the Review of Medicines. Inclusion of a proprietary medicine in this list does not necessarily signify that the ingredients are innocuous or efficacious and reference should be made to the monographs in Parts 1 and 2 for information on the possible adverse effects, abuse potential, contra-indications, and hypersensitivity to the ingredients. It should also be noted that the contents of these preparations are as described by the manufacturers.

Abdine *(Abdine, UK).* Each **Single Strength** powder contains sodium and potassium tartrate 2.75 g, sodium bicarbonate 2.75 g, and citric acid 2.5 g; each **Double Strength** powder contains sodium and potassium tartrate 7 g, sodium bicarbonate 3 g, and citric acid 2.5 g.

Acne-Aid Soap *(Stiefel, UK).* Active ingredient: sulphated surfactant blend 6.3%.

Acriflex *(Evans Medical, UK).* A cream containing chlorhexidine gluconate 0.25% (as a 20% w/v solution).

Actron *(Bayer, UK).* Tablets each containing aspirin 267 mg, paracetamol 133 mg, caffeine 40 mg, sodium bicarbonate 1.606 g, and citric acid 954 mg.

Adult Cough Balsam *(Cupal, UK).* Each 5 mL contains: morphine hydrochloride 0.825 mg, squill vinegar 0.6 mL, acetic acid 0.167 mL, and ammonium acetate 0.175 g.

Aidex Cream *(Cuxson, Gerrard, UK).* Contains aminacrine hydrochloride 0.1%, benzocaine 0.1%, and phenoxyethanol 1.0%.

Aleevex Anti-chill Bath *(Pure Plant Products, UK).* Contains menthol 1%, camphor 1%, and eucalyptus oil 2%.

Algispray *(Kirby-Warrick, UK).* 2-Hydroxyethyl salicylate 5%, diethylamine salicylate 5%, methyl nicotinate 1%.

Alka-Seltzer Tablets *(Bayer, UK).* Each contains aspirin 324 mg, citric acid, anhydrous, 965 mg, and sodium bicarbonate 1.625 g.

Anadin Extra Tablets *(Whitehall, UK).* Each contains aspirin 300 mg, paracetamol 200 mg, and caffeine 45 mg.

Anadin Maximum Strength Capsules *(Whitehall, UK).* Each contains aspirin 500 mg and caffeine 32 mg.

Anadin Paracetamol Tablets *(Whitehall, UK).* Each contains paracetamol 500mg.

Anadin Soluble Tablets *(Whitehall, UK).* Effervescent tablets each containing aspirin 325 mg and caffeine citrate 30 mg.

Anadin Tablets *(Whitehall, UK).* Each contains aspirin 325 mg, caffeine 15 mg, and quinine sulphate 1 mg.

Anbesol *(Whitehall, UK).* Active ingredients: lignocaine hydrochloride 0.9%, chlorocresol 0.1%, and cetylpyridinium chloride 0.02%.

Andrews Answer *(Sterling Health, UK).* Each sachet contains paracetamol 1 g and caffeine 60 mg in an effervescent basis.

Andrews Liver Salt *(Sterling Health, UK).* Contains anhydrous citric acid 19.5%, sodium bicarbonate 22.6%, and magnesium sulphate (dihydrate) 17.4%.

Andrews Liver Salt Diabetic Formula *(Sterling Health, UK).* Contains sodium bicarbonate 45.6%, magnesium sulphate (dihydrate) 17.65%, and anhydrous citric acid 36.7%.

Anestan Tablets *(Crookes Healthcare, UK).* Each contains ephedrine hydrochloride 15 mg and theophylline hydrate 60 mg.

Angiers Junior Paracetamol Tablets *(Bristol-Myers, UK).* Tablets each containing paracetamol 125 mg.

Anodesyn *(Crookes Healthcare, UK).* **Ointment** containing ephedrine hydrochloride 0.25%, lignocaine hydrochloride 0.5%, and allantoin 0.5%. **Suppositories** contain the same active ingredients.

Antipeol *(Medico-Biological Laboratories, UK).* Ointment containing zinc oxide 20%, ichthammol 2.8%, urea 0.1%, and salicylic acid 0.1%.

Antussin Syrup *(Sterling Health, UK).* Each 5 mL contains dextromethorphan hydrobromide 5.28 mg, phenylephrine hydrochloride 3.52 mg, ammonium chloride 44 mg, and ipecacuanha liquid extract 0.005 mL.

Aqua-Ban Tablets *(Thompson Medical, UK).* Each contains ammonium chloride 325 mg and caffeine 100 mg.

Ashton & Parsons Infants Powders *(Beecham Proprietaries, UK).* Contain tincture of matricaria 4 mg and lactose 126 mg.

Askit Powders *(Askit, UK).* Each contains aspirin 530 mg, aloxiprin 140 mg, caffeine citrate 110 mg, and aluminium glycinate 30 mg.

Askit Tablets *(Askit, UK).* Each contains aspirin 230 mg, aloxiprin 110 mg, caffeine 20 mg, and aluminium glycinate 10 mg.

Aspro *(Nicholas, UK).* Each tablet contains aspirin 320 mg. **Aspro Clear.** Each soluble tablet contains aspirin 300 mg or 500 mg.

Ayrtons Antiseptic Cream *(Ayrton, Saunders, UK).* Contains zinc oxide 5% and 2,4-dichlorobenzyl alcohol 0.5%.

Ayrtons Bronchial Emulsion *(Ayrton, Saunders, UK).* Contains liquid paraffin 25%, glycerol 5%, sodium hypophosphite 1%, calcium hypophosphite 1%, compound benzoin tincture 2.5%, squill vinegar 5%, acetic acid 1%, and capsicum tincture 0.25%.

Ayrtons Burn Cream *(Ayrton, Saunders, UK).* Aminacrine hydrochloride 0.1% in a non-greasy basis.

Ayrtons Childrens Cough Syrup *(Ayrton, Saunders, UK).* Each 5 ml contains blackcurrant syrup 0.75 ml, wild cherry syrup 0.5 ml, tolu syrup 0.835 ml, glycerol 0.25 ml, and ipecacuanha liquid extract 0.00625 ml.

Ayrtons Corn and Wart Paint *(Ayrton, Saunders, UK).* Contains salicylic acid 12.5%, zinc chloride 2%, hypophosphorous acid 0.1%, and collodion basis to 100%.

Ayrtons Heart Shaped Indigestion Tablets *(Ayrton, Saunders, UK).* Each contains sodium bicarbonate 55 mg, heavy magnesium carbonate 80 mg, and calcium carbonate 475 mg.

Ayrtons Insect Bite Cream *(Ayrton, Saunders, UK).* Contains antazoline hydrochloride 2%, benzocaine 3%, and cetrimide 0.5%.

Ayrtons Iodised Throat Tablets *(Ayrton, Saunders, UK).* Each contains iodine 0.38%, phenol 8.10%, and menthol 2.50%.

Ayrtons IVY Tablets *(Ayrton, Saunders, UK).* Each contains ferrous gluconate 98 mg, dried yeast 195 mg, vitamin B_1 170 µg, and ascorbic acid 4 mg.

Bactrian Antiseptic Cream *(Loveridge, UK).* Contains cetrimide 1%.

Balto Foot Balm *(Lane, UK).* Contains liquid extract of bladderwrack 1%, camphor 0.5%, oil of pine 1%, menthol 0.2%, precipitated sulphur 3%, potassium iodide 0.25%, salicylic acid 0.187%, zinc oxide 0.47%, and chlorbutol 2%.

Bansor Mouth and Throat Antiseptic *(Thornton & Ross, UK).* Active ingredient: cetrimide 0.01%.

Beecham's Aspirin Tablets *(Beecham Proprietaries, UK).* Each contains aspirin 75 mg.

Beecham's Calcium Supplement Tablets *(Beecham Proprietaries, UK)*. Each contains calcium carbonate 250 mg.

Beecham's Hot Lemon Cold Remedy *(Beecham Proprietaries, UK)*. Each powder contains paracetamol 600 mg, caffeine 50 mg, and ascorbic acid 40 mg. **Beecham's Hot Blackcurrant Cold Remedy** contains the same active ingredients.

Beecham's Pills *(Beecham Proprietaries, UK)*. Each contains aloin 10 mg.

Beecham's Powders *(Beecham Proprietaries, UK)*. Each powder contains aspirin 600 mg and caffeine 50 mg.

Beecham's Powders Capsules *(Beecham Proprietaries, UK)*. Each contains paracetamol 300 mg, caffeine 25 mg and phenylephrine hydrochloride 5 mg.

Beecham's Powders Tablets *(Beecham Proprietaries, UK)*. Each contains aspirin 300 mg and caffeine 25 mg.

Beehive Balsam *(Ayrton, Saunders, UK)*. Contains in each 5 mL: purified honey 0.75 g, glycerol 0.5 mL, ipecac liquid extract 0.015 mL, and terpeneless lemon oil 0.00025 mL.

Belladonna Plaster *(Cuxson, Gerrard, UK)*. Contains belladonna alkaloids 0.25%.

Bemax *(Beecham Bovril, UK)*. Stabilised wheat germ containing in each 100g carbohydrate 35.5 g, protein 24 g, vitamin B_1 1.4 mg, vitamin B_2 560 µg, niacin 5.3 mg, vitamin B_6 810 µg, vitamin E 11.0 mg, manganese 12.5 mg, iron 9 mg, and copper 630 µg.

Bengers *(Fisons, UK)*. Ingredients: partially dextrinised wheaten flour, sodium bicarbonate, and the pancreatic enzymes amylase and trypsin.

Biactol Antibacterial Face Wash *(Richardson-Vicks, UK)*. Active ingredients: sodium lauryl ether sulphate 2.6% and phenoxypropanol 2%.

Birley's Antacid Powder *(Castleowen, UK)*. Contains dried aluminium hydroxide gel 1%, magnesium trisilicate 11.1%, and light magnesium carbonate 87.9%.

Bismag Tablets *(Whitehall, UK)*. Each contains sodium bicarbonate 149 mg, heavy magnesium carbonate 130 mg, and light magnesium carbonate 26 mg.

Bisma-Rex Antacid Powder *(Riker, UK)*. Sodium bicarbonate 65%, calcium carbonate 15%, heavy magnesium carbonate 5%, light kaolin 4%, bismuth carbonate 1%, light magnesium carbonate 10%, peppermint oil 0.12%, vanillin 0.05%, and saccharin sodium 0.05%.

Bisma-Rex Antacid Tablets *(Riker, UK)*. Each contains bismuth carbonate 13 mg, magnesium trisilicate 90 mg, calcium carbonate 460 mg, heavy magnesium carbonate 160 mg, and peppermint oil 2 mg.

BiSoDoL Powder *(Whitehall, UK)*. Each dose contains light magnesium carbonate 345 mg, heavy magnesium carbonate 18 mg, and sodium bicarbonate 532 mg.

BiSoDoL Tablets *(Whitehall, UK)*. Each contains calcium carbonate 522 mg, light magnesium carbonate 68 mg, and sodium bicarbonate 64 mg.

Blisteze *(DDD, UK)*. Cream containing strong ammonia solution 0.2%, aromatic ammonia solution 6.04%, camphor 0.9%, and liquefied phenol 0.49%.

BN Liniment *(3M Health Care, UK)*. Turpentine oil 12%, ammonium chloride 2% and strong ammonia solution 2%.

Bonomint Laxative Chewing Gum *(Intercare, UK)*. Tablets each containing yellow phenolphthalein 97 mg.

Boots Acne Lotion *(Boots, UK)*. Contains benzoyl peroxide 5%.

Boots Antiseptic Cream *(Boots, UK)*. Contains dybenal (2,4-dichlorobenzyl alcohol) 0.5%, cetrimide 0.5%, and allantoin 0.2%.

Boots Antiseptic Lozenges *(Boots, UK)*. Each contains tyrothricin 1 mg and benzocaine 5 mg.

Boots Antiseptic Throat Drops *(Boots, UK)*. Contain amylmetacresol 0.023%.

Boots Bronchial Cough Mixture *(Boots, UK)*. Contains in each 5 mL ammonium chloride 150 mg, ammonium carbonate 100 mg, and guaiphenesin 32.5 mg.

Boots Calamine and Glycerin Cream *(Boots, UK)*. Contains calamine 15%, zinc oxide 5%, glycerol 5%, and liquid phenol 0.5%.

Boots Catarrh Cough Syrup *(Boots, UK)*. Each 10 mL contains codeine phosphate 3 mg, creosote 0.015 mg, and sucrose 7.8 g.

Boots Catarrh Pastilles *(Boots, UK)*. Contain menthol 1%, creosote 0.2%, and pine oil 0.45%.

Boots Catarrh Syrup for Children *(Boots, UK)*. Each 5 mL contains diphenhydramine hydrochloride 12.5 mg and pseudoephedrine hydrochloride 22.5 mg.

Boots Chilblain Cream *(Boots, UK)*. Contains benzyl alcohol 7.5% and eucalyptus oil 1%.

Boots Chilblain Tablets *(Boots, UK)*. Each contains acetomenaphthone 7 mg, nicotinic acid 25 mg, and calcium hydrogen phosphate 320 mg.

Boots Clear Dissolving Pain Relief Tablets *(Boots, UK)*. Each contains paracetamol 500 mg and caffeine 30 mg. **Boots Clear Dissolving Pain Relief Plus Tablets** contain, in addition, codeine phosphate 8 mg.

Boots Cold and Influenza Mixture *(Boots, UK)*. Contains in each 10 mL camphor 0.0015 g, ether spirit 0.062 mL, squill vinegar 0.35 mL, strong ammonium acetate solution 0.16 mL, benzoic acid 0.02 g, anise oil 0.003 mL, and rectified spirit 0.56 mL.

Boots Cold Relief *(Boots, UK)*. Sachets each containing paracetamol 650 mg, sodium citrate 500 mg, and ascorbic acid 50 mg.

Boots Cold Relief Blackcurrant for Children *(Boots, UK)*. Each sachet contains paracetamol 240 mg, sodium citrate 250 mg, and ascorbic acid 50 mg.

Boots Cold Relief Tablets *(Boots, UK)*. Each contains paracetamol 400 mg, ascorbic acid 50 mg, caffeine 30 mg, and phenylephrine hydrochloride 5 mg.

Boots Cold Sore Lotion *(Boots, UK)*. Camphor 3%, menthol 0.2%, dybenal (2,4-dichlorobenzyl alcohol) 0.25%.

Boots Cough Linctus for Children *(Boots, UK)*. Contains in each 5 mL ephedrine hydrochloride 3 mg, ipecacuanha liquid extract 0.00625 mL, tolu syrup 1.4 mL, citric acid monohydrate 50 mg, sodium benzoate 10 mg, and sucrose 2.78 g.

Boots Cough Pastilles for Children *(Boots, UK)*. Contain honey 4.5%, glycerol 6.2%, ipecacuanha liquid extract 0.04%, and squill liquid extract 0.05%.

Boots Cough Relief for Children *(Boots, UK)*. Each 5 mL contains pholcodine 1.5 mg, diphenhydramine hydrochloride 12.5 mg, and absolute alcohol 0.24 mL.

Boots Cream of Magnesia Tablets *(Boots, UK)*. Each contains magnesium hydroxide 300 mg.

Boots Day Cold Comfort *(Boots, UK)*. Linctus containing in each 30 mL pholcodine 10 mg, pseudoephedrine hydrochloride 40 mg, and paracetamol 600 mg.

Boots Day Time Cough Relief *(Boots, UK)*. Each 10 mL contains pholcodine 7.5 mg.

Boots Diarrhoea Mixture *(Boots, UK)*. Each 20 mL contains activated attapulgite 3 g.

Boots Diarrhoea Tablets *(Boots, UK)*. Each white tablet contains codeine phosphate 10 mg and each brown tablet contains activated attapulgite 600 mg.

Boots Double Action Indigestion Mixture *(Boots, UK)*. Each 5 mL contains aluminium hydroxide (calculated as aluminium oxide) 200 mg, magnesium hydroxide 116.5 mg, and activated methylpolysiloxane 25 mg.

Boots Double Action Indigestion Tablets *(Boots, UK)*. Each contains dried aluminium hydroxide gel (calculated as aluminium oxide) 170 mg, magnesium hydroxide 165 mg, and activated polymethylsiloxane 25 mg.

Boots Dual Action Insect Repellent *(Boots, UK)*. Contains diethyltoluamide. **Roll-on** contains diethyltoluamide and permethrin.

Boots Dyspepsia Tablets *(Boots, UK)*. Each contains magnesium trisilicate 100 mg, ginger 5 mg, and sodium bicarbonate 150 mg.

Boots Ear Wax Remover *(Boots, UK)*. Contains docusate sodium 5%.

Boots Embrocation *(Boots, UK)*. Active ingredients: camphor 0.8% and turpentine oil 40%.

Boots Eye Drops *(Boots, UK)*. Contain boric acid 2.5%, sodium borate 0.5%, hamamelis water 5%, and cetrimide 0.01%.

Boots Family Antiseptic *(Boots, UK)*. Contains chloroxylenol 3%, terpineol 5%, and aromatic pine oil 1%.

Boots Foot Cream *(Boots, UK)*. Contains menthol 1%, cetrimide 0.5%, and distearyldimethylammonium chloride 3.75%.

Boots Foot Powder *(Boots, UK)*. Dichlorophen 0.2%, sodium polymetaphosphate 4%, light kaolin 20%.

Boots Glycerin and Blackcurrant Soothing Cough Relief *(Boots, UK)*. Each 5 mL contains glycerol 0.75 mL and sucrose 1.7,g.

Boots Glycerin Honey and Lemon Linctus *(Boots, UK)*. Contains in each 5 mL glycerol 0.75 mL, honey 1.11 g, citric acid monohydrate 50 mg, lemon oil 0.006 mL, and sucrose 1.96 g. **Boots Glycerin Honey and Lemon Linctus with Ipecacuanha** contains, in addition, ipecacuanha liquid extract 0.015 mL.

Boots Glycerin of Thymol Pastilles *(Boots, UK)*. Contain sodium benzoate 0.49%, sodium salicylate 0.3%, sodium carbonate 1%, glycerol 3.8%, menthol 0.02%, thymol 0.03%, pumilio pine oil 0.03%, cineole 0.08%, methyl salicylate 0.02%, and amylmetacresol 0.036%.

Boots Gripe Mixture *(Boots, UK)*. Each 5 mL contains sodium bicarbonate 50 mg, weak ginger tincture 0.025 mL, concentrated caraway water 0.075 mL, concentrated spearmint water (*B.P.C. 1959*) 0.0005 mL, concentrated peppermint water 0.0005 mL, and rectified spirit 0.15 mL.

Boots Headache and Indigestion Tablets *(Boots, UK)*. Each contains paracetamol 500 mg, caffeine 15 mg, citric acid 942 mg, sodium bicarbonate 1390 mg, and anhydrous sodium carbonate 133 mg.

Boots Health Salt *(Boots, UK)*. Sucrose 38.9%, sodium bicarbonate 22.5%, tartaric acid 6.9%, citric acid 6.9%, dried magnesium sulphate 17.3%, and sodium chloride 0.6%.

Boots Herbal Lozenges *(Boots, UK)*. Balsam of tolu 0.7%, menthol 0.2%, anise oil 0.24%, 60% alcoholic extract from 0.06% of capsicum, aqueous extracts from 0.1% of coltsfoot leaf and 0.15% of horehound, liquorice juice 6.3%, basis to 100%.

Boots Indigestion Mixture *(Boots, UK)*. Contains in each 5 mL light magnesium carbonate 225 mg, sodium bicarbonate 225 mg, calcium carbonate 175 mg, peppermint oil 0.005 mL, and chloroform water to 5 mL.

Boots Indigestion Powder *(Boots, UK)*. Each teaspoonful (approximately 2.5 g) contains heavy magnesium carbonate 937.5 mg, sodium bicarbonate 312.5 mg, magnesium trisilicate 234.4 mg, light kaolin 78.1 mg, and prepared chalk 937.5 mg.

Boots Indigestion Tablets *(Boots, UK)*. Each contains calcium carbonate 200 mg, magnesium trisilicate 60 mg, heavy magnesium carbonate 60 mg, sodium bicarbonate 60 mg, and ginger 10 mg.

Boots Iodized Throat Tablets *(Boots, UK)*. Each tablet contains iodophenol 0.4 mg, potassium iodide 0.4 mg, phenol 1.5 mg, and menthol 2 mg.

Boots Iron Tonic Tablets *(Boots, UK)*. Each contains ferrous fumarate 25 mg, dried yeast 300 mg, and thiamine hydrochloride 3 mg.

Boots Medicated Foot Spray *(Boots, UK)*. Chlorhexidine acetate 0.1% and dichlorophen 0.25%.

Boots Medicated Skin Treatment Gel *(Boots, UK)*. Active ingredients: glycerol 3%, allantoin 0.2%, industrial methylated spirit 50%, menthol 0.08%, and dichlorobenzyl alcohol 0.5%.

Boots Medicated Skin Wash *(Boots, UK)*. Active ingredients: cetrimide 0.5% and benzalkonium chloride solution 0.5%.

Boots Medicated Soap *(Boots, UK)*. Contains triclocarban 2%.

Boots Medicated Talc *(Boots, UK)*. Contains allantoin 0.5%.

Boots Menthol and Wintergreen Embrocation *(Boots, UK)*. Active constituents: menthol 2.4%, cineole 2%, cajuput oil 0.5%, eucalyptus oil 1.5%, methyl salicylate 14.2%.

Boots Nappy Rash Cream *(Boots, UK)*. Contains dimethicone 10% and cetrimide 0.5%.

Boots Nasal Spray *(Boots, UK)*. Oxymetazoline hydrochloride 0.05%.

Boots Night Cold Comfort *(Boots, UK)*. Linctus containing in each 30 mL pseudoephedrine hydrochloride 40 mg, pholcodine 10 mg, diphenhydramine hydrochloride 10 mg, paracetamol 600 mg, and absolute alcohol 5.8 mL.

Boots Night Time Cough Relief for Adults *(Boots, UK)*. Each 10 mL contains pholcodine 7.5 mg, diphenhydramine hydrochloride 25 mg, and dehydrated alcohol 0.48 mL.

Boots Oral Antiseptic *(Boots, UK)*. Contains cetylpyridinium chloride 0.025%.

Boots Pain Relief Plus Capsules *(Boots, UK)*. Each contains paracetamol 500 mg and codeine phosphate 8 mg.

Boots Pain Relief Tablets *(Boots, UK)*. Each contains paracetamol 500 mg and caffeine 30 mg.

Boots Pain Relieving Balm *(Boots, UK)*. Contains glycol monosalicylate 7.5%, ethyl nicotinate 1%, and vanillylnonamide 0.015%.

Boots Paracetamol Elixir Paediatric *(Boots, UK)*. Each 5 mL contains paracetamol 120 mg.

Boots Pink Healing Ointment *(Boots, UK)*. Zinc oxide 8%, methyl salicylate 3.6%, liquefied phenol 2%, menthol 0.01%.

Boots Senna Laxative Tablets *(Boots, UK)*. Each contains standardised senna equivalent to 7.5 mg of total sennosides.

Boots Sore Mouth Gel *(Boots, UK)*. Lignocaine 0.6% and cetylpyridinium chloride 0.02%.

Boots Sore Mouth Pastilles *(Boots, UK)*. 2,4-Dichlorobenzyl alcohol 0.1%, alcoholic (90%) extractive from 0.1% of myrrh, glycerol 4.5%, menthol 0.02%.

Boots Sting Relief *(Boots, UK)*. Zinc oxide 2%, benzyl alcohol 1.5%, chloroxylenol 1.5%, eucalyptus oil 1%, borax 1%, menthol 0.5%, camphor 0.25%.

Boots Suppositories for Haemorrhoids *(Boots, UK)*. Each contains zinc oxide 230 mg, glycol monosalicylate 104 mg, benzyl alcohol 52 mg, and methyl salicylate 10 mg.

Boots Syrup of Figs *(Boots, UK)*. Contains in each 5 mL: 45% alcoholic extract from 750 mg of senna fruit, aqueous extract from 550 mg of fig, malt extract 1.87 g, clove oil 0.001 mL, peppermint oil 0.00025 mL, and benzoic acid 10 mg.

Boots Travel Sickness Tablets *(Boots, UK)*. Tablets each containing hyoscine hydrobromide 300 µg.

Boots Vegetable Laxative Tablets *(Boots, UK)*. Each tablet contains compound colocynth extract 60 mg, hyoscyamus dry extract 15 mg, jalap resin 15 mg, and peppermint oil 0.006 mL.

Boots Warming Pain Relief Spray *(Boots, UK)*. Contains methyl salicylate 1.24%, ethyl nicotinate 1.10%, and camphor 0.62%.

Brompton Cough Lozenges *(Ernest Jackson, UK)*. Active ingredients: liquorice extract 13.3% and aniseed oil 2.0%.

Bronal Cough and Catarrh Elixir *(Cupal, UK)*. Contains in each 5 ml dextromethorphan hydrobromide 10 mg, ephedrine hydrochloride 10 mg, menthol 0.5 mg, glycerol 0.25 ml, and alcohol (90%) 1 ml.

Bronalin *(Cupal, UK)*. Each 5 ml contains ammonium chloride 135 mg, diphenhydramine hydrochloride 14 mg, and sodium citrate 57 mg.

Bronalin Dry Cough Elixir *(Cupal, UK)*. Contains in each 5 mL: dextromethorphan hydrobromide 10 mg, ephedrine hydrochloride 10 mg, and alcohol (90%) 1 mL.

Bronalin Paediatric *(Cupal, UK)*. Each 5 ml contains diphenhydramine hydrochloride 7 mg and sodium citrate 28.5 mg.

Bronchipax *(Ashe, UK)*. Extended-action tablets each containing ephedrine resinate equivalent to ephedrine hydrochloride 30 mg and theophylline 40 mg.

Brooklax Chocolate Laxative *(Intercare, UK)*. Tablets each containing yellow phenolphthalein 130 mg.

Brush Off *(Napp, UK)*. Contains povidone-iodine 10% in an alcoholic solution.

Burgess' Lion Ointment *(Burgess, UK)*. Contains yellow soft petroleum jelly 65%, anhydrous lanolin 15%, zinc oleostearate 5%, yellow beeswax 5%, rosin 5%, and methylated spirit 5%.

Burn Aid Cream *(Cupal, UK)*. Aminacrine hydrochloride 0.1% and antazoline hydrochloride 1%.

Burneze *(International Laboratories, UK)*. An aerosol containing benzocaine 1%.

Buttercup Medicated Sweets *(LRC Products, UK)*. **Honey and Lemon Flavour** contain honey 1%, lemon oil 0.68%, menthol 0.15%, and eucalyptus 0.15%. **Original** contain menthol 0.18%.

Buttercup Syrup *(LRC Products, UK)*. Each 5 mL contains squill liquid extract 0.031 mL, stronger capsicum tincture 0.0025 mL, strong ginger tincture 0.005 mL, acetic acid 0.19 mL, and chloroform 0.025 mL.

Buxton Rubbing Bottle *(English Grains, UK)*. Contains capsicum oleoresin 1.1%, turpentine oil 12.2%, camphor 2.65%, and methyl salicylate 2.65%.

Cabdrivers Adult Linctus *(De Witt, UK)*. Each 5 ml contains dextromethorphan hydrobromide 11.5 mg, terpin hydrate 11.5 mg, menthol 7 mg, pumilio pine oil 0.0015 ml, eucalyptus oil 0.0025 ml, glycerol 0.825 ml, glucose syrup 2.83 ml, and alcohol (90%) 0.79 ml.

Cabdrivers Diabetic Linctus *(De Witt, UK)*. Contains in 5 ml ephedrine hydrochloride 6 mg and dextromethorphan hydrobromide 15 mg.

Cabdrivers Junior Glucose Linctus *(De Witt, UK)*. Ephedrine hydrochloride 0.12%, vinegar of ipecacuanha 4.17%, red-poppy syrup 8.33%, anise syrup 4.17%, and glucose syrup 26%.

Calcium Factor 500 *(Intercare, UK)*. Tablets each containing calcium 500 mg derived from calcium carbonate 1.25 g.

Califig *(Sterling Health, UK)*. Contains aqueous extract of senna leaf (1–1) 27.8%.

Calsalettes *(Torbet Laboratories, UK)*. Tablets containing aloin 38 mg.

Cantaba *(Cantassium Co., UK)*. Each tablet contains aminobenzoic acid 100 mg.

Cantarna *(Cantassium Co., UK)*. Each tablet contains ribonucleic acids 450 mg.

Cantassium Discs *(Cantassium Co., UK)*. Each contains ferrous fumarate 2 mg, potassium sulphate 4 mg, potassium iodide 2 mg, and potassium bicarbonate 296 mg.

Carbalax *(Pharmax, UK)*. Suppositories each containing sodium bicarbonate 1.08 g and anhydrous sodium acid phosphate 1.32 g.

Carmil *(Intercare, UK)*. Each 5 ml contains pectin 40 mg, light kaolin 500 mg, morphine hydrochloride 350 µg, and atropine methonitrate 100 µg.

Carnation Callous Caps *(Cuxson, Gerrard, UK)*. Plasters bearing an ointment containing salicylic acid 40%.

Carnation Corn Caps *(Cuxson, Gerrard, UK)*. Plasters bearing an ointment containing salicylic acid 40%.

Carter's Little Pills *(Carter-Wallace, UK)*. Each contains phenolphthalein 16 mg and aloin 8 mg.

Castellan No. 10 Bronchial Pastilles *(Ayrton, Saunders, UK)*. Contain liquorice extract 5.7%, menthol 0.5%, peppermint oil 0.025%, anise oil 0.3%, capsicin 0.001%, benzoin tincture 0.5%, and clove oil 0.05%.

Catarrh-Ex *(Dep, UK)*. Tablets each containing paracetamol 500 mg and pseudoephedrine hydrochloride 60 mg.

Celerub *(Laboratories for Applied Biology, UK)*. Ointment containing methyl salicylate 15%, celery seed oil 5%, clove oil 3.5%, thyme oil 3.5%, pumilio pine oil 3.5%, camphor liniment 20%, menthol 10%, and salicylic acid 2%.

Cephos Powders *(Beecham Proprietaries, UK)*. Each contains aspirin 600 mg and caffeine 50 mg.

Cepton Medicated Clear Gel *(Care, UK)*. Contains chlorhexidine gluconate solution 2.5%.

Cepton Medicated Lotion *(Care, UK)*. Contains chlorhexidine gluconate solution 0.5%.

Cepton Medicated Skin Wash *(Care, UK)*. Contains chlorhexidine gluconate solution 5.0%.

Cetrimax Antiseptic Cream *(Thornton & Ross, UK)*. Contains cetrimide 0.5%.

Chilblain Cream *(Pickles, UK)*. Contains histamine acid phosphate 0.1% and methyl nicotinate 1%.

Christy's Skin Emulsion *(Christy, UK)*. Contains SD alcohol 40, glyceryl stearate, beeswax, synthetic spermaceti, propyl paraben, methyl paraben, lanolin, mineral oil, glycerin, soap flakes, parachlorometaxylenol, aminoacridine hydrochloride, cetyl alcohol, sweet almond oil, F.D. & C. Yellow No. 5, and denatonium benzoate.

Chymol Emollient Balm *(Waterhouse, UK)*. Each 40 g contains terpineol 4%, eucalyptus oil 1.2%, phenol 2.4%, and methyl salicylate 0.8%.

Cidal *(Albion, UK)*. Soap containing Irgasan 0.75%.

Clearasil Cream *(Richardson-Vicks, UK)*. Contains sulphur 8% and triclosan 0.1%.

Clearine Eye Drops *(Optrex, UK)*. Contains: naphazoline hydrochloride, distilled witch hazel, boric acid, borax, glycerol, methyl hydroxybenzoate, propyl hydroxybenzoate, benzalkonium chloride 50% solution, and purified water.

Coda-Med *(Dep, UK)*. Tablets each containing paracetamol 450 mg, caffeine citrate 15 mg, and codeine phosphate 8.1 mg.

Codanin *(Whitehall, UK)*. Tablets each containing paracetamol 500 mg and codeine phosphate 10 mg.

Codella *(Napp, UK)*. Hand cream containing povidone-iodine 0.2%.

Codural Period Pain Tablets *(3M Health Care, UK)*. Each contains caffeine 50 mg, paracetamol 250 mg, and homatropine methylbromide 750 µg.

Cojene *(Fisons, UK)*. Each tablet contains aspirin 300 mg, caffeine citrate 95 mg, and codeine phosphate 8 mg.

Coldrex Granules *(Sterling Health, UK)*. Sachets each containing paracetamol 1 g, phenylephrine hydrochloride 10 mg, and ascorbic acid 60 mg.

Coldrex Tablets *(Sterling Health, UK)*. Each contains paracetamol 500 mg, phenylephrine hydrochloride 5 mg, caffeine 25 mg, terpin hydrate 20 mg, and vitamin C 30 mg.

Collins Elixir *(Collins of Norwich, UK)*. Each 5 mL contains ethylmorphine hydrochloride 1.5 mg, lemon oil 0.016 mL, and sucrose.

Collins Elixir Pastilles *(Collins of Norwich, UK)*. Each contains citric acid 1.65%, lemon oil 0.26%, squill vinegar 0.42%, and glycerol 0.21%.

Collis Browne's (J.) Mixture *(International Laboratories, UK)*. Each 5-ml dose contains anhydrous morphine 1 mg and peppermint oil 0.0015 mL.

Collis Browne's (J.) Tablets *(International Laboratories, UK)*. Each contains light kaolin 750 mg, morphine hydrochloride 350 µg, and calcium carbonate 200 mg.

Colsor Cream *(Pickles, UK)*. Contains tannic acid 5%, camphor 0.1%, menthol 0.5%, and phenol 1%.

Colsor Lotion *(Pickles, UK)*. Contains tannic acid 5%, camphor 5%, phenol 0.5%, and menthol 0.5%.

Coltex Antihistamine Cream *(Thornton & Ross, UK)*. Contains diphenhydramine hydrochloride 2%.

Compound W *(Whitehall, UK)*. A wart remover containing salicylic acid 17%.

Contac 400 *(Wellcome, UK)*. Sustained-release capsules each containing phenylpropanolamine hydrochloride 50 mg and chlorpheniramine maleate 4 mg.

Correctol Tablets *(Kirby-Warrick, UK)*. Dioctyl sodium sulfosuccinate 100 mg, yellow phenolphthalein 65 mg, sodium benzoate 17.65 mg, and calcium gluconate 47.55 mg.

Covonia Bronchial Balsam *(Thornton & Ross, UK)*. Active ingredients: dextromethorphan hydrobromide 0.075%, guaiphenesin 0.5%, and menthol 0.05%.

Cox's Antiseptic Cream *(Cox, UK)*. Contains cetrimide 0.5%.

Cox's Bronchial Balasam *(Cox, UK)*. Each 10 mL contains chloroform and morphine tincture 0.4 mL, ephedrine hydrochloride 16.0 mg, squill liquid extract 0.017 mL, and sucrose 2.2 g.

Cox's Bronchial Mixture, Extra Strong *(Cox, UK)*. Contains in each 10 mL squill liquid extract 0.095 mL, senega liquid extract 0.0475 mL, ipecacuanha tincture 0.15 mL, ammonium bicarbonate 235 mg, and sucrose 3.31 g.

Cox's Digestive Mints *(Cox, UK)*. Each contains dihydroxyaluminium sodium carbonate 300 mg.

Cradocap *(Napp, UK)*. A shampoo containing cetrimide 10%.

Crampex Tablets *(International Laboratories, UK)*. Each contains guaiphenesin 60 mg, nicotinic acid 20 mg, calcium gluconate 200 mg, and ergocalciferol 20 µg.

Cream E45 *(Crookes Healthcare, UK)*. An emollient basis containing white soft paraffin 14.5%, light liquid paraffin 11.6%, and wool fat 1%.

Creds *(Ernest Jackson, UK)*. Contain menthol 0.5%, peppermint oil 0.025%, aniseed oil 0.3%, benzoin tincture 0.5%, capsicin 0.001%, and clove oil 0.05%.

Cremaffin *(Boots, UK)*. A brand of Liquid Paraffin and Magnesium Hydroxide Emulsion.

Cremosan *(Ayrton, Saunders, UK)*. Contains zinc oxide 5.3%, beeswax 10.7%, resin 10.7%, wool fat 22.2%, cresol 2.3%, formaldehyde solution 0.2%, thymol 0.2%, and paraffin basis to 100%.

Crookes Sport Antifungal Foot Foam *(Crookes Healthcare, UK)*. Contains triclosan 0.09%.

Crookes Sport Antiseptic Cream *(Crookes Healthcare, UK)*. Contains 2,4-dichlorobenzyl alcohol 0.5%, cetrimide 0.5%, and allantoin 0.2%.

Crookes Sport Heat Spray *(Crookes Healthcare, UK)*. Contains methyl salicylate 1.24%, ethyl nicotinate 1.1%, and camphor 0.62%.

Crookes Sport Massage Embrocation *(Crookes Healthcare, UK)*. Contains camphor 0.8% and turpentine oil 40%.

Crookes Sport Medicated Foot Powder *(Crookes Healthcare, UK)*. Contains triclosan 0.1%.

Cupal Baby Cough Syrup *(Cupal, UK)*. Each 5 mL contains dilute acetic acid 0.42 mL.

Cupal Cold Sore Lotion *(Cupal, UK)*. Contains tannic acid 5%, salicylic acid 1%, and myrrh 10%.

Cupal Cold Sore Ointment *(Cupal, UK)*. Contains allantoin 1%, diperodon hydrochloride 1%, camphor 1%, and zinc oxide 5%.

Cupal Corn Solvent *(Cupal, UK)*. Contains salicylic acid 13% in a pyroxylin base.

Cupal Insect Bite Cream *(Cupal, UK)*. Contains antazoline hydrochloride 2%.

Cupal Nail Bite Lotion *(Cupal, UK)*. Contains denatonium benzoate 0.256%.

Cupal Verruca Ointment *(Cupal, UK)*. Contains salicylic acid 50%.

Cupal Wart Solvent *(Cupal, UK)*. Contains glacial acetic acid 86.25%.

Cuticura Ointment *(Dep, UK)*. Hard paraffin 18.17%, light liquid paraffin 28.5%, yellow soft paraffin 50.38%, white beeswax 1.94%, pine oil 0.04%, geranium oil 0.17%, chlorophyll 0.08%, hydroxyquinoline 0.05%, sulphur precip. 0.5%, and phenol 0.16%.

Cutinea Foot & Body Powder *(Cupal, UK)*. Active ingredients: chlorphenesin 1% and zinc oxide 10%, in a base of starch and purified talc.

Cymalon *(Sterling Health, UK)*. Sachets each containing sodium citrate 4 g.

Cymex *(De Witt, UK)*. Contains urea 1%, cetrimide 0.5%, dimethicone 9%, and chlorocresol 0.1%.

Cystemme *(Abbott, UK)*. Active ingredients: sodium citrate, sodium bicarbonate, tartaric acid, and citric acid.

Day Nurse *(Beecham Proprietaries, UK)*. Each 20-mL dose contains: paracetamol 500 mg, phenylpropanolamine hydrochloride 25 mg, dextromethorphan hydrobromide 15 mg, and alcohol 3.08 mL.

Day Nurse Capsules *(Beecham Proprietaries, UK)*. Each contains paracetamol 250 mg, phenylpropanolamine hydrochloride 12.5 mg, and dextromethorphan hydrobromide 7.5 mg.

DDD Lotion *(DDD, UK)*. Contains thymol 0.09%, menthol 0.14%, salicylic acid 0.75%, resorcinol 0.75%, chlorbutol 1.13%, methyl salicylate 0.94%, glycerol 7.93%, liquefied phenol 0.98%, and alcohol 34.11%.

DDD Medicated Cream *(DDD, UK)*. Contains thymol 0.09%, menthol 0.15%, methyl salicylate 1.15%, chlorbutol 1.11%, resorcin 0.25%, liquefied phenol 0.98%, and titanium dioxide 0.5%.

De Witt's Analgesic Pills *(De Witt, UK)*. Each contains paracetamol 330 mg and caffeine 30 mg.

De Witt's Antacid Powder *(De Witt, UK)*. Contains magnesium trisilicate 12%, light magnesium carbonate 10%, calcium carbonate 20%, sodium bicarbonate 48.5%, light kaolin 9% and peppermint oil 0.5%.

De Witt's Antacid Tablets *(De Witt, UK)*. Each contains calcium carbonate 324 mg, heavy magnesium carbonate 194.4 mg, magnesium trisilicate 64.8 mg, peppermint oil 3.6 mg, and lactose 129.6 mg.

De Witt's K and B Pills *(De Witt, UK)*. Each contains alcoholic (60%) extract of buchu (1–4) 20 mg, methylene blue 10 mg, aqueous extract of bearberry (2–7) 40 mg, cascara dry extract 15 mg.

De Witt's Throat Lozenges *(De Witt, UK)*. Each contains tyrothricin 1.25 mg, benzocaine 8 mg, and cetylpyridinium chloride 2 mg.

Decongestant Tablets *(Cox, UK)* (Now known as **Mackenzies Decongestant Tablets**). Each contains paracetamol 250 mg, guaiphenesin 50 mg, methylephedrine hydrochloride 15 mg, chlorpheniramine maleate 2 mg, and menthol 1 mg.

Delax *(Boots, UK)*. An emulsion containing in each 5 mL liquid paraffin 2.5 mL, phenolphthalein 45 mg, and benzoic acid 5.5 mg.

Dentinox Colic Drops *(DDD, UK)*. Active ingredient: dimethicone 21 mg per 2.5 mL dose.

Dentinox Infant Cradle Cap Treatment Shampoo *(DDD, UK)*. Contains sodium lauryl ethyl sulphosuccinate 6% and sodium lauryl ether sulphate 2.7%.

Dentinox Teething Gel *(DDD, UK)*. Contains lignocaine hydrochloride 0.33% and cetylpyridinium chloride 0.1%.

Dermidex Cream *(International Laboratories, UK)*. Lignocaine 1.2%, alcloxa 0.25%, chlorbutol 1%, and cetrimide 0.5%.

Digespirin Antacid *(Spencer, UK)*. Tablets each containing dihydroxyaluminium sodium carbonate 300 mg.

Dillex Gripe Mixture *(Optrex, UK)*. Contains sodium bicarbonate 1%, sodium citrate 0.05%, dill oil 0.001%, anise oil 0.006%, caraway oil 0.012%, spearmint 0.003%, rectified spirit 2.4%, and syrup 27%.

Dinneford's Gripe Mixture *(Beecham Proprietaries, UK)*. Each 10-mL dose contains heavy magnesium carbonate 157 mg, citric acid monohydrate 354 mg, sodium bicarbonate 213 mg, sucrose 2.5 g, and alcohol 0.5 mL.

Diocalm Tablets *(Beecham Proprietaries, UK).* Each contains morphine hydrochloride 395 μg, activated attapulgite 312.5 mg, and attapulgite 187.5 mg.

Disprin *(Reckitt & Colman Pharmaceuticals, UK).* Tablets each containing aspirin 300 mg.

Disprol, Junior *(Reckitt & Colman Pharmaceuticals, UK).* **Tablets** each containing paracetamol 120 mg. **Suspension** containing paracetamol 120 mg in each 5 mL.

Disprol, Paediatric *(Reckitt & Colman Pharmaceuticals, UK).* Suspension containing paracetamol 120 mg in each 5 mL.

Doan's Backache Pills Extra Strength *(Ciba Consumer, UK).* Each contains paracetamol 150 mg and sodium salicylate 100 mg.

Do-Do *(Ciba Consumer, UK).* Tablets each containing ephedrine hydrochloride 22 mg, anhydrous caffeine 30 mg, and theophylline sodium glycinate 50 mg.

Do-Do Expectorant Linctus *(Ciba Consumer, UK).* Each 5 mL contains guaiphenesin 100 mg.

Dristan Decongestant Tablets with Antihistamine *(Whitehall, UK).* Each contains phenylephrine hydrochloride 5 mg, chlorpheniramine maleate 2 mg, aspirin 325 mg, and caffeine 16.2 mg.

Dristan Nasal Mist with Oxymetazoline *(Whitehall, UK).* Active ingredient: oxymetazoline hydrochloride 0.05%.

Dusk *(Cupal, UK).* Active ingredients: diethyltoluamide 20%.

Duttons Cough Mixture *(Spencer, UK).* Each 5 mL contains liquorice liquid extract 0.133 mL, acetic acid (80%) 0.133 mL, honey 0.267 mL, chloroform 0.025 mL, glycerol 0.2 mL, capsicum tincture 0.025 mL, treacle 2.275 mL.

Earache Drops *(Ayrton, Saunders, UK).* Cajuput oil 3.12, rosemary oil 3.12, and arachis oil to 100.

Earex *(International Laboratories, UK).* Ear-drops containing arachis oil 33.3%, almond oil 33.3% and rectified camphor oil 33.3%.

Ecdilyn Syrup *(De Witt, UK).* Each 5 mL contains diphenhydramine hydrochloride 14 mg and ammonium chloride 135 mg.

Ectodyne Worm Syrup *(Wigglesworth, UK).* Contains piperazine citrate 12.6%.

Eftab Effervescent Mouthwash Tablets *(Thornton & Ross, UK).* Each contains peppermint oil 0.0019 mL, clove oil 0.0009 mL, spearmint oil 0.00028 mL, menthol 1.87 mg, thymol 0.7 mg, and methyl salicylate 0.00006 mL.

Elkamol *(Kendon, UK).* Tablets each containing paracetamol 500 mg.

Elliman's Embrocation *(Beecham Proprietaries, UK).* Contains turpentine oil 35.41% and acetic acid 10.37%.

Emlab Brewers' Yeast Tablets *(3M Health Care, UK).* Each contains dried yeast 300 mg.

Emlab Iron and Brewers' Yeast Tablets *(3M Health Care, UK).* Each contains dried yeast 300 mg and ferrous fumarate 15 mg.

Endet Teething Powders *(Cullen & Davison, UK).* Contain paracetamol 125 mg, promethazine hydrochloride 5 mg, heavy magnesium carbonate 100 mg, and sucrose 30 mg.

Eno *(Beecham Proprietaries, UK).* Each 5-g dose contains sodium bicarbonate 2.20 g, tartaric acid 1.43 g, citric acid 870 mg, and sodium carbonate 0.50 g.**Sparkling Lemon-Flavoured Eno** contains, in each 5-g dose, sodium bicarbonate 2.17 g, tartaric acid 1.41 g, citric acid 0.86 g, anhydrous sodium carbonate 0.50 g and tartrazine.

Enterosan *(Windsor, UK).* Each tablet contains kaolin 700 mg, morphine hydrochloride 275 μg, and belladonna dry extract 1.8 mg.

Entrotabs *(Wallis, UK).* Tablets each containing attapulgite 360 mg, dried aluminium hydroxide 100 mg, and pectin 50 mg.

Envoy Pastilles *(Ernest Jackson, UK).* Benzalkonium chloride solution 0.06% and hexylresorcinol 0.03%.

EP Tablets *(Pharmax, UK).* Each contains paracetamol 300 mg, caffeine 50 mg, and codeine phosphate 8 mg.

Ex-Lax Pills *(Intercare, UK).* Each contains yellow phenolphthalein 95 mg.

Ex-Lax Tablets *(Intercare, UK).* Each tablet contains yellow phenolphthalein 98 mg in a chocolate basis.

Expelix Worm Elixir *(Cupal, UK).* Consists of Piperazine Citrate Elixir equivalent to piperazine hydrate 750 mg per 5 mL.

Famel Catarrh & Throat Pastilles *(Optrex, UK).* Active ingredients: creosote 0.29%, cinnamon leaf oil 0.21%, lemon oil 0.08%, and menthol 0.34%.

Famel Expectorant *(Optrex, UK).* Linctus containing guaiphenesin 50 mg in each 5 mL.

Famel Honey and Lemon Cough Pastilles *(Optrex, UK).* Each contains guaiphenesin 1%.

Famel Linctus *(Optrex, UK).* Each 5 mL contains pholcodine 5 mg and papaverine hydrochloride 0.5 mg.

Famel Syrup (Original) *(Optrex, UK).* Contains creosote 16.8 mg, codeine phosphate 1.9 mg, and liquid glucose 3.4 mL in each 5 mL.

Fam-Lax Laxative Tablets *(Roberts, UK).* Each contains yellow phenolphthalein 120 mg and powdered rhubarb 27.5 mg.

Femerital *(MCP Pharmaceuticals, UK).* Tablets each containing ambucetamide 100 mg and paracetamol 250 mg.

Feminax *(Nicholas, UK).* Tablets each containing paracetamol 500 mg, codeine phosphate 8 mg, caffeine 50 mg, and hyoscine hydrobromide 100 μg.

Fennings' Adult Cooling Powders *(Fennings, UK).* Each 300-mg powder contains anhydrous caffeine 30 mg and paracetamol 180 mg.

Fennings' Children's Cooling Powders *(Fennings, UK).* Each 200-mg powder contains paracetamol 50 mg.

Fennings' Gripe Mixture *(Fennings, UK).* Each 5 mL contains sodium bicarbonate 50 mg, peppermint oil 0.000625 mL, dill oil 0.00125 mL, and caraway oil 0.00125 mL.

Fennings' Lemon Mixture *(Fennings, UK).* Contains sodium salicylate 5%.

Fennings' Little Healers *(Fennings, UK).* Each tablet contains prepared ipecacuanha 20 mg.

Fenox *(Crookes Healthcare, UK).* Phenylephrine hydrochloride, available as **Nasal Drops** and as **Nasal Spray** each containing 0.5%.

Fiery Jack Rubbing Cream *(Pickles, UK).* Contains capsicin 1.25%, methyl nicotinate 1%, glycol salicylate 5%, and diethylamine salicylate 5%.

Fiery Jack Rubbing Ointment *(Pickles, UK).* Contains capsicum oleoresin 2.15%.

Fisherman's Friend Aniseed Flavoured Cold and Flu Lozenges *(Lofthouse of Fleetwood, UK).* Active ingredients: liquorice powder 7.6%, menthol 0.5%, and anise oil 0.17%.

Fisherman's Friend Extra Strong Throat & Chest Lozenges *(Lofthouse of Fleetwood, UK).* Contain eucalyptus oil 0.153%, capsicum tincture 0.02%, liquorice extract 7.317%, and menthol 0.9%.

Fisherman's Friend Honey Cough Syrup *(Lofthouse of Fleetwood, UK).* Each 5 mL contains honey 1.25 mL, squill vinegar 0.9 mL, citric acid 50 mg, saccharin solution 0.05 mL, anise oil 0.005 mL, benzoic acid 5 mg, peppermint oil 0.0025 mL, menthol 2.5 mg, and cineole 0.001 mL.

Flu-rex *(Cupal, UK).* Each tablet contains paracetamol 400 mg, caffeine 30 mg, phenylephrine hydrochloride 5 mg, and noscapine 7.5 mg.

Flu-rex Capsules *(Cupal, UK).* Each capsule contains paracetamol 150 mg, noscapine 10 mg, terpin hydrate 30 mg, and phenylephrine hydrochloride 5 mg.

Fort-E-Vite *(Lane, UK).* Capsules each containing natural source vitamin E 100, 200, or 500 units.

Fosfor *(Consolidated Chemicals, UK).* Contains phosphorylcolamine 5%.

Franolyn Expect *(WinPharm, UK).* Each 5 mL contains guaiphenesin 25 mg, ephedrine 4.75 mg, and theophylline (anhydrous) 60 mg.

Franolyn Sed *(WinPharm, UK).* Each 5 mL contains dextromethorphan hydrobromide 10 mg.

Franolyn Tablets *(WinPharm, UK).* Each contains ephedrine hydrochloride 11 mg and theophylline 120 mg.

Freezone *(Whitehall, UK).* Active constituents: salicylic acid 17%.

Fynnon Calcium Aspirin *(Beecham Proprietaries, UK).* Each tablet contains aspirin 500 mg and calcium carbonate 150 mg.

Fynnon Salt *(Beecham Proprietaries, UK).* Each 5-g dose contains sodium sulphate 4.8 g, sodium bicarbonate 98 mg, potassium sulphate 103 mg, and lithium sulphate 17 mg.

Galloways Cough Syrup *(LRC Products, UK).* Each 5 mL contains ipecacuanha liquid extract 0.0045 mL, chloroform 0.01 mL acetic acid 0.21 mL, squill vinegar 0.0267 mL, and ether 0.0028 mL.

George's American Marvel Liniment *(Thomas, UK).* Contains alcoholic (60%) capsicum extract (5–1)2.47%, turpentine oil 5.02%, camphor 2.01%, eucalyptus oil 0.2%, rosemary oil 0.3%.

Germolene 2 *(Beecham Proprietaries, UK).* Contains phenol 1.2% and chlorhexidine gluconate solution equivalent to chlorhexidine gluconate 0.25%.

Germolene Footspray *(Beecham Proprietaries, UK).* Contains triclosan 0.03% and dichlorophen 0.1%.

Germolene Ointment *(Beecham Proprietaries, UK).* Contains anhydrous lanolin 35%, yellow soft paraffin 34.80%, light liquid paraffin 7.9%, starch 10%, phenol 1.19%, zinc oxide 6.55%, methyl salicylate 3%, octaphonium chloride 0.3%, and white soft paraffin 1.13%.

Germoloids *(Beecham Proprietaries, UK).* **Ointment** contains zinc oxide 6.6%, methyl salicylate 3.05%, bismuth oxychloride 1.1%, phenol 1%, menthol 0.2%, and chloroxylenol 0.05% in a base containing yellow soft paraffin and anhydrous lanolin. **Suppositories** each contain lignocaine hydrochloride 13.2 mg and zinc oxide 284 mg.

Gerovital H3 Face Cream *(Tudor, UK).* Active constituent: procaine hydrochloride 100 mg in each 27-g pack.

Gerovital H3 Tablets *(Tudor, UK).* Each contains procaine hydrochloride 100 mg, benzoic acid 6 mg, potassium metabisulphite 5 mg, and disodium phosphate 500 μg.

Glacier Cream *(Farillon, UK).* **Green tube:** a non-greasy cream containing ethyl-paradimethylaminobenzoate 1% and titanium dioxide 1%. **Red tube:** a greasy cream containing ethylparadimethylaminobenzoate 1%, titanium dioxide 1%, and zinc oxide 1%.

Glycerin Lemon and Honey *(Waterhouse, UK)*. Each 5 mL contains purified honey 1.5 g, glycerol 0.63 g, and sucrose.

Glycerin Lemon and Honey Melo (with Ipecac) *(Waterhouse, UK)*. Each 5 mL contains purified honey 1.5 g, glycerol 0.5 g, ipecacuanha liquid extract 2.5 mg, and sucrose.

Goddard's Embrocation *(LRC Products, UK)*. Active ingredients: turpentine oil 22%, dilute acetic acid 30%, and dilute ammonia solution 14%.

Grasshopper Ear Drops *(Spencer, UK)*. Docusate sodium 5%.

Grasshopper Ointment *(Spencer, UK)*. Contains colophony 31.68%, yellow beeswax 7.94%, larch oleoresin 23.74%, arachis oil 15.84%, white soft paraffin 19.81%, and copper acetate 0.99%.

Gum-eze *(De Witt, UK)*. Contains myrrh tincture 10%, krameria tincture 2.5%, thymol 0.1%, oil of cloves 0.1%, propylene glycol 50%, glycerol 37.0875%, sodium benzoate 0.1%, cetylpyridinium chloride 0.1%, and saccharin 0.0125%.

Hacks *(Barker Dobson, UK)*. **Original Flavour** contain menthol 0.1%, eucalyptus oil 0.06%, and ascorbic acid 357 mg per 100 g.**Menthol and Eucalyptus Flavour** contain menthol 0.2%, eucalyptus oil 0.12%, and ascorbic acid 357 mg per 100 g.**Blackcurrant** and **Honey and Lemon Flavours** contain menthol 0.06% and ascorbic acid 357 mg per 100 g.

Hactos Chest & Cough Mixture *(Thomas, UK)*. Contains chloroform 0.5%, capsicum extract 0.01%, peppermint oil 0.06%, anise oil 0.05%, clove oil 0.02%.

Haemorex *(Cupal, UK)*. Ointment containing zinc oxide 7.5%, diperodon hydrochloride 1%, allantoin 1%, and basis to 100.

Hedex *(Sterling Health, UK)*. Tablets each containing paracetamol 500 mg. **Hedex Soluble Granules**: Each sachet contains paracetamol 1 g.

Hedex Plus *(Sterling Health, UK)*. Capsules each containing paracetamol 500 mg, codeine phosphate 8 mg, and caffeine 30 mg.

Hedex Seltzer *(Sterling Health, UK)*. Sachets each containing paracetamol 1 g, caffeine 60 mg, sodium bicarbonate 1.54 g, and citric acid 1.24 g.

Heemex *(Lane, UK)*. Contains distilled extract of witch hazel 25.5%, compound tincture of benzoin 8.2%, zinc oxide 5.1%, and emulsified base 61.2%.

Hemocane *(Intercare, UK)*. **Cream** contains lignocaine hydrochloride 0.65%, zinc oxide 10%, bismuth oxide 2%, benzoic acid 0.4%, and cinnamic acid 0.45%. **Suppositories** each contain lignocaine hydrochloride 11 mg, zinc oxide 300 mg, bismuth oxide 25 mg, benzoic acid 8 mg, and cinnamic acid 9 mg.

Hepramist *(DHL Products, UK)*. Non-metered aerosol containing heparin 2 units per mL.

Hewlett's Cream *(Astra, UK)*. Active ingredients: zinc oxide 80 mg and hydrous wool fat 40 mg in each g of cream.

Hill's Adult Expectorant *(Hill's Pharmaceuticals, UK)*. Each 5 mL contains diphenhydramine hydrochloride 13.80 mg, ammonium chloride 136.25 mg, and sodium citrate 56.25 mg.

Hill's Bronchial Balsam for Adults *(Hill's Pharmaceuticals, UK)*. Each 5 mL contains morphine hydrochloride 900 µg, ammonium acetate 180 mg, capsicum tincture 0.0105 mL, compound benzoin tincture 0.3125 mL, ipecacuanha liquid extract 0.025 mL, acetic acid (80%) 0.11 mL, and simple lobelia tincture 0.125 mL.

Hill's Bronchial Balsam Pastilles *(Hill's Pharmaceuticals, UK)*. Contain compound benzoin tincture 0.793%, capsicum oleoresin 0.001%, peppermint oil 0.04%, ipecacuanha liquid extract 0.5%, simple lobelia tincture 2.5%, and menthol 0.11%.

Hill's Junior Balsam *(Hill's Pharmaceuticals, UK)*. Each 5 mL contains compound benzoin tincture 0.156 mL, ipecacuanha liquid extract 0.01 mL, simple lobelia tincture 0.0625 mL, acetic acid (80%) 0.0565 mL, capsicum tincture 0.005 mL, ammonium acetate 90 mg, and squill vinegar 0.156 mL.

Hip-C *(Paines & Byrne, UK)*. Rose hip syrup containing vitamin C not less than 3 mg per mL.

Homocea Ointment *(Mawson & Proctor, UK)*. Contains coconut oil 20%, lard 2%, white beeswax 7.5%, hard paraffin 20%, soft white paraffin 30%, camphor 2%, eucalyptus oil 0.5%, rosemary oil 0.5%, cajuput oil 2.5%, turpentine oil 10%, strong ammonia solution 3%, and water 2%.

Honeytusin Cough Linctus *(Vestric, UK)*. Each 5 mL contains anise oil 0.0078 mL, ipecacuanha liquid extract 0.031 mL, peppermint oil 0.0035 mL, squill vinegar 0.335 mL, tolu syrup 1.888 mL, ether 0.11 mL, chloroform 0.025 mL, potassium iodide 62 mg, liquorice liquid extract 0.292 mL, and squill oxymel 0.310 mL.

Iglodine *(Ayrton, Saunders, UK)*. An antiseptic solution containing the equivalent of phenol 0.089% and combined iodine 0.04%.

Iglodine Ointment *(Ayrton, Saunders, UK)*. Combined iodine 0.14%, zinc oxide 1.43%, phenol 0.32%, bismuth oxychloride 2.86%.

Imps *(Arcadian of Devon, UK)*. Pellets containing liquorice block juice 76%, menthol 1.2%, maize starch, acacia, and capsicin.

Indian Brandee *(Waterhouse, UK)*. Each 5 mL contains cardamom compound tincture 0.187 mL, capsicum tincture 0.125 mL, and concentrated ethyl nitrite solution 0.031 mL.

Iron Jelloids *(Beecham Proprietaries, UK)*. Each contains ferrous fumarate 60 mg, thiamine mononitrate 170 µg, riboflavine 290 µg, nicotinamide 1.67 mg, and ascorbic acid 4.17 mg.

Jaap's Fruit Health Salts *(Askit, UK)*. Active ingredients: sodium potassium tartrate 0.94%, tartaric acid 20.8%, and sodium bicarbonate 21.32%.

Jackson's All Fours Cough Mixture *(Waterhouse, UK)*. Contains in each 5 mL anise oil 0.003 mL, peppermint oil 0.0006 mL, chloroform spirit 0.0125 mL, chloroform 0.0115 mL, ether 0.0031 mL, capsicum tincture 0.023 mL, and treacle 0.5 g.

Jackson's Antiseptic Throat Pastilles *(Ernest Jackson, UK)*. Contain liquorice liquid extract 5.7%, acetic acid 0.9%, menthol 0.12%, camphor 0.03%, terebene 0.05%, benzoic acid 0.01%, thymol 0.003%, methyl salicylate 0.005%, eucalyptol 0.005%, capsicin 0.00001%, and pumilio pine oil 0.2%.

Jackson's Bismuth Dyspepsia Lozenges *(Ernest Jackson, UK)*. Active ingredients: bismuth carbonate 7.2%, sodium bicarbonate 21.7%, and gingerin 0.17%.

Jackson's Bronchial Catarrh Pastilles *(Ernest Jackson, UK)*. Contain creosote 0.15%, menthol 0.6%, aniseed oil 0.02%, peppermint oil 0.02%, capsicin 0.001%, and benzoin tincture 0.5%.

Jackson's Catarrh Pastilles *(Ernest Jackson, UK)*. Contain menthol 0.6%, sylvestris pine oil 0.3%, abietis pine oil 0.3%, and creosote 0.2%.

Jackson's Children's Cough Pastilles *(Ernest Jackson, UK)*. Honey 12%, ipecacuanha liquid extract 0.36%, squill liquid extract 0.73%, and ascorbic acid 0.9%.

Jackson's Eucalyptus & Menthol Pastilles *(Ernest Jackson, UK)*. Contain eucalyptus oil 0.6% and menthol 0.8%.

Jackson's Febrifuge *(Waterhouse, UK)*. Contains in each 5 mL sodium sulphate 209 mg, potassium nitrate 38 mg, ammonium chloride 38 mg, chloroform 0.0065 mL, liquorice liquid extract 0.1 mL, rhubarb liquid extract 0.0095 mL, taraxacum liquid extract 0.033 mL, caramel 0.033 mL, strong ginger tincture 0.023 mL, potassium iodide 0.45 mg, iodine 0.45 mg, capsicum tincture 0.005 mL, camphor 1 mg, alcohol (95%) 0.07 mL, aniseed oil 0.0001 mL, and clove oil 0.0002 mL.

Jackson's Glycerin Thymol Pastilles *(Ernest Jackson, UK)*. Contain sodium benzoate 0.2%, thymol 0.047%, menthol 0.035%, eucalyptol 0.07%, abietis oil 0.024%, methyl salicylate 0.005%, and glycerin 3.53%.

Jackson's Iodised Throat Lozenges *(Ernest Jackson, UK)*. Phenol 0.5%, menthol 0.22%, aqueous iodine solution 0.3%, and methyl salicylate 0.06%.

Jackson's Linseed and Liquorice Lozenges *(Ernest Jackson, UK)*. Active ingredients: liquorice extract 2.86%, mucilage of linseeds 0.35%, peppermint oil 0.02%, aniseed oil 0.02%, capsicum oleoresin 0.0015%, and menthol 0.2%.

Jenners Antacid Suspension *(Savory & Moore, UK)*. Each 5 mL contains magnesium hydroxide mixture 1.29 g, aluminium hydroxide gel 2.56 g, polydimethylsiloxane 7.5 mg, in a flavoured basis.

Joy-rides *(Stafford-Miller, UK)*. Each tablet contains hyoscine hydrobromide 150 µg.

Juno Junipah Salts *(Cox, UK)*. Each 5 g contains anhydrous sodium sulphate 4.41 g, anhydrous sodium phosphate 38.6 mg, sodium bicarbonate 54.8 mg, and juniper oil 0.0028 mL.

Juno Junipah Tablets *(Cox, UK)*. Each contains anhydrous sodium sulphate 450 mg, anhydrous sodium phosphate 60 mg, phenolphthalein 25 mg, juniper oil 0.00025 mL, and sodium chloride 0.25 mg.

Kao-C Adults Diarrhoea Mixture *(Cupal, UK)*. Each 20-mL dose contains light kaolin 2 g and calcium carbonate 1 g.

Kao-C Junior Diarrhoea Mixture *(Cupal, UK)*. Each 5-mL dose contains light kaolin 500 mg and calcium carbonate 250 mg.

KH3 Geriatricum *(Torbet Laboratories, UK)*. Capsules each containing procaine hydrochloride 50 mg and haematoporphyrin base 200 µg.

Koladex Tablets *(Laboratories for Applied Biology, UK)*. Each contains caffeine 21 mg and stabilised kola extract 4.5 mg (equivalent to 80 mg dry kola nuts).

Kompo *(J.F. White, UK)*. Each 5 mL contains catechu 295 mg, clove oil 0.00325 mL, cassia oil 0.0045 mL, and capsicum oleoresin 0.00095 mL.

Kruschen Salts *(Ashe, UK)*. Sodium chloride 10%, anhydrous sodium sulphate 2%, potassium chloride 1%, potassium sulphate 5.5%, citric acid 1.5%, potassium iodide 0.001%, magnesium sulphate, exsiccated ($MgSO_4$,$2.75H_2O$) to 100%.

Kwells *(Nicholas, UK)*. Tablets each containing hyoscine hydrobromide 300 µg. **Junior Kwells**. Tablets each containing hyoscine hydrobromide 150 µg.

Laboprin *(Laboratories for Applied Biology, UK)*. Tablets containing aspirin 300 mg and lysine 245 mg.

Lactocalamine Lotion *(Kirby-Warrick, UK)*. Contains calamine 2%, hamamelis water 5%, phenol 0.2%, and zinc oxide 2%.

Lanacane *(Combe, UK)*. Cream containing benzocaine 3%, resorcinol 2%, and chlorothymol 0.032%.

Lanasting *(Combe, UK).* Contains benzyl alcohol 10% and lignocaine 2%.

Lanes Charcoal Tablets *(Lane, UK).* Each contain charcoal pure vegetable source 125 mg.

Lecigran *(Lane, UK).* Consists of vegetable (soya) lecithin.

Lemonexa Concentrated Hot Lemon Flu Cold Syrup *(Cupal, UK).* Contains in each 5 ml codeine phosphate 5 mg, ephedrine hydrochloride 7.5 mg, and diphenhydramine hydrochloride 5 mg, in a basis containing terpeneless lemon oil 0.01 ml.

Lem-Plus Instant Hot Lemon Drink *(Wallis, UK).* Granules for solution containing paracetamol 650 mg, sodium citrate 500 mg, and ascorbic acid 50 mg.

LemSip *(Reckitt & Colman Pharmaceuticals, UK).* Each sachet contains paracetamol 650 mg, phenylephrine hydrochloride 5 mg, ascorbic acid 10 mg, and sodium citrate 500 mg, in a flavoured basis.

LemSip, Junior *(Reckitt & Colman Pharmaceuticals, UK).* Each sachet contains paracetamol 217 mg, phenylephrine hydrochloride 1.7 mg, ascorbic acid 3.3 mg, and sodium citrate 167 mg.

Lipsavers *(Carter-Wallace, UK).* Active ingredients: 2-ethylhexyl salicylate 4%, sorbic acid 0.5%, and allantoin 0.25%.

Liqufruta Honey and Lemon *(LRC Products, UK).* Each 5 ml contains ipecacuanha liquid extract 13.9 mg, liquid glucose 5.08 g, menthol 1.32 mg, and honey 0.33 g. **Liqufruta Blackcurrant** contains similar active ingredients.

Liqufruta Medica Garlic *(LRC Products, UK).* The water-soluble constituents of linseed 32 mg, irish moss 20 mg, and chamomile 6.05 mg, together with garlic oil 0.00065 mL, peppermint oil 0.0052 mL, anise oil 0.0026 mL, ipecacuanha liquid extract 0.0082 mL, and liquorice juice 37 mg.

Listerine Antiseptic *(Warner-Lambert, UK).* Alcohol (96%) 28.4%, benzoic acid 0.12%, eucalyptol 0.09%, menthol 0.04%, methyl salicylate 0.05%, and thymol 0.06%.

Listermint *(Warner-Lambert, UK).* Contains cetylpyridinium chloride 0.1% and zinc chloride 0.05%.

Lloyd's Cream *(Reckitt & Colman Pharmaceuticals, UK).* Contains diethylamine salicylate 10%.

Lockets Lozenges *(Mars, UK).* **Menthol Eucalyptus Lockets** contain honey 8.2%, glycerol 1.9%, menthol 0.19%, and eucalyptol 0.15%. **Honey and Lemon Lockets** contain honey 8.2%, glycerol 1.9%, menthol 0.22%, and eucalyptol 0.21%.

Loveridge Children's Cherry Bark Cough Syrup *(Loveridge, UK).* Active constituents: acetic acid 33% and ipecacuanha liquid extract 2.2 mg in each 5 mL.

Loveridge Creosote Bronchial Mixture *(Loveridge, UK).* Active constituents: Creosote 0.8%, potassium iodide 2.2%, and liquorice liquid extract 8.0%.

Loveridge Mentholated Balsam *(Loveridge, UK).* Active constituents: Squill oxymel 1.76 g, liquorice liquid extract 209 mg, and capsicum tincture 13 mg, in each 5 mL.

Lucozade *(Beecham Bovril, UK).* Contains glucose syrup, lactic acid, caffeine, and vitamin C.

Luma Bath Salts *(Sestri, UK).* Contain methyl salicylate, capsicum oleoresin, potassium iodide, and sodium carbonate.

Mac Extra *(Beecham Proprietaries, UK).* Each contains hexylresorcinol 2.4 mg.

Mac Medicated Lozenges *(Beecham Proprietaries, UK).* Each lozenge contains amylmetacresol 600µg, sucrose, and glucose syrup solids 2.7 g. **Mac Original**. Contain, in addition, menthol 4 mg.

Macleans Indigestion Powder *(Beecham Proprietaries, UK).* Each 5-g dose contains heavy magnesium carbonate 0.78 g, calcium carbonate 1.86 g, and stabilised aluminium hydroxide equivalent to 0.87 g of dried aluminium hydroxide gel.

Macleans Indigestion Tablets *(Beecham Proprietaries, UK).* Each contains light magnesium carbonate 150 mg, calcium carbonate 400 mg, and stabilised aluminium hydroxide equivalent to 183 mg of dried aluminium hydroxide gel.

Magnesium Complexe *(Lake, UK).* Capsules each containing magnesium chloride 30 mg, magnesium glutamate 50 mg, magnesium glycerophosphate 50 mg, magnesium orotate 100 mg, and magnesium aspartate 150 mg.

Matthews' Fullers Earth Cream *(Ashe, UK).* Contains Matthews' fullers earth 5.3%, zinc oxide 2.9%, calcium carbonate 2.9%, and lanolin 3.4% in an emollient basis.

Medex Elixir *(Savory & Moore, UK).* Each 5 mL contains diphenhydramine hydrochloride 14 mg, ammonium chloride 100 mg, and sodium citrate 44 mg.

Medicaid *(Farillon, UK).* Cream containing cetrimide 0.5% in a hydrophilic basis.

Medicalm *(Savory & Moore, UK).* Each 5 mL contains light kaolin 1.83 g and belladonna tincture 0.1 mL, in an aqueous pectin suspending vehicle.

Medicol Liquid Antiseptic *(Jeyes, UK).* Dichloroxylenol 2.5%, terpineol 5%, and isopropyl alcohol.

Medijel *(DDD, UK).* Contains lignocaine hydrochloride 0.66%, and aminacrine hydrochloride 0.05%.

Medijel Soft Pastilles *(DDD, UK).* Contain lignocaine hydrochloride 0.25% and aminacrine hydrochloride 0.025%.

Medipain *(Savory & Moore, UK).* Tablets each containing paracetamol 500 mg, codeine phosphate 8 mg, and caffeine 30 mg.

Mediquell *(Warner-Lambert, UK).* Chewy squares containing dextromethorphan, 10 mg.

Meggezones *(Kirby-Warrick, UK).* Pastilles each containing menthol 17.3 mg.

Melissin *(Surf Ski International, UK).* Each 5 mL contains guaiphenesin 100 mg, menthol 1 mg, glycerol 1.66 mL, melissa, dried 125 mg, benzoic acid 5 mg, citric acid 50 mg, and aromatic oils.

Meloids *(Crookes Healthcare, UK).* Lozenges each containing liquorice juice 93.3%, menthol 1.5%, cinnamon oil 0.37%, and stronger capsicum tincture 0.12%.

Melrose *(Roberts & Sheppey, UK).* Contains hard paraffin 27.9%, yellow soft paraffin 67.3%, wool fat 1.9%, chloroxylenol 0.1%, and oil of lemon grass.

Meltus Adult Expectorant *(Cupal, UK).* Contains in each 5 mL guaiphenesin 100 mg, cetylpyridinium chloride 2.5 mg, sucrose 1.75 g, and purified honey 500 mg.

Meltus Junior Expectorant *(Cupal, UK).* Contains in each 5 mL guaiphenesin 50 mg, cetylpyridinium chloride 2.5 mg, sucrose 2 g, and purified honey 500 mg.

Mentho Lyptus Extra Strong *(Hall Bros, UK).* Active ingredients: menthol 0.39% and eucalyptus oil 0.14%.

Mentho Lyptus Original *(Hall Bros, UK).* Active ingredients: menthol 0.12% and eucalyptus oil 0.105%. **Blackcurrant Flavour**: menthol 0.04% and eucalyptus oil 0.01%. **Honey and Lemon**: menthol 0.024% and eucalyptus oil 0.021%.

Menthol and Wintergreen Cream *(Cupal, UK).* Contains eucalyptus oil 1.25%, methyl salicylate 11.2%, menthol 0.22%, camphor 0.34%, and volatile mustard oil 0.1%.

Mentholated Balsam *(Savory & Moore, UK).* Each 5 mL contains ipecacuanha tincture 0.1 mL, morphine hydrochloride 0.57 mg, liquorice liquid extract 0.25 mL, squill oxymel 1.25 mL, menthol 2.5 mg, and camphor spirit 0.1 mL.

Mentholated Bronchial Balsam *(Thornton & Ross, UK).* Active ingredients in 5 mL: menthol 4 mg, squill tincture 0.6 mL, and liquorice liquid extract 0.125 mL.

Mentholatum Antiseptic Lozenges *(Mentholatum, UK).* Each contains menthol 16 mg, eucalyptus oil 12 mg, and amylmetacresol 600 µg.

Mentholatum Deep Heat Lotion *(Mentholatum, UK).* Contains menthol 1.58%, methyl salicylate 18.94%, and liquid lanolin 1.9%.

Mentholatum Deep Heat Rub *(Mentholatum, UK).* Contains menthol 5.91%, eucalyptus oil 1.97%, methyl salicylate 12.8% and turpentine oil 1.47%.

Mentholatum Deep Heat Spray *(Mentholatum, UK).* Non-metered aerosol containing 2-hydroxyethyl salicylate 5%, methyl salicylate 1%, methyl nicotinate 1.6%, and ethyl salicylate 5%.

Milk of Magnesia *(Sterling Health, UK).* Each 5 mL contains magnesium hydroxide 415 mg.

Milk of Magnesia Tablets *(Sterling Health, UK).* Each contains magnesium hydroxide 300 mg.

Mil-Par *(Sterling Health, UK).* Each 5 mL contains magnesium hydroxide 300 mg and liquid paraffin 1.25 mL.

Modantis *(Surf Ski International, UK).* Cream containing antazoline hydrochloride 2%, cetrimide 0.5%, titanium dioxide 2%, and allantoin 0.5%, with cetostearyl alcohol, liquid paraffin, and water.

Moorland Indigestion Tablets *(Crookes Healthcare, UK).* Each contains bismuth aluminate 5.4 mg, magnesium trisilicate 29 mg, dried aluminium hydroxide 11.6 mg, heavy magnesium carbonate 94 mg, light kaolin 27 mg, and calcium carbonate 464 mg.

Mrs. Cullen's Powders *(Cullen & Davison, UK).* Contain aspirin 600 mg, caffeine 62 mg, calcium phosphate 34.08 mg, saccharin sodium 3.84 mg, and sodium lauryl sulphate 80 µg.

Mu-Cron Syrup, Junior *(Ciba, UK).* Contains phenylpropanolamine hydrochloride 0.2% and guaiphenesin 0.5%.

Mu-Cron Tablets *(Ciba, UK).* Each contains phenylpropanolamine hydrochloride 25 mg and paracetamol 500 mg.

Mulcets Mouth Ulcer Tablets *(Riker, UK).* Each contains ascorbic acid 25 mg and cetylpyridinium chloride 1 mg.

Murine *(Abbott, UK).* Eye-drops containing naphazoline hydrochloride 0.012%.

N Tonic *(Cupal, UK).* Each 5 mL contains calcium hypophosphite 7.5 mg, potassium hypophosphite 7.5 mg, manganese hypophosphite 2.5 mg, ferric hypophosphite 1.25 mg, thiamine hydrochloride 0.53 mg, potassium citrate 2.2 mg, and phosphoric acid 0.0009 mL.

Napisan *(Richardson-Vicks, UK).* A preparation for cleansing and disinfecting babies' napkins, based on potassium monopersulphate and sodium chloride.

Nasciodine *(Farillon, UK).* Active ingredients: iodine 1.26%, menthol 0.59%, methyl salicylate 3.87%, essential oil of camphor 3.87%, and turpentine oil 3.87%.

Nella Red Oil *(Nella, UK)*. Contains methyl nicotinate 1 g, mustard oil 25 ml, clove oil 1.5 ml, red tax. oil 10 mg, and arachis oil to 100 ml.

Neo Baby Cream *(Neo Laboratories, UK)*. Contains cetrimide 0.2%, benzalkonium chloride solution 0.1%, in a silicone/lanolin basis.

Neo Baby Mixture *(Neo Laboratories, UK)*. Each 5 mL contains sodium bicarbonate 50 mg, essence of ginger 0.01 mL, and dill oil 0.0025 mL.

Nicobrevin Anti-Smoking Capsules *(Intercare, UK)*. Each contains menthyl valerate 100 mg and quinine 15 mg.

Night Nurse *(Beecham Proprietaries, UK)*. Each 20 mL contains promethazine hydrochloride 20 mg, dextromethorphan hydrobromide 15 mg, paracetamol 500 mg, and alcohol 3.08 mL.

Night Nurse Capsules *(Beecham Proprietaries, UK)*. Each contains paracetamol 250 mg, promethazine hydrochloride 10 mg, and dextromethorphan hydrobromide 7.5 mg.

Nirolex Expectorant Linctus *(Boots, UK)*. Contains in each 5 mL guaiphenesin 100 mg, ephedrine hydrochloride 7.5 mg, menthol 1 mg, glycerol 1 mL, and sucrose 2.5 g.

Nirolex for Children *(Boots, UK)*. Each 5 mL contains guaiphenesin 50 mg, sucrose 2.5 g and glycerol 1 mL.

Nirolex Lozenges *(Boots, UK)*. Each contains dextromethorphan hydrobromide 2.5 mg.

Nostroline *(Combe, UK)*. Contains eucalyptol 0.2%, menthol 0.3%, phenol 1.6%, and geranium oil 0.2%.

Novasil Antacid Suspension *(Cupal, UK)*. Contains in each 10 ml sodium bicarbonate 445 mg, light magnesium carbonate 333 mg, and peppermint oil 0.01 ml.

Novasil Antacid Tablets *(Cupal, UK)*. Each contains sodium bicarbonate 15.6 mg, calcium carbonate 220 mg, and heavy magnesium carbonate 220 mg.

Noxacorn Corn Remover *(Cox, UK)*. Contains benzocaine 2.2%, camphor 2.2%, salicylic acid 10.6%, iodine 0.11%, castor oil 2.6%, and phenol 0.31%.

Noxzema Skin Cream *(Ever Ready Personna, UK)*. Contains camphor 0.37%, eucalyptus oil 0.12%, menthol 0.075%, clove oil 0.12%, and phenol 0.32%.

Numark Day Cold Relief *(Independent Chemists Marketing, UK)*. Each 30 mL contains pholcodine 10 mg, pseudoephedrine hydrochloride 40 mg, and paracetamol 600 mg.

Numark Expectorant Cough Relief *(Independent Chemists Marketing, UK)*. Each 5 mL contains diphenhydramine hydrochloride 14 mg, ammonium chloride 100 mg, and sodium citrate 44 mg.

Numark Indigestion Tablets *(Independent Chemists Marketing, UK)*. Each contains calcium carbonate 200 mg, magnesium trisilicate 60 mg, heavy magnesium carbonate 60 mg, sodium bicarbonate 60 mg, and ginger 10 mg.

Numark Night Cold Relief *(Independent Chemists Marketing, UK)*. Each 30 mL contains pholcodine 10 mg, pseudoephedrine hydrochloride 40 mg, diphenhydramine hydrochloride 10 mg, paracetamol 600 mg, and dehydrated alcohol 5.8 mL.

Nurse Harvey's Gripe Mixture *(Harvey-Scruton, UK)*. Contains dill oil 0.035%, caraway oil 0.035%, weak ginger tincture 5.2%, sodium bicarbonate 1%, and syrup 19.5%.

Nurse Sykes Balsam *(Waterhouse, UK)*. Contains in each 5 mL compound benzoin tincture 0.155 mL, capsicum tincture 0.013 mL, camphor 1 mg, acetic acid 0.075 mg, glycerol 0.3125 mL, tolu syrup 1.25 mL, and guaiphenesin 8.75 mg.

Nurse Sykes Powders *(Waterhouse, UK)*. Contain aspirin 165.4 mg, paracetamol 120 mg, caffeine 60 mg, and light kaolin 50 mg.

Nylax Laxative Tablets *(Evans Medical, UK)*. Each contains thiamine hydrochloride 3.9 mg, phenolphthalein 62 mg, cascara dry extract 30 mg, aloin 2 mg, senna leaf 15 mg, and bisacodyl 2 mg.

Opas Indigestion Powder *(Leo, UK)*. Contains sodium bicarbonate 20% calcium carbonate 40%, and heavy magnesium carbonate 40%.

Opas Indigestion Tablets *(Leo, UK)*. Each contains sodium bicarbonate 68 mg, calcium carbonate 136 mg, and heavy magnesium carbonate 136 mg.

Opazimes *(Leo, UK)*. Each tablet contains dried aluminium hydroxide 160 mg, light kaolin 700 mg, morphine hydrochloride 250 µg, and belladonna dry extract 3 mg.

Optabs Eye Lotion Tablets *(Evans Medical, UK)*. Tablets containing phenylephrine hydrochloride 0.05%, adrenaline 0.6%, and acriflavine 0.005%.

Optrex Emergency Eye Wash *(Optrex, UK)*. Contains sterile saline solution (0.9% sodium chloride).

Optrex Eye Drops *(Optrex, UK)*. Distilled witch hazel 12.5%, preserved with benzalkonium chloride 0.005% in a solution buffered with borax and boric acid.

Optrex Eye Lotion *(Optrex, UK)*. Distilled witch hazel 13%, preserved with benzalkonium chloride 0.005% in a solution buffered with borax and boric acid.

Over-Nite *(Cupal, UK)*. Contains in each 20 ml paracetamol 500 mg, diphenhydramine hydrochloride 10 mg, ephedrine hydrochloride 15 mg, and codeine phosphate 10 mg.

Owbridge's *(Chefaro, UK)*. Each 5 mL contains cetylpyridinium chloride 1.25 mg, anise oil 0.0025 mL, clove oil 0.0025 mL, acetic acid 0.06 mL, capsicum tincture 0.025 mL, strong ammonium acetate solution 0.16 mL.

Panacron Decongestant Nasal Spray *(WinPharm, UK)*. Contains oxymetazoline hydrochloride 0.05%.

Panacron Tablets *(WinPharm, UK)*. Each contains phenylpropanolamine hydrochloride 12.5 mg and paracetamol 500 mg.

Pan-A-Gel *(Ursula-Ruth, UK)*. Capsules containing royal jelly. **Pan-B-Gel**. Capsules containing royal jelly.

Panaleve Elixir *(Leo, UK)*. Contains paracetamol 120 mg in each 5 mL.

Panda Baby Cream *(Thornton & Ross, UK)*. Active ingredients: zinc oxide 13.5%, castor oil 9.0%, and lanolin 6.7%.

Panerel *(Cox, UK)*. Tablets each containing paracetamol 450 mg, codeine phosphate 8.1 mg, and caffeine 15 mg.

Panets *(Optrex, UK)*. Each tablet contains paracetamol 500 mg.

Panets Childrens Syrup *(Optrex, UK)*. Each 5 mL contains paracetamol 120 mg in an orange-flavoured basis.

Paracets *(Sussex, UK)*. Tablets each containing paracetamol 500 mg.

Paraclear Tablets *(Nicholas, UK)*. Each contain paracetamol 500 mg. **Junior Paraclear Tablets** each contain paracetamol 120 mg.

Penetrol Catarrh Lozenges *(Crookes Healthcare, UK)*. Each contains menthol 5 mg, ammonium chloride 25 mg, phenylephrine hydrochloride 5 mg, and creosote 1 mg.

Penetrol Inhalant *(Crookes Healthcare, UK)*. Contains menthol 17.5%, cajuput oil 2.5%, lavender oil 8%, eucalyptus oil 7.5%, otto lavender 4%, peppermint oil 0.2%.

Pennine Eye Drops *(Thornton & Ross, UK)*. Contain zinc sulphate 0.05% and distilled witch hazel 5%.

Persomnia *(Ashe, UK)*. Tablets each containing paracetamol 500 mg and codeine phosphate 8 mg.

Pharmacia Dry Skin Treatment *(Vitalia, UK)*. **Face Cream** contains urea 4% and sodium chloride 4%. **Body Lotion** and **Dry Zone Cream** both contain urea 10% and lactic acid 5%.

Phensic *(Beecham Proprietaries, UK)*. Each tablet contains aspirin 325 mg and caffeine 22 mg.

Phillips Iron Tonic *(Phillips Yeast, UK)*. Tablets each containing iron (as saccharated ferrous carbonate) 20 mg, dried yeast 170 mg, vitamin C 10 mg, vitamin B_1 160 µg, vitamin B_2 300 µg, and nicotinic acid 2 mg.

Phillips Tonic Yeast *(Phillips Yeast, UK)*. Each tablet of brewers' yeast contains thiamine hydrochloride 110 µg, riboflavine 200 µg, nicotinic acid 1.4 mg, pyridoxine 9 µg, calcium pantothenate 12 µg, and other vitamins natural to brewers' yeast.

pHiso-Ac *(WinPharm, UK)*. Cream containing colloidal sulphur 6.4% and resorcinol 1.5%.

pHisoDerm *(WinPharm, UK)*. Contains lanolin derivatives.

pHisoHex Lotion *(WinPharm, UK)*. Active ingredients: salicylic acid 0.5%, industrial methylated spirit 25.4%.

pHisoHex Medicated Face Wash *(WinPharm, UK)*. Active ingredient: triclosan 0.5%.

pHisoHex Tissues *(WinPharm, UK)*. Active ingredient: salicylic acid 0.5%.

Pickles Healthy Feet Cream *(Pickles, UK)*. Contains glycerol 5%, menthol 1.5%, undecylenic acid 2.0%, and dibromopropamidine isethionate 0.15%.

Pickles Mouth Treatment *(Pickles, UK)*. Contains iodoform 0.05% and tannic acid 2%.

Pickles Ointment for Corns, Callouses and Hard Skin *(Pickles, UK)*. Contains salicylic acid 50%.

Pickles SCR *(Pickles, UK)*. Contains salicylic acid 1.5%.

Pickles Toothache Tincture *(Pickles, UK)*. Contains lignocaine hydrochloride 0.7% and clove oil 10%.

Placidex *(De Witt, UK)*. Contains paracetamol 240 mg in each 10 mL.

Potter's Catarrh Pastilles *(Booker Health, UK)*. Contain sylvestris pine oil 0.41%, pumilio pine oil 0.41%, eucalyptus oil 0.02%, creosote 0.2%, menthol 0.83%, thymol 0.02%, and aqueous extractive from althaea 0.5%.

Potter's Childrens Cough Pastilles *(Booker Health, UK)*. Honey 6%, glycerol 1.5%, menthol 0.03%, and creosote 0.008%.

Potter's Dermacreme Ointment *(Potter's Herbal Supplies, UK)*. Menthol 0.015%, methyl salicylate 3%, liquefied phenol 1%, starch 8%, zinc oxide 8%, hard paraffin 5%, wool fat 3.25%, and yellow soft paraffin to 100%.

Potter's Glycerin of Thymol Pastilles *(Booker Health, UK)*. Contain thymol 0.04%, menthol 0.03%, cineole 0.06%, pine oil 0.02%, glycerol 3%, and menthyl salicylate 0.004%.

Potter's Menthol and Eucalyptus Pastilles *(Booker Health, UK)*. Contain menthol 0.8% and eucalyptus oil 0.6%.

Potter's Psoriasis Ointment *(Potter's Herbal Supplies, UK)*. Starch 5%, sublimed sulphur 7%, zinc oxide 7%, 35% alcoholic extractive (1–1) from

Poke Root 0.5%, phenols 0.18%, lanolin 28%, and yellow soft paraffin to 100%.

Potter's Skin Clear Ointment *(Potter's Herbal Supplies, UK).* Phenols 0.33%, starch 17%, sulphur sublimed 5%, zinc oxide 23%, and yellow soft paraffin to 100%.

Potter's Varicose Ointment *(Potter's Herbal Supplies, UK).* Cade oil 2.3%, emulsifying wax 2.4%, hamamelis liquid extract 7.4%, hard paraffin 1.85%, wool alcohols 1.48%, zinc oxide 3.57%, and yellow soft paraffin to 100%.

Powerin *(Whitehall, UK).* Tablets each containing paracetamol 200 mg, caffeine 45 mg, and aspirin 300 mg.

PR Tablets *(Boots, UK).* Each tablet contains aspirin 250 mg, paracetamol 125 mg, and caffeine 25 mg.

Preparation H *(Whitehall, UK).* **Ointment** containing the alcohol-soluble extract of 2 g of live yeast cells per g (Bio-Dyne) and shark-liver oil 3%. **Suppositories** each containing the alcohol-soluble extract of 480 mg of live yeast cells and shark-liver oil 72 mg.

Procol *(Wellcome, UK).* Sustained-action capsules each containing phenylpropanolamine hydrochloride 50 mg.

Proctors' Pinelyptus Pastilles *(Ernest Jackson, UK).* Contain menthol 0.548%, eucalyptus oil 0.842%, abietis oil 0.12%, and sylvestris pine oil 0.12%.

Pro-Hyd 50 *(E.C.M. Laboratories, UK).* Capsules each containing procaine hydrochloride 50 mg and haematoporphyrin hydrochloride 200 μg.

Pronel *(Menley & James, UK).* Capsules each containing gelatin 320 mg.

Propa PH Medicated Skin Cleanser *(Christy, UK).* Active constituents: benzethonium chloride 0.05% and benzoic acid 0.1875%.

Pro-Plus Tablets *(Ashe, UK).* Each contains caffeine 50 mg.

Q-Guard Cream *(Cupal, UK).* Active ingredients: cetrimide 0.35% and benzalkonium chloride solution 0.3%.

Q-Panol Elixir *(Cupal, UK).* Contains in each 5 ml paracetamol 120 mg.

Quick Action Cough Cure *(Spencer, UK).* Each dose provides dextromethorphan hydrobromide 3.75 mg and guaiphenesin 25 mg.

Radian-B Liniment *(Fisons, UK).* Contains menthol 1.4%, camphor 0.6%, aspirin 1.2%, and methyl salicylate 0.6% in a spirit base.

Radian-B Rub *(Fisons, UK).* Contains menthol 2.54%, camphor 1.41%, methyl salicylate 0.42%, and camphor oil 0.32%.

Radian-B Warm-up *(Fisons, UK).* Contains capsicum oleoresin 0.1% and methyl salicylate 5% in a cream base.

Ralgex Cream *(Beecham Proprietaries, UK).* Contains methyl nicotinate 1% and capsicin 0.12%.

Ralgex Freeze Spray *(Beecham Proprietaries, UK).* Active ingredients: glycol monosalicylate 4.8%, trichlorofluoromethane 77.35%, and dichlorodifluoromethane 13.65%.

Ralgex Low Odour Spray *(Beecham Proprietaries, UK).* Contains glycol monosalicylate 6% and methyl nicotinate 1.6%.

Ralgex Spray *(Beecham Proprietaries, UK).* Contains glycol monosalicylate 4.8%, ethyl salicylate 4.8%, methyl salicylate 0.96%, and methyl nicotinate 1.6%.

Rayglo BKB *(Cupal, UK).* Each tablet contains buchu extract 10 mg and methylene blue 4 mg.

Red Kooga *(English Grains, UK).* A range of preparations containing Korean panax ginseng.

Reguletts *(Cupal, UK).* Tablets each containing phenolphthalein 120 mg in a chocolate basis.

Rennie *(Nicholas, UK).* Tablets each containing calcium carbonate 680 mg and light magnesium carbonate 80 mg.

Rennie Plus *(Nicholas, UK).* Tablets each containing magnesium hydroxide 100 mg, aluminium hydroxide and magnesium carbonate 275 mg (combined), and activated methylpolysiloxane 250 mg.

Replavite *(Sussex, UK).* Contains pyridoxine hydrochloride 100 mg, magnesium stearate, and starch.

Ress-Q Pastilles *(Ernest Jackson, UK).* Each contains benzalkonium chloride solution 0.094%, tinct. benzoin co. 0.75%, and menthol 0.15%.

Rhuaka Digestive Syrup *(Waterhouse, UK).* Each 5 mL contains cascara liquid extract 0.05 mL, rhubarb concentrated infusion 0.05 mL, compound cardamom tincture 0.018 mL, senna concentrated infusion 0.15 mL, and liquorice liquid extract 0.075 mL.

Rinstead Gel *(Kirby-Warrick, UK).* Contains benzocaine 2% and chloroxylenol 0.106%.

Rinstead Pastilles *(Kirby-Warrick, UK).* Each contains menthol 0.37 mg and chloroxylenol 0.75 mg.

St. James' Balm *(Medico-Biological Laboratories, UK).* Contains zinc oxide 20%, ichthammol 2.8%, urea 0.1%, and salicylic acid 0.1%.

Sanderson's Cough Linctus *(Sandersons, UK).* Contains in each 5 mL compound cardamom tincture 0.2 mL and citric acid 1.4 mg.

Sanderson's Throat Specific *(Sandersons, UK).* **Mixture** contains in each 5 mL squill extract 0.025 mL, capsicum liquid extract 0.025 mL, quassia extract 0.008 mL, and acetic acid 0.113 mL. **Pastilles** each contain honey 145 mg, squill vinegar 96 mg, capsicum oleoresin 19 μg, tolu tincture 3 mg, menthol 1.5 mg, benzoic acid 0.966 mg, eucalyptus oil 0.376 mg, and cinnamic acid 37.5 μg.

Savlon Antiseptic Cream *(Care, UK).* Contains cetrimide 0.5% and chlorhexidine gluconate 0.1%.

Savlon Antiseptic Disinfectant *(Care, UK).* Contains chlorhexidine gluconate 0.3% and cetrimide 3%.

Savlon Baby Cream *(Care, UK).* Contains cetrimide 0.5%.

Savlon Dry First Aid Spray *(Care, UK).* Aerosol containing povidone-iodine 0.5%.

Savlon Nappy Rash Cream *(Care, UK).* Contains cetrimide 10% and dimethicone 0.3%.

Savory & Moore Antihistamine Cream *(Savory & Moore, UK).* Contains diphenhydramine hydrochloride 2% and menthol 1%.

Savory & Moore Antiseptic Cream *(Savory & Moore, UK).* Contains chlorhexidine gluconate 0.05% and cetrimide 0.5%.

Savory & Moore Cherry Cough Linctus *(Savory & Moore, UK).* Each 5 mL contains wild cherry syrup 2.25 mL, squill oxymel 0.5 mL, and ipecacuanha tincture 0.25 mL in a syrup base.

Savory & Moore Cream of Calamine *(Savory & Moore, UK).* Contains calamine 10% and mepyramine maleate 2%.

Scholl Antiseptic Foot Balm *(Scholl, UK).* Active ingredient: halquinol 0.4%.

Scholl Athlete's Foot Gel *(Scholl, UK).* Contains tolnaftate 1%. **Scholl Athlete's Foot Powder, Solution**, and **Spray Liquid** contain the same active ingredient.

Scholl Corn and Callous Salve *(Scholl, UK).* Contains salicylic acid 12.5% and eucalyptus oil 1%.

Scholl Corn Removing Liquid *(Scholl, UK).* Active ingredients: salicylic acid 11.25% and camphor 2.8%.

Scholl Fixo Corn Plasters *(Scholl, UK).* The spread material contains salicylic acid 40%.

Scholl Zino Pads *(Scholl, UK).* Plasters with medicated disks impregnated with salicylic acid 12% or 40%.

Scott's Emulsion *(Beecham Proprietaries, UK).* Each 10 mL contains cod-liver oil to provide vitamin A 1415 I.U. and vitamin D 175 I.U.

Sea-legs *(Evans Medical, UK).* Tablets each containing meclozine hydrochloride 12.5 mg.

Seba Med *(Wellcome, UK).* Soap-free **Liquid Cleanser** contains amino acids, nicotinic acid, nicotinamide, lactic acid, vitamin B_6, vitamin H, and vitamin F. Soap-free **Cleansing Bar** contains amino acids, cholesterol, lecithin, phosphatides, glycerides, and vitamins.

Secaderm Salve *(Fisons, UK).* Active ingredients: phenol 2.4%, terebene 5.25%, melaleuca oil 5.6%, turpentine oil 6%, and resin 26%.

Secron *(De Witt, UK).* Each 5 mL contains ephedrine hydrochloride 6 mg and vinegar of ipecacuanha 208 mg.

Setlers *(Beecham Proprietaries, UK).* **Tablets** each containing calcium carbonate 534 mg and magnesium hydroxide 160 mg. **Extra Strength Tablets** each containing dried aluminium hydroxide 375 mg and magnesium hydroxide 375 mg. **Liquid** contains, in each 5 mL, dried aluminium hydroxide 222 mg and magnesium hydroxide 204 mg.

Seven Seas *(Seven Seas, UK).* Consists of cod-liver oil.

Seven Seas Capsules *(Seven Seas, UK).* Each contains 0.32 mL of cod-liver oil, providing vitamin A 670 units, vitamin D 67 units, and vitamin E 0.3 units.

Seven Seas Orange Syrup *(Seven Seas, UK).* Active ingredients per 10 mL: cod liver oil 2.8 g, vitamin A 4000 units, vitamin B_6 0.7 mg, vitamin C 35 mg, vitamin D 400 units, and vitamin E 3 mg, with concentrated orange juice and polyunsaturates in a syrup base.

Simpkins Bronchial Catarrh Lozenges *(Simpkin, UK).* Contain creosote 0.15%.

Simpkins Throat and Chest Lozenges *(Simpkin, UK).* Contain menthol 0.12% and eucalyptus oil 0.048%.

Simpson's Foot Ointment *(Medico-Biological Laboratories, UK).* Active ingredients: sublimed sulphur 3%, zinc oxide 0.25%, zinc stearate 1.67%.

Sine-Off *(Wellcome, UK).* Each tablet contains aspirin 325 mg, phenylpropanolamine hydrochloride 12.5 mg, and chlorpheniramine maleate 2 mg.

Skintex Medicinal Cream *(Lloyd, Aimee, UK).* Chloroxylenol 0.25%, glycerol 18%, castor oil 10%, and camphor 0.5%.

Slim-Line *(Thompson Medical, UK).* Chewing gum containing benzocaine 6 mg in each tablet.

Sloan's Liniment *(Warner-Lambert, UK).* Contains methyl salicylate 2.65%, camphor 0.63%, pine oil 6.77%, turpentine oil 48.8%, and oleoresin capsicum 0.61%.

Snowfire Healing Tablet *(Pickles, UK).* Contains benzoin 0.02%, citronella oil 0.06%, thyme oil 0.02%, clove oil 0.04%, cade oil 0.04%, and yellow soft paraffin basis 70.33%.

Solarcaine Cream *(Kirby-Warrick, UK)*. Benzocaine 1% and triclosan 0.2%. **Solarcaine Lotion**. Benzocaine 0.5% and triclosan 0.2%. **Solarcaine Spray**. Benzocaine 5% and triclosan 0.1%.

Solprin *(Reckitt & Colman Pharmaceuticals, UK)*. Tablets each containing aspirin 300 mg, calcium carbonate 100 mg, citric acid 30 mg, and saccharin sodium 3 mg.

Solution 41 *(Innoxa, UK)*. Contains salicylic acid 0.07% and triclosan 0.05%.

Soothake *(Pickles, UK)*. Contains benzocaine 7.5% and clove oil 4.0%.

Sovol Liquid *(Carter-Wallace, UK)*. Each 5 mL contains aluminium hydroxide 200 mg, magnesium hydroxide 200 mg, and dimethicone 25 mg.

Sovol Tablets *(Carter-Wallace, UK)*. Each contains aluminium hydroxide-magnesium carbonate co-dried gel 300 mg, magnesium hydroxide 100 mg, and dimethicone 25 mg.

Spreeze *(Tillotts, UK)*. Spray containing dichlorodifluoromethane 15% and trichlorofluoromethane 85%.

Sterotabs *(Boots, UK)*. Tablets each containing sodium dichloroisocyanurate 17 mg.

Stingose *(Chancellor, UK)*. Spray containing aluminium sulphate 20%.

Stomosol Liquid Concentrate *(Thackray, UK)*. Chlorhexidine gluconate 1%, benzalkonium chloride solution (50%) 10%.

Sucrets *(Beecham Proprietaries, UK)*. Throat lozenges each containing hexylresorcinol 2.4 mg.

Sunspot Healing Paint *(Surf Ski International, UK)*. Camphor 8%, benzoin 2%, ethylene glycol 0.02%, benzalkonium chloride 0.1%, allantoin 0.4%, isopropyl alcohol (90%) to 100%.

Sure Shield Adult Travel Tablets *(English Grains, UK)*. Each contains chlorbutol 150 mg.

Sure Shield Antibactic Throat Lozenges *(English Grains, UK)*. Each contains tyrothricin 1 mg and cetylpyridinium chloride 1.5 mg.

Sure Shield Bronchial Mixture *(English Grains, UK)*. Each 5 mL contains ammonium bicarbonate 50 mg, squill liquid extract 0.021 mL, ipecacuanha liquid extract 0.0085 mL, senega liquid extract 0.0145 mL, liquorice extract 0.425 mL, glycerol 310 mg, tolu syrup 0.245 mL, capsicin 0.000125 mL, and treacle 1.75 g.

Sure Shield Children's Travel Tablets *(English Grains, UK)*. Each contains chlorbutol 75 mg.

Sure Shield Diarrhoea Mixture *(English Grains, UK)*. Each 5 mL contains sodium bicarbonate 125 mg, light kaolin 470 mg, compound rhubarb tincture 0.0625 mL, catechu tincture 0.125 mL, chalk 32 mg, and aromatic ammonia solution 0.195 mL.

Sure Shield Iodised Throat Tablets *(English Grains, UK)*. Active constituents: iodine (free and combined) 0.0478%, methyl salicylate 0.0617%, phenol (free and combined) 0.379%, menthol 0.228%, citric acid 0.446%, and cetylpyridinium chloride 0.044%.

Sure Shield Mouth Ulcer Tablets *(English Grains, UK)*. Each contains amylmetacresol 500 μg, ascorbic acid 25 mg, and cetylpyridinium chloride 1.5 mg.

Sure Shield Sure-Lax Tablets *(English Grains, UK)*. Tablets each containing phenolphthalein 90 mg and natural raspberry juice.

Swarm *(Pickles, UK)*. Cream containing dibromopropamidine isethionate 0.15% and calamine 10%.

Tabasan *(Ayrton, Saunders, UK)*. Tablets each containing ephedrine hydrochloride 15 mg, theophylline 30 mg, and paracetamol 250 mg.

Tabmint *(Radiol, UK)*. Chewing gum containing silver acetate 6 mg.

TCP First Aid Antiseptic Cream *(Unicliffe, UK)*. TCP Liquid Antiseptic 25%, chloroxylenol 0.5%, and triclosan 0.3%.

TCP Liquid Antiseptic *(Unicliffe, UK)*. An aqueous solution containing phenol 0.175%, halogenated phenols 0.68%, and sodium salicylate 0.052%.

TCP Ointment *(Unicliffe, UK)*. TCP Liquid Antiseptic 6.4%, iodine 0.2%, methyl salicylate 1.3%, precip. sulphur 1.5%, kaolin 8.5%, with camphor 1.3%, tannic acid 0.4%, salicylic acid 0.4%, and glycerol 2.4%.

TCP Throat Pastilles *(Unicliffe, UK)*. Active ingredients: TCP Liquid Antiseptic 10%.

Tellodont *(Tell, UK)*. Gargle and mouthwash tablets each containing sodium benzoate 5%, peppermint oil 0.9%, thymol 0.3%, menthol 1.2%, cinnamon oil 0.3%, methyl salicylate 0.3%, and saccharin 0.1%, in an effervescent basis.

Tellora *(Tell, UK)*. Powder for preparing mouthwash containing menthol, thymol, sodium benzoate, cetrimide, clove oil, aniseed oil, saccharin, sodium bicarbonate, tartaric acid, and empicol.

Terperoin Elixir *(Savory & Moore, UK)*. Each 5 mL contains codeine phosphate 10.4 mg, menthol 5 mg, terpin hydrate 20 mg, in a flavoured syrup basis.

Thornton & Ross Adults Tonic *(Thornton & Ross, UK)*. Each 5 mL contains caffeine hydrate 12.5 mg, calcium glycerophosphate 45 mg, glycerophosphoric acid 0.125 mL, potassium glycerophosphate 44.9 mg, sodium glycerophosphate 22.8 mg, and thiamine hydrochloride 0.5 mg.

Thornton & Ross Childrens Cherry Cough Syrup *(Thornton & Ross, UK)*. Active ingredients in 5 mL: ipecacuanha tincture 0.156 mL and squill oxymel 0.5 mL.

Thornton & Ross Cold and Influenza Mixture *(Thornton & Ross, UK)*. Active ingredients in 5 mL: ipecacuanha liquid extract 0.0038 mL and ammonium acetate solution strong 0.155 mL.

Thornton & Ross Corn & Wart Solvent *(Thornton & Ross, UK)*. Active ingredients: zinc chloride 1.7% and salicylic acid 12%.

Thornton & Ross Cough Linctus *(Thornton & Ross, UK)*. Active ingredient in 5 mL: squill oxymel 1.66 mL.

Thornton & Ross Fullers Earth Cream *(Thornton & Ross, UK)*. Active ingredients: kaolin, heavy 20.76% and zinc oxide 4.5%.

Thornton & Ross Gargle and Mouthwash *(Thornton & Ross, UK)*. Active ingredients: phenol glycerin 5% and potassium chlorate 2%.

Thornton & Ross Glycerin Ipecacuanha & Squill *(Thornton & Ross, UK)*. Active ingredients in 5 mL: glycerol 0.5 mL, ipecacuanha liquid extract 0.0125 mL, and squill elixir 2.5 mL.

Thornton & Ross Glycerin Lemon and Honey with Glucose *(Thornton & Ross, UK)*. Active ingredients in 5 mL: glycerol 1.11 mL, lemon juice 0.56 mL, purified honey 1.56 g, liquid glucose 280 mg, and citric acid monohydrate 70 mg. **Thornton & Ross Glycerin Lemon and Honey with Glucose and Ipecacuanha** contains in addition ipecacuanha liquid extract 0.01 mL.

Thornton & Ross Gripe Mixture *(Thornton & Ross, UK)*. Active ingredients in 5 mL: strong ginger tincture 0.0063 mL, dill oil 0.005 mL, and sodium bicarbonate 50 mg.

Thornton & Ross Indian Brandee *(Thornton & Ross, UK)*. Contains in each 5 mL rhubarb tincture compound 0.75 mL, capsicum tincture 0.125 mL, and cardamom tincture compound 0.05 mL.

Thornton & Ross Indigestion Mixture *(Thornton & Ross, UK)*. Each 5 mL contains aluminium oxide 150 mg, light magnesium oxide 118 mg, aromatic cardamom tincture 0.05 mL, and peppermint oil 0.0004 mL.

Thornton & Ross Menthol and Wintergreen Cream *(Thornton & Ross, UK)*. Active ingredients: methyl salicylate 12.5% and menthol 1%.

Thornton & Ross Olive Oil and Raspberry Vinegar *(Thornton & Ross, UK)*. Active ingredients in 5 mL: olive oil 2.5 mL, acetic acid 0.1 mL, and raspberry syrup 1.0 mL.

Thornton & Ross Zinc and Castor Oil Cream with Lanolin *(Thornton & Ross, UK)*. Active ingredients: zinc oxide 13.5%, castor oil 9%, wool fat 5%, and purified water 2.25%.

Thornton & Ross Zinc and Castor Oil with Friars Balsam *(Thornton & Ross, UK)*. Active ingredients: friars balsam 1%, zinc oxide 7.4%, and castor oil 49.5%.

Throaties Original Flavour *(Ernest Jackson, UK)*. Active ingredients: benzoin tincture 0.5%, menthol 0.45%, aniseed oil 0.1%, peppermint oil 0.025%, and capsicin 0.001%. **Throaties Catarrh Pastilles.** Active ingredients: menthol 0.6%, abietis pine oil 0.3%, sylvestris pine oil 0.3%, and creosote 0.2%. **Throaties, Lemon Honey & Menthol.** Active ingredients: honey 2.4%, lemon oil 0.3%, and menthol 0.09%. **Throaties, Blackcurrant.** Active ingredients: honey 1.51%, menthol 0.065%, and ascorbic acid 0.2%.

Tiger Balm *(LRC Products, UK)*. Contains paraffin, camphor, menthol, cajuput oil, peppermint oil, and clove oil. **Tiger Balm, Extra Strength** contains, in addition, cinnamon oil.

Tonatexa *(Modern Health Products, UK)*. Contains kola liquid extract, calcium glycerophosphate, ferric chloride tincture, cobalt sulphate, and alcohol.

Top C *(Lane, UK)*. Tablets each containing vitamin C 200 mg.

Topex *(Richardson-Vicks, UK)*. Lotion containing benzoyl peroxide 5%.

Topex Acne Cream *(Richardson-Vicks, UK)*. Contains benzoyl peroxide 5%.

Toptabs *(Sussex, UK)*. Tablets each containing aspirin 350 mg and caffeine 30 mg.

Tramil Capsules *(Whitehall, UK)*. Each contains paracetamol 500 mg and caffeine 32 mg.

Trinity Ointment *(Thornton & Ross, UK)*. Contains zinc oxide 3.75%.

Tunes *(Mars, UK)*. **Blackcurrant Menthol Flavour** contain menthol 0.135%. **Cherry Menthol Flavour** contain menthol 0.135%, tolu balsam 0.03%, camphor 0.007%, and thyme oil 0.002%. **Honey Menthol Flavour** contain menthol 0.135%, anethole 0.114%, cinnamon oil 0.018%, peppermint oil 0.015%, and eucalyptol 0.015%.

Tusana Cough Linctus *(Boots, UK)*. Contains in each 5 mL dextromethorphan hydrobromide 5 mg, ipecacuanha liquid extract 0.025 mg, and tolu syrup 3.71 mL.

Tusana Cough Pastilles *(Boots, UK)*. Contain codeine phosphate 0.13%, cocillana liquid extract 0.2%, ipecacuanha liquid extract 0.4%, squill liquid extract 0.5%, and glycerol 5.8%.

Tussils Cough Lozenges *(Boots, UK)*. Each contains dextromethorphan hydrobromide 2.5 mg and phenylephrine hydrochloride 500 μg.

Tyrobenz Throat Lozenges *(Savory & Moore, UK)*. Each contains benzocaine 5 mg and tyrothricin 1 mg.

Tyrocane Paediatric *(Cupal, UK)*. Lozenges each containing cetylpyridinium chloride 2.5 mg.

Tyrocane Throat Lozenges *(Cupal, UK)*. Tyrothricin 500 µg, cetylpyridinium chloride 2.5 mg, and benzocaine 5 mg.

Ulcaid Tablets *(Cupal, UK)*. Benzocaine 5 mg, cetylpyridinium chloride 2.5 mg, and tyrothricin 0.5 mg.

Unichem Chesty Cough Syrup *(Unichem, UK)*. Each 5 mL contains guaiphenesin 50 mg, liquid glucose 3.18 g, and treacle 1.35 g.

Unichem Childrens Diarrhoea Mixture *(Unichem, UK)*. Each 5 mL contains light kaolin 1 g.

Unichem Cold Relief Capsules *(Unichem, UK)*. Each contains paracetamol 250 mg, phenylpropanolamine hydrochloride 12.5 mg, and dextromethorphan hydrobromide 7.5 mg.

Unichem Day Time Cold Relief *(Unichem, UK)*. Each 30 mL contains pholcodine 10 mg, pseudoephedrine hydrochloride 40 mg, and paracetamol 600 mg.

Unichem Dry Cough Linctus *(Unichem, UK)*. Each 10 mL contains noscapine 15 mg and liquid glucose 8 g.

Unichem Night Time Cold Relief *(Unichem, UK)*. Each 30 mL contains pholcodine 10 mg, pseudoephedrine hydrochloride 40 mg, paracetamol 600 mg and diphenhydramine hydrochloride 10 mg.

Valda Pastilles *(Sterling Health, UK)*. Each contains menthol 3.28 mg, eucalyptol 0.451 mg, thymol 0.016 mg, terpineol 0.016 mg, and guaicol 0.016 mg.

Valderma *(Reckitt & Colman Pharmaceuticals, UK)*. Contains potassium hydroxyquinoline sulphate 0.2% and chlorocresol 0.2%.

Valpeda Foot Balm *(Reckitt & Colman Pharmaceuticals, UK)*. Contains halquinol 0.3%.

Varemoid *(Zyma, UK)*. Each tablet contains hydroxyethylrutosides 100 mg.

Vaseline *(Chesebrough-Pond's, UK)*. Brands of petroleum jelly.

Vaseline Intensive Care *(Chesebrough-Pond's, UK)*. **Cream** contains white petroleum jelly 15% and dimethicones 1%. **Lotion** contains white petroleum jelly 5%, liquid paraffin 4%, and dimethicones 1%.

Veno's Antitussive Cough Mixture *(Beecham Proprietaries, UK)*. Each 10 mL contains noscapine 15 mg and liquid glucose 6 g.

Veno's Expectorant Cough Mixture *(Beecham Proprietaries, UK)*. Each 5-mL dose contains: guaiphenesin 100 mg, liquid glucose 3 g, and treacle 1.35 g, in a base containing aniseed oil, capsicum tincture, and camphor.

Veno's Honey and Lemon *(Beecham Proprietaries, UK)*. Contains in each 5 mL lemon juice 1 mL, honey 250 mg, ammonium chloride 30 mg, and ipecacuanha liquid extract 0.003 mL.

Veno's Night Time *(Beecham Proprietaries, UK)*. Each 5 mL contains chlorpheniramine maleate 2 mg and dextromethorphan hydrobromide 3.75 mg.

Vericap Wart Caps *(Cuxson, Gerrard, UK)*. Plasters bearing an ointment containing podophyllin 20% and linseed oil 20%.

Vicks Coldcare *(Richardson-Vicks, UK)*. Capsules each containing paracetamol 325 mg, dextromethorphan hydrobromide 10 mg, and phenylpropanolamine hydrochloride 12.5 mg.

Vicks Expectorant Cough Syrup *(Richardson-Vicks, UK)*. Each 5 mL contains guaiphenesin 50 mg, sodium citrate 200 mg, and cetylpyridinium chloride 1.25 mg.

Vicks Medinite *(Richardson-Vicks, UK)*. Each 30-mL dose contains ephedrine sulphate 8 mg, doxylamine succinate 7.5 mg, paracetamol 600 mg, dextromethorphan hydrobromide 15 mg, and alcohol 19%.

Vicks Sinex Nasal Spray *(Richardson-Vicks, UK)*. Contains oxymetazoline hydrochloride 0.05%, menthol 0.025%, camphor 0.015%, and eucalyptol 0.0075% in a buffered aqueous solution.

Vicks Vapo-Lem *(Richardson-Vicks, UK)*. Contains paracetamol 500 mg, guaiphenesin 100 mg, phenylephrine hydrochloride 10 mg, and ascorbic acid 50 mg.

Victory V Lozenges *(Barker Dobson, UK)*. Contain menthol 0.08%.

Vitathone Chilblain Cream *(Cupal, UK)*. Contains methyl nicotinate 1.25%, and dimethicone 3%.

Vitathone Chilblain Tablets *(Cupal, UK)*. Each contains acetomenaphthone 7 mg and nicotinic acid 25 mg.

Vocalzone Pastilles *(English Grains, UK)*. Menthol 1%, peppermint oil 0.5%, myrrh 0.25%, and liquorice extract 1.1%.

Wartex Ointment *(Pickles, UK)*. Contains salicylic acid 50% and glycerol 7%.

Wasp-Eze *(International Laboratories, UK)*. An aerosol for insect-bite relief containing mepyramine maleate 0.5% and benzocaine 1%.

Waxaid Ear drops *(Cupal, UK)*. Paradichlorobenzene 2%, chlorbutol 5%, turpentine oil 10%, arachis oil to 100%.

Waxwane Ear Drops *(Thornton & Ross, UK)*. Active ingredients: turpentine oil 15%, terpineol 5%, and chloroxylenol 0.2%.

Witch Doctor *(Ethichem, UK)*. Gel containing witch hazel liquid extract 81.5%.

Witch Stik *(Ethichem, UK)*. Witch hazel extract containing not less than 65% alcohol.

Woodward's Gripe Water *(LRC Products, UK)*. Each 5 mL contains dill water, concentrated 0.18 mL, sodium bicarbonate 50 mg, ginger tincture 0.0625 mL, alcohol (90%) 0.246 mL, and syrup 0.75 mL.

X.89 Geriomar *(Pan-American Pharmaceuticals, UK)*. Capsules each containing para-aminobenzoic acid 25 mg, haematoporphyrin hydrochloride 250 µg, 2-dimethylaminoethanol hydrogen tartrate 15 mg, with traces of minerals and excipients.

Yeast-Vite *(Beecham Proprietaries, UK)*. Each tablet contains caffeine 50 mg, thiamine hydrochloride 167 µg, riboflavine 167 µg, and nicotinamide 1.75 mg.

Zam-Buk *(Fisons, UK)*. Active ingredients: eucalyptus oil 5%, camphor 1.8%, thyme oil 0.5%, and colophony 2.5%.

Zanthine Tablets *(Approved Prescription Services, UK)*. Each contains caffeine 30 mg and dextrose 150 mg.

Zefringe Sachets *(Evans Medical, UK)*. Each contains paracetamol 800 mg and caffeine 60 mg in an effervescent basis.

Zubes Blackcurrant Cough Lozenges *(Roberts, UK)*. Contain aniseed 0.04% and menthol 0.08%. **Zubes Cherry**. Contain aniseed 0.05% and menthol 0.1%. **Zubes Lemon and Honey**. Contain menthol 0.1%, lemon oil 0.22%, citric acid 1.5%, and honey 5%. **Zubes Original**. Contain aniseed 0.2% and menthol 0.3%.

Directory of Manufacturers

The names and addresses of the manufacturers (or distributors) of the products and proprietary medicines mentioned in Martindale are listed below in alphabetical order of the abbreviated names used in the text.

3M Health Care, UK. 3M Health Care Ltd, 1 Morley St, Loughborough, Leics LE11 1EP, England.

3M United Kingdom, UK. 3M United Kingdom PLC, 3M House, Bracknell, Berks RG12 1JV, England.

3M, USA. 3M, 3M Center, St Paul MN 55144, USA.

Aaciphar, Belg. Aaciphar S.A., Ave Marnix 13, 1050 Brussels, Belgium.

Aandersen, Ital. Aandersen Farmaceutisk Institut s.p.a., Viale delle Milizie 12/14, 00192 Rome, Italy.

Abbott, Arg. Abbott S.A., Sarmiento 1113-8° piso, 1041 Buenos Aires, Argentina.

Abbott, Austral. Abbott Australasia Pty Ltd, P.O. Box 101, Cronulla NSW 2230, Australia.

Abbott, Belg. Abbott S.A., Parc Scientifique, rue du Bosquet 2, 1348 Ottignies, Belgium.

Abbott, Canad. Abbott Laboratories Ltd, 6300 ch. Côte de Liesse, Montreal, Quebec H4T 1E3, Canada.

Abbott, Denm. Abbott Laboratories A/S, Bygstubben 15, Trørød, 2950 Vedbaek, Denmark.

Abbott, Fr. Societé Française des Laboratoires Abbott, 6 rue Anatole de la Forge, 75017 Paris, France.

Abbott, Ger. Deutsche Abbott GmbH, Max-Planck-Ring 2, Postfach: 2013, 6200 Wiesbaden-Delkenheim, W. Germany.

Abbott, Ital. Abbott s.p.a., 04010 Campoverde (Latina), Italy.

Abbott, Neth. Abbott B.V., Maalderij 21, 1185 ZB Amstelveen, Netherlands.

Abbott, Norw. Abbott Norge, Nye Vakasv.4, Postboks 85, 1364 Hvalstad, Norway.

Abbott, NZ. Abbott Laboratories (NZ) Ltd, P.O. Box 35-128, Naenae, New Zealand.

Abbott, Philipp. See *Metro, Philipp.*

Abbott, S.Afr. Abbott Laboratories SA (Pty) Ltd, P.O. Box 1616, Johannesburg 2000, S. Africa.

Abbott, Spain. Abbott, Josefa Valcarcel 48, 28027 Madrid, Spain.

Abbott, Swed. Abbott Scandinavia AB, Box 1074, 163 11 Spanga, Sweden.

Abbott, Switz. Abbott SA, Industriestrasse 6, 6301 Zoug, Switzerland.

Abbott, UK. Abbott Laboratories Ltd, Queenborough, Kent ME11 5EL, England.

Abbott, USA. Abbott Laboratories, Pharmaceutical Products Division, North Chicago IL 60064, USA.

ABC, Ital. Istituto Biologico Chemioterapico ABC s.p.a., Viale Thovez 26, 10131 Turin, Italy.

Abdine, UK. Abdine Ltd, 55 Wiltonburn Road, 5th Nitshill Industrial Estate, Glasgow G53 7NY, Scotland.

Abello, Spain. Abello, Julian Camarillo 8, 28037 Madrid, Spain.

Abic, Neth. See *Multi-Pharma, Neth.*

ABM Chemicals, UK. A.B.M. Chemicals Ltd, Poleacre Lane, Woodley, Stockport, Cheshire SK6 1PQ, England.

Acbel, Switz. Lab. Acbel S.A., rue Coulouvrenière 20, 1204 Geneva, Switzerland.

ACF, Neth. ACF Chemiefarma N.V., Straatweg 2, 3604 BB Maarssen, Netherlands.

ACO, Swed. ACO Läkemedel AB, Box 3026, 171 03 Solna, Sweden.

Actipharm, Switz. Actipharm S.àr.l., Case postale 453, 1227 Carouge, Switzerland.

Adam, Austral. See *Nelson, Austral.*

Adams, USA. Adams Laboratories Inc., 3617 Raider Drive, Hurst TX 76053, USA.

Adcock Ingram, S.Afr. Adcock Ingram Laboratories Ltd, Private Bag 1, Industria 2042, S. Africa.

Adenylchemie, Ger. Adenylchemie GmbH Berlin, Salzufer 16, Postfach:100250, 1000 Berlin 10, W. Germany.

Adima, Switz. Adima S.A., Case postale 71, 1211 Geneva 6, Switzerland.

Adria, Canad. Adria Laboratories of Canada Ltd, 4500 Dixie Rd, Mississauga, Ontario L4W 1V7, Canada.

Adria, USA. Adria Laboratories Inc., P.O. Box 16529, Columbus OH 43216, USA.

Adrian-Marinier, Fr. Laboratoires Adrian-Marinier (Adrim), Cedex 29, 92097 Paris-La Defense, France.

Adroka, Neth. See *Hermes, Neth.*

Adroka, Switz. Adroka SA, Case postale, 4123 Allschwil 1, Switzerland.

Adrosanol, Switz. Adrosanol Pharma AG, Industriestrasse 7, 4410 Liestal, Switzerland.

Advanced Care, USA. Advanced Care, USA.

Advanced Medical Nutrition, USA. Advanced Medical Nutrition Inc., P.O. Box 5012, Hayward CA 94540-5012, USA.

Advanced Medical Technologies, Canad. Advanced Medical Technologies Inc., West Royalty Industrial Park, Charlottetown, Prince Edward Island C1E 1B0, Canada.

Aerocid, Fr. Laboratoires de l'Aerocid, 248 bis, rue Gabriel-Peri, 94230 Cachan, France.

Aerosol Marketing & Chemical Co., UK. Aerosol Marketing & Chemical Co., England.

Aesculapius, Ital. Aesculapius Farmaceutici s.r.l., Via Cozzaglio 24, 25128 Brescia, Italy.

AF, Mex. A.F. Laboratorios, Aplicaciones Farmaceuticas S.A., Heriberto Frias No. 1035, Mexico 12 D.F., Mexico.

AFI, Ital. Azienda Farmaceutica Italia, Via A. de Gasperi 47, 21040 Sumirago (VA), Italy.

AFI, Swed. See *Ferring, Swed.*

AFOM, Ital. AFOM Laboratorio Farmacogeno s.r.l. di dott. Bianco & C., Strada Settimo 373, 10156 Turin, Italy.

Agadrian, Spain. Agadrian, Cadiz 5, 03001 Alicante, Spain.

AGIPS, Ital. Azienda Generale Italiana Prodotti Specializzati, Via Amendola 4, 16035 Rapallo (GE), Italy.

AGM, Ger. Aktiengesellschaft für medizinische Produkte (AGM), Sachsenring 37-47, 5000 Cologne 1, W. Germany.

Agpharm, Neth. See *OPG, Neth.*

Agpharm, Switz. Agpharm SA, Reussinsel 28, 6002 Luzern, Switzerland.

Agropharm, UK. Agropharm Ltd, Buckingham House, Church Rd, Penn, High Wycombe, Bucks HP10 8LN, England.

Agua del Carmen, Spain. Agua del Carmen, Avda Estanislao Figueras 4, 43003 Tarragona, Spain.

Aguettant, Fr. Laboratoires Aguettant, 1 ave J.-Carteret, 69007 Lyon, France.

A.H. Marks, UK. A.H. Marks & Co. Ltd, Wyke Lane, Wyke, Bradford, West Yorks BD12 9EJ, England.

Aicardi, Ital. Aicardi Farmaceutici s.r.l., Via Ragazzi del 99 n.5, 40133 Bologna, Italy.

Aima, Ital. Aima derivati s.p.a., 55020 Castelvecchio Pascoli (LU), Italy.

Airkem, USA. Airkem, Division of Airwick Industries Inc., 380 North St, Teterboro NJ 07608, USA.

Ajinomoto, Jpn. Ajinomoto, 1-5-8 Kyobashi, Chuo-ku, Tokyo, Japan.

Akorn, Canad. Akorn Pharmaceuticals Canada Inc., 826 Main St E, Hamilton, Ontario L8M 1L6, Canada.

Akorn, USA. Akorn, Inc., 100 Akorn Drive, Abita Springs LA 70420, USA.

Akzo, UK. Akzo Chemie UK Ltd, Kestrel House, 1-5 Queens Rd, Hersham, Surrey, England.

A.L., Denm. A.L.-Pharma a/s, Emdrupvej 28B, 2100 Copenhagen Ø, Denmark.

A.L., Swed. A.L. Lakemedel AB, Box 260, 131 02 Nacka, Sweden.

Alacan, Spain. Alacan, Capricornio 5, 03006 Alicante, Spain.

Alan Hitchins, UK. Alan Hitchins Pharmaceuticals Ltd, 43 Northside, Clapham Common, London SW4 0AA, England.

Alban, Switz. Alban Pharma SA, St. Albantal 34, 4052 Basel, Switzerland.

Albert, S.Afr. See *Hoechst, S.Afr.*

Albert-Farma, Ital. Albert-Farma s.p.a., Strada Statale 17 Km. 22, 67019 Scoppito (AQ), Italy.

Albert-Pharma, Belg. See *Hoechst, Belg.*

Albert-Roussel, Ger. Albert-Roussel Pharma GmbH, Abraham-Lincoln-Strasse 38-42, Postfach: 1160, 6200 Wiesbaden, W. Germany.

Albion, UK. Albion Group Ltd, 113 Station Rd, Hampton, Middx TW12 2DY, England.

Albofarma, Spain. Albofarma, Raco de San Llorens 6-8, Alboraya, 46010 Valencia, Spain.

Albright & Wilson, Eire. Albright & Wilson, Eire.

Albright & Wilson, Marchon Division, UK. Albright & Wilson Ltd, Detergents Group, P.O. Box 3, Oldbury, Warley, West Midlands B68 0NN, England.

Albula, Arg. Albula S.R.L., Hualfin 829, 1424 Buenos Aires, Argentina.

Alcon, Arg. Alcon S.A., Estados Unidos 1852, 1227 Buenos Aires, Argentina.

Alcon, Austral. Alcon Laboratories (Australia) Pty Ltd, P.O. Box 19, Brookvale NSW 2100, Australia.

Alcon, Canad. Alcon Canada Inc., 6500 Kitimat Rd, Mississauga, Ontario L5N 2B8, Canada.

Alcon, Denm. See *Meda, Denm.*

Alcon, Fr. Laboratoires Alcon, B.P. 1137, 31036 Toulouse Cedex, France.

Alcon, Ger. Alcon Pharma GmbH, Blankreutestr. 1, 7800 Freiburg, Germany.

Alcon, Ital. Alcon Italia s.p.a., V.le della Liberazione 18, 20124 Milan, Italy.

Alcon, Neth. See *Bipharma, Neth.*

Alcon, Norw. See *Meda, Norw.*

Alcon, S.Afr. Alcon Laboratories SA (Pty) Ltd, P.O. Box 75073, Gardenview 2047, S. Africa.

Alcon, Spain. Alcon Iberhis, Aragoneses 7 (Plg Ind.), Alcobendas, 28100 Madrid, Spain.

Alcon, Swed. Alcon Lakemedel Nordiska AB, Box 12233, 102 26 Stockholm, Sweden.

Alcon, Switz. Alcon Pharmaceuticals Ltd, Case postale 80, 6330 Cham, Switzerland.

Alcon, UK. Alcon Laboratories (UK) Ltd, Imperial Way, Watford, Herts WD2 4YR, England.

Alcon Laboratories, USA. Alcon Laboratories Inc., 6201 South Freeway, P.O. Box 1959, Fort Worth TX 76134, USA.

Alcon PR, USA. Alcon (Puerto Rico) Inc., P.O. Box 1959, Fort Worth TX 76101, USA.

Alcon-Couvreur, Belg. Alcon-Couvreur S.A., Rijksweg 6, 2670 Puurs, Belgium.

Alcor, Spain. Alcor, Plg Ind. de Henares, Guadalajara, Spain.

Aldo, Spain. Aldo Union, Angel Guimera 123-5, Esplugas de Llobregat, Barcelona, Spain.

Ale, Spain. Ale, Pasaje Jaime Roig 26-8, 08028 Barcelona, Spain.

Alembic Products, UK. Alembic Products Ltd, Oaklands House, Oaklands Drive, Sale, Manchester M33 1NS, England.

Alet, Arg. C.I.yE. Alet S.A., Dorrego 1068, 1651 San Andres, Buenos Aires, Argentina.

Alfa Farmaceutici, Ital. Alfa Farmaceutici s.p.a., Via Ragazzi del 99 n.5, 40133 Bologna, Italy.

Alfa, UK. Alfa Chemicals Ltd, Broadway House, 7 & 9 Shute End, Wokingham, Berks RG11 1BH, England.

Alfarma, Spain. Alfarma, Ctra Carabanchel-Toledo km 2, 28025 Madrid, Spain.

ALK, Denm. Allergologisk Laboratorium A/S, Ved Amagerbanen 23, 2300 Copenhagen, Denmark.

Alk, Neth. See *Lundbeck, Neth.*

ALK, Norw. See *Lundbeck, Norw.*

Alkaloid, Jug. Alkaloid, Bulevar E. Kardelja 12, PP 572, 91000 Skopje, Jugoslavia.

Alkaloida Chemical Factory, Hung. Alkaloida Chemical Factory, P.O. Box 1, 4441 Tiszavasvari, Hungary.

Allard, Fr. Laboratoires Allard, 10 ave de Messine, 75008 Paris, France.

Allcock, Denm. See *Cosmic, Denm.*

Allcock, Norw. See *Collett, Norw.*

Allen & Hanburys, Austral. See *Glaxo, Austral.*

Allen & Hanburys, Canad. Allen & Hanburys, 1025 The Queensway, Toronto, Ontario M8Z 5S6, Canada.

Allen & Hanburys, S.Afr. See *Glaxo, S.Afr.*

Allen & Hanburys, UK. Allen & Hanburys Ltd, Horsenden House, Oldfield Lane North, Greenford, Middx UB6 0HB, England.

Allergan, Austral. Allergan Pharmaceuticals, P.O. Box 348, Artarmon NSW 2064, Australia.

Allergan, Belg. See *de Bournonville, Belg.*

Allergan, Canad. Allergan Inc., 2255 Sheppard Ave E., Suite 441 West, Willowdale, Ontario M2J 4Y3, Canada.

Allergan, Denm. See *Biofarma, Denm.*

Allergan, Fr. Laboratoires Allergan, B.P. 58, Parc d'activities des Tanneries, 67382 Lingolsheim Cedex, France.

Allergan, Ger. Pharm-Allergan GmbH, Greschbachstr. 1, Postfach: 5180, 7500 Karlsruhe 41, W. Germany.

Allergan, Ital. Allergan s.p.a., Via del Mare 131, 00040 Pomezia (Rome), Italy.

Allergan, Neth. See *Bournonville, Neth.*

Allergan, S.Afr. Allergan Pharmaceuticals, P.O. Box 95101, Grant Park 2051, S. Africa.

Allergan, Swed. Allergan International, Turebergsvagen 5, 191 47 Sollentuna, Sweden.

Allergan, UK. Allergan Ltd, Turnpike Rd, Cressex Industrial Estate, High Wycombe, Bucks HP12 3NR, England.

Allergan, USA. Allergan Pharmaceuticals Inc., 2525 Dupont Dr., Irvine CA 92713, USA.

Allergomed, Switz. Allergomed SA, Drosselstrasse 47, 4059 Basel, Switzerland.

Allergopharma, Ger. Allergopharma Joachim Ganzer KG, Hermann-Korner-Strasse 52, Postfach: 1109, 2057 Reinbek, Germany.

Almirall, Spain. Almirall, Cardoner 68-74, 08024 Barcelona, Spain.

Alpha, Ger. Alpha Therapeutic GmbH, Voltastr. 10, Postfach: 1107, 6070 Langen, Germany.

Alpha, Swed. Alpha Therapeutic Scandinavia, Box 124, 150 13 Trosa, Sweden.

Alpha Laboratories, UK. Alpha Laboratories Ltd, 40 Parham Drive, Eastleigh, Hants SO5 4NU, England.

Alpha Therapeutic, UK. Alpha Therapeutic UK Ltd, Howlett Way, Fison Way Industrial Estate, Thetford, Norfolk IP24 1HZ, England.

Alpha Therapeutic, USA. Alpha Therapeutic Corp., 2410 Lillyvale Ave, Los Angeles CA 90032, USA.

Alphapharm, Austral. Alphapharm Pty Ltd, P.O. Box 144, Camperdown NSW 2050, Australia.

Also, Ital. Also Laboratori, Dr. Sorbini & C. s.a.s., Viale del Ghisallo 16, 20151 Milan, Italy.

Alter, Spain. Alter, Mateo Inurria 30, 28036 Madrid, Spain.

Alto, USA. Alto Pharmaceuticals Inc., P.O. Box 271369, Tampa FL 33688, USA.

Alza, Neth. See *Pharbil, Neth.*

Alza, Norw. See *Astra, Norw.*

Alza, USA. Alza Corporation, 950 Page Mill Rd, Palo Alto CA 94304, USA.

Amacon, Denm. See *Helge Kjelstrup, Denm.*

Amerchol, USA. Amerchol Corporation, A Unit of CPC International Inc., P.O. Box 351, Talmadge Rd, Edison NJ 08817, USA.

Americal, USA. Americal Pharmaceuticals Inc., 20510 Earlgate St, Walnut CA 91789, USA.

American Chicle, USA. American Chicle Sales Division, Warner-Lambert Co., 201 Tabor Rd, Morris Plains NJ 07950, USA.

American Critical Care, Swed. See *Hässle, Swed.*

American Critical Care, USA. American Critical Care, Division of American Hospital Supply Corp., McGaw Park IL 60085, USA.

American Cyanamid, USA. American Cyanamid Co., P.O. Box 400, Princeton NJ 08540, USA.

American Dermal, USA. American Dermal Corp., 12 Worlds Fair Dr., Somerset NJ 08873, USA.

American Hospital Supply, UK. American Hospital Supply (UK) Ltd, Wallingford Rd, Compton, Newbury, Berks RG16 0QW, England.

American Optical, USA. American Optical, USA.

American Urologicals, USA. American Urologicals, USA.

Amersham International, UK. Amersham International PLC, Amersham Place, Little Chalfont, Bucks HP7 9NA, England.

Ames, Austral. See *Miles, Austral.*

Ames, Canad. Ames Co., Division of Miles Laboratories Ltd, 77 Belfield Rd, Rexdale, Ontario M9W 1G6, Canada.

Ames, S.Afr. See *Bayer, S.Afr.*

Ames, UK. Ames Company, Division of Miles Ltd, P.O. Box 37, Stoke Court, Stoke Poges, Slough SL2 4LY, England.

Ames, USA. Ames Division, Miles Laboratories Inc., 1127 Myrtle St, P.O. Box 70, Elkhart IN 46515, USA.

Amfre-Grant, USA. Amfre-Grant Inc., USA.

Amid, USA. Amid, USA.

Amido, Fr. Laboratoires Amido, 65 r. du Dr-Jenner, 59010 Lille Cedex, France.

Amino, Switz. Amino SA, Althofstrasse 12, 5432 Neuenhof, Switzerland.

Amovon, UK. Amovon Ltd, Tree Tops, 208 Seabridge Lane, Newcastle, Staffs ST5 3LS, England.

Ana, Fr. Laboratoires Ana, 171 av. Charles-de-Gaulle, 92521 Neuilly-sur-Seine Cedex, France.

Anabolic, Canad. See *Gordon Piller, Canad.*

Anaquest, Canad. Anaquest, Division of Canadian Oxygen Ltd, 1 Vulcan St, Suite 201, Rexdale, Ontario M9W 1L3, Canada.

Anaquest, UK. Anaquest Ltd, England.

Anaquest, USA. Anaquest, Division of BOC Inc., 2005 W. Beltline Highway, Madison WI 53713, USA.

Anasco, Ger. Anasco GmbH, Aarstrasse 1, Postfach: 1240, 6200 Wiesbaden, Germany.

Anca, Canad. See *Sandoz, Canad.*

Ancalab, Canad. Ancalab, 111 Consumers Dr., Whitby, Ontario L1N 5Z5, Canada.

Andalucia, Spain. Andalucia Farmaceutica, C/Huelma, 5 Polg los Olivares, 23009 Jaen, Spain.

Andard-Mount, UK. Andard-Mount Co. Ltd, West Africa House, Ashbourne Road, Ealing, London, W5 3QP, England.

Andersen, Norw. Jan F. Andersen, Postboks 1132 Flattum, 3501 Hønefoss, Norway.

Anderson, Denm. Karen Hofman Anderson, Karlslunde Parkvej 54, 2690 Karlslunde, Denmark.

Andreu, Spain. Andreu, Moragas 15, 08022 Barcelona, Spain.

Andromaco, Arg. Andromaco S.A.C.I., Ing. Huergo 1145, 1107 Buenos Aires, Argentina.

Andromaco, Spain. Andromaco, Azcona 31, 28028 Madrid, Spain.

Angelini, Ital. Aziende Chimiche Riunite Angelini Francesco s.p.a., Viale Amelia 70, 00181 Rome, Italy.

Angelini, Switz. See *Galenica, Switz.*

Angelopharm, Ger. Angelopharm GmbH, Frohmestrasse 112, 2000 Hamburg 61, Germany.

Anglo-French Laboratories, Canad. Anglo-French Laboratories, 582 rue Orly, Dorval, Quebec H9P 1E9, Canada.

Anphar-Rolland, Fr. Laboratoires Anphar-Rolland, bd de France, 91000 Evry Ville nouvelle, France.

Anstead, UK. D.F. Anstead Ltd, Radford Way, Billericay, Essex CM12 0DE, England.

Antec, UK. Antec AH International Ltd, Windham Rd, Chilton Industrial Estate, Sudbury, Suffolk CO10 6XD, England.

Antibioticos, Spain. Antibioticos, Bravo Murillo 38, 28015 Madrid, Spain.

Antipol, Ital. Laboratorio di Chimica Medica dell' Antipol s.n.c., Via S. Benigno 26, 10154 Turin, Italy.

Antonetto, Ital. Marco Antonetto s.r.l., Via Arsenale 29, 10121 Turin, Italy.

Aplin & Barrett, UK. Aplin & Barrett, England.

Apodan, Denm. Apodan Medicinalvarer, Englandsvej 382A, 2770 Kastrup, Denmark.

Apotex, Canad. Apotex Inc., 150 Signet Dr., Weston, Ontario M9L 1T9, Canada.

Apothekernes Laboratorium, Norw. Apothekernes Laboratorium A.S., Harbitzalleen 3, 0275 Oslo 2, Norway.

Applipharm, Denm. See *A.L., Denm.*

Applipharm, Fr. Laboratoires Applipharm, 468 chemin du Littoral, 13016 Marseille, France.

Applipharm, Neth. See *Pharma-Import, Neth.*

Applipharm, Switz. See *Doetsch, Grether, Switz.*

Approved Prescription Services, UK. Approved Prescription Services Ltd, Whitcliffe House, Whitcliffe Rd, Cleckheaton, West Yorkshire BD19 3BZ, England.

Aprofa, Spain. Aprofa, Plg. Glorias Catalanas, Vial C15, Tarrasa, 08223 Barcelona, Spain.

APS, Ger. APS-Apotheker H. Starke GmbH, Bahnhofstr. 7, Postfach: 11 68, 8130 Starnberg, Germany.

Aqualon, UK. Aqualon, 20 Red Lion St, London WC1R 4PB, England.

Arcadian of Devon, UK. Arcadian of Devon Ltd, Crediton, Devon EX17 3AP, England.

Arcis-Toledano, Fr. Laboratoires Arcis-Toledano, 5 place Gabriel-Peri, 92000 Nanterre, France.

Arco, Norw. See *Remed, Norw.*

Arco, USA. Arco Pharmaceuticals Inc., 105 Orville Dr., Bohemia NY 11716, USA.

Arden, UK. Elizabeth Arden Ltd, 13 Hanover Sq., London W1R 0PA, England.

Arderiu, Spain. Arderiu, Napoles 166, 08013 Barcelona, Spain.

Ardeypharm, Ger. Ardeypharm Heilmittelgesellschaft mbH, Loerfeldstr. 20, Postfach: 107, 5804 Herdecke, Germany.

Ardeypharm, Switz. See *Medipharm, Switz.*

Ardix, Fr. Laboratoires Ardix, 25 rue Eugene Vignat, 45000 Orleans, France.

Arduin, Ital. Lab. Chim. Farm. Arduin s.n.c., Stradone S.Agostino 26/1, 16123 Genoa, Italy.

Areu, Spain. Areu, Ctra Madrid Valencia, KM 235, Arganda del Rey, 28500 Madrid, Spain.

Argentia, Arg. Argentia S.A.C.I.F.I., Larrea 790, 1030 Buenos Aires, Argentina.

Arik, Fr. Laboratoires Arik, 35 av. Saint-Jean, 06400 Cannes, France.

Aristegui, Spain. Aristegui Dr, Alameda de Urquijo 22, Bilbao, 48008 Vizcaya, Spain.

Ariston, Arg. Ariston S.A., O'Connor 555/59, 1704 Ramos Mejia, Buenos Aires, Argentina.

Arkopharma, Fr. Laboratoires Arkopharma, B.P. 28, 06511 Carros Cedex, France.

Arlo, USA. Arlo Interamerican Corporation of Puerto Rico, P.O. Box 1775, Hato Rey PR 00919, Puerto Rico.

Armand-Frappier, Canad. Institut Armand-Frappier, 527 boul. des Prairies, C.P. 310, Laval, Quebec H7N 4Z9, Canada.

Armedic, Denm. Armedic ApS Laegemidler, Islevbrovej 2, 2610 Rodovre, Denmark.

Armour, Belg. See *Christiaens, Belg.*

Armour, Denm. See *Mecobenzon, Denm.*

Armour, Ger. Armour Pharma GmbH, Augustastr. 32, Postfach: 840, 3440 Eschwege, Germany.

Armour, Ital. Armour Medicamenta s.p.a., Viale Europa 11, 21040 Origgio (VA), Italy.

Armour, Neth. See *Tramedico, Neth.*

Armour, S.Afr. See *Berk, S.Afr.*

Armour, Spain. Armour Iberica, Francisco Sancha 8, 28034 Madrid, Spain.

Armour, Switz. See *Pharmakon, Switz.*

Armour, UK. Armour Pharmaceutical Co. Ltd, St Leonard's House, St Leonard's Rd, Eastbourne, East Sussex BN21 3YG, England.

Armour, USA. Armour Pharmaceutical Co., 303 South Broadway, Tarrytown NY 10591, USA.

Armour-Montagu, Fr. See *Rorer, Fr.*

Armstrong, Arg. Armstrong S.A.C.I.F., Joaquín V. Gonzalez 653, 1407 Buenos Aires, Argentina.

Arnaldi, Ital. Arnaldi Emilio, Via Oldoini 55, 19100 La Spezia, Italy.

Arnaldi-Uscio, Ital. Colonia della Salute Carlo Arnaldi s.p.a., 16030 Uscio (GE), Italy.

Aron, Belg. See *Byk, Belg.* and *Lipha, Belg.*

Aron, Fr. S.N.E. des Laboratoires Aron, 116 rue Carnot, 92150 Suresnes Cedex, France.

Aron, Neth. See *Zyma, Neth.*

Arsac, Fr. Laboratoires Arsac, Parc de Sophia-Antipolis, Z.I. Les Croutons, 06600 Antibes, France.

Artesan, Ger. Artesan Pharma GmbH, Wendlandstrasse 1, Postfach: 52, 3130 Lüchow, W. Germany.

Artesan, Switz. See *Lubapharm, Switz.* and *Kogrere, Switz.*

Arther, USA. Arther, Inc., Box 335, Mountain Lakes NJ 07046, USA.

Arun, UK. Arun Products Ltd, The Square, Barnham, Bognor Regis, West Sussex PO22 0HB, England.

Arza, Spain. Arza, Leon XIII 27, Gijon, 33209 Asturias, Spain.

Arznei Müller-Rorer, Ger. See *Rorer, Ger.*

Arzneimittel Huls, Ger. Arzneimittelfabrik Huls Dr. Albin Hense Nachf., Hemelinger Bahnhofstrasse 13, Postfach: 448660, 2800 Bremen 44, Germany.

A.S., Ger. A.S. Biologische und pharmazeutische Produkte GmbH, Kandelstrasse 10, 7815 Kirchzarten, Germany.

AS, Switz. See *Galenica, Switz.*

Asche, Ger. Asche AG, Fischersallee 49, Postfach: 50 0132, 2000 Hamburg 50, W. Germany.

Ascher, USA. B.F. Ascher & Co. Inc., 15501 W 109th St, Lenexa KS 66219, USA.

Ascot, Austral. Ascot Pharmaceuticals Pty Ltd, P.O. Box 518, North Sydney NSW 2060, Australia.

Ascot, USA. Ascot Pharmaceuticals Inc., 7701 N Austin Ave, Skokie IL 60077, USA.

Asens, Spain. Asens, Alava 61, 08005 Barcelona, Spain.

Ashe, Switz. See *Galenica, Switz.*

Ashe, UK. Ashe Consumer Products Ltd, Ashetree Works, Kingston Rd, Leatherhead, Surrey KT22 7JZ, England.

Askit, UK. Askit Laboratories Ltd, 93 Saracen St, Glasgow G22 5HX, Scotland.

Aslan, Neth. See *Bipharma, Neth.*

Associated Hospital Supply, UK. Associated Hospital Supply, P.O. Box 4, Pershore, Worcs, England.

Association Nationale, Fr. Association Nationale pour la distribution des fractions plasmatiques humaines, 37 rue Violet, 75015 Paris, France.

Asta, Belg. See *de Bournonville, Belg.*

Asta, Denm. See *Hermann, Denm.* and *Schering, Denm.*

Asta, Ger. See *Asta Pharma, Ger.*

Asta, Neth. See *Multi-Pharma, Neth.*

Asta, Norw. See *Sunde, Norw.*

Asta Pharma, Ger. Asta Pharma AG, Weismullerstr. 45, Postafch: 100503, 6000 Frankfurt 1, Germany.

Asta-Werke, Swed. See *Degussa, Swed.*

Astier, Fr. Laboratoires du Dr. P. Astier, 42 rue du Dr-Blanche, 75016 Paris, France.

Astier, Switz. See *Uhlmann-Eyraud, Switz.*

Astor, UK. Astor Chemical Ltd, Tavistock Rd, West Drayton, Middx UB7 7RA, England.

Astra, Arg. Astra S.A. Prod. Farm. y Quim., Argerich 536, 1706 Haedo, Buenos Aires, Argentina.

Astra, Austral. Astra Pharmaceuticals Pty Ltd, P.O. Box 131, North Ryde NSW 2113, Australia.

Astra, Canad. Astra Pharmtek/Astra Labs, Divisions of Astra Pharmaceuticals Canada Ltd, 1004 Middlegate Rd, Mississauga, Ontario L4Y 1M4, Canada.

Astra, Denm. Astra-Gruppen A/S, Roskildevej 22, 2620 Albertslund, Denmark.

Astra, Fin. Suomen Astra Oy, Ahventie 4, PL 10, 02171 Espoo, Finland.

Astra, Fr. Laboratoires Astra France, Groupe pharmaceutique Astra Suède, 64 rue du 8 Mai 1945, 92025 Nanterre Cedex, France.

Astra, Ger. Astra Chemicals GmbH, Tinsdaler Weg 183, Postfach: 249, 2000 Wedel (Holstein), W. Germany.

Astra, Neth. Astra Pharmaceutica B.V., De Bruyn Kopsstraat 14, 2288 ED Rijswijk, Netherlands.

Astra, Norw. Astra Farmasøytiske A/S, Skarersletta 50, Postboks 1, 1473 Skårer, Norway.

Astra, NZ. See *Pharmaco, NZ.*

Astra, S.Afr. See *Adcock Ingram, S.Afr.*

Astra, Swed. Astra Läkemedel AB, 151 85 Södertälje, Sweden.

Astra, Switz. Astra Pharmaceutica SA, Buckhauserstrasse 24, 8048 Zurich, Switzerland.

Astra, UK. Astra Pharmaceuticals Ltd, Home Park Estate, Kings Langley, Herts WD4 8DH, England.

Astra, USA. Astra Pharmaceutical Products Inc., 50 Otis St, Westboro MA 01581-4428, USA.

Astra Dental, Ital. Astra Dental s.p.a., Via Valtellina 63, 20159 Milan, Italy.

Astra Meditec, Denm. Astra Meditec A/S, Roskildevej 22, 2620 Albertslund, Denmark.

Astra Meditec, Norw. Astra Meditec A/S, Skarersletta 50, Postboks 160, 1473 Skårer, Norway.

Astra-Meditec, Swed. Astra-Meditec AB, Box 14, 431 21 Molndal, Sweden.

Astra-Ifesa, Spain. See *Ifesa, Spain.*

Astra-Syntex, Denm. Astra-Syntex Laegemidler A/S, C.F. Richsvej 103, 2000 Frederiksberg, Denmark.

Astra-Syntex, Fin. Astra-Syntex Tiedotuskeskus, Koivuvaarankuja 1, PL 13, 01641 Vantaa, Finland.

Astra-Syntex, Norw. Astra-Syntex A/S, Strømsveien 66 C, Postboks 44, 2011 Strømmen, Norway.

Astra-Syntex, Swed. Astra-Syntex Scandinavia AB, Box 9078, 151 09 Sodertalje, Sweden.

Athenstaedt, Ger. Athenstaedt & Redeker KG, Hemelinger Bahnhofstrasse 13, Postfach: 448660, 2800 Bremen 44, W. Germany.

Athrodax, UK. Athrodax Ltd, St Edburys Hall, Priory Rd, Bicester, Oxon, England.

Atlantic, Switz. See *Actipharm, Switz.*

Atlas, UK. Atlas Pharmaceutical Co. Ltd, 20 Abercorn Place, London NW8 9XP, England.

Atmos, Ger. Pharma Atmos GmbH & Co. Arzneimittel, Stresemannallee 6, Postfach: 25, 4040 Neuss 1, W. Germany.

Atzinger, Ger. Dr. Atzinger & Co. KG Pharmazeutische Fabrik, Dr. Atzinger Strasse 5, Postfach: 1129, 8390 Passau, Germany.

Auclair, Fr. See *Ayerst, Fr.*

Auclair, Switz. See *Opopharma, Switz.*

Augot, Fr. Laboratoires Augot, 26 rue de Beauregard, 03400 Yzeure, France.

Auriema, UK. Acal Auriema Ltd, 442 Bath Rd, Slough, Berks SL1 6BB, England.

Ausonia, Ital. Ausonia Farmaceutici s.r.l., Via Laurentina Km. 24.730, 00040 Pomezia (Rome), Italy.

Auspharm, Austral. Auspharm International Ltd, P.O. Box 601, Dandenong Vic. 3175, Australia.

Avebe, Neth. Avebe, Klaas Nieboerweg 12, 9607 PN Foxhol, Netherlands.

Avon, UK. Avon Medicals Ltd, Moons Moat Drive, Redditch, Worcs B98 9HA, England.

Axeltorvs, Denm. Axeltorvs Apotek, Groskenstraede 2A, 3000 Helsingor, Denmark.

Ayerst, Arg. Ayerst Inc., Reconquista 1011 1° piso, 1003 Buenos Aires, Argentina.

Ayerst, Austral. Ayerst Laboratories Pty Ltd, P.O. Box 148, Parramatta NSW 2150, Australia.

Ayerst, Belg. Ayerst Benelux S.A., Beekstraat 46, 9810 Gent, Belgium.

Ayerst, Canad. Ayerst Laboratories, Division of Ayerst, McKenna & Harrison Inc., 1025 boul. Laurentien, St-Laurent Montreal, Quebec H4R 1J6, Canada.

Ayerst, Denm. See *Ferring, Denm.*

Ayerst, Fr. Laboratoires Ayerst, 2 Grande-Rue, 92310 Sevres, France.

Ayerst, Ital. Ayerst Italiana s.p.a., Via dei M. Lepini Km. 50,6, 04100 Latina, Italy.

Ayerst, Neth. Ayerst Benelux N.V., Pilotenstraat 35, 1059 CH Amsterdam, Netherlands.

Ayerst, Norw. See *Nyco, Norw.*

Ayerst, S.Afr. Ayerst Laboratories (Pty) Ltd, P.O. Box 573, Halfway House 1685, S. Africa.

Ayerst, Swed. See *Ferring, Swed.*

Ayerst, Switz. See *Doetsch, Grether, Switz.*

Ayerst, UK. See *Wyeth, UK.*

Ayerst, USA. Ayerst Laboratories, Division of American Home Products Corp., 685 Third Ave, New York NY 10017, USA.

Ayrton, Saunders, UK. Ayrton, Saunders & Co. Ltd, Wilson Road, Huyton, Liverpool L36 6AH, England.

Azienda Farm., Ital. Azienda Farmaceutica Italiana, Via A. de Gasperi 47, 21040 Sumirago (VA), Italy.

Azuchemie, Ger. Azuchemie, Dr med. R. Muller GmbH & Co., Dieselstrasse 5, Postfach : 100126, 7016 Gerlingen, W. Germany.

Azupharma, Ger. See *Azuchemie, Ger.*

Badische, Ger. See *Rhône-Poulenc, Ger.*

Badrial, Fr. See *Boehringer Ingelheim, Fr.*

Baer, Ger. Chemisch-pharmazeutische Fabrik Dr Baer KG GmbH & Co., Ehrwalder Strasse 21, Südmedica-Haus, Postfach:70 16 69, 8000 Munich 70, W. Germany.

Bago, Arg. Bagó S.A., Avda Belgrano 990 3° piso, 1092 Buenos Aires, Argentina.

Bailleul, Fr. Laboratoires Bailleul, 7 rue Michelet, 93360 Neuilly-Plaisance, France.

Bailly, Fr. Laboratoires A. Bailly (S.P.E.A.B.), 7 rue Sabastien-Mercier, 75015 Paris, France.

Bajer, Arg. Felipe Bajer S.A., Alfredo R. Bufano 1265, 1416 Buenos Aires, Argentina.

Baker/Cummins, USA. Baker/Cummins, Dermatological Division of Key Pharmaceuticals Inc., 4400 Biscayne Blvd, Miami FL 33137, USA.

Baldacci, Ital. Laboratori Baldacci s.p.a., Via S. Michele Scalzi 73, 56100 Pisa, Italy.

Baldacci, Spain. Baldacci, Cerdena 322, 08025 Barcelona, Spain.

Baliarda, Arg. Baliarda S.A., Alberti 1283, 1223 Buenos Aires, Argentina.

Bama, Spain. Bama Geve, Bailen 95-97, 08009 Barcelona, Spain.

Banyu, Jpn. Banyu Seiyaku, 2-7 Hon-cho, Nihonbashi, Chuo-ku, Tokyo, Japan.

Barclay & Sons, UK. Barclay & Sons Ltd, Ropery St, Grimsby, S. Humberside DN32 9EL, England.

Bard, UK. C.R. Bard International Ltd, Pennywell Industrial Estate, Sunderland SR4 9EW, England.

Barker Dobson, UK. Barker Dobson Ltd, P.O. Box 49, Huntley Mount Road, Bury, Lancs BL9 6XL, England.

Barnes-Hind, Austral. Barnes-Hind Pty Ltd, 7 Dickson Ave, Artarmon NSW 2064, Australia.

Barnes-Hind, Canad. Barnes-Hind Hydrocurve, 6535 Mill Creek Dr., Unit 67, Mississauga, Ontario L5N 2M2, Canada.

Barnes-Hind, Switz. See *Doetsch, Grether, Switz.* and *Dispersa, Switz.*

Barnes-Hind, UK. Barnes-Hind Ltd, 7 The Bytech Centre, Canada Rd, Byfleet, Surrey KT14 7GX, England.

Barnes-Hind, USA. Barnes-Hind Inc., A Revlon Vision Care Co., 895 Kifer Rd, Sunnyvale CA 94086, USA.

Barnes, Neth. See *Rooster, Neth.*

Barrere, Austral. Barrere Surgical Co., P.O. Box A84, Sydney South NSW 2000, Australia.

Barry, USA. Barry Laboratories Inc., 461 NE 27th St, P.O. Box 1967, Pompano Beach FL 33061, USA.

Bart, USA. A.J. Bart Inc., Gurabo Industrial Park, P.O. Box 813, Gurabo PR 00658, Puerto Rico.

Bartiss, S.Afr. See *Restan, S.Afr.*

BASF, Ger. BASF AG, Carl-Bosch-Strasse 38, 6700 Ludwigshafen, W. Germany.

BASF, UK. BASF (UK) Ltd, P.O. Box 4, Earl Rd, Cheadle Hulme, Cheadle, Cheshire SK8 6QG, England.

BASF Wyandotte, USA. BASF Wyandotte Corporation, 100 Cherry Hill Rd, Parsippany NJ 07054, USA.

Basoderm, Denm. Basoderm a/s, Horkaer 34, 2730 Herlev, Denmark.

Basoderm, Neth. See *Boehringer Ingelheim, Neth.*

Basoderm, Swed. See *Meda, Swed.*

Basotherm, Ger. Basotherm GmbH, Eichendorffweg 5, Postfach: 1254, 7950 Biberach an der Riss 1, W. Germany.

Basotherm, Switz. See *Agpharm, Switz.*

Bastian, Ger. Bastian-Werk GmbH, August-Exeter-Strasse 2-4, Postfach: 600161, 8000 Munich 60, Germany.

Bateman-Jackson, UK. Bateman-Jackson, Tubiton House, Medlock St, Oldham, Lancs OL1 3HS, England.

Bausch & Lomb, USA. Bausch & Lomb Inc., 1400 N. Goodman St, Rochester NY14692, USA.

Bauxili, Spain. Bauxili Dr., Nueva 52, Igualada, 08700 Barcelona, Spain.

Baxter, Ger. Baxter Deutschland GmbH, Edisonstr. 3, Postfach: 1165, 8044 Unterschliessheim bei Munich, Germany.

Baxter, Ital. Laboratori Don Baxter s.p.a., Via Flavia 122, 34147 Trieste, Italy.

Baxter, Spain. See *Farmiberia, Spain.*

Baxter, UK. Baxter Healthcare Ltd, Thorpe Lea Manor, Thorpe Lea Rd, Egham, Surrey TW20 8MY, England.

Baxter Travenol, Belg. See *Christiaens, Belg.*

Bay, USA. Bay Pharmaceuticals Inc., 1111 Francisco Blvd, San Rafael CA 94901, USA.

Bayer, Arg. Bayer Argentina S.A.C.I.F.I.y de M., Gral. Rivas 2466, 1417 Buenos Aires, Argentina.

Bayer, Aust. Bayer-Pharma GmbH, Biberstrasse 15, 1011 Vienna 1, Austria.

Bayer, Austral. Bayer Australia Ltd (Pharmaceutical Division), 46-7 Wilson St, Botany NSW 2019, Australia.

Bayer, Belg. Bayer Belgium S.A., Ave Louise 143, 1050 Brussels, Belgium.

Bayer, Denm. Bayer Danmark A/S, Christian IX's gade 2, 1111 Copenhagen K, Denmark.

Bayer, Fr. Bayer-Pharma, rue Bellocier, 89103 Sens Cedex, France.

Bayer, Ger. Bayer AG, 5090 Leverkusen 12, W. Germany.

Bayer, Ital. Bayer Italia s.p.a., Viale Certosa 126, 20156 Milan, Italy.

Bayer, Neth. Bayer Nederland B.V., divisie Farma, Nijverheidsweg 26, 3641 RR Mijdrecht, Netherlands.

Bayer, Norw. Bayer Kjemi A/S, Granfos Naeringspark, Vollsv. 13, Postboks 311, 1324 Lysaker, Norway.

Bayer, Philipp. See *Metro, Philipp.*

Bayer, S.Afr. Bayer-Miles (Pty) Ltd, P.O. Box 198, Isando 1600, S. Africa.

Bayer, Spain. Bayer, Calabria 268, 08029 Barcelona, Spain.

Bayer, Swed. Bayer (Sverige) AB, Box 5237, 402 24 Goteborg, Sweden.

Bayer, Switz. Bayer Pharma AG, Case postale, 8045 Zurich, Switzerland.

Bayer, UK. Bayer UK Ltd, Pharmaceutical Business Group, Bayer House, Strawberry Hill, Newbury, Berks RG13 1JA, England.

Bayer Agrochem, UK. Bayer UK Ltd, Agrochem Division, Eastern Way, Bury St Edmunds, Suffolk IP32 7AH, England.

Baypharm, UK. See *Bayer, UK.*

Bayropharm, Ger. Bayropharm GmbH, Friedrichstr. 38, 5090 Leverkusen 1 (Manfort), W. Germany.

Bayropharm, Ital. Bayropharm Italiana s.r.l., Via dei Cignoli 9, 20151 Milan, Italy.

BC Lutz, Switz. BC Lutz Company, Case postale, 8702 Zollikon, Switzerland.

BDH Chemicals, UK. BDH Chemicals Ltd, Broom Rd, Poole, Dorset BH12 4NN, England.

BDH Pharmaceuticals, UK. BDH Pharmaceuticals, England.

Be-Tabs, S.Afr. Be-Tabs Pharmaceuticals (Pty) Ltd, P.O. Box 42461, Fordsburg 2033, S.Africa.

Beach, USA. Beach Pharmaceuticals, Division of Beach Products Inc., 5220 S Manhattan Ave, Tampa FL 33611, USA.

Beaufour, Belg. See *de Bournonville, Belg.*

Beaufour, Fr. Laboratoires Beaufour, 18 place Doguereau, 28104 Dreux, France.

Beaufour, Switz. See *Uhlmann-Eyraud, Switz.*

Beautisales, UK. Beautisales Ltd, 65 Loveridge Rd & Mews, London NW6 2DR, England.

Beauty, Canad. Beauty Creations Ltd, 833 Oxford St, Toronto, Ontario M8Z 5X4, Canada.

Beauvais, Denm. Aktieselskabet Beauvais, Horsvinget 1-3, 2630 Tastrup, Denmark.

Becton, Dickinson, Canad. Becton, Dickinson Canada, 2464 South Sheridan Way, Mississauga, Ontario L5J 2M8, Canada.

Beecham, Austral. Beecham Research Laboratories, Private Mail Bag 34, Dandenong Vic. 3175, Australia.

Beecham, Belg. Beecham Pharma S.A., rue de l'Intendant 59, 1210 Brussels, Belgium.

Beecham, Canad. Beecham Laboratories Inc., 115 Brunswick Blvd, Pointe Claire, Quebec H9R 1A4, Canada.

Beecham, Ital. Beecham Italia s.p.a., Via Pirelli 19, 20124 Milan, Italy.

Beecham, Neth. Beecham Farma B.V., Sportlaan 198, 1185 TH Amstelveen, Netherlands.

Beecham, NZ. Beecham (New Zealand) Ltd, P.O. Box 12-442, Penrose, Auckland, New Zealand.

Beecham, S.Afr. Beecham Pharmaceuticals (Pty) Ltd., P.O. Box 347, Bergvlei 2012, S. Africa.

Beecham, Spain. Beecham, Poligono Industrial Toledo, 45007 Toledo, Spain.

Beecham, Swed. See *Meda, Swed.*

Beecham, Switz. Beecham SA, Weltpoststr. 4, 3015 Bern, Switzerland.

Beecham Animal Health, UK. Beecham Animal Health, Beecham House, Brentford, Middx TW8 9BD, England.

Beecham Bovril, UK. Beecham Bovril Brands, Beecham House, Brentford, Middx TW8 9BD, England.

Beecham Laboratories, USA. Beecham Laboratories, Division of Beecham Inc., 501 Fifth St, Bristol TN 37620, USA.

Beecham Products, Fr. Laboratoires Beecham Products France, 7 blvd Romain Rolland, 92128 Montrouge, France.

Beecham Products, USA. Beecham Products, Division of Beecham Inc., P.O. Box 1467, Pittsburgh PA 15230, USA.

Beecham Proprietaries, UK. Beecham Health Care, Beecham House, Great West Rd, Brentford, Middx TW8 9BD, England.

Beecham Research, UK. Beecham Research Laboratories, Beecham House, Great West Rd, Brentford, Middx TW8 9BD, England.

Beecham-Sevigne, Fr. Laboratoires Beecham-Sevigne, 25 bd de l'Amiral Bruix, 75782 Paris Cedex 16, France.

Beecham-Wülfing, Ger. Beecham-Wülfing GmbH & Co. KG, Stresemannallee 6, 4040 Neuss 1, W. Germany.

Behring, Neth. See *Hoechst, Neth.*

Behring, Norw. See *Hoechst, Norw.*

Behring, Spain. Behring, Travesera de Gracia 47-9, 08021 Barcelona, Spain.

Behring, Swed. See *Hoechst, Swed.*

Behring, Switz. See *Hoechst, Switz.*

Behringwerke, Belg. See *Hoechst, Belg.*

Behringwerke, Denm. See *Hoechst, Denm.*

Behringwerke, Ger. Behringwerke AG, Postfach: 1140, 3550 Marburg (Lahn), W. Germany.

Beiersdorf, Ger. Beiersdorf AG, Unnastrasse 48, 2000 Hamburg 20, W. Germany.

Beiersdorf, USA. Beiersdorf Inc., BDF Plaza, P.O. Box 5529, Norwalk CT 06856-5529, USA.

Beige, S.Afr. See *Vesta, S.Afr.*

Belgana, Belg. Laboratoires Belgana S.A., rue Saint-Ghislain 41, 1000 Brussels, Belgium.

Bellon, Belg. See *Wellcome, Belg.*

Bellon, Fr. Laboratoires Roger Bellon, B.P. 105, 159 ave A. Peretti, 92201 Neuilly-sur-Seine Cedex, France.

Bellon, Neth. See *Rhône-Poulenc, Neth.*

Bellon, Switz. See *Rhodia-Pharm, Switz.*

Belphar, Belg. See *Continental Pharma, Belg.*

Bencard, Belg. See *Beecham, Belg.*

Bencard, Canad. Bencard Allergy Service, Division of Beecham Laboratories Inc., 1345 Fewster Dr., Mississauga, Ontario L4W 2A5, Canada.

Bencard, Neth. See *Beecham, Neth.*

Bencard, S.Afr. See *Beecham, S.Afr.*

Bencard, Switz. See *Beecham, Switz.*

Bencard, UK. Bencard, Great West Rd, Brentford, Middx TW8 9BD, England.

Benckiser, UK. Benckiser Ltd, David Murray John Building, Swindon, Wilts SN1 1ND, England.

Bender, Aust. Bender & Co. GmbH, Dr Boehringer-Gasse 5-11, 1121 Vienna XII, Austria.

Bene-Arzneimittel, Switz. See *Max Ritter, Switz.*

Bene, Ger. Bene-Arzneimittel GmbH, Herterichstrasse 1, Postfach: 710269, 8000 Munich 71, W. Germany.

Benedetti, Ital. Benedetti s.r.l., Via Donizetti 52, 50018 Scandicci, Italy.

Bengers, S.Afr. See *Fisons, S.Afr.*

Bengué, UK. Bengué & Co. Ltd, Syntex House, St Ives Rd, Maidenhead, Berks SL6 1RD, England.

Benvegna, Ital. Neoterapici Benvegna s.r.l., Via Liborio Giuffrè 52/B, 90127 Palermo, Italy.

Benzon, Denm. Alfred Benzon Salgsselskab A/S, Halmtorvet 29, 1700 Copenhagen V, Denmark.

Benzon, Neth. Alfred Benzon B.V., Larikslaan 3, 3833 AM Leusden, Netherlands.

Benzon, Norw. Alfred Benzon A/S, Industriv. 8, Postboks 31, 1473 Skarer, Norway.

Benzon, Swed. Alfred Benzon AB, Box 1423, 251 14 Helsingborg, Sweden.

Benzon, UK. Alfred Benzon (UK) Ltd, 47 Bell St, Henley-on-Thames, Oxon RG9 2BA, England.

Berenguer-Beneyto, Spain. Berenguer Beneyto, Trabajo S/N, Sant Just Devern, 08960 Barcelona, Spain.

Bergamon, Ital. Bergamon s.p.a., Via di Cancelliera 60, 0072 Ariccia (Rome), Italy.

Berk, Austral. See *USV, Austral.*

Berk, S.Afr. Berk Pharmaceuticals (SA) (Pty) Ltd, P.O. Box 301, Isando 1600, S. Africa.

Berk Generics, UK. Berk Generics, Division of Rorer Pharmaceuticals, St Leonards House, St Leonards Rd, Eastbourne, Sussex BN12 3YG, England.

Berk Pharmaceuticals, UK. Berk Pharmaceuticals Ltd, St Leonard's House, St Leonard's Rd, Eastbourne, East Sussex BN21 3YG, England.

Berkeley, USA. Berkeley Biologicals, 1831 Second St, Berkeley CA 94710, USA.

Berlex, Canad. Berlex Canada Inc., Subsidiary of Schering AG West Germany, 2260 32e Ave, Lachine, Quebec H8T 3H4, Canada.

Berlex, S.Afr. See *Berlimed, S.Afr.*

Berlex, USA. Berlex Laboratories Inc., 110 East Hanover Ave, Cedar Knolls NJ 07927, USA.

Berlimed, S.Afr. Berlimed (Pty) Ltd, P.O. Box 10259, Johannesburg 2000, S. Africa.

Berna, Ital. Istituto Sieroterapico Berna s.i.r.l., Via Bellinzona 39, 22100 Como, Italy.

Berna, Spain. Berna, Paseo de la Castellana 163, 28046 Madrid, Spain.

Berna, Switz. Institut Serotherapique et Vaccinal Suisse, Case postale 2707, 3001 Berne, Switzerland.

Bernabó, Arg. Bernabó & Cía. S.A.C.I.I.F.A., Terrada 2346/48, 1416 Buenos Aires, Argentina.

Berol Kemi, UK. Berol Kemi (UK) Ltd, 23 Grosvenor Rd, St Albans, Herts AL1 3AN, England.

Berta, Ital. Berta Michele s.a.s. Farmaceutici, Piazza Martelli 7, 20162 Milan, Italy.

Bescansa, Spain. Bescansa, Pl. Inds. Tambre-via Pasteur 8, Santiago de Compostela, La Coruna, Spain.

Besins-Iscovesco, Fr. Laboratoires Besins-Iscovesco, 5 rue du Bourg-l'Abbé, 75003 Paris, France.

Besins-Iscovesco, Switz. See *Golaz, Switz.*

Beta, Arg. Beta S.A., San Juan 2266/74, 1232 Buenos Aires, Argentina.

Beta, Ital. Laboratorio Biologico Chemioterapico Beta s.r.l., Via G. Uberti 8, 25128 Brescia, Italy.

Beta Medical Products, UK. Beta Medical Products Ltd, 5-7 Arkwright Rd, Astmoor, Runcorn, Cheshire, England.

Betafar, Spain. Betafar, Ctra de Andalucia, km 25.8, Valdemoro, 28340 Madrid, Spain.

Beutlich, USA. Beutlich Inc., 7149 North Austin Ave, Niles IL 60648, USA.

Beytout, Fr. Laboratoires Beytout, 10 rue Guynemer, 94160 Saint-Mandé, France.

Beytout, Switz. See *Uhlmann-Eyraud, Switz.*

Biagini, Ital. Farma Biagini s.p.a., 55020 Castelvecchio Pascoli (LU), Italy.

Bicther, Spain. Bicther, Juan XXIII 15-9, Esplugas de Llobregat, 08950 Barcelona, Spain.

Bifarma, Ital. Bifarma Fitoterapici di Bignardi Sergio, Via Pallia 5, 20139 Milan, Italy.

Bilbo, Spain. Bilbo, Andres Isasi 11, Bilbao, 48012 Vizcaya, Spain.

Billerud, Swed. Billerud AB, 663 00 Skoghall, Sweden.

Biobasal, S.Afr. See *Restan, S.Afr.*

Bioceuticals, UK. Bioceuticals Ltd, 26 Zennor Rd, London SW12 0PS, England.

Bio-Chemical Laboratory, Canad. Bio-Chemical Laboratory Inc., 2323 autoroute des Laurentides, Chomedey-Ville de Laval, Quebec H7S 1Z7, Canada.

Biochimica, Switz. Biochimica SA, Schäppistr. 12, 8006 Zurich, Switzerland.

Biochimica Zanardi, Ital. Biochimica Zanardi s.r.l., Via Flavia 10, 00042 Anzio (Rome), Italy.

Biochimici, Ital. Biochimici PSN, Via Viadagola 30, 40127 Quarto Inferiore (BO), Italy.

Biocodex, Fr. Laboratoires Biocodex, 19 rue Barbès, 92126 Montrouge Cedex, France.

Biocodex, S.Afr. See *Restan, S.Afr.*

Biocodex, Switz. See *Sodip, Switz.*

Biocraft, USA. Biocraft Laboratories Inc., 92 Route 46, Elmwood Park NJ 07407, USA.

Biodica, Fr. Laboratoires Biodica, 10 ave du Général-de-Gaulle, B.P. 93, 92164 Antony Cedex, France.

Biodiphar, Belg. Biodiphar S.A., chaussee d'Alsemberg 1001, 1180 Brussels, Belgium.

Biofarma, Denm. Biofarma A/S, Nyvej 16, 1851 Frederiksberg C, Denmark.

Biogal, Hung. Biogal Pharmaceutical Works, P.O. Box 197, 4001 Debrecen, Hungary.

Biogalenique, Fr. Laboratoires Biogalenique, 53 rue de l'Abbe-Carton, 75014 Paris, France.

Bioglan, Austral. Bioglan Laboratories (Aust) Pty Ltd, 25 Gerald St, Marickville NSW 2204, Australia.

Bioglan, UK. Bioglan Laboratories Ltd, 1 The Cam Centre, Wilbury Way, Hitchin, Herts SG4 0TW, England.

Bioindustria, Ital. Bioindustria Farmaceutici s.p.a., Via De Ambrosiis 2, 15067 Novi Ligure (AL), Italy.

Biol, Arg. Biológico Arg. S.A.I.C., J.E. Uriburu 153, 1027 Buenos Aires, Argentina.

Biolax, Denm. Biolax, Sindalsvej 30, 8240 Risskov, Denmark.

Biologia Marina, Spain. See *Cheminova, Spain.*

Biologici Italia, Ital. Laboratori Biologici Italia Petrucci Dr G. & C. s.r.l., Via Sarzanese 160/A, 55100 Lucca, Italy.

Biomarine, Fr. Laboratoires La Biomarine, 19 rue Montigny, B.P. 155, 76204 Dieppe Cedex, France.

Biomed, Switz. Biomed SA, Case postale, 8026 Zurich, Switzerland.

Biomedica Foscama, Ital. Biomedica Foscama Industria Chimico Farmaceutica s.p.a., Via Tiburtina Km. 14.5, 00131 Rome, Italy.

Biomedical, Fr. 3M Biomedical-3M Sante, 40 rue Gabriel-Crie, 92245 Malakoff Cedex, France.

Bio-Medical, UK. Bio-Medical Services Ltd, The White House, Bishopthorpe, York YO2 1QF, England.

Bio-Oil Research, UK. Bio-Oil Research Ltd, The Hawthorns, 64 Welsh Row, Nantwich, Cheshire CW5 5EU, England.

Biopharm, S.Afr. Biopharm (Pty) Ltd, Access City, 32 Stalb St, New Doornfontein, Johannesburg, S. Africa.

Biopharm, UK. Biopharm (UK) Ltd, P.O. Box 5, 2-8 Morfa Rd, Swansea, West Glam SA1 2ET, Wales.

Biopharma, Fr. Laboratoires Biopharmaceutiques de France, 31 rue du Pont, 92200 Neuilly-sur-Seine, France.

Biopharma, Ital. Biopharma Italia s.r.l., Via Bazzini 16, 20131 Milan, Italy.

Bioquim, Arg. Bioquim S.A., Avda Ing. Huergo 1475, 1107 Buenos Aires, Argentina.

Bioresearch, Ital. Bioresearch s.p.a., 20060 Liscate (Milan), Italy.

Biorex, UK. Biorex Laboratories Ltd, Biorex House, Canonbury Villas, London N1 2HB, England.

Biorga, Fr. Laboratoires Biorga, 17 rue St-Mathieu, 78550 Houdan, France.

Bios, Belg. Bios S.A., rue Berkendael 68, 1060 Brussels, Belgium.

Biosedra, Arg. Biosedra S.A.C.I.e 1., Manuela Pedraza 3345, 1429 Buenos Aires, Argentina.

Biosédra, Fr. Laboratoires Biosédra, 42 ave Augustin-Dumont, 92240 Malakoff, France.

Biosedra, Switz. See *Actipharm, Switz.*

Biosint, Ital. Laboratori Farmaco Biologici Biosint s.p.a., Via Zorutti 54, 33030 Campoformido (UD), Italy.

Biostabilex, Fr. Laboratoires Biostabilex, 89 rue Lauriston, 75116 Paris, France.

Bioterax, Spain. Bioterax, Sta Cruz Calafel km 9.7 Ctr Barna, San Baudilio de Llobregat, 08830 Barcelona, Spain.

Biotest, Denm. See *Johnson, Denm.*

Biotest, Ger. Biotest Pharma GmbH, Flughafenstrasse 4, Postfach: 730240, 6000 Frankfurt/Main 73, W. Germany.

Biotest, Swed. See *Design, Swed.*

Biotest, UK. Biotest (UK) Ltd, 171 Alcester Rd, Moseley, Birmingham B13 8JR, England.

Biothera-Asperal, Belg. See *Bio-Therabel, Belg.*

Bio-Therabel, Belg. Bio-Therabel S.A., chaussee d'Alsemberg 1001, 1180 Brussels, Belgium.

Biothérax, Denm. See *Essex, Denm.*

Biothérax, Fr. See *Boehringer Ingelheim, Fr.*

Biotherax, Ger. Biotherax Arzneimittel GmbH, Eckendorfer Str. 91-93, Postfach: 2125 u. 2320, 4800 Bielefeld 1, Germany.

Biotherax, Norw. See *Sentipharm, Norw.*

Biotherax, Swed. See *Pro Medica, Swed.*

Biotrading, Ital. Biotrading Co. s.r.l., Via L. Pogliaghi 1, 20146 Milan, Italy.

Biphar, Fr. Laboratoires Biphar, 34 rue de la Federation, 75015 Paris, France.

Biphar, Switz. Biphar S.A., 102, rue des Eaux-Vives, 1207 Geneva, Switzerland.

Bipharma, Neth. Bipharma B.V., Pilotenstraat 35, 1059 CH Amsterdam, Netherlands.

Bird, USA. Bird, USA.

Biscova, Ger. Biscova Fabrik Pharmaz. Praparate, Guntherstrasse 31, Postfach: 810369, 3000 Hannover 81, Germany.

Bismag, Norw. See *Kobro, Norw.*

Black, UK. S. Black (Import & Export) Ltd, 30 Islington Green, London N1 8DU, England.

Blagden, UK. Blagden Campbell Chemicals Ltd, AMP House, Dingwall Rd, Croydon, Surrey CR9 3QU, England.

Blaine, USA. Blaine Co. Inc., 2700 Dixie Highway, Ft Mitchell, KY 41017, USA.

Blair, USA. Blair Laboratories Inc., 50 Washington St, Norwalk CT 06856, USA.

Blake, UK. Thomas Blake & Co., The Byre House, Fearby, Nr Masham, N. Yorks HG4 4NF, England.

Blakoe, UK. Blakoe Ltd, 225 Putney Bridge Rd, London SW15, England.

Blend-a-med, Ger. Blendax-Werke R. Schneider GmbH & Co., Blend-a-med-Forschung, Rheinallee 88, Postfach: 1580, 6500 Mainz, W. Germany.

Blend-a-pharm, Fr. Laboratoires Blend-a-pharm, 128 rue Marius-Aufan, B.P. 312, 92303 Levallois-Perret, France.

Block, Canad. Block Drug Co. (Canada) Ltd, 36 Northline Rd, Toronto, Ontario M4B 3E3, Canada.

Blood Products Laboratory, UK. Blood Products Laboratory, Dagger Lane, Elstree, Borehamwood, Herts WD6 3BX, England.

Blucher-Schering, Ger. Blucher-Schering & Co., Rademacherstrasse 2, Postfach: 1630, 2400 Lubeck, Germany.

Blue Cross, Ital. Blue Cross s.p.a., Via Calabiana 18, 20139 Milan, Italy.

Blumoller, Denm. a/s Blumoller, Petersmindevej 30, 5100 Odense C, Denmark.

BOC, UK. The BOC Group PLC, Chertsey Rd, Windlesham, Surrey GU20 6HJ, England.

Bock, USA. Bock Pharmacal Co., P.O. Box 29287, St Louis MO 63126, USA.

Bode, Ger. Bode Chemie GmbH & Co., Melanchthonstrasse 27, Postfach: 540709, 2000 Hamburg 54, W. Germany.

Boehringer, Arg. Boehringer Argentina S.A.C.I. e I., Viamonte 2213/15, 1056 Buenos Aires, Argentina.

Boehringer Biochemia, Ital. Boehringer Biochemia Robin s.p.a., Via S. Uguzzone 5, 20126 Milan, Italy.

Boehringer Corp., UK. The Boehringer Corporation (London) Ltd, Bell Lane, Lewes, East Sussex BN7 1LG, England.

Boehringer Ingelheim, Austral. Boehringer Ingelheim Pty Ltd, P.O. Box 219, Lane Cove NSW 2066, Australia.

Boehringer Ingelheim, Belg. Boehringer Ingelheim S.A., rue du Collège St-Michel 17, 1150 Brussels, Belgium.

Boehringer Ingelheim, Canad. Boehringer Ingelheim (Canada) Ltd, 977 Century Drive, Burlington, Ontario L7L 5J8, Canada.

Boehringer Ingelheim, Denm. Boehringer Ingelheim A/S, Hanebred 2, 2720 Vanløse, Denmark.

Boehringer Ingelheim, Fr. Laboratoires Boehringer Ingelheim, 12 rue Henri-Huet, B.P. 292, 51100 Reims, France.

Boehringer Ingelheim, Ger. Boehringer Ingelheim KG, Binger Strasse, Postfach: 200, 6507 Ingelheim am Rhein, W. Germany.

Boehringer Ingelheim, Ital. Boehringer Ingelheim s.p.a., Casella Postale, 50100 Florence, Italy.

Boehringer Ingelheim, Neth. Boehringer Ingelheim B.V., Berenkoog 28, 1822 BJ Alkmaar, Netherlands.

Boehringer Ingelheim, Norw. Boehringer Ingelheim International GmbH, Informasjonskontor Norge, Postboks 405, 1371 Asker, Norway.

Boehringer Ingelheim, Philipp. See *Metro, Philipp.*

Boehringer Ingelheim, Port. Boehringer-Ingelheim, C.H. Boehringer Sohn Lda, Av. Antonio Augusto de Aguiar 104-1, 1063 Lisboa Codex, Portugal.

Boehringer Ingelheim, S.Afr. Boehringer Ingelheim (Pty) Ltd, Private Bag X3032, Randburg 2125, S. Africa.

Boehringer Ingelheim, Spain. Boehringer Ingelheim, Pablo Alcover 31-33, 08017 Barcelona, Spain.

Boehringer Ingelheim, Swed. Boehringer Ingelheim AB, Box 44, 127 21 Skärholmen, Sweden.

Boehringer Ingelheim, Switz. Boehringer Ingelheim GmbH, Peter Merian-Strasse 19/21, 4002 Basel, Switzerland.

Boehringer Ingelheim, UK. Boehringer Ingelheim Ltd, Southern Industrial Estate, Bracknell, Berks RG12 4YS, England.

Boehringer Ingelheim, USA. Boehringer Ingelheim Ltd, 90 East Ridge, P.O. Box 368, Ridgefield CT 06877, USA.

Boehringer Mannheim, Austral. Boehringer Mannheim Australia Pty Ltd, P.O. Box 316, North Ryde NSW 2113, Australia.

Boehringer Mannheim, Belg. See *Boehringer Pharma, Belg.*

Boehringer Mannheim, Canad. Boehringer Mannheim (Canada) Ltd, 11450 ch. Cote-de-Liesse, Dorval, Quebec H9P 1A9, Canada.

Boehringer Mannheim, Ger. Boehringer Mannheim GmbH, Sandhofer Strasse 116, Postfach: 310 120, 6800 Mannheim 31, W. Germany.

Boehringer Mannheim, Neth. Boehringer Mannheim B.V., Markerkant 13-10, 1314 AN Almere, Netherlands.

Boehringer Mannheim, Norw. See *Organon, Norw.*

Boehringer Mannheim, Philipp. See *Marsman, Philipp.*

Boehringer Mannheim, Port. See *Ferraz, Lynce, Port.*

Boehringer Mannheim, S.Afr. Boehringer Mannheim (SA) (Pty) Ltd, P.O. Box 51927, Randburg 2125, S. Africa.

Boehringer Mannheim, Spain. Boehringer Mannheim, Plg. Can Parellada, Les Fonts de Tarrasa, 08194 Barcelona, Spain.

Boehringer Mannheim, Swed. Boehringer Mannheim Scandinavia AB, Box 147, 161 26 Bromma 1, Sweden.

Boehringer Mannheim, Switz. Boehringer Mannheim (Schweiz) SA, Industriestrasse, 6343 Rotkreuz., Switzerland.

Boehringer Mannheim Diagnostics, USA. Boehringer Mannheim Diagnostics Inc., Bio-Dynamics Division, 9115 Hague Rd, Indianapolis IN 46250, USA.

Boehringer Pharma, Belg. Boehringer Pharma S.A., Ave des Croix de Guerre 90, 1120 Brussels, Belgium.

Boehringer Sohn, Arg. C.H. Boehringer Sohn S.R.L., Chile 80, 1098 Buenos Aires, Argentina.

Boehringer Sohn, Switz. C.H. Boehringer Sohn GmbH, Peter-Merian-Strasse 19, Basel, Switzerland.

Bofors, Switz. See *Globopharm, Switz.*

Bohm, Spain. Bohm, Molina Seca 23 (Cobo Calleja), Fuenlabrada, 28940 Madrid, Spain.

Boi, Spain. Boi, Polig Ind Sur, Papiol, 08754 Barcelona, Spain.

Boiron, Fr. Laboratoires Boiron, 20 rue de la Liberation, 69110 Sainte-Foy-les-Lyon, France.

Boizot, Spain. Boizot, Luis Cabrera 63, 28002 Madrid, Spain.

Bolar, USA. Bolar Pharmaceuticals, 130 Lincoln St, Copiague NY 11726, USA.

Bolton, Canad. Bolton Dental Mfg Inc., P.O. Box 757, Sheldon Dr., Unit 5, Cambridge, Ontario N1R 5W6, Canada.

Bonfield, Eire. Bonfield Ltd, Eire.

Boniquet, Spain. Boniquet, Freixa 5-9, 08021 Barcelona, Spain.

Boniscontro & Gazzone, Ital. Lab. Prod. Farm. Boniscontro & Gazzone del Dr M. Pensa & C., Corso Racconigi 23, 10139 Turin, Italy.

Bonmati, Spain. Bonmati, Ampurdan 32, Figueras, 17600 Gerona, Spain.

Bonomelli, Ital. Bonomelli s.p.a., Via Montecuccoli 1, 22042 Dolzago (CO), Italy.

Booker Health, UK. Booker Health Foods Ltd, Canada Rd, Byfleet, Surrey KT14 7JL, England.

Boots, Austral. The Boots Co. (Australia) Pty Ltd, P.O. Box 120, Carlingford NSW 2118, Australia.

Boots, Belg. The Boots Co. Belgium S.A., 't Hofveld 13, 1720 Dilbeek, Belgium.

Boots, Denm. See *Astra, Denm.*

Boots, Neth. The Boots Company (Holland) B.V., De Limiet 24, 4124 PG Hagestein, Netherlands.

Boots, Norw. See *Astra, Norw.*

Boots, S.Afr. The Boots Co. (SA) (Pty) Ltd, P.O. Box 427, Isando 1600, S.Africa.

Boots, Swed. See *Astra, Swed.*

Boots, Switz. See *Doetsch, Grether, Switz.*

Boots, UK. The Boots Co. PLC, 1 Thane Rd West, Nottingham NG2 3AA, England.

Boots, USA. Boots Pharmaceuticals Inc., 6540 Line Ave, Shreveport LA 71106, USA.

Boots Dupont, S.Afr. Boots Dupont, S. Africa.

Boots-Dacour, Fr. Laboratoires Boots-Dacour, 49 rue de Bitche, B.P. 66, 92404 Courbevoie Cedex, France.

Boots-Formenti, Ital. Boots Formenti s.p.a., Via Correggio 28, 20149 Milan, Italy.

Borromeo, Ital. Borromeo Laboratori Farmaco-biologici s.r.l., Via Mac Mahon 45, 20155 Milan, Italy.

Bottger, Ger. Bottger GmbH Pharmazeutische und Kosmetische Praparate, Paulsborner Strasse 2, Postfach: 310320, 1000 Berlin 31, Germany.

Bottu, Belg. See *Roussel, Belg.*

Bottu, Fr. Bottu, 52 ave du Maréchal-Joffre, 92024 Nanterre Cedex, France.

Bottu, Neth. See *Roussel, Neth.*

Bottu, Switz. See *Siegfried, Switz.* and *Uhlmann-Eyraud, Switz.*

Boucard, Belg. See *UPB, Belg.*

Bouchara, Belg. See *Bio-Therabel, Belg.*

Bouchara, Fr. Laboratoires du Dr E. Bouchara, 8 rue Pastourelle, 75003 Paris, France.

Bouchara, Switz. See *Distripharm, Switz.*

Bouchard, Fr. Laboratoires Bouchard, 11 rue de la Loge, 94260 Fresnes, France.

Boucher & Muir, Austral. Boucher & Muir Pty Ltd, P.O. Box 333, North Sydney NSW 2060, Australia.

Bournonville, Neth. Bournonville-Pharma B.V., De Steiger 196, 1351 AV Almere, Netherlands.

Bouteille, Fr. Laboratoires Bouteille, 7 rue des Belges, 87000 Limoges, France.

Bouty, Ital. Italiana Laboratori Bouty, Via Temperanza 6, 20127 Milan, Italy.

Bovit, S.Afr. See *Propan, S.Afr.*

Bowman, USA. Bowman Pharmaceuticals Inc., 119 Schroyer Ave SW, Canton OH 44702, USA.

Box, UK. W.H. Box, 47 Mayflower St, Plymouth, England.

Boxberger, Denm. See *Max Jenne, Denm.*

Boyle, USA. Boyle & Co., 1030 South Arroyo Parkway, Pasadena CA 91105, USA.

BP Chemicals, UK. BP Chemicals Ltd, Belgrave House, 76 Buckingham Palace Rd, London SW1W 0SU, England.

Bracco, Ital. Bracco Industria Chimica s.p.a., Via E. Folli 50, 20134 Milan, Italy.

Bracco, S.Afr. See *SCS, S.Afr.*

Bracco, Switz. See *Opopharma, Switz.*

Bragg, UK. J.L. Bragg (Ipswich) Ltd, 30 Greyfriars Rd, Ipswich, Suffolk IP1 1UP, England.

Braintree, USA. Braintree Laboratories Inc., 285 Washington St, Braintree MA 02184, USA.

Brassovora, Arg. Brassovora S.A., Cerrito 836 8° Piso, 1010 Buenos Aires, Argentina.

Braun & Herberg, Ger. Dr. Braun & Herberg Arzneimittel GmbH & Co. KG, Stockelsdorfer Weg 68, Postfach: 1155, 2407 Bad Schwartau, Germany.

Braun, Belg. B. Braun Belgique S.A., ave Albert Giraud 29-35, 1030 Brussels, Belgium.

Braun, Denm. See *Ottosen, Denm.*

Braun, Norw. B. Braun Medical A/S, Bjellandv. 12, 3103 Vear, Norway.

Braun, UK. B. Braun (Medical) Ltd, Evett Close, Stocklake, Aylesbury, Bucks HP20 1DN, England.

Braun Melsungen, Ger. B. Braun Melsungen AG, Carl-Braun-Strasse 1, Postfach: 110+120, 3508 Melsungen, W. Germany.

Brenner, Ger. Georg A. Brenner, Arzneimittel-Fabrik GmbH, Postfach: 1140, 7297 Alpirsbach, Germany.

Brentchem, UK. Brentchem, England.

Breon, USA. See *Winthrop-Breon, USA.*

Bridge, UK. Bridge Pharmaceuticals, A Division of Smith Kline & French Laboratories Ltd, Welwyn Garden City, Herts AL7 1EY, England.

Bridoux, Fr. Laboratoire Bridoux, 6 rue Salengro, 62160 Bully-les-Mines, France.

Bristol, Belg. Bristol Benelux S.A., chaussée de la Hulpe 185-7, 1170 Brussels, Belgium.

Bristol, Canad. Bristol Laboratories of Canada, Bristol-Myers Canada Inc., 2625 Queensview Dr., P.O. Box 6313, Stn J, Ottowa, Ontario K2A 3Y4, Canada.

Bristol, Fr. Laboratoires Bristol, 32 rue de l'Arcade, 75008 Paris, France.

Bristol, Ger. Bristol-Arzneimittel, Niederlassung der Bristol-Myers GmbH, Hermannstr. 54-56, Postfach: 369, 6078 Neu-Isenburg, W. Germany.

Bristol, Neth. Bristol-Myers B.V., Pampuslaan 188, 1382 JS Weesp, Netherlands.

Bristol, Norw. Bristol-Myers Scandinavia Ltd., Postboks 7603 Skillebekk, 0205 Oslo 2, Norway.

Bristol, NZ. Bristol-Myers (NZ) Ltd, P.O. Box 9175, Newmarket, New Zealand.

Bristol, S.Afr. Bristol/Mead Johnson Pharmaceuticals (Division of B-M Group (Pty) Ltd), P.O. Box 9706, Johannesburg 2000, S. Africa.

Bristol, Swed. Bristol-Myers AB, Box 4081, 171 04 Solna, Sweden.

Bristol, Switz. Bristol-Myers S.A., Riedstrasse 3, 6330 Cham, Switzerland.

Bristol, USA. Bristol Laboratories, Division of Bristol-Myers Co., Thompson Rd, P.O. Box 4755, Syracuse NY 13221, USA.

Bristol Europe, Ital. Bristol Europe s.p.a., Mead Johnson Divisione Farmaceutici, Via Benedetto Croce s.n.c., 00142 Rome, Italy.

Bristol Italiana Sud, Ital. Bristol Italiana (Sud) s.p.a., Via Benedetto Croce s.n.c., 00142 Rome, Italy.

Bristol-Myers, Austral. Bristol-Myers Co. Pty Ltd, P.O. Box 530, Crows Nest NSW 2065, Australia.

Bristol-Myers, Denm. Bristol-Myers, Wilders Plads, Bygning V, 1403 Copenhagen K, Denmark.

Bristol-Myers, Spain. Bristol-Myers, Plg Ind. Isla de Java 1, Fuencarral, 28034 Madrid, Spain.

Bristol-Myers, UK. Bristol-Myers Co. Ltd, Swakeleys House, Milton Rd, Ickenham, Uxbridge UB10 8NS, England.

Bristol-Myers Oncology, USA. Bristol-Myers Oncology Division, Bristol-Myers Co., Thompson Rd, P.O. Box 4755, Syracuse NY 13221, USA.

Bristol-Myers Pharmaceuticals, UK. Bristol-Myers Pharmaceuticals, Swakeleys House, Milton Rd, Ickenham, Uxbridge, Middx UB10 8NS, England.

Bristol-Myers Products, USA. Bristol-Myers Products, Division of Bristol-Myers Co., 1350 Liberty Ave, Hillside NJ 07207, USA.

Britannia Health, UK. Britannia Health Products Ltd, Forum House, 41-75 Brighton Rd, Redhill, Surrey RH1 6YS, England.

Britannia Pharmaceuticals, UK. Britannia Pharmaceuticals Ltd, Forum House, 41-75 Brighton Rd, Redhill, Surrey RH1 6YS, England.

BritCair, UK. BritCair Laboratories Ltd, Progress House, Albert Rd, Aldershot, Hants GU11 1SZ, England.

British Chemotheutic, UK. British Chemotheutic Products Ltd, Kemtheutic House, Grant St, Bradford, W. Yorks BD3 9HF, England.

British Cod Liver Oils, UK. British Cod Liver Oils Ltd, Marfleet, Hull, North Humberside HU9 5NJ, England.

British Pharmaceuticals, Austral. See *Organon, Austral.*

British Traders & Shippers, UK. British Traders & Shippers Ltd, 6-7 Merrielands Crescent, Dagenham, Essex RM9 6SL, England.

Britpharm, UK. Britpharm Laboratories Ltd, Kramer Mews, London SW5 9JL, England.

Brocacef, Neth. Brocacef B.V., Straatweg 2, 3604 BB Maarssen, Netherlands.

Brocades, Belg. Brocades Belga S.A., bd General Jacques 26, 1050 Brussels, Belgium.

Brocades, Ital. Brocades s.p.a., Viale Spagna 45, 20093 Cologno Monzese (MI), Italy.

Brocades, S.Afr. See *Riker, S.Afr.*

Brocades, UK. Brocades (Great Britain) Ltd, Brocades House, Pyrford Rd, West Byfleet, Weybridge, Surrey KT14 6RA, England.

Brocchieri, Ital. Stabilimento Chimico Farmaceutico dr. L. Brocchieri s.r.l., Via Tiburtina Km. 14.4, 00131 Rome, Italy.

Brothier, Fr. Laboratoires Brothier, 41 rue de Neuilly, 92000 Nanterre, France.

Brovar, S.Afr. Brovar S & P (Pty) Ltd, P.O. Box 11434, Johannesburg 2000, S. Africa.

Brown, USA. The Brown Pharmaceutical Co. Inc., 2500 West Sixth St, P.O. Box 57925, Los Angeles CA 90057, USA.

Bruco, Ital. Farmaceutici Bruco s.r.l., Via E. Bazzano 12, 16019 Ronco Scrivia (GE), Italy.

Brum, Spain. Brum, Ramon Asenjo 26, Luarca, 33700 Asturias, Spain.

Bruneau, Fr. Laboratoires Bruneau, 204 ave du Maréchal-Juin, 92107 Boulogne Cedex, France.

Brunel, S.Afr. Brunel Laboratories (Pty) Ltd, P.O. Box 23103, Innesdale 0031, S. Africa.

Brunnengräber, Ger. Dr Christian Brunnengräber GmbH, Ratzeburger Allee 106, Postfach: 2052, 2400 Lübeck, W. Germany.

Bruschettini, Ital. Bruschettini s.r.l., Via Isonzo 6, 16147 Genova Sturla, Italy.

BTP Cocker Chemicals, UK. BTP Cocker Chemicals Ltd, Hayes Rd, Cadishead, Manchester M30 5BX, England.

Bucaneve, Ital. Bucaneve Medicinali s.r.l., Via Sercognani 15, 20156 Milan, Italy.

Bucca, Spain. Bucca, Juan Alvarez Mendizabal 43, 28008 Madrid, Spain.

Buchler, Ger. Buchler GmbH, Harxbutteler Strasse 3, Postfach:1829, 3300 Braunschweig, W. Germany.

Bucopa, Ger. Bucopa Bubenik & Co., Orthstrasse 26, Postafch: 600217, 8000 Munich 60, Germany.

Bull, Austral. David Bull Laboratories Pty Ltd, P.O. Box 170, Mulgrave North Vic. 3170, Australia.

Bull, UK. David Bull Laboratories, Harris Rd, Warwick CV34 5GH, England.

Burgess, UK. Edwin Burgess Ltd, Longwick Rd, Princes Risborough, Aylesbury, Bucks HP17 9RR, England.

Burnus, Ger. Burnus Gesellschaft mbH, Kirschenallee, Postfach: 4241, 6100 Darmstadt, Germany.

Burton Parsons, Austral. See *Alcon, Austral.*

Bush Boake Allen, UK. Bush Boake Allen Ltd, Blackhorse Lane, London E17 5QP, England.

Busto, Spain. Busto Dr., Mendez Alvaro 57, 28045 Madrid, Spain.

Byk, Aust. Byk Chem.-Pharm. Produkte GmbH, Ketzergasse 200, 1235 Vienna, Austria.

Byk, Belg. Byk Belga S.A., rue Anatole France 115-121/Bte 5, 1030 Brussels, Belgium.

Byk, Neth. Byk Nederland B.V., Weerenweg 29, 1161 AG Zwanenburg, Netherlands.

Byk Essex, Ger. See *Essex, Ger.*

Byk Gulden, Denm. See *Nordisk Droge, Denm.*

Byk Gulden, Ger. Byk Gulden Lomberg Chemische Fabrik GmbH, Byk-Gulden-Strasse 2, Postfach: 6500, 7750 Konstanz, W. Germany.

Byk Gulden, Ital. Byk Gulden Italia s.p.a., Via Giotto 1, 20032 Cormano (MI), Italy.

Byk Gulden, Norw. See *Collett, Norw.*

Byk Gulden, S.Afr. Byk Gulden Pharmaceuticals, P.O. Box 51476, Randburg 2125, S. Africa.

Byk Gulden, Swed. See *Ferrosan, Swed.*

Byk Gulden, Switz. See *Iromedica, Switz.*

Byk Liprandi, Arg. Byk Liprandi S.A.C.I., Delgado 1565, 1426 Buenos Aires, Argentina.

Byk-Mallinckrodt, UK. Byk-Mallinckrodt, England.

Byly, Spain. Byly, Aray 2, 08002 Barcelona, Spain.

C & M, USA. C & M Pharmacal Inc., 1519 E Eight Mile Rd, Hazel Park MI 48030-2696, USA.

Caber, Ital. Farmaceutici Caber s.r.l., Via Mazzini 7, 56100 Pisa, Italy.

Cabot, UK. Cabot Ltd, Copyground Lane, High Wycombe, Bucks HP12 3HE, England.

Cadila, Ind. Cadila Laboratories Pvt. Ltd, 244 Ghodasar, P.O. Box 9004, Maninagar, Ahmedabad-380 008, India.

Cahill May Roberts, Eire. Cahill May Roberts Ltd, P.O. Box 1090, Dublin 20, Eire.

Calbiochem, USA. Calbiochem Co., P.O. Box 12087, San Diego CA 92119, USA.

Calmic, Canad. See *Wellcome, Canad.*

Calmic, S.Afr. Calmic, S. Africa.

Calmic, UK. Calmic Medical Division, The Wellcome Foundation Ltd, Crewe Hall, Crewe, Cheshire CW1 1UB, England.

Calor, UK. Calor, England.

Cambden, Austral. See *Auspharm, Austral.*

Cambrian, UK. Cambrian Pharmaceuticals, England.

Cambridge Laboratories, Austral. Cambridge Laboratories Pty Ltd, P.O. Box 690E, Melbourne Vic. 3001, Australia.

Camden, S.Afr. Camden (Pty) Ltd, P.O. Box 781247, Sandton 2146, S. Africa.

Camlab, UK. Camlab Ltd, Nuffield Rd, Cambridge CB4 1TH, England.

Campbell, USA. Campbell Laboratories Inc., 300 East 51st St, New York NY 10022, USA.

Camps, Spain. Camps, Planeta 39, 08012 Barcelona, Spain.

Canderm, Canad. Canderm Pharmacal Ltd, 5353 boul. Thimens, St Laurent, Quebec H4R 2H4, Canada.

Candioli, Ital. Istituto Candioli Profilattico & Farmaceutico s.p.a., Via Manzoni 2, 10092 Torino Beinasco, Italy.

Canizares, Spain. Canizares, Pza del Mercado y Ercilla 27, 46001 Valencia, Spain.

Cantabria, Spain. Cantabria, Plg Ind. Cazona Adarzo s/n, Santander, 39011 Cantabria, Spain.

Cantassium Co., UK. The Cantassium Company, 225 Putney Bridge Rd, London SW15 2PY, England.

Capilares, Spain. Productos Capilares, Plg Ind. Villalonquejar, Burgos, Spain.

Capitol, Spain. See *Nordisk, Spain.*

Care, UK. Care Laboratories Ltd, Badminton Court, Amersham, Bucks, England.

Carlo Erba, Ital. Farmitalia Carlo Erba s.p.a., Gruppo Montedison, Via C. Imbonati 24, 20159 Milan, Italy.

Carlo Erba, Spain. See *Farmitalia, Spain.*

Carlton Laboratories, UK. Carlton Laboratories (UK) Ltd, 4 Manor Parade, Salvington Rd, Durrington, Worthing, West Sussex BN13 2JP, England.

Carnation Foods, UK. Carnation Ltd, St George's House, Croydon CR9 1NR, England.

Carnegie, UK. Carnegie Medical, Loughborough, Leics LE11 1EP, England.

Carnrick, UK. Carnrick Laboratories, Acres Down, Furze Hill, London Rd, Shipston-on-Stour, Warwicks, England.

Carnrick, USA. Carnrick Laboratories Inc., 65 Horse Hill Rd, Cedar Knolls NJ 07927, USA.

Carol, Spain. Carol, Paseo Doctor Bartual Moret 6, Manises, Valencia, Spain.

Carrascal Martin, Spain. Carrascal Martin, Avda de las Camelias 118, Vigo, 36211 Pontevedra, Spain.

Carrion, Fr. Laboratoires Carrion, 30 rue Henri-Régnault, 92400 Courbevoie, France.

Carter Bond, UK. Carter Bond Ltd, Attercliffe Rd, Sheffield S4 7XG, England.

Carter Bros, UK. Carter Bros, England.

Carter-Wallace, Austral. Carter Wallace (Australia) Pty Ltd, P.O. Box 216, Brookvale NSW 2100, Australia.

Carter-Wallace, Switz. See *Doetsch, Grether, Switz.*

Carter-Wallace, UK. Carter-Wallace Ltd, Wear Bay Rd, Folkestone, Kent, England.

Carulla Vekar, Spain. Carulla Vekar, Crta. Nacional I, Km 16200, Alcobendas, 28100 Madrid, Spain.

Casasco, Arg. Casasco S.A.I.C., Boyacá 237/41, 1406 Buenos Aires, Argentina.

Cascan, Ger. Cascan GmbH & Co. KG, Hohenstaufenstr. 7, Postfach: 1907, 6200 Wiesbaden, W. Germany.

Casen Fisons, Spain. Casen Fisons, Autovia de Logrono, KM 13300, Utebo, 50180 Zaragoza, Spain.

Cassella-med, Ger. Cassella-med GmbH, Gereonstrasse 50, 5000 Cologne 1, W. Germany.

Cassella-med, Ital. Cassella-med Italiana s.p.a., P.zza Turr 5, 20149 Milan, Italy.

Cassella Med, S.Afr. Cassella Med., S. Africa.

Cassella-Riedel, Ger. Cassella-Riedel Pharma GmbH, Hanauer Landstrasse 521, 6000 Frankfurt (Main) 61, W. Germany.

Cassella-Riedel, Switz. See *Hoechst, Switz.*

Cassenne, Fr. Laboratoires Cassenne, 3 square Desaix, 75015 Paris, France.

Cassenne, S.Afr. See *Roussel, S.Afr.*

Cassenne-Takeda, Fr. See *Takeda, Fr.*

Castejon, Spain. Castejon, Autopista de Barajas, KM 12 Eq. Bergant, 28022 Madrid, Spain.

Castleowen, UK. Castleowen Ltd, 1347 London Rd, London SW16 4BE, England.

CCD, Fr. Laboratoires C.C.D., 44 rue N.-D. de Lorette, 75009 Paris, France.

CCP, Belg. See *Therabel Pharma, Belg.*

Ceccarelli, Ital. Ceccarelli A. & C. dei F.lli dr. Tanganelli, Via G. Caponsacchi 31, 50126 Florence, Italy.

Cederroth, Spain. Cederroth, Leon 26 (Plg Ind. Cobo Calleja), Fuenlabrada, 28940 Madrid, Spain.

Cedona, Belg. See *Byk, Belg.*

Cedona, Neth. Cedona Haarl. Pharm. Fabriek B.V., Oudeweg 147, 2031 CC Haarlem, Netherlands.

Cedona, Swed. See Astra, *Swed.*

Celaton, UK. Celaton Laboratory Research Ltd, 203 Headstone Lane, Harrow, Middx HA1 6JH, England.

Celtia, Arg. Celtia S.A., B. Mitre 4284, 1201 Buenos Aires, Argentina.

Center Laboratories, USA. Center Laboratories, Division of EM Industries Inc., 35 Channel Dr., Port Washington NY 11050, USA.

Central Pharmaceuticals, USA. Central Pharmaceuticals Inc., 112-128 East Third St, Seymour IN 47274, USA.

Centrallab., Denm. Central Laboratoriet ApS, Kirkevejen 20, Teestrup, 4690 Haslev, Denmark.

Centrapharm, Fr. Laboratoires Centrapharm, 3 rue Onslow, 63000 Clermont-Ferrand, France.

Centrum, Spain. Centrum, Sagitario 12, Llano del Espartal, Alicante, Spain.

Century, USA. Century Pharmaceuticals Inc., 10377 Hague Rd, Indianapolis IN 46256, USA.

CEPA, Spain. CEPA, Paseo Deleite S/N, Aranjucz, 28300 Madrid, Spain.

CERM, Belg. See *Sanders-Probel, Belg.*

Cernep Synthelabo, Fr. Laboratoires Cernep Synthelabo, 22 avenue Galilee, 92350 Le Plessis-Robinson, France.

Cétrane, Fr. See *Unicet, Fr.*

Cetrofarma, Switz. Cetrofarma S.a.g.I., via alla Chiesa 1, 6962 Viganello, Switzerland.

Cetylite, USA. Cetylite Industries Inc., P.O. Box CN6, 9051 River Rd, Pennsauken NJ 08110, USA.

Ceva, UK. Ceva Ltd, P.O. Box 209, 3 Rhodes Way, Watford, Herts WD2 4QE, England.

Chabre, Fr. Laboratoires Chabre, 39 ave de la Resistance, 83055 Toulon Cedex, France.

Chaix et du Marais, Fr. Ste des Laboratoires Chaix et du Marais, 10 rue de la Croix-Faubin, 75011 Paris, France.

Chamberlains, S.Afr. Chamberlains (Pty) (Ltd), 241 Main Road, Retreat, S. Africa.

Chanteaud, Fr. Laboratoires Chanteaud, Quai Jean-Jaures, 07800 La Voulte/Rhone, France.

Chanteaud, Switz. See *Doetsch, Grether, Switz.*

Charoen Bhaesaj, Thai. S. Charoen Bhaesaj Trading Co. Ltd, 209/56, Soi Petchkasem 21, Petchkasem Road, Bangkok, Thailand.

Charpentier, Fr. Laboratoires E. Charpentier, 8 rue Pastourelle, 75003 Paris, France.

Charton, Canad. Charton Laboratories, Division of Herdt & Charton Inc., 9393 boul. Louis-H. Lafontaine, Montreal, Quebec H1J 1Y8, Canada.

Chassot, Switz. Chassot & Cie AG, Sägestrasse 73, 3098 Köniz, Switzerland.

Chatfield Laboratories, UK. Chatfield Laboratories, Kramer Mews, London SW5 9JL, England.

Chauvin-Blache, Fr. Laboratoires Chauvin-Blache, S.A., 104 rue de la Galera, B.P. 1174, 34009 Montpellier Cedex, France.

Chefaro, Belg. Chefaro S.A., ave Marnix 13, 1050 Brussels, Belgium.

Chefaro, Ger. Deutsche Chefaro Pharma GmbH, Wirrigen 25, Postfach: 449, 4355 Waltrop, W. Germany.

Chefaro, Neth. Chefaro International B.V., Keileweg 8, 3029 BS Rotterdam, Netherlands.

Chefaro, UK. Chefaro Proprietaries Ltd, Science Park, Milton Rd, Cambridge CB4 4FL, England.

Chelsea Drug & Chemical, UK. Chelsea Drug & Chemical Co. Ltd, 310 Old Brompton Rd, London SW5 9JQ, England.

Chemedica, Switz. Chemedica SA, Case postale 58, 1896 Vouvry, Switzerland.

Chemfarma, S.Afr. See *Restan, S.Afr.*

Chemia, Denm. Chemia, Postboks 72, 3650 Olstykke, Denmark.

Chemical & Insulating Co., UK. The Chemical & Insulating Co. Ltd, West Auckland Rd, Darlington, Co Durham DL3 0UR, England.

Chemie-Linz, Aust. Chemie-Linz AG, St-Peter-Strasse 25, 4021 Linz, Austria.

Chemie-Linz, Denm. See *Tjellesen, Denm.*

Chemie Linz, Swed. See *Kronans, Swed.*

Chemie-Linz, Switz. See *Opopharma, Switz.*

Chemil, Ital. Chemil Farmaceutici s.r.l., Via Cavour 41/43, 20026 Novate Milanese, Italy.

Cheminex, UK. Cheminex (Sales) Ltd, 30 Imperial Square, Cheltenham, Glos GL50 1QZ, England.

Cheminova, Spain. Cheminova, Emilio Muñoz 15, 28037 Madrid, Spain.

Chemipharm, Ger. Chemipharm GmbH & Co., Chemisch-pharmazeutische Fabrik KG, Sachsenring 37-47, 5000 Cologne 1, W. Germany.

Chemipharm, Switz. See *Diethelm, Switz.*

Chemist Brokers, UK. Chemist Brokers, Division of Food Brokers Ltd, Milburn, 3 Copsem Lane, Esher, Surrey KT10 9EP, England.

Chemi-Tech, USA. Chemi-Tech Labs Inc., 74-80 Marine St, Farmingdale NY 11735, USA.

Chemofux, Switz. See *Searle, Switz.*

Chephasaar, Ger. Chephasaar, Chemisch-Pharmazeutische Fabrik GmbH, Mühlstrasse 50, Postfach: 120, 6670 St Ingbert, W. Germany.

Chesebrough-Pond's, UK. Chesebrough-Pond's Ltd, P.O. Box 1DY, Hesket House, Portman Square, London W1A 1DY, England.

Chibret, Belg. See *Merck Sharp & Dohme, Belg.*

Chibret, Ger. Chibret Pharmazeutische GmbH, Charles-de-Gaulle-Strasse 4, Postfach: 83 09 20, 8000 Munich 83, Germany.

Chibret, Neth. Chibret, divisie van Merck Sharp & Dohme B.V., Waarderweg 39, 2031 BN Haarlem, Netherlands.

Chibret, Switz. See *Merck Sharp & Dohme, Switz.*

Chiesi, Ital. Chiesi Farmaceutici s.p.a., Via Palermo 26/A, 43100 Parma, Italy.

Chinoin, Hung. Chinoin Pharmaceutical and Chemical Works Ltd, P.O. Box 110, 1325 Budapest, Hungary.

Chinoin, Ital. Chinoin s.p.a., Via Zanella 3/5, 20133 Milan, Italy.

Chinosol, Denm. See *Danapharm, Denm.*

Chinosolfabrik, Ger. Chinosolfabrik Zweigniederlassung der Riedel-de Haën (AG), 3016 Seelze 1, W. Germany.

Chinosolfabrik, Switz. See *Doetsch, Grether, Switz.*

Chipman, UK. Chipman Ltd, Station Goods Yard, Nightingale Rd, Horsham, West Sussex, England.

Chlor-Chem, UK. Chlor-Chem Ltd, Mount Pleasant House, Huntingdon Rd, Cambridge CB2 0DA, England.

Choay, Belg. See *de Bournonville, Belg.*

Choay, Fr. Laboratoire Choay, 46 ave Théophile-Gautier, 75782 Paris Cedex 16, France.

Choay, Neth. See *Bournonville, Neth.*

Choay, Switz. See *Panpharma, Switz.*

Choay Lab, S.Afr. See *Script Intal, S.Afr.*

Christiaens, Belg. A. Christiaens S.A., rue de l'Etuve 60, 1000 Brussels, Belgium.

Christy, UK. Thomas Christy Ltd, North Lane, Aldershot, Hants GU12 4QP, England.

Chugai, Jpn. Chugai Seiyaku, 2-1-9 Kyobashi, Chuo-ku, Tokyo, Japan.

Ciba, Arg. Ciba-Geigy Argentina S.A.C.I., Arias 1851, 1429 Buenos Aires, Argentina.

Ciba, Austral. See *Ciba-Geigy, Austral.*

Ciba, Belg. Ciba-Geigy S.A., Noordkustlaan 18, 1720 Groot-Bijgaarden, Belgium.

Ciba, Canad. Ciba Pharmaceuticals, Division of Ciba-Geigy Canada Ltd, 6860 Century Ave, Mississauga, Ontario L5N 2W5, Canada.

Ciba, Denm. Ciba-Geigy A/S, Lyngbyvej 172, 2100 Copenhagen Ø, Denmark.

Ciba, Fr. Laboratoires Ciba-Geigy, Dépt. Ciba, 2 et 4 rue Lionel-Terray, 92506 Rueil-Malmaison, France.

Ciba, Ger. Ciba Pharma Ciba-Geigy GmbH, Öflinger Strasse 44, Postfach: 1160/1180, 7867 Wehr 1, W. Germany.

Ciba, Ital. Ciba Geigy s.p.a., 21040 Origgio, Italy.

Ciba, Neth. Ciba-Geigy B.V., Raapopseweg 1, 6824 DP Arnhem, Netherlands.

Ciba, Norw. Ciba-Geigy A/S, Postboks 6077 Etterstad, 0601 Oslo 1, Norway.

Ciba, NZ. Ciba Pharmaceuticals, Private Bag, Avondale, Auckland, New Zealand.

Ciba, S.Afr. Ciba-Geigy (Pty) Ltd, P.O. Box 92, Isando 1600, S. Africa.

Ciba, Spain. Ciba-Geigy, Paseo Carlos I 206, 08013 Barcelona, Spain.

Ciba, Swed. Ciba-Geigy Läkemedel AB, Box 605, 421 26 V Frölunda, Sweden.

Ciba, Switz. See *Ciba-Geigy, Switz.*

Ciba, UK. Ciba Laboratories, Wimblehurst Rd, Horsham, West Sussex RH12 4AB, England.

Ciba, USA. Ciba Pharmaceutical Co., Division of Ciba-Geigy Corporation, 556 Morris Ave, Summit NJ 07901, USA.

Ciba Consumer, UK. Ciba Consumer Pharmaceuticals, Wimblehurst Rd, Horsham, West Sussex RH12 4AB, England.

Ciba Vision, UK. Ciba Vision, Park West, Hedge End, Southampton, England.

Ciba-Geigy, Arg. Ciba-Geigy Argentina S.A.C.I., Arias 1851, 1429 Buenos Aires, Argentina.

Ciba-Geigy, Austral. Ciba-Geigy Australia Ltd, P.O. Box 4, Wentworthville NSW 2145, Australia.

Ciba-Geigy, Canad. Ciba-Geigy Canada Ltd, 6860 Century Ave, Mississauga, Ontario L5N 2W5, Canada.

Ciba-Geigy, Jpn. Nihon Ciba-Geigy, 10-66 Biko-cho, Takarazuka-shi, Japan.

Ciba-Geigy, Malaysia. Ciba-Geigy (M) Sdn. Bhd., P.O. Box 1005, Jalan Semangat, 46860 Petaling Jaya, Malaysia.

Ciba-Geigy, Singapore. Ciba-Geigy S.E. Asia (Pte) Ltd, 4 Fourth Lok Yang Rd, Singapore S 2262, Singapore.

Ciba-Geigy, Switz. Ciba-Geigy SA, Reinacherstrasse 115, Case postale, 4002 Basel, Switzerland.

Ciba-Geigy, UK. Ciba-Geigy Industrial Chemicals, Tenax Rd, Trafford Park, Manchester M17 1WT, England.

Ciba-Geigy, USA. Ciba-Geigy Corporation, 556 Morris Ave, Summit NJ 07901, USA.

Ciba-Geigy Agrochemicals, UK. Ciba-Geigy Agrochemicals, Whittlesford, Cambridge CB2 4QT, England.

Ciccarelli, Ital. Farmaceutici dott. Ciccarelli s.p.a., Via Clemente Prudenzio 13, 20138 Milan, Italy.

Cidan, Spain. Cidan, Uldecona 69, Benicarlo, 12580 Castellon, Spain.

Cilag, Arg. Cilag Farmaceutica S.A., Artilleros 2218, 1428 Buenos Aires, Argentina.

Cilag, Austral. Cilag Pty Ltd, 5th Floor, 154 Pacific Highway, St. Leonards NSW 2065, Australia.
Cilag, Belg. Cilag S.A., Atealaan 1, Postbus 96, 2410 Herentals, Belgium.
Cilag, Fr. Laboratoires Cilag, 46 rue Lauriston, 75116 Paris, France.
Cilag, Ger. Cilag GmbH, Neue Bergstrasse 9, Postfach: 12 52, 6146 Alsbach-Hahnlein 1, W. Germany.
Cilag, Ital. Cilag s.p.a., V. le Europa 51/53, 20093 Cologno Monzese (MI), Italy.
Cilag, Neth. Cilag N.V., Wetenschappelijke Informatiedienst, Zonnehof 64, 3811 ND Amersfoort, Netherlands.
Cilag, S.Afr. See *Ethnor, S.Afr.*
Cilag, Swed. Cilag AB, Box 7073, 191 07 Sollentuna, Sweden.
Cilag, Switz. Cilag AG, Herblingerstrasse 119, 8207 Schaffhausen, Switzerland.
Cilag-Chemie, Belg. See *Cilag, Belg.*
Cilag-Chemie, Denm. See *Mecobenzon, Denm.*
Cilag-Chemie, Neth. See *Cilag, Neth.*
Cilag-Chemie, Norw. Cilag AB Informasjonskontor, Skiv.200, Postboks 103, 1415 Oppegard, Norway.
Cilco, USA. Cilco, USA.
Cimex, Switz. Cimex SA, Case postale 2546, 4002 Basel, Switzerland.
Cinfa, Spain. Cinfa, Olaz-Chipi 10, Poligono Areta, Huarte, 31620 Navarra, Spain.
Cipharm, Fr. Laboratoires Cipharm, 205 av. du President Wilson, 93210 La Plaine St-Denis, France.
City Chemical Corp., USA. City Chemical Corporation, 132 West 22nd St, New York NY 10011, USA.
Ciurana, Spain. See *Byly, Spain.*
Clarben, Spain. Clarben, Vallermoso 28, 28015 Madrid, Spain.
Clariana, Spain. Clariana Pico, Ctra. Carlet-Valencia km 0.5, Carlet, Valencia, Spain.
Clark, Canad. Clark Laboratories Ltd, 2450 Finch Ave W, Weston, Ontario M9M 2E9, Canada.
Clarke Proprietaries, UK. Clarke Proprietary Medicines Ltd, P.O. Box 3, Pangbourne, Berks, England.
Claudius Ash, UK. Claudius Ash Sons & Co. Ltd, Casco House, Moon Lane, Barnet, Herts EN5 5UA, England.
Climent, Spain. See *Salud, Spain.*
Clin-Comar-Byla, Fr. See *Clin Midy, Fr.*
Clinical Specialities, UK. Clinical Specialities Ltd, 62 Cannock St, Leicester, England.
Clinimed, S.Afr. See *Protea Pharm, S.Afr.*
CliniMed, UK. CliniMed Ltd, Cavell House, Amersham Hill, High Wycombe, Bucks HP13 6NZ, England.
Clin Midy, Fr. Laboratoires Clin Midy, 20 rue des Fossés-St-Jacques, 75005 Paris, France.
Clin-Midy, Spain. See *Labaz, Spain.*
Clin-Midy, Switz. See *Sanofi, Switz.*
Clinod, UK. Clinod Pharmaceuticals, England.
CMW Laboratories, UK. CMW Laboratories Ltd, Bone Cement Division, Cornford Rd, Blackpool, England.
Cob, Belg. Cob & Co. S.A., ave Albert Giraud 115, 1030 Brussels, Belgium.
Co-Caps, UK. Co-Caps (Coded Capsules), 361 Lillie Rd, London SW6 7PA, England.
Codali, Belg. Codali S.A., avenue H. Dunant 31, 1140 Brussels, Belgium.
Colgate-Hoyt, USA. Colgate-Hoyt Laboratories, Division of Colgate-Palmolive Co., 575 University Ave, Norwood MA 02062, USA.
Colgate-Palmolive, UK. Colgate-Palmolive Ltd, 76 Oxford St, London W1A 1EN, England.
Coli, Ital. Farmaceutici Coli s.r.l., Via Campobello 15, 00040 Pomezia (Rome), Italy.
Coll, Spain. Coll Farma, Napoles 166, 08013 Barcelona, Spain.
Collado, Spain. Collado Dr., Varsovia 47-51, 08026 Barcelona, Spain.
Collett, Denm. See *Nordisk Droge, Denm.*
Collett, Norw. Collett-Marwell Hauge A/S, Drammensv. 852, Postboks 205, 1371 Asker, Norway.
Collins of Norwich, UK. Collins of Norwich, 25 Gentleman's Walk, Norwich NR2 1NA, England.
Collins, UK. L.D. Collins & Co. Ltd, Sunray House, 9 Plantagenet Rd, New Barnet, Herts EN5 5JG, England.
Coloplast, UK. Coloplast Ltd, Peterborough Business Park, Peterborough PE2 0FX, England.
Colorcon, UK. Colorcon Ltd, Murray Rd, St Pauls Cray, Orpington, Kent BR5 3QY, England.
Columbia, S.Afr. Columbia Pharmaceuticals (Pty) Ltd, P.O. Box 7026, Bonaero Park 162, S. Africa.
Combe, UK. Combe UK Ltd, AMP House, Dingwall Rd, Croydon, Surrey, England.
Combustin, Ger. Combustin Vertrieb Pharm. Praparate GmbH, Griessberg 2, Postfach: 1116, 8031 Seefeld/Oberbayern, W. Germany.
Combustinwerk, Switz. See *Doetsch, Grether, Switz.*
Commerce Drug, USA. Commerce Drug Co., Division of Del Laboratories Inc., 565 Broad Hollow Rd, Farmingdale NY 11735, USA.
Commonwealth Serum Laboratories, Austral. Commonwealth Serum Laboratories, 45 Poplar Rd, Parkville Vic. 3052, Australia.
Compagnie Rousselot, Fr. Compagnie Rousselet-Department Institut Ronchese, 8 rue Christophe Colomb, 75008 Paris, France.
Comprehensive Pharmaceuticals, UK. Comprehensive Pharmaceuticals Ltd, 95 Frampton St, London NW8 8NA, England.
Comstock, Austral. W.H. Comstock Co. (Aust) Pty Ltd, 17 Grandview St, Pymble NSW 2073, Australia.
Concept Pharmaceuticals, UK. See *Pierre Fabre, UK.*
Connaught, Canad. Connaught Laboratories Ltd, 1755 Steeles Ave West, Willowdale, Ontario M2R 3T4, Canada.
Connaught, USA. Connaught Laboratories Inc., Swiftwater PA 18370, USA.
Connaught Novo, Canad. Connaught Novo Ltd, 1755 Steeles Ave W, Box 3304 Stn D, Willowdale, Ontario M2R 3G6, Canada.
Conpharm, Swed. Conpharm AB, Box 1026, 651 15 Karlstad, Sweden.
Consolidated Chemical, USA. Consolidated Chemical Inc., 3224 S Kingshighway Blvd, St Louis MO 63139, USA.
Consolidated Chemicals, UK. Consolidated Chemicals Ltd, The Industrial Estate, Wrexham, Clwyd LL13 9PS, Wales.
Consolidated Midland, USA. Consolidated Midland Corporation, 195 East Main St, P.O. Box 74, Brewster NY 10509, USA.
Continental Ethicals, S.Afr. Continental Ethicals (Division of S.A. Druggists Ltd), P.O. Box 55307, Northlands 2116, S. Africa.
Continental Pharma, Belg. Continental Pharma S.A., ave Louise 135, 1050 Brussels, Belgium.
Continental Pharma, Neth. See *Int. Med. Prod., Neth.*
Continental Pharma, Switz. See *Cooper, Switz.* and *Pharmos, Switz.*
Cook-Waite, USA. Cook-Waite Laboratories Inc., 90 Park Ave, New York NY 10016, USA.
Coop. Farm., Ital. Cooperativa Farmaceutica Società Cooperativa, Via Passione 8, 20122 Milan, Italy.
Cooper, Austral. Cooper Laboratories Pty Ltd, Locked Bag 957, North Sydney NSW 2060, Australia.
Cooper, Canad. See *Johnson, Canad.*
Cooper, Ger. See *Oral-B, Ger.*
Cooper, Neth. See *Bipharma, Neth.*
Cooper, Spain. See *Oral B, Spain.*
Cooper, Switz. Cooper S.A., Case postale 197, 1701 Fribourg-Moncor, Switzerland.
Cooper, USA. Cooper Laboratories Inc., 305 Fairfield Ave, Fairfield NJ 07006, USA.
Cooper Dermatology, USA. See *Rydelle, USA.*
Cooper Vision, Neth. See *Bournonville, Neth.*
Cooperation Pharmaceutique, Fr. Cooperation Pharmaceutique Francaise, 77020 Melun Cedex, France.
Coopers Animal Health, UK. Coopers Animal Health Ltd, Crewe Hall, Crewe, Cheshire CW1 1UB, England.
Coopervision, Belg. See *de Bournonville, Belg.*
Coopervision, Canad. Coopervision Inc., 100 McPherson St, Markham, Ontario L3R 3V6, Canada.
CooperVision, Swed. See *Kronans, Swed.*
CooperVision, UK. See *Ciba Vision, UK.*
Coopervision, USA. Coopervision Pharmaceuticals Inc., San German PR 00753, Puerto Rico.
Cophar, Switz. Cophar S.A., Case postale 150, 1701 Fribourg-Moncor, Switzerland.
Coquelu, Fr. Laboratoires Coquelu, 71160 Digoin, France.
Cortec, Norw. Cortec medisiner A/S, Postboks 25, 1351 Rud, Norway.
Cortec, Swed. See *Utraco, Swed.*
Cortunon, Canad. Cortunon Inc., 119 ch. Dufferin, Hampstead-Montreal, Quebec H3X 2X8, Canada.
Corvi, Ital. Camillo Corvi s.p.a., Viale dei Mille 3, 29100 Piacenza, Italy.
Cosmic, Denm. Cosmic, Strodamvej 52, 2100 Copenhagen O, Denmark.
Cosmopharma, Neth. Cosmopharma B.V., divisie van Byk Nederland B.V., Weerenweg 29, 1161 AG Zwanenburg, Netherlands.
Cottrell, UK. Cottrell & Co., 15 Charlotte St, London W1P 2AA, England.
Courtaulds, UK. Courtaulds Chemicals & Plastics, P.O. Box 5, Spondon, Derby DE2 7BP, England.
Covan, S.Afr. Covan Pharmaceutical Products (Pty) Ltd, P.O. Box 155, Rosslyn 0200, S. Africa.
Cow & Gate, UK. Cow & Gate Ltd, Cow & Gate House, Trowbridge, Wilts BA14 8YX, England.
Cox, S.Afr. See *Holpro, S.Afr.*
Cox, UK. A.H. Cox & Co. Ltd, Whiddon Valley, Barnstaple, Devon EX32 8NS, England.
CP Pharmaceuticals, S.Afr. See *Fisons, S.Afr.*
CP Pharmaceuticals, UK. CP Pharmaceuticals Ltd, Red Willow Rd, Wrexham Industrial Estate, Wrexham, Clwyd LL13 9PX, Wales.
CPC Foods, Denm. CPC Foods A/S, Skopvlytoften 33, 2840 Holte, Denmark.
CPF, Ger. CPF, Chemisch Pharmazeutische Fabrik GmbH, Heinrich-Bocking-Strasse 6-8, 6600 Saarbrucken, Germany.
Craveri, Arg. Craveri S.A.I.C., Arangreen 830, 1405 Buenos Aires, Argentina.
Crinex, Fr. Laboratoires Crinex, B.P. 337, 92541 Montrouge Cedex, France.
Crinos, Ital. Industria Farmacobiologica Crinos s.p.a., Piazza XX Settembre 2, 22079 Como Villaguardia, Italy.
Crisol, Spain. Crisol, Plg Ind. Can Cuyas, Calle B1, Montcada y Reixach, 08110 Barcelona, Spain.
Croce Bianca, Ital. Laboratorio Biochimico Croce Bianca s.r.l., Via Milano 141, 20021 Baranzate di Bollate (MI), Italy.
Croda, UK. Croda International PLC, Cowick Hall, Snaith, Goole, North Humberside DN14 9AA, England.
Cronofar, Spain. Cronofar, San Cristobal 33, Derio, 48016 Vizcaya, Spain.
Crookes Healthcare, UK. Crookes Healthcare Ltd, P.O. Box 94, 1 Thane Rd West, Nottingham NG2 3AA, England.
Crookes Laboratories, UK. Crookes Laboratories Ltd, Thane Rd, Nottingham NG2 3AA, England.
Crosara, Ital. Lab. Farmaco Biologico Crosara s.p.a., Via Campobello 15, 00040 Pomezia (Rome), Italy.
Crown, UK. Crown Chemical Co. Ltd, Petteridge Lane, Matfield, Tonbridge, Kent TN12 7LZ, England.
Cruz, Spain. Fernandez de la Cruz, Crta Sevilla Malaga Km 9.6, Alcala de Guadaira, 41500 Sevilla, Spain.
Cryosan, USA. Cryosan, USA.
CSL-Novo, Austral. CSL-Novo Pty Ltd, Unit 1/22 Loyalty Rd, North Rocks NSW 2151, Australia.
CT, Ital. C.T., Laboratorio Farmaceutico s.r.l., Via D. Alighieri 69-71, 18038 Sanremo (IM), Italy.
CTS Dental, UK. C.T.S. Dental Supplies, 2 Hardwicke Rd, Reigate, Surrey RH2 9HG, England.
Cuatrecasas-Darkey, Spain. See *Tilfarma, Spain.*
Cullen & Davison, UK. Cullen & Davison Ltd, 52 Lurgan Rd, Portadown, Craigavon, Co Armagh BT63 5QG, Northern Ireland.
Cupal, UK. Cupal Ltd, Pharmaceutical Laboratories, Blackburn, Lancs BB2 2DX, England.
Curarina, Ger. Curarina-Arzneimittel GmbH, Robert-Koch-Strasse 5, Postfach: 61, 8196 Eurasberg/Obb., Germany.
Cusi, Belg. Lab. Cusi S.A., chaussee d'Alsemberg 1001, 1180 Brussels, Belgium.
Cusi, Spain. Cusi, Ctra Nacional II, KM 639, El Masnou, 08320 Barcelona, Spain.
Cussons, UK. Cussons (UK) Ltd, Kersal Vale, Manchester M7 0GL, England.
Cutter, Canad. Cutter Laboratories, Division of Miles Laboratories Ltd, 77 Belfield Rd, Etobicoke, Ontario M9W 1G6, Canada.
Cutter, Norw. See *Bayer, Norw.*
Cutter, Swed. See *Bayer, Swed.*
Cutter, UK. Cutter Laboratories, Division of Miles Ltd, Stoke Court, Stoke Poges, Slough SL2 4LY, England.
Cutter, USA. Cutter Biological, Division of Miles Laboratories Inc., 2200 Powell St, Emeryville CA 94662, USA.

Cuxson, Gerrard, UK. Cuxson, Gerrard & Co. (IMS) Ltd, Oldbury, Warley, West Midlands B69 3BB, England.

C-Vet, UK. C-Vet Ltd, Minster House, Western Way, Bury St Edmunds, Suffolk IP33 3SU, England.

Cyanamid, Belg. Cyanamid Benelux S.A., Parc Scientifique, rue du Bosquet 15, 1348 Mont-St-Guibert, Belgium.

Cyanamid, Ital. Cyanamid Italia s.p.a., Zona Ind. XV Strada, 95030 Catania, Italy.

Cyanamid, Neth. See *Lederle, Neth.*

Cyanamid, Spain. Cyanamid, Ctra Madrid Irun KM 24 BF Algete, San Sebastian de los Reyes, 28700 Madrid, Spain.

Cyanamid, Swed. Cyanamid Nordiska AB, Rissneleden 136, 172 48 Sundbyberg, Sweden.

Cyanamid, UK. Cyanamid of Great Britain Ltd, Fareham Rd, Gosport, Hants PO13 0AS, England.

Cyanamid-Lederle, Ger. Cyanamid GmbH, Abt. Lederle Arzneimittel, Pfaffenrieder Strasse 7, 8190 Wolfratshausen, W. Germany.

Cyanamid-Novalis, Ger. See *Cyanamid-Lederle, Ger.*

Cycloppharma, S.Afr. See *Protea Pharm, S.Afr.*

Dagra, Neth. Dagra N.V., Verrijn Stuartweg 60, 1112 AX Diemen, Netherlands.

Dahl-Hansen, Norw. Advokatfirmaet Schjodt. Advokat Mathias Dahl-Hansen, Postboks 9616 Egertorvet, 0128 Oslo 1, Norway.

Daiichi, Hong Kong. See *Hong Kong Med. Supp., Hong Kong.*

Daiichi, Jpn. Daiichi Seiyaku, 3-14-10 Nihonbashi, Chuo-ku, Tokyo, Japan.

Dainippon, Jpn. Dainippon Seiyaku, 3-25 Doshomachi, Higashi-ku, Osaka, Japan.

DAK, Denm. DAK-Laboratoriet a/s, Lergravsvej 59, 2300 Copenhagen S, Denmark.

Dal-Vita, Austral. Dal-Vita Products Pty Ltd, P.O. Box 670, Brookvale NSW 2100, Australia.

Dalcross, Austral. Dalcross Products Pty Ltd, 10 River Rd, Camden NSW 2570, Australia.

Dales, UK. Dales Pharmaceuticals Ltd, Snaygill Industrial Estate, Keighly Rd, Skipton, North Yorkshire BD23 2RW, England.

Dalin, USA. Dalin, USA.

Dallas, Arg. Dallas S.A., Uriarte 2121/23, 1425 Buenos Aires, Argentina.

Damor, Ital. Farmaceutici Damor s.p.a., Strada S.M. a Cubito 27, 80145 Naples, Italy.

Danapharm, Denm. Danapharm ApS, Horsholmvej 7, 3050 Humlebaek, Denmark.

Danbury, USA. Danbury Pharmacal Inc., 131 West St, P.O. Box 296, Danbury CT 06810, USA.

Daniel-Brunet, Fr. Laboratoires Daniel-Brunet, 112 rue de Silly, 92100 Boulogne-Billancourt, France.

Dansk Dental Depot, Denm. Dansk Dental Depot A/S, Lerso Parkalle 109, 2100 Copenhagen O, Denmark.

Dauelsberg, S.Afr. See *De-Nol, S.Afr.*

Dausse, Fr. See *Synthelabo, Fr.*

Dausse, Switz. See *Pharmac-Service, Switz.*

David Anthony, UK. David Anthony Pharmaceuticals Ltd, Spindus Rd, Speke, Liverpool L24 1YA, England.

Davigo, Belg. Firme Davigo, ave de Broqueville 192/bte 14, 1200 Brussels, Belgium.

Davis & Geck, UK. Davis & Geck, A division of Cyanamid of Great Britain Ltd, Fareham Rd, Gosport, Hants PO13 0AS, England.

Davur, Spain. Davur, Pantoja 14, 28002 Madrid, Spain.

Dayton, USA. Dayton Laboratories, 9424 NW 13th St, Miami FL 33172, USA.

DCG, Swed. DCG Farmaceutica AB, Fack 78, 431 21 Molndal 1, Sweden.

DDD, Ger. DDD Laboratorium Apotheker Gerhard Krauss, Hans-Bockler-Str. 5, Postfach: 468, 6078 Neu-Isenburg, Germany.

DDD, UK. DDD Ltd, 94 Rickmansworth Rd, Watford, Herts WD1 7JJ, England.

DDSA Pharmaceuticals, UK. DDSA Pharmaceuticals Ltd, 310 Old Brompton Rd, London SW5 9JQ, England.

De Angeli, Ital. Istituto De Angeli s.p.a., Via Serio 15, 20139 Milan, Italy.

De Angeli, S.Afr. See *Restan, S.Afr.*

de Angeli, Switz. See *Iromedica, Switz.*

de Bournonville, Belg. Ets A. de Bournonville et Fils S.A., Parc Industriel de la Vallee du Hain, 1420 Braine-l'Alleud, Belgium.

De Witt, UK. De Witt International Ltd, Seymour Rd, London E10 7LX, England.

Debat, Denm. See *Ferring, Denm.* and *GEA, Denm.*

Debat, Fr. Laboratoires Debat, 60 rue de Monceau, 75008 Paris, France.

Debat, Neth. See *Roussel, Neth.*

Debat, Norw. See *Midelfart, Norw.*

Debat, Swed. See *Selena, Swed.*

Debat, Switz. See *Therapia, Switz.*

Deca, Ital. Laboratorio Chimico Deca dr. Capuani & C. s.a.s., Via Balzaretti 17, 20133 Milan, Italy.

Declimed, Ger. Declimed Zweigniederlassung der Desitin Arzneimittel GmbH, Weg beim Jager 214, Postfach: 630120, 2000 Hamburg 63, Germany.

Decon Laboratories, UK. Decon Laboratories Ltd, Conway St, Hove, Sussex BN3 3LY, England.

Dedieu, Fr. Laboratoires Dedieu, av. J.-F.-Kennedy, 33701 Merignac, France.

Defence Medical Equipment Depot, UK. Defence Medical Equipment Depot, Ludgershall, Andover, Hants, England.

Deglaude, Fr. Laboratoires Deglaude, 180 rue de Vaugirard, 75015 Paris, France.

Degussa-Asta, Ger. Asta-Werke Degussa Pharma Gruppe, Artur-Ladeback Strasse 128-152, Postfach: 140129, 4800 Bielefeld, Germany.

Degussa, Ger. Homburg Degussa Pharma Gruppe, Daimlerstrasse 25, Postfach: 100 503, 6000 Frankfurt 1, Germany.

Degussa, Swed. Degussa Norden AB, Kemistvagen 8, 183 34 Taby, Sweden.

Degussa, Switz. Degussa SA, Case postale 2050, 8040 Zurich, Switzerland.

Degussa, UK. Degussa Pharmaceuticals Ltd, The Science Park, Milton Rd, Cambridge CB4 4FY, England.

Deiters, Spain. Deiters, Pasaje de Artemisa 18, 08027 Barcelona, Spain.

Del Saz & Filippini, Ital. Farma.ci Del Saz & Filippini s.r.l., Via P. Diacono 2, 20133 Milan, Italy.

Delagrange, Belg. Delagrange S.A., chaussee de la Hulpe 150/bte 6, 1170 Brussels, Belgium.

Delagrange, Denm. See *Essex, Denm.*

Delagrange, Fr. Laboratoires Delagrange, 1 ave Pierre-Brossolette, 91380 Chilly-Mazarin, France.

Delagrange, Neth. See *Pharmexport, Neth.*

Delagrange, Spain. Delagrange, Avda. de la Industria S/N, Alcobendas, 28100 Madrid, Spain.

Delagrange, Switz. See *Pharmos, Switz.*

Delalande, Belg. Lab. Delalande S.A., rue du Méridien 22, 1030 Brussels, Belgium.

Delalande, Fr. Laboratoires Delalande, 16 rue Henri-Regnault, 92400 Courbevoie, France.

Delalande, Ger. Delalande Arzneimittel GmbH, Aachener Strasse 201-209, Postfach: 410320, 5000 Cologne 41, W. Germany.

Delalande, Ital. Laboratori Delalande s.p.a., Via Torino 19, 10044 Pianezza Torino, Italy.

Delalande, Switz. Lab. Delalande S.A., 20 rue de la Coulouvrenière, 1204 Geneva, Switzerland.

Delamac, Austral. Delamac Pharmaceuticals Pty Ltd, P.O. Box 125, Spring Hill Qld 4000, Australia.

Delandale, Neth. See *ICN, Neth.*

Delandale, UK. Delandale Laboratories Ltd, Delandale House, 37 Old Dover Rd, Canterbury, Kent CT1 3JB, England.

Delmaak, S.Afr. Delmaak Laboratories, S. Africa.

Delmas Perfusion, Fr. Delmas Perfusion, B.P. 241, 37172 Chambray-les-Tours, France.

Delmont, USA. Delmont Laboratories Inc., P.O. Box AA, Swarthmore PA 19081, USA.

Delta Laboratories, Eire. Delta Laboratories Ltd, Fairdale Works, Artane, Dublin 5, Eire.

Demon, S.Afr. See *Propan, S.Afr.*

Dendron, UK. Dendron Ltd, 94 Rickmansworth Rd, Watford, Herts WD1 7JJ, England.

De-Nol, S.Afr. De-Nol Laboratories (SA) (Pty) Ltd, P.O. Box 4857, Johannesburg 2000, S. Africa.

Denolin, Belg. Denolin S.A., rue du Chateau 47, 1420 Braine-l'Alleud, Belgium.

Denolin, Neth. See *Hermes, Neth.*

Denta-Health, Austral. Denta-Health Products Pty Ltd, 54 Mosely St, Strathfield NSW 2135, Australia.

Dental Health Promotion, UK. Dental Health Promotion Ltd, 51 Greencroft Gardens, London NW6 3II, England.

Dentinox, Ger. Dentinox Gesellschaft für Pharmazeutische Präparate Lenk & Schuppan, Nunsdorfer Ring 19, Postfach: 480 369, 1000 Berlin 48, W. Germany.

Denver, S.Afr. See *SCS, S.Afr.*

Denyer, Austral. Denyer Broths Pty Ltd, GPO Box 2533, Sydney NSW 2001, Australia.

Dep, UK. Dep (UK) Ltd, P.O. Box 274, Sterling House, 165 Farnham Rd, Slough SL1 4XJ, England.

Dergo, Belg. Ets Dergo S.A., rue Franz Gailliard 2-2a, 1060 Brussels, Belgium.

Derly, Spain. Derly, Paseo de la Industria s/n, Alcobendas, 28080 Madrid, Spain.

Dermacare, Austral. Dermacare Pty Ltd, GPO Box 2264, Sydney NSW 2001, Australia.

Dermal Laboratories, UK. Dermal Laboratories Ltd, Tatmore Place, Gosmore, Hitchin, Herts SG4 7QR, England.

Dermalex, UK. The Dermalex Co. Ltd, Division of Labaz Sanofi Ltd, Floats Rd, Wythenshawe, Manchester M23 9NF, England.

Dermik, USA. Dermik Laboratories Inc., 500 Virginia Dr., Fort Washington PA 19034, USA.

Dermophil Indien, Fr. Laboratoires du Dermophil Indien, B.P. 30, 61600 La Ferte-Mace, France.

Dermtek, Canad. Dermtek Pharmaceuticals Ltd, 1600 route Transcanadienne, Dorval, Quebec H9P 1H7, Canada.

Desbergers, Canad. Desbergers Ltd, 8480 St Lawrence Blvd, Montreal, Quebec H2P 2M6, Canada.

Design, Swed. Laboratorie Design, Box 1073, 181 21 Lidingo, Sweden.

Desitin, Ger. Desitin Arzneimittel GmbH, Weg beim Jäger 214, Postfach: 63 01 20, 2000 Hamburg 63, W. Germany.

Desitin, Switz. See *Adroka, Switz.* and *Schwarz, Switz.*

Desopharma, Switz. Desopharma SA, Case postale 36, 4020 Basel, Switzerland.

Dessy, Ital. Dessy s.r.l., Via alla Marina 71, 00042 Lavinio-Anzio (Rome), Italy.

Devege, Arg. Devege, Lamadrid esq. Torcuato de Alvear, 1879 Quilmes, Buenos Aires, Argentina.

Deverge, Ital. Deverge Medicina e Medicalizzazione s.r.l., C.so Chieri 11, 10132 Turin, Italy.

Devimy, Fr. Laboratoires Devimy, 104 rue du Fg St-Honore, 75008 Paris, France.

Dexo, Fr. Laboratoires Dexo, 31 rue d'Arras, 92000 Nanterre, France.

Dexo, Switz. See *Serum, Switz.*

Dey, USA. Dey, USA.

DHL Products, UK. DHL Products Ltd, New Mill, New St, Idle, Bradford, West Yorkshire, England.

Diabetylin, Ger. Diabetylin, Gehrn 3, Postfach: 1161, 7902 Blaubeuren, W. Germany.

Diamant, Belg. See *Roussel, Belg.*

Diamant, Fr. Laboratoires Diamant, 1 terrasse Bellini, 92800 Puteaux, France.

Diamed, UK. Diamed Diagnostics Ltd, Mast House, Derby Rd, Bootle, Merseyside, England.

Diasan, Switz. See *Stotzer Zurich, Switz.*

Dibios, Spain. Dibios, Ctra Sabadell-Granollers km 14.5, Llisa de Val, 08185 Barcelona, Spain.

Dicamed, Swed. Dicamed AB, Box 6048, 163 06 Spanga, Sweden.

Dieckmann, Ger. Dieckmann Arzneimittel GmbH, Eckendorfer Str. 91-93, Postfach: 1209, 4800 Bielefeld 1, W. Germany.

Diedenhofen, Belg. See *Madaus, Belg.*

Diephuis, Neth. Diephuis B.V., Moesstraat 34, 9717 JX Groningen, Netherlands.

Dietary Foods, UK. Dietary Foods Ltd, Cumberland House, Brook St, Soham, Cambs CB7 5BA, England.

Dietary Specialities, UK. Dietary Specialities Ltd, DSL House, 159 Mortlake Rd, Kew, Surrey TW9 4AW, England.

Dietetique et Sante, Fr. Laboratoires Dietetique et Sante, B.P. 106, 31250 Revel, France.

Diethelm, Switz. Diethelm & Co. SA, Case postale, 8052 Zurich, Switzerland.

Diethelm, Thai. Diethelm & Co. Ltd, 280 Charoen Krung Rd (New Rd), Bangkok 10100, Thailand.

Dietisa, Spain. Dietisa, Buenaventura Plajas 11, 08028 Barcelona, Spain.

Difa, Ital. Difa-Coopervision s.p.a., Via Milano 160, 21042 Caronno Pertusella (VA), Italy.

Difer, Ital. Difer Industrie Farmaceutiche Triestine s.r.l., Viale XX Settembre 4, 34125 Trieste, Italy.

Difrex, Austral. See *Fisons, Austral.*

Diftersa, Spain. Diftersa, Mallorca 288, 08037 Barcelona, Spain.

Difusora, Spain. See *Diftersa, Spain.*

Diliont, Fr. Laboratoires Diliont, 21 rue Bargue, 75015 Paris, France.

Dinacren, Ital. Dinacren Laboratorio Farmaceutico s.n.c. del Dott. A. Francioni e di M. Gerosa, Via Sempione 72-74, 21018 Sesto Calende (VA), Italy.

Dispersa, Denm. See *Ciba, Denm.*

Dispersa, Ger. Dispersa Baeschlin GmbH, Dornierstrasse 4, Postfach: 1140, 8034 Germering, W. Germany.

Dispersa, Neth. See *Zyma, Neth.*

Dispersa, Norw. See *Andersen, Norw.*

Dispersa, S.Afr. See *Restan, S.Afr.*

Dispersa, Swed. See *Ciba, Swed.*

Dispersa, Switz. Dispersa SA, Case postale, 8442 Hettlingen, Switzerland.

Dispersa, UK. Dispersa (United Kingdom) Ltd, Westhead, 10 West St, Alderley Edge, Cheshire SK9 7XP, England.

Disprovent, Arg. Disprovent S.A.C.I.F. y M., Canalejas 1080, 1405 Buenos Aires, Argentina.

Dissolvurol, Mon. Laboratoires Dissolvurol, Le Minerve, av. Crovetto, B.P. 332 Monte-Carlo, 98006 Monaco Cedex, Monaco.

Dista, Austral. See *Lilly, Austral.*

Dista, Denm. See *Lilly, Denm.*

Dista, S.Afr. See *Lilly, S.Afr.*

Dista, Spain. Dista, Paseo Industria S/N, Alcobendas, 28080 Madrid, Spain.

Dista, Swed. See *Lilly, Swed.*

Dista, Switz. See *Inst. Serother. & Vaccinal, Switz.*

Dista, UK. Dista Products Ltd, Kingsclere Rd, Basingstoke, Hants RG21 2XA, England.

Dista, USA. Dista Products Company, Division of Eli Lilly & Co., Lilly Corporate Center, Indianapolis IN 46285, USA.

Distillers Co., UK. The Distillers Co. (Malt Products) Ltd, Malt Extract Factory, Kirkliston, West Lothian EH29 9DN, Scotland.

Distripharm, Switz. Distripharm SA, 36 route de Grandvaux, 1096 Cully, Switzerland.

Diter, Spain. Diter, Traversera de Dalt 15, 08024 Barcelona, Spain.

Divapharma, Ger. Divapharma-Knufinke Arzneimittel-werk GmbH, Motzener Strasse 41, 1000 Berlin 48, Germany.

Diversey, UK. Diversey Ltd, Weston Favell Centre, Northampton NN3 4PD, England.

Doak, Canad. See *Trans Canaderm, Canad.*

Doak, USA. Doak Pharmacal Co. Inc., 128 Magnolia Ave, Westbury NY 11590, USA.

Doctos, Spain. Doctos, Llorens y Barba 40-6, 08025 Barcelona, Spain.

Doetsch & Grether, Belg. See *Melisana, Belg.*

Doetsch, Grether, Switz. Doetsch, Grether & Cie SA, 4002 Basel, Switzerland.

Dojin Iyaku, Jpn. Dojin Iyaku, 5-2-2 Yayoi-cho, Nakano-ku, Tokyo, Japan.

Dolder, Austral. See *Cambridge Laboratories, Austral.*

Dolorgiet, Ger. Dolorgiet GmbH u. Co. KG, Otto-von-Guericke-Str. 1, Postfach: 3169, 5205 St. Augustin 3/Bonn, W. Germany.

Dolorgiet, Switz. See *Solco, Switz.*

Dome, Denm. See *Bayer, Denm.*

Dome, Neth. See *Bayer, Neth.*

Dome, Swed. See *Bayer, Swed.*

Dome, Switz. See *Diethelm, Switz.*

Dome, USA. Dome Division, Miles Laboratories Inc., 400 Morgan Lane, West Haven CT 06516, USA.

Dome-Hollister-Stier, Austral. See *Bayer, Austral.*

Dome-Hollister-Stier, Fr. Dome-Hollister-Stier Depart. des Laboratoires Miles, Tour Maine-Montparnasse, 75755 Paris Cedex 15, France.

Dome/Hollister-Stier, UK. Dome/Hollister-Stier, Strawberry Hill, Newbury, Berks RG13 1JA, England.

Domenech Garcia, Spain. Domenech Garcia, San Martin 8, Cerdanyolas, 08290 Barcelona, Spain.

Dominguez, Arg. Dominguez S.R.L., Av. La Plata 2552, 1437 Buenos Aires, Argentina.

Dominion, Canad. Dominion Pharmacal, Division of Pharmascience Inc., 8400 ch. Darnley, Montreal, Quebec H4T 1M4, Canada.

Dompè, Ital. Dompè Farmaceutici s.p.a., Via San Martino 12, 20122 Milan, Italy.

Doms, Fr. Laboratoires Doms, B.P. 45, 4 rue Ficatier, 92404 Courbevoie Cedex, France.

Doms, Switz. See *Actipharm, Switz.*

Domus, Arg. Especialidades Comus, Fortbenton Co. Laboratories, Escalada 133, 1407 Buenos Aires, Argentina.

Donini, Ital. Donini A. di Gabbiani G. & C. s.r.l., Via 1 Maggio 42, 37012 Bussolengo (VR), Italy.

Doppel, Ital. Doppel Farmaceutici s.r.l., Strada Regina 2, 29100 Piacenza, Italy.

Dormer, Canad. Dormer Laboratories Inc., 6600 route Transcanadienne, Suite 750, Pointe-Claire, Quebec H9R 4S2, Canada.

Dorsch, Ger. Dorsch GmbH & Co. KG, Postfach: 700480, 8000 Munich 70, Germany.

Dorsey Laboratories, USA. Dorsey Laboratories, Division of Sandoz Inc., P.O. Box 83288, Lincoln NE 68501, USA.

Dow, Canad. Dow Pharmaceuticals, 7777 Keele St, Concord, Ontario L4K 1Y7, Canada.

Dow, Spain. See *Merrell Dow, Spain.*

Dow, USA. See *Merrell Dow, USA.*

Dow Agriculture, UK. Dow Agriculture, Latchmore Court, Brand St, Hitchin, Herts SG5 1HZ, England.

Dow Corning, UK. Dow Corning Ltd, Avco House, Castle St, Reading, Berks RG1 7DZ, England.

Dow Corning, USA. Dow Corning Corporation, Midland MI 48640, USA.

Downs, UK. Downs Surgical Ltd, Church Path, Mitcham, Surrey CR4 3EU, England.

Dox-Al, Ital. Dox-Al Italia s.p.a., Via Fermi 2, 20050 Correzzana (MI), Italy.

Doyle, USA. See *Sandoz Nutrition, USA.*

DRA Pharmedev, Canad. DRA Pharmedev Canada Inc., 135 Place Cote Vertu, Suite 1500, St-Laurent, Quebec H4N 1G4, Canada.

Draco, Denm. See *Astra, Denm.*

Draco, Neth. See *Medicosma, Neth.*

Draco, Norw. See *Astra, Norw.*

Draco, Swed. AB Draco, Box 34, 221 00 Lund, Sweden.

Drag, Spain. Drag, Ctra Villaviciosa Odon a Pinto km 11.1, Fuenlabrada, 28940 Madrid, Spain.

Dreikehl, Spain. Dreikehl, Rafael Batlle 26-8, 08017 Barcelona, Spain.

Dreluso, Ger. Dreluso Pharmazeutika, Dr Elten & Sohn, Markt 5, Postfach: 140, 3253 Hessisch Oldendorf 1, W. Germany.

Drogcentralen, Swed. AB Drogcentralen, Fack 78, 431 21 Molndal 1, Sweden.

Dromicap, Arg. Dromicap S.A., Alte. Brown 611/15, 1704 Ramos Mejia, Buenos Aires, Argentina.

Drossapharm, Switz. Drossapharm SA, Drosselstrasse 47, 4059 Basel, Switzerland.

Drug Houses Austral., Austral. Drug Houses of Australia Pty Ltd, 31-39 Henderson St, Turrella NSW 2205, Australia.

Drug Industries, USA. Drug Industries Co. Inc., 3237 Hilton Rd, Ferndale MI 48220, USA.

Drug Trading, Canad. Drug Trading Co. Ltd, 795 Pharmacy Ave, Scarborough, Ontario M1L 3K2, Canada.

Du Pont, Austral. See *Boots, Austral.*

Du Pont, Belg. Du Pont de Nemours (Belgium) S.A., Mercure Centre, rue de la Fusee 100, 1130 Brussels, Belgium.

Du Pont, Canad. Du Pont Canada Inc., Du Pont Pharmaceuticals, Box 2300, Streetsville, Mississauga, Ontario L5M 2J4, Canada.

Du Pont, Denm. See *Meda, Denm.*

Du Pont, Neth. Du Pont de Nemours (Nederland) B.V. Pharmaceuticals, Helftheuvelweg 1, 5202 CB 's-Hertogenbosch, Netherlands.

Du Pont, Norw. See *Meda, Norw.*

Du Pont, Swed. See *Meda, Swed.*

Du Pont, USA. du Pont Pharmaceuticals, E.I. du Pont de Nemours & Co. Inc., Wilmington DE 19898, USA.

Du Pont de Nemours, Fr. Du Pont de Nemours (France) S.A., 137 rue de l'Universite, 75334 Paris Cedex 07, France.

Du Pont de Nemours, Switz. See *Opopharma, Switz.*

Du Pont Pharmaceuticals, UK. Du Pont (UK) Ltd, Wedgwood Way, Stevenage, Herts SG1 4QN, England.

Dubernard, Fr. Dubernard Hospital S.A., Laboratoire Pharmaceutique, 22 quai de Bacalan, 33075 Bordeaux Cedex, France.

Duchesnay, Canad. Duchesnay Inc. Laboratories, 2925 boul. Industriel, Chomedey-Laval, Quebec H7L 3W9, Canada.

Dukron, Ital. Dukron Italiana s.p.a., 04010 Campoverde (LT), Italy.

Dulcis, Belg. See *UPB, Belg.*

Dulcis, Mon. Laboratoires Dulcis, rue de l'Industrie, MC-Monaco, Monaco.

Dulcis, Neth. See *Bournonville, Neth.*

Dulcis, Switz. See *Interlabo, Switz.*

Dumex, Belg. See *Alcon-Couvreur, Belg.*

Dumex, Denm. A/S Dumex (Dumex Ltd), Prags Boulevard 37, 2300 Copenhagen S, Denmark.

Dumex, Neth. Dumex B.V., Min. Hartsenlaan 11, 1217 LR Hilversum, Netherlands.

Dumex, Norw. A/S Dumex, Nye Vakasv. 8, Postboks 93, 1364 Hvalstad, Norway.

Dumex, Swed. Dumex Läkemedel AB, Box 3501, 250 03 Helsingborg 3, Sweden.

Dumex, Switz. See *Lagap, Switz.*

Duncan, Arg. Duncan S.C.A., Llavallol 4141, 1419 Buenos Aires, Argentina.

Duncan, Ital. Duncan Farmaceutici s.p.a., Via Fleming 2, 37100 Verona, Italy.

Duncan, Flockhart, UK. Duncan, Flockhart & Co. Ltd, 700 Oldfield Lane North, Greenford, Middx UB6 0HD, England.

Dunhall, USA. Dunhall Pharmaceuticals Inc., Highway 59N, P.O. Box 100, Gravette AR 72736, USA.

Duphar, Belg. Duphar & Cie S.N.C., bd E. Bockstael 122, 1020 Brussels, Belgium.

Duphar, Fr. Laboratoires Duphar & Cie, 60 rue de Verdun, 69604 Villeurbanne, France.

Duphar, Ger. Duphar Pharma GmbH & Co. KG, Freundallee 21/23, Postfach: 1605, 3000 Hannover 1, Germany.

Duphar, Neth. Duphar Nederland B.V., Drentestraat 11, 1083 HK Amsterdam, Netherlands.

Duphar, S.Afr. Duphar BV, P.O. Box 10259, Johannesburg 2000, S. Africa.

Duphar, Spain. See *Kali-Farma, Spain.*

Duphar, Swed. See *Solvay, Swed.*

Duphar, Switz. Kali-Duphar Pharma SA, Untermattweg 8, 3027 Berne, Switzerland.

Duphar, UK. Duphar Laboratories Ltd, Gaters Hill, West End, Southampton SO3 3JD, England.

Dupomar, Arg. Dupomar Especialidades Medicinales, Luis Belaustegui 2957, 1416 Buenos Aires, Argentina.

DuPont, Arg. Du-Pont, Div. Ducilo S.A., Av. Eduardo Madero 1020, 1408 Buenos Aires, Argentina.

DuPont, Ger. DuPont (Deutschland) GmbH, Bereich Pharmazeutika, Opernplatz 2, Postfach: 100626, 6000 Frankfurt am Main, Germany.

Dura, USA. Dura Pharmaceuticals Inc., P.O. Box 28331, San Diego CA 92128, USA.

Durachemie, Ger. Durachemie GmbH & Co. KG, Burgermeister-Seidl Str. 7, 8190 Wolfratshausen, W. Germany.

Durascan, Denm. Durascan Medical Products ApS, Klaregade 19, 3., 5000 Odense C, Denmark.

Dutec, Austral. See *Ascot, Austral.*

Dutim, Neth. Pharm. Ind. en Handelsond. Dutim B.V., Handelsweg 8, 2404 CD Alphen a/d Rijn, Netherlands.

Dylade, UK. See *Fresenius, UK.*

Dynamit Nobel, UK. Dynamit Nobel (UK) Ltd, Edinburgh House, 43-51 Windsor Rd, Slough, Berks SL1 2HL, England.

E. Merck, Denm. See *Nordisk Droge, Denm.*

E. Merck, Ger. E. Merck, Frankfurter Strasse 250, Postfach: 4119, 6100 Darmstadt 1, W. Germany.

E. Merck, Neth. E. Merck Nederland B.V., Basisweg 34, 1043 AP Amsterdam, Netherlands.

E. Merck, Norw. Merck A/S, Ulvenv. 92d, 0581 Oslo 5, Norway.

E. Merck, Swed. E. Merck Aktiebolag, Kungsgatan 65, 111 22 Stockholm, Sweden.

E. Merck, Switz. E. Merck SA, Fröbelstrasse 22, 8029 Zurich, Switzerland.

E. Merck, UK. E. Merck Ltd, Winchester Road, Four Marks, Alton, Hants GU34 5HG, England.

Eagle, Austral. Eagle Laboratory Pty Ltd, 39c Church St, Lidcombe NSW 2141, Australia.

Eastman, UK. Eastman Chemical International AG, P.O. Box 66, Kodak House, Station Rd, Hemel Hempstead, Herts HP1 1JU, England.

Eaton, S.Afr. See *Smith Kline & French, S.Afr.*

Eberth, Ger. Dr. Friedrich Eberth Nachf., Kick-Rasel-Strasse 23/25, Postfach: 8, 8454 Schnaittenbach, Germany.

E.C.M. Laboratories, UK. E.C.M. Laboratories, Glebe View, North Rd, Havering-Atte-Bower, Romford, Essex RM4 1PP, England.

Ecobi, Ital. Farmaceutici Ecobi s.p.a., Via E. Bazzano, 16019 Ronco Scrivia (GE), Italy.

Ecological Formulas, USA. Ecological Formulas, Division of Cardiovascular Research Ltd, 1061 Shary Circle, Concord CA 94518, USA.

Econo Med, USA. Econo Med Pharmaceuticals Inc., P.O. Box 3303, Burlington NC 27215, USA.

Edmond Pharma, Ital. Edmond Pharma s.r.l., Via dei Giovi 131, 20037 Paderno Dugnano (MI), Italy.

Edwards, USA. Edwards Pharmacal Inc., P.O. Drawer 129, Osceola AR 72370-9990, USA.

Efamol, Canad. Efamol Research Inc., Annapolis Valley Industrial Park, P.O. Box 818, Kentville, Nova Scotia B4N 4H8, Canada.

Efeka, Ger. Efeka Friedrich & Kaufmann GmbH & Co. KG Arzneimittelfabrik, Siemensstr. 1, Postfach: 100101, 3004 Isernhagen 1, Germany.

Eggochemia, Aust. Eggochemia, Fabrik chemischer u. pharmazeutischer Präparate, Dr Rigobert Plass, Heiligenstädter Strasse Nr. 158, 1195 Vienna XIX, Austria.

Egic, Fr. See *Cernep Synthelabo, Fr.*

Egic, Switz. See *Kramer-Synthelabo, Switz.*

EGIS, Hung. EGIS Pharmaceuticals, P.O. Box 100, 1475 Budapest, Hungary.

Ego, Austral. Ego Pharmaceuticals Pty Ltd, 21-31 Malcolm Rd, Braeside Vic. 3195, Australia.

Eifelfango, Ger. Eifelfango, chemisch pharmazeutische Werke, GmbH & Co. KG, Ringener Strasse 45, Postfach: 100365, 5483 Bad Neuenahr-Ahrweiler, W. Germany.

Eifelfango, Switz. See *Agpharm, Switz.*

Eisai, Indon. Eisai, Jl Pembangunan II/13, Jakarta Pusat, Indonesia.

Eisai, Jpn. Eisai, 4-6-10 Koishikawa, Bunkyo-ku, Tokyo, Japan.

Eisai, Malaysia. Eisai (M) Sdn. Bhd., 4A Jalan 21/22 S.E.A. Park, 46300 Petaling Jaya, Malaysia.

Eisai, Thai. See *Diethelm, Thai.*

Eklow, Swed. Eklow Scandinavia AB, Box 23086, 104 35 Stockholm, Sweden.

Elanco, UK. Elanco Products Ltd, Kingsclere Rd, Basingstoke, Hants RG21 2XA, England.

Elder, Canad. See *ICN, Canad.*

Elder, Neth. See *Tramedico, Neth.*

Elder, S.Afr. See *Propan, S.Afr.*

Elder, USA. Elder Pharmaceuticals Inc., Subsidiary of ICN Pharmaceuticals Inc., 3300 Hyland Ave, Costa Mesa CA 92626, USA.

Elea, Arg. Elea S.A.C.I.F.yA., Saladillo 2450, 1440 Buenos Aires, Argentina.

Electramed, Eire. Electramed Ireland Ltd, 9 Mornington Park, Malahide Rd, Artane, Dublin 5, Eire.

Electrolactil, Spain. Electrolactil, Ciscar 26, 46005 Valencia, Spain.

Elerte, Fr. Laboratoires des Réalisations Thérapeutiques Élerté, 181 rue Andre-Karman, 93303 Aubervilliers Cedex, France.

Elgi, Fr. Laboratoires Elgi, B.P. 432, 69654 Villefranche-sur-Saone Cedex, France.

Elida Gibbs, UK. Elida Gibbs Ltd, P.O. Box 1DY, Portman Square, London W1A 1DY, England.

Elifarma, Ital. Elifarma s.r.l., Via G. Galilei 7, 20016 Pero (MI), Italy.

Elkins-Sinn, USA. Elkins-Sinn Inc., A subsidiary of A.H. Robins Co., 2 Esterbrook Lane, Cherry Hill NJ 08034, USA.

Ellem, Ital. Ellem Industria Farmaceutica s.p.a., Corso di Porta Ticinese 89, 20123 Milan, Italy.

Elmu, Spain. Elmu, Emilio Vargas 2, 28043 Madrid, Spain.

Elvetium, Arg. Elvetium S.A., L.N. Alem 822 13°, Buenos Aires, Argentina.

Emyfar, Spain. Emyfar, Unificacion 22-24, Hospitalet de Llobregat, Barcelona, Spain.

Endo, Austral. See *Du Pont, Austral.*

Endo, Canad. See *Du Pont, Canad.*

Endo, S.Afr. See *Berk, S.Afr.*

Endo, USA. Endo Laboratories Inc., 1000 Stewart Ave, Garden City NY 11530, USA.

Energen, UK. Energen Foods Co., England.

Engelhard, Ger. Karl Engelhard, Fabrik pharmazeutischer Präparate GmbH & Co. KG, Sandweg 94, Postfach: 100824, 6000 Frankfurt am Main 1, W. Germany.

English Grains, UK. English Grains Ltd, Swains Park Industrial Estate, Park Rd, Overseal, Burton-on-Trent, Staffs, England.

Enzypharm, Neth. Enzypharm B.V., Amersfoortsestraat 65, 3769 AE Soesterberg, Netherlands.

Enzypharm, UK. Enzypharm Biochemicals Ltd, P.O. Box 69, Harrogate, N Yorks HG1 2LE, England.

Erba, Norw. See *Farmitalia, Norw.*

Erco, Denm. Ercopharm A/S, Skelstedet 13-15, 2950 Vedbaek, Denmark.

Erco, Norw. See *Organon, Norw.*

Erco, Swed. Erco Läkemedel AB, Box 617, 191 26 Sollentuna, Sweden.

Ercopharm, Neth. See *Multi-Pharma, Neth.*

Ercopharm, Switz. See *Oryx, Switz.*

Eri, Canad. See *ICN, Canad.*

Ern, Spain. Ern, Pedro IV 499, 08020 Barcelona, Spain.

Ernest Jackson, UK. Ernest Jackson & Co. Ltd, Crediton, Devon EX17 3AP, England.

Errekappa, Ital. Errekappa Euroterapici (Linea della Bioresearch s.p.a.), Via C. Menotti 1/A, 20129 Milan, Italy.

Escaned, Spain. Escaned, Tomas Breton 46, 28045 Madrid, Spain.

Espe, Ger. Espe Fabrik pharmazeutischer Praparate GmbH & Co. KG, Griesberg 2, Postfach: 1142, 8031 Seefeld/Oberbayern, Germany.

Esseti, Ital. Esseti s.a.s. Laboratorio Chimico Farmaco Biologico, Via Cavalli di Bronzo 41, 80046 S. Giorgio a Cremona (NA), Italy.

Essex, Arg. Essex Arg. S.A.I.C., Av. San Martin 1750, 1602 Florida, Buenos Aires, Argentina.

Essex, Austral. Essex Laboratories Pty Ltd, P.O. Box 231, Baulkham Hills NSW 2153, Australia.

Essex, Belg. Essex (Belgium) S.A., ave de la Couronne 163, 1050 Brussels, Belgium.

Essex, Denm. Essex Pharma A/S, Hvedemarken 12, 3520 Farum, Denmark.

Essex, Ger. Essex Pharma GmbH, Sonnenstr. 33, Postfach: 330149 (8000 Munich 33), 8000 Munich 2, Germany.

Essex, Ital. Essex Italia s.p.a., Via Ripamonti 89, 20139 Milan, Italy.

Essex, Jpn. Essex, 4-1-20 Tachiuribori, Nishi-ku, Osaka, Japan.

Essex, Neth. Essex (Nederland) B.V., Bankrashof 3, 1183 NP Amstelveen, Netherlands.

Essex, NZ. Essex Laboratories (NZ) Ltd, P.O. Box 22-074, Otahuhu, Auckland 6, New Zealand.

Essex, Spain. Essex, Carretera Burgos S/N, San Agustin de Guadalix, 28750 Madrid, Spain.

Essex, Swed. Essex Läkemedel AB, Box 27190, 102 52 Stockholm, Sweden.

Essex, Switz. Essex Chemie AG, Case postale 2769, 6002 Luzern, Switzerland.

Estebanez, Spain. Estebanez, Ctra Ajalvir Torrejon km 7.5, Ajalvir, 28864 Madrid, Spain.

Estedi, Spain. Estedi, Leopoldo Alas 7, 08012 Barcelona, Spain.

Esterfarm, Ital. Esterfarm Laboratori Farmaceutici, Via Giovannino 7, 95126 Catania, Italy.

Esteve, Spain. Esteve Dr, Avda Virgen Montserrat 221, 28026 Barcelona, Spain.

Ethicals, Denm. See *Helge Kjelstrup, Denm.*

Ethicals, Neth. See *Rhône-Poulenc, Neth.*

Ethicals, Swed. See *Item, Swed.*

Ethichem, UK. Ethichem Ltd, 2 Mansfield Rd, South Croydon, Surrey CR2 6HN, England.

Ethicon, Ger. Ethicon GmbH, Robert-Koch-Strasse 1, 2000 Norderstedt, Germany.

Ethicon, UK. Ethicon Ltd, P.O. Box 408, Bankhead Ave, Edinburgh EH11 4HE, Scotland.

Ethigel, UK. The Ethigel Laboratories Ltd, England.

Ethimed, S.Afr. See *Noristan, S.Afr.*

Ethipharm, Canad. Ethipharm International, 2 boul. Crepeau, St-Laurent, Quebec H4N 1M7, Canada.

Ethitek, USA. Ethitek Pharmaceuticals Co., 8104 N. Lawndale Ave, Skokie IL 60076, USA.

Ethnor, Austral. See *Cilag, Austral.*

Ethnor, S.Afr. Ethnor (Pty) Ltd, P.O. Box 273, Halfway House 1685, Transvaal, S. Africa.

Etris, Fr. Etris S.A.R.L., 14 rue de la Comète, 75007 Paris, France.

Eucomark, UK. Eucomark Distributors Ltd, Glebe View, North Rd, Havering-Atte-Bower, Romford, Essex RM4 1PP, England.

Eurorga, Fr. Eurorga, S.A., 11 rue de la Loge, 94260 Fresnes, France.

Eurospital Pharma, Ital. Eurospital Pharma s.p.a., Via Flavia 122, 34147 Trieste, Italy.

Euroulta, Spain. Euroulta, Gaston de Gotor 4, 50006 Zaragoza, Spain.

Euterapia, Spain. See *Servier, Spain.*

Eutherapie, Belg. Eutherapie Benelux S.A., bd E. Bockstael 93, 1020 Brussels, Belgium.

Eutherapie, Fr. Eutherapie, 41 rue Ybry, B.P. 126, 92201 Neuilly-sur-Seine Cedex, France.

Evans Medical, UK. Evans Medical Ltd, 318 High St North, Dunstable, Beds LU6 1BE, England.

Evans Vanodine, UK. Evans Vanodine International Ltd, Brierley Hill, Walton Summit Centre, Bamber Bridge, Preston, Lancs PR5 8AH, England.

Evening Primrose Oil Co., UK. Evening Primrose Oil Co. Ltd, Unit 1, Jubilee Drive, Loughborough, Leics LE11 0FL, England.

Ever Ready Personna, UK. Ever Ready Personna Ltd, 116 Brent St, Hendon, London NW4 2EL, England.

Everest, Canad. Everest Pharmaceuticals Ltd, 78 St Regis Cr. N., Downsview, Ontario M3J 1Z3, Canada.

Everett, USA. Everett Laboratories Inc., 76 Franklin St, East Orange NJ 07017, USA.

Evident Dental Co., UK. Evident Dental Co. Ltd, 57 Wellington Court, Wellington Rd, London NW8 9TD, England.

Ewe, Arg. Ewe S.A., Pasco 1251, 1251 Buenos Aires, Argentina.

Exa, Arg. Exa Especialidades Medicinates, Division de Impex Ltda. S.A.C.I.F.I.A., Pedro Echague 2437, 1261 Buenos Aires, Argentina.

Exovir, USA. Exovir, USA.

E-Z-EM, Canad. E-Z-EM Canada Inc., 9855 rue Colbert, Ville d'Anjou, Quebec H1J IZ9, Canada.

Ezem, Neth. See *Rooster, Neth.*

Face, Ital. Face Laboratori Farmaceutici s.r.l., Via Albisola 49, 16162 Genova-Balzaneto, Italy.

Fada, Arg. FADA Ind. Com. y Farmaceutica S.R.L., Salquero 560, 1177 Buenos Aires, Argentina.

Fader, Spain. Fader, Castaner 15, 08022 Barcelona, Spain.

Faes, Spain. Faes, Maximo Aguirre 14, Bilbao, 48011 Vizcaya, Spain.

FAIR Laboratories, UK. See *Squibb, UK.*

Falafi, Spain. Falafi, Ramon Llull 6, Consell (Mallorca), 07330 Baleares, Spain.

Falk, Ger. Dr Falk GmbH & Co., Pharm. Praparate KG, Habsburgerstrasse 79, 7800 Freiburg, W. Germany.

Falk, Neth. See *Tramedico, Neth.*

Falk, Switz. See *Phardi, Switz.*

Falqui, Ital. Falqui Prodotti Farmaceutici s.p.a., Via G.R. Carli 2, 20161 Milan, Italy.

FAMA, Ital. F.A.M.A. s.r.l., Istituto Chimico Biologico, Via A. Sauli 21, 20127 Milan, Italy.

Famaco, Swed. Famaco AB, Box 9007, 102 71 Stockholm, Sweden.

Family Planning Sales, UK. Family Planning Sales Ltd, 28 Kelburne Rd, Cowley, Oxford OX4 3SZ, England.

Fandre, Fr. Laboratoires Fandre, rue Lavoisier, 54710 Ludres, France.

Farber-Ref, Ital. Farber Ref s.p.a., Via Imperia 35, 20142 Milan, Italy.

Farco, Belg. See *Melisana, Belg.*

Farco, Denm. See *Tjellesen, Denm.*

Farco-Pharma, Ger. Farco-Pharma GmbH Pharmazeutische Präparate, Mathias-Bruggen-Str. 82, Postfach: 300520, 5000 Cologne 30, W. Germany.

Farco-Pharma, Swed. See *Kronans, Swed.*

Fardi, Spain. Fardi, Grassot 16, 08025 Barcelona, Spain.

Fargal-Pharmasint, Ital. Fargal-Pharmasint s.r.l., Via P. Cavallini 24, 00192 Rome, Italy.

Farge, Ital. Farge, Via Tortona 12, 16139 Genoa, Italy.

Farglo, Spain. Farglo, Bocangel 28, 28028 Madrid, Spain.

Farillon, UK. Farillon Ltd, Ashton Rd, Harold Hill, Romford, Essex RM3 8UE, England.

Farley, Denm. See *Meda, Denm.*

Farma Food, Denm. Farma Food A/S, Vester Farimagsgade 7, 2., 1606 Copenhagen V, Denmark.

Farma-Lepori, Spain. Farma Lepori, Osio 30, 08034 Barcelona, Spain.

Farmabion, Spain. See *Alter, Spain.*

Farmacologico Milanese, Ital. Lab. Farmacologico Milanese s.r.l., Via Monterosso 273, 21042 Caronno Pertusella, Italy.

Farmaconsult, Arg. Farmaconsult S.A. Division Farma, Gandara 3274, 1431 Buenos Aires, Argentina.

Farmades, Ital. Farmades s.p.a., Via di Tor Cervara 282, 00155 Rome, Italy.

Farmadiez, Spain. Farmadiez, Herzegovino 29, 08006 Barcelona, Spain.

Farmaka, Ital. Farmaka s.r.l. Laboratori Farmaceutici, Via Vetreria 1, 22070 Grandate (CO), Italy.

Farmasimes, Spain. Farmasimes, Zamora 46-48, 08005 Barcelona, Spain.

Farmer Hill, Austral. See *Abbott, Austral.*

Farmiberia, Spain. Farmiberia, Mendez Alvaro 57, 28045 Madrid, Spain.

Farmigea, Ital. Farmigea s.p.a., Via Carmignani 2, 56100 Pisa, Italy.

Farmila, Ital. Farmila-Farmaceutici Milano s.p.a., Via E. Fermi 50, 20019 Settimo Milanese (MI), Italy.

Farmitalia, Denm. Farmitalia Carlo Erba Informationskontor, Ny Ostergade 20, 2., 1101 Copenhagen K, Denmark.

Farmitalia, Ger. Farmitalia Carlo Erba GmbH, Merzhauser Strasse 112, Postfach: 480, 7800 Freiburg, W. Germany.

Farmitalia, Ital. Farmitalia Carlo Erba s.p.a., Gruppo Montedison, Via C. Imbonati 24, 20159 Milan, Italy.

Farmitalia, Neth. See *Bournonville, Neth.*

Farmitalia, Norw. Farmitalia Carlo Erba, Montedison group, Roykenv. 70, Postboks 53, 1371 Asker, Norway.

Farmitalia, NZ. See *Pharmaco, NZ.*

Farmitalia, Spain. Farmitalia, Ctra. Mollet a Caldas Km 3, Sta. Perpetua de Moguda, 08130 Barcelona, Spain.

Farmitalia, Thai. Farmitalia Carlo Erba S.p.A. (Thailand Branch), 874 Soi Urupongse 2, Rama 6 Rd, Bangkok 10400, Thailand.

Farmitalia Carlo Erba, Belg. Farmitalia Carlo Erba S.A., rue Colonel Bourg 103/bte 2, 1040 Brussels, Belgium.

Farmitalia Carlo Erba, Fr. Laboratoires Farmitalia Carlo Erba S.A., Tour Franklin, Cedex 11, 92081 Paris-La-Défense, France.

Farmitalia Carlo Erba, S.Afr. Farmitalia Carlo Erba (SA) (Pty) Ltd, P.O. Box 41111, Craighall 2024, S. Africa.

Farmitalia Carlo Erba, Swed. Farmitalia Carlo Erba AB, Box 3511, 183 03 Taby, Sweden.

Farmitalia Carlo Erba, Switz. Farmitalia Carlo Erba SA, Case postale 316, 3000 Berne 25, Switzerland.

Farmitalia Carlo Erba, UK. Farmitalia Carlo Erba Ltd, Italia House, 23 Grosvenor Rd, St. Albans, Herts AL1 3AW, England.

Farmos, Denm. Farmos A/S, Smedeland 20B, 2600 Glostrup, Denmark.

Farmos, Norw. See *Sentipharm, Norw.*

Farmos, Swed. Farmos Group AB, Box 3012, 183 03 Taby, Sweden.

Farmos Finland, Neth. See *Pharbita, Neth.*

Faulding, Austral. Faulding Medical Products, P.O. Box 746, Salisbury SA 5108, Australia.

Faure, Fr. Laboratoires H. Faure (Les Vitacollyres), 07104 Annonay Cedex, France.

Fawns & McAllan, Austral. Fawns & McAllan, P.O. Box 204, Croydon Vic. 3136, Australia.

FBC, UK. FBC Ltd, Nottingham Rd, Stapleford, Nottingham NG9 8AJ, England.

Fecofar, Arg. Fecofar, John F. Kennedy 2742, 1754 San Justo, Buenos Aires, Argentina.

Federico Bonet, Spain. Federico Bonet, Mendez Alvaro 57, San Sebastian de los Reyes, 28045 Madrid, Spain.

Fellows, USA. Fellows-Testagar, Subsidiary of Chromalloy Pharmaceuticals Inc., 12741 Capital Ave, Oak Park MI 48237, USA.

Felo, Denm. Felo ApS, Kirkevejen 20, Teestrup, 4690 Haslev, Denmark.

Fennings, UK. Fennings Pharmaceuticals, 46 London Rd, Horsham, West Sussex RH12 2DT, England.

Fenwal, Canad. Fenwal Laboratories of Canada, Division of Travenol Canada Inc., 6695 Airport Rd, Mississauga, Ontario L4V IT7, Canada.

Fenwal, Denm. See *Travenol, Denm.*

Fernandez y Canivell, Spain. Fernandez y Canivell, Plg el Viso Carabela 4, 29080 Malaga, Spain.

Ferndale, USA. Ferndale Laboratories Inc., 780 West Eight Mile Rd, Ferndale MI 48220, USA.

Ferran, Spain. Ferran, Av. M.J. Verdaguer S/N-P. Font Sta, Sant Joan Despi, 08970 Barcelona, Spain.

Ferraton, Denm. Ferraton A/S, Kirkevejen 20, Teestrup, 4690 Haslev, Denmark.

Ferraz, Lynce, Port. Ferraz, Lynce, LDA, Rua Rosa Araújo 27-31, Apartado 1069, 1002 Lisboa Codex, Portugal.

Ferrer, Spain. Ferrer, Carlos III 94, 08028 Barcelona, Spain.

Ferrer, Switz. See *Adroka, Switz.*

Ferring, Canad. Ferring Laboratories Ltd, 7 Roxville Ave, Toronto, Ontario M4G 3P7, Canada.

Ferring, Denm. Ferring A/S, Indertoften 5, 2720 Vanløse, Denmark.

Ferring, Fr. Laboratoires Ferring, 7 rue des Cordelières, 75013 Paris, France.

Ferring, Ger. Ferring Arzneimittel GmbH, Wittland 11, Postfach: 2145, 2300 Kiel 1, W. Germany.

Ferring, Neth. See *Pharmachemie, Neth.*

Ferring, Norw. See *Nyco, Norw.*

Ferring, Swed. Ferring AB, Box 305 61, 200 62 Malmo, Sweden.

Ferring, Switz. Ferring SA, Schaffhauserstrasse 24, 8006 Zurich, Switzerland.

Ferring, UK. Ferring Pharmaceuticals Ltd, 11 Mount Rd, Feltham, Middx TW13 6JG, England.

Ferrosan, Denm. A/S Ferrosan, Sydmarken 1-5, 2860 Søborg, Denmark.

Ferrosan, Fin. Oy Ferrosan AB, Kutojantie 8, 02630 Espoo, Finland.

Ferrosan, Norw. See *Mekos, Norw.* and *Norfarma, Norw.*

Ferrosan, Swed. AB Ferrosan, Box 839, 201 80 Malmo, Sweden.

FFF, Spain. FFF, Azcona 46, 28028 Madrid, Spain.

Fher, Ital. Fher, Divisione della Boehringer Ingelheim, Casella Postale, 50100 Florence, Italy.

Fher, Spain. Fher, Angli 31, 08017 Barcelona, Spain.

Fibos, Spain. Fibos, Cadaques 30, La Llagosta, 08120 Barcelona, Spain.

Fides, Spain. See *Kabi, Spain.*

Fidia, Ital. Fidia, Farmaceutici Italiani Derivati Industriali e Affini s.p.a., Via Ponte d/ Fabbrica 3/A, 35031 Abano Terme (Padua), Italy.

Fielding, USA. The Fielding Co., 2384 Centerline Industrial Dr., St Louis MO 63146, USA.

Finadiet, Arg. Finadiet S.A.C.I.F.I., Hipólito Yrigoyen 3771, 1208 Buenos Aires, Argentina.

Fine Organics, USA. Fine Organics Inc., 205 Main St, Lodi NJ 07644, USA.

Fink, Ger. Fink GmbH, Daimlerstrasse 3, Postfach: 1160, 7033 Herrenberg, W. Germany.

Fink, Switz. See *Uhlmann-Eyraud, Switz.*

FIRMA, Ital. Fabbr. Ital. Ritrov. Medic. Aff. s.p.a., Via di Scandicci 37, 50143 Florence, Italy.

Fisch-Smith & Nephew, Fr. Laboratoires Fisch-Smith & Nephew S.A., 7 rue Valentin-Hauy, 75015 Paris, France.

Fischer, Israel. Fischer Pharmaceuticals Ltd, P.O. Box 39071, Tel Aviv, Israel.

Fisher, USA. Fisher Scientific Co., 52 Fadem Rd, Springfield NJ 07081, USA.

Fiske, USA. Fiske, USA.

Fisons, Austral. Fisons Pty Ltd, P.O. Box 42, Pennant Hills NSW, Australia.

Fisons, Belg. Fisons S.A., Ambachtelijke Zone Haasrode, Ambachtenlaan 1, 3030 Leuven, Belgium.

Fisons, Canad. Fisons Corporation Ltd, 80 Melford Dr., Scarborough, Ontario M1B 2G3, Canada.

Fisons, Denm. Fisons A/S, Rosenkaeret 22 B, 2860 Søborg, Denmark.

Fisons, Fr. Laboratoires Fisons S.A., Immeuble 'Les 4 M', Chemin du Petit-Bois, 69132 Ecully Cedex, France.

Fisons, Ger. Fisons Arzneimittel GmbH, Max-Planck-Strasse 9-11, Postfach:400224, 5000 Cologne 40, W. Germany.

Fisons, Ital. Fisons s.p.a., V.le Castello d/la Magliana 38, 00148 Rome, Italy.

Fisons, Neth. Fisons B.V., Afd. Pharma, Larikslaan 4, 3833 AM Leusden, Netherlands.

Fisons, Norw. Fisons Norway, A/S, Osterndalen 27, Postboks 24, 1345 Osteras, Norway.

Fisons, S.Afr. Fisons Pharmaceuticals (Pty) Ltd, P.O. Box 84, Chloorkop 1624, S. Africa.

Fisons, Swed. Fisons Sweden AB, Box 42063, 126 12 Stockholm, Sweden.

Fisons, Switz. Fisons SA, Alte Steinhauserstr. 35, 6330 Cham, Switzerland.

Fisons, UK. Fisons PLC, Pharmaceutical Division, 12 Derby Rd, Loughborough, Leics LE11 0BB, England.

Fisons, USA. Fisons Corporation, Pharmaceutical Division, Two Preston Court, Bedford MA 01730, USA.

Fisons Horticultural Division, UK. Fisons Horticultural Division, Paper Mill Lane, Bramford, Ipswich IP8 4BZ, England.

Fitodorfarma, Ital. Fitodorfarma s.a.s., Sezione Erboristeria, Via Genova 28, 21052 Busto Arsizio (VA), Italy.

Fleet, Neth. See *Tramedico, Neth.*

Fleet, USA. C.B. Fleet Co. Inc., 4615 Murray Pl., Lynchburg VA 24502-2235, USA.

Fleming, USA. Fleming & Co., 1600 Fenpark Dr., Fenton MO 63026, USA.

Flint, Canad. Flint Laboratories of Canada, Division of Travenol Canada Inc., 6695 Airport Rd, Mississauga, Ontario L4V 1TL, Canada.

Flint, USA. Flint Laboratories, Division of Travenol Laboratories Inc., Deerfield IL 60015, USA.

Fluoritab, USA. Fluoritab Corp., P.O. Box 381, Flint MI 48501, USA.

FMC Corp., USA. FMC Corporation, 1105 Coleman Ave, San Jose CA 95110, USA.

Foletto, Ital. Foletto Achille, Via Vitt. Emanuele 12, 38060 Pieve di Ledro (Trento), Italy.

Ford, Austral. Ford, Australia.

Ford, Jackson, UK. Ford, Jackson & Co. (Sales) Ltd, 3 Briggate, Leeds LS1 4AF, England.

Forest, Canad. See *Seaway Midwest, Canad.*

Forest, Denm. See *Nordisk Droge, Denm.*

Forest Laboratories, USA. Forest Laboratories Inc., 2510 Metro Blvd, St Louis MO 63043, USA.

Forest Pharmaceuticals, USA. Forest Pharmaceuticals Inc., 2510 Metro Blvd, Maryland Heights MO 63043-9979, USA.

Foret Peroxidos, Spain. Foret Peroxidos, Amigo 65-1-1, 08021 Barcelona, Spain.

Formenti, Ital. Prodotti Formenti s.r.l., Via Correggio 43, 20149 Milan, Italy.

Forrest, Austral. Forrest Pharmaceutical Co. Pty Ltd, 7 Willis St, Arncliffe NSW 2205, Australia.

Fort, Ital. Calmante Fort s.r.l., Via L. Canonica 1, 20154 Milan, Italy.

Fortbenton, Arg. Fortbenton Co. Laboratories, Escalada 133, 1407 Buenos Aires, Argentina.

Forum Chemicals, UK. Forum Chemicals Ltd, Forum House, 41-75 Brighton Rd, Redhill, Surrey RH1 6YS, England.

Fougera, USA. E. Fougera & Co., Division of Altana Inc., 60 Baylis Rd, Melville NY 11747, USA.

Four Macs, Austral. Four Macs, 78 Burns Rd, Wahroonga NSW 2076, Australia.

Fournier Frères, Fr. See *Pharmuka, Fr.*

Fournier S.A., Fr. Laboratoires Fournier S.A., 9 rue Petitot, 21000 Dijon, France.

Fournier, Spain. Fournier, Ctra de Navarra s/n, Hernani, 20120 Guipuzcoa, Spain.

Fox, UK. Charles H. Fox Ltd, 22 Tavistock St, London WC2E 7PY, England.

Foy, USA. Foy, USA.

Français, Fr. See *Boehringer Ingelheim, Fr.*

Francia Farm., Ital. Francia Farmaceutici s.r.l., Via dei Pestagalli 7, 20138 Milan, Italy.

Francisco Durban, Spain. Francisco Durban, Santos Zarate 20, 04004 Almeria, Spain.

Franklin Medical, UK. Franklin Medical Ltd, P.O. Box 138, Turnpike Rd, High Wycombe, Bucks HP12 3NB, England.

Frere, Belg. Frere & Cie S.A., ave des Noisetiers 7, 1170 Brussels, Belgium.

Fresenius, Fr. Laboratoires Fresenius, 8 rue des Pyrenes, Silic 524, 94633 Rungis Cedex, France.

Fresenius, Ger. Fresenius AG, Borkenberg 14, Postfach: 1809, 6370 Oberursel, W. Germany.

Fresenius, Neth. See *Hoechst, Neth.*

Fresenius, S.Afr. See *Saphar, S.Afr.*

Fresenius, Swed. See *Dicamed, Swed.*

Fresenius, Switz. Fresenius SA, Case postale, 6370 Stans, Switzerland.

Fresenius, UK. Fresenius Ltd, 6/7 Christleton Court, Stuart Rd, Manor Park, Runcorn, Cheshire WA7 1ST, England.

Friis, Denm. Friis & Co., Christian, Maltegårdsvej 18, 2820 Gentofte, Denmark.

Frosst, Austral. See *Merck Sharp & Dohme, Austral.*

Frosst, Canad. Frosst, Division of Merck Frosst Canada Inc., C.P. 1005, Pointe Claire-Dorval, Quebec H9R 4P8, Canada.

Frosst, Ger. Frosst Pharma GmbH, Charles-de-Gaulle-Str. 4, Postfach:830960, 8000 Munchen 83, W. Germany.

Frosst, Neth. Frosst, divisie van Merck Sharp & Dohme B.V., Waarderweg 39, 2031 BN Haarlem, Netherlands.

Frosst, S.Afr. See *Merck Sharp & Dohme, S.Afr.*

Frumtost, Spain. Frumtost Zyma, Suiza 9-11, 08023 Barcelona, Spain.

Fuca, Fr. Laboratoires Fuca S.A., 1 bis, rue de Plaisance, 94732 Nogent-sur-Marne Cedex, France.

Fuchs, Switz. Dr med. H. Fuchs, Kurhaus, 6936 Cademario, Switzerland.

Fujisawa, Jpn. Fujisawa Yakuhin, 4-3 Doshomachi, Higashi-ku, Osaka, Japan.

Fujisawa, S.Afr. Fujisawa, S. Africa.

Fujizoki, Jpn. Fuji Zoki Pharmaceutical Co. Ltd, 4-6-7 Shimoochiai, Shinjuku-ku, Tokyo, Japan.

Fulton, Ital. Fulton Medicinali s.r.l., Corso Vercelli 54, 20145 Milan, Italy.

Fumouze, Fr. Laboratoires Fumouze S.A., 1 rue Méchin, 93450 Ile-Saint-Denis, France.

FUNED, Braz. Fundacao Ezequiel Dias (FUNED), Rua Conde Pereira Carneiro, Gameleira, 30000 Belo Horizonte, Minas Gerais, Brazil.

Funk, Spain. Funk, Mallorca 288, 08037 Barcelona, Spain.

Furt, Belg. See *Roussel, Belg.*

Furt, Fr. Laboratoires Furt, 2 rue de Rivière, 33074 Bordeaux Cedex, France.

Furt, Neth. See *Bournonville, Neth.*

Fushimi, Denm. See *PF Medical, Denm.*

Fushimi, Swed. See *Eklow, Swed.*

Fuso, Jpn. Fuso Yakuhin, 2-50 Doshomachi, Higashi-ku, Osaka, Japan.

G & W, USA. G & W Laboratories Inc., 111 Coolidge St, South Plainfield NJ 07080, USA.

Gaba, Neth. Gaba B.V., Bolderweg 1, Industrieterrein de Vaart II, 1332 AX Almere, Netherlands.

Gador, Arg. Dr Gador & Cía S.A.C.I., Florida 868 1^0 y2° Piso, 1005 Buenos Aires, Argentina.

GAF, UK. GAF (Great Britain) Co. Ltd, Tilson Rd, Roundthorn, Wythenshawe, Manchester M23 9PH, England.

Galactina, Switz. Galactina AG, Birkenweg 2-8, 3123 Belp, Switzerland.

Galderma, Fr. Laboratoires Galderma, 2 av. de Stalingrad, 94150 Chevilly-Larue, France.

Galen, UK. Galen Ltd, 19 Lower Seagoe Industrial Estate, Portadown, Craigavon, Armagh BT63 5QD, Northern Ireland.

Galenica, Switz. Galenica Représentations SA, Untermattweg 8, 3001 Bern, Switzerland.

Galenika, Jug. Galenika, Batajnicki put bb, 11080 Zemun, Jugoslavia.

Galenus Mannheim, Ger. Galenus Mannheim GmbH, Sandhofer Str. 116, Postfach: 310105, 6800 Mannheim 31, W. Germany.

Galephar, Belg. See *SMB, Belg.*

Galephar, Neth. See *Multi-Pharma, Neth.*

Galepharma, Spain. Galepharma Iberica, Balmes 127, San Adrian de Vesos, 08930 Barcelona, Spain.

Gallier, Fr. Laboratoires Gallier S.A., 40 rue Lecuyer, 93300 Aubervilliers, France.

Galmeda, Ger. Galmeda GmbH, Ronsdorfer Strasse 4, Postfach: 3404, 4000 Dusseldorf 1, Germany.

Galup, Spain. See *Semar, Spain.*

Gamaprod, Austral. Gamaprod, Australia.

Gambar, Ital. Via Bolognola 45, 00138 Rome, Italy.

Gambro, Swed. Gambro AB, Box 10101, 220 10 Lund, Sweden.

Gamir, Spain. Gamir Aurelio, Ctra Barcelona 2, Almacera, 46132 Valencia, Spain.

Gamma, Spain. See *Laproquifar, Spain.*

Ganassini, Ital. Istituto Ganassini s.p.a. di Ricerche Biochimiche, Via Gaggia 16, 20139 Milan, Italy.

Garcia Suarez, Spain. Garcia Suarez, Cid 3, 28001 Madrid, Spain.

Gayoso Wellcome, Spain. Gayoso Wellcome, Ctra Madrid Barcelona Km 26.3, Alcala de Henares, Madrid, Spain.

Gazzoni, Ital. Gazzoni s.p.a., Via Ilio Barontini 16/20, 40138 Bologna, Italy.

GEA, Denm. A/S GEA, Holger Danskesvej 89, 2000 Frederiksberg, Denmark.

Gea, Neth. See *Multi-Pharma, Neth.*

GEA, Norw. See *KabiVitrum, Norw.*

GEA, Swed. See *Selena, Swed.*

Gebro, Switz. Gebro Pharma SA, Industriestrasse 7, 4410 Liestal, Switzerland.

Gedeon Richter, Hung. Chemical Works of Gedeon Richter Ltd, P.O. Box 27, 1475 Budapest, Hungary.

Gee Lawson, UK. Gee Lawson Chemicals Ltd, 677 Finchley Rd, London NW2 2JP, England.

Geigy, Arg. Ciba Geigy Argentina S.A.C.I., Arias 1851, 1429 Buenos Aires, Argentina.

Geigy, Austral. See *Ciba-Geigy, Austral.*

Geigy, Belg. See *Ciba, Belg.*

Geigy, Canad. Geigy Pharmaceuticals, Division of Ciba-Geigy Canada Ltd, 6860 Century Ave, Mississauga, Ontario L5N 2W5, Canada.

Geigy, Denm. Ciba-Geigy A/S, Lyngbyvej 172, 2100 Copenhagen Ø, Denmark.

Geigy, Eire. Ciba-Geigy Pharmaceuticals Ltd, Franklin House, 140 Pembroke Rd, Ballsbridge, Dublin 4, Eire.

Geigy, Fr. See *Ciba, Fr.*

Geigy, Ger. Geigy Pharmazeutika, Ciba-Geigy GmbH, Öflinger Strasse 44, Postfach: 1160/1180, 7867 Wehr 1, W. Germany.

Geigy, Ital. Ciba-Geigy s.p.a., 21040 Origgio (Varese), Italy.

Geigy, Neth. Ciba-Geigy B.V., Raapopseweg 1, 6824 DP Arnhem, Netherlands.

Geigy, Norw. Ciba-Geigy A/S, Postboks 6077 Etterstad, 0601 Oslo 1, Norway.

Geigy, S.Afr. See *Ciba, S.Afr.*

Geigy, Spain. Ciba-Geigy SA, Paseo Carlos I 206, 08013 Barcelona, Spain.

Geigy, Swed. See *Ciba, Swed.*

Geigy, Switz. See *Ciba-Geigy, Switz.*

Geigy, UK. Geigy Pharmaceuticals, Wimblehurst Rd, Horsham, West Sussex RH12 4AB, England.

Geigy, USA. Geigy Pharmaceuticals, Division of Ciba-Geigy Corporation, Ardsley NY 10502, USA.

Geistlich, Neth. See *Multi-Pharma, Neth.*

Geistlich, Switz. Geistlich-Pharma, 6110 Wolhusen, Switzerland.

Geistlich, UK. Geistlich Sons Ltd, Newton Bank, Long Lane, Chester CH2 3QZ, England.

Gelflex, Austral. Gelflex Australia, 43 Outram St, West Perth WA 6005, Australia.

Gelos, Spain. Gelos, Monistrol 22-4, 08012 Barcelona, Spain.

Gemini, UK. Gemini, England.

Geminis, Spain. See *Dietisa, Spain.*

Gen, Canad. Gen Drug Co. Ltd, 5169 Bradco Blvd, Mississauga, Ontario L4W 2A6, Canada.

Genderm, USA. Genderm Corp., 425 Huehl Rd, Northbrook IL 60062, USA.

Genentech, Canad. Genentech Canada, 977 Century Dr., Burlington, Ontario L7L 5J8, Canada.

Genentech, USA. Genentech Inc., 460 Point San Bruno Blvd, South San Francisco CA 94080, USA.

Genera, Switz. Genera Pharma SA, Case postale, 4501 Soleure, Switzerland.

General Designs, UK. General Designs Ltd, 33 The Manor Dr., Worcester Park, Surrey KT4 7LG, England.

General Diagnostics, UK. General Diagnostics, England.

General Pharm. Prods, USA. General Pharmaceutical Products Inc., 3205 Johnson Rd, Steubenville OH 43952, USA.

Generics, Swed. See *Nobel Medica, Swed.*

Generics, UK. Generics (UK) Ltd, 12 Station Close, Potters Bar, Herts EN6 1TL, England.

Geneva, USA. Geneva Generics, 2599 W Midway Blvd, Broomfield CO 80020, USA.

Génévrier, Fr. Laboratoires Génévrier, 45 rue Madeleine-Michelis, B.P. 149, 92202 Neuilly-sur-Seine, France.

Genifar, Fr. Genifar, 28 rue du Val d'Or, 92150 Sursenes, France.

Genove, Spain. Genove, Prat de la Manta 54, Hospitalet de Llobregat, 08902 Barcelona, Spain.

Gentili, Ital. Istituto Gentili s.p.a., Via Mazzini 112, 56100 Pisa, Italy.

Gerber, USA. Gerber Products Co., Fremont M1 49412, USA.

Gerbiol, Fr. Laboratoires Gerbiol, 5 rue St-Phillipe-du-Roule, 75008 Paris, France.

Gerda, Fr. See *Fisons, Fr.*

Gerhardt, UK. Gerhardt Pharmaceuticals Ltd, Thornton House, Hook Rd, Surbiton, Surrey KT6 5AR, England.

Geriatric Pharm. Corp., USA. Geriatric Pharmaceutical Corp., 1249 North Franklin Pl., Milwaukee WI 53202, USA.

Gerlach, Ger. Eduard Gerlach GmbH, Chemische Fabrik, Backerstrasse 4-8, Postfach: 12 49, 4990 Lubbecke, Germany.

Gerot, Belg. See *Byk, Belg.*

Gerot, Switz. See *Iromedica, Switz.*

Geve, Spain. See *Bama, Spain.*

Gewo, Ger. Gewo Chemie GmbH, Schneidweg 5, Postfach: 110160, 7570 Baden-Baden 11 (Steinbach), W. Germany.

Geymonat, Ital. Geymonat s.p.a., Via S. Anna 2, 03012 Anagni (FR), Italy.

G.F. Dietary Supplies, UK. G.F. Dietary Supplies Ltd, 494 Honeypot Lane, Stanmore, Middx HA7 1JH, England.

Ghimas, Ital. Ghimas s.p.a., Via R. Fucini 2, 40033 Casalecchio di Reno (BO), Italy.

Gibipharma, Ital. Gibipharma s.p.a., Via Carlo Pisacane 7, 20016 Pero (Milan), Italy.

Gifrer Barbezat, Fr. Laboratoires Gifrer Barbezat, B.P. 165, 69151 Decines Cedex, France.

Gilbert, Fr. Laboratoires Gilbert, 43 route de Lion-sur-Mer, 14200 Herouville-Saint-Clair, France.

Gilbert, USA. Gilbert Laboratories, 31 Fairmount Ave, Chester NJ 07930, USA.

Giovanardi, Ital. Laboratorio Farmaceutico Dr. Giovanardi & C. s.a.s., Via Sapeto 28, 16132 Genoa, Italy.

Gipharmex, Ital. Gipharmex s.p.a., Via Palagi 2, 20129 Milan, Italy.

Girol, Switz. Girol AG, Neufrankengasse 6, 8004 Zurich, Switzerland.

Gisand, Switz. Gisand SA, Thunstrasse 163, 3074 Muri, Switzerland.

Gist-Brocades, Austral. See *Astra, Austral.*

Gist-Brocades, Denm. See *Nordisk Droge, Denm.*

Gist-Brocades, Neth. Gist-Brocades Farmaca Nederland B.V., Frijdastraat 7-9, 2288 EX Rijswijk, Netherlands.

Gist-Brocades, Norw. See *Collett, Norw.*

Gist-Brocades, S.Afr. See *Riker, S.Afr.*

Gist-Brocades, Swed. See *Famaco, Swed.*

Gist-Brocades, Switz. See *Doetsch, Grether, Switz.*

Giulani, Ital. Giulani s.p.a., Via Sondrio 12, 20063 Cernusco S/Naviglio (MI), Italy.

Giuliani, Switz. Giuliani SA, via Riviera 21, 6976 Castagnola-Lugano, Switzerland.

Giulini, Denm. See *Meda, Denm.*

Giulini, Ger. Giulini Pharma GmbH, Hans-Böckler-Allee 20, Postfach:220, 3000 Hannover, W. Germany.

Giulini, Neth. See *Schmidt, Neth.*

Giulini, Swed. See *Famaco, Swed.*

Giulini, Switz. See *Hausmann, Switz.*

Giustini, Ital. Istituto Farmacobiologico Giustini s.r.l., Via Cavour 41/43, 20026 Novate Milanese (MI), Italy.

Giusto, Ital. Laboratorio Farmaceutico Giusto s.r.l., Via Cinque Maggio 73-75, 16147 Genova Quarto, Italy.

Givaudan, USA. Givaudan Corporation, 100 Delawanna Ave, Clifton NJ 07014, USA.

Glaxo, Arg. Glaxo (Arg.) S.A.C.eI., J.J. Castelli 6701, 1605 Munro, Pcia. Buenos Aires, Argentina.

Glaxo, Austral. Glaxo Australia Pty Ltd, P.O. Box 168, Boronia Vic. 3155, Australia.

Glaxo, Belg. Glaxo Belgium S.A., rue Blanche 15/bte 5, 1050 Brussels, Belgium.

Glaxo, Canad. Glaxo Laboratories, 1025 The Queensway, Toronto, Ontario M8Z 5S6, Canada.

Glaxo, Denm. Glaxo Laegemidler A/S, Lerso Parkallé, 2100 Copenhagen O, Denmark.

Glaxo, Fr. Laboratoires Glaxo, 43 rue Vineuse, 75764 Paris, France.

Glaxo, Ger. Glaxo Pharmazeutika GmbH, Industriestrasse 32, Postfach: 1460, 2060 Bad Oldesloe, Germany.

Glaxo, Ind. Glaxo Laboratories (India) Ltd, Dr Annie Besant Rd, Worli, Bombay-400 018, India.

Glaxo, Ital. Glaxo s.p.a., Via A. Fleming 2, 37135 Verona, Italy.

Glaxo, Neth. Glaxo B.V., Wattbaan 51, 3439 ML Nieuwegein, Netherlands.

Glaxo, Norw. Glaxo A/S, Sandakerv.72, Postboks 4312 Torshov, 0402 Oslo 4, Norway.

Glaxo, NZ. Glaxo New Zealand Ltd, Private Bag, Palmerston North, New Zealand.

Glaxo, S.Afr. Glaxo (Pty) Ltd, P.O. Box 485, Germiston 1400, Transvaal, S. Africa.

Glaxo, Spain. Glaxo, Plza de Carlos Trias Bertran 4, 28020 Madrid, Spain.

Glaxo, Swed. Glaxo Lakemedel AB, Box 263, 431 23 Molndal, Sweden.

Glaxo, Switz. Glaxo SA, Giacomettistrasse 3, Case postale, 3000 Berne 31, Switzerland.

Glaxo, UK. Glaxo Laboratories Ltd, Greenford Rd, Greenford, Middx UB6 0HE, England.

Glaxo, USA. Glaxo Inc., Five Moore Dr., Research Triangle Park NC 27709, USA.

Glaxo Animal Health, UK. Glaxo Animal Health Ltd, Breakspear Rd South, Harefield, Uxbridge, Middx UB9 6LS, England.

Glaxovet, UK. Glaxovet Ltd, Breakspear Rd South, Harefield, Uxbridge, Middx UB9 6LS, England.

Glenbrook, USA. Glenbrook Laboratories, Division of Sterling Drug Inc., 90 Park Ave, New York NY 10016, USA.

Glenden, Switz. See *Imal, Switz.*

Glenfair, S.Afr. Glenfair Pharmaceuticals Ltd, P.O. Box 20031, Alkantrant 0005, S. Africa.

Glenwood, Canad. Glenwood Laboratories Canada Ltd, 1195 Meyerside Dr., Unit 4, Mississauga, Ontario L5T 1H3, Canada.

Glenwood, Switz. See *Galenica, Switz.*

Glenwood, UK. Glenwood Laboratories Ltd, 19 Wincheap, Canterbury, Kent CT1 3TB, England.

Glenwood, USA. Glenwood Inc., 83 North Summit St, Tenafly NJ 07670, USA.

Globechem, Hong Kong. Globechem (HK) Ltd, Rm 1209, Penninsula Centre, 67 Mody Road, TST East Kowloon, Hong Kong.

Globopharm, Belg. See *Labaz, Belg.*

Globopharm, Switz. Globopharm SA, 8700 Küsnacht, Switzerland.

Glover, UK. G.D.S., Glover Dental Supplies Ltd, Lancaster Rd, Shrewsbury SY1 3NF, England.

Glower, Spain. Glower, San Pablo 74, 08001 Barcelona, Spain.

Glycinia, Spain. Glycinia, San Gamin 17, 08006 Barcelona, Spain.

GMP, S.Afr. GMP Pharmaceuticals, P.O. Box 1682, Johannesburg 2000, S. Africa.

Gobbi-Novag, Arg. Gobbi-Novag S.A.I.C., F. Onsari 498, 1875 Wilde, Buenos Aires, Argentina.

Gödecke, Ger. Gödecke Aktiengesellschaft, Salzufer 16, Postfach:10 02 50, 1000 Berlin 10, W. Germany.

Gohl, Switz. Gohl Pharma SA, Case postale 2366, 1211 Geneva 2, Switzerland.

Golaz, Switz. Laboratoire Golaz SA, Ch. du Devent, 1024 Ecublens VD, Switzerland.

Gold Cross, UK. Gold Cross Pharmaceuticals, P.O. Box 53, Lane End Rd, High Wycombe, Bucks HP12 4HL, England.

Goldschmidt, Ger. Th. Goldschmidt AG, Goldschmidtstrasse 100, Postfach: 101461, 4300 Essen 1, W. Germany.

Goldschmidt, UK. Th. Goldschmidt Ltd, Tego House, Victoria Rd, Ruislip, Middx HA4 0YL, England.

Goldschmidt, USA. Goldschmidt Chemical Corporation, P.O. Box 1299, Hopewell VA 23860, USA.

Gomenol, Fr. Laboratoires du Gomenol, 48 rue des Petites-Écuries, 75010 Paris, France.

Gønget, Denm. F.F. Gønget & Co., Englandsvej 382 A, 2770 Kastrup, Denmark.

Gonnon, Fr. Laboratoires Gonnon, 16 rue François-Dauphin, 69002 Lyon, France.

Goodrich, UK. B F Goodrich Chemical (UK) Ltd, The Lawn, 100 Lampton Rd, Hounslow, Middx TW3 4EB, England.

Gordon Piller, Canad. Gordon Piller Inc., 2175 Dunwin Dr., Unit 2, Mississauga, Ontario L5L 1X2, Canada.

Goupil, Fr. Laboratoires Goupil S.A., 30 ave du Président-Wilson, 94230 Cachan, France.

Goupil, Ital. Goupil Italia s.p.a., Via Barigozzi 6, 20138 Milan, Italy.

G.P. Laboratories, Austral. See *Pfizer, Austral.*

GPL, Switz. Ginsana Products Lugano SA, Case postale, 6903 Lugano, Switzerland.

Grace, UK. W.R. Grace Ltd, Northdale House, North Circular Rd, Park Royal, London NW10 7UH, England.

Graesser, Denm. See *PF Medical, Denm.*

Graino, Spain. Graino Dr., Mina 6, Alcobendas, 28100 Madrid, Spain.

Gramon, Arg. Gerardo Ramón y Cía. S.A.I.yC., Int. Amaro Avalos 4208, 1605 Munro, Buenos Aires, Argentina.

Granata, Ital. Laboratori Chimico Biologici Granata s.p.a., Strada Padana Superiore 32, 20063 Cernusco (Milan), Italy.

Granelli, Ital. Lab. Chim. Farm. E. Granelli s.p.a., Via Castelvetro 17/23, 20154 Milan, Italy.

Granions, Mon. Laboratoires des Granions, 14 av. Crovetto-Freres, Monaco.

Gray, USA. Gray Pharmaceutical Co., Affiliate The Purdue Frederick Co., 100 Connecticut Ave, Norwalk CT 06854, USA.

Great Southern, USA. Great Southern, USA.

Greeff, USA. Greeff, USA.

Green Cross Corp., Jpn. The Green Cross Corporation, 1-15-1 Imahashi, Higashi-ku, Osaka, Japan.

Green Cross, Thai. See *Osothsapha, Thai.*

Greiter, Switz. Greiter Distribution AG, Postfach 128, 9450 Alstätten, Switzerland.

Gremy-Longuet, Belg. See *UPB, Belg.*

Grémy-Longuet, Fr. See *Smith Kline & French, Fr.*

Grifols, Spain. Grifols, Via Levante 40, Parets del Valles, 08150 Barcelona, Spain.

Grossmann, Switz. Dr Grossmann SA, Binningerstrasse 95, Case postale, 4123 Allschwil 1, Switzerland.

Grünenthal, Ger. Grünenthal GmbH, Steinfeldstrasse 2, Postfach:129, 5190 Stolberg, W. Germany.

Grünenthal, S.Afr. Grünenthal (SA) Pty Ltd, P.O. Box 41298, Craighall 2024, S. Africa.

Grünenthal, Switz. See *Protochemie, Switz.*

Gry, Ger. Gry-Pharma GmbH, Kandelstr. 10, 7815 Kirchzarten, Germany.

GS, S.Afr. GS Pharmaceuticals, P.O. Box 1123, Halfway House 1685, S. Africa.

Guardian, Canad. See *Omega, Canad.*

Guardian, USA. Guardian Chemical, A division of United-Guardian Inc., 230 Marcus Blvd, P.O. Box 2500, Smithtown NY 11787, USA.

Guerbet, Denm. See *Lindeburg, Denm.*

Guerbet, Fr. Laboratoires Guerbet, 16 rue Jean-Chaptal, B.P. 15, F 93601 Aulnay-sous-Bois Cedex, France.

Guerbet, Neth. See *Byk, Neth.*

Guerbet, Norw. See *Plesner, Norw.*

Guerbet, Swed. See *Nobel Medica, Swed.*

Guerbet, Switz. See *Max Ritter, Switz.*

Guidotti, Ital. Laboratori Guidotti s.p.a., Via Trieste 40, 56100 Pisa, Italy.

Guieu, Ital. Laboratori Guieu s.p.a., Via Lomellina 10, 20133 Milan, Italy.

Gunnar Kjems, Denm. Cand. Pharm. Gunnar Kjems ApS, Peder Huitfeldts Straade 12, 1173 Copenhagen K, Denmark.

Gustin, Spain. Gustin Dr., Mallorca 313, 08037 Barcelona, Spain.

Haedensa, Neth. See *Nicholas, Neth.*

Hall Bros, UK. Hall Brothers, Dumers Lane, Radcliffe, Manchester, England.

Hall, Canad. Hall Laboratories, 120 Glacier St, Unit 4, Coquitlam, British Columbia V3K 5Z6, Canada.

Hall Forster, UK. Hall Forster & Co. Ltd, P.O. Box 1DB, Pooley Close, Newcastle-upon-Tyne NE99 1DB, England.

Halocarbon, Denm. See *Friis, Denm.*

Halty, Fr. See *Pierre Fabre, Fr.*

Hameln, Ger. Pharma Hameln GmbH, Langes Feld 30-38, Postfach: 100863, 3250 Hameln 1, Germany.

Hamilton, Austral. Hamilton Laboratories Pty Ltd, G.P.O. Box 7, Adelaide SA 5001, Australia.

Hammer Pharma, Ital. Hammer s.r.l. società collegata al gruppo Lepetit s.p.a., Via Vetreria 1, 22070 Grandate (CO), Italy.

Harimex-Ligos, Neth. Harimex-Ligos BV, Kieveen 20, 7371 GD Loenen, Netherlands.

Harkers, UK. Harkers Ltd, Minster House, Western Way, Bury St Edmunds, Suffolk IP33 3SU, England.

Hartmann, Ger. Paul Hartmann AG Verbandstoff-Fabriken, Paul-Hartmann-Strasse, Postfach: 14 20, 7920 Heidenheim (Brenz), Germany.

Harvard, S.Afr. See *Restan, S.Afr.*

Harvey, Switz. See *Mundipharma, Switz.*

Harvey, USA. Harvey Laboratories Inc., 113 West Wyoming Ave, Philadelphia PA 19140, USA.

Harvey-Scruton, UK. Harvey-Scruton Ltd, 4 Baker Lane, York, England.

Hässle, Denm. See *Astra, Denm.*

Hassle, Fin. See *Astra, Fin.*

Hässle, Norw. See *Astra, Norw.*

Hässle, Swed. AB Hässle, 431 83 Mölndal, Sweden.

Hauck, USA. W.E. Hauck Inc., P.O. Box 1065, Roswell GA 30075, USA.

Hauser, Denm. See *Tjellesen, Denm.*

Hausmann, Denm. See *Meda, Denm.*

Hausmann, Norw. See *Andersen, Norw.*

Hausmann, S.Afr. See *Swisspharm, S.Afr.*

Hausmann, Switz. Laboratoires Hausmann SA, Case postale, 9001 St Gallen, Switzerland.

Health & Diet Food Co., UK. Health & Diet Food Co. Ltd, Seymour House, South Street, Godalming, Surrey GU7 1BZ, England.

Health Care, UK. Health Care Products Ltd, Half-Acre House, The Mount, Highclere, Newbury RG15 9PW, England.

Heath & Heather, UK. Heath & Heather Ltd, Division of Associated Health Foods, Canada Road, Byfleet, Surrey KT14 7JL, England.

Hefa-Frenon, Ger. Hefa-Frenon Arzneimittel GmbH & Co. KG, Am Bahnhof 1-3, Postfach:220, 4712 Werne, W. Germany.

Hefti, Switz. Hefti AG, 8048 Zurich, Switzerland.

Heilit, Ger. Heilit Arzneimittel GmbH, Danziger Strasse 5, Postfach:1248, 2057 Reinbek, W. Germany.

Heineking, Switz. L. Heineking & Cie, alte Landstrasse 32, 8800 Thalwil, Switzerland.

Hek, Ger. Hek Pharma GmbH, Hinter den Kirschkaten 49, Postfach: 2095, 2400 Lubeck 1, Germany.

Helge Kjelstrup, Denm. Helge Kjelstrup ApS, Vangede Bygade 138, 2820 Gentofte, Denmark.

Helixor, Ger. Helixor Heilmittel GmbH & Co., Postfach:8, 7463 Rosenfeld, W. Germany.

Helopharm, Ger. Helopharm W. Petrik GmbH & Co. KG, Waldstrasse 23-25, 1000 Berlin 51, Germany.

Helopharm, Switz. See *Schönenberger, Switz.*

Helvepharm, Switz. Helvepharm AG, Bahnhofstr., 3185 Schmitten, Switzerland.

Hemofarm, Jug. Hemofarm, Beogradski put bb, 26300 Vrsac, Jugoslavia.

Henk, Ger. Emil Henk oHG Chemisch-Pharmazeutische Praparate, Handelsstrasse 15, Postfach: 102720, 6904 Eppelheim/u Heidelberg, Germany.

Henkel, Ger. Henkel KGaA, Henkelstrasse 67, Postfach:1100, 4000 Düsseldorf 1, W. Germany.

Henleys, UK. Henleys Medical Supplies Ltd, Alexandra Works, Clarendon Rd, London N8 0DL, England.

Hennig, Ger. Hennig Arzneimittel GmbH & Co. KG, Liebigstrasse 1-2, Postfach: 1240, 6093 Florsheim am Main, W. Germany.

Henning Berlin, Ger. Henning Berlin GmbH, Chemie- und Pharmawerk, Komturstrasse 58-62, Postfach: 420732, 1000 Berlin 42, W. Germany.

Henning, Denm. See *Gønget, Denm.*

Henning, Switz. See *Oryx, Switz.*

Henry Christenson, Norw. Henry Christenson & Co., Brenneriv. 7, Postboks 108 Ankertorget, 0133 Oslo 1, Norway.

Hepatoum, Fr. Ste d'Exploitation du Laboratoires Hepatoum, 03270 Saint-Yorre, France.

Herbal Laboratories, UK. Herbal Laboratories (UK) Ltd, Copse Rd, Fleetwood, Lancs FY7 7PF, England.

Herbert, Ger. Apotheker A. Herbert GmbH, Fabrik pharmazeutischer Praparate, Am Wolsfeld 17, Postfach: 3080, 6200 Wiesbaden 1, 6200 Wiesbaden-Bierstadt, Germany.

Herbert, USA. Herbert Laboratories, Dermatology Division of Allergan Pharmaceuticals Inc., 2525 Dupont Dr., Irvine CA 92713, USA.

Herbrand, Ger. Dr Herbrand KG, chem.-pharm. Werk, Nollenstrasse 54, Postfach:1107, 7614 Gengenbach, W. Germany.

Herbrand, Switz. See *Panpharma, Switz.*

Hercules, UK. Hercules Ltd, 20 Red Lion St, London WC1R 4PB, England.

Herdel, Ital. Herdel s.r.l., Via Porpora 132, 20131 Milan, Italy.

Herli, S.Afr. Herli Pharma (Pty) Ltd, P.O. Box 4325, Johannesburg 2000, S. Africa.

Hermal, Ger. Hermal Kurt Herrmann, Scholtzstr. 3, Postfach: 1228, D-2057 Reinbek b. Hamburg, W. Germany.

Hermal, Neth. See *Bipharma, Neth.*

Hermal, Norw. See *E. Merck, Norw.*

Hermal, Swed. See *E. Merck, Swed.*

Hermal, Switz. See *Allergomed, Switz.* and *Lubapharm, Switz.*

Hermal, USA. Hermal Pharmaceutical Laboratories Inc., Route 145, Oak Hill NY 12460, USA.

Hermann, Denm. C.C. Hermann, Ryvangs Alle 54, 2900 Hellerup, Denmark.

Hermes, Ger. Hermes Arzneimittel GmbH, Georg-Kalb-Strasse 5-8, 8023 Grosshesselohe, Germany.

Hermes, Neth. Hermes & Co. B.V., Tasmanstraat 92-94, 2518 VP 's-Gravenhage, Netherlands.

Hermes, Spain. See *Organon, Spain.*

Hesperia, Spain. See *Travenol, Spain.*

Hetty, Arg. Hetty S.R.L., Cabrera 3156, 1186 Buenos Aires, Argentina.

Heumann, Ger. Heumann Pharma & Co. GmbH, Heideloffstrasse 18, Postfach:2260, 8500 Nürnberg, W. Germany.

Heumann, Switz. See *Desopharma, Switz.*

Hevert, Ger. Hevert-Arzneimittel GmbH & Co. KG, Eckweiler Strasse 10-12, Postfach: 61, 6553 Sobernheim/Nahe, Germany.

Hexcel, USA. Hexcel, USA.

Heyden, Ger. von Heyden GmbH, Volkartstrasse 83, 8000 Munich 19, W. Germany.

Heyden, Norw. See *Kobro, Norw.*

Heyden, Swed. See *Meda, Swed.*

Heyden, Switz. See *Biomed, Switz.*

Heyl, Ger. Heyl chem.-pharm. Fabrik GmbH & Co. KG, Goerzallee 253, 1000 Berlin 37, W. Germany.

Hi-Eisai, Philipp. Hi-Eisai Pharmaceutical Inc., MCPO Box 1045, Makati, Metro Manila, The Philippines.

Hickam, USA. Dow B. Hickam Inc., P.O. Box 2006, Sugar Land TX 77478, USA.

High Chemical, USA. High Chemical Co., Division Day & Frick Inc., 1760 N Howard St, Philadelphia PA 19122, USA.

High Noon, Pakistan. High Noon Laboratories Ltd, P.O. Box 3318, Gulberg-Lahore-11, Pakistan.

Hill, USA. Hill Dermaceuticals Inc., P.O. Box 19283, Orlando FL 32814, USA.

Hill's Pharmaceuticals, UK. Hill's Pharmaceuticals Ltd, Talbot St, Briercliffe, Burnley, Lancs BB10 2JY, England.

Hindustan Antibiotics, Ind. Hindustan Antibiotics Ltd, Sir JJ Road, Sasoon Hospital Compound, Pimpri, Pune-411 001, India.

Hisamitsu, Jpn. Hisamitsu Seiyaku, 408 Tashiro Daikan-cho, Torisu-shi, Saga-ken, Japan.

Hishiyama, Jpn. Hishiyama Seiyaku, 2-37 Doshomachi, Higashi-ku, Osaka, Japan.

Hobein, Ger. Dr Hobein & Co. Nachf. GmbH, Grenzstrasse 2, 5309 Meckenheim-Merl, W. Germany.

Hoechst Animal Health, UK. Hoechst Animal Health, A Division of Hoechst UK Ltd, Walton Manor, Walton, Milton Keynes, Bucks MK7 7AJ, England.

Hoechst, Arg. Química Hoechst S.A., 25 de Mayo 460 3° Piso, 1002 Buenos Aires, Argentina.

Hoechst, Austral. Hoechst Australia Ltd, P.O. Box 4300, Melbourne Vic. 3001, Australia.

Hoechst, Belg. Hoechst Belgium S.A., chaussée de Charleroi 111-113, 1060 Brussels, Belgium.

Hoechst, Braz. Hoechst do Brasil Quimica e Farmaceutica S.A., Braulio Gomes 36, 01047 Sao Paulo, Brazil.

Hoechst, Canad. Hoechst Canada Inc., Pharmaceutical Division, 4045 Côte Vertu Blvd, Montreal, Quebec H4R 1R6, Canada.

Hoechst, Denm. Hoechst Danmark A/S, Islevdalvej 110, 2610 Rødovre, Denmark.

Hoechst, Fr. Laboratoires Hoechst, Tour Roussel-Hoechst, 92080 Paris-La Defense Cedex 3, France.

Hoechst, Ger. Hoechst Aktiengesellschaft, Brüningstrasse 50, Postfach: 800320, 6230 Frankfurt (Main) 80, W. Germany.

Hoechst, Ital. Hoechst Italia Sud, Strada Statale 17-Km. 22, 67019 Scoppito (AQ), Italy.

Hoechst, Jpn. Hoechst Japan, 8-10-16 Akasaka, Minato-ku, Tokyo, Japan.

Hoechst, Neth. Hoechst Holland N.V., divisie Pharma, Hogehilweg 21, 1101 CB Amsterdam, Netherlands.

Hoechst, Norw. Norske Hoechst A/S, Økernvn. 145, Postboks 177 Økern, Oslo 5, Norway.

Hoechst, S.Afr. Hoechst Pharmaceuticals (Pty) Ltd, P.O. Box 8692, Johannesburg 2000, S. Africa.

Hoechst, Spain. Hoechst, Travesera de Gracia 47-9, 08021 Barcelona, Spain.

Hoechst, Swed. Svenska Hoechst AB, Läkemedelsdivisionen, Box 42026, 126 12 Stockholm, Sweden.

Hoechst, Switz. Hoechst-Pharma SA, Herostrasse 7, 8048 Zurich, Switzerland.

Hoechst, UK. Hoechst UK Ltd, Pharmaceutical Division, Hoechst House, Salisbury Rd, Hounslow, Middx TW4 6JH, England.

Hoechst, USA. Hoechst-Roussel Pharmaceuticals Inc., Route 202-206 North, Somerville NJ 08876, USA.

Hokuriku, Jpn. Hokuriku Seiyaku, 1-3-14 Tachikawa-cho, Katsuyama-shi, Fukui-ken, Japan.

Hollister-Stier, Canad. Hollister-Stier Canada, Division of Miles Laboratories Ltd, 77 Belfield Rd, Etobicoke, Ontario M9W 1G6, Canada.

Holloway, USA. Holloway Pharmaceuticals Inc., 230 Oxmoor Circle, Suite 1111, Birmingham AL 35209, USA.

Holphar, Ger. Holphar Arzneimittel GmbH, Justus-von-Liebig-Strasse 16, Postfach: 1145, 6603 Sulzbach-Neuweiler, W. Germany.

Holpro, S.Afr. Holpro Pharmaceuticals (Pty) Ltd, P.O. Box 7868, Johannesburg 2000, S. Africa.

Homburg, Belg. See *de Bournonville, Belg.*

Homburg, Ger. See *Asta Pharma, Ger.*

Homburg, Neth. See *Multi-Pharma, Neth.*

Homburg, S.Afr. See *Remedia, S.Afr.*

Home, Ital. Home Products Italiana s.p.a., C.so Sempione 75, 20149 Milan, Italy.

Homme de Fer, Fr. Laboratoires de l'Homme de Fer, 2 pl. de l'Homme de Fer, 67000 Strasbourg, France.

Hommel, Ger. Chemische Werke Hommel GmbH, Postfach: 1263, 7840 Müllheim/Baden 1, W. Germany.

Hommel, Switz. Hommel SA, 1260 Nyon, Switzerland.

Honeyrose, UK. Honeyrose Products Ltd, Creeting Rd, Stowmarket, Suffolk, England.

Honeywill & Stein, UK. Honeywill & Stein Ltd, Greenfield House, 69-73 Manor Rd, Wallington, Surrey SM6 0BP, England.

Hong Kong Med. Supp., Hong Kong. Hong Kong Medical Supplies Ltd, Room 1302, Hua Qin International Bldg, 340 Queens Road, Central, Hong Kong.

Hopkin & Williams, UK. Hopkin & Williams, England.

Hormocor, S.Afr. Hormocor Ltd, P.O. Box 201, Howard Place 7450, S. Africa.

Hormonchemie, Ger. Hormon-Chemie München GmbH, Freisinger Landstrasse 74, Postfach: 45 03 61, 8000 Munich 45, W. Germany.

Hormosan, Ger. Hormosan-Kwizda GmbH, Wilhelmshoher Strasse 106, Postfach: 600340, 6000 Frankfurt/Main 60, Germany.

Horner, Canad. Frank W. Horner Inc., 5485 Ferrier St, Town of Mount Royal, Quebec H4P 1M6, Canada.

Hortel, Spain. Hortel, Avda de Cieza 58, Abaran, 30550 Murcia, Spain.

Horwell, UK. Arnold R. Horwell Ltd, 73 Maygrove Rd, London NW6 2BP, England.

Hosbon, Spain. Hosbon, Montana 83-7, 08026 Barcelona, Spain.

Hotta, Jpn. Hotta Yakuhin, 3-88 Uchiyama-cho, Senju-ku, Nagoya-shi, Japan.

Hotz, Ger. Dr. W. Hotz & Co. KG, Wielandstrasse 11b, Postfach: 2104, 7053 Kernen i. R. (2), Germany.

Houde, Belg. See *Roussel, Belg.*

Houdé, Fr. Laboratoires Houdé, 1 Terrasse Bellini, 92800 Puteaux, France.

Hough, Hoseason, UK. Hough, Hoseason & Co. Ltd, 22 Chapel St, Levenshulme, Manchester M19 3PT, England.

Howard Lloyd, UK. Howard Lloyd & Co. Ltd, Clerk Green, Batley, West Yorkshire WF17 5RU, England.

Howmedica, UK. Howmedica (UK) Ltd, 622 Western Ave, London W3 0TF, England.

Hoyer, Ger. Hoyer GmbH & Co., Siemensstrasse 14, Postfach: 210355, 4040 Neuss 21, W. Germany.

Hoyt, UK. Hoyt Laboratories, Division of Colgate-Palmolive Ltd, 76 Oxford St, London W1A 1EN, England.

HR Health Care, UK. HR Health Care Ltd, 135 Eign St, Hereford HR4 0AJ, England.

HSL Vaccine Laboratory, UK. HSL Vaccine Laboratory, 55 Wimpole St, London W1M 7DF, England.

Hubber, Spain. Hubber, Berlin 38-48, 08029 Barcelona, Spain.

Hubner, Ger. Anton Hubner GmbH, Schloss-Strasse 11-17, Postfach: 49, 7801 Ehrenkirchen 1, Germany.

Huffman, USA. Huffman Laboratories, 7356 N.W. 35th Terrace, Miami FL 33122, USA.

Hughes & Hughes, UK. Hughes & Hughes Ltd, Elms Industrial Estate, Church Rd, Harold Wood, Romford, Essex RM3 0HR, England.

Human-Pharm, Fr. Laboratoires Human-Pharm, 52 av. du Marechal Joffre, 92024 Nanterre Cedex, France.

Hyland, Canad. Hyland Therapeutics, Division of Travenol Canada Inc., 6695 Airport Rd, Mississauga, Ontario L4V 1T7, Canada.

Hyland, Denm. See *KabiVitrum, Denm.*

Hyland, USA. Hyland Therapeutics Division, Travenol Laboratories Inc., 444 W Glenoaks Blvd, Glendale CA 91202, USA.

Hyland Terapeutici, Ital. Laboratori Travenol s.p.a., Divisione Hyland Terapeutici, Viale Tiziano 25, 00196 Rome, Italy.

Hynson, Westcott & Dunning, Canad. See *Beauty, Canad.*

Hynson, Westcott & Dunning, USA. Hynson, Westcott & Dunning, Division of Becton Dickinson & Co., Charles & Chase Sts, Baltimore MD 21201, USA.

Hynson, Westcott & Dunning Diagnostics, Canad. See *Becton, Dickinson, Canad.*

Hypoguard, UK. Hypoguard (UK) Ltd, Dock Lane, Melton, Woodbridge, Suffolk IP12 1PE, England.

Hyrex, USA. Hyrex Pharmaceuticals, 3494 Democrat Rd, Memphis TN 38118, USA.

Hythe, UK. See *BP Chemicals, UK.*

IBE, Spain. IBE, Afueras S/N 29.5, Villalba Saserra, Barcelona, Spain.

Ibi, Ital. Ibi, Istituto Biochimico Italiano Giovanni Lorenzini s.p.a., Via G. Lorenzini 2-4, 20139 Milan, Italy.

Ibi Sud, Ital. Ibi Sud s.p.a., Via di Fossignano 2, 04011 Aprillia (Latina), Italy.

Ibirn, Ital. Istituto Bioterapico Nazionale s.r.l., Via Vittorio Grassi 9/11, 00155 Rome (Tor Sapienza), Italy.

IBIS, Ital. IBIS, Istituto Biochimico Sperimentale s.p.a., Viale Machiavelli 31/33, 50125 Florence, Italy.

IBP, Ital. Istituto Biochimico Pavese s.p.a., Viale Certosa 10, 27100 Pavia, Italy.

IBS, Ital. Istituto Biochimico Sardo s.p.a., Via Dante-de Gioannis 1, 09100 Cagliari, Italy.

Ibsa, Switz. Institut Biochimique SA, Via al Ponte 13, 6903 Lugano, Switzerland.

Ibse, Spain. Ibse, Pedro IV 499, 08020 Barcelona, Spain.

IBYS, Spain. IBYS, Antonio Lopez 111, 28026 Madrid, Spain.

Ichthyol, Ger. Ichthyol-Gesellschaft Cordes, Hermanni & Co., Sportallee 85, Postfach: 630380, 2000 Hamburg 63, W. Germany.

Ichthyol, Switz. See *Diethelm, Switz.*

ICI, Austral. ICI Australia Operations Pty Ltd, P.O. Box 4311, Melbourne Vic. 3001, Australia.

ICI, Belg. ICI-Pharma S.A., Schaessestraat 15, 9120 Destelbergen, Belgium.

ICI, Canad. ICI Pharma, 16 Falconer Dr., Mississauga, Ontario L5N 3M1, Canada.

ICI, Denm. ICI-Pharma AS, Islands Brygge 41, 2300 Copenhagen S, Denmark.

ICI, Ger. ICI-Pharma, Otto-Hahn-Strasse, 6831 Plankstadt, Germany.

ICI, Neth. ICI-Farma, farmaceutische afd. van ICI Holland B.V., Wijnhaven 107, 3011 WN Rotterdam, Netherlands.

ICI, Norw. A/S ICI-Pharma, Drammensv. 126A, Postboks 173 Skøyen, 0212 Oslo 2, Norway.

ICI, S.Afr. ICI SA (Pharmaceuticals) Ltd, P.O. Box 11270, Johannesburg 2000, S. Africa.

ICI, Spain. ICI Farma, La Relva S/N (Apartado 17), Porrino, 36400 Pontevedra, Spain.

ICI, Swed. ICI-Pharma AB, Stora Badhusgatan 20, 411 21 Göteborg, Sweden.

ICI, Switz. ICI-Pharma, Landenbergstr. 34, 6002 Lucerne, Switzerland.

ICI Mond, UK. Imperial Chemical Industries PLC, Mond Division, P.O. Box 13, The Heath, Runcorn, Cheshire WA7 4QF, England.

ICI Organics, UK. Imperial Chemical Industries PLC, Organics Division, P.O. Box 42, Hexagon House, Blackley, Manchester M9 3DA, England.

ICI Petrochemicals, UK. Imperial Chemical Industries PLC, Petrochemicals & Plastics Division, P.O. Box 6, Bessemer Rd, Welwyn Garden City, Herts AL7 1HD, England.

ICI Pharmaceuticals, UK. ICI Pharmaceuticals (UK), Mereside, Alderley Park, Macclesfield, Cheshire SK10 4TG, England.

ICI Plant Protection, UK. Imperial Chemical Industries PLC, Plant Protection Division, Woolmead House East, Woolmead Walk, Farnham, Surrey GU9 7UB, England.

ICI Speciality Chemicals, UK. Imperial Chemical Industries PLC, Speciality Chemicals, Northern Operations Group, Cleeve Rd, Leatherhead, Surrey KT22 7SW, England.

ICI-Farma, Arg. ICI-Farma, División de Duperial S.A.I.C., Paseo Colón 285, 1330 Buenos Aires, Argentina.

I.C.I.-Pharma, Fr. I.C.I.-Pharma, Le Galien, 1 rue des Chauffours, B.P. 127, 95022 Cergy Cedex, France.

ICI-Pharma, Ital. ICI-Pharma, Divisione Farmaceutici, Imperial Chemical Industries (Italia) s.p.a., Viale Isonzo 25, 20135 Milan, Italy.

ICN, Canad. ICN Canada Ltd, 1956 Bourdon St, Montreal, Quebec H4M 1V1, Canada.

ICN, Neth. ICN Pharmaceuticals Holland B.V., Stephensonstraat 1, 2723 RM Zoetermeer, Netherlands.

ICN, USA. ICN Pharmaceuticals Inc., ICN Plaza, 3300 Hyland Ave, Costa Mesa CA 92626, USA.

ICT-Lodi, Ital. Istituto Chemioterapico di Lodi s.p.a., Via Borsa 11, 20073 Codogno (MI), Italy.

Iderne, Fr. Laboratoires Michel Iderne, Dpt Unipharm, 4 rue de Girlenhirsch, 67400 Illkirch-Graffenstaden, France.

IDI, Ital. IDI Farmaceutici s.p.a., Via dei Castelli Romani 83/85, 00040 Pomezia (Rome), Italy.

Iema, Ital. Iema Industria Farmaceutica s.r.l., Via Adelasio 33, 24020 Ranica (BG), Italy.

IFCI, Ital. Industria Farmaceutica Cosmetica Italiana s.p.a., Via Magnanelli 2, 40033 Casalecchio di Reno (BO), Italy.

Ifesa, Spain. Ifesa, San Salvador 2-14, Esplugues de Llobregat, 08950 Barcelona, Spain.

IFI, Ital. Istituto Farmacoterapico Italiano s.p.a., Via Paolo Frisi 23, 00197 Rome, Italy.

Igoda, Spain. See *Merck Igoda, Spain.*

Ika-Pharm, Swed. See *Serono, Swed.*

Ikapharm, Israel. Ikapharm (Teva Ltd), Hashikma St Industrial Zone, Kfar-Saba, Israel.

Iketon, Ital. Iketon Farmaceutici s.r.l., Via Clemente Prudenzio 16, 20138 Milan, Italy.

Ilon Laboratories, UK. Ilon Laboratories (Hamilton) Ltd, Lorne St, Hamilton, Strathclyde ML3 9AB, Scotland.

Ima, Arg. Ima S.A.I.C., Cramer 1030, 1426 Buenos Aires, Argentina.

Imal, Switz. Imal Pharmaceutica AG, Postfach, 8053 Zurich, Switzerland.

Imba, Spain. Imba, Paseo Padre Feijoo 14, Ceuta, Spain.

Imeco, Swed. IMECO Astra Agency Co AB, 151 85 Sodertalje, Sweden.

Immuno, Arg. Immuno S.A.C.I.F.I.A., Sarmiento 329, 1041 Buenos Aires, Argentina.

Immuno, Canad. Immuno Canada Ltd, 5647 Yonge St, Suite 1727, Toronto, Ontario M2M 4E9, Canada.

Immuno, Denm. Immuno Danmark ApS, Strandboulevarden 96, 2100 Copenhagen O, Denmark.

Immuno, Ger. Immuno GmbH, Slevogtstrasse 3, Postfach: 103080, 6900 Heidelberg, W. Germany.

Immuno, Ital. Immuno s.p.a., Via A. Vespucci 119, 56100 Pisa, Italy.

Immuno, Spain. Immuno, San Just Desvern s/n, 28002 Barcelona, Spain.

Immuno, Swed. Immuno Sweden AB, Rasundavagen 166, 171 30 Solna, Sweden.

Immuno, Switz. Immuno SA, Case postale 168, 8034 Zurich, Switzerland.

Immuno, UK. Immuno Ltd, Arctic House, Rye Lane, Dunton Green, Nr Sevenoaks, Kent TN14 5HB, England.

IMS, UK. International Medication Systems (UK) Ltd, 11 Royal Oak Way South, Daventry, Northants NN11 5PJ, England.

Inava, Fr. Laboratoires Inava, département médical de Pierre-Fabre Medicament, 125 rue de la Faisanderie, 75116 Paris, France.

Indelfar, Spain. See *Serono, Spain.*

Independent Chemists Marketing, UK. Independent Chemists Marketing Ltd, 51 Boreham Rd, Warminster, Wilts BA12 9JU, England.

Industrial Pharmaceutical, UK. Industrial Pharmaceutical, England.

Inexfa, Spain. Inexfa, Ctra Nacional 340, KM 28, Orihuela, 03300 Alicante, Spain.

Infale, Spain. Infale, Mallorca 216, 08008 Barcelona, Spain.

Infar Nattermann, Spain. Infar Nattermann, Plg Malpica, Calle C4, 50016 Zaragoza, Spain.

Infar, Port. Infar, Industria Farmaceutica Lda, P.O. Box 8, Venda Nova, 2701 Amadora Codex, Portugal.

Ingasetter, UK. Ingasetter Ltd, Royal Deeside, 391 Union St, Aberdeen, Grampian AB1 2BX, Scotland.

Ingram & Bell, Canad. Ingram & Bell Inc., 20 Bond Ave, Don Mills, Ontario M3B 1L9, Canada.

Inibsa, Spain. Inibsa, Ctra Sabadell Granollers KM 14, Llissa de Vall, 08185 Barcelona, Spain.

Inkey, Spain. Inkey, Juan XXIII 15, Esplugas de Llobregat, 08950 Barcelona, Spain.

Innothéra, Fr. Laboratoires Innothéra (Chantereau), 10 ave P.-Vaillant-Couturier, B.P. 35, 94117 Arcueil Cedex, France.

Innothera, Switz. See *Uhlmann-Eyraud, Switz.*

Innoxa, UK. Innoxa (England) Ltd, 202 Terminus Rd, Eastbourne, East Sussex BN21 3DF, England.

Inofar, Arg. Inofar S.A., Parana 755, 1017 Buenos Aires, Argentina.

Inofarma, Spain. Inofarma, Plg Ind. Los Angeles Fundidores, Getafe, 28900 Madrid, Spain.

Inpharzam, Belg. Inpharzam S.A., ave R. Vandendriessche 18/bte 1, 1150 Brussels, Belgium.

Inpharzam, Ger. Inpharzam GmbH, Kirchenholzl 11, Postfach: 1602, 8032 Grafelfing, W. Germany.

Inpharzam, Neth. Inpharzam Nederland B.V., De Paal 41, 1351 JH Almere, Netherlands.

Inpharzam, Swed. See *Ciba, Swed.*

Inpharzam, Switz. Inpharzam S.A., PO Box 200, 6814 Cadempino, Switzerland.

Inquinasa, Spain. Inquinasa, Avda de Arostegui s/n, Echavacoiz, Navarra, Spain.

Inst. Serother. & Vaccinal, Switz. See *Berna, Switz.*

Institut Merieux, Fr. Institut Merieux, 58 av. Leclerc, 69007 Lyon, France.

Institut Merieux, Ger. Institut Merieux GmbH, Muhlenweg 131, 2000 Norderstedt, Germany.

Institut Pasteur, Fr. Institut Pasteur, 28 rue du Dr Roux, 75724 Paris Cedex, France.

Instituto Farmacologico, Spain. Instituto Farmacologico, Ramallosa Teo, Santiago de Compostela, La Coruna, Spain.

Int. Med. Prod., Neth. International Medical Products B.V., Gerritsenweg 5, 7202 BP Zutphen, Netherlands.

Interbras, Braz. Interbras, Petrobras, Commercio International SA, Rua do Rosario 90, 20041 Rio de Janeiro, Brazil.

Intercare, UK. Intercare Products Ltd, Fishponds Rd, Wokingham, Berks RG11 2QD, England.

Interdelta, Switz. Interdelta SA, Case postale 460, 1701 Fribourg, Switzerland.

Interfalk, Canad. Interfalk Canada Inc., 587 Place Choquette, Mont St-Hilaire, Quebec J3H 3Z6, Canada.

Interfalk, Ital. Interfalk Italia s.r.l., Div. Gephar, Via Isimbardi 22, 20141 Milan, Italy.

Interlabo, Switz. Interlabo SA, Case postale 453, 1227 Carouge, Switzerland.

Intermed, S.Afr. See *Pharmco, S.Afr.*

Internationaal Laboratorium, Belg. See *Cob, Belg.*

International Laboratories, UK. International Laboratories Ltd, Charwell House, Wilsom Rd, Alton, Hants GU34 2TJ, England.

International Pharmaceutical, USA. International Pharmaceutical Corporation, Subsidiary of Marion Laboratories Inc., 10236 Bunker Ridge Rd, Kansas City MO 64137, USA.

Interox, UK. Interox Chemicals Ltd, P.O. Box 7, Warrington, Cheshire WA4 6HB, England.

Interpharm, Canad. Interpharm Pharmaceutical Products Inc., 2323 autoroute des Laurentides, Laval, Quebec H7S 1Z7, Canada.

Interpharma, Spain. Interpharma, Santa Rosa 6, Santa Coloma de Gramanet, 08921 Barcelona, Spain.

Intersan, Ger. Intersan, Institut fur pharmazeutische und klinische Forschung GmbH, Einsteinstrasse 30, Postfach: 1404, 7505 Ettlingen, Germany.

Intersan, Switz. See *Uhlmann-Eyraud, Switz.*

Intervet, UK. Intervet Laboratories Ltd, Science Park, Milton Rd, Cambridge CB4 4BH, England.

Inter-Yeda, Israel. Inter-Yeda Ltd, Science-Based Industrial Park, Kiryat Weizmann, Nes Ziona 76110, Israel.

INTES, Ital. INTES, Industria Terapeutica Splendore, Oftalmoterapica ALFA, Via F.lli Bandiera 26, 80026 Casoria 8NA9, Italy.

Intradal, Neth. Intradal N.V., Brabantsestraat 17, 3812 PJ Amersfoort, Netherlands.

Inverni della Beffa, Ital. Inverni della Beffa s.p.a., Via Ripamonti 99, 20141 Milan, Italy.

Inwood, USA. Inwood Laboratories Inc., Division of Forest Laboratories Inc., Prospect St, Inwood NY 11696, USA.

Ioquin, Austral. See *Alcon, Austral.*

IPA, Ital. International Pharm Associated s.r.l., Via Casale Cavallari 53, 00156 Rome, Italy.

IPFI, Ital. I.P.F.I., Industria Farmaceutica s.r.l., Via Strambio 26, 20133 Milan, Italy.

IPIT, Ital. Ist. Profil. Ital. s.r.l., Via P.C. Boggio 79/81, 10138 Turin, Italy.

I.P.R.A.D., Fr. Laboratoires I.P.R.A.D., 4 rue Galvani, 75017 Paris, France.

IPSEN, Fr. Institut de Produits de Synthèse et d'Extraction Naturelle, 30 rue Cambronne, 75737 Paris Cedex 15, France.

Iquinosa, Spain. Iquinosa, Alpedrete 24, 28045 Madrid, Spain.

IRBI, Ital. IRBI s.p.a., S.S. Pontina 28, 00040 Pomezia (Rome), Italy.

IRFI, Ital. Istituto Richerche Farmacobiologiche Internationale s.p.a., Via Morolese 87, 03013 Ferentino (FR), Italy.

Irmesan, Spain. See *Upsamedica, Spain.*

Iromedica, Switz. Iromedica SA, Haggenstrasse 45, 9014 St Gallen, Switzerland.

ISC Chemicals, UK. ISC Chemicals Ltd, St Andrew's Rd, Avonmouth, Bristol BS11 9HP, England.

ISC, Swed. See *Triplus, Swed.*

Isdin, Spain. Isdin, Tucuman 4, 08030 Barcelona, Spain.

ISF, Ital. ISF s.p.a., Via Leonardo da Vinci 1, 20090 Trezzano s/Naviglio (MI), Italy.

ISI, Ital. Istituto Sierovaccinogeno Italiano s.p.a., 55020 Castelvecchio Pascoli, Italy.

ISM, Ital. Ist. Sieroterapico Milanese S. Belfanti, Via Darwin 22, 20143 Milan, Italy.

Ismunit, Ital. Ismunit s.r.l., Istituto Immunologico Italiano, Via Castagnetta 7, 00040 Pomezia (Rome), Italy.

Isnardi, Ital. Pietro Isnardi & C. s.p.a., Via XXV Aprile 69, 18100 Imperia Oneglia, Italy.

Isola-Ibi, Ital. Isola Ibi, Istituto Bioterapico Internazionale, Viale Pio VII 50, 16148 Genova Quarto, Italy.

ISOM, Ital. I.S.O.M. s.p.a., Via Bisceglie 96, 20152 Milan, Italy.

Ist. Chim. Inter., Ital. Istituto Chimico Internazionale Dr. Giuseppe Rende s.r.l., Via Salaria 1240, 00138 Rome, Italy.

Istituto Behring, Ital. Istituto Behring s.p.a., S.S. 17, Km.22, 67019 Scoppito (AQ), Italy.

Istituto Wassermann, Ital. Istituto Wassermann s.p.a., Contrada Sant'Emidio, 65020 Alanno (PE), Italy.

ITA, Ital. Istituto Terapeutico Ambrosiano s.r.l., Via del Lavoro 20, 20032 Ospitaletto di Cormano (MI), Italy.

Ital Suisse, Ital. Ital Suisse Co. s.a.s. di Giancarlo Ceroni & C., Via Binasco 54, 20080 Casarile (MI), Italy.

Italchimici, Ital. Italchimici s.p.a., Viale Tiziano 25, 00196 Rome, Italy.

Italfarmaco, Ital. Italfarmaco s.p.a., Viale F. Testi 330, 20126 Milan, Italy.

Italfarmaco, Switz. See *Pharnova, Switz.*

Item, Norw. Inger Asen, ITEM Development A/S, Postboks 89, 6016 Hatlane, Norway.

Item, Swed. Item Development AB, Box 65, 182 71 Stocksund, Sweden.

Itherapia, Ger. Itherapia Pharmavertrieb GmbH, Westendstr. 195, Postfach: 210446, 8000 Munich 21, W. Germany.

Itting, Ger. Franz Itting KG, Lauensteiner Strasse 41/42, Postfach: 40, 8642 Ludwigsstadt, W. Germany.

Ives, USA. See *Wyeth, USA.*

IVP, Ital. Istituto Vaccinogeno Pozzi s.p.a., V. Cassia Nord La Tognazza 21B, 53100 Siena, Italy.

Jacobus, USA. Jacobus Pharmaceutical Co. Inc., 37 Cleveland Lane, P.O. Box 5290, Princeton NJ 08540, USA.

Jamieson, Canad. C.E. Jamieson & Co. (Dom.) Ltd, 2051 Ambassador Dr., Windsor, Ontario N9C 2R5, Canada.

Jamieson-McKames, USA. Jamieson-McKames Inc., 3227 Morganford Rd, St Louis MO 63116, USA.

Jamol, USA. Jamol Laboratories Inc., 13 Ackerman Ave, Emerson NJ 07630, USA.

Jan, Canad. Jan Distributing, P.O. Box 623, Thornhill, Ontario L3T 4A5, Canada.

Janssen, Arg. Janssen Farmaceutica S.A., Julian Alvarez 148, 1414 Buenos Aires, Argentina.

Janssen, Aust. Janssen Pharmazeutika GmbH, Inzersdorfer Strasse 64, 1102 Vienna, Austria.

Janssen, Austral. Janssen Pharmaceutica Pty Ltd, P.O. Box 100, Frenchs Forest NSW 2086, Australia.

Janssen, Belg. Janssen Pharmaceutica N.V., Turnhoutseweg 30, 2340 Beerse, Belgium.

Janssen, Canad. Janssen Pharmaceutica Inc., 6535 Millcreek Dr., Mississauga, Ontario L5N 2M2, Canada.

Janssen, Denm. Janssenpharma A/S, Hammerbakken 21, 3460 Birkerød, Denmark.

Janssen, Fr. Laboratoires Janssen, 5 rue de Lübeck, 75116 Paris, France.

Janssen, Ger. Janssen GmbH, Raiffeisenstrasse 8, Postfach: 210440, 4040 Neuss 21, W. Germany.

Janssen, Ital. Janssen Farmaceutici s.p.a., V.le Castello d/Magliana 38, 00148 Rome, Italy.

Janssen, Neth. Janssen Pharmaceutica B.V., Nieuwkerksedijk 21, 5051 HS Goirle, Netherlands.

Janssen, Norw. Janssen Pharma, Skiv. 200, Postboks 113, 1415 Oppegard, Norway.

Janssen, S.Afr. Janssen Pharmaceutica (Pty) Ltd, Private Bag 3014, Randburg 2125, S. Africa.

Janssen, Spain. Janssen Farmaceutica, Serrano 23-1p, 28001 Madrid, Spain.

Janssen, Swed. See *Famaco, Swed.*

Janssen, Switz. Janssen Pharmaceutica SA, Sihlbruggstrasse 111, 6340 Baar, Switzerland.

Janssen, UK. Janssen Pharmaceutical Ltd, Grove, Wantage, Oxon OX12 0DQ, England.

Janssen, USA. Janssen Pharmaceutica Inc., 40 Kingsbridge Rd, Piscataway NJ 08854, USA.

Janssen Pharmaceutica, Swed. Janssen Pharma AB, Box 5052, 421 05 Vastra Frolunda, Sweden.

Janssen-le Brun, Belg. See *Therapeutica, Belg.*

Janus, Ital. Janus Farmaceutici s.r.l., Via Flavia 10, 00042 Anzio (Rome), Italy.

Jayco, USA. Jayco Pharmaceuticals, 895 Poplar Church Rd, Camp Hill PA 17011, USA.

J.B. Williams, USA. The J.B. Williams Co. Inc., 750 Walnut Ave, Cranford NJ 07016, USA.

Jean-Marie, Hong Kong. Jean-Marie Pharmacal Co. Ltd, Jing Ho Industrial Bldg, 17th Floor, 78-84 Wang Lung St, Tsuen Wan, Hong Kong.

Jenks Brokerage, UK. Jenks Brokerage, Castle House, 71-5 Desborough Rd, High Wycombe, Bucks HP11 2HS, England.

Jessel, Belg. See *UPB, Belg.*

Jeyes, UK. Jeyes UK Ltd, Brunel Way, Thetford, Norfolk, England.

J.F. White, UK. Dr J.F. White's Kompo Ltd, 25 Fulwith Dr., Harrogate HG2 8HW, England.

Johnson & Johnson, Fr. Johnson et Johnson S.A., 29 av. MacMahon, 75017 Paris, France.

Johnson & Johnson, Ger. Johnson & Johnson GmbH, Kaiserswerther Str. 270, Postfach: 3820, 4000 Dusseldorf 30, Germany.

Johnson & Johnson, S.Afr. Johnson & Johnson (Pty) Ltd, 7th Floor, Barclays Bank Building, Union St, East London, S. Africa.

Johnson & Johnson, Spain. Johnson Johnson, Crta Madrid-Valencia km 24.7, Arganda del Rey, 28500 Madrid, Spain.

Johnson & Johnson, Switz. Johnson & Johnson SA, Rotzenbühlstrasse 55, 8957 Spreitenbach 1, Switzerland.

Johnson & Johnson, UK. Johnson & Johnson Ltd, Brunel Way, Slough, Berks SL1 4EA, England.

Johnson & Johnson, USA. Johnson & Johnson Products Inc., 501 George St, New Brunswick NJ 08903, USA.

Johnson & Johnson Orthopaedic, UK. Johnson & Johnson Orthopaedic, England.

Johnson, Arg. Johnson & Johnson de Arg. S.A., Darwin 471, 1414 Buenos Aires, Argentina.

Johnson, Canad. S.C. Johnson and Son Ltd, 1 Webster st, Brantford, Ontario N3T 5R1, Canada.

Johnson, Denm. A. Johnson & Co. A/S, Jaegersborg Alle 14, 2920 Charlottenlund, Denmark.

Johnsons, UK. Johnson's Veterinary Products Ltd, Reddicap Trading Estate, Sutton Coldfield, West Midlands B75 7DF, England.

Jorba, Spain. Jorba, Josefa Valcarcel 30, 28027 Madrid, Spain.

Jossa-Arznei, Ger. Jossa-Arznei Kurt Merz GmbH, Bruder-Grimm-Strasse 62, Postfach: 1169, 6497 Steinau an der Strasse 1, Germany.

Jouveinal, Canad. Jouveinal Laboratories Inc., 5450 ch. Cote des Neiges, Suite 230, Montreal, Quebec H3T 1Y6, Canada.

Jouveinal, Fr. Jouveinal Laboratoires, 1 rue des Moissons, 94260 Fresnes, France.

Juanola, Spain. Juanola, Marti 131, 08024 Barcelona, Spain.

Jugoremedija, Jug. Jugoremedija, 23101 Zrenjanin, Jugoslavia.

Jungle Formula Co., UK. The Jungle Formula Co., Cwm Crawnon Rd, Llangynidr, Crickhowell, Powys NP8 1LS, Wales.

Juste, Spain. Juste, Julio Camba 7, 28028 Madrid, Spain.

Juventus, Spain. Juventus, Valentin Beato 44, 28037 Madrid, Spain.

K & K-Greeff, UK. K & K-Greeff Ltd, Suffolk House, George St, Croydon CR9 3QL, England.

K/L Pharmaceutical, UK. K/L Pharmaceuticals Ltd, 25 Macadam Place, South Newmoor Industrial Estate, Irvine KA11 4HP, Scotland.

Kabi, Ger. Deutsche KabiVitrum GmbH, Levelingstrasse 18, Postfach: 800468, 8000 Munich 80, W. Germany.

Kabi, Neth. See *KabiVitrum, Neth.*

Kabi, Norw. See *KabiVitrum, Norw.*

Kabi, S.Afr. See *Keatings, S.Afr.*

Kabi, Spain. Kabi-Fides, Conception Arenal 23-7, 08027 Barcelona, Spain.

Kabi, Swed. KabiVitrum AB, 112 87 Stockholm, Sweden.

KabiVitrum, Belg. KabiVitrum S.A., rue des 3 Arbres 54, 1180 Brussels, Belgium.

KabiVitrum, Denm. KabiVitrum A/S, Borgergade 10, 1300 Copenhagen K, Denmark.

Kabivitrum, Fr. Kabivitrum S.A., 12 rue du Centre, 93160 Noisy-le-Grand, France.

KabiVitrum, Neth. KabiVitrum B.V., Ingelandenweg 1, 1069 WE Amsterdam, Netherlands.

KabiVitrum, Norw. A/S KabiVitrum, Nesbruvn. 33, Postboks 22, 1362 Billingstad, Norway.

KabiVitrum, S.Afr. See *Saphar, S.Afr.*

KabiVitrum, Switz. KabiVitrum SA, 8700 Kusnacht, Switzerland.

KabiVitrum, UK. KabiVitrum Ltd, KabiVitrum House, Riverside Way, Uxbridge, Middx UB8 2YF, England.

Kabivitrum, USA. Kabivitrum Inc., 1131 Harbor Bay Parkway, Alameda CA 94501, USA.

Kade, Belg. See *de Bournonville, Belg.*

Kade, Ger. Dr Kade Pharmazeutische Fabrik GmbH, Rigigstrasse 2, Postfach: 48209, 1000 Berlin 48, W. Germany.

Kade, S.Afr. See *Nattermann, S.Afr.*

Kade, Switz. See *Doetsch, Grether, Switz.*

Kaigai, Jpn. Kaigai Koeki, 2-2-2 Hon-cho, Nihonbashi, Chuo-ku, Tokyo, Japan.

Kairon, Spain. Kairon, Marmoles 10 Bis, 41004 Sevilla, Spain.

Kaken, Jpn. Kaken Seiyaku, 2-28-8 Honkomagome, Bunkyo-ku, Tokyo, Japan.

Kali, Belg. See *Triosol, Belg.*

Kali-Chemie, Denm. See *Meda, Denm.*

Kali-Chemie, Ger. Kali-Chemie Pharma GmbH, Hans-Böckler-Allee 20, Postfach: 220, 3000 Hannover 1, W. Germany.

Kali-Chemie, Neth. See *Schmidt, Neth.* and *VSM, Neth.*

Kali-Chemie, Norw. See *Meda, Norw.*

Kali-Chemie, Swed. See *Meda, Swed.*

Kali-Chemie, Switz. See *Duphar, Switz.*

Kali-Farma, Spain. Kali-Farma, Ctra Barcelona a Ribas, Parets del Valles, 08150 Barcelona, Spain.

Kalopharma, Ital. Kalopharma s.p.a., Via IV Novembre 76, 20019 Settimo Milanese (Milan), Italy.

Kanebo, Jpn. Kanebo, 1-3-12 Motoakasaka, Minato-ku, Tokyo, Japan.

Kanoldt, Ger. Kanoldt Arzneimittel GmbH, Oberer Weberberg 11, Postfach: 1160, 8884 Höchstädt (Donau), W. Germany.

Kanto Isei, Jpn. Kanto Isei, 2-1-1 Nishishinjuku, Shinjuku, Tokyo, Japan.

Karibion, Spain. Karibion, Gran Via 318, Barcelona, Spain.

Karlspharma, Ger. Karlspharma Pharmazeutische Produkte GmbH, Greschbachstr. 4, 7500 Karlsruhe 41, W. Germany.

Kasdorf, Arg. Kasdorf, S.A., Loria 117, 1173 Buenos Aires, Argentina.

Katwijk, Neth. Katwijk Farma B.V., Prins Hendrikkade 11, 2225 TZ Katwijk aan Zee, Netherlands.

Kayaku, Jpn. Kayaku Kosei, 2-16-23 Mejiro, Toshima-ku, Tokyo, Japan.

Keatings, S.Afr. See *Adcock Ingram, S.Afr.*

Keene, USA. Keene Pharmaceuticals Inc., 333 S. Mockingbird, P.O. Box 7, Keene TX 76059, USA.

Keimdiät, Ger. Keimdiät GmbH - Vertrieb Synpharma GmbH, Pfladergasse 7, Postfach: 111 649, 8900 Augsburg, W. Germany.

Kelco International, UK. Kelco International Ltd, Westminster Tower, 3 Albert Embankment, London SE1 7RZ, England.

Kelco, USA. Kelco, Division of Merck & Co. Inc., 8355 Aero Dr., San Diego CA 92123, USA.

Kelemata, Ital. Kelemata s.p.a., Via G. Reiss Romoli 10, 10155 Turin, Italy.

Keller, Switz. E. Keller Erben AG, 6901 Lugano, Switzerland.

Kemi-Intressen, Swed. See *Nobel Medica, Swed.*

Kemiflor, Swed. Kemiflor AB, Box 7245, 103 89 Stockholm, Sweden.

Kendon, UK. Kendon International Ltd, 8-14 Orsman Rd, London N1 5QJ, England.

Kenral, Canad. Kenral Inc., P.O. Box 4444, Don Mills, Ontario M3C 2T9, Canada.

Kenwood, USA. Kenwood Laboratories Inc., Division of Bradley Pharmaceuticals Inc., 383 Route 46 West, Fairfield NJ 07006-2402, USA.

Kerfoot, UK. Thomas Kerfoot & Co. Ltd, Vale of Bardsley, Ashton-under-Lyne, Lancs OL7 9RR, England.

Kettelhack Riker, Ger. Kettelhack Riker Pharma GmbH, Wilbecke 12-14, Postfach: 1340, 4280 Borken, W. Germany.

Key, Austral. Key Pharmaceuticals Pty Ltd, A Muir & Neil Co., P.O. Box 121, Concord West NSW 2138, Australia.

Key, Denm. See *Smith Kline & French, Denm.*

Key, USA. Key Pharmaceuticals Inc., 4400 Biscayne Blvd, Miami FL 33137, USA.

Kin, Spain. Kin, San Mario 53-55, 08022 Barcelona, Spain.

Kingswood, Canad. Kingswood Canada Inc., 50 Venture Dr., Scarborough, Ontario M1B 3L6, Canada.

Kinney, USA. Kinney & Co. Inc., 1307 12th St, Columbus IN 47201, USA.

Kirby, Neth. See *Medica, Neth.*

Kirby-Warrick, Eire. See *Cahill May Roberts, Eire.*

Kirby-Warrick, UK. Kirby-Warrick Pharmaceuticals Ltd, Mildenhall, Bury St Edmunds, Suffolk IP28 7AX, England.

Kissei, Jpn. Kissei Yakuhin Kogyo, 19-48 Yoshino, Matsumoto-shi, Japan.

Klein, Ger. Dr Gustav Klein, Steinenfeld 3, Postfach: 1165, 7615 Zell-Harmersbach, W. Germany.

Klinge, Ger. Klinge Pharma GmbH, Berg-am-Laim-Str. 129, Postfach: 801063, 8000 Munich 80, W. Germany.

Klinge, Switz. See *Ridupharm, Switz.*

Klinge-Nattermann, Ger. See *Klinge, Ger.*

Kneipp, Ger. Kneipp-Werke, Steinbachtal 43, Postfach: 5960, 8700 Würzburg, W. Germany.

Knickerbocker, Spain. Knickerbocker, Conde de Borell 158, 08015 Barcelona, Spain.

Knoll, Arg. Knoll Arg. S.A., Guemes 3475, 1425 Buenos Aires, Argentina.

Knoll, Austral. See *Schering, Austral.*

Knoll, Belg. See *Searle, Belg.*

Knoll, Canad. Knoll Pharmaceuticals Canada Inc., 26-825 Denison St, Markham, Ontario L3R 5E4, Canada.

Knoll, Denm. See *Meda, Denm.*

Knoll, Ger. Knoll AG, Knollstrasse (Eingang Sudermannstrasse), Postfach: 210805, 6700 Ludwigshafen, W. Germany.

Knoll, Ital. Knoll s.p.a., Via Soperga 37-39, 20127 Milan, Italy.

Knoll, Neth. Knoll B.V., Afd. Farma, Markerkant 13-10, 1314 AN Almere, Netherlands.

Knoll, Norw. See *Meda, Norw.*

Knoll, S.Afr. See *Holpro, S.Afr.*

Knoll, Swed. See *Meda, Swed.*

Knoll, Switz. Knoll SA, Case postal 631, 4410 Liestal, Switzerland.

Knoll, UK. Knoll Ltd, The Brow, Burgess Hill, West Sussex RH15 9NE, England.

Knoll, USA. Knoll Pharmaceutical Co., 30 North Jefferson Rd, Whippany NJ 07981, USA.

Knoll-Made, Spain. Knoll-Made, Avda. de Burgos 91, 28050 Madrid, Spain.

Knox, UK. Knox Laboratories Ltd, England.

Kobro, Norw. Kobro & Co. A/S, Sørkedalsvn. 10 A, Postboks 5295 Majorstua, 0303 Oslo 3, Norway.

Koch-Light, UK. Koch-Light, England.

Kodama, Jpn. Kodama, 2-5 Ogawa-machi, Kanda, Chiyada-ku, Tokyo, Japan.

Kogrere, Switz. Kogrere SA, Case postale 273, 8033 Zurich, Switzerland.

Köhler, Ger. Dr Franz Köhler Chemie GmbH, Neue Bergstrasse 3-7, Postfach: 1117, 6146 Alsbach-Hähnlein 1, W. Germany.

Kohler, Neth. See *Tramedico, Neth.*

Kolassa, Aust. Dr Kolassa, Arzneimittel GmbH, Gastgebgasse 5-13, Postfach 27, 1231 Vienna, Austria.

Korn Pharma, Denm. Korn Pharma, Brogade 19 (P.O.Box 107), 4300 Holbaek, Denmark.

Kowa, Jpn. Kowa, 3-6-29 Nishiki, Naka-ku, Nagoyashi, Japan.

Kramer-Synthelabo, Switz. Kramer-Synthelabo SA, Case Postale 45, 1000 Lausanne 21, Switzerland.

Kramer, USA. Kramer Pharmacal Inc., 8778 SW 8th St, Miami FL 33174, USA.

Kremers-Urban, USA. See *Rorer, USA.*

Kreussler, Denm. See *Felo, Denm.*

Kreussler, Ger. Chemische Fabrik Kreussler & Co. GmbH, Rheingaustrasse 87-93, Postfach: 120454, 6200 Wiesbaden 12, W. Germany.

Kreussler, Neth. See *Multi-Pharma, Neth.*

Kreussler, Swed. See *Imeco, Swed.*

Kreussler, Switz. See *Globopharm, Switz.*

Krewel, Ger. Krewel-Werke GmbH, Krewelstrasse 2, Postfach: 260, 5208 Eitorf, Germany.

Kronans, Swed. Kronans Farm. & Kem. Laboratorium, Box 33, 170 11 Drottningholm, Sweden.

Krugmann, Ger. Krugmann GmbH, Mundipharma Strasse 4, Postfach: 1350, 6250 Limburg (Lahn), W. Germany.

Kwizda, Switz. See *Schwarz, Switz.*

Kyorin, Jpn. Kyorin Seiyaku, 2-5 Surugadai, Kanda, Chiyoda-ku, Tokyo, Japan.

Kyowa, Denm. See *Pharmavit, Denm.*

Kyowa, Ital. Kyowa Italiana Farmaceutici s.r.l., Via Gian Battista Vico 14, 20123 Milan, Italy.

Kyowa, Jpn. Kyowahakko, 1-6-1 Ote-machi, Chiyoda-ku, Tokyo, Japan.

Kyowa Hakko Kogyo, Belg. See *Christiaens, Belg.*

Laake, Norw. See *Farmitalia, Norw.*

Laakefarmos, Fin. Laakefarmos, PL 425, 20101 Turku, Finland.

Laakefarmos, Swed. See *Farmos, Swed.*

Laaketukku, Fin. Laaketukku Oy, Vattuniemenkuja 1, PL 52, 00211 Helsinki, Finland.

Lab. de Serocytologie, Switz. Laboratoire de Sérocytologie SA, Beau-Rivage 6, 1006 Lausanne, Switzerland.

Lab. Francais Ther., Belg. See *Therapeutica, Belg.*

LAB, Switz. See *Schönenberger, Switz.*

Labatec-Pharma, Switz. Labatec-Pharma S.A., 36 rue du 31-Décembre, 1211 Geneva 6, Switzerland.

Labaz, Belg. Labaz-Sanofi S.A., ave de Béjar 1, 1120 Brussels, Belgium.

Labaz, Fr. Laboratoires Labaz, 39 ave Pierre-1er-de-Serbie, 75008 Paris, France.

Labaz, Ger. Labaz GmbH, Pharmaz. Präparate, Augustenstrasse 10, Postfach: 201708, 8000 Munich 2, W. Germany.

Labaz, Neth. See *Sanofi Labaz, Neth.*

Labaz, S.Afr. See *Reckitt & Colman, S.Afr.*

Labaz, Spain. Labaz, Beethoven 9, 08021 Barcelona, Spain.

Labaz, Switz. See *Sanofi, Switz.*

Labaz Sanofi, UK. See *Sanofi, UK.*

Labcatal, Fr. Laboratoires Labcatal, 7 rue Roger-Salengro, 92120 Montrouge, France.

Labcatal, Switz. See *Panpharma, Switz.*

Labinca, Arg. Labinca S.A., Cramer 4130, 1429 Buenos Aires, Argentina.

Labopharma, Ger. Labopharma, Chemische-pharmazeutische Fabrik GmbH, Nordhauser Strasse 30, 1000 Berlin 10, W. Germany.

Laboratoire Européen du Médicament, Fr. See *Pierre Fabre, Fr.*

Laboratoires Biologiques de l'Île-de-France, Fr. Laboratoires Biologiques de l'Île-de-France S.A., 45 rue de Clichy, 75009 Paris, France.

Laboratoires de l'Hémédonine, Fr. Laboratoires de l'Hémédonine, 117 rue Félix-Faure, 59110 La Madeleine, France.

Laboratories de l'Hepatrol, Switz. See *Pharmos, Switz.*

Laboratories for Applied Biology, UK. Laboratories for Applied Biology Ltd, 91 Amhurst Park, London N16 5DR, England.

Lacefa, Arg. Lacefa S.A.I.C.A., Ladines 2263/67, 1419 Buenos Aires, Argentina.

Lacer, Spain. Lacer, Cerdena 350, 08025 Barcelona, Spain.

Lactaid, USA. Lactaid Inc., 600 Fire Rd, P.O. Box 111, Pleasantville NJ 08232-0111, USA.

Lacteol du Dr Boucard, Fr. Laboratoires du Lacteol du Dr Boucard S.A., Route de Bu, B.P. 41, 78550 Houdan, France.

Laevosan, Aust. Laevosan GmbH & Co. KG, Estermannstrasse 17, 4020 Linz, Austria.

Laevosan, Norw. See *Med-Kjemi, Norw.*

Laevosan, Swed. See *Kemiflor, Swed.*

Laevosan, Switz. See *Boehringer Mannheim, Switz.*

Lafage, Arg. Lafage S.R.L., José E. Uriburu 61, 1027 Buenos Aires, Argentina.

Lafar, Ital. La Far s.r.l., Via Noto 7, 20141 Milan, Italy.

Lafare, Ital. Laboratorio Farmaceutico Reggiano s.n.c., Via S.B. Cozzolino 77, 80056 Ercolano Resina (NA), Italy.

Lafarge, Fr. Laboratoires Lafarge, 19 rue Reaumur, 75003 Paris, France.

Lafarquim, Spain. Lafarquim, Avd. Aragon 18, 28027 Madrid, Spain.

Lafayette, USA. Lafayette Pharmacal Inc., 4200 South Hulen St, Fort Worth TX 76109, USA.

Lafon, Fr. Laboratoires Lafon, 19 ave du Professeur Cadiot, B.P. 22, 94701 Maisons-Alfort Cedex, France.

Lafran, Fr. Laboratoires Lafran, 1 route de Stains, 94380 Bonneuil-sur-Marne, France.

Lagamed, S.Afr. Lagamed (Pty) Ltd, P.O. Box 533, Isando 1600, S. Africa.

Lagap, Ital. Lagap Italiana s.r.l., Via Doberdo 16, 20126 Milan, Italy.

Lagap, Switz. Lagap S.A., P.O. Box 7, 6943 Vezia, Switzerland.

Lagap, UK. Lagap Pharmaceuticals Ltd, Woolmer Way, Bordon, Hants GU35 9QE, England.

Lagrol, Spain. Lagrol, Menendez Pelayo 100, Santander, 39006 Cantabria, Spain.

Lainco, Spain. Lainco, Avda Bizet 8-12, Rubi, 08191 Barcelona, Spain.

Laing-National, UK. Laing-National Ltd, Ashburton Rd, Trafford Park, Manchester M17 1BJ, England.

Lake, UK. Lake Pharmaceuticals Ltd, 36 Haven Green, Ealing Broadway, London W5 2NX, England.

Lakeside, USA. Lakeside Pharmaceuticals, Division of Merrell Dow Pharmaceuticals Inc., P.O. Box 429553, Cincinnati OH 45242-9553, USA.

Laleuf, Fr. Societe d'exploitation des Laboratoires Laleuf S.A., 6 rue Laugier, 95100 Argenteuil, France.

Lambda Pharmacal, USA. See *Bart, USA.*

Lampugnani, Ital. Lampugnani Farmaceutici s.p.a., Via Gramsci 4, 20014 Nerviano (Milan), Italy.

Lancet, Austral. See *Boots, Austral.*

Lancet, UK. Lancet Pharmaceuticals Ltd, England.

Landerlan, Spain. Landerlan, Agastia 67, 28043 Madrid, Spain.

Lane & Stedman, UK. Lane & Stedman Ltd, 100 Western Rd, Hove, E. Sussex BN3 1GA, England.

Lane, UK. G.R. Lane Health Products Ltd, Sisson Rd, Gloucester GL1 3QB, England.

Langdale, UK. Langdale Webb Ltd, Vulcan Way, New Addington, Surrey CR9 0BS, England.

Langly, Austral. Langly Laboratories Pty Ltd, 64 Rose St, Chippendale NSW 2008, Australia.

Lannacher, Aust. Lannacher Heilmittel GmbH, 8502 Lannach 1-3, Steiermark, Austria.

Lannacher, Denm. See *Ringsted & Semler, Denm.*

Lannacher, Swed. See *Kronans, Swed.*

Lannett, USA. The Lannett Co. Inc., 9000 State Rd, Philadelphia PA 19136, USA.

Lansberg, Neth. See *Bipharma, Neth.*

Lantigen, Belg. See *Cob, Belg.*

Lanzas, Spain. Lanzas, Doctor Blanco Soler 1, 28044 Madrid, Spain.

Laphal, Fr. Laboratoires Laphal, 13190 Allauch, France.

Laporte, UK. Laporte Industries Ltd, P.O. Box 8, Kingsway, Luton, Beds, England.

Lappe, Ger. See *Bristol, Ger.*

Laproquifar, Spain. Laproquifar, Las Carolinas 13, 08012 Barcelona, Spain.

Laquifal, Spain. Laquifal, Ayala 99, 28006 Madrid, Spain.

L'Arguenon, Fr. L'Arguenon (s.a.r.l.) - S.E.R.B. Laboratoires, 53 rue Villiers de l'Isle Adam, 75020 Paris, France.

Lariviere, Neth. See *Bipharma, Neth.*

Larkhall Laboratories, UK. Larkhall Laboratories, 225 Putney Bridge Rd, London SW15 2PY, England.

Laroche Navarron, Belg. S.A. Belge Laroche Navarron, ave Louise 326/bte 4, 1050 Brussels, Belgium.

Laroche Navarron, Fr. Laboratoires Laroche Navarron, 20 rue Jean-Jaurès, 92800 Puteaux, France.

Laroche-Navarron, Neth. See *Bournonville, Neth.*

Laroche Navarron, Switz. See *Uhlmann-Eyraud, Switz.*

Lasa, Spain. Lasa, Laurea Miro 385, San Feliu de Llobregat, 08980 Barcelona, Spain.

Lasalle, USA. Lasalle Laboratories Inc., Subsidiary of Mallard Inc., 3021 Wabash Ave, Detroit MI 48216, USA.

Laser, USA. Laser Inc., 2000 N. Main St, P.O. Box 905, Crown Point IN 46307, USA.

Latema, Belg. See *Triosol, Belg.*

Latema, Denm. See *Meda, Denm.*

Latéma, Fr. See *L.T.M., Fr.*

Latema, Neth. See *Nourypharma, Neth.* and *Vemedia, Neth.*

Latema, Swed. See *Meda, Swed.*

Latéma, Switz. See *Duphar, Switz.*

Laurentian, Canad. Laurentian Agencies, a division of Laurentian Laboratories Ltd, C.P. 4444, Pointe-Claire, Dorval, Quebec H9R 4R1, Canada.

Laves, Ger. Laves-Arzneimittel GmbH, Barbarastrasse 14, Postfach: 100352, 3003 Ronnenberg/Hannover, W. Germany.

Lawrence Industries, UK. Lawrence Industries, Mitcham Industrial Estate, Streatham Rd, Mitcham, Surrey CR4 2AP, England.

Lazar, Arg. Dr Lazar & Cía S.A., Av. Vélez Sarsfield 5855, 1605 Munro, Pcia Buenos Aires, Argentina.

Le Marchand, Fr. Laboratoires Le Marchand, 24 av. M. Maunoury, 28600 Luisant, France.

Lederle, Arg. Lederle, Division de Cyanamid de Arg. S.A., Charcas 5051, 1425 Buenos Aires, Argentina.

Lederle, Austral. Lederle Laboratories, Division of Cyanamid Australia Pty Ltd, 5 Gibbon Rd, Baulkham Hills NSW 2153, Australia.

Lederle, Belg. See *Cyanamid, Belg.*

Lederle, Canad. Lederle Cyanamid Canada Inc., 2255 Sheppard Ave E., Willowdale, Ontario M2J 4Y5, Canada.

Lederle, Denm. Lederle Cyanamid Danmark, St. Kongensgade 68, 1264 Copenhagen K, Denmark.

Lederle, Fr. Laboratoires Lederle, 74 rue d'Arcueil, Immeuible lena, Silic 275, 94578 Rungis Cedex, France.

Lederle, Jpn. Nihon Lederle, 1-10-3 Kyobashi, Chuo-ku, Tokyo, Japan.

Lederle, Neth. Lederle Nederland B.V., Stationsplein 23, 4872 XL Etten-Leur, Netherlands.

Lederle, Norw. Lederle Informasjonskontor, Skippergt. 30, Postboks 138 Sentrum, 0102 Oslo 1, Norway.

Lederle, S.Afr. Lederle Laboratories (Division of S.A. Cyanimid (Pty) Ltd), P.O. Box 7552, Johannesburg 2000, S. Africa.

Lederle, Spain. See *Cyanamid, Spain.*

Lederle, Swed. See *Cyanamid, Swed.*

Lederle, Switz. See *Opopharma, Switz.*

Lederle, UK. Lederle Laboratories, Fareham Rd, Gosport, Hants PO13 0AS, England.

Lederle, USA. Lederle Laboratories, Division of American Cyanamid Co., Pearl River NY 10965, USA.

Lee-Adams, Canad. Lee-Adams Laboratories, Division of Pharmascience Inc., 8400 ch. Darnley, Montreal, Quebec H4T 1M4, Canada.

Leeming, USA. Leeming Division, Pfizer Inc., 100 Jefferson Rd, Parsippany NJ 07054, USA.

Leerbeck & Holms, Denm. Leerbeck & Holms kermiske Fabrikker, Ingemannsvej 3, 1964 Frederiksberg C, Denmark.

Lefrancq, Fr. Laboratoires Lefrancq, 36 ave de Metz, 93230 Romainville, France.

Legere, USA. Legere Pharmaceuticals Inc., 7326 E. Evans Rd, Scottsdale AZ 85260, USA.

Leiras, Denm. See *Nordisk Droge, Denm.*

Leiras, Fin. Leiras, PL 415, 20101 Turku 10, Finland.

Leiras, Swed. See *Roussel, Swed.*

Lemmon, USA. Lemmon Co., Ethical Division, P.O. Box 630, Sellersville PA 18960, USA.

Lemoine, Fr. Laboratoires Lemoine, 36 rue du Magasin, 59000 Lille, France.

Lenau, Denm. Lenau & Co., Gammel Kongevej 98, 1850 Frederiksberg C, Denmark.

Lennon, S.Afr. Lennon Ltd, P.O. Box 52316, Saxonwold 2132, S. Africa.

Lensa, Spain. Lensa, Estadella 12 Bis, 08030 Barcelona, Spain.

Lentheric Morny, UK. Lentheric Morny Ltd, Vale Rd, Camberley, Surrey GU15 3AX, England.

Lenza, Ital. Farmaceutici Lenza s.r.l., Via Padula (Racc. Autos), 80026 Casoria (Naples), Italy.

Leo, Aust. Leo-Arzneimittel GmbH, Brigittagasse 22-26, Postfach: 201, 1201 Vienna, Austria.

Leo, Belg. Leo Pharmaceutical Products Belgium S.A., chaussee de Waterloo 1359 I, 1180 Brussels, Belgium.

Leo, Canad. Leo Laboratories Canada Ltd, 1305 Pickering Parkway, Suite 704, Pickering, Ontario L1V 3P2, Canada.

Leo, Denm. Løvens kemiske Fabrik, Industriparken 55, 2750 Ballerup, Denmark.

Leo, Fr. Laboratoires Leo, 6 rue J.-P.-Timbaud, 78180 Montigny-le-Bretonneux, France.

Leo, Neth. See *Leo Pharm., Neth.* and *UCB, Neth.*

Leo, Norw. Løvens kemiske Fabrik, Hegdehaugsv. 36, Postboks 7186 Homansbyen, 0307 Oslo 3, Norway.

Leo, S.Afr. Leo Laboratories (Pty) Ltd, P.O. Box 76237, Wendywood 2144, S. Africa.

Leo, Spain. Leo, Avda Pio XII 99, 28036 Madrid, Spain.

Leo, Swed. Leo Lakemedel AB, Box 941, 251 09 Helsingborg, Sweden.

Leo, Switz. Leo Pharmaceutical Products Sarath Ltd, Eggbühlstrasse 20, 8052 Zurich, Switzerland.

Leo, UK. Leo Laboratories Ltd, Longwick Rd, Princes Risborough, Aylesbury, Bucks HP17 9RR, England.

Leo Pharm., Neth. Leo Pharmaceutical Products B.V., Van Houten Industriepark 11, 1381 MZ Weesp, Netherlands.

Leo Rhodia, Swed. Leo Rhodia, Box 945, 251 09 Helsingborg, Sweden.

Leo Suede, Switz. Leo SA, Case postale, 8051 Zurich, Switzerland.

Leopold Charles, UK. Leopold Charles & Co. Ltd, England.

Lepetit, Arg. Lepetit S.A., L.N. Alem 896, 1001 Buenos Aires, Argentina.

Lepetit, Fr. See *Merrell, Fr.*

Lepetit, Ital. Gruppo Lepetit s.p.a., Via Murat 23, 20159 Milan, Italy.

Lepetit, Spain. See *Merrell Dow, Spain.*

Lepetit, UK. See *Merrell, UK.*

Lersa, Spain. Lersa, Plg Ind. la Red Jota 181, Alcala de Guadaira, 41500 Sevilla, Spain.

Lerta, Fr. Laboratoires Etudes et Recherches-Therapeutiques Aristegni, 44 cours Camou, B.P. 205, 64002 Pau Cedex, France.

Lerta, Switz. See *Interlabo, Switz.*

Lesourd, Fr. Laboratoires Gabriel Lesourd, 6 rue Sainte-Isaure, 75018 Paris, France.

Lesvi, Spain. Lesvi, Plg Ind. Can Pelegri S/N, San Andres de la Barca, 08740 Barcelona, Spain.

Letap, UK. Letap Pharmaceuticals, Celtic House, 17-19 Grove Vale, London SE22 8EQ, England.

Leti, Spain. Leti, Parraco Triado 62, 08014 Barcelona, Spain.

Leurquin, Fr. Laboratoires Leurquin, 22 rue du Capitaine-Ferber, 75960 Paris Cedex 20, France.

Level, Spain. Level, Pedro IV 499, 08020 Barcelona, Spain.

Lever Industrial, UK. Lever Industrial, P.O. Box 208, Lever House, St James's Rd, Kingston-on-Thames, Surrey KT1 2BB, England.

Lexalabs, USA. Lexalabs, USA.

Liade, Spain. Liade, Ctra Barcelona km 28.6, Alcala de Henares, Madrid, Spain.

Liberman, Spain. Liberman, Pedro IV 84, 08005 Barcelona, Spain.

LIC, Swed. LIC, Hygien, Box 173, 578 00 Aneby, Sweden.

Licardy, Fr. Laboratoire Licardy, 35 av. Carnot, 21340 Nolay, France.

Lifasa, Spain. See *Sabater, Spain.*

Lifepharma, Ital. Lifepharma s.r.l., Via Principe Eugenio 48, 20155 Milan, Italy.

Lilly, Arg. See *Lepetit, Arg.*

Lilly, Austral. Eli Lilly (Australia) & Co., Wharf Rd, West Ryde NSW 2114, Australia.

Lilly, Belg. Eli Lilly Benelux S.A., rue de l'Etuve 52/bte 1, 1000 Brussels, Belgium.

Lilly, Canad. Eli Lilly Canada Inc., 3650 Danforth Ave, Scarborough, Ontario M1N 2E8, Canada.

Lilly, Denm. Eli Lilly and Company Denmark ApS, Tømmerup Stationsvej 10, 2770 Kastrup, Denmark.

Lilly, Fr. Lilly France S.A., 203 bureaux de la Colline, 92213 Saint-Cloud, France.

Lilly, Ger. Eli Lilly GmbH, Saalburgstr. 153, Postfach: 1441, 6380 Bad Homburg, W. Germany.

Lilly, Ital. Eli Lilly Italia s.p.a., Via Gramsci 731/733, 50019 Sesto Fiorentino (FI), Italy.

Lilly, Neth. Eli Lilly Nederland, Kantoor van Duvenborch, Stationsplein 97, 3511 ED Utrecht, Netherlands.

Lilly, Norw. Eli Lilly S.A. Informasjonsavdeling Norge, Enebakkv. 287, Postboks 45 Abelso, 1105 Oslo 11, Norway.

Lilly, NZ. Lilly Industries (NZ) Ltd, P.O. Box 23-398, Papatoetoe, New Zealand.

Lilly, S.Afr. Eli Lilly (SA) (Pty) Ltd, P.O. Box 98, Isando 1600, S. Africa.

Lilly, Spain. Lilly, Paseo Industria S/N, Alcobendas, 28080 Madrid, Spain.

Lilly, Swed. Eli Lilly Sweden AB, Box 30037, 104 25 Stockholm, Sweden.

Lilly, Switz. See *Inst. Serother. & Vaccinal, Switz.*

Lilly, UK. Eli Lilly & Co. Ltd, Kingsclere Rd, Basingstoke, Hants RG21 2XA, England.

Lilly, USA. Eli Lilly & Co., Lilly Corporate Center, Indianapolis IN 46285, USA.

Lindeburg, Denm. Lindeburg Farma ApS, Naerum Hovedgade 2, 2850 Naerum, Denmark.

Lindopharm, Ger. Lindopharm GmbH, Neustrasse 82, Postfach: 560, 4010 Hilden, W. Germany.

Linton, UK. Linton, England.

Linz, Neth. See *Bipharma, Neth.*

Lion, Jpn. Lion, 1-3-7 Honjyo, Sumida-ku, Tokyo, Japan.

Lionelle, Hong Kong. Lionelle Pharmaceuticals Hong Kong Ltd, Apt. B-1136, 24 Salisbury Rd, Tsimshatsui, Kowloon, Hong Kong.

Lipha, Belg. Lipha, rue Katteput 10 bis, 1080 Brussels, Belgium.

Lipha, Denm. See *Meda, Denm.*

Lipha, Ger. Lipha Arzneimittel GmbH, Zeche Katharina 6, Postfach: 130326, 4300 Essen 13, W. Germany.

Lipha, Ital. Lipha s.p.a., Via G. Garibaldi 80/82, 50041 Calenzano (FI), Italy.

Lipha, Norw. See *Meda, Norw.*

Lipha, Swed. See *Meda, Swed.*

Lipha, Switz. See *Biochimica, Switz.* and *Uhlmann-Eyraud, Switz.*

Lipha, UK. Lipha Pharmaceuticals Ltd, Harrier House, High St, Yiewsley, West Drayton, Middx UB7 7QG, England.

Lipomed, UK. Lipomed Ltd, 19 London End, Beaconsfield, Bucks HP9 2HN, England.

Lirca, Ital. L.I.R.C.A. Synthelabo s.p.a., Via Rivoltana 35, 20090 Limito (MI), Italy.

Lisapharma, Ital. Lisapharma s.p.a., Via Licinio 11-13-15, 22036 Erba (Como), Italy.

Lister, UK. Lister Institute of Preventive Medicine, Royal National Orthopaedic Hospital, Brockley Hill, Stanmore, Middx, England.

Llano, Spain. Llano Dr, Ctra Ajalvir Daganzo km 1.5, Ajalvir, 28864 Madrid, Spain.

Llorens, Spain. Llorens, Ciudad de Balaguer 7-11, 08022 Barcelona, Spain.

Llorente, Spain. Llorente, General Rodrigo 6, 28003 Madrid, Spain.

Lloyd, Swed. See *Meda, Swed.*

Lloyd, Aimee, UK. Lloyd, Aimee & Co. Ltd, Kingsend House, 44 Kingsend, Ruislip, Middx HA4 7DA, England.

Lloyd Wood, Canad. W. Lloyd Wood Co. Ltd, Division of Beauty Creations Ltd, 833 Oxford St, Toronto, Ontario M8Z 5X4, Canada.

Lloyd-Hamol, Reckitt & Colman Pharm., UK. Lloyd-Hamol Ltd, Reckitt & Colman Pharmaceutical Division, Clerk Green, Batley, W Yorks WF17 5RU, England.

Lloyds Pharmaceuticals, Reckitt & Colman Pharm., UK. Lloyds Pharmaceuticals Ltd, Reckitt & Colman Pharmaceutical Division, Clerk Green, Batley, W Yorks WF17 5RU, England.

LOA, Arg. Laboratorio Oftalmol Arg. S.A.I.C.I.F., Dr J.F. Aranguren 344, 1405 Buenos Aires, Argentina.

Locatelli, Ital. Farmaceutici Locatelli, s.r.l., Via Campobello 15, 00040 Pomezia (Rome), Italy.

Loders & Nucoline, UK. Loders & Nucoline Ltd, Civic Way, Burgess Hill, West Sussex, England.

Lofarma, Ital. Lofarma Allergeni s.r.l., Viale Cassala 40, 20143 Milan, Italy.

Lofthouse of Fleetwood, UK. Lofthouse of Fleetwood Ltd, Maritime St, Fleetwood, Lancs FY7 7LP, England.

Logeais, Fr. Laboratoires Jacques Logeais, 71 ave du Général-de-Gaulle, 92130 Issy-les-Moulineaux, France.

Logeais, Switz. See *Biphar, Switz.* and *Interdelta, Switz.*

Logifarm, Ital. Logifarm s.r.l., Via L. da Vinci 168, 20090 Trezzano S.N. (MI), Italy.

Lomapharm, Ger. Lomapharm, Rudolf Lohmann GmbH KG, Langes Feld 5, Postfach:1210, 3254 Emmerthal 1, W. Germany.

Longuet, Belg. See *Bio-Therabel, Belg.*

Lorex, Denm. See *Searle, Denm.*

Lorex, Neth. See *Searle, Neth.*

Lorex, UK. Lorex Pharmaceuticals Ltd, Old Bank House, 39 High St, High Wycombe, Bucks HP11 2AG, England.

Lövens, Swed. Lövens Läkemedel AB, Box 404, 201 24 Malmo, Sweden.

Loveridge, UK. J.M. Loveridge PLC, Southbrook Rd, Southampton SO9 3LT, England.

Loxley, UK. Loxley Medical, Bessingby Estate, Bridlington, North Humberside YO16 4SU, England.

LPB, Ital. LPB Istituto Farmaceutico s.p.a., Via dei Lavoratori 54, 20092 Cinisello Balsamo (MI), Italy.

LRC Products, UK. LRC Products Ltd, North Circular Rd, London E4 8QA, England.

L.T.M., Fr. Laboratoires de Therapeutique Moderne, 42 rue Rouget de Lisle, 92151 Sursenes Cedex, France.

Lubapharm, Switz. Lubapharm SA, Drosselstrasse 47, 4002 Basel, Switzerland.

Lucchini, Ital. Lucchini Italiana s.r.l., Via Trionfale 6909, 00136 Rome, Italy.

Lucchini, Switz. Lab. Lucchini S.A., 20 rue Coulouvrenière, 1204 Geneva, Switzerland.

Lucien, Fr. Laboratoires Lucien, 3 rue des Écoles, 92704 Colombes Cedex, France.

Lugaresi, Ital. Lugaresi & C., Via B. da Carpi 15, 4041 Bologna, Italy.

Luitpold, Austral. See *Organon, Austral.*

Luitpold, Belg. See *Will-Pharma, Belg.*

Luitpold, Denm. See *GEA, Denm.*

Luitpold, Ger. Luitpold-Werk, GmbH & Co., Chemisch-pharmazeutische Fabrik, Zielstattstrasse 9, Postfach: 70 12 09, 8000 Munich 70, W. Germany.

Luitpold, Ital. Luitpold s.r.l., Via Bernardino Alimena 126, 00173 Rome, Italy.

Luitpold, Norw. See *Nyco, Norw.*

Luitpold, S.Afr. Luitpold, S. Africa.

Luitpold, Switz. Luitpold-Werk, Industriestrasse 7, 8117 Fällanden, Switzerland.

Luitpold-Werk, Swed. See *Selena, Swed.*

Lundbeck, Belg. Lundbeck S.A., blvd du Midi 33/bte 7, 1000 Brussels, Belgium.

Lundbeck, Denm. H. Lundbeck A/S, Ottiliavej 7, 2500 Valby, Denmark.

Lundbeck, Fin. Oy H. Lundbeck AB, Komeetankatu 1, PL 45, 02211 Espoo, Finland.

Lundbeck, Neth. Lundbeck B.V., Kabelweg 55, 1014 BA Amsterdam, Netherlands.

Lundbeck, Norw. H. Lundbeck A/S, Drammensv. 342, Postboks 188, 1324 Lysaker, Norway.

Lundbeck, Philipp. See *Marsman, Philipp.*

Lundbeck, S.Afr. See *SCS, S.Afr.*

Lundbeck, Swed. H. Lundbeck AB, Djäknegatan 21, 211 35 Malmo, Sweden.

Lundbeck, Switz. Lundbeck SA, Case postale, 8051 Zurich, Switzerland.

Lundbeck, UK. Lundbeck Ltd, Lundbeck House, Hastings St, Luton, Beds LU1 5BE, England.

Lusofarmaco, Ital. Istituto Luso Farmaco D'Italia s.p.a., Via Carnia 26, 20132 Milan, Italy.

Lusty, UK. Lusty's Natural Products Ltd, Sisson Rd, Gloucester GL1 3OB, England.

Lyka, Ind. Lyka Labs Private Ltd, 77 Nehru Rd, Vile Parle (East), Bombay-400 099, India.

Lyocentre, Fr. Laboratoires Lyocentre, 63203 Riom Cedex, France.

Lyphomed, Canad. Lyphomed Canada Inc., 6600 Goreway Dr., Mississauga, Ontario L4V 1S6, Canada.

Lyphomed, USA. Lyphomed Inc., 2020 Ruby St, Melrose Park IL 60160, USA.

Lysoform, Ger. Lysoform Dr. Hans Rosemann GmbH, Kaiser-Wilhelm-Strasse 133, Postfach: 460120, 1000 Berlin 46, Germany.

Lyssia, Switz. See *Priorin, Switz.*

Mabo, Spain. Mabo, Rocio 7, Castellar, 46026 Valencia, Spain.

MacAndrews & Forbes, UK. MacAndrews & Forbes Ltd, Pembroke House, 44 Wellesley Rd, Croydon CR9 3QE, England.

Macarthys, UK. Macarthys Medical Ltd, Chesham House, Chesham Close, Romford RM1 4JX, England.

Macfarlan Smith, UK. Macfarlan Smith Ltd, Wheatfield Rd, Edinburgh EH11 2QA, Scotland.

Mack, Belg. See *de Bournonville, Belg.*

Mack, Neth. See *Multi-Pharma, Neth.*

Mack, Switz. Mack Pharma, Flüelastrasse 7, Case postale, 8048 Zurich, Switzerland.

Mack, Illert., Ger. Heinrich Mack Nachf., Chemisch-Pharmazeutische Fabrik, Heinrich-Mack-Strasse 35, Postfach: 2064, 7918 Illertissen, W. Germany.

Macro Vitamin, Austral. Macro Vitamin Distributors Pty Ltd, Box A420, Sydney South NSW 2000, Australia.

MacroChem, USA. MacroChem, USA.

Macsil, USA. Macsil Inc., 1326 Frankford Ave, Philadelphia PA 19125, USA.

Madariaga, Spain. Madariaga, Bocangel 19-21, 28028 Madrid, Spain.

Madaus, Belg. Madaus Pharma S.A., chaussee d'Alsemberg 1001, 1180 Brussels, Belgium.

Madaus, Ger. Dr Madaus GmbH & Co., Ostmerheimer Strasse 198, Postfach: 910555, 5000 Cologne 91, W. Germany.

Madaus, Neth. See *Byk, Neth.*

Madaus, S.Afr. Madaus Pharmaceuticals (Pty) Ltd, P.O. Box 76246, Wendywood 2144, S. Africa.

Madaus, Swed. See *Pro Medica, Swed.*

Madaus, Switz. See *Biomed, Switz.*

Madaus Cerafarm, Spain. Madaus Cerafarm, Fuego S/N, 08004 Barcelona, Spain.

Made, Spain. See *Knoll-Made, Spain.*

Maggioni, Switz. See *Galenica, Switz.*

Maggioni-Winthrop, Ital. Maggioni-Winthrop S.p.A., Via G. Colombo 40, 20133 Milan, Italy.

Magis, Ital. Magis Farmaceutici s.p.a., Via Cacciamali 34-36-38, Zona Ind. (Loc. Noce), 25128 Brescia, Italy.

Magistra, Switz. Laboratoires Magistra SA, 28 Chemin du Grand-Puits, Case postale 122, 1217 Meyrin 2/GE, Switzerland.

Mago, Ger. Mago Dr. Bischoff, Magdalinski & Co. Herstellung u. Vertrieb pharm. Spezialitaten GmbH & Co. KG, Manteuffelstrasse 7, Postfach: 1605, 4690 Herne 1, Germany.

Maipe, Spain. Maipe, Pintor Moreno Carbonero 5, 28028 Madrid, Spain.

Maizena, Ger. Maizena Diat GmbH, Knorrstrasse 1, Postffach: 2760, 7100 Heilbronn, Germany.

Major, USA. Major, USA.

Makapharm, Switz. Makapharm s.a.r.l., Case postale 73, 5037 Muhen, Switzerland.

Makara, Ger. Makara GmbH, Koppelskamp 23, Postfach: 340265, 4000 Dusseldorf 31, Germany.

Makara, Neth. See *Bournonville, Neth.*

Malam, UK. Malam Laboratories Ltd, 37 Oakwood Rise, Heaton, Bolton BL1 5EE, England.

Malesci, Ital. Malesci Istituto Farmacobiologico s.p.a., Via Porpora 22/24, 50144 Florence, Italy.

Mallard, USA. Mallard Inc., 3021 Wabash Ave, Detroit MI 48216, USA.

Mallinckrodt, Austral. Mallinckrodt Australia Pty Ltd, 2 Eskay Rd, South Oakleigh Vic. 3167, Australia.

Mallinckrodt, Canad. Mallinckrodt Canada Inc., 600 av. Delmar, Pointe-Claire, Quebec H9R 4A8, Canada.

Mallinckrodt, Switz. See *Oryx, Switz.*

Mallinckrodt, USA. Mallinckrodt Pharmaceuticals, Division Mallinckrodt Inc., 675 Brown Rd, St Louis MO 63134, USA.

Manceau, Fr. Laboratoires Manceau, 25 blvd de l'Amiral Bruix, 75782 Paris Cedex 16, France.

Manchem, UK. Manchem Ltd, Ashton New Rd, Manchester M11 4AT, England.

Mandri, Spain. Mandri, Provenza 277, 08037 Barcelona, Spain.

Manetti Roberts, Ital. L. Manetti H.Roberts & C. per Azioni, Via Antonio da Noli 4, 50127 Florence, Italy.

Mann, Belg. Lab. Mann S.A., Antwerpsesteenweg 65, 2630 Aartselaar, Belgium.

Mann, Ger. Dr Gerhard Mann, Chemisch-pharmazeutische Fabrik GmbH, Brunsbütteler Damm 165-173, Postfach: 200456, 1000 Berlin 20, W. Germany.

Mann, Neth. See *Tramedico, Neth.*

Mann, S.Afr. See *Restan, S.Afr.*

Manushi, Denm. See *Friis, Denm.*

Manzoni, Ital. Lab. Manzoni Giulio & C. s.r.l., Via V. Vela 5, 20133 Milan, Italy.

Marco Viti, Ital. Marco Viti Industria Farmaceutica s.r.l., Via Riccione 8, 20156 Milan, Italy.

Marcofina, Fr. Laboratoires Marcofina, 48 bis, rue des Belles-Feuilles, 75116 Paris, France.

Marcopharma, Denm. Marcopharma Laboratories Ltd, Molestien 1, 2450 Copenhagen SV, Denmark.

Marion, Belg. See *Christiaens, Belg.*

Marion Laboratories, S.Afr. See *Script Intal, S.Afr.*

Marion Laboratories, USA. Marion Laboratories Inc., Pharmaceutical Division, Marion Industrial Park, Marion Park Dr., Kansas City MO 64137, USA.

Marion Scientific, USA. Marion Scientific, Division of Marion Laboratories Inc., P.O. Box 8480, Kansas City MO 64114, USA.

Marlyn, USA. Marlyn Pharmaceutical Co. Inc., 350 Pauma Place, Escondido CA 92025, USA.

Mars, UK. Mars Ltd, Dundee Rd, Slough, Bucks, England.

Marshall's Pharmaceuticals, UK. Marshall's Pharmaceuticals, England.

Marsman, Philipp. Marsman & Co. Inc., MCPO Box 467, Makati, Metro Manila, The Philippines.

Martin, Fr. Laboratoires Martin, Le Comte, 03340 Bessay-sur-Allier, France.

Martin, Switz. See *Schönenberger, Switz.* and *Uhlmann-Eyraud, Switz.*

Martindale Pharmaceuticals, UK. Martindale Pharmaceuticals Ltd, Chesham House, Chesham Close, Romford RM1 4JX, England.

Martinet, Fr. Laboratoires Martinet, 222 blvd Pereire, 75848 Paris Cedex 17, France.

Martinez Llenas, Spain. Martinez Llenas, Pujadas 77, Planta 5, 08005 Barcelona, Spain.

Maruishi, Neth. See *Rooster, Neth.*

Mason, Hong Kong. Mason International Ltd, 304 Watson's Estate, Block B, 6 Watson Rd, Hong Kong.

Mason, USA. Mason Pharmaceuticals Inc., 1201 Dove St, Suite 520, Newport Beach CA 92660, USA.

Mastar, USA. Mastar Pharmaceutical Co. Inc., P.O. Box 3144, Bethlehem PA 18017, USA.

Mastelli, Ital. Lab. Biol. Dott. Mastelli s.a.s. di V. Dogliotti & C., Via Armea 90, 18038 Sanremo (IM), Italy.

Master Pharma, Ital. Master Pharma s.r.l., Via S. Leonardo 96, 43100 Parma, Italy.

Material Clinico, Spain. See *Palex, Spain.*

Matthews & Wilson, UK. Matthews & Wilson, Larkhall Laboratories, Mouliniere House, Putney Bridge Rd, London SW15 2PY, England.

Maurer, Ger. Maurer-Pharma GmbH, Ursulinenstrasse 55, 6600 Saarbrucken, Germany.

Mawson & Proctor, UK. Mawson & Proctor Pharmaceuticals Ltd, Kingsway South, Gateshead NE8 1YX, England.

Max Factor, UK. Max Factor Ltd, P.O. Box 7, Frances Ave, West Howe, Bournemouth BH11 8NZ, England.

Max Jenne, Denm. A/S Max Jenne, Skolevej 1, 6200 Åbenrå, Denmark.

Max Ritter, Switz. Max Ritter Pharma SA, Case postale, 8039 Zurich, Switzerland.

May & Baker Agrochemicals, UK. May & Baker Agrochemicals, Regent House, Hubert Rd, Brentwood, Essex CM14 4QQ, England.

May & Baker, Austral. May & Baker Australia Pty Ltd, 19-23 Paramount Rd, West Footscray Vic. 3012, Australia.

May & Baker, Neth. See *Rhône-Poulenc, Neth.*

May & Baker, S.Afr. Maybaker (SA) (Pty) Ltd, P.O. Box 1130, Port Elizabeth 6000, S. Africa.

May & Baker, UK. May & Baker Pharmaceuticals, Rhone Poulenc Ltd, Rainham Rd South, Dagenham, Essex RM10 7XS, England.

Mayoly-Spindler, Fr. Laboratoires Mayoly-Spindler, B.P. 206, 92502 Rueil-Malmaison, France.

Mayoly-Spindler, Switz. See *Uhlmann-Eyraud, Switz.*

Mayrand, USA. Mayrand Inc., 4 Dundas Circle, P.O. Box 8869, Greensboro NC 27419, USA.

Mazuelos, Spain. Mazuelos, Medina y Galnares 52, 41015 Sevilla, Spain.

McGaw, Canad. McGaw Laboratories, Division of AHS Canada, 2390 Argentia Rd, Mississauga, Ontario L5N 3P1, Canada.

McGaw, USA. American McGaw Laboratories, American Hospital Supply Corp., 2525 McGaw Ave, Irvine CA 92714, USA.

McGloin, Austral. J. McGloin Pty Ltd, P.O. Box 294, Kings Grove NSW 2208, Australia.

McGregor, USA. McGregor Pharmaceuticals, 32580 Grand River Ave, Farmington MI 48024, USA.

McNeil, Canad. McNeil Pharmaceutical (Canada) Ltd, 600 Main St W., Stouffville, Ontario L0H 1L0, Canada.

McNeil, Norw. See *Cilag-Chemie, Norw.*

McNeil, Swed. See *Cilag, Swed.*

McNeil Consumer, USA. McNeil Consumer Products Co., McNeilab Inc., Fort Washington PA 19034, USA.

McNeil Pharmaceutical, USA. McNeil Pharmaceutical, McNeilab Inc., Spring House PA 19477, USA.

MCP Pharmaceuticals, UK. MCP Pharmaceuticals Ltd, Simpson Parkway, Kirkton Campus, Livingston, West Lothian, Scotland.

Mead Johnson, Austral. See *Bristol-Myers, Austral.*

Mead Johnson, Belg. Mead Johnson Benelux S.A., chaussée de la Hulpe 185/187, 1170 Brussels, Belgium.

Mead Johnson, Canad. Mead Johnson Canada, Division of Bristol-Myers Canada Inc., 2625 Queensview Dr., P.O. Box 6313, Stn J, Ottawa, Ontario K2A 3Y4, Canada.

Mead Johnson, S.Afr. See *Bristol, S.Afr.*

Mead Johnson, UK. Mead Johnson, Division of Bristol-Myers Co. Ltd, Swakeleys House, Milton Rd, Ickenham, Uxbridge, Middx UB10 8NS, England.

Mead Johnson Laboratories, USA. Mead Johnson Laboratories, Mead Johnson & Co., 2404 West Pennsylvania St, Evansville IN 47721, USA.

Mead Johnson Nutritional, USA. Mead Johnson Nutritional Division, Mead Johnson & Co., 2404 W Pennsylvania St, Evansville IN 47721, USA.

Mead Johnson Pharmaceutical, USA. Mead Johnson Pharmaceutical Division, Mead Johnson & Co., 2404 W Pennsylvania St, Evansville IN 47721, USA.

Mecobenzon, Denm. Mecobenzon A/S, Halmtorvet 29, 1503 Copenhagen V, Denmark.

Med Fabrik, Ger. Med Fabrik chemisch-pharmazeutische Praparate J. Carl Pfluger GmbH & Co., Neukollnische Allee 146/148, Postfach: 440358, 1000 Berlin 44, Germany.

Med. Prod. Panam., USA. Medical Products Panamericana Inc., P.O. Box 771, Coral Gables FL 33134, USA.

Med. y Prod. Quím., Spain. Medicamentos y Productos Quimicos, Sepulveda 125, 08015 Barcelona, Spain.

Meda, Denm. Meda AS, Dynamovej 11, 2730 Herlev, Denmark.

Meda, Norw. Meda A/S, Bjerkas Industriomrade, 3470 Slemmestad, Norway.

Meda, Swed. Meda AB, Box 138, 401 22 Göteborg, Sweden.

Medac, Ger. Medac Gesellschaft fur klinische Spezialpraparate mbH, Fehlandstrasse 3, Postfach: 303629, 2000 Hamburg 36, Germany.

Medea, Spain. Medea, Santa Carolina 53-59, 08025 Barcelona, Spain.

Medefield, Austral. Medefield Pty Ltd, 19 Dickson Ave, Artarmon NSW 2064, Australia.

Medex, Austral. Medex Laboratories Pty Ltd, 44-46 Chippen St, Chippendale NSW 2008, Australia.

Medexport, UK. Medexport Ltd, P.O. Box 25, Arundel, West Sussex BN18 0SW, England.

Medexport, USSR. Medexport, 31 Kakhovka, Building 2, 113461 Moscow, USSR.

Medi-Star, Denm. Medi-Star A/S, Trorodvej 59, 2950 Vedbaek, Denmark.

Medic, Canad. Medic Laboratory Ltd, 2925 boul. Industriel, Laval, Quebec H7L 3W9, Canada.

Medica, Fin. Medica, Teollisuuskatu 23-25, 00510 Helsinki, Finland.

Medica, Neth. Medica B.V., Lederstraat 1, 5223 AW 's-Hertogenbosch, Netherlands.

Medica, Swed. See *Selena, Swed.*

Medical, Arg. Medical Argentina, Mercedes 1529, 1407 Buenos Aires, Argentina.

Medical, Spain. Medical, Virgen de las Angustias 2, 14006 Cordoba, Spain.

Medical Market, USA. Medical Market Specialities Inc., P.O. Box 307, Cedar Grove NJ 07009, USA.

Medical Research, Austral. Medical Research (Marketing) Pty Ltd, 6 Lenton Place, North Rocks NSW 2151, Australia.

Medical Wire, UK. Medical Wire & Equipment Co. (Bath) Ltd, Potley, Corsham, Wilts SN13 9RT, England.

Medice, Ger. Medice, Chem.-pharm. Fabrik Putter GmbH & Co. KG, Kuhloweg 37, Postfach: 2063, 5860 Iserlohn, Germany.

Medice, Switz. See *Doetsch, Grether, Switz.*

Medichemie, Neth. See *Bipharma, Neth.*

Medichemie, Switz. Medichemie SA, Case postale 3650, 4002 Basel, Switzerland.

Medici Domus, Ital. Medici Domus s.r.l., Via Parini 1-3, 20028 S. Vittore Olona (MI), Italy.

Medici, Ital. Lab. Farm. Dr Medici s.r.l., Via F.lli Ruspoli 14, 00198 Rome, Italy.

Médicia, Fr. Laboratoires Médicia, 34 rue Saint-Romain, 69008 Lyon, France.

Medico-Biological Laboratories, UK. Medico-Biological Laboratories Ltd, Kingsend House, 44 Kingsend, Ruislip, Middx HA4 7DA, England.

Medico, S.Afr. See *Propan, S.Afr.*

Medicone, USA. Medicone Co., 225 Varick St, New York NY 10014, USA.

Medicosma, Neth. See *Roussel, Neth.*

Medicoteknik, Denm. Palle Medicoteknik A/S, Troldkaervej 14, 2610 Rødovre, Denmark.

Medikema, Swed. Medikema AB, Box 169, 282 00 Tyringe, Sweden.

MediMar, UK. MediMar Laboratories, Sarum House, 17 The Queensway, Chalfont St Peter, Bucks SL9 8NB, England.

Medimpex, Hung. Medimpex, Hungarian Trading Co. for Pharmaceutical Products, 4 Vorosmarty Ter, 1808 Budapest, Hungary.

Medinex, Canad. Medinex Ltd, 2 boul. Crepeau, Ville Saint-Laurent, Quebec H4N 1M7, Canada.

Medinfar, Port. Laboratorio Medinfar, Rua Particular a Rua Henrique Paiva Couceiro Nos 15 e 16, Venda Nova, 2700 Amadora, Portugal.

Medinova, Switz. Medinova SA, Eggbühlstrasse 14, 8052 Zurich, Switzerland.

Medinsa, Spain. Medinsa, Carr Vicalvaro 37, 28022 Madrid, Spain.

Mediolanum, Ital. Mediolanum Farmaceutici s.r.l., Via S.G. Cottolengo 31, 20143 Milan, Italy.

Mediolanum, Switz. See *Lucchini, Switz.*

Medipharm, Switz. Medipharm SA, Case postale 48, 1636 Broc, Switzerland.

Medipharma, Ger. Medipharma Saar, Dr. Becker & Cie KG, Mainzer Str. 201-209, 6600 Saarbrucken, Germany.

Medipolar, Fin. Medipolar, 90650 Oulu, Finland.

Medipolar, Swed. See *Farmos, Swed.*

Mediscan, Denm. Mediscan, Knuden 21, 9260 Gistrup, Denmark.

Medix, Spain. Medix, avda de Aragon 13, 28027 Madrid, Spain.

Med-Kjemi, Norw. Med-Kjemi A/S, Kirkeveien 230, Postboks 413, 1371 Asker, Norway.

Medo, UK. Medo Pharmaceuticals Ltd, East St, Chesham, Bucks HP5 1DG, England.

Medopharm, Ger. Medopharm Arzneimittelwerk, Dr. Zillich GmbH & Co., Drosselgasse 5, Postfach: 1380, 8032 Grafelfing, Germany.

Medosan, Ital. Medosan, Industrie Biochimiche Riunite S.p.A., Via di Cancelliera 12, 00040 Cecchina (RM), Italy.

Meiji, Jpn. Meiji Seika, 2-4-16 Kyobashi, Chuo-ku, Tokyo, Japan.

Meiji, Philipp. See *Hi-Eisai, Philipp.*

Mein, Spain. Mein, Dr. Ferran s/n, Vilassar de Dalt, 08339 Barcelona, Spain.

Mekos, Norw. A/S Mekos, Sandviksv. 26, 1322 Hovik, Norway.

Mekos, Swed. AB Mekos, Box 944, 251 09 Helsingborg, Sweden.

Melisana, Belg. Melisana S.A., ave du Four a Briques 1, 1140 Brussels, Belgium.

Melusin, Ger. Melusin Schwarz GmbH, Mittelstrasse 11-13, Postfach: 100662, 4019 Monheim/Rhld., W. Germany.

Menadier, Ger. Menadier Heilmittel GmbH, Fischers Allee 49-59, Postfach: 501004, 2000 Hamburg 50, Germany.

Menarini, Belg. Menarini Belgium S.A., ave E. Demolder 128, 1030 Brussels, Belgium.

Menarini, Ital. A. Menarini s.a.s., Via Sette Santi 3, 50131 Florence, Italy.

Menarini, Spain. Menarini, Alfonso XII 587, Badalona, 08913 Barcelona, Spain.

Mendelejeff, Ital. Mendelejeff, Stabilimento Chimico Farmaceutico s.r.l., Via Aurelia 58, 00165 Rome, Italy.

Mendell, USA. EMCO International Corporation, Route 52, Carmel NY 10512, USA.

Menley & James, Canad. Menley & James, 1940 Argentia Rd, Mississauga, Ontario L5N 2V7, Canada.

Menley & James, Switz. See *Diethelm, Switz.*

Menley & James, UK. Menley & James Laboratories, Welwyn Garden City, Herts, England.

Menley & James, USA. Menley & James Laboratories, A SmithKline Beckman Co., P.O. Box 8082, Philadelphia PA 19101, USA.

Mentholatum, Neth. See *Bipharma, Neth.*

Mentholatum, UK. The Mentholatum Co. Ltd, Longfield Rd, Twyford, Berks, England.

Mepha, Switz. Mepha SA, Case postale 137, 4143 Dornach 1, Switzerland.

Mer-National, S.Afr. Mer-National (Division of Dow Chemical Africa (Pty) Ltd), P.O. Box 2432, Randburg 2125, S. Africa.

Méram, Fr. Laboratoires Méram, 4 blvd Malesherbes, 75008 Paris, France.

Merchant, USA. W.F. Merchant Pharmaceutical Co. Inc., P.O. Box 2600, Laurel MD 20811, USA.

Merck, Arg. Merck Química Argentina S.A.I.C., Rosetti 1084, 1427 Buenos Aires, Argentina.

Merck, Aust. Austro-Merck GmbH, Zimbagasse 5, 1147 Vienna, Austria.

Merck, Belg. Merck S.A., Brusselsesteenweg 288, 1900 Overijse, Belgium.

Merck, S.Afr. Merck Pharmaceuticals (SA) (Pty) Ltd, P.O. Box 3497, Johannesburg 2000, S. Africa.

Merck Igoda, Spain. Merck Igoda, Ctra. N-152 Km 19 Can Mollet, Mollet del Valles, 08100 Barcelona, Spain.

Merck-Clévenot, Fr. Laboratoires Merck-Clévenot, 5 rue Anquetil, B.P. 8, 94731 Nogent-sur-Marne Cedex, France.

Merck-Clévenot, Switz. See *Diethelm, Switz.*

Merck Sharp & Dohme, Arg. Merck Sharp & Dohme (Argentina) Inc., Av. Libertador 1410, 1638 Vte Lopez, Buenos Aires, Argentina.

Merck Sharp & Dohme, Austral. Merck Sharp & Dohme (Australia) Pty Ltd, P.O. Box 79, Granville NSW 2142, Australia.

Merck Sharp & Dohme, Belg. Merck Sharp & Dohme, chaussee de Waterloo 1135, 1180 Brussels, Belgium.

Merck Sharp & Dohme, Canad. Merck Sharp & Dohme Canada, Division of Merck Frosst Canada Inc., P.O. Box 1005, Pointe Claire, Dorval, Quebec H9R 4P8, Canada.

Merck Sharp & Dohme, Denm. Merck Sharp & Dohme, Marielundvej 46 C, 2730 Herlev, Denmark.

Merck Sharp & Dohme, Ger. MSD Sharp & Dohme GmbH, Charles-de-Gaulle-Str. 4, Postfach: 830960, 8000 Munich 83, W. Germany.

Merck Sharp & Dohme, Ital. Merck Sharp & Dohme (Italia) s.p.a., Via G. Fabbroni 6, 00191 Rome, Italy.

Merck Sharp & Dohme, Neth. See *Chibret, Neth.* and *MSD, Neth.*

Merck Sharp & Dohme, Norw. MSD (Norge) A/S, Solbakken 1, 3011 Drammen, Norway.

Merck Sharp & Dohme, Port. Merck Sharp & Dohme LDA, Rua Barata Salgueiro 37-1, 1200 Lisbon, Portugal.

Merck Sharp & Dohme, S.Afr. Merck Sharp & Dohme (Pty) Ltd, Private Bag 3, Halfway House 1685, S. Africa.

Merck Sharp & Dohme, Spain. Merck Sharp & Dohme, Ctra Barcelona KM 32.16, Alcala de Henares, Madrid, Spain.

Merck Sharp & Dohme, Swed. Merck Sharp & Dohme (Sweden) AB, Box 20520, 161 20 Bromma, Sweden.

Merck Sharp & Dohme, Switz. Merck Sharp & Dohme-Chibret SA, Case postale 937, 8034 Zurich, Switzerland.

Merck Sharp & Dohme, UK. Merck Sharp & Dohme Ltd, Hertford Rd, Hoddesdon, Herts EN11 9BU, England.

Merck Sharp & Dohme, USA. Merck Sharp & Dohme, Division of Merck & Co. Inc., West Point PA 19486, USA.

Merck Sharp & Dohme-Chibret, Belg. See *Merck Sharp & Dohme, Belg.*

Merck Sharp & Dohme-Chibret, Fr. Laboratoires Merck Sharp & Dohme-Chibret, 3 ave Hoche, 75008 Paris, France.

Merckle, Ger. Merckle GmbH, Gehrn 3, Postfach: 1161, 7902 Blaubeuren, W. Germany.

Merckle, Neth. See *Hermes, Neth.*

Mericon, USA. Mericon Industries Inc., 8819 N Pioneer Rd, Peoria IL 61615, USA.

Merieux, Arg. Merieux Argentina S.A., Moreno 957 7° Piso, 1091 Buenos Aires, Argentina.

Merieux, Belg. Institut Merieux Benelux S.A., ave Jules Bordet 13, 1140 Brussels, Belgium.

Merieux, Ital. Istituto Merieux Italia s.p.a., Via di Villa Troili 56, 00163 Rome, Italy.

Merieux, Neth. See *Rhône-Poulenc, Neth.*

Merieux, Swed. See *Rhone-Poulenc, Swed.*

Merieux, Switz. See *Rhone-Poulenc, Switz.*

Merieux, UK. Merieux UK Ltd, Clivemont House, Clivemont Rd, Maidenhead, Berks SL6 7BU, England.

Merieux, USA. Merieux Institute Inc., P.O. Box 52-3980, Miami FL 33152, USA.

Merrell, Fr. Merrell Dow France, Division Merrell, 47 rue de Villiers, 92203 Neuilly-sur-Seine Cedex, France.

Merrell, Ger. Merrell Dow Pharma, Eisenstrasse 40, Postfach: 1639, 6090 Russelsheim, W. Germany.

Merrell, Ital. Merrell s.p.a., Via Murat 23, 20159 Milan, Italy.

Merrell, UK. Merrell Dow Pharmaceuticals Ltd, Stana Place, Fairfield Ave, Staines, Middx TW18 4SX, England.

Merrell Dow, Austral. Merrell-Dow Pharmaceuticals Australia Pty Ltd, P.O. Box 384, North Sydney NSW 2060, Australia.

Merrell Dow, Belg. Merrell Dow Belgium S.A., Hilton Tower, blvd de Waterloo 38, 1000 Brussels, Belgium.

Merrell Dow, Canad. Merrell Dow Pharmaceuticals (Canada) Inc., 7777 Keele St, Concord, Ontario L4K 1Y7, Canada.

Merrell Dow, Spain. Merrell Dow, Ctra. Madrid Barcelona Km 25.8, Alcala de Henares, Madrid, Spain.

Merrell Dow, Switz. Merrell Dow Pharmaceuticals SA, Case postale, 8036 Zurich, Switzerland.

Merrell Dow, USA. Merrell Dow Pharmaceuticals Inc., Subsidiary of The Dow Chemical Co., Cincinnati OH 45242-9553, USA.

Merrell-National, USA. See *Merrell Dow, USA.*

Mertens, Arg. Mertens S.A., California 1728, 1289 Buenos Aires, Argentina.

Merz, Denm. See *Meda, Denm.*

Merz, Ger. Merz & Co., GmbH & Co., Eckenheimer Landstrasse 100, 6000 Frankfurt (Main) 1, W. Germany.

Merz, Neth. See *Roussel, Neth.*

Merz, Switz. See *Adroka, Switz.*

Metro Med, USA. Metro Med Inc., 2201 Denton Drive, Austin TX 78758, USA.

Metro, Philipp. Metro Drug Corp., MC PO Box 465, Makati, Metro Manila, The Philippines.

Meuse, Belg. Laboratoires de la Meuse S.A., rue Hanesse 38, 5220 Andenne, Belgium.

Meyer, Fr. Laboratoires Meyer, 54510 Tomblaine-Nancy, France.

Miba, Ital. Miba Prodotti Chimici e Farmaceutici s.p.a., Via Falzarego 8, 20021 Ospiate di Bollate (MI), Italy.

Michels, Fr. See *Lefrancq, Fr.*

Micro-Biologicals, UK. Micro-Biologicals Ltd, Fordingbridge, Hants SP6 1AE, England.

Microsules, Arg. Microsules Argentina S.A. de S.C.I.I.A., Carlos Pellegrini 331, 1009 Buenos Aires, Argentina.

Midelfart, Norw. Midelfart & Co. A/S, Amtmannsvingen 2, Postboks 356, 3001 Drammen, Norway.

Midy, Fr. See *Clin Midy, Fr.*

Midy, Ger. Midy Arzneimittel GmbH, Augustenstrasse 10, Postfach: 201708, 8000 Munich 2, Germany.

Midy, Ital. Midy s.p.a., Via Piranesi 38, 21037 Milan, Italy.

Midyfarm, Fr. Midyfarm, rue A. Durouchez, 80003 Amiens Cedex, France.

Midysan, Switz. See *Sanofi, Switz.*

Migra, Arg. Migra, Argerich 265, 1406 Buenos Aires, Argentina.

Miguez, Spain. Miguez, General Pingarron 5, Getafe, 28902 Madrid, Spain.

Milance, USA. Milance, USA.

Milanfarma, Ital. Milanfarma s.p.a., Via G. Frua 26, 20146 Milan, Italy.

Miles, Austral. Miles Laboratories Australia Pty Ltd, Private Bag 5, Mulgrave Vic. 3170, Australia.

Miles, Canad. Miles Pharmaceuticals, Division of Miles Laboratories Ltd, 77 Belfield Rd, Etobicoke, Ontario M9W 1G6, Canada.

Miles, Neth. See *Bayer, Neth.*

Miles, Swed. See *Bayer, Swed.*

Miles, Switz. See *Bayer, Switz.*

Miles Laboratories, USA. Miles Laboratories Inc., P.O. Box 340, Elkhart IN 46515, USA.

Miles Martin, Spain. Miles Martin, Plaza de Espana 10, 28008 Madrid, Spain.

Miles Pharmaceuticals, USA. Miles Pharmaceuticals, Division of Miles Laboratories Inc., 400 Morgan Lane, West Haven CT 06516, USA.

Milex-Budlong, Canad. Milex-Budlong Ltd, 400 Madison bd. E., Unit 26, Mississauga, Ontario L4Z 1N8, Canada.

Milex, USA. Milex Products Inc., 5915 Northwest Highway, Chicago IL 60631, USA.

Miller of Golden Square, UK. Miller of Golden Square Ltd, 14 Golden Square, London W1R 3AG, England.

Miller, USA. Miller, USA.

Millet, Arg. Millet S.A.C.el., Montevideo 160, 1019 Buenos Aires, Argentina.

Millipore, UK. Millipore (UK) Ltd, 11-15 Peterborough Rd, Harrow, Middx HA1 2YH, England.

Millot-Solac, Belg. See *Therapeutica, Belg.*

Millot-Solac, Fr. Laboratoires Millot-Solac, 16 ave George-V, 75008 Paris, France.

Millot-Solac, Switz. See *Lucchini, Switz.*

Milo, Spain. Milo, Av. Constitucion, Nave 6, Cuarte de Huerva, 50410 Zaragoza, Spain.

Milupa, Canad. Milupa Co., 1312 Blundell Rd, Mississauga, Ontario L4Y 1M5, Canada.

Milupa, UK. Milupa Ltd, Milupa House, Uxbridge Rd, Hillingdon, Middx UB10 0NE, England.

Minden, Ger. Minden Pharma GmbH, Karlstrasse 42-44, Postfach: 1180, 4950 Minden, W. Germany.

Miquel, Spain. Miquel, Santany 16, 08016 Barcelona, Spain.

Mirren, S.Afr. See *Glenfair, S.Afr.*

Misemer, USA. Misemer Pharmaceuticals Inc., 4553 South Campbell St, Springfield MO 65804, USA.

Mission Pharmacal, USA. Mission Pharmacal Co., 1325 East Durango, P.O. Box 1676, San Antonio TX 78296, USA.

Mitchell, Denm. See *Tjellesen, Denm.*

Mitchum, UK. Mitchum Thayer Ltd, 86 Brook St, London W1Y 2BA, England.

Mitim, Ital. Mitim s.r.l., Via Cipro 50, 25125 Bresciano, Italy.

Mitsui, Jpn. Mitsui Seiyaku, Asahi Building, 3-12-2 Nihonbashi, Chuo-ku, Tokyo, Japan.

Mochida, Jpn. Mochida Seiyaku, 1-7 Yotsuya, Shinjuku-ku, Tokyo, Japan.

Modern Health Products, UK. Modern Health Products Ltd, Davis Rd, Chessington, Surrey KT9 1TH, England.

Molimin, Ger. Molimin Arzneimittel GmbH, Emil-Kemmer Strasse 33, 8605 Hallstadt/Ofr., Germany.

Molina Vinas, Spain. Molina Vinas, Rambla de las Flores 90, 08002 Barcelona, Spain.

Molnlycke, Swed. Molnlycke Sjukhusprodukter AB, Fabriksvagen 1, 43501 Molnlycke, Sweden.

Molteni, Ital. Molteni L. & C. dei F.lli Alitti Società Esercizio s.p.a., Via Pisana 458, 50018 Scandicci (FI), Italy.

Monal, Fr. Laboratoires Monal, 5 rue Salvador-Allende, 91120 Palaiseau, France.

Monal, Switz. See *Golaz, Switz.*

Monico, Ital. Monico Jacopo, Casa Fondata nel 1883, Via Orlanda, Ponte P. 10, 30173 Venezia-Mestre (VE), Italy.

Monik, Spain. Monik, Avda de la Playa 1, Conil de la Frontera, 11140 Cadiz, Spain.

Monoclonal Antibodies, USA. Monoclonal Antibodies, Inc., 2319 Charleston Rd, Mountain View CA 94043, USA.

Monot, Fr. Laboratoires Monot, 21801 Quetigny-les-Dijon, France.

Monsanto, UK. Monsanto PLC, Monsanto House, Chineham Court, Chineham, Basingstoke, Hants RG24 0UL, England.

Monsanto, USA. Monsanto Chemical Co., 800 North Lindbergh Blvd, St Louis MO 63166, USA.

Montavit, Switz. See *Lucchini, Switz.*

Montedison, Arg. Montedison Farmaceutica S.A.C.I.F.I.A., Arcos 2626, 1428 Buenos Aires, Argentina.

Montedison, Norw. See *Farmitalia, Norw.*

Montedison, Spain. See *Farmitalia, Spain.*

Montefarmaco, Ital. Montefarmaco s.p.a., Via G. Galilei 7, 20016 Pero (MI), Italy.

Montpellier, Arg. Montpellier S.A., Virrey Liniers 667, 1220 Buenos Aires, Argentina.

Morgens, Spain. Morgens, Vizconde de Matamala 7, 28028 Madrid, Spain.

Morishita, Jpn. Morishita Seiyaku, 4-29 Doshu-cho, Higashi-ku, Osaka, Japan.

Morrith, Arg. Morrith S.A. Argentina, Dr J.F. Aranguren 2955, 1406 Buenos Aires, Argentina.

Morrith, Spain. Morrith, Miguel Juste 45, 28037 Madrid, Spain.

Morson, UK. Thomas Morson Pharmaceuticals, Hertford Rd, Hoddesdon, Herts EN11 9BU, England.

MPS Lab., S.Afr. MPS Laboratories (Pty) Ltd, P.O. Box 260778, Excom 2023, S. Africa.

MSD, Neth. Merck Sharp & Dohme B.V., Waarderweg 39, 2031 BN Haarlem, Netherlands.

MSD, Swed. See *Merck Sharp & Dohme, Swed.*

Much, Swed. See *Famaco, Swed.*

Mucos, Ger. Mucos Pharma GmbH & Co., Alpenstrasse 29, Postfach: 1380, 8192 Geretsried 1, W. Germany.

Mucos, Neth. See *van Oven, Neth.*

Muir & Neil, Austral. See *Key, Austral.*

Müller/Göppingen, Ger. Chemische-Pharmazeutische Fabrik Göppingen Carl Müller, Apotheker, GmbH u. Co. KG, Bahnhofstrasse 33-35 u. 40, Postfach: 869, 7320 Göppingen, W. Germany.

Mulli, Ger. Dr Kurt Mulli Nachf. GmbH & Co. KG, Otto-Hahn-Str. 2, Postfach: 1252, 7844 Neuenberg, W. Germany.

Multilan, Denm. See *Organon, Denm.*

Multilan, Switz. See *Organon, Switz.*

Multipax, UK. Multipax Laboratories Ltd, England.

Multi-Pharma, Neth. Multi-Pharma B.V., Eemmeerlaan 3, 1382 KA Weesp, Netherlands.

Multipharmax, Switz. Multipharmax Ets., Case postale 12, 1211 Grange-Canal, Switzerland.

Mundipharma, Ger. Mundipharma GmbH, Mundipharma-Strasse 2, Postfach: 1350, 6250 Limburg (Lahn), Germany.

Mundipharma, Neth. See *Dagra, Neth.*

Mundipharma, S.Afr. See *Keatings, S.Afr.*

Mundipharma, Switz. Mundipharma Pharmazeutika, St Alban-Vorstadt 91, 4006 Basel, Switzerland.

Munoz, Spain. Munoz, Queipo de Llano 32, 21720 Huelva, Spain.

Muro, USA. Muro Pharmaceutical Inc., 890 East St, Tewksbury MA 01876, USA.

Murphy Chemical, UK. Murphy Chemical Co. Ltd, Paper Mill Lane, Bramford, Ipswich IP8 4BZ, England.

Nadeau, Canad. Nadeau Laboratory Ltd, 8480 boul. Saint-Laurent, Montreal, Quebec H2P 2M6, Canada.

NAF, Norw. NAF-Laboratoriene A/S, Sven Oftedals vei 8, 0950 Oslo 9, Norway.

Napa, UK. Napa Products Ltd, Barmston House, Barmston Rd, Beverley, E. Yorks HU17 0LA, England.

Napp, Austral. See *Sigma, Austral.*

Napp, UK. Napp Laboratories Ltd, Cambridge Science Park, Milton Rd, Cambridge CB4 4GW, England.

National Dermaceutical, USA. National Dermaceutical Products Inc., 8749 Surrey Place, Maineville OH 45039, USA.

National Institutes of Health, USA. National Institutes of Health, Bethesda MD 20205, USA.

National Pharm., USA. National Pharmaceutical Manufacturing Co., Barre-National Inc., 7502 Windsor Blvd, Baltimore MD 21207, USA.

Nativelle, Belg. Nativelle S.A., ave Franklin Roosevelt 138, 1050 Brussels, Belgium.

Nativelle, Fr. Laboratoires Nativelle S.A., 34 rue de la Federation, 75015 Paris, France.

Nativelle, Ital. Istituto Farmochimico Nativelle s.p.a., Via G. Bechi 3, 50141 Florence, Italy.

Nativelle, Switz. See *Interdelta, Switz.*

Natrapharm, Ger. Natrapharm Arzneimittel GmbH, Nattermannallee 1, Postfach: 350120, 5000 Cologne 30, W. Germany.

Natterman, Neth. See *Nicholas, Neth.*

Nattermann, Ger. A. Nattermann & Cie. GmbH, Nattermannallee 1, Postfach: 350120, 5000 Cologne 30, W. Germany.

Nattermann, Ital. Nattermann Farmaceutici s.r.l., Via C. Conti Rossini 26, 00147 Rome, Italy.

Nattermann, S.Afr. Nattermann (SA) (Pty) Ltd, P.O. Box 41298, Craighall 2024, S. Africa.

Nature's Bounty, USA. Nature's Bounty Inc., 90 Orville Drive, Bohemia NY 11716, USA.

Navarro, Spain. Navarro, J., Azcona 31, 28028 Madrid, Spain.

ND & K, Denm. See *Nordisk Droge, Denm.*

NDF, Neth. See *ACF, Neth.*

Neda, Ger. Neda Arzneimittel GmbH & Co. KG, Rudolf-Diesel-Ring 21, Postfach: 208, 8029 Sauerlach, Germany.

Nefro-Pharma, Ger. Nefro-Pharma Arzneimittel GmbH, Munchnerstrasse 6, Postfach: 1424, 8202 Bad Aibling, Germany.

Negma, Fr. Laboratoires Negma, rue Fourny, 78530 Buc, France.

Nella, UK. Nella Pharmaceutical Products Ltd, 63 Jenkin Rd, Sheffield S9 1DS, England.

Nelson, Austral. Nelson Laboratories (Sales) Pty Ltd, P.O. Box 210, Ermington NSW 2115, Australia.

Neo Laboratories, UK. Neo Laboratories Ltd, 1a Frognal, London NW3 6AN, England.

Neolab, Canad. Neolab Inc., 5476 Upper Lachine Rd, Montreal, Quebec H4A 2A4, Canada.

Neomed, Switz. Neomed AG, Bahnhofstrasse, 3185 Schmitten, Switzerland.

Neopharmed, Ital. Neopharmed s.p.a., Via Pordoi 18, 20021 Baranzate di Bollate (MI), Italy.

Neos-Donner, Ger. Neos Donner KG, Erkelenzdamm 11-13, 1000 Berlin 36, Germany.

Nessa, Spain. Nessa, Juan Gamper 19-23, 08014 Barcelona, Spain.

Nestle, Arg. Nestle S.A. de Productos Alimenticios, Carlos Pelligrini 887, 1009 Buenos Aires, Argentina.

Nestle, Austral. Nestle Australia Ltd, 60 Bathurst St, Sydney NSW 2000, Australia.

Nestle, Denm. Nestle Danmark A/S, Masnedogade 20, 2100 Copenhagen 0, Denmark.

Nestlé, Norw. A/S Nestlé Norge, Postboks 595, 1301 Sandvika, Norway.

Nestle, Switz. Société des Produits Nestlé SA, Hofwiesenstrasse 370, 8050 Zurich, Switzerland.

Nestlé, UK. The Nestlé Co. Ltd, St George's House, Croydon CR9 1NR, England.

Neusc, Spain. Neusc, Ctra de Sant Hipolit km 1, Gurb-Vic, 08519 Barcelona, Spain.

Neutrogena Dermatologics, USA. Neutrogena Dermatologics, Division of Neutrogena Corp., 5755 West 96th St, P.O. Box 45036, Los Angeles CA 90045, USA.

Neutrogena, UK. Neutrogena (UK) Ltd, 2 Mansfield Rd, South Croydon, Surrey CR2 6HN, England.

Newport, USA. Newport Pharmaceuticals International Inc., P.O. Box 1990, Newport Beach CA 92660-0147, USA.

Newton, UK. Newton Chemical Ltd, 2 Mansfield Rd, South Croydon, Surrey CR2 6HN, England.

Nezel, Spain. Nezel, av. Diagonal 507, 08029 Barcelona, Spain.

NIBSC, UK. National Institute of Biological Standards and Control (NIBSC), Blanche Lane, South Mimms, Potters Bar, Herts, England.

Nichiiko, Jpn. Nichiiko, 1-6-21 Sokyokuwa, Toyama-shi, Japan.

Nicholas, Austral. Nicholas Kiwi (Pacific) Pty Ltd, P.O. Box 1, Chadstone Vic. 3148, Australia.

Nicholas, Belg. Nicholas Laboratories S.A., rue de Normandie 14, 1080 Brussels, Belgium.

Nicholas, Denm. See *Meda, Denm.*

Nicholas, Fr. Laboratoires Nicholas S.A., 74240 Gaillard, France.

Nicholas, Ger. Nicholas GmbH, Otto-Volger Str. 11, Postfach: 1240, 6231 Sulzbach/Ts., W. Germany.

Nicholas, Neth. Nicholas-Mepros B.V., Industrieweg 1, 5531 AD Bladel, Netherlands.

Nicholas, Norw. See *Henry Christenson, Norw.*

Nicholas, Swed. See *Famaco, Swed.*

Nicholas, Switz. See *Galenica, Switz.* and *Sauter, Switz.*

Nicholas, UK. Nicholas Laboratories Ltd, P.O. Box 17, Slough SL1 4AU, England.

Nikken, Jpn. Nikken Kagaku, 5-4-14 Tsukiji, Chuo-ku, Tokyo, Japan.

Nion, S.Afr. See *Vernleigh, S.Afr.*

Nipa, UK. Nipa Laboratories Ltd, Llantwit Fardre, Pontypridd, Mid Glam CF38 2SN, Wales.

Nippon, Philipp. See *Marsman, Philipp.*

Nippon Kayaku, Jpn. Nippon Kayaku, 1-2-1 Marunouchi, Chiyoda-ku, Tokyo, Japan.

Nippon Roussel, Jpn. Nippon Roussel, 4-5 Muro-machi, Nihonbashi, Chuo-ku, Tokyo, Japan.

Nippon Shinyaku, Jpn. Nippon Shinyaku, Hachijyo Sagaru, Nishioji-dori, Minami-ku, Kyoto, Japan.

Nirvana, Spain. Nirvana, Caidos 23, Soto del Real, 28791 Madrid, Spain.

NLH, Norw. See *NAF, Norw.*

Nobel Medica, Swed. Nobel Medica AB, Box 6018, 172 06 Sundbyberg, Sweden.

Norcliff Thayer, Swed. See *ACO, Swed.*

Norcliff Thayer, USA. Norcliff Thayer Inc., 303 South Broadway, Tarrytown NY 10591, USA.

Nordic, Canad. Nordic Laboratories Inc., 16700 route Transcanadienne, Kirkland, Quebec H9H 4M7, Canada.

Nordic, UK. Nordic Pharmaceuticals Ltd, 11 Mount Rd, Feltham, Middx TW13 6JG, England.

Nordisk, Fr. Nordisk-France, S.A., tour Berkeley, 19 av. du Capitaine-Guy-nemer, 92081 Paris-la Defense, France.

Nordisk, Neth. Nordisk Nederland, Information-office of Nordisk Insulin Laboratorium, Verrijn Stuartlaan 27, 2288 EK Rijswijk, Netherlands.

Nordisk, Norw. Nordisk Norge, Eiksv. 115, 1345 Osteras, Norway.

Nordisk, S.Afr. See *Leo, S.Afr.*

Nordisk, Spain. Nordisk, General Oraa 70, 28006 Madrid, Spain.

Nordisk, Swed. See *Leo, Swed.*

Nordisk, Switz. Nordisk-Schweiz c/o SA Leo, Case postale, 8051 Zurich, Switzerland.

Nordisk Droge, Denm. Nordisk Droge Afdl., Ragnagade 9, 2100 Copenhagen Ø, Denmark.

Nordisk Gentofte, Denm. Nordisk Gentofte A/S, Niels Steensenvej 1, 2820 Gentofte, Denmark.

Nordisk Insulin, Belg. See *Lundbeck, Belg.*

Nordisk Insulin, Canad. See *Horner, Canad.*

Nordisk-UK, UK. Nordisk-UK, Highview House, Tattenham Crescent, Epsom, Surrey KT18 5QJ, England.

Nordisk-USA, USA. Nordisk-USA, 6500 Rock Spring Dr., Suite 304, Bethesda MD 20817, USA.

Nordmark, Ger. Nordmark Arzneimittel GmbH, Pinnau-Allee, Postfach: 1244, 2082 Uetersen/Holstein 1, W. Germany.

Nordmark, Swed. See *Famaco, Swed.*

Nordmark, Switz. See *Sanofi, Switz.*

Norfarma, Norw. Norfarma A/S, Treschowsg. 2b, 0477 Oslo 4, Norway.

Norgan, Fr. Laboratoires Norgan, 21 rue de Madrid, 75008 Paris, France.

Norgan, Neth. See *Tramedico, Neth.*

Norgine, Austral. Norgine Pty Ltd, Suite 5, 532 Hampton St, Hampton Vic. 3188, Australia.

Norgine, Belg. Norgine S.A., rue Defacqz 78-80, 1050 Brussels, Belgium.

Norgine, Ger. Norgine GmbH, Im Schwarzenborn 4, Postfach:1840, 3550 Marburg 1, W. Germany.

Norgine, Neth. See *Tramedico, Neth.*

Norgine, Switz. See *Panpharma, Switz.*

Norgine, UK. Norgine Ltd, 116 London Rd, Headington, Oxford OX3 9BA, England.

Norgine, USA. Norgine Laboratories Inc., 2 Overhill Rd, Scarsdale NY 10583, USA.

Noristan, S.Afr. Noristan Laboratories (Pty) Ltd, Private Bag X516, Silverton 0127, S. Africa.

Norit, Neth. Norit N.V. (Pharm. dept.), Nijverheidsweg-Noord 74, 3812 PM Amersfoort, Netherlands.

Norma, UK. Norma Chemicals Ltd, 1a Frognal, London NW3 6AN, England.

Normon, Spain. Normon, Nierenberg 10, 28002 Madrid, Spain.

Northia, Arg. Northia, Madero 135, 1408 Buenos Aires, Argentina.

Norton, UK. H.N. Norton & Co. Ltd, Patman House, George Lane, South Woodford, London E18 2LY, England.

Norwich-Eaton, Austral. Norwich Eaton Pharmaceuticals Pty Ltd, 1408 Centre Rd, Clayton Vic. 3168, Australia.

Norwich-Eaton, Canad. Norwich-Eaton Pharmaceuticals Inc., A Procter & Gamble Co., 210 Sheldon Dr., P.O. Box 819, Cambridge, Ontario N1R 5W6, Canada.

Norwich Eaton, Denm. See *A.L., Denm.*

Norwich Eaton, Neth. Norwich Eaton, Europalaan 101, 3526 KR Utrecht, Netherlands.

Norwich-Eaton, UK. Norwich-Eaton Ltd, Hedley House, St. Nicholas Ave, Gosforth, Newcastle-upon-Tyne NE3 1LR, England.

Norwich Eaton, USA. Norwich Eaton Pharmaceuticals Inc., P.O. Box 191, Norwich NY 13815, USA.

Nourypharma, Ger. Nourypharma GmbH, Mittenheimer Strasse 62, Postfach: 60, 8042 Oberschleissheim, W. Germany.

Nourypharma, Neth. Nourypharma B.V., Wethouder van Eschstraat 1, 5342 AV Oss, Netherlands.

Nourypharma, Switz. See *Oryx, Switz.*

Nova Argentia, Ital. Nova Argentia Industria Farmaceutica s.r.l., Via G. Pascoli 1, 20064 Gorgonzola (MI), Italy.

Novag, Spain. Novag, Gran Via de Carlos III 94, 08028 Barcelona, Spain.

Novo, Austral. Novo Laboratories Pty Ltd, P.O. Box 46, Parramatta NSW 2150, Australia.

Novo, Belg. Novo Industrie S.A., ave Charles-Quint 345, 1080 Brussels, Belgium.

Novo, Denm. Novo Industri A/S, Gl. Koge Landevej 117, 2500 Valby, Denmark.

Novo, Fr. Novo Industrie Pharmaceutique, 103 rue La Boetie, 75008 Paris, France.

Novo, Ger. Novo Industrie GmbH Pharmaceutika, Kantstrasse 2, Postfach: 2840, 6500 Mainz, W. Germany.

Novo, Ital. Novo Farmaceutici Italia s.r.l., Via Trebazia 30(Appia Antica), 00179 Rome, Italy.

Novo, Neth. Novo Industri B.V., De Klencke 4, 1083 HH Amsterdam, Netherlands.

Novo, Norw. Novo Industri A/S, Hauger Skolev. 16, Postboks 24, 1351 Rud, Norway.

Novo, S.Afr. Novo Industries (Pharmaceuticals) (Pty) Ltd, P.O. Box 783155, Sandton 2146, S. Africa.

Novo, Spain. Novo Espana, Rufino Gonzalez 14, 28037 Madrid, Spain.

Novo, Swed. Novo Industri AB, Box 69, 201 20 Malmo 1, Sweden.

Novo, Switz. Novo Industrie SA, Case postale 235, 8032 Zurich, Switzerland.

Novo, UK. Novo Laboratories Ltd, Ringway House, Bell Rd, Daneshill East, Basingstoke, Hants RG24 0QN, England.

Novofarma, Spain. See *Merck Igoda, Spain.*

Novopharm, Canad. Noropharm Ltd, 1290 Ellesmere Rd, Scarborough, Ontario M1P 2Y1, Canada.

Novopharma, Switz. Novopharma S.A., ch. Grand-Puits 28, 1217 Meyrin 2/Geneva, Switzerland.

Noxell, UK. Noxell Corporation (UK) Ltd, North House, 9 St Edwards Way, Romford, Essex RM1 1UJ, England.

Nubilo-Landman, Neth. Nubilo-Landman B.V., Bronsstraat 2, 1411 AV Naarden, Netherlands.

Nuovo, Ital. Nuovo Consorzio Sanitario Nazionale di Malizia Dr Paolo, Via Svetonio 6, 00136 Rome, Italy.

Nutricia, Denm. Nutricia Nordica A/S, Sdr. Ringvej 39 (postbox 21), 2605 Brondby, Denmark.

Nutrition Control Products, USA. Nutrition Control Products, Division of Pharmex Inc., 2113 Lincoln St, P.O. Box 151, Hollywood FL 33022, USA.

Nyal, Austral. See *Winthrop, Austral.*

Nyco, Denm. NycoMed A/S, Mose Alle 10 A, 2610 Rødovre, Denmark.

Nyco, Norw. Nycomed A/S. Division Internasjonal, Nycov. 2, Postboks 4220 Torshov, 0401 Oslo 4, Norway.

Nycomed, Swed. Nycomed AB, Box 1215, 181 24 Lidingo, Sweden.

Nycomed, UK. Nycomed (UK) Ltd, Nycomed House, 2111 Coventry Rd, Sheldon, Birmingham B26 3EA, England.

Nyegaard, Belg. Nyegaard S.A., ave A. Giraud 1/bte 6, 1030 Brussels, Belgium.

Nyegaard, Neth. See *Pharmachemie, Neth.*

O'Neal, Canad. See *Seaway Midwest, Canad.*

Oberlin, Fr. Laboratoires Conseil Oberlin, 128 rue Danton, 92500 Rueil-Malmaison, France.

Oberval, Fr. Laboratoires Oberval, 34 rue Saint-Romain, 69008 Lyon, France.

Ocumed, USA. Ocumed Inc., 109 Kinderkamack Rd, Montvale NJ 07645, USA.

Odan, Canad. Odan Laboratories Ltd, 8235 av. Mountain Sights, Suite 103, Montreal, Quebec H4P 2B4, Canada.

Odopharm, Fr. Laboratoires Odopharm, 83 bis, rue Thiers, 92100 Boulogne-Billancourt, France.

OFF, Ital. Officina Farmaceutica Fiorentina S.r.l. Istituto Biochimico, Quart. Varignano 12/13/14, 55049 Viareggio (Lucca), Italy.

OFL, Ital. OFL, Officine Farmacologiche Lombarde di Antonio Meli e C. s.n.c., Via F. De Sanctis 73, 20141 Milan, Italy.

OFT, Ital. Officina Farmaceutica Tiberina s.r.l., Via Oslavia 34, 00195 Rome, Italy.

Oftalmiso, Spain. Oftalmiso, Estacion 6, Beniajan, 30570 Murcia, Spain.

Ogna, Ital. Giovani Ogna & Figli s.p.a., Via C. Farini 63, 20159 Milan, Italy.

Olin, USA. Olin Corporation, 120 Long Ridge Rd, Stamford CT 06904, USA.

Oluf Mork, Denm. Oluf Mork Bio-Chemie A/S, Rodovrevej 251-253, 2610 Rodovre, Denmark.

Om, Switz. Laboratoire Om S.A., rue du Bois-du-Lan 22, 1217 Meyrin 2/Geneva, Switzerland.

Omega, Arg. Esp. Med. Omega, Serrano 985, 1414 Buenos Aires, Argentina.

Omega, Canad. Omega Laboratories Ltd, 11450 rue Hamon, Montreal, Quebec H3M 3A3, Canada.

Ondee, Canad. Ondee Limitee (Laboratoire), 280 rue Milice, Longueuil, Quebec J4L 4J2, Canada.

Ono, Jpn. Ono Yakuhin, 2-14 Doshomachi, Higashi-ku, Osaka, Japan.

Onyx Chemical Co., USA. Onyx Chemical Co., USA.

Opfermann, Ger. Opfermann Arzneimittel GmbH, Robert-Koch-Strasse 2, Postfach: 1420, 5276 Wiehl, W. Germany.

OPG, Neth. De Cooperatieve Apothekers Vereeniging 'De Onderlinge Pharmaceutische Groothandel' UA, Europalaan 2, 3526 KS Utrecht, Netherlands.

Opocalcium, Fr. Laboratoires de l'Opocalcium, 7 rue de l'Industrie, 95310 St-Ouen l'Aumone, France.

Opodex, Denm. See *Axeltorvs, Denm.*

Opodex, Fr. Opodex-SLS, 18 rue Raymond-Ridel, 92250 La Garenne-Colombes, France.

Opopharma, Switz. Opopharma SA, Case postale 315, 8025 Zurich, Switzerland.

Oppenheimer, UK. Oppenheimer, Son & Co. Ltd, England.

Optrex, UK. Optrex Ltd, P.O. Box 94, Nottingham NG2 3AA, England.

Oral-B, Austral. Oral-B Laboratories Pty Ltd, P.O. Box 957, North Sydney NSW 2060, Australia.

Oral-B, Canad. Oral-B Laboratories Inc., 974 Lakeshore Rd E., Mississauga, Ontario L5E 1E4, Canada.

Oral-B, Denm. See *Blumoller, Denm.*

Oral-B, Ger. Oral-B Laboratories GmbH, Russelsheimer Str. 22, Postfach: 190340, 6000 Frankfurt/M. 1, Germany.

Oral B, Spain. Oral B, Avda de la Constitucion 240, Torrejon de Ardoz, 28850 Madrid, Spain.

Oral-B, UK. Oral-B Laboratories Ltd, Gatehouse Rd, Aylesbury, Bucks HP19 3ED, England.

Oramon, Ger. Oramon Arzneimittel GmbH, Mittelstrasse 18, Postfach: 320, 7958 Laupheim 1, Germany.

Orapharm, Austral. Orapharm, 55 Fitzgerald St, South Yarra Vic. 3141, Australia.

Ordesa, Spain. Ordesa, Ctra Nacional 152, km 22.6, San Baudilio de Llobregat, 08830 Barcelona, Spain.

Orfi, Spain. Orfi, Baronesa de Malda 73, Esplugas de Llobregat, 08950 Barcelona, Spain.

Organon, Arg. Organon Argentina S.A., Charcas 3673, 1425 Buenos Aires, Argentina.

Organon, Austral. Organon (Australia) Pty Ltd, Private Bag 25, Lane Cove NSW 2066, Australia.

Organon, Belg. Organon Belge S.A., ave Marnix 13, 1050 Brussels, Belgium.

Organon, Canad. Organon Canada Ltd, 565 Coronation Drive, West Hill, Ontario M1E 4S2, Canada.

Organon, Denm. Organon AS, Literbuen 9, 2740 Skovlunde, Denmark.

Organon, Fin. Oy Organon AB, Ruokolahdenkatu 23 B, PL 254, 00181 Helsinki, Finland.

Organon, Fr. Organon S.A., B.P. 144, 93204 Saint-Denis Cedex 01, France.

Organon, Ger. Organon GmbH, Mittenheimer Strasse 62, Postfach: 60, 8042 Oberschleissheim, W. Germany.

Organon, Jpn. Nihon Organon, 1-13-13 Ginza, Chuo-ku, Tokyo, Japan.

Organon, Neth. Organon Nederland B.V., Wethouder van Eschstraat 1, 5342 AV Oss, Netherlands.

Organon, Norw. Organon A/S, Postboks 325, 1371 Asker, Norway.

Organon, Peru. Organon Internacional BV, Camana 993-A, Oficina 404, Lima, Peru.

Organon, S.Afr. Organon (Pty) Ltd, P.O. Box 65463, Benmore 2010, S. Africa.

Organon, Spain. Organon, Plg Salinas, Ctra de Enlace B 20, San Baudilio de Llobregat, 08830 Barcelona, Spain.

Organon, Swed. Organon AB, Box 5076, 421 05 V Frölunda, Sweden.

Organon, Switz. Organon SA, Case postale 129, 8808 Pfäffikon SZ, Switzerland.

Organon, UK. Organon Laboratories Ltd, Cambridge Science Park, Milton Rd, Cambridge CB4 4FL, England.

Organon, USA. Organon Pharmaceuticals, 375 Mount Pleasant Ave, West Orange NJ 07052, USA.

Organon Teknika, Canad. Organon Teknika Inc., 2200 Eglinton Ave E., Scarborough, Ontario M1K 5C9, Canada.

Organon Teknika, Neth. Organon Teknika Nederland B.V., Wethouder van Eschstraat 1, 5342 AV Oss, Netherlands.

Organon Teknika, Switz. Organon Teknika AG, Case postale 129, 8808 Pfäffikon SZ, Switzerland.

Organon Teknika, UK. Organon-Teknika Ltd, Cambridge Science Park, Milton Rd, Cambridge CB4 4FL, England.

Orion, Denm. See *Erco, Denm.*

Orion, Eire. See *Electramed, Eire.*

Orion, Fin. Orion Laaketehdas, PL 65, 02101 Espoo, Finland.

Orion, Norw. See *Organon, Norw.*

Orion, Swed. See *Erco, Swed.*

Orion, Switz. See *Oryx, Switz.*

Ormed, S.Afr. Ormed, S. Africa.

Orravan, Spain. Orravan, Marco Aurelio 18, 08006 Barcelona, Spain.

Ortega, USA. Ortega, USA.

Orthana, Denm. See *Nyco, Denm.*

Ortho, Canad. Ortho Pharmaceutical (Canada) Ltd, 19 Green Belt Dr., Don Mills, Ontario M3C 1L9, Canada.

Ortho, Swed. See *Cilag, Swed.*

Ortho Dermatological, USA. Ortho Pharmaceutical Corp., Dermatological Division, P.O. Box 300, Raritan NJ 08869, USA.

Ortho Diagnostic, Belg. Ortho Diagnostic Systems N.V., Antwerpseweg 19-21, 2340 Beerse, Belgium.

Ortho Diagnostic, USA. Ortho Diagnostic Systems Inc., Route 202, Raritan NJ 08869, USA.

Ortho Diagnostics, UK. Ortho Diagnostic Systems Ltd, Enterprise House, Station Rd, Loudwater, High Wycombe, Bucks HP10 9UF, England.

Ortho Pharmaceutical, USA. Ortho Pharmaceutical Corp., Raritan NJ 08869, USA.

Ortho-Cilag, UK. Ortho-Cilag Pharmaceutical Ltd, P.O. Box 79, Saunderton, High Wycombe, Bucks HP14 4HJ, England.

Oryx, Switz. Oryx Pharmazeutika SA, Case postale 244, 8025 Zurich, Switzerland.

Osiris, Arg. Osiris S.A.I.C.F.I., Canalejas 1647, 1406 Buenos Aires, Argentina.

Osothsapha, Thai. Osothsapha (Teck Heng Yoo) Co. Ltd, 2100 Ram Khamhaeng Rd, Huamark-Bangkapi, Bangkok 10240, Thailand.

Österreichische Stickstoffwerke, Switz. See *Globopharm, Switz.*

Ostlund, Swed. See *Alpha, Swed.*

OTC, Spain. OTC-Iberica, President Lluis Companys 16, Santa Coloma de Gramanet, 08921 Barcelona, Spain.

Otifarma, Ital. Otifarma s.p.a., Via Martiri d/la Liberta 34, 43058 Sorbolo (PR), Italy.

Otsuka, Jpn. Otsuka Seiyaku, 2-9 Tsukasa-cho, Kanda, Chiyoda-ku, Tokyo, Japan.

Otsuka, Thai. See *Charoen Bhaesaj, Thai.*

Otto Broe, Denm. Otto Broe A/S, Formervangen 9, 2600 Glostrup, Denmark.

Otto Jann, Switz. See *Doetsch, Grether, Switz.*

Ottolenghi, Ital. Dr. Ottolenghi & C. s.r.l., Via Lanfranchi 6, 10131 Turin, Italy.

Ottosen, Denm. G.R. Ottosen, Romancevej 31, 2730 Herlev, Denmark.

OTW, Ger. Organotherapeutische Werke GmbH (OTW), Roonstrasse 23a, Postfach: 2940, 7500 Karlsruhe 1, Germany.

Owen, Austral. See *Alcon, Austral.*

Owen, USA. Owen, USA.

Oxoid, UK. Oxoid Ltd, Wade Rd, Basingstoke, Hants RG24 0PW, England.

Ozothine, Fr. See *S.C.A.T., Fr.*

Pacific, Canad. Pacific Pharmaceuticals Ltd, a subsidiary of The Terry Fox Medical Research Foundation, 1176 W. Georgia St, Suite 1130, Vancouver, British Columbia V6E 4A2, Canada.

Paddock, USA. Paddock, USA.

Padil, Ital. Farmaco Italiano Padil s.p.a., Via Calabiana 18, 20139 Milan, Italy.

Padma, Switz. Padma SA, Rieterstrasse 18, 8002 Zurich, Switzerland.

Padro, Spain. Padro, Paseo Carlos I 208, 08013 Barcelona, Spain.

Paillusseau, Fr. Laboratoires Paillusseau, 11 rue de la Loge, 94260 Fresnes, France.

Paines & Byrne, UK. Paines & Byrne Ltd, Pabyrn Laboratories, 177 Bilton Rd, Perivale, Greenford, Middx UB6 7HG, England.

Palex, Spain. Palex, Ctra. Tarrasa s/n Km 21.6, Rubi, Barcelona, Spain.

Palisades, USA. Palisades Pharmaceuticals Inc., 219 County Rd, Tenafly NJ 07670, USA.

Pan-American Pharmaceuticals, UK. Pan-American Pharmaceuticals Ltd, Glebe View, North Rd, Havering-Atte-Bower, Romford, Essex RM4 1PP, England.

Pan Britannica, UK. Pan Britannica Industries Ltd, Britannica House, Waltham Cross, Herts EN8 7DY, England.

Pan Medica, Fr. Laboratoires Pan Medica, 1re avenue 2065 m-L.I.D., 06516 Carros Cedex, France.

Pan Química Farmac., Spain. Pan Química Farmacéutica, Rufino Gonzalez 30, 28037 Madrid, Spain.

Pannoc, Belg. Pannoc Chemie S.A., Stationstraat 2/1, B.P. 77, 2410 Herentals, Belgium.

Panpharma, Switz. Panpharma SA, Untermattweg 8, 3001 Bern, Switzerland.

Panpharma, UK. Panpharma Ltd, Hayes Gate House, 27 Uxbridge Rd, Hayes, Middx UB4 0JN, England.

Panray, USA. Panray, USA.

Panthox & Burck, Ital. Panthox & Burck s.p.a., Istituto Biochimico Italo Svizzero, Via Beldiletto 1, 20142 Milan, Italy.

Par, USA. Par, USA.

Paramed, Switz. See *Amino, Switz.*

Para-Pharma, Switz. Para-Pharma AG, Löwenstrasse 59, 8021 Zurich, Switzerland.

Parergerm, Fr. Paragerm, Z.I., 3^{e} rue, 06510 Carros, France.

Parisis, Spain. Parisis, Juan de Juanes 8, 28007 Madrid, Spain.

Parkdale, USA. Parkdale, San Antonio, USA.

Parke, Davis, Arg. Parke, Davis & Cía. de Arg. S.A.I.C., Sarmiento 3401, 1196 Buenos Aires, Argentina.

Parke, Davis, Austral. Parke Davis Pty Ltd, P.O. Box 42, Caringbah NSW 2229, Australia.

Parke, Davis, Canad. Parke, Davis Canada Inc., P.O. Box 2200, Station A, Scarborough, Ontario M1K 5C9, Canada.

Parke, Davis, Denm. Parke-Davis, Emdrupvej 28B, 2100 Copenhagen O, Denmark.

Parke, Davis, Fr. See *Substantia, Fr.*

Parke, Davis, Ger. Parke, Davis & Co., Mooswaldallee 1-9, Postfach: 5620, 7800 Freiburg, W. Germany.

Parke, Davis, Ital. Parke Davis s.p.a., Via C. Colombo 1, 20020 Lainate (Milan), Italy.

Parke, Davis, Neth. See *Substantia, Neth.*

Parke, Davis, Norw. See *Collett, Norw.*

Parke, Davis, NZ. Parke Davis Pty Ltd, C.P.O. Box 4275, Auckland, New Zealand.

Parke, Davis, Philipp. See *Warner-Lambert, Philipp.*

Parke, Davis, S.Afr. Parke-Davis Laboratories, Division of Chamberlains (Pty) Ltd, Private Bag X6, Tokai 7966, S. Africa.

Parke, Davis, Spain. Parke Davis, Plg Manso Mateu s-n, Prat de Llobregat, 08820 Barcelona, Spain.

Parke, Davis, Swed. See *Warner-Lambert, Swed.*

Parke, Davis, Switz. See *Warner-Lambert, Switz.*

Parke, Davis, UK. Parke-Davis Medical, Mitchell House, Southampton Rd, Eastleigh, Hants SO5 5RY, England.

Parke, Davis, USA. Parke-Davis, Division Warner-Lambert Co., 201 Tabor Rd, Morris Plains NJ 07950, USA.

Parmentier, Belg. Lab. Parmentier S.A., ave Brugmann 425d, 1180 Brussels, Belgium.

Pasadena Research Labs, USA. Pasadena Research Labs Inc., 2107 E. Villa St, Pasadena CA 91107, USA.

Pascoe, Ger. Pascoe Pharmazeutische Präparate GmbH, Schiffenberger Weg 55, Postfach:6140, 6300 Giessen, W. Germany.

Passauer, Ger. Herbert J Passauer, Chemisch-Pharmazeutische Fabrik, Kirchhainer Damm 62, Postfach: 490248, 1000 Berlin 49, Germany.

Pasteur, Belg. See *Labaz, Belg.*

Pasteur Vaccins, Fr. Pasteur Vaccins, 1 bd Raymond-Poincare, 92430 Marnes-la-Coquette, France.

Pasteur Vaccins, Switz. See *Sanofi, Switz.*

Patentex, Denm. See *Helge Kjelstrup, Denm.*

Patentex, Ger. Patentex GmbH, Marschnerstr. 10, 6000 Frankfurt (Main) 1, Germany.

Patentex, Switz. See *Adroka, Switz.*

Paton, UK. F.C. Paton (Southport) Ltd, 43a Old Park Lane, Southport, Merseyside PR9 7BC, England.

Paul Maney, Canad. Paul Maney Laboratories, a division of Technilab Inc., 1490 rue Beaulac, St-Laurent, Quebec H4R 1R7, Canada.

Paylos, Arg. Paylos S.R.L., Dardo Rocha 202, 1870 Avellaneda, Buenos Aires, Argentina.

Pearson, Ger. Pearson & Co., Marienstrasse 149, 5000 Cologne 30, W. Germany.

Pearson, UK. William Pearson Ltd, Clough Rd, Hull, North Humberside HU6 7QA, England.

Pech, Fr. Laboratoires Pech, 14 rue de Belfort, 11100 Narbonne, France.

Pechiney, UK. Pechiney World Trade London, 359-61 Euston Rd, London NW1 3AW, England.

Pedemonte, Spain. Pedemonte, San Vicente 21, 08001 Barcelona, Spain.

Pedersen, Norw. O. Chr. Pedersen A/S Farm. Kjemisk Laboratorium, Trondheimsvn. 139, 0570 Oslo 5, Norway.

Pediatric, S.Afr. Pediatric, P.O. Box 1682, Johannesburg 2000, S. Africa.

Pedinol, USA. Pedinol Pharmacal Inc., 30 Banfi Plaza North, Farmingdale NY 11735, USA.

Pelayo, Spain. Pelayo, Tallers 16, 08001 Barcelona, Spain.

Penn, UK. Penn Pharmaceuticals Ltd, Buckingham House, Church Rd, Penn, High Wycombe, Bucks HP10 8LN, England.

Pennwalt, Canad. Pennwalt Inc., Pharmaceutical Division, 1851 Sandstone Manor, Pickering, Ontario L1W 3R9, Canada.

Pennwalt, Eire. Pennwalt Ireland Ltd, 57 Merrion Square, Dublin 2, Eire.

Pennwalt, USA. Pennwalt Prescription Divsion, Pennwalt Corp., 755 Jefferson Rd, Rochester NY 14623, USA.

Pensa, Spain. Pensa, Literato Azorin 20, 46006 Valencia, Spain.

Pentafarm, Spain. Pentafarm, La Cuesta 71, 08023 Barcelona, Spain.

Pentagone, Canad. See *Berlex, Canad.*

Pental, Spain. See *Cederroth, Spain.*

Pentapharm, Switz. Pentapharm SA, Engelgasse 109, 4002 Basle, Switzerland.

Pereira, Spain. See *Inkey, Spain.*

Perez Jimenez, Spain. Perez Jimenez, Plg Chinales, Parcela 16, 14080 Cordoba, Spain.

Perga, Spain. Perga, Providencia 42, 08024 Barcelona, Spain.

Perkins, Ital. Perkins Chimical Co. s.a.s., Via Passo Buole 166, 10135 Turin, Italy.

Permamed, Switz. Permamed SA, Drosselstrasse 47, 4002 Basel, Switzerland.

Peroxidos, Spain. See *Foret Peroxidos, Spain.*

Person & Covey, USA. Person & Covey Inc., 616 Allen Ave, Glendale CA 91201, USA.

Perstorp, Swed. Perstorp Pharma, Perstorp AB, 284 80 Perstorp, Sweden.

Peter Hand, UK. Peter Hand (GB) Ltd, 15-19 Church Rd, Stanmore, Middx HA7 4AR, England.

Petersen, S.Afr. Petersen Ltd, P.O. Box 5787, Johannesburg, S. Africa.

Petri, Denm. Chr. F. Petri's Eftf. I/S Kemisk Fabrik, Apollovej 33, 2720 Vanløse, Denmark.

PF Medical, Denm. PF Medical, Julivej 28, 8210 Arhus V, Denmark.

Pfanstiehl, USA. Pfanstiehl Laboratories Inc., 1219 Glen Rock Ave, Waukegan IL 60085, USA.

Pfipharmecs, USA. Pfipharmecs Division, Pfizer Inc., 235 E 42nd St, New York NY 10017, USA.

Pfister Chemical, USA. Pfister Chemical Inc., Linden Ave, Ridgefield NJ 07657, USA.

Pfizer, Arg. Pfizer S.A.C.I., Miñones 2177, 1428 Buenos Aires, Argentina.

Pfizer, Aust. Pfizer Corporation Austria GmbH, Mondscheingasse 16, 1071 Vienna VII, Austria.

Pfizer, Austral. Pfizer Pty Ltd, P.O. Box 57, West Ryde NSW 2114, Australia.

Pfizer, Belg. Pfizer S.A., rue Léon Théodor 102, 1090 Brussels, Belgium.

Pfizer, Braz. Pfizer S.A., P.O. Box 143, Rodovia Presidente Dutra Km 225, 07000 Guarulhos, Brazil.

Pfizer, Canad. Pfizer Canada Inc., P.O. Box 800, Pointe Claire, Dorval, Quebec H9R 4V2, Canada.

Pfizer, Denm. Pfizer A/S, Vestre Gade 18, 2650 Hvidovre, Denmark.

Pfizer, Fr. Laboratoires Pfizer, 86 rue de Paris, B.P. 60, 91400 Orsay, France.

Pfizer, Ger. Pfizer GmbH, Pfizerstrasse 1, Postfach: 4949, 7500 Karlsruhe 1, W. Germany.

Pfizer, Hong Kong. Pfizer Corp., 8/F Citicorp Centre, 18 Whitfield Road, Causeway Bay, Hong Kong.

Pfizer, Ital. Pfizer Italiana s.p.a., Via del Fornetto 85, 00149 Rome, Italy.

Pfizer, Neth. Pfizer B.V., Koningslaan 200, 3067 TG Rotterdam, Netherlands.

Pfizer, Norw. Pfizer A/S, Sofiesg. 60, 0168 Oslo 1, Norway.

Pfizer, S.Afr. Pfizer Laboratories (Pty) Ltd, P.O. Box 783720, Sandton 2146, S. Africa.

Pfizer, Spain. Pfizer, Ctra Nacional KM 26.2, San Sebastian de los Reyes, 28700 Madrid, Spain.

Pfizer, Swed. Pfizer AB, Box 501, 183 25 Täby, Sweden.

Pfizer, Switz. Pfizer SA, Case postale, 8048 Zurich, Switzerland.

Pfizer, Thai. Pfizer International Corp. (S.A.), 17th Floor, Ocean Building, 163 Surawongse Rd, Bangkok 10500, Thailand.

Pfizer, UK. Pfizer Ltd, Sandwich, Kent CT13 9NJ, England.

Pfizer, USA. Pfizer Laboratories Division, Pfizer Inc., 235 East 42nd St, New York NY 10017, USA.

Pfizer Taito, Jpn. Pfizer Taito, P.O. Box 226, 2-1-1 Nishishinjuku, Shinjuku-ku, Tokyo, Japan.

Pfleger, Ger. Dr R. Pfleger Chemische Fabrik GmbH, Dr-Robert-Pfleger-Strasse 12, Postfach: 2240, 8600 Bamberg 1, W. Germany.

P.F.M., Fr. Laboratoires Department medical de Pierre Fabre Medicament, 75116 Paris, France.

Pfrimmer, Austral. Pfrimmer & Co., 180 Bay St, Port Melbourne Vic. 3207, Australia.

Pfrimmer, Belg. See *de Bournonville, Belg.*

Pfrimmer, Denm. See *Otto Broe, Denm.*

Pfrimmer, Ger. Pfrimmer & Co., Pharmazeutische Werke Erlangen GmbH & Co. KG, Hofmannstrasse 26, Postfach: 2840, 8520 Erglangen, W. Germany.

Pfrimmer, Neth. See *Bournonville, Neth.*

Pfrimmer, Norw. See *Meda, Norw.*

Pfrimmer, Spain. Pfrimmer, Les Escomes s/n, Argentona, Barcelona, Spain.

Phagogene, Fr. Laboratoire Phagogene, Z.I. de Carros, B.P. 128, 06513 Carros Cedex, France.

Pharbil, Belg. Pharbil-Rorer S.A., rue des Palais 112, 1210 Brussels, Belgium.

Pharbil, Neth. Pharbil-Rorer B.V., Wijnhaven 44, 3011 WS Rotterdam, Netherlands.

Pharbita, Neth. B.V. Pharbita, Corn. van Uitgeeststraat 2, 1508 EH Zaandam, Netherlands.

Phardi, Switz. Phardi AG, Case postale 3650, 4002 Basel, Switzerland.

Pharkos, Ital. Pharkos s.r.l., Via Appia Km.54,700, 04012 Cisterna di Latina (LT), Italy.

Pharma 2000, Fr. Laboratoires Pharma 2000, 584 rue Fourny, 78530 Buc, France.

Pharma-Import, Neth. Pharma-Import B.V., Oudeweg 147, 2031 CC Haarlem, Netherlands.

Pharma-Medica, Denm. pHarma-Medica a-s, Farmaceutisk-teknisk laboratorium, Vesterlundvej 19, 2730 Herlev, Denmark.

Pharma-Medica, Norw. See *Sentipharm, Norw.*

Pharma-medica, Switz. See *Globopharm, Switz.*

Pharma-Schwarz, Switz. See *Adrosanol, Switz.*

pHarma, Swed. See *Pro Medica, Swed.*

Pharma-Vinci, Denm. pharma-Vinci A/S, Undalsvej 6, 3300 Frederiksvaerk, Denmark.

Pharmac-Service, Switz. Pharmac-Service S.A., rue Micheli-du-Crest 4, 1205 Geneva, Switzerland.

Pharmacare, USA. Pharmacare Generic Drugs Inc., 3227 Morganford Rd, St Louis MO 63116, USA.

Pharmaceutical Mfg, UK. Pharmaceutical Manufacturing Co., Home Park Estate, Kings Langley, Herts WD4 8DH, England.

Pharmachemie, Neth. Pharmachemie B.V., Nijverheidsweg 48-50, 2031 CP Haarlem, Netherlands.

Pharmachim, Bulg. Pharmachim, 16 Iliensko Chaussee, Sofia, Bulgaria.

Pharmacia Arzneimittel, Ger. Pharmacia Arzneimittel GmbH, Siemensstr. 9-11, 4030 Ratingen 4, Germany.

Pharmacia, Austral. Pharmacia (Australia) Pty Ltd, P.O. Box 175, North Ryde NSW 2113, Australia.

Pharmacia, Belg. Pharmacia S.A., rue de la Fusee 62/bte 2, 1130 Brussels, Belgium.

Pharmacia, Canad. Pharmacia (Canada) Inc., 2044 boul. Saint-Regis, Dorval, Quebec H9P 1H6, Canada.

Pharmacia, Denm. Pharmacia AS, Herredsvejen 2, 3400 Hillerød, Denmark.

Pharmacia, Fr. Pharmacia France S.A., B.P. 210, 78051 Saint-Quentin-en-Yvelines Cedex, France.

Pharmacia, Ger. Pharmacia GmbH, Munzinger Strasse 9, Postfach: 5480, 7800 Freiburg, W. Germany.

Pharmacia, Ital. Pharmacia s.p.a., Via A. Volta 16, 20093 Cologno Monzese (MI), Italy.

Pharmacia, Neth. Pharmacia Nederland B.V., Ohmweg 12, 3442 AA Woerden, Netherlands.

Pharmacia, Norw. Pharmacia Norge A/S, Sandviksv. 26, 1322 Hovik, Norway.

Pharmacia, S.Afr. See *Keatings, S.Afr.*

Pharmacia, Swed. Pharmacia AB, 751 82 Uppsala, Sweden.

Pharmacia, Switz. Pharmacia SA, Lagerstrasse 14, Case postale, 8600 Dübendorf, Switzerland.

Pharmacia, UK. Pharmacia Ltd, Pharmacia House, Midsummer Blvd, Milton Keynes MK9 3HP, England.

Pharmacia, USA. Pharmacia Laboratories, Division of Pharmacia Inc., 800 Centennial Ave, Piscataway NJ 08854, USA.

Pharmaco, NZ. Pharmaco (NZ) Ltd, P.O. Box 4079, Auckland, New Zealand.

Pharmacraft, USA. Pharmacraft Division, Pennwalt Corp., 755 Jefferson Rd, Rochester NY 14623, USA.

Pharmador, S.Afr. Pharmador (Pty) Ltd, P.O. Box 422, East London 5200, S. Africa.

Pharmadrug, Ger. Pharmadrug Production GmbH, P.O. Box 4, 7204 Wurmlingen, W. Germany.

Pharmafair, USA. Pharmafair Inc., 110 Kennedy Dr., Hauppauge NY 11788, USA.

Pharmagen, UK. Pharmagen Ltd, Church Road, Perry Barr, Birmingham B42 2LD, England.

Pharmagene, Switz. Pharmagène SA, Case postale 762, 1211 Geneva 1, Switzerland.

Pharmainvesti, Spain. Pharmainvesti, avda Castilla 19-B Pol. Industr., San Fernando de Henares, Madrid, Spain.

Pharmakon, Switz. Pharmakon SA, Bürglistrasse 39, 8304 Wallisellen, Switzerland.

Pharmasal, Ger. Pharmasal Chem.-Pharm. Fabrik H. Franzke KG, Drosselgasse 5, Postfach: 1380, 8032 Grafelfing, Germany.

Pharmascience, Canad. Pharmascience Inc., 8400 ch. Darnley, Montreal, Quebec H4T 1M4, Canada.

Pharmascience, Fr. Laboratoires Pharmascience, 73 blvd de la Mission-Marchand, 92400 Courbevoie, France.

Pharmastra, Fr. Pharmastra, 40 rue du Canal, 67460 Souffelweyersheim, France.

Pharmatec, Neth. See *Multi-Pharma, Neth.*

Pharmaton, S.Afr. See *Swisspharm, S.Afr.*

Pharmaton, Switz. Pharmaton S.A., 6934 Bioggio, Switzerland.

Pharmavit, Denm. Pharmavit, Fredsholmvej 10, 3460 Birkerod, Denmark.

Pharmax, Belg. See *Wellcome, Belg.*

Pharmax, Denm. See *Nordisk Droge, Denm.*

Pharmax, Norw. See *KabiVitrum, Norw.*

Pharmax, S.Afr. See *Script Intal, S.Afr.*

Pharmax, UK. Pharmax Ltd, Bourne Rd, Bexley, Kent DA5 1NX, England.

Pharmco, S.Afr. Pharmco, S. Africa.

Pharmelac, Fr. Laboratoires Pharmelac, 45 rue de Lourmel, 75015 Paris, France.

Pharmeurop, Fr. Laboratoires Pharmeurop, 22 rue de Marignan, 75008 Paris, France.

Pharmeurop, Switz. See *Uhlmann-Eyraud, Switz.*

Pharmexport, Neth. Pharmexport B.V., Oudeweg 147, 2031 CC Haarlem, Netherlands.

Pharminter, Fr. Laboratoires Pharminter, B.P. 8481, 34 rue St-Romain, 69359 Lyon Cedex, France.

Pharmos, Switz. Pharmos S.A., Case postale 411, 1211 Geneva 11, Switzerland.

Pharmuka, Fr. Pharmuka S.F., 35 quai du Moulin de Cage, 92231 Gennevilliers, France.

Pharnova, Switz. Pharnova S.A., Petit-Chêne 36, 1003 Lausanne, Switzerland.

Phenolaine, UK. Phenolaine Co., England.

Philip Harris, UK. Philip Harris Medical Ltd, Hazelwell Lane, Birmingham B30 2PS, England.

Philips-Duphar, Belg. See *Duphar, Belg.*

Phillips Yeast, UK. Phillips Yeast Products Ltd, Park Royal Rd, London NW10 7JX, England.

Phoenix, Arg. Phoenix S.A.I.C.F., Humahuaca 4065, 1192 Buenos Aires, Argentina.

Phoenix, UK. Phoenix Pharmaceuticals, Unit 2, Glevum Works, Upton St, Gloucester GL1 4LA, England.

Phosma, Fr. Laboratoires Phosma S.A., 59 rue Bourbon, 33028 Bordeaux Cedex, France.

Phyteia, Switz. Phyteia AG, Postfach 17, 9102 Herisau, Switzerland.

Piam, Ital. Vecchi & Piam di G. Assereto, E. Maragliano e C. s.a.p.a., Via Padre G. Semeria 5, 16131 Genoa, Italy.

Pickles, UK. J. Pickles & Sons, Beech House, 62 High St, Knaresborough, North Yorkshire HG5 0EA, England.

Picot, Fr. Laboratoires des Produits Picot, 189 quai Lucien-Lheureux, B.P. 83, 62102 Calais Cedex, France.

Pierre Fabre, Fr. Laboratoires Pierre Fabre, Department medical de Pierre Fabre Medicament, 125 rue de la Faisanderie, 75116 Paris, France.

Pierre Fabre, Spain. Pierre Fabre, Santander 25C, 08020 Barcelona, Spain.

Pierre Fabre, UK. Pierre Fabre Ltd, The Old Coach House, Amersham Hill, High Wycombe, Bucks HP13 6NQ, England.

Pierrel Hospital, Ital. Pierrel Hospital s.p.a., Via Cavriana 14, 20134 Milan, Italy.

Pierrel, Ital. Pierrel s.p.a., Via Bisceglie 96, 20152 Milan, Italy.

Piette, Belg. Lab. Piette International S.A., Groot-Bijgaardenstraat 128, 1620 Drogenbos, Belgium.

Pilsworth, UK. Pilsworth Manufacturing Co. Ltd, 252 Newchurch Rd, Bacup, Lancs OL13 0UE, England.

Pinewood, Eire. Pinewood Laboratories Ltd, Ballymacarbry, Clonmel, Co. Tipperary, Eire.

Plan, Switz. Laboratoires Plan SA, Chemin des Sellières, 1219 Aïre-Geneva, Switzerland.

Plantier, Fr. Laboratoires du Dr Plantier, av. J.-F. Kennedy, 33701 Merignac, France.

Plantier, Neth. See *Dagra, Neth.*

Plantorgan, Ger. Plantorgan Werk KG Chemisch-pharmazeutische Fabrik, Hornbusch 1, Postfach: 1463, 2903 Bad Zwischenahn, Germany.

Plantorgan, Neth. See *Bipharma, Neth.*

Plesner, Norw. Plesner Farmasoytisk A/S, Postboks 77 Leirdal, 1008 Oslo 10, Norway.

Plos, Arg. Plos S.A.C.I.F., Santa Fe 2618, 1425 Buenos Aires, Argentina.

Plough, Austral. Plough (Australia) Pty Ltd, P.O. Box 130, North Ryde NSW 2113, Australia.

Plough, UK. Plough UK, SP Consumer Products Ltd, 182-204 St. John St, London EC1P 1DH, England.

Plough, USA. Plough Inc., 3030 Jackson Ave, Memphis TN 38108, USA.

Poen, Arg. Poen S.A.C.I.F.I., Av. Gaona 5120/24, 1407 Buenos Aires, Argentina.

Pohl-Boskamp, S.Afr. See *Script Intal, S.Afr.*

Pohl-Boskamp, Swed. See *Hässle, Swed.*

Pohl-Boskamp, Switz. See *Lubapharm, Switz.*

Pohl, Denm. See *A.L., Denm.*

Pohl, Ger. G. Pohl-Boskamp GmbH & Co. KG, Kieler Strasse 11, Postfach: 80, 2214 Hohenlockstedt, W. Germany.

Pohl, Neth. See *Tramedico, Neth.*

Pohl, Norw. See *Med-Kjemi, Norw.*

Polcopharma, Austral. Polcopharma Polley F & Co. Pty Ltd, P.O. Box 100, Epping NSW 2121, Australia.

Polcrome, UK. Polcrome Ltd, 11 Mount Rd, Feltham, Middx TW13 6JG, England.

Polfa, Pol. Polfa Scientific Information Centre, Warynskiego 8, 00631 Warsaw, Poland.

Poli, Ital. Poli Industria Chimica s.p.a., Via Volturno 48, 20089 Quinto De Stampi-Rozzano (MI), Italy.

Poli, Switz. See *Galenica, Switz.*

Polifarma, Ital. Polifarma s.p.a., Via Tor Sapienza 138, 00155 Rome, Italy.

Pons, Spain. Pons, Mayor 27, 25007 Lerida, Spain.

Porcher-Lavril, Fr. See *Clin Midy, Fr.*

Porton, UK. Porton Products Ltd, CAMR, Porton Down, Salisbury, Wilts SP4 0JG, England.

P.O.S., Fr. Laboratoires P.O.S., 68240 Kaysersberg, France.

Potter & Clarke, UK. Potter & Clarke, England.

Potter's Herbal Supplies, UK. Potter's (Herbal Supplies) Ltd, Leyland Mill Lane, Wigan, Lancs WN1 2SB, England.

Poythress, USA. Poythress Laboratories Inc., 16 North 22nd St, P.O. Box 26946, Richmond VA 23261, USA.

Prats, Spain. Prats, Travesera del Dalt 44, 08024 Barcelona, Spain.

Precision-Cosmet, USA. Precision-Cosmet Co. Inc., 11140 Bren Rd West, Minnetonka MN 55343, USA.

Princeton, USA. Princeton Pharmaceutical Products (A Squibb Co.), P.O. Box 4000, Princeton NJ 08543-4000, USA.

Princhipharm, Switz. See *Distripharm, Switz.*

Priorin, Switz. Priorin SA, Case postale, 9001 St-Gall, Switzerland.

Pro Doc, Canad. Pro Doc (Laboratories) Ltd, 2925 boul. Industriel, Laval, Quebec H7L 3W9, Canada.

Pro Medica, Swed. Pro Medica AB, Box 27206, 102 53 Stockholm, Sweden.

Procemsa, Ital. Farmaceutici Procemsa s.r.l., Via Pinerolo 12, 10152 Turin, Italy.

Procter & Gamble, Canad. See *Norwich-Eaton, Canad.*

Procter & Gamble, Switz. See *Galenica, Switz.*

Procter & Gamble, USA. Procter & Gamble, P.O. Box 171, Cincinnati OH 45201, USA.

Proctor & Gamble, UK. Proctor & Gamble Ltd, P.O. Box 1 EE, Gosforth, Newcastle Upon Tyne NE99 1EE, England.

Prodes, Spain. Prodes, Trabajo s/n, San Justo de Desvern, 08960 Barcelona, Spain.

Prof. Hlth Prod., USA. Professional Health Products, USA.

Prof. Pharm. Corp., Canad. Professional Pharmaceutical Corporation, 9200 ch. Cote-de-Liesse, Lachine, Quebec H8T 1A1, Canada.

Prof. Pharmacal, USA. Professional Pharmacal Co., Ketchum Laboratories Inc., 369 Bayview Ave, Amityville NY 11701, USA.

Profarmi, Ital. Profarmi s.r.l., Via C. Imbonati 85, 20159 Milan, Italy.

Promeco, Arg. Promeco S.A., Av. del Libertador 7208, 1429 Buenos Aires, Argentina.

Promedica, Fr. Laboratoires Promedica, 41 rue Camille-Pelletan, 92305 Levallois-Perret, France.

Promedica, Neth. See *Multi-Pharma, Neth.*

Promedica, Switz. See *Pharmac-Service, Switz.*

Promesa, Spain. Promesa, Los Cedros, s/n Polg. Industrial, Paracuellos del Jarama, 28860 Madrid, Spain.

Promonta, Belg. See *Byk, Belg.*

Promonta, Ger. Chemische Fabrik Promonta GmbH, Hammer Landstrasse 162, Postfach: 261755, 2000 Hamburg 26, W. Germany.

Propan, S.Afr. Propan-Lipworth, P.O. Box 83, Germiston 1400, S. Africa.

Prophin, Ital. Prophin s.p.a., Via A. Binda 21, 20143 Milan, Italy.

Propper, UK. Chance Propper Ltd, Spon Lane, Smethwick, Warley, West Midlands, England.

Prosana, Austral. Prosana Laboratories, P.O. Box 76, Revesby NSW 2212, Australia.

Prospa, Belg. Prospa S.A., blvd Lambermont 140/bte 5, 1030 Brussels, Belgium.

Prospa, Switz. Prospa SA, Case postale 284, 1401 Yverdon-les-Bains, Switzerland.

Protea, Austral. Protea Pharmaceuticals, A Division of Fisons Pty Ltd, P.O. Box 42, Pennant Hills NSW 2120, Australia.

Protea Pharm, S.Afr. Protea Pharm (Pty) Ltd, P.O. Box 1682, Johannesburg 2000, S. Africa.

Proter, Ital. Proter s.p.a., Via Lambro 38, 20090 Opera (Milan), Italy.

Protexine, Fr. Laboratoires de la Protexine, 29 rue David d'Angers, 75019 Paris, France.

Protina, Ger. Protina, Chemische GmbH, Adalperostr. 30, Postfach: 1253, 8045 Ismaning, W. Germany.

Protochemie, Switz. Protochemie AG, 8756 Mitlödi/Glarus, Switzerland.

Provita, Switz. Provita S.A., La Route-Neuve, 1920 Martigny, Switzerland.

Puerto Galiano, Spain. Puerto Galiano, Cea Bermudez 16, 28003 Madrid, Spain.

Pulitzer, Ital. Pulitzer Italiana s.p.a., Via Tiburtina 1004, 00156 Rome, Italy.

Purdue Frederick, Canad. Purdue Frederick Inc., 123 Sunrise Ave, Toronto, Ontario M4A 1A9, Canada.

Purdue Frederick, USA. The Purdue Frederick Co., 100 Connecticut Ave, Norwalk CT 06854, USA.

Pure Plant Products, UK. Pure Plant Products, Grosvenor Rd, Hoylake, Wirral, Merseyside, England.

Purissimus, Arg. Purissimus S.A., Juan F. Seguí 4635, 1425 Buenos Aires, Argentina.

Puropharma, Ital. Puropharma s.r.l., Galleria del Corso 2, 20122 Milan, Italy.

PVO International, USA. PVO International Inc., 416 Division St, Boonton NJ 07005, USA.

QDL, Austral. QDL Pty Ltd, 160 Wecker St, Upper Mount Gravatt Qld 4122, Australia.

Quaker, USA. Quaker City Pharmacal Co., 129 North 4th St, Philadelphia PA 19106, USA.

Qualiphar, Belg. Lab. Qualiphar S.A., Rijksweg 9, 2680 Bornem, Belgium.

Quantum, USA. Quantum, USA.

Quesada, Arg. Quesada S.A., Saavedra 363/77, 1704 Ramos Mejia, Pcia Buenos Aires, Argentina.

Quest, UK. Quest Vitamins (UK) Ltd, Unit 1, Premier Trading Estate, Dartmouth Middleway, Birmingham B7 4AT, England.

Quimica Medica, Spain. La Quimica Medica, San Juan Bosco 63, 08017 Barcelona, Spain.

Quimpe, Spain. Quimpe, Cruz 49, Alhaurin el Grande, 29120 Malaga, Spain.

Quinoderm, Switz. See *Golaz, Switz.*

Quinoderm, UK. Quinoderm Ltd, Manchester Rd, Oldham, Lancs OL8 4PB, England.

R. Rius, Spain. R. Rius, Mahon 19, 08022 Barcelona, Spain.

Rabi & Solabo, Fr. Laboratoires Rabi & Solabo, 20 av. Foucard, 87006 Limoges Cedex, France.

Rachelle, Neth. See *Pharbil, Neth.*

Rachelle, USA. Rachelle, USA.

Radhuslab., Denm. Radhusapoteket, Smedegade 6-8, 4200 Slagelse, Denmark.

Radiol, UK. Radiol Chemicals Ltd, Stepfield, Witham, Essex CM8 3AG, England.

Radiumfarma, Ital. Radiumfarma s.r.l., Laboratori Farmaco Biologici, Via Cavour 57, 20063 Cernusco S/N (Milan), Italy.

Raffo, Arg. Raffo S.A., Agustín Alvarez 4185, 1603 Villa Martelli, Buenos Aires, Argentina.

Ragionieri, Ital. Dr R.R. Ragionieri s.p.a, Via Corsi Salviati 27, 50019 Sesto Fiorentino (FI), Italy.

Ragusan, Spain. See *Pfrimmer, Spain.*

Ralay, Spain. Ralay, Fernando Puig 58-60, 08023 Barcelona, Spain.

Ram, USA. Ram Laboratories Corp., P.O. Box 559071, Miami FL 33255, USA.

Ramon Sala, Spain. Ramon Sala, Paris 174, 08036 Barcelona, Spain.

RAN, Ger. RAN-Pharm Novesia-Arzneimittel GmbH, Hurtgener Strasse 6, Postfach: 101 243, 4040 Neuss/Rhein 1, Germany.

Ranbaxy, Ind. Ranbaxy Laboratories Ltd, Okhla Industrial Estate, New Delhi-110 020, India.

Rapide, Spain. Rapide, Artistas 12-4, 28020 Madrid, Spain.

Rappai, Switz. Dr F. Rappai, Case postale, 8952 Schlieren-Zurich, Switzerland.

Ratiopharm, Ger. Ratiopharm GmbH Arzneimittel, Im Gehrn 3, 7902 Blaubeuren, W. Germany.

Ratje, Denm. W. Ratje froskaller ApS, Postbox 1900 (Oxford alle 60), 2300 Copenhagen S, Denmark.

Ravasini, Ital. Ravasini Organon Dr R. & C.ia s.p.a., Via Ostilia 15, 00184 Rome, Italy.

Ravensberg, Ger. Ravensberg GmbH Chemische Fabrik, Schneckenburgstrasse 46, Postfach: 1228, 7750 Constance, W. Germany.

Ravizza, Belg. See *Therapeutica, Belg.*

Ravizza, Ital. Ravizza s.p.a., Via Europa 35, 20053 Muggiò (MI), Italy.

Ravizza, Switz. See *Uhlmann-Eyraud, Switz.*

Raway, USA. Raway, USA.

RBS Pharma, Ital. RBS Pharma (Roger Bellon Schoum) s.p.a., Via A. Kuliscioff 6, 20152 Milan, Italy.

Reckitt & Colman, Austral. Reckitt & Colman (Pharmaceutical Division), P.O. Box 138, West Ryde NSW 2114, Australia.

Reckitt & Colman, Belg. Reckitt & Colman S.A., rue de la Bienvenue 7-9, 1070 Brussels, Belgium.

Reckitt & Colman, Denm. See *Meda, Denm.*

Reckitt & Colman, Norw. See *Collett, Norw.*

Reckitt & Colman, S.Afr. Reckitt & Colman Pharmaceuticals (Pty) Ltd, P.O. Box 31069, Merebank 4059, S. Africa.

Reckitt & Colman, Swed. See *Meda, Swed.*

Reckitt & Colman, Switz. See *Desopharma, Switz.*

Reckitt & Colman Pharmaceuticals, UK. Reckitt & Colman, Pharmaceutical Division, Dansom Lane, Hull HU8 7DS, England.

Reckitt Products, UK. Reckitt Products Household Division, Reckitt House, Stoneferry Rd, Hull HU8 8DD, England.

Recofarma, Ital. Recofarma s.r.l., Via Mediana Cisterna 4, 04010 Campoverde di Aprilia (LT), Italy.

Recordati, Belg. See *de Bournonville, Belg.*

Recordati, Ital. Recordati Industria Chimica e Farmaceutica s.p.a., Via Civitali 1, 20148 Milan, Italy.

Recordati, Switz. See *Galenica, Switz.*

Reddish Savilles, UK. Reddish Savilles Ltd, Stanley Rd, Cheadle Hulme, Cheadle, Cheshire SK8 6RB, England.

Redel, Ger. Julius Redel Cesra-Arzneimittelfabrik GmbH & Co., Braunmattstr. 20, Postfach: 20 20, 7570 Baden-Baden, W. Germany.

Reder, Spain. Reder, Cayetano Pando 4, 28047 Madrid, Spain.

Reed & Carnrick, Canad. Reed & Carnrick, Division of Block Drug Co. (Canada) Ltd, 36 Northline Rd, Toronto, Ontario M4B 3E3, Canada.

Reed & Carnrick, Denm. See *Searle, Denm.*

Reed & Carnrick, Neth. See *Pharma-Import, Neth.*

Reed & Carnrick, USA. Reed & Carnrick, 1 New England Ave, Piscataway NJ 08854, USA.

Regal, Canad. Regal Pharmaceutical and Surgical Supply Co. Ltd, 900 Harrington Ct, Burlington, Ontario L7N 3N4, Canada.

Regent Laboratories, UK. Regent Laboratories Ltd, Cunard Rd, London NW10 6PN, England.

Reid-Provident, USA. See *Reid-Rowell, USA.*

Reid-Rowell, USA. Reid-Rowell Inc., 640 Tenth St NW, Atlanta GA 30318, USA.

Reig Jofré, Spain. Reig Jofré, Encarnacion 126, 08024 Barcelona, Spain.

Reiss, Ger. Dr Rudolf Reiss Chemische Werke GmbH & Co. KG, Sachsenring 37-47, 5000 Cologne 1, W. Germany.

Remed, Norw. A/S Remed Inpharma, Tollbug 68, Postboks 2093, 300 Drammen, Norway.

Remedia, S.Afr. Remedia Medical (Pty) Ltd, P.O. Box 42128, Fordsburg 2033, S. Africa.

Remedica, Cyprus. Remedica Ltd, Aharnon St, Industrial Estate, P.O. Box 1706, Limassol, Cyprus.

Renapharm, Switz. Renapharm S.A., Case postale 48, 1636 Broc, Switzerland.

Rendell, UK. W.J. Rendell Ltd, Ickleford Manor, Hitchin, Herts SG5 3XE, England.

Rentokil, UK. Rentokil Ltd, Products Division, Felcourt, East Grinstead, West Sussex RH19 2JY, England.

Rentschler, Ger. Dr. Rentschler Arzneimittel GmbH & Co., Mittelstrasse 18, Postfach: 320, 7958 Laupheim 1, Germany.

Rentschler, Switz. See *Agpharm, Switz.*

Requa, USA. Requa Manufacturing Co. Inc., P.O. Box 4008, Greenwich CT 06830, USA.

Research Industries Corp., USA. Research Industries Corporation, Pharmaceutical Division, 1847 West 2300 South, Salt Lake City UT 84119, USA.

Resfar, Ital. Resfar s.r.l., Via Gradisca 8, 20151 Milan, Italy.

Restan, S.Afr. Restan Laboratories (Pty) Ltd, P.O. Box 41286, Craighall 2024, S. Africa.

Revlon, UK. Revlon International Corporation, 86 Brook St, London W1Y 2BA, England.

Rewo, UK. Rewo Chemical Ltd, 9th Floor, Crown House, London Rd, Morden, Surrey SM4 5DU, England.

Rexar, USA. Rexar Pharmacal Corp., 396 Rockaway Ave, Valley Stream NY 11581, USA.

Rh Institute, Canad. See *Winnipeg Rh Institute, Canad.*

Rhein-Pharma, Ger. Rhein-Pharma Arzneimittelwerk GmbH, Brauereistrasse, 6831 Plankstadt, W. Germany.

RHM Foods, UK. RHM Foods Ltd, Victoria Rd, London NW10 6NU, England.

Rhodia, Arg. Rhodia Argentina Química y Textil S.A.I.C. y F., Primera Junta 525, 1879 Quilmes, Buenos Aires, Argentina.

Rhodia-Pharm, Switz. Rhodia-Pharm S.A., rue du Lièvre 2-4, 1211 Geneva, Switzerland.

Rhone, Spain. Rhone, Plg Ind. Urtinsa s/n, Alcorcon, Madrid, Spain.

Rhone-Poulenc, Belg. Rhone-Poulenc Belgique S.A., av. Carton de Wiart 128, 1090 Brussels, Belgium.

Rhône-Poulenc, Canad. Rhône-Poulenc Pharma Inc., 8580 Esplanade Ave, Montreal, Quebec H2P 2R9, Canada.

Rhone-Poulenc, Denm. Rhone-Poulenc Pharma Norden A/S, Topstykket 12, 3460 Birkerød, Denmark.

Rhône-Poulenc, Ger. Rhône-Poulenc Pharma GmbH, Nattermannallee 1, Postfach: 350120, 5000 Cologne 30, W. Germany.

Rhone-Poulenc, Ital. Rhone-Poulenc Pharma Italia s.p.a., Via A. Kuliscioff 6, 20152 Milan, Italy.

Rhône-Poulenc, Neth. Rhône-Poulenc Nederland B.V., Draaistroom 1, 1181 VT Amstelveen, Netherlands.

Rhône-Poulenc, Norw. Rhône-Poulenc, Medisinsk Informasjonskontor, Industriv. 2, 1481 Hagan, Norway.

Rhone-Poulenc, Swed. Rhone-Poulenc Sverige AB, Box 4189, 102 62 Stockholm 4, Sweden.

Rhone-Poulenc, Switz. Rhône-Poulenc Pharma (Suisse) SA, Case postale 336, 1213 Petit-Lancy 1, Switzerland.

Richard, Fr. Laboratoires Richard, Sauzet, 26740 Montelimar, France.

Richard Daniel, UK. Richard Daniel & Son Ltd, Mansfield Rd, Derby DE1 3RE, England.

Richards & Appleby, UK. Richards & Appleby Ltd, Gerrard Place, East Gillibrands, Skelmersdale, Lancs WN8 9SF, England.

Richardson, Switz. See *Doetsch, Grether, Switz.*

Richardson-Vicks, Austral. Richardson-Vicks Pty Ltd, P.O. Box 95, Villawood NSW 2163, Australia.

Richardson-Vicks, Belg. Richardson-Vicks S.A., chee de Waterloo 868-870, 1180 Brussels, Belgium.

Richardson-Vicks, Canad. Richardson-Vicks Ltd, 2 Norelco Dr., Weston, Ontario M9L 1R9, Canada.

Richardson-Vicks, Neth. Richardson-Vicks B.V., Vanadiumweg 16, 3812 PZ Amersfoort, Netherlands.

Richardson-Vicks, Swed. See *Famaco, Swed.*

Richardson-Vicks, UK. Richardson-Vicks Ltd, Rusham Park, Whitehall Lane, Egham, Surrey TW20 9NW, England.

Richardson-Vicks, USA. Richardson-Vicks Inc., 10 Westport Rd, Wilton CT 06897, USA.

Richelet, Fr. Laboratoires Richelet, 33 rue de Liege, 75008 Paris, France.

Richet, Arg. Richet S.A., Terrero 1251/59, 1416 Buenos Aires, Argentina.

Richmond, Canad. Richmond Pharmaceuticals Inc., 12285 Yonge St, P.O. Box 417, Richmond Hill, Ontario L4C 4Y6, Canada.

Richter, Denm. See *Lenau, Denm.*

Richter, Ital. Ormonoterapia Richter (Gruppo Lepetit s.p.a.), Via Murat 23, 20159 Milan, Italy.

Rida, Spain. Rida, Matias Perello 55, 46005 Valencia, Spain.

Riddell, UK. Riddell, England.

Ridupharm, Switz. Ridupharm, Emil Frey-Strasse 99, 4142 Münchenstein, Switzerland.

Riker 3M, Switz. Riker Laboratories 3M, Case postale, 8803 Rüschlikon, Switzerland.

Riker, Arg. Riker S.A., Av. del Trabajo 5820, 1439 Buenos Aires, Argentina.

Riker, Austral. Riker Laboratories Pty Ltd, P.O. Box 122, Hornsby NSW 2077, Australia.

Riker, Belg. Riker Benelux S.A., Roekhout 47, 1720 Dilbeek, Belgium.

Riker, Canad. Riker Canada Inc., P.O. Box 5757, London, Ontario N6A 4T1, Canada.

Riker, Denm. Riker a/s, Fabriksparken 15, 2600 Glostrup, Denmark.

Riker, Fr. Laboratoires Riker 3M, 40 rue Gabriel Crie, 92245 Malakoff Cedex, France.

Riker, Neth. Riker/3M (Nederland) B.V., Industrieweg 24, 2382 NW Zoeterwoude, Netherlands.

Riker, Norw. Riker Laboratories, Informasjonskontoret for Norge, Hvamvn. 6, Postboks 100, 2013 Skjetten, Norway.

Riker, S.Afr. Riker Laboratories (Africa) (Pty) Ltd, P.O. Box 10465, Johannesburg 2000, S. Africa.

Riker, Swed. 3M Riker Laboratories, Staffans vag 4, 191 89 Sollentuna, Sweden.

Riker, UK. Riker Laboratories, Morley St, Loughborough, Leics LE11 1EP, England.

Riker, USA. Riker Laboratories Inc., Subsidiary of 3M, 225-1S-07 3M Center, St Paul MN 55144, USA.

Ringsted & Semler, Denm. Ringsted & Semler A/S, N. Farimagsgade 13, 1364 Copenhagen K, Denmark.

Rio, S.Afr. See *Adcock Ingram, S.Afr.*

Riom, Fr. Riom Laboratoires-C.E.R.M., 63203 Riom Cedex, France.

Ripari-Gero, Ital. Istituto Farmaco Biologico Ripari Gero s.r.l., Via Chiantigiana 84, 53035 Monteriggioni (SI), Italy.

RIT, Belg. See *Smith Kline-RIT, Belg.*

Ritsert, Ger. Dr. E. Ritsert GmbH & Co. KG, Klausenweg 12, Postfach: 1254, 6390 Eberbach, Germany.

Riva, Canad. Riva Ltee Laboratories, 1905 rue Gutenberg, Chomedey-Laval, Quebec H7S 1A1, Canada.

Rivero, Arg. Rivero & Cía. S.A.I.C., Av. Boyacá 419, 1406 Buenos Aires, Argentina.

RMB Animal Health, UK. RMB Animal Health Ltd, Rainham Rd South, Dagenham, Essex RM10 7XS, England.

Robapharm, Belg. See *de Bournonville, Belg.*

Robapharm, Fr. Laboratoires Robapharm S.A.R.L., 1 av. du Quebec, Z.A. de Courtaboeuf, 91945 Les Ulis, France.

Robapharm, Ger. Deutsche Robapharm GmbH, Langmatten 10, 7801 Pfaffenweiler b. Freiburg, Germany.

Robapharm, Neth. See *Bournonville, Neth.*

Robapharm, Switz. Robapharm SA, St Alban-Rheinweg 174, 4006 Basel, Switzerland.

Robeco Chemicals, USA. Robeco Chemicals Inc., 99 Park Ave, New York NY 10016, USA.

Robert et Carrière, Fr. See *Synthelabo, Fr.*

Robert et Carrière, Switz. See *Actipharm, Switz.*

Robert, Spain. Robert, Avda. San Antonio M. Claret 158, 08025 Barcelona, Spain.

Robert, Switz. See *Adroka, Switz.*

Roberts & Sheppey, UK. Roberts & Sheppey, Melrose Skin Products, Manor Farm House, Ickford, Aylesbury, Bucks HP18 9JB, England.

Roberts, UK. Roberts Laboratories Ltd, Burnden Rd, Bolton, Lancs BL3 2RB, England.

Robertson/Taylor, USA. Robertson/Taylor, USA.

Robilliart, Fr. See *Millot-Solac, Fr.*

Robin, Ital. Boehringer Biochemia Robin s.p.a., Via S. Uguzzone 5, 20126 Milan, Italy.

Robins, Austral. A.H. Robins Pty Ltd, Private Bag 1, Punchbowl NSW 2196, Australia.

Robins, Canad. A.H. Robins Canada Inc., 2360 Southfield Rd, Mississauga, Ontario L5N 3R6, Canada.

Robins, Denm. See *Meda, Denm.*

Robins, Neth. See *Pharbil, Neth.*

Robins, Norw. See *Andersen, Norw.*

Robins, Swed. See *Famaco, Swed.*

Robins, Switz. A.H. Robins S.à.r.l., Case postale, 6300 Zoug 2, Switzerland.

Robins, UK. A.H. Robins Co. Ltd, Sussex Manor Business Park, Gatwick Rd, Crawley, West Sussex RH10 2NH, England.

Robins, USA. A.H. Robins Co., Pharmaceutical Division, 1407 Cummings Dr., Richmond VA 23220, USA.

Robins Consumer Products, UK. A.H. Robins Consumer Products, Sussex Manor Business Park, Gatwick Rd, Crawley, West Sussex RH10 2NH, England.

Robugen, Ger. Robugen GmbH Pharmazeutische Fabrik, Alleenstrasse 22, Postfach: 266, 7300 Esslingen-Zell 1, W. Germany.

Robugen, S.Afr. See *Vernleigh, S.Afr.*

RoC, Fr. RoC, 50 rue de Seine, 92704 Colombes Cedex, France.

Roc, UK. Laboratoires RoC UK Ltd, 13 Grosvenor Crescent, London SW1X 7EE, England.

Rocador, Spain. Rocador, Ctra. Hospitalet a Cornella 35, 08027 Barcelona, Spain.

Roche, Arg. Roche S.A.Q. e I., Fray Justo Sarmiento 2350, 1636 Olivos, Buenos Aires, Argentina.

Roche, Austral. Roche Products Pty Ltd, P.O. Box 255, Dee Why NSW 2099, Australia.

Roche, Belg. Produits Roche S.A., rue Dante 75, 1070 Brussels, Belgium.

Roche, Braz. Produtos Roche Quimicos e Farmaceuticos S.A., Rua General Canabarro 666, P.O. Box 329, Maracana, 20272 Rio de Janeiro, Brazil.

Roche, Canad. Hoffmann-La Roche Ltd, 401 The West Mall, Suite 700, Etobicoke, Ontario M9C 5J4, Canada.

Roche, Denm. Roche A/S, Industriholmen 59, 2650 Hvidovre, Denmark.

Roche, Fr. Produits Roche S.A., 52 blvd du Parc, 92521 Neuilly-sur-Seine Cedex, France.

Roche, Ger. Hoffmann-La Roche Aktiengesellschaft, Emil-Barell-Strasse 1, Postfach: 1380, 7889 Grenzach-Wyhlen 1, W. Germany.

Roche, Ital. Prodotti Roche s.p.a., Piazza Durante 11, 20131 Milan, Italy.

Roche, Jpn. Nihon Roche, 3-2-3 Marunouchi, Chiyoda-ku, Tokyo, Japan.

Roche, Neth. Hoffmann-La Roche B.V., Nijverheidsweg 36-38, 3641 RR Mijdrecht, Netherlands.

Roche, Norw. Roche Norge A/S, Kristoffer Robinsv. 13, Postboks 41 Haugenstua, 0915 Oslo 9, Norway.

Roche, Port. Roche Farmaceutica Quimica Lda, Avenida Fontes Pereira de Melo 6-6, 1098 Lisboa Codex, Portugal.

Roche, S.Afr. Roche Products (Pty) Ltd, P.O. Box 4589, Johannesburg 2000, S. Africa.

Roche, Spain. Roche, Ctra. Carabanchel Andalucia s/n, 28025 Madrid, Spain.

Roche, Swed. Roche-Produkter AB, Box 250, 127 25 Skärholmen 1, Sweden.

Roche, Switz. F. Hoffmann-La Roche & Co. SA, Grenzacherstrasse 124, 4002 Basel, Switzerland.

Roche, UK. Roche Products Ltd, P.O. Box 8, Welwyn Garden City, Herts AL7 3AY, England.

Roche, USA. Roche Laboratories, Division of Hoffmann-La Roche Inc., Nutley NJ 07110, USA.

Rodeca, Canad. Rodeca Inc., 8480 St Lawrence Blvd, Montreal, Quebec H2P 2M6, Canada.

Roemmers, Arg. Roemmers S.A.I.C.F., México 1661, 1100 Buenos Aires, Argentina.

Roerig, Belg. See *Pfizer, Belg.*

Roerig, Neth. See *Pfizer, Neth.*

Roerig, Swed. Roerig AB, Box 501, 183 25 Taby, Sweden.

Roerig, USA. Roerig, Division of Pfizer Pharmaceuticals, 235 East 42nd St, New York NY 10017, USA.

Roger, Spain. Roger, Corcega 541-3, 08025 Barcelona, Spain.

Roger, USA. Roger Pharmacal Inc., P.O. Box 011022, Miami FL 33010, USA.

Roha, Ger. Roha Arzneimittel GmbH, Rockwinkeler Heerstrasse 100, Postfach: 330 340, 2800 Bremen 33, Germany.

Röhm, Ger. Röhm Pharma GmbH, Dr-Otto-Röhm-Strasse 2-4, Postfach: 4347, 6100 Darmstadt 1, W. Germany.

Rohm, Neth. See *Rooster, Neth.*

Rohm & Haas, UK. Rohm & Haas (UK) Ltd, Lennig House, 2 Mason's Ave, Croydon CR9 3NB, England.

Rohm Pharma, S.Afr. See *Noristan, S.Afr.*

Rolab, S.Afr. Rolab (Pty) Ltd, P.O. Box 57129, Springfield 2137, S. Africa.

Roland, Ger. Roland Arzneimittel GmbH, Bargkoppelweg 66, Postfach: 730 820, 2000 Hamburg 73, W. Germany.

Roland-Marie, Fr. See *Millot-Solac, Fr.*

Roland-Marie, Neth. See *Servier, Neth.*

Rolland, Belg. See *Lipha, Belg.*

Rolland, Switz. See *Pharmos, Switz.*

Ronchèse, Fr. See *Compagnie Rousselot, Fr.*

Ronsheim & Moore, UK. Ronsheim & Moore, Division of Hickson & Welch Ltd, Ings Lane, Castleford, West Yorkshire WF10 2JT, England.

Rontag, Arg. Rontag S.A., Franklin Roosevelt 2157, 1428 Buenos Aires, Argentina.

Rooster, Neth. J.H. Rooster & Zn. B.V., Industrieweg 24, 2921 LB Krimpen a/d IJssel, Netherlands.

Roques, Fr. Laboratoires Roques, 31 rue Jules-Guesde, 92130 Issy-les-Moulineaux, France.

Roquette, UK. Roquette (UK) Ltd, Pantiles House, 2 Nevill St, Tunbridge Wells, Kent TN2 5TT, England.

Rorer, Canad. Rorer Canada Inc., 130 East Dr., Bramalea, (Toronto), Ontario L6T 1C3, Canada.

Rorer, Denm. See *KabiVitrum, Denm.*

Rorer, Fr. Rorer, s.a., 4 rue de la Gare, 92300 Levallois-Perret, France.

Rorer, Ger. Rorer GmbH, Stieghorster Strasse 86-90, Postfach: 70 10, 4800 Bielefeld 1, W. Germany.

Rorer, Ital. Rorer s.p.a., Industria Chimica Farmaceutica Biologica, Viale Europa 11, 21040 Origgio (VA), Italy.

Rorer, Mex. Rorer de Mexico S.A.deC.V., Av. Division del Norte No. 3315, Mexico 21 D.F., Mexico.

Rorer, Neth. See *Pharbil, Neth.*

Rorer, Swed. See *Kabi, Swed.*

Rorer, Switz. See *Biochimica, Switz.* and *Panpharma, Switz.*

Rorer, UK. Rorer Pharmaceuticals, St Leonards House, St Leonards Rd, Eastbourne, East Sussex BN21 3YG, England.

Rorer, USA. William H. Rorer Inc., 500 Virginia Dr., Fort Washington PA 19034, USA.

Rosa-Phytopharma, Fr. Laboratoires Rosa-Phytopharma S.A., 55 rue Jules-Auffret, 93502 Pantin, France.

Rosco, Denm. A/S Rosco, Farmaceutisk Industri, Tåstrupgårdsvej 30, 2630 Tåstrup, Denmark.

Rosco, Norw. See *Andersen, Norw.*

Rosco, Swed. See *Selena, Swed.*

Rosell, Canad. Institut Rosell Inc., 8480 boul. Saint-Laurent, Montreal, Quebec H2P 2M6, Canada.

Rosken, Austral. Rosken Division of Fisons Pty Ltd, 6 Chilvers Rd, Thornleigh NSW 2120, Australia.

Ross, Austral. See *Abbott, Austral.*

Ross, Canad. Ross Laboratories, Division of Abbott Laboratories Ltd, 6300 ch. Cote-de-Liesse, Montreal, Quebec H4T 1E3, Canada.

Ross, USA. Ross Laboratories, Division of Abbott Laboratories, Columbus OH 43216, USA.

Roter, Neth. Pharm. Fabr. Roter B.V., Arendstraat 3, 1223 RE Hilversum, Netherlands.

Roter, Switz. See *Galenica, Switz.*

Roterpharma, UK. Roterpharma Ltd, Littleton House, Littleton Rd, Ashford, Middx, England.

Rotex, USA. Rotex Pharmaceuticals Inc., P.O. Box 19283, Orlando FL 32814, USA.

Rottapharm, Ital. Rottapharm s.p.a., Via Valosa di Sopra 9, 20050 Monza (MI), Italy.

Rougier, Canad. Rougier Inc., 8480 St Lawrence Blvd, Montreal, Quebec H2P 2M6, Canada.

Roussel, Arg. Roussel-Lutetia S.A.C.I., Avellaneda 2202, 1636 Olivos, Buenos Aires, Argentina.

Roussel, Austral. Roussel Pharmaceuticals Pty Ltd, P.O. Box 193, Castle Hill NSW 2154, Australia.

Roussel, Belg. Roussel S.A., ave Adolphe Lacomblé 59/bte 5, 1040 Brussels, Belgium.

Roussel, Canad. Roussel Canada Inc., 4045 ch. Côte Vertu, Montreal, Quebec H4R 2E8, Canada.

Roussel, Denm. See *Hoechst, Denm.*

Roussel, Fr. Laboratoires Roussel, 97 rue de Vaugirard, 75279 Paris Cedex 06, France.

Roussel, Neth. Roussel B.V., Bijenvlucht 30, 3871 JJ Hoevelaken, Netherlands.

Roussel, Norw. See *Hoechst, Norw.*

Roussel, S.Afr. Roussel Laboratories (Pty) Ltd, P.O. Box 39110, Bramley 2018, S. Africa.

Roussel, Spain. Roussel Iberica, San Rafael 3, Alcobendas, 28100 Madrid, Spain.

Roussel, Swed. Roussel Nordiska AB, Box 42058, 126 12 Stockholm 42, Sweden.

Roussel, Switz. Roussel Suisse, Herostrasse 9, 8048 Zurich, Switzerland.

Roussel, UK. Roussel Laboratories Ltd, Broadwater Park, North Orbital Rd, Uxbridge, Middx UB9 5HP, England.

Roussel Maestretti, Ital. Roussel Maestretti s.p.a., Viale Gran Sasso 18, 20131 Milan, Italy.

Roussel-UCLAF, USA. Roussel-UCLAF, USA.

Roux-Ocefa, Arg. Roux Ocefa S.A., Montevideo 79/81, 1019 Buenos Aires, Argentina.

Rovafarm, Arg. See *Sidus, Arg.*

Rovi, Spain. Rovi, Julian Camarillo 35, 28037 Madrid, Spain.

Rowa, Canad. See *Anglo-French Laboratories, Canad.*

Rowa, Eire. Rowa Pharmaceuticals Ltd, Bantry, Co. Cork, Eire.

Rowa, S.Afr. See *Holpro, S.Afr.*

Rowa-Wagner, Ger. Rowa-Wagner KG, Arzneimittelfabrik, Frankenforster Strasse 77, Postfach: 100556, 5060 Bergisch Gladbach 1, W. Germany.

Rowell, USA. See *Reid-Rowell, USA.*

Roxane, USA. Roxane Laboratories Inc., 330 Oak St, Columbus OH 43216, USA.

Roy, Canad. C.A. Roy Ltd, 330 Marwood Dr., Oshawa, Ontario L1H 8B4, Canada.

R.P. Drugs, UK. R.P. Drugs Ltd, R.P.D. House, Yorkdale Industrial Park, Braithwaite St, Leeds LS11 9XE, England.

RP-LABO, Fr. RP-LABO, 6 rue Beffroi, 92200 Neuilly-sur-Seine, France.

Rubio, Spain. Rubio, Berlines 39, 08022 Barcelona, Spain.

Rudolphs, Swed. Rudolphs Kemiska Fabrik HB, Setterwalls Vag 7, 131 36 Nacka, Sweden.

Rugby, USA. Rugby Laboratories Inc., 20 Nassau Ave, Rockville Center, New York NY 11570, USA.

Russ, USA. Russ Pharmaceuticals Inc., P.O. Box 20507, Birmingham AL 35216, USA.

Rutin Products, UK. Rutin Products Ltd, 10 Central Ave, Airfield Estate, Pocklington, York YO4 2NR, England.

Rybar, UK. Rybar Laboratories Ltd, 30 Sycamore Rd, Amersham, Bucks HP6 5DR, England.

Rycovet, UK. Rycovet Ltd, 127 Houldsworth St, Glasgow G3 8JT, Scotland.

Rydelle, USA. Rydelle Laboratories Inc., Subsidiary of S.C. Johnson & Son Inc., 1525 Howe St, Racine WI 53403, USA.

Rystan, USA. Rystan Co. Inc., 47 Center Ave, P.O. Box 214, Little Falls NJ 07424, USA.

S & B, Neth. See *Multi-Pharma, Neth.*

S. Chobet, Arg. Soubeiran Chobet S.R.L., Iberó 5055, 1431 Buenos Aires, Argentina.

Saarstickstoff-Fatol, Ger. Saarstickstoff-Fatol GmbH, Robert-Koch-Strasse, Postfach: 12 60, 6685 Schiffweiler, W. Germany.

Saarstickstoff-Fatol, S.Afr. See *Script Intal, S.Afr.*

Saba, Ital. Saba, Via Salbertrand 21, 10146 Turin, Italy.

Sabater, Spain. J. Sabater, Los Centelles 7, 46006 Valencia, Spain.

Sabex, Canad. Sabex International (1980) Ltd, 977 boul. Pierre-Duprey, Longueuil, Quebec J4K 1A1, Canada.

Sagitta, Ger. Sagitta Arzneimittel GmbH, Frühlingstrasse 7, Postfach: 1262, 8152 Feldkirchen, W. Germany.

Sainsbury, UK. J. Sainsbury PLC, Stamford House, Stamford St, London SE1 9LL, England.

Salf, Ital. Salf Laboratorio Farmacologico s.p.a., Via G. d'Alzano 12, 24100 Bergamo, Italy.

Salfa, Ital. Salfa, Biochimici dr. Ferranti s.a.s., Piazza Rosselli 2, 60100 Ancona, Italy.

Salmon, Switz. Salmon Pharma GmbH, St. Jakobs-Strasse 96, Case postale, 4002 Basel, Switzerland.

Salmond & Spraggon, Austral. Salmond & Spraggon (Aust) Pty Ltd, 14 Loyalty Rd, North Rocks NSW 2151, Australia.

Salsbury, UK. Salsbury Laboratories, Animal Health Division, Solvay House, Flanders Rd, Hedge End, Southampton SO3 4QH, England.

Salt, UK. Salt & Son Ltd, 220 Corporation St, Birmingham B4 6QR, England.

Salud, Spain. Salud, La Explanada 8, 28040 Madrid, Spain.

Salus, Ital. Salus Researches, Sarm s.p.a., Via Aurelia 58, 00165 Rome, Italy.

Salusa, S.Afr. Salusa (Pty) Ltd, Private Bag X516, Silverton 0127, S. Africa.

Salushaus, Ger. Salus-Haus Dr. med. Otto Greither, Inh. Otto Greither, Bahnhofstrasse 24, Postfach: 1180, 8206 Bruckmuhl/Mangfall (Obb.), Germany.

Salvat, Spain. Salvat, Gallo 30, Esplugas de Llobregat, 08950 Barcelona, Spain.

Samil, Ital. Samil s.p.a., Via Gerano 5, 00156 Rome, Italy.

San Carlo, Ital. S. Carlo Farmaceutici s.p.a., Tor Maggiore, 00040 S. Palomba Pomezia (Rome), Italy.

San Roque, Arg. Linea San Roque, Dupomar Esp. Med., Luis Belaustegui 2957, 1416 Buenos Aires, Argentina.

Sanal, Switz. Laboratorium Sanal, Warlin, Philippe & Cie, Leimenstrasse 57, 4011 Basel, Switzerland.

Sanbolagen, Swed. San-bolagen AB, Box 839, 201 80 Malmo, Sweden.

Sanders-Probel, Belg. Sanders-Probel S.A., rue H. Wafelaerts 47/51, 1060 Brussels, Belgium.

Sandersons, UK. Sandersons (Chemists) Ltd, 37 Oakwood Rise, Heaton, Bolton BL1 5EE, England.

Sandoz, Arg. Sandoz Argentina S.A.I.C., Hipolito Yrigoyen 1628 14° Piso, 1344 Buenos Aires, Argentina.

Sandoz, Aust. Sandoz GmbH, Brunnerstrasse 59, Objekt 4, 1235 Wien-Liesing, Austria.

Sandoz, Austral. Sandoz Australia Pty Ltd, P.O. Box 101, North Ryde NSW 2113, Australia.

Sandoz, Canad. Sandoz Canada Inc., 385 Bouchard Blvd, Dorval, Quebec H9S 1A9, Canada.

Sandoz, Denm. Sandoz A.S., Titangade 9 A, 2200 Copenhagen N, Denmark.

Sandoz, Eire. Sandoz Products (Ireland) Ltd, Airton Rd, Off Greenhills Rd, Tallaght, Co. Dublin, Eire.

Sandoz, Fr. Laboratoires Sandoz S.A.R.L., 14 blvd Richelieu, 92500 Rueil-Malmaison, France.

Sandoz, Ger. Sandoz AG, Deutschherrnstrasse 15, 8500 Nürnberg, W. Germany.

Sandoz, Greece. Sandoz (Hellas) S.A.C.I., 57 rue Deligiorgi, Place Karaiskaki, Athens 107, Greece.

Sandoz, Ital. Sandoz Prodotti Farmaceutici s.p.a., Via C. Arconati 1, 20135 Milan, Italy.

Sandoz, Neth. Sandoz B.V., Loopkantstraat 25, 5405 AC Uden, Netherlands.

Sandoz, Norw. Sandoz-informasjon, Økernveien 121, Boks 237 Økern, 0510 Oslo 5, Norway.

Sandoz, NZ. Sandoz Pharma Ltd, P.O. Box 56-055, Dominion Rd, Auckland 3, New Zealand.

Sandoz, S.Afr. Sandoz Products (Pty) Ltd, P.O. Box 50371, Randburg 2125, S. Africa.

Sandoz, Spain. Sandoz, Gran Via Corts Catalanes 764, 08013 Barcelona, Spain.

Sandoz, Swed. Sandoz AB, Box 122, 183 22 Täby, Sweden.

Sandoz, Switz. Sandoz Produkte (Schweiz) SA, Missionsstrasse 60/62, 4012 Basel, Switzerland.

Sandoz, UK. Sandoz Products Ltd, Sandoz House, 98 The Centre, Feltham, Middx TW13 4EP, England.

Sandoz, USA. Sandoz Pharmaceuticals, Division of Sandoz Inc., Route 10, East Hanover NJ 07936, USA.

Sandoz Agrochem, UK. Sandoz Agrochem, Norwich Union House, 16-18 Princes St, Ipswich IP1 1QT, England.

Sandoz Nutrition, USA. Clinical Nutrition Division, Sandoz Nutrition Corp., 5320 West 23rd St, P.O. Box 370, Minneapolis MN 55440, USA.

Sandoz-Wander, Belg. Sandoz S.A., chaussee de Haecht 226, 1030 Brussels, Belgium.

Sands, Canad. Sands Pharmaceuticals, Division of Novopharm Ltd, 575 Hood Rd, Markham, Ontario L3R 4E1, Canada.

Sanico, Belg. Sanico S.A., Industrieterrein, Veedijk 4, 2300 Turnhout, Belgium.

Sanitas, Arg. Sanitas Argentina S.A., Teodoro Vilardebó 2855/65, 1417 Buenos Aires, Argentina.

Sanitas, Ital. Lab. Chim. Farm. Sanitas, Via Tanzi 39/D, 70121 Bari, Italy.

Sankyo, Jpn. Sankyo, 2-7-12 Ginza, Chuo-ku, Tokyo, Japan.

Sanofi, Denm. See *Meda, Denm.*

Sanofi, Philipp. See *Zuellig, Philipp.*

Sanofi, Switz. Sanofi Pharma SA, Case postale, 4002 Basel, Switzerland.

Sanofi, UK. Sanofi UK Ltd, Floats Rd, Wythenshawe, Manchester M23 9NF, England.

Sanofi Labaz, Neth. Sanofi Labaz, Govert van Wijnkade 48, 3144 EG Maassluis, Netherlands.

Sanofi Midy, Neth. Sanofi Midy, Govert van Wijnkade 48, 3144 EG Maassluis, Netherlands.

Sanol, Ger. Sanol GmbH, Mittelstrasse 11-13, Postfach: 100662, 4019 Monheim, W. Germany.

Sanol Schwarz, UK. Schwarz Pharmaceuticals Ltd, East St, Chesham, Bucks HP5 1DG, England.

Sanorania, Ger. Sanorania, Dr Gerhard Strohscheer, Düsterhauptstrasse 30, 1000 Berlin 28, W. Germany.

Sanorania, Switz. See *Medipharm, Switz.*

Santen, Jpn. Santen Seiyaku, 3-9-19 Shimoshinjyo, Higashiyodogawa-ku, Osaka, Japan.

Santiveri, Spain. Santiveri, Troquel 8, 08004 Barcelona, Spain.

Santos, Spain. Santos, Regalada 5, 28007 Madrid, Spain.

Saphar, S.Afr. See *Adcock Ingram, S.Afr.*

Sapos, Neth. See *Roussel, Neth.*

Sapos, Switz. Sapos S.A., rue G. Moynier 5, Case postale 762, 1211 Geneva 1, Switzerland.

Sarbach, Fr. See *L.T.M., Fr.*

Sarbach, Switz. See *Duphar, Switz.*

Sarein, Fr. See *Vaillant-Defresne, Fr.*

Sarep, Belg. See *de Bournonville, Belg.*

Sarep-Pharmeurop, Fr. See *Pharmeurop, Fr.*

Sarget, Fr. Laboratoires Sarget, ave J.-F. Kennedy, 33701 Mérignac, France.

Sarget, Spain. Sarget, Avda de Fuentemar 25 (Plg Ind.), Coslada, 28820 Madrid, Spain.

Sarm, Ital. Sarm s.r.l., Soc. An. Ritrovati Medicinali, Via Tiburtina Km 18,300, 00012 Guidonia (Rome), Italy.

Saron, USA. Saron Pharmacal Corporation, 1640 Central Ave, St Petersburg FL 33712, USA.

Sarva, Belg. See *Sarva-Syntex, Belg.*

Sarva, Neth. Sarva-Syntex Nederland, Limpergstraat 4, 2288 AD Rijswijk, Netherlands.

Sarva-Syntex, Belg. Sarva-Syntex S.A., av. Louise 326/bte 48, 1050 Brussels, Belgium.

Sas, UK. Sas Pharmaceuticals Ltd, Sas Group House, 45 Wycombe End, Beaconsfield, Bucks HP9 1LZ, England.

Sasse, Ger. Dr Friedrich Sasse, Zweigniederlassung der Gödecke AG Berlin, Mooswaldallee 1-9, Postfach: 569, 7800 Freiburg, W. Germany.

Sauba, Fr. Laboratoires Sauba, 260 rue de Rosny, 93104 Montreuil, France.

Sauflon, UK. Sauflon Pharmaceuticals Ltd, 16 Childs Place, London SW5 9RX, England.

Saunier-Daguin, Belg. See *de Bournonville, Belg.*

Saunier-Daguin, Fr. Laboratoires Saunier-Daguin, 89 rue Lauriston, 75116 Paris, France.

Sauter, Austral. See *Roche, Austral.*

Sauter, Switz. Lab. Sauter S.A., Case postale 224, 1211 Geneva 28, Switzerland.

Savage, USA. Savage Laboratories, Division of Byk-Gulden Inc., 60 Baylis Road, P.O. Box 2006, Melville NY 11747, USA.

Savio, Ital. Istituto Biochimico Nazionale Savio s.p.a., Via E. Bazzano 14, 16019 Ronco Scrivia (GE), Italy.

Savoma, Ital. Savoma Medicinali s.p.a., Via Baganza 2, 43100 Parma, Italy.

Savory & Moore, UK. Savory & Moore Ltd, 31 Hockliffe St, Leighton Buzzard LU7 8EZ, England.

Savoy Laboratories, UK. Savoy Laboratories (International) Ltd, Prosper House, 146-154 Kilburn High Rd, London NW6, England.

Sawai, Jpn. Sawai Seiyaku, 1-4-25 Akagawa, Higashi-ku, Osaka, Japan.

SBL, Swed. Statens bakteriologiska laboratorium, 105 21 Stockholm, Sweden.

SCA, Ital. Stablimento Chimici dell'Adda s.p.a., Via G. Ripamonti 89, 20139 Milan, Italy.

Scania, Swed. Scania Dental AB, Box 5, 741 00 Knivsta, Sweden.

S.C.A.T., Fr. Societe de Conception et d'Applications Therapeutique division Ozothine, 92003 Nanterre Cedex, France.

Schabru, Denm. See *Mediscan, Denm.*

Schaper & Brümmer, Ger. Schaper & Brümmer GmbH & Co. KG, Bahnhofstrasse 35, Postfach: 61 1160, 3320 Salzgitter 61 (Ringelheim), W. Germany.

Scharper, Ital. Scharper s.p.a., Via Fabio Filzi 41, 20124 Milan, Italy.

Schattner, USA. The R. Schattner Co., Pharmaceutical Division, 4000 Massachusetts Ave NW, Washington DC 20016, USA.

Schein, USA. Schein Pharmaceutical Inc., 5 Harbor Park Dr., Port Washington NY 11050, USA.

Scherag, S.Afr. Scherag (Pty) Ltd, P.O. Box 46, Isando 1600, S. Africa.

Scherax, Ger. Scherax Arzneimittel GmbH, Elbchaussee 336, D-2000 Hamburg 52, Germany.

Scherer, Canad. R.P. Scherer (Canada), Division of R.P. Scherer Hardcapsule Ltd, P.O. Box 2370, Windsor, Ontario N8Y 4S2, Canada.

Scherer, Ital. R.P. Scherer s.p.a., Via Nettunese Km. 20,100, 04011 Aprilia (Latina), Italy.

Scherer, Neth. See *Medicosma, Neth.*

Scherer, USA. Scherer Laboratories Inc., 14335 Gills Rd, P.O. Drawer 400009, Dallas TX 75240, USA.

Schering, Arg. Schering Argentina S.A.I.C., Monroe 1378, 28 Buenos Aires, Argentina.

Schering, Austral. Schering Pty Ltd, 9-10 Wood St, Tempe NSW 2044, Australia.

Schering, Belg. Schering S.A., J.E. Mommaertslaan 14 B.P.8, 1920 Machelen, Belgium.

Schering, Canad. Schering Canada Inc., 3535 Trans-Canada, Pointe Claire, Quebec H9R 1B4, Canada.

Schering, Denm. Schering AS, Fjeldhammervej 8, 2610 Rodovre, Denmark.

Schering, Fr. Schering, rue de Toufflers, B.P. 69, 59452 Lys-lez-Lannoy, France.

Schering, Ger. Schering AG, Müllerstrasse 170, Postfach: 650311, 1000 Berlin 65, W. Germany.

Schering, Ital. Schering s.p.a., Via Cassanese ang. V. Marconi, 20090 Segrate (MI), Italy.

Schering, Neth. Schering Nederland B.V., Flevolaan 28, 1382 JZ Weesp, Netherlands.

Schering, Norw. See *Schering AG, Norw.* and *Sentipharm, Norw.*

Schering, NZ. See *Essex, NZ.*

Schering, S.Afr. See *Berlimed, S.Afr.*

Schering, Spain. Schering, Mendez Alvaro 55, 28045 Madrid, Spain.

Schering, Swed. See *Essex, Swed.* and *Schering Nordiska, Swed.*

Schering, Switz. Schering Zürich SA, Case postale, 8010 Zurich, Switzerland.

Schering, UK. Schering Health Care Ltd, The Brow, Burgess Hill, West Sussex RH15 9NE, England.

Schering, USA. Schering Corporation, Galloping Hill Rd, Kenilworth NJ 07033, USA.

Schering AG, Norw. Schering Norsk A/S,, Gamle Drammensv. 48, Postboks 180, 1321 Stabekk, Norway.

Schering AG, NZ. Schering (NZ) Ltd, P.O. Box 65-051, Auckland 10, New Zealand.

Schering Corp., Denm. See *Essex, Denm.*

Schering Nordiska, Swed. Schering Nordiska AB, Box 152, 131 06 Nacka, Sweden.

Schering-Prebbles, UK. Schering-Prebbles Ltd, Schering Hospital Supplies Division, The Brow, Burgess Hill, West Sussex RH15 9NE, England.

Scheurich, Ger. E. Scheurich, Pharmwerk GmbH, Strassburger Strasse 77, Postfach: 1140, 7604 Appenweier, W. Germany.

Schiapparelli, Ital. Schiapparelli Farmaceutici s.p.a., P.za Duca D'Aosta 12, 20124 Milan, Italy.

Schieffer, Neth. See *Nicholas, Neth.*

Schieffer, S.Afr. See *Nattermann, S.Afr.*

Schiwa, Ger. Schiwa GmbH, Averfehrdener Str. 57, Postfach: 1180, 4519 Glandorf, Germany.

Schmid, USA. Schmid Products Co., Division of Schmid Laboratories Inc., Route 46 West, Little Falls NJ 07424, USA.

Schmidgall, Switz. See *Iromedica, Switz.*

Schmidt, Neth. C.N. Schmidt B.V., Jan Rebelstraat 8, 1069 CB Amsterdam, Netherlands.

Scholl, UK. Scholl (UK), 182 St John St, London EC1P 1DH, England.

Schönenberger, Switz. H. Schönenberger & Cie SA, Case postale, 5037 Muhen bei Aarau, Switzerland.

Schoum, Fr. Laboratoires Schoum, 38 rue de Silly, 92100 Boulogne, France.

Schoum, Spain. Schoum, Escolta Real 32, San Sebastian, 20008 Guipuzcoa, Spain.

Schulke & Mayr, Ger. Schulke & Mayr GmbH Applikationshilfen, Postfach: 630230, 2000 Hamburg 63, Germany.

Schur, Ger. Schur Pharmazeutika GmbH & Co. KG, Emanuel-Leutze-Strasse 1, 4000 Dusseldorf 11, Germany.

Schur, Switz. See *Panpharma, Switz.*

Schürholz, Ger. Schürholz Arzneimittel GmbH, Fritz-Berne-Strasse 47, Postfach: 600761, 8000 Munich 60, W. Germany.

Schwab, Ger. Dr Schwab GmbH, Berg-am-Laim-Strasse 129, Postfach: 801507, 8000 Munich 80, W. Germany.

Schwabe, Ger. Dr Willmar Schwabe GmbH & Co., Willmar-Schwabe-Strasse 4, Postfach: 410925, 7500 Karlsruhe 41, W. Germany.

Schwabe, Neth. See *VSM, Neth.*

Schwabe-Farmasan, Ger. Dr. Willmar Schwabe GmbH & Co., Abt Farmasan Arzneimittel, Pforzheimer Str. 5, Postfach: 410440, 7500 Karlsruhe 41, Germany.

Schwarz, Belg. See *Byk, Belg.*

Schwarz, Ger. Schwarz-Pharma GmbH, Mittelstrasse 11, Postfach: 100662, 4019 Monheim, W. Germany.

Schwarz, Ital. Schwarz Italia s.p.a., Via Emilia 99, 20075 S. Grato-Lodi (MI), Italy.

Schwarz, Switz. Schwarz AG, Industriestrasse 7, 4410 Liestal, Switzerland.

Schwarzhaupt, Ger. Schwarzhaupt KG, GmbH & Co., Sachsenring 37, 5000 Cologne 1, W. Germany.

Schwarzhaupt, Neth. See *van Oven, Neth.*

Schweiz. Serum & Impfinstitut, Switz. Schweiz. Serum & Impfinstitut, Postfach 2707, 3001 Bern, Switzerland.

Schwulst, S.Afr. Geo Schwulst Laboratories (Pty) Ltd, P.O. Box 38481, Booysens 2016, S. Africa.

Scientific Hospital Supplies, Denm. See *Meda, Denm.*

Scientific Hospital Supplies, UK. Scientific Hopsital Supplies Ltd, 38 Queensland St, Liverpool L7 3JG, England.

Sclavo, Ital. Sclavo s.p.a., Via Fiorentina 1, 53100 Siena, Italy.

Sclavo, USA. Sclavo Inc., 5 Mansard Court, Wayne NJ 07470, USA.

Scot-Tussin, USA. Scot-Tussin Pharmacal Co. Inc., 50 Clemence St, P.O. Box 8217, Cranston RI 02920-0217, USA.

Scotia, UK. Scotia Pharmaceutical Products, 558 Cathcart Rd, Glasgow G42 8YG, Scotland.

Script Intal, S.Afr. See *Propan, S.Afr.*

SCS, S.Afr. SCS Pharmalab (Pty) Ltd (Member of The Noristan Group), Private Bag X516, Silverton 0127, S. Africa.

SCT, Ital. S.C.T. s.n.c. di G. Boccheni & C., Via Liberta 21, 10095 Grugliasco (TO), Italy.

Seaford, UK. Seaford Laboratories Ltd, Cradle Hill Industrial Estate, Seaford, Sussex BN25 3JE, England.

Seamless Hosp. Prod., USA. Seamless Hospital Products Co., Division of Dart Industries, P.O. Box 828, Barnes Industrial Park, Wallingford CT 06492, USA.

Searle, Arg. Searle Argentina S.A.C.I., Pedro Echague 2437, 1261 Buenos Aires, Argentina.

Searle, Austral. Searle Australia Pty Ltd, P.O. Box 1380, Crows Nest NSW 2065, Australia.

Searle, Belg. Lab. Searle S.A., Digue du Canal 112-3, 1070 Brussels, Belgium.

Searle, Canad. G.D. Searle and Co. of Canada Ltd, 400 Iroquois Shore Rd, Oakville, Ontario L6H 1M5, Canada.

Searle, Denm. G.D. Searle A/S, H.C. Ørstedsvej 4, 5., 1879 Frederiksberg C, Denmark.

Searle, Fr. Laboratoires Searle, 7 blvd Romain-Rolland, 92128 Montrouge, France.

Searle, Ger. G.D. Searle GmbH, Philipp-Reis-Str. 14, Postfach: 102048, 6072 Dreieich, W. Germany.

Searle, Ital. Searle Italia s.p.a., Via L. da Vinci 1, 20090 Trezzano S/N (MI), Italy.

Searle, Mex. Searle de Mexico S.A.deC.V., Calzada del Hueso No. 859, Mexico 22 D.F., Mexico.

Searle, Neth. Searle Farmaca, Pampuslaan 1, 1382 JM Weesp, Netherlands.

Searle, Norw. Searle Norge A/S, Trondheimsvn. 137, Postboks 6594 Rodeløkka, 0501 Oslo 5, Norway.

Searle, S.Afr. G.D. Searle (SA) (Pty) Ltd, P.O. Box 391157, Bramley 2018, S. Africa.

Searle, Spain. Searle Iberica, La Granja 23 (Plg Ind), Alcobendas, 28100 Madrid, Spain.

Searle, Swed. G.D. Searle AB, Sodra Forstadsgatan 34, 211 43 Malmo, Sweden.

Searle, Switz. Searle SA, 1170 Aubonne, Switzerland.

Searle, UK. Searle Pharmaceuticals, P.O. Box 53, Lane End Rd, High Wycombe, Bucks HP12 4HL, England.

Searle, USA. G.D. Searle & Co., 4901 Searle Pkwy, Skokie IL 60077, USA.

Seatrace, USA. The Seatrace Co., P.O. Box 363, Gadsden AL 35902, USA.

Seaway Midwest, Canad. Seaway Midwest Ltd, 1255 Fewster Dr., Mississauga, Ontario L4W 1A3, Canada.

Seber, Spain. See *Sigma Tau, Spain.*

Seclo, Fr. Laboratoires Seclo, 3 Impasse Dumur, 92110 Clichy, France.

Sedaph, Fr. See *Pharmuka, Fr.*

Sedifa, Mon. Sedifa, Le Thales, rue du Stade, MC 98000 Monaco, Monaco.

Seid, Spain. Seid, Ctra. Sabadell Granollers Km 15, Llissa de Vall, 08185 Barcelona, Spain.

Selena, Swed. Selena Lakemedel AB, Torggatan 15, 171 54 Solna, Sweden.

Sella, Ital. Sella A. Lab. Chim. Farm. s.r.l., Via Vicenza 2, 36015 Schio (Vicenza), Italy.

Selvi, Ital. Selvi 3M s.p.a., Via Gallarate 184, 20151 Milan, Italy.

Selvi, S.Afr. See *Vernleigh, S.Afr.*

Semar, Spain. Semar, Padilla 353-5, 08025 Barcelona, Spain.

Semper, Norw. See *Collett, Norw.*

Sempio, Ital. Farmaceutici Sempio, Via Nino Bixio 1, 21040 Carnago (VA), Italy.

Senju, Jpn. Senju Seiyaku, 3-6-1 Hirano-cho, Higashi-ku, Osaka, Japan.

Sentipharm, Norw. Sentipharm AG, Informasjonsavdelingen Norge, Aslakvn. 14, 0753 Oslo 7, Norway.

Septa, Spain. Septa, Arroyo de la Elipa 9, 28017 Madrid, Spain.

Serag-Wiessner, Ger. Serag-Wiessner GmbH & Co. KG, Kugelfang 8-12, Postfach: 1150, 8674 Naila, Germany.

Seres, USA. Seres Laboratories Inc., 3331 Industrial Dr., P.O. Box 470, Santa Rosa CA 95402, USA.

Serono, Arg. Serono de Argentina S.A., Santiago del Estero 2455/85, 1640 Martinez, Buenos Aires, Argentina.

Serono, Belg. See *Zyma-Galen, Belg.*

Serono, Denm. See *Anderson, Denm.*

Serono, Fr. Laboratoires Serono, 84 rue Edouard-Vaillant, 92300 Levallois-Perret, France.

Serono, Ger. Serono Pharm. Praparate GmbH, Merzhauserstr. 134, 7800 Freiburg, W.Germany.

Serono, Hong Kong. See *Globechem, Hong Kong.*

Serono, Ital. Industria Farmaceutica Serono s.p.a., Via Casilina 125, 00176 Rome, Italy.

Serono, Neth. See *Pharma-Import, Neth.*

Serono, S.Afr. See *Script Intal, S.Afr.*

Serono, Spain. Serono, Pedro IV, 78, 08005 Barcelona, Spain.

Serono, Swed. Svenska AB Serono, Box 22114, 104 22 Stockholm, Sweden.

Serono, Switz. Laboratoires Serono SA, Frobenstrasse 55, 4053 Basel, Switzerland.

Serono, UK. Serono Laboratories (UK) Ltd, 2 Tewin Court, Welwyn Garden City, Herts AL7 1AU, England.

Serono, USA. Serono Laboratories Inc., 280 Pond St, Randolph MA 02368, USA.

Serono O.T.C., Ital. Serono O.T.C. s.p.a., Piazzetta M. Bossi 3, 20121 Milan, Italy.

Serozym, Fr. Laboratoires Serozym, 30 rue Armand-Silvestre, 92400 Courbevoie, France.

Serpero, Ital. Serpero, Industria Galenica Milanese s.p.a., Viale L. Maino 40, 20129 Milan, Italy.

Serra Pamies, Spain. Serra Pamies, Ctra de Castellvell s/n, Reus, 43206 Tarragona, Spain.

Serravallo, Ital. J.Serravallo s.n.c., Via del Cerreto 20, 34136 Trieste Barcola, Italy.

Serum, Switz. Serum SA, 20 rue de la Coulouvrenière, 1204 Geneva, Switzerland.

Servier, Austral. Servier Laboratories (Aust.) Pty Ltd, P.O. Box 196, Hawthorne Vic. 3122, Australia.

Servier, Belg. Servier Benelux S.A., bd E. Bockstael 93, 1020 Brussels, Belgium.

Servier, Canad. Servier Canada Inc., 2155 rue Guy, Suite 1120, Montreal, Quebec H3H 2L9, Canada.

Servier, Denm. See *Armedic, Denm.*

Servier, Fr. Laboratoires Servier, 45400 Gidy, France.

Servier, Ital. Servier Italia s.p.a., Via degli Aldobrandeschi 13, 00163 Rome, Italy.

Servier, Neth. Servier Nederland B.V., Storkstraat 5, 2722 NN Zoetermeer, Netherlands.

Servier, S.Afr. Servier Laboratories (SA) (Pty) Ltd, P.O. Box 39493, Bramley 2018, S. Africa.

Servier, Spain. Servier, Avda. de Madronos 33, 28043 Madrid, Spain.

Servier, Switz. Servier S.A., rue Hugo de Senger 10, 1205 Geneva, Switzerland.

Servier, UK. Servier Laboratories Ltd, Fulmer Hall, Windmill Rd, Fulmer, Slough, Bucks SL3 6HH, England.

Servipharm, Switz. Servipharm SA, Case postale, 4002 Basel, Switzerland.

Sestri, UK. Sestri (Sales) Ltd, Kingsend House, 44 Kingsend, Ruislip, Middx HA4 7DA, England.

Seton, Swed. See *Smith & Nephew Scandinavia, Swed.*

Seton, UK. Seton Products Ltd, Tubiton House, Medlock St, Oldham, Lancs OL1 3HS, England.

Seven Seas, UK. Seven Seas Health Care Ltd, Marfleet, Kingston-Upon-Hull HU9 5NJ, England.

Sévenet, Fr. Laboratoires Sévenet, 8 rue de Choiseul, 75002 Paris, France.

Sharpe, Austral. Sharpe Laboratories Pty Ltd, P.O. Box 432, Artarmon NSW 2064, Australia.

Shear/Kershman, USA. Shear/Kershman Laboratories Inc., 14500 South Outer 40 Rd, Chesterfield MO 63017, USA.

Shell Chemicals, UK. Shell Chemicals UK Ltd, 1 Northumberland Ave, Trafalgar Square, London WC2N 5LA, England.

Shionogi, Jpn. Shionogi Seiyaku, 3-12 Doshomachi, Higashi-ku, Osaka, Japan.

Shire, UK. Shire Pharmaceuticals Ltd, 13-17 Bridge St, Andover, Hants SP10 1BE, England.

Sidel, Fr. Laboratoires Sidel, 12 av. Ste-Anne, 92609 Asnieres, France.

Sidmak, USA. Sidmak, USA.

Sidus, Arg. Sidus S.A., Larrea 926, 1117 Buenos Aires, Argentina.

Siegfried, Belg. See *Triosol, Belg.*

Siegfried, Ger. Siegfried GmbH, Fabrik für chemisch-pharmazeutische Produkte, Mumpfer Fährstrasse 68, Postfach: 1141, 7880 Bad Säckingen, W. Germany.

Siegfried, Switz. Siegfried SA, département Pharma, 4800 Zofingen, Switzerland.

Sifarma, Ital. Sifarma s.r.l., Via N.A. Porpora 132, 20131 Milan, Italy.

SIFI, Ital. Società Industria Farmaceutica Italiana s.p.a., Via N. Coviello 15/B, 95128 Catania, Italy.

SIFRA, Ital. Societa Italiana Farmaceutici Ravizza s.p.a., Via Camagre 41/43, 37063 Isola della Scala (VR), Italy.

Sigamed, Switz. Sigamed SA, 4800 Zofingen, Switzerland.

Sigma, Austral. Sigma Pharmaceuticals Pty Ltd, P.O. Box 144, Clayton Vic. 3168, Australia.

Sigma, UK. Sigma Chemical Co. Ltd, Fancy Rd, Poole, Dorset BH17 7NH, England.

Sigma Tau, Spain. Sigma Tau, Pl. Ind. Azque, Parcelas 13-4, Alcala de Henares, 28013 Madrid, Spain.

Sigmatau, Ital. Sigma Tau s.p.a., Via Pontina Km. 30.400, 00040 Pomezia, Italy.

Sigma-Tau, USA. Sigma-Tau Inc., 723 North Beers St, Holmdel NJ 07733, USA.

Sigurtà, Ital. Sigurtà s.r.l., Viale Certosa 210, 20156 Milan, Italy.

Simanite, Austral. Simanite Medical Preparations, William Pearce & Co. Pty Ltd, P.O. Box 69, Strawberry Hills NSW 2012, Australia.

Simcare, UK. Simcare, Peter Rd, Lancing, West Sussex BN15 8TJ, England.

Simes, Austral. Simes (Aust) Pty Ltd, 5 George St, Stepney SA 5069, Australia.

Simes, Ital. Simes s.p.a., Via della Chimica 9, 37100 Vicenza, Italy.

Simpkin, UK. A.L. Simpkin & Co. Ltd, Pharmaceutical Laboratories, Hunter Rd, Sheffield S6 4LD, England.

Simpla, UK. Simpla Plastics Ltd, Phoenix Estate, Caerphilly Rd, Cardiff CF4 4XG, Wales.

Sinbio, Fr. Laboratoires Sinbio, Pierre Fabre Medicament, 192 rue Lecoubre, 75015 Paris, France.

Sinclair, UK. Sinclair Pharmaceuticals Ltd, Borough Rd, Godalming, Surrey GU7 2AB, England.

Singer, Neth. The Singer Import B.V., Ambachtsweg 22, 3831 KB Leusden, Netherlands.

Sintesa, Belg. Sintesa S.A., chaussee d'Alsemberg 1001, 1180 Brussels, Belgium.

Sintetica, Switz. Sintetica S.A., San Martino, 6850 Mendrisio, Switzerland.

Sintyal, Arg. Sintyal Chemotécnica S.A., Carlos Berg 3669, 1437 Buenos Aires, Argentina.

Sis-Ter, Ital. Sis-Ter, Sistemi Terapeutici S.p.A., Via Crema 8, 26020 Palazzo Pignano (CR), Italy.

Sisu, Canad. Sisu Enterprises Ltd, 6-1734 West Broadway, Vancouver, British Columbia V6J 1Y1, Canada.

SIT, Ital. Specialità Igienico Terapeutiche s.p.a., C.so Cavour 70, 27035 Mede (Pavia), Italy.

SK & F, Swed. See *Smith Kline & French, Swed.*

Skelskor, Denm. Skaelskor Frugtplantage A/S, 4230 Skaelskor, Denmark.

Smaller, Spain. Smaller, Azcona 25, 28028 Madrid, Spain.

SMB, Belg. Lab. S.M.B.-Galephar S.A., rue de la Pastorale 26-28, 1080 Brussels, Belgium.

Smith, USA. Smith Laboratories Inc., 2211 Sanders Rd, P.O. Box 3044, Northbrook IL 60062, USA.

Smith & Hill, UK. Smith & Hill (Chemists) Ltd, P.O. Box 110, Cresswell Rd, Darnell, Sheffield S9 4LZ, England.

Smith & Nephew, Austral. Smith & Nephew (Australia) Pty Ltd, P.O. Box 150, Clayton Vic. 3168, Australia.

Smith & Nephew, Canad. Smith & Nephew Inc., 2100 52e Ave, Lanchine, Quebec H8T 2Y5, Canada.

Smith & Nephew, Denm. Smith & Nephew Scandinavia A/S, Naerum Hovedgade 2, 2850 Naerum, Denmark.

Smith & Nephew, Neth. See *Bournonville, Neth.*

Smith & Nephew, Norw. See *Weiders, Norw.*

Smith & Nephew, S.Afr. Smith & Nephew Pharmaceuticals (Pty) Ltd, P.O. Box 92, Pinetown 3600, S.Africa.

Smith & Nephew, Swed. See *Meda, Swed.*

Smith & Nephew, UK. Smith & Nephew Medical Ltd, P.O. Box 81, 101 Hessle Rd, Hull HU3 2BN, England.

Smith & Nephew Pharmaceuticals, UK. Smith & Nephew Pharmaceuticals Ltd, Bampton Rd, Harold Hill, Romford, Essex RM3 8SL, England.

Smith & Nephew Scandinavia, Swed. Smith & Nephew Scandinavia AB, Box 2365, 403 16 Goteborg, Sweden.

Smith & Walker, UK. Smith & Walker Ltd, Linby St, Bulwell, Nottingham, England.

Smith Kendon, UK. Smith Kendon Ltd, Waterton, Bridgend, Mid Glam CF31 3DJ, Wales.

Smith Kline & French, Arg. See *Essex, Arg.*

Smith Kline & French, Austral. Smith Kline & French Laboratories (Australia) Ltd, P.O. Box 90, Brookvale NSW 2100, Australia.

Smith Kline & French, Canad. Smith Kline & French Canada Ltd, 1940 Argentia Rd, Mississauga, Ontario L5N 2V7, Canada.

Smith Kline & French, Denm. Smith Kline & French, Bygning O Wilders Plads, 1403 Copenhagen K, Denmark.

Smith Kline & French, Fr. Laboratoires Smith Kline & French, 12 place de la Defense Cedex 26, 92090 Paris-La Defense, France.

Smith Kline & French, Ital. Smith Kline & French s.p.a., Viale Ortles 12, 20139 Milan, Italy.

Smith Kline & French, Neth. Smith Kline & French B.V., Jaagpad 1, 2288 AB Rijswijk, Netherlands.

Smith Kline & French, Norw. Smith Kline & French, Astrids vei 3, 1473 Skårer, Norway.

Smith Kline & French, S.Afr. Smith Kline & French Laboratories, P.O. Box 38, Isando 1600, S. Africa.

Smith Kline & French, Spain. Smith Kline & French, Juan Bravo 3, 28006 Madrid, Spain.

Smith Kline & French, Swed. Smith Kline & French AB, Box 4092, 171 04 Solna, Sweden.

Smith Kline & French, Switz. Smith Kline & French SA, Obergrundstrasse 70, 6003 Lucerne, Switzerland.

Smith Kline & French, UK. Smith Kline & French Laboratories Ltd, Welwyn Garden City, Herts AL7 1EY, England.

Smith Kline & French, USA. Smith Kline & French Laboratories, Division of SmithKline Beckman Corp., 1500 Spring Garden St, P.O. Box 7929, Philadelphia PA 19101, USA.

Smith Kline Animal Health, UK. Smith Kline Animal Health Ltd, Cavendish Rd, Stevenage, Herts SG1 2EJ, England.

Smith Kline Dauelsberg, Ger. Smith Kline Dauelsberg GmbH, Hildebrandstrasse 10-12, Postfach: 3333, 3400 Gottingen, W. Germany.

Smith Kline-RIT, Belg. Smith Kline-R.I.T. S.A., rue du Tilleul 13, 1320 Genval, Belgium.

SmithKline Diagnostics, USA. SmithKline Diagnostics Inc., A SmithKline Beckman Co., P.O. Box 61947, Sunnyvale CA 94086, USA.

Sobio, Fr. Laboratoires Sobio, 25 blvd de l'Amiral Bruix, 75782 Paris Cedex 16, France.

Sobio, Switz. See *Sodip, Switz.*

Soca, Mon. Laboratoires Soca, 19 av. Crovetto-Freres, Monaco (Pte), Monaco.

Society for Cancer Research, Switz. Society for Cancer Research, Arlesheim, Switzerland.

Sodip, Switz. Sodip S.A., rue Alphonse Large 11, 1217 Meyrin 1, Switzerland.

Soekami, Fr. Laboratoires Soekami Pharmaceutical Research, 94 rue Ed. Vaillant, 92300 Levallois-Perret, France.

Sofar, Ital. Sofar Farmaceutici s.p.a., Via Ramazzini 5, 20129 Milan, Italy.

Sokatarg, Spain. Sokatarg, Ter 16, 08026 Barcelona, Spain.

Solac, Switz. See *Sanofi, Switz.*

Solco, Belg. See *Christiaens, Belg.*

Solco, Ger. Solco GmbH, Pharm. Spezialitäten, Salzwerkstrasse 7, Postfach: 110, 7889 Grenzach-Wyhlen 2, W. Germany.

Solco, Neth. See *Dagra, Neth.*

Solco, Switz. Solco Basel SA, Rührbergstrasse 21, 4127 Birsfelden, Switzerland.

Solgar, USA. Solgar Vitamin Co. Inc., P.O. Box 330, Lynbrook NY 11563, USA.

Solvay, Swed. Solvay Svenska AB, Strandvagen 5A, 114 51 Stockholm, Sweden.

Sopar, Belg. Sopar S.A., rue de Thyle 3a, 6328 Sart-Dames-Avelines, Belgium.

Sopar, Neth. See *Bournonville, Neth.*

Sopharga, Switz. See *Distripharm, Switz.*

Sorel, Ital. Sorel Farmaceutici s.a.s., Via del Corno 10, 40069 Zola Predosa (BO), Italy.

Sorex, UK. Sorex Ltd, St Michael's Industrial Estate, Hale Rd, Widnes, Cheshire WA8 8TJ, England.

Sorin-Maxim, Fr. Laboratoires Sorin-Maxim S.A., 14 rue A-Briand, B.P. 19, 44130 Blain, France.

Southon-Horton, UK. Southon-Horton, England.

SPA, Ital. Società Prodotti Antibiotici s.p.a., Via Biella 8, 20143 Milan, Italy.

Spa, Spain. Spa, Moratin 2, Mataro, 08302 Barcelona, Spain.

Spearhead, UK. Spearhead Ltd, 258 Vauxhall Bridge Rd, London SW1V 1BS, England.

Specia, Fr. Specia S.A., 16 rue Clisson, 75636 Paris Cedex 13, France.

Specia, Neth. See *Rhône-Poulenc, Neth.*

Spedrog-Caillon, Arg. Spedrog Caillon S.A.I.C., Venezuela 1600, 1095 Buenos Aires, Argentina.

Spemsa, Ital. Spemsa, Specialità Medicinali s.p.a., Via G. Garibaldi 80/82, 50041 Calenzano, Italy.

Spencer, UK. Brian G. Spencer Ltd, Common Lane, Fradley, Lichfield, Staffs WS13 8LA, England.

Speywood, UK. Speywood Laboratories Ltd, Ash Rd, Wrexham Industrial Estate, Wrexham, Clwyd, Wales.

Spiphar, Belg. Spiphar S.P.R.L., ave de la Couronne 116, 1050 Brussels, Belgium.

Spirig, Switz. Spirig SA, 4622 Egerkingen, Switzerland.

Spitzner, Ger. W. Spitzner, Arzneimittelfabrik GmbH, Bunsenstrasse 6-10, Postfach: 1654, 7505 Ettlingen, W. Germany.

Spodefell, UK. Spodefell Ltd, 5 Inverness Mews, London W2 3QJ, England.

Spofa, Cz. Spofa, Stare Mesto, Dlouha tr. 11, Prague, Czechoslovakia.

Spraylab, Canad. Spraylab Inc., 3025 mtee Saint-Aubin, Chomedey-Laval, Quebec H7L 4E4, Canada.

Spret-Mauchant, Fr. See *Pharmuka, Fr.*

Springbok, USA. Springbok Pharmaceuticals Inc., 12502 South Garden St, Houston TX 77071, USA.

Spyfarma, Spain. Spyfarma, Ctra Sevilla-Malaga Km 9.500, Alcala de Guadaira, 41500 Sevilla, Spain.

Squibb, Austral. E.R. Squibb & Sons Pty Ltd, 556 Princes Highway, Noble Park Vic. 3174, Australia.

Squibb, Belg. Squibb S.A., ave Louise 130a/bte 4, 1050 Brussels, Belgium.

Squibb, Canad. Squibb Canada Inc., 2365 Côte de Liesse Rd, Montreal, Quebec H4N 2M7, Canada.

Squibb, Denm. See *Novo, Denm.*

Squibb, Fr. Laboratoires Squibb, Tour Generale, Cedex 22, 92088 Paris-La Defensee, France.

Squibb, Hong Kong. See *Mason, Hong Kong.*

Squibb, Ital. Squibb s.p.a., Via Paolo di Dono 73, 00142 Rome, Italy.

Squibb, Neth. Squibb B.V., J.C. van Markenlaan 3, 2285 VL Rijswijk, Netherlands.

Squibb, NZ. E.R. Squibb & Sons (NZ) Ltd, P.O. Box 8453, Auckland 1, New Zealand.

Squibb, S.Afr. Squibb Laboratories (Pty) Ltd, P.O. Box 48, Isando 1600, S. Africa.

Squibb, Spain. Squibb, Jose Anselmo Clave 95-101, Esplugas De Llobregat, 08950 Barcelona, Spain.

Squibb, Swed. Squibb AB, Box 925, 181 09 Lidingo, Sweden.

Squibb, Switz. Squibb SA, Militärstrasse 90, Case postale, 8021 Zurich, Switzerland.

Squibb, UK. E.R. Squibb & Sons Ltd, Squibb House, 141 Staines Rd, Hounslow, Middx TW3 3JA, England.

Squibb, USA. E.R. Squibb & Sons Inc., P.O. Box 4000, Princeton NJ 08540, USA.

Squibb Surgicare, UK. Squibb Surgicare Ltd, Squibb House, 141 Staines Rd, Hounslow, Middx TW3 3JA, England.

Squibb-Novo, USA. Squibb-Novo Inc., 120 Alexander St, Princeton NJ 08540, USA.

S.S. Pharmaceuticals, Jpn. S.S. Pharmaceuticals, 2-12-4, Hama-cho, Nihonbashi, Chuo-ku, Tokyo, Japan.

S.S.I., Neth. See *Bipharma, Neth.*

Stada, Ger. Stada-Arzneimittel AG, Stada-Strasse 2-18, Postfach: 1260, 6368 Bad Vilbel 4, W. Germany.

Stadapharm, Ger. Stadapharm GmbH, Stada-Strasse 2-18, Postfach: 1260, 6368 Bad Vilbel 4, W. Germany.

Stafford-Miller, Austral. Stafford Miller Ltd, P.O. Box 185, Revesby NSW 2212, Australia.

Stafford-Miller, Denm. See *Searle, Denm.*

Stafford-Miller, Fr. Laboratoires Stafford-Miller, 18 rue Hoche, 92130 Issy-les-Moulineaux, France.

Stafford-Miller, Norw. See *Nyco, Norw.*

Stafford-Miller, S.Afr. See *Searle, S.Afr.*

Stafford-Miller, Swed. See *Famaco, Swed.*

Stafford-Miller, Switz. See *Doetsch, Grether, Switz.*

Stafford-Miller, UK. Stafford-Miller Ltd, Stafford-Miller House, The Common, Hatfield, Herts AL10 0NZ, England.

Stago, Fr. See *Merck-Clévenot, Fr.*

Stallergenes, Switz. See *Actipharm, Switz.*

Standard Laboratories, UK. Standard Laboratories Ltd, Windmill Rd, Sunbury-on-Thames, Middx TW16 7DT, England.

Standard Process, USA. Standard Process Laboratories Inc., 2023 West Wisconsin Ave, Milwaukee WI 53233, USA.

Stanley, Canad. Stanley Drug Products Ltd, 1353 Main St, N. Vancouver, British Columbia V7J 1C5, Canada.

Stansen, Austral. A.E. Stansen & Co. Pty Ltd, P.O. Box 118, Mount Waverley Vic. 3149, Australia.

Star, Swed. See *Pharmacia, Swed.*

Star, USA. Star Pharmaceuticals Inc., 1990 NW 44th St, R.R. 2, Box 904J, Pompano Beach FL 33067-9802, USA.

Statens Seruminstitut, Denm. Statens Seruminstitut, Amager Boulevard 80, 2300 Copenhagen S, Denmark.

Statens Seruminstitut, Swed. See *SBL, Swed.*

STD Pharmaceutical Products, UK. STD Pharmaceutical Products Ltd, Fields Yard, Plough Lane, Hereford HR4 0EL, England.

Stecker, USA. Stecker, USA.

Steetley Berk, UK. Steetley Berk Ltd, P.O. Box 56, Basing View, Basingstoke, Hants RG21 2EG, England.

Steigerwald, Ger. Steigerwald Arzneimittelwerk GmbH, Havelstrasse 5, Postfach: 4335, 6100 Darmstadt, Germany.

Steiner, UK. Steiner Ltd, Steiner House, 66 Grosvenor St, Mayfair, London W1X 0AX, England.

Steinhard, UK. M.A. Steinhard Ltd, 32 Minerva Rd, London NW10 6HJ, England.

Stella, Belg. Lab. Stella S.A., rue des Pontons 25, 4600 Liege, Belgium.

Steriseal, UK. Steriseal Ltd, 26-7 Thornhill Rd, North Moons Moat, Redditch, Worcs B98 9NL, England.

Sterling, Austral. See *Winthrop, Austral.*

Sterling, Canad. Sterling Products, Division of Sterling Drug Ltd, Aurora, Ontario L4G 3H6, Canada.

Sterling, USA. Sterling Drug Inc., 90 Park Ave, New York NY 10016, USA.

Sterling Health, UK. Sterling Health, Sterling-Winthrop House, Onslow St, Guildford, Surrey GU1 4YS, England.

Sterling Industrial, UK. Sterling Industrial, 10 Churchfield Court, Churchfield, Barnsley, S. Yorks S70 2LL, England.

Sterling Research, UK. Sterling Research Laboratories, Sterling-Winthrop House, Onslow St, Guildford, Surrey GU1 4YS, England.

Sterling-Winthrop, Denm. See *Winthrop, Denm.*

Sterling Winthrop, Fr. Sterling Winthrop S.A., 92 blvd Victor-Hugo, 92115 Clichy, France.

Sterling Winthrop, Neth. Sterling Winthrop B.V., Prins Bernhardlaan 2, 2032 HA Haarlem, Netherlands.

Sterling-Winthrop, Swed. Sterling-Winthrop AB, Box 1403, 171 27 Solna, Sweden.

Sterobiotics, Canad. Sterobiotics Inc., P.O. Box 926, Streetsville Postal Station, Mississauga, Ontario L5M 2C5, Canada.

Sterwin, Spain. Sterwin-Winthrop, Avda. General Peron 27-4, 28020 Madrid, Spain.

Stholl, Ital. Stholl Farmaceutici s.p.a., Via Giardini 1271, 41100 Modena, Italy.

Stickley, Canad. E.L. Stickley & Co. Ltd, P.O. Box 1748, Brantford, Ontario N3T 5V7, Canada.

Stiefel, Austral. Stiefel Laboratories Pty Ltd, P.O. Box 1081, Crows Nest NSW 2065, Australia.

Stiefel, Canad. Stiefel Canada Inc., 6635 boul. Henri-Bourassa Ouest, Montreal, Quebec H4R 1E1, Canada.

Stiefel, Fr. Laboratoires Stiefel S.A.R.L., Z.I. du Petit Nanterre, 15 rue des Grands Pres, 92000 Nanterre, France.

Stiefel, Ger. Stiefel Laboratorium GmbH, Muhlheimer Strasse 231, 6050 Offenbach am Main, Germany.

Stiefel, Neth. Stiefel Laboratories B.V., Nieuwstraat 1, 2161 PM Lisse, Netherlands.

Stiefel, S.Afr. Stiefel Laboratories SA (Pty) Ltd, P.O. Box 7553, Johannesburg 2000, S. Africa.

Stiefel, Swed. See *Erco, Swed.*

Stiefel, Switz. See *Desopharma, Switz.*

Stiefel, UK. Stiefel Laboratories (UK) Ltd, Holtspur Lane, Wooburn Green, High Wycombe, Bucks HP10 0AU, England.

Stiefel, USA. Stiefel Laboratories Inc., 2801 Ponce de Leon Blvd, Coral Gables FL 33134, USA.

Stockhausen, Ger. Chemische Fabrik Stockhausen GmbH Stockhausen Pharma, Bakerpfad 25, Postfach: 570, 4150 Krefeld 1, Germany.

Stockli, Switz. Dr J. Stöckli SA, Leimenstrasse 57, 4011 Basel, Switzerland.

Stotzer, Switz. Stotzer AG, Postfach, 3000 Bern 22, Switzerland.

Stotzer Zurich, Switz. Stotzer AG Zurich, Postfach, 8023 Zurich, Switzerland.

Strenol, UK. Strenol Products Ltd, Pearl House, 746 Finchley Rd, London NW11 7TH, England.

Streuli, Switz. G. Streuli & Co. SA, 8730 Uznach, Switzerland.

Stroder, Ital. Ist. Farmaco Biologico Stroder s.r.l., Via di Ripoli 207/V, 50126 Florence, Italy.

Stroschein, Ger. Pharma Stroschein GmbH, Frohmestrasse 110, 2000 Hamburg 61, W. Germany.

Stuart, S.Afr. Stuart Pharmaceuticals (S.A.) (Pty) Ltd, P.O. Box 32616, Braamfontein 2017, S. Africa.

Stuart, UK. Stuart Pharmaceuticals Ltd, Stuart House, 50 Alderley Rd, Wilmslow, Cheshire SK9 1RE, England.

Stuart Pharmaceuticals, USA. Stuart Pharmaceuticals, Division of ICI Americas Inc., Wilmington DE 19897, USA.

Stulln, Neth. See *Bipharma, Neth.*

Stulln, Switz. See *Galenica, Switz.*

Substantia, Fr. Substantia Division Sante, 11 ave Dubonnet, 92407 Courbevoie Cedex, France.

Substantia, Neth. B.V. Substantia, Oderweg 1, 1043 AG Amsterdam, Netherlands.

Substantia, Swed. See *Famaco, Swed.*

Südmedica, Ger. Südmedica GmbH, Chemisch-pharmazeutische Fabrik, Ehrwalder Strasse 21, Postfach: 701669, 8000 Munich 70, W. Germany.

Sumitomo, Jpn. Sumitomo Seiyaku, 5-15 Kitahama, Higashi-ku, Osaka, Japan.

Sunde, Norw. Hoyesterettsadvocat Jens A. Sunde, Akersg. 16, 0158 Oslo 1, Norway.

Sundrychem, S.Afr. Sundrychem, S. Africa.

Superol, S.Afr. Superol, S. Africa.

Superpharm, Canad. Superpharm, 317 boul. Sir Wilfrid-Laurier, Saint-Lambert, Quebec J4R 2L1, Canada.

Supramed, S.Afr. Supramed, P.O. Box 201, Howard Place 7450, S. Africa.

Sur De Espana, Spain. Sur De Espana, Cuarteles 29, 29002 Malaga, Spain.

Surf Ski International, UK. Surf Ski International Ltd, Atlantique, Grande Route Des Mielles, St Ouen, Jersey, Channel Islands.

Surgikos, UK. Surgikos Ltd, Kirkton Campus, Livingston, Scotland.

Surinach, Spain. Surinach, Aribau 180, 08036 Barcelona, Spain.

Survival Technology, USA. Survival Technology Inc., 8101 Glenbrook Rd, Bethesda MD 20814, USA.

Sussex, UK. Sussex Pharmaceutical Ltd, Charlwoods Rd, East Grinstead, Sussex RH19 2HL, England.

Svenska Dental, Swed. Svenska Dental Instrument AB, Box 420, 194 04 Upplands Vasby, Sweden.

Swaab, Neth. See *Roter, Neth.*

Swe FARM, Swed. Swe FARM Lakemedels och Utvecklings AB, Erick Dahlbergsallen 9, 115 24 Stockholm, Sweden.

Sween, USA. Sween Corp., Sween Building, P.O. Box 980, Lake Crystal MN 56055, USA.

Swiss Herbal, Canad. Swiss Herbal Remedies Ltd, 181 Don Park Rd, Markham, Ontario L3R 1C2, Canada.

Swisspharm, S.Afr. Swisspharm (Pty) Ltd, P.O. Box 260132, Excom 2023, S. Africa.

Swiss-Pharma, Ger. Swiss-Pharma GmbH, Basler Strasse 56, 7850 Lörrach, W. Germany.

Syncare, Canad. Syncare, a division of Syntex Inc., 2100 Syntex Ct, Mississauga, Ontario L5N 3X4, Canada.

Synchemicals, UK. Synchemicals Ltd, 44 Grange Walk, London SE1 3DY, England.

Syncro, Arg. Syncro (Arg.) S.A.Q.I.C.I.F., Sarmiento 1230 Pisos 7°-9°, 1041 Buenos Aires, Argentina.

Synlab, Fr. Laboratoires Synlab, 209 rue de Bercy, 75585 Paris Cedex 12, France.

Synmedic, Switz. Synmedic AG, Postfach 338, 8036 Zurich, Switzerland.

Synpharma, Switz. Synpharma SA, Case postale, 9240 Uzwil, Switzerland.

Syntetic, Denm. A/S Syntetic, Edwin Rahrs Vej, 8220 Brabrand, Denmark.

Syntex, Austral. Syntex Australia Ltd, P.O. Box 370, Milsons Point NSW 2061, Australia.

Syntex, Belg. See *Sarva-Syntex, Belg.*

Syntex, Canad. Syntex Inc., 2100 Syntex Court, Mississauga, Ontario L5N 3X4, Canada.

Syntex, Denm. Astra-Syntex Laegmidler A/S, C.F. Richsvej 103, 2000 Frederiksberg, Denmark.

Syntex, Fr. Laboratoires Syntex, 20 rue Jean-Jaures, 92807 Puteaux Cedex, France.

Syntex, Ger. Syntex Arzneimittel GmbH, Viktoriaallee 3-5, Postfach: 1287, 5100 Aachen, Germany.

Syntex, Mex. Syntex S.A., Division Farmaceutica, Cerrada de Bezares No. 9, Mexico 10 D.F., Mexico.

Syntex, Neth. See *Pharbil, Neth.*

Syntex, S.Afr. Syntex Pharmaceuticals, P.O. Box 89566, Lyndhurst 2106, S. Africa.

Syntex, Swed. See *Astra-Syntex, Swed.*

Syntex, Switz. Syntex Pharm SA, Case postale, 4123 Allschwil 1, Switzerland.

Syntex, UK. Syntex Pharmaceuticals Ltd, Syntex House, St Ives Rd, Maidenhead, Berks SL6 1RD, England.

Syntex, USA. Syntex Laboratories Inc., 3401 Hillview Ave, P.O. Box 10850, Palo Alto CA 94303, USA.

Syntex-Latino, Spain. Syntex-Latino, Severo Ochoa 13, Leganes, 28914 Madrid, Spain.

Synthelabo, Belg. Synthelabo Benelux S.A., ave de Schiphol 2, 1140 Brussels, Belgium.

Synthelabo, Fr. Laboratoires Synthelabo France, 58 rue de la Glaciere, 75013 Paris, France.

Synthelabo, Philipp. See *Zuellig, Philipp.*

Synthelabo, Switz. See *Kramer-Synthelabo, Switz.*

Synthol, Spain. Synthol, Roca Umbert 17, Hospitalet de Llobregat, 08907 Barcelona, Spain.

Szama, Arg. Dr Herbert Szama S.A.C.I., Lafuente 161, 1406 Buenos Aires, Argentina.

Taco, Ger. Taco GmbH, Chem.-Pharm. Fabrik, Alte Heerstrasse 76, Postfach: 2146, 5205 St. Augustin 2, Germany.

TAD, Ger. TAD Pharmazeutisches Werk GmbH, Heinz-Lohmann-Strasse 5, Postfach: 720, 2190 Cuxhaven, W. Germany.

TAD, Switz. See *Wiedenmann, Switz.*

Tafir, Spain. Tafir, Trifon Pedrero 4-6, 28019 Madrid, Spain.

Taiho, Jpn. Taiho Yakuhin, 2-9 Tsukasa-cho, Kanda, Chiyoda-ku, Tokyo, Japan.

Taisho, Jpn. Taisho Seiyaku, 3-24-1 Takada, Toshima-ku, Tokyo, Japan.

Takeda, Fr. Laboratoires Takeda, 3 square Desaix, 75015 Paris, France.

Takeda, Ger. Takeda Pharma GmbH, Schellerweg 3, Postfach: 1949, 5190 Stolberg, Germany.

Takeda, Jpn. Takeda Yakuhin, 2-27 Doshomachi, Higashi-ku, Osaka, Japan.

Takeda, Philipp. See *Metro, Philipp.*

Tambrands, UK. Tambrands Ltd, Dunsbury Way, Havant, Hants PO9 5DG, England.

Tambrands, USA. Tambrands Inc., 10 Delaware Dr., Lake Success NY 11042, USA.

Tanabe, Jpn. Tanabe Seiyaku, 3-21 Doshomachi, Higashi-ku, Osaka, Japan.

Tanabe, S.Afr. See *Noristan, S.Afr.*

Tanabe, Switz. See *Biochimica, Switz.*

Tantallon, Austral. See *Cambden, Austral.*

Tap, Canad. See *Abbott, Canad.*

TAP, USA. TAP Pharmaceuticals, 1400 Sheridan Rd, North Chicago IL 60064, USA.

Taro, Canad. Taro Pharmaceuticals Inc., 305 Supertest Rd, Downsview, Ontario M3J 2M4, Canada.

T.E. Williams, USA. T.E. Williams Pharmaceuticals Inc., P.O. Box 1860, Edmond OK 73083, USA.

Tebib, Spain. Tebib, Plg Balconcillo, Parcela 47, 19000 Guadalajara, Spain.

Tecfar, Spain. See *Bohm, Spain.*

Technicon, S.Afr. Technicon Laboratories, P.O. Box 1554, Randburg 2125, S. Africa.

Technilab, Canad. Technilab Inc., 1490 rue Beaulac, Ville Saint-Laurent, Quebec H4R 1R7, Canada.

Techni-Pharma, Mon. Techni-Pharma, 7 rue del'Industrie, MC 98000 Monaco (Pte), Monaco.

Teikoku, Jpn. Teikoku Zoki, 2-5-1 Akasaka, Minato-ku, Tokyo, Japan.

Teknofarma, Ital. Teknofarma s.p.a., S. Bertolla Abb. Stura 14, 10156 Turin, Italy.

Tell, UK. Tell Products Ltd, 93 Cobbold Rd, London NW10 9SU, England.

Temis-Lostalo, Arg. Temis-Lostalo S.A., Zepita 3178, 1285 Buenos Aires, Argentina.

Temmler, Denm. See *Nordisk Droge, Denm.*

Temmler, Ger. Temmler Pharma GmbH, Temmlerstrasse 2, Postfach: 2269, 3550 Marburg/Lahn, W. Germany.

Temmler, Switz. See *Doetsch, Grether, Switz.*

Tendo-Haco, Neth. Tendo-Haco Farmacie B.V., Kloosterweg 3, 8191 JA Wapenveld, Netherlands.

Tenneco, UK. Tenneco Organics Ltd, Rockingham Works, Avonmouth, Avon BS11 0YT, England.

Terapeutico M.R., Ital. Labor. Terapeutico M.R. s.r.l., Via Domenico Veneziano 13int., 50143 Florence, Italy.

Terapia, Roum. The Terapia Medicinal Drugs Enterprise, Cluj-Napoca, Roumania.

Terme di Chianciano, Ital. Terme di Chianciano s.p.a., Via delle Rose 12, 53042 Chianciano Terme (Siena), Italy.

Terme di Montecatini, Ital. Terme di Montecatini s.p.a., Viale Marconi 7, 51016 Montecatini Terme (PT), Italy.

Terme di Salsomaggiore, Ital. Terme di Salsomaggiore s.p.a., Via Roma 9, 43039 Salsomaggiore Terme (Parma), Italy.

Terumo, Denm. See *Meda, Denm.*

Terumo, Swed. See *Pharmacia, Swed.*

Teva, Israel. Teva Pharmaceuticals Ltd, P.O. Box 1142, Jerusalem, Israel.

Teva, Neth. See *ICN, Neth.*

Thackray, UK. Thackraycare Ltd, 45-47 Great George St, Leeds LS1 3BB, England.

Thames, UK. Thames Laboratories Ltd, The Old Blue School, 5 Lower Square, Isleworth, Middx TW7 6RL, England.

Thames Genelink, UK. Thames Genelink Ltd, 50 Occam Rd, Surrey Research Park, Guildford, Surrey GU2 5YN, England.

Thepenier, Fr. Laboratoires Thepenier, 10 rue Clapeyron, 75008 Paris, France.

Therabel Pharma, Belg. Therabel Pharma S.A., chaussee d'Alsemberg 1001, 1180 Brussels, Belgium.

Théramex, Fr. Laboratoires Théramex, 2 blvd Charles III, B.P. 59, MC 98007 Monaco Cedex, France.

Théranol, Fr. Laboratoires Théranol, 180 rue de Vaugirard, 75015 Paris, France.

Therapeutica, Belg. Therapeutica S.A., rue de Geneve 512, 1030 Brussels, Belgium.

Therapeutique-Splenodex, Fr. Laboratoires Recherche Therapeutique-Splenodex, 4 av. Maurice-Leroy, 77310 Ponthierry, France.

Therapex, Canad. Therapex Inc., Division of E-Z-EM Canada Inc., 9855 rue Colbert, Ville d'Anjou, Quebec H1J 1Z9, Canada.

Therapia, Switz. Thérapia SA, Monséjour 2, Case postale 878, 1701 Fribourg, Switzerland.

Théraplix, Fr. Théraplix S.A., 46 rue Albert, 75640 Paris Cedex 13, France.

Théraplix, Neth. See *Rhône-Poulenc, Neth.*

Therica, Fr. Laboratoires Therica, 15 av. Henry Dunant, 27400 Louviers, France.

Thiemann, Ger. Thiemann Arzneimittel GmbH, Wirrigen 25, Postfach: 440, 4355 Waltrop, W. Germany.

Thiemann, Switz. See *Diethelm, Switz.*

Thilo, Belg. See *de Bournonville, Belg.*

Thilo, Ger. Dr Thilo & Co. GmbH Chem.-pharm. Fabrik, Rudolf-Diesel-Ring 21, Postfach: 260, 8029 Sauerlach, W. Germany.

Thilo, Neth. See *Bournonville, Neth.*

Thomae, Ger. Dr Karl Thomae GmbH, Chemisch-pharmazeutische Fabrik, Birkendorfer Strasse 65, Postfach: 1755, 7950 Biberach, W. Germany.

Thomas, UK. Hubert A.C. Thomas & Co., Copperworks Rd, New Dock, Llanelli, Dyfed, Wales.

Thompson, USA. Thompson Medical Co. Inc., 919 Third Ave, New York NY 10022, USA.

Thompson Medical, UK. Thompson Medical Co. Ltd, Kew Bridge House, Kew Bridge Rd, Brentford, Middx TW8 0EJ, England.

Thomson & Joseph, UK. Thomson & Joseph Ltd, T & J House, 119 Plumstead Rd, Norwich, Norfolk, England.

Thor, Spain. Thor, Rodriguez Arango s/n, 09001 Burgos, Spain.

Thornton & Ross, UK. Thornton & Ross Ltd, Linthwaite Laboratories, Huddersfield HD7 5QH, England.

Thylmer, Belg. Thylmer S.A., chaussee d'Alsemberg 1001, 1180 Brussels, Belgium.

Thylmer, Switz. See *Galenica, Switz.*

Tiber, Ital. Tiber s.r.l., Prodotti Chimico Biologici, Via Tiburtina 1496, 00131 Rome, Italy.

Ticen, Eire. Ticen, Eire.

Tidebrook, UK. Tidebrook Chemical Products Ltd, 46 Parkside Rd, Leeds LS6 4QG, England.

Tika, Denm. See *Astra, Denm.*

Tika, Norw. See *Astra, Norw.*

Tika, Swed. AB Tika, Box 2, 221 00 Lund, Sweden.

Tilfarma, Spain. Tilfarma, Bruc 9, Badalona, 08915 Barcelona, Spain.

Tillotts, UK. Tillotts Laboratories, Unit 24, Henlow Trading Estate, Henlow, Beds SG16 6DS, England.

Tissot, Fr. Laboratoires du Dr Tissot S.A., 34 blvd de Clichy, 75018 Paris, France.

Tjellesen, Denm. E. Tjellesen A/S, Blokken 81, 3460 Birkerød, Denmark.

Toa Eiyo, Jpn. Toa Eiyo, 3-1-2 Kyobashi, Chuo-ku, Tokyo, Japan.

Tobishi, Jpn. Tobishi Yakuhin, 1-10-1 Yuraku-cho, Chiyoda-ku, Tokyo, Japan.

Togal, Neth. See *Multi-Pharma, Neth.*

Toho, Jpn. Toho Yakuhin, 1-14 Awaju-cho, Higashi-ku, Osaka, Japan.

Topfer, Denm. See *Max Jenne, Denm.*

Topfer, Ger. Topfer GmbH, Heisingerstrasse 6, Postfach: 1180, 8969 Dietmannsried, Germany.

Torbet Laboratories, UK. Torbet Laboratories, Boughton Lane, Maidstone, Kent ME25 9QQ, England.

Torch Laboratories, USA. Torch Laboratories Inc., USA.

Torii, Jpn. Torii Yakuhin, 3-3-14 Hon-cho, Nihonbashi, Chuo-ku, Tokyo, Japan.

Torlan, Spain. Torlan, Ballester 46, 08023 Barcelona, Spain.

Torre, Ital. Dr. A. Torre Farmaceutici s.r.l., Viale E. Forlanini 15, 20134 Milan, Italy.

Torrens, Spain. Torrens, Via Agusta 59, 08006 Barcelona, Spain.

Torres Munoz, Spain. Torres Munoz, Ctra de Fuenlabrada Pinto, Madrid, Spain.

Tosara, UK. Tosara Products (UK) Ltd, P.O. Box 5, 70 Picton Rd, Liverpool L15 4NS, England.

Tosi, Ital. Istituto Franco Tosi s.p.a., Via Bertola da Novate 14, 20157 Milan, Italy.

Tosi-Novara, Ital. Tosi Dr A. Farmaceutici s.r.l., C.so della Vittoria 12/B, 28100 Novara, Italy.

Tosse, Ger. E. Tosse & Co. mbH, Friedrich-Ebert-Damm 101, Postfach: 70 16 48, 2000 Hamburg 70, W. Germany.

Toulade, Fr. Laboratoires Toulade, 18 rue Andre-Doucet, 92000 Nanterre, France.

Towa, Swed. See *Eklow, Swed.*

Townendale, UK. Townendale Pharmaceuticals, P.O. Box 53, Harrogate, North Yorkshire HG1 5BD, England.

Toyama, Jpn. Toyama Kagaku, 3-2-5 Nishishinjuku, Shinjuku-ku, Tokyo, Japan.

Toyo Jozo, Jpn. Toyo Jozo, 4-5-13 Shibaura, Minato-ku, Tokyo, Japan.

Toyo Seika, Jpn. Toyo Seika, 3-15-3 Doshomachi, Higashi-ku, Osaka, Japan.

Tramedico, Neth. Tramedico B.V., Flevolaan 19C, 1382 JX Weesp, Netherlands.

Trans Canaderm, Canad. Trans Canaderm Inc., 5353 blvd Thimens, Saint-Laurent, Quebec H4R 2H4, Canada.

Travenol, Austral. Travenol Laboratories Pty Ltd, P.O. Box 88, Toongabbie NSW 2146, Australia.

Travenol, Belg. Travenol Laboratories S.A., Industrielaan 6, 1740 Ternat, Belgium.

Travenol, Canad. Travenol Canada Inc., 6695 Airport Rd, Mississauga, Ontario L4V 1T8, Canada.

Travenol, Denm. Travenol A/S, Hovegaden 49, 3460 Birkerod, Denmark.

Travenol, Ital. Laboratori Travenol s.p.a., Viale Tiziano 25, 00196 Rome, Italy.

Travenol, Spain. Travenol, Del's Gremis 7, 46014 Valencia, Spain.

Travenol, Swed. Travenol AB, Box 20115, 161 20 Bromma, Sweden.

Travenol, UK. Travenol Laboratories Ltd, Caxton Way, Thetford, Norfolk IP24 3SE, England.

Travenol, USA. Travenol Laboratories Inc., One Baxter Parkway, Deerfield IL 60015, USA.

Trenka, Aust. F. Trenka, Chem.-pharm. Fabrik, Goldeggasse 5, 1040 Vienna, Austria.

Trenka, Denm. See *Tjellesen, Denm.*

Trenka, Switz. See *Uhlmann-Eyraud, Switz.*

Trenker, Belg. Lab. Pharm. Trenker S.A., ave Dolez 480-482, 1180 Brussels, Belgium.

Trentham, UK. Trentham Laboratories Ltd, Seymour Rd, London E10 7LX, England.

Treupha, Switz. Treupha SA, Zürcherstrasse 59, 5401 Baden, Switzerland.

Trianon, Canad. Trianon Laboratories Inc., 1905 rue Gutenberg, Laval, Quebec H7S 1A1, Canada.

Triasic, Canad. Triasic Pharmaceuticals Inc., 1865-128 St, Surrey, British Columbia V4A 3V5, Canada.

Tricum, Swed. See *Cyanamid, Swed.*

Trimen, USA. Trimen Laboratories Inc., 80-26th St, Pittsburgh PA 15222, USA.

Triomed, S.Afr. Triomed, P.O. Box 309, Bellville 7530, S. Africa.

Triosol, Belg. Triosol S.A., ave Louise 176, 1050 Brussels, Belgium.

Triplus, Swed. Triplus Sjukvardsprodukter AB, Box 10152, 434 01 Kungsbacka, Sweden.

Trofield, Denm. See *Danapharm, Denm.*

Trommsdorff, Ger. H. Trommsdorff GmbH & Co. Arzneimittel, Trommsdorffstrasse 2-6, Postfach: 1420, 5110 Alsdorf, W. Germany.

Tropon, Ger. Troponwerke GmbH & Co. KG, Berliner Strasse 156, Postfach: 80 10 60, 5000 Cologne 80, W. Germany.

Tropon-Cutter, Ger. See *Tropon, Ger.*

Truw, Ger. Truw Arzneimittel GmbH, Tonisberger Strasse 67, Postfach: 1360, 4150 Krefeld 29-Huls, Germany.

Tubi Lux, Ital. Tubi Lux Farma, Istituto Farmaco Oftalmico, Via del Mare 131, 00040 Pomezia (Rome), Italy.

Tudor, UK. Tudor Trading Co., P.O. Box 94, Edgware, Middx HA8 0JP, England.

Tunnel Avebe, UK. Tunnel Avebe Starches Ltd, Avebe House, Otterham Quay, Rainham, Gillingham, Kent ME8 7UU, England.

Turimed, Switz. Turimed SA, Hertistrasse 8, 8304 Wallisellen, Switzerland.

Turon, Spain. Turon, Lauria 96, 08009 Barcelona, Spain.

Tuta, Austral. Tuta Laboratories (Australia) Pty Ltd, P.O. Box 166, Lane Cove NSW 2066, Australia.

Tutag, USA. Tutag Pharmaceuticals, Division of Reid-Provident, 640 Tenth St, Atlanta GA 30318, USA.

Tuypens, Belg. Lab. Tuypens S.A., August De Boeckstraat 1, 2700 Sint-Niklaas, Belgium.

Typharm, UK. Typharm Ltd, 14 Parkstone Rd, Poole, Dorset, England.

Tyson, USA. Tyson & Associates Inc., 1661 Lincoln Blvd, Suite 300, Santa Monica CA 90404, USA.

UAD, USA. UAD Laboratories Inc., 6635 Highway 18 West, Jackson MS 39209, USA.

UCB, Arg. Unión Científica Belgo-Argentina S.A., Av. V. Sarsfield 5855, 1605 Munro, Buenos Aires, Argentina.

UCB, Belg. UCB S.A., rue Berkendael 68, 1060 Brussels, Belgium.

UCB, Denm. See *Nordisk Droge, Denm.*

UCB, Fr. UCB, 21 rue de Neuilly, 92003 Nanterre, France.

UCB, Ger. UCB Chemie GmbH, Hüttenstrasse 205, Postfach: 1340, 5014 Kerpen, W. Germany.

UCB, Ital. Laboratori UCB s.p.a., Via S. Clemente 8, 10143 Turin, Italy.

UCB, Neth. UCB Farma Nederland B.V., Druivenstraat 3/Nieuwe Kadijk, 4816 KB Breda, Netherlands.

UCB, Norw. See *Mekos, Norw.*

UCB, S.Afr. UCB (Pty) Ltd, P.O. Box 30136, Braamfontein 2017, S. Africa.

UCB, Spain. UCB, Santiago Ramon y Cajal 6, Molins de Rei, 08750 Barcelona, Spain.

UCB, Swed. UCB Pharma AB, Box 946, 251 09 Helsingborg, Sweden.

UCB, Switz. UCB-Pharma SA, Eggbühlstr. 14, 8052 Zurich, Switzerland.

UCM-Difme, Ital. Unione Chimica Medicamenti Difme s.p.a., Via Sabaudia 44, 10095 Grugliasco (TO), Italy.

Uhlmann-Eyraud, Switz. F. Uhlmann-Eyraud S.A., ch. du Grand-Puits 28, 1217 Meyrin 2/Geneva, Switzerland.

Ulmer, USA. Ulmer Pharmacal Co., 2440 Fernbrook Lane, Minneapolis MN 55441, USA.

Ultra, UK. Ultra Laboratories Ltd, Trinity Trading Estate, Tribune Drive, Sittingbourne, Kent ME10 2PG, England.

Ultra, USA. Ultra, USA.

Ultrapharm, UK. Ultrapharm Ltd, Kenton House, 21 New St, Henley-on-Thames, Oxon RG9 2PB, England.

Unibios, Spain. Unibios, Avda. Pedro Diez 33, 28019 Madrid, Spain.

Unicet, Fr. Laboratoires Unicet, 92 rue Baudin, 92307 Levallois-Perret Cedex, France.

Unichem, UK. Unichem Ltd, Unichem House, Cox Lane, Chessington, Surrey, England.

Unichema, UK. Unichema Chemicals Ltd, Bebington, Wirral, Merseyside L62 4UF, England.

Unicliffe, UK. Unicliffe, England.

Unifa, Arg. Unifa S.A.Q.eI., Av. San Martin 1750, 1602 Florida, Buenos Aires, Argentina.

Unifarma, Spain. Unifarma, Guillermo Tell 51, 08006 Barcelona, Spain.

Unigreg, UK. Unigreg Ltd, Spa House, 15-17 Worple Rd, Wimbledon, London SW19 4JS, England.

Unilabo, Fr. See *Unicet, Fr.*

Unimed, Canad. Unimed Canada Inc., 626 rue Meloche, Dorval, Quebec H9P 2P4, Canada.

Unimed, S.Afr. See *Keatings, S.Afr.*

Unimed, UK. Unimed Pharmaceuticals Ltd, 24 Steynton Ave, Bexley, Kent DA5 3HP, England.

Unimed, USA. Unimed Inc., 35 Columbia Rd, Somerville NJ 08876, USA.

Union Carbide, UK. Union Carbide UK Ltd, Union Carbide House, High St, Rickmansworth, Herts WD3 1RB, England.

Union Carbide, USA. Union Carbide Corporation, USA.

Unipath, UK. Unipath Ltd, Norse Rd, Bedford MK41 0QG, England.

Unipharma, Switz. Unipharma S.A., 6911 Barbengo, Switzerland.

United, USA. United, Division of Pfizer Hospital Products Group, 1175 Starkey Rd, Largo FL 33543, USA.

Unitex, Spain. Unitex, Castanos 79, Mataro, 08302 Barcelona, Spain.

Univet, UK. Univet Ltd, Wedgwood Rd, Bicester, Oxon OX6 7UL, England.

UPB, Belg. Union Pharmaceutique Belge S.P.R.L., Parc Industriel de la Vallee du Hain, 1420 Braine-l'Alleud, Belgium.

UPB, Neth. See *Bournonville, Neth.*

Upjohn, Austral. Upjohn Pty Ltd, P.O. Box 138, Parramatta NSW 2150, Australia.

Upjohn, Belg. Upjohn S.A., Lichterstraat, 2670 Puurs, Belgium.

Upjohn, Canad. The Upjohn Co. of Canada, 865 York Mills Rd, Don Mills, Ontario M3B 1Y6, Canada.

Upjohn, Denm. Upjohn, Ericavej 149, 2820 Gentofte, Denmark.

Upjohn, Eire. Upjohn Ltd, Unit 31, Airways Industrial Estate, Cloghran, Co. Dublin, Eire.

Upjohn, Fr. Laboratoires Upjohn, Tour Franklin, Cedex 11, 92081 Paris La Défense, France.

Upjohn, Ger. Upjohn GmbH, Humboldstrasse 10, Postfach: 449, 6148 Heppenheim, W. Germany.

Upjohn, Ital. Upjohn s.p.a., Via G.E. Upjohn 2, 20040 Caponago (MI), Italy.

Upjohn, Neth. Upjohn-Nederland, Morsestraat 15, 6716 AH Ede, Netherlands.

Upjohn, Norw. Upjohn Informasjon, Postboks 10, 1310 Blommenholm, Norway.

Upjohn, S.Afr. Upjohn (Pty) Ltd, P.O. Box 246, Isando 1600, S. Africa.

Upjohn, Spain. Upjohn, C-100 a Base Torrejon km 15, Alcala de Henares, Madrid, Spain.

Upjohn, Swed. Upjohn AB, Box 289, 433 25 Partille, Sweden.

Upjohn, Switz. Upjohn SA, Case postale 208, 8033 Zurich, Switzerland.

Upjohn, UK. Upjohn Ltd, Fleming Way, Crawley, West Sussex RH10 2NJ, England.

Upjohn, USA. The Upjohn Co., 7000 Portage Rd, Kalamazoo MI 49001, USA.

UPSA, Fr. UPSA, 128 rue Danton, 92500 Rueil-Malmaison, France.

UPSA, Switz. See *Pharmagene, Switz.*

Upsamedica, Belg. Lab. Upsamedica S.A., Centre International Rogier 402/bte 6, 1210 Brussels, Belgium.

Upsamedica, Spain. Upsamedica, Carretera General de Ulia S/N, Villa de la Carabela, Guipuzcoa, Spain.

Upsher-Smith, USA. Upsher-Smith Laboratories Inc., 14905 23rd Ave North, Minneapolis MN 55441, USA.

Uquifa, Spain. Uquifa, Cartella 87, 08031 Barcelona, Spain.

Urca, Spain. Urca, Matilde Hernandez 34, 28019 Madrid, Spain.

Uriach, Spain. Uriach, Decano Bahi 59-67, 08026 Barcelona, Spain.

U.R.P.A.C., Fr. Unitc dc Recherche Pharmaceutique et d'Application Clinique, 40 rue de la Faisanderie, 75116 Paris, France.

Ursapharm, Ger. Ursapharm, Bernhard, Buxmann & Co. GmbH, Industriestrasse, Postfach: 8, 6601 Bubingen, Germany.

Ursula-Ruth, UK. Ursula-Ruth, 73 Church Rd, London NW4 4DP, England.

US Ethicals, Norw. See *Item, Norw.*

US-Ethicals, Switz. See *Doetsch, Grether, Switz.*

US Ethicals, USA. US Ethicals Inc., 37-02 48th Ave, Long Island City NY 11101, USA.

US Pharmaceutical, USA. US Pharmaceutical Corp., 2500 Park Central Blvd, Decatur GA 30035, USA.

US Products, USA. US Products, USA.

USV, Austral. USV Australia Pty Ltd, P.O. Box 110, Arncliffe NSW 2205, Australia.

USV, Canad. See *Rorer, Canad.*

USV Pharmaceutical Corp., USA. USV Pharmaceutical Corporation, 303 South Broadway, Tarrytown NY 10591, USA.

Utraco, Swed. Utraco Aktiebolag, Box 5073, 200 71 Malmo, Sweden.

Utus, UK. Utus Pharmaceutical Co. Ltd, England.

Vaillant, Ital. Laboratori Italiani Vaillant s.r.l., Via Melzi d'Eril 32, 20154 Milan, Italy.

Vaillant-Defresne, Fr. Laboratoires Vaillant-Defresne, 65 rue Falguière, 75739 Paris Cedex 15, France.

Vaillant-Defresne, Switz. See *Uhlmann-Eyraud, Switz.*

Valda, Ital. Valda Laboratori Farmaceutici s.p.a., Via Riva di Trento 13, 20139 Milan, Italy.

Valda, Spain. Valda, Gaudi 28, La Llagosta, 08120 Barcelona, Spain.

Vale, USA. The Vale Chemical Co. Inc., 1201 Liberty St, Allentown PA 18102, USA.

Valeas, Ital. Valeas s.p.a., Via Vallisneri 10, 20133 Milan, Italy.

Valles Mestre, Spain. Valles Mestre, Av. Generalitat 181, Viladecans, 08840 Barcelona, Spain.

Valpan, Fr. Laboratoires Valpan, B.P. 8, 77350 Le Mée-sur-Seine, France.

Van Dyk, USA. Van Dyk & Co. Inc., Main and William Sts, Belleville NJ 07109, USA.

van Oven, Neth. Laboratorium Dr. A. van Oven B.V., Zoutkeetsingel 139-140, 2512 HS Den Haag, Netherlands.

Vandenbroeck, Belg. Vandenbroeck S.A., chaussee de Wavre 362, 5980 Grez-Doiceau, Belgium.

Vandenbussche, Belg. Lab. Vandenbussche, Hogeweg 16, 8600 Menen, Belgium.

Vanderbilt, USA. R.T. Vanderbilt Co. Inc., 30 Winfield St, Norwalk CT 06855, USA.

Vandos, Austral. Vandos, Australia.

Vangard, USA. Vangard, USA.

Vectem, Spain. Vectem, Wagner 12, Rubi, 08191 Barcelona, Spain.

Vemedia, Neth. Vemedia B.V., Drentestraat 11, 1083 HK Amsterdam, Netherlands.

Venture Chemicals, UK. Venture Chemicals Ltd, England.

Vera, Spain. Vera, Lope de Rueda 42, 28009 Madrid, Spain.

Verex, USA. Verex Laboratories Inc., 8925 East Nichols Ave, Englewood CO 80112, USA.

Verkos, Spain. Verkos, Ctra Zaragoza Logrono km 20.2, Pinseque, 50298 Zaragoza, Spain.

Verla, Ger. Verla-Pharm, Arzneimittelfabrik, Apotheker H.J. v. Ehrlich GmbH & Co. KG, Hauptstrasse 98, Postfach: 1261, 8132 Tutzing, W. Germany.

Verla-Pharm, Switz. See *Biomed, Switz.*

Vernin, Fr. Laboratoires Vernin, 311 ave du Colonel-Fabien, 77190 Dammarie-les-Lys, France.

Vernleigh, S.Afr. Vernleigh Pharmaceuticals (Pty) Ltd, P.O. Box 9027, Johannesburg 2000, S. Africa.

Vessen, UK. Vessen Ltd, Mansen House, 320 London Rd, Hazel Grove, Stockport, Cheshire SK7 4RF, England.

Vesta, S.Afr. Vesta Medicines (Pty) Ltd, P.O. Box 4325, Johannesburg 2000, S.Africa.

Vestric, UK. Vestric Ltd, West Lane, Runcorn, Cheshire WA7 2PE, England.

Veyron-Froment, Fr. Laboratoires Veyron-Froment, 72 rue Monte-Cristo, 13248 Marseille Cedex 04, France.

Vicente, Spain. Vicente Dr., Cartagena 113, 28002 Madrid, Spain.

Vick International, Ital. Vick International s.p.a., Via Cavriano 14, 20134 Milan, Italy.

Vidal Sanz, Spain. Vidal Sanz, Conde de Altea 53, 46005 Valencia, Spain.

Viderfarm, Spain. Viderfarm, Avda Republica Argentina 54-6, 08023 Barcelona, Spain.

Vifor, Neth. See *Roussel, Neth.*

Vifor, Switz. Vifor S.A., rte d'Annecy 48, 1227 Carouge/GE, Switzerland.

Vilardel, Spain. Vilardel, San Gabriel 16, Esplugas de Llobregat, 08950 Barcelona, Spain.

Villette, Fr. Villette-Department des laboratoires Pharmascience, 73 blvd de la Mission Marchand, 92400 Courbevoie, France.

Villette, Neth. See *Bipharma, Neth.*

Vinas, Spain. Vinas, Torrente Vidalet 29, 08012 Barcelona, Spain.

Vinco, Spain. See *Reig Jofré, Spain.*

Vine Chemicals, UK. Vine Chemicals Ltd, Lugsdale Rd, Widnes, Cheshire WA8 6ND, England.

Vine Products, UK. Vine Products and Whiteways Ltd, The Winery, Villiers Rd, Kingston Upon Thames, Surrey KT1 3AS, England.

Vines Biocrin, UK. Vines Biocrin Ltd, 111 Clarence Rd, London E5 8EE, England.

Vinsi, Spain. Vinsi, Aragon 68, Palma de Mallorca, 07005 Baleares, Spain.

Vinyals, Spain. Vinyals, Granada 21-5, Sant Andreu de la Barca, 08740 Barcelona, Spain.

Viobin, USA. Viobin Corp., A Subsidiary of A.H. Robins Co., 226 W Livingston St, Monticello IL 61856, USA.

Viogarlo, Spain. Viogarlo, Doctor Zamenhof 28, 46008 Valencia, Spain.

Vir, Spain. Vir, Cardenal Mendoza 42, 28011 Madrid, Spain.

Vis, Ital. Vis Farmaceutici s.p.a., Istituto Scientifico delle Venezie, Viale dell'industria 54, 35100 Padua, Italy.

Vister, Ital. Vister s.p.a., Via C. Columbo 1, 20020 Lainate (Milan), Italy.

Vita, Ital. Vita Farmaceutici s.p.a., Via Boucheron 14, 10122 Turin, Italy.

Vita, Spain. Vita, Avda de Barcelona-51, San Juan Despi, 08970 Barcelona, Spain.

Vita-Valu, Austral. See *Winthrop, Austral.*

Vitabiotics, UK. Vitabiotics Ltd, 122 Mount Pleasant, Alperton, Middx HA0 1UG, England.

Vitalia, UK. Vitalia Ltd, Paradise, Hemel Hempstead, Herts HP2 4TF, England.

Vitaline, USA. Vitaline Formulas, P.O. Box 6757, Incline Village NV 89450, USA.

Vitamin Supplies, Austral. See *Vitaplex, Austral.*

Vitapharm, Spain. Vitapharm, Alto de los Robles 12, Barrio de Loyola, 20014 Guipuzcoa, Spain.

Vitaplex, Austral. Vitaplex Pty Ltd, P.O. Box 652, Chatswood NSW 2067, Australia.

Vitrum, Norw. See *KabiVitrum, Norw.*

Vitrum, Swed. See *Kabi, Swed.*

Vivan, USA. Vivan Pharmacol Inc., 1000 Bennett Blvd, Lakewood NJ 08701, USA.

Viviar, Spain. Viviar, Pista de Adenurz km 9.4, Paterna, 46980 Valencia, Spain.

Vogalia, Spain. Vogalia, Martin Martinez 4, 28002 Madrid, Spain.

Voigt, Ger. Dr med. Hans Voigt, Pharmazeutische Fabrik GmbH, Mundipharma-Strasse 4, Postfach: 1350, 6250 Limburg/Lahn, W. Germany.

Volpino, Arg. Volpino S.A.C.I., Posadas 1564 1^0 Piso, 1112 Buenos Aires, Argentina.

Von Boch, Ital. Von Boch Arzneimittel s.r.l. Istituto Farmacobiologico, Via Rovigo 1, 00161 Rome, Italy.

Vortech, USA. Vortech, USA.

Voxsan, UK. Voxsan Ltd, Wellfield Rd, Hatfield, Herts AL10 0BT, England.

VSM, Neth. VSM Geneesmiddelen B.V., Berenkoog 35, 1822 BH Alkmaar, Netherlands.

Wacker Chemicals, UK. See *Hoechst, UK.*

Wahl, USA. Wahl, USA.

Walker, Corp, USA. Walker, Corp & Co. Inc., P.O. Box 1320, Syracuse NY 13201, USA.

Walker Pharmacal, USA. Walker Pharmacal Co., 4200 Laclede Ave, St Louis MO 63108, USA.

Wallace, USA. Wallace Laboratories, Division of Carter-Wallace Inc., P.O. Box 1, Cranbury NJ 08512, USA.

Wallace, Cameron, UK. Wallace, Cameron & Co. Ltd, Ultra House, Drakemire Drive, Castlemilk Industrial Estate, Glasgow G45 9SU, Scotland.

Wallace Mfg Chem., UK. Wallace Manufacturing Chemists Ltd, 1a Frognal, London NW3 6AN, England.

Wallis, UK. Wallis Laboratory, 11 Camford Way, Sundon Park, Luton, Beds LU3 3AN, England.

Wampole, Canad. Wampole Inc., Perth, Ontario K7H 3E6, Canada.

Wander, Austral. Wander (Australia) Pty Ltd, 1/1761 Pittwater Rd, Mona Vale NSW 2103, Australia.

Wander, Belg. See *Sandoz-Wander, Belg.*

Wander, Ger. Wander Pharma GmbH, Deutschherrnstrasse 15, Postfach: 4124, 8500 Nürnberg, W. Germany.

Wander, Ital. Wander s.p.a., Via Meucci 39, 20128 Milan, Italy.

Wander, Neth. Wander Pharma, afdeling van Sandoz B.V., Loopkantstraat 25, 5405 AC Uden, Netherlands.

Wander, Norw. See *Dahl-Hansen, Norw.*

Wander, S.Afr. See *Sandoz, S.Afr.*

Wander, Spain. Wander, Corts Catalanes 766-8, 08013 Barcelona, Spain.

Wander, Swed. See *Sandoz, Swed.*

Wander, Switz. Wander SA, Case postale 2747, 3001 Bern, Switzerland.

Wander, UK. Wander Pharmaceuticals, Division of Sandoz Products Ltd, P.O. Horsforth Box 4, Calverley Lane, Horsforth, Leeds LS18 4RP, England.

Wander Dietetique, Switz. See *Wander, Switz.*

Warne, UK. E.E. Warne & Co., White Lion Rd, Amersham, Bucks, England.

Warner, Austral. See *Parke, Davis, Austral.*

Warner, Ger. W.R. Warner & Co. GmbH, Mooswaldallee 1-9, Postfach: 569, 7800 Freiburg im Breisgau, W. Germany.

Warner, NZ. Warner-Lambert (NZ) Ltd, (incorporating Wm R. Warner & Co. Ltd), P.O. Box 430, Auckland, New Zealand.

Warner, S.Afr. Warner Pharmaceuticals, Division of Chamberlains (Pty) Ltd, Private Bag X6, Tokai 7966, S. Africa.

Warner, UK. William R. Warner & Co. Ltd, Mitchell House, Southampton Rd, Eastleigh, Hants SO5 5RY, England.

Warner-Lambert, Philipp. Warner-Lambert (Phil.) Inc., MCPO Box 65, Makati, Metro Manila, Philippines.

Warner-Lambert, Swed. Warner-Lambert Scandinavia AB, Box 4130, 171 04 Solna, Sweden.

Warner-Lambert, Switz. Warner-Lambert SA, Case postale, 8040 Zurich, Switzerland.

Warner-Lambert, UK. Warner-Lambert Health Care, Mitchell House, Southampton Rd, Eastleigh, Hants SO5 5RY, England.

Warner-Lambert, USA. Warner-Lambert Co., 201 Tabor Rd, Morris Plains NJ 07950, USA.

Warrick, Denm. Warrick Laegemidler (Essex Pharma A/S), Hredemarken 12, 3520 Farum, Denmark.

Warrick, Neth. Warrick (Nederland) B.V., Bankrashof 3, 1183 NP Amstelveen, Netherlands.

Wassen, S.Afr. See *Script Intal, S.Afr.*

Wassen, UK. Wassen International Ltd, 14 The Mole, Business Park, Leatherhead, Surrey KT22 7BA, England.

Wasserman, Spain. Wasserman, Avda. San Antonio M. Claret 173, 08026 Barcelona, Spain.

Waterhouse, UK. J. Waterhouse & Co. Ltd, Unit C, Shepley Industrial Estate South, Shepley Rd, Audenshaw, Lancs M34 5DW, England.

Watson, USA. T.E. Watson Co., P.O. Box 3829, Sarasota FL 33578, USA.

WB Pharmaceuticals, UK. See *Boehringer Ingelheim, UK.*

Webber, Canad. Webber Inc., Division of Sterisystems Ltd, 3909 Nashua Dr., Unit 9, Mississauga, Ontario L4V 1P3, Canada.

Webcon, USA. Webcon Pharmaceuticals, Division of Alcon (Puerto Rico) Inc., P.O. Box 6380, Fort Worth TX 76115, USA.

Weddel, Austral. Weddel Pharmaceuticals, A Division of Fisons Pty Ltd, P.O. Box 42, Pennant Hills NSW 2120, Australia.

Weiders, Norw. Weiders Farmasøytiske A/S, Hausmannsgt. 6, Postboks 9113 Vaterland, 0134 Oslo 1, Norway.

Weimer, Ger. Waldemar Weimer chem.-pharm. Fabrik Gmbh, Steingerust 30, Postfach: 2454, 7550 Rastatt, W. Germany.

Welbeck, UK. Welbeck, England.

Welcker-Lyster, Canad. Welcker-Lyster Ltd, 8480 St Lawrence Blvd, Montreal, Quebec H2P 2M6, Canada.

Weleda, Fr. Laboratoire Weleda, 9 rue Eugene-Jung, 68330 Huningue, France.

Weleda, Ger. Weleda AG, Mohlerstrasse 3, Postfach: 1309/1320, 7070 Schwabisch Gmund, Germany.

Weleda, UK. Weleda (UK) Ltd, Heanor Rd, Ilkeston, Derbyshire DE7 8DR, England.

Welfare Foods, UK. Welfare Foods (Stockport) Ltd, 63 London Road South, Poynton, Stockport, Cheshire SK12 1LA, England.

Wellcome, Arg. Wellcome Argentina Ltda, Av. Leandro N Além 619 2° Piso, 1001 Buenos Aires, Argentina.

Wellcome, Austral. Wellcome Australia Ltd, P.O. Box 12, Concord NSW 2137, Australia.

Wellcome, Belg. Wellcome S.A., Industriezone III, 9440 Aalst, Belgium.

Wellcome, Canad. Burroughs Wellcome Inc., Wellcome Medical Division, 16751 route Transcanadienne, Kirkland, Quebec H9H 4J4, Canada.

Wellcome, Denm. The Wellcome Foundation Ltd, Nyvej 16, 1851 Frederiksberg C, Denmark.

Wellcome, Fr. Laboratoires Wellcome S.A., 159 rue Nationale, 75640 Paris Cedex 13, France.

Wellcome, Ger. Deutsche Wellcome GmbH, Felde 5, Postfach: 1352, 3006 Burgwedel 1, Germany.

Wellcome, Ital. Wellcome Italia s.p.a., Via del Mare 36, 00040 Pomezia (Rome), Italy.

Wellcome, Neth. Wellcome Nederland B.V., IJsselmeerlaan 2, 1382 JT Weesp, Netherlands.

Wellcome, Norw. The Wellcome Foundation Ltd, Informasjonsavdeling i Norge, Gamle Drammensvn. 107, 1322 Hovik, Norway.

Wellcome, S.Afr. Wellcome (Pty) Ltd, P.O. Box 653, Kempton Park 1620, S. Africa.

Wellcome, Swed. The Wellcome Foundation Ltd, Box 2118, 183 02 Taby, Sweden.

Wellcome, Switz. Wellcome SA, Holeestrasse 87, 4015 Basel, Switzerland.

Wellcome, UK. Wellcome Medical Division, The Wellcome Foundation Ltd, Crewe Hall, Crewe, Cheshire CW1 1UB, England.

Wellcome, USA. Burroughs Wellcome Co., 3030 Cornwallis Rd, Research Triangle Park NC 27709, USA.

Wellcome Diagnostics, UK. Wellcome Diagnostics, A Division of The Wellcome Foundation Ltd, Temple Hill, Dartford DA1 5AH, England.

Wellcome Reagents, UK. Wellcome Reagents, England.

Wellcopharm, Ger. See *Wellcome, Ger.*

Welt, Arg. Welt S.A., Tronador 3030, 1430 Buenos Aires, Argentina.

Wesley, USA. The Wesley Pharmacal Co. Inc., 9984 Gantry Rd, Philadelphia PA 19115, USA.

Westbrook, UK. Westbrook Lanolin Co., Argonaut Works, Laisterdyke, Bradford BD4 8AU, England.

WestCan, Canad. Western Canadian Custom Pharmaceutical Co., Division of Vita Health Co. Ltd, 150 Beghin Ave, Winnipeg, Manitoba R2J 3R4, Canada.

Westmont, Philipp. Westmont Pharmaceuticals Inc., P.O. Box 3594, Manila, The Philippines.

Westone, UK. Westone Products Ltd, 104 Marylebone Lane, London W1M 5FU, England.

Westwood, Canad. Westwood Pharmaceuticals, 420 College St E., Belleville, Ontario K8N 5E9, Canada.

Westwood, USA. Westwood Pharmaceuticals Inc., 100 Forest Ave, Buffalo NY 14213, USA.

Whaley, UK. Whaley Pharmaceuticals, 7 Sheep St, Rugby, Warwicks CV21 3BU, England.

Wharton, Ital. Wharton s.r.l., Via Ragazzi del 99 n.5, 40133 Bologna, Italy.

Wharton, USA. Wharton Laboratories Inc., 37-02 48th Ave, Long Island City NY 11101, USA.

Whatman, S.Afr. See *Riker, S.Afr.*

White, Belg. See *Essex, Belg.*

White, J.F., UK. See *J.F. White, UK.*

Whitehall, Canad. Whitehall Laboratories Ltd, 1060 Middlegate Rd, Mississauga, Ontario L4Y 1M3, Canada.

Whitehall, UK. Whitehall Laboratories Ltd, Chenies St, London WC1E 7ET, England.

Whitehall, USA. Whitehall Laboratories Inc., Division of American Home Products Corp., 685 Third Ave, New York NY 10017, USA.

Whitelaw, UK. Robert Whitelaw (Newcastle) Ltd, England.

Widmer, Switz. Laboratoires Louis Widmer & Co, 8048 Zurich, Switzerland.

Wiedenmann, Switz. Wiedenmann SA, Hardstrasse 25, 4127 Birsfelden, Switzerland.

Wigglesworth, UK. Wigglesworth (1982) Ltd, Cunard Rd, North Acton, London NW10 6PN, England.

Wilcox, UK. Wilcox Laboratories Ltd, 20 Essex St, London WC2, England.

Wild, Switz. Dr Wild & Co. SA, Lange Gasse 4, 4002 Basel, Switzerland.

Will-Pharma, Belg. Will-Pharma S.A., ave Monplaisir 33, 1030 Brussels, Belgium.

Willen, USA. Willen Drug Co., 18 North High St, Baltimore MD 21202, USA.

Willows Francis, UK. Willows Francis, England.

Willows Francis Veterinary, UK. Willows Francis Veterinary, Sussex Manor Business Park, Gatwick Rd, Crawley RH10 2NH, England.

Wilson, Pakistan. Wilson's Pharmaceuticals, 387-388, Sector 1/9, Industrial Area, Islamabad, Pakistan.

Windsor, UK. Windsor Pharmaceuticals, Ellesfield Ave, Bracknell, Berks RG12 4YS, England.

Wingfield, UK. Wingfield, England.

Winnipeg Rh Institute, Canad. Winnipeg Rh Institute Inc., University of Manitoba, Winnipeg, Manitoba R3T 2N2, Canada.

WinPharm, UK. WinPharm, 1 Onslow St, Guildford, Surrey GU1 4YS, England.

Winston, USA. Winston, USA.

Winthrop, Arg. Winthrop Est. Med., Av. del Libertador 6796, 1429 Buenos Aires, Argentina.

Winthrop, Austral. Winthrop Laboratories, Division of Sterling Pharmaceuticals Pty Ltd, P.O. Box 3, Ermington NSW 2115, Australia.

Winthrop, Belg. Lab. Winthrop S.A., rue Franz Merjay 103, 1060 Brussels, Belgium.

Winthrop, Canad. Winthrop Laboratories, Division of Sterling Drug Ltd, Yonge St S., Aurora, Ontario L4G 3H6, Canada.

Winthrop, Denm. Sterling-Winthrop A/S, Østerbrogade 165 B, 2100 Copenhagen Ø, Denmark.

Winthrop, Fr. See *Sterling Winthrop, Fr.*

Winthrop, Ger. Winthrop GmbH, Heidbergstrasse 100, 2000 Norderstedt, Germany.

Winthrop, Neth. See *Sterling Winthrop, Neth.*

Winthrop, Norw. See *Nyco, Norw.*

Winthrop, S.Afr. Winthrop, Division of Sterling Drug (SA) (Pty) Ltd, P.O. Box 32074, Mobeni 4060, S. Africa.

Winthrop, Switz. Winthrop SA, Case postale, 4002 Basel, Switzerland.

Winthrop, UK. Winthrop Laboratories, Sterling-Winthrop House, Onslow St, Guildford, Surrey GU1 4YS, England.

Winthrop, USA. See *Winthrop-Breon, USA.*

Winthrop-Breon, USA. Winthrop-Breon Laboratories, 90 Park Ave, New York NY 10016, USA.

Winzer, Ger. Dr Winzer, Chem.-pharm. Fabrik, Mainaustrasse 146, Postfach: 5126, 7750 Constance, W. Germany.

Wisconsin Pharmacal, USA. Wisconsin Pharmacal Co., USA.

Witco, UK. Witco Chemical Ltd, Union Lane, Droitwich, Worcs WR9 9BB, England.

Woelm, Denm. See *Dansk Dental Depot, Denm.*

Woelm, Ger. Woelm Pharma GmbH, Stresemannstr. 7, Postfach: 840, 3440 Eschwege, W. Germany.

Woelm, Norw. See *Remed, Norw.*

Woelm, Switz. See *Adroka, Switz.*

Woelm-Pharma, Swed. See *Scania, Swed.*

Wolfer, Ger. Otto A.H. Wolfer GmbH, Kluvensiek, 2371 Bovenau, Germany.

Wolff, Ger. Dr. August Wolff Chem.-pharm. Fabrik GmbH & Co. KG, Sudbrackstrasse 56, Postfach: 9540, 4800 Bielefeld 1, Germany.

Wolins, USA. Wolins Pharmacal Corporation, 75 Marcus Dr., Melville NY 11746, USA.

Wolo, Switz. Wolo SA, Eggbühlstrasse 20, 8052 Zurich, Switzerland.

Wood's Dispensary, Canad. Wood's Dispensary Ltd, 2931 20th Ave S., Lethbridge, Alberta T1K 3M5, Canada.

Woods, Austral. H.W. Woods Pty Ltd, P.O. Box 5, Huntingdale Vic. 3166, Australia.

Woodward, UK. G.O. Woodward & Co. Ltd, Larkhall Laboratories, Mouliniere House, Putney Bridge Rd, London SW15 2PY, England.

Worwag, Ger. Worwag Pharma GmbH, Lindenbachstr. 74, 7000 Stuttgart 31, Germany.

Wulfing, Belg. See *Beecham, Belg.*

Wyeth, Arg. John Wyeth Laborat. S.A., Reconquista 1011 1° piso, 1003 Buenos Aires, Argentina.

Wyeth, Austral. Wyeth Pharmaceuticals Pty Ltd, P.O Box 148, Parramatta NSW 2150, Australia.

Wyeth, Belg. Wyeth S.A., bd de la Cambre 33-39/bte 10-11, 1050 Brussels, Belgium.

Wyeth, Canad. Wyeth Ltd, P.O. Box 370, Downsview, Ontario M3M 3A8, Canada.

Wyeth, Denm. See *Ferrosan, Denm.*

Wyeth, Fin. See *Laaketukku, Fin.*

Wyeth, Ger. Wyeth-Pharma GmbH, Schleebruggenkamp 15, Postfach:8807, 4400 Munster, W. Germany.

Wyeth, Ital. Wyeth s.p.a., Via Nettunense 90, 04011 Aprilia (LT), Italy.

Wyeth, Neth. Wyeth Laboratoria B.V., Daalmeerstraat 24, 2131 HC Hoofddorp, Netherlands.

Wyeth, Philipp. See *Marsman, Philipp.*

Wyeth, S.Afr. Wyeth (Pty) Ltd, P.O. Box 42, Isando 1600, S. Africa.

Wyeth, Switz. Wyeth SA, Dufourstrasse 49, 4052 Basel, Switzerland.

Wyeth, UK. Wyeth Laboratories, Huntercombe Lane South, Taplow, Maidenhead, Berks SL6 0PH, England.

Wyeth, USA. Wyeth Laboratories, Division of American Home Products Corp., P.O. Box 8299, Philadelphia PA 19101, USA.

Wyeth-Byla, Fr. Laboratoires Wyeth-Byla, 117 rue du Chateau des Rentiers, 75013 Paris, France.

Xttrium, USA. Xttrium, USA.

Yamanouchi, Jpn. Yamanouchi Seiyaku, 2-5 Hon-cho, Nihonbashi, Chuo-ku, Tokyo, Japan.

Yer, Spain. Yer, Pablo Alcover 31, 08017 Barcelona, Spain.

York, Arg. York S.A., México 1477, 1097 Buenos Aires, Argentina.

Yoshitomi, Jpn. Yoshitomi Seiyaku, 3-35 Hirano-cho, Higashi-ku, Osaka, Japan.

Youngs, USA. Youngs, USA.

Ysatfabrik, Ger. Johannes Bürger Ysatfabrik GmbH, Herzog-Julius-Strasse 83, Postfach: 167, 3388 Bad Harzburg 1, W. Germany.

Zambeletti, Ital. Dr. L. Zambeletti s.p.a., Via Zambeletti, 20021 Baranzate (MI), Italy.

Zambeletti, Spain. Zambeletti, Carriles s/n (Plg Ind), Coslada, Madrid, Spain.

Zambon, Ital. Zambon Farmaceutici s.p.a., Via Lillo del Duca 10, 20091 Bresso (MI), Italy.

Zambon, Spain. Zambon, Ctra. Madrid Barcelona km 607.3, San Vicente dels Horts, 08620 Barcelona, Spain.

Zenith, USA. Zenith Laboratories Inc., 140 LeGrand Ave, Northvale NJ 07647, USA.

Zeta, Ital. Zeta Farmaceutici s.p.a., Via Galvani 10, 36066 Sandrigo (VI), Italy.

Zila, USA. Zila, USA.

Zilliken, Ital. Zilliken & Co. s.a.s., Via F. Nullo 23, 16147 Genova Quarto, Italy.

Zoecon, UK. See *Sandoz Agrochem, UK.*

Zoecon, USA. Zoecon Corporation, Palo Alto, USA.

Zoja, Ital. Zoja Giorgio s.p.a., Viale Lombardia 20, 20131 Milan, Italy.

Zuellig, Philipp. Zuellig Pharma Corp., PO Box 604, Manila 2800, The Philippines.

Zyma, Arg. See *Elvetium, Arg.*

Zyma, Austral. See *Ciba-Geigy, Austral.*

Zyma, Denm. See *Ciba, Denm.*

Zyma, Fr. Laboratoires Zyma, Tour Albert 1er, 65 av. de Colmar, 92507 Rueil-Malmaison Cedex, France.

Zyma, Ger. Zyma GmbH, Zielstattstrasse 40, Postfach: 701980, 8000 Munich 70, W. Germany.

Zyma, Ital. Zyma s.p.a., Corso Italia 13, 21047 Saronno (VA), Italy.

Zyma, Neth. B.V. Zyma-Nederland, Energieweg 4, 3641 RT Mijdrecht, Netherlands.

Zyma, Norw. See *Ciba, Norw.*

Zyma, S.Afr. See *Ciba, S.Afr.*

Zyma, Spain. See *Frumtost, Spain.*

Zyma, Swed. See *Ciba, Swed.*

Zyma, Switz. Zyma S.A., 1260 Nyon, Switzerland.

Zyma, UK. Zyma (UK) Ltd, Westhead, 10 West St, Alderley Edge, Cheshire SK9 7XP, England.

Zyma-Galen, Belg. Zyma-Galen S.A., rue de Wand 209-213, 1020 Brussels, Belgium.

Index to Clinical Uses
Mentioned in Parts 1 and 2

This index is only a guide to the uses described in the text; it is not a comprehensive therapeutic index. The drugs or groups of drugs under each heading are arranged alphabetically and not by order of preference.
Synonyms for diseases are given where these may be helpful. However, in some cases related conditions are also given because they may be treated similarly.

of the individual antidote or antagonist. More information is provided in the relevant Treatment of Adverse Effects sections.

ALCOHOL.—Fructose, 1264.

ANTICHOLINESTERASES.—See Cholinesterase Inhibitors; Parasympathomimetics.

ANTICOAGULANTS.—Phytomenadione, 1286; Protamine Sulphate (*heparin*), 852.

ANTIMONY.—Dimercaprol, 840.

ANTIMUSCARINIC AGENTS.—Physostigmine, 1334.

ARSENIC.—Dimercaprol, 840; Succimer, 855.

BENZODIAZEPINES.—Flumazenil, 841.

BISMUTH.—Dimercaprol, 840.

CALCIUM-CHANNEL BLOCKING AGENTS.—Calcium Gluconate, 1030.

CARBON MONOXIDE.—Oxygen, 1070.

CHOLINESTERASE INHIBITORS (Organophosphorus Insecticides).—Atropine, 525; Obidoxime Chloride, 847; Pralidoxime, 851. See also Parasympathomimetics.

COPPER.—Penicillamine, 849.

CYANIDE.—Amyl Nitrite, 1493; Dicobalt Edetate, 839; 4-Dimethylaminophenol Hydrochloride, 840; Oxygen, 1071; Sodium Nitrite, 854; Sodium Thiosulphate, 855.

DIGITALIS (Digoxin).—Digoxin-specific Antibody Fragments, 839.
Prophylaxis.—Potassium Chloride, 1037.

GOLD.—Dimercaprol, 840.

IODINE.—Starch, 1275.

IRON.—Desferrioxamine Mesylate, 838.

LEAD.—Dimercaprol, 840; Penicillamine, 849; Succimer, 855; Sodium Calciumedetate, 852.
Diagnosis.—Sodium Calciumedetate, 853.

MANGANESE.—Levodopa, 1018.

MERCURY (Acrodynia; Pink Disease).—Dimercaprol, 840; Penicillamine, 849; Succimer, 855; Unithiol, 856.

METALS, HEAVY.—Dimercaprol, 840; Penicillamine, 849; Sodium Calciumedetate, 853; Unithiol, 856. See also individual metals.

MUSCLE RELAXANTS, COMPETITIVE (Non-depolarising Muscle Relaxants).—Atropine, 525; Glycopyrronium Bromide, 532; Neostigmine, 1333; Tacrine Hydrochloride, 1337.

NICKEL CARBONYL.—Sodium Diethyldithiocarbamate, 853.

OPIATES (Narcotic Analgesics; Opioid Analgesics).—Levallorphan Tartrate, 842; Nalmefene, 844; Nalorphine, 844; Naloxone Hydrochloride, 845; Naltrexone Hydrochloride, 846; Potassium Permanganate (*lavage*), 1607.

ORGANOPHOSPHORUS COMPOUNDS.—See Cholinesterase Inhibitors.

PARACETAMOL.—Acetylcysteine, 903; Cysteamine Hydrochloride, 837; Methionine, 843.

PARAQUAT.—Fuller's Earth, 842.

PARASYMPATHOMIMETICS.—Atropine, 525.

PHOSPHORUS.—Copper Sulphate, 1259.

STRYCHNINE.—Potassium Permanganate (*lavage*), 1607.

THALLIUM.—Dimercaprol, 840; Prussian Blue, 852; Sodium Diethyldithiocarbamate, 853.

TUBOCURARINE.—See Curare.

VITAMIN D.—Calcitonins, 1339.

Poliomyelitis Prophylaxis.—Poliomyelitis Vaccines, 1174.

Polyarteritis Nodosa.—See Arteritis.

Polyarthritis, Juvenile.—See Rheumatic Disorders.

Polycythaemia (Polycythaemia Rubra Vera).—Antineoplastic Agents and Immunosuppressants, 580–657, **585**; Phosphorus-32, 1381.

Polymyalgia Rheumatica.—See Arteritis.

Polymyositis.—Corticosteroids, 875.

Polyneuropathies.—See Neuropathies.

Polyserositis, Paroxysmal.—See Fever, Mediterranean, Familial.

Polyuria.—See Diabetes Insipidus.

Porphyria.—Activated Charcoal, 836; Chlorpromazine, 724; Desferrioxamine Mesylate, 839; Haematin, 1577; Propranolol Hydrochloride (*tachycardia and hypertension*), 807.

Porphyria Cutanea Tarda.—See Photosensitivity.

Potassium Depletion.—See Hypokalaemia.

Precocious Puberty.—See Puberty, to Delay.

Pregnancy Diagnosis.—Pregnancy and Fertility Tests, 944.

Pregnancy, Termination of.—See Abortion, to Induce.

Premedication.—See Anaesthetics, Premedication.

Premenstrual Syndrome; Premenstrual Tension.—See Tension, Premenstrual.

Proctitis.—Acetarsol, 659; Hydrocortisone, 895; Sulphasalazine, 1110. See also Constipation: Lubricants; Haemorrhoids.

Prolactinoma.—See Neoplasms: Pituitary.

Prostatic Hypertrophy.—See Hypertrophy, Prostatic.

Prostatitis.—Antibacterial Agents, 94–337; Phenazopyridine Hydrochloride (*pain*), 35; Rifampicin, 576.

Protoporphyria, Erythropoietic.—See Photosensitivity.

Pruritus (Itching; Prurigo).—Activated Charcoal, 836; Antihistamines, 443–65; Cholestyramine (*biliary obstruction*), 1198; Crotamiton, 918; Local Anaesthetics, 1205–27; Menthol, 1586; Titanium Dioxide, 935.

Psittacosis.—See Infections, Chlamydial.

Psoriasis.—Allantoin, 916; Cade Oil, 917; Chrysarobin, 918; Coal Tar, 934; Corticosteroids, 876; Dithranol, 919; Etretinate, 921; Methotrexate, 639; Methoxsalen, 927; Pyrogallol, 930; Razoxane, 649; Salicylic Acid, 931; Tar, 933; Tretinoin, 935.

Psychoneuroses.—See Neuroses.

Psychoses.—Anxiolytic Sedatives Hypnotics and Neuroleptics, 706–76; Carbamazepine, 402.

Pterygium.—Thiotepa, 653.

Puberty, Delayed.—

FEMALE.—Buserelin Acetate, 1142; Danazol, 1396; Gonadorelin, 1143.

MALE.—Chorionic Gonadotrophin, 1144; Sex Hormones (Androgens), 1383–1415, **1383**; Gonadorelin, 1396.

Puberty, to Delay (Precocious Puberty).—Danazol, 1396; Gonadorelin, 1142.

Pudendal Block.—See Anaesthetics, Regional Block.

Pulmonary Oedema.—See Oedema, Pulmonary.

Purpura, Thrombocytopenic.—See Thrombocytopenia.

Pyelography.—See Organ, Tissue, and Tumour Delineation: Kidney and Urinary Tract.

Pyelonephritis.—See Urinary-tract Infections.

Pylorospasm and Pyloric Stenosis.—Atropine, 524.

Pyoderma.—Loflucarban, 429.

Pyrexia.—See Fever, to Reduce.

Q Fever.—See Infections, Rickettsial.

Rabies Prophylaxis.—Rabies Antisera, 1175; Rabies Immunoglobulins, 1175; Rabies Vaccines, 1176.

Radiation Sickness.—See Nausea and Vomiting.

Radioprotection.—

THYROID.—Potassium Iodate, 1186; Potassium Perchlorate, 686.

Rat-bite Fever.—See Fever, Rat-bite.

Raynaud's Disease.—See Vascular Diseases, Occlusive.

Reiter's Disease.—Phenylbutazone, 37; Tetracycline, 321.

Relapsing Fever.—See Fever, Relapsing.

Renal Failure.—See Kidney Disorders: Kidney Failure.

Renal Osteodystrophy.—See Kidney Disorders: Kidney Failure.

Renography.—See Organ, Tissue, and Tumour Delineation: Kidney and Urinary Tract.

Respiratory Depression.—See Depression, Respiratory.

Respiratory Diseases, Acute (Respiratory-tract Infections).—Antibacterial Agents, 94–337, **99**; Corticosteroids, 880; Natamycin, 431. See also Asthma and Bronchitis; Alveolitis; Respiratory Distress Syndrome.

Respiratory Distress Syndrome.—

ADULT.—Alprostadil, 1367; Corticosteroids, 880; Oxygen, 1071.

NEONATAL.—Frusemide, 991; Lecithin, 1583; Orgotein, 1045; Oxygen, 1071; Pancuronium Bromide, 1237; Theophylline, 1534.
Prophylaxis.—Betamethasone, 884; Lecithin, 1583; Theophylline, 1534.

Respiratory Failure.—See Depression, Respiratory.

Respiratory Insufficiency.—See Depression, Respiratory.

Respiratory-tract Infections.—See Respiratory Diseases, Acute.

Restless Legs Syndrome.—Carbamazepine, 402; Clonazepam, 402; Disopyramide, 78.

Reticulum Cell Sarcoma; Reticulosarcoma.—See Neoplasms: Lymphoma, Non-Hodgkin's.

Index to Martindale Identity Numbers

Each monograph and chapter introduction has an identity number. This index lists the identity number followed by the relevant monograph or chapter title and the page on which it appears.

General Index

Entries are arranged alphabetically in word-by-word order. Where an entry is followed by more than one page reference, the principal reference is printed in bold type.